Textbook of Rheumatology

SECOND EDITION

WILLIAM N. KELLEY, M.D.

John G. Searle Professor and Chairman,
Department of Internal Medicine, and
Professor, Department of Biological Chemistry,
University of Michigan Medical Center,
Ann Arbor, Michigan

EDWARD D. HARRIS, JR., M.D.

Professor and Chairman, Department of Medicine,
UMDNJ - Rutgers Medical School,
New Brunswick, New Jersey

SHAUN RUDDY, M.D.

Professor of Medicine, Microbiology and Immunology,
Chairman, Division of Immunology and
     Connective Tissue Diseases,
Medical College of Virginia, Health Sciences Division,
Virginia Commonwealth University,
Richmond, Virginia

CLEMENT B. SLEDGE, M.D.

John B. and Buckminster Brown Professor
     of Orthopedic Surgery, Harvard Medical School,
Orthopedic Surgeon-in-Chief,
Brigham and Women's Hospital,
Boston, Massachusetts

W.B. SAUNDERS COMPANY

Philadelphia □ London □ Toronto □ Mexico City □ Rio de Janeiro □ Sydney □ Tokyo

W. B. Saunders Company: West Washington Square
                           Philadelphia, PA 19105

                           1 St. Anne's Road
                           Eastbourne, East Sussex BN21 3UN, England

                           1 Goldthorne Avenue
                           Toronto, Ontario M8Z 5T9, Canada

                           Apartado 26370–Cedro 512
                           Mexico 4, D.F., Mexico

                           Rua Coronel Cabrita, 8
                           Sao Cristovao Caixa Postal 21176
                           Rio de Janeiro, Brazil

                           9 Waltham Street
                           Artarmon, N.S.W. 2064, Australia

                           Ichibancho, Central Bldg., 22-1 Ichibancho
                           Chiyoda-Ku, Tokyo 102, Japan

Library of Congress Cataloging in Publication Data
Main entry under title:

Textbook of rheumatology.

  1. Rheumatism. 2. Collagen diseases. I. Kelley,
William N. [DNLM: 1. Arthritis. 2. Rheumatism. WE 544
T355]
RC927.T49 1985   616.7'23   83-20114
ISBN 0-7216-5362-6

Textbook of Rheumatology

Single Volume ISBN   0-7216-5362-6
     Volume I ISBN   0-7216-5363-4
    Volume II ISBN   0-7216-5364-2
Two Volume Set ISBN   0-7216-5365-0

Last digit is the print number: 9   8   7   6   5   4   3   2

We wish to dedicate this edition of the
Textbook of Rheumatology to our wives and children.

Lois Kelley and children:
Paige Kelley, Ginger Kelley, Lori Kelley and Mark Kelley.

Mary Ann Harris and children:
Ned Harris, Tom Harris, and Chandler Harris.

Millicent Ruddy and children:
Christi Ruddy and Candace Ruddy.

Georgia Sledge and children:
Mego Sledge, John Sledge, Matthew Sledge, and Claire Sledge.

Contributors

Margaret A. Alspaugh, Ph.D.
Associate Professor of Medicine and Pathology, University of Missouri; Associate Scientist, Cancer Research Center, Columbus, Missouri
Sjögren's Syndrome

Roy D. Altman, M.D.
Professor of Medicine, University of Miami School of Medicine; Chief, Arthritis Division, Miami Veterans Administration Medical Center, Miami, Florida
Hypertrophic Osteoarthropathy

Ronald J. Anderson, M.D.
Associate Professor of Medicine, Harvard Medical School; Director of Clinical Training, Department of Rheumatology and Immunology, Brigham and Women's Hospital, Boston, Massachusetts
Polyarticular Arthritis

William J. Arnold, M.D., F.A.C.P.
Clinical Associate Professor of Medicine, Abraham Lincoln School of Medicine, University of Illinois at The Medical Center; Director, Section of Rheumatology, Lutheran General Hospital, Park Ridge, Illinois
The Rheumatic Manifestations of Sarcoidosis

Dianna Ausprunk, Ph.D.
Assistant Professor, Department of Anatomy, Harvard Medical School; Research Associate, Children's Hospital Medical Center, Boston, Massachusetts
Connective Tissue: Small Blood Vessels and Capillaries

Lloyd Axelrod, M.D.
Associate Professor of Medicine, Harvard Medical School; Associate Physician, Massachusetts General Hospital; Chief, Medical Unit, Massachusetts Eye and Ear Infirmary, Boston, Massachusetts
Glucocorticoids

Barbara Figley Banwell, M.A., P.T.
Program Leader in Physical Therapy, University of Michigan Multipurpose Arthritis Center, University Medical Center, Ann Arbor, Michigan
Psychological and Sexual Health in Rheumatic Disease

Alan J. Barrett, Ph.D., Sc.D.
Head of Department of Biochemistry, Strangeways Laboratory, Cambridge, England
Proteinases in Joint Disease

J. Claude Bennett, M.D.
Professor and Chairman, Department of Medicine, and Director, Multipurpose Arthritis Center, University of Alabama in Birmingham; Physician, University of Alabama Hospitals, Birmingham, Alabama
The Etiology of Rheumatoid Arthritis

Robert M. Bennett, M.D., M.R.C.P., F.A.C.P.
Professor of Medicine, Oregon Health Sciences University; Head, Division of Rheumatic Diseases, Oregon Health Sciences University Hospital and Clinics; Consultant, Portland Veterans Administration Medical Center, Portland, Oregon
Mixed Connective Tissue Disease and Other Overlap Syndromes

A.G. Björkengren, M.D.
New York, New York
Surgery for Arthritis of the Cervical Spine

George L. Blackburn, M.D., Ph.D.
Associate Professor of Surgery, Harvard Medical School; Director, Nutrition Support Service, New England Deaconess Hospital, Boston, Massachusetts
Nutrition and Rheumatic Diseases

R. Michael Blaese, M.D.
Chief, Cellular Immunology Section, Metabolism Branch, National Cancer Institute, National Institutes of Health; Attending Physician, Clinical Center, National Institutes of Health, Bethesda, Maryland
Immunodeficiency Diseases

Arthur L. Boland, Jr., M.D.
Assistant Clinical Professor of Orthopedic Surgery, Harvard Medical School; Associate in Orthopedic Surgery, Brigham and Women's Hospital; Staff Orthopedic Surgery, New England Baptist Hospital; Staff Orthopedic Surgery, Harvard Community Health Plan Hospital, Boston, Massachusetts
Recreational Musculoskeletal Injuries

Alfred Jay Bollet, M.D.
Clinical Professor of Medicine, Yale University School of Medicine New Haven, Connecticut; Adjunct Professor of Medicine, New York Medical College; Chairman, Department of Medicine, Danbury Hospital, Danbury, Connecticut
Nonsteroidal Anti-inflammatory Drugs

Walter G. Bradley, D.M., F.R.C.P.
Professor and Chairman, Department of Neurology, University of Vermont College of Medicine and Medical Center Hospital of Vermont, Burlington, Vermont
Structure and Function of the Motor Unit; Muscle Weakness; Diagnostic Tests in Neuromuscular Diseases; Inflammatory Diseases of Muscle

Kenneth D. Brandt, M.D.
Professor of Medicine and Chief, Rheumatology Division, Indiana University School of Medicine; Attending Physician, University Hospital, Indiana University Medical Center; Consulting Physician, Richard L. Roudebush Veterans Administration Medical Center, Indianapolis, Indiana
Glycosaminoglycans; Pathogenesis of Osteoarthritis; Osteoarthritis: Clinical Patterns and Pathology; Management of Osteoarthritis

Joel N. Buxbaum, M.D.
Professor of Medicine, New York University Medical Center; Chief, Rheumatology Section, Department of Medicine, New York Veterans Administration Medical Center, New York, New York
Immunoglobulins and Their Genes

David S. Caldwell, M.D.
Assistant Professor of Medicine, Duke University School of Medicine; Attending Rheumatologist, Duke University Hospital, Durham, North Carolina, Consulting Rheumatologist, Fayetteville Veterans Administration Hospital, Fayetteville, North Carolina; Consulting Rheumatologist, The Memorial Hospital, Danville, Virginia
Musculoskeletal Syndromes Associated with Malignancy

Andrei Calin, M.D., M.R.C.P.
Consultant Rheumatologist, Royal National Hospital for Rheumatic Diseases, Bath, England
Ankylosing Spondylitis; Reiter's Syndrome

Dennis A. Carson, M.D.
Associate Member, Department of Basic and Clinical Research, Scripps Clinic and Research Foundation, La Jolla, California
Rheumatoid Factor

James T. Cassidy, M.D.
Professor and Chairman, Department of Pediatrics, Creighton University School of Medicine, Omaha, Nebraska
Juvenile Rheumatoid Arthritis

John E. Castaldo, M.D.
Instructor of Clinical Medicine, Section of Neurology, Dartmouth Medical School, Hanover, New Hampshire; Attending Neurologist, Lehigh Valley Hospital Center, Allentown, Pennsylvania
Peripheral Nerve: Structure, Function, and Dysfunction

Edgar S. Cathcart, M.D., D.Sc.
Professor of Medicine, Boston University School of Medicine, Boston; Chief, Arthritis Gerontology Center, Edith Nourse Rogers Memorial Veterans Administration Hospital, Bedford, Massachusetts
Amyloidosis

Zanvil A. Cohn, M.D.
Professor and Senior Physician, Laboratory of Cellular Physiology and Immunology, The Rockefeller University; Senior Physician, The Rockefeller University Hospital, New York, New York
Cellular Components of Inflammation: Monocytes and Macrophages

Robert O. Cone, III, M.D.
Assistant Professor, Department of Radiology, University of Texas Health Science Center, and Medical Center Hospital, San Antonio, Texas
Radiographic Evaluation of Articular Disorders

Doyt L. Conn, M.D.
Professor of Medicine, Mayo Medical School; Chairman, Division of Rheumatology, and Consultant in Rheumatology and Internal Medicine, Mayo Clinic, Rochester, Minnesota
Necrotizing Vasculitis; Giant Cell Arteritis and Polymyalgia Rheumatica

E. Dayer, M.D.
Research Associate, Transfusion Center, Department of Medicine, Hôpital Cantonal Universitaire, Genève, Switzerland
Immune Complexes

Frederick C. Ewald, M.D.
Associate Clinical Professor, Orthopedic Surgery, Harvard Medical School; Orthopedic Surgeon, Brigham and Women's Hospital; Consultant, West Roxbury Veterans Administration Hospital and New England Baptist Hospital, Boston, Massachusetts
Reconstructive Surgery and Rehabilitation of the Elbow

Anthony S. Fauci, M.D.
Chief, Laboratory of Immunoregulation, National Institute of Allergy and Infectious Diseases, National Institutes of Health, Bethesda, Maryland
Cytotoxic and Other Immunoregulatory Agents

Jerry Fenenbaum, M.D. F.R.C.P. (C.), F.A.C.P.
Assistant Professor, University of Toronto Faculty of Medicine; Consultant Rheumatologist, Mount Sinai Hospital, Baycrest Geriatric Centre, and Toronto General Hospital, Toronto, Ontario
Hypertrophic Osteoarthropathy

Andrew P. Ferry, M.D., F.A.C.S.
Professor and Chairman, Department of Ophthalmology, and Professor of Pathology, Medical College of Virginia of Virginia Commonwealth University; Ophthalmic Surgeon-in-Chief, Medical College of Virginia Hospitals; Consultant, Veterans Administration Hospital, Richmond, Virginia
Ocular Manifestations of Rheumatic Diseases

J. William Fielding, M.D., F.R.C.S.(C.)
Clinical Professor of Orthopaedic Surgery, Columbia University College of Physicians and Surgeons; Clinical Professor of Orthopaedic Surgery, New York University School of Medicine; Attending Orthopaedic Surgeon, New York University Medical Center and Bellevue Hospital; Director, Department of Orthopaedic Surgery, St. Luke's–Roosevelt Center Hospital, New York, New York
Surgery for Arthritis of the Cervical Spine

Judah Folkman, M.D.
Julia Dyckman Andrus Professor of Pediatric Surgery and Professor of Anatomy, Harvard Medical School; Director of The Surgical Research Laboratories, Children's Hospital, Boston, Massachusetts
Connective Tissue: Small Blood Vessels and Capillaries

Irving H. Fox, M.D., C.M.
Professor, Department of Internal Medicine, and Associate Professor, Department of Biological Chemistry, University of Michigan; Director, Clinical Research Center, University Hospital, Ann Arbor, Michigan
Gout and Related Disorders of Purine Metabolism; Arthropathy with Iron Storage Disease

Blas Frangione, M.D., Ph.D.
Professor of Pathology, New York University Medical Center, New York, New York
Immunoglobulins and Their Genes

James F. Fries, M.D.
Associate Professor of Medicine, Stanford University School of Medicine and Stanford University Hospital, Palo Alto; Attending Physician, Palo Alto Veterans Administration Hospital, Palo Alto, and Santa Clara Valley Medical Center, Santa Clara, California
General Approach to the Rheumatic Disease Patient

Lynn H. Gerber, M.D.
Chief, Department of Rehabilitation Medicine, National Institutes of Health; Adjunct Associate Professor of Medicine, George Washington University; Physician, Arthritis and Rheumatism Branch, NIADDK, National Institutes of Health, Bethesda, Maryland
Rehabilitation of Patients with Rheumatic Diseases

William W. Ginsburg, M.D.
Assistant Professor of Internal Medicine, Mayo Foundation; Consultant, Rochester Methodist Hospital and St. Marys Hospital, Rochester, Minnesota
Multicentric Reticulohistiocytosis

Edward J. Goetzl, M.D.
Professor of Medicine, University of California, San Francisco; Director, Division of Allergy and Immunology, Moffitt-Long Hospitals of the University of California, San Francisco, California
Cellular Components of Inflammation: Granulocytes

Ira M. Goldstein, M.D.
Professor of Medicine, University of California, San Francisco; Chief, Division of Rheumatology, San Francisco General Hospital, San Francisco, California
Cellular Components of Inflammation: Granulocytes

Armin E. Good, M.D.
Professor of Medicine, University of Michigan; Chief, Arthritis Section, Ann Arbor Veterans Administration Medical Center, Ann Arbor, Michigan
Enteropathic Arthritis

Paul F. Good
Research Technologist, Department of Pathology, University of Vermont College of Medicine, Burlington, Vermont
Structure and Function of the Motor Unit

John L. Gordon, Ph.D.
Head of Vascular Biology, Clinical Research Centre, Medical Research Council; Head of Vascular Biology, Northwick Park Hospital, Harrow, England
Cellular Components of Inflammation: Platelets

Norman L. Gottlieb, M.D.
Professor of Medicine, University of Miami School of Medicine, Miami, Florida
Gold Compounds

Norbert Gschwend, Prof. Dr. Med.
Medical Faculty, University of Zürich; Chief Orthopaedic Surgeon, Klinik Wilhelm Schulthess, Zürich, Switzerland
Synovectomy

Virgil Hanson, M.D.
Professor of Pediatrics, University of Southern California, School of Medicine; Head, Division of Rheumatology, Childrens Hospital of Los Angeles, Los Angeles, California
Systemic Lupus Erythematosus, Dermatomyositis, Scleroderma, and Vasculitides in Childhood

Edward D. Harris, Jr., M.D.
Professor and Chairman, Department of Medicine, UMDNJ–Rutgers Medical School;

Chief of Medical Services, Middlesex General–University Hospital, New Brunswick, New Jersey
Biology of the Joint; Pathogenesis of Rheumatoid Arthritis; Rheumatoid Arthritis: The Clinical Spectrum

Brian L. Hazleman, M.B.
Associate Lecturer, Faculty of Clinical Medicine, University of Cambridge; Consultant Physician, Department of Rheumatology, Addenbrooke's Hospital, Cambridge, England
Giant Cell Arteritis and Polymyalgia

Peter M. Henson, D.V.M., Ph.D.
Professor, Department of Pathology and Medicine, University of Colorado School of Medicine; Vice-President for Biomedical Affairs, National Jewish Hospital and Research Center/National Asthma Center, Denver, Colorado
Cellular Components of Inflammation: Platelets

Jerome H. Herman, M.D.
Professor of Medicine, University of Cincinnati, College of Medicine; Attending Physician, University Hospital and Holmes Division of the University of Cincinnati; Consultant (Immunology/Rheumatology), Veterans Administration Hospital, Cincinnati, Ohio
Polychondritis

Gary S. Hoffman, M.D., F.A.C.P.
Associate Professor of Clinical Medicine, Columbia University College of Physicians and Surgeons, New York; Attending Physician, The Mary Imogene Bassett Hospital, Cooperstown, New York
Mycobacterial and Fungal Infections of Bones and Joints

Edward W. Holmes, M.D.
Professor of Medicine, Duke University School of Medicine; Chief, Division of Metabolism, Endocrinology, and Genetics, Duke University Medical Center, Durham, North Carolina
Antihyperuricemic Drugs

David S. Howell, M.D.
Professor of Medicine, and Director, Arthritis Division, Department of Medicine, University of Miami School of Medicine; Attending Staff, Veterans Administration Medical Center and Jackson Memorial Hospital, Miami, Florida
Diseases Due to the Deposition of Calcium Pyrophosphate and Hydroxyopatite

Gene G. Hunder, M.D.
Professor of Medicine, Mayo Medical School; Consultant in Rheumatology and Internal Medicine, Mayo Clinic, Rochester, Minnesota
Examination of the Joints; Giant Cell Arteritis and Polymyalgia; Necrotizing Vasculitis

David S. Hungerford, M.D.
Associate Professor of Orthopaedics, The Johns Hopkins University School of Medicine; Chief, Orthopaedic Surgery, Good Samaritan Hospital, Baltimore, Maryland
Osteonecrosis

Thomas F. Ignaczak, M.D.
Memphis, Tennessee
Amyloidosis

John N. Insall, M.D.
Professor of Orthopaedic Surgery, Cornell University Medical College, Ithaca; Attending Orthopaedic Surgeon, Hospital for Special Surgery and New York Hospital; Chief of Knee Service, Hospital for Special Surgery, New York, New York
Reconstructive Surgery and Rehabilitation of the Knee

Israeli A. Jaffe, M.D.
Professor of Clinical Medicine, Columbia University College of Physicians and Surgeons; Attending Physician, The Presbyterian Hospital, New York, New York
D-Penicillamine

Andrew H. Kang, M.D.
Professor and Chairman, Department of Medicine, University of Tennessee College of Medicine; Physician-in-Chief, Regional Medical Center of Memphis; Staff Physician, Veterans Administration Medical Center, Memphis, Tennessee
Structural Proteins: Collagen, Elastin, and Fibronectin; Localized Fibrotic Disorders

Allen P. Kaplan, M.D.
Professor of Medicine and Head, Division of Allergy, Rheumatology, and Clinical Immunology, State University of New York at Stony Brook; Attending Physician, SUNY–Stony Brook Hospital, Veterans Administration Medical Center, Stony Brook, New York
The Intrinsic Coagulation, Fibrinolytic, and Kinin–Forming Pathways of Man

William N. Kelley, M.D.
John G. Searle Professor and Chairman, Department of Internal Medicine, Professor, Department of Biological Chemistry, University of Michigan Medical Center, Ann Arbor, Michigan
Purine and Deoxypurine Metabolism; Approach to the Patient with Hyperuricemia; Antihyperuricemic Drugs; Gout and Related Disorders of Purine Metabolism

William J. Koopman, M.D.
Professor of Medicine and Director, Division of Clinical Immunology and Rheumatology, University of Alabama in Birmingham Medical School; Attending Physician, University of Alabama in Birmingham Hospitals, Birmingham, Alabama
Genetic Control of Immune Responses

Brian L. Kotzin, M.D.
Assistant Professor of Medicine, University of Colorado Health Sciences Center; Chief, Rheumatology Section, Veterans Administration Medical Center, Denver, Colorado
Immunologic Aspects of Inflammation: Lymphocyte Populations

Irving Kushner, M.D.
Professor of Medicine, Case Western Reserve University; Director, Division of Rheumatology, and Associate Director, Department of Medicine, Cleveland Metropolitan General Hospital, Cleveland, Ohio
The Acute Phase Reactants

P.H. Lambert, M.D.
Head, World Health Organization/Immunology Research and Training Center, Lausanne and Geneva; Blood Transfusion Center, Hôpital Cantonal Universitaire, Genève Switzerland
Immune Complexes

Robert Langer, Sc.D.
Dorothy Poitras Associate Professor of Biochemical Engineering, Massachusetts In-

stitute of Technology, Cambridge; Research Associate in Surgery, Children's Hospital, Boston, Massachusetts
Connective Tissue: Small Blood Vessels and Capillaries

E. Carwile LeRoy, M.D.
Professor of Medicine, Professor of Physical Medicine and Rehabilitation, and Professor of Basic and Clinical Immunology and Microbiology, Medical University of South Carolina; Attending Physician, Medical University Hospital, Veterans Administration Medical Center, St. Francis Hospital, and Charleston Memorial Hospital, Charleston, South Carolina
Scleroderma (Systemic Sclerosis)

Peter H. Levine, M.D.
Professor of Medicine, University of Massachusetts Medical School; Chief of Medicine, Worcester Memorial Hospital, Worcester, Massachusetts
Hemophilia and Arthritis

Robert W. Lightfoot, Jr., M.D., F.A.C.P.
Associate Professor of Medicine and Chief, Rheumatology Section, Medical College of Wisconsin; Director, Rheumatology Service, and Senior Attending Physician, Milwaukee County Medical Complex; Director, Veterans Administration Pilot Rheumatology Program, Wood Veterans Administration Medical Center, Milwaukee, Wisconsin
Cryoglobulinemia and Other Dysproteinemias

Stephen J. Lipson, M.D.
Assistant Professor of Orthopedic Surgery, Harvard Medical School; Orthopedic Surgeon, Brigham and Women's Hospital, Boston, Massachusetts
Low Back Pain

Carlo L. Mainardi, M.D.
Associate Professor of Medicine and Chief, Rheumatology Division, UMDNJ–Rutgers Medical School, University of Medicine and Dentistry of New Jersey; Physician, Middlesex General–University Hospital, New Brunswick, New Jersey
Localized Fibrotic Disorders; Hemophilia and Arthritis

Stephen E. Malawista, M.D.
Professor of Medicine, Department of Internal Medicine, and Chief, Section of Rheumatology, Yale University School of Medicine, New Haven, Connecticut
Lyme Disease

Edward A. Mascioli, M.D.
Clinical Fellow in Medicine, Harvard Medical School; Nutrition Support Service, New England Deaconess Hospital, Boston, Massachusetts
Nutrition and Rheumatic Diseases

John B. McGinty, M.D.
Clinical Professor of Orthopaedic Surgery, Tufts University School of Medicine, Boston; Chief of Orthopaedic Surgery, Newton-Wellesley Hospital, Newton, Massachusetts
Arthroscopy

James L. McGuire, M.D.
Assistant Professor of Medicine, University of Massachusetts Medical School, Worcester, Massachusetts
Arthropathies Associated with Endocrine Disorders

Clement J. Michet, M.D., M.P.H.
Assistant Professor of Medicine, Mayo Medical School, Division of Rheumatology,
Department of Internal Medicine, Mayo Clinic, Rochester, Minnesota
Examination of the Joints

Lewis H. Millender, M.D.
Clinical Professor of Orthopedic Surgery, Tufts University School of Medicine; Assistant Chief, Hand Surgery Service, New England Baptist Hospital, Boston, Massachusetts
Reconstructive Surgery and Rehabilitation of the Hand

G. James Morgan, Jr., M.D., F.A.C.P.
Assistant Professor of Clinical Medicine, Dartmouth Medical School; Acting Chief,
Section of Rheumatology, and Staff Rheumatologist, Mary Hitchcock Memorial Hospital, Hanover, New Hampshire
Panniculitis and Erythema Nodosum

Allen R. Myers, M.D.
Professor and Acting Chairman, Department of Medicine, Temple University School
of Medicine, Philadelphia, Pennsylvania
Septic Arthritis Caused by Bacteria

Kenneth K. Nakano, M.D., M.P.H., S.M., F.R.C.P.(C.), F.A.A.N.A.O.S.-C.
Former Assistant Professor of Neurology, Harvard Medical School; Neurologist,
Straub Clinic and Hospital, Honolulu, Hawaii
Neck Pain; Entrapment Neuropathies

Edward A. Nalebuff, M.D.
Clinical Professor of Orthopedic Surgery, Tufts University School of Medicine; Chief,
Hand Surgery Service, New England Baptist Hospital, Boston, Massachusetts
Reconstructive Surgery and Rehabilitation of the Hand

Thomas C. Namey, M.D., F.A.C.P.
Associate Professor of Medicine and Radiology and Chief, Division of Rheumatology,
Medical College of Ohio; Adjunct Professor, Department of Electrical Engineering,
University of Toledo; Attending Physician and Director of Rheumatology Clinics,
Medical College of Ohio Hospital, Toledo, Ohio
*Nuclear Medicine and Special Radiologic Imaging and Technique in the Diagnosis of
Rheumatic Diseases*

Carl F. Nathan, M.D.
Associate Professor, Rockefeller University; Adjunct Associate Professor, Cornell
University Medical Center, Ithaca, New York
Cellular Components of Inflammation: Monocytes and Macrophages

Charles S. Neer, II, M.D.
Professor of Clinical Orthopaedic Surgery, College of Physicians and Surgeons, Columbia University; Attending Orthopaedic Surgeon and Chief of Adult Reconstruction
Service, New York Orthopaedic Hospital–Columbia-Presbyterian Medical Center;
Chief of Shoulder and Elbow Clinic, New York Orthopaedic Hospital–Columbia-
Presbyterian Medical Center, New York, New York
Reconstructive Surgery and Rehabilitation of the Shoulder

Jose L. Ochoa, M.D., D.Sc.
Professor of Neurology, University of Wisconsin-Madison; Neurologist, University
Hospital and Clinics, Madison, Wisconsin
Peripheral Nerve: Structure, Function, and Dysfunction

J. Desmond O'Duffy, M.D.
Professor of Medicine, Mayo Medical School; Consultant in Medicine, Mayo Clinic; Staff, Methodist Hospital and St. Marys Hospital, Rochester, Minnesota
Behçet's Disease; Multicentric Reticulohistiocytosis

Duncan S. Owen, Jr., M.D.
Professor of Medicine, Medical College of Virginia, Virginia Commonwealth University; Attending Physician, Medical College of Virginia Hospitals and McGuire Veterans Administration Hospital, Richmond, Virginia
Aspiration and Injection of Joints and Soft Tissues

Thomas D. Palella, M.D.
Assistant Professor of Internal Medicine, University of Michigan Medical School; Director of Education and Evaluation, Multipurpose Arthritis Center, University Medical Center, Ann Arbor, Michigan
Purine and Deoxypurine Metabolism

Robert S. Pinals, M.D.
Professor of Medicine and Director, Division of Connective Tissue Diseases, University of Tennessee Center for the Health Sciences; Attending Physician, University of Tennessee Hospital, Veterans Administration Medical Center, Regional Medical Center, and Le Bonheur Childrens Medical Center, Memphis, Tennessee
Felty's Syndrome

Paul H. Plotz, M.D.
Chief, Connective Tissue Diseases Section, Arthritis and Rheumatism Branch National Institute of Arthritis, Diabetes, Digestive, and Kidney Diseases, National Institutes of Health, Bethesda, Maryland
Aspirin and Salicylate

Robert Poss, M.D.
Associate Professor, Orthopedic Surgery, Harvard Medical School; Orthopedic Surgeon, Brigham and Women's Hospital, Boston, Massachusetts
Surgery of the Hip in Rheumatoid Arthritis and Ankylosing Spondylitis

Morris Reichcin, M.D.
Member and Head, Arthritis and Immunology Laboratory, Oklahoma Medical Research Foundation; Professor and Chief, Combined Immunology Section, Department of Medicine, University of Oklahoma Health Sciences Center, Oklahoma City, Oklahoma
Antinuclear Antibodies

Donald Resnick, M.D.
Professor, University of California, San Diego, School of Medicine; Chief of Radiology, San Diego Veterans Administration Hospital; Staff, University Hospital, San Diego, California
Radiographic Evaluation of Articular Disorders

Donald S. Robinson, M.D.
Professor of Pharmacology and Medicine and Chairman, Department of Pharmacology, Marshall University School of Medicine; Attending Physician, Veterans Administration Hospital, Cabell-Huntington Hospital and St. Mary's Hospital, Huntington, West Virginia
Principles of Pharmacodynamics and Pharmacokinetics

Dwight R. Robinson, M.D.
Associate Professor of Medicine, Harvard Medical School; Physician, Massachusetts General Hospital, Boston, Massachusetts
Low Molecular Weight Mediators of Inflammation: Prostaglandins, Leukotrienes, and Cyclic Nucleotides

Naomi Rothfield, M.D.
Professor of Medicine and Chief, Division of Rheumatic Diseases, University of Connecticut School of Medicine; Attending Physician, University Hospital, Farmington, and Veterans Administration Hospital, Newington, Connecticut
Clinical Features of Systemic Lupus Erythematosus

David W. Rowe, M.D.
Associate Professor of Pediatrics, University of Connecticut School of Medicine; Attending Pediatrician, John Dempsey Hospital, University of Connecticut Health Center, Farmington, Connecticut
Heritable Disorders of Connective Tissue

Shaun Ruddy, M.D.
Professor of Medicine, Microbiology and Immunology, and Chairman, Division of Immunology and Connective Tissue Diseases, Medical College of Virginia, Virginia Commonwealth University, Richmond, Virginia
Process and Principles of Inflammation; Plasma Effectors of Inflammation: Complement; The Management of Rheumatoid Arthritis; Complement Deficiencies and the Rheumatic Diseases

Richard I. Rynes, M.D.
Professor of Medicine, Albany Medical College; Attending Physician, Albany Medical Center Hospital, Albany, New York
Antimalarials

Jeremy Saklatvala, Ph.D.
Strangeways Laboratory, Cambridge, England
Proteinases in Joint Disease

Alan L. Schiller, M.D.
Associate Professor of Pathology, Harvard Medical School; Chief, Autopsy, Pathology, and Bone Laboratory, Massachusetts General Hospital; Consultant Pathologist, Brigham and Women's Hospital; Visiting Assistant in Orthopedic Surgery, Children's Hospital Medical Center, Boston, Massachusetts
Tumors and Tumor-like Lesions Involving Joints

Frank R. Schmid, M.D.
Professor of Medicine and Chief, Section of Arthritis–Connective Tissue Diseases, Northwestern University Medical School; Attending Physician, Northwestern Memorial Hospital; Consultant, Rehabilitation Institute of Chicago, Veterans Administration Lakeside Medical Center, and Children's Memorial Hospital, Chicago, Illinois
Approach to Monarticular Arthritis

Thomas J. Schnitzer, M.D., Ph.D.
Associate Professor, University of Michigan Medical School; Attending Physician, University Hospital, Ann Arbor, Michigan
Viral Arthritis

H. Ralph Schumacher, Jr., M.D.
Professor of Medicine, University of Pennsylvania School of Medicine; Director, Rheumatology–Immunology Center, Veterans Administration Medical Center; Staff Rheumatologist, Hospital of the University of Pennsylvania, Philadelphia, Pennsylvania
Synovial Fluid Analysis; Synovial Biopsy and Pathology; Arthritis Associated with Sickle Cell Disease and Other Hemoglobinopathies

Richard D. Scott, M.D.
Assistant Clinical Professor of Orthopedic Surgery, Harvard Medical School; Surgeon, Brigham and Women's Hospital, New England Baptist Hospital, Children's Hospital Medical Center, Boston, Massachusetts
The Surgery of Juvenile Rheumatoid Arthritis

Jerome M. Seyer, Ph.D.
Professor of Biochemistry, University of Tennessee Center for the Health Sciences, Memphis, Tennessee
Structural Proteins: Collagen

Jay R. Shapiro, M.D.
Director, Pratt Diagnostics, Tufts University Medical Center, Boston, Massachusetts; Consultant in Endocrinology, Washington Hospital Center, Seattle, Washington
Heritable Disorders of Connective Tissue

Sheldon R. Simon, M.D.
Associate Professor of Orthopaedics, Harvard Medical School; Director, Rehabilitation Service, Brigham and Women's Hospital; Associate in Orthopedic Surgery, Brigham and Women's Hospital and Children's Hospital; Director, Gait Analysis Laboratory, Children's Hospital, Boston, Massachusetts
Biomechanics of Joints

Frederick R. Singer, M.D.
Professor of Medicine and Orthopaedic Surgery, University of Southern California School of Medicine; Associate Program Director, USPHS General Clinical Research Center, Los Angeles County/University of Southern California Medical Center; Director, Endocrine Laboratory, Orthopaedic Hospital/University of Southern California Bone and Connective Laboratories, Los Angeles, California
Metabolic Bone Disease

Clement B. Sledge, M.D.
John B. and Buckminster Brown Professor of Orthopedic Surgery, Harvard Medical School; Orthopedic Surgeon-in-Chief, Brigham and Women's Hospital, Boston, Massachusetts
Formation and Resorption of Bone; Introduction to the Surgical Management of Arthritis; The Surgery of Juvenile Rheumatoid Arthritis; Surgery of the Hip in Rheumatoid Arthritis and Ankylosing Spondylitis

Hugh A. Smythe, M.D., F.R.C.P.(C.)
Professor and Director, Division of Rheumatology, University of Toronto; Director, Rheumatic Disease Unit, Wellesley Hospital, Toronto, Ontario, Canada
"Fibrositis" and Other Diffuse Musculoskeletal Syndromes

Nicholas A. Soter, M.D.
Professor of Dermatology, New York University School of Medicine; Medical Director, Skin and Cancer Unit, and Attending Physician, University Hospital, New York University Medical Center, New York, New York
Cutaneous Manifestations of Rheumatic Disorders

Steven K. Spencer, M.D.
Associate Professor of Clinical Medicine (Dermatology), Dartmouth Medical School; Staff Physician, Mary Hitchcock Memorial Hospital, Hanover, New Hampshire; Consulting Staff, Veterans Administration Medical Center, White River Junction, and Gifford Memorial Hospital, Randolph, Vermont
Localized Scleroderma–Morphea

Allen C. Steere, M.D.
Associate Professor of Medicine, Department of Internal Medicine, Yale University School of Medicine, New Haven, Connecticut
Lyme Disease

Alfred D. Steinberg, M.D.
Chief, Cellular Immunology Section, Arthritis and Rheumatism Branch, NIADDK, National Institutes of Health, Bethesda, Maryland
Management of Systemic Lupus Erythematosus

Gene H. Stollerman, M.D.
Professor of Medicine, Boston University School of Medicine; Chief, Section of General Medicine, University Hospital, Boston, Massachusetts
Rheumatic Fever

Samuel Strober, M.D.
Professor of Medicine and Chief, Division of Clinical Immunology, Stanford University School of Medicine, Palo Alto, California
Immunologic Aspects of Inflammation: Lymphocyte Populations

William H. Thomas, M.D.
Associate Clinical Professor of Orthopedic Surgery, Harvard Medical School; Orthopedic Surgeon, Brigham and Women's Hospital; Consultant Orthopedic Surgeon, New England Baptist Hospital, Boston, Massachusetts
Reconstructive Surgery and Rehabilitation of the Ankle and Foot

Thomas S. Thornhill, M.D.
Assistant Clinical Professor, Harvard Medical School; Orthopedic Surgeon, Brigham and Women's Hospital and New England Baptist Hospital, Boston, Massachusetts
The Painful Shoulder

Peter D. Utsinger, M.D.
Professor of Clinical Medicine, Temple University School of Medicine; Chief, Immunology, and Director, Research and Development, Germantown Hospital and Medical Center, Philadelphia, Pennsylvania
Enteropathic Arthritis

Stanley L. Wallace, M.D.
Professor of Medicine and Director of the Division of Internal Medicine, State University of New York Downstate Medical Center; Attending Physician, Kings County Hospital and State University Hospital; Rheumatology Consultant, Brooklyn Veterans Administration Hospital, Brooklyn, New York
Colchicine

Barbara N.W. Weissman, M.D.
Associate Professor of Radiology, Harvard Medical School; Director, Bone Radiology Service, Brigham and Women's Hospital, Boston, Massachusetts
Radiographic Evaluation of Total Joint Replacement

Keith Whaley, M.D., Ph.D., F.R.C.P., M.R.C. Path.
Professor of Immunopathology, Department of Pathology, University of Glasgow;
Honorary Consultant in Immunopathology, Western Infirmary, Glasgow, Scotland
Sjögren's Syndrome

Robert J. Winchester, M.D.
Professor of Medicine, Mount Sinai School of Medicine, City University of New York;
Director, Department of Rheumatic Diseases, Hospital for Joint Diseases, Orthopaedic
Institute, New York, New York
The Major Histocompatibility Complex

Bruce Wood, D.P.M.
Associate in Orthopedics (Podiatry), Harvard Medical School; Associate in Orthopedics (Podiatry), Brigham and Women's Hospital; Staff Podiatrist, New England Deaconess Hospital, Boston, Massachusetts
The Painful Foot

Virgil L. Woods, Jr., M.D.
Assistant Professor of Medicine in Residence, School of Medicine, University of
California, San Diego; Physician, University of California Medical Center, San Diego,
California
Etiology and Pathogenesis of Systemic Lupus Erythematosus

V. Wright, M.D., F.R.C.P.
Professor of Rheumatology, University of Leeds Medical School; Consultant Physician
in Rheumatology, Leeds Area Health Authority and Yorkshire Regional Health
Authority, Harrogate, England
Psoriatic Arthritis

Beth Ziebell, Ph.D.
Tucson, Arizona
Psychological and Sexual Health in Rheumatic Disease

Thomas M. Zizic, M.D.
Associate Professor of Medicine, The Johns Hopkins University School of Medicine;
Associate Director, NIADDK Multipurpose Arthritis Center, The Johns Hopkins
University; Assistant Professor of Medicine, Department of Medicine, University of
Maryland; Physician, The Johns Hopkins Hospital and University of Maryland; As-
sociate Director, Rheumatic Disease Unit, The Good Samaritan Hospital; Rheuma-
tology Consultant, Loch Raven Veteran's Administration Hospital and United States
Public Health Service Hospital, Baltimore, Maryland
Osteonecrosis

Nathan J. Zvaifler, M.D.
Professor of Medicine, School of Medicine, University of California, San Diego; Phy-
sician, University of California Medical Center, San Diego, California
Etiology and Pathogenesis of Systemic Lupus Erythematosus

Preface

The field of rheumatology continues to show remarkable progress. An impressive transition has occurred from the empiric approach practiced in spas of the nineteenth century to the multidisciplinary specialty of today. Indeed, the discipline spans the monumental advances in immunogenetics and immunoregulation to the modern miracle of total joint replacement. There are many critical elements in this evolutionary process. Pathologists and orthopedic surgeons such as Goldthwaite, Smith-Peterson, and Wilson began their important work early in this century. In the 1930s, internists such as Bauer, Cecil, Hench, Holbrooke, and Pemberton contributed their creative, scientific, and organizational skills to the embryonic discipline. Societies were created to stimulate the exchange of ideas. The explosion of federal funding for research and the resultant expansion of new scientific information began; remarkable progress occurred.

Over the past three decades, consolidation of efforts in diverse disciplines has provided a truly scientific basis for rheumatology. The basic structure and function of immunoglobulins is now clarified, not only at the protein but also at the gene level. Highly sophisticated techniques have allowed the careful study of specific lymphocyte subpopulations and their role in control of the immune response. A multitude of effectors and the target cells that respond to them as part of the inflammatory process have been defined. The genes coding for these effectors are now being cloned, as are the genes for the receptors on the target cells. Such studies will allow not only an improved understanding of their specific structure but may also eventually allow for the production of effectors in pharmacologic quantities. The relevance of the biochemistry of connective tissue, proteolytic enzymes, glycosaminoglycans, and purines to rheumatology has become increasingly apparent. Critical breakthroughs in bioengineering, matched with sophisticated surgical approaches, have made use of metal and polymer prostheses as replacements for destroyed joints a major factor in reduction of morbidity of these diseases. The exciting breakthroughs in molecular biology highlight the possibility that many of the lymphokines will be available for therapeutic purposes at some point in the near future. Finally, we have come to understand the epidemiology, pathogenesis, and in some cases, etiology of certain connective tissue diseases; the outlook for progress is bright.

In the first edition, the editors paid particularly careful attention to the organization and content. The principal goal was to include a complete spectrum of information necessary for the understanding, differential diagnosis, and management of the patient with the rheumatic complaint. This led to the inclusion of chapters in areas not covered by existing reference books in rheumatology such as the scientific basis of rheumatology, a large section on the general approach to the patient, a full evaluation of the diagnostic tests utilized in the evaluation of patients with rheumatic diseases, as well as extensive coverage of rehabilitation and reconstructive surgery as they relate to rheumatology.

The overall organization of the second edition is very similar to the first in terms of the major sections in the Textbook. The first section deals with the scientific basis of rheumatology and includes a detailed consideration of immunology, immunogenetics, the inflammatory process, the structure and function of connective tissue, the physiology of bones and joints, and purine and deoxypurine metabolism. The second section describes the approach to the patient presenting with rheumatic complaints or with a problem possibly related to an underlying rheumatic disease. Although chapters dealing with this subject matter are difficult to write, they are especially useful to the clinician. In the third section, we review the more important diagnostic tests used in the evaluation of the patient with rheumatic complaints. The clinical pharmacology of the drugs used most often in rheumatology is provided in section four. The next seventeen sections deal with specific diseases. The last three sections of the book focus on medical orthopedics, rehabilitation, and reconstructive surgery. In these latter chapters we have chosen to cover not only the current indications for the various surgical procedures but a brief description of the relevant surgical techniques, potential complications, and appropriate postoperative rehabilitation.

The editors continue to be well aware that the quality of a book such as this relates to the quality of the contributions and, hence, the contributors. We also recognize the importance of a regular turnover of contributors for a book such as this to ensure over a period of several editions that even the best chapters will be updated extensively. In the second edition, we strictly follow this deliberate policy of asking new authors to contribute a substantial fraction of the chapters in the book. This allowed us to cover certain areas with a different approach, including immunogenetics, the biology of inflammation, the major histocompatibility complex, the use of cytotoxic agents, and the understanding of immune complex diseases. In addition, we were able to consolidate several areas of cellular physiology to improve the flow of the text. Even in those chapters where new authors were not selected, we were pleased to see a substantial updating and, where possible, on improvement in quality. The editors are highly pleased with the final product.

The expertise of the professionals with whom we worked at W. B. Saunders throughout the preparation of this book continued to be impressive to us. We benefited from the assistance of Mr. Jack Hanley, who as President and Publisher helped us to conceive of the second edition aboard the sloop Windlove off the Maine coast near Damariscove during the summer of 1982. Subsequently we worked closely with Mr. Dereck Jeffers. Further work on the book required several site visits to places such as the "R Lazy S" Dude Ranch in Jackson Hole, Wyoming. Others of considerable help to us included Mr. Robert Butler, Production Supervisor, and Mr. William Donnelly, Designer. Their help was obviously necessary and deeply appreciated. We also wish to express our thanks to our teachers and to our students from whom we have learned as well as to our colleagues at our institutions for their patience and understanding with respect to the time demands that the development of this textbook placed upon us. Finally, we wish to thank our secretaries and editorial assistants, including Candace Johnson, Linda Newman, Ollie May Lee, and Phyllis White, who have been of unmeasurable value.

WILLIAM N. KELLEY, M.D.

EDWARD D. HARRIS, JR., M.D.

SHAUN RUDDY, M.D.

CLEMENT B. SLEDGE, M.D.

Contents

Contents

Figure 26-1A

Figure 26-1B

Figure 26-1C

PLATE 1

Figure 26–1. Bunnel's sign. This sign is used to distinguish synovitis of the proximal interphalangeal joint from spasm of the intrinsic muscles due to metacarpophalangeal synovitis as the cause of decreased motion of the proximal interphalangeal joint. *A,* With the metacarpophalangeal joint extended, decreased flexion of the proximal interphalangeal joint is noted. If normal flexion is noted (i.e., the tip of the finger can touch the volar pad), then involvement of all three joints (metacarpophalangeal, proximal interphalangeal, and distal intraphalangeal) is excluded. *B,* With the metacarpophalangeal joint flexed, the contracted intrinsic muscles are relaxed. Restricted motion with the metacarpophalangeals flexed therefore is indicative of proximal interphalangeal involvement. *C,* Normal proximal interphalangeal motion when the metacarpophalangeal joints are flexed indicates that the prior proximal interphalangeal restriction was due to intrinsic muscle contracture, presumably caused by metacarpophalangeal synovitis.

Figure 35–1

Figure 35–4

Figure 35–1. Keratoconjunctivitis sicca. Intense hyperemia of the conjunctival vessels accounts for the prominent redness. Dryness of the corneal epithelium causes the reflection from the photographic flash to be dull and irregular rather than normally sharp and highly polished.

Figure 35–4. Severe episcleritis involving the temporal aspect of the right eye in the region of the interpalpebral fissure. Congestion of the episcleral vessels accounts for the bright red appearance.

Figure 35–5. Necrotizing scleritis. *B,* Same patient as shown in *A* (p. 516), 2 weeks later. The eye is adducted and slightly elevated. Further destruction of sclera has rendered visible the underlying ciliary body, which has a bluish-gray color.

Figure 35–15. Wegener's granulomatosis. Deep ring ulcer in corneal periphery supratemporally in patient with previously undiagnosed Wegener's granulomatosis. Note also the episcleritis adjacent to the corneal lesion. Necrotizing scleritis developed in this area within several weeks after the photograph was made.

Figure 35–20. Amyloidosis of the vitreous body. On ophthalmoscopic examination the retina inferonasal to the left optic nerve head is partially obscured by a grayish-white, veil-like, opaque accumulation of amyloid in the vitreous body.

Figure 35–5B

Figure 35–15

Figure 35–20

PLATE 2

Figure 36-10B

Figure 36-11

Figure 59-16

Figure 59-23

PLATE 3

Figure 36–10. Necrotizing venulitis. *B.* Close-up view of the lesions.

Figure 36–11. Necrotizing venulitis. Circumscribed area of edema (urticaria).

Figure 59–16. The collagen matrix of cartilage at this pannus/cartilage junction stains darkly. The pale area represents destroyed cartilage in the perimeter around an invasive cell which has many thin cell processes (accentuated by a modification of a trichrome stain), which may be the "in vivo equivalent" of stellate cells seen on cell cultures of dissociated rheumatoid synovial tissue. (Courtesy of Fred Meyer, M.D.)

Figure 59–23. Trichrome stain of a micronodule within a larger rheumatoid nodule. Radially arranged strands of collagen separate large histiocytes. The central necrotic area is composed of cellular debris, fibrin, and collagen fragments.

Figure 38-4

Figure 38-2

Figure 38-2. Synovial fluid rice bodies containing fibrin and debris from degenerated villi are especially common in rheumatoid arthritis but can also be seen in other conditions such as tuberculous arthritis.

Figure 38-4. Shards of golden or ochre cartilage fragments embedded in detached synovium found floating in synovial fluid in a patient with ochronotic arthropathy.

Figure 38-5. Monosodium urate crystals from a gouty synovial fluid as viewed with compensated polarized light. The crystals are yellow parallel to the axis of slow vibration marked on the compensator (negative birefringence).

Figure 38-6. CPPD crystals can be needle, rod, or rhomboid shaped but usually have blunt ends (*A*). They often have fainter birefringence than is seen with urates (*B*). CPPD are blue when aligned longitudinally with the axis of slow vibration of the compensator (positive birefringence).

Figure 38-5

Figure 38-6 A

Figure 38-6 B

PLATE 4

Figure 38–7

Figure 38–8

Figure 38–9

Figure 38–10

PLATE 5

Figure 38–7. Triamcinolone acetonide (Aristospan) crystals phagocytized by synovial fluid cells after intra-articular injection.

Figure 38–8. Cholesterol crystals from a chronic rheumatoid olecranon bursal effusion. These are most often flat plates with notched corners.

Figure 38–9. Synovial lining cell. The prominent homogeneous blue cytoplasm is typical of type B or synthetic cells. Other large cells with nucleus:cytoplasm ratio of less than 50 percent have vacuolated cytoplasm and are either phagocytic lining cells or large monocytes (macrophages).

Figure 38–10. Synovial fluid small lymphocytes with one activated lymphocyte, the larger cell with nucleus filling most of the cytoplasm.

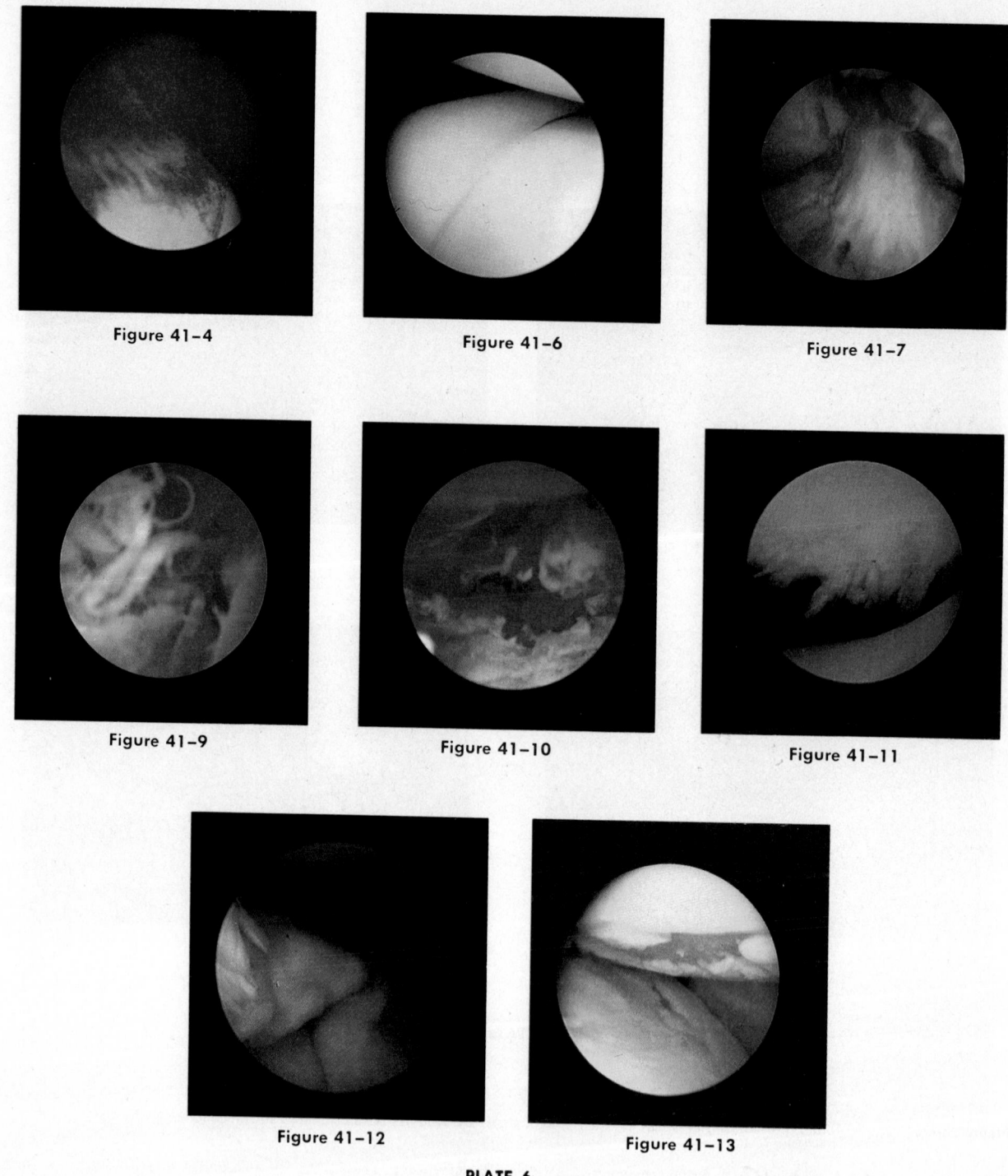

Figure 41–4

Figure 41–6

Figure 41–7

Figure 41–9

Figure 41–10

Figure 41–11

Figure 41–12

Figure 41–13

PLATE 6

Figure 41–4. Normal synovium. Note details of vascular pattern.

Figure 41–6. Normal medial meniscus, left knee. Femoral condyle above, tibia below.

Figure 41–7. Anterior cruciate ligament in intercondylar notch, proximal attachment above.

Figure 41–9. Rheumatoid arthritis with proliferative, injected synovial villi.

Figure 41–10. Acute pyogenic arthritis with fibrous debris, granular exudate in superior surface of meniscus, and loss of articular cartilage on femur.

Figure 41–11. Chondromalacia patellae.

Figure 41–12. Bucket handle tear of medial meniscus looking into apex of tear where torn fragment leaves rim.

Figure 41–13. Chondromalacia. Medial femoral condyle with exposed subchondral bone. Note changes on tibia. These changes represent a postmeniscectomy degenerative change in the medial compartment.

Figure 42–4

Figure 42–5

Figure 42–6

Figure 42–8

Figure 42–9

PLATE 7

Figure 42–4. Normal synovial membrane of the knee. There is a single layer of flattened synovial cells overlying areolar connective tissue. Note the small synovial vessels immediately under the lining layer and the larger vessel in the lower right corner. × 100. Hematoxylin and eosin stain.

Figure 42–5. Rheumatoid arthritis synovium showing many layers of synovial lining cells on the left and infiltration of lymphocytes and plasm cells on the right. × 100. Hematoxylin and eosin stain.

Figure 42–6. Synovial membrane in early scleroderma shows massive superficial fibrin, loss of lining cells, and infiltration with lymphocytes and plasma cells. × 100. Hematoxylin and eosin stain.

Figure 42–8. Granuloma in superficial synovium in tuberculous arthritis. Some superficial granulomas such as this one do not show caseation. There is also scattered chronic inflammatory cell infiltration. × 100. Hematoxylin and eosin stain.

Figure 42–9. Tophus-like deposits in synovium containing positively birefringent crystals in pseudogout. × 100. Hematoxylin and eosin stain.

Figure 42–10

Figure 42–11

Figure 42–12

Figure 42–13

PLATE 8

Figure 42–10. Amyloid arthritis as seen here in a patient with multiple myeloma is characterized by Congo red staining on the surface and sparing the synovial vessels (V). × 100. Congo red stain.

Figure 42–11. Dark, angular cartilage shards pigmented brown with homogentisic acid polymer are embedded in ochronotic synovium. Note also a giant cell (arrow) and mild proliferation of synovial lining cells. × 400. Hematoxylin and eosin stain.

Figure 42–12. Iron stain of synovial membrane in idiopathic hemochromatosis shows blue (dark) staining predominantly in the lining cells. × 100. Prussian blue stain.

Figure 42–13. Pigmented villonodular synovitis is characterized by golden brown hemosiderin in deep macrophages, giant cells (marked by arrows), monotonous proliferation of deep cells with pale nuclei, and, not illustrated here, foam cells, lining cell hyperplasia (dark), and villous proliferation. × 400. Hematoxylin and eosin stain. (Courtesy of Schumacher, H.R.: Sem. Arthritis Rheum. 12:32, 1982.)

Figure 69–2

Figure 69–3

Figure 69–5

Figure 69–9

Figure 69–12

Figure 69–2. Extensive discoid lesion in the scalp. The lesion is inactive. Note hyperpigmented margins.

Figure 69–3. Active hyperkeratotic discoid lesion, which may be confused with hypertrophic psoriasis or lichen planus.

Figure 69–5. Vasculitic lesions. Note periungual involvement and vasculitic lesions on tip of the fourth finger.

Figure 69–9. Large superficial mucosal ulcer on hard palate.

Figure 69–12. Green granules in the dermal-epidermal junction of nonlesional skin from an SLE patient, stained with anti-IgG conjugated to fluorescein isothiocyanate. Dermis (top) has pinkish autofluorescence.

PLATE 9

Figure 74–1

Figure 74–2

Figure 74–3

Figure 74–4

Figure 77–1

Figure 74–1. Painful oral aphtha of the upper lip; an erythematous border surrounds a necrotic yellow ulcer. (Photo provided by Dr. R. Rogers III.)

Figure 74–2. Vaginal aphthous ulcer. This asymptomatic vaginal ulcer was discovered on routine pelvic examination of a patient presenting with polyarthritis, oral aphthae, and visual symptoms. (From O'Duffy, J.D., et al.: Ann. Intern. Med. 75:561, 1971.)

Figure 74–3. Hypopyon, or pus in the anterior chamber, is clearly shown as a yellow segment in front of the iris at 6 o'clock. Previously common in Behçet's disease, anterior uveitis of this severity is now uncommon. (Courtesy of Dr. Dennis Robertson.)

Figure 74–4. Ocular fundus demonstrating inflammation of the optic nerve head with retinal infarction and hemorrhage. The medium is cloudy because of vitreous cellular infiltration associated with posterior uveitis. (Courtesy of Dr. M. Colvard.)

Figure 77–1. Localized plaque of morphea, showing ivory-colored center with wrinkled surface and surrounding telangiectasia and hyperpigmentation.

PLATE 10

xliv

Figure 79–8

Figure 79–9C

Figure 95–1

Figure 122–14C

Figure 79–8. The eye of the patient in Figure 79–7 (p. 1235) 2½ years after the previous photograph, showing a severe relapse of the skin rash and ulceration of the skin.

Figure 79–9. *C,* View of a 15-year-old boy with severe dermatomyositis, showing a very extensive skin rash of the knuckles in the characteristic distribution despite 3 months of treatment with prednisone.

Figure 95–1. Reddish-brown nodules on dorsum of hands and around nail folds.

Figure 122–14. Subtraction technique. *C,* Color subtraction (different patient from *A* and *B* (p. 1952)). Contrast fills a normal pseudocapsule. Filling of the trochanteric bursa suggests trochanteric bursitis. There is no evidence of component loosening.

PLATE 11

Section I
Scientific Bases of Rheumatology

Chapter 1
Process and Principles of Inflammation

Shaun Ruddy

INTRODUCTION

Although rheumatologists are occupied with lessening the redness, heat, pain, and swelling of inflammation, the ability of an organism to recognize a foreign or injurious stimulus and to defend against it is essential to survival. As every physician quickly learns, the more aggressive and potent is the pharmacologic attempt to suppress this reaction, the more defenseless is the resulting host. The widespread prescription of nonspecific anti-inflammatory agents substitutes for the use of specific remedies based on knowledge of the proximate or ultimate causes of rheumatic diseases. The availability of antimicrobials significantly diminished the fervor with which antipyretics were administered to patients with pneumonia. As knowledge about the etiologies of the rheumatic diseases increases and specific treatments directed at the causes are developed, the use of nonspecific anti-inflammatory agents will also wane.

Different kinds of inflammation and repair produce widely disparate manifestations. Time courses range from the few hours required for the development of florid acute gouty or septic arthritis to the many years involved in the chronic progressive fibrosis of scleroderma. Distribution in space may range from the single distal interphalangeal joint involved in psoriatic arthritis to the life-threatening multisystem involvement with which systemic lupus erythematosus may present. While it might be argued that such variations and complexities preclude any useful summary of inflammation, the process may be subjected to systematic analysis. This chapter will provide that analysis, a framework within which to place the detailed descriptions of the components of inflammation contained in the next 20 chapters.

THE PROCESS OF INFLAMMATION

The components of the inflammatory process are diagrammed in Figure 1–1. These include the *selectors,* which serve to locate the abnormal area of injury or invasion, and the *detectors,* which transduce the signal from a selector to one or more *delivery* vehicles. *Effector* systems delivered to the selected area catalyze reactions that are almost exclusively hydrolytic in nature—the addition of a water molecule to a covalent bond such as the peptide of a protein (Fig.1–2), the ester of a lipid (Fig. 1–3), or glycoside of a polysaccharide (Fig. 1–4).[1] Though not central to the process of inflammation, inhibiting or *controlling* factors that retard the rate and extent of the process[2] are of sufficient importance to warrant being shown in Figure 1–1. Similarly, the *resynthesis* phase, in which the hydrolyzed materials are replaced either appropriately (repair) or inappropriately (fibrosis), is not integral to inflammation but an important consequence. Since the final effectors are chiefly enzymes that catalyze hydrolytic reactions, an energy source for the process is also required. Normal body heat, which is often increased locally in the area of inflammation due to increased rate of blood flow, is one energy source. Mechanical pressure in tissues, also increased because of loss of vascular integrity with flow of water, proteins, and other solutes into the extravascular space in the area of tissue inflammation, is another potential source. Finally, nutrients and oxygen, normally used by cells that localize to the inflamed area, are most important. Inflammatory cells require energy for locomotion, phagocytosis, and synthesis of reactive metabolites.[3] In some instances, especially in body cavities not adequately supplied with blood vessels, evidence of anaerobiosis, such as increased lactate and reduced pH, or evidence of nutrient depletion, such as low glucose levels, may be found.[4]

Selectors. These elements specify the area in which the inflammation will occur. Some examples are listed in Table 1–1. While the most obviously specific are antibody, or the antibody-like antigen-binding sites on the surface of T lymphocytes (see Chapters 2 and 3), a number of nonimmunologic elements may select the area of inflammation. Contact of the plasma protein Hageman factor with negatively charged surfaces initiates the

Figure 1–1. The inflammatory process.

kinin-forming, coagulation, and fibrinolytic cascades (see Chapter 8). Recognition by the alternative pathway for complement activation of bacterial polysaccharides or other foreign materials involves assembly of the complement enzymes on the activating surface so that they are protected from dissociation by the control protein, Factor H (see Chapter 7). Mechanical or ischemic damage may specify the locale for inflammation by releasing materials from cells resident in the damaged area. Degranulation of tissue mast cells with release of low molecular weight mediators into the surrounding area is responsible for the wheal and flare that follows stroking of the skin. Intracellular proteases liberated following ischemic death of myocardial cells are capable of acting on plasma substrates, e.g., the fifth complement component, to form chemotactic factors.[5] Although inflammation may occur in a totally denervated extremity or organ, areas of inflammation may be specified by neurologic control, perhaps by regulating or perturbating vascular dynamics or by altering chemical or electrical potentials.

Antibodies or other immunologic selectors may specify not only the locale but also the character of the reaction that ensues. Union of antigen with IgE antibody molecules bound to the surface of a basophil results in the secretion of mediators of the immediate allergic reaction. Union of antigen with IgG or IgM antibody to form immune complexes may trigger the complement system and cause the changes of subacute tissue damage and vasculitis. Union of antigen with antibody-like antigen-binding sites on the surface of T lymphocytes initiates the formation and secretion of lymphokines, which signal the development of a delayed hypersensitivity reaction. Similar effects of the selector on the nature of the inflammation that follows seem likely for the nonimmunologic selecting elements, but these have not been as thoroughly studied.

Detectors. These elements monitor the status of the selectors—which may be viewed as a set of switches—

detect those that are "turned on," and transduce this signal to the delivery system. A clear example of a detector is the C1q subunit of the first complement component. This protein has six sites which are capable of weak interactions with native IgG or IgM; such binding has no effect on the remainder of the C1 complex or the complement system.[6] If the IgG or IgM is combined with antigen or in an aggregated state, however, then the multivalent binding of the C1q subunit results in the internal proteolysis of C1 and activation of the remaining components.[7] Receptors for plasma proteins or their fragments present on cell membranes constitute a large class of detectors.[8] Only recently have some of the mechanisms by which these membrane proteins function been elucidated. For example, the receptor sites on mast cells for IgE antibodies signal the "triggered" state when they are aggregated. Usually this occurs when antibody molecules occupying the receptor sites are bridged by antigen, but direct cross-linking of the detectors by antireceptor antibody also opens a calcium channel and results in mediator secretion.[9] Other cell membrane receptors that serve as detectors are those for the Fc end of IgG and for fragments of complement proteins. There must also be proteins in the membranes of lymphocytes that detect the union of antigen with specific binding sites on these cells and trigger the release of lymphokines or other events. Finally, plasma protein substrates of such activatable selectors as Hageman factor may transduce the signal to the delivery system (Chapter 8).[10]

Delivery. Ultimately the means of delivery of the effectors of inflammation is the vasculature (Chapter 13). Avascular tissues such as cornea, sclera, or articular cartilage do not manifest florid inflammatory reactions until they have been invaded by vascular granulation tissue. Locally, delivery involves the movement of cells and plasma proteins or other solutes from within the intravascular compartment into the extravascular one. A large number of parallel mechanisms have evolved for accomplishing these movements into areas specified by the selectors. The mechanisms are triggered by the detectors.

Observations of the microvasculature identify alterations in blood flow through an inflamed area as one of the earliest changes.[11] The total blood flow through the tissue is increased, chiefly owing to opening of preferential channels connecting arterioles and venules. Flow through the capillaries, however, becomes stagnated, owing to a generalized relaxation of capillary sphincters. Normal laminar streaming is disrupted and leukocytes that usually roll along the endothelium slow down, so that the vessel wall becomes coated with these cells, thus further slowing capillary flow. Simultaneous with these changes, increased permeability of the vessels occurs, allowing egress of plasma proteins and resulting in the loss of oncotic pressure within the vessel lumen due to the normal intravascular location of these proteins; egress of water and other solutes also ensues.[12] These initial steps in delivery are usually attributed to the low molecular weight mediators of inflammation, including histamine, serotonin (in some species), bradykinin, and

PROTEOLYSIS

Figure 1–2. A general equation for the hydrolysis of peptide bonds.

Figure 1–3. An example of lipolysis: the hydrolysis of phospholipid.

Table 1–1. Selectors of the Inflammatory Process

Immunologic
  Antibody (IgG, IgM, IgA, or IgE)
  Antigen-binding sites on surfaces of cells
Nonimmunologic
  Hageman factor
  β1H globulin
  Tissue cells which secrete mediators
  Tissue cells which release proteases
  Nerve cells or smooth muscle of vasculature(?)

arachidonate metabolites, including prostaglandins and leukotrienes.[13] The primary site of action of many of these materials within the vasculature appears to be the small venule. Sequential action of these mediators appears likely, since in many experimental models antihistaminics block permeability changes seen within the first few minutes, whereas inhibitors of prostaglandin synthesis suppress changes observed from 1 to 24 hours later.

The same opening-up of clefts between endothelial cells that allows escape of plasma proteins, water, and solutes also permits the delivery of leukocytes into the inflamed area.[14] In contrast to the egress of proteins, which may be viewed as a passive phenomenon conse-

quent to change in pore size and pressure, the emigration of leukocytes is an active process. A variety of chemotactic factors (Chapter 9) attract leukocytes into the area. These include bacterial products, active enzymes of the complement and kinin-forming systems, fragments of complement components, and peptides released by mast cells or lymphocytes. Some of these factors attract a number of different types of cells, whereas others tend to specify a particular type, such as eosinophils.[16] All have in common the property of inducing migration of their target cells in the direction of the chemical gradient of the chemotactic factor. Once located in the area of inflammation, the cells may be induced to remain there either by the absence of any further chemotactic factor gradient or by other proteins, such as macrophage migration inhibition factor,[17] which actively reduce their mobility.

Effectors. With the exception of the amphipathic terminal complement component complex[18] and reactive oxygen metabolites, which can cause damage by nonenzymatic means, all effects of inflammation can be reduced to hydrolysis of proteins, lipids, or carbohydrates. An example of each of these is diagrammed in Figures 1–2, 1–3, and 1–4. The enzymes that catalyze these reactions are usually brought to the inflammatory site

HYDROLYSIS OF POLYSACCHARIDES

Figure 1–4. An example of the hydrolysis of glycosidic bonds: hyaluronic acid digestion by hyaluronidase.

packaged within cells. Although such hydrolytic reactions are effective in defense against the invading parasite, they may destroy host tissues as well. Proteolysis of collagen, elastin, and other structural proteins is central to the destruction of supporting tissues such as bone cartilage and basement membrane seen in many rheumatic diseases (Chapters 12 and 14). The hydrolysis of lipids, e.g., phospholipids of cell membranes, with the mobilization of arachidonic acid and formation of prostaglandins, leukotrienes, and related agents, is clearly important to the destructive changes observed with inflammation. Secondary damage mediated by lysophosphatides formed during the process of lipolysis may also contribute. Finally, disruption of glycosidic linkages, which contributes to the destruction of cartilage, may also have direct effects on cell function when the carbohydrates being hydrolyzed are parts of membrane glycoproteins.

All the hydrolyses catalyzed by the effector enzymes are essentially irreversible; proteins, for example, are not reassembled by condensation reactions among the polypeptides into which they have been hydrolyzed. The same is true of the lipids and carbohydrates. De novo resynthesis of the hydrolyzed molecule is, therefore, required for repair of tissue damage consequent to inflammation. The extent of the damage in part governs the success of the reparative resynthesis in reproducing the original tissue. In particular, loss of framework or structural molecules appears important. In viral hepatitis, for example, extensive hepatocellular necrosis may occur, but complete repair ensues provided the underlying reticulin and collagen framework of the lobules has not been destroyed. Once collapse of the framework has occurred, the disorganized and fibrotic reaction of postnecrotic cirrhosis is the consequence.[19] Similarly, once the hyaline cartilage lining a joint is lost, "resynthesis" implies replacement by fibrocartilage. In some diseases, such as scleroderma, an uncontrolled or exuberant fibrotic reparative process appears to be the major pathogenic feature.

COMMON THEMES IN THE INFLAMMATORY PROCESS

Although the intensity, extent, and even the pathways involved may vary greatly from one rheumatic disease to another, a systematic view of inflammation as a process immediately makes apparent certain principles that apply to every form, whether it be an acute allergic response or a chronic granulomatous process. Some of these principles are listed in Table 1-2. The knowledge that the final effects of inflammation are almost exclusively hydrolytic and irreversible implies that these effector mechanisms must exist in a *precursor or protected form*. The alternative would be rampant proteolysis, lipolysis, and hydrolysis of saccharides. Two general mechanisms for maintaining this inactive precursor state exist. In the first, the enzyme in question circulates as an inactive proenzyme which is cleaved by a limited

Table 1–2. General Principles of Inflammation

1. Effectors exist in precursor form—
   activated by proteolysis in fluid phase
   packaged in intracellular vesicles and released
2. Controls modulate the process—
   at the level of delivery mechanisms
   at the level of effectors
3. Alternative pathways reach the same biologic end (redundancy)
4. Feedback loops amplify detection or delivery
5. Interactive network is representative

proteolytic reaction to form an active protease. This mechanism is especially prevalent in delivery cascades such as complement, kinin-forming, and coagulation systems. The second, and more common, involves the "packaging" of hydrolytic enzymes within intracellular vesicles, or lysosomes (Chapter 9).[20]

A second principle implicit in effector function is the existence of *controlling or modulating influences,* which serve to dampen the inflammatory effects and to limit their extent. A number of different plasma proteins that inhibit the delivery cascades have been described.[21] Not infrequently deficiency of such a protein leads to undesirable spontaneous activation of the delivery system. Other plasma proteins inhibit the hydrolytic effector proteolytic enzymes. Deficiency of alpha-1 antitrypsin, the plasma protein effective in inhibiting leukocyte elastase, is associated with premature pulmonary emphysema and other effects that have been attributed to uncontrolled digestion of the structural protein elastin.[22]

The existence of multiple factors, all of which attract leukocytes, is an excellent example of the *multiplicity of pathways* leading to a common biologic event. There are many others, such as the duplicate pathways leading to activation of the coagulation cascade, or the two pathways, classic and alternative, leading to activation of the terminal complement sequence. The survival value of such duplication is readily apparent, and the existence of apparently healthy individuals with isolated deficiencies of a single pathway constituent bears witness to its usefulness (Chapter 85).

The existence of *feedback loops* is by no means unique to the process of inflammation, but their multiplicity and their tendency to have a positive or amplifying effect in inflammation are remarkable. At the level of the delivery systems, the feedback effects within the Hageman factor-dependent systems are extremely complex. The alternative complement pathway is primarily an amplification loop.[23] Interactions between cellular products and fluid-phase constituents also frequently have positive feedback effects. The number and variety of amplifying loops in the inflammatory process make especially clear the importance of the controlling or modulating influences mentioned above.

Finally, the foregoing analysis of the inflammatory process (Fig. 1–1) tends to give the impression of a simple linear system with a beginning, a middle, and an end. It should already be clear from the multiple pathways, the modulation by controls, the feedbacks, and the precursor forms that the process of inflammation is much more correctly represented by a complex interactive multilevel network. Although many of these interactions have been defined, the rate constants or other parameters allowing quantification or precise representation of the most important interactions are not yet available, even for a single segment of the system. The complexities of this interactive network will become readily apparent as the next 20 chapters are read.

References

1. Weissmann, G., Serhan, C., Korchak, H.M., and Smolen, J.E.: Neutrophils: Release of mediators of inflammation with special reference to rheumatoid arthritis. Ann. N.Y. Acad. Sci. 389:11, 1982.
2. Ruddy, S.: Function of the control proteins of the classical and alternative complement activation pathways. *In* Thompson, R.A. (ed.): Recent Advances in Clinical Immunology. London, Churchill Livingstone, 1980, pp. 91–111.
3. Weisdorf, D.S., Craddock, P.R., and Jacob, H.S.: Granulocytes utilize different energy sources for movement and phagocytosis. Inflammation 6:245, 1982.
4. Falchuk, K.H., Goetzl, E.J., and Kulka, J.P.: Respiratory gases of synovial fluids. Am. J. Med. 49:223, 1970.
5. Hugli, T.E.: The structural basis for anaphylatoxin and chemotactic functions of C3a, C4a, and C5a C.R.C. Crit. Rev. Immunol. 1:321, 1981.
6. Reid, K.B.M.: Proteins involved in the activation and control of the two pathways of human complement. Biochem. Soc. Trans. 11:1, 1983.
7. Ziccardi, R.J., and Cooper, N.R.: Activation of C1r by proteolytic cleavage. J. Immunol. 116:504, 1976.
8. Bianco, C., and Nussenzweig, V.: Complement receptors. Contemp. Top. Mol. Immunol. 68:145, 1977.
9. Ishizaka, T., Ishizaka, K., Conrad, D.H., and Froese, A.H.: A new concept of triggering mechanisms of IgE-mediated histamine release. J. Allergy Clin. Immunol. 61:320, 1978.
10. Kaplan, A.P., Silverberg, M., Dunn, J.P., and Ghebrehiwet, B.: Interaction of the clotting, kinin-forming, complement and fibrinolytic pathways in inflammation. Ann. N.Y. Acad. Sci. 389:25, 1982.
11. Cotran, R.S., and Majno, G.: A light and electron microscopic analysis of vascular injury. Ann. N.Y. Acad. Sci. 116:750, 1964.
12. Intaglietta, M., Pawula, R.F., and Tompkins, W.R.: Pressure measurements in the mammalian microvasculature. Microvasc. Res. 2:212, 1970.
13. Samuelsson, B.: Leukotrienes: mediators of allergic reactions and inflammation. Int. Arch. Allergy Appl. Immunol. 66(Suppl. 1):98, 1981.
14. Marchesi, V.T., and Florey, H.W.: Electron microscopic observations on the emigration of leukocytes. Quart. J. Exp. Physiol. 45:343, 1960.
15. Ward, P.A.: Leukotactic factors in health and disease. Am. J. Pathol. 64:521, 1971.
16. Kay, A.B., Stechschulte, D.J., and Austen, K.F.: An eosinophil leukocyte chemotactic factor of anaphylaxis. J. Exp. Med. 133:602, 1971.
17. David, J.R.: Lymphocyte mediators and cellular hypersensitivity. N. Engl. J. Med. 288:143, 1973.
18. Mayer, M.M., Hammer, C.H., Michaels, D.W., and Shin, M.I.: Immunologically mediated membrane damage: The mechanism of complement action and the similarity of lymphocyte-mediated cytotoxicity. Immunochemistry 15:813, 1978.
19. Boyer, J.L., and Klatskin, G.: Pattern of necrosis in acute viral hepatitis: Prognostic value of bridging (subacute hepatic necrosis). N. Engl. J. Med. 283:1063, 1970.
20. Goldstein, I.: Lysosomal hydrolases and inflammatory materials. *In* Weissman, G. (ed.): The Plasma Proteins. New York, Academic Press, 1975, p. 51.
21. Laurell, C.B., and Jeppsson, J.: Protease inhibitors in plasma. *In* Putnam, F.W. (ed.): The Plasma Proteins. New York, Academic Press, 1975, p. 229.
22. Janoff, A., and Carp, H.: Proteases, antiproteases and oxidants: Pathways of tissue injury during inflammation. Monogr. Pathol. 23:163, 1982.
23. Kazatchkine, M.D., and Nydegger, U.E.: The human alternative complement pathway: Biology and immunopathology of activation and regulation. Prog. Allergy 30:193, 1982.

Chapter 2
Immunoglobulins and Their Genes

Blas Frangione and Joel N. Buxbaum

INTRODUCTION

The elucidation of the molecular mechanisms responsible for the origin of antibody diversity has been a scientific challenge of long standing. The answer to this problem resides in the genes that code for the polypeptide chains of which antibody molecules are composed. For many years scientists who were looking for the answer had to examine the structure of a large number of myeloma proteins and then reason backward to work out the genetic arrangements that could best explain the structures. In the last few years, as a result of the development of techniques for probing genes, nucleotide sequence analysis, and more efficient determination and comparison of the amino acid sequence of proteins, investigators are acquiring the kind of information they need to unravel the mystery of antibody diversity: how is a single animal able to make more than a million different antibodies. This chapter discusses the structure and function of immunoglobulin molecules and explains how antibody diversity is generated.

HUMAN IMMUNOGLOBULINS: NOMENCLATURE AND CLASSIFICATION

The symbol Ig is used to designate immunoglobulins. There are five classes of immunoglobulin molecules in man (Table 2–1): IgG, IgA, IgM, IgD, and IgE. They have the same basic four-chain structure: two heavy (H) and two light (L) chains (H_2L_2). The H chain in each immunoglobulin is class specific, and it is designated by the corresponding Greek letter, as shown in Table 2–1. They differ in length, disulfide bridge pattern, number of domains, degree of polymerization, amino acid sequence, and number and kind of oligosaccharides. IgG and IgA can be further divided into subclasses based on specific antigenic determinants present on the H chains. Subclasses are indicated by arabic numerals following the letter denoting the class. The corresponding H chains are named γ_1, γ_2, γ_3, γ_4, and α_1 and α_2, respectively.

Table 2-1. Human Immunoglobulins

Isotypes	Molecular Weight	Serum Level (mg/ml)	Carbohydrate (%)	Half-life (days)	L Chain (common)	H Chain (unique)	Subclasses of H Chain	Genetic Markers (alleles)*	
								C+	N, M
IgG	150,000	12	2.5	25	κ or λ	γ(gamma)	γ1 γ2 γ3 γ4	Za · fa⁻ n⁻ : n g : b 4a · 4b	Za n⁻ b 4a
IgA	160,000–350,000	2	8	6	κ or λ	α(alpha)	α1 α2	A2m(1) · A2m(2)	A2m(2)
IgM	900,000	1	10	5	κ or λ	μ(mu)			
IgD	160,000	0.03	10	3	κ or λ	δ(delta)			
IgE	180,000	0.0003	12	2	κ or λ	ε(epsilon)			

+C: Caucasian; N: Negro; M: Mongoloid

*Alternative nomenclature (1,2)

Gm z,a	= G1m (17,1)	Gm fa⁻	= G1m (3,N1)
Gm n	= G2m (23)		
Gm g	= G3m (21)	Gmb	= G3n (5)
Gm 4a	= G4m (N4a)	Gm4b	= G4m (N4b)

L chains exist in two different types, kappa (κ) and lambda (λ), which can be readily distinguished immunologically. They are not class specific, and both types occur in all classes. In human serum, the number of immunoglobulins containing κ chains is approximately twice that of those bearing λ chains. Subclasses have been found only for the λ type, and at present they are identified in terms of the specific markers that distinguish them.[1,2]

The different classes, subclasses, and types of immunoglobulin polypeptide chains are called *isotypes*. They are present in all individuals, and they are the products of different structural genes. Two of the Ig classes contain other nonhomologous chains. IgA in external secretions is dimeric and contains a chain not present in serum IgA. The additional polypeptide chain is called secretory component (SC), and the entire molecule is termed secretory IgA (sIgA).[3] Furthermore, polymeric immunoglobulins (IgM, IgA, and sIgA molecules) contain an antigenically and physicochemically distinctive polypeptide termed the J chain.[4]

VARIABLE AND CONSTANT REGIONS

Each immunoglobulin chain consists of two regions. One is designated the variable (V) region; the other, the constant (C) region. The V region is the amino terminal portion of the L and H chain (about 110 to 120 residues) and is made up of many different amino acid sequences, even within one class or subclass. On the other hand, the C region is the carboxyl terminal portion of the chain and has the same primary structure as all other chains of the same class, subclass, and type. The particular immunoglobulin chain in which these regions are studied is designated by subscripts, e.g., V_L, C_L, V_H, C_H. The C regions of κ and λ chains contain 110 residues; the C regions of γ, α, and δ chains are three times larger; and the C regions of μ and ϵ chains are four times larger. The various V and C regions are homologous in structure and evolutionarily related. Owing to their amino acid sequence and the presence of one intrachain disulfide bond, each homology region folds in a somewhat similar conformation, a compact globular

domain. The average amount of homology of all domains is about 25 percent, although the degree of homology varies from domain to domain. This shows that individual domains of L and H chains evolved with different mutation rates from a common primordial gene.

β_2 Microglobulin

β_2Microglobulin ($\beta_2 M$) is a protein of low molecular weight (11,800 daltons) present in small amounts in normal urine, serum, and other biological fluids. It is synthesized by all nucleated cells and is present on their surfaces. Its biological role remains unclear. Several reports indicate that in patients with a variety of malignant tumors, serum $\beta_2 M$ levels may be abnormally elevated[5] when compared with controls (normal values range from 900 to 2800 μg per liter[6]). The elevation of serum $\beta_2 M$ in malignancies of the B lymphocyte type has helped to differentiate idiopathic benign monoclonal gammapathies from B lymphocyte neoplasms.[5] Certain inflammatory diseases involving polyclonal lymphocyte activation are also associated with increased $\beta_2 M$ synthesis. Elevated serum $\beta_2 M$ levels have been reported in rheumatoid arthritis, Sjögren's syndrome, systemic lupus erythematosus, sarcoidosis, Crohn's disease, and angioimmunoblastic lymphadenopathy.[7] $\beta_2 M$ was the first nonantibody molecule that could be shown to be homologous with immunoglobulins. The $\beta_2 M$ protein can be readily aligned with a single Ig domain.[8] $\beta_2 M$ was subsequently found to be the smaller of two noncovalently associated polypeptides that constitute the class I major histocompatibility antigens (HLA-A, B, and C antigens).[9] The H chain of the HLA-A, B, and C antigens contains two disulfide bonded loops, each of which shows homology with C domains.[10] Very recently, two other molecules, class II histocompatibility antigens (or D antigens) and Thy-1 antigen, a surface glycoprotein characteristic of murine T lymphocytes, have also been shown to be homologous to Ig, although less so (Fig. 2–1). These findings have led to a provocative hypothesis about the genetics and evolution of Ig superfamily genes.[11–12]

V regions sharing certain similarities in their amino acid sequence can be classified as belonging to a single

LYMPHOCYTE SURFACE MOLECULES SHARING HOMOLOGIES WITH IMMUNOGLOBULIN DOMAINS

Figure 2–1. Lymphocyte surface molecules sharing homologies with Ig domains (represented by loops). IgD (m); MHC, major histocompatibility complex, class I antigens consist of a heavy (H) variable chain and a light chain, β_2 microglobulin. MHC class II antigens are composed of two chains, α and β. Thy-1 antigen is a surface glycoprotein characteristic of T lymphocytes.

subgroup (Table 2–2). Within a subgroup, a number of subdivisions can be made such that V regions of any one subgroup resemble one another more closely than they do members of other subgroups. Four subgroups of κ chains and six subgroups of λ chains are identified. The V regions of H chains also can be classified into at least three subgroups, which are not class specific, i.e., they can be expressed in any of the Ig classes. Certain positions in the variable region are highly conserved; in fact, 65 percent of this region shows limited sequence variation. Within a subgroup, most variations involve amino acid interchanges due to single base replacements in the corresponding codons. Other V region positions vary to a greater extent. These are clustered in three areas of both chains (amino acids 24–34, 50–56, and 89–97 in the light chains and residues 31–35, 50–65, and 95–102 in the heavy chains), which are called the hypervariable or complementarity-determining regions (CDR). These broad regions of sequence hypervariability are believed to be related to the antigen-binding site.[13,14] They are surrounded by relatively invariant framework (FR) regions.

IMMUNOGLOBULIN G

IgG molecules consist of identical pairs of H and L chains (MW = 50,000 and 25,000, respectively) linked by disulfide bridges (Fig. 2–2). A proteolytic enzyme (papain) splits IgG into three fragments, which retain biologic activity: two Fab (for antigen binding) fragments and one Fc (for crystallizable).[15] Each Fab fragment contains one antigen-combining site and consists of one L chain and the amino terminal half of the H

Table 2–2. Subgroups of the Light Chain (V_L) and Heavy Chain (V_H) Variable Regions

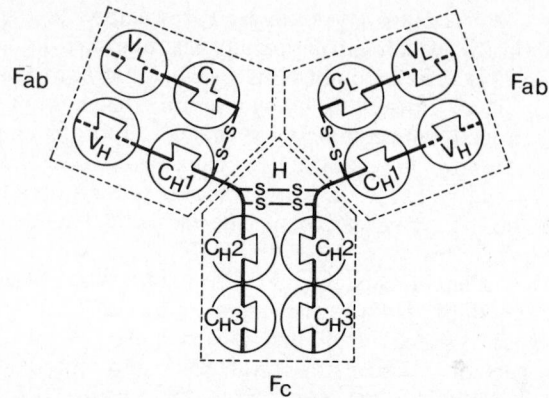

Figure 2–2. Diagram of a human IgG molecule. The L chains are divided into two domains, V_L and C_L. The H chains are divided into four domains, V_H, C_H1, C_H2, and C_H3. The heavy chains are joined by disulfide bridges in the hinge region (H). Cleavage of IgG by papain generates Fab fragments and an Fc fragment.

chain, termed the Fd fragment. The remaining carboxy-terminal halves of the two H chains, including the inter-H chain disulfide bonds (or hinge region), are the Fc fragment, which contains the sites responsible for the mediation of most biologic functions (Table 2–3). Pepsin cleaves the basic unit at the carboxyl end of the hinge region and thus liberates a bivalent section comparable to two papain-derived Fab fragments termed $F(ab')_2$ and a smaller Fc fragment (pFc'), which contains the C_H3 domain.[14]

In 1969, the first complete amino acid sequence of a human $IgG_{1\kappa}$ myeloma protein was reported.[16] One of the most striking features of the immunoglobulin molecule was the demarcation of its chains into connected regions that are associated with different biological functions.[17]

Normal human IgG contains a mixture of different subclasses of H chains: γ_1, γ_2, γ_3, and γ_4. IgG activates complement by the classic pathway, with IgG_1 and IgG_3 subclasses being most effective (Table 2–3). IgG_4 does not fix complement in the native state but does so after proteolytic cleavage. This property appears to be associated primarily with the C_H2 domain. IgG is the only class of immunoglobulin that provides passive immunity to the newborn, since the four gamma subclasses are the only immunoglobulins that cross the placenta. IgG proteins also interact with cell receptors for the Fc fragment on polymorphonuclear cells, monocytes, macrophages, and platelets. This property is important in initiating the inflammatory response, and it is associated predominantly with the C_H3 domain. IgG has a slow catabolic rate; its half-life is approximately 3 weeks, with only IgG_3 being degraded more rapidly. However, the rates vary directly with the serum concentration.

In most species immunologic memory resides primarily in the IgG fraction, with certain antigens eliciting preferential responses of one or another of the subclasses. Amino acid sequence studies of different subclasses of γ chains provide additional evidence that the immu-

Table 2–3. Biological Properties (Effector Functions) of Human Immunoglobulins

Property	IgG 1	IgG 2	IgG 3	IgG 4	IgM	IgA	IgE	Domain Localization
Antigen-Dependent								
Complement Fixation — Classical Pathway	+	+	+		+			C_H2(IgG) C_H4(IgM)
Complement Fixation — Alternate Pathway						+	+	
Opsonic Activity (neutrophils and monocytes)	+		+			+		
Antigen-Independent								
Mast Cell and Basophil Binding							+	
Macrophage Binding	+		+					C_H3
Lymphocyte Binding	+		+		+			C_H3
Placental Passage	+	+	+	+				Fc
Immunoglobulin Catabolism	+	+	+	+	+	+	+	C_H2
Passive Cutaneous Anaphylaxis	+		+					C_H3
Interaction with Protein "A"	+	+	+					C_H2, C_H3
Antigenic Target for Rheumatoid Factor	+	+	+	+	+	+	+	Fc

noglobulin molecule evolved by the successive duplication of a precursor gene of about 300 nucleotides and that a loop of approximately 60 residues is a fundamental subunit that is repeated 12 times in an IgG molecule. The γ subclasses are almost identical in this primary structure (over 95 percent amino acid sequence homology). The main subclass-related differences are in the hinge segment.[18] The hinge region varies from 15 to 60 residues; it is rich in proline and cysteine residues. The latter are involved in the disulfide bridges linking both H chains.

IgG_1 and IgG_4 proteins contain four interchain bridges. Two such bonds join the H chains to each other, and two bonds join H to L chains. IgG_2 proteins are crosslinked by six interchain bonds, two joining H to L chains and the other four binding both H chains. It has recently become evident that human IgG_3 has structural and biologic features not shared by the other three subclasses. IgG_3 does not bind to staphylococcal protein A, which tightly binds the other subclasses; it has a more rapid turnover; and it is the most potent subclass in activating the first component of complement. Structurally, the γ_3 chain has a higher molecular weight than other human chains, owing to an extended hinge region. This region is four times larger than the same region in the three other subclasses. This is due to a quadruplication of a 45-nucleotide DNA segment, resulting in a γ_3 hinge region that is 62 amino acid residues long and consists of an NH_2-terminal 17-residue segment followed by a 15-residue segment, which is identically and consecutively repeated three times.[19] Very recently, an IgG_3 protein carrying a rare allotype G3m (s,t) has been shown to bind staphylococcal protein A.[20] A histidine residue at the carboxyl end of the H chain (position 435) has been implicated in the binding of the protein.[21] It has been suggested that protein-A-binding IgG_3-like molecules comprise a fifth subclass of IgG, since they appear to be present in normal sera.[20]

IMMUNOGLOBULIN M

The IgM molecule is a pentamer composed of five identical subunits and one nonimmunoglobulin chain, the J chain. The J chain and a disulfide interchanging enzyme facilitate the formation of the polymer.[4,22] IgM appears to fill a special role in the primary immune response, and certain antigens such as the I antigen, aggregated immunoglobulins, and other red cell antigens stimulate a persistent IgM response. However, most antigenic stimuli result in a switch to other immunoglobulins after the initial burst of IgM. IgM is located predominantly in the intravascular space; its turnover is fast; and it cannot cross the placenta. It can however, initiate complement activation. While the valence of the IgM pentamer is 10 for small antigens, it may not exceed 5 for larger antigens, presumably as a consequence of steric hindrance.

Of great interest is the finding in recent years that the monomer of an IgM appears to be, together with IgD, the major protein on the surface of B lymphocytes. The V regions of both surface H chains (μ and δ) appear to be identical on the same cell. It has been suggested that both molecules act as receptors for antigens.[23,24]

Structural analyses of IgM were performed primarily with proteins obtained from patients suffering from Waldenström's macroglobulinemia. The availability of these homogeneous products of monoclonal lymphoid populations allowed the detailed study of IgM, just as myeloma proteins and Bence Jones proteins served as models for IgG antibodies and light chains, respectively. A disulfide-bonded model for human IgM is shown in Figure 2–3. Four bonds are interchain; ten, intrachain. The interchain disulfide bridges are arranged as follows: one joins H to L; one joins H to H in the monomer subunit; one is intersubunit; and the fourth cysteine apparently joins either the J chain or the homologous cysteine of the next monomer subunit, that is, it behaves as a J

Figure 2–3. Schematic diagram of the pentameric structure of the Fc fragment of human IgM. A two-domain structure for J chain is indicated.[37] One J chain is attached per pentameric IgM, through the C-terminal cysteine of μ chains and the amino terminal domain of the J chain.

bond or as a second intersubunit bond. The μ chain (MW = 70,000) contains five domains instead of the four present in γ chains: V_H, $C_\mu 1$, $C_\mu 2$, $C_\mu 3$, and $C_\mu 4$. Most of $C_\mu 2$ is degraded to peptides after trypsin digestion, suggesting that there is an exposed and flexible region resembling the hinge region in other Ig molecules.[25]

B lymphocyte membranes contain immunoglobulins that act as receptors for antigen. Membrane-bound IgM (IgM_m) is present as a four-chain monomer and differs from the secreted molecule (IgM_s) only near the C-terminal end of the μ chain. The last 20 amino acid residues of the secreted chain (μ_s) are missing from μ_m and are replaced by a different sequence of 41 residues (21 residues longer than μ_s). The extended μ_m includes a stretch of about 26 hydrophobic residues which is responsible for the insertion of IgM into the cell membrane.[26] A hydrophobic C-terminal region is present in the membrane-bound forms of all immunoglobulin H chains.

IMMUNOGLOBULIN A

In lower vertebrates, including fish, reptiles, and amphibians, IgM in tetrameric and pentameric configurations, represents the predominant immunoglobulin in serum as well as external secretions.[27] IgA first appears in birds and mammals, and secretory IgM is replaced by polymeric secretory IgA (sIgA). In man, IgA is produced in large quantities in areas adjacent to secretory surfaces. Mucosal B lymphocyte follicles in the intestinal and respiratory tracts have been implicated in the generation of cells enriched in precursors for IgA plasma cells. The precursors of the IgA plasma cells are first recognizable as bone-marrow-derived B lymphocytes in

the Peyer's patches (PP), where they can encounter antigens entering from the gut by way of epithelial cells. The precursors may initiate DNA synthesis in the PP, but eventually they leave by way of lymphatics draining into the mesenteric lymph nodes (MLN) where they proliferate further and eventually mature into IgA-containing blast cells. These blasts are capable of leaving the MLN and migrating to the small intestine and by the afferent and thoracic duct lymph entering into the bloodstream, from which they emerge at mucosal sites. This process is called the IgA-cell cycle.[28-32] Polymeric IgA interacts specifically with epithelial cells by means of the membrane glycoprotein secretory component (SC), which acts as a receptor and mediates its selective transport into secretions.

Unlike the other classes of immunoglobulins, IgA tends to be polydisperse in size. In normal human sera most of the IgA is monomeric, i.e., composed of a single four-chain unit, $\alpha_2 L_2$; about 10 percent consists of dimer or higher oligomers. Recognition of antigenic heterogeneity among IgA myelomas has led to the detection of two subclasses, IgA_1 and IgA_2. The genetic locus coding for IgA_2 heavy-chain constant region (α_2) has two allelic forms, $A_2m_{(1)}$ and $A_2m_{(2)}$, with some linkage to the Gm system of IgG. Unlike other immunoglobulins, $A_2m_{(1)}$ molecules lack covalent links between H and L chains, and their L chains are instead covalently linked to one another. In the α_1 and α_2 chains the major chemical differences lie in the hinge region and in the number, locations, and types of oligosaccharides. The hinge region of the α_1 chain contains a triplicated octapeptide that is lacking in α_2 chains; instead α_2 chains have a deletion and an unusual pentaproline sequence. In addition, there are a number of other amino acid substitutions that correlate with subclass or allotype. About 90 percent of the IgA in serum is IgA_1; but external secretions contain a more equal division.[34]

Secretory Component. sIgA is a special form of IgA, found predominantly in gastrointestinal and respiratory secretions, and represents a first line of local defense against environmental pathogens.[33] Its consists of two monomeric IgA subunits, a J chain and the SC, or transport piece, which has a molecular weight of approximately 70,000 daltons. SC is synthesized by the epithelial cells of the glands that secrete IgA polymer. More than 85 percent of the plasma cells in the intestinal lamina propria elaborate IgA, and there are high concentrations of sIgA in all secretions. In addition to the functions it shares with serum IgA (such as complement activation by the alternative pathway and viral neutralization), sIgA appears to prevent bacterial adherence to the intestinal mucosal surface and inhibits uptake of some proteins by the gut and other surfaces.

Oral immunization produces higher levels of sIgA antibodies. This reaction is of great practical significance, as orally administered polio vaccines are more effective than systemic vaccines, which fail to induce production of IgA antipoliovirus antibodies. After local stimulation, lymphocytes of the lamina propria of the intestines and other secretory organs develop into mature plasma cells and synthesize IgA molecules, which are dimerized by the presence of J chain on lymphocyte membranes. The SC synthesized by the epithelial cells combines with IgA antibodies and facilitates the entrance of the complete sIgA molecule into the intracellular space and secretion into intestinal lumen. The precise site and the mechanism by which SC accomplishes this function are not known.

The SC is linked to the H chains of one IgA subunit by a disulfide bridge,[34] which appears to protect it against proteolytic digestion. Normal feces contain a proteolytic enzyme that cleaves serum and sIgA to yield Fab and Fc fragments. The enzyme was termed IgA protease because enzymatic activity has thus far been found only against IgA. IgA protease can be obtained from centrifuged suspensions of feces or from culture fluids of *Streptococcus sanguis, Neisseria gonorrhoeae, N. meningitidis,* and *Haemophilus influenzae.* The specificity of the enzyme is quite restricted. It cleaves the Pro-Thr or Pro-Ser peptide bond in the hinge region of IgA_1. It does not cleave IgA_2, since the target dipeptide is absent in this class. The presence of α_1 Fc fragments in normal feces suggests a role for this enzyme in the secretory immune system. Of considerable interest is the observation that the enzyme is produced in those regions of the alimentary tract populated by bacteria, mainly the mouth and the colon. The increased ratio of $IgA_2:IgA_1$ detected in secretions may represent an evolutionary adaptation of man to what has become the normal flora of the gastrointestinal tract.[35,36]

J Chain. J chain is structurally unrelated to L and H chains and evolved independently of them. It combines covalently with the H chains of IgA and IgM in the unusual stoichiometric proportion of one J chain per polymeric molecule regardless of the size of the polymer. J chain is linked by the disulfide bond to a cysteine that is the penultimate residue in human μ and α chains. The similarity in location is not surprising because the carboxyl terminal ends of μ and α chains are homologous. J chain is thought to initiate polymerization by sequential disulfide exchange with the C-terminal intrachain S–S bond of monomeric IgA or IgM. Because the stoichiometry indicates one J chain per polymer, the mode of attachment poses a problem. Recent results favor the "clasp" model, in which the J chain acts as a disulfide clasp between two monomers and the polymer is closed by disulfide bonds between the other monomer units (Fig. 2–3). Human J chain consists of a single polypeptide chain, with a molecular weight of 15,000, and a single oligosaccharide. Unlike L and H chains, J chain appears to have a unique sequence; there is no evidence for variation, and J_α and J_μ appear to be identical both chemically and antigenically. Little progress has been made in correlating the structure and function of the J chain, owing to the lack of mutant forms of J chain with altered function. It has also been difficult to isolate sufficient J chain for detailed chemical analysis, since J chain is highly susceptible to enzymatic degradation. Very recently, comparison of the primary structure of the human polypeptide with the murine J chain

sequence deduced from nucleotide analysis of cloned cDNA suggested that the J chain possesses two domains having different characteristics. It would appear that the polymerization function resides in its amino terminal half.[37]

IMMUNOGLOBULIN D

IgD was described 20 years ago; nonetheless a distinct functional role for this class remains an enigma.[38] The most striking aspect of IgD is its distribution. It is present in normal serum in very low quantities and yet is found on the surface of most B lymphocytes as a membrane Ig, usually in association with another Ig class (most frequently IgM), sharing the same V_H-V_L regions.[39] Early findings, not surprisingly therefore, focused on the possibility that IgD might be the antigen receptor for B cells. A wealth of evidence now suggests that IgD is not the sole Ig serving a receptor function.

Structural studies of the IgD protein were greatly hindered by several factors. First, concentrations of normal serum IgD are low, and IgD myeloma proteins are rare. Second, IgD is very susceptible to spontaneous enzymatic degradation either in serum or during preparation. The antigenic distinctiveness of IgD, as in other immunoglobulins, lies in its δ chain. Human IgD myeloma proteins are predominantly of λ chain type, although this is not true of cells expressing surface IgD. IgD has a molecular weight of approximately 160,000 and contains about 10 percent carbohydrate, all bound to the δ chain. The complex sugars consist of three large glucosamine oligosaccharides linked to the Fc region and four or five galactosamine trisaccharides in close proximity in the hinge. The glucosamine is always N-linked to an asparagine in the obligatory tripeptide acceptor sequence Asn-X-Thr/Ser, where X may be any amino acid.[40] In the serum the protein may be degraded almost completely to fragments similar to Fc and Fab in several days, even at 4°C. This may be retarded by addition of ϵ-aminocaproic acid (EACA) at a final concentration of 0.02M immediately after the plasma is collected. IgD is crosslinked by three interchain bridges, two H-L and one H-H. The presence of only a single inter-H chain bond is unique among human immunoglobulins, although it has also been found in rabbit IgG. IgD from lymphocyte membranes has an apparently higher molecular weight (a property shared with membrane IgM). There has also been a suggestion of different subclasses of IgD; however, in view of the lack of any chemical evidence, it would be premature to conclude that such is the case.

IMMUNOGLOBULIN E

This quantitatively minor class of Ig contains most of the molecules bearing the biologic and immunochemical characteristics of reaginic antibodies. IgE antibodies have the ability to bind reversibly with high affinity to specific membrane receptors on basophils and mast cells. The combination of specific cell-bound antibody with antigens triggers a series of events that ultimately lead to the release of vasoactive amines and other pharmacologically active substances responsible for the clinical manifestations of hypersensitivity. One can confidently state that without myeloma proteins much of the information we now have about IgE would not exist. This is because the level of IgE, even in the most severely allergic individual, seldom exceeds 1 μg per ml. Myeloma protein IgE has been used to prepare radiolabeled anti-IgE; and together with allergen coupled to an insoluble adsorbent it is used in the radioallergosorbent test (RAST) to measure antibodies to a specific allergen in the serum of atopic patients. It also seems possible that IgE antibodies play a protective role in parasitic infections, perhaps by increasing vascular permeability and thus allowing other antibodies to arrive at the site of inflammation.

IgE has a molecular weight of 180,000, of which approximately 12 percent is accounted for by carbohydrate. The molecule has the same basic four-chain structure found in other immunoglobulins. A comparison of the molecular size of the H chain (ϵ) with that of the H chains of the other classes shows it to be greater (11,000 daltons greater) than γ, δ, or α but about the same as μ. The ϵ chain consists of 547 amino acid residues, organized into the V region, and four constant homology regions ($C_\epsilon 1$, $C_\epsilon 2$, $C_\epsilon 3$, and $C_\epsilon 4$). Thus, both IgE and IgM possess an extra domain and lack a hinge region. Of the 15 half-cystine residues present on the ϵ chain, 10 participate in the formation of intrachain disulfide bridges, one in each of the five homology regions. Only three interchain bonds are present: one inter-H-L chain bond and two inter-H chain bonds. The two remaining half-cystines are engaged in the formation of an additional intrachain bond located in the $C_H 1$ region. The high carbohydrate content in IgE is explained by the presence of six oligosaccharide chains attached to the ϵ chain. The ability of IgE to bind to specific receptors is mediated through sites localized within the Fc region. Thermal inactivation of IgE is correlated with structural changes involving both the $C_\epsilon 3$ and $C_\epsilon 4$ domains, but not the $C_\epsilon 2$ region; on the other hand the loss of cytotropic activity accompanying reduction of IgE seems to correlate with the cleavage of one interchain disulfide bond between the paired $C_H 2$ domains. The current interpretation is that reduction of this bond alters the quaternary structure of Fc, leading to inactivation.[41-43]

GENETIC POLYMORPHISM OR ALLOTYPES

Allotypes are genetic variants of immunoglobulins and are inherited according to simple Mendelian laws. These genetic markers are detected by intraspecies antisera, as obtained in humans after inadvertent immunization by transfusion of whole blood or after pregnancy.

In humans, allotypes appear to be the product of a single autosomal codominant gene.[44] Three sets of allotypic markers are recognized in human immunoglobulins, the closely linked Gm and Am factors and the independently inherited km system. Genetic markers have been shown to reside mainly in the constant region of human H chain (Table 2–1). So far, no clear cut allotypic differences have been demonstrated for the μ, δ, and ϵ chains. The km factors are associated with κ type Bence Jones proteins and L chains. Since L chains are common to all classes of Ig, km antigens can be found in IgG, A, M, D, and E proteins.

Km markers are inherited through a series of three alleles $km^{1,2}$, km^1, and km^3. The serologic allotypic specificities are due to amino acid sequence differences that involve interchanges at one or two contiguous positions that are not critical to the overall structure of function of the antibody molecule. $Km^{1,2}$ is associated with a leucine residue in the C region of κ chain (position 191), and km^3 is associated with a valine at the same position. When the rare antigen km^1 is present, valine is in position 153 instead of alanine. Gm factors are associated with IgG molecules and are located on the C_γ region. Some of them have been structurally defined.[44] The A2m(2) allotype is predominant in the human A_2 subclass and is characterized by the absence of the H-L interchain disulfide bonds. Studies of allotypic markers in the constant and variable regions in conjunction with amino acid sequence data have been of major importance in the understanding of the polygenic control of immunoglobulin polypeptide synthesis. These genetic differences have also proved to be of use in serology, rheumatology, and forensic medicine.

IDIOTYPES AND THE COMBINING SITE

Idiotypes are antigenic determinants localized on the V region and correspond to the antigen-binding specificity of a given antibody molecule. Antibody specificity results from the molecular complementarity between determinant groups on the antigen molecule and amino acid residues in the active site. H and L chains contribute to the combining site, as shown by reassociation experiments. In general, most studies have come to the same general conclusion, namely that both H and L chains can bind specifically to the antigen to which the antibody is directed, although binding to the H chain is invariably stronger.

Antigen binding by antibodies involves weak noncovalent associations, including electrostatic bonding, hydrogen bonding, and van der Waals interactions. The specific sites are predominantly nonpolar niches. Evidence obtained from amino acid sequence analysis and affinity labeling studies has been used to identify the segments of polypeptide chains involved in the antibody combining sites (hypervariable regions, or CDRs). These findings led to the hypothesis that CDRs contributed in some way to the conformation of the antibody active sites. Definitive evidence was obtained by x-ray crystallographic studies of Fab fragments obtained from two myeloma proteins.[45,46] Their combining sites extended over a large area surrounding a central groove or pocket, which was 15 Å long, 6 Å wide, and 6 Å deep, the walls of which were composed of hypervariable segments. CDRs contain insertions, deletions, and amino acid substitutions. Sequence modifications of this type have a very significant effect on the size and shape of the combining site and consequently on the specificity. Moreover, extensive binding-site diversity can be generated by the combinatorial properties of L-H chain association. It is further increased by the ability of a single antibody molecule to combine with a spectrum of different antigens (multispecificity). Thus, every antibody will react with the inducing antigen, but each antibody will differ in the spectrum of disparate antigens it can bind (crossreactivity).

IMMUNOGLOBULIN GENES

The structures we recognize as immunoglobulin heavy and light chains are the products of genes organized into three discrete families, each located on a separate chromosome. One of the major insights into the structure of Ig genes was the demonstration that the elements coding for the variable and constant regions of the heavy and light polypeptides were not contiguous on their respective chromosomes. In the germ line, V and C gene families are separated by many thousands of nucleotides, although the distance has not yet been defined.[47]

Kappa Chain Germ Line Genes. In man the kappa gene family has been localized to chromosome 2.[48] The variable region complex is the most 5′ of the elements (Fig. 2–4). It appears that there are between 15 and 30 V_κ genes in humans, which is about 10 percent of the number found in mouse DNA, an observation consistent with amino acid sequence data showing that there are four human kappa subgroups compared to many in the mouse.[49]

The genes are generally homologous in the two species, with DNA segments from human easily hybridizable with mouse and vice versa.[50] Each of the V_κ genes examined has a fairly well conserved 5′ sequence which contains a promoter site and a CAP (or ribosome-binding) site.[51] The spatial relationships between these two functionally important regions and the initiation codon (ATG) seem to be well preserved and analogous to those found in most eukaryotic proteins. The initiation codon is followed by a run of some 45 to 75 bases, which code for a hydrophobic amino acid sequence. This structure has been shown to play a role in the binding of the polyribosomes synthesizing immunoglobulins to the endoplasmic reticulum.[52] After most of the polypeptide has been synthesized, these N-terminal residues are proteolytically cleaved and are not found on the mature cytoplasmic or secreted immunoglobulin.[53] Immediately 3′ (or downstream) from the leader exon (or coding sequence) is an intervening sequence (intron), which varies from 85 to 105 base pairs. The major single exon of the V region follows, with the bases specifying the last 4 or 5 amino acids of the leader and the 95 amino acids coded by the V_κ gene. The V gene terminates with a sequence CACAGTG, a heptamer, followed by a 12-base spacer, TTACACACCCGA, followed by a nanomer, ACATAAACC. These sequences and their spatial configuration have a functional importance in the recombinations between gene segments.

Within the coding sequence, the greatest differences among members of the same family of V sequences are found in those regions coding for the CDRs 1, 2, and 3. Amino acid residues 89 to 95 represent most of CDR 3. The remaining residues in the expressed light chain are not encoded in the V region exon per se but are derived from one of four J_κ (or joining) segments, each of 85 bases separated one from the other by 300 base-

THE BIOGENESIS OF KAPPA LIGHT CHAIN

Figure 2–4. The biogenesis of a kappa light chain. The transition from germ line to B-lymphocyte configuration is accomplished by translocation and deletion (see text). Nuclear processing removes the transcribed introns to generate a mature mRNa.

intervening sequences.[54] The amount of germ line DNA between the Vs and the Js is not known. The single kappa constant region exon is located 2.5 kilobases (kb) 3′ to the 4th J_κ segment. Each J_κ contains the 39 nucleotides sufficient to code for the amino acids comprising the c-terminal portion of CDR 3, framework region 4, and some 30 nucleotides of flanking sequence on either side. The constant region segment codes for the remaining amino acids (109–214), the termination codon, and a 3′ untranslated region of 180 bases followed by a polyadenylation signal AATAAA.[55] This germ line organization of the kappa locus is found in the DNA of sperm, oocytes, and all nonlymphoid tissues (Fig. 2–4). The changes that occur in the course of B lymphocyte differentiation will be described below.

Lambda Chain Germ Line Genes. The lambda chain locus on chromosome 22 has a similar general configuration in the germ line but has certain attributes that are distinct.[56] First, its constellation of V genes is uniquely its own. Amino acid sequence analysis has indicated that there are at least six V_λ subgroups[57] (versus four V_κ subgroups). It is likely that the greatest differences between human and mouse Ig genes will be found at this locus, since λ-chain-containing molecules comprise only 5 percent of the total murine antibody population but 30 to 40 percent of human immunoglobulins. There is little experimental data currently available concerning the makeup of the V_λ complex in humans. The J_λ constant region segment has been the subject of intense investigation in both species. In contrast to the C_κ locus, which contains only one gene, the human C_λ locus contains at least six nonallelic genes, which are spread over approximately 50 kb of DNA.[58] One of these genes has been shown to have its own J segment, a feature likely to be shared by all the functional C_λ genes.[59] This structural feature has also been noted in murine lambda genes. Thus, in contrast to the kappa locus, there is no discrete J_λ cluster. In the center of the C_λ cluster is a region that seems to be particularly predisposed to undergo recombination. This predisposition has created considerable technical difficulty in the elucidation of the details of C_λ structure. Its significance in vivo is uncertain. Interestingly, a nonfunctional, or pseudo, λ gene is found elsewhere in the genome, unlinked to the functional locus. It appears to represent an integrated copy of a processed λ mRNA.[60] As with κ, the differentiation

of a cell along the B lymphocyte pathway to become a λ-expressing lymphocyte or plasma cell is associated with alterations in the germ line gene configuration.

Heavy Chain Germ Line Genes. The heavy chain locus on chromosome 14 exhibits a germ line composition similar to, but more complex than, those coding for the two light chain classes[61] (Fig. 2–5). Again, the most 5′ portion of the heavy chain complex is the V region cluster. Protein sequence data have suggested that there are three V_H subgroups, hence three V_H gene families. There is considerable homology between human and mouse V_H gene families; the same DNA probes have been used to determine the size of particular V_H groups in both species.[62] These experiments suggested that there might be 2- to 3-fold more members of the human V_{HIII} gene subgroup.[63] Additional studies in the mouse have indicated that the V_H genes of different subgroups were not intermingled. Within the subgroups it has been found that V_H genes may be separated from each other by 8 to 16 kb of noncoding sequence.[64]

The structure of individual V_H genes is quite similar to that of V_L. There is an exon that codes for most of the hydrophobic signal sequence followed by an intron of 84 (V_{HI}) or 104 (V_{HIII}) base pairs (depending on the particular V_H subgroup). This is followed by an exon containing the remainder (usually four or five amino acids) of the leader sequence and V region amino acids 1 to 94, followed by two base pairs, then the consensus recombination sequence CACAGTG–21 base pair spacer–GACACAAACC.

The first major organizational departure of the heavy chain locus from that of the light chains is the presence of a region containing at least three and perhaps more families of D (diversity) segments.[65] To date, families have been described which contain from 2 to 9 D segments. The segments themselves contain about 30 nucleotides and are flanked on both sides by the heptamer–12 or 13 base pair spacer–nanomer consensus recombination signal. The families thus far described have been spread over 30 to 60 kb of sequence. These codons contribute to the amino acids comprising the heavy chain CDR 3 (vide infra).[66] 3′ to the bulk of the D segment region is the J_H cluster. Included in the cluster is a single, presumably functional D segment, three pseudo J_H genes, and six bona fide J_H segments[67] (Fig. 2–5). Each functional J is comprised of the nanomer–

HUMAN IMMUNOGLOBULIN HEAVY CHAIN GENES

Figure 2–5. *A*, Tentative gene order for the human heavy chain locus. The broken lines indicate that the amount of DNA encompassed by the region is not known (see text). The regions of known length are not drawn to scale. The areas designated by -●- or -○- represent sequences involved in class switching. *B*, Ig heavy chain locus in plasma cells synthesizing IgA₁. V, D and J_H have been translocated, and the germ line genes 5′ to the expressed α_1 gene have been deleted from the productively rearranged chromosome. The constant region genes 3′ to the expressed α_1 gene have been retained. The intron 5′ to the $C_\alpha1$ exon now contains a switch region comprised partially of the germ line μ switch region and partially of sequences from the homologous area of the germ line α_1 gene (-◐-).

21-23 base pair spacer-heptamer, 45 to 60 base pairs of coding sequence followed by a consensus splice site (vide infra). From the 3' end of J_H6 is a region of 2000 base pairs extending approximately 3 kb that is involved in the class switch. It consists of multiple tandem repeats of the sequence GGCCTGAGCTGAGCTGAACT, with some variation in the repeats, and is 90 percent homologous with the murine sequence that has been demonstrated to be utilized in the switching of the cell from the synthesis of one class of Ig to another, e.g., from IgM to IgG (vide infra).[68]

Approximately 1.5 kb further downstream is the first exon of the μ constant region gene.[67-70] The C_μ gene is the most 5' of the heavy chain constant region genes. It contains 5 exons. The first four of these code for the four μ chain domains found in serum IgM. $C_\mu1$ contains *306* bases; it is followed by an intron of 130 bases, $C_\mu2$ (330 bases), an intervening sequence (IVS) of 242 bases, $C_\mu3$ (317 bases), an IVS of approximately 150 nucleotides, and $C_\mu4$, 387 bases coding for the carboxy-terminal domain of the μ chain. This is followed by 101 bases of 3' untranslated DNA and the polyadenylation signal (AATAAA). At 1.9 kb 3' to the end of $C_\mu4$ are 2 exons separated by a small intron. They encode a protein segment of 39 amino acids that is hydrophobic and represents the portion of the μ chain that is anchored in the cell membrane when the cell expresses IgM as a cell-bound receptor[68,71] (Fig. 2–6).

The general structure, comprising separate exons coding for each protein domain with consensus splice signals at the 5' and 3' termini of each exon, is characteristic of all the human heavy chain genes. Further, the presence of small "membrane" exons at a distance 3' to the carboxy-terminal coding exon has been demonstrated to be characteristic of each γ class in the mouse and is probably true in humans.[72] C_μ and C_ϵ have four relatively equally sized exons, while the C_δ, C_γ, and C_α genes have three similar exons coding for C_H1, C_H2, and C_H3 but, between the first and second domains, we find a small separate exon coding for the hinge segment[73] (Fig. 2–7). The exons in all the genes are separated by introns. The intron sequences, apart from the intron-exon borders, show much less conservation of sequence than the exons.

In humans, C_δ is located some 5000 bases 3' to the end of $C_\mu4$ and approximately 3000 nucleotides 3' to $C_{\mu m}$, a spacing quite similar to that in the mouse. The human and mouse IgD heavy chains vary considerably, and little more is known about the human genes. The murine δ gene has been fully sequenced.[74] It is likely that the human gene will share some but not all of its features. All of the intron-exon borders in both are marked by consensus splice sequences.[75] The distance between the δ gene and the next heavy chain gene in the human genome is not known, while in the mouse, δ and $C_\gamma3$ have been linked with an intervening segment of 55,000 bases.[76] Although the general structure of the remaining individual heavy chain constant region genes is similar in the two species, their organization and number appear to differ. Hence, the distances between the μ and δ genes and the γ, ϵ, α complex may not be comparable.

The available data suggest that in the human genome the presently identified heavy chain genes 3' of μ and δ exist as two separate clusters.[77] The most 5' of the clusters consists of $C_\gamma3$, 26 kb of intervening sequence; $C_\gamma1$, a 19-kb IVS; a pseudo-ϵ gene; a 13-kb IVS; and the α_1 gene. The cluster is separated by an undetermined interval from a second homologous cluster containing $C_\gamma2$, an 18-kb intron; $C_\gamma4$, 23 kb of intervening DNA; C_ϵ, a 10-kb IVS, followed by $C_\alpha2$ (Fig. 2–5). This type of genomic structure, deduced in part from the analysis of the DNA of individuals showing a germ line deletion of the γ_1, γ_2, γ_4, and α genes, suggests that not only did the individual Ig genes evolve by duplication of an original domain-sized unit but that an entire cluster of relatively mature constant region genes may have duplicated in the period after the primate and murine lineages separated.[78]

Each of the genes in the two human clusters exhibit the prototypic exon-intron structure plus the presence of a region 5' to the C_H1 exon which participates in the class switching process. It comprises approximately 2.7 kb located about 2 kb 5' to the C_H1 exon, which is homologous to a similar region 5' to $C_\mu1$ and highly conserved between mouse and human. Similar sequences have been identified 5' to the constant region genes for

Figure 2–6. Different transcripts yield an mRNA coding for a membrane or secreted μ chain. It has not yet been determined if the transcript coding for μ_s results from termination at the first polyadenylation signal or from alternative processing of a single transcript extending from V to μ_m.

Figure 2–7. The exon-intron structure of a rearranged γ_1 heavy chain gene. Each domain is coded by a single exon. The introns are removed from the primary transcript in the nucleus. Splice junctions, sites from which introns have been removed, generally have the dinucleotide GT on the 5' (donor) side and AG on the 3' (acceptor) side. The rearranged heavy chain gene contains six exons derived from two genes.

the remaining γ, ϵ, and α heavy chains. The pseudo-ϵ gene between $C_\gamma 1$ and $C_\alpha 1$ lacks sequences coding for $C_H 1$ and $C_H 2$ and cannot be expressed.[79] A second human pseudo-ϵ gene has been identified unlinked to either cluster and localized to chromosome 9.[80]

As expected, all four identified C_γ genes have similar structures. $C_\gamma 3$ shows the only departure in that its hinge region is coded by four exons of 59 bases (H1) and 53 bases (H2, H3, H4) separated by IVS (not shown).[81] Such a structure was predicted on the basis of amino acid sequence analysis of human heavy chain disease proteins in which the heavy chain deletions seemed to end at hinge segment borders.[82] A pseudo-γ_1 gene has also been identified, but its location in the cluster has not been established.[81] The presence of at least one additional gamma gene has been hypothesized on the basis of amino acid sequence data; however, since it has not yet been isolated, its existence remains putative.[83]

B LYMPHOCYTE DIFFERENTIATION

Given these gene structures, which are present in all cells, how do B lymphocytes manage to produce up to 10^6 different antibody specificities, which can be expressed either on the cell surface or as secreted molecules with different biologic functions, without totally reconstructing the system in every generation? Evolution appears to have resulted in the employment of a combination of molecular mechanisms to resolve the problem. Specific DNA rearrangements are utilized early in the preparation of B lymphocytes for activation and again in the serologic maturation of the immune response. Differential splicing of primary RNA transcripts allows the utilization of the same genes for different functions at the same time. Finally, a multiplicity of devices, including multiple germ line V genes, complex combinatorial associations to form CDR 3's, and somatic mutation have been used to insure adequate antibody diversity.

The observation that V and C genes are located at an enormous distance from each other in embryonic DNA was followed by experiments indicating that the

distance is much smaller in immunoglobulin-expressing lymphocytes and plasma cells.[84] T lymphocyte DNA in general, with some exceptions, and the DNA of nonlymphoid organs are maintained in the germ line configuration with respect to immunoglobulin genes.[85]

Gene Rearrangements. It appears that the first recognizable event occurring in the Ig genes of a cell of B lineage is the rearrangement of a D segment to a J_H segment.[67] The coupling is mediated by the heptamer-spacer-nanomer sequences. It has been established that the spacer length is critical, in that an element with a 12 base pair (bp) spacer can only recombine with an element containing a 23–25 base pair spacer.[86] Hence, the 5' spacer sequence of each J_H has a 25 bp sequence while the D segment has a 12 bp spacer on both the 3' and 5' sides. The DNA between the recombining D and J segments may be deleted during the process, while the DNA between the utilized J and C_μ is retained. The recombined D still has a free recombination site with a 12 bp spacer present on its 5' side. This site is now available for recombination with a V_H gene. All the V_H genes have a recombination signal with a 23–25 bp spacer at their 3' termini; therefore, VDJ–μ joining can readily occur. The VDJ junction is reflected in the amino acid sequence of CDR 3. Hence, the protein product of the same germ line V_H gene can vary in its CDR 3 depending upon which D and J are involved in the recombination. Further, there is imprecision in the D segment joining, which may result in variability in the number of D segment bases included in the site.

If the bases can be read in frame with the V_H gene, i.e., in triplets with each codon specifying a given amino acid, the recombination will be successful and yield a functional heavy chain gene; if not, the rearrangement will be nonproductive. It appears that if a nonproductive heavy chain gene rearrangement occurs, the heavy chain locus on the other copy of chromosome 14 can rearrange. The presence of both a successfully and a nonproductively rearranged heavy chain gene is very common in B lymphocyte DNA.[87] During V_H rearrangement all the V genes and D segments between the recombining V and D may be deleted from that chromosome. A cell that has successfully rearranged its heavy chain genes may also be identified as a pre-B lymphocyte by the presence of μ or, less commonly, other heavy chain polypeptide chains in the cytoplasm.[88]

Light chain gene rearrangement appears to follow successful heavy chain rearrangement, although it is not clear what signals the light chain chromosome to rearrange. The process is simpler, since only V_L and J_L have to recombine. Again the process is mediated by the consensus recombination sequence, with V carrying a 12 bp spacer and J a 23 bp spacer. The intervening DNA between the rearranging V and J is deleted.[89] The third CDR varies with the choice of J segment utilized in the recombination.

In most B lymphocytes, from data obtained in normal and leukemic human lymphocytes, it appears that after H chain rearrangement, κ chain genes rearrange first; if neither of the κ chromosomes is successfully rearranged, λ genes are free to rearrange until a successful event occurs.[85-87,89-91] At present, the data suggest that the apparent κ, λ hierarchy is stochastic rather than mechanistic, reflecting the larger V_κ repertoire.[87] In either case the biologic signals that initiate and control the process have not been identified.

Allelic Exclusion. It has been noted for many years that immunoglobulin-producing cells exhibit what has been termed allelic exclusion. Each B lymphocyte expresses the immunoglobulin genes coded by only one of the pair of parental chromosomes. The term "allelic exclusion" implied a positive genetic mechanism controlling the utilization of only one of two available alleles. From the foregoing, it appears that allelic exclusion is a result, rather than a cause, of a mechanism giving each B lymphocyte precursor the greatest possible chance to express its V region repertoire. It is evident on all three Ig-coding chromosomes and implies that there must be regulatory elements that can sense when successful rearrangements have occurred. The first productive heavy chain gene rearrangement should turn off the translocation mechanism at the allelic locus. The evidence to date suggests that it also initiates rearrangement of one copy of the κ locus (chromosome 2) without activating the other copy or the similar λ locus on chromosome 22. The stimulus to each of these events may be the protein product itself (i.e., the synthesized μ chain), its mRNA, the conformation of the rearranged gene, or some other molecule, either protein or nucleic acid, coded by the rearranged gene.

Differential Processing of Immunoglobulin Gene Transcripts. The successfully rearranged heavy and light chain genes must be transcribed and translated in order to be expressed as proteins. The primary transcripts include both the exons and the intervening sequences. Processing then occurs that utilizes consensus splice sequences found at each intron–exon border to remove the nonstructural RNA[75] (Figs. 2–4 and 2–5). This process is not specific for immunoglobulin molecules, since almost all eukaryotic protein coding genes contain introns that must be spliced out after transcription. All the intron sequences are removed, leaving only coding sequences in the final cytoplasmic mRNA. Similarly,

the transcription termination signal for all genes appears to be the AATAA site, which specifies that adenylic acid residues (poly-A) should be added to the transcript within 20 to 30 bases downstream.[55]

The B lymphocyte uses these mechanisms in the same way as other cells; however, it also uses them to segregate heavy chains within the cell (Fig. 2–6). Studies utilizing murine B lymphocyte tumors indicate that if the μ chain is to be expressed on the cell surface, the transcript includes the large intervening sequence 3' to $C_\mu 4$ and the two membrane exons and recognizes the polyadenylation site 3' to the gene segment encoding the hydrophobic membrane insertion site. During processing, the usual introns are excised, as is the sequence between $C_\mu 4$ and $C_{\mu m}$, and a protein with a carboxy terminus appropriate to interact with the cell membrane is available. If a cytoplasmic or secreted type μ chain is to be produced, an mRNA with a poly-A tail just 3' to the end of the $C_\mu 4$ exon is found in the cytoplasm.[92,93] No explanation was given as to how the differential polyadenylation would be controlled, but the fact is that the same specificity can be expressed on both the cell surface and as secreted antibody. The signals that allow cells to choose between membrane and secreted transcripts are not understood; however, it is likely that cells producing other immunoglobulin classes utilize the same scheme to produce membrane and secreted molecules.

The successful rearrangement of the heavy and light chain loci identify a B lymphocyte as having specificity and as being capable of responding to the appropriate antigen. Many early B lymphocytes express both IgM and IgD of the same specificity on the cell surface. If only IgM is synthesized, the C_δ gene is fully methylated.[94] In the mouse, and presumably the human, if both chains are to be expressed, neither is methylated and a single long transcript encompassing VDJ–C_μ, the IVS between the μ and δ genes, and the VDJ–C_δ introns and exons is produced. The expressed proteins reflect the differential splicing patterns. A cell expressing both μ and δ on the cell surface will have processed transcripts encompassing VDJ–$C_{\mu m}$ and some encompassing VDJ–$C_{\delta m}$, each of which has the introns and inappropriate exons spliced out. The primary transcript will also include the exons coding for the secretory c-termini of both proteins. If only SIgD is expressed, then the VDJ–$C_{\delta s}$ will be dominant. Differential processing is thus utilized to express a new class of immunoglobulin bearing the same antigen-binding specificity in its V region.[74] It is possible that the simultaneous expression of two other classes of Ig heavy chains (e.g., α and γ) on the surface of small numbers of normal human B lymphocytes may reflect the use of differential splicing of a long transcript.[95] However, this hypothesis has not been tested.

Heavy Chain Class Switching. The maturation of the immune response is characterized by the expression of the same binding specificity on immunoglobulins of different heavy chain classes with a variety of biologic effector functions. Murine myeloma cells synthesizing a given Ig heavy chain, e.g., γ_{2b}, were found to have one chromosome unrearranged or with its J_H nonproductively rearranged and the other missing its μ and some γ genes.[96] When the germ line genes were cloned and placed in order on the chromosome, it was found that on the productively rearranged chromosome the heavy chain genes 5' to the expressed gene were deleted up to the switch sequences adjacent to that constant region gene.[97] Observations in human lymphoid cells are consistent with those in the mouse. Further analysis of rearranged genes showed that the intervening sequence between the rearranged VDJ and C_H1 contained some sequences derived from the germ line μ gene, i.e., those 3' to the J, including the region of tandem repeats, and some from the similar sequences 5' to the germ line C_H1 sequence. A model was proposed suggesting that heavy chain class switching was accomplished by recombination between switch sites with deletion of the intervening DNA[96] (Fig. 2–7). It implied that switching should occur in a 5' to 3' order and could never go 3' to 5'. However, one or two instances of the latter have been reported (e.g., murine γ_{2b} to γ_{2a}), resulting in the further proposal that sister chromatid exchange might be a mechanism whereby switching could go in either direction with or without deletion, but with the 5' to 3' direction dominant.[98]

It is not clear whether the development of each B lymphocyte is characterized by a phase in which each heavy chain class is transiently expressed. It is also unclear what makes the switching stop, or whether potential sequences can be skipped (i.e., can a cell go directly from μ to α?).

Phenotypic analysis indicates that switching does not take place prior to exposure to antigen and that it may be under specific T lymphocyte control.[99] Other studies, analyzing Ig class expression in human pre-B lymphocyte leukemias, suggest that switching is stochastic, a hypothesis based on the fact that the frequency of expression of the heavy chains roughly corresponds to the 5' to 3' order of the genes.[88] The latter type of argument is weakened by the necessarily limited sample size from which the frequency distribution was determined.

Isotype Exclusion. It has thus emerged that the general observations that each antibody-producing cell expresses only one heavy chain and one light chain bearing specificity for only one antigen (apart from considerations of crossreactivity) have a basis in the DNA coding for the polypeptides. The cell does not choose to express κ or λ. It can only rearrange a λ gene if it has failed to successfully activate κ.

With respect to the heavy chain chromosome, it is apparent that the deletional mechanism precludes cellular expression of two heavy chains simultaneously. Genes coding for μ and δ may be a special case because of their proximity and their relatively specialized function on the cell surface. However, it appears that when IgD is expressed as a secreted protein, as in IgD myeloma, the 5' μ gene is deleted.[100] Recent data in the mouse have also suggested that IgE-bearing cells have not deleted their 5' genes.[101] Hence, it may be that the deletional mechanism is active in all Ig secretory plasma cells but not necessarily in B lymphocytes with primarily surface Ig expression. The cloned or single human B lymphocytes that have been reported to express two classes of Ig other than IgM and IgD on the cell surface may be the result of differential splicing of long transcripts.[95]

ANTIBODY DIVERSITY

The immune system is capable of expressing the same antigen-binding specificity coded in the V region as an antibody of any heavy chain class expressed either as a membrane or secreted molecule. Much of the diversity found in the V-region repertoire can be accounted for by a large number of germ line V_H and V_L genes coupled with the enormous variability in CDR3 generated by the various types of combinatorial joining, i.e., V_LJ_L and V_HDJ_H. However, there are two other mechanisms utilized to expand the variability of response. One is the selection of different pairs of activated heavy and light chains, which may generate diversity in the tertiary structure of the binding site. While there is much circumstantial evidence suggesting specific interactions between heavy and light chain coding genes, particularly in the regulation of rearrangement and synthesis, there is little knowledge of how these events take place.

Recent data, obtained primarily in the mouse, have clearly demonstrated that somatic mutation in rearranged heavy and light chain V region genes can add substantially to the diversity of the antibody response.[102,103] Much of the mutational activity seems to localize to CDRs 1 and 2, although some has also been noted in CDR3. It has been suggested that somatic mutation in V_H regions is more likely to occur in γ and α proteins than in IgM antibodies, i.e., after the class switch.[104]

A small number of germ line V genes have now been subjected to nucleotide sequencing, and it is striking that almost 40 percent of the analyzed genes appear to be pseudogenes, that is, incapable of coding for a functional V gene.[63] Nonetheless, some of them may be available for recombination events and could be responsible for some of the nonproductive gene rearrangements noted so frequently.

EVOLUTIONARY CONSIDERATIONS

DNA analysis has added substantially to our concepts of how the Ig loci have evolved. While protein sequences certainly indicate that the basic unit of evolution was the single protein domain, nucleic acid studies have shown unequivocally that even in the heavy chain polypeptides, which are the result of multiple duplications, a domain-sized unit, the exon, is retained as the basic genomic structure. The conservation of regions, not expressed at the protein level, which are required for the expression of complete functional immunoglobulins, e.g., 5' regulatory sequences, switch sequences, and splice junctions, suggests that polymorphism is poorly tolerated at some sites.

The phenomenon of gene conversion among tandemly arranged homologous Ig genes has only been appreciated recently with the observations that different alleles at the murine IgG_{2a} locus differ not only by mutation but by the substitution of an exon-length segment from the adjacent IgG_{2b} gene for the original IgG_{2a} exon.[105] A similar process has been suggested for the genesis of the human γ_3 gene.[81] While the mechanism of gene conversion is not understood, the ability of tandem genes, each bearing regions of homology, to recombine in a variety of locations with either its paired chromosome, its sister chromatid, or even itself can allow for both expansion and contraction of the size of a gene family and yet retain the structural features necessary for the protein products of the locus.[106]

A good example of this phenomenon, with respect to immunoglobulins, are the γ chain subclasses. The mouse and human both have four γ subclasses identified to date. In each species the homology among the classes is greater than that between any combination of human and mouse subclasses, suggesting that in each species the four classes arose independently, yet the complex appears to have evolved similarly in the two species. The analyses above imply that gene conversion has occurred between members of the group in both man and mouse, presumably responding to the same evolutionary pressures.

IMPLICATIONS FOR DISEASE

Humans, as an outbred experimental species, would be expected to show substantial polymorphism. Many of the analyses of human Ig genes have noted so-called restriction enzyme polymorphism in the human Ig loci. These are characterized by the presence of differently sized pieces of DNA carrying identifiable Ig genes when germ line (unrearranged) DNA is digested by a given enzyme. Some of these have been noted around the switch site of the μ gene and appear to be inherited in a Mendelian fashion linked to Gm loci.[107] In addition, recent data from experiments utilizing inbred mouse strains strongly suggest that V_H gene families may be inherited linked to heavy chain loci.[108] None of this should be terribly surprising, since the linkage analysis confirms what we already know from looking at the DNA of the chromosome. However, if specific human V_H families containing the structural genes for certain antibodies are either increased or diminished in some individuals, they may be at greater or lesser risk for disease states characterized by enhanced or reduced production of those antibodies.

While most of the markers that have shown increased associations with rheumatic diseases have been on chromosome 6, i.e., the MHC locus (see Chapters 4 and 5), it is possible that investigations of the Ig loci may prove fruitful and that analysis of V_H polymorphic profiles may be informative with respect to the pathogenesis of rheumatic diseases.[109]

The genetic mechanisms responsible for retaining the structural features of the immunoglobulin proteins over the centuries have managed to amplify a relatively limited amount of genetic information by employing recombinational events among various elements, posttranscriptional differential processing, somatic mutation, and combinatorial association between gene products to simultaneously generate common structures with enormous variation in specificity and families of proteins with the same or similar specificities and multiple biologic effector functions. The present Ig genes represent one set of constraints under which the B-lymphocyte arm of the immune response operates. The role of these genes in T lymphocyte function has not been established. While there is much circumstantial evidence indicating that Ig V_H gene products function in T lymphocytes, attempts to demonstrate functional rearrangements of Ig genes in these cells have failed. Recently, work from several laboratories has established that the T-lymphocyte antigen receptor is composed of two nonimmunoglobulin polypeptide chains.[110-113] The gene family coding for one of these chains has been identified and shown to have a structure similar to that coding for Ig heavy chains with V, D, J, and C segments, which appear to rearrange by translocation to yield the active genes. Hence the generation of T-lymphocyte specificity seems to involve the same general process as does that of B lymphocytes but an independent set of similar gene segments carried on different chromosomes.

References

1. World Health Organization: WHO Bul. J. Immunol. 35:953, 1966; 38:151, 1968; 41:975, 1969; 108:1733, 1972. Eur. J. Immunol. 6:599, 1976.
2. Natvig, J.B., and Kunkel, H.G.: Human immunoglobulins: Classes, subclasses, genetic variants, and idiotypes. Adv. Immunol. 16:1, 1973.
3. Lamm, M.D.: Cellular aspects of immunoglobulin A. Adv. Immunol. 22:223, 1976.
4. Koshland, M.E.: Structure and function of the J chain. Adv. Immuno. 20:41, 1975.
5. Caserto, J.P., and Kress, B.P.: β_2M, a tumor marker of lymphoproliferative disorders. Lancet 2:108, 1978.
6. Ervin, P.E., and Wibell, L.: The serum levels and urinary excretion of β_2-microglobulin in apparently healthy subjects. Scand. J. Clin. Lab. Invest. 29:69, 1982.
7. Poulik, M.D., and Reisfeld, R.A.: β_2-Microglobulins. In Inman, F.P., and Mandy, W.J. (eds.): Contemporary Topics in Molecular Immunology. Vol. 4. New York, Plenum Press, 1975.
8. Peterson, P.A., Cunningham, B.A., Berggard, I., and Edelman, G.M.: β_2-microglobulin: A free immunoglobulin domain. Proc. Natl. Acad. Sci. (USA) 69:1697, 1972.
9. Snell, G.D., Dausset, J., and Nathenson, S.G.: Histocompatibility. New York, Academic Press, 1976.
10. Ploegh, H.L., Orr, H.T., and Strominger, J.L.: Major histocompatibility antigens: The human (HLA-A, -B, -C) and murine (H-2K, H-2D) class I molecules. Cell 24:287, 1981.
11. Klein, J., Juretic, A., Baxevanis, C.N., and Nagy, Z.A.: The traditional and a new version of the mouse H-2 complex. Nature 291:455, 1981.
12. Williams, A.F., and Gagnon, J.: Neuronal cell Thy-l glycoprotein: Homology with immunoglobulins. Science 216:696, 1982.
13. Kabat, E.A., Wu, T.T., and Bilofsky, H.: Variable regions of immunoglobulin chains. Tabulations and analyses of amino acid sequence. Bethesda, Maryland, National Institutes of Health, 1983.
14. Capra, J.D., and Kehoe, J.M.: Hypervariable regions, idiotype and the antibody combining site. Adv. Immunol. 20:1, 1975.
15. Porter, R.R.: The combining sites of antibodies. Harvey Lect. 65:157, 1971.
16. Edelman, G.M., Cunningham, W.E., Gall, P.D., Gottlieb, H., Rutishau-

ser, U., and Waxdal, M.J.: The covalent structure of entire IgG₁ immunoglobulin molecule. Proc. Natl. Acad. Sci. (USA) 63:78, 1969.

17. Spiegelberg, H.: Biological activities of immunoglobulins of different classes and subclasses. Adv. Immunol. 19:259, 1974.

18. Frangione, B., Milstein, C., and Franklin, E.C.: Chemical typing of immunoglobulins. Nature 221:149, 1969.

19. Michaelsen, T.E., Frangione, B., and Franklin, E.C.: Primary structure of the "hinge" region of human IgG3. J. Biol. Chem. 253:883, 1977.

20. Recht, B., Frangione, B., Franklin, E.C., and van Loghem, E.: Structural studies of a human γ_3 myeloma protein (GOE) that binds staph protein A. J. Immunol. 127:917, 1981.

21. Haake, D.A., Franklin, E.C., and Frangione, B.: The modification of human immunoglobulin binding to staphylococcal protein A using diethylpyrocarbonate. J. Immunol. 129:190, 1982.

22. Mestecky, J., and Schrohenloher, R.E.: Site of attachment of J chain to human immunoglobulin M. Nature 249:650, 1974.

23. Fu, S.M., Winchester, R.J., and Kunkel, H.G.: Occurrence of surface IgM, IgD, and free light chains on human lymphocytes. J. Exp. Med. 139:1451, 1974.

24. Vitetta, E.A., and Uhr, J.W.: Immunoglobulin-receptors revisited. A model for the differentiation of bone marrow-derived lymphocytes is described. Science 189:964, 1975.

25. Putnam, F.: Immunoglobulins. I. Structure. In Putnam, F.W. (ed.): The Plasma Proteins: Structure, Function and Genetic Control. New York, Academic Press, 1977.

26. Rogers, J., Early, P., Carter, C., Calame, K., Bond, M., Hood, L., and Wall, R.: Two mRNA's with different 3′ ends encode membrane-bound and secreted forms of immunoglobulin μ chain. Cell 20:303, 1980.

27. Lobb, C.J., and Clem, L.W.: Phylogeny of immunoglobulin structure and function XII. Secretory immunoglobulins in the bile of the marine teleost Archosargus probatocephalus. Mol. Immunol. 18:615, 1981.

28. Gowans, J.L., and Knight, E.J.: The route of recirculating lymphocytes in the rat. Proc. Royal Soc. (Series B) 159:257, 1964.

29. Craig, S.W., and Cebra, J.J.: Rabbits' Peyer's patches, appendix and popliteal lymph node lymphocytes: A comparative analysis of their membrane immunoglobulin components and plasma cell precursor potential. J. Immunol. 114:492, 1975.

30. McWilliams, M., Phillips-Quagliata, J., and Lamm, M.E.: Mesenteric node B lymphoblasts which home to the small intestine are precommitted to IgA synthesis. J. Exp. Med. 145:866, 1977.

31. McDermott, M.R., and Bienenstock, J.: Evidence for a common mucosal immunological system. I. Migration of B immunoblasts into intestinal, respiratory and genital tissues. J. Immunol. 122:1892, 1979.

32. Roux, M.E., McWilliams, M., Phillips-Quagliata, J., and Lamm, M.E.: Differentiation pathway of Peyer's patch precursors of IgA plasma cells in the secretory immune system. Cell. Immunol. 61:141, 1981.

33. Tomasi, T.B., Jr.: The gamma A globulins. First line of defense. In Good, R.A., and Fisher, D.W. (eds.): Immunobiology. Stamford, Connecticut, Sinauer, 1971.

34. Garcia-Pardo, A., Lamm, M.E., Plaut, A.G., and Frangione, B.: Secretory component is covalently bound to a single subunit in human secretory IgA. Immunochemistry 16:477, 1979.

35. Plaut, A.G., Genco, R.J., and Tomasi, T.B., Jr.: Isolation of an enzyme from Streptococcus sanguis which specifically cleaves IgA. J. Immunol. 113:289, 1974.

36. Mulks, M.H., Plaut, A.G., Feldman, H.A., and Frangione, B.: IgA proteases of two distinct specificities are released by Neiseria Meningitidis. J. Exp. Med. 152:1442, 1980.

37. Cann, G.M., Zaritsky, A., and Koshland, M.E.: Primary structure of the immunoglobulin J chain from the mouse. Proc. Natl. Acad. Sci. (USA) 79:6656, 1982.

38. Rowe, D.S., and Fahey, J.L.: A new class of human immunoglobulins. I. A unique myeloma protein. J. Exp. Med. 121:171, 1965.

39. Rowe, D.S., Hug, K., Forni, L., and Pernis, B.: Immunoglobulin D as a lymphocyte receptor. J. Exp. Med. 138:965, 1973.

40. Takahashi, N., Tetaert, D., Debuire, B., Lin, L.C., and Putnam, F.W.: Complete amino acid sequence of the heavy chain of human immunoglobulin D. Proc. Natl. Acad. Sci. (USA) 79:2850, 1982.

41. Ishizaka, K., Ishizaka, T., and Lee, E.H.: Biologic function of the Fc fragments of E myeloma protein. Immunochemistry 7:687, 1970.

42. Dorrington, K.J., and Bennich, H.: Structure-function relationship in human immunoglobulin E. Immunol. Rev. 41:3, 978.

43. Holowka, D., and Metzger, H.: Further characterization of the B-component of the receptor for immunoglobulin E. Molec. Immunol. 19:219, 1982.

44. Kunkel, H.G., and Kindt, T.: Allotypes and idiotypes. In Benaceraff, B. (ed.): Immunogenetics and Immunodeficiency. Lancaster, England, Medical and Technical Publishing Company, 1975.

45. Poljak, R.J., Amzel, L.M., Avey, H.P., Chen, B.L., Phizackerley, R.P., and Saul, F.: Three-dimensional structure of the Fab′ fragment of a human immunoglobulin at 2.8Å resolution. Proc. Natl. Acad. Sci. (USA) 70:3305, 1973.

46. Davies, D.R., Padlan, E.A., and Segal, D.M.: Immunoglobulin structures at high resolution. In Inman, F.P., and Mandy, W.J. (eds.): Contemporary Topics in Molecular Immunology. Vol. 4. New York, Plenum Press, 1975.

47. Hozumi, N., and Tonegawa, S.: Evidence for somatic rearrangement of immunoglobulin genes coding for variable and constant region. Proc. Natl. Acad. Sci. (USA) 73:3628, 1976.

48. Malcolm, S., Barton, P., Murphy, C., Ferguson-Smith, M.A., Bentley, D.L., and Rabbitts, T.H.: Localization of human immunoglobulin κ light gene variable region genes to the short arm of chromosome 2 by in situ hybridization. Proc. Natl. Acad. Sci. (USA) 79:4957, 1982.

49. Bentley, D.L., and Rabbitts, T.H.: Human V_κ immunoglobulin gene number: Implications for the origin of antibody diversity. Cell 24:613, 1981.

50. Rabbitts, T.H., Matthyssens, G., and Hamlyn, P.H.: Contribution of immunoglobulin heavy-chain variable region genes to antibody diversity. Nature 284:238, 1980.

51. Bentley, D.L., and Rabbitts, T.H.: Human immunoglobulin variable region genes: DNA sequences of two V_κ genes and a pseudogene. Nature 288:730, 1980.

52. Blobel, G., and Dobberstein, B.: Transfer of proteins across membranes. I. Presence of proteolytically processed and unprocessed nascent immunoglobulin light chains on membrane-bound ribosomes of murine myeloma. J. Cell Biol. 67:834, 1975.

53. Milstein, C., Brownlee, G.G., Harrison, T.M., Mathews, M.B.: A possible precursor of immunoglobulin light chains. Nature (New Biol.) 239:117, 1972.

54. Hieter, P.A., Max, E.E., Seidman, J.G., Maizel, J.V., Jr., Leder, P.: Cloned human and mouse kappa immunoglobulin constant and J region genes conserve homology in functional segments. Cell 22:197, 1980.

55. Proudfoot, N.J., and Brownlee, G.G.: 3′ Non-coding region sequences in eukaryotic messenger RNA. Nature 263:211, 1976.

56. Erikson, J., Martinis, J., and Croce, C.M.: Assignment of the genes for human λ immunoglobulin chains to chromosome 22. Nature 294:173, 1981.

57. Kabat, E.A., Wu, T.T., Bilofsky, H., Reid-Miller, M., Perry, H.: Sequences of proteins of immunological interest. U.S. Dept. of Health and Human Services, Public Health Service, National Institutes of Health, p. 14, 1983.

58. Hieter, P.A., Hollis, G.F., Korsmeyer, S.J., Waldmann, T.A., Leder, P.: Clustered arrangement of immunoglobulin λ constant region genes in man. Nature 294:536, 1981.

59. Taub, R.A., Hollis, G.F., Hieter, P.A., Korsmeyer, S., Waldmann, T.A., and Leder, P.: Variable amplification of immunoglobulin λ light chain genes in human populations. Nature 304:172, 1983.

60. Hollis, G.F., Hieter, P.A., McBride, O.W., Sloan, D., Leder, P.: Processed genes: A dispersed human immunoglobulin gene bearing evidence of RNA-type processing. Nature 296:321, 1982.

61. Croce, C.M., Shander, M., Martinis, J., Cicurel, L., D'Ancona, G., Dolby, T.W., and Koprowski, H.: Chromosomal location of the genes for human immunoglobulin heavy chain. Proc. Natl. Acad. Sci. (USA) 76:3416, 1979.

62. Matthyssens, G., and Rabbitts, T.H.: Structure and multiplicity of genes for the human immunoglobulin heavy chain variable region. Proc. Natl. Acad. Sci. (USA) 77:6561, 1980.

63. Rechavi, G., Bienz, B., Ram, D., Ben-Neriah, Y., Cohen, J.B., Zakut, R., and Givol, D.: Organization and evolution of immunoglobulin V_H subgroups. Proc. Natl. Acad. Sci. (USA) 79:4405, 1982.

64. Rechavi, G., Ram, D., Glazer, L., Zakut, R., Givol, D.: Evolutionary aspects of immunoglobulin heavy chain variable region (V_H) gene subgroups. Proc. Natl. Acad. Sci. (USA) 80:855, 1983.

65. Siebenlist, U., Ravetch, J.V., Korsmeyer, S., Waldmann, T., and Leder, P.: Human immunoglobulin D-segments encoded in tandem multigenic families. Nature 294:631, 1981.

66. Schilling, J., Clevinger, B., Davie, J.M., and Hood, L.: Amino acid sequence of homogeneous antibodies to dextran and DNA rearrangements in heavy chain V-region gene segments. Nature 283:35, 1980.

67. Ravetch, J.V., Siebenlist, U., Korsmeyer, S., Waldmann, T., and Leder, P.: Structure of the human immunoglobulin μ locus: Characterization of embryonic and rearranged J and D genes. Cell 27:583, 1981.

68. Rabbitts, T.H., Forster, A., and Milstein, C.P.: Human immunoglobulin heavy chain genes: Evolutionary comparisons of C_μ, C_δ, and C_γ genes and associated switch sequences. Nucleic Acids Res. 9:4509, 1981.

69. Ravetch, J.V., Kirsch, I.R., and Leder, P.: Evolutionary approach to the question of immunoglobulin heavy chain switching. Evidence from cloned human and mouse genes. Proc. Natl. Acad. Sci. (USA) 77:6734, 1980.

70. Takahashi, N., Nakai, S., Honjo, T.: Cloning of human immunoglobulin μ gene and comparison with mouse μ gene. Nucleic Acids Res. 8:5983, 1980.

71. Williams, P.B., Kubo, R.T., and Grey, H.M.: μ-Chains from a nonsecretor B-cell line differ from secreted μ chains at the C-terminal end. J. Immunol. 121:2435, 1978.

72. Rogers, J., Choi, E., Souza, L., Carter, C., Word, C., Kuehl, M., Eisenberg, D., and Wall, R.: Gene segments encoding transmembrane carboxy termini of immunoglobulin γ_1 chains. Cell 26:19, 1981.

73. Ellison, J., Buxbaum, J., and Hood, L.: The nucleotide sequence of a human immunoglobulin gamma 4 constant region gene. DNA 1:11, 1981.

74. Cheng, H.L., Blattner, F.R., Fitzmaurice, L., Mushinski, J.F., and Tucker, P.W.: Structure of genes for membrane and secreted murine IgD heavy chains. Nature 296:410, 1982.

75. Breathnach, R., and Chambon, P.: Organization and expression of eukaryotic split genes coding for proteins. Ann. Rev. Biochem. 50:349, 1981.

76. Shimizu, A., Takahashi, N., Yaoita, Y., and Honjo, T.: Organization of the constant-region gene family of the mouse immunoglobulin heavy chain. Cell 28:499, 1982.

77. Flanagan, J.G., and Rabbitts, T.H.: Arrangement of human immunoglobulin heavy chain constant region genes implies evolutionary duplication of a segment containing γ, ϵ and α genes. Nature 300:709, 1982.

78. Lefranc, M., Lefranc, G., and Rabbitts, T.H.: Inherited deletion of immunoglobulin heavy chain constant region genes in normal human individuals. Nature 300:760, 1982.

79. Max, E.E., Battey, J., Neu, R., Kirsch, I.R., and Leder, P.: Duplication and deletion in the human immunoglobulin ϵ genes. Cell 29:691, 1982.

80. Battey, J., Max, E.E., McBride, W.O., Swan, D., and Leder, P.: A processed human immunoglobulin ϵ gene has moved to chromosome 9. Proc. Natl. Acad. Sci. (USA) 79:5956, 1982.

81. Takahashi, N., Ueda, S., Obata, M., Nikaido, T., Nakai, S., and Honjo, T.: Structure of human immunoglobulin gamma genes: Implications for evolution of a gene family. Cell 29:671, 1982.

82. Franklin, E.C., and Frangione, B.: Structural variants of human and murine immunoglobulins. In Inman, F.P., and Mandy, W.J. (eds.): Contemporary Topics in Molecular Immunology, Vol. 4, New York, Plenum Press, 1975.

83. Alexander, A., Steinmetz, M., Barritault, D., Frangione, B., Franklin, E.C., Hood, L., and Buxbaum, J.: Gamma heavy chain disease in man: cDNA sequence supports partial gene deletion model. Proc. Natl. Acad. Sci. (USA) 79:3260, 1982.

84. Matthyssens, G., and Tonegawa, S.: V and C parts of immunoglobulin κ-chain genes are separate in myeloma. Nature 273:763, 1978.

85. Korsmeyer, S.J., Hieter, P.A., Sharrow, S.O., Goldman, C.K., Leder, P., and Waldmann, T.: Normal human B cells display ordered light chain gene rearrangements and deletions. J. Exp. Med. 156:975, 1982.

86. Early, P., Huang, H., Davis, M., Calame, K., and Hood, L.: An immunoglobulin heavy chain variable region gene is generated from three segments of DNA: V_H, D and J_H. Cell 19:981, 1980.

87. Coleclough, C., Perry, R.P., Karjalainen, K., and Weigert, M.: Aberrant rearrangements contribute significantly to the allelic exclusion of immunoglobulin gene expression. Nature 290:372, 1981.

88. Kubagawa, H., Mayumi, M., Crist, W.M., and Cooper, M.D.: Immunoglobulin heavy-chain switching in pre-B leukemias. Nature 301:340, 1983.

89. Sakano, H., Hüppi, K., Heinrich, G., and Tonegawa, S.: Sequences at the somatic recombination sites of immunoglobulin light chains. Nature 280:288, 1979.

90. Korsmeyer, S.J., Hieter, P.A., Ravetch, J.V., Poplack, D.G., Waldmann, T.A., and Leder, P.: Developmental hierarchy of immunoglobulin gene arrangements in human leukemic pre-B cells. Proc. Natl. Acad. Sci. (USA) 78:7096, 1981.

91. Hieter, P.A., Korsmeyer, S.J., Waldmann, T.A., and Leder, P.: Human immunoglobulin κ light chain genes are deleted or rearranged in λ-producing B-cells. Nature 290:368, 1981.

92. Early, P., Rogers, J., Davis, M., Calame, K., Bond, M., Wall, R., and Hood, L.: Two mRNA's can be producing from a single immunoglobulin μ gene by alternative RNA processing pathways. Cell 20:313, 1980.

93. Kemp, D.J., Morahan, G., Cowman, A.F., and Harris, A.W.: Production of RNA for secreted immunoglobulin μ chains does not require transcriptional termination 5' to the μ_M exons. Nature 301:84, 1983.

94. Rogers, J., and Wall, R.: Immunoglobulin heavy chain genes: Demethylation accompanies class switching. Proc. Natl. Acad. Sci. (USA) 78:7497, 1981.

95. Vessiere-Louveauz, F.M.Y.R., Hijmans, W., and Schuit, H.R.E.: Multiple heavy chain isotypes on the membrane of the small B-lymphocytes in human blood. Clin. Exp. Immunol. 43:149, 1981.

96. Honjo, T., and Kataoka, T.: Organization of immunoglobulin heavy chain genes and allelic deletion model. Proc. Natl. Acad. Sci. (USA) 75:2140, 1978.

97. Yaoita, Y., and Honjo, T.: Deletion of immunoglobulin heavy chain genes from expressed allelic chromosome. Nature 286:850, 1980.

98. Obata, M., Kataoka, T., Nakai, S., Yamagishi, H., Takahashi, N., Yamawaki-Kataoka, Y., Nikaido, T., Shimizu, A., and Honjo, T.: Structure of a rearranged γ_1 chain gene and its implication to immunoglobulin class-switch mechanism. Proc. Natl. Acad. Sci. (USA) 78:2437, 1981.

99. Isakson, P.C., Pure, E., Vitetta, E.A., and Kramer, P.H.: T-cell derived B-cell differentiation factors. J. Exp. Med. 155:734, 1982.

100. Moore, K.W., Rogers, J., Hunkapiller, T., Early, P., Nottenburg, C., Weissman, I., Bazin, H., Wall, R., and Hood, L.E.: Expression of IgD may use both DNA rearrangement and RNA splicing mechanisms. Proc. Natl. Acad. Sci. (USA) 78:1800, 981.

101. Yaoita, Y., Kimagai, Y., Okumura, J., and Honjo, T.: Expression of lymphocyte surface IgE does not require switch recombination. Nature 297:697, 1982.

102. Selsing, E., and Storb, U.: Somatic mutation of immunoglobulin light chain variable region genes. Cell 25:47, 1981.

103. Crews, S., Griffin, J., Huang, H., Calame, K., and Hood, L.: A single V_H gene segment encodes the immune response to phosphoryl choline: Somatic mutation is correlated with the class of antibody. Cell 25:59, 1981.

104. Kim, S., Davis, M., Sinn, E., Patten, P., and Hood, L.: Antibody diversity: Somatic hypermutation of rearranged V_H genes. Cell 27:573, 1981.

105. Ollo, R., and Rougeon, F.: Gene conversion and polymorphism: Generation of mouse immunoglobulin γ_{2a} chain alleles by differential gene conversion by γ_{2b} chain gene. Cell 32:515, 1983.

106. Baltimore, D.: Gene conversion: Some implications for immunoglobulin genes. Cell 24:592, 1981.

107. Migone, N., Feder, J., Cann, H., van West, B., Hwang, H., Takahashi, N., Honjo, T., Piazza, A., and Cavalli-Sforza, L.L.: Multiple DNA fragment polymorphisms associated with immunoglobulin μ chain switch-like regions in man. Proc. Natl. Acad. Sci. (USA) 80:467, 1983.

108. Ben-Neriah, Y., Cohen, J.B., Rechavi, G., Zakut, R., Givol, D.: Polymorphism of germline immunoglobulin V_H genes correlates with allotype and idiotype markers. Eur. J. Immunol. 11:1017.

109. Rechavi, G., Givol, D., and Geltner, D.: Human V_H restriction length polymorphism: A possible association with autoimmune disease. Arth. Rheum. 26:S23, 1983.

110. Yanagi, Y., Yasunobo, Y., Leggett, K., Clark, S.P., Aleksander, I., and Mak, T.W.: A human T-cell specific cDNA clone encodes a protein having extensive homology to immunoglobulin chains. Nature 308:145, 1984.

111. Hedrick, S.M., Nielsen, E.A., Kavaler, J., Cohen, D.I., and Davis, M.M.: Sequence relationships between putative T-cell receptor polypeptides and immunoglobulins. Nature 308:153, 1984.

112. Chien, Y., Gascoigne, N.R.J., Kavaler, J., Lee, N.E., and Davis, M.M.: Somatic recombination in a murine T-cell receptor gene. Nature 309:322, 1984.

113. Siu, G., Clark, S.P., Yoshikai, Y., Malissen, M., Yanagi, Y., Strauss, E., Mak, T.W., and Hood, L.: The human T-cell antigen receptor is encoded by variable, diversity and joining gene segments that rearrange to generate a complete V-gene. Cell 37:393, 1984.

Acknowledgments

The authors gratefully acknowledge the secretarial expertise of Beverly Coopersmith, Randi Klein, and Carol O'Brien. Work from the authors' laboratories was supported by NIH grants AM01431, AM02594 and research funds from the Veterans Administration.

Chapter 3
Immunologic Aspects of Inflammation: Lymphocyte Populations

Brian L. Kotzin and Samuel Strober

INTRODUCTION

Although a variety of cell populations participate in the inflammatory response, the specificity of the immune response for antigen resides within the lymphocytes. Only lymphocytes have surface receptors that allow specific recognition of foreign substances and the development of antigen-specific immunologic memory. Differences in lymphocyte populations were initially defined by differences in function and organs of origin. Recently major technological advances have allowed the development of specific reagents (including monoclonal antibodies) that identify surface markers on distinct lymphocyte subpopulations. There has ensued a rapid accumulation of experimental data. Events in lymphocyte differentiation before and after antigen stimulation have been further clarified, and in addition, a series of complex lymphocyte interactions that control the immune response have been defined.

TWO SYSTEMS OF IMMUNITY

Studies of immunity in chickens demonstrated a clear dichotomy in the immune system.[1-3] Removal of the thymus gland shortly after hatching resulted in the elimination of immune responses mediated by cells but, not those mediated by serum antibodies in irradiated birds. On the other hand, neonatal removal of the bursa of Fabricius rendered the birds agammaglobulinemic and unable to develop serum antibody responses after antigenic challenge. Cell-mediated immune responses in these bursectomized birds remained intact.

This dichotomy is also seen in two congenital immunodeficiency syndromes in humans (Table 3–1). Children with X-linked agammaglobulinemia (Bruton's syndrome) appear to have deficits similar to those of bursectomized chickens. Humoral immunity is lacking, as judged by the marked reduction in the concentration of serum immunoglobulins (~1 percent of normals), by the absence of isohemagglutinins, and by the inability to make serum antibodies to the usual vaccines (e.g., DPT vaccine). However, cell-mediated immunity is intact in these patients, as judged by the ability to reject skin allografts and to mediate delayed hypersensitivity responses to the intradermal injection of certain antigens (e.g., dinitrochlorobenzene [DNCB], streptokinase-streptodornase [SKSD], and tuberculin [PPD]). Children with Bruton's syndrome become increasingly susceptible to bacterial infections (i.e., sinusitis, pneumonia, furunculosis, meningitis) after 6 months of age when maternal antibodies begin to disappear. Viral exanthems and superficial fungal infections are generally not major threats to these children.

Children born without a thymus gland, resulting from improper development of the fourth pharyngeal pouch during embryogenesis (DiGeorge syndrome), show immune deficits similar to those of thymectomized birds. Thus, allograft rejection and delayed hypersensitivity reactions are absent, but the concentration of serum immunoglobulins is near normal. These children frequently succumb to viral infection and can develop disseminated fungal infections after superficial skin involvement.

The two systems of immunity were subsequently shown to be mediated by two different lines of lymphocytes.[4-6] Thus, B ("bursa-equivalent") lymphocytes are capable of developing from cells in the bone marrow independent of the influence of the thymus, and give rise to antibody-producing cells. The other line of cells, which requires the thymus for development, is called T (thymus-derived) lymphocytes. T and B lymphocytes are morphologically similar, although some differences have been described by electron microscopy. With the development of reagents that identify surface markers, B lymphocytes were shown to carry immunoglobulin on the cell surface. This appears to be true for all mammals studied thus far. The mouse was the first animal to be extensively studied for T lymphocyte surface antigens. Raff and his colleagues showed that nearly all cells in the thymus and the progeny of thymus cells in peripheral lymphoid tissues (spleen and lymph nodes) could be identified by antisera directed against θ (Thy-1) antigen.[5] This antigen is the product of a single genetic locus called the Thy-1 locus, which is known to have different alleles. Although all mouse T lymphocytes are recognized by anti-Thy-1 antisera, this antigen is not expressed on B lymphocytes or other hematolymphoid cells. There is no crossreactivity of this antisera with human T lymphocytes, which are recognized by their surface receptors for sheep red blood cells and more recently by surface determinants recognized by a variety of monoclonal antibodies (see below).[6]

Table 3–1. Dichotomy of the Immune System

	Humoral Immunity	Cellular Immunity
Effector Cell:	B lymphocyte	T lymphocyte
Defense Against:	Extracellular organisms (e.g., pyogenic bacterial infections)	Intracellular organisms (e.g., viral, fungal, and opportunistic bacterial infections)
Examples of Immunodeficiency:	X-linked agammaglobulinemia (Bruton's syndrome) Acquired hypogammaglobulinemia	Congenital thymic aplasia (DiGeorge syndrome) Acquired immunodeficiency syndrome (AIDS)
Laboratory Findings:	Decreased serum Ig levels Low to absent isohemagglutinins	Decreased delayed hypersensitivity reaction (e.g., PPD, SKSD, DNCB)
	Decreased antibody response to injected antigens (e.g., DPT vaccine)	Decreased allograft rejection
	Decreased Ig production by peripheral blood cells after in vitro stimulation (e.g., with pokeweed mitogen)	Decreased proliferative response of peripheral blood cells to mitogens (e.g., phytohemmagglutin [PHA] and conanavalin A [ConA])

LYMPHOCYTE MIGRATION AND HOMING

Studies by Everett and his co-workers[7] suggested that small lymphocytes in mammals could be divided into two major categories: long-lived cells with a life span greater than 2 weeks and short-lived cells with a life span of less than 2 weeks (usually a few days). Their work showed that small lymphocytes in the thymus and

bone marrow had a life span of approximately 48 hours, and that these cells were probably renewed in these organs from rapidly dividing precursors. On the other hand, over 90 percent of thoracic duct and lymph node cells had a life span measured in weeks to months. Gowans showed that the long-lived cells in the thoracic duct continually recirculate from the blood to the lymph (Fig. 3–1) and that small lymphocytes from thymus and bone marrow are not members of the recirculating pool.[8] These findings indicated that the physiologic characteristics of small lymphocytes could be used to divide them into two major categories—(1) recirculating long-lived cells and (2) nonrecirculating short-lived cells.

Speculation that the recirculating long-lived cells were T lymphocytes and that the nonrecirculating short-lived cells were B lymphocytes was proved incorrect. Experiments clearly demonstrated that B lymphocytes can recirculate in rats and that a portion of B lymphocytes had a life span of at least several weeks.[9,10] Several studies using both surface markers and immune function to identify T and B lymphocytes indicated that both populations contain mixtures of long- and short-lived cells and that these mixtures depend upon the lymphoid tissue investigated.[11] The thymus and bone marrow contain almost exclusively short-lived T and B lymphocytes, respectively, and the thoracic duct lymph contains mainly long-lived T and B lymphocytes.

Studies of the relationship between nonrecirculating, short-lived B lymphocytes and recirculating, long-lived B lymphocytes suggested that antigen is the signal that transforms the former cells into the latter. Strober and colleagues showed that B lymphocytes that have not seen antigen previously ("virgin B lymphocytes") are unable to recirculate from the blood to the lymph and are replaced through cell division approximately every 48 hours.[9] On the other hand, B lymphocytes that have encountered antigen previously ("memory B lymphocytes") continuously recirculate and have a long life span.[9] Thus virgin B lymphocytes are ordinarily destined

Figure 3–1. Lymphocyte recirculation. Arrows indicate pathway of lymphocyte migration through arterial system, postcapillary venule, lymph node cortex and medulla, efferent lymphatics, thoracic duct, and major veins leading back to the heart. (Adapted from Douglas, S.D.: Development and structure of cells in the immune system. *In* Fudenberg, H.H., Stites, D.P., Caldwell, J.L., and Wells, J.V. (eds.): Basic and Clinical Immunology. 3rd ed. Los Altos, Lange Medical Publications, 1980.)

for a short life in the peripheral lymphoid tissues, unless their lives are "saved" by the chance encounter with antigen, which transforms them into memory cells.

A similar transformation may occur with T lymphocytes. The earliest migrants to arrive in the peripheral lymphoid tissues from the thymus appear to be short-lived T lymphocytes. On the other hand, memory T lymphocytes have been shown to be recirculating, long-lived cells.[12] It is possible that antigen is the signal that triggers this transformation. However, it is not clear that antigen is the only signal that mediates this process, since there are instances in which T lymphocytes recirculate without obvious prior exposure to antigen.

Although T and B lymphocytes are similar in some of the physiologic characteristics discussed above, they differ in their migratory and homing characteristics within the peripheral lymphoid tissues.[13] T lymphocytes injected intravenously into laboratory animals home to the periarteriolar sheaths in the splenic white pulp and to the paracortex of lymph nodes (Fig. 3–2). The latter

are "T lymphocyte areas" of the lymphoid tissues. B lymphocytes take the same initial migration pathway as T lymphocytes in leaving the central arterioles of the spleen and postcapillary venules of the lymph nodes. However, they eventually home to the primary follicles or mantle areas near the germinal centers in the spleen and to the primary follicles in the nodes (Fig. 3–2). The latter are "B lymphocyte areas" of the lymphoid tissues and are thus compartmentalized by virtue of splenic and lymph node architecture from the "T lymphocyte areas." Germinal centers contain both T and B lymphocytes and are thought to contain recently activated cells from both populations which may contribute to the memory cell pool.

There is also evidence for organ specificity of lymphocyte migration.[14-16] For example, lymphocytes isolated from intestinal lymphoid tissues (Peyer's patches) will migrate back to intestinal lymphoid tissues, while lymphocytes isolated from peripheral lymph nodes return preferentially to the peripheral nodes. This organ

Figure 3–2. *A*, Lymph node structure. Within the cortex, the primary follicles are the major B cell area while the paracortex (diffuse cortex) is the major T cell area. The secondary follicle is composed of the mantle (with lymphocytes similar to the primary follicle) and the germinal center, composed of large and small B and T cells. Both T and B lymphocytes migrate to their respective domains after exiting from the postcapillary venule. *B*, Structure of a segment of spleen. White pulp is shown in both longitudinal and cross section. Primary follicles are the major B cell area. The periarteriolar lymphoid sheath, an accumulation of small lymphocytes surrounding the central arteriole, is the major T cell area. Secondary follicles are similar to those described in lymph nodes. The marginal areas receive much of the blood entering the spleen and are the major areas of T and B cell entry. (Adapted from Hood, L.E., Weissman, I.L., and Wood, W.B. (eds.): Immunology. Menlo Park, Benjamin/Cummings Publishing Company; 1978.)

specificity of lymphocyte migration seems to be determined by a selective interaction of lymphocytes with the specialized endothelial cells of the postcapillary high endothelial venules in lymph nodes (Fig. 3–2).[16] When in lymphocyte development organ specificity develops is unclear. Selective migration to different lymphoid organs occurs in the absence of antigenic stimulation, and may determine the distribution of functionally distinct lymphocyte populations (i.e., B versus T lymphocytes) in mucosal versus nonmucosal lymphoid tissues. Blast cells (i.e., after antigenic stimulation) initially lose the ability to migrate but may demonstrate homing specificity later after a period of local proliferation and differentiation.

T LYMPHOCYTES

Maturation of T Lymphocytes. As noted above, neonatal thymectomy results in the failure of T lymphocyte surface markers and T lymphocyte function to develop.[17] The cellular deficits can be restored by transplantation of a thymus gland. Surprisingly the cells repopulating the thymus graft and the T lymphocytes repopulating the peripheral lymphoid tissues after thymic transplantation are of host rather than donor origin.[18] This suggests that cells that migrate from the thymus to the T lymphocyte areas of the peripheral lymphoid tissues are not generated de novo in the thymus. Instead, it appears that there is a traffic of cells that enter and then leave the thymus. More recent chromosomal marker studies indicate that the bone marrow is the source of cells entering the thymus. These cells are called pre-T lymphocytes, since they do not have the surface or functional characteristics of mature T lymphocytes but are thought to be the precursors of the latter cells.[19]

The actual conversion of pre-T into T lymphocytes appears to occur in the thymus by virtue of interactions between the former cells and the thymic epithelial cells.[19] The contribution of thymic hormones to T lymphocyte maturation in mammals remains controversial (reviewed in ref. 20). It is not clear to what extent maturation of T lymphocytes occurs within the thymus and to what extent maturation occurs after T lymphocytes migrate out of the thymus and into the peripheral tissues. Furthermore, it is uncertain that the in-migration of bone marrow cells to the thymus contributes significantly to the out-migration of thymus cells in the adult, since the thymus may develop the capacity for self-renewal after it is initially populated by pre-T lymphocytes from the marrow. The precise role of the thymus and thymus cell maturation in adult animals remains to be elucidated, since adult thymectomy produces few acute changes in the number and function of T lymphocytes in the peripheral tissues. The lack of reported immunologic deficits after removal of the thymus gland during open heart surgery in children suggests that the role of the thymus gland in the maintenance of cellular immunity in man may be minimal after the first few years of life. This may be due in part to the long life span of mature T

lymphocytes, to the self-renewing capacity of T lymphocytes in the periphery, and possibly to the extrathymic maturation of some T lymphocyte precursors (i.e., without physically entering the thymus).[21]

Profound changes in cell surface antigens mark the various stages of T lymphocyte maturation in both mouse and man (Fig. 3–3).[22-25] In the differentiation of mouse T lymphocytes, pre-T lymphocytes do not express the membrane glycoprotein Thy-1 antigen but do have surface major histocompatibility (H-2) antigens (which continue to be expressed during cell differentiation). These cells are induced in the thymus to express Thy-1 as well as TL and Lyt antigens. The TL antigen is expressed on greater than 95 percent of normal thymocytes and is present on most thymic leukemia (TL) cell lines.[23,26] However, nearly all peripheral T lymphocytes are Thy-1+ but TL negative. Thus, TL is an example of a surface antigen that defines an intrathymic differentiation stage. Lyt antigens (Lyt-1, 2, and 3) are *all* expressed on greater than 90 percent of thymocytes and on less than 50 percent of peripheral T lymphocytes.[22-24] Cytotoxic depletion studies suggested that the majority of peripheral T lymphocytes carry either the Lyt-1 antigen alone (Lyt-1+,23−) or a combination of the Lyt-2 and Lyt-3 antigens without the Lyt-1 antigen (Lyt-1−,23+). The two different phenotypes define functionally distinct peripheral T lymphocyte subsets (see below). More sensitive immunofluorescence techniques have shown that Lyt-1 is found on all peripheral T lymphocytes but is present in lower levels on those cells previously identified as Lyt-1−,23+.[27]

A series of monoclonal antibodies have been developed that are reactive with human thymocyte and/or peripheral T lymphocyte cell surface antigens. As proposed by Reinherz and Schlossman (Fig. 3–3),[25] using the OKT series of monoclonal antibodies, the earliest thymocytes bear OKT9 and OKT10, and this stage defines the minority (10 percent) of thymocytes. With further maturation, human thymocytes concurrently express OKT6, OKT4, OKT5, and OKT8 (accounting for more than 70 percent of the thymic population). With further maturation, thymocytes lose OKT6 reactivity, acquire OKT3 and OKT1, and segregate into OKT4 and OKT5/T8 subsets. As the thymocyte is exported into the peripheral T lymphocyte compartment, it loses the T10 marker. The OKT4 (or Leu-3, using the analagous Leu series of monoclonal antibodies) and OKT5/OKT8 (or Leu-2) subsets appear to be nonoverlapping, relatively functionally distinct populations in the peripheral lymphoid tissues (see below).

T Lymphocyte Subpopulations. Table 3–2 summarizes some distinctive surface markers present on two major peripheral lymphoid T lymphocyte subpopulations in mice and humans.[22-25,28-38] Included in the "helper/inducer" subset are T lymphocytes that help in the differentiation of B lymphocytes into immunoglobulin-secreting cells (help antibody production), T lymphocytes that help in the development of cell-mediated lymphocytotoxicity (CML), and T lymphocytes that are effectors for delayed hypersensitivity. The other major subset

Figure 3–3. Differentiation of mouse and human T lymphoctytes showing acquisition of cell surface antigens within the thymus. (Adapted from Hood, L.E., Weissman, I.L., and Wood, W.B. (eds.): Immunology. Menlo Park, Benjamin/Cummings Publishing Company, 1978; and Reinherz, E.L., and Schlossman, S.F.: The differentiation and function of human T lymphoctytes. Cell 19:821, 1980.)

ilarities exist, there is no crossreactivity between the murine and human T lymphocyte antigens when staining with either anti-Leu or anti-Lyt antibodies. The maintenance of these surface structures through evolution suggests that these molecules perform essential functions for the cells on which they are found. Some evidence for this has been provided in studies showing that both anti-Leu-2 and anti-Lyt-2 (in the absence of complement) can block cell-mediated cytotoxicity.[35,39] This observed blocking, however, could also be due to a tendency for the Leu or Lyt molecules to associate with other molecules relevant to the killing activity.

Some differences in function of the two major human T lymphocyte subsets are presented in Table 3–3.[25,32-37] Some of these are discussed below. It should be emphasized that the broad classification of lymphocyte subsets by surface phenotype does not imply that all lymphocytes with a given surface phenotype have the same function. Indeed, examples of OKT4 cells with suppressor or cytotoxic functions exist.[40,41] However, when OKT4 (Leu-3) lymphocytes are isolated from peripheral blood, they mediate predominantly helper/inducer functions in a variety of assay systems, and similarly, when OKT5 or OKT8 (Leu-2) cells are isolated, they mediate predominantly suppressor or cytotoxic functions. Recently, it has been suggested that these surface markers primarily determine the class of major histocompatibility antigens that are recognized (especially in association with antigens) rather than function.[37,41] Leu-3 (OKT4) cells recognize class II HLA antigens, whereas Leu-2 (OKT8) cells recognize class I HLA antigens (in association with antigen).

The mature T lymphocyte populations can be further divided into functional subpopulations based on differences in the display of major histocompatibility (MHC)-encoded determinants. This has allowed further delineation of T lymphocyte interactions in immunoregulatory circuits (see below).

Human T lymphocytes have also been separated into functionally distinct subsets by the specificity of their Fc receptors for either IgG (Tγ cells) or IgM (Tμ cells).[42-45] Tγ lymphocytes mediate suppression of in vitro immunoglobulin production while Tμ lymphocytes

contains T lymphocytes that suppress B lymphocyte differentiation and other T lymphocyte functions, as well as those that mediate CML (T cytotoxic cells). Monoclonal antibodies to all of the surface determinants in Table 3–2 now exist. The Leu-1 (OKT1) antigen is present on nearly all human peripheral blood T lymphocytes but is present in lower amounts on those 20 to 30 percent of T lymphocytes that carry Leu-2a and Leu-2b (OKT5) antigens. Leu-3 (or OKT4) antigens are present on 60 percent of peripheral blood T lymphocytes.

The human T lymphocyte antigens Leu-1, Leu-2a, and Leu-2b appear to have strong analogies to the mouse Lyt-1, Lyt-2, and Lyt-3 antigens, respectively.[38] This is based on studies of tissue distribution, molecular weight, subunit composition, and sensitivity to proteolysis of the respective cell surface antigens. Although these sim-

Table 3–2. Surface Determinants of the Major T Lymphocyte Subpopulations in Mouse and Man

	Human Surface Ag	Murine Surface Ag
All T Lymphocytes	SRBC Receptor	
	OKT1, OKT3	Thy-1
	Leu-1, Leu-4	Lyt-1*
Suppressor/Cytotoxic Lymphocytes	OKT5, OKT8	Lyt-2, 3
	Leu-2a, Leu-2b	
Helper/Inducer Lymphocytes	OKT4	L3T4*
	Leu-3	(Lyt-1+,23−)*

*By immunofluorescence techniques, the Lyt-1 antigen is present on all mature mouse T lymphocytes, although present in lower density on suppressor/cytotoxic cells. By cytotoxic depletion techniques, the Lyt-1 antigen is present on the the helper/inducer subset but not on the suppressor/cytotoxic subset. The murine helper/inducer subset can be recognized by the *absence* of Lyt-2 and Lyt-3 antigens. The L3T4 antigen has been recently described as the murine homologue of the human Leu-3/OKT4 molecule.[124]

Table 3–3. Immunologic Functions of the Two Major Human T Lymphocyte Subsets

	Leu-3 OKT4	Leu-2 OKT5, OKT8
Proliferative Responses (In Vitro)		
To Phytohemagglutin	+	+
Concanavalin A (ConA)	+	+
Allogeneic non-T cells	+	+
Autologous non-T cells	+	−
Soluble Antigens	+	−
Helper/Inducer Function (T-T, T-B,)	+	−
Delayed Hypersensitivity	+	−
Cytotoxic Effector Function	−	+
Suppressor Function (T-T, T-B)	−	+

mediate helper function. Unlike the subsets identified by monoclonal antibodies, Tγ lymphocytes may not maintain cell surface phenotype stability. For example, after incubation with immune complexes, the Fc-IgG receptor can be irreversibly lost and later Fc-IgM expression has been observed.[44,45] Some groups have compared T lymphocyte subsets defined by Fc receptors and by reactivity with monoclonal antibodies, and suggest that all Tγ lymphocytes may not even be of the T lymphocyte lineage (i.e., carry the OKT3 or Leu-1 antigens).[46,47] Other studies concluded that the majority of Tγ lymphocytes are T lymphocytes but that correlation with the OKT8 or Leu-2 subset (suppressor/cytotoxic cells by monoclonal antibodies) was poor.[48] Unlike subsets defined by monoclonal antibodies, subsets defined by Fc receptors are not analogous to functionally distinct murine T lymphocyte subsets. Thus, the Fc receptor T lymphocyte classification system has considerable disadvantages compared with the monoclonal antibody classification scheme defined above, especially in the study of autoimmune diseases such as SLE.

T Helper (T_H)–T Cytotoxic (T_c) Cell Interactions. In the allogeneic mixed leukocyte reaction (MLR), T lymphocytes are stimulated in vitro to proliferate by the MHC determinants on stimulator non-T cells. In addition, T lymphocytes are induced to differentiate into cytotoxic cells (T_c cells), which are capable of lysing allogeneic target cells without added antibody or complement.[23] It was demonstrated in murine MLR systems that the T lymphocytes mediating cytotoxicity were surface Lyt-1⁻,23⁺ (determined by cytotoxic depletion studies). However, collaboration between an Lyt-1⁺,23⁻ (T helper/inducer cell) subset and the Lyt-1⁻,23⁺ subset was necessary for optimum development of cytotoxicity (Fig. 3–4).[28,29] In the absence of Lyt-1⁺ cells (T_H cells), little cytotoxicity was generated. Interestingly these T_H lymphocytes were shown to recognize predominantly antigens on the surface of the stimulatory cells coded for by the I gene region of the H-2 locus (analogous to the D region in man; class II MHC antigens). In contrast, the T_c lymphocytes recognized target cell antigens coded for by K and D gene regions of H-2 (analogous to A and B regions in man, class I MHC antigens).[23,29,49,50] Thus, two stimulatory signals are required for the most efficient development of cytotoxicity. As shown in Figure 3–4, there is now evidence that the helper effect is mediated in large part by a soluble T lymphocyte product, T lymphocyte growth factor (interleukin II).[51,52]

The above in vitro system may relate to immune events that occur in tissue transplantation such as graft rejection or the graft-versus-host reaction. However, the

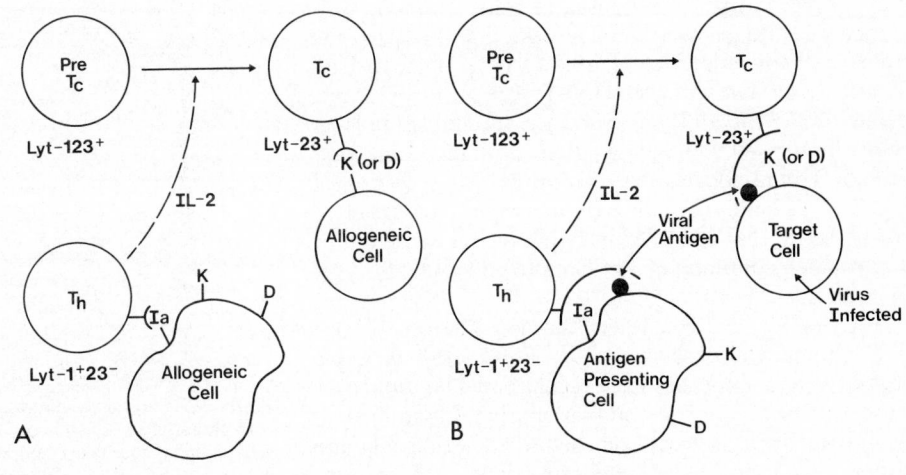

Figure 3–4. Cellular interactions involved in the generation of cell-mediated cytotoxicity both for allogeneic cells and virus infected cells. T_h, T helper cell; T_c, T cytotoxic cell; Pre-T_c, precursor of the T cytotoxic cell; *IL-2*, interleukin 2 or T cell growth factor. *A*, In the generation of cytotoxicity for allogeneic cells, T_h cells recognize allogeneic I region determinants, whereas T_c cells recognize allogeneic K or D region determinants. *B*, In the generation of cytotoxicity for virus-infected cells, all cells depicted are autologous, and T_h cells recognize viral antigens in the context of *self* I region determinants, whereas T_c cells recognize viral antigens in the context of *self* K or D region determinants (see text for details).

response to allogeneic cells is not likely to be required during everyday living. The allogeneic system does have strong analogies to the T lymphocyte interactions required to kill virus-infected cells (Fig. 3–4).[23,53-55] Thus, in the mouse, T_H(Lyt-1+,23-) lymphocytes can only recognize viral or virus-encoded surface antigens when presented on cells that express *self* I region determinants. The T_H lymphocyte must therefore recognize both viral antigens *and* I region cell surface products, and the T_H response is said to be restricted for I region determinants. The T_c cell (Lyt-1-,23+) recognizes viral antigens in association with *self* K and D antigens (restricted to K and D). Although T_H–T_c cooperation in man has not been elucidated in the same detail as in mice, studies suggest that similar mechanisms are operative.

T Suppressor (T_s) Lymphocytes. The preceding discussion focused on the T_H–T_c interaction. The systems that induce cell-mediated cytotoxicity are also regulated by suppressor T lymphocytes (T_s cells). These cells have a function opposite that of the helper cells and therefore decrease the amount of cytotoxicity generated. Different types of suppressor T lymphocytes have been described in the MLR-CML system.[23,56-63] For example, some suppressor cells suppress responder cell proliferation while others suppress only the development of cytotoxicity. Suppressor cells can function at the level of T_c precursor at initiation of cytotoxicity (afferent suppressor cell) or at the level of cytotoxic effector events (efferent suppressor cell). Suppressor cells can also be specific for the alloantigen stimulating cell (antigen specific) or suppress any MLR combination (antigen nonspecific).

The existence of suppressor T lymphocytes was actually first shown for antibody production by Gershon and his colleagues.[28] These investigators induced tolerance to sheep red blood cells (SRBC) in mice. Thus, these mice were unable to generate a normal antibody response after immunization with SRBC. The tolerant state was then passed to other mice by transferring lymphoid cells from the tolerant donors to otherwise immunocompetent recipients. The recipients of the tolerant cells became tolerant themselves and were unable to mount an immune response to SRBC. However, they had normal antibody responses to other antigens (tolerance was antigen specific). The cells that mediated the transfer of tolerance were shown to be antigen-specific T suppressor lymphocytes (Lyt-1-,23+) (by cytotoxic depletion).[28,31] In addition to antigen-specific suppressor cells of antibody production, there are nonspecific suppressor T lymphocytes that can inhibit the secretion of immuno-globulins by all B lymphocytes, or other T lymphocytes that can selectively inhibit the secretion of a particular immunoglobulin class (e.g., IgA), allotype, or even idiotype.[23,64-67]

T Lymphocyte Regulatory Circuits. The complexity of T lymphocyte subsets increases enormously when one studies interactions between regulatory T lymphocyte subpopulations. Several complex murine T lymphocyte suppressor circuits have been described which regulate either T-lymphocyte-mediated functions (delayed hypersensitivity) or B-lymphocyte-mediated functions (antibody production).[68] These amplification circuits have numerous similarities and apparently serve to maintain a finely balanced expression of immunity. In these circuits, surface markers that have additionally helped in determining subsets of functional T lymphocytes are related to the expression of determinants encoded by the MHC (e.g., I-J locus) and closely related loci (e.g., Qa).

Figure 3–5 depicts a suppressor pathway that is activated concomitantly with normal immunization to the T-lymphocyte-dependent antigen SRBC.[68-71] If Lyt-1+, 23- T lymphocytes are isolated from a mouse previously immunized to SRBC and then combined in vitro with B lymphocytes in the presence of SRBC, an in vitro anti-SRBC antibody response can be measured. Immunization also activates an inducer cell (Lyt-1+,23-, Qa-1+,I-J+), which acts on a nonprimed (no previous antigen stimulation required) Lyt-123+, I-J+, Qa-1+ target cell (feedback suppressor cell), which eventually results in an Lyt-1-,23+ suppressor effector cell. The suppressor effector cell mediates suppression of anti-SRBC antibody production in an antigen (SRBC)-specific, MHC-restricted fashion at the level of the T_H lymphocyte. This suppression has been known to be mediated by suppressor factors. Another T lymphocyte circuit is also induced, which actually decreases the amount of feedback suppression (contrasuppression) (not shown in Fig. 3–5).[72]

Analogous but less detailed "suppressor amplifier" circuits have been described using human peripheral

Figure 3–5. Suppressor pathway activation when mice are immunized with an antigen such as sheep red blood cells (SRBC). The resulting generation of "feedback suppression" negatively regulates the production of anti-SRBC antibodies (see text for details).

blood lymphocytes.[73-76] Various methods of in vitro B lymphocyte activation that are T_H lymphocyte dependent (require Leu-3 [OKT4] cells for antibody production) have been employed. In these systems, activation of the Leu-2 (OKT8) (suppressor amplifier) cell requires a Leu-3 (OKT4) inducer cell.

T Lymphocyte Clones and the Nature of the T Lymphocyte Receptor. The functions of the different T lymphocyte subpopulations described in the preceding section were studied using whole lymphocyte populations isolated by their respective surface markers. The heterogeneity of these populations must be continually emphasized. The ability to obtain pure populations of immunocompetent T lymphocytes (T lymphocyte clones) in vitro has been a recent major advance in the study of T lymphocytes. One technique of T lymphocyte cloning takes advantage of the lymphokine T lymphocyte growth factor (interleukin II), which causes the continued in vitro proliferation of activated T lymphocytes.[77-79] Thus, cells from an immunized animal with a particular antigen specificity and function (e.g., T helper, T delayed hypersensitivity, T cytotoxic, or T suppressor) can be propagated as cell lines and then cloned at the single cell level. Another technique is analogous to that used to produce monoclonal antibodies. However, instead of fusing antigen-stimulated B lymphocytes to malignant myeloma cells to "immortalize" cells secreting the desired antibody, immunocompetent T lymphocytes are fused to malignant thymoma cell lines.[79,80] The T lymphocyte hybridomas that result are screened for the desired antigen specificity and functions and then expanded into large numbers from a single cell.

T lymphocyte cloning has considerably increased our understanding of the molecular nature of the T lymphocyte receptor.[78-83] As alluded to previously, observations suggest that during antigen presentation, most T lymphocytes recognize both the antigen and the MHC region gene products expressed by the antigen-presenting cell. T_H lymphocytes and those lymphocytes that mediate delayed hypersensitivity recognize antigen in the context of I region (class II) gene products. T_H lymphocytes do not bind soluble antigens nor do they bind to I region determinants alone. T_c lymphocytes recognize antigen in the context of class I MHC determinants. In contrast to T_H and T_c lymphocytes, T suppressor lymphocytes have been noted to bind free antigen and thus might be activated by free antigen alone. This might have important consequences in those situations in which Ia-positive antigen-presenting cells are absent (e.g., in the early neonatal period), blocked (e.g., by anti-Ia antisera), or saturated (e.g., by high concentrations of antigen). The result might be selective suppressor cell activation with net immunologic unresponsiveness. Some T lymphocyte receptors have been noted to bear crossreactive idiotypes with antibodies directed at the same antigenic determinants.[78-86] However, studies have demonstrated that T lymphocyte receptors do not carry conventional immunoglobulin light chains nor immunoglobulin heavy chain constant region determinants.

T Lymphocyte Soluble Mediators—Lymphokines. T lymphocytes and especially activated T lymphocytes produce a wide variety of soluble mediators called lymphokines. These lymphokines are critically important for T lymphocyte communication with other cell types and for the generation and amplification of the inflammatory response. For example, it is thought that much of the recruitment of immunologically uncommitted cells in the delayed hypersensitivity reaction is mediated by lymphokines. A partial list of lymphokines with their functions is shown in Table 3–4.[87-93] While these substances exert marked biologic effects, they are produced in only minute quantities by activated lymphocytes. Some of the mediators have been purified sufficiently for determination of their structure, but most have not been, and

Table 3–4. T Lymphocyte Lymphokines

Lymphokine	Function
Affecting Macrophages	
Macrophage activation factor (MAF)	Activates macrophage to increase bacteriocidal and tumorcidal activity
Migration inhibition factor (MIF)	Inhibits macrophage movement; localizes macrophages in area of antigen-lymphocyte interaction
Macrophage chemotactic factor	Attracts macrophages and monocytes to site of inflammation
Macrophage Ia-Inducing Factor	Induces and increases expression of Ia on macrophage cell surface; important for antigen presenting function
Affecting Polymorphonuclear Leukocytes	
Leukocyte inhibitory factor (LIF)	Analagous to MIF
Chemotactic factor	Analagous to macrophage chemotactic factor
Affecting T Lymphocytes	
T Cell Growth factor (interleukin II)	Induces stimulated T cells to proliferate
Other mitogen factors	Induce T cells to proliferate
Gamma interferon	Inhibits viral replication; increases T cell cytotoxicity; suppresses lymphocyte proliferation induced by alloantigens and mitogens; enhances natural killer function; regulates antibody production
Transfer factor	Induces lymphocytes to become antigen specific effector cells in delayed hypersensitivity reactions
Affecting B Lymphocytes	
B cell growth factor (BCGF)	Induces B cells to proliferate after initial stimulation
T cell replacing factor	Induces B cells to differentiate into antibody producing cells after initial stimulation
Gamma interferon	See above
Affecting Other Cell Types	
Lymphotoxin (LT)	Cytotoxin released in area of antigen-lymphocyte interactions

they are identified by their different biologic functions. The number of chemically distinct humoral substances is not known, and one molecule may serve more than one function.

B LYMPHOCYTES

Maturation of B Lymphocytes. Early work in chickens showed that the first B lymphocytes appear in the bursa of Fabricius at about the time of hatching.[23,94] After hatching, the bursa involutes, and B lymphocyte precursors are thought to leave the bursa to populate the bone marrow and perhaps other lymphoid tissues. A bursalike organ has not been found in mammals. However, the mammalian fetal liver may have a function similar to that of the bursa, since pre-B lymphocytes and B lymphocytes appear first in this organ during embryogenesis.[95,96]

Maturation of B lymphocytes continues after embryogenesis and throughout the life of the adult. The continuous generation of B lymphocytes from precursors in the adult bone marrow is similar to that of the other blood elements. Indeed, B lymphocytes are derived from the same pluripotent hematopoietic stem cells in the marrow that generate erythrocytes, granulocytes, megakaryocytes, and monocytes.[97] Similarly, B lymphocytes are constantly replaced through cell division from precursor cells in the marrow every few days.[98] Many of the small lymphocytes produced in the marrow are immature cells of the B lymphocyte lineage. The maturation of B lymphocytes differs from that of the other blood elements in that the B lymphocytes have an antigen-independent and an antigen-dependent maturation scheme (Fig. 3–6).

Pre-B lymphocytes in the marrow are identified by cytoplasmic immunoglobulin without surface immunoglobulin expression.[98,99] The heavy chain of IgM is the first immunoglobulin molecule to appear in the cytoplasm, followed later by light chain expression. The first surface immunoglobulin to appear on the developing B lymphocyte is also IgM (Fig. 3–6).[98] Unlike secreted IgM, surface IgM is monomeric and has an additional hydrophobic addition on the carboxy-terminal portion of the μ chain, which apparently allows for insertion into the membrane.[100] After surface IgM expression, the B lymphocyte acquires other surface markers, including Ia antigens and both surface receptors for complement and the Fc region of immunoglobulin (not shown in Fig. 3–6).[23,101,102] Subsequently, the cell acquires surface IgD or other immunoglobulin isotypes, or both, and can be identified as the mature virgin B lymphocyte.[98,103]

Although Ig-bearing small lymphocytes are constantly generated in the marrow from rapidly dividing cells that bear no surface immunoglobulin, the last part of the antigen-independent maturation sequence may take place after B lymphocytes have migrated to the periphery. Surface IgD may be gained after migration to the periphery (i.e., to lymph nodes or spleen), since almost

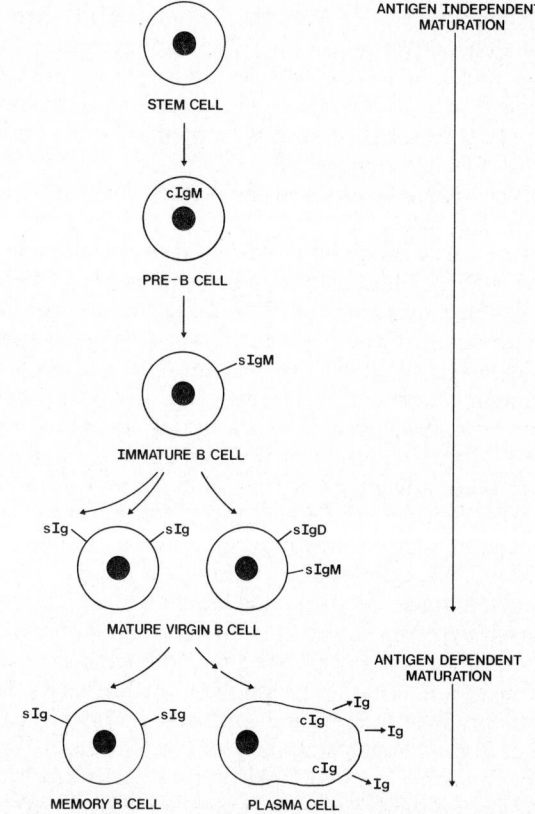

Figure 3–6. *B* lymphocyte development and differentiation. The maturation from stem cell through pre-B cell (recognized by cytoplasmic IgM without surface immunoglobulin) to mature virgin *B* cell occurs without interaction with antigen. The differentiation of the virgin *B* cell to either memory *B* cell or immunoglobulin-producing cell requires activation by antigen (see text for details).

all B lymphocytes in the marrow express surface IgM without IgD, but the majority of IgM-bearing cells in the periphery also express IgD.[103] The marrow thus contains few mature virgin B lymphocytes. The weight of evidence favors the notion that the diversity of Ig classes found on the B lymphocyte surface (i.e., IgM, IgD, IgG, IgA) is gained during antigen-independent maturation. Although individual B lymphocytes can express more than one Ig heavy chain isotype, they express only one Ig heavy chain variable region and one light chain, and thus only one idiotype.

The antigen-dependent scheme includes those differentiation steps after the virgin B lymphocyte is stimulated by antigen to give rise to (1) antibody-secreting cells or to (2) memory B cells or to (3) both (Fig. 3–6). The memory B lymphocytes differ from the virgin B lymphocytes in several important ways, including their migration pattern and life span.[9] The former cells are nonrecirculating, short-lived cells and are found in highest concentrations in the thoracic duct lymph. The marrow contains few memory B lymphocytes.

Recently, B lymphocyte differentiation antigens were described as a result of studies of mice with an X-linked immunodeficiency syndrome (CBA/N mice).[104-110] These mice are unable to generate an antibody response to one group of thymic-independent antigens (T lymphocyte help not required for the antibody response). These mice do produce antibodies to other thymic-independent antigens and to thymic-dependent antigens. The defect appears to result from the absence of a particular subset of B lymphocytes, and alloantisera were prepared that recognized distinct antigens on this subset, including the Lyb-5 antigen. The Lyb-5$^+$ B lymphocytes, which are absent in these defective mice, appear later in ontogeny, are not present in high numbers in bone marrow, have a high density of surface IgD, are difficult to tolerize, and are responsible for the antibody response to the thymic-independent antigens to which CBA/N mice cannot respond. The B lymphocytes that do not bear Lyb-5 appear early in ontogeny, are the predominant B lymphocytes in adult bone marrow, have a high density of surface IgM with little surface IgD, and are easy to tolerize. Both subsets are found in the adult spleen, although Lyb-5$^+$ B lymphocytes predominate. Interestingly, although both subsets can produce antibody to T-dependent antigens, the T lymphocyte–B lymphocyte interactions appear to be different. Thus, T lymphocyte help for the Lyb-5$^-$ B lymphocytes is MHC (I region) restricted for both the accessory (antigen-presenting) cell and B cell, while help for the Lyb-5$^+$ B cells is only MHC restricted for the accessory cell. Furthermore the Lyb-5$^+$ but not the Lyb-5$^-$ subset can be activated by soluble products from activated T helper cells. It is as yet unclear whether the Lyb-5$^+$ and Lyb-5$^-$ subsets represent further differentiation of the same B lymphocyte line, or two separate B lymphocyte lineages.

B Lymphocyte Subpopulations. B lymphocytes exist as a heterogeneous population in the peripheral lymphoid tissues, which includes cells at distinct stages of development. For example, peripheral blood B lymphocytes appear to be a variable mixture of early marrow migrants, mature virgin B lymphocytes, and memory B lymphocytes, which enter from the lymph. Studies of B lymphocyte subpopulations have been hampered by the relative lack of reagents (compared with those for T lymphocytes) that detect surface markers on functionally distinct subsets. For example, there continue to be no surface markers that easily distinguish virgin and memory B lymphocytes.

Subpopulations of B lymphocytes can, of course, be recognized by their different expression of surface immunoglobulin. The majority of B lymphocytes in mouse and man express both IgM and IgD on the cell surface.[103,107,111] The minority of cells express surface IgG.[112] Most of the IgG-bearing cells in the mouse spleen express an additional class of surface immunoglobulin (either IgM or IgD). The functional significance of having the same antigen-combining site (idiotype) associated with more than one immunoglobulin heavy chain on the surface of a single B lymphocyte is not well understood at present. However, some investigators have theorized that IgM receptors on the cell surface bind antigen and provide a tolerizing or "off" signal and that antigen interaction with IgD receptors provides a triggering or

"on" signal.[112-115] Thus, the first B lymphocytes to appear during embryogenesis bear only IgM and are tolerized after antigenic challenge. More mature B lymphocytes, which have acquired IgD receptors, are stimulated to give rise to antibody-forming cells after antigenic challenge. This may play an important role in eliminating B lymphocyte clones that recognize "self" antigens, since all young B lymphocytes come in contact with the latter antigens during early stages of differentiation.

There is evidence that the subpopulation of IgG-bearing cells contains memory cells that give rise to a rapid secondary IgG antibody response after rechallenge with antigen.[116,117] However, there appears to be no simple correlation between memory cells and surface IgG. In addition, there is no clear correlation between the expression of a given class of Ig on the surface of a B lymphocyte and the class of antibody secreted by its progeny. For example, Strober and his colleagues have shown that virgin and memory B lymphocytes bearing surface IgM but little or no IgG give rise to an early IgM antibody response followed by an IgG response.[118] This "switching" of immunoglobulin classes by B lymphocyte clones has been shown to take place during the secretory phase of immunoglobulin synthesis.

B lymphocytes have been commonly identified by other surface markers in addition to immunoglobulins. These include the receptor for the Fc piece of immunoglobulins, the receptor for the C3 component of complement, and surface antigens coded for by the I gene region in the mouse (D region in man).[23,101,102] These other B lymphocyte markers (Fc receptor, C3 receptor, Ia antigen) are present on the majority of, but not all, mature B lymphocytes. The subpopulations of B lymphocytes carrying these markers may differ in their function from those which do not. However, the role of these markers or receptors in the function of B lymphocytes in the immune response is unclear.

B Lymphocyte Activation. Studies suggest that for T lymphocyte dependent antibody production, B lymphocytes require at least two signals to become antibody-secreting cells.[23,89,92,93,119,120] One signal involves the interaction between antigen and B lymphocyte immunoglobulin receptors. Another signal is provided by the T helper lymphocyte and B lymphocyte interaction. As emphasized above, T helper lymphocytes require the presence of accessory cells (antigen-presenting cells) in order to augment the triggering of B lymphocytes into antibody-forming cells. While the T helper and accessory cell interaction is restricted to the I region, the T helper restriction for B lymphocytes may vary (see previous discussion of Lyb-5 antigen). T helper lymphocytes also elaborate factors necessary for B lymphocyte activation. After antigen exposure or appropriate initial stimulus, B lymphocytes express receptors for a B lymphocyte growth factor. This factor seems capable of maintaining proliferation of activated B lymphocytes in the absence of differentiation. These cells go on to express receptors for another T lymphocyte factor (T lymphocyte replacing factor or B lymphocyte differentiation factor), which drives B lymphocytes to terminal differentiation.

NULL LYMPHOCYTES

A small proportion of lymphocytes (~10 percent) in the peripheral tissues bear no surface markers for either T lymphocytes or B lymphocytes and are referred to as null lymphocytes. Two in vitro functions mediated by subpopulations of these cells have gained widespread interest and have been extensively studied.[121,122] Natural killer (NK) cells kill certain cell targets, especially tumor cells, in the absence of antibodies to the target cells and without prior immunization. The cells that mediate antibody-dependent cellular cytotoxicity (ADCC) are able to kill target cells that are coated with specific antibody. Again, no prior immunization of the effector cell is necessary. Thus, these null-cell-mediated functions show no recognition of specific antigens. Although the in vitro assays of natural killing generally use tumor cell targets, NK cells may also be involved in killing of virus-infected cells, foreign tissue, altered cellular self-antigens, or even other normal lymphoid cells. It has been theorized that NK cells may be involved in a primitive host defense and may perhaps be the front line of defense against malignancy.

Recent evidence has demonstrated that human null cells that mediate natural killing activity and ADCC against tumor target cells are large granular lymphocytes.[121,122] These cells are morphologically distinct from most T and B lymphocytes. The cells that mediate natural killing appear to be quite heterogeneous with regard to surface markers, and the exact lineage of these cells is still controversial. Most, but not all, carry the Fc receptor for the heavy chain of IgG. Although large granular lymphocytes do not carry the usual array of pan-T surface markers, and NK cells are actually increased in thymectomized animals, NK cells share characteristics of some T lymphocytes, such as reactivity with certain monoclonal anti-T lymphocyte antibodies. Some investigators have also noted the presence of surface markers characteristic of monocytes-macrophages. However, NK cells are nonphagocytic and nonadherent, and their enzyme pattern is in line with that of lymphoid cells. Recently, several reagents (including monoclonal antibodies) have become available for identifying major subpopulations of NK cells, and cell clones with natural killing activity have been developed. These studies should greatly increase our understanding of the NK cell.

EXPERIMENTAL METHODS FOR STUDYING HUMAN LYMPHOCYTE SUBPOPULATIONS

Assays for Enumeration and Separation of B and T Lymphocytes. Assays for B and T lymphocytes in man are generally confined to those contained in peripheral blood lymphocytes. Peripheral blood mononuclear leukocytes (PBL), which include both lymphocytes and monocytes, are separated from red blood cells and granulocytes on the basis of buoyant density (Table 3–5). The most commonly used technique is the Ficoll-Hypaque separation procedure.

Human B lymphocytes are most often identified by the presence of cell surface immunoglobulin. Heterologous antisera made against whole human immunoglobulin molecules or purified light chains can be used to detect all B lymphocytes. Antisera (heterologous or monoclonal) directed against the heavy chains of purified myeloma proteins can be used to detect only those B lymphocytes that bear μ, δ, γ, or α heavy chains. These antisera are generally used in direct or indirect immunofluorescence assays. In the former assay, the antihuman antisera is directly conjugated with a fluorochrome (i.e., fluorescein). PBL are incubated with this reagent and then the number of fluorescent-positive cells are counted. In the latter assay, PBL are first incubated with the appropriate antihuman antisera (unconjugated), washed, and then reacted with a fluorochrome-conjugated antibody directed against the first step reagent (i.e., a fluorescein conjugated goat antirabbit immunoglobulin if the first step antisera was raised in rabbits, or a fluorescein conjugated antimouse immunoglobulin if the first reagent was a mouse monoclonal antibody).

The number of positively staining cells can be determined by fluorescence microscopy or by cytofluorograph machines such as the fluorescence-activated cell sorter (FACS).[123] These machines have become powerful tools for the immunologist in both enumerating and separating lymphocyte subpopulations. After cells are stained as described above, the machine can arrange them as single cells in a row, each enclosed within a microdroplet. The cells are then passed in front of a laser beam, and those cells that fluoresce are recognized by photoelectric receivers. The number of positive-staining cells and the intensity of fluorescence, as well as

Table 3–5. Approximate Percentage of T and B Lymphocytes in Normal Human Peripheral Blood Mononuclear Cells Purified on a Ficoll-Hypaque Gradient

	T Lymphocytes	B Lymphocytes	Null (Non-T,Non-B) Lymphocytes	Monocytes and Myeloid Cells
% Lymphocytes	77	11	12	–
% Total Cells	64	9	10	17

other cellular parameters, are electronically recorded. The machine can routinely count 10^4 cells in a few seconds, separate live from dead cells, accurately and quantitatively determine the intensity of fluorescence, and separate the positive cells from the negative cells (see below).

Human T lymphocytes and their subsets can be identified by distinct surface markers using several techniques. A commonly used method for enumerating all T lymphocytes is based on the ability of human peripheral blood T lymphocytes to bind to sheep red blood cells. These erythrocyte-rosette-forming cells are counted in a standard hematocytometer. More recently, T lymphocytes and T lymphocyte subpopulations have been identified using monoclonal antibodies that recognize all T lymphocytes or a particular T lymphocyte subset. Generally, indirect immunofluorescence techniques are employed (as described above) using a second step fluorochrome-conjugated antimouse immunoglobulin reagent. Positively stained cells are enumerated as described above. T lymphocytes can also be enumerated by complement-dependent cytotoxicity methods using the same monoclonal antihuman antibodies (provided they are complement fixing). Cells are incubated with antibody and complement, and the percentage of dead cells is determined.

Similar techniques can be used to separate B and T lymphocytes from human PBL. T lymphocytes are generally isolated by their ability to bind to sheep red blood cells. After the formation of T lymphocyte-erythrocyte rosettes, the T lymphocytes can be separated from other nonrosetting mononuclear cells by buoyant density. After lysis of the attached sheep red blood cells, nearly pure T lymphocytes are obtained. The non-T (nonrosetting) cells contain a mixture of B lymphocytes, null lymphocytes, and monocytes. The monocytes can be removed by a variety of techniques (e.g., plastic or glass adherence), resulting in a greatly enriched B lymphocyte population.

B lymphocytes can also be "positively" isolated by using antisera directed against surface immunoglobulin, and either adherence or immunofluorescence techniques.

CONCLUSIONS

A striking variety of lymphocyte subpopulations have been detected during the past several years. Each population appears to play an important function in the ever increasing complexity of control of the immune system. There are cells that augment the immune response, those that suppress it, those that specialize in antibody secretion, those that specialize in killing, and those that specialize in the production of different lymphokines. Given the complexity of cell populations, it is not surprising that there is a wide variety of congenital and acquired defects in the immune system in man. Elucidation of the characteristics and function of these cell populations in health and disease continues to pro-

vide a firm scientific basis for the diagnosis and treatment of both immunodeficiency and autoimmune diseases.

References

1. Szenberg, A., and Warner, N.L.: Immunological function of thymus and bursa of Fabricius. Dissociation of immunological responsiveness in fowls with a hormonally arrested development of lymphoid tissues. Nature 194:145, 1962.
2. Cooper, M.D., Peterson, R.D.A., and Good, R.A.: Delineation of thymic and bursal lymphoid systems in the chicken. Nature 205:143, 1965.
3. Cooper, M.D., Peterson, R.D.A., South, M.A. and Good, R.A.: The functions of the thymus system and the bursa system in the chicken. J. Exp. Med. 123:75, 1966.
4. Miller, J.F.A.P., and Mitchell, G.F.: Thymus and antigen-reactive cells. Transplant. Rev. 1:3, 1969.
5. Raff, M.C.: Surface antigenic markers for distinguishing T and B lymphocytes in mice. Transplant. Rev. 6:52, 1971.
6. Moller, G.(ed.): T and B Lymphocytes in Humans. Transplant Rev. 15:1, 1973 (entire volume).
7. Everett, N.B., and Tyler, R.W.: Lymphopoiesis in the thymus and other tissues: Functional implications. Int. Rev. Cytol. 22:205, 1967.
8. Gowans, J.L., and McGregor, D.D.: The immunological activities of lymphocytes. Prog. Allergy 9:1, 1965.
9. Strober, S.: Immune function, cell surface characteristics, and maturation of B cell subpopulations. Transplant. Rev. 24:84, 1975.
10. Howard, J.C., Hunt, S.V., and Gowans, J.L.: Identification of marrow-derived and thymus-derived small lymphocytes in the lymphoid tissue and thoracic duct lymph of normal rats. J. Exp. Med. 135:200, 1972.
11. Sprent, J., and Basten, A.: Circulating T and B lymphocytes of the mouse. II. Lifespan. Cell. Immunol. 7:40, 1973.
12. Strober, S., and Dilley, J.: Biological characteristics of T and B memory lymphocytes in the rat. J. Exp. Med. 137:1275, 1973.
13. Weissman, I.L., Gutman, G.A., and Friedberg, S.H.: Tissue localization of lymphoid cells. Ser. Haematol. 7:482, 1974.
14. Guy-Grand, D., Griscelli, C., and Vassalli, P.: The mouse gut T lymphocyte, a novel type of T cell. Nature, origin, and traffic in mice in normal and graft-versus-host conditions. J. Exp. Med. 148:1661, 1978.
15. Hall, J.G., Hopkins, J., and Orlans, E.: Studies on the lymphocytes of sheep. III. Destination of lymph born immunoblasts in relation to their tissue of origin. Eur. J. Immunol. 7:30, 1979.
16. Butcher, E.C., Scollay, R.G., and Weissman, I.L.: Organ specificity of lymphocyte migration: Mediation by highly selective lymphocyte interaction with organ-specific determinants on high endothelial venules. Eur. J. Immunol. 10:556, 1980.
17. Miller, J.F.A.P.: Role of the thymus in transplantation immunity. Ann. N.Y. Acad. Sci. 99:340, 1962.
18. Haris, J.E., and Ford, C.E.: Cellular traffic of the thymus: Experiments with chromosome markers. Nature 201:884, 1964.
19. Cantor, H., and Weissman, I.L.: Development and function of subpopulations of thymocytes and T lymphocytes. Prog. Allergy 20:1, 1976.
20. Freidman, H.(ed.): Thymus factors in immunity. Ann. N.Y. Acad. Sci. 249:1, 1975.
21. Kruisbeek, A.M., Sharrow, S.O., and Singer, A.: Differences in the MHC-restricted self-recognition repertoire of intrathymic and extra-thymic cytotoxic T lymphocyte precursors. J. Immunol. 130:1027, 1983.
22. Cantor, H., and Boyse, E.A.: Functional subclasses of T lymphocytes bearing different Ly antigens 1. The generation of functionally distinct T-cell subclasses is a differentiative process independent of antigen. J. Exp. Med. 141:1376, 1975.
23. Katz, D.A.: Lymphocyte Differentiation Recognition, and Regulation. Academic Press, New York, 1977.
24. Hood, L.E., Weissman, I.L., Wood, W.B. (eds.): Immunology. Menlo Park, California, Benjamin/Cummings Pub. Co., Menlo Park, 1978, p. 13.
25. Reinherz, E.L., and Schlossman, S.F.: The differentiation and function of human T lymphocytes. Cell 19:821, 1980.
26. Boyse, E.A., Old, L.J., and Stockert, E.: The TL (thymus leukemia) antigen: A review. In Grabar, P., and Miescher, P.A. (eds.): Immunopathology. IV. International Symposium. Basel, Switzerland, Schwabe and Co., 1967, p. 23.
27. Ledbetter, J.A., Rouse, R.V., Micklem, H.S., and Herzenberg, L.A.: T cell subsets defined by expression of Lyt-1, 2, 3 and Thy-1 antigens. Two-parameter immunofluorescence and cytotoxicity analysis with monoclonal antibodies modifies current views. J. Exp. Med. 152:280, 1980.

28. Gershon, R.K.: T cell suppression. Contemp Top. Immunobiol. 3:1, 1974.
29. Cantor, H., and Boyse, E.A.: Functional subclasses of T lymphocytes bearing different Ly antigens. II. Cooperation between subclasses of Ly+ cells in the generation of killer activity. J. Exp. Med. 141:1390, 1975.
30. Jandinski, J., Cantor, H., Tadakuma, T., Peavy, D.L., and Pierce, C.W.: Separation of helper T cells from suppressor T cells expressing different Ly components. 1. Polyclonal activation: suppressor and helper activities are inherent properties of distinct T-cell subclasses. J. Exp. Med. 143:1382, 1976.
31. Cantor, H., Shen, F.W., and Boyse, E.A.: Separation of helper T cells from suppressor T cells expressing different Ly components. II. Activation by antigen: after immunization, antigen-specific suppressor and helper activities are mediated by distinct T-cell subclasses. J. Exp. Med. 143:1391, 1976.
32. Reinherz, E.L., Kung, P.C., Goldstein, G., and Schlossman, S.F.: Further characterization of the human inducer T cell subset defined by monoclonal antibody. J. Immunol. 123:2894, 1979.
33. Reinherz, E.L., Kung, P.C., Goldstein, G., and Schlossman, S.F.: A monoclonal antibody reactive with the human cytotoxic suppressor T cell subset previously defined by a heteroantiserum termed TH2. J. Immunol. 124:1301, 1980.
34. Reinherz, E.L., Morimoto, C., Penta, A.C., and Schlossman, S.F.: Regulation of B cell immunoglobulin secretion by functional subsets of T lymphocytes in man. Eur. J. Immunol. 10:570, 1980.
35. Evans, R.L., Wall, D.W., Platsoucas, C.D., Siegal, F.P., Fikrig, S.M., Testa, C.M., and Good, R.A.: Thymus-dependent membrane antigens in man: Inhibition of cell-mediated lympholysis by monoclonal antibodies to the TH2 antigen. Proc. Natl. Acad. Sci. (USA) 78:544, 1981.
36. Kotzin, B.L., Benike, C.J., and Engleman, E.G.: Induction of immunoglobulin-secreting cells in the allogeneic mixed leukocyte reaction: regulation by helper and suppressor lymphocyte subsets in man. J. Immunol. 127:931, 1981.
37. Engleman, E.G., Benike, C.J., Grumet, F.C., and Evans, R.L.: Activation of human T lymphocyte subsets: Helper and suppressor/cytotoxic T cells recognize and respond to distinct histocompatibility antigens. J. Immunol. 127:2124, 1981.
38. Ledbetter, J.A., Evans, R.L., Lipinski, M., Cunningham-Rundles, C., Good, R.A., and Herzenberg, L.A.: Evolutionary conservation of surface molecules that distinguish T lymphocyte helper/inducer and T cytotoxic/suppressor subpopulations in mouse and man. J. Exp. Med. 153:310, 1981.
39. Moller, G. (ed.): Effects of anti-membrane antibodies on killer T cells. Immunol. Rev. 68:1, 1982 (entire volume).
40. Thomas, Y., Rogozinski, L., Irigoyen, O., Friedman, M., Kung, P.C., Goldstein, G., and Chess, L.: Functional analysis of human T cell subsets defined by monoclonal antibodies. IV. Induction of suppressor cells within the OKT4+ population. J. Exp. Med. 154:459, 1981.
41. Krensky, A.M., Clayberger, C., Reiss, C.S., Strominger, J.L., and Burakoff, S.J.: Specificity of OKT4+ cytotoxic T lymphocyte clones. J. Immunol. 129:2001, 1982.
42. Moretta, L., Ferrarini, M., Mingari, M.C., Moretta, A., and Webb, S.R.: Subpopulations of human T cells identified by receptors for immunoglobulins and mitogen responsiveness. J. Immunol. 117:2171, 1976.
43. Moretta, L., Webb, S.R., Grossi, C.E., Lydyard, P.M., and Cooper, M.D.: Functional analysis of two human T-cell subpopulations: Help and suppression of B-cell responses by T cells bearing receptors for IgM or IgG. J. Exp. Med. 146:184, 1977.
44. Moretta, L., Moretta, A., Canonica, G.W., Bacigalupo, A., Mingari, M.C., and Cerottini, J-C.: Receptors for immunoglobulins on resting and activated human T cells. Immunol. Rev. 56:141, 1981.
45. Pichler, W.J., and Broder, S.: In vitro functions of human T cells expressing Fc-IgG or Fc-IgM receptors. Immunol. Rev. 56:163, 1981.
46. Reinherz, E.L., Moretta, L., Roper, M., Breard, J.M., Mingari, M.C., Cooper, M.D., and Schlossman, S.F.: Human T lymphocyte subpopulations defined by Fc receptors and monoclonal antibodies: A comparison. J. Exp. Med. 151:969, 1980.
47. Kay, H.D., and Horwitz, D.A.: Evidence by reactivity with hybridoma antibodies for a probable myeloid origin of peripheral blood cells active in natural cytotoxicity and antibody dependent cell mediated cytotoxicity. J. Clin. Invest. 66:847, 1980.
48. Fox, R.I., Thompson, L.F., and Huddlestone, J.F.: Tγ cells express T-lymphocyte-associated antigens. J. Immunol. 126:2062, 1981.
49. Alter, B.J., Schendel, D.J., Bach, M.L., Bach, F.J., Klein, J., and Stimpfling, J.H.: Cell-mediated lympholysis: Importance of serologically defined H-2 regions. J. Exp. Med. 137:1303, 1973.
50. Bach, F.H., Bach, M.L., and Sondel, P.M.: Differential function of major histocompatibility complex antigens in T-lymphocyte activation. Nature 259:273, 1976.
51. Plate, J.M.D.: Soluble factors substitute for T-T cell collaboration in generation of T killer lymphocytes. Nature 260:329, 1976.
52. Wagner, H., Hardt, C., Heeg, K., Pfizenmaier, K., Solbach, W., Bartlett, R., Stockinger, H., and Rollinghoff, M.: T-T cell interactions during

cytotoxic T lymphocyte (CTL) responses: T cell-derived helper factor (Interleukin 2) as a probe to analyze CTL responsiveness and thymic maturation of CTL progenitors. Immunol. Rev. 51:215, 1980.
53. Zinkernagel, R.M., and Doherty, P.C.: MHC-restricted cytotoxic T cells: Studies on the biological role of polymorphic major transplantation antigens determining T-cell restriction-specificity, function, and responsiveness. Adv. Immunol. 27:51, 1979.
54. Finberg, R., and Benacerraf, B.: Induction, control, and consequences of virus specific cytotoxic T cells. Immunol. Rev. 58:157, 1981.
55. Reiss, C.S., and Burakoff, S.J.: Specificity of the helper T cell for the cytolytic T lymphocyte response to influenza viruses. J. Exp. Med. 154:541, 1981.
56. Gershon, R.K.: Suppressive interactions between different MLR loci. In Katz, D.H., and Benacerraf, B. (eds.): The Role of Products of the Histocompatibility Gene Complex in Immune Responses. New York, Academic Press, 1976, p. 193.
57. Rich, S.S., and Rich, R.R.: Regulatory mechanisms in cell-mediated immune responses. 1. Regulation of mixed lymphocyte reactions by alloantigen-activated thymus-derived lymphocytes. J. Exp. Med. 140:1588, 1974.
58. Nadler, L.M., and Hodes, R.J.: Regulatory mechanisms in cell-mediated immune responses. II. Comparison of culture-induced and alloantigen-induced suppressor cells in MLR and CML. J. Immunol. 118:1886, 1977.
59. Truitt, G.A., Dennison, D.K., Rich, R.R., and Rich, S.S.: Interaction between T cells and non-T cells in suppression of cytotoxic lymphocyte responses. J. Immunol. 123:745, 1979.
60. Sasportes, M., Wollman, E., Cohen, D., Carosella, E., Bensussan, A., Fradelizi, D., and Dausset, J.: Suppression of the human allogeneic response in vitro with primed lymphocytes and suppressor supernates. J. Exp. Med. 152:270S, 1980.
61. Chaout, G., Mathieson, B.J., and Asofsky, R.: Regulatory mechanisms in the mixed lymphocyte reaction: evidence for the requirement of two T cells to interact in the generation of effective suppression. J. Immunol. 129:502, 1982.
62. Okada, S., and Strober, S.: Spleen cells from adult mice given total lymphoid irradiation or from newborn mice have similar regulatory effects in the mixed leukocyte reaction. 1. Generation of antigen-specific suppressor cells in the mixed leukocyte reaction after the addition of spleen cells from adult mice given total lymphoid irradiation. J. Exp. Med. 156:522, 1982.
63. Susskind, B.M., Merluzzi, V.J., Faanes, R.B., Palladino, M.A., and Choi, Y.S.: Regulatory mechanisms in cytotoxic T lymphocyte development. 1. A suppressor T cell subset that regulates the proliferative stage of CTL development. J. Immunol. 130:527, 1983.
64. Waldman, T.A., Blaese, R.M., Broder, S., and Krakauer, R.S.: Disorders of suppressor immunoregulatory cells in the pathogenesis of immunodeficiency and autoimmunity. Ann. Intern. Med. 88:226, 1978.
65. Herzenberg, L.A., Okumura, K., and Metzler, C.M.: Regulation of immunoglobulin and antibody production by allotype suppressor T cells in mice. Transplant. Rev. 27:57, 1975.
66. Eichmann, K.: Idiotype suppression. II. Amplification of a suppressor T cell with anti-idiotypic activity. Eur. J. Immunol 5:511, 1975.
67. Bona, C., and Paul, W.E.: Cellular basis of regulation of expression of idiotype. I. T-suppressor cells specific for MOPC 460 idiotype regulate the expression of cells secreting anti-TNP antibodies bearing 460 idiotype. J. Exp. Med. 149:592, 1979.
68. Germain, R.N., and Benacerraf, B.: A single major pathway of T-lymphocyte interactions in antigen specific immune suppression. Scand. J. Immunol. 13:1, 1981.
69. Gershon, R.K.: Immunoregulation circa 1980: Some comments on the state of the art. J. Allergy Clin. Immunol. 66:18, 1980.
70. Cantor, H., Hugenberger, J., McVay-Boudreau, L., Eardley, D.D., Kemp, J., Shen, F.W., and Gershon, R.K.: Immunoregulatory circuits among T-cell subsets: Identification of a subpopulation of T-helper cells that induces feedback inhibition. J. Exp. Med. 148:871, 1979.
71. Eardley, D.D., Murphy, D.B., Kemp, J.D., Shen, F.W., Cantor, H., and Gershon, R.K.: Ly-1 inducer and Ly-1,2 acceptor T cells in the feedback suppression circuit bear an I-J-subregion controlled determinant. Immunogenetics 11:549, 1980.
72. Gershon, R.K., Eardley, D.D., Durum, S., Green, D.R., Shen, F,W., Yamauchi, K., Cantor, H., and Murphy, D.B.: Contrasuppression: A novel immunoregulatory activity. J. Exp. Med. 153:1533, 1981.
73. Thomas, Y., Sosman, J., Origoyen, O., Friedman, S.M., Kung, P.C., Goldstein, G., and Chess, L.: Functional analysis of human T cell subsets defined by monoclonal antibodies. 1. Collaborative T-T interactions in the immunoregulation of B cell differentiation. J. Immunol. 125:2402, 1980.
74. Gatenby, P.A., Kotzin, B.L., Kansas, G.S., and Engleman, E.G.: Immunoglobulin secretion in the human autologous mixed leukocyte reaction. Definition of a suppressor-amplifier circuit using monoclonal antibodies. J. Exp. Med. 156:55, 1982.
75. Morimoto, C., Distaso, J.A., Borel, Y., Schlossman, S.F., and Reinherz,

E.L.: Communicative interactions between subpopulations of human T lymphocytes required for generation of suppressor effector function in a primary antibody response. J. Immunol. 128:1645, 1982.

76. Yachie, A., Miyawaki, T., Yokoi, T., Nagaoki, T., and Taniguchi, N.: Ia-positive cells generated by PWM-stimulation within OKT4+ subset interact with OKT8+ cells for inducing active suppression on B cell differentiation in vitro. J. Immunol. 129:103, 1982.

77. Gillis, S., and Smith, K.A.: Long-term culture of tumor-specific cytotoxic T cells. Nature 268:154, 1977.

78. Moller, G. (ed.): T cell clones. Immunol. Rev. 54:1, 1981 (entire volume).

79. Fitch, F., and Fathman, C.G. (eds.): Isolation, Characterization, and Utilization of T Lymphocyte Clones. Academic Press, New York, 1982.

80. Kappler, J.W., Skidmore, B., White, J., and Marrack, P.: Antigen-inducible, H-2 restricted, interleukin-2-producing T cell hybridomas. Lack of independent antigen and H-2 recognition. J. Exp. Med. 153:1198, 1981.

81. Infante, A.J., Infante, P.D., Gillis, S., and Fathman, C.G.: Definition of T cell idiotypes using anti-idiotypic antisera produced by immunization with T cells. J. Exp. Med. 155:1100, 1982.

82. Marrack, P., and Kappler, J.: Use of somatic cell genetics to study chromosomes contributing to antigen plus I recognition by T cell hybridomas. J. Exp. Med. 147:404, 1983.

83. Haskins, K., Kubo, R., White, J., Pigeon, M., Kappler, J., Marrack P.: The major histocompatibility restricted antigen receptor on T cells. 1. Isolation with a monoclonal antibody. J. Exp. Med. 157:1149, 1983.

84. Eichmann, K.: Expression and function of idiotypes on lymphocytes. Adv. Immunol. 26:195, 1978.

85. Binz, H., and Wigzell, H.: Idiotypic, alloantigen-reactive T lymphocyte receptors and their use to induce specific transplantation tolerance. Prog. Allergy 23:154, 1977.

86. Germain, R.N., Ju, S-T., Kipps, T.J., Benacerraf, B., and Dorf, M.E.: Shared idiotypic determinants on antibodies and T-cell-derived suppressor factor specific for the random terpolymer L-glutamic acid-L-alanine-L-tyrosine. J. Exp. Med. 149:613, 1979.

87. Rocklin, R.E., Bendtzen, K., and Greineder, D.: Mediators of immunity: Lymphokines and monokines. Adv. Immunol. 29:55, 1980.

88. Smith, K.A., and Ruscetti, F.W.: T cell growth factor and the culture of cloned functional T cells. Adv. Immunol. 31:137, 1981.

89. Moller, G. (ed.): Interleukins and lymphocyte activation. Immunol. Rev. 63:1, 1982 (entire volume).

90. Beller, D.I., and Ho, K.: Regulation of macrophage populations V. Evaluation of the control of macrophage Ia expression in vitro. J. Immunol. 129:971, 1982.

91. Fleisher, T.A., Attallah, A.M., Tosato, G., Blaese, R.M., and Greene, W.C.: Interferon-mediated inhibition of human polyclonal immunoglobulin synthesis. J. Immunol. 129:1099, 1982.

92. Muraguchi, A., and Fauci, A.S.: Proliferative responses of normal human B lymphocytes. Development of an assay system for human B cell growth factor (BCGF). J. Immunol. 129:1104, 1982.

93. Okada, M., Sakaguchi, N., Yoshimura, N., Hara, H., Shimizu, K., Yoshida, N., Yoshizaki, K., Kishimoto, S., Yamamura, Y., and Kishimoto, T.: B cell growth factors and B cell differentiation factor from human T hybridomas: Two distinct kinds of B cell growth factor and their synergism in B cell proliferation. J. Exp. Med. 157:583, 1983.

94. Kincade, P.W., and Cooper, M.D.: Development and distribution of immunoglobulin-containing cells in the chicken: An immunofluorescent analysis using purified antibodies to μ, γ, and light chains. J. Immunol. 106:371, 1971.

95. Owen, J.J.T., Cooper, M.D., and Raff, M.C.: In vitro generation of B lymphocytes in mouse foetal liver, a mammalian bursa equivalent. Nature 249:361, 1974.

96. Melchers, F., Von Boehmer, H., and Phillips, R.A.: B lymphocyte subpopulations in the mouse: Organ distribution and ontogeny of immunoglobulin-synthesizing and of mitogen sensitive cells. Transplant. Rev. 25:26, 1975.

97. Abramson, S., Miller, R.G., and Phillips, R.A.: The identification in adult bone marrow of pluripotent and restricted stem cells of the myeloid and lymphoid systems. J. Exp. Med. 145:1567, 1977.

98. Cooper, M.D.: Ontogeny and differentiation of B cells. In Cooper, M.D., Mosier, D.E., Scher, I., and Vitetta, E.S. (eds.): B Lymphocytes in the Immune Response. New York, Elsevier/North-Holland, 1979, p. 61.

99. Raff, M.C., Megson, M., Owen, J.J.T., and Cooper, M.D.: Early production of intracellular IgM by B lymphocyte precursors in mouse. Nature (Lond.) 259:224, 1975.

100. Grey, H.: Surface markers on B cells. In Cooper, M.D., Mosier, D.E., Scher, I., and Vitetta, E.S. (eds.): B Lymphocytes in the Immune Response. New York, Elsevier/North-Holland, 1979, p. 1.

101. Kearney, J.F., Cooper, M.D., Klein, J., Abney, E.R., Parkhouse, R.M.E., and Lawton, A.R.: Ontogeny of Ia and IgD on IgM-bearing B lymphocytes in mice. J. Exp. Med. 146:297, 1977.

102. Rosenberg, Y.J., and Parish, C.R.: Ontogeny of the antibody-forming cell line in mice. IV. Appearance of cells bearing Fc receptors, complement receptors, and surface immunoglobulin. J. Immunol. 118:612, 1977.

103. Vitetta, E.S., Melcher, U., McWilliams, M., Lamm, M.E., Phillips-Quagliata, J.M., and Uhr, J.W.: Cell surface immunoglobulin. XI. The appearance of an IgD-like molecule on murine lymphoid cells during ontogeny. J. Exp. Med. 141:206, 1975.

104. Scher, I., Ahmed, A., Strong, D.M., Steinberg, A.D., and Paul, W.E.: X-linked B lymphocyte immune defect in CBA/N mice. 1. Studies of the function and composition of spleen cells. J. Exp. Med. 141:788, 1975.

105. Scher, I., Steinberg, A.D., Berning, A.K., and Paul, W.E.: X-linked B lymphocyte immune defect in CBA/N mice. II. Studies of the mechanisms underlying the immune defect. J. Exp. Med. 142:637, 1975.

106. Ahmed, A., Scher, I., Sharrow, S.O., Smith, A.H., Paul, W.E., Sachs, D.H., and Sell, K.W.: B lymphocyte heterogeneity: Development and characterization of an alloantiserum which distinguishes B lymphocyte differentiation alloantigens. J. Exp. Med. 145:101, 1977.

107. Scher, I., Titus, J.A., and Finkelman, F.D.: The ontogeny and distribution of B cells in normal and mutant immunedefective CBA/N mice: Two-parameter analysis of surface IgM and IgD. J. Immunol. 130:619, 1983.

108. Singer, A., Morrissey, J., Hathcock, K.S., Ahmed, A., Scher, I., and Hodes, R.J.: Role of the major histocompatibility complex (MHC) in T cell activation of B cell subpopulations. Lyb5− and Lyb5+ B cell subpopulations differ in their requirement for MHC restricted T cell recognition. J. Exp. Med. 145:501, 1977.

109. Klinman, N., Mosier, D.E., Scher, I., and Vitetta, E.S. (eds.): B Lymphocytes in the Immune Response: Functional, Developmental, and Interactive Properties. New York, Elsevier/North-Holland, 1981, p. 295.

110. Moller, G. (ed.): Genetic models of B cell differentiation. Immunol. Rev. 64:1, 1982 (entire volume).

111. Gathings, W.E., Lawton, A.R., and Cooper, M.D.: Immunofluorescent studies of the development of pre-B cells, B lymphocytes, and immunoglobulin isotype diversity in humans. Eur. J. Immunol. 7:804, 1977.

112. Vitetta, E.S., and Uhr, J.W.: Immunoglobulin-receptors revisited: A model for the differentiation of bone marrow-derived lymphocyte is described. Science 189:964, 1975.

113. Metcalf, E.S., and Klinman, N.R.: In vitro tolerance induction of neonatal murine B cells. J. Exp. Med. 143:1327, 1976.

114. Raff, M.C., Owen, J.J.T., Cooper, M.D., Lawton, A.R., Megson, M., and Gathings, W.E.: Differences in susceptibility of mature and immature mouse B lymphocytes to anti-immunoglobulin-induced immunoglobulin suppression in vitro: Possible implications for B-cell tolerance to self. J. Exp. Med. 142:1052, 1975.

115. Vitetta, E.S., Cambier, J.C., Ligler, F.L., Kettman, J.R., Zan-Bar, I., Strober, S., and Uhr, J.W.: The role of surface immunoglobulins in triggering and tolerance of B cells. In Cooper, M.D., Mosier, D.E., Scher, I., Vitetta, E.S. (eds.): B Lymphocytes in the Immune Response. New York, Elsevier/North-Holland, 1979, p. 233.

116. Okumura, K., Julius, M.H., Tsu, T., Herzenberg, L.A., and Herzenberg, L.A.: Demonstration that IgG memory is carried by IgG-bearing cells. Eur. J. Immunol. 6:467, 1976.

117. Mason, D.W.: The class of surface immunoglobulin on cells carrying IgG memory in rat thoracic duct lymph: The size of the subpopulation mediating IgG memory. J. Exp. Med. 143:1122, 1976.

118. Zan-Bar, I., Vitetta, E.S., Assisi, F., and Strober, S.: The relationship between surface immunoglobulin isotype and immune function of murine B lymphocytes. III. Expression of a single predominant isotype on primed and unprimed B cells. J. Exp. Med. 147:1374, 1978.

119. Moller, G. (ed.): Concepts of B lymphocyte activation. Immunol. Rev. 23:1, 1975 (entire volume).

120. Falkoff, R.J., Zhu, L.P., and Fauci, A.S.: Separate signals for human B cell proliferation and differentiation in response to Staphylococcus aureus: evidence for a two-signal model of B cell activation. J. Immunol. 129:97, 1982.

121. Herberman, R.B., (ed.): Natural Cell-Mediated Immunity Against Tumors. Academic Press, New York, 1980.

122. Moller, G. (ed.): Natural killer cells. Immunol. Rev. 44:1, 1979 (entire volume).

123. Herzenberg, L.A., and Herzenberg, L.A.: Analysis and separation using the fluorescence activated cell sorter (FACS). In Weir, D.M. (ed.): Handbook of Experimental Immunology. 3rd ed. Oxford, Blackwell, 1978, p. 22.1.

124. Dialynas, D.P., Wilde, D.B., Marrack, P., Pierres, A., Wall, K.A., Havran, W., Otten, G., Loken, M.R., Pierres, M., Kappler, J., and Fitch, F.W.: Characterization of the murine antigenic determinant, designated L3T4a, recognized by monoclonal antibody GK1.5: Expression of L3T4a by functional T cell clones appears to correlate primarily with class II MHC antigen-reactivity. Immunol. Rev. 74:29, 1983.

Chapter 4

The Major Histocompatibility Complex

R. J. Winchester

INTRODUCTION

The segment on the short arm of the sixth chromosome that is usually termed the major histocompatibility complex (MHC) contains the genetic determinants for a number of characteristics that have regulation of the immune response as their principal focal point. These gene products achieve this regulation in part by controlling the differentiation and proliferation of T lymphocytes and B lymphocytes induced by contact with antigen.

One of the most interesting aspects of this control is that recognition of conventional antigens by T lymphocytes occurs in a context of "self" that is provided by the MHC molecules. This molecular definition of biologic individuality derives from the products of the extremely large number of alternative MHC genes found in the population. A second aspect of control is that the functional capabilities of the immune response differ according to the MHC alleles an individual inherits. As a consequence of this variation, the MHC genes have a profound influence on resistance or susceptibility to certain diseases, particularly a number of those that are rheumatic in character. The survival of allografts is also determined by this variation because the different alternative molecules are in themselves intensely antigenic. Indeed it was this property of histocompatibility that first directed attention to the existence of the MHC long before its central role in immune regulation was known. Understanding the basis of the biologic impetus to development of this genetic diversity is one of the tantalizing challenges in the study of the MHC.

A distinctive feature of many genes of the MHC is that their products are expressed on the cell membrane and appear to mediate cell-to-cell interactions. These cell surface molecules occur in two entirely distinct varieties. The first class, sometimes designated class I, consists of the HLA-A, B, and C molecules (Table 4–1). These molecules are encoded by genes located at the most distal position of the MHC (Fig. 4–1). The genes encoding the class II products, or Ia/DR molecules, are present at the centromeric end of the major histocompatibility complex. There are two additional classes of MHC gene products: the class III molecules, which comprise the C3 convertase systems of the classic and alternative complement pathways, and are located between the class I and class II genes; and the class IV cytoplasmic molecules, about which relatively little is known in the human. The class III complement component molecules will be discussed in Chapter 7.

The basic structure of the class I molecule consists of two chains. One chain, the heavy or α chain is an intrinsic membrane component of several distinct regions or domains. The molecule extends across the entire membrane (Fig. 4–2). The much smaller light or β chain is β^2 microglobulin and is an extrinsic membrane component and is present only on the exterior of the membrane. It is shown as a shaded structure associated by noncovalent interactions with the α-2 and α-3 domains. The gene encoding the β chain is located on chromosome 15.

The basic structure of the class II or Ia molecules consists of two different chains more nearly equivalent in size that are both intrinsic membrane components (Fig. 4–2). Both chains are encoded by genes that are located in the same region of chromosome 6, designated "class II" in Fig. 4–1. Each chain is organized into two intracellular domains, a transmembrane portion and a small intercellular portion.

The total size of the MHC is considerable, and it has been calculated that there is sufficient space for several hundred genes. Thus, to the dismay of some but the joy of others, it is evident that there are large areas of ignorance despite the fact that the MHC is perhaps the most intricate biologic response to have been analyzed in man. In this context the disease associations may result in the appreciation of entirely unsuspected elements in the MHC.

Because of the astonishing rapidity with which knowledge concerning disease associations is unfolding, coupled with the promise of its immediate practical application, the content of this chapter has been oriented to provide much of the background that is necessary to gain access to the current literature, with primary emphasis on the markers that constitute the reference points for these disease associations.

HISTORICAL ORIENTATION

Knowledge regarding the human MHC spans a period of less than three decades. The early history was dominated by the clinical problem of transplantation and aimed at defining the population genetics of the allodeterminants. The initial studies began with the observation that sera from multiply transfused patients contained antibodies termed "leukoagglutinins," which agglutinated a suspension of donor leukocytes.[1,2] Subsequently, pregnancy sera were found to be a source of

Table 4–1. Comparison of the Two Classes of Cell Surface Glycoproteins Encoded by Genes of the Major Histocompatibility Complex

	Class I	Class II
Terminology	HLA-A, B, C	Ia(DR)
Expression	Essentially all cells except mature RBC trophoblast, early embryonic tissue (?)	Certain cells of immune system B, monocyte, dendritic stimulated T cells plus a few other cell types
Structure		
α chain	44 kD	34 kD
β chain	11.5 kD	29 kD
Membrane Relationship		
α chain	intrinsic	intrinsic
β chain	extrinsic	intrinsic
Location of polymorphisms		
α chain	α1 and α2 domains	α1 domains of DS and SB
β chain	−	β1 domains of DR, DS, and SB
Site of gene		
α chain	chromosome 6	chromosome 6
β chain	chromosome 15	chromosome 6
Number of loci		
α chain	3 (HLA-A, B, C)	1DR, 2DS, 2SB
β chain	1(?)	3DR, 2DS, 2SB

the leukoagglutinins. This finding simplifed the recognition of discrete alloantigen specificities because of the more limited antigenic challenge provided by the paternal MHC antigens expressed in the fetus. The delineation of specificities in these reagent sera for various leukocyte antigens was further assisted by the introduction of analytic approaches that enabled clusters of related specificities to be recognized.[3] In 1964, the complement-mediated cytotoxic assay using lymphocytes was introduced, and its superiority over the agglutination technique was clearly demonstrated.[4] By the end of the first decade of studies, two leukocyte antigen segregant series, now designated HLA-A and B, were characterized. Furthermore, an international collaborative arrangement for assigning specificities was established. At that time all observations were concerned with the class I MHC molecules.

Subsequent progress has moved in three main directions. First, there has been continual refinement of the A and B locus specificities, especially among non-Caucasian populations. In addition, a third locus, C, was also described. Secondly, one of the biologic roles of the class I molecules was found to be participation as a component of the structures recognized by cytotoxic T lymphocytes when they attack target cells expressing viral antigens.[5] Thirdly, the entry of this field of knowl

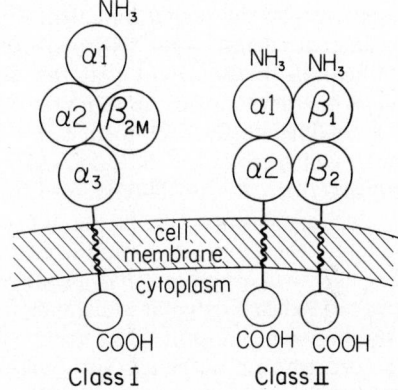

Figure 4–2. Domain structure of class I and class II MHC molecules.

edge into the mainstream of internal medicine began in 1973 with the observations on the association between the HLA-B27 allele and susceptibility to ankylosing spondylitis.[6,7]

The focus of the field shifted further from histocompatibility to the significance of these gene products in the biology of the individual during the mid 1970s with the recognition of the class II molecules and their central role of regulating the immune response. Indeed, some emphasize this change in perspective by referring to the MHC as the MIC, the *major immunogene complex*. In the latter years of the 1970s the importance of the class II or IA/DR alleles in influencing susceptibility to nearly all rheumatic diseases with immunologic features provided a further dimension of clinical significance to the biology of the MHC. Lastly, the concept of the MHC as the site of other loci was expanded by the finding that genes for the complement component C2 mapped within it.

A dominant characteristic of all research on the MHC has been the interchange of information between inves-

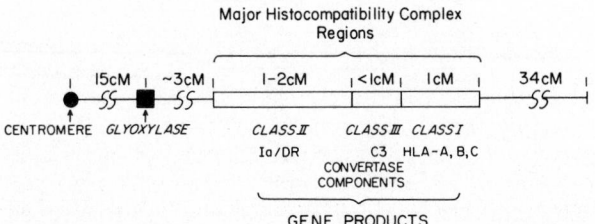

Figure 4–1. Schematic representation of the short arm of the 6th chromosome illustrating the location of the major histocompatibility complex.

tigators primarily concerned with different species, particularly research performed using the mouse.[8] Insights obtained in one species can often be readily transferred to another because of the intriguing biologic fact that the MHC of each species is organized in a homologous manner.

GENETIC PRINCIPLES

Terminology. The basic unit of genetic information is the *gene*. The segment of chromosome that contains the gene and codes for all or part of a specific single polypeptide chain is a *locus*. A *region* is the portion of the chromosome where the locus is situated. Other *traits* can map in this region without necessarily inferring that they are specified by the same locus or gene. Alternative forms of genes are termed *alleles*. These arise by mutation. An individual with different alleles (A_1 and A_2) of the same gene is a *heterozygote*, with each allelic gene on a different homologous chromosome of either maternal or paternal origin. The offspring of this individual illustrate Mendel's first law that these alleles will segregate. Mendel's second law—that nonallelic traits, determined by different genes, will sort independently—requires modification to the extent that the genes are located close to one another on the same chromosome in *linkage*. Or, defined in the reciprocal sense, linkage is the degree to which genes on the same chromosome are inherited together. *Recombination* resulting from crossing over during meiosis occurs in rough proportion to the distance that the genes are separated on the chromosome. This is the mechanism that produces independent sorting of genes located at a distance from one another on the same chromosome. The group of linked alleles of loci located on a single chromosome of either maternal or paternal origin is a *haplotype*. The concept of haplotype is important because the haploid chromosome is the vehicle of inheritance of the genome, and thus the haplotype represents the basic unit of inheritance. The various genes under consideration define the *genotype* of an individual. The expression of the genotype is the *phenotype* of an individual. This can take the form of a trait or of a specific structurally defined component. The Mendelian concepts of *dominance* and *recessivity* primarily apply to the expression of traits. In contrast, the genes of each haplotype that have structurally recognized products are almost always both expressed, and this pattern of gene expression is termed *codominance*.

Usually, as a result of natural selection, the number of alleles in a population is limited and mutant forms are present at low frequencies. For certain loci, an unusual situation exists in which there are two or more alleles that are each present at a frequency higher than can be accounted for by mutation. This state of multiple allelic forms is a *polymorphism*, and most of the loci of the MHC are composed of highly polymorphic series.[9,10]

The term *complex* refers to two or more loci. The "complexity" of the MHC is very real, but progress can be materially aided by always recalling there are only two families or classes of MHC molecules and that each family varies in only two ways. One dimension of this variation consists of duplicated genes, by which an individual is endowed with several loci on one chromosome that encode similar but not identical gene products, each with somewhat different functions. For example, there are three loci on each chromosome 6 that encode slightly different types of class I molecules (Fig. 4–3). This can be thought of as complexity or diversity at the level of the *locus*. It presumably serves to multiply the roles of the MHC molecules within an individual, since the independently segregating genes of each locus can undergo separate evolutionary routes. The second dimension of this variation is evident in the species but not necessarily in all individuals. It involves the development of alternative gene forms for each of the duplicated loci. These new alleles become the property of the species, endowing different individuals with regulatory molecules that have different properties. This second dimension of *allele diversity* results in a biologic individuality that presumably is the substrate for fitness to a particular environment. This strategy is unlike that found in the immunoglobulin system, where each individual is provided with an immense repertoire of alternative variable regions and there is very little difference among individuals. The existence of the MHC gene cluster on one chromosome in all higher species suggests that in some way the products interact to maintain this association. Most duplicated genes, such as the hemoglobin α and β genes, are not located in proximity to one another.

Genetic Relationships Within a Family. In the case of a typical polymorphic MHC gene with a product that is codominantly expressed on the cell surface, a situation would frequently be found in which each parent will not share any MHC gene product with the other parent. If the alleles, or their haplotypes that result from meiotic division in the parent, are designated a, b, c, d, the kinds of genotypes found in the family and their interrelationships can be designated as in Figure 4–4. If the genotypes of the father and mother are a/b and c/d, respectively, the children, according to Mendel's first law, will be a/c, a/d, b/c, or b/d. Thus, a total of six genotypes are present in such a family (Fig.4–4). Note that individuals II-1 and II-5 are identical.

Figure 4–3. Complexity of the MHC occurs at two levels: (1) at the locus, where duplication of primordial gene results in a multi-gene family and (2) at the generation of a family of alleles for each locus by mutation, conversion, and so on.

I

1   a/b   2   c/d

Figure 4–4. Genotype of idealized family illustrating inheritance of a polymorphic gene with four alleles: a, b, c, and. d.

II

1	2	3	4	5
a/c	a/d	b/c	b/d	a/c

There are three types of genetic relationship among various members of the family: (1) identity (0 haplotype difference), (2) complete dissimilarity (2 haplotype difference), and (3) partial sharing or haplo-identity (1 haplotype difference). Among the siblings of a sufficiently large family, all three relationships will be found. The relationship of parent to child, however, always involves a one allele difference.

Genes in a Population. The task of measuring gene frequency is simplified in the case of class I and class II molecules to counting alternative gene products in a population because of the codominant expression of all the products encoded by genes at each locus of each chromosome 6. This works particularly well in families in which haplotypes are easily defined. Since the unit of inheritance is the haploid chromosome, it is convenient to approach the idea of studying the gene pool by considering first the frequency of genes on gametes. For example, if the frequency of the HLA-A1 allotype in a population is p and the frequency of the HLA-A3 allotype is q, then among individuals of the entire population, p gametes will contain the HLA-A1 gene and q gametes will contain the HLA-A3 gene. If there are no restrictions on mating choice, and the presence of the gene is neutral with respect to survival, the combination of male and female gametes in the fertilized zygote will occur in the proportions of $(p + q) \times (p + q)$ or p^2, $2pq$, and q^2. These describe the expected frequencies of homozygotes for HLA-A1, heterozygotes expressing HLA-A1 and HLA-A2, and homozygotes for HLA-A3 (Table 4–2). Again assuming random mating

generation, since there has not been any change in the frequency of gametes bearing the A1 or A3 alleles, the same proportion of individuals heterozygous or homozygous for A1 or A3 will result. This is the basic concept of Hardy-Weinberg equilibrium.

By rearranging terms, a useful expression for calculating gene frequency can be derived as follows:

$$\text{Gene frequency} = 1 - \sqrt{1 - \text{phenotype frequency}}$$

where the phenotype frequency is expressed as a decimal fraction. Although these concepts are widely used in this field, in a strict sense it is not likely that the genes of the human MHC are in perfect Hardy-Weinberg equilibrium, because certain combinations confer a selective advantage or disadvantage on individuals.

The observed frequencies and proportions of heterozygotes and homozygotes would be tested against those expected on the basis of genetic theory, assuming that the population is at equilibrium. This test would support the hypothesis that the measurement of the allelic products was exact and unbiased from a genetic view. The reader is referred to the field of population genetics for a full treatment of this area.[9]

A bias is particularly likely for genes determining disease susceptibility because of the problem in deciding whether an affected individual is homozygous or heterozygous. Therefore, in practice, it is usually best to estimate gene frequency directly by counting haplotypes in families.

Linkage and Recombination. When two loci are located close together, as within the histocompatibility

Table 4–2. Terminology*

Prefix	Meaning	Noun	Adjective	Immunogenetic Relationship
Auto-	Self	Autoantigen Autoantibody	Autologous Autochthonous	Self to self
Iso-(syn-)	Same	Isograft Isotype†	Syngeneic Isogeneic	Same species, genetically identical
Allo-(homo)	Other	Allotype Alloantigen Alloantibody	Allogeneic	Same species, genetically different
Hetero-(xeno-)	Foreign	Heteroantigen Heteroantibody	Heterologous Xenogeneic	Different species

*After Cunningham, A.J.: Understanding Immunology, New York, Academic Press, 1978.
†In certain situations, blood group antibodies have been termed "isoantibodies." The term isotype is also applied to the different classes of immunoglobulin present in an individual.

complex, the linked genes are usually inherited as a unit. Linkage can be deduced only from analyses of family pedigrees. In a population, for the most part, the alleles have become separated by recombination events and behave as independent entities. An example of linkage is illustrated in Figure 4–5. Here the linked genes in the first parent are designated a-b and c-d, comprising two haplotypes. The degrees of genetic relationships among the family members are 0, 1, and 2 haplotype differences.

A recombination event occurring during meiosis in the father gave rise to the recombinant haplotype a-d seen in the fifth child. This occurs in about 1 percent of families. Recombination ultimately leads to genetic equilibrium, where the expected frequency of finding a and b on the same haplotype is simply the product of the frequencies of the a and the b gene in the population.

$$p(a,b) = p(a) \cdot p(b)$$

It is a matter of very great interest, however, that among unrelated individuals certain alleles of one locus are found together on a haplotype with particular alleles of a second locus much more frequently than expected. This indicates that for this pair of alleles, normal recombination has not occurred and a state of non-or disequilibrium exists. The two alleles are said to be in positive *linkage disequilibrium*. This is measured mathematically by the following formula:

$$\text{Observed frequency} - \text{expected frequency} = \Delta$$

Since the value of Δ is the difference between two frequencies, it is expressed either as a decimal or, more conveniently, as an integer after multiplication by 1000. If the sign of Δ is positive, the alleles occur together more frequently than expected by chance, and the linkage disequilibrium is said to be positive. If the alleles are encountered together less frequently than expected, the linkage disequilibrium is negative. It should be stressed that the nonrandom recombination evident as linkage disequilibrium is only a property of pairs of alleles in a haplotype and not a general property of the locus. The origin of this disequilibrium results either from the recent introduction into the gene pool of particular gene combinations from genetically isolated individuals or from a selective advantage resulting from the presence of the two alleles in one individual. An alternative designation for this phenomenon is gametic association, because it appears that certain pairs of alleles are seen in association at high frequency.

NOMENCLATURE OF RELATIONSHIPS

Another set of distinctions and terms arises through the close relationship of transplantation to the topic of this chapter. Table 4–2 summarizes the categories of relationship that one's "self" can have, and the terms that describe and name them.

Perhaps the most important set of these terms derives from the concept of an allele. Allotype refers to the genetically determined alternative form of the same molecule. Most commonly, these structural differences are demonstrated as allotypic antigenic determinants or simply alloantigens that are recognized by alloantibodies. Classically, an alloserum is prepared by immunizing one member of a species with cells from another. This occurs during pregnancy or transplantation. More recently, monoclonal antibodies obtained from mice immunized with human materials have begun to replace the human antihuman alloreagents. It should be stressed that the distinction between allele and allotype, one between gene and gene product, should be carefully maintained. By convention, when one refers to the locus or allotypic gene, the term is italicized or underlined.

SEROLOGIC ANALYSIS OF MHC ANTIGENS

Serologic Specificity. The delineation of an alloantigen through the use of a reagent serum containing alloantibodies is a central theme in analysis of the histocompatibility complex. The use of an alloantiserum implicitly assumes that a genetic difference is responsible for the recognition of the alternative form of the products of one locus. The origin of this immunogenetic approach came from observations on blood groups, and the basic principles established apply to histocompatibility testing. The primary sources of reagent sera are from pregnant women, organ transplant and transfusion recipients, and, less commonly, intentionally immunized normal donors. In each instance, the alloantiserum recognizes foreign histocompatibility determinants on the

Figure 4–5. Genotype of a family illustrating linkage and recombination. Two loci are depicted: the first with alleles a, c, e, and g; the second with alleles b, d, f, and h. The pairs of alleles form haplotypes a-b and c-d in the father, and e-f and g-h in the mother. In all but one of the offspring the linked genes (haplotypes) are inherited as a unit. In individual II-5, the paternal haplotype (a-d) reflects a recombination occurring during meiosis.

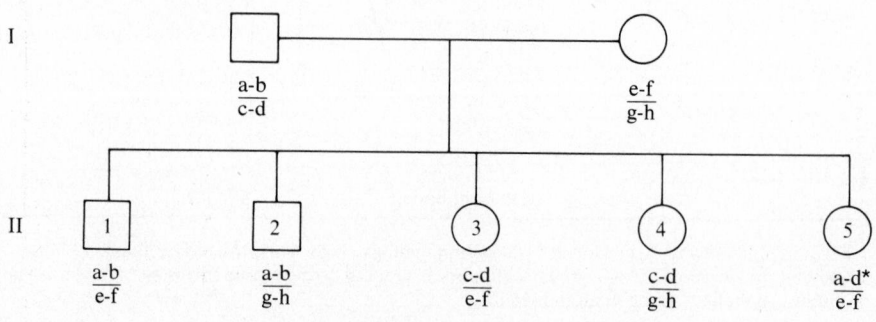

immunizing cells that, in the case of the fetus, are of paternal origin.

HLA Specificities. The path taken in serologic analysis involves first, the recognition that various allosera define a HLA specificity, and second, the application of these sera to determine whether an individual has the particular specificity. An example of the approach used in establishing serologic specificity of a system is illustrated in Table 4–3. The situation involves a family similar to that of Figure 4–4 in which an alloantibody appeared after the birth of a third child. The antibody reacts with lymphocytes from the father and the third and fourth children, suggesting it detects antigen b.

In practice the events would occur in opposite sequence: the serum typing reaction would be performed first and the phenotype of the individual would be thereby assigned. Then by consideration of the pattern of antigens in the family that reflects the genotype of the individuals, the haplotype assignments would be made.

The central problem in serologic analysis is the development of methods to arrive at the conclusion that a discrete and generally testable specificity is being detected. The first step in this process could be the demonstration that a number of different alloantisera recognize the same determinants. To return to the example, further testing of this serum with a panel of 100 unrelated individuals yields a 20 percent frequency of positive reactions. Testing of a second serum on the same 100 individuals reveals a 24 percent frequency of positive reactions. The relationship of the specificities of the two sera can be seen in a 2 × 2 table in which each of the 100 individuals is scored as positive or negative for the presence of the alloantigen (Fig. 4–6). The use of a 2 × 2 table is an important analytic tool because through the comparison, reagent sera with similar but not precisely identical specificities can be identified. In this example 20 individuals expressed an antigen detected by both sera, and 76 lacked these determinants. There were no individuals positive for serum 1 who were not also positive for serum 2, but the reciprocal case was differ-

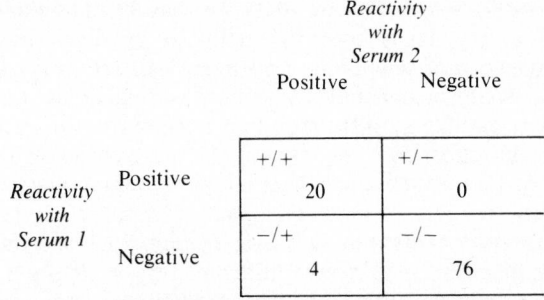

Figure 4–6. 2 × 2 table illustrating analysis of a serum cluster for coincidence of reactivity of 100 patients. Chi square = 79,167. Chi square (Yates = 74.044; p < <0.001 that the sera have unrelated specificities.

ent. Four persons bore an antigen detected only by serum 2. These are "extra" reactions; however, serum 2 might still be useful for indicating the presence of the antigen detected by both sera.

Statistical Analysis. The statistic applied to testing the hypothesis that the two sera react with the same determinant is the chi square (χ^2).[9] If the sample size were smaller, a modification of the chi square statistic, such as the Yates correction for continuity, should be used. For still smaller samples, the exact probability can be calculated by the method of Fisher. In the case of the example given for serum 1 and serum 2, the χ^2 is 79.167 and the corrected χ^2 (Yates) is 74.044. Since the degree of freedom is one, reference to χ^2 tables shows the probability that serum 1 and serum 2 react with independent antigens to be very much less than 1 in 1000. This suggests the interpretation that the two sera detect the same or closely related specificities.

A further refinement is the calculation of a modified coefficient of correlation, usually designated "r", by the formula $r = \sqrt{\chi^2/N}$. This provides an index that is independent of the sample size. This statistic in effect measures the extent of the similarity between the two sera, and is 0.89 in this example. The sign of r is obtained by comparing the products of the two diagonals. It is taken as positive when $(+/+)$ $(-/-)$ exceeds $(+/-)$ $(-/+)$. It is evident that other sera, when tested on the same 100 individuals, can have one of three categories of relationship that reflect the value and sign of the coefficient of correlation. A high positive value indicates similar specificities; a value near zero indicates a lack of relationship; a negative number is interpreted as describing a reciprocal repulsion relationship between the specificities such as would exist for an allelic alloantigen.

For statistical analyses it is necessary that the immunization event that yields the alloantiserum be between two "outbred" individuals who might potentially differ for many alloantigens. This would result in a reagent that contains minor interfering specificities. At early stages in the delineation of an alloantigenic system, the reagents have frequently been complex, and the mathematical treatments were essential.

The same mathematical analysis can be applied to the situation in which other facts are known about the mem-

Table 4–3. Relation of Genotype to Phenotype: Detection of Phenotypes by Alloantibodies Appearing in Pregnancy Serum Induced by Paternal MHC Antigens

Lympho-cyte Source	Genotype	Lymphocytes Killed After Addition of Complement (%)		
		Control Serum	Mother I-2 Pregnancy Serum	Presumed Phenotype
Sib 1 II-1	a/c	<5	<5	—
Sib 2 II-2	a/d	<5	<5	—
Sib 3 II-3	b/c	<5	100	b
Sib 4 II-4	b/d	<5	100	b
Father I-1	a/b	<5	100	b
Mother I-2	c/d	<5	<5	—

bers of the panel. If it were known that 18 individuals were of the HLA type B7, it could be determined whether or not sera 1 and 2 detected HLA-B7 (Fig. 4–7). It would be concluded that both sera have, as their major specificity, alloantibodies that react with the HLA-B7 alloantigen but that both sera have extra reactions that presumably reflect minor contaminant specificities.

Practical Aspects of Serologic Typing. Each specificity is determined by several different sera to assure accurate typing results. Sometimes, combinations of sera, each with more than one specificity, must be used to detect certain antigens. In practice a large number of sera are used in HLA typing because of the great variety of MHC alloantigens (Table 4–4). Usually 120 sera or more are used for typing an individual. In order to conserve lymphocytes and reagent sera, each reaction is performed with 0.001 ml volumes of serum and cells. Binding of antibodies is most commonly detected by complement-dependent cytotoxicity, and dyes are used to determine cell death. The entire reaction is performed on a 60-well "Terasaki tray" filled with oil to prevent evaporation.

Typing for Class I or Class II Alloantigens. The evaluation of the two classes of MHC molecules is simply performed by taking advantage of the fact that class I molecules are expressed on all lymphocytes and monocytes, while class II molecules are usually restricted to B lymphocytes and monocytes. The analysis of alleles of the class I loci is carried out using whole mononuclear cell preparations, while the class II Ia allodeterminants are defined with mononuclear cells that have been depleted of T lymphocytes, yielding a "B cell" preparation that contains some monocytes and various other cells. Since B lymphocytes also contain class I molecules the reagent allosera that define Ia allodeterminants must be freed of antibodies to class I molecules by absorption. Platelets, since they only express class I alloantigens, are usually used for this purpose.

Class I Allodeterminants. The class I alloantigens form three segregant series designated HLA-A, HLA-B, and HLA-C, and the respective genetic loci receive the same designation but are italicized.[11–13] The alloantigens of the *HLA-A, B,* and *C* series are highly polymorphic.[11–13] This is illustrated in Table 4–4. There are at least 18 distinct alloantigenic forms comprising HLA-A and 24 comprising HLA-B. The *C* locus is less well

defined, and considerably fewer alleles are known. The terminology that refers to the different alloantigens reflects an extensive international collaborative effort. The first term is a letter referring to the locus; the second, a number that is simply assigned when the specificity is delineated. The prefix "w" before a number signifies that the specificity is recognized but still requires additional definition. In general, typing results include the alloantigen phenotype of the HLA-A and B segregant series as well as the specification of the individual as Bw4 or Bw6. *C* locus typing is not as advanced, in part because of the difficulty of obtaining good typing sera. This is so because the antigens appear to be poorly immunogenic, and the problem is compounded by the tight linkage with the HLA-B locus.

The specificities previously termed "4a" and "4b" and now designated "Bw4" and "Bw6" are an incompletely understood alloantigenic system. Recent chemical evidence supports the prevailing view that these are "supratypic specificities" of various HLA-B antigens. They have practical value in permitting the assignment of certain difficult HLA specificities because of characteristics in their association, and their matching is reported to be relevant to renal transplant survival.

The interpretation of the results of HLA typing should be made with attention to class, locus or allelic series, and particular allele. For example, a report of *HLA-A1-B8 and B7* signifies that all three alleles are of class I, and that for the *A* locus only one allelic product is detected. This could mean that the individual is homozygous for the *A1* allele or that an uncharacterized allelic product is encoded by the *A* locus gene of one chromosome 6. The two *B* locus alleles are located on the two different 6 chromosomes. If the individual were Caucasian, it would be likely that the *A1* and the *B8* alleles were present on the same chromosome by virtue of their linkage disequilibrium.

Certain *A* and *B* locus alleles are found together on the same chromosome more frequently than would be expected by the product of their respective gene frequencies. This nonrandom distribution of certain alleles is an example of linkage disequilibrium (Table 4–5).[9,14]

DETERMINANTS DEFINED BY LYMPHOCYTE RESPONSES

In contrast to the antigens detected by serologic means, there is another category of MHC determinants that are recognized directly by lymphocytes. The recognition event is detected either by killing of the target cell by a lymphocyte, e.g., cell-mediated lympholysis (CML), or by proliferation of the responding lymphocyte, e.g., mixed lymphocyte culture (MLC) or primed lymphocyte test (PLT). Proliferation is usually assayed by incorporation of radiolabeled thymidine into the newly synthesized DNA.[15–17]

The MHC determinants recognized by these lymphocyte responses are relatively restricted to class I molecules in the case of cell-mediated lympholysis and to

SERUM 1

		Positive +	Negative −
Anti-HLA-B7	Positive	+/+ 17	+/− 0
	Negative	−/+ 3	−/− 80

Figure 4–7. Identification of specificity of serum 1 as related to HLA-B7. Chi square=81,928. Chi square (Yates) = 76.014; p < <0.001 that serum 1 and an anti-HLA-B7 serum have unrelated specificities.

class II molecules for the MLC and PLT reaction. This restriction is paralleled by the fact that T lymphocytes belonging to different T lymphocyte lineages primarily mediate either reactivity to class I molecules, the Leu 2+,T8+ suppressor-cytotoxic cell or reactivity to class II molecules, the Leu 3+,T4+ helper-inducer cell. Exceptions to this generalization exist, such as Leu 3+,T4+ cells that have class II antigens as the target of their cytotoxicity.

The MLC reaction is of special historical interest because it was used to define the existence of the class II gene products. As a practical test for typing an individual it has been supplanted by the simpler serologic determination of Ia allotype. However, the reaction still is of very considerable importance in defining subspecificities among Ia allodeterminants and in situations such as transplantation, where histocompatibility is critical.

Table 4–4. HLA Gene Frequencies in Different Populations*

	North American Caucasoids	American Blacks	African Blacks	Japanese	American Indians
A Locus Alleles:					
A1	16.1	8.1	3.9	1.2	2.5
A2	28.0	16.3	9.4	25.3	45.3
A3	14.1	7.0	6.4	0.7	0.6
A9 ⎰ Aw23	1.9	10.6	10.8	37.2	23.2
⎱ Aw24	7.3	5.1	2.4		
A10 ⎰ Aw25	2.6	0.4	3.5	12.7	0.6
⎱ Aw26	3.4	2.3	4.5		
A11	5.1	2.8	—	6.7	—
A28	4.2	5.8	8.9	—	2.8
A29	3.6	2.3	6.4	0.2	0.6
Aw30	2.9	13.0	22.1	0.5	1.1
Aw31	4.5	2.8	4.2	8.7	19.9
Aw32	3.7	1.9	1.5	0.5	1.1
Aw33	1.2	5.1	1.0	2.0	0.6
Aw43	—	—	4.0	—	—
Blank	1.3	16.5	11.0	4.2	1.8
B Locus Alleles:					
B5	5.9	4.9	3.0	20.9	14.0
B7	10.5	12.6	7.3	7.1	0.6
B8	10.4	5.5	7.1	0.2	1.7
B12 Bw6	13.8	14.0	12.7	6.5	1.7
B13	2.6	0.4	1.5	0.8	—
B14	5.1	4.6	3.6	0.5	—
B15	5.9	4.7	3.0	9.3	13.7
Bw16 ⎰ Bw38	2.5	0.4	—	1.8	14.5
⎱ Bw39	1.4	0.4	1.5	4.7	
B17	4.9	11.2	16.1	0.6	—
B18	3.1	3.6	2.0	—	0.6
Bw21	3.8	4.4	1.5	1.5	
Bw22	2.3	3.9	—	6.5	0.6
B27	5.6	0.8	—	0.3	6.2
Bw35	8.6	12.5	7.2	9.4	22.1
B37	1.7	1.2	—	0.8	—
B40	9.2	3.9	2.0	21.8	16.6
Bw41	—	—	1.5	—	—
Bw42	—	—	12.3	—	—
Blank	2.8	11.0	17.9	7.6	7.8
C Locus Alleles:					
Cw1	3.7	1.9	—	11.1	10.1
Cw2	6.0	9.2	11.4	1.4	4.6
Cw3	11.4	8.8	5.5	26.3	16.6
Cw4	10.2	12.9	14.2	4.3	23.4
Cw5	5.2	1.4	1.0	1.2	1.1
Cw6	11.3	—	17.7	2.1	—
Blank	52.1	65.8	50.2	53.5	44.2

Alleles marked with a minus sign (−) are not present in this population.

*In the B Locus, Bw4 brackets B5 through Bw16, and Bw6 brackets B12 through B40, as indicated by the vertical groupings in the original.

*From data of the VII Workshop on histocompatibility testing. *In* Bodmer, W.F., et al. (eds.): Histocompatibility Testing 1977. Copenhagen, Munksgaard, 1978.

Table 4–5. Some Haplotypes in Different Populations*

HLA-A, B Haplotypes:

North American Caucasoid		Linkage Disequilibrium	Haplotype Frequency
A1	B8	59.2	67.9
A3	B7	27.6	38.0
A3	B14	14.5	19.3
A28	B14	12.7	13.3
A26	B38	9.2	10.0
A26	B5	8.8	9.7
A25	B18	7.5	8.3
Japanese			
Aw24	B7	34.9	55.1
A26	Bw35	16.6	25.8
Aw33	B12	11.5	11.5
A1	B37	7.6	7.7
American Indian			
Aw24	Bw35	69.2	103.2
A1	B8	10.8	11.3
African Black			
Aw30	Bw42	44.6	61.6
Aw32	Bw35	13.0	13.5

HLA-B, D Haplotypes:

North American Caucasoid			
B27	Dw1	8.4	11.4
Bw35	Dw1	13.4	20.4
B12	Dw2	30.0	41.1
B7	Dw2	23.2	30.9
B8	Dw3	56.9	57.6
Bw44	Dw4	19.4	24.4
B12	Dw4	19.0	22.4
B15	Dw4	9.3	13.1
B14	Dw5	15.3	16.5
Bw51	Dw5	10.6	12.9
B5	Dw5	9.7	12.6
Bw22	Dw6	11.7	12.9

*From data of the VII Workshop on histocompatibility testing. *In* Bodmer, W.F., et al. (eds.): Histocompatibility Testing 1977. Copenhagen, Munksgaard, 1978.

The Mixed Lymphocyte Culture Reaction. The basic elements of the MLC are the co-culture of responder lymphocytes from one individual with stimulator lymphocytes from another. The stimulator lymphocytes are treated by γ-irradiation or alkylating agents, rendering them incapable of DNA synthesis. This reaction is a one-way MLC. By the fifth day of culture, a vigorous proliferative response of the responder cells in the culture indicates that foreign histocompatibility determinants are present. Conversely, compatibility or "MLC identity" is signaled by the absence of a significant response. This implies that the stimulator and responder cells share certain genetic markers.

The components in the cell membrane responsible for inducing stimulation are not yet precisely defined on a molecular basis. They clearly involve the class II or Ia/DR allodeterminants. For this reason B lymphocytes, dendritic cells, and monocytes are considered to be the principal stimulators in the MLC. Conversely, the responding lymphocytes are T cells.

The mixed lymphocyte culture reaction has deeper biologic aspects that are only beginning to be understood. Several distinctive features of the reaction are as follows: The number of T lymphocytes that respond is greater than the response to conventional antigens such as tetanus toxoid. Furthermore, the response to allodeterminants is greater than that to heterodeterminants on lymphocytes from other species, a pattern that contrasts with antibody responses. Lastly, the responding T lymphocytes elaborate factors that interact with autologous B lymphocytes and provide a supplemental stimulus to the B lymphocytes' response to an antigen.

A curious phenomenon that may be of considerable biologic significance is termed the autologous MLC. This proliferative response of T lymphocytes is initiated by *isolated* autologous cells that bear class II molecules.[19]

However, B lymphocytes and monocytes are relatively inefficient as stimulators in the autologous reaction, reflecting an interesting divergence between cells capable of presenting antigen and those most capable of initiation in an autologous MLC.

Genetic Control of the Mixed Lymphocyte Culture Response. The major genetic control of the stimulating determinants in the classic allogeneic MLC maps at one locus, termed *HLA-D*.[17] This locus is located very near *HLA-B*. Evidence exists for a second minor locus near *HLA-A*, but less information is available about this.

A representative experiment illustrating the relationships among family members as revealed by the MLC reaction is given in Figure 4–8. The results of this experiment demonstrate that the two siblings that share the same haplotype are compatible, as is indicated by the absence of a mixed lymphocyte culture response. In about 1 to 2 percent of HLA-A and B identical individuals the expected compatibility is not observed. This is due to recombination, and these results provide the evidence that the *D* locus is distinct from the *B* locus.

Homozygous Typing Cells. The fact that compatibility requires identity between heterozygous individuals necessarily limited the application of MLC analysis as a tool of genetic analysis. The solution to the use of MLC reaction as a practical analytic method was the introduction of homozygous stimulator lymphocytes as a typing reagent. A MLC homozygous individual must fulfill the criterion that neither parent be significantly stimulated by their child.

Table 4–6 illustrates the typing of the individuals of the family illustrated in Figure 4–8 using homozygous typing cells. The presence of compatibility of stimulator and responder cells is illustrated by a low level of DNA

synthesis. This implies that the individual shares the MHC-stimulating determinants with the cells of the homozygous stimulator.

Through the identification of a number of different homozygous individuals in an extensive international effort, a series of lymphocyte-defined allodeterminants that comprise a segregant series were found. These alleles are designated HLA-D1, 2, and so on. Certain of these *D* locus alleles exhibit linkage disequilibrium forming haplotypes; for example, A1-B8-D3 and A3-B7-D2.[11-13]

Newer approaches using lymphocytes primed to respond in an enhanced secondary manner (PLT) to determinants involving HLA-D components appear to offer considerable simplification in regard to performance. The reader is referred to the histocompatability literature for a detailed explanation.[11-13,17]

THE IA SYSTEM

The genes encoding the class II gene products form a chromosomal region, the presumed organization of which was summarized in Figure 4–1. The β chains are of special interest because they appear to contain the determinants responsible for all of the allo variation of the molecules. In addition to the β chain polymorphisms the α chain genes of the DS and SB molecules are polymorphic. In recognition of the terminology initially developed in the murine system that names homologous molecules with emphasis on their role in regulating the immune response, the general designation of the class II gene products used in this chapter will be "Ia antigens" or "Ia molecules."

The DR Allotypes. A relatively imperfect relationship

Pedigree (same as in Fig. 4–4):

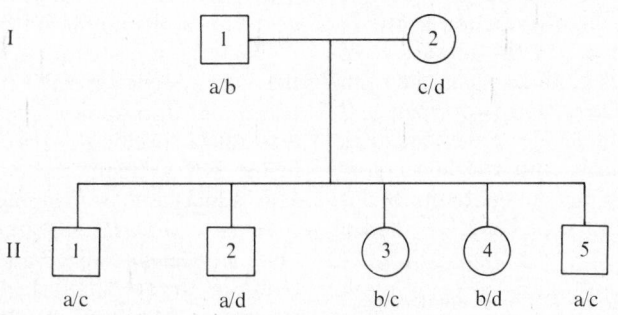

Representative MHC Testing Results:

Haplotype Difference	Stimulator (Irradiated)	Responder	Stimulation DNA Synthesis cpm ^{3}H Thymidine Incorporated
2	I: 1 (a/b)	I: 2 (c/d)	45,000
2	II: 1 (a/c)	II: 4 (b/d)	42,000
1	II: 1 (a/c)	II: 2 (a/d)	30,000
0	II: 1 (a/c)	II: 5 (a/c)	300

Figure 4–8. Relationships among family members revealed by MHC testing.

Table 4–6. MHC Results Using a Homozygous Typing Cell (in Family of Fig. 4–8)

Stimulator (Irradiated)	Responder	Stimulation DNA Synthesis CPM 3H Thymidine Incorporated	Interpre- tations
a/a	I 1 (a/b)	400	Type a
a/a	I 2 (c/d)	41,000	
a/a	II 1 (a/c)	450	Type a
a/a	II 3 (b/c)	39,000	

between certain allospecificities of the class II molecules and particular MLC determinants resulted in the designation of certain of the class II alloantigens as "DR" (*D* Related antigens).[19] Evidence has been gathered that at least 10 serologically Ia allospecificities form a segregant series that has been assumed to map to a single locus designated *DR*. Table 4–7 lists the frequencies of the major DR specificities in different populations. The population variation is of great interest and will be discussed later. These DR specificities are, however, still in the process of being defined, and the use of DR to designate a segregant series is only an operational one, since tests, such as the existence of a Hardy-Weinberg equilibrium, are not met for this series of alloantigens; moreover, there is chemical evidence of increased complexity. This chemical evidence has revealed, for example, that the serologic specificity DR[4] is present on five molecularly differentiable species that are each a distinct allele. Since the Ia molecule consists of two chains, then according to this greatly oversimplified early model, there was a single MHC locus that encoded α chains and a second locus for the multiple alternative β chain alleles, one for each DR specificity.

This simple model serves as an introduction to the Ia system but is not at all accurate. In the Ia system of the mouse, the two main types of Ia antigens are each composed of two types of α chains and two types of β chains, and all four types of molecules are encoded in two subregions designated *I-E/C* and *I-A*. The most frequent amino acid structure of the human Ia molecules was found to be homologous to the sequence of α chain

Table 4–7. Frequencies of Some Major Ia Alleles in Different Races*

Designation	Phenotype (Alloantigen) Frequency (%)		
	Caucasoid	*Negroid*	*Mongoloid*
DR1	16	13	12
DR2	25	32	36
DR3	21	32	3
DR4	21	10	41
DR5	20	28	4
DR7	24	20	1
DR8	4	8	9

*VIII Workshop Data.[13]

and β chain molecules encoded by the murine *I-E/C* subregion (Table 4–8).[20-22] For this reason the structure of the DR allodeterminants are referred to as *I-E/C*-like.

However, biochemical and immunologic studies have demonstrated that in man there are three DR β chains that have a very similar but not identical *I-E/C*-like amino acid sequence.[21-23] The inter-relationships of these gene products are illustrated in Figure 4–9, which emphasizes the distinctness of each of the Ia species on the cell surface. These new data raise two challenging problems. The first is the nature of the basis of the DR specificities in terms of the multiple β chains. Are the polyclonal anti-DR allosera actually directed to a number of distinct but generally similar gene products that are too closely linked to be separated by recombination? Secondly, what is the genetic basis of these molecules and allospecificities? The conventional view might be summarized as "one distinct alloantigen implies one molecule under the control of one gene." Alternatively, in view of the revolution in eukaryotic molecular biology, there could be a more intricate system involving lateral gene transfer and movable genetic elements such as "mini genes" that encode only the particular segment of the allodeterminant. These genes would be inserted into one or several basic β chain genes to result in a large variety of molecules bearing distinct allodeterminants. Furthermore, there is the potential for additional diversity being generated by post-translational events such as α and β chain combination or modification by the addition of complex carbohydrates. Of course, the resolution of these questions is of critical importance in determining the precise genetic basis of disease susceptibility influenced by these gene products. The resolution of this will have to await further studies involving monoclonal allotypic reagents or recombinant DNA technology.

The DS/DC System of Non-DR Ia Specificities. Evidence for a second major locus analogous to the murine *I-A* subregion has come forward (Fig. 4–9). Well before the DR system assumed its present degree of characterization, information began to accumulate about additional Ia specificities that were not able to be included in the DR system. The initial evidence for these non-DR Ia loci came from studies on susceptibility to certain rheumatic diseases: Sjögren's syndrome and systemic lupus erythematosus[24,25] and rheumatoid arthritis.[26] For example, the specificity Ia $4\times7\times10$ that would now be designated MT3 was shown, by co-capping studies and segregation analysis, to be distinct from the allele of the DR series DR4.[19,26]

More recently a number of the non-DR allospecificities of the Ia system were grouped into DC, MB, and MT and other related segregant series.[27-29] The relationship of these newer specificities to those of the DR system is summarized in Table 4–9. There were two contradictory views of the nature of this relationship. In one view, for example, the sera defining the MB3 specificity would be considered to recognize a "public" or supratypic antigen expressed on the DR4 and DR5

Table 4–8. Amino Acid Sequence Comparison of Murine I-E, I-A, and Human DR, DS, and IVD12 Allodeterminants

Alpha Chains

Position:	1	3	4	6	7	8	1	12	13	14	15	16	19	22	24	29
I-E	Ilu	–	–	–	Ilu	Ilu	–	Phe	Tyr	–	–	–	–	Phe	Phe	–
DR	Ilu	–	–	Val	Ilu	Ilu	–	Phe	Tyr	Leu	–	–	–	Phe	Phe	–
I-A	–	Ilu	–	–	–	Val	Tyr		–	–	Val	Tyr	–	–	–	Phe
DS	–	Ilu	Val	–	–	Val	Tyr		Val	–	Leu	Tyr	Tyr	–	–	Phe
IVD12	–	Ilu	Val	–	–	Val	Tyr	–	Val	–	Leu	Tyr	Tyr	–	–	Phe

Beta Chains

Position:	7	8	9	10	11	14	16	17	18	24	26	27	30	31	32
I-E	Phe	Leu	–	Tyr	Val	–	–	Phe	Tyr	–	Phe	Leu	Phe	–	–
DR	Phe	Leu	–	–	–	–	–	Phe	Phe	Val	Phe	Leu	Tyr	Phe	Tyr
I-A	Phe	Val	Tyr	Tyr	Phe	Phe	Tyr	Phe	–	–	Tyr	–	Tyr	–	–
DS	Phe	Val	–	–	Phe	–	Tyr	Phe	–	–	–	–	–	–	–
IVD12	Phe	Val	Tyr	–	Phe	–	Tyr	Phe	–	Val	Val	Val	Tyr	–	Tyr

47

Figure 4–9. Working model of chromosomal region coding for Ia antigens. Based on analysis of known gene products, recent advances in molecular biology reveal an additional β and α gene in the SB region and another α gene in the DS region.

β chains. This supratypic antigen would signify an evolutionary relationship of these two alleles to a common ancestral antecedent. For example, the presence of the MB3 specificity might be taken as an indication that the genes encoding DR4 and DR5 arose by mutation from an MB3+ precursor. Immediately, however, it is evident that the MT3 specificity would argue for a different ancestry. No simple scheme was advanced to explain the systems in this way.

In another view, for which considerable evidence is emerging, the non-DR specificities of the Ia system belong to entirely distinct molecules and hence define alleles of a new segregant series, tentatively designated DS,[23,28,30-33] that involves the MB and possibly some of the MT specificities. The MT determinants are primarily expressed on one or two of the DR β chains. The amino acid sequence of the Ia molecules bearing MB determinants resembles that of the murine I-A molecules[34] (Table 4–8). These data, along with those derived from recombinant DNA technology, provide firm evidence for the existence of a second Ia locus entirely unrelated to DR. These other loci presumably arose by gene duplication of an original Ia locus, giving daughter loci that developed their separate allelic series by further mutational events. The alleles of this locus are still under investigation.

The current view of the DS region is that it contains two genes encoding α chains and two genes encoding β chains, all of which are polymorphic. The possibility of 16 different combinational products arising from trans and cis interactions emphasizes the complexity of the resulting determinants.

The amino acid sequence of the MT system is at present difficult to harmonize with a simple origin at either an *I-A* or *I-E/C*-like locus. Even with the use of monoclonal antibodies the MT specificities are present on molecules that have curious mixtures of amino acid sequences resembling both DR and DS molecules. This latter fact adds support to the nonclassical genetic mechanisms involving gene transfer. The evidence that the β chains of the MT and MB specificities are encoded by different genes, at least in the DR4 haplotype, is provided by co-capping experiments.

Monoclonal Antibodies. An important methodologic advance that is revolutionizing this field has been the application of monoclonal antibody technology to the problem of detecting alloantigens. Until this advance, polyclonal human alloantisera were used which, although they were operationally monospecific typing reagents, contained a variety of alloantibodies resulting from the immune response to closely linked genes encoding the foreign histocompatibility antigens. Monoclonal antibodies, in contrast, can be selected so that they can be used as probes for the presence of a single alloantigenic determinant.

The SB Subregion. The third well-documented subregion of the human Ia system is termed SB and encodes α and β chains that are distinct from both DS and DR α and β chains.[35] The recognition of the alleles of this locus is made largely by primed lymphocyte typing, and these alleles are not related to any of the DR, MT, or MB specificities. The genetic organization here resembles that of DS with two α and two β chains. There is no homologue of this subregion in the mouse. Monoclonal antibodies have been identified that react with the SB molecules.

Ia Antigens as Markers of Differentiation. The Ia alloantigen-bearing molecules have been most extensively studied, in part because of the simplicity with which heteroantisera can be raised to isolated preparations of the Ia molecules.[19] These antisera are of considerable value in the examination of the distribution of the Ia molecule on different cell types.

Within the B lymphocyte lineage, Ia molecules, while present on the earliest recognizable stage, are progressively lost from the B lymphocyte when entering the

Table 4–9. DR Specificity Associations

DR:	1	2	3	4	5	6	7	6Y	8	9
MT 1	x	x						x		
MT 2			x		x	x			x	
MT 3				x			x			x
MT 4				x	x				x	
MT 5	x	x								
MT 6			x			x				
MB 1	x	x				x			x	
MB 2			x			x				
MB 3				x	x	x				x
TE 21	x	x								
TE 22				x	x					
TE 23	x			x						
TE 24			x			x				

terminal phase of differentiation as plasma cells. While all but a few percent of unstimulated T lymphocytes lack detectable Ia antigens, after mitogen or antigen stimulation a major proportion of the T lymphocytes can be found to express Ia antigen determinants. This implies a considerable degree of control over the activation of genes that specify the Ia molecules.

The monocyte is the most frequent cell in the blood that expresses Ia antigens. The level of Ia antigens is independently controlled on monocytes. One example of this is that in most individuals the incubation of monocytes with lipopolysaccharide-endotoxin preparations results in suppression of Ia synthesis and expression. Monocytes are also distinctive in that certain Ia antigens primarily associated with the MT specificities are found at higher levels on monocytes compared with B cells. This lack of coordinate expression of different Ia species is another example of the special control of Ia synthesis and expression on this lineage that perhaps relates to the role of these cells in antigen presentation to T lymphocytes.

Among other Ia antigen-bearing cells are the dendritic cells. These cells lack detectable membrane antigens of the monocyte lineage and are highly efficient stimulators in the autologous MLC. The dendritic cells also appear to be capable of presenting soluble protein antigens. Similarly present in the blood are small numbers of committed hematopoietic progenitor cells that are Ia(+).

Ia antigens are also found as a major cell membrane glycoprotein during the early stages of differentiation in each of the principal hematopoietic cell lineages. In the granulocyte series, Ia molecues are demonstrable on the committed progenitor cell through the myeloblast stage. In the erythrocyte series, the erythropoietin sensitive burst and colony forming progenitor cells, as well as pronormoblasts, have readily demonstrable Ia antigens. In both these lineages, the disappearance of Ia at an early stage contrasts with the persistence of this molecule on the surface membrane of B lymphocytes and monocytes until a more terminal stage.[19]

The presence of Ia antigens on analogous stages of murine hematopoietic cells has not been identified, and this fact suggests that in man Ia molecules serve an additional function outside that of the immune system. Possibly this function relates to the control of proliferative hematopoietic differentiation.

Function. The functions of the class I and II molecules are known only to a limited degree. Both classes of molecules have central roles in controlling immunologic defense mechanisms. The class I molecules have their best defined function in the effector phase of T lymphocyte cytotoxic reactions. Antigen recognition and killing of the target cell is restricted to T lymphocyte–target cell systems that are compatible for specific class I locus alleles. The functions of the class II molecules that have been recognized are primarily in the afferent limits of the immune response. Through antigen presentation to T lymphocytes, the specific immmune response to T-lymphocyte-dependent antigens is controlled by the class II molecules. It appears that the T lymphocyte by itself is incapable of responding to an antigen unless the antigen is presented to the T lymphocyte in the context of class II molecules on the surface of a monocyte or dendritic cell. A second element of the function of class II molecules is apparent in the various antigen-dependent interactions among cell subpopulations during the immune response. This is especially evident in circuits involving suppressor cells and their factors. Other kinds of class II molecule functions suggest that they have a direct role in determining cellular interactions. In terms of the Niels Jerne view of clonal selection, the particular MHC allodeterminants also influence the T lymphocyte antigen receptor repertoire by causing the elimination of any strongly autoreactive T cell clones. These deleted T lymphocyte clones leave gaps in the recognition of certain antigens. Each of these functions, along with those to be discovered, are relevant for their potential derangement and subsequent role in influencing susceptibility to disease.

DISEASE ASSOCIATIONS

With the emerging knowledge concerning the association of certain diseases with genes that map in the MHC, the MHC has acquired a relevance to the practice of medicine that will be substantial in its implications.[19,36] This is particularly the case in the rheumatic diseases, of which a number have been demonstrated to have this association. Among the implications of these associations are the following: (1) the potential for improved diagnostic accuracy, (2) an enhanced knowledge of the pathogenetic mechanisms through which a genetic predisposition is turned into a disease process, (3) an improvement in the nosologic classifications of the rheumatic diseases as an outgrowth of the increase in knowledge, and (4) perhaps the most novel, the ability to define in precise terms who is at risk for the development of a disease. Here there is the potential for a new area of specific preventative medical therapy directed to altering the disease predisposition state.

Background. The initial assertion of an association between the MHC and human disease was made in patients with Hodgkin's disease. While the exact nature of this particular relationship has remained difficult to characterize until very recently, the subsequent finding that HLA-B27 was associated with axial arthropathies has galvanized attention to this area of investigation. The presence or absence of HLA-B27 has proved itself to be an important practical diagnostic test in the evaluation of a patient with perplexing back pain or rheumatoid factor-negative arthritis, and the application of the test facilitated an enlargement of the concept of a family of axial arthropathies and their extra-articular manifestations. Furthermore, the puzzling limited inheritance of ankylosing spondylitis was clarified by the ability to identify the haplotype that conferred susceptibility.

While other diseases were found that had associations to particular HLA-A or B alleles, notably Behçet's syndrome and psoriasis (see Chapters 66 and 74), the emphasis has switched to studies on diseases primarily associated with the more newly described determinants of histocompatibility, including those relating to the HLA-D alleles. Studies on multiple sclerosis led this line of investigation when in 1973 the strong association with HLA-D2 was reported and in 1975 when the first association of a B lympocyte alloantigen with disease was made in patients with multiple sclerosis. The previously reported weak association of multiple sclerosis with HLA-A3 and B7 was shown to be simply a reflection of the linkage disequilibrium of these determinants with the B lymphocyte alloantigens associated with the DR2 specificity.[19]

More recently, a number of rheumatic diseases have been found that are associated with B lymphocyte alloantigens or, to a slightly lesser extent, with HLA-D alleles. In these diseases, the linkage disequilibrium with the HLA-A and B alloantigens was usually insufficient to provide a clue to the presence of the disease association. Thus, there now exist two main categories of MHC disease associations within the rheumatic diseases: (1) The constellations of arthritides associated with HLA-B27 and other alleles involved in susceptibility to psoriasis. These will be discussed in detail elsewhere in this book. (2) Those that are related to the B lymphocyte alloantigens, including, in part, rheumatoid arthritis,[26,37-40] systemic lupus erythematosus,[39,41,42] Sjögren's syndrome,[43] and rheumatic fever.[44]

Genetics. From the perspective of genetics, the acquisition of one of these diseases can be considered as a trait determined by a polymorphic gene mapping within the MHC. However, the common denominator in all these associations is that the MHC phenotype associated with a disease does not automatically confer the disease on all individuals who receive the particular allele. It is, rather, susceptibility or predisposition that is inherited, and it is evident that some additional factors—either inherited or acquired from the environment—are necessary in order to result in the disease.

Mendelian inheritance of a disease is readily recognized by the simple patterns of dominance or recessivity of either autosomal or sex chromosome genes. In contrast, the diseases under discussion are characterized by a more elusive mode of inheritance in which the disease, while occasionally appearing to be familial, lacks a well-defined genetic pattern (Fig. 4–10).

In general, a number of distinct events can account for non-Mendelian inheritance. These include a basic heterogeneity in the disease under study, reflecting several distinct types of disease, each with a separate gene. Alternatively, the disease can vary in detectability so that subclinical cases go unnoticed and obscure proper patient ascertainment. Lastly, the occurrence of the disease may be the result of the action of two independent events, with the second event being either the presence of a second gene or a particular environmental circumstance. This latter situation is referred to as incomplete penetrance. In each of these explanations of non-Mendelian inheritance, the existence of a genetic marker that

NUMBER OF INDIVIDUALS (2 × 2 TABLE)

Figure 4–10. Calculation of association of rheumatoid arthritis with presence of an alloantigen detected by a B cell alloantiserum. Chi square (Yates) = 18.9. p < 0.001.

characterized the individual at risk for development of the disease would provide a method for deciding among the possibilities.

Methods of Procedure. In practice, the determination that a gene mapping within the MHC determines susceptibility to a particular disease involves two levels of investigation. In the first, a significant association with an allele of the MHC is determined. In the second, the mode of inheritance of the disease trait in relation to the locus of the MHC allele is defined by examination of family pedigrees.

Two statistics are used to determine the association between the MHC allele and disease. The intensity of the association is measured by the relative risk.[45,46] This is simply calculated by the formula:

$$RR = \frac{\text{Patients positive for allele}}{\text{Patients negative for allele}} \times \frac{\text{Controls negative for allele}}{\text{Controls positive for allele}}$$

The ratio has an expectation of 1 if there is no association between the presence of the allele and the occurrence of the disease. A positive association results in an increasing positive number that is the ratio of the odds of developing the illness if the particular allele is present compared with its likelihood when the allele is absent. Because a negative association or protection from acquiring the disease has an expectation of less than 1, it is difficult to compare values ranging between 0 and 1 with those that range above 1 without limit. These fractional or protective relative risks are frequently represented as the reciprocal of the relative risk preceded by a negative sign. For smaller samples the calculation recommended by Haldane is preferable and results in a less biased value.[46] Independent of the RR, which measures the intensity of the disease association, the standard χ^2 statistic is used to determine the significance of the association. Both RR and χ^2 can be conveniently calculated from a simple 2 × 2 tabular presentation of data (Fig. 4–11).

An idea of the intensity of the association of certain diseases with particular alleles depicted in Table 4–10 can be obtained by considering that the classic relative

Figure 4–11. SLE in two siblings who share D/DRw3 (3^m) through a recombination event.

risk of the association between blood group O and duodenal ulcer disease was only 1.3.[45] It is obvious that the percentage of patients expressing the marker is also of major importance. A significant association with a marker that is present on only a proportion of patients implies either that the disease is heterogeneous with only one form associated with a MHC determinant or, alternatively, that the MHC determinant identified is a clue to the presence of an allele of another locus with which the disease has a more complete and perhaps mechanistic relation.

Ethnic Relationships of MHC Alleles. It is of very considerable interest that different races and ethnic groups vary markedly with respect to the composition of their pools of MHC alleles (Tables 4–4, 4–5, and 4–7). For example, *DR3* is infrequent among Mongoloids yet common among central and northern European Caucasians, where it is often present as a haplotype, *HLA A1-B8-DR3*. A second haplotype found in this same region, and especially in the North, is the haplotype *HLA-A3-B7-DR2*. Neither of these haplotypes is frequent among other populations. Among Caucasians they are uncommon among those of the Mediterranean basin. *HLA-B27* is distributed more evenly among all Caucasians, achieving its greatest frequency among some American Indian tribes, yet it is rare among the Mongoloid races from which these Indians were derived.

In a practical sense the calculation of a relative risk requires that the control population and the disease population be identical with respect to their ethnic composition. For example, there would be a major bias in such data derived from a disease associated with Mediterranean origin, such as familial Mediterranean fever if the control group were composed of randomly selected North American Caucasians.

The origins of the ethnic differences are still not well understood. Certain ones reflect relatively recent migrations: The *HLA-A3-B7-DR2* haplotype is Nordic in origin, and its presence correlates well with the extent of the Viking sphere of influence approximately 1000 years ago. Similarly, the distribution of the *HLA-A1-B8-DR3* haplotype suggests that it is Indo-European in origin, possibly having been introduced into Europe by invasions along this route (Fig. 4–12).

However, if mixing of populations were the only factor responsible for the linkage disequilibrium, one should not encounter the high values for Δ in the outbred human population. A difference in gene frequency of Δ = 0.1 would take approximately 200 generations or 4000 years to fall to the insignificant value of 0.02. The presence of the elevated Δ values suggests that a positive survival value could be associated with certain haplotypes. Similarly, the associations of disease with haplotypes or allotypes appear to reflect a much more fundamental event than a historical accident. Certain diseases, such as the spondyloarthropathies, are closely associated with HLA-B27 in all populations. Other categories of diseases shift their associations even within

Table 4–10. Contrasting Activities of B Lymphocyte Alloantisera in Patients with Systemic Lupus Erythematosus, Rheumatic Fever, or Rheumatoid Arthritis

Reagent	HLA-DR Specificity	Normal (n = 40) %	Systemic Lupus Erythematosus (n = 24) %	p^*	$RR^†$	Rheumatic Fever (n = 21) %	p	RR	Rheumatoid Arthritis (n = 45) %	p	RR
7AO	1	28	28	0.55	1.0	26	0.50	−1.1	9	0.02	−3.6
1239	2	28	46	0.11	2.0				13	0.09	−2.5
1146	2	26	50	0.04	2.8	25	0.59	−1.1	12	0.08	−2.5
CH	2 + 3 + ?	40	72	0.02	3.7				34	0.34	−1.3
1033	3	24	55	0.02	3.7	20	0.43	−1.2	14	0.14	−1.9
2134	3	26	56	0.02	3.5				14	0.14	−2.1
1283	4 × 7 × 10 (MT3)	28	12	0.14	−2.6				80	$<1×10^{-5}$	9.6
1038	4 × 7 × 10 (MT3)	24	6	0.03	−3.9	24	0.59	1.0	76	$<1×10^{-5}$	9.4
191	4 × 10 (DR4)	22	4	0.049	−4.8	26	0.57	1.3	60	$4.6×10^{-4}$	5.1
1995	5	12	8	0.47	−1.4	11	0.54	−1.0	4	0.17	−2.8
883	Undefined	17	0	0.03	−10.6	71	$5×10^{-5}$	10.8	4	0.054	−4.1

*p = Fisher exact probability.
†RR = relative risk (defined in text), calculated, according to Haldane.

Figure 4–12 A map of Europe with the circles illustrating the basic geographic distribution of MHC haplotypes, presumably established at the time when agriculture stablized the peoples of this area. Two subsequent major migrations are illustrated by the branching lines with arrows. The "Nordic" haplotype HLA-A3-B7-DR2 and the "Indo-European" haplotype HLA-A1-B8-DR3 may have been introduced by military conquest. (Courtesy of Professor J. Dausset.)

different Caucasian ethnic subsets. For example, among Eastern Mediterraneans the Ia alloantigen associations of multiple sclerosis and rheumatoid arthritis are different from those in the main Caucasian population. An explanation of these associations is one of the challenges of current medical research.

Rheumatic Disease Associations. The analysis of B lymphocyte alloantigens in patients with rheumatoid arthritis or systemic lupus erythematosus, summarized in Table 4–10, demonstrates that both diseases are related to B cell alloantigens; however, the profile of alloantigens in each disease is entirely different. This indicates that while there are certain autoimmune features in common between these two diseases, the MHC determinants for susceptibility to either one are entirely contrasting.

The fact that patients with systemic lupus erythematosus have two DR allospecificities has several interpretations, and it is not yet possible to choose among them: (1) That there are two clinically similar but pathogenetically distinct categories of patients. (2) That the primary association is with disease resistance, e.g., possibly mediated by the allele bearing MT3. (3) That susceptibility is associated with an as yet unrecognized allele that occurs most commonly with DR2 and DR3.

Of further interest in regard to the presence of DR2 in patients with systemic lupus erythematosus is the presence of DR2 in two disease states usually considered to have some interrelationship: the atypical lupus like syndrome associated with C2 deficiency, and idiopathic thrombocytopenic purpura.[47] In the case of C2 deficiency, the association is most frequently with a special haplotype—A10, B18, D2, DR2.[48] These observations suggest that the findings of an association with DR2 could be considered as evidence that these diseases have a nosologic relationship.

Family studies are the most reliable method of defining the relationship of disease susceptibility to genetic factors. The study illustrated in Figure 4–11 serves to illustrate several aspects of this approach. Two siblings, aged 24 and 28, presented with classic SLE. Conventional HLA testing of A, B, and C alleles revealed that they appeared not to share any haplotype. MHC studies and typing for B lymphocyte alloantigens, however, cast a different perspective on the family. Both siblings typed for the presence of D/DR3. Since the assignment of D/DR could be verified among other family members not illustrated, it appears that a maternal recombination occurred, with the major portion of the sixth chromosome bearing *HLA A1, B8, D/DR3* losing its distal short arm between *HLA B* and *HLA D* and exchanging this segment for one bearing HLA A24,B16, manifested as the haplotype 24-16-3[m.] The susceptibility to disease presumably maps in the vicinity of the D/DR locus in association with the D/DR3 specificity. A similar association with the *HLA-A1-B8-DR3* haplotype in families with multiple instances of males with lupus erythematosus has been reported.[49]

Hypothetical Mechanisms of Disease Associations. If indeed the association of the B27 arthropathy complex remains maximal with the B locus and is not related to another determinant of histocompatibility that maps at a nearby locus, then the disease mechanisms of this group would most likely relate to the specific functions of the class I MHC antigens. These relate to the recognition phase in cytotoxic effector functions and could include B locus allele linked differences in the efficiency of eliminating particular targets. The concept of a mimetic relationship between pathogen and cell receptor is also an attractive one. Alternatively, the role of the MHC in immune functions may not be involved, and it is possible that other aspects of MHC function, such as cell interactions or differentiation, could result in the disease state.

The second category of diseases that relate to alleles of class II molecules raises an entirely different spectrum of possibilities, as a reflection of the presumed functions of genes in this region. The dominant hypotheses would relate to the role of these gene products in the positive or negative control of the immune response. These take two general forms: one in which the determinants controlling the selective response to a pathogenic agent such as a virus are absent or abnormal; and the other in which the immune system is disregulated because of imperfect receptor-acceptor interactions, without any particular pathogen or inciting organism. The influence of the MHC alloantigens on the T cell antigen repertoire could also result in a deficiency of T cell clones necessary to recognize an antigen on a pathogenic organism. Here, as in the previous HLA-B locus mechanisms, an excessive reliance on immune phenomena may be unwarranted. The fact that the same diseases in different ethnic groups are stongly associated with entirely distinct MHC specificities, depending on the ethnic group,[19] serves to highlight the challenge of understanding the biologic significance of the disease associations and their potential role in determining human evolution. A recent survey of some aspects of disease associations provides additional access to the current literature.[50]

CONCLUSION

The manner in which the MHC is intertwined with many of the rheumatic diseases is a logical reflection of the participation of the immune system in their pathogenesis, as well as the multiple organ involvement that characterizes them. Mastery of this aspect of basic rheumatology is complicated by the inherent intricacy of the subject matter, as well as its dependence upon genetics and a basically subtle methodology. This difficulty is tempered by the potential for imminent application of this knowledge. Already, assays for B27 have been of practical diagnostic assistance in patients and have served to enhance the understanding of several categories of arthritic disease. Very much the same is now occurring in the area of B lymphocyte alloantigen measurements for a larger sphere of diseases. At the next level of application, the ability of the MHC determinants to identify individuals at risk for these diseases should serve as an additional stimulus for the development of preventive measures. Finally, it is very likely that the study of mechanisms of these diseases will contribute major insights into the basic biologic knowledge of what is an extraordinary adaptive mechanism.[51]

References

1. Payne, R.: The association of febrile transfusion reactions with leukoagglutinins. Vox Sang. 2:233, 957.
2. Dausset, J.: Iso-leuco-corps. Acta Haematol. 20:156, 1958.
3. Van Rood, J.J., and van Leeuwen, A.: Leukocyte grouping: A method and its application. J. Clin. Invest. 42:1382, 1963.
4. Terasaki, P.I., and McClelland, J.D.: Microdroplet assay of human serum cytotoxins. Nature 204:998, 1964.
5. Zinkernagel, R.M., and Doherty, P.C.: Major transplantation antigens, viruses, and specificity of surveillance T-cells: The "altered self" hypothesis. Contemp. Topics Immunobiol. 7:179, 1977.
6. Brewerton D.A., Hart, F.D., Nicholls, A., Caffrey, M., James, D.C.O., and Sturrock, R.D.: Ankylosing spondylitis and HL-A 27. Lancet 1:904, 1973.
7. Schlosstein, L., Terasaki, P.I., Bluestone, R., and Pearson, C. M.: High association of an HLA antigen, W27, with ankylosing spondylitis. N. Engl. J. Med. 288:704, 1973.
8. Klein, J.: Biology of the Mouse Histocompatibility-2 Complex. New York, Springer, 1975.
9. Cavalli-Sforza, L.L., and Bodmer, W.F.: The Genetics of Human Populations. San Francisco, W.H. Freeman, 1971.
10. Bodmer, W.F.: Evolutionary significance of the HL-A system. Nature 237:139, 1972.
11. Kissmeyer-Nielsen, F.: Histocompatibility Testing, 1975. Copenhagen, Munksgaard, 1975.
12. Bodmer, W.F., Batchelor, J.R., Bodmer, J.G., Festenstein, H., and Morris, P.J.: Histocompatibility Testing, 1977 Copenhagen, Munksgaard, 1978.
13. Terasaki, P.I. (ed.): Histocompatibility Testing. Los Angeles, UCLA Press, 980.
14. Albert, E.D.: The major histocompatibility complex (MHC) in man. Clin. Rheum. Dis. 3:175, 1977.
15. van Rood, J.J., de Vries, R.P., Bradley, B.A.: Genetics and biology of the HLA System. In Dorf, M.E. (ed.): The Role of the Major Histocompatibility Complex in Immunology. New York, Garland Press, 1981, p. 59.
16. Bruakoff, S.J.: Specificity of cytolytic T-cell responses. In Dorf, M.E. (ed.): The Role of the Major Histocompatibility Complex in Immunology. New York, Garland Press, 1981, p. 343.
17. Bach, F.H., and van Rood, J.J.: The major histocompatibility complex. Genetics and biology. N. Engl. J. Med. 295:806, 872, 927, 1976.
18. Green, S.S., and Sell, K.W.: Mixed leukocyte stimulation of normal peripheral leukocytes by autologous lymphoblastoid cells. Science 170:989, 1970.
19. Winchester, R., and Kunkel, H.G.: The human Ia system. Advances in Immunology. New York, Academic Press, 1979, p. 221.
20. Korman, A.J., Auffray, C., Schamboeck, A., and Strominger, J.L.: The amino acid sequence and gene organization of the heavy chain of the HLA-DR antigen: Homology to immunoglobulins. Proc. Natl. Acad. Sci. USA 79:6013, 1982.
21. Kratzin, H., Yang, C., Gotz, H., Pauly, E., Kolbel, S., Egert, G., Thinnes, F.P., Wernet, P., Altevogt, P., and Hilschmann, N.: Primärstruktur menschlicher Histokompatibilitätsantigene der Klasse II. I. Mitteilung: Aminosäuresequenz der N-terminalen 198 Reste der beta-Kette des HLA-Dw2,2; DR2,2-Alloantigens. Hoppe Seylers Z. Physiol. Chem. 362:1665, 1981 (English Abstr.).
22. Hurley, C.K., Nunez, G., Winchester, R., Finn, O.J., Levy, R., and Capra, J.D.: The human HLA-DR antigens are encoded by multiple beta chain loci. J. Immunol 129:2103, 1982.
23. Karr, W.R., Kannapell, C.C., Stein, J.A, Fuller, T.C., Duquesnoy, R.J., Rodey, G.E., Mann, D.L., Gebel, H.M. and Schwartz, B.D.: Demonstration of a third structurally distinct human Ia beta chain by two dimensional gel electrophoresis. J. Exp. Med. 156:652, 1982.
24. Moutsopoulos, H.M., Mann, D.L., Johnson, A.H., and Chused, T.M.: Genetic differences between primary and secondary sicca syndrome. N. Engl. J. Med. 302:761, 1979.
25. Reinertsen, J.L., Klippel, J.H., Johnson, A.H., Steinberg, A.D., Decker, J.L., and Mann, D.L.: B-lymphocyte alloantigens associated with systemic lupus erythematosus. N. Engl. J. Med. 299:515, 1978.
26. Gibofsky, A., Winchester, R., Hansen, J., Patarroyo, M., Dupont, B., Paget, S., Lahita, R., Halper, J., Fotino, M., Yunis, E., and Kunkel, H.G.: Contrasting patterns of newer histocompatibility determinants in patients with rheumatoid arthritis and systemic lupus erythematosus. Arthritis Rheum. 21:S123, 1978.
27. Duquesnoy, R.J., Marrari, M., and Annen, K.: Identification of an HLA-DR associated system of B cell alloantigens. Trans. Proc. 11:1757, 1979.
28. Corte, G., Calabi, F., Damiani, G., Bargellesi, A., Tosi, R., and Sorrentino, R.: Human Ia molecules carrying DC1 determinants differ in both A- and B-subunits from Ia molecules carrying DR determinants. Nature 292:357, 1981.
29. Park, M.S., Teresaki, P.I., Nakata, S., and Adki, D.: Supertypic DR groups: MT1, MT2 and MT3. In Teraski, P.I. (ed.): Histocompatibility Testing 1980. Los Angeles, UCLA Press, 1980, p. 854.
30. Goyert, S.M., Shively, J.E., and Silver J.: Biochemical characterization of a second family of human Ia molecules, HLA-DS, equivalent to murine I-A subregion molecules. J. Exp. Med. 156:550, 1982.
31. Bona, M.R., and Strominger, J.L.: Direct evidence of homology between human DC-1 antigen and murine I-A molecules. Nature 299:836, 1982.

32. Tanigaki, N., and Tosi, R.: The genetic control of human Ia alloantigens: A three-locus model derived from the immunochemical analysis of "supertypic specificities. Immunol. Rev. 66:5, 1982.
33. Schackelford, D.A., Kaufman, J.F., Korman, A.J. and Strominger, J.L., HLA-DR antigens: structure, separation of subpopulations, gene and cloning and function. Immunol. Rev. 66:133, 1982.
34. Giles, R.C., Nunez, G., Hurley, C.K., Nunez-Roldan, A., Winchester, R., Stastny, P., and Capra, J.D.: Structural analysis of a human I-A homologue using a monoclonal antibody which recognizes an MB3-like specificity. J. Exp. Med. 157:1461, 1981.
35. Shaw, S., Kavathas, P., Pollack, M.S., Charmot, D., and Mawas, C.: Family studies define a new histocompatibility locus, SB, between HLA-DR and GLO. Nature (Lond.) 293:745, 1981.
36. Sasazuki, T., McDevitt, H.O., and Grumet, F.C.: The association between genes in the major histocompatibility complex and disease susceptibility. Ann Rev. Med. 28:425, 1977.
37. Winchester, R.J.: B-lymphocyte allo-antigens, cellular expression, and disease significance with special reference to rheumatoid arthritis. Arthritis Rheum. 20:159s, 1977.
38. Stastny, P.: Association of the B-cell alloantigen DRw4 with rheumatoid arthritis. N. Engl. J. Med. 298:869, 1978.
39. Gibofsky, A., Winchester, R.J., Patarroyo, M., Fotino, M., and Kunkel, H.G.: Disease associations of the Ia like human alloantigens. Contrasting patterns in rheumatoid arthritis and systemic lupus erythematosus. J. Exp. Med. 148:1728, 1978.
40. Winchester, R.J.: Genetic aspects of rheumatoid arthritis, Springer Semin. Immunopathol. (Springer-Verlag) 4:89, 1981.
41. Ahearn, J.M., Provost, T.T., Dorsch, C.A., Stevens, M.B., Bias, W.B. and Arnett, F.C.: Interrelationships of HLA-DR, MB, and MT phenotypes, autoantibody expression, and clinical features in systemic lupus erythematosus. Arthritis Rheum. 25:1031, 1982.
42. Winchester, R.J., and Nunez-Roldan, A.: Some genetic aspects of systemic lupus erythematosus. Arthritis Rheum. 25:833, 1982.
43. Chused, T.M., Kassan, S.S., and Opelz, G.: Sjögren's syndrome associated with HLA-Dw3. N. Engl. J. Med. 296:895, 977.
44. Patarroyo, M.E., Winchester, R.J., Veherano, A., Gibofsky, A., Chalem, F., Zabriskie, J.B., and Kunkel, H.G.: Association of a particular B cell alloantigen with susceptibility to rheumatic fever. Nature 278:173, 1979.
45. Woolf, B.: On estimating the relation between blood group and disease. Ann. Hum. Genet. 19:251, 1955.
46. Haldane, J.B.S.: The estimation and significance of the logarithm of a ratio of frequencies. Ann. Hum. Genet. 20:309, 1955.
47. Karpatkin, S., Fotino, M., Gibofsky, A., and Winchester, R.J.: Association of HLA DRw2 with auto-immune thrombocytopenic purpura. J. Clin. Invest. 63:1085, 1979.
48. Fu, S.M., Kunkel, H.G., Brussman, H.P., Allen, F.H., Jr., and Fotino, M.: Evidence for linkage between HL-A histocompatibility genes and those involved in the synthesis of the second component of complement. J. Exp. Med. 140:1108, 1974.
49. Lahita, R.G., Chiorazzi, N., Gibofsky, A., Winchester, R.J., and Kunkel, H.G.: Familial SLE in males. Arthritis Rheum. 26:39, 1983.
50. Moller, G. (ed.): HLA and disease susceptibility. Immunol. Rev. 70:1, 1983.
51. Bodmer, W.F.: Evolution and function of the HLA system. Br. Med. Bull. 34:309, 1978.

Chapter 5
Genetic Control of Immune Responses

William J. Koopman

GENES REGULATE IMMUNE RESPONSES AT SEVERAL LEVELS— AN OVERVIEW

It has long been recognized that individual animal strains differ considerably in their capacity to mount specific humoral and/or cellular immune responses against a variety of immunogens. More recently, genetically related differences in immune response characteristics have also been documented in man. While the precise mechanism(s) underlying genetically determined immune response characteristics has not yet been elucidated, it has become increasingly clear that distinct genetic loci are capable of influencing specific immune responses. A major role(s) for genes residing within the major histocompatibility complex (MHC) and for genes linked to immunoglobulin (Ig) structural genes, particularly immunoglobulin heavy chains (IgH), has been well established for responses to several immunogens. That other loci also influence responses to particular antigens seems certain; however, the nature of these loci is less well defined at this time.

More generalized effects of certain genetic factors on immune responses have also been identified. In this regard genetically determined cell surface differentiation antigens (markers) have facilitated identification of functionally (and antigenically) distinct lymphoid cell subpopulations. The interactions among these distinct cell types play a critical role in determining the quality and quantity of an ensuing immune response. In several instances, these genetically determined differentiation markers have been implicated as contributing to the functional properties of these distinct cell populations.

In discussing the influence of genetic factors on immune responses, it seems appropriate to focus on two distinct groups of genes: (1) major histocompatibility complex (MHC) genes and (2) Ig-linked genes. Interest in genes that influence immune responses has been heightened by increasing evidence that closely related, if not identical, genes also influence susceptibility to a variety of diseases in which immune events appear to play a critical role. Most striking in this regard is the significant association of enhanced susceptibility to several rheumatic diseases with genes residing within the MHC. An important role(s) for genes associated with immune response characteristics is further suggested by studies in which genes linked to Ig structural loci, particularly IgH loci, have been demonstrated to associate with an increased prevalence of several autoimmune diseases. Moreover, parallel analysis of MHC and IgH genetic markers has convincingly established that these genetic loci situated on separate chromosomes exert more than additive effects with regard to susceptibility to some of these diseases. Taken together, these observations suggest that genes regulating immune responses concurrently influence predisposition to certain diseases.

In approaching the subject of genetic control of immune responses, familiarity with basic genetic concepts is helpful. A glossary of relevant terms is provided in Table 5–1.

GENES OF THE MAJOR HISTOCOMPATIBILITY COMPLEX

The MHC consists of a cluster of genes residing on the short arm of the human chromosome 6 (chromosome 17 in the mouse) that encodes three distinct classes of proteins of immunologic importance (Fig. 5–1). Class I MHC proteins are heterodimers consisting of a highly polymorphic heavy chain (MW $\sim$ 45,000) encoded by MHC genes which is noncovalently associated with β_2 microglobulin (β_2M, MW $\sim$ 12,000), an essentially invariant polypeptide encoded by a non-MHC locus.[1-3] These antigens are expressed on the cell surfaces of all nucleated cells and platelets and serve as restriction elements in the recognition of target cells by cytotoxic T lymphocytes.[4] HLA-A, HLA-B, and HLA-C antigens in man[3] and H-2K, H-2L, and H-2D antigens in the mouse[5] are class I MHC proteins. Class II MHC molecules are polymorphic bimolecular complexes consist-

ing of an α heavy chain and a smaller β polypeptide chain, with the β chains accounting for most of the polymorphism of these antigens.[6-10] These antigens, also referred to as Ia antigens, are encoded by I region genes of the mouse and the corresponding D region genes of man. Ia antigens have a more restricted tissue distribution than class I antigens and are found on B lymphocytes, monocyte/macrophages, activated T lymphocytes, Langerhans' cells, dendritic cells, some endothelial cells, sperm, and a population of thymic epithelial cells. Class II antigens function as restriction elements in the recognition of antigen on monocyte/macrophages of B lymphocytes by T lymphocytes.[11] Furthermore, genes controlling the magnitude of immune responses to a variety of antigens (immune response (Ir) genes)[12] have been mapped to the I region of the mouse, specifically the I-A and I-E subregions.[13] Ia antigens appear to be equivalent to Ir gene products.[14] Finally, class III proteins constitute complement components encoded by genes residing within the MHC (C4, C2, and B in man). A detailed discussion of the MHC is presented in Chapter 4. Attention in this chapter is directed primarily toward the Ir genes of the MHC, in view of their evident role in regulation of immune responses.

Immune Response (Ir) Genes

Location of Ir Genes in the MHC. *Murine Ir Genes.* As previously mentioned, experimental data strongly suggest that Ir genes reside within the I region of the mouse. The murine I region has been subdivided into five subregions on the basis of recombinational analysis: I-A, I-B, I-J, I-E, and I-C.[15,16] In mice, two well characterized groups of Ia antigens (the putative products of Ir genes) have been identified: I-A and I-E. I-A subregion molecules consist of an Aα and Aβ bimolecular complex with both α and β chains encoded by genes residing entirely within the I-A subregion. In contrast, I-E antigens consist of an Eα polypeptide chain encoded within the I-E subregion and an Eβ chain derived from the I-A subregion[17] (Fig. 5–2). The I-J subregion was initially defined by antisera that recognized determinants on suppressor T cells[18] and soluble antigen-specific suppressor factors.[19] Although characterization studies are in progress,[20-22] the structure of I-J molecules remains considerably less certain than that of I-A and I-E antigens. The precise location of the I-J subregion is also unclear at present in view of recent observation of Steinmetz and colleagues.[23] These workers have analyzed segments of DNA totaling 200 kilobases in the I region, and their results limit the I-B and I-J subregions to a segment of DNA no longer than 3.4 kilobases in length, raising the possibility that I-J products may be encoded by genes located outside the I region. The status of I-B also appears to be uncertain, since no Ia specificity has been exclusively localized to I-B.[24]

Human Ir Genes. Although evidence for specific immune response genes in man is less substantial than in the mouse, there is, nonetheless, strong evidence indicating that the D region in man is equivalent to the

Table 5–1. Glossary of Genetic Terms

Gene	a segment of DNA (the basic unit of inheritance) that directs the transcription of a specific messenger RNA, which directs the translation of a specific polypeptide chain.
Locus	the location of a gene on a chromosome.
Allele	alternative forms of the same gene, having usually arisen by some mutational event. Within the major histocompatibility complex (MHC) each locus possesses multiple alleles. When this occurs with considerable frequency within a given population, it is said to represent polymorphism.
Genotype	the description of the combination of genes inherited by an individual from both parents.
Phenotype	the genetically determined expressed characteristics of an individual, which reflect the summation of all of his genes and thereby give him a descriptive identity.
Haplotype	a combination of closely linked genes on the same chromosome.
Linkage	the tendency of genes located near each other on the same chromosome to segregate together.
Allogeneic	a description for the genetic relationship of two individuals from the same species possessing different allelic forms of a particular gene.
Syngeneic	a description for the genetic relationship of two individuals from the same species possessing the same allelic forms of a particular gene.
Congenic	two strains bred in such a way that they differ genetically only at a particular locus (and generally at a segment of the chromosome surrounding or adjacent to that particular locus).

Figure 5–1. Comparison of the major histocompatibility complex (MHC) of mouse and man. (Reproduced, with permission, from the Annual Review of Immunology, Volume 1. ©1983 by Annual Reviews Inc.)

murine I region, including (1) comparable structure of protein products encoded by the two regions,[6] (2) homology of amino acid sequence between human D and murine I region products,[25] and (3) homology in sequences between human D and murine I region genes.[23]

Structure of Ir Gene Products. *Murine Ia Antigens.* As alluded to previously, two groups of murine Ia molecules encoded by genes located within the I region have been identified and characterized, the I-A and I-E molecules. These molecules have both been demonstrated to be integral cell membrane glycoproteins[26] and can be

Figure 5–2. Gene organization and expression of the murine I-A and I-E antigens. The heavy chain (α) of the I-A antigen is encoded by the gene Aa, whereas the polymorphic β chain is encoded by the gene Aβ. Both I-A chains are therefore encoded for by genes residing in the I-A subregion of the MHC. In contrast, the α heavy chain of the I-E antigen is encoded by the Ea gene, which resides in the I-E (or I-C) subregion, while the lighter β chain is encoded by the Eβ gene, which resides in the I-A subregion. (From Uhr, J.W., et al.: Science 206:292, 1979, Copyright 1979 by the AAAS.)

immunoprecipitated from solubilized membrane preparations utilizing antibodies generated by immunizing mice with cells from congenic strains of mice differing only at the I-A or I-E subregion of the MHC.[27] I-A antigens consist of a disulfide-bonded αβ dimer with an approximate molecular weight of 55,000. Under reducing conditions, the Aα and Aβ chains can be separated and demonstrate apparent molecular weights of 35,000 and 26,000, respectively.[25] Similarly, I-E antigens also consist of two polypeptide chains designated Eα and Eβ of approximate molecular weights of 32,000 and 29,000, respectively.[6] Also associated with both I-A and I-E molecules is a third polypeptide (Mr ∼ 31,000), designated (Ii), that is not encoded by MHC genes and appears to be invariant in structure.[28] Although I-A and I-E molecules are both heterodimers of similar molecular size, finer structural analysis has clearly demonstrated the two molecules to be distinct. In this regard, differences between the α and β chains of the two groups of molecules have been identified utilizing both N-terminal amino acid sequencing[29-31] and peptide mapping[32,17] techniques. Since the Ia molecules are obviously quite polymorphic[33] it has been important to delineate the structural basis of this polymorphism. Comparison of Ia molecules isolated from different congenic strains differing only at the I region has clearly demonstrated that the β chain is highly polymorphic whereas the α chain is more conserved.[6,34,35] Further heterogeneity may be introduced as a result of differences in glycosylation.[10] Heterogeneity may also result from the random association of Aα and Aβ chains in heterozygotes.[6] Furthermore, expression of Eα and Eβ chains has also been demonstrated in situations in which the genes are trans to each other.[36]

It should be stressed that other murine Ia antigens may exist. Utilizing Eα and human DCβ cDNA probes, Southern blot analyses of the murine I region suggest the existence of at least two α and four to six β genes.[23] The existence of additional class II genes, which may not be sufficiently homologous to the probes to be identified, cannot be excluded.

Progress has been made in the analysis of the structure of murine class II genes. Analyses of cDNA and genomic clones of the Aα and Eα genes have been reported.[37,38] Interestingly, the exon-intron organization of the Eα gene appears quite similar to the human DRα gene.[39-41] Furthermore, the deduced amino acid sequence of Eα exhibits 76 percent homology with DRα,[38] thus confirming the earlier hypothesis that DRα and Eα are homologous genes.[25] The exon organization of the Eα gene corresponds with the domains of the protein product. Specifically, two external domains (N-terminal and membrane proximal) and the transmembrane and cytoplasmic domains are encoded by four distinct exons. The second external domain (i.e., membrane proximal) of both Eα and Aα exhibits strong homology with immunoglobulin constant regions.[37]

Human Ia Antigens. Serologic analysis of human Ia antigens has been pursued utilizing heteroantisera, alloantisera, and, more recently, monoclonal reagents. At least three groups of human Ia antigens have been identified utilizing these serologic reagents in conjunction with mixed leukocyte reaction testing or discriminatory recognition of the antigens utilizing cytotoxic T lymphocytes. Human DR antigens consist of a bimolecular complex of α "heavy chain" of approximately 34,000 molecular weight associated with a β "light chain" of molecular weight 29,000.[6] A third polypeptide, the Ia-associated invariant chain (Ii), has also been identified in immunoprecipitates containing human DR antigens.[42] N-terminal amino acid analysis indicates close homology between DRα and murine Eα chains and between DRβ and murine Eβ chains.[25] The polymorphism of human DR antigens is predominantly determined by the β chain subunit.[8,6,10,9,43] Shaw and colleagues have identified another group of Ia molecules, designated SB,[44,45] which consists of two chains that resemble the α and β chains of DR antigens with regard to molecular weight.[46] This set of antigens is encoded by an HLA-D subregion distinct from DR. While limited N-terminal sequence data indicate that SBα and SBβ chains differ from DRα and DRβ chains,[47] SBα appears to be related to murine Eα, suggesting that SB antigen may also be homologous to murine I-E molecules.[47]

A third group of polymorphic Ia molecules, termed DC antigens, has been identified. It differs from DR molecules in both α and β subunits by two-dimensional gel analysis[48] and by peptide mapping.[49] Amino acid sequence analysis suggests that DC antigens are homologous to murine I-A molecules.[50] The DS molecules described by Goyert and colleagues[51] appear to belong to the DC Ia group, and, indeed, limited sequence analysis of these molecules indicates homology with the murine I-A group. The SB locus appears to be localized

centromeric to the DR locus in the D region on the basis of recombinational analysis[45] and study of deletion mutants.[52] The precise location of the DC locus has not been determined.

Human class II α and β genes have recently been cloned and characterized; sequencing has provided important insights into the structure of the corresponding protein products.[39,53-56] The predicted amino acid sequence of DRα chains suggests that α chains consist of two external domains similar to murine Eα chains; moreover, sequence homology between immunoglobulin constant regions and the second external domain (membrane proximal) of the α chain has been identified.[39,57] Partial DRβ chain amino acid sequence data indicate that the membrane proximal external domain of these chains is also homologous to immunoglobulin constant regions.[58-60] As mentioned previously, the homology between DRα and Eα genes is supported by the similar exon-intron structure of the two genes in addition to the deduced amino acid sequences of the two α chains.[38]

Ir Genes Regulate Immune Responses to Antigens. *Animal Studies.* Although individual differences in immune responses to particular antigens had been previously recognized by immunologists, Levine and colleagues first demonstrated genetic control of such responses. These workers observed that humoral and cellular immune responses by outbred guinea pigs to the antigen DNP-poly-L-lysine (DNP-PLL) were controlled by a single autosomal dominant gene.[61,62] "Responders" possessed the gene that was therefore designated an immune response or Ir gene. Ir genes were subsequently demonstrated in inbred strains of guinea pigs for several synthetic antigens[63] and for conventional antigens, particularly at low concentrations (presumably related to selection for response to a limited number of dominant determinants).[64,65] Moreover, Ir genes were documented in several other species, including mice,[66] rats,[67] and monkeys.[68] The availability of inbred strains of mice permitted rapid progress in the localization of Ir genes in the genome. These genes were shown to map to the murine MHC (H-2 complex).[69,70] Similar linkage of Ir genes with the MHC was subsequently demonstrated in other species, including guinea pigs,[71] rats,[67] and monkeys.[68] Analysis of immune response characteristics of recombinant and congenic strains of mice permitted more precise localization of Ir genes to the I region of the murine MHC.[72] Additional studies indicated that Ir genes for some antigens mapped strictly to the I-A subregion of the I region whereas others mapped to both the I-A and I-E subregions.[73,74] The latter Ir genes were of considerable interest, since "responder" status for these antigens was dependent upon inheritance of both I-A and I-E-linked Ir genes (termed α and β, respectively) located either cis or trans to each other.[73,74] Referred to as gene complementation, this phenomenon later facilitated identification of cell surface Ia antigens as the likely products of Ir genes.

Immunization of mice with lymphoid cells from strains differing only at the I region elicits production of antibodies in the recipient strain that recognize characteristic cell surface glycoproteins (Ia antigens) expressed particularly on B lymphocytes, macrophages, dendritic cells, and activated T lymphocytes. Considerable evidence suggests that these Ia antigens are the products of Ir genes: (1) Ia molecules are encoded by genes residing in the same location of the I region as Ir genes; (2) antibodies directed against I-A molecules are able to block specific immune responses governed by Ir genes mapping to the same I-A subregion;[75] (3) antibodies directed against either I-A or I-E products block immune responses to antigens under dual Ir gene control in which the two genes map to the I-A and I-E subregions;[75] (4) the dual genetic control of expression of I-E antigens by genes residing in the I-A subregion (Eβ) and I-E subregion (Eα) correlates with the dual Ir gene complementation observed for certain antigens; (5) response to antigens under dual Ir gene control correlates with cell surface levels of relevant E$\alpha\beta$ complexes,[76,77] and (6) the predicted amino acid sequence of protein products encoded by genes residing in the I region agrees with limited sequence data obtained for isolated Ia molecules[57] (Table 5–2). Taken together, these observations provide convincing evidence that Ia antigens are encoded by structural genes located within the I region and are indistinguishable from Ir genes.

In contrast to the positive influence of Ir genes on immune responses to several antigens, unresponsiveness to some antigens appears to be related to negative influences of immune suppressor (Is) gene(s) residing in the I region. For example, the synthetic terpolymer GAT (poly[L-glu^{60}-L-ala^{30}-L-tyr^{10}])[78] and hen egg lysozyme[79] elicit predominantly T suppressor cell responses when injected into certain nonresponder strains of mice. The

Is genes have not yet been precisely localized in the I region, and the relationship of these genes to the I-J subregion has not been determined. Genes tentatively assigned to the I-J subregion had been previously demonstrated to direct the expression of I-J antigens present on the cell surface of T suppressor lymphocytes[18,19] and on antigen-specific suppressor factors produced by T suppressor lymphocytes.[19,80] The precise localization of these putative I-J subregion genes is uncertain at present in view of difficulties in identifying a corresponding suitable length of DNA in the I region for the postulated I-J subregion.[23]

Human Studies. Demonstration of specific Ir genes in man has been predictably more difficult to achieve than in animal models. Several studies have established a statistical association between the presence of particular HLA antigens and immune responsiveness (or unresponsiveness) to specific antigens, including ragweed allergen Ra5,[81,82] collagen,[83] streptococcal antigens,[84] influenza A antigens,[85] vaccinia virus,[86] and tetanus toxoid.[87] In some cases antigen responsiveness was shown to associate with particular D region specificities.[81-83] Such an association would, of course, be expected in view of overwhelming evidence demonstrating homology between the murine I region and the human D region. Mechanisms underlying the association of HLA antigens and immune responsiveness have received limited attention. Responsiveness to collagen in vitro was shown to correlate with HLA-DR4 positivity and was attributed to absence of OKT 8$^+$ suppressor T lymphocyte activity for collagen otherwise present in DR4 negative individuals.[88]

While these studies have provided circumstantial evidence of MHC-linked Ir (or Is) genes in man, family studies are clearly required to establish linkage between particular HLA antigens and immune responsiveness and to determine the mode of inheritance of these gene(s). Toward this end, Sasazuki and colleagues[89,90] have analyzed T lymphocyte proliferative responses to streptococcal cell wall (SCW) antigen(s) in Japanese families and have reported evidence for a single dominant immune suppression gene for SCW linked to HLA in these families. Thus, despite the experimental constraints of analyzing antigen specific responses in man, the available data strongly supports the existence of MHC-linked Ir (or Is) genes in man. With the recent development of serologic reagents for the detection of distinct Ia antigen groups in man (e.g., DC, DR, and SB), additional progress is anticipated in the precise localization of Ir genes in the human D region.

Association of Ir Genes with Disease Susceptibility. In recent years many human diseases have been demonstrated to associate with the presence of particular HLA specificities (see Chapter 4). For several of these diseases the primary association appears to be with D region antigens[91] (Table 5–3). Although family studies are required to determine the precise location of susceptibility gene(s) for these diseases, it is tempting to speculate that diseases associated with class II MHC (i.e., D region) antigens reflect the inheritance of specific

Table 5–2. Evidence That ρDR-α-1 Is the Structural Gene of the HLA-DR α Chain*

ρDR-α-1	Ile-Ile-Gln-Ala-
	5 10
Raji α chain	Ile-Lys-Glu-Asp-His-Val-Ile-Ile-Gln-Ala-
ρDR-α-1	Glu-Phe-Tyr-Leu-Asn-Pro-Asp-Gln-Ser-Gly-
	15 20
Raji α chain	Glu-Phe-Tyr-Leu-Asn-Pro-Asp-Gln-Ser-Gly-
ρDR-α-1	Glu-Phe-Met-Phe-Asp-Phe-Asp-Gly-Asp-Glu-
	25 30
Raji α chain	Glu-Phe-Met-Phe-Asp-Phe-Asp-Gly-Asp-Glu-
ρDR-α-1	Ile-Phe-His-Val-Asp-
	35
Raji α chain	Ile-Phe-His-Val-Asp-

*adapted from Larhammar, D., et al.: Cell 30:153, 1982, Copyright MIT Press. Comparison of the predicted amino acid sequence obtained from the 5′ end of the coding strand of the cDNA clone ρDR-α-1 and the actual amino-terminal amino acid sequence of the alpha chain (Raji) of the HLA-DR antigen. Since the latter contained more than one amino acid at some positions, only the dominant amino acid obtained at any position is indicated.

Table 5–3. Associations of Some Diseases with HLA-D/DR Antigens*

Disease	Race	HLA-D/DR	Relative Risk†
Grave's disease	Cau	DR3	5.5–4.1
Hashimoto's with goiter	Cau	DR5	3.7–3.2
Multiple sclerosis	Cau	DR2	4.8
Giant cell arteritis	Cau	DR4	8.2
Rheumatoid arthritis	Cau	DR4	6.0
Juvenile arthritis, systemic	Cau	DR2	3.6
Systemic lupus erythematosus	Cau	DR3	5.7–3.0
		DR2	3.6
Subacute cutaneous lupus erythematosus	Cau	DR3	11.8
Dermatomyositis	Cau	DR3	3.9
Scleroderma	Cau	DR5	5.0
CREST syndrome	Cau	DR3	6.2
Sjögren's syndrome, primary	Cau	DR3	3.9
Sjögren's syndrome with arthritis	Cau	DR4	4.7

*Adapted from Stastny, P., et al.: Immunol. Rev. 70:113, 1983.
†Where appropriate, the range of published values is indicated.

Ir (or Is) genes that predispose an individual to disease development. Recent evidence indicating that expression of certain autoantibodies correlates with D region specificities strengthens this possibility. In this regard, previous studies have demonstrated an association between susceptibility to systemic lupus erythematosus (SLE) and D region antigens, particularly DR3.[92-95] It is therefore of interest that the presence of anti-native DNA antibodies also significantly associates with DR3 not only in patients with SLE but also in patients with other diagnoses.[96] A similar association between DR3 and anti-Ro (SS-A) antibodies has been demonstrated by Bell and Maddison.[97]

In view of evidence that distinct profiles of autoantibodies characterize various rheumatic diseases,[99] these data raise the possibility that expression of particular autoantibodies is regulated by Ir genes residing in the D region and that acquisition of such gene(s) constitutes one mechanism underlying disease susceptibility. Genetic studies of inbred autoimmune strains of mice have provided some support for this possibility. For example, at least six genes appear to be responsible for the SLE syndrome manifested by the autoimmune NZB mouse strain,[99] and some of these genes appear to govern expression of specific autoantibodies (e.g., anti-nDNA).[100] Although genes associated with specific autoantibody expression have been localized to the murine chromosome 17, linkage of these genes with the MHC (H-2) region has not been demonstrable with recombinant inbred lines.[101] It is evident that further studies are required to determine whether Ir (or Is) genes contribute to autoantibody expression in murine or human autoimmune disease.

Theories of Ir Gene Function. Considerable progress has been achieved in the elucidation of mechanisms underlying Ir gene regulation of immune responses. These genes have been demonstrated to regulate T lymphocyte dependent responses to a variety of antigens, including T lymphocyte dependent antibody responses, delayed hypersensitivity reactions, lymphokine production, and antigen-induced T lymphocyte proliferation. An initial

dilemma concerning Ir gene function related to the cell types involved. Specifically, it was difficult to reconcile the influence of Ir genes on T lymphocyte responses with the restricted cellular distribution of Ia antigens, the apparent products of Ir genes. These antigens could be easily identified on the surfaces of B lymphocytes, macrophage/monocytes, and dendritic cells but were generally present on only a small fraction of T lymphocytes. The initial observation that T lymphocyte activation required simultaneous recognition of antigen and MHC-encoded products suggested an explanation for how Ia antigens present on antigen-presenting cells (APC) might influence subsequent T lymphocyte responses. It was clearly demonstrated that antigen-primed T lymphocytes from guinea pigs[102] and mice[103] proliferated in response to antigen presented on syngeneic but not allogeneic APC. These studies established that the presence of antigen on APC was not sufficient for T lymphocyte activation but that genetic restrictions also existed. Shevach and Rosenthal extended these observations by demonstrating that T lymphocytes from (nonresponder × responder)F$_1$ guinea pigs only responded to antigen when presented on F$_1$ or responder APC but not on nonresponder APC.[104] Evidence that Ia antigens on APC were the restricting genetic elements in these T lymphocyte responses included the demonstration that APC possessing I-A and I-E antigens were required for murine T lymphocyte proliferation[105] and that function of APC could be blocked by treatment with appropriate anti-Ia antisera.[106] Taken together with evidence that I antigens are the products of Ir genes, these observations provided strong support for the view that Ir genes are expressed on APC and that activation of T lymphocytes by antigen requires co-recognition of antigen and the Ir gene product (Ia antigen) on the APC by the responding T lymphocyte. It should be stressed that the responding T lymphocytes in these Ia-restricted responses bear the Ly1+ phenotype.[107] Similarly, cytotoxic T lymphocytes that bear the Ly2+ phenotype also exhibit MHC restrictions in their recognition of antigen on target cells, but in this case class I MHC gene products (K or D antigens) are generally the responsible restricting elements(s).[4,108,109] Thus, cytotoxic T lymphocyte recognition of antigen is blocked by appropriate anti-K or anti-D reagents but not anti-Ia antisera.

Less extensive studies in man have strongly suggested that the HLA-D region encoded antigens present on APC restrict antigen-specific human T lymphocyte responses also. Antigen-induced T lymphocyte proliferative responses have been demonstrated to require HLA-DR compatible APC.[110] Similar requirements for antigen presentation by HLA-D compatible APC for long-term proliferation of antigen-specific T lymphocytes have been observed.[111] Further evidence indicating that HLA-D-antigen-bearing APC are involved in T lymphocyte activation comes from experiments indicating that cytolytic treatment of APC with anti-Ia antisera eliminated the capacity of these cells to support antigen-specific T lymphocyte proliferation.[112] More recently, antigen-specific human T lymphocyte clones have been generated that recognize specific antigen only in the context of HLA-DR compatible APC.[113]

The precise nature of the HLA-D encoded restriction elements required for antigen recognition by T lymphocytes has not been fully elucidated. In this regard, tetanus-toxoid-induced T lymphocyte proliferative responses were prevented by treatment of APC with monoclonal anti-DR but not anti-DC antibodies.[114] Interestingly, anti-DC antibody did block generation of cytotoxic effector T lymphocytes in MLC reactions despite having no effect on antigen-specific (tetanus toxoid) T lymphocyte proliferative responses.[114] In view of evidence that both I-A and I-E antigens may serve as restriction elements for antigen-induced murine T lymphocyte responses,[75] it would be anticipated that human antigens homologous to murine I-A antigens (e.g., DC [DS] molecules) are also involved in T lymphocyte recognition for at least some antigens. Recent studies have suggested that this is indeed the case. Using antigen-primed T lymphocyte blasts, Berle and Thorsby have provided evidence that DC antigens may function as restriction elements in T lymphocyte responses to herpes simplex virus.[115] Furthermore, APC bearing both DR and DS (i.e., DC) antigens were shown to be necessary for induction of antigen-induced (Candida albicans) T lymphocyte proliferation whereas macrophages bearing DR antigens alone were ineffective.[116] In this system monoclonal anti-DS antibody also effectively blocked T lymphocyte proliferation in response to Candida, further suggesting a role for these class II molecules as restriction elements in T lymphocyte antigen recognition.[116] These observations closely parallel previously discussed observations in the mouse and suggest that: (1) Ir genes in man are expressed at the APC level; (2) class II antigens homologous to murine I-E and I-A antigens are products of Ir genes; and (3) these Ia antigens function by serving as restriction elements for T lymphocyte recognition of antigen.

While evidence for MHC-restricted antigen recognition by T lymphocytes has been well established, the mechanism(s) underlying actual antigen recognition by T cells has not been elucidated. Specifically, do T lymphocytes possess distinct receptors for Ia antigens and nominal antigen (dual receptor recognition), or does a single receptor recognize an Ia antigen-nominal antigen complex on the APC surface? Conclusive evidence for physical linkage of Ia antigens and nominal antigen has not yet been obtained. Nonetheless, the elegant somatic cell hybridization experiments of Kappler and colleagues indicate that recognition of Ia and antigen could not be dissociated, suggesting that antigen recognition was mediated either by linked receptors for Ia and antigen or by a single receptor recognizing the Ia antigen-nominal antigen complex.[117] Regardless of the precise mechanism(s) underlying antigen recognition by T lymphocytes (dual receptor recognition versus single receptor recognition), the basis of Ir-gene-controlled immune responsiveness remains unclear. Several hypotheses have been advanced; however, current evidence suggests that two theories are most plausible: (1) the determinant selection hypothesis[118,119] and (2) the clonal deletion theory.[120,121]

The Determinant Selection Hypothesis of Ir Gene Function. The determinant selection theory of Ir gene function provides that antigen processing by the APC results in selective display of restricted portions of the nominal antigen to the responding T lymphocyte. Presumably, Ia antigens on the APC interact with the nominal antigen such that a specific orientation of the antigen on the cell surface of the APC ensues. Ir gene-linked unresponsiveness would presumably result either from failure of the nominal antigen to associate with APC Ia molecules or because of failure of Ia-antigen interaction to result in display of a particular antigenic determinant. Thus, this theory attributes Ir-linked unresponsiveness to inability of the APC to present the antigen (determinants) to responding cells.

Recent studies that suggest an important role for the T lymphocyte in Ir gene function have provided strong evidence against this theory. After depleting alloreactive T lymphocytes, Ishii and colleagues were able to induce T lymphocyte responses to poly(glu^{40}ala^{60}) (GA) and poly(glu^{51}lys^{34}tyr^{15}) (GLT) despite presentation of the antigens on nonresponder APC.[122] Clark and Shevach were able to generate antigen-specific guinea pig strain 2 T lymphocyte colonies capable of proliferating to the synthetic copolymer L-glutamic acid, L-lysine when it was presented by APC from nonresponder strain 13 guinea pigs.[123] More recently, APC from strain 2 guinea pigs (bovine insulin B chain nonresponders) were clearly shown to be capable of displaying the B chain of bovine insulin to T lymphocytes derived from strain 13 guinea pigs, which are normally responsive to the insulin B chain.[124] Taken together, these results cast doubt on the determinant selection theory and suggest that APC per se are not solely responsible for Ir gene-linked antigen unresponsiveness.

Clonal Deletion Model of Ir Gene Function. According to this theory, T lymphocyte unresponsiveness to a particular antigen mediated by Ir genes is attributable to the deletion of T lymphocyte clones reactive with complexes of self Ia molecules and the specific antigen.[120] This "hole" in the T lymphocyte repertoire results from the elimination of T lymphocytes strongly reactive with self Ia molecules and/or complexes of self Ia with self antigens. Presumably, antigen unresponsiveness occurs in situations in which the Ia antigen-nominal antigen complex mimics self closely enough such that T lymphocytes that might have been capable of recognizing the complex have previously been eliminated during development because of their strong reactivity to self (Fig. 5–3). While the clonal deletion theory places the expression of Ir gene products at the APC level, responsiveness ultimately reflects the presence (or absence) of T lymphocytes capable of recognizing the complex of self Ia and nominal antigen presented on the APC surface. Thus, the Ia-negative T lymphocyte plays a critical role in Ir gene-linked antigen unresponsiveness according to this theory.

Emerging evidence that antigen presented by nonresponder haplotype APC is capable of triggering T lymphocyte responses by allogeneic responder T lymphocytes is compatible with this view. Furthermore, the observation that autologous insulin presented on allogeneic APC but not autologous APC is capable of eliciting T lymphocyte responses against autologous insulin further supports this model[124] (Table 5–4). Evidence that self antigens presented in the context of foreign (or altered) Ia molecules are capable of inducing "anti-self" responses is particularly provocative and raises the possibility that alterations of self Ia antigens could trigger responses to a variety of self antigens by virtue of activation of autologous T lymphocytes capable of reacting with altered Ia antigen–self antigen complexes present on APC.

In summary, strong evidence suggests that Ir gene expression occurs at the APC level. Ir gene-linked antigen responsiveness does not appear to be solely attributable to the APC, since nonresponder APC are capable of presenting the relevant antigen to allogeneic T lymphocytes. Considerable evidence indicates that T lymphocytes must recognize both Ia antigen and nominal antigen on the APC (either separately or as a complex) in order to respond to the particular antigen. The hypothesis that Ir gene-linked unresponsiveness reflects the deletion of T lymphocytes capable of reacting with

Figure 5–3. Schematic diagram of the type of complex antigenic determinants that might be formed as a result of interaction of a self antigen (A) or foreign antigen (B) with an I region product of the haplotype x(Ix) or y(Iy). The interaction of the self antigen A or foreign antigen B with the Ix product results in complex antigenic determinants, which have identical shape. In this case, the deletion of T cells reactive with the self-Ix complex would be associated with unresponsiveness to the foreign antigen B. In contrast, interaction of self antigen A and foreign antigen B with the Iy product leads to the formation of complexes with differing shapes. In this case, deletion of T cells reactive with the A-Iy complex would not be associated with lack of response to B-Iy. (From Schwartz, R.H.: Scand. J. Immunol. 7:3, 1978.)

a particular Ia antigen–nominal antigen complex is compatible with the available data, but further studies to test this model are clearly required.

IMMUNOGLOBULIN GENES

Introduction

A fundamental characteristic of the vertebrate immune system is the capacity for discriminant recognition of the incredible array of different molecules (antigens) routinely encountered in the environment by the host. It is therefore not surprising that this requirement for diverse (but specific) immune recognition is reflected at the B lymphocyte level by the capacity of an individual to elaborate an estimated 10^6 to 10^8 different antibody molecules. Genes responsible for the generation of antibody diversity clearly must be considered in a discus-

Table 5–4. Strain 13 T Lymphocyte Colonies Recognize a Determinant Present on the Autologous Guinea Pig Insulin B Chain (5–16) Peptide Sequence Presented by Strain 2 Accessory Cells*

| T Lymphocyte Stimulation By | ([3H]TdR Incorporation by Colony | | | |
	I-30-D4	I-32-F5	I-32-D8	I-32-D9
Strain 13 accessory cells alone (peritoneal exudate cells)	628	330	340	573
Strain 13 accessory cells + guinea pig insulin B chain (5–16)	228	550	531	442
Strain 2 accessory cells alone	1,496	1,012	644	638
Strain 2 accessory cells + guinea pig insulin B chain (5–16)	16,546	6,242	4,115	4,342

*Adapted from Dos Reis, G.A., and Shevach, E.M.: J. Exp. Med. 157:1287, 1983, by copyright permission of the Rockefeller University Press.

sion of genetic regulation of immune responses. An obvious question in this regard relates to the precise role that inherited immunoglobulin genes play in determining individual differences in antibody responses evoked by a particular antigen. Approaches to this question have taken advantage of the realization that antibody specificity is due to the chemical structure of the binding or variable (V) region of the antibody molecule. Hence, antibody molecules bear antigenic determinants related to the binding specificity of the molecules, a property known as *idiotypy*. Idiotypes therefore serve as useful markers for analyzing immunoglobulin diversity and for examining the genetic control of specific immunoglobulin expression.

In this section we briefly discuss the genetic mechanisms underlying expression of the antibody repertoire (see Chapter 2 for additional details) and consider the evidence that inherited immunoglobulin genes influence specific immune responses. It should be stressed that specific recognition structures are also clearly expressed at the T lymphocyte level and that genes governing expression of these T lymphocyte recognition structures appear to be distinct from immunoglobulin heavy chain variable region (V_H) genes. Unfortunately these genes have yet to be identified, and, therefore, the genetic mechanisms contributing to establishment of the T lymphocyte repertoire are not yet clear.

Organization of Immunoglobulin Genes

The structure of the immunoglobulin protein provided important clues with regard to genetic mechanisms underlying the generation of antibody diversity. Specifically, both heavy (H) and light (L) chains possessed constant region domains that were identical for all antibody molecules of the same isotype, subclass, and light chain type present in the same individual. Moreover, H and L chains also contained a variable region domain that varied among different antibody molecules and therefore accounted for the tremendous diversity of immunoglobulins encountered in each individual. These properties led Dreyer and Bennett[125] to postulate that multiple genes contributed to the expression of variable

region diversity whereas only single genes were necessary for the expression of constant regions of light chains (C_L) or of each heavy chain isotype (C_H). This radical "two gene–one polypeptide" hypothesis predicted that joining between a constant region gene (C_L or C_H) and one of many available variable region genes (V_H or V_L) accounted for the peculiar structural features of the immunoglobulin molecule. Subsequent studies in several laboratories have confirmed and amplified this hypothesis such that the tremendous diversity of the B lymphocyte repertoire is now understandable at a molecular level.

Heavy Chain Genes. Located on chromosome 14 in humans,[126] immunoglobulin heavy (H) chain genes in the germ line consist of four linked multigene families arranged sequentially in the following order on the chromosome (5'end → 3'end): variable (V_H), diversity (D), joining (J_H) and constant (C_H) gene segments (Fig. 5–4). While the precise number of V_H gene segments remains to be elucidated, there appear to be several groups of V_H genes, with the members of each group exhibiting homologous sequences. Although presumably closely related, the members of each V_H group do not necessarily encode for the same antigen-binding specificity. This has been demonstrated in the antiphosphorylcholine antibody system in the mouse in which only one of the four members of the so-called T15 group of V_H genes is used for antiphosphorylcholine antibody.[127] Multiple D gene segments are located in clusters close to the 5' end of J_H genes. Although the precise location of these gene segments is under investigation, a germ line D gene segment has been identified 750 nucleotide base pairs (bp) to the 5' end of the initial mouse J_H segment.[128] D region gene segments vary in both base sequence and length (18 to 41 bp in the mouse).[129,130] Situated approximately 8 kilobases (kb) to the 5' side of $C\mu$, the J_H group of genes in humans consists of a 3.2 kb nucleotide segment that contains six complete J_H genes and three incomplete (or pseudo) J_H genes.[131] The last group of H genes are the C_H genes, which determine the class of the H-chain polypeptide. Five classes of H chain (α, δ, ϵ, γ, and μ), four γ subclasses (γ_1, γ_2, γ_3, and γ_4), and two α subclasses (α_1 and α_2) occur in humans. The

Figure 5–4. A schematic diagram of the germ-line organization and subsequent assembly of the human immunolglobulin heavy chain gene. The immunoglobulin heavy chain genes consist of multiple V_H regions, each preceded by its own leader (L) sequence; six functional J_H segments; families of D segments; and one constant $C\mu$ gene per chromosome. Initially, a single V_H, D, J_H region must be successfully recombined at the DNA level to form an active gene. The remaining intervening sequence (IVS) is then removed at the RNA level by splicing, thereby producing a complete μ-mRNA, which is subsequently translated to a complete μ heavy chain. (From Korsmeyer, S.J., et al.: J. Clin. Invest. 71:301, 1983, by copyright permission of The American Society for Clinical Investigation.)

order of these C_H genes has recently been determined in man to be 5'end$\rightarrow J_H \rightarrow$ 8kb$\rightarrow$ $C\mu \rightarrow$ 5kb$\rightarrow$ $C\delta \rightarrow$ $C\gamma 3 \rightarrow$ 26kb$\rightarrow$ $C\gamma 1 \rightarrow$ 19kb$\rightarrow$ pseudoC$\epsilon \rightarrow$ 13kb$\rightarrow$ $C\alpha 1 \rightarrow$ $C\gamma 2 \rightarrow$ 18kb$\rightarrow$ $C\gamma 4 \rightarrow$ 23kb$\rightarrow$ $C\epsilon \rightarrow$ 10kb$\rightarrow$ $C\alpha 2 \rightarrow$ 3' end.[132] This arrangement of human C_H genes suggests a duplication of a γ-γ-ϵ-α multigene segment.[132]

Light Chain Genes. Genes for human κ and λ light (L) chains are located on chromosomes 2 and 22, respectively.[132] L chain genes consist of three multigene families (V_L, J_L, and C_L). In the case of κ chain genes, 15 to 20 $V\kappa$ genes have been estimated to be present in the human germ line, situated in a cluster 5' to the $J\kappa$ gene family.[134] The human $J\kappa$ gene family consists of five complete $J\kappa$ genes located in a cluster approximately 2.5 kb 5' to the single $C\kappa$ gene.[135] Lambda chain genes are arranged differently then κ chain genes. The precise number of $V\lambda$ genes has not been determined, but several are assumed to exist.[136] In contrast to the single $C\kappa$ gene in man, at least six human $C\lambda$ genes have been identified.[137] As demonstrated in the mouse, each human $C\lambda$ gene is assumed to be associated with its own $J\lambda$ segment.[138,139]

Assembly of Variable Region Gene Segments—the Generation of Variable Region Diversity. The complete variable region of the immunoglobulin H polypeptide chain is encoded by a DNA segment created by the recombinational joining of a V_H, D, and J_H gene with associated deletion of the DNA previously separating these segments in the germ line gene configuration (Fig. 5–4). In the case of L chains, a V_L and a J_L gene segment are joined. Investigation of DNA rearrangement mechanisms underlying V-(D)-J joining have yielded important insights into the generation of immunoglobulin variable region diversity. At least five mechanisms contribute to the generation of antibody diversity:[136] (1) the large number of germ line V_H and V_L genes; (2) random joining of V, (D), and J genes; (3) imprecisions (flexibility) in the precise site of recombination of these gene segments; (4) somatic mutations arising in V genes; and (5) random association of H and L chains. Further studies are required to delineate the precise relative contributions of each of these mechanisms to variable region diversity; however, theoretical calculations of the possibilities arising from these processes indicate that one need not invoke additional explanations.

It should be noted that the occurrence of V-(D)-J joining at the pre-B lymphocyte level implies that the generation of antibody diversity largely occurs independent of antigen stimulation, since these immature cells do not exhibit surface Ig. On the other hand, observations that somatic mutation is frequently expressed in the variable regions (H or L) of IgA or IgG molecules, but not IgM molecules, raises the possibility that isotype switching may trigger somatic mutational processes.[140,141] A role for antigen in influencing somatic mutation (perhaps via triggering B lymphocyte proliferation and differentiation) cannot be excluded at this time.

Genetic Basis of Heavy Chain "Switching"—the Generation of Isotype Diversity. The formation of a partic-

ular V_H-D-J_H combination at the pre-B lymphocyte level is necessary before the expression of μ heavy chains in the cytoplasm of the cell.[142,143] This is accomplished by the transcription of an RNA segment containing the $V_H DJ_H$ segment and the $C\mu$ gene followed by deletion of the intervening RNA (RNA splicing) resulting in μ mRNA (Fig. 5–4). The $V_H DJ_H$ may be subsequently expressed in combination with a different C_H gene, a process referred to as "switching."

Pre-B lymphocytes, the earliest recognizable stage of B lymphocyte differentiation, are characterized by the expression of cytoplasmic μ heavy chains without light chains. At the DNA level, these cells exhibit a productive arrangement of heavy chain gene segments (V-D-J joining). Combination of this V-D-J segment with $C\mu$ at the mRNA level as a result of RNA splicing events results in a μ polypeptide H chain being translated (Figs. 5–4 and 5–5). It is now clear that subsequent differentiation of the pre-B cell is associated with an orderly sequence of immunoglobulin L chain rearrangements.[143,145] Initially a rearrangement of κ genes occurs on one chromosome 2, with resultant joining of a V_κ and J_κ gene and subsequent formation of a κ chain mRNA with synthesis of intact κ chains. However, the flexibility or imprecision of V-J joining events leads to frequent nonproductive arrangements (null genes), which are excluded from expression and which may actually be deleted at the DNA level (Fig. 5–6). In this case, rearrangement of κ chain genes on the other chromosome 2 occurs. Should this also prove to be ineffective, rearrangements of λ chain genes are then attempted on one chromosome 22, followed by DNA rearrangements on the other chromosome 22 if the first try also proves unproductive. This model of B lymphocyte differentiation in which H chain rearrangements are followed by κ gene rearrangements and then, if necessary, by λ gene recombinations has been observed in both transformed and normal human B lymphocytes.[144,145]

In addition to intact surface IgM molecules, B lymphocytes may also express other surface immunoglobulins. At least two mechanisms for the expression of

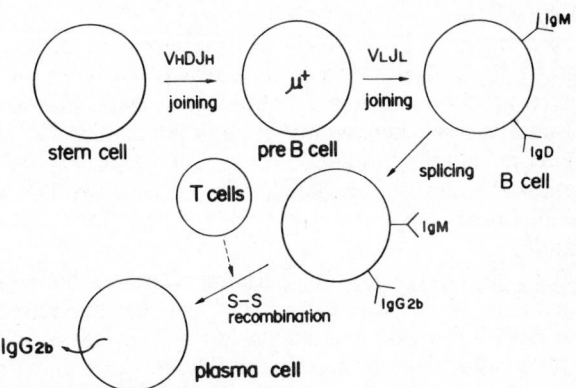

Figure 5–5. Schematic diagram of the order of DNA rearrangements during B cell development from the pre-B to the plasma cell level. (Reproduced, with permission, from the Annual Review of Immunology, Volume 1. ©1983 by Annual Reviews Inc.)

Figure 5–6. Diagram of the two types of DNA rearrangements that occur in the H chain gene locus. In V-J recombination, V_H, D, and J_H segments are joined together at the DNA level and the intervening sequence between the active $V_H DJ_H$ gene and the $C\mu$ gene is removed at the RNA level by splicing. In S-S recombination, DNA between two switch (S) sites is deleted, with subsequent movement of the $C\gamma 2b$ gene adjacent to the $V_H DJ_H$ complex. (From Honjo, T., et al.: Immunol. Rev. 59:33, 1981.)

immunoglobulin isotypes other than μ have been delineated. In the case of lymphocytes expressing both IgM and IgD on the surface, $C\mu$ and $C\delta$ genes appear not to be rearranged, suggesting that RNA splicing mechanisms account for the dual expression of IgM and IgD.[146,147] Presumably, a large RNA transcript containing a V-D-J sequence in addition to $C\mu$ and $C\delta$ would be variably spliced in such a way that mRNAs for both μ and δ could be produced. A similar mechanism has been proposed to account for lymphocytes co-expressing IgM and IgE in the absence of demonstrable C_H gene rearrangements.[148] On the basis of such observations it has been postulated that class switching may be initially accomplished by RNA splicing mechanisms before C_H gene rearrangements occur.[148,136] Direct evidence for the existence of the large RNA transcripts predicted by this theory has not yet been obtained.

The second mechanism responsible for isotype switching involves rearrangement of C_H genes at the DNA level. Sequencing studies of the C_H genes have revealed the presence of long stretches of homologous nucleotide sequences (S regions), which are repeated in tandem and located to the 5' of each C_H gene.[149-152] Interestingly, the length of the S region preceding each C_H gene in the mouse varies and correlates with the serum concentration of the isotype.[150] Rearrangement of C_H genes involved in isotype switching observed in some plasmacytomas is associated with deletion of intervening DNA sequence between S-S regions (Fig. 5–7). Thus, the formation of a complete H chain involves at least two DNA recombinational events: V-D-J joining and S-S recombination.

A particularly important question relates to the regulation of isotype expression, i.e., what are the forces that govern expression of isotype? In this regard, strong evidence indicates that diversity of B lymphocyte surface isotype expression is observed during B lymphocyte ontogeny and that this isotype switching occurs independently of antigen and T lymphocyte influence.[153] Indeed, heavy chain switching has been observed at the pre-B

lymphocyte level preceding the expression of surface Ig.[154] On the other hand, additional evidence suggests that isotype diversity can be influenced by T lymphocytes. Cloned T lymphocyte lines obtained from murine Peyer's patches, a rich source of IgA-committed B lymphocytes,[155] have been demonstrated to induce isotype switching in B lymphocytes from surface IgM+ to surface IgA+ cells. Moreover, soluble factors released by T lymphocyte hybridomas have been shown to influence the subclass of IgG produced by lipopolysaccharide (LPS)-stimulated B lymphocytes.[157] Pure and coworkers have been able to separate two soluble B lymphocyte differentiation factors (BCDF): a high molecular weight BCDFμ (MW 30,000 to 60,000), which

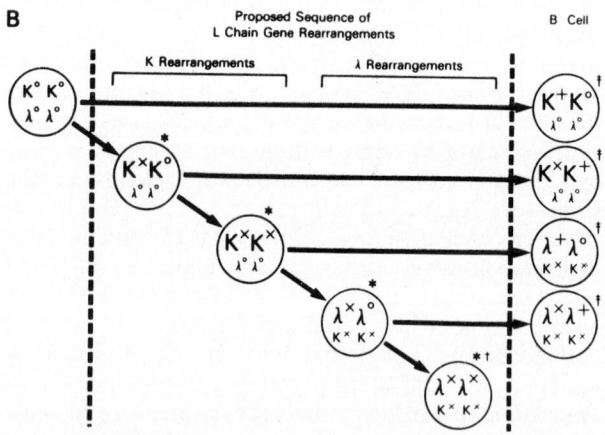

Figure 5–7. Proposed sequence of human L chain gene rearrangements which occur following H chain gene rearrangement in the course of early B cell development.. In general, L chain rearrangements begin with first one κ gene, then the other if the first attempt is ineffective (x). If both κ gene rearrangement attempts are unsuccessful, then λ rearrangements would follow. Cells with effectively rearranged κ or λ genes could become mature B cells (‡) if prior H chain rearrangements were successful. Cells with ineffectively rearranged L chain genes (*) would lack L chain production and therefore be unable to synthesize intact immunoglobulin molecules. Theoretically, a population of B cells with totally ineffective κ and λ gene rearrangements (†) could exist. (From Korsmeyer, S.J., et al.: J. Clin. Invest. 71:301, 1983, by copyright permission of The American Society for Clinical Investigation.)

preferentially induces IgM secretion by B cells, and a smaller BCDFγ (MW < 20,000), which induces predominant IgG1 secretion in LPS-stimulated B lymphocytes.[158] Further evidence for T lymphocyte regulation 41of isotype expression has come from studies in mice indicating that T lymphocytes are capable of enhancing IgG2 responses to the type 2 T-independent antigens TNP-Ficoll and TNP-Levan.[159] Certainly these data strongly suggest a role for T lymphocytes in regulation of the isotype profile of specific immune responses. Whether this is accomplished by means of triggering of switching events or through selective amplification of already committed ("preswitched") B lymphocytes has not been unequivocally established.

The T Lymphocyte Antigen Receptor and Immunoglobulin Heavy Chain Genes. The structural basis for T lymphocyte antigen specificity remains uncertain. Observations that anti-idiotypic and anti-V_H framework reagents were capable of interfering with T lymphocyte function and binding to soluble antigen by specific T lymphocyte factors suggested that V_H genes encoded for at least a portion of the T lymphocyte antigen receptor.[160-162] Linkage of these serologically recognized T lymphocyte receptor determinants to immunoglobulin H chain genes supported this view.[163-166] Moreover, the identification of T lymphocyte surface alloantigens and mapping of the responsible genes to murine chromosome 12 between the C_H gene cluster and the prealbumin gene (Pre-1)[167-169] raised the possibility that these structures represented the constant region portion of the T lymphocyte antigen receptor. Evidence for this association was obtained from studies in which anti-T lymphocyte allotype reagents blocked the binding of idiotypic-specific suppressor T lymphocytes to idiotype-bearing Ig.[169] More recently Tokuhisa and colleagues have successfuly raised monoclonal antibodies that recognize constant region determinants present on both antigen-specific helper and suppressor T lymphocyte factors.[170] Taken together, these observations suggest that the T lymphocyte antigen receptor consists of a constant region encoded by C_H-linked genes and an antigen-binding variable region encoded by V_H-like genes. Efforts to directly demonstrate a role for V_H genes in determining the variable region portion of the T lymphocyte receptor, however, have been unsuccessful. Indeed, Kronenberg and colleagues were unable to find evidence of RNA transcripts in three T lymphocyte hybridomas (one helper; two suppressor) that contained V_H gene sequences.[171] Analysis of B and T lymphocytes sharing the same antigen-binding specificity and cell surface idiotypic determinants revealed that the T lymphocytes did not transcribe the same V_H gene segment as the B lymphocytes.[172] The evidence indicates therefore that the antigen-binding variable region of the T lymphocyte receptor is encoded by V genes distinct from the V_H genes.

Relationship of Immunoglobulin Genes to Immune Response Characteristics. Since Ig genes determine the potential for variable region diversity expressed in antibody molecules, it is not surprising that these genes have been demonstrated to control specific immune re-

sponses. Two Ig gene markers have been primarily utilized to investigate the relationship between immune responses and inherited Ig genes: *allotypes* and *idiotypes.*

Immunoglobulin allotypes are genetic variants of immunoglobulins and are inherited by simple Mendelian genetics. These variants reflect the presence of alleles for C_H and C_L genes. In man, alleles for V_H or V_L genes have not been clearly demonstrated (although this does occur in the rabbit). Allotypic differences resulting from slight amino acid sequence differences in the constant regions of H or L chains can be recognized by serologic reagents. Utilizing this approach, allotypes for κ light chains and for IgG and IgA heavy chains have been identified in man (Table 5–5). These allotype-specific reagents have provided useful tools for analyzing the relationship between immune response characteristics and inherited Ig genes.

While allotypes reflect allelic heterogeneity of C_H and C_L genes, idiotypes are encoded by V region genes. Idiotypes can be defined as a group of determinants (idiotopes) expressed in the V region of an antibody or in the V regions of antibodies with similar specificity.[173,174] Serologic reagents reactive with particular idiotypes (anti-idiotypes) can be prepared and have been quite helpful in examining genetic mechanisms underlying antibody diversity. Idiotypes shared by antibodies (or T lymphocyte receptors) possessing similar antigen-binding specificity are referred to as crossreactive idiotypes. The structural basis of idiotype expression is under intense investigation. Current evidence indicates that im-

Table 5–5. Human Immunoglobulin Allotypes*

Class and Subclass or Light Chain Type	Allotype (Numerical Designation)		Location of Determinant
IgG1	G1m	(1)	C_H3
		(2)	C_H3
		(3)	C_H1
		(17)	C_H1
IgG2	G2m	(23)	C_H2
IgG3	G3m	(11)	C_H3
		(5)	C_H2
		(13)	C_H3
		(14)	C_H2
		(10)	C_H3
		(6)	
		(24)	
		(21)	
		(15)	
		(16)	
		(26)	
		(27)	
IgA2	A2m	(1)	
	A2m	(2)	
κ	Km	(1)	
		(2)	
		(3)	

*Adapted from WHO Committee Report: J. Immunogenet. 3:357, 1976.

munoglobulin idiotypes generally reflect amino acid sequences of immunoglobulin complementarity-determining regions (CDR). Thus, sequences determined by V, D, and J genes appear to be responsible for the expression of idiotypic determinants in immunoglobulin molecules.

It has become evident that the expression of a particular idiotype is under genetic control. This has been clearly shown in mice responding to α(1-3) dextran (DEX), in which the expression of a dominant idiotype (IdX) on anti-DEX antibodies correlates with the inherited allotype of the strain.[175,176] Mice bearing the Igh-C^a allotype are high IdX responders to DEX whereas mice of the Igh-C^b allotype do not produce detectible concentrations of IdX in response to DEX. Molecular analysis of specific immune responses dominated by a particular IdX has revealed that these responses are associated with inheritance of a single (or few) relevant V_H and V_L genes in the germ line. Examples of this phenomenon include the responses to arsonate,[177] phosphorylcholine,[178,179] and (4-hydroxy-3-nitrophenyl) acetyl groups (NP).[180,181] Thus, the responses to these particular antigens appear to be restricted because of the limited number of relevant or expressible V genes available in the germ line. A critical question then relates to whether the expressed idiotype repertoire is entirely dependent upon the nature of inherited V genes or whether other genetically determined influences are operative.

Linkage of IdX responses with particular IgH genes (allotypes) has been interpreted as evidence for the former hypothesis. In this regard, recent studies in normal mice and T lymphocyte deficient nude mice have shown linkage between allotype background and the frequency of IdX$^+$ precursor B lymphocytes.[182] These data appear to support the view that selection and maintenance of the B lymphocyte V region repertoire is encoded by germ line genes and that its expression is independent of T lymphocytes. However, several investigators have succeeded in inducing expression of IdX-bearing antibodies of desired antigenic specificites in mice of "nonresponder" allotypes by administration of anti-idiotypic antibodies.[183-186] These results suggest that regulatory influences contribute to the expression of particular idiotypes, and, indeed, evidence for suppressor T cell participation in idiotype expression is convincing in some systems.[187,184] A role for helper T lymphocytes in governing idiotype expression is also suggested by other studies.[188,186,189] Presumably these regulatory influences are heavily dependent upon idiotype–anti-idiotype interactions, the so-called "network theory" of immune regulation initially proposed by Jerne.[190] The precise role of V_H genes and T lymphocyte V genes in these complementary interactions is not clear.

Taken together, these results indicate that the expressed V region repertoire is restricted by the inherited germ line V gene repertoire. In addition, regulatory influences (T lymphocyte and ?other) contribute to the pattern of immunoglobulin V region determinants (idiotypes) expressed in response to a particular antigen. The well-documented linkage of allotype background with idiotype expression could reflect an association of allotype with a particular set of germ line V region genes and/or linkage of IgH genes with regulatory genes that restrict the pattern of V gene expression (through T lymphocytes or other mechanisms).

Immunoglobulin Genes and Disease Susceptibility. Evidence for an association between immunoglobulin genes (allotype) and responsiveness to specific antigens in man has been obtained for some antigens, including bacterial flagellin[191,192] and various bacterial polysaccharides.[193,194] That certain diseases are also associated with inheritance patterns of immunoglobulin genes is not surprising in view of the apparent relationship of these genes to immune response characteristics of the individual. These associations have most frequently been established through an analysis of immunoglobulin allotype patterns. Associations of particular Gm allotypes with several diseases have been recently identified, including myasthenia gravis,[195] chronic active hepatitis,[196] Grave's disease,[195,197] SLE[195,198] multiple sclerosis,[199] and Hashimoto's thyroiditis.[195] In each of these diseases it appears that both MHC-linked and immunoglobulin-linked genes contribute to disease susceptibility. The precise mechanisms underlying apparent dual gene control of disease susceptibility remain uncertain. Recent evidence that MHC-linked genes are capable of influencing idiotypic interactions suggests at least one mechanism underlying interaction between MHC-linked and Ig-linked genes.[200]

CONCLUSIONS

Immune responses to specific antigens are controlled by several distinct genetic loci. Moreover, genes residing in (or near) these loci also appear to influence susceptibility to a variety of diseases in which immune mechanisms have been implicated. Presumably, at least some of these putative disease susceptibility genes function through regulation of specific immune responses critical to expression of the disease in question. Elucidation of mechanisms underlying gene regulation of immune response characteristics should furnish important insights into pathogenetic mechanisms operative in these diseases.

Two major gene groups, MHC and Ig, have been clearly implicated in the regulation of specific immune responsiveness. The available evidence suggests that MHC genes operate at the level of antigen recognition by T lymphocytes. Thus, MHC-linked unresponsiveness to a particular antigen appears to result from the inability of T lymphocytes to recognize the antigen presented in the context of self MHC antigens. In some cases, suppressor T lymphocytes, which contribute to the lack of antigen responsiveness, may be preferentially induced. Evidence that modification of self MHC antigens may promote development of enhanced reactivity to self antigens is provocative and clearly warrants further investigation as a plausible mechanism underlying susceptibility to autoimmune conditions. Moreover, reversal of antigen unresponsive states by alteration of relevant self MHC antigens may prove to be feasible.

The role(s) of Ig genes in controlling specific immune responses appears to be complex. The pattern of inherited immunoglobulin V region genes restricts the potential repertoire of the antibody response; however, closely linked genes also appear to regulate the pattern of immunoglobulin V region products ultimately expressed. The precise identity of these putative regulatory genes is unclear but there is reason to suspect that T lymphocyte V genes, which appear to be distinct from B lymphocyte V_H genes, are likely to be involved. Indeed, immunoregulatory T lymphocyte circuits that modulate B lymphocyte function have been demonstrated to be dependent upon genes closely linked to IgH genes for their function. The availability of techniques for cloning human T lymphocytes of desired specificity should provide opportunities for in vivo manipulation of immune responses. The implications with regard to interruption of potentially harmful immune responses (e.g., autoimmune phenomena) are clear.

References

1. Vitetta, E.S., and Capra, J.D.: The protein products of the murine 17th chromosome. Genetics and structure. Adv. Immunol. 26:147, 1978.
2. Klein, J., Figueroa, F., and Nagy, Z.A.: Genetics of the major histocompatibility complex: The final act. Ann. Rev. Immunol. 1:119, 1983.
3. Ploegh, H.L., Orr, H.T., and Strominger, J.L.: Major histocompatibility antigens: The human (HLA-A,-B,-C) and murine (H-2K, H-2D) class I molecules. Cell 24:287, 1981.
4. Zinkernagel, R.M., and Doherty, P.C.: Immunological surveillance against altered self components by sensitized T lymphocytes in lymphocytic choriomeningitis. Nature 251:547, 1974.
5. Klein, J.: Biology of the Mouse Histocompatibility-2 Complex. New York, Springer, 1975.
6. Silver, J., Walker, L.E., Reisfield, R.A., Pellegrino, M.A., and Ferrone, S.: Structural studies of murine I-E and human DR antigens. Mol. Immunol. 16:37, 1979.
7. Ferrone, S., Allison, J.P., and Pellegrino, M.A.: Human DR (Ia-like) antigens: Biological and molecular profile. Contemp. Top. Mol. Immunol. 7:239, 1978.
8. Tosi, R., Tanigaki, N., Centis, G., Ferrara, D.B., and Pressman, D.: Immunological dissection of human Ia molecules. J. Exp. Med. 148:1592, 1978.
9. Charron, D.J., and McDevitt, H.O.: Characterization of HLA-D region antigens by two-dimensional gel electrophoresis. J. Exp. Med. 152:18s, 1980.
10. Shackelford, D.A., and Strominger, J.L.: Demonstration of structural polymorphism among HLA-DR light chains by two-dimensional gel electrophoresis. J. Exp. Med. 151:144, 1980.
11. Nagy, Z., Baxevanis, C., Ishii, N., and Klein, J.: Ia antigens as restriction molecules in Ir-gene controlled T cell proliferation. Immunol. Rev. 60:59, 1981.
12. McDevitt, H.O., and Benacerraf, B.: Genetic control of specific immune response. Adv. Immunol. 11:31, 1969.
13. Shreffler, D., David, C., Cullen, S., Frelinger, J., and Niederhuber, J.: Serological and functional evidence for further subdivision of the I regions of the H-2 gene complex. Cold Spring Harbor Symp. Quant. Biol. 41:477, 1976.
14. Klein, J., Juretic, A., Baxevanis, C.N., and Nagy, Z.A.: The traditional and the new version of the mouse H-2 complex. Nature 291:455, 1981.
15. Dorf, M.E.: The Role of the Major Histocompatibility Complex in Immunobiology. New York, Garland Publishing, 1980.
16. Shreffler, D.C., and David, C.S.: The H-2 major histocompatibility complex and the I immune response region. Genetic variation, function and organization. Adv. Immunol. 20:125, 1975.
17. Silver, J.: Genetic and structural organization of murine Ia and human DR antigens. CRC Crit. Rev. Immunol. 2:225, 1981.
18. Murphy, D.B., Herzenberg, L.A., Okumura, K., and McDevitt, H.O.: A new I subregion (I-J) marked by a locus (Ia-4) controlling surface determinants on suppressor lymphocytes. J. Exp. Med. 144:699, 1976.
19. Tada, T., Taniguchi, M., and David, C.S.: Properties of the antigen specific suppressive T cell factor in the regulation of antibody response in the mouse. IV. Special subregion assignment of the gene(s) that code for the suppressive T cell factor in the H-2 histocompatibility complex. J. Exp. Med. 144:713, 1976.
20. Taniguchi, M., Tokuhisa, T., Kanno, M., Yaoita, Y., Shimizu, A., and Honjo, T.: Reconstitution of antigen-specific suppressor activity with translation products of mRNA. Nature 298:172, 1982.
21. Krupen, K., Araneo, B.A., and Brink, L.: Purification and characterization of a monoclonal T cell suppressor factor specific for poly(L-Glu^{60}L-Ala^{30}L-Tyr^{10}). Proc. Natl. Acad. Sci. USA 79:1254, 1982.
22. Wieder, K.J., Araneo, B.A., Kapp, J.A., and Webb, D.R.: Cell-free translation of a biological active, antigen-specific suppressor T cell factor. Proc. Natl. Acad. Sci. USA 79:3599, 1982.
23. Steinmetz, M., Minard, K., Horvath, S., McNicholas, J., Frelinger, J., Wake, C., Long, E., Mach, B., and Hood, L.: A molecular map of the immune response region from the major histocompatibility complex of the mouse. Nature 300:35, 1982.
24. McKenzie, I.F.C., and Potter, T.: Murine lymphocyte surface antigens. Adv. Immunol. 27:179, 1979.
25. Allison, J.P., Walker, L.E., Russell, W.A., Pellegrino, M.A., Ferrone, S., Reisfield, R.A., Frelinger, J.A., and Silver, J.: Murine Ia and DR antigens. Homology of amino terminal sequences. Proc. Natl. Acad. Sci. USA 75:3953, 1978.
26. Cullen, S.E., Freed, J.H., and Nathenson, S.G.: Structural and serological properties of murine Ia alloantigens. Transplant. Rev. 30:236, 1976.
27. Cullen, S.E., Kindle, C.S., and Littman, D.R.: Structural comparison of murine Ia antigens determined by the I-A and I-E subregions. J. Immunol. 122:855, 1979.
28. Jones, P., Murphy, D., Hewgill, D., and McDevitt, H.O.: Detection of a common polypeptide chain in I-A and I-E subregion immunoprecipitates. Immunochemistry 16:51, 1978.
29. Cecka, J., McMillon, M., Murphy, D., McDevitt, H.O., and Hood, L.: Partial N-terminal amino acid sequence analyses and comparative tryptic peptide maps of murine Ia molecules encoded by the I-A subregion. Eur. J. Immunol. 9:955, 1979.
30. Cook, R.G., Siegelman, M.H., Capra, J.D., Uhr, J.W., and Vitetta, E.S.: Structural studies on the murine Ia alloantigens. IV. NH$_2$-terminal sequence analysis of allelic products of the I-A and E/C subregions. J. Immunol. 122:2232, 1979.
31. Uhr, J.W., Capra, J.D., Vitetta, E.S. and Cook, R.G.: Organization of the immune response genes. Science 206:292, 1979.
32. Freed, J.H., David, C.S., Shreffler, D.C., and Nathenson, S.G.: Structural studies of the protein portion of the H-2-linked Ia glycoprotein antigens of the mouse. Tryptic peptide comparison of products from the I-A and I-C subregions of B10.HTT. J. Immunol. 121:91, 1978.
33. Klein, J., and Figueroa, F.: Polymorphism of the mouse H-2 loci. Immunol. Rev. 60:23, 1981.
34. Silver, J., and Russell, W.A.: Genetic mapping of the component chains of Ia molecules. Immunogenetics 8:339, 1979.
35. Cook, R.G., Vitetta, E.S., Uhr, J.W., and Capra, J.D.: Structural studies on the murine Ia alloantigens. V. Evidence that the structural gene for the E/C β polypeptide is encoded within the I-A subregion. J. Exp. Med. 149:981, 1979.
36. Silver, J.: Transgene complementation of I-E subregion antigens. J. Immunol. 123:1423, 1979.
37. Benoist, C.O., Mathis, D.J., Kanter, M.R., Williams, V.E., and McDevitt, H.O.: The murine Ia α chains, Eα and Aα, show a surprising degree of sequence homology. Proc. Natl. Acad. Sci. USA 80:534, 1983.
38. Mathis, D.J., Benoist, C.O., Williams, V.E., Kanter, M.R., and McDevitt, H.O.: The murine Eα immune response gene. Cell 32:745, 1983.
39. Lee, J., Trowsdale, J., Travers, P., Carey, J., Grosveld, F., Jenkins, J., and Bodmer, W.: Sequence of an HLA-DR α chain cDNA clone and intron-exon organization of the corresponding gene. Nature 299:750, 1982.
40. Korman, A., Auffray, C., Schamboeck, A., and Strominger, J.: The amino acid sequence and gene organization of the heavy chain of the HLA-DR antigens. Homology to immunoglobulins. Proc. Natl. Acad. Sci. USA 79:6013, 1982.
41. Das, H., Lawrance, S., and Weissman, S.: The structure and nucleotide sequence of the heavy chain gene of HLA-DR. Proc. Natl. Acad. Sci. USA, in press.
42. Charron, D.J., and McDevitt, H.O.: Analysis of HLA-D region-associated molecules with monoclonal antibody. Proc. Natl. Acad. Sci. USA 76:6567, 1979.
43. Corte, G., Damiani, G., Calabi, F., Fabbi, M., and Bargellesi, A.: Analysis of HLA-DR polymorphism by two-dimensional peptide mapping. Proc. Natl. Acad. Sci. USA 78:534, 1981.
44. Shaw, S., Johnson, A.H., and Shearer, G.M.: Evidence for a new segregant series of B cell antigens which are encoded in the HLA-D region and stimulate secondary allogeneic proliferative and cytotoxic responses. J. Exp. Med. 152:565, 1980.
45. Shaw, S., Kavathas, P., Pollack, M.S., Charmot, D., and Mawas, C.:

Family studies define a new histocompatibility locus, SB, between HLA-DR and GLO. Nature 293:745, 1981.

46. Nadler, L.M., Stashenko, P., Hardy, R., Tomaselli, K.J., Yunis, E.J., Schlossman, S.F., and Pesando, J.M.: Monoclonal antibody identifies a new Ia-like (p29,34) polymorphic system linked to the HLA-D/DR region. Nature 290:591, 1981.

47. Hurley, C.K., Shaw, S., Nadler, L., Schlossman, S., and Capra, J.D.: Alpha and beta chains of SB and DR antigens are structurally distinct. J. Exp. Med. 156:1557, 1982.

48. Shackelford, D.A., Mann, D.C., van Rood, J.J., Ferrara, G.B., and Strominger, J.L.: Human B cell alloantigens DC1, MT1 and LB12 are identical to each other but distinct from the HLA-DR antigens. Proc. Natl. Acad. Sci. USA 78:4566, 1981.

49. Corte, G., Calabi, F., Damiani, G., Bargellesi, A., Tosi, R., and Sorrentino, R.: Human Ia molecules carrying DC1 determinants differ in both alpha and beta subunits from Ia molecules carrying DR determinants. Nature 292:357, 1981.

50. Bono, R., and Strominger, J.L.: Direct evidence of homology between DC-1 antigen and murine I-A molecules. Nature 299:836, 1982.

51. Goyert, S.M., Shively, J.E., and Silver, J.: Biochemical characterization of a second family of human Ia molecules, HLA-DS, equivalent to murine I-A subregion molecules. J. Exp. Med. 156:550, 1982.

52. Kavathas, P., Demars, R., Bach, F.H., and Shaw, S.: SB: A new HLA-linked human histocompatibility gene defined using HLA-mutant cell lines. Nature 293:747, 1981.

53. Korman, A., Knudsen, P.J., Kaufman, J.F., and Strominger, J.L.: cDNA clones for the heavy chain of HLA-DR antigens obtained after immunization of polysomes by monoclonal antibody. Proc. Natl. Acad. Sci. USA 79:1844, 1982.

54. Larhammar, D., Schenning, L., Gustafsson, K., Wiman, K., Claesson, L., Rask, L., and Peterson, P.A.: The complete amino acid sequence of an HLA-DR antigen-like β chain as predicted from the nucleotide sequence. Similarities with immunoglobulins and HLA-A,B,C antigens. Proc. Natl. Acad. Sci. USA 79:3687, 1982.

55. Stetler, D., Das, H., Nunberg, J., Saiki, R., Shen-Dong, R., Mullis, K.B., Weissman, S.M., and Erlich, H.A.: Isolation of a cDNA clone for the human HLA-DR antigen α chain by using a synthetic oligonucleotide as a hybridization probe. Proc. Natl. Acad. Sci. USA 79:5966, 1982.

56. Wiman, K., Larhammar, D., Claesson, L., Gustafsson, K., Schenning, L., Bill, P., Bohme, J., Denaro, M., Dobberstein, B., Hammerling, U., Kvist, S., Servenius, B., Sundelin, J., Peterson, P.A., and Rask, L.: Isolation and identification of a cDNA clone corresponding to an HLA-DR antigen β chain. Proc. Natl. Acad. Sci. USA 79:1703, 1982.

57. Larhammar, D., Gustafsson, K., Claesson, L., Bill, P., Wiman, K., Schenning, L., Sundelin, J., Widmark, E., Peterson, P.A., and Rask, L.: Alpha chain of HLA-DR transplantation antigens is a member of the same protein superfamily as the immunoglobulins. Cell 30:153, 1982.

58. Kratzin, H., Yang, C.-Y., Götz, H., Pauly, E., Kölbel, S., Egert, G., Thinnes, F.P., Wernet, P., Altevogt, P., and Hilschmann, N.: Primary structure of class II human histocompatibility antigens. Hoppe-Seyler's Z. Physiol. Chem. 362:1665, 1981.

59. Larhammar, D., Wiman, K., Schenning, L., Claesson, L., Gustafsson, K., Peterson, P.A., and Rask, L.: Evolutionary relationship between HLA-DR antigen β chains, HLA-A,B,C antigen subunits and immunoglobulin chains. Scand. J. Immunol. 14:617, 1981.

60. Kaufman, J.F., and Strominger, J.L.: HLA-DR light chain has a polymorphic N-terminal region and a conserved Ig-like C-terminal region. Nature 297:694, 1982.

61. Levine, B.B., Ojeda, A., and Benacerraf, B.: Studies on artificial antigens. III. The genetic control of the immune response to hapten poly-L-lysine conjugates in guinea pigs. J. Exp. Med. 118:953, 1963.

62. Levine, B.B., and Benacerraf, B.: The genetic control of the immune response to hapten polylysine conjugates in guinea pigs. Science 147:517, 1965.

63. Bluestein, H.G., Green, I., and Benacerraf, B.: Specific immune response genes of the guinea pig. I. Dominant genetic control of immune responsiveness to co-polymers of L-glutamic acid and L-alanine and L-glutamic acid and L-tyrosine. J. Exp. Med. 134:458, 1971.

64. Vaz, N.M., deSouza, C.M., and Maia, L.C.S.: Genetic control of immune responsiveness in mice. Responsiveness to ovalbumin in (C57BL x DBA/2)F₁ mice. Int. Arch. Allergy 46:275, 1974.

65. Green, I., and Benacerraf, B.: Genetic control of immune responsiveness to limiting doses of proteins and hapten protein conjugates in guinea pigs. J. Immunol. 107:374, 1971.

66. McDevitt, H.O., and Sela, M.: Genetic control of the antibody response. I. Demonstration of determinant-specific differences in response to synthetic polypeptide antigens in two strains of inbred mice. J. Exp. Med. 122:517, 1965.

67. Günther, R., Rüde, E., and Stark, O.: Antibody response in rats to the synthetic polypeptide (T,G)-A–L genetically linked to the major histocompatibility system. Eur. J. Immunol. 2:151, 1972.

68. Dorf, M.E., Balner, H., and Benacerraf, B.: Mapping of the immune response genes in the major histocompatibility complex of the rhesus monkey. J. Exp. Med. 142:673, 1975.

69. McDevitt, H.O., and Benacerraf, B.: Genetic control of specific immune response. Adv. Immunol. 11:31, 1969.

70. Benacerraf, B., and McDevitt, H.O.: The histocompatibility-linked immune response genes. Science 175:273, 1972.

71. Ellman, L., Green, I., Martin, W.J., and Benacerraf, B.: Linkage between the PLL gene and the locus controlling the major histocompatibility antigens in strain 2 guinea pigs. Proc. Natl. Acad. Sci. USA 66:322, 1970.

72. McDevitt, H.O., Deak, B.D., Shreffler, D.C., Klein, J., Stimpfling, J.H., and Snell, G.D.: Genetic control of the immune response. Mapping of the Ir.1 locus. J. Exp. Med. 135:1259, 1972.

73. Dorf, M.E., and Benacerraf, B.: Complementation of H-2 linked Ir genes in the mouse. Proc. Natl. Acad. Sci. USA 72:3671, 1975.

74. Benacerraf, B., and Germain, R.N.: The immune response genes of the major histocompatibility complex. Immunol. Rev. 38:70, 1978.

75. Schwartz, R.H., David, C.S., Dorf, M.E., Benacerraf, B., and Paul, W.E.: Inhibition of dual Ir gene-controlled T-lymphocyte proliferative response to poly(Glu⁵⁶Lys³⁵Phe⁹)n with anti-Ia antisera directed against products of either I-A or I-C subregion. Proc. Natl. Acad. Sci. USA 75:2387, 1978.

76. McNicholas, J.M., Murphy, D.B., Matis, L.A., Schwartz, R.H., Lerner, E.A., Janeway, C.A., and Jones, P.P.: Immune response gene function correlates with the expression of an Ia antigen. I. Preferential association of certain Ae and Eα chains results in a quantitative deficiency in expression of an Ae:Eα complex. J. Exp. Med. 155:490, 1982.

77. Matis, L.A., Jones, P.P., Murphy, D.B., Hedrick, S.M., Lerner, E.A., Janeway, C.A., McNicholas, J.M., and Schwartz, R.H.: Immune response gene function correlates with the expression of an Ia antigen. II. A quantitative deficiency in Ae:Eα complex expression causes a corresponding defect in antigen-presenting cell function. J. Exp. Med. 155:508, 1982.

78. Kapp, J.A., Pierce, C.W., Schlossman, S., and Benacerraf, B.: Genetic control of immune responses in vitro. V. Stimulation of suppressor T cells in nonresponder mice by the terpolymer L-glutamic acid⁶⁰-L-alanine³⁰-L-tyrosine¹⁰ (GAT). J. Exp. Med. 140:648, 1974.

79. Adorini, L., Miller, A., and Sercarz, E.E.: The fine specificity of regulatory cells. I. Hen-egg-white lysozyme-induced suppressor T cells in a genetically non-responder mouse strain do not recognize a closely related immunogeneic lysozyme. J. Immunol. 122:871, 1979.

80. Theze, J., Waltenbaugh, C., Dorf, M.E., and Benacerraf, B.: Immunosuppressive factors specific for L-glutamic acid⁵⁰-L-tyrosine⁵⁰(GT). II. Presence of I-J determinants on the GT suppressive factor. J. Exp. Med. 146:287, 1977.

81. Marsh, D.G., Hsu, S.H., Roebber, M., Ehrlich-Kautsky, E., Freidhoff, L.R., Meyers, D.A., Pollard, M.K., and Bias, W.B.: HLA-Dw2: A genetic marker for human immune response to short ragweed pollen allergen Ra5. I. Response resulting primarily from natural antigenic exposure. J. Exp. Med. 155:1439, 1982.

82. Marsh, D.G., Meyers, D.A., Freidhoff, L.R., Erhlich-Kautzky, E., Roebber, M., Norman, P.S., Hsu, S.H., and Bias, W.B.: HLA-Dw2: A genetic marker for human immune response to short ragweed pollen allergen Ra5. II. Response after ragweed immunotherapy. J. Exp. Med. 155:1452, 1982.

83. Solinger, A.M., Bhatnagar, R., and Stobo, J.D.: Cellular, molecular, and genetic characteristics of T cell reactivity to collagen in man. Proc. Natl. Acad. Sci. USA 78:3877, 1981.

84. Greenberg, L.J., Gray, E.D., and Yunis, E.J.: Association of HLA-5 and immune responsiveness in vitro to streptoccocal antigens. J. Exp. Med. 141:953, 1975.

85. Spencer, M.J., Cherry, J.D., and Terasaki, P.I.: HL-A antigens and antibody response after influenza A vaccination. Decreased response associated with HL-A type w/6. N. Engl. J. Med. 294:13, 1976.

86. DeVries, R.R.P., Kreeftenberg, H.G., Loggen, H.G., and van Rood, J.J.: In vitro immune responsiveness to vaccinia virus and HLA. N. Engl. J. Med. 297:692, 1977.

87. Sasazuki, T., Kohno, Y., Iwamoto, I., Tanimuro, M., and Naito, S.: Association between an HLA haplotype and low responsiveness to tetanus toxoid in man. Nature 272:359, 1978.

88. Solinger, A.M., and Stobo, J.D.: Immune response gene control of collagen reactivity in man. Collagen unresponsiveness in HLA-DR4 negative nonresponders is due to the presence of T-dependent suppressive influences. J. Immunol. 129:1915, 1982.

89. Sasazuki, T., Kaneoka, H., Nishimura, Y., Kaneoka, R., Hayama, M., and Ohkuni, H.: An HLA-linked immune suppression gene in man. J. Exp. Med. 152:297s, 1980.

90. Sasazuki, T., Nishimura, Y., Muto, M., and Ohta, N.: HLA-linked genes controlling immune response and disease susceptibility. Immunol. Rev. 70:51, 1983.

91. Stastny, P., Ball, E.J., Dry, P.J., and Nunez, G.: The human immune response region (HLA-D) and disease susceptibility. Immunol. Rev. 70:113, 1983.

92. Reinertsen, J.L., Klippel, J.H., Johnson, A.H., Steinberg, A.D., Decker, J.L., and Mann, D.L.: Lymphocyte alloantigens associated with systemic lupus erythematosus. N. Engl. J. Med. 299:515, 1978.

93. Gibofsky, A., Winchester, R.J., Patarroyo, M., Fotino, M., and Kunkel, H.G.: Disease associations of the Ia-like human alloantigens. Contrasting patterns in rheumatoid arthritis and systemic lupus erythematosus. J. Exp. Med. 148:1728, 1978.

94. Celada, A., Barras, C., Benzonana, G., and Jeannet, M.: Increased frequency of HLA-DR3 in systemic lupus erythematosus. New Engl. J. Med. 301:1398, 1979.

95. Scherak, O., Smolen, J.S., and Mayr, W.R.: HLA-DRw3 and systemic lupus erythematosus. Arth. Rheum. 23:954, 1980.

96. Griffing, W.L., Moore, S.B., Luthra, H.S., McKenna, C.H., and Fathman, C.G.: Associations of antibodies to native DNA with HLA-DRw3. A possible major histocompatibility complex-linked human immune response gene. J. Exp. Med. 152:319s, 1980.

97. Bell, D.A., and Maddison, P.J.: Serologic subsets in systemic lupus erythematosus: An examination of autoantibodies in relationship to clinical features of disease and HLA antigens. Arth. Rheum. 23:1268, 1980.

98. Notman, D.D., Kurata, N., and Tan, E.M.: Profiles of antinuclear antibodies in systemic rheumatic diseases. Ann. Intern. Med. 83:464, 1975.

99. Raveche, E.S., Novotny, E.A., Hansen, C.T., Tjio, J.H., and Steinberg, A.D.: Genetic studies in NZB mice. V. Recombinant inbred lines demonstrate that separate genes control autoimmune phenotype. J. Exp. Med. 153:1187, 1981.

100. Shirai, T.: The genetic basis of autoimmunity in murine lupus. Immunol. Today 3:187, 1982.

101. Bocchieri, M.H., Cooke, A., Smith, J.B., Weigert, M., and Riblet, R.J.: Independent segregation of NZB autoimmune abnormalities in NZBxC58 recombinant inbred mice. Eur. J. Immunol. 12:349, 1982.

102. Rosenthal, A.S., and Shevach, E.M.: Function of macrophages in antigen recognition by guinea pig T lymphocytes. I. Requirements for histocompatible macrophages and lymphocytes. J. Exp. Med. 138:1194, 1973.

103. Yano, A., Schwartz, R.H., and Paul, W.E.: Antigen presentation in the murine T-lymphocyte proliferative response. I. Requirements for genetic identity at the major histocompatibility complex. J. Exp. Med. 146:828, 1977.

104. Shevach, E.M., and Rosenthal, A.S.: Function of macrophages in antigen recognition by guinea pig T lymphocytes. II. Role of the macrophage in the regulation of genetic control of the immune response. J. Exp. Med. 138:1213, 1973.

105. Cowing, C., Pincus, S.H., Sachs, D.H., and Dickler, H.B.: A subpopulation of adherent accessory cells bearing both I-A and I-E or C subregion antigens is required for antigen specific murine T lymphocyte proliferation. J. Immunol. 121:1680, 1978.

106. Schwartz, R.H., David, C.S., Sachs, D.H., and Paul, W.E.: T lymphocyte-enriched murine peritoneal exudate cells. III. Inhibition of antigen-induced T lymphocyte proliferation with anti-Ia antisera. J. Immunol. 117:531, 1976.

107. Cantor, H., and Boyse, E.A.: Functional subclasses of T lymphocytes bearing different Ly antigens. J. Exp. Med. 141:1376, 1975.

108. Shearer, G.M.: Cell mediated cytotoxicity to trinitrophenyl modified syngeneic lymphocytes. Eur. J. Immunol. 4:527, 1974.

109. Bevan, M.J.: The major histocompatibility complex determines susceptibility to cytotoxic T-cells directed against minor histocompatibility antigens. J. Exp. Med. 142:1349, 1975.

110. Bergholtz, B.O., and Thorsby, E.: HLA-D restriction of the macrophage-dependent response of immune human T lymphocytes to PPD in vitro. Inhibition by anti-HLA-DR antisera. Scand. J. Immunol. 8:63, 1978.

111. Kurnick, J.T., Altevogt, P., Lindblom, J., Sjöberg, O., Danneus, A., and Wigzell, H.: Long-term maintainance of HLA-D restricted T cells specific for soluble antigens. Scand. J. Immunol. 11:131, 1980.

112. Breard, J., Fuks, A., Friedman, S.M., Schlossman, S.F., and Chess, L.: The role of p23,30 bearing human macrophages in antigen induced T lymphocyte responses. Cell. Immunol. 45:108, 1979.

113. Sredni, B., Volkman, D., Schwartz, R.H., and Fauci, A.S.: Antigen-specific human T-cell clones. Development of clones requiring HLA-DR-compatible presenting cells for stimulation in presence of antigen. Proc. Natl. Acad. Sci. USA 78:1858, 1981.

114. Corte, G., Moretta, A., Cosulich, M.E., Ramarli, D., and Bargellesi, A.: A monoclonal anti-DC1 antibody selectively inhibits the generation of effector T cells mediating specific cytolytic activity. J. Exp. Med. 156:1539, 1982.

115. Berle, E.J., and Thorsby, E.: Both DR and MT class II HLA molecules may restrict proliferative T-lymphocyte responses to antigen. Scand. J. Immunol. 16:543, 1982.

116. Gonwa, T.A., Picker, L.J., Raff, H.V., Goyert, S.M., Silver, J., and Stobo, J.: Antigen-presenting capabilities of human monocytes correlates with their expression of HLA-DS, an Ia-determinant distinct from HLA-DR. J. Immunol. 130:706, 1983.

117. Kappler, J.W., Skidmore, B., White, J., and Marrack, P.: Antigen-inducible, H-2 restricted, IL-2-producing T cell hybridomas. Lack of independent antigen and H-2 recognition. J. Exp. Med. 153:1198, 1981.

118. Rosenthal, A.S.: Determinant selection and macrophage function in genetic control of the immune response. Immunol. Rev. 40:136, 1978.

119. Benacerraf, B.: A hypothesis to relate the specificity of T-lymphocytes and the activity of I region-specific Ir genes in macrophages and B lymphocytes. J. Immunol. 120:1809, 1978.

120. Schwartz, R.H.: A clonal deletion model for Ir gene control of the immune response. Scand. J. Immunol. 7:3, 1978.

121. Singer, A., Hathcock, K.S., and Hodes, R.J.: Self recognition in allogeneic radiation bone marrow chimeras. A radiation-resistant host element dictates the self specificity and immune response gene phenotype of T-helper cells J. Exp. Med. 153:1286, 1981.

122. Ishii, N., Baxevanis, C.N., Nagy, Z.A., and Klein, J.: Responder T cells depleted of alloreactive cells react to antigen presented on allogeneic macrophages from nonresponder strains. J. Exp. Med. 154:978, 1981.

123. Clark, R.B., and Shevach, E.M.: Generation of T cell colonies from responder strain 2 guinea pigs that recognize the copolymer L-glutamic acid, L-lysine in association with nonresponder strain 13 Ia antigens. J. Exp. Med. 155:635, 1982.

124. Dos Reis, G.A., and Shevach, E.M.: Antigen-presenting cells from nonresponder strain 2 guinea pigs are fully competent to present bovine insulin B chain to responder strain 13 T cells. Evidence against a determinant selection model and in favor of a clonal deletion model of immune response gene function. J. Exp. Med. 157:1287, 1983.

125. Dreyer, W.J., and Bennett, J.C.: The molecular basis of antibody formation. A paradox. Proc. Natl. Acad. Sci. USA 54:854, 1965.

126. Croce, C.M., Shandler, M., Martinis, J., Cicurel, L., D'Ancona, G.G., Dolby, T.W., and Koprowski, H.: Chromosomal location of the genes for human immunoglobulin heavy chains. Proc. Natl. Acad. Sci. USA 76:3416, 1979.

127. Crews, S., Griffin, J., Huang, H., Calame, K., and Hood, L.: A single V_H gene segment encodes the immune response to phosphorylcholine: Somatic mutation is correlated with the class of the antibody. Cell 25:59, 1981.

128. Sakano, H., Kurosawa, Y., Weigert, M., and Tonegawa, S.: Identification and nucleotide sequence of a diversity DNA segment (D) of immunoglobulin heavy-chain genes. Nature 290:562, 1981.

129. Kurosawa, Y., von Boehmer, H., Haas, W., Sakano, H., Trauneker, A., and Tonegawa, S.: Identification of D segments of immunoglobulin heavy-chain genes and their rearrangement in T lymphocytes. Nature 290:565, 1981.

130. Kurosawa, Y., and Tonegawa, S.: Organization, structure, and assembly of immunoglobulin heavy chain diversity DNA segments. J. Exp. Med. 155:201, 1982.

131. Ravetch, J.V., Siebenlist, U., Korsmeyer, S., Waldmann, T., and Leder, P.: Structure of the human immunoglobulin μ locus. Characterization of embryonic and rearranged J and D genes. Cell 27:583, 1981.

132. Flanagan, J.G., and Rabbitts, T.H.: Arrangement of human immunoglobulin heavy chain constant region genes implies evolutionary duplication of a segment containing γ, ε and α genes. Nature 300:709, 1982.

133. McBride, O.W., Hieter, P.A., Hollis, G.F., Swan, D., Otey, M.C., and Leder, P.: Chromosomal location of human kappa and lambda immunoglobulin light chain constant region genes. J. Exp. Med. 155:1480, 1982.

134. Bentley, D.L., and Rabbitts, T.H.: Human V_K immunoglobulin gene number. Implication for the origin of antibody diversity. Cell 24:613, 1981.

135. Hieter, P.A., Maizel, J.V., and Leder, P.: Evolution of human immunoglobulin κ J region genes. J. Biol. Chem. 257:1516, 1982.

136. Honjo, T.: Immunoglobulin genes. Ann. Rev. Immunol. 1:499, 1983.

137. Hieter, P.A., Hollis, G.F., Korsmeyer, S.J., Waldmann, T.A., and Leder, P.: Clustered arrangement of immunoglobulin λ constant region genes in man. Nature 294:536, 1981.

138. Miller, J., Selsing, E., and Storb, U.: Structural alterations in J regions of mouse immunoglobulin λ genes are associated with differential gene expression. Nature 295:428, 1982.

139. Blomberg, B., and Tonegawa, S.: DNA sequences of the joining regions of mouse λ light chain immunoglobulin genes. Proc. Natl. Acad. Sci. USA 79:530, 1982.

140. Gearhart, P.J.: Generation of immunoglobulin variable region diversity. Immunol. Today 3:107, 1982.

141. Bothwell, A.L.M., Paskind, M., Reth, M., Imanishi-Kari, T., Rajewsky, K., and Baltimore, D.: Somatic variants of murine immunoglobulin λ light chains. Nature 298:380, 1982.

142. Early, P., Huang, H., Davis, M., Calame, K., and Hood, L.: An immunoglobulin heavy chain variable region gene is generated from three segments of DNA: V_H, D and J_H. Cell 19:981, 1980.

143. Korsmeyer, S.J., Hieter, P.A., Ravetch, J.V., Poplack, D.G., Waldmann, T.A., and Leder, P.: Developmental hierarchy of immunoglobulin gene

rearrangements in human leukemic pre-B-cells. Proc. Natl. Acad. Sci. USA 78:7096, 1981.

144. Hieter, P.A., Korsmeyer, S.J., Waldmann, T.A., and Leder, P.: Human immunoglobulin κ light-chain genes are deleted or rearranged in λ-producing B cells. Nature 290:368, 1981.

145. Korsmeyer, S.J., Arnold, A., Bakhshi, A., Ravetch, J.V., Siebenlist, U., Hieter, P., Sharrow, S.O., LeBien, T.W., Kersey, J.H., Poplack, D.G., Leder, P., and Waldmann, T.A.: Immunoglobulin gene rearrangement and cell surface antigen expression in acute lymphocytic leukemias of T cell and B cell precursor origins. J. Clin. Invest. 71:301, 1983.

146. Moore, K.W., Rogers, J., Hunkapiller, T., Early, P., Nottenburg, C., Weissman, I., Bazir, H., Wall, R., and Hood, L.E.: Expression of IgD may use both DNA rearrangement and RNA splicing mechanisms. Proc. Natl. Acad. Sci. USA 78:1800, 1981.

147. Maki, R., Roeder, W., Traunecker, A., Sidman, C., Wabl, M., Rasehke, W., and Tonegawa, S.: The role of DNA rearrangement and alternative RNA processing in the expression of immunoglobulin delta genes. Cell 24:353, 1981.

148. Yaoita, Y., Kumagai, Y., Okumura, K., and Honjo, T.: Expression of lymphocyte surface IgE does not require switch recombination. Nature 297:697, 1982.

149. Nikaido, T., Nakai, S., and Honjo, T.: The switch (S) region of the immunoglobulin Cμ gene is composed of simple tandem repetitive sequences. Nature 292:845, 1981.

150. Nakaido, T., Yamawaki-Kataoka, Y., and Honjo, T.: Nucleotide sequences of switch regions of immunoglobulin Cε and Cγ genes and their comparison. J. Biol. Chem. 257:7322, 1982.

151. Kataoka, T., Miyata, T., and Honjo, T.: Repetitive sequences in class-switch recombination regions of immunoglobulin heavy chain genes. Cell 23:357, 1981.

152. Dunnick, W., Rabbitts, T.H., and Milstein, C.: An immunoglobulin deletion mutant with implications for the heavy chain switch and RNA splicing. Nature 286:669, 1980.

153. Kincade, P.W., and Cooper, M.D.: Development and distribution of immunoglobulin-containing cells in the chicken. An immunofluorescent analysis using purified antibodies to μ, γ and light chains. J. Immunol. 106:371, 1971.

154. Vogler, L.B., Gathings, W.E., Preud'homme, J.L., Bollum, F.J., Crist, W.M., Seligmann, M., and Cooper, M.D.: Diversity of immunoglobulin expression in leukaemic cells resembling B lymphocyte precursors. Nature 290:339, 1981.

155. Craig, S.W., and Cebra, J.J.: Peyer's patches. An enriched source of precursors for IgA-producing immunocytes in the rabbit. J. Exp. Med. 134:188, 1971.

156. Kawanishi, H., Saltzman, L.E., and Strober, W.: Mechanisms regulating IgA class-specific immunoglobulin production in murine gut-associated lymphoid tissues. I. T cells derived from Peyer's patches that switch sIgM B cells to sIgA B cells in vitro. J. Exp. Med. 157:433, 1983.

157. Isakson, P.C., Pure, E., Vitetta, E.S., and Krammer, P.H.: T cell derived B cell differentiation factor(s). Effect on the isotype switch of murine B cells. J. Exp. Med. 155:734, 1982.

158. Pure, E., Isakson, P.C., Kappler, J.W., Marrack, P., Krammer, P.H., and Vitetta, E.S.: T cell derived B cell growth and differentiation factors. Dichotomy between the responsiveness of B cells from adult and neonatal mice. J. Exp. Med. 157:600, 1983.

159. Mongini, P.K., Paul, W.E., and Metcalf, E.S.: T cell regulation of immunoglobulin class expression in the antibody response to trinitrophenyl-Ficoll. Evidence for T cell enhancement of the immunoglobulin class switch. J. Exp. Med. 155:884, 1982.

160. Binz, H., and Wigzell, H.: Antigen-binding, idiotypic T-lymphocyte receptors. Contemp. Top. Immunobiol. 7:113, 1977.

161. Rajewski, K.: Genetics, expression, and function of idiotypes. Ann. Rev. Immunol. 1:569, 1983.

162. Krammer, P.H.: The T cell receptor problem. Curr. Top. Microbiol. 91:179, 1981.

163. Binz, H., Wigzell, H., and Bazin, H.: T-cell idiotypes are linked to immunoglobulin heavy chain genes. Nature 264:639, 1976.

164. Bach, B.A., Greene, M.I., Benacerraf, B., and Nisonoff, A.: Mechanisms of regulation of cell-mediated immunity. IV. Azobenzenearsonate-specific suppressor factor(s) bear cross-reactive idiotypic determinants the expression of which is linked to the heavy-chain allotype linkage group of genes. J. Exp. Med. 149:1084, 1979.

165. Mozes, E., and Haimovich, J.: Antigen specific T-cell helper factor cross reacts idiotypically with antibodies of the same specificity. Nature 278:56, 1979.

166. Suzan, M., Boned, A., Lieberkind, J., Valsted, F., and Rubin, B.: The 5936 Ig-idiotype(s): Genetic linkage to Ig-C_H loci, T cell-dependence of synthesis and possible specificities. Scand. J. Immunol. 14:673, 1981.

167. Owen, F.L., Finnergar, A., Gates, E.R., and Gottlieb, P.D.: A mature T lymphocyte subpopulation marker closely linked to the Igh-1 allotype C_H locus. Eur. J. Immunol. 9:948, 1979.

168. Spurll, G.M., and Owen, F.L.: A family of T cell alloantigens linked to Igh-1. Nature 293:742, 1981.

169. Owen, F.L., Riblet, R., and Taylor, B.A.: The T suppressor cell alloantigen Tsu^d maps near immunoglobulin allotype genes and may be a heavy chain constant region marker on a T cell receptor. J. Exp. Med. 153:801, 1981.

170. Tokuhisa, T., Komatsu, Y., Uchida, Y., and Taniguchi, M.: Monoclonal alloantibodies specific for the constant region of T cell antigen receptors. J. Exp. Med. 156:888, 1982.

171. Kronenberg, M., Kraig, E., Siu, G., Kappa, J.A., Kappler, J., Marrack, P., Pierce, C.W., and Hood, L.: Three T-cell hybridomas do not contain detectable heavy chain variable gene transcripts. J. Exp. Med., in press.

172. Kraig, E., Kronenberg, M., Kapp, J.A., Pierce, C.W., Abruzzini, A.F., Sorensen, C.M., Samelson, L.E., Schwartz, R.H., and Hood, L.E.: GAT-specific T and B cells do not transcribe similar heavy chain variable region gene segments. J. Exp. Med., in press.

173. Kunkel, H.G., Mannik, M., and Williams, R.C.: Individual antigenic specificity of isolated antibodies. Science 140:1218, 1963.

174. Oudin, J., and Michel, M.: Une nouvelle forme d'allotypie des globulines du sérum de lapin, apparemment liée à la fonction et la spécifité anticorps. Compt. Rend. Acad. Sci. 257:805, 1963.

175. Blomberg, B., Geckelev, W.R., and Weigert, M.: Genetics of the antibody response to dextran in mice. Science 177:178, 1972.

176. Riblet, R., Blomberg, B., Weigert, M., Lieberman, R., Taylor, B.A., and Potter, M.: Genetics of mouse antibodies. I. Linkage of the dextran response locus, V_H-Dex, to allotype. Eur. J. Immunol. 5:775, 1975.

177. Nisonoff, A., Ju, S.-T., and Owen, F.L.: Studies of structure and immunosuppression of a cross-reactive idiotype in strain A mice. Immunol. Rev. 34:89, 1977.

178. Lieberman, R., Potter, M., Mushinski, E.B., Humphrey, W. Jr., and Rudikoff, S.: Genetics of a new IgV_H (T15 idiotype) marker in the mouse regulating natural antibody to phosphorylcholine. J. Exp. Med. 139:983, 1974.

179. Cosenza, H., Julius, M.H., and Augustin, A.A.: Idiotypes as variable region markers: Analogies between receptors on phosphorylcholine-specific T and B lymphocytes. Immunol. Rev. 34:3, 1977.

180. Jack, R.S., Imanishi-Kari, T., and Rajewsky, K.: Idiotypic analysis of the response of C57BL/6 mice to the (4-hydroxy-3-nitrophenyl) acetyl group. Eur. J. Immunol. 7:559, 1977.

181. Mäkelä, O., and Karjalainen, K.: Inherited immunoglobulin idiotypes of the mouse. Immunol. Rev. 34:119, 1977.

182. Juy, D., Primi, D., Sanchez, P., and Cazenave, P.-A.: The selection and maintenance of the V region determinant repertoire is germ-line encoded and T cell-independent. Eur. J. Immunol. 13:326, 1983.

183. LeGuern, C., BenAissa, F., Juy, D., Mariamé, B., Buttin, G., and Cazenzve, P.A.: Expression and induction of MOPC-460 idiotypes in different strains of mice. Ann. Immunol. (Paris) 130C:193, 1979.

184. Bona, C., Hooghe, R., Cazenave, P.A., LeGuern, C., and Paul, W.E.: Cellular basis of regulation of expression of idiotype. II. Immunity to anti-MOPC-460 idiotype antibodies increases the level of anti-trinitrophenyl antibodies bearing 460 idiotypes. J. Exp. Med. 149:815, 1979.

185. Bona, C., Heber-Katz, E., and Paul, W.E.: Idiotype-anti-idiotype regulation. I. Immunization with a levan-binding myeloma protein leads to the appearance of auto-anti-(anti-idiotype) antibodies and to the activation of silent clones. J. Exp. Med. 153:951, 1981.

186. Miller, G.G., Nadler, P.I., Hodes, R.J., and Sachs, D.H.: Modification of T cell antinuclease idiotype expression by in vivo administration of anti-idiotype. J. Exp. Med. 155:190, 1982.

187. Juy, D., Primi, D., Sanchez, P., and Cazenave, P.A.: Idiotype regulation. Evidence for the involvement of Igh-C-restricted T cells in the M-460 idiotype suppressive pathway. Eur. J. Immunol. 12:24, 1982.

188. Rubinstein, L.J., Yeh, M., and Bona, C.: Idiotype-anti-idiotype network. II. Activation of silent clones by treatment at birth with idiotypes is associated with the expansion of idiotype specific helper T-cells. J. Exp. Med. 156:506, 1982.

189. Eichmann, K., Falk, I., and Rajewsky, K.: Recognition of idiotypes in lymphocyte interactions. II. Antigen-dependent cooperation between T-and B-lymphocytes that possess similar and complementary idiotypes. Eur. J. Immunol. 8:853, 1978.

190. Jerne, N.K.: Towards a network theory of the immune response. Ann. Immunol. (Paris) 125C:373, 1974.

191. Wells, J.V., Fudenberg, H.H., and MacKay, I.R.: Relation of the human antibody response to flagellin to Gm genotype. J. Immunol. 107:1505, 1971.

192. Whittingham, S., Mathews, J.D., Schanfield, M.S., Matthews, J.V., Tait, B.D., Morris, P.J., and MacKay, I.R.: Interactive effect of Gm allotypes and HLA-B locus antigens on the human antibody response to a bacterial antigen. Clin. Exp. Immunol. 40:8, 1980.

193. Pandey, J.P., Fudenberg, H.H., Virella, G., Kyong, C.U., Loadholt, C.B., Galbraith, R.M., Gotschlich, E.C., and Parke, J.C.: Association between immunoglobulin allotypes and immune responses to Haemophilus influenza and meningococcus polysaccharides. Lancet I:190, 1979.

194. Pandey, J.P., Zollinger, W.D., Fudenberg, H.H., and Loadholt, C.B.:

Immunoglobulin allotypes and immune responses to meningococcal group B polysaccharide. J. Clin. Invest. 68:1378, 1981.

195. Nakao, Y., Matsumoto, H., Miyazaki, T., Nishitani, H., Takatsuki, K., Kasukawa, R., Nakayama, S., Izumi, S., Fujita, T., and Tsuji, K.: IgG heavy chain allotypes (Gm) in autoimmune diseases. Clin. Exp. Immunol. 42:20, 1980.

196. Whittingham, S., Mathews, J.D., Schanfield, M.S., Tait, B.D., and MacKay, I.R.: Interaction of HLA and Gm in autoimmune chronic active hepatitis. Clin. Exp. Immunol. 43:80, 1980.

197. Uno, H., Sasazuki, T., Tamai, H., and Matsumoto, H.: Two major genes, linked to HLA and Gm, control susceptibility to Grave's disease. Nature 292:768, 1981.

198. Whittingham, S., Mathews, J.D., Schanfield, M.S., Tait, B.D., and MacKay, I.R.: HLA and Gm genes in systemic lupus erythematosus. Tissue Antigens 21:50, 1983.

199. Pandey, J.P., Goust, J.-M., Salier, J.-P., and Fudenberg, H.H.: Immunoglobulin G heavy chain (Gm) allotypes in multiple sclerosis. J. Clin. Invest. 67:1797, 1981.

200. Holmberg, D., Ivars, F., and Coutinho, A.: An example of major histocompatibility complex-linked control of idiotype interactions. Eur. J. Immunol. 13:82, 1983.

Chapter 6

Low Molecular Weight Mediators of Inflammation: Prostaglandins, Leukotrienes, and Cyclic Nucleotides

Dwight R. Robinson

INTRODUCTION

The numerous and varied events that constitute an inflammatory reaction involve several soluble mediators influencing cellular activity. Vasodilatation, vascular permeability, chemotaxis, cell proliferation, phagocytosis, and other functions may be modified by a number of chemical and hormonal agents or messengers. In any particular inflammatory reaction, however, it may be difficult to determine the relative importance of any given agent acting as a mediator or regulator. It becomes important to know which mediators are of greatest significance, since the inhibition or stimulation of these agents may provide a basis for the rational design or choice of anti-inflammatory drugs. Prostaglandins, leukotrienes, and cyclic nucleotides have a wide variety of physiologic effects involving essentially all human tissues. Some of these effects appear to be important factors in the development of inflammatory reactions and in the mechanisms of action of anti-inflammatory drugs. In this chapter we will briefly review certain aspects of prostaglandin, leukotriene, and cyclic nucleotide biochemistry and physiology and their possible contributions to the pathogenesis of the inflammatory rheumatic diseases.

PROSTAGLANDIN BIOCHEMISTRY

Prostaglandins (PGs) and thromboxanes and their metabolites comprise a large number of compounds, and only a few of the most important of these will be con-

sidered here (Fig. 6–1). The prostaglandins are 20-carbon fatty acid derivatives characterized by a 5-membered ring. They are designated alphabetically (e.g., PGE and PGF) depending upon the structure and substituents on the 5-membered ring and further by numerical subscripts (e.g., PGE_1, PGE_2), which refer to the number of double bonds in the aliphatic limbs of each compound. The compounds shown in Figure 6–1 are all of the 2 series, containing two double bonds in their aliphatic side chains, and these appear to be the most important, although compounds of the 1 and 3 series also occur in nature. Thromboxane A_2 differs from prostaglandins by possessing a 6-membered ring structure. The subscript α, in $PGF_{2\alpha}$, refers to the steric configuration of the two hydroxy substituents on the 5-membered ring.[1-3]

The pathway of synthesis of PGs is also briefly outlined in Figure 6–1. Prostaglandins are not stored in tissues to any appreciable extent. Their precursors, arachidonic acid in the case of compounds of the 2 series, are stored in cell membranes in the form of complex lipids, primarily phospholipids (I). Under the

$$H_2COOCR_1$$
$$|$$
$$HCOOCR_2$$
$$|$$
$$H_2COPO_3R_3$$

I

influence of certain stimuli, such as tissue injury, activation of the phospholipase enzymes occurs, hydrolyzing

Figure 6–1. Formation of prostaglandins and thromboxane A_2 from arachidonic acid in phospholipids.

arachidonic acid from its ester linkage, on the two position of glycerol in phospholipids (I, R_2).

Having been released from phospholipids through the action of phospholipase, arachidonic acid becomes available for the first reaction on the pathway of PG and thromboxane synthesis, catalyzed by the enzyme cyclooxygenase. This is a complex reaction involving the addition of two molecules of oxygen to arachidonic acid, with closure of the 5-membered ring to form PGG_2. Subsequently the peroxy group at the 15 position is reduced to the 15 hydroxy group to form PGH_2.[1-3]

The endoperoxide PGH_2 is a key intermediate in PG synthesis because the other prostaglandins arise from PGH_2 by the action of enzymes generally termed isomerases. The amount of each PG or thromboxane produced is determined by the activities of these different isomerase enzymes present in each tissue. For example, platelets produce primarily thromboxane A_2 and only small quantities of the classic prostaglandins PGE_2 and $PGF_{2\alpha}$; vascular tissues, predominantly PGI_2 (prostacyclin);[4] and rheumatoid synovial tissue, mainly PGE_2.[5]

METABOLISM

Prostaglandins are generally labile in tissues. Some, such as the classic PGs, PGE_2 and $PGF_{2\alpha}$, are chemically stable but are rapidly hydrolyzed to inactive metabolites in the circulation. Others, including the prostaglandin endoperoxides, thromboxane A_2 and prostacyclin, are chemically labile, with half-lives ranging from about 30 seconds to a few minutes under physiologic conditions.[6-8] In addition, the breakdown of these labile compounds to inactive metabolites may be further accelerated by enzyme action.

The classic PGs are metabolized rapidly, having a half-life in the circulation of less than 30 seconds. Some of the major metabolites of PGE_2 are shown in Figure 6–2, and similar products are formed from metabolism of $PGF_{2\alpha}$. Most of the biological activities of PGE_2 are reduced or eliminated by the first metabolic step, the formation of 15-keto-PGE_2 by the oxidation of the 15-hydroxy group of PGE_2 catalyzed by the enzyme 15-hydroxy-prostanoate dehydrogenase utilizing NAD or NADH coenzymes. This compound is reduced by the Δ_{13}-reductase to form 13,14-dihydro-15-keto-PGE_2. After several steps a major portion of PGE_2 released into the blood is converted to the 16-carbon decarboxylic acid PGE-M and excreted in the urine. Several other compounds are formed in smaller amounts and will not be considered here. Measurements of the PGE-M levels in urine have been used as a measure of total PGE synthesis. Measurements of the 13,14-dihydro-15-keto metabolites of $PGF_{2\alpha}$ and PGE_2 in blood have similarly been used as a measure of PG synthesis, since these compounds are more stable than their parent PGs and are not formed artifactually during sampling of blood.[3,9]

Thromboxane A_2 is rapidly hydrolyzed to thromboxane B_2, giving a half-life of thromboxane A_2 of about 30 seconds under physiologic conditions. Thromboxane B_2 is reasonably stable in biologic fluids, and its levels may provide a good estimate of thromboxane A_2 production. Finally, prostacyclin (PGI_2) is also labile, with a half-life of about 2 minutes under physiologic conditions. It is hydrolyzed to 6-keto-$PGF_{1\alpha}$ in an acid-catalyzed reaction with loss of most biologic activity.[3,9]

These and other observations of the synthesis and metabolism of PGs lead to some general conclusions relating to the functions of these compounds in tissues. Nearly all cells and tissues are capable of synthesizing PGs. They are not stored in tissues but are synthesized in response to certain stimuli. The PGs synthesized are released to interact with neighboring cells, possibly through contact with specific PG receptors on cell surfaces. Because of the lability of PGs it seems unlikely that they often have effects at sites distant from their cells of origin, especially by way of the circulation.

CYCLIC NUCLEOTIDE BIOCHEMISTRY

The cyclic nucleotides also have a widespread distribution throughout the animal kingdom and are present in nearly all human tissues. They have a wide variety of physiologic effects and are regulated by a large number of hormones and other agents. Two cyclic nucleotides are important in human biology, adenosine 3',5'-cyclic monophosphate (cAMP) and guanosine 3',5'-cyclic monophosphate (cGMP).

The levels of cyclic nucleotides in tissues are regulated

Figure 6–2. Major metabolic products of prostaglandin E_2.

by their rates of synthesis and degradation. Cyclic AMP is synthesized from adenosine triphosphate by the enzyme adenylate cyclase (Fig. 6–3). This enzyme consists of regulatory and catalytic subunits and is located within the plasma membrane of cells. The regulatory subunit is exposed to the cell surface and contains receptors for several different hormones. Interaction of hormones at the cell surface with receptors on the regulatory subunit modulates the activity of the catalytic subunit near the interior of the plasma membrane. Adenylate cyclase is subject to multivalent regulation by many hormones, but the specificity for the hormones recognized varies with different tissues.[10]

Degradation of cAMP is accomplished by phosphodiesterases catalyzing the hydrolysis of the cyclic phosphate diester linkage of cAMP to form 5'-adenosine monophosphate (5'-AMP).[11] These enzymes are also widely distributed in human tissues and are present in both soluble and membrane fractions of cells. Regulation of cAMP levels in cells could result from control of either synthesis or degradation steps. In general, regulation of cAMP levels by hormones is accomplished primarily by changes in adenylate cyclase activity rather than by changes in phosphodiesterase. Changes in phosphodiesterase activity may also be responsible for changes in cAMP levels. For example, many of the effects of methylxanthines such as theophylline have been attributed to inhibition of phosphodiesterase, leading to elevations in tissue levels of cAMP.[11]

The other cyclic nucleotide of importance is cyclic GMP, although its biological functions are not well established at present. It has effects on tissues which are often opposite or antagonistic to those of cAMP. Cyclic GMP is synthesized from guanosine triphosphate in a reaction resembling the synthesis of cAMP. The reaction is catalyzed by the enzyme guanylate

$$\text{GTP} \xrightarrow[\text{Mn}^{++}]{\genfrac{}{}{0pt}{}{\text{Guanylate}}{\text{cyclase}}} \text{cGMP} \xrightarrow{\genfrac{}{}{0pt}{}{\text{Phospho-}}{\text{diesterase}}} \text{5'-GMP} \qquad (1)$$

$$+$$

$$\text{pyrophosphate}$$

Figure 6–3. Synthesis and degradation of adenosine 3',5'-cyclic monophosphate (cAMP).

cyclase with the cofactor, manganous ion (Eq. 1). The enzyme is distinct from adenylate cyclase and differs in several of its properties. Guanylate cyclase is widely distributed in tissues and is present in both soluble and membrane fractions. One of the major differences between adenylate and guanylate cyclases is the lack of sensitivity of isolated guanylate cyclase in cell fractions to hormonal and other agents, although many of these same agents elevate cGMP levels in intact cells and tissues. The degradation of cGMP is catalyzed by phosphodiesterases, which in some cases are specific for the guanyl moiety and have little or no activity on cAMP. Other phosphodiesterases exist which are active toward both cyclic nucleotides. Cyclic GMP phosphodiesterases are also inhibited by methylxanthines.[11]

FUNCTIONS OF CYCLIC NUCLEOTIDES

Cyclic AMP probably acts as a mediator of the actions of a wide variety of hormones and other agents in essentially all tissues. A few of these hormonal agents are adrenergic agents, glucagon, parathyroid hormone, ACTH, prostaglandins E_1, E_2, D_2, I_2, and the PG endoperoxides. $PGF_{2\alpha}$ is essentially inactive toward adenylate cyclase. The specificity of hormone effects appears to be related to the presence of specific hormone receptors on the regulatory subunits of adenylate cyclase in the cell membranes of appropriate tissues, leading to activation of cell functions in response to adenylate cyclase activation and elevation of cellular cAMP levels. There may be multivalent regulation of adenylate cyclase brought about by receptors for several hormones on each adenylate cyclase enzyme, at least in some tissues.[10]

The biologic effects of changes in cAMP levels in cells are thought to be a consequence of the activation of various cyclic AMP dependent protein kinases, leading in turn to specific protein phosphorylation. The formation of these phosphoproteins may be the basis for the physiologic effects of cAMP.[10,12]

Many tissue functions have been associated with changes in levels of cGMP, although they are not as varied as functions influenced by cAMP. Some of the changes associated with elevations of cGMP levels include the stimulation of secretion of lysosomal enzymes, enhancement of cardiac contractility, stimulation of neuronal excitability, and promotion of inflammatory responses. The biochemical events following changes in cGMP have not been as well characterized, but evidence indicates that similar reactions to those following cAMP stimulation occur. Cyclic GMP activates certain protein kinases that are independent of cAMP, and these could provide the basis for physiologic effects of cGMP.[13,14]

Numerous factors are known to elevate cGMP levels in tissues, including certain hormonal agents, oxidants or substances with oxidizing potential, free radicals, and fatty acids, especially arachidonic acid. Prostaglandin stimulation of cGMP is usually limited to $PGF_{2\alpha}$, or possibly also to PGG_2 because of the oxidizing potential of the latter. The E prostaglandins are ineffective toward cGMP.[14]

Observations with several systems have shown that cAMP and cGMP frequently act antagonistically. It was proposed by Goldberg that the cyclic nucleotides act as opposite limbs of a bidirectional regulatory system in many tissues. For example, cyclic GMP or cholinergic agents leading to elevations of tissue cGMP levels suppress contraction of cardiac muscles, whereas cAMP or β-adrenergic agents stimulating cAMP levels augment cardiac contractility. Other examples will be described below when considering inflammation. The opposing effects of stimulating cAMP and cGMP have been referred to as the Yin-Yang hypothesis, but the role of this mechanism of control of biologic functions remains controversial.[14]

LEUKOTRIENES AND OTHER LIPOXYGENASE PRODUCTS

Several other products besides PGs are formed from reactions of polyunsaturated fatty acids with oxygen. Molecular oxygen may react at one of several positions of arachidonic acid to form hydroperoxy- and hydroxy-derivatives, catalyzed by lipoxygenase enzymes. An example is the reaction shown in Figure 6–4, in which oxygen reacts at the 12 position of arachidonic acid to form 12-hydroperoxyeicosatetraenoic acid (HPETE). A subsequent peroxidase-catalyzed reaction reduces HPETE to 12-hydroxytetraenoic acid (HETE), and as a by-product forms an oxygen free radical, most likely a hydroxyl radical. Oxygen-free radicals are highly reactive and have been postulated to contribute to tissue injury during inflammatory reactions.[15] A similar peroxidase reaction occurs on the pathway of PG synthesis during the conversion of PGG_2 to PGH_2 (Fig. 6–1). Therefore some contributions to events occurring in inflammatory reactions may be mediated by free radical by-products as well as by the PGs and LTs themselves.

Inhibition of the peroxidase reaction converting 12-HPETE to 12-HETE (Fig. 6–4) has been described for aspirin, indomethacin, and sodium salicylate, and it was suggested that the anti-inflammatory effects of these drugs may be accounted for by inhibition of this peroxidase reaction.[16] However, the concentrations required for inhibition of this reaction were greater than concentrations required to inhibit PG synthesis, and whether peroxidase inhibition contributes significantly to the effects of nonsteroidal anti-inflammatory drugs remains unclear.

The most important lipoxygenase products are derived from the 5-lipoxygenase pathway leading to the biosynthesis of leukotrienes (Fig. 6–5). The name of these compounds is related to their synthesis by leukocytes (leuko) and to the presence of three conjugated or alternating double bonds (triene), which leads to characteristic optical and chemical properties. Each LT derived from arachidonic acid also has a fourth double bond, indicated by the subscript 4, and the letters A through E refer to the nature of substituents on the fatty acid backbone. The first LT on the 5-lipoxygenase pathway is LTA_4. It contains a reactive three-member ring,

Figure 6–4. Formation of 12-hydroperoxyeicosatetraenoic acid (HPETE) and 12-hydroxyeicosatetraenoic acid. These compounds are representative of several hydroperoxy and hydroxy derivatives of arachidonic acid.

an epoxide, which may react either with water at the 12 position to give LTB$_4$, a potent chemotactic agent, or with glutathione at the 6 position, leading to three thionylpeptide derivatives, LTC$_4$, LTD$_4$, and LTE$_4$. The latter three compounds account for the activity of slow-reacting substance of anaphylaxis (SRS-A) and are therefore important mediators of immediate hypersensitivity reactions and other inflammatory processes.[17]

Although the PGs and LTs described thus far have been derived from AA and are quantitatively the most important of these compounds, two other polyunsaturated fatty acids give rise to PGs and lipoxygenase products. These are 20-carbon fatty acids differing from AA in the number of double bonds they possess (Fig. 6–6). Production of the 1 series of PGs (e.g., PGE$_1$) is quantitatively unimportant compared with the 2 series, probably because of the small amounts of its precursor, dihomo-γ-linolenic acid, in tissues. Furthermore, the absence of the double bond in the 5 position of dihomo-γ-linolenic acid eliminates the possibility of forming 5-lipoxygenase products, and for the same reason a prostacyclin analogue cannot be formed. On the other hand, eicosapentaenoic acid, a fatty acid plentiful in marine animals, gives rise to PGs and LTs that are analogues of the AA products but contain an additional double bond at the 17 position (3 carbon atoms from the methyl terminal end of the molecule) (Fig. 6–6). Some of these

compounds have been examined and found to be biologically active, e.g. PGE$_3$, PGI$_3$, TBX$_3$, and LTD$_5$, although usually less active than their AA analogues. These considerations are of some importance in view of recent studies demonstrating that alterations in dietary fatty acids may lead to changes in tissue fatty acid composition and in the biosynthesis of eicosanoids (vide infra).

FUNCTIONS OF PROSTAGLANDINS AND LEUKOTRIENES

The properties and functions of most PGs are well known, although their role in inflammation is incompletely understood. The LTs and HETEs have for the most part been studied recently, and while they have several more potent biologic effects, much remains to be learned about the functions of many of these compounds. The PGs are ubiquitous compounds, produced by every tissue and every cell with the exception of erythrocytes. LTs have been less extensively studied, but are also widespread. Neither class of compounds is stored in cells but is rapidly synthesized and released following appropriate stimuli, including certain hormones, drugs, and cell injury. The life span of most PGs is transient in the circulation. They are rapidly converted

Figure 6–5. The 5-lipoxygenase pathway leading to formation of leukotrienes (LTs). LTA$_4$ reacts with glutathione to form LTC$_4$, LTD$_4$ and LTE$_4$. These three LTs account for the activity of slow-reacting substance of anaphylaxis (SRS-A). Reaction of LTA$_4$ with water forms LTB$_4$, an active chemotactic factor.

ARACHIDONIC ACID

DIHOMO - γ - LINOLENIC ACID

EICOSAPENTAENOIC ACID

Figure 6–6. Structures of all-*cis* polyunsaturated fatty acids which are precursors of prostaglandins and leukotrienes.

to inactive metabolites by dehydrogenase and reductase enzymes, leading to almost complete inactivation, for example, of PGE_2 during one passage through the pulmonary vascular bed.[6] Prostacyclin and thromboxane A_2 are labile compounds and decompose, with half-lives ranging from 30 seconds to a few minutes, respectively, under physiologic conditions.[6-8] However, prostacyclin is not readily inactivated in the pulmonary circulation, in contrast to other PGs.[18] It was thus postulated that prostacyclin may act as a circulating hormone and maintain a continuous antithrombotic effect, but more recent studies have shown that circulating levels of PGE_1 are below the range capable of significant effects on platelet aggregation.[19] It has been difficult to measure PGs by assays of body fluids or tissues. Circulating levels of some PGs have been estimated to be extremely low, on the order of 10^{-11} M, generally below the range of convenient analytical techniques such as radioimmunoassay. Levels of LTs and their metabolites have only recently been investigated and little information is available.

The physiologic effects of PGs and LTs are numerous, with potent action on every organ system. Both families of compounds have effects on smooth muscle in many tissues, and different PGs may act antagonistically. We cannot review the functions of these compounds in any comprehensive way but will outline some that appear to be important for inflammation and for the actions of anti-inflammatory drugs. Several PGs, (PGE_2, PGE_1, PGD_2, PGI_2) are potent vasodilators and probably contribute to the vascular phase of inflammatory reactions. Others, $PGF_{2\alpha}$ and the thromboxane A_2, are vasoconstrictors, the latter being the most potent vasoconstrictor known. The vasodilator PGs, especially PGE_2, potentiate the vasodilatation and increased vascular permeability produced by other mediators, including bradykinin, histamine, the complement component anaphylatoxin, C5a, and LTB_4.[20] Effects of TBA_2 and PGI_2 as regulators of platelet aggregation may also contribute to inflammation under some conditions by modulating the release of mediators from platelets.

The leukotrienes are undoubtedly important mediators of inflammation, and their roles are currently under active investigation. It is clear that the LTs are highly potent agents; for example, LTC_4 aerosol was found to be over 1000-fold more active than histamine in promoting bronchoconstriction in human volunteers.[21] LTC_4, LTD_4, and LTE_4 produce vasoconstriction of small arterioles but are more potent than histamine in increasing permeability of capillaries and venules.[17] The latter property may contribute to the edema of inflammation. Inflammatory cells are the major sources of LTs. Neutrophils produce large quantities of LTB_4, whereas monocyte/macrophages produce large quantities of LTC_4, LTD_4, and LTE_4.[22,23] Many other lipoxygenase products, especially hydroxyl and hydroperoxyl derivatives of arachidonic acid, are produced in tissues, but little is known of their functions at this time.

INFLAMMATION

The arachidonate metabolites and cyclic nucleotides are potentially capable of participating in the pathogenesis of inflammatory reactions of various types, but the actual functions of these substances in inflammation have not been resolved. Several lines of evidence have indicated that prostaglandins, primarily PGE_2 and PGI_2, may act as mediators of inflammatory processes.[24-28] (1) These PGs cause inflammation on injection. They are vasodilators in most systems, and they potentiate the formation of edema induced by other agents. They sensitize tissue to stimulation of pain. They cause fever when injected into the central nervous system of experimental animals. (2) As implied above, the prostaglandins not only act by themselves to produce inflammation but also potentiate several effects of other mediators of inflammation such as bradykinin and histamine.[20] (3) Prostaglandins E_1, E_2, and I_2 have been found in elevated concentrations in inflammatory exudates. (4) The biosynthesis of prostaglandins is strongly inhibited by anti-inflammatory drugs.

Leukotrienes may also contribute to the pathogenesis of inflammation. LTB_4 is a potent chemotactic agent toward leukocytes, including neutrophils, eosinophils, and monocytes. It may act synergistically with vasodilator PGs to increase vascular permeability.[20] The SRS-A LTs (LTC_4, LTD_4, and LTE_4) may contribute to the edema of inflammation by their ability to increase the permeability of the microvascular bed.[17]

In spite of the evidence that certain PGs may promote inflammatory reactions, other evidence indicates that the E prostaglandins may have anti-inflammatory properties. This has most often been proposed for immune reactions and their regulation by cyclic nucleotides. Many immune reactions are suppressed by cAMP or its derivatives, or by agents that elevate levels of cAMP in tissues, such as β-adrenergic agents, methylxanthines, PGE_1, or PGE_2.[29] We will briefly review some of the evidence, examining the effects of cyclic nucleotides and their interactions with PGs on immune reactions and immune-induced inflammation. At the outset it might be noted that many of the effects of PGs may be mediated by their effects on cyclic nucleotides, especially cAMP, since PGE_1 and PGE_2 stimulate adenylate cyclase in many systems. However, it does not necessarily follow that all effects of PGs are mediated through effects on cyclic nucleotides, and in fact, examples have been described in which alterations in cell functions by PGE are not accompanied by changes in cAMP levels.[30,31] Even in systems in which exposure to PGE leads to elevations in cAMP levels, it may be hard to prove (or disprove) that the PG effects are mediated by changes in the cyclic nucleotide.

Several classes of immune reactions are influenced by PGs and/or cyclic nucleotides. Certain reactions of immediate hypersensitivity are suppressed by cAMP derivatives or agents, leading to elevation of cAMP levels in intact animals and in tissue preparation. Antigen-induced histamine and SRS-A release from sensitized human leukocytes and lung preparations are inhibited by cAMP.[29]

A large number of investigations have been carried out examining the effects of PGs and cyclic nucleotides on various aspects of cellular immunity. Elevation of levels of cyclic AMP invariably suppresses in vitro manifestations of cellular immunity.[29] In some systems elevation of cGMP has been shown to augment these reactions.[13] Prostaglandin E_1 or E_2 generally suppresses cellular immunity, often in association with elevation of cAMP.[29] Some of the systems demonstrating these effects are briefly summarized here.

Antibody-dependent lymphocyte-mediated cytotoxicity (K cells) is suppressed by PGE_1 and other agents associated with increased levels of cAMP. A derivative of cGMP augmented this cytotoxic effect.[32] Another form of cellular cytotoxicity, lymphocyte(T cell)-mediated cytotoxicity toward alloantigen-bearing target cells, was inhibited by agents leading to elevation of cAMP and augmented by agents elevating cGMP.[33] Lymphocyte proliferation induced by lectin stimulation is modified by cyclic nucleotides. The effects on B cell mitogenesis in mixed populations of mononuclear cells are indirect, apparently mediated through macrophages. Macrophage-rich preparations release a nondialyzable factor (lymphocyte-activating factor or interleukin 1) that stimulates mitogenesis in the presence of lectins. The release of the lymphocyte-activating factor is suppressed by cAMP and enhanced by cGMP.[34,35] Prostaglandins E_1 and E_2 reduced the antigen-stimulated secretion of macrophage inhibitory factor by lymphocytes. It was not determined whether these effects were associated with changes in cyclic nucleotides.[36]

Several investigators have reported studies of PGs (and cyclic nucleotides) on T lymphocyte mitogenesis. In the studies of Goodwin and colleagues on suppression of lectin-induced mitogenesis of human peripheral blood mononuclear cells, the T lymphocyte mitogen phytohemagglutinin induced mitogenesis, which was suppressed by added PGE_2 at concentrations as low as 10^{-8}M.[37] It was also demonstrated that other mono-

nuclear cells in these preparations secreted sufficient PGE_2 to partially inhibit lectin-induced mitogenesis. Other studies by these investigators have demonstrated a higher degree of suppression of T cell mitogenesis in vitro by the population of prostaglandin E_2-producing mononuclear cells in the peripheral blood of patients with Hodgkin's disease. It was suggested that the deficiency of cellular immunity in patients with Hodgkin's disease may be related to increased activity of PGE_2-producing suppressor cells.[38]

It is not clear whether or not these effects of PGE_2 are mediated through changes in cAMP, since nucleotide levels in these cells were not determined. Earlier work in similar systems has shown that cyclic AMP levels in human lymphocytes are elevated after exposure to phytohemagglutinin, so it is possible that cAMP elevation is associated with PGE_2-induced suppression of lymphocyte mitogenesis in the previous experiments.[39]

Studies directed toward the regulation of antibody production have led to the conclusion that B lymphocyte mitogenesis and antibody production may be regulated by cyclic nucleotides, with cAMP suppression and cGMP stimulation. The effects of B lymphocyte mitogens may be inhibited directly by cyclic AMP elevation in B lymphocytes, whereas B lymphocyte stimulation by antigens may involve T lymphocyte regulation, which is in turn influenced by cyclic nucleotides.[40]

On the other hand, T lymphocyte reactivity may be enhanced by PGE_1, as measured by enhanced production of the lymphokine, osteoclast-activating factor,[41] and by enhanced blastogenic responses of a certain subpopulation of T lymphocytes exposed to PGE_1.[42] Since T lymphocyte subpopulations may either augment (helper-inducer) or inhibit (suppressor) immune reactions, the consequence of an overall suppression of T lymphocyte function on any given immune reaction may be difficult to predict. Recently others have shown that IgM rheumatoid factor production in vitro is inhibited by nonsteroidal anti-inflammatory drugs (NSAIDs), an effect attributed to the reduction of PGE_2-inhibited T helper cell influence on rheumatoid-factor-producing B lymphocytes.[43] Whether this mechanism is important in vivo is unknown at the present time.

There are other in vitro phenomena influenced by PGs and cyclic nucleotides, and these effects may contribute to modification of immune-induced as well as other forms of inflammation. It has been demonstrated that lysosomal enzyme release from polymorphonuclear leukocytes undergoing phagocytosis is influenced by these agents. Elevation of cAMP associated with exposure of cells to PGE_1 or other agents is accompanied by significant reduction in the release of lysosomal enzymes, and cholinergic stimulation leads to elevation of cGMP and augmentation of lysosomal enzyme release.[44,45] Another system is the chemotactic response of polymorphonuclear leukocytes. These cells exposed to chemotactic stimuli have their responsiveness inhibited by cAMP and augmented by cGMP.[46] It is also of interest that the opposite responses are observed with human monocytes; cAMP stimulates chemotaxis and cGMP is inhibitory. The differences between the influences of cyclic nucleotides on the responses of polymorphonuclear leukocytes and monocytes to chemotactic stimuli have been suggested to account for the sequential accumulation of these cell types at sites of inflammation.[47]

It is obvious from even a brief review that there are a large number of laboratory observations indicating that cyclic nucleotides may modulate the inflammatory response. In addition, the consistent observations that the E prostaglandins stimulate cAMP in many (but not all) systems suggest that PGE_1 and PGE_2 may inhibit inflammatory responses under some circumstances. This may seem contradictory to the observations previously described indicating that the E prostaglandins act to promote inflammation. It is possible that PGs may have opposing effects on inflammation under different circumstances or at different times during an inflammatory response.[48,49] It has also been shown that certain forms of inflammation in experimental animals are suppressed by injection of PGE_1. Both adjuvant arthritis in rats and the glomerulonephritis of NZB/NZW hybrid mice are suppressed by repeated injections of PGE_1. Although the mechanisms of these effects are not known, Zurier and co-workers have suggested the hypothesis that in the NZB/NZW mice adenylate cyclase stimulation by PGE_1 may promote thymocyte maturation and thereby relieve a deficiency of suppressor T lymphocytes in these animals.[50-52]

It should be pointed out that most if not all of the experiments discussed here pertaining to effects of cyclic nucleotides on immune and other systems have utilized concentrations of PGs which are pharmacologic, certainly greatly exceeding concentrations of PGs achieved in biologic fluids. It is possible, therefore, that many of the observed phenomena in vitro are irrelevant to events that occur in vivo. At present it is not possible to *prove* that PGs have a role in the pathogenesis of any form of clinical inflammation. While it seems likely that PGs do modulate inflammatory reactions, their functions may be varied and complex.

ANTI-INFLAMMATORY DRUGS

Nonsteroidal Compounds. In 1971 it was first reported that aspirin and related drugs inhibited the synthesis of PGs.[53-55] Since that time a large body of evidence has accumulated in support of the hypothesis of Vane and co-workers that the major effects of these drugs can be accounted for by PG synthesis inhibition.[56] This hypothesis largely rests on correlations that have been established in many tissues between the relative potency of series of compounds as anti-inflammatory agents and their potency as inhibitors of PG synthesis. An example of this kind of correlation is shown in Table 6–1. Here, the relative effectiveness of three drugs on four different forms of experimental inflammation is compared with a microsomal prostaglandin synthesizing system from bovine seminal vesicle. Although the correlation is not exact, the order of effectiveness of the three anti-inflammatory drugs on experimental inflammation and on in vitro PGE_2 synthesis is the same. Furthermore, the specificity of these effects is demonstrated by the lack of effectiveness of the 1-stereoisomer of naproxen either on inflammation or on PG synthesis.[57] Many other similar correlations have been made utilizing a wide variety of tissues with similar results.[58]

Other evidence that PG synthesis inhibition may account for the pharmacologic effects of anti-inflammatory drugs is that the concentrations of these drugs that inhibit PG synthesis are similar to concentrations achieved in plasma during therapy. An example is given in Table 6–2. Rheumatoid synovial fragments in tissue culture produce large quantities of PG, primarily PGE_2, and many anti-inflammatory drugs have been shown to strongly inhibit PG synthesis. The data in Table 6–2 compare concentrations of the drugs required to suppress rheumatoid synovial PGE_2 synthesis by 50 percent (IC_{50}) with plasma concentrations of the same drugs achieved in patients taking therapeutic doses. The total drug concentrations have been corrected for plasma protein binding to give peak free drug concentrations. The concentrations of drugs giving 50 percent inhibition of PGE_2 synthesis by rheumatoid synovium in tissue culture is similar to or lower than the levels of these drugs achieved in plasma.[5] Therefore, it is reasonable to assume that therapeutic doses of these drugs actually inhibit PGE_2 in urine (see Metabolism, above).[59]

Finally, it is worth noting that there is no other persuasive explanation for the mechanism of action of these anti-inflammatory drugs. At present, the most reasonable mechanism appears to be their suppression of PG synthesis, although it is possible that other as yet undiscovered mechanisms may exist.[56]

It has also been found that certain other drugs used for their anti-inflammatory effects in treatment of rheu-

Table 6–1. Pharmacologic Effects of Anti-Inflammatory Drugs Compared with Prostaglandin Synthesis Inhibition*

Compound	Adjuvant Arthritis	Carrageenan	Antipyretic	Analgesic	PGE_2 Synthesis Inhibition BSVM
Indomethacin	2000	48	18	58	2140
Naproxen(d)	200	33	22	7	150
Naproxen(1) (inactive enantiomer)	–	≥1.5		≥0.5	
Aspirin	1	1	1.5	1	2
			1		1

*From Tomlinson, R. W., et al.: Biochem. Biophys. Res. Commun. 46:552, 1972. Relative activity of aspirin set at 1.

Table 6–2. Comparison of Plasma Concentrations of Anti-Inflammatory Drugs During Therapy with Concentrations Inhibiting Prostaglandin Synthesis by Rheumatoid Synovial Cultures*

	Approximate Peak Plasma Concentration In Man (μM)	Plasma Protein Binding (%)	Peak Free Plasma Concentration (μM)	IC_{50}[†] (μM)
Indomethacin	5.0	90	0.5	0.005
Flufenamic acid	53.0	90	5.3	0.2
Ibuprofen	155.0	99	1.6	2.0
D-Naproxen	305.0	99.4	1.8	6.0
Phenylbutazone	320.0	98.0	6.4	10.0
Acetylsalicylic acid	110.0	0	110.0	20.0

*From Robinson, D.R., et al.: Prostaglandins and Medicine 1:461, 1978.
[†]IC_{50} is the concentration of drug giving 50 percent reduction of PGE_2 production by rheumatoid synovial organ cultures.

matic diseases have weak or absent effects on rheumatoid synovial tissue in culture and on other in vitro systems. These drugs include antimalarials, gold, sodium thiomalate, penicillamine, and colchicine. These drugs are relatively specific and have clinical properties differing from the nonsteroidal drugs considered in Table 6–2 and related compounds. These differences suggest that the previous group of drugs acts by different mechanisms, and their lack of potent effects on PG synthesis indicates that PGs are not involved in their mechanisms of action.[5]

Thus far, it can be concluded that NSAIDs have no important effects on LT biosynthesis in the low concentration ranges at which PG synthesis inhibition is observed. The development of effective LT synthesis inhibitors should yield agents with important clinical usefulness in inflammatory, allergic, and other disease states.

Corticosteroids. Recently it has been discovered that anti-inflammatory corticosteroids are also potent inhibitors of PG synthesis in many cells and tissues.[60-63] Effects of corticosteroids on PGE_2 synthesis by rheumatoid synovial tissue culture are summarized in Table 6–3. The inhibitory effects of glucocorticoids are potent, with IC_{50} values in the range of 10^{-8} M. The order of effectiveness in inhibiting PGE_2 synthesis—dexamethasone > prednisolone > hydrocortisone—is the same as the relative anti-inflammatory potency of these drugs. The ability to inhibit PG synthesis is limited to glucocorticoids, since the two mineralocorticoids are inactive, in parallel with their lack of anti-inflammatory effects. While glucocorticoids have many biologic effects that might be related to their anti-inflammatory properties, it seems likely that their ability to inhibit PG synthesis may contribute to their anti-inflammatory effects.

MECHANISMS OF PG SYNTHESIS INHIBITION

It is well established that aspirin and other nonsteroidal anti-inflammatory drugs inhibit PG synthesis by interacting with the enzyme cyclooxygenase.[64,65] Aspirin has been found to irreversibly inactivate cyclooxygenase in human platelets by acetylating a serine residue of the enzyme.[66] The platelet enzyme is sensitive to low doses of aspirin; as little as 160 mg per day is sufficient to inactivate essentially all platelet enzyme in man.[67,68] Other nonsteroidal drugs have been shown also to act by a direct interaction with cyclo-oxygenase, although the mechanism of inhibition is unclear. A variety of chemical structures are active inhibitors, including indomethacin, phenylbutazone, fenamates, and the phenylalkanoic acid derivatives such as ibuprofen, naproxen, tolmetin, and many others. Although the activity includes a wide variety of different chemical structures, the interaction is also specific in that many similar structures, including stereoisomers of these compounds (lacking anti-inflammatory effects), are inactive as inhibitors of cyclo-oxygenase.[58,69] The mechanism of inhibition of PG synthesis by corticosteroids is less clear than the mechanism of nonsteroidal drugs. It seems clear that in some tissues, including rheumatoid synovia, the steroids actually inhibit synthesis rather than accelerate PG catabolism or modify transport of PGs from cells.[61-63] However, there is no direct effect of steroids on isolated subcellular preparations of cyclo-oxygenase enzyme.[53-55] Evidence in some systems suggests that steroids inhibit the release of the precursor of PGs, arachidonic acid, from phospholipids by inhibiting the enzyme phospholipase.[70-72] In both cases, the steroids as well as nonsteroidal drugs inhibit at an early step in PG synthesis, and therefore the formation of all cyclo-oxygenase products is reduced. If glucocorticoids inhibit the release of arachidonic acid from phospholipids, it might be expected that these steroids would also inhibit the synthesis of lipoxygenase products, HETEs and leukotrienes. This possibility has not yet been studied in detail.

Table 6–3. Effects of Corticosteroids on Prostaglandin E_2 Synthesis by Rheumatoid Synovial Cultures

Steroid	IC_{50} (μM)
Dexamethasone	0.0030
Prednisolone	0.010
Hydrocortisone	0.030
Deoxycorticosterone	>1.0
Aldosterone	>1.0

PROSTAGLANDINS AND BONE RESORPTION

Prostaglandins E_1 and E_2 stimulate osteoclastic activity and resorption of bone when added in vitro to bone culture systems. Other PGs have negligible activity, with the exception of moderate activity of a PGE_2 metabolite.[73-76] It was found by Tashjian and co-workers, and later by others, that two experimental transplantable tumors, a mouse fibrosarcoma and the rabbit VX_2 carcinoma, cause hypercalcemia in tumor-bearing animals on the basis of secretion of large quantities of PGE_2 by the tumor cells. The PGE_2 secreted from the implanted tumors appears to cause hypercalcemia on a humoral basis, with stimulation of osteoclast activity by circulating PGE_2.[74,77,78] It remains possible that a metabolite of PGE_2 retains some ability to stimulate bone resorption, since PGE_2 is rapidly metabolized in the circulation, but this possibility has not been resolved.[77]

A similar role for PGE_2 has been postulated in hypercalcemia associated with human neoplastic disease. A group of patients has been described with hypercalcemia that returned to or toward normal on treatment with aspirin or indomethacin. Hypercalcemia was associated with elevated excretion of a major metabolite of the E prostaglandins, PGE-M, in the urine, a measure of total production of the E prostaglandins, PGE, by these individuals. Levels of PGE-M were markedly reduced in association with aspirin or indomethacin therapy. Levels of parathyroid hormone in plasma were normal by radioimmunoassay. This study and similar observations by others suggest that hypercalcemia associated with malignancy in some patients may develop because of excessive circulating PGE produced by the neoplasm. In particular, this mechanism may account for the hypercalcemia in the absence of demonstrable bone metastases.[79,80]

Prostaglandin-induced bone resorption has also been postulated to be of significance in rheumatoid arthritis. Explants of rheumatoid synovium and isolated synovial cells in tissue culture produce large quantities of PGE_2.[81] It was demonstrated that rheumatoid synovial tissue also releases potent bone resorption stimulating activity in tissue culture media. In a model system utilizing mouse calvarial bone cultures, potent bone resorption stimulating activity was found secreted into culture media by rheumatoid synovial tissue. As shown in Figure 6–7, stimulation of osteoclastic bone resorption in culture was detected by release of bone calcium into culture medium. Addition of small volumes of rheumatoid synovial culture media caused maximal release of bone calcium, shown in the cross-hatched bars. Evidence that this bone resorption stimulating activity is prostaglandin induced includes the following points: (1) The activity is completely recovered in an ether extract of the rheumatoid synovial culture media (clear bars). (2) The activity is completely suppressed by indomethacin in doses shown to completely (> 99 percent) suppress PGE_2 synthesis. (3) The concentration of PGE_2 in several rheumatoid synovial cultures determined by radioimmu-

Figure 6–7. Bone resorption stimulating activity in rheumatoid synovial culture media (tissue R37). Aliquots of synovial culture media were added to groups of three or four bone cultures at each dosage level. The elevation in medium calcium concentrations from treated bone cultures above that obtained in control bones is the calcium concentration. A portion of the synovial culture media was extracted with ether, and the reconstituted ether extracts were also assayed (▨) and compared to unextracted media (▨). Each bar represents the mean calcium elevation from duplicate synovial cultures (six to eight bones), with standard errrors. Replicate synovial cultures were treated with indomethacin (5 μg per milliliter), which reduced PGE_2 levels to < 1 percent of controls. (From Robinson, D. R., et al.: Trans. Assoc. Am. Physicians 88:146, 1975. Reproduced with the permission of the publisher.)

noassay was sufficient to account for the observed effects, based on the known response of the bone cultures to PGE_2.[82,83]

We have suggested, based on this model system, that PGE_2 secreted by the invading rheumatoid synovial pannus may stimulate osteoclastic bone resorption, leading to erosions of juxta-articular bone. Because of the close proximity of the synovial pannus to subchondral bone and the localization of bone destruction to areas of pannus invasion, the PGE_2 may be released from the pannus in close apposition to bone. It may therefore escape exposure to degradative enzymes as it passes from synovial cells to osteoclasts, or their precursors. The model system further suggests that adequate therapy with anti-inflammatory drugs that inhibit PGE_2 synthesis should prevent or retard the development of juxta-articular bone erosions in rheumatoid arthritis.

AN EXPERIMENTAL NUTRITIONAL APPROACH TO MODIFICATION OF PG SYNTHESIS

Since PGs and related compounds are derived from polyunsaturated fatty acids in tissues, it may seem reasonable that PG and LT production may be manipulated by changing the fatty acid composition of tissues. Long chain fatty acids may be synthesized from fatty acid precursors or may be directly incorporated into tissues from dietary sources. Epidemiologic studies have demonstrated that, in fact, the fatty acid composition of the diet is capable of altering tissue fatty acid composition in man, and subsequent experimental studies have provided further confirmation. Eskimos in northwestern Greenland ingest a diet almost completely derived from marine sources, which contain a high content of $\omega 3$ fatty acids, which are compounds each having a double bond between carbons 17 and 18, near the methyl end of the molecule. Analyses of serum and platelet lipids have shown that Greenland Eskimos have high levels of $\omega 3$ fatty acids, primarily eicosapentaenoic (EPA) acid (C20:5), an analogue of arachidonic acid, and docosahexaenoic acid (C22:6).[84,85] Studies of Greenland Eskimos, as well as short-term (2 to 3 weeks) feeding of fish oil to human volunteers, have demonstrated that there is a mild bleeding time prolongation and defective platelet aggregation accompanying the ingestion of a marine diet and associated with alterations in PG synthesis and changes in fatty acid composition in tissues.[85-88]

Although EPA may be converted to cyclo-oxygenase products, including thromboxane A_3, which may have some effects similar to the AA product thromboxane A_2, many studies have demonstrated that EPA is a poor substrate for cyclo-oxygenase in cells and therefore the end result of enrichment of tissue lipids with EPA is an inhibition of AA-derived cyclo-oxygenase products, without formation of significant quantities of products derived from EPA.[89] Ingestion of diets containing a high content of fish oils then may lead to inhibition of the usual PGs formed from AA, and marine diets may thus provide a form of cyclo-oxygenase inhibition. The effects of marine diets on lipoxygenase products, including leukotrienes, have not been studied extensively, but initial investigations indicate that marine diets may lead to production of lipoxygenase products derived from EPA.[90-92] It has been suggested that the marine diet-induced antiplatelet effect may be responsible, at least in part, for the reduced incidence of coronary thrombosis in Greenland Eskimos, although these diets are also associated with lower levels of serum cholesterol and triglycerides than are Western diets.[84,85]

The ability of dietary lipids to alter PG formation and induce abnormal platelet functions suggested to us that similar dietary programs could alter other functions attributed to PGs, especially in inflammatory reactions. Studies investigating the effects of dietary fish oils on inflammatory states in experimental animals have demonstrated a striking protection from glomerulonephritis in the New Zealand black-white hybrid mouse (NZB $\times$ NZW)F_1 or (NZB/W), a model for human systemic lupus erythematosus.[93] Previous work by other investigators had demonstrated that essential fatty acid deficiency prolonged the life span of these animals.[94] Other investigators had also shown that essential fatty acid deficiency could reduce the intensity of certain inflammatory reactions, and this anti-inflammatory effect has been postulated to be secondary to inhibition of PG synthesis, due to reduction of fatty acid precursors of PGs in tissues.[95] Another series of experiments initially carried out by Zurier and colleagues and subsequently confirmed in several laboratories demonstrated that the NZB/W mouse and other strains developing murine

lupus could also be protected by daily injections of the E PGs.[51,52]

It may seem paradoxical at first that essential fatty acid deficiency, a disorder leading to deficiency of polyunsaturated fatty acids and PGs derived from these substances, should lead to protection from renal disease in NZB/W mice, and at the same time, that administration of PGs should also lead to similar beneficial effects. One possible explanation is that protection from murine lupus by administration of PGs requires large doses of PGs. Furthermore, the parenteral administration of PGs requires absorption and transport of the PGs to sites through the circulation, whereas endogenous PGs and LTs exert their physiologic effects on tissues near their sites of synthesis rather than at distant sites via the circulation. Therefore it is possible that repeated administration of large doses of PGs may produce effects that differ from effects of endogenously synthesized PGs. Of course, it is also possible that essential fatty acid deficiency or other alterations in tissue fatty acid composition may produce effects that are mediated by factors independent of PGs or related compounds.

The mechanism of the protective effect of essential fatty acid deficiency or a fish oil-containing diet on murine lupus glomerulonephritis is unknown. These diets could produce alterations in PG and LT synthesis that might change the course of the disease, but other possibilities exist. Alterations in cell fatty acid composition itself could affect cell functions in many ways. Regardless of the mechanisms involved, these experiments suggest that dietary approaches may be effective therapy for renal disease in human systemic lupus and possibly in other inflammatory diseases. Manipulation of tissue fatty acid by dietary means, referred to as polyenoic acid competition by Lands, and its effect on human disease are in the early stages of investigation.[96] Preliminary indications suggest that $\omega 3$ fatty acid substitution may hold promise as a therapeutic approach to some inflammatory disease states as well as in vascular diseases. We may speculate that many diseases in which PGs and/or LTs are involved may be influenced by suitable alterations in ingested lipids, but the clinical usefulness of this approach remains to be determined.

References

1. Adv. Prostaglandin, Thromboxane, Leukotriene Res. 1976–1983. Volumes 1–12. New York, Raven Press.
2. Nelson N.A., Kelly R.C., and Johnson R.A.: Prostaglandins and the arachidonic acid cascade. Chem. Eng. News (August 16):30, 1982.
3. Samuelsson, B., Goldyne, M., Granstrom, E., Hamberg, M., Hammarström, S., and Malmsten, C.: Prostaglandins and thromboxanes. Ann. Rev. Biochem. 47:997, 1978.
4. Bunting, S., Gryglewski, R., Moncado, S., and Vane, J.R.: Arterial walls generate from prostaglandin endoperoxides a substance (prostaglandin X) which relaxes strips of mesenteric and coeliac arteries and inhibits platelet aggregation. Prostaglandins 12:897, 1976.
5. Robinson, D.R., McGuire, M.B., Bastian, D., Kantrowitz, F., and Levine, L.: The effects of antiinflammatory drugs on prostaglandin production by rheumatoid synovial tissue. Prostaglandins and Medicine 1:461, 1978.
6. Ferreira, S.H., and Vane, J.R.: Prostaglandins: Their disappearance from and release into the circulation. Nature (Lond.) 216:868, 1967.
7. Johnson, R.A., Morton, D.R., Kinner, J.H., Gorman, R.R., McGuire,

J.C., and Sun, F.F.: The chemical structure of prostaglandin X (pros-tacyclin). Prostaglandins 12:915, 1976.

8. Hamberg, M., Svensson, J., and Samuelsson, B.: Thromboxanes: a new group of biologically active compounds derived from prostaglandin endoperoxides. Proc. Natl. Acad. Sci. USA 72:2994, 1975.

9. Samuelsson, B., Granstrom, E., Green, K., Hamberg, M., and Ham-marström, S.: Prostaglandins. Ann. Rev. Biochem. 44:669, 1975.

10. Perkins, J.P.: Adenyl cyclase. In Greengard, P., and Robison, G.A. (eds.): Advances in Cyclic Nucleotide Research. Vol. 3. New York, Raven Press, 1973.

11. Appleman, M.M., Thompson, W.J., and Russell, T.R.: Cyclic nucleotide phosphodiesterases. In Greengard, P., and Robison, G.A. (eds.): Advances in Cyclic Nucleotide Research. Vol. 3. New York, Raven Press, 1973.

12. Ingebritsen, T.S., and Cohen, P.: Protein phosphatases: Properties and role in cellular regulation. Science 221:331, 1983.

13. Goldberg, N.D., O'Dea, R.F., and Haddox, M.K.: Cyclic GMP. In Greengard, P., and Robison, G.A. (eds.): Advances in Cyclic Nucleotide Research. Vol. 3. New York, Raven Press, 1973.

14. Goldberg, N.D., and Haddox, M.K.: Cyclic GMP metabolism and involvement in biological regulation. Ann. Rev. Biochem. 46:823, 1977.

15. Fridovich, I.: The biology of oxygen radicals. Science 201:875, 1978.

16. Siegel, M.I., McConnell, R.T., and Cuatrecasas, P.: Aspirin-like drugs interfere with arachidonate metabolism by inhibition of the 12-hydro-peroxy-5,8,10,14-eicosatetraenoic acid peroxidase activity of the lipox-ygenase pathway. Proc. Natl. Acad. Sci. USA 76:3774, 1979.

17. Lewis, R.A., and Austen, K.F.: Mediation of local homeostasis and inflammation by leukotrienes and other mast cell-dependent compounds. Nature 293:103, 108, 1981.

18. Armstrong, J.M., Lattimer, N., Moncada, S., and Vane, J.R.: Comparison of the vasodepressor effects of prostacyclin and 6-oxo-prostaglandin $F_{1\alpha}$ with those of prostaglandin E_2 in rats and rabbits. Br. J. Pharmacol. 62:125, 1978.

19. Fitzgerald, G.A., Brash, A.R., Falardeau, P., and Oates, J.A.: Estimated rate of prostacyclin secretion into the circulation of normal man. J. Clin. Invest. 68:1272, 1981.

20. Wedmore, C.V., and Williams, T.J.: Control of vascular permeability by polymorphonuclear leukocytes in inflammation. Nature 289:646, 1981.

21. Weiss, J.W., Drazen, J.M., Coles, N., McFadden, E.R., Jr., Weller, P.F., Corey, E.J., Lewis, R.A., and Austen, K.F.: Bronchoconstrictor effects of leukotriene C in humans. Science 216:196, 1982.

22. Borgeat, P., and Samuelsson, B.: Arachidonic acid metabolism in polymorphonuclear leukocytes: effects of ionophore A23187. Proc. Natl. Acad. Sci. USA 76:2148, 1979.

23. Scott, W.A., Pawlowski, N.A., Murray, H.W., Andreach, M., Zrike, J., and Cohn, Z.: Regulation of arachidonic acid metabolism by macrophage activation. J. Exp. Med. 155:1148, 1982.

24. Vane, J.R.: Prostaglandins as mediators of inflammation. In Samuellson, B., and Paoletti, R. (eds.): Advances in Prostaglandin and Thromboxane Research. Vol. 2. New York, Raven Press, 1976.

25. Komoriya, K., Ohmori, H., Azuma, A., Kurozumi, S., and Hashimoto, Y.: Prostaglandin I_2 as a potentiator of acute inflammation in rats. Prostaglandins 15:557, 1978.

26. Ferreria, S.H., Nakamura, M., and deAbreu Castro, M.S.: The hyperalgesic effects of prostacyclin and prostaglandin E_2. Prostaglandins 16:31, 1978.

27. Ford-Hutchinson, A.W., Walker, J.R., Davidson, E.M., and Smith, M.J.H.: PGI_2: A potential mediator of inflammation. Prostaglandins 16:253, 1978.

28. Higgs, E.A., Moncada, S., and Vane, J.R.: Inflammatory effects of prostacyclin (PGI_2) and 6-OXO-$PGF_{1\alpha}$ in the rat paw. Prostaglandins 16:153, 1978.

29. Bourne, H.R., Lichtenstein, L.M., Melmon, K.L., Henney, C.S., Weinstein, Y., and Shearer, G.M.: Modulation of inflammation and immunity by cyclic AMP. Science 184:19, 1974.

30. Polgar, P., and Taylor, L.: Effects of prostaglandin on substrate uptake and cell division in human diploid fibroblasts. Biochem. J. 162:1, 1977.

31. Feher, I., and Gidaili, J.: Prostaglandin E_2 as a stimulator of haemopoietic stem cell proliferation. Nature 247:550, 1974.

32. Garavoy, M.R., Strom, B.T., Kaliner, M., and Carpenter, C.B.: Antibody-dependent lymphocyte mediated cytotoxicity mechanism and modulation by cyclic nucleotides. Cell. Immunol. 20:197, 1975.

33. Strom, T., Deisseroth, A., Morganroth, J., Carpenter, C., and Merriel, J.: Alteration of the cytotoxic action of sensitized lymphocytes by cholinergic agents and activators of adenylate cyclase. Proc. Natl. Acad. Sci. USA 69:2995, 1972.

34. Diamantstein, T., and Ulmer, A.: Stimulation by cyclic AMP of lymphocytes mediated by soluble factor released from adherent cells. Nature 256:418, 1975.

35. Diamantstein, T., and Ulmer, A.: The antagonistic action of cGMP and cAMP on proliferation of B and T lymphocytes. Immunology 28:113, 1975.

36. Gordon, D., Bray, M.A., and Morley, J.: Control of lymphokine secretion by prostaglandins. Nature 262:401, 1976.

37. Goodwin, J.S., Bankhurst, A.D., and Messner, R.P.: Suppression of human T-cell mitogenesis by prostaglandin: Existence of a prostaglandin-producing suppressor cell. J. Exp. Med. 146:1719, 1977.

38. Goodwin, J.S., Messner, R.P., Bankhurst, A.D., Peake, G.T., Saiki, J.H., and Williams, R.G.: Prostaglandin producing suppressor cells in Hodgkin's disease. N. Engl. J. Med. 297:963, 1977.

39. Smith, J.W., Steiner, A.L., Newberry, W., Jr., and Parker, C. W.: Cyclic adenosine 3'5'-monophosphate in human lymphocytes. Alterations after phytohemagglutinin stimulation. J. Clin. Invest. 60:432, 1971.

40. Watson J.: Cyclic nucleotides as intracellular mediators of B cell activation. Transplant. Rev. 23:223, 1975.

41. Yoneda, T., and Mundy, G.R.: Monocytes regulate osteoclast activating factor production by releasing prostaglandin. J. Exp. Med. 150:338, 1979.

42. Stobo, J.D., Kennedy, M.S., and Goldyne, M.E.: Prostaglandin E modulation of the mitogenic response of human T cells. J. Clin. Invest. 64:1188, 1979.

43. Ceuppens, J.L., Rodriguez, M.A., and Goodwin, J.S.: Non-steroidal anti-inflammatory agents inhibit the synthesis of IgM rheumatoid factor in vitro. Lancet I:528, 1982.

44. Weissmann, G., Goldstein, I., Hoffstein, S., Chauvet, G., and Robineaux, R.: Yin/Yang modulation of lysosomal enzyme release from polymorphonuclear leukocytes by cyclic nucleotides. Ann. N.Y. Acad. Sci. 256:222, 1975.

45. Weissmann, G., Goldstein, I., Hoffstein, S., and Tsung, P.K.: Reciprocal effects of cAMP and cGMP on microtubule-dependent release of lysosomal enzymes. Ann. N.Y. Acad. Sci. 253:750, 1975.

46. Hill, H.R., Estensen, R.D., Quie, P.G., Hogan, N.A., and Goldberg, N.D.: Modulation of human neutrophil chemotactic responses by cyclic 3',5'-guanosine monophosphate and cyclic 3',5'-adenosine monophosphate. Metabolism 24:447, 1975.

47. Genta, G.E., and Hill, H.R.: Paradoxical influence of cyclic AMP on human monocyte chemotactic responses. Clin. Res. 24:180A, 1976.

48. Bonta, I.L., Parnham, M.J., and Van Vliet, L.: Combination of theophylline and prostaglandin E_1 as inhibitors of the adjuvant-induced arthritis syndrome of rats. Ann. Rheum. Dis. 37:212, 1978.

49. Parnham, M.J., Bonta, I.L., and Adolfs, M.J.P.: Cyclic AMP and prostaglandin E in perfusates of rat hind paws during the development of adjuvant arthritis. Ann. Rheum. Dis. 37:218, 1978.

50. Zurier, R.B., and Quagliata, F.: Effect of prostaglandin E_1 on adjuvant arthritis. Nature 234:304, 1971.

51. Zurier, R.B., Sayadoff, D.M., Torrey, S.B., and Rothfield, N.F.: Prostaglandin E_1 treatment of NZB/W mice. I. Prolonged survival of female mice. Arthritis Rheum. 20:723, 1977.

52. Zurier, R.B., Damjanov, I., Sayadoff, D.M., and Rothfield, N.F.: Prostaglandin E_1 treatment of NZB/W mice. II. Prevention of glomerulonephritis. Arthritis Rheum. 20:1449, 1977.

53. Vane, J.R.: Inhibition of prostaglandin synthesis as a mechanism of action for aspirin-like drugs. Nature New Biol. 231:232, 1971.

54. Smith J.B., and Willis, A.L.: Aspirin selectively inhibits prostaglandin production in human platelets. Nature New Biol. 231:235, 1971.

55. Ferreira, S.H., Moncada, S., and Vane J.R.: Indomethacin and aspirin abolish prostaglandin release from the spleen. Nature New Biol. 231:237, 1971.

56. Ferreira, S.H., and Vane, J.R.: New aspects of the mode of action of nonsteroid anti-inflammatory drugs. Ann. Rev. Pharmacol. 14:57, 1974.

57. Tomlinson, R.W., Ringold, H.J., Qureshi, M.C., and Forchielli, E.: Relationship between inhibition of prostaglandin synthesis and drug efficacy: Support for the current theory on mode of action of aspirin-like drugs. Biochem. Biophys. Res. Commun. 46:552, 1972.

58. Flower, R.J.: Drugs which inhibit prostaglandin biosynthesis. Pharmacol. Rev. 26:33, 1974.

59. Hamberg, M.: Inhibition of prostaglandin synthesis in man. Biochem. Biophys. Res. Commun. 49:720, 1972.

60. Lewis, G.P., and Piper, P.J.: Inhibition of release of prostaglandins as an explanation of some of the actions of anti-inflammatory corticosteroids. Nature 254:308, 1975.

61. Gryglewski, R.J., Panczenko, B., Korbut, R., Grodzinska, L., and Ocet-kiewcz, A.: Corticosteroids inhibit prostaglandin release from perfused mesenteric blood vessels of rabbit and from perfused lungs of sensitized guinea pig. Prostaglandins 10:343, 1975.

62. Kantrowitz, F., Robinson, D.R., McGuire, M.B., and Levine, L.: Corticosteroids inhibit prostaglandin production by rheumatoid synovia. Nature 258:737, 1975.

63. Tashjian, A.H., Jr., Voelkel, E.F., McDonough, J., and Levine, L.: Hydrocortisone inhibits prostaglandin production by mouse fibrosarcoma cells. Nature 258:739, 1975.

64. Roth, G.J., Stanford, N., and Majerus, P.W.: Acetylation of prostaglandin synthase by aspirin. Proc. Natl. Acad. Sci. USA 72:3073, 1975.

65. Roth, G.J., and Majerus, P.W.: The mechanism of the effect of aspirin on human platelets. I. Acetylation of a particulate fraction protein. J. Clin. Invest. 56:624, 1975.

66. Van Der Ouderaa, F.J., Buytenhek, M., Nugeren, D.H., and Van Dorp, D.A.: Acetylation of prostaglandin endoperoxide synthetase with acetylsalicyclic acid. Eur. J. Biochem. 109:1, 1980.

67. Patrignani, P., Filabozzi, P., and Patrono, C.: Selective cumulative inhibition of platelet thromboxane production by low-dose aspirin in healthy subjects. J. Clin. Invest. 69:1366, 1982.

68. Weksler, B.B., Pett, S.B., Alonso, D., Richter, R.C., Stelzer, P., Subramanian, V., Tack-Goldman, K., and Gay, W.A., Jr.: Differential inhibition by aspirin of vascular and platelet prostaglandin synthesis in atherosclerotic patients. N. Engl. J. Med. 308:800, 1083.

69. Rome, L.H., and Lands, W.E.: Structural requirements for time-dependent inhibition of prostaglandin biosynthesis by anti-inflammatory drugs. Proc. Natl. Acad. Sci. USA 72:4863, 1975.

70. Hong, S.-C., and Levine, L.: Inhibition of arachidonic acid release from cells as the biochemical action of anti-inflammatory corticosteroids. Proc. Natl. Acad. Sci. USA 73:1730, 1976.

71. Blackwell, G.J., Carnuccio, R., DiRosa, M., Flower, R.J., Parente, L., and Persico, P.: Macrocortin: a polypeptide causing the anti-phospholipase effect of glucocorticoids. Nature 287:147, 1980.

72. Hirata, F.: The regulation of lipomodulin, a phospholipase inhibitory protein, in rabbit neutrophils by phosphorylation. J. Biol. Chem. 256:7730, 1981.

73. Klein, D.C., and Raisz, L.G.: Prostaglandins: Stimulation of bone resorption in tissue culture. Endocrinology 86:1436, 1970.

74. Tashjian, A.H., Jr., Voelkel, E.F., Levine, L., and Goldhaber, P.: Evidence that the bone resorption stimulating factor produced by mouse fibrosarcoma cells is prostaglandin E_2. J. Exp. Med. 36:1329, 1972.

75. Dietrich, J.W., Goodson, J.M., and Raisz, L.G.: Stimulation of bone resorption by various prostaglandins in organ culture. Prostaglandins 10:231, 1975.

76. Tashjian, A.H., Jr., Tice, J.E., and Sides, K.: Biological activities of prostaglandin analogs and metabolites on bone in organ culture. Nature 266:645, 1977.

77. Seyberth, H.W., Hubbard, W.C., Oelz, O., Sweetman, B.J., Watson, J.T., and Oates, J.A.: Prostaglandin-mediated hypercalcemia in the VX_2 carcinoma-bearing rabbit. Prostaglandins 14:319, 1977.

78. Tashjian, A.H., Jr., Voelkel, E.F., and Levine, L.: Plasma concentrations of 13,14-dihydro-15-keto-prostaglandin E_2 in rabbits bearing the VX_2 carcinoma: Effects of hydrocortisone and indomethacin. Prostaglandins 14:309, 1977.

79. Seyberth, H.W., Segre, G.V., Morgan, J.L., Sweetman, B.J., Potts, J.T., Jr., and Oates, J.A.: Prostaglandins as mediators of hypercalcemia associated with certain types of cancer. N. Engl. J. Med. 293:1278, 1975.

80. Seyberth, H.W., Segre, G.V., Hamet, P., Sweetman, G.J., Potts, J.T., Jr., and Oates, J.A.: Characterization of the group of patients with the hypercalcemia of cancer who respond to treatment with prostaglandin synthesis inhibitors. Trans. Assoc. Am. Physicians 89:93, 1976.

81. Robinson, D.R., and McGuire, M.B.: Prostaglandins in the rheumatic diseases. Ann. N.Y. Acad. Sci. 256:318, 1975.

82. Robinson, D.R., Tashjian, A.H., Jr., and Levine, L.: Prostaglandin-induced bone resorption by rheumatoid synovia. Trans. Assoc. Am. Physicians 88:146, 1975.

83. Robinson, D.R., Tashjian, A.H., Jr., and Levine, L.: Prostaglandin-stimulated bone resorption by rheumatoid synovia. J. Clin. Invest. 56:1181, 1975.

84. Dyerberg, J., Bang, H.O., and Hjorne, N.: Fatty acid composition of the plasma lipids in Greenland Eskimos. Am. J. Clin. Nutr. 28:958, 1975.

85. Dyerberg, J., Bang, H.O., Stoffersen, E., Moncada, S., and Vane, J.R.: Eicosapentaenoic acid and prevention of thrombosis and atherosclerosis? Lancet II:117, 1978.

86. Goodnight, S.H., Jr., Harris, W.S., and Connor, W.E.: The effects of dietary $\omega 3$ fatty acids on platelet composition and function in man: A prospective, controlled study. Blood 58:880, 1981.

87. Thorngren, M., and Gustafson, A.: Effects of 11-week increase in dietary eicosapentaenoic acid on bleeding time, lipids, and platelet aggregation. Lancet I:1190, 1981.

88. Hay, C.R.M., Saynor, R., and Durber, A.P.: Effect of fish oil on platelet kinetics in patients with ischaemic heart disease. Lancet I:1269, 1982.

89. Whitaker, M.O., Wyche, A., Fitzpatrick, F., Sprecher, H., and Needleman, P.: Triene prostaglandins: prostaglandin D_3 and eicosapentaenoic acid as potential antithrombotic substances. Proc. Natl. Acad. Sci. USA 76:5919, 1979.

90. Hammarström, S.: Conversion of ^{14}C-labeled eicosapentaenoic acid (n-3) to leukotriene C_5. Biochim. Biophys. Acta 663:575, 1981.

91. Murphy, R.C., Pickett, W.C., Culp, B.R., and Lands, W.E.M.: Tetraene and pentaene leukotrienes: selective production from murine mastocytoma cells after dietary manipulation. Prostaglandins 22:613, 1981.

92. Hammarström, S.: Conversion of 5,8,11-eicosatrienoic acid to leukotrienes C_3 and D_3. J. Biol. Chem. 256:2275, 1981.

93. Prickett, J.D., Robinson, D.R., and Steinberg, A.D.: Effects of dietary enrichment with eicosapentaenoic acid upon autoimmune nephritis in female NZB × NZW/F_1 mice. Arthritis Rheum. 26:133, 1983.

94. Hurd, E.R., Johnston, J.M., Okita, J.R., MacDonald, P.C., Ziff, M., and Gilliam, J.N.: Prevention of glomerulonephritis and prolonged survival in New Zealand black/New Zealand white F_1 hybrid mice fed an essential fatty acid-deficient diet. J. Clin. Invest. 67:476, 1981.

95. Bonta, I.L., Bult, H., Vincent, J.E., and Zijlstra, F.J.: Acute anti-inflammatory effects of aspirin and dexamethasone in rats deprived of endogenous prostaglandin precursors. J. Pharm. Pharmacol. 29:1, 1977.

96. Lands, W.E.M.: manuscript in preparation.

Chapter 7

Plasma Protein Effectors of Inflammation: Complement

Shaun Ruddy

INTRODUCTION

Originally defined as the heat-labile serum factor required to "complete" the killing of bacteria coated with antibody, complement is now known to be a system of 18 plasma proteins that act together to mediate many inflammatory effects.[1-4] Like the other groups of plasma proteins that deliver inflammatory effects—the coagulation, kinin-forming, and fibrinolytic sequences (Chapter 8)—complement is characterized by the underlying principle of latent, recurrent, limited proteolysis. At several steps in the sequence a precursor or zymogen is activated to a protease, which cleaves a plasma protein substrate. This liberates an activation peptide and generates a new protease or modifies the specificity of an already active protease. In its turn, this new proteolytic enzyme cleaves yet another plasma protein, forming a new proteolytic activity, and the process recurs in cascade fashion. Products of the proteolysis have biologic activities, including the alteration of vascular permeability, the attraction of leukocytes and enhancement of their ability to ingest coated particles, the immobilization of these cells at the site of inflammation, and the assembly in cell membranes of the cytolytic membrane attack complex. Binding of complement cleavage products to specific receptors on the surface of erythrocytes, mast cells, macrophages or monocytes, lymphocytes, and platelets triggers additional biologic effects. Included among these may be the facilitation of cell-cell interactions required for the processing of antigen, for the initiation of an immune response, or for the control of an effective response.

All the complement proteins have been obtained in chemically homogeneous form (Table 7–1), and their functions are now well understood. Recognition of activating agents by either of two proteolytic pathways leads to a final common pathway, which assembles the membrane attack complex. The "classic" pathway for activation is so named because it was discovered first, but phylogenetic studies indicate that the "alternative" activation pathway is probably the older and more primitive.[5] The classic pathway is triggered by immune complexes formed from the union of IgG or IgM antibodies with their antigens, and such antibodies are found later in evolution than are analogues of alternative pathway factors. Animals without antibodies have plasma proteins that can be activated by repeating polysaccharides or other polymeric structures in the absence of specific antibody. Activation by either pathway generates endopeptidases with identical specificity: Both the alternative and classic pathway enzymes cleave the third complement component, C3, at arginine number 77 on the α-chain. The events that follow—assembly of the membrane attack complex—are also identical.

Proteins of the classic activation pathway and the terminal sequence are called "components" and are symbolized by the letter "C" followed by a number, e.g.,

C1, C4, C2, C3, C5, C6, C7, C8, and C9. Proteins of the alternative activation pathway are termed "factors" and are symbolized by letters, e.g., B, D, and P. Enzymatically active forms are indicated by a bar over the letter or number, e.g., $\overline{C1}$, $\overline{D}$; and cleavage fragments are denoted with suffixed lower case letters, e.g., C3a, C3b, C3c, and C3d. Polypeptide subunit chains are suffixed with Greek letters, starting with the largest chain, e.g., C3α, C3β. Control proteins are symbolized with contractions of their trivial names, e.g., $\overline{C1}$ inhibitor ($\overline{C1}$ INH), C3b inactivator (I), β1H globulin (H), C4 binding protein (C4BP).

CHEMISTRY AND REACTION MECHANISMS

Classic Activation Pathway (Fig. 7–1). Immune complexes containing antibodies of either the IgG or IgM class induce the internal proteolysis of C1 and thereby convert the precursor form of C1 to an active enzyme, $\overline{C1}$.[6-8] The first component comprises three glycoprotein molecules, C1q, C1r, and C1s, held together in a calcium-dependent complex.[9] In normal human serum these three subunits are present in equimolar concentrations.[10] The C1q subunit contains the binding site for immunoglobulins, and the C1r and C1s subunits are proteases. In agreement with physical measurements indicating that the valence of C1q for IgG is 6, electron microscopic studies of C1q find a hexamer structure with six globular "heads" joined together by fibrillar "stalks" (Fig. 7–2).[7,11] The heads interact with immunoglobulin; and the "stalks," which resemble collagen in their content of repeating glycines, hydroxylated lysines and prolines, and glucosylgalactose disaccharide, bind to C1r and C1s.

Table 7–1. Physicochemical Characteristics of Proteins of the Complement System

	Molecular Weight	Electro-phoretic Mobility	Serum Concentration (μg/ml)	Cleavage Fragments
Classic activation pathway				
C1q	385,000	γ_2	70	
C1r	190,000	β	34	
C1s	174,000	α_2	31	
C4	209,000	β_1	430	C4a, C4b, C4c, C4d
C2	117,000	β_2	30	C2a, C2b
Alternative activation pathway				
Properdin	220,000	γ_2	25	
D	23,500	α	2	
B	100,000	β_2	240	Bb, Ba
C3	180,000	β_1	1300	C3a, C3b, C3c, C3d, C3g
Terminal sequence				
C5	206,000	β_1	75	C5a, C5b
C6	128,000	β_2	60	
C7	121,000	β_2	55	
C8	153,000	γ	80	
C9	79,000	α	160	
Combined proteins				
$\overline{C1}$INH	105,000	α_2	150	
I	88,000	β_2	35	
H	150,000	β_1	360	
C4BP	590,000	β_2	400	

Figure 7–1. The classic pathway for complement activation.

C1q binds to immunoglobulins in the Fc region; F(ab')₂ fragments prepared by pepsin digestion do not interact with C1q (although they activate complement via the alternative pathway). Multivalent interaction of C1q with IgG is required for activation, since monomeric IgG has no effect, but IgG that has been aggregated either artificially or in an immune complex does activate. Complexes of polycations with polyanions such as protamine with heparin, or C polysaccharide with C-reactive protein are also capable of binding C1q and activating C1.[12]

C1r and C1s are both serine proteases with very similar structures and mechanisms of action. Both are non-covalently linked dimers of two identical polypeptide chains.[13,14] C1r binds to C1q in the presence of calcium and forms a physical link between C1q and C1s. During activation both polypeptide chains of C1r and C1s are cleaved one third of the way from the N-terminus, and the resulting two pieces of each chain remain linked by disulfide bonds. The active proteolytic sites on both molecules are on the lighter of the two pieces, as judged by the binding of diisopropylfluorophosphidate, which reacts with a serine in the active site and blocks further enzymatic activity. Amino acid sequences of peptides containing the reactive serine residue in C1s are closely homologous with those in C1r as well with other serine

proteases such as trypsin, thrombin, plasmin, and factor D̄.[7] Activation involves the apposition of one chain of the C1r protease to the other chain and internal proteolysis. Subsequent cleavage of C1s by C1r is highly specific; thus far no other protein substrates for this protease have been found.

The fourth component is a glycoprotein of 209,000 molecular weight composed of three polypeptide chains of 90,000, 80,000 and 30,000 each.[15] C1s, whether bound to immune complexes in intact C1̄ or free in solution, cleaves a peptide bond in the α-chain, releasing a 6000 molecular weight activation peptide, C4a. The remaining fragment, C4b, is transiently able to bind covalently to immune complexes or other acceptors. Another more stable site on the C4b molecule allows its interaction in a magnesium-dependent complex with C2a.[8] A third site binds C4b to complement receptors on a variety of cell types.[16]

The presence of C4b greatly enhances the rate at which C1̄s cleaves its other natural substrate, C2̄.[17] This component, a glycoprotein of 117,000 molecular weight, is split into a catalytically active fragment, C2a, of 85,000 molecular weight and an activation peptide, C2b, of 35,000 molecular weight.[18] C2a becomes incorporated in a magnesium-dependent complex with C4b, forming C4̄2̄, the classic pathway C3 convertase. C4̄2̄ is unstable: At 37° C it decays with a half-life of a few minutes, losing C3 convertase activity and leaving C4b, which is capable of regenerating active C4̄2̄ in the presence of fresh C2. A glycoprotein in the membranes of human erythrocytes accelerates this decay rate.[19]

Inhibition of C1̄. Normal serum contains an α-2 neuraminoglycoprotein of 105,000 molecular weight that forms an equimolar complex with both C1̄s and C1̄r, irreversibly blocking the activities of these proteases and preventing activation of C1s or cleavage of C4 and C2.[20-22] This C1̄ inhibitor functions as a "false substrate," entering the active site of the protease, forming an acyl intermediate, but then failing to be cleaved and to dissociate out of the active site. Direct binding studies have shown that the interaction between C1̄s and C1̄INH occurs on the light peptide chain of C1̄s, which contains the active proteolytic site. The complex thus formed is stable under conditions that normally dissociate non-covalent bonds.[22] C1̄INH also inhibits the activity of kallikrein in the kinin-forming system, factor XI of the intrinsic clotting pathway, plasmin of the fibrinolytic pathway, and activated Hageman factor or its fragments. Plasmin cleaves C1̄INH, producing lower molecular weight fragments, which retain the ability to interact with C1̄s.[22] Individuals with congenital partial deficiency of C1̄INH experience unopposed spontaneous activation of C1 with consequent hypercatabolism of C4 and C2; clinically, they have the syndrome of hereditary angioedema (Chapter 85).[23]

Degradation of C4b. Control of the assembly of active C4̄2̄ is effected by the further cleavage of C4b into two inactive fragments, C4c and C4d, with molecular weights of approximately 150,000 and 47,000, respectively. This is the result of the cooperative effect of two

Figure 7–2. Comparison of the C1q model proposed by Reid and Porter with the three-dimensional structure of an IgG protein as determined by x-ray crystallography. (Courtesy of Dr. Manuel Navia, National Institutes of Health.)

plasma proteins: the C4 binding protein (C4BP)[24] and the C3b inactivator (I).[25] C4BP is a glycoprotein that consists of six to eight identical subunits of 70,000 daltons linked by disulfide bridges. Binding of C4b to C4BP renders it susceptible to attack by I. Proteolysis at two points in the α-chain of C4b yields three peptides with molecular weights of 47,000, 25,000, and 17,000. The first of these is C4d, which is released from the molecule; the other two remain bridged by disulfide linkages to the intact β- and γ-chains in the form of C4c. In the case of C4b bound to complexes, C4c is released into the fluid phase, indicating that the site by which C4b binds covalently is located on the C4d portion of the α-chain. C4b that has been degraded by I in the presence of C4BP is incapable of interacting with C2 to form active $\overline{C42}$. Complexes bearing only C4d on their surfaces do not react in immune adherence with C4b receptors present on human erythrocytes or leukocytes.[26]

The Alternative Pathway: Activation and Amplification (Fig. 7–3). The addition of polysaccharides such as yeast cell wall zymosan or gram-negative bacterial endotoxin to the serum of animals congenitally deficient in either C4 or C2 leads to cleavage of C3 and assembly of the membrane attack complex by a mechanism that is independent of the classic activation pathway. The reaction sequence resembles that of the classic pathway, with factor $\overline{D}$ functioning as the homologous protein for $\overline{C1s}$, C3 for C4, and factor B for C2. An extra protein, properdin, serves to stabilize the magnesium-dependent complex enzyme C3 convertase, $\overline{C3bBb}$, which like its classic homologue, $\overline{C42}$, decays rapidly at 37° C. Like the classic pathway, activation of the alternative pathway produces an enzyme that cleaves C3 and C5 and initiates the terminal sequence.

A pathway for C3 inactivation that was independent of antibody and the early classic components was attributed to a single isolatable nonspecific substance termed "properdin."[27] This material was thought to be involved in numerous biologic systems, including the killing of gram-negative bacteria, the neutralization of certain viruses, the lysis of erythrocytes in paroxysmal nocturnal hemoglobinuria, and protection against the lethal effects of whole-body radiation.[28] As evidence for specificity of the system appeared, and its effects were reproduced by small amounts of antibody and the early complement components,[29] the entire properdin system was discredited. The important report that properdin

was a unique protein present in normal serum and immunochemically distinct from immunoglobulin[30] was virtually ignored by the scientific community. Only the weight of evidence obtained from a number of converging lines of research served to establish the existence of the alternative (properdin) pathway separate and distinct from the classic one.

Four factors participate in the formation of the alternative pathway C3 convertase. Of these, C3 is by far the most important, since it serves as a link between the classic, alternative, and terminal pathways and is involved in the positive feedback or amplification loop. C3 is a glycoprotein composed of two polypeptide chains of 115,000 and 75,000 molecular weight linked by disulfide bridges.[31] With a plasma concentration of 1 mg per ml, it is also the most plentiful of the complement proteins. Cleavage of the α-chain of C3 at arginine 77 by either the classic or alternative pathway C3 convertases releases an 8000 molecular weight activation peptide, C3a, and exposes a labile internal thioester bond on the α-chain formed between the gamma carboxyl group of a glutamic acid residue and the thiol group on a neighboring cysteine. The resulting activated carbonyl on the major fragment, C3b, forms covalent ester or amide linkages with appropriate acceptors, such as sugar residues on polysaccharides or immunoglobulin oligosaccharides.[32] As in the case of C4b, failure to react promptly with an appropriate acceptor surface results in irreversible inactivation of the C3b in the fluid phase, presumably by reaction of the carbonyl group with water. Just as cleavage of C4 to C4b reveals a stable site for interaction with C2, cleavage of C3 to C3b permits C3b to develop the ability to participate in a magnesium-dependent complex with factor B.[33-36]

Factor B is the alternative pathway homologue of C2. Linkage studies locate C2 and B in the major histocompatibility complex in such close proximity that gene duplication is virtually certain.[37] B is a single polypeptide chain of 102,000 molecular weight. The catalytic site of B is present on the native form as judged by its esterase activity and by weak C3 convertase activity found in the complex of C3b and native B.[38] Cleavage of C3b-bound B by $\overline{D}$ to form $\overline{C3bBb}$ greatly enhances the activity of the B-derived enzyme.[39] As in the case of C2, the major Bb fragment, of molecular weight 65,000, has the active site; magnesium ions are required for formation of the C3 convertase; and the complex enzyme $\overline{C3bBb}$ is unstable at 37° C. Decay leads to loss of activity, release of an inactive fragment, and regeneration of C3b in a form capable of interacting with fresh B in the presence of $\overline{D}$ to form additional C3 convertase.

Factor $\overline{D}$ is a serine protease of 23,500 molecular weight and has amino acid sequence homologies, both in the active site and at the N-terminus, with other serine proteases, including thrombin and C1s, its classic pathway homologue.[40] In the case of factor $\overline{D}$, however, the enzyme already exists in plasma in its active form. Control of proteolysis is exerted by the limited availability of substrate: $\overline{D}$ acts only on B that has complexed with C3b, and not on free or unbound B.[41]

Figure 7–3. The alternative pathway for complement activation.

Properdin is not required for alternative pathway activation, but it increases the efficiency of the other proteins in the system. Properdin is a 220,000 molecular weight gamma globulin consisting of four identical subunits of 53,000 each.[42,43] In free solution it binds to polymeric C3b. Interaction of properdin with surface-bound C3b probably involves more than one molecule of C3b in close proximity.[44] Following binding, there occurs a reversible conformational change from native P to an activated form, which binds much more avidly to C3.[45] The function of properdin appears to be that of stabilizing the C3bBb interaction; a dose-dependent increase in the half-life of this enzyme occurs upon the introduction of properdin.[46]

An autoantibody with specificity for antigenic determinants unique to the assembled alternative pathway C3 convertase (C3bBb) appears in the serum of patients with membranoproliferative glomerulonephritis and mimics the action of properdin.[47-49] The immunoglobulin nature of C3 nephritic factor (C2NeF) was confirmed when a mother with nephritis and C3NeF in her plasma gave birth to an infant with C3NeF in his plasma as well.[50] Like properdin, C3NeF functions by binding to the C3bBb enzyme and stabilizing it.[51] Although C3NeFs may be of any IgG subclass and either light chain type, and are usually heterogeneous in these attributes,[52] some C3NeF proteins have restricted heterogeneity and abnormal heavy chains.[53] Like properdin, C3NeF greatly increases the efficiency of the alternative pathway proteins, and it is not absolutely required for alternative pathway activation.

Control Proteins of the Alternative Pathway. Agents that trigger the alternative pathway do so by protecting the newly formed C3bBb enzyme from dissociation and degradation by the control proteins, H and I. Activators shift the proteolytic activity from the fluid phase to the solid state and accelerate the assembly of the particle-bound C3 and C5 convertases. Factor I was initially recognized by its ability to inhibit the reactivity of C3b-coated erythrocytes with cells bearing receptors for them in the immune adherence phenomenon.[54] Subsequently, the proteolytic activity of I for C3b was identified, and cleavage of C3b into C3c and C3d was recognized.[55] Later studies have shown that the degradation of C3b occurs in several steps and involves the action of other proteins in addition to I.

The first protein shown to cooperate in the inactivation of C3b was Factor H, a 150,000 molecular weight glycoprotein that physically binds to C3b and thereby greatly increases its susceptibility to cleavage by I.[56-58] H is required for the cleavage of fluid phase C3b by I,[59] but surface-bound C3b is susceptible to slow digestion by I alone.[57] The first cleavage of the α'-chain of C3b by factor I results in NH$_2$-terminal 68,000-dalton and COOH-terminal 46,000-dalton peptides. A second cleavage releases a 3000-dalton peptide from the 46,000-dalton fragment.[60] The product C3bi consists of the two major α-chain fragments, which remain disulfide-bonded to the intact β-chain. It has no activity in binding to C3b receptors on human erythrocytes but does

adhere to C3bi receptors on the surfaces of glomerular epithelial cells and certain leukocytes.[61] C3bi has no activity in continuing the cytolytic sequence by modifying the C3 convertases so that they can attack C5, nor can it complex with B to form an alternative pathway convertase.

The third cleavage of the α'-chain of C3bi occurs at a site 27,000 daltons from the amino terminus and yields C3c (140,000 daltons) and C3dg (40,000 daltons).[60] The latter fragment contains the thioester region by which C3b is covalently linked to acceptors, so that if acceptor-bound C3bi is being cleaved, C3dg remains bound and C3c is released into the fluid phase. The cofactor for factor I in production of C3c and C3dg is the C3b receptor present on the surface of human erythrocytes.[62] Elastase purified from human polymorphonuclear leukocytes is active at nanogram concentrations and also fragments the α'-chain of C3b.[63]

In addition to its ability to enhance the rate at which I digests C3b, H physically binds to C3b, competes with B for binding to C3b, and accelerates decay of the C3bBb and C3bBbP enzymes.[64] Once the B has been stripped from the complex by accelerated decay-dissociation induced by H, the C3b becomes available for cleavage by I. As will be seen below, the "activating" capacity of polysaccharides and certain cell membranes reflects the extent to which they provide a microenvironment that protects the complexed C3bBb from this action of H.

Mechanism of Activation: Solid-State Amplification. Since a role for immunoglobulins as an enhancing factor is demonstrable for activation of the alternative pathway under certain circumstances, and activation by polysaccharides clearly occurs independently of antibody, it is likely that there is more than one set of events leading to such activation. Activating agents increase the formation of alternative pathway convertase by transforming an inefficient fluid phase reaction into a fruitful solid-state assembly of the enzyme complex. In the fluid phase a small amount of C3 is continuously being hydrolyzed at its internal thioester bond, permitting B to complex with it and become susceptible to cleavage by D.[65] This generates small amounts of C3 convertase and produces small amounts of C3b. In the fluid phase, these small amounts of C3b are effectively controlled by I and H before the C3b fragment can cycle through the positive feedback loop and result in the amplification phase whereby a product of C3 cleavage induces the formation of more C3-cleaving enzyme. Surfaces that activate the alternative pathway provide a haven for the small amount of C3b produced by the fluid phase reactions, where it can be deposited and be protected from the action of the control proteins. Such surface-bound C3b is, however, capable of interacting with B in the presence of D to form C3bBb and with properdin to form C3bBbP, both of which are also protected from the control proteins. The slow fluid phase reaction is thus shifted to an amplified solid state cleavage. "Activators" thus exist in name only; initiation is a spontaneous event occurring continuously in the fluid phase. The "activating" surfaces might better be termed "protectors," since their function appears to be one of affording a microenvironment in which C3b and complex enzymes containing C3b are protected from inactivation by I and decay dissociation by H.[66]

At least one chemical characteristic of the protecting surface has been identified: sialic acid content.[67,68] Cells that do not normally provide surfaces for alternative pathway amplification acquire this capacity after membrane sialic acid residues have been removed by treatment with sialidase or modified by chemical treatment. Among inbred strains of mice, there is an inverse relationship between the capacity to activate the human alternative complement pathway and membrane sialic acid content.[69] Comparative binding studies with radiolabeled B and H indicate that these two proteins compete for a single binding site on C3b. Decreases in sialic acid content do not affect the ability of B to bind to C3b located on the particle surface, but they greatly reduce the number and affinity of C3b sites available for binding and inhibition by H.

THE TERMINAL SEQUENCE (Fig. 7–4)

Cleavage of additional C3 by either the $\overline{C42}$ or $\overline{C3bBb}$ convertases results in the development of C5 convertase activity. While the C3b was once thought to be incorporated into the enzyme complex, thereby modifying its substrate specificity, more recent data indicate that C3b provides a binding site for native C5 and makes it susceptible to the action of the convertase.[70] Only surface-bound C3b functions to promote C5 cleavage, and the C3b molecule that is involved in C5 binding and subsequent cleavage must be free of other ligands such as B, P, or H. In the case of the alternative pathway, therefore, this means that at least two molecules of C3b are involved in C5 cleavage: one to interact with B and form the cleaving enzyme and another to interact with C5 and support the cleavage reaction.[71]

C5 is remarkably similar both in structure and reaction mechanism to C3.[72] It is a β-glycoprotein of 206,000 molecular weight, consisting of two nonidentical peptide chains of 80,000 and 130,000 daltons. Cleavage

of C5 by its convertase occurs at an argininyl-leucine bond between residues 74 and 75 on the α-chain (versus arginine 77 for C3 cleavage), releasing an 11,000-dalton peptide, C5a.[73] C5a and C3a, which represent the N-terminal ends of the α-chains of the corresponding parent molecules, have extensive sequence homology, including the conservation of three disulfide bridges,[72] and nearly equal contents of regular secondary structure as judged by circular dichroism studies. A major difference is the carbohydrate (25 percent) present in C5a but not in C3a.[73]

Both C6 and C7 are single polypeptide chains, with molecular weights of 128,000 and 121,000 daltons, respectively, and both have identical electrophoretic mobilities.[74] Both show genetic polymorphism, and the loci for these are closely linked.[75] An individual with combined deficiency of C6 and C7 has been found, and inheritance of these two deficiencies within his family behaves as a single genetic characteristic.[76] It seems likely that C6 and C7 are, like C2 and B, products of tandem gene duplication.

C8 has an unusual structure: It contains three polypeptide chains of 77,000, 63,000, and 13,700 daltons, termed α, β, and γ. These subunits occur as a disulfide-linked α-γ dimer which is noncovalently associated with β. Interaction of C8 with C5b-7 complexes is mediated through β, whereas interaction with the membrane bilayer occurs primarily through the α-chain of α-γ. Failure of the α-chain to label with radioactive iodine suggests that it may be relatively hydrophobic and sequestered within the interior of the molecule, a formulation that is attractive in view of the function of C8 within the C5-9 cytolytic complex.[77] The last component to react, C9, is an α-globulin of 79,000 molecular weight.

Assembly of the Membrane-Damaging C5b-9 Complex. Activated C5b has a specific metastable binding site for C6, as well as exposed hydrophobic sites. It combines with C6 in a reversible complex[78,79] to form C56, which reacts with C7. The product is the highly labile C5b,6,7 complex, which, if generated in the fluid phase, is capable of reacting with lipid membranes in its immediate vicinity. If the interaction occurs between C7 and C5b,6 bound to a cell membrane (favored by interaction of C5b with binding sites provided by C3b), more efficient binding of the C5b,6,7 complex to the target membrane occurs. In either case, binding of the C5b,6,7 complex to the membrane is the first step in assembling the membrane attack complex. It has been shown to occur on the membranes of bacteria and nucleated cells as well as on the sheep erythrocytes usually used in model systems. Even liposomes, synthetic vesicles prepared from mixtures of phospholipid and cholesterol, have been shown to bind C5b,6,7. Reaction with C8 initiates membrane damage, and C5b-8 complexes have been shown to penetrate membranes of about 6 nm thickness.[80] A stable transmembrane channel is formed by the addition of multiple molecules of C9, possibly in polymeric form, to the complex. Evidence obtained from enzymatic stripping experiments, from studies of planar lipid concentration, from electron mi-

Figure 7–4. The terminal sequence leading to membrane damage.

croscopy, and from the structure of the C5b-9 complex itself supports the notion that the complex forms a tunnel or channel inserted through the lipid bilayer, with hydrophobic residues on the exterior in contact with the lipid bilayer and a hydrophilic interior allowing the passage of ions and water.[81-84] The loss of control over ion flux dooms the cell to the imbibition of water from isosmotic media with eventual swelling and rupture of the cell.

BIOLOGIC CONSEQUENCES OF COMPLEMENT ACTIVATION
(Table 7–2)

Although assembly of the C5b-9 complex and membrane damage is the most well known effect of complement activation, a variety of other inflammatory events also ensue. Changes in vascular permeability have been attributed to the cleavage of C4 and C2 by C$\bar{1}$ and may explain the pathogenesis of the angioedema associated with C$\bar{1}$INH deficiency,[85] but the peptide(s) responsible for inducing the permeability change have not yet been fully characterized, and even the existence of a kinin-like fragment derived from C2 is in doubt.[86] Biologic activities have been identified for products of the alternative activation pathway. Specifically, the active enzyme C3bBb is chemotactic for polymorphonuclear neutrophils.[87] The Bb fragment of factor B induces rapid spreading and increase in surface area of unstimulated

Table 7–2. Biologic Activities of the Products of Complement Activation

Product	Activity
C4, C2 kinin	Increase in vascular permeability; putative mediator of edema in hereditary angioedema
C3bBb	Chemotaxis of polymorphonuclear leukocytes
Bb	Spreading of monocytes
C3a	Anaphylatoxin; releases histamine from basophils and mast cells, serotonin from platelets, possibly direct cytotoxic effect, possibly chemotactic, suppresses lymphocytes
C5a	Anaphylatoxin; same activities as C3a on mast cells, marked chemotactic effect for monocytes and polymorphonuclear leukocytes
C3b	Multiple effects, depending on cell-bearing receptor: phagocytosis enhancement, triggers cycling of alternative pathway amplification loop (Fig. 7–3)
C3bi	Binding to glomerular, monocyte complement receptors
C3d	Binding to lymphocyte complement receptors
C567	Active complex capable of binding to "innocent bystander" cell membranes and initiating formation of C5b-9
C5b-9	Membrane attack complex: forms transmembrane channels leading to cytolysis

peritoneal macrophages[88] and inhibits their migration in the capillary tube assay used to measure macrophage migration inhibitory factor.[89] The enzymatic site on Bb is required for these activities, since they are inhibited by chemicals or monoclonal antibodies that react with the active site. Since macrophages can synthesize C3, factor B and factor $\bar{D}$,[90] the relation of these factors to migration inhibition observed following antigen stimulation of mixed mononuclear cells requires further investigation.

The activation peptides C3a and C5a are anaphylatoxins capable of inducing the secretion of histamine by mast cells and basophils.[91-93] The degranulating effects on skin mast cells are observable at a concentration of 10^{-12} and 10^{-15} M for C3a and C5a, respectively. Both peptides also possess some smooth muscle contractile activity that is independent of histamine release. The anaphylatoxic activities are blocked by scission of the terminal arginine from either C3a or C5a by carboxypeptidase N, a magnesium-dependent enzyme, which also has been termed the anaphylatoxin inactivator.[94]

C5a is responsible for most of the chemotactic activity in plasma after activation of the complement system.[95] It attracts neutrophils, eosinophils, and monocytes and also releases lysosomal enzymes of polymorphonuclear neutrophils into phagocytic vacuoles or the surrounding medium.[96] Aggregation of granulocytes is observable after exposure to C5a.[97] Unlike the anaphylatoxic activity, which requires the terminal arginine, these other activities of C5a persist following its removal, so that C5a$_{des\ arg}$ is fully chemotactic.[98] C3a does not appear to have chemotactic activity,[99] but C3e, a polypeptide derived from the α-chain of C3, produces an initial leukopenia followed by a leukocytosis.[100] C3e also causes release of leukocytes from the perfused rat femur and has been termed leukocyte-mobilizing factor.[101]

The fragment C3b has several different biologic activities, specified by the type of cell bearing the C3b receptor to which it binds. Perhaps the most important of these, judging from the clinical features of C3 deficiency in which sepsis with pyogenic organisms is prominent,[102] is the enhancement of phagocytosis by polymorphonuclear neutrophils and monocytes. Binding of C3b-coated immune complexes to polymorphonuclear leukocytes enhances phagocytosis of the complexes by these cells, provided the complexes contain IgG antibody that interacts with the Fc receptors also present on the polys; C3b by itself promotes adherence but not ingestion. A marked synergy between the effects of IgG and C3b on phagocytosis has been demonstrated.[103] In contrast, "activated" macrophages elicited by intraperitoneal injection of thioglycollate or bacterial endotoxin or by antigen in the sensitized animal both bind *and* ingest complexes coated only with C3b; unstimulated monocytes are not active in this regard and require IgG, as do neutrophils.[104] Receptors for both C3b and for C3bi are present in the renal glomerulus and on the Kupffer cells of the hepatic sinusoids.[105,106] Receptors for C3d are present on some human lymphocytes and lymphoblastoid cell lines.[106,107] Although a close association between the presence of C3d receptors and receptors for the Epstein-Barr virus was described,[108] this was found to be due to co-selection of the two receptors, and they are separate and distinct entities.[109]

Although the existence of C3bi or C3d receptors on monocytes or B lymphocytes has been known for a long time, the functional significance of these receptors remains incompletely understood. Interpretation of some experiments may be confused by the capacity of these cells to synthesize C3 and other complement proteins during the course of the culture experiment. C3 has been implicated in such functions as lymphokine production,[110] lymphocyte proliferation,[111] and prostaglandin release from monocytes.[112] In vivo, depletion of C3 prevents the development of a primary antibody response to T-dependent antigens[113] but not a secondary response. The failure of this response and the generation of B memory cells have been attributed to the role of activated C3 in binding antigen-containing complexes to dendritic antigen-processing cells in the lymphoid follicle. In the absence of C3 there is a failure of normal interaction between the antigen-processing cells and virgin B lymphocytes.[114] Experiments demonstrating that the lymphocyte response to antigens or mitogens is inhibited by other fragments of C3 may indicate direct effects on lymphocytes as well.[115]

METABOLISM OF COMPLEMENT PROTEINS

In vitro culture studies have detected synthesis of C4, C2,[116] C3, B, D, and P by peritoneal macrophages[90] and synthesis of C3, C5, and C9 by hepatoma cells.[116] By contrast, in vivo studies have tended to identify the liver as the primary, if not sole, source of synthesis. Patients with severe hepatic failure have marked depressions of the serum levels of C4 and C3, and impaired synthesis of C3 has been measured directly in metabolic turnover studies.[117] Following hepatic allografting, the electrophoretic polymorphic types of C3 and C6 change from that of the recipient to those of the donor.[118] Although immunofluorescent studies indicate synthesis of C3 by hepatic parenchymal cells, examination of inflammatory synovium from rheumatoid arthritis identifies cells in this tissue that appear to be synthesizing C3.[119] Explants of inflamed rheumatoid synovial tissue incorporate ^{14}C-amino acids into complement protein.[119] Such complement synthesis during immune inflammation may be induced by the lymphokine, monocyte complement stimulator. This substance, produced by sensitized T lymphocytes when exposed to antigen, stimulates the synthesis of C2 by human peripheral blood monocytes.[120]

Measurements of the fractional catabolic rates of C4, C3, C5, and B from the turnover of purified and radiolabeled proteins indicate that complement proteins are among the most rapidly metabolized of all plasma proteins.[121] The mean fractional catabolic rates in normals are in the range of 50 percent of the plasma pool per 24 hours. Synthetic rates are significantly correlated with serum levels, indicating that in normal individuals the rate of synthesis is the major determinant of plasma concentration. Considering the highly positive correlation between levels of C3, B, and P and those of the two proteins that control their interaction, I and H,[122] it is possible that normal catabolism of the alternative pathway proteins is accounted for by their participation in continuous low level activation of the pathway, much as the catabolic route of fibrinogen may involve normal in vivo activation of the coagulation sequence.

Biosynthetic studies in cell-free systems indicate that both C4 and C3 are synthesized as single polypeptide chains and post-translationally cleaved into the three and two polypeptide chains, respectively, in which they appear in plasma.[123,124] Small amounts of the single chain precursor molecules may be found in normal plasma.[125] Genomic clones coding for the major portions of C3, C4, and factor B have been isolated and partly sequenced (Chapter 85).

CLINICAL SIGNIFICANCE OF COMPLEMENT MEASUREMENTS

Methods of Measurement. Since the complement proteins have hemolytic activity, assays based on the ability of a test specimen to lyse cells afford a sensitive assay technique. The traditional method for the determination of complement in serum or other body fluids measures the ability of the test specimen to lyse 50 percent of a standard suspension of sheep erythrocytes coated with rabbit antibody in a reaction that includes the entire classic reaction sequence.[126] This test, the "CH50" (for "complement hemolytic 50 percent") is widely available and has been in use for more than 30 years, so that it has the advantage that many of the observations relating complement levels to human disease are based on it. The CH50 continues to be a useful screening procedure, particularly when deficiency states are suspected or when the measurement is performed on a body fluid, e.g., synovial or pleural fluid, where failure of normal clearance mechanisms may have allowed the persistence of hemolytically inactive but immunoreactive complement protein. Specific hemolytic assays for each of the classic and alternative pathways and the terminal sequence are available, but their difficulty of performance has restricted them to the research laboratory.[127]

Concentrations of complement proteins may also be measured by their reactivities in immunoassays based on reaction with antibody specific for the protein in question.[128] These are the most inexpensive and widely available of assays because materials required for their performance are offered by commercial suppliers in the form of kits for use in the clinical pathology laboratory. Physicians interpreting the results of tests should keep in mind the following caveats:

1. Under the best conditions, the coefficient of variation of immunoassays such as the commonly available

radial immunodiffusion is likely to be of the order of 8 percent, well above that which applies to most other results obtained from the clinical pathology laboratory.

2. There are no agreed-upon international standards, so that considerable variation in absolute values obtained by kits from different suppliers or even in lots of kits from the same supplier may be observed. The clinical pathology laboratory must maintain independent checks of the "range of normal" and of the lot-to-lot variation rather than uncritically accepting the standards and normal ranges provided by the supplier. This "normal range" should be provided with the test result.

3. As is the case for other plasma proteins, the range of normal for complement proteins is quite broad, often of the order of $\pm$ 50 percent of the mean value for the population. Thus, serial changes in levels for a given patient over a period of time may often be more informative than comparison with an absolute range of normal. Furthermore, since plasma levels of many of the complement proteins tend to rise during acute inflammation, a "normal" value may actually reflect a marked fall from a previous level and indicate an active disease process. A striking example of this occurs in systemic lupus erythematosus, in which levels of C9 in patients with relatively quiescent disease are two to three times the normal mean; with activity, levels fall dramatically by 50 or 75 percent—into the "normal" range.[129]

4. The most widely available test for a complement component (C3) is not necessarily the most useful. Because C3 is the most plentiful of the complement components, it was the first to be purified and measured in immunoassays. Measurements of C4 are more sensitive to minor episodes of in vivo complement activation. Most workers agree that a useful routine complement screen includes measurements of C4 and C3 by immunoassay and total hemolytic activity by CH50.

Interpretation of Complement Abnormalities. As a consequence of their participation in complement activation, the complement proteins become recognizable as "altered" and are rapidly cleared from the plasma space.[130] Clearance from extravascular spaces such as pleural, synovial, or cerebrospinal proceeds more slowly.[131] Although some compensatory increases in synthesis may occur, the result is usually a fall in the plasma level of one or more of the complement proteins. In reverse fashion, as the complement-activating stimulus or disease abates, there may be a parallel return of the complement level toward normal. Virtually any disease that gives rise to circulating immune complexes may result in hypocomplementia, provided the complexes contain IgG or IgM antibodies capable of activating complement. A list of such diseases is contained in Table 7–3. In systemic lupus erythematosus, complement depressions are associated with increased severity of disease, and particularly with renal involvement.[132] Serial observations have revealed decreased levels in advance of clinical exacerbations; reductions in C4 usually precede those of C3 or CH50.[129] As attacks subside, levels

Table 7–3. Hypocomplementemic States

Hyposynthesis
  Congenital deficiencies (see Chapter 85)
  Severe hepatic failure
  Severe malnutrition
  Glomerulonephritis*
  Systemic lupus erythematosus*
Hypercatabolism
  Deficiency of control proteins
    C1 inhibitor deficiency: Hereditary angioedema
    C3b inactivator deficiency
  Rheumatic diseases with immune complexes
    Systemic lupus erythematosus
    Rheumatoid arthritis (with extra-articular disease)
    Systemic vasculitis
    Essential mixed cryoglobulinemia
  Infectious diseases
    Subacute bacterial endocarditis
    Infected atrioventricular shunts
    Pneumococcal sepsis
    Gram-negative sepsis
    Viremias, e.g., hepatitis B surface antigenemia, measles, dengue
    Parasitemias, e.g., trypanosomiasis, malaria, babesiosis
  Glomerulonephritis
    Post-streptococcal
    Membranoproliferative
    Idiopathic proliferative or focal sclerosing

*Usually associated with simultaneous and marked hypercatabolism.

return toward normal in reverse order. Discoid lupus or drug-induced lupus is not ordinarily associated with hypocomplementemia.

Any cause of chronic antigenemia is likely to be associated with acquired hypocomplementemia, including, for example, subacute bacterial endocarditis,[133] hepatitis B surface antigenemia,[134] pneumococcal infections,[135] gram-negative sepsis,[136] viremias such as measles,[137] or recurrent parasitemias such as malaria.[138] Other diseases of unknown etiology may be associated with hypocomplementemia, such as essential mixed cryoglobulinemia[139] or certain kinds of nephritis.[140] In contrast to all the diseases mentioned previously, which usually have evidences of classic pathway activation such as low C4, type II membranoproliferative glomerulonephritis patients usually have only low C3, indicating direct activation of the alternative pathway, perhaps as a consequence of circulating C3NeF, which stabilizes the C3bBb enzymes and favors positive feedback into the amplification loop[141] (Fig. 7–3).

Inactive complement fragments may persist in joint or pleural spaces, so that radial immunodiffusion determinations of C3 or C4 in synovial or pleural fluid detect only spent fragments. Functional assays such as CH50 are required to detect evidence of local complement activation in diseases such as rheumatoid arthritis.[142,143] Although one report has indicated that depressed levels of C4 in cerebrospinal fluid correlated with central nervous system involvement,[144] another study has failed to confirm these findings, except in patients from whom serial specimens of cerebrospinal fluid are analyzed in a prospective fashion.[145]

Serum complement levels are elevated in rheumatoid arthritis, except in patients with systemic rheumatoid vasculitis, which usually is accompanied by a high titer of rheumatoid factor and the clinical finding of multiple subcutaneous nodules. Synovial fluid levels are frequently profoundly depressed, especially in patients with positive tests for rheumatoid factor.[142,143] Although both functional and immunodiffusion tests have demonstrated depressions of C1 in some patients and marked reductions in C4 and C2 in most, immunodiffusion results may not be reliable, because they detect complement protein that has already participated in an ongoing in vivo complement activation process but that has not yet been cleared from the joint space. An additional source of confusion arises from the local synthesis of complement proteins occurring in or near the joint space.[119] Thus, the abundant evidence for intra-articular activation of the complement system in rheumatoid arthritis is helpful in understanding the pathogenesis of the disease process, but it is rarely of value as a discriminating diagnostic test.

References

1. Atkinson, J.P., and Frank, M.M.: Complement. In Parker, C.W. (ed.): Clinical Immunology. Philadelphia, W.B. Saunders Co., 1980. p. 219.
2. Ruddy, S., Gigli, I., and Austen, K.F.: The complement system of man. N. Engl. J. Med. 287:489, 545, 592, 642, 1972.
3. Mayer, M.M.: The complement system. Sci. Am. 229:54, 1973.
4. Müller-Eberhard, H.I.: Chemistry and function of the complement system. Hosp. Pract. 12:33, 1978.
5. Colten, H.R., and Goldberger, G.: Ontogeny of serum complement proteins. Pediatrics 64(5 Pt. 2 Suppl.):775, 1979.
6. Reid, K.B., and Porter, R.R.: The proteolytic activation systems of complement. Ann. Rev. Biochem. 50:433, 1981.
7. Porter, R.R.: The Croonian Lecture, 1980. The complex proteases of the complement system. Proc. R. Soc. Lond. (Biol.) 210:477, 1980.
8. Kerr, M.A.: The human complement system: Assembly of the classical pathway C3 convertase. Biochem. J. 189:173, 1980.
9. Ziccardi, R.J.: Nature of the metal ion requirement for assembly and function of the first component of human complement. J. Biol. Chem. 258:6187, 1983.
10. Ziccardi, R.J., and Cooper, N.R.: The subunit composition and sedimentation properties of human C1. J. Immunol. 118:2047, 1977.
11. Knobel, H.R., Villiger, W., and Isliker, H.: Chemical analysis and electron microscopy studies of human C1q prepared by different methods. Eur. J. Immunol. 5:78, 1975.
12. Claus, D.R., Siegel, J., Petras, K., Skor, D., Osmand, A.P., and Gewurz, H.: Complement activation by interaction of polyanions and polycations. III. Complement activation by interaction of multiple polyanions and polycations in the presence of C-reactive protein. J. Immunol. 118:83, 1977.
13. Valet, G., and Cooper, N.R.: Isolation and characterization of the proenzyme form of the C1s subunit of the first complement component. J. Immunol. 112:339, 1974.
14. Ziccardi, R.J., and Cooper, N.R.: Physiochemical and functional characterization of the C1r subunit of the first complement component. J. Immunol. 116:496, 1976.
15. Schreiber, R.D., and Müller-Eberhard, H.J.: Fourth component of human complement. Description of a three polypeptide chain structure. J. Exp. Med. 140:1324, 1974.
16. Dykman, T.R., Cole, J.L., Iida, K., and Atkinson, J.P.: Polymorphism of human erythrocyte C3b/C4b receptor. Proc. Natl. Acad. Sci. USA 80:1698, 1983.
17. Gigli, I., and Austen, K.F.: Fluid phase destruction of C2hu by C1hu. II. Unmasking by C4ihu of C1−hu specificity for C2.hu J. Exp. Med. 130:833, 1969.
18. Polley, M.J., and Müller-Eberhard, H.J.: The second component of human complement: Its isolation, fragmentation by C'1 esterase, and incorporation into C'3 convertase. J. Exp. Med. 128:533, 1968.
19. Nicholson-Weller, A., Burge, J., Fearon, D.T., Weller, P.F., Austen, K.F.: Isolation of a human erythrocyte membrane glycoprotein with decay-accelerating activity for C3 convertases of the complement system. J. Immunol. 129:184, 1982.
20. Pensky, J., Levy, L.R., and Lepow, I.H.: Partial purification of a serum inhibitor of C'1-esterase. J. Biol. Chem. 236:1674, 1961.
21. Sim, R.B., and Reboul, A.: Preparation and properties of human C1 inhibitor. Methods Enzymol. 80:43, 1981.
22. Harpel, P.C., and Cooper, N.R.: Studies on human plasma C1 inactivator enzyme interactions. I. Mechanisms of interaction with C1s, plasmin, and trypsin. J. Clin. Invest. 55:593, 1975.
23. Donaldson, V.H., and Evans, R.R.: A biochemical abnormality in hereditary angioneurotic edema. Absence of serum inhibitor of C'1-esterase. Am. J. Med. 35:37, 1963.
24. Scharfstein, J., Ferreira, A., Gigli, I., and Nussenzweig, V.: Human C4-binding protein. I. Isolation and characterization. J. Exp. Med. 147:207, 1978.
25. Cooper, N. R.: Isolation and analysis of the mechanism of action of an inactivator of C4b in normal human serum. J. Exp. Med. 141:890, 1975.
26. Dobson, N.J., Lambris, J.D., Ross, G.D.: Characteristics of isolated erythrocyte complement receptor type one (CR1, C4b-C3b receptor) and CR1-specific antibodies. J. Immunol. 126:693, 1981.
27. Pillemer, L., Blum, L., Lepow, I.H., Ross, D.A., Todd, E.W., and Wardlaw, A.C.: The properdin system and immunity: I. Demonstration and isolation of a new serum protein, properdin, and its role in immune phenomena. Science 120:279, 1954.
28. Pillemer, I.: The nature of the properdin system and its interactions with polysaccharide complexes. Ann. N.Y. Acad. Sci. 66:233, 1956.
29. Nelson, R.A., Jr.: Alternative mechanism for properdin system. J. Exp. Med. 108:515, 1958.
30. Pensky, J., Hinz, C.F., Jr., Todd, E.W., Wedgwood, R.J., Boyer, J.T., and Lepow, I.H.: Properties of highly purified human properdin. J. Immunol. 100:142, 1968.
31. Bokisch, V.A., Dierich, M.P., and Müller-Eberhard, H.J.: Third component of complement (C3): Structural properties in relation to functions. Proc. Natl. Acad. Sci. 72:1989, 1975.
32. Law, S.K., and Levine, R.P.: Interaction between the third complement protein and cell surface macromolecules. Proc. Natl. Acad. Sci. 74:2701, 1977.
33. Müller-Eberhard, H.J., and Götze, O.: C3 proactivator convertase and its mode of action. J. Exp. Med. 135:1003, 1972.
34. Fearon, D.T., and Austen, K.F.: Properdin: Initiation of alternative complement pathway. Proc. Natl. Acad. Sci. 72:3220, 1975.
35. Schreiber, R.D., Medicus, R.G., Götze, O., and Müller-Eberhard, H.J.: Properdin- and nephritic factor-dependent C3 convertases: Requirement of native C3 for enzyme formation and the function of bound C3b as properdin receptor. J. Exp. Med. 142:760, 1975.
36. Schreiber, R.D., Pangburn, M.K., Lesavre, P.H., and Müller-Eberhard, H.J.: Initiation of the alternative pathway of complement: Recognition of activators by bound C3b and assembly of the entire pathway from six isolated proteins. Proc. Natl. Acad. Sci. 75:3848, 1978.
37. Raum, D., Glass, D., Carpenter, C.B., Alper, C.A., and Schur, P.H.: The chromosomal order of genes controlling the major histocompatibility complex, properdin factor B, and deficiency of the second component of complement. J. Clin. Invest. 58:1240, 1976.
38. Medicus, R.G., Götze, O., and Müller-Eberhard, H.J.: The serine protease nature of the C3 and C5 convertases of the classical and alternative complement pathways. Scand. J. Immunol. 5:1049, 1976.
39. Fearon, D.T., Austen, K.F., and Ruddy, S.: Formation of a hemolytically active cellular intermediate by the interaction between properdin factors B and D and the activated third component of complement. J. Exp. Med. 138:1305, 1973.
40. Davis, A.E., III: Active site amino acid sequence of human factor D. Proc. Natl. Acad. Sci. USA 77:4938, 1980.
41. Lesavre, P.H., and Müller-Eberhard, H.J.: Mechanism of action of factor D of the alternative complement pathway. J. Exp. Med. 148:1498, 1978.
42. Götze, O., and Müller-Eberhard, H.J.: The role of properdin in the alternate pathway of complement activation. J. Exp. Med. 139:44, 1974.
43. Müller-Eberhard, H.J., and Schreiber, R.D.: Molecular biology and chemistry of the alternative pathway of complement. Adv. Immunol. 29:1, 1980.
44. Chapitis, J., and Lepow, I.H.: Multiple sedimenting species of properdin in human serum and interaction of purified properdin with the third component of complement. J. Exp. Med. 143:241, 1976.
45. Götze, O., Medicus, R.G., and Müller-Eberhard, H.J.: Alternative pathway of complement: Non-enzymatic reversible transition of precursor to active properdin. J. Immunol. 118:525, 1977.
46. Fearon, D.T., and Austen, K.F.: Properdin: Binding to C3b and stabilization of the C3b-dependent C3 convertase. J. Exp. Med. 142:856, 1975.
47. Spitzer, R.E., Vallota, E.H., Forristal, J., Sudora, E., Stitzel, A., Davis, N.C., and West, C.D.: Serum C'3 lytic system in patients with glomerulonephritis. Science 164:436, 1969.
48. Thompson, R.A.: C3 inactivating factor in the serum of a patient with

chronic hypocomplementemic proliferative glomerulonephritis. Immunology 22:147, 1972.

49. Whaley, K., Ward, D., and Ruddy, S.: Modulation of the properdin amplification loop in membranoproliferative and other forms of glomerulonephritis. Clin. Exp. Immunol. 35:101, 1979.

50. Davis, A.E., III, Arnaout, M.A., Alper, C.A., and Rosen, F.S.: Transfer of C3 nephritic factor from mother to fetus. N. Engl. J. Med. 297:144, 1977.

51. Daha, M.R., Fearon, D.T., and Austen, K.F.: Isolation of alternative pathway C3 convertase containing uncleaved B and formed in the presence of C3 nephritic factor (C3NeF). J. Immunol. 116:568, 1976.

52. Daha, M.R., Austen, K.F., and Fearon, D.T.: Heterogeneity, polypeptide chain composition and antigenic reactivity of C3 nephritic factor. J. Immunol. 120:1389, 1978.

53. Scott, D.M., Amos, N., Sissons, J.G.P., Lachmann, P.J., and Peters, D.K.: The immunoglobulin nature of nephritis factor (NeF). Clin. Exp. Immunol. 32:12, 1978.

54. Tamura, N., and Nelson, R.A., Jr.: Three naturally occurring inhibitors of components of complement in guinea pig and rabbit serum. J. Immunol. 99:582, 1967.

55. Ruddy, S., and Austen, K.F.: C3b inactivator of man. II. Fragments produced by C3b inactivator cleavage of cell-bound or fluid phase C3b. J. Immunol. 107:742, 1971.

56. Whaley, K., and Ruddy, S.: Modulation of C3b hemolytic activity by a plasma protein distinct from C3b inactivator. Science 193:1011, 1976.

57. Whaley, K., and Ruddy, S.: Modulation of the alternative complement pathway by β1H globulin. J. Exp. Med. 144:1147, 1977.

58. Weiler, J.M., Daha, M.D., Austen, K.F., and Fearon, D.T.: Control of the amplification convertase of complement by the plasma protein β1H. Proc. Natl. Acad. Sci. 73:3268, 1976.

59. Pangburn, M.K., Schreiber, R.D., and Müller-Eberhard, H.J.: Human complement C3b inactivator: Isolation, characterization, and demonstration of an absolute requirement for the serum protein β1H for cleavage of C3b and C4b in solution. J. Exp. Med. 146:257, 1977.

60. Law, S.K., Fearon, D.T., and Levine, R.P.: Action of the C3b inactivator on cell bound C3b. J. Immunol. 122:759, 1979.

61. Carlo, J., Conrad, D.H., and Ruddy, S.: Complement receptor binding of C3b-coated cells treated with C3b inactivator, β1H globulin and trypsin. J. Immunol. 123:523, 1979.

62. Medicus, R.G., Melamed, J., and Arnaout, M.A.: Role of human factor I and C3b receptor in the cleavage of surface-bound C3bi molecules. Eur. J. Immunol. 13:465, 1983.

63. Carlo, J.R., Spitznagel, J.K., Studer, E.J., Conrad, D.H., and Ruddy, S.: Cleavage of membrane bound C3bi, an intermediate of the third component of complement, to C3c and C3d-like fragments by crude leucocyte lysosomal lysates and purified leucocyte elastase. Immunology 44:381, 1981.

64. Conrad, D.H., Carlo, J.R., and Ruddy, S.: Interaction of β1H-globulin with cell-bound C3b: Quantitative analysis of binding and influence of alternative pathway components on binding. J. Exp. Med. 122:523, 1978.

65. Pangburn, M.K., Schreiber, R.D., and Müller-Eberhard, H.J.: Formation of the initial C3 convertase of the alternative complement pathway. Acquisition of C3b-like activities by spontaneous hydrolysis of the putative thioester in native C3. J. Exp. Med. 154:856, 1981.

66. Fearon, D.T., and Austen, K.F.: Activation of the alternative complement pathway due to resistance of zymosan-bound amplification convertase to endogenous regulatory mechanisms. Proc. Nat. Acad. Sci. 74:1683, 1977.

67. Fearon, D.T.: Regulation by membrane sialic acid of β1H-dependent decay-dissociation of amplification C3 convertase of the alternative complement pathway. Proc. Natl. Acad. Sci. 75:1971, 1978.

68. Kazatchkine, M.D., Fearon, D.T., and Austen, K.F.: Human alternative complement pathway: Membrane-associated sialic acid regulates the competition between B and β1H for cell bound C36. J. Immunol. 122:75, 1979.

69. Nydegger, U.E., Fearon, D.T., and Austen, K.F.: Autosomal locus regulates inverse relationship between sialic acid content and capacity of mouse erythrocytes to activate human alternative complement pathway. Proc. Natl. Acad. Sci. 75:6078, 1978.

70. Vogt, W., Schmidt, G., von Buttlar, B., and Dieminger, L.: A new function of the activated third component of complement: Binding to C5, an essential step for C5 activation. Immunology 34:29, 1978.

71. Daha, M.R., Fearon, D.T., and Austen, K.F.: C3 requirements for formation of alternative pathway C5 convertase. J. Immunol. 117:630, 1976.

72. Fernandez, H.N., and Hugli, T.E.: Chemical evidence for common genetic ancestry of complement components C3 and C5. J. Biol. Chem. 252:1826, 1977.

73. Fernandez, H.N., and Hugli, T.E.: Partial characterization of human C5a anaphylatoxin. I. Chemical description of the carbohydrate and polypeptide portions of human C5a. J. Immunol. 117:1688, 1976.

74. Podack, E.R., Kolb, W.P., and Müller-Eberhard, H.J.: Purification of the sixth and seventh component of human complement without loss of hemolytic activity. J. Immunol. 116:263, 1976.

75. Hobart, M.J., Joysey, V., and Lachmann, P.J.: Inherited structural variation and linkage relationships of C7. J. Immunogenet. 5:157, 1978.

76. Lachmann, P.J., Hobart, M.J., and Woo, P.: Combined genetic deficiency of C6 and C7 in man. Clin. Exp. Immunol. 33:193, 1978.

77. Kolb, W.P., and Müller-Eberhard, H.J.: The membrane attack mechanism of complement: The three polypeptide chain structure of the eighth component (C8). J. Exp. Med. 143:1131, 1976.

78. Thompson, R.A., and Lachmann, P.J.: Reactive lysis: The complement-mediated lysis of unsensitized cells. I. The characterization of the indicator factors and its identification as C7. J. Exp. Med. 131:629, 1970.

79. Goldman, J.N., Ruddy, S., and Austen, K.F.: Reaction mechanisms of nascent C567 (reactive lysis). I. Reaction characteristics for production of EC567 and lysis by C8 and C9. J. Immunol. 109:353, 1972.

80. Mayer, M.M., Hammer, C.H., Michaels, D.W., and Shin, M.L.: Immunologically mediated membrane damage: The mechanism of complement action and the similarity of lymphocyte-mediated cytotoxicity. Immunochemistry 15:813, 1978.

81. Green, H., Barrow, P., and Goldberg, B.: Effect of antibody and complement on permeability control in ascites tumor cells and erythrocytes. J. Exp. Med. 110:699, 1959.

82. Podack, E.R., Kolb, W.P., and Müller-Eberhard, H.J.: The C5b-9 complex: Subunit composition of the classical and alternative pathway-generated complex. J. Immunol. 116:1431, 1976.

83. Bhakdi, S., and Tranum-Jensen, J.: Membrane damage by complement. Biochim. Biophys. Acta. 737:343, 1983.

84. Steckel, E.W., Welbaum, B.E., and Sodetz, J.M.: Evidence of direct insertion of terminal complement proteins into cell membrane bilayers during cytolysis. Labeling by a photosensitive membrane probe reveals a major role for the eighth and ninth components. J. Biol. Chem. 258:4318, 1983.

85. Donaldson, V.H., Ratnoff, O.D., Dias da Silva, W., and Rosen, F.S.: Permeability-increasing activity in hereditary angioneurotic edema plasma. II. Mechanism of formation and partial characterization. J. Clin. Invest. 48:642, 1969.

86. Fields, T., Ghebrehiwet, B., and Kaplan, A.P.: Kinin formation in hereditary angioedema plasma: Evidence against kinin derivation from C2 and in support of "spontaneous" formation of bradykinin. J. Allergy Clin. Immunol. 72:54, 1983.

87. Ruddy, S., Austen, K.F., and Goetzl, E.J.: Chemotactic activity derived from interaction of factors D and B of the properdin pathway with cobra venom factor or C3b. J. Clin. Invest. 55:587, 1975.

88. Götze, O., Bianco, C., and Cohn, Z.A.: The induction of macrophage spreading by factor B of the properdin system. J. Exp. Med. 149:372, 1979.

89. Bianco, C., Götze, O., and Cohn, Z.A.: Regulation of macrophage migration by products of the complement system. Proc. Natl. Acad. Sci. 76:888, 1979.

90. Bentley, C., Fries, W., and Brade, V.: Synthesis of factors D, B and P of the alternative pathway of complement activation, as well as of C3, by guinea-pig peritoneal macrophages in vitro. Immunology 35:971, 1978.

91. Cochrane, C.G., and Müller-Eberhard, H.J.: The derivation of two distinct anaphylatoxin activities from the third and fifth components of human complement. J. Exp. Med. 122:99, 1968.

92. Becker, S., Meuer, S., Hadding, U., and Bitter-Suermann, D: Platelet activation: A new biological activity of guinea-pig C3a anaphylatoxin. Scand. J. Immunol. 7:173, 1978.

93. Ferluga, L., Schorlemmer, H., Baptista, L.C., and Allison, A.C.: Cytolytic effects of the complement cleavage product, C3a. Br. J. Cancer 34:626, 1976.

94. Bokisch, V.A., Müller-Eberhard, H.J., and Cochrane, C.G.: Isolation of a fragment (C3a) of the third component of human complement containing anaphylatoxin and chemotactic activity and description of an anaphylatoxin inactivator of human serum. J. Exp. Med. 129:1109, 1969.

95. Ward, P.A., and Newman. L.J.: A neutrophil chemotactic factor from human C'5. J. Immunol. 102:93, 1969.

96. Goldstein, I.M., and Weissmann, G.: Generation of C5-derived lysosomal enzyme-releasing activity (C5a) by lysates of leukocyte lysosomes. J. Immunol. 113:1583, 1974.

97. Craddock, P.R., Hammerschmidt, D., White, J.G., Dalmasso, A.P., and Jacob, H.S.: Complement (C5a)-induced granulocyte aggregation in vitro. J. Clin. Invest. 60:260, 1977.

98. Fernandez, H.N., Henson, P.M., Otani, A., and Hugli, T.E.: Chemotactic response to human C3a and C5a anaphylatoxins. I. Evaluation of C3a and C5a leukotaxis in vitro and under simulated in vivo conditions. J. Immunol. 120:109, 1978.

99. Damerau, B., Grünefeld, E., and Vogt, W.: Chemotactic effects of the complement derived peptides C3a, C3a, and C5a (classical anaphyla-

toxin) on rabbit and guinea pig polymorphonuclear leukocytes. Arch. Pharmacol. 305:181, 1978.

100. McCall, C.E., de Chatelet, L.R., Brown, D., and Lachmann, P.: New biological activity following intravascular activation of the complement cascade. Nature 249:841, 1974.

101. Rother, K.: Leukocyte mobilizing factor: A new biological activity derived from the third component of complement. Eur. J. Immunol. 2:550, 1972.

102. Alper, C.A., Propp, R.P., Klemperer, M.R., and Rosen, F.S.: Inherited deficiency of the third component of human complement (C'3). J. Clin. Invest. 48:533, 1969.

103. Ehlenberger, A.G., and Nussenzweig, V.: The role of membrane receptors for C3b and C3d in phagocytosis. J. Exp. Med. 145:357, 1977.

104. Bianco, C., Griffin, F.M., and Silverstein, S.C.: Studies of the macrophage complement receptor. Alteration of receptor function upon macrophage activation. J. Exp. Med. 141:1278, 1975.

105. Shin, M.L., Gelfand, M.C., Nagle, R.B., Carlo, J.R., Green, I., and Frank, M.M.: Localization of receptors for activator complement on visceral epithelial cells of the human renal glomerulus. J. Immunol. 118:869, 1977.

106. Inada, S., Brown, E.J., Gaither, T.A., Hammer, C.H., Takahaski, T., and Frank, M.M.: C3d receptors are expressed on human monocytes after in vitro activation. Proc. Nat. Acad. Sci. 80:2351, 1983.

107. Lay, W.H., and Nussenzweig, V.: Receptors for complement on leukocytes. J. Exp. Med. 128:941, 1968.

108. Jondal, M., Klein, G., Oldstone, M.B.A., Bokish, V., and Yefenof, E.: Surface markers on human B and T lymphocytes: VIII. Association between complement and Epstein-Barr virus receptors on human lymphoid cells. Scand. J. Immunol. 5:401, 1976.

109. Hutt-Fletcher, L.M., Fowler, E., Lambris, J.D., Feighny, R.J., Simmons, J.G., and Ross, G.D.: Studies of the Epstein-Barr virus receptor found on Raji cells. II. A comparison of lymphocyte binding studies for Epstein-Barr virus and C3d. J. Immunol. 130:1309, 1983.

110. Sandberg, A.L., Wahl, S.M., and Mergenhagen, S.E.: Lymphokine production by C3b-stimulated B cells. J. Immunol. 116:139, 1975.

111. Hartman, K-V, and Bokisch, V.A.: Stimulation of murine B lymphocytes by isolated C3b. J. Exp. Med. 145:600, 1975.

112. Rutherford, B., and Schenkein, H.: C3 cleavage products stimulate release of prostaglandins by human mononuclear cells in vitro. J. Immunol. 130:874, 1983.

113. Pepys, M.B.: Role of complement in the induction of the immunological responses. Transplant. Rev. 32:157, 1976.

114. Klaus, G.G.B., and Humphrey, J.H.: The generation of memory cells. I. The role of C3 in the generation of B memory cells. Immunology 33:31, 1977.

115. Ballas, Z.K., Feldbush, T.L., Needleman, B.W., and Weiler, J.M.: Complement inhibits immune responses: C3 preparations inhibit the generation of human cytotoxic T lymphocytes. Eur. J. Immunol. 13:274, 1983.

116. Colten, H.R.: Biosynthesis of complement. Adv. Immunol. 22:67, 1976.

117. Petz, L.D.: Variable mechanisms for low serum complement in liver disease. Lancet 2:1033, 1971.

118. Alper, C.A., Johnson, A.M., Birtch, A.G., and Moore, F.D.: Human C'3: Evidence for the liver as the primary site of synthesis. Science 163:286, 1969.

119. Ruddy, S., and Colten, H.R.: Rheumatoid arthritis: Biosynthesis of complement proteins by synovial tissues. N. Engl. J. Med. 290:1284, 1974.

120. Littman, B.H., and Ruddy, S.: Production of the second component of complement by human monocytes: Stimulation by antigen-activated lymphocytes or lymphokines. J. Exp. Med. 145:1344, 1977.

121. Ruddy, S., Carpenter, C.B., Chin, K.W., Knostman, J.N., Soter, N.A., Götze, O., Müller-Eberhard, H.J., and Austen, K.F.: Human complement metabolism: An analysis of 144 studies. Medicine 54:165, 1975.

122. Whaley, K., Widener, H., and Ruddy, S.: Modulation of the alternative pathway amplification loop in rheumatic diseases. In Opferkuch, W., Rother, K., and Schultz, D.R. (eds.): Clinical Aspects of the Complement System, Proceedings of an International Symposium held in Bochum, Germany. Stuttgart, George Thieme Publishers, 1978, p. 99.

123. Sakiyama, U., Hall, R.E., and Colten, H.R.: Translation of precursors of C4 and albumin by isolated guinea pig M-RNA. J. Immunol. 120:1795, 1978.

124. Patel, F., and Minta, J.O.: In vitro studies on the biosynthesis of rabbit C3: Evidence for the synthesis of a nascent single chain precursor C3. J. Immunol. 122:1582, 1979.

125. Gorski, J.P., and Müller-Eberhard, H.J.: Single-chain C4 from human plasma. J. Immunol. 120:1775, 1978.

126. Mayer, M.M.: Complement and complement fixation. In Kabat, E.A., and Mayer, M.M. (eds.): Experimental Immunochemistry. Springfield, Ill., Charles C Thomas, 1961, p. 133.

127. Ruddy, S., and Austen, K.F.: Complement and its components. In Cohen, A. (ed.): Laboratory Diagnostic Procedures in the Rheumatic Diseases. 2nd ed. Boston, Little, Brown & Company, 1975, p. 131.

128. Ruddy, S., Carpenter, C.B., Müller-Eberhard, H.J., and Austen, K.F.: Complement component levels in hereditary angioneurotic edema and isolated C'2 deficiency in man. In Miescher, P.A., and Grabar, P. (eds.): Mechanisms of Inflammation Induced by Immune Reactions. Vth International Immunopathology Symposium. Basel, Schwabe and Company, 1968, p. 231.

129. Ruddy, S., Everson, L.K., Schur, P.H., and Austen, K.F.: Hemolytic assay of the ninth complement component: Elevation and depletion in rheumatic diseases. J. Exp. Med. 134:259S, 1971.

130. Alper, C.A., and Rosen, F.S.: Studies in the in vivo behavior of human C'3 in normal subjects and patients. J. Clin. Invest. 46:2021, 1967.

131. Rynes, R.I., Ruddy, S., Schur, P.H., Spragg, J., and Austen, K.F.: Levels of complement components, properdin factors, and kininogen in patients with inflammatory arthritides. J. Rheumatol. 1:413, 1974.

132. Schur, P.H.: Complement studies of sera and other biologic fluids. Hum. Pathol. 14:338, 1983.

133. Williams, R.C., Jr., and Kunkel, H.G.: Rheumatoid factor, complement and conglutinin aberrations in patients with subacute bacterial endocarditis. J. Clin. Invest. 41:666, 1962.

134. Alpert, E., Isselbacher, K.J., and Schur, P.H.: Pathogenesis of arthritis associated with viral hepatitis. N. Engl. J. Med. 285:185, 1971.

135. Reed, W.P., Davidson, M.S., and Williams, R.C., Jr.: Complement system in pneumococcal infections. Infect. Immun. 13:1120, 1976.

136. Fearon, D.T., Ruddy, S., Schur, P.H., and McCabe, W.R.: Activation of the properdin pathway of complement in patients with gram-negative bacteremia. N. Engl. J. Med. 292:937, 1975.

137. Charlesworth, J.A., Pussell, B.A., Roy, L.P., Robertson, M.R., and Beveridge, J.: Measles infection: Involvement of the complement system. Clin. Exp. Immunol. 24:401, 1976.

138. Ward, P.A., and Kibukamusoke, J.W.: Evidence for soluble immune complexes in the pathogenesis of the glomerulonephritis of quartan malaria. Lancet 1:283, 1969.

139. Riethmuller, G., Meltzer, M., Franklin, E., and Miescher, P.A.: Serum complement levels in patients with mixed (IgM-IgG) cryoglobulinemia. Clin. Exp. Immunol. 1:337, 1966.

140. West, C.D., Northway, J.D., and Davis, N.C.: Serum levels of β_{1c} globulin, a complement component, in the nephritides, lipoid nephrosis and other conditions. J. Clin. Invest. 43:1507, 1964.

141. Hunsicker, L.G., Ruddy, S., Carpenter, C.B., Schur, P.H., Merrill, J.P., Müller-Eberhard, H.J., and Austen, K.F.: Metabolism of third complement component (C3) in nephritis involvement of the classic and alternate (properdin) pathways for complement activation. N. Engl. J. Med. 287:835, 1972.

142. Pekin, T.J., Jr., and Zvaifler, N.J.: Hemolytic complement in synovial fluid. J. Clin. Invest. 43:1372, 1964.

143. Ruddy, S., and Austen, K.F.: Activation of the complement system in rheumatoid synovitis. Fed. Proc. 32:134, 1973.

144. Petz, L.D., Sharp, G.C., Cooper, N.R., et al.: Serum and cerebrospinal fluid complement and serum autoantibodies in systemic lupus erythematosus. Medicine 50:259, 1971.

145. Hadler, N.M., Gerwin, R.D., Frank, M.M., Whitaker, J.N., Baker, M., and Decker, J.L.: The fourth component of complement in the cerebrospinal fluid in systemic lupus erythematosus. Arthritis Rheum. 16:507, 1973.

Chapter 8

The Intrinsic Coagulation, Fibrinolytic, and Kinin-Forming Pathways of Man

Allen P. Kaplan

INTRODUCTION

During the past decade, considerable progress has been made in understanding the mechanism by which the intrinsic coagulation and fibrinolytic pathways are activated and defining their relationship to the generation of the vasoactive peptide, bradykinin.

In Figure 8–1 is shown a simplified section scheme for bradykinin formation which subdivides it into three critical steps. First, Hageman factor is activated, a reaction dependent upon interaction with certain negatively charged surfaces. Next, activated Hageman factor converts prekallikrein to kallikrein, and then kallikrein digests high molecular weight (HMW) kininogen to generate bradykinin. In addition, activated Hageman factor also converts coagulation factor XI to factor XIa, and factor XIa then continues the intrinsic coagulation pathway. Although this scheme is technically correct, it does not indicate the complex manner in which those proteins interact so as to link the initiation of coagulation with kinin formation. In fact, the three proteins of the plasma kinin-forming system, Hageman factor, prekallikrein, and HMW kininogen, are all required for contact activation of plasma. In addition, we have learned that prekallikrein and factor XI each circulate as a complex with HMW kininogen and are bound to surfaces where they then interact with surface-bound Hageman factor. Methods have been developed for the purification of each of these reactants; their mechanism of activation has been determined; and considerable progress has been made in understanding their interactions. In this review I will present a detailed analysis of our present concept of the early events of these pathways and attempt to relate such events to the inflammatory reactions that are characteristic of connective tissue disorders.

Identification of the Factors Required for Contact Activation of Plasma. The intrinsic coagulation pathway is initiated by interaction of plasma with certain negatively charged surfaces;[1-4] thus activation proceeds upon contact with glass or kaolin when a clotting time or partial thromboplastin time (PTT) is determined. In 1955, Ratnoff and Colopy described a patient named Hageman[5] who had a markedly prolonged PTT and appeared to lack a plasma factor, designated Hageman factor, which bound to the surface and was active at the initiating step of the coagulation cascade.[6] The protein was partially purified from normal plasma[7,8] and was found to be a β globulin with a sedimentation coefficient of approximately 5S.[9] In addition, Hageman factor deficient plasma was subsequently shown to possess a profound abnormality of surface-dependent fibrinolysis[10,11] and generated no bradykinin upon incubation with glass beads or kaolin.[12-15]

In 1965, a new coagulation abnormality was discovered in a family named Fletcher,[16] which was characterized as having a prolonged PTT that autocorrected as the time of incubation with surfaces was increased.[16,17] This latter property suggested that it possessed an abnormal *rate* of contact activation. In addition, the abnormality could be corrected upon addition of small quantities of normal plasma, and the corrective factor was partially purified.[18] It was clearly distinguishable from Hageman factor, and, although it appeared in fractions containing factor XI, chromatographic separation of the Fletcher factor from factor XI was achieved.[18] Subsequently Wuepper identified the Fletcher factor to be prekallikrein.[19] A detailed analysis of the functional abnormalities associated with prekallikrein deficiency revealed a diminished rate of Hageman factor dependent fibrinolysis,[20-22] which was corrected upon prolonged incubation with surfaces,[21] and an inability to generate any bradykinin regardless of the incubation time.[20-22] Fletcher trait plasma not only lacked functional prekallikrein, but possessed no detectable antigenic prekallikrein.[18-22] Weiss and colleagues[21] observed that the addition of preparations of activated Hageman factor to prekallikrein deficient plasma corrected the diminished rate of intrinsic coagulation and fibrinolysis but not the inability to generate bradykinin. These data suggested that the plasma possessed an abnormal rate of formation of activated Hageman factor and thereby implicated prekallikrein as a factor required for contact activation. The autocorrection with time, in the absence of prekallikrein, suggested that a slower, alternative mechanism existed that could also lead to the formation of activated Hageman factor. Reconstitution with prekallikrein, however, was an absolute requirement for kinin generation, as suggested by earlier work in which kallikrein was identified to be the plasma enzyme that digests kininogen to generate bradykinin (Fig. 8–1).

The next development in the identification of the plasma factors required for contact activation was ob-

Figure 8–1. Scheme indicating those proteins required for initiation of the coagulation-kinin forming system.

servations by Webster and Pierce[24] and by Schiffman and Lee[25] indicating that the combination of a surface, Hageman factor, and prekallikrein was not sufficient to initiate kinin generation or factor XI activation. Evidence that an additional plasma factor is required for contact activation was presented, and the latter workers called it the "contact activation cofactor." Soon thereafter, three different patients possessing unique abnormalities of contact activation were reported; two of these patients, named Williams and Fitzgerald, were reported at an international "kallikrein-kinin" meeting,[26,27] and the third patient, named Flaujeac, was reported at a coagulation meeting in France.[28] Each plasma was shown to possess a markedly prolonged PTT that did not autocorrect with time, diminished surface-dependent fibrinolysis, and absent kinin formation.[26,28-30] Flaujeac trait plasma was then shown to possess only 8 percent of normal plasma kininogen, and the functional abnormalities were each corrected upon addition of plasma fractions containing HMW kininogen.[31,32] Williams trait plasma was found to be completely devoid of functional or antigenic kininogen,[26,33] and the abnormality was attributed to a new coagulation factor[33] that was also identified to be HMW kininogen.[34] These observations were confirmed when Fitzgerald trait was identified as HMW kininogen deficiency in a fourth patient (Washington) possessing the identical functional abnormalities.[35] HMW kininogen was also shown to be the same protein whose function had been observed using partially purified plasma fractions,[24,25] and the contact activation cofactor was shown to be lacking in Fitzgerald trait plasma[36] and then to be identical to HMW kininogen.[37,38]

The triad of abnormal coagulation, fibrinolysis, and kinin generation appears to be a property of each abnormal plasma that functions at the initial step of the cascade. Thus, although factor XI was shown to be a substrate of Hageman factor,[39] factor XI deficient plasma has a normal initial rate of kaolin-activatable fibrinolysis and normal kinin generation. Factor XI deficient plasma does not, therefore, possess an abnormal rate of Hageman factor activation or function. A time course of surface dependent activation of the intrinsic coagulation pathway is shown in Figure 8–2 and demonstrates the marked abnormality present in both Hageman factor deficient plasma and HMW kininogen deficient plasma as well as the abnormal rate of activation of prekallikrein deficient plasma.

Interaction of Prekallikrein, Factor XI, and HMW Kininogen in Plasma. It is clear that Hageman factor, prekallikrein, HMW kininogen, factor XI, and plasminogen are intimately related functionally, but they clearly represent different plasma proteins that are antigenically unrelated and are represented in the genome by distinct structural genes. However, reports suggesting that kallikrein can be purified as a complex with another plasma protein[40] and that prekallikrein appears to circulate in plasma as a complex[41] prompted the studies of Mandle and colleagues[42] and Thompson and associates,[43] in which prekallikrein and factor XI were each shown to circulate bound to HMW kininogen.

When normal human plasma was fractionated on Sephadex G-200, the apparent molecular weight of each of the aforementioned proteins could be determined. Factor XI was found at a molecular weight of 380,000, prekallikrein was found at 260,000, Hageman factor fractionated at 115,000, and plasminogen was located at 95,000. However, when the molecular weights of purified factor XI and prekallikrein were assessed by gel filtration, values of 175,000 and 100,000, respectively, were obtained, a discrepancy of approximately 200,000. Purified Hageman factor and plasminogen fractionated at the same position as they did when whole plasma was assessed, and therefore did not appear to circulate as part of a complex. When the molecular weight of prekallikrein and factor XI was determined in plasma that was deficient in HMW kininogen, factor XI was found at 175,000 and prekallikrein was found at 100,000, suggesting that each protein normally circulates bound to HMW kininogen. Reconstitution of HMW kininogen deficient plasma with purified HMW kininogen followed by fractionation by Sephadex G-200 gel filtration reproduced the chromatographic pattern of factor XI and prekallikrein in normal plasma.[42,43] In addition, direct binding of purified prekallikrein to HMW kininogen[42] and direct binding of partially purified factor XI to HMW kininogen[43] have been demonstrated. Normal plasma contains approximately twice the concentration of HMW kininogen as the sum of the factor XI and prekallikrein concentrations; thus complete binding of

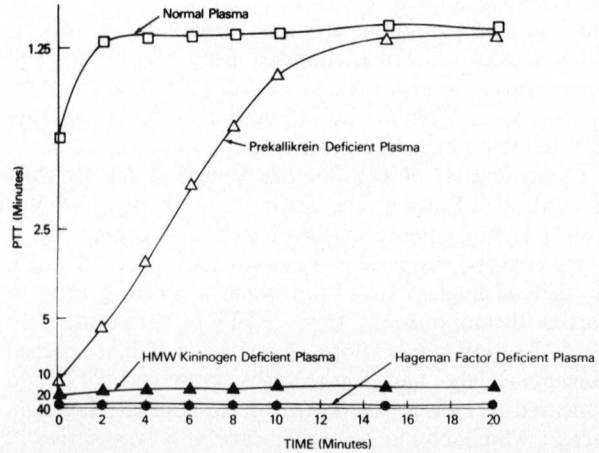

Figure 8–2. Time course of activation of the Hageman factor–dependent coagulation pathway.

factor XI and prekallikrein results, and the major peak of HMW kininogen seen represents uncomplexed protein.[43] No complex has been observed containing prekallikrein, factor XI, and HMW kininogen as a single entity; prekallikrein and factor XI appear to circulate bound to different molecules of HMW kininogen. Binding to HMW kininogen also appears to be a specific property of the Hageman factor substrates, and the complexes of prekallikrein–HMW kininogen and factor XI–HMW kininogen are each adsorbed to surfaces where they then interact with surface-bound Hageman factor. A schematic diagram showing the critical constituents bound to the surface is shown in Figure 8–3.

Identification of Surfaces upon Which Activation Can Proceed. The materials that serve as initiators of the intrinsic coagulation pathway include a diverse array of substances, such as silicon dioxide, glass, kaolin, talc, diatomaceous earth, celite, supercel, barium carbonate, cellulose sulfate, dextran sulfate (molecular weight 500,000), carrageenan, and ellagic acid.[15,44-49] In addition certain biologic materials can initiate the cascade; for example, crystals of sodium urate,[50] calcium pyrophosphate,[50] or L-homocysteine,[51] which are produced by patients with gout, pseudogout, and homocystinuria, respectively, may act as appropriate surfaces. Exposure of human plasma to articular cartilage also yields kininlike activity that appears to be Hageman factor dependent,[52] while skin contact[53] and interaction with fatty acids[54-56] may also lead to Hageman factor activation. Activation of Hageman factor has been reported to occur upon contact with certain bacterial lipopolysaccharides[57] in which the lipid A fraction containing negatively charged phosphate groups appears to be the functional moiety. Evidence of Hageman factor activation during episodes of endotoxic shock has been reported,[58-64] and the products of this reaction may contribute to the intravascular coagulation and hypotension seen. Of particular interest is the observation that endotoxic shock in monkeys was not inhibited by prior complement depletion, although much of the tissue inflammatory reaction was diminished.[63] It is possible that the generation of vasoactive peptides such as bradykinin is responsible for the vasodilatation and pooling of fluid into tissues that is characteristic of endotoxic shock. Immune complexes have been thought to be capable of initiating the Hageman factor dependent pathways.[64-70] However, incubation of purified Hageman factor with immune complexes or aggregated immunoglobulins did not lead to activation of Hageman factor, and binding of Hageman factor to the complexes was not observed.[71] It is possible that the positive results reported may have been attributable to traces of kallikrein contaminating immunoglobulin preparations, or that activation was observed by a pathway independent of Hageman factor.

It would be of obvious interest and importance to identify connective tissue components that can act as appropriate surfaces for binding the critical reactants in order to initiate the Hageman factor dependent pathways. Crude preparations of collagen[72-74] or vascular basement membrane[74] appear to be capable of initiating the cascade, and the carboxyl groups of collagen have been reported to be required for the reaction to proceed. In addition, insoluble bovine collagen preparations have been shown to bind kallikrein, and such binding was dependent upon the availability of both carboxyl and amino groups.[75] However, one study reported no activation of Hageman factor when purified Hageman factor was incubated with purified triple helical soluble collagen.[76] In addition, Meier and Kaplan[77] have reported that preparation of purified type I, II, and III collagens, chondroitin sulfates A and C, dermatan sulfate, bovine nasal cartilage proteoglycans, and collagen fibrils formed with incorporated proteoglycans all failed to initiate kinin formation when incubated with normal plasma. Thus we have not yet been able to identify the specific component or combination of components present in connective tissue that can initiate Hageman factor dependent coagulation, fibrinolysis, and kinin formation.

HAGEMAN FACTOR

Properties of Human Hageman Factor. Hageman factor was found to be a single chain β globulin of molecular weight 80,000 and was present in plasma at concentrations ranging from 23 to 47 μg per milliliter (mean, 29 μg per milliliter).[78] The peak isoelectric point of human Hageman factor was reported to be between 6.1 and 6.5; however, considerable charge heterogeneity was observed with a pH range of 5.9 to 7.0.[71]

Assays of Unactivated and Activated Hageman Factor. Hageman factor can be assayed by a modification of the PTT,[79] utilizing Hageman factor deficient plasma as the substrate. This method is routinely utilized in coagulation laboratories and consists of an initial incubation of the deficient plasma with the Hageman factor source, kaolin, and cephalin for 2 minutes at 37° C. Calcium is added, and the time of formation of a clot is recorded. A 1:10 dilution of pooled normal human plasma is serially diluted, each dilution is assayed for Hageman factor, and a standard dose-response curve is constructed. The Hageman factor content of samples can then be expressed as a percentage of normal plasma Hageman factor or in units per milliliter if 1 unit represents the quantity of Hageman factor in pooled plasma. This method is reliable only for the determination of unactivated Hageman factor. Upon activation,

Figure 8–3. Schematic diagram depicting the interaction of surface-bound Hageman factor (HF) with complexes of HMW kininogen and prekallikrein and complexes of HMW kininogen and factor XI.

Hageman factor readily fragments, resulting in considerable loss of coagulant activity.[80,81] The presence of activated Hageman factor can be detected using a coagulation assay by clotting the sample in the absence of kaolin.[81] If a sample shortens the PTT of Hageman factor deficient plasma but has no effect upon factor XI deficient plasma, it is likely to contain activated Hageman factor. However, the assay does not distinguish the particular form of activated Hageman factor present; e.g., one might have an active but nonfragmented form of Hageman factor or one or more active fragments of Hageman factor. Since the various fragments differ in specific activity, the assay cannot be used in a quantitative fashion.

A sensitive, specific, primary assay for activated Hageman factor is not available; thus most assays require at least one incubation with a second plasma protein. Activated Hageman factor has been shown to digest D-pro-phe-arg-p-nitro-anilide[82] and this is particularly useful when assaying the purified protein. It does not distinguish the various activated forms of Hageman factor (all are equally reactive), and it cannot be used in plasma, since this substrate is cleaved by a variety of proteases, particularly kallikrein. Utilizing a very different approach we have recently developed a double antibody ELISA assay which measures the circulating complex of activated HF and its inhibitor, C$\overline{1}$ INH.[82a] In this assay IgG antihuman HFa is bound to a microtiter plate, and the sample is added, incubated, and washed. We then incubate with (Fab')$_2$ antihuman C$\overline{1}$ INH to which alkaline phosphatase is covalently coupled. p-Nitrophenyl phosphate is then added as an alkaline phosphatase substrate, which when cleaved, yields p-nitrophenol, a yellow component whose absorbance is read at O.D.405 nm. The color formation is dependent upon reaction with bound C$\overline{1}$ INH, which in turn is directly proportional to the amount of activated HF present. The assay does not distinguish HFa from HFf but does detect both since the antibody to HFa also detects HFf. This assay is presently being utilized as a sensitive and specific measure of initiation of the Hageman factor dependent pathways, but there are no data available as yet for specific disease entities. Similar assays are now available for the determination of kallikrein[83] and plasmin.[84]

Activated Hageman factor can also be determined by its ability to convert prekallikrein to kallikrein. This approach has the advantage of detecting all the various forms of activated Hageman factor (although it does not distinguish one from the other), and the kallikrein generated can be accurately determined. A purified "standard" prekallikrein preparation can be used and its rate of conversion to kallikrein determined. Alternatively, the Hageman factor sample can be added directly to normal plasma anticoagulated with EDTA and the kallikrein generated assayed, using synthetic substrates that are specific for kallikrein[85] (see Prekallikrein, below, for details of these assays). A major limitation of such assays is that activated Hageman factor exists for only a short period of time and it is inactivated by binding to C$\overline{1}$

INH. Thus the aforementioned assay for the activated Hageman factor-C$\overline{1}$ INH complex is a more reliable assessment of activation.

Hageman factor protein can be assayed immunologically using monospecific antisera. By radial immunodiffusion, its concentration in plasma has been estimated to be 27 to 45 μg per milliliter,[74] and a sensitive radioimmunoassay for Hageman factor has been reported.[86] Immunologic assays do not, of course, give any information regarding the state of activation of the protein and can yield erroneous results if the Hageman factor is fragmented. For example, if an antiserum is reactive with the Hageman factor fragments, the more rapid diffusion of the fragments can yield falsely elevated results by immunodiffusion. A radioimmunoassay may also give spurious results, depending upon the relative ability of the Hageman factor fragments and the standard Hageman factor preparation to compete for binding to the antiserum.

Activation and Fragmentation of Hageman Factor: The Role of the Surface, HMW Kininogen, and Prekallikrein. The activation of Hageman factor differs from that observed with the other proenzymes to be described herein because two different proteolytic steps are involved; the first consists of a cleavage without obvious fragmentation, and the second, a cleavage that liberates one or more active fragments. The discovery of the active fragments of Hageman factor by Kaplan and Austen[80] provided the first evidence that activation could be performed enzymatically.[81] The final product, a prealbumin fragment observed as two closely migrating bands upon alkaline disc gel electrophoresis, functioned as a potent prekallikrein activator but retained only 2 to 5 percent of the coagulant activity of the unfragmented Hageman factor. These fragments are designated HFf. Subsequently, plasmin was shown to be capable of directly digesting Hageman factor to yield these fragments.[81] Similar prealbumin activities described in the rabbit,[86] guinea pig,[87] and man[88,89] were subsequently shown to be derived from Hageman factor,[90,91] and the ability of plasmin to activate and fragment Hageman factor was confirmed.[92] Although not purified, an activated preparation of Hageman factor was also described whose molecular weight upon gel filtration was identical to that of unactivated Hageman factor, yet it readily clotted Hageman factor deficient plasma in the absence of kaolin. This preparation was designated intact activated Hageman factor or HFa.[81] In addition, at least two active fragments were described whose molecular weight was intermediate between that of HFf and HFa.

The discovery of prekallikrein deficient plasma led to an examination of the ability of kallikrein to activate and fragment Hageman factor. Kallikrein was found to function in a similar manner to plasmin; however, it was approximately 10 times as effective[94] and could act upon either surface bound or fluid phase Hageman factor. When Hageman factor was iodinated, digested, and examined by SDS gel electrophoresis, trypsin, plasmin, and kallikrein were found to yield similar patterns.[78] The molecular weight of Hageman factor was 90,000 in un-reduced gels and 80,000 after reduction; upon digestion it was converted to HFf, and a 50,000-dalton fragment remained. Further digestion converted the 50,000-dalton fragment to fragments of 40,000 and 10,000. However, the formation of HFa was not detected. The 50,000-dalton fragment was subsequently shown to be the por-tion of the molecule that binds to surfaces.[95]

These studies suggested that activated Hageman fac-tor converts prekallikrein to kallikrein and kallikrein enzymatically activates Hageman factor, i.e., they acti-vate each other. With the discovery of HMW kininogen deficiency, it became clear that such a reciprocal mech-anism was an oversimplification. For example, addition of HFa to Hageman factor deficient plasma causes co-agulation in the absence of kaolin by activation of factor XI. Addition of factor XIa to factor XI deficient plasma causes coagulation in the absence of kaolin by activation of factor IX. However, addition of kallikrein to pre-kallikrein deficient plasma, in the absence of a surface, did not result in appreciable coagulation.[96] Thus the surface appeared to be required for this function of kal-likrein to be expressed. Furthermore, the addition of activated Hageman factor to HMW kininogen deficient plasma, even in the presence of a surface, did not sig-nificantly shorten its partial thromboplastin time.[97,98] HMW kininogen therefore appeared to be required for the activation of Hageman factor and/or the expression of Hageman factor activity. When the role of HMW kininogen was further examined, it was found to enhance both the function of activated Hageman factor and the formation of activated Hageman factor.[97-101] For a fixed amount of surface-bound Hageman factor, the subse-quent activation of prekallikrein and factor XI appeared proportional to the quantity of HMW-kininogen added.[97,101] Such an experiment could be performed uti-lizing HFf in the absence of a surface[100] or limited trypsin treatment of surface-bound Hageman factor (presum-ably HFa),[97] indicating that the effect of HMW kinin-ogen observed was upon the function of activated Hage-man factor, i.e., it facilitated its ability to activate prekallikrein and factor XI. However, these observations do not preclude an effect upon the activation of Hage-man factor. Griffin and Cochrane reported that the rate of cleavage of Hageman factor by kallikrein appeared to be enhanced by HMW kininogen,[97] suggesting an effect upon Hageman factor activation. Meier and col-leagues assessed this reaction functionally and demon-strated that the ability of kallikrein to activate Hageman factor was markedly augmented by HMW kininogen.[101] When the presence of activated Hageman factor was assessed functionally, formation of new active sites was determined by incorporation of ^{3}H-DFP.[101] In the pres-ence of HMW kininogen, the function of each of these sites could then be fully expressed. Figure 8–4 is a sche-matic diagram of this reciprocal interaction of surface-bound Hageman factor and prekallikrein, indicating that the reaction rate in each direction is augmented by HMW kininogen.

It should be emphasized that the surface and the active

Figure 8–4. Schematic diagram of the reciprocal activation of surface-bound Hageman factor and prekallikrein that is catalyzed by HMW kininogen.

site of kallikrein were required for this activation of Hageman factor[99,101] to proceed. Thus kallikrein did not correct prekallikrein deficient plasma in the absence of a surface,[96,101] DFP-kallikrein did not correct prekalli-krein deficient plasma in the presence of a surface,[99,101] and DFP-kallikrein would not activate purified surface-bound Hageman factor.[101] The surface has been esti-mated to augment the rate of cleavage of Hageman factor by kallikrein by as much as 50-fold.[102] Thus the surface appears to augment the rate of interaction of the reac-tants, and, in particular, render the Hageman factor a better substrate for plasma kallikrein. The ability of HMW kininogen to augment the function of activated Hageman factor has been estimated to be 3- to 4-fold, while its effect upon the activation of Hageman factor yields a 40-fold enhancement.[101] When combined with the surface, the rate is augmented 6000-fold. It is likely that changes observed upon binding of Hageman factor to surfaces or ellagic acid[103] may relate to the increased rate of cleavage of Hageman factor rather than the gen-eration of a new active site in the Hageman factor.

More recent studies have attempted to further delin-eate the molecular mechanism by which HMW kin-inogen affects both the activation of Hageman factor as well as the effect of HFa upon its substrates. Wiggins and colleagues[104] determined that the quantity of pre-kallikrein and factor XI bound to the surface in HMW kininogen deficient plasma is diminished and that the rate of cleavage by surface bound Hageman factor was abnormal. These data appear consistent with Figure 8–3, in which HMW kininogen is the "bridge" by which prekallikrein and factor XI are attached to surfaces. However, using purified proteins in aqueous solution and a kaolin surface, Silverberg and colleagues[105] have shown that prekallikrein and factor XI bind to kaolin equally well in the presence or absence of HMW kinin-ogen but that activation is markedly diminished when HMW kininogen is absent. These results indicate that with a surface such as kaolin, HMW kininogen binding of prekallikrein and factor XI allow them to attach to the surface in a conformation that facilitates cleavage by HFa. The fact that the quantity of prekallikrein and factor XI bound in plasma is indeed less than normal in the absence of HMW kininogen was reproduced but appears less important than the way in which binding occurs. Other data have further delineated the role of HMW kininogen upon the activation of Hageman factor by kallikrein. Once prekallikrein is converted to kallikrein, a fraction of the kallikrein can dissociate from the HMW kininogen,[106] and it is then able to interact with Hageman factor molecules bound to other sites or to adjacent particles.[105,107] Interestingly, when prekallikrein is bound directly to kaolin, it does not dissociate. In this fashion, the activation of Hageman factor is markedly amplified. This dissociation is consistent with observations that the binding constant of the prekallikrein–HMW kininogen complex is such that at plasma concentration, about 10 percent of prekallikrein should be free,[106] and other studies have demonstrated this small fraction of unbound prekallikrein.[108] In the presence of a surface with an equilibrium between bound and unbound prekallikrein, some of the kallikrein formed would be expected to dissociate. Thus the effect of HMW kininogen upon Hageman factor activation is indirect, since it does not augment the intrinsic activity of kallikrein, nor does it directly affect the rate at which Hageman factor is cleaved. It appears to maximize the effective ratio of kallikrein to Hageman factor, thereby facilitating the enzymatic reaction. This is accomplished by its cofactor function for conversion of prekallikrein to kallikrein and then allowing dissociation of kallikrein to sites of bound Hageman factor.[105]

Activation of Hageman Factor: Autoactivation upon Negatively Charged Surfaces. One of the enigmas faced when considering the initiation of contact activation is the fact that all of the enzymes involved exist in the circulation in a precursor form. Thus, it is unclear how the first active site is created to initiate the cascade. Studies pertaining to this issue generally focus upon Hageman factor as the starting point of the cascade, as depicted in Figure 8–1. Earlier studies presented evidence to suggest that when Hageman factor is bound to a surface, it undergoes a conformational change[103,109] and exposes an active site. Other studies failed to demonstrate active site formation in the absence of proteolysis.[97,99,101,102,110] On the other hand, some publications have presented data to suggest that rabbit, bovine,[111–113] and human[114] Hageman factor possess significant intrinsic enzymatic activity when surface bound in the absence of any cleavage and proposed the possibility of a substrate-induced conformational change in Hageman factor that facilitates the process.[112] In fact, data using bovine Hageman factor indicated that HFa is only 3- to 4-fold better than native, uncleaved HF in activating prekallikrein and factor XI.[111,112] Our own studies of human Hageman factor indicate that a different mechanism of initiation is involved. This was first suggested by observations made in rabbit[110] and human[115] Hageman factor in which purified Hageman factor slowly

appeared to autoactivate upon binding to surfaces. For example, with time and in the absence of any identifiable contaminants, the Hageman factor was digested to yield both HFa and HFf, and incorporation of ^{3}DFP into these activated forms was demonstrated.[115] Then in an attempt to prove that an autoactivation mechanism is operative, it was shown that the kinetics of the reaction indicate an accelerating reaction, i.e., a continuously increasing velocity as the concentration of activated enzyme increases[82] and that HFa can digest native HF to form more HFa[82] and then HFf.[116] When a careful estimate was made to quantitate the activity present in native, uncleaved Hageman factor it was found to be not greater than $^1/_{4000}$ the activity of HFa.[117] Thus, if native HF possesses any intrinsic activity it is exceedingly small, and we suspect that putative intrinsic activity reported by others when the HF was not treated with potent HFa inactivators was due to traces of HFa present. Results similar to ours have been recently reported in preliminary form.[118]

The initial cleavage of human Hageman factor has been reported to occur within a disulfide bridge in such a way that the product is the same size as the starting material.[119,120] This is shown in Figure 8–5 as cleavage at site 1. A second cleavage occurs at site 2 and then at site 3 to yield the 28,500 and 30,000 molecular weight forms of HFf.[116,121] Although cleavage at sites 2 and 3 occur in sequence, i.e., 2 precedes 3, we usually obtain a mixture of these two forms in which a 28,000-dalton heavy chain (the same as the light chain of HFa) is disulfide linked to light chains of either 2000 or 500. Since the rate of autoactivation is much slower than the rate of Hageman factor activation by kallikrein,[116] most HFa and HFf formed are dependent upon the reciprocal activation by kallikrein. But we envision the autoactivation mechanism as the initiating reaction, and both are depicted in Figure 8–6. When the products of autoactivation are examined in the absence of any prekallikrein, an additional active enzyme of molecular weight 40,000 is seen[116,121] in quantities about equal to that of HFf. This represents one of the intermediate-sized active moieties originally described.[81] However, it is either not formed by kallikrein digestion of Hageman factor, or it is further degraded to HFf so rapidly that it is not seen when normal plasma is examined. Theoretically, it should be one of the products evident when prekallikrein deficient plasma is activated; it is thought that the gradual autocorrection of the partial thromboplastin time seen in this plasma is a reflection of Hageman factor autoactivation.

Identification of Permeability Factor of Dilution

Figure 8–5. Cleavage sites in Hageman factor required for activation. HFa is formed by cleavage at site 1 within the disulfide bridge, while the two molecular forms of HFf are formed by cleavage at sites 2 and 3.

Figure 8–6. Diagram of the Hageman factor–dependent pathways, indicating the two-step process for HF activation. An autoactivation step is followed by reciprocal interaction with prekallikrein (kallikrein) for which HMW-kininogen acts as a cofactor. Digestion of HMW kininogen then generates bradykinin.

(PF/dil) as Activated Hageman Factor. Dilution of normal plasma obtained from several animal species in a glass vessel led to the formation of a permeability factor that was detected when the diluted plasma was injected into guinea pig skin.[13,14,122–125] The factor was found in a globulin-containing fraction of plasma; therefore the increase in vascular permeability was not attributable to the direct injection of bradykinin into the skin. Generation of PF/dil was shown to require the presence of Hageman factor;[14,126,127] thus neither dilution of normal plasma in a plastic vessel nor dilution of Hageman factor deficient plasma in a glass vessel generated permeability enhancing activity. Furthermore antiserum to human Hageman factor appeared to inhibit the formation of PF/dil when added prior to dilution, but did not inhibit PF/dil activity once it had formed.[128] Thus Hageman factor was required for the formation of PF/dil but did not appear to be identical to PF/dil. It was proposed that a precursor molecule (pro-PF/dil) exists that is activated by Hageman factor to PF/dil and that PF/dil could in turn convert prekallikrein to kallikrein.[14,15,126–130] When attempts to isolate PF/dil were initially made, a β globulin fraction of human plasma was identified which could increase vascular permeability when injected into guinea pig skin. It could also generate bradykinin upon incubation with fresh plasma but not heat-inactivated plasma (plasma that is heated to 61° C for 2 hours destroys prekallikrein but not HMW kininogen).[131,132] PF/dil was therefore thought to be a prekallikrein activator. Subsequently, Kaplan and Austen attempted to purify PF/dil[133] and thereby isolated the Hageman factor fragments.[80] It therefore appeared that activated Hageman factor could directly convert prekallikrein to kallikrein and that PF/dil was, in fact, a form of activated Hageman factor.[80] Subsequently an anti-Hageman factor immunoadsorbent was used to remove PF/dil activity from diluted human plasma.[134] However, neither of these studies identified the particular molecular form of HFa present in diluted plasma, and it was suggested that a mixture of active fragments was present.[70,80] A later study by Oh-Ishi and Webster[135] confirmed the association of PF/dil activity with multiple molecular forms of activated Hageman factor.

It is likely that Hageman factor is activated in diluted plasma in the fluid phase as well as at the surface, and that dilution minimizes inhibition of the various Hageman factor fragments formed. Consistent with the conclusion that PF/dil is a form of activated HF are observations that both prekallikrein in HMW kininogen deficient plasmas possess an abnormality in the surface-dependent generation of PF/dil.[19,20,22,27,31] Each of these plasmas has also been shown to possess a diminished rate of liberation of Hageman factor fragments from the surface.[119] When PF/dil is injected into the skin of an animal, the generation of bradykinin locally might account for the enhanced vascular permeability. However, PF/dil activity has been shown to be expressed normally upon injection into the skin of a prekallikrein deficient patient, suggesting that plasma prekallikrein is not required at this stage of the assay and that bradykinin may not be the mediator of the enhanced permeability.[136,137] Identification of other permeability factors that may be generated and an examination of the direct effect of activated HF upon blood vessels may lead to new concepts relating the activation of the intrinsic coagulation pathway to the inflammatory response.

PREKALLIKREIN

Properties of Human Prekallikrein. The molecular weights reported for human prekallikrein as assessed by gel filtration have ranged from 100,000 to 127,000. However, when purified prekallikrein was examined by SDS gel electrophoresis, two molecular variants were identified at 88,000 and 85,000 daltons and have been designated prekallikrein I and II, respectively. Upon immunoelectrophoresis, in 1 percent agar at pH 8.3, prekallikrein migrated as a fast γ globulin, and its isoelectric point was determined to be between 8.5 and 9.0 (peak value at 8.7), utilizing ampholytes that ranged from pH 7 to 10.

Assays of Prekallikrein and Kallikrein. The correction of the abnormal partial thromboplastin time of prekallikrein deficient plasma can provide a very sensitive assay for prekallikrein, since reconstitution to a level of only 5 percent of normal plasma prekallikrein fully corrects the coagulation defect.[19,20] The prekallikrein concentration can be expressed as a percent of normal plasma concentration by comparison with the partial thromboplastin time obtained, using diluted plasma as a source of prekallikrein. If a purified prekallikrein preparation is available, it can be serially diluted to generate a standard curve, and unknowns can then be expressed on a weight basis. The limitations of this assay are as follows: (1) active coagulation factors that might contaminate the sample (e.g., factor XIa) will give false positives, although they can be controlled for by coagulation assays using other deficient plasmas; (2) since a level of only 5 percent of normal prekallikrein completely corrects the deficiency, the dose-response range is narrow and accurate quantitation is difficult; and (3) the assay does not distinguish prekallikrein from kallikrein. Prekallikrein deficiency appears to be an autosomal recessive trait, and both homozygotes and heterozygotes can be detected using a coagulation assay if celite or kaolin (rather than ellagic acid) is used as the surface.[138] The cold dependent activation of factor VII can also be used as an assay for prekallikrein[139] if one has ruled out Hageman factor deficiency. The requirement for HMW kininogen in the performance of this last test, however, has not been defined.

Synthetic substrates that are specific for kallikrein are available and can be utilized to assay for either kallikrein or prekallikrein. For example, α-benzoyl-L-prolyl-L-phenylalanyl-L-arginyl-p-nitroanilide can be used in a simple and rapid colorimetric assay.[85] Quantitative assessment of kallikrein activity with this assay appears to correlate with proteolytic activity. The potential contribution by contaminating enzymes is small, since the substrate is highly specific for kallikrein. However, when assaying plasma samples, the kallikrein-α_2 macroglobulin complex retains significant activity for low molecular weight substrates;[140,141] thus a falsely elevated estimate may result.

Using H-D-pro-phe-arg-p-nitroanilide and dextran sulfate as the plasma activator, assays that measure prekallikrein by its conversion to kallikrein have been reported using varying conditions of time and temperature.[142,143] More recently an assay for prekallikrein was devised utilizing kaolin activation of chloroform-treated plasma, and 78 percent of the absolute amount of prekallikrein in plasma was actually measured,[143] which compared favorably with other assays utilizing synthetic substrates and was more accurate than coagulation assays.

The synthetic substrate tosyl-arginine methyl ester (TAME)[145] has been used to quantitate preparations of partially purified kallikrein or to assess kallikrein generated upon kaolin activation of human plasma.[146–148] Kallikrein accounted for virtually all the TAME-esterase activity generated during the first few minutes of incubation of plasma with kaolin, and the kinetics of bradykinin generation, as assessed by radioimmunoassay,[149] paralleled the rate of ester hydrolysis.[150] Nevertheless, this substrate is not specific for kallikrein, and it is less sensitive than the assay utilizing synthetic p-nitroanilides. ^{3}H-TAME has been utilized to improve the sensitivity as well as the ease of performance of the assay;[151] the ^{3}H-methanol liberated is extracted with scintillation fluid and directly counted.

Kallikrein or prekallikrein antigen can be determined by radial immunodiffusion using a monospecific antiserum,[152] and a radioimmunoassay for prekallikrein has been reported.[153] The latter assay is sensitive and specific; however, it does not distinguish between prekallikrein and kallikrein. Further studies are needed to determine whether kallikrein bound to either $\overline{CI}$ INH[154] or α_2 macroglobulin[155] is detected before such an assay could be applied to activated plasma.

Nevertheless such an assay can be utilized to determine the total antigen content of plasma[156] and has been used to determine that some patients with Fletcher trait (prekallikrein deficiency) contain a nonfunctional but immunologically reactive form of prekallikrein.[157] Similar molecular heterogeneity of patients with Hageman factor deficiency has been shown using anti-Hageman factor antibody,[158] and the protein in one patient has been shown to be noncleavable using the usual enzymes.[159] Another potential complication with regard to both immunochemical and functional determination of prekallikrein/kallikrein is that binding to HMW kininogen affects the prekallikrein determination;[108] thus determination of prekallikrein in plasma deficient in HMW kininogen requires reconstitution with HMW kininogen. Similar results were obtained using Laurell rocket electroimmunodiffusion,[160] although there is lack of agreement regarding the quantitation of prekallikrein in HMW kininogen deficient plasma.[108,160,161]

Kallikrein can also be determined by its ability to liberate bradykinin from kininogen. Kallikrein or Hageman factor fragment-activated prekallikrein is incubated for 5 minutes either with heat-inactivated plasma prepared at 61° C for 2 hours[162] or with a source of purified HMW kininogen. The bradykinin generated can then be assayed by its ability to contract a smooth muscle such as a guinea pig ileum.[163] If the kininogen source is incubated with kallikrein ranging from 0.1 to 5 percent by weight, a proportionate increase in the bradykinin liberated results. This assay is sensitive (can detect as little as 2 ng bradykinin), is not affected by most buffer constituents, and is highly specific for kallikrein. However, it is only semiquantitative. Use of a radioimmunoassay for bradykinin[149] can improve the reproducibility of the method. This approach is quite useful for following kallikrein (or prekallikrein) activity during isolation procedures but cannot be utilized as an assay for plasma kallikrein or prekallikrein.

The Mechanism of Activation of Human Prekallikrein. Activation of human prekallikrein by HFa proceeds by limited proteolytic digestion. Each of the molecular forms of prekallikrein seen at 88,000 and 85,000 daltons is cleaved, and upon reduction a two-chain disulfide-linked enzyme results. A heavy chain of 52,000 daltons is linked to a light chain of either 36,000 or 33,000 daltons corresponding to the two forms of the starting material.[164] When activation was carried out in the presence of ^{3}H-DFP, all the ^{3}H was seen in the light chains, indicating that this portion of the molecule contains the active site of kallikrein.[145] The evidence that both molecular weight forms represent prekallikrein include the following: (1) both were cleaved by Hageman factor fragments and yielded similar activation patterns, (2) they were not interconvertible upon activation by Hageman factor or incubation or prekallikrein with kallikrein, (3) they contained the same antigenic determinants, (4) DFP was incorporated into the light chains of each molecular form of the active enzymes, and (5) neither band was seen when prekallikrein deficient plasma was fractionated.[164] Similar results have been reported by other workers,[165] and kinetic studies of the activation of purified prekallikrein by HFf[166] have been reported. The heavy and light chains of reduced and alkylated kallikrein have been recently purified; the heavy chain was shown to possess the binding site for HMW kininogen, while the light chain retained enzymatic activity characteristic of kallikrein.[167]

Prekallikrein has been purified in other species, and its mechanism of activation has been examined. Bovine prekallikrein[168-170] was shown to be a single chain proenzyme that was digested by bovine Hageman factor to yield a two-chain disulfide-linked enzyme in a fashion analogous to that seen in man. Guinea pig prekallikrein is activated similarly.[171] Rabbit prekallikrein was found to be a β globulin with a molecular weight of 90,000 daltons and an isoelectric point of 5.9.[172] Upon conversion to kallikrein, not only was a kinin-generating enzyme formed but the kallikrein was found to shorten the PTT of rabbit plasma and human kallikrein behaved similarly.[173] Thus the function of kallikrein as a coagulation factor can be detected in rabbit plasma. Addition of kallikrein to human plasma or to congenitally deficient plasmas (other than Fletcher trait) has no effect. When the mechanism of conversion of rabbit prekallikrein to kallikrein was examined, activation was associated with the loss of an 8000-dalton peptide.[172] However, when the mechanism was examined in greater detail, activation in the presence of trasylol yielded conversion to a two-chain disulfide-linked enzyme without any change in molecular weight.[174] Since trasylol inactivates kallikrein but not Hageman factor,[93] it appeared that the peptide released was secondary to digestion of prekallikrein (or kallikrein) by the kallikrein produced. This phenomenon has also been observed for human prekallikrein. Digestion of ^{125}I prekallikrein with 5 percent nonradiolabeled kallikrein followed by SDS gel electrophoresis and autoradiography resulted in the formation of a prekallikrein that was diminished in size by approximately 10,000 daltons.[164] The molecule remained as a single chain, and no conversion to kallikrein was detected.

The enzyme kallikrein has at least three substrates in plasma that are relevant to coagulation, fibrinolysis, and kinin formation, as shown in Figure 8–7. The interaction with Hageman factor has been discussed above, and the interaction of kallikrein with HMW kininogen and plasminogen will be described presently.

HMW KININOGEN

Plasma Kininogens. The number of kininogens circulating in plasma had been a controversial issue; it was resolved largely as a consequence of the discovery of

Figure 8–7. Diagram of the interaction of kallikrein with three of its substrates—Hageman factor, HMW kininogen, and plasminogen.

plasmas deficient in HMW kininogen. In 1966, two highly purified human kininogens (I and II) were isolated which had a molecular weight of approximately 50,000 as estimated by gel filtration and sucrose density ultracentrifugation.[175] Kininogen I appeared to have the bradykinin moiety at the C-terminus because its kinin-forming capacity was inactivated by carboxypeptidase B. However, kininogen II was not inactivated by exopeptidases and appeared to have the bradykinin located within the molecule. Given our present information, both these kininogens would be considered low molecular weight kininogen, and kininogen I might represent a partially degraded form. Soon thereafter, Jacobsen demonstrated the presence of two different kininogens in various mammalian plasmas.[176-178] These consisted of a high molecular weight form of about 200,000 daltons that was rapidly cleaved by plasma kallikrein, and a low molecular weight kininogen of 60,000 daltons that was slowly cleaved by plasma kallikrein. Tissue kallikreins appeared to digest both forms of kininogen at the same rate. Several investigators subsequently reported finding only the low molecular weight form in human plasma,[90,179-181] while others have found both high and low molecular weight forms in human[182-186] and bovine plasmas.[187,188] The discovery of plasmas that are deficient in kininogen (particularly HMW kininogen) has demonstrated that the two molecular weight forms do indeed exist in plasma, and confirmed earlier observations that HMW kininogen represents approximately 15 to 20 percent of the total plasma kininogen.[189] Furthermore, careful analysis of the kinetics of cleavage of high and low molecular weight kininogens demonstrated that high molecular weight kininogen is clearly the preferred substrate for plasma kallikrein.[189] The Km and k/cat for the cleavage of HMW kininogen by plasma kallikrein were 115 to 2.7, respectively, while the Km and k/cat for the cleavage of low molecular weight kininogen were 3.7 and 3.2, respectively.[189]

Properties of Human HMW Kininogen. Purified HMW kininogen[189a] had a molecular weight of 210,000 upon Sephadex G-200 gel filtration, an isoelectric point of 4.3, and a molecular weight of 120,000 when assessed by SDS gel electrophoresis. Over 90 percent of the material remained at 120,000 daltons after reduction, indicating that the HMW kininogen isolated was a single chain. When a time course of digestion of human HMW-kininogen by kallikrein was performed and the mixture reduced and alkylated, separation into a heavy and light chain was observed. When the isolated heavy and light chains were examined for their ability to correct the coagulation defect in HMW kininogen deficient plasma, all of the activity was found in the light chain.[189a] The light chain was then shown to bind prekallikrein and factor XI[106] and attach them to negatively charged surfaces.[105] Similar results have been observed by others;[192-196] however, the molecular weight of the light chain obtained has varied while there is agreement that the heavy chain is approximately 62,000 to 66,000. Schiffman and colleagues[196] presented evidence that following the initial cleavage, both heavy and light chains are of equal size at 65,000. Then the light chain is further digested to yield a 54,000 light chain. Other workers have not observed a light chain equal in size to a heavy chain but have reported a light chain of 56,000 that is then further degraded to 45,000,[193] while some have found the light chain to be yet smaller, between 37,000 and 44,000.[189a,194] All forms of the light chain isolated possess the same functional capability, and it is clear that once HMW kininogen is initially cleaved to liberate bradykinin, further digestion of the light chain occurs to yield products of differing molecular weight. These observations are consistent with earlier work demonstrating that kallikrein cleavage of human HMW kininogen does not diminish its coagulant activity.[33,37] However, excessive in vitro digestion of the light chain by kallikrein can destroy such activity.[184]

Studies of bovine HMW kininogen have conclusively demonstrated that bradykinin is located at the center of the molecule; thus two cleavages by plasma kallikrein are necessary in order to liberate bradykinin.[198,199] An illustration of the cleavages in HMW kininogen observed upon digestion by kallikrein are shown in Figure 8–8. Early studies of bovine HMW kininogen have suggested that a partially cleaved form of HMW kininogen in which only one of the two bond cleavages needed to liberate bradykinin has occurred may be a superior cofactor to that of the native molecule or the isolated light chain.[200,201] The degree to which this is important in man is unclear, but some evidence to suggest that cleavage of HMW kininogen augments its activity has been presented.[202] Further, the ability of HMW kininogen to displace fibrinogen from the surface may relate to such activity.[203]

Antibody to HMW kininogen has been prepared and used to determine the distinguishing features of HMW kininogen and LMW kininogen. A sheep was immunized with kininogen and the sheep plasma adsorbed with Williams trait plasma to yield an antibody that reacts with both high and low molecular weight kininogens. When the sheep antiserum was adsorbed with Fitzgerald trait plasma (which has significant quantities of LMW kininogen), an antiserum that was monospecific for HMW kininogen resulted. When each of these antisera was reacted with normal plasma, the pattern shown in Figure 8–9 was seen. Two arcs that fuse at one end are seen with the antikininogen serum, indicating a reaction

Figure 8–8. Steps by which HMW kininogen is cleaved by plasma kallikrein. Digestion at two sites within a disulfide bridge is required for release of kinin, and two chains of approximately equal size are left disulfide linked. Rapid further cleavage of one chain yields the 56,000 light chain (the major product) followed by a second slower cleavage to a 45,000 final product. The function of this light "chain" is as indicated.

of partial antigenic identity (upper trough). When normal plasma was reacted against the anti-HMW kininogen serum placed in the lower trough, only the inner arc was seen. When this latter antiserum was then reacted with the isolated HMW kininogen heavy and light chains, a precipitin was obtained only with the light chain. Thus the light chain appeared to possess the major antigenic determinants that distinguish HMW kininogen from LMW kininogen.[189a,195] Furthermore, the data demonstrated that the antigens they share were associated with the heavy chain, as has been reported when the chains of bovine kininogens were compared.[204-206]

Assay of HMW Kininogens. The presence of HMW kininogen can be assessed by cleavage with plasma kallikrein, urinary kallikrein,[207,208] or trypsin. The enzyme is inactivated by boiling[209] or by further incubation with soybean trypsin inhibitor. In each instance, the bradykinin generated is determined by either bioassay or radioimmunoassay. This method, however, does not distinguish HMW kininogen from LMW kininogen, and the known difference in their rate of cleavage by plasma kallikrein cannot be readily used to construct a simple assay. Clearly the ability of HMW kininogen to correct the prolonged partial thromboplastin time of HMW kininogen deficient plasma provides a specific and readily performed assay. Since reconstitution of this plasma with 10 to 12 percent of normal HMW kininogen completely

Figure 8–9. Immunoelectrophoresis of normal plasma reacted against antibody to human kininogens (upper trough) and against antibody rendered specific for HMW kininogen (lower trough). A line of partial identity is seen.

corrects the functional abnormality, significant dilution of normal plasma must be made in order to obtain a dose response between 0 and 12 percent of normal so that a standard curve can be constructed. Unknowns can be diluted and compared with the standards and expressed as a percent of normal HMW kininogen or in units per milliliter if the quantity of HMW kininogen present in plasma is set at 1.0 unit. If purified HMW kininogen is available, the HMW kininogen content of normal plasma can be expressed in μg per milliliter based upon either functional or antigenic analysis. We have found close agreement between the functional and antigenic determinations of plasma HMW kininogen and estimate the normal plasma level to be between 70 and 90 μg per milliliter. Since HMW kininogen is relatively plentiful in plasma and monospecific antisera can be prepared, HMW kininogen antigen could be measured by radial immunodiffusion, counterimmunoelectrophoresis, or radioimmunoassay.[160,210] Recently, an assay for HMW kininogen antigen using hemagglutination inhibition has been reported,[161] which is both sensitive and specific.

FACTOR XI

Properties of Purified Factor XI. Factor XI[211] is a γ globulin of molecular weight 158,000[19,96] as assessed by SDS gel electrophoresis and has an isoelectric point of 9.1.[212]

Assays for Factor XI. The standard assay of factor XI is a coagulation assay in which the partial thromboplastin time of factor XI deficient plasma is corrected. It is performed essentially as described above for either Hageman factor or HMW kininogen. Factor XIa appears to have weak esterolytic activity;[19] however, there is no known synthetic substrate that is specifically digested by factor XIa. The concentration of factor XI in plasma is only about 4 to 7 ng per milliliter,[19,96] which limits the ability to see precipitin lines when whole plasma is reacted with monospecific antisera to factor

XI. Thus radial immunodiffusion or electroimmunodiffusion assays may not be feasible. A radioimmunoassay for factor XI has been described,[213] which represents the most sensitive way of determining factor XI; it does not, however, distinguish factor XI from factor XIa, and it is therefore not useful as a measure of activation. Nevertheless antisera to human factor XI have been prepared[96,214,215] and used to distinguish the homozygous from the heterozygous deficiency by functional inhibition of coagulant activity.[215]

Activation of Human Factor XI. Purified preparations of human factor XI have a molecular weight of 155,000 to 160,000 upon SDS gel electrophoresis; however, upon reduction, the molecular weight is 80,000 to 82,000,[19,215,216] and only a single band is seen. Thus it appears that factor XI is a two-chain molecule and the two constituent chains are virtually the same size. A similar observation was made when highly purified bovine factor XI was examined,[217] and thus far incorporation of high concentrations of benzamidine and DFP into the isolation procedure has not resulted in the formation of a single-chain form of factor XI.

Cleavage of human factor XI by trypsin,[19,218,219] Hageman factor fragments,[96,98,212] or surface-bound activated Hageman factor[220,221] resulted in cleavage of the 80,000 dalton chains within a disulfide bridge. Thus in the absence of reduction, the molecular weights of factor XI and factor XIa were essentially the same.[70,214,218,222] However, upon reduction, the two 80,000 chains of the starting material appeared to be cleaved to chains of 50,000 and 30,000. Factor XIa has been shown to be a serine protease[223] that can be inhibited by DFP. When factor XI was activated by Hageman factor, inactivated by ^{3}H-DFP, and reduced, ^{3}H-DFP was incorporated into the 30,000-dalton light chain.[220] When binding of antithrombin III-heparin by factor XIa was quantitated, two moles of antithrombin III appeared to be found by each mole of factor XIa, suggesting that there are two active sites in factor XIa, one for each light chain present.[221]

Factor XI circulates as a complex with HMW kininogen,[43] the rate of conversion of factor XI to factor XIa is augmented by HMW kininogen,[37,97–101] and the rate of formation of activated Hageman factor (and factor XIa) is dependent upon prekallikrein.[20–22,97–99,101] Yet prekallikrein circulates complexed to different HMW kininogen molecules from those of factor XI;[43] thus a mechanism must exist in which Hageman factor that is activated by kallikrein can interact with the factor XI–HMW kininogen complex. Binding of factor XI to surfaces is augmented by HMW kininogen in a plasma milieu,[104,105] and, as is the case for prekallikrein,[105] the HMW kininogen appears to counteract competing plasma proteins that inhibit factor XI binding.[224] Factor XIa attachment to the HMW kininogen appears to reside in the heavy chain.[225] A case of acquired factor XI deficiency has been reported in which an IgG antifactor XI was shown to inhibit its interaction with HMW kininogen and its ability to be activated and cleaved by HFa.[226]

The ability of factor XIa to completely correct the

coagulation defect of Hageman factor, prekallikrein, or HMW kininogen deficient plasmas, and the normal rate of generation of plasmin and bradykinin upon activation of factor XI deficient plasma, indicate that in a practical sense activation of factor XIa represents the second step in the intrinsic coagulation pathway. It may, however, play an alternative role in the initial step when prekallikrein is absent.[227]

THE ROLE OF THE EARLY STEPS OF THE INTRINSIC COAGULATION PATHWAY IN FIBRINOLYSIS

Hageman factor dependent conversion of plasminogen to plasmin is readily demonstrable in whole plasma.[10,11,228] Since prekallikrein and HMW kininogen are required for optimal activation and function of Hageman factor, they are also required for activation of the Hageman factor dependent fibrinolytic pathway. However, identification of the molecule or molecules that directly convert plasminogen to plasmin has been the subject of numerous investigations, and the results have not been clear. Colman[229] first reported that incubation of kallikrein with plasminogen leads to the generation of plasmin, and the kinetics of the reaction appeared to be stoichiometric. Ogston and colleagues[230] demonstrated a cofactor required for Hageman factor dependent fibrinolysis that appeared to be distinguishable from kallikrein and factor XIa. However, it was clearly present in plasma fractions containing these factors. The assay for this protein was dependent upon reconstitution of glass-adsorbed plasma from which the fibrinolytic factor had been depleted. This "Hageman factor cofactor" had a molecular weight of 160,000, and it migrated with the γ globulins. Kaplan and Austen subsequently demonstrated a Hageman factor–activatable plasma factor called plasminogen proactivator, which, upon activation, was able to directly convert plasminogen to plasmin.[231] These authors proposed that the plasminogen activator derived was responsible for the plasminogen-converting activity in kallikrein preparations. The demonstration of plasminogen proactivator activity in the γ globulin fraction of prekallikrein deficient plasma appeared to confirm their interpretation.[231] This postulate was challenged by Laake and Vennerod based upon their inability to separate prekallikrein from plasminogen proactivator, and they concluded that kallikrein and plasminogen-activating activities are functions of the same molecule.[232] When these authors examined the γ globulin effluent obtained from prekallikrein deficient plasma, no plasminogen activator or proactivator activity was observed.[233]

The successful purification of human prekallikrein has shed further light upon this question. First, when human prekallikrein was isolated in the presence of proteolytic inhibitors, the prekallikrein and plasminogen proactivator activities coincided and the two-banded pattern was shown to represent prekallikrein heterogeneity rather than two separate Hageman factor substrates.[164]

Second, kallikrein was shown to cleave prekallikrein and decrease its molecular weight by 10,000 daltons; this difference in size corresponded to the previously reported difference in size between prekallikrein and plasminogen proactivator.[234] Finally, fractionation of prekallikrein deficient plasma demonstrated that the plasminogen proactivator activity seen associated with prekallikrein was absent.[164] Hence the conclusion was reached that prekallikrein is a plasminogen proactivator and that the previous reported activity was a property of prekallikrein and/or the prekallikrein degradation product. However, plasminogen-activating activity was again found in the γ globulin fraction of normal plasma[235] which was not attributable to prekallikrein, and this same activity was found in prekallikrein deficient plasma. Further fractionation of this material demonstrated that the activity was superimposed upon factor XI.[164] Isolation of the plasminogen proactivator activity present in prekallikrein plasma was then identified as factor XI, and factor XIa was shown to directly convert plasminogen to plasmin.[236]

The observation that plasminogen-activating activity does indeed reside in the γ globulin effluent of prekallikrein deficient plasma has been confirmed;[237] however, these authors did not demonstrate that the activity was Hageman factor activatable and considered prekallikrein to be the only plasminogen proactivator. Clearly, the gradual conversion of plasminogen to plasmin observed in prekallikrein deficient plasma is secondary to a Hageman factor dependent enzyme that is not kallikrein. When the fibrinolytic activity of factor XI deficient plasma was examined, its rate of activation was normal, but it failed to generate a normal amount of plasmin. Reconstitution with purified factor XI corrected this abnormality.[238] A single report has presented evidence that activated Hageman factor itself can function as a weak plasminogen activator;[239] however, when experiments are performed in which the fibrinolytic capacity of prekallikrein is assessed (i.e., Hageman factor fragments plus plasminogen), the contribution of HFf is less than 5 percent of the activity seen with kallikrein.[236] Thus larger quantities of activated Hageman factor may be required for this effect to reach significant levels. It appears clear that prekallikrein is a plasminogen proactivator, factor XI may function as a second proactivator, and HFa or HFf may directly contribute to plasminogen activation.

The identity of the Hageman factor cofactor is not clear; however, the function these authors observed does not appear to be distinguishable from that of the known Hageman factor substrates. Glass adsorbed plasma, used in the assay for the Hageman factor cofactor, has been shown to be depleted of prekallikrein;[240] thus the kallikrein present in Hageman factor cofactor preparations may contribute to the fibrinolysis observed by its effect upon Hageman factor activation. Yet the molecular weight reported for this factor was quite different from kallikrein, and the factor appeared to be separable from the bulk of kallikrein but not from factor XI.[230,241] The active factor was also inhibited by α_1 antitrypsin, a property it shares with factor XIa.[242] The molecular properties of this cofactor most closely resemble the activity we have observed with our factor XI preparation; thus it is possible that the activity being measured was a function of more than one protein.

Further studies in whole plasma are needed to distinguish the effect of kallikrein upon fibrinolysis via its ability to activate Hageman factor from its ability to convert plasminogen to plasmin. It is of interest that one estimate of the direct contribution of kallikrein to the conversion of plasminogen to plasmin was approximately 50 percent[241] of the total Hageman factor dependent fibrinolytic activity present in plasma.

A summary of the known interactions leading to coagulation, fibrinolysis, and kinin formation is shown in Figure 8–10.

CONTROL MECHANISMS

The binding of Hageman factor to surfaces is markedly inhibited by the presence of plasma, and the effect is attributable to many plasma fractions and does not, therefore, appear to be specific.[243] Nevertheless, such inhibition would serve to limit in vivo activation at the very first step. In vitro studies of Hageman factor activation have demonstrated that excess HMW kininogen also appears to be inhibitory.[102, 103] There is approximately twice the plasma concentration of HMW kininogen needed to bind all the prekallikrein and factor XI.[42,43,106] Since HMW kininogen is normally present in excess, activation in plasma may be suboptimal. This possibility has not, however, been examined. Once activation proceeds beyond the initial cleavage of Hageman factor, fragmentation of the Hageman factor occurs and the prealbumin fragment is liberated from the surface[119] and can continue to function as a prekallikrein activator in the fluid phase. The consequence of this step would be to divert the pathway from coagulation to fibrinolysis and kinin generation, as originally proposed by Kaplan and Austen.[81] The major inhibitor of activated Hageman factor[244] and Hageman factor fragments[245] is the inhibitor of the activated first component of complement (C$\bar{1}$ INH). The C$\bar{1}$ INH has been shown to bind[95] and irreversibly inactivate the Hageman factor fragments. Antithrombin III has also been shown to bind and inactivate HFa and HFf as well as an unfragmented form of Hageman factor in which the active site was available; however, the inactivation observed was slower than that obtained with comparable concentrations of C$\bar{1}$ INH.[246] Heparin markedly accelerated the binding and inactivation of Hageman factor by antithrombin III such that the reaction was virtually complete within 30 seconds. There was no inhibition of activated Hageman factor by α_2 macroglobulin, α_1 antitrypsin, α_1 antichymotrypsin, and·inter α trypsin inhibitor.

The major inhibitor of plasma kallikrein also appears to be C$\bar{1}$ INH, which has been shown to bind to the active site of the enzyme such that all esterase and proteolytic activities were inhibited[154,247] and a 1:1 stoichiometric complex was formed.[248] α_2 Macroglobulin functions as a second kallikrein inhibitor,[155] although complete inactivation does not result; most of the esterase activity and a small fraction of residual proteolytic activity remain.[140] It is likely that α_2 macroglobulin inhibits by sterically interfering with the function of the active site without actually binding to it. Of particular

Figure 8–10. Diagram of the known interactions leading to Hageman factor dependent coagulation, fibrinolysis, and the generation of bradykinin.

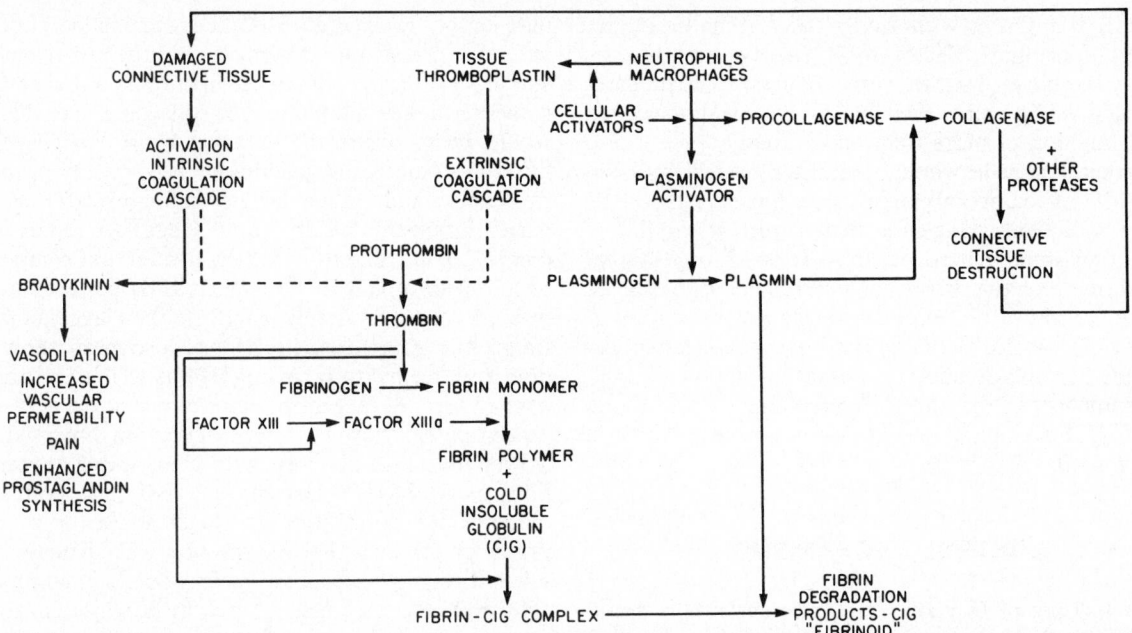

Figure 8–11. Diagram depicting the roles of the coagulation cascades in inflammation. The extrinsic pathway appears to be recruited by release of tissue factor from activated cells and interaction of coagulation, and fibrinolytic proteases yield deposition of "fibrinoid." Damaged connective tissue can serve as a surface upon which initiation of the intrinsic coagulation pathway can occur with formation of bradykinin.

interest is that the residual activity of the kallikrein–α_2 macroglobulin complex resists further inactivation by C$\overline{1}$ INH; thus if there is continual activation of this pathway under normal conditions, this is one form in which a trace quantity of active enzyme could persist in plasma. Antithrombin III can also function as an inhibitor of plasma kallikrein,[249] although there is not agreement regarding the magnitude of augmentation in the presence of heparin.[250,251] Under conditions in which antithrombin III–heparin rapidly inactivated Hageman factor, little inhibition of plasma kallikrein was obtained.[246] Although α_1 antitrypsin had been thought to inhibit plasma kallikrein,[247] recent studies utilizing purified α_1 antitrypsin failed to demonstrate any effect.[212] Recent studies of the contribution of various plasma inhibitors to the inactivation of kallikrein have demonstrated that C$\overline{1}$ INH and α_2 macroglobulin together account for about 90 percent of the inhibitory activity of plasma.[252, 253]

The major plasma inhibitor of factor XIa was initially shown to be α_1 antitrypsin,[212] and this observation has been recently confirmed by determination of the second-order rate constants for inhibition of factor XIa by plasma proteases.[254] Other plasma inhibitors that may contribute include C$\overline{1}$ INH[244] and antithrombin III.[255] The latter activity is markedly increased by the addition of heparin while α_2 macroglobulin, α_1 antichymotrypsin, and inter-α trypsin inhibitor have no effect.[212]

Although α_2 macroglobulin had long been considered to be the major plasma inhibitor of plasmin,[141, 256, 257] it is clear that a newly described proteolytic inhibitor called α_2 antiplasmin is the major plasmin inactivator.[258-260] Since the concentration of plasminogen exceeds that of the inhibitor, only when excess plasmin is gen-

erated does significant binding to α_2 macroglobulin result.[261,262] Other inhibitors of plasmin demonstrable in vitro include α_1 antitrypsin[257] and C$\overline{1}$ INH;[263,264] however, it is clear that these contribute little in whole plasma. Antithrombin III can also function as a plasmin inhibitor; however, its effect is not significant unless it is assayed in the presence of heparin.[265] An extensive review of the inhibitory effect of α_2 macroglobulin and antithrombin III upon activated coagulation factors has been published.[266] The inhibitory spectrum of α_2 plasmin inhibitor includes weak activity upon HFf, kallikrein, and factor XIa,[267] but its contribution to the inactivation of these enzymes in whole plasma is small. Of particular interest is the observation that congenital deficiency of this protein leads to excessive plasma fibrinolysis and a bleeding diathesis,[268-271] thus demonstrating its critical function as a regulator of fibrinolysis in blood. In order to manifest its in vivo effect as a plasmin inhibitor α_2 antiplasmin may be crosslinked to fibrin by fibrin-stabilizing factor (factor XIIIa), and the bound inhibitor then interacts within plasmin that is also bound along the surface of the clot.[272] The major plasma inhibitors of each enzyme of the Hageman factor dependent pathways are shown in Table 8–1.

EFFECTS OF THE HAGEMAN FACTOR DEPENDENT PATHWAYS UPON OTHER SYSTEMS AND THEIR POTENTIAL ROLE IN RHEUMATIC DISEASES (Fig. 8–11)

Patients who are deficient in Hageman factor, prekallikrein, and HMW kininogen have little or no evidence of a hemostatic defect, although their plasmas

Table 8–1. Inhibitors of Enzymes of the Hageman Factor Dependent Pathways

Enzyme	Inhibitors
HFa, HFf	C̄l INH
Kallikrein	C̄l INH
	α_2 Macroglobulin
Factor XIa	C̄l INH
	α_1 Antitrypsin
Plasmin	α_2 Antiplasmin
	α_2 Macroglobulin

possess profound in vitro abnormalities. Since these are the only deficiencies in which there is simultaneous impairment of coagulation, fibrinolysis, and kinin generation, it is possible that the latter defects are somehow protective and diminish the incidence of bleeding. It is also possible that the normal function of this pathway is not to produce a blood clot but to regulate blood flow via the vasodilator activity of bradykinin and/or to contribute to the body's ability to respond to injury and generate an inflammatory response. Bradykinin not only acts as a vasodilator but also increases vascular permeability, causes a burning sensation upon contact with sensory nerve endings, and in high concentrations can cause hypotension.[273] Kallikrein has been shown to aggregate neutrophils[274] and to possess chemotactic activity for human neutrophils and monocytes[275,276] and could thereby act to recruit these cells into sites of tissue injury. Consistent with this possibility is the observation that the chemotactic activity seen in serum was diminished when prekallikrein deficient plasma was examined.[21] Surprisingly, skin windows placed in HMW kininogen deficient plasma revealed a markedly augmented infiltration with neutrophils,[277] suggesting that HMW kininogen or a fragment derived from HMW kininogen functions to inhibit cellular infiltration. The Hageman factor dependent pathways may also play a role in the complement pathways. Thus Hageman factor deficient plasma had an abnormal rate of activation of the alternative complement pathway.[278] In addition, patients with hereditary angioedema who lack C̄l INH have "spontaneous" activation of Cl, which appears to be dependent upon Hageman factor.[279] Studies by Ghebrehiwet and colleagues[280,281] have demonstrated that HFf can directly activate Cl by cleavage of the Clr subcomponent. Thus in the absence of C̄l INH, not only is Cl more likely to autoactivate[282,283] but further enzymatic digestion by HFf (and perhaps other enzymes) may lead to the profound consumption of C4 and C2 seen during attacks of swelling. Other possible interactions between these cascades, whose importance is less clear, include the ability of kallikrein to activate factor B[284] and the ability of plasmin to activate C1s[285] and cleave C3.[286] Numerical evidence regarding the pathogenesis of hereditary angioedema is of particular note; induced skin blisters in such patients have been shown to possess elevated levels of kallikrein[287] and spontaneous generation of bradykinin has been observed upon

incubating such plasma in nonactivating surfaces[288] while massive activation of only the complement cascade failed to generate a contractile or vasoactive factor.[288]

The role of the Hageman factor dependent pathways in rheumatic diseases has not been systematically explored, and much work in this area is required. It is not likely that it is the primary mediator pathway activated in such disorders, since immune complexes do not directly initiate the cascade, and at least one patient with Hageman factor deficiency has been reported with rheumatoid arthritis.[289] Although uric acid and pyrophosphate crystals can initiate Hageman factor activation in vitro,[50] this potential contribution to the joint inflammation seen in gout and pseudogout has not been quantitated relative to the other effects of such crystals upon the complement cascade[290,291] and phagocytosis. Recently the activation of Hageman factor by sodium urate crystals has been examined in plasma and joint fluid. Hageman factor cleavage was shown to be dependent upon the presence of prekallikrein and HMW kininogen, and both HFa and HFf were generated.[292]

The observation that exposure to connective tissue elements can initiate the Hageman factor dependent pathways requires confirmation, and the specific connective tissue element responsible for such activity needs to be identified. Certainly, if damaged connective tissue secondary to inflammation initiated by immune complexes and complement or by cellular immune reactions can then lead to recruitment of these pathways, perpetuation of the inflammatory process might result. Thus the ability of bradykinin to increase vascular permeability would increase swelling and augment the local deposition of immune complexes and complement. Bradykinin would also increase the pain perceived by interaction with pain receptors. Plasmin has been identified as an enzyme that can convert a synovial procollagenase to a collagenase;[293] thus the fibrinolytic pathway may thereby augment connective tissue destruction. It is possible that activated Hageman factor or kallikrein might have additional effects upon the enzymes present in connective tissue or perhaps direct effects upon connective tissue itself. Kallikrein might also contribute to the influx of neutrophils and monocytes seen. In addition, local coagulation and fibrinolysis undoubtedly are responsible for the presence of fibrin degradation products or "fibrinoid" that is routinely seen in the lesions of virtually all the connective tissue disorders. Yet the relative contributions of the intrinsic and extrinsic coagulation pathways to the deposition of "fibrinoid" is unknown.

The critical components of the Hageman factor dependent pathways have been identified, their major interactions have been elucidated, and we actually possess sensitive functional assays for each component but also possess monospecific antisera that can be utilized to quantitate each component as a protein. In addition, further studies can be performed by radiolabeling purified preparations of each factor. Thus the reagents and techniques are now available with which to evaluate the possible contribution of these pathways to virtually any disorder, and future studies should be specifically focused upon the rheumatic diseases.

Acknowledgment

The excellent typing and editing of this manuscript by Ms. Madeline Lee, Ms. Mavis Bolotsky, and Ms. Barbara Sykes are gratefully acknowledged.

References

1. Bordet, J., and Genou, O.: Recherches sur la coagulation du sang et les serums anticoagulants. Ann. Inst. Pasteur 15:129, 1901.
2. Shafrir, E., and de Vries, A.: Studies on the clot-promoting activity of glass. J. Clin. Invest. 35:1183, 1956.
3. Margolis, J.: Glass surface and blood coagulation. Nature 178:805, 1956.
4. Hubbard, D., and Lucas, G.L.: Ionic charges of glass surfaces and other materials and their possible role in the coagulation of blood. J. Appl. Physiol. 15:265, 1960.
5. Ratnoff, O.D., and Colopy, J.E.: A familial hemorrhagic trait associated with a deficiency of clot-promoting fraction of plasma. J. Clin. Invest. 34:602, 1955.
6. Ratnoff, O.D., and Rosenblum, J.M.: Role of Hageman factor in the initiation of clotting by glass: Evidence that glass frees Hageman factor inhibition. Am. J. Med. 25:160, 1958.
7. Ratnoff, O.D., and Davie, E.W.: The purification of activated Hageman factor (activated XII). Biochemistry 1:967, 1962.
8. Speer, R.J., Ridgway, H., and Hill, J.M.: Activation of human Hageman factor (XII). Thromb. Diath. Haemorrhag. 14:1, 1965.
9. Donaldson, V.H., and Ratnoff, O.D.: Hageman factor: Alterations in physical properties during activation. Science 150:754, 1965.
10. Niewiarowski, S., and Prow-Wartelle, O.: Role du facteur contact (Facteur Hageman) dans la fibrinolyse. Thromb. Diath. Haemorrhag. 3:593, 1959.
11. Iatridis, S.G., and Ferguson, J.H.: Active Hageman factor. A plasma lysokinase of the human fibrinolytic system. J. Clin. Invest. 41:1277, 1962.
12. Margolis, J.: Plasma pain-producing substance and blood clotting. Nature 180:1464, 1957.
13. Margolis, J.: Activation of a permeability factor in plasma by contact with glass. Nature 180:635, 1958.
14. Margolis, J.: Activation of plasma by contact with glass. Evidence for a common reaction which releases plasma kinin and initiates coagulation. J. Physiol. 144:1, 1959.
15. Margolis, J.: The interrelationship of coagulation of plasma and release of peptides. Ann. N.Y. Acad. Sci. 104:133, 1963.
16. Hathaway, W.E., Belhausen, L.P., and Hathaway, H.S.: Evidence of a new plasma coagulation factor. I. Case report, coagulation studies and physiochemical properties. Blood 26:521, 1965.
17. Hattersley, P.G., and Hayse, D.: Fletcher factor deficiency. A report of three unrelated cases. Br. J. Haematol. 18:411, 1970.
18. Hathaway, W.E., and Alsever, J.: The relation of "Fletcher factor" to factors XI and XII. Br. J. Haematol. 18:161, 1970.
19. Wuepper, K.D.: Biochemistry and biology of components of the plasma kinin-forming system. In Lepow, I.H., and Ward, A. (eds.): Inflammation: Mechanisms and Control. New York, Academic Press, 1972, pp. 93–117.
20. Wuepper, K.D.: Prekallikrein deficiency in man. J. Exp. Med. 138:1345, 1973.
21. Weiss, A.S., Gallin, J.I., and Kaplan, A.P.: Fletcher factor deficiency. Abnormalities of coagulation, fibrinolysis, chemotactic activity, and kinin generation attributable to absence of prekallikrein. J. Clin. Invest. 53:622, 1974.
22. Saito, H., Ratnoff, O.D., and Donaldson, V.H.: Defective activation of clotting, fibrinolytic, and permeability enhancing systems in human Fletcher trait plasma. Circ. Res. 34:641, 1974.
23. Webster, M.E.: Human plasma kallikrein, its activation and pathologic role. Fed. Proc. 27:84, 1968.
24. Webster, M.E., and Pierce, J.V.: Activators of Hageman factor (factor XII): Identification and relationship to kallikrein-kinin system. Fed. Proc. 32:845, 1973.
25. Schiffman, S., and Lee, P.: Preparation, characterization, activation of a highly purified factor XI. Evidence that a hitherto unrecognized plasma activity participates in the interaction of factors XI and XII. Br. J. Haematol. 27:101, 1974.
26. Colman, R.W., Bagdasarian, A., Talamo, R.C., and Kaplan, A.P.: Williams trait: A new deficiency with abnormal levels of prekallikrein, plasminogen proactivator, and kininogen. In Pisano, J.J., and Austen,

K.F. (eds.): The Chemistry and Biology of the Kallikrein-Kinin System in Health and Disease. Fogarty International Proceedings No. 27. Washington, D.C., U.S. Government Printing Office, 1974, pp. 65–72.
27. Saito, H., and Ratnoff, O.D.: Fitzgerald trait: An asymptomatic disorder with impaired blood coagulation, fibrinolysis, kinin generation, and generation of permeability factor of dilution. In Pisano, J.J., and Austen, K.F. (eds.): The Chemistry and Biology of the Kallikrein-Kinin System in Health and Disease. Fogarty International Proceedings No. 27. Washington, D.C., U.S. Government Printing Office, 1974, pp. 73–74.
28. LaCombe, M.J.: Déficit constitutionnel en un nouveau facteur de la coagulation intervenant au niveau de contact: Le facteur "Flaujeac." C. R. Acad. Sci. (D) 280:1039, 1975.
29. Waldman, R., and Abraham, J.: Fitzgerald factor: A heretofore unrecognized coagulation factor. Blood 46:761, 1975.
30. Saito, H., Ratnoff, O.D., Waldmann, R., and Abraham, J.P.: Fitzgerald trait. Deficiency of a hitherto unrecognized agent, Fitzgerald factor, participating in surface-mediated reactions of clotting, fibrinolysis, generation of kinins, and the property of diluted plasma enhancing vascular permeability (PF-dil). J. Clin. Invest. 55:1082, 1975.
31. Wuepper, K.D., Miller, D.R., and LaCombe, M.J.: Flaujeac trait: Deficiency of kininogen in man. Fed. Proc. 34:859, 1975.
32. Wuepper, K.D., Miller, D.R., and LaCombe, M.J.: Flaujeac trait. Deficiency of human plasma kininogen. J. Clin. Invest. 56:1663, 1975.
33. Colman, R.W., Bagdasarian, A., Talamo, R.C., Seavey, M., Scott, C.F., and Kaplan, A.P.: Williams trait: Combined deficiency of plasma plasminogen proactivator, kininogen, and a new procoagulant factor. Fed. Proc. 34:859, 1975.
34. Colman, R.W., Bagdasarian, A., Talamo, R.C., Scott, C.F., Seavey, M., Guimaraes, J.A., Pierce, J.V., and Kaplan, A.P.: Williams trait. Human kininogen deficiency with diminished levels of plasminogen proactivator and prekallikrein associated with abnormalities of the Hageman factor-dependent pathways. J. Clin. Invest. 56:1650, 1975.
35. Donaldson, V.H., Glueck, H.I., Miller, M.A., Movat, H.Z., and Habal, F.: Kininogen deficiency in Fitzgerald trait: Role of high molecular weight kininogen in clotting and fibrinolysis. J. Lab. Clin. Med. 87:327, 1976.
36. Schiffman, S., Lee, P., and Waldmann, R.: Identity of contact activation cofactor and Fitzgerald factor. Thromb. Res. 6:451, 1975.
37. Schiffman, S., and Lee, P.: Partial purification and characterization of contact activation cofactor. J. Clin. Invest. 56:1082, 1975.
38. Schiffman, S., Lee, P., Feinstein, D.I., and Pecci, R.: Relationship of contact activation cofactor (CAC) procoagulant activity to kininogen. Blood 49:935, 1977.
39. Ratnoff, O.D., Davie, E.W., and Mallet, D.L.: Studies on the action of Hageman factor: Evidence that activated Hageman factor in turn activates plasma thromboplastin antecedent. J. Clin. Invest. 40:803, 1961.
40. Wendel, U., Vogt, W., and Seidel, G.: Purification and some properties of a kininogenase from human plasma activated by surface contact. Hoppe Seylers Z. Physiol. Chem. 353:1591, 1972.
41. Nagasawa, S., and Nakayasu, T.: Human plasma prekallikrein as a protein complex. J. Biochem. 74:401, 1973.
42. Mandle, R., Jr., Colman, R.W., and Kaplan, A.P.: Identification of prekallikrein and HMW-kininogen as a circulating complex in human plasma. Proc. Natl. Acad. Sci. USA 73:4179, 1976.
43. Thompson, R.E., Mandle, R., Jr., and Kaplan, A.P.: Association of factor XI and high molecular weight kininogen in human plasma. J. Clin. Invest. 60:1376, 1977.
44. Ratnoff, O.D.: The biology and pathology of the initial stages of blood coagulation. Prog. Hematol. 5:204, 1966.
45. Margolis, J.: The effect of colloidal silica on blood coagulation. Aust. J. Exp. Biol. Med. Sci. 39:249, 1961.
46. Ratnoff, O.D., and Crum, J.D.: Activation of Hageman factor by solutions of ellagic acid. J. Lab. Clin. Med. 63:359, 1964.
47. Schwartz, H.J., and Kellermeyer, R.W.: Carrageenan and delayed hypersensitivity. II. Activation of Hageman factor by carrageenan and its possible significance. Proc. Soc. Exp. Biol. Med. 132:1021, 1969.
48. Kellermeyer, W.F., Jr., and Kellermeyer, R.W.: Hageman factor activation and kinin formation in human plasma induced by cellulose sulfate solutions. Proc. Soc. Exp. Biol. Med. 130:1310, 1969.
49. Kluft, C.: Assay for prekallikrein levels and prekallikrein activation in human plasma using dextran sulphate as a soluble activator. Thromb. Haemostasis 38:220, 1977.
50. Kellermeyer, R.W., and Breckenridge, R.T.: The inflammatory process in acute gouty arthritis. I. Activation of Hageman factor by sodium urate crystals. J. Lab. Clin. Med. 65:307, 1965.
51. Ratnoff, O.D.: Activation of Hageman factor by L-homocysteine. Science 29:1007, 1968.
52. Moskowitz, R.W., Schwartz, H.J., Michel, B., Ratnoff, O.D., and Astrup, T.: Generation of kinin-like agents by chondroitin sulfate, heparin, chitin sulfate, and human articular cartilage: Possible pathophysiologic implications. J. Lab. Clin. Med. 76:790, 1970.

53. Nossel, H.L.: Activation of factors XII (Hageman) and XI (PTA) by skin contact. Proc. Soc. Exp. Biol. Med. 122:16, 1966.
54. Margolis, J.: Activation of Hageman factor saturated fatty acids. Aust. J. Exp. Biol. Med. Sci. 40:505, 1962.
55. Botti, R.E., and Ratnoff, O.D.: The clot-promoting effect of soaps of long chain saturated fatty acids. J. Clin. Invest. 42:1569, 1963.
56. Didisheim, P., and Mibashan, R.S.: Activation of Hageman factor (factor XII) by long chain saturated fatty acids. Thromb. Diath. Haemorrh. 9:346, 1963.
57. Morrison, D.C., and Cochrane, C.G.: Direct evidence for Hageman factor (factor XII) activation by bacterial lipopolysaccharides (endotoxins). J. Exp. Med. 140:787, 1974.
58. McKay, D.G., Muller-Berghaus, G., and Gruse, V.: Activation of Hageman factor by ellagic acid and the generalized Shwartzman reaction. Am. J. Pathol. 54:393, 1969.
59. Pettinger, W.A., and Young, R.: Endotoxin-induced kinin (bradykinin) formation: Activation of Hageman factor and plasma kallikrein in human plasma. Life Sci. 9:313, 1970.
60. Kimball, H.R., Melmon, K.L., and Wolff, S.M.: Endotoxin-induced kinin production in man. Proc. Soc. Exp. Biol. Med. 139:1078, 1972.
61. Mason, J.W., Kleeberg, U., Dolan, P., and Colman, R.W.: Plasma kallikrein and Hageman factor in gram-negative bacteremia. Ann. Intern. Med. 73:545, 1970.
62. Rodriguez-Erdmann, F.: Studies on the pathogenesis of the generalized Schwartzman reaction. III. Trigger mechanism for the activation of the prothrombin molecule, Thromb. Diath. Haemorrh. 12:471, 1964.
63. Ulevitch, R.J., Cochrane, C.G., Henson, P.M., Morrison, D.C., and Doe, W.I.: Mediation systems in bacterial lipopolysaccharide-induced hypotension and disseminated intravascular coagulation. I. The role of complement. J. Exp. Med. 142:1570, 1975.
64. Eisen, V., and Smith, H.G.: Plasma kinin formation by complexes of aggregated γ-globulins and serum proteins. Br. J. Exp. Pathol. 51:328, 1970.
65. Movat, H.Z., and DiLorenzo, N.L.: Activation of the plasma kinin system by antigen-antibody aggregates. I. Generation of permeability factor in guinea pig serum. Lab. Invest. 19:187, 1968.
66. Movat, H.Z., DiLorenzo, N.L., and Treloar, M.P.: Activation of the plasma kinin system by antigen-antibody aggregates. II. Isolation of permeability enhancing and kinin releasing fractions from activated guinea pig serum. Lab. Invest. 19:201, 1968.
67. Movat, H.Z., Treloar, M.P., and Takeuchi, Y.: A small molecular weight permeability factor in guinea pig serum: Adsorption to antigen-antibody aggregates. J. Immunol. 103:875, 1969.
68. Epstein, W.V., Tan, M., and Melman, K.L.: Rheumatoid factor and kinin generation. Ann. N.Y. Acad. Sci. 168:173, 1969.
69. Cochrane, C.G., and Wuepper, K.D.: The kinin-forming system: Delineation and activation. In Miescher, P. (ed.): Immunopathology. Basel, Schwabe and Company, 1972, pp. 220–235.
70. Kaplan, A.P., Spragg, J., and Austen, K.F.: The bradykinin-forming system in man. In Austen, K.F., and Becker, E.L. (eds.): Biochemistry of the Acute Allergic Reaction. Oxford, Blackwell Scientific Publications Ltd., 1971, pp. 279–298.
71. Cochrane, C.G., Wuepper, K.D., Aiken, B.S., Revak, S.D., and Spiegelberg, H.L.: The interaction of Hageman factor and immune complexes. J. Clin. Invest. 51:2736, 1972.
72. Niewiarowski, S., Bankowski, E., and Rogowicka, J.: Studies on the adsorption and activation of Hageman factor (factor XII) by collagen and elastin. Thromb. Diath. Hemorrhag. 14:387, 1965.
73. Wilner, G.D., Nossel, H.L., and LeRoy, E.C.: Activation of Hageman factor by collagen. J. Clin. Invest. 47:2608, 1968.
74. Cochrane, C.G., Revak, S.D., Aiken, B.S., and Wuepper, K.D.: The structural characteristics and activation of Hageman factor. In Lepow, I.H., and Ward, P.A.: Inflammation: Mechanisms and Control. New York, Academic Press, 1972, pp. 119–138.
75. Harpel, P.C.: Studies on the interaction between collagen and a plasma kallikrein-like activity. Evidence for a surface-active enzyme system. J. Clin. Invest. 51:1813, 1972.
76. Griffin, J.H., Harper, A., and Cochrane, C.G.: Studies on the activation of human blood coagulation factor XII (Hageman factor) by soluble collagen. Fed. Proc. 34:860, 1975.
77. Meier, H.L., and Kaplan, A.P.: Evaluation of potential initiators of the Hageman factor (HF) dependent pathways. Fed. Proc. 37:12, 1978.
78. Revak, S.D., Cochrane, C.G., Johnston, A., and Hugli, T.: Structural changes accompanying enzymatic activation of Hageman factor. J. Clin. Invest. 54:619, 1974.
79. Proctor, R.R., and Rapaport, S.I.: The partial thromboplastin time with kaolin: A simple screening test for first stage plasma clotting deficiencies. Am. J. Clin. Pathol. 35:212, 1961.
80. Kaplan, A.P., and Austen, K.E.: A prealbumin activator of prekallikrein. J. Immunol. 105:802, 1970.
81. Kaplan, A.P., and Austen, K.F.: A prealbumin activator of prekallikrein. II. Derivation of activators of prekallikrein from active Hageman factor by digestion with plasmin. J. Exp. Med. 133:672–712, 1971.
82. Silverberg, M., Dunn, J.T., Garen, L., and Kaplan, A.P.: Autoactivation of human Hageman factor: Demonstration utilizing a synthetic substrate. J. Biol. Chem. 255:7281, 1980.
82a. Kaplan A.P., and Harpel, P.C.: Activation of the intrinsic coagulation-kinin system: Quantitation of activated Hageman factor-C1 INH complexes by an enzyme-linked immununosorbent assay. Clin. Res. 31:483a, 1983.
83. Lewin, M.F., Kaplan, A.P. and Harpel P.C.: Studies of C1 inactivator-plasma kallikrein complexes in purified systems and in plasma. Quantification by an enzyme-linked differential antibody immunosorbant assay. J. Biol. Chem. 258:6415, 1983.
84. Harpel, P.C.: α2 Plasmin inhibitor and α2 macroglobulin-plasmin complexes in plasma. Quantitation by an enzyme-linked differential antibody immunosorbent assay. J. Clin. Invest. 68:46, 1981.
85. Amandsen, E., Svendsen, L., Vennerod, A.M., and Laake, K.: Determination of plasma kallikrein with a new chromogenic tripeptide derivative. In Pisano, J.J., and Austen, K.F.: Chemistry and Biology of the Kallikrein-Kinin System in Health and Disease. Fogarty International Proceedings No. 27. Washington, D.C., U.S. Government Printing Office, 1974, pp. 215–220.
86. Saito, H., Ratnoff, O.D., and Pensky, J.: Radioimmunoassay of human Hageman factor (factor XII). J. Lab. Clin. Med. 88:506, 1976.
87. Wuepper, K.D., Tucker, E.S., III, and Cochrane, C.G.: Plasma kinin system: Proenzyme components. J. Immunol. 105:1307, 1970.
88. Treloar, M.P., and Movat, H.Z.: Isolation of two small molecular activators of the plasma kinin system in the guinea pig. Fed. Proc. 59:576, 1970.
89. Movat, H.Z., Poon, M.C., and Tukeuchi, Y.: The kinin system of human plasma. I. Isolation of a low molecular weight activator of prekallikrein. Int. Arch. Allergy Appl. Immunol. 40:89, 1971.
90. Wuepper, K.D., and Cochrane, C.G.: Isolation and mechanism of activation of components of the plasma kinin-forming system. In Austen, K.F., and Becker, E.L. (eds.): The Biochemistry of the Acute Allergic Reactions—Second International Symposium. Oxford, Blackwell Scientific Publications Ltd., 1971, pp. 299–320.
91. Cochrane, C.G., and Wuepper, K.D.: The first component of the kinin-forming system in human and rabbit plasma. Its relationship to clotting factor XII (Hageman factor). J. Exp. Med. 134:986, 1971.
92. Soltay, M.J., Movat, H.Z., and Ozge-Anwar, A.H.: The kinin system of human plasma. V. The probable derivative of prekallikrein activator from activated Hageman factor. Proc. Soc. Exp. Biol. Med. 138:952, 1972.
93. Burrowes, C.E., Movat, H.Z., and Soltay, M.J.: The kinin system of human plasma. VI. The action of plasmin. Proc. Soc. Exp. Biol. Med. 135:959, 1975.
94. Cochrane, C.G., Revak, S.D., and Wuepper, K.D.: Activation of Hageman factor in solid and fluid phases. J. Exp. Med. 138:1564, 1973.
95. Revak, S.D., and Cochrane, C.G.: The relationship of structure and function in human Hageman factor. The association of enzymatic and binding activities with separate regions of the molecule. J. Clin. Invest. 57:852, 1976.
96. Kaplan, A.P., Meier, H.L., Yecies, L.D., and Heck, L.W.: Hageman factor and its substrates: The role of factor XI (PTA), prekallikrein, and plasminogen proactivator in coagulation, fibrinolysis, and kinin-generation. In Pisano, J.J., and Austen, K.F. (eds.): Chemistry and Biology of the Kallikrein-Kinin System in Health and Disease. Fogarty International Center Proceedings No. 27. Washington, D.C., U.S. Government Printing Office, 1974, pp. 237–254.
97. Griffin, J.H., and Cochrane, C.G.: Mechanism for the involvement of high molecular weight kininogen in surface-dependent reactions of Hageman factor. Proc. Natl. Acad. Sci. USA 73:2559, 1976.
98. Kaplan, A.P., Meier, H.L., and Mandle, R., Jr.: The Hageman factor dependent pathways of coagulation, fibrinolysis, and kinin-generation. Semin. Thromb. Haemostasis 3:1, 1976.
99. Meier, H.L., Scott, C.F., Mandle, R., Jr., Webster, M.E., Pierce, J.V., Colman, R.W., and Kaplan, A.P.: Requirements for contact activation of human Hageman factor. Ann. N.Y. Acad. Sci. 283:93, 1977.
100. Liu, C.Y., Scott, C.F., Bagdasarian, A., Pierce, J.V., Kaplan, A.P., and Colman, R.W.: Potentiation of the function of Hageman factor fragments by high molecular weight kininogen. J. Clin. Invest. 60:7, 1977.
101. Meier, H.L., Pierce, J.V., Colman, R.W., and Kaplan, A.P.: Activation and function of human Hageman factor. The role of high molecular weight kininogen and prekallikrein. J. Clin. Invest. 60:18, 1977.
102. Griffin, J.H.: Role of surface in surface-dependent activation of Hageman factor (blood coagulation factor XII). Proc. Natl. Acad. Sci. 75:1998, 1978.
103. McMillin, C.R., Saito, H., Ratnoff, O.D., and Walton, A.G.: The secondary structure of human Hageman factor (Factor XII) and its alteration by activating agents. J. Clin. Invest. 54:1312, 1974.
104. Wiggins, R.C., Bouma, B.N., Cochrane, C.G., and Griffin, J.H.: Role of

high molecular weight kininogen in surface-binding and activation of coagulation factor XI and prekallikrein. Proc. Natl. Acad. Sci. 77:4636, 1977.

105. Silverberg, M., Nicoll, J.E., and Kaplan, A.P.: The mechanism by which the light chain of cleaved HMW-kininogen augments the activation of prekallikrein, factor XI, and Hageman factor. Thromb. Res. 20:173, 1980.

106. Thompson, R.E., Mandle, R., Jr., and Kaplan, A.P.: Studies of the binding of prekallikrein and factor XI to high molecular weight kininogen and its light chain. Proc. Natl. Acad. Sci. 76:4862, 1979.

107. Cochrane, C.G., and Revak, S.D.: Dissemination of contact activation in plasma by plasma kallikrein. J. Exp. Med. 152:608, 1980.

108. Scott, C.F., and Colman, R.W.: Function and immunochemistry of prekallikrein-high molecular weight kininogen complex in plasma. J. Clin. Invest. 65:413, 1980.

109. Fair, B.D., Saito, H., Ratnoff, O.D., and Rippon, W.B.: Detection by fluorescence of structural changes accompanying the activation of Hageman factor (factor XII). Proc. Soc. Exp. Biol. Med. 55:199, 1977.

110. Wiggins, R.C., and Cochrane, C.G.: The autoactivation of rabbit Hageman factor. J. Exp. Med. 150:1122, 1979.

111. Kurachi, K., Fujikawa, K., and Davie, E.W.: Mechanism of activation of bovine factor XI by factor XII and factor XIIa. Biochemistry 19:1330, 1980.

112. Heimark, R.L., Kurachi, K., Fujikawa, K., and Davie, E.W.: Surface activation of blood coagulation, fibrinolysis, and kinin formation. Nature 456, 1980.

113. Sugo, T., Hamaguchi, A., Shimada, J., Kato, H., and Iwanaga, S.: Mechanism of surface-mediated activation of bovine factor XII and plasma prekallikrein. J. Biochem. 92:689, 1982.

114. Ratnoff, O.D., and Saito, H.: Amidolytic properties of single-chain activated Hageman factor. Proc. Natl. Acad. Sci. 76:1461, 1979.

115. Miller, G., Silverberg, M., and Kaplan, A.P.: Autoactivatability of human Hageman factor (factor XII). Biochem. Biophys. Res. Commun. 52:803, 1980.

116. Dunn, J.T., Silverberg, M., and Kaplan, A.P.: The cleavage and formation of activated human Hageman factor by autodigestion and by kallikrein. J. Biol. Chem. 275:1779, 1982.

117. Silverberg, M., and Kaplan, A.P.: Enzymatic activities of activated and zymogen forms of human Hageman factor (factor XII). Blood 60:64, 1982.

118. Tankersley, D.L., and Finlayson, J.S.: Kinetics of activation and autoactivation of factor XII (Hageman factor). Circ. Supp. II. 66:296, 1982.

119. Revak, S.D., Cochrane, C.G., and Griffin, J.H.: The binding and cleavage characteristics of human Hageman factor during contact activation. A comparison of normal plasma with plasmas deficient in factor XI, prekallikrein, or high molecular weight kininogen. J. Clin. Invest. 59:1167, 1977.

120. Revak, S.D., Cochrane, C.G., Bouma, B.N., and Griffin, J.H.: Surface and fluid phase activities of two forms of activated Hageman factor produced during contact activation of plasma. J. Exp. Med. 147:719, 1978.

121. Dunn, J.T., and Kaplan, A.P.: Formation and structure of human Hageman factor fragments. J. Clin. Invest. 70:627, 1982.

122. Mackay, M.E., Miles, A.A., Schacter, C.B., and Wilhelm, D.L.: Susceptibility of the guinea pig to pharmacological factors from its own serum. Nature 172:714, 1953.

123. Stewart, P.B., and Bliss, J.Q.: The permeability increasing factor in diluted human plasma. Br. J. Exp. Path. 38:462, 1957.

124. Mill, P.J., Elder, J.M., Miles, A.A., and Wilhelm, D.L.: Enzyme-like globulins from serum reproducing the vascular phenomena of inflammation. VI. Isolation and properties of permeability factor and its inhibition in human plasma. Br. J. Exp. Path. 39:343, 1958.

125. Elder, J.M., and Wilhelm, D.L.: Enzyme-like globulins from serum producing the vascular phenomena of inflammation. V. Active permeability factor in human serum. Br. J. Exp. Path. 39:23, 1958.

126. Ratnoff, O.D., and Miles, A.A.: Activation of a vascular permeability increasing factor in human plasma incubated with purified activated Hageman factor. J. Lab. Clin. Med. 60:1009, 1962.

127. Ratnoff, O.D., and Miles, A.A.: The induction of permeability increasing activity in human plasma by activated Hageman factor. Br. J. Exp. Path. 45:328, 1964.

128. Kellermeyer, R.W., and Ratnoff, O.D.: Abolition of the permeability-enhancing properties of Hageman factor by specific antiserum. J. Lab. Clin. Med. 70:356, 1967.

129. Webster, M.E., and Ratnoff, O.D.: Role of Hageman factor in the activation of vasodilator activity in human plasma. Nature 192:180, 1961.

130. Webster, M.E., and Pierce, J.V.: Studies on the enzymes involved in the activation of human plasma kallikrein. In Rocha e Silva, M., and Rothschild, H.A. (eds.): International Symposium on Vasoactive Polypeptides: Bradykinin and Related Kinins. New York, Plenum Publishing Company, 1967, pp. 155–160.

131. Kagen, L.J., Leddy, J.P., and Becker, E.L.: Isolation of two permeability globulins from human plasma. Nature 197:693, 1963.

132. Kagen, L.J., Leddy, J.P., and Becker, E.L.: The presence of two permeability globulins in human serum. J. Clin. Invest. 42:1353, 1963.

133. Kaplan, A.P., Spragg, J., Gigli, I., and Austen, K.F.: Purification of kallikrein and PF/dil and their interaction with kininogen and with C1 Inhibitor (C1 INH). Fed. Proc. 29:491, 1970.

134. Johnston, A.R., Cochrane, C.G., and Revak, S.D.: The relationship between PF/dil and activated Hageman factor. J. Immunol. 113:103, 1974.

135. Oh-Ishi, S., and Webster, M.E.: Vascular permeability factors PF/nat and PF/dil: Their relationship to Hageman factor and the kallikrein-kinin system. Biochem. Pharm. 24:591, 1975.

136. Wuepper, K.D.: Plasma prekallikrein: Its characterization, mechanism of activation, and inherited deficiency in man. In Pisano, J.J., and Austen, K.F. (eds.): Chemistry and Biology and the Kallikrein-Kinin System in Health and Disease. Fogarty International Center Proceedings No. 27, Washington, D.C., U.S. Government Printing Office, 1974, pp. 37–51.

137. Hathaway, W.E., Wuepper, K.D., Weston, W.L., Hambert, J.R., Rivers, R.P.A., Genton, E., August, C.S., Montgomery, R.R., and Moss, M.F.: Clinical and physiologic studies of two siblings with prekallikren (Fletcher factor) deficiency. Am. J. Med. 60:654, 1976.

138. Abildgaard, C.F., and Harrison, J.: Fletcher factor deficiency: Family study and detection. Blood 43:641, 1974.

139. Stormorken, H., and Abildgaard, C.F.: The Fletcher factor—prekallikrein deficiency: A diagnostic test which identifies heterozygotes. Thromb. Res. 5:375, 1974.

140. Harpel, P.C.: Studies on human plasma α_2 macroglobulin enzyme interactions. Evidence for proteolytic modification of the subunit chain structures. J. Exp. Med. 138:508, 1973.

141. Harpel, P.C., and Mosesson, M.W.: Degradation of human fibrinogen by plasma α_1-macroglobulin-enzyme complexes. J. Clin. Invest. 52:2175, 1973.

142. Kluft, C.: Determination of prekallikrein in plasma: Optional condition for activation of prekallikrein. J. Lab. Clin. Med. 91:83, 1978.

143. Friberger, P., Eriksson, E., Constavsson, S., and Cleson, G.: Determination of prekallikrein in plasma by means of a chromogenic tripeptide substrate for plasma kallikrein. In Fugii, S., Moriya, H., and Suzuki, T. (eds.): Kinins II—Biochemistry, Pathophysiology, and Clinical Aspects. New York, Plenum Press, 1979, pp. 67–82.

144. Fisher, C.A., Schmaier, A.H., Addonizio, P., and Colman, R.W.: Assay of prekallikrein in human plasma: Comparison of amidolytic, esterolytic, coagulation, and immunochemical assays. Blood 59:963, 1982.

145. Webster, M.E., and Pierce, J.V.: Action of kallikreins on synthetic ester substrates. Proc. Soc. Exp. Biol. Med. 107:186, 1961.

146. Colman, R.W., Mason, J.W., and Sherry, S.: The kallikreinogen-kallikrein enzyme system of human plasma: Assay of components and observations in disease states. Ann. Intern. Med. 71:763, 1969.

147. Colman, R.W., Mattler, L., and Sherry, S.: Studies on the prekallikrein (kallikreinogen)-kallikrein enzyme system of human plasma. I. Isolation and purification of plasma kallikreins. J. Clin. Invest. 48:11, 1969.

148. Colman, R.W., Mattler, L., and Sherry, S.: Studies on the prekallikrein (kallikreinogen)-kallikrein enzyme system of human plasma. II. Evidence relating the kaolin-activated arginine esterase to plasma kallikrein. J. Clin. Invest. 48:23, 1969.

149. Talamo, R.C., Haber, E., and Austen, K.F.: A radioimmuno-assay for bradykinin in plasma and synovial fluid. J. Lab. Clin. Med. 74:816, 1969.

150. Gireg, G.J.D., Talamo, R.C., and Colman, R.W.: The kinetics of the release of bradykinin by kallikrein in normal human plasma. J. Lab. Clin. Med. 80:496, 1972.

151. Imanari, T., Kaizu, T., Yoshida, H., Yates, K., Pierce, J.V., and Pisano, J.J.: Radiochemical assay for human urinary, salivary, and plasma kallikreins. In Pisano, J.J., and Austen, K.F. (eds.): Chemistry and Biology of the Kallikrein-Kinin System in Health and Diseases. Fogarty International Center Proceedings No. 27. Washington, D.C., U.S. Government Printing Office, 1974, pp. 205–213.

152. Bagdasarian, A., Lahiri, B., Talamo, R.C., Wong, P., and Colman, R.W.: Immunochemical studies of plasma kallikrein. J. Clin. Invest. 54:1444, 1974.

153. Saito, H., and Poon, M.C.: Radioimmunoassay for a human plasma prekallikrein (Fletcher factor). Fed. Proc. 36:329, 1977.

154. Gigli, I., Mason, J.W., Colman, R.W., and Austen, K.F.: Interaction of plasma kallikrein with C1 Inhibitor. J. Immunol. 104:574, 1970.

155. Harpel, P.C.: Human plasma α_2 macroglobulin. An inhibitor of plasma kallikrein. J. Exp. Med. 132:329, 1970.

156. Saito, M., Poon, M.C., Vivic, W., Goldsmith, G.H., Jr., and Menitove, J.E.: Human plasma prekallikrein (Fletcher factor) clotting activity and antigen in health and disease. J. Lab. Clin. Med. 92:84, 1978.

157. Saito, H., Goodnough, L.T., Soria, J., Soria, C., Aznar, J., and Espana, F.: Heterogeneity of human prekallikrein deficiency (Fletcher trait).

Evidence that five of 18 cases are positive for cross-reacting material. N. Engl. J. Med. 305:910, 1981.

158. Saito, H., Ratnoff, O. D., and Pensky, J.: Radioimmunoassay of human Hageman factor (factor XII) J. Lab. Clin. Med. 88:506, 1976.

159. Saito, H., and Scialla S.J.: Isolation and properties of an abnormal Hageman factor (factor XII) molecule in a cross-reacting material-positive Hageman trait plasma. J. Clin. Invest. 68:1028, 1981.

160. Bouma, B.N., Kerbiriou, D.M., Vlooswijk, R.A.A., and Griffin, J.H.: Immunochemical studies of prekallikrein, kallikrein, and high-molecular weight kininogen in normal and deficient plasmas and in normal plasmas after cold-dependent activation. J. Lab. Clin. Med. 96:693, 1980.

161. Donaldson, V.M., Kleniewski, J., Saito, H., and Sayed, J.K.: Prekallikrein deficiency in a kindred with kininogen deficiency and Fitzgerald trait clotting defect. Evidence that high molecular weight kininogen and prekallikrein exist as a complex in normal human plasma. J. Clin. Invest. 60:571, 1977.

162. Jonasson, O., and Becker, E.L.: Release of kallikrein from guinea pig lung during anaphylaxis. J. Exp. Med. 123:509, 1966.

163. Rocha e Silva, M., Beraldo, W.T., and Rosenfeld, G.: Bradykinin, hypotensive and smooth muscle stimulating factor released from plasma globulin by snake venom and trypsin. Am. J. Physiol. 156:261, 1949.

164. Mandle, R., Jr., and Kaplan, A.P.: Hageman factor substrates. Human plasma prekallikrein. Mechanism of activation by Hageman factor and participation in Hageman factor-dependent fibrinolysis. J. Biol. Chem. 252:6097, 1977.

165. Bouma, B.N., Miles, L.A., Baretta, G., and Griffin, J.H. Human plasma prekallikrein. Studies of its activation by activated factor XII and of its inactivation by diisopropyl phosphofluoridate. Biochemistry 19:1151, 1980.

166. Tankersley, D.I., Fournel, M.A., and Schroeder, D.D. Kinetics of activation of prekallikrein by prekallikrein activator. Biochemistry 19:3121, 1980.

167. Van der Graff, F., Tans, G., Bouma, B.N., and Griffin, J.H.: Isolation and functional properties of the heavy and light chains of human plasma kallikrein. J. Biol. Chem. 257:14300, 1982.

168. Nagasawa, S., Takahashi, H., Koida, M., and Suzuki, T.: Partial purification of bovine plasma kallikreinogen, its activation by the Hageman factor. Biochem. Biophys. Res. Commun. 32:644, 1968.

169. Takahashi, H., Nagasawa, S., and Suzuki, T.: Studies on prekallikrein of bovine plasma. I. Purification and properties. J. Biochem. 71:471, 1972.

170. Takahashi, H., Nagasawa, S., and Suzuki, T.: Studies on prekallikrein of bovine plasma II. Activation of prekallikrein with proteinases and properties of kallikrein activated by bovine Hageman factor. J. Biochem. 87:23, 1980.

171. Yamamoto, T., Kozono, K., Okamoto, T., Kato, H., and Kamabara, T.: Purification of guinea-pig plasma prekallikrein. Activation by prekallikrein activator derived from guinea pig skin. Biochem. et Biophys. Acta 614:511, 1980.

172. Wuepper, K.D., and Cochrane, C.G.: Plasma prekallikrein: Isolation, characterization and mechanism of activation. J. Exp. Med. 135:1, 1972.

173. Wuepper, K.D., and Cochrane, C.G.: Effect of plasma kallikrein on coagulation in vitro. Proc. Soc. Exp. Biol. Med. 141:271, 1972.

174. Johnson, A.R., Ulevitch, R.J., and Ryan, K.: Biochemical and biological properties of rabbit prekallikrein. Fed. Proc. 35:693, 1976.

175. Pierce, J.V., and Webster, M.E.: The purification and some properties of two different kallidinogens. In Erdos, E.G., Back, N., and Sicuteri, F. (eds.): Hypotensive Peptides. New York, Springer-Verlag, 1966, pp. 130–138.

176. Jacobsen, S.: Substrates from plasma kinin-forming enzymes in human, dog, and rabbit plasmas. Br. J. Pharmacol. 26:403, 1966.

177. Jacobsen, S.: Substrates for plasma kinin-forming enzymes in rat and guinea pig plasma. Br. J. Pharmacol. 28:64, 1966.

178. Jacobsen, S., and Kriz, M.: Some data on two purified kininogens from human plasma. Br. J. Pharmacol. 29:25, 1967.

179. Spragg, J., Haber, E., and Austen, K.F.: The preparation of human kininogen and the elicitation of antibody for use in a radial immunodiffusion assay. J. Immunol. 104:1348, 1970.

180. Spragg, J., and Austen, K.F.: The preparation of human kininogen. II. Further characterization of purified human kininogen. J. Immunol. 107:1512, 1971.

181. Spragg, J., and Austen, K.F.: Preparation of human kininogen. III. Enzymatic digestion and modification. Biochem. Pharmacol. 23:781, 1974.

182. Pierce, J.V.: Purification of mammalian kallikreins, kininogens and kinins. In Erdos, E.G. (ed.): Handbook of Experimental Pharmacology. New York, Springer-Verlag, 1970, Vol. 25, pp. 21–51.

183. Habal, F.M., and Movat, H.Z.: Kininogens of human plasma. Res. Commun. Chem. Path. Pharmacol. 4:477, 1972.

184. Habal, F.M., Movat, H.Z., and Burrowes, C.E.: Isolation of two functionally different kininogens from human plasma—separation from proteinase inhibitors and interaction with plasma kallikrein. Biochem. Pharmacol. 23:2291, 1974.

185. Habal, F.M., and Movat, H.Z.: Some physicochemical and functional differences between low and high molecular weight kininogens of human plasma. In Pisano, J.J., and Austen, K.F. (eds.): The Chemistry and Biology of the Kallikrein-Kinin System in Health and Disease. Fogarty International Center Proceedings No. 27. Washington, D.C., U.S. Government Printing Office, 1974, pp. 129–131.

186. Habal, F.M., Underdown, B.J., and Movat, H.Z.: Further characterization of human plasma kininogens. Biochem. Pharmacol. 24:1241, 1975.

187. Suzuki, T., Mizushima, Y., Sato, T., and Iwanaga, S.: Purification of bovine bradykininogen. J. Biochem. 57:14, 1965.

188. Yano, M., Nagasawa, S., Hairuchi, K., and Suzuki, T.: Separation of a new substrate, kininogen I, for plasma kallikrein in bovine plasma. J. Biochem. 62:504, 1967.

189. Pierce, J.V., and Guimaraes, J.A.: Further characterization of highly purified human plasma kininogens. In Pisano, J.J., and Austen, K.F. (eds.): Chemistry and Biology of the Kallikrein-Kinin System in Health and Disease. Fogarty International Center Proceedings No. 27. Washington, D.C., U.S. Government Printing Office, 1974, pp. 121–127.

189a. Thompson, R.E., Mandle R.J., and Kaplan, A.P.: Characterization of human high molecular weight kininogen: Procoagulant activity associated with the light chain of kinin-free high molecular weight kininogen, J. Exp. Med. 147:488, 1978.

190. Saito, H.: Purification of high molecular weight kininogen and the role of this agent in blood coagulation. J. Clin. Invest. 60:584, 1977.

191. Nakayasa, T., and Nagasawa, S.: Studies on human kininogens I. Isolation characterization, and cleavage by plasma kallikrein of high molecular weight (HMW) kininogen. J. Biochem. 85:249, 1979.

192. Mori, K., and Nagasawa, S.: Studies on human high molecular weight (HMW) kininogen II. Structural change of HMW-kininogen by the action of human plasma kallikrein. J. Biochem. 89:1465, 1981.

193. Mori, K., Sakamoto, W., and Nagasawa, S.: Studies on human high molecular weight (HMW) kininogen III. Cleavage of HMW kininogen by the action of human salivary kallikrein. J. Biochem. 90:503, 1981.

194. Kerbiriou, D.M., and Griffin, J.H.: Human high molecular weight kininogen. Studies of structure-function relationships and of proteolysis of the molecule occurring during contact activation of plasma. J. Biol. Chem. 254:12020, 1979.

195. Kerbiriou, D.M., Bouma, B.N., and Griffin, J.H.: Immunochemical studies of human high molecular weight kininogen and of its complexes with plasma prekallikrein or kallikrein. J. Biol. Chem. 255:3952, 1980.

196. Schiffman, S., Mannhalter, C., and Tynerk, D.: Human high molecular weight kininogen. Effects of cleavage by kallikrein on protein structure and procoagulant activity. J. Biol. Chem. 255:6433, 1980.

197. Chan, J.Y.C., Habal, F.M., Burrowes, C.C., and Movat, H.Z.: Interaction between factor XII (Hageman factor), high molecular weight kininogen and prekallikrein. Thromb. Res. 9:423, 1976.

198. Han, Y.N., Kato, H., Iwanaga, S., and Suzuki, T.: Primary structure of bovine high molecular weight kininogen. The amino acid sequence of a glycopeptide (fragment) following the C-terminus of the bradykinin moiety. J. Biochem. 79:1201, 1976.

199. Han, Y.N., Kato, M., Iwanaga, S., and Suzaki, T.: Bovine plasma high molecular weight kininogen; the amino acid sequence of fragment 1 (glycopeptide) released by the action of plasma kallikrein and its location in the precursor molecule. FEBS Lett 67:197, 1976.

200. Scicli, A.G., Waldmann, R., Guimaraes, J.A., Scicli, G., Carretero, O.A., Kato, H., Han, Y.N., and Iwanaga, S.: Relationship between structure and correcting activity of bovine high molecular weight kininogen upon the clotting time of Fitzgerald-trait plasma. J. Exp. Med. 145:847, 1979.

201. Sugo, T., Kato, H., Iwanaga, S., and Fujii, S.: The accelerating effect of bovine plasma HMW kininogen on the surface-mediated activation of factor XII: Generation of a derivative form (active kininogen) with maximal cofactor activity by limited proteolysis. Thromb. Res. 24:329, 1981.

202. Sugo, T., Kato H., Iwanaga, S., and Fujii, S.: The accelerating effect of bovine plasma HMW kininogen on the surface-mediated activation of factor XII: Generation of a derivative form (active kininogen) with maximal cofactor activity by limited proteolysis. Thromb. Res. 24:329, 1981.

203. Vroman, L., Adams A.L., Fischer, G.C., and Munoz, P.C.: Interaction of high molecular weight kininogen, factor XII, and fibrinogen in plasma at interfaces. Blood 55:156, 1980.

204. Kato, H., Han, Y.N., Iwanaga, S., Suzuki, T., and Komiya, M.: Bovine plasma HMW and HMW kininogens. Structural differences between heavy and light chains derived from the kinin-free proteins. J. Biochem. 80:1299, 1966.

205. Komiya, M., Kato, H., and Suzuki, T.: Homology between bovine high molecular weight and low molecular weight kininogens. Biochem. Biophys. Res. Commun. 49:1438, 1972.

206. Komiya, M., Kato, H., and Suzuki, T.: Bovine plasma kininogens III. Structural comparison of high molecular weight and low molecular weight kininogens. J. Biochem. 76:833, 1974.

207. Prado, E.S., Prado, J.L., and Brandi, C.M.W.: Further purification and some properties of horse urinary kallikrein. Arch. Int. Pharmacodyn. 137:358, 1962.

208. Webster, M.E., and Prado, E.S.: Glandular kallikreins from horse and human urine and from hog pancreas. Methods Enzymol. 19:681, 1970.

209. Diniz, C.R., and Carvalho, I.F.: A micromethod for determination of bradykininogen under several conditions. Ann. N.Y. Acad. Sci. 104:77, 1963.

210. Proud, D., Pierce, J.V., and Pisano, J.J.: Radioimmunoassay of human high molecular weight kininogen in normal and deficient plasmas. J. Lab. Clin. Med. 95:563, 1980.

211. Rosenthal, R.L., Dreskin, O.H., and Rosenthal, N.: New hemophilia-like disease caused by deficiency of a third plasma thromboplastin factor. Proc. Soc. Exp. Biol. Med. 82:171, 1953.

212. Heck, L.W., and Kaplan, A.P.: Substrates of human Hageman factor. I. Isolation and characterization of PTA (Factor XI) and its inhibition by α₁ antitrypsin. J. Exp. Med. 140:1615, 1630, 1974.

213. Saito, H., and Goldsmith, G.H., Jr.: Plasma thromboplastin antecedent (PTA, factor XI): A specific and sensitive radioimmunoassay. Blood 50:377, 1977.

214. Forbes, C.D., and Ratnoff, O.D.: Studies on plasma thromboplastin antecedent (factor XI), PTA deficiency, and inhibition of PTA by plasma, pharmacologic inhibitors, and specific antiserum. J. Lab. Clin. Med. 79:113, 1972.

215. Rimon, A., Schiffman, S., Feinstein, D.I., and Rapaport, S.I.: Factor XI activity and factor XI antigen in homozygous and heterozygous factor XI deficiency. Blood 48:165, 1976.

216. Chan, J.Y.C., and Movat, H.Z.: Purification of factor XII (Hageman factor) from human plasma. Thromb. Res. 8:337, 1976.

217. Kaode, T., Hermodson, M.A., and Davie, E.W.: Active site of bovine Hageman factor XI (plasma thromboplastin antecedent). Nature 266:729, 1977.

218. Saito, H., Ratnoff, O.D., Marshall, J.S., and Pensky, J.: Partial purification of plasma thromboplastin antecedent (factor XI) and its activation by trypsin. J. Clin. Invest. 52:850, 1973.

219. Mannhalter, C., Schiffman, S., and Jacobs, A.: Trypsin activation of human factor XI. J. Biol. Chem. 255:2667, 1980.

220. Bouma, B.N., and Griffin, J.H.: Human blood coagulation factor XI: Purification, properties and mechanism of activated Factor XII. J. Biol. Chem. 252:6432, 1977.

221. Kurachi, K., and Davie, E.W.: Activation of human factor XI (plasma thromboplastin antecedent) by factor XIIa (activated Hageman factor). Biochemistry 16:5831, 1977.

222. Ratnoff, O.D.: Studies on the product of the reaction between activated Hageman factor (factor XII) and plasma thromboplastin antecedent. J. Lab. Clin. Med. 80:704, 1972.

223. Kingdon, H.S., Davie, E.W., and Ratnoff, O.D.: The reaction between activated plasma thromboplastin antecedent and diisopropyl-phosphofluoridate. Biochemistry 3:166, 1964.

224. Schiffman, S., and Margalit, R.: Factor XI adsorption to surface: Interaction of high molecular weight kininogen (HMWK) and a plasma adsorption inhibitor. Blood 56:168, 1980.

225. Schiffman, S., and Mannhalter, C.: Surface adsorption of factor XI. Association of adsorption sites with the heavy chain of activated factor XI.

226. Stern, D.M., Nossel, H.L., and Owen, J.: Acquired antibody to factor XI in a patient with congenital factor XI deficiency. J. Clin. Invest. 69:1270, 1982.

227. Meier, M.L., Thompson, R.E., and Kaplan, A.P.: Ativation of Hageman factor by factor XIa-HMW-kininogen. Thromb. Haemostasis 38:14, 1977.

228. McDonagh, K.S., and Ferguson, J.H.: Studies on the participation of Hageman factor in fibrinolysis. Thromb. Diath. Haemorrh. 24:1, 1970.

229. Colman, R.W.: Activation of plasminogen by human plasma kallikrein. Biochem. Biophys. Res. Commun. 351:273, 1969.

230. Ogston, D., Ogston, C.M., Ratnoff, O.D., and Forbes, C.O.: Studies on a complex mechanism for the activation of plasminogen by kaolin and by chloroform: The participation of Hageman factor and additional cofactors. J. Clin. Invest. 48:1786, 1969.

231. Kaplan, A.P., Goetzl, E.J., and Austen, K.F.: The fibrinolytic pathway of human plasma. II. Generation of chemotactic activity by activation of plasminogen proactivator. J. Clin. Invest. 52:2591, 1973.

232. Laake, K., and Vennerod, A.M.: Factor XII-induced fibrinolysis. Studies on the separation of prekallikrein, plasminogen proactivator, and factor XI in human plasma. Thromb. Res. 4:285, 1974.

233. Vennerod, A.M., and Laake, K.: Prekallikrein and plasminogen proactivator: Absence of plasminogen proactivator in Fletcher factor deficient plasma. Thromb. Res. 8:519, 1976.

234. Kaplan, A.P., and Austen, K.F.: The fibrinolytic pathway of human plasma. Isolation and characterization of the plasminogen proactivator. J. Exp. Med. 136:1378, 1972.

235. Mandle, R., Jr., and Kaplan, A.P.: Plasminogen proactivators of human plasma: Relationship to prekallikrein and factor XI. Fed. Proc. 36:329, 1977.

236. Mandle, R., Jr., and Kaplan, A.P.: Hageman factor-dependent fibrinolysis: Generation of fibrinolytic activity by the interaction of human activated factor XI and plasminogen. Blood 54:850, 1979.

237. Bouma, B.N., and Griffin, J.H.: Human prekallikrein (plasminogen proactivator): Purification, characterization and activation by activated factor XII. Thromb. Haemostasis 38:136, 1977.

238. Saito, H.: The participation of plasma thromboplastin antecedent (Factor XI) in contact-activated fibrinolysis. Proc. Soc. Exp. Biol. Med. 164:153, 1980.

239. Goldsmith, G.H., Saito, H., and Ratnoff, O.D.: The activation of plasminogen by Hageman factor (factor XII) and Hageman factor fragments. J. Clin. Invest. 62:54, 1978.

240. Wuepper, K.D.: Prekallikrein–Hageman factor cofactor–Fletcher factor: Are they identical? Clin. Res. 21:484, 1973.

241. Kluft, C.: An inventory of plasminogen activators in human plasma. Thromb. Haemostasis 38:134, 1977.

242. Robyn, J.C., Ogston, D., and Douglas, A.T.: Further purification and properties of Hageman factor cofactor. Biochim. Biophys. Acta 271:371, 1972.

243. Saito, H., Ratnoff, O.D., Donaldson, V.H., Haney, G., and Pensky, J.: Inhibition of the adsorption of Hageman factor (factor XII) to glass by normal plasma. J. Lab. Clin. Med. 84:62, 1974.

244. Forbes, C.O., Pensky, J., and Ratnoff, O.D.: Inhibition of activated Hageman factor and activated plasma thromboplastin antecedent by purified CĪ inactivator. J. Lab. Clin. Med. 76:809, 1970.

245. Schreiber, A.D., Kaplan, A.P., and Austen, K.F.: Inhibition by CĪ INH of Hageman factor fragment activation of coagulation, fibrinolysis, and kinin-generation. J. Clin. Invest. 52:1402, 1973.

246. Stead, N.W., Kaplan, A.P., and Rosenberg, R.D.: The inhibition of human activated Hageman factor (HF) by human antithrombin-heparin cofactor (AT). J. Biol. Chem. 251:6481, 1976.

247. McConnell, D.J.: Inhibitors of kallikrein in human plasma. J. Clin. Invest. 51:1611, 1972.

248. Harpel, P.C.: Circulating inhibitors of human plasma kallikrein. In Pisano, J.J., and Austen, K.F. (eds.): Chemistry and Biology of the Kallikrein-Kinin System in Health and Disease. Fogarty International Center Proceedings No. 27. Washington, D.C., U.S. Government Printing Office, 1974, pp. 169–177.

249. Lahiri, B., Rosenberg, R., Mitchell, R.C., Bagdasarian, A., and Colman, R.W.: Antithrombin III. An inhibitor of plasma kallikrein. Fed. Proc. 33:642, 1974.

250. Burrowes, C.E., Habal, F.M., and Movat, H.Z.: The inhibition of human plasma kallikrein by antithrombin III. Thromb. Res. 7:175, 1975.

251. Vennerod, A.M., Laake, K., Solberg, A.K., and Stromland, S.: Inactivation and binding of human plasma kallikrein by antithrombin III. Thromb. Res. 9:457, 1976.

252. Schapira, M., Scott, C.F., and Colman, R.W.: Contribution of plasma protease inhibitor to the inactivation of kallikrein in plasma. J. Clin. Invest. 65:462, 1982.

253. Van der Graaf, F., Koedam, J.A., and Bouma, B.N.: Inactivation of kallikrein in human plasma. J. Clin. Invest. 71:149, 1983.

254. Scott, C.F., Schapira, M., James, H.L., Cohen, A.B., and Colman, R.W.: Inactivation of factor XIa by plasma protease inhibitor. Predominant role of α₁ proteinase inhibitor and protective effect of high molecular weight kininogen. J. Clin. Invest. 69:844, 1982.

255. Damus, P.S., Hicks, M., and Rosenberg, R.D.: Anticoagulant action of heparin. Nature 246:355, 1973.

256. Ganrot, P.O.: Inhibition of plasmin activity by α₂ macroglobulin. Clin. Chim. Acta 16:328, 1967.

257. Schreiber, A.D., Kaplan, A.P., and Austen, K.F.: Plasma inhibitors of the components of the fibrinolytic pathway in man. J. Clin. Invest. 52:1394, 1973.

258. Collen, D.: Identification and some properties of a new fast-reacting plasmin inhibitor in human plasma. Eur. J. Biochem. 69:209, 1976.

259. Moroi, M., and Aoki, N.: Isolation and characterization of α₂ plasmin inhibitor from human plasma. J. Biol. Chem. 251:5956, 1976.

260. Mullertz, S., and Clemmensen, I.: The primary inhibitor of plasmin in human plasma. Biochem. J. 159:545, 1976.

261. Harpel, P.C.: Plasmin inhibitor interactions. The effectiveness of α₂ plasmin inhibitor in the presence of α₂ macroglobulin. J. Exp. Med. 146:1033, 1977.

262. Aoki, N., Moroi, M., Matsuda, M., and Tachiya, K.: The behavior of α₂ plasmin inhibitor in fibrinolytic states. J. Clin. Invest. 60:361, 1977.

263. Harpel, P.C.: CĪ inactivator inhibition by plasmin. J. Clin. Invest. 49:569, 1970.

264. Harpel, P.C., and Cooper, N.R.: Studies on human plasma CĪ inactivator-enzyme interactions. I. Mechanisms of interaction with CĪs, plasmin, and trypsin. J. Clin. Invest. 55:593, 1975.

265. Highsmith, R.F., and Rosenberg, R.D.: The inhibition of human plasmin by human antithrombin-heparin cofactor. J. Biol. Chem. 249:4335, 1974.

266. Harpel, P.C., and Rosenberg, R.D.: α_2-Macroglobulin and antithrombin-heparin cofactor. In Spaet, T.H. (ed.): Modulators of Hemostatic and Inflammatory Reactions. New York, Grune & Stratton, 1976, pp. 145–191.
267. Saito, H., Goldsmith, G.H., Moroi, M., and Aoki, N.: Inhibitory spectrum of α_2 plasmin inhibitor. Proc. Natl. Acad. Sci. 76:2013, 1979.
268. Koie, K., Ogata, K., Kamiya, T., and Takamatsu, J.: α_2-Plasmin-inhibitor deficiency. Lancet 2:1334, 1978.
269. Aoki, N., Saito, H., Kamiya, T., Koie, K., Sakata, Y., and Kobakura, M.: Congenital deficiency of α_2 plasmin inhibitor associated with severe hemorrhagic tendency. J. Clin. Invest. 63:877, 1979.
270. Kluft, C., Vellenga, E., Brommer, E.J.P., and Wijngaards, G.: A familial hemorrhagic diathesis in a Dutch family: An inherited deficiency of α_2 antiplasmin. Blood 59:1169, 1982.
271. Miles, L.A., Plow, E.F., Donnelly, K.J., Hougie, C., and Griffin, J.H.: A bleeding disorder due to deficiency of α_2-antiplasmin. Blood 59:1246, 1982.
272. Sakata, Y., and Aoki, N.: Significance of cross-linking of α_2 plasmin inhibitor to fibrin in inhibition of fibrinolysis and in hemostasis. J. Clin. Invest. 69:536, 1982.
273. Rocha e Silva, M.: The kinin trail: Possible significance of bradykinin and related kinins to autopharmacology. In Maxwell, R.A., and Acheson, G. (eds.): Pharmacology and the Future of Man. Vol. 5. Basel, S. Karger, 1972, pp. 250–266.
274. Schapira, M., Despland, E., Scott, C.F., Boxer, L.A., and Colman, R.W.: Purified human kallikrein aggregates human blood neutrophils. J. Clin. Invest. 69:1199, 1982.
275. Kaplan, A.P., Kay, A.B., and Austin, K.F.: A prealbumin activator of prekallikrein III. Appearance of chemotactic activity in human neutrophils by the conversion of human prekallikrein to kallikrein. J. Exp. Med. 135:81, 1972.
276. Gallin, J.I., and Kaplan, A.P.: Mononuclear cell chemotactic activity of kallikrein and plasminogen activator and its inhibition by C1 INH and α_2 macroglobulin. J. Immunol. 113:1928, 1974.
277. Waldmann, R., Rebuck, J.W., Saito, H., Abraham, J.P., Caldwell, J., and Ratnoff, O.D.: Fitzgerald factor: A hitherto unrecognized coagulation factor. Lancet 1:949, 1975.
278. Gigli, I., Koethe, S., and Austen, K.F.: Participation of an early component of complement and Hageman factor in C3 destruction by zymosan. Clin. Immunol. Immunopathol. 4:189, 1975.
279. Donaldson, V.H.: Mechanism of activation of C'1 esterase in hereditary angioneurotic edema in vitro. The role of Hageman factor, a clot-promoting agent. J. Exp. Med. 127:411, 1967.
280. Ghebrehiwet, B., Silverberg, M., and Kaplan, A.P.: Activation of the classical pathway of complement by Hageman factor fragment. J. Exp. Med. 153:665, 1981.
281. Ghebrehiwet, B., Randazzo, B.P., Dunn, J.T., Silverberg, M., and Kaplan, A.P.: Mechanisms of activation of the classical pathway of complement by Hageman factor fragment. J. Clin. Invest. 71:1450, 1983.
282. Ziccardi, R.J.: Spontaneous activation of the first component of human complement (C1) by an intramolecular autocatalytic mechanism. J. Immunol. 128:2500, 1982.
283. Ziccardi, R.J.: A new role for C1-inhibitor in homeostasis: Control of activation of the first component of human complement. J. Immunol. 128:2505, 1982.
284. DiScipis, R.G.: The activation of the alternative pathway C3 convertase by human plasma kallikrein. Immunology 45:587, 1982.
285. Ratnoff, O.D., and Naff, G.B.: The conversion of C1s and C'1 esterase by plasmin and trypsin. J. Exp. Med. 125:337, 1961.
286. Ward, P.A.: A plasmin-split fragment of C3 as a new chemotactic factor. J. Exp. Med. 126:189, 1967.
287. Curd, J.G., Prograis, L.J., Jr., and Cochrane, C.G.: Detection of active kallikrein in induced blister fluids of hereditary angioedema patients. J. Exp. Med. 152:742, 1980.
288. Fields, T., Ghebrehiwet, B., and Kaplan, A.P.: Kinin formation in hereditary angioedema plasma: Evidence against kinin derivation from C2 and in support of "spontaneous" formation of bradykinin. J. Allergy Clin. Immunol. 72:54, 1983.
289. Donaldson, V.H., Glueck, H.I., and Fleming, T.: Rheumatoid arthritis in a patient with Hageman trait. N. Engl. J. Med. 286:529, 1972.
290. Giclas, P.C., Ginsberg, M.H., and Cooper, N.R.: Immunoglobulin G independent activation of the classical complement pathway by monosodium urate crystals. J. Clin. Invest. 63:759, 1979.
291. Fields, T.R., Abramson, S.P., Weissman, G., Kaplan, A.P., and Ghebrehiwet, B.: Activation of the alternative pathway of complement by monosodium urate crystals. Clin. Immunol. Immunopathol 26:249, 1983.
292. Ginsberg, M., Jaques, B., Cochrane, C.G., and Griffin, J.H.: Urate crystal-dependent cleavage of Hageman factor in human plasma and synovial fluid. J. Lab. Clin. Med. 95:497, 1980.
293. Ward, Z., Mainardi, C.L., Vater, C.A., and Harris, E.D., Jr.: Endogenous activation of collagenase by rheumatoid synovial cells: Evidence for the role of plasminogen activator. N. Engl. J. Med. 296:1017, 1977.

Chapter 9

Cellular Components of Inflammation: Granulocytes

Edward J. Goetzl and Ira M. Goldstein

INTRODUCTION

The influx and participation of granulocytes are constant features of acute, subacute, and some forms of chronic inflammation. Granulocytes play a central role in host defense, but if they accumulate in excessive numbers, persist, and are activated in an uncontrolled manner, the result may be deleterious to host tissues. Neutrophils can ingest and destroy bacteria, but they also mediate some types of necrotizing vasculitis. Similarly, eosinophils appear to contain parasitic invasion but may contribute to the endocardial fibrosis associated with sustained hypereosinophilia. The capacity of basophil mediators to increase the local delivery of antibodies and complement by increasing vascular permeability is still hypothetical in most instances, and the basophil continues to be identified principally with allergic reactions and some delayed cutaneous hypersensitivity states. This chapter will delineate the cellular characteristics and unique biochemical capabilities of the different subclasses of granulocytes, which account for both general and specialized functions. Deficiencies in function that may underlie increased susceptibility of some patients to infections will be discussed. The possible involvement of granulocytes in some rheumatic diseases will be explored by considering their roles in tissue damage.

THE ORIGIN, DISTRIBUTION, AND FATE OF GRANULOCYTES

Granulocytes are derived in adults from pluripotential cells of the bone marrow, which are termed stem cells. Stem cells have the potential for both self-renewal and differentiation into the progenitors of granulocytes. The initial phases of differentiation in the bone marrow commit the cells to development into one type of granulocyte and lead to specific sensitivity to principles that regulate the production and terminal differentiation of that line of granulocytes. The results of studies of the capacity of bone marrow cells to form hematopoietic colonies in the spleens of lethally irradiated mice[1] and of human bone marrow cells to form clonal colonies of hematopoietic cells in agarose and other gelled media in vitro[2] have elucidated some characteristics of the progenitor cells of colony-forming units (CFUs). For example, each type of granulocyte is derived from a different subclass of progenitor cells, which are stimulated to proliferate and differentiate by structurally and functionally distinct glycoprotein colony-stimulating activities from several cellular sources.[1,3]

The terminal stages of proliferation and development of granulocytes in the bone marrow consist of a series of cell divisions that lead to the appearance of class-specific nuclear morphology and unique cytoplasmic granules, which distinguish the mature nonmitotic members of each subclass of granulocytes. All granulocyte precursors during the late blast and promyelocyte stages synthesize enzymes, other proteins, and smaller factors that are stored in the cytoplasmic secretory granules. Other cellular properties critical to the effector functions of granulocytes also develop during the later stages of maturation. Receptors appear for the Fc portion of immunoglobulin molecules, for complement components, and for lectins, and Ia antigens disappear during neutrophil differentiation.[4,5] Neutrophils and eosinophils acquire or increase their ability to phagocytize and respond to specific chemotactic factors.[6]

The apparent morphologic and constitutive differences among subclasses of granulocytes are accompanied by a striking divergence of cellular kinetics, tissue distribution, and function. While the knowledge of human granulocytes is incomplete, several studies have revealed a marrow storage compartment, intravascular circulating and marginated pools, and tissue representation for both neutrophils and eosinophils. Mature neutrophils and eosinophils remain in the marrow compartment for approximately 5 and 3 to 4 days, respectively, and circulate for about 10 and 12 hours, respectively, before entering the tissues.[7,8] A high percentage of the mature eosinophils and a smaller number of the basophils are located normally in tissues, while neutrophils are found in tissues only in relation to foci of irritation or infection. The tissue eosinophils are distributed in lymphoid organs and below the epithelial surfaces of the skin, lungs, intestines, and genitourinary tract.[8,9] Despite the differences in normal tissue representation, any significant influx of neutrophils, eosinophils, or basophils requires recruitment from the circulating pools. While some data suggest that eosinophils and basophils persist in tissue for much longer periods than neutrophils, the mechanism of the elimination of granulocytes is still unknown. However, recirculation of tissue granulocytes appears to be an uncommon and quantitatively insignificant phenomenon.

CELLULAR FUNCTIONS OF GRANULOCYTES

Regulation of Granulocyte Migration. Granulocyte chemotaxis is initiated by the presentation to the cells of a concentration gradient of a specific stimulus and leads to the accumulation of granulocytes at tissue sites of inflammation.[10] Chemokinesis is the enhancement of random migration of granulocytes that is evoked as a function of stimulus concentration irrespective of a gradient. Both the development of in vitro methods for the quantitation of granulocyte migration and the availability of purified and synthetic principals have fostered intensive investigations of the stimulation of migration, have permitted the distinction between chemokinesis and chemotaxis, and have led to the understanding of several types of inhibitory mechanisms. In those assays that are modifications of Boyden's technique,[11] one or more micropore filters are employed to separate the granulocytes from the stimulus. Following routine fixation, a variety of granulocyte stains can be used, and the response is quantified by microscopically enumerating the cells within the filter. For the techniques that utilize radiolabeled granulocytes and a pair of micropore filters, quantification is based on counting the cell-associated radioactivity in the filter farther from the source of granulocytes. With the former approach, the use of selective stains precludes the necessity for prior purification of the target granulocytes,[12] and the cells can be counted at multiple levels within the micropore filter to establish the distance traveled by the "leading front."[13] The modifications using cells prelabeled with ^{51}Cr or other isotopes are highly objective and especially well suited to clinical studies of cellular migration defects as the granulocytes must migrate through the first filter to be counted in the second filter, a distance greater than that of conventional assays.[14] However, the radioassays require essentially total purification of cells in order to allow the radioactivity to be equated with a given population of granulocytes.[15] The newly developed agarose well assays[16] are also dependent on the use of purified cells, unless the agarose is removed to permit the staining and identification of the granulocytes that have migrated out of the wells. The need for only a relatively small number of granulocytes per assay and the ease of macroscopic assessment of maximal migratory responses are the primary advantages of the agarose well techniques.

The initial event in the stimulation of granulocyte chemotaxis involves the activation of the pathways for generation of specific chemotactic factors. Alterations of basement membrane or collagen structure activate Hageman factor,[17] which subsequently converts prekallikrein to kallikrein, a kinin-generating enzyme with chemotactic activity.[18] Activation by immune complexes of the classic complement pathway and by microbial polysaccharides of the alternative complement pathway elaborates chemotactic fragments, most notably the minor fragment of the fifth component, C5a,[19] or complexes such as C$\overline{567}$,[20] while the alternative pathway alone contributes the chemotactic factor C3bBb.[21] IgE-dependent activation of human mast cell–rich tissues releases both the eosinophil chemotactic factor of anaphylaxis (ECF-A),[22,23] which is composed in part of two acidic tetrapeptides,[24] and neutrophil chemotactic activities, consisting of high molecular weight proteins. The IgE-directed stimulation of mast cells also results in the elaboration of lipid chemotactic and chemokinetic factors, the most potent of which are lipoxygenase products of arachidonic acid.[25-27] Chemotactic factors for granulocytes and other leukocytes can be classified according to their structural properties (Table 9–1). While many of the protein complexes or fragments with chemotactic

activity are derived from the complement pathways, large peptides and proteins liberated as a result of the proteolysis of fibrin and collagen also attract granulocytes in vitro.[28,29] The expression of chemotactic activity by the enzymatic factors is dependent on the integrity of their active site, as exemplified by the chemotactic inactivity of prekallikrein, which does not possess the capacity to generate bradykinin, and by the comparable degree of inhibition of both the chemotactic and kinin-generating activities of kallikrein by increasing concentrations of diisopropylfluorophosphate.[30] The peptides of ECF-A and other low molecular weight peptides and amines are cellular products released upon specific activation of the host cells or, in the case of bacterial factors,[31] during phases of rapid bacterial growth. Numerous chemotactic lymphokines have been described, which are proteins that vary in heat stability, size, and charge.[32] The lipid chemotactic factors that have been defined are either components of bacterial cell walls[33]

Table 9–1. The Structural Diversity and Specificity of Natural Factors Chemotactic for Human Granulocytes and Monocytes

Class	Factor	Source	Molecular Weight	Structural Characteristics	Cellular Preference	Other Functions
I. Protein fragments or complexes	C5a	Complement pathways C5 proteolysis	17,000	Basic protein	N,E,B,M	Chemotactic deactivation Mast cell degranulation Smooth muscle contraction
	C$\overline{567}$	Complement pathways	435,000	Protein complex	N,E	Lysis of bacteria
	Fibrin fragments	Fibrinolysis	30,000-50,000	Proteins	N,E,M	Chemotactic deactivation
	Collagen fragments	Collagenolysis	300-1000	Peptides	M,N	Fibroblast attraction
II. Enzymes	Plasma kallikrein	Kinin-generating sequence	108,000	γ-globulin	N	Bradykinin generation Chemotactic deactivation
	C3bBb	Alternative complement pathway	234,000	Protein complex	N	Chemotactic deactivation
III. Cellular peptides or amines	ECF-A peptides	Mast cells	360-390	Acidic peptides	E > N	Chemotactic deactivation Increase in eosinophil C3b receptors
	Histamine	Mast cells	111	Amine	E > N	Chemotactic facilitation and deactivation Increase in eosinophil C3b receptors
	Bacterial soluble factors	Bacteria	300-1000	Peptides	N	—
IV. Lymphokines		Lymphocytes	20,000-60,000	Protein	E,N	—
		Lymphocytes	12,500	Protein	M	—
		Lymphocytes	12,500	?	B	—
V. Lipids	LTB$_4$	Arachidonate lipoxygenase	340		E > N	Chemokinetic stimulation Chemotactic deactivation
	HHT	Arachidonate cyclooxygenase	280	—	E > N	Chemokinetic stimulation Chemotactic deactivation
	Bacterial lipids	Bacteria	—	Lipoproteins and lipids	N,M	—

N = Neutrophil. E = Eosinophil. B = Basophil. M = Mononuclear leukocyte. LT = Leukotriene. HHT = 12-L-OH-5,8,10-heptadecatrienoic acid.

or lipoxygenase metabolites of arachidonic acid or related fatty acids.[34-36] The latter pathways are of special
significance as the generation of the potent chemotactic
fatty acid designated 5(S),12(R)-dihydroxy-eicosa-6,14
cis-8,10 trans-tetraenoic acid (leukotriene B_4)[26,27] by 5-
lipoxygenases is not inhibited by the currently available
nonsteroidal anti-inflammatory drugs.

The second aspect of the modulation of chemotaxis
is the potency and leukocyte specificity of each stimulus.
While for many chemotactic factors the potential range
of responder leukocytes has not been explored, the cellular preference of some principals has been delineated.
C5a attracts eosinophils, neutrophils, basophils, and
monocytes with comparable activity.[37,38] In contrast,
kallikrein preferentially attracts neutrophils and monocytes,[30] leukotriene B_4 is more active for neutrophils
and eosinophils than monocytes, and ECF-A is most
chemotactic for eosinophils, although it has some activity for neutrophils.[24,39] This aspect of regulation of chemotaxis and some of the other effects of chemotactic factors on granulocytes are functions of the properties of
specific subsets of receptors, each of which is committed
to one chemotactic factor.[10] A third regulatory dimension encompasses inactivators and inhibitors of chemotactic factors (Fig. 9-1). The anaphylatoxin inactivator
acts to diminish the chemotactic potential of C5a[19,40]
and leads to a dependence on a serum protein, termed
the C5a des Arg "cochemotaxin," for the expression of
maximal chemotactic activity.[19] The chemotactic factor
inactivator, which is composed of at least two aminopeptidases, irreversibly destroys a variety of chemotactic
factors.[41,42] Lysosomal proteases of granulocytes themselves inactivate C5a and possibly other protein chemotactic factors.[43] The inhibitor of the activated first component of complement, C̄1INH, and α_2-macroglobulin
reversibly suppress the chemotactic activity of kallikrein.[30] The fourth level of regulation is granulocyte-
directed and includes noncytotoxic factors which specifically influence the responsiveness of the stimulated
population of cells irrespective of the nature of the chemotactic factor (Fig. 9-1). The chemotactic principals
themselves reduce responsiveness through a process
which has been designated chemotactic deactivation.[31,44,45] Chemotactic deactivation by any factor has a
leukocyte specificity comparable to its chemotactic specificity,[39] but the biochemical mechanisms have not been
elucidated. Concentrations of several chemotactic stimuli that are equal to or greater than maximally chemotactic levels induce a state of relative chemotactic unresponsiveness, which is not restricted to the initial
stimulus and is mediated by an increase in granulocyte
adherence.

A wide range of nonchemotactic agents specifically
influence the chemotactic responses of granulocytes with
or without affecting other functions (Fig. 9-1). At noncytotoxic concentrations, colchicine and cytochalasin B
inhibit both chemotaxis and phagocytosis by actions on
the microtubules and actin filaments, respectively.[46-49] In
contrast, the release of lysosomal enzymes from granulocytes that are engaged in phagocytosis or are stim-

Figure 9–1. Regulation of granulocyte chemotaxis. N = Neutrophil.
E = Eosinophil. Lym = Lymphocyte. Plt = Platelet. NIF = Neutrophil immobilizing factor. LIF = Leukocyte inhibition factor. ⤳
= Inhibitory effect. CF = Chemotactic factor. CFI = Chemotactic
factor inactivator. AC = Adenylate cyclase. GC = Guanylate cyclase.
MT = Microtubule. MF = Actin microfilament.▨▨▨ = Chemotaxis. ⟶ = Release or generation. ---⟶ = Enhancing effect.

ulated by the introduction of some chemotactic factors
is inhibited by colchicine and markedly enhanced by
cytochalasin B.[48-50] Amphotericin inhibits granulocyte
chemotaxis, presumably by disorganizing the structure
of plasma membrane sterols, but only inhibits phagocytosis at much higher concentrations than would be
attainable in vivo during antifungal therapy.[51] Exogenous 3',5'-adenosine monophosphate (cyclic AMP) and
agonists that elevate intracellular levels of cyclic AMP
in granulocytes, including β-adrenergic agents, prostaglandins of the E series, and histamine acting through
an H_2 receptor, inhibit chemotaxis with far less effect
on phagocytosis.[52,53] Although ascorbic acid, serotonin,
and prostaglandin $F_{2\alpha}$ ($PGF_{2\alpha}$) enhance both the random
and chemotactic migration of granulocytes at concentrations known to raise the intracellular levels of 3',5'-
guanosine monophosphate (cyclic GMP) in mononuclear leukocytes, comparable elevations of cyclic GMP
levels have not been demonstrable in granulocytes.[53,55]
Of the few principles which have been recognized to
directly facilitate migration in vitro, ascorbic acid is of
special interest. Levels of ascorbic acid ranging from 10-
to 50-fold the normal plasma concentration induce a
several-fold enhancement of random and directed migration of granulocytes and mononuclear leukocytes and
a concomitant stimulation of hexose monophosphate
shunt activity, without affecting phagocytosis.[54] Ascorbic acid has reversed the chemotactic and other functional deficiencies in granulocytes of patients with the
Chédiak-Higashi syndrome[56] and the Quie-Hill syndrome[57] both in vitro and in vivo. Several naturally
occurring peptides and proteins modulate granulocyte
migration with both cellular and functional specificity,
but the mechanisms of their effects are unknown. The
neutrophil immobilizing factor (NIF) is composed of
two basic lysosomal peptides of approximately 4000 daltons that are derived from human neutrophils or mononuclear leukocytes.[58] NIF lacks chemotactic activity, but
suppresses the random and directed migration of neu-

trophils and eosinophils without influencing their metabolism, phagocytic capacity, or adherence to surfaces, and is without any action on monocytes.[59,60] Plasma proteins with other recognized humoral functions, such as α_1-antitrypsin and α_2-macroglobulin, can directly influence neutrophil random migration and chemotactic responsiveness, but do not alter phagocytosis.[61]

The interest in granulocyte migration has been heightened by observations of the modulatory effects of numerous other relevant cell types and by the evolving evidence for activities of chemotactic factors which bear on granulocyte functions other than migration. Proteases released upon stimulation of human platelets degrade C5 in a manner which releases chemotactic fragments.[62] Platelet aggregation, which activates the arachidonate oxygenases and provides a supply of substrate,[63] leads not only to the release of the chemotactic principal, 12-L-hydroxy-eicosatetraenoic acid (12-HETE), but also to the elaboration of $PGF_{2\alpha}$ and PGE_2 which are positively and negatively chemokinetic for granulocytes, respectively.[10] The interaction of human lymphocytes with mitogens or specific antigen generates and releases a 23,000 molecular weight esterase, termed the leukocyte inhibitory factor (LIF), which suppresses neutrophil but not mononuclear leukocyte migration from capillary tubes[64,65] and inhibits the random and chemotactic migration of neutrophils in modified Boyden micropore filter chambers.[66] Incubation of neutrophils with LIF releases additional inhibitory activity (Fig. 9–1), which resembles NIF by virtue of its molecular weight, susceptibility to inactivation by trypsin, and noncytotoxic preferential inhibition of granulocyte migration, as compared to that of mononuclear leukocytes.[66] Thus a spectrum of lymphokines may stimulate leukocyte chemotaxis, directly inhibit leukocyte responses to chemotactic factors, and induce the release of chemotactic inhibitors from the target granulocytes. Chemotactic factors not only are capable of evoking chemotactic and chemokinetic responses and of inducing chemotactic deactivation, but also stimulate neutrophil adherence, aggregation[67] and release of lysosomal enzymes,[68] and modulate the expression of plasma membrane C3b receptors on human eosinophils.[69] Treatment of eosinophils with chemotactic concentrations of the tetrapeptides of ECF-A led to a significant increase in the number of C3b receptors per eosinophil, an effect that was also observed upon the addition of histamine but was not reproduced by other mediators.[69]

CHARACTERISTICS OF GRANULOCYTE INTERACTIONS WITH PARTICULATE STIMULI

Recognition—Neutrophil Receptors for Immunoglobulins and Complement

Wright and Douglas,[70] in 1903, observed that fresh serum greatly enhanced ingestion and killing of bacteria by peripheral blood neutrophils. Numerous investigators

subsequently established that there are two major constituents of serum (i.e., opsonins) that act upon certain bacteria, fungi, and other particles to increase their palatability. One is heat stable (56° C for 30 minutes) and present primarily in immune serum. The other is heat labile and present in fresh normal serum. The heat-stable constituent is recognized now as immunoglobulin (i.e., antibody) of the IgG class. The Fc regions of IgG immunoglobulins that have been altered as a consequence of either aggregation or binding to antigen attach to specific receptors ("Fc receptors" or "IgG recptors") on the plasma membrane of neutrophils (Table 9–2). Thus, neutrophils "recognize" particles sensitized with IgG antibody.

Heat-labile opsonic activity is attributable primarily to a fragment of the third component of complement. When complement is activated by either the classical or the alternative pathways, C3 is cleaved into two fragments, C3a and C3b. The larger of these fragments, C3b, is capable of becoming attached to the surfaces of cells and other particles (including bacteria and fungi).[71] C3b renders the particles to which it is attached recognizable by neutrophils and mediates firm particle–neutrophil adherence through interactions with "C3b receptors" (Table 9–2). The nature of the neutrophil receptors for IgG and C3b, as well as the consequences of receptor-ligand binding, are discussed in sections that follow.

IgG Receptors. After it was established that antigen-antibody complexes and antibody-coated particles are recognized by mononuclear phagocytes,[72] evidence appeared of receptors for immunoglobulins on the surface of neutrophils.[73,75] Henson,[73] for example, demonstrated that sheep erythrocytes sensitized with IgG antibody adhere to human, rabbit, and guinea pig neutrophils. Minimal adherence was noted when IgM antibody was used. Messner and Jelinek[76] extended these findings and provided evidence that receptors for the Fc regions of human IgG antibodies exist on both human neutrophils

Table 9–2. Properties of Human Neutrophil Immunoglobulin and Complement Receptors

Immunoglobulin Receptor	Complement Receptor
Recognizes Fc regions of IgG (and some IgA immunoglobulins)	Recognizes C3b fragment of native C3
Present on 75 to 90 percent of neutrophils in peripheral blood	Present on greater than 90 percent of neutrophils in peripheral blood
Not affected by trypsin	Trypsin-sensitive
Receptor-mediated functions unaffected by reduced temperatures, EDTA, H_2O_2, and hydrocortisone	Receptor-mediated functions inhibited by reduced temperatures, EDTA, H_2O_2, hydrocortisone, and trypsin blue
Mobile in plane of neutrophil surface membrane	Distributed uniformly in clusters on the neutrophil surface
"Macromolecule(s)" with a molecular weight of 52,000 to 64,000	Glycoprotein with a molecular weight of 205,000

and monocytes. They demonstrated that adherence of sensitized human erythrocytes to monolayers of neutrophils could be inhibited by native IgG, myeloma globulins of the IgG_1 and IgG_3 subclasses, and isolated Fc (but not Fab) fragments. Subsequent studies have established that 75 to 90 percent of human peripheral blood neutrophils bear receptors on their surface for IgG-coated particles.[77,78] Attachment of IgG-coated particles to human neutrophils does not require divalent cations,[73,74] nor is it influenced by reduced temperatures (e.g., 4° C) or prior treatment of cells with trypsin.[77]

The specificity of the immunoglobulin receptor on neutrophils has been confirmed in several studies. Sajnani and colleagues,[79,80] for example, demonstrated by fluorescence microscopy that human neutrophils bind isolated Fc fragments as well as intact IgG. Attempts to demonstrate binding of IgM to human neutrophils generally have not been successful.[73,74,76] Similarly, neutrophils appear to lack receptors for IgE and IgD.[73,81] Evidence has been provided recently that some phagocytic cells possess different receptors for monomeric immunoglobulins and for aggregated (or complexed) immunoglobulins.[82] This could explain the finding that whereas neutrophils bind unaggregated immunoglobulins only of the IgG_1 and IgG_3 subclasses[81] aggregated IgG of all four subclasses can bind to and stimulate these cells.[83]

As indicated above, binding to neutrophils of antigen-antibody complexes, immunoglobulin-coated particles, and aggregated immunoglobulins depends upon the integrity of the Fc regions of the immunoglobulin molecules. Binding to neutrophils of either aggregated or antigen-complexed immunoglobulins exceeds that of the corresponding monomeric immunoglobulin molecules. At least two hypotheses have been formulated to account for these observations. One hypothesis assumes that although monomeric immunoglobulins have an exposed binding site on their Fc regions available for attachment to neutrophils, univalent binding is unstable. More stable, and therefore detectable, binding results only from the formation of complexes with mulitple sites. Thus, stable binding of polyvalent antigen-antibody complexes or of immunoglobulin aggregates would result from cooperative binding to Fc receptors of several molecules (which exponentially increases binding of the whole complex).[75] The alternative hypothesis suggests that either aggregation of immunoglobulins or interactions between antibodies and antigens produce changes in the conformation of immunoglobulin molecules.[84] Such conformational changes would expose sites capable of interacting with the neutrophil surface. Thus, the tertiary structure of intact immunoglobulins may influence binding to neutrophils.

Fc receptors on human neutrophils have been visualized indirectly by fluorescence microscopy as well as by electron microscopy and shown to be mobile in the plane of the neutrophil plasma membrane.[79,80,85] Interestingly, a very close correlation was observed between Fc receptor redistribution and immune complex–induced neutrophil responses, suggesting a relationship between activation of neutrophils and surface receptor mobility.

Macromolecules with Fc receptor activity have been isolated from leukocytes of several species.[86,87] Kulczycki and colleagues,[87] for example, subjected solubilized, radiolabeled surface proteins of human neutrophils and mononuclear cells to repetitive affinity chromatography and succeeded in purifying material capable of binding specifically to Fc fragments of IgG. Neither Fab fragments nor IgM bound to the isolated receptorlike macromolecules. Analysis of the purified Fc-binding material by sodium dodecylsulfate polyacrylamide gel electrophoresis revealed a single, broad, 52,000 to 64,000 molecular weight band.

Complement Receptors. Although it was appreciated for many years that complement components on the surfaces of antibody-sensitized particles facilitated phagocytosis by neutrophils,[88,89] it was not until 1968 that evidence was reported of a complement receptor on the neutrophil surface membrane. Lay and Nussenzweig[74] observed that sheep erythrocytes sensitized with rabbit IgM antibodies did not adhere to isolate mouse peripheral blood neutrophils unless they were first incubated with fresh mouse serum for 30 minutes at 37° C. Adherence to neutrophils of sheep erythrocytes sensitized with IgG antibody also was enhanced after incubation with fresh mouse serum. Subsequent studies in the mouse, rabbit, guinea pig, and man have established that neutrophils possess receptors on their surface for fragments of the third component of complement (primarily C3b).[73,77,90–94] In man, such receptors can be demonstrated on greater than 90 percent of neutrophils in peripheral blood.[94] Binding to human neutrophils of particles coated with fragments of C3 is inhibited by treating cells with trypsin[73,74] and by reduced temperatures (4° C).[74,77] Binding can also be modulated by divalent cations (particularly Mg^{2+}).[95,96]

The function of C3 receptors on human neutrophils can be influenced by other agents. Boxer and colleagues,[77] for example, were able to inhibit attachment of complement-coated particles to human neutrophils by exposing these cells to the sulfhydryl-blocking agent N-ethylmaleimide as well as to hydrogen peroxide and hydrocortisone. Results similar to these were obtained by Guckian and associates[97] when human neutrophils were exposed to the vital dye trypan blue. The precise mechanisms whereby these compounds interfere with the function of neutrophil complement receptors are unknown.

Structurally specific receptors for C3b have been identified on the surface of neutrophils and have been isolated from these cells.[98–100] The human neutrophil C3b receptor is a glycoprotein with an apparent molecular weight of 205,000.[98] It appears to be similar to, or identical with, C3b receptors on human erythrocytes, B lymphocytes, and monocytes.[98] When examined at 0° C by indirect immunofluorescence, C3b receptors on human neutrophils appeared to be distributed in a random fashion in small clusters on the plasma membrane.[99] Interestingly, rapid receptor-mediated endocytosis of soluble ligands was observed when neutrophils were warmed to 37° C. It is not known yet whether aggregation of C3b receptors is a prerequisite for C3-dependent cytoadherence. More work is required to elucidate the mechanisms whereby receptor–ligand interactions promote specific neutrophil functions, such as adherence to particles or surfaces, phagocytosis, alterations in oxidative metabolism, and degranulation (see below).

It should not be concluded from the foregoing discussion that neutrophils only recognize particles or surfaces coated with fragments of C3 and/or IgG. It also should not be concluded that recognition is mediated only by structurally specific surface membrane receptors. Indeed, the term "receptor" need only imply an ability of neutrophils to recognize a given molecule and to be activated by it. Whereas molecular entities within (or on) the neutrophil surface membrane are presumed to mediate these functions, the presence of some of these only can be inferred. Receptors for some ligands have neither been identified nor isolated. Consequently, it is best to consider neutrophil surface membrane receptors as "recognition units," which may or may not be represented by specific single molecules or even by complex intramembranous structures. Recognition units, by necessity, would be linked to "effector units" (of similarly vague composition), which trigger or initiate specific cellular functions.

Phagocytosis

When contact is established between a neutrophil and a suitable particle, the particle is ingested by the cell, a process termed phagocytosis. Direct observations of phagocytosis by light microscopy and by electron microscopy have revealed that attachment of a neutrophil to a suitable small particle results in the formation, at the site of attachment, of pseudopodia, which surround the particle and ultimately fuse at its distal pole.[101] The process of particle engulfment by neutrophils requires energy (supplied by anaerobic glycolysis) as well as complex interactions between cytoplasmic contractile proteins (i.e., actin and myosin) and the plasma membrane.[102,103]

Whereas neutrophils appear capable of ingesting seemingly "inert" particles (e.g., polystyrene latex beads), particularly under conditions in which particle-cell contact is maximized, opsonins such as C3b or IgG clearly increase the rate and extent of particle uptake. Stossel,[95] for example, found that particle-bound C3 fragments markedly accelerated maximal rates of ingestion by human neutrophils of albumin-coated paraffin oil particles. Interestingly, whereas opsonically active C3 and IgG increased the V_{max} of the ingestion rate, only IgG altered the apparent K_m of the reaction (markedly decreasing it). It was concluded that while both C3 and IgG increase the rate of ingestion, only IgG increases the affinity of the particle for some "catalytic site" that activates internalization. In a subsequent study, Stossel and colleagues[104] demonstrated that human peripheral blood neutrophils ingest lipopolysaccharide-coated par-

Table 9–3. Roles Played by Neutrophil Immunoglobulin and Complement Receptors in Adherence and Phagocytosis*

	Adherence	Phagocytosis
EA (IgM)	−	−
EA (IgG)	+	+
EA (IgM-C3b)	+++	−
EA (IgG-C3b)	+++	+++

*Adapted from Ehlenberger and Nussenzweig.[24] Sheep erythrocytes (E) sensitized with IgM or IgG antibodies (A) with or without complement (C3b).

affin oil droplets only if fragments of C3 are attached to the surfaces of these particles. Binding of radiolabeled C3 to these particles correlated precisely with their ingestibility.

More recent work has shed additional light on the roles played by C3 fragments and IgG in promoting particle recognition and phagocytosis by neutrophils. By using erythrocytes coated with IgG and/or C3b, several investigators have demonstrated that the neutrophil C3b receptor is involved primarily in recognition and attachment and only inefficiently promotes ingestion of bound or adherent particles. In contrast, particle binding to the neutrophil IgG receptor, while less efficient, appears necessary for the induction of optimal phagocytosis.[90,92,93] Thus, C3b and IgG have separate but synergistic roles in phagocytosis (Table 9–3). Depending upon the experimental conditions, the presence of particle-bound C3b is able to reduce by 100-fold the amount of IgG required to promote engulfment of particles. Under certain conditions, C3b receptors may serve to overcome electrostatic repulsion and permit contact between the neutrophil surface and moieties on particles that promote engulfment. The role of C3b in opsonization is mainly one of establishing contact between particles and phagocytes.

Neutrophils are capable of ingesting certain particles in the complete absence of complement or immunoglobulins. It is likely that such particles have chemical moieties on their surfaces that not only permit attachment by neutrophils but also behave as "surrogate immunoglobulins" and promote ingestion. Indeed, it has been demonstrated that particles requiring only C3b on their surfaces for optimal ingestion by neutrophils are ingestible in the native state if particle–cell contact is enhanced.[95]

How does IgG promote ingestion of particles? Although it has been suggested that phagocytosis occurs as a consequence of perturbation of the neutrophil cell membrane,[105] there is no direct evidence relating the ability of "altered" IgG to perturb artificial lipid bilayers with the ability to promote ingestion of particles.[106] Indeed, there is evidence to suggest that membrane perturbation may not be sufficient to induce phagocytosis. Stendahl and associates,[107] for example, demonstrated that whereas opsonized *Salmonella typhimurium* 395 MS and nonopsonized *S. typhimurium* 395 MR 10 are ingested by neutrophils to the same extent, only the opsonized bacteria perturb liposomal membranes. An alternative explanation for the role that IgG plays in promoting phagocytosis has been proposed by Griffin and co-workers.[108] These investigators suggested that phagocytosis results only from a sequential interaction of ligands and receptors around the surface of a particle (the "zipper" theory). They would suggest that the distribution of C3b moieties on the surface of a sensitized erythrocyte and C3b receptors on the surface of a neutrophil would not permit sufficient interactions of ligands and receptors around the entire particle. Cooperation with Fc receptors, however, would permit optimal ligand–receptor interactions and engulfment of the particle. A great deal more must be learned of the mechanisms whereby attachment of particles to the neutrophil surface membrane ultimately leads to phagocytosis.

Lysosomes and Neutrophil Degranulation

Lysosomes are a class of subcellular organelles that contain various hydrolytic enzymes, predominantly with acid pH optima, bound in latent form within a relatively impermeable membrane.[109] Lysosomal granules of phagocytic cells constitute their vacuolar system, or internal digestive system. Human neutrophils contain two major types of lysosomal granules, distinguishable by their morphology, staining characteristics, and enzyme content. Azurophil granules, which contain peroxidase and other lysosomal hydrolases, appear in the cytoplasm of neutrophils during the promyelocyte stage of development and arise from the concave surface of the Golgi complex. Specific granules, on the other hand, are formed from the convex face of the Golgi complex during the myelocyte stage of development and contain predominantly lysozyme and the iron-binding protein lactoferrin.[110,111] Alkaline phosphatase is not a granule associated enzyme in human neutrophils but is associated only with the plasma membrane.[112,113] In rabbit neutrophils, however, 90 percent of total cellular alkaline phosphatase sediments with specific granules.[114]

Zonal sedimentation, velocity sedimentation, and isopycnic equilibration techniques have enabled investigators to localize more precisely most of the granule-associated enzymes of human neutrophils. It has been established, for example, that azurophil granules contain

all of the myeloperoxidase and β-glucuronidase found in these cells.[112,113] Azurophil granules also contain all of the elastase and cathepsin G,[115] the bulk of other acid glycosidases, and approximately 50 percent of the lysozyme in human neutrophils.[112,113] Specific granules, on the other hand, contain all of the lactoferrin in these cells and the remainder of their lysozyme.[112,116] Specific granules also contain latent collagenase[117] and vitamin B12-binding protein.[118] Less well-defined human neutrophil granules contain N-acetyl-β-glucosaminidase and a latent, neutral gelatinase.[113] Human neutrophils, therefore, contain granule-associated enzymes capable of hydrolysing a wide variety of both natural and synthetic substrates, including simple and complex polysaccharides, oligopeptides, and phosphate esters (Table 9–4). The roles played by these enzymes in maintaining normal host defenses and in mediating inflammation have been the subject of several reviews[119–123] and are discussed elsewhere in this volume (Chapter 12).

Degranulation. As indicated in previous sections, phagocytosis by neutrophils entails recognition of the particle to be ingested, binding of the particle to the cell surface, and finally, engulfment of the particle within a vacuole and closure of the plasma membrane. Shortly after, or coincident with these events, lysosomal granules fuse with those portions of the plasma membrane that constitute the phagocytic vacuole (or "phagosome").[124] Membrane fusion leads to the discharge of lysosomal enzymes and other granule constituents into the newly formed, or forming, phagosome (the process of "degranulation")[125] (Fig. 9–2). The resultant structure has been termed a phagolysosome.[124] Phagolysosomes, therefore, contain not only acid hydrolases but also substrate. In phagocytic cells, formation of phagolysosomes is crucial for normal host defenses.[126] It is within phagolysosomes, for example, that killing and digestion of microorganisms take place.[125] Stossel and colleagues[127] isolated phagolysosomes from human and guinea pig neutrophils and confirmed biochemically that degranulation occurs coincidentally with ingestion. Based on the kinetics of particle uptake and translocation of granule constituents into phagolysosomes, these investigators concluded that the "triggering" mechanisms for both phagocytosis and degranulation may be similar or identical.

Degranulation of neutrophils is not a uniform process. Azurophil and specific granules discharge their contents at different rates during phagocytosis.[127–129] Bainton[129]

Table 9–4. Some Lysosomal Constituents of Human Neutrophils

Azurophil Granules	Specific Granules	Others
Myeloperoxidase	Lactoferrin	Latent gelatinase
β-Glucuronidase (other glycosidases)	Vitamin B12-binding protein	N-acetyl-β-glucosaminidase
Lysozyme (50 percent)	Lysozyme (50 percent)	
Phospholipase	Latent collagenase	
Ribonuclease		
Elastase		
Cathepsin G		

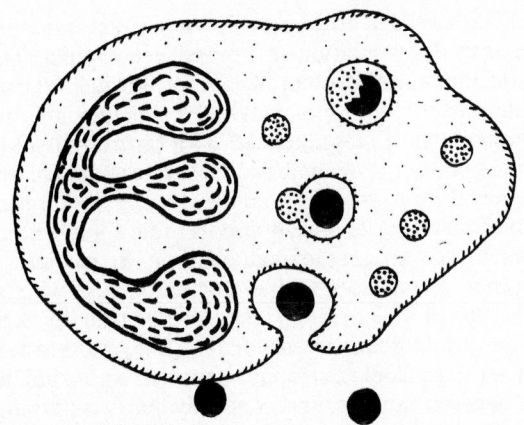

Figure 9–2. Neutrophil degranulation. Following phagocytosis, membrane fusion leads to the discharge of lysosomal constituents into newly formed, or forming, phagosomes.

found that specific granules of rabbit neutrophils fuse with phagosomes and discharge their contents more rapidly than azurophil granules. In addition, although azurophil and specific granules discharge their contents during phagocytosis, specific granule constituents appear to be more accessible for extracellular release.[128,130,131] Finally, based on the responses of neutrophils to mechanical and other nonphagocytic stimuli, it has been suggested that specific granules actually may be secretory granules and that their contents function extracellularly rather than intracellularly.[130,132,133] The precise mechanism whereby specific granules fuse so readily with portions of the neutrophil plasma membrane has not been elucidated. It has been found, however, that azurophil and specific granules differ with respect to their content of cholesterol, phospholipid, and protein.[134]

Extracellular Release of Neutrophil Lysosomal Constituents. Whereas the contents of neutrophil granules most often are discharged intracellularly into phagosomes, under certain circumstances they can be released extracellularly. One mechanism whereby granule con-

stituents are extruded from neutrophils is simply "cell death" (Fig. 9–3A). When neutrophils are exposed to a variety of toxins, injury to the plasma membrane is an early consequence, and ultimately, all intracellular materials are released from the injured cells, including those ordinarily sequestered within azurophil and specific granules. Biologic detergents, for example, act in this manner to cause primary lysis of cell membranes and, only subsequently, disruption of cytoplasmic granules.[135] Under these circumstances, cytoplasmic enzymes and other cellular constituents, in addition to lysosomal hydrolases, are released into the medium surrounding dead and dying neutrophils.

Another mechanism by which lysosomal constituents can be released from neutrophils conforms to the "suicide sac" hypothesis of de Duve and Wattiaux.[136] Under some circumstances, materials gain access to the interior of the cells' vacuolar system wherein they cause membranes of lysosomes to rupture (Fig. 9–3B). Such damage of lysosomal membranes subsequently leads to release from neutrophils of cytoplasmic enzymes and other intracellular constituents as the cells die as a consequence of "perforation from within" of their vacuolar system.[137,138] Crystalline substances, such as monosodium urate and silica, act on neutrophils (and other phagocytic cells) in this fashion.[137-141]

Yet another mechanism of enzyme release from neutrophils involves the discharge of lysosomal constituents into the medium surrounding intact cells engaging in phagocytosis. Such release is not accompanied by leakage of cytoplasmic enzymes and appears to be due to the extrusion of lysosomal granule contents from incompletely sealed phagosomes, open at their external borders to the extracellular space but already joined at their internal borders by lysosomal granules actively discharging their contents (Fig. 9–3C). The cell engaging in phagocytosis remains viable, but its released lysosomal enzymes are free to act extracellularly. This probably is a common mechanism whereby neutrophils provoke tissue injury in a variety of disease states.[120,123]

Figure 9–3. Extracellular release of neutrophil lysosomal constituents. A, Cell death. B, Perforation from within. C, Regurgitation during feeding. D, Reverse endocytosis.

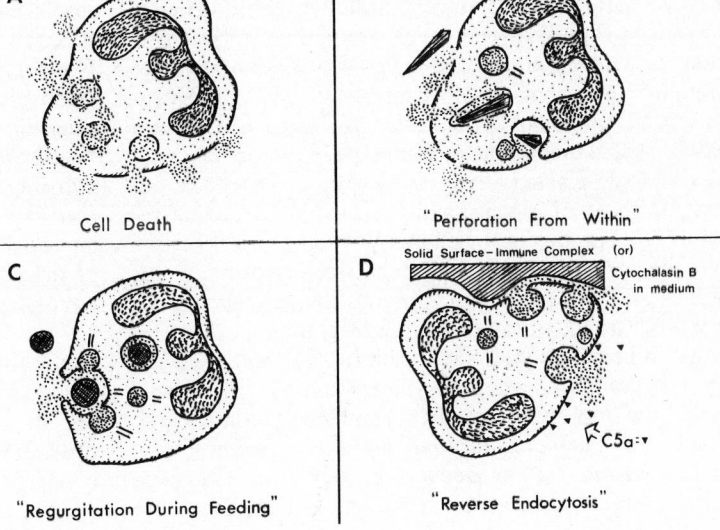

Biochemical and morphologic evidence for this mechanism, which has been termed "regurgitation during feeding,"[137,138] has been presented for several experimental systems involving particle ingestion by neutrophils.[83,137,138,142–148]

Phagocytosis per se is not an absolute prerequisite for degranulation by neutrophils. In fact, there is a substantial amount of evidence indicating that degranulation of neutrophils can be provoked not only by appropriate ligand–surface membrane receptor interactions but also by "nonspecific" membrane perturbation. For example, when neutrophils encounter either immune complexes or aggregated immunoglobulins deposited on solid surfaces (e.g., micropore filters, collagen membranes), the cells adhere to these surfaces and selectively release a portion of their granule contents[138,142–145,148–150] (Fig. 9–3D). A similar phenomenon occurs when adherent cells encounter some soluble stimuli, such as the complement component, C5a.[50] Lysosomal enzyme release under these conditions occurs by a process of "reverse endocytosis"[138] or "frustrated phagocytosis,"[150] during which merger of granules with the plasma membrane results in discharge of granule constituents directly to the outside of cells as though into phagosomes. Phagocytosis per se does not occur, and the viability of adherent cells is not altered. This mechanism of granule constituent release from neutrophils very likely is relevant to the pathogenesis of tissue injury in a variety of diseases in which immune complexes are deposited on cell surfaces or extracellular structures, such as vascular basement membranes and articular cartilage.[120,123,149]

Lysosomal enzyme release from neutrophils by the mechanism of "reverse endocytosis" is facilitated greatly when cells are treated with the fungal metabolite cytochalasin B. Cytochalasin B interferes with the function of cytoplasmic microfilaments and inhibits membrane transport of sugars and nucleosides in cultured cells.[151–154] Cytochalasin B-treated neutrophils are unable to ingest particles, but nevertheless, release, or secrete, lysosomal but not cytoplasmic constituents (i.e., degranulate) when appropriate particles or soluble stimuli come into contact with their surfaces[48–50,68,148,154–157] (Fig. 9–3D). With some soluble stimuli (e.g., complement-derived and synthetic peptide chemotactic factors), treatment of neutrophils with cytochalasin B is an absolute prerequisite for maximal degranulation.[68,155,156] Ultrastructural studies of cytochalasin B-treated neutrophils have revealed membrane fusion between lysosomal granules and the plasma membrane as the morphologic accompaniment of biochemically measurable enzyme release.[49,156] The precise mechanism is unknown whereby cytochalasin B facilitates fusion between lysosmal membranes and the plasma membranes of stimulated neutrophils leading to the discharge of granule contents.

As indicated above, cytochalasin B-treated neutrophils degranulate when they are exposed to the soluble, low molecular weight complement component, C5a.[50,146,156] Such cells respond similarly to other chemotactic factors, e.g., products of bacteria, synthetic peptides, and oxygenation products of arachidonic acid.[50,155,158,159] Yet other soluble stimuli are capable of provoking degranulation of normal neutrophils. These include the tumor-promoting agent phorbol myristate acetate (specific granules only),[160,161] calcium ions with or without the ionophore, A23187 (azurophil and/or specific granules),[162,163] and the cell surface-reactive lectin concanavalin A (specific granules only).[164,165] Degranulation of neutrophils in response to these soluble stimuli occurs in the absence of cytochalasin B, particles, or adherence to surfaces and is not associated with any alterations of cell viability. The mechanism by which specific granule constituents (e.g., lysozyme) are selectively released from neutrophils exposed to phorbol myristate acetate, calcium, and concanavalin A is unknown. Some data, however, suggest that the limiting membranes of specific granules have unique physical and/or chemical properties that facilitate fusion with the neutrophil plasma membrane.[134]

OXIDATIVE METABOLISM

Cellular and Biochemical Aspects

Encounters between phagocytic leukocytes and appropriate particulate stimuli lead to increased consumption by the leukocytes of molecular oxygen.[102,121] The bulk of oxygen that is consumed is reduced to water through the formation of several highly reactive intermediates. Oxygen, in its ground state, contains two unpaired electrons with parallel spins. Since these present a "barrier" to the insertion of additional pairs of electrons, ground state oxygen "prefers" to be reduced by univalent, or single electron steps. When oxygen accepts a single electron, it is converted to the superoxide anion radical. In human neutrophils, a pyridine nucleotide-dependent oxidase, localized to either an intracellular granule fraction or the plasma membrane,[165–167] appears to catalyze this reaction. It has been demonstrated conclusively that the bulk of oxygen that is consumed by stimulated neutrophils is converted directly to superoxide anion radicals.[168] In addition to superoxide, stimulated neutrophils generate hydrogen peroxide,[169] hydroxyl radicals,[170] and, perhaps, singlet oxygen.[171] Concomitantly, there is stimulation of the hexose monophosphate shunt pathway of glucose oxidation and iodination of protein (mediated by the granule enzyme myeloperoxidase).[172,173] The increased ability of phagocytosing neutrophils to reduce nitroblue tetrazolium (NBT) dye is a reflection of the enhanced generation of superoxide anion radicals[174] (Fig. 9–4). The importance of these metabolic events to the microbicidal activity of neutrophils has been reviewed extensively.[102,121,175]

As is the case with degranulation, enhanced oxidative metabolism by neutrophils can be stimulated in the absence of phagocytosis. For example, neutrophils adherent to certain nonphagocytizable surfaces have been observed to increase their oxidative metabolism, particularly if the surfaces are coated with immune complexes, aggregated IgG, or the opsonic fragment of the third

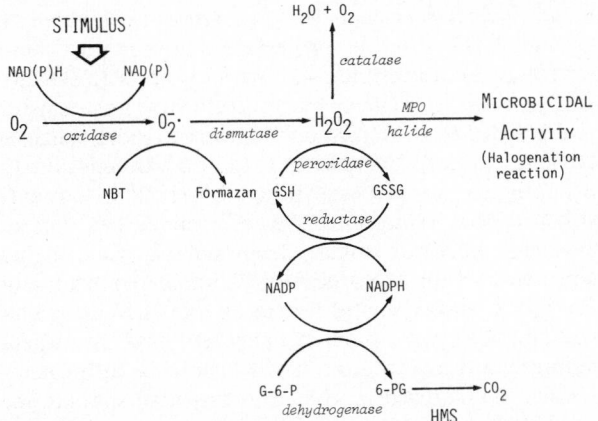

Figure 9–4. Changes in oxidative metabolism following stimulation of neutrophils. *NBT* = Nitroblue tetrazolium. *MPO* = Myeloperoxidase. *GSH* = Reduced glutathione. *G-6-P* = Glucose-6-phosphate. *HMS* = Hexose monophosphate shunt.

component of complement (C3b).[145,149] Similarly, neutrophils exposed to certain soluble stimuli have been demonstrated to increase their oxygen uptake, production of superoxide anion, hexose monophosphate shunt activity, and nitroblue tetrazolium dye reduction. These soluble stimuli include immune complexes, aggregates of IgG, and chemotactic factors (e.g., C5a) as well as a variety of surface-reactive compounds, such as phospholipase *c*, phorbol myristate acetate, concanavalin A, and digitonin.[145,146,165,176-180] The metabolic responses of neutrophils to these soluble stimuli require intact, viable cells and resemble closely those observed during phagocytosis.

It appears that cell surface stimulation of neutrophils is sufficient, in the absence of phagocytosis, to provoke the degranulation and the burst of oxidative metabolism that ordinarily accompany ingestion of particles. What is the relation between these two responses of neutrophils to stimulation? Whereas it is true that when normal neutrophils are allowed to ingest particles, the two responses appear to be inseparable, studies with non-phagocytic stimuli indicate that they can occur independently. For example, it has been demonstrated that there is no significant correlation between the ability of various stimuli to provoke lysosomal enzyme release from neutrophils (i.e., degranulation) and their ability to enhance generation of superoxide anion.[146]

Measurements of extracellular superoxide anion, as performed in most studies of stimulated neutrophils, presumably reflect not only the production of this radical but also the activity of endogenous superoxide dismutase and, possibly, the rate of release of superoxide from the cytoplasm to the extracellular fluid. The demonstration that neutrophils contain superoxide dismutase in their cytosol satisfied the requirement for a protective mechanism against the potentially injurious effects of superoxide anion radicals and led to the suggestion that production of superoxide takes place on the outer surface of the cell membrane as well as in phagocytic vacuoles that are formed by invaginations of this

membrane[165,181] (Fig. 9–5). The hypothesis that the neutrophil superoxide-generating system is localized to the plasma membrane is attractive. Surface generation of superoxide would allow for its concentration within phagocytic vacuoles and provides a convenient explanation for the extracellular recovery of this highly reactive free radical. By conversion to freely diffusible hydrogen peroxide, extracellular or intraphagosomal superoxide anion radicals can mediate all of the biochemical events that ordinarily accompany particle contact, phagocytosis, and microbial killing.

Oxygen-Derived Free Radicals as Mediators of Inflammation

Some recent observations have led to the suggestion that oxygen-derived free radicals are important mediators of inflammation and tissue injury. First, oxygen-derived free radicals injure tissues (e.g., damage lipid membranes) and irreversibly alter macromolecules (Table 9-5). Second, superoxide dismutase and other scavengers of oxygen-derived free radicals prevent tissue injury in vitro and possess anti-inflammatory activity in vivo. Further, some commonly used anti-inflammatory drugs either scavenge oxygen-derived free radicals directly (i.e., exhibit superoxide dismutase-like activity) or inhibit production of oxygen-derived free radicals by phagocytic cells.

Oxygen-Derived Free Radicals Injure Tissues and Irreversibly Alter Macromolecules. A role for oxygen-derived free radicals in the injury of biomembranes has been demonstrated in several experimental systems. Target cells have included human erythrocytes,[182] human neutrophils,[183] and cultured human endothelial cells.[184] The precise nature of the reactive molecules that mediate injury to biomembranes is unknown. Results of most studies, however, indicate roles for both superoxide anion radicals and hydrogen peroxide or, more specifically, for products of their interaction such as hydroxyl radicals and singlet oxygen. These reactive species can produce lipid peroxides, and it is likely that lipid peroxidation is responsible for altering membrane integrity.

Figure 9–5. Generation of superoxide at the surface of a human neutrophil: response to particulate stimuli (from Goldstein, I.M.: Curr. Topics Hematol. 2:145, 1979.)

Table 9–5. Macromolecules Altered by
Oxygen-Derived Free Radicals

Hyaluronic acid
Collagen and tropocollagen
α-1-Proteinase inhibitor
Arachidonic acid
DNA

In addition to damaging cells and tissues directly, oxygen-derived free radicals may provoke inflammation and tissue injury indirectly by irreversibly altering macromolecules. Several observations are particularly relevant to the possible roles played by oxygen-derived free radicals in provoking tissue injury in patients with arthritis. A number of investigators,[185-189] for example, have demonstrated that oxygen-derived free radicals, generated by the aerobic action of xanthine oxidase on either xanthine or hypoxanthine,[190] "degrade" bovine synovial fluid as well as purified hyaluronic acid. "Degradation" was manifested by a marked reduction in relative viscosity and by the inability of the treated synovial fluid to form a mucin clot. Depolymerization of hyaluronic acid also was demonstrated.[188] Addition of either catalase or superoxide dismutase provided protection against the "degradation," indicating that both hydrogen peroxide and superoxide were participants in the reaction. Normal synovial fluid was found to contain barely detectable levels of catalase and approximately 1 nanogram per milliliter of superoxide dismutase.[185] Interestingly, superoxide dismutase activity could not be detected at all in synovial fluids from patients with rheumatoid arthritis.[191] Furthermore, Rister and colleagues[192] reported that neutrophils from children with rheumatoid arthritis contain less superoxide dismutase activity than neutrophils from normal controls.

Another macromolecule that can be altered by oxygen-derived free radicals is collagen. Collagen solutions fail to gel normally and exhibit a slightly lower intrinsic viscosity after exposure to a superoxide-generating system (i.e., xanthine oxidase and hypoxanthine).[193] Soluble tropocollagen also does not gel properly (when heated) after exposure to chemically generated singlet oxygen.[194] After exposure to singlet oxygen, tropocollagen has a lower intrinsic viscosity and an apparently altered subunit composition. These findings support the hypothesis that the loss of synovial fluid viscosity and some changes in connective tissue observed in patients with inflammatory arthritides are mediated by the unrestrained action of oxygen-derived free radicals produced by stimulated leukocytes.[185]

Effects of Oxygen-Derived Free Radicals on Antiproteinases. Another way in which oxygen-derived free radicals may provoke inflammation and tissue injury is by altering the function of naturally occurring antiproteinases. Carp and Janoff[195] reported recently that superoxide anion radicals and hydrogen peroxide, produced by stimulated human neutrophils, were capable of inactivating α_1-proteinase inhibitor. Inactivation was attributed to oxidation of methionine thioether residues

(to sulfoxides) in or near the active site of the proteinase inhibitor.[196] Oxidized α_1-proteinase inhibitor was found to be incapable of forming stable complexes with elastase and, consequently, incapable of influencing the elastolytic activity of the enzyme.[196] A recent report suggests that altered antiproteinase function may be relevant to the pathogenesis of tissue injury observed in patients with arthritis. Wong and Travis[197] found that the α_1-proteinase inhibitor isolated from synovial fluid of patients with rheumatoid arthritis contained residues of methionine sulfoxide and was incapable of forming stable complexes with porcine pancreatic elastase. These findings confirmed that naturally occurring antiproteinases can be oxidized in vivo, and provided support for the hypothesis that oxygen-derived free radicals released from phagocytic leukocytes may mediate inflammation and tissue injury by altering the balance between proteinases (also released from these cells) and naturally occurring antiproteinases. Such an imbalance could render adjacent tissues and/or other macromolecules more susceptible to proteolytic attack.

Effects of Oxygen-Derived Free Radicals on Lipids— Generation of Chemoattractants. As indicated above, it appears that oxygen-derived free radicals alter the integrity of biomembranes by provoking lipid peroxidation. Hydroxyl radicals, for example, are capable of abstracting hydrogen atoms from allylic positions of unsaturated lipids to yield hydroperoxides.[198] Hydroperoxides also may be formed by the direct action of singlet oxygen on polyunsaturated fatty acids.[199] Peroxidation of unsaturated fatty acids after their exposure to simple superoxide-generating systems also has been demonstrated.[200]

As discussed elsewhere in this volume (Chapter 6), oxidized fatty acids have attracted a great deal of attention recently because of the roles they may play in provoking inflammation. It is possible, for example, that hydroxy and dihydroxy derivatives of arachidonic acid with chemotactic activity are responsible, in part, for provoking the accumulation of neutrophils in inflamed joints.[201] Since conversion of arachidonic acid to chemotactically active hydroxy derivatives proceeds through the formation of hydroperoxides, it is not surprising that similar derivatives can be generated nonenzymatically by free radical-mediated reactions. Turner and colleagues,[34,202] for example, found that exposure of arachidonic acid either to air for 24 hours or to ultraviolet irradiation resulted in the generation of oxidized lipids that were chemotactic for human neutrophils.

Recently, Perez and colleagues[203] described another mechanism whereby arachidonic acid could be converted nonenzymatically to biologically active products. These investigators found that chemotactic activity for human neutrophils was generated upon exposure of arachidonic acid to a superoxide-generating system consisting of xanthine oxidase and acetaldehyde. Generation of chemotactic activity in this experimental system was time dependent and could be inhibited significantly by scavengers of singlet oxygen, as well as by scavengers of superoxide, hydrogen peroxide, and hydroxyl radicals.

Silica gel thin-layer radiochromatography demonstrated a product with chemotactic activity that was distinct from that of unaltered arachidonic acid and 12-hydroxyeicosatetraenoic acid (12-HETE). The isolated product was chemotactic for human neutrophils at a concentration (approximate) of 3.0 ng per ml and chemokinetic at concentrations of 0.75 to 1.5 ng per ml.

Another chemoattractant formed by the action of oxygen-derived free radicals was described recently by Petrone and colleagues.[204] These investigators found that potent chemotactic activity for human neutrophils could be generated in vitro by exposing normal human plasma to a source of superoxide anion radicals (i.e., xanthine oxidase and xanthine). Generation of chemotactic activity in this system was inhibited by superoxide dismutase but not by catalase. When plasma that had been exposed to superoxide anion radicals was injected intradermally into rats, large numbers of neutrophils accumulated at the injection sites. A similar response was observed when rats were injected intradermally with xanthine oxidase and xanthine. No leukocyte infiltration was observed, however, if superoxide dismutase was injected simultaneously with the enzyme and substrate.

The chemotactic activity that was formed by exposing plasma to superoxide was heat labile (56° C for 30 minutes), nondialyzable, and stable to lyophilization. The bulk of the activity was recovered after gel filtration and ion exchange chromatography of superoxide-treated plasma in fractions containing albumin. Albumin itself, however, was not chemotactic. Rather, the chemotactic factor appeared to consist of a chloroform-extractable component (i.e., lipid) that was bound to albumin. Since the nature of the lipid was not determined, it is intriguing to speculate that it may be a hydroperoxy or hydroxy derivative of arachidonic acid.

Superoxide Dismutase and Other Scavengers of Oxygen-Derived Free Radicals Possess Anti-Inflammatory Activity. For organisms to survive in an aerobic environment, they must be protected from the potentially toxic effects of oxygen-derived free radicals and singlet oxygen. Protection of cells from the potentially injurious superoxide anion radical is provided primarily by superoxide dismutases, intracellular enzymes that catalyze dismutation of superoxide to hydrogen peroxide and oxygen. Eukaryotic organisms contain two distinct types of superoxide dismutases: a manganese-containing mitochondrial enzyme and a copper- and zinc-containing cytoplasmic enzyme.[205] By scavenging superoxide and thereby preventing either spontaneous dismutation or reactions between superoxide and hydrogen peroxide, superoxide dismutase also prevents the formation of toxic hydroxyl radicals and singlet oxygen.

In 1968, Huber and colleagues[206] reported the isolation and purification from bovine liver of an anti-inflammatory, copper-containing protein. This protein, termed orgotein, exhibited potent anti-inflammatory activity in several animal models of acute and chronic inflammation.[207] When administered subcutaneously to either rats or mice, orgotein effectively suppressed carrageenan-induced paw edema, abscess formation, and pleurisy. In guinea pigs, orgotein inhibited the vascular damage and neutrophil infiltration of skin observed as a consequence of reversed passive Arthus reactions. Orgotein also inhibited adjuvant-induced paw edema and arthritis in rats. Finally, orgotein suppressed anti-DNA antibody formation, as well as autoimmune glomerulonephritis, in NZB $\times$ NZW F_1 hybrid mice. It is appreciated now that orgotein is identical with bovine liver superoxide dismutase.[190,207]

Other studies in experimental animals have confirmed some of the seemingly remarkable anti-inflammatory effects of superoxide dismutase. Oyanagui,[208] for example, found that native superoxide dismutase from bovine liver, when administered intravenously to rats, completely suppressed carrageenan-induced paw edema. McCormick and colleagues[209] found that superoxide dismutase blocked immune complex–induced dermal vascular injury (i.e., Arthus reactions) in rats, as well as the early phases of immune complex–induced lung injury (i.e., edema, hemorrhage, and neutrophil accumulation). Neither heat-inactivated superoxide dismutase nor catalase affected the Arthus reactions in skin and lung, suggesting that the enzymatic activity of native superoxide dismutase was required for its anti-inflammatory effects.

Since superoxide dismutase (i.e., orgotein) was reported to be effective in the treatment of periostitis and arthritis in horses and dogs,[210,211] attention naturally was directed at the possibility that it might also be effective in the treatment of arthritis in man. Lund-Oleson and Menander[212] reported that treatment with multiple intra-articular injections of orgotein produced beneficial effects (e.g., decreased pain and swelling, increased range of motion and overall functional status) in 16 of 22 patients with osteoarthritis. It is noteworthy that Rosner and colleagues[213] found that intra-articular injections of orgotein did not ameliorate experimentally induced osteoarthritis in rabbits. In a very recent study, Goebel and colleagues[214] found that intra-articular injections of orgotein (4 mg per week for 6 weeks) in patients with classical rheumatoid arthritis resulted in significant improvement of several clinical parameters, including pain, morning stiffness, and range of motion. Orgotein also depressed significantly the levels in synovial fluid of rheumatoid factors, prostaglandin E_2, and lactate dehydrogenase. It should be emphasized that in all of the studies that have been reported to date of the effects of superoxide dismutase therapy in man, insufficient data preclude critical analysis of the results. Consequently, results of more rigorously controlled prospective clinical trials are required before any conclusions can be reached concerning the efficacy in man of treatment with superoxide dismutase.

One mechanism whereby superoxide dismutase may inhibit inflammatory reactions is through effects on other anti-inflammatory substances (e.g., protection of naturally occurring antiproteinases from oxidant-induced inactivation).[195] Another mechanism involves free radical-mediated generation of chemotactic activity for neutrophils. By preventing formation of chemotactic products by the action of oxygen-derived free radicals on either arachidonic acid[203] or substrates in plasma,[204] superoxide dismutase could prevent accumulation of neutrophils at foci of inflammation. Such an effect would serve to limit amplification of inflammatory reactions.

Effects of Anti-Inflammatory Drugs on Oxygen-Derived Free Radicals. Some commonly used potent anti-inflammatory drugs can influence oxygen-derived free radicals in two general ways (which may account for at least some of their anti-inflammatory effects). First, several drugs have been found capable of inhibiting production of oxygen-derived free radicals by appropriately stimulated phagocytic cells. Goldstein and colleagues,[215] for example, demonstrated that anti-inflammatory adrenal corticosteriods inhibit production of superoxide anion radicals by human neutrophils exposed to aggregated human IgG, opsonized zymosan particles, and the complement component C5a. Lehmeyer and Johnston[216] found that adrenal corticosteroids also were capable of inhibiting generation of superoxide anion radicals by human neutrophils and monocytes exposed to nonphagocytizable surfaces coated with aggregated IgG (an in vitro model of immunologically induced inflammation).

Another way in which commonly used anti-inflammatory drugs may influence oxygen-derived free radicals is by directly scavenging these reactive molecules. A number of drugs, for example, have been found capable of preventing the loss of relative viscosity that occurs when synovial fluid is exposed to xanthine oxidase and hypoxanthine.[189,217] Copper (II) chelates of salicylates, for example, have been demonstrated to possess superoxide dismutase-like activity,[218] as have low molecular weight cupric peptides.[219] In the absence of copper, these compounds do not exhibit superoxide-scavenging activity. It is of some interest that copper chelates of some commonly used drugs appear to have greater anti-inflammatory potency in vivo than the native compounds.[220] Whether this is due to their superoxide dismutase-like activity has not been determined.

GRANULOCYTES AS SOURCES OF PEPTIDE AND LIPID MEDIATORS OF INFLAMMATION

The full range of functional capabilities of each class of granulocytes is developed fully by the generation of an array of fatty acid and phospholipid mediators, and by the liberation of peptide mediators from plasma protein precursors by granulocyte proteinases. The activity of many of the neutrophil proteinases is regulated by α-globulin inhibitors. Although α_1-proteinase inhibitor plays a relatively restricted role in the control of the plasma enzymes of coagulation, kinin generation, and fibrinolysis,[30] in comparison to the other α-globulin inhibitors, it is a critical inhibitor of a wide spectrum of neutrophil-derived proteases. The α_1-proteinase-inhibitable enzymes of neutrophils that are granule associated include the neutral proteases,[221] elastase,[221,222] and a family of cationic proteins with chymotrypsinlike, bactericidal, and phagocytosis-enhancing activities.[223] Inhibition of neutrophil elastase by α-globulins is associated with the formation of complexes that exhibit an enzyme to inhibitor ratio of 1:1 for α_1-proteinase inhibitor and 2:1 for α_2 macroglobulin.[224] However, the quantitative predominance of α_1-proteinase inhibitor over α_2 macroglobulin in normal serum suggests that it is the dominant inhibitor. The overall significance of this regulatory role of α_1-proteinase inhibitor is emphasized by the observation that one half of the elastase-inhibiting capacity of serum from individuals with homozygous deficiency of α_1-proteinase inhibitor (PiZZ), containing less than 15 percent of the normal levels of α_1-proteinase inhibitor, was nonetheless attributable to the residual α_1-proteinase inhibitor.[224]

In addition to the lysosomal proteinases with broad activity, neutrophils possess proteinases that express specific activity for the liberation of potent peptide mediators from plasma proteins. Angiotensin II, assessed by both radioimmunoassay and smooth muscle contractile activity, is generated directly from plasma angiotensinogen by neutrophil cathepsin G, without the appearance of angiotensin I or the participation of angiotensin-converting enzyme.[225,226] Neutrophils also possess enzymatic pathways for the production of bradykinin and other kinins, which may be important fluid-phase mediators in some types of inflammation.[227,228] The generation of angiotensin II and kinins by neutrophils is controlled by two normally occurring classes of plasma proteins: α_1-proteinase inhibitor and other α-globulins, which block the activity of cathepsin G and kininogenases, and plasma inactivators that enzymatically degrade the peptide mediators.[225-227] Highly purified cathepsin G and the native cathepsin G in neutrophils are exquisitely sensitive to the inhibitory effect of α_1-proteinase inhibitor. Less than 1 percent of the α_1-proteinase inhibitor in 1 ml of normal human blood totally inhibits the expression of the cathepsin G of the 3 to 5 $\times 10^6$ neutrophils that would be present in the 1 ml portion of blood. The plasma inactivator of angiotensin II resembles kininase I and the anaphylatoxin inactivator in that it has a molecular weight of 300,000 to 350,000 and its activity is heat labile and calcium dependent.[227] As α_1-proteinase inhibitor regulates both general and specific proteases of neutrophils, it is of considerable interest that a deficiency in serum α_1-proteinase inhibitor is associated with the premature development of severe pulmonary emphysema and hepatic cirrhosis.[229,230] The increased incidence of the diseases noted suggests that a depression in the local tissue concentrations of α_1-proteinase inhibitor accompanied the serum deficiency and resulted in a relative excess of free protease activities in some tissues, which led to proteolytic tissue damage and the secondary development of fibrosis. Evidence has emerged that extends the relevance of these findings to the rheumatic diseases, as a higher incidence of rheumatoid arthritis and juvenile rheumatoid arthritis was found in some groups of subjects who are severely deficient in α_1-proteinase inhibitor.[231]

The recognition of the roles played by oxygenation products of arachidonic acid in inflammation led to the definition of the structures of several such products of granulocytes. The principal products and the quantities of each vary significantly for the different types of granulocytes. Prostaglandin E_2 (PGE_2) is the major cyclooxygenase metabolite of neutrophils and eosinophils, while PGD_2 predominates for basophils.[232] The 5-lipoxygenase pathway is the most active in neutrophils and basophils, but the distribution of leukotrienes (LTs) differs substantially. Neutrophils generate LTB_4, which is a potent stimulus of PMN leukocyte function and may endogenously amplify neutrophil chemotaxis and protein secretion elicited by other agonists.[26,27] LTB_4 is also an immunosuppressive factor, which stimulates suppressor T-lymphocyte function.[27,233] Basophils secrete large quantities of LTB_4 and the C-6 peptide leukotriene LTD_4, which is a potent mediator of smooth muscle contraction and increased vascular permeability, which appear to be important in allergic reactions and asthma.[234] In contrast, the 15-lipoxygenase predominates in eosinophils, with the generation of a series of 14,15-di-HETEs, 8,15-di-HETEs, and 5,15-di-HETEs,[235] which demonstrate effects on PMN leukocytes similar to those of LTB_4 but are far less potent.[236] Basophils and neutrophils are, in addition, capable of synthesizing and secreting 1-O-hexadecyl-2-acetyl-sn-glyceryl-3-phosphorylcholine, which is a platelet-activating factor (PAF) that induces platelet aggregation and the release of granule constituents from human and rabbit platelets in vitro[237] and rabbit platelets in vivo.[238] Thus granulocytes have the capacity to contribute to inflammation not only by cellular activities but also by the elaboration of a wide range of peptide and lipid mediators.

GENERATION AND RELEASE OF CHEMICAL MEDIATORS OF THE BASOPHIL

The bridging of basophil membrane–bound IgE by specific antigen or anti-IgE, or the exposure of basophils to fluid phase immunological principals such as C5a or platelet factor 4 leads to the intracellular generation of unstored mediators and their release along with the preformed chemical mediators of the basophil.[239-241] Basophils differ from mast cells with respect to origin, tissue distribution, some cellular constituents, and their patterns of involvement in hypersensitivity reactions. Both cell types, however, may serve a central role in immediate-type hypersensitivity reactions by virtue of the brief interval required for mobilization of their full capacity to secrete a wide array of chemical mediators. Less is known for basophils than for mast cells of the biochemical events of activation, the structures of some of the mediators, and the mechanisms of cellular regulation of immediate hypersensitivity reactions.[242] The release of histamine from human basophils by IgE-dependent mechanisms and by C5a differs with respect to temperature optimum, time course, and the desensitizing activity of each stimulus, but both pathways of activation share with mast cell mechanisms a dependence on extracellular calcium.[240] Further, the immunological release of basophil mediators is inhibited by agents that elevate the intracellular levels of cyclic AMP in a manner comparable to cyclic AMP inhibition of mast cell activation.[243,244] Morphologic studies of human basophils that were challenged in various reactions revealed two patterns of degranulation.[245] One pattern, which is characteristic of anaphylactic reactions, exhibited prominent fusion of the membranes of adjacent granules and of granule membranes with the plasma membrane. The other pattern, typically seen in human allergic contact dermatitis, consisted of multiple cytoplasmic membrane–bound vesicles that were presumably derived from the granules and in many instances were in communication with the plasma membrane, suggesting "piecemeal" release of mediators without granule movement or loss of integrity. The primary mediators of the basophil, like those of the mast cell, may be viewed as belonging to two classes, namely those that are present totally preformed prior to challenge and those that are unstored and must be generated from inactive precursors subsequent to immunological activation (Table 9–6). Histamine, heparin,[246] and several leukocyte chemotactic factors[247] are in the former category, while LTD_4, LTB_4, phospholipid platelet-activating factor (PAF),[248] and other leukocyte chemotactic factors[249] cannot be detected in unchallenged basophils. The histamine content and the fraction of total proteoglycans accounted for by heparin both appear to be lower in the basophil than in the mast cell. Esterases of varying specificities have been identified in the granules of guinea pig basophils.[250] Both high and low molecular weight preformed leukocyte chemotactic factors have been extracted from human leukemic basophils,[247] but neither has been characterized structurally or functionally beyond its chemotactic preference for neutrophils and eosinophils, respectively. The SRS-A activity generated by basophils is attributable to LTD_4, as contrasted with LTC_4 or a mixture of LTC_4 and LTD_4 for different types of mast cells.[251] PAF from rabbit or human basophils results in platelet aggregation, stimulates the platelet release reaction, and appears to be the low molecular weight phospholipid 1-O-hexadecyl-2-acetyl-sn-glyceryl-3-phosphorylcholine, which is susceptible to inactivation by several phospholipases,[248,252] as is the case for some PAFs of mast cell origin.[253] A chemotactic factor which preferentially attracts eosinophils is generated from human basophils by immunological challenge, as well as from other human leukocytes during phagocytosis or exposure to the calcium ionophore A23187.[249,254] The major lipid chemotactic agent secreted by basophils is LTB_4.

Delayed hypersensitivity responses are recognized to be heterogeneous reactions that involve predominantly lymphocytes and macrophages, but basophils are substantial components in some instances.[255] Infiltrates of basophils that appear with a delayed time course are especially prominent in cutaneous contact reactions, Jones-Mote reactions to proteins, some instances of al-

Table 9–6. Chemical Mediators of the Basophilic Granulocyte

Type	Mediator	Structural Characteristics	Assay(s)	Other Functions	Inactivation
Preformed	Histamine	β-Imidazolyl-ethylamine, molecular weight 111	Contraction of guinea pig ileum	Increased vascular permeability	Histaminase Histamine N-methyltransferase
			Radiolabeling by histamine N-methyltransferase	Enhancement of eosinophil migration	
	Leukotactic activities	Molecular weight > 150,000	Chemotactic attraction of granulocytes (N > E)*	Chemotactic deactivation of granulocytes	–
		Molecular weight ≃ 300–1000	Chemotactic attraction of granulocytes (E > N)	Chemotactic deactivation of granulocytes	–
	Heparin	Acidic proteoglycan, molecular weight ≃ 1 million	Antithrombin III activation	Anticoagulation	–
	Chymase	–	Hydrolysis of synthetic esters	–	–
	Tryptase	–	Hydrolysis of synthetic esters	–	–
Unstored	Slow reacting substance of anaphylaxis (SRS-A)	LTD$_4$	Contraction of antihistamine-treated guinea pig ileum	Contraction of human bronchiole	Peroxidase
	Leukotactic activity	LTB$_4$	Chemotactic attraction of granulocytes (E > N)	Increased vascular permeability	
	Platelet activating factor (PAF9)	1-O-hexadecyl-2-acetyl-sn-glyceryl-3-phosphoryl-choline	Release of ^{14}C-5-OH-tryptamine from platelets	Platelet aggregation	Phospholipases

*Abbreviations used are the same as in Table 9–1.

lograft rejection, and many tissue responses to tumors as well as viral and parasitic infections.[256] That basophil mediators may modulate mononuclear leukocyte function in such reactions has been suggested by a relative deficiency of macrophages in basophil-rich infiltrates and, in some cases, by lower concentrations of lymphokines than are found associated with classic delayed hypersensitivity reactions.[257] Both mast cells and basophils are common in subsynovial connective tissues, but any role in synovial inflammation remains speculative. The predominant possibilities are based on the observations that the chemical mediators that alter microvascular permeability enhance the local deposition of immune complexes,[258] and that mast cells and basophils release factors that are chemotactic for lymphocytes as well as granulocytes.

ABNORMALITIES OF NEUTROPHIL FUNCTION IN HUMAN DISEASE

Neutrophils of some subjects predisposed to an increased incidence of bacterial infections may exhibit severe isolated defects in phagocytosis, in the absence of other functional abnormalities. Such defects may be considered in terms of the stages of the phagocytic process, and accordingly classified as predominantly ineffective opsonization, disordered ingestion, or deficient degranulation and/or metabolic activation.[259] These phagocytic abnormalities are largely congenital disorders or transient states, and none is associated with excessive spontaneous inflammation or rheumatic disease-like syndromes. In contrast, abnormalities in neutrophil chemotaxis with or without defects in random migration, phagocytosis, or other functions are linked both to defects in host defense against infections and to the de-

velopment of a variety of inflammatory diseases. As such in vitro abnormalities have been reviewed recently,[260,261] this chapter will cover only illustrative examples and conditions relevant to the rheumatic diseases (Tables 9–7 and 9–8). Defects in chemotaxis resulting from intrinsic cellular disorders are subdivided into the permanent types, which are largely congenital, and the transient types, which include states of bone marrow development, viral and overwhelming bacterial infections, and some of the rheumatic diseases (Table 9–7). The neutrophils in the permanent states exhibit numerous functional abnormalities, and the patients are universally more susceptible to pyogenic infections. Neutropenia may occur as well, which presumably reflects in part abnormal migration and efflux from the bone marrow. It is of special interest that neutrophil migration in some cases of both the Chédiak-Higashi and the Quie-Hill syndromes may respond in vitro and in vivo to ascorbic acid.[56,57] The mechanism of enhancement of migration by ascorbic acid is unknown in the latter condition, but in the Chédiak-Higashi leukocytes ascorbic acid depresses the abnormally high intracellular level of cyclic AMP and concomitantly restores microtubule function to normal.[262] In the category of transient defects, the neutrophil abnormalities generally only respond to successful management of the basic disease. One notable exception is in viral infections, in which mononuclear leukocyte and, in some cases, neutrophil defects in migration are strikingly reversed by levamisole.[263]

Discrepancies exist among the results of several studies of neutrophil migration and other functions in the rheumatic diseases. Differences in in vitro methodology may be the basis for some of the discrepant results, as a double filter radiomigration assay, which requires that the neutrophils migrate farther than in single filter assays, has proved to be more sensitive than the conven-

Table 9–7. Defects In Neutrophil In Vitro Chemotaxis in Human Diseases

Level of Defect	Disorder	Other Leukocyte-Related Abnormalities	Clinical Features
Cellular Permanent	Lazy leukocyte syndrome	Neutropenia, decreased neutrophil mobilization from bone marrow, depressed random migration of neutrophils	Recurrent upper respiratory infections, gingivitis, stomatitis
	Chédiak-Higashi syndrome	Neutropenia, defective bactericidal activity and decreased deformability of neutrophils, defective monocyte chemotaxis	Recurrent pyogenic infections, lymphoma-like phase
	Quie-Hill syndrome	Depressed random migration of neutrophils, defective monocyte random and chemotactic migration	Respiratory, cutaneous and ocular staphylococcal and *Candida* infections; eczema, peripheral eosinophilia, elevated serum IgE level
	Defective actin poly-merization	Depressed neutrophil random migration and phagocytosis, but enhanced degranulation	Recurrent infections
Transient or episodic	Viral infections	—	Measles, influenza
	Septicemia	Depressed random migration and phagocytosis, morphologic abnormalities	Overwhelming bacterial infection
	Bone marrow transplantation	—	Subjects exhibiting graft-vs.-host reactions and treated with anti-thymocyte sera
	Neonatal period	Decreased neutrophil deformability, defective monocyte chemotaxis	
	Rheumatoid arthritis	Depressed phagocytosis, serum inhibitors of chemotaxis in some patients	
	Felty's syndrome	Neutropenia, immunoglobulin inclusions	—
	Systemic lupus erythematosus	Neutropenia, anti-leukocyte antibodies, serum may not generate a normal level of chemotactic activity	—
Fluid phase Inadequate generation of chemotactic activity	Clr deficiency	Delayed generation of serum chemotactic activity	Systemic lupus erythematosus and dermato-myositis-like states, necrotizing angiitis
	C4 deficiency	Delayed generation of serum chemotactic activity	Systemic lupus erythematosus and dermato-myositis-like states, necrotizing angiitis
	C2 deficiency	Delayed generation of serum chemotactic activity	Systemic lupus erythematosus and dermato-myositis-like states, necrotizing angiitis
	C3 deficiency	Serum also lacks opsonic and bactericidal activity	Recurrent gram-positive and gram-negative infections
	C5 deficiency	May be co-existent inhibitors of chemotaxis	Systemic lupus erythematosus–like state and recurrent infections
	C7 deficiency	—	Scleroderma-like syndrome
	Mucocutaneous candidiasis, Wiskott-Aldrich syndrome	Decreased generation of lymphocyte-derived chemo-tactic activity: inhibitors of monocyte migration; deficient delayed hypersensitivity	Frequent infections
Excessive chemotactic factor inactiva-tion or inhibition	Hodgkin's disease	High serum levels of normally occurring α-globulin aminopeptidases	Recurrent infections
	Lepromatous leprosy	High serum levels of normally occurring α-globulin aminopeptidases	Recurrent infections
	Sarcoidosis	High serum levels of normally occurring α-globulin aminopeptidases	Recurrent infections
	Hypogamma-globulinemia	High serum levels of normally occurring α-globulin aminopeptidases	Recurrent infections
	Cirrhosis in alcoholics	High serum levels of normally occurring α-globulin aminopeptidases	Recurrent infections
	Hypocomplementemic nephritis	Serum inhibitor of complement-derived factors	—
Leukocyte-directed inhibition	Elevated levels of IgA polymers	Leukocytosis, absent cutaneous delayed hypersen-sitivity	Recurrent respiratory and cutaneous infections
	Recurrent infections in childhood	Reversible inhibitor of chemotaxis	Respiratory and cutaneous infections

tional Boyden assays in detecting the intrinsic abnormalities of neutrophils in rheumatic diseases.[14,264] The relationship of the neutrophil defects in rheumatic diseases to circulating antileukocyte antibodies or other inhibitors or to the prior in vivo phagocytosis of immune complexes by the neutrophils is not fully understood.[265] However, it appears that such qualitative abnormalities rather than coexisting neutropenia are the major determinant of the increased rate of infections in such patients.[266]

ABNORMAL NEUTROPHIL FUNCTIONS ASSOCIATED WITH RHEUMATIC DISEASES

Systemic Lupus Erythematosus. Among patients with rheumatic diseases, those with systemic lupus erythematous (SLE) suffer most frequently from severe bacterial infections.[267] Although therapy with adrenal corticosteroids (and other immunosuppressive and/or cytotoxic drugs) very likely is a contributory factor,[268] there is

Table 9–8. Excessive Neutrophil In Vitro Chemotaxis in Human Diseases

Level of Defect	Disorder	Other Leukocyte-Related Abnormalities	Special Clinical Features
Cellular			
Permanent	–		
Transient or episodic	Acute bacterial infections	Leukocytosis	Moderately severe infections with host compensation
	Behçet's disease		
	Reactive arthritis (HLA-B27 positive)		
Fluid phase			
Increased generation of chemotactic activity	Cold urticaria	Mast cell–derived chemotactic factors, in vivo chemotactic deactivation of neutrophils	Chemotactic activity observed only in blood from cold-challenged area
	Bullous pemphigoid	In vivo chemotactic deactivation of eosinophils, lymphocyte migration–enhancing factors in bullous fluid	–
	Psoriasis	Arachidonic acid and complement-derived chemotactic factors	–
	Gout	Chemotactic glycoprotein of 8400 molecular weight derived from neutrophils phagocytosing crystals	–
	Rheumatoid arthritis	C5-derived chemotactic factor and LTB_4 in synovial fluid	–
Deficient chemotactic factor inactivation	Alpha$_1$-antitrypsin deficiency	Decreased serum levels of chemotactic factor–inactivating α-globulin aminopeptidase	Pulmonary and hepatic tissue damage and fibrosis
Leukocyte-directed enhancement	Pyoderma gangrenosum	Plasma protein migration–enhancing factor of 160,000 molecular weight	Joint and cutaneous necrotizing inflammation
	Corticosteroid therapy	Neutrophil migration–enhancing factor derived from mononuclear leukocytes	–

ample evidence that the disease itself is associated with altered host defenses against infection. Several functions of neutrophils have been found to be abnormal in patients with SLE. Goetzl,[264] for example, found neutrophils from four untreated patients with SLE less responsive to a standard chemotactic stimulus than cells from either normal controls or patients with other rheumatic diseases (i.e., rheumatoid arthritis, Felty's syndrome). A similar abnormality of neutrophil migration was reported by Landry[269] in six of 14 untreated patients with SLE. In yet another study, Clark and colleagues[266] found reduced amounts of complement-derived chemotactic activity (25 to 58 percent of controls) in endotoxin-activated serum from 10 of 24 patients with SLE. Neutrophils from all but one patient, however, migrated normally toward a standard, complement-derived chemotactic stimulus. Patients with the apparent abnormality in chemotactic factor generation were generally younger, had an earlier age of onset of SLE, and had a history of serious pyogenic infections. The precise nature of the abnormality observed in sera from these patients was not determined. It is likely, however, that these sera contained the inhibitor of complement (C5)-derived chemotactic activity described subsequently by Perez and colleagues.[270] This inhibitor does not act directly on neutrophils and does not affect the chemotactic activity exhibited by either synthetic peptides or filtrates prepared from cultures of *Escherichia coli* (bacterial chemotactic factors). Rather, it acts specifically and reversibly to inhibit the chemotactic activity exhibited by "complexes" of C5a des Arg and a naturally occurring serum protein, termed the cochemotaxin.[271,272] The inhibitor was isolated and purified from SLE serum and was found to be a heat stable (56° C for 30 minutes) cationic protein with a molecular weight of approximately 69,000.[271] Interestingly, patients with SLE whose serum contains the inhibitor have more active disease clinically and appear

to have more frequent bacterial infections than patients whose serum does not contain the inhibitor.[273] It is possible, therefore, that this inhibitor of C5-derived chemotactic activity contributes, in part, to the increased susceptibility of patients with SLE to severe bacterial infections.

Neutrophils from some patients with SLE also exhibit abnormalities involving recognition and phagocytosis. Landry,[269] for example, found subnormal rates of particle ingestion by neutrophils from six of 25 untreated patients with SLE. In another report, Brandt and Hedberg[274] found that neutrophils from seven patients with SLE (receiving steroid therapy) had reduced phagocytic activity when compared with neutrophils from 12 normal controls and seven patients with rheumatoid arthritis. Phagocytosis was not reduced when normal cells were suspended in SLE plasma. In contrast to these findings, Zurier[275] reported that serum from 22 of 30 patients with SLE interfered significantly with particle uptake by normal neutrophils. Inhibitory activity in serum did not correlate with disease activity, levels of complement (CH_{50} and C3), or corticosteroid therapy and was not influenced by mixing with normal serum. The nature of this "inhibitor" was not determined. It is of interest that Temple and Loewi[276] found that sera from SLE patients significantly inhibited the uptake by human blood monocytes of sheep erythrocytes coated with antibody. This effect was attributed to immune complexes in the sera that presumably were capable of binding preemptively to Fc receptors on the normal cells.

Support for the possibility that phagocytic cells in patients with SLE have impaired surface receptor function has been provided by the studies of Frank and colleagues.[277] These investigators measured the in vivo clearance of isologous erythrocytes coated with either C3b or IgG in patients with SLE. Four of eight patients were found to have a major defect in clearance mediated by Fc receptors. These four had the highest levels of circulating immune complexes as assessed by Clq-serum binding activity. Several patients also had defects in clearance mediated by C3b receptors. It should be noted that these experiments did not establish whether the defects were a cause or a consequence of circulating immune complexes (e.g., pre-emptive binding of ligands to receptors). Three groups of investigators reported recently that erythrocytes from patients with SLE possess decreased numbers of surface receptors for C3b.[278-280] Whereas one group concluded that this abnormality was acquired (as a consequence of disease activity),[278] the other two presented evidence that it was inherited.[279,280] It was suggested that the occurrence of SLE in individuals having reduced numbers of erythrocyte C3b receptors results from an impairment in complement-dependent clearance of potentially pathogenetic immune complexes.

Whereas detailed studies of the oxidative metabolism of neutrophils from patients with SLE have not been reported, abnormal nitroblue tetrazolium dye reduction by these cells has been observed.[281] Insofar as this may be an indicator of abnormal superoxide anion generation,[174] this finding suggests that the oxidative metabolism of neutrophils from some patients with SLE may be impaired. Degranulation of neutrophils from patients with SLE also has not been studied in detail. Zurier,[275] however, did find that SLE sera that inhibited particle ingestion by normal neutrophils also suppressed extracellular release of lysosomal enzymes.

Rheumatoid Arthritis. Patients with rheumatoid arthritis (RA) also exhibit an unusual susceptibility to bacterial infections,[282] as well as abnormalities of neutrophil function. Several investigators[283-285] have reported that neutrophils from the peripheral blood of some patients with RA have an impaired ability to respond to chemotactic stimuli and to ingest suitably opsonized particles in vitro. Mowat and Baum,[283] for example, found that the mean chemotactic index measured with neutrophils from 24 patients with definite RA was significantly less than that measured with cells from an equal number of normal controls matched for age and sex. As an explanation for this abnormality, it has been observed that incubation of normal neutrophils with serum from some patients with RA impairs their capacity to migrate randomly and/or in a directed fashion.[283,285,286] Identical results have been obtained when normal neutrophils were exposed to preformed immune complexes, particularly complexes containing rheumatoid factor.[283] Exposure of normal neutrophils to either RA serum or immune complexes also impairs phagocytosis and killing of bacteria.[287-289] Turner and colleagues[289] observed that phagocytosis of yeast particles by normal peripheral blood neutrophils was decreased if the cells were preincubated with complexes prepared with aggregated human IgG and sera from patients with high-titer rheumatoid factor. In fact, there was a significant correlation between the log of the reciprocal of the rheumatoid factor titer in sera used to prepare complexes and the phagocytic capacity exhibited by test neutrophils. Thus, it appears that the functional abnormalities exhibited by neutrophils from patients with RA occur largely as a consequence of encounters with immune complexes either in vivo or in vitro. Since such encounters are most likely to occur in the inflamed rheumatoid joint, it is not surprising that synovial fluid neutrophils from patients with RA exhibit the most severe abnormalities of chemotaxis and phagocytosis.[289-291] RA synovial fluid also interferes with ingestion of opsonized particles by normal leukocytes.[276,289] These findings may be relevant to the fact that septic arthritis is a particularly common complication of RA.[292]

The abnormalities of neutrophil functions observed in patients with Felty's syndrome also appear to be attributable to encounters with circulating immune complexes. Neutrophils from patients with Felty's syndrome exhibit abnormal chemotaxis in vitro[293] as well as abnormal phagocytosis and bacterial killing.[294] Immunoglobulin-containing inclusions have been seen in these cells by immunofluorescence and electron microscopy.[294] Normal neutrophils develop similar inclusions when they are incubated with serum from patients with Felty's syndrome.[265] It has been suggested that phagocytosis of circulating immune complexes by neutrophils may not only interfere with the function of these cells in combating infection, but also may render them susceptible to removal from the circulation.[265] It is noteworthy that bacterial infections in patients with Felty's syndrome are not always associated with decreased numbers of circulating neutrophils.[295]

Not all of the abnormalities of neutrophil function observed in patients with RA are attributable to encounters in vivo with immune complexes.[296,297] Hanlon and colleagues,[297] for example, described deficient generation of chemotactic activity in RA serum after incubation with *E. coli* lipopolysaccharide. This abnormality was associated with the presence of a heat stable (56° C for 30 minutes) inhibitor of chemotaxis, the potency of which was inversely related to the level of chemotactic activity generated in the rheumatoid sera.

It should be mentioned that some investigators have failed to detect abnormalities of neutrophil function in patients with RA.[274,281] Notably, van de Stadt and colleagues[298] found that if precautions were taken to prevent phagocytosis of immune complexes during the isolation of neutrophils from either peripheral blood or synovial fluid of patients with RA, the cells functioned in vitro quite normally. Oxygen uptake, extracellular release of lysosomal enzymes, and the granule enzyme content of RA neutrophils were comparable to that of peripheral blood neutrophils from healthy volunteer blood donors.

OTHER RHEUMATIC SYNDROMES AND INFLAMMATORY STATES ASSOCIATED WITH ABNORMALITIES OF NEUTROPHIL FUNCTION

With the exception of a single report describing impaired directed migration of neutrophils from patients with juvenile rheumatoid arthritis,[283] most investigators have failed to detect defective neutrophil functions in patients with rheumatic diseases other than SLE and RA.[299-302] In fact, the chemotactic responsiveness of neutrophils has been found to be enhanced in some children with chronic arthritis,[299] patients with Behçet's disease,[300] and some patients with reactive arthritis following yersinia infections.[302] Interestingly, enhanced neutrophil migration (both chemokinesis and chemotaxis) was observed only with cells from patients with reactive arthritis who were HLA-B27 positive. Furthermore, enhanced chemokinetic and chemotactic responses to zymosan-activated serum were observed with neutrophils from HLA-B27 positive individuals irrespective of whether they suffered from either yersinia infections or arthritis. Finally, when activated with zymosan, sera from HLA-B27 positive patients and controls were significantly more chemokinetic than zymosan-activated sera from HLA-B27 negative individuals. These results suggest that the responsiveness of neutrophils to complement-derived chemotactic stimuli is regulated in some fashion by genes associated with the major histocompatibility complex. The increased chemokinetic activity of activated serum from HLA-B27 positive individuals, as well as the enhanced ability of neutrophils from these individuals to migrate in a directed fashion, may contribute to the pathogenesis of "B27-associated" inflammatory arthritides.

An inadequate capacity to generate chemotactic activity in serum, with no demonstrable intrinsic neutrophil defect, is frequently associated with a rheumatic disease-like syndrome, most notably in the cases attributable to a deficiency of a complement component (Table 9–7). Patients lacking an early component of the classic pathway, namely Clr, C4, or C2, are subject to an increased incidence of an SLE-like illness or, more rarely, a dermatomyositis-like syndrome or necrotizing angiitis.[303,304] Patients lacking one of the terminal components, C5, C6, or C7, occasionally present with either an SLE-like disease or, in one instance, Raynaud's syndrome with scleroderma-like features.[305,306] C6-deficient serum develops normal chemotactic activity, however, in contrast to the abnormality in C5- or C7-deficient serum. As the defect in chemotactic activity in C7-deficient serum was originally presumed to reflect the decreased formation of the $\overline{C567}$ chemotactic factor, the normal chemotactic activity of C6-deficient sera, which would also fail to generate $\overline{C567}$, lends substantial credence to those reports of the generation of normal chemotactic activity in C7-deficient serum. Patients deficient in C3, a component critical to both the classic and alternative pathways, have a more pronounced serum abnormality relative to neutrophil function than individuals deficient in other complement components. C3-deficient patients are predisposed to recurrent severe infections, but do not develop rheumatic syndromes at an increased frequency.[307] Children with Wiskott-Aldrich syndrome and mucocutaneous candidiasis exhibit a variety of lymphocyte abnormalities, including decreased generation of chemotactic lymphokines, a defect that may possibly be related to their frequent incidence of infections.[308] A diverse group of diseases, previously related only by a common predisposition to frequent infections, characteristically leads to elevated serum levels of one or more aminopeptidases normally present in serum and known to degradatively inactive numerous chemotactic factors.[309,310] In several other conditions associated with recurrent infections or the occurrence of spontaneous inflammatory disease, serum factors have been detected which either inhibit the activity of chemotactic stimuli or suppress the chemotactic responsiveness of the neutrophils. A serum principal in hypocomplementemic nephritis appears to be a relatively selective inhibitor of complement-derived chemotactic activity.[311] Neutrophil-directed inhibitors have been found in rare children with multiple episodes of pulmonary and cutaneous infections, and the effect of these inhibitors was reversible upon washing the neutrophils.[312] Polymeric IgA is a neutrophil-directed inhibitor of chemotaxis[313] and has been related to in vivo defects in the neutrophil chemotactic responses of a group of patients with elevated serum levels of polymeric IgA in association with neutrophilic leukocytosis and absent cutaneous delayed hypersensitivity.

In comparison with the human diseases that are characteristically associated with defects in neutrophil chemotaxis, those conditions related to excessive neutrophil chemotactic activity in vitro are largely inflammatory disorders without deficiencies of host resistance (Table 9–8). The only subjects documented to have intrinsically hyperactive neutrophils have been those mounting an appropriate response to acute bacterial infections,[314] and some patients with Behçet's disease[300] or reactive arthritis in association with HLA-B27 antigen.[302] For other patients with chemotactically hyperactive neutrophils, the abnormalities have been predominantly in the fluid phase. The local generation of mast cell–derived chemotactic factors in quantities exceeding an apparent physiological need has been observed in acute cold urticaria and in bullous pemphigoid.[315,316] In both instances, eosinophil and neutrophil chemotactic activities were detected in association with the lesions, and the granulocytes exposed to the elevated local concentrations of the stimuli were chemotactically hyporesponsive in vitro, suggesting that in vivo chemotactic deactivation had occurred. High local concentrations of specific granulocyte chemotactic factors also have been found in samples of skin or synovial tissues of patients with psoriasis, gout, and rheumatoid arthritis, and the characteristics of these principals will be presented below. Defects in the in vitro modulation of chemotaxis have been recorded in α_1-proteinase inhibitor deficiency, in which a concomitant deficiency exists in the α-globulin chemotactic factor inactivator,[317] but the clinical significance of this finding is uncertain. Neutrophils in mixed leukocyte suspensions are chemotactically hyperactive following corticosteroid therapy as a result of the elaboration of a mononuclear leukocyte–derived factor that enhances the chemotactic responsiveness of neutrophils.[318] A naturally occurring leukocyte migration–enhancing principal has been found in sera of rare patients with pyoderma gangrenosum, characterized by episodes of sterile pyarthrosis and cutaneous inflammation.[319] This migration-enhancing factor was recovered from serum by Sephadex G-200 gel filtration and found to have a molecular weight of approximately 160,000. The partially purified principal enhanced the random migration of purified normal human neutrophils and mononuclear leukocytes by up to 200 percent without specifically influencing chemotaxis. Trauma or other stimuli which alter microvascular permeability may lead to an accumulation of this serum factor in tissues of such patients, with resultant excessive influx of leukocytes and heightened local activity of neutrophils and mononuclear leukocytes in the inflammatory exudate.

SPECIFIC CHEMOTACTIC FACTORS IN RHEUMATIC DISORDERS

The possibility that one pathway for the generation of chemotactic activity may predominate in a given disease has been explored using relevant biological fluids or cell extracts for the absorption of known chemotactic principals with specific antisera and for the purification of the existing chemotactic activities. Initial efforts indicated that the major chemotactic factors for neutrophils in rheumatoid synovial fluid and in extracts of cutaneous lesions in a rat model for vasculitis were fragments of C5 of approximately 17,000 molecular weight that were analogous to C5a, while fragments of C3 appeared to account for the bulk of the neutrophil chemotactic activity in synovial fluid of some nonrheumatoid arthritides and in pericardial fluid following limited myocardial infarctions in rats.[320] Analyses of fluid phase and tissue enzymes capable of cleaving C5 and C3 suggested that the major protease that generated chemotactic fragments from C5 in rheumatoid synovial fluid was derived from the neutrophils themselves,[321] while in nonrheumatoid effusions the C3-directed protease was from the synovial tissue.[322] In other analyses, LTB_4 and C5a were the principal chemotactic factors of synovial fluid from patients with rheumatoid arthritis, while LTB_4 predominated in the spondyloarthritis.[201] Despite the demonstration of additional specific chemotactic factors and inhibitors in synovial fluid and tissue from patients with rheumatoid arthritis, in vitro studies have not provided an adequate explanation for the preferential accumulation of neutrophils in the synovial fluid and of mononuclear leukocytes in synovial tissue. The task of explaining the basis for the neutrophil infiltration in psoriatic skin has led to the discovery of at least two classes of factors which may stimulate neutrophil chemotaxis into the cutaneous lesions. Lipid analyses of extracts of psoriatic plaques have revealed increased levels of arachidonic acid and its lipoxygenase metabolites, especially the chemotactic factors 12-HETE and LTB_4, as compared to uninvolved skin of psoriasis patients and to normal skin.[323] Further, the levels of lipoxygenase metabolites and other arachidonate derivatives were suppressed by topical therapy with corticosteroids. A second neutrophil chemotactic factor identified in psoriatic scales was a protein of molecular weight 12,500 by Sephadex G-75 filtration.[324] The expression of the chemotactic activity of this principal was dependent on the presence of C3 or C5, which suggested it was a protease capable of generating chemotactic fragments from the complement components. This factor may be a portion of the 28,000 molecular weight neutral protease of human skin since the intact protease is present at higher concentrations in psoriatic skin than in normal skin, and has the capacity to generate C5-dependent chemotactic activity by a reaction that is blocked by some esterase inhibitors such as diisopropyl fluorophosphate, soybean trypsin inhibitor, and α_2-macroglobulin.[325]

The chemotactic activity that appears rapidly in synovial fluid during acute gouty attacks is derived largely from the neutrophils phagocytizing monosodium urate crystals. Both human and rabbit granulocytes exposed to monosodium urate or calcium pyrophosphate crystals release an 8400 molecular weight glycoprotein that is chemotactic for neutrophils and mononuclear leukocytes.[326] The factor is not preformed, but appears in the lysosomal granular fraction during phagocytosis. The production and release of the factor require endocytosis of the crystals and are blocked by actinomycin D, colchicine, cytochalasin B, indomethacin, phenylbutazone, and some protease-esterase inhibitors including trasylol and epsilon-aminocaproic acid.[327] This neutrophil-derived factor, like other chemotactic principals, induces chemotactic deactivation and augments the release of lysosomal enzymes from neutrophils in the presence of cytochalasin B. Injection of the purified factor into rabbit joints led to the influx of neutrophils into the synovial tissues, without a significant increase in vascular permeability, as assessed by the rate of transport of circulating ^{125}I-albumin into the joint space. The leukocyte infiltration of the joints injected with the purified chemotactic factor that had been generated in vitro was comparable in magnitude to that seen in joints injected with monosodium urate crystals, but the peak response was achieved at 90 minutes in contrast to over 300 minutes with the crystals.

SPECIAL FUNCTIONS OF THE EOSINOPHIL AND THE SPECTRUM OF HYPEREOSINOPHILIC DISEASES

The eosinophil is a characteristic constituent of the tissue response evoked by immunological reactions of various types. Eosinophils are especially prominent in both the early and late cellular infiltrates of immediate-type hypersensitivity reactions,[328,329] which presumably reflects the release of numerous mast cell–derived eosinophilotactic factors. Eosinophils possess many of the general functional capabilities of neutrophils, which are often expressed at reduced levels relative to those of neutrophils.

Eosinophil granules contain a wide array of enzymes generally comparable to those found in lysosomes of neutrophilic leukocytes, although the human eosinophil lacks lysozyme.[8,9] A number of constituents of the eosinophil, however, are not present in the neutrophil. Eosinophil peroxidase, found in the large granule of the cell, differs physiochemically and functionally from neutrophil myeloperoxidase.[330] The enzyme lysophospholipase, prominent in the eosinophil and associated with eosinophil membranes, is the sole constituent of the distinctive dipyramidal Charcot-Leyden crystals, found in human tissues and fluids, such as sputum and feces, in a number of eosinophilic disease processes.[331,332] Lysophospholipase, which is found in eosinophils and basophils, is absent from neutrophils. In addition, several unique cationic proteins are present in the large granule of the eosinophil, including the major basic protein in the crystalloid core of the granule, eosinophil cationic protein, and another basic protein with neurotoxic properties.[333,334]

Membrane receptors for immunoglobulins and complement components are expressed on the surface of the eosinophil. Receptors for immunoglobulins G and E and for the components of complement C3b and C3d are demonstrable on the plasma membrane of eosinophils.[8,9] In addition, tissue eosinophils also fulfill at least two unique roles in defending the sensitized host. The eosinophil is specially endowed with high concentrations of a range of specific enzymes capable of degrading mediators released by immunologically activated mast cells and basophils. Eosinophil histaminase, like that of the neutrophil, is a diamine oxidase that oxidatively deaminates histamine with a pH optimum of 6.0 to 8.0.[335] Phospholipase D, which is preferentially contained in eosinophils as compared to neutrophils and mononuclear leukocytes degrades some forms of phospholipid PAF with the same pH optimum of 4.5 to 6.0 at which it most efficiently cleaves synthetic phospholipids.[253] Eosinophil-derived peroxidase inactivates LTC_4 by conversion to LTC_4-sulfone and to two 6-trans isomers of LTB_4, in the presence of H_2O_2 and chloride ion.[336] The peroxidatic inactivation of LTC_4 by intact eosinophils is dependent on the stimulation of maximum oxidative activity and is suppressed by sodium azide or catalase. The rate of degradation of LTC_4 by intact eosinophils is far greater than that for the isolated peroxidase, suggesting that intracellular peroxidation may account for the conversion of LTC_4 in vivo. In contrast, the actions of histaminase and phospholipase D on mediators are believed to be dependent on prior degranulation of the eosinophils.

As a further mechanism for the containment of immediate-type hypersensitivity reactions, eosinophils apparently preferentially phagocytose extruded mast cell granules,[337] which avidly retain both macromolecular heparin and a cationic chymotrypsin-like protease that is active while still in the granule.[338] A recently recognized additional capacity of the eosinophil, which bridges its activities in the traditional immune response[339] and its direct functions in host defense, is the IgG antibody–dependent destruction of schistosomulae[340] and schistosoma eggs[341] in vitro that is appreciated as enhanced helminthicidal activity in vivo.[342] The special ability of eosinophils to damage nonphagocytosable parasites may be related to their substantial concentrations of various phospholipases, some of which are associated with the plasma membrane, and to the sustained production and release of high levels of superoxide anion.[343] Other special functions have been proposed for the eosinophil, including preferential phagocytosis of Mycoplasma and soluble immune complexes, predominantly those containing IgE, binding and inactivation of estrogens, and participation in fibrinolytic reactions.[344]

Marked peripheral blood and tissue eosinophilia commonly accompanies allergic and parasitic diseases.[345-348] Eosinophilia in the absence of these precipitating factors, however, is less well defined and has been classified either according to the affected organ system or in terms of the overall clinical presentation. The term hypereosinophilic syndrome[349,350] has been applied to the range of entities within this spectrum which present with involvement of critical organs (Table 9–9). The pulmonary eosinophilias are the most common form and vary from the transient pulmonary infiltrates of Löffler's syndrome to the more chronic lesions associated with endomyocardial fibrosis and cardiac failure.[351,352] In general, Löffler's syndrome, bronchopulmonary aspergillosis, and tropical eosinophilia are responsive to therapy, whereas chronic eosinophilic pneumonitides with substantial abnormalities in pulmonary function, pulmonary eosinophilias with endomyocardial fibrosis, and polyarteritis with pulmonary involvement are more resistant to drug treatment.[350-353]

The extraction of tumor tissues obtained from three subjects with anaplastic squamous cell carcinoma of the lung, associated with peripheral blood hypereosinophilia and eosinophil infiltration of the tumors and surrounding normal lung tissue, led to the recognition of a low molecular weight eosinophil chemotactic peptide which is apparently unique to the tumors.[354] The approximate content of low molecular weight eosinophil chemotactic activity per milligram of tumor tissue was 2 to 35 times the level of activity in normal human lung tissue and far exceeded that in tumors not associated with eosinophilia. Further purification of the tumor-related eosinophil chemotactic factor, obtained from tissue extracts and cell culture supernatants, showed it to be comparable in size to the ECF-A tetrapeptides, but less acidic. Eosinophils from one of the patients were chemotactically unresponsive in vitro during the entire course, while those from a second patient exhibited normal chemotaxis initially but became hyporesponsive to C5 fragments and the tumor-derived factor at a time when the peripheral blood eosinophilia achieved a maximal level and the tumor eosinophil chemotactic factor first was detected in the urine. As the migration of eosinophils from both patients was enhanced by ascorbate, the selective chemotactic unresponsiveness was attributed to in vivo deactivation. In the disseminated hypereosinophilic syndromes and the rare cases of eosinophilic leukemia, the eosinophils exhibit profound morphological abnormal-

Table 9–9. Hypereosinophilic Syndromes

Category	Organ Involvement	Pathological and Clinical Features	Morphological Characteristics of Eosinophils	Therapy
Löffler's syndrome	Transient pulmonary infiltrates	No vascular involvement, bronchospasm in some patients	Normal	Corticosteroids
Chronic eosinophilic pneumonitis	Pulmonary eosinophilic infiltrates	Altered pulmonary mechanics, impaired gas exchange	Normal	Corticosteroids
Tropical eosinophilia	Pulmonary eosinophilic infiltrates	Nocturnal bronchospasm, may be altered pulmonary mechanics	May be vacuolization	Diethylcarbamazine
Pulmonary eosinophilic angiitis	Pulmonary and usually systemic angiitis	Necrotizing granulomatous angiitis with vascular and parenchymal fibrosis; bronchospasm common	Normal	Generally resistant to anti-inflammatory therapy
Löffler's endomyocardial fibrosis	Cardiac and pulmonary eosinophilic infiltrates	Subendocardial eosinophilic infiltration and fibrosis, myocardial failure with early dyskinesis	May be vacuolization and hypogranulation	No specific treatment, related to level and duration of eosinophilic states
Other localized eosinophilias	Diffuse fasciitis with eosinophilia	Fibrosis and chronic inflammation of deep fascia of legs, arms, and trunk, large joint contractures, peripheral blood and variable tissue eosinophilia	Normal	Corticosteroids
Eosinophilia with large cell bronchogenic carcinoma	Tumor, normal pulmonary and cardiac tissue	Local tumor extension, pulmonary and endomyocardial fibrosis	May be vacuolization and hypogranulation	No specific treatment
Disseminated hypereosinophilic syndrome	Cutaneous, lymph node, liver, spleen, cranial and peripheral nerves, pulmonary and cardiac infiltrates	Predominantly adult males, neurological disease and endomyocardial fibrosis frequently fatal	Generally abnormal mature eosinophils	Hydroxyurea
Eosinophilic leukemia	Similar to disseminated hypereosinophilic syndrome	Thrombocytopenia	Increased bone marrow and circulating blasts, eosinophil chromosomal abnormalities	Insufficient experience with any drug

ities and the prognosis for survival of such patients is poor.[350,351] Some of the eosinophil degranulation and vacuolization that have been observed may be secondary to therapy,[355] but studies of eosinophil function have not been performed systematically. Recent evidence supports the use of hydroxyurea as the drug of choice in aggressive hypereosinophilic syndromes.[356]

In the rheumatic diseases, substantial eosinophilia has been found in rheumatoid arthritis, in association with an increased incidence of extra-articular manifestations of disease,[357] polyarteritis with pulmonary involvement,[353] and occasional other states in an acute or accelerated phase. Eosinophilic fasciitis[358] is a localized infiltration of the connective tissues of the upper and lower extremities which may lead to fibrosis and significant functional losses. Thus, while eosinophils predominantly fulfill a protective role, they apparently are capable of injuring host tissues in some inflammatory reactions. As eosinophils, unlike neutrophils, are largely located in tissue spaces below the body surfaces both normally and in allergic and other transient reactive states, their capacity to damage autologous tissues and lead to fibrosis must be dependent not on redistribution, but on special conditions or pathways of activation which are not fully understood.

References

1. Price, G.B., and McCulloch, E.A.: Cell surfaces and the regulation of hemopoiesis. Semin. Hematol. 15:283, 1978.
2. Bradley, T.R., and Metcalf, D.: The growth of mouse bone marrow cells in vitro. Aust. J. Exp. Biol. Med. Sci. 44:287, 1966.
3. Metcalf, D.: Studies on colony formation in vitro by mouse bone marrow cells. I. Continuous cluster formation and relation of clusters to colonies. J. Cell Physiol. 74:323, 1969.
4. Ross, G.D., Jarowski, C.I., Rabellino, E.M., and Winchester, R.J.: The sequential appearance of Ia-like antigens and two different complement receptors during the maturation of human neutrophils. J. Exp. Med. 147:730, 1978.
5. Bainton, D.F.: Differentiation of human neutrophilic granulocytes: Normal and abnormal. In Greenwalt, T.J., and Jamieson, G.A. (eds.): Progress in Clinical and Biological Research. Vol. 13. New York, Alan R. Liss, Inc., 1977.
6. Lichtman, M.A.: Cellular deformability during maturation of the myeloblast. Possible role in marrow egress. N. Engl. J. Med. 283:943, 1970.
7. Cronkite, E.P., and Vincent, P.: Granulocytopoiesis. Ser. Haem. II:3, 1969.
8. Weller, P.F., and Goetzl, E.J.: The regulatory and effector roles of eosinophils. Adv. Immunol. 27:339, 1979.
9. Weller, P.F., and Goetzl, E.J.: The human eosinophil: Roles in host defense and tissue injury. Am. J. Pathol. 100:791, 1980.
10. Snyderman, R., and Goetzl, E.J.: Molecular and cellular mechanisms of leukocyte chemotaxis. Science 213:830, 1981.
11. Boyden, S.: The chemotactic effect of mixtures of antibody and antigen on the polymorphonuclear leukocytes. J. Exp. Med. 115:453, 1962.
12. Wilkinson, P.C., and Allan, R.B.: Assay systems for measuring leukocyte locomotion: An overview. In Gallin, J.I., and Quie, P.G. (eds.): Leukocyte Chemotaxis: Methods, Physiology, and Clinical Implications. New York, Raven Press, 1978.
13. Zigmond, S.H., and Hirsch, J.G.: Leukocyte locomotion and chemotaxis: New methods for evaluation and demonstration of a cell-derived chemotactic factor. J. Exp. Med. 137:387, 1973.
14. Gallin, J.I., Clark, R.A., and Goetzl, E.J.: Radioassay of leukocyte locomotion: A sensitive technique for clinical studies. In Gallin, J.I., and Quie, P.G. (eds.): Leukocyte Chemotaxis: Methods, Physiology, and Clinical Implications. New York, Raven Press, 1978.
15. Goetzl, E.J., and Austen, K.F.: A method for assessing the in vitro chemotactic response of neutrophils utilizing ^{51}Cr-labeled human leukocytes. Immunol. Commun. 1:142, 1972.
16. Nelson, R.D., Quie, P.G., and Simmons, R.L.: Chemotaxis under agarose: A new and simple method for measuring chemotaxis and spontaneous migration of human polymorphonuclear leukocytes and monocytes. J. Immunol. 115:1650, 1975.
17. Revak, S.D., and Cochrane, C.G.: The relationship of structure and

function in human Hageman factor. The association of enzymatic and binding activities with separate regions of the molecule. J. Clin. Invest. 57:852, 1976.

18. Kaplan, A.P., Kay, A.B., and Austen, K.F.: A prealbumin activator of prekallikrein, III. Appearance of chemotactic activity for human neutrophils by the conversion of human prekallikrein to kallikrein. J. Exp. Med. 135:81, 1972.

19. Fernandez, H.N., Henson, P.M., Otani, A., and Hugli, T.E.: Chemotactic response to human C3a and C5a anaphylatoxins. I. Evaluation of C3a and C5a leukotaxin in vitro and under simulated in vivo conditions. J. Immunol. 120:109, 1978.

20. Lachmann, P.J., Kay, A.B., and Thompson, R.A.: The chemotactic activity for neutrophil and eosinophil leukocytes of the trimolecular complex of the fifth, sixth, and seventh components of human complement (C567) prepared in free solution by the "reactive lysis" procedure. Immunology 19:985, 1970.

21. Ruddy, S., Austen, K.F., and Goetzl, E.J.: Chemotactic activity derived from interaction of factors D̄ and B of the properdin pathway with cobra venom factor or C3b. J. Clin. Invest. 55:587, 1975.

22. Kay, A.B., Stechschulte, D.J., and Austen, K.F.: An eosinophil leukocyte chemotactic factor of anaphylaxis. J. Exp. Med. 133:602, 1971.

23. Kay, A.B., and Austen, K.F.: The IgE-mediated release of an eosinophil leukocyte chemotactic factor from human lung. J. Immunol. 107:899, 1971.

24. Goetzl, E.J., and Austen, K.F.: Purification and synthesis of eosinophilotactic tetrapeptides of human lung tissue: Identification as eosinophil chemotactic factor of anaphylaxis. Proc. Natl. Acad. Sci. USA 72:4123, 1975.

25. Valone, F.H., and Goetzl, E.J.: Immunological release in the rat peritoneal cavity of lipid chemotactic and chemokinetic factors for polymorphonuclear leukocytes. J. Immunol. 120:102, 1978.

26. Goetzl, E.J.: Oxygenation products of arachidonic acid as mediators of hypersensitivity and inflammation. Med. Clin. North Am. 65:809, 1981.

27. Goetzl, E.J.: Leukocyte recognition and metabolism of leukotrienes. Fed. Proc., 42:3128, 1983.

28. Richardson, D.L., Pepper, D.S., and Kay, A.B.: Chemotaxis for human monocytes by fibrinogen-derived peptides. Br. J. Haematol. 32:507, 1976.

29. Postlethwaite, A.E., and Kang, A.H.: Collagen- and collagen peptide-induced chemotaxis of human blood monocytes. J. Exp. Med. 143:1299, 1976.

30. Goetzl, E.J., Schreiber, A.D., and Austen, K.F.: Chemotactic activity of components of the kallikrein-kinin and fibrinolytic sequences. *In* Pisano, J. (ed.): Chemistry and Biology of the Kallikrein-Kinin System in Health and Disease, Bethesda, Md., National Institute of Health, 1977.

31. Becker, E.L.: The relationship of the chemotactic behavior of the complement-derived factor C3a, C5a, and C567 and a bacterial factor to their ability to activate the proesterase 1 of rabbit polymorphonuclear leukocytes. J. Exp. Med. 135:376, 1972.

32. Altman, L.C.: Chemotactic lymphokines: A review. *In* Gallin, J.I., and Quie, P.G. (eds.): Leukocyte Chemotaxis: Methods, Physiology, and Clinical Implications. New York, Raven Press, 1978.

33. Tainer, J.A., Turner, S.R., and Lynn, W.S.: New aspects of chemotaxis: Specific target cell attraction by lipid and lipoprotein fractions of *Escherichia coli* chemotactic factor. Am. J. Pathol. 81:401, 1975.

34. Turner, S.R., Tainer, J.A., and Lynn, W.S.: Biogenesis of chemotactic molecules by the arachidonic lipoxygenase system of platelets. Nature 257:680, 1975.

35. Goetzl, E.J., Woods, J.M., and Gorman, R.R.: Stimulation of human eosinophil and neutrophil polymorphonuclear leukocyte chemotaxis and random migration by 12-L-hydroxy-5,8,10,14-eicosatetraenoic acid (HETE). J. Clin. Invest. 59:179, 1977.

36. Goetzl, E.J., and Gorman, R.R.: Chemotactic and chemokinetic stimulation of human eosinophils and neutrophil polymorphonuclear leukocytes by 12-L-hydroxy-5,8,10-heptadecatrienoic acid (HHT). J. Immunol. 120:526, 1978.

37. Goetzl, E.J.: Modulation of human eosinophil polymorphonuclear leukocyte migration and function. Am. J. Pathol. 95:419, 1976.

38. Kay, A.B., and Austen, K.F.: Chemotaxis of human basophil leukocytes. Clin. Exp. Immunol. 11:557, 1972.

39. Goetzl, E.J., Wasserman, S.I., and Austen, K.F.: Modulation of the eosinophil chemotactic response in immediate hypersensitivity. *In* Brent, L., and Holborow, J. (eds.): Progress in Immunology II. Vol. 4. Amsterdam, North-Holland Publishing Company, 1974.

40. Valotta, E.H., and Müller-Eberhard, H.J.: Formation of C3a and C5a anaphylatoxins in whole serum after inhibition of the anaphylatoxin inactivator. J. Exp. Med. 137:1109, 1973.

41. Berenberg, J.L., and Ward, P.A.: The chemotactic factor inactivator in normal human serum. J. Clin. Invest. 52:1200, 1973.

42. Till, G., and Ward, P.A.: Two distinct chemotactic factor inactivators in normal human serum. J. Immunol. 114:843, 1975.

43. Wright, D.G., and Gallin, J.I.: Modulation of the inflammatory response by products released from human polymorphonuclear leukocytes during phagocytosis: Generation and inactivation of the chemotactic factor C5a. Inflammation 1:23, 1975.

44. Ward, P.A., and Becker, E.L.: The deactivation of rabbit neutrophils by chemotactic factor and the nature of the activatable esterase. J. Exp. Med. 127:693, 1968.

45. Ward, P.A., and Becker, E.L.: Biochemical demonstration of the activatable esterase of the rabbit neutrophil involved in the chemotactic response. J. Immunol. 105:1057, 1970.

46. Caner, J.E.Z.: Colchicine inhibition of chemotaxis. Arthritis Rheum. 8:757, 1965.

47. Becker, E.L., Davis, A.T., Estensen, R.D., and Quie, P.G.: Cytochalasin B: IV, Inhibition and stimulation of chemotaxis of rabbit and human polymorphonuclear leukocytes. J. Immunol. 108:396, 1972.

48. Zurier, R.B., Weissman, G., Hoffstein, S., Kammerman, S., and Tai, H.H.: Mechanism of lysosomal enzyme release from human leukocytes. II. Effects of cyclic AMP and cyclic GMP, autonomic agents, and agents which affect microtubule function. J. Clin. Invest. 53:297, 1974.

49. Zurier, R.B., Hoffstein, S., and Weissman, G.: Cytochalasin B: Effect on lysosomal enzyme release from human leukocytes. Proc. Natl. Acad. Sci. USA 70:844, 1973.

50. Becker, E.L., Showell, H.J., Henson, P.M., and Hsu, L.S.: The ability of chemotactic factors to induce lysosomal enzyme release: I. The characteristics of the release, the importance of surfaces and the relation of the enzyme release to chemotactic responsiveness. J. Immunol. 112:2047, 1974.

51. Björksten, B., Ray, C., and Quie, P.G.: Inhibition of human neutrophil chemotaxis and chemiluminescence by amphotericin B. Infect. Immun. 14:315, 1976.

52. Hatch, G.E., Nichols, W.K., and Hill, H.R.: Cyclic nucleotide changes in human neutrophils induced by chemoattractants and chemotactic modulators. J. Immunol. 119:450, 1976.

53. Hill, H.R., Estensen, R.D., Quie, P.G., Hogan, N.A., and Goldberg, N.D.: Modulation of human neutrophil chemotactic responses by cyclic 3',5' guanosine monophosphate and cyclic 3',5' adenosine monophosphate. Metabolism 24:447, 1975.

54. Goetzl, E.J., Wasserman, S.I., Gigli, I., and Austen, K.F.: Enhancement of random migration and chemotactic response of human leukocytes by ascorbic acid. J. Clin. Invest. 53:813, 1974.

55. Sandler, J.A., Gallin, J.I., and Vaughan, M.: Effects of serotonin, carbamylcholine, and ascorbic acid on leukocyte cyclic GMP and chemotaxis. J. Cell Biol. 67:480, 1975.

56. Boxer, L.A., Watanage, A.M., Rister, M., Besch, H.R., Jr., Allen, J., and Baehner, R.L.: Correction of leukocyte function in Chédjak-Higashi syndrome by ascorbate. N. Engl. J. Med. 295:1041, 1976.

57. Foster, C.S., and Goetzl, E.J.: Impaired neutrophil and monocyte chemotaxis in a patient with atopy, hyperimmunoglobulinemia E and recurrent infection: Effects of ascorbate therapy. Arch. Ophthalmol. 96:2069, 1978.

58. Watt, K.W.K., Brightman, I.L., and Goetzl, E.J.: Isolation of two polypeptides comprising the neutrophil-immobilizing factor of human leukocytes. Immunology 48:79, 1983.

59. Goetzl, E.J., and Austen, K.F.: A neutrophil immobilizing factor derived from human leukocytes. I. Generation and partial characterization. J. Exp. Med. 136:1564, 1972.

60. Goetzl, E.J., Gigli, I., Wasserman, S.I., and Austen, K.F.: A neutrophil immobilizing factor derived from human leukocytes. II. Specificity of action on polymorphonuclear leukocyte mobility. J. Immunol. 111:938, 1973.

61. Goetzl, E.J.: Modulation of human neutrophil polymorphonuclear leukocyte migration of human plasma alpha-globulin inhibitors and synthetic esterase inhibitors. Immunology 29:1419, 1973.

62. Weksler, B.B., and Coupal, C.E.: Platelet-dependent generation of chemotactic activity in serum. J. Exp. Med. 137:1419, 1973.

63. Samuelsson, B., Hamberg, M., Malmsten, C., and Svensson, J.: The role of prostaglandin endoperoxides and thromboxanes in platelet aggregation. *In* Samuelsson, B., and Paoletti, R. (eds.): Advances in Prostaglandin and Thromboxane Research, Vol. 2. New York, Raven Press, 1976.

64. Rocklin, R.E.: Products of activated lymphocytes: Leukocyte inhibitory factor (LIF) distinct from migration inhibitory factor (MIF). J. Immunol. 112:1461, 1974.

65. Rocklin, R.E.: Partial characterization of leukocyte inhibitory factor by concanavalin A–stimulated human lymphocytes (LIF con A). J. Immunol. 114:1161, 1975.

66. Goetzl, E.J., and Rocklin, R.E.: Amplification of the activity of human leukocyte inhibitory factor (LIF) by the generation of a low molecular weight inhibitor of PMN leukocyte chemotaxis, J. Immunol. 121:891, 1978.

67. Craddock, P.R., White, J.G., and Jacob, H.S.: Potentiation of complement

(C5a)-induced granulocyte aggregation by cytochalasin B. J. Lab. Clin. Med. 91:490, 1978.

68. Showell, H.J., Freer, R.J., Zigmond, S.H., Shiffman, E., Aswanikumar, S., Corcoran, B., and Becker, E.L.: The structure-activity relations of synthetic peptides as chemotactic factors and inducers of lysosomal enzyme secretion of neutrophils. J. Exp. Med. 143:1154, 1976.

69. Anwar, A.R.E., and Kay, A.B.: The ECF-A tetrapeptides and histamine selectivity enhance human eosinophil complement receptors. Nature 269:522, 1977.

70. Wright, A.E., and Douglas, S.R.: An experimental investigation of the role of blood fluids in connection with phagocytosis. Proc. R. Soc. Lond. Biol. 72:357, 1903.

71. Bokisch, V.A., Dierich, M.P., and Müller-Eberhard, H.J.: Third component of complement (C3): Structural properties in relation to functions. Proc. Natl. Acad. Sci. USA 72:1989, 1975.

72. Cline, M.J., and Lehrer, R.I.: Phagocytosis by human monocytes. Blood 32:423, 1968.

73. Henson, P.M.: The adherence of leukocytes and platelets induced by fixed IgG antibody or complement. Immunology 16:107, 1969.

74. Lay, W.H., and Nussenzweig, V.: Receptors for complement on leukocytes. J. Exp. Med. 128:991, 1968.

75. Phillips-Quagliata, J.M., Levine, B.B., and Uhr, J.W.: Studies on the mechanism of binding of immune complexes to phagocytes. Nature (Lond.) 222:1290, 1969.

76. Messner, R.P., and Jelinek, J.: Receptors for human γG globulin on human neutrophils. J. Clin. Invest. 49:2165, 1970.

77. Boxer, L.A., Richardson, S.B., and Baehner, R.L.: Effects of surface-active agents on neutrophil receptors. Infect. Immun. 21:28, 1978.

78. Klempner, M.S., and Gallin, J.I.: Separation and functional characterization of human neutrophil subpopulations. Blood 51:659, 1978.

79. Sajnani, A.N., Ranadive, N.S., and Movat, H.Z.: The visualization of receptors for the Fc portion of the IgG molecule on human neutrophil leukocytes. Life Sci. 14:2427, 1974.

80. Sajnani, A.N., Ranadive, N.S., and Movat, H.Z.: Redistribution of immunoglobulin receptors on human neutrophils and its relationship to the release of lysosomal enzymes. Lab. Invest. 35:143, 1976.

81. Lawrence, D.A., Weigle, W.O., and Spiegelberg, H.L.: Immunoglobulins cytophilic for human lymphocytes, monocytes, and neutrophils. J. Clin. Invest. 55:368, 1975.

82. Walker, W.S.: Separate Fc receptors for immunoglobulin IgG2a and IgG2b on an established cell line of mouse macrophages. J. Immunol. 116:911, 1976.

83. Henson, P.M., Johnson, H.B., and Spiegelberg, H.L.: The release of granule enzymes from human neutrophils stimulated by aggregated immunoglobulins of different classes and subclasses. J. Immunol. 109:1182, 1972.

84. Schlessinger, J., Steinberg, I.Z., Givol, D., Hochman, J., and Pecht, I.: Antigen-induced conformational changes in antibodies and their Fab fragments studies by circular polarization of fluorescence. Proc. Natl. Acad. Sci. USA 72:2775, 1975.

85. An, T.: Fc receptors on human neutrophils: electron microscopic study of natural surface distribution. Immunology 40:1, 1980.

86. Loube, S.R., McNabb, T.C., and Dorrington, K.J.: Isolation of an Fc γ-binding protein from the cell membrane of a macrophage-like cell line (P388D₁) after detergent solubilization. J. Immunol. 120:709, 1978.

87. Kulczycki, A. Jr., Solanki, L., and Cohen, I.: Isolation and partial characterization of Fc γ-binding proteins of human leukocytes. J. Clin. Invest. 68:1558, 1981.

88. Ward, H.K., and Enders, J.F.: An analysis of the opsonic and tropic action of normal and immune sera based on experiments with the pneumococcus. J. Exp. Med. 57:527, 1933.

89. Nelson, D.S.: Immune adherence. In Wolstenholme, G.E.W., and Knight, J. (eds.): Ciba Foundation Symposium: Complement. Boston, Little, Brown and Co., 1965.

90. Mantovani, B.: Different roles of IgG and complement receptors in phagocytosis by polymorphonuclear leukocytes. J. Immunol. 115:15, 1975.

91. Gigli, I., and Nelson, R.A.: Complement dependent immune phagocytosis. I. Requirements for C'1, C'4, C'2, C'3. Exp. Cell Res. 51:45,1968.

92. Scribner, D.J., and Fahrney, D.: Neutrophil receptors for IgG and complement: Their roles in the attachment and ingestion phases of phagocytosis. J. Immunol. 116:892, 1976.

93. Ehlenberger, A.G., and Nussenzweig, V.: The role of membrane receptors for C3b and C3d in phagocytosis. J. Exp. Med. 145:357, 1977.

94. Pross, S.H., Hallock, J.A., Armstrong, R., and Fishel, C.W.: Complement and Fc receptors on cord blood and adult neutrophils. Pediatr. Res. 11:135, 1977.

95. Stossel, T.P.: Quantitative studies of phagocytosis. Kinetic effects of cations and heat-labile opsonin. J. Cell Biol. 58:346, 1973.

96. Stossel, T.P., Alper, C.A., and Rosen, F.S.: Serum-dependent phagocytosis of paraffin oil emulsified with bacterial lipopolysaccharide. J. Exp. Med. 137:690, 1973.

97. Guckian, J.C., Christensen, W.D., and Fine, D.P.: Trypan blue inhibits

complement-mediated phagocytosis by human polymorphonuclear leukocytes. J. Immunol. 120:1580, 1978.

98. Fearon, D.T.: Identification of the membrane glycoprotein that is the C3b receptor of the human erythrocyte, polymorphonuclear leukocyte, B lymphocyte and monocyte. J. Exp. Med. 152:20, 1980.

99. Fearon, D.T., Kaneko, I., and Thomson, G.G.: Membrane distribution and adsorptive endocytosis by C3b receptors on human polymorphonuclear leukocytes. J. Exp. Med. 153:1615, 1981.

100. Ross, G.D., and Lambris, J.D.: Identification of a C3bi specific membrane complement receptor that is expressed on lymphocytes, monocytes, neutrophils, and erythrocytes. J. Exp. Med. 155:96, 1982.

101. Moore, P.L., Bank, H.L., Brissie, N.T., and Spicer, S.S.: Phagocytosis of bacteria by polymorphonuclear leukocytes. A freeze-fracture, scanning electron microscope, and thin-section investigation of membrane structure. J. Cell Biol. 76:158, 1978.

102. Karnovsky, M.L.: The metabolism of leukocytes. Semin. Hematol. 5:156, 1968.

103. Boxer, L.A., and Stossel, T.P.: Interactions of actin, myosin and an actin-binding protein of chronic myelogenous leukemia granulocytes. J. Clin. Invest. 56:964, 1976.

104. Stossel, T.P., Field, R.J., Gitlin, J.D., Alper, C.A., and Rosen, F.S.: The opsonic fragment of the third component of human complement (C3). J. Exp. Med 141:1329, 1975.

105. Patriarca, P., Cramer, R., Moncalvo, S., Rossi, F., and Romeo, D.: Enzymatic basis of metabolic stimulation in leukocytes during phagocytosis: the role of activated NADPH oxidase. Arch. Biochem. Biophys. 145:255, 1971.

106. Tagesson, C., Magnusson, K.-E., and Stendahl, O.: Physicochemical consequences of opsonization: perturbation of liposomal membranes by Salmonella typhimurium 395 MS opsonized with IgG antibodies. J. Immunol. 119:609, 1977.

107. Stendahl, O., Hed, J., Kihlstrom, E., Magnusson, K.-E., and Tagesson, C.: Phagocytic internalization and the requirement for membrane perturbation. FEBS Lett. 81:118, 1977.

108. Griffin, F.M. Jr., Griffin, J.A., Leider, J.E., and Silverstein, S.C.: Studies on the mechanism of phagocytosis. I. Requirements for circumferential attachment of particle-bound ligands to specific receptors on the macrophage plasma membrane. J. Exp. Med. 142:1263, 1975.

109. de Duve, C., Pressman, B.C., Gianetto, R., Wattiaux, R., and Appelmans, F.: Tissue fractionation studies. 6. Intracellular distribution patterns of enzymes in rat liver tissue. Biochem. J. 60:604, 1955.

110. Bainton, D.F., Ullyot, J.L., and Farquhar, M.G.: The development of neutrophilic polymorphonuclear leukocytes in human bone marrow. Origin and content of azurophil and specific granules. J. Exp. Med. 134:907, 1971.

111. Spitznagel, J.K., Dalldorf, M.G., Leffell, M.S., Folds, J.D., Welsh, I.R.H., Conney, M.H., and Martin, L.E.: Character of azurophil and specific granules purified from human polymorphonuclear leukocytes. Lab. Invest. 30:774, 1974.

112. West, B.C., Rosenthal, A.S., Gelb, N.A., and Kimball, H.R.: Separation and characterization of human neutrophil granules. Am. J. Pathol. 77:41, 1974.

113. Dewald, B., Bretz, U., and Baggiolini, M.: Release of gelatinase from a novel secretory compartment of human neutrophils. J. Clin. Invest. 70:518, 1982.

114. Zeya, H.I., and Spitznagel, J.K.: Characterization of cationic protein-bearing granules of polymorphonuclear leukocytes. Lab. Invest. 24:229, 1971.

115. Folds, J.D., Welsh, I.R.H., and Spitznagel, J.K.: Neutral proteases confined to one class of lysosomes of human polymorphonuclear leukocytes. Proc. Soc. Exp. Biol. Med. 139:461, 1972.

116. Leffell, M.S., and Spitznagel, J.K.: Association of lactoferrin with lysozyme in granules of human polymorphonuclear leukocytes. Infect. Immun. 6:761, 1972.

117. Murphy, G., Bretz, U., Baggiolini, M., and Reynolds, J.J.: The latent collagenase and gelatinase of human polymorphonuclear neutrophil leukocytes. Biochem. J. 192:517, 1980.

118. Kane, S.P., and Peters, T.J.: Analytical subcellular fractionation of human granulocytes with reference to the localization of vitamin B₁₂-binding proteins. Clin. Sci. Mol. Med. 49:171, 1975.

119. Goldstein, I.M.: Lysosomal hydrolases and inflammatory materials. In Weissmann, G.(ed.): Mediators of Inflammation. New York, Plenum Press, 1973.

120. Goldstein, I.M.: Polymorphonuclear leukocyte lysosomes and immune tissue injury. Prog. Allergy 20:301, 1976.

121. Babior, B.M.: Oxygen-dependent microbial killing by phagocytes. N. Engl. J. Med. 298:659, 1978.

122. Weissmann, G., Smolen, J.E., and Korchak, H.M.: Release of inflammatory mediators from stimulated neutrophils. N. Engl. J. Med. 303:27, 1980.

123. Weissmann, G.: Activation of neutrophils and the lesions of rheumatoid arthritis. J. Lab. Clin. Med. 100:322, 1982.

124. Straus, W.: Occurrence of phagosomes and phagolysosomes in different segments of the nephron in relation to the reabsorption, transport, digestion, and extrusion of intravenously injected horseradish peroxidase. J. Cell Biol. 21:295, 1964.

125. Hirsch, J.G., and Cohn, Z.A.: Degranulation of polymorphonuclear leukocytes following phagocytosis of microorganisms. J. Exp. Med. 112:1005, 1960.

126. Densen, P., and Mandell, G.L.: Gonococcal interactions with polymorphonuclear neutrophils. Importance of the phagosome for bactericidal activity. J. Clin. Invest. 62:1161, 1978.

127. Stossel, T.P., Pollard, T.D., Mason, R.J., and Vaughan, M.: Isolation and properties of phagocytic vesicles from polymorphonuclear leukocytes. J. Clin. Invest. 50:1745, 1971.

128. Leffell, M.S., and Spitznagel, J.K.: Intracellular and extracellular degranulation of human polymorphonuclear azurophil and specific granules induced by immune complexes. Infect. Immun. 10:1241, 1974.

129. Bainton, D.F.: Sequential degranulation of the two types of polymorphonuclear leukocyte granules during phagocytosis of microorganisms. J. Cell Biol. 58:249, 1973.

130. Leffell, M.S., and Spitznagel, J.K.: Fate of human lactoferrin and myeloperoxidase in phagocytizing human neutrophils: effects of immunoglobulin G subclasses and immune complexes on latex beads. Infect. Immun. 12:813, 1975.

131. Bentwood, B.J., and Henson, P.M.: The sequential release of granule constituents from human neutrophils. J. Immunol. 124:855, 1980.

132. Wright, D.G., Bralove, D.A., and Gallin, J.I.: The differential mobilization of human neutrophil granules. Effects of phorbol myristate acetate and ionophore A23187. Am. J. Pathol. 87:273, 1977.

133. Wright, D.G., and Gallin, J.I.: Secretory responses of human neutrophils: exocytosis of specific (secondary) granules by human neutrophils during adherence in vitro and during exudation in vivo. J. Immunol. 123:285, 1979.

134. Nachman, R., Hirsch, J.G., and Baggiolini, M.: Studies on isolated membranes of azurophil and specific granules from rabbit polymorphonuclear leukocytes. J. Cell Biol. 54:133, 1972.

135. Weissmann, G., Hirschhorn, R., and Krakauer, K.: Effect of mellitin upon cellular and lysosomal membranes. Biochem. Pharmacol. 18:1771, 1969.

136. de Duve, C., and Wattiaux, R.: Functions of lysosomes. Annu. Rev. Physiol. 28:435, 1966.

137. Weissmann, G., Zurier, R.B., Spieler, P.J., and Goldstein, I.M.: Mechanisms of lysosomal enzyme release from leukocytes exposed to immune complexes and other particles. J. Exp. Med. 134:148s, 1971.

138. Weissmann, G., Zurier, R.B., and Hoffstein, S.: Leukocytic proteases and the immunologic release of lysosomal enzymes. Am. J. Pathol. 68:539, 1972.

139. Weissmann, G., and Rita, G.A.: Molecular basis of gouty inflammation: interaction of monosodium urate crystals with lysosomes and liposomes. Nature New Biol. 240:167, 1972.

140. Schumacher, H.R., and Phelps, P.: Sequential changes in human polymorphonuclear leukocytes after urate crystal phagocytosis. An electron microscopic study. Arthritis Rheum. 14:513, 1971.

141. Allison, A.C., Harrington, J.S., and Birbeck, M.: An examination of the cytotoxic effects of silica on macrophages. J. Exp. Med. 124:141, 1968.

142. Hawkins, D.: Neutrophilic leukocytes in immunological reactions. Evidence for the selective release of lysosomal constituents. J. Immunol. 108:310, 1972.

143. Henson, P.M.: Interaction of cells with immune complexes. Adherence, release of constituents, and tissue injury. J. Exp. Med. 134:114s, 1971.

144. Henson, P.M.: Pathologic mechanisms in neutrophil-mediated injury. Am. J. Pathol. 68:593, 1972.

145. Henson, P.M., and Oades, Z.G.: Stimulation of human neutrophils by soluble and insoluble immunoglobulin aggregates. Secretion of granule constituents and increased oxidation of glucose. J. Clin. Invest. 56:1053, 1975.

146. Goldstein, I.M., Roos, D., Weissmann, G., and Kaplan, H.: Complement and immunoglobulins stimulate superoxide production by human leukocytes independently of phagocytosis. J. Clin. Invest. 56:1155, 1975.

147. Wright, D.G., and Malawista, S.E.: The mobilization and extracellular release of granular enzymes from human leukocytes during phagocytosis. J. Cell Biol. 53:788, 1972.

148. Zurier, R.B., Hoffstein, S., and Weissmann, G.: Mechanisms of lysosomal enzyme release from leukocytes. I. Effect of cyclic nucleotides and colchicine. J. Cell Biol. 58:27, 1973.

149. Johnston, R.B. Jr., and Lehmeyer, J.E.: Elaboration of toxic oxygen byproducts by neutrophils in a model of immune complex disease. J. Clin. Invest. 57:836, 1976.

150. Henson, P.M.: The immunologic release of constituents from neutrophil leukocytes. I. The role of antibody and complement on nonphagocytosable surfaces or phagocytosable particles. J. Immunol. 107:1535, 1971.

151. Carter, S.B.: Effects of cytochalasin on mammalian cells. Nature (Lond.) 213:261, 1967.

152. Hartwig, J.H., and Stossel, T.P.: Interactions of actin, myosin, and an actin-binding protein of rabbit pulmonary macrophages. III. Effects of cytochalasin B. J. Cell Biol. 71:295, 1976.

153. Plagemann, P.G.W., and Estensen, R.D.: Cytochalasin B. VI. Competitive inhibition of nucleotide transport by cultured Novikoff rat hepatoma cells. J. Cell Biol. 55:179, 1972.

154. Zigmond, S.H., and Hirsch, J.G.: Effects of cytochalasin B on polymorphonuclear leukocyte locomotion, phagocytosis, and glycolysis. Exp. Cell Res. 73:383, 1972.

155. Becker, E.L.: Some interrelationships of neutrophil chemotaxis, lysosomal enzyme secretion, and phagocytosis as revealed by synthetic peptides. Am. J. Pathol. 85:385, 1976.

156. Goldstein, I., Hoffstein, S., Gallin J., and Weissmann, G.: Mechanisms of lysosomal enzyme release from human leukocytes: microtubule assembly and membrane fusion induced by a component of complement. Proc. Natl. Acad. Sci. USA 70:2916, 1973.

157. Hawkins, D.: Neutrophilic leukocytes in immunologic reactions in vitro. Effect of cytochalasin B. J. Immunol. 110:294, 1973.

158. Stenson, W.F., and Parker, C.W.: Monohydroxyeicosatetraenoic acids (HETEs) induce degranulation of human neutrophils. J. Immunol. 124:2100, 1980.

159. O'Flaherty, J.T., Wykle, R.L., Lees, C.J., Shewmake, T., McCall, C.E., and Thomas, M.J.: Neutrophil degranulating action of 5,12-dihydroxy-6,8,10,14-eicosatetraenoic acid and 1-O-alkyl-2-O-acetyl-sn-glycero-3-phosphocholine. Am. J. Pathol. 105:264, 1981.

160. Estensen, R.D., White, J.G., and Holmes, B.: Specific degranulation of human polymorphonuclear leukocytes. Nature (Lond.) 248:347, 1974.

161. Goldstein, I.M., Hoffstein, S.T., and Weissmann, G.: Mechanisms of lysosomal enzyme release from human polymorphonuclear leukocytes. Effects of phorbol myristate acetate. J. Cell Biol. 66:647, 1975.

162. Goldstein, I.M., Horn, J.K., Kaplan, H.B., and Weissmann, G.: Calcium-induced lysozyme secretion from human polymorphonuclear leukocytes. Biochem. Biophys. Res. Commun. 60:807, 1974.

163. Goldstein, I.M., Hoffstein, S.T., and Weissmann, G.: Influence of divalent cations upon complement-mediated enzyme release from human polymorphonuclear leukocytes. J. Immunol. 115:665, 1975.

164. Hoffstein, S., Soberman, R., Goldstein, I., and Weissmann, G.: Concanavalin A induces microtubule assembly and specific granule discharge in human polymorphonuclear leukocytes. J. Cell Biol. 68:781, 1976.

165. Goldstein, I.M., Cerqueira, M., Lind, S., and Kaplan, H.B.: Evidence that the superoxide generating system of human leukocytes is associated with the cell surface. J. Clin. Invest. 59:249, 1977.

166. Iverson, D., DeChatelet, L.R., Spitznagel, J.K., and Wang, P.: Comparison of NADH and NADPH oxidase activities in granules isolated from human polymorphonuclear leukocytes with a fluorometric assay. J. Clin. Invest. 59:282, 1977.

167. Tauber, A.I., and Goetzl, E.J.: Structural and catalytic properties of the solubilized superoxide-generating activity of human polymorphonuclear leukocytes. I. Solubilization, stabilization in solution, and partial characterization. Biochemistry 18:5576, 1979.

168. Root, R.K., and Metcalf, J.A.: H_2O_2 release from human granulocytes during phagocytosis. Relationship to superoxide anion formation and cellular catabolism of H_2O_2: studies with normal and cytochalasin B-treated cells. J. Clin. Invest. 60:1266, 1977.

169. Root, R.K., Metcalf, J., Oshino, N., and Chance, B.: H_2O_2 release from human granulocytes during phagocytosis. I. Documentation, quantitation, and some regulating factors. J. Clin. Invest. 55:945, 1975.

170. Tauber, A.I., and Babior, B.M.: Evidence for hydroxyl radical production by human neutrophils. J. Clin. Invest. 60:374, 1977.

171. Krinsky, N.I.: Singlet excited oxygen as a mediator of the antibacterial action of leukocytes. Science 186:363, 1974.

172. Root, R.K., and Stossel, T.P.: Myeloperoxidase-mediated iodination by granulocytes. Intracellular site of operation and some regulating factors. J. Clin. Invest. 53:1207, 1974.

173. Klebanoff, S.J.: Iodination of bacteria: a bactericidal mechanism. J. Exp. Med. 126:1063, 1967.

174. Baehner, R.L., Boxer, L.A., and Davis, J.: The biochemical basis of nitroblue tetrazolium reduction in normal human and chronic granulomatous disease polymorphonuclear leukocytes. Blood 48:309, 1976.

175. DeChatelet, L.R.: Oxidative bactericidal mechanisms of polymorphonuclear leukocytes. J. Infect. Dis. 131:295, 1975.

176. Goetzl, E.J., and Austen, K.F.: Stimulation of human neutrophil leukocyte aerobic glucose metabolism by purified chemotactic factors. J. Clin. Invest. 53:591, 1974.

Goldstein, I.M., Kaplan, H.B., Radin, A., and Frosch, M.: Independent effects of IgG and complement upon human polymorphonuclear leukocyte function. J. Immunol. 117:1282, 1976.

178. Kaplan, S.S., Finch, S.C., and Basford, R.E.: Polymorphonuclear leukocyte activation: effects of phospholipase c. Proc. Soc. Exp. Biol. Med. 140:540, 1972.

179. DeChatelet, L.R., Shirley, P.S., and Johnston, R.B., Jr.: Effect of phorbol myristate acetate on the oxidative metabolism of human polymorphonuclear leukocytes. Blood. 47:545, 1976.
180. Cohen, H.J., and Chovaniec, M.E.: Superoxide generation by digitonin-stimulated guinea pig granulocytes. A basis for a continuous assay for monitoring superoxide production for the study of the activation of the generating system. J. Clin. Invest. 61:1081, 1978.
181. Salin, M.C., and McCord, J.M.: Superoxide dismutases in polymorphonuclear leukocytes. J. Clin. Invest. 54:1005, 1974.
182. Lynch, R.E., and Fridovich, I.: Effects of superoxide on the erythrocyte membrane. J. Biol. Chem. 253:1838, 1978.
183. Salin, M.C., and McCord, J.M.: Free radicals and inflammation. Protection of phagocytosing leukocytes by superoxide dismutase. J. Clin. Invest. 56:1319, 1975.
184. Sacks, T., Moldow, C.F., Craddock, P.R., Bowers, T.K., and Jacob, H.S.: Oxygen radicals mediate endothelial cell damage by complement-stimulated granulocytes: An in vitro model of immune vascular damage. J. Clin. Invest. 62:1161, 1978.
185. McCord, J.M.: Free radicals and inflammation: protection of synovial fluid by superoxide dismutase. Science 185:529, 1974.
186. Moore, J.S., Phillips, G.O., Davies, J.V., and Dodgson, K.S.: Reactions of connective tissue and related polyanions with hydrated electrons and hydroxyl radicals. Carbohyd. Res. 12:253, 1970.
187. Halliwell, B.: Superoxide-dependent formation of hydroxyl radicals in the presence of iron salts. Its role in degradation of hyaluronic acid by a superoxide-generating system. FEBS Lett. 96:238, 1978.
188. Greenwald, R.A., and Moy, W.W.: Effect of oxygen-derived free radicals on hyaluronic acid. Arthritis Rheum. 23:455, 1980.
189. Puig-Parellada, P., and Planas, J.M.: Synovial fluid degradation induced by free radicals: in vitro action of several free radical scavengers and anti-inflammatory drugs. Biochem. Pharmacol. 27:535, 1978.
190. McCord, J.M., and Fridovich, I.: Superoxide dismutase. An enzymic function for erythrocuprein (hemocuprein). J. Biol. Chem. 244:6049, 1969.
191. Blake, D.R., Hall, N.D., Treby, D.A., Halliwell, B., and Gutteridge, J.M.C.: Protection against superoxide and hydrogen peroxide in synovial fluid from rheumatoid patients. Clin. Sci. 61:483, 1981.
192. Rister, M., and Bauermeister, K.: Superoxide-dismutase and superoxide-radical-release in rheumatoid arthritis. Klin. Wochenschr. 60:561, 1982.
193. Greenwald, R.A., and Moy, W.W.: Inhibition of collagen gelation by action of the superoxide radical. Arthritis Rheum. 22:251, 1979.
194. Venkatasubramanian, K., and Joseph, K.T.: Action of singlet oxygen on collagen. Ind. J. Biochem. Biophys. 14:217, 1977.
195. Carp, H., and Janoff, A.: Potential mediator of inflammation. Phagocyte-derived oxidants suppress the elastase-inhibitory capacity of α_1-proteinase inhibitor in vitro. J. Clin. Invest. 66:987, 1980.
196. Johnson, D., and Travis, J.: The oxidative inactivation of human α-1-proteinase inhibitor: further evidence for methionine at the reactive center. J. Biol. Chem. 254:4022, 1979.
197. Wong, P.S., and Travis, J.: Isolation and properties of oxidized α-1-proteinase inhibitor from human rheumatoid synovial fluid. Biochem. Biophys. Res. Commun. 96:1449, 1980.
198. Tien, M., Svingen, B.A., and Aust, S.D.: An investigation into the role of hydroxyl radical in xanthine oxidase–dependent lipid peroxidation. Arch. Biochem. Biophys. 216:142, 1982.
199. Rawls, H.R., and van Santen, P.J.: A possible role for singlet oxygen in the initiation of fatty acid autoxidation. J. Am. Oil Chem. Soc. 47:121, 1969.
200. Kellogg, E.W. III, and Fridovich, I.: Superoxide, hydrogen peroxide, and singlet oxygen in lipid peroxidation by a xanthine oxidase system. J. Biol. Chem. 250:8812, 1975.
201. Klickstein, L.B., Shapleigh, C., and Goetzl, E.J.: Lipoxygenation of arachidonic acid as a source of polymorphonuclear leukocyte chemotactic factors in synovial fluid and tissue in rheumatoid arthritis and spondyloarthritis. J. Clin. Invest. 66:1166, 1980.
202. Turner, S.R., Campbell, J.A., and Lynn, W.S.: Polymorphonuclear leukocyte chemotaxis toward oxidized lipid components of cell membranes. J. Exp. Med. 141:437, 1975.
203. Perez, H.D., Weksler, B.B., and Goldstein, I.M.: Generation of a chemotactic lipid from arachidonic acid by exposure to a superoxide-generating system. Inflammation 4:313, 1980.
204. Petrone, W.F., English, D.K., Wong, K., and McCord, J.M.: Free radicals and inflammation: superoxide-dependent activation of a neutrophil chemotactic factor in plasma. Proc. Natl. Acad. Sci. USA 77:1159, 1980.
205. Fridovich, I.: Superoxide dismutases. Annu. Rev. Biochem. 44:147, 1975.
206. Huber, W., Schulte, T.L., Carson, S., Goldhamer, R.E., and Vogin, E.E.: Some chemical and pharmacological properties of a novel antiinflammatory protein. Toxicol. Appl. Pharmacol. 12:308, 1968.
207. Huber, W., and Saifer, M.G.P.: Orgotein, the drug version of bovine Cu-Zn superoxide dismutase: I. A summary account of safety and pharmacology in laboratory animals. In Michelson, A.M., McCord, J.M.,

and Fridovich, I. (eds.): Superoxide and Superoxide Dismutases. London, Academic Press, 1977.
208. Oyanagui, Y.: Participation of superoxide anions at the prostaglandin phase of carrageenan foot-oedema. Biochem. Pharmacol. 25:1465, 1976.
209. McCormick, J.R., Harkin, M.M., Johnson, K.J., and Ward, P.A.: Suppression by superoxide dismutase of immune-complex-induced pulmonary alveolitis and dermal inflammation. Am. J. Pathol. 102:55, 1981.
210. Cushing, L.S., Decker, W.E., Santos, F.K., Schutle, T.L., and Huber, W.: Orgotein therapy for inflammation in horses. Mod. Vet. Pact. 54:17, 1973.
211. Breshears, D.E., Brown, C.D., Riffel, D.M., Cobble, R.J., and Cheesman, S.F.: Evaluation of orgotein in treatment of locomotor dysfunction in dogs. Mod. Vet. Pract. 55:85, 1974.
212. Lund-Oleson, K., and Menander, K.B.: Orgotein: a new anti-inflammatory metalloprotein drug: preliminary evaluation of clinical efficacy and safety in degenerative joint disease. Curr. Therap. Res. 16:706, 1974.
213. Rosner, I.A., Goldberg, V.M., Getzy, L., and Moskowitz, R.W.: A trial of intraarticular orgotein, a superoxide dismutase, in experimentally-induced osteoarthritis. J. Rheumatol. 7:24, 1980.
214. Goebel, K.M., Storck, U., and Neurath, F.: Intrasynovial orgotein therapy in rheumatoid arthritis. Lancet 1:1015, 1981.
215. Goldstein, I.M., Roos, D., Weissmann, G., and Kaplan, H.B.: Influence of corticosteroids on human polymorphonuclear leukocyte function in vitro. Reduction of lysosomal enzyme release and superoxide production. Inflammation 1:305, 1976.
216. Lehmeyer, J.E., and Johnston, R.B. Jr.: Effect of anti-inflammatory drugs and agents that elevate intracellular cyclic AMP on the release of toxic oxygen metabolites by phagocytes. Clin. Immunol. Immunopathol. 9:482, 1978.
217. Greenwald, R.A.: Effects of oxygen-derived free radicals on connective tissue macromolecules: inhibition by copper-penicillamine complex. J. Rheumatol. 8:9, 1981.
218. Younes, M., Lengfelder, E., Zienau, S., and Weser, U.: Pulse radiolytically generated superoxide and Cu (II)-salicylates. Biochem. Biophys. Res. Commun. 81:576, 1978.
219. Weinstein, J., and Bielski, B.H.J.: Reaction of superoxide radicals with copper (II)-histidine complexes. J. Am. Chem. Soc. 102:4916, 1980.
220. Sorenson, J.R.J.: Some copper coordination compounds and their anti-inflammatory and antiulcer activities. Inflammation 1:317, 1976.
221. Ohlsson, K.: Neutral leucocyte proteases and elastase inhibited by plasma α_1-antitrypsin. Scand. J. Lab. Invest. 28:251, 1971.
222. Janoff, A.: Neutrophil proteases in inflammation. Ann. Rev. Med. 23:177, 1972.
223. Venge, P., Olsson, I., and Odeberg, H.: Cationic proteins of human granulocytes. V. Interaction with plasma protein inhibitors. Scand. J. Lab. Invest. 35:737, 1975.
224. Ohlsson, K., and Olsson, I.: Neutral proteases of human granulocytes. III. Interaction between human granulocyte elastase and plasma protease inhibitors. Scand. J. Clin. Lab. Invest. 34:349, 1974.
225. Wintroub, B.U., Goetzl, E.J., and Austen, K.F.: A neutrophil-dependent pathway for the generation of a neutral peptide mediator: Partial characterization of components and control by α_1-antitrypsin. J. Exp. Med. 140:812, 1974.
226. Wintroub, B.U., Klickstein, L.B., and Watt, K.W.K.: A human neutrophil-dependent pathway for generation of angiotensin II. Purification of the product and identification as angiotensin II. J. Clin. Invest. 68:484, 1981.
227. Wintroub, B.U., and Austen, K.F.: Interaction of neutrophil-bound enzymes with plasma protein substrates. In Miescher, P.A. (ed.): Immunopathology. Vol. VII. Basel, Schwabe & Company, 1977.
228. Greenbaum, L.M.: Leukocyte kininogenases and leukokinins from normal and malignant cells. Am. J. Pathol. 68:613, 1972.
229. Eriksson, S.: Studies in α_1-antitrypsin deficiency. Acta Med. Scand. (Suppl.)432:1, 1965.
230. Eriksson, S., and Larson, C.: Purification and partial characterization of PAS-positive inclusion bodies from the liver in alpha$_1$-antitrypsin deficiency. N. Engl. J. Med. 292:176, 1975.
231. Sjöblom, K.G., and Wolheim, F.A.: α_1-Antitrypsin phenotypes and rheumatic diseases. Lancet 2:41, 1977.
232. Jakschik, B.A., Lee, L.N., Shuffer, G., Parker, C.W.: Arachidonic acid metabolism in rat basophilic leukemia (RBL-1) cells. Prostaglandins 16:733, 1978.
233. Payan, D.G., and Goetzl, E.J.: Specific suppression of human T-lymphocyte function by leukotriene B$_4$. J. Immunol. 131:551, 1983.
234. Lewis, R.A., and Austen, K.F.: Mediation of local homeostasis and inflammation by leukotrienes and other mast cell-dependent compounds. Nature 293:103, 1982.
235. Turk, J., Maas, R.L., Brash, A.R., Roberts, L.J., and Oates, J.A.: Arachidonic acid 15-lipoxygenase products from human eosinophils. J. Biol. Chem. 257:7068, 1982.

236. Shak, S., Perez, H.D., Goldyne, M., Gold, W., and Goldstein, I.M.: A novel dioxygenation product of arachidonic acid possesses potent chemotactic activity for human polymorphonuclear leukocytes. Clin. Res. 31:47A, 1983.

237. Hanahan, D.J., Demopoulos, C.A., Liehr, J., and Pinckard, R.N.: Identification of platelet activating factor isolated from rabbit basophils as acetyl glyceryl ether phosphorylcholine. J. Biol. Chem. 255:5514, 1980.

238. McManus, L.M., Morley, C.A., Levine, S.P., and Pinckard, R.N.: Platelet activating factor (PAF) induced release of platelet factor 4 (PF4) in vitro and during IgE anaphylaxis in the rabbit. J. Immunol. 123:2835, 1979.

239. Osler, A.G., Lichtenstein, L.M., and Levy, D.A.: In vitro studies of human reaginic allergy. Adv. Immunol. 8:183, 1968.

240. Siraganian, R.P., and Hook, W.A.: Complement-induced histamine release from human basophils. II. Mechanisms of the histamine release reaction. J. Immunol. 116:639, 1976.

241. Brindley, L.L., Sweet, J.M., and Goetzl, E.J.: Stimulation of histamine release from human basophils by human platelet factor 4. J. Clin. Invest. 72:1218, 1983.

242. Goetzl, E.J.: Mast cell-mediated reactions of host defense and tissue injury: The regulatory role of epsinophil polymorphonuclear leukocytes. Inflammation 2:239, 1977.

243. Lichtenstein, L.M., and Gillespie, E.: Inhibition of histamine release by histamine is controlled by an H_2 receptor. Nature 244:287, 1973.

244. Lichtenstein, L.M., and Margolis, S.: Histamine release in vitro: Inhibition by catecholamines and methylxanthines. Science 161:902, 1968.

245. Dvorak, A.M., Mihm, M.C., Jr., and Dvorak, H.F.: Degranulation of basophilic leukocytes in allergic contact dermatitis reactions in man. J. Immunol. 116:687, 1976.

246. Olsson, I., Berg, B., Fransson, L.A., and Norden, A.: The identity of the metachromatic substance of basophilic leukocytes. Scand. J. Haemaetol. 7:440, 1970.

247. Lewis, R.A., Goetzl, E.J., Wasserman, S.I., Valone, F.H., Rubin, R.H., and Austen, K.F.: The release of four mediators of immediate hypersensitivity from human leukemic basophils. J. Immunol. 114:87, 1975.

248. Benveniste, J., Henson, P.H., and Cochrane, C.G.: Leukocyte-dependent histamine release from rabbit platelets. J. Exp. Med. 136:1365, 1972.

249. Czarnetski, B.M., König, W., and Lichtenstein, L.M.: Antigen-induced eosinophil chemotactic factor (ECF) release by human leukocytes. Inflammation 1:201, 1976.

250. Orenstein, N.S., Hammand, M.E., Dvorak, H.F., and Feder, J.: Esterase and protease activity of purified guinea pig basophil granules. Biochem. Biophys. Res. Commun. 72:230, 1976.

251. Payan, D.G., Goldman, D.W. and Goetzl, E.J.: Biochemical and cellular characteristics of the regulation of human leukocyte function by lipoxygenase products of arachidonic acid. In Chakrin, L.W., and Bailey, D.M., (eds.): Biochemical and Cellular Characteristics of the Regulation of Human Leukocyte Function by Lipoxygenase Products of Arachidonic Acid. New York, Academic Press, Inc., in press.

252. Benveniste, J.: Platelet activating factor, a new mediator of anaphylaxis and immune complex deposition from human and rabbit basophils. Nature 249:581, 1974.

253. Kater, L.A., Goetzl, E.J., and Austen, K.F.: Isolation of human eosinophil phospholipase D. J. Clin. Invest. 57:1173, 1976.

254. Czarnetski, B., König, W., and Lichtenstein, L.M.: Eosinophil chemotactic factor (ECF). I. Release from polymorphonuclear leukocytes by the calcium inophore A23187. J. Immunol. 117:229, 1976.

255. Richerson, H.A., Dvorak, H.F., and Leskowitz, S.: Cutaneous basophil hypersensitivity. I. A new look at the Jones-Mote reaction, general characteristics. J. Exp. Med. 132:546, 1970.

256. Dvorak, H.F., and Dvorak, A.M.: Cutaneous basophil hypersensitivity. In Brent, L., and Holborow, J. (eds.): Progress in Immunology II, Vol. 3. Amsterdam, North-Holland Publishing Company, 1974.

257. Bast, R.C., Jr., Simpson, B.A., and Dvorak, H.F.: Heterogeneity of the cellular immune response. II. The role of adjuvant. Lymphocyte stimulation in cutaneous basophil hypersensitivity. J. Exp. Med. 133:202, 1971.

258. Cochrane, C.G., and Koffler, D.: Immune complex disease in experimental animals. Adv. Immunol. 16:185, 1973.

259. Stossel, T.P.: Phagocytosis. N. Engl. J. Med. 290:717, 774, 833, 1974.

260. Quie, P.G., and Cates, K.L.: Chemical conditions associated with defective polymorphonuclear leukocyte chemotaxis. Am. J. Pathol. 88:711, 1977.

261. Clark, R.A.: Disorders of granulocyte chemotaxis. In Gallin, J.I., and Quie, P.G. (eds.): Leukocyte Chemotaxis: Methods, Physiology, and Clinical Implications. New York, Raven Press, 1978.

262. Oliver, J.M., and Zurier, R.B.: Correction of characteristic abnormalities of microtubule function and granule morphology in Chédiak-Higashi syndrome with cholinergic agonists. J. Clin. Invest. 57:1239, 1976.

263. Pike, M.C., Daniels, C.A., and Snyderman, R.: Influenza induced depression of monocyte chemotaxis: Reversal by levamisole. Cell. Immunol. 32:234, 1977.

264. Goetzl, E.J.: Defective responsiveness to ascorbic acid of neutrophil random and chemotactic migration in Felty's syndrome and systemic lupus erythematosus. Ann. Rheum. Dis. 35:510, 1976.

265. Hurd, E.R., Andreis, and Ziff, M.: Phagocytosis of immune complexes by polymorphonuclear leukocytes in patients with Felty's syndrome. Clin. Exp. Immunol. 28:413, 1977.

266. Clark, R.A., Kimball, H.R., and Decker, J.L.: Neutrophil chemotaxis in systemic lupus erythematosus. Ann. Rheum. Dis. 33:167, 1974.

267. Perez, H.D., and Goldstein, I.M.: Infection and host defenses in systemic lupus erythematosus. In Franklin, E.C. (ed.): Clinical Immunology Update. New York, Elsevier, 1979.

268. Staples, P.J., Gerding, D.N., Decker, J.L., and Gordon, R.S.: Incidence of infection in systemic lupus erythematosus. Arthritis Rheum. 17:1, 1974.

269. Landry, M.: Phagocyte function and cell-mediated immunity in systemic lupus erythematosus. Arch. Dermatol. 113:147, 1977.

270. Perez, H.D., Lipton, M., and Goldstein, I.M.: A specific inhibitor of complement (C5)-derived chemotactic activity in serum from patients with systemic lupus erythematosus. J. Clin. Invest. 62:29, 1978.

271. Perez, H.D., Goldstein, I.M., Chernoff, D., Webster, R.O., and Henson, P.M.: Chemotactic activity of C5a des Arg: evidence of a requirement for an anionic peptide "helper factor" and inhibition by a cationic protein in serum from patients with systemic lupus erythematosus. Mole. Immunol. 17:163, 1980.

272. Perez, H.D., Goldstein, I.M., Webster, R.O., and Henson, P.M.: Enhancement of the chemotactic activity of human C5a des Arg by an anionic polypeptide ("cochemotaxin") in normal human serum and plasma. J. Immunol. 126:800, 1981.

273. Perez, H.D., Andron, R.I., and Goldstein, I.M.: Infection in patients with systemic lupus erythematosus. Association with a serum inhibitor of complement-derived chemotactic activity. Arthritis Rheum. 22:1326, 1979.

274. Brandt, L., and Hedberg, H.: Impaired phagocytosis by peripheral blood granulocytes in systemic lupus erythematosus. Scand. J. Haematol. 6:348, 1969.

275. Zurier, R.B.: Reduction of phagocytosis and lysosomal enzyme release from human leukocytes by serum from patients with systemic lupus erythematosus. Arthritis Rheum. 19:73, 1976.

276. Temple, A., and Loewi, G.: The effect of sera from patients with connective tissue diseases on red cell binding and phagocytosis by monocytes. Immunology 33:109, 1977.

277. Frank, M.M., Hamburger, M.I., Lawley, T.J., Kimberly, R.P., and Plotz, P.H.: Defective reticuloendothelial system Fc-receptor function in systemic lupus erythematosus. N. Engl. J. Med. 300:518, 1979.

278. Iida, K., Mornaghi, R., and Nussenzweig, V.: Complement receptor (CR_1) deficiency in erythrocytes from patients with systemic lupus erythematosus. J. Exp. Med. 155:1427, 1982.

279. Miyakawa, Y., Yamada, A., Kosaka, K., Tsuda, F., Kosugi, E., and Mayumi, M.: Defective immune-adherence (C3b) receptor on erythrocytes from patients with systemic lupus erythematosus. Lancet 2:493, 1981.

280. Wilson, J.G., Wong, W.W., Schur, P.H., and Fearon, D.T.: Mode of inheritance of decreased C3b receptors on erythrocytes of patients with systemic lupus erythematosus. N. Engl. J. Med. 307:981, 1982.

281. Wenger, M.E., and Bole, G.G.: Nitroblue tetrazolium dye reduction by peripheral blood leukocytes from rheumatoid arthritis and systemic lupus erythematosus patients measured by a histochemical and spectrophotometric method. J. Lab. Clin. Med. 82:513, 1973.

282. Baum, J.: Infection in rheumatoid arthritis. Arthritis Rheum. 14:135, 1971.

283. Mowat, A.G., and Baum, J.: Chemotaxis of polymorphonuclear leukocytes from patients with rheumatoid arthritis. J. Clin. Invest. 50:2541, 1971.

284. Hallgren, R., Hakansson, L., and Venge, P.: Kinetic studies of phagocytosis. I. The serum independent particle uptake by PMN from patients with rheumatoid arthritis and systemic lupus erythematosus. Arthritis Rheum. 21:107, 1978.

285. Attia, W.M., Clark, H.W., Brown, T.M., Ali, M.K.H., and Bellanti, J.A.: Inhibition of polymorphonuclear leukocyte migration by sera of patients with rheumatoid arthritis. Ann. Allergy 48:21, 1982.

286. Kemp, A.S., Roberts-Thomson, P., Neoh, S.H., and Brown, S.: Inhibition of neutrophil migration by sera from patients with rheumatoid arthritis. Clin. Exp. Immunol. 36:423, 1979.

287. Attia, W.M., Shams, A.H., Ali, M.K.H., Clark, H.W., Brown, T.M., and Bellanti, J.A.: Studies of phagocytic cell function in rheumatoid arthritis. I. Phagocytic and metabolic abnormalities of neutrophils. Ann. Allergy 48:279, 1982.

288. Attia, W.M., Shams, A.H., Ali, M.K.H., Jang, L.W., Clark, H.W., Brown, T.M., and Bellanti, J.A.: Studies of phagocytic cell functions in rheumatoid arthritis. II. Effects of serum factors on phagocytic and metabolic activities of neutrophils. Ann. Allergy 48:283, 1982.

289. Turner, R.A., Schumacher, H.R., and Myers, A.R.: Phagocytic function

of polymorphonuclear leukocytes in rheumatic diseases. J. Clin. Invest. 52:1632, 1973.

290. Bodel, P.T., and Hollingsworth, J.W.: Comparative morphology, respiration and phagocytic function of leucocytes from blood and joint fluid in rheumatoid arthritis. J. Clin. Invest. 45:580, 1966.

291. Kemp, A.S., Brown, S., Brooks, P.M., and Neoh, S.H.: Migration of blood and synovial fluid neutrophils obtained from patients with rheumatoid arthritis. Clin. Exp. Immunol. 39:240, 1980.

292. Karten, I.:Septic arthritis complicating rheumatoid arthritis. Ann. Intern. Med. 70:1147, 1969.

293. Zivkovic, M., and Baum, J.: Chemotaxis of polymorphonuclear leukocytes from patients with systemic lupus erythematosus and Felty's syndrome. Immunol. Commun. 1:39, 1972.

294. Gupta, R.C., Laforce, F.M., and Mills, D.M.: Polymorphonuclear leukocyte inclusions and impaired bacterial killing in patients with Felty's syndrome. J. Lab. Clin. Med. 88:183, 1976.

295. Ruderman, M., Miller, L.M., and Pinals, R.S.: Clinical and serologic observations on 27 patients with Felty's syndrome. Arthritis Rheum. 11:37, 1968.

296. Walker, J.R., Smith, M.J.H., and James D.W.: A comparison of two *in vitro* methods for studying a defect in leucocyte movement in rheumatoid arthritis. Int. Arch. Allergy Appl. Immunol. 59:343, 1979.

297. Hanlon, S.M., Panayi, G.S., and Laurent, R.: Defective polymorphonuclear leucocyte chemotaxis in rheumatoid arthritis associated with a serum inhibitor. Ann. Rheum. Dis. 39:68, 1980.

298. van de Stadt, R.J., van de Voorde-Vissers, E., and Feltkamp-Vroom, T.M.: Metabolic and secretory properties of peripheral and synovial granulocytes in rheumatoid arthritis. Arthritis Rheum. 23:17, 1980.

299. Trung, P.H., Prieur, A.M., and Griscelli, C.: Neutrophil chemotaxis in juvenile chronic arthritis. Ann. Rheum. Dis. 39:481, 1980.

300. Djawari, D., Hornstein, O.P., and Schotz, J.: Enhancement of granulocyte chemotaxis in Behçet's disease. Arch. Dermatol. Res. 270:81, 1981.

301. Mowat, A.G.: Neutrophil chemotaxis in ankylosing spondylitis, Reiter's disease, and polymyalgia rheumatica. Ann. Rheum. Dis. 37:9, 1978.

302. Leirisalo, M., Repo, H., Tiilikainen, A., Kosunen, T.U., and Laitinen, O.: Chemotaxis in yersinia arthritis. HLA-B27 positive neutrophils show high stimulated motility in vitro. Arthritis Rheum. 23:1036, 1980.

303. Day, N.K., Gieger, H., Stroud, R., DeBracco, M., Manacado, B., Windhorst, D., and Good, R.A.: Cr deficiency: An inborn error associated with cutaneous and renal disease. J. Clin. Invest. 51:1102, 1972.

304. Glass, D., Raum, D., Stillman, J.S., and Schur, P.H.: Inherited deficiency of the second component of complement. Rheumatic disease associations. J. Clin. Invest. 58:853, 1976.

305. Rosenfeld, S.I., Kelly, M.D., and Leddy, J.P.: Hereditary deficiency of the fifth component of complement in man. I. Clinical, immunochemical and family studies. J. Clin. Invest. 57:1626, 1976.

306. Wellek, B., and Opferkuch, W.: A case of deficiency of the seventh component of complement in man. Clin. Exp. Immunol. 19:223, 1975.

307. Ballow, M., Shira, J.E., Harden, Yang, S.Y., and Day, N.K.: Complete absence of the third component of complement in man. J. Clin. Invest. 56:703, 1975.

308. Altman, L.C., Snyderman, R., and Blaese, R.M.: Abnormalities of chemotactic lymphokine synthesis and mononuclear leukocyte chemotaxis in Wiskott-Aldrich syndrome. J. Clin. Invest. 54:486, 1974.

309. Maderazo, E.G., Ward, P.A., Woronick, C.L., Kubik, J., and DeGraff, A.C.: Leukotactic dysfunction in sarcoidosis. Ann. Intern. Med. 84:414, 1976.

310. Ward, P.A., Goralnick, S., and Bullock, W.E.: Defective leukotaxis in patients with lepromatous leprosy. J. Lab. Clin. Med. 87:1025, 1976.

311. Gewurz, H., Page, A.R., Pickering, R.J., and Good, R.A.: Complement activity and inflammatory neutrophil exudation in man. Int. Arch. Allergy Appl. Immunol. 32:64, 1967.

312. Ward, P.A., and Schlegel, R.A.: Impaired leucotactic responsiveness in a child with recurrent infections. Lancet 2:344, 1969.

313. Van Epps, D.E., and Williams, R.C., Jr.: Suppression of leukocyte chemotaxis by human IgA myeloma components. J. Exp. Med. 144:1227, 1976.

314. Hill, H.R., Gerrard, J.M., Hogan, N.A., and Quie, P.G.: Hyperactivity of neutrophil leukotactic responses during active bacterial infection. J. Clin. Invest. 53:996, 1974.

315. Soter, N.A., Wasserman, S.I., and Austen, K.F.: Cold urticaria: Release into the circulation of histamine and eosinophil chemotactic factor of anaphylaxis during cold challenge. N. Engl. J. Med. 294:687, 1976.

316. Wintroub, B.U., Mihm, M.C., Jr., Goetzl, E.J., Soter, N.A., and Austen, K.F.: Morphologic and functional evidence for the release of mast cell products in bullous pemphigoid. N. Engl. J. Med. 298:417, 1978.

317. Ward, P.A., and Talamo, R.C.: Deficiency of the chemotactic factor inactivator in human sera with α_1-antitrypsin deficiency. J. Clin. Invest. 52:516, 1973.

318. Stevenson, R.D.: Effect of steroid therapy on in vitro polymorph migration. Clin. Exp. Immunol. 23:285, 1976.

319. Jacobs, J.C., and Goetzl, E.J.: "Streaking leukocyte factor," arthritis, and pyoderma gangrenosum. Pediatrics 56:570, 1975.

320. Ward, P.A.: Leukotactic factors in health and disease. Am. J. Pathol. 64:521, 1971.

321. Ward, P.A., and Hill, J.H.: C5 chemotactic fragments produced by an enzyme in lysosomal granules of neutrophils J. Immunol. 104:535, 1970.

322. Hill, J.H., and Ward, P.A.: C3 leukotactic factors produced by a tissue protease. J. Exp. Med. 103:505, 1969.

323. Hammarstrom, S., Hamberg, M., Samuelsson, B., Duell, E.A., Stawiski, M., and Voorhees, J.J.: Increased concentration of nonesterified arachidonic acid. 12L-hydroxy-5,8,10,14-eicosatetraenoic acid, prostaglandin E_2 and prostaglandin F_{2n} in epidermis of psoriasis. Proc. Natl. Acad. Sci. USA 72:5130, 1975.

324. Jagani, H., and Ofugi, S.: Characterization of a leukotactic factor derived from psoriatic scale. Br. J. Dermatol. 97:509, 1977.

325. Lazarus, G.S., Yost, F.J., Jr., and Thomas, C.A.: Polymorphonuclear leukocytes: Possible mechanism of accumulation in psoriasis. Science 198:1162, 1977.

326. Spilberg, I., Gallacher, A., Mehta, J.M., and Mandell, B.: Urate crystal induced chemotactic factor: Isolation and partial characterization. J. Clin. Invest. 58:815, 1976.

327. Spilberg, I., Gallacher, A., Mandell, B., and Rosenberg, D.: A mechanism of action for non-steroidal anti-inflammatory agents in calcium pyrophosphate dihydrate (CPPD) crystal induced arthritis. Agents Actions 7:153, 1977.

328. Dolovich, J., Hargreave, F.E., Chalmers, R., Shier, K.J., Gauldie, J., and Bienenstock, J.: Late cutaneous allergic responses in isolated IgE-dependent reactions. J. Allergy Clin. Immunol. 49:43, 1972.

329. Hargreave, F.E., and Pepys, J.: Allergic respiratory reactions in bird fanciers provoked by allergen inhalation provocation test. Relation to clinical features and allergic mechanism. J. Allergy Clin. Immunol. 50:157, 1973.

330. Klebanoff, S.J., Jong, E.C., and Henderson, Jr., W.R.: The eosinophil peroxidase: Purification and biologic properties. *In* Mahmoud, A.F., and Austen, K.F. (eds.): The Eosinophil in Health and Disease, New York, Grune & Stratton, 1980.

331. Weller, P.F., Goetzl, E.J., and Austen, K.F.: Identification of human eosinophil lysophospholipase as the constituent of Charcot-Leyden crystals. Proc. Natl. Acad. Sci. 77:7440, 1980.

332. Gleich, G.J., Loegering, D.A., Mann, K.G., and Maldonado, J.E.: Comparative properties of the Charcot-Leyden crystal protein and the major basic protein from human eosinophils. J. Clin. Invest. 57:633, 1976.

333. Olsson, I., Venge, P., Spitznagel, J.K., and Lehrer, R.I.: Arginine-rich cationic proteins of human eosinophil granules. Comparison of the constituents of eosinophilic and neutrophilic leukocytes. Lab. Invest. 36:493, 1977.

334. Venge, P., Dahl, R., Fredens, K., Hällgren, R., and Peterson, C.: Eosinophil cationic proteins (ECP and EPX) in health and disease. *In* Yoshida, T., and Torisu, M., (eds.): Immunobiology of the Eosinophil, New York, Elsevier Science Publishing Co., Inc., 1983.

335. Zeiger, R.S., Yurdin, D.L., and Colten, H.R.: Histamine metabolism. II. Cellular and subcellular localization of the catabolic enzymes, histaminase and histamine methyl transferase in human leukocytes. J. Allergy Clin. Immunol. 58:172, 1976.

336. Goetzl, E.J.: The conversion of leukotriene C_4 to isomers of leukotriene B_4 by human eosinophil peroxidase. Biochem. Biophys. Res. Commun. 106:270, 1982.

337. Welsh, R.A., and Geer, J.C.: Phagocytosis of mast cell granules by the eosinophilic leukocyte in the rat. Am. J. Pathol. 35:103, 1959.

338. Yurt, R.W., and Austen, K.F.: Cascade events in mast cell activation and function. *In* Lepow, I. (ed.): Proteolysis, Demineralization and Other Degradative Processes. New York, Academic Press, 1978.

339. Litt, M.: Studies in experimental eosinophilia. VII. Eosinophils in lymph nodes during the first 24 hours following primary antigenic stimulation. J. Immunol. 93:807, 1964.

340. Butterworth, A.E., David, J.R., Franks, D., Mahmoud, A.A.F., David, R.H., Sturrack, R.F., and Houba, V.: Antibody-dependent eosinophil-mediated damage to ^{51}Cr labeled schistosomula of *Schistosoma mansoni*: Damage by purified eosinophils. J. Exp. Med. 145:136, 1977.

341. James, S.L., and Colley, D.G.: Eosinophil-mediated destruction of *Schistosoma mansoni* eggs. J. Reticuloendothel. Soc. 20:359, 1976.

342. Mahmoud, A.A.F., Warren, K.S., and Peters, P.A.: A role for the eosinophil in acquired resistance to *Schistosoma mansoni* infection as determined by anti-eosinophil serum. J. Exp. Med. 142:805, 1975.

343. Tauber, A.I., Goetzl, E.J., and Babior, B.M.: Unique characteristics of superoxide production by human eosinophils in eosinophilic states. Inflammation 3:261, 1979.

344. Goetzl, E.J., Wasserman, S.I., and Austen, K.F.: Eosinophil polymorphonuclear leukocyte function in immediate hypersensitivity. Arch. Pathol. 99:1, 1975.

345. Ansari, A., and Williams, J.F.: The eosinophilic response of the rat to infection with *Taenia taeniaeformis*. J. Parasitol. 62:728, 1976.

346. Gelfand, M., and Bernberg, H.: Tropical eosinophilic syndrome: A clinical description of the disorder as seen in S. Rhodesia. Cent. Afr. J. Med. 5:405, 1959.
347. Lowell, F.C.: Clinical aspects of eosinophilia in atopic disease. JAMA 202:875, 1967.
348. Zolov, D.M., and Levine, B.B.: Correlation of blood eosinophilia with antibody classes. Int. Arch. Allergy 35:179, 1969.
349. Hardy, W.R., and Anderson, R.E.: The hypereosinophilic syndromes. Ann. Intern. Med. 68:1220, 1968.
350. Chusid, M.J., Dale, D.C., West, B.C., and Wolff, S.M.: The hypereosinophilic syndrome: Analysis of fourteen cases with review of the literature. Medicine 54:1, 1975.
351. Zucker-Franklin, D.: Eosinophil function and disorders. Adv. Intern. Med. 19:1, 1974.
352. Brockington, T.F., and Olsen, E.G.J.: Löffler's endocarditis and Davies' endomyocardial fibrosis. Am. Heart J. 85:308, 1973.
353. Crofton, J.W., and Douglas, A.C.: Pulmonary eosinophilia, polyarteritis nodosa, and Wegener's granulomatosis. In Crofton, J.W., and Douglas, A.C. (eds.): Respiratory Diseases. Oxford, Blackwell Scientific Publications, 1969.
354. Goetzl, E.J., Tashjian, A.H., Jr., Rubin, R.H., and Austen, K.F.: Production of a low molecular weight eosinophil polymorphonuclear leukocyte chemotactic factor by anaplastic squamous cell carcinomas of human lung. J. Clin. Invest. 61:770, 1978.
355. Kelenyi, G., Nemeth, A., Istvan, L., and Mohay, A.: Effect of corticosteroids on eosinophil leukocytes in hypereosinophilic syndromes. Acta Haematol. 49:235, 1973.
356. Parrillo, J.E., Fauci, A.S., and Wolff, S.M.: The hypereosinophilic syndrome: Dramatic response to therapeutic intervention. Trans. Am. Assoc. Physicians 90:135, 1977.
357. Panush, R.S., Franco, A.E., and Schur, P.H.: Rheumatoid arthritis associated with eosinophilia. Ann. Intern. Med. 75:199, 1971.
358. Shulman, L.E.: Diffuse fasciitis with eosinophilia: A new syndrome. Trans. Am. Assoc. Physicians 88:80, 1975.

Chapter 10

Cellular Components of Inflammation: Monocytes and Macrophages

Carl F. Nathan and Zanvil A. Cohn

INTRODUCTION

Metchnikoff discovered phagocytosis in 1880, and soon thereafter designated one type of large phagocyte the macrophage.[1] A century later, phagocytosis remains central to our understanding of the physiology of this cell. Indeed, phagocytosis by macrophages is crucial to survival of the organism, for such diverse functions as remodeling tissue during normal growth and wound healing, clearance of senescent erythrocytes and neutrophils, and destruction of invading microbes.

Nonetheless, after 80 years in which phagocytosis received most of the attention in investigations on macrophages, the last 20 years have introduced entirely new concepts of macrophage function. First, it has become clear that the ability of macrophages to secrete soluble factors is as important as their ability to ingest particulates. Macrophage secretory products are more numerous and diverse in composition and function than those known for any other cell of the immune system. They endow the macrophage with the capacity to exert potent effects of both pro- and anti-inflammatory nature and to regulate the function of other cells. Prominent among these secretory factors are hydrolytic enzymes, products of oxidative metabolism (the reactive oxygen intermediates and the oxygenated derivatives of arachidonic acid), and the protein interleukin-1, which affects lymphocytes, hepatocytes, fibroblasts, synoviocytes, and cells in the hypothalamus.

Second, the classical notion that macrophages are involved in delayed-type hypersensitivity remains valid but too restrictive; macrophages have the capacity to participate in immediate hypersensitivity reactions as well. Third, the distribution of macrophages in pathologic sites is broader than earlier believed. It is now appreciated that macrophages are prominent not only in granulomas but also in the lesions of atherosclerosis and glomerulonephritis. Macrophages line not only the hepatic and splenic sinusoids but also the renal tubules and the surfaces of bone.

Other recent advances include the identification of molecules secreted by lymphocytes that regulate macrophage function, and the definition of mechanisms by which macrophages kill other cells, both microbial and mammalian. Sharper tools, especially monoclonal antibodies, have allowed us to dissect away from macrophages some of the functions to which they once laid exclusive claim, such as initiating T lymphocyte activation, a role now known to belong primarily to dendritic cells. Monoclonal antibodies and related techniques are throwing the macrophage surface into a relief of ligand-binding receptors and differentiation antigens. The function of purified receptors is under analysis at the biophysical level. Finally, for the first time since Metchnikoff observed phagocytosis in the starfish, studies of the macrophages of man now rival reports on cells from laboratory animals.

What follows is a brief summary of macrophage ontogeny, structure, and function. Many facts and citations in an enormous literature have been omitted. The reader seeking these will have to turn both to older books[2-7] and to the most recent volumes of journals of immunology, cell biology, biochemistry, pathology, and medicine.

THE LIFE CYCLE OF MONONUCLEAR PHAGOCYTES

When colloidal dyes are injected intravenously, they are taken up by histiocytes, fibrocytes, and endothelial cells. Beginning with Aschoff in the 1920s, histologists grouped such cells together as the reticuloendothelial system (RES). In 1970, however, appreciation that the RES comprises cells of different lineages led to a more restricted definition of the mononuclear phagocyte system, based on appropriate morphology, an avid phagocytic capacity for antibody-coated particles, and a common origin in the bone marrow.[8] The cells that make up the mononuclear phagocyte system are listed in Table 10–1. In the 1980s, there has been a return to staining patterns in tissues as an aid in identifying mononuclear phagocytes. This time, however, the stains are not colloidal dyes, but reagents that detect monoclonal antibodies binding specifically to macrophages in tissue sections. Such techniques are continuing to yield new information about the distribution of macrophages in normal and inflamed organs.[9,10]

The Marrow Progenitors. Monocytes arise from precursors in the bone marrow.[11,12] It is not yet certain whether there is a separate or shared stem cell for monocytes and granulocytes. Murine monoblasts grown in liquid culture appear as round cells, 10 to 12 microns in diameter, with a small rim of basophilic cytoplasm containing few granules. Like their progeny, monoblasts ruffle their membranes, adhere to glass, phagocytize, display Fc receptors, and stain positively for nonspecific esterase and peroxidase. Murine monoblasts divide once, giving rise to two promonocytes, with a cycle time of about 12 hours.[13,14]

Compared to the monoblast, the murine promonocyte is larger (14 to 20 microns), with an indented nucleus and more vigorous phagocytic activity. Its pool size (5 $\times 10^5$) is only twice that of the monoblast, representing 0.25 percent of nucleated marrow cells. Its cycle time is about 16 hours.[13,15,16] In man, promonocytes represent some 2.9 percent of nucleated marrow cells, with a pool size of 6 $\times 10^8$ per kg.[17-21]

The Circulating Monocyte. In contrast to neutrophils, the marrow reserve of preformed monocytes is small. Just 2 hours (in the mouse)[22] or 19 to 60 hours (in man)[18,19] after they are formed, monocytes are released in G1 phase[18] into the blood, where they circulate with a half-life of 22 hours in the mouse[16] and from 8 to 71 hours in man.[18,20] Monocytes leave the circulating pool at random[16] by marginating in capillaries, the marginating pool being some 3.5 times the size of the circulating pool.[21] Monocytes emigrate[23] into an extravascular pool, which is vast compared to that in the blood[24] and from which re-entry into the blood is rare.[19]

During inflammation, monocyte production is increased by several adaptations. The promonocyte pool expands, the proportion of promonocytes in cycle increases, the promonocyte cycle time decreases, and monocytes are released into the circulation more promptly after their formation. In this manner, the monocyte birth rate may increase 2- to 4-fold within 12 to 15 hours of an inflammatory stimulus.[16,25]

Thus, compared to granulocytes, monocytes have a much smaller marrow reserve, a more limited capacity to augment production under stress, a longer intravascular half-life, and a relatively larger extravascular compartment. During experimentally induced inflammation, up to 70 percent of the marrow production of monocytes may emigrate to the inflamed site, so that there may be insufficient reserve to supply subsequent inflammatory foci.

In culture, monocytes increase in size, display more mitochondria and lysosomes, and develop enhanced receptor-mediated phagocytic activity and diminished production of reactive oxygen intermediates, thereby coming to resemble tissue macrophages.[26-31]

The Tissue Macrophage. Tissue macrophages arise in two ways: by emigration from the blood and by proliferation of precursors in local sites. The relative predominance of these two sources in the steady state is difficult to establish, since the cells that proliferate locally themselves arise in the marrow. Most studies favor a primarily hematopoietic origin not only for peritoneal macrophages[23,32,33] but also for those of skin,[34] lung,[35] liver,[36,37] and brain.[38] In the mouse in the normal steady state, 56 percent of blood monocytes settle in the liver as Kupffer cells, 15 percent exit to the pulmonary alveoli, 8 percent emigrate into the peritoneal cavity, and 21 percent distribute to other tissues.[39]

With local inflammation, both the influx of blood monocytes and the local proliferation of tissue precursors may increase dramatically.[12,40-43] In chronic inflammatory foci, granulomas arise with both local replication and hematogenous replenishment of their constituent cells,[44,45] sometimes with a high turnover, as in tuberculous lesions. During long-term culture, monocyte-derived macrophages take on the appearance of "epithelioid cells," with a decreased vacuolar apparatus (suggesting less endocytic activity) and increased rough endoplasmic reticulum (suggesting increased secretory activity).[26,44,46] During prolonged culture, monocyte-derived macrophages also fuse to form multinucleated giant cells.[26,46,47] Giant cell formation is augmented by mediators from antigen- or mitogen-stimulated lymphocytes.[47] Epithelioid cells and multinucleated giant cells arising from monocytes in vitro closely resemble the mononuclear phagocytes of granulomas.[48]

In the tissues, in response to lymphocyte mediators and complement components, macrophages may become "activated," a process leading to dramatic structural and functional changes, of which over 50 have been enumerated. Macrophage activation is discussed more fully at the end of this chapter.

In rodents in the steady state, the turnover time of

Figure 10–1. The morphologic heterogeneity of mononuclear phagocyte populations. Phase contrast × 2000. *A*, Human blood monocyte shortly after isolation and attachment to glass substrate. The reniform nucleus, small numbers of phase dense lysosomes in the nuclear "hof," and ruffled peripheral membrane are all typical of this class of cell. *B*, Resident macrophage obtained from the unstimulated peritoneal cavity of the mouse. The cell has spread on its substrate and in many ways is similar to the blood monocyte. The short, dense organelles surrounding the nucleus are largely mitochondria. *C*, A serous cavity macrophage which has accumulated large numbers of phase dense lysosomes. These are relatively uniform in size as a consequence of their pinocytic origin. Macrophages which interiorize large particles, such as the alveolar cell, exhibit a much more heterogeneous array. *D*, A macrophage obtained from an inflamed peritoneum some days after the acute insult. This cell is larger in size, and exhibits an extensive perinuclear vacuolar apparatus filled with endocytic vesicles and phagolysosomes.

Table 10-1. Mononuclear Phagocytes: Pools and Populations*

Bone Marrow	Blood	Tissue (Resident Populations)

Multipotential stem cell
Committed stem cell
Monoblast
Promonocyte $\Big\} \sim 10^6$
Monocyte
	Monocyte	Bone (osteoclasts)?
		Bone marrow
		CNS (CSF, microglia?)
		Liver (Kupffer cell)
		Lung (Alveolar macrophage,
		       Interstitial macrophage)
		Lymph node
		Perivascular connective tissue
		Serous cavities—peritoneum
		                        pleura
		                        synovium
		Spleen
		Skin connective tissue
		Synovial membrane (type A cell)

Production rate: 1–2×10^6/day	1–2×10^6 T½ 24–30 hours in circulation	Tissue pool $> 10^8$ Survival time 15–> 60 days

*Murine

tissue macrophages ranges from 20 to 60 days.[23] The fate of senescent macrophages is not clear. The lung and gut may represent important routes of their loss.

Control Mechanisms. Products of antigen-stimulated lymphocytes, injected in vivo, increase the number of peritoneal macrophages synthesizing DNA.[49] Injection of irritants into nonsensitized animals results in the appearance in the serum of a protein of 18,000 to 24,000 daltons molecular mass, which elicits a brisk and selective monocytopoiesis when injected into normal hosts.[50] In vitro, glycoproteins from stimulated lymphocytes and fibroblasts trigger the replication of cells that give rise to colonies of macrophages or of macrophages and granulocytes (colony-stimulating factors).[51-53] Factors such as these may regulate the kinetics of mononuclear phagocytes. However, more work is needed to establish their physiologic role.

DYNAMIC ASPECTS OF MACROPHAGE STRUCTURE

The Plasma Membrane. The capacity of the macrophage to recognize foreign or damaged autologous materials upon contact, the dramatic responses triggered by such recognition, and the large flux of membrane during endocytosis have directed the interest of many biologists to the macrophage plasma membrane. Fruitful approaches have included study of membrane proteins and lipids, transport systems, ectoenzymes, antigens, and receptors.

Exogenous proteins found on the surface of peritoneal macrophages include immunoglobulin[54] and fibrinogen-fibrin.[55] Procoagulant activity appears on the surface of mononuclear phagocytes after exposure to endotoxin, antigen-antibody complexes, and C3b or after phagocytosis.[56]

The intrinsic membrane proteins of macrophage mem-

branes turn over rapidly even in the absence of phagocytosis, with a half-life of about 7 hours.[57] During phagocytosis, ectoenzymes are internalized and inactivated even faster.[58] For example, the half-life for 5'-nucleotidase falls to about 2 hours.[59] Macrophages taken from inflammatory sites have lower levels of 5'-nucleotidase[60] and alkaline phosphodiesterase[61] than those from uninflamed sites, probably reflecting their greater pinocytic activity,[62] with faster turnover of these ectoenzymes. During phagocytosis and pinocytosis, individual proteins are represented in the endocytic vacuoles with little alteration from their distribution on the plasma membrane itself. With immunologic activation of macrophages, major protease-sensitive surface glycoproteins of 160,000 daltons (gp160 in the guinea pig and probably F4/80 in the mouse) are dramatically decreased.[63,64]

The membrane lipids are in a state of dynamic equilibrium, which is well illustrated by cholesterol. The mouse macrophage does not synthesize cholesterol, but takes it up from serum lipoproteins into a rapidly exchanging plasma membrane compartment, and a smaller, slowly exchanging lysosomal membrane compartment.[65] While there is little increased turnover of phospholipids during phagocytosis, and no net increase, membrane cholesterol and phospholipids do begin to increase 4 to 8 hours later, to an extent proportionate to the phagocytic load.[65,66] The fatty acid composition of the macrophage plasma membrane influences its viscosity, as reflected in the activation energy for phagocytosis. Thus, a high level of saturated fatty acids in the culture medium leads to corresponding changes in the membrane, which then behaves as if it were stiffer.[67] A major membrane component is arachidonate, which in the mouse represents up to 25 percent of total macrophage fatty acid in phospholipid and serves as an important reservoir for the formation of cyclo-oxygenase and lipoxygenase products, both by the macrophage itself and perhaps also by neighboring granulocytes, as discussed later in this chapter.

A large number of antigens have recently been characterized on the macrophage surface with the aid of monoclonal antibodies. Many of these are shared with other cells, such as class I products of the major histocompatibility complex (e.g., HLA-A, B, and C antigens),[68] class II products (Ia and HLA-DR antigens),[69,70] and various antigens common to macrophages and certain other cells such as granulocytes and natural killer cells,[71] neurons,[72] or T lymphocytes.[73] Another group of antigens, partially overlapping with those just mentioned, are displayed by the plasma membrane receptors described below.[74] Of special interest, however, are the apparently macrophage-specific antigens, such as F4/80 in the mouse[75] and 3C10 in man,[10] as well as the differentiation antigens that mark subsets of macrophages, such as those that have undergone immunologic activation.[76] The antibodies of the last two categories represent powerful tools that are likely to provide considerable new information in the next few years.

Plasma Membrane Receptors. The macrophage continually samples and senses its environment through specific receptors. In turn, engagement of the receptors can trigger the secretion of numerous products, described below, through which the macrophage influences its environment. While some macrophage receptors are intracellular, like those for steroids, most are located on the plasma membrane. Macrophage receptors are listed in Table 10–2.

Receptors for the Fc portion of immunoglobulin permit the macrophage to ingest antibody-coated particles[77-80] and to secrete reactive oxygen intermediates,[81,82] oxidation products of arachidonic acid,[83] and lysosomal hydrolases.[84] In the mouse, macrophages display three different receptors for IgG.[80] In other species,

Fc receptors for IgE have also been described on mononuclear phagocytes.[85-87] The trypsin-sensitive Fc receptor on mouse macrophages binds IgG2a monomers as cytophilic antibody, that is, antibody that binds to the cell without first reacting with antigen. Normal mouse peritoneal macrophages have about 1×10^5 such receptors. The number of receptors quadruples after injection of mice with certain inflammatory agents.[80] In vivo, ambient IgG could rapidly displace any given molecule of monomer from this Fc receptor, suggesting that it may not efficiently mediate phagocytosis so much as help localize antigen to the surface. Firm attachment and subsequent ingestion are probably mediated by the trypsin-resistant Fc receptor, which binds antigen-antibody complexes as well as IgG1 and IgG2b monomers. Mouse macrophages display about 5 to 8×10^5 such sites per cell,[80] although the number falls with macrophage activation.[82] In man, the monocyte displays an Fc receptor with the same specificity as that on the neutrophil. As the cell matures into a macrophage, a receptor analogous to the trypsin-resistant mouse macrophage receptor appears.[88] The latter receptor can be induced on both myeloid cells and on monocytes by gamma-interferon.[89]

The trypsin-resistant mouse macrophage Fc receptor has been purified through the use of a monoclonal antibody.[90] The purified receptor, a glycoprotein with a molecular mass of about 55,000 daltons, orients in lipid bilayers in such a manner that it specifically binds immune complexes added to the same side of the artificial membrane. Upon binding ligand, the lipid-moored receptor behaves as a ligand-dependent cation channel. That is, it permits a brief flux of cations (especially Na^+) to cross the membrane.[91] It remains to be demonstrated whether this cation flux is in fact responsible for triggering ingestion and secretion in macrophages.

There are at least three types of complement receptors

Table 10–2. Ligands for Macrophage Receptors

Immunoglobulin and Complement	Lipoproteins
IgG1, IgG2b (murine)	LDL (apo-E)
IgG2a (murine)	Modified LDL
IgG3 (murine)	β-VLDL
IgG1, IgG3 monomers (human)	Peptides
IgG complexes (human)	Neuropeptides (enkephalins, endorphins)
IgE	Arginine vasopressin
C3b, C4b	N-formylated peptides from bacteria, mitochondria
C3bi	Polysaccharides
C3d	Lipopolysaccharide endotoxin
C5a	Carbohydrates on certain cells
Other Proteins	Other
Mannosyl-, fucosyl-, N-acetylglucosaminyl-terminal glycoproteins	Adrenergic agents
α2-macroglobulin–protease complexes	Cholinergic agents
Fibronectin	Phorbol diesters
Fibrin	Histamine
Lactoferrin	
Colony-stimulating factors	
Migration inhibitory and macrophage activation factors	
Insulin	
Factors VII, VIIa	
Interferons	

on mononuclear phagocytes.[74,79,92-96] They are under complex regulation. For example, complement-coated particles bind to resident mouse peritoneal macrophages without triggering ingestion.[94] In this setting, their function may be to enhance the capacity of limiting amounts of antibody to mediate ingestion through the Fc receptor. However, as macrophages phagocytize, they release a factor that stimulates T lymphocytes to release another factor. Within seconds, the latter factor capacitates the macrophage complement receptor to mediate not only attachment but ingestion as well.[97] Macrophages taken from inflammatory sites already have this capacity. Macrophages derived from culture of human monocytes, like resident mouse peritoneal macrophages, bind but do not efficiently ingest complement-coated particles. However, exposure to a fibronectin-coated surface or to certain amyloid-related proteins quickly capacitates their complement receptors for ingestion.[98,99]

Binding of C5a anaphylatoxin to its receptor on macrophages triggers the release of interleukin-1,[96] which in turn enhances T-lymphocyte proliferation and the development of antibody-forming cells. Numerous other effects of interleukin-1, including pyrogenicity, are described later.

While galactose-terminal asialoglycoproteins are cleared from the circulation by hepatocytes, glycoproteins terminating in mannose, fucose, or N-acetylglucosamine are cleared by Kupffer cells and other macrophages through specific receptors.[100] Complexes of proteases with α_2-macroglobulin are rapidly taken up by macrophages, even though proteases alone and the inhibitor alone are not.[101] Such a mechanism could be important for in vivo clearance of thrombin, plasmin, kallikrein, and active complement components.

Macrophages have receptors for the lymphokines that affect their behavior, such as migration inhibitory factor (MIF),[102] colony-stimulating factor,[103] and interferons. The MIF receptor appears to be a glycolipid[102] with a terminal fucose[104] important for its function.

Macrophage receptors for lipoproteins are of great interest in view of the monocyte or macrophage origin of many lipid-laden foam cells found in atheromatous plaques. Macrophages ingest low density lipoproteins (LDL) poorly,[105] but avidly ingest modified LDL.[106,107] This was first demonstrated with acetylated, maleylated, or malondialdehyde-treated LDL. It is doubtful that such LDL are physiologic. However, endothelial cells modify LDL in such a way that they are taken up by macrophages through the modified LDL receptor.[108] Foam cells can be generated in vitro by presenting macrophages either with modified LDL[106-108] or with β-migrating very low density lipoproteins from hyperlipidemic subjects.[109-111] It is of interest that maleylated bovine serum albumin, which may interact with the modified LDL receptor on macrophages, triggers the secretion of proteases, including plasminogen activator.[112] The pathophysiologic consequences of receptor-mediated macrophage interaction with lipoproteins remain to be fully explored.

Macrophage receptors for cholinergic agents[113] and for histamine[114] have been demonstrated only by pharmacologic criteria and are not yet characterized physicochemically. Nonetheless, they illustrate the responsiveness of the cell to the rapidly shifting environment of inflammatory sites.

The Vacuolar Apparatus. Through its vacuolar system, the macrophage both samples and modifies its environment at a prodigious rate. Combined morphometric and functional studies indicate that an unstimulated mouse peritoneal macrophage cultured in 20 percent fetal bovine serum forms at least 125 pinocytic vacuoles per minute, representing 0.43 percent of the cell volume of 395 cubic microns and 3.1 percent of the surface area of 825 square microns. Thus, even in the absence of a phagocytic load, the macrophage interiorizes the equivalent of its entire surface area every 33 minutes.[115] During phagocytosis, the cell can wrap in membrane each of some 150 to 200 latex beads with a diameter of 1 micron, thus interiorizing nearly its entire initial surface area in the form of phagosomes.[116]

Pinosomes flow through the cell, apparently guided by microtubules radiating from the centrioles, toward the perinuclear region. Here, lysosomes (see Chapter 9) have been formed by budding off the Golgi saccules, after being filled with acid hydrolases synthesized in the

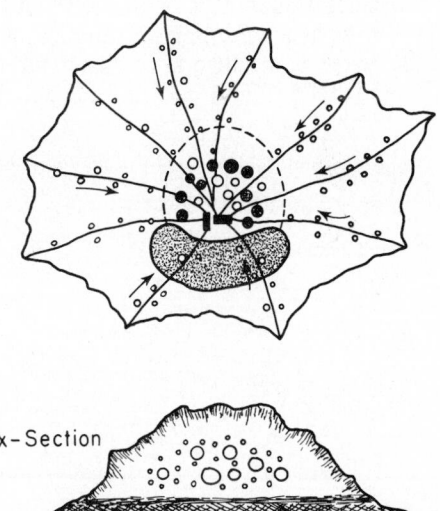

x-Section

Figure 10–2. Organization and polarization of the macrophage cytoplasm. *Upper,* Schematic representation of a mononuclear phagocyte. Microtubules radiate from the two centrioles, spreading into the peripheral cytoplasm like spokes on a wheel and ending in proximity to the plasma membrane. These structures form a matrix along which endocytic vesicles, generated from the plasma membrane, flow centripetally (arrow) and congregate in the centrosphere area (outlined by the dotted line). Here, in the perinuclear region, fusion between endocytic vesicles and primary and secondary lysosomes takes place. This fusion of organelle membranes mixes exogenous substrates and acid hydrolases, leading to the intracellular digestion of most naturally occurring macromoles. *Lower,* A cross section through a spread macrophage pseudopod to illustrate the organization of contractile elements. On the superior surface, amorphous actin filaments decorate the inner surface of the plasma membrane and adjacent cytoplasm. In the central region microtubule bundles and the larger endocytic vesicles are mixed. Cells which attach to a substrate often demonstrate bundles of microfilament parallel to the cell membrane.

rough endoplasmic reticulum. These primary lysosomes fuse with incoming endosomes, the pH of which has already become acidic,[117] to form secondary lysosomes.[118-120] Both primary and secondary lysosomes may fuse with phagosomes. During pinocytosis, the size of the secondary lysosome compartment remains constant at about 2.5 percent of the cell's volume; yet, each hour, the secondary lysosome compartment accommodates a flux of incoming vesicles 10 times its own volume.[115] This implies that there is a recycling mechanism by which most of the pinocytosed fluid is expelled from the cell and the vesicles are reincorporated into the plasma membrane. Recycling of membrane proteins from phagolysosomes to plasma membrane has indeed been demonstrated, and is extremely rapid.[121]

In 1963, phase contrast cinemicrographs dramatically demonstrated the fusion of macrophage lysosomes with incoming vacuoles containing bacteria, and the discharge of lysosomal contents into the space around the microbes.[122] Lysosomes have been shown to contain over 40 hydrolytic enzymes. It became clear that this was the manner in which macrophages degrade endocytosed foreign matter. Tracer studies revealed that within about 2 hours, bacterial macromolecules were degraded to acid-soluble fragments.[123] Proteins, for example, were broken down into amino acids and dipeptides, which then escaped into the cytoplasm.[124]

The Cytoskeletal Apparatus. The muscles of the macrophage lie in the hyaline ectoplasm beneath the plasma membrane, where a meshwork of filaments excludes most other organelles[125] and undergoes regional sol-gel

Selected Properties and Dynamics of the Vacuolar Apparatus of Macrophages

Figure 10–3. Exogenous solutes and particulates, which are either recognized and bound by plasma membrane receptors (adsorption) or free in the medium (fluid phase), are internalized via plasma-membrane-derived vesicles and vacuoles. The major portion of these organelles traverses the cytoplasm and fuses with secondary lysosomes. Selected contents remain within the lysosome. The membrane pinches off and the resulting vesicle returns to the cell surface. In such a manner membrane is reutilized for multiple bouts of endocytosis and maintains the volume and surface of the cell without the need for extensive membrane synthesis.

transitions and contractions. These appear to be responsible for membrane ruffling, pseudopod formation, and locomotion.[126] The main constituent of the microfilaments is actin, the most abundant protein of macrophages, accounting for 12 percent of cellular protein.[127] The globular form (G-actin) is a 42-kilodalton monomer that tends to polymerize into the F (filament) form until restrained by two factors; acumentin, a 65-kilodalton globular protein that caps the pointed end of the nascent chain in a calcium-insensitive manner;[128] and gelsolin, a 91-kilodalton globular protein that caps the barbed end of the filament only after binding Ca^{++} in the micromolar range. When the concentration of Ca^{++} falls, gelsolin releases F-actin and polymerization can proceed.[129] Actin filaments alone produce a weak meshwork. A rigid gel ensues when the filaments are crosslinked by actin-binding protein, which constitutes about 1 percent of macrophage protein. The 270-kilodalton monomers of the actin-binding protein dimer are joined to each other head-to-head, leaving two tails, each of which is free to bind an actin filament with high affinity,[130] resulting in branching and crosslinking. Contraction of actin filaments is the function of macrophage myosin, a Mg^{++}-ATPase hexamer of two 200-kilodalton heavy chains and two pairs of light chains of 20 kilodaltons and 15 kilodaltons, representing about 0.7 to 1.5 percent of macrophage protein.[127] Thus, local transients in Ca^{++} concentration appear to control the length, branching, and rigidity of the filaments that form the skeleton upon which myosin contracts.

The role of microtubules in macrophages is less clear. When the microtubules are disrupted by colchicine, pinocytic vacuoles move about the cell in a disorderly manner, but phagocytosis can proceed.[131] Likewise, colchicine-treated cells lose directionality of migration in a chemotactic gradient but retain motility. Thus, microtubules may serve in part to provide polarity to the cell.

THE CONGREGATION OF MACROPHAGES IN INFLAMMATORY SITES

Model in Man: The Skin Window. For macrophages to accumulate in an inflammatory focus, circulating monocytes must adhere to nearby endothelium, penetrate between cells and through the basement membrane, emigrate into the perivascular space, migrate to the tissue site, and remain there, where they are likely to become activated, and where a proportion of them may proliferate. The technique most often applied in man to assess the adequacy of macrophage mobilization in inflammatory sites is the skin window popularized by Rebuck and Crowley.[132] Sterile glass coverslips, applied sequentially to an area of abraded skin, with or without soluble antigen, permit direct visualization of the accumulation of monocytes and their maturation into macrophages, from about the sixth through the fortieth hour. However, to study separately each phase of the congregation of macrophages in inflammatory sites, it has been necessary to resort to in vitro models.

Sticking and Spreading. Macrophages both stick and spread rapidly on surfaces coated with antigen-antibody complexes, polyanions, or certain lectins. On uncoated glass or plastic and on collagen, sticking is rapid, but spreading occurs more slowly, requiring up to 24 hours for normal mouse peritoneal macrophages. Spreading can be enhanced by adding a variety of agents to the medium, including ATP and certain proteases.[133]

Unlike normal mouse peritoneal macrophages, macrophages from inflammatory exudates spread almost immediately on glass or plastic. This is probably related to the fact that activation of either the coagulation or the complement cascades generates activities in plasma or serum that promote rapid and dramatic spreading when added to normal macrophages.[136] Purified plasmin and complement component fragment Bb both cause macrophages to spread on glass.[135] The mechanism of this reaction is not understood.

Macrophage receptors for fibronectin[136] mediate the adherence of the cells to fibronectin-coated surfaces. Blood vessels produce fibronectin in response to injury.[137] In vivo, receptor-mediated adherence of monocytes to fibronectin or fibrin[138] may play a role in adherence within the vessels in inflamed tissue.

Migration Through Tissues. How mononuclear phagocytes make or find a path through connective tissue is not certain. This remarkable ability to wander, which macrophages share with malignant cells, is probably mediated by neutral proteases. Plasminogen activator is secreted by both macrophages[139] and malignant cells and is required for their ability to migrate in vitro. Macrophage elastase[140] and collagenases[141,142] are also active at extracellular pH. Unlike granulocyte elastase, macrophage elastase is resistant to inhibition by α_1-protease inhibitor, and in fact, cleaves the inhibitor.[143] Macrophage elastase also degrades fibronectin, laminin, proteoglycans, and denatured collagen.[144] One macrophage collagenase is active against collagen types I, II, and III; another degrades type V collagen. In vitro, macrophages digest the extracellular matrix around them to lucent zones.[145,146] Similar events probably accompany the migration of the cells through tissue in vivo.

Chemotaxis. No less remarkable than the ability of macrophages to penetrate tissue is the directionality and speed that can be imparted to their movement. Numerous substances generated during the inflammatory response have the capacity both to enhance the speed of macrophage movement (chemokinesis) and to orient movement in the direction of increasing concentration of the agent (chemotaxis). Such factors are derived from plasma, from connective tissue, and from other cells (Table 10–3).

Among factors derived from plasma, the foremost chemotaxin for macrophages is C5a.[147] Macrophages have specific receptors for this anaphylatoxin,[148] which may be released as a consequence of complement activation by antigen-antibody complexes, by bacterial lipopolysaccharides, or by thrombin-coated platelets,[149] as

Table 10–3. Factors Chemotactic for Macrophages

From Plasma
  C5a
  Thrombin*
  Kallikrein
  Denatured albumin
From Connective Tissue
  Fibronectin fragments*
  Elastin fragments*
  Collagen and collagen fragments*
  Desmosine
  Fluids from resorbing bone*
From Host Cells
  Lymphocytes: chemotactic factor*
  Phagocytes: lipoxygenase products
  Platelets: platelet factor 4
  Fibroblasts: fibroblast-derived factor
  Erythrocytes: denatured hemoglobin
  Tumor cells: chemotactic polypeptides*
  Many cells: formylated mitochondrial peptides†
From Bacteria
  N-formylmethionyl peptides
  Phospholipids*
  Others

*Relatively selective for macrophages rather than neutrophils.
†Chemotactic activity demonstrated only for neutrophils but expected for macrophages as well.

well as by the direct action of cell-derived proteases on C5.[147] Such proteases may be released from damaged cells, from granulocytes,[150] or from macrophages themselves.[147] Other plasma-derived chemotactic factors for macrophages include thrombin,[151] a factor arising during the conversion of prekallikrein to kallikrein,[152] and denatured albumin.[153]

Proteolytic fragments of fibronectin are chemotactic for monocytes, whereas intact fibronectin is not.[154] Proteases that can cleave fibronectin include thrombin, macrophage elastase, and plasmin. Macrophages, of course, can promote the generation of plasmin by secreting plasminogen activator. Fibronectin fragments are also chemotactic for fibroblasts.[158] Other components of connective tissue with chemotactic activity for macrophages include fragments derived from the action of neutrophil elastase on vascular and tendinous elastin,[156,157] desmosine,[157] and collagen and its collagenase fragments.[158] In addition, culture fluids from resorbing bone are chemotactic for monocytes.[159]

Lymphocytes, neutrophils, platelets, erythrocytes, fibroblasts, tumor cells, and other cells can each release chemotaxins for macrophages. For example, lymphocytes release a chemotactic protein when encountering an antigen to which the host has been sensitized,[160] or when B lymphocytes are stimulated by bacterial lipopolysaccharide, antigen-antibody complexes, or aggregated immunoglobulin.[161] Lymphocyte-derived chemotactic factor appears to be the major chemotaxin produced in vivo when antigen is injected into the peritoneal cavity of immunized guinea pigs.[162] Neutrophil granules appear to be important. Thus, a patient with an apparently isolated deficiency of the specific granules of neutrophils failed to accumulate monocytes normally in skin windows, although the monocytes themselves responded even better than normally to standard test agents in vitro.[163] Platelet factor 4 is a monocyte chemotaxin.[164] The chemotactic activity of denatured hemoglobin has been related to the hydrophobicity of the unfolded chains.[153] The ability of tumor cells to secrete chemotaxins in vitro correlates with the content of macrophages in the tumors in vivo.[165]

Bacteria produce a variety of chemotaxins for macrophages. *Corynebacterium* and *Listeria* are of special interest, because they are intracellular pathogens of macrophages.[153] Formylation of terminal methionyl residues on peptides appears to be restricted to microbes and mitochondria. Macrophages have receptors for formylated peptides and respond to them chemotactically.[166] This may provide a detection system both for bacterial invasion and for tissue destruction that has resulted in spillage of mitochondrial contents.[167].

At least eight of the known chemotaxins attract macrophages much more efficiently than neutrophils. These are thrombin, collagen, fibronectin fragments, elastin fragments, fluids from resorbing bone, the lymphocyte-derived factor, tumor factors,[168] and a phospholipid from *C. parvum*. The specificity exhibited by these factors raises but does not adequately answer the important question of what controls the orderly succession of cell types in an inflammatory focus.

Factors influencing macrophage responsiveness to chemotactic stimuli are beginning to be recognized. Peritoneal macrophages from mice injected with BCG are more chemotactically responsive in vitro than resident peritoneal macrophages or blood monocytes.[169] Not only do tumor cells make chemotaxins, but they also release factors that decrease the chemotactic responsiveness of macrophages to other stimuli in vivo and in vitro.[170-172] Some such factors are immunologically related to envelope proteins of retroviruses, even when derived from human[173] or murine[174] tumors not shedding virus. Finally, tumor cells sometimes inactivate other chemotaxins directly.[175]

Retention of Macrophages. Antigen- or mitogen-stimulated lymphocytes release not only a chemotactic factor for macrophages but also physicochemically distinct substances[176] that inhibit macrophage migration (MIFs).[177,178] It has been suggested that MIF might serve to retain macrophages at the site of delayed hypersensitivity reactions. In addition, activation of complement produces factors, such as Bb, which inhibit migration of macrophages in vitro in a manner like that of MIF.[179] Finally, macrophages in delayed hypersensitivity lesions are invested in a basket of fibrin strands, which may also favor their retention at the site.[180]

Thus, proteases, complement and coagulation components, lymphocyte-derived factors, bacterial products, and substances released by tumor cells all have the direct or indirect potential both to enhance and to retard macrophage migration. It remains enigmatic how these are regulated to yield the reproducible, coordinated accumulation of cells seen in the skin window. Equally obscure are the messages, if any, that retract these commands to congregate.

INTAKE: ENDOCYTOSIS

Recognition and Attachment. One of the most fascinating aspects of phagocytosis is the cell's ability to discriminate between normal self components on the one hand and damaged self or foreign particles on the other.[181,182] The recognition process is subserved in part by receptors. As discussed earlier, there are at least three classes of receptors for opsonized particles, that is, receptors for immunoglobulin, complement, or fibronectin. In addition, there are receptors that bind ligands without the mediation of opsonins, such as the receptor for mannose-terminal glycoproteins and the receptors for lipoprotein particles. Beyond this, there are particles that are avidly ingested, for which neither an opsonin nor a receptor is known. Examples are polystyrene latex beads and aldehyde-treated erythrocytes.[183] No single physicochemical feature of such particles seems adequate to explain their recognition. Some bacteria are phagocytized without opsonins, while others have antiphagocytic proteins that must be neutralized by opsonins before ingestion will occur. Other particles, such as mycoplasma, will attach to macrophages without triggering ingestion. When antimycoplasma antibody is added, the microbes are promptly engulfed.[184] Some ligand-receptor systems may interact synergistically in promoting ingestion. Illustrations involving antibody and complement, as well as fibronectin and complement, were discussed above. Thus, many mechanisms have evolved for the recognition of particles for phagocytosis, not all of which are yet understood.

Triggering of Ingestion. The macrophage surface response to a phagocytic stimulus is segmental, not global. This has been demonstrated by adding both C3b-coated and IgG-coated particles to resident mouse peritoneal macrophages in the cold. The C3 receptors on such cells mediate attachment but not ingestion. When the cells were warmed, they engulfed only the IgG-coated particles, while excluding the others.[185] When particles were coated with IgG on only one hemisphere, phagocytic vacuoles enclosed such particles only as far as the margin of opsonization. When the naked hemisphere was then opsonized, the macrophages completed enclosure.[186,187] Thus, ingestion is not triggered by point attachment, but requires continuous approximation, or "zippering," of receptors to opsonized sites over the entire surface of the particle. When the number of ligands per unit area of the opsonized surface is high, the apposition of the macrophage to the particle is so close that soluble proteins of molecular mass about 60 kilodaltons are excluded.[188] Thus, in the case of particles whose uptake is dependent on Fc receptors, tight surface-to-surface apposition proceeds under finely regulated local control until the macrophage membrane fuses over the top of the particle. It is unknown how these events are regulated, what restricts the diffusible signals, if any, to such a short range of action during ligand-receptor interaction, and whether the same sequence operates in the case of other ligand-receptor combinations that lead to ingestion.

Metabolism During Phagocytosis. Particle ingestion

by macrophages is usually accompanied by a respiratory burst similar to that in neutrophils and eosinophils (Fig. 10–4).[189] That is, there is a dramatic increase in oxygen consumption, during which a reduced nicotinamide adenine dinucleotide phosphate-dependent, flavoprotein-dependent oxidase, probably with a cytochrome b cofactor and a ubiquinone, reduces molecular oxygen to superoxide in or near the plasma membrane. Superoxide anion dismutates, in large part, to hydrogen peroxide. A portion of the peroxide diffuses from the cell, but some of it is catabolized either by catalase or by glutathione peroxidase. Glutathione is regenerated in reduced form by glutathione reductase in concert with NADPH. The NADPH for this last step, as well as that responsible for the initial reduction of oxygen, derives from the hexose monophosphate shunt, whose cycling of glucose to CO_2 spins faster to accommodate the increased reduction of oxygen. Meanwhile, superoxide and hydrogen peroxide can interact to give rise to hydroxyl radical. In monocytes, which contain myeloperoxidase, hypohalous ions are also formed.

A second, much smaller respiratory burst is initiated with similar kinetics by many of the same stimuli. It is immediately preceded by activation of phospholipases, which release arachidonic acid from cellular phospholipids. The free arachidonate is then oxygenated by either of two enzymes, cyclo-oxygenase or lipoxygenase, whose products are then further metabolized to produce a shower of pharmacologically active products.

Historically, the respiratory burst has been intimately linked to phagocytosis. However, the two processes are now known to be dissociable. Thus, there are many soluble agents that trigger the respiratory burst without phagocytosis, although they may lead to vacuole formation. These include antigen-antibody complexes, C5a, lectins, fatty acids, ionophores, and tumor promoters.[190] The respiratory burst can also be triggered by opsonized particles, when phagocytosis is blocked with microfilament-disrupting cytochalasins. Moreover, phagocytosis can proceed without the respiratory burst. This is seen with certain particles, like some preparations of latex, or with certain phagocytes, like those from patients with chronic granulomatous disease, which often lack the cytochrome cofactor of the oxidase.[191] Thus, the respiratory burst is a normal but by no means essential accompaniment of phagocytosis. It is more important for the microbicidal or inflammatory consequences of ingestion than for translocation of the particle into the cell.

If the extra respiration of phagocytosis is thus not devoted to recovery of utilizable chemical energy, what does fuel the musclelike movements that phagocytosis entails? It now appears that glycolysis generates ATP, which in turn maintains a large pool of creatine phosphate. The high energy bond in creatine phosphate is probably the proximate energy source for phagocytosis in macrophages.[192]

OUTPUT: THE SECRETIONS OF MACROPHAGES

The inflammatory response is subject to influence at nearly every point by one or another macrophage secretory product, acting over a range as short as a few microns, or in the case of endogenous pyrogen, at a distance as great as two meters.

The enormous secretory repertoire is under complex regulation. Some products are secreted constitutively, others almost instantaneously following ligand-receptor

Figure 10–4. Metabolic pathways in the respiratory burst. These pathways appear to be the same in mononuclear phagocytes as in neutrophils, except that the activities of the various enzymes vary greatly in mononuclear phagocytes, depending on their source, manner of elicitation, maturity, and level of activation. Singlet oxygen could theoretically be produced at many points, such as by the reaction of hypochlorous ion with hydrogen peroxide; superoxide with hydrogen peroxide; hydrogen peroxide with hydrogen peroxide; or hydroxyl radical with superoxide. The overall effect is the consumption of glucose and oxygen and the production of carbon dioxide and water, with the generation of reactive metabolites of oxygen as intermediates.

Exocytosis
Vesicular Mechanisms

Figure 10–5. Possible mechanisms for the release and secretion of macromolecular products. *Left,* Small secretory vesicles derived from the endoplasmic reticulum-Golgi network fuse with the plasma membrane, liberating their contents to the extracellular space. This is analogous to secretion in the hepatocyte. *Superior,* Preformed secondary lysosomes or digestive bodies fuse with an unclosed phagocytic vacuole, thereby liberating their acid hydrolases. This may occur when the cell attaches to an irregular surface or following the phagocytosis of large, unusually shaped particles. *Right,* Secondary lysosomes fuse directly with the plasma membrane. This event occurs rarely under normal circumstances but is enhanced by agents which interfere with the distribution of contractile elements and allow these organelles closer access to the membrane.

interaction, still others only days after a stimulus. These patterns are illustrated in Table 10–4. In addition, the state of macrophage activation profoundly affects secretory capacity, but differently for different products. The macrophage itself is subject to influence by many of its own secretions, which can interact with macrophage receptors or which can generate other substances that do so. Finally, some macrophage products can interact with each other, or can regulate the function of cells, which in turn affect macrophage activation and secretion. A partial listing of macrophage secretory products is furnished in Table 10–5. Some of the individual products are highlighted below.

Complement. Complement components can affect the locomotive, endocytic, metabolic, and secretory behav-

ior of the macrophage. Yet, the macrophage itself secretes many of the factors of the classical and alternative pathways and their regulators, omitting only the terminal components.[193-198] Perhaps through the action of other proteases on macrophage-derived complement components, macrophage culture supernatants may also contain cleavage products such as Bb, C3b, and C3a.[193] As noted earlier, Bb inhibits macrophage migration. C3b stimulates monocyte release of prostaglandins.[199] Prostaglandins, in turn, inhibit the secretion of C2 by monocytes.[200] In contrast, antigen-stimulated lymphocytes release a factor that enhances monocyte secretion of C2.[201] This is of considerable interest, because the low level of C2 in serum and the instability of the C42 complex may make C2 rate-limiting for classical pathway activation in extravascular sites. Finally, the C3a anaphylatoxin stimulates thromboxane release from guinea pig macrophages.[202] C3a also suppresses the ability of human helper T lymphocytes to release certain lymphocyte mediators.[203] It is not yet known whether the mediators whose release is suppressed include the one that enhances monocyte C2 synthesis.

Coagulation Factors. Several coagulation factors are secreted by macrophages,[204,205] as is an enzyme that promotes thrombolysis (plasminogen activator)[139] and inhibitors of thrombolytic enzymes (plasmin inhibitors).[206,207] Perhaps of equal importance, however, are surface activities involved in coagulation which are not secreted. These include inducible tissue factor activity (binding and activation of factor VII)[208] and a prothrombinase activity.[209] The prothrombinase is rapidly induced 10,000-fold when antigen-antibody complexes or bacterial lipopolysaccharides interact with lymphocytes that share Ia-like antigens with the monocytes.[209] The procoagulant activities of stimulated monocytes may account for the deposition of fibrin in delayed hypersensitivity sites.[210] It is the fibrin that appears to account in large part for the induration and swelling characteristic of such reactions.[180]

Lysozyme. Quantitatively, lysozyme is one of the major macrophage secretory products.[211] Its synthesis, which is constitutive, accounts for up to 2.5 percent of cellular protein per day. Lysozyme is a cationic protein of 14 kilodaltons that hydrolyzes a specific glucosidic link in bacterial cell walls. It is not known what advantage accrues to the host by committing such a large portion of the biosynthetic capacity of the macrophage to this enzyme in a noninducible manner, other than its well-known role in lysing a number of Gram-positive bacteria. These organisms are not usually regarded as pathogenic, but this may be thanks to the efficiency of lysozyme. Markedly elevated levels of the enzyme in the blood and urine are characteristic of the monocytic and myelomonocytic leukemias and may play a role in the hyperkaliuretic tubulopathy that sometimes accompanies them.

Plasminogen Activator. The secretion of plasminogen activator[139] is of special interest because of the numerous effects of the enzyme itself (it may, for example, act as a mitogen for lymphocytes) and of plasmin, whose for-

Table 10–4. Regulation of Secretion from Macrophages

Stimuli	Lag*	Products
None (constitutive)	—	Lysozyme, lipoprotein lipase
Phorbol myristate acetate	Seconds	Reactive O_2 intermediates
Immune complexes	Seconds	Reactive O_2 intermediates
	Minutes	Arachidonate metabolites
Endocytosis	Hours	Plasminogen activator
Redox agents, endocytosis, C'-activators without added complement	Days	Lysosomal hydrolases
Lymphocyte mediators	Days	Lysosomal hydrolases

*Influenced by assay sensitivity.

Table 10–5. Secretory Products of Mononuclear Phagocytes

Complement Components	Binding Proteins	Factors Regulating Synthesis of Substances by Other Cells
C1	Transferrin	Hepatocytes
C4	Transcobalamin II	Serum amyloid A
C2	Fibronectin	Serum amyloid P
C3	95K Gelatin-binding protein	Haptoglobin
C5	Apolipoprotein E	Synovial lining cells
Factor B	*Oligopeptides*	Collagenase
Factor D	Glutathione	Plasminogen activator
Properdin	*Bioactive Lipids*	Prostaglandins
C3b inactivator	Arachidonate metabolites	Chondrocytes
β1H	Prostaglandin E_2	Prostaglandins
Coagulation Factors	Prostaglandin $F_{2\alpha}$	Adipocytes
X	6-keto-Prostaglandin $F_{1\alpha}$ (from prostacyclin)	Lipoprotein lipase
IX	Thromboxane B_2 (from A_2)	Acetyl Co-A carboxylase
VII	Leukotrienes B, C, D, E	Fatty acid synthetase
V	Monohydroxyeicosatetraenoic acids (5-; 12-; 15-)	*Factors Promoting Replication of*:
Thromboplastin	Dihydroxyeicosatetraenoic acids	Lymphocytes (including interleukin-1)
Prothrombin	Platelet-activating factors (including 1-O-alkyl-2-acetyl-*sn*-glyceryl-3-phosphorylcholine)	Myeloid precursors (including colony-stimulating factors; factor inducing monocytopoiesis)
Other Enzymes	*Nucleosides and Metabolites*	Erythroid precursors (including erythropoietin)
Lysozyme	Thymidine	Fibroblasts
Neutral proteases	Uracil	Smooth muscle cells
Plasminogen activator	Uric acid	Microvasculature
Collagenase	*Reactive Metabolites of Oxygen*	*Factors Inhibiting Replication of*:
Elastase	Superoxide	Lymphocytes
Angiotensin-convertase	Hydrogen peroxide	Myeloid precursors
Acid hydrolases	Hydroxyl radical	Mesangial cells
Proteases	Hypohalous acids	Tumor cells
Lipases	*Chemotactic Factors*	Viruses (interferon)
(deoxy) Ribonucleases	For neutrophils	*Listeria monocytogenes*
Phosphatases	For eosinophils	*Other Hormonelike Factors*
Glycosidases	For fibroblasts	Endogenous pyrogens
Sulfatases		Insulin-like activity
Arginase		Thymosin B4
Lipoprotein lipase		
Phospholipase A_2		
Enzyme Inhibitors		
Plasmin inhibitors		
α_2-Macroglobulin		
α_1-Antiprotease		
Phospholipase A_2 inhibitor (steroid-induced)		

mation it catalyzes. Plasmin not only lyses fibrin but activates C1 and C3 and cleaves activated Hageman factor to subunits that promote the conversion of pre-kallikrein to kallikrein. Plasmin degrades glycoprotein in extracellular matrix and accelerates degradation by elastase.[144-146] Macrophages secrete plasminogen activator continuously after exposure to mediators from antigen-stimulated T lymphocytes.[212,213] Activated macrophages secrete even more plasminogen activator during phagocytosis;[214] secretion subsides as the phagocytic particles are degraded. However, nonphagocytizable immune complexes fixed to a surface shut off plasminogen activator release from human monocytes.[215]

Collagenase and Elastase. Macrophages secrete another group of proteases, which like plasminogen activator are active at neutral pH and which are likely to play a role in degradation of connective tissue. This group includes collagenases,[141,142,216] elastase,[140,217-219] gelatinase,[218] azocaseinase,[218] and others. The various enzymes are secreted following phagocytosis,[142] exposure to endotoxin,[220] interaction with immune complexes,[215] or incubation in lymphocyte mediators. Macrophage

elastase, a metalloenzyme distinct from the neutrophil serine enzyme, degrades not only elastin but also α_1-protease inhibitor,[143] immunoglobulin,[221] plasminogen, fibrinogen, fibrin, fibronectin, laminin, and proteoglycans.[144-146] Destruction of α_1-protease inhibitor by macrophage elastase would favor the action of neutrophil elastase in the same site.

Acid Hydrolases. A large number of hydrolases, active at acid pH, are present in macrophage lysosomes,[118] and increase in amount with activation of the cells.[119,217] The type-specific polysaccharide and peptidoglycans of streptococcal cell walls, which induce chronic inflammatory lesions in vivo, lead both to augmentation of lysosomal enzyme levels in cultured macrophages and to the discharge of such enzymes into the culture medium.[222] A large number of other microbial materials or polysaccharides have a similar effect, including endotoxin, BCG, *C. parvum*, yeast cell walls, dental plaque, carrageenan, and dextran sulfates. Such substances are also capable of activating complement by the alternative pathway, and with a similar rank order of potency.[223] Lysosomal enzyme release is also triggered by engagement of Fc[84] and complement[223] receptors and by incubation in lymphocyte mediators.[216]

Thus, lysosomal acid hydrolases may contribute to tissue breakdown when there is a sufficiently low pH extracellularly, or when portions of the matrix are ingested by macrophages[146] into phagolysosomes, which have an acid milieu.[224] Among the substances susceptible to degradation by macrophage acid hydrolases are collagen, cartilage, basement membrane, proteoglycans, immunoglobulin, kininogen, and complement components.[225]

Protease Inhibitors. Plasminogen activator, plasmin, collagenase, elastase, thrombin, kallikrein, and a variety of other proteases are all inhibited by α_2-macroglobulin.[226] Alpha$_2$-macroglobulin also enhances the ability of lymphocyte-derived migration inhibitory factor to retard macrophage motility.[227] Human monocytes synthesize and secrete substantial amounts of this protein in culture (about 50 ng per 10^6 cells per day),[228] as do human alveolar macrophages.[229] Recently, macrophages have also been found to synthesize and secrete α_1-protease inhibitor.[230-232] It may seem paradoxical that macrophages secrete not only elastase[140,217-219] but also two protease inhibitors, one of which is a substrate for elastase[143] and one of which is an inhibitor of it.[226]

Bioactive Lipids. Engagement of Fc receptors, ingestion of particles, or exposure to other membrane-active agents trigger the rapid release from macrophages of a variety of oxygenation products of arachidonic acid that are likely to be of critical importance in the inflammatory response.[233-249]

This assertion rests on the following points. First, the proportion of phospholipid fatty acid that is arachidonate is much higher in macrophages (about 26 percent in the mouse) than in most other cell types. The mouse macrophage is capable of putting 45 percent of this fatty acid at the disposal of cyclo-oxygenase and lipoxygenase within minutes of a membrane stimulus without suffering a loss of viability.[236,238,242] As a consequence, the quantities of arachidonate oxygenation products secreted by mouse macrophages (e.g., 33 nmol per mg cell protein) are enormous in comparison with other cells, such as guinea pig neutrophils (e.g., 0.044 nmol per mg cell protein in one comparable study; see Table 10–6). Second, the spectrum of arachidonate metabolites secreted by macrophages is wide and includes such important mediators as leukotriene C,[237,239,242,244] one of the slow-reacting substances of anaphylaxis, in quantity, as well as leukotriene B,[243] a potent chemotactic factor. Third, this secretory spectrum is profoundly influenced by the state of immunologic activation of the macrophage,[249] which suggests possible mechanisms of control during the evolution of an inflammatory response. Finally, macrophages are distributed in submucosal and perivascular sites, in the pulmonary alveoli and interstitium,[242] in the renal interstitium and juxtaglomerular apparatus,[9] and in other control points under normal steady-state conditions. Thus, it is plausible that macrophages could play a role as sentinels in the earliest stages of inflammation, releasing products that regulate vasodilation, constriction, and permeability, bronchial smooth muscle contractility, neutrophil and monocyte motility, lymphocyte function,[246,247] myeloid stem cell proliferation,[248] hepatic release of acute phase reactants,[249] and nociception. The fact that complexes of antigen with IgE are potent triggers of macrophage leukotriene release[239] supports the idea that macrophages may play a role in immediate hypersensitivity reactions.

Table 10–6. Metabolism of 20:4* from Endogenous Phospholipids of Mouse Tissue Macrophages in Response to a Triggering Agent (Zymosan)[†]

Feature	Peritoneal Macrophages		Pulmonary Macrophages		Guinea pig PMN with A23187[‡]
	Resident	Activated	Tissue	Alveolar	
Fatty acid					
Percentage of phospholipid	26	25	23	ND	
Percentage 20:4 released	45	17	14	5.5	
Percentage of released 20:4 oxygenated	95	30	80	75	
Pmol products/ µg protein	33	6	15	6	0.004
Cyclooxygenase products					
PGE$_2$	18 (54)[§]	4 (65)	2 (12)	0.8 (13)	0.002
PGI$_2$	6 (20)	0.02 (0.3)	0.9 (6)	0	0.001
TXA$_2$	0	0.7 (17)	1.2 (8)	0.6 (10)	0.010
PGF$_2$	0	0	0	0	0.001
Lipoxygenase products					
HETES	3 (10)	1 (15)	5 (32)	2 (39)	0.030
LTC	5 (16)	0.13 (2)	3 (23)	1 (13)	

*20:4 = arachidonic acid.
[†]Compiled from Scott and colleagues, refs. 236, 238, and 242.
[‡]From ref. 245.
[§]Numbers in parentheses are percentage of released 20:4.

Table 10–6 presents quantitative data for arachidonate metabolites produced by tissue macrophages in the mouse. These data reflect only one of two major pathways utilized by these cells, that is, the endogenous pathway in which the substrate is derived from the phospholipid pool of the producing cell in response to a membrane-perturbing agent.[236] However, free arachidonate, such as might be released from damaged cells by phospholipases, is also rapidly oxygenated by macrophages in the absence of a stimulus.[240,241] This pathway is not demonstrably saturable when macrophages are repeatedly provided with free arachidonic acid at nontoxic concentrations in vitro. Thus, it could be quantitatively important. The distribution of products formed by the exogenous pathway is given in Table 10–7. In addition, the free arachidonate released by macrophages may markedly augment the production of leukotriene B by neutrophils in the same site.

The influence of immunologic activation on the secretion of arachidonate metabolites by murine macrophages is summarized in Table 10–8. Of note is the marked decrease in PGE$_2$, PGI$_2$, hydroxyeicosatetraenoic acids, and leukotriene C and the appearance of significant amounts of thromboxane. In the guinea pig, macrophage activation increases rather than decreases PGE$_2$ release.[250] It is of interest that activation also has opposite effects on the secretion of complement components by macrophages in these two species. The reasons for these differences are not understood.

In man, leukotriene B$_4$ is a prominent product of the stimulated alveolar macrophage[243] and probably represents one of the major sources of alveolar macrophage chemotactic activity for neutrophils.[251] Study of the human blood monocyte has been complicated by the rosetting of platelets to monocytes during most isolation procedures. Recent techniques have overcome this prob-

lem and have permitted the demonstration that the human blood monocyte is a potent source of thromboxane, fully equivalent to the platelet on a protein basis, and much higher than the neutrophil.[244] Depending on the stimulus, human blood monocytes also release substantial amounts of lipoxygenase products, including leukotrienes B and C.[244] Studies with other populations of human mononuclear phagocytes should soon be forthcoming.

Reactive Oxygen Intermediates. As already noted, macrophages respond to immune complexes, phagocytic particles, and other membrane-active agents by secreting superoxide anion, hydrogen peroxide, hydroxyl radical, and in the case of monocytes, hypohalous acid, into phagosomes and into the extracellular space.[190] Immunologic activation markedly increases the ability of macrophages to secrete these products, both in laboratory animals[190,252-254] and in man.[225,256] In the mouse, many malignant cells and some nonmalignant cells secrete a product that selectively down-regulates the capacity of macrophages to secrete reactive oxygen intermediates.[257]

These products can inactivate thiol groups in enzymes, rearrange and break bonds in proteins, lipids, and nucleic acids, and initiate radical chain reactions capable of inflicting further damage of the same kind.[258] The primary evolutionary role of the leukocyte-derived reactive oxygen intermediates is probably microbicidal. However, their other pro- and anti-inflammatory effects are legion, as summarized in Table 10–9. In addition to cytotoxicity toward malignant and normal cells,[190] reactive oxygen intermediates can regulate the function of neutrophils, platelets, and lymphocytes in a noncytotoxic manner, which is not yet fully understood. Oxidation of critical methionyl residues can inactivate a number of humoral mediators or regulators of inflammation, including leukotriene C and α_1-protease inhibitor.

It has already been noted that macrophages undergo two respiratory bursts simultaneously in response to many of the same stimuli: incomplete reduction of molecular oxygen to produce reactive intermediates, and oxygenation of arachidonic acid. In an immunologically activated mouse peritoneal macrophage, about 100 times more oxygen is consumed in the former path than in the latter. The two respiratory bursts may interact at the levels of initiation, radical formation and utilization, and glutathione oxidation and consumption, in ways not yet fully analyzed. It is of interest that the activities of these two respiratory bursts are often under reciprocal control during immunologic activation in the mouse.[238,252]

Regulatory Factors for Other Cells. One of the most rapidly growing areas in the study of macrophage secretory function concerns factors that regulate synthesis by or growth of other types of cells. Many of these factors have been identified only as bioactivities and may be chemically similar to each other or to macrophage products whose composition is already known. An example is the remarkable protein interleukin-1,[259] whose purification has been achieved.[260] Interleukin-1 appears

Table 10–7. Metabolism of 20:4 by Mouse Peritoneal Macrophages Utilizing Exogenous Free Fatty Acid Without a Triggering Stimulus*

Feature	Resident Macrophages	Activated Macrophages
Percentage 20:4 incorporated into cell phospholipid†	34	70
Percentage 20:4 oxygenated†	65	17
Metabolites (as percentage of 20:4 oxygenated)†		
Cyclooxygenase products		
PGE$_2$	8	6
PGI$_2$	26	1
TXA$_2$	0	2
PGF$_{2\alpha}$	0	4
Lipoxygenase products		
HETES	42‡	4
LTC	3	0

*Compiled from ref. 241.

†Within 5 minutes of supplying cells with up to 1 μM 20:4 in serum-free medium.

‡Within 60 minutes 50 percent of released or exogenously supplied mono-hydroxyeicosatetraenoic acids (mono-HETES) are metabolized to di-HETES.[240]

Table 10–8. Possible Shifts in Mouse Macrophage 20:4* Metabolites During an Inflammatory Response

Metabolites	Early Inflammation: Resident Cells		Late Inflammation: Activated Cells	
	From Endogenous Phospholipid 20:4 With Trigger	From Exogenous Free Fatty Acid 20:4 Without Trigger[†]	From Endogenous Phospholipid 20:4 With Trigger	From Exogenous Free Fatty Acid 20:4 Without Trigger[†]
PGE$_2$	18[‡]	0.6	4	0.03
PGI$_2$	6	1.6	0.02	0.01
TXA$_2$	0	0	0.7	0.01
PGF$_2$	0	0	0	0.02
HETES	3	4.4	1	0.08
LTC	5	0.02	0.13	0

*20:4 = arachidonic acid.
[†]Assuming 1 μM exogenous 20:4 in serum-free conditions.
[‡]pmol per μg cell protein.

to be a major macrophage product involved in stimulation of thymocyte proliferation (lymphocyte-activating factor);[261] B lymphocyte proliferation;[262] hyperthermia (endogenous pyrogen);[263] synovial cell synthesis of prostaglandins, collagenase, and plasminogen activator;[264] fibroblast growth[265] and collagenase production;[266] and perhaps hepatocyte synthesis of acute phase reactants.[267,268] However, there are clearly different factors made by macrophages that promote the growth of myeloid cells and of erythrocytes,[269] including erythropoietin.[270] The nature of other macrophage growth factors for fibroblasts, smooth muscle cells, and endothelial cells[271,272] remains to be defined.

Macrophages release both an insulinlike activity[273] and a factor that inhibits the action of insulin on adipocytes, suppressing their activity of lipoprotein lipase,[274] acetyl Co-A carboxylase, and fatty acid synthetase.[275] The latter factor is secreted by macrophages challenged with endotoxin and may contribute to the

hypertriglyceridemia of acute phase responses and the insulin resistance of chronic infection. Even though this macrophage product inhibits lipoprotein lipase in adipocytes, macrophages themselves spontaneously secrete lipoprotein lipase into the medium.[276,277]

Factors from macrophages that suppress the replication of other cells include tumor necrosis factor,[278] interferon,[279] arginase (which depletes arginine from the medium),[280] reactive oxygen intermediates,[281] prostaglandins,[247] and thymidine.[282] The interferon secreted by macrophages is probably usually of the alpha type, but secretion of gamma interferon has also been reported.[283,284] The question has not yet been settled whether the latter is in fact acid-labile alpha-interferon. The issue is of interest, because gamma-interferon is a potent macrophage-activating factor.[256]

ANTIMICROBIAL FUNCTIONS

Spectrum. Presumably, one of the functions of macrophages providing the greatest evolutionary pressure for their representation throughout the phyla is that of inactivating invading microbes. In general, the antimicrobial spectrum of macrophages exceeds that of neutrophils, although neutrophils kill many organisms more rapidly than macrophages. However, the chief distinction between the antimicrobial ability of macrophages and neutrophils consists in the inducibility of this function in macrophages. Thus, normal macrophages will often support or succumb to viruses, *Chlamydia, Rickettsia, Listeria, Legionella, Corynebacterium, Salmonella, Brucella, Pasteurella, Nocardia, Mycobacteria, Leishmania, Toxoplasma, Trypanosoma, Cryptococcus,* or *Aspergillus.* With "activation," however, macrophages can inhibit or destroy many of the same organisms.[285] In addition, macrophages can damage multicellular parasites such as schistosomula[286] and microfilariae[287] through attachment that does not lead to phagocytosis.

If macrophages are not sufficiently microbicidal, however, they may provide certain microbes with a sanctuary within which to replicate. *Legionella pneumophila* is such a pathogen.[288] In fact, some parasites exist in the tissues

Table 10–9. Effects of Reactive Oxygen Intermediates

On Cells	On Extracellular Factors
Killing of viruses, bacteria, fungi, protozoa, nematodes, trematodes	Depolymerization of ground substance
Mutagenesis of bacteria	Aggregation of immunoglobulin
Killing of tumor cells	Inactivation of chemotactic peptides
Killing of erythrocytes, endothelial cells, fibroblasts, lung parenchyma, spermatazoa, platelets, leukocytes	Inactivation of leukotrienes and prostaglandins
	Activation of chemotactic lipids
	Inactivation of met-enkephalin
Inhibition of leukocyte lysosomal enzyme release	Inactivation of α_1-antiprotease
Noncytolytic triggering of platelet and mast cell secretion	Inactivation of leukocyte lysosomal hydrolases
	Inactivation of bacterial toxins
Suppression of lymphocyte responses, directly or through oxidation of soluble immune response suppressor from T cells	
Suppression of natural killer cells	

almost exclusively within macrophages. *Leishmania* is an important example.

Mechanisms. One of the major antimicrobial mechanisms of macrophages is the production of reactive oxygen intermediates (ROI).[190,289] This is true both for monocytes, which are richly endowed with myeloperoxidase, and for tissue macrophages, which are not. For *Toxoplasma, Leishmania, Trypanosoma, Candida,* and *Mycobacterium,* there is a close correlation between the antimicrobial activity of a given macrophage population and its capacity to secrete ROI. Similarly, there is a correlation between the ability of a pathogen to trigger the secretion of ROI during its ingestion and its susceptibility to killing by macrophages. The susceptibility of a microbe to killing by ROI often correlates with the susceptibility of the same organisms to killing by macrophages, and this in turn can be inversely related to the levels of antioxidant defense pathways in the parasites. Finally, experimental interventions that decrease the level of ROI within macrophages also decrease killing, and interventions that augment the level or the cytotoxic efficiency of ROI enhance killing. Thus there is abundant evidence (reviewed in ref. 289) to support the importance of oxygen-dependent antimicrobial mechanisms.

However, oxygen-independent antimicrobial mechanisms also function within macrophages.[289] This seems assured from the fact that the monocytes of patients with chronic granulomatous disease, which produce very little ROI during ingestion of parasites, have reduced but definite antimicrobial activity.[290] Chronic granulomatous disease macrophages can be activated by lymphocyte products to display enhanced antimicrobial activity, and this is not accompanied by increased secretion of ROI, nor is it impeded by interventions designed to lower the intracellular concentration of ROI.[291] Indeed, fibroblasts and endothelial cells can kill some of the same pathogens as macrophages without evidence for secretion of ROI.[291]

The nature of the oxygen-independent antimicrobial mechanisms of macrophages is not yet firmly established.[289,293] Contributory factors may include acidification of the phagosome, the action of cationic peptides and lysosomal hydrolases, the production of complement components and interferon, depletion of arginine by secretion of arginase, and sequestration of iron by iron-binding proteins. Finally, the possibility has been raised that withholding of a trophic factor, rather than provision of a toxic one, may contribute to the ability of activated macrophages to inhibit the replication of certain organisms that depend on parasitization of macrophages for their survival in the mammalian host.[289]

The importance of individual antimicrobial mechanisms can be inferred from the evasions employed by parasites during successful infection of macrophages. For example, *Toxoplasma gondii* enters nonactivated macrophages without triggering the usual production of ROI, although the macrophages are fully capable of being triggered by other agents. When the macrophages are activated, or when the parasite is coated with antibody, then its ingestion elicits a normal respiratory burst, and survival of the parasite is impaired.[290] *Brucella abortus* secretes an unusual adenylate cyclase, which is taken up by macrophages, acutely raises their cyclic adenosine monophosphate levels, and suppresses their ability to secrete ROI in response to any stimulus, including the ingestion of the bacterium.[294] *Mycobacterium tuberculosis* frustrates the ability of the macrophage to empty its lysosomes into the phagosome, apparently by means of sulfolipids, which prevent fusion of the membranes of these organelles.[295] *M. lepraemurium,* however, permits fusion of phagosomes and lysosomes to occur and survives nonetheless.[296] *Trypanosoma cruzi* breaks out of its phagolysosome to replicate within the cytoplasm.[297] The complexity of the behavior of parasites during and after their ingestion by macrophages testifies to the variability of antimicrobial mechanisms that may be paramount in individual macrophage–parasite combinations.

ANTITUMOR FUNCTION

One of the most dramatic performances of the macrophage on the stage of the microscope is the destruction of malignant cells. Through a reaction resembling a receptor-ligand interaction, activated macrophages form a firm attachment with tumor cells and secrete a cytolytic factor whose action includes a proteolytic step.[298] Nonmalignant cells and nonactivated macrophages appear unable to participate in this form of binding and lysis.[6] Small amounts of hydrogen peroxide released from activated macrophages may interact synergistically with the cytolytic factor.[299] The actual basis of cytotoxicity is not yet clear but appears to involve damage to tumor cell mitochondria at specific sites in the respiratory chain in a pattern typical of peroxidative damage.[300]

Compared with the spontaneous cytolysis described above, even more rapid and extensive lysis of tumor cells can result from triggering the respiratory burst of the activated macrophage.[281] Antibody-coated tumor cells interacting with Fc receptors on the macrophage sometimes elicit their own destruction in this manner.[301] Oxidative injury also appears to account for the rapid lysis of tumor cells coated with eosinophil peroxidase and exposed to activated macrophages in the absence of any known stimulus of the macrophage respiratory burst.[302]

There are numerous lines of evidence to indicate that macrophages can kill tumor cells in vivo.[303] Recent attention has focused on the role of macrophages in the therapeutic effects of monoclonal antitumor antibodies[304] and of adjuvant-laden liposomes.[305]

Just as many microbes have found ways to evade destruction by macrophages, so do tumor cells suppress macrophage-mediated cytotoxicity. For example, tumor cell products have been found both in the mouse and in man that inhibit the ability of macrophages to accumulate in tumors.[173,174] A product of malignant cells selectively suppresses the ability of macrophages to se-

crete hydrogen peroxide[257] and to kill intracellular protozoa.[306] Finally, tumor cells catabolize macrophage cytotoxic factors and repair their lesions. Pharmacologic
agents that interfere with these processes enhance macrophage-mediated cytotoxicity.[307,308]

IMMUNOREGULATORY FUNCTIONS

Helper Effects. T and B lymphocytes are highly dependent on adherent mononuclear cells for many of their
functions. Initial reports attributed this accessory cell
activity solely to macrophages, a view that now requires
revision. Most macrophage-rich populations, including
those from human blood, contain small numbers of dendritic cells, which are also mononuclear, adherent, bone
marrow-derived, and rich in Ia antigens in the mouse
or in the homologous antigens in other species.[309] It has
been clearly shown, however, that dendritic cells are
distinct from macrophages. Indeed, these two populations are segregated from each other anatomically in
lymph nodes, spleen, and dermis, although they circulate
together in blood.[10] Almost all procedures used to deplete macrophages (including anti-Ia antibodies) also
deplete dendritic cells and do not clarify which cell may
be required. However, selective elimination of dendritic
cells with specific monoclonal antibody plus complement removes nearly all accessory activity for mixed
leukocyte reactions, generation of cytotoxic T lymphocytes, proliferation of T lymphocytes in response to per-
iodate-treated cells or antigen, and development of antibody-secreting B lymphocytes.[310] Highly enriched
populations of dendritic cells reconstitute the same responses. The numbers of dendritic cells needed to do so
are consistent with their number in the unseparated
lymphoid cell populations. In contrast, using monoclonal antibodies which spare dendritic cells, specific
depletion of monocytes has little or no effect on the
same immune responses.[311]

Nonetheless, macrophages or their secretory products
clearly can promote lymphocyte viability and proliferation. Reconstitution of macrophage-depleted cultures
with 2-mercaptoethanol and/or interleukin-1 often re-
establishes much of the response. 2-Mercaptoethanol
may substitute for glutathione, a macrophage secretory
product;[312] interleukin-1 is also a macrophage product
and has been discussed above.

One somewhat speculative way of viewing accessory
cell function is as follows. Resting T lymphocytes require
contact with both antigen and dendritic cells in order
to initiate secretion of interleukin-2. After the onset of
interleukin-2 secretion, dendritic cells are no longer required.[313] The magnitude of the ensuing response will
be much greater in the presence of trophic factors derived
from macrophages, especially interleukin-1, which augments interleukin-2 secretion by T lymphocytes.[314] In
the presence of the antigen alone (without need for dendritic cells), antigen-responsive T lymphocytes express
interleukin-2 receptors. Binding of interleukin-2 to these
receptors drives proliferation. If some T lymphocytes

are already activated at the time the experiment begins
(that is, they are secreting interleukin-2), a dendritic cell
requirement may not be evident, and the only accessory
cell still augmenting the response may be the macrophage (or another cell that produces interleukin-1).

Another area of controversy concerns the presentation
and processing of antigen by macrophages. In several
experimental systems, optimal immunologic responses
have occurred with 3 to 4 logs less antigen when the
antigen was added in association with macrophage-rich
populations than when added alone.[315] In part, this may
represent the contribution of the trophic macrophage
products discussed above, but additional factors are
likely to be involved and are not yet fully understood.
The ability to partially degrade antigens and select determinants under immune response gene control was
also attributed to macrophages. That is, it was thought
that macrophages from a nonresponder animal failed to
present the appropriate determinant to T cells. Recently,
further data obtained in the original experimental system
have supported alternative interpretations.[316] Thus, portions of antigen indeed seem to be associated with macrophages, but it is doubtful that IR genes act by determining how macrophages catabolize a given antigen.

Suppressor Effects. Many of the same immunologic
functions that are impaired by depleting adherent cells
are also suboptimal when the number of adherent cells
is higher than normal or when the macrophages among
them are activated.[317] Depressed immunologic responses
in vitro using lymphocytes from patients with myeloma,
Hodgkin's disease, other malignancies, or fungal infections appear to be due to adherent suppressor cells,
which in many cases are probably monocytes or macrophages.[318] The mechanism of suppression often seems
to involve prostaglandin secretion by the adherent
cells.[247,318] In some cases, inhibitory effects can be attributed to the secretion of hydrogen peroxide[318] or arginase.[280]

SELECTIVE REMOVAL OF
AUTOLOGOUS CELLS

Removal of senescent, damaged, and perhaps aberrant
cells is one of the chief functions of macrophages. The
process has been best studied with erythrocytes, which
are subject to at least three kinds of changes that lead
to their selective removal. These mechanisms, while imperfectly understood, can serve as models for the means
by which macrophages may be signaled to remove other
kinds of autologous cells.

Senescent Cells. Aged red cells are opsonized by an
immunoglobulin present in normal human serum and
are ingested by autologous macrophages.[319] This may be
the mechanism by which macrophages, mostly in the
spleen, daily remove some 3×10^{11} red cells from the
circulation, a meal of 2.7 kg of hemoglobin per year.[81]
The antigen recognized on senescent red cells appears
to be related to the transmembrane protein, band 3. It
is not known how senescence leads to autoantigenicity

of a tiny portion of band 3 sites per cell.[319] Macrophages also ingest senescent neutrophils.[320] The basis of recognition in this case is unknown. There are natural antibodies in man to desialyated cells[321] as well as antibody-independent receptors on monocytes for some desialylated erythrocytes.[322] Thus, loss of sialic acid may also provide a signal.[323]

Cells Targeted by Autoimmune Reactions. In immune hemolytic anemias, red cells are opsonized, pulled from the circulation by macrophages, and ingested or destroyed extracellulary. Spherocytes, the morphologic hallmark of such anemias, are red cells from which opsonized pieces of membrane have been plucked, reducing the surface-to-volume ratio. In a similar manner, ingestion of opsonized platelets by macrophages underlies autoimmune thrombocytopenia.[324]

Metabolically Defective Cells. Red cells that are abnormally susceptible to oxidant stress are removed by splenic and hepatic macrophages. For example, during infection, leukocytes engaged in phagocytosis release hydrogen peroxide, which depletes the glutathione of glucose-6-phosphate dehydrogenase–deficient red cells and leads to their destruction in the liver and spleen.[325]

Wound Healing. The rate of removal of fibrin, neutrophils, erythrocytes, and other debris from wounds and the local ingrowth of fibroblasts and vascular buds are markedly impaired when monocytopenia is induced.[326]

EFFECTS OF ANTI-INFLAMMATORY DRUGS ON MACROPHAGES

Glucocorticoids. In man, intravenous hydrocortisone induces a profound monocytopenia, with a nadir at 4 to 7 hours and restoration of normal counts in 24 hours.[327] This time course suggests that redistribution of cells may be partly responsible for the changes. Prednisone depresses both the blood monocyte count and the accumulation of monocytes in skin windows. Both features normalize with alternate-day administration of the drug.[328] Epicutaneous application of glucocorticoids retards accumulation of monocytes in skin windows at the same site.[329] In the mouse, hydrocortisone causes a 35 percent drop in the number of marrow promonocytes. Mitotic activity is unaffected, and the monocyte production rate falls only 20 percent. However, the release of newly formed monocytes from the marrow is sharply curtailed, and peripheral monocytopenia is marked.[330]

Monocytes from prednisone-treated volunteers are subnormal in killing of *Staphylococcus* and *Candida* despite normal phagocytosis.[331] Macrophages from hydrocortisone-treated mice are 1000-fold more susceptible to murine hepatitis virus in vitro than those from untreated animals.[332]

In vitro, glucocorticoids retard the increases in size and lysosomal enzyme content that normally accompany the differentiation of monocytes into macrophages.[333] If the monocytes are exposed continuously to hydrocortisone for 4 days, their ability to release hydrogen peroxide is suppressed by over 90 percent. The 50 percent inhibitory concentration of hydrocortisone is only about 0.2 micromolar. However, if continuous exposure is limited to 2 days, there is no suppressive effect even from 10 micromolar hydrocortisone.[334] Thus, diurnal peaks of endogenous glucocorticoids, or alternate-day administration of the drugs, would not be expected to have the same effect as continuous maintenance of high blood levels. In vitro treatment of human monocytes with cortisone also suppressed their ability to bind erythrocytes opsonized with immunoglobulin or complement.[335]

In the mouse, treatment of macrophages in vitro with glucocorticoids suppresses glucose utilization and overall protein synthesis.[336] Thus it is not surprising that there is depressed expression or secretion of Ia antigens,[337] interleukin-1,[337] plasminogen activator, collagenase, elastase, and other neutral proteases.[338] In contrast, low-dose treatment of rat peritoneal macrophages with cortisol reportedly enhances their protein synthesis and their ability to resorb bone in vitro.[339] Glucocorticoids also inhibit macrophage spreading on glass[274] and response to migration inhibitory factor from lymphocytes.[341]

While not anti-inflammatory, the estrogenic steroids also affect macrophages. Phagocytic activity of the fixed macrophages, as measured by clearance studies, is increased by estrogenic but not androgenic hormones.[342] Changes in phagocytic activity attend the fluctuations in estrogenic levels during the menstrual cycle and pregnancy. Ovariectomy reduces the capacity of mice to resist virulent infections.[342]

Gold Salts. Gold salts accumulate in macrophage lysosomes, where they inhibit a number of enzymes.[343] The chemotactic response of human monocytes to formylated peptides is also inhibited by these agents.[344] Of considerable interest is the ability of therapeutically attained concentrations of gold salts to block the ability of lymphocyte mediators to enhance monocyte production of complement component C2 in the absence of demonstrable toxicity to the monocytes. Monocytes that are already activated by lymphokine are unaffected.[345] This raises the possibility that the delayed therapeutic benefits of gold salts in vivo could have to do, in part, with the time it takes activated macrophages in the joint to be replaced by new cells that have yet to be activated. In murine models, treatment with gold salts impairs the virucidal[346] and tumoricidal activity of macrophages.[347]

D-Penicillamine. The enhanced mitogen responses of lymphocytes from arthritic animals treated with D-penicillamine have been attributed in part to diminished suppressor activity of their macrophages.[348] The drug also seems to stimulate the uptake of aggregated immunoglobulin by macrophages.[349] In addition, this agent seems to protect α_1-antiprotease from oxidative inactivation.[350] The mechanisms of these effects and their possible relevance to the anti-inflammatory action of D-penicillamine remain to be worked out.

Cytotoxic Agents. Azathioprine blocks mouse promonocytes in late S or G2 phase, resulting in a severe drop in monocyte production and failure of monocytes to accumulate in inflammatory exudates.[351] Cyclophosphamide also reduces marrow colony-forming cells, circulating monocyte levels, and accumulation of macrophages in inflammatory exudates.[352,353]

Other Nonsteroidal Anti-Inflammatory Agents. Many of these agents have the expected effect on macrophage synthesis of arachidonic acid metabolites, which may account in part for some of their beneficial effects in vivo.[354]

AN OVERVIEW: MACROPHAGE ACTIVATION

Almost every structural or functional feature of macrophages has been reported to change when the hosts or the cells are treated in some way. This accounts for much of the fascination these cells hold for many investigators, and also for some of the difficulty the investigators have in communicating with each other. For example, any gradual augmentation may be called "activation," or the term may be used to refer to the effect of any stimulus, however prompt. However, there is a more restricted usage of the term, which forms a central thread in the study of macrophages from the time of Metchnikoff to the present day. It is fitting to conclude a description of macrophage physiology by retracing this thread.[289]

Metchnikoff observed that macrophages in infected hosts often responded more vigorously to the introduction of phagocytic particles. In 1939, Lurie clearly demonstrated that the macrophages from tuberculous animals were larger and more phagocytic than those from controls. In the 1960s, Mackaness and his colleagues revealed both the immunologic basis and the protective function of macrophage activation. They demonstrated that in the later stages of infection or after the host recovers, its lymphocytes, when encountering the antigens of the original infecting organism, confer upon macrophages an enhanced capacity to inhibit the intracellular replication of the same or unrelated pathogens. That is, induction of macrophage activation is immunologically specific, while its expression is nonspecific and consists, in its essence, of enhanced antimicrobial capacity.

At the same time that macrophages acquire enhanced antimicrobial capacity, they undergo innumerable other changes, such as increased spreading on glass and alterations in phagocytic activity, surface receptor function, and the content of organelles and enzymes. These changes, for a time, were also referred to as macrophage activation. In the mid and late 1970s, however, it became apparent that such changes could be induced by a variety of means in macrophages that did not express enhanced antimicrobial activity, that not all the changes appear concordantly, that macrophages with enhanced antimicrobial activity often exhibit decreases rather than increases in other functions, or that these other functions may change in different ways under different experimental conditions, without relation to antimicrobial ac-

tivity. By the end of the decade, the only biochemical feature that could be firmly correlated with antimicrobial capacity was the ability to secrete hydrogen peroxide. This surely reflects the prominent role of reactive oxygen intermediates in the killing of intracellular pathogens by macrophages. However, it has become increasingly apparent that oxygen-independent antimicrobial mechanisms are important under certain conditions, and in these cases, peroxide-secretory capacity and antimicrobial activity can be dissociated.

Just as some workers use macrophage "activation" in the sense introduced by Mackaness, and others use it to refer to enhanced antitumor activity, or to enhanced peroxide-secretory capacity, or to any altered function, so there is divergence in usage of the term "macrophage activating factor." Recent evidence indicates that in the case of oxidative metabolism, killing of intracellular protozoal pathogens, and killing of extracellular tumor cells, the primary T-lymphocyte product that activates macrophages is gamma-interferon.[256] However, other macrophage-activating factors may remain to be defined in the same or other assays. What about activation of macrophages by non-T lymphocytes, by nonlymphoid cells, by humoral agents like complement, or by bacterial products like lipopolysaccharide and muramyl dipeptide? It is conceivable that these involve secretion of alpha- or beta-interferon, or act through the induction of interferon secretion by the macrophages themselves.[355] In this view, there would be a final common pathway for macrophage activation. Alternatively, there may be many ways to activate a macrophage. The consequences of activation are so dramatic for numerous functions of this ubiquitous cell that this question remains an area of intense research 100 years after it was raised.

References

1. Metchnikoff, E.: Immunity in Infective Diseases. F.G. Binnie, trans. London, Cambridge University Press, 1905.
2. van Furth, R. (ed.): Mononuclear Phagocytes. Oxford, Blackwell Scientific Publications, 1970.
3. van Furth, R. (ed.): Mononuclear Phagocytes in Immunity, Infection and Pathology. Oxford, Blackwell Scientific Publications, 1975.
4. van Furth, R. (ed.): Mononuclear Phagocytes: Functional Aspects. The Hague, Martinus Nijhoff, 1980.
5. Nelson, D.W. (ed.): Immunobiology of the Macrophage. New York, Academic Press, 1976.
6. Fink, M.A. (ed.): The Macrophage in Neoplasia. New York, Academic Press, 1976.
7. Zweifach, B.W., Grant, L., and McCluskey, R.T. (eds.): The Inflammatory Process. 2nd ed. New York, Academic Press, 1973.
8. Langevoort, H.C., Cohn, Z.A., Hirsch, J.G., Humphrey, J.H., Spector, W.G., and van Furth, R.: The nomenclature of mononuclear phagocytes: Proposal for a new classification. In van Furth, R. (ed.): Mononuclear Phagocytes. Oxford, Blackwell Scientific Publications, 1970, p. 1.
9. Hume, D.A., and Gordon, S.: The mononuclear phagocyte system of the mouse defined by immunohistochemical localisation of antigen F4/80. Identification of resident macropahges in renal medullary and cortical interstitium and the juxtaglomerular complex. J. Exp. Med. 157:1704, 1983.
10. van Voorhis, W.C., Steinman, R.M., Hair, L.S., Luban, J., Witmer, M.D., Koide, S., and Cohn, Z.A.: Specific antimononuclear phagocyte monoclonal antibodies. Application to the purification of dendritic cells and the tissue localization of macrophages. J. Exp. Med. 158:126, 1983.
11. Volkman, A., and Gowans, J.L.: The origin of macrophages from bone marrow in the rat. Br. J. Exp. Pathol. 46:62, 1965.
12. van Furth, R., and Cohn, Z.A.: The origin and kinetics of mononuclear phagocytes. J. Exp. Med. 128:415, 1968.

13. Goud, T.J.L.M., Schotte, C., and van Furth, R.: Identification and characterization of the monoblast in mononuclear phagocyte colonies grown in vitro. J. Exp. Med. 142:1180, 1975.

14. Goud, T.J.L.M., and van Furth, R.: Proliferative characteristics of monoblasts grown in vitro. J. Exp. Med. 142:1200, 1975.

15. van Furth, R., Hirsch, J.G., and Fedorko, M.E.: Morphology and peroxidase cytochemistry of mouse promonocytes, monocytes, and macrophages. J. Exp. Med. 132:794, 1970.

16. van Furth, R.: Origin and kinetics of mononuclear phagocytes. Ann. N.Y. Acad. Sci. 278:161, 1976.

17. Meuret, G., Batara, E., and Furste, H.O. Monocytopoiesis in normal man: Pool size, proliferation activity and DNA synthesis time of promonocytes. Acta Haematol. 54:261, 1975.

18. Meuret, G., Bammert, J., and Hoffman, G.: Kinetics of human monocytopoiesis. Blood 44:801, 1974.

19. Whitelaw, D.M., and Batho, H.F.: Kinetics of monocytes. In van Furth, R. (ed.): Mononuclear Phagocytes in Immunity, Infection and Pathology. Oxford, Blackwell Scientific Publications, 1975, p. 175.

20. Whitelaw, D.M.: Observations on human monocyte kinetics after pulse labelling. Cell Tissue Kinet. 5:311, 1972.

21. Meuret, G., and Hoffmann, G.: Monocyte kinetic studies in normal and disease states. Br. J. Haematol. 24:275, 1973.

22. van Furth, R., and Diesselhoff-den Dulk, M.C.: The kinetics of promonocytes and monocytes in the bone marrow. J. Exp. Med. 132:813, 1970.

23. Ebert, R.H., and Florey, H.W.: The extravascular development of the monocyte observed in vivo. Br. J. Exp. Pathol. 20:342, 1939.

24. van Furth, R.: Origin and kinetics of monocytes and macrophages. Semin. Hematol. 7:125, 1970.

25. Meuret, G., Detel, U., Kilz, H.P., Senn, H.J., and van Lessen, H.: Human monocytopoiesis in acute and chronic inflammation. Acta Haematol. 54:328, 1975.

26. Lewis, M.R.: The formation of macrophages, epithelioid cells and giant cells from leukocytes in incubated blood. Am. J. Pathol. 1:91, 1925.

27. Bennett, W.E., and Cohn, Z.A.: The isolation and selected properties of blood monocytes. J. Exp. Med. 123:145, 1966.

28. Johnson, W.D., Jr., Mei, B., and Cohn, Z.A.: The separation, long-term cultivation, and maturation of the human monocyte. J. Exp. Med. 146:1613, 1977.

29. Musson, R.A., Shafran, H., and Henson, P.M.: Intracellular levels and stimulated release of lysosomal enzymes from human peripheral blood monocytes and monocyte-derived macrophages. J. Reticuloendothel. Soc. 28:249, 1980.

30. Newman, S.L., Musson, R.A., and Henson, P.M.: Development of functional complement receptors during in vitro maturation of human monocytes into macrophages. J. Immunol. 125:2236, 1980.

31. Nakagawara, A., Nathan, C.F., and Cohn, Z.A.: Hydrogen peroxide metabolism in human monocytes during differentiation in vitro. J. Clin. Invest. 68:1243, 1981.

32. Volkman, A.: Disparity in origin of mononuclear phagocyte populations. J. Reticuloendothel. Soc. 19:249, 1976.

33. Shands, J.W., and Axelrod, B.J.: Mouse peritoneal macrophages: Tritiated thymidine labelling and cell kinetics. J. Reticuloendothel. Soc. 21:69, 1977.

34. Volkman, A.: Monocyte kinetics and their changes in infection. In Nelson, D.S. (ed.): Immunobiology of the Macrophage. New York, Academic Press, 1976, p. 294.

35. Pinkett, M.O., Cordrey, C.R., and Nowell, P.C.: Mixed hematopoietic and pulmonary origin of 'alveolar macrophages' as demonstrated by chromosome markers. Am. J. Pathol. 48:859, 1966.

36. Crofton, R.W., Martina, M.C., Diesselhoff-den Dulk, M.M.C., and van Furth, R.: The origin, kinetics, and characteristics of the Kupffer cells in the normal steady state. J. Exp. Med. 148:1, 1978.

37. Gale, R.P., Sparkes, R.S., and Golde, D.W.: Bone marrow origin of hepatic macrophages (Kupffer cells) in humans. Science 201:937, 1978.

38. Oehmichen, M.: Monocytic origin of microglia cells. In van Furth, R. (ed.): Mononuclear Phagocytes in Immunity, Infection and Pathology. Oxford, Blackwell Scientific Publications 1975, p. 223.

39. Blussé van Oud Ablas, A., and van Furth, R.: Origin, kinetics, and characteristics of pulmonary macrophages in the normal steady state. J. Exp. Med. 149:1504, 1979.

40. Evans, J.J., Cabral, L.J., Stephens R.J., and Freeman, G.: Cell division of alveolar macrophages in rat lung following exposure to NO_2. Am. J. Pathol. 70:199, 1973.

41. Steward, C.C., Lin, H.S., and Adles, C.: Proliferation and colony-forming ability of peritoneal exudate cells in liquid culture. J. Exp. Med. 141:1114, 1975.

42. Volkman, A., and Gowans, J.L.: The production of macrophages in the rat. Br. J. Exp. Pathol. 46:50, 1965.

43. North, R.J.: The mitotic potential of fixed phagocytes in the liver as revealed during the development of cellular immunity. J. Exp. Med. 130:315, 1969.

44. Spector, W.G., and Mariano, M.: Macrophage behaviour in experimental granulomas. In van Furth, R. (ed.): Mononuclear Phagocytes in Immunity, Infection and Pathology. Oxford, Blackwell Scientific Publications, 1975, p. 927.

45. Dannenberg, A.M., Ando, M., Shima, K., and Tsuda, T.: Macrophage turnover and activation in tuberculous granulomata. In van Furth, R. (ed.): Mononuclear Phagocytes in Immunity, Infection and Pathology. Oxford, Blackwell Scientific Publications, 1975, p. 959.

46. Sutton, J.S.: Ultrastructural aspects of in vitro development of monocytes into macrophages, epithelioid cells, and multinucleated giant cells. Natl. Cancer Inst. Monograph 26:71, 1967.

47. Postlethwaite, A.E., Jackson, B.K., Beachey, E.H., and Kang, A.H.: Formation of multinucleated giant cells from human monocyte precursors. Mediation by a soluble protein from antigen- and mitogen-stimulated lymphocytes. J. Exp. Med. 155:168, 1982.

48. Lewis, W.H.: The formation of giant cells in tissue cultures and their similarity to those in tuberculous lesions. Am. Rev. Tuberculosis 15:616, 1927.

49. Izumi, S., Penrose, J.M., More, D.G., and Nelson, D.S.: Further observation on the immunological induction of DNA synthesis in mouse peritoneal macrophages. Int. Arch. Allergy App. Immunol. 49:573, 1975.

50. van Waarde, D., Hulsing-Hesselink, E., and van Furth, R.: Properties of a factor increasing monocytopoiesis (FIM) occurring in serum during the early phase of an inflammatory reaction. Blood 50:727, 1977.

51. Chervenick, P., and Lobuglio, A.F.: Human blood monocytes: Stimulators of granulocyte and mononuclear colony formation in vitro. Science 78:164, 1972.

52. Parker, J.W., and Metcalf, D.: Production of colony-stimulating factor in mitogen-stimulated lymphocyte cultures. J. Immunol. 112:502, 1974.

53. Stanley, E.R., and Guilbert, L.J.: Regulation of macrophage production by a colony stimulating factor. In van Furth, R. (ed.): Mononuclear Phagocytes: Functional Aspects. The Hague, Martinus Nijhoff, 1980, p. 417.

54. Loor, kF., and Roelants, G.E.: The dynamic state of the macrophage plasma membrane. Attachment and fate of immunoglobulin, antigen, and lectins. Eur. J. Immunol. 4:649, 1974.

55. Colvin, R.B., and Dvorak, H.F.: Fibrinogen/fibrin on the surface of macrophages: Detection, distribution, binding requirements, and possible role in macrophage adherence phenomena. J. Exp. Med. 142:1337, 1975.

56. van Ginkel, C.J.W., and van Akan, W.G.: Generation of tissue thromboplastin by human monocytes. In van Furth, R. (ed.): Mononuclear Phagocytes: Functional Aspects. The Hague, Martinus Nijhoff, 1980, p. 1351.

57. Nachman, R.L., Ferris, B., and Hirsch, J.G.: Macrophage plasma membrane. II. Studies on synthesis and turnover of protein constituents. J. Exp. Med. 133:807, 1971.

58. Werb, Z., and Cohn, Z.A.: Plasma membrane synthesis in the macrophage following phagocytosis of polystyrene latex particles. J. Biol. Chem. 247:2439, 1972.

59. Edelson, P.J., and Cohn, Z.A.: 5'-Nucleotidase activity of mouse peritoneal macrophages. II. Cellular distribution and effects of endocytosis. J. Exp. Med. 144:1596, 1976.

60. Edelson, P.J., and Cohn, Z.A.: 5'-Nucleotidase activity of mouse peritoneal macrophages. I. Synthesis and degradation in resident and inflammatory populations. J. Exp. Med. 144:1581, 1976.

61. Edelson, P.J., and Erbs, C.: Plasma membrane localization and metabolism of alkaline phosphodiesterase I in mouse peritoneal macrophages. J. Exp. Med. 147:77, 1978.

62. Edelson, P.J., Zweibel, R., and Cohn, Z.A.: The pinocytic rate of activated macrophages. J. Exp. Med. 142:1150, 1975.

63. Ezekowitz, R.A.B., Austyn, J., Stahl, P.D., and Gordon, S.: Surface properties of bacillus Calmette-Guerin-activated mouse macrophages. Reduced expression of mannose-specific endocytosis, Fc receptors, and antigen F4‖80 accompanies induction of Ia. J. Exp. Med. 154:60, 1981.

64. Remold-O'Donnell, E., and Lewandrowski, K.: Decrease of the major surface glycoprotein gp160 in activated macrophages. Cell. Immunol. 70:85, 982.

65. Werb, Z., and Cohn, Z.A.: Cholesterol metabolism in the macrophages. I. The regulation of cholesterol exchange. J. Exp. Med. 134:1545, 1971.

66. Werb, Z.: Macrophage membrane synthesis. In van Furth, R. (ed.): Mononuclear Phagocytes in Immunity, Infection and Pathology. Oxford, Blackwell Scientific Publications, 1975, p. 331.

67. Mahoney, E.M., Hamill, A.L., Scott, W.A., and Cohn, Z.A.: Response of endocytosis to altered fatty acyl composition of macrophage phospholipids. Proc. Natl. Acad. Sci. USA 74:4895, 1977.

68. Shreffler, D.C., and David, C.S.: The H-2 major histocompatibility complex and the I immune response gene region: Genetic variation, function and organization. Adv. Immunol. 20:125, 1975.

69. Steeg, P.S., Moore, R.N., and Oppenheim, J.J.: Regulation of macrophage

Ia-antigen expression by products of activated spleen cells. J. Exp. Med. 152:1734, 1980.

70. Steinman, R.M., Nogueira, N., Witmer, M.D., Tydings, J.D., and Mellman, I.S.: Lymphokine enhances the expression and synthesis of Ia antigens on cultured mouse peritoneal macrophages. J. Exp. Med. 152:1248, 1980.

71. Todd, R.F., III, and Schlossman, S.F.: Analysis of antigenic determinants of human monocytes and macrophages. Blood 59:775, 1982.

72. Hogg, N., Slusarenko, M., Cohen, J., and Reiser, J.: Monoclonal antibody with specificity for monocytes and neurons. Cell 24:875, 1981.

73. LeBien, T.W., Kersey, J.H.,: A monoclonal antibody (TA-1) reactive with human T lymphocytes and monocytes. J. Immunol. 125:2208, 1980.

74. Beller, D.P., Springer, T.A., and Schreiber, R.D.: Anti-Mac-1 selectively inhibits the mouse and human type three complement receptor. J. Exp. Med. 156:1000, 1982.

75. Austyn, J.M., and Gordon S.: F4∥80, a monoclonal antibody directed specifically against the mouse macrophage. Eur. J. Immunol. 11:805, 1981.

76. Taniyama, T., and Watanabe, T.: Establishment of hybridoma secreting a monoclonal antibody specific for activated tumoricidal macrophages. J. Exp. Med. 156:1286, 1982.

77. Berken, A., and Benacerraf, B.: Properties of antibodies cytophilic for macrophages. J. Exp. Med. 123:119, 1966.

78. Lobuglio, A.F., Cotran, R.S., and Jandl, J.H.: Red cells coated with immunoglobulin G: Binding and sphering by mononuclear cells in man. Science 158:1582, 1967.

79. Huber, H., Polley, M.J., Linscott, W.D., Fudenberg, H.H., and Muller-Eberhard, H.J.: Human monocytes: Distinct receptor sites for the third component of complement and for immunoglobulin G. Science 162:1281, 1968.

80. Unkeless, J.C., Fleit, H., and Mellman, I.S.: Structural aspects and heterogeneity of immunoglobulin Fc receptors. Adv. Immunol. 31:247, 1981.

81. Johnston, R.B., Jr., Lehmeyer, J., and Guthrie, L.: Generation of superoxide anion and chemiluminescence by human monocytes during phagocytosis and by contact with surface-bound immunoglobulin G. J. Exp. Med. 143:1551, 1978.

82. Ezekowitz, R.A.B., Bampton, M., and Gordon, S.: Macrophage activation selectively enhances expression of Fc receptors for IgG2a. J. Exp. Med. 157:807, 983.

83. Bonney, R.J., Naruns, P., Davies, P., and Humes, J.L.: Antigen-antibody complexes stimulate the synthesis and release of prostaglandins by mouse peritoneal macrophages. Prostaglandins 18:605, 1979.

84. Cardella, C.J., Davies, P., and Allison, A.C.: Immune complexes induce selective release of lysosomal hydrolases from macrophages. Nature 247:46, 1974.

85. Melewicz, F.M., and Spiegelberg, H.L.: Fc receptors for IgE on a subpopulation of human peripheral blood monocytes. J. Immunol. 125:1026, 1980.

86. Finbloom, D.S., and Metzger, H.: Binding of immunoglobulin E to the receptor on rat peritoneal macrophages. J. Immunol. 129:2004, 1982.

87. Joseph, M., Tonnel, A.-B., Torpier, G., and Capron, A.: Involvement of immunoglobulin E in the secretory processes of alveolar macrophages from asthmatic patients. J. Clin. Invest. 71:221, 1983.

88. Fleit, H.B., Wright, S.D., and Unkeless, J.C.: Human neutrophil Fc receptor distribution and structure. Proc. Natl. Acad. Sci. USA 79:3275, 1982.

89. Perussia, B., Dayton, E.T., Lazarus, R., Fanning, V., and Trinchieri, G.: Immune interferon induces the receptor for monomeric IgG1 on human monocytic and myeloid cells. J. Exp. Med., 158:1092, 1983.

90. Mellman, I.S., and Unkeless, J.C.: Purification of a functional mouse Fc receptor through the use of a monoclonal antibody. J. Exp. Med. 152:1048, 1980.

91. Young, J.D., Unkeless, J.C., Kaback, H.R., and Cohn, Z.A.: Mouse macrophage Fc receptor for IgG 2bγ1 in artificial and plasma membrane vesicles functions as a ligand-dependent ionophore. Proc. Natl. Acad. Sci. USA 80:1636, 1983.

92. Griffin, F.M., Jr., Bianco, C., and Silverstein, S.C.: Characterization of the macrophage receptor for complement and demonstration of its functional independence from the receptor for the Fc portion of immunoglobulin G. J. Exp. Med. 141:1269, 1975.

93. Ehlenberger, A.G., and Nussenzweig, V.: The role of membrane receptors for C3b and C3d in phagocytosis. J. Exp. Med. 145:357, 1977.

94. Bianco, C., Griffin, F.M., Jr., and Silverstein, S.C.: Studies of the macrophage complement receptor. Alteration of receptor function upon macrophage activation. J. Exp. Med. 141:1278, 1975.

95. Rabellino, E.M., Ross, G.D., and Polley, M.J.: Membrane receptors of mouse leukocytes. Two types of complement receptors for different regions of C3. J. Immunol. 120:879, 1978.

96. Goodman, M.G., Chenoweth, D.E., and Weigle, W.O.: Induction of interleukin 1 secretion and enhancement of humoral immunity by binding of human C5a to macrophage surface C5a receptors. J. Exp. Med. 156:912, 1982.

97. Griffin, J.A., and Griffin, F.M.: Augmentation of macrophage complement receptor function in vitro. I. Characterization of the cellular interactions required for the generation of a T-lymphocyte product that enhances macrophage complement receptor function. J. Exp. Med. 150:653, 1979.

98. Pommier, C.G., Inada, S., Fries, L.F., Takahashi, T., Frank, M.M., and Brown, E.J.: Plasma fibronectin enhances the phagocytosis of opsonized particles by human peripheral blood monocytes. J. Exp. Med. 157:1844, 1983.

99. Wright, S.D., Craigmyle, L., and Silverstein, S.C.: Fibronectin and serum amyloid P-component stimulate C3b- and C3bi-mediated phagocytosis in cultured human monocytes. J. Exp. Med., 158:1338, 1983.

100. Stahl, P.D., Rodman, J.S., Miller, M.J., and Schlesinger, P.H.: Evidence for receptor-mediated binding of glycoproteins, glycoconjugates and lysosomal glycosidases by alveolar macrophages. Proc. Natl. Acad. Sci. USA 75:1399, 1978.

101. Debanne, M.T., Bell, R., and Dolovich, J.: Uptake of proteinase-macroglobulin complexes by macrophages. Biochim. Biophys. Acta 411: 295, 1975.

102. Liu, D.Y., Petschek, K.D., Remold, H.G., and David, J.R.: Isolation of a guinea pig macrophage glycolipid with the properties of the putative migration inhibitory factor receptor. J. Biol. Chem. 257:159, 1982.

103. Guilbert, L.J., and Stanley, E.R.: Specific interaction of murine colony-stimulating factor with mononuclear phagocytic cells. J. Cell Biol. 85:153, 1980.

104. Remold, H.G.: Requirement for α-L-fucose on the macrophage membrane receptor for MIF. J. Exp. Med. 138:1065, 1973.

105. Traber, M.G., and Kayden, H.J.: Low density lipoprotein receptor activity in human monocyte-derived macrophages and its relation to atheromatous lesions. Proc. Natl. Acad. Sci. USA 77:5466, 1980.

106. Goldstein, J.L., Ho, Y.K., Basu, S.K., and Brown, M.S.: Binding site on macrophages that mediates uptake and degradation of acetylated low density lipoprotein, producing massive cholesterol deposition. Proc. Natl. Acad. Sci. USA 76:33, 1979.

107. Fogelman, A.M., Shechter, I., Seager, J., Hokom, M., Child, J.S., and Edwards, P.A.: Malondialdehyde alteration of low density lipoproteins leads to cholesteryl ester accumulation in human monocyte-macrophages. Proc. Natl. Acad. Sci. 77:2214, 1980.

108. Henriksen, T., Mahoney, E.M., and Steinberg, D.: Enhanced macrophage degradation of low density lipoprotein previously incubated with cultured endothelial cells: recognition by receptors for acetylated low density lipoproteins. Proc. Natl. Acad. Sci. USA 78:6499, 1981.

109. Goldstein, J.L., Ho, Y.K., Brown, M.S., Innerarity, T.L., and Mahley, R.W.: Cholesteryl-ester accumulation in macrophages resulting from receptor-mediated uptake and degradation of hypercholesterolemic canine β-very low density lipoproteins. J. Biol. Chem. 255:1839, 1980.

110. Gianturco, S.H., Bradley, W.A., Gotto, A.M., Jr., Morrisett, J.D., and Peavy, D.L.: Hypertriglyceridemic very low density lipoproteins induce tryglyceride synthesis and accumulation in mouse peritoneal macrophages. J. Clin. Invest. 70:168, 1982.

111. van Lenten, B.J., Fogelman, A.M., Hokom, M.M., Benson, L., Haberland, M.E., and Edwards, P.A.: Regulation of the uptake and degradation of β-very low density lipoprotein in human monocyte macrophages. J. Biol. Chem. 258:5151, 1983.

112. Johnson, W.J., Pizzo, S.V., Imber, M.J., and Adams, D.O.: Receptors for maleylated proteins regulate secretion of neutral proteases by murine macrophages. Science 218:574, 1982.

113. Whaley, K., Lappin, D., and Barkas, T.: C2 synthesis by human monocytes is modulated by a nicotinic cholinergic receptor. Nature 293:580, 1981.

114. Diaz, P., Jones, D.G., and Kay, A.B.: Histamine receptors on guinea-pig alveolar macrophages: chemical specificity and the effects of H1- and H2-receptor agonists and antagonists. Clin. Exp. Immunol. 35:462, 1979.

115. Steinman, R.M., Brodie, S.E., and Cohn, Z.A.: Membrane flow during pinocytosis: A stereologic analysis. J. Cell Biol. 68:665, 1976.

116. Steinman, R.M., and Cohn, Z.A.: Endocytosis and the vacuolar apparatus. In Cook, J.A. (ed.): Biogenesis and Turnover of Membrane Macromolecules. New York, Raven Press, 1976, p. 1.

117. Galloway, C.J., Dean, G.E., Marsh, M., Rudnick, G., and Mellman, I.: Acidification of macrophage and fibroblast endocytic vesicles in vitro. Proc. Natl. Acad. Sci. USA 80:3334, 1983.

118. Cohn, Z.A., and Wiener, E.: The particulate hydrolases of macrophages. I. Comparative enzymology, isolation and properties. J. Exp. Med. 118:991, 1963.

119. Cohn, Z.A., and Wiener, E.: The particulate hydrolases of macrophages. II. Biochemical and morphological response to particle ingestion. J. Exp. Med. 118:1009, 1963.

120. Cohn, Z.A., Fedorko, M.E., and Hirsch, J.G.: The in vitro differentiation of mononuclear phagocytes. V. The formation of macrophage lysosomes. J. Exp. Med. 123:757, 1966.

121. Steinman, R.M., Mellman, I.S., Muller, W.A., and Cohn, Z.A.: Endo-

cytosis and the recycling of the plasma membrane. J. Cell Biol. 96:1, 1983.

122. Cohn, Z.A., Hirsch, J.G., and Wiener, E.: The cytoplasmic granules of phagocytic cells and the degradation of bacteria. In de Reuck, A.V.S., and Cameron, M.P. (eds.): Ciba Foundation Symposium on Lysosomes. London, J. and A. Churchill, 1963, p. 126.

123. Cohn, Z.A.: The fate of bacteria within phagocytic cells. I. The degradation of isotopically labelled bacteria by polymorphonuclear leukcoytes and macrophages. J. Exp. Med. 117:27, 1963.

124. Ehrenreich, B.A., and Cohn, Z.A.: The fate of peptides pinocytosed by macrophages in vitro. J. Exp. Med. 129:227, 1969.

125. Reaven, E.P., and Axline, S.G.: Subplasmalemmal microfilaments and microtubules in resting and phagocytizing cultivated macrophages. J. Cell Biol. 59:12, 1973.

126. Hartwig, J.H., and Stossel, T.P.: Macrophages: their use in elucidation of the cytoskeletal roles of actin. Meth. Cell Biol. 25:201, 1982.

127. Hartwig, J.H., and Stossel, T.P.: Isolation and properties of actin, myosin, and a new actin-binding protein in rabbit alveolar macrophages. J. Biol. Chem. 250:5696, 1975.

128. Southwick, F.S., and Hartwig, J.H.: Acumentin, a protein in macrophages which caps the 'pointed' end of actin filaments. Nature 297:303, 1982.

129. Yin, H.L., Hartwig, J.H., Maruyama, K., and Stossel, T.P.: Ca^{2+} control of actin filament length. Effects of macrophage gelsolin on actin polymerization. J. Biol. Chem. 256:9693, 1981.

130. Brotschi, E.A., Hartwig, J.H., and Stossel, T.P.: The gelation of actin by actin-binding protein. J. Biol. Chem. 253:8988, 1978.

131. Bhisey, A.N., and Freed, J.J.: Altered movement of endosomes in colchicine-treated cultured macrophages. Exp. Cell Res. 64:430, 1971.

132. Rebuck, J.W., and Crowley, J.H.: A method of studying leukocytic functions in vivo. Ann. N.Y. Acad. Sci. 59:757, 1955.

133. Rabinovitch, M.: Macrophage spreading in vitro. In van Furth, R. (ed.): Mononuclear Phagocytes in Immunity, Infection and Pathology. London, Blackwell Scientific Publications, 1975, p. 369.

134. Bianco, C., Eden, A., and Cohn, Z.A.: The induction of macrophage spreading: Role of coagulation factors and the complement system. J. Exp. Med. 144:1531, 1976.

135. Götze, O., Bianco, C., Sundsmo, J.S., and Cohn, Z.A.: The stimulation of mononuclear phagocytes by components of the classical and the alternative pathways of complement activation. In van Furth, R. (ed.): Mononuclear Phagocytes: Functional Aspects. The Hague, Martinus Nijhoff, 1980, p. 1421.

136. Bevilacqua, M.P., Amrani, D., Mosesson, M.W., and Bianco, C.: Receptors for cold-insoluble globulin (plasma fibronectin) on human monocytes. J. Exp. Med. 153:42, 1981.

137. Clark, R.A.F., Quinn, J.H., Winn, H.J., Lanigan, J.M., Dellepella, P., and Colvin, R.B.: Fibronectin is produced by blood vessels in response to injury. J. Exp. Med. 156:646, 1982.

138. Sherman, L.A., and Lee, J.: Specific binding of soluble fibrin to macrophages. J. Exp. Med. 145:76, 1977.

139. Unkeless, J.C., Gordon, S.C., and Reich, E.: Secretion of plasminogen activator by stimulated macrophages. J. Exp. Med. 139:834, 1974.

140. Werb, Z., and Gordon, S.: Elastase secretion by stimulated macrophages. J. Exp. Med. 142:345, 1975.

141. Wahl, L.M., Wahl, S.M., Mergenhagen, S.E., and Martin, G.R.: Collagenase production by lymphokine-activated macrophages. Science 187:261, 1975.

142. Werb, Z., and Gordon, S.: Secretion of a specific collagenase by stimulated macrophages. J. Exp. Med. 142:345, 1975.

143. Banda, M.J., Clark, E.J., and Werb, Z.: Limited proteolysis by macrophage elastase inactivates human α_1-protease inhibitor. J. Exp. Med. 152:1563, 1980.

144. Werb, Z., Banda, M.J., and Jones, P.A.: Degradation of connective tissue matrices by macrophages. I. Proteolysis of elastin, glycoproteins, and collagen by proteinases isolated from macrophages. J. Exp. Med. 152:1340, 1980.

145. Jones, P.A., and Werb, Z.: Degradation of connective tissue matrices by macrophages. II. Influence of the matrix composition on proteolysis of glycoproteins, elastin, and collagen by macrophages in culture. J. Exp. Med. 152:1527, 1980.

146. Werb, Z., Bainton, D.F., and Jones, P.A.: Degradation of connective tissue matrices by macrophages. III. Morphological and biochemical studies on extracellular, pericellular, and intracellular events in matrix proteolysis by macrophages in culture. J. Exp. Med. 152:1537, 1980.

147. Snyderman, R., and Mergenhagen, S.E.: Chemotaxis of macrophages. In Nelson, D.S. (ed.): Immunobiology of the Macrophage. New York, Academic Press, 1976, p. 323.

148. Chenoweth, D.E., Goodman, M.G., and Weigle, W.O.: Demonstration of a specific receptor for human C5a anaphylatoxin on murine macrophages. J. Exp. Med. 156:68, 1982.

149. Polley, M.J., and Nachman, R.: The human complement system in thrombin-mediated platelet function. J. Exp. Med. 147:1713, 1978.

150. Ward, P.A.: Chemotaxis of mononuclear cells. J. Exp. Med. 128:1201, 1968.

151. Bar-Shavit, R., Kahn, A., Fenton, J.W., II, and Wilner, G.D.: Chemotactic response of monocytes to thrombin. J. Cell Biol. 96:282, 1983.

152. Gallin, J.I., and Kaplan, A.P.: Mononuclear cell chemotactic activity of kallikrein and plasminogen activator and its inhibition by C1 inhibitor and α_2-macroglobulin. J. Immunol. 113:1928, 1974.

153. Wilkinson, P.C.: Cellular and molecular aspects of chemotaxis of macrophages and monocytes. In Nelson, D.S. (ed.): Immunobiology of the Macrophage. New York, Academic Press, 1976. p. 350.

154. Norris, D.A., Clark, R.A.F., Swigart, L.M., Huff, J.C., Weston, W.L., and Howell, S.E.: Fibronectin fragment(s) are chemotactic for human peripheral blood monocytes. J. Immunol. 129:1612, 1982.

155. Postlethwaite, A.E., Keski-Oja, J., Balian, G., and Kang, A.H.: Induction of fibroblast chemotaxis by fibronectin. Localization of the chemotactic region to a 140,000-molecular weight non-gelatin-binding fragment. J. Exp. Med. 153:494, 1981.

156. Hunninghake, G.W., Davidson, J.M., Rennard, S., Szapeil, S., Gadek, J. E., and Crystal, R.G.: Elastin fragments attract macrophage precursors to diseased sited in pulmonary emphysema. Science 212:925, 1981.

157. Senior, R.M., Griffin, G.L., and Mecham, R.P.: Chemotactic activity of elastin-derived peptides. J. Clin. Invest. 66:859, 1980.

158. Postlethwaite, A.E., and Kang, A.H.: Collagen- and collagen peptide-induced chemotaxis of human blood monocytes. J. Exp. Med. 143:1299, 1976.

159. Mundy, G.R., Varani J., Orr, W., Gondek, M.D., and Ward, P.A.: Resorbing bone is chemotactic for monocytes. Nature 275:132, 1978.

160. Ward, P.A., Remold, H.G., and David, J.R.: Leukotactic factor produced by sensitized lymphocytes. Science 163:1079, 1969.

161. Wahl, S.M., Iverson, G.M., and Oppenheim, J.J.: Induction of guinea pig B-cell lymphokine synthesis by mitogenic and nonmitogenic signals to Fc, Ig and C3 receptors. J. Exp. Med. 140:1631, 1974.

162. Postlethwaite, A.E., Arnold, E., and Snyderman, R.: Characterization of chemotactic activity produced in vivo by a cell-mediated immune reaction in the guinea pig. J. Immunol. 114:274, 1975.

163. Gallin, J.I., Fletcher, M.P. Seligmann, B.E., Hoffstein, S., Cehrs, K., and Mounessa, N.: Human neutrophil-specific granule deficiency: A model to assess the role of neutrophil-specific granules in the evolution of the inflammatory response. Blood 59:1317, 1982.

164. Deuel, T.F., Senior, R.M., Chang, D., Griffin, G.L., Heinrikson, R.L., and Kaiser, E.T.: Platelet factor 4 is chemotactic for neutrophils and monocytes. Proc. Natl. Acad. Sci. USA 78:4584, 1981.

165. Bottazzi, B., Polentaratti, N., Balsari, A., Boraschi, D., Ghezzi, P. Salmona, M., and Mantovani, A.: Chemotactic activity for mononuclear phagocytes of culture supernatants from murine and human tumor cells: Evidence for a role in the regulation of the macrophage content of neoplastic tissues. Int. J. Cancer 31:55, 1983.

166. Schiffman, E., Corcoran, B.A., and Wahl, S.M.: N-formylmethionyl peptides as chemoattractants for leukocytes. Proc. Natl. Acad. Sci. USA 72:1059, 1975.

167. Carp, H.: Mitochondrial N-formylmethionyl proteins as chemoattractants for neutrophils. J. Exp. Med. 155:264, 1982.

168. Meltzer, M.S., Stevenson, M.M., and Leonard E.J.: Characterization of macrophage chemotaxins in tumor cell cultures and comparison with lymphocyte-derived chemotactic factors. Cancer Res. 37:721, 1977.

169. Meltzer, M.S., Jones, E.E., and Boetcher, D.A.: Increased chemotactic response of macrophages from BCG-infected mice. Cell. Immunol. 17:268, 1975.

170. Boetcher, D.A., and Leonard, E.J.: Abnormal monocyte chemotactic response in cancer patients. J. Natl. Cancer Inst. 52:1091, 1974.

171. Snyderman, R., Pike, M.C., Blaylock, B.L., and Weinstein, P.: Effects of neoplasms on inflammation: Depression of macrophage accumulation after tumor implantation. J. Immunol. 116:585, 1976.

172. Stevenson, M.M., and Meltzer, M.S.: Depressed chemotactic responses in vitro of peritoneal macrophges from tumor-bearing mice. J. Natl. Cancer Inst. 57:847, 1976.

173. Cianciolo, G., Hunter, J., Silva, J., Haskill, J.S., and Snyderman, R.: Inhibitors of monocyte responses to chemotaxins are present in human cancerous effusions and react with protein of retroviruses. J. Clin. Invest. 68:831, 1981.

174. Cianciolo, G., Lostrom, M., Tam, M., and Snyderman, R.: Murine malignant cells synthesize a 19,000-dalton protein that is physicochemically and antigenically related to the immunosuppressive retroviral protein, P15E. J. Exp. Med. 158:885, 1983.

175. Brozna, J.P., and Ward, P.A.: Antileukotactic properties of tumor cells. J. Clin. Invest. 56:616, 1975.

176. Remold, H.G., McCarthy, P.L., Jr., and Mednis, A.D.: Purification of guinea pig pH 3 migration inhibitory factor. Proc. Natl. Acad. Sci. USA 78:4088, 1981.

177. David, J.R.: Delayed hypersensitivity in vitro: Its mediation by cell-free substances formed by lymphoid cell-antigen interaction. Proc. Natl. Acad. Sci. USA 56:72, 1966.

178. Bloom, B.R., and Bennet, B.: Mechanism of a reaction in vitro associated with delayed-type hypersensitivity. Science 153:80, 1966.

179. Bianco, C., Gotze, O., and Cohn, Z.A.: Complement, coagulation, and

mononuclear phagocytes. *In* van Furth, R. (ed.): Mononuclear Phagocytes: Functional Aspects. The Hague, Martinus Nijhoff, 1980, p. 1443.

180. Hopper, K.E., Geczy, C.L., and Davies, W.A.: A mechanism of migration inhibition in delayed-type hypersensitivity reactions. I. Fibrin deposition on the surface of elicited peritoneal macropahges in vivo. J. Immunol. 126:1052, 1981.

181. Silverstein, S.C., Steinman, R.M., and Cohn, Z.A.: Endocytosis. Ann. Rev. Biochem. 46:669, 1977.

182. Stossel, T.P.: Phagocytosis. N. Engl. J. Med. 209:717, 774, 833, 1974.

183. Rabinovitch, M.: Phagocytic recognition. *In* van Furth, R. (ed.): Mononuclear Phagocytes. Oxford, Blackwell Scientific Publications, 1970, p. 299.

184. Jones, T.C., and Hirsch, J.G.: The interaction in vitro of Mycoplasma pulmonis with mouse peritoneal macrophages and L-cells. J. Exp. Med. 133:231, 1971.

185. Griffin, F.M., Jr., and Silverstein, S.C.: Segmental response of the macrophage plasma membrane to a phagocytic stimulus. J. Exp. Med. 139:323, 1974.

186. Griffin, F.M., Jr., Griffin, J.A., Leider, J.E., and Silverstein, S.C.: Studies on the mechanism of phagocytosis. I. Requirements for circumferential attachment of particle-bound ligands to specific receptors on the macrophage plasma membrane. J. Exp. Med. 142:1263, 1975.

187. Griffin, F.M., Jr., Griffin, J.A., and Silverstein, S.C.: Studies on the mechanism of phagocytosis. II. The interaction of macrophages with anti-immunoglobulin IgG-coated bone marrow-derived lymphocytes. J. Exp. Med. 144:788, 1976.

188. Wright, S.D., and Silverstein, S.C.: Phagocytosing macrophages exclude soluble macromolecules from the zone of contact with ligand-coated targets. J. Cell Biol. 95:443a, 1982.

189. Babior, B.M.: Oxygen-dependent microbial killng by phagocytes. N. Engl. J. Med. 298:659, 1978.

190. Nathan, C.F.: Secretion of oxygen intermediates: role in effector functions of activated macrophages. Fed. Proc. 41:2206, 1982.

191. Segal, A.W., Cross, A.R., Garcia, R.C., Borregaard, N., Valerius, N. H., Soothill, J.F., and Jones, O.T.G.: Absence of cytochrome b245 in chronic granulomatous disease: A multicenter European evaluation of its incidence and relevance. N. Engl. J. Med. 308:245, 1983.

192. Loike, J.D., Kozler, V.F., and Silverstein, S.C.: Increased ATP and creatine phosphate turnover in phagocytosing mouse peritoneal macrophages. J. Biol. Chem. 254:958, 1979.

193. Brade, V., and Bentley, C.: Synthesis and release of complement components by macrophages. *In* van Furth, R. (ed.): Mononuclear Phagocytes: Functional Aspects. The Hague, Martinus Nijhoff, 1980, p.1385.

194. Bentley, C., Fries, W., Brade, V.: Synthesis of factors D, B, and P of the alternative pathway of complement activation, as well as of C3, by guinea pig peritoneal macrophages in vitro. Immunology. 35:971, 1978.

195. Whaley, K.: Biosynthesis of the complement components and the regulatory proteins of the alternative pathway by human peripheral blood monocytes. J. Exp. Med. 151:501, 1980.

196. Zimmer, B, Hartung, H.-P., Scharfenberger, G., Bitter-Suermann, D., and Hadding, U.: Quantitative studies of the secretion of complement component C3 by resident, elicited and activated macrophages. Comparison with C2, C4 and lysosomal enzyme release. Eur. J. Immunol. 12:426, 1982.

197. Einstein, L.P., Hansen, P.J., Ballow, M., Davis, A.E., III, Davis, J.S., IV, Alper, C.A., Rosen, F.S., and Colten, H.R.: Biosynthesis of the third component of complement (C3) in vitro by monocytes from both normal and homozygous C3-deficient humans. J. Clin. Invest. 60:963, 1977.

198. Einstein, L.P., Schneeberger, E.E., and Colten, H.R.: Synthesis of the second component of complement by long-term primary cultures of human monocytes. J. Exp. Med. 143:114, 1976.

199. Rutherford, B., and Schenkein, H.A.: C3 cleavage products stimulate release of prostaglandins by human mononuclear phagocytes in vitro. J. Immunol. 130:874, 1983.

200. Lappin, D.F., and Whaley, K.: Prostaglandins and prostaglandin synthetase inhibitors regulate the synthesis of complement components by human monocytes. Clin. Exp. Immunol. 49:623, 1982.

201. Littman, B.H., and Ruddy, S.: Production of the second component of complement by human monocytes: Stimulation by antigen-activated lymphocytes or lymphokines. J. Exp. Med. 145:1344, 977.

202. Hartung, H.-P., Bitter-Suermann, D., and Hadding, U.: Induction of thromboxane release from macrophages by anaphylatoxin peptide C3a of complement and synthetic hexapeptide C3a 72-77. J. Immunol. 130:1345, 1983.

203. Payan, D.G., Trentham, D.E., and Goetzl, E.J.: Modulation of human lymphocyte function by C3a and C3a (70-77). J. Exp. Med. 156:756, 1982.

204. Osterud, B., Lindahl, U., and Seljelid, R.: Macrophages produce blood coagulation factors. FEBS Lett. 120:41, 1980.

205. Osterud, B., Bogwald, J., Lindahl, U., and Seljelid, R.: Production of

206. Klimetzek, V., and Sorg, C.: The production of fibrinolysis inhibitors as a parameter of the activation state in murine macrophages. Eur. J. Immunol. 9:618, 1979.

207. Chapman, H.A., Jr., Vavrin, Z., and Hibbs, J.B., Jr.: Macrophage fibrinolytic activity: Identification of two pathways of plasmin formation by intact cells and of a plasminogen activator inhibitor. Cell 28:653, 1982.

208. Broze, G.J., Jr.: Binding of human factor VII and VIIa to monocytes. J. Clin. Invest. 70:526, 1982.

209. Schwartz, B.S., Levy, G.A., Fair, D.S., and Edgington, T.S.: Murine lymphoid procoagulant activity induced by bacterial lipopolysaccharide and immune complexes is a monocyte prothrombinase. J. Exp. Med. 155:1464, 1982.

210. Hogg, N.: Human monocytes are associated with the formation of fibrin. J. Exp. Med. 157:473, 1983.

211. Gordon, S., Todd, J., and Cohn, Z.A.: In vitro synthesis and secretion of lysozyme by mononuclear phagocytes. J. Exp. Med. 139:1228, 1974.

212. Klimetzek, V., and Sorg, C.: Lymphokine-induced secretion of plasminogen activator by murine macrophages. Eur. J. Immunol. 7:185, 1977.

213. Vassalli, J.-D., and Reich, E.: Macrophage plasminogen activator: Induction by products of activated lymphoid cells. J. Exp. Med. 145:429, 1977.

214. Gordon, S., Unkeless, J.C., and Cohn, Z.A.: Induction of macrophage plasminogen activator by endotoxin stimulation and phagocytosis. J. Exp. Med. 140:995, 1975.

215. Ragsdale, C.G., and Arend, W.P.: Neutral protease secretion by human monocytes. Effect of surface-bound immune complexes. J. Exp. Med. 149:954, 1979.

216. Pantalone, R., and Page, R.C.: Enzyme production and secretion by lymphokine-activated macrophages. J. Reticuloendothel. Soc. 21:343, 1977.

217. Schnyder, J., and Baggiolini, M.: Secretion of lysosomal hydrolases by stimulated and nonstimulated macrophages. J. Exp. Med. 148:435, 1978.

218. Gordon, S., and Werb, Z.: Secretion of macrophage neutral proteinases is enhanced by colchicine. Proc. Natl. Acad. Sci. USA 73:872, 1976.

219. Levine, E.A., Senior, R.M., and Butler, J.V.: The elastase activity of alveolar macrophages: Measurements using synthetic substrates and elastin. Amer. Rev. Respir. Dis. 113:25, 1976.

220. Wahl, L.M., Wahl, S., Mergenhagen, S.E., and Martin, G.E.: Collagenase production by endotoxin-activated macrophages. Proc. Natl. Acad. Sci. USA 71:3598, 1974.

221. Banda, M.J., Clark, E.J., and Werb, Z.: Selective proteolysis of immunoglobulins by mouse macrophage elastase. J. Exp. Med. 157:1184, 1983.

222. Davies, P., Page, R.C., and Allison, A.C.: Changes in cellular enzyme levels and extracellular release of lysosomal acid hydrolases in macrophages exposed to group A streptococcal cell wall substance. J. Exp. Med. 139:1262, 1974.

223. Schorlemmer, H.V., Bitter-Suermann, D., and Allison, A.C.: Complement activation by the alternative pathway and macrophage enzyme secretion in the pathogenesis of chronic inflammation. Immunology 32:929, 1977.

224. Ohkuma, S., and Poole, B.: Fluorescence probe measurement of the intralysosomal pH in living cells and the perturbation of pH by various agents. Proc. Natl. Acad. Sci. 75:3327, 1978.

225. Davies, P., and Allison, A.C.: Secretion of macrophage enzymes in relation to the pathogenesis of chronic inflammation. *In* Nelson, D.S. (ed.): Immunobiology of the Macrophage. New York, Academic Press, 1976, p. 428.

226. Barrett, A.J., and Starkey, P.M.: The interaction of α₂-macroglobulin with proteinases. Characteristics and specificity of the reaction, and a hypothesis concerning its molecular mechanism. Biochem. J. 133:709, 1973.

227. Remold, H., and Rosenberg, R.D.: Enhancement of migration inhibitory factor activity by plasma esterase inhibitors. J. Biol. Chem. 250:6608, 1975.

228. Hovi, T., Mosher, D., and Vaheri, A.: Cultured human monocytes synthesize and secrete α₂-macroglobulin. J. Exp. Med. 145:1580, 1977.

229. White, R., Janoff, A., and Godfrey, H.P.: Secretion of α₂-macroglobulin by human alveolar macrophages. Lung 158:9, 1980.

230. Wilson, G.B., Walker, J.H., Watkins, J.H., Jr., and Wolgroch, D.: Determination of subpopulations of leukocytes involved in the synthesis of α₁-antitrypsin in vitro. Proc. Soc. Exp. Biol. Med. 164:105, 1980.

231. White, R., Lee, D., Habicht, G.S., and Janoff, A.: Secretion of α₁-proteinase inhibitor by cultured rat alveolar macrophages. Am Rev. Resp. Dis. 123:447, 1981.

232. Boldt, D.H., Chan, S.K., and Keaton, K.: Cell surface α₁-protease inhibitor on human peripheral mononuclear cells in culture. J. Immunol. 129:1830, 1982.

233. Humes, J.L., Bonney, R.J., Pelus, L., Dahlgren, M.E., Sadowski, S.J.,

Kuehl, F.A., Jr., and Davies, P.: Macrophages synthesize and release prostaglandins in response to inflammatory stimuli. Nature 269:149, 1977.

234. Kurland, J.I., and Bockman, R.: Prostaglandin E production by human blood monocytes and mouse peritoneal macrophages. J. Exp. Med. 147:952, 1978.

235. Bonney, R.J., Wightman, P.D., Davies, P., Sadowski, S.J., Kuehl, F.A., Jr., and Humes, J.L.: Regulation of prostaglandin synthesis and of the selective release of lysosomal hydrolases by mouse peritoneal macrophages. Bioch. J. 176:433, 1978.

236. Scott, W.A., Zrike, J.M., Hamill, A.L., Kempe, J., and Cohn, Z.A.: Regulation of arachidonic acid metabolites in macrophages. J. Exp. Med. 152:324, 1980.

237. Rouzer, C.A., Scott, W.A., Hamill, A.L., and Cohn, Z.A.: Dynamics of leukotriene C production by macrophages. J. Exp. Med. 152:1236, 1980.

238. Scott, W.A., Pawlowski, N.A., Murray, H.W., Andreach, M., Zrike, J., and Cohn, Z.A.: Regulation of arachidonic acid metabolism by macrophage activation. J. Exp. Med. 155:1148, 1982.

239. Rouzer, C.A., Scott, W.A., Hamill, A.L., Liu, F.-T., Katz, D.H., and Cohn, Z.A.: Secretion of leukotriene C and other arachidonic acid metabolites by macrophages challenged with immunoglobulin E immune complexes. J. Exp. Med. 156:1077, 1982.

240. Pawlowski, N.A., Scott, W.A., Andreach, M., and Cohn, Z.A.: Uptake and metabolism of monohydroxyeicosatetraenoic acids by macrophages. J. Exp. Med. 155:1653, 1982.

241. Scott, W.A., Pawlowski, N.A., Andreach, M., and Cohn, Z.A.: Resting macrophages produce distinct metabolites from exogenous arachidonic acid. J. Exp. Med. 155:535, 1982.

242. Rouzer, C.A., Scott, W.A., Hamill, A.L., and Cohn, Z.A.: Synthesis of leukotriene C and other arachidonic acid metabolites by mouse pulmonary macrophages. J. Exp. Med. 155:720, 1982.

243. Fels, A.O.S., Pawlowski, N.A., Cramer, E.B., King, T.K.C., Cohn, Z.A., and Scott, W.A.: Human alveolar macrophages produce leukotriene B4. Proc. Natl. Acad. Sci. USA 79:7866, 1982.

244. Pawlowski, N.A., Kaplan, G.A., Hamill, A.L., Cohn, Z.A., and Scott, W.A.: Arachidonic acid metabolism by human monocytes. Studies with platelet-depleted cultures. J. Exp. Med., 158:393, 1983.

245. Bokoch, G.M., and Reed, P.W.: Stimulation of arachidonic acid metabolism in the polymorphonuclear leukocyte by an N-formylated peptide. J. Biol. Chem. 255:10223, 1980.

246. Kurland, J.I., Kincade, P.W., and Moore, M.A.S.: Regulation of B-lymphocyte clonal proliferation by stimulatory and inhibitory macrophage-derived factors. J. Exp. Med. 146:1420, 1977.

247. Goodwin, J.S., Bankhurst, A.D., and Messner, R.P.: Suppression of human T-cell mitogenesis by prostaglandin. Existence of a prostaglandin-producing suppressor cell. J. Exp. Med. 146:1719, 1977.

248. Kurland, J.I., Broxmeyer, H.E., Pelus, L.M., Bockman, R.S., and Moore, M.A.S.: Role of monocyte-macrophage-derived colony-stimulating factor and prostaglandin E in the positive and negative feedback control of myeloid stem cell proliferation. Blood 52:388, 1978.

249. Voelkel, E.F., Levine, L., Alper, C.A., and Tashjian, A.H., Jr.: Acute phase reactants ceruloplasmin and haptoglobin and their relationship to plasma prostaglandins in rabbits bearing the VX_2 carcinoma. J. Exp. Med. 147:1078, 1978.

250. Friedman, S.A., Remold-O'Donnell, E., and Piessens, W.F.: Enhanced PGE production by MAF-treated peritoneal exudate macrophages. Cell. Immunol. 42:213, 1979.

251. Hunninghake, G.W., Gadek, J.E., Fales, H.M., and Crystal, R.G.: Human alveolar macrophage-derived chemotactic factor for neutrophils. Stimuli and partial characterization. J. Clin. Invest. 66:473, 1980.

252. Nathan, C.F., and Root, R.K.: Hydrogen peroxide release from mouse peritoneal macrophages. Dependence on sequential activation and triggering. J. Exp. Med. 146:1648, 1977.

253. Johnson, R.B., Jr., Godzik, C.A., and Cohn, Z.A.: Increased superoxide anion production by immunologically activated and chemically elicited macrophages. J. Exp. Med. 148:115, 1978.

254. Nathan, C., Nogueira, N., Juangbhanich, C., Ellis, J., and Cohn, Z.: Activation of macrophages in vivo and in vitro: Correlation between hydrogen peroxide release and killing of Trypanosoma cruzi. J. Exp. Med. 149:1056, 1979.

255. Nakagawara, A., DeSantis, N.M., Nogueira, N., and Nathan, C.F.: Lymphokines enhance the capacity of human monocytes to secrete reactive oxygen intermediates. J. Clin. Invest. 70:1042, 1982.

256. Nathan, C.F., Murray, H.W., Wiebe, M.E., and Rubin, B.Y.: Identification of interferon-γ as the lymphokine which activates human macrophage oxidative metabolism and antimicrobial activity. J. Exp. Med. 158:670, 1983.

257. Szuro-Sudol, A., and Nathan, C.F.: Suppression of macrophage oxidative metabolism by products of malignant and nonmalignant cells. J. Exp. Med. 156:945, 1982.

258. Slater, T.F.: Free Radical Mechanisms in Tissue Injury. London, Pion Ltd, 1972.

259. Oppenheim, J.J., and Gery, I.: Interleukin 1 is more than an interleukin. Immunol. Today 3:113, 1982.

260. Mizel, S.B., and Mizel, D.: Purification to apparent homogeneity of murine interleukin 1. J. Immunol. 126:834, 1981.

261. Gery, I., Gershon, R.K., and Waksman, B.H.: Potentiation of the T lymphocyte response to mitogens. I. The responding cell. J. Exp. Med. 136:128, 1972.

262. Howard, M., Mizel, S.B., Lachman, L., Ansel, J., Johnson, B., and Paul, W.E.: Role of interleukin-1 in anti-immunoglobulin-induced B cell proliferation. J. Exp. Med. 157:1529, 1983.

263. Murphy, P.A., Simon, P.L., and Willoughby, W.F.: Endogenous pyrogens made by rabbit peritoneal exudate cells are identical with lymphocyte-activating factors made by rabbit alveolar macrophages. J. Immunol. 124:2498, 1980.

264. Mizel, S.B., Dayer, J.-M., Krane, S.M., and Mergenhagen, S.E.: Stimulation of rheumatoid synovial cell collagenase and prostaglandin production by partially purified lymphocyte-activating factor (interleukin 1). Proc. Natl. Acad. Sci. USA 78:2474, 1981.

265. Schmidt, J.A., Mizel, S.B., Cohen, D., and Green, I.: Interleukin 1, a potential regulator of fibroblast proliferation. J. Immunol. 128:2177, 1982.

266. Postlethwaite, A.E., Lachman, L.B., Mainardi, C.L., and Kang, A.H.: Interleukin 1 stimulation of collagenase production by cultured fibroblasts. J. Exp. Med. 157:801, 1983.

267. Sipe, J.D., Vogel, S.N., Ryan, J.L., McAdam, K.P.W.J., and Rosenstreich, D.L.: Detection of a mediator derived from endotoxin-stimulated macrophages that induces the acute phase serum amyloid A response in mice. J. Exp. Med. 150:597, 1979.

268. Le, P.T., Muller, T., and Mortensen, R.F.: Acute phase reactants of mice. I. Isolation of serum amyloid P-component (SAP) and its induction by a monokine. J. Immunol. 129:665, 1982.

269. Kurland, J.I., Meyers, P.A., and Moore, M.A.S.: Synthesis and release of erythroid colony- and burst-potentiating activities by purified populations of murine peritoneal macrophages. J. Exp. Med. 151:838, 1980.

270. Rich, I.N., Heit, W., and Kubanck, B.: Extrarenal erythropoietin production by macrophages. Blood 60:1007, 1982.

271. Leibovich, S.J., and Ross, R.: A macrophage-dependent factor that stimulates the proliferation of fibroblasts in vitro. Am. J. Pathol. 84:501, 1976.

272. Polverini, P.J., Cotran, R.S., Gimbrone, M.A., Jr., and Unanue, E.R.: Activated macrophages induce vascular proliferation. Nature 269:804, 1977.

273. Filkins, J.P.: Endotoxin-enhanced secretion of macrophage insulin-like activity. J. Reticuloendothel. Soc. 27:507, 1980.

274. Kawakami, M., and Cerami, A.: Studies of endotoxin-induced decrease in lipoprotein lipase activity. J. Exp. Med. 154:631, 1981.

275. Pekala, P.H., Kawakami, M., Angus, C.W., Lane, M., and Cerami, A.: A selective inhibition of the synthesis of the enzymes for de novo fatty acid biosynthesis by an endotoxin-induced mediator from exudate cells. Proc. Natl. Acad. Sci. USA 80:2743, 1983.

276. Mahoney, E.M., Khoo, J.C., and Steinberg, D.: Lipoprotein lipase secretion by human monocytes and rabbit alveolar macrophages in culture. Proc. Natl. Acad. Sci. USA 79:1639, 1982.

277. Chait, A., Iverius, P.-H., and Brunzell, J.D.: Lipoprotein lipase secretion by human monocyte-derived macrophages. J. Clin. Invest. 69:490, 1982.

278. Kull, F.C., Jr., and Cuatrecasas, P.: Preliminary characterization of the tumor cell cytotoxin in tumor necrosis serum. J. Immunol. 126:1279, 1981.

279. Smith, T.J., and Wagner, R.R.: Rabbit macrophage interferons. I. Conditions for biosynthesis by virus-infected and uninfected cells. J. Exp. Med. 125:559, 1967.

280. Kung, J.T., Brooks, S.B., Jakway, J.P., Leonard, L.L., and Talmage, D.W.: Suppression of in vitro cytotoxic response by macrophages due to induced arginase. J. Exp. Med. 146:665, 1977.

281. Nathan, C.F., Silverstein, S.C., Brukner, L.H., and Cohn, Z.A.: Extracellular cytolysis by activated macrophages and granulocytes. II. Hydrogen peroxide as a mediator of cytotoxicity. J. Exp. Med. 149:100, 1979.

282. Stadecker, M.J., Calderon, J., Karnovsky, M.L., and Unanue, E.R.: Synthesis and release of thymidine by macrophages. J. Immunol. 119:1738, 1977.

283. Neumann, C., and Sorg, C.: Immune interferon. I. Production by lymphokine-activated murine macrophages. Eur. J. Immunol. 7:719, 1977.

284. Olstad, R., Degre, M., and Seljelid, R.: Production of immune interferon (Type II) in cocultures of mouse peritoneal macrophages and syngeneic tumor cells. Scand. J. Immunol. 13:605, 1981.

285. Krahenbuhl, J.L., Remington, J.S., and McLeod, R.: Cytotoxic and microbicidal properties of macrophages. In van Furth, R. (ed.): Mononuclear Phagocytes: Functional Aspects. The Hague, Martinus Nijhoff, 1980, p. 1631.

286. Mahmoud, A., Peters, P.A.S., Civil, R.H., and Remington, J.S.: In vitro killing of schistosomula of Schistosoma mansoni by BCG and C. parvum-activated macrophages. J. Immunol. 122:1655, 1979.

287. Haque, A., Ouaissi, A., Joseph, M., Capron, M., and Capron, A.: IgE antibody in eosinophil- and macrophage-mediated in vitro killing of Dipetalonema viteae microfilariae. J. Immunol. 127:716, 1981.

288. Horwitz, M.A., and Silverstein, S.C.: Legionnaires' disease bacterium (Legionella pneumophila) multiplies intracellularly in human monocytes. J. Clin. Invest. 66:445, 1980.

289. Nathan, C.F.: Mechanisms of macrophage antimicrobial activity. Trans. Roy. Soc. Trop. Med. Hyg., 77:620, 1983.

290. Wilson, C.B., Tsai, V., and Remington, J.S.: Failure to trigger the oxidative metabolic burst by normal macrophages: Possible mechanism for survival of intracellular pathogens. J. Exp. Med. 151:328, 1980.

291. Murray, H.W., Byrne, G.I., Rothermel, C.D., and Cartelli, D.M.: Lymphokine enhances oxygen-independent activity against intracellular pathogens. J. Exp. Med. 158:234, 1983.

292. Wisseman, C.L., Jr., and Waddell, A.: Interferonlike factors from antigen- and mitogen-stimulated human leukocytes with antirickettsial and cytolytic actions of Rickettsia prowazekii. Infected human endothelial cells, fibroblasts, and macrophages. J. Exp. Med. 157:1780, 1983.

293. Klebanoff, S.J., and Hamon, C.B.: Antimicrobial systems of mononuclear phagocytes. In van Furth (ed.): Mononuclear Phagocytes in Immunity, Infection, and Pathology. Oxford, Blackwell Scientific Publications, 1975, p. 507.

294. Confer, D.L., and Eaton, J.W.: Phagocyte impotence caused by an invasive bacterial adenylate cyclase. Science 217:948, 1982.

295. Draper, P, and D'Arcy Hart, P.: Phagosomes, lysosomes, and mycobacteria: cellular and microbial aspects. In van Furth, R. (ed.): Mononuclear Phagocytes in Immunity, Infection, and Pathology. Oxford, Blackwell Scientific Publications, 1975, p. 575.

296. Goren, M.B.: Phagocyte lysosomes: Interactions with infectious agents, phagosomes and experimental perturbations in function. Ann. Rev. Microbiol. 31:507, 1977.

297. Nogueira, N., and Cohn, Z.A.: Trypansosoma cruzi: In vitro induction of macropahge microbicidal activity. J. Exp. Med. 148:288, 1978.

298. Adams, D.O., Johnson, W., and Marino, P.: Mechanisms of target recognition and destruction in macrophage-mediated tumor cytotoxicity. Fed. Proc. 41:2212, 1982.

299. Adams, D.O., Johnson, W.J., Fiorito, E., and Nathan, C.F.: Hydrogen peroxide and cytolytic factor can interact in effecting cytolysis of neoplastic targets. J. Immunol. 127:1973, 1981.

300. Granger, D.L., and Lehninger, A.L.: Sites of inhibition of mitochondrial electron transport in macrophage-injured neoplastic cells. J. Cell Biol. 95:527, 1982.

301. Nathan, C., and Cohn, Z.: Role of oxygen-dependent mechanisms in antibody-induced lysis of tumor cells by activated macrophages. J. Exp. Med. 152:198, 1980.

302. Nathan, C.F., and Klebanoff, S.J.: Augmentation of spontaneous macrophage-mediated cytolysis by eosinophil peroxidase. J. Exp. Med. 155:1291, 1982.

303. Nathan, C.F., Murray, H.W., and Cohn, Z.A.: Current concepts: the macrophage as an effector cell. N. Engl. J. Med. 303:622, 1980.

304. Herlyn, D., and Koprowski, H.: IgG2a monoclonal antibodies inhibit human tumor growth through interaction with effector cells. Proc. Natl. Acad. Sci. USA 79:4761, 1982.

305. Kleinerman, E.S., Erickson, K.L., Schroit, A.J., Fogler, W.E., and Fidler, I.J.: Activation of tumoricidal properties in human blood monocytes by liposomes containing lipophilic muramyl tripeptides. Cancer Res. 43:2010, 1983.

306. Szuro-Sudol, A., Murray, H.W., and Nathan, C.F.: Suppression of macrophage antimicrobial activity by a tumor cell product. J. Immunol. 131:384, 1983.

307. Nathan, C.F., Arrick, B.A., Murray, H.W., DeSantis, N.M., and Cohn, Z.A.: Tumor cell antioxidant defenses: Inhibition of the glutathione redox cycle enhances macrophage-mediated cytolysis. J. Exp. Med. 153:766, 1981.

308. Arrick, B.A., Nathan, C.F., Griffith, O.W., and Cohn, Z.A.: Glutathione depletion sensitizes tumor cells to oxidative cytolysis. J. Biol. Chem. 257:1231, 1982.

309. Steinman, R.M., and Nussenzweig, M.C.: Dendritic cells: features and functions. Immunol. Rev. 53:127, 1980.

310. Steinman, R.M., Gutchinov, B., Witmer, M.D., and Nussenzweig, M.C.: Dendritic cells are the principal stimulators of the primary mixed leukocyte reaction in mice. J. Exp. Med. 157:613, 1983.

311. van Voorhis, W.C., Valinsky, J., Hoffman, E., Luban, J., Hair, L.S., and Steinman, R.M.: Relative efficacy of human monocytes and dendritic cells as accessory cells for T cell replication. J. Exp. Med. 158:174, 1983.

312. Rouzer, C.A., Scott, W.A., Griffith, O.W., Hamill, A.L., and Cohn, Z.A.: Glutathione metabolism in resting and phagocytizing peritoneal macrophages. J. Biol. Chem. 257:2002, 1982.

313. Austyn, J.M., Steinman, R.M., Weinstein, D.E., Granelli-Piperno, A., and Palladino, M.: Dendritic cells initiate a two-stage mechanism for T lymphocyte proliferation. J. Exp. Med. 157:1101, 1983.

314. Smith, K.A., Lachman, L.B., Oppenheim, J.J., and Favata, M.F.: The functional relationship of the interleukins. J. Exp. Med. 151:1551, 1980.

315. Unanue, E.R.: The regulatory role of macrophages in antigenic stimulation. Adv. Immunol. 15:95, 1972.

316. Dos Reis, G.A., and Shevach, E.M.: Antigen-presenting cells from nonresponder strain 2 guinea pigs are fully competent to present bovine insulin chain B to responder strain 13 T cells. Evidence against a determinant selection model and in favor of clonal deletion. J. Exp. Med. 157:1287, 1983.

317. Kirchner, H., Holden, H.T., and Herberman, R.B.: Splenic suppressor macrophages induced in mice by injection of Corynebacterium parvum. J. Immunol. 115:1212, 1975.

318. Fisher, R.I., and Bostick-Bruton, F.: Depressed T cell proliferation responses in Hodgkin's disease: role of monocyte-mediated suppression via prostaglandins and hydrogen peroxide. J. Immunol. 129:1770, 1982.

319. Kay, M.M.B., Goodman, S.R., Sorensen, K., Whitfield, C.F., Wong, P., Zaki, L., and Rudloff, V.: Senescent cell antigen is immunologically related to band 3. Proc. Natl. Acad. Sci. USA 80:1631, 1983.

320. Newman, S.L., Henson, J.E., and Henson, P.M.: Phagocytosis of senescent neutrophils by human monocyte-derived macrophages and rabbit inflammatory macrophages. J. Exp. Med. 154:430, 1982.

321. Rosenberg, S.A., and Rogentine, N.: Natural human antibodies to "hidden" membrane components. Nature New Biol. 239:203, 1972.

322. Czop, J.K., Fearon, D.T., and Austen, K.F.: Membrane sialic acid on target particles modulate their phagocytosis by a trypsin-sensitive mechanism on human monocytes. Proc. Natl. Acad. Sci. USA 75:3831, 1978.

323. Aminoff, D., Bruegge, W.F.V., Bell, W.C., Sarpolis, K., and Williams, R.: Role of sialic acid in survival of erythrocytes in the circulation: interaction of neuraminidase-treated and untreated erythrocytes with spleen and liver at the cellular level. Proc. Natl. Acad. Sci. USA 74:1521, 1977.

324. Ahn, Y.S., Byrnes, J.J., Harrington, W.J., Cayer, M.L., Smith, D.S., Bruskill, D.E., and Pall, L.M.: The treatment of idiopathic thrombocytopenia with vinblastine-loaded platelets. N. Engl. J. Med. 298:1101, 1978.

325. Baehner, R.L., Nathan, D.G., and Castle, W.B.: Oxidant injury of Caucasian glucose-6-phosphate dehydrogenase-deficient red blood cells by phagocytosing leukocytes during infection. J. Clin. Invest. 50:2466, 1971.

326. Leibovich, S.J., and Ross, R.: The role of the macrophage in wound repair. A study with hydrocortisone and anti-macrophage serum. Am. J. Path. 78:71, 1975.

327. Fauci, A.S., and Dale, D.C.: The effect of in vivo hydrocortisone on subpopulations of human lymphocytes. J. Clin. Invest. 53:240, 1974.

328. Dale, D.C., Fauci, A.S., and Wolff, S.M.: Alternate-day prednisone. Leukocyte kinetics and susceptibility to infections. N. Engl. J. Med. 291:1154, 1974.

329. Norris, D.A., Capin, L., Weston, W.L.: The effect of epicutaneous glucocorticoids on human monocyte and neutrophil migration in vivo. J. Invest. Dermatol. 78:386, 1982.

330. Thompson, J., and van Furth, R.: The effect of glucocorticoids on the proliferation and kinetics of promonocytes and monocytes of the bone marrow. J. Exp. Med. 137:10, 1973.

331. Rinehart, J.J., Sagone, A.L., Balcerzak, S.P., Ackerman, G.A., and Lobuglio, A.F.: Effects of corticosteroid therapy on human monocyte function. N. Engl. J. Med. 292:236, 1975.

332. Taylor, C.E., Weiser, W.Y., and Bang, F.B.: In vitro macrophage manifestation of cortisone-induced decrease in resistance to mouse hepatitis virus. J. Exp. Med. 153:732, 1981.

333. Rinehart, J.J., Wuest, D., and Ackerman, G.A.: Corticosteroid alterations of human monocyte to macrophage differentiation. J. Immunol. 129:1436, 1982.

334. Nakagawara, A., DeSantis, N.M., Nogueira, N., and Nathan, C.F.: Lymphokines enhance the capacity of human monocytes to secrete reactive oxygen intermediates. J. Clin. Invest. 70:1042, 1982.

335. Schreiber, A.D., Parsons, J. McDermott, P., and Cooper, R.A.: Effect of corticosteroids on the human monocyte IgG and complement receptors. J. Clin. Invest. 56:1189, 1975.

336. Norton, J.M., and Munck, A.: In vitro actions of glucocorticoids on murine macrophages: effects on glucose transport and metabolism, growth in culture, and protein synthesis. J. Immunol. 125:259, 1980.

337. Snyder, D.S., and Unanue, E.R.: Corticosteroids inhibit murine macrophage Ia expression and interleukin 1 production. J. Immunol. 129:1803, 1982.

338. Werb, Z.: Biochemical actions of glucocorticoids on macrophages in culture. Specific inhibition of elastase, collagenase, and plasminogen activator secretion and effects on other metabolic functions. J. Exp. Med. 147:1695, 1978.

339. Teitelbaum, S.L., Malone, J.D., and Kahn, A.J.: Glucocorticoid enhancement of bone resorption by rat peritoneal macrophages in vitro. Endocrinology 108:795, 1981.

340. Fauve, R.M., and Pierce-Chase, C.H.: Comparative effects of corticosteroids on host resistance to infection in relation to chemical structure. J. Exp. Med. 125:807, 1967.

341. Balow, J.E., and Rosenthal, A.S.: Glucocorticoid suppression of macrophage migration inhibitory factor. J. Exp. Med. 137:1031, 1973.

342. Vernon-Roberts, B.: The effect of steroid hormones on macrophage activity. Int. Rev. Cytol. 25:131, 1969.

343. Persellin, R.H., and Ziff, M.: The effect of gold salts on lysosomal enzymes of the peritoneal macrophage. Arthr. Rheum. 9:56, 1966.

344. Ho, P.P.K., Young, A.L., and Southard, G.L.: Chemotactic responses of human blood monocytes to the methyl ester of N-formylmethionylleucylphenylalanine and its inhibition by gold compounds. J. Cell Biol. 75:95a, 1977.

345. Littman, B.H., and Schwartz, P.: Gold inhibition of the production of the second complement component by lymphokine-stimulated human monocytes. Arthr. Rheum. 25:288, 1982.

346. Oaten, S.W., Jagelman, S., and Webb, H.E.: Further studies of macrophages in relationship to avirulent semliki forest virus infections. Br. J. Exp. Path. 61:150, 1980.

347. Ghaffar, A., McBride, W.H., and Cullen, R.T.: Interaction of tumor cells and activated macrophages in vitro: Modulation by Corynebacterium and gold salts. J. Reticuloendothel. Soc. 20:283, 1976.

348. Binderup, L., Bramm, E., and Arrigoni-Martelli, E.: Immunological effects of D-penicillamine during experimentally induced inflammation in rats. Scand. J. Immunol. 12:239, 1980.

349. Binderup, L., Bramm, E., and Arrigoni-Martelli, E.: Effect of D-penicillamine in vitro and in vivo on macrophage phagocytosis. Biochem. Pharmacol. 29:2273, 1980.

350. Skosey, J.L., Chow, D.C., Lichon, F., and Hinckley, C.C.: Drug interference with inactivation of serum alpha-1-proteinase inhibitor by oxygen radicals. In Greenwald, R.A., and Cohen, G. (eds.): Oxygen Radicals and Their Scavenger Systems. Vol. II. Cellular and Medical Aspects. New York, Elsevier, 1983, p. 264.

351. van Furth, R., Gassmann, E., and Diesselhoff-den Dulk, M.M.C.: The effect of azathioprine (Imuran) on the cell cycle of promonocytes and the production of monocytes in the bone marrow. J. Exp. Med. 141:531, 1975.

352. Buhles, W.C., Jr, and Shifrine, M.: Effects of cyclophosphamide on macrophage numbers, fucntions and progenitor cells. J. Reticuloendothel. Soc. 21:285, 1977.

353. Mantovani, A.: The interaction of cancer chemotherapy agents with mononuclear phagocytes. Adv. Pharmacol. Chemother. 19:35, 1982.

354. Schnyder, J., Dewald, B., and Baggiolini, M.: Effects of cyclooxygenase inhibitors and prostaglandin E_2 on macrophage activation in vitro. Prostaglandins 22:411, 1981.

355. Schultz, R.M., and Chirigos, M.A.: Selective neutralization by antiinterferon globulin of macrophage activation by L-cell interferon, *Brucella abortus* ether extract, *Salmonella typhimurium* lipopolysaccharide, and polyanions. Cell. Immunol. 48:52, 1979.

Chapter 11

Cellular Components of Inflammation: Platelets

Peter M. Henson and John L. Gordon

INTRODUCTION

Because of their size, platelets, which are the smallest circulating element in mammalian blood, were discovered much later than the other blood cells. They were first described in the mid-nineteenth century, but even in the early years of the twentieth century their existence was not universally recognized.[1,2] During the first half of this century, most of the research on platelets was connected with their role in the clotting process, but in the past 20 years or so there has been an enormous upsurge of interest in platelet biology. This is partly because they are easily obtainable as a virtually homogeneous population and exhibit a wide variety of cellular reactions, e.g., adhesion, aggregation, active transport, degranulation, and prostaglandin synthesis. They are thus valuable cellular models for studying such processes. Equally important, however, is their participation in many biologic events apart from coagulation. Their paramount role in the cellular aspects of hemostasis and thrombosis is now well recognized, and they have been implicated in the maintenance of capillary integrity, in wound healing, in atherosclerosis, in transplant rejection, in the clearance of particles from the blood, and in inflammation.[3] It is their role in inflammation with which this chapter is concerned.

Because studies on platelets have developed so rapidly,

it will not be possible to provide a comprehensive review of all the literature in this area. Accordingly we will use more general reviews or representative papers to illustrate a number of points in this discussion. For a more detailed analysis see reference 3. In addition it is important to emphasize at the outset that although platelets seem to participate in many aspects of inflammation, and certainly possess many properties that are consistent with a potential role in these processes, nevertheless proof of a requirement for these cells in inflammation and in rheumatic diseases is not yet available. Therefore, while platelets should certainly be considered as likely contributors to the pathogenesis of inflammation, they do not appear to be sufficient by themselves to induce an inflammatory response, nor are they necessary for one to occur. Futhermore, there is no evidence that platelets can penetrate intact vascular walls. Therefore one must presume that their activation is confined to the intravascular compartment. This is not to exclude the possibility that platelet-derived mediators might act extravascularly but suggests that the parent cell remains within the blood vessel.

Platelet Constituents and Structural Organization. Platelets are anucleate, discoid fragments of megakaryocyte cytoplasm, about 2 μm in diameter, formed by megakaryocyte pseudopodia extruding in the bone marrow and budding off platelets from the periphery. In healthy subjects 250,000 to 400,000 platelets per cubic millimeter circulate in peripheral blood, and platelet production is about 35,000 per cubic millimeter per day, although these values can vary greatly in disease states, including arthritis. The life span of platelets is around 10 days in man, circulating cells being removed either by the reticuloendothelial system when effete or by incorporation into hemostatic plugs or intravascular aggregates when exposed to stimuli. Specific glycoprotein receptors on the platelet membrane form the recognition sites for many such stimuli, and changes in other membrane glycoproteins regulate the removal of "spent" platelets. The composition of the platelet membrane changes with age,[4] and removal of up to 10 percent of the sialic acid in the membrane results in the immediate clearance of the cells from the circulation, although their response to stimuli is virtually unaffected.[5]

Beneath the platelet membrane is a peripheral bundle of microtubules, running in the equatorial plane (Fig. 11–1), which apparently acts as a cytoskeleton and helps to maintain the characteristic shape of platelets (microtubules are disorganized in stimulated platelets that have lost their discoid form). The contractile proteins actin and myosin are abundant in platelets and seem to play a vital role in responses to stimuli[6] (see below). Most of the major platelet organelles are shown in Figure 11–1. Dense granules (dg) contain vasoactive amines (chiefly serotonin), adenine nucleotides (chiefly ATP), and bivalent cations (Ca^{2+}, Mg^{2+}). Alpha granules (αg) are less osmiophilic than dense granules, are numerous, and contain fibrinogen, heparin-binding proteins such as β-thromboglobulin and platelet factor 4, fibronectin, and platelet-derived growth factor (PDGF).[7,8] True lysosomes are present in small numbers and contain a conventional array of acid hydrolases. Glycogen granules (gg) are abundant, but mitochondira (m) are sparse, with few cristae, which is consistent with the platelet's energy being derived mainly from glycolysis rather than oxidative phosphorylation. Finally, the apparently empty vesicles (v) frequently seen in platelets are usually not enclosed vacuoles but parts of a complex, surface-connected canalicular system that is apparently involved in uptake and secretory processes (see below). Intimately involved with this canalicular system (but not evident in Fig. 11–1) is a network of dense tubules that are apparently the site of prostaglandin synthesis. A more detailed description of platelet ultrastructure and cytochemistry is given by White.[3,9]

The energy required to support the platelet's response to stimuli is supplied by a metabolic pool of ATP in the cytoplasm, which is in very slow equilibrium with the storage pool of ATP in the dense granules. The review by Holmsen[10] provides a detailed account of platelet metabolism.

PLATELET BIOLOGY

Shape Change. The first detectable response of platelets to most stimulants is extrusion of pseudopodia, with consequent loss of discoid shape (Fig. 11–2). This change

Figure 11–1. Platelet isolated from rabbit citrated platelet-rich plasma. × 45,000. αg = Alpha granules; dg = dense granules; gg = glycogen granules; m = mitochondria; mt = microtubules; v = vesicles. (From MacIntyre, D.E., et al.: J. Cell Sci. 28:211, 1977.)

in shape is extremely rapid and is not associated with any significant change in platelet volume. The intracellular events that accompany the shape change may represent a triggering mechanism, which leads in turn to the more profound cellular changes that regulate the processes of aggregation and secretion.[11] The mechanism of the shape change is unknown, but it is of interest that granulocytes also undergo profound alteration in shape as a very early step in stimulus-response coupling processes.[12]

Adhesion. Platelets adhere to many artificial surfaces, and, indeed, the production of surfaces that are "passive" to platelets is of considerable importance in the development of vascular prostheses and other appliances that must come in contact with blood. Of greater importance, particularly with regard to the inflammatory process, is the adhesion of platelets to biologic macromolecules. Most biopolymers (e.g., fibrin, proteoglycans, gelatin, elastin) are not good substrates for platelet adhesion, but platelets readily adhere to polymeric collagen[13] and other connective tissue elements, and this adhesion stimulates platelet secretion and aggregation. Platelet-collagen interaction may be biologically significant because the subendothelial region of the vascular wall contains these proteins; hence, when endothelial cells are

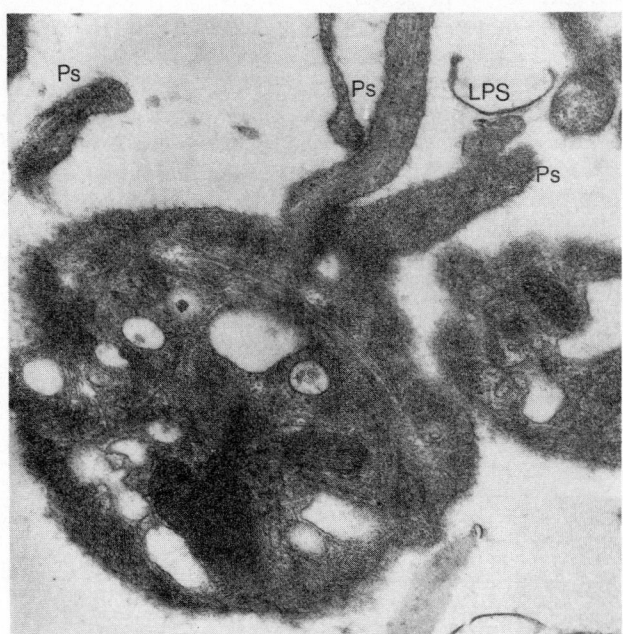

Figure 11–2. Rabbit platelets showing change in shape after exposure to bacterial endotoxin lipopolysaccharide. × 40,000. *LPS* = Lipopolysaccharide; *Ps* = pseudopodia. (From MacIntyre, D.E., et al.: J. Cell Sci. 28:211, 1977.)

damaged (or separated by vasodilation or by endothelial contraction), platelets can adhere to the exposed subendothelium (Fig. 11–3). This phenomenon of platelet accumulation at sites of vascular damage is fundamental to the physiologic and pathologic role of platelets and was recognized over a century ago[14] in studies with frog thrombocytes (the amphibian equivalent of the mammalian platelet). However, there has been some controversy as to which subendothelial constituent the platelets actually adhere to. Part of this confusion comes from the fact that adhesion and aggregation (stimulation) are separate events. Thus, aggregation of platelets in a test tube by collagen types I and III but not by type IV (basement membrane collagen) requires that there first be adhesion to the polymeric collagen and then secretion of aggregating constituents (ADP and/or thromboxane) (see below). More recently the importance of von Willebrand's factor in the interaction of platelet surface glycoprotein Ib and subendothelial constituents has been recognized.[15] Fibronectin, which is expressed on platelet surfaces following activation,[16] could also play a role in this process,[17] although others have questioned such a mechanism[18] and have implicated a separate collagen receptor on the platelet surface.

Aggregation. Several soluble biologic stimuli (e.g., ADP, serotonin, some prostaglandins, catecholamines, thrombin) can induce platelet aggregation. This is usually preceded by the extrusion of pseudopodia, and the aggregation response to the stimulant can be followed (if the stimulant concentration is high enough) by a secondary aggregation response caused by constituents (such as ADP or thromboxane A_2) secreted from the platelets initially stimulated. Aggregation requires extracellular Ca^{2+} and fibrinogen, and the secretory response that results in secondary aggregation may be mediated by an increase in ionized calcium concentration in the platelet cytoplasm (see below). Consequently, aggregation and secretion can be induced by calcium ion-

Figure 11–3. Platelet adhering to subendothelial basement membrane exposed between two endothelial cells. Bar indicates 1 μm. *Ec* = Endothelial cell; *Er* = erythrocyte; *L* = lumen of blood vessel; *P* = platelet; *S* = suendothelial basement membrane. (From Tranzer, J.P., and Baumgartner, H.R.: Nature 216:1126, 1967.)

ophores.[19] Particulate stimuli such as collagen and bacterial endotoxin also induce aggregation (Fig. 11–4), but the aggregation reaction follows initial adhesion between the platelets and the stimulant and depends on the secretion of aggregatory constituents from the platelets.

Platelet aggregation is the process mainly responsible for the early development of a hemostatic plug or thrombus, and because of its association with secretion it is also important in regulating the local concentrations in plasma or tissue of platelet constituents, some of which are powerful inflammatory agents (see Platelet Products with Potential Inflammatory Actions, below).

Recent work on the process of aggregation has begun to define its mechanism. Activated platelets develop binding sites for fibrinogen, which appear to involve in part the major surface glycoprotein Gp IIb-IIIa complex.[20,21] Additional work has suggested the involvement of an alpha granule–derived lectin termed thrombospondin, which may crosslink the fibrinogen molecules.[22]

Secretion. When stimulated, platelets can selectively release the contents of their dense granules and alpha granules and under some conditions, particularly with higher concentrations of stimulus, their lysosomal constituents. The adenine nucleotides and serotonin stored in the dense bodies can be released by stimulants such as ADP without significant secretion of alpha granule contents.[23] Stimulatory prostanoids evoke a similar pattern of secretion,[24] whereas "stronger" stimuli such as thrombin and collagen induce secretion of lysosomal hydrolases as well.[25-27] Blockade of platelet thromboxane

Figure 11–4. Platelet aggregation induced by bacterial endotoxin lipopolysaccharide (*LPS*). *A*, × 30,000. *B*, × 40,000. Note whorls of LPS between platelets and closely approximated platelet plasma membranes that retain their integrity. Granules and disrupted microtubules are visible within platelets. (From MacIntyre, D.E., et al.: J. Cell Sci. 28:211, 1977.)

synthesis by drugs such as aspirin can inhibit the secretion of platelet constituents by collagen, implying that here thromboxane synthesis is necessary for the secretory response.[27]

The cellular mechanisms regulating platelet secretion are not yet fully known, but the events seem to be very similar to those seen in other cells.[28] The process is initiated by a stimulant that binds to specific receptors on the platelet surface. This probably induces ionic alterations and depolarization[29] accompanied by an increase in cytoplasmic calcium ion concentration.[30] The platelet's contractile proteins (actin and myosin) are likely involved as well as a process of fusion of the granule membranes with the platelet plasma membrane (or some derivative of this) that results in extrusion of the granule contents. The exact morphologic mechanism for the discharge of dense bodies has not yet been clarified. Alpha granules on the other hand are thought to fuse first with each other to form a compound granule and then with the plasma membrane or the open canalicular system.[31] At least one intrinsic inhibitory pathway also exists: degranulation is readily inhibited if the level of cyclic AMP in platelets is raised,[32] either by stimulating the adenylate cyclase that forms cAMP or by inhibiting the phosphodiesterase that degrades it.

Arachidonate Metabolism. When platelets are exposed to a stimulus sufficiently powerful to induce degranulation, the arachidonic acid biosynthetic pathways are activated. Some of the products of this pathway have inflammatory activity (see below) and/or promote platelet aggregation and secretion. The main features of the pathway are outlined in Figure 11–5. General synthetic

pathways and biologic activities of arachidonate derivatives are reviewed in Chapter 6. Briefly, activation of a phospholipase(s) associated with the platelet membrane liberates arachidonic acid from membrane phospholipids. This 20-carbon fatty acid is converted by a membrane-bound cyclo-oxygenase into labile intermediate compounds, the endoperoxides PGG_2 and PGH_2. These compounds, which can themselves induce platelet aggregation and secretion, are converted mainly to thromboxane $(Tx)A_2$, which is highly labile (half-life about 30 seconds) but is an extremely potent platelet stimulant[33] and vasoconstrictor. The metabolic product of TxA_2, known as TxB_2, is stable and readily measurable by radioimmunoassay but inactive on platelets. Small amounts of PGD_2, PGE_2, and $PGF_{2\alpha}$ are also formed from the endoperoxides. Although all are vasoactive, the only one with a powerful effect on platelets is PGD_2, which can inhibit platelet responses by stimulating adenylate cyclase,[34] thus elevating cyclic AMP. Through the lipo-oxygenase pathway, 12-hydroxytetraenoic acid (12-HETE) is produced in platelets. Interestingly, it has been suggested that platelets (12-lipo-oxygenase) and neutrophils (5-lipo-oxygenase) can cooperate to produce the important phlogistic agent LTB_4 (5,12-DiHETE) from arachidonic acid.[35] As we shall see later, cooperative interactions such as this between leukocytes and platelets may contribute significantly to inflammation. Finally, 12-hydroxy-5-*cis*,8,10-*trans*-heptadecatrienoic acid (HHT), together with the three-carbon fragment malondialdehyde (MDA), is produced from the endoperoxides. Although HHT and MDA are without effect on platelets, MDA can easily be measured either colorimetrically or fluorimetrically after combination with thiobarbituric acid, thus serving as a simple indicator of PG synthesis by platelets.

Nonsteroidal anti-inflammatory drugs such as aspirin and indomethacin block the cyclo-oxygenase and thus inhibit the platelet responses mediated by TxA_2 and the endoperoxides. The production of HHT, MDA, and the stable prostaglandins D_2, E_2 and $F_{2\alpha}$ is also prevented by these drugs, but they do not interfere with the formation of 12-HETE.

Phospholipid Metabolism. Stimulation of platelets by ligand–receptor interactions produces profound alteration in phospholipid metabolism, and it has been suggested that this participates in the stimulus-response coupling mechanism. Liberation of arachidonate has already been mentioned, and this appears to be derived from both phosphatidyl inositol and phosphatidyl choline, probably as as result of action of phospholipases C and A_2, respectively.[36,37] The so-called phosphoinositol (PI) cycle is activated, and both diacylglycerol (DAG) and phosphatidic acid (PA) are formed very early in the activation sequence. PA has been suggested to act as an ionophore, i.e., a molecule that promotes redistribution of calcium,[38] but this has been challenged.[37] DAG, on the other hand, acts as a cofactor for a unique protein kinase (protein kinase C), which is now felt to be important in cell activation.[36] By contrast, the arachidonate for thromboxane generation may well be derived via an

Figure 11–5. Schematic outline of prostaglandin (PG) synthetic pathways in platelets.

as yet unidentified phospholipase A_2 (PLA_2) from other phospholipids, probably phosphatidyl choline. Interestingly, some of this substrate may have an ether-linked alkyl chain in the sn-1 position. The removal of arachidonate from this alkyl-acyl-glycero-phosphoryl choline would yield the precursor for the synthesis of platelet-activating factor (PAF) (see below). It should be emphasized, however, that platelet activation can proceed (following the appropriate stimuli) without participation of endogenous arachidonate derivatives and probably without the generation of PAF. However, these two lipid derivatives may significantly contribute to the amplification of the overall platelet response and thus lead to an explosive reaction, which can generate a significant thrombus, for example, before inhibitory processes take over.

Uptake by Active Transport. Platelets accumulate by active transport several vasoactive amines, which are then stored in the dense granules. The most striking example is serotonin, whose uptake by platelets has been studied for many years.[39] The transport process is highly efficient (see Fig. 11–6), and under normal circumstances all the serotonin in blood is carried in the platelet dense granules, which effectively isolates it from the vascular cells. The same system is used to transport dopamine, though with much lower affinity,[40] and norepinephrine is also transported into the platelet by the serotonin carrier, with even lower affinity (Olverman and Gordon, unpublished work).

Platelets also actively transport other vasoactive substances such as amino acids and adenosine, which provide fuel for the platelet's energy requirements. Adenosine is incorporated into the metabolic pool of adenine nucleotides, as is adenine.[41] The platelet's capacity to remove vasoactive agents such as adenosine from the plasma, though possibly important in inflammation, is subordinate to that of the vascular endothelial cells.[42]

Uptake by Endocytosis. Individual platelets, and platelet aggregates, can take up particulate materials of many kinds, such as lipid droplets, carbon particles, latex beads, and micro-organisms.[43] Whether this uptake represents genuine pinocytosis and phagocytosis, trapping of particles within the canalicular system, or in some cases merely incorporation of material within a platelet aggregate, is open to question. It is clear, however, that this is not just an in vitro phenomenon of academic interest; platelets can and do play an important role in removing some kinds of particulate material from the bloodstream.[44] This therefore merits further investigation, particularly with respect to the interaction of platelets and micro-organisms, a potentially important event in inflammation.

PLATELET PRODUCTS WITH POTENTIAL INFLAMMATORY ACTIONS

Amines. The amine content of human platelets is virtually all serotonin, although rabbit platelets are apparently unique in having a substantial content of histamine also.[45] These amines (as well as the small amounts of catecholamines also present in platelets) are stored in the dense granules, which possess an uptake mechanism capable of concentrating the amines transported from the extracellular medium into the platelet cytoplasm by the carrier on the plasma membrane. The amine content of platelets varies widely in different species, from about 3 to 60 nmole per mg cell protein, with values in man near the lower end of the range.[46]

Because the contents of dense granules are readily secreted by platelets, exposure of platelets to stimuli results in a high local concentration of serotonin in the plasma, which can have profound effects on vascular tone and permeability (Chapter 8). In addition, serotonin is a fibrogenic agent[47] and may therefore affect the connective tissue composition at sites of chronic inflammation. It is instructive to calculate the plasma concentration of serotonin that might be achieved around a human platelet aggregate; assuming 1×10^9 platelets form an aggregate at a site of local endothelial damage and release 50 percent of their serotonin (about 0.2 μg), then the serotonin concentration in the plasma (say, 0.1 ml in volume) around the aggregate is over 10 μM. In making this calculation it should be remembered that 10^9 platelets are derived from about 3 ml blood, that an aggregate of 10^9 platelets occupies only about 10 μl, and that platelets often release more than 50 percent of their serotonin.

Arachidonate Products. These have already been discussed above (see Arachidonate Synthesis). Thromboxane A_2 is a potent vasoconstrictor. Its role in inflam-

Figure 11–6. Uptake of [³H]-5-hydroxytryptamine (serotonin; 5HT) by rat platelets in plasma. Samples of supernatant plasma were taken at the times shown for assay of total 5HT (closed symbols) and measurement of radioactivity (open symbols). Initial [³H]-5HT concentrations added were (○) 2 μm. (△) 1μM. (□) 0.5 μM. (From Drummond, A.H., and Gordon, J.L.: Br. J. Pharmacol. 56:417, 1976.)

matory processes is not clear. Nevertheless (as outlined below) hemodynamic alterations are so important in inflammation that one cannot disregard the potential contribution of TxA_2. On the other hand, prostaglandins are secreted in such small amounts by platelets that although these molecules participate in inflammatory processes, the platelet does not seem to be an important source.

As indicated above, 12-HETE may have some chemotactic potential of its own but can be converted to LTB_4 by neutrophils. LTB_4 is an extremely potent chemoattractant and neutrophil stimulus and thus must be considered as a candidate for a platelet contribution to inflammation.

These mediators are all discussed in more detail in Chapter 6.

Enzymes. It has been known for some years that platelets contain acid hydrolases, such as β-glucuronidase, in lysosomal granules (see above). In addition to lysosomal glycosidases and acid phosphatase, platelets contain acid proteinases. Cathepsins A, C, D, and E have been described.[48] Cathepsin D is apparently the most prominent proteinase in human platelets, but, as with other platelet constituents, there are substantial interspecies variations. Neutral proteinases in platelets have been less well characterized; elastase, collagenase, and other neutral proteinases have been described, but the amounts of elastase and collagenase present per milligram of cell protein are very small compared with those in other cells such as neutrophils or those produced by macrophages. Indeed, some of these enzyme activities measured in "platelet" preparations may have been due to contaminating neutrophils,[48] although in the case of elastase there is apparently a small amount of activity in the platelets themselves.[49] This enzyme is not, however, readily detectable with substrates (including [³H]-elastin) conventionally used to characterize the elastase in other cells, such as neutrophils.

The roles of the hydrolytic enzymes released by platelets remain to be determined. Most (if not all) of them are released when platelets are exposed to powerful stimuli such as thrombin and collagen. The ability of the acid hydrolases to attack components of connective tissue is presumably severely limited by the buffering action of the plasma surrounding platelets, which keeps the milieu around the platelets at a pH too alkaline for significant activity of acid hydrolases. Likewise, the platelet neutral proteinases would be affected by inhibitors such as α_1-antitrypsin and α_2-macroglobulin in the surrounding plasma. Therefore, it seems that such enzymes could only be effective in the immediate pericellular environment, where the access of plasma constituents might be restricted.

However, platelet neutral proteinases may play a role in generating phlogistic factors. For example, biologically active fragments of C5 are generated when platelets are activated in plasma.[50] This was shown to result from liberation of a platelet neutral proteinase. Such C5 fragments can themselves initiate a complete inflammatory reaction with both cellular infiltration and increased permeability.[51] Local production of such factors at the site of platelet–vessel wall interaction should therefore be considered as a candidate for initiation of some types of inflammatory reactions.

Platelet-Derived Growth Factor. Ross[52,53] described a low molecular weight protein from platelet granules that promoted proliferation of vascular smooth muscle cells. This molecule, platelet-derived growth factor (PDGF) has since been studied extensively. It has been purified, cloned, and sequenced and shows a fascinating homology in primary structure with an oncogene product.[54] Its receptors and growth-promoting effect on mesenchymal cells have also been well described,[55] and it may represent an important contribution to the repair processes following inflammation.

INTERACTION OF PLATELETS WITH COMPONENTS OF THE INFLAMMATORY SYSTEM

Purines. There are three main aspects to the interactions between platelets and purines. First, ADP induces platelet aggregation (and a modest secretory response in human platelets) by combining with a specific receptor.[56] Second, adenosine inhibits platelet responses by interacting with another receptor[56] that is coupled to adenylate cyclase and thus elevates cyclic AMP in platelets. Finally, the ATP and ADP secreted during platelet degranulation are powerful vasoactive agents, largely because of their capacity to induce endothelium-dependent vasodilation,[57,58] a phenomenon in which endothelial cells are stimulated to release a mediator that relaxes the subjacent vascular smooth muscle. It should be emphasized that although ATP stimulates the release of PGI_2 from endothelial cells, PGI_2 is not the mediator of endothelium-dependent vasodilation.[60] Nucleotides can be released from cells other than platelets in response to a damaging stimulus—e.g., from erythrocytes and vascular endothelium[61]—and these extracellular nucleotides affect platelet function and vascular tone (see above); however, their effects are localized and transient, because nucleotides released into the plasma are rapidly metabolized, mainly by ectoenzymes located on the luminal surface of endothelial cells.[62] Adenosine, one of the products of such metabolism, induces vasodilation through a direct action on vascular smooth muscle, as well as by inhibiting platelet responsiveness.[56]

It may seen unusual to classify purines as components of the inflammatory system, but their powerful effects on vasoregulation suggest that their role in the inflammatory process may have been underrated (see also Chapter 21).

Amines. Amines are an important class of inflammatory mediators, chief among which are histamine and serotonin; catecholamines are also important because of their effects on blood flow. Platelets are unaffected by histamine but can be stimulated to aggregate and secrete by serotonin, epinephrine, norepinephrine, and (weakly) dopamine. Catecholamines induce aggregation with little or no shape change in human platelets. Serotonin is regarded as a weak platelet stimulant but is very sensitive to calcium ion concentration, and therefore anticoagulation with citrate can give a false picture.[63] Also aggregation is greatly potentiated when serotonin and a catecholamine are present together (Fig. 11–7). This is important because the circulating levels of catecholamines (in the nanomolar range) are too low to induce aggregation directly but can potentiate platelet responses to other stimuli. For example, platelet responsiveness is increased in subjects under stress,[64] and this may be correlated with increases in circulating catecholamines.

Arachidonate Derivatives. The arachidonate product that is the most powerful platelet stimulant is TxA_2, and the most potent inhibitory product is PGI_2 (prostacyclin). Both of these were discovered using platelets.[33,65] TxA_2 has already been discussed. PGI_2 and, to a lesser extent, PGE_2 inhibit platelet responses by activating adenylate cyclase and increasing the intracellular levels of cyclic AMP. PGI_2 has been suggested to contribute to the nonthrombogenic surface of the vascular endothelium, although other factors may also play a role in this important endothelial function.[66,67] Interestingly, as with platelets and neutrophils combining to synthesize LTB_4, platelet endoperoxides have been suggested to be "used" by endothelial cells to synthesize PGI_2.[68] Thus, cooperation between cells in the modulation of vascular responses is implied. Prostaglandins such as PGI_2 and PGE_2 are vasodilators in some vascular beds and thus may enhance vascular permeability and neutrophil migration in inflammation.

Platelet-Activating Factor (PAF). This phospholipid was first described as a platelet activator but is now known to have much broader biologic activities. The breadth is well illustrated in the recently published proceedings of the first international symposium on this molecule.[69] The structure of the PAF that is derived from rabbit basophils is 1-0-alkyl-2-acetyl-*sn*-glycero-3-phosphorylcholine. Molecule(s) derived from neutrophils, mononuclear phagocytes, endothelial cells, and the renal medulla are very similar, but their exact structure has not yet been determined.[69,70] As well as acting as a potent platelet stimulus, PAF (or acetyl-glyceryl-ether-phosphorylcholine [AGEPC] or [PAF acether][72]) contracts smooth muscle in a slow and prolonged fashion, activates neutrophils, and causes increased vascular permeability. Its actions in vivo also include induction of pulmonary hypertension and systemic hypotension.[70] Some of these effects are apparently mediated via its action on platelets; some, by other means. PAF is derived from ubiquitous membrane ether lipids. It is an extremely potent molecule (a few micrograms are lethal), and mammalian tissues and plasma contain a highly specific acetylhydrolase that inactivates the molecule.[72] These observations suggest that we may have to pay considerable attention to this group of compounds as inflammatory mediators in the future.

Thrombin. Thrombin is one of the most important physiologic activators of platelets and also plays a role in the inflammatory response around fibrin-cell clots. Lower concentrations of thrombin are needed to induce platelet secretion and aggregation than to clot fibrinogen, but despite many studies on the effect of thrombin on platelets no fully accepted explanation of its mechanism of action has yet emerged. The proteolytic action of thrombin is probably important for platelet stimulation, but the molecule also binds to receptors on the platelet surface.[71] The protein with which thrombin interacts to stimulate platelets is not fibrinogen; thrombin induces platelet secretion when fibrinogen is absent or blocked by antibodies,[72,73] although fibrinogen is a necessary cofactor for platelet aggregation.

Other Coagulation Factors. Platelets exhibit an intricate and intimate relationship with the process of coagulation. Additionally, the coagulation process is probably involved in inflammation; for example, fibrin deposition is a common occurrence. Nevertheless, the exact contribution of these elements to inflammation is as yet unclear, and, since coagulation is discussed in more detail in Chapter 8, it is only mentioned herein for completeness.

Immune Stimuli and Complement Components. For a recent review of immunologic reactions of platelets see reference 7. Platelets can be stimulated or damaged by several immunologic reactions (some complement mediated) in which the stimulus is not directed at the platelet in an immunologically specific sense. These immunologic reactions, in which the platelet is a "bystander," can be separated into two main classes, depending on whether the platelets are able to bind the third complement component C3b (i.e., are immune adherence positive) (see Chapter 7). Immune adherence is species dependent; platelets from many nonprimate species (e.g., rabbit, rat, mouse, guinea pig) are immune adherence positive and are consequently attracted to particles and surfaces that have fixed C3b.[74]

Immune adherence negative platelets (e.g., human)

Figure 11–7. Platelet aggregation induced by 5-hydroxytryptamine (5HT) and by norepinephrine (noradrenaline [NA]), alone and in combination.

react with aggregated gamma globulin, with IgG-coated surfaces, or with immune complexes containing IgG. This induces platelet secretion and, under appropriate conditions, aggregation, but not lysis. Complement activation is apparently not essential; indeed, the reactions proceed in platelet suspensions free of serum or plasma.[75] IgG stimulates platelets by interacting with a typical Fc receptor on the platelet membrane that is not one of the major glycoproteins.[76] This process can be markedly enhanced by the presence of lipopolysaccharide (endotoxin).[7] Activated zymosan (i.e., with C3b attached via the alternative pathway) also induces aggregation and secretion (but not lysis) in human platelets, whereas endotoxin alone does not,[77] but because zymosan readily accumulates IgG as well as C3b, and the attached C3b progressively decays to C3d (which is inactive), there is still some doubt about the mechanisms responsible for zymosan-induced stimulation of human platelets.

An interesting observation in relation to the interaction of platelets with complement components is that part of the Clq molecule is structurally similar to part of the collagen molecule, and Clq can inhibit platelet stimulation by collagen.[78,80] It has been suggested that complement activation is involved in platelet stimulation by collagen,[79] although this hypothesis now seems unlikely.

Polly and associates have studied another way in which platelets may interact with the complement system.[81] Assembly of components on the surface of the thrombin-activated platelet was suggested to represent a unique and perhaps important activating pathway for complement. Certainly various investigators have detected complement components on the surface of washed platelets (see reference 74), although whether this represented molecules trapped in the canalicular system is not clear.

Platelets participate in several immunologic reactions that result in inflammatory lesions (e.g., the Arthus and local Shwartzman reactions), and although their presence is apparently not always essential, there is no doubt that they often contribute to the biologic consequences.[82]

Vascular Cells. Changes in the vasculature (especially in the microcirculation) are central to the inflammatory process, as emphasized by Cohnheim almost a century ago. Since the participation of platelets in the body's response to a stimulus (whether "inflammatory" or otherwise) is necessarily an intravascular event, the interaction of platelets with vascular cells is of primary importance. The vascular cells involved are those of the endothelium and the underlying smooth muscle layer.

Under normal circumstances, platelets do not adhere to endothelial cells. This is partly because endothelium apparently does not present a surface "attractive" to platelets, and partly because endothelial cells synthesize and secrete prostacyclin (PGI_2) which, like PGD_2 and PGE_1, is a powerful adenylate cyclase stimulant and thus inhibits platelet secretion, aggregation, and adhesion.[66,67,83] In contrast to endothelium, vascular smooth muscle cells or fibroblasts readily induce platelet aggregation and secretion in vitro, possibly because of the connective tissue elements on their surface.[84] These in vitro findings are consistent with observations made in vivo; namely, that as long as the endothelial lining is maintained intact, platelets do not adhere in large numbers, but when endothelial damage occurs and the underlying connective tissue is exposed, then platelets adhere and form aggregates at these sites.

It is important to note that the preferential adhesion of platelets to vascular smooth muscle rather than endothelium is not a phenomenon observed with other cells such as leukocytes; granulocytes readily adhere to endothelial cells in vitro but have a lesser affinity for smooth muscle cells.[85]

Mononuclear Phagocytes. It has been established that platelet aggregates in vivo are eventually invaded by monocytes, and resolution of the thrombus is achieved by the monocytes phagocytizing platelet debris.[86] The signal for this phagocytosis has not yet been determined but may be similar to the mechanism by which senescent platelets are recognized as being ready for removal from the circulation; this recognition apparently involves a small reduction in platelet membrane sialic acid.[4,5] Interestingly, platelets appear to have some affinity for blood monocytes and may contribute to their adhesion to surfaces.[87]

The biochemical aspects of platelet-monocyte interactions have also been neglected. For example, although it seems likely that platelet constituents could affect the migration and endocytic activity of mononuclear phagocytes, this possibility has apparently not been investigated.

Neutrophils. Platelet aggregates that form in vivo or in vitro in a system with white cells present are frequently surrounded by PMN leukocytes in the form of "halos"[88] or "rosettes"[89] (Fig. 11–8). Similarly, the adhesion of platelets to blood vessels stripped of endothelial cells in vivo is followed by the attachment of leukocytes, and the leukocyte adhesion is a consequence of the presence of activated platelets rather than the loss of endothelium per se.[90] The leukocytes are apparently attracted by factors derived from the platelets, and the most likely candidates are C5a (formed in the plasma by the platelet proteinases)[50] or prostanoid products such as HETE and HHT or LTB_4.

The possible cooperation of platelets and neutrophils in synthesizing LTB_4 has already been mentioned. LTB_4 is an important neutrophil stimulant. In the other direction, neutrophils synthesize and secrete PAF, which can activate the platelets. This reciprocal activation may play an important role in the explosive early stages of inflammation. In addition, a recent report implicates platelet products in the enhancement of neutrophil-endothelial interactions,[91] i.e., the putative first step in leukocyte emigration.

It is clear that platelets may also interact with other circulating leukocytes. However, detailed mechanisms need further investigations.

Fibroblasts. Platelet-derived growth factor has already been mentioned and could contribute to fibroblast proliferation in the reparative phases of inflammation.

Figure 11–8. Platelet aggregates formed in vitro by rotating samples of recalcified citrated blood in plastic tubes. Aggregates are surrounded by "halos" of polymorphonuclear leukocytes. *A,* × 100. *B.* × 250.

However, like many aspects of platelet function, the in vivo involvement remains to be clarified.

THE INFLAMMATORY PROCESS—A ROLE FOR PLATELETS?

Inflammation could be defined as a beneficial, nonspecific response of tissues to injury, which generally leads to resolution of the injury. As such, chronic inflammatory diseases might represent examples of continued or repetitive stimuli and/or abnormalities of the resolution process. In this context, chronic disease resulting from inflammatory processes might include persistent inflammation, permanent tissue destruction, or fibrosis. The last could be seen as a resolution that is inappropriate for the tissue, a last-ditch effect to repair the site of injury but one that does not allow restitution of normal tissue function. The inflammatory process can therefore be considered in three phases: initiation; resolution of the inflammation; and, lastly, resolution of the injury.

Initiation of inflammation involves alterations in blood vessel functions, emigration of leukocytes, and increased vascular permeability. Despite all the investigative efforts over the last 100 years, we still know surprisingly little about the details of these three processes. The contribution of hemodynamic alterations to inflammation has been known since the nineteenth century but has received a resurgence of interest following the recent suggestion that vasodilator prostaglandins (PGE_2, PGI_2) can enhance vascular permeability and increase neutrophil emigration.[92,93] Whether these effects are solely hemodynamic or whether they are the direct effects of the prostaglandins on the vessel wall and/or the leukocytes is not yet clear. The data do, however, suggest one area in which nonsteroidal anti-inflammatory cyclo-oxygenase inhibitors might be effective.

The emigration of leukocytes is also an area fraught with surprising mystery. Initial adhesion of leukocytes to the vascular endothelium is followed by migration between these cells and then across the barrier of the basement membrane (or basal lamina). The major site of emigration appears to be the postcapillary venules, but neutrophils can migrate through the walls of large arteries, veins, and capillaries.[94,95] Chemotactic factors apparently induce the expression of adhesive properties on the leukocytes, which induce the initial interaction with the endothelium. Subsequent events can be described only superficially, however. We[96] and Liotta's[97] group have suggested that cells migrate across basal laminae by digesting components of the connective tissue following release of proteases, but this hypothesis has not yet been proved in vivo. Additionally, the true nature and function of the putative chemotactic factors in these systems remain to be elucidated.

Increased permeability is also an integral component of inflammation. It has often been associated with the leukocytic phases of the inflammation,[92,95] but experiments have also suggested that leukocyte emigration and increased permeability are separable events.[96] While the suggested mechanisms for the permeability changes are beyond the scope of this chapter, it is noteworthy that leukocytes may "open" tight junctions between cells by release of neutral proteases or oxygen radicals (Parsons, Cott, Mason, and Henson, unpublished). This is an area of intense investigation in many centers, and evidence for specific mechanisms should be forthcoming in the near future.

Since most of the aforementioned processes occur in the blood vessels, platelets are potential candidates for contributing to these events. As indicated throughout this chapter, there is great *potential* for such platelet involvement but very little evidence that it actually occurs. Platelet depletion studies did not seem to alter significantly the induction of an Arthus reaction in the rabbit (Henson and Cochrane, 1969, unpublished). However, we know so much more about the systems involved now that it would seem appropriate to repeat this type of study with more detailed quantitative analysis of the effects of the depletion on the inflammatory process. Certainly platelets accumulate at sites of inflammation,[98,99] though whether as participants or as a consequence of the process is unclear.

With regard to termination of the inflammation itself (the shut-off mechanisms) we know even less, and the mechanisms involved in resolution and repair also require much more investigation. In these two areas, the role of platelets is largely unknown. Hints of a contribution come from the secretion and known effects of PDGF, but it may be that this molecule exerts its influence in vivo primarily on the blood vessel wall.

Future studies of the contribution of platelets to specific inflammatory processes should include the following:

1. Quantitative evidence of platelet accumulation
2. Morphologic evidence of platelet presence and secretion
3. The presence of platelet products
4. Prevention of effects by specific platelet inhibition or depletion
5. Prevention of effects by inhibition of the action of platelet products
6. Reproduction of the given effect by administration of platelets or the platelet product to the platelet-depleted system
7. Studies in animals or man with genetically malfunctioning platelets.

Clearly such investigations are easier in acute reactions, but even then they suffer from problems of specificity. Inflammation is a highly redundant process with many "collateral" mechanisms. Elimination of one component of the system often has little effect on the overall process because other cells and systems can take over, hence, the difficulty and fascination of research in this area.

SUMMARY

The potential contributions of platelets to the inflammatory process are considerable, but their actual participation has not been established. Intravascular accumulation of platelets at sites of tissue injury has been clearly demonstrated,[99] and there have also been claims that platelets were present in inflammatory exudates,[100] but further investigations in the same laboratory revealed that these claims were incorrect.[101] It therefore appears that intact platelets are not found extravascularly at inflammatory sites. Indeed this might be expected, since the rapidity with which they adhere to vascular collagen would preclude their migration out of blood vessels. Nevertheless platelet constituents released intravascularly at an injury site may diffuse across the vessel wall[102] and could affect tissues in this manner.

It therefore appears that platelets may influence extravascular events in the inflammatory process to a limited extent through the actions of their secreted constituents, but their role in this respect would normally be subordinate to that of leukocytes. In intravascular events, however, platelets may play an important role, as the evidence summarized in this chapter demonstrates. This should be borne in mind when considering the vascular aspects of inflammation, as platelets can interact with many components of the inflammatory response. But as well as revealing potential biologic consequences, the study of such interactions can increase our understanding of the processes involved; as emphasized earlier in this chapter, platelets have been and will continue to be valuable cellular models for the biologist interested in adhesion, degranulation, and prostaglandin synthesis, and in the receptors and mediators that regulate these events.

REFERENCES

1. Buckmaster, G.A.: The blood platelets. Sci. Prog. 1:73, 1906.
2. Robb-Smith, A.H.T.: Why the platelets were discovered. Br. J. Haematol. 13:618, 1967.
3. Gordon, J.L. (ed.): Platelets in Biology and Pathology 2. Amsterdam, Elsevier-North Holland-Biomedical Press, 1981.
4. George, J.N., and Lewis, P.C.: Studies on platelet plasma membranes. J. Lab. Clin. Med. 91:301, 1978.
5. Greenberg, J., Packham, M.A., Cazenave, J.P., Reimers, H.J., and Mustard, J.F.: Effects on platelet function of removal of platelet sialic acid by neuraminidase. Lab. Invest. 32:476, 1975.
6. Lind, S.E., and Stossel, T.P.: The microfilament network of the platelet. Prog Hemost. Thromb. 6:63, 1982.
7. Henson, P.M., and Ginsberg, M.H.: Immunological reactions of platelets. In Gordon, J.L. (ed): Platelets in Biology and Pathology 2. Amsterdam, Elsevier-North Holland-Biomedical Press, 1981.
8. Packham, M.A., and Mustard, J.F.: In vitro methods and the study of platelet mechanisms. Vox Sang. 40(Suppl. 1):22, 1981.
9. White, J.G.: Platelet morphology. In Johnson, S.A. (ed): The Circulating Platelet. New York, Academic Press. 1971.
10. Holmsen, H.: Energy metabolism in platelets. Vox Sang. 40(Suppl. 1):1, 1981.
11. Frojmovic, M.M., and Milton, J.G.: Human platelet size, shape and related functions in health and disease. Physiol. Rev. 62:185, 1982 .
12. Smith, C.W. and Hollens, J.C.: Motility and adhesiveness in human neutrophils: Redistribution of chemotactic factor induced adhesion sites. J. Clin. Invest. 65:804, 1980.
13. Gordon, J.L., and Dingle, J.T.: Binding of radiolabelled collagen to blood platelets. J. Cell Sci. 16:157, 1976.
14. Wharton-Jones, W.T.: On the state of the blood and blood vessels in inflammation. Guy's Hospital. Rep. Ser. 2 7:1, 1851.
15. Coller, B.S., Peerschke, E.I., Scudder, L.E., and Sullivan, C.A.: Studies with a murine monoclonal antibody that abolishes ristocetin-induced binding of von Willebrand factor to platelets: Additional evidence in support of GPIb as a platelet receptor for von Willebrand factor. Blood 61:99, 1983.
16. Ginsberg, M.H.. Forsyth, J., Lightsey, A., Chediak, J., and Plow, E.F.: Reduced surface expression and binding of fibronectin by thrombin-stimulated thrombasthenic platelets. J. Clin. Invest. 71:619, 1983.
17. Bensusan, H.B., Koh, T.L., Henry, K.G., Murray, B.A., and Culp L.A.: Evidence that fibronectin is the collagen receptor on platelet membranes. Proc. Natl. Acad. Sci. 75:5864, 1978.
18. Chiang, T.M. and Kang, A.H.: Isolation and purification of collagen α 1(I) receptor from human platelet membrane. J. Biol. Chem. 257:7581, 1982.
19. Feinman, R.D., and Detwiler, T.C.: Platelet secretion induced by divalent calcium ionophores. Nature 249:172, 1974.
20. Di Minno, G., Thiagarajan, P., Perussia, B., Martinez, J., Shapiro, S., Trinchieri, G., and Murphy, S.: Exposure of platelet fibrinogen-binding sites by collagen, arachidonic acid, and ADP: Inhibition by a monoclonal antibody to the glycoprotein IIb-IIIa Complex. Blood 61:140, 1983.
21. Bennett, J.S., Hoxie, J.A., Leitman, S.F., Vilaire, G., and Cines, D.B.: Inhibition of fibrinogen binding to stimulated human platelets by a monoclonal antibody. Proc. Natl. Acad. Sci. 80:2417, 1983.
22. Jaffe, E.A., Leung, L.L.K., Nachman, R.L., Levin, R.I. and Mosher, D.F.: Thrombospondin is the endogenous lectin of human platelets. Nature 295:246, 1982.
23. Mills, D.C.B., Robb, I.A., and Roberts, G.C.K.: The release of nucleotides, 5-hydroxytryptamine and enzymes from human blood platelets during aggregation. J. Physiol. 195:715, 1968.
24. MacIntyre, D.E., Salzman, E.W., and Gordon, J.L.: Prostaglandin receptors on human platelets. Structure-activity relationships of stimulatory prostaglandins. Biochem. J. 174:921, 1978.
25. Holmsen, H., and Day, H.J.: The selectivity of the thrombin-induced platelet release reaction: Subcellular localization of released and retained constituents. J. Lab. Clin. Med. 75:840, 1970.
26. Gordon, J.L.: Blood platelet lysosomes and their contribution to the pathophysiological role of platelets. In Dingle, J.T., and Dean, R.T. (eds.): Lysosomes in Biology and Pathology, Vol. 4. Amsterdam, North-Holland, 1975.
27. MacIntyre, D.E., McMillan, R.M., and Gordon, J.L.: Secretion of lysosomal enzymes by platelets. Biochem. Soc. Trans. 5:1181, 1977.
28. Henson, P.M., Ginsberg, M.H. and Morrison, D.C.: Mechanisms of mediator release by inflammatory cells. In Poste, G. and Nicolson, G.L. (eds.): Membrane Fusion. Amsterdam, Elsevier-North Holland-Biomedical Press, 1978.
29. Friedhoff, L.T., and Sonenberg, M.: The membrane potential of human platelets. Blood 61:180, 1983.
30. Feinstein, M.B.: The role of calmodulin in hemostasis. Prog. Hemost. Thromb. 6:25, 1982.
31. Ginsberg, M.H., Taylor, L. and Painter R.G.: The mechanism of thrombin-induced platelet factor 4 release. Blood 55:661, 1980.
32. Haslam, R.J.: Roles of cyclic nucleotides in platelet function. In Biochemistry and Pharmacology of Platelets. Amsterdam, Elsevier, 1975.
33. Hamberg, M., Svensson, J., and Samuelsson, B.: Thromboxanes: A new group of biologically active compounds derived from prostaglandin endoperoxides. Proc. Natl. Acad. Sci. USA 72:2994, 1975.
34. Smith, J.B., Ingerman, C.M., and Silver, M.J.: Formation of prostaglandin D2 during endoperoxide-induced platelet aggregation. Thromb. Res. 9:413, 976.
35. Marcus, A.J., Brockman, M.J., Safier, G., Ullman, H.C., Islam, N., Sherman, C.N., Rutherford, L.E., Korchak, H.M., Weissmann, G.: Formation of leukotrienes and other hydroxy acids during platelet-neutrophil interactions in vitro. Biochem. Biophys. Res. Comm. 109:130, 1982.
36. Rittenhouse, S.E.: Inositol lipid metabolism in the responses of stimulated platelets. Cell Calcium 3:311, 1982.
37. Majerus, P.W., Prescott, S.M., Hoffman, S.C., Neufeld, E.J. and Wilson, D.B.: Uptake and release of arachidonate by platelets. Adv. Prostaglandin Thromboxane Leukotriene Res. 11:45, 1983.
38. Serhan, C., Anderson, P., Goodman, E., Dunham, P., and Weissmann, G.: Phosphatidate and oxidized fatty acids are calcium ionophores. J. Biol. Chem. 256:2736, 1981.
39. Sneddon, J.M.: Blood platelets as a model for mono-amine containing neurons. In Kerkut, G.A., and Phillis, J.W. (eds.): Progress in Neurobiology, Vol. 1. Oxford, Pergamon Press, 1973.
40. Gordon, J.L., and Olverman, H.J.: 5-Hydroxytryptamine and dopamine transport by rat and human platelets. Br. J. Pharmacol. 62:219, 1978.
41. Holmsen, H.: Platelet adenine nucleotide metabolism and platelet malfunction. In Caen, J. (ed): Platelet Aggregation. Paris, Masson, 1971.
42. Pearson, J.D., Carleton, J.S., Hutchings, A., and Gordon, J.L.: Uptake and metabolism of adenosine by pig aortic endothelial and smooth muscle cells in culture. Biochem. J. 170:265, 1978.
43. Mustard, J.F., and Packham, M.A.: Platelet phagocytosis. Ser. Haematol. 1:168, 1968.
44. Donald, K.J., and Tennent, R.J.: The relative roles of platelets and macrophages in clearing particles from the blood: the value of carbon

clearance as a measure of reticuloendothelial phagocytosis. J. Pathol. 117:235, 1975.

45. Humphrey, J.H., and Jacques, R.: The histamine and serotonin content of the platelets and polymorphonuclear leukocytes in various species. J. Physiol. 124:305, 1954.

46. DaPrada, M., Richards, J.R., and Kettler, R.: Amine storage organelles in platelets. In Gordon, J.L. (ed.): Platelets in Biology and Pathology 2. Amsterdam, Elsevier-North Holland Biomedical Press, 1981.

47. Aalto, M., and Kulonen, E.: Effects of serotonin, indomethacin and other antirheumatic drugs on the synthesis of collagen and other proteins in granulation tissue slices. Biochem. Pharmacol. 21:2835, 1972.

48. Ehrlich, H.P., and Gordon, J.L.: Proteinases and platelets. In Gordon, J.L. (ed.): Platelets in Biology and Pathology. Amsterdam, Elsevier-North Holland-Biomedical Press, 1976.

49. Homebeck, W., Starkey, P.M., Gordon, J.L., Legrand, Y., Pignaud, G., Robert, L., Caen, J.P., Ehrlich, H.P., and Barrett, A.J.: The elastase-like enzyme of platelets. Thrombos. Haemostas. 42:1681, 1980.

50. Weksler, B.B., and Coupal, C.E.: Platelet-dependent generation of chemotactic activity in serum. J. Exp. Med. 137:1419, 1973.

51. Larsen, G.L. and Henson, P.M.: Mediators in Inflammation. In Brass, A. (ed.): Annual Review of Immunology. Vol. 1. Palo Alto, Annual Reviews, Inc., 1983.

52. Ross, R., Glomset, J., Kariya, B., and Harker, L.: A platelet-dependent serum factor that stimulates the proliferation of arterial smooth muscle cells in vitro. Proc. Natl. Acad. Sci. USA 71:1207, 1974.

53. Ross, R., and Vogel, A.: The platelet-derived growth factor. Cell 14:203, 1978.

54. Doolittle, R.F., Hunkapiller, M.W., Hood, L.E., Devare, S.G., Robbins, K.E., Aaronson, S.A., and Antoniades, H.N.: Simian sarcoma virus onc gene, v-sis, is derived from the gene (or genes) encoding a platelet-derived growth factor. Science 221:275, 1983.

55. Stiles, C.D.: The molecular biology of platelet-derived growth factor. Cell 33:653, 1983.

56. Mills, D.C.B., Macfarlane, D.E., Lemmex, B.W.G., and Haslam, R.J.: Receptors for nucleosides and nucleotides on blood platelets. In Berne, R.M., Rall, T.W., and Rubio, R. (eds.): Regulatory Function of Adenosine. Boston, Marinus Nishoff, 1981.

57. Furchgott, R.F., and Zawadski, J.V.: The obligatory role of endothelial cells in the relaxation of arterial smooth muscle by acetylcholine. Nature 288:373, 1980.

58. DeMey, J.D., and Vanhoutte, P.M.: Role of the intima in cholinergic and purinergic relaxation of isolated canine femoral arteries. J. Physiol. 316:347, 1981.

59. Pearson, J.D., Slakey, L.L., and Gordon, J.L.; Stimulation of prostaglandin production through purinaceptors on cultured porcine endothelial cells. Biochem. J. 214:273, 1983.

60. Gordon, J.L., and Martin, W.: Stimulation of endothelial prostacyclin production plays no role in endothelium-dependent relaxation of the pig aorta. Br. J. Pharmacol. 80:179, 1983.

61. Pearson, J.D., and Gordon, J.L.: Vascular endothelial and smooth muscle cells in culture selectively release adenine nucleotides. Nature 281:384, 1979.

62. Gordon, J.L.: Vessel wall metabolism and vasoactive agents. In Woolf, N. (ed.): Biology and Pathology of the Vessel Wall. Eastbourne, Praeger, 1983.

63. Gordon, J.L., and Drummond, A.H.: Irreversible aggregation of pig platelets and release of intracellular constituents induced by 5-hydroxytryptamine. Biochem. Pharmacol. 24:33, 1975.

64. Gordon, J.L., Bowyer, D.E., Evans, D.W., and Mitchinson, M.J.: Human platelet reactivity during stressful diagnostic procedures. J. Clin. Pathol. 26:958, 1973.

65. Moncada, S., Gryglewski, R., Bunting, S., and Vane, J.R.: An enzyme isolated from arteries transforms prostaglandin endoperoxides to an unstable substance that inhibits platelet aggregation. Nature 263:663, 1976.

66. Gimbrone, M.A., and Buchanan, M.R.: Interactions of platelets and leukocytes with vascular endothelium: In vitro studies. Ann. N.Y. Acad. Sci. 401:171, 1982.

67. Weksler, B.B.: Prostacyclin Prog. Hemost. Thromb. 6:13, 1982.

68. Marcus, A.J., Weksler, B.B., Jaffe, E.A., and Brockman, M.J.: Synthesis of prostacyclin from platelet-derived endoperoxides by cultured human endothelial cells. J. Clin. Invest. 66:979, 1980.

69. First International Symposium on Platelet Activation Factor. J. Benveniste, editor. In press.

70. Lynch, J.M., Worthen, G.S., and Henson, P.H.: Mediators and the mechanism of their release: PAF. In Buckle, D.R., and Smith, H. (eds.): The Development of Antiasthma Drugs. In press.

71. Gordon, J.L. (ed.): Platelets in Biology and Pathology 2. In Dingle, J.T., and Gordon, J.L. (eds.): Research Monographs in Cell and Tissue Physiology. Vol. 5. Amsterdam. Elsevier/North-Holland, 1981.

72. Keenen, J.P., and Solum, N.O.: Quantitative studies on the release of platelet fibrinogen by thrombin. Br. J. Haematol. 23:461, 1972.

73. Tollefsen, D.M., and Majerus, P.W.: Inhibition of human platelet aggregation by monovalent antifibrinogen antibody fragments. J. Clin. Invest. 55:1259, 1975.

74. Henson, P.M.: The adherence of leukocytes and platelets induced by fixed IgG antibody or complement. Immunology 16:107, 969.

75. Pfueller, S.L., and Luscher, E.F.: The effects of aggregated immunoglobulins on human blood platelets in relation to their complement-fixing abilities. J. Immunol. 109:517, 526, 1972.

76. Pfueller, S.L., Jenkins, C.S.P., and Luscher, E.F.: A comparative study of the effect of modification of the surface of human platelets on the receptors for aggregated immunoglobulins and for ristocetin-von Willebrand factor. Biochim. Biophys. Acta 465:614, 1977.

77. Pfueller, S.L., and Luscher, E.F.: Studies of the mechanisms of the human platelet release reaction induced by immunologic stimuli. II. The effects of zymosan. J. Immunol. 112:1211, 1974.

78. Csako, G., and Suba, E.A.: A physiologic regulator of collagen-induced platelet aggregation: Inhibition by Clq. Thromb. Haemost. 45:110, 1981.

79. Chater, B.V.: The role of membrane-bound complement in the aggregation of mammalian platelets by collagen. Br. J. Haematol. 32:515, 1976.

80. Wautier, J.L., Legrand, Y.J., Fauvel, F. and Caen, J.P.: Inhibition of platelet collagen interactions by the Cls subcomponent of the first component of complement. Thromb. Res. 21:2, 1981.

81. Chater, B.V. The role of membrane-bound complement in the aggregation of mammalian platelets by collagen. Br. J. Haematol. 32:515, 1976.

82. Clark, W.F., Friesen, M., Linton, A.L., and Lindsay, R.M.: The platelet as a mediator of tissue damage in immune complex glomerulonephritis. Clin. Nephrol. 6:287, 1976.

83. Best, L.C., Martin, T.J., Russell, R.G.G., and Preston, F.E.: Prostacyclin increases cyclic AMP levels and adenylate cyclase activity in platelets. Nature 267:850, 1978.

84. MacIntyre, D.E., Pearson, J.D., and Gordon, J.L.: Localization and stimulation of prostacyclin production by vascular cells. Nature 271:549, 1978.

85. Beesley, J.E., Pearsons, J.D. Carleton, J.S., Hutchings, A., and Gordon, J.L.: Interaction of leukocytes with vernacular cells in culture. J. Cell Sci. 33:85, 1978.

86. Jorgensen, L., Rowsell, H.C., Hovig, T., and Mustard, J.F.: Resolution and organization of platelet-rich mural thrombi in carotid arteries of swine. Am. J. Pathol. 51:681, 1967.

87. Musson, R.A. and Henson, P.M.: Humoral and formed elements of blood modulate and response of peripheral blood monocytes. I. Plasma and serum inhibit and platelets enhance monocyte adherence. J. Immunol. 122:2026, 1979.

88. Sharp, A.A.: Platelet structure and function in relation to blood coagulation and haemostasis. In Chalmers, D.G., and Gresham, G.A. (eds.): Biological Aspects of Occlusive Vascular Disease. Cambridge, Cambridge University Press, 1964.

89. Giordano, N.D., Radivoyevitch, M., and Goodsitt, E.: Thrombus formation time in hemophilia: An in vitro study. Thromb. Diathes. Haemorrh. 20:596, 1968.

90. Baumgartner, H.R., and Muggli, R.: Adhesion and aggregation: Morphological demonstration and quantitation in vivo and in vitro. In Gordon, J.L. (ed.): Platelets in Biology and Pathology. Amsterdam, Elsevier-North Holland-Biomedical Press, 1976.

91. Boogaerts, M.A., Yamado, O., Jacob, H.S., Moldow, C.F.: Enhancement of granulocyte-endothelial cell adherence and granulocyte-induced cytotoxicity by platelet release products. PNAS 79:7019, 1982.

92. Williams, T.J. Jose, P.J., Wedmore, C.V., Peck, M.J., and Forrest, M.J.: Mechanisms underlying inflammatory edema. Adv. Prostaglandin Thromboxane Leukotriene Res. 11:33, 1983.

93. Larsen, G.L., and Henson, P.M.: Mediators of inflammation. In Brass, A. (ed.): Annual Review of Immunology. Volume 1. Palo Alto, Annual Reviews, Inc., 1983.

94. Issekutz A.C.: Effect of vasoactive agents on polymorphonuclear leukocyte emigration in vivo. Lab. Invest. 45:234, 1981.

95. Lipscomb, M.F., Onofrio, J.M., Nash, E.J., Pierce, A.K., and Toews, G.B.: A morphological study of the role of phagocytes in the clearance of Staphylococcus aureus from the lung. J. Reticuloendothel. Soc. 33:429, 1983.

96. Tonnesen, M., Smedly, L., Goins, A., and Henson, P.M.: Interaction between neutrophils and vascular endothelial cells. In Parnham, M.J., and Winkelmann, J. (eds.): Agents and Actions Supplements. Volume 11. 1st Cologne Atherosceloriosis Conference. Basel, Birkhauser Verlag, 1982.

97. Russo, R.G., Liotta, L.A., Thorgeirsson, U., Brundage, R., and Schiffmann, E.: Polymorphonuclear leukocyte migration through human amnion membrane. J. Cell Biol. 91:459, 1981.

98. Henson, P.M., Larsen, G.L., Henson, J.E., Newman, S.L., Musson, R.A., and Leslie, C.C.: Resolution of pulmonary inflammation. In press.

99. Kravis, T.C., and Henson, P.M.: Accumulation of platelets at sites of

antigen-antibody-mediated injury: A possible role for IgE antibody and mast cells. J. Immunol. 118:1569, 1977.

100. Cotran, R.S.: The delayed and prolonged vascular leakage in inflammation. II. An electron microscopic study of the vascular response after thermal injury. Am. J. Pathol. 46:589, 1965.

101. Smith, M.J.H., Walker, J.R., Ford-Hutchinson, A.W., and Penington, D.G.: Platelets, prostaglandins and inflammation. Agents Actions 6:701, 1976.

102. Bolam, J.P., and Smith, M.J.H.: Platelets in inflammatory exudates. J Pharm. Pharmacol. 29:674, 1977.

Acknowledgments

Supported in part by NIH Grants HL21565, HL28520, and GM24834.

Chapter 12
Proteinases in Joint Disease

Alan J. Barrett and Jeremy Saklatvala

INTRODUCTION

Proteinases may be involved in several aspects of joint disease. For example, the formation of antibodies to immunoglobulins and collagen in rheumatoid arthritis may depend upon the formation of products of limited degradation of these proteins by extracellular proteinases.[1,2] Proteinases in the joints may also activate precursors of the complement and kinin systems to liberate polypeptide mediators of inflammation responsible for leukocyte chemotaxis, increased vascular permeability, and pain.[3,4] The formation of fibrin in the synovial fluid that is commonly seen in rheumatoid arthritis may arise from the action of proteinases other than thrombin on fibrinogen, or from the activation of prothrombin by an unusual mechanism. There is no doubt, however, that the aspect of joint pathology in which proteolytic enzymes are most strongly implicated by evidence currently available is that of the tissue damage that so often accompanies joint disease, and this will form the main topic of the present chapter.

THE PROTEINASES OF THE JOINT

The proteases that are most important in the pathologic degradation of the extracellular structural proteins of connective tissues are those that cleave peptide bonds in the body of the protein chains, rather than simply releasing terminal residues; these are the *proteinases* or *endopeptidases*.[6,7] The enzymologist classifies the proteinases on the basis of the chemical groups responsible for catalytic activity. Four classes of proteinase are distinguished in this way: the *aspartic* (previously "acid" or "carboxyl"), *cysteine* (previously "thiol"), *serine*, and *metallo*-proteinases[5] (Table 12–1). Newly discovered proteinases can usually be assigned to one of these groups according to their response to appropriate active-site–directed inhibitors. Inhibitors also provide the most direct approach to identifying the proteinases active in biologic systems.

Aspartic Proteinases—Cathepsin D. It was recognized long ago that the stomach contains a proteinase, pepsin, capable of digesting proteins under the very acidic conditions of the stomach contents. Subsequently, it was discovered that many protozoa use intracellular "stomachs," or digestive vacuoles, to break down food particles, also under acidic conditions, and much more recently it has become clear that many mammalian cells carry out intracellular digestive processes at low pH. The most conspicuous of the acid-acting proteinases in cells is cathepsin D, an enzyme with many similarities to pepsin and evolved from the same primitive precursor. The vacuolar digestive system of mammalian cells is, of course, the lysosomal system, and several lines of evidence implicate this system in the pathology of inflammation. All nucleated cells seem to contain lysosomes, and all mammalian cells examined have been found to contain an enzyme with the properties of cathepsin D. Cathepsin D is the only aspartic proteinase likely to occur in the rheumatoid joint.

Cathepsin D[8-10] is an enzyme of molecular weight about 42,000 that is most active in the degradation of hemoglobin (a convenient test substrate) at about pH 3.5. Degradation of cartilage proteoglycan is most rapid at pH 5, but the enzyme shows little action on this or any other substrate above pH 6, and none at or above pH 7.

The mechanism of catalysis of the aspartic proteinases remains somewhat mysterious, but it is clear that there are at least two active groups, both being β-carboxyl groups of aspartic acid residues. The most useful reagent in the attribution of acid proteinase activity to aspartic proteinases is pepstatin.[11-13] This pentapeptide is produced by various species of *Streptomyces* and is a powerful and highly specific inhibitor of the aspartic proteinases. It has low toxicity and is suitable for inhibition of extracellular aspartic proteinase activity in biologic systems. Still more specific inhibition of cathepsin D can be produced with antibodies, however.[14]

The specificity of peptide bond cleavage by cathepsin D is relatively broad but shows a distinct preference for

Table 12–1. Classes of Proteinase (Endopeptidase) and Some of Their Characteristics

	Aspartic	Cysteine	Serine	Metallo-
Examples	Pepsin Cathepsin D Renin	Cathepsin B Cathepsin L	Trypsin Chymotrypsin Plasmin Kallikrein Elastases Cathepsin G	Collagenase Macrophage elastase Gelatinase
pH range for activity	3–6	3–7	6–10	6–9
Test inhibitors	Pepstatin	E-64, leupeptin, thiol-blocking reagents	Dip-F, Pms-F	1,10-phenanthroline
Major plasma inhibitors		$\alpha_2 M$ αCPI	α_1-PI $\alpha_2 M$ $\alpha_2 M$	$\alpha_2 M$

Abbreviations: $\alpha_2 M$: α_2-macroglobulin; α_1-PI: α_1-proteinase inhibitor; Dip-F: diisopropyl fluorophosphate; Pms-F: phenylmethylsulfonyl-fluoride.

bonds flanked by hydrophobic amino acid residues. A sequence of at least five residues is generally required in a substrate, and no test substrate of really low molecular weight is available for routine use in the laboratory.

The degradation of cartilage proteoglycan by human cathepsin D has been characterized at the molecular level.[5-17] The enzyme cleaves the hyaluronic acid-binding region from the molecule and splits the polysaccharide-attachment region into rather large fragments (Fig. 12–1).

The structural integrity of collagen type II fibers is not detectably affected by cathepsin D, although some other types of collagen may have a few susceptible peptide bonds.[18-20]

In the body, any extracellular activity of cathepsin D is likely to be severely restricted by pH conditions, although it is possible that production of carbon dioxide and lactic acid by a cell creates pericellular regions of sufficiently low pH to allow the action of acid proteinases.[21] α_2-Macroglobulin is capable of binding cathepsin D,[22] but little other inhibitory activity exists in mammalian tissues.

Cysteine Proteinases—Cathepsins B and L. Part of the acid proteinase activity of mammalian cells is expressed only in the presence of low molecular weight thiol compounds (e.g., glutathione, cysteine) and is destroyed by reagents that react with thiol groups (e.g., iodoacetate). This activity is attributable to the cysteine proteinases, the best known of which is lysosomal cathepsin B.

Human cathepsin B has been isolated and characterized.[3-5] It is a protein of about 25,000 molecular weight, with less activity against hemoglobin than cathepsin D but much more against collagen and gelatin. The optimum pH for the action of cathepsin B on its synthetic substrates is 6, but maximal activity against proteins may occur at a pH as low as 3, probably because the acidity sensitizes the substrate. Cathepsin B loses activity irreversibly above pH 7.

Cathepsin B is evolutionarily homologous with papain[26] and undoubtedly has a catalytic site in which the side chains of cysteine and histidine are active. The enzyme is best assayed fluorimetrically with the synthetic substrate benzyloxycarbonyl-arginyl-arginyl-methylcoumarylamide.[25]

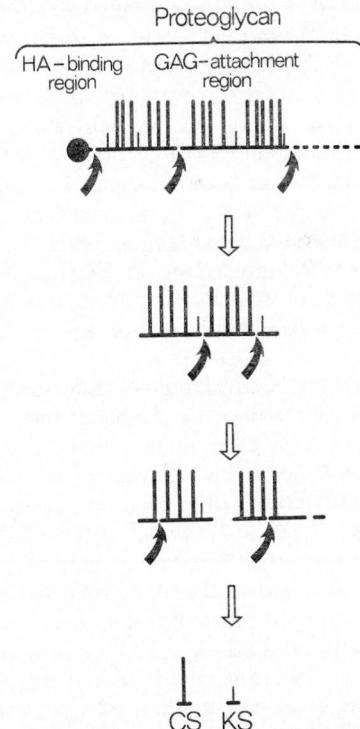

Figure 12–1. A diagrammatic representation of the cartilage proteoglycan molecule, showing the distinct hyaluronic acid-binding and glycosaminoglycan-attachment regions, the latter bearing groups of chondroitin sulfate chains with occasional (shorter) keratan sulfate chains. The arrows indicate points of proteolytic attack in the progressive degradation of the molecule. The sequence of events is the same for most proteinases, but some are able to take the process much further than others. Very early on, the hyaluronic acid-binding region is split off. Then large groups of polysaccharide chains are liberated, and these are further fragmented, but with no liberation of single polysaccharide chains until very late (and then only with the few proteinases of broadest specificity). (Redrawn from Roughley, P.J.: Biochem. J. 167:639, 1977).

In human tissues, the cysteine proteinase with greatest activity against collagen and proteoglycan is cathepsin L. Like cathepsin B, cathepsin L is a lysosomal enzyme, is active at acid pH, and is irreversibly denatured at neutral pH. At present, no convenient specific assay for cathepsin L has been discovered, but benzyloxycarbonyl-phenylalanyl-arginyl-methycoumarylamide is a sensitive substrate, and results can be corrected for the contribution from cathepin B.[25] Molar concentrations of active cathepsin B and cathepsin L can be determined by active site titration.[25] Cathepsins B and L both cleave the N-terminal peptides of collagen that contain the covalent crosslinks within and between molecules (see Chapter 12 and Fig. 12–2), but cathepsin L is very much the more active of the two.[27,28]

Cathepsin B cleaves the hyaluronic acid-binding region from cartilage proteoglycan and degrades the glycosaminoglycan-attachment region to rather small fragments.[15-17] Action on this substrate is rapid at pH 5 to 6.

Cathepsins B and L are inactivated by thiol-blocking reagents in general, but more selective inhibitors usable in biologic systems are leupeptin, E-64, and certain chloromethanes. Leupeptin is propionyl-leucyl-leucyl-L-argininaldehyde; it is a tight-binding reversible inhibitor of cathepsin B[29,30] (and cathepsin L). E-64, which is L-trans-epoxysuccinyl-leucylamido(4-guanidino) butane, is a very rapidly reacting irreversible inhibitor of these enzymes.[31] The synthetic peptidyl chloromethanes are notable for offering the potential of some selectivity of inhibition of cathepsin B or cathepsin L,[32] but the sensitivity of cathepsin B to benzyloxycarbonyl-phenyl-alanyl-phenylalanyl-chloromethane varies greatly between species, the human and rat enzymes being little affected. The lysosomal cysteine proteinases are also inhibited by protein inhibitors of the cystatin family.[32a,32b]

Serine Proteinases. The family of endopeptidases with a catalytically essential serine residue at their active site is by far the largest class of mammalian proteinases, and this may relate to the fact that these enzymes are ideally suited to acting in the conditions most common within cells and tissues: they are most active at about neutral pH and require no special co-factors. Their physiologic importance seems also to be reflected in the fact that 10 percent of the plasma protein is represented by serine proteinase inhibitors!

The serine proteinases include many of the proteins of the "cascades" of coagulation, fibrinolysis, complement, and kinins in the plasma, such as thrombin, plasmin, Cls, Clr, and kallikrein, as well as trypsin, chymotrypsin, and elastase from the exocrine pancreas. Of particular note to rheumatology are plasmin and the plasminogen activators, plasma kallikrein and the serine proteinases of the polymorphonuclear leukocytes, the lysosomal elastase and cathepsin G, both of which are major components of the azurophile granules of these cells (see Chapter 9).

Plasmin. The inactive precursor of plasmin, plasminogen, occurs in the plasma at a concentration of about 20 mg per deciliter. Activation of the precursor can be brought about by a plasminogen activator system in the plasma, by bacterial components such as streptokinase, or by activators (which are themselves serine proteinases) produced by stimulation of various cells, including macrophages, synovial cells, and neutrophil leukocytes.[33-35] Activation by any of these agents is inhibited by 6-aminohexanoic acid and related antifibrinolytic compounds.[36]

Plasmin preferentially cleaves lysyl bonds. The enzyme seems to have evolved for the function of breaking down fibrin clots; not only is plasmin itself very active in degrading fibrin, but plasminogen has a high affinity for fibrin, so that a clot forms with a built-in mechanism for its own dissolution. (This may represent a common pattern for proteinases acting on insoluble proteins: elastase and collagenase also bind to their respective substrates.) Plasmin certainly has the capacity to degrade cartilage proteoglycan,[37] but it has little action on collagen, although it activates latent collagenase (see below).The major plasma inhibitors of plasmin are the α_2-plasmin inhibitor and α_2-macroglobulin.[38]

Plasma Kallikrein. There are two distinct enzymes called kallikrein: tissue kallikrein and plasma kallikrein.[7] Plasma kallikrein is generated from the inactive precursor prokallikrein, by the action of coagulation factor XII (Hageman factor), or kallikrein itself.[39] Plasma kallikrein acts on high molecular weight kininogen to yield bradykinin, and the consequences of this are considered fully in Chapter 8.

Kallikrein also has the capacity to activate latent collagenase, and although active kallikrein is normally present in rheumatoid synovial fluid only at very low concentrations, it may be a significant activator.[40]

Leukocyte Elastase. Elastin, the crosslinked structural protein important for the elastic strength of the arterial walls, the joint capsule, and skin, is highly resistant to proteolytic degradation, but it is attacked by the elastases of the pancreas and polymorphonuclear leukocytes. Unlike the collagenases, the elastases are by no means specific for the substrate after which they are named but have very broad proteolytic activity.

The polymorphonuclear leukocyte (lysosomal) elastase has not yet been positively detected in any other cells. It is a protein of about 28,000 molecular weight[41] that acts on cartilage proteoglycan to remove the hyaluronic acid–binding region, and then to fragment the glycosaminoglycan attachment region.[16,17,42]

The route by which leukocyte elastase degrades collagen fibers is illustrated diagrammatically in Figure 12–2.[43,44] The N-terminal peptides are degraded, with the elimination of the crosslinks that play a crucial part in the stabilization of collagen fibers. The individual molecules then separate and, if solubilized, denature in a few hours at 37° C, and are degraded to small peptides and amino acids by further proteolytic activity. Interestingly, the leukocyte elastase is several times more active against cartilage collagen (type II) than against type I collagen, whereas the reverse is true of the specific collagenases. The enzyme also degrades the type IV

Figure 12–2. The mode of action of the neutrophil serine proteinases in the degradation of articular cartilage collagen. The initial proteolysis affects the terminal nonhelical peptides, and thus eliminates almost all cross-links. The link shown is the CB 4 × 9 link common in cartilage collagen. The solubilization of the uncross-linked molecules presumably occurs spontaneously, although it can be accelerated in vivo by high ionic strength. The subsequent thermal denaturation of the modified tropocollagen also would be spontaneous, since the body is close to the denaturation temperature (especially at a site of inflammation). (The soluble collagen would also be a favourable substrate for the specific collagenase, or might be taken into cells for lysosomal degradation). The final degradation of the denatured polypeptide chains would be rapid, since they are very sensitive to both extracellular and intracellular proteinases. (Redrawn from Barrett, A.J.: Agents Actions 8:11, 1978).

collagen of basement membranes, which seems resistant to the specific collagenases.[45,46]

Inhibitors of leukocyte elastase include diisopropyl fluorophosphate and phenylmethylsulfonylfluoride (general inhibitors of the serine proteinases), but also specific reagents such as methyl-*N*-succinyl-dialanyl-prolyl-valyl-chloromethane,[47] which can be used experimentally in vivo. Two drugs used in rheumatology, gold sodium thiomalate and pentosan polysulfate also inhibit leukocyte elastase.[48] In the body, extracellular activity is likely to be controlled by α_1-proteinase inhibitor (previously known as α_1-antitrypsin) and α_2-macroglobulin.[49]

Cathepsin G. Cathepsin G, the "chymotrypsin-like" enzyme of neutrophil leukocytes, shows distinct similarities to the pancreatic chymotrypsins, especially chymotrypsin C,[50] and also to the chymases of mast cell granules,[51] but it is clearly a separate enzyme. Like the elastase, cathepsin G seems to occur only in the azurophile granules of the neutrophil granulocytes. Cathepsin G is normally assayed with substrates originally

used for chymotrypsin A such as benzyloxycarbonyl-tyrosine nitrophenyl ester.[47] The general inhibitors of serine proteinases are effective against cathepsin G, and a rather specific chloromethyl ketone inhibitor has been described.[47]

The action of cathepsin G on cartilage proteoglycan is somewhat more restricted than that of the elastase,[16,42] and the enzyme has little or no action on elastin or type I collagen. Cathepsin G is effective in solubilizing collagen from cartilage, however,[43] and may generate physiologically active products from complement components.[52]

Physiologic inhibitors of cathepsin G include α_1-antichymotrypsin, α_1-proteinase inhibitor, and α_2-macroglobulin.[53]

Metalloproteinases—Collagenase and Others. The fourth class of proteinases contains the enzymes that are dependent on metal ions for activity. The indications are that Zn^{2+} is essential for the catalytic activity of all of these, and they are additionally stabilized and perhaps activated by Ca^{2+}. There are several metalloproteinases in human tissues, but the one most studied is of particular concern to rheumatology, the specific collagenase.

Collagenase. The mammalian collagenases[54,55] are specific for collagen as substrate and cleave all three chains of the triple helix at one susceptible point, about three quarters of the way along the molecule from the N-terminus (Fig. 12–3).[56] The bonds cleaved are between residues of glycine and isoleucine or leucine (Fig. 12–4), but many similar bonds occur in collagen, and it is not clear why this region of the helix is particularly sensitive to proteolysis.[57,58]

There is little agreement as to how many distinct human collagenases exist, but there are at least two, since the neutrophil granulocyte has an enzyme[59] different from those produced by cells of tissues such as the synovium. Tissue collagenase is produced by many types of cells, including fibroblasts and macrophages.[69-71] The neutrophil collagenase is stored in the specific, or primary, granules of the leukocytes,[59,72] and secreted in response to appropriate stimuli.

Rheumatoid synovial collagenase is about fivefold more active against type I collagen than the type II cartilage collagen, when both are in solution.[60] Covalent crosslinking of the molecules in fibrils makes them far more resistant to the action of collagenase than is soluble collagen,[61,62] and cartilage collagen is particularly highly crosslinked. The polymorphonuclear leukocyte collagenase occurs in much smaller amounts in the cells than elastase and cathepsin G,[56] and it has yet to be shown that it is active enough to be significant in collagen degradation.

No really useful synthetic substrate for the vertebrate collagenases is available, so assays are made with collagen. The common form of assay involves measurement of the solubilization of radioactivity from fibrils of labeled collagen formed in vitro at 37° C.[63,64]

There is evidence that the molecule of collagenase contains an atom of zinc, and the enzyme is both stabilized and activated by Ca^{2+} ions.[65] In vitro, collagenase

Figure 12–3. Diagram of the helical type I tropocollagen (TC) molecule and its cleavage into 75 percent (TCᴬ) and 25 percent (TCᴮ) fragments by collagenase. In this particular molecule, the intramolecular crosslink occurs between the two α1 chains forming a β1, 1 component; however, the crosslink may occur between α1 and α2 chains, giving rise to the other type of β component, β1, 2. On either side are photographs of sodium dodecylsulfate polyacrylamide gels on which the denatured components of the collagen have been run. On the left is undigested collagen, showing the two types of α and β components (the alternative forms to those depicted in the diagram are shown in brackets). On the right is shown the pattern of cleavage products of these chains, the TCᴬ and TCᴮ pieces. The differing mobilities of the α1 and α2 chains (and the β components) in sodium dodecylsulfate gel electrophoresis are anomalous, not reflecting any appreciable difference in molecular weight. (Redrawn from Harris, E.D., Jr., and Cartwright, E.C.: In Barrett, A.J. [ed.]: Proteinases in Mammalian Cells and Tissues. Amsterdam, North-Holland Publishing Company, 1977, pp. 249–283.

                    Collagenase
                         ↓

α1(I)ᴮ bovine   GLY⫶ILE-ALA-GLY-GLN-ARG-GLY-VAL-VAL-GLY-LEU-HYP-GLY-GLN-ARG-GLY-GLU-ARG-GLY

α1(I)ᴮ chick   GLY⫶ILE-ALA-GLY-GLN-ARG-GLY-VAL-VAL-GLY-LEU-HYP-GLY-GLN-ARG-GLY-GLU-ARG-GLY

α1(II)ᴮ human   GLY⫶ILE-ALA-GLY-GLN-ARG-GLY-_LEU_-VAL-GLY-LEU-HYP-GLY-GLN-ARG-GLY-GLU-ARG-GLY
                    *

α1(III)ᴮ human   GLY⫶ILE*-ALA-GLY-_LEU_-ARG-GLY-_ALA_-_ARG_-GLY-LEU-_ALA_-GLY-_PRO_-_HYP_-GLY-_MET_-_HYP_-GLY
                    *

α2ᴮ chick   GLY⫶_LEU_-ALA-GLY

Residue number 772 ⫶773   775   780   785   790

Figure 12–4. The primary structure of homologous regions of α1 (I), α1 (II), α (III) and α2 chains immediately adjacent on the carboxyl side to the sites of cleavage by collagenase. The site of cleavage at residues 772–773 is depicted by the arrows. The underlined residue in the α1 (II)ᴮ sequence denotes an amino acid substitution relative to the α1 (I)ᴮ. The underlined residues in the α1 (III)ᴮ sequence denote amino acid substitution relative to both α1 (I)ᴮ and α1 (II)ᴮ sequences. The residue at the right of the cleavage site in the α1 (III) chain (marked *) was originally identified as -LEU-, but new results suggest that it is -ILE- (E.D. Harris, Jr., personal communication). (Redrawn from Miller, E.J., et al.: Biochemistry 15:787, 1976).

is powerfully inhibited by chelating agents such as 1,10-phenanthroline, but these are too toxic for use in biologic systems. Some thiol compounds (e.g., thiorphan[65a] are effective inhibitors, and these might be applicable to biologic test systems. In rheumatology, it may be of interest that penicillamine (another thiol compound) is somewhat inhibitory.[66]

About 95 percent of the inhibitory capacity of plasma for collagenase is due to α_2-macroglobulin, which reacts more slowly with the leukocyte collagenase than with that from other cells.[67] The lower molecular weight β_1-anticollagenase[68] and the closely related TIMP (tissue inhibitor of metalloproteinases) probably can enter cartilage matrix (unlike α_2-macroglobulin) and might therefore be of significance in the control of collagenolysis.

Collagenase (like most of the other mammalian metalloproteinases) is commonly encountered in culture media and tissue preparations in an inactive or "latent" form. Typically, the latent collagenase can be activated by treatment with trypsin (or various other proteinases) or a mercurial compound such as aminophenylmercuric acetate. Probably, the latent collagenases are proenzymes requiring proteolytic activation. Evidence supporting this view comes from the synthesis of a single-chain latent collagenase in a cell free system with mRNA from synovial cells.[73] The mechanism of activation by the mercurial compounds remains to be explained, but the view that latent collagenase is an enzyme-inhibitor complex dissociable by the various activators is no longer widely held.

Macrophage Elastase. Stimulated macrophages secrete a metalloproteinase that degrades elastin, proteoglycan, and also protein inhibitors of other proteinases, including α_1-proteinase inhibitor.[74-76a] If this enzyme is produced by the macrophage-like cells of the synovial lining, it certainly has the potential to contribute to tissue damage, but it is inhibited by α_2-macroglobulin.

Other Metalloproteinases. In culture many types of cell have been shown to produce metalloproteinases in latent forms similar to those of collagenase. The enzymes are of two main types, a "gelatinase" active on denatured collagens and native collagen of types IV and V, and a general proteinase or "proteoglycanase" that readily hydrolyzes proteoglycan.[77] Neutrophil leukocytes contain a gelatinase in their "C particles" in addition to the collagenase of the specific granules.[72,78]

ENDOGENOUS PROTEINASE INHIBITORS

Any assessment of the activities of proteinases in vivo must obviously take into account the naturally occurring inhibitors of the enzymes. In the context of the destruction of extracellular matrix components, the important inhibitors are those that derive from the plasma and those that are secreted by tissue cells.

α_2-**Macroglobulin.** In general, the protein inhibitors of proteinases are easily classified as inhibitors of aspartic, cysteine, or serine proteinases or metalloproteinases, but α_2-macroglobulin (α_2M) is exceptional in inhibiting enzymes from all four groups, and the mechanism by which it does so is a unique form of protein–protein interaction. Each of the four identical subunits of α_2M has near the center of its polypeptide chain a short sequence of amino acids that is highly sensitive to attack by the great majority of proteinases. When a proteinase cleaves this "bait region," it triggers a change in the shape of the α_2M molecule, such that the proteinase molecule is physically trapped within it. The complexed enzyme molecule remains reactive with low molecular weight substrates and inhibitors that are able to diffuse to the interior of the trap but has little or no reactivity with large molecules, whether they be protein substrates, inhibitors, or antibodies. Since the original proposal of this remarkable mechanism of action by Barrett and Starkey,[22] a great deal more has been learned about the protein.[79,81,82] Particularly interesting has been the discovery that α_2M contains a thiol ester group (formed between side-chains of neighboring cysteine and glutamic acid residues) that becomes chemically highly reactive in response to cleavage of the bait region and forms covalent links to the trapped proteinase molecule or other molecules that may be in the vicinity. This is a very similar reaction to that by which complement components C3 and C4 become linked to cell surfaces and immune complexes after their proteolytic activation, and indeed, they also contain thiol esters in sequences homologous with that of α_2M. The covalent linking reaction of α_2M does not contribute to its inhibition of proteinases, however, and the biologic significance of that reaction is not known.

In the course of its reaction with a proteinase, the α_2M molecule acquires recognition sites for high affinity receptors on macrophages and some other cells. These cause the proteinase–α_2M complexes to be removed from the plasma extremely rapidly.[83] α_2M occurs in plasma at a concentration of about 250 mg per deciliter, but its molecular weight of 725,000 prevents it from escaping into the synovial fluid of a normal joint. In inflammation, however, it does escape, and rheumatoid synovial fluid holds about the same concentration as plasma. A difference is that α_2M-proteinase complexes have a greater tendency to accumulate in synovial fluid than in plasma.

Cysteine Proteinase Inhibitors. The major extracellular inhibitor of the cysteine proteinases is α_2M, but in addition these enzymes are specifically inhibited by a more minor plasma protein, α-cysteine proteinase inhibitor (αCPI).[84] αCPI occurs in several forms of molecular weight 60,000 and greater; presumably it diffuses into the joint space from the circulation about as readily as albumin. αCPI would probably enter cartilage matrix, whereas the α_2M molecule is much too large to do so.

In human cells, there are two cytoplasmic inhibitors of cysteine proteinases, both of molecular weight about 13,000.[32b] Inhibitory activity corresponding to these was extracted from human articular cartilage,[86] but it was not shown whether it originated from the chondrocytes or the matrix.

Serine Proteinase Inhibitors. The inhibitors of serine proteinases in the joint are primarily those brought in in the plasma, which have been the subject of a recent review.[87] α_2M is an important inhibitor of plasmin, kallikrein, leukocyte elastase, and cathepsin G, but plasmin is also powerfully inhibited by α_2-antiplasmin, and kallikrein by C1 inhibitor.

The leukocyte enzymes are inhibited by α_1-proteinase inhibitor and for cathepsin G, α_1-antichymotrypsin. These plasma proteins also enter the synovial fluid and penetrate cartilage to some extent.

Metalloproteinase Inhibitors. By far the major inhibitor of the collagenases and the other metalloproteinases in plasma and rheumatoid synovial fluid is α_2M. A lower molecular weight inhibitor of collagenase ("β_1-anticollagenase") is present at very low concentrations in plasma.[68,88]

Various connective tissue cells produce a 30,000 molecular weight inhibitor of collagenase and other metalloproteinases (TIMP).[89]

ARTICULAR TISSUE DAMAGE: THE MOLECULAR PROCESSES

As was mentioned above, the role of proteinases in causing damage to the articular cartilage and its underlying bone, with the likelihood of permanent impairment of joint function, is by far the most studied aspect of proteinases in rheumatology. Cartilage, bone, and tendon have each evolved to serve their physiologic functions by the development of extracellular matrices that comprise a large proportion of the mass of the tissue, but the matrices are chemically quite different and are subject to different forms of enzymic attack. None of these tissues has the capacity to repair itself with the full restoration of the original tissue structure.

Cartilage. In the remarkable extracellular matrix of cartilage, multimolecular assemblies of proteoglycan and collagen molecules interact to produce a rigid gel with very special physical properties, on which normal joint function depends.[90,91] Degradation of the molecules of either proteoglycan or collagen destroys this system, and the way in which this occurs is now understood in some detail.

Proteoglycan. Since the cartilage proteoglycan is approximately 90 percent polysaccharide (see Chapter 15) it would be perfectly possible, in principle, for the degradation of the molecule to be mediated by polysaccharidases, but in fact, examination of the degradation products has tended to show the size of the polysaccharide chains to be unaltered, whereas the protein backbone is fragmented by the proteolytic attack. The backbone or "core protein" includes two regions, the glycosaminoglycan-attachment region, bearing clusters of covalently linked chondroitin sulfate and keratan sulfate chains, and the hyaluronic acid–binding region, which binds noncovalently to hyaluronic acid to assemble the multimolecular aggregates (Fig. 12–1). The binding to hyaluronic acid is stabilized by the participation

of one or two "link proteins." The retention of proteoglycan in the matrix depends on the proteoglycan being assembled into these aggregate molecules, which are trapped within the three-dimensional meshwork of collagen fibers.[92]

The assay of enzymes active against proteoglycan is not an easy matter, since the physicochemical properties of the early products are not very different from those of the substrate. Model systems can be constructed, however, by trapping proteoglycan in polyacrylamide gels, which to some extent mimic the natural matrix.[93] Sensitive assays with reasonable quantitation can then be made with beads of this "synthetic matrix," in which the proteoglycan substrate is radiolabeled. The products are small enough to diffuse out of the gel and appear as radioactivity free in solution after removal of the beads.[94] Alternatively, release of nonradioactive proteoglycan from beads.[95] or from cartilage in culture is conveniently quantified by use of the metachromatic reaction of dimethylmethylene blue.[96]

The hyaluronic acid–binding region of the cartilage proteoglycan molecule is very susceptible to proteolysis, so that molecules in which there has been minimal degradation of the polysaccharide-attachment region often lack the capacity to bind to form aggregates. It is probable that loss of the hyaluronic acid–binding region is sufficient degradation to allow a proteoglycan molecule to diffuse out of the cartilage matrix, and thus make no further contribution to functional integrity of the tissue, and certainly very little degradation of the glycosaminoglycan-attachment region is required to allow this. Degradation of the polysaccharide-attachment region proceeds to different degrees with different proteinases; for example, cathepsin D liberates only rather large fragments bearing several polysaccharide chains, whereas cathepsin B takes the degradation further.[15-17] It is unclear as yet whether proteolysis of the link proteins occurs and, if so, what effect it has on the strength of the matrix.

The contribution made to the strength of cartilage matrix by the proteoglycan element is demonstrated by the effect of cathepsin D, which acts selectively on the proteoglycan. The enzyme causes a decrease in the resistance of the tissue to compression but not in the tensile stiffness at high stress. These changes in mechanical properties are explicable in terms of the model for the structure of cartilage matrix in which proteoglycan provides the resilient resistance to compression, whereas collagen is responsible for the tensile stiffness.[91]

Collagen. The destruction of collagen is a process of especial interest in pathologic tissue damage for two reasons. First, it has seemed that the degradation of collagen is such a specific function of highly specialized enzymes that it may well be a rate-limiting process in tissue destruction. Second, there are strong indications that the capacity of a tissue to replace damaged collagenous elements with retention of the proper organization and structure may be so limited that the destruction of collagen is virtually irreparable. In particular, articular cartilage is irreversibly destroyed when the collagen component (type II) is degraded.

Collagen is largely polypeptide in nature, with some short carbohydrate side-chains. There is evidence for at least three distinct routes of proteolytic degradation (summarized in Fig. 12–5). Among the factors that will determine the relative importance of the various routes is the type of collagen involved; thus type II collagen (predominant in cartilage) is more resistant to the collagenases than is type I (present in tendon and bone) but more sensitive to the leukocyte elastase. Degradation of mature collagen must begin extracellularly, but it is thought to be completed intracellularly, and the uptake into the cells may occur at an early or late stage.

Mature collagen of adult cartilage exists as a network of fibers, each a bundle of collagen fibrils in which the molecules are aligned in the "quarter-stagger" array and covalently crosslinked (see Chapter 14). The intermolecular crosslinks of collagen are of great significance to its properties, conferring increased physical strength, raising the temperature for denaturation from 37° to above 50° C, and decreasing sensitivity to attack by collagenase 10-fold to 100-fold.[61,62]

Woolley and co-workers[60] have reported one of the few direct demonstrations that collagenase from rheumatoid synovium will degrade fibrous cartilage collagen, although more slowly than tendon collagen. If collagenase were to initiate the degradation of mature collagen fibers in vivo, it would be by cleavage of the helical regions of crosslinked molecules. Although the resulting A and B fragments would first be attached to other molecules, they would soon denature and become susceptible to nonspecific proteinases, including elastase, plasmin, and gelatinase.

An alternative form of attack on the collagen fibers may be mediated by the leukocyte elastase, or possibly by other nonspecific proteinases acting similarly.[43,44] The terminal, nonhelical peptides are cleaved by the elastase in such a way that the crosslinks are eliminated. The modified tropocollagen molecules then represent a highly susceptible substrate for the specific collagenase. Uncrosslinked molecules are more easily solubilized than crosslinked ones, and once solubilized, they denature quite rapidly at 37° C to give gelatin, which is rapidly degraded by almost any proteinase. Biomechanical measurements have shown that treatment of articular cartilage with leukocyte elastase markedly reduces its tensile stiffness and tensile strength.[97]

It is clear that there exists the third possibility of fragments of collagen fibers being taken up by cells and digested within the lysosomal system. The process has been studied in detail with the electron microscope for the fibroblasts of mouse periodontal ligament[98] and other cells and has been observed in a case of rheumatoid arthritis.[99] The lysosomal degradation of collagen would occur at the characteristic acid pH of these organelles and would be mediated by cysteine proteinases, cathepsin B, and cathepsin L, followed by exopeptidases, completing the degradation to very small peptides and amino acids. Even for the pathways of degradation initiated extracellularly by collagenase or elastase-like enzymes it is probable that the fragments are eventually taken into cells, either in the connective tissue itself or elsewhere in the body, for the final stages of breakdown.

Bone. The strength of bone is largely due to its mineral component, but the organic matrix of collagen, glycoprotein, and proteoglycan is formed first as the tissue develops, and is generally destroyed last as the tissue is broken down, since the mineral protects the organic component from enzymatic attack.[100] Thus it seems that dissolution of the inorganic components of bone may be rate controlling in its resorption, and yet very little is known of the molecular mechanism by which this is brought about. Although bone cells or bone fragments in culture produce specific collagenase, some studies suggest that bone resorption in vitro is related more to activity of cysteine proteinases (e.g., cathepsin B or L) than to the classic metalloproteinases.

Figure 12–5. A diagrammatic representation of three possible routes for the degradation of collagen. The steps marked 37° C are those in which the thermally unstable modified tropocollagen and TC[A] and TC[B] fragments are considered to be denatured at body temperature.

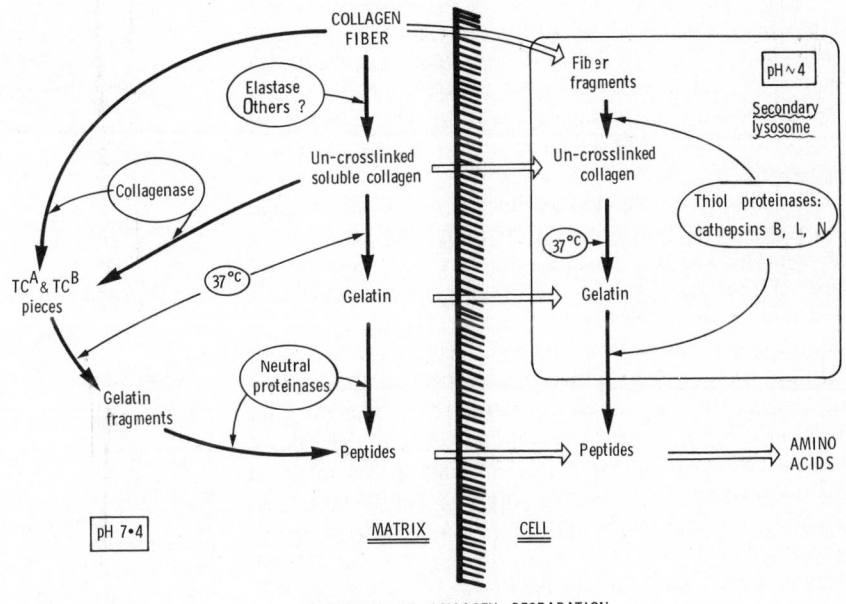

PATHWAYS OF COLLAGEN DEGRADATION

Tendon. In rheumatoid arthritis, degradation of tendons can be a serious problem. The tendon is very largely composed of type I collagen in fiber bundles aligned parallel to the tensile stress; breakdown of the collagen leads to virtually complete destruction of the tissue and loss of its function.

DEGRADATIVE PROTEINASES IN JOINT DISEASE: THEIR CELLULAR ORIGINS AND CONTROL PROCESSES

Since the various types of cells forming the articular tissues differ in the range of proteinases that they can produce, the questions of the identity of the proteinases responsible for tissue damage and their anatomic origin are closely linked. Two main lines of evidence may be considered in attempting to answer these questions: the anatomic locations of damage in the joint, and the capacity of the cells of each tissue within the joint to produce effective enzymes and to get them to the target tissues in an active state.

The Anatomy of Joint Damage. Much is written elsewhere in the present volume about the anatomy of joint damage, but certain points are of particular relevance to the questions of the identity and source of the degradation proteinases. In rheumatoid arthritis, the inflammatory changes affect the joint generally, and it is possible to argue in favor of the degradative enzymes originating from almost any of the cells that are present (Fig. 12–6). The apparent erosion of cartilage and bone at the margins of the articulating surface has suggested to many that the destructive enzymes arise from the adjacent soft tissue in a genuinely invasive process. That is to say that the enzymes are *extrinsic,* arising outside the target tissues, rather than *intrinsic.* This view seems to be supported by the demonstration of cathepsin D and collagenase at the pannus–cartilage junction.[101-103] Alternatively, it can be argued that the pannus is a form of granulation tissue produced in an attempt to heal areas of cartilage lysed by intrinsic enzymes. In this view, collagenase might arise from the pannus cells in the course of the (abortive) repair process, just as it has been reported that collagenase is produced, presumably for the remodeling of collagen, in the healing of dermal wounds.[104]

Besides the destruction at the margin of the articular surface that is associated with pannus, there is evidence of damage to other parts of the cartilage. Generalized loss of proteoglycan can be observed histologically.[105] Large areas of ulceration of the cartilage surface are commonly found remote from the pannus, and surface damage can be seen under the electron microscope in areas that are macroscropically normal.[106] The enzymes responsible for these types of damage may arise from within the cartilage itself or from cells in the synovial fluid in which it is bathed. Both cartilage and fluid contain enzymes and inhibitors (see below), and the arguments for intrinsic and extrinsic origins of the enzymes seem about equally balanced. Of course, a com-

bination of the two is perfectly possible. The arguments relating to cartilage seem equally applicable to bone and tendon.

In osteoarthrosis, the lack of cellular infiltration of the synovium or synovial fluid makes an intrinsic mechanism of breakdown by enzymes from the chondrocytes themselves seem much more likely than an extrinsic attack by enzymes from outside the tissue. Normal cartilage matrix is known to show a slow but definite rate of turnover,[107] and it seems reasonable that the organized growth of cartilage would require the tissue cells to have the capacity to break down as well as to form the matrix in which they are embedded. It may well be that in osteoarthrosis one sees enhanced activity of the normal breakdown process.

Proteinases and Their Inhibitors in Articular Cells and Tissues. *Cartilage.* The major proteinases extractable from cartilage are the lysosomal acid proteinases cathepsin D and cathepsin B, both of which are highly effective in the degradation of cartilage proteoglycan in the range of pH 5 to 6.[108,109] Osteoarthrotic and osteophytic cartilage contains abnormally large amounts of both cathepsin D and cathepsin B.[109,110] Cathepsin D and other lysosomal enzymes are synthesized and secreted in greatly increased amounts by cartilage organ cultures stimulated to resorb with slight excess of retinol.[111] Attempts to block the breakdown of living cartilage in culture by inhibition of cathepsin D with pepstatin or antibodies have so far been unsuccessful, however, and this despite clear evidence that the pepstatin was present in the matrix at high concentration.[112]

Traces of a neutral proteinase have been detected in cartilage, and the enzyme has been characterized.[113] Extracts of cartilage contain inhibitors of cysteine, serine and metalloproteinases.[86] Articular cartilage explanted in organ culture produces collagenase[114] and other neutral metalloproteinases.[115] Chondrocytes in culture produce a spectrum of proteinases: collagenase, other

Figure 12–6. A schematic depiction of the possible tissue origins for degradative enzymes in the rheumatoid joint. The arrows indicate the possibilities of release of degradative enzymes from the cells. As is discussed in the text, enzymes released into the synovial fluid probably mainly form inhibitor complexes.

metalloproteinases[116,117] and plasminogen activator.[118] Cultured cartilage and chondrocytes also produce an inhibitor of metalloproteinases (TIMP).[119]

Synovium. Rheumatoid synovium ex vivo contains a variety of proteinases that reflect its cellular heterogeneity; these include cathepsin D,[101,120,121] cathepsin G, elastase, unidentified serine proteinases,[122] and small amounts of collagenase.[123] Collagenase is secreted into the medium in quantity by rheumatoid synovium in culture, and this led to the first observation of a mammalian collagenase.[124] Subsequently, culture experiments have shown the production of collagenase by synovium from other arthritides, and from normal joints.[54,55]

The rheumatoid synovium collagenase has been purified,[60] and immunohistochemical studies have shown it to be present at some areas of the synovium–cartilage junction in some rheumatoid joints.[103] It is not known which cell type produces the collagenase at the junction, but collagenase can be secreted by both fibroblastic cells and macrophages (see above). Cultures of adherent cells obtained by enzymic disaggregation of rheumatoid synovium produce collagenase,[125] and immunofluorescent localization of the enzyme shows large amounts of it associated with small cells with long dendritic processes. These dendritic cells are morphologically different from any cells observed in the tissue.[126]

Relatively little attention has been paid to the occurrence of neutral proteinases other than collagenase in rheumatoid synovium, although they could well be important in cartilage breakdown. Removal of proteoglycan by such proteinases would render the collagen accessible to collagenase, and there is good reason to believe that proteoglycan is lost from the cartilage before the collagen. A gelatinase has been described in the culture medium of rheumatoid synovial tissue,[127] and two types of metalloproteinase have been detected from rabbit synovial fibroblasts[69] and from macrophages.[128] Synovial fibroblasts also make plasminogen activator.[129-131] Besides making proteinases, organ cultures of synovium also make the ubiquitous metalloproteinase inhibitor.[119]

Synovial Fluid. In rheumatoid arthritis and other inflammatory joint diseases, large numbers of leukocytes may enter the synovial fluid. The human polymorphonuclear leukocyte is unusual among cells in having lysosomes containing neutral proteinases with only traces of acid proteinases. (Most cell types have acid proteinases in their lysosomes, and some species, e.g., rabbits, have predominantly acid proteinases in their polymorphonuclear cell granules.)[132] In human neutrophils, the azurophilic granules contain the serine enzymes, leukocyte elastase and cathepsin G,[133] and the specific granules contain two neutral metalloproteinases, a collagenase and a gelatinase, both being found in latent form.[59,78,134]

The leukocyte proteinases are released from the cells during phagocytosis. Elastase and collagenase are released on uptake of aggregated IgG,[135] and neutral proteinases are released when the cells are incubated with pieces of articular cartilage coated with IgG.[136] In the

rheumatoid joint, release could accompany phagocytosis of immune complexes or tissue debris, or contact with a cartilage surface bearing immune complexes.

Proteinases of lymphocytes, monocytes, and macrophages have been little studied in man or animals. Human lymphocytes are known to contain a small amount of acid proteinase, probably cathepsin D,[137] and cathepsin D is present in rabbit macrophages.[138] Mouse macrophages have been shown to secrete collagenase, metalloproteinase and plasminogen activator in tissue culture,[33,71,74,76] and rabbit macrophages secrete a neutral metalloproteinase and collagenase.[75] Human platelets contain acid proteinases but not significant amounts of elastase or collagenase.[139-141]

Almost certainly there is release of proteinases into the synovial fluid in rheumatoid arthritis. Complexes of leukocyte elastase with α_1-proteinase inhibitor have been found by crossed immunoelectrophoresis, and collagenase–α_2M complexes have also been demonstrated.[142,143] The enhanced vascular permeability of the rheumatoid synovium allows even the high molecular weight plasma proteins such as α_2M to equilibrate into the synovial fluid, so the fluid has essentially the same proteinase inhibitors as plasma. It has been calculated that the large numbers of neutrophils entering the synovial fluid (where they die and disintegrate within hours) could bring in large amounts of leukocyte proteinase,[44] but direct tests for active proteinases in rheumatoid synovial fluids have revealed only a small percentage (those with leukocyte counts exceeding 50,000 per cubic millimeter) with some collagenase activity.[144] Since it must be recognized that some findings of either free collagenase or proteinase-inhibitor complexes in synovial fluid could be due to breakage of cells during withdrawal of the fluid from the patient or subsequent storage, we feel that there is room for doubt as to whether proteinases are in excess over their inhibitors frequently enough to be of any real significance to the disease process. It is therefore uncertain whether any proteinases from cells of the synovial fluid or the synovial lining can traverse the fluid and damage the cartilage. It is conceivable, however, that membrane-bound or latent forms of the enzymes might escape synovial fluid inhibitors and then adhere to the cartilage surface and be activated locally. A proteinase-like metal-dependent enzyme associated with lipid, probably membrane fragments, is regularly found in rheumatoid synovial fluid.[145]

Another way in which the enzymes may evade the inhibitors is by direct release onto the cartilage surface by cells adherent to it. Such a process of "frustrated phagocytosis" might well be promoted by the presence of immune complexes at the cartilage surface,[146,147] and the effectiveness of this mechanism of circumventing proteinase inhibitors has been demonstrated directly in a model system.[148] Direct microscopic observations pointing strongly to a role for neutrophil leukocytes adherent to the cartilage surface in the erosion of the tissue have been reported.[149,150]

So far we have discussed enzymes originating from the cellular phase of the synovial fluid, but there are proenzymes of plasma proteinases in the bulk phase also. Plasminogen could be converted to plasmin by activators from synovial cells, and in septic arthritis activation might be by streptokinase or analogous bacterial products. Plasmin is a potent proteinase that will hydrolyze proteoglycan, and the possibility that it might play a role in cartilage degradation has been discussed.[37,129,151,152] Two considerations cast some doubt on the possibility of plasmin acting in the joint. (1) The synovial fluid contains very potent inhibitors derived from the plasma (notably the α_2-plasmin inhibitor). (2) It is difficult to see why fibrin, the substrate for which plasmin has such high affinity, is abundant in rheumatoid joints if they contain the active enzyme.

There is some evidence for a proteinase activator in rheumatoid synovial fluid. As was mentioned earlier, the specific granules of the neutrophil contain latent forms of a collagenase and a gelatinase. A protein of about 35,000 molecular weight that will activate the latent forms of both collagenase and gelatinase has been isolated from rheumatoid synovial fluid.[153] Rheumatoid synovial cultures apparently produce an activator of the leukocyte gelatinase and collagenase that has similar properties to that in synovial fluid.[154] In other hands it has been shown that plasma kallikrein has the capacity to activate latent collagenase, and that the major activator in some samples of rheumatoid synovial fluid is identifiable as plasma kallikrein.[155]

CONTROL PROCESSES

The current, widely held view is that resorption of connective tissues is brought about by the release of collagenase and other proteinases from cells. Various agents have been found to stimulate or inhibit release of collagenase. Anti-inflammatory steroids such as dexamethasone inhibit its production by synovial fibroblasts,[125] as do retinoids.[156] Agents stimulating collagenase production by synovial fibroblasts are phorbol myristate acetate,[157] cytochalasin B, vinblastine, aminophylline[158] and collagen.[159] Colchicine (10^{-7} M) has a stimulatory effect on synovial organ cultures.[160]

Ingestion of nondigestible particles (mimicked experimentally with polystyrene latex) increases collagenase production by rabbit synovial fibroblasts and mouse peritoneal macrophages.[69,71]

To obtain collagenase from macrophages in culture it has been found necessary to stimulate them in some way. Thioglycolate has been used for mouse peritoneal macrophages; and the lipid A component of bacterial endotoxin, for cells from guinea pig peritoneum.[69-71] Whether or not these agents have similar effects in vivo is unknown.

Macrophages,[161] synovial fibroblasts,[162] and chondrocytes[116] are stimulated in vitro to produce collagenase by products of mononuclear leukocytes. The synovial cells and chondrocytes also make increased amounts of prostaglandin E_2[163-165] and plasminogen activator.[131] The "lymphokines" or "monokines" responsible for this

stimulation have not been purified, but the activity is associated with a small protein (or proteins) of about 14,000 molecular weight called mononuclear cell factor.[163,166] Production of this mononuclear cell factor is stimulated in vitro by aggregated IgG, the Fc portion of IgG, concanavalin A,[167] native human collagens,[168] and products of activated lymphocytes.[169,170] There is now strong evidence that the activity of mononuclear cell factor is at least partly attributable to the monocyte-macrophage product interleukin I.[171,172] Interleukin I is a protein that enhances blastic stimulation of lymphocytes and was formerly called lymphocyte activating factor (LAF).[173] Another protein that may well be similar to interleukin I is catabolin, which is defined by its ability to induce resorption of cartilage matrix proteoglycans in vitro. It is made by synovium in organ culture,[174] by synovial fibroblasts[175] (especially if stimulated by phorbol myristate acetate), and by lectin-stimulated mononuclear leukocytes.[176] Pig catabolin is of 20,000 molecular weight and has a pI of 4.8[176a]; human catabolin is of similar size but has a pI of 5.2.[177] Leukocyte and fibroblast catabolins seem to be the same protein. The human catabolin is a more acid protein than human interleukin I, which has an isoelectric point of pH 6.8.[178] Purification of these proteins will enable their relationships and possible role in tissue resorption to be established.

Besides the secreted enzymes such as collagenase, the other group of proteinases that have been considered to be important in degradation are the lysosomal proteinases. Unlike the secreted proteinases, lysosomal hydrolases are stored in the cells and are normally discharged into intracellular digestive organelles, phagosomes. However, the neutral proteinases of polymorphonuclear leukocytes may be released extracellularly during phagocytosis and by interaction of the cell with complement cleavage products (C5a).[179] Similarily the lysosomal enzymes of macrophages are released during phagocytosis and by C3a.[180]

The rheumatoid synovial cells in culture produce mainly latent enzymes, and the latent collagenase tends to bind to collagen.[181] Presumably the enzymes are initially latent in vivo, too, so their activation is obviously a potential control process. A variety of proteinases will activate latent collagenase, and plasmin has been proposed to play a significant role in rheumatoid arthritis, since the synovial fluid may contain large amounts of plasminogen, and rheumatoid synovial cells can produce plasminogen activators.[129-131] Plasma kallikrein may act in a similar way.[40] The latent collagenase does not interact with α_2M but does bind to collagen (though less strongly than active enzyme). Latent collagenase could therefore evade α_2M, bind to its substrate, and then be activated locally by plasmin.[129]

CONCLUSIONS

Although we are not yet able to reach any definite conclusions as to the identity of proteinases important in joint diseases, there is reason for confidence that the foundation of knowledge at the molecular level that has been established during the past decade will form the basis for progress in the future.

One can speculate about the areas of current research that may prove particularly productive. The elucidation of the complex chemistry of the important structural molecules of connective tissues and the isolation of the major cellular proteinases are already allowing a clearer understanding of the precise way in which the proteinases could contribute to joint disease. The detailed characterization of degradation products formed in vivo may lead to the positive identification of some of the important enzymes.

Purification of the cellular proteinases has permitted the raising of specific antisera against them. The resulting immunochemical methods clearly have much to offer. Already antisera are being used to show which cells release particular enzymes; they are potentially useful also for specific immunoinhibition, ultrasensitive immunoassays, and study of synthesis and turnover of the enzymes. Further use of these techniques may follow from refinement of methods for raising specific antisera with very small amounts of pure immunogen, or with only partially purified immunogen. Such advances should allow more work with enzymes from diseased human tissues, for the small amounts of human articular tissues available usually preclude the complete purification of enzymes from this source, although cultivation of the tissue in vitro has been helpful.

The discovery of better substrates and inhibitors has a crucial role to play in the study of the physiologic functions of proteinases. The specificity and sensitivity of assays with synthetic substrates are becoming greater, and the extent to which these can be used in place of less convenient assays with complex substrates is becoming clearer. A powerful armory of proteinase inhibitors of microbial and synthetic origin has now become available and awaits full exploitation in appropriately designed biologic test systems.

A major area for future work is that of the natural regulation of the catabolic enzymes, including controls of synthesis and translocation. The question of the nature of latent collagenase will presumably be answered following the complete purification of greater amounts of material, but the larger question of the reactivity or otherwise of masked forms of the cellular proteinases with inhibitors may remain for some time. There are interesting indications of ways in which proteinases in the extracellular fluid can escape binding by the proteinase inhibitors and subsequently show activity perhaps after adsorption to collagen or proteoglycan.

Another topic of major interest is the possibility that regions of low pH around cells are sufficiently acid to allow extracellular activity of the lysosomal acid proteinases. Conversely, further evidence as to the part played by endocytosis and intracellular digestion in catabolism of connective tissue matrices will be welcome.

These, then, seem to be some of the important directions for future research into the role of cellular proteinases in joint disease.

References

1. Fehr, K., Velvart, M., Böni, A., Watanabe, H., Spycher, M.A., and Rüttner, J.R.: Experimental arthritis of rabbits caused by intra-articular injection of autologous Fab2 produced by digestion of IgG with cathepsin D. 1. Microscopical and immunohistochemical findings in short-term experiments. Ann. Rheum. Dis. 35:85, 1976.
2. Trentham, D.E., Townes, A.S., and Kang, A.H.: Autoimmunity to type II collagen: An experimental model of arthritis. J. Exp. Med. 146:857, 1977.
3. Ward, P.A.: Complement-dependent phlogistic factors in rheumatoid synovial fluids. Ann. N.Y. Acad. Sci. 256:169, 1975.
4. Hayashi, H.: The intracellular neutral SH-dependent protease associated with inflammatory reactions. Int. Rev. Cytol. 40:101, 1975.
5. Barrett, A.J.: Introduction: the classification of proteinases. In Evered, D., and Whelan, J. (eds.): Protein Degradation in Health and Disease (Ciba Foundation Symposium 75). Amsterdam, Excerpta Medica, 1980, pp. 1–13.
6. Barrett, A.J. (ed.): Proteinases in Mammalian Cells and Tissues. Amsterdam, North-Holland Publishing Co., 1977.
7. Barrett, A.J., and McDonald, J.K.: Mammalian Proteases. A Glossary and Bibliography. London, Academic Press, 1980.
8. Barrett, A.J.: Cathepsin D and other carboxyl proteinases. In Barrett A.J. (ed.): Proteinases of Mammalian Cells and Tissues. Amsterdam, North-Holland Publishing Company, 1977, pp. 209–248.
9. Barrett, A.J.: Cathepsin D. Purification of isoenzymes from human and chicken liver. Biochem. J. 117:601, 1970.
10. Takahashi, T., and Tang, J.: Cathepsin D from porcine and bovine spleen. Methods Enzymol. 80:565, 1981.
11. Barrett, A.J., and Dingle, J.T.: The inhibition of tissue acid proteinases by pepstatin. Biochem. J. 127:439, 1972.
12. Dingle, J.T., Barrett, A.J., Poole, A.R., and Stovin, P.: Inhibition by pepstatin of human cartilage degradation. Biochem. J. 127:443, 1972.
13. Knight, C.G., and Barrett, A.J.: Interaction of human cathepsin D with the inhibitor pepstatin. Biochem. J. 115:117, 1975.
14. Dingle, J.T., Barrett, A.J., and Weston, P.D.: Cathepsin D. Characteristics of immunoinhibition and the confirmation of a role in cartilage breakdown. Biochem. J. 123:1, 1971.
15. Morrison, R.I.G., Barrett, A.J., Dingle, J.T., and Prior, D.: Cathepsins B1 and D. Action on human cartilage proteoglycans. Biochim. Biophys. Acta 302:411, 1973.
16. Roughley, P.J., and Barrett, A.J.: The degradation of cartilage proteoglycans by tissue proteinases. Proteoglycan structure and its susceptibility to proteolysis. Biochem. J. 167:629, 1977.
17. Roughley, P.J.: The degradation of cartilage proteoglycans by tissue proteinases. Proteoglycan heterogeneity and the pathway of proteolytic degradation. Biochem. J. 167:639, 1977.
18. Harris, E.D., Jr., Lock, S., and Lin, T.-Y.: Limited degradation of gelatin substrate by cathepsin D. Conn. Tiss. Res. 1:103, 1972.
19. Burleigh, M.C., Barrett, A.J., and Lazarus, G.S.: Cathepsin B1. A lysosomal enzyme that degrades native collagen. Biochem. J. 137:387, 1974.
20. Scott, P.G., and Pearson, C.H.: Cathepsin D—cleavage of soluble collagen and cross-linked peptides. FEBS Lett. 88:41, 1978.
21. Dingle, J.T.: The secretion of enzymes into the pericellular environment. Phil. Trans. R. Soc. Lond. B 271:315, 1975.
22. Barrett, A.J., and Starkey, P.M.: The interaction of α_2-macroglobulin with proteinases. Characteristics and specificity of the reaction and a hypothesis concerning its molecular mechanism. Biochem. J. 133:709, 1973.
23. Barrett, A.J.: Human cathepsin B1. Purification and some properties of the enzyme. Biochem. J. 131:809, 1973.
24. Barrett, A.J.: Cathepsin B and other thiol proteinases. In Barrett, A.J. (ed.): Proteinases of Mammalian Cells and Tissues. North-Holland Publishing Company, Amsterdam, 1977, pp. 181–208.
25. Barrett, A.J., and Kirschke, H.: Cathepsin B, cathepsin H and cathepsin L. Methods Enzymol. 80:535, 1981.
26. Pohl, J., Baudys, M., Tomasek, V., and Kostka, V.: Identification of the active site cysteine and of the disulphide bonds in the N-terminal part of bovine spleen cathepsin B. FEBS Lett. 142:23, 1982.
27. Burleigh, M.C., Barrett, A.J., and Lazarus, G.S.: Cathepsin B1. A lysosomal enzyme that degrades native collagen. Biochem. J. 137:387, 1974.
28. Kirschke, H., Kembhavi, A.A., Bohley, P., and Barrett, A.J.: Action of rat liver cathepsin L on collagen and other substrates. Biochem. J. 201:367, 1982.
29. Knight, C.G.: Human cathepsin B. Application of the substrate N-benzyloxycarbonyl-L-arginyl-L-arginine 2-naphthylamide to a study of the inhibition by leupeptin. Biochem. J. 189:447, 1980.
30. Baici, A., and Gyger-Marazzi, M.: The slow, tight-binding inhibition of cathepsin B by leupeptin. A hysteretic effect. Eur. J. Biochem. 129:33, 1982.
31. Barrett, A.J., Kembhavi, A.A., Brown, M.A., Kirschke, J., Knight, C.G., Tamai, M., and Hanada, K.: L-Trans-epoxysuccinyl-leucyl-amino(4-

guanidino)butane (E-64) and its analogues as inhibitors of cysteine proteinases including cathepsins B, H and L. Biochem. J. 201:189, 1982.

32. Shaw, E., and Green, G.D.J.: Inactivation of thiol proteases with peptidyl diazomethyl ketones. Methods Enzymol. 80:820, 1981.

32a. Anastasi, A., Brown, M.A., Kembhavi, A.A., Nicklin, M.J.H., Sayers, C.A., Sunter, D.C., and Barrett, A.J.: Cystatin, a protein inhibitor of cysteine proteinases. Improved purification from egg white, characterization, and detection in chicken serum. Biochem. J. 211:129, 1983.

32b. Green, G.D.J., Kembhavi, A.A., Davies, M.E., and Barrett, A.J.: Biochem. J. in press, 1984.

33. Unkeless, J.C., Gordon, S., and Reich, E.: Secretion of plasminogen activator by stimulated macrophages. J. Exp. Med. 139:834, 1974.

34. Granelli-Piperno, A., Vassalli, J.-D., and Reich, E.: Secretion of plasminogen activator by human polymorphonuclear leukocytes. Modulation by glucocortoids and other effectors. J. Exp. Med. 146:1693, 1978.

35. Werb, Z., and Aggeler, J.: Proteases induce secretion of collagenase and plasminogen activator by fibroblasts. Proc. Natl. Acad. Sci. USA 75:1839, 1978.

36. Okamoto, S., Oshiba, S., Mihara, H., and Okamoto, U.: Synthetic inhibitors of fibrinolysis: In vitro and in vivo mode of action. Ann. N.Y. Acad. Sci. 146:414, 1968.

37. Lack, C.H., and Rogers, H.J.: Action of plasmin on cartilage. Nature 182:948, 1958.

38. Harpel, P.C.: Plasmin inhibitor reactions. The effectiveness of α_2-plasmin inhibitor in the presence of α_2-macroglobulin. J. Exp. Med. 146:1033, 1977.

39. Heimark, R.L. and Davie, E.W.: Bovine and human plasma prekallikrein. Methods Enzymol. 80:157, 1981.

40. Nagase, H., Cawston, T.E., DeSilva, M. and Barrett, A.J.: Identification of plasma kallikrein as an activator of latent collagenase in rheumatoid synovial fluid. Biochim. Biophys. Acta 702:133, 1982.

41. Barrett, A.J.: Leukocyte elastase. Methods Enzymol. 80:581, 1981.

42. Keiser, H., Greenwald, R.A., Feinstein, G., and Janoff, A.: Degradation of cartilage proteoglycan by human leukocyte neutral proteases—a model of joint injury. II. Degradation of isolated bovine nasal cartilage proteoglycan. J. Clin. Invest. 57:625, 1976.

43. Starkey, P.M., Barrett, A.J., and Burleigh M.C.: The degradation of articular collagen by neutrophil proteinases. Biochim. Biophys. Acta 483:386, 1977.

44. Barrett, A.J.: The possible role of neutrophil proteinases in damage to articular cartilage. Agents Actions 8:11, 1978.

45. Davies, M., Barrett, A.J., Travis, J., Sanders, E., and Coles, G.A.: The degradation of human glomerular basement membrane with purified lysosomal proteinases: Evidence for the pathogenic role of the polymorphonuclear leucocyte in glomerulonephritis. Clin. Sci. Mol. Med. 54:233, 1978.

46. Mainardi, C.L., Dixit, S.N., and Kang, A.H.: Degradation of type IV (basement membrane) collagen by a proteinase isolated from human polymorphonuclear leukocyte granules. J. Biol. Chem. 255:5435, 1980.

47. Powers, J.C., Gupton, B.F., Harley, A.D., Nishono, N., and Whitely, R.J.: Specificity of porcine pancreatic elastase, human leucocyte elastase and cathepsin G. Inhibition with peptide chloromethyl ketones. Biochim. Biophys. Acta 485:156, 1977.

48. Baici, A., Salgam, P., Fehr, K., and Böni, A.: Inhibition of human elastase from polymorphonuclear leucocytes by gold sodium thiomalate and pentosan polysulfate (SP-54®). Biochem. Pharmacol. 30:703, 1981.

49. Ohlsson, K., and Ohlsson, L.: Neutral proteases of human granulocytes. III. Interaction between granulocyte elastase and plasma protease inhibitors. Scand. J. Clin. Lab. Invest. 34:349, 1974.

50. Barrett, A.J.: Cathepsin G. Methods Enzymol. 80:561, 1981.

51. Woodbury, R.G., Everitt, M.T., and Neurath, H.: Mast cell proteases. Methods Enzymol. 80:588, 1981.

52. Venge, P.: PMN proteases and their effects on complement components and neutrophil function. In Havermann, K. (ed.): Neutral Proteases of Human Polymorphonuclear Leukocytes. Baltimore, Urban & Schwartzenberg, 1978.

53. Venge, P., Ohlsson, I., and Odeberg, H.: Cationic proteins of human granulocytes. V. Interaction with plasma protease inhibitors. Scand. J. Clin. Lab. Invest. 35:737, 1975.

54. Harris, E.D. Jr., and Krane, S.M.: Collagenases. N. Engl. J. Med. 291:557, 605, 652, 1974.

55. Woolley, D.E., and Evanson, J.M. (eds.): Collagenase in Normal and Pathological Connective Tissues. New York, John Wiley and Sons, 1980.

56. Miller, E.J., Harris, E.D. Jr., Finch, J.E. Jr., Chung, E., McCroskery, P.A., and Butler, W.T.: Cleavage of type II and III collagens with mammalian collagenase: Site of cleavage and primary structure at the NH$_2$-terminal portion of the smaller fragment released from both collagens. Biochemistry 15:787, 1976.

57. Gross, J., Highberger, J.H., Johnson-Wint, B., and Biswas, C.: Mode of action and regulation of tissue collagenases. In Woolley, D.E., and Evanson, J.M. (eds.): Collagenase in Normal and Pathological Connective Tissues. New York, John Wiley & Sons, 1980, p. 11.

58. Welgus, H.G., Jeffrey, J.J., Stricklin, G.P., and Eisen, A.Z.: The gelatinolytic activity of human skin fibroblast collagenase. J. Biol. Chem. 257:11534, 1982.

59. Christner, P., Damato, D., Reinhart, M., and Abrams, W.: Purification of human neutrophil collagenase and production of a monospecific antiserum. Biochemistry 21:6005, 1982.

60. Woolley, D.E., Lindberg, K.A., Glanville, R.W., and Evanson, J.M.: Action of rheumatoid synovial collagenase on cartilage collagen. Different susceptibilities of cartilage and tendon collagen to collagenase attack. Eur. J. Biochem. 50:437, 1975.

61. Harris, E.D. Jr., and Farrell, M.E.: Resistance to collagenase. A characteristic of collagen fibrils crosslinked by formaldehyde. Biochim. Biophys. Acta 278:133, 1972.

62. Vater, C.A., Harris, E.D. Jr., and Siegel, R.C.: Native cross-links in collagen fibrils induce resistance to human synovial collagenase. Biochem. J. 181:639, 1979.

63. Cawston, T.E., and Barrett, A.J.: A rapid and reproducible assay for collagenase using [1-^{14}C]acetylated collagen. Anal. Biochem. 99:340, 1979.

64. Cawston, T.E., and Murphy, G.: Mammalian collagenases. Methods Enzymol. 80:711, 1981.

65. Cawston, T.E., and Tyler, J.A.: Purification of pig synovial collagenase to high specific activity. Biochem. J. 183:647, 1979.

65a. Dr G. Murphy, personal communication, 1983.

66. François, J., Cambie, E., and Fehr, J.: Collagenase inhibition by penicillamine. Ophthalmologica 166:222, 1973.

67. Werb, Z., Burleigh, M.C., Barrett, A.J., and Starkey, P.M.: The interaction of α_2-macroglobulin with proteinases. Binding and inhibition of mammalian collagenase and other metal proteinases. Biochem. J. 139:359, 1974.

68. Wooley, D.E., Roberts, D.R., and Evanson, J.M.: Small molecular weight β_1 serum protein which specifically inhibits human collagenase. Nature 261:325, 1976.

69. Werb, Z., and Reynolds, J.J.: Purification and properties of a specific collagenase from rabbit fibroblast. Biochem. J. 151:645, 1975.

70. Wahl, L.M., Wahl, S.M., Mergenhagen, S.E., and Martin, G.R.: Collagenase production by endotoxin-activated macrophages. Proc. Natl. Acad. Sci. USA 71:3598, 1974.

71. Werb, Z., and Gordon, S.: Secretion of a specific collagenase by stimulated macrophages. J. Exp. Med. 1420:346, 1975.

72. Murphy, G., Reynolds, J.J., Bretz, U., and Baggiolini, M.: Collagenase is a component of the specific granules of human neutrophil leucocytes. Biochem. J. 162:195, 1977.

73. Nagase, H., Jackson, R.C., Brinckerhoff, C.E., Vater, C.A., and Harris, E.D. Jr.: A precursor form of latent collagenase produced in a cell-free system with mRNA from rabbit synovial cells. J. Biol. Chem. 256:11951, 1981.

74. Werb, Z., and Gordon, S.: Elastase secretion by stimulated macrophages. Characterization and regulation. J. Exp. Med. 142:361, 1975.

75. Hauser, P., and Vaes, G.: Degradation of cartilage proteoglycans by neutral proteinase secreted by rabbit bone-marrow macrophages in culture. Biochem. J. 172:275, 1978.

76. Banda, M.J., and Werb, Z.: Mouse macrophage elastase. Purification and characterization as a metalloproteinase. Biochem. J. 193:589, 1981.

76a. Banda, M.J., and Werb, Z.: Limited proteolysis by macrophage elastase inactivates human α_1-proteinase inhibitor. J. Exp. Med. 152:1563, 1980.

77. Galloway, W.A., Murphy, G., Sandy, J.D., Gavrilovic, J., Cawston, T.E., and Reynolds, J.J.: Purification and characterization of a rabbit bone metalloproteinase that degrades proteoglycan and other connective tissue components. Biochem. J. 209:741, 1983.

78. Sopata, I.: Further purification and some properties of a gelatin-specific proteinase of human leucocytes. Biochim. Biophys. Acta 717:26, 1982.

79. Starkey, P.M., and Barrett, A. J.: α_2-Macroglobulin: inhibitor of endopeptidase? In Barrett, A.J. (ed.): Proteinases in Mammalian Cells and Tissues. Amsterdam, North-Holland Publishing Company, 1977, pp. 663–696.

81. Starkey, P.M., and Barrett, A.J.: α_2-Macroglobulin, A Remarkable Proteinase Inhibitor. London, Academic Press, in press, 1984.

82. Feinman, R. (ed.): α_2-Macroglobulin. Ann. N.Y. Acad. Sci., in press, 1983.

83. Imber, M.J., and Pizzo, S.V.: Clearance and binding of two electrophoretically "fast" forms of human α_2-macroglobulin. J. Biol. Chem. 256:8134, 1981.

84. Sasaki, M., Taniguchi, K., and Minakata, K.: Multimolecular forms of thiol proteinase inhibitor in human plasma. J. Biochem. 89:169, 1981.

85. Green, G.D.J., Kembhavi, A.A., Davies, M.E., and Barrett, A.J.: Biochem. J. in press, 1984.

86. Killackey, J.J., Roughley, P.J., and Mort, J.S.: Proteinase inhibitors of human articular cartilage. Collagen Ref. Res. 3:419, 1983.

87. Travis, J., and Salvesen, G.S.: Plasma proteinase inhibitors. Ann. Rev. Biochem., 52:655, 1983.
88. Macartney, H.W., and Tschesche, H.: Interaction of β_1-anticollagenase from human plasma with collagenase from various tissues and competition with α_2-macroglobulin. Eur. J. Biochem. 130:93, 1983.
89. Cawston, T.E., Galloway, W.A., Mercer, E., Murphy, G., and Reynolds, J.J.: Purification of rabbit bone inhibitor of collagenase. Biochem. J. 195:159, 1981.
90. Harris, E.D. Jr., Parker, H.G., Radin, E.L., and Krane, S.M.: Effects of proteolytic enzymes on structural and mechanical properties of cartilage. Arthritis Rheum. 15:497, 1972.
91. Kempson, G.E., Tuke, M.A., Dingle, J.T., Barrett, A.J., and Horsefield, P.H.: The effects of proteolytic enzymes on the mechanical properties of adult human articular cartilage. Biochim. Biophys. Acta 428:741, 1976.
92. Pottenger, L.A., Lyon, N.B., Hecht, J.D., Neustadt, P.M., and Robinson, R.A.: Influence of cartilage particle size and proteoglycan aggregation on immobilization of proteoglycans. J. Biol. Chem. 257:11479, 1982.
93. Barrett, A.J.: Chondromucoprotein-degrading enzymes. Nature (London) 211:1188, 1966.
94. Dingle, J.T., Blow, A.M.J., Barrett, A.J., and Martin, P.E.N.: Proteoglycan-degrading enzymes. A radiochemical assay method and the detection of a new enzyme, cathepsin F. Biochem. J. 167:775, 1977.
95. Nagase, H., and Woessner, J.F.: An improved assay for proteases and polysaccharidases employing a cartilage proteolglycan substrate entrapped in polyacrylamide beads. Anal. Biochem. 107:385, 1980.
96. Farndale, R.W., Sayers, C.A., and Barrett, A.J.: A direct spectrophotometric microassay for sulphated glycosaminoglycans. Conect. Tissue Res. 9:247, 1982.
97. Bader, D.L., Kempson, G.E., Barrett, A.J., and Webb, W.: The effect of leucocyte elastase on the mechanical properties of adult articular cartilage in tension. Biochim. Biophys. Acta 677:103, 1981.
98. Garant, P.R.: Collagen resorption by fibroblasts—a theory of fibroblastic maintenance of the periodontal ligament. J. Periodont. 47:380, 1976.
99. Harris, E.D. Jr., Glauert, A.M., and Murley, A.H.G.: Intracellular collagen fibres at the pannus-cartilage junction in rheumatoid arthritis. Arthritis Rheum. 20:657, 1977.
100. Stern, B., Golub, L., and Goldhaber, P.: Effects of demineralization and parathyroid hormone on the availability of bone collagen to degradation by collagenase. J. Periodont. Res. 5:116, 1970.
101. Poole, A.R.: Immunocytochemical studies of the secretion of a proteolytic enzyme, cathepsin D, in relation to cartilage breakdown. In Burleigh, P.M.C., and Poole, A.R. (eds.): Dynamics of Connective Tissue Macromolecules. Amsterdam, North-Holland Publishing Company, 1975, pp. 357–383.
102. Poole, A.R., Hembry, R.M., and Dingle, J.T.: Cathepsin D in cartilage: The immunohistochemical demonstration of extracellular enzyme in normal and pathological conditions. J. Cell Sci. 14:139, 1974.
103. Woolley, D.E., Crossley, M.J., and Evanson, J.M.: Collagenase at sites of cartilage erosion in the rheumatoid joint. Arthritis Rheum. 20:1231, 1977.
104. Donoff, R.B., McLennan, J.E., and Grillo, H.C.: Preparation and properties of collagenase from epithelium and mesenchyme of healing mammalian wounds. Biochim. Biophys. Acta 277:639, 1971.
105. Hamerman, D.: Cartilage change in the rheumatoid joint. Clin. Orthopaed. 64:91, 1969.
106. Kimura, H., Tateishi, H., and Ziff, M.: Surface ultrastructure of rheumatoid articular cartilage. Arthritis Rheum. 20:1085, 1977.
107. Maroudas, A.: Glycosaminoglycan turnover in articular cartilage. Proc. Roy. Soc. B. 271:293, 1975.
108. Sapolsky, A.I., Howell, D.S., and Woessner, J.F. Jr.: Neutral proteases and cathepsin D in human articular cartilage. J. Clin. Invest. 53:1044, 1974.
109. Bayliss, M.T., and Ali, S.Y.: Studies on cathepsin B in human articular cartilage. Biochem. J. 171:149, 1978.
110. Sapolsky, A.I., Altman, R.D., Woessner, J.F. Jr., and Howell, D.: The action of cathepsin D in human articular cartilage on proteoglycans. J. Clin. Invest. 52:624, 1973.
111. Fell, H.B., and Dingle, J.T.: Studies on the mode of action of excess of vitamin A. Lysosomal protease and the degradation of cartilage matrix. Biochem. J. 87:403, 1963.
112. Hembry, R.M., Knight, C.G., Dingle, J.T. and Barrett, A.J.: Evidence that cathepsin D is not responsible for the resorption of cartilage matrix in culture. Biochim. Biophys. Acta 714:307, 1982.
113. Sapolsky, A.I., and Howell, D.S.: Further characterization of a neutral metalloproteinase isolated from human articular cartilage. Arthritis Rheum. 25:981, 1982.
114. Ehrlich, M.G., Mankin, J.H.J., Jones, H., Wright, R., Crispen, C., and Vigliani, G.: Collagenase and collagenase inhibitors in osteoarthritis and normal human cartilage. J. Clin. Invest. 59:226, 1977.
115. Murphy, C., McGuire, M.B., Russell, R.G.G., and Reynolds, J.J.: Characterization of collagenase, other metallo-proteinases and an inhibitor

116. Deshmukh-Phadke, K., Nanda, S., and Lee, K.: Macrophage factor that induces neutral protease secretion by normal rabbit chondrocytes. Eur. J. Biochem. 104:175, 1980.
117. Morales, T.I., and Kuettner, K.E.: The properties of the neutral proteinase released by primary chondrocyte cultures and its action on proteoglycan aggregate. Biochim. Biophys. Acta 705:92, 1982.
118. Meats, J.E., McGuire, M.B., and Russell, R.G.G.: Human synovium releases a factor which stimulates chondrocyte production of PGE_2 and plasminogen activator. Nature 286:891, 1980.
119. Murphy, G., Cambray, G.J., Virani, N., Page-Thomas, D.P., and Reynolds, J.J.: The production in culture of metalloproteinases and an inhibitor by joint tissues from normal rabbits and from rabbits with a model arthritis. I. Synovium. Rheumatol. Int. 1:11, 1981.
120. Luscombe, M.: Acid phosphatase and catheptic activity in rheumatoid synovial tissue. Nature 197:1010, 1963.
121. Barrett, A.J.: The enzymic degradation of cartilage matrix. In Burleigh, P.M.C., and Poole, A.R. (eds.): Dynamics of Connective Tissue Macromolecules. Amsterdam, North-Holland Publishing Company, 1975, pp. 189–226.
122. Saklatvala, J., and Barrett, A.J.: Identification of proteinases in rheumatoid synovium. Detection of leukocyte elastase, cathepsin G and another serine proteinase. Biochim. Biophys. Acta 615:167–177, 1980.
123. Nagai, Y., and Hori, H.: Vertebrate collagenase: Direct extraction from animal skin and human synovial membrane. J. Biochem. 72:1147, 1972.
124. Evanson, J.M., Jeffrey, J.J., and Krane, S.M.: Studies on collagenase from rheumatoid synovium in tissue culture. J. Clin. Invest. 47:2639, 1968.
125. Dayer, J.-M., Krane, S.M., Russell, R.G.G., and Robinson, D.R.: Production of collagenase and prostaglandins by isolated adherent rheumatoid synovial cells. Proc. Natl. Acad. Sci. USA 73:945, 1976.
126. Woolley, D.E., Harris, E.D. Jr., Mainardi, C.L., and Brinckerhoff, C.E.: Collagenase immunolocalization in cultures of rheumatoid synovial cells. Science 200:773, 1978.
127. Harris, E.D. Jr., and Krane, S.M.: An endopeptidase from rheumatoid synovial tissue culture. Biochim. Biophys. Acta 258:566, 1972.
128. Hauser, P., and Vaes., G.: Degradation of cartilage proteoglycans by a neutral proteinase secreted by rabbit bone-marrow macrophages in culture. Biochem. J. 172:275, 1978.
129. Werb, Z., Mainardi, C.L., Vater, C.A., and Harris, E.D. Jr.: Endogeneous activation of latent collagenase by rheumatoid synovial cells. N. Engl. J. Med. 296:1017, 1977.
130. Berger, H.: Secretion of plasminogen activator by rheumatoid and nonrheumatoid synovial cells in culture. Arthritis Rheum. 20:1198, 1977.
131. Hamilton, J.A., and Slywka, J.: Stimulation of human synovial fibroblast plasminogen activator production by mononuclear cell supernatants. J. Immunol. 126:851, 1981.
132. Folds, J.D., Welsh, I.R.H., and Spitznagel, J.K.: Neutral proteases confined to one class of lysosomes of human polymorphonuclear leukocytes. Proc. Soc. Exp. Biol. Med. 139:461, 1972.
133. Dewald, B., Rindler-Ludwig, R., Bretz, U., and Baggiolini, M.: Subcellular localisation and heterogeneity of neutral proteases in neutrophilic polymorphonuclear leucocytes. J. Exp. Med. 141:709, 1975.
134. Tschesche, H., and Macartney, H.W.: A new principle of enzyme regulation of enzymic activity. Activation and regulation of human polymorphonuclear leukocyte collagenase via disulfide-thiol exchange as catalysed by the glutathione cycle in a peroxidase-coupled reaction to glucose metabolism. Eur. J. Biochem. 120:183, 1981.
135. Oronsky, A.L., Perper, R.J., and Schroder, H.C.: Phagocytic release and activation of human leukocyte procollagenase. Nature 246:417, 1973.
136. Oronsky, A., Ignarro, L., and Perper, R.: Release of cartilage mucopolysaccharide-degrading neutral protease from human leucocytes. J. Exp. Med. 138:461, 1973.
137. Stiles, M.A., and Fraenkel-Conrat, J.: Subcellular distribution of human leukocytic cathepsins. Blood 32:119, 1968.
138. Rojas-Espinosa, O., Dannenberg, A.M., Murphy, P.A., Straat, P.A., Huang, P.C., and James, S.P.: Purification and properties of the cathepsin D type proteinase from beef and rabbit lung and its identification in macrophages. Infect. Immun. 8:100, 1973.
139. Ehrlich, H.P., and Gordon, J.L.: Proteinases in platelets. In Gordon, J. (ed.): Platelets in Biology and Pathology. Amsterdam, North-Holland Publishing Company, 1976, pp. 353–372.
140. Starkey, P.M., Gordon, J., Ehrlich, H.P., and Barrett, A.J.: Do platelets contain elastase? Haemostasis 39:542, 1978.
141. Hornebeck, W., Starkey, P.M., Gordon, J.L., Legrand, Y., Pignaud, G., Robert, L., Caen, J.P., Ehrlich, H.P., and Barrett, A.J.: The elastase-like enzyme of platelets. Thromb. Haemostas. 42:1681, 1981.
142. Ohlsson, K.: α_1-Antitrypsin and α_2-macroglobulin. Interactions with human neutrophil collagenase and elastase. Ann. N.Y. Acad. Sci. 256:409, 1975.
143. Abe, S., and Nagai, Y.: Evidence for the presence of a complex of collagenase with α_2-macroglobulin in human rheumatoid synovial fluid:

(TIMP) produced by human synovium and cartilage in culture. Clin. Sci. 61:711, 1981.

A possible regulatory mechanism of collagenase activity in vivo. J. Biochem. 73:897, 1973.

144. Harris, E.D. Jr., DiBona, D.R., and Krane, S.M.: Collagenases in human synovial fluid. J. Clin. Invest. 48:2104, 1969.

145. Saklatvala, J.: Hydrolysis of elastase substrate succinyltrialanine nitroanalide by a metal-dependent enzyme in rheumatoid synovial fluid. J. Clin. Invest. 59:794, 1977.

146. Henson, P.M.: Mechanisms of release of granulocyte enzymes from human neutrophils phagocytosing aggregated immunoglobulin. An electron microscopic study. Arthritis Rheum. 16:208, 1973.

147. Cochrane, C.G.: Role of granulocytes in immune complex-induced tissue injuries. Inflammation 2:319, 1977.

148. Campbell, E.J., Senior, R.M., McDonald, J.A., and Cox, D.L.: Proteolysis by neutrophils. Relative importance of cell-substrate contact and oxidative inactivation of proteinase inhibitors in vitro. J. Clin. Invest. 70:845, 1982.

149. Mohr, W., and Menninger, H.: Polymorphonuclear granulocytes at the pannus-cartilage junction in rheumatoid arthritis. Arthritis Rheum. 23:1413, 1980.

150. Mohr, W., Wessinghage, D., and Kohley, G.: The role of neutrophil granulocytes in the rheumatoid tissue destruction. I. Light microscopic demonstration of neutrophil polymorphonuclear cells in rheumatoid nodules. Z. Rheumatol. 39:322, 1980.

151. Lack, C.H.: Chondrolysis in arthritis. J. Bone Joint. Surg. 41:384, 1959.

152. Christman, O.D., Southwick, W.O., and Fessel, J.M.: Plasmin and articular cartilage. Yale J. Bio. Med. 34:524, 1962.

153. Wize, J., Sopata, I., Wojtecka-Lukasik, E., Ksiezny, S., and Dancewicz, A.M.: Isolation, purification and properties of a factor from rheumatoid synovial fluid activating the latent forms of collagenolytic enzymes. Acta Biochim. Polon. 22:239, 1975.

154. Wize, J., Abgarowicz, T., Wojtecka-Lukasik, E., Ksiezny, S., and Dancewicz, A.M.: Activation of human leucocyte procollagenase by rheumatoid synovial tissue culture medium. Ann. Rheum. Dis. 34:520, 1975.

155. Nagase, H., Cawston, T.E., DeSilva, M., and Barrett, A.J.: Identification of plasma kallikrein as an activator of latent collagenase in rheumatoid synovial fluid. Biochim. Biophys. Acta 702:133, 1982.

156. Brinckerhoff, C.E., and Harris, E.D. Jr.: Modulation by retinoic acid and corticosteroids of collagenase production by rabbit synovial fibroblasts treated with phorbol myristate acetate or polyethylene glycol. Biochim. Biophys. Acta. 677:424, 1981.

157. Brinckerhoff, C.E., McMillan, R.M., Fahey, J.V., and Harris, E.D. Jr.: Collagenase production by synovial fibroblasts treated with phorbol myristate acetate. Arthritis Rheum. 22:1109, 1979.

158. Harris, E.D. Jr., Reynolds, J.J., and Werb, Z.: Cytochalasin B increases collagenase production by cells in vitro. Nature 257:243, 1975.

159. Biswas, C., and Dayer, J.-H.: Stimulation of collagenase production by collagen in mammalian cell cultures. Cell 18:1035, 1979.

160. Harris, E.D. Jr., and Krane, S.M.: Effects of colchicine on collagenase in cultures of rheumatoid synovium. Arthritis Rheum. 14:669, 1971.

161. Wahl, L.M., Wahl, S.M., Mergenhagen, S.E., and Martin, G.R.: Collagenase production by lymphokine-activated macrophages. Science 187:261, 1975.

162. Dayer, J.-M., Russell, R.G.G., and Krane, S.M.: Collagenase production by rheumatoid synovial cells. Stimulation by a human lymphocyte factor. Science 195:181, 1977.

163. Dayer, J.-M., Breard, J., Chess, L., and Krane, S.M.: Participation of monocyte-macrophages and lymphocytes in the production of a factor which stimulates collagenase release by rheumatoid synovial cells. J. Clin. Invest. 64:1386, 1979.

164. Dayer, J.-M., Robinson, D.R., and Krane, S.M.: Prostaglandin produc-

tion by rheumatoid synovial cells. Stimulation by a factor from human mononuclear cells. J. Exp. Med. 145:1399, 1977.

165. Meats, J.E., McGuire, M.B., and Russell R.G.G.: Human synovium releases a factor which stimulates chondrocyte production of PGE and plasminogen activator. Nature 286:891, 1980.

166. Dayer, J.-M., Stephenson, M.L., Schmidt, E., Karge, W., and Krane, S.M.: Purification of a factor from blood monocyte-macrophages which stimulates the production of collagenase and prostaglandin E$_2$ by cells cultured from rheumatoid synovial tissues. FEBS Lett. 124:253, 1981.

167. Dayer, J.-M., Passwell, J.H., Schneeberger, E.E., and Krane, S.M.: Interactions among rheumatoid synovial cells and monocyte-macrophages: production of collagenase stimulating factor by human monocytes exposed to Con A or immunoglobulin Fc fragments. J. Immunol. 124:1712, 1980.

168. Dayer, J.-M., Trentham, D.E., and Krane, S.M.: Collagens act as ligands to stimulate human monocytes to produce mononuclear cell factor (MCF) and prostaglandins (PGE$_2$). Collagen Rel. Res. 2:523, 1982.

169. Amento, E.P., Kurnick, J.T., Epstein, A., and Krane, S.M.: Modulation of synovial cell products by a factor from a human cell line: T lymphocyte induction of a mononuclear cell factor. Proc. Natl. Acad. Sci. USA 79:5307, 1982.

170. Huybrechts-Godin, G., Hauser, P., and Vaes, G.: Macrophage-fibroblast interactions in collagenase production and cartilage degradation. Biochem. J. 184:643, 1979.

171. Mizel, S.B., Dayer, J.-M., Krane, S.M., and Mergenhagen, S.E.: Stimulation of rheumatoid synovial cell collagenase and prostaglandin production by partially purified lymphocyte activating factor (interleukin 1). Proc. Natl. Acad. Sci. USA 78:2474, 1981.

172. Postlethwaite, A.E., Lachman, L.B., Mainardi, C.L., and Kang, A.H.: Interleukin 1 stimulation of collagenase production by cultured fibroblasts. J. Exp. Med. 157:801, 1983.

173. Mizel, S.B., and Mizel, D.: Purification to apparent homogeneity of murine interleukin 1. J. Immunol. 126:834, 1981.

174. Saklatvala, J.: Characterization of catabolin, the major product of pig synovial tissue that induces resorption of cartilage proteoglycan in vitro. Biochem. J. 199:705, 1981.

175. Pilsworth, L.M., and Saklatvala, J.: The cartilage resorbing protein catabolin is made by synovial fibroblasts and its production is enhanced by phorbol myristate acetate. Biochem. J. 216:481, 1983.

176. Saklatvala, J., and Sarsfield, S.J.: Lymphocytes induce resorption of cartilage by producing catabolin. Biochem. J. 202:275, 1982.

176a. Saklatvala, J. Curry, V.A., and Sarsfield, S.J.: Purification to homogeneity of pig leucocyte catabolin, a protein that causes cartilage resorption in vitro. Biochem. J. 215:385, 1983.

177. Saklatvala, J., Sarsfield, S.J., and Pilsworth, L.M.C.: Characterization of proteins from human synovium and mononuclear leucocytes that induce resorption of cartilage proteoglycan in vitro. Biochem. J. 209:337, 1983.

178. Lachman, L.B., Hacker, M.P., and Handschumacher, R.E.: Partial purification of human lymphocyte activating factor (LAF) by ultrafiltration and electrophoretic techniques. J. Immunol. 119:2019, 1977.

179. Goldstein, I.M., Hoffstein, S., Gallin, J., and Weissmann, G.: Mechanisms of lysosomal enzyme release from human leukocytes. Microtubule assembly and membrane fusion induced by a component of complement. Proc. Natl. Acad. Sci. USA. 70:2916, 1973.

180. Schorlemmer, H.-U., Davies, P., and Allison, A.C.: Ability of activated complement components to induce lysosomal enzyme release from macrophages. Nature 261:48, 1976.

181. Vater, C.A., Mainardi, C.L., and Harris, E.D. Jr.: Binding of latent rheumatoid synovial collagenase to collagen fibrils, Biochim. Biophys. Acta 539:238, 1978.

Chapter 13

Connective Tissue: Small Blood Vessels and Capillaries

Judah Folkman, Dianna Ausprunk, and Robert Langer

INTRODUCTION

Proliferation and regression of vascular endothelium play important roles in a variety of biologic processes. These include wound healing, inflammatory granulation tissue, some immunologic reactions, organization of thrombi, and growth of tumors. Vascular proliferation may determine the rate of progression of certain diseases, e.g., diabetic retinopathy, rheumatoid arthritis, and neoplasia.

Vascular endothelium throughout the body is generally of at least two types: (1) large vessel endothelium such as in the aorta and vena cava, and (2) capillary endothelium. Only recently has it been appreciated that there are some functional differences between these two kinds of endothelium. For example, in cell culture, there are differences in growth rate and response to specific growth factors, and morphologic differences. Here we will be concerned primarily with capillary endothelium.

EMBRYOLOGY

It is not appropriate in this chapter to examine in detail the developmental biology of the vascular system. However, one general theme seems to have some bearing on capillary proliferation and arthritis. In the embryo, many organs do not originally contain or develop their own vessels. Instead, the anlage of such an organ is "invaded" by capillaries that later establish arterial and venous patterns unique to that organ. The vessels and their vascular endothelium, however, arise as a completely separate tissue[1] from primitive cells in the yolk sac that quickly differentiate into hematopoietic cells and vascular endothelial cells. Capillary tubes form. The capillaries grow, migrate, and invade the various organs. For example, the kidney of the mouse embryo is an avascular island of mesenchyme until day 11, when it is invaded by new capillary blood vessels. This has been elegantly confirmed by Ekblom's experiments in which mouse renal primordium was transplanted to the chorioallantoic membrane of the chick embryo.[2]

The liver anlage also begins as an avascular field of mesenchyme that is invaded by capillary sprouts. The same pattern is seen with the limb bud and bone.[3] Vessels enter the limb bud at a time when it is a small clump of cartilage cells. Chondrolysis occurs in the path of the advancing capillary tips. Bone formation follows. Vessel advance is finally halted at the end of the limb at the future joint cartilage. In certain cartilages, such as the human mandibular condyle, vascular canals and their contained vessels do not regress until the neonatal period.[4]

The development of mammalian joints is described in detail by O'Rahilly and Gardner[5] (see also Chapter 16). By the time the limb bud center contains mostly chondrocytes that have developed from mesenchyme, the synovial mesenchyme develops and is itself soon vascularized. Cavitation then takes place beneath the synovial membrane. Under normal conditions, once the joint cavity is formed, the vessels in the synovial membrane never contact the joint cartilage. However, in progressive stages of arthritis, these vessels generate the new capillaries that eventually contact and invade cartilage.

MAINTENANCE OF NORMAL VASCULAR ENDOTHELIUM DURING ADULT LIFE

In the adult, vascular endothelium occupies an estimated 2 kg of the body weight. It is a ubiquitous tissue and represents a population of cells that undergo a very slow renewal. Mitoses are rarely encountered in adult endothelium, and autoradiographic studies with ^{3}H-labeled thymidine have confirmed the rarity of cell division. However, there is considerable variability in the normal rate of endothelial labeling among different tissues. For example, the labeling index with ^{3}H-thymidine was 0.13 percent in myocardial capillaries, while it was only 0.01 percent in the retina.[6] In fact, retinal vessels may be the most resistant to an angiogenic stimulus of any vascular bed. Most published ^{3}H-thymidine labeling indices of capillary endothelium have been less than 1 percent, being most often in the vicinity of 0.1 percent.

Against this background of sluggish turnover, the capillary endothelium in some organs undergoes slow waves of proliferation in response to physiological stimuli. For example, endothelial proliferation occurs in the endometrium during the menstrual cycle and has been induced experimentally by diethylstilbestrol.[7] Also, capillaries around hair follicles undergo cyclic changes during the hair growth cycle.[8] It is not known what factors are responsible for the normal level of maintenance that keeps the whole vascular network coated with a monolayer of endothelium. Nor is it clear if certain diseases like scleroderma, in which capillaries appear to be disintegrating, result from diminution of some "maintenance" factor or appearance of a factor harmful to endothelial cells (see Chapter 76).

NEOVASCULARIZATION

The term neovascularization is used for convenience to categorize those conditions in which capillary proliferation occurs beyond the normal requirements for maintenance. Examples are the capillary proliferation that takes place in the healing of large wounds; granulation tissue that follows necrotizing inflammation; delayed hypersensitivity reaction; diabetic retinopathy; retrolental fibroplasia; rheumatoid arthritis; and neoplasia.

Angiogenesis is the term generally used to describe the phenomenon that eventually generates new capillary blood vessels. The proliferation of capillaries has been studied extensively in such systems as the rabbit ear chamber, the hamster cheek pouch, and the cremaster muscle. The light and electron microscopic sequence of events in the formation of new capillary blood vessels has been well described.[9] In all these systems, wounds were used as the vascularization stimulus.

The study of tumor angiogenesis and the mechanisms of angiogenesis in general required the development of new techniques that could be quantitated. Also, methods were needed that would permit the study of biochemical compounds that would stimulate angiogenesis or inhibit it. Four methods, developed over the past decade, are now used by most investigators who study angiogenesis.

New Methods of Studying Angiogenesis

The Corneal Micropocket. This technique permits the linear measurement of individual growing capillaries. Tumor implants (1 mm³) are inserted into a pocket made in the cornea of a rabbit at a distance of 1 to 2 mm from the edge of the cornea and the normal vascular bed[10] (Fig. 13–1). New capillaries grow at right angles from the edge of the cornea and elongate toward the tumor at approximately 0.2 mm per day (Fig. 13–2). They are measured with a slit-lamp stereoscope. Tissues or biochemical compounds can be interposed between the tumor and its vascular bed. For example, the angiogenesis inhibitory property of protamine was demonstrated in this way.[11] The rabbit cornea has some unique anatomic features: It is avascular; new vessels grow into it in a two-dimensional plane; accurate measurements of vessel growth can be made; and, finally, the anatomic separation of the angiogenic stimulus from the responding vascular bed ensures easy identification of new vessels because they arise at right angles to the preexisting limbal vasculature. A disadvantage is that heterologous tumors, once vascularized, may excite an immune response. Subsequent immunologic neovascularization superimposed on tumor neovascularization may be confusing. This problem can be avoided by the implantation of mouse tumor into the cornea of inbred

Figure 13–1. Method of implanting a sustained-release polymer pellet in the cornea. Through a small incision in the cornea, an intracorneal pocket is made with a spatula. The rabbit has been anesthetized. A slow-release polymer pellet is then implanted into the cornea.

mice.[12] Nonspecific inflammation is another problem of this assay. Inflammatory agents can often be defined by their ability to attract leukocytes (mainly polymorphonuclear neutrophils, lymphocytes, or macrophages).[13] These cells then migrate rapidly into the cornea and may themselves elicit or enhance neovascularization. For example, solutions that are hyperosmotic or of abnormally low or high pH are inflammatory. Whenever a new substance is tested for angiogenic activity, histologic sections are essential to determine if the angiogenesis has been induced directly or indirectly.

Sustained-Release Polymer Implants. After the corneal micropocket technique was developed, the testing

Figure 13–2. Rabbit cornea viewed through a slit-lamp stereoscope. A sustained-release pellet of ethylene vinyl acetate copolymer containing tumor-derived angiogenic activity has been implanted approximately 2 mm from the periphery of the cornea (limbus). New capillaries have grown toward the implant at a mean rate of approximately 0.2 mm/per day.

of fractions for angiogenesis activity required that they be released over a sustained period of time so that a concentration gradient could be established within the cornea. Two polymeric systems were developed that could release proteins and other macromolecules at approximately zero-order kinetics for periods of weeks to months.[14-16] These polymers are poly-hydroxyethyl methacrylate and ethylene-vinyl acetate co-polymer. They are not inflammatory when implanted as small pellets (1 mm³) in the cornea.

Chick Embryo–Chorioallantoic Membrane. As biochemists attempted to purify angiogenic fractions from tumor and normal tissues, a need arose for a rapid screening assay for large numbers of test fractions that would be less expensive than rabbits and would avoid the problem of immunologic reactions. A method of dropping the chorioallantoic membrane and opening the eggshell to reveal a large expanse of chorioallantoic vascular membrane was previously described by Leighton.[17] We learned that the vessels of the chorioallantoic membrane grow rapidly until day 11, after which endothelial proliferation rapidly decreases.[18] Tumors or tumor fractions implanted on day 9 gave the most reproducible angiogenic response within 48 to 72 hours. This response could be recognized under a 6× stereoscope as new capillary loops converging on the implant.[18,19]

Cloned Capillary Endothelial Cells. Recently it has been possible to isolate cloned capillary endothelial cells and passage them in vitro for long periods of time.[20] This method is being used to test for endothelial cell mitogens. It has also confirmed in vivo observations implying that capillary growth is a multistep phenomenon that unfolds as an orderly sequence of events.

Sequential Steps of Capillary Growth

By studying angiogenesis with these techniques, it has become clear that capillary growth takes place by a series of steps that are much the same regardless of the type of angiogenic stimulus. These steps can be summarized as follows: (i) New capillaries originate from small venules. Larger vessels with layers of smooth muscle do not usually give rise to capillary sprouts. (ii) Local degradation of the basement membrane on the side of the venule closest to the angiogenic stimulus[21] is one of the earliest events. Capillary endothelial cells stimulated in vitro by angiogenic substances secrete high concentrations of collagenase and plasminogen activator.[22,23] Also, fetal aortic endothelial cells degrade types IV and V collagen as they migrate when the stimulus for migration is an angiogenic factor.[24] These findings suggest that the local degradation of basement membrane in vivo is carried out directly by endothelial cells once they receive an angiogenic stimulus. (iii) Through this opening in the basement membrane, leader endothelial cells begin to migrate toward the angiogenic stimulus.[21] (iv) Endothelial cells that follow the leaders align in a bipolar fashion as the first sprout begins to form. (v) Lumen formation begins. In most examples of postembryonic angiogenesis, a lumen appears to be produced by a cur-

vature that develops in the capillary endothelial cell, as if the cytoskeleton itself were responsible. This phenomenon has been observed in vivo in the cornea[21] and also in vitro.[25,26] However, during early embryonic angiogenesis lumen formation may take place by vacuole formation. This has also been observed in vivo[27] and in vitro.[25] (vi) Endothelial cells in the mid-section of the sprout begin to undergo mitosis. The leading capillary endothelial cells at the very tip of the sprout continue to migrate, but usually do not divide. (vii) Loop formation occurs next as individual sprouts join or anastomose with each other. These loops then elongate and may be the origin of additional sprouts. The loops continue to converge upon the angiogenic target. (viii) Flow begins sluggishly after loops have formed. (ix) Pericytes emerge along the length of the capillary sprouts. (x) Synthesis of new basement membrane follows.

When cloned capillary endothelial cells are cultured, i.e. "angiogenesis in vitro," most of these same events occur. Tubes form, branches appear, and whole capillary networks develop.[25] Maciag has shown that these in vitro "tubes" can also form from umbilical vein endothelial cells and that they are hollow and will carry fluid.[26] Fetal aortic endothelial cells can also generate tubes in culture.[28] Pericytes are absent in vitro. When these in vitro findings are taken together with in vivo observations, they suggest that all of the information necessary to form tubular structures and build an entire capillary network can be expressed by vascular endothelial cells. The program that is expressed seems to be similar for each type of angiogenic stimulus, whether the source of the stimulus is inflammatory, immunologic, or neoplastic.

Modulation of the Rate of Capillary Growth

While the instructions for generating a capillary network originate from the vascular endothelial cell (once it is stimulated), the *rate* at which this endothelial cell program is revealed is modulated by several nonendothelial components. Two of these that have recently been studied in some detail are matrix components and mast cells.

Matrix Components Modulate Endothelial Proliferation and Differentiation. *Collagen.* When rat capillary endothelial cells are cultured on interstitial collagens (i.e., types I, III), they proliferate rapidly until a confluent monolayer is formed.[29] They form tubes only after very long periods of culture (i.e., 2 to 4 weeks). By contrast, when these cells are grown on basement membrane collagens (types IV and V), the cells do not proliferate but aggregate and form tubes early, i.e., after 4 days. Also, cells grown on basement membrane collagen produced more basement membrane constituents than did endothelial cells grown on interstitial collagen. In a confirmatory experiment, capillary endothelial cells were grown on either side of an amniotic membrane which was itself acellular. On the basement membrane surface these cells formed early tubelike structures and did not

Figure 13–3. *A*, Electron micrograph of an endothelial cell (*E*) in a nonstimulated quiescent venule at the edge of the cornea, 2 days after implanting heat-killed tumor in a corneal pocket. The flattened cell has smooth contours, makes junctional contact with a neighboring cell (arrow), and is covered by a continuous basal lamina. (*B*). The vessel lumen contains erythrocytes (*R*). × 12,000. *B*, Endothelial cell (*E*) in a blood vessel at edge of cornea, 1 day after implanting live tumor in the cornea. The cell exhibits increased thickness, luminal projections (*P*), an increase in cytoplasmic organelles, and fragmentation of the basal lamina (arrow). × 13,500. (From Ausprunk, D.H., and Folkman, J.: Microvasc. Res. 14:53, 1977. With permission of the publisher.)

Figure 13–4. Limbal endothelial cell 2 days after tumor implant in cornea. A larger cytoplasmic extension (*E*) protudes into the perivascular connective tissue in the direction of the tumor implant. This pseudopod is mostly devoid of basal lamina. Carbon particles (arrows) have escaped from the vessel lumen (*L*) through a large intercellular gap (*G*). × 7700. (From Ausprunk, D.H., and Folkman, J.: J. Microvasc. Res. 14:53, 1977. With permission of the publisher.)

migrate through the basement membrane. In contrast, on the stromal surface (i.e., interstitial collagen) the endothelial cells proliferated and migrated into the stromal surface of the amnion. Tubelike structures occurred only occasionally and formed much later (21 days) and not until high cell densities were present. Taken together, these studies show that different collagenous components of extracellular matrix direct endothelial cells either toward proliferation and migration or toward tube formation. These collagenous components may have a similar role in vivo. Their relevance to neovascularization of the joint (as, for example, in rheumatoid arthritis) may be as follows: While vascular endothelium within the joint could be activated by angiogenic activity from macrophages or immune lymphocytes, whether or not they "invade" joint tissues may depend upon the state of collagen in the extravascular matrix.

Glycosaminoglycans. In mature resting (nonproliferating) capillaries, the basement membrane is rich in glycosaminoglycans, of which heparan sulfate is the most prominent. Highly sulfated glycosaminoglycans produced by vascular endothelial cells and incorporated in their matrix appear to help maintain the nonproliferative state of capillary endothelium. In contrast, proliferating capillaries have little or no basement membrane. Endothelial cells synthesize primarily nonsulfated glycosaminoglycans, mainly hyaluronate, which remain associated with the cells and are not secreted into the matrix. This GAG pattern has been observed during embryonic

angiogenesis[30] and also in inflammatory and tumor angiogenesis.[31,32]

Whether the extent of GAG sulfation and collagen type act independently on capillary growth and maturation, or together, is unknown.

Mast Cells Promote Angiogenesis But Cannot Initiate It. Mast cells have been observed to accumulate around many types of solid tumors.[33] These cells are especially conspicuous in the neighborhood of in situ tumors prior to vascularization. In experimental studies with the chick embryo, mast cells accumulated at the site of the tumor extract within 24 hours after implantation and increased to 40-fold above normal mast cell density. Furthermore, mast cells preceded the new vessel sprouts that were converging upon the tumor site. However, mast cells added to the chorioallantoic membrane could not initiate angiogenesis.[34]

These findings suggested that mast cells might play an amplifying or a promoting role in the growth of new capillaries.

It has recently been reported that mast cells are significantly increased in the synovial membranes of patients with rheumatoid arthritis, and that mast cell counts were directly related to the intensity of clinical synovitis in the affected joint.[85]

Heparin Is the Mediator by Which Mast Cells Amplify Capillary Growth. After it became possible to grow capillary endothelial cells in long-term culture,[20] an assay was developed to measure their migration in vitro (chemokinesis).[35] This method was based upon phagokinetic

Figure 13–5. *A* A new lumen (*IU*) formed within the wall of an existing venule. It is the origin of a new capillary sprout, and is surrounded by two endothelial cells (*EI, E2*) that retain contact with the lumen (*L*) of the parent vessel. Two days after tumor implant. × 31,000. (From Ausprunk, D.H., and Folkman J.: Microvasc. Res. 14:53, 1977. With permission of the publisher.) *B*, A capillary sprout (*C*) adjacent to a preformed limbal venule (*V*) four days after tumor implant. The pseudopods (arrows) extending from the endothelial cells of the capillary suggest that the section is near the tip of this sprout. The double layer of active-appearing endothelial cells (*E*) in the venule indicates that the new capillary has probably budded from this vessel. × 6000.

Figure 13–6. A later step in capillary formation. Endothelial cells align with each other, end to end, to form a sprout. The leading tip of such a sprout extends through collagen of the rabbit cornea. A lumen is beginning to form in the mid-section of this sprout. (Scanning electron micrograph × 2300.)

tracks, which cells make as they travel over colloidal gold and ingest it.[36] Culture medium conditioned by rat mast cells stimulated *migration* of capillary endothelial cells in vitro in a dose-dependent manner, but it did not stimulate proliferation[37] (Fig. 13–8).

These results suggest that mast cells may enhance angiogenesis by increasing the rate of directional migration of capillary endothelial cells toward an angiogenic stimulus such as tumor. When many mast cell products were tested, only heparin was found to significantly stimulate capillary endothelial cell migration.[37] Heparin could completely substitute for mast-cell-conditioned medium. Heparin antagonists such as protamine and heparinase blocked the stimulatory effect of heparin on capillary endothelial cell migration. When heparin was applied to the chorioallantoic membrane of the chick embryo at the time of implantation of tumor or tumor extract, angiogenesis was enhanced.[11] There was intense neovascularization at the site of tumor extracts within 1 day instead of 3 days as previously. Also, lower concentrations of tumor angiogenesis activity were detectable. Nonanticoagulant heparin lacking antithrombin III activity (supplied by Dr. Robert Rosenberg) also enhanced angiogenesis. Furthermore, neither heparin nor its nonanticoagulant subcomponents could initiate angiogenesis over a wide range of concentrations up to 500 times the enhancing dose.

Figure 13–7. New capillary loop in cornea, showing beginning of another capillary sprout (arrow). × 160. India ink injection after implant of TAF pellet in cornea.

Figure 13–8. The effect of mast cell products on migration of bovine capillary endothelial cells. The mast cell products were dissolved in DMEM 10% calf serum and tested at log dose intervals from 10 ng to 1 mg/per ml. Heparin (solid circle); chondroitin sulfate A,B,C, (solid square); eosinophilic chemotactic factor-A (open square); and histamine phosphate (solid triangle). Each point represents the mean area of 100 phagokinetic tracks ± SEM. (Reprinted from *The Journal of Experimental Medicine* 152:931–944, 1980, with permission of the publisher.)

Angiogenesis Factors from Non-neoplastic Cells

There are some recently discovered inducers of vascularization that may have an important role in mediating the neovascularization of the synovium in rheumatoid arthritis. Under certain conditions, lymphocytes and also macrophages have been found to liberate such substances.

Lymphocytes. Certain immune reactions are followed by neovascularization. The present experimental evidence suggests that white cells precede capillary invasion into the target tissue and then send back a diffusible signal that stimulates capillary proliferation. The best evidence so far comes from the studies of Sidky and Auerbach.[38] Originally Auerbach found that a rabbit's own lymph node implanted into its own cornea elicited neither neovascularization nor any other reaction. However, a lymph node implant from another outbred rabbit caused a weak vascular response after some delay. In contrast, a lymph node from a mouse produced a strong neovascular response. However, a lymph node from a nude mouse (thymic deficient) was unable to stimulate neovascularization in the rabbit eye.

Therefore, more extensive studies were undertaken using inbred mouse spleen cells. Those cells were injected intradermally into recipient normal animals that had been irradiated a few hours previously with 800 roentgens. After 2 to 3 days the animals were sacrificed, and the injection sites exposed by dissection. The number of new vessels was counted in the vascular response. No vascular response was seen in syngeneic combinations, i.e., donor spleen cells from the same animal strain. In contrast, allogeneic spleen cells inoculated into an irradiated normal recipient gave a typical vascular response.[39] Recent studies support these findings.[40] In other studies, an increase in capillary density[41] and extensive proliferation of postcapillary venular endothelium[42] were found in lymph nodes that were undergoing strong immunologic reactions.

Macrophages. Macrophages also appear capable of stimulating capillary endothelium under certain conditions. The first hint of this came from the observation that significant vascular endothelial proliferation and delayed hypersensitivity reactions occurred in the skin of guinea pigs at the time of maximal mononuclear cell infiltration.[43] It was further found that macrophages activated in vivo or in vitro and the medium conditioned by these cells were capable of inducing vascular proliferation in the guinea pig cornea.[44] Macrophages obtained from guinea pigs previously injected with paraffin oil or thioglycolate induced neovascularization in the cornea. Furthermore, macrophage-conditioned medium that had been dialyzed, concentrated, and impregnated into the cornea induced vessel growth. The microvascular responses were not associated with an acute inflammatory response. Also, the neovascularization could not be attributed solely to an immunologic reaction, because it was produced in a completely syngeneic cell system. In these and other studies, only activated macrophages (achieved either in vivo or in vitro) had the capacity to induce formation of new vessels, findings that parallel studies of enzymes and stimulatory factors released by macrophages (see Chapter 10).

Macrophages may play a key role as stimulators of blood vessel growth during wound healing.[45-47] Macrophages obtained from wounds have been shown to release angiogenic activity.[48] An angiogenic factor from wound fluid has been partially purified and found to be chemotactic for endothelial cells in vitro. It is a polypeptide with a molecular weight of approximately 10,000.[49] Furthermore, release of angiogenesis activity by wound macrophages was increased as local oxygen tension fell.

The increasing understanding about the angiogenic capacity of immune lymphocytes and activated macrophages may have important implications for arthritis. Synovial fluid from joints with rheumatoid arthritis contains angiogenic activity[50] and often has decreased oxygen tension. However, the cellular source of angiogenic activity in rheumatoid arthritis joint fluid has not been determined.

A factor has been discovered in the supernatant of proliferating fat cells (adipocytes) that stimulates capillary proliferation in vitro and angiogenesis in the chorioallantoic membrane. The adipocytes originated from 3T3 fibroblasts[51] that had differentiated in culture. Angiogenic activity was not found in the precursor cells.

At least six normal tissues have been reported to elicit angiogenesis during brief periods of their adult life. These are corpus luteum,[52,53] retina,[54,55] testicle,[56] skin,[57,58] salivary gland,[59] and kidney.[60] However, for each tissue, the cell or cells responsible for expressing angiogenic activity are unknown.

Regression of Capillaries

Newly formed capillaries are not static but undergo remodeling. Some differentiate to form arterioles and venules, whereas others regress and disappear completely.[61] For example, certain vascular networks in the embryo seem to be intrinsically programmed for regression.[62] By contrast, tumor-induced vessels seem to depend for their maintenance upon the continuous presence of angiogenic activity at appropriate concentrations. By taking advantage of this short "half-life" of tumor-induced vessels, it has become possible to initiate capillary regression at will in the vascularized rabbit cornea. In this way, the topographic, histologic, and ultrastructural changes that occur in regressing capillaries can be precisely timed and sequenced.[63]

Pellets of ethylene-vinyl acetate co-polymer[63] were impregnated with partially purified tumor extracts that were angiogenic and implanted in corneal pockets 1.5 mm from the limbal vascular plexus. The polymer pellets were set to release up to 1 μg of this angiogenic protein per day for as long as 3 months. Four or 5 days after the implant, small capillaries penetrated the corneas and grew toward the polymer pellets at a rate of approximately 0.2 mm per day. They surrounded the polymers

POLYMER
REMOVED

(a) (b)

FIRST WEEK

(c) (d)

THIRD WEEK   TENTH WEEK

Figure 13-9. Diagram of the slit-lamp appearance of blood vessels in the cornea during regression. *a*, Before removing the TAF containing polymer, which had been implanted 10 to 12 days earlier. *b*, One week after polymer removal; only the largest vessels remain. *c*, These are thinner by the third week. *d*, Only two or three bloodless vessels persist to 10 weeks. (From Ausprunk, D.H., et al.: Lab. Invest. 38: 284, 1978. With permission of the publisher.)

by 10 to 12 days. Vessels then stopped growing but persisted in the cornea for at least 2 months if the polymer implants remained in place. However, if the pellets were removed 2 to 3 weeks after implantation, capillaries began to regress. The gross appearance in the slit-lamp stereoscope is shown schematically in Figure 13-9.

During regression, capillaries gradually narrow; by the end of the first week, the small distal branches disappear. Intravenously injected fluorescein appears rapidly in corneal vessels until 3 weeks after the onset of regression. Thereafter, vessels are not perfusable, as fluorescein cannot be detected by slit-lamp microscopy. At the microscopic level, the following sequence of morphologic changes occurs in the regressing vessels, regardless of vessel diameter or location within the vascular tree:

1. Endothelial cell changes and platelet sticking. One to 2 days after the removal of the stimulus, endothelial cells lining the distal corneal vessels contain swollen mitochondria and irregular cytoplasmic projections along their luminal surfaces (Fig. 13-10). Some cells become very thin or exhibit fenestrations. Fenestrated endothelium has never been observed in nonregressing corneal capillaries. Simultaneously, platelets adhere to the vessel wall (Fig. 13-11).

2. Stasis. Distal capillary branches become plugged with erythrocytes 1 to 2 days after removal of tumor angiogenesis pellets. However, larger, more proximal vessels are still perfused.

3. Endothelial cell degeneration. After stasis occurs, endothelial cells began to degenerate and lyse.

4. Removal of vessel debris. Dying endothelial cells are removed by macrophages. These mononuclear clear cells accumulate in the perivascular tissue of the cornea during the first week of regression (Fig. 13-12). They surround the degenerating capillaries and ingest the cell

debris. By 6 to 10 weeks, only lipid-filled macrophages and some fibroblasts remain in most corneas.

Throughout the blood vessel regression, only an occasional polymorphonuclear neutrophil or mast cell is seen. The same sequence is observed when vessels regress after removal of different kinds of angiogenic stimuli, such as a sodium hydroxide pellet (e.g., vessels induced by an inflammatory stimulus instead of by tumor).

This corneal study has particular implications for cartilage, because both are avascular tissues that can be invaded by proliferating capillaries during certain pathologic states. The similar regressive behavior of blood vessels in these studies, whether induced by a neoplastic stimulus or an inflammatory stimulus, suggests that the fate of proliferating vessels is determined by a balance between the local environment and the continued presence of the vascularization stimulus. In normally vascularized tissue, such as a healed wound, regenerated blood vessels do not all regress.[64] Many are remodeled to restore the microvascular bed of the healed tissue. By contrast, the disappearance of *all* corneal vessels suggests that, whatever the stimulus for initiating vascularization, it must be continuously present to maintain the newly formed vessels and that it may be acting to overcome an inhibitor of angiogenesis in the cornea. The mechanism of regression is still unclear. That endothelial cells degenerate so soon after removal of the angiogenic stimulus implies that a humoral signal (in this case angiogenic activity from tumors) acts as a critically essen-

Figure 13-10. Sick endothelial cell in corneal capillary sprout, 1 day after removal of TAF polymer. Mitochondria are swollen, and the plasma membrane exhibits surface projection. × 19,500. *Inset:* Cell cytoplasm is attenuated and displays fenestrations. × 29,000. (From Ausprunk, D.H., et al.: Lab. Invest 38:284, 1978. With permission of the publisher.)

Figure 13–11. Platelets (*P*) accumulating in a small corneal blood vessel 2 days after removing a TAF polymer. Gaps (arrows) have formed between endothelial cells, permitting extravasation of vessel contents. The larger vessel is more normal in appearance except for a few platelets which adhere to the endothelium closest to the small vessel. × 9000. (From Ausprunk, D.H., et al.: Lab. Invest. 38:284, 1978. With permission of the publisher.)

Figure 13–12. Regressing corneal vessels three days after removal of the TAF polymer. Monocytic cells (*C*) have infiltrated the perivascular stroma and are differentiating into macrophages (*M*). The smallest capillaries are plugged with erythrocytes × 900. (From Ausprunk, D.H., et al.: Lab. Invest. 38:284, 1978. With permission of the publisher.)

tial growth factor with a short half-life. Once there is blood stasis and macrophages have moved in, the process of regression appears to be irreversible.

Angiogenesis Inhibitors

The term "antiangiogenesis" was proposed in 1972 to describe a potential therapy based on compounds that might specifically inhibit capillary proliferation.[65]

At that time, no such "angiogenesis inhibitor" existed. Clinical clues suggested that cartilage might contain such an inhibitor. For example, in mice, carcinomas induced in the ear by chemical carcinogens rarely infiltrate the cartilage but grow instead only in the surrounding tissues.[66] Furthermore, in certain human tumors, the field of neovascularization around the tumor stops at a cartilage interface. An example is squamous cell carcinoma of the trachea in which the tumor is unable to induce vascularization from the zone around the cartilage ring. Another example is osteogenic sarcoma, in which the tumor rarely enters the epiphyseal plate or the joint cartilage. Also, developmental studies on limb formation in the embryo have shown that vessels invade the field of chondrocytes that occupy the future central portion of a long bone. This is followed by chondrolysis and bone formation. However, zones of articular cartilage emerge in the neonatal period in an avascular state.[67]

The first experimental evidence for this inhibitor came from implants of cartilage in the chick embryo. It was reported that pieces of cartilage placed on the chorioallantoic membrane of the chick embryo did not become vascularized.[68] The general idea was proposed that cartilage may be resistant to "invasion" by a variety of tissues such as inflammatory cells, new vessels, and tumor cells, because cartilage contains certain protease inhibitors. In subsequent papers,[69,70] Kuettner and colleagues reported isolation of a trypsin inhibitor and a collagenase inhibitor from cartilage. Quantitation of the angiogenesis inhibiting capacity of cartilage was obtained by implanting 1-mm^3 pieces of fresh neonatal rabbit or calf cartilage into the cornea of the rabbit eye.[71,72]

The cartilage was positioned between the normal vascular bed of the limbus and a tumor implant in the cornea. In this experiment, vessels induced by the tumor had to pass through the zone of the cartilage before reaching the tumor. Fresh cartilage was capable of inhibiting new vessel growth for up to 3 months. In contrast, boiled cartilage or pieces of bone or other "control" tissues had no inhibitory effects; neovascularization continued unabated. Large vascularized tumors formed, and the rabbits had to be sacrificed by 3 weeks.

A partially purified angiogenesis inhibitor has been isolated from cartilage.[73] The active fraction contained several different proteins; the major one had a molecular weight of 16,000. It strongly inhibited proteinase activity. When impregnated into a sustained-release polymer pellet of ethylene-vinyl acetate co-polymer and implanted into the cornea, this fraction produced no detectable reaction by itself. However, when tumor was implanted behind the slow-release pellet, vessels induced by the tumor stopped growing as they approached the polymer implant containing the cartilage inhibitor.[73] In contrast, various controls and heat-degraded inhibitor had no effect. The active inhibitor fraction has been further purified. Infusion of this cartilage-derived inhibitor into the carotid artery of rabbits at concentrations of 1 mg per day inhibited tumor-induced vessels in the eye, with no detectable toxicity.[74]

The most potent inhibitor of neovascularization prepared by this method inhibits both trypsin and collagenase (type I) and shows two proteins with pKs of approximately 4.6 and 6.5 by isoelectric focusing. A second fraction with inhibitory activity toward trypsin can be isolated from cartilage by affinity chromatography and preparative gel electrophoresis or high pressure liquid chromatography.[75] However, this fraction does not have antiangiogenesis activity. The collagenase inhibitor has been purified several thousand–fold by ion exchange chromatography, molecular sieve chromatography, heparin-sepharose chromatography, and concanavalin A chromatography. While not enough of this material has been isolated to test its antiangiogenic activity, preliminary results show that it effectively inhibits cell migration in tissue culture in response to tumor-conditioned media or other growth factors.[76] It is possible that a mechanism of vessel inhibition involves the neutralization of proteolytic or collagenolytic activity found in blood vessels.

A recent study has shown that sharks, whose entire endoskeleton is cartilage and does not undergo ossification, have up to 100,000 times more angiogenesis inhibitor on a per organism basis than calf cartilage.[77] It is interesting to note that elasmobranchs such as sharks, in contrast to mammals, bony fishes, reptiles, and amphibians, rarely exhibit neoplasms.[78,79]

Another demonstration that normal cartilage can resist invasion by vascular endothelial cells has been made by Pauli and colleagues.[80] Small discs of bovine articular cartilage are used as a substratum for culturing vascular endothelial cells. The cartilage is extracted with guanidine hydrochloride to deplete the tissue of the soluble proteoglycan pool as well as the factor that inhibits neovascularization. Endothelial cells adhere to this devitalized cartilage and form a monolayer.[81] After 6 days of incubation, a basement-membrane-like matrix forms between the endothelial cells and the cartilage. The few microvilli on the basal surface of the endothelial cells do not reach the cartilage matrix. However, addition of heparin or tumor extract (Walker 256 carcinoma cells) to the medium stimulates the endothelial cells to penetrate the cartilage matrix with numerous microvilli.[82] The observation that salt-extracted, devitalized cartilage can be penetrated by stimulated endothelial cells yet remain impermeable to fibroblastic ingrowth further supports the hypothesis of Kuettner and colleagues that hyaline cartilage contains extractable components that specifically inhibit the invasive apparatus of potentially invasive cells.[81]

Figure 13–13. A method of using the chick embryo for detecting angiogenesis inhibitors. Embryonated embryos are grown in petri dishes. A 10 μl pellet of 0.5 percent methylcellulose is placed on the yolk sac vascular membrane at day 4, and an avascular zone appears at day 6 if the pellet contains an angiogenic inhibitor (in this case 100 μg cortisone acetate and 12 μcg hexasaccharide fragment of heparin). Another method is to use 50 μg of hydrocortisone, implant the methylcellulose pellet on the 6 day chorioallantoic membrane, and look for an avascular zone 48 hours later.

No one has yet completely purified the cartilage-derived angiogenesis inhibitor. Nonetheless, the presence of angiogenesis-inhibiting activity in cartilage provided a clue that angiogenesis inhibitors might also be found in other tissues or natural products.

Subsequently, protamine was found to be a potent angiogenesis inhibitor.[11] This discovery was made during experiments carried out to demonstrate that heparin could enhance or promote tumor angiogenesis. Protamine is a known antagonist of heparin, and it blocked the ability of mast cells or heparin to stimulate migration of capillary endothelial cells in vitro.[37] Protamine is an arginine-rich basic protein, with a relative molecular weight of 4300, found only in sperm. Protamine also reversed the heparin enhancement of tumor angiogenesis when it was mixed in a 2:1 ratio (wt/wt) with the heparin. When protamine concentrations were increased further, all angiogenesis in the chick embryo was inhibited, even in the absence of exogenous heparin. Further studies showed that protamine could inhibit angiogenesis regardless of whether the angiogenic source was embryologic, inflammatory, immunogenic, or neoplastic. When protamine was administered systemically, it in-

hibited angiogenesis in lung metastases, restricting these lesions to the avascular phase and markedly limiting their size. However, the toxic side effects of protamine, unrelated to its antiangiogenic activity (hypocalcemia and anaphylaxis), did not permit the use of sufficiently high doses to treat large primary tumors.

Recently, a more potent method of angiogenesis inhibition has been discovered (Fig. 13–13). During an experiment in which heparin was added to the chorioallantoic membrane to enhance tumor-induced angiogenesis, cortisone was also added. The rationale was that tumor angiogenesis, enhanced by heparin, might be made more conspicuous in the chick embryo bioassay if cortisone were added to suppress background inflammation on the membrane (usually due to eggshell dust). The result was unexpected. While heparin alone enhanced tumor angiogenesis and cortisone alone had little or no effect, angiogenesis was inhibited by the combination of heparin and cortisone.[83] Further experiments showed that heparin and cortisone, when administered together, abolished angiogenesis regardless of the type of angiogenic stimulus. Inflammatory, immunologic, embryologic, and neoplastic forms of angiogenesis were strongly inhibited. Furthermore, a nonanticoagulant fragment of heparin could substitute for whole heparin in this synergism. This fragment is a hexasaccharide with a molecular weight of about 1600. It has been further found that heparin administered orally is degraded into nonanticoagulant fragments that have similar antiangiogenic effects in the presence of cortisone. When mice bearing large tumor masses of B16 melanoma, Lewis lung carcinoma, or reticulum cell sarcoma were allowed to drink heparin and cortisone, the tumors regressed and in the majority of animals were completely eradicated. Metastases were so markedly reduced that the majority of animals remained tumor free after the angiogenesis inhibition was discontinued. Several further experiments showed that the tumor regression was specifically the result of angiogenesis inhibition and not the effect of cytotoxicity. In fact, cortisone alone increased the number of metastases while heparin had little effect. And, the combination of cortisone and heparin in tissue culture increased the proliferation rate of all these tumor lines.

The mechanism of angiogenesis inhibition by this heparin fragment in the presence of cortisone is unknown. Nevertheless, the potent angiogenesis inhibition that can be obtained when these two compounds are administered either locally or systemically raises the possibility of their use against the destructive neovascularization in the joints of certain patients with rheumatoid arthritis.

Unanswered Questions

If an angiogenesis inhibitor as potent as the combination of hexa-saccharide and cortisone were available, could cartilage destruction be prevented? This and many other fundamental questions must be addressed before we can learn the full role of angiogenesis in diseases

CORTISONE

HEPARIN

CORTISONE + HEPARIN   CORTISONE + HEXASACCHARIDE

Figure 13–14. Inhibition of angiogenesis in the chorioallantoic membrane (CAM) of the chick embryo. Histologic cross-sections of 8 days CAMs. Test substances were implanted in a methylcellulose disc (10 μl) on day 6 and the histologic sections were made through this area on day 8. *A*, Cortisone alone: Ectoderm, vascular mesoderm and endoderm are normally developed. *B*, Heparin alone: All three layers are normally developed. *C*, Heparin plus cortisone: New vessel proliferation is inhibited in the mesoderm, leaving an avascular zone. *D* Hexasaccharide fragment of heparin plus cortisone: Similar avascular zone as produced in *C* and as viewed from above as seen in Figure 13–13. (From Folkman, et al.: Science 221:719, 1983, with permission of the publisher.)

such as rheumatoid arthritis. Some of these questions form the basis of investigations in other fields, such as tumor biology and diabetes research. For example: What are the requirements for the maintenance of endothelium in the normal microvasculature? How does a capillary, thinner than a hair, invade a tissue as tough as the cornea? What accounts for the directional growth of capillaries toward an angiogenic stimulus? Is there some undiscovered "chemotactic" mechanism for capillary endothelial cells that guides their migration? What is the role of fibrin? Could fibrin strands exuding from these capillary tips also help guide the migration of endothelium? Are angiogenesis inhibitors distributed in other normal tissues that parallel the angiogenesis inhibitor of cartilage? Finally, what are the signals that initiate capillary proliferation in the synovium, even before the formation of the pannus? Are these being secreted from activated macrophages or from sensitized lymphocytes? Once the angiogenesis stimulators from these cells have been identified, will they be detectable in the joint fluid

in early phases of arthritis? Is there a vascular permeability factor in inflammatory fluid similar to the one reported from certain tumor cells?[84] Regardless of which field of investigation leads to explanations of these questions, at least one basic mechanism that is common to several chronic diseases may be revealed.

References

1. Harr, J.A., and Ackerman, G.A.: A phase and electron microscopic study of vasculogenesis and erythropoiesis in the yolk sac of the mouse. Anat. Rec. 170:199, 1971.
2. Ekblom, P., Sariola, H., Karkinen, M., and Saxen, L.: The origin of the glomerular endothelium. Cell Differ. 11:35, 1982.
3. Smith, P.E., and Copenhaver, W.M.: Bailey's Textbook of Histology. Baltimore, Williams & Wilkins Company, 1953, p. 125.
4. Blackwood, H.J.J.: Vascularization of the condylar cartilage of the human mandible. J. Anat. 99:551, 1965.
5. O'Rahilly, R., and Gardner, E.: The embryology of movable joints. *In* Sokoloff, L. (ed.): The Joints and Synovial Fluid. Vol. I. New York, Academic Press, 1978.
6. Engerman, R.L., Pfaffenbach, D., and David, M.D.: Cell turnover of capillaries. Lab. Invest. 17:738, 1967.
7. Widman, J., and Cotran, R.S.: Personal communication.

8. Durward, A., and Randall, K.M.: Vascularity and patterns of growth of hair follicles. *In* Montagna, W, and Ellis, R.A. (eds.): The Biology of Hair Growth. New York, Academic Press, 1968.
9. Schoefl, G.I.: Growing capillaries: Their structure and permeability. Arch. Path. Anat. Physiol. 337:97, 1963.
10. Gimbrone, M.A., Jr., Cotran, R.S., Leapman, S.B., and Folkman, J.: Tumor growth and neovascularization: An experimental model using the rabbit cornea. JNCI 52:413, 1974.
11. Taylor, S., and Folkman, J.: Protamine is an inhibitor of angiogenesis. Nature 297:307, 982.
12. Muthukkaruppan, V., and Auerbach, R.: Angiogenesis in the mouse cornea. Science 205:1416, 1980.
13. Fromer, C.H., and Klinworth, G.K.: An evaluation of the role of leukocytes in the pathogenesis of experimentally induced corneal neovascularization. II. Studies on the effect of leukocytic elimination on corneal neovascularization. Am. J. Pathol. 81:531, 1975.
14. Langer, R.S., and Folkman, J.: Polymers for the sustained release of proteins and other macromolecules. Nature 263:797, 1976.
15. Rhine, W.D., Hseih, D.S., and Langer, R.S.: Polymers for sustained release of macromolecules. Procedure to fabricate reproducible delivery systems and control release kinetics. J. Pharm. Sci. 69:265, 1980.
16. Murray, J.B., Brown, L., Langer, R.S., and Klagsbrun, M.: A micro sustained release system for epidermal growth factor. In Vitro 19:743, 1983.
17. Leighton, J.: The Spread of Cancer. New York, Academic Press.
18. Knighton, D.R., Ausprunk, D., Tapper, D., and Folkman, J.: Avascular and vascular phases of tumour growth in the chick embryo. Br. J. Cancer 35:347, 1977.
19. Klagsbrun, M., Knighton, D., and Folkman, J.: Tumor angiogenesis activity in cells grown in tissue culture. Cancer Res. 36:110, 1976.
20. Folkman, J., Haudenschild, C.C., and Zetter, B.: Long-term culture of capillary endothelial cells. Proc. Natl. Acad. Sci. USA 76:5217, 1979.
21. Ausprunk, D.H., and Folkman, J.: Migration and proliferation of endothelial cells in preformed and newly formed blood vessels during tumor angiogenesis. Microvasc. Res. 14:53, 1977.
22. Rifkin, D.B., Gross, J.L., Moscatelli, D., and Jaffee, E.: Proteases and angiogenesis: Production of plasminogen activator and collagenase by endothelial cells. *In* Nosel, H., and Vogel, H.J. (eds.): Pathobiology of the Endothelial Cell. New York, Academic Press, 1982, p. 191.
23. Gross, J.L., Moscatelli, D., Jaffe, E.A., and Rifkin, D.B.: Plasminogen activator and collagenase production by cultured capillary endothelial cells. J. Cell Biol. 95:974, 1982.
24. Kalebio, T., Garbisa, S., Glaser, B., and Liotta, L.: Basement membrane collagen: Degradation by migrating endothelial cells. Science 221:281, 1983.
25. Folkman, J., and Haudenschild, C.: Angiogenesis in vitro. Nature 288:551, 1980.
26. Maciag, T., Hoover, G.A., van der Spek, J., Stemerman, M.B., and Weinster, R.: Growth and differentation of human umbilical-vein endothelial cells in culture. In Sato, G.H., Pardee, A.B., and Sirbasku, D.A. (eds.): Growth of Cells in Hormonally Defined Media. Book A (Cold Spring Harbor Conferences on Cell Proliferation). New York, Cold Spring Harbor Laboratories, 1982, p. 525.
27. Bar, T., and Wolff, J.R.: The formation of capillary basement membranes during internal vascularization of the rat's cerebral cortex. Z. Zellforsch. 133:231, 1972.
28. Feder, J., Marasa, J.C., and Olander, J.: The formation of capillary-like tubes by fetal calf aortic endothelial cells grown in vitro. In Vitro 18:303, 1982.
29. Madri, J.A., Williams, S.K., Wyatt, T., and Mezzio, C.: Capillary endothelial cell cultures: Pheontypic modulation by matrix components. J. Cell Biol. 97:153, 1983.
30. Ausprunk, D.H.: Synthesis of glycoproteins by endothelial cells in embryonic blood vessels. Dev. Biol. 90:79, 1982.
31. Ausprunk, D.H., and Boudreau, C.: Proteoglycans in the microvasculature. I. Histochemical localization in microscopic vessels of rabbit eyes. Am. J. Pathol. 103:353, 1981.
32. Ausprunk, D.H., and Boudreau, C.: Proteoglycans in the microvasculature. II. Proliferating capillaries of the rabbit cornea. Am. J. Pathol. 103:367, 1981.
33. Selye, H.: The Mast Cells. Washington, Butterworth Inc., 1965.
34. Kessler, D.A., Langer, R.S., Pless, N.A., and Folkman, J.: Mast cells and tumor angiogenesis. Int. J. Cancer 18:703, 1976.
35. Zetter, B.R.: Migration of capillary endothelial cells is stimulated by tumour-derived factors. Nature 285:41, 1980.
36. Albrecht-Buehler, G.: The phagokinetic tracks of 3T3 cells. Cell 11:395, 1977.
37. Azizkhan, R.G., Azizkhan, J.C., Zetter, B.R., and Folkman, J.: Mast cell heparin stimulates migration of capillary endothelial cells in vitro. J. Exp. Med. 152:931, 1980.
38. Sidky, Y., and Auerbach, R.: Lymphocyte-induced angiogenesis: A quantitative and sensitive assay of the graft-vs.-host reaction. J. Exp. Med. 141:1084, 1975.
39. Auerbach, R.: Angiogenesis-inducing factors: A review. Lymphokines 4:69, 1981.
40. Kaminski, M., Kaminski, G., and Majewski, S.: Local graft-versus-host reaction in mice evoked by Peyer's patch and other lymphoid tissue cells tested in a lymphocyte-induced angiogenesis assay. Folia Biol. 24:104, 1978.
41. Herman, P.G., Yamamoto, I., and Mellins, H.Z.: Blood microcirculation in the lymph node during the primary immune response. J. Exp. Med. 136:697, 1972.
42. Anderson, N.D., Anderson, A.O., and Wyllie, R.G.: Microvascular changes in lymph nodes during skin allografts. Am. J. Pathol. 81:131, 1975.
43. Polverini, P.J., Cotran, R.S., and Sholley, M.M.: Endothelial proliferation in the delayed hypersensitivity reaction: An autoradiographic study. J. Immunol. 118:529, 1977.
44. Polverini, P.J., Cotran, R.S., Gimbrone, M.A., Jr., and Unanue, E.R.: Activated macrophages induce vascular proliferation. Nature 269:804, 1977.
45. Clark, R.A., Stone, R.D., Leung, D.Y., Silver, I., Hohn, D.C., and Hunt, T.K.: Role of macrophages in wound healing. Surg. Forum 27:16, 1976.
46. Greenberg, G.B., and Hunt, T.K.: The proliferation response in vitro of vascular endothelial and smooth muscle cells exposed to wound fluids and macrophages. J. Cell Physiol. 97:353, 1978.
47. Thakral, K.K., Goodson, W.H., III, and Hunt, T.K.: Stimulation of wound blood vessel growth by wound macrophages. J. Surg. Res. 26:430, 1979.
48. Knighton, D.R., Silver, I.A., and Hunt, T.K.: Regulation of wound-healing angiogenesis—effect of oxygen gradients and inspired oxygen concentration. Surgery 90:262, 981.
49. Banda, M., Knighton, D.R., Hunt, T.K., and Werb, Z.: Isolation of a nonmitogenic angiogenesis factor from wound fluid. Proc. Natl. Acad. Sci. USA 79:7773, 1982.
50. Brown, R.A., Weiss, J.B., Tomlinson, I.W., Phillips, P., and Kumar, S.: Angiogenic factor from synovial fluid resembling that from tumours. Lancet 1:682, 1980.
51. Castellot, J.J., Jr., Karnovsky, M.J., and Spiegelman, B.M.: Potent stimulation of vascular endothelial cell growth by differentiated 3T3 adipocytes. Proc. Natl. Acad. Sci. USA 77:6007, 1980.
52. Jakob, W., Jentzsch, K.D., Mauersberger, B., and Oehme, P.: Demonstration of angiogenesis-activity in the corpus luteum of cattle. Exp. Pathol. (Jena) 13:321, 1977.
53. Gospodarowicz, D., and Thakral, K.K.: Production of a corpus luteum angiogenic factor responsible for proliferation of capillaries and neovascularization of the corpus luteum. Proc. Natl. Acad. Sci. USA 75:847, 1978.
54. Glaser, B.M., D'Amore, P., Michels, R., Patz, A., and Fenselau, A.: Demonstration of vasoproliferation activity from mammalian retina. J. Cell Biol. 84:298, 1980.
55. D'Amore, P., Glaser, B.M., Brunson, S.K., and Fenselau, A.H.: Angiogenic activity from bovine retina: Partial purification and characterization. Proc. Natl. Acad. Sci. USA 78:3068, 1981.
56. Huseby, R.A., Currie, C., Lagerborg, V.A., and Garb, S.: Angiogenesis about and within grafts of normal testicular tissue: A comparison with transplanted neoplastic tissue. Microvas. Res. 10:396, 1975.
57. Nishioka, K., and Ryan, T.J.: The influence of the epidermis and other tissues on blood vessel growth in the hamster cheek pouch. J. Invest. Dermatol. 58:33, 1972.
58. Wolf, J.E., and Harrison, R.G.: Demonstration and characterization of an epidermal angiogenic factor. J. Invest. Dermatol. 61:130, 1973.
59. Hoffman, H., McAuslan, B., Robertson, D., and Burnett, E.: An endothelial growth-stimulating factor from salivary glands. Exp. Cell Res. 102:269, 1976.
60. Warren, B.A., Greenblatt, M., and Kommineni, V.R.C.: Tumour angiogenesis: Ultrastructure of endothelial cells in mitosis. Br. J. Exp. Pathol. 53:215, 1972.
61. Jack, R.L.: Regression of the hyaloid vascular system. Am. J. Ophthalmol. 74:261, 1972.
62. Clark, E.R., and Clark, E.L.: Microscopic observations on the growth of blood capillaries in the living mammal. Am. J. Anat. 64:251, 939.
63. Ausprunk, D.H., Falterman, K., and Folkman, J.: The sequence of events in the regression of corneal capillaries. Lab. Invest. 38:284, 1978.
64. Jennings, M.A., and Florey, H.W.: Healing. *In* Florey, H.W. (ed.): General Pathology. Philadelphia, W. B. Saunders Company, 1970.
65. Folkman, J.: Anti-angiogenesis: New concept for therapy of solid tumors. Ann. of Surg. 175:409, 1972.
66. Dontenwill, W., Chevalier, H.J., and Reckzeh, G.: Growth of carcinomas in the region of the cartilage. JNCI 50:291, 1973.
67. Haraldson, S.: The vascular pattern of a growing and full-grown human epiphysis. Acta Anat. 48:156, 1962.
68. Eisenstein, R., Sorgente, N., Soble, L.W., Miller, A., and Kuettner, K.E.: The resistance of certain tissues to invasion. Am. J. Pathol. 73:675, 1973.
69. Kuettner, K.E., Croxen, R.L., Eisenstein, K., and Sorgente, N.: Proteinase inhibitor activity in connective tissues. Experientia 30:595, 1974.
70. Kuettner, K.E., Hiti, J., Eisenstein, R., and Harper, E.: Collagenase in-

hibition by cationic proteins derived from cartilage and aorta. Biochem. Biophys. Res. Commun. 72:40, 1976.

71. Brem, H., Arensman, R., and Folkman, J.: Inhibition of tumor angiogenesis by a diffusible factor from cartilage. In Slavkin, H.C., and Greulich, R.C. (eds.): Extracellular Matrix Influences on Gene Expression. New York, Academic Press, 1975.

72. Brem, H., and Folkman, J.: Inhibition of tumor angiogenesis mediated by cartilage. J. Exp. Med. 141:427, 1975.

73. Langer, R., Brem, H., Falterman, K., Klein, M., and Folkman, J.: Isolation of a cartilage factor that inhibits tumor neovascularization. Science 193:70, 1976.

74. Langer, R., Conn, H., Vacanti, J., Haudenschild, J., and Folkman, J.: Control of tumor growth in animals by infusion of an angiogenesis inhibitor. Proc. Natl. Acad. Sci. USA 77:4331, 1980.

75. Langer, R., and Murray, J.: Angiogenesis inhibitors and their delivery systems. Appl. Biochem. Biotech. 8:9, 1983.

76. Murray, J., Krochin, N., Hill, C., Zetter, B., and Langer, R.: Partial purification of a cartilage-derived collagenase inhibitor. Fed. Proc. 42:1889, 1983.

77. Lee, A., and Langer, R.: Shark cartilage contains inhibitors of tumor angiogenesis. Science, 221:1185, 1983.

78. Harshbarger, J.C.: Activities Report of Registry of Tumors in Lower Animals 1965–1973, Washington, D.C., Smithsonian Institute, 1974.

79. Prier, D.J., Fenstermacher, J.K., and Guarino, A.M.: A choroid plexus papilloma in an elasmobranch (Squalus carcanthias). JNCI 56:1207, 1976.

80. Pauli, B.U., Memoli, V.A., and Kuettner, K.E.: Regulation of invasion by cartilage-derived anti-invasion factor. JNCI 67:65, 1981.

81. Pauli, B.U., and Kuettner, K.E.: Vascularity of cartilage. In Hall, B.K. (ed.): Cartilage, Vol. 1. New York, Academic Press, 1983.

82. Kuettner, K.E., Memoli, V.A., Croxen, R.L., Madesen, L., and Pauli, B.U.: Anti-invasion factor mediates avascularity of hyaline. Semin. Arthritis Rheum. 11:67, 1981.

83. Folkman, J., Langer, R., Linhardt, R.J., Haudenschild, C., and Taylor, S.: Angiogenesis inhibition and tumor regression caused by a heparin or a heparin fragment in the presence of cortisone. Science, 221:719, 1983.

84. Senger, D.R., Galli, S.J., Dvorak, A.M., Perraszi, C.A., Harvey, V.S., and Dvorak, H.F.: Vascular permeability factor: A protein secreted by tumors that can cause ascites fluid accumulation. Fed. Proc. 41:4058, 1982.

85. Crisp, A.J., Chapman, C.M., Kirkham, S.E., Schiller, A.L., and Krane, S.M: Articular mastocytosis in rheumatoid arthritis. Arthritis Rheum., 1984, in press.

Chapter 14

Structural Proteins: Collagen, Elastin, and Fibronectin

Jerome M. Seyer and Andrew H. Kang

INTRODUCTION

The connective tissues are those tissues that support and bind together the specialized elements of the body into functional, anatomic units. Thus, connective tissue is present in all internal organs, dermis, and blood vessels, and, in addition, forms the structural lattice of the bony skeleton and its attachments such as cartilage, ligaments, tendons, and fasciae. The most readily appreciated function of the tissue is to provide mechanical support and maintain structural integrity. However, it may also serve many other functions. For example, it plays an important role in regenerative and healing processes and is involved in inflammation. In the cornea, it must maintain transparency in addition to its supportive, structural role. In the kidney, the basement membrane of the renal glomerulus may function as a filtration barrier.

The connective tissues consist of cells and extracellular protein fibers, with an amorphous ground substance occupying the intercellular, interfibrillar space. Three kinds of fibers have been described: collagen, elastin, and reticulin, although the last may be closely related or identical chemically to collagen. The amorphous ground substance consists of acidic proteoglycans, glycoproteins such as fibronectin, laminin, chondronectin, and so on, and other less well characterized matrix components. Metabolism of these fibrous components as well as ground substance is governed by connective tis-sue cells, such as fibroblasts, chondroblasts, osteoblasts, and other cells extrinsic to the tissue.

COLLAGEN

Collagen is the most ubiquitous and abundant protein in the animal kingdom. In most vertebrates, including humans, it comprises aproximately one third of total body proteins. It is also unique among proteins in that it undergoes a series of modifications in both primary and tertiary structure after the molecule is synthesized and excreted into the extracellular space. These changes have profound influence on the properties of the protein and, therefore, the extracellular tissues. Implicit in this is that these post-translational steps in collagen metabolism might be one of the sites of biologic control of the properties of connective tissue as well as the potential sites of pathologic processes.

Structure of Collagen

The collagen molecule, which is the basic building unit of collagen fibers, has a highly asymmetric, rigid, rodlike structure. It is 1.5 nm in width and 300 nm in length and has a molecular weight of 285,000.[1-3] Amino acid composition of collagen from tissues of many different animals, including humans, has been well documented.[4-8] The composition of collagen from some of

Table 14–1. Compositional Characteristics of Different Collagens*

Amino acid	Major Interstitial Collagens				Basement Membrane Collagen		Pericellular Collagen		
	α1(I)	α2(I)	α1(II)	α1(III)	α1(IV)	α2(IV)	α1(V)	α2(V)	α3(V)
3 OH-proline	1.1	1.2	1.1	0	1	1	2.9	2.5	2.2
4 OH-proline	114	105	96	126	122	107	109	109	92
Aspartic acid	46	45	36	42	45	50	50	51	42
Threonine	18	18	22	13	19	28	19	26	19
Serine	35	30	27	38	38	30	36	31	34
Glutamic acid	77	70	95	71	78	64	91	84	98
Proline	118	114	106	107	85	73	118	97	99
Glycine	330	331	334	352	334	328	344	341	332
Alanine	119	105	108	95	30	47	46	52	49
Cystine/2	0	0	0	2	0	3	0	0	1
Valine	19	35	19	15	33	25	25	24	29
Methionine	7	8	11	8	15	14	8	11	8
Isoleucine	8	16	11	13	32	19	19	11	8
Leucine	20	33	27	23	52	56	39	35	20
Tyrosine	2	3	1	3	5	6	2	2	56
Phenylalanine	13	11	13	8	27	36	12	14	2
Hydroxylysine	10	12	18	6	50	39	35	24	9
Lysine	27	20	20	29	6	3	20	18	43
Histidine	4	10	2	6	6	5	8	11	15
Arginine	49	51	52	48	22	42	45	50	14
Glucose	1	1	5	1	44	29	18	10	42
Galactose	1	2	10	2	46	31	30	14	17

*Residues per 1000 total residues.

the representative tissues is presented in Table 14–1. Most striking is the constancy of the content of glycine (approximately one third of total residues) and imino acids (proline plus 3- and 4-hydroxyproline comprise approximately 20 percent). The amino acids 4-hydroxyproline and hydroxylysine occur exclusively in collagen, the Clq component of serum complement[9] and acetylcholinesterase.[10] A small amount of 4-hydroxyproline is also present in elastin (see Table 14–3). However, over 99 percent of total hydroxyproline in the body is found in collagen. Thus, studies on the turnover of the imino acids have been a convenient and useful tool in providing information on the metabolism of the protein.

The complete amino acid sequence of two genetically distinct collagen polypeptide chains, α1(I)[11] and α1(III),[12] have now been determined, and sufficient information is available on the remaining chains to indicate that collagen polypeptide chains consist of repeating triplet sequences of (Gly-X-Y)n (Fig. 14–1) where X and Y can be any amino acid but frequently are proline and 4-hydroxyproline, respectively. Short regions at each end of the molecule are nonhelical and differ markedly in amino acid content from the rest of the molecule. The significance of these regions will be discussed later in connection with crosslinking.

Chemical, physicochemical, and x-ray diffraction studies have established that the whole collagen molecule consists of three polypeptide chains, each of molecular weight 95,000 and each composed of approxi-

mately 1050 amino acid residues.[13-16] At least five different types of collagen have been identified in vertebrates (Table 14–2). Type I collagen is the principal form of collagen present in interstitial tissues, dermis, tendon, and bone.[1,4,6] It is composed of two identical polypeptide chains, designated α1(I), and one α2(I) chain, which differ from each other in amino acid composition and chromatographic behavior. Type I collagen, then, has the chain composition $[\alpha1(I)]_2\alpha2(I)$ In most of these tissues, an additional species of collagen, type III, is also found, though the proportion of type I and type III varies, depending on the tissue and the age of the animal.[6] The type III molecule is composed of three identical α chains, $[\alpha1(III)]_3$, which differ in amino acid composition from the chains of type I collagen. Collagen present in hyaline cartilage and vitreous of the eye (type II) is composed of three identical but distinct α chains $[\alpha1(II)]_3$.[5] The collagen present in basement membranes is referred to as type IV, which is composed of two nonidentical polypeptide chains α1(IV) and α2(IV) (for review see refs. 17 and 18). Both polypeptide chains have predominantly a Gly-X-Y sequence similar in length to the interstitial collagens with occasional interruptions. In addition, type IV molecules contain additional collagenous and noncollagenous segments at the amino and carboxyl ends in a manner similar to a procollagen molecule (see below). The molecular structure is still controversial at this time, but a heteropolymer $[\alpha1(IV)]_2\alpha2(IV)$ is favored. The large noncollagenous

A. TYPICAL SEQUENCE

-Gly-Pro- Y — Gly-Pro-Hypro-Gly-X-Hypro-Gly-X — Hylys-Gly-X — Y—

B. MINOR HELIX

C. MAJOR (TRIPLE) HELIX

D. MICROFIBRIL PACKING

Figure 14–1. Diagrammatic representation of collagen structure. *A* shows that glycine occurs in every third position, and there are large amounts of proline and hydroxyproline in the other two positions. X and Y represent any amino acid. *B* shows an individual α chain in helix. *C* shows the triple helix. The individual α chains are left-handed helixes with approximately three residues per turn. *D* shows a stained microfibril of collagen exhibiting characteristic cross-striations with a regular repeat period (*D*) of approximately 68 nm, and a two-dimensional representation of the packing arrangement of collagen molecules in the microfibril. As discussed in the text, each collagen molecule has large numbers of darkly staining bands, and five of these separated by a regular distance of 68 nm account for the repeat period in the microfibril. (Adapted from similar presentations by Grant, M.E., and Prockop, D.J.: N. Engl. J. Med. 286:194, 1972, and Nimni, M.E.: Semin. Arthritis Rheum. 4:95, 1974, with permission of the authors and the publishers).

protein portion contains a heteropolysaccharide and many disulfide intrachain crosslinks.[19]

Type V collagen has recently been identified as a minor component of most tissues, including skin, liver, lung, placenta, and blood vessels, and has been referred to as possibly the exocytoskeleton of connective tissue cells.[20-22] It represents the major collagen product of certain smooth muscle cells in culture, but its biologic function remains uncertain. The type V collagen molecule consists of three polypeptide chains, α1(V), α2(V), and α3(V), and has a molecular structure of $[\alpha1(V)]_2$ α2(V) as the major form plus either $[\alpha3(V)]_3$ or $[\alpha1(V)$ α2(V) α3(V)] as a minor form. The major tissue source from which type V collagen has been obtained is the amnion/chorionic membrane, which contains only the α1(V) and α2(V) polypeptide chains. The placenta, in contrast, contains all three polypeptide chains. Hyaline cartilage, which, as stated previously, has type II collagen as its major interstitial collagen component, also contains minor amounts of a type-V-like collagen species, referred to as 1α, 2α, and 3α collagen polypeptide chains. While these polypeptide chains are similar to the α1(V), α2(V), and α3(V) collagen chains, some differences exist in amino acid composition and therefore in their amino acid sequence. It appears, therefore, that three clearly different collagen families may exist in vertebrate tissues. These may be classified as interstitial collagens (type I, II, and III), the basement membrane collagen (type IV), and the minor cytoskeleton collagens (type V and 1α, 2α, 3α). Type V collagen represents less than 6 percent of the total collagen in most tissues.

The search for additional, unidentified collagenous components in connective tissue continues, and many other less abundant collagen-like species will most likely be found. The complement component Clq, for example, contains a 72 amino acid, triple-helical segment of [Gly-X-Y] structure with 4-hydroxyproline occasionally in the Y position.[9] Acetylcholinesterase also has a short, less defined triple helical collagenous segment in the molecule.[10] More relevant to connective tissues, however, is the discovery of small quantities of high molecular weight collagenous complexes (HMC), which, with reduction of their disulfide bonds, yield three collagenous polypeptide chains of 45,000 to 55,000 molecular weight.[23] These short collagen polypeptide chains are genetically distinct from all of the above collagen types. Yet, it is clear that HMC exists as an intrinsic collagenous component of many tissues, including skin, liver, lung and placenta. A similar, but different, high molecular weight complex occurs in hyaline cartilage.[24] The tissue localization and functional significance of these unusual collagens remain uncertain, but it has been proposed that they may function as connecting or link proteins with collagens and other macromolecules.

As mentioned previously, the collagen chains contain a high content of the imino acids proline and hydroxyproline. The stereochemical configuration of the imino acid forces each of the α chains to assume a left-handed helical conformation (minor helix), with a residue repeat distance of 0.291 nm and a relative twist of 110 degrees, making the number of residues per turn of the helix 3.27 and the distance between each third glycine 0.87 nm (Fig. 14–1).[15] Thus, the minor helix of the collagen chains

Table 14–2. Distribution of Different Collagen Types

Type	Molecular Structure	Location
I	$[\alpha1(I)]_2\alpha2(I)$	This is the most abundant collagen found in the body. It is the major protein component of bone, tendon, and skin, but it is also ubiquitous in the body. Most of the initial knowledge of collagen chemistry was based on this collagen. A minor variant, type I trimer, $[\alpha1(I)]_3$, has been found in embryonic tissue and some experimental systems.
II	$[\alpha1(II)]_3$	This is a cartilage-specific collagen, found also in certain eye structures and the vitreous. It is in the sole collagen of hyaline cartilage but is mixed with type I in certain fibrocartilage structures.
III	$[\alpha1(III)]_3$	This collagen was formerly considered to be reticulum, although this relationship remains circumstantial. It is generally found whenever type I is present but in increasing amounts in flexible tissues such as blood vessels, lung, and liver. It is also elevated in proliferating tissues, such as in fetal development, bone marrow, and early wound healing. A disulfide intramolecular crosslink is present in the COOH-terminal triple-helical region.
IV	$[\alpha1(IV)]_2\alpha2(IV)$	This is a basement membrane–specific collagen. It is located in the lamina densa of basement membrane with high concentrations in the anterior lens capsule, glomerulus of the kidney, and placenta. Other structures such as $[\alpha1(IV)]_3$ have not been ruled out. Segments of the polypeptide chain do not have a repeating [Gly-X-Y] sequence and are therefore subject to nonspecific proteolytic cleavage.
V	$[\alpha1(V)]_2\alpha2(V)$ and $\alpha1(V), \alpha2(V), \alpha3(V)$ or $[\alpha3(V)]_3$	This collagen is thought to be a cell surface collagen or to be associated with the plasma membrane cells. It has been localized as the exocytoskeleton of connective tissue cells and is found throughout the body, with high concentrations in smooth muscle tissues such as amnionic/chorionic membranes and in capillary vasculature. The major structure is $[\alpha1(V)]_2\alpha2(V)$; but varying amounts of $[\alpha3(V)]_3$ are also present. The presence of a different $\alpha1(V)$, $\alpha2(V)$, or $\alpha3(V)$ molecule has been suggested in cartilage.
Unusual collagens	Disulfide-bonded high molecular weight aggregates of 45,000 to 55,000 daltons collagen chains	These high molecular weight collagenous complexes are widespread in connective tissue but generally represent less than 1 percent of the total collagen. Although they represent clearly distinct entities apart from the above collagen chains, their functional significance and molecular structure remain unsure.

is nearly fully stretched, unlike the α helix found in most other proteins, which characteristically has an axial residue distance of 0.15 nm. The collagen chain minor helix also differs in that there are no hydrogen bonds between amino acids in the same chain due to the relatively large separation of the residues. Instead, the minor helix formed by each chain is stabilized by hydrogen bonds between it and the other two chains in the same collagen molecule.

The presence of glycine (which has no bulky side chain attached to its α carbon atom) at every third residue then allows three of the α chains to wind around a common axis, forming a right-handed super helix (Fig. 14–1). A cross-sectional visualization of the triple-helical structure would reveal only glycine in the central core, with the X and Y amino acid side-chains radiating away from the core. The three strands are stabilized by regularly occurring interchain hydrogen bonds. Hydroxyproline is known to exert a major stabilizing force in the triple helix presumably through hydrogen bond formation with its hydroxyl group. The exact number of hydrogen bonds used to maintain the triple helical structure is not known for certain. Two molecular models

have been proposed, one containing two hydrogen bonds per triplet, and the other, one per triplet. Thus, the collagen monomer is a thin, long, rigid, three-stranded ropelike structure with a right-handed twist. Each of the strands itself is a left-handed helix.[15]

Sufficient information is built into the primary structure so that, under physiologic conditions of ionic strength, pH, and temperature, collagen molecules spontaneously aggregate into fibrils of the native type seen in tissues.[1,3] Examined with an electron microscope, each fibril can be seen to bear a characteristic repeating pattern of cross-striations of about 68 nm periodicity (Fig. 14–2). The periodicity of the cross-striations is explained by the fact that each collagen molecule (300 nm in length) has five charged regions 68 nm apart, which, using appropriate stains, appear as bands on electron microscopy, and by the highly ordered and regular way in which the collagen molecules are aligned within fibrils. As schematically depicted in Figure 14-1D, each neighboring row of collagen molecules is displaced along the long axis by a distance of 68 nm (a value of D in Fig. 14-1D). In addition, within the same row, there is a gap or "hole" of about 41 nm between the end of one mol-

Figure 14–2. Native collagen fibril. Shadow-cast with platinum. The bar represents 0.2 μ × 70,000. (Courtesy of Dr. Jerome Gross.)

ecule and the beginning of the next (Fig. 14-1*D*). The "hole" created by this longitudinal displacement of the ends has attracted attention, because it may serve as a nidus for the deposition of hyroxyapatite crystals of bone.[25]

Biosynthesis of Collagen

Ribosomal Synthesis of Pro-α Chains on Polyribosomes. As with all other known proteins, the peptide bonds linking the amino acids in the polypeptide chains of collagen are synthesized on ribosomal complexes containing mRNA (Fig.14–3).[26] Studies on the ribosomal clusters operating in collagen synthesis in fibroblasts indicate that associations of 23 to 60 ribosomes are involved and function with a monocistronic mRNA coding for single polypeptide chains larger than the α chains.[25,26] Recent evidence also has shown that the polypeptide chains of collagen synthesized by cells are indeed larger than the α chains with an estimated molecular weight of approximately 160,000.[26,27] This would require a 6 kilobase mRNA molecule. Each of the polypeptide

Figure 14–3. Biosynthesis of collagen. Each pro α chain is a distinct gene product. Messenger RNA is translated on membrane-bound ribosomes. As the pro α chains are being assembled and fed into the cisternae of the rough endoplasmic reticulum, certain prolyl and lysyl residues become hydroxylated by the action of prolyl and lysyl hydroxylases, and some of the susceptible hydroxylysyl residues are glycosylated by the action of glycosyl transferases. Following completion of the chain synthesis, chains align and disulfide bonds form at the COOH-terminal extension peptides. Helix formation then follows, and the assembled procollagen molecules are secreted to the extracellular space.

chains contains extensions of "noncollagenous" peptides at the NH_2- and COOH-termini.[28,29] These biosynthetic precursors of the collagen α chains have been designated pro-α chains. The role of the noncollagenous extension peptides is not known with certainty. Since the pro-α chains contain several residues of cystine in the extension peptides, it has been suggested that they facilitate the association of the three chains into a triple-helical structure (procollagen) by providing interchain disulfide bonds.[26,30] Since the NH_2-terminal end of a polypeptide chain is synthesized first,[31] association of these extensions on three separate pro-α chains might initiate the formation of a triple helix while the growing chains are still attached to ribosomes. Another role suggested for the extension peptides is that they render the procollagen molecule more soluble under physiologic conditions of pH, ionic strength, and temperature and keep the molecules from polymerizing into fibrils until transported into the extracellular space.[32] The NH_2-terminus of the procollagen polypeptide chain contains, in addition, a pre-pro segment (signal sequence), as do other newly synthesized proteins. This hydrophobic segment binds the molecule to the ribosome and is rapidly cleaved as the polypeptide chain passes through the membrane of the endoplasmic reticulum into the cisternae.[33]

The Collagen Genes. The five different collagen types thus far identified in mammalian systems are made up of nine genetically distinct collagen polypeptide chains, which therefore require a minimum of nine structural genes. Recombinant DNA technology has now made possible a partial characterization of the α1(I) and α2(I) genes (for review see refs. 34 and 35). The α2(I) collagen gene has been the most extensively characterized, and this discussion will be limited to its structure. The entire α2(I) gene consists of a 38-kilobase pair (kbp) segment, which codes for the helical region containing 338 Gly-X-Y triplets, short nonhelical telopeptide regions at the NH_2-terminal and COOH-terminal ends of the helical molecule, the 125-amino-acid NH_2-terminal procollagen α2(I) end-piece and the 264 COOH-terminal procollagen α2(I) end-piece representing 1442 amino acid residues, not including the signal peptide of the pre-procollagen polypeptide chain. The 38-kbp DNA has approximately eight times the number of base pairs required to code for the protein (Fig. 14–4). The RNA transcribed from this 38-kbp genomic DNA, like most other eukaryotic transcript RNAs thus far studied, contains numerous noncoding sequences (introns) that interrupt their coding sequences (exons).

The intron-exon structure was first identified using electron microscopic pictures of mRNA-DNA hybrids (Fig. 14–4) and was confirmed with the partial DNA sequence analysis. Utilizing the established amino acid sequence of α2(I), the DNA coding only the exon regions could be determined as well as the exact intron-exon junctions. Each exon is a multiple of the 9 bp, the required number of a single collagen triplet (Gly-X-Y), and begins by coding for Gly. An estimated 41 or 42 exons code for the complete triple-helical region; an additional 4 exons, for the COOH-terminal procollagen

end-piece; and 2 or 3 exons, for the NH_2-terminal procollagen end-piece (Fig. 14–5). This suggests there must be at least 50 coding exons and an equal number of intervening introns. The DNA sequence of the introns segmenting the triple-helical coding exons has no repeating Gly-X-Y sequence; in fact little homology is found between intron and exon DNA sequences. The introns range in size from 86 bp to 2000 bp, and the length of the exons varies from 45 to 108 bp. Seven of the 14 exons thus far identified contain 54 bp each, and two contain 108 bp (multiple of 54), indicating a certain degree of repetition (Gly-X-Y)$_6$. The latter structure may represent a primordial gene which grew through duplication and recombination. Recombination between two exons at nonidentical positions within the 9 bp coding for the Gly-X-Y repeat is not possible, since it would result in disruption of the helical structure of collagen and thus be fatal. Therefore, the exon size must always be a multiple of 9 bp, and it is most frequently a 54-bp segment.

There are no definite exon-intron junctions separating either the triple-helical region, the telopeptides, or the initial segments of the procollagen end-piece. For example, the exon at the NH_2-terminal helical end codes for a COOH-terminal segment of the procollagen end-piece, all of the telopeptide, and the first three residues of the helical region. A somewhat similar situation occurs at the COOH-terminal helical region. These inclusive regions within one exon structure suggest that these segments of the nonhelical region are also highly conserved regions, especially around the procollagen peptidase cleavage sites.

In summary, the total amino acid sequence of the procollagen α2(I) molecule requires a 6-kb mRNA molecule for translation. This mRNA molecule is transcribed from a 38-kbp genomic DNA segment, which also codes approximately 50 interrupting intron segments. The excision of these multiple noncoding segments from the primary transcript RNA with subsequent splicing to form a 6-kb mRNA molecule requires complex nuclear multistep assembly process with possibly a nuclear control mechanism prior to the cytosol translation and post-translational control mechanisms of collagen synthesis.

Protocollagen Hydroxylases. As mentioned previously, the two characteristic amino acids of collagen are hydroxyproline and hydroxylysine. Neither of them, however, is genetically coded. Exogenously administered labeled hydroxyproline and hydroxylysine are not incorporated into collagen, and there is no clear evidence for the existence of hydroxyprolyl-tRNA or hydroxylysyl-tRNA. Isotopic experiments have established that the two amino acids are biosynthetically formed from precursor residues of proline and lysine in peptide chains, respectively, by the action of two specific oxygenases, *protocollagen proline hydroxylase* and *protocollagen lysine hydroxylase.*[26,36,37]

Protocollagen hydroxylases have now been isolated from various connective tissues in a highly purified state, and their requirements for the cofactors and the se-

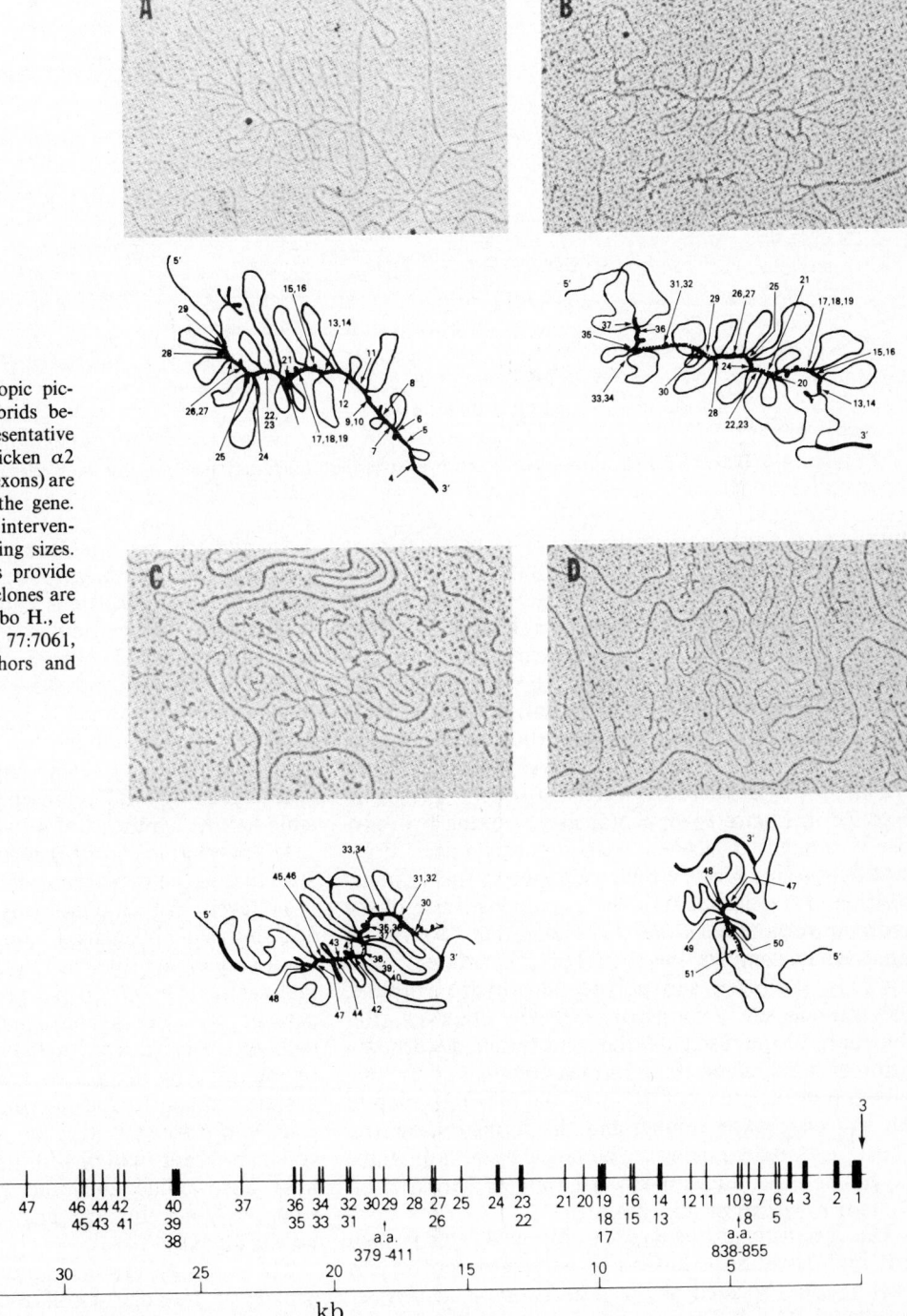

Figure 14–4. Electron microscopic pictures and diagrams of the hybrids between the DNAs of four representative overlapping clones and the chicken α2 mRNA. The coding sequences (exons) are numbered from the 3' end of the gene. The loops and nodes represent intervening sequences (introns) of varying sizes. Measurements of these lengths provide evidence that the recombinant clones are truly overlapping. (From Ohkubo H., et al.: Proc. Natl. Acad. Sci. USA 77:7061, 1980, with permission of authors and publisher.)

Figure 14–5. Graphic representation of measurements of coding and intervening sequences of the chicken α2 gene. The measurements were based on electromicroscopic pictures of DNA-mRNA hybrids (Fig. 14–4). Each vertical band represents the coding sequence or exon, and the lines between the bars correspond to intervening sequences or introns. Note that the coding information of the α2 collagen chain is divided into approximately 50 coding segments, which are separated by intervening sequences of various lengths. The length of the noncoding sequences varies but in general is much greater than the coding sequences. (From Ohkubo H., et al.: Proc. Natl. Acad. Sci. USA 77:7061, 1980, with permission of authors and publisher.)

Figure 14–6. Biosynthesis of hydroxyproline and hydroxylysine. Unhydroxylated pro α chain is referred to as protopro α chain.

quence of the substrate prolyl and lysyl peptides have been characterized.[26,33] The enzyme systems require molecular oxygen (Km $= 1 \times 10^{-5}$ M), Fe^{2+} ions (Km $= 1 \times 10^{-6}$ M) and α-ketoglutarate (Km $= 5 \times 10^{-6}$ M) for their activity. The requirements for these substances are absolute and specific. The systems also require the presence of a reducing agent, but this agent is not specific and may be ascorbic acid or other reducing compounds. The mechanism of action of protocollagen proline and lysine hydroxylases has been proposed as depicted in Figure 14–6; protocollagen lysine hydroxylase is thought to act via a similar mechanism. Polypeptidyl proline forms a hydroperoxide at the 4 (trans) position of the proline residue. The anionic form of the hydroperoxide attacks the α-ketoglutarate to form an intermediate complex; this then is decarboxylated, yielding CO_2, succinate, and polypeptidyl hydroxyproline. This mechanism is consistent with the observed stoichiometry of the reactants, the concomitant decarboxylation of α-ketoglutarate to form succinate, and the distribution of the atoms of $^{18}O_2$ between the OH-group of the hydroxyproline residue and the formed succinate. Thus, these hydroxylases are among the class of unique oxygenases that utilize α-ketoglutarate and transfer an O atom to succinate and substrate.

The specificity of the enzymes for substrates is such that hydroxylation is limited to only those prolyl and lysyl residues located at position Y of the triplet sequence of (Gly-X-Y)n and never at position X.[14,26,36] Substrates of (Gly-X-Y)n in smaller than 50 triplets are poorly hydroxylated or not hydroxylated at all. Further, hydroxylation is possible only if the substrates are denatured and the triple-helical structure abolished. Although the precise intracellular site at which hydroxylation takes place is controversial, the major site of hydroxylation is probably the nascent chains, concurrent with translation on ribosomes.[26,36]

In addition to 4-hydroxyproline, there are smaller amounts of 3-hydroxyproline in various collagens (see Table 14–1). Very little is known about its biosynthesis or function. In the only case in which the residue is located in the type I collagen sequence, 3-hydroxyproline follows glycine and precedes 4-hydroxyproline.[12] No 3-hydroxyproline is found in type III collagen, but bovine type IV collagen contains up to 10 residues per chain in certain tissues. Evidence indicates that its synthesis is catalyzed by a different enzyme than the one responsible for the synthesis of 4-hydroxyproline.

Glycosylation. Another interesting feature of collagen structure is the occurrence of covalently bound hexoses in collagen. The amounts vary, depending on the types and source of collagens. In most type I and III collagens from vertebrates, the carbohydrate content is 1 percent or less; in type II, it is 5.5 percent; and in type IV, 12 percent. All the carbohydrates in type I, II, and III collagens consist of either the monosaccharide galactose or the disaccharide glucosylgalactose bound via O-glycosidic linkage to the δ-hydroxy group of hydroxylysine.[1,2] The same is true for the basement membrane collagen except that, in addition, small amounts of mannose, hexosamine, and other sugars may be bound covalently;[19] their linkage structure, however, remains to be elucidated.

The enzymes responsible for the glycosylation of hydroxylysyl residues of collagen have been isolated from various connective tissues, including kidney cortex, cartilage, and uterus.[26,39,40] Both *glucosyl-* and *galactosyl-transferases* have been prepared. The UDP-galactose:hydroxylysine-collagen galactosyl transferase can transfer a galactose unit to a hydroxylysine residue of collagen. It cannot transfer galactose to free hydroxylysine or to small peptides containing hydroxylysine. The UDP–glucose:galactosyl–hydroxylysine–collagen glucosyl–transferase can transfer a glucose unit to hydroxylysine-linked galactose in either high or low molecular weight compounds. Both enzymes require a divalent cation, particularly Mn^{2+}, and they act in sequence so that galactose is added to hydroxylysine, and then glucose. It is not clear where these glycosyl transferases are located, and seemingly conflicting evidence locates these enzymes in either the cytoplasm or plasma membrane of cells.

Secretion by the Cells. Finally, the completed triple-stranded procollagen molecule is secreted by cells into the extracellular space, where the NH_2- and COOH-terminal extension peptides are proteolytically removed by the action of specific procollagen peptidases, yielding the triple helical collagen molecule (Fig. 14–7). Separate amino and carboxyl procollagen endopeptidases cleave pro $\alpha1(I)$ and pro $\alpha2(I)$ chains at specific sites.[41] The same excision of procollagen end-pieces occurs with type II, type III, and type V collagen, although different propeptidases are required. With type IV collagen, there is no evidence that any such processing of the procollagen molecule occurs, and it appears that the intact procollagen molecule may in fact be deposited in the tissue. The above procollagen peptidases are inhibited by EDTA but not by serine protease inhibitors.[42]

In summary, the biosynthesis of collagen has many similarities with that of other proteins, but it is distinguished by at least three prominent features: (1) the genomic structure is extremely large, i.e., eight times larger than necessary to code for the mRNA, (2) the protein is first synthesized in a precursor form known as procollagen, and (3) the biosynthesis involves several unusual post-translational modifications after assembly of amino acids into polypeptide chains. These include

hydroxylation of certain prolyl and lysyl residues, glycosylation of certain hydroxylysyl residues, and the formation of disulfide linkages in the peptide extensions of procollagen. These post-translational changes are necessary for some of the biologic functions of collagen. In particular, the hydroxylation of peptidyl proline is essential for folding of the three polypeptide chains into the "correct" triple-helical structure. Hydroxylation of lysyl residues and glycosylation of the hydroxylysyl residues may influence the subsequent formation of interchain crosslinks (discussed below). The importance of these post-translational reactions has been further emphasized by the demonstration that if one or more of the reactions is interfered with, the secretion of procollagen by cells is markedly altered so that either it is not secreted or it is secreted at a reduced rate.

Collagen Fibrillogenesis. The mechanism for the formation of fibrils from the triple-helical molecules (Fig. 14–1) still remains unclear. At present, the process appears to involve formation of smaller aggregates from simple monomeric units (triple-helical molecules) with subsequent growth to intermediate size aggregates (for review see ref. 43). The collagen fibril formation then involves a stepwise formation from intermediate aggregates rather than from monomeric molecules. These monomeric procollagen molecules begin to aggregate in the secretory vacuoles of the cells. It is probably during this initial compartmentalization that other macromolecules such as proteoglycans exert influence on the aggregation state and ultimately fibrillogenesis. In this manner of using the same secretory vacuoles, the cell may regulate the stoichiometry of mixing of various connective tissue components and ultimately effect dif-

Figure 14–7. Secreted procollagen is acted on by procollagen peptidases(s) to cleave off the NH_2- and the COOH-extension peptides. The resulting collagen molecules then self-assemble into native-type fibrils. Certain of the lysyl and hydroxylysyl residues located at the NH_2- and COOH-terminal, nonhelical regions are converted to allysine and hydroxyallysine by the action of lysyl oxidase (see Fig. 14–8), and crosslinks form (see Fig. 14–9).

ferent morphologies of collagen fibrils. The formation of the small aggregates is most likely initiated through amino terminal–carboxyl terminal attachment of monomeric units by charge-charge interactions, since this process is dependent on the pH and ionic strength. This process sets up the 4D staggered dimers and trimers (Fig. 14–1). Lateral aggregation occurs subsequently by means of both hydrophobic and electrostatic interactions, with the basic unit being a stabilized 5-membered lateral fibril packing assembly. The aggregates then grow in length by the addition of other intermediate aggregates at the end of the subfibril and in width by lateral wrapping of subfibrils. The effects of other collagens and connective tissue macromolecules such as glycoproteins and proteoglycans continue to influence the process of these subassemblies. Ultrastructural data suggest that the latter assembly and fibril growth occur near the cell surface within its indentations. The process of fibrillogenesis therefore remains under continued cellular regulation and influence, since these recesses may act as a microenvironment of the cell surface.

Intracellular Degradation. Current evidence suggests that connective tissue cells may be highly inefficient in producing collagen molecules. Variable amounts (10 to 60 percent) of the newly synthesized collagen may be degraded intracellularly prior to secretion (for review, see ref. 44). The appearance of intracellular small peptide fragments of hydroxyproline and hydroxylysine provides unique markers for this process, since hydroxylation of these amino acidly occurs only after polypeptide chain synthesis. One source of this degraded collagen understandably comes from removal of abnormal collagen molecules or errors during synthesis. This is shown when cells are grown without ascorbic acid, which is needed for full hydroxylation, or when a proline analogue such as azetidine is incorporated into the polypeptide chains. It may also be an attempt by the cells to regulate the amount and type of collagen secreted by the cells. For instance, any agent that causes an elevation in the intracellular cAMP can increase intracellular degradation and consequently decrease collagen deposition by lung and skin fibroblasts. This appears to affect type I collagen production more than type III collagen. In this manner, the intracellular degradation of newly synthesized collagen may be an additional mechanism by which cells regulate both the quality and quantity of the collagen secreted in normal and disease states.

Turnover of Collagen

Metabolic turnover of collagen, as measured in a whole animal or even in a whole tissue such as skin, is very low; $t^{1/2}$ is measured in years. This extremely slow metabolic turnover is compatible with the function of collagen as a structural protein. However, this generalization should not obscure the fact that in several specific physiologic situations the metabolic turnover in a particular region of the body is extremely active. For example, during metamorphosis the collagenous tissue present in the tails of tadpoles is rapidly removed and that of back skin swiftly remodeled. Likewise, there must be an active turnover of the collagenous matrix during remodeling of bone. In patients with Paget's disease, in which there is markedly enhanced synthesis and resorption of bone, a marked increase in the urinary secretion of hydroxyproline, hydroxylysine, and its glycosides has been observed.[45-48] Since most hydroxyproline, hydroxylysine, and its glycosides in the blood are of collagenous origin, the urinary excretion of these compounds has been used as an index of collagen metabolism. Various metabolic studies have demonstrated that in states in which there is an increased breakdown of collagen, such as metastatic diseases of bone, hyperparathyroidism, and hyperthyroidism, the urinary excretion of the imino acid in the form of both free imino acid and oligopeptides and hydroxylysine glycosides is markedly increased; but that in states in which there is an increased synthesis of collagen, such as during growth, the urinary excretion of hydroxyproline in polypeptide form is increased.[46] Thus, an increase in the ratio of nondialyzable to low molecular weight hydroxyproline is found in states in which synthesis of collagen exceeds breakdown.

The mechanism of the resorption of collagen has been the subject of considerable interest, since collagen in the native state is resistant to attack by most proteolytic enzymes at physiologic pH and temperature, although it is degraded by a wide variety of proteolytic enzymes once the molecule is denatured (or the helical structures disrupted). It has recently been shown that physiologic breakdown of collagen is accomplished by the action of specific collagenases produced in extremely small amounts in situ where needed. Such specific collagenase activity has been demonstrated in many physiologic and pathologic situations, and the enzyme has been purified from several different sources.[49-51] Their molecular characteristics and mechanisms of action are detailed in Chapter 13.

Maturational Changes and Crosslinking

After the deposition of collagen in the extracellular matrix, covalent bridges or crosslinks among the polypeptide α chains form both within the molecule and between the adjacent molecules.[52,53] There is much similarity in the crosslinking mechanism of collagen and elastin in that the crosslinks are derived from lysyl residues through the formation of reactive aldehydes by the action of *lysyl oxidase*,[54] and that some of the crosslink compounds are common to both. However, there are major differences. The first is the prominent involvement of the hydroxylysyl residues in collagen crosslinking rather than the lysyl residues solely as seen in elastin. The second is the functional difference in the crosslinkages formed. Collagen utilizes the crosslinking compounds for interchain bridges, whereas the crosslinks in elastin serve as both intra- and interchain bridges.

The knowledge of collagen crosslinking has been derived mostly from studies on type I collagen, which predominates in dermis, tendon, and bone. Specific lysyl and hydroxylysyl residues located in the nonhelical NH_2-

Figure 14–8. Oxidative deamination of peptide bound lysine and hydroxylysine by the action of lysyl. Allysine is formed both in collagen and elastin. Hydroxyallysine is found only in collagen.

and COOH-terminal regions of the α chains are converted to aldehydes, α-amino adipic-δ-semialdehyde (allysine, Fig. 14–8) and δ-hydroxy-α-amino adipic-δ-semialdehyde, respectively (hydroxyallysine, Fig. 14–8). These are catalyzed by the action of lysyl oxidase,[54] which is pyridoxal dependent and requires Cu^{2+} for action. Apparently only the residues in the nonhelical portions of the collagen molecule are oxidatively deaminated, and the similar residues in the more rigid triple-helical region are not affected. Whether this is a result

of enzyme specificity for a certain amino acid sequence present only in the NH_2- and COOH-termini, or a result of steric inaccessibility of the triple-helical region to the enzymes, is not known.

Once the aldehydes are formed, they undergo two basic types of reactions.[52,53] The first is the formation of aldamine bonds (Schiff bases) with ε-amino groups of lysine or hydroxylysine from an adjacent polypeptide chain, thus forming $\Delta^{6,7}$ dehydrolysinonorleucine, $\Delta^{6,7}$ dehydrohydroxylysinonorleucine, or $\Delta^{6,7}$ dehydrohydroxylysinohydroxynorleucine (Fig. 14–9). These compounds are unstable during acid hydrolysis and have been isolated from tissues in their reduced forms following chemical reduction with borohydride. The relative proportions of these aldamine crosslinks vary according to the source of tissues. Thus, hydroxylysinonorleucine predominates in dermal collagen, whereas hydroxylysinohydroxynorleucine represents the major aldamine crosslink in the more insoluble collagen present in bone and tendon. Lysinonorleucine is usually a minor component in normal collagenous tissues. Tissue differences in these aldamine crosslinks appear, therefore, to be controlled by the degree of post-translational lysyl hydroxylation.

Figure 14–9. Aldamine crosslinks of collagen. Natural reduction of the double bond between N and C of the dehydro compounds apparently does not occur in collagen. In elastin, both dehydrolysinonorleucine and its reduced form lysinonorleucine are found. Hydroxylysine-containing crosslinks in collagen become stabilized by the formation of ketoimine structures by Amadori rearrangement. The proposed condensation of two ketoimine structures yields a hydroxypyridinium residue and free hydroxylysine.

These aldamine compounds apparently undergo Amadori rearrangement reactions to form keto-imine structures (Fig. 14–9), which are much more stable than the Schiff base forms and probably help explain the stability of the tissues to heat and dilute acid. A more stable trifunctional crosslink has recently been isolated from tendon, bone, and cartilage.[55] This crosslink, named hydroxypyridinoline (Fig. 14–9), appears to originate by the condensation of three amino acid side-chains (one hydroxylysine and two hydroxyallysine) to form a cyclic 3-hydroxypyridinoline. This crosslink compound, which links three collagen chains, increases in amount with age of the tissue and does not require prior borohydride reduction for its isolation. Its specific position within the collagen polypeptide chains remains undetermined.[55] The hexose-linked hydroxylysyl residues also participate as the amino donors to the aldamine bonds, especially in tissues of older animals. The compounds glucosyl-galactosyl dehydrohydroxylysinohydroxynorleucine and galactosyl dehydrohydroxylysinohydroxynorleucine have been identified in mature dermis. What effects the sugar moiety imparts to the individual crosslinks are unknown.

The second basic type of crosslink compounds found in collagen originates from an aldol condensation reaction of two allysine residues with the formation of the corresponding dehydrated aldol (Fig. 14–10). This type of lysine-derived aldol crosslink has been identified in soft tissue collagens of dermis and tendon (and in elastin). The aldol condensate can undergo a further series of reactions with hydroxylysine and histidine to give rise to tri- and tetra-functional crosslinks, dehydrohydroxymerodesmosine, aldolhistidine, and histidinohydroxymerodesmosine.[2,56] These crosslinks link together three or four α chains.

It should be mentioned that although allysine and hydroxyallysine formation is enzymatically mediated, once these functional groups have been formed, the subsequent aldamine and aldol condensation as well as the histidine addition can proceed spontaneously in vitro. Whether this is also true in vivo is not known. It seems unnecessary, however, to hypothesize the existence of a separate enzyme system mediating these latter reactions.

In any case, the result of crosslinking of collagen is that it becomes then an enormous complex of macromolecules covalently linked together, giving rise to tissue of high tensile strength and great insolubility.

The physiologic significance of the relative distributions of these various crosslinks in collagens of various tissues cannot be fully appreciated at present. Available data suggest that the more insoluble tissues such as bone and tendon tend to contain a higher proportion of dehydrohydroxylysinohydroxynorleucine, and hydroxypyridinoline, whereas the tissues such as dermis, the collagen of which is slightly more soluble, contain a higher content of relatively less stable dehydrohydroxylysinonorleucine. Likewise, scar tissue of skin tends to contain a higher content of the more stable dehydrohydroxylysinohydroxynorleucine as compared with the normal skin.

The nature of crosslinks in type II, III, IV, and V collagens has not been investigated to the same extent as that of type I collagen. Presumably similar crosslinks will be found but with tissue-specific and age-specific variations. For instance, cartilage contains predominantly the more stable hydroxyallysine- and hydroxylysine-derived crosslinks. Type III collagen contains two cysteine residues at the COOH-terminus of the triple helix, and these participate in intramolecular crosslinks. Type IV contains numerous inter- and intrachain disulfide crosslinks, providing this collagen with even greater crosslinking capabilities. The high molecular weight complexes discussed earlier contain many cysteine residues, which may bind noncollagenous proteins to this poorly understood collagenous complex.[23,24]

Relationship of Structure and Biologic Function of Collagen

In order for collagen to function as a structural protein in a mechanical and supportive role, several properties are essential or at least desirable; it must be insoluble in the kind of solutions encountered under physiologic conditions in living tissue; it must have a low overall metabolic turnover rate; and its tensile strength must be high. The preceding discussion on the structure of collagen should make it clear that collagen meets these requirements eminently well. Throughout the animal kingdom the rigid preservation of the general structure of the protein further attests to the suitability of its structural characteristics.

On the other hand, since collagen serves different functions in different tissues such as in bone, tendon, skin, and basement membrane, many variations in its structure must also be possible. Knowledge of the relationship between the biologic properties and the salient features of the molecular structure is of utmost importance in understanding structural bases for functional abnormalities found in pathologic states. In connective tissue it has been particularly difficult to obtain this type of information, largely because of the enormous complexity of the constituent macromolecules. Nevertheless, data are beginning to accumulate which have bearing

Figure 14–10. Aldol condensation product between two residues of allysine. This crosslink is found in both collagen and elastin.

Figure 14–11. Schematic diagram of the epidermal basement membrane zone. Bullous pemphigoid antigen is localized to the lamina lucida by immunoelectron microscopy and is also closely associated with the basal cell plasma membrane. Laminin is localized to the lamina lucida as well and consists of three short chains as a long chain (molecular weights, 200,000 and 400,000). The basement membrane proteoglycan appears to be localized to both edges of the lamina densa. Type IV collagen is probably in a reticular pattern in the electron dense zone, the lamina densa. (From Stanley, J.R., et al.: J. Invest. Dermatol. 79:685, 1982, with permission of authors and publisher.)

basement membrane structures such as renal glomeruli and anterior lens capsule have been the major source of information on type IV collagen.[60-63] Two procollagen chains are synthesized by partial yolk sac cells, i.e., $\alpha 1(IV)$ and $\alpha 2(IV)$. Their molecular weights are 180,000 and 165,000, which are consistent with those of other procollagens. All of the post-translational modifications described above are necessary, except possibly for procollagen peptidase cleavage.

Evidence now suggests that the entire procollagen molecule is deposited into a loosely woven matrix unlike that observed with the interstitial collagens (Fig. 14–12). Both intermolecular disulfide and lysine-derived

BASEMENT MEMBRANE
TYPE IV COLLAGEN

Figure 14–12. The model proposed for the arrangement of type IV collagen molecules in basement membrane. Type IV collagen molecules are incorporated into a netlike structure with the like ends of the molecule in apposition and presumably crosslinked. The 7S region refers to the part of the net where the NH₂-terminus of four triple-helical molecules align and form a very stable structure with both lysine-derived and disulfide inter- and intramolecular crosslinks. The COOH-terminal ends of the type IV molecules are "ball" shaped and presumably globular structures with uncertain crosslinks. (From Stanley, J.R., et al: J. Invest. Dermatol. 79:70s, 1982, with permission of authors and publisher.)

crosslinks contribute to its extreme insolubility. Most of the information on the structure of type IV collagen has been derived from limited pepsin digestion to produce α chain size molecules, $\alpha 1(IV)$ and $\alpha 2(IV)$, with amino acid compositions shown in Table 14–1. This pepsin-derived basement membrane collagen contains nearly one third glycine and has secondary and tertiary structures similar to other collagens.[61] The content of hydroxylysine is elevated, as is that of carbohydrate. Higher amounts of 3-hydroxyproline are present in bovine but not human placenta type IV collagen. One unusual characteristic is that in some cases, glycine does not appear at every third residue. Therefore, a less compact helix is present and nonspecific protease digestion can occur, such as with pepsin, to yield a heterogeneous mixture of collagenous components varying from >220,000 to 25,000 molecular weight. Amino acid sequence analyses have confirmed these "flaws" in the triplet sequence in type IV collagen chains, especially the $\alpha 2(IV)$ polypeptide chain. At present, it is uncertain whether the molecular structure consists of $[\alpha 1(IV)]_2$-$\alpha 2(IV)$ or two molecular forms having identical subunits. Quantitation is difficult because of the extreme susceptibility of the $\alpha 2(IV)$ polypeptide chain to nonspecific proteolysis even in its native state.

As stated previously, the type IV collagen appears to be deposited in the tissue as a large procollagen-like molecule. Immunofluorescent staining has pinpointed the location of this collagen in the lamina densa of the basement membrane. With milder extraction procedures and the use of a mouse tumor, several salient features have been demonstrated. The NH₂-terminal propeptide portion of the procollagen molecule contains collagenous regions rich in cysteine in addition to noncollagenous segments. Multiple disulfide and lysine-derived crosslinks are present in this domain, from which a highly crosslinked aggregate (referred to as 7S based on its sedimentation coefficient) can be obtained. In this complex, a minimum of 4 triple-helical molecules are densely crosslinked (see Fig. 14–12). The carboxyl-terminal region of the type IV procollagen molecule contains "ball-like" structures when visualized by rotary shadowing techniques. This, therefore, must contain a globular, non-triple-helical region as seen with the procollagen end-pieces of interstitial collagens.

In summary, several features of type IV collagn distinguish it from the interstitial collagens. Whether or not the entire procollagen molecule is indeed deposited in the tissue or an even larger polypeptide chain is synthesized remains a controversy. Regardless, previous dogma concerning strict structural characteristics of interstitial collagen does not hold true for type IV. The departure from or substitution of glycine at every third residue in limited areas of the triple-helical region of the polypeptide chain renders the native molecule susceptible to nonspecific protease cleavage by enzymes such as mast cell protease and elastase and enzymes from tumor cells, the latter being perhaps important in tumor invasion through basement membrane structures.[17,63]

Reticulin. Reticulin is primarily a histologic phenomenon describing particular kinds of fibers that are abundantly seen in embryonic connective tissues and in some tissues of adults. In contrast to collagen fibers, which are in nonbranching coarse bundles, reticular fibers form a delicate network of freely branching fibers that stain black by a silver impregnation technique. It has long been assumed that during development these fine argyrophilic fibers are somehow transformed into the coarse strands of collagen fibers and lose argyrophilia, although in some tissues such as spleen, lymph nodes, liver, and bone marrow they persist throughout life.

The chemical and structural relationship between reticulin and collagen has long been controversial. A major problem has been to obtain reticulin in quantities sufficient for purification and analysis in a rigorous manner. Biochemical analysis[64,65] on the material obtained by microdissection showed that it has amino acid composition not dissimilar to that of collagen. In addition, a relatively large amount of carbohydrate was detected. It is, however, difficult to interpret the analytic data obtained from impure preparations. Ultrastructural studies with the electron microscope have demonstrated that reticulin possesses the same fine structure as collagen, with typical 64 nm periodicity. Since the cross-striation pattern as seen with the electron microscope is a reflection of the charged group distribution of the constituent amino acid side-chains, this suggests that reticulin has a primary structure very similar to or identical with collagen. Although the biologic function of reticulin is unknown, it seems reasonable to consider the possibility that reticulin may represent an embryonic form of collagen analogous to hemoglobin F. Reticulin is the first fibrous element to appear in embryonic connective tissue, which, in most tissues but not all, gives way to adult collagen during subsequent development. Although it is tempting to speculate on the possibility that reticulin may represent type III collagen, proof of the relationship has not been established.

Immunochemistry of Collagens and Procollagen. The complex structure of collagen is reflected by the different types of antigenic determinants that have been identified on the molecule. These can be defined as follows.[66,67]

1. *Helical determinants* depend on conformational factors inherent in the quaternary structure of the triple helix.

2. *Terminal determinants* are nonhelical and are different on both the NH_2-terminus and COOH-terminus of the molecule. Procollagen, with additional peptides on both ends of the molecule, produces different antibodies to the nonhelical portions from those of collagen itself.

3. *Central determinants* are unmasked after disruption of the helical structure and are a function of the primary sequence of the molecules. There is much interspecies cross-reaction of antibodies to these determinants but not of antibodies to the helical or terminal determinants.

Current data indicate that in mice the immune response to calf skin collagen is controlled by at least two genes.[68] One is the H-2 gene and represents a T-lymphocyte-dependent response. Another locus appears to be T-lymphocyte independent and responsible, in association with H-2, for high responsiveness to collagen.

Radioimmunoassay has been adapted to antibodies directed to the procollagen end-pieces of type I and type III collagen. After labeling the end-pieces with [125]iodine, nanogram quantites of procollagen end-pieces were detected in serum.[69,70] Up to 200 ng of the procollagen end-pieces from type I collagen were detected, presumably being derived from normal bone remodeling. Five to 7 ng of type III procollagen end-pieces were detected, and this level was elevated in certain diseases with elevated collagen synthesis, namely alcoholic liver disease.[71]

The remainder of the collagen-like material in plasma represents the first component of complement, Clq.[9] Initial studies using this method have indicated that increased amounts of immunoreactive collagen can be found circulating (and in other body fluids) in patients with a number of other different disorders involving increased turnover of collagen.[72]

Studies of cell-mediated immunity to collagen and the role of this response in pathogenesis of inflammatory diseases of joints are described below.

Biological Considerations. Detailed clinical descriptions and some of the known defects of the collagen biosynthesis[73,74] and structure found in heritable disorders of connective tissues in humans are given in Chapter 105. In the present chapter, discussion will be confined to some of the animal disorders involving collagen that have been useful in our understanding of the human diseases, and to selected facets of collagen metabolism and structure in acquired disorders of humans.

Animal Disorders. Lathyrism. Lathyrism is an experimental disease state in animals caused by administering β-aminopropionitrile, $H_2N\text{-}CH_2\text{-}CH_2\text{-}C\equiv N$, a constituent of the sweet pea, *Lathyrus odoratus*. Administration of this agent to a wide variety of mammals and birds results in gross skeletal deformities as well as widely scattered abnormalities in the structure of connective tissue and an apparent failure in tensile strength. These include weakness of blood vessel walls with aneurysm formation or even rupture, slipped epiphyseal plates, avulsed tendons and ligaments, and weakness of fascial planes with subsequent hernia formation. The mechanism of action by β-aminopropionitrile in producing this remarkable disease state is now understood in detail.[75,76] It results from interference with aldehyde formation from the specific lysyl and hydroxylysyl residues by competitive inhibition of lysyl oxidase. Thus, there is an acquired failure of crosslinking of collagen in these animals resulting in marked diminution in tensile strength of the collagenous tissues, explaining the clinical abnormalities noted above. This conclusion is further supported by the observation that the state of lathyrism can be mimicked by agents such as D-penicillamine (Fig. 14–13), which also interfere with crosslinking but at a later step in the process.[77] The latter agent binds to the aldehydes already formed, preventing them from undergoing Schiff base formation or aldol condensation (Fig. 14–13). Thus, the importance of crosslinking to the proper functioning of collagen is established through

Figure 14–13. Schematic drawing of the mode of action of D-penicillamine. This compound interacts with aldehydes of collagen and prevents their subsequent aldamine or aldol condensation reactions. (From Nimni, M.E.: Semin. Arthritis Rheum. 4:95, 1974, with permission of author and publisher.)

our understanding of the biochemical pathogenesis of this disease state. The possible clinical importance of this is suggested by reports of side effects on connective tissues associated with the use of D-penicillamine in various situations. The side effects include poor wound healing,[78] hyperelastic skin, premature aging of skin, and other skin abnormalities.[79] An infant with widely scattered connective tissue malformation was born to a mother receiving penicillamine therapy for cystinuria during her pregnancy.[80] In homocystinuria (see Chapter 104), there is also an apparently acquired defect in collagen.[81] The mechanism of this defect may be similar to that produced by D-penicillamine, since both are structurally similar with adjacent aminothiol groups.

Dermatosparaxis. Dermatosparaxis, an inherited disease observed in cattle and sheep, is characterized by extreme fragility of skin and connective tissues. Morphologic studies have shown that there is a gross disorganization in the collagenous fibrils in connective-tissues with pseudofiber formation. Biochemically, collagen molecules extracted from the tissues of the affected animals contain a bulk of nonhelical NH_2-terminal extension peptides which have not been cleaved off from procollagen molecules. Called pN-collagen, these molecules have a molecular weight intermediate between that of procollagen and collagen, and cannot form native-type fibrils in vitro under conditions that favor polymerization of normal collagen. The defect has been shown to be the deficient activity of procollagen peptidase(s).[83] A similar enzymatic defect has been demonstrated in some patients with Ehlers-Danlos syndrome.[84]

Acquired Disorders. In many acquired human diseases, the pathologic processes seem to involve predominantly connective tissue, and the resultant destruction or alteration of the tissue plays a significant role in the genesis of morbid states. These include wound healing and its abnormal forms, including keloids, scurvy, several inflammatory diseases such as scleroderma and rheumatoid arthritis, corneal ulceration secondary to trauma or infection, and degenerative diseases of joints and several other unrelated diseases.

Wound Healing. Wound healing,[95] although not "pathologic," deserves a special consideration here because of the importance the metabolism of collagen plays in the process. If a wound is a break in the continuity of tissue, healing is the restoration of continuity of tissue. The process of wound healing may be divided into three phases: initial or lag phase, the phase of fibroplasia, and the phase of contraction of scar.

Following an injury, the hemostatic mechanism immediately comes into play, leading to the formation of clot. A firmly retracted clot not only stops bleeding but also provides support for the wound's edges, allowing proliferation and migration of capillary endothelial cells, fibroblasts, and epithelial cells. During this period of initial phase, there is active removal of cellular and other tissue debris, both within and outside the phagocytic cells. Of particular interest is the secretion of active collagenase by the epithelial cells and fibroblasts at the wound edge.[49]

The fibroblastic proliferation, which begins during the initial phase, reaches a maximum during the second phase (2 to 10 days after injury) and the cells begin to synthesize and secrete collagen. It is the collagen deposition that provides strength to the wound. After an adequate amount of collagen is deposited (10 to 14 days after injury), the fibroblasts begin to disappear from the scar, with gradual diminution and cessation of further collagen synthesis. Meanwhile, progressive crosslinking of the newly deposited collagen proceeds. This last phase is associated with increasing tensile strength of the wound, which reaches a maximum some 3 weeks following the initiation of healing.

The process of wound healing described above requires adequate general nutrition, blood supply, and control of infection. The precise factors that control the process are, however, not well understood. What is the message that attracts the fibroblast to the injured site? What messages do fibroblasts recognize to initiate and terminate the synthesis of collagen and collagenase? What is the biochemical event that transpires to bring about the contraction of the scar and the increase of tensile strength? The answers to these important questions must await further studies.

Evidence, however, is compelling for the crucial role of collagen metabolism in normal healing. Administration of β-aminopropionitrile (see Lathyrism, above) leads to marked weakness in tensile strength of wounds.[75] Presumably, this effect is mediated by its interference with crosslinking of collagen, discussed previously. This effect of the compound has been utilized for the treatment of conditions in which excessive contraction of scars in itself may be harmful, such as esophageal strictures following chemical or physical injuries and adhesions of tendons to tendon sheaths following repair of tendon disruption.

Likewise, scurvy, a state induced by a deficiency of ascorbic acid, is associated with poor wound healing as well as marked vascular fragility. As indicated previously, ascorbic acid probably serves as as cofactor in hydroxylation of proline and lysine during in vivo collagen biosynthesis. In vitro studies indicate that there is a marked diminution in collagen synthesis and secretion, and that extensively underhydroxylated collagen accumulates within cells in the absence of ascorbic acid.[96,97]

Lastly, an abnormality in collagen biosynthesis and/or degradation leads to defective wound healing such as keloid and hypertrophic scar. The precise defect or defects in these conditions, however, remain to be elucidated.

Inflammation. Recent studies have also implicated collagen and its degradative products in the process of inflammation. Evidence suggests that collagen and its breakdown products are directly chemotactic for blood monocytes and fibroblasts.[98,99] Since collagen is ubiquitous in all tissues, its chemotactic property may play a significant role in calling for monocytes and fibroblasts to clean up the tissue debris at the injury site during the early phase of inflammation, and begin to effect the synthesis of the extracellular matrix for healing.

In addition, data have been presented indicating that immunity against collagen or its fragments may play a role in the pathogenesis of chronic inflammation seen in scleroderma and rheumatoid arthritis,[93,94,100,101] in which there is a widespread inflammatory process taking place in various connective tissues with lymphocytic and monocytic infiltration. The histologic features observed in these diseases are quite compatible with cellular immune-mediated inflammation. Thus, the discovery that the patients with these diseases possess evidence of cell-mediated immunity against collagen is of extreme interest in our understanding of the pathogenesis of these vexing conditions. There is also evidence that humoral immunity to collagen or its degradative products may be associated with the pathogenesis of rheumatoid arthritis.[93,94] In this connection, recent studies demonstrating induction of polyarthritis in rodents by immunization with purified type II collagen are of particular interest, and therefore the experimental model will be briefly described.

Collagen-Induced Arthritis. Chronic polyarthritis can be induced by immunization with heterologous or homologous type II collagen in susceptible animals.[85-88] This property appears to be unique for type II as opposed to type I, III, IV, or V collagen. Its triple-helical structure is also required, since denatured collagens are ineffective. Antibodies to type II collagen are normally not present in the animal but appear after immunization, and arthritis occurs when antibody levels are high. The major clinical manifestation of collagen-induced arthritis in rats and mice is an erosive, inflammatory polyarthritis affecting the peripheral joints.[89] Additionally, auricular chondritis[90] and sensory hearing loss[91] with vestibular dysfunction occur occasionally. The arthritic joints show proliferative synovitis with erosion of cartilage and bone resembling that seen in humans with chronic inflammatory arthritis.

A strong correlation exists between immunity to type II collagen and arthritis (for review, see ref. 92). Arthritis

is associated with high levels of circulating IgG anticollagen antibodies. Purified IgG antibodies from arthritic donors, when injected into a naive rat, can passively transfer the disease. In addition to the humoral immunity, the rats demonstrated an increased T-lymphocyte proliferative response suggesting a possible role for cell-mediated immunity in the disease. Subcutaneous injection of spleen cells containing covalently linked type II collagen induces cell-mediated immunity in the donor animal without antibody production or arthritis.[88] Immune tolerance to collagen-induced arthritis can also be developed using a single large intravenous injection of type II collagen either before or immediately after the primary immunization. The role of autoimmunity to collagen as a potential cause of inflammatory arthritis in man is less well understood. Many patients with rheumatoid arthritis have circulating antibodies to collagen in their serum.[93,94] It is unclear whether these autoantibodies are involved in the pathogenesis of arthritis or are the result of arthritis. Regardless, autoantibodies produced after the onset of arthritis may attack cartilage type II collagen, thus contributing to the inflammation and joint destruction.

More recently, several clones of monoclonal antibodies to type II collagen have been developed. At least one of the monoclonal antibodies can passively transfer arthritis in naive recipients, while others can protect the recipients from arthritis induction by active immunization. Taken together, these observations indicate that immune response directed to type II collagen can induce and perpetuate chronic polyarthritis in experimental animals.(see Chapter 58),

In addition, in patients with rheumatoid arthritis, an inflammatory disease that often results in severe destruction and deformities of joints, it has been found that the synovial tissue produces active collagenase capable of degrading native collagen (see Chapter 12). Although the primary cause of the disease is not known, it might be expected that inhibition of the collagenolytic enzyme may prevent or retard the destruction of the articular tissues. As yet, no attempt has been made to treat this condition with agents that inhibit the enzyme, such as EDTA, cysteine, macroglobulins, or other tissue-derived inhibitors.

In vitamin D–deficient rickets, it has been reported that the osteoid collagen is abnormally overglycosylated.[102] Whether this is a direct result of the deficiency of vitamin D per se or an indirect effect of the associated hypocalcemia is not known. Nonetheless, the common assumption that the defective bone formation in rickets is attributable to inadequate availability of mineral must be modified to include a defect in collagen structure as a factor.

Other biochemical alterations of connective tissue have been reported such as increased glycosylation of the renal basement membrane collagen in patients with diabetic nephropathy.[103] and alterations in the specific types of collagen deposited in liver cirrhosis and pulmonary fibrosis.[104,105] Although it is still premature to evaluate these findings, they do suggest a widespread involvement of the connective tissues in many pathologic states.

ELASTIN

Distribution and Mechanical Properties of Elastin

Elastin is the other major fibrous protein component of the extracellular connective tissue matrix. The yellow elastic ligaments such as the ligamenta flava of man or the ligamentum nuchae of grazing animals are largely composed of elastic fibers in close association with collagen and amorphous ground substance. Elastin also predominates in the media of large blood vessels. In contrast, the elastin content of other connective tissues such as dermis, tendon, and bone is low.

Elastin fiber exhibits some of the properties of an elastomer in that it has a high extensibility (i.e., the degree of elongation without irreversible changes per unit force applied to unit cross-sectional area is high). However, the tensile strength of elastin fibers is considerably less than that of collagen fibers. This is similar to the mechanical properties of rubber and is consistent with the function of elastin in relation to its distribution in arterial walls and ligaments. From consideration of its mechanical properties together with the ultrastructural and wide-angle x-ray diffraction studies showing no evidence of any repeating fine structure, it has been suggested that elastin is a three-dimensional network of randomly coiled polypetides joined together by covalent crosslinks.[2]

Structure

Elastin is a highly insoluble protein and has been loosely defined as that protein material which remains after all other connective tissue components are removed. Virtually all the isolation methods for elastin for biochemical analyses have utilized the aforementioned principles.[2] The methods used to remove the nonelastin components have been variable but most commonly involve extracting the tissue with boiling water and/or hot alkali (0.1N NaOH at 95°) until no further protein components are solubilized. In an attempt to avoid these rather harsh treatments, other methods have also been tried in which the other connective tissue components are removed by the use of enzymes (trypsin, collagenase, and α-amylase) that do not attack elastin, in conjunction with various extracting solvents such as salt solutions, organic acids, or guanidine hydrochloride solutions.

Regardless of the method of preparation, the final products have an amino acid composition that is reasonably reproducible and constant (Table 14–3). The composition is unusual in several respects. As in collagen, glycine is one third of the total residues. The proline content is also similar. In contrast to collagen,

Table 14–3. Amino Acid Composition of Elastin, Tropoelastin, and Fibronectin*

	Porcine Aortic Elastin[†]	Porcine Tropoelastin[†]	Fibronectin[‡]
4-Hydroxyproline	15	11	0
Aspartic acid	9	3	94
Threonine	7	14	100
Serine	8	9	74
Glutamic acid	21	18	118
Proline	94	109	77
Glycine	329	334	106
Alanine	233	218	47
Valine	125	121	66
Methionine	2	—	13
Isoleucine	20	19	38
Leucine	57	46	55
Tyrosine	17	16	37
Phenylalanine	32	28	19
1/4 Isodesmosine	8	0	—
1/4 Desmosine	8	0	—
Tryptophan	0	0	36
Lysine	8	48	34
Histidine	1	0	16
Arginine	7	7	53

*Residues per 1000 total residues.
[†]From Sandberg, L.B., et al.: Biochemistry 8:2940, 1969.
[‡]From Yamata, K.M., et al.: Biochemistry 16:5532, 1977.

there is very little hydroxyproline and no hydroxylysine and a preponderance of the nonpolar amino acids, alanine, valine, isoleucine, and leucine. The polar amino acids, aspartic and glutamic acids, lysine, and arginine, are present in very small amounts, as are the hydroxyl amino acids.

Since elastin is insoluble, physicochemical studies to probe the molecular structure have been impossible to perform. Solubilization has been achieved only through limited disruption of the peptide bonds either by the use of weak acids or by the action of specific enzymes such as pancreatic elastase. Limited hydrolysis of elastin from bovine ligamentum nuchae by hot, dilute oxalic acid yields two fractions of solubilized polypeptides. On the basis of NH_2-terminal residue analyses and molecular weight determinations of these two fractions, it has been suggested that a considerable number of interchain crosslinks must be present in elastin.[2] This is not surprising, since it is well known among the polymer chemists that a rubber-like elastomer must contain a reasonable number of crosslinks in its structure. These crosslinks impose a mechanical restriction on the elastomer, so that while stretching under stress one chain does not slip completely past another, preserving the ability of the elastomer to return to its original size when the stress is removed.

Crosslinks

There is a great deal of similarity between crosslinks of collagen and elastin. The basic difference is that no

Figure 14–14. Structure of elastin crosslinks, merodesmosine and desmosine. An isomer of desmosine, isodesmosine, and their reduced and oxidized forms are also found in elastin.

hydroxylysine is present in elastin, so that all crosslinks in elastin are lysine derived. A second major difference is that in elastin, reduction of several of the crosslinks occurs spontaneously by unknown mechanisms. A final difference is the quantity of the crosslinks: collagen, for example, contains one to two lysine- or hydroxylysine-derived crosslinks per 1000 residues of amino acids, whereas elastin may have as many as 40 lysine-derived crosslinks per 1000 residues.[2]

Four basic types of compounds have been identified in elastin.[2] These are dehydrolysinonorleucine and its reduced form, lysinonorleucine (Fig. 14–9); the aldol condensation product of two residues of allysine (Fig. 14–10); dehydromerodesmosine and its reduced form, merodesmosine (Fig. 14–14); and desmosine (Fig. 14–14). Biosynthetically, all these compounds are derived from lysyl residues through allysine. The mechanism of formation of the aldol condensate and dehydrolysinonorleucine in elastin is identical with that described for collagen. Unlike collagen, in elastin some of the dehydro compound is reduced in vivo to lysinonorleucine. Presumably, this is catalyzed in vivo by an enzyme system, but such a system has not been characterized.

The biosynthetic origin of dehydromerodesmosine appears to be through aldamine bond formation between a residue each of the aldol condensate and lysine. The precise biosynthetic pathway for desmosine is less certain and has not been characterized.

The maturation of elastin, therefore, represents another case in which post-translational modifications of the protein are involved in determining the ultimate properties of the tissues. In comparison to collagen, elastin utilizes a much larger number of crosslinkages, both within and between the polypeptide chains.

Tropoelastin

Unlike collagen, no soluble precursors of elastin can be found in extracts of normal tissues. This presumably is because of the low rate of synthesis and the rapidity with which the precursor forms are converted to mature, highly crosslinked elastin fibers via the enzyme lysyl oxidase. However, a soluble protein regarded by most investigators as the elastin precursor has been isolated

from the aorta of piglets with copper deficiency,[106] a state in which there is a generalized inhibition of crosslinking in elastin. Since lysyl oxidase is a copper metalloenzyme, presumably copper deficiency leads to deficient biosynthesis of allysine so that normal crosslinking of elastin is prevented. Tropoelastin has also been isolated from animals treated with β-aminopropionitrile.[107]

The soluble protein, termed tropoelastin, has been purified and partially characterized.[2,106,107] It has a molecular weight of 67,000 daltons. Its amino acid composition is presented in Table 14–3, together with that of insoluble elastin prepared from normal animals. The composition is similar, except that tropoelastin lacks the normal crosslinks described previously, but instead has a much higher content of lysine. This is consistent with the fact that the crosslink compounds of mature elastin are derived from lysyl residues. The observed lysyl residue content of 47 in tropoelastin is compatible with the observed values (approximately 40 per 1000 residues) of various lysyl-derived crosslinks in mature elastin.

Much of the structural information of elastin has been derived from analyses of this tropoelastin molecule (for review, see ref. 108). The approximately 800 amino acid polypeptide precursor contains large segments of hydrophobic amino acid residues which are interrupted with shorter segments of polyalanine sequence and clusters of lysine residues. The shorter segments are in alpha helix, but the larger hydrophobic regions possess a beta spiral structure with elastomeric properties. Within the hydrophobic regions a repeating pentapeptide (Pro-Gly-Val-Gly-Val) has been identified, which presumably imparts some unusual folding properties to the molecule. From this, it is evident that a collagen-like sequence [Gly-Val-Pro-Gly] occurs rather frequently. This would explain certain collagen-like properties of tropoelastin, such as its limited susceptibility to bacterial collagenase (Pro-Gly-X-Y) and also the observation of small amounts of hydroxyproline in tropoelastin. The sequence (Gly-X-Pro-Gly) is recognized by the enzyme prolyl hydroxylase. Only a small percentage of the proline residues, however, become hydroxylated.

The other unusual segments are the polyalanine regions. Each begins with tyrosine and exists as repeats

1 Ala-Lys-Ala-Ala-Lys-Tyr-Ala-(Ala)-(Pro)-Gly

    Des

Ala-Ala-Lys-Ala-Ala-Ala-Lys-Ala-Ala-(Glu)-Phe

2 Ala-Ala-Ala-Ala-Lys-Ala-Ala-Lys-Tyr-Gly-(X)-(X)-(X)-

    Des

Ala-Ala-Ala-Lys-Ala-Ala-Ala-Lys-Ala-Ala-Glu-Phe-

Figure 14–15. Amino acid sequence of two enzymatic fragments derived from mature elastin. (From Foster, J.A., et al.: J. Biol. Chem. 249:6191, 1974, with permission of authors and publisher.)

of two sequences, Ala-Ala-Lys and Ala-Ala-Ala-Lys.[109] This is of particular interest in view of the data describing the sequence of two crosslink peptides obtained from mature elastin from enzymatic digestion. Their sequence is shown in Figure 14–15. The clustering of alanyl residues adjacent to desmosine is noteworthy. The use of space-filling atomic models indicates that lysines separated by two or three alanyl residues in α helical conformation protrude on the same side of the helix. Hence, the sequence Lys-Ala-Ala-Lys allows the formation of dehydrolysinonorleucine, whereas the sequence Lys-Ala-Ala-Ala-Lys accommodates either aldol condensate or dehydrolysinonorleucine. Condensation of the two intrachain crosslinks could result in the formation of the interchain desmosine crosslinkages.

Metabolism. Ultrastructural studies indicate that the fibroblasts are the cell type producing elastin in most tissues. However, in the case of the arterial wall, the smooth muscle cells seem to be responsible for biogenesis of elastin. Elastin is synthesized on polysomes with a short leader sequence of about 25 residues[108] which is removed before tropoelastin is secreted. Regulation of elastin synthesis appears to be controlled at the pretranslational level, since the amount of elastin mRNA available is proportional to the level of elastin synthesis.[110] Utilizing a cDNA clone, a 3.5-kb mRNA was isolated and quantitated from chick aorta. The relative amount of elastin mRNA compared favorably with the functional elastin mRNA measured by elastin cell-free translation. Age-dependent changes in elastin synthesis also correlated with elastin mRNA content of the aorta.[111]

Very little is known about turnover of elastin. Even the existence of a physiologic elastolytic enzyme in connective tissue is not proved. The mammalian enzymes known to degrade elastin include polymorphonuclear leukocyte and pancreatic elastase (see Chapter 12).

Although little is known about the control in vivo of elastin turnover, there is a possible relationship between the absence of circulating elastase inhibitors and the development of destructive pulmonary disease seen in hereditary α_1-proteinase inhibitor (formerly called α_1-antitrypsin) deficiency.[112] In this disorder, the affected

individuals suffer from gradual but progressive destruction of connective tissue of the lung, leading to a marked distortion in the architecture of the lung at a relatively young age. These patients are deficient in antielastase and α_1-antitrypsin activity. The administration of elastase via aerosol therapy in mammals produces disordered pulmonary architecture similar to that seen in emphysema.[11] Since elastin is a major functional connective tissue component of the lung, it is possible that the pathologic process may be in some way related to the deficiency of the antienzyme activites. No large vessel disease is seen in this syndrome. Patients with rheumatoid arthritis carry normal amounts of this inhibitor in serum.

Biologic Considerations, Copper Deficiency, and Lathyrism

Chick and swine fed a diet deficient in copper develop a clinical syndrome in which the main manifestation is vascular fragility with subcutaneous and internal hemorrhage.[114] Histologically, there is fragmentation of the elastic elements of the arterial wall and minute breaks in the internal elastic membrane of the arteries. Dissecting aneurysm of the aorta is usually observed. Elastin isolated from the diseased animals has been shown to be deficient in the content of the crosslink compounds but high in lysyl content as compared with the control.[107] In addition, there is evidence that collagen in these animals may be deficient in the content of collagen crosslinks.[115] It is now known that the defect in these animals is a failure of conversion of the lysyl residues to allysyl residues, thus blocking the crosslinking of elastin and collagen. The enzyme system involved in this deamination requires copper for action.

FIBRONECTIN

Fibronectin is a high molecular weight glycoprotein that has rapidly gained prominence due to its cell surface interaction with extracellular matrix proteins. Its potential role in the control of cellular functions such as replication, motility, and differentiation has stimulated extensive studies from a variety of scientific disciplines (for review, see refs. 116 to 118). The name fibronectin (*fibra* [Lat.] = fiber; *nectene* [Lat.] = connect, link) is now accepted and replaces many others, such as cold insoluble globulin (plasma fibronectin), LETS protein, SF antigen, CSP, galactoprotein, and cell attachment factor. As early as 1940 it was identified as a cryoprecipitate of plasma; hence the early name was cold insoluble globulin. In connective tissue, its prominence became apparent as a cell attachment factor from serum which, in tissue culture, promoted binding of fibroblasts to collagen-coated surfaces.[119] It was later found to be a biosynthetic product of many different cell types in vitro. The multifaceted binding properties of this protein has led to identification of specific binding domains within its polypeptide structure. The rapid explosion of information on fibronectin has revealed its function in cell adhesion, connective tissue matrix formation, opsonization, blood coagulation and malignant transformation.

Chemical Properties

Fibronectin exists as a 450,000-dalton, disulfide-linked dimer in plasma and tissue. With reduction, two equal- or nearly equal-sized polypeptide chains are released, with apparent molecular weights of 220,000 daltons each. Pyroglutamic acid was identified as the single NH_2-terminal amino acid of the intact dimer, and peptide maps of each of the individual polypeptide chains from plasma fibronectin monomers were identical, leading to the conclusion that it is a dimer of two identical polypeptides.[120] The amino acid composition of the intact fibronectin is presented in Table 14–3.

The precise relationship between plasma fibronectin, fibronectins on various cell surfaces, and tissue fibronectin remains unclear. All fibronectins examined thus far are immunochemically indistinguishable, even though the gel electrophoretic mobility may vary with species and source; and the extensive crossreactivity of antisera to fibronectin of widely diverse species further indicates its primary structure has been highly conserved during evolution.[121]

Interactions of Fibronectin

Most of the proposed biologic functions of fibronectin deal with its ability to adhere to cells and/or the extracellular matrix proteins, hence its role as an anchor protein in the extracellular matrix. This protein has been shown to interact with collagens, glycosaminoglycans, fibrinogen, actin, and certain gram-positive bacteria (Table 14–4). As more information is obtained, the list will

Figure 14–16. A model for the structure and interactions of fibronectin. Only a single subunit of fibronectin is shown, although identical sites are present with the other subunit. The specific molecules that interact are tabulated in Table 14–4. The free SH may be involved in certain interactions, and the X represents the site of covalent crosslinking via transglutaminase (Factor XIII of complement), which also crosslinks fibrin. The additional interaction of glycosaminoglycans to both fibronectin and collagen serve to stabilize this multimolecular complex. (From Rouslahti E., et al.: Coll. Res. 1:104, 1981, with permission of authors and publisher.)

presumably grow considerably, but, even now, the magnitude of the fibronectin involvement as a biologically active molecule in extracellular matrices must be appreciated. The adhesion is rapid, requires divalent cations, and is temperature-dependent, and cell adhesion is inhibited by cytochalasin B. The specific binding regions of the polypeptide structure have been classified as domains of the polypeptide chain (Fig. 14–16).

Collagen. The binding properties of fibronectin with collagen have been studied in the greatest detail.[114] It was initially identified as a factor responsible for the attachment of cells in culture to collagen-coated surfaces. This cell adhesion was greatly enhanced by addition of serum or culture media now known to contain fibronectin. With time, cells can produce sufficient fibronectin to promote their own attachment.

All genetic types of collagen have been shown to bind fibronectin.[122] In fact, Clq of complement, which also contains a Gly-X-Y repeating structure, has affinity for fibronectin.[123] Several important observations have emerged from these collagen binding studies. Denatured collagens have a much greater affinity for fibronectin compared with their native counterparts. While this gelatin binding has been very exciting to cell attachment studies, its significance in connective tissue in vivo is uncertain, since gelatin is not a normal component of the extracellular matrix. The fact remains, however, that native collagens do bind fibronectin, and other macromolecules, such as hyaluronic acid and heparin sulfate, stabilize this attachment. From studies with denatured collagen and fragments from their chains, it appears that

Table 14–4. Molecular Interactions of Fibronectin*

Binding Site	Ligand	Comment
1	Collagen Fibrin(ogen) Actin	The same or adjacent binding sites in fibronectin
2	Heparin Heparin sulfate DNA Dextran sulfate	A shared binding site
3	Hyaluronic acid	A binding site separate from the heparin binding site?
4	Staphylococci	A separate binding site in the N-terminal end of the fibronectin molecule
5	Cell surfaces	A separate binding site. Interacts with oligosaccharide portion of cell surface gangliosides?

*From Rouslahti, E., et al.: Coll. Res. 1:98, 1981, with permission of authors and publisher.

numerous binding sites may exist along the unfolded collagen backbone. One site in particular may have a great affinity, namely, CB-7 of the α1(I) collagen chain or CB-5 of α1(III).[117] These cyanogen bromide peptides occur in homologous regions of their respective polypeptide chains, which also contain the single mammalian collagenase cleavage site of the collagen molecule. In the native collagen molecule, this specific region contains fewer imino acids and more bulky hydrophobic amino acids. Hypothetically, this yields a less compact triple helix and is more accessible to disruptive forces.[124] In fact, polymorphonuclear elastase has been shown to cleave native type III collagen[125] in this region. Extrapolating from these data, the binding site of fibronectin to native collagen has been relegated primarily to the cleavage region of the collagen chain. It is therefore notsurprising that type III collagen (native) has a greater affinity for fibronectin than the other collagens.

Fibrinogen. Fibrinogen has long been known to coprecipitate with fibronectin (cold insoluble globulin) in the cold. It also becomes incorporated into a blood clot and becomes covalently crosslinked to fibrin via transglutaminase, the enzyme that crosslinks fibrin.[126] On the basis of these facts and the known cell attachment property of fibronectin, it has been proposed that fibronectin bound to a fibrin clot could provide an adhesive temporary matrix for cells to grow in. This would provide a scaffold then for early wound healing. This binding is inhibited by gelatin; hence the fibrinogen binding domain must be at or near the collagen binding domain. Although fibrinogen binding is very weak, the covalent linking of fibrin to fibronectin via the transglutaminase enzyme (Factor XIII) would provide a stable bond.[127]

Glycosaminoglycans. A number of polyanionic macromolecules bind to fibronectin. Heparin, heparin sulfate, dextran sulfate, and DNA compete with each other for binding to the fibronectin molecule, suggesting they all share the same binding site.[116] Hyaluronic acid also interacts but at a different domain of the fibronectin molecule.[129] Other polyanionic macromolecules such as chondroitin sulfates and dermatan sulfate do not bind, thereby demonstrating a certain degree of specificity.

Polyanionic binding can be augmented by gelatin-coated beads. In the presence of *both* fibronectin and glycosaminoglycan, the gelatin-coated beads agglutinated. Addition of heparin sulfate or hyaluronic acid to fibronectin-coated gelatin-Sepharose columns enhanced the stability of fibronectin-gelatin binding. This combined interaction of the three major components of extracellular matrix, fibronectin, glycosaminoglycan, and collagen, may serve as a model for the formation of extracellular matrix as an insoluble complex. In the presence of heparin, fibronectin will also precipitate native type I and type III collagen. Alone, neither fibronectin or heparin is effective. Therefore, this cooperative effect utilizing two distinct binding domains on the fibronectin molecule with enhancement of the binding affinity of native collagen to fibronectin makes this precipitation possible.

A similar situation occurs with fibrinogen. The addition of heparin to a solution of fibrinogen and fibronectin causes precipitation at low temperatures. Since fibrinogen occupies a site on the fibronectin molecule similar to that of collagen, a similar mechanism presumably exists. Therefore, the trimolecular complex may be a more physiologic situation to examine when studying the biologic significance of fibronectin in tissue matrix (Fig. 14–16).

Cell Surfaces. It is well-established that cell suspensions preferentially attach to surfaces in the presence of fibronectin. Furthermore, fibronectin provides a divalent cation-dependent linkage between collagen-coated surfaces and specific cells (Fig. 14–17). The presence of a specific cell attachment domain on the fibronectin molecule therefore comes as no surprise, and this domain is located at a distant site from the collagen, fibrinogen, and polyanionic macromolecular domain. The specific component of the cell membrane that is recognized by fibronectin has not been fully established. The current evidence based on binding inhibition studies with various gangliosides suggests that certain widely distributed cell surface oligosaccharides serve as these receptor sites.[129]

Actin. Fibronectin has been shown to bind directly to actin, and this binding can be inhibited by collagen, suggesting that the actin binding site is located in close proximity to the collagen and fibrin binding domain. Since actin is an intracellular protein, the significance of this specific binding remains unclear. The interaction of fibronectin with actin, an insoluble intracellular protein, may perhaps play a role in elimination of remnants of dead cells by utilizing the nonimmune opsonization ability of fibronectin. Alternatively, since both actin and fibronectin play a role in cell spreading, a possible communication between these two molecules through the cell membrane has been postulated (Fig. 14–17).

Bacteria. Another binding site on the fibronectin molecule has an affinity for specific gram-positive bacteria. Thus far, *Staphylococcus aureus*,[131] *Streptococcus pyogenes*,[132] and *Streptococcus pneumoniae*,[133] bind to a similar receptor on fibronectin at regions distinct from the collagen binding domain. The mucosal cell surface fibronectin serves as a receptor for the lipoteichoic acid–

Figure 14–17. Schematic model of cell adhesion to fibronectin and collagen. Fibronectin contains a specific binding site for collagen and another for the cell surface. Collagen contains a specific binding region for fibronectin and a glycoconjugate, possibly a glycolipid in the cell membrane is recognized by fibronectin. Proteoglycans are also present and stabilize the interaction. The interaction, if any, between actin (intracellular) and fibronectin remains uncertain. (From Kleinman, H.K., et al.: J. Cell. Biol. 88:479, 1981, with permission of authors and publisher.)

mediated binding of Group A streptococci. This affinity is through the lipid region of the lipoteichoic acid to a fatty acid binding site on fibronectin. The binding of bacteria to fibronectin has been shown to enhance opsonization by circulating phagocytic cells. Gram-negative bacteria do not bind to fibronectin, but interestingly, *E. coli* does bind to laminin, the fibronectin counterpart in basement membrane tissue.[134]

The amount of information on fibronectin binding to proteins and cells has grown enormously in recent years, but with the complex nature of biologic systems, this information is probably far from complete. Already, fibronectin appears to be the "molecular fly paper" for many complex molecular structures. This ability to link molecules and cells via separate domains of the molecule alters the physical characteristics of these complexes and hence biologic properties of these unrelated components.

Binding Sites on the Fibronectin Molecule

The designation of specific binding domains on fibronectin has been derived primarily by competitive inhibition of the various molecules in solution or on Sepharose affinity columns (for review, see ref. 118). Recent procedures have utilized large proteolytic fragments of fibronectin to pinpoint these areas. A 30,000 to 40,000 molecular weight NH₂-terminal fragment, which contains the collagen-binding region, has been isolated by gelatin-Sepharose affinity chromatography.[136] This was confirmed by the Dintzis procedure of short-term pulse labeling cells during polypeptide chain elongation.[137]

A tentative model for the fibronectin molecule has been presented in Figure 14–18. In this molecule, two similar 220,000 dalton subunits are linked via a disulfide bond near the COOH-terminus. The binding site for staphylococci occurs in the 27,000-dalton NH₂-terminal

domain of fibronectin and may be obtained with mild tryptic digestion. This fragment was identified as the NH₂-terminal fragment by pulse labeling and by the fact that it contains a blocked NH₂-terminal (pyroglutamic acid). This fragment also contains the glutamic residue which becomes crosslinked to fibrin via the transglutaminase enzyme (Factor XIII) that crosslinks fibrin. The next binding domain is the collagen binding site. This was confirmed by isolation of a 72,000 MW fragment with a blocked NH₂-terminal which contains the gelatin-binding site. This fragment was further cleaved into two peptides, a 29,000 MW component (block NH₂-terminal) and a 43,000 MW fragment, which binds gelatin. The smallest fragment known to contain both the gelatin-binding domain and the cell attachment region was 130,000 MW. From this, it is assumed that these latter two domains must be considerably distant from each other. The smallest fragment known to contain the heparin-binding site, the cell attachment site, and the gelatin-binding domain is 200,000 MW, thereby placing the heparin-binding region near the COOH-terminus of the polypeptide chain. At least one and possibly two free SH groups are available. The free SH group at a position of about 170,000 MW from the NH₂-terminus of the polypeptide chain seems to participate in disulfide bond formation with the insoluble matrix at the cell surface. The location of the carbohydrate on the fibronectin molecule has been identified on a 40,000 MW gelatin-binding fragment in the hamster fibroblast fibronectin. However, as stated above, the degree of glycosylation is variable among species, and other carbohydrate regions may be found.

Cell Origin and Tissue Distribution

Fibronectin, as stated previously, occurs as a circulating plasma fibronectin (soluble) and as that which is present in extracellular spaces (insoluble) (for review,

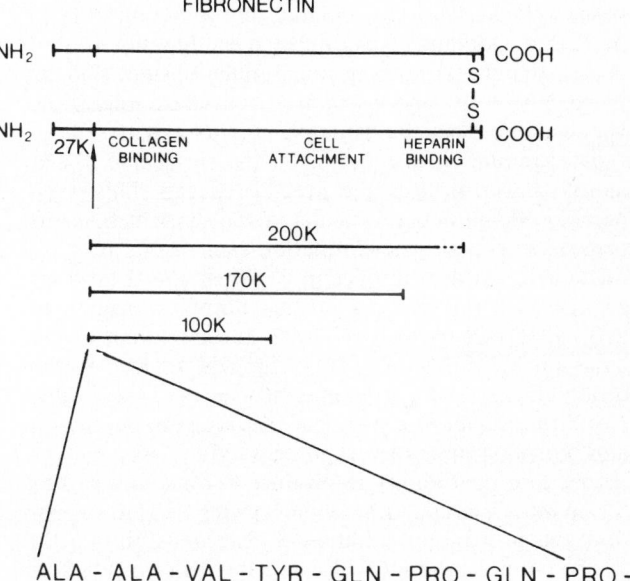

Figure 14–18. Schematic representation of plasmin-derived fragments from fibronectin and their localization in the fibronectin polypeptide. (From Ruoslahti E., et al.: J. Invest. Dermatol. 76:65s, 1982, with permission of authors and publisher.)

see ref. 116). Fibronectin levels in the plasma are quite high (300 μg per ml). Tissue fibronectin was first identified in fibroblast culture medium (up to 50 μg per ml at confluency). The cells of liver, kidney, gut, breast, and amnionic membranes produce fibronectin as do Schwann cells, macrophages, melanoma cells, endothelial cells, and undifferentiated chondrocytes. Endothelial cells and liver cells appear to be the source of plasma fibronectin. With cell cultures, fibronectin is found in the medium, at the cell surface, and in the extracellular matrix. An important fraction of the cell surface fibronectin is located at sites where the cells make contact with the substratum (Fig. 14–17). The cells may be detached by chelating agents and leave behind material that contains fibronectin and proteoglycans involved in cell attachment. Little is known about the physiologic significance of the culture medium fibronectin or the insoluble matrix fibronectin. These two latter fibronectin compartments appear to be in equilibrium with each other. In the same manner, when radiolabeled plasma fibronectin is injected into the same species, it becomes incorporated into the tissue matrix, indicating equilibration between body fluid and extracellular matrix fibronectin. The fibronectin in the tissue appears throughout loose connective tissues, with higher amounts at the interface between basement membrane and the cells. It is not, however, a component of basement membranes.

Biologic Function and Significance of Fibronectin

The functional characteristics of fibronectin are derived primarily from its interaction properties (Table 14–4). It promotes cell attachment and spreading in vitro and presumably in vivo. The attachment of cells to an insoluble matrix is required for cell spreading and replication.

The circulating plasma fibronectin has been assigned a variety of roles in the cascade of wound healing events. It promotes adhesion and spreading of platelets on exposed collagen surfaces, binding of circulating cells to the fibrin clot and exposed collagen, binding to cell debris, thereby promoting nonimmune opsinization by phagocytic cells, and promoting fibroblast migration, via chemotaxis, to the damaged area for repair.[117]

The amount of fibronectin on the surface of malignantly transformed cells is greatly reduced. This is especially evident in experimental systems in which a shift of conditions to a transformation also results in a reduction in surface fibronectin.[116] When the conditions are reversed, the cells regain their normal morphology and cell surface fibronectin. The reduced amount of cell adhesion by malignant cells is thought to lead to increased invasive properties and metastases of these cells.

Fibronectin may play a role in directing differentiation and morphogenesis of certain cells. Myoblasts, for example, lose their ability to produce fibronectin prior to fusion into myotubules.[116] Chondrocytes also fail to produce this protein, but addition of exogenous fibronectin to the culture medium will cause the cells to dedifferentiate, assume a fibroblastic phenotype with lowered production of proteoglycans and cartilage-specific type II collagen, and induce the synthesis of endogenous fibronectin.[117]

There has been little conclusive information on abnormalities of fibronectin in diseased connective tissues. Skin lesions of scleroderma contain increased amounts of fibronectin as judged by immunofluorescent staining. Changes in fibronectin distribution are seen in various diseases affecting the skin. One must assume more alterations in matrix fibronectin will be identified as methodologies in this area improve.[116] Fibronectin has long been known to cause an enhancement of phagocytosis (opsonization) of gelatin-coated particles. More information is needed to determine the extent of this opsonization.

As alluded to earlier, some cells do not require fibronectin for attachment to native collagen. For example, baby hamster kidney (BHK) and BALB 3T3 cells attach more efficiently when fibronectin is added, but this requirement of fibronectin is not absolute. A controversy remains over whether these cells utilize exogenously added fibronectin or rapidly produce their own fibronectin or whether a different mechanism of cell attachment is possible for direct binding to native collagen or other surfaces. Additional unidentified glycoproteins may also mediate some cell attachment. These may be cell-specific and matrix-specific such as in cartilage.

Chondrocytes use another glycoprotein, chondronectin, to promote adherence. This protein has a molecular weight of 180,000 daltons, contains disulfide-linked chains, is present in serum, and is produced by cultured chondrocytes.[113] Although only a limited amount of information is available to date, it is presumed to be analogous in function to fibronectin.

Epithelial cells attach preferentially to type IV collagen in basement membrane. This adhesion is slow and not stimulated by fibronectin. In this case, laminin, another glycoprotein is apparently the attachment factor for these cells. Laminin is an 800,000-dalton glycoprotein found in basement membranes, and like fibronectin, apparently binds to the substrate (type IV collagen), and then the cells bind to the laminin–type IV collagen complex (Fig. 14–11). Some cells, such as regenerating rat liver hepatocytes, produce both laminin and fibronectin and may perhaps use both mechanisms for cell adhesions.[116] With metastatic cells, the target organ of a specific cell invasion and tumorigenicity may be dependent on the genetically programmed specific attachment protein of the metastatic cell. Clearly, the role of fibronectin and other adherence-promoting glycoproteins in biologic systems is exceedingly complex due to its multivalent capabilities and their widely diverse biologic activities.

REFERENCES

1. Traub, W., and Piez, K.A.: The chemistry and structure of collagen. Adv. Prot. Chem. 25:243, 1971.
2. Gallop, P.M., Blumenfeld, O.O., and Seifter, S.: Structure and metabolism of connective tissue proteins. Ann. Rev. Biochem. 41:617, 1972.

3. Gross, J., Highberger, J.H., and Schmitt, F.O.: Collagen structures considered as states of aggregation of a kinetic unit. The tropocollagen particle. Proc. Natl. Acad. Sci. USA 40:679, 1954.
4. Epstein, E.H., Scott, R.D., Miller, E.J., and Piez, K.A.: Isolation and characterization of the peptides derived from soluble human and baboon skin collagen after CNBr cleavage. J. Biol. Chem. 246:1718, 1971.
5. Miller, E.J., and Lunde, L.G.: Isolation and characterization of the CNBr peptides from the $\alpha1(II)$ chain of bovine and human cartilage collagen. Biochemistry 12:3153, 1973.
6. Chung, E., Keele, E.M., and Miller, E.J.: Isolation and characterization of CNBr peptides from $\alpha1(II)$ chain of human collagen. Biochemistry 13:3463, 1974.
7. Kefalides, N.A.: Isolation of a collagen from basement membranes containing three identical α chains. Biochem. Biophys. Res. Commun. 45:226, 1971.
8. Bornstein, P., and Traub, W.: The chemistry and biology of collagen. In Neurath. H. (ed.): The Proteins. Vol. 4. 3rd ed. New York, Academic Press, 1979.
9. Reid, K.: A collagen-like amino acid sequence in a polypeptide chain of human Clq (a subcomponent of the first component of complement). Biochem. J. 141:189, 1974.
10. Rosenberry, T., and Richardson, J.: Structure of 18S and 14S acetylcholinesterase. Biochemistry 16:3550, 1977.
11. Seyer, J.M., and Kang, A.H.: Covalent structure of collagen: Amino acid sequence of $\alpha1(III)$-CB9 from type III collagen of human liver. Biochemistry 20:2621, 1981.
12. Highberger, J.H., Corbett, C., Dixit, S.N., Yu, W., Seyer, J.M., Kang, A.H., and Gross, J.: The amino acid sequence of chick skin collagen $\alpha1(I)$-CB8 and the complete primary structure of the helical portion of the chick skin collagen $\alpha1(I)$ chain. Biochemistry 21:2048, 1982.
13. Piez, K.A.: Primary structure (of collagen). In Ramachandran, G.N., and Reddi, A.H. (eds.): Biochemistry of Collagen. New York and London, Plenum Press, 1976.
14. Hulmes, D.J.S., and Miller, A., Parry, D.A.D., Piez, K.A., and Woodhead-Galloway, J.: Analysis of the primary structure of collagen for the origins of molecular packing. J. Mol. Biol. 79:137, 1973.
15. Ramachandran, G.N., and Ramakrishnan, C.: Molecular structure (of collagen). In Ramachandran, G.N., and Reddi, A.H. (eds.): Biochemistry of Collagen. New York and London, Plenum Press, 1976.
16. Piez, K.A., Eigner, E.A., and Lewis, M.S.: The chromatographic separation and amino acid composition of the subunits of several collagens. Biochemistry 2:58, 1963.
17. Bornstein, P., and Sage, H.: Structurally distinct collagen types. Ann. Rev. Biochem. 49:957, 1980.
18. Burgeson, R.E.: Genetic heterogeneity of collagens. J. Invest. Dermatol. 79:25, 1982.
19. Kefalides, N.A.: Structure and biosynthesis of basement membranes. Int. Rev. Conn. Tissue Res. 6:63, 1973.
20. Chung, E., Rhodes, R.K., and Miller, E.J.: Isolation of three collagenous components of probable basement membrane origin from several tissues. Biochem. Biophys. Res. Commun. 71:1167, 1976.
21. Burgeson, R.E., El Adli, F.A., Kaitila, I.I., and Hollister, D.W.: Fetal membrane collagens: Identification of two new collagen α chains. Proc. Natl. Acad. Sci. USA 73:2579, 1976.
22. Gay, S., Rhodes, R.K., Gay, R.E., and Miller, E.J.: Collagen molecules composed of $\alpha1(V)$ chains (B-chains): An apparent localization in the excytoskeleton. Coll. Res. 1:53, 1981.
23. Furato, D.K., and Miller, E.J.: Isolation of a unique collagenous fraction from limited pepsin digests of human placental tissue. J. Biol. Chem. 255:290, 1980.
24. Reese, C.A., and Mayne, R.: Minor collagens of chick hyaline cartilage. Biochemistry 20:918, 1981.
25. Glimcher, M.J., and Krane, S.M.: The organization and structure of bone and the mechanism of calcification. In Gould, B.S., and Ramachandran, G.N. (eds.): A Treatise on Collagen, Vol. II. London and New York, Academic Press, 1968.
26. Prockop, D.J., Berg, R.A., and Kivirrikko, K.: Intracellular steps in the biosynthesis of collagen. In Ramachandran, G.N., and Reddi, A.H. (eds.): Biochemistry of Collagen. New York and London, Plenum Press, 1976.
27. Bornstein, P.: The biosynthesis of collagen. Ann. Rev. Biochem. 43:567, 1974.
28. Monson, J.M., Click, E.M., and Bornstein, P.: Further characterization of procollagen. Purification and analysis of the pro $\alpha1$ chain of chick bone procollagen. Biochemistry 14:4088, 1975.
29. Morris, N.P., Fessler, L.I., Weinstock, A., and Fessler, J.H.: Procollagen assembly and secretion in embryonic chick bone. J. Biol. Chem. 250:5719, 1975.
30. Uitto, J., and Prockop, D.J.: Rate of helix formation by intracellular procollagen and protocollagen. Evidence for a role for disulfide bonds. Biochem. Biophys. Res. Commun. 55:904, 1973.
31. Vuust, J., and Piez, K.A.: A kinetic study of collagen biosynthesis. J. Biol. Chem. 247:856, 1972.
32. Layman, D.L., McGoodwin, E.B., and Martin, G.R.: The nature of collagen synthesized by cultured human fibroblasts. Proc. Natl. Acad. Sci., USA 68:454, 1971.
33. Graves, P.N., Olsen, B.R., Fietzek, P.P., Prockop, D.J., and Monson, J.M.: Comparison of the NH_2-terminal sequence of chick type I preprocollagen chains synthesized in an mRNA-dependent reticulocyte lysate. Eur. J. Biochem. 118:363, 1981.
34. Wozney, J., Hanahaw, D., Tate, V., Boedtker, H., and Doty, P.: Structure of the pro $\alpha2(I)$ collagen gene. Nature 294:129, 1981.
35. Tolstoshev, P., and Crystal, R.G.: The collagen alpha-2 chain gene. J. Invest. Dermatol. 79:60, 1982.
36. Grant, M.E., and Prockop, D.J.: The biosynthesis of collagen. N. Engl. J. Med. 286:194, 242, 291, 1972.
37. Cardinale, G.J., and Udenfriend, S.: Prolyl hydroxylase. Adv. Enzymol. 41:245, 1974.
38. Kuutti, E.R., Tuderman, L., and Kivvirikko, K.I.: Human prolyl hydroxylase. Purification, characterization, and preparation of antiserum to the enzyme. Eur. J. Biochem. 57:181, 1975.
39. Myllylä, R., Risteli, L., and Kivvirikko, K.I.: Assay of collagen galactosyltransferase and collagen glucosyltransferase activities and characterization of enzyme reactions with transferases from chick embryo cartilage. Eur. J. Biochem. 52:401, 1975.
40. Myllylä, R., Risteli, L., and Kivvirrikko, K.I.: Collagen glucosyltransferase. Partial purification and characterization of the enzyme from whole chick embryos and chick-embryo cartilage. Eur. J. Biochem. 61:59, 1976.
41. Tuderman, L., Kivvirikko, K., and Prockop, D.J.: Partial purification and characterization of neutral protease which cleaves the N-terminal propeptides from procollagen. Biochemistry 17:2948, 1978.
42. Leung, M.K.K., Fessler, L.I., Greenberg, D.B., and Fessler, J.H.: Separate amino acid carboxyl procollagen peptidases in chick embryo tendon. J. Biol. Chem. 254:224, 1979.
43. Trelstad, R.L., Birk, D.E., and Silver, F.H.: Collagen fibrillogenesis in tissues, in solution, and from modeling: A synthesis. J. Invest. Dermatol. 79:109, 1982.
44. Rennard, S.E., Steir, L.E., and Crystal, R.G.: Intracellular degradation of newly synthesized collagen. J. Invest. Dermatol. 79:77, 1982.
45. Kivvirikko, K.I.: Urinary excretion of hydroxyproline in health and disease. Int. Rev. Conn. Tissue Res. 5:93, 1970.
46. Krane, S.M., Munoz, A.J., and Harris, E.D., Jr.: Urinary polypeptides related to collagen synthesis. J. Clin. Invest. 49:716, 1970.
47. Askenasi, R.: Urinary hydroxylysine and hydroxylysyl glycoside excretions in normal and pathologic states. J. Lab. Clin. Med. 83:673, 1974.
48. Krane, S.M., Kantrowitz, F.G., Byrne, M., Pinnell, S.R., and Singer, F.R.: Urinary excretion of hydroxylysine and its glycosides as an index of collagen degradation. J. Clin. Invest. 59:819, 1977.
49. Gross, J.: Aspects of the animal collagenase. In Ramachandran, G.N., and Reddi, A.H. (eds.): Biochemistry of Collagen. New York and London, Plenum Press, 1976.
50. Harris, E.D., and Krane, S.M.: Collagenases. N. Engl. J. Med. 291:557, 605, 652, 1974.
51. Evanson, J.M., Jeffrey, J.J., and Krane, S.M.: Studies on collagenase from rheumatoid synovium in tissue culture. J. Clin. Invest. 47:2639, 1968.
52. Tanzer, M.L.: Cross-linking (of collagen). In Ramachandran, G.N., Reddi, A.H. (eds.): Biochemistry of Collagen. New York and London, Plenum Press, 1976.
53. Gallop, P.M., and Paz, M.A.: Posttranslational protein modifications with special attention to collagen and elastin. Physiol. Rev. 55:418, 1975.
54. Siegel, R.C.: Collagen crosslinking; Purification and substrate specificity of lysyl oxidase. J. Biol. Chem. 251:5779, 1976.
55. Fujimoto, D., Moriguchi, T., Ishida, T., and Hayashi, H.: The structure of pyridinoline: a collagen crosslink. Biochem. Biophys. Res. Commun. 84:52, 1978.
56. Bornstein, P.H., and Mechanic, G.L.: A natural histidine-based imminium crosslink in collagen and its location. J. Biol. Chem. 255:10414, 1980.
57. Epstein, E.H., and Munderloh, N.H.: Isolation and characterization of CNBr peptides of human $[\alpha1(IV)]_3$ collagen and tissue distribution of $[\alpha1(I)]_2\alpha2$ and $[\alpha1(III)]_3$ collagens J. Biol. Chem. 250:9304, 1975.
58. Bailey, A.J., Bazin, S., Sims, T.J., Lelous, M., Nicoletis, C., and Dalauncy, A.: Characterization of the collagen of human hypertrophic and normal scars. Biochim. Biophys. Acta 405:412, 1975.
59. Miller, E.J.: A review of biochemical studies on the genetically distinct collagens of the skeletal system. Clin. Orthop. Relat. Res. 92:260, 1973.
60. Foidant, J.M., and Yaar, M.: Type IV collagen, laminin, and fibronectin at the dermal-epidermal junction. Front Matrix Biol. Vol. 8. Basel, S. Karger, 1981, pp. 175–188.
61. Kresina, T.F., and Miller, E.J.: Isolation and characterization of basement membrane collagen from human placental tissue: Evidence of the pres-

ence of two genetically distinct collagen chains. Biochemistry 18:3089, 1979.

62. Timpl, R., Wiedemann, H., von Delden, V., Furthmayr, H., and Kühn, K.: A network model for the organization of type IV collagen molecules in basement membranes. Eur. J. Biochem. 120:203, 1981.

63. Sage, H.: Collagen of basement membranes. J. Invest. Dermatol. 79:51, 1982.

64. Valdrighi, L., and Vidol, B.C.: Silver impregnation: Collagenic and reticular fibers and the ground substance. Ann. Histochim. 16:29, 1971.

65. Windrum, G.M., Kent, P.W., and Eastoe, J.E.: Constitution of human renal reticulin. Br. J. Exp. Path. 36:49, 1955.

66. Furthmayer, H., and Timpl, R.: Immunochemistry of collagens and procollagens. In Hall, D.A., and Jackson, D.S. (eds.): International Review of Connective Tissue Research, Volume 7. New York, Academic Press, 1976, pp.61–99.

67. Beil, W., Timpl, R., and Furthmayer, H.: Conformation dependence of antigenic determinants on the collagen molecule. Immunology 24:13, 1973.

68. Nowack, H., Hahn, E., David, C.S., Timpl, R., and Götze, D.: Immune response to calf collagen Type I in mice: A combined control of Ir-1A and H-2 linked genes. Immunogenetics 2:331, 1975.

69. Taubman, M.B., Goldberg, B., and Sherr, C.J.: Radioimmunoassay for human procollagen. Science 186:1115, 1974.

70. Keiser, H., LeRoy, E.C., Udenfriend, S., and Sjoerdsma, A.: Collagen-like protein in human plasma. Science 142:1678, 1963.

71. Rohde, H., Vargas, L., Hahn, E., Kalbfleisch, H., Brugeura, M., and Timpl, R.: Radioimmunoassay for type III procollagen peptide and its application to human liver disease. Eur. J. Clin. Invest. 9:451, 1979.

72. Taubman, M.B., Kammerman, S., and Goldberg, B.: Radioimmunoassay of procollagen in serum of patients with Paget's disease of bone. Proc. Soc. Exp. Biol. Med. 152:284, 1976.

73. McKusick, V.A.: Heritable Disorders of Connective Tissue. 4th ed. St. Louis, C.V. Mosby Company, p. 192.

74. Pinnell, S.R.: Disorders of collagen. In Stanbury, J.B., Wyngaarden, J.B., and Fredrickson, D.S. (eds.): The Metabolic Basis of Inherited Disease. 4th ed. New York, McGraw-Hill Book Company, 1978.

75. Gross, J.: Collagen biology: Structure, degradation and disease. Harvey Lect. 68:351, 1974.

76. Narayanan, A.S., Siegel, R.C., and Martin, G.R.: On the inhibition of lysyl oxidase by β-aminopropionitrile. Biochem. Biophys. Res. Commun. 46:745, 1972.

77. Nimni, M.E., and Deshmukh, G.N.: Collagen defect induced by penicillamine. Nature 240:220, 1972.

78. Burry, H.C.: Penicillamine and wound healing: A potential hazard? Postgrad. Med. J. (Suppl.) 50:75, 1974.

79. Scheinberg, I.H.: Uses and usefulness of penicillamine. N. Engl. J. Med. 292:1080, 1975.

80. Mjolerod, I.K., Rasmussen, K., Dommerud, S.A., and Gjeruldsen, S.T.: Congenital connective tissue defect probably due to D-penicillamine treatment in pregnancy. Lancet 1:673, 1971.

81. Kang, A.H., and Trelstad, R.L.: A collagen defect in homocystinuria. J. Clin. Invest. 52:2571, 1973.

82. Helbe, O., and Ness, N.N.: A hereditary skin defect in sheep. Acta Vet. Scand. 13:443, 1972.

83. Lenaers, A., Ansay, M., Nusgens, B.V., and Lapiere, C.M.: Collagen made of extended α chains: Procollagen in genetically defective dermatosparaxic calves. Eur. J. Biochem. 23:533, 1971.

84. Lichtenstein, J.R., Kohn, L.D., Martin, G.R., Byers, P., and McKusick, V.A.: Procollagen peptidase deficiency in a form of the Ehlers-Danlos syndrome. Trans. Assoc. Am. Physicians 86:333, 1973.

85. Trentham, D.E., Townes, A.S., and Kang, A.H.: Autoimmunity to type II collagen: An experimental model of arthritis. J. Exp. Med. 146:857, 1977.

86. Trentham, D.E., Townes, A.S., Kang, A.H., and David, J.R.: Humoral and cellular sensitivity to collagen in type II collagen-induced arthritis in rats. J. Clin. Invest. 61:89, 1978.

87. Stuart, J.M., Cremer, M.A., Townes, A.S., and Kang, A.H.: Collagen-induced arthritis in rats: Evaluation of early immunologic events. Arthritis Rheum. 12:1344, 1979.

88. Trentham, D.E., Dynesius, R.A., and David, J.R.: Passive transfer by cells of type II collagen-induced arthritis in rats. J. Clin. Invest. 62:359, 1978.

89. Cremer, M.A., Pitcock, J.A., Stuart, J.M., Kang, A.H., and Townes, A.S.: Auricular chondritis in rats: An experimental model of relapsing polychondritis induced with type II collagen. J. Exp. Med. 154:535, 1981.

90. Yoo, T.J., Stuart, J.M., Kang, A.H., Townes, A.S., and Tomoda, K.: Type II collagen autoimmunity in otosclerosis and Meniere's disease. Science 217:1153, 1982.

91. Yoo, T.J., Tomoda, K., Stuart, J.M., Cremer, M.A., Kang, A.H., and Townes, A.S.: Type II collagen induced autoimmune sensorineural hearing loss and vestibular dysfunction in rats. Ann. Otol. Rhinol. Larynol., in press, 1983.

92. Stuart, J.M., Townes, A.S., and Kang, A.H.: The role of collagen autoimmunity in animal models and human diseases. J. Invest. Dermatol. 79:121, 1982.

93. Postlethwaite, A.E., and Kang, A.H.: Collagen and collagen peptide-induced chemotaxis of human blood monocytes. J. Exp. Med. 143:1299, 1976.

94. Postlethwaite, A.E., Seyer, J.M., and Kang, A.H.: Induction of fibroblast chemotaxis by type I, II, and III collagens and collagen degradation peptides. Proc. Natl. Acad. Sci. USA 75:871, 1978.

95. Peacock, E., and Van Winkle, W.V.: Wound Repair. 2nd ed. Philadelphia, W.B. Saunders Company, 1976.

96. Fernandez-Madrid, F.: Collagen biosynthesis. Clin. Orthop. 68:163, 1970.

97. Blanck, T.J., and Peterkofsky, B.: Stimulation of collagen secretion by ascorbic acid in fibroblasts. Arch. Biochem. Biophys. 17:259, 1975.

98. Stuart, J.M., Postlethwaite, A.E., and Kang, A.H.: Evidence for cell-mediated immunity to collagen in progressive systemic sclerosis. J. Lab. Clin. Med. 88:601, 1976.

99. Trentham, D.E., Dynesius, R.A., Rocklin, R.E., and David, J.R.: Cellular sensitivity to collagen in rheumatoid arthritis. N. Engl. J. Med. 299:327, 1978.

100. Andriopoules, N.A., Mestecky, J., Miller, E.J., and Bradley, E.L.: Antibodies to native and denatured collagens in sera of patients with rheumatoid arthritis. Arthritis Rheum. 19:613, 1976.

101. Cracchiolo, A., Michaeli, D., Goldberg, L.S., and Fudenberg, H.H.: The occurrence of antibodies to collagen in synovial fluids. Clin. Immunol. Immunopathol. 3:567, 1975.

102. Toole, B.P., Kang, A.H., Trelstad, R.L., and Gross, J.: Collagen heterogeneity within different growth regions of long bones of rachitic and nonrachitic chicks. Biochem. J. 127:715, 1972.

103. Beisswenger, P.J., and Spiro, R.G.: Studies on the human glomerular basement membrane: Composition, nature of carbohydrate units and chemical changes in diabetes mellitus. Diabetes 22:180, 1973.

104. Seyer, J.M., Hutcheson, E.T., and Kang, A.H.: Collagen polymorphism in idiopathic pulmonary fibrosis. J. Clin. Invest. 57:1498, 1976.

105. Seyer, J.M., Hutcheson, E.T., and Kang, A.H.: Collagen polymorphism in normal and cirrhotic human liver. J. Clin. Invest. 59:241, 1977.

106. Sandberg, L.B., Weissman, N., and Smith, D.W.: The purification and partial characterization of a soluble elastin-like protein from copper-deficient porcine aorta. Biochemistry 8:2940, 1969.

107. Foster, J.A., Shapiro, R., Voynow, P., Crombie, G., Faris, B., and Franzblau, C.: Isolation of soluble elastin from lathyritic chicks: Comparison of tropoelastin from copper deficient pigs. Biochemistry 14:5343, 1975.

108. Sandberg, L.B., Soskel, N.J., and Wolt, M.S.: Structure of the elastic fiber: An overview. J. Invest. Dermatol. 79:128, 1982.

109. Foster, J.A., Bruenger, E., Gray, W.R., and Sandberg, L.: Isolation and amino acid sequences of tropoelastin peptides. J. Biol. Chem. 248:2876, 1973.

110. Burnett, W., Yoon, K., Finnigan-Bunick, A., and Rosenbloom, J.: Control of elastin synthesis. J. Invest. Dermatol. 79:138, 1982.

111. Burnett, W., Yoon, K., and Rosenbloom, J.: Construction, identification and characterization of a chick elastin cDNA clone. Biochem. Biophys. Res. Commun. 99:364, 1981.

112. Stevens, P.M., Hrilica, V.S., Johnson, P.C., and Bell, R.L.: Pathophysiology of hereditary emphysema. Ann. Intern. Med. 74:672, 1971.

113. Kühn, C., Yu, S., Chraplyvy, M., Lander, H.E., and Senior, R.M.: The induction of emphysema with elastase. II. Changes in connective tissue. Lab. Invest. 34:372, 1976.

114. Carnes, W.H.: Role of copper in connective tissue metabolism. Fed. Proc. 30:995, 1971.

115. Chou, W.S., Savage, J.E., and O'Dell, B.L.: Role of copper in biosynthesis of intramolecular crosslinks in chick tendon collagen. J. Biol. Chem. 244:5785, 1969.

116. Ruoslahti, E., Engvall, E., and Jayman, E.G.: Fibronectin: Current concepts of its structure and function. Coll. Res. 1:95, 1981.

117. Kleinman, H.K., Klebe, R.J., and Martin, G.R.: Role of collagenous matrices in the adhesion and growth of cells. J. Cell Biol. 88:473, 1981.

118. Ruoslahti, E., Pierschbacher, M., Engvall, E., Oldberg, A., and Hayman, E.G.: Molecular and biological interactions of fibronectin. J. Invest. Dermatol. 79:65, 1982.

119. Klebe, R.J.: Isolation of a collagen-dependent cell attachment factor. Nature 250:248, 1974.

120. Mosesson, M.W., Chen, A.B., and Huseby, R.M.: The cold-insoluble globulin of human plasma: Studies of its essential structural features. Biochim. Biophys. Acta 386:509, 1975.

121. Ruoslahti, E., and Engvall, E.: Immunochemical and collagen-binding properties of fibronectin. Ann. N.Y. Acad. Sci. 312:198, 1978.

122. Engvall, E., and Ruoslahti, E., and Miller, E.J.: Affinity of fibronectin to collagen of different genetic types and to fibronectin. J. Exp. Med. 147:1584, 1978.

123. Porter, R.R., and Reid, K.B.M.: The biochemistry of complement. Nature 285:699, 1978.

124. Highberger, J.H., Corbett, C., and Gross, J.: Isolation and characterization of a peptide containing the site of cleavage of the chick skin

collagen αl(I) chain by animal collagenases. Biochem. Biophys. Res. Commun. 89:202, 1979.

125. Mainardi, C.L., Hasty, D.L., Seyer, J.M., and Kang, A.H.: Specific cleavage of human type III collagen by human polymorphonuclear leukocyte elastase. J. Biol. Chem. 255:12006, 1980.

126. Mosher, D.F.: Crosslinking of cold insoluble globulin by fibrin stabilizing factor. J. Biol. Chem. 250:6614, 1975.

127. Grinnell, F., Feld, M., and Minter, D.: Fibroblast adhesion to fibronectin and fibrin substrate: Requirement for cold-insoluble globulin (plasma fibronectin). Cell 19:517, 1980.

128. Yamata, K.M., Kennedy, D.W., Kimato, K., and Pratt: Characterization of fibronectin interaction with glycosaminoglycans and identification of active proteolytic fragments. J. Biol. Chem. 255:6055, 1980.

129. Kleinman, H.K., Martin G.R., and Fishman, P.H.: Ganglioside inhibition of the fibronectin-mediated cell adhesion to collagen. Proc. Natl. Acad. Sci. USA 76:3367, 1979.

130. Keski-Oja, J., Sen, A., and Todara, G.J.: Direct association of fibronectin and actin molecules in vitro. J. Cell Biol. 85:527, 1980.

131. Kuersela, P.: Fibronectin binds to *Staphylococcus aureus*. Nature 276:718, 1978.

132. Simpson, W.A., Hasty, D.L., Mason, J.M., and Beachey, E.H.: Fibronectin mediates the binding of streptocococci to human polymorphonuclear leukocytes. Infect. Immun. 37:805, 1982.

133. Simpson, W.A., and Beachey, E.H.: Adherence of group A streptococci to fibronectin on oral epithelial cells. Infect. Immun. 39:275, 1983.

134. Speziale, P., Höök, M., Wadström, T., Timpl, R.: Binding of the basement membrane protein laminin to *Escherichia coli*. FEBS Lett. 146:55, 1982.

135. Balian, G., Click, E.M., Crouch, E., Davidson, J.M., and Bornstein, P.: Isolation of a collagen-binding fragment from fibronectin and cold-insoluble globulin. J. Biol. Chem. 254:1429, 1979.

136. Wagner, D.D., and Haynes, R.O.: Topological arrangement of the major structural features of fibronectin. J. Biol. Chem. 255:4304, 1980.

137. Hewitt, A.T., Varner, H.H., and Martin, G.H.: Isolation of chondronectin. *In* Furthmayr, H. (ed.): Immunochemistry of Collagen. Vol. I: Methods. Boca Raton, Florida, CRS Press, 1982.

138. Terranova, V.P., Rohrback, D.H., and Martin, G.R.: Role of laminin in the attachment of PAM 212 (epithelial) cell to basement membrane collagen. Cell, 22:719, 1980.

Chapter 15

Glycosaminoglycans

Kenneth D. Brandt, M.D.

NOMENCLATURE

"Glycosaminoglycan" (GAG) is the term currently used to designate members of the class of compounds formerly called "acid mucopolysaccharides." It represents a shortening of "glycosaminoglucuronoglycan," the designation proposed by Jeanloz[1] for these long-chain, unbranched carbohydrate polymers (-glycans) composed of repeating disaccharide units, one constituent of which is an aminosugar (glycosamino-) and the other a hexuronic acid (glucurono-). Since keratan sulfate contains galactose instead of hexuronic acid, it is not a glycosamino*glucurono*glycan and hence is an exception to this rule of generic structure. Glycosaminoglycan, therefore, is both a simpler and more accurate designation for this class of compounds.

GAG COMPOSITION AND STRUCTURE

Several clear, concise reviews of GAG structure have been published.[2-4] The relevant features will be summarized here. Seven GAGs have been characterized: (1) hyaluronic acid, (2) chondroitin 4-sulfate, (3) chondroitin 6-sulfate, (4) dermatan sulfate, (5) heparan sulfate, (6) heparin, and (7) keratan sulfate. The current nomenclature, which has evolved as the molecular structures of these GAGs have become known, and their old synonyms, are shown in Table 15–1. Each GAG is distinguished by the composition of its disaccharide repeating units, the location and number of its sulfate groups, and the position and configuration of its glycosidic linkages (Table 15–2; Fig. 15–1). Hyaluronic acid and the chondroitin sulfates are homogeneous chains,

showing unvarying repetition of their basic disaccharide units, whereas other GAGs, for example, heparin, heparan sulfate, and dermatan sulfate, contain variations in their repeating units, either in block structures or in a less well-ordered fashion.

GAGs are very widely distributed in animal tissues. They do not normally occur in vivo as free polymers, however, but as protein-carbohydrate complexes (proteoglycans:protein-polysaccharides), i.e., complex molecules in which many GAG chains are linked covalently to protein via an intercalated specific linkage region involving the terminal reducing sugar of the chain. Proteoglycans differ structurally from glycoproteins; in the latter the carbohydrate exists as heteropolysaccharides rather than as homogeneous disaccharide repeating units.

GAGs are synthesized and secreted by connective tissue cells (e.g., fibroblasts and chondrocytes) and play an essential role in maintaining the structural integrity

Table 15–1. Current and Old Nomenclature of Glycosaminoglycans

New Term	Old Term
Hyaluronic acid	Hyaluronic acid
Chondroitin 4-sulfate	Chondroitin sulfate A
Chondroitin 6-sulfate	Chondroitin sulfate C
Dermatan sulfate	Chondroitin sulfate B
Heparan sulfate	Heparitin sulfate; heparin monosulfate
Heparin	Heparin
Keratan sulfate	Keratosulfate
Glycosaminoglycan	Acid mucopolysaccharide
Proteoglycan	Chondromucoprotein; protein-polysaccharide complex

Table 15–2. Composition, Structure and Occurrence of Glycosaminoglycans

Compound	Monosaccharides in Disaccharide Repeating Unit	Molecular Weight ($\times 10^{-3}$)	N-Acetyl Groups	O-Sulfate Groups	N-Sulfate Groups	Sulfate (Moles per Disaccharide Unit)	Examples of Sites of Occurrence
Hyaluronic acid	D-glucosamine + D-glucuronic acid	4–8	+	–	–	0	Synovial fluid, umbilical cord, vitreous humor, skin cartilage
Chondroitin 4-sulfate	D-galactosamine + D-glucuronic acid	5–50	+	+	–	0.1–1.3	Cartilage, cornea, skin, bone
Chondroitin 6-sulfate	D-galactosamine + D-glucuronic acid	5–50	+	+	–	0.1–1.3	Arterial wall, leukocytes, platelets
Dermatan sulfate	D-galactosamine + L-iduronic acid or D-glucuronic acid	15–40	+	+	–	1.0–3.0	Skin, heart valve, arterial wall, tendon
Heparan sulfate	D-glucosamine + L-iduronic acid or D-glucuronic acid	50	+	+	+	0.4–2.0	Lung, arterial wall
Heparin	D-glucosamine + L-iduronic acid or D-glucuronic acid	4–25	+	+	++	1.6–3.0	Mast cells (lung, liver, skin, intestinal mucosa)
Keratan sulfate	D-glucosamine + galactose	4–19	+	+	–	0.9–1.8	Cartilage, cornea, intervertebral disc

of connective tissue. In addition, some GAGs are synthesized and stored within specialized cells in the circulation, e.g., platelets and leukocytes,[5] where they may have an intracellular structural role. Heparan sulfate, which is present on the cell surface, mediates fibroblast adhesion,[6] and the heparan sulfate proteoglycan on the surface of endothelial cells functions as an anticoagulant[7] and, by binding lipoprotein lipase, may help regulate removal of triacylglycerol fatty acids from the circulation.[8] Heparin is synthesized and stored in tissue mast cells and hence is not a component of connective tissue. It is, however, secreted into the connective tissue where it is an anticoagulant and perhaps has other functions, but no structural role.

Hyaluronic Acid. Hyaluronic acid preparations vary greatly in chain length and, therefore, in molecular weight, depending on the tissue of origin (Table 15–2).[9] Their disaccharide repeating units contain one molecule of N-acetyl-D-glucosamine and one of D-glucuronic acid in $1 \rightarrow 3$ glycosidic linkage (Fig. 15–1). The repeating unit undergoes no further modification. Hyaluronic acid is the predominant GAG in synovial fluid, vitreous humor, and umbilical cord, and occurs in lesser proportions in most tissues of the body, and in all cartilage,

where it serves as an integral part of proteoglycan aggregates (see below).

Chondroitin 4- and Chondroitin 6-Sulfate. The repeating disaccharides of the chondroitin sulfate 4- and 6- isomers are identical except for the position of their substituent sulfate moieties. The chondroitin sulfates are the most abundant of the GAGs in the body and occur in both skeletal and soft connective tissues; they are the predominant GAGs of articular cartilage. The 4-sulfate isomer is characteristic of embryonic and immature cartilage, while the tissue content of chondroitin 6-sulfate increases with maturation. Chondroitin 4-sulfate has also been identified in leukocytes and platelets.[5]

Chondroitin sulfate chains are shorter than those of hyaluronic acid, and consist of some 20 to 100 repeating units, which account for average molecular weights of about 5000 to 50,000 (Table 15–2). Each repeating unit consists of N-acetyl-D-galactosamine and D-glucuronic acid in $1 \rightarrow 3$ glyosidic linkage. The sulfate groups are situated on the galactosamine (Fig. 15–1). In some cases chondroitin sulfate chains may be hybrids, with some galactosamine residues bearing sulfate in the 4- position and others in the 6- position.[10] Occasionally, the glucuronic acid moiety also may contain ester sulfate.

Dermatan Sulfate. Dermatan sulfate differs from chondroitin sulfate in that it contains predominantly L-iduronic acid rather than D-glucuronic acid. (Iduronic acid is the carbon-5 epimer of glucuronic acid). The uronosyl linkage is $1 \rightarrow 3$, as in hyaluronic acid and the chondroitin sulfates. Since the purified GAG chain invariably contains some D-glucuronic acid residues,[11] which are in disaccharide units identical to those of chondroitin sulfate, dermatan sulfate can be regarded as a hybrid molecule, or a co-polymer of chondroitin sulfate. Dermatan sulfate is found chiefly in skin, heart valves, tendon, and arterial wall. In the skin, dermatan sulfate is copolymerized with chondroitin 4-sulfate, whereas the dermatan sulfate in umbilical cord is copolymerized with chondroitin 6-sulfate.[11] In some cases dermatan sulfate may contain more than one sulfate group per disaccharide unit.[12]

In vitro, dermatan sulfate proteoglycans exhibit a strong ability to precipitate tropocollagen from solution at physiologic pH and ionic strength, which is not seen with chondroitin sulfate proteoglycans.[13] It has been suggested that the main function of dermatan sulfate may be related to the formation of collagen fibers.[14] In vivo, dermatan sulfate is very closely associated with collagen.[15]

Heparan Sulfate. Heparan sulfate is found in significant quantities in lung and in blood vessel walls, where it probably plays a structural role, and is associated with amyloid fibrils in the connective tissue.[16] Heparan sulfate occurs predominantly in the microenvironment of the cell. It is present at the external surface of a number of cell types grown in vitro,[17] and in the extracellular matrix synthesized by fibroblast-like cells in culture.[18] It is also a constituent of the glomerular basement membrane,[19,20] but it is not a constituent of skeletal tissue.

Heparan sulfate contains some disaccharide repeating units comprised of D-glucosamine and D-glucuronic acid, and others composed of D-glucosamine and L-iduronic acid. It differs from all of the GAGs mentioned previously with respect to its glycosidic linkage, since its uronosyl linkages are $1 \rightarrow 4$, rather than $1 \rightarrow 3$. Heparan sulfate and heparin uniquely contain N-sulfate groups in addition to O-sulfate groups on the glucosamine residues (Table 15-2).

Heparin. Heparin bears close structural similarity to heparan sulfate, and it has been considered that these two GAGs make up a family of related molecules. There is evidence to suggest that heparan sulfate may be a normal precursor in the biosynthesis of heparin.[21,22] Thus, heparin consists of disaccharide repeating units containing D-glucosamine and either D-glucuronic or L-iduronic acid. The uronosyl linkage is $1 \rightarrow 4$, with an α-configuration, which distinguishes it from the chondroitin sulfates and keratan sulfate, which contain β $1 \rightarrow 3$ uronosyl linkages. In contrast to heparan sulfate, nearly all of the glucosamine residues of heparin are N-sulfated and many of the uronic acid moieties also bear sulfate groups.[23] Furthermore, while heparan sulfate exists in

Figure 15-1. Disaccharide repeating units of glycosaminoglycans. The sulfate shown in parentheses on C2 of the glucuronic acid residue of the heparan sulfate disaccharide is variably present. In keratan sulfate, a sulfate moiety may be present on C6 of galactose as well as on the glucosamine.

extracellular locations, heparin is stored in the specific granules of the tissue mast cell.

Keratan Sulfate. Keratan sulfate contains a repeating disaccharide unit made up of galactose linked in a β-configuration 1 → 3 to N-acetylglucosamine. Sulfate may be present at C-6 of the glucosamine and also on the galactose residues. Keratan sulfate has been reported to show a good amount of compositional heterogeneity, and to contain small amounts of mannose, fucose, sialic acid, xylose, and N-acetyl galactosamine.[24,25] More recent data, however, indicate that these sugars are not components of the GAG chain itself but constituents of oligosaccharides situated in the keratan sulfate–rich region of the proteoglycan[26] (see below).

Two types of keratan sulfate have been characterized: Type I occurs in cornea, and Type II in cartilage and nucleus pulposus.[27,28] In cartilage proteoglycans, keratan sulfate and chondroitin sulfate are covalently linked to the same protein core. The linkage to protein of Type I and Type II keratan sulfate, however, is not the same. In cornea the link appears to be N-glycosidic, involving N-acetyl glucosamine and asparagine.[29] In cartilage, however, the linkage is O-glycosidic and involves the hydroxyaminoacids, threonine or serine,[30] and N-acetyl galactosamine.[31]

LINKAGE OF GAGs TO PROTEIN

There is now clear evidence that most of the GAGs in cartilage exist as proteoglycans, covalently linked to protein,[32,33] although the question of whether hyaluronic acid is covalently bound to protein has not been conclusively answered.

Hyaluronate-Proteoglycan. Most of the protein can be removed from synovial fluid hyaluronic acid by centrifugation under associative conditions in a cesium chloride density gradient.[34] Synovial fluid hyaluronate purified by this method, without exposure to proteolytic enzymes, still contains some 2 to 4 percent protein, and hyaluronate from rooster comb about 0.35 percent protein.[35] Evidence has been presented that suggests that this protein may be covalently linked to the hyaluronate in synovial fluid.[36] If this is the case, since hyaluronate is an essentially linear, unbranched polymer,[37] it differs in structure from the other proteoglycans, which consist of multiple GAG chains attached to a common peptide.

On the other hand, when cultures of Swarm rat chondrosarcoma were labeled with ^{3}H-lysine, no ^{3}H-labeled molecules, and therefore no core protein, was found to be associated with the hyaluronate.[38]

Chondroitin Sulfate–Keratan Sulfate Proteoglycans. The most extensively studied proteoglycan is the chondroitin 4-sulfate–keratan sulfate protein of cartilage. The demonstration of a covalent linkage between the GAG and protein was provided by Muir,[39] who noted that after exhaustive treatment with proteolytic enzymes, purified chondroitin sulfate preparations retained an abundance of serine. The structure of the chondroitin 4-sulfate linkage region was subsequently worked out[40,41] and was shown to consist of serine, xylose, galactose, and glucuronic acid, in molar ratios of 1:1:2:1. The chondroitin sulfate is covalently attached via an O-glycosidic bond between xylose and the hydroxyl group of serine on the protein core of the proteoglycan (Fig. 15–2). About 50 percent of the total serine of the proteoglycan is occupied in linkage of chondroitin sulfate chains.[42] A linkage structure identical to that described above for 4-sulfate proteoglycans has been described for proteoglycans of chondroitin 6-sulfate, dermatan sulfate, heparan sulfate, and heparin.[43,44]

The protein core of a typical cartilage proteoglycan has a molecular weight of approximately 200,000 daltons. It constitutes about 5 to 10 percent of the total weight of the molecule, and contains approximately 100 chondroitin sulfate chains and 60 keratan sulfate chains covalently bound to the protein. The complete proteoglycan molecule thus averages 1 to 4 × 10^6 daltons in molecular weight.[33] However, very low molecular weight (approximately 7.6 × 10^4 daltons) proteoglycans, containing only 1 to 2 large chondroitin sulfate chains, have also been identified in cartilage extracts.[45] The average molecular weight of hyaline cartilage proteoglycans varies with their source. Thus, sedimentation coefficients (S_{20}^w,S) of proteoglycans from nasal, tracheal, and articular cartilage were found to be 25, 20, and 16S, respectively.[46] The structural model for chondroitin sulfate-proteoglycans is that of a molecule with a bottle-brush configuration, in which the protein core is situated internally, with the GAG chains extending outward[47,48] (Fig. 15–3). Recent work suggests, however, that proteoglycans are not rigid molecules, but exhibit considerable flexibility over at least 80 percent of the core protein backbone.[49] The molecular structure of

glucuronic acid   galactose   galactose   xylose   serine

Figure 15–2. Structure of the common linkage region of proteoglycans.

———— = Chondroitin sugar
– – — = Keratan sulfate
● = O-linked
    oligosaccharides
□ = N-linked
    oligosaccharides

Figure 15–3. Proteoglycan molecule, depicting bottle-brush configuration and heterogeneity of the core protein with respect to attachment sites for chondroitin sulfate and keratan sulfate, and hyaluronate-binding region.

the proteoglycan renders it especially vulnerable to degradation by proteolytic enzymes, so that cleavage of only one or two peptide bonds on the protein core will destroy the molecule.[39]

The GAGs are not homogeneously distributed along the protein core of the proteoglycan, but most of the chondroitin sulfate chains are attached near the C-terminal end, while the N-terminal portion is devoid of polysaccharide and constitutes a hyaluronate-binding region whose integrity is crucial for aggregation[50,51] (Fig. 15–1). Most of the keratan sulfate is attached to the protein near the hyaluronate-binding region, in a region proximal to the attachment sites of most of the chondroitin sulfate chains.

The hyaluronate-binding region appears to have the same structure whenever present, and it is found on most proteoglycans. However, some nonaggregating proteoglycans with a high molecular weight appear to lack the hyaluronate-binding region and the adjacent keratan-sulfate–rich segment.[52] The very low molecular weight (7.6×10^4 daltons) proteoglycan mentioned above also does not interact with hyaluronate.[45] Its protein core (apparent molecular weight = 1.5×10^4 daltons) has an amino acid composition that is different from that of other cartilage proteoglycans, but similar to that found in low molecular weight proteoglycans from sclera, tendon, aorta, and cornea.

The polysaccharide attachment region of the aggre-

gating proteoglycans varies in length; proteoglycans from young cartilage appear to have a longer chondroitin sulfate attachment region than those from older cartilage.[53]

Recently, small oligosaccharide chains containing sialic acid have been shown to be integral constituents of cartilage proteoglycans.[26] Two classes of oligosaccharides have been described: the first, which is of larger size, contains mannose, galactose, glucosamine, and sialic acid and is linked to an asparagine molecule on the core protein via an *N*-glycosidic bond. The second class of oligosaccharide contains galactosamine, galactose, and glucosamine, in addition to sialic acid, and is linked to serine or threonine on the core protein via an *O*-glycosidic bond involving *N*-acetylgalactosamine.

The structure of the *O*-linked oligosaccharides markedly resembles that of the keratan sulfate linkage region, and it is likely, therefore, that they represent a biosynthetic precursor of keratan sulfate. Consistent with this possibility is the observation that an inverse relationship exists between the number of *O*-linked oligosaccharides and the number of keratan sulfate chains at various ages and in various cartilages.[26,54] Furthermore, in view of the evidence that the uptake of glycoproteins, including lysosomal enzymes, by cells is mediated by receptors that recognize specific monosaccharide markers carried on the oligosaccharide chains of the glycoproteins,[55-58] it is possible that the oligosaccharides on proteoglycans serve similarly as markers to facilitate their uptake by cells.

Indeed, studies indicate that sulfated proteoglycans are internalized by skin fibroblasts by endocytosis, following their association with binding sites on the cell surface.[59] GAGs and other anionic macromolecules inhibit the endocytosis of sulfated proteoglycans noncompetitively, and do not interact with the cell surface receptors for the sulfated proteoglycans, suggesting that the core protein is required for binding to the cell surface. The data suggest also that a recycling of the receptors occurs between the endocytotic vesicles and/or lysosomes and the cell surface.[59]

The molecular structure of the proteoglycans accounts for some of the unique biological properties of articular cartilage. Due to their high carboxylate and sulfate content GAGs are polyanions, possessing a high negative charge density. Adjacent GAG chains on the proteoglycan, therefore, strongly repel each other. Because of this charge repulsion, the protein core and the GAG chains tend to be fully extended in the cartilage so that each proteoglycan, in attempting to occupy the largest possible molecular domain, encompasses a very large volume of water. The hydroxyl groups on the GAGs, furthermore, are highly hydrophilic. These factors thus account for the very high water content of articular cartilage (some 70 to 80 percent of the total weight), and its elastic resistance to compression.

Articular cartilage proteoglycans inhibit fibroblast spreading and adhesion to collagenous substrates.[60] On the basis of this data it has been hypothesized that loss of proteoglycans from the cartilage in rheumatoid arthritis may be necessary for invasion of the surface by the cells in the pannus.

In normal articular cartilage about 75 percent of the proteoglycans exist in aggregates, in which many individual molecules are noncovalently associated with a long, chainlike molecule of hyaluronic acid[61,62] (Fig. 15–4). Link proteins, which constitute about 3 percent of the weight of the complex, stabilize the proteoglycan-hyaluronate interaction.[50] Two link proteins, with molecular weights of approximately 44,000 and 48,000 daltons, respectively, have been identified. The larger contains 9.5 percent carbohydrate while the smaller, whose amino acid composition is similar, contains only 3 percent carbohydrate and is presumed to be a degradation product of the larger.[63,64] These molecular interactions account for sedimentation coefficients ($S_{20^{\circ}w}$) of 60 to 70 S and molecular weights of 1×10^8 daltons exhibited by the aggregates. Recent evidence suggests that the interaction of link with hyaluronate may induce a structural change in the latter, leading to a larger aggregate than that seen with equimolar concentrations of proteoglycans and of hyaluronate in the absence of link.[65]

The proteoglycan-hyaluronate interaction has been examined in detail[66] by viscometry and molecular sieve chromatography. From these studies, on the basis of average molecular weights of proteoglycans and hyaluronate (approximately 0.5×10^6 daltons), a model for the aggregate was derived.[67] The dimensions of the model closely approximate those calculated from electron photomicrographs of aggregates.[68] Figure 15–5 shows the ultrastructure of a PG aggregate, published by Rosenberg and associates.[68] Weaving through the structure is the backbone of the aggregate, the chain of hyaluronic acid. The "side chains" represent individual proteoglycan molecules (monomers) noncovalently linked to the hyaluronate backbone. The cartilage hy-

Figure 15–5. Dark-field electron photomicrograph of a proteoglycan aggregate. The central core is comprised of a molecule of hyaluronic acid. The appended "side chains" represent individual proteoglycans. The length of the white bar in the lower right hand corner represents 0.5 m (magnification = 120,000). (From Rosenberg, L., Hellmann, W., Kleinschmidt, A.K.: J. Biol. Chem. 250:1877, 1975.)

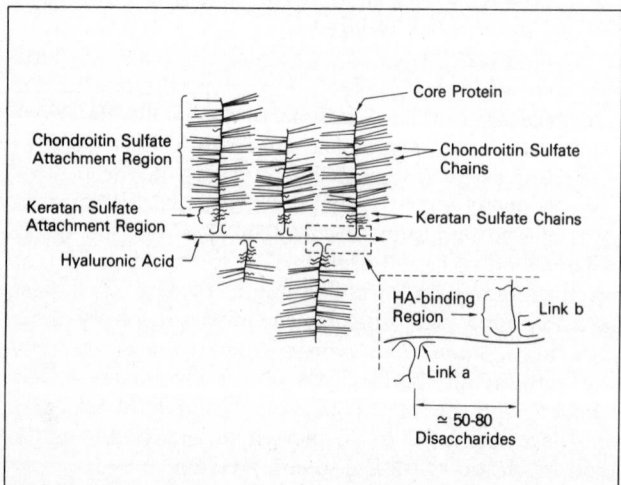

Figure 15–4. Schematic model for structure of cartilage proteoglycans and for a portion of a proteoglycan aggregate. (From Hascall, V.C.: J. Supramolecular Struct. 7:101, 1977.)

aluronate molecules range from about 4000 to 40,000 Å in length, and the number of proteoglycan subunits per aggregate is roughly proportional to the length of the hyaluronate. Some 30 to 60 repeating disaccharide units of hyaluronic acid are present between adjacent proteoglycans. The binding region for each proteoglycan occupies some 5 to 10 disaccharide units of the hyaluronate.[68,69] Decasaccharides of hyaluronic acid compete strongly with high molecular weight hyaluronic acid and effectively inhibit the interaction, whereas smaller oligosaccharides have little effect on aggregation.[69,70]

The aggregation phenomenon is phenotypic of cartilage and is highly specific. Cartilage proteoglycans will interact only with hyaluronate and not with other GAGs.[71] Aggregation presumably helps constrain individual proteoglycans (which themselves may have molecular weights greater than 1×10^6 daltons) in the collagen meshwork. Although proteoglycan monomers interact more extensively among themselves than aggregates, interactions among aggregates are much stronger than those among monomers. Furthermore, the stiffening of an interacting network of monomers produced by shear forces relaxes much more quickly than the shear stiffening of a network of interacting aggregates.[72] In addition, aggregation may help protect proteoglycans from proteolytic degradation.[50]

Aggregation may also modulate cartilage metabolism, since hyaluronic acid, if free and not combined with proteoglycans, inhibits proteoglycan synthesis in chondrocyte cultures.[71,73] There is also evidence that proteoglycan aggregates inhibit calcification of cartilage,[74] presumably by shielding minute crystal particles and preventing their further growth.[75] Proteoglycan aggregates may prevent urate, as well as calcium, from precipitating in cartilage, since they retard precipitation of monosodium urate from supersaturated solutions, whereas equimolar concentrations of nonaggregated proteoglycans do not.[76]

Recently, a chondroitin-sulfate proteoglycan that inhibits Clq, the first component of complement, has been identified in serum.[77] This molecule contains less than 1 percent glucosamine and presumably lacks keratan sulfate. Since it does not form a complex with hyaluronic acid or contain any chondroitin 6-sulfate, its origin is presumably noncartilaginous. Interaction between the inhibitor and Clq was evident in 0.15M NaCl, suggesting that it may have some importance under physiologic conditions.

Heparin-Proteoglycan. Studies of heparin-proteoglycans have yielded seemingly contradictory results. Heparin is synthesized by mast cells, which store it in specific cytoplasmic granules. In some tissues, e.g., bovine liver capsule, heparin occurs as free GAG chains, with a molecular weight less than 1×10^4 daltons,[78] a value comparable to that of the commercial heparin used as an anticoagulant. Heparin isolated from rat peritoneal mast cells, in contrast, has a molecular weight of about 7.5×10^5 daltons and appears to consist of multiple GAG chains joined to a protein core.[79] This complex is notably resistant to proteolysis. It is possible that single-chain forms of heparin represent reaction products resulting from cleavage of peptide-bound chains by specific endoglycosidases.[80]

GAG BIOSYNTHESIS

Present information suggests that the protein core is synthesized in a conventional manner on a ribosomal template, and the carbohydrate chains are assembled post-translationally,[81,82] one sugar at a time, starting with the attachment of xylose to serine in a structurally specific linkage region. Sulfation takes place after the appropriate monosaccharide has been linked into the growing chain. The sugars and the sulfate residues each are derived from "activated" precursors, i.e., uridine sugar nucleotides and phosphoadenosine-5'-phosphosulfate, respectively. Elongation of the GAG chain, and its sulfation, occur in the endoplasmic reticulum and Golgi complex as the core protein progresses from the polyribosomes to the exterior of the cell.

The requisite sugar nucleotides that serve as monosaccharide precursors of the growing chain of repeating disaccharides are synthesized from D-glucose, as shown in Figure 15–6. Details of the enzymatic steps involved have been reviewed.[2,3] The UDP-sugars are then transferred sequentially to the growing GAG chain (or its linkage region).

Intracellular levels of UDP derivatives are controlled to some extent by feedback inhibition. For example, increasing levels of UDP-xylose inhibit UDP-glucose dehydrogenase, which converts UDP-glucose to UDP-glucuronic acid, the immediate precursor of UDP-xylose.[3] Similarly, excessive levels of UDP-N-acetylglucosamine inhibit formation of glucosamine 6-phosphate from fructose 6-phosphate and glutamine[3] (Fig. 15–6). Since xylose is the initial sugar to be added to protein in GAG chain synthesis, a deficiency of acceptor protein will lead to accumulation of UDP-xylose which, by the negative feedback mechanism described above, can suppress formation of UDP-glucuronic acid, inhibiting further GAG chain synthesis.

For the biosynthesis of a chondroitin sulfate chain several transferase steps are required, involving a variety of glycosyltransferases and one sulfotransferase (Fig. 15–7). The first reaction involves xylosyltransferase, which

Figure 15–6. Nucleotide sugars involved in biosynthesis of GAGs and relevant sugar interconversions. Dotted lines indicate sites of feedback inhibition.

- Serine (on core protein) -
|
① Xylosyl transferase
|
② Galactosyl transferase
|
③ Galactosyl transferase
|
④ Glucuronic acid transferase
|
⑤ N-acetylgalactosamine transferase
|
⑥ Sequential action of No. 4 and No. 5 for lengthening of chain
|
⑦ Sulfotransferase

Figure 15–7. Enzymes involved in biosynthesis of a chrondroitin sulfate chain and its specific linkage region on a proteoglycan. The glycosyl transferases act on UDP-sugars and the sulfotransferase on PAPS.

effects the transfer of xylose from UDP-xylose to serine on the protein core.[83] The next two reactions involve galactosyltransferase, which transfers two moles of galactose from UDP-galactose.[84] This is followed by the addition of the first N-acetylglucuronic acid residue, which is covalently bound to the second galactose residue by the action of O-glucuronic acid transferase on UDP-N-acetylglucuronic acid. Growth of the chondroitin sulfate chain then occurs by alternating transfer of N-acetylgalactosamine and D-glucuronic acid residues from their respective UDP-derivatives, mediated by their specific transferases (Fig. 15–7).

Sulfation of the GAG, which occurs during or after growth of the chain, requires 3-phosphoadenosyl-5-phosphosulfate (PAPS) as an intermediate.[85] Sulfate is then transferred from PAPS to the GAG chain in a reaction catalyzed by sulfotransferase (Fig. 15–8). There is no evidence that sulfated polymers can be synthesized from sulfated monosaccharide nucleotide precursors. Thus, UDP-N-acetylgalactosamine sulfate was not incorporated into chondroitin sulfate in epiphyseal cartilage.[86] The N-sulfate groups of heparan sulfate and of heparin are synthesized by displacement of pre-existing N-acetyl groups.[87] The chondroitin sulfate chains within a single proteoglycan molecule are heterogeneous with

respect to chain length, degree of sulfation, and the location of the sulfate groups (position 4 or 6 of the galactosamine), but the factors that account for these differences are not entirely clear. It has been suggested that differences in molecular size of GAGs may be due to partial degradation of the chains.[88]

Whether the sulfotransferases lack specificity or whether different enzymes are involved in sulfation of the 4- and 6- positions of the galactosamine in chondroitin sulfate remains uncertain. The conformation of the acceptor monosaccharides and the adjacent sugar residues may influence the position of sulfation. For example, dermatan sulfate from umbilical cord contains 6-sulfate on galactosamine groups situated next to glucuronic acid residues, and chiefly 4-sulfate on those near iduronic residues.[89] Other evidence suggests the presence of specific sulfatases in embryonic chick cartilage that catalyze sulfation of specific hydroxyl groups of hexosamine residues. Robinson and Dorfman[90] found that the proportions of chondroitin 4-sulfate and 6-sulfate varied with the stage of development of the embryo, and that the proportion of the isomeric chondroitin sulfates synthesized in vitro was similar to that found in ovo at the same stage of development. A cell-free system synthesized both isomers in the presence of PAPS, but the proportion of chondroitin 4-sulfate was affected by pH and length of incubation, suggesting the presence of two sulfotransferases.[91]

GAG DEGRADATION

Degradation of the PG involves breakdown of the GAG chain, desulfation of the sugars, and proteolysis. The loss of cartilage matrix that results from intravenous injection of the proteolytic enzyme papain[92] illustrates the importance of the protein core to the structural integrity of the proteoglycan. Rupture of only one or two peptide bonds will cause the molecule to fall apart.[39] Cartilage contains lysosomal acid proteases, which degrade proteoglycans (e.g., cathepsin D),[93] but which have an acid pH optimum and are not active at pH 7, i.e., the pH of the extracellular ground substance. It is likely, therefore, that these acid proteases play a role in digestion of proteoglycans intracellulary, and in the immediate vicinity of the cell, but not in the expanse of matrix between the chondrocytes. On the other hand, neutral proteases are present in cartilage and will degrade proteoglycans at neutral pH 7,[94] and are presumably responsible for the normal turnover of proteoglycans in the territory between the cells. The neutral proteases appear to be controlled by potent inhibitors, which have been demonstrated in normal cartilage.[95,96]

Studies of newly synthesized cartilage proteoglycans, labeled simultaneously with ^{14}C-lysine and ^{35}S-sulfate, have shown that the protein and GAG moieties of the proteoglycan turn over concomitantly.[97] Degradation of the GAG chains of proteoglycans occurs principally in the lysosomes.[98,99] The most well-defined GAG lyase is the hyaluronidase from testes, which degrades hyalu-

sulfate + ATP $\xrightarrow{①}$ adenosine-5' phosphosulfate (APS) + PPi

APS + ATP $\xrightarrow{②}$ 3' phosphoadenosine-5' phosphosulfate (PAPS) + ADP

chondroitin + PAPS $\xrightarrow{③}$ chondroitin sulfate + phospho AMP

① = ATP: sulfate adenyltransferase

② = ATP: adenylsulfate-3' phosphotransferase

③ = sulfotransferase

Figure 15–8. Enzymatic reactions in sulfation of chondroitin.

ronic acid to a family of even-numbered oligosaccharides, with tetrasaccharides predominating.[100] The enzyme is an endo-β-N-acetylhexosaminidase, and thus degrades chondroitin, chondroitin 4-sulfate, and chondroitin 6-sulfate, yielding oligosaccharide products similar in size to those that result from its action on hyaluronic acid.[101,102] Since dermatan sulfate is a chondroitin sulfate copolymer, it will also be partially degraded by these enzymes.

Endoglycosidases that degrade the iduronic acid–containing portions of dermatan sulfate or heparan sulfate, or that break down keratan sulfate, have not yet been identified in mammalian tissues. Heparin and heparan sulfate, however, are degraded by an enzyme produced by adapted strains of *Flavobacterium heparinum.*[102] This enzyme specificity may explain why chondroitin sulfate, even when injected in large amounts, is extensively degraded, whereas other mucopolysaccharides can be largely recovered in an unaltered state from the tissues and urine.[103] On the other hand, normal urine contains small quantities of GAGs, about two thirds of which are derived from chondroitin sulfate, and the remainder from chondroitin, heparan sulfate, dermatan sulfate, hyaluronic acid, and keratan sulfate.[104] The chondroitin sulfate in urine has a lower molecular weight and less sulfate than that in tissue, and is bound to a smaller protein fragment, indicative of its degraded state.

Hyaluronidase has been demonstrated in a variety of mammalian tissues in addition to testis, including liver, skin, and synovium,[105] although earlier studies failed to find evidence of hyaluronidase in articular cartilage.[105] Recently, by use of a viscometric technique more sensitive than the previously employed colorimetric methods, hyaluronidase activity was demonstrated in normal articular cartilage.[106] The activity, which had a pH optimum around 3, appeared to be specific (it could not be demonstrated when chondroitin was employed as substrate) and was related to the concentration of cyclic adenosine monophosphate in the tissue.

Other glycosidases, i.e., exoglycosidases, are required to complete the breakdown to monosaccharides of the oligosaccharides resulting from the action of hyaluronidase on GAGs. Glucuronidase and N-acetylhexosaminidases are lysosomal exo-enzymes, capable of cleaving terminal nonreducing glucuronic acid or hexosamine residues, respectively, from oligo- or polysaccharides. Lysosomes also contain β-xylosidase, β-galactosidase, and α-iduronidase.[107] As indicated above, xylose and galactose occur in minor and major amounts, respectively, in keratan sulfate and also in the GAG-protein linkage region common to these proteoglycans; α-L-iduronic acid is a constituent of dermatan sulfate, heparan sulfate, and heparin.

Lysosomal sulfatases are responsible for the desulfation of GAGs. Activity of sulfatases against intact GAG chains has not been demonstrated, but they may act on the terminal nonreducing end of sulfated oligosaccharides, or monosaccharides. A deficiency of sulfoiduronate sulfatase is the basic defect in Hurler's syndrome and deficiency of a sulfamidase specific for terminal hexosaminyl residues has been identified in another mucopolysaccharidosis, Sanfilippo A disease.

GAGs IN THE GENETIC MUCOPOLYSACCHARIDOSES

While the excessive breakdown of GAGs in articular cartilage is important in the pathogenesis of various joint diseases (e.g., osteoarthritis, rheumatoid arthritis), incomplete degradation of GAGs is the essence of another group of disorders—the genetic mucopolysaccharidoses. A detailed description of the clinical features of these diseases is beyond the scope of this chapter but may be found elsewhere.[108] This section will review the specific biochemical abnormalities in the mucopolysaccharidoses and emphasize the relationship of these disorders to normal GAG catabolism.

The mucopolysaccharidoses are storage disorders in which the lysosomal breakdown of GAGs is incomplete, so that partially degraded GAGs are retained in lysosomes[109] within the tissues and excreted in elevated amounts in the urine. Since the demonstration by Danes and Bearn that fibroblasts cultured from the skin of patients with Hurler's syndrome show metachromasia and accumulate GAGs,[110] tissue culture has been widely applied to the study of the mucopolysaccharidoses. It was subsequently shown, on the basis of kinetics of $^{35}SO_4$ accumulation in cultured fibroblasts from patients with Hurler's and Hunter's syndromes, that the GAG accumulation was due to defective degradation[111] rather than to abnormalities in GAG synthesis or secretion. Furthermore, it was found that cocultivation of Hurler and Hunter cells resulted in mutual correction of the excessive GAG accumulation.[112] Correction of the metabolic defect in the fibroblasts could also be achieved by use of culture medium, tissue extracts, or urine from patients with any genotype except that of the patient from whom the fibroblasts were derived;[113] thus, material from patients with various mucopolysaccharidoses cross-corrected each other's defects. This led to the recognition that the various mucopolysaccharidoses were each associated with deficiencies in specific lysosomal hydrolases involved in normal GAG catabolism.

Except for the Morquio syndrome, which involves a defect in breakdown of keratan sulfate, all the other presently classified mucopolysaccharidoses involve a disturbance in the breakdown of dermatan sulfate and/or heparan sulfate by lysosomal exoenzymes, i.e., glycosides and sulfatases. These exoenzymes cleave the chains from their nonreducing termini and sequentially remove sulfate groups and sugar residues as they become exposed. For complete degradation of a GAG chain, multiple enzymes are thus required. If any are missing, the degradative sequence is blocked. Some further degradation may occur through the action of lysosomal endoglycosidases (e.g., hyaluronidase), but in the absence of the exoenzyme complete degradation cannot occur. Thus, in patients with a mucopolysaccharidosis, elevated levels of degradation fragments of the GAGs are found in urine and within lysosomes. Figure 15–9 schematically depicts portions of GAG chains and indicates the specific defects in lysosomal degradative enzymes that have been identified in the mucopolysaccharidoses.

The "corrective factors" described above have proved to be the lysosomal hydrolases missing from the fibroblasts.[114,115] Uptake of the missing enzyme by the cell does not occur simply by endocytosis, but the enzyme is taken up selectively by the cells, which appear to have a specific receptor on their surface that recognizes a specific marker associated with the carbohydrate portion of lysosomal enzymes.

In I-cell (inclusion cell) disease (mucolipidosis II) and pseudo-Hurler dystrophy (mucolipidosis III)[116] glycosidases, sulfatases, and cathepsins required for GAG degradation, as well as a number of enzymes associated with sphingolipid metabolism, are not packaged into lysosomes, but are secreted extracellularly. The clinical features of I-cell disease resemble those of Hurler's syndrome (i.e., retarded psychomotor development, progressive organomegaly, skeletal abnormalities, restricted joint mobility). Most patients die by age 6. Pseudo-Hurler polydystrophy resembles the Maroteaux-Lamy syndrome (mucopolysacchidosis VI), in which the lysosomal enzyme N-acetylgalactosamine 4-sulfatase is deficient.[108] In contrast to the mucopolysaccharidoses, however, in which the primary abnormality is a genetic defect in the synthesis of a specific lysosomal enzyme, in I-cell and the pseudo-Hurler disorder the enzymes are synthesized normally. Many of them are present in strikingly large amounts in plasma and other body fluids in vivo, and in the tissue culture medium when fibroblasts from afflicted individuals are cultured in vitro.

The basic defect in these disorders lies in the post-

Figure 15–9. Enzyme defects in mucopolysaccaridoses.

Enzyme	Substrate	Deficiency Disease
① α-L-iduronidase	heparan sulfate; dermatan sulfate	Hurler's and Scheie's syndromes
② iduronate sulfatase	heparan sulfate; dermatan sulfate	Hunter's syndrome
③ N-acetylgalactosamine 4-sulfatase	dermatan sulfate; chondroitin sulfate	Maroteaux-Lamy syndrome
④ β-glucuronidase	chondroitin sulfate; heparan sulfate; dermatan sulfate	Glucuronidase deficiency
⑤ heparan N-sulfatase (sulfamidase)	heparan sulfate	Sanfilippo's A syndrome
⑥ α-N-acetylglucosaminidase	heparan sulfate	Sanfilippo's B syndrome
⑦ N-acetylhexosamine 6-sulfatase	keratan sulfate; chonroitin 6-sulfate	Morquio's syndrome

translational modification of the acid hydrolases, and is marked by a deficiency of the mannose-6-phosphate receptor, which is present on normal hydrolases and is essential for mediating the uptake of the hydrolase by lysosomes.[55] The biochemical defect resides in the enzymatic pathway that phosphorylates mannose residues on the oligosaccharide chains of the newly synthesized hydrolases. In normal fibroblasts, this is accomplished by initial transfer of phosphate together with N-acetyl-glucosamine from UDP-N-acetylglucosamine, resulting in formation of a mannose-P-N-acetylglucosamine diester,[117] which is subsequently cleaved, leaving the mannose phosphate.[118] Patients with I-cell disease lack the specific UDP-N-acetylglucosamine phosphotransferase involved in this process,[119,120] while in fibroblasts from patients with pseudo-Hurler dystrophy the reaction proceeds at a very low rate.[120]

PHYSICAL PROPERTIES OF GAGs IN RELATION TO THEIR STRUCTURE

How do GAGs subserve a structural role in connective tissue? There is considerable evidence that GAGs in certain tissues, such as cartilage and umbilical cord, exist not as solutions but as gels.[121] In hyaline cartilage and intervertebral disc, for example, GAGs may account for as much as 10 percent of the wet weight of the tissue. Because of their enormous hydrodynamic volumes (Fig. 15–10) (which, for hyaluronate and cartilage proteoglycan are 1000 and 100 times, respectively, larger than the volumes occupied by the dehydrated molecules) their solute domains are very large. For this reason, at concentrations of approximately 1 mg per cm^3 and 10 mg per cm^3, respectively, which are achieved in vivo, hyaluronate and cartilage proteoglycan molecules will begin to entangle with themselves; at higher concentrations a continuous overlapping molecular network will exist. The entanglement will tend to immobilize the proteoglycans in the tissues, achieving physical stability. The

Figure 15–10. Molecular domains of hyaluronic acid and some other common macromolecules. (From Comper, C.W., and Laurent, T.C.: Physiological function of connective tissue polysaccharides. Physiol. Rev. 58:255, 1978.)

specific association of cartilage proteoglycans with hyaluronic acid, leading to formation of aggregates stabilized by link glycoproteins,[50,61] also may provide mechanical stability to cartilage. The entangled and/or aggregated proteoglycans are further constrained physically by the fibrous network of connective tissue (collagen, elastin). The proteoglycan gels prevent the gross flow of water through the tissues, although individual water molecules and small solutes diffuse readily through the gel. Large molecules, however, such as proteins, are excluded from the domain of the proteoglycan.[121,122] The diffusion of larger molecules through cartilage is limited by size and steric configuration, as well as by charge.[123] Larger molecules, therefore, such as albumin, are effectively excluded from the tissue, as reflected by studies of Maroudas showing that the partition coefficients for albumin, transferrin, and IgG were only about 0.01, in comparison with a value of 1 for proline.[123]

Because of their polyanionicity and the localization of sulfate and carboxyl groups within the molecule, the negative charge concentration within the domain of a proteoglycan is very high. The proteoglycan thus is able to participate extensively in intermolecular electrostatic interactions with adjacent molecules, such as collagen. In addition, transport of ions through connective tissue, osmotic pressure effects, and the distribution of other ions (Donnan effect) are affected considerably by the composition and concentration of the proteoglycans in tissue, and their macromolecular organization. Detailed discussion of these aspects of connective tissue physiology may be found in reference 121.

ROLE OF HYALURONATE IN SKELETAL MORPHOGENESIS

GAGs appear to play an essential role in embryologic differentiation. For example, during morphogenesis of the limb bud at a stage characterized by extensive cell migration, hyaluronic acid accumulates in the tissues. For cell differentiation to occur the hyaluronate must be removed. Hyaluronidase can be detected, in association with a fall in GAG content of the tissue, at the onset of differentiation, as marked by the appearance of metachromasia and increase in synthesis of chondroitin sulfate.[124,125]

Hyaluronic acid, when added at an appropriate stage, can inhibit the normal formation of cartilage nodules in cultures of cells from chick embryo somites,[126] although chondroitin sulfates, heparin, or other biologic polyanions (e.g., nucleic acids) do not have this effect. A hyaluronate surface coat may regulate cell-cell interactions. Thus, in vitro, hyaluronidase digestion of endogenous surface-bound hyaluronate inhibits receptor-mediated aggregation of simian virus 40–transformed 3T3 cells.[127] The same effect was observed upon addition of a large excess of exogenous hyaluronate, which presumably caused all receptor sites to be occupied, thereby preventing crossbridging and inhibiting cell aggregation.[127] It has been considered possible that a similar phenomenon might affect embryonic cells in vivo. Thus, the hyaluronate concentrations present in the pathways of migration of embryonic cells may prevent cells from adhering to one another, thereby facilitating movement by preventing interactions that would immobilize the cells.[128] In addition, since cell movement requires sequential attachments and detachments of localized areas of the cell surface, hyaluronate interposed between the cell and the substratum may facilitate detachment, and hence cell migration. Hyaluronate has been shown to be a component of cell "foot pads"[129] and to interact specifically with fibronectin, another component of these structures.[130]

Hyaluronate is an extremely potent inhibitor of proteoglycan synthesis[131] by chondrocytes; as little as 0.005 μg per ml decreases $^{35}SO_4$ incorporation into chondroitin sulfate, whereas other polyanions have no effect even at much higher concentrations.[132] Furthermore, this inhibitory effect of hyaluronic acid on GAG synthesis is specific for chondrocytes, since synthesis of sulfated GAGs by fibroblasts is unaffected by concentrations of hyaluronic acid as high as 10 μg per ml.

^{14}C-labeled hyaluronic acid is taken up by cells, and this uptake can be diminished by unlabeled hyaluronate. Since the label and the inhibition of GAG synthesis can be removed by mild trypsinization, it appears to be associated with the surface of the chondrocyte.[133] The inhibitory effect of hyaluronate can be abolished by benzyl-β-D-xyloside (an exogenous initiator of GAG chain polymerization), suggesting that hyaluronate acts by interfering with initiation of the GAG chain (and thus the proteoglycan) by specifically inhibiting formation of the core protein or, perhaps, of the xylosyl transferase that initiates synthesis of chondroitin sulfate chains on the protein. In contrast to hyaluronic acid, sulfated GAGs stimulate GAG synthesis by chondrocytes, although relatively high concentrations are required and no evidence for a receptor-mediated mechanism has been noted.[134] Thus, the GAG composition and concentration in the extracellular matrix appear to influence cell differentiation in the skeleton, and the metabolism of mature cells in connective tissue.

GAGs AS REGULATORS OF CARTILAGE MINERALIZATION

Chains of chondroitin sulfate have been shown to bind Ca^{+2}, but Ca^{+2} binding is much greater when the chondroitin sulfate is present in cartilage proteoglycan,[135,136] suggesting that individual calcium ions were each bound by two sulfate groups, located on adjacent GAG chains of the proteoglycan. Endochondral calcification is accompanied by a sharp decrease in the chondroitin sulfate content of the tissue.[137] It has been proposed that the binding of calcium by proteoglycans raises the local calcium concentration in the cartilage, increasing the local pH and thereby causing an influx of phosphate

and hydroxyl ions, leading to precipitation of calcium salts.[138] On the other hand, proteoglycans, especially when present as very large aggregates, may inhibit the sedimentation of precipitating calcium phosphate.[139] The inhibitory effect of aggregates, as opposed to nonaggregated proteoglycans, on calcification is not due to differential calcium binding affinity. It has been suggested that the aggregate provides a physical shield to prevent growth of minute calcium crystals.[140] Evidence indicates that in vivo the onset of calcification in cartilage is associated with disaggregation of proteoglycans. It is unlikely that disaggregation in these circumstances is effected by proteolytic enzymes, since there is no indication that individual proteoglycans are degraded, and it seems unlikely that a protease in calcifying cartilage would selectively attack proteoglycans in aggregates. Lysozyme, a low molecular weight cationic protein that is present in cartilage in large amounts,[141] has been shown to cause disaggregation of proteoglycans in vitro. The mechanisms of calcification in fracture callus may be similar to those of endochondral calcification in skeletal growth. Thus, in healing of rat tibial fractures a rise in lysozyme was associated with a decrease in proteoglycan aggregation prior to mineralization of the callus.[142]

BINDING OF GAGs TO LYSOSOMAL ENZYMES

Because of the pre-eminent role of lysosomal enzymes as mediators of tissue damage in rheumatic disease, it is relevant that GAGs have been identified as components of primary lysosomes and have been shown to affect the activity of lysosomal enzymes. When chondroitin sulfate, dermatan sulfate, and heparin were added to lysosomal hydrolases the activity of the latter was augmented or decreased. The increase in acid hydrolase activity was proposed to be due to protection of the enzyme from degradation by lysosomal proteases.[143] Lysosomal enzymes in polymorphonuclear leukocytes have been shown to interact with GAGs in pH-dependent reversible electrostatic binding.[144] It has been postulated that the enzymes contained in primary lysosomes exist in complexes with GAGs in a protected, inactive form. During phagocytosis, fusion of the primary lysosome with phagosome would lead to an influx of extracellular fluid, diluting the intralysosomal fluid and raising its pH, causing dissociation of the enzyme-GAG complex and release of intact active hydrolases.

Based on a rationale stemming from observations such as the above, attempts have been made to utilize GAGs in treatment of arthritis. When Arteparon, a glycosaminoglycan polysulfate, was administered to animals with experimentally induced osteoarthritis, the extent of cartilage damage appeared to be less than that in controls.[145,146] The efficacy of such therapy in human arthritis, however, remains to be demonstrated.[147]

FUNCTION OF GAGs IN THE CLOTTING OF BLOOD

Anticoagulant Function of Heparin. Heparin is synthesized and stored within mast cells in the connective tissue, in the vicinity of blood vessels. Despite the ability of exogenous heparin to inhibit clotting of blood, whether it is present in the plasma under physiological conditions is not resolved.[148] Thus, the function of endogenous heparin in anticoagulation is not entirely clear. Notably, native heparin possessed only about 10 percent of the anticoagulant activity of commercial heparin.[149]

The molecular mechanisms underlying heparin's activity as an anticoagulant have recently been reviewed in detail.[150] The action of heparin as an anticoagulant appears to be indirect. It binds to a plasma protease inhibitor, antithrombin (antithrombin III), and markedly accelerates the rate at which the latter forms stable, equimolar complexes with serine proteases of the hemostatic cascade, neutralizing their activity.[151] Antithrombin, which is an α-globulin (molecular weight = about 5.5×10^4 daltons), inactivates thrombin stoichiometrically.[150] The interaction involves an attack by thrombin of a specific Arg-Ser bond on the inhibitor. In the presence of heparin, formation of the antithrombin-thrombin complex is accelerated up to 2000-fold, preventing formation of fibrin. Other serine proteases in the coagulation system (Factors IX_a, X_a, XI_a, XII_a) are similarly inactivated by antithrombin, by reactions that are also greatly increased by the presence of heparin.

Heparin catalyzes the antithrombin-protease reaction. Since it is not consumed during the reaction, upon release from the antithrombin-protease complex it is available again for binding to another molecule of antithrombin.[150] Plasmin, a component of the fibrinolytic system, appears to be inactivated in the same way. Evidence indicates that heparin binds to lysine residues in antithrombin, inducing a conformational change in the inhibitor, which makes its reactive site more accessible to the active center of thrombin and the other serine proteases.[151]

Heparin preparations vary considerably with respect to molecular size, glucuronic acid:iduronic acid molar ratios, degrees of N-acetylation, and amounts of ester and N-sulfation. However, changes in none of these molecular parameters have shown a high degree of correlation with the anticoagulation activity of the molecule, suggesting that a highly defined, specific molecular structure may not be required for anticoagulant activity.[152] Recently, however, highly purified commercial heparin was shown to contain two distinct forms, separable by sucrose density gradient centrifugation: about one third of the molecules bound to antithrombin and had potent anticoagulant activity; the remaining two thirds could not form a stable complex with antithrombin and had minimal anticoagulant activity.[152] Similar results have been obtained with heparin from a murine mastocytoma.[153] The antithrombin-binding region in heparin contains a pentasaccharide with a unique glucosamine-3-0-sulfate group, which is not present in other regions of the molecule, or in heparin with low affinity for antithrombin.[151] Also, the biological function of the majority of the heparin molecules (which are poor anticoagulants), and whether the heparin that binds to antithrombin has other (nonanticoagulant) function in vivo, remain to be determined.[154]

Procoagulant Function of Platelet Factor 4-Proteoglycan Complex. Platelets contain a chondroitin 4-sulfate proteoglycan[5] in their cytoplasmic granules, where it exists in a complex with platelet factor 4 (PF4).[155] The latter has the ability to neutralize the anticoagulant effect of heparin in plasma after release from the platelets and, therefore, may be of clinical significance in relation to heparin therapy. Its physiologic role, however, is not clear.

The proteoglycan-PF4 complex is dissociable at high ionic strength into the proteoglycan carrier (MW = 59,000 daltons) and PF4 (MW = 29,000 daltons). The proteoglycan contains four chains of chondroitin 4-sulfate (MW = 12,000 daltons each), covalently linked to a single polypeptide. When fully saturated with PF4, the molecular weight of the complex is about 350,000 daltons, indicating that it occurs as a dimer, with each monomer comprised of 4 molecules of PF4 and one molecule of proteoglycan.[149]

Other GAGs are able to displace PF4 from the proteoglycan carrier. Heparin has the highest, and hyaluronic acid the lowest, affinity from the protein; in general, binding appears to be promoted by high charge density and by L-iduronic acid residues. Thus, heparan sulfate and dermatan sulfate, which are present in blood vessel walls, could, by displacing PF4 from its proteoglycan carrier, serve to control its deposition locally on the vessel wall.

Anticoagulant Function of Heparan Sulfate. While the above interaction between heparan sulfate and the PF4-proteoglycan complex would imply a potential coagulation-promoting role for this GAG, heparan sulfate proteoglycans on the surface of vascular endothelial cells have been shown also to interact with one of the enzymes of the thromboplastin pathway, thereby inhibiting conversion of prothrombin to thrombin.[7] This action could have some importance in vivo in maintaining the fluidity of the blood within the vascular tree.

The heparan sulfate proteoglycan on the surface of endothelial cells of aorta has been shown also to bind lipoprotein lipase, the extrahepatic enzyme that is responsible for hydrolysis of plasma triacylglycerol.[8] A recent study showed that at saturation 1.24×10^{11} molecules of lipoprotein lipase were bound per cm of intact porcine aortic endothelium.[8] Binding was reduced by prior trypsinization, which would have degraded the heparan-sulfate proteoglycan, and was reversed by exogenous heparin. (It is well known that heparin administration releases the lipase into the circulation in vivo.) The porcine endothelium was shown to have available at its surface approximately 5.4×10^{11} chains of heparan sulfate per cm^2, suggesting that lipoprotein lipase may interact with approximately 25 percent of the available GAG chains.[8]

Studies of the heparan sulfate proteoglycan–cell interaction indicate that binding of the proteoglycan to the surface of hepatocytes requires intact GAG chains.[17] Since exogenous heparin displaces about two thirds of the endogenous heparan sulfate proteoglycans from the cell, the polysaccharide receptor is involved also in their association with the cell surface. Furthermore, the ability of heparin to displace endogenous heparan sulfate was proportional to the molecular weight.

POSSIBLE ROLE OF HEPARIN IN INFLAMMATION

The mast cell is an important effector of inflammation via release of the biologically active substances (histamine, serotonin, eosinophilic chemotactic factor of anaphylaxis, and so on) contained in its cytoplasmic granules. Since these granules also contain its heparin, it is relevant to examine the possible functions of this GAG that may be unrelated to its effects on clotting. Several lines of evidence point to the likelihood that heparin has such functions.

Commercial heparin has been shown to be anticomplementary, and it inhibits both the classical and alternative pathways.[156,157] Heparin enhances the activity of the inhibitor of the first component of the complement (C1 INH) on activated C1.[157] Commercial heparin also inhibits the binding of C1q to immune complexes,[156] the interaction of C1s with C4 and C2,[158] the binding of C2 to the C4b receptor,[159] and formation, or binding, of the trimolecular complex C567.[160]

In addition, native heparin has been shown to mask the active site of chymase,[161] a chymotrypsin-like enzyme contained in the mast cell granules, which is released upon degranulation of the cell induced by immunologic or nonimmunologic stimuli. Additional evidence indicates that heparin suppresses the in vitro assay for macrophage-inhibitor factor (MIF).[162]

Recently, it has been shown that macrophages, which occur in association with mast cells in the tissues, produce and secrete coagulation enzymes.[163] Mouse peritoneal macrophages produce the proteinase precursors needed for formation of fibrin via the extrinsic pathway (factor VII, factor X, prothrombin) and also tissue thromboplastin and factor V, which are required for activation of the enzymes.[150] Thromboplastin production, which triggers the extrinsic pathway, results from interaction of macrophages with activated T lymphocytes.[164,165] Thus, the coagulation mechanism of the macrophage may be activated in the course of a cellular immune response, and may explain synovial fibrin deposition in joint diseases such as rheumatoid arthritis. This fibrin-generating system is susceptible to inhibition by heparin.[150]

From the foregoing it is apparent that heparin may possess a potential for modulating immediate hypersensitivity reactions, complement-mediated immunologic reactions (involving both classical and alternative pathways), and delayed hypersensitivity.

HEPARIN-INDUCED OSTEOPOROSIS

In 1965, Griffith and associates reported spontaneous vertebral and/or rib fractures in 6 of 10 patients treated with 15,000 to 30,000 units of heparin for 6 months or longer.[166] Marked osteopenia was noted radiologically, and serum concentrations of calcium, phosphorus, and alkaline phosphatase, and renal tubular resorption of phosphate, were normal. The complication appeared to be dose related, since no symptoms of osteoporosis were noted in 107 patients who received 10,000 units of heparin or less daily for up to 15 years. Several subsequent reports have confirmed that osteoporosis and fractures may occur as a result of high-dose heparin therapy.[167-171] The true frequency of heparin-induced osteopenia is unknown, but x-ray changes and clinical evidence of fracture appear to be much less common than the 60 percent prevalence reported initially.[166]

The mechanism(s) underlying the effect of heparin on bone are unclear; data suggest that heparin may interfere with osteoblastic activity, or with bone crystal nucleation and enchondral ossification.[172] Other data suggest that heparin may act as a cofactor for the action of parathyroid hormone on bone.[173] The calcium-mobilizing effect of heparin on bone may also be direct, and may occur even in the absence of parathyroid hormone.[174] Mast cells are associated with the multinucleated cells (osteoclasts) that resorb bone, and heparin may be an *endogenous* cofactor in bone resorption in normal individuals. Consistent with this possibility, protamine was recently shown to decrease the resorption of devitalized bone particles implanted subcutaneously in normal rats.[175]

References

1. Jeanloz, R.W.: The nomenclature of acid mucopolysaccharides. Arthritis Rheum. 3:323, 1960.
2. Lamberg, S.I., and Stoolmiller, A.C.: Glycosaminoglycans. A biochemical and clinical review. J. Invest. Derm. 63:433, 1974.
3. Silbert J.E.: Structure and metabolism of proteoglycans and glycosaminoglycans. J. Invest. Derm. 79:31s, 1982.
4. Lindahl, U., and Hook, M.: Glycosaminoglycans and their binding to biological macromolecules. Ann. Rev. Biochem. 47:385, 1978.
5. Olsson, I., and Gardell, S.: The isolation and characterization of glycosaminoglycans from human leukocytes and platelets. Biochim. Biophys. Acta 141:348, 1967.
6. Laterra, J., Silbert, J.E., and Culp, L.A.: Cell surface heparan sulfate mediates some adhesive responses to glycosaminoglycan-binding matrices, including fibronectin. J. Cell Biol. 96:112, 1983.
7. Buonassisi, V., and Colburn, P.: Biological significance of heparan sulfate proteoglycans. Ann. N.Y. Acad. Sci. 401:76, 1982.
8. Williams, M.P., Streeter, H.B., Wusteman, F.S., and Cryer, A.: Heparan sulphate and the binding of lipoprotein lipase to porcine thoracic aorta endothelium. Biochim. Biophys. Acta 756:83, 1983.
9. Mathews, M.B.: Macromolecular evolution of connective tissue. Biol. Rev. 42:499, 1967.
10. Antonopoulos, C.A., Engfeldt, B., Gardell, S., Hjertquist, S., and Solheim, K.: Isolation and identification of the glycosaminoglycans from fracture callus. Biochim. Biophys. Acta 101:150, 1965.
11. Fransson, L.A., and Roden, L.: Structure of dermatan sulfate. II. Characterization of products obtained by hyaluronidase digestion of dermatan sulfate. J. Biol. Chem. 242:4170, 1967.
12. Suzuki, S., Saito, H., Yamagata, I., Anno, K., Seno, N., Kawai, Y., and

Furuhashi, T.: Formation of three types of disulfated disaccharides from chondroitin sulfates by chondroitinase digestion. J. Biol. Chem. 243:1543, 1968.

13. Toole, B.P., and Lowther, D.: Dermatan sulphate protein: Isolation from and interaction with collagen. Arch Biochem. 128:567, 1968.

14. Mathews, M.B., and Decker, L.: The effect of acid mucopolysaccharide proteins on fibril formation from collagen solutions. Biochem. J. 109:517, 1968.

15. Toole, B.P., and Lowther, D.: The isolation of dermatan sulphate protein complex from bovine heart valves. Biochim. Biophys. Acta 101:364, 1965.

16. Brandt, K.D., Skinner, M., and Cohen, A.S.: Characterization of the mucopolysaccharides associated with fractions of guanidine-denatured amyloid fibrils. Clin. Chim. Acta 55:295, 1974.

17. Kjellen, L., Oldberg, A., and Hook, M.: Cell-surface heparan sulfate. Mechanisms of proteoglycan-cell association. J. Biol. Chem. 255:10407, 1980.

18. Rollins, B.J., and Culp, L.A.: Glycosaminoglycans in the substrate adhesion sites of normal and virus-transformed murine cells. Biochemistry 18:141, 1979.

19. Kanwar, Y.S., and Farquhar, M.G.: Presence of heparan sulfate in the glomerular basement membranes. Proc. Natl. Acad. Sci. U.S.A. 76:1303, 1979.

20. Kanwar, Y.S., and Farquhar, M.G.: Isolation of glycosaminoglycans (heparan sulfate) from glomerular basement membranes. Proc. Natl. Acad. Sci. U.S.A. 76, 4493, 1979.

21. Lindahl, U., and Backstrom, G.: Biosynthesis of L-iduronic acid in heparin: Epimerization of D-glucuronic acid on the polymer level. Biochem. Biophys. Res. Commun. 46:985, 1972.

22. Helting, T., and Lindahl, U.: Occurrence and biosynthesis of β-glucuronidic linkages in heparin. J. Biol. Chem. 246:5442, 1971.

23. Foster, A.B., Hanison, R., Inch, T.D., Stacey, M., and Webber, J.M.: Amino sugars and related compounds. IX. Periodate oxidation of heparin and some related substances. J. Chem. Soc. pp. 2279–2287, 1963.

24. Hirano, S., Hoffman, P., and Meyer, K.: The structure of keratosulfate of bovine cornea. J. Org. Chem. 26:5064, 1961.

25. Baldini, G., Brovelli, A., and Castellani, A.A.: Gas chromatography identification of neutral sugars in keratan sulfates from different sources. Ital. Biochem. J. 17:257, 1968.

26. Lohmander, L.S., DeLuca, S., Nilsson, B., Hascall, V.C., Caputo, C.B., Kimura, J.H., and Heinegard, D.K.: Oligosaccharides on proteoglycans from the Swarm rat chondrosarcoma. J. Biol. Chem. 255:6084, 1980.

27. Bhavanandan, V.P., and Meyer, K.: Studies on keratosulfates: Methylation, desulfation and acid hydrolysis studies in old human cartilage keratosulfate. J. Biol. Chem. 243:1052, 1968.

28. Bhavanandan, V.P., and Meyer, K.: Studies on keratosulfates: Methylation and partial acid hydrolysis of bovine corneal keratosulfate. J. Biol. Chem. 242:4352, 1967.

29. Nilsson, B., Nakazawa, K., Hassell, J.R., Newsome, D.A., and Hascall, V.G.: Structure of oligosaccharides and the linkage region between keratan sulfate and the core protein on proteoglycans from monkey cornea. J. Biol. Chem. 258:6056, 1983.

30. Seno, N., Meyer, K., Anderson, B., and Hoffman, P.: Variations in keratosulfates. J. Biol. Chem. 240:1005, 1965.

31. Bray, B., Lieberman, R., and Meyer, K.: Structure of human skeletal keratosulfate. The linkage region. J. Biol. Chem. 242:3373, 1967.

32. Muir, H., and Hardingham, T.E.: Structure of proteoglycans. In Whelan, W.J. (ed.): Biochemistry of Carbohydrates. MTP International Review of Science. Vol. 5. London, Butterworths, 1975, pp. 153–222.

33. Mathews, M.B.: Connective Tissue. Macromolecular Structure and Evolution. New York, Springer, 1975, p. 318.

34. Silpanata, P., Dunstone, J.R., and Ogston, A.G.: Fractionation of a hyaluronic acid preparation in a density gradient. Biochem. J. 109:43, 1968.

35. Swann, D.A.: Studies of hyaluronic acid. I. The preparation and properties of rooster comb hyaluronic acid. Biochim. Biophys. Acta 156:17, 1968.

36. Scher, I., and Hamerman, D.: Isolation of human synovial fluid hyaluronate by density-gradient ultracentrifugation and evaluation of its protein content. Biochem. J. 126:1073, 1972.

37. Fessler, J.H., and Fessler, L.I.: Electron microscopic visualization of the polysaccharide hyaluronic acid. Proc. Natl. Acad. Sci. USA 56:141, 1966.

38. Mason, R.M., d'Arville, C., Kimura, J.H., and Hascall, V.C.: Absence of covalently linked core protein from newly synthesized hyaluronate. Biochem. J. 207:445, 1982.

39. Muir, H.: The nature of the link between protein and carbohydrate of a chondroitin sulphate complex from hyaline cartilage. Biochem. J. 69:195, 1958.

40. Lindahl, U., and Roden, L.: The chondroitin 4-sulfate-protein linkage. J. Biol. Chem. 241:2113, 1966.

41. Roden, L., and Smith, R.: Structure of the neutral trisaccharide region of the chondroitin 4-sulfate protein linkage region. J. Biol. Chem. 241:5949, 1966.

42. Baker, J.R., Roden, L., and Stoolmiller, A.C.: Biosynthesis of chondroitin sulfate proteoglycan: Xylosyl transfer to Smith-degraded cartilage proteoglycan and other exogenous acceptors. J. Biol. Chem. 247:3838, 1972.

43. Roden, L.: Linkage of acid mucopolysaccharides to protein. In Rossi, E. and Stahl, E. (eds.): Biochemistry of Glycoproteins and Related Substances. Basel, Karger, 1968, pp. 185–202.

44. Lindahl, U.: The structures of xyloserine and galactosyl-xyloserine from heparin. Biochim. Biophys. Acta 130:361, 1966.

45. Heinegard, D., Paulsson, M., Inerot, S., and Carlstrom, C.: A novel low-molecular-weight chondroitin sulphate proteoglycan isolated from cartilage. Biochem. J. 197:355, 1981.

46. Rosenberg, L.: Structure of cartilage proteoglycans. In Burleigh, P.M.C., and Poole, A.R. (eds.): Dynamics of Connective Tissue Macromolecules. Amsterdam, North Holland Publishers, 1975, p. 105.

47. Mathews, M.B., and Lozaityte, I.: Sodium chrondroitin sulfate-protein complexes of cartilage. I. Molecular weight and shape. Arch. Biochem. Biophys. 74:158, 1958.

48. Partridge, S.M., Davis, H.F., and Adair, G.S.: The chemistry of connective tissue and the constitution of the chondroitin sulphate protein complex in cartilage. Biochem. J. 79:15, 1961.

49. Torchia, D.A., Hason, M.A., and Hascall, V.C.: ^{13}C Nuclear magnetic resonance suggests a flexible proteoglycan core protein. J. Biol. Chem. 256:7129, 1981.

50. Heinegard, D., and Hascall, V.S.: Aggregation of cartilage proteoglycans. III. Characteristics of the proteins isolated from trypsin digests of aggregates. J. Biol. Chem. 249:4250, 1974.

51. Brandt, K.D., Palmoski, M., and Perricone, E.: Aggregation of cartilage proteoglycans. II. Evidence for the presence of a hyaluronate-binding region on proteoglycans from osteoarthritic cartilage. Arthritis Rheum. 19:1308. 1976.

52. Heinegard, D., and Hascall, V.: Characteristics of the nonaggregating proteoglycans isolated from bovine nasal cartilage. J. Biol. Chem. 254:927, 1979.

53. Heinegard, D., Paulsson, M., and Sonmarin, Y.: Proteoglycans and matrix proteins in cartilage. Prog. Clin. Biol. Res. 110B:35, 1983.

54. Sweet, M.B.E., Thonar, E.J.-M.A., and Marsh, J.: Age-related changes in proteoglycan structure. Arch. Biochem. Biophys. 198:439, 1979.

55. Willingham, M.C., Pastan, I.H., Sahagian, G.G., Jourdian, G.W., and Neufeld, E.F.: Morphologic study of the internalization of a lysosomal enzyme by the mannose 6-phosphate receptor in cultured Chinese hamster ovary cells. Proc. Natl. Acad. Sci. 78:6967, 1981.

56. Ashwell, G., and Morell, A.G.: The role of surface carbohydrates in the hepatic recognition and transport of circulating glycoproteins. Adv. Enzymol. 41:99, 1974.

57. Hudgin, R.L., Pricer, W.E., Jr., Ashwell, G., Stockert, R.J., and Morell, A.G.: The isolation of properties of a rabbit liver binding protein specific for asialoglycoproteins. J. Biol. Chem. 249:5536, 1974.

58. Lunney, J., and Ashwell, G.: A hepatic receptor of avian origin capable of binding specifically modified glycoproteins. Proc. Natl. Acad. Sci. U.S.A. 73:341, 1976.

59. Prinz, R., Schwermann, J., Buddecke, E., and von Figura, K.: Endocytosis of sulphated proteoglycans by cultured skin fibroblasts. Biochem. J. 176:671, 1978.

60. Rich, A.M., Pearlstein, E., Weissmann, G., and Hoffstein, S.: Cartilage proteoglycans inhibit fibronectin-mediated adhesion. Nature 293:224, 1981.

61. Hascall, V.C., and Heinegard, D.: Aggregation of cartilage proteoglycans. I. The role of hyaluronic acid. J. Biol. Chem. 249:4232, 1974.

62. Hardingham, T.E., and Muir, H.: Hyaluronic acid in cartilage and proteoglycan aggregation. Biochem. J. 139:565, 1974.

63. Baker, J., and Caterson, B.: The isolation and characterization of the link proteins from proteoglycan aggregates of bovine nasal cartilage. J. Biol. Chem. 254:2387, 1979.

64. Baker, J. and Caterson, B.: The link proteins. Glycoconjugate Res. 1:329, 1979.

65. Pita, J.C., Howell, D.S., Goldberg, V.M., and Moskowitz, R.W.: Proteoglycan aggregation in normal and experimental osteoarthritic articular cartilage. Trans. Orthop. Res. Soc. 8:171, 1983.

66. Hardingham, T.E., and Muir, H.: The specific interaction of hyaluronic acid with cartilage proteoglycans. Biochim. Biophys. Acta 279:401, 1972.

67. Hardingham, T.E., and Muir, H.: The function of hyaluronic acid in proteoglycan aggregation. In Ali, S.Y., Elves, M.W., and Leaback, D.H. (eds.): Normal and Osteoarthrotic Articular Cartilage. London, Institute of Orthopaedics, 1974, pp. 51–63.

68. Rosenberg, L., Hellmann, W., and Kleinschmidt, A.K.: Electron microscopic studies of proteoglycan aggregates from bovine articular cartilage. J. Biol. Chem. 250:1877, 1975.

69. Hardingham, T.E., and Muir, H.: Binding of oligosaccharides of hyaluronic acid to proteoglycans. Biochem. J. 135:905, 1973.

70. Hascall, V.C., and Heinegard, D.: Aggregation of cartilage proteoglycans. II. Oligosaccharide competitors of the proteoglycan-hyaluronic acid interaction. J. Biol. Chem. 249:4242, 1974.

71. Wiebkin, O.W., Hardingham, T.E., and Muir, H.: The interaction of proteoglycans and hyaluronic acid and the effect of hyaluronic acid on proteoglycan synthesis by chondrocytes of adult cartilage. In Burleigh, P.M.C., and Poole, A.R. (eds.): Dynamics of Connective Tissue Macromolecules. Amsterdam, North-Holland, 1975, pp. 81–104.

72. Mak, A.F., Mow, V.C., and Lai, W.M.: Predictions of the number and strength of the proteoglycan-proteoglycan interactions from viscometric data. Trans. Orthop. Res. Soc. 10:3, 1983.

73. Toole, B.P.: Hyaluronate and hyaluronidase in morphogenesis and differentiation. Am. Zool. 13:1061, 1973.

74. Howell, D.S., Pita, J.C., Marquez, J.F., et al.: Demonstration of macromolecular inhibitor(s) of calcification and nucleaton factor(s) in fluid from calcifying sites in cartilage. J. Clin. Invest. 48:630, 1969.

75. Cuervo, L.A., Pita, J.C., and Howell, D.S.: Inhibition of calcium phosphate mineral growth by proteoglycan aggregate fractions in a synthetic lymph. Calcif. Tiss. Res. 13:1, 1973.

76. Perricone, E., and Brandt, K.: Enhancement of urate solubility by connective tissue. I. Effect of proteoglycan aggregates and buffer cation. Arthritis Rheum. 21:453, 1978.

77. Silvestri, L., Baker, J.R., Roden, L., and Stroud, R.M.: The Clq inhibitor in serum is a chondroitin 4-sulfate proteoglycan. J. Biol. Chem. 256:7383, 1981.

78. Jansson, L., Ogren, S., and Lindahl, U.: Macromolecular properties and end-group analysis of heparin isolated from bovine liver capsule. Biochem. J. 145:53, 1975.

79. Yurt, R.W., Leid, R.W., Austen, K.F., and Silbert, J.E.: Native heparin from rat peritoneal mast cells. J. Biol. Chem. 252:518, 1977.

80. Robinson, H.C., Horner, A.A., Höök, M., Ögren, S., and Lindahl, U.: A proteoglycan form of heparin and its degeneration to single chain molecules. J. Biol. Chem. 253:6687, 1978.

81. Telser, A., Robinson, H.C., and Dorfman, A.: The biosynthesis of chondroitin-sulfate protein complex. Proc. Natl. Acad. Sci. USA 54:912, 1965.

82. Cole, N.N., and Lowther, D.A.: The inhibition of chondroitin sulfate protein synthesis by cycloheximide. FEBS Lett. 2:351, 1969.

83. Stoolmiller, A.C., Horwitz, A.L., and Dorfman, A.: Biosynthesis of the chondroitin sulfate proteoglycan. Purification and properties of xylosyltransferase. J. Biol. Chem. 247:3525, 1972.

84. Helting, T., and Rodin, L.: Biosynthesis of chondroitin sulfate. I. Galactosyl transfer in the formation of the carbohydrate-protein linkage region. J. Biol. Chem. 244:2790, 1968.

85. Robbins, P.W., and Lippmann, F.: Isolation and identification of active sulfate. J. Biol. Chem. 229:837, 1957.

86. Picard, J., Gardais, A., and Dubernand, L.: Presence of sulphated nucleotides in the epiphyseal growth cartilage of the rat. Nature 202:1213, 1964.

87. Silbert, J.E.: Biosynthesis of heparin. IV. N-Deacetylation of a precursor glycosaminoglycan. J. Biol. Chem. 242:5153, 1967.

88. Olssen, I.: The intracellular transport of glycosaminoglycans (mucopolysaccharides) in human leukocytes. Exp. Cell. Res. 54:318, 1969.

89. Fransson, L-A.: Structure of dermatan sulfate. III. The hybrid structure of dermatan sulfate from umbilical cord. J. Biol. Chem. 243:1504, 1968.

90. Robinson, H.C., and Dorfman, A.: The sulfation of chondroitin sulfate in embryonic chick cartilage epiphyses. J. Biol. Chem. 244:348, 1969.

91. Robinson, H.C.: The sulphation of chondroitin sulphate in embryonic chicken cartilage. Biochem. J. 113:543, 1969.

92. Thomas, L.: The effect of papain, vitamin A and cortisone on cartilage matrix in vivo. Biophys. J. 4(Suppl.):207, 1964.

93. Sapolsky, A.I., Altman, R.D., and Howell, D.S.: Cathepsin D activity in normal and osteoarthritic human cartilage. Fed. Proc. 32:1489, 1973.

94. Sapolsky, A.I., Howell, D.S., and Woessner, J.F., Jr.: Neutral proteases and cathepsin D in human articular cartilage. J. Clin. Invest. 53:1044, 1974.

95. Kuettner, K.E., Harper, E., and Eisenstein, R.: Protease inhibitors in cartilage. Arthritis Rheum. 20(Suppl.):S124, 1977.

96. Knight, J.A., Stephens, R.W., Bushell, G.R., Ghosh, P., and Taylor, T.K.F.: Neutral protease inhibitors from human intervertebral disc and femoral head articular cartilage. Biochim. Biophys. Acta 584:304, 1979.

97. Gross, J.I., Mathews, M.B., and Dorfman, A.: Sodium chondroitin sulfate-protein complexes of cartilage. J. Biol. Chem. 235:2889, 1960.

98. Hutterer, F.: Degradation of mucopolysaccharides by hepatic lysosomes. Biochim. Biophys. Acta 115:312, 1966.

99. Aronson, N.N., and Davidson, E.A.: Lysosomal hyaluronidase from rat liver. I. Preparation. J. Biol. Chem. 242:437, 1967.

100. Weissmann, B., Meyer, K., Sampson, P., and Linker, A.: Isolation of oligosaccharides enzymatically produced from hyaluronic acid. J. Biol. Chem. 208:417, 1954.

101. Hoffman, P., Meyer, K., and Linker, A.: Transglycosylation during the mixed digestion of hyaluronic acid and chondroitin sulfate by testicular hyaluronidase. J. Biol. Chem. 219:653, 1956.

102. Linker, A., and Hovingh, P.: The enzymic degradation of heparin and heparitin sulfate. I. The fractionation of crude heparinase from flavobacteria. J. Biol. Chem. 240:3724, 1965.

103. Kaplan, D., and Meyer, K.: The fate of injected mucopolysaccharides. J. Clin. Invest. 41:743, 1962.

104. Varadi, D.P., Cifonelli, J.A., and Dorfman, A.: The acid mucopolysaccharides in normal urine. Biochim. Biophys. Acta 141:103, 1967.

105. Bollet, A.J., Bonner, W.M., and Nance, J.L.: The presence of hyaluronidase in various mammalian tissues. J. Biol. Chem. 238:3522, 1963.

106. Stack, M.T., and Brandt, K.D.: Identification and characterization of articular cartilage hyaluronidase. Arthritis Rheum. 25:S100, 1982.

107. van Hoof, F., and Hers, H.G.: The abnormalities of lysosomal enzymes in mucopolysaccharidoses. Eur. J. Biochem. 7:34, 1968.

108. McKusick, V.A. and Neufeld, E.F.: The mucopolysaccharide storage diseases. In Stanbury, J.B., Wyngaarden, J.B., Fredrickson, D.S., Goldstein, J.L., and Brown, M.S. (eds.): The Metabolic Basis of Inherited Disease. 5th ed. New York, McGraw-Hill Book Company, 1983, p. 751.

109. van Hoof, F., and Hers, H.G.: L'ultrastructure des cellules hepatiques dans la maladie de Hurler. Compt. Rend. Acad. Sci. 259:1281, 1964.

110. Danes, B.S., and Bearn, A.G.: Hurler's syndrome: Demonstration of an inherited disorder of connective tissue in cell culture. Science 149:987, 1965.

111. Fratantoni, J.C., Hall, C.W., and Heufeld, E.F.: The defect in Hurler's and Hunter's syndromes: Faulty degradation of mucopolysaccharides. Proc. Natl. Acad. Sci. USA 60:699, 1968.

112. Fratantoni, J.C., Hall, C.W., and Neufeld, E.F.: Hurler and Hunter syndromes: Mutual correction of the defect in cultured fibroblasts. Science 162:570, 1968.

113. Neufeld, E.F., and Cantz, M.J.: Corrective factors for inborn errors of mucopolysaccharide metabolism. Ann. N.Y. Acad. Sci. 179:580, 1970.

114. Neufeld, E.F.: The biochemical basis for mucopolysaccharidoses and mucolipidoses. Prog. Med. Genet. 10:81, 1974.

115. Neufeld, E.F.: The enzymology of inherited mucopolysaccharide storage disorders. Trends Biochem. Sci. 2:25, 1977.

116. Neufeld, E.F., and McKusick, V.A.: Disorders of lysosomal enzyme synthesis and localization: I-cell disease and pseudo-Hurler polydystrophy. In Stanbury, J.B. Wyngaarden, J.B., Fredrickson, D.S., Goldstein, J.L., and Brown, M.S. (eds.): The Metabolic Basis of Inherited Disease. 5th ed. New York, McGraw-Hill Book Company, 1983, p. 778.

117. Hasilik, A., Klein, U., Waheed, A., Strecker, G., and von Figura, K.: Phosphorylated oligosaccharides in lysosomal enzymes: Identification of α-N-acetylglucosamine (1) phospho (6) mannose diester groups. Proc. Natl. Acad. Sci. USA 77:7074, 1980.

118. Varki, A., and Kornfeld, S.: Identification of a rate liver α-N-acetylglucosaminyl phosphodiesterase capable of removing "blocking" α-N-acetylglucosamine residues from phosphorylated high mannase oligosaccharides of lysosomal enzymes. J. Biol. Chem. 255:8398, 1980.

119. Hasilik, A., Waheed, A., and von Figura, K.: Enzymatic phosphorylation of lysosomal enzymes in the presence of UDP-N-acetylglucosamine. Absence of the activity in I-cell fibroblasts. Biochem. Biophys. Res. Commun. 98:761, 1981.

120. Reitman, A.L., Varki, A., and Kornfeld, S.: Fibroblasts from patients with I-cell disease and pseudo-Hurler polydystrophy are deficient in uridine 5'-diphosphate-N-acetylglucosamine: Glycoprotein N-acetylglucosaminylphosphotransferase activity. J. Clin. Invest. 67:1574, 1981.

121. Comper, C.W., and Laurent, T.C.: Physiological function of connective tissue polysaccharides. Physiol. Rev. 58:255, 1978.

122. Ogston, A.G., and Phelps, C.F.: The partition of solutes between buffer solutions containing hyaluronic acid. Biochem. J. 78:827, 1961.

123. Maroudas, A.: Physical chemistry of articular cartilage and the intervertebral disc. In Sokoloff, L. (ed.): The Joints and Synovial Fluid. Vol. II. New York, Academic Press, 1980, p. 239.

124. Toole, B.P.: Hyaluronate turnover during chondrogenesis in the developing chick limb and axial skeleton. Dev. Biol. 29:321, 1972.

125. Toole, B.P., and Linsenmayer, T.F.: Newer knowledge of skeletogenesis. Clin. Orthop. 129:258, 1977.

126. Toole, B.P., Jackson, G., and Gross, J.: Hyaluronate in morphogenesis: Inhibition of chondrogenesis in vitro. Proc. Natl. Acad. Sci. USA 69:1384, 1972.

127. Underhill, C.B., and Dorfman, A.: The role of hyaluronic acid in intercellular adhesion of cultured mouse cells. Exp. Cell Res. 117:155, 1978.

128. Toole, B.P.: Developmental role of hyaluronate. Conn. Tiss. Res. 10:93, 1982.

129. Culp, L.A.: Molecular composition and origin of substrate-attached material from normal and virus-transformed cells. J. Supramol. Struct. 5:239, 1976.

130. Yamada, K., Kennedy, D.W., Kimata, K., and Pratt, R.M.: Characterization of fibronectin interactions with glycosaminoglycans and identification of active proteolytic fragments. J. Biol. Chem. 255:6055, 1980.

131. Solursh, M., Vaerewyck, S.A., and Reiter, R.S.: Depression by hyaluronic acid of glycosaminoglycan synthesis by chick cultured embryo chondrocytes. Dev. Biol. 41:233, 1974.

132. Wiebkin, O.W., Hardingham, T.E., and Muir, H.: The interaction of proteoglycans and hyaluronic acid and the effect of hyaluronic acid on proteoglycan synthesis by chondrocytes of adult cartilage. In Burleigh, P.M.C., and Poole, A.R. (eds.): Dynamics of Connective Tissue Macromolecules. Amsterdam, North-Holland, 1975, p. 81.

133. Wiebkin, O.W., Hardingham, T.E., and Muir, H.: Hyaluronic acid-proteoglycan interaction and the influence of hyaluronic acid on proteoglycan synthesis by chondrocytes from adult cartilage. In Slavkin, H., and Greulich, R.C. (eds.): Extracellular Matrix Influences on Gene Expression. New York, Academic Press, 1975, pp. 209–223.

134. Nevo, Z., and Dorfman, A.: Stimulation of chondromucoprotein synthesis in chondrocytes by extracellular chondromucoprotein. Proc. Natl. Acad. Sci. USA 69:2069, 1972.

135. Farber, S.J., and Schubert, M.: The binding of cations by chondroitin sulfate. J. Clin. Invest. 36:1715, 1957.

136. Woodward, C., and Davidson, E.A.: Structure-function relationships of protein polysaccharide complexes: Specific ion-binding properties. Proc. Natl. Acad. Sci. USA 60:201, 1968.

137. DeBarnard, B., Stagni, N., Colautti, I., et al.: Glycosaminoglycans and endochondral calcification. Clin. Orthop. 126:285, 1977.

138. Waddell, W.J.: A molecular mechanism for biological calcification. Biochem. Biophys. Res. Commun. 49:127, 1972.

139. Howell, D.S., Pita, J.C., Marquez, J.F., et al.: Demonstration of macromolecular inhibitor(s) of calcification and nucleation factor(s) in fluid from calcifying sites in cartilage. J. Clin. Invest. 48:630, 1969.

140. Cuervo, L.A., Pita, J.C., and Howell, D.S.: Inhibition of calcium phosphate mineral growth by proteoglycan aggregate fractions in a synthetic lymph. Calcif. Tiss. Res. 13:1, 1973.

141. Pita, J.C., Muller, F., and Howell, D.S.: Disaggregation of proteoglycan aggregate during endochondral calcification. Physiological role of cartilage lysozyme. In Burleigh, P.M.C., and Poole, A.R. (eds.): Dynamics of Connective Tissue Macromolecules. Cambridge, North-Holland, 1974, p. 247.

142. Greenwald, R.A., and Lane, J.M.: Proteoglycan and lysozyme content of healing fracture callus. Trans. Orthop. Res. Soc. 3:33, 1978.

143. Kint, J.A., Dacremont, G., Carton, D., Orye, E., and Hooft, C.: Mucopolysaccharidosis: Secondarily induced abnormal distribution of lysosomal isoenzymes. Science 181:352, 1973.

144. Avila, J.L., and Convit, J.: Inhibition of leukocytic lysosomal enzymes by glycosaminoglycans in vitro. Biochem. J. 152:57, 1975.

145. Ueno, R.: Ergebnisse der behandlung mit einem mucopolysaccharid-polyschwefelsaureester bei der experimentellen arthrose des kniegelenks. Z. Orthop. 111:886, 1973.

146. Dustmann, H.O., Puhl, W., and Martin, K.: Der Einfluss intraartikularer arteparoninjektionen bei arthrose. Z. Orthop. 112:1188, 1974.

147. Fife, R.S., and Brandt, K.D.: Experimental modes of therapy in osteoarthritis. In Moskowitz, R.W., Howell, D.S., Goldberg, V.M., and Mankin, H.J. (eds.): Osteoarthritis Diagnosis and Management. In Press.

148. Horner, A.A.: Demonstration of endogenous heparin in rat blood. Adv. Exp. Med. Biol. 52:85, 1975.

149. Lindahl, U., and Hook, M.: Glycosaminoglycans and their binding to biological macromolecules. Ann. Rev. Biochem. 47:385, 1978.

150. Bjork, I., and Lindahl, U.: Mechanism of the anticoagulant action of heparin. Molecular and Cellular Biochemistry 48:161, 1982.

151. Rosenberg, R.D., and Damus, P.S.: The purification and mechanism of action of human antithrombin-heparin cofactor. J. Biol. Chem. 248:6490, 1973.

152. Lam, L.H., Silbert, J.E., and Rosenberg, R.D.: The separation of active and inactive forms of heparin. Biochem. Biophys. Res. Commun. 69:570, 1976.

153. Lewis, R.G., Spencer, A.F., and Silbert, J.E.: Biosynthesis of glycosaminoglycans by cultured mastocytoma cells. Biochem. J. 134:455, 1973.

154. Jacques, L.B.: Heparin: An old drug with a new paradigm. Science 206:528, 1979.

155. Barber, A.J., Kaser-Glanzmann, R., Jakabova, M., and Luscher, E.F.: Characterization of a chondroitin 4-sulfate proteoglycan carrier for heparin neutralizing activity (platelet factor 4) released from human blood platelets. Biochim. Biophys. Acta 286:312, 1972.

156. Raepple, E., Hill, H., and Loos, M.: Mode of interaction of different polyanions with the first (Cl,Cl̄), the second (C2) and the fourth (C4) component of complement. I. Immunochemistry 13:251, 1976.

157. Rent, R., Myhrman, R., Fiedel, B.A., and Gewurz, H.: Potentiation of Cl-esterase inhibitor activity by heparin. Clin. Exp. Immunol. 23:264, 1976.

158. Loos, M., Volanakis, J.E., and Stroud, R.M.: Mode of interaction of different polyanions with the first (Cl,Cl̄), the second (C2) and the fourth (C4) component of complement. III. Immunochemistry 13:789, 1976.

159. Loos, M., Volanakis, J.E., and Stroud, R.M.: Mode of interaction of different polyanions with the first (Cl,Cl̄), the second (C2) and the fourth (C4) component of complement. II. Immunochemistry 13:257, 1976.

160. Baker, P.J., Liat, T.F., McLeod, B.C., Behrends, C.L., and Bewurz, H.: Studies on the inhibition of C56-induced lysis (reactive lysis). VI. Modulation of C56-induced lysis by polyanions and polycations. J. Immunol. 114:554, 1975.

161. Yurt, R.W., and Austen, K.F.: Preparative purification of the rat mast cell chymase. Characterization and interaction with granule components. J. Exp. Med. 146:1405, 1977.

162. Makinen, I., Totterman, T.H., Gordin, A., and Weber, T.H.: Migration inhibition factor and the blood clotting system: Effects of defibrination, heparin and thrombin. Clin. Exp. Immunol. 29:181, 1977.

163. Oslerud, B., Bogwald, J., Lindahl, U., and Seljelid, R.: Production of blood coagulation factor V and tissue thromboplastin by macrophages in vitro. FEBS Lett. 127:154, 1981.

164. Levy, G.A., and Edgington, T.S.: Lymphocyte cooperation is required for amplification of macrophage procoagulant activity. J. Exp. Med. 151:1232, 1980.

165. Greczy, C.L., and Hopper, K.E.: A mechanism of migration inhibition in delayed-type hypersensitivity reactions. J. Immunol. 126:1059, 1981.

166. Griffith, G.C., Nichols, G., Jr., Asher, J., and Flanegan, B.: Heparin osteoporosis. JAMA 193:91, 1965.

167. Miller, W.E., and deWolfe, V.G.: Osteoporosis resulting from heparin therapy. Cleveland Clin. Quart. 33:31, 1966.

168. Sackler, J.P., and Liu, L.: Heparin-induced osteoporosis. Br. J. Radiol. 46:548, 1973.

169. Squires, J.W., and Pinch, L.W.: Heparin-induced spinal fractures. JAMA 241:2417, 1979.

170. Wise, P.H., and Hall, A.J.: Heparin-induced osteopenia in pregnancy. Br. Med. J. 11:110, 1980.

171. Rupp, W.M., McCarthy, H.B., Rohde, T.D., Blackshear, P.J., Goldenberg, F.J., and Buchwald, H.: Risk of osteoporosis in patients treated with long-term intravenous heparin therapy. Curr. Surg. 39:419, 1982.

172. Avioli, L.: Heparin-induced osteopenia: an appraisal. Adv. Exp. Med. Biol. 52:375, 1975.

173. Goldhaber, P.: Heparin enhancement of factors stimulating bone resorption in tissue culture. Science 147:407, 1965.

174. Jowsey, J., Adams, P., and Schlein, A.P.: Calcium metabolism in response to heparin administration. Calc. Tiss. Res. 6:249, 1970.

175. Glowacki, J.: Heparin's role in bone resorption. Calcif. Tiss. Int. 35:641, 1983.

Chapter 16
Biology of the Joint

Edward D. Harris, Jr.

INTRODUCTION

Joints hold the end or the periphery of bone in apposition to an adjacent bone. Joints that have essentially no motion (e.g., the fibrous joints in the skull vault) are of no concern to rheumatologists. An increase in the potential for motion of joints is accompanied by an increased potential for trauma; motion also accentuates inflammation when it occurs in the joint, hastening deterioration. Thus, for the rheumatologist and orthopedic surgeon, the study of joints must link biology to motion.

CLASSIFICATION OF JOINTS

The function of each joint is closely linked to its structure. Some joints have a wide range of motion but little intrinsic stability (e.g., the knee, shoulder). Others have minimal movement and need little if any stabilization from overlying muscle groups (e.g., the sacroiliac joints). It is useful for students of joint disease to recognize two basic types of articulation: (1) *synovial or diarthrodial joints* (Fig. 16–1), which are articulations

Figure 16–1. A diagram of a normal human interphalangeal joint in sagittal section, as an example of a synovial or diarthrodial joint. The "tidemark" represents the calcified cartilage which bonds articular cartilage to the subchondral bony plate. (From Sokoloff, L., and Bland, J.H.: The Musculoskeletal System. Baltimore, Williams & Wilkins Company, 1975).

254

with free movement, with synovial membrane lining a joint cavity, and (2) *synarthroses*, which have very little movement. There are four subclassifications of synarthroses: (a) *Symphyses*: a fibrocartilaginous disc separates bone ends that are joined by firm ligaments (e.g., symphysis pubis and intervertebral joints). (b) *Synchondroses*: bone ends are covered with articular cartilage, but there is no synovium or significant joint cavity (e.g., sternomanubrial joint). (c) *Syndesmoses*: bones are joined directly by fibrous ligaments without a cartilagenous interface (e.g., the distal tibiofibular articulation, the only joint of this type outside the cranial vault). (d) *Synostoses*: bone bridges between bones, producing ankylosis.

Among synovial joints there are great differences in structure, and therefore function. For instance, the humeroulnar joint is a true hinge joint limited to motion in one plane, whereas the spherical hip joint, a ball (the femoral head) and socket (the acetabulum) joint, has motion in all directions and rotations. Accompanying the relative restrictions upon planes of motion of the elbow there is an intrinsic stability; the hinge construction needs little surrounding muscle to stablize it. Conversely, the freedom of motion inherent in the structure of a ball-and-socket joint such as the hip or shoulder demands that a very powerful musculature be developed to provide stability and to prevent frequent subluxation.

Details of structure and range of motion of individual joints are discussed in detail in Chapter 24.

DEVELOPMENTAL BIOLOGY OF THE DIARTHRODIAL JOINT

Extensive histochemical studies of embryonic human specimens have provided much data about the sequence of joint development in the fetus[1] (Fig. 16–2). Experimental work to supplement these descriptive studies has been done in other vertebrate species, especially the chick.

Genetic information controlling the development of joints is expressed by cells in the *apical ectodermal* ridge of the embryo.[2] Excision of this ridge prevents normal joint development by removing competence of the distal mesenchyme to form organized limb components.[3]

The normal sequences following induction of limb bud formation are described very well by O'Rahilly and Gardner.[1] A summary follows.

1. Condensation. Condensation of mesenchyme by cellular aggregation forms a blastema. This occurs shortly after limb buds appear[4] and is believed to occur before a cartilaginous matrix is formed (i.e., chondrification).

Figure 16–2. Diagram of the development of a synovial joint. Joints develop from the blastema, not the surrounding mesenchyme. Chondrification has occurred in *B.* The *interzone* remains avascular and highly cellular. The *synovial mesenchyme* develops from the periphery of the interzone (*C*) and becomes vascularized. Following shortly after differentiation of synovial membrane is *cavitation*, which may begin centrally in the interzone or peripherally (*D*) and merge to form the joint cavity. (From O'Rahilly, R., and Gardner, E.,: In Sokoloff, L. [ed.]: The Joints and Synovial Fluid, Vol. 1, New York, Academic Press, 1978.)

2. Chondrification (Fig. 16–3). This begins in the regions of future bones and effectively divides the blastema. Intercellular sulfated material accumulates, and this can be demonstrated by radioautography.[6] In the human, chondrification can be detected when the emryo is as small as 11.7 mm (stage 17 of embryologic development).[5]

3. Interzones, the Future Joints. The space between segments undergoing chondrification remains as avascular, homogeneous, densely cellular areas that secrete material staining intensely for polysaccharides (probably chondroitin sulfate).[7] This extracellular material appears almost to force the interzone cells apart. The border of each interzone is continuous at the periphery of this evolving joint with perichondrium and serves as an appositional growth zone for the preskeletal segments.

4. Formation of Synovial Mesenchyme. The synovium differentiates from the periphery of the interzone. It probably orginates from the blastema and not from the surrounding general mesenchyme.[7,8] In addition to the synovial lining, joint capsule, intracapsular ligaments, menisci, and tendons all develop from the synovial mesenchyme. Unlike the central interzone or its chondrogenous borders, the synovial mesenchyme becomes vascularized. A dense capillary network develops in the subsynovial tissue. The tough joint capsule evolves as a structural continuum from the more cellular and vascular subsynovial tissue.[9]

This vascularization is the critical point of development of synovial tissue. Among other phenomena it permits delivery of extrablastemal cells to the developing synovium. These extrablastemal cells include *mast cells* (appearing when the embryo is approximately 80 mm in crown-rump length) and *macrophages* that become histiocytes.[9] The macrophages have been identified by the presence of cytoplasmic granules that stain for acid phosphatase or esterases and by their signs of motility. Although not proved, it is presumed that these macrophages arise from primitive endothelial cells, are released into the lumen of primitive vessels, and move to the surrounding tissue.[10]

5. Formation of the Joint Cavity. Cavitation occurs at about the time the synovial mesenchyme differentiates into a membrane (Fig. 16–4). The precise mechanisms causing cavitation have not been completely defined. Extracellular matrix destruction by enzymes is probably the final pathway, and the interzone cells are probably programmed to release the enzymes that degrade the extracellular material. In chick embryos it has been shown that movement of the limb is essential for normal cavitation,[11,12] but similar experiments in developing human embryonic joints have yielded conflicting views.[13,14]

The cavity begins in the central interzone, which is, in effect, absorbed into each adjacent chondrogenous zone, which evolves into the underlying articular cartilage surface. Thus, when the joint cavity has formed, the joint is lined at all surfaces either by hyaline cartilage or by synovial membrane. These two very different tissues merge at the periphery of the joint, where the cartilage melds into bone. A potential space in the body has developed without any basement membrane below the lining cell surface. This absence of any epithelial tissue is a major determinant of joint physiology.

Direct experimental evidence is lacking as to when sodium hyaluronate (characteristic of joint fluid) first appears in the newly formed cavity. Synovial fibroblasts synthesize and release hyaluronate which is admixed with a protein-rich filtrate of blood to form synovial fluid. It is assured, therefore, that true synovial fluid cannot form until the synovial mesenchyme has vascularized and cellular differentiation in lining cells has progressed sufficiently to result in hyaluronate synthesis.

The entire development from a cellular but undifferentiated blastema to structures resembling an adult joint occurs in the human from about 4½ to 7 weeks after fertilization.[1] By this time all large synovial joints have recognizable cavities and are, functionally, true joints. Formation of joints occurs prior to many other crucial phases of musculoskeletal development, including vascularization of epiphyseal cartilage (8 to 12 weeks), appearance of villous folds in synovium (10 to 12 weeks), evolution of bursae (after 3 or 4 months), and appearance of fat pads (4 to 5 months).

In contrast to other joints, the temporomandibular joint develops slowly, with cavitation at a crown-rump length of 57 to 75 mm (i.e., well into the fetal stage).[15,16] This retardation may be related to the fact that this joint

Figure 16–3. Coronal section of the hand at 11.7 mm (stage 17). The blastema with its increased cellularity serves to outline the form of the hand. Faint lightening in the region of the third and fourth metacarpals indicates very early chondrification. The radius and ulna are further along in chondrification. (From O'Rahilly, R.: Irish J. Med. Sci. 6:456, 1957).

Figure 16–4. The embryonic joint developing between the femur and tibia at 31 mm (stage 23). The lateral meniscus is outlined by cavitation on the femoral side. Cavitation will subsequently spread in a medial direction as well as developing spontaneously at other foci. (From Gardner, E., and O'Rahilly, R.: J. Anat. 102:289, 1968)

develops in the absence of a continuous blastema and that its completion is related to insertion of a fibrocartilaginous disc between bone ends[15,17] derived from muscular and mesenchymal derivatives of the first pharyngeal arch.[16]

Synostoses (cartilaginous and fibrous joints) are presumed to evolve similarly, with the important exceptions that synovial mesenchyme is not formed and cavitation does not occur. Indeed, the "fused" peripheral joints induced in chicken embryos by paralyzing their limbs[18] resemble symphyses, with fibrocartilaginous plates developing between hyaline cartilage at the ends of bones. It may be that these joints develop as they do because there is relatively little motion during their development.

Human vertebrae and intervertebral discs probably develop as units from material arising from somites that form a homogeneous blastema.[19] The embryonic intervertebral discs serve as chondrogenous zones (both rostral and caudal) for the evolving vertebral bodies. The embryonic "disc" is replaced after it ceases chondrifying by the annulus fibrosus[20,21] (Fig. 16–5). It seems possible that since the nucleus pulposus contains proteoglycans as well as type II (cartilaginous) collagen,[22-24] it may represent segmented inclusions of the original embryonic disc still active in chondrification.

ORGANIZATION OF THE MATURE JOINT

The mature joint is a complex structure. Understanding it demands consideration of biomechanics (see Chapter 20) and analysis of the different function of each joint, which is determined in turn by the anatomy peculiar to each joint.

In the following section, components of the "typical" synovial joint will be described.

Muscles, Tendons, and Ligaments. The physiology of muscle is described in detail in Chapter 18. It is sufficient here to emphasize only the direct correlation between muscle mass around a joint relative to its normal motion in different planes, such as the hip and shoulder. The shoulder, for example, is surrounded by bulky musculature with multiple components. This is essential to allow control of its many arcs of motions: forward flexion, 160 degrees; backward extension, 50 degrees; abduction, 170 degrees; adduction, 50 degrees; rotation (internal, 70 degrees; external, 70 to 90 degrees). In contrast, peripheral joints are not stablized by contracting muscle mass but rather by their anatomy, which restricts planes of normal motion, and by dense ligaments, which are structurally a part of the joint capsule.

Figure 16–5. At 50 mm human fetal development, the body of the second and third cervical vertebrae has completed chondrification. The anulus fibrosus is beginning to differentiate at the periphery of the interzone (which in this section contains a nub of persisting notochord). (From O'Rahilly, R., and Gardner, E.: In Sokoloff, L. [ed.]: The Joint and Synovial Fluid, New York, Academic Press, 1978.)

The ankle, for example, moves in one plane through limited arcs: flexion, 50 degrees, and extension, 20 degrees. Muscle mass is directly proportional to stability of certain joints such as the knee. Joint effusions produce reflex inhibition of muscle contraction,[25] and muscle atrophy around a painful (and therefore hypomobile) joint occurs within days. It is unusual for the muscle/tendon apparatus to fail, but when it does, it is secondary to enormous, quickly generated forces across a joint. The site of failure is usually at the tendinous insertion into bone.

Individual variability in passive joint motion has a broad range, from the muscled athlete often at risk for muscle "pulls and strains" to the "loosed-jointed" asthenic person who suffers frequent joint sprains, who may have a predisposition to develop osteoarthritis,[26] and who may resemble those with Ehlers-Danlos type III syndromes (see Chapter 105).

Tendons act as functional and anatomic bridges between muscle and bone. As described by Canoso,[27] in addition to focusing the force of a large mass of muscle into a localized area on bone, tendons can, by splitting to form numerous insertions on different bones, transmit the force of a single muscle to different bones (e.g., the multiple distal insertions of the tibialis posterior). In development, muscle is not necessary for early differentiation of tendons, but without muscle (and muscle contraction?) sustained development of tendons fails.[28] Tendons are formed of logitudinally arranged type I collagen bundles interlaced by a delicate reticular network of type III collagen blood vessels, lymphatics, and possibly thin cellular processes of fibroblasts which can provide cell to cell contact.[29] The principal cell product for export from tendon fibroblasts is type I collagen, although they also synthesize proteoglycans (always a part of the connective tissue matrix) and other proteins (e.g., inhibitor[s] of metalloproteinases and collagenases, which have potential for degrading tendon components).

Most tendon attachments to bone are a highly specialized complex of tiers through which collagen fibers blend into fibrocartilage; then mineralized fibrocartilage merges into bone.[30] "Sharpey's perforating fibers," the tendon fibrils that have been seen to run through the periosteum and become continuous with outer bone lamellae (i.e., a functional staple), may be important at tendon insertions where there are no intervening tiers of fibrocartilage. An example of this type is the insertion of the pectoralis major tendon into the humerus.[31]

Many tendons, particularly those with a large range of motion, run through vascularized, discontinuous sheaths of collagen lined with mesenchymal cells resembling synovium. Tendon sheaths provide gliding function, which probably is enhanced by hyaluronic acid produced by the lining cells.[32] Loss of gliding function by formation of fibrous adhesions between tendons and their sheaths occurs when inflammation or surgical scar is followed by long periods of immobilization.

Pain of tendinous origin, tendinous calcification, and tendon rupture are complex pathophysiologic processes that have not been thoroughly evaluated. Factors in-

volved at different times to a greater or lesser degree are (1) ageing processes, including loss of extracellular water and an increase in intermolecular crosslinks of collagen; (2) traumatically induced ischemic areas in tendon; (3) iatrogenic factors, including intratendon injection of glucocorticoids; (4) deposition of calcium hydroxyapatite crystals (perhaps enhanced by presence of the calcium-binding amino acid γ-carboxyglutamic acid [Gla]).[33]

There are few anatomic and structural differences between ligaments and tendons. The obvious one is that one set of the end of tendon collagen fibrils are intertwined and braided among the fibrillar endomysium that surrounds each individual muscle fiber, whereas both ends of ligaments insert into bone on either side of a joint. Often the latter are recognized only as hypertrophied components of the fibrous joint capsule. Some ligaments have a much higher ratio of elastin to collagen (1:4) than do tendons (1:50).[27] The ligamentum flavum, which holds adjacent vertebral laminae in place, is an example of these. The ligament that sustains the greatest stress during normal function is the plantar ligament of the foot, which has a large functional role in keeping the longitudinal arch of the foot raised. Ligaments and tendons synthesize substances that regulate connective tissue metabolism locally. In addition to collagen, for instance, tendon cells produce collagenase in latent form as well as inhibitors of collagenolytic enzymes.

The stabilization of joints is in part a function of ligaments, capsule, and menisci of joints. In the knee (the most studied of all joints), the medial collateral ligaments and anterior cruciate ligaments form a resistant couple for stability when there is little or no load upon the joint. During load-bearing conditions there is an increasing contribution to stability from the joint surfaces themselves as compressive load increases. The components that provide surface stability are friction (minimal) between the joint surfaces, deformation of the cartilage, and geometrical conformity of the condyles.

Bursae. The many bursae in the human body serve to facilitate gliding function much as a tendon sheath facilitates movement of the tendon within, enabling low friction motion of one tissue over another. Bursae are closed sacs, lined sparsely with mesenchymal cells similar to synovial cells. Although most bursae differentiate concurrently with synovial joints during embryogenesis, during life new bursae may develop in response to stress and previously existing ones may become hypertrophied.[34] During life, again in response to stress (i.e., inflammation or trauma), deep bursae often develop communications with joints.[27] Examples of this include (1) iliopsoas bursa—hip joint; (2) subacromial bursae—glenohumeral joint; these develop secondary to degenerative or inflammatory involvement of the rotator cuff tendons; and (3) gastrocnemius or semimembranous bursae—knee joint. It is unusual for subcutaneous bursae (e.g., the prepatellar bursa or olecranon bursa) to develop communication with the underlying joint. Bursal fluid, even when the bursa is infected or host to an attack of gout, rarely generates an inflammatory response (measured by numbers of PMN leukocytes) that a similar process does within a joint.[35] This may be related to a lesser degree of vascularization of bursae.

Vascular and Nerve Supply to the Joint. Arterial and venous networks of the joint are complex and are characterized by arteriovenous anastomoses that communicate freely with the vascular supply to periosteum and to periarticular bone.[36] As large synovial arteries enter the deep layers of the synovium near the capsule, they give off branches, which branch again to form "microvascular units" in the subsynovial layers. As in other tissues, precapillary arterioles probably play a major role in controlling circulation to the lining layer. The surface area of the synovial capillary bed is very large and, as it runs only a few cell layers deep to the surface, it has a role in trans-synovial exchange of molecules that may explain the propensity of diarthrodial joints to develop effusions and hemarthroses.

Heat (up to an intra-articular temperature of 40° C) increases blood flow through synovial capillaries.[37] Exercise, although resulting in an increase in periarticular muscle blood flow, may actually result in a decrease in the clearance rate of small molecules.[38] Immobilization, in experimental animals, actually decreases the number of capillary plexi as well as blood flow in joints.[37] Pressure also has an effect on blood flow. Effusions can act to tamponade blood supply, and it is possible that large effusions could virtually shut off blood flow to superficial lining layers.

Synovial capillaries are fenestrated; they contain small pores covered by a thin membrane[38,39] (Fig. 16–6). These fenestrations may facilitate rapid exchange of small molecules (e.g., glucose, lactate, and so on) with the synovial fluid.

Dissection studies have shown that each joint has a dual nerve supply: (1) specific articular nerves that penetrate the capsule as independent branches of adjacent peripheral nerves and (2) articular branches that arise from related muscle nerves.[39] The definition of joint position and the detection of joint motion are monitored separately and by a combination of multiple inputs from different receptors in varied systems. Dee has summarized data indicating that nerve endings in muscle as well as in the joint capsule are involved in articular kinesthetic sensation.[40] Patients who have had capsulectomy along with total hip replacement[41] or surgical removal of proximal interphalangeal or metacarpophalangeal joints of the hand[42] still retain good joint position sensation.

The Subchondral Bone. The microstructure of bone in the plate beneath the calcified base of articular cartilage may have many effects upon the cartilage above it. The subchondral bone of the knee is formed from a meshwork of fine trabeculae of less than 0.2 mm diameter and in a density of fewer than 2 per mm of bone. The stiffness of subchondral bone, and thus the impact transmitted to cartilage during weight bearing or effort, may be a factor in the health of normal articular cartilage.[43]

Articular Cartilage—the Unique Functional Struc-

Figure 16–6. Fenestrated blood capillary in human synovium. This capillary is situated just beneath the lining layer. Pores in endothelium are indicated by the arrow. A red blood cell lies in the lumen of the capillary. × 11,000. (From Bassleer, R., et al.: Histological structure and functions of synovium. In Franchimont, P. [ed.]: Articular Synovium: Anatomy, Physiology, Pathology, Pharmacology, and Therapy. Basel, Karger, 1982, pp. 1–26.)

ture of Joints. Articular cartilage is highly differentiated and has physical properties that no other tissue or synthetic product of bioengineering laboratories can equal. Articular cartilage must provide a smooth, resilient surface for joint motion under conditions of either intense pressure or high velocity, or both. At the same time the cartilage must retain capacity for maintenance without morphologic change and in the absence of any blood vessels to carry in nutrients and remove products of chondrocyte metabolism and matrix turnover. While endowed with a capacity for maintenance, articular cartilage cannot effectively regenerate itself, and this imposes a limitation on the organism—a need to protect articular cartilage from destruction.

Articular cartilage is composed principally of collagen and proteoglycans. The structure and biology of these components are discussed in detail in Chapters 14 and 15.

ORGANIZATION OF ARTICULAR CARTILAGE

Intensive study of the articular cartilage from the metacarpophalangeal joints of young steers has provided the most recent and precise data on the organization of this tissue.[44,45] Figure 16–7 is a diagrammatic representation of the various zones and regions of cartilage.

The *superficial zone* (5 to 10 percent of total thickness) has a reduced metachromatic staining for glycosaminoglycans and a rich content of immunoreactive proteoglycan core protein and link protein. Called the lamina splendens, this is probably composed of hyaluronic acid and/or absorbed glycoproteins.[46] The superficial zone is covered at the cartilage surface by a layer of thin fibrils (4 to 10 μm in diameter), which are arranged in

BOVINE METACARPAL CONDYLAR CARTILAGE (~10 Months)

Figure 16–7. Diagrammatic representation of the zones and regions of bovine articular cartilage (From Poole, A. R. et al.: J. Cell Biol. 93:921, 1982.)

Figure 16–8. Scanning electron microscopic view of the "pits" found on the surface of articular cartilage. This view is of adult rabbit cartilage at ~500 magnification. It is not known whether the depressions are present in vivo or whether they represent artifacts produced by desiccation and shrinkage during preparation for microscopy. Prominent ridgings of the surface of articular cartilage reported by earlier investigators are probably true cutting artifacts. Surface irregularity of some magnitude is essential for the full development of hypothesis of squeeze-film lubrication in which, during weight-bearing, interstitial fluid from cartilage matrix would be trapped in surface depressions (or between ridges) and prevent direct cartilage-cartilage contact. (From Ghadially, F. N., et al.: J. Anat. 121:119, 1976).

a random fashion up to several microns in depth. Early studies using scanning electron microscopy showed ridges and undulations in the cartilage surface.[47,48] Other investigators believe that these undulations are artifacts of cutting and fixation.[49,50] Instead, there is evidence[51-53] that there are shallow pits or round undulations in the surface contour (10 to 40 μm in diameter and 1 to 6 μm deep), which may represent underlying lacunae of chondrocytes (Fig. 16–8). It is not known whether these depressions exist in vivo, although those who study joint lubrication have often used the existence of undulations as evidence of crucial "trapped" reservoirs for squeeze-film lubrication.

Collagen fibril diameters in this and the other zones are listed in Table 16–1. In pericellular areas collagen fibril diameters are much less than in territorial and interterritorial areas. Type II collagen represents approximately 85 to 90 percent of the total tissue collagen in articular cartilage. Type V collagen also is found in cartilage, primarily in a pericellular location near chondrocytes.[54] Thus, the narrow diameter pericellular fibrils probably represent type V collagen.

Proteoglycan and link proteins are organized in territorial and pericellular regions of the deep zone in a manner similar to that of comparable regions in the superficial and middle zones.[44,45] Immunoelectron mi-

Table 16-1. Collagen Fibril Diameters*

Zone/Region	Diameter (nm)
	mean ± SD (n)
Superficial zone	
1. Pericellular	15.4 ± 8.3 (18)
2. Territorial	29.2 ± 5.4 (22)
Middle zone	
3. Pericellular	21.5 ± 12.7 (18)
4. Territorial	31.8 ± 5.0 (23)
Deep zone	
5. Pericellular	19.0 ± 4.4 (23)
6. Territorial	48.5 ± 7.0 (23)
7. Interterritorial	57.5 ± 7.6 (25)

*From Poole, A.R. et al.: J. Cell Biol. 93:921, 1982.

All measurements were made from one experiment (BC14). Student's t test analyses revealed that the following were significantly different from each other ($P < 0.001$): *1* and *2, 3* and *4, 5* and *6, 6* and *7, 4* and *6, 4* and *7.*

croscopic studies have revealed that the interterritorial regions of the deep zone differ markedly in organization from the territorial regions of the deep zone. The territorial regions revealed minimal evidence for link protein, whereas only the interterritorial regions of the deep zone revealed staining patterns consistent with structural organization of hyaluronate, link protein, proteoglycan core protein, and glycosaminoglycans as large aggregates.

These large aggregates and the large amount of H_2O bound to them form a massive polyanionic complex that has a large domain and the capacity to resist compressive force; compression shrinks the domain of each aggregate, increasing the electronegative repellent force. In addition, the charge effects cause a resistance to bound water flow. The effect, in biomechanical terms, is to make the cartilage elastic, so that after compression is released, the aggregated proteoglycans return to their fully extended state from forces generated by mutual repulsion of negatively charged groups.

It has been suggested that since the interterritorial regions have widely spaced, thick collagen fibrils and large amounts of link-stabilized proteoglycans, it is this area of cartilage that has the greatest compressibility.[44,45] The nature of the association of proteoglycans and hyaluronic acid with collagen is complex.[55] Certain fractions of proteoglycans may affect the formation of fibrils,[56] while others may inhibit calcification in articular cartilage.[57] Significantly, fractions of proteoglycans capable of inhibiting mineral crystal formation are absent from calcifying cartilage.[58]

Cartilage Glycoproteins. Glycoproteins are present in collagen in a concentration inverse to that of collagen.[59] Lysozyme and other cationic glycoproteins of low molecular weight are present in cartilage, probably synthesized by chondrocytes. Some of these cationic proteins have the capacity to inhibit proteolytic enzymes[60-62] and tumor neovascularization[63] and retard the development of osteoclasts.[64] These factors are of particular interest because avascular cartilage is generally resistant to invasion by tumors. The proteinase (trypsin) inhibi-

tors in cartilage appear to be identical to the well-known bovine pancreatic trypsin inhibitor described by Kunitz.[62] The collagenase inhibitor found in cartilage is a molecular species separate from the serine or thiol proteinase inhibitors.[65]

Cartilage Water and Small Solutes. Amidst collagen fibers is a heterogeneous collection of water and ground substance. Water content is about 70 to 75 percent of the wet weight,[66] and in many cases this rises to over 80 percent near the surface.

Micropuncture studies of articular cartilage have revealed an electrolyte concentration in this extracellular fluid similar to that in plasma except for a pH of 7.1 to 7.2.[67] Interestingly, at the growth area of articular cartilage around hypertrophic cells the pH is higher, a factor that may facilitate the mechanism of calcification near the tidemark.

As reviewed by Mankin[68] most of the water of articular cartilage is bound loosely within the matrix and exchanges readily with water in synovial fluid. The cartilage glycosaminoglycan do not appear to be essential for water binding; in osteoarthritis, when proteoglycans content is decreased, water content in cartilage can be increased by as much as 8 percent[69] due to loss of restraint of GAG and to collagen network defects.

It is of interest that movement of uncharged small solutes, such as glucose, is not impaired by diffusion through matrices containing large amounts of glycosaminoglycans, and Hadler has reviewed studies indicating that diffusivity of small molecules through hyaluronate is actually enhanced.[70] If applicable to articular cartilage in vivo, this phenomenon would facilitate nutrient exchange during compressive force on cartilage.

Chondrocytes. Chondrocytes exist in relative isolation, living singly or in pairs or with a few other cells in clusters. In addition, they are highly specialized and express the capacity to synthesize matrix components (e.g., collagen, proteoglycans, noncollagenous acidic glycoproteins, chondronectin, small cationic polypeptides, and other glycoproteins) as well as enzymes (e.g., collagenase, neutral proteinases, and cathepsins) capable of breaking down matrix components. Chondrocytes lie in a zone of finely textured matrix containing abundant ground substance but only a few collagen fibers.[71] Taking into consideration mean cell size and density, Stockwell and Meachim[72] have estimated that the volume of cartilage occupied by cells is between 0.4 and 2.0 percent of total cartilage volume. The "lacunae" seen around chondrocytes prepared for light microscopy are probably shrinkage artifacts.[73] Preparations of articular cartilage prepared for transmission electron microscopy show cells with rounded or oval nuclei that sometimes contain fibrous laminae (up to 95 nm thick, particularly in chondrocytes involved, apparently, in repair of tissue defects).[74] Rough endoplasmic reticulum and the Golgi complex are most developed in chondrocytes of zones II and III. Short cell processes are seen on all chondrocytes but are better developed in cells of deeper zones[75] and may play a role in transport of cellular enzymes to the extracellular space and/or in pinocytotic

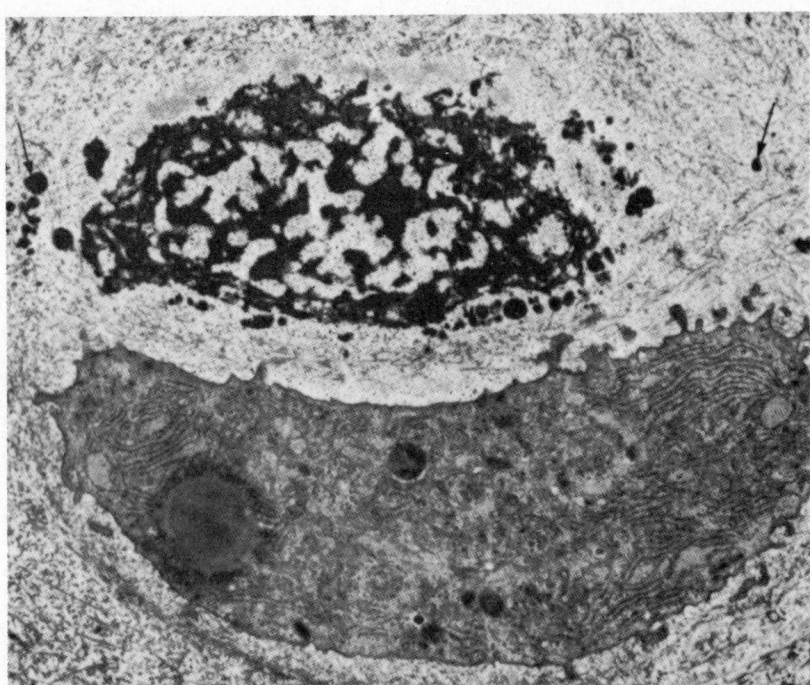

Figure 16–9. In situ necrosis and disintegration of one of two chondrocytes in articular cartilage. Such finds indicate that chondrocytes do replicate in normal cartilage, because despite the findings of dead or effete chondrocytes in cartilage sections it is recognized that the cell concentration in human articular cartilage does not change during aging. (From Ghadially, F. N.: In Sokoloff, L. [ed.]: The Joints and Synovial Fluid, Vol. 1, New York, Acadamic Press, 1978.)

function. Chondrocytes certainly have a phagocytic function and can be shown to take up red blood cell products in chronic hemarthrosis[76] (see Chapter 100). Cartilage cells die in situ from time to time. Necrotic remnants of cells are found adjacent to healthy cells(Fig. 16–9). Since data by Stockwell[77] have shown that the cell density of the full thickness of human adult femoral condylar cartilage is $14.5 \pm 3.0 \times 10^3$ cells per cubic millimeter from age 20 through 80 years, it follows that new chondrocytes arise by mitosis to replace dead ones. Despite this logical extrapolation of data, mitoses are not observed in normal adult articular cartilage.[78]

Since William Hunter's observations in 1743 that adult articular cartilage contains no blood vessels,[79] there has been debate about how chondrocytes receive nutrients, although numerous studies have confirmed an early study by Bywaters[80] that articular cartilage principally utilizes anaerobic glycolysis for energy production.

In the growing child, active enchondral ossification occurs at the base of articular cartilage just as it does at the growth plate (primary epiphysis). Here, in the hypertrophic zone of cartilage, blood vessels penetrate between columns of chondrocytes. The cartilage is calcified and subsequently is replaced by true bone. It is likely that diffusion from these tiny end capillaries through matrix to chondrocytes occurs. This mechanism is unlikely in the adult, although there is an argument over whether the "tidemark" (the dense calcified plate of articular cartilage) is or is not bridged by capillaries. Some studies[81,82] have described partial defects in the osteocartilaginous barrier. Collins[83] has suggested that the existence of this calcified barrier characterizes a "stable" contact, which, whether in a joint, rib, or inter-

vertebral disc, prevents passage of anything across the barrier.

In contrast, morphologic, physiologic, and pathologic studies have confirmed that solutes pass easily from the synovial fluid into cartilage and that cartilage does not survive without contact with synovial fluid in vivo. Strangeways provided early support for the concept of nutrition by diffusion by noting that loose bodies of cartilage in joints actually grow in size.[84] In experimental systems it has been shown that sufficient agitation of synovial fluid results in nourishment of even the deepest layers of articular cartilage.[85]

There are three potential mechanisms for nutrient transfer within cartilage matrix: diffusion, active transport by chondrocytes, and pumping by intermittent compression of cartilage matrix. Maroudas and coworkers[86] have demonstrated that molecules the size of hemoglobin (Mr 65,000) are the largest that can diffuse through normal articular cartilage. Fortunately, the molecular weight of solutes needed for cellular metabolism is small enough to permit adequately diffusion within the cartilage of mobilized, healthy joints.

Intermittent compression serving as a pump mechanism for solute exchange in cartilage is a concept that has arisen from observations that joint immobilization[87] or dislocation[88] or other events that interfere with normal movement of one articular surface upon its counterpart lead to degenerative changes in cartilage. Exercise, in contrast, increases solute penetration into cartilage in experimental systems.[85] Pressing filter paper against cartilage squeezes out liquid that has the ionic composition of extracellular fluid.[89] McCutchen[90] suggested that during weight bearing, fluid escapes from the load-bearing region by flow to other cartilage sites and into grooves in the slightly irregular cartilage surface. When the load was removed, cartilage would re-expand and draw back fluid. Nutrients could be exchanged with waste materials during such a process. Whether diffusion, even boosted by pressure, could occur fast enough for this weeping lubrication to facilitate solute exchange and penetration is hotly debated but is supported by studies showing free exchange of water between cartilage and synovial fluid and the enchanced diffusivity of solutes in a matrix of hyaluronate.

Characteristics of Chondrocytes in Vitro. The specialized nature of chondrocytes is emphasized when these cells are separated from their matrix environment and grown in cell culture. The expression of the chondrogenic phenotype in vitro has been shown to be susceptible to many environmental factors.

In general, chondrocytes placed in monolayer culture shift from synthesis of type II to type I collagen[91] and produce a different amount and type of glycosaminoglycans[92] than they do in vivo or in organ culture. If placed into suspension (spinner) cultures from monolayer cultures, rabbit chondrocytes begin to express once again the capability of synthesizing type II collagen[93] as well as cartilage-specific proteoglycans.[94] If cultured in soft agar in low density,[95] chondrocytes thrive and continue to express their capability to produce type II collagen and large amounts of glycosaminoglycans, which appear as a "lake" around the chondrocytes (Fig. 16–10). Addition to the agar cultures of growth factors (e.g., epidermal growth factor) results in a proliferation of chondrocytes, which aggregate as balls of cells, although the surrounding lake of glycosaminoglycans becomes much smaller when expressed as area per cell.[95] Thus, the growth and the extracellular matrix production of these cells in culture can be dissociated by the addition of exogenous agents.

Joint Lubrication. This complicated subject has been reviewed effectively for physicians by Wright and Dowson[96] and in more detail by McCutchen[97] and Swanson.[98]

Although there have been at least 12 distinct mechanisms put forth to explain part or all of joint lubrication, most fall into two basic categories: (1) *fluid-film lubrication,* in which cartilage surfaces are separated by a fluid film, and (2) *boundary lubrication,* in which surface-to-surface contact exists, with protection and a decreased coefficient of friction offered by special molecules attached to cartilage surfaces. Variants of these may evolve as follows: (a) squeeze film lubrication, in which, as discussed above, a film of fluid is trapped between opposing cartilage surfaces and, because the fluid film is noncompressible, prevents the surfaces from touching.[99] This is very similar, of course, to weeping lubrication;[100] (b) boosted lubrication,[101,102] in which pools of synovial fluid are compressed, as in weeping lubrication, but at high load the low molecular weight solute is driven back into cartilage or to non-weight-bearing fluid, leaving hyaluronate ("mucin") concentrates to bear weight; and (c) elastohydrodynamic lubrication,[103] in which the viscosity and shear rate (hence,

Figure 16–10. Chondrocytes in organ culture. This represents a 21 day culture pf rabbit articular condrocytes that had been dissociated into a single cell suspension and cultured in 0.25% agar and F-12 medium with 10 percent fetal calf serum as described by Benya and Straffer (Cell 30:215, 1982). Note the "islands" of chondrocytes surrounded by "lakes" of glycosaminoglycans (proteoglycans) that have been stained by alcian blue dye. × 100. (From Skantze, K. A. et al. in press.)

the coefficient of friction) is reduced because cartilage surfaces are deformable by a combination of tangential stretching and compression of the opposing surfaces.

In reality, several of these mechanisms and mixtures of them are involved in lubrication at both high and low loads and velocity imposed by daily activities. While walking, the load on weight-bearing joints (hip and knee) rises to three or four times body weight, yet is reduced to a fraction of body weight moments later. Thus, during the walking cycle,[96] three distinct modes may lubricate the knee: (1) As the heel hits the walking surface, impact is high and load maximal. Squeeze-film lubrication could protect the surfaces from direct contact and attenutate the force of impact. (2) As the point of contact shifts from heel to toe, a combination of many mechanisms may apply. Cartilage may be deformed by sheer forces which minimize surface-surface motion (elastohydrodynamic lubrication). Boundary lubrication is always available if cartilage surfaces approximate each other sufficiently, although the evidence suggests that boundary mechanisms fail during high load (see below). (3) After toe-off, the knee is in a minimal load situation, and the simplest of hydrodynamic lubrication mechanisms may be useful.

In Figure 16–11 a mechanism is portrayed for both enhanced perfusion and lubrication of cartilage-cartilage surfaces during weight bearing; this is "squeeze-film" lubrication.

Hyaluronate, the extremely large and viscous molecule found in abundance in synovial fluid, is probably not involved in cartilage-cartilage lubrication. Hyalu-

Figure 16–11. A scheme of a possible mechanism for both cartilage lubrication and provision of nutrition to chondrocytes. Two opposing articular surfaces are shown at rest and during weight bearing. The lines indicate collagen fibrils within cartilage. The circles represent solute, the interstitial fluid. Proteoglycans are not included for sake of clarity. During weight bearing the cartilage is compressed. Fluid is driven out of the cartilage into the intercondylar space. When weight bearing is released, solute (presumably having exchanged cellular metabolites for nutrients) is resorbed as cartilage re-expands.[90]

ronidase treatment did not inhibit lubrication capability of synovial fluid at low load, while trypsin (with the capability of digesting glycoproteins) in synovial fluid did eliminate lubricating ability.[104] The compound responsible for cartilage-cartilage lubrication has been purified. It is glycoprotein of molecular weight of 225,000 daltons and has been named *lubricin*. This molecule, synthesized by synovial cells, is 200 nm in length and 1 to 2 nm in diameter. The exact structure-function relationships of this molecule remain unknown,[105] but it appears to be the primary boundary lubricant in mammalian joints. Another boundary lubricant may be fat. Lipid is reported to comprise 1 to 2 percent of dry weight of cartilage,[106] and experimental treatment of cartilage surfaces with fat solvents has impaired lubrication qualities of the tissue.[107]

It is also important to realize that articular surfaces are protected by other mechanisms not involving lubrication. During impact loading, muscles and bone absorb the great majority of force and energy, leaving only a small amount to be absorbed by cartilage itself.[108] Finely tuned neuromuscular reflexes are essential for this system to work effectively. It is possible that small failures in these reflex arcs may lead to insufficient attenuation of impact loading resulting in degenerative changes in joints and subchondral bone (i.e., Charcot's arthropathy).

Mechanical Properties of Cartilage During Load. The most important function of cartilage—its ability to be

compressed by a load and recover from this deformity—has been an object of research since Bar's studies in 1926[109] (Fig. 16–12). When a load is applied to cartilage, there is a rapid ("instantaneous") indentation, followed by a time-dependent creep phase during which indentation increases while load remains constant. On removal of the load there is an initial immediate recovery, followed by a long, sustained recovery to normal volume. The initial rapid deformation results from a bulk movement of water and compression of collagen fibers. In the second, time-dependent compression (called "creep"), water flows through the matrix.

From studies of the bone-bone contact in the absence of cartilage, it has become apparent that a function of cartilage, in addition to providing low-friction movement at high speeds, may be to absorb some of the energy of impact loading by deforming and effectively spreading a load over a broad area. Freeman and Kempson[110] have put forth the argument that in normal cartilage both collagen and proteoglycans contribute to load carriage. Tensile strength of the collagen resists deformation and maintains the basic structural framework to allow proteoglycans to remain in place. The proteoglycans, through strong charge interactions with water, control solute flow and therefore the absolute and time-dependent deformation by weight bearing.

Studies of matrix-depleted cartilage have helped clarify the relative roles of collagen and proteoglycans in the function of cartilage. Using canine articular cartilage slices, it was demonstrated that cartilage incubated with collagenase became filmy, flimsy, and transparent (Fig. 16–13); it was devoid of tensile strength.[111] Similar slices incubated with trypsin sufficient to deplete matrix proteoglycans did not change in gross appearance; however, the physical qualities changed. Control slices were relatively rigid, while trypsin-treated slices were easily bent

Figure 16–12. A typical curve of deformation of articular cartilage by a load as a function of time. The four phases expressed as a function of time are as follows: 1 = instantaneous deformation coincident with application of the load; 2 = slow deformation which gradually slows in rate of deformation; 3 = instantaneous recovery; 4 = time-dependent recovery to normal cartilage thickness. (After Bär[83] and Kempson.[88])

Figure 16–13. Effect of collagenase and trypsin on canine patellar cartilage slices. Each piece was incubated separately; buffer was 0.1 M Tris-HCl, 0.005 M in CaCl₂, pH 7.6 *a*, Buffer only; *b*, trypsin, 15 μg in buffer; *c*, trypsin, 10 μg in buffer; *d*, synovial coll agenase (partially purified) in buffer. Approximately 35 percent of the collagen was removed from the collagenase-treated sample, < 5 percent from the trypsin-treated samples, and none from the control sample. (From Harris, E.D., Jr., et al.: Excerpta Medica International Congress Series No. 229 , Immunopathology of Inflammation, 1970.)

in half. More detailed studies to measure deformation revealed that proteoglycan-depleted cartilage had lost its ability to rebound from a deforming load; it had lost compressive stiffness.[112,113] In similar experiments, using cathepsin D, British investigators[114] freed 50 percent of tissue uronic acid without releasing any hydroxyproline (a collagen marker). This produced a 50 percent reduction in compressive stiffness.

Repair of Cartilage. Healing of cartilage defects that do not penetrate the subchondral bone plate is dependent entirely on surviving chondrocytes near the margins of injury. In man, essentially no repair is generated by these cells.[115] Occasionally, the chondrocytes proliferate to form clones in "brood capsules," but the clefts in cartilage do not heal. Defects will remain without progression so long as the subchondral bony plate remains intact.

In deeper injury through the subchondral plate there is extensive fibroblastic proliferation in the defect, but seldom is true hyaline cartilage produced. More often a fibrocartilaginous scar results from this extrinsic repair effort.[115,116] Thus, repair of articular cartilage is not programmed well in human biologic systems; the emphasis is on protection from damage. In the early stages of osteoarthritis, however, there is considerable increase in new matrix synthesis, which may retard progression of destructive disease (see Chapter 88).

Aging of Articular Cartilage. The thickness of articular cartilage in mammalian limbs has been found to be related to body weight, to hip-to-shoulder length, and to the area of the tibial plateau.[117] Cartilage thickness is asymmetrical over the surface of weight-bearing joints.[118] On the surface of the human femoral head, cartilage is thickest on the anterosuperior surface of the femoral head and increases with age. The increased thickness has not been related to fibrillation of the cartilage[119] and cannot be interpreted as a change associated with early osteoarthrosis.

The overall cellularity of cartilage does not change with age nor does the fluid content or total amounts of collagen and glycosaminoglycan.[120] Changes in color appear; adult cartilage develops a yellow tinge, but there is no evidence that this pigment has any functional significance. As mentioned above, cartilage collagen fibers in aged articular cartilage are thicker than those in cartilage of younger people.

In contrast to the lack of change in normal cartilage with age, it must be recognized that cartilage fibrillation is an age-related process.[121] Fibrillation, however, cannot be considered as necessarily leading to osteoarthritis, and may best be considered a "regressive change." It often occurs first at the periphery of joint surfaces.[119,122] Fibrillation is initially confined to the superficial layers of cartilage. The cartilage shows foci of mild splitting and fraying. Surface "pits" develop, and grossly the surface develops a "matte" appearance instead of a "gloss" appearance. It has been suggested that clefts develop at the base of small splits in the surface.

Chemical analysis of fibrillated areas of cartilage has shown a depletion of glycosaminoglycans with normal collagen concentration.[123,124] Comparative stiffness of the cartilage is decreased. If fibrillation progresses into deeper layers of cartilage, an abnormal multicellular cluster of chondrocytes that stain intensely for glycosaminoglycans is found at the base of clefts.[125] The fibrillated areas by this time are noticeably softer or malacic. Freeman and Meachim[120] have presented a reasonable argument for the hypothesis that fibrillation begins with fatigue fracture of superficial collagen bundles. This results in superficial clefts, which deepen if the process continues. See Chapter 88 for a detailed discussion of the A's in osteoarthritis.

SYNOVIUM

The synovial membrane covers all intra-articular structures except for articular cartilage and the central portions of fibrocartilaginous menisci,[83] and for localized "bare areas" where bone is exposed. As mentioned in the discussion of embryologic development of joints, the synovium has at least two unusual features. (1) It develops from the blastema from which the skeleton evolves and not from the general mesenchyme. (2) Although it lines a closed space in the body, there is no epithelial tissue in the synovium and therefore no basement membrane or structural barrier between synovial fluid and synovial blood vessels.

Organization of the Synovium. The absence of a basement membrane assures a continuation of morphology as well as of function. Although the outer layers of the joint capsule are relatively acellular and formed of thick interwining bands of collagen fibers that do not resemble the highly cellular synovial lining, the change from one to the other is not abrupt. The cells below the lining layers resemble lining cells, but there is more connective tissue. Continuing centrifugally, the cells appear more as fibroblasts. Fat cells increase in number, larger blood

Figure 16–14. *A*, Type A human synovial cell with many undulations in the cell membrane, vacuoles, and inclusions. This cell presumably has phagocytic capabilities and is thought of as a macrophage × 11,200. (Courtesy of Donald Gates.) *B*, Type B human synovial cell with a very well-developed endoplasmic reticulum. This cell presumably has capabilities for snythesis of protein × 17,500. (Courtesy of Donald Gates.) It must be emphasized that there are many synovial cells with organelles developed for both synthetic and phagocytic function. In addition, it is possible that individuals cells may be modulated from cel ls with synthetic to ones with phagocytic function.

Synovial Lining Cells. Barland and colleagues defined two principal types of synovial lining cells[127] (Fig.16–14), and their existence has been confirmed by others.[128] *Type A cells* (macrophage-like) contain a prominent Golgi complex and many microvesicles, various and heterogeneous inclusions (residual bodies), and lysosomes. The nucleus contains dense chromatin. Microfilaments are abundant, lying in the long axis of the cell. Frequent thin cell processes stretching into the adjacent matrix are seen. *Type B cells* (fibroblast-like) have a prominent, rough endoplasmic reticulum with few cell processes and vacuoles. Nuclear chromatin is less dense, and nucleoli are more developed. Cytoplasmic vacuoles and vesicles are rare.

It has been natural to ascribe phagocytic and, therefore, macrophage-like function to type A cells and synthetic or fibroblast-like function to type B cells.[129,130] This, however, may be a naive assumption. It ignores the facts that one cell may have more than one function and that, in response to different stimuli, cells can modulate their internal structure as their function changes. A number of observations support this. (1) Type C cells or intermediate synovial cells have been described which have endoplasmic reticulum and Golgi complexes and vacuoles.[130] (2) Using stains for RNA on ribosomes (an acceptable index of synthetic function in cells), only a few cells stain positively in normal synovium. Staining increases in intensity and appears in increased numbers of cells if a joint has been traumatized;[131] in severe inflammatory states no cells without a developed endoplasmic reticulum are observed. Synovial cells that appear morphologically to be fibroblasts nevertheless demonstrate macrophage-like function in response to certain stimuli. Rabbit synovial "fibroblasts," for example, actively phagocytose latex particles[132] (Fig. 16–15). Gold salts injected into the synovial cavity are rapidly taken up in pinocytotic vesicles,[133] and iron pigment is readily engulfed after intra-articular hemorrhage in hemophilia[134] (also see Chapter 100). Evidence is mounting that type A cells may synthesize and secrete

vessels are seen, and dense bands of collagen appear. The ligaments that span joints and confer stability on them are continuous with the outer layers of capsule in many joints. With this concept of a structural continuum established, however, it is convenient to divide the lining into (1) the intima or synovial lining, (2) subsynovial tissue, and (3) the joint capsule.

The synovial lining layer is discontinuous. In some areas where the synovium is subjected to pressure and over ligaments and tendons, the cells are widely separated; at these loci, the extracellular connective tissue, not synovial cells, constitutes the lining layer.[126] Intra-articular fat pads are usually covered by a single layer of synovial cells. In other areas not subject to trauma, the synovial cells often accumulate in layers three to four cells deep (Fig. 16–14). Viewed under a tangential light source, a faint pebbling can be seen, which represents microvilli.

Figure 16–15. Rabbit synovial fibroblasts in cell culture have the capacity to phagocytose latex particles (these are 0.05 to 0.15 μm in diameter). The patchy uptake is apparent in this photograph (×400); some cells have phagocytosed particles, while other have not. Yet, all appeared the same on microscopic examination prior to being exposed to latex. These cell populations, having been exposed to latex, or other inert but phagocytosable substance, produce and release large amounts of collagenase.[105]

hyaluronic acid. The firmest data are the demonstrations by ultrastructural studies that hyaluronic acid is found both in the Golgi complex and in large secretory vacuoles of these "phagocytic cells."[135]

It may be reasonable to consider the synovial lining cell as one with multiple phenotypic possibilities and to resist categorizing it by its morphologic resemblance at certain stages to other, better characterized cells. As noted by Ghadially, "[Type A and B may be cells] whose difference in morphology reflects the function they are performing at a given moment."[136]

Fibronectin[137] and probably laminin[138] are secreted by synovial cells. These glycoproteins may aid in attachment of cells to underlying matrix.[138-141] In cell culture, synovial cells synthesize collagen (types I and III), latent collagenase, latent proteinases, an activator of collagenase, inhibitors of neutral metalloproteinases, hyaluronic acid, proteoglycans, and many other minor and non-identified matrix constituents. Normal synovium in culture can be induced to produce a substance named "catabolin," which appears to stimulate chondrocytes to release enzymes that degrade the proteoglycans matrix in cartilage.[142,143] A similar messenger molecule(s) is found in human rheumatoid synovium.

Synovial Fluid. Fluid in normal joints is present in small quantities sufficient to coat multiple folds of synovial membrane. Small pools collect in recesses in the joint, but in the normal state there is never sufficient volume to distend the joint or to separate redundant surfaces of synovium one from the other.

As in other systems, more is known about abnormal synovial fluid than normal because there is an excess of the former. Truly normal synovial fluid is rarely analyzed. The largest accumulation of data was by Ropes and Bauer,[144] and their treatise is still a valuable reference. Synovial fluid is a filtrate of plasma that passes through the fenestrations of subsynovial capillary endothelium into the extracellular space, where it joins with hyaluronic acid that is secreted by synovial cells and achieves an equilibrium with free fluid in the joint space. Rates of transfer from capillaries to the interstitial fluid and of diffusion through this tissue are affected by many factors. Each component of synovial fluid must be considered separately. (The procedure for aspiration and analysis of synovial fluid is outlined in Chapters 37 and 38.)

Components of Synovial Fluid Originating in Plasma. Small Molecules. Most of small molecules pass through synovial interstitium by a process of free diffusion.[145] The concentration of electrolytes is the same as in plasma. Cations that bind significantly to protein are present in concentrations consistent with the lower concentrations of serum proteins present in synovial fluid (see below). The concentration of glucose in synovial fluid is close to that of plasma.[146] However, in the non-steady state glucose enters the joint space at a rate faster than expected from its molecular size,[145] indicating facilitated diffusion or active transport of this molecule into (but not out of) joints. It seems likely, therefore, that to explain low levels of glucose in sepsis or severe

inflammation one must invoke both impaired delivery and increased utilization by synovial components.

Large Molecules. Proteins are present in synovial fluid in concentration inversely proportional to molecular size.[147] The cause of this selective retardation of large molecule flux into synovial fluid is due in part to regulation by the extracellular matrix of synovium; when plasma is filtered through hyaluronic acid, an ultrafiltrate is produced with a composition similar to that found in normal synovial fluid.[148] Hyaluronic acid in interstitial tissues probably acts as a molecular filter; by its large domain it excludes large solute molecules from passing through into synovial fluid. Because of their large size, molecules such as α_2-macroglobulin (the principle proteinase inhibitor of plasma), fibrinogen, and IgM are present in only small quantities in noninflammatory synovial fluid. In inflammatory synovial fluids this selective exclusion is altered,[147] perhaps because of increased size of endothelial cell fenestrations or because interstitial hyaluronate-protein complexes are fragmented by enzymes associated with the inflammatory process. Thus, larger proteins enter synovial fluid, enabling it to form fibrin clots and to have higher concentrations of proteinase inhibitors. Details of the structure of hyaluronic acid are found in Chapter 15.

Removal of Material from Synovial Fluid. The synovial lining cells phagocytize debris presented at the fluid-cell interface. In addition, the lymphatic system can enhance removal of synovial fluid macromolecules. All large molecules appear to leave the joint at equivalent rates, unlike the rate (inversely proportional to molecular weight) at which they enter the joint space.[149] There is indirect evidence to suggest that this clearing mechanism is inadequate to the task presented in severe inflammation of joints. For instance, the synovial fluid appears to act as a "sink" for complement components in rheumatoid arthritis.[150] In severe inflammation, proteinases released by leukocytes drawn by chemotactic factors accumulate within the joint fluid and soon saturate the inhibitors present there.[151,152]

Other Aspects of Synovial Physiology. Intra-Articular Temperature. The vascular system of the extremities acts as a countercurrent distribution system for temperature of tissues. Although core body temperature in most human beings varies little from the mean of 37° C, it is likely that temperatures reflect more the temperature of overlying soft tissues. For example, the metacarpophalangeal joint, one with very little overlying insulation of fat or muscle, has intra-articular temperatures that parallel those of skin closely between the resting temperatures and 39 to 40° C created by insertion of the hand into an electric mitten[153] (Fig. 16–16). The knee joint temperature is not so simple a function. Although intra-articular temperatures are always below 36° C (at ambient temperatures of around 20° C), there are wide variations noted between joint and skin temperature.[154] In addition, cold or hot packs reflexly change knee joint temperatures in the opposite direction.[155] Similarly, painful stimuli (e.g., apprehension, alarm, or smoking) lower the skin temperature and elevate the joint temperature.

Figure 16-16. A sterile needle temperature probe was inserted into the left second metacarpophalangeal joint of a physician (E. D. Harris, Jr.) without joint disease. Skin and intra-articular temperatures were monitored by a Thermalert (Bailey Instruments, Saddle Brook, N.J.). An electric mitten was put on at the time indicated and removed 30 minutes later. □-□ Body core temperature: •——• = intra-articular temperature; •——• = skin temperature over the same joint. (See ref. 157.)

Non-weight-bearing active movements increase intra-articular temperature as much as 1° C, a phenomenon probably best explained by an increased subsynovial tissue blood flow.

The reason for interest in these data is that rates of enzyme action are a direct function of temperature. Connective tissue metabolism is generally studied in vitro at 37° C, yet tissues in joints do not reach this temperature except during inflamed states. Biochemical reactions that proceed vigorously at 37° C may at 32° be altered sufficiently so that the net effect would be movement of a metabolic pathway in the opposite direction, or retardation of rates of reaction. For instance, the rate of destruction of articular cartilage collagen fibers by synovial collagenase is significant at 37° C; at 32° it is imperceptible.[156] In addition, large increases in the rate of hyaluronic acid synthesis occur over an 8° C temperature change (30 to 38° C) in both normal and rheumatoid cell lines in culture, whereas glucose utilization and lactate production increase only slightly.[157]

Intra-articular Pressure. The joint cavity is a potential space. The small amount of synovial fluid present lines synovial surfaces but does not separate them. Indeed, the pressure within normal joints may be a negative one compared with ambient atmospheric pressure.[158] Negative pressure must be very large within finger joints during the "knuckle-cracking" process, which is a nervous (and/or aggravating) habit of some persons. During this procedure of pulling rapidly on a relaxed phalanx, a gas bubble is created within the joint, which cavitates with a cracking sound, liberating energy in the form of heat and sound.[159] This cavitation is the same process that destroys propellers of steamships; presumably, if repeated frequently enough, it could destroy a joint. The normal negative pressure in the joint plays a role in stabilizing articular surfaces against one another.

The presence of a synovial effusion changes all this. Intra-articular pressure becomes positive, and roentgenograms may show a widening of the apparent joint space as the articulating surfaces are forced apart. Pressure within a joint is perceived by humans as an uncomfortable sensation; a patient with a knee effusion rests it in a position of slight flexion, the position at which pressure is minimal[160] (see Chapter 29). Full flexion or extension increases pressures within joints containing effusions and may be sufficient to rupture a joint capsule.[161] High intra-articular pressure may compromise synovial blood flow. Inflamed, chronic proliferative synovitis generates a thickened joint capsule, which gradually, perhaps secondary to increased joint pressure, becomes redundant and stretched and demonstrates decreased compliance.[162] Pressure in these joints may be minimal until a critical volume at which the noncompliant capsule stretches no more and intra-articular pressure soars to produce rupture or even penetration through weakened bone to form subchondral cysts.[163,164] It is likely that increased intra-articular pressure in the presence of effusions affects synovial blood flow.[165]

References

1. O'Rahilly, R., and Gardner, E.: The embryology of movable joints. *In* Sokoloff, L. (ed.): The Joints and Synovial Fluid. Vol I. New York, Academic Press, 1978, pp. 49–97.
2. Saunders, J.W.: Developmental control of three-dimensional polarity in the avian limb. Ann. N.Y. Acad. Sci. 193:29, 1972.
3. Stocum, D.L.: Outgrowth and pattern formation during limb ontogeny and regeneration. Differentiation 3:167, 1975.
4. O'Rahilly, R.: The development of joints. Irish J. Med. Sci. 6:456, 1957.
5. Thorogood, P.V., and Hinchcliffe, J.R.: An analysis of the condensation process during chondrogenesis in the embryonic chick hind limb. J. Embryol. Exp. Morphol. 33:581, 1975.
6. Friberg, V., and Ringertz, N.R.: An autoradiographic study on the uptake of radiosulfate in the rat embryo. J. Embryol. Exp. Morphol. 4:313, 1956.
7. Anderson, H., and Bro-Rasmussen, F.: Histochemical studies on the

histogenesis of the joints in human fetuses with special reference to the development of the joint cavities in the hand and foot. Am. J. Anat. 108:111, 1961.

8. Warsilev, W.: Elektronenmikroskopische und histochemische Untersuchungen zur Entwicklung des Kniegelenkes der Ratte. Z. Anat. Entwicklungsgesh. 137:221, 1972.
9. Anderson, H.: Development morphology and histochemistry of the early synovial tissue in human foetuses. Acta Anat. 58:90, 1964.
10. Bloom, W., and Fawcett, D.W.: A Textbook of Histology. 8th ed. Philadelphia, W.B. Saunders Company, 1972.
11. Drachman, D.B., and Sokoloff, L.: The role of movement in embryonic joint development. Dev. Biol. 14:401, 1966.
12. Murray, P.D.F., and Drachman, D.B.: The role of movement in the development of joints and related structures: The head and neck in the chick embryo. J. Embryol. Exp. Morphol. 22:349, 1969.
13. Yasuda, Y.: Differentiation of human limb buds in vitro. Anat. Rec. 175:561, 1973.
14. Rajan, K.T., and Merker, H.J.: Joint formation in culture. Ann. Rheum. Dis. 34:200, 1975.
15. Symons, N.B.B.: The development of the human mandibular joint. J. Anat. 86:326, 1952.
16. Moffett, B.C.: The prenatal development of the human temporomandibular joint. Contrib. Embryol. Carnegie Inst. 36:19, 1957.
17. Levy, B.M.: Embryological development of the temporomandibular joint. In Sarnat, B.G. (ed.): The Temporomandibular Joint. 2nd ed. Springfield, Ill., Charles C Thomas, 1964, pp. 59–70.
18. Bradley, S.J.: An analysis of self-differentiation of chick limb buds in chorio-allantoic grafts. J. Anat. 107:479, 1970.
19. Bauer, R.: Zur Problem der Neugliederung der Wurbelsaule. Acta Anat. 72:321, 1969.
20. Peacock, A.: Observations on the pre-natal development of the intervertebral disc in man. J. Anat. 85:260, 1951.
21. Walmsley, R.: The development and growth of the intervertebral disc. Endinburgh Med. J. 60:341, 1953.
22. Eyre, D.R., and Muri, H.: Collagen polymorphism: Two molecular species in pig intervertebral discs. FEBS Lett. 42:192, 1974.
23. Linsenmeyer, T.F., Trelstad, R.L., and Gross, J.: The collagen of chick embryonic notochord. Biochem. Biophys. Res. Commun. 53:39, 1973.
24. Herbert, C.M., Lindberg, K.A., Jayson, M.I.V., and Bailey, A.J.: Changes in the collagen of human intervertebral discs during aging and degenerative joint disease. J. Mol. Med. 1:79, 1975.
25. Jayson, M.I.V.: Inter-articular pressure. Clin. Rheum. Dis. 7:149, 1981.
26. Bird, H.A., Tribe, C.R., and Bacon, P.A.: Joint hypermobility leading to osteoarthritis and chondrocalcinosis. Ann. Rheum. Dis. 37:203, 1978.
27. Canoso, J.J.: Bursae, tendons and ligaments. Clin. Rheum. Dis. 7:189, 1981.
28. Kieny, M. and Chevallier, A.: Autonomy of tendon development in the embryonic duck wing. J. Embryol. Exp. Morphol. 49:153, 1979.
29. Gay, S., and Miller, E.J.: Collagen in the Physiology and Pathology of Connective Tissue. Stuttgart and New York, Gustav Fisher, 1978.
30. Cooper, R.R., and Misol, S.: Tendon and ligament insertion. A light and electron microscopic study. J. Bone Joint Surg. 52A:1, 1970.
31. Dorfl, J.: Vessels in the region of tendinous insertions. Chondroapophyseal insertion. Folia Morphol. 17:74, 1969.
32. Swann, D.A.: Macromolecules of synovial fluid. In Sokoloff, L. (ed): The Joints and Synovial Fluid. New York, Academic Press, 1978, pp. 407–435.
33. Glimcher, M.J., Brickley-Parsons, D., and Kossiva, D.: Phosphopeptides and γ-carboxyglutamic acid-containing peptides in calcified turkey tendon: Their absence in uncalcified tendon. Calcif. Tissue Int. 27:281, 1979.
34. Kuhns, J.G.: Adventitious bursa. Arch. Surg. 46:687, 1943.
35. Canoso, J.J., and Yood, R.A.: Reaction of superficial bursae to specific disease stimuli. Arthritis Rheum. 22:1361, 1979.
36. Liew, M., and Dick, C.: The anatomy and physiology of blood flow in a diarthrodial joint. Clin. Rheum. Dis. 7:131, 1981.
37. Lindstrom, J.: Microvascular anatomy of synovial tissue. Acta Rheum. Scand. (Suppl.) 7:1, 963.
38. Suter, J., and Majno, G.: Ultrastructure of the joint capsule in the rat: Presence of two kinds of capillaries. Nature 202:920, 1964.
39. Schumacher, H.R.: The microvasculature of the synovial membrane of the monkey: Ultrastructural studies. Arthritis Rheum. 112:387, 1969.
40. Dee, R.: Structure and function of hip joint innervation. Ann. R. Coll. Surg. Engl. 45:357, 1969.
41. Griff, P., Finerman, G.A., and Riley, L.H.R.: Joint position sense after total hip replacement. J. Bone Joint Surg. 55A:1016, 1973.
42. Cross, M.J., and McCloskey, D.I.: Position sense following surgical removal of joints in man. Brain Res. 55:443, 1973.
43. Pugh, J.W., Radin, E.L., and Rose, R.M.: Quantitative studies of human subchondral cancellous bone. J. Bone Joint Surg. 56A:313, 1974.
44. Poole, A.R., Pidoux, I., Reiner, A., Tang, L.-H., Choi, H., and Rosenberg, L.: Localization of proteoglycan monomer and link protein in the

matrix of bovine articular cartilage: An immunohistochemical study. J. Histochem. Cytochem. 28:621, 1980.
45. Poole, A.R., Pidoux, I., Reiner, A., and Rosenberg, L.: An immuno-electron microscope study of the organization of proteoglycan monomer, link protein, and collagen in the matrix of articular cartilage. J. Cell. Biol. 93:921, 1982.
46. Balacz, E.A., Bloom, G.D., and Swann, D.A.: Fine structure and glycosaminoglycan content of the surface layer of articular cartilage. Fed. Proc. 25:1813, 966.
47. Redler, I., and Zimmy, M.L.: Scanning electron microscopy and abnormal articular cartilage and synovium. J. Bone Joint Surg. 52A:1395, 1970.
48. Gardner, D.L.: The influence of microscopic technology on knowledge of cartilage surface structure. Ann. Rheum. Dis. 31:235, 1972.
49. Clarke, I.C.: Human articular surface contours and related surface depression frequency studies. Ann. Rheum. Dis. 30:15, 1971.
50. Clarke, I.C.: Surface characteristics of human articular cartilage—a scanning electron microscope study. J. Anat. 108:23, 1971.
51. Gardner, D.L., and McGilliwray, D.C.: Living articular cartilage is not smooth. Ann. Rheum. Dis. 30:3, 1971.
52. Clarke, I.C.: Human articular surface contours and related surface depression frequency studies. Ann. Rheum. Dis. 30:15, 1971.
53. Ghadially, F.N., Ghadially, J.A., Oryschak, A.F., and Yong, N.K.: Experimental production of ridges on rabbit articular cartilage: A scanning electron microscopic study. J. Anat. 121:119, 1976.
54. Burgeson, R.E., Hebda, P.A., Morris, N.P., and Hollister, D.W.: Human cartilage collagens. Comparison of cartilage collagens with human type V collagen. J. Biol. Chem. 257:7852, 1982.
55. Hardingham, T.E., and Muir, H.: The specific interaction of hyaluronic acid with cartilage proteoglycans. Biochim. Biophys. Acta 279:401, 1972.
56. Poole, B.P., and Lowther, D.A.: The effect of chondroitin sulfate protein on the formation of collagen fibrils in vitro. Biochim. J. 109:857, 1968.
57. DiSalvo, J., and Schubert, M.: Specific interaction of some cartilage protein polysaccharides with freshly precipitating calcium phosphate. J. Biol. Chem. 242:705, 1967.
58. Howell, D.S., Pita, J.C., Marquez, J.F., and Galtes, R.A.: Demonstration of macromolecular inhibitors of calcification and nucleation factor(s) in fluid from calcifying sites in cartilage. J. Clin. Invest. 48:630, 1969.
59. Muir, H., Bullough, P., and Maroudas, A.: The distribution of collagen in human articular cartilage with some of its physiological implications. J. Bone Joint Surg. 52B:554, 1970.
60. Kuettner, K.F., Hiti, J., Eisenstein, R., and Harper, E.: Collagenase inhibition by cationic proteins derived from cartilage and aorta. Biochem. Biophys. Res. Commun. 72:40, 1976.
61. Keuttner, K.E., Soble, L., Croxen, R.L., Marczynska, B., Hiti, J., and Harper, E.: Tumor cell collagenase and its inhibitions by a cartilage-derived protease inhibitor. Science 196:653, 1977.
62. Rifkin, D.B., and Crowe, R.M.: Isolation of a protease inhibitor from tissues resistant to tumor invasion. Hoppe Seyler's Z. Physiol. Chem. 358:1525, 1977.
63. Langer, R., Brem, H., Flaterman, K., Klein, M., and Folkman, J.: Isolation of a cartilage factor that inhibits tumor neovascularization. Science 193:70, 1976.
64. Horton, J.E., Wezeman, F.H., and Kuettner, K.E.: Inhibition of bone resorption in vitro by a cartilage-derived anticollagenase factor. Science 199:1342, 1978.
65. Roughley, P.J., Murphy, G., and Barrett, A.J.: Proteinase inhibitors of bovine nasal cartilage. Biochem. J. 169:721, 1978.
66. Linn, F.C., and Sokoloff, L.: Movement and composition of interstitial fluid of cartilage. Arthritis Rheum. 8:481, 1965.
67. Pita, J.C., and Howell, D.S.: Micro-biochemical studies of cartilage. In Sokoloff, L. (ed.): The Joints and Synovial Fluid. Vol. 1. New York, Academic Press, 1978, pp. 273–330.
68. Mankin, H.J.: The water of articular cartilage. In Simon, W.H. (ed.): The Human Joint in Health and Disease. Philadelphia, University of Pennsylvania Press, 1978, pp. 37–42.
69. Bollet, A.J., and Nance, J.L.: Biochemical findings in normal and osteoarthritic articular cartilage. II. Chondroitin sulfate concentration and chain length, water and ash content. J. Clin. Invest. 45:1170, 1966.
70. Hadler, N.M.: The biology of the extracellular space. Clin. Rheum. Dis. 7:71, 1981.
71. Ghadially, F.N.: Fine structure of joints. In Sokoloff, L. (ed.): The Joints and Synovial Fluid. Vol. I. New York, Academic Press, 1978, pp. 105–176.
72. Stockwell, R.A., and Meachim, G.: The chondrocytes. In Freeman, M.A.R. (ed.): Adult Articular Cartilage. London, Pitman Medical, 1979, pp. 69–145.
73. Davies, D.V., Barnett, C.H., Cochrane, W., and Palfrey, A.J.: Electron microscopy of articular cartilage in the young adult rabbit. Ann. Rheum. Dis. 21:11, 1962.
74. Ghadially, F.N.: Waxing and waning of nuclear fibrous lamina. Arch. Pathol. 94:303, 1972.
75. Ghadially, F.N., Meachim, G., and Collins, D.H.: Extracellular lipid in

the matrix of human articular cartilage. Ann. Rheum. Dis. 24:136, 1965.

76. Ghadially, F.N., Oryshak, A.F., Ailsby, R.L., and Mehta, P.N.: Electron-probe X-ray analysis of siderosomes in haemarthrotic articular cartilage. Virchows Arch. B. 16:43, 1974.

77. Stockwell, R.A.: The cell density of human articular and costal cartilage. J. Anat. 101:753, 1967.

78. Stockwell, R.A., and Meachim, G.: The chondrocytes. In Freeman, M.A.R. (ed.): Adult Articular Cartilage. New York, Grune & Stratton, 1974, pp. 51–99.

79. Hunter, W.: On the structure and diseases of articulating cartilage. Philos. Trans. 42:514, 1743.

80. Bywaters, E.G.L.: The metabolism of joint tissues. J. Pathol. Bact. 44:247, 1937.

81. Woods, G.C., Greenwald, A.J., and Haynes, D.W.: Subchondral vascularity in the human femoral head. Ann. Rheum. Dis. 29:138, 1970.

82. Mitul, M.A., and Millington, P.F.: Osseous pathway of nutrition to articular cartilage of the human femoral head. Lancet 1:842, 1970.

83. Collins, D.H.: The Pathology of Articular and Spinal Diseases. London, Arnold, 1949.

84. Strangeways, T.S.P.: The nutrition of articular cartilage. Br. Med. J. 1:661, 1920.

85. Maroudas, A., Bullough, P., Swanson, S.A.V., and Freeman, M.A.R.: The permeability of articular cartilage. J. Bone Joint Surg. 50B:166, 1968.

86. Maroudas, A.: Physico-chemical properties of articular cartilage. In Freeman, M.A.R. (ed.): Adult Articular Cartilage. New York, Grune & Stratton, 1974, pp. 131–170.

87. Sood, S.C.: A study of the effects of experimental immobilization on rabbit articular cartilage. J. Anat. 108:497, 1971.

88. Bennett, G., and Baner, W.: Joint changes resulting from patellar displacement and their relation to degenerative hip disease. J. Bone Joint Surg. 19A:667, 1937.

89. Lewis, P.R., and McCutchen, C.W.: Experimental evidence for weeping lubrication in mammalian joints. Nature 184:1285, 1959.

90. McCutchen, C.W.: An approximate equation for weeping lubrication, solved with an electrical analogue. Ann. Rheum. Dis. 34 (Suppl. 2):85, 1975.

91. Layman, D.L., Sokoloff, L., and Miller, E.J.: Collagen synthesis by articular chondrocytes in monolayer culture. Exp. Cell. Res. 73:107, 1972.

92. Srivastava, V.M.L., Malemud, C.J., and Sokoloff, L.: Chondroid expression by lapine articular chondrocytes in spinner culture following monolayer growth. Connect. Tissue Res. 2:127, 1974.

93. Norby, D.P., Malemud, C.J., and Sokoloff, L.: Differences in the collagen types synthesized by lapine articular chondrocytes in spinner and monolayer cultures. Arthritis Rheum. 20:709, 1977.

94. Wiebkin, O.W., and Muir, H.: Synthesis of cartilage-specific proteoglycan by suspension cultures of adult chondrocytes. Biochem. J. 164:269, 1977.

95. Skantze, K.A., Brinckerhoff, C.E., Collier, J.P., and Harris, E.D., Jr.: Modulation of chondrocyte function in agar culture. Abstr. Arthritis Rheum. 26:41, 1983.

96. Wright, V., and Dowson, D.: Lubrication and cartilage. J. Anat. 121:107, 1976.

97. McCutchen, C.W.: Lubrication of joints. In Sokoloff, L. (ed.): The Joints and Synovial Fluid. Vol I. New York, Academic Press, 1978, pp. 437–477.

98. Swanson, S.A.V.: Lubrication. In Freeman, M.A.R. (ed.): Adult Articular Cartilage. New York, Grune & Stratton, 1977, pp. 247–277.

99. Fein, R.S.: Are synovial joints squeeze-film lubricated? Proc. Inst. Mech. Eng. London 181:125, 1967.

100. McCutchen, C.W.: Animal joints and weeping lubrication. New Scientist 15:412, 1962.

101. Dowson, D., Unsworth, A., and Wright, V.: Analysis of boosted lubrication in human joints. J. Mech. Eng. Sci. 12:364, 1970.

102. Walker, P.S., Dowson, D., Longfield, M.D., and Wright, V.: "Boosted lubrication" in synovial joints by fluid entrapment and enrichment. Ann. Rheum. Dis. 27:512, 1968.

103. Dintenfass, L.: Lubrication in synovial joints. Nature 197:496, 1963.

104. Radin, E.L., Swann, D.A., and Weisser, P.A.: Separation of hyaluronate-free lubricating fraction from synovial fluid. Nature 288:377, 1970.

105. Swamm, D.A.: Structure and function of lubricin, the glycoprotein responsible for the boundary lubrication of articular cartilage. In Franchimont, P. (ed.): Articular Synovium. Basel, Karger, 1982, pp. 45–58.

106. Stockwell, R.A.: Lipid content of human costal and articular cartilage. Ann. Rheum. Dis. 26:481, 1967.

107. Little, T., Freeman, M.A.R., and Swanson, S.A.V.: Experiments on friction in the human hip joint. In Wright, V. (ed.): Lubrication and Wear Joints. London, Sector, 1969, p. 110.

108. Radin, E.L., and Paul, I.L.: A consolidated concept of joint lubrication. J. Bone Joint Surg. 54A:607, 1972.

109. Bar, E.: Elasticitätsprüfungen der Gelenkknorpel. Arch. J. Entwicklungsmech. Organ. 108:739, 1926.

110. Freeman, M.A.R., and Kempson, G.E.: Load carriage. In Freeman, M.A.R. (ed.): Adult Articular Cartilage. New York, Grune & Stratton, 1974, pp. 228–246.

111. Harris, E.D., Jr., DiBona, D.R., and Krane, S.M.: A mechanism for cartilage destruction in rheumatoid arthritis. Trans. Assoc. Am. Physicians. 83:267, 1970.

112. Harris, E.D., Jr., Parker, H.G., Radin, E.L., and Krane, S.M.: Effects of proteolytic enzymes on structural and mechanical properties of cartilage. Arthritis Rheum. 15:497, 1972.

113. Kempson, G.E., Muir, H., Swanson, S.A.V., and Freeman, M.A.R.: Correlations between stiffness and the chemical constituents of cartilage on the human femoral head. Biochim. Biophys. Acta 215:70, 1970.

114. Kempson, G.E.: Mechanical properties of articular cartilage. In Freeman, M.A.R. (ed.): Adult Articular Cartilage. New York, Grune & Stratton, 1974, p. 196.

115. Landelles, J.W.: The reactions of injured human articular cartilage. J. Bone Joint Surg. 39B:548, 1957.

116. Meachim, G., and Osborne, G.V.: Repair at the femoral articular cartilage surface in osteoarthritis of the hip. J. Pathol. 102:1, 1970.

117. Simon, W.H.: Scale effects in animal joints. I. Articular cartilage thickness and compressive stress. Arthritis Rheum. 13:244, 1970.

118. Armstron, C.G., and Gardner, D.L.: Thickness and distribution of human femoral head articular cartilage. Changes with age. Ann. Rheum. Dis. 36:407, 1977.

119. Byers, P.D., Contepomi, C.A., and Farker, T.A.: A postmortem study of the hip joint. Ann. Rheum. Dis. 29:15, 1970.

120. Freeman, M.A.R., and Meachim, G.: Aging, degeneration and remodeling of articular cartilage. In Freeman, M.A.R. (ed.): Adult Articular Cartilage. New York, Grune & Stratton, 1973, pp. 287–330.

121. Collins, D.H., and Meachim, G.: Sulphate ($^{35}SO_4$) fixation by human articular cartilage compared in the knee and shoulder joints. Ann. Rheum. Dis. 20:117, 1961.

122. Meachim, G.: Light microscopy of Indian ink preparations of fibrillated cartilage. Ann. Rheum. Dis. 31:457, 1972.

123. Bollet, A.J., and Nance, J.L.: Biochemical findings in normal and osteoarthritic articular cartilage. II. Chondroitin sulfate concentration and chain length, water, and ash content. J. Clin. Invest. 45:1170, 1966.

124. Mankin, H.J., and Lippiello, L.: Biochemical and metabolic abnormalities in articular cartilage from osteoarthritic human hips. J. Bone Joint Surg. 52A:424, 1970.

125. Collins, D.H., and McElliggott, T.F.: Sulfate ($^{35}SO_4$) uptake by chondrocytes in relation to histological changes in osteoarthritic human articular cartilage. Ann. Rheum. Dis. 19:318, 1960.

126. Bassleer R, Lhoest-Ganthier, M.-P., Renard, A-M., Heinen, E., and Goessins, G.: Histological structure and functions of synovium. In Franchimont, P. (ed.): Articular Synovium, Basel, Karger, 1982, pp. 1–26.

127. Barland, P., Novikoff, A.B., and Hamerman, D.: Electron microscopy of the human synovial membrane. J. Cell. Biol. 14:207, 1962.

128. Ghadially, F.N., and Roy, S.: Ultrastructure of synovial joints, in health and disease. London, Butterworth, 1969.

129. Hirobata, H., and Kobayaski, I.: Fine structure of the synovial tissue in rheumatoid arthritis. Kobe J. Med. Sci. 10:195, 1964.

130. Krey, P.R., Cohen, A.S., Smith, C.B., and Finland, M.: The human fetal synovium. Histology, fine structure and changes in organ culture. Arthritis Rheum. 14:319, 1971.

131. Roy, S., Ghadially, F.N., and Crane, W.A.J.: Synovial membrane in traumatic effusion. Ultrastructure and autoradiography with tritiated leucine. Ann. Rheum. Dis. 25:259, 1966.

132. Werb, Z., and Reynolds, J.J.: Stimulation by endocytosis of the secretion of collagenase and neutral proteinases from rabbit synovial fibroblasts. J. Exp. Med. 140:1482, 1976.

133. Norton, W.L., Lewis, D.C., and Ziff, M.: Electron-dense deposits following injection of gold sodium thiomalate and thiomalic acid. Arthritis Rheum. 11:436, 1968.

134. Ghadially, F.N., Ailsby, R.L., and Yong, N.K.: Ultrastructure of the hemophilic synovial membrane and electron-probe X-ray analysis of haemosiderin. J. Pathol. 120:201, 1976.

135. Roy, S., and Ghadially, F.N.: Synthesis of hyaluronic acid by synovial cells. J. Pathol. Bacteriol. 93:555, 1967.

136. Ghadially, F.N.: Fine structure of joints. In Sokoloff, L. (ed.): The Joints and Synovial Fluid. New York, Academic Press, 1978, p. 140.

137. Hynes, R.O.: Cell surface proteins and malignant transformation. Biochim. Biophys. Acta 458:73, 1976.

138. Clemmensen, I., Holund, B., and Andersen, R.B.: Fibrin and fibronectin in rheumatoid synovial membrane and rheumatoid synovial fluid. Arthritis Rheum. 26:497, 1983.

139. Ali, I.V., Mautner, V., Lanza, R., and Hynes, R.O.: Restoration of normal morphology, adhesion and cytoskeleton sensitive surface protein. Cell 11:115, 1977.

140. Yamada, K.M., and Weston, J.A.: Isolation of a major cell surface glycoprotein from fibroblasts. Proc. Natl. Acad. Sci. USA 71:3492, 1974.

141. Hynes, R.O.: Alteration of cell-surface proteins by viral transformation and proteolysis. Proc. Natl. Acad. Sci. USA 70:3170, 1973.

142. Fell, H.B., and Jubb, R.W.: The effect of synovial tissue on the breakdown of articlar cartilage in organ culture. Arthritis Rheum. 20:1359, 1977.

143. Dingle, J.T., Saklatvata, J., Hembry, R., Tyler, J.: A cartilage catabolic factor from synovium. Biochem. J. 184:177, 1979.

144. Ropes, M.W., and Bauer, W.: Synovial Fluid Changes in Joint Diseases. Cambridge, Harvard University Press, 1953.

145. Simkin, P.A., and Pizzoro, J.E.: Transynovial exchange of small molecules in normal human subjects. J. Appl. Physiol. 36:581, 1974.

146. Ropes, M.W., Muller, A.F., and Bauer, W.: The entrance of glucose and other sugars into joints. Arthritis Rheum. 3:496, 1960.

147. Kushner, I., and Somerville, J.A.: Permeability of human synovial membrane to plasma proteins. Arthritis Rheum. 14:560, 1971.

148. Nettelbladt, E., Sundblad, L., and Jonsson, E.: Permeability of the synovial membrane to proteins. Acta. Rheum. Scand. 9:28, 1963.

149. Brown, D.L., Cooper, A.G., and Bluestone, R.: Exchange of IgM and albumin between plasma and synovial fluid in rheumatoid arthritis. Ann. Rheum. Dis. 29:644, 1969.

150. Ruddy, S.: Synovial fluid: Mirror of the inflammatory lesion in rheumatoid arthritis. *In* Harris, E.D., Jr. (ed.): Rheumatoid Arthritis. New York, Medcom Press, 1974, pp. 58–71.

151. Harris, E.D., Jr., Faulkner, C.S., II, and Brown, F.E.: Collagenolytic systems in rheumatoid arthritis. Clin. Orthop. 110:303, 1975.

152. Abe, S., and Nagai, Y.: Evidence for the presence of a complex of collagenase with α_2-macroglobulin in human rheumatoid synovial fluid: A possible regulatory mechanism of collagenase activity in vivo. J. Biochem. 73:897, 1973.

153. Mainardi, C.L., Walter, J.M., Spiegel, P.K., Goldkamp, O.G., and Harris, E.D., Jr.: The lack of effect of daily heat therapy on the progression of rheumatoid arthritis. Arch. Phys. Med. Rehab. 60:390, 1979.

154. Horvath, S.M., and Hollander, J.L.: Intra-articular temperature as a measure of joint reaction. J. Clin. Invest. 28:469, 1949.

155. Hollander, J.L., and Horvath, S.M.: The influence of physical therapy procedures on the intra-articular temperature of normal and arthritic subjects. Am. J. Med. Sci. 218:543, 1949.

156. Harris, E.D., Jr., and McCroskery, P.A.: The influence of temperature and fibril stability on degradation of cartilage collagen by rheumatoid synovial collagenase. N. Engl. J. Med. 290:1, 1974.

157. Castor, C.W., and Yaron, M.: Connective tissue activation. VIII. The effects of temperature studied in vitro. Arch. Phys. Med. Rehab. 57:5, 1976.

158. Mueller, W.: Über den negativen Luftdruck im Gelenkram. Dtsch. Z. Chirurgie 218:395, 1929.

159. Unsworth, A., Dowson, D., and Wright, V.: "Cracking Joints." A bioengineering study of cavitation in the metacarpophalangeal joint. Ann. Rheum. Dis. 30:348, 1971.

160. Jayson, M.I.V., and Dixon, A.St.J.: Intra-articular pressure in rheumatoid arthritis of the knee. III. Pressure changes during joint use. Ann. Rheum. Dis. 29:401, 1970.

161. Jayson, M.I.V., and Dixon, A.St.J.: Valvular mechanisms in juxta-articular cyts. Ann. Rheum. Dis. 29:415, 1970.

162. Myers, D.B., and Palmer, D.G.: Capsular compliance and pressure-volume relationships in normal and arthritic knees. J. Bone Joint Surg. 54B:710, 1972.

163. Jayson, M.I.V., Rubenstein, D., and Dixon, A.St.J.: Intra-articular pressure and rheumatoid geodes (bone 'cysts'). Ann. Rheum. Dis. 29:496, 1970.

164. Magyer, E., Talerman, A., Feher, M., and Wonters, H.W.: The pathogenesis of the subchondral pseudocysts in rheumatoid arthritis. Clin. Orthop. 100:341, 1974.

165. Jayson, M.I.V., and Dixon, A.St.J.: Intra-articular pressure in rheumatoid arthritis of the knee. II. Effect of intra-articular pressure on blood circulation to the synovium. Ann. Rheum. Dis. 29:266, 1970.

Chapter 17

Formation and Resorption of Bone

Clement B. Sledge

INTRODUCTION

The skeleton serves both a mechanical and a metabolic role. As an internal, articulated strut it provides the framework of the body, protects vital organs, and facilitates locomotion. Although these functions are important, especially in relation to arthritis, they are clearly secondary to the homeostatic role of the skeleton. As an ion-reservoir, the skeleton contains 99 percent of the total body calcium, 85 percent of the phosphorus, and 66 percent of the magnesium.[1] The maintenance of serum calcium ion concentration is vital to survival; it is therefore the role of the skeleton as a source of reserve calcium that occupies primary importance. Diseases that produce excessive loss of calcium (e.g., hyperparathyroidism, renal disease) may weaken the skeleton to the point of mechanical failure while serum calcium levels are maintained within a close range. A skeletal system that is mechanically inadequate (osteogenesis imperfecta, severe osteoporosis, multiple fractures) will continue its metabolic role and maintain a normal serum (Ca^{++}).

Paradoxical features of bone are its hardness and its ability to heal without a scar. Hardness suggests an inert character, which belies the constant turnover and internal remodeling that eventually result in the obliteration of the scars left by fractures, infections, and loss of blood supply.

The word bone is used to describe both the tissue and the organ. In the former sense it denotes a special mineralized connective tissue; in the latter it includes cartilage and hematopoietic and adipose tissues. Bones, as organs, are the structural elements of the body and as such are dealt with in standard textbooks of orthopedics. This chapter is devoted to a brief review of mechanisms of bone *tissue* formation and resorption, to provide a background for the discussion of metabolic bone disease and the alterations in bone structure that accompany rheumatoid arthritis.

BONE AS A TISSUE

Bone Cells. Osteogenic cells (osteoblasts, osteoclasts, and osteocytes) cover all bone surfaces except those of

Figure 17–1. Polyhedral osteoblasts lying on the surface of newly formed bone matrix. (From Jowsey, J.: Metabolic Diseases of Bone. Philadelphia, W.B. Saunders Company, 1977. Courtesy of Dr. B. Boothroyd.)

the sinuses of the adult skull.[2] Thus, all interactions of the skeleton with the body in general are mediated by these cells, which constitute a functional continuum resembling a membrane.[3] Young[4] stated that "each problem in bone physiology may be considered in the light of the relative distribution of bone cells among their various functional roles, for this system of cells acts as the 'final common path' through which the great variety of stimuli affecting bone must pass."

All the osteogenic cells are felt to arise from a common stem cell, a mononuclear blood cell, which, when identified by its spatial relation to bone, is termed an "osteo-progenitor cell."[5] Reacting to mechanical, chemical, or hormonal stimuli, these pleuripotent cells "modulate" to a functional-blast or -clast. The term modulation indicates that this change in functional state is only temporary, as opposed to permanent change or "differentiation." Numerous studies have shown conversion from one functional type to another within the osteogenic series.[6-9] The naming of these cells therefore depends upon location and presumed function or upon demonstration of specific cytoplasmic elements.

Osteoblasts. These are plump cuboidal cells usually seen as a layer, one cell thick, applied to the surface of bone (Fig. 17–1). These features help distinguish the osteoblasts from osteo-progenitor cells, which are not polygonal but flattened and are not found in sheets or applied to bone surfaces.[10] The osteoblasts are linked to one another by tight junctions, so that the environment of bone surface can be altered from that of the general extracellular fluid space.[11] This ability of the osteoblast to produce a localized change in environment may be important in the formation of new bone and/or its mineralization. Electron microscopy reveals an extremely abundant rough endoplasmic reticulum with cisternae

and a well developed Golgi body as well as abundant free ribosomes.[12] The Golgi body may be visible by light microscopy, and the ribosomes produce the basophilia seen in hematoxylin and eosin section.

The major function of the osteoblast is to produce osteoid,[13] composed chiefly of collagen and proteoglycans. The former is classified as a type I collagen and appears to be similar to that found in skin and tendon.[14,15] The formation and secretion of this collagen appears identical to collagen formation in other cells, with formation on the rough endoplasmic reticulum of a procollagen which is secreted from the dilated cisternae into the extracellular space on the bone side of the osteoblast.[16] Extracellular modification, with removal of terminal regions and the formation of inter- and intramolecular cross-links, results in fibril deposition. The collagen fibrils are deposited as sheets about 3 to 10 μm in thickness, with the individual fibrils oriented in parallel array within each sheet.[17] These sheets, or lamellae, tend to lie parallel to the long axis of the bone, with adjacent lamellae alternating about 30 degrees from this axis.[18,19] The collagen bundles thus alternate by about

Figure 17–2. Ground section of bone photographed with polarized light showing the concentric lamellar structure of the basic unit of mature bone, the osteon. The central vascular canal (empty in this preparation) is surrounded by multiple lamellae of bone. The adjacent lamellae are composed of collagen bundles with differing orientations, giving rise to alternating light and dark bands in polarized light.

60 degrees from lamella to lamella, providing tensile strength and a characteristic appearance under polarized light microscopy (Fig. 17–2).

The "functional life" of the osteoblast in man is unknown. Estimates vary from 3 days in young rabbits[7,20] to 54 days in aged mice.[21] Jowsey[22] estimates that each osteoblast produces a seam of osteoid about 15 μm thick, at a rate of 1 μm per day. The functional life in man would thus be 15 days. During this span, each osteoblast has produced 1500 cubic μm of new bone matrix.

Osteocytes. As new osteoid is laid down, osteoblasts become encased within the lacunae of the new bone, becoming osteocytes. At one time these cells were considered effete and unresponsive. It is now known that under stress conditions (e.g., PTH stimulation, calcium deprivation) the osteocyte participates in resorption of the surrounding bone.[23-25] This process, termed osteocytic osteolysis, is probably responsible for the moment-to-moment maintenance of serum calcium, since it can be evoked rapidly, rather than depending upon the induction of new multinucleated osteoclasts. When the period of stress is over, the osteocyte replaces the lost bone around its lacuna and returns to a resting state. The osteocyte, therefore, rather than being effete, is capable of both bone resorption and formation, but quantitative data are lacking.[26]

Each osteocyte in its lacuna is connected to adjacent osteocytes by way of cytoplasmic extensions extending through tunnels (canaliculi) radiating outward from the central vascular canal (Fig. 17–3). These provide a pathway of nutrition through the dense bone matrix and connect each osteocyte via gap junctions.[27] The volume of bone occupied by this system has been estimated at 4 to 6 percent for canaliculi and 1 to 2 percent for lacunae.[28] The surface area of the lacunar and canalicular system has been estimated to be at least 250 sq meters per liter of calcified bone matrix and communicates with a submicroscopic, interfibrillar space representing 35,000 sq mm per cubic millimeter. Exchange of mineral across this enormous surface is very rapid and is under the control of the osteocyte.[29]

Osteoclasts. Where bone is being removed or internally remodeled, large multinucleate cells are seen lying in irregular resorption cavities known as Howship's lacunae (Fig. 17–4). These cells vary in size from 200 to 200,000 sq μm, with from 2 to 100 or more nuclei.[30] The cell surface applied to bone is characterized by a brush or ruffled border where active bone resorption occurs.[31] The cytoplasm is often foamy, owing to the large number of digestive vacuoles and vesicles. There are numerous lysosomal bodies, which contain histochemically demonstrable acid hydrolases.[32,33] In remodeling bone, there are normally many more osteoblasts than osteoclasts (22 to 1 in the growing rabbit),[34] suggesting much greater efficiency on the part of the osteoclast. Figures for humans are lacking, but Jowsey[35] suggests that it is reasonable to multiply osteoclast nuclei by 6 to estimate the activity equivalent of the osteoblast. These ratios are of interest, since they allow an estimate of metabolic activity in histologic sections of bone. Because of osteocytic osteolysis and variable resorption rates by individual osteoclasts,[36] however, the method is only semiquantitative.

Osteoclasts are seen in increased numbers during rapid remodeling, as in the metaphysis of growing bone, and in response to parathyroid hormone. Even when bone resorption is produced by other factors, such as hyperoxia or vitamin A, osteoclasts are seen, suggesting that they participate in bone resorption even though the process may be initiated by mononuclear cells.[37]

The origin, functional span, and fate of the osteoclast have been debated for years. Three theories of origin suggest that osteoclasts arise from specific "pre-osteo-

Figure 17–3. Ground section of bone photographed in normal light showing empty osteocyte lacunae (OL) connected by fine darkly stained canaliculi. The central haversian canal (HC) is seen in the upper left hand corner; the reversal line (*) marking the junction between two adjacent osteons and the cement line (→ ←) separating adjacent lamellae are seen.

Figure 17–4. *A*, Paragon-stained mineralized section with large multinucleate osteoclasts lying along the pale staining bone surface. *B*, Microradiograph of the same area showing Howship's lacunae in the areas of osteoclastic resorption. (From Jowsey, J., and Gordan, G.: *In* Bourne, G.H. [ed.]: The Biochemistry and Physiology of Bone. Vol. III. 2nd ed. New York, Academic Press, 1972, pp. 201–238.)

clasts" found on bone surfaces as resting mononuclear cells;[34,38] arise from the same pool of undifferentiated "osteo-progenitor cells" that gives origin to osteoblasts;[8] or arise from wandering phagocytes.[39,40] A recent convincing review of available information gives strong support to the concept that osteoclasts arise from mononuclear lymphoid cells of the monocyte-macrophage series.[41] Whatever their origin, increased numbers of osteoclasts can be seen within 17 to 24 hours after injection of parathyroid hormone into experimental animals.[42]

The life span and ultimate fate of the osteoclast are also obscure. Tissue culture experiments suggest a life span of from 48 to 72 hours[43] to 3 days.[5] No convincing evidence has been found to suggest that osteoclasts can give rise to mononuclear cells. They thus appear to arise from mononuclear cells in response to various stimuli, carry out bone resorption, and then shed nuclei and finally disappear when stimuli to resorption (PTH, OAF, etc.) are removed or when there is no bone matrix left to be resorbed.[41]

Mast cells are seen in increased numbers in direct contact with resorbing bone surfaces in a number of conditions (lathyrism, PTH excess, mast cell disease), leading to the suggestion that they too can produce bone resorption.[44-46] Since heparin can enhance the resorptive response to parathyroid hormone[47] and produce osteoporosis after chronic administration,[48-50] it is interesting to speculate on the role, if any, of the mast cell content of this polysaccharide in bone resorption.

Myeloma cells also appear to resorb bone directly, as do some other malignant cells.[51] In addition, leukocytes produce a factor called osteoclast-activating factor (OAF) that stimulates osteoclastic activity and bone resorption.[52]

Thyroxin stimulates both bone formation and resorption, especially the latter.[53,54] Glucocorticoids have complex effects on bone formation and resorption, depending on the model used[55] and method of stimulation, whether PTH[56] or vitamin D metabolites[57] or prostaglandins.[58]

In clinical situations such as corticosteroid treatment of asthma[56] or rheumatoid arthritis,[56,57] bone loss may be severe, owing to a primary decrease in bone formation accompanied by hypercalciuria that leads to secondary hyperparathyroidism with increased bone resorption.[59]

Prostaglandins probably do not play a role in normal bone turnover,[60] but may be influential in pathological bone resorption by tumors[61] and inflammatory processes such as rheumatoid arthritis.[62,63] For a more detailed discussion of the role of hormones and other factors affecting bone growth and remodeling see Chapter 106 and reference 64.

Organization of Bone. Bone can be classified in a number of ways: (1) by its gross appearance (cortical or cancellous); (2) by its microscopic appearance (lamellar, woven, or haversian); or (3) on the basis of its origin (endochondral or intramembranous).[17]

Classification based on gross appearance has only limited usefulness, and that based on developmental origin suggests differences which do not exist since both endochondral and intramembranous bone are usually intermixed and indistinguishable. For our purposes, therefore, a system of classification based on microscopic appearance will be used.[65]

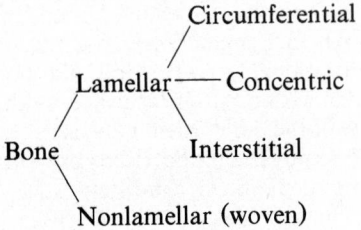

Nonlamellar or woven bone is the result of rapid bone formation. It is characteristic of embryonic and fetal development, but when seen in the adult is always pathological (i.e., tumor bone or fracture healing).

Lamellar bone can be packed tightly to form the cortex of a bone or loosely, as in cancellous bone[66,67] (Fig. 17–5).

After formation of the periosteal cuff surrounding the primary center of ossification, bone grows in diameter by one of two methods. During rapid growth, spicules of new bone are formed perpendicular to the surface, allowing maximal radial expansion with minimal material. Later, the gaps between the spicules are filled in by lamellar bone surrounding individual periosteal blood vessels which parallel the long axis of the bone (Fig. 17–6). These systems of lamellar bone surrounding a blood vessel are known as haversian systems or osteons.[68] An osteon that is formed de novo is referred to as a primary osteon, while one that is formed to replace a pre-existing bone structure is known as a secondary osteon.

When slow diametric growth occurs, seams of new bone are laid on the existing surface (Fig. 17–7A). These *circumferential* lamellae resemble the layers of an onion and provide a strong laminated structure like plywood. Indeed, the collagen bundles in adjacent lamellae alternate in direction from layer to layer, maximizing strength in all planes.[69] Later, for maximal strength, the circumferential lamellae are replaced by individual concentric lamellar systems; when these replace pre-existing bone (lamellar, woven, or earlier osteonal bone), they are

Figure 17–5. Diagrammatic representation of the structure of human cortical bone.

Figure 17–6. Outer cortex of bone showing the results of rapid periosteal bone formation producing woven bone, followed by the slower formation of primary osteons surrounding blood vessels.

termed secondary osteons and constitute the bulk of adult bone[70] (Fig. 17–7B). Remnants of pre-existing osteons and circumferential lamellae persist between newer, complete osteons. These fragments are called interstitial lamellae (Fig. 17–8).

The mechanical strength of fully mature osteonal bone is greater than that of immature bone composed of circumferential lamellae with only a few osteons.[71,72] The analogy of a bundle of straws compared to a solid stick has been used; as bending forces are applied to each, they bend. The solid stick breaks at fairly low bending loads, while the bundle of straws with the same mass will continue to deform rather than break. Each twig of straw slips, relative to adjacent bundles, thereby dissipating applied forces and avoiding excessive tensile forces and ultimate failure. In the same manner, individual lamellae have been observed to slip relative to adjacent lamellae, dissipating energy and allowing the entire system to react in a more elastic manner rather than sustain brittle failure or fracture.[18,71]

In order to replace pre-existing bone, it must first be resorbed. If the structural function of bone is to be preserved during this remodeling, it must be carried out little by little with the simultaneous removal of bone from one location and its deposition elsewhere. The most common stimulus for this remodeling is physical stress. If excessive demand is placed upon a bone (or the direction of application of force is changed), the bone remodels to meet the increased demand.[73,74] The first response is the formation of a "cutting cone" composed of a group of osteoclasts that bore into the old bone, creating a resorption cavity (Fig. 17–7B). In the wake

of this resorptive process, a capillary grows in, surrounded by osteoblasts constructing a new haversian system.[75,76] In the absence of unusual physical demands, the process of conversion and remodeling of immature bone is quite orderly and predictable. Indeed, Kerley[70] has quantified the percentage of the cross section of the tibia that has been converted into mature osteonal bone and has related this percent conversion to the age of the individual. The resulting graph of percent osteonal bone versus age has been useful in forensic medicine and archeology in determining the age at death of skeletal remains.

When bone is being resorbed, osteoclasts are seen lying in irregular Howship's lacunae, the irregular margins of which allow one to recognize resorption even if the osteoclasts themselves are not seen (microradiographs, ground sections). When resorption is completed, these irregularities are smoothed out before new bone formation begins. This process leaves a boundary, which is visible in histologic sections as a "reversal line." If the resorbed bone is to be replaced by new bone, the reversal line clearly demarcates the junction between old and new bone. A similar line, called a "cement line," is seen between the adjacent lamellae of bone (Fig. 17–3).

During growth in diameter new bone is added peripherally (appositional growth) and old bone is resorbed on the inner or parallel surface (endosteal resorption). Some of the old cortical bone is spared during the process of removal on the endosteal surface and becomes a component of the cancellous structure. The appearance of these trabeculae of cancellous bone reflects this origin, and fragments of osteons as well as new lamellae and abundant cement lines are seen (Fig. 17–9). In places, trabeculae are covered with osteoblasts making new bone, while in other places osteoclasts are seen eroding the surface. By this process of resorption and formation, orientation of the trabeculae is changed to meet the altered forces produced by longitudinal growth or change in alignment secondary to disease or fracture.[74]

Composition of Bone. Newly synthesized bone matrix, before calcification, is called osteoid. The precise chemical composition is unknown, since the material normally exists as thin seams scattered throughout the skeleton, mixed with mineralized bone, cells, and marrow elements. Separation has been attempted by fragmentation of bone followed by density separation based on the fact that osteoid is less dense than mineralized bone (1.46 vs. 2.2 grams per milliliter).[77] Analysis of material obtained by this technique is shown in Table 17–1.

Bone collagen is classified as type I[78] and resembles other type I collagens found in skin and tendon. It differs from the collagen of cartilage (type II) in several salient aspects, primarily in that the latter contains much more glycosylated hydroxylysine. Cartilage collagen is also more resistant to degradation by collagenase than is bone collagen. More subtle, but important, differences exist between bone collagen and other type I collagens,[79,80] and these are discussed below.

Figure 17–7. *A*, Microradiograph of the full thickness of cortical bone showing outer (+) and inner (*) circumferential lamellae with concentric (osteonal) bone in the center. *B*, Enlarged section of a portion of *A*, Showing a resorption cavity (→) with irregular margins, "burrowing" into the older circumferential lamellar bone.

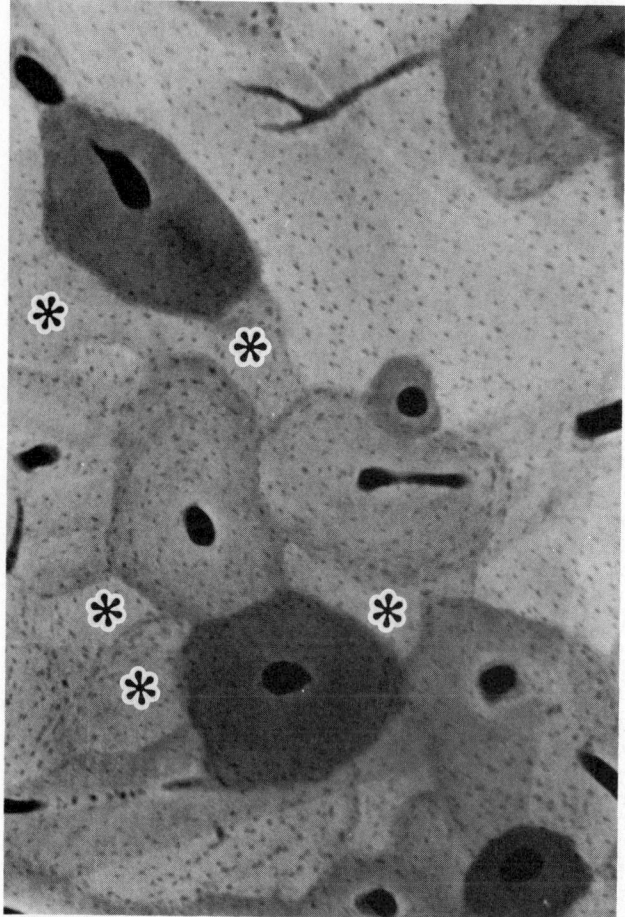

Figure 17–8. Microradiograph of cortical bone showing osteons in varying degrees of mineralization with numerous interstitial fragments (*).

The polysaccharides of bone have been difficult to analyze.[81,82] Chondroitin sulfate linked to protein and resembling the proteoglycan of cartilage has been identified by Herring,[83] who has also isolated a glycoprotein that represents the majority of the noncollagenous portion of bone matrix. A fraction rich in sialic acid, sialoprotein, has been characterized and is thought to be unique to bone. Lipids and phospholipids have also been identified but poorly characterized.[83,84]

Bone mineral is referred to as hydroxyapatite $[Ca_{10}(PO_4)_6 \cdot (OH)_2]$ but is quite different from naturally occuring apatite, containing a number of impurities, including sodium, fluorine, strontium, lead, and radium. The initial deposits of bone mineral may not be hydroxyapatite but amorphous calcium phosphate (ACP)[85] or octacalcium phosphate (OCP),[86] which are gradually transformed to more crystalline hydroxyapatite. The enormous surface area of ACP, with its hydration shell, provides an immense surface for exchange. This is reflected in the greater avidity of new bone for "bone-seeking" isotopes (technetium, fluorine, strontium) and the greater rate of calcium exchange in young as opposed to old subjects. Vaughan estimates that 100 percent of

bone surfaces are available for exchange at the age of 1 year compared with 1 to 2 percent in adults.[87]

Mineralization. The process by which unmineralized bone matrix is converted to calcified bone remains incompletely understood. There are two leading theories. The first suggests a central role for collagen as a "nucleator," with proteoglycans and other minor constituents serving as inhibitors, protecting noncalcifying tissues.[88,89] The second theory suggests that mineral-rich lipid vesicles are produced by calcifying tissues (cartilage and bone) and that these vesicles serve as the initial foci of mineralization, which then spreads to permeate the entire structure.[90,91] Current evidence points to a role for these vesicles in the calcification of growth cartilage,[92] but supports the principal role of collagen in bone mineralization.[93]

Body fluids are supersaturated with respect to hydroxyapatite. If type I collagen is capable of nucleating crystals of hydroxyapatite from such solutions, why do not ligaments, skin, and tendon normally calcify? Convincing evidence has been accumulated that the proteoglycans found in these noncalcifying collagenous structures prevent mineral deposition (see reference 93 for review). Enzymatic removal of these blocking substances would allow mineral deposition. An abrupt loss of sulfated proteoglycan at the calcification front has been shown,[89] confirming earlier, in vitro demonstrations that collagen "contaminated" with proteoglycan did not include mineralization as effectively as did purified type I collagen.

There is general agreement that early in the mineralization process crystals of hydroxyapatite are seen within collagen fibrils, reproducing the 640 Å periodicity and apparently lying in "holes" in the collagen fibril.[94] The initial localization of mineral to these "hole" regions is presumably due to both spatial and chemical factors. The water that is displaced during mineralization (Table 17–1) presumably is concentrated in the holes, and the organic phosphate groups, which institute crystal nucleation, are concentrated nearby.[95] As crystal growth occurs, mineralization spreads beyond the hole region but remains largely or wholly within the fibrils, which are held together by strong interfibrillar and interfiber

Table 17-1. Composition of Bone*

	Osteoid	"New" Bone	"Old" Bone
Density	1.460	2.005	2.211
Collagen	31.99%	25.85%	23.63%
Other protein	12.87	11.31	1.56
Mucopolysaccharides	1.64	0.83	0.75
Mineral	11.07	39.25	54.59
Water	20.15	15.15	17.45
Total	77.7%	92.4%	98%

*Composition given as percent dry weight. After Herring, G.M.: *In* Bourne, G.H. (ed.): The Biochemistry and Physiology of Bone, Vol. I. 2nd ed. New York, Academic Press, 1972, p. 127. Data from Pugliarello, M.C., et al.: Calc. Tissue Res. 5:108, 1970.

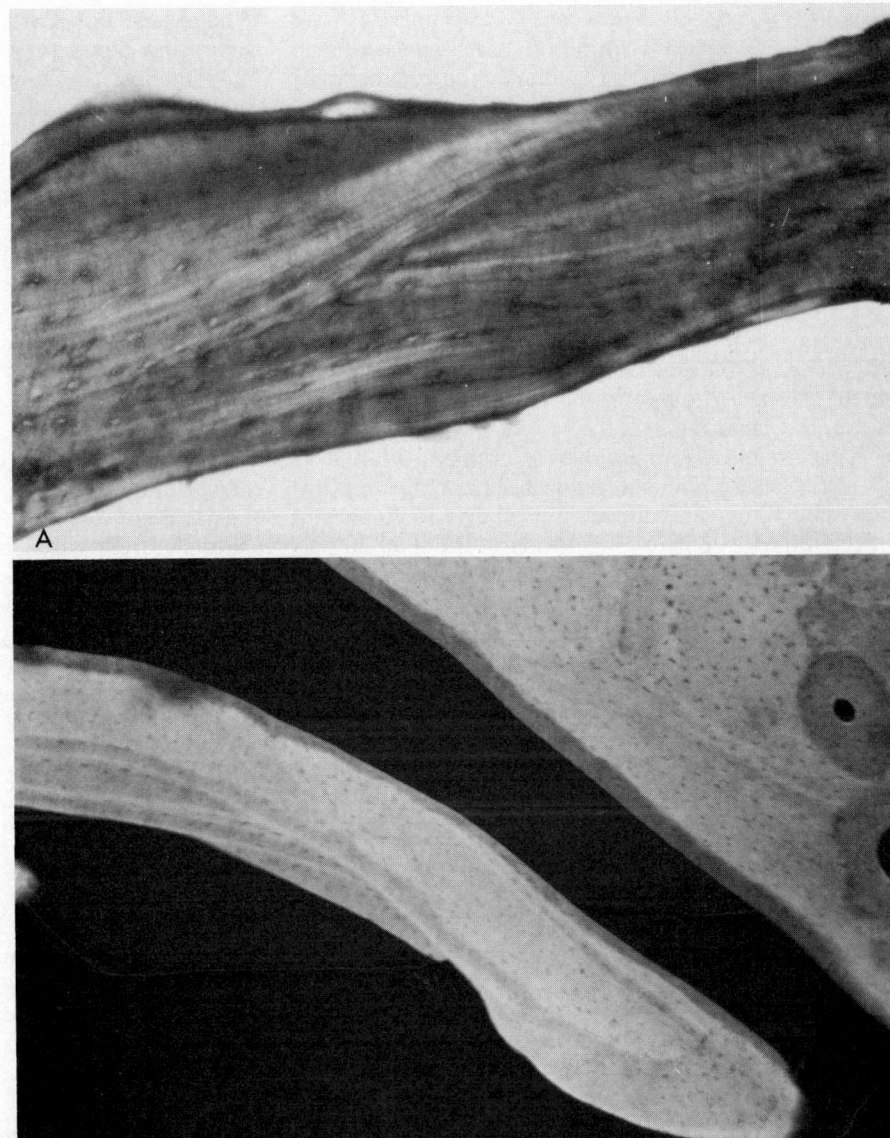

Figure 17–9. *A,* Ground section of cancellous bone showing a single trabecula composed of multiple lamellae of bone and numerous osteocytes. *B,* Microradiograph of a trabecula adjacent to the inner cortex of bone. Growth of the trabecula by the addition of new seams of lamellar bone is clearly seen.

bonds. The total amount of mineral that can be accommodated by this theory—two thirds of the weight of the tissue—is the amount measured in mature, fully calcified bone. In tissues that do not normally calcify, the "holes" are smaller, but the lack of strong inter- and intramolecular bonds allows more mineral to be deposited outside of the fibrils. Thus, these structures may contain more mineral than bone, and the mineral is both within and outside the fibril.[93] It has been postulated that in calcific "bursitis" or tendinitis, the inflammatory process produces enzymatic loss of the protective proteoglycan, allowing the exposed collagen fibrils to nucleate hydroxyapatite from the supersaturated interstitial fluid.

A vitamin K–dependent calcium-building amino acid residue, γ-carboxyglutamic acid, has been identified in bone, calcifying cartilage, and various pathologic calcifications.[96,97] The parent protein, named osteocalcin, constitutes only 0.5 to 1 percent of total bone protein (20 percent of the noncollagenous protein) but may represent a critical regulatory mechanism in the mineralization of tissues.[98]

After osteoid is formed, there is normally a lag of 10 to 15 days before mineralization begins. Following this lag, mineral increases almost immediately to 70 percent of the ultimate content. Deposition of the final 30 percent may take several months.[99] In undemineralized ground sections, microradiography demonstrates differences in the calcium content of various osteons, thus allowing separation into "old" or "new" osteons based on mineral content (Fig. 17–7). In addition, very young osteons, in the process of formation, have large central vascular canals which narrow with maturity. Remodeling rates can thus be inferred from morphological characteristics.[99]

BONES AS ORGANS

General Considerations. Bones are remarkably well suited for their structural role. As hollow tubes, they combine maximal strength with minimal weight. This strength-to-weight ratio is further enhanced by the microscopic arrangement of the collagen within the bone and the two-phase composition of collagen and mineral. The tensile strength of the bone approximates that of cast iron; its bending strength is between that of oak and cast iron, while its weight is only one third the weight of the latter.

Because of its strength, the shaft of a bone can be quite narrow for its length. In order to distribute forces on the articular cartilage, thereby minimizing wear and the deleterious effects of excessive force on the articular chondrocyte, the end of the bone flares to a larger diameter. The type and distribution of material also change to minimize weight and protect the articular cartilage (see discussion in Chapter 18) (Fig. 17–10). Additionally, bone responds to the physical demands placed upon it, not only by changes in size but by changes in shape and internal structure. The skeleton

also reconstitutes itself after fracture in such a way that its form-function relationship is maintained. In order to meet these demands, bone is constantly being internally remodeled by a complex and interrelated sequence of resorption and formation which is never entirely quiescent and is capable of responding to metabolic demands without loss of structural integrity.

As organs, bones are composed of marrow, cartilage, nerves and blood vessels, and the periosteal covering. Functionally, the origins and insertions of muscles should also be included.

In childhood and early adult life, marrow is hematopoietic in most of the bones. With advancing age, this red marrow retreats from the appendicular skeleton and occupies the flat bones, vertebral bodies, and epiphyseal ends of the larger tubular bones such as the humerus and femur. As hematopoietic red marrow is lost, it is replaced by fatty yellow marrow. This process begins at about the sixth year and is complete by the eighteenth. Since the red marrow is much more vascular than the fatty marrow, the ends of the long bones, the vertebra, and the flat bones are metabolically more responsive, and it is here that the changes of systemic disease are usually first apparent.

For ease of discussion, the long bones are divided into anatomic areas based on the zones of growing bones: the juxta-articular or epiphyseal area (on the articular side of the growth plate), the metaphysis (the tapered portion from the epiphysis to the straight tubular midsection), and the diaphysis (the shaft). Although these regions are imprecise and are used somewhat differently by anatomists and radiologists, they are useful for descriptive purposes.

Most of the bones of the skeleton are first formed in the embryo as cartilaginous models, which are later resorbed and replaced by bone tissue. The cartilage model (anlage) is formed by the condensation of mesenchymal cells in the developing limb bud. The shape of the anlage resembles that of the adult bone and is genetically determined. The bone that replaces it, however, is greatly influenced by physical factors (e.g., weight bearing, muscle pull), and remodels constantly as these forces change (Wolff's law).[73]

At the stage of the cartilage anlage, bone as an organ is composed entirely of cartilage.[1] The anlage expands and elongates by interstitial growth in which chondrocytes divide, enlarge, and surround themselves with a new matrix.[100] As growth continues, the limits of diffusion are reached and materials can no longer diffuse into the avascular cartilage model. The oldest and most centrally placed cells become hypertrophic, and the matrix surrounding them becomes encrusted with mineral deposits (the "primary center of ossification"). At about the same time, cells in the connective tissues surrounding the anlage (perichondrium) begin to lay down bone tissue and form a collar of bone around the center of the cartilage model. At about the time it is formed, it is pierced by a capillary, which invades the calcified cartilage matrix and begins to hollow out the center of the anlage, replacing the excavated cartilage with bone and

Figure 17–10. *A,* Macerated preparation of the human knee showing the trabecular structure which supports the flared articular surface. *B,* Radiograph of the specimen shown in *A.*

creating the primitive marrow space. This process of vascular invasion of the cartilage model, followed by bone deposition, is referred to as endochondral ossification. The process continues until the entire shaft of the anlage is replaced by marrow and bone, confining the growth process of chondrocyte multiplication to the epiphyseal ends of the bone. As these enlarge, the centrally placed chondrocytes again find themselves too far removed from a blood supply to exist by diffusion. The process of chondrocyte death followed by vascular invasion and bone formation is repeated, this time producing the "secondary center of ossification" in the epiphysis. The growth process continues between these two centers of ossification, confined to a relatively thin disc of cartilage called the physis, growth plate, or epiphyseal plate. A similar zone of proliferating cells exists under the articular cartilage as a "microepiphyseal plate." Both areas respond to growth hormone (via somatomedin) and provide longitudinal growth of the bone and enlargement of the articular end to maintain an appropriate size and shape for the weight-bearing surface (Fig. 17–11).

While growth in length occurs at the growth plate, growth in diameter occurs by the centrifugal deposition of bone by cells on the surface—so-called periosteal osteoblasts.[101]

This process of adding new bone to the exterior surface and resorbing bone from the inner surface continues throughout life. When "rate-linked," the mass and strength of the skeleton remain constant; however, aging and hormonal changes lead to alterations in shape and strength. "The outer, subperiosteal surface undergoes lifelong apposition, more in the male than in the female, with a classic 'adolescent spurt' and with a slower rate of gain thereafter, through to the end of life. The inner, endosteal bone surface undergoes resorption from childhood until adolescence, an appositional phase from mid-

dle adolescence through the end of the fourth decade, and then a second resorptive phase thereafter—demonstrably larger in the female and of greater consequence."[102]

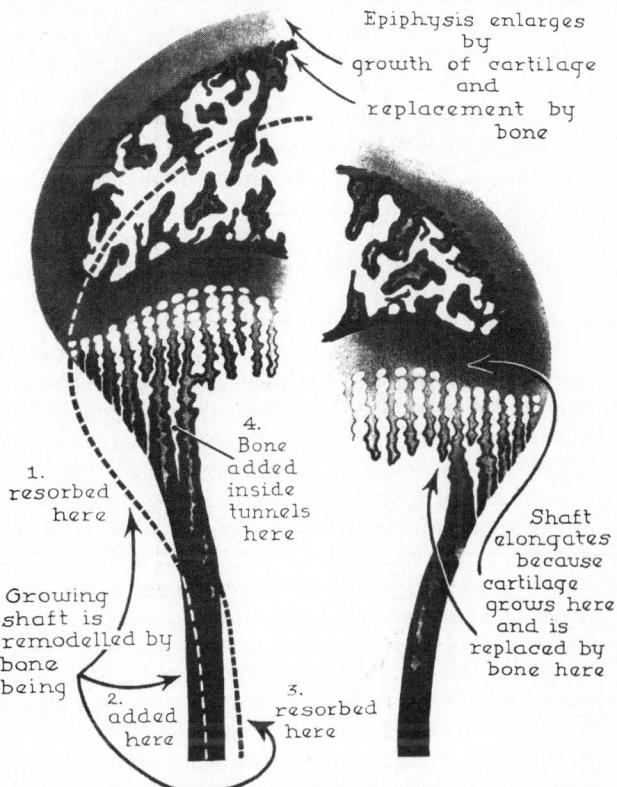

Epiphysis enlarges by growth of cartilage and replacement by bone

1. resorbed here

4. Bone added inside tunnels here

Growing shaft is remodelled by bone being

2. added here

3. resorbed here

Shaft elongates because cartilage grows here and is replaced by bone here

Figure 17–11. Diagram of the articular end of the bone showing the process of addition of new bone and removal of old bone which allows the articular end to increase in size while maintaining its shape during longitudinal growth. (From Ham, A.W.: J. Bone Joint Surg. 34A:701, 1952.)

Figure 17–12. Endosteal capillary penetrating the inner cortex to communicate with two haversian canals, providing an anastomotic communication between the nutrient artery, periosteal arteries, and capillaries traveling longitudinally within the haversian canal.

Periosteum. When enlargement of the cartilaginous anlage first begins, a condensed layer of mesenchyme develops around it as a membrane of cells and collagen. While this tissue surrounds the cartilage model, it is called *perichondrium.* As cartilage is replaced by bone, the membrane is renamed *periosteum.* In the growing skeleton, this periosteum is rather clearly divided into an inner cellular layer and an outer fibrous layer which merges gradually into the surrounding muscle. Muscles take origin from the periosteum and tendons insert into it. Collagen bundles can be traced from the tendon, through periosteum, and directly into bone as Sharpey's fibers.[103]

Blood Supply of Bone. Bone is extremely vascular, both as an organ and as a tissue, and receives approximately 10 percent of the cardiac output.[104]

Blood supply to the cortical diaphysis is derived from the nutrient artery and the periosteal vessels. The nutrient artery (or arteries) represents the original capillary which pierced the cartilaginous anlage to form the primitive marrow cavity. With continued longitudinal and circumferential growth, this vessel enlarges and arborizes to supply the marrow and inner two thirds of the cortex. The outer one third of the cortex is supplied by numerous vessels which perforate the periosteum and cortex.[105] These *periosteal capillaries* are especially abundant at sites of tendon and ligament insertion and muscle origin (Fig. 17–12). In the metaphyseal ends of the bone, where metabolism is most active, the periosteal vessels are large and abundant and they are also referred to as *metaphyseal arteries,* although they are entirely analogous to the periosteal capillaries. The third set of vessels, the *epiphyseal arteries,* supply the subarticular ends of the bones and assume special importance because of the growth process in this area and the vulnerability of these vessels to injury (Fig. 17–13).

During infancy and adolescence, the epiphyseal (growth) plate serves as a barrier separating the epiphysis from the metaphysis. Although a few vessels crossing the plate have been described, it is widely accepted that there is no effective circulation across the plate. The epiphyses therefore exist with an isolated blood supply via the epiphyseal arteries. In most joints, there are abundant soft tissue attachments to the epiphyses (muscles, ligaments, capsule), so that numerous vessels supply the bone through these attachments (Fig. 17–14*A*). In a few locations, such as the proximal femur, the entire epiphysis may be intraarticular and therefore covered by articular cartilage. Since neither this cartilage nor the growth cartilage is penetrated by vessels, the few epiphyseal arteries must pass alongside the growth plate, covered by a thin layer of periosteum, to perforate the epiphysis[106] (Fig. 17–14*B*). The route of blood supply is extremely vulnerable to trauma (fractures through the growth plate), increased intra-articular pressure (joint infections or bleeding into the joint), or idiopathic interruption (Legg-Perthes disease in children, avascular necrosis in adults).

Epiphyseal vessels arborize within the bony nucleus to supply the marrow, cancellous bone, and the crucial dividing chondrocytes in the microepiphyseal plates in the depths of the articular cartilage and the growth plate itself (Fig. 17–14*C*). Because of this, interruption of the vessels leads to cessation of longitudinal growth and loss of further diametric growth of the epiphysis and joint surface.

In contrast to the critical role of epiphyseal vessels during growth, the metaphyseal vessels are responsible only for resorption of the growth plate prior to its replacement by bone. Interruption of these vessels therefore will lead only to temporary loss of this function with increased thickness of the growth plate owing to

Figure 17–13. Diagrammatic representation fo the circulation of bone emphasizing the multiple communications seen at the site of heavy fascial attachment contrasted with the sparse communication in other areas. (From Rhinelander, F.W.: *In* Bourne, G.H. [ed.]: The Biochemistry and Physiology of Bone. Vol. II. 2nd ed. New York, Academic Press, 1972.)

function, estimates of skeletal metabolic activity can be made by morphologic techniques that assess the amount of either bone or mineral. The simplest technique is a visual assessment of mineral quantity on routine clinical radiographs. The technique is insensitive (30 percent of vertebral mass must be removed before it is detected by this technique[108]) and inaccurate (varying technical factors such as kilovoltage and exposure change the radiographic appearance[109]). The use of a densitometer, multiple scans of the same bone, and inclusion of a reference aluminum step wedge increase the accuracy of the technique and have allowed useful estimates of bone loss caused by bed rest[110] and the weightlessness of space flight.[111]

Estimates of cortical thickness, either metacarpal or vertebral body, have been used to follow age-related and pathological loss of bone mass and the response to therapy in osteoporosis.[112,113] The most useful of these techniques involves the determination of the combined cortical thickness of a reference bone, usually a metacarpal, although the humerus, clavicle, and phalanges have been used.[114] The thickness of the two cortices is measured

accumulation of chondrocytes and matrix. Upon re-establishment of the metaphyseal blood supply, the thickened plate is resorbed to its normal thickness and growth is not affected.[107]

Even in growing bones there is an abundant system of anastomoses between metaphyseal, periosteal, and nutrient arteries. Interruption of a single system results in limited changes in bone. With termination of longitudinal growth and obliteration of the growth plate, anastomoses are established between the metaphyseal system and the epiphyseal system, thereby interconnecting the entire blood supply of the bone. For this reason, elevation of the periosteum (dissecting infection or surgical approaches) or obliteration of the nutrient artery (intra-articular fixation devices or infection) have only limited effects on the blood supply to the entire bone.[105]

Within the cortex of bone, capillaries travel primarily in the longitudinal direction within haversian canals. Occasional branching is seen, and lateral communications with the periosteal vessels through Volkmann's canals provide collateral circulation.[68] The usual haversian system is 100 μm or less in diameter; thus individual osteocytes are not more than 50 μm from their blood supply. The rich system of canaliculi radiating out from the central canal enhances microcirculation to the most distant osteocytes.

Although the periosteum and marrow have long been known to be innervated with sensory and autonomic fibers, nerves within the haversian canals have only recently been described.[19]

Neural, hormonal, and metabolic factors affecting the blood supply to bone have been discussed by Shim,[104] and the effects of loss of blood to cortical and cancellous bone are discussed in Chapter 107.

Assessment of Bone Formation and Resorption. Because of the close relationship between bone form and

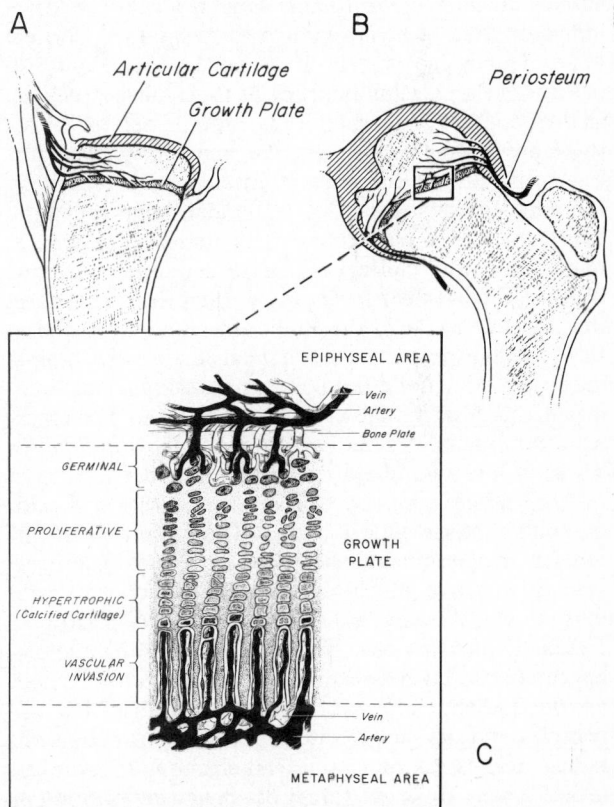

Figure 17–14. Epiphyseal blood supply of growing bone. *A*, The blood supply of most secondary centers of ossification is abundant by virtue of the numerous soft tissue attachments. *B*, Certain secondary centers, such as the proximal femur, are devoid of soft tissue attachments, and the blood supply therefore follows a tenuous route through the joint where it is liable to injury. *C*, Diagrammatic representation of the blood supply to the growth plate showing the contribution of the epiphyseal artery to the germinal portion of the growth plate. (From Sledge, C.B.: *In* Cave, E.F., et al. [eds.]: Trauma Management. Chicago, Year Book Medical Publishers, 1974.)

Figure 17–15. Singh index of trabecular patterns, illustrating the progressive stages of trabecular loss in osteoporosis. (From Jowsey, J.: Metabolic Diseases of Bone. Philadelphia, W.B. Saunders Company, 1977.)

and expressed as a ratio of that thickness to the diameter of the bone. Although having the advantage of simplicity, this technique is not as accurate as the quantitative radiographic technique discussed in the preceding paragraph.[109]

Because both bone formation and bone resorption are surface phenomena, trabecular bone is a more sensitive indicator of bone turnover than are changes in cortical bone. Trabeculae of cancellous bone occupy only 20 percent of the skeleton but present the same surface area as does cortical bone, roughly 5.5 square meters.[115] Furthermore, decreases in trabecular bone mass occur primarily by loss of the entire trabecula, rather than by thinning.[116] Thus, losses of trabecular bone are more easily detected in radiographs than are losses of cortical bone. Singh and colleagues[117] have developed an index of femoral trabecular patterns based on the observation that the trabeculae of the femoral neck are arranged in three predominant groups: a vertical compressive bundle in the medial femoral head, a curved vertial tensile bundle in the lateral head and neck region, and an interconnecting bundle lying more horizontally (Fig. 17–15). These groups of trabeculae are lost in reverse order in osteoporosis, giving rise to a sequential series of radiographic patterns graded 1 to 7. The usefulness of this index is in determining when bone loss, or osteoporosis, reaches a degree which endangers the mechanical stability of the skeleton and produces a risk of fracture.

Kinetic analyses of bone turnover, based on the disappearance of bone-seeking isotopes from the blood, provided useful information in early studies, but are complex and difficult to interpret. The information obtained relates to mineral metabolism and turnover, rather than to new rates of bone deposition or loss.[118-120]

Gamma-emitting bone-seeking isotopes that can be imaged with a gamma camera can provide visual and quantitative information on bone turnover. It is not clear to what degree bone formation and blood supply contribute to localization of the isotope; therefore these techniques are largely qualitative (see Chapter 40).

Total body bone mass can be determined by neutron activation analysis whereby stable body calcium (^{48}Ca)

is converted to ^{49}Ca, which emits gamma rays with a half-life of 8.8 minutes. Quantitative determination of bone mass with an accuracy of 1 percent has been reported using this technique.[121] Comparison between this technique and the photon absorption method (see below) suggests the latter is less precise in measuring small changes in bone mass.[122,123]

Variations in the characteristics of x-ray emissions and film processing gave imprecision to radiographic techniques of bone mass measurement and led to the development of mono-energetic sources of gamma rays and quantitative determinations of their absorption. Called photon absorption, the technique is fairly rapid and inexpensive but relatively insensitive.[124] The use of two different isotope sources allows subtraction of the soft tissue absorption and improved accuracy.[125]

New developments in computerized axial tomography have largely supplanted both total body neutron activation and photon absorption as methods of determining bone mineral content. Multiple "cuts" through one or more vertebral bodies can be averaged by the computer, obviating many of the sampling problems inherent in other methods, and giving calcium content with an accuracy of ± 3 percent.[126,127]

The unique nature of bone collagen has given rise to other techniques of estimating skeletal turnover based on analysis of urinary hydroxyproline[128] and glycosylated hydroxylysines.[129] Because it is not entirely possible to distinguish between fragments of collagen resulting from bone breakdown and those resulting from increased but faulty synthesis, these techniques are only semi-quantitative, but their simplicity and noninvasiveness are attractive.

Bone Biopsy. The techniques of determination of skeletal and/or mineral mass described above are useful and accurate to varying degrees but produce results that are largely "net effects." They do not clearly discern between decreased formation and increased resorption; nor do they separate changes in matrix metabolism from those of mineral balance. In osteomalacia, for example, bone mass and bone mineral changes may be masked by coexisting osteoporosis.[130] Bone biopsy, in addition to providing material for the usual histological evaluation of disease processes in the skeleton, has been developed into an extremely useful and accurate method of measuring bone metabolism.[131] The interested reader is referred to the excellent monograph by Jowsey,[10] the discussion by Byers,[132] and a monograph on noninvasive bone measurements edited by Dequeker and Johnston.[133]

References

1. Krane, S.M., and Potts, J.T., Jr.: Skeletal remodeling and factors influencing bone and bone mineral metabolism. *In* Thorn, G.W., Adams, R.D., Braunwald, E., Isselbacher, K.J., and Petersdorf, R.G. (eds.): Harrison's Principles of Internal Medicine. New York, McGraw-Hill Book Company, 1972.
2. Vaughan, J.M.: Osteogenic cells. *In* The Physiology of Bone. Oxford, Oxford University Press, 1970, p. 23.
3. Neuman, W.F., and Ramp, W.K.: The concept of a bone membrane: Some implications. *In* Nichols, G., Jr., and Wasserman, R.H. (eds.): Cellular Mechanisms for Calcium Transfer and Homeostasis. New York, Academic Press, 1971, p. 197.

4. Young, R.W.: Nucleic acids, protein synthesis and bone. Clin. Orthop. 26:147, 1963.

5. Young, R.W.: Cell proliferation and specialization during endochondral osteogenesis in young rats. J. Cell Biol. 14:357, 1962.

6. Tonna, E.A., and Cronkite, E.P.: Histochemical and autoradiographic studies on the effects of aging on the mucopolysaccharides of the periosteum. J. Biophys. Biochem. Cytol. 6:171, 1959.

7. Owen, M.E.: Cell population kinetics of an osteogenic tissue. J. Cell Biol. 19:19, 1963.

8. Young, R.W.: Autoradiographic studies on postnatal growth of the skull in young rats injected with tritiated glycine. Anat. Rec. 143:1, 1962.

9. Young, R.W.: Specialization of bone cells. In Frost, H.M. (ed.): Bone Biodynamics. Boston, Little, Brown & Company, 1964.

10. Jowsey, J.: Metabolic Disease of Bone. Philadelphia, W.B. Saunders Company, 1977, p. 59.

11. Weinger, J.M., and Holtrop, M.E.: An ultrastructural study of bone cells: the occurrence of microtubules, microfilaments and tight junctions. Calcif. Tissue Res. 14:15, 1974.

12. Pritchard, J.J.: The osteoblast. In Bourne, G.H. (ed.): The Biochemistry and Physiology of Bone, Vol. I. 2nd ed. New York, Academic Press, 1972, p. 21.

13. Carneiro, J., and Leblond, C.P.: Role of osteoblasts and odontoblasts in secreting the collagen of bone and dentin, as shown by radioautography in mice given tritium-labelled glycine. Exp. Cell Res. 18:291, 1959.

14. Miller, E.J., Martin, G.R., Piez, K.A., and Powers, M.J.: Characterization of chick bone collagen and compositional changes associated with maturation. J. Biol. Chem. 242:5481, 1967.

15. Miller, E.J.: A review of biochemical studies on the genetically distinct collagens of the skeletal system. Clin. Orthop. 91:260, 1973.

16. Prockop, D.J., Kivirikko, K.I., Tuderman, L., and Guzman, N.A.: The biosynthesis of collagen and its disorders. N. Engl. J. Med. 301:13, 77, 1979.

17. Pritchard, J.J.: General histology of bone. In Bourne, G.H. (ed.): The Biochemistry and Physiology of Bone, Vol. I. 2nd ed. New York, Academic Press, 1972, p. 15.

18. Gebhardt, W.: Über funktionel wichtige Anordnungsweisen der feineren und grosseren Bauelemente des wirbeltier Knockens. 2. Spezieller Teil. Der Bau Der Haversischen Lamellen Systeme und seine functionelle Bedeutung. Arch. Entwicklungsmech. Organismen. 20:187, 1906.

19. Cooper, R.R., James, M.D., Milgram, J.W., and Robinson, R.A.: Morphology of the osteon. J. Bone Joint Surg. 48A:1239, 1966.

20. Owen, M.: Cellular dynamics of bone. In Bourne, G.H. (ed.): The Biochemistry and Physiology of Bone, Vol. III. 2nd ed. New York, Academic Press, 1972, p. 271.

21. Tonna, E.A.: A study of osteocyte formation and distribution in aging mice complemented with ^{3}H-proline autoradiography. J. Gerontol. 21:124, 1966.

22. Jowsey, J.: Metabolic Diseases of Bone. Philadelphia, W.B. Saunders Company, 1977, p. 61.

23. Ruth, E.B.: Further observations on histological evidence of osseous tissue resorption (abstract). Anat. Rec. 118:347, 1954.

24. Bélanger, L.F.: Osteocytic resorption. In Bourne, G.H. (ed.): The Biochemistry and Physiology of Bone, Vol. III. 2nd ed. New York, Academic Press, 1972, p. 239.

25. Duriez, J.: Les modifications calciques péri-ostéocytaires; étude microradiographique à l'analyseur automatique d'images. Nouv. Presse Med. 3:2007, 1974.

26. Liu, C.C., Baylink, D.J., and Wergedahl, J.: Vitamin D—enhanced osteoclastic bone resorption at vascular canals. Endocrinology 95:1011, 1974.

27. Holtrop, M.E., and Weinger, J.M.: Ultrastructural evidence for a transport system in bone. In Talmage, R.V., and Munson, P.L. (eds.): Calcium, Parathyroid Hormone and the Calcitonins. Excerpta Medica International Congress Series No. 243. Amsterdam, Excerpta Medica Foundation, 1972, p. 365.

28. Robinson, R.A.: Observations regarding compartments for tracer calcium in the body. In Frost, H.M. (ed.): Bone Biodynamics. Boston, Little, Brown & Company, 1964.

29. Baud, C.A.: The fine structure of normal and parathormone-treated bone cells. In Galliard, P.J., Van Den Hoof, A., and Steendijk, R. (eds.): Fourth European Symposium on Calcified Tissues. Excerpta Medica International Congress Series No. 120. Amsterdam, Excerpta Medica Foundation, 1966, p. 4.

30. Hancox, N.M.: The Osteoclast. In Bourne, G.H. (ed.): The Biochemistry and Physiology of Bone, Vol. I. 2nd ed. New York, Academic Press, 1972, p. 45.

31. Holtrop, M.E., Raisz, L.G., and Simmons, H.: The effects of PTH, colchicine and calcitonin on the ultrastructure and activity of osteoclasts in organ culture. J. Cell Biol. 60:346, 1974.

32. Walker, D.G.: Enzymatic and electron microscopic analysis of isolated osteoclasts. Calcif. Tissue Res. 9:296, 1972.

33. Vaes, G.: Lysosomes and the cellular physiology of bone resorption. In

Dingle, J.T., and Fell, H.B. (eds.): Lysosomes in Biology and Pathology, Vol. 1. Amsterdam, North-Holland Publishers, 1969, p. 217.

34. Owen, M.: The origin of bone cells. Int. Rev. Cytol. 28:213, 1970.

35. Jowsey, J.: Metabolic Diseases of Bone. Philadelphia, W.B. Saunders Co., 1977, p. 73.

36. Jaworski, Z.F.G., and Lok, E.: The rate of osteoclastic bone erosion in Haversian remodeling sites of adult dog's rib. Calcif. Tissue Res. 10:103, 1972.

37. Sledge, C.B.: Biochemical events in the epiphyseal plate and their physiological control. Clin. Orthop. Rel. Res. 61:37, 1968.

38. Scott, B.L.: The occurrence of specific cytoplasmic granules in the osteoclast. J. Ultrastruct. Res. 19:417, 1967.

39. Fischman, D.A., and Hay, E.D.: Origin of osteoclasts from mononuclear leukocytes in regenerating newt limbs. Anat. Rec. 143:329, 1962.

40. Jee, W.S.S., and Nolan, P.D.: Origin of osteoclasts from the fusion of phagocytes. Nature 200:225, 1963.

41. Bonucci, E.: New knowledge on the origin, function and fate of osteoclasts. Clin. Orthop. Rel. Res. 158:252, 1981.

42. Bingham, P.J., Brazell, I.A., and Owen, M.: The effect of parathyroid extract on cellular activity and plasma calcium levels in vivo. J. Endocrinol. 45:387, 1969.

43. Hancox, N.M.: The osteoclast. In Willmer, E.N. (ed.): Cells and Tissues in Culture, Vol. 2. New York, Academic Press, 1965, p. 261.

44. Frame, B., and Nixon, R.K.: Bone marrow mast cells in osteoporosis of aging. N. Engl. J. Med. 279:626, 1968.

45. Severson, A.R.: Mast cells in areas of experimental bone resorption and remodeling. Br. J. Exp. Pathol. 50:17, 1969.

46. Camus, J.P., Prier, A., Lièvre, J.A., Stephañ, J.C., and Laveant, C.: L'ostéoporose mastocytaire. Rev. Rhumat. 46:29, 1979.

47. Goldhaber, P.: Heparin enhancement of factors stimulating bone resorption in tissue culture. Science 147:407, 1965.

48. Griffith, G.C., Nichols, G., Jr., Asher, J.D., and Flanagan, B.: Heparin osteoporosis. JAMA 193:91, 1965.

49. Squires, J.W., and Pinch, L.W.: Heparin-induced spinal fractures. JAMA 241:2417, 1979.

50. Henderson, R.G., Russell, R.G.G., Earnshaw, M.J., Ledingham, J.G.G., Oliver, D.O., and Woods, C.G.: Loss of metacarpal and iliac bone in chronic renal failure: Influence of haemodialysis, parathyroid activity, type of renal disease, physical activity and heparin consumption. Clin. Sci. 56:317, 1979.

51. Mundy, G.R., Raisz, L.G., Cooper, R.A., Schechter, G.P., and Salmon, S.E.: Evidence for the secretion of an osteoclast stimulating factor in myeloma. N. Engl. J. Med. 21:1041, 1974.

52. Raisz, L.G., Luben, R.A., Mundy, G.R., Dietrich, J.W., Horton, J.E., and Trummel, C.L.: Effect of osteoclast activating factor from human leukocytes on bone metabolism. J. Clin. Invest. 56:408, 1975.

53. Krane, S.M., Brownell, G.L., Stanbury, J.B., and Corrigan, H.: The effect of thyroid disease on calcium metabolism in man. J. Clin. Invest. 35:874, 1956.

54. Mundy, G.R., Shapiro, J.L., Bandelin, J.G., Canalis, E.M., and Raisz, L.G.: Direct stimulation of bone resorption by thyroid hormones. J. Clin. J. Invest. 58:529, 1976.

55. Adinoff, A.D., and Hollister, J.R.: Steroid-induced fractures and bone loss in patients with asthma. N. Engl. J. Med. 309:265, 1983.

56. Hahn, T.J.: Corticosteroid-induced osteopenia. Arch. Intern. Med. 138:882, 1978.

57. Gluck, O.S., Murphy, W.A., Hahn, T.J., and Hahn, B.: Bone loss in adults receiving alternate day glucocorticoid therapy: A comparison with daily therapy. Arthritis Rheum. 24:892, 1981.

58. Chyun, Y.S., and Raisz, L.G.: Opposing effects of prostaglandin E_2 and cortisol on bone growth factor in organ culture. Clin. Res. 30:387A, 1982.

59. Suzuki, Y., Ichikawa, Y., Saito, E., and Homma, M.: Importance of increased urinary calcium excretion in the development of secondary hyperparathyroidism of patients under glucocorticoid therapy. Metabolism 32:151, 1983.

60. Klein, D.C., and Raisz, L.G.: Prostaglandin: Stimulation of bone resorption in tissue culture. Endocrinology 86:1436, 1970.

61. Tashjian, A.H., Jr., Voelkel, E.F., Levine, L., and Goldhaber, P.: Evidence that the bone resorption-stimulating factor produced by mouse fibrosarcoma cells is prostaglandin E_2: A new model for the hypercalcemia of cancer. J. Exp. Med. 136:1329, 1972.

62. Raisz, L.G., Sandberg, A., Goodson, J.M., Simmons, H.A., and Mergenhagen, S.E.: Complement-dependent stimulation of prostaglandin synthesis and bone resorption. Science 185:789, 1974.

63. Robinson, D.R., McGuire, M.B., and Levine, L.: Prostaglandins in the rheumatic diseases. Ann. N.Y. Acad. Sci. 256:318, 1975.

64. Raisz, L.G., and Kream, B.E.: Regulation of bone formation: N. Engl. J. Med. 309:29 (Part I), 309:83 (Part II), 1983.

65. Weidenreich, F.: Das Knochengewebe. In von Möllendorff, W. (ed.): Handbuch der mikroskopischen Anatomie des Menschen, Vol. 2. Berlin and New York, Springer-Verlag, 1930, p. 408.

66. Boyde, A., and Hobdell, M.H.: Scanning electron microscopy of lamellar bone. Z. Zellforsch. 93:213, 1969.

67. Dyson, E.D., Jackson, C.K., and Whitehouse, W.J.: Scanning electron microscope studies of human trabecular bone. Nature 225:957, 1970.

68. Cohen, J., and Harris, W.H.: The three-dimensional anatomy of haversian systems. J. Bone Joint Surg. 40A:419, 1958.

69. Boyde, A.: Scanning electron microscopic studies of bone. In Bourne, G.H. (ed.): The Biochemistry and Physiology of Bone, Vol. I. 2nd ed. New York, Academic Press, 1972, p. 259.

70. Kerley, E.R.: The Microscopic Determination of Age in Human Bone. University of Michigan, Ph.D. Anthropology, 1962.

71. Tischendorf, F.: Die mechanische Reaktion der haversschen Systeme und ihrer Lamellen auf experimentelle Belastung (nebst Bemerkungen zur Histogenese des lamellaren Knochengewebes). Wilhelm Roux Arch. Entwicklungsmechanik 146:661, 1954.

72. Ascenzi, A., and Bell, G.H.: Bone as a mechanical engineering problem. In Bourne, G.H. (ed.): The Biochemistry and Physiology of Bone, Vol. I. 2nd ed. New York, Academic Press, 1972, p. 311.

73. Wolff, J.: Das Gesetz der Transformation der Knochen. Berlin, Hirschwald, 1892.

74. Koch, J.C.: The laws of bone architecture. Am. J. Anat. 21:177, 1917.

75. Lacroix, P.: The internal remodeling of bones. In Bourne, G.H. (ed.): The Biochemistry and Physiology of Bone, Vol. III. 2nd ed. New York, Academic Press, 1972, p. 119.

76. Johnson, L.C.: Morphologic analysis in pathology: The kinetics of disease and general biology of bone. In Frost, H.M, (ed.): Bone Biodynamics. Boston, Little, Brown & Company, 1964, p. 543.

77. Pugliarello, M.C., Vittur, F., de Bernard, B., Bonucci, E., and Ascenzi, A.: Chemical modifications in osteones during calcification. Calc. Tissue Res. 5:108, 1970.

78. Miller, E.J., and Matukas, V.J.: Chick cartilage collagen: A new type of alpha-1 chain not present in bone or skin of the species. Proc. Natl. Acad. Sci. 64:1264, 1969.

79. Glimcher, M.J.: Studies of the structure, organization and reactivity of bone collagen. In Gibson, T. (ed.): Proceedings of the International Symposium on Wound Healing. Montreaux Found. Intern. Coop. Med. Sci., 1975, p. 253.

80. Pinnell, S.R., Fox, R., and Krane, S.M.: Human collagens: Differences in glycosylated hydroxylysines in skin and bone. Biochim. Biophys. Acta. 229:119, 1971.

81. Herring, G.M.: The chemical structure of tendon cartilage, dentin and bone matrix. Clin. Orthop. 60:261, 1968.

82. Castellani, A.A.: Protein-polysaccharides from ossifying cartilage and cornea. In Fitton-Jackson, S., Harkness, R.D., Partridge, S.M., and Tristram, G.R. (eds.): Structure and Function of Connective and Skeletal Tissue. London, Butterworths, 1965, p. 131.

83. Herring, G.M.: The organic matrix of bone. In Bourne, G.H. (ed.): The Biochemistry and Physiology of Bone, Vol. I. 2nd ed. New York, Academic Press, 1972, p. 127.

84. Shapiro, I.M., Wuthier, R.E., and Irving, J.T.: A study of the phospholipids of bovine dental tissues. I. Arch. Oral Biol. 11:501, 1966.

85. Posner, A.S.: Crystal chemistry of bone mineral. Physiol. Rev. 49:760, 1969.

86. Brown, W.E.: Crystal growth of bone mineral. Clin. Orthop. 44:205, 1966.

87. Vaughan, J.M.: Osteogenic cells. In The Physiology of Bone. Oxford, Oxford University Press, 1970, p. 110.

88. Glimcher, M.J., and Krane, S.M.: The organization and structure of bone and the mechanism of calcification. In Ramachandran, G.N., and Gould, B.S. (eds.): Treatise on Collagen, Vol. IIB, Biology of Collagen. New York, Academic Press, 1968, p. 68.

89. Baylink, D., Wergedal, J., and Thompson, E.: Loss of protein polysaccharides at sites where bone mineralization is initiated. J. Histochem. Cytochem. 20:279, 1972.

90. Anderson, H.C.: Vesicles associated with calcification in the matrix of epiphyseal cartilage. J. Cell Biol. 41:59, 1969.

91. Bonucci, E.: The locus of initial calcification in cartilage and bone. Clin. Orthop. 78:108, 1971.

92. Ali, S.Y., Sajdera, S.W., and Anderson, H.C.: Isolation and characterization of calcifying matrix vesicles from epiphyseal cartilage. Proc. Natl. Acad. Sci. 67:1513, 1970.

93. Glimcher, M.J.: Composition, structure and organization of bone and other mineralized tissues and the mechanism of calcification. Handbook of Physiology: Endocrinology, VII. Baltimore, Williams & Wilkins Company, 1976, p. 25.

94. Hodge, A.J., and Petruska, J.A.: Recent studies with the electron microscope on ordered aggregates of the tropocollagen macromolecule. In Ramachandran, G.N. (ed.): Aspects of Protein Structure. New York, Academic Press, 1963, p. 289.

95. Krane, S.M., Stone, M.J., Francois, C.J., and Glimcher, M.J.: Collagens and gelatins as phosphoryl acceptors for protein phosphokinase. Biochim. Biophys. Acta III:562, 1965.

96. Gallop, P.M., Lian, J.B., and Hauschka, P.Z.: Carboxylated calcium-binding proteins and vitamin K. N. Engl. J. Med. 302:1460, 1980.

97. Lian, J.B., Pachman, L.M., Gundberg, C.M., Partridge, R.E., and Maryjowski, M.C.: Gamma-carboxyglutamate excretion and calcinosis in juvenile dermatomyositis. Arthritis Rheum. 25:1094, 1982.

98. Gundberg, C.M., Lian, J.B., and Gallop, P.M.: Measurements of gamma-carboxyglutamate and circulating osteocalcin in normal children and adults. Clin. Chem. Acta 128:1, 1983.

99. Jowsey, J.: Microradiography: A morphologic approach to quantitating bone turnover. Excerpta Medica International Congress Series No. 270. Amsterdam, Excerpta Medica Foundation, 1972, p. 114.

100. Gardner, E.: Osteogenesis in the human embryo and fetus. In Bourne, G.H. (ed.): The Biochemistry and Physiology of Bone, Vol. III, 2nd ed. New York, Academic Press, 1972.

101. Sissons, A.: The growth of bone. In Bourne, G.H. (ed.) :The Biochemistry and Physiology of Bone, Vol. III. 2nd ed. New York, Academic Press, 1972.

102. Garn, S.M.: The course of bone gain and the phases of bone loss. Orthop. Clin. North Am. 3:503, 1972.

103. Cooper, R.R., and Misol, S.: Tendon and ligament insertion: A light and electron microscopic study. J. Bone Joint Surg. 52A:1, 1970.

104. Shim, S.S.: Physiology of blood circulation of bone. J. Bone Joint Surg. 50A:812, 1968.

105. Rhinelander, F.W.: Circulation of bone. In Bourne, G.H. (ed.): The Biochemistry and Physiology of Bone, Vol. II. 2nd ed. New York, Academic Press, 1972.

106. Sledge, C.B.: Epiphyseal injuries. In Cave, E.F., Burke, J.F. and Boyd, R.J. (eds): Trauma Management. Chicago, Year Book Medical Publishers, 1974.

107. Trueta, J.: Studies of the Development and Decay of the Human Frame. Philadelphia, W.B. Saunders Company, 1968.

108. Reifenstein, E.C., Jr.: Definitions, terminology and classification of metabolic bone disorders. Clin. Orthop. 9:30, 1957.

109. Shimmins, J., Anderson, J.B., Smith, D.A., and Aitken, M.: The accuracy and reproducibility of bone mineral measurements "in vivo." Clin. Radiol. 23:42, 1972.

110. Donaldson, C.L., Hulley, S.B., Vogel, J.M., Hattner, R.S., Bayers, J.H., and McMillan, D.E.: Effect of prolonged bedrest on bone mineral. Metabolism 19:1071, 1970.

111. Mack, P.B., LaChance, P.A., Vose, G.P., and Vogt, F.B.: Bone demineralization of foot and hand of Gemini-Titan IV, V, and VII astronauts during orbital flight. Am. J. Roentgenol. Rad. Ther. Nucl. Med. 100:503, 1967.

112. Barnett, E., and Nordin, B.E.C.: The radiological diagnosis of osteoporosis: A new approach. Clin. Radiol. 11:166, 1960.

113. Meema, H.E.: Cortical bone atrophy and osteoporosis as a manifestation of aging. Am. J. Roentgenol. Rad. Ther. Nucl. Med. 89:1287, 1963.

114. Meema, H.E., and Meema, S.: Prevention of postmenopausal osteoporosis by hormone treatment of the menopause. Can. Med. Assoc. J. 99:248, 1968.

115. Jowsey, J.: Metabolic Diseases of Bone. Philadelphia, W.B. Saunders Company, 1977, p. 45.

116. Wakamatsu, E., and Sissons, H.A.: The cancellous bone of the iliac crest. Calcif. Tissue Res. 4:147, 1969.

117. Singh, M., Riggs, B.L., Beabout, J.W., and Jowsey, J.: Femoral trabecular pattern index for evaluation of spinal osteoporosis: A detailed methodologic description. Mayo Clin. Proc. 48:184, 1973.

118. Heaney, R.P., and Whedon, G.D.: Radiocalcium studies of bone formation rate in human metabolic bone disease. J. Clin. Endocrinol. Metabol. 18:1246, 1958.

119. Neer, R., Berman, M., Fisher, L., and Rosenberg, L.E.: Multicompartmental analysis of calcium kinetics in normal adult males. J. Clin. Invest. 46:1364, 1967.

120. Marshall, J.H.: Measurements and models of skeletal metabolism. In Comar, C.L., and Bronner, F. (eds.): Mineral Metabolism, Vol. III. New York, Academic Press, 1969.

121. Cohn, S.H., Shukla, K.K., Dombrowski, C.S., and Fairchild, R.G.: Design and calibration of a "broad-beam" ^{238}Pu, Be neutron source for total body neutron activation analysis. J. Nucl. Med. 13:487, 1972.

122. Aloia, J.F., Ellis, K., Zanzi, I., and Cohn, S.H.: Photon absorptimetry and skeletal mass in the treatment of osteoporosis. J. Nucl. Med. 16:196, 1975.

123. Goldsmith, N.E., Johnston, J.O., Ury, H., Vose, G., and Colbert, C.: Bone mineral estimation in normal and osteoporotic women: A comparability trial of four methods and seven bone sites. J. Bone Joint Surg. 53A:83, 1971.

124. Cameron, J.R., and Sorenson, J.: Measurement of bone mineral in vivo: An improved method. Science 142:230, 1963.

125. Hansson, T.H., Ross, R.O., and Nachemson, A.: Development of osteopenia in the fourth lumbar vertebra during prolonged bed rest after operation for scoliosis. Acta Orthop. Scand. 46:621, 1975.

126. Genant, H.K., and Body, D.: Quantitative bone mineral analysis using dual energy computed tomography. Invest. Radiol. 12:545, 1977.
127. Genant, H.K., Turski, P.A., and Moss, A.A.: Advances in CT assessment of metabolic and endocrine disorders. Adv. Intern. Med. 28:409, 1983.
128. Krane, S.M., Munoz, A.J., and Harris, E.D., Jr.: Urinary polypeptides related to collagen synthesis. J. Clin. Invest. 49:716, 1970.
129. Nagant de Deuxchaisnes, C., and Krane, S.M.: The treatment of adult phosphate diabetes and Fanconi syndrome with neutral sodium phosphate. Am. J. Med. 43:508, 1967.
130. Chalmers, J., Conacher, W.D.H., Gardner, D.L., and Scott, P.: Osteo-malacia—a common disease in elderly women. J. Bone Joint Surg. 49B:403, 1967.
131. Jowsey, J., Kelly, P.J., Riggs, B.L., Bianco, A.J., Scholz, D.A., and Gershon-Cohen, J.: Quantitative microradiographic studies of normal and osteoporotic bone. J. Bone Joint Surg. 47A:785, 1965.
132. Byers, P.D.: The diagnostic value of bone biopsies. In Avioli, L.V., and Krane, S.M. (eds.): Metabolic Bone Disease, Vol. I. New York, Academic Press, 1977.
133. Dequeker, J., and Johnston, C.C., Jr.: Non-invasive Bone Measurements: Methodological Problems, Oxford, Eng., Wash. D.C., IRL Press, 1982.

Chapter 18

Structure and Function of the Motor Unit

Walter G. Bradley and Paul F. Good

INTRODUCTION

The function of the muscles is to produce force and movement. Their structure and biochemistry are intimately directed to this end, and the control of their activity is achieved through the motor nerves. This chapter provides a brief outline of current knowledge of neuromuscular function.

ANATOMY

The motor unit is the functional unit of striated muscle activity. It consists of an alpha motoneuron in the anterior horn of the spinal cord or the motor nuclei of the brainstem, its peripheral axon, and the muscle fibers on which it synapses. The number of muscle fibers in a motor unit ranges from the tens in the extraocular muscles to the thousands in the large proximal limb muscles. The domain of one motor unit is intermingled with the domains of other units and covers an area of 5 to 10 mm in transverse section. Motor units are of three distinct functional and biochemical types: slow twitch (S, type 1), fast twitch, fatigue resistant (FR, type 2A), and fast twitch, easily fatigued (FF, type 2B). The slow twitch fibers rely predominantly on mitochondrial oxidative metabolism for energy production. They have slower rates of contraction and relaxation, and their motoneuron fires more tonically than in type 2 units. The FF (type 2B) fibers rely predominantly on glycolysis and intracellular stores of glycogen for energy supply, fire phasically in short bursts, and are rapidly fatigued. The type 2A fibers are fast-contracting fibers and have both high glycolytic and high mitochondrial activity; they are thus fatigue resistant. Though it is standard to teach that slow motor units are used for maintaining posture and that fast motor units are used for rapid movements, recent evidence indicates that in man this distinction is less than absolute.

The myosin ATPase, which is responsible for the transduction of biochemical energy to contractile force, is different in type 1 and type 2 fibers with regard to pH optima and stability. These differences form the basis of the myosin ATPase stains used for the histochemical typing of muscle fibers.

A single muscle *fiber* (Fig. 18–1) is the cellular unit of the muscle. Each fiber is a syncytium of postmitotic myoblasts. Each fiber has a basal lamina which surrounds it and is bound together with other fibers into bundles of *fascicles* by a thin layer of collagen, the *endomysium*. Thicker sheets of collagen, the *perimysium*, bind fascicles together and surround the entire muscle (*epimysium*). The muscle fibers can course the entire length of a muscle (up to 34 cm in the human sartorius muscle) or can insert laterally into tendons (pennate muscles) or, rarely, can make muscle-muscle attachments. Muscle fibers vary in diameter from 10 to 100 μm, with a mean diameter in normal muscle of about 50 μm. The collagen of the tendon (or other connective tissue) is physically attached to the basal lamina of the muscle fiber. Muscle is invested with a capillary bed, intramuscular nerves, and a specialized sensory organ, the *spindle*, composed of 4 to 12 *intrafusal* muscle fibers and associated with γ motor and sensory nerve fibers.

The extrafusal muscle fibers contain up to thousands of postmitotic nuclei, which were the original nuclei of the mononucleated myoblasts. They are oriented longitudinally beneath the muscle fiber plasma membrane (the *sarcolemma*) and are called sarcolemmal nuclei.

CONTRACTILE PROTEINS

The predominant constituents (about 75 percent) of the muscle fiber cytoplasm (*sarcoplasm*) are the myofibrils, which consist predominantly of the contractile proteins, actin and myosin.

Actin (Figure 18-2) is a globular single-chain protein

SKELETAL MUSCLE

Figure 18–1. Diagram of the organization of skeletal muscle from the gross to the molecular level. *F, G, H,* and *I* are cross sections of the levels indicated. (From Bloom, W., and Fawcett, D.W.: A Textbook of Histology. 10th ed. Philadelphia, W. B. Saunders Co., 1975.)

(G-actin) with a molecular weight of about 42,000 daltons and a diameter of 5.5 nm. It will polymerize into a double-stranded helical filament (F-actin). This helix has a half pitch or repeating distance of 38.5 nm. Each molecule of G-actin can bind to the head of a myosin molecule. Associated with each strand of F-actin is one molecule of *tropomyosin* extending along seven molecules of G-actin and one molecule of *troponin* at the end of each tropomyosin molecule. These are regulatory proteins involved in the control of muscular contraction and relaxation.

Myosin (Fig. 18–3) is a large, elongated molecule of about 460,000 daltons. It is about 160 nm long with a globular head at one end. It is composed of two identical heavy chains that are predominantly α helical and are supercoiled around each other. At one end, the heavy chains are folded into globular structures, which, along with four light chains, form the head. The myosin mol-

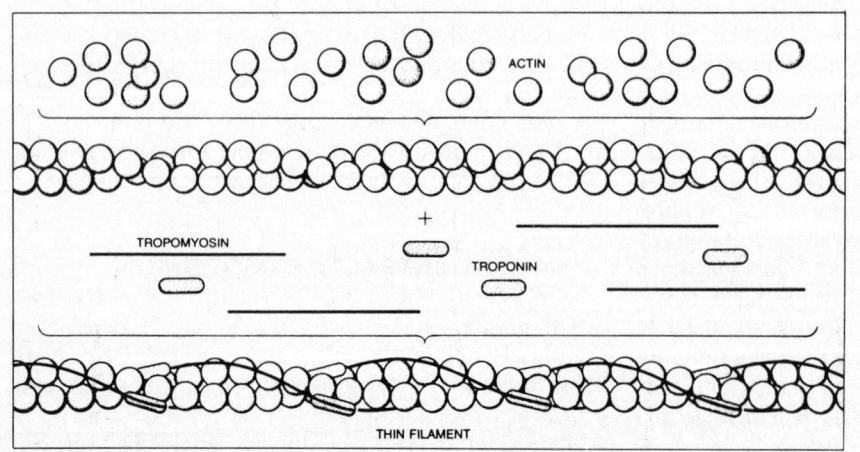

Figure 18–2. A thin filament contains actin, tropomyosin, and troponin molecules, assembled as shown schematically here. The spherical actin molecules are arranged like a double string of beads twisted to form a helix. A tropomyosin molecule extends along seven actin molecules, and there is one troponin molecule near the end of each tropomyosin. (From Murray, J.M., and Weber, A.: The cooperative action of muscle proteins. Copyright © 1974 by Scientific American, Inc. All rights reserved.)
batch 18 p. 288

Figure 18–3. *A*, A diagram of the myosin molecule with its two identical sub-units. The enzyme trypsin preferentially cleaves the molecule in two between the parts labeled as heavy meromyosin (HMM) and light meromyosin (LMM) because of their relative molecular weights. Further enzymatic digestion of HMM produces subfragments S_1 and S_2. *B*, A diagram showing the arrangement of myosin molecules in a filament. The heads of the molecules are oriented towards the two ends, while the tails of the molecules are oriented towards the center. *C*, X-ray diffraction patterns indicate that the filament in part *B* is twisted into a helix with a spacing of about 43 nm. The heads of the myosin molecules, here indicated by pegs, would then be spaced just above 14 nm apart and rotated 120 degrees from each other. *D*, Cross-sectional diagram showing that over a distance of 43 nm crossbridges from each thick filament will project toward all six neighboring thin filaments in the hexagonal array. (From Stein, R.B.: Nerve and Muscle: Membranes, Cells, and Systems. New York, Plenum Press, 1980.)
p. 289

Figure 18–4. Longitudinal section of frog sartorius muscle (top) together with diagram showing the overlap of filaments that gives rise to the band pattern. The A band is most dense in its lateral zones, where the thick and thin filaments overlap. The central zone of the A band (the H zone) is less dense, since it contains thick filaments only. The I bands are less dense still because they contain only thin filaments. The sarcomere length here is about 2.5 μm. (From Huxley, H.E.: Molecular basis of contraction in cross striated muscle. *In*, The Structure and Function of Muscle. Vol. 1. Bourne, G.H.: New York, Academic Press, 1972.)
p. 289

ecule can be split by trypsin into a part containing about 96 nm of the tail, called light meromyosin (LMM), and the remainder, including the head, called heavy meromyosin (HMM). The HMM can be further split by papain into the head (S_1) and the rest of the tail (S_2). The subunits form functional parts of the myosin molecule. The myosin head has the enzymatic activity of ATPase (myosin ATPase).

Myosin molecules will aggregate to form a myosin filament. They begin with a tail-to-tail association and add additional molecules with heads all pointing away from the initiation point, toward the end of the filament (Fig. 18–3). This central initiation point therefore has no myosin heads (forming the M line, described below). The myosin filament is constructed so that myosin heads are paired on opposite sides of a filament and each additional pair is rotated 120 degrees, at a distance of 14.3 nm. This causes the repeat distance to be three sets of pairs, or 42.9 nm. Neither of these distances is an integral multiple of the G-actin size or the F-actin repeat distance, which has significance for the smooth contraction of muscle (see below).

ULTRASTRUCTURE OF THE MUSCLE FIBER

The contractile filaments are bound together in parallel bundles to form a *myofibril*. The actin filaments are bound together at the Z line and interdigitate in a hexagonal pattern with the myosin filaments, which are bound together at their central zone (the M line). The area from one Z line to the next, a *sarcomere* (Figs. 18–1 and 18–4), is composed of the region of actin filaments alone (the I [isotropic] *band*, which is about 1 μm at rest), the region of myosin filaments with or without interdigitating actin (the A [anisotropic] *band*, which is about 1.6 μm at rest), and the region on either side of the M line with no actin (*the H zone*).

In addition to the contractile proteins there are two sets of tubules running among the myofibrils (Fig. 18–5). There is a transverse system (the *T tubules*). Each T tubule is an invagination of sarcolemma, which runs to the interior of the fiber at the A-I band junction. The other set of tubules, the *sarcoplasmic reticulum* (SR), is derived from the cellular endoplasmic reticulum. The

Figure 18–5. Schematic representation of the distribution of the sarcoplasmic reticulum around the myofibrils of skeletal muscle. The longitudinal sarcotubules are confluent with transverse elements called the terminal cisternae. A slender transverse tubule (T tubule) extending inward from the sarcolemma is flanked by two terminal cisternae to form the so-called triads of the reticulum. The location of these with respect to the cross banded pattern of the myofibrils varies from species to species. In frog muscle, depicted here, the triads are at the Z line. In mammalian muscle there are two to each sarcomere, located at the A-I junctions. (From Bloom, W., and Fawcett, D.W., A Textbook of Histology. 10th ed., Philadelphia, W.B. Saunders Co., 1975.)

Labels on figure: Myofibrils; Sarcolemma; Triad of the reticulum; Z line; Transverse tubule; A band; Sarcoplasmic reticulum; Mitochondrion; I band; Transverse tubule; Terminal cisternae; Sarcotubules

Figure 18–6. Vertebrate neuromuscular junction showing relationship of axon (*B*) and axon terminals (A₁, A₂, A₃) with Schwann cells (*S*) and perineural cells (*P*). Fibrocyte (*F*) lies adjacent to a Schwann cell. Basement lamina covering the muscle fiber and within the subneurial clefts is indicated by dots and Schwann cell basement lamina by crosshatching. Note presence of mitochondria, coated vesicles, and synaptic vesicles in all terminals. (From Hubbard, J.I.: Microphysiology of vertebrate neuromuscular transmission. Physiol. Rev. 53:674, 1973.)

SR runs essentially longitudinally, surrounds the myofibrils, and abuts the T tubules in a specialized structure, the *triad.* Also among the myofibrils are mitochondria, glycogen granules, lipid droplets, etc.

THE NEUROMUSCULAR JUNCTION

The sarcolemma has a specialization at the location of the motoneuron axon terminal, the *motor endplate* (Fig. 18– 6). This is a complex folding of the sarcolemma into the *primary synaptic cleft,* which conforms to the axon surface and from which project the *secondary synaptic clefts.* On the apex of each fold between the secondary synaptic clefts lie the *acetylcholine receptors (AChR),* which are proteins embedded in the plasma membrane. These AChR bind acetylcholine (ACh), the neurotransmitter of the neuromusclar junction.

Approximately 1 to 1.5 μm from the neuromuscular junction the nerve fiber loses its perineurial sheath, and the myelin is lost from the Schwann cell as well. A thin layer of Schwann cell cytoplasm continues until it meets the sarcolemma, where its basal lamina fuses with that of the muscle fiber. This fused basal lamina continues between the axon terminal and the sarcolemma. There is a 40- to 60-nm gap between the axon and the muscle fiber, the *synaptic gap.* Bound to the basal lamina of the synaptic gap is the enzyme *acetylcholinesterase (AChE),* which hydrolyzes the transmitter ACh.

The axon terminal contains unit membrane–bound *synaptic vesicles,* 40 to 50 nm in diameter, containing ACh, large coated vesicles about 100 nm in diameter, mitochondria, neurotubules, and neurofilaments.

PHYSIOLOGY OF THE MOTOR UNIT

The internal and external environments of nerve and muscle cells are quite different. Internally the concentration of potassium is high, and there is an electrical potential or voltage difference (polarization) of 70 to 90 mV negative with respect to the outside. Externally there is a high concentration of sodium, chloride, and calcium with respect to the inside. The resting potential (-70 mV) corresponds to the potassium equilibrium potential, since the cell membrane is freely permeable to potassium ion. The positive external potential resists the tendency for the potassium ion to flow outward toward its chemical equilibrium point. The resting membrane potential is created and maintained by the presence internally of large impermeable negative ions and the sodium pump, which extrudes sodium from the cell.

The sarcolemma contains voltage-dependent sodium channels, which run from the outside of the sarcolemma to the inside. At rest these are mainly closed (i.e., there is only a small resting permeability to sodium). A small depolarization opens some channels, increasing the sodium permeability, and thus tending to increase the depolarization. Below a threshold (about 20 to 30 mV) of depolarization this influx will be balanced by the efflux of the much more highly permeable potassium ion. At the *critical membrane depolarization potential* (that potential required to generate an action potential), the inward sodium current becomes regenerative, opening all the sodium channels, leading to depolarization of the sarcolemma to the sodium equilibrium potential of 20 mV positive internally. The sodium channels have an active closure mechanism, which terminates the influx of sodium. Repolarization is achieved by the opening of separate potassium channels, which allow the potassium ions to flow outward, restoring the resting membrane potential. The sodium is extruded by the sodium pump.

In the motoneuron the action potential is initiated in the cell body and propagated down the axon to the axon terminal. There the action potential opens specific calcium channels, which allow the entry into the axon terminal of calcium ions. The increase in intraterminal calcium concentration initiates release of the synaptic vesicles containing ACh. ACh is synthesized by the acetylation of choline by acetylcoenzyme A catalyzed by choline acetyltransferase (ChAT). There are about 10^4 molecules of ACh in each synaptic vesicle. Random events will allow the occasional discharge of one synaptic vesicle of ACh (*one quantum*). The ACh diffuses across the synaptic gap and binds to the AChR on the motor endplate membrane. This binding changes the physical conformation of the receptor and opens an ion channel permeable to sodium and other ions. Subsequently, the ACh is released from the receptor and hydrolyzed by AChE in the synaptic gap into choline and acetate. The choline is then taken up by the axonal terminal and synthesized to acetylcholine.

The depolarization of the motor endplate produced by one quantum of ACh (*miniature endplate potential*) is about 0.5 mV. The action potential reaching the axon terminal causes the release of 100 to 300 synaptic vesicles into the synaptic gap. This will depolarize the postsynaptic muscle membrane by about 50 mV, which is greater than the critical depolarization potential of the muscle membrane.

EXCITATION-CONTRACTION COUPLING

Activation of the muscle contractile mechanism is achieved by the propagation of an action potential along the muscle fiber and into the T-tubule system. The depolarization of the T-tubules induces the release of calcium ion from the SR into the sarcoplasm. The mechanism is not completely understood, but the coupling between the T-tubules and SR is mediated either by depolarization of the SR or, more likely, by influx of calcium from the extracellular to the intracellular space at the T-tubules, which induces further release of calcium from the SR (calcium-mediated calcium release).

The increased sarcoplasmic calcium binds to the troponin molecule on the actin filament, exposing the binding site on the G-actin monomer for the head of the myosin molecule. This process, from T-tubule depolarization to contraction, is termed *excitation-contraction coupling*.

THE BIOCHEMISTRY OF CONTRACTION

In the resting state (Fig. 18–7) the myosin head has a molecule of ATP bound to it. The entry of calcium into the sarcoplasm from the longitudinal sarcoplasm reticulum produces a calcium-troponin complex, the formation of which exposes the actin binding site and pro-

Figure 18–7. *A* Interactions between the head of a myosin molecule and a thin filament during one contraction cycle. The parts of the cycle are numbered and described in more detail in the text. *B*, For analysis of the overall kinetics of the cycle, it can be simplified, perhaps to as few as three rate-limiting steps. (From Stien, R. B. Nerve and Muscle: Membranes, Cells and Systems. New York, Plenum Press, 1980.), *C* Suggested behavior of myosin molecules in the thick filaments. The light meromyosin (LMM) of the molecule is bonded into the backbone of the filament, while the linear portion of the heavy meromyosin (HMM) component can tilt further out from the filament (by bending at the HMM–LMM junction), allowing the globular part of HMM (that is, the SI fragment) to attach to actin over a range of different side spacings while maintaining the same orientation. (From Huxley, H.E.: Molecular basis of contraction in cross striated muscle. *In* Bourne, G.H. (ed.): The Structure and Function of Muscle. Vol. 1. New York, Academic Press, 1972.)

duces an activated actin-myosin-ATP complex. The myosin molecule is bent away from the myosin filament at the HMM-LMM junction to reach the actin filament and achieve this binding. The myosin ATPase of the myosin head cleaves the ATP, yielding energy that rotates the myosin head about the S_1-S_2 junction. This moves the actin and myosin relative to one another (*sliding filaments*), producing muscle contraction. Dissociation from the myosin head of ADP and inorganic phosphate produces the low energy *rigor complex* (also found in rigor mortis). The binding of a molecule of ATP allows the dissociation of actin and myosin and the spontaneous return of the myosin head to its resting position. If calcium ions remain in high concentration in the sarcoplasm from repeated muscle action potentials, the actin and myosin filaments continue to slide past each other, producing further muscle contraction. The previously discussed lack of matching between the repeat distances of the action and myosin monomers allows a continuous application of force rather than a saltatory effect, which would result from the cross-bridges all lining up and rotating together.

The nerve and muscle action potentials can arrive at a higher frequency than the contraction cycling of actin-myosin, allowing a continuous contraction of the muscle fibers.

ATP-dependent reabsorption of sarcoplasmic calcium ions into the longitudinal SR occurs when the muscle action potentials cease. This allows regenerated ATP to remain bound to the myosin heads and removes the trigger for activation of actin and myosin. The tension produced by sliding of the filaments is removed, and the filaments return to their preactivated position. Thus, relaxation as well as contraction is an energy-dependent process.

MUSCLE ENERGY METABOLISM

The high energy compound ATP is replenished by the transfer of high-energy phosphate to ADP from *creatine phosphate*. This transfer is catalyzed by the enzyme *creatine kinase (CK)*. Rapid muscle contraction, as in sprinting, depends on the *glycolytic pathway* for the anaerobic production of ATP by conversion of glycogen to lactate (see Fig. 18–8). More sustained exertion depends on the oxidative metabolism initially of pyruvate produced by glycolysis (see Fig. 18–8), and later of *free fatty acids* derived from lipid droplets in the muscle fibers and fat depots of the body (see Fig. 18–9). Long-chain fatty acids cannot enter mitochondria. They must first be activated to fatty acylcoenzyme A, which is then converted to fatty acylcarnitine by carnitine palmityl transferase. The fatty acylcarnitine then enters the mitochondria and is reconverted to fatty acylcoenzyme A. It is then subject to beta oxidation for the production of ATP via the Krebs cycle and the mitochondrial electron transport chain.

Figure 18–8. Scheme of glycogen metabolism and glycolysis. Roman numerals refer to glycogen storage diseases and indicate the sites of metabolic block due to deficiency of the following enzymes: I, glucose-6-phosphatase; II, acid maltase; III, debrancher; IV, brancher; V, muscle phosphorylase; VI, liver phosphorylase; VII, muscle phosphofructokinase; VIII, liver dephosphophosphorylase kinase (G-1-P—glucose-1-phosphate; G-6P—glucose-6-phosphate; F-6-P—fructose-6-phosphate; F-1, 6-P—fructose-1, 6-diphosphate; UDPG—uridine diphosphate-glucose; PLD—phosphorylase limit dextrin). (From DiMauro, S.D., Metabolic myopathies. *In* Vinken, P.J., and Bruyn, G.W. (eds.): Handbook of Clinical Neurology. Vol. 41. North-Holland Publishing Co., Amsterdam, 1979.)

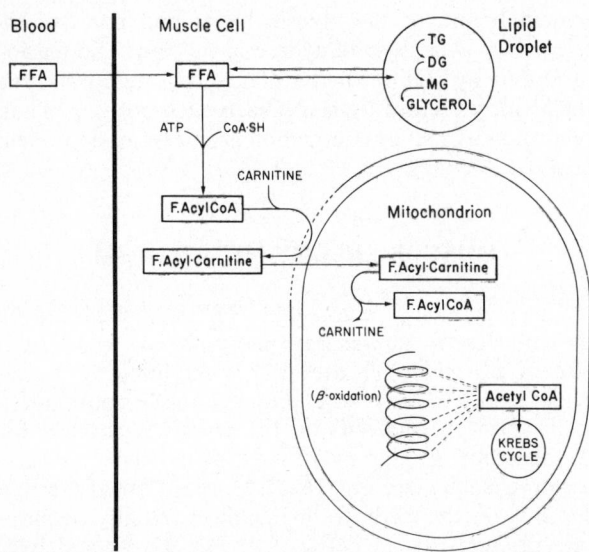

Figure 18–9. Scheme of intracellular long-chain fatty acid metabolism (FAA—free fatty acids; TG—triglyceride; DG—diglyceride; MG—monoglyceride). (From DiMauro, S.D.: Metabolic Myopathies. *In* Vinke, P.J., and Bruyn, G.W. (eds.); Handbook of Clinical Neurology. Vol. 41. North-Holland Publishing Co., Amsterdam, 1979.)

THE PHARMACOLOGY OF THE MOTOR UNIT

The nerve and muscle membranes are extremely sensitive to external ionic concentrations. As mentioned previously, ACh release requires external calcium as does excitation-contraction coupling. Therefore, removal of external calcium or high external magnesium concentrations will block ACh release.

If the external concentration of potassium falls below 2.5 mEq or rises above 7 mEq per liter, action potential initiation and conduction are compromised and muscle weakness results. Hypercalcemia (above 12 mg per ml), as in vitamin D intoxication, hyperparathyroidism, and carcinomatosis, will also cause lethargy and weakness, due mainly to central nervous system effects.

Certain drugs can inhibit the synthesis of ACh by blocking the uptake of choline into the nerve terminal. The major group of these compounds are quaternary ammonium ions, the best known being hemicholinium-3 (HC-3). They compete with choline for choline carrier sites. Other drugs can inhibit the synthesis of ACh by directly blocking choline acetyltransferase. These generally are analogs of choline or acetylcoenzymes, which bind to ChAT and modify the enzyme.

There are many animal venoms and toxins that have their effect on the nerve terminal as well as on the postsynaptic membrane (see below). The release of ACh is blocked by botulinum toxin, probably by reduction of the sensitivity of the ACh release mechanism to intracellular calcium. Beta-bungarotoxin has an effect similar to botulinum toxin. The venom of the black widow spider produces paralysis by causing the uncontrolled release of all the synaptic vesicles into the synaptic gap. Puffer fish toxin (tetrodotoxin) and paralytic shellfish poison (saxitoxin) selectively block sodium channels in nerve and muscle membranes, abolishing excitability. Local anesthetic drugs such as procaine and lidocaine block both sodium and potassium channels.

Other drugs act on the postsynaptic muscle membrane. Compounds such as decamethonium and succinylcholine depolarize the membrane by binding to the AChR, opening the ion channel, but are not hydrolyzed by AChE. Curarelike drugs and the α-bungarotoxin (cf. above) fraction of the venom of the Taiwan multibanded krait (*Bungarus multicinctus*) bind to the AChR without depolarization, thus preventing acetylcholine from binding and initiating an endplate potential.

In myasthenia gravis the body has produced immune antibodies against the acetylcholine receptor, which attack it and vastly reduce the number of receptors available for binding ACh. This large loss of ion channels diminishes the muscle's ability to produce an endplate potential, leading to rapid fatigability and weakness. *Anticholinesterases* such as neostigmine (Prostigmin), pyridostigmine (Mestinon), edrophonium (Tensilon), physostigmine (Eserine), as well as some "nerve gases" and organophosphorus insecticides, allow the accumulation of acetylcholine and therefore the increased function of the remaining AChR, partially reversing the effects of the lost AChR. In the healthy individual these lead to paralysis by continuous depolarization of the muscle membrane by nonhydrolysis of acetylcholine.

References

1. Katz, B.: Nerve, Muscle and Synapse. New York, McGraw Hill, 1966.
2. Bourne, G.H. (ed.): The Structure and Function of Muscle. New York, Academic Press, 1972.
3. Stein, R.B.: Nerve and Muscle: Membranes, Cells and Systems. New York, Plenum Press, 1980.
4. Hubbard, J.I.: Microphysiology of vertebrate neuromuscular transmission. Physiol. Rev. 53:674, 1973.
5. Pepe, R.A., Sanger, J.W., and Nachmias, V.T. (eds.): Motility in Cell Function. New York, Academic Press, 1979.
6. Squire, J.: The Structural Basis of Muscular Contraction. New York, Plenum Press, 1981.
7. Bowman, W.C.: Pharmacology of Neuromuscular Function. Baltimore, University Park Press, 1980.

Chapter 19

Peripheral Nerve: Structure, Function, and Dysfunction

John E. Castaldo and José Ochoa

INTRODUCTION

Disorders of the nerve fiber may affect the peripheral motor, sensory, or autonomic units in various combinations to produce muscle weakness, atrophy, skin numbness, paresthesias, pain, or dysautonomia. The specific constellation of symptoms and signs, and the tempo of evolution of neural dysfunction, judiciously interpreted in the light of nerve pathophysiology, provide useful preliminary evidence on the kind of pathology and the types of nerve fibers affected. Clinical electrophysiology sharpens detection of subclinical damage while clarifying the kind of primary nerve fiber pathology and its extent, if diffuse, as well as its precise location, if focal. Finally, neuromuscular biopsy endorses the indirect clinical and neurophysiological criteria for the type of fiber affected and the kind of nerve fiber pathology while potentially disclosing an etiology. What follows is an attempt to correlate normal and abnormal structure and function of peripheral nerve in order to optimize the clinical evaluation, diagnosis, and early treatment of peripheral neuropathy.

GENERAL ORGANIZATION OF THE PERIPHERAL NERVOUS SYSTEM

The peripheral nervous system is functionally organized into sensory, motor, and autonomic components. *Motor* nerve fibers emerge from anterior horn cell bodies in the spinal cord and from analogous brainstem nuclei. They exit via specific cranial nerves and anterior roots in the spinal cord to innervate extrafusal and intrafusal striated muscle fibers. The cell bodies of bipolar primary *sensory* neurons reside in dorsal root or cranial nerve ganglia. Sensory neurons give rise to fibers that innervate sensory receptors in skin, muscle, and deep tissues. Preganglionic sympathetic *autonomic* nerve cell bodies reside in the intermediolateral gray columns of the thoracic and first and second lumbar segments of the spinal cord. Preganglionic fibers emerge with ventral roots and enter the sympathetic chain as white rami to synapse with multipolar sympathetic ganglion cells. These neurons then give rise to postganglionic unmyelinated axons, which emerge from the ganglia as gray rami and innervate sweat glands and smooth muscle of blood vessels, hair, and other effector organs. Preganglionic neurons of the parasympathetic system reside in the brainstem, integrating functions of cranial nerves III, VII, IX, and X and in the S2 through S4 segments of the spinal cord. Axons from these cell bodies synapse in ganglia in close proximity to the smooth muscle, heart muscle, and glandular tissue they innervate.

GROSS STRUCTURE OF NERVE TRUNKS

Nerve trunks are composed of groups of macroscopic nerve fascicles bound together in a connective epineurial sheath. Within a laminated cellular perineurium, fascicles contain microscopic myelinated and unmyelinated fibers suspended amid collagen, at pressures of 0.4 to 2.9 mm Hg[1,2] (Fig. 19–1). Polygonal perineurial cells, linked by tight junctions and layered in concentric sleeves, constitute the major diffusion barrier within nerve.[3-5] This structure is instrumental in protecting the endoneurial fascicular contents from microorganisms and macromolecular substances, in particular, toxins and antigens.[6] While perineurial permeability may be altered in mechanical crush injuries to nerve, it is remarkably resistant to ischemia[7] and to mediators of the inflammatory response. Perineurium is also an effective barrier to pus cells, even when it is contiguous to tissue abscesses.[8]

Peripheral nerves are abundantly vascularized throughout their length by a widely anastomotic network of longitudinal and segmental arteries.[9,10] Nutrient arteries penetrate perineurium and form an endoneurial plexus composed largely of capillaries, which supply longitudinal segments of nerves. Small vessel occlusive disease with resultant damage to peripheral nerve most commonly occurs at the level of the epineurial arterioles and may occur in conjunction with a number of systemic diseases, including diabetes, polyarteritis, rheumatoid arthritis (RA), and systemic lupus erythematosus (SLE) as well as the cryoglobulinemic states. Intrafascicular capillaries are the site of the blood-nerve barrier (Fig. 19–2). Nutrients and metabolites that ultimately reach endoneurium must meet permeability requirements of the capillary endothelium.[11] Integrity of the endoneurium is fundamental for efficient nerve fiber regeneration of axons subsequent to wallerian degeneration. In particular, continuity of the basal lamina tubes of damaged nerve fibers allows regenerating nerve fibers to elongate through their original Schwann cell columns to be paired eventually with their target muscle fibers or sensory end organs.

Figure 19–1. Light micrograph of part of a normal human nerve in cross section. Abundant myelinated fibers are seen within two nerve fascicles, which are defined by thin perineurial sheaths. Connective tissue and fat globules intervene (glutaraldehyde-Epon-toluidine blue).

Figure 19–2. Electron-micrograph of cross section at the periphery of a normal human nerve fascicle. Slender perineurial cell processes course diagonally at top right. A capillary shows section across endothelial cell nucleus its lumen is filled with amorphous (plasma) material. The capillary as well as the perineurial cell surface are dressed by basal lamina. (glutaraldehyde-Epon-toluidine blue).

NERVE FIBER POPULATIONS AND SOME OF THEIR SELECTIVE DISORDERS

Most peripheral nerves contain mixtures of myelinated and unmyelinated fibers. Nothing in the fiber structure distinguishes sensory myelinated fibers from motor myelinated fibers or sensory unmyelinated fibers from autonomic unmyelinated fibers. In nerves to human skin, unmyelinated fibers are three to four times more numerous than myelinated fibers. In terms of fiber diameters, most nerves contain two populations of myelinated fibers and a single one of unmyelinated fibers (Fig. 19–3A). The fact that nerve conduction velocity is a function of axonal diameter (and degree of myelination) is reflected in the compound nerve action potential (NAP). When a nerve trunk is supramaximally stimulated at one point, the compound nature of the propagated wave can be displayed oscillographically by recording at a suitable conduction distance. The different elevations reflect more or less synchronous conduction along nerve fibers of the different populations.[12]

The modern classification of the components in the sensory NAP includes A-alpha (30 to 72 meters per second), A-delta (4 to 30 meters per second), and C (0.4 to 2 meters per second).[13] In human nerves, the fastest component of the sensory NAP can be comfortably recorded through the skin with surface electrodes.[14] All three components can be recorded in vitro following nerve biopsy[15] (Fig. 19–3B).

In nerves to skin, the large diameter myelinated fibers connect with low threshold mechanoreceptor units (RA, SA-I,SA-II) while A-delta fibers connect with cold units and with nociceptive units for sharp, "first" pain. Within the unmyelinated population and together with efferent sympathetic fibers are represented two categories of afferent cutaneous units: the high threshold nociceptive units for dull, "second" (C-type) pain and units for warmth.[16]

In nerves to muscle, the largest diameter myelinated fibers are proprioceptive spindle afferents, whereas the smallest are the fusimotor fibers destined for the end plates of intrafusal muscle. Unmyelinated fibers connected to muscle are sympathetic efferent or sensory afferent; the latter are probably concerned mostly with pain rather than with thermal sensation.

Diseases causing selective loss of unmyelinated fibers abolish C-type pain and itch and warmth sensations and also cause dysautonomia.[17] These diseases erase the C elevation in the compound NAP recorded in vitro, without affecting maximal motor conduction velocity or the fast component of the sensory nerve action potentials. On the other hand, selective block of myelinated fiber activity (for example, through the ischemic block induced by placing a pneumatic cuff around a limb at suprasystolic pressure for about 30 minutes) causes paralysis and sensory loss, except for warmth and C-type pain.[18,19] Acute local nerve lesions caused by mechanical trauma tend to affect all nerve fiber types. "Neurapraxia" from acute local nerve compression is an exception in that it causes a specific pathologic lesion with conduction block of large diameter myelinated fibers only.[20]

AXONS AND AXOPLASM

Ultrastructurally, *axoplasm* contains smooth endoplasmic reticulum, mitochondria, and numerous microtubules and neurofilaments. Microtubules are well categorized as 240-Å (24-nm) diameter helical chains of dimer proteins with a central core of about 14 nm. These cytoskeletal structures probably play key roles as conduits for subcellular particle movements.[21] That particle movements occur in axons has been accepted for years. Weiss and Hiscoe[22] showed that placing a ligature around an axon or regenerating nerve resulted in focal distention of the axon proximal to the constricting band. They concluded that a continuous cellulofugal flow of axonal contents arises from neuronal perikaryon and is essential for maturation, maintenance, and regeneration of distal nerve fibers. Proteins and nutrients stored within the neuronal cell body must be conveyed along the nerve fiber; this is accomplished by *fast* and *slow axoplasmic transport mechanisms*. In addition to the anterograde trophic influences of the cell bodies on nerve fibers, Schwann cells, and effector organs, axoplasmic transport is also channeled in a *retrograde* manner, al-

Figure 19–3. *A,* Trimodal caliber spectrum (fiber size–frequency histogram) of normal human cutaneous (sural) nerve. Nerve fibers increase in number as they decrease in diameter. (Modified from Ochoa, J. and Mair, W.G.P. Acta Neuropathol. 13:197, 1969.) *B,* Diagrammatic representation of compound action potential of normal human sural nerve recorded in vitro, showing Aα, Aβ and C fiber potentials. (Modified from Dyck, P.J. et al.: Arch. Neurol. 20:490, 1969.)

lowing the periphery to feed back to the soma. Nerve growth factor is one example of a substance carried by retrograde transport; it is believed that feedback suppression due to axonal injury might trigger the necessary cellular reactions for nerve regeneration (chromatolysis).[23] Other substances carried by retrograde transport include tetanospasmin (tetanus toxin), herpes virus, and the useful cytologic marker, horseradish peroxidase.

Definitive measurements of axoplasmic flow were obtained in the 1960s from studies using isotope labeled tracers. Calculated flow rates of 1 to 3 mm per day were in keeping with the known rates of elongation of regenerating axons and with the simple early idea of "perpetual" bulk translocation of axoplasm. This slow transport system, however, did not account for why wallerian degeneration occurred so rapidly within a nerve only a few days after its transection. Interruption of a "fast" axoplasmic transport system was soon postulated and, in the late 1960s, transport systems attaining flow rates of 50 to 2000 mm per day were documented in different animal models.[24-26]

The mechanism underlying *fast axoplasmic transport* is incompletely understood. It is not dependent on propulsive force exerted in the neuronal cell body, but is dependent on local supplies of energy. The "transport filament" theory of Ochs proposes that the ATP activates crossbridges between bits of filaments that carry the transported material on axonal microtubules[27] (Fig. 19-4). The "sliding vesicle" theory also implicates microtubules as the guiding framework for fast transport.[24] These theories are supported by observations that colchicine and vinca alkaloid agents, which arrest mitosis by binding to microtubular subunits, also block fast transport in low doses. However, higher doses of these agents block *slow axonal transport* and electron microscopic studies of nerve after treatment with these agents have shown microtubules to be intact.[28] This evidence, along with critical studies of fast axoplasm recovery time after rewarming from cold injury, suggests that colchicine and vinblastine may exert their effects in some way other than through disaggregation of microtubular systems.[29] Other subcellular organelles may be crucial to the system of particle transport. Droz and colleagues have emphasized the importance of the longitudinal smooth endoplasmic reticulum in *fast axoplasmic transport* and demonstrated the passage of substances from axon to myelin by direct diffusion and by distribution via Schmidt-Lanterman clefts.[30]

As to the *slow axoplasmic displacement*, its physical mechanism also remains unknown; peristaltic waves have not been demonstrated in vivo in undisturbed nerve fibers. While a portion of the substances transported are "absorbed" as they pass down the axon or are used for renewal of material at the axon terminals, a portion are *"turned around"* and channeled in retrograde manner.

Defects in neuronal synthesis or axonal transport of materials cause various grades of atrophy or frank disintegration of the motor, sensory, and autonomic nerve fibers and target organs. The worst example is *wallerian*

Figure 19–4. Injection and sampling technique showing transport. The L7 ganglion shown in the insert contains T-shaped neurons with one branch ascending in the dorsal root, the other descending in the sciatic nerve. A pipette containing ^{3}H-leucine is passed into the ganglion; after its injection and the incorporation of precursor, the downflow of labeled components in the fibers is sampled at various times by sacrificing the animal and sectioning the nerve. Each segment is placed in a vial and solubilized; scintillation fluid is added; and the activity is counted. The outflow pattern is displayed on the ordinate log scale; the abscissa is in millimeters, taking the distance from the center of the ganglion as zero. A high level of activity is seen remaining in the ganglion region; more distally, a plateau rises to a crest before abruptly falling at the front of the crest to baseline levels. For motoneurons the left-hand side of the cord undergoes an injection of the precursor into the L7 cell body region followed by removal of ventral root and sciatic nerve at a later time for a similar treatment and display of outflow. (Reproduced by permission from Ochs, S. and Worth, R.M.: In Waxman, S.G.: Physiology and Pathobiology of Axons. New York, Raven Press, 1978, pp. 251–264.)

degeneration, by which anatomic interruption of the axon leads to fragmentation and resorption of axons and myelin in the distal stump and "denervation atrophy" of target organs. Empty Schwann cell columns (bands of Büngner), well characterized by electron microscopy, testify to past degeneration of myelinated and unmyelinated fibers, a useful pathologic criterion (Fig. 19-5).[31]

In a large number of neurologic diseases, a "dyingback" pattern of structural decay is observed, affecting first the most distal parts of the longest nerve fibers and spreading centripetally.[32] It is attributable to defective synthesis or flow of "trophic" material. Such a pattern explains distal emphasis of weakness, wasting, sensory loss, and reflex change. More recently, the expression *central-peripheral distal axonopathy* has been used to emphasize that often there is simultaneous involvement of the central and peripheral nervous systems[33] (Fig. 19-6). Important refinements in the concept of dying-back have been made as the result of experiments with neurotoxic agents that interfere with neuronal cell processing and axoplasmic transport.[34-42]

Axonal Regeneration. Even during the administration of toxic substances that cause axonal damage and degeneration, axonal *regeneration* may occur. In general,

Figure 19–5. Electron micrograph of cross-section through "denervated" or "empty" Schwann cell bands from human sural nerve. Large isolated, irregular band on the left (*Xm*) is typically ex-myelinated. On the right, smaller, grouped, more regularly shaped bands, one of which still contains a surviving unmyelinated axon (*u*), two of which contain probably axonal sprouts (arrows), while the remaining three are "denervated." (× 11,600) (Reproduced by permission from Ochoa, J.: Proceedings of the VIth International Congress of Neuropathology, p. 589, Masson et Cie, Paris, 1970.)

regeneration of an axon involves a number of steps, including (a) synthesis of new structural material; (b) its transport down the axon; (c) elongation of the new sprouts (at about 1 mm per day) consequent to locomotion of the growth cone and insertion of new material at the tip; (d) guidance of the sprouts to a peripheral target to re-establish a functional connection; and (e) myelination and maturation in diameter.

Predictably, in the dying-back axonopathies, the process of regeneration is upset,[43] and interference of growth cone dynamics may arrest elongation of new axons, at least as seen in tissue culture experimentation.[44] Regenerating axons that fail to establish functional connections with a peripheral target remain immature, and excess numbers of them are produced. Immature axon sprouts may behave abnormally as impulse generators.[45,46] In cross sections of nerves, regenerating myelinated axons are often grouped in characteristic "clusters" (Fig. 19–7), whereas regenerating unmyelinating axons distort the unimodal size-frequency histogram of axon diameters. These are further pathologic criteria substantiating past axonal degeneration.[47]

Schwann Cells and Myelin. There is a single kind of Schwann cell. Nevertheless, axons may be myelinated or unmyelinated. This is dependent upon the message given by the axon to its satellite cell. Groups of unmyelinated axons are packaged communally within Schwann cell chains, each axon separated from the others by enveloping Schwann cell cytoplasm whose cell tongues interdigitate to define the *mesaxon* (Fig. 19–8).

Individualization of a single axon in an exclusive Schwann cell is a prerequisite for myelination. During development, axons destined to become large in diameter myelinate first and more abundantly. Such early, short myelin segments are more exposed to developmental

stretch, especially in the limbs. As a result, in the adult, large diameter axons have thicker and longer myelin segments than small axons. New myelin segments laid on axons that regenerate in nerves of adults remain short. This constitutes yet another useful pathologic criterion[48,49] (Fig. 19–9).

Schwann cell cytoplasm is found internal to (adaxonal) and external to myelin sheaths. The adaxonal cytoplasm is traversed by the inner mesaxon and communicates with Schwann cell cytoplasm external to myelin through the Schmidt-Lanterman clefts. The *internode* (or segment) is that section of a nerve fiber subserved by a single Schwann cell bounded at its extremities by nodes of Ranvier. The node is enveloped by contiguous Schwann cells which interdigitate multiple fingerlike projections from cytoplasm external to myelin. External to Schwann cell plasma membrane lies a continuous *basement membrane (basal lamina) sleeve* to which collagen is intimately attached.

Within spinal roots, a short distance from the spinal cord, Schwann cells are abruptly replaced by oligodendroglia at nodes of Ranvier.[50,51] At this level, epineurium becomes dura mater, but endoneurium persists as far as the junction of roots with central nervous tissue. Inner layers of perineurium merge with the root sheath, which is in continuity with the subarachnoid space.

The myelin sheath is a compound unit membrane appendage and arises after cytoplasmic resorption of a Schwann cell process that has wrapped about an axon.[52,53] The concentric lamellae of the myelin spiral have a periodicity of 150 to 180 Å between *major dense lines.* These are separated by a less electron dense *intraperiod line* (Fig. 19–10). The darker staining, major dense line is formed by a fusion of the internal cytoplasmic faces of Schwann cell membrane, while the fain-

Figure 19–6. Cellular target sites of some neurotoxic chemicals illustrated by upper (*1*) and lower (*2*) motor neurons, dorsal root ganglion cells (*3*), and second order sensory neurons (*4*) in the gracile nucleus of the medulla oblongata. The central nervous system (CNS) is represented above the sloping horizontal line; the peripheral nervous system (MNS), below. The peripheral receptors on fibers *A–C* are Pacinian corpuscles. Fibers *D–F* innervate extrafusal muscle fibers. *A*, Neuronopathy: The excitotoxin alanosine acts as a false transmitter at neuron 4, causing maintained depolarization leading to cellular damage. *B*, Neuronopathy: Doxorubicin irreversibly damages neuron *3*, resulting in a rapid anterograde (arrows) pattern of total axonal breakdown and myelin loss. *C*, Central distal axonopathy: Clioquinol induces retrograde degeneration of the central axonal process of the dorsal root ganglion cell (*3*) but leaves the cell and peripheral process intact. *D*, Central-peripheral distal axonopathy: 2,5-hexanedione causes retrograde axonal degeneration (*a*) to develop slowly in long and large central and peripheral axons. Muscle atrophy will occur unless axons regenerate and sprouts reinnervate the muscle. The anterior horn cell (*2*) is left intact, and eventually (after months to years) a secondary demyelination in the ventral root ensues (*d*). *E*, IDPN causes a giant axonal swelling (*a*) to develop in the intraspinal portion of the axon; the distal axon at the distal axon attenuates but does not degenerate. *F*, Myelinopathy: AETT causes myelin bubbling (*d*) focally along the axon of large diameter central (*1*) and peripheral (*2*) axons. Axonal denudation is followed by remyelination: this is occurring in the ventral roots (*r*) and medulla oblongata when demyelination (*d*) is in progress in the peripheral nerve and elsewhere. A similar process would occur in a primary disease of the myelinating cell except that remyelination might not occur during intoxication. (Reproduced by permission from Spencer, P., and Schaumburg, H., (ed.): Experimental and Clinical Neurotoxicology. Baltimore, Williams & Wilkins, 1980, pp. 92–99.)

ter staining, intraperiod line represents its paired apposed external surfaces.

Peripheral myelin is composed of water (40 percent net weight), lipids (75 percent dry weight), and protein (25 percent).[54] It is structurally quite different from central myelin, containing less glycolipid and more sphingomyelin in polyunsaturated fatty acid than its central counterpart. Myelin proteins and lipids are interesting in that they are immunogenic and may play a role in experimental "allergic neuritis" in animals and in idiopathic inflammatory demyelinating neuropathy in man.[55]

Axolemma. Like the surface membranes of other electrically excitable cells, the unit membrane enveloping the axon is specialized to generate all-or-nothing action potentials in response to adequate excitation. A differ-

ence of -15 to -100 mV electrochemical potential exists between the inside of any cell and the extracellular fluid of warm-blooded animals. This is generated largely by selective permeability features of the resting membrane and by the fact that various species of ions (chiefly sodium, potassium, chloride, and large protein anions) are unequally distributed across the plasma membrane. Intracellular potassium and large impermeable protein anions exceed extracellular concentrations of these ions by a ratio of 50:1. At rest, the axolemma is selectively permeable to potassium ions, which tend to diffuse outward along their chemical concentration gradient. Net potassium efflux leads to the progressive development of a transmembrane voltage that apposes further outward potassium movement. Such is the *potassium equilibrium potential* (E_k); it largely determines the value of

Figure 19–7. Cross section of a cluster of regenerated fibers from the sural nerve of a patient with isoniazid neuropathy. Within the unit there are small myelinated fibers and axons devoid of myelin (arrows) suspended in their Schwann cells. A "growth cone" (*gc*) also occurs. The various subunits and the fibroblast (*F*) fit to complement an oval pattern. (Osmium tetroxide immersion fixation, × 7200.) (Reproduced by permission from Ochoa, J.: In Dyck, P.J., et al. (eds.): Peripheral Neuropathy. Philadelphia, W.B. Saunders Co., 1975, pp. 131–150.)

the membrane potential at rest. The resting membrane is to some extent also permeable to sodium ions. Since the concentration of sodium is higher outside the cell than inside the cell, sodium passively "leaks" into the cell, propelled there by electrochemical forces. This inward flow of positive charges tends to balance the ionic disequilibrium and to decrease the resting membrane

Figure 19–8. Electron micrograph across normal human unmyelinated fibers. Multiple axons devoid of myelin congregate in space, wrapped individually or in subgroups by Schwann cell processes which separate the axons from the collagen-rich endoneurial spaces.

potential established by the potassium leak outward. Maintenance of the steady concentration gradient across the membrane is secured by active transport of sodium ions outward and potassium ions inward against their concentration gradients at the expense of ATP.

The above description concerns the axolemma at rest. But this electrically excitable membrane contains ion-specific, voltage-dependent channels through which ions can move to generate action potentials. These channels may be opened or closed depending on the electrical potential across the membrane. At resting membrane potential (polarized negatively inside to about −80 mV), the channels are closed but available for activation. Depolarization of the membrane may occur by application of cathode current to the nerve membrane, by mechanical deformation of axolemma, or naturally by the arrival of positive charges to the inside of the axon during propagation of action potentials. At an intracellular potential difference of about −50 mV, threshold is reached for opening (activation; m) of voltage-dependent sodium channels in the axolemma. This permits the sudden influx of sodium along its concentration and electrochemical gradients in a positive feedback fashion. Indeed, the rapid influx of sodium further depolarizes the membrane, which activates more voltage-dependent sodium channels, thus accelerating the course of the all-or-none depolarizing shift, which eventually overshoots zero potential. After a few milliseconds, sodium influx is interrupted by voltage-dependent closure (h) of sodium channels. During this same period, there is opening of voltage-regulated potassium channels. This allows for rapid efflux of positive charges, which repolarize the membrane potential down toward its original potassium (resting) equilibrium potential. The system remains *refractory* (unexcitable) for 2 to 4 msec, since sodium

Figure 19–9. *A,* Thinly remyelinated segment intercalated in fiber microdissected from baboon sciatic nerve during repair of paranodal invagination and demyelination (bar = 10 μm). *B,* Low-power electron micrograph after ultrathin sectioning of the fiber above. It shows detail of the node on the left. (× 5500) (Reproduced by permission from Ochoa, J.: J. Neurol. Sci. 17:103, 1972.)

inactivation gates will remain shut until the membrane fully repolarizes. This absolute refractory period sets the limit for the maximum firing rates that can be triggered in nerve fibers (Fig. 19–11). It is more prolonged in unmyelinated than in myelinated fibers. Prolonged inactivation of the sodium conductance may occur if the membrane does not repolarize, a recognized cause being the chronic extracellular accumulation of potassium ions.[56]

The density of sodium and potassium channels can in principle be estimated through the use of labeled neurotoxins that bind specifically to either.[57-59] Unmyelinated axons have relatively few scattered sodium channels and relatively abundant potassium channels. Myelinated axons have abundant sodium channels concentrated at the nodes of Ranvier and at the initial segment of the axon. This is probably the basis for special cytochemical reactivity of the axolemma at those sites.[60] The potassium channels in myelinated axons are hidden under the myelin. Such channel formulae may explain why myelinated axons (particularly sensory axons) *accommodate* little and are easily induced into spontaneous impulse generation.[46,59]

Decreased membrane excitability may result from deviations in the resting membrane potential related to abnormal ionic concentration. It may also result from blocking activation of sodium channels, for example, by certain specific neurotoxins or by local anesthetic drugs. As mentioned earlier, the membrane may remain unexcitable if the inactivation gates are not reopened after an action potential.

Spontaneous impulse generation from nerve fibers may produce a variety of abnormal sensory phenomena, inclusive of paresthesias and perhaps neuralgic pains. Ectopic impulse generation is thought to result from membrane insults, such as the abolition of sodium inactivation caused by certain neurotoxins or drugs, or the blocking of potassium channels by similar means,

Figure 19–10. Electron micrograph across normal human myelinated fiber. Sector of nucleus (*N*) is seen to the left of sector of myelinated axon. Regular myelin periodicity is disturbed by a partial Schmidt-Lanterman cleft (*SL*). Note external and internal mesaxons (arrowed) and tubular and filamentous contents of axoplasm. A basal lamina (*BL*) separates the Schwann cell membrane from endoneurial collagen fibrils (*C*).

Figure 19–11. Time course of the action potential and of the associated changes in sodium and potassium permeabilities. (Modified from Dudel, J.: *In* Schmidt, R. F.: Fundamentals of Neurophysiology. New York, Springer, 1978.)

or deviations in the time or voltage dependence of subpopulations of sodium channels, allowing the extemporaneous channel opening (m-h overlap).[46] One form of spontaneous impulse generation, postischemic paresthesia, is less readily elicited in patients with certain neuropathies. One explanation for this observation is that potassium channels become exposed through paranodal myelin defects, thus increasing accommodation.

Propagation of the action potential occurs along the membrane owing to the fact that influx of ions moves longitudinally within the axon. If axons acted as though they were inert cables, the propagated longitudinal current would fall off exponentially with distance, owing to outward current leakage. However, the potential change propagates along the whole length of unmyelinated axons without decreasing in amplitude. This is because the positively charged longitudinal current brings to threshold neighboring points in the excitable membrane. Indeed, upon turning outward through the membrane, the internal longitudinal current initiates voltage-dependent excitation of ion channels in every point visited. This in turn supplies fresh inward current for further depolarization for neighboring regions of the membrane. The velocity of propagation of the action potential is dependent upon several factors:

a. It increases together with the magnitude of the sodium (sodium channel density), since a greater internal longitudinal current will accelerate the excitation of adjacent membrane.

b. It increases markedly with increased membrane resistance (for example, myelin), since the longitudinal

current will hardly weaken with distance. Thus, conduction time along the internodal portions of the myelinated axons is negligible but is delayed at the naked nodal portions. Here the progressive depolarization comparatively slowly builds up to the threshold for channel opening. The term "saltatory" conduction expresses such excitation jumping from node to node (Fig 19–12*A*).

c. It increases with the diameter of the axon, since the resistance to the flow of internal longitudinal current is inversely proportional to the square of the axon diameter.

Pathologically, conduction of the action potential is slowed along thin regenerated axons. Nerve conduction is also slowed in partially demyelinated axons and in nerves with presumably abnormal membrane composition. Slowing of conduction in demyelinated axons may either reflect abnormally delayed "saltation" or the development of internodal voltage-dependent channels and continuous conduction, as occurs normally in unmyelinated fibers[62-64] (Fig. 19–12*B*). Slowing of conduction may also occur in severe axonopathies such as acute intermittent porphyria, uremia, and certain heavy metal poisonings. This is not necessarily due to drop out of fast conducting axons; it may be due to secondary demyelination in these disorders. Conduction of the action potential may be completely blocked in severe demyelination. A few layers of remyelination may transform conduction block into slowed conduction and hence restore strength to a nerve-muscle preparation (see Fig. 19–9). Patchy demyelination affecting many nerve fibers slows their conduction to different extents. Functions requiring synchronous conduction of nerve volleys, as in tendon reflexes and vibration sense, are selectively upset. Equally, compound nerve action potentials recorded locally become dispersed and are ultimately unobtainable from desynchronization of impulses.

THE CLINICAL SYNDROME OF PERIPHERAL NEUROPATHY

Peripheral nerve disorders may be broadly categorized into two groups based on their clinical pattern of extent.

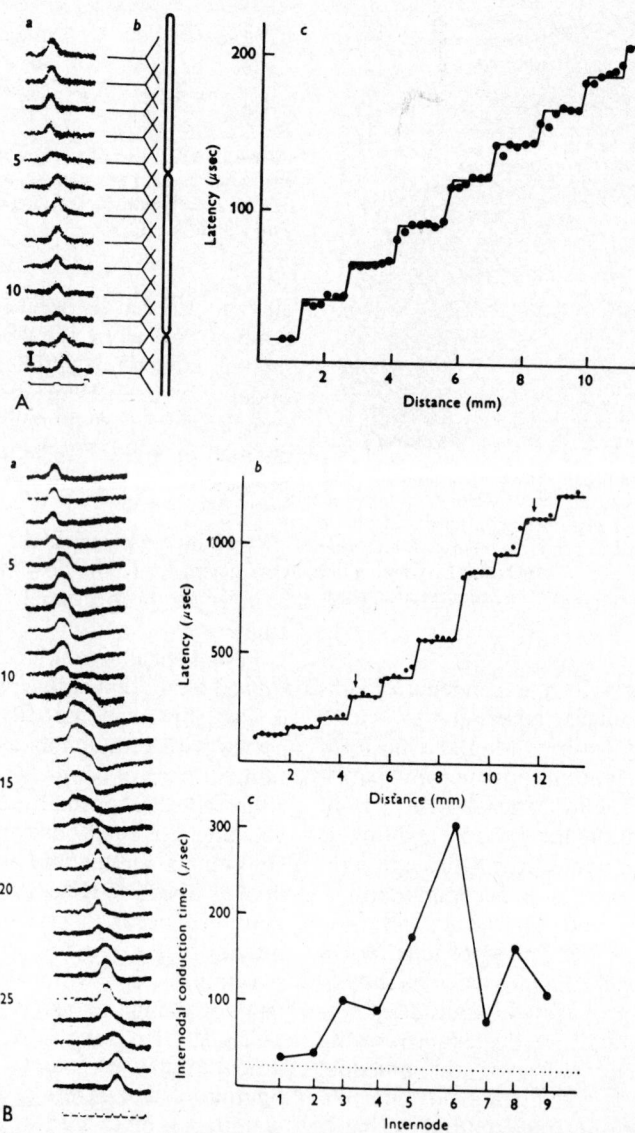

Figure 19–12. *A,* Normal single fiber from intact ventral root. (*a*) Superimposed records of longitudinal current from a single fiber as electrode pair was moved along ventral root in steps of 200 μm. Time scale = 100 μsec/division. Vertical bar = 100 μV. Upward deflection represents current flowing in a direction opposite that of propagation. (*b*) Lines from each record indicate positions of the electrode with respect to the diagrammatic fiber. Sites of nodes of Ranvier are inferred from records. (*c*) Latency to peak of longitudinal current as a function of distance along the fiber. *B,* Records and plotting (*a* and *b*) from a single fiber from a demyelinated ventral root. (*c*) Data of *b* replotted as internodal conduction time for each of nine successive internodes examined. (Reproduced with permission from Rasminsky, M., and Sears, T.A.: J. Physiol. 227:323, 1972.)

They are either more or less symmetrical polyneuropathies or a focal injury of a single nerve trunk, designated mononeuropathy. Polyneuropathies are diffuse disorders of peripheral nerves presenting as muscle weakness, with or without wasting, areflexia, and sensory and autonomic disturbance, in a distal-greater-than-proximal distribution, usually in the feet and legs before the hands and arms. The term polyradiculoneuropathy is used to emphasize symmetrical involvement of spinal roots as well as nerve trunks. Polyneuropathies may be genetically inherited or acquired from a host of metabolic, toxic, infectious, or nutritional insults. As shown in Table 19–1, it is possible to subclassify polyneuropathies as primarily due to axonal degeneration or as primarily due to demyelination of nerve fibers. Useful and usually accurate insights into the kind of pathology affecting nerve fibers can be derived from measurements of nerve conduction velocity.[65] Even morphologically, however, this distinction is not pure in many disease states. Chronic axonal degenerations may be preceded by axonal atrophy accompanied by secondary demyelination. Similarly, primary demyelinating diseases, especially if chronic, may be associated with some degree of secondary axonal degeneration.

Mononeuropathies may occur from chronic entrapment or acute mechanical compression, from ischemia, from neoplastic infiltration, or from granulomatous disease. At times, multiple mononeuropathies (often termed mononeuritis multiplex) may become so widespread and confluent in an individual as to resemble polyneuropathy. In these cases thorough electrophysiologic study may differentiate the two and may precisely localize the sites of the lesions, thus calling for appropriate tissue biopsy and medical or surgical intervention when indicated.

Neuropathies may present as acute (less than one week), subacute (less than one month), or chronic (greater than one month) disorders and they may be predominantly motor, sensory, autonomic, or mixed, depending on the type of function involved at presentation. Weakness with minor sensory complaint is often seen in idiopathic inflammatory demyelinating polyneuropathy (Guillain-Barré syndrome), lead intoxication, porphyria, diphtheritic neuropathy, and in some forms of hereditary peroneal muscular atrophy.[66,67] Minor sensory symptoms are often neglected and may be elicited only by careful questioning. A genuinely pure motor neuron syndrome of a subacute or chronic nature is rarely due to polyneuropathy and, after appropriate screening tests, most often proves to be a form of anterior horn cell disease.

Predominant sensory involvement is a common feature of many polyneuropathies, including leprosy, diabetes, amyloid neuropathy, uremia, vitamin B_6 and B_{12}

Table 19–1. Common Causes of Polyneuropathy in Man

Marked Axonal Degeneration	Marked Demyelination
Acquired	
Metabolic	*Metabolic*
Vitamin deficiency (B_1, B_6, B_{12}, folic acid, nicotinic acid)	Carcinoma (remote effect)
Diabetes	Lymphoma, myeloma, dysproteinemias
Uremia	Diabetes
	Hypothyroidism
	Liver failure
Toxic	*Toxic*
Heavy metals (lead, arsenic, mercury, thallium, gold, etc.)	Diphtheria
Inorganic compounds (nitrous oxide, etc.)	Buckthorn toxin
Organic compounds (alcohol, organomercury, organophosphorus (TOCP), hexacarbons (*n*-hexane, MnBK, kepone, etc.), acrylamide, carbon disulfide, hexachlorophene, dietary cyanides)	*Inflammatory*
	Guillain-Barré syndrome (autoimmune and variants)
Drugs (vincristine, vinblastine, isoniazid (B6), nitrogen mustards, cliquinol, thalidomide, nitrofurantoin, phenytoin, dapsone, disulfiram, perhexiline)	
Collagen vascular disease and sarcoidosis	
Leprosy	*Leprosy*
Genetic	
Degenerative	*Degenerative*
Porphyria	Hypertrophic Charcot-Marie-Tooth disease
Neuronal-type Charcot-Marie-Tooth disease	H.N. of Dejerine-Sottas type
Friedreich's ataxia	Refsum's disease
Ataxia telangiectasia	Metachromatic leukodystrophy
Bassen-Kornzweig syndrome (abetalipoproteinemia)	Adrenomyeloneuropathy
Primary amyloidosis	Krabbe's disease
Hereditary sensory neuropathies	Liability to pressure palsies
Tangier disease (alphalipoproteinemia)	
Fabry's disease	
Leigh's disease	
Familial dysautonomia	
Giant axonal neuropathy (?)	
	Dysgenetic (?)
	Arrested myelinogenesis

deficiencies, arteritis, alcoholic neuropathy, hereditary sensory neuropathy, and a form of carcinomatous neuropathy.

Symptoms and Signs of Neuropathy. Paresthesias of "burning," "pins and needles," and "tingling" qualities, pain (aching, brief stabbing, etc.), and numbness in a stocking-glove distribution are common symptoms of polyneuropathy. The sensation of a bandlike constriction about a limb or a feeling of swelling in the limb is sometimes volunteered. "Restless legs," a nondescript discomfort in the calves, which usually occurs while sitting or during sleep and is relieved with movement of the legs, may herald early polyneuropathy. Atypically, sensory manifestations may occur in a proximal distribution. This has been described in acute intermittent porphyria,[68,69] Tangier disease,[70] and leprosy. In lepromatous leprosy, the pattern of sensory loss can be related to the fact that bacilli proliferate in nerves of cooler tissues, thus sparing midline, palms, axillae, and the warm regions of the face.[71]

On examination, weakness is greater in a distal rather than proximal distribution in most forms of polyneuropathy and is usually seen in feet before hands. There are several notable exceptions to this rule, however. In lead neuropathy, wrist drop from radial nerve dysfunction classically is reputed to precede onset of weakness in the lower limbs. Proximal weakness greater than distal is commonly encountered in cases of inflammatory demyelinating polyneuropathy and in acute intermittent porphyria. The explanation for this is unclear. Thomas suggests this may be due to the fact that proximal portions of limbs are supplied by nerve fibers of greater diameter than those supplying distal extremities. Hence, the myelin of these fibers may be more susceptible to certain metabolic or immunogenic injury.[72]

Cranial nerve involvement in polyneuropathy is uncommon on the whole. Ophthalmoplegia, in particular when in combination with global areflexia and ataxia, should be considered to be the Miller-Fisher variant of inflammatory polyneuropathy until proven otherwise.[73] Patchy involvement of mixed motor and sensory cranial nerves, as well as the nerves in the extremities, may be seen in diabetes, sarcoidosis, carcinomatosis, Tangier's disease, leprosy, and in various forms of arteritis.

Muscle wasting is not to be expected in pure demyelinating neuropathy or in axonal neuropathies of recent onset. The deformities associated with chronic muscle wasting may be characteristically revealing. For example, pes cavus, usually signifying inherited axonal neuropathy and, of course, the various clawhands point to lesions of particular isolated nerves. Fasciculations from involuntary contraction of individual motor units are commonly found in motor neuropathies by careful scrutiny of skin overlying muscle groups. These may be identified as spontaneous, fine, irregular twitches of muscle that occur at rest and are usually not strong enough to displace a joint. It is now generally agreed that the origin of fasciculations may be the ectopic generation of nerve impulses propagated from anywhere along the motor neuron.[74,75] The abnormal mechanisms responsi-

ble for development of ectopic impulse generation in nerve fibers have been analyzed by Diamond and colleagues.[46]

Intact tendon (stretch) reflexes require the normal functioning of spindle afferent nerve fibers and alpha motor neuron fibers to extrafusal muscle. In addition, these reflexes require gamma motor neuron output for appropriate tuning of the intrafusal spindle apparatus. In polyneuropathy, reflexes are most often lost or diminished following the axonal dying-back pattern of sensorimotor dysfunction or as a result of demyelination with desynchronization of the nerve volleys required for the compound muscle response. Similarly, in mononeuropathies, reflexes are diminished in a focal pattern that often clarifies the exact root or nerve involved. Brisk reflexes in the setting of a polyneuropathy should suggest concurrent damage of spinal cord and peripheral nerves, as may be seen in vitamin B_{12} deficiency,[76,77] porphyric neuropathy,[69,78] adrenomyeloneuropathy,[79] and in some neuropathies caused by toxic agents, for example, triorthocresyl phosphate[80] and nitrous oxide.[81] It should be remembered that *joint deformity* might be a consequence of peripheral neuropathy. Indeed, Charcot joints, thought to result from loss of joint nociception, can be a dramatic manifestation of chronic sensory neuropathies, inclusive of diabetic neuropathy and Charcot-Marie-Tooth disease.

NEUROPATHIES OF SPECIAL INTEREST TO RHEUMATOLOGISTS

Neuropathies Associated with the Arteritides. *Rheumatoid Arthritis.* Peripheral neuropathy may be a particularly vexing complication to patients already weakened and disabled from rheumatoid arthritis (RA). While its precise incidence in the rheumatoid population is unknown, peripheral neuropathy, excluding entrapment syndromes, has been reported in 1.2 to 9.8 percent of cases.[82,83] Electrophysiologic examination of muscle and nerve shows abnormalities in 85 percent of patients with RA who have no specific neurologic complaints.[84]

The neuropathy usually presents insidiously as a symmetrical, predominantly sensory abnormality with numbness, tingling, or burning of distal extremities. Subtle motor deficits are difficult to quantitate in patients with joint pain or deformity, but a degree of muscle wasting and weakness is usually present.[82,85] The clinical picture is characterized by a distal loss of vibration sense and proprioception, although all modalities are affected to some degree.[86-88] Less commonly, abrupt painful asymmetric mononeuropathy or a fairly symmetric chronic sensorimotor neuropathy may arise as a complication of systemic arteritis in RA. The distal sensorimotor polyneuropathy resembling infectious polyneuritis may present abruptly or with stuttering progression over several months.[82,85] Most commonly this type of neuropathy is seen in patients with severe, long-standing disease who are on steroids or experiencing rapid change in steroid doses. Commonly, these patients demonstrate severe joint deformities, rheumatoid nodules, high titers of rheumatoid factor, diminished serum complement, high ESR, anemia, anorexia, and fever.[85,87,89,90]

There is now considerable evidence indicating that these deficits are a result of axonal degeneration of nerve fibers due to occlusion of vasa nervorum and resultant ischemia of nerve trunks. Perivascular mononuclear infiltrates, fibrinoid necrosis of media with polymorphonuclear infiltrates, arteriolar intimal proliferation, perivascular hemorrhages, fibrosis, and small vessel occlusions are documented evidence of diffuse necrotizing angiopathy of peripheral nerve in these patients.[91,92] Ischemia occurs most commonly in the middle of the upper arm and thigh, with a striking central fascicular pattern of maximal nerve fiber damage. Between axilla and elbow and between hip and thigh, portions of nerve receive relatively few nutrient arteries; hence, there are diminished systems of collateral circulation.[9] Under conditions of widespread inflammation and occlusion of vasa nervorum, these regions of nerve may represent watershed zones of selective ischemic vulnerability.[91,93] Electrophysiologic and histologic studies have documented axonal degeneration with some segmental demyelination.[86] Myelinated fibers sustain most of the damage with relatively less involvement of smaller unmyelinated fibers.[94] This may reflect a greater vulnerability of myelinated fibers to ischemia.[95-98]

The etiology of rheumatoid vasculitis is unknown, although its correlation with high titers of rheumatoid factor, low serum complement, and the presence of 7S IgM suggests it may be immune mediated. The definitive diagnosis may be aided by skin, rectal, muscle, or nerve biopsy.[90,94,99] The overall mortality of patients with rheumatoid neuropathy due to vasculitis approaches 30 to 50 percent, and aggressive management with steroids, cyclophosphamide, penicillamine, and/or plasmapheresis has been advocated.[88,92,99]

Polyarteritis Nodosa. This disorder is a systemic vasculitis of small and medium-sized arteries, occurring throughout the body. Peripheral neuropathy is common in this disorder and has been reported in up to 52 percent of cases.[100] While mononeuritis multiplex (with the onset of weakness, pain, numbness, and paresthesia radiating down an arm or a leg) is often described as the classic form of neuropathy in this disorder,[101] polyneuropathy may indeed be more common.[90] Mononeuritis multiplex may, however, become so extensive and confluent as to resemble a symmetrical "pseudo"-polyneuropathy. Electrophysiologic testing will identify subclinical polyneuropathy in a substantial number of neurologically asymptomatic patients with systemic vasculitis and thus aid in the early recognition and treatment of this disorder.

The clinical features of neuropathy due to polyarteritis nodosa are largely similar to those secondary to the arteritis of RA, though differences have been described. Polyarteritis neuropathy has been cited as more commonly asymmetrical, primarily motor, and rarely pure sensory, while rheumatoid neuropathy is commonly a symmetrical, distal, predominantly sensory polyneurop-

athy.[89] These characteristics are unreliable in differentiating the two diseases, however, and nerve biopsy of either may give similar pathologic appearances. Nevertheless, peripheral neuropathy as a presenting complaint is uncommon in RA but common in polyarteritis nodosa, and should initiate a careful search for other signs of systemic vasculitis.

Peripheral neuropathy due to vasculitis may be seen in a variety of other connective tissue diseases including Churg-Strauss' arteritis, systemic lupus erythematosus, Sjögren's syndrome, cranial arteritis, and Wegener's granulomatosis.[82] The clinical features commonly take the form of mononeuritis multiplex or symmetrical sensory polyneuropathy. The frequency of peripheral neuropathy in Sjögren's syndrome may approach 60 percent of cases,[102] and has recently been shown to correlate with high titers of anti-Ro (SSA) antibodies in these patients.[103] Electrophysiologic studies and neuropathology document ischemic centrofascicular nerve lesions with axonal degeneration likely due to vasculitic changes in vasa nervorum.[94]

Peripheral Neuropathy and Dysimmunoglobulinemia. Neuropathy may develop in association with dysimmunoglobulinemia in a number of systemic disorders, including myeloma, cryoglobulinemic states, Waldenström's macroglobulinemia, solitary plasmacytoma, amyloidosis, and "benign" monoclonal gammopathies, unaccompanied by cancer or systemic illness. The pathophysiology of neuropathy in these illnesses is disputed. Theories have incriminated subperineurial immunoglobulin deposition, serum hyperviscosity due to paraproteins, direct infiltration of nerve by tumor cells, and metabolic or immunologic injury of nerve.[104]

Peripheral neuropathy may be seen in association with systemic *amyloidosis* in approximately 15 percent of cases.[105] Typically, it presents as a moderate to severe sensorimotor-autonomic neuropathy which comes on in the late decades of life and is associated with systemic cardiac, renal, hematologic, or gastrointestinal involvement in approximately one half of cases.[106] The polyneuropathy usually begins with positive sensory symptoms in lower limbs described as a stabbing, prickling, piercing, burning, or "painful" numbness. The dysesthesias predominate over sensory loss and, in some cases, may be incapacitating enough to prohibit weight bearing and may require narcotics. Pain, cold, and warm sensations are disproportionately affected early in the disease, beginning in the distal extremities and progressing proximally.[107] Disturbances of proprioception and light touch may follow in similar fashion and are accompanied by symmetrical distal weakness, usually beginning in extensor muscles of the feet and progressing to complete disability in some cases.[108]

Autonomic dysfunction typified by postural hypotension, diarrhea, impotence, and bladder incontinence in men is common. Serum protein electrophoresis may be abnormal in 50 percent of cases, and monoclonal proteins may be found in 90 percent when urine and serum are examined simultaneously. The diagnosis is often made by rectal biopsy, but when neuropathy is present, amyloid may be identified by sural nerve biopsy in virtually all cases.[106]

Electromyographic studies usually confirm primary distal axonal degeneration, though the mechanism of neural injury is uncertain.[106,108] Amyloid deposits within epineural arteries may lead to small vessel occlusion and nerve ischemia.[109] This by itself would not explain the selective small fiber dropout witnessed early in the course of the disease.

Macroglobulinemia. The term macroglobulinemia was first coined by Waldenström and categorizes a group of patients with hepatosplenomegaly, anemia, weight loss, malaise, bleeding diathesis, and an elevated level of 19S IgM found on immunoelectrophoresis of plasma[110] (see Chapter 84). Commonly, these patients have an elevated ESR and lymphoid proliferation of bone marrow, lymph nodes, spleen, and other tissues. Peripheral neuropathy occurs in up to 25 percent of cases of macroglobulinemia[111,112] and may be associated with chronic lymphocytic leukemia, lymphosarcoma, carcinoma, cirrhosis of the liver, and a variety of connective tissue disorders.[113]

A heterogenous pattern of peripheral nerve dysfunction may occur, including mononeuropathy, mononeuritis multiplex, and pure sensory, sensorimotor, and predominantly motor (resembling Guillain-Barré) and cranial neuropathies.[112,114,115] Most commonly, however, patients suffer a symmetrical distal sensory syndrome, involving spontaneous pain, paresthesias, and numbness, which usually precedes the onset of weakness and muscle cramps and occasionally antedates other protean manifestations of the disease.[116,117]

Histopathologic examination of involved nerves shows partial demyelination of nerve fibers. Often scattered lymphocytic infiltrates are seen around small and medium-sized vessels. Ultrastructural examination of nerve may reveal occasional plasma cells within endoneurium.[118] Amyloid deposits within nerve fascicles may be identified on Congo red stain in a small percentage of patients with macroglobulinemia and neuropathy.

The pathogenesis of peripheral neuropathy is uncertain, but to date much evidence has been collected implying that IgM paraproteins may be directed against peripheral myelin. Iwashita and colleagues[104] identified IgM paraprotein deposits in perineurium and vasa nervorum in a patient with Waldenström's macroglobulinemia. Others have demonstrated large deposits of macroglobulin in the myelin sheath of nerve fibers associated with a marked distortion of myelin lamellae and swelling of the mesaxon.[118-120] More recently, Latov and colleagues[120] demonstrated abnormal activity of IgM immunoglobulin against peripheral nerve myelin using complement fixation and immunoglobulin techniques in a patient with IgM monoclonal gammopathy and demyelinating peripheral neuropathy. In this case, marked clinical improvement was obtained through reduction of serum paraprotein by means of plasmapheresis, prednisone, and chlorambucil, suggesting that IgM-mediated demyelination is the primary pathophysiology

in this disorder. Using the immunoperoxidase technique, Abrams and colleagues[121] later demonstrated immunohistochemical binding of IgM paraproteins in 10 patients with peripheral neuropathy and plasma cell dyscrasia. Binding of IgM paraprotein to peripheral myelin and to axons was seen in seven cases. Subsequently, myelin-associated glycoprotein was demonstrated as the likely antigen in patients with antimyelin IgM antibodies.[122]

Multiple Myeloma. This is a disease characterized by malignant proliferation of plasma cell lines that infiltrate bone marrow and other tissues and commonly produce abnormal quantities of immunoglobulins in serum and urine. Evidence of peripheral neuropathy is reported in 5 to 13 percent of cases[123,124] and may be found histologically or electrophysiologically in 40 to 60 percent of cases when neurologically asymptomatic patients are included in studies.[124,125] The neuropathy may occur in the disorder with or without amyloidosis and, in both forms, has been associated with axonal degeneration and segmental demyelination.[126,127] However, amyloid deposition in nerve is rarely found and is thought to play no role in the development of neuropathy.[114,128]

The neuropathy of myeloma without amyloidosis is not stereotyped and may present as a pure sensory, mild sensorimotor, or subacute relapsing polyneuropathy. Neuropathy in myeloma may also be associated with systemic amyloidosis and has the same features of amyloid neuropathy described earlier. Long-term survival of patients is uncommon in this disease but most often is seen in patients with a good response to chemotherapy.[129] The use of alkylating agents and other forms of chemotherapy in this disease, however, does not seem to alter the continuous progression of neuropathy in patients who suffer from it.

Osteosclerotic Myeloma. A rare form of myeloma seen in younger, healthier individuals, osteosclerotic myeloma is associated with peripheral neuropathy in 50 percent of cases.[126,130,131] In these patients, polyneuropathy is characterized by a predominantly symmetrical distal motor weakness, which overshadows sensory loss and may mimic the presentation of chronic inflammatory demyelinating neuropathy.[130] The abnormal monoclonal "spike" may be missed on routine serum protein electrophoresis; for this reason, skeletal survey and serum immunoelectrophoresis are recommended for definitive diagnosis in selected patients. Surgical extirpation of a solitary plasmacytoma may be curative.[131] Tumoricidal radiation therapy and chemotherapy are associated with improvement of polyneuropathy in some patients.[132,133] The exact role that monoclonal antibody plays in the pathogenesis of polyneuropathy in this disorder is unknown.

Cryoglobulinemia. Cryoglobulins are immunoglobulins that precipitate at 4°C and redissolve upon rewarming (see Chapter 84). They may be characterized as either monoclonal IgM or IgG in patients with plasma cell dyscrasia, or as mixed polyclonal comprised of two or more immunoglobulins, usually IgM and IgG; this latter group is associated with infection, liver disease, and collagen vascular diseases such as rheumatoid arthritis, systemic lupus erythematosus, and polyarteritis nodosa.[134]

Peripheral neuropathy has been reported to occur in up to 15 percent of cases of cryoglobulinema and is usually characterized by symmetrical, subacute motor-sensory polyneuropathy or mononeuritis multiplex.[112,135] Electrophysiology of muscle and nerve may show evidence for axonal degeneration. On nerve biopsy, vasculitis of medium and small size epineurial arteries and perivascular infiltration of lymphocytes in plasma cells may be seen.[136] Abnormal immunoglobulin deposits in perineurial capillaries and throughout subperineurial and endoneurial subspaces have been demonstrated.[135,137,138]

While the pathogenesis of axonal degeneration in cryoglobulinemic states is uncertain, the evidence for an ischemic factor is attractive and plasmapheresis may be beneficial in some patients.[137]

Sarcoid Neuropathy. Sarcoidosis is a systemic granulomatous disease of unknown etiology that most commonly involves lung, lymph nodes, parotid glands, spleen, skin, and eyes (see Chapter 93). A wide variety of central and peripheral nervous system disturbances are reported in about 5 percent of cases.[139-141] Of these, the most remarkable feature of neurologic sarcoid is the occurrence of multiple relapsing and remitting cranial nerve palsies, involvement of the VII cranial nerve being the single most common.[141-144] Polyneuropathy is a rare development but may present as a subacute or chronic symmetrical sensorimotor disturbance or as an acute mononeuritis or Guillain-Barré syndrome.[145-148]

The pathogenesis of sarcoid neuropathy is not well categorized, and there have been few histopathologic studies.[142,146,147] Electrophysiologic data has shown evidence for axonal degeneration with[146,149] or without[141,147] segmental demyelination. Panarteritis in sarcoid neuropathy has been documented by others and has been cited as a possible underlying etiology to the neuropathy.[147] Frank infiltration of nerve by granuloma, however, has also been documented on nerve biopsy in this disorder and may play a role in subsequent nerve injury.[142,146,147,149]

The natural history of sarcoid neuropathy is difficult to establish. Most patients with peripheral neurologic symptoms and sarcoidosis are treated with high-dose glucocorticoids, and the general prognosis is favorable in most cases. Whether a good prognosis is due to the self-limiting nature of the disease or the use of corticosteroids is currently unknown.[140,142,143]

Leprosy of the Peripheral Nervous System. Leprosy is a chronic, disabling disease of superficial body parts caused by the acid-fast bacillus *Mycobacterium leprae*. The disease is of relatively low contagiousness and is common to tropical and subtropical areas of the world, with endemic foci in India, Spain, Portugal, Mexico, and portions of the southern United States.[150] In part as a result of the increasing influx of Hispanic and Southeast Asian immigrants, the incidence of leprosy has risen sharply in the United States, particularly in the cities of New York, San Francisco, and Los Angeles.[151] Since the disease is not readily recognized by many physicians, it may go undiagnosed for many years, mimicking a variety of neurologic, rheumatologic, and dermatologic syndromes.[152]

A wide clinical pathologic spectrum of the disease is seen, ranging from the well circumscribed, slowly progressive tuberculoid form to the rapidly proliferating, widely disseminating lepromatous type. The form of leprosy that develops depends, to a large extent, on host response factors. Patients with lepromatous leprosy display abnormalities of cellular immunity characterized by delayed hypersensitivity reactions and impaired lymphocyte transformation while retaining normal humoral response mechanisms.[153-156] Inability to contain the infection results in unchecked proliferation of bacilli and extensive hematogenous spread to skin, mucous membranes, eyes, upper respiratory tract, and peripheral nerves.

In all forms of leprosy, sensory loss is the hallmark of neurologic involvement and is commonly the first manifestation of the disease.[157-160] In lepromatous leprosy, the pattern of neurologic deficit can be shown to occur in tissues of cooler body temperature where bacilli tend to reproduce most readily.[158] The pinnae of the ears, dorsal surfaces of the hands and feet, dorsomedial surfaces of the forearm, and anterolateral aspects of the legs are the areas most commonly involved. The precise sequence of sensory modality loss is disputed.[157] Commonly, however, patients retain the ability to differentiate sharp from blunt sensation while demonstrating a remarkable insensitivity to pain. The skin is marked by numerous deep lacerations, abrasions, contusions, and burns in various stages of healing, suffered, without comment or notice, while performing the routine chores of life. Modalities of light touch, proprioception, and vibration sense may be variably lost as the disease progresses. Motor strength and deep tendon reflexes are typically preserved well into advanced stages of the illness.

Hypertrophic nerves are common in leprosy and predispose the patient to a variety of compression neuropathy syndromes. Motor and sensory nerve conduction studies may reveal mononeuropathy multiplex with focal slowing in several nerves at common sites of nerve entrapment and enlargement. Electromyography may show evidence of chronic denervation of involved muscle groups.[157,161,162]

Peripheral neuropathy in leprosy results from direct invasion of nerve by the bacillus, an unusual but consistent characteristic of infection with *Mycobacterium leprae*. The histopathology of nerve lesions is usually diagnostic. Typically there is marked proliferation of perineurium and intraneural fibrous tissue, with an increased number of endoneurial collagen fibrils seen. There is hypertrophy of Schwann cells with the formation of multiple cytoplasmic protrusions. *Mycobacterium leprae* may be seen singly or in aggregates within

Schwann cells as well as within scattered foamy macrophages and other inflammatory cells throughout an involved nerve. Foamy degeneration of Schwann cells associated with myelinated and unmyelinated axons may be seen, with little or no involvement of axoplasm and myelin.[163] In lepromatous leprosy, acid-fast stains may reveal large numbers of bacilli invading epineurium, perineurium, and occasionally endoneurial blood vessels, even in asymptomatic patients with the disease.[157,159,163] It has been speculated that these bacilli may gain access to peripheral nerves by primary invasion of Schwann cell cytoplasm. Sporadic Schwann cell degeneration from bacterial infestation could ultimately lead to focal demyelination and secondary axonal degeneration, thus explaining focal slowing of nerve conduction in these patients.[161,163,164] When erythema nodosum is associated with lepromatous leprosy, the histopathology of nerve lesions shows foci of an acute angiitis, largely of small arteries and arterioles within perineurium. Inflammatory infiltrates, vascular occlusions, and subsequent intraneural edema may result in segmental infarction of neural elements or multiple microabscesses of neural trunks.[165]

Treatment of leprosy with adequate doses of diaminodiphenylsulfone, rifampin, or both is the mainstay of therapy. When antibacterial therapy is provided early in the course of the disease, it will halt the progression of the destructive process and promote natural recovery of the neuropathy.[151,157] Surgical intervention for cosmesis, stabilization of joints, transposition, and drainage of entrapped or infected nerves is often beneficial.[166]

MECHANICAL INJURIES OF NERVE

Mechanical injuries of nerve are a common complication of rheumatologic illness. The degree, character, and duration of neuropathy in these patients depend on the type of nerve fiber damage and the efficiency of repair processes, when they occur. Nerve injury may be broadly classified as acute or chronic, with the type of structural damage differing dramatically in each. The histopathologic features of acute and chronic compressive neuropathies, as studied in animal models, provide insight into their nature and mechanism and thus a scientific approach to their management.

Acute Nerve Compression. Acute compressive nerve injury may result in sensorimotor deficit or paresthesias, which may be completely and rapidly reversible or virtually permanent. Early clinical manifestations of nerve dysfunction (numbness, paralysis, paresthesia, and pain) may provide little clue as to the nature of the underlying pathology or the possibility of recovery. Short-lasting compression of peripheral nerve above systolic pressure results in a *rapidly reversed physiologic block* of nerve conduction. Lewis, Pickering, and Rothschild, in pneumatic tourniquet experiments conducted on themselves, elegantly demonstrated that this is a result of nerve ischemia rather than the direct effect of high pressure on nerve.[18] In addition, they established the sequence of

sensory modality loss during progressive nerve ischemia and described in detail the quality of paresthesia perceived during recovery from the ischemic insult.

Typically, if a pneumatic cuff is placed proximally on an arm at suprasystolic pressures, numbness is detected in the fingertips within 13 to 15 minutes. Loss of light touch and pressure modalities spreads centripetally toward the tourniquet at about 3 to 4 cm per minute. Pain, cold, and warm modalities are later lost in a similar fashion within 30 to 40 minutes. Weakness starts distally and spreads centrally soon after anesthesia, with complete paralysis occurring by 30 to 40 minutes of limb ischemia. If the tourniquet is removed at this point, recovery is normally always accompanied by tingling paresthesias, which may become uncomfortably intense and last for some four to six minutes. Sensory deficits are usually fully restored within 30 seconds and full muscle power some time after 10 minutes.

That this sequence of sensorimotor nerve disturbance is due to ischemia and not direct pressure on nerve was established by placing a second pneumatic cuff on the extremity, proximal to the first, just before the time of distal cuff release. Release of the distal cuff and hence release of local nerve compression without restoration of blood supply, failed to result in recovery of neural deficits. The stereotyped sequence of sensory modality loss suggested to Lewis and colleagues that the excitable membrane function of myelinated nerve fibers may be more vulnerable to ischemia; this has recently been corroborated by others.[95,167-169]

Regarding the pathophysiology of postischemic paresthesia, there is much evidence favoring nerve fibers as their site of origin.[170-172] Torebjörk and colleagues[172] and Ochoa and colleagues,[173] using intraneural microelectrode recording from sensory fascicles, concluded that the paroxysmal discharges recorded from single sensory units during postischemic paresthesias are generated ectopically along nerve fibers and not primarily from skin receptors.

As early as 1876, Erb described a type of nerve dysfunction that is more prolonged than the typical reversible physiologic block yet less severe than that resulting from nerve section.[174] Seddon called this *neurapraxia* (Saturday night paralysis) and noted the absence of muscle atrophy and the usually rapid recovery.[175] Denny-Brown and Brenner[176] demonstrated that neurapraxia could be produced in experimental animals with the use of a pneumatic cuff, and the end result was segmental demyelination of nerve. They erroneously concluded, however, that this lesion was ischemic in nature—a complication of the ischemic paralysis described earlier by Lewis, Pickering, and Rothschild.[18] Gilliatt and associates showed later that the demyelinating lesions occurred only in portions of nerve corresponding to the edges of the cuff, where pressure gradients are greatest. The mechanical nature of the neurapraxic lesion nerve was elucidated by Ochoa and colleagues[177] and is depicted in Figure 19–13A through D. Axoplasm and myelin are displaced outwardly from sites of compression, corresponding to cuff edges. Nodes ent cell body, some degree of retrograde axonal degeneration, and target tissue atrophy. After three to five days, electrodiagnostic tests will distinguish this lesion from neurapraxia in that wallerian degeneration leads to total inexcitability of distal nerve segments.

Nerve regeneration is preceded by Schwann cell proliferation to form cellular columns, known as bands of Büngner, within the basal lamina tubes. Nerve sprouts from the tips of proximal stump axons slowly advance through these columns to regenerate the distal axons at a rate of approximately 1 mm per day.[178] Myelination proceeds centrifugally down nerve fibers soon after Schwann cells reorganize, to establish one satellite cell per internode segment.[179,180]

Prognosis for functional recovery is favorable in axonotmesis with preservation of original basal lamina tubes because guidance of regenerating axons to their original peripheral targets is accurate. If a mechanical injury is sufficient to disrupt the normal architecture of nerve fibers, with destruction of the anatomic integrity of endoneurium, the term *neurotmesis* is used. In contrast to axonotmesis, regeneration of axons to their original targets is unlikely and the functional outcome is poor. In addition, regenerating fibers may be unable to proceed beyond the site of injury and, instead, ball-up and entwine to form a painful neuroma.[181-183]

Chronic Nerve Compression. If a nerve fiber is chronically constricted or entrapped, there may be slowing or a block of nerve impulse conduction through the area of compression and histologic evidence for demyelination. Single nerve fiber histopathology of this type of nerve injury, however, demonstrates a physical distortion of fiber architecture quite unlike that of acute injuries. Dr. Nakano discusses the various nerve entrapment syndromes in Chapter 110. In this section we will describe the fine structural pathology in these lesions which, to a large degree, explains the pathophysiology of nerve dysfunction.

A naturally occurring animal model for chronic compressive nerve lesions was identified in elderly guinea pigs in the 1960s by Fullerton and Gilliatt.[184,185] They found that these animals had a high incidence of carpal tunnel syndrome at the wrist and that the severity of the entrapment could be predicted from the results of nerve conduction studies. Conduction delay and, eventually, conduction block were associated with progressively severe focal demyelinating nerve lesions extending a few millimeters in length under the flexor retinaculum. In severe cases, there was gross narrowing of the nerve trunk with evidence of wallerian degeneration of myelinated fibers at the level of compression.

Ochoa and Marotte[186] studied these animals at very early stages of nerve entrapment when nerve conduction studies were still normal. They found that along stretches of several millimeters proximal and distal to the entrapment, myelin internodes were distorted into tapered "tadpole"-appearing segments with bulbous ends always polarized away from the site of compression. A schematic illustration of how chronic compression appears at different stages in its development is shown

Figure 19–13. *A,* Normal myelinated fiber microdissected from baboon tibial nerve after fixation in buffered glutaraldehyde and postfixation in osmium tetroxide. Note myelin gap at node of Ranvier. *B,* Occlusion of nodal gap with invagination (intussusception) of adjacent myelin segments. Myelin has stretched beyond original site of node marked by indentation *j* to reach *n.* Fiber was microdissected from baboon tibial nerve soon after acute compression with pneumatic cuff, leading to neurapraxia. Bar = 20 μm. *C,* Low-power electron micrograph of abnormal myelinated fiber from baboon ulnar nerve soon after compression, leading to neurapraxia. Original site of node is marked by indentation at site of Schwann cell junction *j.* Note new position of node covered by infolded myelin, *n. D,* Diagram describing primary lesion of myelinated fibers underlying neurapraxia. Myelin segment on right has partially invaginated segment on left. (*B* and *C* from Rudge, P., Ochoa, J., and Gilliatt, R.W.: J. Neurol. Sci. 23:403, 1974; *D* from Ochoa, J., Fowler, T.J., and Gilliatt, R.W.: In Desmedt, J.E. (ed.): New Developments in Electromyography and Clinical Neurophysiology. Vol. 2. Karger, Basel, 1973).

of Ranvier prolapse into paranodal regions a considerable distance from their normal anatomic sites.

More severe forms of nerve injury may result in significant disruption of endoneurial elements. The term *axonotmesis* is used to indicate that the distal portion of the axon is physically separated from the neuronal cell body. Unlike neurapraxic lesions, in axonotmesis, disruption of axonal transport at the site of the lesion results in wallerian degeneration, chromatolysis of par-

Figure 19–14. *A,* Diagram showing distorted myelin segments from median nerve of young guinea pig. Note reversal of polarity at the wrist. *B,* Further distortion and exposure of the axon proximal and distal to the site of entrapment. The median nerve under the carpal tunnel has lost its original myelin segments. Multiple, short remyelinated internodes repair the lesion. *C,* Advanced lesion with massive bulbs and axonal wallerian degeneration and regeneration. (Reproduced by permission from Ochoa, J.: In Omer, G.E., and Spinner, M. (eds.): Management of Peripheral Nerve Problems. Philadelphia, W.B. Saunders Co., 1980, pp. 487–501.)

in Figure 19–14*A* to *C*. The more prolonged the nerve injury, the more pronounced is the demyelination under the carpal band, with abnormal segments heading away from the entrapment site. In severe lesions, wallerian degeneration and regeneration are identified (Figure 19–14*C*).

Examination of these abnormal myelin segments by electron microscopy reveals the pathophysiology. Internal myelin lamellae normally attached to the axolemma at the node of Ranvier are retracted along the fiber at tapered ends of the "tadpole" segment, resulting in buckling of redundant myelin at the bulbous ends (Fig. 19–15). The likely sequence of demyelination, then, is through progressive retraction of unattached myelin, followed by complete demyelination of the axon at one end of the internode.

Ultrastructural examination of entrapment neuropathies in man corroborate the histopathology obtained in animal models.[187] Ochoa has suggested that detachment of terminal loops and subsequent myelin deformation may be due to repeated longitudinal stretching or fric-

Figure 19–15. *A,* Low-power electron micrograph of a moderately abnormal fiber taken from a guinea pig median nerve above the wrist. The paranode on the left is tapered. The bulbous paranode on the right shows inturning of a group of inner lamellae. (*R* = node of Ranvier.) (× 7000.) *B,* Enlargement of the area enclosed in the rectangle in *A.* Six myelin lamellae end in cytoplasmic loops between the arrows. (× 48,000.) *C,* Detail of the bulbous paranode. (× 20,000.) (Reproduced by permission from Ochoa and Marotte: J. Neurol. Sci. 19:491, 1973.)

tion against flexor tendons, producing pressure waves that propagate away from the entrapment.[61]

AGING OF THE PERIPHERAL NERVOUS SYSTEM

A variety of age-related changes in the peripheral nervous system are commonly seen in uncomplicated senesence.[188-190] Beginning at 50 years of age, there is diminished appreciation of vibratory sense (128 cps tuning fork) in the lower extremities, particularly at the great toe, with no appreciable loss in upper extremities.[191-194] Less dramatic changes in perception of light touch, proprioception, pain, and thermal sense may be expected with increasing age.[193-195,196] Muscle wasting, particularly of thigh, calf, and dorsal interossei, not associated with much weakness, fasciculation, or fibrillation, is common in the elderly and not necessarily related to disuse.[197,198] Reduction or loss of ankle jerks with normal or diminished knee and upper extremity reflexes in aging individuals is a common finding.[193,199,200]

The histopathologic changes associated with these clinical findings are multivariable.[189] The causes of the age-related changes in the peripheral nervous system are largely unknown and await futher study.

LABORATORY INVESTIGATIONS

Complete neurologic and electrodiagnostic evaluation should precede indiscriminate laboratory investigation of peripheral neuropathy. The history, neurologic examination, and neurophysiology should help broadly categorize the neuropathy as acquired versus inherited, axonal versus demyelinating, mononeuropathy multiplex versus polyneuropathy. In acquired neuropathies, those clues should guide the physician toward an appropriate laboratory search for uremia, diabetes, vitamin B_{12} deficiency, heavy metal poisoning, collagen vascular disease, dysproteinemia, sarcoidosis, or other likely entities. Following inconclusive neurologic and electrodiagnostic studies and a negative routine laboratory screen, further investigation may include the following in selected patients: (a.) special assays for serum vitamin, enzyme, or metabolite levels (e.g., phytanic acid deficiency in Refsum's disease); (b.) detection of porphyrin metabolites; (c.) serum and cerebrospinal fluid examination with focus on protein electrophoresis and immunoelectrophoresis when indicated; (d.) bone marrow microscopy; (e.) urine screen for metachromatic material and serum lysosomal analysis for inborn errors of metabolism; (f.) organ function tests (liver, thyroid, adrenal, pituitary); and (g.) appropriate screens for occult malignancy.

The search for toxic etiologies to peripheral neuropathy should rely more heavily on epidemiologic data than on laboratory investigation. Heavy metal screening in blood and urine should be complemented by assays of nail and hair for toxic exposure.

Finally, nerve biopsy can firmly establish the diagnosis in a number of neuropathies. These include leprosy, primary amyloidosis, metachromatic leukodystrophy, Fabry's disease, familial liability to pressure palsies, and the vasculitides.

References

1. Low, P.A., Marchand F., and Dyck, P.J.: Measurement of endoneurial fluid pressure with polyethylene matrix capsules. Brain Res. 122:373, 1977.
2. Low, P.A., Dyck P.J., and Schmelzer, J.D.: Mammalian peripheral nerve sheath has unique responses to chronic elevations of endoneurial fluid pressure. Exp. Neurol. 70:300, 1980.
3. Thomas, P.K.: The connective tissue of peripheral nerve: An electron microscope study. J. Anat. 97:35, 1963.
4. Olsson, Y., Kristensson K., and Klatzo, J.: Permeability of blood vessels and connective tissue sheath in the peripheral nervous system to exogenous protein. Acta Neuro. Pathol. (Supplement) 5:61, 1971.
5. Olsson, Y., and Reese, T.S.: Permeability of vasa nervorum and perineurium in mouse sciatic nerve studied by fluorescence and electron microscopy. J. Neuropathol. Exp. Neurol. 30:105, 1971.
6. Waggener, J.P., Bunn, S.M., and Beggs, J.: The diffusion of ferritin within the peripheral nerve sheath: An electron microscopy study. J. Neuropathol. Exp. Neurol. 24:430, 1965.
7. Lundborg, G., Nordborg, C., Rydevik, B., and Olsson, Y.: The effect of ischemia on the permeability of the perineurium to protein tracers in rabbit tibial nerve. Acta Neurol. Scand. 49:287, 1973.
8. Denny-Brown, P.: Importance of neural fibroblasts in the regeneration of nerve. Arch. Neurol. Psychiatry 55:171, 1946.
9. Adams, W.E.: The blood supply of nerves. 1. Historical review. J. Anat. 76:323, 1942.
10. Sunderland, S.: Nerve and Nerve Injuries. Edinburgh, London, and New York, Churchill Livingstone, 1978.
11. Olsson, Y.: Vascular permeability in the peripheral nervous system. In Dyck, P.J., Thomas, P.K., and Lambert, E.H. (eds.): Peripheral Neuropathy. Philadelphia, W.B. Saunders Company, 1975, pp. 190–200.
12. Erlanger, J., and Gasser, H.S.: The compound nature of the action current of nerve as disclosed by the cathode ray oscillograph. Am. J. Physiol. 70:624, 1924.
13. Burgess, P.R., and Perl, E.R.: Cutaneous mechanoreceptors and nocireceptors. In Iggo, A. (ed.): Handbook of Sensory Physiology. Vol. 2. Berlin, Springer Verlag, 1973, pp. 29–78.
14. Dawson, G.D.: The relative excitability and conduction velocity of sensory and motor nerve fibers in man. J. Physiol. 131:436, 1956.
15. Lambert, E.H., and Dyck, P.J.: Compound action potentials of sural nerve in vitro in peripheral neuropathy. In Dyck, P.J., Thomas, P.K., and Lambert, E.H. (eds.): Peripheral Neuropathy. Philadelphia, W.B. Saunders Company, 1975, pp. 427–441.
16. Vallbo, A.B., Hagbarth, K.-E., Torebjörk, H.E., and Wallin, B.G.: Somatosensory, proprioceptive, and sympathetic activity in human peripheral nerves. Physiol. Rev. 59:920, 1979.
17. Dyck, J.P., and Lambert, E.H.: Dissociated sensation in amyloidosis. Arch. Neurol. 20:490, 1969.
18. Lewis, T., Pickering, G.W., and Rothschild, P.: Centripetal paralysis arising out of arrested blood flow to the limb, including notes on a form of tingling. Heart 16:1, 1931.
19. Kugelberg, E.: Accommodation in human nerves. Acta Physiol. Scand. 8(Suppl. 24):105, 1944.
20. Ochoa, J., Fowler, T.J., and Gilliatt, R.W.: Anatomical changes in peripheral nerves compressed by pneumatic tourniquet. J. Anat. 113:433, 1972.
21. Tsukita, S., and Ishikawa, H.: The cytoskeleton in myelinated axons: Serial section study. Biomed. Res. 2:424, 1981.
22. Weiss, P., and Hiscoe, H.B.: Experiments on the mechanism of nerve growth. J. Exp. Zool. 107:315, 1948.
23. Levi-Montalcini, R., and Angeletti, P.U.: Essential role of the nerve growth factor in the survival and maintenance of dissociated sensory and sympathetic embryonic nerve cells in vitro. Dev. Biol. 7:653, 1963.
24. Schmitt, F.O.: Fibrous proteins—neuronal organelles. Proc. Natl. Acad. Sci. USA 60:1092, 1968.
25. Dahlström, A.: Axoplasmic transport (with particular respect to adrenergic neurons). Philos. Trans. R. Soc. Lond. (Biol.) 261:1325, 1971.
26. Schmitt, F.O., and Samson, F.E.: Neuronal fibrous proteins. Neurosci. Res. Program Bull. 6:113, 1968.
27. Ochs, S.: Fast axoplasmic transport-energy metabolism and mechanism. In Hubbard, J.I. (ed.): The Vertebrate Peripheral Nervous System. New York, Plenum Press, 1974.
28. Samson, F.E.: Mechanism of axoplasmic transport. J. Neurobiol. 2:347, 1971.

29. Ochs, S.: Axoplasmic transport—a basis for neural pathology. *In* Dyck, P.J., Thomas, P.K., and Lambert, E.H. (eds.): Peripheral Neuropathy. Philadelphia, W.B. Saunders Company, 1975, pp. 213–230.

30. Droz, B., and Barondes, S.H.: Nerve endings: Rapid appearance of labeled protein shown by electron microscopic radioautography. Science 165:1131, 1969.

31. Ochoa, J., and Mair, W.G.P.: The normal sural nerve in man. II. Changes in axons and Schwann cells due to age. Acta Neuropathol. 13:217, 1969.

32. Cavanagh, J.B.: The significance of the "dying-back" process in experimental and human neurological disease. Int. Rev. Exp. Pathol. 3:219, 1964.

33. Spencer, P.S., and Schaumburg, H.H.: Ultrastructural studies of the dying-back process. IV. Differential vulnerability of PNS and CNS fibers in experimental central-peripheral distal axonopathies. J. Neuropathol. Exp. Neurol. 36:300, 1977.

34. Mendell, J.R., and Sahenk, Z.: Interference of neuronal processing and axoplasmic transport by toxic chemicals. *In* Spencer, P.S., and Schaumburg, H.H. (eds.): Experimental and Clinical Neurotoxicology. Baltimore, Williams and Wilkins Co., 1980.

35. Cho, E.-S., Schaumburg, H.H., and Spencer, P.S.: Adriamycin produces ganglioradiculopathy in rats. J. Neuropathol. Exp. Neurol. 36:597, 1977.

36. Cavanagh, J.B., and Chen, F.C.K.: The effect of methyl-mercury-decyandiamide on the peripheral nerves and spinal cord of rats. Acta Neuropathol. 19:208, 1971.

37. Chou, S.-M., and Hartmann, H.A.: Electron microscopy of focal neuroaxonal lesions produced by B, B-iminodipropionitrile (IDPN) in rats. Acta Neuropathol. 4:590, 1965.

38. Prineas, J.W.: The pathogenesis of dying-back polyneuropathies. Part II. An ultrastructural study of experimental acrylamide intoxication in the cat. J. Neuropathol. Exp. Neurol. 28:598, 1969.

39. Schaumburg, H.H., and Spencer, P.S.: Degeneration in central and peripheral nervous systems produced by pure n-hexane: An experimental study. Brain 99:183, 1976.

40. Clark, A., Griffin, J.W., Price, D.L., Carroll, P., and Hoffman, P.: Pathogenesis of neurofilamentary swellings in B, B-iminodipropionitrile (IDPN): Role of slow axonal transport. Neurology 28a:357, 1978.

41. Sahenk, Z., and Mendell, J.R.: Abnormal retrograde axoplasmic transport in the pathogenesis of the experimental dying-back neuropathy of BOTZ. Neurology 28a:357, 1978.

42. Thomas, P.K.: The selective vulnerability of the centripetal axons of primary sensory neurons. Lecture: Physiologic approaches to neuromuscular disease. Presented at the Mayo Clinic, Department of Neurology, Rochester, Minnesota, April 25, 1982.

43. Morgan-Hughes, J.A., Sinclair, S., and Durston, J.H.: The pattern of peripheral nerve regeneration induced by crush in rats with severe acrylamide neuropathy. Brain 97:235, 1974.

44. Yamada, K.M., Spooner, B.S., and Wessells, N.K.: Axon growth: Roles of microfilaments and microtubules. Proc. Natl. Acad. Sci. USA 66:1206, 1970.

45. Wall, P.D., and Gutnick, M.: Properties of afferent nerve impulses originating from a neuroma. Nature 248:740, 1974.

46. Diamond, J., Ochoa, J., and Culp, W.J.: An introduction to abnormal nerves and muscles as impulse generators. *In* Culp, W.J., and Ochoa, J. (eds.): Abnormal Nerves and Muscles As Impulse Generators. New York, Oxford University Press, 1982.

47. Ochoa, J.: Isoniazid neuropathy in man: Quantitative electron microscope study. Brain 93:831, 1970.

48. Fullerton, P., Gilliatt, R., Lascelles, R., and Morgan-Hughes, J.: The relationship between fiber diameter and internodal length in chronic neuropathy. J. Physiol. 178:26P, 1965.

49. Vizoso, A.D., and Young, J.Z.: Internodal length and fiber diameter in developing and regenerating nerves. J. Anat. 82:110, 1948.

50. Steer, J.M.: Some observations on the fine structure of rat dorsal spinal nerve roots. J. Anat. 109:467, 1971.

51. Maxwell, D.S., Kruger, L., and Pineda, A.: The trigeminal nerve root with special reference to the central peripheral transition zone: An electron microscope study in macaques. Anat. Rec. 164:113, 1969.

52. Geren, B.B.: The formation from the Schwann cell surface of myelin in the peripheral nerves of chick embryos. Exp. Cell Res. 7:558, 1954.

53. Robertson, J.D.: The ultrastructure of adult vertebrate peripheral myelinated nerve fibers in relation to myelinogenesis. J. Biophys. Biochem. Cytol. 1;271, 1955.

54. Bradley, W.G.: Disorders of Peripheral Nerves. Oxford, Blackwell Scientific Publications, 1974.

55. Waksman, B.H., and Adams, R.D.: Allergic neuritis: An experimental disease of rabbits induced by the injection of peripheral nervous tissue and adjuvant. J. Exp. Med. 102:213, 1955.

56. Rogart, R.B., and Stampfli, R.: Voltage clamp studies of mammalian myelinated nerve. *In* Culp, W.J., and Ochoa, J. (eds.): Abnormal Nerves and Muscles as Impulse Generators. New York, Oxford University Press, 1982, pp. 193–210.

57. Ritchie, J.M., and Rogart, R.B.: The density of sodium channels in mammalian myelinated nerve fibers and the nature of the axonal membrane under the myelin sheath. Proc. Natl. Acad. Sci. USA 74;211, 1977.

58. Barchi, R.L., Weigele, J.B., and Cohen, S.A.: Biochemical approaches to the sodium channel: Saxitoxin binding component from mammalian excitable membrane. *In* Culp, W.J., and Ochoa, J., (eds.): Abnormal Nerves and Muscles as Impulse Generators. New York, Oxford University Press, 1982, pp. 130–151.

59. Culp, W.J.: Scorpion neurotoxins as affinity reagents for voltage-dependent sodium channel components. *In* Culp, W.J., and Ochoa, J., (eds.): Abnormal Nerves and Muscles as Impulse Generators. New York, Oxford University Press, 1982, pp. 151–162.

60. Waxman, S.G.: Variations in axonal morphology and their functional significance. *In* Waxman, S.G. (ed.): Physiology and Pathobiology of Axons. New York, Raven Press, 1978.

61. Ochoa, J.: Nerve fiber pathology in acute and chronic compression. *In* Omer, G.E., and Spinner, M. (eds.): Management of Peripheral Nerve Problems. Philadelphia, W.B. Saunders Company, 1980, p. 47.

62. Rasminsky, M.: Physiology of conduction in demyelinated axons. *In* Waxman, S.G. (ed.): Physiology and Pathobiology of Axons. New York, Raven Press, 1978, p. 361.

63. Bostok, H., and Sears, T.A.: The internodal axon membrane: Electrical excitability and continuous conduction in segmental demyelination. J. Physiol. 280:273, 1978.

64. Bostok, H.: Conduction changes in mammalian axons following experimental demyelination. *In* Culp, W.J., and Ochoa, J. (eds.): Abnormal Nerves and Muscles as Impulse Generators. New York, Oxford University Press, 1982, pp. 236–252.

65. Gilliatt, R.W.: Nerve conduction in human and experimental neuropathies. Proc. R. Soc. Med. 59:989, 1966.

66. Dyck, P.J., and Lambert, E.H.: Lower motor and primary sensory neuron diseases with peroneal muscular atrophy. I. Neurologic, genetic and electrophysiologic findings in hereditary polyneuropathies. Arch. Neurol. 18:603, 1968.

67. Dyck, P.J., and Lambert, E.H.: Lower motor and primary sensory neuron diseases with peroneal muscular atrophy. II. Neurologic, genetic and electrophysiological findings in various neuronal degenerations. Arch. Neurol. 18:619, 1968.

68. Ridley, A.: The neuropathy of acute intermittent porphyria. Q. J. Med. 38:307, 1969.

69. Cavanagh, J.B., and Mellick, R.S.: On the nature of the peripheral nerve lesions associated with acute intermittent porphyria. J. Neurol. Neurosurg. Psychiatry 28:320, 1965.

70. Kocen, R.S., Thomas, P.K., Kink, R.H.M., and Haas, L.F.: Nerve biopsy findings in two cases of Tangier disease. Acta Neuropathol. 26:317, 1973.

71. Sabin, T.D.: Temperature-linked sensory loss: A unique pattern in leprosy. Arch. Neurol. 20:257, 1969.

72. Thomas, P.K.: Symptomatology and differential diagnosis of peripheral neuropathy. Clinical features and differential diagnosis. *In* Dyck, P.J., Thomas, P.K., and Lambert, E.H. (eds.): Peripheral Neuropathy. Philadelphia, W.B. Saunders Company, 1975, pp. 495–512.

73. Fisher, M.: An unusual variant of acute idiopathic polyneuritis (syndrome of ophthalmoplegia, ataxia and areflexia). N. Engl. J. Med. 255:57, 1956.

74. Wertstein, A.: The origin of fasciculations in motor neuron disease. Ann. Neurol., 5:295, 1979.

75. Roth, G.: The origin of fasciculations. Ann. Neurol. 12:542, 1982.

76. Woltmann, H.W.: The nervous symptoms in pernicious anemia: An analysis of 150 cases. Am. J. Med. Sci. 173:400, 1919.

77. Victor, M.: Polyneuropathy due to nutritional deficiency and alcoholism. *In* Dyck, P.J., Thomas, P.K., and Lambert, E.H. (eds.): Peripheral Neuropathy. Philadelphia, W.B. Saunders Company, 1975, pp. 1030–1066.

78. Ridley, A.: Porphyric neuropathy. *In* Dyck, P.J., Thomas, P.K., and Lambert, E.H. (eds.): Peripheral Neuropathy. Philadelphia, W.B. Saunders Company, 1975, pp. 942–955.

79. Griffin, J.W., Goren, E., Schaumburg, H., Engel, W.K., and Loriaux, L.: Adrenomyeloneuropathy: A probable variant of adrenoleukodystrophy. I. Clinical and endocrinologic aspects. Neurology 27:1107, 1977.

80. Cavanagh, J.B.: Peripheral nerve changes in orthocresyl phosphate poisoning of the cat. J. Pathol. Bacteriol. 87:365, 1964.

81. Layzer, R.B.: Myeloneuropathy after prolonged exposure to nitrous oxide. Lancet 2:1227, 1978.

82. Conn, D.L., and Dyck, P.J.: Angiopathic neuropathy in connective tissue diseases. In Dyck, P.J., Thomas, P.K., and Lambert, E.H. (eds.): Peripheral Neuropathy. Philadelphia, W.B. Saunders Company, 1975, pp. 1149–1165.

83. Johnson, R.L., Smyth, C.J., Holt, G.W., Lubckenco, A., and Valentine, E.: Steroid therapy and vascular lesions in rheumatoid arthritis. Arthritis Rheum. 2:224, 1959.

84. Good, A.F., Christopher, R.P., Koepke, G.H., Bender, L.F., and Tarter, M.: Peripheral neuropathy associated with rheumatoid arthritis: A clinical and electrodiagnostic study of 70 consecutive rheumatoid arthritis patients. Ann. Intern. Med. 63:87, 1965.

85. Pallis, C.A., and Scott, J.T.: Peripheral neuropathy in rheumatoid arthritis. Br. Med. J. I:1141, 1965.

86. Weller, R.O., Bruckner, F.E., and Chamberlain, M.A.: Rheumatoid neuropathy: A histological and electrophysiological study. J. Neurol. Neurosurg. Psychiatry 33:592, 1970.

87. Irby, R., Adams, R.A., and Toone, E.C.: Peripheral neuritis associated with rheumatoid arthritis. Arthritis Rheum. 1:44, 1958.

88. Ferguson, R.H., and Slocumb, C.H.: Peripheral neuropathy in rheumatoid arthritis. Bull. Rheum. Dis. II:251, 1961.

89. Hart, F.D., and Golding, J.R.: Rheumatoid neuropathy. Br. Med. J. 1:1594, 1960.

90. Wees, S.J., Sun Woo, I.N., and Joong Oh, S.: Sural nerve biopsy in systemic necrotizing vasculitis. Am. J. Med. 71:525, 1981.

91. Dyck, P.J., Conn, D.L., and Okazaki, H.: Necrotizing angiopathic neuropathy: Three-dimensional morphology of fiber degeneration related to sites of occluded vessels. Mayo Clin. Proc. 47:461, 1972.

92. Conn, D.L., McDuffee, F.C., and Dyck, P.J.: Immunopathologic study of sural nerves in rheumatoid arthritis. Arthritis Rheum. 15:135, 1972.

93. Moore, P.M., and Fauce, A.S.: Neurologic manifestations of systemic vasculitis. A retrospective and prospective study of the clinicopathologic features and responses to therapy in 25 patients. Am. J. Med. 71:517, 1981.

94. Peyronnard, J.M., Charron, L., Beaudet F., and Couture, F.: Vasculitic neuropathy in rheumatoid disease and Sjögren's syndrome. Neurology 32:839, 1982.

95. Fox, J.D., and Kenmore, P.I.: The effect of ischemia on nerve conduction. Exp. Neurol. 17:403, 1967.

96. Garven, H.S.D., Gairns, F.W., and Smith, G.: The nerve fiber populations of the nerves of the leg in chronic occlusive arterial disease in man. Scott. Med. J. 7:250, 1962.

97. Hess, K., Eames, R.A., Darveniza, P., and Gilliatt, R.W.: Acute ischemic neuropathy in the rabbit. J. Neurol. Sci. 44:19, 1979.

98. Korthals, J.K., and Wisnuwski, H.M.: Peripheral nerve ischemia. I. Experimental model. J. Neurol. Sci. 24:65, 1975.

99. Scott, D.G., Bacon, P.A., and Tribe, C.R.: Systemic rheumatoid vasculitis: A clinical and laboratory study of 50 cases. Medicine 60:288, 1981.

100. Frohner, P.P., and Sheps, S.G.: Long-term follow-up study of periarteritis nodosa. Am. J. Med. 43:8, 1967.

101. Lovelace, R.E.: Mononeuritis multiplex in polyarteritis nodosa. Neurology 14:434, 1964.

102. Alexander, E.L., Provost, T., Stevens, M.B., and Alexander, G.: Neurologic complications of primary Sjögren's syndrome. Medicine 61:247, 1982.

103. Alexander, G.E., Provost, T.T., Stevens, M.B., and Alexander, E.L.: Sjögren's syndrome: Central nervous system manifestations. Neurology 31:1391, 1981.

104. Iwashita, H., Argyrakis, A., Lowetzseh, K., and Spaar, F.-W.: Polyneuropathy in Waldenström's macroglobulinemia. J. Neurol. Sci. 21:341, 1974.

105. Kyle, R.A., and Bayrd, E.D.: Amyloidosis: A review of 236 cases. Medicine (Baltimore) 54:271, 1975.

106. Kelly, J., Kyle, R., and O'Brien, P.: The natural history of peripheral neuropathy in primary systemic amyloidosis. Ann. Neurol. 6:1, 1979.

107. Dyck, P.J., and Lambert, E.H.: Dissociated sensation in amyloidosis. Arch. Neurol. 20:490, 1969.

108. Blom, S., Steen, L., and Zetterlund, B.: Familial amyloidosis with polyneuropathy-Type I: A neurophysiological study of peripheral nerve function. Acta Neurol. Scand. 63:99, 1981.

109. Cohen, A.S., and Benson, M.: Amyloid neuropathy. In Dyck, P.J., Thomas, P.K., and Lambert, E.H. (eds.): Peripheral Neuropathy. Philadelphia, W.B. Saunders Company, 1975, pp. 1012–1029.

110. Waldenström, J.: Incipient myelomatosis or "essential" hyperglobulinemia with fibrinogenia-A new syndrome? Acta Med. Scand. 117:216, 1944.

111. Fahey, J.L., Barth, W.F., and Solomon, A.: Serum hyperviscosity syndrome. JAMA 192:464, 1965.

112. Logothetis, J.P., Silverstein, P., and Coe, J.: Neurologic aspects of Waldenström's macroglobulinemia. Arch. Neurol. 5:564, 1960.

113. Waldenström, J.: Studies on "abnormal" serum globulins (M-components) in myeloma macroglobulinasemia and related disease: Clinical diagnosis and biochemical finding in material of 296 sera with M type marrow Y globulins. Acta Med. Scand. 170(Suppl. 367):110, 1961.

114. McLeod, J.G., and Walsh, J.C.: Neuropathies associated with paraproteinemias and dysproteinemias. In Dyck, P.J., Thomas, P.K., and Lambert, E.H. (eds.): Peripheral Neuropathy. Philadelphia, W.B. Saunders Company, 1975, pp. 1012–1029.

115. Kreindler, A., and Macover-Patrichi, M.: Recurrent cranial nerve palsies of dysglobulinaemic origin. J. Neurol. Sci. 6:117, 1968.

116. Darnley, J.D.: Polyneuropathy in Waldenström's macroglobulinemia. Neurology 12:617, 1962.

117. Aarseth, S., Ofstad, E., and Torvek, A.: Macroglobulinaemia Waldenström: A case with haemolytic syndrome and involvement of the nervous system. Acta Med. Scand. 169:691, 1961.

118. Vital, C., Valeat, J., Deminiere, C., et al.: Peripheral nerve damage during multiple myeloma and Waldenström's macroglobulinemia. An ultrastructural and immunopathologic study. Cancer 50:1491, 1982.

119. Propp, R.P., Means, E., Derbel, R., et al.: Waldenström's macroglobulinemia and neuropathy. Deposition of M component in myelin sheaths. Neurology 25:980, 1975.

120. Latov, N., Sherman, W., Nemni, R., Galassi, G., Shyong, J., Penn, A., Chess, L. Olarte, M., Rowland, L., and Osserman, E.: Plasma-cell dyscrasia and peripheral neuropathy with monoclonal antibody to peripheral nerve myelin. N. Engl. J. Med. 303:618, 1980.

121. Abrams, G., Latov, N., Hays, A., Shermann, W., and Zimmerman, E.: Immunocytochemical studies of human peripheral nerve with serum from patients with polyneuropathy and paraproteinemia. Neurology 32:821, 1982.

122. Braun, P.E., Latov, N., and Freil, M.D.: MAG is the antigen for a monoclonal antibody in patients with a demyelinating neuropathy. Trans. Am. Soc. Neurochem. 13:230, 1982.

123. Silverstein, A., and Doniger, D.E.: Neurologic complications of myelomatosis. Arch. Neurol. 9:534, 1963.

124. Walsh, J.C.: The neuropathy of multiple myeloma: An electrophysiological histological study. Arch. Neurol. 25:404, 1971.

125. Hesselvik, M.: Neuropathological studies on myelomatosis. Acta Neurol. Scand. 45:95, 1969.

126. Kelly, J.J., Kyle, R.A., Miles, J.M., O'Brien, P.C., and Dyck, P.J.: The spectrum of peripheral neuropathy in myeloma. Neurology 31:24, 1981.

127. Victor, M., Banker, B.Q., and Adams, R.D.: The neuropathy of multiple myeloma. J. Neurol. Neurosurg. Psychiatry 21:73, 1958.

128. Campbell, A.M., and Halford, M.: Syndrome of diarrhoea and peripheral nerve changes due to generalized vascular disease. Br. Med. J. 2:1509, 1964.

129. Kyle, R.: Long-term survival in multiple myeloma. N. Engl. J. Med. 308:314, 1983.

130. Kelly, J.J., Kyle, R.A., Miles, J.M., and Dyck, P.J.: Osteosclerotic myeloma and peripheral neuropathy. Neurology 33:202, 1983.

131. Waldenström, J.G., Adner, A., Gydell, K., and Zettervall, O.: Osteosclerotic "plasmacytoma" with polyneuropathy, hypertrichosis, and diabetes. Acta Med. Scand. 203:297, 1978.

132. Morley, J.B., and Schwieger, A.C.: The relation between chronic polyneuropathy and osteosclerotic myeloma. J. Neurol. Neurosurg. Psychiatry 30:432, 1967.

133. Read, D., and Warlow, C.: Peripheral neuropathy and solitary plasmacytoma. J. Neurol. Neurosurg. Psychiatry 41:177, 1978.

134. Brouet, J.C., Clauvel, J.P., Danon, F., Klein, M., and Seligman, M.: Biologic and clinical significances of cryoglobulins: A report of 86 cases. Am. J. Med. 57:775, 1974.

135. Konesi, T., Saida, K., Ohnishi, A., and Nishitani, H.: Perineuritis in mononeuritis multiplex with cryoglobulinemia. Muscle Nerve 5:173, 1982.

136. Cream, J.J., Hern, J.E.C., Hughes, R., and MacKenzie, I.: Mixed or immune complex cryoglobulinaemia and neuropathy. J. Neurol. Neurosurg. Psychiatry 37:82, 1974.

137. Chad, D., Parisher, K., Bradley, W., et al.: The pathogenesis of cryoglobulinemic neuropathy. Neurology 32:725, 1982.

138. Vallat, J.M., Desproges-Gotteron, R., Leboutet, M., Loubet, A., Gaulde, N., and Treves, R.: Cryoglobulinemic neuropathy: A pathological study. Ann. Neurol. 8:179, 1980.

139. Maycock, R.L., Bertrand, P., Morrison, C.E., and Scott, J.: Manifestations of sarcoidosis. Am. J. Med. 35:67, 1963.

140. Delaney, P.: Neurologic manifestations in sarcoidosis. Review of the literature, with a report of 23 cases. Ann. Intern. Med. 87:336, 1977.

141. Silverstein, A., Feur, M.M., and Seltzbach, L.E.: Neurologic sarcoidosis. Arch. Neurol. 12:1, 1965.

142. Matthews, W.B.: Sarcoid neuropathy. In Dyke, P.J., Thomas, P.K., and Lambert, E.H. (eds.): Peripheral Neuropathy. Philadelphia, W.B. Saunders Company, 1975, pp. 1199–1226.

143. Jefferson, M.: Sarcoidosis of the nervous system. Brain 80:540, 1957.

144. Tharp, B.R., and Pfeiffer, J.B.: Sarcoidosis and the acoustic nerve. Arch. Otolaryngol. 90:360, 1969.

145. Strickland, G.T., and Moser, K.M.: Sarcoidosis with a Landry-Guillain-Barré syndrome and clinical response to corticosteroids. Am. J. Med. 43:131, 1967.

146. Nemni, R., Galassi, G., Cohen, M., Hays, A., Gould, R., Singh, N., Bressman, S., and Gamboa, E.: Symmetric sarcoid polyneuropathy: Analysis of a sural nerve biopsy. Neurology 31:1217, 1981.

147. Oh, S.J.: Sarcoid polyneuropathy: A histologically proven case. Ann. Neurol. 7:178, 1980.

148. Colover, J.: Sarcoidosis with involvement of the nervous system. Brain 71:451, 1948.
149. Wells, C.E.C.: The natural history of neurosarcoidosis. Proc. R. Soc. Med. 60:1172, 1967.
150. Bechelli, L.M., and Martinez, D.V.: The leprosy problem in the world. Bull. WHO 34:811, 1966.
151. Levis, W.R., and Hedrick, J.L.: Rising incidence of leprosy in the United States. N. Engl. J. Med. 304:363, 1981.
152. Sabin, T.B.: Neurologic features of lepromatous leprosy. Am. Fam. Physician 4:84, 1971.
153. Sheagren, J.N., Block, J.B., Trautman, J.R., and Wolff, S.M.: Immunologic reactivity in patients with leprosy. Ann. Intern. Med. 70:295, 1969.
154. Nath, I., and Singh, R.: The suppressive effect of M. leprae. Clin. Exp. Immunol. 41:406, 1980.
155. Bullock, W.E.: Studies of immune mechanisms in leprosy. I. Depression of delayed allergic response to skin test antigens. N. Engl. J. Med. 278:298, 1968.
156. Turk, J.L., and Waters, M.E.R.: Cell-mediated immunity in patients with leprosy. Lancet 2:243, 1969.
157. Sabin, T.D., and Swift, T.R.: Leprosy. In Dyck, P.J., Thomas, P.K., and Lambert, E.H. (eds.): Peripheral Neuropathy. Philadelphia, W.B. Saunders Company, 1975, pp. 1166–1199.
158. Sabin, T.D., and Ebner, J.D.: Patterns of sensory loss in lepromatous leprosy. Int. J. Lepr. 37:239, 1969.
159. Pedley, J.C., Harman, D.J., Waudy, H., and McDougall, A.C.: Leprosy in peripheral nerves: Histopathological findings in 119 untreated patients in Nepal. J. Neurol. Neurosurg. Psychiatry 43(3):198, 1980.
160. Dastur, D.K.: Cutaneous nerve in leprosy: The relationship between histopathology and cutaneous sensitivity. Brain 78:615, 1955.
161. Rosenberg, R.N., and Lovelace, R.E.: Mononeuritis multiplex in lepromatous leprosy. Arch. Neurol. 19:310, 1968.
162. Kopell, H.P., and Thompson, W.A.C.: Peripheral Entrapment Neuropathies. Baltimore, Williams and Wilkins, 1965.
163. Job, C.K.: Mycobacterium leprae in nerve lesions in lepromatous leprosy. An electron microscopic study. Arch. Pathol. 89:195, 1970.
164. Dastur, D.K.: Lepromatous leprosy as a model of Schwann cell pathology and lysosomal activity. Clin. Exp. Neurol. 16:277, 1979.
165. Enna, C.D., and Brand, P.W.: Peripheral nerve abscess in leprosy. Lepr. Rev. 41:175, 1970.
166. Brand, P.W.: Treatment of leprosy: The role of surgery. N. Engl. J. Med. 254:64, 1956.
167. Behse, F., and Buckthal, F.: Slowing in maximum nerve conduction velocity during acute hypoxia due to block of large fibers or to slowing along all fibers. 21st Scandinavian Congress of Neurology, Stockholm, June 1975.
168. Caruso, G., Labianca, O., and Ferrannini, E.: Effects of ischemia on sensory protential of normal subjects of different ages. J. Neurol. Neurosurg. Psychiatry 36:455, 1973.
169. Caruso, G., Santoro, L., Perretti, A., and Amantin, B.: Recovery of sensory potentials after ischemic block by pneumatic compression of varying duration. Proceedings of the International Symposium on Peripheral Neuropathies, Milan, June 1978.
170. Kugelberg, E., and Cobb, W.: Repetitive discharges in human motor nerve fibers during the postischemic state. J. Neurol. Neurosurg. Psychiatry 14:88, 1951.
171. Merrington, W.R., and Nathan, P.W.: A study of postischemic paresthesiae. J. Neurol. Neurosurg. Psychiatry 12:1, 1949.
172. Torebjörk, H.E., Ochoa, J.L., and McCann, F.V.: Paresthesiae: Abnormal impulse generation in sensory nerve fibers in man. Acta Physiologica Scand. 105:518, 1979.
173. Ochoa, J.L., and Torebjörk, H.E.: Paresthesiae from ectopic impulse generation in human sensory nerves. Brain 103:835, 1980.

174. Erb, W.: Diseases of the peripheral cerebrospinal nerves. In Ziemssen, H. Von (ed.): Cyclopedia of the Practice of Medicine. Vol. XI. London, Samson, Low, Marston, Searle and Rivington, 1876.
175. Seddon, H.J.: Three types of nerve injury. Brain 66:237, 1943.
176. Denny-Brown, D., and Brenner, C.: Paralysis of nerve induced by direct pressure and by tourniquet. Arch. Neurol. Psychiatry 51:1, 1944.
177. Ochoa, J., Danta, G., Fowler, T.J., and Gilliatt, R.W.: Nature of the nerve lesion caused by pneumatic tourniquet. Nature 233:265, 1971.
178. Lubinska, L.: Axoplasmic streaming in regenerating and in normal nerve fibers. In Singer, M., and Schade, J.P. (eds.): Progress in Brain Research. Vol. 13, Mechanisms of Neural Regeneration. Amsterdam, Elsevier Publishing Co., 1964, pp. 1–77.
179. Hiscoe, H.B.: Distribution of nodes and incisurae in normal and regenerated nerve fibers. Anat. Rec. 99:447, 1947.
180. Lubinska, L.: Demyelination and remyelination in the proximal parts of regenerated nerve fiber. J. Comp. Neurol. 117:275, 1961.
181. Seddon, H.J.: Peripheral nerve injuries in Great Britain during World War II: A review. Arch. Neurol. Psychiatry 63:171, 1950.
182. Seltzer, C.A., and Sevor, M.: Ephaptic transmission in chronically damaged peripheral nerves. Neurology 29:1061, 1979.
183. Ochoa, J.: Pain in local nerve lesions. In Culp, W., and Ochoa, J. (eds.): Abnormal Nerves and Muscles as Impulse Generators. New York, Oxford University Press, 1982.
184. Fullerton, P.M.: The effect of ischemia on nerve conduction in carpal tunnel syndrome. J. Neurol. Neurosurg. Psychiatry 26:385, 1963.
185. Fullerton, P.M., and Gilliatt, R.W.: Median and ulnar neuropathy in the guinea pig. J. Neurol. Neurosurg. Psychiatry 30:393, 1967.
186. Ochoa, J., and Marotte L.: Nature of the nerve lesion underlying chronic entrapment. J. Neurol. Sci. 19:49, 1973.
187. Neary, D., Ochoa, J., and Gilliatt, R.W.: Subclinical entrapment neuropathy in man. J. Neurol. Sci. 24:283, 1975.
188. Schaumburg, H.H., Spencer, P.S., and Ochoa, J.: The aging human peripheral nervous system. In Katzman, R., and Terry, R.D. (eds.): The Neurology of Aging, Philadelphia, F.A. Davis Co., 1983.
189. Spencer, P.S., and Ochoa, J.: The mammalian peripheral nervous system in old age. In Johnson, J.E., Jr. (ed.): Aging and Cell Structure. Vol. I. New York, Plenum Press, 1981.
190. Jenkyn, L.R., and Reeves, A.G.: Neurologic signs in uncomplicated aging (senescence). Semin. Neurol. 1:21, 1981.
191. Steiness, I.: Vibration perception in normal subjects. Acta Med. Scand. 158:315, 1957.
192. Pearson, G.H.: Effect of age on vibratory sensibility. Arch. Neurol. Psychiatry 20:482, 1928.
193. Critchley, M.: The neurology of old age. Lancet 1:1221, 1931.
194. Goldberg, J.M., and Lindblom, U.: Standardized method of determining vibratory perception thresholds for diagnosis and screening in neurological investigation. J. Neurol. Neurosurg. Psychiatry 42:793, 1979.
195. Potvin, A.R., Syndulko, K., Tourtellotte, W.W., Lemman, J.A., and Potvin, J.H.: Human neurologic function and the aging process. J. Am. Geriatr. Soc. 28:1, 1980.
196. Dyck, P.J., Curtis, D.J., Bushek, W., and Offord, K.: Description of "Minnesota thermal discs" and normal values of cutaneous thermal discrimination in man. Neurology 24:325, 1974.
197. Prakash, C., and Stern, G.: Neurological signs in the elderly. Age Ageing 2:24, 1973.
198. Carter, A.B.: The neurologic aspects of aging. In Rossman, I. (ed.): Clinical Geriatrics. Second edition. Philadelphia, J.B. Lippincott, 1979.
199. Jenkyn, L.R., Walsh, D.B., Walsh, B.T., Culver, C.M., and Reeves, A.G.: The nuchocephalic reflex. J. Neurol. Neurosurg. Psychiatry 38:561, 1975.
200. Klawans, H.L., Tupo, H.M., Ostfeld, A.M., Shekelli, R.B., and Killridge, J.A.: Neurologic examination in an elderly population. Dis. Nerv. Syst. 32:374, 1971.

Chapter 20
Biomechanics of Joints

Sheldon R. Simon

INTRODUCTION

Webster's Third New International Dictionary defines that specialized organ system of the body called a joint as the "point of contact between elements of an animal skeleton . . . with the parts . . . that surround and support it." It continues to describe a joint in more general terms as "an area at which two ends, surfaces, or edges are *attached,*" "the junction of two or more members of a *framed structure,*" "a fracture or crack in rock *not accompanied by dislocation,*" and "a part or *space* included between two articulations" (emphasis added). Mechanics is defined as that "branch of physical science that deals with energy and forces" and their effect on bodies, and the "practical application of mechanics to the design, construction, or operation of machines," and "of the nature of or resembling a machine especially in routine or automatic performance." In describing the biomechanics of joints how many of these definitions apply? The answer is simpler than the explanation: all of them and more.

All joints in the body exist as the point, place, crack, or junction where at least two skeletal members attach, and all joints essentially consist of the same elements of the space between the members and the parts that surround, support, and stabilize it. However, the location of each joint in its proximal or distal, upper or lower position sufficiently alters the mechanics to make it uniquely distinct (e.g., hip joint, knee joint, elbow joints, or finger joints).[1-7]

Animal joints are classified into groups according to the biologic nature of the materials and the amount of relative motion between the articular ends of the bones. In general three types of joints exist:[8] (1) fibrous joints or synarthroses: joints with no relative motion; (2) cartilaginous joints or amphiarthroses: joints with little or no relative motion; and (3) diarthrodial or synovial joints: joints with large degrees of motion.[9-15] Whether mechanical conditions have created distinct individual joint constructs or biological design has designated their uniquely specified mechanics is not known; but as we shall see, when joint destruction is present and treatment is attempted, the outcome of the situation is heavily dependent upon the mechanics.

BIOMECHANICS OF NORMAL JOINTS

Joint Stability. All joints have the potential to move. True joint movement is the relative change in position of one skeletal member in relation to its adjacent one. When we pick up a glass and bring it to our mouth, our wrist moves from a position on the table to one adjacent to our face. This type of movement may be considered extremity movement and total joint displacement, rather than true joint movement. There are six possible types of motion about three perpendicular axes: three rotational and three translational (Fig. 20–1). In general most joint motion is only minimally translational and is primarily rotational.[9-17] If the motion were solely rotational, at any instant, the center of the radius of the arc of motion would repeatedly be at the same point. However, there exists a small component of translational movement, and the deviation from absolute rotatory motion may be noted by the changes in the path of the joint's "instantaneous centers of rotation" (Fig. 20–2). These centers have been measured for the shoulder, elbow, wrist, knee, and ankle and found to vary only slightly from true arcs of rotation.[18-28] However, this minimal translation or deviation from it may be detrimental to the joints.

The inability of the structures making up a joint to limit translational motions and to restrict some rotational arcs of motion is considered subluxation or dislocation of the joint. To stabilize joints and maintain them moving principally in rotational arcs, three anatomical structures are utilized: bones, ligaments, and muscles. These three structures contribute to different extents at different joints.

The first structure to be considered is bone. The contours of the ends of each bone are unique for each joint and each side of a joint. No two are alike. Although in general one side of a joint may be considered concave in shape and the other side convex, at each joint significant deviations exist in each of the three rotational planes in the radius of curvature, and in the amount of the arc of curvature that is present. Since bone is the most rigid anatomical structure, in any rotational plane the greater the arc of motion enclosed by bone, the greater the amount of inherent stability that exists. For example, at the hip the spherical head of the femur is almost enclosed by a hemispherical arc of bony acetabulum, whereas the shoulder, with a similar shape but a much flatter radius of curvature and a less enclosed humeral head is markedly different in the ease with which it can be subluxed or dislocated (Fig. 20–3).[19,30]

If stability is desired and the contour of the bone is inadequate to achieve it, a second structure is available—ligaments. The ability of ligaments to restrict displacement absolutely is not as good as that of bone but is perfectly adequate under most circumstances and situations. The intrinsic properties of ligaments are different from those of bone in several aspects. Unlike bone, ligament cannot provide stability against translational mo-

Figure 20-1. All motions of two adjacent bodies relative to each other consist of translational motions along three mutually perpendicular axes and three rotational motions about these same three axes.

Figure 20-3. Both the hip and shoulder joints have no rotational restrictions and have similar ball-in-socket shapes. The glenoid socket does not stabilize the humeral head as well as the acetabulum stabilizes the femoral head.

tions in any direction which is across or perpendicular to its major axis—it is not "solid enough." The medial collateral ligament of the knee, for example, will not prevent anterior-posterior (AP) or medial-lateral translational motions by itself (Fig. 20-4). Ligaments resist motions that are situated in the plane in which the ligament lies. Furthermore, when ligaments are called upon to resist displacement in such a direction, they are not only weaker than bone in being able to do so, but also will yield or stretch.[31-37] In certain circumstances this feature seems to be a desirable one, as ligaments are commonly used throughout the body as structural joint stabilizers.[38-54] Most often they complement the effect of bony contouring by limiting the degree of *allowable* rotatory motion rather than by preventing translation. The control of translational motions, which can lead to subluxation or dislocation, is left in most cases for bone.[38-41,48,49] At the ankle, the deltoid and lateral ligaments limit varus-valgus rotation in the same plane as the tibial-fibular ankle mortise limits medial-lateral translation (Fig. 20-5). In other circumstances bone and ligaments function in different planes. For example, at the elbow, bony contouring in the AP plane limits AP translation, while ligaments in the medial-lateral plane limit varus-valgus rotation.

At certain joints the forces in a given rotational plane are minimal and a single ligament may act alone. If the forces are high, several ligaments, or a markedly thickened or structurally modified and strengthened ligament, or even the complementary action of a third structural member, muscle, may be present.[58-69] For example, to control varus-valgus and internal-external rotation in the medial-lateral plane of the knee, bone and ligaments are complemented by multiple muscles such as the hamstrings (Fig. 20-6).[42-69] Another example is the spine, where the posterior ligamentous elements are multiple, with each one having a different basic structure and anatomic size, and they work in combination with the extensor paraspinal muscle group to prevent excessive flexion.

The muscle-tendon complex, similar to ligaments in the manner in which it stabilizes a joint, is unlike either bone or ligament in its capability to respond, as it first must be activated. Of all three structural "stabilizers," muscle is the only one which can be controlled during the immediate action. It can thus act as a stabilizer and resist rotatory motions created by external forces or can itself create unstable rotatory motions.[58-69]

Figure 20-2. If a body rotates in place, the center of its rotation does not move. If the body translates as it rotates, movement of the center of rotation reflects this motion.

Figure 20-4. At the knee the medial collateral ligament can only restrict the valgus rotational motions—i.e., motions parallel to the ligament's length. It cannot restrict anterior-posterior or medial-lateral translational or flexion-extension rotational motions of the joint, motions which are perpendicular to its axis.

Figure 20–5. Ankle stability in the medial-lateral plane is maintained by a combination of bony contouring limiting translational movements and ligaments limiting rotational movements.

Figure 20–6. At the knee, bony contouring (tibial spine) only stabilizes medial-lateral translational motion. To control all the other motions that this joint undergoes, multiple ligaments of different sizes and shapes as well as muscles in many planes are needed.

The intricate balance among the three structural stabilizers, bone, ligament, and muscle, is best illustrated by the spine. To protect the spinal cord while still allowing rotatory motions of the trunk to occur, a sophisticated mechanical stabilizing arrangement has evolved. Each intervertebral segment has unique modification of all three structures to satisfy differing mechanical conditions yet maintain balance. The intervertebral unit is composed of two joints (one disc, an amphiarthritic joint, and two diarthrodial facet joints), multiple ligaments (anterior and posterior longitudinal ligaments, ligamentum flavum, and interspinous ligaments), and paraspinal muscles. The disc, unlike other amphiarthritic joints, is a very important joint, being the major supporting unit between the vertebral bony units and maintaining the vertical rigidity of the entire system.[70,71] This biological structure with its central nucleus pulposus and surrounding ligamentous anulus fibrosus may be compared to a hydrostatic balloon set in a coffee can; the nucleus is resistant to being vertically deformed because no significant sideways displacement is permitted by the anulus fibrosus (Fig. 20–7A). Although the disc will stabilize vertical loads and prevent vertical translation, it does not stabilize horizontal translation.[72] When a person sits, stands, or bends forward, whether to tie a shoelace or pick up a weight, the body's weight is located anterior to the spine. This configuration would not only compress the disc but would also topple the spine by creating forces tending to tilt and slide one vertebral unit over the one below it. To prevent the sliding, "slipping" motions, each vertebral body must overhang the one below it. This arrangement is provided by the facet joints, located posteriorly and laterally. They provide little vertical support for body weight but prevent AP and medial-lateral translational motions (Fig. 20–7B). However, movements in rotational arcs whose axes cross at the posterior central portion of the disc are still allowed. Depending on the degree to which the translational sliding motions in any direction need be restricted, the joints are oriented differently in the atlantoaxial region, cervical spine region, and thoracic and lumbar spine regions. Within the planes and motions so allowed, the ligaments and muscles then limit the *extent* and control the degree and speed with which such motions occur, acting as the major source of stability to rotation (Fig. 20–7C).[72-89] However, a price is paid for the use of muscle effort. To control forward trunk flexion the erector spinae muscles must exert large forces

Figure 20–7. The intervertebral unit of the spine has multiple structures contributing to its stability. The disc (A) prevents vertical translational motions, like a balloon placed in a coffee can. The facet joints (B) prevent forward translation, permitting the more proximal vertebrae only to rotate about the more distal one in a prescribed arc. Multiple ligaments and paraspinal muscles control the speed and extent within this arc of movement through their "clamping" effect on the posterior elements (C).

to counterbalance body weight. These forces cause large compression forces, ranging from 600 to 1500 lbs, to be exerted across the disc.[86,90,91] The intervertebral discs cannot routinely be subjected to these extreme pressures, as they would not be able to withstand them. Thus investigators suspected that another structure besides the spine might play a role in trunk stability. At first sight it seems unreasonable to assume any pressure transfers through the trunk other than through the spine, because all the other structures are soft. However, a soft material can be arranged in such a way that use is made of its tensile strength, rather than its rigidity, to transmit pressures.[92] In a manner similar to the way the disc controls and withstands the vertical pressures imposed upon it, intra-abdominal pressure may play a significant role in trunk stability (Fig. 20–8).[86-94] Although the abdominal muscle is potentially a source to reduce the load across the disc regardless of its strength, in certain situations it may not be utilized, and its effect in reducing disc loads has therefore been disputed.[89,93,94]

Joint Motions. As a consequence of bone, ligaments, and muscles contributing to joint stability to various degrees and in various planes, each joint in the body is distinct with regard to both the types of motions that exist and the degree to which each is allowed.[95-98] While some joints have grossly similar movements, for example, hip and shoulder, knee and elbow, ankle and wrist, the combinations of the three structural units comprising them are different and appear related to the external force demands and functional requirements imposed upon them.

The spine, while providing support for the body above it and protecting the spinal cord within it, must have some degree of flexibility to allow proper sensing of the head and proper coordination between the head, upper extremities, and lower extremities for the vital functions of daily living. Although motions at any given joint cannot and need not be large (as this would place too great a strain on the spinal cord at any individual level), they are different at different levels of the spine owing to the functions that must be performed.[75,99-102]

In the human, the primary function of the upper extremities is to transport and manipulate objects; that of the lower extremities is to facilitate locomotion. To provide for the wide sphere of influence an extremity can encompass, the most proximal joint must have the widest range of motion and allow rotatory motions of large degrees in all three planes (Fig. 20–9).[103,104] Because most of the external forces on the extremity are exerted at some distance from the joint, controlling muscle forces about the joint must be high. One can liken this situation to that existing on a seesaw. If even a light weight is placed far out on one side of the fulcrum, it must be balanced by another, much larger weight close in on the other side of the fulcrum. Further, the fulcrum must be sufficiently stable that the plank does not slide from side to side.

In vertebrate animals, the joint established at the shoulder to suit these demands is a ball-and-socket joint—large enclosing stable bony contours with large muscle masses that obviate the need for intricate ligamentous systems. In the human the hip maintains the same functional characteristics as in other animals, namely that of balancing a large mass (body weight) at very frequent intervals, and also maintains the same

Figure 20–8. The fluid-filled abdomen and the abdominal musculature around it, in a manner similar to the way the discs support loads, can act to support the trunk above and reduce the forces and loads the disc must feel. However, unlike the anulus fibrosus, the abdominal muscles must contract for this mechanism to operate, such as when a Valsalva maneuver is performed.

Figure 20–9. The shoulder joint provides rotational motions in all planes, allowing the arm to be placed in many locations. To provide such freedom while still maintaining joint stability, shoulder muscles must be large; they are situated close to the fulcrum of balance while the weight that they control is so far away.

bone and muscle characteristics. The shoulder, however, reduced in its demand of weight and repetitive use, relies less on bony stability but retains its muscle mass.[104-106]

In order for an extremity to cover all areas within the range allowed, a means must be provided to alter its length. It would not be advisable to have the bones of the upper and lower arm or leg extend and shorten in piston-like manner, as a number of repetitions in combination with high imposed loads would place too great a strain on the bony structures.[107,108] The rotational motion of the elbow or knee joint allows overall limb length changes only if both adjacent limb segments move (Fig. 20–10). This movement can occur only if motion at another, more proximal joint occurs simultaneously and coordination and synchronization between the two joints are maintained. In some circumstances the existing mechanism for this process is a passive one. During the initiation of the swing phase of walking or while climbing stairs, hip flexors flex the hip, while the knee flexes passively; the inertia of the shank lagging behind that of the actively mobile femur creates knee flexion and a relative shortening of the limb's length to provide floor or step clearance. In other circumstances muscles must be utilized.[107-110] Although neurologic control could coordinate separate muscles about each joint to perform the task, it is often more efficient to provide control with a single muscle which spans two joints. Such muscles are used when a repetitive act of limb shortening or lengthening occurs in which one joint does not move or is moving in a direction to stretch the muscle and the other rotates in an opposite direction to take advantage of the active contraction of the muscle. The two-joint muscles act to move one joint while the other remains in a stable position or is controlled by other forces.[110,111]

Joint Forces. Control of movement by muscles has several distinguishing features that are important to joint mechanics. Because all muscle-tendon systems cross a joint, their contraction creates a force at the joint regardless of whether their effort is for the purpose of causing active rotation or for inhibiting the movement that might be created by body inertia. No muscle goes through a joint; rather, all known biological muscle systems span the periphery of the joint. A major advantage is thereby obtained in controlling rotational motion. The torque or force causing rotational motion is not merely the contractile force produced by the muscle but is the product of this force multiplied by the distance between the joint's center of rotation and the tendon (Figs. 20–9 and 20–11). The tendon placed at the periphery of the joint gives the muscle a mechanical advantage in creating the greatest torque with the least effort.[1-7,112-125]

In addition to the torque that rotates the joint, muscle contraction produces additional types of forces at the joint. One is compression, which tends to squeeze the joint together (Fig. 20–12). This force is considerable, and in most of the weight-bearing joints of the lower extremities it can be up to three to four times body weight.[113-122] As will be discussed below (joint lubrication), the joint takes advantage of this situation for the purposes of its own lubrication. This force also maintains stability against forces that might pivot a joint open (Figs. 20–6, 20–7C, 20–9, 20–11, and 20–13). However, in so doing it creates relatively high forces that the joint

Figure 20–11. When one-legged support is required, the abductor muscles contract to produce a rotational force about the hip joint opposite to that produced by body weight. The farther away the muscle-tendon complex is from the center of the joint, the lower the muscle force needs to be to create the same rotational force. In most cases the muscle-tendon complex's distance from the center of the joint is less than that of the weight it is trying to counteract. This produces a larger force in the muscles than the weight it balances. As a consequence during the functional activities of daily living the major muscles about the hip typically produce forces two to four times body weight.

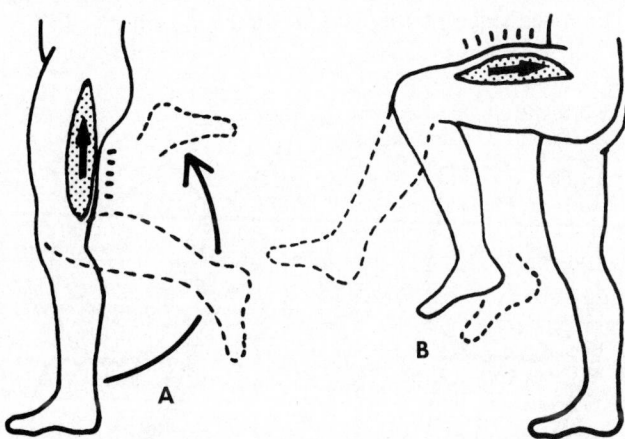

Figure 20–10. If the femur is stationary (A), knee motions alone are not an effective means of producing limb shortening. Under such circumstances the foot can move only in a single prescribed 180 degrees arc behind the knee. However, if at the same time the thigh is allowed to move by rotatory motions produced about the hip (B), the limb can be shortened or placed within a wide spherical volume.

Figure 20–12. The force that a muscle produces tends to squeeze or compress the joint it spans.

Figure 20–14. In many areas, the muscles placed on the concave, medial, or lateral sides of the joint become more parallel to the surface of the joint as the joint is flexed. Joint compressive forces are reduced but shear forces arise.

surface must withstand. Further, in certain movements as the joint is rotated to positions of greater flexion, the muscles become more parallel to the joint surface (Fig. 20–14). In many cases the shear force or rotational torque parallel to the joint line is helpful in stabilizing the joint against inertial or weight-bearing forces that tend to translate the two sides of the joint apart.[118-125] Rotational torque produced about the knee of a skier traversing a mountain, twisting outward over his planted ski, is but one example. However, as will be discussed below, in cases of joint instability shear forces can be detrimental.[126-133] In other cases, such as the flexor ten-

dons of the fingers, pulleys are provided to maintain a constant direction of pull across the joint (Fig. 20–15).

Joint Control. If muscles were to act continuously with the same degree of forceful contraction, the nature of stresses placed upon the joint would merely depend upon the angular position of the joint relative to the direction of muscle pull. But such is not the case. Joint motions allow multiple functional body activities. The neurologic control system and muscle physiology that could dictate such continuous constant force situations would not be efficient, either in performing the activity or in preserving energy. Rather, the total magnitude of the forces as well as the time that the joint feels them in compression or shear fluctuates and depends on what the specific functional activity is, how the activity is performed, how fast it is completed, and when in the time sequence of the act the forces are observed.[134-150]

Figure 20–13. Being eccentrically placed, a muscle will produce compressive force that will prevent a joint from pivoting open. At the knee the vastus lateralis assists knee ligaments (*A*), preventing body weight medially placed from opening up the lateral side of the joint during one-legged support (*B*).

Figure 20–15. At certain joints pulleys located proximal to the joint maintain flexor tendons at fixed distances and orientation to the joint's surface.

Figure 20–16. The muscle activity of the quadriceps will depend upon the type of activity that is being performed—i.e., the early stance phase of walking (*A*), running (*B*), going up stairs (*C*), and the early wing phase of walking or running (*D*).

At the knee joint, while walking, 15 to 20 degrees of knee flexion occurs in the early stance phase. The quadriceps muscle attempts to prevent collapse of the leg under the body's weight as the leg is decelerating. Most of the force exerted at this joint is compressive in nature. If the individual walks faster, greater muscle activity is needed for deceleration with the knee in a relatively similar position, thereby creating higher compressive loads across the joint (Fig. 20–16).[141-145] Quadriceps activity increases even further during the act of running, where again it is needed for decelerative purposes. It also increases in rising from a chair or climbing stairs to lift the body to a greater height rather than to control deceleration.[146,147] In the latter case, the knee is in greater flexion and, in addition to compression forces, higher shear forces arise. In contrast, during the swing phase of walking an equal and even greater degree of flexion occurs, but no significant muscle activity is present about the knee and joint forces are thus minimal. The activity of the quadriceps and the consequent forces at the knee joint during such highly repetitive activities are relatively the same from person to person, appearing to be dictated by single, fixed, preprogrammed neurological responses. Other joints engaged in repetitive activities in which overall efficiency and energy are prime considerations function in a manner similar to the knee.

In activities involving less repetitive motions, the consistency in the manner in which such activities are performed varies from person to person and from time to time in the same person. As an example, activities involving joints of the spine, such as bending or lifting, are dictated by factors in addition to a single, fixed, preprogrammed, neurologic response. These factors seem to be related to the fact that activities that require the involvement of the low back region can also require the participation of one or more joints of the upper or lower extremities.

One factor relates to an individual's *potential* to perform a task in a chosen manner. This ability depends on the strength of various muscle groups in different parts of the body. For example, a person wishing to bend over and pick something up may accomplish this task by keeping the legs straight and bending from the back and hips (Fig. 20–17*A*). The person may pick up the object in this manner because of habit, but he or she must also have the appropriate strength in the back

muscles to withstand the brunt of the lifting that will be required of these tissues. Alternatively, the person may desire to bend at the hips, knees, and ankles, keeping the back straight, and therefore lift the object by utilizing the leg muscles (Fig. 20–17*B*). If this method is chosen, there must exist sufficient strength in the leg muscles.[149,150] A person may also chose to utilize a combination of these two methods, employing both back and lower extremity muscles (Fig. 20–17*C*).

Another factor relates to the "psychological bent" of the person. Because of overall temperament and manner, each individual can perform the same task in a unique way (Figs. 20–17 to 20–19).[101,110] If a specific function (bending) is performed utilizing lower extremity segment motions and upper extremity segment motions in combination with the back "correctly," less stress may be placed on the lower lumbar region. One might liken this to "good or bad form" observed on the part of someone playing an individual sport. Proper form not only utilizes other joints but relates to the speed and frequency with which a movement at any particular joint occurs (Figs. 20–18 and 20–19). Alterations in the speed the limbs move during any given interval time in which a given function occurs will place certain stresses on the muscular tissues and/or the joints at various intervals owing to the fact that large acceleration and deceleration forces will occur. One could liken this situation to viewing someone swinging a golf club or tennis racket. One might note that the person may not be using his or her body to the extent required for proper form. The person might be swinging rapidly at the onset of stroke prior to hitting the ball, and minimizing the follow-up after the ball is

Figure 20–17. A person attempting to lift a box off the floor may utilize hip, trunk, and arm motions (*A*), hip, knee, and ankle motions (*B*), or a combination of all of these (*C*). Muscles needed, and the magnitude of the force from each that is required, will be dependent upon which method the individual chooses.

Figure 20–18. Whatever muscles a person chooses to utilize when lifting a box off the floor, nonpurposeful movement may be employed, such as overshooting the table and then setting the box back down. Muscles needed for such unnecessary movements create additional forces and stresses across respective joints.

hit. This type of movement would cause increased stresses in certain muscles and at certain arcs of joint motion in the initial part of the stroke, while reducing those which would occur normally in the latter part of the stroke. Thus, the same function utilizing relatively the same neurologic controlling programs can produce different forces in different joints in the same individual

Figure 20–19. Whatever method a person chooses to utilize when lifting a box off the floor, different speeds may be employed during different intervals of the act. Changes in speed require muscles to control body weight and inertial acceleration and decelerations, creating additional, often unnecessary forces and stresses across the joints if "improper form" is used.

at different times and in different individuals acting at the same time.

Joint Structure. Body movements and the muscular effort needed to control them, both constrained by joints, combine to create a multitude of joint stresses that mandate a specialized construct for the joint itself to prevent its failure.[151] As an example, it is estimated that in 1 year each joint in the lower extremity undergoes approximately two million oscillatory cycles solely in the act of walking. Each cyclical movement occurs over a period of approximately 1 second or less, and the loads imposed upon the joint are not only three to four times body weight but are of very brief duration (three tenths of a second), making these loads impulsive and of more potential damage than a constant steady load alone. Such conditions of heavy loads and pressures (up to 5 times body weight and 5 MN per square meter), low speeds (sliding speeds of less than 65 mm per second), and intermittent oscillatory motion (about 1 to 2 cycles per second) are extremely severe for weight-bearing joints; yet animal joints last longer than any man-made joint thus far devised (wear rate about 2 μg per hour). The way in which these joints function mechanically seems to have dictated a specific structure, anatomic form, and mechanism to ensure their survival. Over the past 50 years considerable investigation has led to the understanding that all aspects of a joint structure are related and that each serves a specific need for the mechanical survival of the joint—be it synovial fluid and articular cartilage surfaces to withstand the interfacial frictional forces created, the biochemical composition and geometrical distribution of water and organic matrix within the articular cartilage to provide "micromovement" and conformational load bearing, or the highly specialized subchondral trabecular bone arrangement to absorb some of the shock of impulsive loading. Each aspect of the joint structure appears to be optimized to allow joint movement to occur, reduce the mechanical forces that it must withstand, and provide some way to nourish and protect the cells needed for self-repair.

Minimization of Frictional Forces. The rotational movements of a joint, constrained by bony contours and ligamentous tissues, create a sliding motion of one articular surface on another. Such a motion should create shearing or frictional forces between the two surfaces which would be expected to cause joint breakdown, yet joints do not wear down by rubbing.

Frictional force is defined as the resistance one surface exerts on the other to impede its progress.[152] Such resistance depends upon the compressional load that is imposed across the two surfaces, the nature of the material and smoothness of the surfaces themselves, and the presence and characteristics of any material interposed between the two surfaces (a lubricant) which prevents the two sides from coming in contact with each other (Fig. 20–20). Under a standard load and a standard force to move one surface over another, the resistance to movement may be quantitated by a unitless number called the "coefficient of friction." The lower this number is, the more slippery is the movement of

Figure 20–20. The ease with which one surface may be slid over another is dependent upon the compressive load, the characteristics of the two opposing materials and their surfaces, and the nature of the material interposed between the two surfaces.

the two surfaces, and the lower the shear forces created between them. Good man-made joints, such as steel-on-steel lubricated by oil, operate at coefficients of friction between 0.1 and 0.5, whereas an ice skate moving on ice with a film of water between the two is about 0.01. Biological joints operate at coefficients of friction between 0.02 and 0.002, nearly one tenth to one hundredth that of what humans can at present design![153-155] Thus, if a 70-kilogram man walks and creates a 200-kilogram compressive force across the joint, the shear or frictional force felt at the joint would only be 0.2 kilogram.

The low frictional forces minimizing surface wear appear to be related to a number of biological constructs of the joint which are present at the surface, above the surface in the intervening fluid, and below the surface.

The porous deformable collagen surface is arranged with its fibers parallel to the surface of the joint. This layer has the highest concentration of collagen fibers in the joint,[156] and this factor plus its orientation may be considered ideal for preserving surface integrity.[156-160] Any shear forces generated may disrupt the surface by pulling the material apart (tensile stretch). Collagen is strongest in the direction parallel to its fiber length and more resistant to breaking when it is pulled apart rather than squeezed together along this axis. However, this structural feature resists only the shear forces that might be imposed.[161,162] It does little to reduce the overall magnitude of the shear forces the joint must bear.

Articular cartilage, with an intact surface layer but without any fluid imbibed within it, has a coefficient of friction of 0.3. If saline is added, the cartilage imbibes this fluid like a sponge; when the surfaces are now slid against each other, the coefficient of friction is reduced to 0.1 to 0.02.[163,164] If a glycoprotein fraction[165] molecule in the concentrations found in synovial fluid is added to the saline, the coefficient of friction is further reduced to 0.02 to 0.002.[164-167] (It appears that the exact coeffi-

cient of friction at any given time depends on the loading configuration, joint position, and magnitude and speed of the joint's motion.) The porosity of the cartilage soaked with fluid and an active lubricant in the synovial fluid are both major features that *reduce* the shear forces that the articular surface feels. How they interact to produce this low level of frictional resistance is still a matter of controversy, and many theories have been proposed.[167-179] Common to all theories is the movement of fluid in and out of the porous cartilage. McCutchen[164] postulated that as the cartilage is compressed, the fluid from within seeps out and forms a layer separating the two surfaces, thereby lubricating the joint. This theory is called weeping lubrication. In contrast, Walker and co-workers[167] postulated that when compression exists across the joint, it causes the fluid at the surface where compression is occurring to move into the articular cartilage; the fluid inside then moves sideways to areas that are not compressed; and the central cartilage, which is compressed, deforms. Because of their size, the "slippery" synovial fluid macromolecules[180-184] are trapped and concentrated in pools on the surface, thereby lowering the coefficient of friction.[170,172-175] This mechanism is called boosted lubrication. The accumulating evidence seems to indicate that under different loading conditions and movement speeds, one of the two fluid flow mechanisms dominates and that in most circumstances a combination of these two mechanisms may exist. While no one denies the existence of either mechanism, the two theories are somewhat contradictory as to how the fluid moves in the area of compression. Recent theoretical evidence and in vitro tests from Mow and co-workers[177-179] suggest that, in general, in the trailing area of compression, fluid is imbibed into articular surface, while at the same time at the leading edge where compression is developing, fluid is expressed (Fig. 20–21).

Figure 20–21. To minimize the resistance of moving one cartilage surface over another, the porous cartilaginous surface is layered with viscous macromolecules, but primarily weeps synovial fluid dialysate at the leading edge, absorbs this fluid in the trailing area, and deforms in the "area of contact," allowing the two cartilaginous surfaces to be kept apart.

FORCE   VS.   PRESSURE

Figure 20–22. An individual's response to a tack pressed into a finger is dependent upon the pressure of stress that tack exerts at the skin. The force may be the same whether the point of the tack or the head of the tack is pressed against the skin, but the skin will feel worse when the same force is exerted over a smaller area (point).

Regardless of how this controversy is resolved, it is clear that each component of the joint surface appears to be important in determining the final reduction in shear forces. The mechanism is so efficient that in normal joints such forces do not appear to be the major cause of surface breakdown.

Maximization of Contact Area. As with shear forces, the joint handles the compressive forces it receives by having a structure which both minimizes and withstands these loads. One important feature is contact area. The breakdown of any structure depends not only upon the total force it receives but also upon the size of the area that receives it. For example, if a tack is pressed into a person's finger, there is a big difference in the individual's reaction to it, depending upon whether the needle point of the tack or the flat part of the tack comes in contact with the skin (Fig. 20–22). In the former case, a given force is distributed over a very small area and the stress created (force per unit area) is much greater than in the latter case when the force is distributed over a larger area. Despite the wide variation in the shapes and sizes of distal and proximal joints, their gross structures are designed to provide a contact surface commensurate with the magnitude of the imposed forces, thereby maintaining approximately the same level of stress at all joints. At the hip, knee, and ankle joints, although joint shapes are markedly different, the loads imposed upon them are approximately the same and the maximal potential surface contact areas are of a similar size.

Each of these joints provides this contact area in different ways.[185-187] Under conditions of low loads the hip does not utilize the entire hemisphere of the acetabulum to provide contact; rather, a small portion in a peripheral horseshoe shape is utilized.[188-190] The knee, although appearing to have a large potential cartilaginous contacting area, actually has a small one, owing to the convex nature of the surfaces of both the femoral and tibial articulations. Recent evidence, however, has shown that the load-bearing contact area is greater owing to the fact that the meniscus plays an important function in transmitting loads.[191-194] At the ankle the contact area of the tibial-talar joint is potentially smaller than that of the hip but is increased by the load-sharing properties of the fibular-talar joint.[195] This latter joint can bear up to one sixth of the compressive forces transmitted from the joint to the shank.[196] In the small joints of the hands and feet, although the joint contact areas are smaller, it has been found that the forces they must bear are less, and recent evidence has shown again that compressive stresses of the joint are roughly in the same range of magnitude as those found in the larger "weight-bearing joints," approximately 5.0 MN per square meter.[197]

To reduce the frequency with which any part of the joint might feel such compressive loads, at any joint the potential contacting area is not always completely utilized. The deforming properties of cartilage and the surrounding subchondral bone allow the total potential contacting surfaces to exist only under high loads. At lower loads less surface area is in contact. Furthermore, the location of the contact area changes, dependent upon the angular position of the joint. Studies have shown that a changing contact area allows for continued circulation of fluid along the surface interface and the entrance and exit of synovial fluid into cartilage, thereby permitting all aspects of the articular cartilage to be nourished.[198,199] The changing areas of contact along the surface also provide a mechanism to entrap fluid under high loads when it is most needed for lubrication purposes. Lest one believe that this design is perfect, it is to be emphasized that at best the stress levels achieved appear to be relatively the same in all joints only within a certain range. Different joints do appear to have different ratios of maximal force to contacting area, and this fact may explain why certain joints are more susceptible to degenerative arthritis.[197]

Resistance to Compressive Stresses. Alterations in the contact area tend to reduce the stresses in articular cartilage, and cartilage is constructed in an ideal way to withstand the final compressive stress level.[201] It has two components: a liquid and a solid. The liquid is a dialysate of synovial fluid and possesses the mechanical property of incompressibility.[202,203] However, for this property to be effective and withstand the compressive loads that joints sustain, like the nucleus pulposus of the disc, this liquid must be contained. The cartilage matrix, as previously described, grossly resembles a sponge with multiple pores. The small diameter (60 Å) of these pores and their arrangement in random circuitous "tunnels" prevent large molecules from entering the cartilage, and offer considerable resistance to the direct flow in and out of the cartilage and from side to side within the cartilage (Fig. 20–23).[204-210] These characteristics provide the mechanism for the fluid to support the load.

At any instant, only a part of the whole joint is load bearing or compressed. If one part is in compression, an adjacent area is being stretched and pulled apart. This situation places high stresses of both compression and tension on the organic matrix of cartilage. The organic matrix of cartilage is a fiber-reinforced composite consisting primarily of collagen and proteoglycans and is designed to resist compression and tension. Collagen is distributed throughout the tissue with definite ultrastructure, while the proteoglycans are dispersed and immobilized in the interfibular space. Many of the proteoglycan subunits (PGS) are found in aggregates (PGA) associated with hyaluronic acid, which immobilize and anchor the subunits. Although the nature of the interaction between collagen and PGA is not known, recent evidence indicates that these interactions are responsible for the structural integrity of the tissues and the ability of cartilage to function as a bearing material. The matrix component of articular cartilage has greater mechanical resistance to being stretched apart[209,210] in a direction parallel to the oscillating direction of movement and perpendicular to the orientation of surface collagen bundles. Although many recent scanning electron microscope studies have shown that the distribution of collagen fibers in the middle and deep zones is random when the joint is unloaded,[211,212] in vitro studies have clearly indicated that their mechanical properties and the fluid flow through them are not uniform in all directions and at all levels.[213] Further, the collagen fibers of the midzone, although randomly distributed when the joint is unloaded, alter their alignment under compression to provide maximal resistance against load.[214] Such changes not only allow the matrix itself to accommodate the imposed loads better but also decrease the pore size and increase resistance to fluid flow through the cartilage. Recent studies have shown that the permeability of the tissue (ease of fluid flow) decreases exponentially[207] and the mechanical strength of cartilage increases as greater loads are imposed.[215] Such findings are dependent on age and on the depth of the cartilage layer examined, for the greater the depth the larger these factors become.[216,217]

The electrical properties of the proteoglycans and their interaction with the surrounding substances also con-tribute to the mechanical strength of cartilage. The carboxyl and sulfate groups of the glycosaminoglycan are endowed with highly polyanionic charge characteristics.[218-221] This charge correlates with the negative fixed charge density found in articular cartilage, which increases with the depth from the articular surface. At the surface the content of hexosamine is 3 to 8.5 percent of the dry weight of cartilage; with increasing depth it increases to 35 percent, and then gradually decreases to approximately 5.5 percent at the tidemark.[222] The large proteoglycan molecules are fixed and highly charged and hold a large volume of water. Under compressive loads these molecules "open up," exposing a greater charge to the surrounding fluid and offering increasing electrical resistance to the flow of such fluid away from it, thereby increasing the mechanical strength of the cartilage. Further, the synovial fluid dialysate itself consists of charged particles, and their movement is impeded by the repelling electrical barriers they encounter (known as streaming potential).[223-236]

Both the fluid and the organic matrix of cartilage are uniquely designed to complement each other in maintaining the integrity of the structure in the face of repeated compressive stresses. Yet ultimately, as a consequence of various arthritis diseases, cartilage in most cases weakens and tears apart.[237-241]

Additional Resistance to Compressive Loads. It has long been recognized that subchondral bone has a lattice arrangement with a specific orientation at each joint with respect to the surface. Subchondral bone in certain areas shows a high concentration of trabeculae, while in others the trabeculae may occupy a broader total cross-sectional area with its outer cortical margins "flaring" out. Over the past decade Radin and others investigating the mechanical properties of the subchondral bone appear to have confirmed the ideas of earlier clinical workers that this specialization provides a means for absorbing some of the compressible impulses the

Figure 20–23. Cartilage is composed of a liquid and a multi-component solid, consisting of collagen and hydrophilic proteoglycan molecules. In the middle layer (*A*) the mechanical and electrical properties and architectural design of the solid "contain" the fluid, preventing it from being compressed, while still allowing fluid flow providing nourishment for cartilage cells. In the deepest zone (*B*), though the content of proteoglycans decreases, the collagen is secured tightly to subchondral bone similar to liquid-solid properties.

Figure 20–24. At the hip, trabecular bone in the femoral head is concentrated along an axis 160 degrees to the vertical where the greatest concentration of forces occurs. In contrast, the trabecular bone on the acetabular side flares out to occupy a greater area than the joint's contacting surface, distributing the same forces over a wide area, thereby reducing the stresses and allowing some of the stresses to be absorbed by bone deformation.

joint receives.[242-253] This mechanism can be viewed in the following way. If a hardball hits one's hand, the shock of impact can be reduced if the hand moves away from the ball; some of the energy of the shock is dissipated by the motion produced. The trabeculae arranged in a lattice-like array provide micromotion to absorb the impact. The greater the amount of material present (in areas of trabecular concentration) or the greater the ability of any one area to deform (areas of bone flaring), the more energy can be absorbed.

Perhaps no better example of this system exists than that seen at the hip (Fig. 20–24). The acetabulum is concave, and under low loads contact with the femur is made about its periphery; thus as the load is increased, the surface tends to flare out. This plus the fact that more bone is present allows the acetabulum to absorb some of the compressive load. The femur is convex, and thus in its peripheral contact with the acetabulum it is "clamped" and "squeezed" from all sides. To absorb the load, trabeculae are present in greater concentration along the lines of greatest force.

The ability of the subchondral bone to absorb compressive loads provides added protection for the cartilage. Although cartilage is very compliant, it is thin and is limited in its ability to absorb impulsive loads; one would not like to fall 10 feet onto a mattress 1 inch thick laid on a concrete floor, no matter how soft the mattress is!

BIOMECHANICS OF JOINT DEGENERATION

Under normal conditions joints last. The fact that an individual can get at least 40 to 50 years of good service from almost all the joints is ample tribute to nature's grand design and marvelous mechanical structural architecture. Yet under certain conditions these structures do "wear out," and their loss is markedly disabling. To provide for their proper restoration requires therapeutic modalities which take into account how the entire mechanical system has broken down.

Normal function of any joint requires that all structures (cartilage, bone, ligaments, and muscles) act in combination to allow smooth steady motion while still maintaining stability. However, since this system is so delicately balanced and since relatively low safety factors exist within any given structure, alteration of any individual component alters the balance and often leads to mechanical breakdown of the entire joint system. Although many different factors may initiate joint destruction, it is the mechanical factors which lead to chronic joint dysfunction, and it is the total system that must be repaired. Knowledge of how this mechanical breakdown occurs and how the body can compensate for it leads to a better understanding of why function at some joints is more readily restored than at others and what must or can be done to any aspect of the system to prevent total joint destruction. An examination of different types of "joint disease" and their effects on various joints illustrate this concept.

Hip Degeneration—Chemical Breakdown of the Organic Matrix of Cartilage. Over one million persons over the age of 60 have impaired locomotion because of hip dysfunction. Symptoms may be present for many years before the dysfunction becomes disabling. When the cause is rheumatoid arthritis, the initial symptoms may be due to a synovitis or the earliest onset of direct enzymatic destruction of the organic matrix of the cartilage. The chemical effect clearly is aggravated even by normal external mechanical stresses that the body imposes upon the weakened bearing surface. Often when the disease is "burned out" or, as in juvenile rheumatoid arthritis, quiescent for many years, cartilage destruction continues to progress because of the alteration in balance between the forces sustained and the structure which is present to withstand them. Pain while walking or moving the hip implies that this imbalance is too great. Since little biochemical "repair" is possible, the body must use compensatory mechanisms to reduce the forces across the hip joint and to overcome lost hip motion.[253,254] As most of the forces across the joint or any joint arise from muscle action, such action must be reduced in magnitude, duration, and frequency. At the hip the greatest muscle forces in walking arise during the stance phase and are needed to counteract the body's weight and the body's inertial forces as the trunk moves over and around the involved hip. The body weight is medial to the hip joint on a long fulcrum (Fig. 20–11).[139] To balance this weight with minimal abductor effort, the trunk may shift so that the weight is brought closer to the center of the fulcrum over the hip joint itself.[258,259] To balance the inertial forces which occur in slowing down and speeding up the leg during the various aspects of the gait cycle, and to minimize the muscular effort about the hip, an individual may reduce the walking speed. But this reduction will increase the duration of the muscle's action in any given cycle, unless the stance phase on that side is shortened; thus, an asymmetric gait is produced. These factors—trunk shift, pelvic drop, slower walking speed, and a shortened stance phase on the involved side—are the characteristics of a Trendelenburg antalgic gait. The greater the number of these factors that are present and the more severe they are, the greater need to lower the forces across the joint and the more severe the state of joint degeneration. If forces are to be reduced further, the entire body weight cannot be transmitted through the leg; a substitute "peg leg" must be utilized, i.e., transmission to the ground via the arm by use of a cane or crutch.[259]

Although such mechanisms can reduce the forces, motions, and, therefore, pain, significant consequences result. With decreased stimulation muscles atrophy, and subchondral bone resorption and joint contractures (secondary to decreased motion) will progress even when the disease itself is quiescent. If pain is dramatically eliminated (disease remission or successful use of medications or surgical replacement of the joint), limitations to normal functional ability are eliminated without rapid concomitant restoration of bone structure, muscle strength, or loss of contractures.[260] Improvement in function occurs, with increased walking speed and greater joint forces.[261] This situation, over time, may be detrimental in that subchondral bone collapse may occur and the protective influence that this bone has upon the cartilage is lost. The problem is further compounded by the fact that weak muscles and/or joint contractures in the face of subchondral weakness may alter the locus, direction, and distribution of the forces across the joint, concentrating the stresses in some areas and possibly increasing the stresses in other areas not designed to cope with them. This situation may lead to further cartilage breakdown and to preferential breakdown in particular locations leading to lateral or medial femoral displacement (femoral subluxation or protrusion) (Fig. 20–25). Although localized areas of breakdown are often seen at the hip, they do not lead to a significant loss of stability and dislocation. Nevertheless, progressive joint destruction can be viewed as a vicious spiral. Each cycle is initiated by cartilage breakdown, causing compensa-

Figure 20–25. Two radiographic examples of moderate arthritis at the hip joint. Loss of cartilage can preferentially occur on the lateral side of the joint (*A*) or on the medial side (*B*).

tory body reactions; total joint changes occur which eventually stop because of medical intervention or disease quiescence; function consequently improves with a relative increase in "abnormal" forces over unprotected weakened surfaces, leading to further mechanical joint destruction.

Although the example cited above illustrates the situation if rheumatoid arthritis is the initiating factor, the consequent mechanical-biological steps in the cycle leading to joint destruction occur in a variety of other diseases leading to hip arthritis. In degenerative arthritis, whose cause is still unknown but is currently viewed as an initial weakening of the mechanical structure of cartilage or bone (owing to congenital microstructural abnormalities, normal aging, or impulsive, repetitive overstressing), the delicate balance of imposed stresses and structural resistance is altered and the cycle is initiated (see Chapter 88). From the onset of symptoms to final complete hip dysfunction can take many years. Thus, the cycle may not be rapid, and the individual and his or her practitioner can keep the imbalance small enough to prevent rapid acceleration of the process. How severe and chronic the initiating cause is, how effectively medical treatments produce disease remission, whether available compensatory mechanisms are adequate, whether an individual can sufficiently invoke such mechanisms or is limited by physical, psychological, or social factors, and how well the practitioner can understand and relate to the patient what is necessary to slow down the process are all important in the rapidity with which joint disability progresses.

The practitioner can control only some of these factors but must be aware of all of them and understand their interaction. In a patient who already has arthritic changes, the achievement of relief of pain or reduction in inflammatory reaction with medications does not imply that the patient can return to a full, active life. The need for caution and an awareness of the detrimental effects that activities such as sports can have must be understood by the practitioner and conveyed to the patient. Individuals who are in active jobs—e.g., are on their feet all day—may still need some reduction in their normal functional activities; they may require continued use of a cane or a reduction in the total number of "poundings" the joint will feel in a given day, month, or year. The physician must ensure that a proper range of motion is present and that muscle strength is maintained at the involved joints and about all other joints for proper compensations to occur.

Knee Arthritis—Instability and Ligamentous Injury. Arthritis of the knee constitutes almost as great an incidence of locomotion disability as does that of the hip.[262] A comparison of the biomechanics of these two joints illustrates (1) how different joints have different safety factors in the balance between the stresses imposed on them and the structural resistance to the stresses and (2) how damage to structures in the joint system other than cartilage can cause joint degeneration.

In most cases the cause of joint degeneration is the same in the knee as it is in the hip—idiopathic degen-

erative joint disease or rheumatoid arthritis. Unlike the hip, cartilage destruction in its initial stages often is not uniform over the entire cartilage surface of the knee. In degenerative joint disease the medial compartment is usually more involved; in rheumatoid arthritis it is the lateral compartment. This fact has three consequences: (1) As cartilage breakdown occurs, a varus-valgus angle forms which concentrates the force in the area of cartilage degeneration and further enhances the tendency toward mechanical breakdown. (2) Differential compartment destruction may be associated, with the joint surfaces losing their parallelism with the horizontal plane when the body is upright. Vertical body loads will then begin to have a greater tendency to create high shear or translational forces, which themselves are potentially highly damaging to the cartilage. (3) Such changes, by their effect on the surrounding ligaments, may indirectly affect the cartilage by stretching and weakening the ligaments. Since the knee is so dependent on ligaments for stability, ligamentous laxity eventually can allow even greater abnormally directed shear motions and forces.

As with degeneration at the hip, an individual's attempt to compensate for knee joint damage is aimed primarily at reducing joint load. During walking an individual can reduce the joint load by decreasing walking speed to decrease quadriceps activity.[263,264] Joint stability (maintenance of knee extension) may still be retained by leaning the trunk forward over the knee in the stance phase. However, in so doing the posterior capsule is abnormally stretched and the muscle, relatively little used, becomes weakened. The deficiency of bony contouring in the sagittal plane to stabilize the knee can eventually lead to increased AP translational motion with consequent abnormal shear forces that further aggravate cartilage damage. In the coronal plane the major compensatory action would be a shift of the trunk in a direction away from the compartment most involved. Because of the trunk's position this shift can only be made to a very limited degree. Ligamentous contractures can further nullify this compensating attempt.

On the concave side of a varus-valgus angulation (medial collateral ligament when the joint goes into varus, lateral collateral ligament when it goes into valgus) a contracture may result. Such contractures will even further limit the individual's compensatory attempt to redistribute the forces more appropriately.[265,266] If sufficiently severe, this lack of compensatory mechanisms, added to the aforementioned factors, may be accompanied by rapid, unremitting joint destruction, created not by the basic underlying disease but by the consequent superimposed mechanical conditions.

Thus, in contrast to the stabilizing effect of bony contours at the hip, the use of ligamentous constraints in normal knees to stabilize and limit certain motions, and the use of muscles to stabilize the joint in other directions, places the joint in an extremely precarious situation which tends to amplify even the most minimal joint damage.

These conditions also make the knee more susceptible to arthritis from those traumatic incidents which, by their nature, damage only ligaments and other soft tissues.[50-52,267-270] Increasingly, ligamentous injuries are becoming a larger cause of knee joint dysfunction. Often, after an injury to the knee that affects only the ligaments, laxity may remain despite proper medical management. Because the fibers have stretched or scarred, weaker ligaments result and their stabilizing effect is diminished. If the medial collateral ligament is damaged, varus-valgus rotational motions can occur, allowing the joint to open and close and thereby creating more severe impact on the cartilage bed. If the posterior or anterior cruciate ligaments or posterior medial or lateral capsular ligaments are damaged, AP or internal-external rotational translational motions can now occur with a magnitude which the femoral-tibial cartilage was not designed to withstand. Meniscal injuries will increase the stresses the joint surface feels by concentrating the load transmitted through the joint to a smaller area. Commonly, when such injuries exist (ligaments and menisci) even without direct cartilage damage, the eventual outcome is the same—cartilage destruction and arthritis.[271]

Low Back Pain—Total System Destruction. If knee arthritis illustrates how the various components of the joint system are affected when any single element is damaged, and how difficult it therefore is to compensate mechanically, low back problems epitomize this situation. When one considers how each component of this joint system—disc, facet joints, ligaments, and muscles—is so specifically designed to control a given aspect of joint stability and motion, it is not hard to see why back problems are so difficult for the patient and the clinician to manage. Many different diseases cause low back problems; one of these, "disc degeneration," will be used as an illustration. (See also Chapter 30.)

Disc degeneration constitutes the leading cause of morbidity in middle age.[272-280] The initial symptom is back pain.[281-286] Such pain must be compensated for by reducing the forces across the disc and reducing the movements of the joint. Again, as in the hip or knee joint, as the major load is not body weight but muscle activity, use of paraspinal muscles must be decreased in frequency and/or lessened in magnitude. However, to reduce motion while an individual is upright, the muscles must function as an internal brace. So long as the patient attempts to function, a vicious cycle is established: the upright position leads to back pain, back pain leads to muscle spasm, muscle spasm leads to increased disc pressure, and disc pressure leads to more back pain. Unlike the hip or knee, as long as a vertical position is maintained, muscle activity will be present as long as the body's center of gravity is in front of the disc and pressure will exist across the disc.

The patient's ability to compensate for back pain is extremely limited because, in the upright position, loads must remain across the disc. Medications, besides being directed toward the original source of pain, must be given to break ths cycle. Since the trunk does not have another side to help compensate for its disability, if medication proves ineffective, two additional measures can be tried: bed rest, which eliminates all vertical loading on the back; or bracing, which allows the abdomen to work like a disc to support the spine or restrict motion. Each of these measures has the detrimental effect of causing muscle atrophy, and prolonged use can have a markedly adverse effect on the long-term prognosis. If atrophy is present, support is lost; and although the total force across the disc may be decreased, the stability of the intervertebral joint is also decreased. This loss must be taken up by high strains on the disc, facet joints, or ligaments.

Since low back disorders are such a common disability, many attempts have been made to reduce their rate of occurrence in industrial settings. Since the middle 1930s, it has generally been recommended that all lifting activities be carried out with the back near vertical and the knees and hips bent.[287] The advocates of this method have been so enthusiastic and persistent in regard to training programs that nearly every major industry has adopted this method to the exclusion of any other method regardless of the size, shape, or weight of the object to be lifted, the person's ability to lift, or the desire to do it in the proper fashion.[288] In view of the popularization of the theory of correct lifting methods, it was expected that the incidence of low back injury would be significantly reduced. However, studies conducted in Britain and Canada offer clear evidence that there is no such reduction in the number of back injuries due to lifting and handling activities.[89]

A skepticism regarding the proper way to lift emerged from these and similar studies, and some investigators sought the reasons for the apparent failure of the instructional programs that had been designed to promote correct lifting. A photographic study of the actual lifting techniques of industrial workers showed that a wide variety of lifting methods were employed, and that the prescribed manner of lifting with a straight back and bent knees was seldom used.[89] Results indicated either that the indoctrination was insufficient or that the workers preferred to use another method even though they understood the "proper" lifting technique. In any case, the proper lifting method was not used consistently, so it could not be expected to contribute to a reduction in the incidence of low back injuries even if it were a truly superior technique.

A study that attempted to calculate the forces in the lower trunk during various acts of lifting was reported by Park and Chaffin.[287] This study indicated that the proper lifting method increased the compressive load on the lumbosacral disc by over 50 percent of that incurred by the "improper" method under certain specific conditions. Generally the straight-back, bent-knees method induced larger compressive forces whenever the object to be lifted was sufficiently heavy, and was too large to be lifted "between the knees," thus preventing the efficiency of a near vertical positioning of the upper extremities.

Brown[288] found that the greatest energy cost occurs with the straight-back, bent-knees method; this result is not unexpected, since the proper method requires an additional mass, i.e., the thighs and lower trunk, to be moved against gravity. Thus, if a person must continually perform this manner of lift throughout the working day, a great deal of unnecessary fatigue would develop, and therefore this method is not appropriate for prolonged repetitive tasks.

Since the training of individuals to lift "properly" has not been effective in reducing the incidence of low back problems,[288,289] studies were carried out to determine the maximal load acceptable to industrial workers during various lifting tasks.[290,291] The amount of weight to be lifted was adjusted according to the subject's assessment after the individual was informed of the duration, frequency, and conditions of the task at hand. With such facts, it was found that an ergonomic approach by "designing the job to fit the worker"[292] can reduce the incidence of low back disorders. Further, a study of pre-employment static strength testing showed that a correlation exists between the type of job that a person has to do, the incidence of low back pain, and the static strength that a person has.[293-300]

If such techniques are not utilized or are ineffective, since joint destruction has begun, and although both the clinician and the patient are aware of it, little compensation is invoked and the delicate balance between stresses imposed and joint resistance to them has been tipped in the wrong direction. With time, even when nerve root irritation does not intervene, there frequently occurs a gradual loss of disc height, which further upsets the balance among disc, facet, ligaments, and muscle function. With disc narrowing, facet joint subluxation can result, causing higher stresses in the area of the joint still in contact and eventually leading to facet arthritis. With loss of disc height, normal ligament length is also reduced. The ligaments either can maintain a lax position, in which case they offer less protection to the disc, or can contract and be put on stretch, thereby becoming a source of pain themselves. Similarly, muscles may become slightly lax or operate at the lower end of their length-tension curve and be unable to control movement properly. Such lack of control creates abnormally high accelerative or decelerative forces in the disc, facet joints, or ligaments, thereby adding to the forces imposed upon these structures. Although such disc height loss, facet joint subluxation, ligamentous laxity, or muscle laxity may seem small in absolute magnitude, one must realize that in comparison to the total normal length of these structures, such changes may constitute a 25 to 50 percent difference.

References

1. Morris, J.M.: Biomechanics of the spine. Arch. Surg. 107:418, 1973.
2. Lucas, D.B.: Biomechanics of the shoulder joint. Arch. Surg. 107:425, 1973.
3. Morris, J.M.: Biomechanical aspects of the hip joint. Orthop. Clin. North Am. 2:33, 1971.
4. Radin, E.L.: Biomechanics of the knee joint. Its implication in the design of replacements. Orthop. Clin. North Am. 4:539, 1973.
5. Frankel, V.H.: Biomechanics of the knee. Orthop. Clin. North Am. 2:175, 1971.
6. Kaufer, J.: Mechanical function of the patella. J. Bone Joint Surg. 53A:155, 1971.
7. Frankel, V.H.: Biomechanics of the musculoskeletal system. Introduction. Arch. Surg. 107:405, 1973.
8. Goss, C.M.: Gray's Anatomy of the Human Body. Philadelphia, Lea & Febiger, 1973, Chapter 4.
9. Walmsley, T.: On the form of the surface of diarthroses. Proc. Anat. Soc., Great Britain and Ireland, 1918.
10. Walmsley, T.: The articular mechanism of the diarthroses. J. Bone Joint Surg. 10:40, 1928.
11. MacConaill, M.A.: The movements of bones and joints. J. Bone Joint Surg. 31B:100, 1949.
12. Barnett, C.H., Davies, D.V., and MacConaill, M.A.: Synovial Joints—Their Structure and Mechanics. London, Longmans, 1961.
13. Steindler, A.: Kinesiology of the Human Body. Springfield, Ill., Charles C Thomas, 1955.
14. Langa, G.S.: The morphology and function of the human joint. Acta Anat. 55:16, 1963.
15. Landsmeer, J.M.F.: Power grip and precision handling. Ann. Rheum. Dis. 21:164, 1962.
16. Goodfellow, J., and O'Connor, J.: The mechanics of the knee and problems in reconstructive surgery. J. Bone Joint Surg. 60:358, 1978.
17. Frigerio, N.A., Stowe, R.S., and Howe, J.W.: Movement of the sacroiliac joint. Clin. Orthop. 100:379, 1974.
18. Poppen, N.K., and Walker, P.S.: Normal and abnormal motion of the shoulder. J. Bone Joint Surg. 58A:195, 1976.
19. Morrey, B.F., and Chao, E.Y.S.: Passive motion of the elbow joint. J. Bone Joint Surg. 58A:501, 1976.
20. Chao, E.Y.S., and Morrey, B.F.: Three-dimensional rotation of the elbow. J. Biomechanics 11:57, 1978.
21. Youm, Y., Dryer, R.F., Thambyrajah, K., et al.: Biomechanical analysis of forearm pronation-supination and elbow flexion-extension. J. Biomechanics 12:245, 1979.
22. McMurty, R.Y., Youm, Y., and Flatt, A.E., et al: Kinematics of the wrist. II. Clinical applications. J. Bone Joint Surg. 60A:955, 1978.
23. Youm, Y., McMurty, R.Y., Flatt, A.E., et al.: Kinematics of the wrist. I. An experimental study of radial ulnar deviation and flexion-extension. J. Bone Joint Surg. 60A:423, 1978.
24. Youm, Y., Gillespie, T.E., Flatt, A.E., et al.: Kinematic investigation of normal MCP joint. J. Biomechanics 11:109, 1978.
25. Frankel, V.H., Burstein, A.H., and Brooks, D.B.: Biomechanics of internal derangement of the knee. Pathomechanics as determined by analysis of the instant centers of motion. J. Bone Joint Surg. 53A:945, 1971.
26. Walker, P.S., Shoji, J., and Erkman, M.J.: The rotational axis of the knee and its significance to prosthesis design. Clin. Orthop. 89:160, 1972.
27. Soudan, K., Auderkercke, and Martens, M.: Methods, difficulties and inaccuracies in the study of human joint kinematics and pathokinematics by the instant axis concept. Example: The knee joint. J. Biomechanics 12:27, 1979.
28. Laurin, C., and Mathiev, J.: Sagittal mobility of the normal ankle. Clin. Orthop. 108:99, 1975.
29. Rothman, R.H., Marvel, J.P., Jr., and Heppenstall, R.B.: Anatomic considerations in glenohumeral joint. Orthop. Clin. North Am. 6:341, 1975.
30. Clark, I.C., and Amstutz, H.C.: Human hip geometry and hemiarthroplasty selection. Proceedings of the Hip Society, 1975. In The Hip. St. Louis, C. V. Mosby Company, 1975.
31. Benedict, J.V., Walker, L.B., and Harris, E.H.: Stress-strain characteristics and tensile strength of unembalmed human tendon. J. Biomechanics 1:53, 1968.
32. Blanton, P.L., and Biggs, N.L.: Ultimate tensile strength of fetal and adult human tendons. J. Biomechanics 3:181, 1970.
33. Crisp, J.D.C.: Properties of tendon and skin. In Fung, Y.C., Perrone, N., and Anliker, M. (eds.): Biomechanics, Its Foundations and Objectives. Englewood Cliffs, N.J., Prentice-Hall, 1972.
34. Noyes, F.R., DeLucas, J.L., and Torvik, P.J.: Biomechanics of anterior cruciate ligament failure: An analysis of strain rate sensitivity and mechanisms of failure in primates. J. Bone Joint Surg. 56A:236, 1974.
35. Kennedy, J.C., Hawkins, R.J., Willis, R.B., et al.: Tension studies of human knee ligaments. J. Bone Joint Surg. 58A:350, 1977.
36. Noyes, F.R., Torvik, P.J., Hyde, M.S., et al.: Biomechanics of ligament failure. J. Bone Joint Surg. 56A:1406, 1974.
37. Noyes, F.R., and Groud, E.S.: The strength of the anterior cruciate ligament in humans and Rhesus monkeys. J. Bone Joint Surg. 58A:1074, 1976.
38. Rosenorn, M., and Pederson, E.B.: The significance of the coracoclavicular ligament in experimental dislocation of the acromioclavicular joint. Acta Orthop. Scand. 45:346, 1974.
39. Ogden, J.A.: The anatomy and function of the proximal tibiofibular joint. Clin. Orthop. 101:186, 1974.
40. Ogden, J.A.: Subluxation and dislocation of the proximal tibiofibular joint. J. Bone Joint Surg. 56A:145, 1974.

41. Moseley, H.F., and Overgaard, B.: The anterior capsule mechanism in recurrent anterior dislocation of the shoulder. J. Bone Joint Surg. 44B:913, 1962.

42. Brantigan, O.C., and Voshell, A.F.: The mechanics of the ligaments and menisci of the knee joint. J. Bone Joint Surg. 23:44, 1941.

43. Trent, P.S., Walker, P.S., and Wolf, B.: Ligament length patterns, strengths and rotational axes of the knee joint. Clin. Orthop. 117:263, 1976.

44. Hsieh, H-H., and Walker, P.S.: Stabilizing mechanisms of the loaded and unloaded knee joint. J. Bone Joint Surg. 58A:87, 1976.

45. Fowler, P.J.: Medial and anterior instability of the knee. An anatomical and clinical study using stress machines. J. Bone Joint Surg. 53A:1257, 1971.

46. Kennedy, J.C., Weinberg, H.W., and Wilson, A.S.: The anatomy and function of the anterior cruciate ligament. As determined by clinical and morphological studies. J. Bone Joint Surg. 56A:223, 1974.

47. Shaw, J.A., and Murray, D.G.: The longitudinal axis of the knee and the role of the cruciate ligaments in controlling transverse rotation. J. Bone Joint Surg. 56A:1603, 1974.

48. Girgis, F.G., Marshall, J.L., and Monajem, A.R.S.: The cruciate ligaments of the knee joint. Anatomical, functional and experimental analysis. Clin. Orthop. 106:216, 1975.

49. Furman, W., Marshall, J.L., and Girgis, F.G.: The anterior cruciate ligament. J. Bone Joint Surg. 58A:179, 1976.

50. Hughston, J.C., Cross, M.J., and Andrews, J.R.: Classification of lateral ligament instability of the knee. J. Bone Joint Surg. 56A:1539, 1974.

51. Hughston, J.C., Andrews, J.R., Cross, M.J., et al.: Classification of knee ligament instabilities. Part I: The medial compartment and cruciate ligaments. J. Bone Joint Surg. 58A:159, 1976.

52. Hughston, J.C., Andrews, J.R., Cross, M.J., et al.: Classification of knee ligament instabilities. Part II: The lateral compartment. J. Bone Joint Surg. 58A:173, 1976.

53. Wang, C.J., and Walker, P.S.: Rotatory laxity of the human knee joint. J. Bone Joint Surg. 56A:161, 1974.

54. Warren, L.A., Marshall, J.L., and Griggs, F.: The prime static stabilizer of the medial side of the knee. J. Bone Joint Surg. 56A:665, 1974.

55. Noyes, F.R., Grood, E.S., Butler, D.L., and Malek, M.: Clinical laxity tests and functional stability of the knee: Biomechanical concepts. Clin. Orthop. 146:84, 1980.

56. Grood, E.S., Noyes, F.R., Butler, D.L., and Suntay, W.S.: Ligamentous and capsular restraints preventing straight medial and lateral laxity in intact human cadaver knees. J. Bone Joint Surg. 63A:1257, 1981.

57. Noyes, F.R., Grood, E.S., Butler, D.L., and Paulos, L.E.: Clinical biomechanics of the knee-ligament restraints and functional stability. *In* The American Academy of Orthopaedic Surgeons: Symposium on the Athlete's Knee: Surgical Repair and Reconstruction. St. Louis, C. V. Mosby, 1980.

58. White, A.A., III, and Raphael, I.G.: The effect of quadriceps loads and knee position on strain measurements of the tibial collateral ligament. An experimental study on human amputation specimens. Acta Orthop. Scand. 43:176, 1972.

59. Bose, K., and Chong, K.C.: The clinical manifestations and pathomechanics of contracture of the extensor mechanism of the knee. J. Bone Joint Surg. 58B:478, 1976.

60. Sylvia, L.E.: A more exact measurement of the sagittal stability of the knee joint. Acta Orthop. Scand. 46:1008, 1975.

61. Basmajian, J.V., and Bazant, F.J.: Factors preventing downward dislocation of the adducted shoulder—an electromyographic and morphological study. J. Bone Joint Surg. 41A:1182, 1959.

62. Linscheid, R.L., Dobyns, J.H., Beabout, J.W., et al.: Traumatic instability of the wrist. Diagnosis, classification, and pathomechanics. J. Bone Joint Surg. 54A:1612, 1972.

63. Smith, R.J.: Post-traumatic instability of the metacarpophalangeal joint of the thumb. J. Bone Joint Surg. 59A:14, 1977.

64. Coventry, M.B., and Tapper, E.M.: Pelvic instability: A consequence of removing iliac bone for grafting. J. Bone Joint Surg. 54A:83, 1972.

65. Marshall, J.L., Girgis, F.G., and Zelko, R.R.: The biceps femoris tendon and its functional significance. J. Bone Joint Surg. 54A:1444, 1972.

66. Noyes, F.R., and Sonstegard, D.G.: Biomechanical function of the pes anserinus at the knee and the effect of its transplantation. J. Bone Joint Surg. 55A:1225, 1973.

67. Poe, M.H., Johnson, R.J., and Brown, D.W.: The role of the musculature in injuries to the medial collateral ligament. J. Bone Joint Surg. 61A:398, 1979.

68. Symeonides, P.P.: The significance of the subscapularis muscle in the pathogenesis of recurrent anterior dislocation of the shoulder. J. Bone Joint Surg. 54B:476, 1972.

69. Weisman, H.J., Simon, S.R., Ewald, F.C., et al.: Total hip replacement with and without osteotomy of the greater trochanter: Clinical and biomechanical comparisons in the same patients. J. Bone Joint Surg. 60A:203, 1978.

70. Parke, W.W., and Schiff, D.C.M.: The applied anatomy of the intervertebral disc. Orthop. Clin. North Am. 2:309, 1971.

71. Markolf, K.L., and Morris, J.M.: The structural components of the intervertebral disc. A study of their contributions to the ability of the disc to withstand compressive forces. J. Bone Joint Surg. 56A:675, 1974.

72. MacNab, I.: The traction spur. An indicator of segmental instability. J. Bone Joint Surg. 53A:663, 1971.

73. Palacios, E., Brackett, C.E., and Leary, D.J.: Ossification of the posterior longitudinal ligament associated with a herniated intervertebral disk. Radiology 100:313, 1971.

74. Markolf, K.L.: Deformation of the thoracolumbar intervertebral joints in response to external loads: A biomechanical study using autopsy material. J. Bone Joint Surg. 54A:511, 1972.

75. White, A.A., III, and Panjabi, J.M.: Clinical Biomechanics of the Spine. Philadelphia, J. B. Lippincott Company, 1978.

76. Radin, E.L., Simon, S.R., and Rose, R.M.: Practical Biomechanics for the Orthopedic Surgeon. New York, John Wiley & Sons, 1978.

77. Fielding, J.W., Gehran, G., Van, B., et al.: Tears of the transverse ligament of the atlas. A clinical and biomechanical study. J. Bone Joint Surg. 56A:1683, 1974.

78. Callahan, R.A., Johnson, R.M., Margolis, R.N., et al.: Cervical facet fusion for control of instability following laminectomy. J. Bone Joint Surg. 59A:991, 1977.

79. Bauze, R.J., and Ardran, G.M.: Proceedings: The mechanism of forward dislocation in the human cervical spine. J. Bone Joint Surg. 57B:253, 1975.

80. White, A.A., III, and Hirsch, C.: The significance of the vertebral posterior elements in the mechanics of the thoracic spine. Clin. Orthop. 81:2, 1971.

81. Panjabi, M.M., Brand, R.A., Jr., and White, A.A., III: Mechanical properties of the human thoracic spine as shown by three-dimensional load-displacement curves. J. Bone Joint Surg. 58A:642, 1976.

82. Lin, H.S., Liu, Y.K., and Atems, K.H.: Mechanical response of the lumbar intervertebral joint under physiological loading (complex). J. Bone Joint Surg. 60A:41, 1978.

83. Howes, R.G., and Isdale, I.C.: The loose back: An unrecognized syndrome. Rheumatol. Phys. Med. 11:72, 1971.

84. Liu, Y.K., Ray, G., and Hirsch, C.: The resistance of the lumbar spine to direct shear. Orthop. Clin. North Am. 1:33, 1975.

85. Floyd, W.F., and Silver, P.H.: The function of the erectors spinae muscles in certain movements and postures in man. J. Physiol. 129:184, 1955.

86. Morris, J.M., Lucas, D.B., and Bresler, B.: Role of the trunk in stability of the spine. J. Bone Joint Surg. 43A:327, 1961.

87. Morris, J.M., Benner, G., and Lucas, D.G.: An electromyographic study of the intrinsic muscles of the back in man. J. Anat. 96:509, 1962.

88. Asmussen, E.: The functions of the back muscles in standing and while holding weights. Prog. Phys. Ther. 1:87, 1979.

89. Asmussen, E., Dahlerup, J.V., and Fredsted, A.: Quantitative Evaluation of the Activity of the Back Muscles in Lifting. Communications from the Danish National Association for Infantile Paralysis, p. 21, 1965.

90. Nachemson, A., and Morris, J.M.: In vivo measurements of intradiscal pressure. J. Bone Joint Surg. 45A:1077, 1964.

91. Nachemson, A.: The effect of forward leaning on lumbar intradiscal pressure. Acta Orthop. Scand. 35:314, 1965.

92. Bartelink, D.L.: Role of abdominal pressure in relieving the pressure on the lumbar intervertebral discs. J. Bone Joint Surg. 39B:718, 1957.

93. Eie, N., and When, P.: Measurements of the intra-abdominal pressure in relation to weight bearing of the lumbosacral spine. J. Oslo City Hosp. 12:205, 1962.

94. Asmussen, E., and Poulsen, E.: On the Role of Intraabdominal Pressure in Relieving the Back Muscles While Holding Weights in a Forward Inclined Position. Communications from the Danish National Association for Infantile Paralysis, p. 28, 1968.

95. American Academy of Orthopaedic Surgeons: Joint Motion: Method of Measuring and Recording. Chicago, American Academy of Orthopaedic Surgeons, 1965.

96. Kapandji, I.A.: The Physiology of Joints. 2nd ed. Edinburgh, E.R.S. Livingstone, 1970.

97. Boone, D.C., and Azen, S.P.: Normal range of motion of joints in male subjects. J. Bone Joint Surg. 61A:756, 1979.

98. Plagenhoff, S.: Patterns of Human Motion. Englewood Cliffs, N.J., Prentice-Hall, 1971.

99. Panjabi, M.M.: Experimental determination of spinal motion in segment behavior. Orthop. Clin. North Am. 8:169, 1977.

100. Pennal, G.F., Conn, G.S., McDonald, G., et al.: Motion studies of the lumbar spine: A preliminary report. J. Bone Joint Surg. 54B:442, 1972.

101. Davis, P.R., Troup, J.D., and Barnard, J.H.: Movements of the thoracic and lumbar spine when lifting: A chronocyclophotographic study. J. Anat. 99:13, 1965.

102. Kulak, R.F., Schultz, A.B., Belytschko, T., et al.: Biomechanical characteristics of vertebral motion segments and intervertebral discs. Orthop. Clin. North Am. 6:121, 1975.

103. Cleland, J.: The shoulder-girdle and its movements. Lancet, Feb. 19, 1881, p. 283.

104. Saha, A.K.: Theory of Shoulder Mechanism. Springfield, Ill., Charles C Thomas, 1961.

105. Saha, A.K.: Dynamic stability of the glenohumeral joint. Acta Orthop. Scand. 42:491, 1971.

106. Saha, A.K.: Mechanics of elevation of glenohumeral joint. Its application in rehabilitation of flail shoulder in upper brachial plexus injuries and poliomyelitis and in replacement of the upper humerus by prosthesis. Acta Orthop. Scand. 44:668, 1973.

107. Blacharski, P.A., Somerset, JH., and Murray, D.G.: A three-dimensional study of the kinematics of the human knee. J. Biomechanics 8:375, 1975.

108. Hallen, L.G., and Lindahl, O.: The "screw-home" movement in the knee joint. Acta Orthop. Scand. 37:97, 1966.

109. Murray, M.P.: Gait as a total pattern of movement—including a bibliography on gait. Am. J. Phys. Med. 46:290, 1967.

110. Eberhart, H.D., Inman, V.T., et al.: Fundamental Studies of Human Locomotion and Other Information Relating to Design of Artificial Limbs. Report to the Committee on Artificial Limbs, National Research Council. Washington, D.C., 1945–47.

111. Waters, R.L., Perry, J., McDaniels, J.M., et al.: The relative strength of the hamstrings during hip extension. J. Bone Joint Surg. 56A:1592, 1974.

112. Brand, P.W.: Biomechanics of tendon transfer. Orthop. Clin. North Am. 5:205, 1974.

113. Denham, R.A.: Hip mechanics. J. Bone Joint Surg. 41B:550, 1959.

114. McLeish, R.D., and Charnley, J.: Abduction forces in the one-legged stance. J. Biomechanics 3:191, 1970.

115. Johnston, R.C.: Mechanical considerations of the hip joint. Arch. Surg. 107:411, 1973.

116. Rydell, N.: Forces in the hip joint. II. Intravital studies. In Kenedi, R.M. (ed.): Biomechanics and Related Bioengineering Topics. London, Pergamon Press, 1965.

117. Rydell, N.: Biomechanics of the hip-joint. Clin. Orthop. 92:6, 1973.

118. Morrison, J.B.: Function of the knee joint in various activities. Med. Biol. Eng. 4:573, 1969.

119. Morrison, J.B.: The mechanics of the knee joint in relation to normal walking. J. Biomechanics 3:51, 1970.

120. Paul, J.P.: Force actions transmitted in the knee of normal subjects and by prosthetic joint replacements. Institute of Mechanical Engineering Conference on Total Knee Replacement, London, September, 1974.

121. Sammarco, G.J., Burstein, A.H., and Frankel, V.H.: Biomechanics of the ankle: A kinematic study. Orthop. Clin. North Am. 4:75, 1973.

122. Brewster, R.C., Chao, E.Y., and Stauffer, R.N.: Force analysis of the ankle joint during the stance phase of gait. 27th Proceedings of the Annual Conference on Engineering in Medicine and Biology, Philadelphia, 1974, p. 368.

123. DeLuca, C.J., and Forrest, W.F.: Force analysis of individual muscles acting simultaneously on the shoulder joint during isometric abduction. J. Biomechanics 6:385, 1973.

124. Dvir, Z., and Berme, N.: The shoulder complex in elevation of the arm: A mechanism approach. J. Biomechanics 11:219, 1978.

125. Cooney, W.P., III, and Chao, E.Y.S.: Biomechanical analysis of static forces in the thumb during hand function. J. Bone Joint Surg. 59A:27, 1977.

126. Swanson, A.B., and Swanson, G.D.: Pathogenesis and pathomechanics of rheumatoid deformities in the hand and wrist. Orthop. Clin. North Am. 4:1039, 1973.

127. Hakstian, R.W., and Tubiana, R.: Ulnar deviation of the fingers. J. Bone Joint Surg. 49A:299, 1967.

128. Flatt, A.E.: The pathomechanics of ulnar drift. Social and Rehabilitation Services Final Report. Grant No. RD, 226M, 1971.

129. Wise, K.S.: The anatomy of the metacarpo-phalangeal joints, with observations of the aetiology of ulnar drift. J. Bone Joint Surg. 57B:485, 1975.

130. Smith, R.J.: Balance and kinetics of the fingers under normal and pathological conditions. Clin. Orthop. 104:92, 1974.

131. Hueston, J.T., and Wilson, W.F.: The role of the intrinsic muscles in the production of metacarpophalangeal subluxation in the rheumatoid hand. Plast. Reconstr. Surg. 52:342, 1973.

132. Pieron, A.P.: The mechanism of the first carpometacarpal (CMC) joint. An anatomical and mechanical analysis. Acta Orthop. Scand. (Suppl.) 48:1, 1973.

133. Hirsch, D., Page, D., Miller, D., Dumbleton, J.G., and Miller, E.H.: A biomechanical analysis of the metacarpophalangeal joint of the thumb. J. Biomechanics 7:343, 1974.

134. Johns, R.J., and Draper, I.T.: The control of movement in normal subjects. Bull. Johns Hopkins Hosp. 115:447, 1964.

135. Haffajee, D., Moritz, U., and Svantesson, G.: Isometric knee extension strength as a function of joint angle, muscle length and motor unit activity. Acta Orthop. Scand. 43:138, 1972.

136. Basmajian, J.V., and Latif, A.: Integrated actions and functions of the chief flexors of the elbow. J. Bone Joint Surg. 39A:1106, 1957.

137. Landsmeer, J.M.F.: The coordination of finger-joint motions. J. Bone Joint Surg. 45:1654, 1963.

138. Basmajian, J.V., and Travill, A.: Electromyography of the pronator muscles in the forearm. Anat. Rec. 139:45, 1961.

139. Barnett, C.H., and Harding, D.: The activity of antagonist muscles during voluntary movement. Ann. Phys. Med. 2:290, 1955.

140. Basmajian, J.V.: Muscles Alive—Their Functions Revealed by Electromyography. Baltimore, Williams & Wilkins Company, 1974.

141. Basmajian, J.V., and Bentzon, J.W.: An electromyographic study of certain muscles of the leg and foot in the standing position. Surg. Gynecol. Obstet. 98:662, 1954.

142. Elftman, H.: Biomechanics of muscle with particular application to studies of gait. J. Bone Joint Surg. 48A:363, 1966.

143. Mann, R.A., Hagy, J.L., and Simon, S.R.: Biomechanics of Gait. A Critical Visual Analysis. Instructional Course Lectures, The American Academy of Orthopaedic Surgeons, March 1975.

144. Bigland, B., and Lippold, O.J.C.: The relation between force, velocity and integrated activity in human muscles. J. Physiol. 123:214, 1954.

145. Stern, J.T.: Investigations concerning the theory of spurt and shunt muscles. J. Biomechanics 4:437, 1971.

146. Joseph, J., and Watson, R.: Telemetering electromyography of muscles used in walking up and down stairs. J. Bone Joint Surg. 49B:774, 1967.

147. Andriacchi, T.P., Andersson, G.B.J., Fermier, R.W., et al.: A study of lower limb mechanics during stair climbing. J. Bone Joint Surg. (in press).

148. Andersson, B.J., Ortengren, R., Nachemson, A.L., Elfstrom, G., and Broman, H.: The sitting posture: An electromyographic and discometric study. Orthop. Clin. North Am. 6:105, 1975.

149. Farfan, H.F.: Muscular mechanism of the lumbar spine and the position of power and efficiency. Orthop. Clin. North Am. 6:135, 1975.

150. Davis, P.R.: Posture of the trunk during the lifting of weights. Br. Med. J. 5114:87, 1959.

151. Mow, V.C., and Lai, W.M.: Selected unresolved problems in synovial joint biomechanics. ASME, 1979 Biomechanics Symposium, AMD-32, p. 19.

152. Naylor, H.: Bearings and lubrication. Chart. Mech. Eng. 12:642, 1965.

153. Archard, J.F., and Hirst, W.: The wear of metals under unlubricated conditions. Proc. R. Soc. London, 236A:397, 1956.

154. Unsworth, A., Dowson, D., and Wright, V.: The frictional behavior of human synovial joints. Part I. Natural joints. J. Lubrication Tech. 97F:369, 1975.

155. Simon, S.R., Paul, I.L., Rose, R.M., and Radin, E.L.: "Stiction-friction" of total hip prostheses and its relationship to loosening. J. Bone Joint Surg. 57A:226, 1975.

156. Muir, H., Bullough, P., and Maroudas, A.: The distribution of collagen in human articular cartilage with some of its physiological implications. J. Bone Joint Surg. 52B:554, 1970.

157. Sayles, R.S., Thomas, T.R., Anderson, J., Haslock, I., and Unsworth, A.: Measurement of the surface microgeometry of articular cartilage. J. Biomechanics. 12:257, 1979.

158. Gardner, D.L., and McGillivray, D.C.: Living articular cartilage is not smooth. Ann. Rheum. Dis. 30:3, 1971.

159. Gardner, D.L., and McGillivray, D.C.: Surface structures of articular cartilage. Ann. Rheum. Dis. 30:10, 1971.

160. Clarke, I.C.: Human articular surface contours and related surface depression frequency studies. Ann. Rheum. Dis. 30:15, 1971.

161. Archard, J.F.: Surface topography and tribology. Tribology 7:213, 1974.

162. Archard, J.F., and Kirk, M.T.: Influence of elastic modulus on the lubrication of point contacts. Lubrication and Wear Convention. Proc. Inst. Mech. Engrs., London 117:181, 1963.

163. Jones, E.S.: Joint lubrication. Lancet 226:1426, 1934.

164. McCutchen, C.W.: The frictional properties of animal joints. Wear 5:1, 1962.

165. Linn, F.C.: Lubrication of animal joints. J. Bone Joint Surg. 49A:1079, 1967.

166. Linn, F.C., and Radin, E.L.: Lubrication of animal joints. Arthritis Rheum. 2:674, 1968.

167. Walker, P.S., Dowson, D., Longfield, M.D., et al.: Boosted lubrication in synovial joints by fluid entrapment and enrichment. Ann. Rheum. Dis. 27:512, 1968.

168. MacConaill, M.A.: The movements of bones and joints. II. The synovial fluid and its assistants. J. Bone Joint Surg. 32B:244, 1950.

169. McCutchen, C.W., and Lewis, P.R.: Mechanism of animal joints. Nature 184:1284, 1959.

170. Dintenfass, L.: Rheology of synovial fluid and its role in joint lubrication. In Copley, A.L. (ed.): Proceedings of the International Congress on Rheology, Part IV. New York, Wiley Interscience, 1963, pp. 489–503.

171. McCutchen, C.W.: Boundary lubrication by synovial fluids: Demonstration and possible osmotic explanation. Fed. Proc. 25:1061, 1966.

172. Dowson, D.: Modes of lubrication in human joints. Symposium on Lubrication and Wear in Living and Artificial Human Joints. Proc. Inst. Mech. Engrs., London 181:45, 1967.

173. Linn, F.C.: Lubrication of animal joints. II. The mechanism. J. Biomechanics 1:193, 1968.
174. Longfield, M.D., Dowson, D., Walker, P.S., et al.: Boosted lubrication of human joints by fluid enrichment and entrapment. Bio-Med. Engr. 4:517, 1969.
175. Walker, P.S., Unsworth, A., Dowson, D., et al.: Modes of aggregation of hyaluronic acid protein complex on the surface of articular cartilage. Ann. Rheum. Dis. 29:591, 1970.
176. Radin, E.L., and Paul, I.L.: A consolidated concept of joint lubrication. J. Bone Joint Surg. 54A:607, 1972.
177. Ling, F.F.: A new model of articular cartilage in human joints. J. Lubrication Tech. 96:449, 1974.
178. Torzilli, P.A., and Mow, V.C.: On the fundamental fluid transport mechanisms through normal and pathological articular cartilage during function. II. The analysis, solution and conclusions. J. Biomechanics 9:587, 1976.
179. Mansour, J.M., and Mow, V.C.: On the natural lubrication of synovial joints: Normal and degenerate. J. Lubrication Tech. 99:163, 1977.
180. Ogston, A.G., and Stanier, J.E.: The physiological function of hyaluronic acid in synovial fluid; viscous elastic and lubricant properties. J. Physiol. 119:244, 1953.
181. Laurent, T.C.: Physico-chemical Studies on Hyaluronic Acid. Uppsala, Sweden, Almquist & Wiksell, 1957, pp. 1–28.
182. Balazs, E.A., Watson, D., Duff, I.F., et al.: Hyaluronic acid in synovial fluid. I. Molecular parameters of hyaluronic acid in normal and arthritic human fluids. Arthritis Rheum. 10:357, 1967.
183. Davis, D.V., and Palfrey, A.F.: Some of the physical properties of normal and pathological synovial fluids. J. Biomechanics 1:79, 1968.
184. Maroudas, A.: Studies on the formation of hyaluronic acid films. In Wright, V. (ed.): Lubrication and Wear in Joints. Philadelphia, J.B. Lippincott Company, 1969.
185. Bullough, P.G., Goodfellow, J.B., Greenwald, A.S., et al.: Incongruent surfaces in the human joint. Nature 217:1290, 1968.
186. Oberlander, W.: On biomechanics of joints. The influence of functional cartilage swelling on the congruity of regular curved joints. J. Biomechanics 11:151, 1978.
187. Simon, W.H., Friedenberg, S., and Richardson, S.: Joint congruence. A correlation of joint congruence and thickness of articular cartilage in dogs. J. Bone Joint Surg. 55A:1614, 1973.
188. Greenwald, A.S., and Haynes, D.W.: Weight-bearing areas in the human hip joint. J. Bone Joint Surg. 54B:157, 1972.
189. Day, W.H., Swanson, S.A.V., and Freeman, M.A.R.: Contact pressures in the loaded human cadaver hip. J. Bone Joint Surg. 57B:302, 1975.
190. Armstrong, C.G., Bahrani, A.S., and Gardner, D.L.: In vitro measurement of articular cartilage deformation in the intact human hip joint under load. J. Bone Joint Surg. 61A:744–755, 1979.
191. Walker, P.S., and Hajek, J.V.: The load-bearing areas in the knee joint. J. Biomechanics 5:581, 1972.
192. Kettlkamp, D.B., and Jacobs, A.W.: Tibiofemoral contact area—determination and implications. J. Bone Joint Surg. 54A:349, 1972.
193. Maquet, P.G., Van de Berg, A.J., and Simoret, J.C.: Femorotibial weight-bearing areas. Experimental determination. J. Bone Joint Surg. 57A:766, 1975.
194. Walker, P.S., and Erkman, J.J.: The role of the menisci in force transmission across the knee. Clin. Orthop. 109:184, 1975.
195. Greenwald, A.S., and Matejczyk, M-B.: A contact area study of the human ankle joint. Orthop. Rev. 6:85, August 1967.
196. Lambert, K.L.: The weight-bearing function of the fibula. A strain gauge study. J. Bone Joint Surg. 53A:507, 1971.
197. Walker, P.S.: Human Joints and Their Artificial Replacements. Springfield, Ill., Charles C Thomas, 1977.
198. Salter, R.B., and Field, P.: The effects of continuous compression on living articular cartilage. J. Bone Joint Surg. 42A:31, 1960.
199. Mankin, H., and Thrasher, A.Z.: Water content and binding in normal and osteoarthritic human cartilage. J. Bone Joint Surg. 57A:76, 1975.
200. Radin, E., Paul, I., and Rose, R.: Role of mechanical factors in the pathogenesis of primary osteoarthritis. Lancet 1:519, 1972.
201. Freeman, M.A.R.: Articular Cartilage. New York, Grune & Stratton, 1974.
202. MacConaill, M.A.: The movement of bones and joints. IV. The mechanical structure of articulating cartilage. J. Bone Joint Surg. 33B:251, 1951.
203. Linn, F.C., and Sokoloff, L.: Movement and composition of interstitial fluid of cartilage. Arthritis Rheum. 8:481, 1965.
204. Eisenfeld, J., Mow, V.C., and Lipshitz, H.: The mathematical analysis of stress relaxation in articular cartilage during compression. Math. Biosci. 39:97, 1978.
205. Mow, V.C.: Biphasic rheological properties of cartilage. Bull. Hosp. Joint Dis. 38:121, 1977.
206. Hayes, W.C., and Mockros, L.F.: Viscoelastic properties of human articular cartilage. J. Appl. Physiol. 31:562, 1971.
207. Mansour, J.M., and Mow, V.C.: The permeability of articular cartilage under compressive strain and at high pressures. J. Bone Joint Surg. 58A:509, 1976.
208. Camosso, M.E., and Marotti, G.: The mechanical behavior of articular cartilage under compressive stress. J. Bone Joint Surg. 44A:699, 1962.
209. Kempson, G.E.: Mechanical properties of articular cartilage. In Freeman, M.A.R. (ed.): Adult Articular Cartilage. New York, Grune & Stratton, 1979, p. 197.
210. Woo, S.L-Y., Akeson, W.H., and Jemmott, C.F.: Measurement of non-homogeneous, directional mechanical properties of articular cartilage in tension. J. Biomechanics 9:785, 1976.
211. Redler, I.: A scanning electron microscopic study of human normal and osteoarthritis articular cartilage. Clin. Orthop. 103:262, 1974.
212. Redler, I., and Zimmy, M.: Scanning electron microscopy of normal and abnormal articular cartilage and synovium. J. Bone Joint Surg. 52A:1395, 1970.
213. Lane, J.M., and Weiss, C.: Review of articular cartilage collagen research. Arthritis Rheum. 18:553, 1975.
214. Roth, V., and Mow, V.C.: Finite element analysis of contact problems for indentation of articular cartilage. In Grood, E.S., and Smith, C.R. (eds.): Advances in Bioengineering. New York, American Society of Mechanical Engineers, 1977, pp. 47–48.
215. Maroudas, A.: Physico-chemical properties of articular cartilage. In Freeman, M.A.R. (ed.): Adult Articular Cartilage. New York, Grune & Stratton, 1974.
216. Bullough, P.G., and Goodfellow, J.: The significance of the fine structure of articular cartilage. J. Bone Joint Surg. 50B:852, 1968.
217. Roth, V., Wirth, C., Mow, V.C., et al.: Variation of tensile properties of articular cartilage with age. Transactions, 24th Annual Meeting of the Orthopedic Research Society, Dallas, Texas, 3:9, 1978.
218. Mathews, M.B., and Lozaityte, I.: Sodium chondroitin sulfate-protein complexes of cartilage. I. Molecular weight and shape. Arch. Biochem. Biophys. 74:158, 1978.
219. Muir, H.: The nature of the link between protein and carbohydrate of a chondroitin sulphate complex from hyaline cartilage. Biochem. J. 69:195, 1958.
220. Partridge, S.M., Davis, H.F., and Adair, F.S.: The chemistry of connective tissues. 6. The constitution of the chondroitin sulphate-protein complex in cartilage. Biochem. J. 79:15, 1961.
221. Rosenberg, L.: Cartilage proteoglycans. Fed. Proc. 32:1467, 1973.
222. Lipshitz, H., Etheridge, R., and Glimcher, M.J.: Changes in the hexosamine content and swelling ratio of articular cartilage as a function of depth from the surface. J. Bone Joint Surg. 58A:1149, 1976.
223. Lipshitz, H., Etheridge, R., and Glimcher, M.J.: In vitro wear of articular cartilage. J. Bone Joint Surg. 57A:527, 1975.
224. Maroudas, A., Muir, H., and Wingham, J.: The correlation of fixed negative charge with glycosaminoglycan content of human articular cartilage. Biochim. Biophys. Acta 177:492, 1969.
225. Maroudas, A.: Physiochemical properties of cartilage in the light of ion-exchange theory. Biophys. J. 8:575, 1968.
226. Maroudas, A.: Biophysical chemistry of cartilaginous tissues with special reference to solute and fluid transport. Biorheology 12:233, 1975.
227. Gordon, S.S., Mow, V.C., Lee, R., et al.: Permeability and transport properties of articular cartilage. Proceedings, 3rd International Congress of Biorheology, La Jolla, California, 1978, p. 175.
228. Sokoloff, L.: Elasticity of articular cartilage: Effect of ions and viscous solutions. Science 141:1055, 1963.
229. Picheny, M.A., and Grodzinsky, A.J.: Method for measurement of charge in collagen and polyelectrolyte composite materials. Biopolymers 15:1845, 1976.
230. Nussbaum, J.H., and Grodzinsky, A.J.: H^+ binding and diffusion-reaction rates in collagen electromechanics. In Ostrander, L.E. (ed.): Proceedings, 7th New England (Northeast) Bioengineering Congress, 1979, pp. 61–64.
231. Grodzinsky, A.J., and Shoenfeld, N.A.: Tensile forces induced in collagen by means of electromechanochemical transductive coupling. Polymer 18:421, 1977.
232. Grodzinsky, A.J., Lipschitz, H., and Glimcher, M.J.: Electromechanical properties of articular cartilage during compression and stress relaxation. Nature 275:448, 1978.
233. Grodzinsky, A.J., Roth, V., Fox, P., et al.: The influence of electrochemical transduction on matrix interactions in articular cartilage. Transactions, 25th Annual Meeting, Orthopedic Research Society, San Francisco, 4:141, 1979.
234. Grodzinsky, A.J., and Eisenberg, S.R.: Double layer mediated energy conversion with a protein membrane using an imposed frequency and wavelength. J. Electrostatics 5:33, 1978.
235. Grodzinsky, A.J., and Melcher, J.R.: Electromechanical transduction with charged polyelectrolyte membranes. IEEE Trans. Biomed. Eng. 23:421, 1976.
236. Lotke, P.A., Black, J., and Richardson, S.: Electromechanical properties in human articular cartilage. J. Bone Joint Surg. 56A:1040, 1974.
237. Meachim, G., Ghadially, F., and Collins, D.M.: Regressive changes in

the superficial layer of human articular cartilage. Ann. Rheum. Dis. 24:23, 1965.

238. Goodfellow, J.W., and Bullough, P.G.: The pattern of aging of the articular cartilage of the elbow joint. J. Bone Joint Surg. 49B:175, 1967.

239. Mankin, H.J.: The reaction of articular cartilage to injury and osteoarthritis (first of two parts). N. Engl. J. Med. 291:1285, 1974.

240. Krane, S.M.: Joint erosion in rheumatoid arthritis. Arthritis Rheum. 17:206, 1974.

241. Muir, H.: Molecular approach to understanding of osteoarthrosis. Ann. Rheum. Dis. 36:199, 1977.

242. Radin, E.L., Paul, I.L., and Lowy, M.: A comparison of the dynamic force-transmitting properties of subchondral bone and articular cartilage. J. Bone Joint Surg. 52A:444, 1970.

243. Radin, E.L., and Paul, L.: Importance of bone in sparing articular cartilage from impact. Clin. Orthop. 78:342, 1971.

244. Chamay, A., and Tschantz, P.: Mechanical influences in bone remodeling. Experimental research on Wolff's law. J. Biomechanics 5:173, 1972.

245. Dickson, R.A.: The assessment of hand function. II. Forces and bone density, a relationship in the hand. Hand 5:15, 1973.

246. Pugh, J.W., Rose, R.M., and Radin, E.L.: Elastic and viscoelastic properties of trabecular bone: Dependence on structure. J. Biomechanics 6:475, 1973.

247. Pugh, J.W., Rose, R.M., and Radin, E.L.: A possible mechanism of Wolff's law: Trabecular microfractures. Arch. Intern. Physiol. Biochim. 81:27, 1973.

248. Behrens, J.C., Walker, P.S., and Shoji, H.: Variations in strength and structure of cancellous bone at the knee. J. Biomechanics 7:201, 1974.

249. Pugh, J.W., Radin, E.L., and Rose, R.M.: Quantitative studies of human subchondral cancellous bone. Its relationship to the state of its overlying cartilage. J. Bone Joint Surg. 56A:313, 1974.

250. Leriem, P., et al.: Hardness of the subchondral bone of the tibial condyles in the normal state and in osteoarthritis and rheumatoid arthritis. Acta Orthop. Scand. 45:614, 1974.

251. Raux, P., Townsend, P.R., Meigel, R., et al.: Trabecular architecture of the human patella. J. Biomechanics 8:1, 1975.

252. Bullough, P., Goodfellow, J., and O'Connor, J.: The relationship between degenerative changes and load-bearing in the human hip. J. Bone Joint Surg. 55B:746, 1973.

253. F. Pauwel's Der Schenkelhalsbruch: Ein mechanisches Problem: Grundlagen Heilungsvorganges. Prognose und kausale Therapie: Zeitchrift für orthopadische Chirurgie, Vol. 63. Stuttgart, Enke, 1935.

254. Murray, M.P., Gore, D.R., and Clarkson, B.H.: Walking patterns of patients with unilateral hip pain due to osteoarthritis and avascular necrosis. J. Bone Joint Surg. 53A:259, 1971.

255. Murray, M.P., Brewer, B., and Zuege, R.C.: Kinesiologic measurements of functional performance before and after McKee-Farrar total hip replacement. A study of thirty patients with rheumatoid arthritis, osteoarthritis, or avascular necrosis of the femoral head. J. Bone Joint Surg. 54A:237, 1972.

256. Gord, D.R., Murray, M.P., and Sepic, S.B.: Walking patterns of men with unilateral surgical hip fusion. J. Bone Joint Surg. 57A:759, 1975.

257. Hauge, M.F.: The knee in patients with hip joint ankylosis. Clinical survey and bio-mechanical aspects. Acta Orthop. Scand. 44:485, 1973.

258. Johnston, R.C., Brand, R.A., and Crowinshield, R.D.: Reconstruction of the hip. A mathematical approach to determine optimum geometric relationships. J. Bone Joint Surg. 61A:639, 1979.

259. Blount, W.: Don't throw away the cane. J. Bone Joint Surg. 38A:695, 1956.

260. Gore, D.R., Murray, M.P., Gardner, G.M., et al.: Roentgenographic measurements after Muller total hip replacement. J. Bone Joint Surg. 59A:948, 1977.

261. Stauffer, R.N., Smidt, G.L., and Wadsworth, J.B.: Clinical and biomechanical analysis of gait following Charnley total hip replacement. Clin. Orthop. 99:70, 1974.

262. Cracchiolo, A. (ed.): Statistics of total knee replacement. Clin. Orthop. Rel. Res. 120:2085, 1976.

263. Reilly, D.T., and Martens, M.: Experimental analysis of the quadriceps muscle force and patello-femoral joint reaction force for various activities. Acta Orthop. Scand. 43:126, 1972.

264. Zdravkovic, D., and Damholt, V.: Knee and quadriceps function after fracture of the femur. Acta Orthop. Scand. 42:460, 1971.

265. Kostuik, J.P., Schmidt, O., Harris, W.R., and Wooldridge, C.: A study of weight transmission through the knee joint with applied varus and valgus loads. Clin. Orthop. 108:95, 1975.

266. Kellelkamp, D.B.: Clinical implications of knee biomechanics. Arch. Surg. 107:406, 1973.

267. Hughston, J.C., and Eilers, A.F.: The role of the posterior oblique ligament in repairs of acute medial (collateral) ligament tears of the knee. J. Bone Joint Surg. 55:923, 1973.

268. Harrington, K.: Degenerative arthritis of the ankle secondary to longstanding lateral ligament instability. J. Bone Joint Surg. 61A:347, 1979.

269. Lew, W.D., and Lewis, J.L.: An anthropometric scaling method with application to the knee joint. J. Biomechanics 10:171, 1977.

270. Lewis, J.L., and Lew, W.D.: A method for locating an optimal "fixed" axis of rotation for the human knee joint. J. Biomech. Eng. 100:187, 1978.

271. Krause, W.R., Pope, M.H., Johnson, R., et al.: Mechanical changes in the knee after meniscectomy. J. Bone Joint Surg. 58A:599, 1976.

272. Snook, S.H., and Ciriello, V.M.: Low back pain in industry. ASSE J. 17:17, 1972.

273. Bond, M.B.: Low back injuries in industry. Indust. Med. Surg. 39:204, 1970.

274. National Center for Health Statistics: Prevalence of chronic skin and musculo-skeletal conditions, United States 1969. Series 10, No. 92, 1974.

275. Rowe, M.L.: Low back pain in industry. J. Occup. Med. 11:161, 1969.

276. National Center for Health Statistics: Limitation of Activity Due to Chronic Conditions, United States, 1969 and 1970. Series, 10, No. 80, 1973.

277. National Center for Health Statistics: Types of Injuries. Incidence and Associated Disability, United States, July 1965–1967. Series 10, No. 57, 1969.

278. Rowe, M.L.: Low back disability in industry: Updated position. J. Occup. Med. 13:476, 1971.

279. Horal, J.: The clinical appearance of low back disorders in the city of Gothenburg, Sweden. Acta Orthop. Scand. Suppl. No. 118, 1969.

280. Kosiak, M., Aurelius, J.R., and Hatfield, W.F.: Backache in industry. J. Occup. Med. 8:51, 1966.

281. Hirsch, C.: Etiology and pathogenesis of low back pain. Israel J. Med. Sci. 2:362, 1966.

282. Farfan, H.F., Huberdeau, R.M., and Dubow, H.I.: Lumbar intervertebral disc degeneration: The influence of geometrical features on the pattern of disc degeneration—a post mortem study. J. Bone Joint Surg. 54A:492, 1972.

283. Fahrni, W.H.: Conservative treatment of lumbar disc degeneration: Our primary responsibility. Orthop. Clin. North Am. 6:93, 1975.

284. Nachemson, A.: Towards a better understanding of low-back pain: A review of the mechanics of the lumbar disc. Rheumatol. Rehabil. 14:129, 1975.

285. Cailliet, R.: Lowback Pain Syndrome. Philadelphia, F. A. Davis, 1962.

286. Magora, A.: Investigation of the relationship between low back pain and occupation. Indust. Med. Surg. 39:504, 1970.

287. Park, K.S., and Chaffin, D.B.: Methods of manual load lifting: A biomechanical evaluation of an old problem. Technical report, University of Michigan, Department of Industrial and Operations Engineering, Ann Arbor, Michigan, 1973.

288. Brown, J.R.: Manual Lifting and Related Fields: An Annotated Bibliography. Labour Safety Council of Ontario. Ontario, Ministry of Labour, 1972.

289. Snook, S.H.: The design of manual handling tasks. Ergonomics 21:963, 1978.

290. Snook, S.H., and Ciriello, V.M.: Maximum weights and work loads acceptable to female workers. J. Occup. Med. 16:527, 1974.

291. Snook, S.H., and Irvine, C.H.: Maximum acceptable weight of lift. Am. Indust. Hyg. Assoc. J. 28:322, 1967.

292. Snook, S.H., Campanelli, R.A., and Hart, J.W.: A study of three preventive approaches to low back injury. J. Occup. Med. 20:478, 1978.

293. Chaffin, D.B., Herrin, C.D., Keyerling, W.M., et al.: Preemployment strength testing in selecting workers for materials handling jobs. NIOSH Contract No. CDC-99-74-62, May 1977.

294. Chaffin, D.B.: Human strength capability and low-back pain. J. Occup. Med. 16:248, 1974.

295. Chaffin, D.B.: Biomechanics of manual materials handling and lowback pain. In Zenz, C. (ed.): Occupational Medicine: Principles and Practical Applications. Chicago, Year Book Medical Publishers, 1975, Chapter 19.

296. Chaffin, D.B., and Park, K.S.: A longitudinal study of lowback pain as associated with occupational weight lifting factors. Am. Indust. Assoc. J. 34:513, 1973.

297. Chaffin, D.B., Herrin, C.D., Keyserling, W.M., et al.: Preemployment Strength Testing in Selecting Workers for Manual Handling Jobs. Washington, D.C., U.S. Department of Health, Education and Welfare, CDC-99-74-72, 1976.

298. Pedersen, O.F., Petersen, R., and Staffeldt, E.S.: Back pain and isometric back muscle strength of workers in a Danish factory. Scand. J. Rehabil. Med. 7:125, 1975.

299. Poulsen, E.: Prediction of maximum loads in lifting from measurements of muscular strength. Communications from the Danish National Association for Infantile Paralysis, 1970, 31.

300. Chaffin, D.B., Herrin, G.D., and Keyserling, W.M.: Preemployment strength testing, an updated position. J. Occup. Med. 20:No. 6, 403, 78.

Chapter 21
Purine and Deoxypurine Metabolism

Thomas D. Palella and William N. Kelley

Recognition of the role of purines in human disease began with the observation that uric acid, a purine base, was a component of some renal calculi,[1] and in its ionized form, monosodium urate, was (1) a major constituent of tophi,[2] (2) elevated in the serum of gouty patients,[3] and (3) present, in its crystalline form, in synovial fluid during the acute attack of gouty arthritis.[4] In more recent years the role in human disease of other purines such as xanthine, hypoxanthine, adenine, and 2,8-dihydroxyadenine, as well as the potential role of the deoxypurines, deoxyguanosine and deoxyadenosine, has become increasingly apparent. In this chapter we will trace (1) the reactions by which purine compounds are synthesized, interconverted, salvaged, degraded, and eventually oxidized to uric acid; (2) the mechanisms by which these pathways are controlled in man; (3) the mechanisms by which the final degradative product of the pathway, uric acid, is excreted and/or degraded; and (4) the physical properties of uric acid.

BIOCHEMISTRY OF PURINE COMPOUNDS

The parent compound, the purine base, is composed of a six-membered pyrimidine ring fused to the five-membered imidazole ring. The origins of individual atoms of the purine ring are as follows: carbon atoms 4 and 5 and nitrogen atom 7 come from glycine;[5-7] carbon atoms 2 and 8 come from formate;[7,8] carbon atom 6 comes from CO_2;[6,9] nitrogen atoms 3 and 9 come from the amide nitrogen of glutamine;[10-12] and nitrogen atom 1 comes from aspartic acid.[11] These precursor-product relationships are shown in Figure 21-1.

The most important purine bases are adenine, guanine, hypoxanthine, xanthine, and uric acid (Fig. 21-2). The purines all show lactam-lactim isomerism and may be written in either form, as shown for uric acid in Figure 21-2B.

Purine nucleosides are composed of a purine base plus a pentose joined to the base by a β-N-glycosyl bond between carbon atom 1 of the pentose and nitrogen atom 9 of the purine base. There are two series of nucleosides: the ribonucleosides, which contain D-ribose as the sugar component, and the deoxyribonucleosides, which contain 2-deoxy-D-ribose (Fig. 21-3).

Purine nucleotides and deoxynucleotides consist of a nucleoside or deoxynucleoside with a phosphate group in ester linkage with carbon 5 of the pentose (Fig. 21-

Figure 21–1. Origins of atoms of the purine ring.

Adenine

Guanine

Hypoxanthine

Xanthine

(Lactam) (Lactim)

Uric acid

Figure 21–2. Structures of the purine bases, adenine, guanine, hypoxanthine, xanthine, and uric acid. All purine bases may exist in the lactam form in a reversible manner as shown for uric acid.

Figure 21–3. Structures of adenosine and 2'-deoxyadenosine as examples of nucleosides and 2'-deoxynucleosides, respectively.

Figure 21–5. Comparison of the structures of nucleoside, mono-, di-, and triphosphates.

4). The nucleosides and deoxynucleosides may exist as 5'-monophosphates, 5'-diphosphates, and 5'-triphosphates (Fig. 21-5). The phosphoric acid residues of these compounds are designated by the symbols α, β, and γ. These compounds serve (1) as building blocks for RNA and DNA; (2) as precursors of the cyclic nucleotides, adenosine 3',5'-cyclic phosphate, and guanosine 3',5'-cyclic phosphate; (3) as a source of chemical energy; and (4) as precursors of various purine cofactors and coenzymes such as nicotinamide adenine dinucleotide (NAD).

Biosynthesis of the Purine Ring. A key intermediate in the synthesis of purine is 5-phosphoribosyl-1-pyrophosphate (PP-ribose-P) (Fig. 21-6). This high-energy compound is involved in purine synthesis in two types of reactions: in one it is a substrate, together with L-glutamine, for the first specific reaction of purine synthesis de novo;[13] in the other it participates in salvage of purine bases which are reconverted to ribonucleotides by a condensation reaction with liberation of inorganic pyrophosphate.[14,15] PP-ribose-P is formed by transfer of the terminal pyrophosphate group of ATP to carbon 1 of ribose 5-phosphate:[16,17]

$$\text{Ribose-5-phosphate} + \text{ATP} \xrightarrow{\text{Mg}^{2+}}$$
$$\text{PP-ribose-P} + \text{AMP} \qquad (1)$$

Inorganic phosphate is a required allosteric activator of PP-ribose-P synthetase.[18] The enzyme is subject to met-

abolic regulation by purine and pyrimidine ribonucleotides and certain other compounds.[19]

The first specific step of purine synthesis de novo is that in which the highly labile amino sugar, 5-β-phospho-D-ribosyl-1-amine, is generated. There are three known reactions for synthesis of phosphoribosylamine. In the best studied of the three,[12,13,20] the amide group of glutamine is transferred to PP-ribose-P and inorganic pyrophosphate is displaced. There is simultaneously an inversion of substituents at carbon 1 with formation of the β linkage characteristic of the glycosidic bond of all naturally occurring ribonucleotides (Fig. 21-7).[13]

$$\alpha\text{-PP-ribose-P} + \text{glutamine} + \text{H}_2\text{O} \xrightarrow{\text{Mg}^{2+}}$$
$$\beta\text{-phosphoribosylamine} + \text{glutamic acid} + \text{PP}_i \qquad (2)$$

This reaction which is catalyzed by anidophasphoribosyltransferase, is irreversible, and an important site of feedback control of purine synthesis. Other potential pathways for the synthesis of phosphoribosylamine include the direct reaction of PP-ribose-P with ammonia and a direct reaction of ribose-5-phosphate with ammonia. The contribution of this latter reaction in mammalian cells is probably insignificant. Cultured mammalian cell lines deficient in the first two synthetic reactions for phosphoribosylamine are auxotrophic for purines, despite the presence of the direct condensation of ammonia and ribose-5-phosphate.[21,22,23] The aminotransferase reaction, whereby ammonia and PP-ribose-P condense enzymatically, has been shown to contribute to de novo purine synthesis in human lymphocytes. In these same studies, the inhibitory effects of purine nucleotides were independent of the origin of the amine nitrogen.[24]

Figure 21–4. General structures of nucleoside and deoxynucleoside 5'-monophosphates.

$\alpha - 5 - \text{phospho} - \text{D} - \text{ribosyl} - 1 - \text{pyrophosphate}$

Figure 21–6. Structure of α-5-phospho-D-ribosyl-1-pyrophosphate (PP-ribose-1').

Figure 21-7. Biosynthesis of the purine ring. The encircled numbers in this figure refer to numbered reactions in the text. (From Wyngaarden, J.B., and Kelley, W.N.: Gout and Hyperuricemia. New York, Grune and Stratton, 1976.)

The stepwise synthesis of the purine ring is shown in Figure 21-7. Phosphoribosylamine is conjugated with glycine to yield 5'-phosphoribosylglycineamide, the first intermediate in which one finds the fundamental components of a nucleotide—namely, the combination of base, sugar, and phosphoric acid. ATP is involved in this reaction as an energy source.[12,25,26] Nucleotides of adenine and guanine show no inhibitory effects upon the enzyme catalyzing this reaction.[27]

$$\text{Phosphoribosylamine + glycine + ATP} \xrightarrow{\text{Mg}^{2+}}$$
$$\text{5'-phosphoribosylglycineamide (PRG)}$$
$$\text{+ADP+P}_i \qquad (3)$$

Phosphoribosylglycineamide receives a one-carbon "formyl" unit from N^5,N^{10}-methenyltetrahydrofolic acid (N^5,N^{10}-methenyl-THFA).[28,29] The transformylase activity has been shown to proceed through a direct displacement mechanism involving only formyl donor (10-CHO-H$_4$ folate) and formyl acceptor.[30]

$$\text{Phosphoribosylglycineamide}$$
$$+ N^5,N^{10}\text{-methenyl-THFA}$$
$$+ \text{H}_2\text{O} \rightarrow \text{phosphoribosyl-}\alpha\text{-}N\text{-formylglycineamide}$$
$$+ \text{THFA + H}^+ \qquad (4)$$

Next, the amide group of glutamine is transferred to phosphoribosylglycineamide to form the corresponding amidine compound,[31-33] following which ring closure generates the five-membered imidazole ring.[34] Each of these reactions requires ATP as an energy source and magnesium. The ring-closure reaction requires potassium as well.

$$\text{5'-Phosphoribosyl-}\alpha\text{-}N\text{-formylglycineamide}$$
$$+ \text{glutamine + ATP + H}_2\text{O} \xrightarrow{\text{Mg}^{2+}}$$
$$\text{5'-phosphoribosyl-}\alpha\text{-}N\text{-formylglycineamidine}$$
$$+ \text{glutamic acid + ADP + P}_i \qquad (5)$$

$$\text{5'-phosphoribosyl-}\alpha\text{-}N\text{-formylglycineamidine}$$
$$+ \text{ATP} \xrightarrow{\text{Mg}^{2+}, \text{K}^+}$$
$$\text{5'-phosphoribosyl-5-aminoimidazole}$$
$$+ \text{ADP + P}_i \qquad (6)$$

5'-Phosphoribosyl-5-aminoimidazole now receives a carboxyl group at carbon 4 by a reversible CO$_2$ fixation reaction that requires a high concentration of bicarbonate.[35] The carboxyl serves as a point for condensation of this intermediate with aspartic acid through an amide linkage involving another ATP as source of energy.[35] Hydrolysis of the intermediate yields 5'-phosphoribosyl-

5-amino-4-imidazolecarboxamide, a compound lacking only carbon 2 of a complete purine ribonucleotide.

$$5'\text{-Phosphoribosylaminoimidazole} + CO_2 \longrightarrow$$
$$5'\text{-phosphoribosyl-5-amino-} \quad (7)$$
$$4\text{-imidazolecarboxylate}$$

$$5'\text{-Phosphoribosyl-5-amino-4-imidazole-}$$
$$\text{carboxylate} + \text{aspartate} + ATP \xrightarrow{Mg^{2+}}$$
$$5'\text{-phosphoribosyl-5-amino-4-imidazole-}$$
$$\text{succinocarboxamide} + ADP + P_i \quad (8)$$

$$5'\text{-Phosphoribosyl-5-amino-4-imidazole-}$$
$$\text{succinocarboxamide} \longrightarrow \text{fumarate} + 5'\text{-}$$
$$\text{phosphoribosyl-5-amino-4-imidazole-}$$
$$\text{carboxamide} \quad (9)$$

Phosphoribosylaminoimidazolecarboxamide receives a formyl group from N^{10}-formyl-THFA.[36,37] AICAR transformylase probably exists in a multienzyme complex with other transformylase enzymes and a "trifunctional" protein. The actual carbon donor may be formate directly through this complex.[38] Ring closure completes the biosynthesis of the purine structure by forming inosine 5'-monophosphate (IMP):[37]

$$5'\text{-Phosphoribosyl-5-amino-4-imidazolecarboxamide}$$
$$+ N^{10}\text{-formyl-THFA} \xrightarrow{K^+} + \text{THFA} \quad (10)$$
$$5'\text{-phosphoribosyl-5-formamido-4-inudazole-}$$
$$\text{carboxamide } 5'\text{-Phosphoribosyl-5-formamido-4-}$$
$$\text{imidazolecarboxamide} \longrightarrow IMP + H_2O \quad (11)$$

Biosynthesis of Other Nucleotides. Inosinic acid may be considered the parent purine compound. It is an intermediate in the formation of adenylic acid (adenosine 5'-monophosphate, AMP) and guanylic acid (guanosine 5'-monophosphate, GMP), the major purine nucleotide components of nucleic acids. Conversion of inosinic acid to adenylic acid occurs in two steps. There is an initial condensation of inosinic acid with aspartic acid to form adenylosuccinic acid (AMP-S).[39,40] Energy for this reaction is derived from guanosine triphosphate.[41-44] Cleavage of adenylosuccinic acid yields adenylic acid and fumaric acid. This reaction is freely reversible;[41] it is analogous to cleavage of phosphoribosylaminoimidazole-succinocarboxamide (reaction 9) and is probably catalyzed by the same enzyme, adenylosuccinate lyase.

$$IMP + \text{L-asparate} + GTP \xrightarrow{Mg^{2+}}$$
$$AMP\text{-}S + GDP + P_i \quad (12)$$

$$AMP\text{-}S \longrightarrow AMP + \text{fumarate} \quad (13)$$

Conversion of inosinic acid to guanylic acid also occurs in two steps. There is first an irreversible oxidation of inosinic acid to xanthosine 5'-monophosphate (XMP), with nicotinamide adenine dinucleotide (NAD) as hydrogen acceptor.[45-47] The second reaction involves amination of XMP at the 2 position, and the specific donor is the amide group of glutamine.[48,49] The second step

requires ATP. These reactions proceed according to the following overall schemes:

$$IMP + NAD^+ H_2O \xrightarrow{K^+} XMP$$
$$+ NADH + H^+ \quad (14)$$

$$XMP + \text{glutamine} + ATP \xrightarrow{Mg^{2+}} GMP$$
$$+ \text{glutamic acid} + AMP + P_i \quad (15)$$

These pathways as well as those described below are summarized in Figure 21-8.

Salvage Pathways. Purine ribonucleosides and bases result from catabolism of endogenous or ingested ribonucleotides, or from administration of purine compounds. Conversion of purine bases to ribonucleotides may occur by one of two mechanisms. Purine bases may be conjugated with PP-ribose-P to form ribonucleotides in one step, or the bases may react with ribose 1-phosphate to form ribonucleosides, which may then be phosphorylated in the presence of ATP to ribonucleotides.

The phosphoribosyltransferase reaction has the following general form:

$$\text{Base} + \text{PP-ribose-P} \longrightarrow$$
$$\text{base-ribosephosphate} + P_i \quad (16)$$

This reaction is responsible for the conversion of purines,[14,15] pyrimidines,[50] nicotinamide,[51] and certain other nitrogenous bases to their respective ribonucleotides. Two different mammalian purine phosphoribosyltransferases (formerly termed ribonucleotide pyrophosphorylases) have been identified: one, ademine phosphoribosyltransferase (APRT), acting on AIC and adenine (Reaction 4, Fig. 21-8),[14,52] the other, hypoxanthine-guanine phosphoribosyltransferese (HPRT), acting on hypoxanthine and guanine (Reaction 2, Fig. 21-8).[15,53] APRT will also accept adenine analogues such as 2,6-diaminopurine and 8-azadenine. HPRT will catalyze the

Figure 21–8. Outline of purine metabolism. (1) Amidophosphoribosyltransferase; (2) hypoxanthine-guanine phosphoribosyltransferase; (3) PRPP synthetase; (4) adenine phosphoribosyltransferase; (5) adenosine deaminase; (6) purine nucleoside phosphorylase; (7) 5'-nucleotidase; (8) xanthine oxidase. (From Seegmiller, J.E. et al.: Science 155:1682, 1967.)

conversion of xanthine to XMP, but at only about 0.3 percent of the rate of the reaction with hypoxanthine or guanine.[54] HPRT will also catalyze the conversion of 6-thiopurine,[15] 6-thioguanine, 8-azaguanine, allopurinol,[55] and oxipurinol[56] to their respective ribonucleotides. In man, HPRT activity is widely distributed and is especially rich in brain, where activity is greatest in basal ganglia.[57] Activity is low in muscle and bone marrow.[57] The K_{eq} of both phosphoribosyltransferases is far toward the ribonucleotide; a value of 290 has been estimated for APRT.[52] Both phosphoribosyltransferases are inhibited by purine ribonucleoside monophosphates. Adenine phosphoribosyltransferase is inhibited by adenylic acid.[52] Hypoxanthine- guanine phosphoribosyltransferase is inhibited by inosinic acid and guanylic acid whether the substrate is hypoxanthine or guanine.[53] The inhibitions are formally competitive against PP-ribose-P, but appear to involve mutually exclusive binding rather than product inhibition at the substrate site.[58]

The two-step pathway has the following general form:

$$\text{Base} + \text{(deoxy)ribose 1-phosphate} \longrightarrow$$
$$\text{base-(deoxy)ribose} + P_i \qquad (17)$$

$$\text{Base} - \text{(deoxy)ribose} + \text{ATP} \longrightarrow$$
$$\text{base-(deoxy)ribosephosphate} + \text{ADP} \qquad (18)$$

Reaction 17 is catalyzed by purine nucleoside phosphorylase, an enzyme widely distributed in mammalian tissue and active with guanine, with hypoxanthine, and, to a lesser extent, with xanthine (Reaction 6, Fig. 21-8). Deoxyribose 1-phosphate may substitute for ribose 1-phosphate. The erythrocyte enzyme does not accept adenine,[59,60] but adenosine appears to be cleaved by the purine nucleoside phosphorylase of liver.[61] In the case of hypoxanthine, the equilibrium point is far toward the ribonucleoside. The phosphorylase has been extensively studied in human erythrocytes.[60,62]

Reaction 18 is catalyzed by a nucleoside or deoxynucleoside kinase. Kinases capable of catalyzing the phosphorylation of inosine or guanosine have been described in animal tissues,[63] and labeled inosine is incorporated into adenine and guanine nucleotides in liver of both normal and HPRT-deficient subjects.[64] These kinases appear to be absent in human fibroblasts.[65] In contrast, deoxyguanosine and deoxyinosine are readily converted to their respective monophosphates in a reaction that appears to be catalyzed by deoxycytidine kinase.[66] Adenosine kinase is an active enzyme, widely distributed in mammalian tissues, that is capable of catalyzing the phosphorylation of both adenosine and deoxyadenosine.[67,68] Adenosine kinase is inhibited by AMP and ADP, both of which are products of the reaction. Inhibition constants are of the order of the physiologic concentrations of each and may thus indicate a regulatory role for the adenine nucleotides.[69] The phosphorylation of deoxyadenosine may also be catalyzed by kinases other than adenosine kinase.[70-74]

Studies in subjects who lack activity of HPRT, and of their cells in culture, indicate that HPRT is normally responsible for a much more extensive recycling of purine bases into nucleotide pools than was initially appreciated. By contrast, recycling of hypoxanthine and guanine via the nucleoside phosphorylase-nucleoside kinase route is not very active. While this two-step pathway does not appear to be important in the normal salvage of purine nucleosides or bases, salvage of deoxynucleosides by the appropriate kinase appears to occur in patients lacking adenosine deaminase[75,76] or purine nucleoside phosphorylase.[77]

Nucleic Acid Catabolism. Enzymatic hydrolysis of polynucleotide chains of nucleic acid occurs through the action of various nucleases.[78] The major products released by ribonuclease a and b and by deoxyribonuclease I and II are oligonucleotides. The oligonucleotides are further cleaved by phosphodiesterases to yield 5'- and 3'-mononucleotides.

The mononucleotides are split by group-specific 5'-nucleotidases,[79] as well as by nonspecific phosphatases,[80] to yield the corresponding purine or pyrimidine nucleoside and orthophosphate. At least one form of 5'-nucleotidase is localized in the external surface of the plasma membrane (ecto-5'-nucleotidase). This enzyme is selectively present on the surface of B lymphocytes. In diseases associated with low levels of B lymphocytes (e.g., hypogammaglobulenemia) it appears to be deficient when mixed lymphocyte populations are studied.[81,82] Ecto-5'-nucleotidase appears to have little role in the regulation of intracellular nucleotide metabolism.[83] The purine nucleoside or deoxynucleoside is then split by purine nucleoside phosphorylase to yield a free purine base and ribose 1-phosphate or deoxyribose 1-phosphate as described above.

$$\text{Purine(deoxy)mononucleotide} \longrightarrow$$
$$\text{purine(deoxy)nucleoside} + P_i \qquad (19)$$

$$\text{Purine(deoxy)nucleoside} + P_i \longrightarrow$$
$$\text{purine base} + \text{(deoxy)ribose 1-phosphate} \qquad (20)$$

In addition to these general reactions, adenylic acid and adenosine are acted upon by specific deaminating enzymes. Adenylic acid is converted to inosinic acid by adenylic acid deaminase (Fig. 21-8)[84] and adenosine or deoxyadenosine to inosine or deoxyinosine by adenosine deaminase (Reaction 5, Fig. 21-8).[85] Guanylic acid may be deaminated to inosinic acid in bacteria. These various reactions and their controls may serve to provide the cell with the proper balance of adenyl and guanyl ribonucleotides, and also allow for replenishment of one from the other when necessary.

Formation of Uric Acid. The free purine bases that result from nucleoside cleavage are adenine, guanine, hypoxanthine, and xanthine. Since purine nucleoside phosphorylase acts most readily on inosine and guanosine,[59] the major bases generated are very likely hypoxanthine and guanine. Guanine is deaminated to xanthine by guanase (Fig. 21-8). Hypoxanthine is oxidized to xanthine by xanthine oxidase and then further oxidized to uric acid by the same enzyme (Reaction 8, Fig. 21-8).[86] Thus, whereas adenine, hypoxanthine, and guanine arise exclusively by cleavage of the corresponding nucleoside, xanthine potentially has three direct precursors—namely, xanthosine (or deoxyxanthosine), hypoxanthine, and guanine.

In man, xanthine oxidase is found in high activity only in liver and small intestinal mucosa.[87,88] Because of this restricted distribution of xanthine oxidase, uric acid synthesis appears largely to be a hepatic process in man. Presumably purine degradation products of other tissues are transported to the liver for further oxidation. Plasma contains small quantities of xanthine and hypoxanthine, together amounting to about 0.1 to 0.3 mg per 100 ml,[89,90] but no other uric acid precursors have been detected in normal plasma in significant quantity, with the possible exception of IMP following anoxic muscle injury.[91]

REGULATION OF
PURINE METABOLISM

Nucleotide Synthesis de Novo. Data obtained in bacterial,[92] avian,[93,94] and mammalian[95-98] systems indicate that adenylic acid (AMP) and guanylic acid (GMP) inhibit amidophosphoribosyltransferase (Reaction 1, Fig. 21-8), the initial and rate-limiting step of de novo purine biosynthesis, by interacting at separate sites on the enzyme termed the 6-amino and 6-hydroxy sites, respectively. Inhibition of the human enzyme by purine nucleotides is competitive with respect to PP-ribose-P, and the kinetics of the reaction shift from a hyperbolic to a sigmoidal function when PP-ribose-P is the variable substrate. Adenylic acid and guanylic acid are also inhibitors of formylglycinamide ribonucleotide (FGAR) amidotransferase, although the importance of this feedback site to the control of the rate of purine synthesis de novo is not established.[99]

A regulatory role of PP-ribose-P was suggested by several observations in human cell culture as well as in man in vivo.[100-103] Under normal conditions depletion of PP-ribose-P in vitro and in vivo decreases the rate of purine biosynthesis de novo.[100-103] Elevation of PP-ribose-P by several different mechanisms is associated with an increased rate of purine biosynthesis de novo.[101,104,105] In addition, when PP-ribose-P concentrations are initially elevated and then reduced to levels that are still supranormal, there is no inhibitory effect on purine biosynthesis de novo.[100] Finally, the normal intracellular concentration of PP-ribose-P is considerably less than the Michaelis constant established for amidophosphoribosyltransferase in lower organisms[92,106-108] or in mammalian cells.

The mechanism by which PP-ribose-P and purine ribonucleotides interact to regulate the activity of amidophosphoribosyltransferase was provided by direct study of the enzyme from a human source, and, in subsequent studies, from Chinese hamster fibroblasts and mouse liver.[109,110] Two forms of human amidophosphoribosyltransferase are apparent following gel filtration; the small form has a molecular weight of about 133,000, and the large form has a molecular weight of

about 270,000.[98] The larger species appears to be catalytically inactive, while the smaller species appears to be catalytically active. Purine ribonucleotides shift the active smaller species to the inactive larger molecular species: PP-ribose-P converts the large inactive species back to the small active species (Fig. 21-9). Direct in vivo conformation of this model has now been obtained in mouse liver.[110]

Regulation of Purine Ribonucleotide Interconversions. The first branch point in the pathway leading to the synthesis de novo of adenylic acid and guanylic acid occurs with the synthesis of inosinic acid (Fig. 21-8). In bacterial systems each nucleotide appears to regulate its own de novo formation by inhibiting the appropriate nucleotide interconversion; guanylic acid inhibits inosinic acid dehydrogenase that catalyzes the formation of xanthylic acid (XMP) from inosinic acid,[47,111] adenylic acid inhibits the formation of adenylosuccinic acid (AMP-S) from inosinic acid that is catalyzed by adenylosuccinic acid synthetase.[42] An analysis, however, of the regulation of adenylosuccinic acid synthetase[44] and inosinic acid dehydrogenase[112] from a human source suggests that the utilization of inosinic acid by each of the alternative pathways may be governed by the intracellular concentration of GTP. GTP is a substrate of adenylosuccinate synthetase with a K_m ranging from 31 to $72\mu M$[44] and an inhibitor of inosinic acid dehydrogenase.[112] While those observations cannot be applied directly to the setting in vivo, they suggest that as inosinic acid is formed, it is utilized for the synthesis of XMP, guanylic acid (GMP), GDP, and GTP. As GTP reaches a critical concentration in the cell, probably in the micromolar range, it may then increase the activity of AMP-S synthetase, allowing inosinic acid to be effectively utilized in the synthesis of adenylic acid. As GTP reaches an even higher level, not only can it promote the flux of inosinic acid in the direction of adenylic acid, but it can then function as a direct inhibitor of the conversion of inosinic acid to XMP and thus guanylic acid. Indirect evidence in support of this mode of regulation derives from studies with cultured murine lymphoma cells partially deficient in adenylosuccinic acid synthetase. AMP synthesis is maintained at the expense of elevated GTP and IMP.[113]

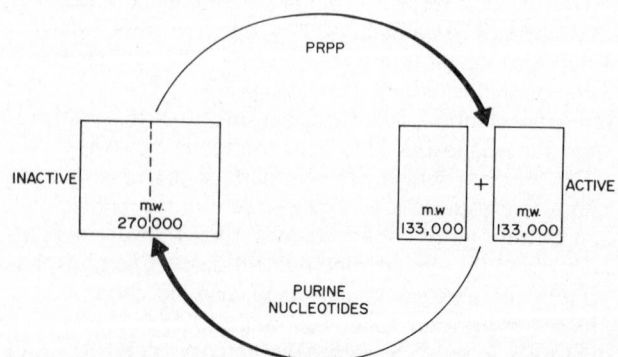

Figure 21-9 Model of interconversion of small (active) and large (inactive) forms of amidophosphoribosyltransferase. (From Kelley, W.N., et al.: Arthritis Rheum. 18:673, 1975.)

Ribonucleotide Cleavage. In circumstances in which accelerated purine biosynthesis de novo results in production of a surfeit of inosinic acid, there is a rapid conversion of the excess ribonucleotide to uric acid. The controls that lead to this result rather than to continual expansion of pools of adenyl and guanyl nucleotides, are not well characterized, but may depend on tight regulation of nucleotide biosynthetic pathways plus improved competition of 5'-nucleotidase for inosinic acid as its concentration is raised.

A comparison of the K_m values of cytoplasmic 5'-nucleotidases with reactions of inosinic acid leading to synthesis of adenylic acid or guanylic acid suggest that increasing concentrations of inosinic acid will saturate adenylosuccinic acid synthetase and inosinic acid dehydrogenase first and then activate the 5'-nucleotidase reaction. The latter will lead to hydrolysis of inosinic acid to inosine, which can then be cleaved by phosphorolysis to form hypoxanthine, followed by oxidation to xanthine and uric acid. Adenylic acid and guanylic acid may be relatively protected from this fate by their higher K_m values and slower rates of hydrolysis in the 5'-nucleotidase reaction and by their conversions to triphosphates, which are poor 5'-nucleotidase substrates.[114,115,116]

Purine Salvage. As described earlier, the purine phosphoribosyltransferases are inhibited by the nucleoside monophosphate products of each reaction. Whether such product inhibition is of any physiologic significance in the control of these pathways remains uncertain.

ORIGIN OF URIC ACID IN MAN

The Exogenous Contribution. Unless an individual is in a total fast or ingesting a highly artificial purine-free diet, there is a significant exogenous contribution to the body load and urinary excretion of uric acid. The magnitude of this contribution depends on both the amount and type of purine in the diet, but it is often considerable. For example, when Griebsch and Zollner[117] placed healthy young males on an isocaloric purine-free formula diet, serum urate values declined in 10 days from about 4.9 mg per 100 ml to 3.1 ± 0.4 mg per 100 ml, and urinary excretion of uric acid declined from 500 to 600 mg per day to 336 ± 39 mg per day. Roughly 50 percent of the RNA purines and 25 percent of DNA purines are absorbed and excreted in the urine as uric acid.[118] The difference between amounts of purine administered and excreted may be due to partial hydrolysis, incomplete absorption, enteric decomposition, suppression of purine synthesis de novo, or a combination of some or all of these factors.[117]

Endogenous Formation of Uric Acid. Urinary uric acid excretion declines to constant low values after 5 to 7 days of dietary purine elimination or severe restriction. Mean values then range from 336 ± 39 to 426 ± 81 mg per 24 hours. These values reflect the continued synthesis and turnover of endogenous purines. However, the urinary uric acid excretion accounts for only a part of the daily disposition of uric acid. Another part is disposed of by extrarenal routes. Thus, the true rate of endogenous purine turnover cannot be accurately determined by measurement of urinary uric acid excretion but requires the use of isotope dilution techniques in subjects in whom the exogenous contribution has been reduced to a minimum by severe dietary purine restriction.

EXTRARENAL DISPOSITION OF URIC ACID

Recovery Studies. Urinary recoveries of intravenously administered uric acid are incomplete in normal subjects. Over 50 years ago Folin and colleagues[119] and Koehler[120] reported urinary recoveries of unlabeled uric acid that ranged from 28 to 91 percent, and averaged about 50 percent. More recently recoveries of infused ^{15}N-uric acid or 2-^{14}C-uric acid ranging from 55 to 95 percent have been reported.[121-124] The average of 14 studies with ^{15}N-uric acid was 75.6 percent. These studies suggested extrarenal disposal of 25 to 50 percent of infused uric acid.

Studies of the turnover of uric acid in normal man have uniformly shown that the quantity of uric acid turning over each day exceeds the quantity appearing in urine. Surplus amounts have ranged from 100 to 365 mg per day.[125-127] Thus, these studies also indicate that a significant quantity of uric acid is disposed of by routes other than the kidney. In fact, in comparative studies the fraction of the turnover appearing in urine is essentially the same as the fraction of injected isotopic uric acid recovered in urine.[57,128,129]

Sorensen[126] estimated that 100 mg or more of uric acid enters the alimentary tract in saliva, gastric juice, and bile. An equal quantity may enter in pancreatic and intestinal juices. These quantities of uric acid are larger than once thought[130,131] and are sufficient to account for the degradation of one third of the uric acid normally turned over each day.

The total amount of uricolysis that can be attributed to human tissues is unknown but has been estimated to be less than 2 percent of the turnover of the uric acid pool.[132] Thus, for all practical purposes, extrarenal disposal of uric acid is synonymous with intestinal uricolysis.

RENAL HANDLING OF URIC ACID IN NORMAL MAN

Initially it was thought that renal excretion of uric acid in man occurred by glomerular filtration followed by extensive, though incomplete, tubular reabsorption.[133] Next, a three-component system was proposed on the basis of evidence for tubular secretion of uric acid in animals and man.[134] More recently several investigators have proposed a four-component model: of glomerular filtration, early proximal tubular reabsorption, tubular secretion, and finally postsecretory tubular reabsorption. Within the vertebrate phylum there is an impressive variety of patterns for the renal disposition of uric acid. In some animals net secretion of urate is the rule—e.g., birds,[135] reptiles,[136,137] guinea pigs,[138] Dalmatian coach hounds,[139] and certain species of monkeys.[140] In others net reabsorption is the rule—e.g., rats,[141,142] non-Dalmatian dogs,[139] cats,[138] several species of New World monkeys,[140] the great apes,[140] and man.[133] In many of these species there is evidence for bidirectional transport. In some species in which net secretion occurs, clearance ratios (i.e., C_{urate}/C_{inulin}) fall below 1.0 in the presence of inhibitors of urate secretion.[138,143,144] In almost all animals exhibiting net reabsorption, there is evidence that secretion of urate also occurs but is normally masked by extensive reabsorption.[144-152]

The species most nearly comparable to man in the renal handling of urate is the chimpanzee, and next the *Cebus* monkey. The ratio, C_{urate}/GFR, is about 0.07 to 0.11 in these species,[145,146,153] as in man. Both species respond appropriately to substances that are uricosuric in man.[153-156] The discussion to follow will emphasize studies performed in man or in these lower primates.

Glomerular Filtration of Uric Acid. Glomerular ultrafiltration of uric acid was first conclusively demonstrated by micropuncture studies of Bowman's space in the snake and frog in which urate concentrations in the glomerular fluid were the same as in plasma.[157] Although comparable studies have not been performed with a mammalian glomerulus, micropuncture of the earliest portion of the proximal tubule of the rat also discloses urate concentrations of tubular fluid equal to those of plasma.[147] It is reasonable to assume that ultrafiltration of uric acid also occurs in man.

Whether all urate in plasma is freely filterable at the glomerulus is uncertain. While some urate may be bound to plasma protein, this fraction is currently thought to be small, perhaps less than 5 percent. If the fraction is larger, as some studies suggest, binding could result in the incomplete filtration of urate at the glomerulus.

Reabsorption of Uric Acid. Comparisons of renal clearance of uric acid with those of inulin or creatinine disclose a mean ratio of about 0.07 to 0.10 in normal human subjects. If complete glomerular ultrafiltration of plasma urate is assumed, such clearance ratios indicate tubular reabsorption of at least 90 to 93 percent of filtered urate.

Almost all studies of uric acid reabsorption indicate that the process takes place in the proximal tubule. Most localizations have been made with the stop-flow technique in lower animals. Results of free-flow micropuncture studies in *Cebus albifrons* are essentially in accord with results of stopflow experiments in specifying that most urate reabsorption occurs in the proximal tubule.[158] However, distal tubular fluid contains a greater fraction of filtered urate than does final urine. This finding, confirmed in additional animals,[159] may signify reabsorption of a small fraction of filtered or secreted urate in collecting ducts. Thus, although net urate reabsorption occurs largely in proximal tubules in all animals in which the process has been localized (with the exception of the rat, in which it may take place in the loop of Henle),

the possibility exists of reabsorption in more distal segments, at least in certain animals.

Available evidence suggests that urate reabsorption occurs by a mechanism of *active transport.* In lower animals ouabain and metabolic poisons inhibit urate reabsorption.[152,160] In rats, the net urate reabsorption in the proximal tubule is an active transport process, although passive movement of urate into and out of the proximal tubule has been demonstrated.[161] This active transport mechanism has been shown to have saturable kinetics, indicating that urate reabsorption in the rat proximal tubule is probably carrier mediated.[162] By way of contrast, urate reabsorption in the rabbit proximal tubule has been shown to consist of both passive and facilitated mechanisms. In these studies, it appeared that the net absorptive flux in the rabbit proximal tubule was passive.[163] In nonhuman primates and in man the concentration of uric acid in urine may approach one tenth the concentration in plasma during diuresis and inhibition of urate secretion with pyrazinoate.[164] In free-flowing micropuncture samples in the chimpanzee and monkey, the concentrations of urate average 0.6 of the concentrations in plasma, and in individual samples may be as low as 0.2. Thus, urate reabsorption may occur against a concentration gradient. According to Weiner and Fanelli[159] the transepithelial potential difference in the proximal tubule is too small to account for this phenomenon by passive forces.

There is a close link between reabsorption of sodium and reabsorption of a number of other components of the glomerular filtrate such as glucose,[165] phosphate,[166] calcium,[167] and bicarbonate,[168] and also uric acid.[167,169,170] In conditions associated with an increase in proximal reabsorption of sodium the clearance of uric acid is reduced (Table 21-1); in conditions leading to decreased proximal reabsorption of sodium the clearance of uric acid is increased (Table 21-2). In addition, sodium reabsorption per nephron is decreased[171] and uric acid excretion per nephron is increased[172] in chronic renal failure in man.

The responses of proximal sodium reabsorption to changes in extracellular fluid volume or filtration fraction have been attributed to changes of hydrostatic and effective oncotic pressure ("physical factors") in the peritubular capillaries.[173] Tubular reabsorption of many solutes in addition to sodium is affected.[167] Uric acid is among the solutes that respond to changes in "physical factors."[170]

The pH of the fluid in the proximal tubule is approximately the same as that of plasma.[174] Since the pK_{a1} of uric acid is 5.75, over 98 percent of this compound will be in the form of the monovalent urate ion in the proximal tubule. Excretion of uric acid is largely independent of changes of pH of urine,[175] but acidification is a distal tubular function, and would not be expected to affect proximal processes. In highly acidified distal tubular fluid, uric acid will be minimally ionized. One might anticipate that uric acid would then undergo reabsorption by nonionic diffusion. If so, the contribution to urate reabsorption is too small to be readily

Table 21-1. Conditions Associated with Hyperuricemia or Reduced Renal Uric Acid Clearance*

Condition	Δ Serum Urate	Δ Uric Acid Clearance	Δ Extracellular Fluid Volume	Δ Filtration Fraction	Predicted Δ Proximal Tubular Sodium Reabsorption†
Salt restriction	↑	↓	↓	—	↑
Diuretic therapy without salt replacement	↑	↓	↓	—	↑
Diabetes insipidus	↑	↓	↓	↑	↑
Hypertension	↑	↓	—	↑	↑
Angiotensin infusion (without increased lactate or ketones)	—	↓	—	↑	↑
Norepinephrine (without increased lactate or ketones)	—	↓	—	↑	↑

*From Holmes, E. W., et al.: Kidney Int. 2:115, 1972. Reproduced with permission.
†Proximal tubular sodium reabsorption was not evaluated directly in the reported studies; the changes listed represent a prediction from the observed changes in extracellular fluid volume and filtration fraction.

detected, for unlike other weak organic acids, the overall process of uric acid reabsorption does not follow principles of nonionic diffusion.[159]

Secretion of Uric Acid. The first evidence for uric acid secretion in man was published in 1950, when Praetorius and Kirk[176] reported the case of a young man with a plasma urate concentration of less than 0.6 mg per 100 ml, and a urate/inulin clearance ratio of 1.46. Subsequently, Gutman and coworkers[148] achieved urate/inulin clearance ratios as high as 1.23 in normal subjects following urate loading, mannitol diuresis, and large doses of probenecid. Each of these studies indicated net tubular secretion of urate in man under these special conditions. The biphasic effects of salicylate upon uric acid excretion were interpreted as representing inhibition of urate secretion with urate retention at low salicylate doses plus inhibition of urate reabsorption with urate diuresis at higher salicylate doses.[177] More recently Diamond and colleagues[178] have suggested that this apparent paradoxical effect of salicylate on uric acid excretion is due to inhibition of reabsorption by salicylate itself with inhibition of secretion due to a metabolite, salicylurate. Irrespective of the mechanism, bidirectional transport of uric acid is apparent.

The site within the nephron of man where uric acid secretion occurs is not definitely established. In the only study of this process in man, the proximal nephron transported uric acid from plasma to tubular fluid but the distal nephron was unable to do so.[179]

In animals in which net secretion occurs, urate moves into the proximal lumen against an electrical potential difference. Thus, the process qualifies as an active transport mechanism. In animals in which net movement of urate is reabsorptive, secretory flux of urate normally proceeds in the direction of a favorable concentration gradient. However, the process can be inhibited by certain chemicals[151,152,180,181] and possesses specificity; it cannot therefore represent simple diffusion. Weiner and Fanelli[159] have evidence that the mechanism is capable of transport against a gradient and is therefore active. In the chimpanzee,[182] the mercurial diuretic mersalyl is sufficiently uricosuric to unmask net secretion of urate. These results suggest a model involving two oppositely oriented active transport systems in the proximal tubule.

Although a number of authors have expressed the view that urate is secreted by the same mechanism responsible for the secretion of other organic anions, e.g., p-aminohippurate (PAH),[151,183] there is reason to consider an alternative hypothesis—namely, that urate and PAH are secreted by different transport systems. Two types of observation support this concept. In the reptile, transport of PAH and urate is not strictly coextensive along the nephron. In the chimpanzee[164,165] and man,[184] pyrazinoate reduces urate excretion to very low levels at concentrations that do not influence clearance or T_m of PAH.

A number of organic acids will inhibit uric acid excretion in animals and man. These include lactate,[185,186]

Table 21-2. Conditions Associated with Reduction in Serum Urate Levels*

Condition	Δ Serum Urate	Δ Uric Acid Clearance	Δ Extracellular Fluid Volume	Δ Filtration Fraction	Predicted Δ Proximal Tubular Sodium Reabsorption
Salt	↓	↑	↑	—	↓
Diuretic therapy with salt replacement	↓	↑	↑	—	↓
Inappropriate secretion of ADH	↓	↑	↑	—	↓
Pregnancy (early)	↓	↑	↑	—	↓

*From Holmes, E. W., et al.: Kidney Int. 2:115, 1972. Reproduced with permission.

β-hydroxybutyrate,[187] acetoacetate,[187] and branched-chain keto acids.[188] These effects have been interpreted as representing inhibition of tubular secretion of urate,[177,189] for which there is evidence in micropuncture studies.[190]

Postsecretory Reabsorption. A number of observations have proved difficult to accommodate within the model of filtration, early proximal reabsorption, and later proximal secretion. In patients with Wilson's disease[191] or Hodgkin's disease,[192] and hypouricemia associated with raised renal urate clearance values, pyrazinamide suppresses the hyperuricosuria. In both chimpanzee[146] and man[134,193] the uricosuric response to probenecid is virtually abolished by pretreatment with pyrazinamide or pyrazinoate. Finally, the uricosuric responses to intravenous chlorothiazide[134] or volume expansion with hypertonic sodium chloride[194] are substantially diminished by pretreatment with pyrazinamide. If these effects were to be interpreted within the three-component model, one would need to conclude that the renal tubular dysfunctions of Wilson's and Hodgkin's diseases, and the administration of probenecid, chlorothiazide, and saline, resulted in enhanced tubular secretion of urate which was suppressible by pyrazinamide.

In 1973, Steele and Boner,[193] Steele,[195] and Diamond and Paolino[196] proposed a more tenable model to account for these observations, in which extensive postsecretory reabsorption of urate was postulated. In this model the effects of pyrazinamide are explained in terms of reduced secretory delivery to the late reabsorptive sites. The location of the postsecretory reabsorptive process could be coextensive with the secretory mechanism, or separate and distal to it, or both. Fanelli and Weiner have attempted to demonstrate that the observations upon which this model is based are consistent with coextensive secretion and reabsorption.[197] The latter possibilities are supported in some animals by evidence for urate reabsorption beyond the proximal tubule, as cited above. A patient with renal urate wasting, presumably on the basis of a defect in postsecretory reabsorption, has now been described.[198] Additionally, in two kindreds with familial hyperuricemia due to diminished renal clearance of urate it was proposed that the defect was due to increased postsecretory reabsorption.[199] Thus postsecretory reabsorption may be more important than previously recognized.

Quantitative Estimates of Reabsorption and Secretion. The existence of bidirectional uric acid transport in man is certain from the evidence cited above. However, the relative contributions of tubular reabsorption and tubular secretion have been difficult to ascertain. In man mean urate/inulin (or creatinine) ratios of 1.23 to 1.46 have been observed in unusual situations[148,176] In the chimpanzee a ratio of 1.78 was observed following administration of mersalyl.[159] These figures provide minimal estimates of unidirectional urate secretion, for there is no evidence in any of these studies that urate reabsorption was reduced to zero or that secretion was unimpaired by the drugs or procedures employed. The data

suggest that secretion may be of the same order of magnitude as filtration, and therefore, that reabsorption may be very much greater than might be deduced from control clearance periods.

Additional Factors Controlling Renal Clearance of Uric Acid in Normal Subjects. Urine Flow. In 1940, Brochner-Mortensen[200] observed that uric acid excretion and clearance were increased at high rates of urine flow in man. He reported an augmentation limit of 2 ml per minute, above which further increases of rates of urine flow did not affect uric acid clearance. Others have reported that uric acid excretion in dogs is also dependent on the rate of urine flow.[144,150]

More recently, Diamond and colleagues[201] found that uric acid excretion increased from 290 to 410 μg per minute as urine flow increased from 2.7 to 6.4 ml per minute in response to oral and intravenous fluid loading in man. The effects of flow may be difficult to distinguish from those of osmotic diuresis.[202] Nevertheless, both the basal uric acid excretion and the increment accompanying diuresis were greatly reduced by pyrazinamide. Diamond and Meisel[203] suggest that the uricosuria of water diuresis can be attributed to diminished postsecretory reabsorption of urate, perhaps in the collecting duct.

Estrogens. The serum urate concentration is relatively low in children; increases in males and to a lesser extent also in females at puberty; and in females increases again at the menopause. Changes in renal urate clearance are at least partly responsible. Wolfson and colleagues[204] and Scott and Pollard[205] observed that the mean clearance of uric acid was 2.3 and 1.2 ml per minute higher in females than in males. Nicholls and associates[206] found that exogenous estrogens produced a significant increase in mean C^{urate} values from 6.3 to 9.1 ml per minute in 22 transsexual males.

Surgery. Snaith and Scott[207] observed an increase in the excretion of uric acid, and in the urinary uric acid-to-creatinine ratio, in 10 patients undergoing abdominal surgery. Little or no change in serum urate concentration occurred. Factors such as anesthetics, increased endogenous steroids, intravenous fluids, intestinal manipulation, and vagotomy were suggested as possibly affecting urate clearance. The only patient not exhibiting a postoperative increase in uric acid excretion was one of two who did not have a vagotomy.

Autonomic Nervous System. In 1937, Grabfield[208] noted that the uricosuric effect of cincophen depended on an intact renal nerve supply in the dog. Denervation increased the renal clearance of uric acid to values attained with cincophen in the intact dog. Cincophen had no additional uricosuric effect in the denervated dog. The effects of cincophen were blocked by ergotamine but not by atropine. Excretion of allantoin, which is cleared by glomerular filtration without subsequent tubular reabsorption, was unchanged by denervation.

Postlethwaite and colleagues[209] noted that several anticholinergic agents increased renal clearance of uric acid in some subjects. One interpretation is that the parasympathetic nervous system plays a role in controlling the renal excretion of uric acid, perhaps through an effect on peritubular blood flow.

Physical Properties of Uric Acid

Ionization and Salt Formation. The weakly acidic nature of uric acid is due to ionization of hydrogen atoms at position 9 ($pK_a = 5.75$) and position 3 ($pK_a = 10.3$).[210] The hydrogen atoms at positions 1 and 7 do not ionize significantly. The ionized forms of uric acid readily form salts such as mono- and disodium or potassium urates. In extracellular fluids in which sodium is the principal cation, about 98 percent of uric acid is in the form of the monosodium salt at pH 7.4. When the solubility limits of body fluids are exceeded, the crystals that occur in the synovial fluid or the tophi of gouty patients are composed of monosodium urate monohydrate.

Solubility in Water. Monosodium urate is soluble in water to the extent of 120 mg per 100 ml, compared with the much more limited solubility of uric acid in water of only 6.5 mg per 100 ml.[210] The solubility product of monosodium urate is 4.9×10^{-5}. Based on this value, aqueous solutions having the sodium content of serum, 0.13 M, are saturated with urate at 6.4 mg per 100 ml at 37° C.[210] Allen and colleagues[211] and Loeb[212] have found that urate solubility in solutions of 140 mEq per liter sodium content is markedly temperature dependent, with a two-fold drop in solubility between 37 and 25° C (Table 21-3). Wilcox and colleagues[213] have carefully reinvestigated the solubility of uric acid and monosodium urate, and have found that both are dependent on pH; with increasing pH uric acid is more soluble, whereas monosodium urate is less. The solubility of monosodium urate is dependent on sodium concentration and ionic strength as well. No stoichiometric relationship between urate and sodium (or potassium) exists. Binding of monovalent cations is a complex function of crystal shape, ion concentration, time, pH, and ion competition.[214]

Solubility in Plasma. The solubility of urate in plasma is somewhat greater than the saturation value in aqueous solutions of 0.13 M sodium. Actual determinations of solubility of monosodium urate in human plasma (or serum) indicate that saturation occurs at concentrations of about 7 mg per 100 ml.[215,216] Considerably higher concentrations of monosodium urate in plasma can be achieved in supersaturated solutions. Concentrations approaching 400 mg per 100 ml can be obtained by dissolving free uric acid in serum at 38° C.[215] These solutions are unstable, and monosodium urate readily precipitates out. At somewhat lower concentrations of 100 to 200 mg per 100 ml the solution may remain in a stable supersaturated state for longer periods of time, and no crystallization may occur for 24 hours or more, or until a seed crystal of monosodium urate is added. Stable supersaturated solutions of monosodium urate ranging

up to 40 to 90 mg per 100 ml have been observed in patients with leukemia or lymphoma following aggressive therapy with cytotoxic drugs in the absence of allopurinol therapy.[217,218] The factors responsible for enhanced urate solubility in such patients are not clear, and may include both the natural tendency for urate to form stable supersaturated solutions and an increase in plasma of substances capable of solubilizing urate.[219] However, even at these remarkable plasma concentrations, all urate is digestible by uricase.[217]

The physicochemical state of urate in plasma has been a controversial subject for decades. Some early investigators claimed substantial binding of urate to nondiffusible elements of plasma,[220] whereas others concluded that all urate was in true solution because it was readily ultrafilterable[221] and dialyzable.[222] Even studies of urate localization following filter paper electrophoresis of serum yielded conflicting data in different laboratories.[223] In one laboratory a careful study of urate binding[225] disclosed no more than 4 to 5 percent of urate bound to plasma protein, a figure agreeing with results of earlier studies in vitro using equilibrium dialysis,[222] as well as with more recent studies in vivo.[226] These studies confirm that the binding of uric acid to plasma proteins at 37° C is small and probably of little physiological significance.

Solubility in Urine. As the urine is acidified along the renal tubule a portion of urinary urate is converted to uric acid. The solubility of uric acid in aqueous solutions is substantially less than that of urate. At pH 5 urine is saturated with uric acid at 15 mg per 100 ml, whereas at pH 7 urine will accommodate 158 to 200 mg per 100 ml in solution.[210,216] The limited solubility of uric acid in urine of pH 5 is of particular significance in patients with gout, many of whom display a tendency toward excretion of unusually acidic urine.

At any pH value human urine will dissolve more urate than can be carried in water. The solubilizing effects of urine have been attributed to urea,[227] proteins, and a mucopolysaccharide that resembles the Tamm-Horsfall mucopolysaccharide.[228,229] It was initially anticipated

Table 21-3. Solubility of Urate Ion (U−) as a Function of Temperature in the Presence of 140 mM Na+ *

Temperature (°C)	Maximal Equilibrium Concentration of U− in the Presence of 140 mM Na+ (mg/100 ml)
37	6.8
35	6.0
30	4.5
25	3.3
20	2.5
15	1.8
10	1.2

*From Loeb, J. N.: Arthritis Rheum. 8:1123, 1965. Reproduced by permission.

that habitual uric acid stone formers would show deficits of this mucopolysaccharide, but this could not be demonstrated.[229]

Crystalline Forms. Monosodium urate occurs as a monohydrate and forms crystals that are needle- or bar-shaped in a monoclinic or triclinic system. When rapidly crystallized from pure solutions, the crystals are very fine and appear amorphous.

Free uric acid crystallizes from pure solutions in an orthorhombic system, forming rhombic plates. Crystals formed in urine incorporate pigments and exist in a variety of crystalline forms. Tissue deposits are composed of monosodium urate monohydrate, and urinary stones largely of uric acid.[230,231] Both urate and uric acid crystals show strong negative birefringence when viewed under polarized light. With the use of a red compensator, urate cyrstals are yellow when oriented in parallel with the axis of polarization, and blue when perpendicular (see Chapter 38). These features permit ready identification of urate cyrstals in synovial fluid, leukocytes, or tissue deposits, and thus constitute an important diagnostic aid.[232,233]

The clinical features of gout and related disorders are reviewed in Chapter 86.

References

1. Scheele, K.W.: Examen chemicum calculi urinarii. Opuscula 2:73, 1776.
2. Wollaston, W.H.: On gouty and urinary concretions. Philos. Trans. R. Soc. Lond. 87:386, 1797.
3. Garrod, A.B.: Observations on certain pathological conditions of the blood and urine in gout, rheumatism and Bright's disease. Trans. M-Chir. Soc. Edinburgh 31:83, 1848.
4. Freudweiler, M.: Experimentelle Untersuchungen über das Wesen der Gichtknoten. Deutsch. Arch. Klin. Med. 63:266, 1899.
5. Shemin, D., and Rittenberg, D.: On the utilization of glycine for uric acid synthesis in man. J. Biol. Chem. 167:875, 1947.
6. Buchanan, J.M., Sonne, J.C., and Delluva, A.M.: Biologic precursors of uric acid. II. The role of lactate, glycine, and carbon dioxide as precursors of the carbon chain and nitrogen atom 7 of uric acid. J. Biol. Chem. 173:81, 1948.
7. Karlson, J.L., and Barker, H.A.: Biosynthesis of uric acid labeled with radioactive carbon. J. Biol. Chem. 177:597, 1949.
8. Sonne, J.C., Buchanan, J.M., and Delluva, A.M.: Biological precursors of uric acid. I. The role of lactate, acetate and formate in synthesis of the ureido groups of uric acid. J. Biol. Chem. 173:69, 1948.
9. Heinrich, M.R., and Wilson, D.W.: Biosynthesis of nucleic acid components studied with C[14]. I. Purines and pyrimidines in the rat. J. Biol. Chem. 186:447, 1950.
10. Sonn, J.C., Lin, I., and Buchanan, J.M.: Biosynthesis of the purines. IX. Precursors of the nitrogen atoms of the purine ring. J. Biol. Chem. 220:369, 1956.
11. Levenberg, B., Hartman, S.C., and Buchanan, J.M.: Biosynthesis of the purines. X. Further studies in vitro on the metabolic origin of nitrogen atoms 1 and 3 of the purine ring. J. Biol. Chem. 220:379, 1956.
12. Goldthwait, D.A., Peabody, R.A., and Greenberg, G.R.: On the mechanism of synthesis of glycinamide ribotide and its formyl derivative. J. Biol. Chem. 221:569, 1956.
13. Hartman, S.C., and Buchanan, J.M.: Biosynthesis of the purines. XXI. 5-phosphoribosylpyrophosphate-amidotransferase. J. Biol. Chem. 233: 451, 1958.
14. Flaks, J.G., Erwin, M.J., and Buchanan, J.M.: Biosynthesis of the purines. XVI. The synthesis of adenosine 5'-phosphate and 5'-amino-4-imidazolecarboxamide ribotide by a nucleotide pyrophosphorylase. J. Biol. Chem. 228:201, 1957.
15. Lukens, L.N., and Herrington, K.A.: Enzymic synthesis and properties of 6-mercaptopurine ribotide. Biochim. Biophys. Acta 24:432, 1957.
16. Kornberg, A., Lieberman, I., and Simms, E.S.: Enzymatic synthesis and properties of 5-phosphoribosylpyrophosphate. J. Biol. Chem. 215:389, 1955.
17. Remy, C.N., Remy, W.T., and Buchanan, J.M.: Biosynthesis of the purines. VIII. Enzymatic synthesis and utilization of 5-phosphoribosyl-prophosphate. J. Biol. Chem. 217:855, 1955.
18. Switzer, R.L.: Regulation and mechanism of phosphoribosylpyrophosphate synthetase. I. Purification and properties of the enzyme from *Salmonella typhimurium*. J. Biol. Chem. 244:2854, 1959.
19. Fox, I.H., and Kelley, W.N.: Human phosphoribosylpyrophosphate synthetase: Kinetic mechanism and endproduct inhibition. J. Biol. Chem. 247:2126, 1972.
20. Goldthwait, D.A.: 5-Phosphoribosylamine, a precursor of glycinamide ribotide. J. Biol. Chem. 222:1051, 1956.
21. Feldman, R.I., and Taylor, M.W.: Purine mutants of mammalian cell lines. II. Identification of a phosphoribosylpyrophosphate amidotransferase deficient mutant of Chinese hamster lung cells. Biochem. Genet. 13:227, 1975.
22. Holmes, E.W., King, G.L., Leyva, A., and Singer, S.C.: A purine auxotroph deficient in phosphoribosylpyrophosphate amidotransferase and phosphoribosylpyrophosphate amidotransferase activities with normal activity of ribose-5-phosphate aminotransferase, Proc. Natl. Acad. Sci. (Wash.) 73:2458, 1976.
23. Oates, D.C., and Patterson, D.: Biochemical genetics of Chinese hamster cell mutants with deviant pruine metabolism: Characterization of Chinese hamster call mutants defective in phosphoribosylpyrophosphate amidotransferase and phosphoribosylglycinamide sythetase and an examination of alternatives to the first step of purine biosynthesis. Somatic Cell Genet. 3:561, 1977.
24. McCarvus, E., Fahey, D., Sauer, D., and Rowe, P.B.: De novo purine synthesis in human lymphocytes: Partial co-purification of the enzymes and some properties of the pathway. J. Biol. Chem. 258:1983, 1983.
25. Harman, S.C., Levenberg, B., and Buchanan, J.M.: Biosynthesis of the purines. XI. Structure, enzymatic synthesis, and metabolism of glycinamide ribotide and (α-N-formyl) glycinamide ribotide. J. Biol. Chem. 221:1057. 1956.
26. Hartman, S.C., and Buchanan, J.M.: Biosynthesis of the purines. XXII. 2-Amino-N-ribosylacetamide-5'-phosphate kinosynthetase. J. Biol. Chem. 223:456, 1958.
27. Nierlich, D.P., and Magasanik, B.: Phosphoribosylglycinamide synthetase of *Aerobacter aerogenes*. J. Biol. Chem. 240:366, 1965.
28. Warren, L., and Buchanan, J.M.: Biosynthesis of the purines. XIX. 2-Amino-N-ribosylacetamide-5'-phosphate (glycinamide ribotide) transformylase. J. Biol. Chem. 229:613, 1957.
29. Warren, L., Flaks, J.G., and Buchanan, J.M.: Biosynthesis of the purines. XX. Integration of enzymatic transformylation reactions. J. Biol. Chem. 229:627, 1957.
30. Smith, G.K., Mueller, W.T., Slieker, L.J., et al.: Direct transfer of one-carbon units in the transformylations of de novo purine biosynthesis. Biochemistry 21:2870, 1982.
31. Mizobuchi, K., and Buchanan, J.M.: Biosynthesis of the purines: Purification and properties of formylglycinamide ribonucleotide amidotransferase from chicken liver. J. Biol. Chem. 243:4842, 1968.
32. Mizobuchi, K., and Buchanan, J.M.: Biosynthesis of the purines: Isolation and characterization of formylglycinamide ribonucleotide amidotransferase-glutamyl complex. J. Biol. Chem. 243:4853, 1968.
33. Mizobuchi, K., Kenyon, G.L., and Buchanan, J.M.: Binding of formylglclinamide ribonucleotide and adenosine triphosphate to formylglycinamide ribonucleotide amidotransferase. J. Biol. Chem. 243:4863, 1968.
34. Levenberg, B., and Buchanan, J.M.: Biosynthesis of the purines. XII. Structure enzymatic, synthesis, and metabolism of 5-aminoimidazole ribotide. J. Biol. Chem. 224:1005, 1957.
35. Lukens, L.N., and Buchanan, J.B.: Further intermediates in the biosynthesis of inosinic acid de novo. J. Am. Chem. Soc. 79:1511, 1957.
36. Flaks, J.G., Warren, L., and Buchanan, J.M.: Biosynthesis of the purines. XVII. Further studies of the inosinic acid transformylase system. J. Biol. Chem. 228:215, 1957.
37. Flaks, J.G., Erwin, M.J., and Buchanan, J.M.: Biosynthesis of the purines. XVII. 5-Amino-1-ribosyl-4-imidazole-carboxamide 5'-phosphate transformylase and inosinicase. J. Biol. Chem. 229:603, 1957.
38. Smith, G.K., Mueller, W.T., Wasserman, G.F., et al.: Characterization of the enzyme complex involving the folate-requiring enzymes of de novo purine biosynthesis. Biochemistry 19:4313, 1980.
39. Carter, C.E., and Cohen, C.H.: The preparation and properties of adenylosuccinase and adenylosuccinic acid. J. Biol. Chem. 222:17, 1956.
40. Joklik, W.K.: Adenine succinic acid and adenylosuccinic acid from mammalian liver: Isolation and identification. Biochem. J. 66:333, 1957.
41. Lieberman, I.: Enzymatic synthesis of adenosine 5'-phosphate from inosine 5'-phosphate. J. Biol. Chem. 223:327, 1956.
42. Wyngaarden, J.B., and Greenland, R.A.: The inhibition of succinoadenylate kinosynthetase of *Escherichia coli* by adenosine and guanosine 5'-monophosphates. J. Biol. Chem. 238:1054, 1963.
43. Murihead, K.M., and Bishop, S.H.: Purification of adenylosuccinate synthetase from rabbit skeletal muscle. J. Biol. Chem. 249:459, 1974.
44. Van Der Weyden, M., and Kelley, W.N.: Human adenylosuccinate synthetase. Partial purification kinetic and regulatory properties of the enzyme. J. Biol. Chem. 249:7282, 1974.
45. Magasanik, B., Moyed, H.S., and Gehring, L.B.: Enzymes essential for

the biosynthesis of nucleic acid guanine: Iinosine-5'-phosphate dehydrogenase of *Aerobacter aerogenes.* J. Biol. Chem. 226:339, 1957.

46. Lagerkvist, U.: Biosynthesis of guanosine 5'-phosphate. I. Xanthosine 5'-phosphate as an intermediate. J. Biol. Chem. 223:138, 1958.

47. Mager, J., and Magasanik, B.: Guanosine 5'-phosphate reductase and its role in the interconversion of purine nucleotides. J. Biol. Chem. 235:1474, 1960.

48. Lagerkvist, U.: Biosynthesis of guanosine 5'-phosphate. II. Amination of xanthosine 5'-phosphate by purified enzymes from pigeon liver. J. Biol. Chem. 223:143, 1958.

49. Abrams, R., and Bentley, M.: Biosynthesis of nucleic acid purines. III. Guanosine 5'-phosphate formation from xanthosine 5'-phosphate and L-glutamine. Arch. Biochem. 79:91, 1959.

50. Lieberman, I., Kornberg, A., and Simms, E.S.: Enzymatic synthesis of pyrimidine nucleotides: Orotidine-5'-phosphate and uridine-5'phosphate J. Biol. Chem. 215:403, 1955.

51. Preiss, J., and Handler, P.: Enzymatic synthesis of nicotinamide mononucleotide. J. Biol. Chem. 255:759, 1957.

52. Hori, M., and Henderson, J.F.: Kinetic studies of adenine phosphoribosyltransferase. J. Biol. Chem. 241:3304, 1966.

53. Henderson, J.F., Brox, L.W., Kelley, W.N., et al.: Kinetic studies of hypoxanthine-guanine phosphoribosyltransferase. J. Biol. Chem. 243:2514, 1968.

54. Kelley, W.N., Rosenbloom, F.M., Henderson, J.F., et al.: Xanthine phosphoribosyltransferase in man. Relationship of hypoxanthine-guanine phosphoribosyltransferase. Biochem. Biophys. Res. Commun. 28:340, 1967.

55. McCollister, R.J., Gilbert, W.R., Jr., Ashton, D.M. et al.: Pseudofeedback inhibition of purine synthesis by 6-mercaptopurine ribonucleotide and other purine analogues. J. Biol. Chem. 239:1560, 1964.

56. Krenitsky, T.A., Papaioannou, R., and Elion, G.B.: Human hypoxanthine phosphoribosyltransferase. J. Biol. Chem. 244:1263, 1969.

57. Kelley, W.N., Greene, M.L., Rosenbloom, F.M., et al.: Hypoxanthineguanine phosphoribosyltransferase deficiency in gout. Ann. Intern. Med. 70:155, 1969.

58. Henderson, J.K.: Kinetic properties of hypoxanthine-guanine and adenine phosphoribosyltransferases. Fed. Proc. 27:1053, 1968.

59. Friedkin, N., and Kalckar, H.: Nucleoside phosphorylases. *In* Boyer, P.D., Lardy, H., and Myrback, K. (eds.): The Enzymes, Vol. 5. New York, Academic Press, 1961, p. 237.

60. Krenitsky, T.A., Elion, G.B., Henderson, A.M., et al.: Inhibition of human purine nucleoside phosphorylase: Studies with intact erythrocytes and the purified enzyme. J. Biol. Chem. 243:2876, 1968.

61. Zimmerman, T.P., Gersten, N., and Miech, R.P.: Adenine and adenosine metabolism in liver. Proc. Am. Assoc. Cancer Res. 11:87, 1970.

62. Sandberg, A.A., Lee, G.R., Cartwright, G.E., et al.: Purine nucleoside phosphorylase activity of blood. I. Erythrocytes. J. Clin. Invest. 34:1823, 1955.

63. Pierre, K.J., and LePage, G.A.: Formation of inosine-5'-monophosphate by a kinase in cell-free extracts of Ehrlich ascites cells in vitro. Proc. Soc. Exp. Biol. Med. 127:342, 1968.

64. Wada, Y., Arakawa, T., and Koizumi, K.: Lesch-Nyhan syndrome: Autopsy findings and in vitro study of incorporation of 14C-8-inosine into uric acid, guanosine-monophosphate and adenosine-monophosphate in the liver. Tohoku J. Exp. Med. 95:253, 1968.

65. Friedman, T., Seegmiller, J.E., and Subak-Sharpe, J.H.: Evidence against the existence of guanosine and inosine kinases in human fibroblasts in tissue culture. Exp. Cell Res. 56:425, 1969.

66. Gudas, L.J., Allman, B., Cohen, A., and Martin, D.W.: Deoxyguanosine toxicity in a mouse T lymphoma: Relationship to purine nucleoside phosphorylase-associated immune dysfunction. Cell 14:531, 1978.

67. Capputo, R.: The enzymatic synthesis of adenylic acid. Adenosine kinase. J. Biol. Chem. 189:801, 1951.

68. Kornberg, A., and Pricer, W.E., Jr.: Enzymatic phosphorylation of adenosine and 2,6-diaminopurine riboside, J. Biol. Chem. 193:481, 1951.

69. Palella, T.D., Andres, C.M., and Fox, I.H.: Human placental adenosine kinase: Kinetic mechanism and inhibition. J. Biol. Chem. 255:5264, 1980.

70. Streeter, D.G., Simon, L.N., Robins, R.K., and Miller, J.P.: The phosphorylation of ribavirin by deoxyadenosine kinase from rat liver. Differentiation between adenosine and deoxyadenosine kinase. Biochemistry 13:4543, 1974.

71. Krygier, V., and Momparler, L.: Mammalian deoxynucleoside kinase. II. Deoxyadenosine kinase: Purification and properties. J. Biol. Chem. 246:2745, 1971.

72. Krygier, V., and Momparler, L.: Mammalian deoxynucleoside kinase. III. Deoxyadenosine kinase. Inhibition by nucleotides and kinetic studies. J. Biol. Chem. 246:2752, 1971.

73. Carson, D.A., Kaye, J., and Seegmiller, J.E.: Lymphospecific toxicity in adenosine deaminase deficiency and purine nucleoside phosphorylase deficiency: Possible role of nucleoside kinase(s). Proc. Natl. Acad. Sci. USA 74:5677, 1977.

74. Fox, I.H., and Kelley, W.N.: The role of adenosine and 2'-deoxyadenosine in mammalian cells. Ann. Rev. Biochem. 47:566, 1978.

75. Coleman, M.A., Donofrio, J., Hutton, J.J., and Hahn, L.: Identification and quantitation of adenine deoxynucleotides in erythrocytes of a patient with adenosine deaminase deficiency and severe combined immunodeficiency. J. Biol. Chem. 253:1619, 1978.

76. Cohen, A., Hirschhorn, R., Horowitz, S.D., Rubinstein, A., Polmar, S.H., Hong, R., and Martin, D.W.: Deoxyadenosine triphosphate as a potentially toxic metabolite in adenosine deaminase deficiency. Proc. Natl. Acad. Sci. USA 75:472, 1978.

77. Martin, W.D., Gudas, L.J., Cohen A., and Ammann, A.J.: The common molecular mechanism of immune dysfunction in the inherited deficiencies of adenosine deaminase and purine nucleoside phosphorylase. Clin. Res. 26:501A, 1978.

78. Heppel, L.A., and Rabinowitz, J.C.: Enzymology of nucleic acids, purines, and pyrimidines. Ann. Rev. Biochem. 27:613, 1958.

79. Heppel, L.A., and Hilmoe, R.J.: Purification and properties of 5'-nucleotidase. J. Biol. Chem. 188:665, 1951.

80. Schmidt, G.: Nucleases and enzymes attacking nucleic acid components. *In* Chargaff, E., and Davidson J.N. (eds.): The Nucleic Acids, Vol. 1. New York, Academic Press, 1955, p. 555.

81. Johnson, S.M., Asherson, G.L., Watts, R.W.E., et al.: Lymphocyte purine 5'-nucleotidase deficiency in primary hypogammaglobulinemia. Lancet 1:168, 1977.

82. Edwards, N.L., Magilavy, D.B., Cassidy, J.T., and Fox, I.H.: Lymphocyte ecto-5'-nucleotidase deficiency in agammaglobulinemia. Science 201:628, 1978.

83. Edwards, N.L., Recker, D., Montredi, J., et al.: Regulation of purine metabolism by plasma membrane and cytoplasmic 5'-nucleotidoses. Am. J. Physiol. 243:C270, 1982.

84. Nikiforuk, G., and Colowick, S.P.: The purification and properties of 5-adenylic acid deaminase from muscle. J. Biol. Chem. 219:119, 1956.

85. Kalckar, H.M.: Differential spectrophotometry of purine compounds by means of specific enzymes. III. Studies of the enzymes of purine metabolism. J. Biol. Chem. 167:461, 1947.

86. Bergmann, F., and Dikstein, S.: Studies on uric acid and related compounds. III. Observations on the specificity of mammalian xanthine oxidase. J. Biol. Chem. 223:765, 1956.

87. Engleman, K., Watts, R.W.E., Klinenberg, J.R., et al.: Clinical physiological and biochemical studies of a patient with xanthinuria and pheochromocytoma. Am. J. Med. 37:839, 1964.

88. Watts, R.W.E., Watts, J.E.M., and Seegmiller, J.E.: Xanthine oxidase activity in human tissues and its inhibition by allopurinol (4-hydroxypyrazolo(3,4-d)pyrimidine). J. Lab. Clin. Med. 66:688, 1965.

89. Segal, S., and Wyngaarden, J.B.: Plasma glutamine and oxypurine content in patients with gout. Proc. Soc. Exp. Biol. Med. 88:342, 1955.

90. Jorgensen, S., and Poulsen, H.E.: Enzymatic determination of hypoxanthine and xanthine in human plasma and urine. Acta Pharmacol. 11:223, 1955.

91. Hoffman, G.T., Rottino, A., and Albaum, H.G.: Levels of nucleotide in the blood during shock. Science 114:188, 1951.

92. Nierlich, D.P., and Magasanik, B.: Regulation of purine ribonucleotide synthesis by end product inhibition: The effect of adenine and guanine ribonucleotides on the 5'-phos-phoribosylpyrophosphate amidotransferase of *Aerobacter aerogenes.* J. Biol. Chem. 240:358, 1965.

93. Wyngaarden, J.B., and Ashton, D.M.: The regulation of activity of phosphoribosylpyrophosphate amidotransferase by purine ribonucleotides: A potential feedback control of purine biosynthesis. J. Biol. Chem. 234:1492, 1959.

94. Caskey, C.T., Ashton, D.M., and Wyngaarden, J.B.: The enzymology of feedback inhibition of glutamine phosphoribosylpyrophosphate amidotransferase by purine ribonucleotides. J. Biol. Chem. 239:2570, 1964.

95. Henderson, J.F.: Feedback inhibition of purine biosynthesis in ascites tumor cells. J. Biol. Chem. 237:2631, 1962.

96. Holmes, E.W., McDonald, J.A., McCord, M.M., Wyngaarden, J.B., and Kelley, W.N.: Human glutamine phosphoribosylpyrophosphate amidotransferase: Kinetic and regulatory properties. J. Biol. Chem. 248:144, 1973.

97. Wood, A.W., and Seegmiller, J.E.: Properties of 5-phosphoribosyl-1-pyrophosphate amidotransferase from human lymphoblasts. J. Biol. Chem. 248:138, 1973.

98. Holmes, E.W., Wyngaarden, J.B., and Kelley, W.N.: Human glutamine phosphoribosylpyrophosphate amidotransferase: Two molecular forms interconvertible by purine ribonucleotide and phosphoribosylpyrophosphate. J. Biol. Chem. 248:6035, 1973.

99. Howard, W.J., and Appel, S.I.: Control of purine biosynthesis: FGAR amidotransferase (abstr.) Clin. Res. 16:344, 1968.

100. Kelley, W.N., Fox, I.H., and Wyngaarden, J.B.: Regulation of purine biosynthesis in cultured human cells. I. Effects of orotic acid. Biochim. Biophys. Acta 215:512, 1970.

101. Kelley, W.N., Fox, I.H., and Wyngaarden, J.B.: Essential role of phos-

phoribosylpyrophosphate (PRPP) in regulation of purine biosynthesis in cultured human fibroblasts. Clin. Res. 18:457, 1970.

102. Fox, I.H., and Kelley, W.N.: Phosphoribosylpyrophosphate in man: Biochemical and clinical significance. Ann. Intern. Med. 74:424, 1971.

103. Kelley, W.N., Greene, M.L., Fox, I.H., Rosenbloom, F.M., Levy, R.H., and Seegmiller, J.E.: Effects of orotic acid on purine and lipoprotein metabolism in man. Metabolism 19:1025, 1970.

104. Henderson, J.F., and Khoo, M.K.Y.: Synthesis of 5-phosphoribosyl-1-pyrophosphate from glucose in Ehrlich ascites tumor cells in vitro. J. Biol. Chem. 240:2349, 1965.

105. Lindsay, R.H., Cash, A.G., and Hill, J.B.: TSH stimulation of orotic acid conversion of pyrimidine nucleotides and RNA in bovine thyroid. Endocrinology 84:534, 1969.

106. Rottman, F., and Guarino, A.J.: The inhibition of phosphoribosylpyrophosphate amidotransferase activity by cordecepin monophosphate. Biochim. Biophys. Acta 89:465, 1964.

107. Nagy, M.: Regulation of biosynthesis of purine nucleotides in *Schizosaccharomyces pombe*. I. Properties of the phosphoribosylpyrophosphate glutamine amidotransferase of the wild strain and of a mutant desensitized towards feedback modifiers. Biochim. Biophys. Acta 198:471, 1970.

108. Rowe, P.B., Coleman, M.D., and Wyngaarden, J.B.: Glutamine phosphoribosylpyrophosphate amidotransferase: Catalytic and conformational heterogeneity of the pigeon liver enzyme. Biochemistry 9:1498, 1970.

109. King G., Meade, J.C., Borinous, C.G. and Holmes, E.W.: Demonstration of ammonia utilization for purine biosynthesis by the intact cell and characterization of the enzymatic activity catalyzing this reaction. Metabolism 28:348, 1979.

110. Itakura, M., Sabina, R., Heald, P. and Holmes, E.W.: Basis for the control of purine biosynthesis by purine ribonucleotides. J. Clin. Invest, 67:994, 1981.

111. Magasanik, B., and Karibian, D.: Purine nucleotide cycles and their metabolic role. J. Biol. Chem. 235:2672, 1960.

112. Holmes, E.W., Pehlke, D.M., and Kelley, W.N.: The role of human inosinic acid dehydrogenase in the control of purine biosynthesis de novo. Biochim. Biophys. Acta 364:209, 1974.

113. Ullman, B., Wormsloud, M.A., Cohen, M.B., and Martin, D.W.: Purine oversecretion in cultured murine lymphoma cells deficient in adenylosuccinate synthetase: Genetic model for hyperuricemia and gout. Proc. Natl. Acad. Sci. (USA) 79:2673, 1982.

114. Wyngaarden, J.B., and Kelley, W.N.: Gout and Hyperuricemia. New York, Grune & Stratton, 1976.

115. Fox, I.H.: Metabolic basis for disorders of purine nucleotide degradation. Metabolism 30:616, 1981.

116. Bagnora, A.S., and Hershfield, M.S.: Mechanism of deoxyadenosine-induced catabolism of adenine ribonucleotides in adenosine deaminase-inhibited human T lymphoblastoid cells.: Proc. Natl. Acad. Sci. (USA) 79:2673, 1982.

117. Griebsch, A., and Zollner, N.: Effect of ribonucleotides given orally on uric acid production in man. In Sperling, O., de Vries, A., and Wygaarden, J.B. (eds.): Purine Metabolism in Man, Vol. 41B. New York, Plenum Press, 1974, p. 443.

118. Zollner, N.: Influence of various purines on uric acid metabolism. Bibl. "Nutr. Diet." No. 19. Basel, Karger, 1973, pp.34–43.

119. Folin, O., Berglund, H., and Derick, C.: The uric acid problem: An experimental study on animals and man, including gouty subjects. J. Biol. Chem. 60:361, 1924.

120. Koehler, A.E.: Uric acid excretion. J. Biol. Chem. 60:721, 1924.

121. Buzard, J., Bishop, C., and Talbott, J.H.: Recovery in humans of intravenously injected isotopic uric acid. J. Biol. Chem. 196:179, 1952.

122. Wyngaarden, J.B.: The effect of phenylbutazone on uric acid metabolism in two normal subjects. J. Clin. Invest. 34:256, 1955.

123. Sorensen, L.B.: The elimination of uric acid in man studies by means of C¹⁴-labeled uric acid. Scand. J. Clin. Lab. Invest. 12(Suppl. 54):1, 1960.

124. Spilman, E.L.: Uric acid synthesis in the nongouty and gouty human (abstr.) Fed. Proc. 13:302, 1954.

125. Benedict, J.D., Forsham, P.H., and Stetten, DeW., Jr.: The metabolism of uric acid in the normal and gouty human studied with the aid of isotopic uric acid. J. Biol. Chem. 18:183, 1949.

126. Sorensen, L.B.: Degradation of uric acid in man. Metabolism 8:687, 1959.

127. Scott, J.T., Holloway, V.P., Glass, H.I., et al.: Studies of uric acid pool size and turnover rate. Ann. Rheum. Dis. 28:366, 1969.

128. Seegmiller, J.D., Grayzel, A.I., Laster, L., et al.: Uric acid production in gout. J. Clin. Invest. 40:1304, 1961.

129. Kelley, W.N., Rosenbloom, F.M., Seegmiller, J.E., et al.: Excessive production of uric acid in type I glycogen storage disease. J. Pediat. 72:488, 1968.

130. Lucke, H.: Das Harnsaureproblem und seine klinische Bedeutung. Ergeb. Inn. Med. Kinderheilk. 44:499, 1932.

131. Kurti, L.: Untersuchungen uber den Harnsaurestoffwechsel bei Nierenkranken. Z. Klin. Med. 122:585, 1932.

132. Wyngaarden, J.B.: Gout. In Stanbury, J.B., Wyngaarden, J.B., and Fredrickson, D.S., (eds.): The Metabolic Basis of Inherited Disease. New York, McGraw-Hill Book Company, 1960, p. 728.

133. Berliner, R.W., Hilton, J.G., Yu, T-F., et al.: The renal mechanism for urate excretion in man. J. Clin. Invest. 29:296, 1950.

134. Gutman, W.B., and Yu, T-F.: A three-component system for regulation of renal excretion of urate in man. Trans. Assoc. Am. Physicians 74:353, 1961.

135. Shannon, J.A.: The excretion of uric acid by the chicken. J. Cell. Comp. Physiol. 11:135, 1938.

136. Dantzler, W.H.: Comparison of renal tubular transport of urate and PAH in water snakes. Evidence for differences in mechanisms and sites of transport. Comp. Biochem. Physiol. 34:609, 1970.

137. Dantzler, W.H.: Characteristics of urate transport by isolated perfused snake proximal renal tubules. Am. J. Physiol. 224:445, 1973.

138. Mudge, G.H., McAlary, B., and Berndt, W.O.: Renal transport of uric acid in the guinea pig. Am. J. Physiol. 214:875, 1969.

139. Kessler, R.H., Hierholzer, K., and Gurd, R.S.: Localization of urate transport in the nephron of mongrel and Dalmatian dog kidney. Am. J. Physiol. 197:601, 1959.

140. Fanelli, G.M., Bohn, D., and Russo, H.F.: Renal clearance of uric acid in non-human primates. Comp. Biochem. Physiol. 33:459, 1970.

141. Boudry, J.F.: Mécanismes de l'excretion d'acide urique chez le rat. Pfluegers Arch. Ges. Physiol. 328:265, 1971.

142. Boudry, J.F.: Effet d'inhibiteurs des transports transtubulaires sur l'execretion renale d'acide urique chez le rat. Pfluegers Arch. Ges. Physiol. 328:279, 1971.

143. Berger, L., Yu, T-F., and Gutman, A.B.: Effects of drugs that alter uric acid excretion in man on uric acid clearance in the chicken. Am. J. Physiol. 198:575, 1960.

144. Yu, T-F., Berger, L., Kupfer, S., et al.: Tubular secretion of urate in the dog. Am. J. Physiol. 199:1199, 1960.

145. Fanelli, G.M., Jr., Bohn, D., and Stafford, S.: Functional characteristics of renal urate transport in the *Cebus* monkey. Am. J. Physiol. 218:627, 1970.

146. Fanelli, G.M., Jr., Bohn, D.L., and Reilly, S.S.: Renal urate transport in the chimpanzee. Am. J. Physiol. 220:613, 1971.

147. Greger, R., Lang, F., and Deetjen, P.: Handling of uric acid by the rat kidney. I. Microanalysis of uric acid in proximal tubular fluid. Eur. J. Physiol. 324:279, 1971.

148. Gutman, A.B., Yu, T-F., and Berger, L.: Tubular secretion of urate in man. J. Clin. Invest. 39:1778, 1959.

149. Lathem, W., Davis, B.B., and Rodnan, G.P.: Renal tubular secretion of uric acid in the mongrel dog. Am. J. Physiol. 199:9, 1960.

150. Mudge, G.H., Cucchi, J., Platts, M., et al.: Renal excretion of uric acid in the dog. Am. J. Physiol. 215:404, 1968.

151. Nolan, R.P., and Foulkes, E.C.: Studies on renal urate secretion in the dog. J. Pharmacol. Exp. Ther. 179:429, 1971.

152. Zins, G.R., and Weiner, I.M.: Bidirectional urate transport limited to the proximal tubule in dogs. Am. J. Physiol. 215:411, 1968.

153. Blanchard, K.C., Maroske, D., May, D.G., et al.: Uricosuric potency of 2-substituted analogs of probenecid. J. Pharmacol. Exp. Ther. 180:397, 1972.

154. Fannelli, G.M., Jr., Bohn., D.L., and Reilly, S.S.: Renal effects of uricosuric agents in the *Cebus* monkey. J. Pharmacol. Exp. Ther. 175:259, 1970.

155. Fanelli, G.M., Jr., Bohn, D.L., and Reilly, S.S.: Renal effects of uricosuric agents in the chimpanzee. J. Pharmacol. Exp. Ther. 177:591, 1971.

156. Fanelli, G.M., Jr., Bohn, D.L., Reilly, S.S., et al.: Renal excretion and uricosuric properties of halofenate, a hypolipidemic uricosuric agent, in the chimpanzee. J. Pharmacol. Exp. Ther. 180:377, 1972.

157. Bordley, J., III, and Richards, A.N.: Quantitative studies of the composition of glomerular urine. VIII. The concentration of uric acid in glomerular urine of snakes and frogs, determined by an ultramicro adaption of Folin's method. J. Biol. Chem. 101:193, 1933.

158. Roch-Ramel, F., and Weiner, I.M.: Excretion of urate by the kidneys of *Cebus* monkeys: A micropuncture study. Am. J. Physiol. 224:1369, 1973.

159. Weiner, I.M., and Fanelli, G.M., Jr.: Renal urate excretion in animal models. Nephron 14:33, 1975.

160. Berndt, W.O., and Beechwood, E.C.: Influence of inorganic electrolytes and ouabain on urate transport. Am. J. Physiol. 208:642, 1965.

161. Weinman, E.J., Senekjian, H.O., Sansom, S.C. et al.: Evidence for active and passive urate transport in the rate proximal tubule. Am. J. Physiol. 240:F90, 1981.

162. Sansom, S.C., Senekjian, H.O., Knight, T.F. et al.: Determination of the apparent transport constants for urate absorption in the rate proximal tubule. Am. J. Physiol. 240:F406, 1981.

163. Senekjian, H.O., Knight, T.F., and Weinman, E.J.: Urate transport by the isolated perfused S₂ segment of the rabbit. Am. J. Physiol. 240:F530, 1981.

164. Fanelli, G.M., Jr., and Weiner, I.M.: Pyrazinoate excretion in the chim-

panzee. Relation to urate disposition and the actions of uricosuric drugs. J. Clin. Invest. 52:1946, 1973.

165. Robson, A.M., Srivastave, P.L., and Bricker, N.S.: The influence of saline loading on renal glucose reabsorption in the rat. J. Clin. Invest. 47:329, 1968.

166. Bricker, N.S.: On the pathogenesis of the uremic state: The "trade-off hypothesis." N. Engl. J. Med. 286:1093, 1972.

167. Cannon, P.J., Svahn, D.S., and DeMartini, F.E.: The influence of hypertonic saline infusion upon the fractional reabsorption of urate and other ions in normal and hypertensive man. Circulation 41:97, 1970.

168. Kurtzman, N.A.: Regulation of renal bicarbonate reabsorption by extracellular volume. J. Clin. Invest. 49:586, 1970.

169. Holmes, E.W., Kelley W.N., and Wyngaarden, J.B.: The kidney and uric acid excretion in man. Kidney Int. 2:115, 1972.

170. Weinman, E.J., Eknoyan, G., and Suki, W.N.: The influence of the extracellular fluid volume on the tubular reabsorption of uric acid. J. Clin. Invest. 55:283, 1975.

171. Kahn, T., Mohammed, G., and Stein R.M.: Alterations in renal tubular sodium and water reabsorption in chronic renal disease in man. Kidney Int. 2:164, 1972.

172. Steele, T.H., and Rieselbach, R.E.: The contributions of residual nephrons within the chronically diseased kidney to urate homeostasis in man. Am. J. Med. 43:876, 1967.

173. Martino J.A., and Earley, L.E.: Demonstration of a role of physical factors as determinants of the natriuretic response to volume expansion. J. Clin. Invest. 56:1963, 1967.

174. Malnic, G., Aires, M.M., and Giebisch, G.: Micropuncture study of renal tubular hydrogen ion transport in the rat. Am. J. Physiol. 222:147, 1972.

175. Weiner, I.M., and Mudge, F.H.: Renal tubular mechanisms for excretion of organic acids and bases. Am. J. Med. 36:743, 1964.

176. Praetorius, D., and Kirk, J.E.: Hypouricemia: With evidence for tubular elimination of uric acid. J. Lab. Clin. Med. 35:865, 1950.

177. Yu, T-F., and Gutman, A.B.: Study of the paradoxical effects of salicylate in low, intermediate and high dosage on the renal mechanisms for excretion of urate in man. J. Clin. Invest. 38:1298, 1959.

178. Diamond, H.S., Sterba, G., Jayadeven, K., and Meisel, A.D.: On the mechanism of the paradoxical effect of salicylate on urate excretion. In Ropado, A. Watts, R.W.E., and DeBruyn, C.H.M. (eds.): Third International Symposium on Purine Metabolism in Man. New York, Plenum Publishing Co., 1980, pp. 221–225.

179. Podevin, R., Ardaillou, R., Paillar, F., et al.: Étude chez l'homme de la cinétique d'apparition dans l'urine de l'acide urique-2^{14}C. Nephron 5:134, 1968.

180. Nechay, B.R., and Nechay, L.: Effects of probenecid, sodium lactate, 2, 4-dinitrophenol, and pyrazinamide on renal secretion of uric acid in chickens. J. Pharmacol. Exp. Ther. 126:291, 1959.

181. Moller, J.V.: The tubular site of urate transport in the rabbit kidney and the effect of probenecid on urate secretion. Acta Pharmacol. Toxicol. 23:329, 1965.

182. Fanelli, G.M., Jr., Bohn, D.L., Reilly, S.S., et al.: Effects of mercurial diuretics on renal transport of urate in the chimpanzee. Am. J. Physiol. 224:985, 1973.

183. Moller, J.V.: The relation between secretion of urate and p-aminohippurate in the rabbit kidney. J. Physiol. 192:505, 1967.

184. Boner, G., Steele, T.H.: Relationship of urate and p-aminohippurate secretion in man. Am. J. Physiol. 225:100, 1973.

185. Yu, T-F., Sirota, J.H., Berger, L., et al.: Effect of sodium lactate infusion on urate clearance in man. Proc. Soc. Exp. Biol. Med. 96:809, 1957.

186. Reem, G.H., and Vanamee, P.: Effect of sodium lactate on urate clearance in the Dalmatian and mongrel dog. Am. J. Physiol. 207:113, 1964.

187. Goldfinger, S., Klinenberg, J.R., and Seegmiller, J.E.: Renal retention of uric acid induced by infusion of betahydroxybutyrate and acetoacetate. N. Engl. J. Med. 272:351, 1965.

188. Schulman, J.F., Lustberg, T.J., Kennedy, J.L., et al.: A new variant of maple syrup urine disease (branched chain ketoaciduria). Clinical and biochemical evaluation. Am. J. Med. 49:118, 1970.

189. Gutman, A.B., and Yu, T-F.: Renal mechanisms for regulation of uric acid excretion, with special reference to normal and gouty man. Semin. Arthritis Rheum. 2:1, 1972.

190. Greger, R., Lang, R., and Deetjen, P.: Handling of uric acid by the rat kidney. II. Microperfusion studies on bidirectional transport of uric acid in the proximal tubule. Eur. J. Physiol. 335:257, 1972.

191. Wilson, D.M., and Goldstein, N.P.: Renal urate excretion in patients with Wilson's disease. Kidney Int. 4:331, 1973.

192. Bennet, J.S., Bond, J., Singer, J., et al.: Hypouricemia in Hodgkin's disease. Ann. Intern. Med. 76:751, 1972.

193. Steele, T.H., and Boner G.: Origins of the uricosuric response, J. Clin. Invest. 52:1368, 1973.

194. Manuel, M.A., and Steele, T.H.: Pyrazinamide suppression of the uricosuric response to sodium chloride infusion. J. Lab. Clin. Med. 83:417, 1974.

195. Steele, T.H.: Urate secretion in man: The pyrazinamide suppression test. Ann. Intern. Med. 79:734, 1973.

196. Diamond, H.S., and Paolino, J.S.: Evidence for a postsecretory reabsorptive site for uric acid in man. J. Clin. Invest. 52:1491, 1973.

197. Fanelli, G.M. Jr., and Werner, I.M.: Urate excretion: Drug interactions. J. Pharmacol. Exp. Therap. 210:186, 1979.

198. Tofuku, Y., Mitsuhiko, K. and Takeda, R.: Hypouricemia due to renal urate wasting. Nephron 30:39, 1982.

199. Stapleton, F.B., Nyhan, W.L., et al.: Renal pathogenesis of familial hyperuricemia: Studies in two kindreds. Pediatr. Res. 15:1447, 1981.

200. Brochner-Mortensen, K.: The uric acid content in blood and urine in health and disease. Medicine 19:161, 1940.

201. Diamond, H.S., Lazarus, R., Kaplan, E., et al.: Effect of urine flow rate on uric acid excretion in man. Arthritis Rheum. 15:338, 1972.

202. Skeith, M.D., Healy, L.A., and Cutler, R.E.: Urate excretion during mannitol and glucose diuresis. J. Lab. Clin. Med. 70:213, 1967.

203. Diamond, H.S., and Meisel, A.D.: Collecting duct urate reabsorption in man. Program abstracts, 39th Annual Meeting of American Rheumatism Association, Section of Arthritis Foundation, New Orleans, June 4–6, 1977.

204. Wolfson, W.Q., Hunt, H.D., Levine, R., et al.: The transport and excretion or uric acid in man; sex difference and urate metabolism with note on clinical and laboratory findings in gouty women. J. Clin. Endocrinol. Metab. 9:749, 1949.

205. Scott, J.T., and Pollard, A.D.: Uric acid excretion in the relatives of patients with gout. Ann. Rheum. Dis. 29:397, 1970.

206. Nicholls, A., Snaith, M.L., and Scott, J.T.: Effect of oestrogen therapy on plasma and urinary levels of uric acid. Br. Med. J. 1:449, 1973.

207. Snaith, M.L., and Scott, J.T.: Uric acid excretion and surgery. Ann. Rheum. Dis. 31:162, 1972.

208. Grabfield, B.P.: A pharmacologic study of the mechanism of gout. Ann. Intern. Med. 11:651, 1937.

209. Postlethwaite, A.E., Ramsdell, C.M., and Kelley, W.N.: Uricosuric effect of an anticholinergic agent in hyperuricemic subjects. Arch. Intern. Med. 134:270, 1974.

210. Peters, J.P., and Van Slyke, K.K.: Quantitative Clinical Chemistry, Vol. 1. 2nd ed. Baltimore, Williams & Wilkins Company, 1946, p. 937.

211. Allen, D.J., Milosovich, G., and Mattocks, A.M.: Inhibition of monosodium urate crystal growth. Arthritis Rheum. 8:1123, 1965.

212. Loeb, J.N.: The influence of temperature on the solubility of monosodium urate. Arthritis Rheum. 15:189, 1972.

213. Wilcox, W.R., Khalaf, A., Weinberger, A., et al.: The solubility of uric acid and monosodium urate. Med. Biol. Eng. 10:522, 1972.

214. McNabb, R.A., and McNabb, F.M.A.: Physiological chemistry of uric acid: solubility, colloid and ion-binding properties. Comp. Biochem. Physiol. 67A:27, 1980.

215. Seegmiller, J.E.: The acute attack of gouty arthritis. Arthritis Rheum. 8:714, 1965.

216. Klinenberg, J.R., Goldfinger, S.E., and Seegmiller, J.E.: The effectiveness of a xanthine oxidase inhibitor on the treatment of gout. Ann. Intern. Med. 62:639, 1965.

217. Gold, G.L., and Fritz, R.D.: Hyperuricemia associated with the treatment of acute leukemia. Ann. Intern. Med. 47:428, 1957.

218. Kjellstrand, C.M., Campbell, D.C., III, von Hartizseh, B., et al.: Hyperuricemic acute renal failure. Arch. Intern. Med. 133:349, 1974.

219. Alvsaker, J.O.: Uric acid in human plasma. V. Isolation and identification of plasma proteins interacting with urate. Scand. J. Clin. Lab. Invest. 18:228, 1966.

220. Adlersberg, D., Grishman, E., and Sobotka, H.: Uric acid partition in gout and hepatic disease. Arch. Intern. Med. 70:101, 1942.

221. Yu, T-F., and Gutman, A.B.: Ultrafilterability of plasma urate in man. Proc. Soc. Exp. Biol. Med. 84:21, 1953.

222. Wyngaarden, J.B.: Uric acid. In Piersol, G.M. (ed.): The Cyclopedia of Medicine, Surgery. Specialties. Philadelphia, F.A. Davis Company, 1955, p. 341.

223. Morris, J.E.: The transport of uric acid in serum. Am. J. Med. Sci. 235:43, 1958.

224. Villa, L., Robecchi, A., and Ballabio, C.B.: Physiopathology clinical manifestations, and treatment of gout. Part I. Physiopathology and pathogenesis. Ann. Rheum. Dis. 17:9, 1958.

225. Kovarsky, J., Holmes, E., and Kelley, W.N.: Absence of significant urate binding to human serum proteins. J. Lab. Clin. Med. 93:85, 1979.

226. Postlethwaite, A.E., Gutman, R.A., and Kelley, W.N.: Salicylate-mediated increase in urate removal during hemodialysis: Evidence of urate binding to protein in vivo. Metabolism 23:771, 1974.

227. Medes, G.: Solubility of calcium oxalate and uric acid in solutions of urea. Proc. Soc. Exp. Biol. Med. 30:281, 1932.

228. Atsmon, A., De Vries, A., and Frank, M.: Uric Acid Lithiasis. Amsterdam, Elsevier, 1963, p. 63.

229. Sperling, O., De Vries, A., and Kedem, O.: Studies on the etiology of uric acid lithiasis. IV. Urinary non-dialyzable substances in idiopathic uric acid lithiasis. J. Urol. 94:286, 1965.

230. Prien, E.L., and Prien, E.L., Jr.: Composition and structure of urinary stone. Am. J. Med. 45:654, 1968.
231. Howell, R.R., Eanes, E.D., and Seegmiller, J.E.: X-ray diffraction studies on the tophaceous deposits in gout. Arthritis Rheum. 6:97, 1963.
232. McCarty, D.J., Jr., and Hollander, J.L.: Identification of urate crystals in gouty synovial fluid. Ann. Intern. Med. 54:452, 1961.
233. Zwaifler, N.J., and Pekin, T.J.: Significance of urate crystals in synovial fluids. Arch Intern. Med. 111:99, 1963.
234. Seegmiller, J.E., Rosenbloom, F.M., and Kelley, W.N.: An enzyme defect associated with a sex-linked human neurological disorder and excessive purine synthesis. Science 155:1682, 1967.
235. Kelley, W.N., Holmes, E.W., and van der Weyden, M.B.: Current concepts on the regulation of purine biosynthesis de novo in man. Arthritis Rheum. 18:673, 1975.

Chapter 22
Nutrition and Rheumatic Diseases

Edward A. Mascioli and George L. Blackburn

INTRODUCTION

Nutrition is an important science interacting with rheumatic diseases. A major focus of nutrition deals with nutrient intake to preserve and sustain immune competence and the host's defenses to inflammatory insults. In turn, a primary role of the body's response to inflammation involves the breakdown of various body tissues to effect a redistribution of nutrients, which, if unrecognized and untreated, can lead to nutritional deficiencies and malnutrition and subsequent morbidity and mortality.

Given the recent development of techniques for measuring the metabolic response to inflammation, the development of biometric parameters to assess nutritional deficiencies, and the development of new nutritional support techniques, it is possible to utilize the science of nutrition in the treatment of rheumatic diseases. Nutritional intervention in the area of rheumatology need not be restricted to correcting deficiencies that result from anorexia and catabolism associated with rheumatologic conditions; very promising work is being done in treating and palliating the inflammatory response to rheumatologic disease by altering the inflammatory response, particularly by way of dietary manipulation to alter ptostaglandin production and by the administration of vitamin A derivatives.

The main focus of this chapter will be the indications and requirements for nutritional support of the rheumatology patient. Included is a discussion of various metabolic changes that occur with inflammation. Changes in specific nutrients will also be addressed as well as the therapeutic trials designed to restore the normal concentrations of nutrients following inflammation and arthritis. Direct potential therapeutic interventions involving nutritional therapies will be addressed, followed by the role of overnutrition (obesity) and its impact on rheumatologic diseases.

NUTRITION ASSESSMENT AND BODY COMPOSITION

The various tissues of the body are not equivalent with regard to their water, fat, protein and mineral composition. More importantly, in starvation, with and without added inflammation, there are significant differences as to what tissues account for the observed weight losses. After adaptation to simple starvation, adipose tissue accounts for most (90 percent) of the loss. However, an inflammatory disease process coupled with anorexia will lead to proportionately much greater losses of lean tissues (50 percent), those metabolically functioning tissues containing most of the body's protein, such as skeletal muscle (Fig. 22–1). Before making a diagnosis of malnutrition, a nutritional assessment is performed with normal body composition in mind (Table 22–1).

The patient's weight for height is a traditional approach. Standardized tables have been assembled (Table 22–2) to help gauge the adequacy of the patient's weight. A more discerning parameter is the recent involuntary loss of weight. As a rule, loss of 5 percent of the patient's normal weight over a 1-month interval or loss of 10

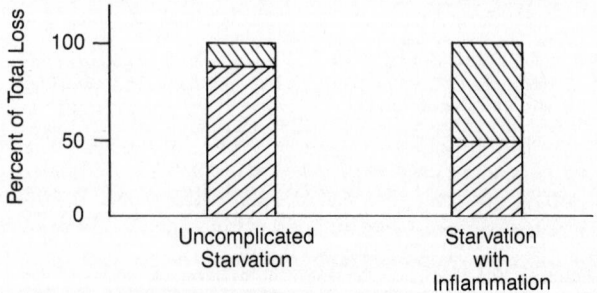

Figure 22–1. Differential tissue losses from uncomplicated starvation and starvation associated with inflammation. ▨ denotes fat loss; ▨ denotes lean tissue loss.

Table 22–1. The Major Parameters for the Assessment of Nutritional Status, With Corresponding Components of Body Composition*

Body Composition	Percent Body Weight	Protein (kg) (Total = 13 kg)	Nutritional Assessment
Fat (160,000 calories)	20		Triceps skin fold (mm)
Skin; Skeleton	9	6.3	
Extracellular Fluid	20	0.7	
Viscera	11	1.5	Albumin, total lymphocyte count, delayed hypersensitivity
Skeletal muscle	40	4.5	Arm muscle circumference (cm)

*Adapted from Moore, F.D., and Brannan, M.F.: Manual of Surgical Nutrition. American College of Surgeons. Philadelphia, W. B. Saunders Co., 1975.

percent over a 6-month interval should be considered significant weight loss. As discussed later, this weight loss puts the patient at increased risk.

Other parameters that are conveniently available in the clinical setting and have utility in a nutritional assessment include serum albumin, the total lymphocyte count, and cutaneous delayed hypersensitivity to common antigens. The serum albumin level, although affected by several factors, is a very good indicator of the adequacy of the patient's protein intake over the prior 2 to 3 weeks. In addition, it serves as an indicator of the degree of catabolic stress the patient is undergoing. The total lymphocyte count, obtained as the product of the total white blood cell count and the percentage of lymphocytes, often mirrors albumin as an indicator of malnutrition. Measuring the patient's ability to mount appropriate type 4 immunologic reactions to intradermally placed skin test antigens is a third approach to assessing the impact malnutrition has had on the functioning tissues of the body. These parameters are needed to diagnose the type of malnutrition and are powerful predictors of subsequent morbidity and mortality.

Protein-calorie malnutrition (PCM) has two major subcategories. Marasmus is defined by the patient's weight being less than 80 percent of the standard for his height. Marasmus is usually the result of starvation or semistarvation without added catabolic stresses such as infections, surgery, or inflammatory processes. Since most of this weight loss has been at the expense of adipose tissue, albumin, total lymphocyte count, and skin test reactivity are usually at normally expected values. Hypoalbuminemic malnutrition or adult kwashiorkor gives a reverse picture. Body weight for height is often at or above the standard. However, significant deficits in serum albumin, total lymphocyte count, and skin test reactivity are found. The albumin level is below 3 g/dl, the total lymphocyte count is less than 1200 per mm³, and the patient fails to react to intradermally placed antigens such as Candida, mumps, or tetanus. Hypoalbuminemic malnutrition carries a higher mortality than does marasmus. The difference in pathogenesis of this form of malnutrition is the concomitant presence of a catabolic stress such as inflammation or infection.

There are other parameters that are utilized in the more complete nutritional assessment.[1] However,

Seltzer[2-4] has popularized an abbreviated assessment consisting of serum albumin, total lymphocyte count, and involuntary weight loss of 10 pounds or more in the prior 6 months. This assessment was performed in surgical patients on admission to the hospital, and a 19-fold increase in mortality was found among the malnourished patients. How nutritional assessment can help to have an impact on the patient's course will become more evident after a discussion of protein-calorie malnutrition.

Table 22–2. Ideal Weight for Height

Males					
Height (cm)	Weight (kg)	Height (cm)	Weight (kg)	Height (cm)	Weight (kg)
145	51.9	159	59.9	173	68.7
146	52.4	160	60.5	174	69.4
147	52.9	161	61.1	175	70.1
148	53.5	162	61.7	176	70.8
149	54.0	163	62.3	177	71.6
150	54.5	164	62.9	178	72.4
151	55.0	165	63.5	179	73.3
152	55.6	166	64.0	180	74.2
153	56.1	167	64.6	181	75.0
154	56.6	168	65.2	182	75.8
155	57.2	169	65.9	183	76.5
156	57.9	170	66.6	184	77.3
157	58.6	171	67.3	185	78.1
158	59.3	172	68.0	186	78.9

Females					
Height (cm)	Weight (kg)	Height (cm)	Weight (kg)	Height (cm)	Weight (kg)
140	44.9	150	50.4	160	56.2
141	45.4	151	51.0	161	56.9
142	45.9	152	51.5	162	57.6
143	46.4	153	52.0	163	58.3
144	47.0	154	52.5	164	58.9
145	47.5	155	53.1	165	59.5
146	48.0	156	53.7	166	60.1
147	48.6	157	54.3	167	60.7
148	49.2	158	54.9	168	61.4
149	49.8	159	55.5	169	62.1

This table corrects the 1959 Metropolitan Standards to nude weight without shoe heels. Adapted from Jelliffe, D.B.: The Assessment of the Nutritional Status of the Community. Geneva, W.H.O., 1966.

METABOLIC RESPONSE TO
INFLAMMATION

With any systemic metabolic insult to the body, whether it be infection, trauma, surgery, or inflammatory process, there is a remarkably consistent and universal metabolic and hormonal response. Any stimulus leading to a sufficient amount of inflammatory activity involving white blood cells serves as the initiator of this process. Stimulated mononuclear phagocytes release a polypeptide, variously called leukocyte pyrogen (LP), interleukin 1(IL 1), or leukocyte endogenous mediator (LEM).[5] This polypeptide then acts on many tissues, causing fever, modulation of the immune response, and a redirection of tissue proteins (to name just a few). We shall concern ourselves with the metabolic and nutritional consequences of inflammation. The reader is referred to the earlier chapters of this text for more detail on the other processes present with inflammation.

Inflammatory arthritides, although not eliciting the same magnitude of a metabolic response as trauma or a burn, for example, can be nutritionally as detrimental because of their chronicity. Increased energy expenditure occurs early, in part to support a fever, and is supported by catecholamine-mediated lipolysis and glycogenolysis. Hyperglycemia, hypoinsulinemia, and high free fatty acid levels due to release from adipose tissue serve to increase the energy substrate availability for increased energy expenditure. This is termed the acute phase response to injury.[6] After the acute phase, lasting from 1 to 3 days, comes the adaptive phase. Since the inflammatory insult has persisted, other hormonal inputs occur. This phase is dominated by increased endogenous glucocorticosteroid secretion. This leads to hyperglycemia, hyperinsulinemia, and increased protein catabolism (especially in skeletal muscle), leading to protein breakdown. The increased amino acids exiting from skeletal muscle as well as connective tissue serve as precursors for new hepatic synthesis of the so-called acute phase reactants. Among these are fibrinogen, ceruloplasmin, α_1-antitrypsin, and other plasma globulins.

The redistributed amino acids also serve as carbon skeletons in gluconeogenesis, which is augmented owing to the glucocorticoid effect. The consequently increased ureagenesis accounts for the excessive nitrogen loss seen in periods of catabolic stress. Exogenously supplied protein, either from the diet or given intravenously, is used much less efficiently for protein synthesis because of the enhanced gluconeogenesis. Therefore the patient's protein requirement, for the maintenance of a net protein balance, is increased. Convalescence can only begin after the inflammatory stimulus lessens sufficiently to allow glucocorticoid secretion to approach the normal diurnal pattern, thereby restoring protein utilization efficiency. The obvious inciting event is IL 1–mediated inflammation, but an understanding of the ensuing metabolic response can lead to more rational nutritional therapy until the inflammation is eliminated. An unfortunate accompaniment to this response is anorexia, serving to thwart the physician's attempts at nutritional manage-

ment. Pragmatic approaches to solutions of this problem are discussed later in this chapter.

Several nutrients have been specifically investigated because of observed changes related directly or inversely to the activity of the underlying rheumatologic disease. Most of the work has been done in patients with rheumatoid arthritis, and most therapeutic interventions have been equivocal at best. This is perhaps explained by the changes being a consequence of the metabolic response to inflammation, rather than being etiologic in nature.

Histidine. Many studies have shown a decreased histidine concentration in the blood of patients with rheumatoid arthritis. Gerber[7] reviews these reports and documents statistically significant correlations with more conventional clinical parameters used to monitor disease activity. Direct correlations were found between hypohistidinemia and hematocrit and grip strength, whereas inverse correlations were found with erythrocyte sedimentation rate, duration of morning stiffness, walking time, rheumatoid factor, and the duration of arthritis. Other patients, defined only as a group without rheumatoid arthritis, had normal histidine levels. A subsequent report demonstrated that patients with rheumatoid arthritis normalized their serum histidine concentrations within 1 hour of an oral dose of histidine.[8] This implies that the defect is not due to a malabsorption disorder. Comparing relatives of patients with rheumatoid arthritis, Kirkham and co-workers showed that hypohistidinemia was an acquired feature of the disease and not predictive of risk. Histidine levels were followed in patients receiving drug therapy.[10,11] In spite of clinical improvement there were no changes in histidine levels after treatment with gold, prednisone, or hydroxychloroquine. However, coincident with clinical improvement, normalization of hypohistidinemia was seen following D-penicillamine therapy. This discrepancy further calls into question any role histidine could play in the pathogenesis of rheumatoid arthritis or as a form of therapy in this disorder. Gerber has proposed a mechanism for hypohistidinemia in the pathogenesis of rheumatoid arthritis,[12] but clinical evaluation is lacking.

Iron. It is well-known that a hypoferremic anemia (also known as the anemia of chronic disease) often accompanies active rheumatoid arthritis.[13] The anemia is also characterized by occasional hypochromia, a decrease in the total iron-binding capacity, a reduced ratio of iron to total iron-binding capacity, decreased marrow sideroblasts, and an increase in marrow reticuloendothelial iron. The anemia has been shown to have normal or even slightly increased erythropoiesis, increased ineffective erythropoiesis and a decreased mean red cell life span.[14] The shortened life span is due to some as yet unexplained hemolysis. The anemia is also due to some degree of failure of the marrow to respond sufficiently to the hemolysis. This may be related to inadequate release of iron from the reticuloendothelial cells.

It is very important to differentiate the anemia of chronic disease from that of iron deficiency. This is because the anemia of iron deficiency, unlike that of chronic disease, is responsive to iron administration. Establishing a firm diagnosis of iron deficiency anemia in the rheumatoid arthritis patient can be difficult. Because of the coexisting anemia of chronic disease, serum iron, total iron-binding capacity, the ratio of iron to total iron-binding capacity, and red blood cell indices are not specific. The serum ferritin level, normally low in iron deficiency (reflecting minimal or absent iron stores), rises with concomitant inflammation.[15] The lower end of the normal range is 12 μg per liter, but in patients with rheumatoid arthritis and no iron stores demonstrable on bone marrow biopsy, the mean value is 38 μg per liter.[16] This highlights the lack of sensitivity but enhanced specificity of a low serum ferritin in patients with rheumatoid arthritis. If the serum ferritin is normal or elevated, iron deficiency is not ruled out, since the ferritin may be spuriously elevated owing to inflammation. In this case, a bone marrow biopsy and Prussian blue staining for iron should be performed to directly assess iron stores.

Zinc. Serum zinc levels have been shown to be low in patients with rheumatoid arthritis.[17] They have also been shown to correlate inversely with osteoporosis associated with rheumatoid arthritis.[18] Balogh and colleagues found zinc levels to correlate directly with serum albumin and inversely with the erythrocyte sedimentation rate and serum globulins but not to correlate with joint tenderness.[19] Simkin argued that the changes in zinc levels were more than changes merely associated with the inflammation of rheumatoid arthritis.[20] He felt that oral supplementation with zinc, given its anti-inflammatory properties, would favorably affect the course of patients with rheumatoid arthritis. In a double-blind trial of 24 patients, positive results were seen in the treatment group for some clinical parameters but not in the erythrocyte sedimentation ratio or hematocrit. Kennedy, Bessent, and Reynolds divided 14 rheumatoid arthritis patients into two equal groups depending on their respective whole-body zinc amounts.[21] The half with the lowest zinc amounts were treated with zinc, while the other half received penicillamine. Neither group showed any statistically significant changes in clinical or laboratory parameters nor in whole-body zinc over the course of the 8-week trial. Despite large differences in whole-body zinc amounts between the two groups before the trial, there were no differences in severity of disease. Further negative evidence of a beneficial effect from zinc supplementation in rheumatoid arthritis came from Job and colleagues[22] and Mettingly and Mowat.[23] The trials lasted 4 and 6 months, respectively, and no statistically significant differences were detected in clinical or laboratory parameters between the treatment and placebo groups. In sum, the published reports to date relate changes in plasma zinc levels to the inflammation of rheumatoid arthritis and attribute no convincing etiologic nor therapeutic role to zinc.

Copper. It has been discovered that serum copper levels rise in patients with rheumatoid arthritis.[24] Since 90 percent of the serum copper is complexed to ceruloplasmin, an acute phase reactant protein, these levels rise as well in rheumatoid arthritis patients.[25] Direct correlations with disease activity, articular index, erythrocyte sedimentation rate, and antioxidant activity of the serum were found with serum copper and ceruloplasmin, whereas inverse correlations were found with serum iron and serum zinc.[26-28] In patients with severe disease, values twice normal can be found, a range similar to that seen with estrogen administration. Antirheumatic drugs that are associated with a lowering of copper levels include glucocorticosteroids, gold, and penicillamine. Because of ceruloplasmin's role as an antioxidant, it has been hypothesized to act as a free-radical scavenger in rheumatoid synovial effusions.[29] Other workers, however, have not found enhanced levels of ceruloplasmin in synovial fluid.[30] It must again be concluded that the changes observed in this nutrient, copper, are secondary to systemic inflammation and not nutritional aberrations.

SURVEYS OF MALNUTRITION

For the practitioner unfamiliar with currently accepted nutritional standards, the prevalence of malnutrition among hospitalized patients will seem astounding. Many different surveys have been done by various groups, all with similar results. Bistrian and colleagues surveyed the entire surgical patient population of an urban municipal hospital on one day.[31] Using the anthropometric measures of triceps skin fold and arm muscle circumference and serum albumin levels, the prevalence rate for protein-calorie malnutrition was 50 percent. In a similar survey conducted among medical patients in the same hospital, a rate of protein-calorie malnutrition comparable to that found in the surgical patients was found.[32] Differences were more depletion on a calorie basis (less weight/height and smaller triceps skin folds) and less depletion on a protein basis (greater arm muscle circumference and greater serum albumin levels) among medical patients as compared with surgical patients. In surveys done on orthopedic patients specifically, similar results were obtained. Dreblow and colleagues found a prevalence of 48 percent among 82 consecutively admitted orthopedic patients.[33] McFarlane studied 65 consecutively admitted fractured hip patients to a community hospital.[34] Although the prevalence of protein-calorie malnutrition was not as great as in the studies cited above, it was still noteworthy. Over one third of the group was anergic to skin test antigens on admission and 20 percent of those initially positive became negative over 1 week after surgery. The only statistically significant difference between those patients who developed anergy and those who remained immunocompetent was age; most of the patients in the former group were older than 85 years. One third of the total series had measurements less than 85 percent of the standard for arm muscle circumference, whereas 10 percent were less than a comparable value for weight for height. This discrepancy probably reflects the age-associated decline in muscle mass with its replacement by adipose tissue.

Lom-Orta and colleagues reported on five patients

with systemic lupus erythematosus as well as concomitant, severe protein-calorie malnutrition.[35] They speculated that the origin of the observed hypocomplementemia in these patients may have been due to poor production rather than increased utilization. In work done with young women suffering from anorexia nervosa, multiple complement proteins of the alternate pathway were observed to rise from deficient to normal levels coincident with feeding.[36] This highlights the need to consider two possible causes for hypocomplementemia in the rheumatologic patient—decreased synthesis secondary to malnutrition as well as increased utilization due to an inflammatory process. In 24 patients with classic rheumatoid arthritis or rheumatoid spondylitis, Pettersson and colleagues showed either malnutrition or malabsorption or both in over one half of the cases.[37] Folic acid deficiency, abnormal D-xylose absorption tests, and intestinal amyloidosis demonstrated by biopsy were among their criteria. In 1963, Eising summarized much earlier literature concerning arthritis and nutrition and remarked on the equivocal nature of the studies taken as a whole.[38] The weights and dietary intakes of patients with rheumatoid arthritis and degenerative arthritis were also analyzed. The only statistically significant differences were in body weight and acidic residues of the respective diets. The rheumatoid arthritis patients were shown to average 10 pounds below their recommended weights, whereas the patients with degenerative arthritis averaged 15 pounds above their recommended weights. The above studies all support a finding of malnutrition among the rheumatologic patient to varying degrees. It is reasonable to ask ourselves what impact malnutrition has on the subsequent course of the patient.

Malnutrition and Prognosis. In studies done on general surgical patients, mortality during the hospital stay was directly related to the presence of protein-calorie malnutrition. Meakins and colleagues found a mortality rate of 74 percent among anergic patients, whereas for immunocompetent patients, mortality was only 5 percent.[39] In a similar study, albumin levels, transferrin levels, and immunocompetence were found to be the only statistically significant predictors of complications among 16 factors studied.[40]

Other nutritional and anthropometric measures as well as in vivo and in vitro immunologic tests did not reliably predict outcome. In a study of orthopedic patients, the patients with three abnormal nutritional markers had longer hospital stays than those without.[33] These reports all point to an etiologic role for malnutrition and complications. The primary complications are an increased incidence of infection or sepsis and poor wound healing.

Nutritional Intervention. Given the malnourished patient's increased risk for complications, work has been done to evaluate preoperative nutritional support in decreasing predicted risk. Three studies have recently shown quite striking benefits of total parenteral nutrition among malnourished patients facing surgery, chemotherapy, or radiation therapy.[41-43] Nutritional therapy was shown to effect a three- to sixfold reduction in morbidity and mortality.[41] Although no comparable

trials have yet been published on rheumatologic patients not undergoing surgery, given our understanding of the metabolic response to a catabolic insult, we would expect a similar benefit of nutritional support in the rheumatologic patient, though perhaps not of the same magnitude because the insult is less. A potential mechanism through which this effect may occur is enhanced production of leukocyte endogenous mediator (LEM). As shown by Hoffman-Goetz and colleagues, production of LEM was impaired in leukocytes from malnourished patients but was restored after a period of nutritional support.[44] Conceivably the normalized production of LEM could be the route through which enhanced survival has been seen with nutritional support, by allowing the patient to optimally mobilize energy and protein stores to meet the catabolic, inflammatory insult. Whatever the mechanism, it is clear that full nutritional support is indicated wherever and whenever the physician encounters a malnourished patient.

NUTRITIONAL REQUIREMENTS

Nearly 40 individual substances are required by adults for a healthy nutritional intake. We will discuss some of the requirements, but the reader is referred to other sources for more detailed discussions of the various nutrients required for an adequate diet.[45]

Energy. Many factors affect the energy requirement of the individual. Age, sex, physical activity, weight, and degree of systemic inflammation all interact to help determine energy needs. Some factors change, often on a daily basis. Nevertheless, estimates can and should be made so that proper amounts of calories can be given. The basal energy expenditure (BEE) is the amount of energy the patient would burn at rest, free of illness, in 24 hours. A reasonable estimate of the BEE for an individual patient can be made from the Harris-Benedict equation.[46] For men the kilocaloric requirement is estimated by the following:

$$BEE = 655 + 13.8 \times Weight$$
$$+ 5.0 \times Height - 6.8 \times Age$$

For women it is as follows:

$$BEE = 655 + 9.6 \times Weight$$
$$+ 1.8 \times Height - 4.7 \times Age$$

Weight is in kilograms, height is in centimeters, and age is in years.

For a patient for whom enteral intake is feasible, approximately 125 percent of their calculated BEE should be given if weight maintenance is the goal of nutritional therapy. If weight gain is needed, then 150 percent of the BEE should be ingested by the patient. Since energy sources delivered parenterally are utilized less efficiently, 175 percent of the BEE is needed for anabolism to occur by this route.[46] A quicker, less accurate method, but one which is certainly justifiable in the clinical situation, is to estimate the patient's caloric requirement using 25 to 30 kilocalories per kilogram of body weight. Since the figures are approximate, this approach gives an adequate estimate.

Protein. The Food and Nutrition Board set, as a safe estimate of protein requirements, a value of 0.8 gram protein per kilogram of body weight per day.[45] Owing to the enhanced gluconeogenesis occurring in the metabolic response to injury, greater amounts of protein than normal are oxidized. Therefore more protein should be ingested to keep the patient in a state of no net protein loss. Consequently the protein requirement should be based on a factor of 1.0 to 1.5 grams of dietary protein per kilogram of body weight per day. Given adequate energy intakes, this is sufficient to keep all but the most catabolic patients in nitrogen balance. For a reference 70-kg man, this is approximately 90 grams of protein per day, which is the amount in the typical American diet.

Additional nutrients, such as vitamins, minerals, and trace elements, are vitally important in a complete nutritional intake. Other than specific reference to a few nutrients in regard to rheumatologic diseases, no further mention of these nutrients will be made in this chapter. The interested reader is referred to other sources for further discussion.[45]

NUTRITIONAL THERAPY APPROACHES

The start of any nutritional therapy depends on an accurate assessment of the nutritional status of the patient as well as the establishment of nutritional goals.

If the patient is not depleted nutritionally or has normal levels of serum albumin and is immunocompetent, then maintenance of the nutritional state is indicated. However, if the patient has suffered recent weight loss, is anergic or has a low serum albumin level, and is facing an additional catabolic insult such as surgery, then full nutritional repletion is warranted. Elective surgery should be delayed, if possible, until immunocompetence is restored. This usually necessitates a week of nutritional intervention.

Choice of Feeding Approach. Significant advances have been made in methods of feeding patients. No longer is it justified to allow a patient to starve if voluntary oral intake is insufficient. Many products and techniques have become available, allowing the physician many means for the successful treatment of malnutrition.

Once the patient's nutritional status is assessed, therapeutic goals outlined, and nutritional requirements estimated, daily counts of the caloric and protein contents of the food ingested are made by a dietitian. If consistently below requirements, nutritional intervention is in order (Fig. 22–2). Oral supplements are first used in an attempt to reach calculated requirements. These are available in innumerable flavors and formulations and are "complete" nutritionally; that is, they contain protein, carbohydrate, fat, and micronutrients.[47] Other more specialized formulas exist and are used depending on the inadequacy of the patient's gastrointestinal tract or the presence of renal, hepatic, or cardiac failure. The invaluable aid of a dietitian is essential in situations such as these.

If the patient is unable or unwilling to eat sufficient

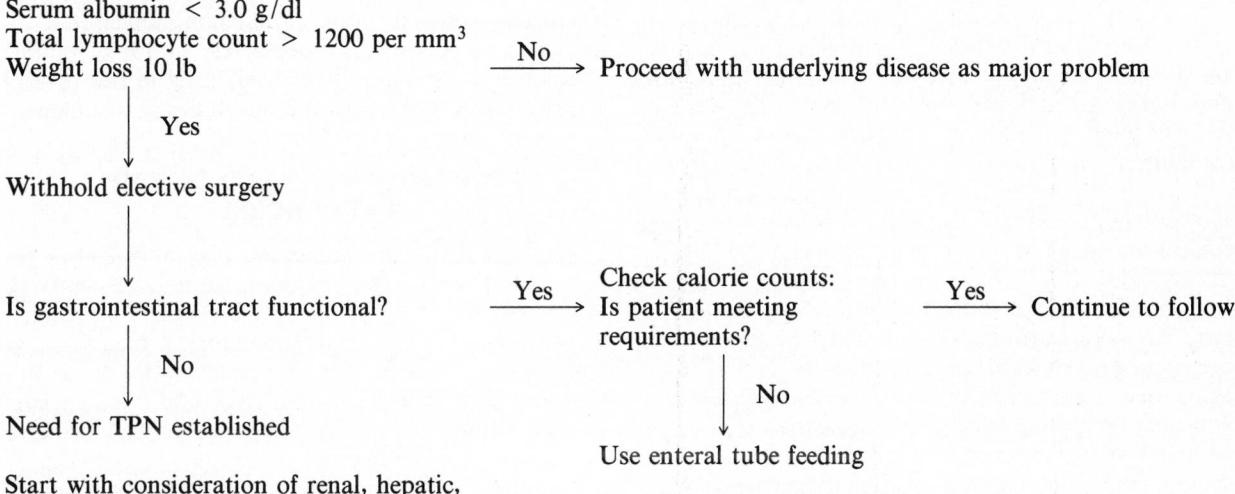

Figure 22–2. Algorithm for nutritional management.

amounts and has a functioning gastrointestinal tract, then a nasoenteral feeding tube should be passed. There are many available, but common features include a small diameter and pliability for optimal patient comfort. These are easily and rapidly passed with little or no trauma, which is quite in contrast to the experience with a larger, stiff tube for nasogastric aspiration. The use of nasoenteral tubes has been reviewed recently.[48] This simple technique should be utilized for many patients at risk for malnutrition.

For those patients whose gastrointestinal tract is unable to accommodate their nutritional requirements, a parenteral route must be used. Fortunately the delivery of total parenteral nutrition (TPN) has developed into a readily available technique whereby patients can be maintained in near optimal health for years in spite of no oral intake. TPN supplies the patient with all nutritional requirements, including water, calories, protein, fat, vitamins, minerals, and salts. Since the final solution is hypertonic, it must be infused through a large, high-flow central vein. Given the mechanical, metabolic, and infectious complications that can arise with TPN, it is strongly advised that only those physicians familiar with the procedure administer it.[49]

FURTHER NUTRITIONAL CONSIDERATIONS

Ascorbic Acid. Severe deficiency of dietary ascorbic acid, vitamin C, results in the clinical syndrome known as scurvy. One biochemical role ascorbic acid has is as a coenzyme in collagen biosynthesis. The clinical manifestations of scurvy are thought to be due to a defect in collagen synthesis. Signs and symptoms include recurrent hemarthroses, bleeding gums, perifollicular hemorrhages, and purpura and ecchymoses.[50] Today in the United States scurvy is usually seen in the elderly who subsist on processed foods or in alcoholics.

Since patients with scurvy are often suffering from multiple nutritional deficiencies, hemarthroses secondary to scurvy should be easily differentiated from other non-nutritional arthritides. If the diagnostic work-up leads to joint aspiration, the diagnostic possibilities are certainly narrowed.

Selenium. Selenium, a trace mineral, has recently been shown to be an essential nutrient for humans.[51,52] Among clinical the symptoms of selenium deficiency are arthritis, myalgias, and a congestive cardiomyopathy mostly seen in children. An individual patient maintained on total parenteral nutrition was reported to have developed debilitating myalgias and muscle tenderness in her lower extremities.[53] Examination of her nervous system and upper extremities revealed no abnormalities. Coincident with this syndrome was a very low blood level of selenium. The symptoms resolved after one week of intravenous selenium supplementation.

The amount of selenium in the diet is dependent upon the amount found in the soil on which the food was grown. Large geographic areas with deficient soil selenium include New Zealand and a large area of China. Keshan disease, originally thought to be caused by food toxins, is now believed due to selenium deficiency.[54] Keshan disease, endemic in the area of China with low soil selenium, is characterized by a congestive cardiomyopathy in children and an episodic, recurring arthritis over the years involving the spine and peripheral joints, leading to a disabling premature osteoarthritis. In a large-scale trial involving dietary supplementation of selenium in Chinese children, the incidence of cardiomyopathy was drastically reduced; but to date, there has been no published report of changes in the incidence of the arthritis.[55,56]

Pyridoxine. Vitamin B_6 (pyridoxine) levels have been found to be low in patients suffering from rheumatoid arthritis.[57-60] The question of whether this is, through some unknown mechanism, an etiology of rheumatoid arthritis has been investigated by the use of therapeutic trials. Ellis and Presley did find some improvement with arthritis of the hands and in carpal tunnel syndrome.[61] However, other trials have not shown this effect. Bruckner and co-workers failed to see any improvement in neuropathies due to rheumatoid disease.[62] In a double-blind trial of 21 patients, no change in clinical parameters or in erythrocyte sedimentation rate was seen in vitamin B_6 deficient patients, in spite of tripling of pre-treatment plasma pyridoxine levels.[60] The conclusion that we can draw from these studies is that in spite of the high prevalence of nutritional deficiencies in arthritis patients, correction of the deficits is indicated from a nutritional viewpoint and not from a rheumatologic one.

Retinoic Acid. Retinoic acid is the acid form of retinol, or vitamin A. It has been shown recently that the all-*trans* as well as the 13-*cis* isomers of retinoic acid can inhibit collagenase and prostaglandin E_2 production from cultures of rheumatoid synovial cells.[63] A mechanism thought responsible for the beneficial effect of corticosteroids in rheumatoid arthritis is the inhibition of collagenase and prostaglandin E_2 production by synovial cells; in contrast nonsteroidal anti-inflammatory drugs block only prostaglandin production. Given the remarkable success and relative safety of 13-*cis* retinoic acid in severe acne, the use of this drug in rheumatoid arthritis patients may prove to be clinically justifiable.[64]

PROSTAGLANDINS AND DIETARY FATTY ACIDS

The central role prostaglandins play in mediating inflammation (see Chapter 6) has recently led to research in this area on the possible development of nutritional interventions to modify inflammatory processes. It is important to keep in mind the many different prostaglandins, each with its own specific effects on specific tissues, including those that enhance as well as those that suppress inflammation.

Zurier and colleagues demonstrated prolongation of survival and prevention of anemia and glomerulonephritis in NZB/NZW F_1 hybrid mice (a strain that spontaneously develops a disease pathologically similar to human systemic lupus erythematosus) when treated with daily subcutaneous prostaglandin E_1 (PGE_1).[65,66] Oral administration of a stable analog of PGE_1,15-(S)-15-

methyl prostaglandin E_1, has been shown to ameliorate the damage from immune complex–induced vasculitis as well as adjuvant-induced polyarthritis.[67,68] This experimental rat model has led to further experiments with dietary manipulations of essential fatty acid content, because essential fatty acids serve as the precursors of prostaglandins.

Humoral immunity in mice was found to be significantly impaired when the animals were made deficient in essential fatty acids.[69] In the murine lupus model, Hurd and co-workers found a striking increase in survival and prevention of glomerulonephritis among essential-fatty-acid-deficient mice.[70,71] The treated mice were shown to develop antibodies to double-stranded DNA, but at a later age than the control animals. Mice treated with PGE_1 fared better than controls but not as well as the essential-fatty-acid-deficient animals. In a different approach, Prickett and colleagues treated NZB/NZW mice with diets enriched with eicosapentaenoic acid.[72] This fatty acid is a precursor of prostaglandin E_3 and is thought to interfere with the metabolism of arachidonic acid, an essential fatty acid, to other prostaglandins and thromboxanes. The treated animals did have lower levels of arachidonic acid but were not deficient in essential fatty acids. Probably the effect of eicosapentaenoic acid is exerted through prostaglandin metabolism but other than through depletion of arachidonic acid, as occurs in essential fatty acid deficiency. Dihomo-gamma-linolenic acid is a fatty acid that serves as a precursor of prostaglandin E_1. A rich source of this fatty acid is the oil of the evening primrose plant. Kunkel and associates have shown a beneficial effect from dietary supplementation of this oil, using an adjuvant-induced polyarthritis model in rats.[73] The mechanism thought to be operative in this situation is enhanced endogenous production of PGE_1 due to increased precursor concentration, leading to a less enhanced inflammatory response to the injected adjuvant.

No in vivo work in this area for humans has been published as yet; but in vitro data do exist, and they show that the synovium of patients with rheumatoid arthritis produces significant amounts of prostaglandins.[74] It has been recently shown that the dietary mix of fatty acids can significantly alter the fatty acid profile seen in plasma phospholipids, triglycerides, sterol esters, and platelet lipids.[75,76] These studies show that adults fed diets enriched with fish oils, abundant sources of eicosapentaenoic acid, demonstrated changes in lipid profiles within four weeks of the new diet. These studies and the work to date in animal models set the stage for therapeutic dietary trials in patients with arthritis.

OBESITY

Gout. Gout and obesity are directly associated. In the Framingham Heart Study, over 5000 patients were followed longitudinally. The study revealed that patients with gout or hyperuricemia were on the average 10 percent heavier than nongouty or nonhyperuricemic subjects.[78] The relationship was linear; that is, the greater the degree of obesity, the greater the chance of gout.

With weight loss, uric acid levels tend to decrease.[79] However, in diets sufficiently restrictive in calories as to allow starvation ketosis to occur, transient hyperuricemia may result from renal tubular excretion competition between urate and ketone bodies.[80] When starvation ketosis is abolished, urate levels return to baseline values. (See Chapters 21 and 86 for further discussion.)

Degenerative Joint Disease. A direct correlation exists between obesity and osteoarthritis of weight-bearing joints.[38] There is also an increased prevalence of osteoarthritis in non-weight-bearing joints of obese patients.[81] The prevalence of osteoarthritis among the obese is approximately twice that for the normal-weighted individual, for both weight-bearing as well as non-weight-bearing joints. The mechanism for this increase is thought to be mechanical in origin, but this certainly cannot be the process in non-weight-bearing joints.

References

1. Blackburn, G.L., Bistrian, B.R., Maini, B.S., Schlamm, H.T., and Smith, M.F.: Nutritional and metabolic assessment of the hospitalized patient. JPEN 1:11, 1977.
2. Seltzer, M.H., Bastidas, J.A., Cooper, D., Engler, P., Slocum, B., and Fletcher, H.S.: Instant nutritional assessment. JPEN 3:157, 1979.
3. Seltzer, M.H., Fletcher, H.S., Slocum, B.A., and Engler, P.E.: Instant nutritional assessment in the intensive care unit. JPEN 5:70, 1981.
4. Seltzer, M.H., Slocum, B.A., Cataldi-Betcher, E.L., Fileti, C., and Gerson, N.: Instant nutritional assessment: absolute weight loss and surgical mortality. JPEN 6:218, 1982.
5. Dinarello, C.A., and Wolff, S.M.: Molecular basis of fever in humans. Am. J. Med. 72:799, 1982.
6. Blackburn, G.L., and Bistrian, B.R.: Nutritional care of the injured and/or septic patient. Surg. Clin. North Am. 56:1195, 1976.
7. Gerber, D.A.: Low free serum histidine concentration in rheumatoid arthritis. J. Clin. Invest. 55:1164, 1975.
8. Gerber, D.A., Tanenbaum, L., and Ahrens, M.: Free serum histidine levels in patients with rheumatoid arthritis and control subjects following an oral load of free L-histidine. Metabolism. 25:655, 1976.
9. Kirkham, J., Lowe, J., Bird, H.A., and Wright, V.: Serum histidine in rheumatoid arthritis: a family study. Ann. Rheum. Dis. 40:501, 1981.
10. Pickup, M.E., Dixon, J.S., Lowe, J.R., and Wright, V.: Serum histidine in rheumatoid arthritis: changes induced by antirheumatic drug therapy. J. Rheumatol. 7:71, 1980.
11. Gerber, D.A.: Antirheumatic drugs, the ESR and the hypohistidinemia of rheumatoid arthritis. J. Rheumatol. 4:40, 1977.
12. Gerber, D.A.: Inhibition of denaturation of human gamma globulin by a mixture of L-histidine, L-cystine, and copper and its clinical implications in rheumatoid arthritis. Arthritis Rheum. 19:593, 1976.
13. Cartwright, G.E.: The anemia of chronic disorders. Semin. Hematol. 3:351, 1966.
14. Dinant, H.J., and DeMaat, C.E.M.: Erythropoiesis and mean red-cell lifespan in normal subjects and in patients with the anemia of active rheumatoid arthritis. Br. J. Hematol. 39:437, 1978.
15. Blake, D.R., and Bacon, P.A.: Serum ferritin and rheumatoid disease. Br. Med. J. 282:1273, 1981.
16. Bentley, D.P. and Williams, P.: Serum ferritin concentration as an index of storage iron in rheumatoid arthritis. J. Clin. Pathol. 27:786, 1974.
17. Niedermeier, W., Prillaman, W.W., and Griggs, J.H.: The effect of chrysotherapy on trace metals in patients with rheumatoid arthritis. Arthritis Rheum. 14:533, 1971.
18. Kennedy, A.C., Fell, G.S., Rooney, P.J., Stevens, W.H., Dick, W.C., and Buchanan, W.W.: Zinc: its relationship to osteoporosis in rheumatoid arthritis. Scand. J. Rheumatol. 4:243, 1975.
19. Balogh, Z., El-Ghobarey, A.F., Fell, G.S., Brown, D.H., Dunlop, J., and Dick, W.C.: Plasma zinc and its relationship to clinical symptoms and drug treatment in rheumatoid arthritis. Ann. Rheum. Dis. 39:329, 1980.
20. Simkin, P.A.: Oral zinc sulfate in rheumatoid arthritis. Lancet 2:539, 1976.
21. Kennedy, A.C., Bessent, R.G., and Reynolds, P.M.G.: Effect of oral zinc sulfate and penicillamine on zinc metabolism in patients with rheumatoid arthritis. J. Rheumatol. 7:639, 1980.
22. Job, C., Menkes, C.J., and Delbarre, F.: Zinc sulfate in the treatment of rheumatoid arthritis. Arthritis Rheum. 23:1408, 1980.
23. Mattingly, P.C., and Mowat, A.G.: Zinc sulfate in rheumatoid arthritis. Ann. Rheum. Dis. 41:456, 1982.
24. Scudder, P.R., Al-Timimi, D., McMurray, W., White, A.G., Zoob, B.C.,

and Dormandy, T.L.: Serum copper and related variables in rheumatoid arthritis. Ann. Rheum. Dis. 37:67, 1978.

25. Scudder, P.R., McMurray, W., White, A.G., and Dormandy, T.L.: Synovial fluid copper and related variables in rheumatoid and degenerative arthritis. Ann. Rheum. Dis. 37:71, 1978.

26. Pryzanski, W., Russell, M.L., Gordon, D.A., and Ogryzlo, M.A.: Serum and synovial fluid proteins in rheumatoid arthritis and degenerative joint diseases. Am. J. Med. Sci. 265:483, 1973.

27. Brown, D.H., Buchanan, W.W., El-Ghobarey, A.F., Smith, W.E., and Teape, J.: Serum copper and its relationship to clinical symptoms in rheumatoid arthritis. Ann. Rheum. Dis. 38:174, 1979.

28. Banford, J.C., Brown, D.H., Hazelton, R.A., McNeil, C.J., Sturrock, R.D., and Smith, W.E.: Serum copper and erythrocyte superoxide dismutase in rheumatoid arthritis. Ann. Rheum. Dis. 41:458, 1982.

29. Lunec, J., Halloran, S.P., White, A.G., and Dormandy, T.L.: Free-radical oxidation (peroxidation) products in serum and synovial fluid in rheumatoid arthritis. J. Rheumatol. 8:233, 1981.

30. Blake, D.R., Hall, N.D., Treby, D.A., Halliwell, B., and Gutteridge, J.M.C.: Protection against superoxide and hydrogen peroxide in synovial fluid from rheumatoid patients. Clin. Sci. 61:483, 1981.

31. Bistrian, B.R., Blackburn, G.L., Hallowell, E., and Heddle, R.: Protein status of general surgical patients. JAMA 230:858, 1974.

32. Bistrian, B.R., Blackburn, G.L., Vitale, J., Cochran, D., and Naylor J.: Prevalence of malnutrition in general medical patients. JAMA 235:1567, 1976.

33. Dreblow, D.M., Anderson, C.F., and Moxness, K.: Nutritional assessment of orthopedic patients. Mayo Clin. Proc. 56:51, 1981.

34. McFarlane, D.S.: The role of nutrition in the metabolic response to trauma and in the production of endogenous pyrogen. Master's Thesis, University of Edinburgh, Scotland, 1982.

35. Lom-Orta, H., Diaz-Jouanen, E., and Alarcon-Segovia, D.: Protein calorie malnutrition and systemic lupus erythematosus. J. Rheumatol. 7:178, 1980.

36. Wyatt, R.J., Farrell, M., Berry, P.L., Forristal, J., Maloney, M.J., and West, C.D.: Reduced alternative complement pathway control protein levels in anorexia nervosa: response to parenteral alimentation. Am. J. Clin. Nutr. 35:973, 1982.

37. Pettersson, T., Wegelius, O., and Skrifvars, B.: Gastro-intestinal disturbances in patients with severe rheumatoid arthritis. Acta. Med. Scand. 188:139, 1970.

38. Eising, L.: Dietary intake in patients with arthritis and other chronic diseases. J. Bone Joint Surg. 45:69, 1963.

39. Meakins, J.L., Pietsch, J.B., Bubenick, O., Kelly, R., Rode, H., Gordon, J., and MacLean, L.D.: Delayed hypersensitivity: indicator of acquired failure of host defenses in sepsis and trauma. Ann. Surg. 186:241, 1977.

40. Mullen, J.L., Gertner, M.H., Buzby, G.P., Goodhart, G.L., and Rosato, E.F.: Implications of malnutrition in the surgical patient. Arch. Surg. 114:121, 1979.

41. Mullen, J.L., Buzby, G.P., Matthews, D.C., Smale, B.F., and Rosato, E.F.: Reduction of operative morbidity and mortality by combined preoperative and postoperative nutritional support. Ann. Surg. 192:604, 1980.

42. Daly, J.M., Dudrick, S.J., and Copeland, E.M.: Intravenous hyperalimentation: effect on delayed cutaneous hypersensitivity in cancer patients. Ann. Surg. 192:587, 1980.

43. Smale, B.F., Mullen, J.L., Buzby, G.P., and Rosato, E.F.: The efficacy of nutritional assessment and support in cancer surgery. Cancer 47:2375, 1981.

44. Hoffman-Goetz, L., McFarlane, D., Bistrian, B.R., and Blackburn, G.L.: Febrile and plasma iron responses of rabbits injected with endogenous pyrogen from malnourished patients. Am. J. Clin. Nutr. 34:1109, 1981.

45. Food and Nutrition Board, National Research Council: Recommended Dietary Allowances, 9th ed. Washington, D.C., National Academy of Science, 1980.

46. Rutten, P., Blackburn, G.L., Flatt, J.P., Hallowell, E., and Cochran, D.: Determination of optimal hyperalimentation infusion rate. J. Surg. Res. 18:477, 1975.

47. Bothe, A., Wade, J.E., and Blackburn, G.L.: Enteral nutrition—an overview. In Hill, G.L. (ed.): Nutrition and the Surgical Patient. London, Churchill Livingstone, 1981.

48. Orr, G., Wade, J., Bothe, A., and Blackburn, G.L.: Alternatives to total parenteral nutrition in the critically ill patient. Crit. Care Med. 8:29, 1980.

49. Blackburn, G.L., Maini, B.S., and Pierce, E.C.: Nutrition in the critically ill patient. Anesthesiology 47:181, 1977.

50. Hodges, R.E., Hood, J., Canham, J.E., Sauberlich, H.E., and Baker, E.M.: Clinical manifestations of ascorbic acid deficiency in man. Am. J. Clin. Nutr. 24:432, 1971.

51. Young, V.R.: Selenium: a case for its essentiality in man. N. Engl. J. Med. 304:1228, 1981.

52. Johnson, R.A., Baker, S.S., Fallon, J.T., Maynard, E.P., Ruskin, J.N., Wen, Z., Ge, K., and Cohen, H.J.: An occidental case of cardiomyopathy and selenum deficiency. N. Engl. J. Med. 304:1210, 1981.

53. VanRij, A.M., Thomson, C.D., McKenzie, J.M., and Robinson, M.F.: Selenium deficiency in total parenteral nutrition. Am. J. Clin. Nutr. 32:2076, 1979.

54. Keshan Disease Research Group of the Chinese Academy of Medical Sciences, Beijing: Epidemiologic studies on the etiologic relationship of selenium and Keshan Disease. Chinese Med. J. (Engl.) 92:477, 1979.

55. Keshan Disease Research Group of the Chinese Academy of Medical Sciences, Beijing: Observations on effect of sodium selenite in prevention of Keshan disease. Chinese Med. J. (Engl.) 92:471, 1979.

56. Anonymous. Prevention of Keshan cardiomyopathy by sodium selenite. Nutr. Rev. 38:278, 1980.

57. Houpt, J.B., Ogryzlo, M.A., and Hunt, M.: Tryptophan metabolism in man (with special reference to rheumatoid arthritis and scleroderma). Semin. Arthritis Rheum. 2:333, 1973.

58. Jaffe, I.A., and Altman, K.: The effect of pyridoxine on the abnormal tryptophan metabolism in rheumatoid arthritis. Arthritis Rheum. 7:319, 1964.

59. Anderson, B.B., Peart, M.D., and Fulford Jones, C.E.: The measurement of serum pyridoxal by a microbiological assay using Lactobacillus casei. J. Clin. Pathol. 23:232, 1970.

60. Schumacher, H.R., Bernhart, F.W., and György, P.: Vitamin B_6 levels in rheumatoid arthritis: effect of treatment. Am. J. Clin. Nutr. 28:1200, 1975.

61. Ellis, J.M., and Presley, J.: Vitamin B_6: The Doctor's Report. New York, Harper & Row, 1973, p. 39.

62. Bruckner, F.E., Smith, H.G., Lakatos, C., and Chamberlain, M.H.: Tryptophan metabolism in rheumatoid neuropathies. Ann. Rheum. Dis. 31:311, 1972.

63. Brinckerhoff, C.E., McMillan, R.M., Dayer, J.M., and Harris, E.D.: Inhibition by retinoic acid of collagenase production in rheumatoid synovial cells. N. Engl. J. Med. 303:432, 1980.

64. Peck, G.L., Olsen, T.G., Yoder, F.W., Strauss, J.S., Downing, D.T., Pandya, M., Butkus, D., and Arnaud-Battandien, J.: Prolonged remissions of cystic and conglobate acne with 13-cis-retinoic acid. N. Engl. J. Med. 300:329, 1979.

65. Zurier, R.B., Sayadoff, D.M., Torrey, S.B., and Rothfield, N.F.: Prostaglandin E_1 treatment of NZB/NZW mice. Prolonged survival of female mice. Arthritis Rheum. 20:723, 1977.

66. Zurier, R.B., Damjanov, I., Sayadoff, D.M., and Rothfield, N.F.: Prostaglandin E_1 treatment of NZB/NZW F_1 hybrid mice. Prevention of glomerulonephritis. Arthritis Rheum. 20:1449, 1977.

67. Kunkel, S.L., Thrall, R.S., Kunkel, R.G., McCormick, J.R., Ward, P.A., and Zurier, R.B.: Suppression of immune complex vasculitis in rats by prostaglandin. J. Clin. Invest. 64:1525, 1979.

68. Kunkel, S.L., Ogawa, H., Conran, P.B., Ward, P.A., and Zurier, R.B.: Suppression of acute and chronic inflammation by orally administered prostaglandins. Arthritis Rheum. 24:1151, 1981.

69. De Wille, J.W., Fraker, P.J., and Romsos, D.R.: Effects of essential fatty acid deficiency, and various levels of dietary polyunsaturated fatty acids, on humoral immunity in mice. J. Nutr. 109:1018, 1979.

70. Hurd, E.R., Johnston, J.M., Okita, J.R., McDonald, P.C., Ziff, M., and Gilliam, J.N.: Prevention of glomerulonephritis and prolonged survival in New Zealand Black/New Zealand White F_1 hybrid mice fed an essential fatty acid deficient diet. J. Clin. Invest. 67:476, 1981.

71. Hurd, E.R., and Gilliam, J.N.: Beneficial effect of an essential fatty acid deficient diet in NZB/NZW F_1 mice. J. Invest. Dermatol. 77:381, 1981.

72. Prickett, J,D., Robinson, D.R., and Steinberg, A.D.: Dietary enrichment with the polyunsaturated fatty acid eicosapentaenoic acid prevents proteinuria and prolongs survival in NZB × NZW F_1 mice. J. Clin. Invest. 68:556, 1981.

73. Kunkel, S.L., Ogawa, H., Ward, P.A., and Zurier, R.B.: Suppression of chronic inflammation by evening primrose oil. Prog. Lipid Res. 20:885, 981.

74. Sturge, R.A., Yates, D.B., Gordon, D., Franco, M., Paul, W., Bray, A., and Morley, J.: Prostaglandin production in arthritis. Ann. Rheum. Dis. 37:315, 1978.

75. Bronsgeest-Schoute, H.C., Van Gent, C.M., Luten, J.B., and Ruiter, A.: The effect of various intakes of ω3 fatty acids on the blood lipid composition in healthy human subjects. Am. J. Clin. Nutr. 34:1752, 1981.

76. Goodnight, S.H., Harris, W.S., and Connor, W.E.: The effects of dietary ω3 fatty acids on platelet composition and function in man: a prospective, controlled study. Blood 58:880, 1981.

77. Acheson, R.M., and O'Brien, W.M.: Dependence of serum uric acid on hemoglobin and other factors in the general population. Lancet 2:777, 1966.

78. Hall, A.P., Barry, P.E., Dawber, T.R., and McNamara, P.M.: Epidemiology of gout and hyperuricemia. A long-term population study. Am. J. Med. 42:27, 1967.

79. Nicholls, A., and Scott, J.T.: Effect of weight-loss on plasma and urinary levels of uric acid. Lancet 2:1223, 1972.

80. Lecoq, F.R., and McPhaul, J.J.: The effects of starvation, high fat diets and ketone infusions on uric acid balance. Metabolism 14:186, 1965.

81. Kellgren, J.H.: Osteoarthrosis in patients and populations. Br. Med. J. 2:1, 1961.

Section II
General Approach to the Patient

Chapter 23
General Approach to the Rheumatic Disease Patient

James F. Fries

INTRODUCTION

The intrinsic nature of the rheumatic diseases poses an ultimate challenge to the skill and humanity of the managing physician. The chronicity of disease processes, their variability, their tendency to exacerbate and remit, their biochemical and immunologic complexity, their unknown pathogenesis, their variable response to specific treatment, and the myriad ways in which the diseases affect the patient's life style, family relationships, self-image, and employability combine to complicate the therapeutic equation. Complex therapeutic decisions must be made for the most part without adequate experimental justification and evaluated against a poorly understood natural history.

Within the complicated mixture of fact and opinion which constitutes the literature of rheumatic disease lies a strategy which forms the basis for contemporary management of the rheumatic disease patient. Essentially, this strategy requires quite simply that the rheumatic disease patient be treated as an individual and that therapeutic decisions be based upon individual circumstances.[1,2] Further, decisions are modified in a continuing feedback between application of treatment and observed response. Decisions evolve and change with time as appropriate to the trends, tempo, and previous response of the disease in the particular patient. The broad principles underlying this strategy are set forth in this chapter. Despite the generalizations required by this topic, it is hoped that the reader will find a structure which will aid in understanding the specific chapters to follow.

In the old view, arthritis was a single disease, about which "nothing much could be done" and for which aspirin was the best, perhaps the only, medication. The inadequacy of this perception should be too obvious to merit mention, but even today it is shared by large segments of the lay community, a surprising number of physicians in practice, and many members of policy-making political bodies. Its lingering effects are found in hospitals whose laboratories offer an "arthritis profile" and in management approaches based upon monolithic "pyramids." The following paragraphs develop an approach to selective individualized management based upon six major management questions.

WHAT IS WRONG WITH THIS PATIENT?

Diagnosis in the rheumatic diseases has been overemphasized. On the one hand, current classifications frequently contain patients with features of several diagnostic entities, often termed "overlap" patients, with no absolute diagnosis possible. On the other hand, patients with the same diagnosis often should be managed very differently. Modern management individualizes therapy within diagnostic categories, based upon subgroups of patients with differing prognoses and therapeutic requirements.

Management in the rheumatic diseases is more closely linked to the underlying pathophysiologic process than to the specific disease entity. Simple decision aphorisms, such as, "Do not use an anti-inflammatory agent if there is no evidence of inflammation," can be obscured by excessive reliance upon a link between diagnostic category and treatment. Even such a basic concept as "inflammation" has different therapeutic implications, depending upon the underlying pathophysiology. The inflamed synovial membrane typical of rheumatoid arthritis responds to a different spectrum of anti-inflammatory agents than does the inflammation of ligamentous insertions typical of ankylosing spondylitis, or the inflammation within the joint space induced by crystals.

Eight specific types of musculoskeletal pathology are distinguished by history and physical examination in most patients[3] and provide a framework for pathophysiologic categorization. These categories are not entirely mutually exclusive, but correct categorization of the predominant pathophysiology in a given patient is usually straightforward. The eight categories are discussed below and are listed in Table 23–1, together with the prototype disease of the category, examples of the most useful laboratory tests for that category, and typical treatments required. The management implications for each category are surprisingly distinct, and provide guidelines for the ordering of laboratory investigations and the selection of initial treatment.

Synovitis. Inflammation of the synovial membrane with eventual damage to surrounding joint structures is most strikingly manifested in the disease rheumatoid arthritis. The synovium is tender, thickened, and palpable, and often may demonstrate heat and, less often, redness. Joint destruction is presumed to be caused by the enzymatic products of inflammation and may occur slowly over many years. Management is based upon reducing the inflammation and thereby reducing the rate of damage to joint structures. In the laboratory, the sedimentation rate is consistently elevated with significant synovitis, and the latex fixation or other tests for rheumatoid arthritis are often useful for further categorization. A wide range of pharmacologic and other treatments may be required, and many patients require sequential trial with a variety of agents. Some useful drugs, such as gold, penicillamine, and hydroxychloroquine, appear to be therapeutically ineffective in any other disease category, and others, such as aspirin, find their greatest use here.

Enthesopathy. Inflammation here is most marked at the enthesis, that transition region where ligament attaches to bone.[4] Such inflammation is the hallmark of a family of rheumatic diseases of which the most common is ankylosing spondylitis. The distribution of musculoskeletal involvement follows the location of regions of enthesis throughout the body. The marked predilection for the sacroiliac joints, heels, and spine illustrates involvement of areas characterized by ligament and tendon attachment rather than synovium. This pathophysiology has been recognized only in the last several years and provides a unifying observation upon which to base the observed clinical features of the diseases and their typical response to specific therapy. Nonsteroidal anti-inflammatory agents, in particular indomethacin, phenylbutazone, and naproxen, are therapeutically effective and are well tolerated over the long term. The spectrum of effective anti-inflammatory drugs is different from that used for synovitis.

Cartilage Degeneration. Degenerative and other processes can cause fraying and destruction of the articular cartilage, with injury to the underlying subchondral bone. This occurrence is usually termed osteoarthritis or osteoarthrosis, and a group of specific syndromes is recognized within this category. Narrowing of the apparent joint space and development of spurs make radiography the most useful investigation; other laboratory aids are predictably negative. Few patients have significant inflammation, and it is not surprising that anti-inflammatory treatment is not frequently useful. The analgesic effects of aspirin or nonsteroidal anti-inflammatory agents may be helpful; doses required for optimal effect are often considerably less than doses required for anti-inflammatory effects with the same compound. Treatment is symptomatic and seldom dramatically effective.

Crystal-Induced Synovitis. Microcrystalline arthritis occurs when crystals forming in the synovial fluid (or injected therein) induce an inflammatory reaction in the joint fluid and the surrounding synovium. Gout is the prototypic disease, with inflammation induced by crystals of sodium urate. Similar syndromes may occur with crystals of several other types. The rapid, acute inflammatory response creates a rather sudden onset, increasing to very intense inflammation within a period of hours, with slow resolution without treatment over a period of a few days to a few weeks. The physical factors underlying crystal formation ensure that only one or at most a few joints are involved at a time. The crucial laboratory observation is inspection of aspirated joint fluid for crystals under polarized light. Drugs inhibiting the mobilization of polymorphonuclear leukocytes are particularly effective, as exemplified by colchicine, a drug with little effect in any other rheumatic disease category.

Joint Infection. The synovium encloses a body space that can be the site of direct infection by microorganisms. Critical to investigation of the patient with suspected joint infection are aspiration and culture of the joint fluid and, in many instances, culture of other body fluids as well. Treatment, obviously, consists of a specific antibiotic.

Myositis. Inflammation of muscle occurs in two closely related diseases, dermatomyositis and polymyositis, and in a distant relative, polymyalgia rheumatica. Determination of muscle enzymes and histologic examination of involved muscle are the critical labora-

Table 23–1. Categories of Rheumatic Disease

Pathology	Prototype	Most Useful Tests	Typical Treatment
Synovitis	Rheumatoid arthritis	Latex, erythrocyte sedimentation rate	Acetylsalicylic acid, gold
Enthesopathy	Ankylosing spondylitis	Sacroiliac radiographs, B27	Indomethacin
Cartilage degeneration	Osteoarthritis	Radiographs of affected areas	Analgesic
Crystal-induced synovitis	Gout	Joint fluid crystal examination	Colchicine
Joint infection	Staphylococcal	Joint fluid culture	Antibiotics
Myositis	Dermatomyositis	Muscle enzymes, muscle biopsy	Corticosteroids
Focal conditions	Tennis elbow	None, radiographs of affected area	Localized
Generalized conditions	Fibrositis	Erythrocyte sedimentation rate	Conservative

tory observations. In polymyalgia, the sedimentation rate separates this disease from the final category below. Corticosteroids are almost always required and, in contrast to every other rheumatic disease category, are usually required at the outset.

Focal Conditions. A wide variety of conditions affecting the musculoskeletal system do not truly warrant the term "disease." Tendinitis, bursitis, low back strain, calcific tendinitis, and a variety of others can affect almost any area of the body and are among the most common medical problems of the population. Laboratory aids are few, although radiography may be occasionally useful in locating calcium deposits or spurs. The therapeutic approach, unfortunately often neglected, is to apply localized treatment measures. Treatment of the entire organism when the problem exists only in one small area is seldom rewarding. Splints, slings, heat, or local injection constitutes the most reasonable initial approach.

Generalized Conditions. A variety of poorly defined entities fall into this poorly defined category. Terms such as "fibrositis" or the "chronic muscle contraction syndrome" are sometimes used to indicate the likelihood of organic disease. The terms "psychogenic rheumatism" or "nonarticular rheumatism" or "depressive equivalent" are frequently used to suggest an emotional component to such complaints. These patients are rich in symptoms but poor in objective pathology. The conditions may be extremely troublesome for the individual but are not progressive and do not result in physical crippling. Laboratory aids, such as the sedimentation rate, are normal and are employed only to rule out other categories. Treatment is best termed "conservative." The therapeutic approaches listed for other categories are unlikely to help, and the physician who attempts major pharmacologic intervention rather than reassurance, life style counseling, and support often ends up with a drug-dependent patient who gets no better.

These eight categories and the brief descriptions above are supported by generalizations that will find some exceptions. However, Table 23–1 suggests quite specific directions in which laboratory investigation and the therapeutic approach may begin. The experienced physician will soon move far beyond this table, but it has provided for us an extraordinarily useful framework upon which to build the clinical knowledge of the young physician.

WHAT INVESTIGATIONS, IF ANY, ARE REQUIRED?

One in six visits by a patient to a health professional is for a musculoskeletal complaint.[3] The great majority of such physician visits occur for the category of "focal conditions" and do not pose a major hazard to the health of the patient. The overwhelming majority of such complaints are easily identified as self-limited. Optimal management includes the ruling out of significant illness, advice about activity or rest, reassurance, occasionally symptomatic medication, and transmission of the ex-

pectation that the natural healing process will resolve the difficulty. The usual healing period for minor musculoskeletal problems requires 2 to 6 weeks, depending on the magnitude of the often inapparent injury, with the healing process beginning again from the start if there is reinjury during this period. Healing cannot be pharmacologically accelerated. Thus, optimal treatment requires "masterly inactivity," with confident reliance upon the natural healing process. Inappropriate management can lead to investigative mishaps, therapeutic side reactions, and an intensity of focus upon the problem entirely inappropriate to its magnitude.

Ulysses, it is said, went off to fight the Trojan War. Battle completed, he attempted to return home but found it necessary to pass through a series of dramatic crises and often unpleasant adventures in order finally, after 20 years, to arrive once again at his starting point. The "Ulysses syndrome" in medicine consists of a series of adverse events stemming from a procedure or a therapy that should never have been undertaken, and sometimes requiring heroic measures just to get back to the starting point. The careful rheumatic disease clinician uses *time* to establish the trends and tempo of the condition in the individual, and to remove the self-limited condition from the hazard of inappropriate response.

A critical clinical decision, therefore, is whether the problem requires immediate investigation and action, or whether the decision to investigate or treat can be postponed with profit until the course of the disease and the magnitude of the appropriate response may be better estimated.[5]

The algorithm of Figure 23–1 displays the major con-

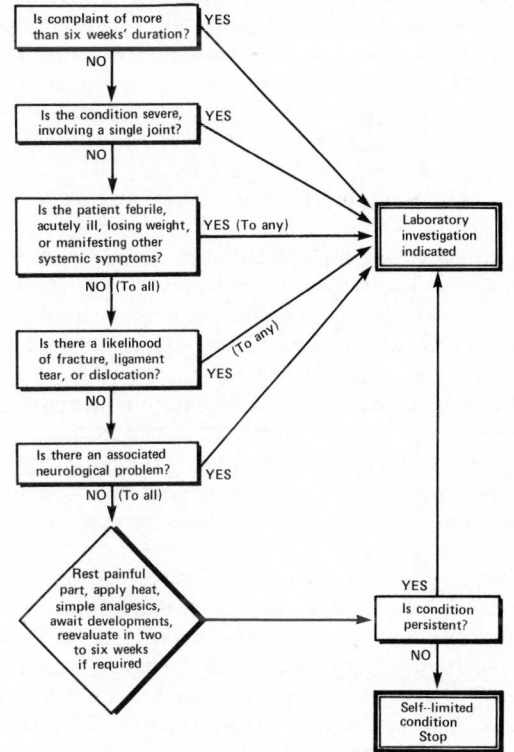

Figure 23–1. The initial approach to the patient.

siderations that determine the need for immediate investigation. Chronicity is the most frequent indication for more elaborate investigation and management. For most complaints, an observation period of approximately 6 weeks is appropriate. Four major exceptions obtain. First, a condition that is severe and involves a single joint or at most a few joints is much more likely, paradoxically, to require immediate attention than is a widespread arthritis. Acute gouty arthritis and infections of the joint space each require immediate attention. In contrast, in rheumatoid arthritis a period of 6 weeks is required before the criteria for diagnosis can even be met, and management in the first days of disease is most appropriately conservative. Many "possible rheumatoid arthritis" patients or patients with a "rheumatoid arthritis-like" illness will have minor problems that disappear as the viral or minor hypersensitivity reaction subsides.

Second, a patient who is febrile, systemically ill, and otherwise showing signs of major disease of multiple organs deserves immediate attention. Endocarditis, neoplasm, tuberculosis, and other major illnesses are frequently identified at this stage through musculoskeletal clues, and a connective tissue disease with systemic manifestations deserves immediate attention. Third, if the problem is associated with significant trauma, the possible need for immediate orthopedic management should be considered. And fourth, an associated neurologic problem such as carpal tunnel syndrome, sciatic nerve pain radiation, or cervical nerve root compression syndromes is benefited by immediate attention. These indications are relatively unusual in practice. When this algorithm is applied, the large majority of patients with initial complaints of "joint pain" or "arthritis" will be found not to have serious conditions requiring immediate evaluation.

WHAT ARE THE GOALS OF MANAGEMENT FOR THIS PATIENT?

With increasing sophistication in laboratory aids and biochemical knowledge, there has been a tendency for management goals to be defined in terms of easily measured, numerically expressed test results. The level of autoantibodies, titer of rheumatoid factor, number of radiographic erosions, and sedimentation rate have often become the criteria for therapeutic success. Such measurements of medical process have value only to the extent that they correlate with illness perceived eventually by the patient, and unfortunately the correlations in each instance are poor.

The patient and the patient's family are more directly interested in survival, in normal mobility and function, in absence from pain and other symptoms, in freedom of toxicity from the therapeutic regimen, and in the ability to remain solvent through the duration of a chronic disease. ARAMIS (The American Rheumatism Association Medical Information System) and several

multipurpose arthritis centers have recently employed the five "D's" (death, disability, discomfort, drug toxicity, and dollar cost) as dimensions for describing patient outcome (Fig. 23-2). The disability dimension is meant to include psychological disability as well as physical, and the discomfort dimension to include functional symptoms as well as physical ones.[6] Carefully validated instruments, usually self-administered patient questionnaires, now allow accurate and reproducible measurement of the "quality of life" dimensions.[7] New patient record formats allow serial notation of these values over time. Figure 23-3A and B reproduces the disability and pain sections of the Health Assessment Questionnaire (HAQ) of the Stanford Arthritis Center together with scoring conventions.[7]

Patients have very individual preferences for the values which they place upon one outcome dimension relative to others. Thus, a treatment strategy expected to minimize disability but with a small potential hazard of iatrogenic death will be embraced enthusiastically by some patients and shunned by others. In some disease areas, such as oncology, the single outcome dimension of death suffices to dominate most clinical decisions. In the rheumatic diseases, value trade-offs between outcome dimensions must be predicated upon the values of the patient after informed explanation, with the expectation that these values will not always perfectly match the physician's view.[8]

The setting of goals logically must precede development of the individual management strategy.[9] In some instances a limited goal, such as regaining the ability to walk, may be dramatically useful to the patient and far more valuable than a modest reduction in the general severity of the disease. Some very worthy goals may not be achievable in the particular instance, and their pursuit will only increase the dimension of therapeutic toxicity. The question "What is desirable?" is subordinate to "What is achievable?" for the individual patient.

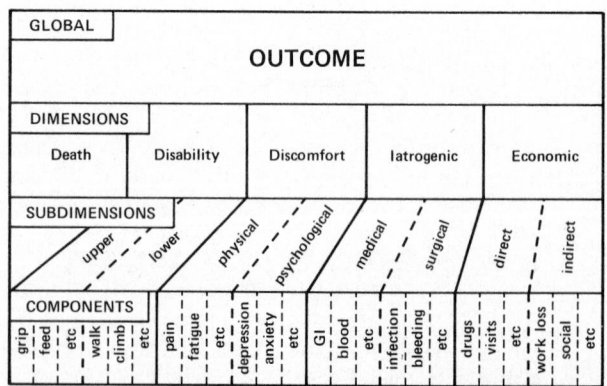

Figure 23-2. Conceptualization of "outcome" as a hierarchy of dimensions, subdimensions, and components which collectively include all patient concerns allows particular observations to be placed in the context of other relevant events, provides perspective on the role of a specific assessment, and permits the investigator to select appropriate measures for each study while maintaining some comparability with the results of others.

OVER WHAT TIME PERIOD SHOULD THE GOALS BE ACHIEVED?

A chronic disease can be psychologically as well as physically devastating, and the difficulties of adjustment are difficult to overstate. In general, management strategies are designed to provide the most favorable outcomes across each outcome dimension, and also along the time dimension representing the duration of the illness. Frequently, agents dramatically effective over the short term are available. Corticosteroids, narcotic analgesics, and intra-articular injections often have this characteristic. Unfortunately, the agent that provides the best initial response may not provide the best long-term outcome.

The experienced clinician spends a great deal of time discussing with the patient the time period for response as well as the expected magnitude of response. In general, simple and nontoxic measures are used first and hazardous medications withheld unless the simpler approaches fail. But the individual patient frequently poses special considerations requiring modification of such rational progressions. Thus, the tempo of disease may be such that serious joint destruction appears likely over a short period of months and the therapeutic progression thus requires acceleration. A major therapeutic attempt with an agent such as gold, penicillamine, or an immunosuppressant may require many months until the expected date of response; meanwhile, the patient may have exhausted sick leave, leading to a forced retirement because of disability. Additional use of a more immediately effective agent, such as prednisone, might well be indicated under such circumstances. In a patient of advanced age, concern about eventual hazard of malignancy secondary to a drug might well be smaller. In a vigorous and active male patient, concern about corticosteroid osteopenia over long administration of such a drug might be less. In a young patient, the expectation for patient outcome might be integrated over 20 to 30 years. In the older patient, both the risks and the benefits of treatment might be reduced, but not by the same amount. Again, the necessity for the individual program is seen.

The inexperienced clinician is often trapped by taking the short view of a chronic illness. The quack practitioner more intentionally follows the strategy of attempting to maximize immediate benefits at the expense of future problems. A chronic disease cannot be managed by tactics; it requires a long-term strategy, shared and negotiated with the patient.

This strategy requires tactical modification at nearly every physician-patient encounter. At each visit, new information is always present, even if it is only the information about what has transpired in response to the last set of decisions. Decision is thus followed by observation, then by further decision, and then by another period of observation. The decision strategy is flexible and, in the final analysis, frequently empiric.

WHAT THERAPEUTIC STRATEGY IS MOST LIKELY TO ACHIEVE THE GOALS?

Treatment is frequently discussed only in terms of available pharmacologic agents. This myopic view neglects the dominant contributions often afforded by reconstructive surgical procedures, by the use of appliances and devices to allow handicapped individuals to function more normally, or by personal interaction designed to increase the motivation and self-image of the patient.

A drug-based strategy tends to find its greatest use in early, systemic, inflammatory disease processes. Orthopedic approaches tend to have greatest utility if the number of joints or regions involved is small, if major problems are concentrated in a single anatomic region, or if the inflammatory process has "burned out." Improvement after occupational therapy intervention is often seen in individuals with moderate to major disability who require adaptive devices to render the environment somewhat more friendly. The will of the patient to live normally sometimes can be more important to outcome than any specific therapy. Indeed, medical therapy that interferes with mental or emotional adaptation frequently appears to make things worse.

The novice at managing rheumatic diseases employs only a limited therapeutic repertoire. Typically, the patient requires a diverse program individualized to specific needs and frequently making use of a variety of individuals and skills in the community as well as within the medical establishment. Development of rational strategies requires intimate knowledge of the strengths and weaknesses of all available therapeutic modalities. The physician cannot manage rheumatic disease patients effectively without having either direct knowledge of community resources and the techniques of adjacent disciplines or a good working relationship and individuals who possess these skills.

DOES THE PATIENT UNDERSTAND ENOUGH TO ACHIEVE THE GOALS?

The partnership between physician and patient, often eulogized but seldom practiced, is of particular importance in management of a difficult chronic disease. The informed patient brings tremendous strength to the therapeutic encounter. Transmission of knowledge about the disease process to the patient, appropriately individualized to the particular situation, is a therapeutic imperative.[10]

Consider some of the outside factors that operate if the partnership is not well established and the patient is told to take aspirin. Frequent reports in the lay media describe the hazards of aspirin, advertisements suggest that you don't need a doctor for aspirin, colloquialisms associate aspirin with neglect on the part of the physi-

HEALTH ASSESSMENT QUESTIONNAIRE

OFFICE USE ONLY

Name _____

Date _____

TOR NO: _____

In this section we are interested in learning how your illness affects your ability to function in daily life. Please feel free to add any comments on the back of this page.

- **Please check the one response which best describes your usual abilities OVER THE PAST WEEK:**

	Without ANY Difficulty	With SOME Difficulty	With MUCH Difficulty	UNABLE To Do
					(246) _____

DRESSING & GROOMING

Are you able to:
—Dress yourself, including tying shoelaces and doing buttons?

—Shampoo your hair?

ARISING   (217) _____

Are you able to:
—Stand up from an armless straight chair?

—Get in and out of bed?

EATING   (235) _____

Are you able to:
—Cut your meat?

—Lift a full cup or glass to your mouth?

—Open a new milk carton?

WALKING   (220) _____

Are you able to:
—Walk outdoors on flat ground?

—Climb up five steps?

- **Please check any AIDS OR DEVICES that you usually use for any of these activities:**

_____ Cane

_____ Walker

_____ Crutches

_____ Wheelchair

_____ Devices Used for Dressing (button hook, zipper pull, long-handled shoe horn, etc.)

_____ Built Up or Special Utensils

_____ Special or Built Up Chair

_____ Other (Specify: _____)

- **Please check any categories for which you usually need HELP FROM ANOTHER PERSON:**

_____ Dressing and Grooming

_____ Arising

_____ Eating

_____ Walking

– 1 –   Stanford Arthritis Center Disability and Discomfort Scales, 1981

Figure 23–3. *A*, Page 1, The Health Assessment Questionnaire (HAO), Disability Dimension. *B*, Page 2, Disability and Pain Dimensions. Columns are scored 0, 1, 2, 3, and are parallel in structure to ARA Functional Class scores of I, II, III, and IV. The highest score for each component is used. A notation of use of aids, devices, or help from another requires a minimal score of 2 for the corresponding component. Component scores are added, then divided by 8 in order to calculate the Disability Index.

OFFICE USE ONLY

● Please check the one response which best describes your usual abilities OVER THE PAST WEEK:

	Without ANY Difficulty	With SOME Difficulty	With MUCH Difficulty	UNABLE To Do

(251) _____

HYGIENE

Are you able to:
—Wash and dry your entire body?

—Take a tub bath?

—Get on and off the toilet?

REACH (210) _____

Are you able to:
—Reach and get down a 5 pound object (such as a bag of sugar) from just above your head?

—Bend down to pick up clothing from the floor?

GRIP (216) _____

Are you able to:
—Open car doors?

—Open jars which have been previously opened?

—Turn faucets on and off?

ACTIVITIES (368) _____

Are you able to:
—Run errands and shop?

—Get in and out of a car?

—Do chores such as vacuuming or yardwork?

● Please check any AIDS OR DEVICES that you usually use for any of these activities:

_____ Raised Toilet Seat　　　　　_____ Bathtub Bar

_____ Bathtub Seat　　　　　　　_____ Long-Handled Appliances for Reach

_____ Jar Opener (for jars previously opened)　_____ Long-Handled Appliances in Bathroom

　　　　　　　　　　　　　　　_____ Other (Specify _____)

● Please check any categories for which you usually need HELP FROM ANOTHER PERSON:

_____ Hygiene　　　　　　　　　_____ Gripping and Opening Things

_____ Reach　　　　　　　　　　_____ Errands and Chores

We are also interested in learning whether or not you are affected by pain because of your illness.

● How much pain have you had because of your illness IN THE PAST WEEK ? (700) _____

PLACE A MARK ON THE LINE TO INDICATE THE SEVERITY OF THE PAIN

NO PAIN　　　　　　　　　　　　　　　　　　　　　VERY SEVERE PAIN

├───┤

0　　　　　　　　　　　　　　　　　　　　　　　　100

— 2 —　Stanford Arthritis Center Disability and Discomfort Scales, 1981 cian, and the lack of requirement for prescription suggests a minor and ineffective remedy. For anti-inflammatory treatment with aspirin the physician may aim for a rather narrow therapeutic range just below toxicity and far above the doses to which the public is accustomed. During the establishment of dosage the patient is almost certain to run into one or another side effect even though the drug later may be well tolerated over the long term. The informed patient must know that anti-inflammatory and analgesic activities of aspirin are different, that a particular therapeutic range is desired, that the drug will be active against the inflammatory process itself, that many weeks may be required to see the full effects of the drug, and so forth. In the absence of such information, it is extremely unusual for a patient to do well on acetylsalicylic acid; patient education becomes a prerequisite for therapeutic success.

The patient with arthritis is under intense psychologic pressures. Self-image is threatened by diseases that may cripple or prevent remunerative employment. The possibility of dependence upon others in the future is often present. The patient's expectations for the future are frequently drawn from the most unfortunate individuals whom the patient has encountered. Recognition that every patient with arthritis has significant fears is essential to good management. Direct discussion of expectation is essential. For the most part, positive expectations are the most realistic. Only 15 per cent of patients with rheumatoid arthritis, for example, actually experience severe "crippling," and many of these instances are probably preventable. A patient should almost never be told to expect to become housebound, wheelchair bound, or bedridden. The expectation for gradually increasing disease activity is likewise unfortunate, since the disease activity will usually subside, even after many years. Most clinicians believe that the patient with positive expectations comes to a better outcome. While direct inference of causality is not warranted from this association, it is reasonable to assume as an operational principle that restoration of hope and a positive self-image are beneficial therapeutic adjuncts.

The informed patient is more likely to comply with a particular therapeutic regimen and will report more reliably the effects, good or bad, of that regimen. The physician making a series of clinical decisions with the patient over a long period is heavily influenced by the patient's report of success or failure with a previous regimen. This report must be as accurate as possible, and the accuracy depends upon the directness of the patient-physician communication.

Advice for living is frequently requested of the physician. While it is well known that splinting, hospitali-

zation, bed rest, and other techniques of resting inflamed joints decrease inflammation temporarily, it is not clear that these effects persist beyond the period of rest. Costs incurred by such treatment in terms of muscle wasting, osteopenia, and loss of social image detract from the temporary gain. As a general rule, we find employment preferred to disability retirement by our patients, and attempt in the therapeutic relationship to guide the patient into activities consistent with a normal or nearly normal life.

Unrealistic expectations and inadequate patient education are probably the major causes of a burgeoning business in quack treatment of arthritis. The charlatan promises a quick and easy response to a difficult and chronic disease. The patient must be armed to recognize the intrinsic falsity of such superficially attractive claims and the losses in courage, independence, and money that may result. The obscenity of the quack who makes a living by defrauding patients with arthritis focuses the attention of most physicians upon the outrage. At a more basic level, however, the patient susceptible to the claims of the quack does not have a confident and informed relationship with his personal physician.

We do not like to think of patients with arthritis as "victims." Illness of some type at some point is a universal human occurrence. The various forms of arthritis may be worse than some illnesses and less bad than others. The repressed hostility emanating from "Why did this have to happen to me?" is not constructive to an optimal life adjustment. Most persons with arthritis are independent and healthy despite the arthritis. This independence is the final goal of the individualized management strategy.

References

1. Urowitz, M.B.: SLE subsets—divide and conquer. J. Rheumatol. 4:332, 1977.
2. Fries, J.F., and Holman, H.R.: Systemic Lupus Erythematosus: A Clinical Analysis. Philadelphia, W.B. Saunders Company, 1975.
3. Fries, J.F., and Mitchell, D.M.: Joint pain or arthritis. JAMA 235:199, 1976.
4. Calin, A.C., and Fries, J.F.: Ankylosing Spondylitis; Discussions in Patient Management. Garden City, N.Y., Medical Examination Publishing Company, 1978.
5. Vickery, D.F., and Fries, J.F.: Take Care of Yourself: A Consumer's Guide to Medical Care. Reading, Massachusetts, Addison-Wesley Publishing Company, 1976.
6. Fries, J.F.: Education for outcome. J. Rheumatol. 5:1, 1978.
7. Fries, J.F.: Toward an understanding of patient outcome measurement. Arthritis Rheum. 26:697–704, 1983.
8. Murphy, E.A.: The Logic of Medicine. Baltimore, Johns Hopkins University Press, 1976.
9. Feinstein, A.R.: Clinical Judgment. Baltimore, Waverly Press, 1967.
10. Tumulty, P.A.: The Effective Clinician. Philadelphia, W.B. Saunders Company, 1973.

Chapter 24
Examination of the Joints

Clement J. Michet and Gene G. Hunder

HISTORY IN THE PATIENT WITH MUSCULOSKELETAL DISEASE

A detailed description of symptoms related to the musculoskeletal system will provide much of the information necessary to making a diagnosis. The goal of the interview is to understand precisely what the patient means by what is said about symptoms. In obtaining a history of the patient's illness the physician must probe for details of the sequence and severity of symptoms and patterns of progression, exacerbation, or remission. The effects of the previous therapy, associated diseases, and stress must be elucidated. The impact of the disease on the patient must be defined.

The effects of current or previous therapy on the course of the illness are important. Frequently, these are not volunteered by the patient. Assessment of compliance is extremely important; even an ideal therapeutic regimen will fail if the patient does not comply with the outlined program.

The patient's behavior usually provides clues to the nature of the illness and the patient's response to it. It is important to determine whether the patient is reacting appropriately to an illness or is overly concerned or has ignored the joint symptoms. The patient's understanding of his illness will affect his response to it.

Pain. Pain is the complaint that most commonly brings the patient with musculoskeletal disease to the physician. Pain is a complex subjective sensation that is often difficult to define, explain, or measure. It has different meanings to different people and even to the same person at different times. Response to pain is affected by the patient's current emotional status as well as previous experiences, including observations of others in pain.

Pain must be localized anatomically. If the pain is in a joint, an articular disorder is likely to be present. Pain between joints may suggest bone or muscle disease or referred pain. Pain in bursal areas, fascial planes, or along tendons, ligaments, or nerve distributions suggests disease in these structures. Pain arising from deeper structures is often less focal than pain originating from superficial tissues. Pain in small joints of the hand or feet tends to be more accurately localized than pain in larger more proximal joints such as the shoulder, hip, or spine. Pain from the hip joint, for example, may be felt in the groin, buttock, or over the greater trochanter or referred to the anterior portion of the thigh or knee. When pain is diffuse, variable, poorly described, or unrelated to anatomic structures, a functional problem or fibromyalgia may be suspected.

Although variable from one patient to another, the character of the pain often helps in understanding the patient's illness. For example, "aching" in a joint area suggests an arthritic disorder, whereas "burning" or "prickling" in an extremity may indicate a neuropathy. An "intolerable" or "excruciating" pain in a patient who otherwise is able to carry out normal activities suggests that emotional factors may be amplifying symptoms.

The presence or absence of pain at rest usually helps the evaluation. Joint pain present both at rest and with movement is more suggestive of an inflammatory process, whereas pain mainly or only during motion often indicates a mechanical disorder such as degenerative arthritis or traumatic arthritis. However, many patients with more advanced degenerative joint disease of the hip or spine also have pain at night.

Swelling. An important finding in rheumatic diseases is swelling. Patients vary in their perception of swelling and ability to describe it. The interviewer needs to determine where and when the swelling occurs; it is helpful to learn whether the swelling is visible to others. Description of the exact location of the swelling helps in understanding whether the swelling conforms to an anatomically discrete area such as a particular joint, bursa, or other specific extra-articular area. An obese person may interpret normal collections of adipose tissue over the medial aspects of the elbow or knee and lateral aspect of the ankle as swellings.

Information about the onset, persistence, and influencing factors help define the nature of the swelling. Discomfort with use of the swollen part may indicate synovitis or bursitis because of tension on these tissues during motion of a joint. However, when inflamed tissues are not put under stress during joint movement, pain is minimal; for example, movement of the knee is generally painless in cases of prepatellar bursitis. Swelling in a confined area such as a synovial sac or bursa is most painful when it has developed acutely. In such instances, even light palpation may be intolerable. In chronic swelling when the synovial sac has stretched or when the distention has developed gradually, pain is generally less severe.

Limitation of Motion. Patients with rheumatic disorders frequently complain of limitation of motion. Determination of the extent of disability resulting from lack of motion is important. The length of time restrictions of motion have been present can be helpful in predicting reversibility of the disability. It is helpful also to know whether the limitation of motion began abruptly, as with a tendon rupture or onset of psychogenic episode, or gradually as in slowly progressive inflammatory disease.

Stiffness. Stiffness is a word that has different meanings to different patients. Some equate it with pain or fatigue; others equate it with soreness, weakness or restrictions of movement; and still others use the term without being able to tell clearly what they feel. Most rheumatologists define stiffness as discomfort perceived by the patient attempting to move joints after a period of inactivity. When it occurs, stiffness or "gelling" usually develops after inactivity of one or more hours. Mild stiffness may resolve within a few minutes. When severe, as in rheumatoid arthritis or polymyalgia rheumatica, the stiffness may improve only over one to several hours.

Morning stiffness can be a prodromal symptom of arthritis, and it is a criterion of the American Rheumatism Association for the diagnosis of rheumatoid arthritis. (See Chapter 60.) It should be differentiated from the discomfort associated with movement of a mechanically damaged joint. Morning stiffness associated with noninflammatory joint diseases is almost always of short duration, usually less than one-half hour, and of less severity than stiffness of inflammatory joint disease. In addition, in mechanical, degenerative, or other destructive joint disease, the degree of stiffness is related to the extent of overuse of the damaged joint and responds usually within a few days to adequate limitation of the use of the affected joint. In degenerative joint disease stiffness may be more noticeable during the day after resting an hour or more than it is in the morning.

The absence of stiffness does not exclude the possibility of the presence of systemic inflammatory rheumatic diseases such as rheumatoid arthritis, but its absence is uncommon. Stiffness from neurologic disorders of the Parkinsonism type, without a recognized inflammatory basis, also occurs and sometimes is conspicuous, although the "limbering up" component is lacking.

Weakness. When present, a loss of motor power or muscular strength is nearly always objectively demonstrable during the examination, at least in relation to what a patient was formerly able to do. True weakness can be noted only when muscles are actively being used. In musculoskeletal disorders weakness is usually persistent rather than intermittent. Muscle weakness as a result of inflammatory myopathies occurs typically in proximal portions of the extremities, whereas weakness caused by most neuropathies is found in a distal or peripheral parts.

Fatigue. A common and important complaint of many patients with musculoskeletal disease, fatigue is nonetheless an imprecise term. It can be defined as an inclination to rest even though pain and weakness are not limiting factors. It implies exhaustion and depletion of energy. Fatigue is a normal phenomenon after variable degrees of activity but resolves after rest. In rheumatic diseases fatigue may be prominent even when the patient has not been active physically. If the arthritis improves, fatigue tends to lessen. In the absence of organic disease, anxiety and muscular tension or related emotional states are prominent factors in producing chronic fatigue. Patients with an inflammatory arthritis may complain of weakness when they are experiencing stiffness. The differentiation from stiffness and weakness may be facili-

tated by remembering that stiffness is a discomfort during movement and weakness is an inability to move normally against resistance. Fatigue may be sensed when the patient is resting and is an aversion to activity.

CLASSIFICATION OF THE JOINTS

Joints are of three main types: synarthroses (immobile articulations), such as suture joints between the bones of the skull; amphiarthroses (slightly movable joints), such as those between the vertebral bodies and the inferior tibial-fibular articulation; and diarthroses (freely movable articulations), such as the knee.

Diarthrodial joints are the most common joints of the body and damage to them by disease causes most disability. The articulating ends of the bones forming a diarthrodial joint are covered by cartilage and are enclosed in a capsule of fibrous tissue (Fig. 24–1). The structure and physiology of diarthrodial joints are discussed in detail in Chapter 16.

Diarthrodial joints have been classified further according to the shapes of the surfaces that articulate. The shape of the articulating surface along with the supporting ligaments determines the type and the extent of motion in the joint. *Plane joints* allow only gliding movements. Articular surfaces of this type of joint are planar or flat or slightly curved. Carpal and tarsal joints are of this type. *Spheroidal joints*, also called ball and socket joints, are formed by the articulation of a rounded convex surface with a cuplike cavity. The distal bone is thus capable of a wide variety of movements, including rotation and circumduction. The shoulder and hip joint are examples of spheroidal joints. *Cotylic joints* are sim-

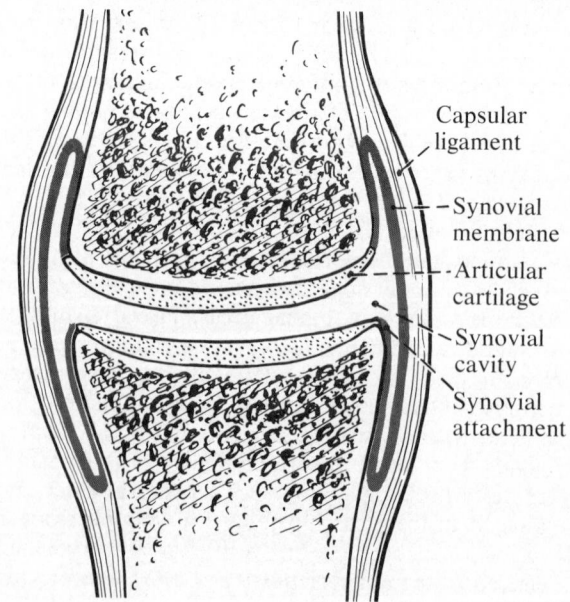

Figure 24–1. Schematic diagram of a diathrodial joint. (From Polley, H.F., and Hunder, G.G.: Rheumatologic Interviewing and Physical Examination of the Joints. Philadelphia, W.B. Saunders Company, 1978.)

Labels on figure:
Capsular ligament
Synovial membrane
Articular cartilage
Synovial cavity
Synovial attachment

ilar to spheroidal joints, but the articular surfaces resemble an ellipse rather than a circle. Movement is less free than in spheroidal joints, since rotation is not permitted. The metacarpophalangeal joints of the hand and radiocarpal joint are examples of cotylic joints. *Hinge joints* permit motion in only one plane, namely flexion and extension. Examples are interphalangeal joints of the hand and the humeral-ulnar joint. *Condylar joints* articulate by two distinct articular surfaces whose movements are not dissociable. Each of the surfaces is referred to as a condyle. The knee is an example and has two femoral condyles and two tibial condyles. *Trochoid* or *pivot joints* move in rotation only. The proximal radioulnar and atlanto-odontal (medial atlantoaxial) joints are examples. *Sellar joints* have saddle-shaped articular surfaces. All motions are permitted except axial rotation. The carpometacarpal joint of the thumb is an example.

SYSTEMIC METHOD OF EXAMINATION

As with the general physical examination, a systematic method of examining joints is the quickest and easiest way of obtaining a thorough assessment of the status of the joints. Many rheumatologists begin with the joints of the upper extremities and proceed to the joints of the trunk and lower extremity, but each examiner should establish his or her own routine. Gentle handling of tender and painful joints will enhance cooperation by the patient and allow an accurate evaluation of the joints.

Important Physical Signs of Arthritis. The general aim of the examination of the joints is to detect abnormalities in structure and function of joints. Some of the more common signs of articular disease are swelling, tenderness, limitation of motion, and instability.

Swelling. Swelling about a joint may be caused by intra-articular effusion; synovial thickening; periarticular soft tissue inflammation, such as bursitis or tendinitis; bony enlargement; or extra-articular fat pads. All need to be differentiated from each other. Familiarity with the anatomic configuration of the synovial membrane in various joints aids in differentiating soft tissue swelling due to synovitis (articular effusion or synovial thickening) from swelling of periarticular tissues. The presence of an effusion of a joint is often visible or palpable as bulging of the joint capsule. The presence of palpable fluid in a joint in the absence of immediately preceding trauma usually indicates synovitis. The normal synovial membrane is too thin to palpate, whereas the thickened synovial membrane in rheumatoid arthritis may have a "doughy" or "boggy" consistency. In some joints the extent of the synovial cavity can be delineated on physical examination by compressing the fluid into one of the extreme limits of synovial reflection. The edge of the resulting bulge may thus be palpated more easily. If this palpable edge is within the anatomic confines of the synovial membrane and disappears on release of the compression, the distention may be regarded as representing synovial effusion; if it persists, it is an indication

of a thickened synovial membrane. Reliable differentiation between synovial membrane thickening and effusion is not always possible by physical examination. Occasional intrasynovial loose bodies or fibrin clots may be palpated.

Localization of tenderness by palpation should help determine whether the reaction is intra-articular or in a periarticular structure such as a fat pad, tendon attachments, ligaments, bursae, muscles, or skin.

Limitation of Motion. Since *limitation of motion* is a common manifestation of articular disease, it is important to know the normal type and range of motion of each joint in order to detect restriction resulting from abnormalities of the joint or adjacent structures. In patients with joint disease, passive range of motion is often greater than active motion, providing the patient is relaxed during the examination. This may be due to pain, weakness, or the state of the articular or periarticular structures.

Crepitation. A palpable or audible grating or crunching sensation produced by motion, crepitation may or may not be accompanied by discomfort. Crepitation occurs when roughened articular or extra-articular surfaces are rubbed together, either by active motion or by manual compression. Fine crepitation is often palpable over joints involved by chronic inflammatory arthritis and usually indicates roughening of the opposing cartilage surfaces as a result of erosion or the presence of granulation tissue. Coarse crepitation is also due to irregularity of the cartilage surfaces caused by either inflammatory or noninflammatory arthritis. Bone-on-bone crepitus produces a higher frequency palpable and audible "squeak." Crepitation from within the joints should be differentiated from cracking sounds caused by the slipping of ligaments or tendons over bony surfaces during motion. The latter are usually less significant to the diagnosis of joint disease and may be heard over many normal joints. In scleroderma a peculiar coarse, creaking, leathery crepitation may be palpable or audible about various joints and tendon sheaths.

Deformity. A deformity is a malalignment of the joint and may occur as a bony enlargement, articular subluxation, contracture, or ankylosis in abnormal positions. Deformed joints do not function normally, usually restrict activities, and may be associated with pain when put under stressful use.

Instability. Joint instability is present when the joint has greater than normal movement in any plane. Subluxation is defined as a partial displacement of the articular surfaces with some persistent joint surface-to-surface contact, whereas a dislocated joint has lost all cartilage surface contact. Instability is best determined by supporting the joint between the examiner's two hands and stressing the adjacent bones in directions in which the normal joint does not move.

Muscle testing is covered in Chapters 18 and 27.

Recording the Joint Examination. A permanent record of examination of the joints is of importance in determining the status and following the progress of arthritic diseases. A variety of methods have been described. To avoid a cumbersome chart, suitable abbreviations for joints can be used such as TM for temporomandibular or SC for sternoclavicular. In recording the degree of swelling (S), tenderness (T), and limitation of motion (L) of a joint, a quantitative estimate of gradation based on a system of grades from 0 (normal) to 4 (highly abnormal) is convenient. The abbreviation S refers to synovial effusion, thickening, or a combination of these. Tenderness of structures other than joints should be specifically described. In the case of limitation of motion, L, grade 1 may be used to indicate about 25 percent loss of motion; grade 2, about 50 percent loss; grade 3, about 75 percent loss; and grade 4, 100 percent loss or ankylosis. In most instances, when more accuracy is desired, it is preferable to record degrees of motion in one or more joints using a goniometer. A table can be constructed with a column for each S, T, and L and the findings recorded for each joint.

A still more abbreviated, narrative form of recording the joint examination may be used, especially when a limited number of joints are involved. An example is as follows: Lt Sh S_0, T_2, L_1; Rt Wr S_2, T_2, L_1; Lt-MCP$_{1 \text{ and } 2}$ S_1, T_0, L_1; Rt knee S_1 (bulge), T_0, L_1 (lacks 10° of extension).

Alternative methods include the following: the use of a schematic skeleton with marked articulations that may be used to record the status of individual joints (Fig. 24–2); determination of the total number of tender and/ or swollen joints and the use of this number as a joint count or joint index; measurement of the size of joints

Figure 24–2. Skeleton diagram for recording joint examination findings. (From Polley, H.F., and Hunder, G.G.: Rheumatologic Interviewing and Physical Examination of the Joints. Philadelphia, W.B. Saunders Company, 1978.)

by use of a tape measure or jeweler's ring; determination of the degree of warmth by use of thermography; and measurement of the amount of tenderness by use of a dolorimeter. Grip strength can be measured by asking a patient to squeeze a partially inflated (20 mm Hg) sphygmomanometer cuff. The use of joints can be assessed by determining the speed and the ability to perform other specified coordinated functions.

EXAMINATION OF SPECIFIC JOINTS

Temporomandibular Joint. The temporomandibular joint is formed by the condyle of the mandible and the fossa of the temporal bone just anterior to the external auditory canal. It is uncommon for this joint to be visibly swollen. The joint is palpated by placing a finger just anterior to the external auditory canal and asking the patient to open and close the mouth and to move the mandible from side to side. Because of normal differences in soft tissue thickness, the presence of synovial thickness or swelling of minimal or moderate degree can be detected most easily if the synovitis is unilateral or asymmetrical. Vertical movement of the temporomandibular joint can be measured by determining the space between the upper and lower incisor teeth with the patient's mouth open maximally. This distance is normally 3 to 6 cm. Lateral movement can be determined by using incisor teeth as landmarks.

Many forms of arthritis affect the temporomandibular joints. Juvenile rheumatoid arthritis commonly affects these joints and may produce arrest of bone growth of the mandible with resultant micrognathia. Audible or palpable crepitus or clicking occur frequently in those without evidence of severe arthritis.

Cricoarytenoid Joint. The paired cricoarytenoid joints are formed by the articulation of the base of the small pyramidal arytenoid cartilage and the upper posterolateral border of the cricoid cartilage. The vocal ligaments (cords) are attached to the arytenoid cartilages. The cricoarytenoid joints are normally very mobile diarthrodial joints that move both medially and laterally and rotate during opening and closing of the vocal cords.

Examination of these joints is performed by direct or indirect laryngoscopy. Erythema, swelling, and lack of mobility during phonation may result from inflammation of the joints.

The cricoarytenoid joints may be affected in rheumatoid arthritis, trauma, and infection. Involvement in rheumatoid arthritis is more common than clinically apparent. Early symptoms include a sense of fullness or discomfort in the throat that is worse upon speaking or swallowing. Hoarseness may occur, and significant airway obstruction has been reported.

Sternoclavicular, Manubriosternal, and Sternocostal Joints. The medial ends of the clavicles articulate on each side of the sternum at its upper end to form the sternoclavicular joints. The articulations of the first ribs and the sternum (sternocostal joints) are immediately caudad. The articulation of the manubrium and body of the sternum is at the level of the attachment of the second costal cartilage to the sternum. The third through seventh sternocostal joints articulate distally along the lateral borders of the sternum. The sternoclavicular joints are the only articulations in this group that are always diarthrodial in form. The others may be amphiarthroses or synchondroses. The sternoclavicular joints are the only true points of articulation of the shoulder girdle with the trunk. These joints lie beneath the skin, and thus any synovitis is visible and easily palpated. Movement of these joints is slight and cannot be measured accurately.

Involvement of the sternoclavicular joints is common in ankylosing spondylitis, rheumatoid arthritis, and degenerative arthritis but is frequently overlooked. The sternoclavicular joint also may be the site of septic arthritis, especially in drug abusers. Tenderness of the manubriosternal or costosternal joints is much more frequent than actual swelling. Many older patients with no systemic rheumatic disorder may be found to have tender sternocostal joints or costal cartilages (costochondritis). Actual swelling of the upper costal cartilages or areas of the costochondral junctions (Tietze's syndrome) is uncommon.

Acromioclavicular Joint. The acromioclavicular joint is formed by the lateral end of the clavicle and medial margin of the acromion process of the scapula. Bony enlargement of this joint is often seen in middle-aged or older persons, but soft tissue swelling is not usually visible or palpable. Local tenderness, or pain with adduction of the arm across the front of the chest, helps pinpoint the involvement to this joint. Arthritis of the acromioclavicular joint is usually secondary to trauma lending to degenerative disease. It is not usually severely affected in rheumatoid arthritis. Movement occurs at this joint during shoulder motion, but actual measurements need not be made in the routine joint examination.

Shoulder. The glenohumeral joint is formed by the articulation of the head of the humerus and the shallow glenoid cavity of the scapula (glenoid fossa). Details of shoulder anatomy are presented in Chapter 29. Two outpouchings of synovium perforate the shoulder capsule; one contains the long head of the biceps along the bicipital groove of the humerus, and the other is located under the subscapularis tendon.

The rotator cuff of the shoulder is the term used for the broad, flat, conjoined tendons of the supraspinatus, infraspinatus, teres minor, and subscapularis muscles. Tendons of the first three muscles insert into the superior and posterolateral surface of the greater tubercle (tuberosity) of the humerus as a group. When the shoulder is passively extended, a portion of the rotator cuff moves out from under the anterolateral border of the acromion where this portion of the rotator cuff may be palpated. Alternatively, the posterior portion of the rotator cuff can be palpated inferior to the posterolateral border of the acromion when the patient adducts the arm across the chest.

The subacromial bursa lies under the acromion process and extends anterolaterally beyond the edge of the acromion under the deltoid muscle. It overlies the rotator cuff. The bursa facilitates movement of the greater tuberosity of the humerus beneath the acromion during abduction of the arm.

The shoulders should be inspected for evidence of swelling, muscular atrophy, and muscle fasciculations. Alteration of normal bony landmarks should be noted. If the shoulder is dislocated anteriorly, as is most common, the rounded lateral aspect of the shoulder is lost and it appears flattened. To cause visible distention of the articular capsule, a moderate to large effusion must be present. In such cases, distention usually occurs over the anterior aspect of the joint. Lesser effusions may be palpated by alternate ballottement of the anterior and lateral aspects of the shoulder. Large effusions of the subacromial bursa may produce a localized swelling under the deltoid that may be confused with swelling of the shoulder joint.

A systematic examination of the shoulder includes palpation of the acromioclavicular joint, rotator cuff, region of the subacromial bursa, the bicipital (intertubercular) groove, and the anterior, lateral and posterior aspects of the glenohumeral joint and articular capsule. Details of this examination in specific disease states are given in Chapter 29.

Normally motion of the shoulder and arm is a combination of shoulder girdle and shoulder joint movement. The ball and socket glenohumeral joint is capable of movement in any direction, as is the shoulder girdle on the chest wall. The overall motion of the shoulder can be assessed by moving the shoulder through a full range of motion actively or passively. Shoulder motion can be considered normal if the patient can make a full circle of the arms from the sides of the body anteriorly up over the head at 180 degrees and back down to the original position. To test glenohumeral motion, the examiner fixes the scapula with one hand or prevents the shoulder girdle from moving upward by placing one hand over the top of the acromion while the shoulder again is put through an active and passive range of motion. Normally the glenohumeral joint can be abducted to 90 degrees and rotated internally and externally 90 degrees. Many conditions of the shoulder or periarticular structures may cause restriction of shoulder motion (Fig. 24–3).

In most cases, the muscles of the shoulders can be tested adequately with the patient sitting. Muscle function can be assessed by testing flexion, extension, abduction, adduction, and rotation. Prime movers of flexion are the anterior portion of the deltoid muscles (C5 and 6) and the coracobrachialis muscles (C5 and 6). The latissimus dorsi (C5 and 6), teres major (C5 and 6), and deltoid (C5 and 6) muscles are the prime movers of shoulder extension. Abduction is carried out by the middle fibers of the deltoid (C5 and 6) and supraspinatus (C5) muscles. Prime movers of adduction are the pectoralis major (C5-8, T1) and latissimus dorsi (C5, 6) and teres minor (C5, 6) muscles. The prime movers of medial rotation are the subscapularis, pectoralis major, and teres major muscles.

Figure 24–3. Attempted abduction of the right arm in a patient with a rotator cuff tear. (From Polley, H.F., and Hunder, G.G.: Rheumatologic Interviewing and Physical Examination of the Joints. Philadelphia, W.B. Saunders Company, 1978.)

Many diseases cause referred pain to the shoulder area and thereby mimic shoulder joint disease. Heart disease, pleural involvement, and hiatal hernia may produce pain referred to the shoulder. Subphrenic inflammation may affect the diaphragm and, through this, cause referred pain to the shoulder or neck. Conditions of the cervical portion of the spinal column, nerve roots, or peripheral nerves in the upper extremity may be frequent sources of shoulder pain and disability. When pain in the shoulder is not related to use of the shoulder and when the examination indicates a completely normal shoulder, referred pain should be considered as a possible cause of the symptoms.

Elbow. The elbow joint (see also Chapter 115) is composed of three bony articulations. The principal one is the humeroulnar joint, which is a hinge joint. The radiohumeral and proximal radioulnar articulations allow rotation of the forearm.

To examine the elbow joint, the examiner's thumb is placed between the lateral epicondyle and the olecranon process in the lateral para-olecranon groove and one or two fingers are placed in the corresponding groove medial to the olecranon (Fig. 24–4). The elbow should be relaxed and moved passively through flexion, extension, and rotation. Limitation of motion and crepitus may thus be noted. Synovial swelling is most easily palpated as it bulges under the examiner's thumb when the elbow is passively extended fully. At times synovial membrane can be palpated over the posterior aspect of the joint between the olecranon process and distal humerus. Synovitis is commonly associated with limitation of extension of the joint.

The olecranon bursa overlies the olecranon process of the ulna. Olecranon bursitis is common after repeated or chronic local trauma or occurs in rheumatic diseases such as rheumatoid arthritis and tophaceous gout.

The medial and lateral epicondyles of the humerus and tendinous attachments are common sites of tenderness (tennis elbow, lateral or medial epicondylitis).

Muscle function of the elbow can be assessed by testing flexion and extension. The prime movers of flexion are the biceps brachii (C5, 6), brachialis (C5, 6) and brachioradialis (C5, 6) muscles. The prime mover of extension is the triceps brachii muscle (C7, 8).

Wrist and Carpal Joints. The wrist is a complex joint (see also Chapter 114). The true wrist or radiocarpal articulation is formed proximally by the distal end of the radius and the articular disc and distally by a row of three of the carpal bones, the scaphoid, the lunate, and the triangular. The distal radioulnar joint is usually separated from the wrist joint. The mid-carpal joints are formed by the junction of the proximal and distal rows of the carpal bones, which are, from radial to the ulnar side, the trapezium, trapezoid, capitate, and ha-

Figure 24–4. Palpation of the paraolecranon grooves of the elbow joint. (From Polley, H.F., and Hunder, G.G.: Rheumatologic Interviewing and Physical Examination of the Joints. Philadelphia, W.B. Saunders Company, 1978.)

mate. The mid-carpal and carpometacarpal articular cavities often communicate.

The long flexor tendons of the muscles of the forearm cross the front of the wrist and are enclosed in a flexor tendon sheath under the flexor retinaculum (transverse carpal ligament). The flexor retinaculum and the underlying carpal bones form the carpal tunnel. The median nerve also runs through the carpal tunnel superficial to the flexor tendons. The extensor tendons of the forearm pass under the extensor retinaculum (dorsal carpal ligament) enclosed in a synovial sheath.

The palmar aponeurosis (fascia) spreads out into the palm from the flexor retinaculum. In *Dupuytren's contracture* the palmar aponeurosis becomes thickened and contracted drawing one or more fingers into flexion at the metacarpophalangeal joint. The fourth finger is usually affected earliest, then the fifth and the third. The first two digits are rarely involved. The skin frequently feels adherent to the palmar fascia.

A *ganglion* is a cystic enlargement arising from a joint capsule; it characteristically occurs on the dorsum of the wrist between the tendons of the common extensors of the digits and the radial extensors at the base of the second metacarpal bone.

Subluxation of the ulna occurs secondary to chronic inflammatory arthritis. The subluxed ulna appears as a prominence on the dorsolateral wrist and presses against the extensor digitorum communis tendons, especially those of the fourth and fifth digits. Attrition may result in rupture of these tendons. The long extensor tendon of the thumb is also particularly vulnerable to wear and fraying as a result of its course over bony prominences.

Swelling of the wrist may be due to involvement of the sheaths of the tendons crossing the wrist and/or the wrist joint itself. When swelling is due to tenosynovitis, the outpouching tends to be more localized and is altered by flexing and extending the fingers (Fig. 24–5). Articular swelling is more diffuse and protrudes anteriorly and posteriorly from under the tendons.

Figure 24–5. Localized swelling of the dorsal wrist tenosynovium in a patient with rheumatoid arthritis. (From Polley, H.F., and Hunder, G.G.: Rheumatologic Interviewing and Physical Examination of the Joints. Philadelphia, W.B. Saunders Company, 1978.)

Synovitis of the wrist joint is detected most reliably by palpating over the dorsal surface (Fig. 24–6). Because of structures overlying both the dorsal and palmar aspects of the wrist, accurate localization of the margins of the synovial membrane may be difficult. To examine the wrist the physician should palpate or pinch this joint gently between the thumbs and fingers to detect abnormalities of bony and soft tissue structures. Swelling in hypertrophic osteoarthropathy, if present, extends proximal to the wrist and does not have the typical consistency of either synovial fluid swelling or pitting edema. In addition, clubbing may be present.

Tenosynovitis and *trigger finger* can be detected by palpating crepitus or nodules along the tendons in the palm while the patient slowly flexes and extends the fingers. Tendon nodules causing triggering usually occur at the level of the metacarpal heads, where a thickening

Figure 24–6. Illustration of the relationship of the synovial membranes of the wrist and carpal and metacarpal joints to the surrounding bony structures. (From Polley, H.F., and Hunder, G.G.: Rheumatologic Interviewing and Physical Examination of the Joints. Philadelphia, W.B. Saunders Company, 1978.)

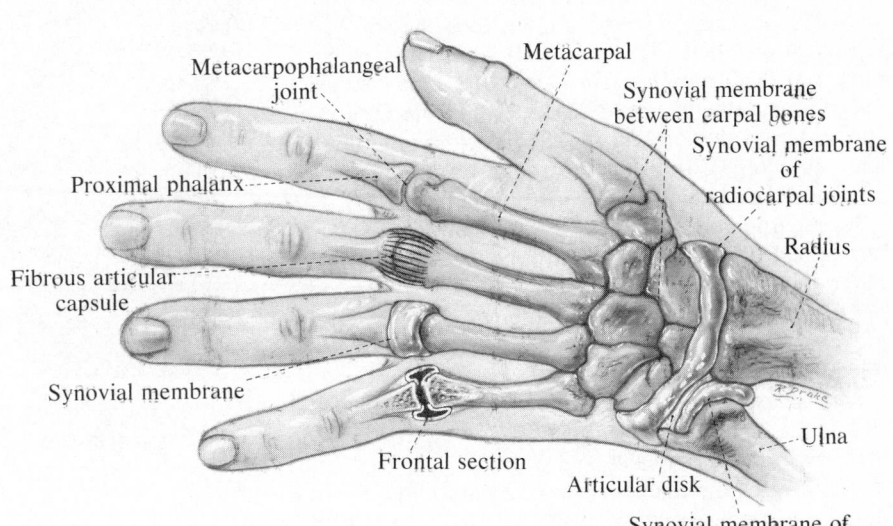

of the deep fascia forms the proximal annular ligament in the sheath of the flexor tendons (proximal pulley).

Movements of the wrist include palmar flexion (flexion), dorsiflexion (extension), radial deviation, ulnar deviation, and circumduction. Pronation and supination of the hand and forearm occur primarily at the proximal and distal radioulnar joints. The only carpometacarpal joint that moves to any degree is the carpometacarpal joint of the thumb, which possesses the movements of a sellar joint. Crepitus at this joint is commmon in degenerative arthritis.

The wrist can normally be extended to about 70 degrees and flexed to 80 or 90 degrees. Ulnar deviation averages 50 degrees and radial deviation 20 to 30 degrees. Loss of dorsiflexion is the most incapacitating functional impairment of wrist motion.

Stenosing tenosynovitis at the radial styloid process (de Quervain's tenosynovitis) characteristically involves the long abductor and short extensor tendons of the thumb. Tenderness near the radial styloid process can be localized to these tendons by having the patient make a fist with the thumb in the palm of his hand. The examiner then moves the patient's wrist into ulnar deviation. The development of severe pain over the radial styloid is a positive Finkelstein's test and is caused by stretching the thumb tendons in the stenosed sheath.

Carpal tunnel syndrome results from pressure on the median nerve in the carpal tunnel and is discussed in detail in Chapter 110.

Muscle function of the wrist can be measured by testing flexion and extension, and supination and pronation of the forearm. Prime movers in wrist flexion are the flexor carpi radialis (C6, 7) and flexor carpi ulnaris (C8, T1) muscles. Each of these two muscles can be tested separately. This can be accomplished if the examiner provides resistance to flexion at the base of the second metacarpal bone in the direction of extension and ulnar deviation in the case of the flexor carpi radialis and resistance at the base of the fifth metacarpal in the direction of extension and radial deviation in the case of the flexor carpi ulnaris. The prime extensions of the wrist are the extensor carpi radialis longus (C6, 7), extensor carpi radialis brevis (C6, 7), and extensor carpi ulnaris (C7, 8) muscles. The radial and ulnar extensor muscles can also be tested separately. Prime movers in supination of the forearm are the biceps brachii (C5, 6) and supinator (C6). Prime movers in pronation are the pronator teres (C6, 7) and pronator quadratus (C8, T1).

Metacarpophalangeal, Proximal, and Distal Interphalangeal Joints. The metacarpophalangeal joints are hinge joints. Lateral collateral ligaments that are loose in extension tighten in flexion, thereby preventing lateral movement of the digits. The extensor tendons that cross the dorsum of each joint strengthen the articular capsule. When the extensor tendon of the digit reaches the distal end of the metacarpal head, it is joined by fibers of the interossei and lumbricales and expands over the entire dorsum of the metacarpophalangeal joint and on to the dorsum of the adjacent phalanx. This expansion of the extensor mechanism is known as the extensor hood.

The proximal and distal interphalangeal joints are also hinge joints. The ligaments of the interphalangeal joints resemble those of the metacarpophalangeal joints. When the fingers are flexed, the bases of the proximal phalanges slide toward the palmar side of the heads of the metacarpal bones. The metacarpal heads form the rounded prominences of the knuckles with the metacarpal joint spaces lying about 1 cm distal to the apices of the prominences.

The skin on the palmar surface of the hand is relatively thick and covers a fat pad between it and the metacarpophalangeal joint. This makes palpation of the palmar surface of the joint more difficult than the dorsal surfaces.

Swelling of the fingers may result from articular or periarticular causes. Synovial swelling produces symmetrical enlargement of a joint itself, whereas extra-articular swelling may be diffuse, extending beyond the joints, or asymmetrical, involving only one side of the digit or joint (Fig. 24–7). Chronic swelling and distention of the metacarpophalangeal joints tends to produce stretching and laxity of the articular capsule and ligaments. This laxity, combined with muscle imbalance and other forces, results in the extensor tendons of the digits slipping off the metacarpal heads to the ulnar sides of the joints. The abnormal pull of the displaced tendons is one of the factors that causes ulnar deviation of the fingers in chronic inflammatory arthritis.

"*Swan-neck*" deformity describes the appearance of a finger in which there is a flexion contracture of the metacarpophalangeal joint, hyperextension of the proximal interphalangeal joint, and flexion of the distal interphalangeal joint. These changes are produced by contraction of the interossei and other muscles that flex the metacarpophalangeal joints and extend the proximal interphalangeal joints. This deformity is characteristic of

Figure 24–7. Symmetrical proximal interphalangeal joint swelling in a patient with systemic lupus erythematosus.

rheumatoid arthritis but may be seen in other chronic arthritides such as lupus erythematosus (Fig. 24–8).

The term *"boutonnière"* deformity is used to describe a finger with a flexion contracture of the proximal interphalangeal joint associated with hyperextension of the distal interphalangeal joint. The deformity is relatively common in rheumatoid arthritis and results when the central slip of the extensor tendon of the proximal interphalangeal joint becomes detached from the base of the middle phalanx, allowing palmar dislocation of the lateral bands. The dislocated bands cross the fulcrum of the joint and then act as flexors instead of extensors of the joint.

Another abnormality is "telescoping" or shortening of the digits produced by resorption of the ends of the phalanges secondary to destructive arthropathy. Shortening of the fingers is associated with wrinkling of the skin over involved joints and also is called "opera-glass hand" or "la main en lorgnette." Bony hypertrophic or osteophytic articular nodules on the distal interphalangeal joints are called *Heberden's nodes*, and when they are located on the proximal interphalangeal joints are called *Bouchard's nodes*.

The metacarpophalangeal joints are palpated on the dorsal aspect of the metacarpal heads on each side of the extensor tendons (Fig. 24–9) with the proximal phalanges flexed 20 to 30 degrees. Small amounts of swelling in one or more joints can best be detected by comparing the joints in question with others. Synovitis of metacarpophalangeal joints is often associated with lateral compression tenderness, which can be elicited by gently squeezing the patient's hand at the level of the joints.

The proximal and distal interphalangeal joints are best examined by palpating gently over the lateral and medial aspects of the joint where the flexor and extensor tendons do not interfere with assessment of the synovial membrane. Alternatively, the joint can be compressed anteroposteriorly by the thumb and index finger of one of the examiner's hands while the other thumb and index finger palpate for synovial distention medially and laterally (Fig. 24–10).

The presence of clubbing of the fingernails can be detected by repeated gentle palpation of the distal nail

Figure 24–9. Palpation of the metacarpophalangeal joints. The examiner's thumbs palpate the dorsal aspect of the joint while the index fingers palpate the volar aspect of the metacarpal head. (From Polley, H.F., and Hunder, G.G.: Rheumatologic Interviewing and Physical Examination of the Joints. Philadelphia, W.B. Saunders Company, 1978.)

edge with one hand while using the other hand to palpate the proximal edge of the nail for elevation from the nail bed. Alternatively, the examiner can palpate the proximal edge of the patient's nail with the tip of one or more fingers or thumbs pointing distally (same direction as the patient's fingers). When clubbing is present, the proximal edge of the nail "floats" in its bed.

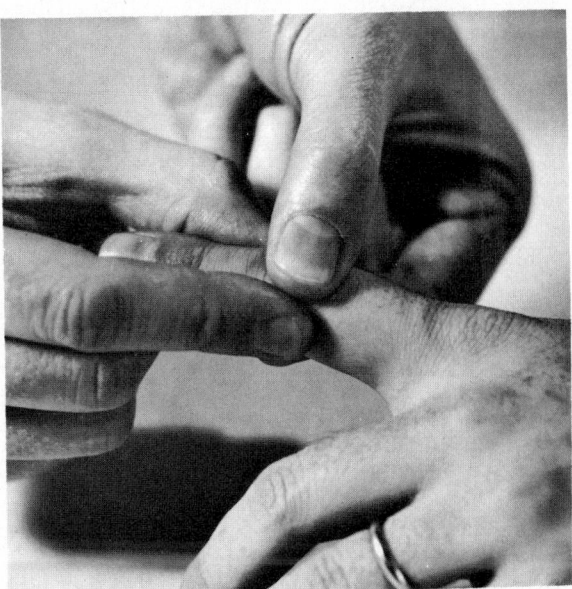

Figure 24–10. Palpation of the proximal interphalangeal joint. Anteroposterior compression of the joint by the examiner's thumb and index finger while the other thumb and index finger palpate for medial and lateral synovial distention. (From Polley, H.F., and Hunder, G.G.: Rheumatologic Interviewing and Physical Examination of the Joints. Philadelphia, W.B. Saunders Company, 1978.)

Figure 24–8. Swan neck deformities in a patient with chronic Reiter's syndrome.

A general assessment of the strength of the hands can be made when the patient makes a tight fist by gripping two or more of the examiner's fingers. A more accurate measure, which can be used in comparative studies, is obtained having the patient squeeze a partially inflated sphygmomanometer (at 20 mm Hg).

It is often helpful to test strength of the fingers separately. The prime movers of flexion of the second through fifth metacarpophalangeal joints are the dorsal and palmar interosseus muscles (C8, T1). The lumbrical muscles (C6, 7, 8) flex the metacarpophalangeal joints when the proximal phalangeal joints are extended. The flexors of the proximal interphalangeal joints are the flexor digitorum superficialis muscles (C7, 8, T1) and the flexor of the distal interphalangeal joints is the flexor digitorum profundus muscle (C7, 8, T1).

The prime extensors of the metacarpophalangeal joints and interphalangeal joints of the second through fifth fingers are the extensor digitorum communis (C6, 7, 8), the extensor indicis proprius (C6, 7, 8), and the extensor digiti minimi (C7) muscles. The interossei and lumbrical muscles simultaneously flex the metacarpophalangeal joints and extend the interphalangeal joints. The dorsal interosseus muscles (C8, T1) and abductor digiti minimi (C8) abduct the fingers, whereas the palmar interosseus muscles adduct the fingers.

The thumb is moved by a number of muscles. Prime flexor of the first metacarpophalangeal joint is the flexor pollicus brevis muscle (C6, 7, 8, T1). The prime flexor of the first interphalangeal joint is the flexor pollicus longus muscle (C8, T1). The metacarpophalangeal joint of the thumb is extended by the extensor pollicus brevis muscle, and the prime extensor of the interphalangeal joint is the extensor pollicus longus muscle (C6-8).

The prime abductors of the thumb are the abductor pollicis longus (C6, 7) and the abductor pollicis brevis (C6, 7) muscles. Motion takes place primarily at the carpometacarpal joint. The prime mover in thumb adduction is the adductor pollicis muscle (C8, T1). Motion takes place primarily at the carpometacarpal joint. The prime movers in opposition of the thumb and fifth fingers are the opponens pollicis muscles (C6, 7) and opponens digiti minimi muscle (C8, T1).

Spine and Sacroiliac Joints. In conjunction with muscles and ligaments, the bony structure of the spinal column allows for upright posture and provides for flexion of the trunk and rotation of the head. The spine has four normal curves, including the two anterior convexities in the cervical and lumbar region and the two posterior convexities in the thoracic and sacrococcygeal regions. Each vertebra consists of two segments, the anterior portion, including the vertebral body and disc, and the posterior portion or vertebral arch. Details of spinal anatomy are found in Chapters 28 and 30.

The sacroiliac joints are of particular interest to rheumatologists. At the caudal end of the spine the triangular-shaped sacral segment of the vertebral column articulates with the bony pelvis via the sacroiliac joints. The sacroiliac joints function to transmit the upper body weight to the pelvis and legs. The upper two thirds of the joint is in an oblique plane and the tuberosities of the posterior iliac crests project medially beyond the joints and overlie them. The lower one third of the joint articulates in the anteroposterior plane with the ilium. Because of the bony shape of the joint and the strong ligaments there is essentially no motion across the sacroiliac joint in adults.

Additional stability of the vertebral column is provided for by ligaments. The strong anterior longitudinal ligament supplies reinforcement to the anterior annulus fibrosus and also limits spine extension. The posterior longitudinal ligament provides less support. Limitation of spinal flexion and lateral bending are provided by the interspinous ligaments. Between the laminae are the elastic ligamenta flava, which help return the vertebral column to its initial position after movement.

Motion of the spine is dependent upon multiple muscle groups. The intrinsic back muscles, including the long sacrospinalis, act as spine extensors. The abdominal wall muscles, including the internal and external obliques and the rectus abdominous, are the major flexors of the spine. They are assisted by muscles anterior to the spine, including the quadratus lumborum and the psoas muscles. Lateral bending and rotation occur with unilateral contraction of the abdominal and intrinsic back muscles with contralateral simultaneous relaxation.

The landmark surface anatomy of the back is important in order to localize the site of pathologic involvement. It is best appreciated with the patient standing with the entire back, posterior shoulder, and legs exposed to the examiner. The subject should stand in a relaxed manner with the feet slightly separated and the hips and knees fully extended. Arms should be at the sides. In the midline, the seventh cervical and first thoracic spinous processes are prominent at the base of the neck. Because of the caudal sloping projection of the thoracic spinous processes, the tips of the spinous processes overlie the adjacent inferior thoracic vertebral body. In the lumbar region, the spinous processes overlie the corresponding vertebral body. With the arms relaxed and held at the sides, the inferior angles of the scapulae lie in the horizontal line that intersects the spine of the seventh thoracic vertebra. The horizontal line between the highest point of each iliac crest intersects the fourth lumbar vertebra. The sacral dimples overlie the posterior superior iliac spines and mark the level of the second sacral vertebra. Medial to the posterior superior iliac spine is the mid portion of the sacroiliac joint.

Inspection of the spine from behind includes notation of scars, asymmetry of shoulder elevation, scapular prominence, height of iliac crests, and gluteal creases. The examiner should draw an imaginary vertical line from the first thoracic process to the sacrum. If the line does not fall on the sacral midline, a lateral list of spinal tilt is present. A compensatory scoliosis may obscure a lateral tilt.

If a scoliosis is present, it is described by the direction of the convexity. A functional versus structural scoliosis should be differentiated by examining the patient in a forward bending position. While a functional scoliosis will disappear, a structural scoliosis will not, and may actually be accentuated. A rotational thoracic scoliosis will create a prominent hump on the side of the convexity. At times, a very mild curvature may not be appreciated unless the thorax is observed with the examiner seated in front of the patient who bends forward with the arms extended in front of the body. Similarly, while a lumbar scoliosis may cause prominence of the sacrospinalis muscle on the side of the convexity, a mild curve may be appreciated only by careful palpation of the spinous processes.

Pelvic tilt may accompany a scoliosis. This is identified by noting one superior iliac crest higher than the other. The scoliotic convexity will be toward the lower side. If the pelvic tilt and scoliosis are related to an anatomic leg length discrepancy, they should be abolished by leveling the pelvis with support under the short leg. With the pelvis leveled, a persistent scoliosis is related to spinal column disease.

Additional spinal deformities are noted by observing the patient from the side. Thoracic kyphosis may be either structural or postural. In young persons, elimination of postural kyphosis may be observed with the patient lying in the prone position of hyperextending the spine or with the patient standing with the shoulders back. In older adults with postural kyphosis correction may not be possible. In addition, a postural kyphosis tends to cause a smooth symmetrical forward curve of the spine with forward bending, while a structural kyphosis may appear to originate at a specific segmental level. Hyperlordosis, loss of lordosis, forward pelvic tilt, and head protrusion are also best observed from the side.

Muscle spasm may be recognized by prominent paravertebral musculature, usually asymmetrical. While palpation can be performed with the patient erect, fixed spasm is best appreciated with the patient prone with a pillow under the abdomen. Palpation should begin at a site distant to the location of pain and discomfort, as indicated by the patient. This will allow assessment of general muscle tone and the overall level of the patient's reactivity and pain tolerance. To localize areas of tenderness, it is important to use a systematic approach to palpation, beginning with the spinous processes. Localized levels of bony tenderness should be noted, as well as levels of step-off as observed in spondylolisthesis. Bony palpation is then followed by palpation of the paravertebral musculature. Additional sites of tenderness, such as fatty nodules or ligaments, should be noted. The buttock is palpated for areas of gluteus muscle attachment tenderness, trochanteric bursitis, ischial tuberosity bursitis, and sciatic notch tenderness. Percussion of tender areas may help localize the painful structures. Tenderness elicited by reflex hammer or fingertip percussion over a vertebral body suggests disease in that specific spinal segment.

Observation of lumbar spine range of motion is performed with the examiner standing to the side of and behind the patient. With the knees kept straight, the patient is instructed to bend forward to attempt to touch the floor. Normally, a flattening of the lumbar lordosis will occur; persistence of lordosis suggests paravertebral muscle spasm or intrinsic spine deformity. Although the recording of the finger-to-floor distance is often cited as a method of estimating lumbar spine flexion, it is inaccurate, since the majority of motion measured is due to hip flexion. The contribution made by hip flexion may be eliminated by grasping the patient around the hips to stabilize the pelvis. Lumbar flexion is normally up to 45 degrees.

The *Schober test*, as used by Moll and Wright, is another method for reproducibly measuring lumbar flexion.[3] It is commonly employed to evaluate spondylitis. A skin mark is placed in the midline at the level of the sacral dimples. Two additional marks are placed 10 cm above and 5 cm below the first mark. The patient is then instructed to bend forward as far as possible. The distance between the upper and lower marks is measured and the difference between the resting 15 cm and flexion measurement is calculated. Normal distraction of the marks is 5 cm. Movement of the marks less than 5 cm indicates abnormally decreased lumbar spine flexion secondary to enthesopathy or to hyperostosis or severe muscle spasm.

With forward flexion, the ease with which the patient moves should be observed. "Corkscrewing," with rotation to one side during flexion, suggests muscle spasm. A break in the normal rhythm of motion should be noted, such as a catch with resuming the upright position, in which the patient completes the motion of standing upright by bending the hips and knees to move the pelvis under the spine, rather than to further extend a painful spine. Corkscrew motion and catching are most often seen in lumbar disc disease. Lateral bending is observed with the examiner standing behind the patient. The patient should stand with feet apart and bend by sliding the hand down the lateral thigh. Lateral bending is estimated by observing the degrees of distraction from vertical of an imaginary line from the lumbosacral level to the occiput. Motion may be estimated in degrees, with normal to 30 degrees or more.

Extension is performed with the physician stabilizing the pelvis with one hand firmly over the sacrum and the other over the upper anterior thigh. With extension, the normal lordosis should increase. Motion is estimated in degrees, and the normal is up to 30 to 40 degrees from the vertical.

Thoracolumbar spine motion may be estimated by the degree of spine rotation. With the physician stabilizing the pelvis, motion is recorded in degrees; normal rotation is 30 degrees or more. With the exception of rotation, the use of goniometer usually does not provide any improvement in estimation of degrees of spinal motion.[4]

Costovertebral motion, often reduced in ankylosing spondylitis, is estimated by the change in chest circumference with inspiration and expiration. The usual site for measuring chest motion is at the nipple line in males and just above the line in females. The extent of chest expansion from full expiration to full inspiration is measured with a tape measure. Normally, there is at least a 5 to 6 cm difference in healthy young adults.

The sacroiliac joint is first evaluated by identifying the joint with palpation. The joint is under the sacral dimple or is found by palpating medially to the posterior iliac spine. The *Gaenslen test* is performed as the patient lies at the edge of the table. In this test the leg and thigh closest to the edge are hyperextended over the side of the table by lowering toward the floor. The other leg is held in a knee chest position by the patient in order to fix the pelvis. If the sacroiliac joint is the origin of the patient's back pain, the maneuver will elicit pain in the joint on the hyperextended side. The maneuver is repeated by hyperextending the other leg over the other side of the table. The sacroiliac joint can also be stressed by applying pelvic compression. The patient is instructed to lie on his side. The examiner places downward compression against the lateral iliac crest. Caution should be exercised in the interpretation of these maneuvers to examine the sacroiliac joints. A recent prospective study has shown that they lack specificity and are not capable of distinguishing sacroiliac pathology from other causes of low back pain.[5]

Examination of the patient with back pain should always include a neurologic examination, including reflexes, straight leg raising, muscle strength, and sensory testing. In performing the tests for straight leg raising, the examiner should not interpret the occurrence of all lumbosacral pain as a positive test, since pelvic rotation with leg raising will cause pain in a diseased lumbosacral segment. In addition, pain in the posterior thigh caused by tight hamstrings should not be confused with a positive test. Pain aggravated by ankle dorsiflexion and relieved by knee flexion supports a positive straight leg test. The bowstring test is good supporting evidence for root tension: With the knee flexed and the pain relieved, firm pressure applied by the thumbs into the popliteal space may reproduce the pain. The crossed straight leg test, in which the elevation of the uninvolved leg causes pain in the opposite affected leg, is a reliable sign of nerve root tension.

Because low back pain is often a social problem involving medical-legal or work disability issues, the examiner should be aware of signs during the examination that suggest a nonorganic basis to the patient's complaints. A group of five standardized nonorganic signs has been suggested in which the presence of three or more is thought to be significant.[6] First, tenderness over a wide area of skin to light pinching, as well as extensive deep tenderness over more than one anatomic structure, suggests nonorganic tenderness. Second, simulation of movements that created pain during the examination should be performed in a manner by which the actual structure does not move. These include painful axial loading of the lumbar spine by placing downward pressure on the patient's skull, and the provocation of back pain by rotating both the shoulders and pelvis in the

same plane. Third, the examiner should use distraction testing, in which a painful part of the examination is repeated in another painless manner. Fourth, regional weakness and sensory changes in a nonanatomic distribution are important to note, as well as cogwheel giving way on muscle testing. Fifth, overreaction to minimal stimuli should be noted.

No examination of the patient with low back pain is complete without an abdominal examination for masses and aortic aneurysms and a pelvic-rectal examination. The supine lithotomy position is best for providing an adequate rectal examination of the coccyx, sacrum, and surrounding tissues. Tenderness of the piriformis muscle, as seen in pelvic floor myalgias or the piriformis syndrome, should be noted.[7] The coccyx may be palpated for tenderness and mobility with the index finger in the rectum and the thumb outside.

Cervical spine motion is measured by observing flexion and extension (nodding), supplied primarily by the atlantooccipital joint; rotation, primarily the atlantoaxial joint; and lateral bending motion from the C2-7. Flexion of the chin towards the chest is normally about 45 degrees; rotation of the chin towards the shoulder is about 60 to 90 degrees and extension is about 50 to 60 degrees. Lateral bending with the head towards the shoulder should be performed without elevation of the ipsilateral shoulder girdle. Pain occurring on the ipsilateral side of the neck with lateral bending suggest apophyseal joint disease, while the presence of contralateral pain suggests a muscular or ligamentous origin.

The cervical spinous processes can be palpated from C2 to C7. C1 is not palpable. The surrounding soft tissue should be palpated for tenderness and spasm. Palpation should extend to include the trapezius muscles, interscapular musculature, and sternocleidomastoid muscles. It is important to palpate for greater occipital nerve tenderness at the base of the occiput in patients with occipital headaches or pain.

In evaluating patients with possible cervical radicular symptoms, the *foramen compression test*, or *Spurling maneuver*, is used. This examination should only be done after radiographic examination of the cervical spine has been performed and fractures or lytic lesions of the vertebrae or odontoid are known to be absent. The patient's head is placed in hyperextension or tilted toward the side of the radicular symptoms. Pressure is placed on the top of the patient's skull for 10 seconds. The test is positive if the symptoms are reproduced or aggravated by the maneuver.

Atlantoaxial subluxation may be observed at times by noticing a change in the smooth rhythm of flexion and extension. The patient may be aware of a clicking or jerking sensation. The jerking motion may be observed or palpated in the upper cervical spine. The subluxation may be palpated using a finger to examine the patient's posterior pharyngeal wall while the neck moves in flexion and extension. Radiographic analysis of the cervical spine in flexion and extension remains the most accurate means of assessing subluxation.

The occiput-to-wall measurement as well as overall

height of the patient is a useful test for following upper spine involvement in ankylosing spondylitis. The patient is instructed to stand with the back against the wall and heels as close to the wall as possible. With the chin level, the neck is extended to bring the occiput to the wall. The distance remaining between the head and the wall is measured in centimeters.

Hip. The hip joint is a spheroidal or ball and socket joint consisting of the rounded head of the femur and the cup-shaped acetabulum (see also Chapter 120). Stability of the joint is ensured by the fibrocartilaginous rim of the glenoid labrum and the dense articular capsule and surrounding ligaments, including the iliofemoral, pubofemoral, and ischiocapsular ligaments that reinforce the capsule. The hip joint is also surrounded by powerful muscle groups. The primary hip flexor is the iliopsoas muscle assisted by the sartorius and the rectus femoris muscles. Hip adduction is accomplished by the three adductors, the longus, brevis, and magnus plus the gracilis and pectineus muscles. The gluteus medius is the major hip abductor, while the gluteus maximus and hamstrings extend the hip. There are several clinically important bursae about the hip joint. Anteriorly, the iliopsoas bursa lies between the psoas muscle and the joint surface. The trochanteric bursa lies between the gluteus maximus muscle and the posterolateral greater trochanter, and the ischiogluteal bursa overlies the ischial tuberosity.

Examination of the hip begins by observing the patient's stance and gait. The patient should stand in front of the examiner so that the anterior iliac spines are visible. If pelvic tilt or obliquity is present, it may be related to a structural scoliosis, anatomic leg length discrepancy, or hip disease. Hip contractures may result in abduction or adduction deformities. To compensate for an adduction contracture, the pelvis is tilted upward on the side of the contracture. This allows the legs to be parallel during walking and weight bearing. With a fixed abduction deformity, the pelvis becomes elevated on the normal side during standing or walking. This causes an apparent shortening of the normal leg and forces the patient to stand or walk on the toes of the normal side or to flex the knee on the abnormal leg.

Viewed from the rear, with the legs parallel, the patient with hip disease and an adducted hip contracture may have asymmetrical gluteal folds due to pelvic tilt with the diseased side elevated. In this situation, the patient is unable to stand with the foot of the involved leg flat on the floor. In abduction contracture, the findings are reversed; with both legs extended and parallel the uninvolved side is elevated.

A hip flexion deformity commonly occurs in diseases of the hip but is often overlooked. Unilateral flexion of the hip in the standing position reduces weight bearing on the involved side, and relaxes the joint capsule, causing less pain. This posture may be noted when observing the patient from the side. There is a hyperlordotic curve of the lumbar spine to compensate for lack of full hip extension.

The patient with possible hip disease should be observed walking. With a normal gait, the abductors of the weight-bearing leg contract to hold the pelvis level or elevate the non-weight-bearing side slightly. Two abnormalities of gait may be observed in hip disease. With a painful hip, the most common abnormality is the antalgic gait. In this gait, the person leans over the diseased hip during the phase of weight bearing on that hip, placing the body weight directly over the joint to avoid painful contraction of the hip abductors. Alternatively, a Trendelenburg gait may develop. Here, with weight bearing on the affected side, the pelvis drops and the trunk shifts to the normal side. While the antalgic gait is said to be seen with painful hips and the Trendelenburg gait in conditions with weak hip abductors, neither gait is specific and either accompanies a painful hip.

The *Trendelenburg test* is a measure of the gluteus medius hip abductor weakness. The patient is asked to stand bearing weight only on the involved side. Normally, the abductors will hold the pelvis level or the nonsupported side slightly elevated. If the non-weight-bearing side drops, the test is positive for weakness of the weight-bearing gluteus medius. This test is nonspecific and may be observed in primary neurologic or muscle disorders or in a variety of hip diseases, leading to weakness of the abductors, including coxa vara, congenital dislocation, slipped capital femoral epiphysis, or femoral neck fracture. A mild Trendelenburg gait is seen commonly in normal persons.

The patient is next examined in the supine position. The presence of a hip flexion contracture is suggested by persistence of lumbar lordosis and pelvic tilt, masking the contracture by allowing the involved leg to remain in contact with the examination table. The *Thomas test* will demonstrate the flexion contracture. In this test the opposite hip is fully flexed, to flatten the lumbar lordosis and fix the pelvis. The involved leg should then be extended towards the table as far as possible. The diseased hip's flexion contracture will become more obvious and can be estimated in degrees from full extension. While the patient is supine, measurement for leg length discrepancy is performed with the legs fully extended. To detect true leg length discrepancy, each leg is measured from the anterior superior iliac spine to the medial malleolus. A difference of 1 cm or less is unlikely to cause any abnormality of gait. An apparent leg length discrepancy may result from pelvic tilt or abduction or adduction contractures of the hip.

The hip joint range of motion includes flexion, extension, abduction, adduction, and internal and external rotation and circumduction. The degree of flexion permitted varies with the manner in which it is assessed. When the knee is held flexed 90 degrees, the hip normally flexes to an angle of 120 degrees between the thigh and long axis of the body. If the knee is held in extension, the hamstrings limit the hip flexion to about 90 degrees. Abduction is measured with the patient still supine with the leg in an extended position perpendicular to the pelvis. Pelvic stabilization is achieved by placing one arm across the pelvis with the hand on the opposite anterior iliac spine. With the other hand, the examiner grasps the patient's ankle and abducts the leg until the pelvis is noted to begin moving. Normally, abduction is to approximately 45 degrees. The maneuver is repeated on the other side. The examiner may also stand at the foot of the table, grasp both ankles and simultaneously abduct the legs. Differences between the two hips can be appreciated, and the intermalleolar distance is measured. Abduction is commonly limited in hip joint disease. Adduction is tested by grasping the ankle and raising the leg off the examination table by flexing the hip enough to allow the tested leg to cross over the opposite leg. Normal adduction is to about 20 to 30 degrees. Hip rotation may be tested with both hip and knee flexed to 90 degrees or with the leg extended. In the flexed position, external rotation is performed by moving the foot medially and internal rotation is performed by moving the foot laterally.

Normal hip external rotation is to 45 degrees, and internal rotation is to 40 degrees. These figures vary somewhat in normals. There is also a difference in rotation between the flexed and extended hip. Owing to the increased stabilization of the joint by the surrounding ligaments in the extended position, rotation decreases with extension. To test hip rotation, the extended leg is grasped above the ankle and rotated externally and internally from the neutral position. Limitation of internal rotation of the hip is a very sensitive indicator of hip joint disease.

Extension is tested with the patient in the prone position. Estimating actual hip joint extension can be difficult, since some of the apparent motion arises from hyperextension of the lumbar spine, pelvis rotation, motion of the buttock soft tissue, and flexion of the opposite hip. The pelvis and lumbar spine are partially immobilized by placing one arm across the posterior iliac crest and lower lumbar spine. The examiner places the other hand under the thigh with the knee flexed and hyperextends the thigh. Normal extension ranges up to 10 to 20 degrees. Limitation of extension is most often secondary to a hip flexion contracture.

The iliotibial band is a part of the fascia lata extending from the iliac crest, sacrum, and ischium over the greater trochanter to the lateral femoral condyle, tibial condyle, and fibular head and along the lateral intermuscular system, separating the hamstrings from the vastus lateralis. The tensor fascia lata may cause an audible snap as it slips over the greater trochanter if the weight-bearing leg moves from hip flexion and adduction to a neutral position, as in climbing stairs. Most commonly observed in young women, the "snapping" hip usually does not cause any significant degree of pain.

In patients complaining of lateral hip pain, the soft tissues over the greater trochanter should be palpated for tenderness. The lateral surface of the trochanter is tender in cases of trochanteric bursitis. Swelling occasionally may be palpable and helps to differentiate actual bursitis from gluteus tendinitis or attachment tenderness in which there is posterolateral trochanteric tenderness without swelling. If lateral tenderness without swelling is present, differentiation between the two conditions

can be difficult. The pain of trochanteric bursitis is aggravated by actively resisted abduction of the hip.

Patients complaining of anterior hip or groin pain should be examined for iliopsoas bursitis. Swelling and tenderness may be noted in the middle one third of the inguinal ligament lateral to the femoral pulse. The pain is aggravated by hip extension and reduced by flexion. The bursitis may be a localized problem or represent extension of hip synovitis to the bursa, since there is communication between the two structures in approximately 15 percent of cases. In the latter instance, the bursitis actually represents a synovial cyst. It is impossible to differentiate a bursitis from a cyst on examination. If the patient is tender in the region of the iliopsoas bursa but no swelling is palpable, it is not possible to differentiate this condition from an overlying tendonitis of the iliopsoas muscle. The inguinal region should be carefully palpated for other abnormalities such as hernias, femoral aneurysms, adenopathy, tumor, and psoas abscess masses.

Muscle strength testing should include the hip flexors, extensors, abductors, and adductors. The primary hip flexor is the iliopsoas muscle (L2, L3). Flexion may be tested with the patient sitting at the end of the table. The pelvis is stabilized by placing one hand on the ipsilateral iliac crest while the patient actively flexes the hip. The examiner uses the other hand to exert downward pressure against the thigh proximal to the knee. A second approach is to have the patient assume the supine position and hold the leg to be tested in 90 degrees of flexion at the hip while the examiner attempts to straighten the hip. Hip extension is tested with the patient lying prone. The primary hip extensor is the gluteus maximus muscle (L5, S1). With the knee flexed to remove hamstring action, the patient is instructed to extend the hip and thigh off the surface of the table as the examiner places one forearm across the posterior iliac crest to stabilize the pelvis while the other hand presses down against the thigh. The major hip abductor is the gluteus medius (L4, L5). Hip abductor strength is tested with the patient lying on his side. The upper abducting leg should be slightly extended to eliminate contribution from the hip flexors and tensor fascia lata. The examiner must stabilize the pelvis by placing one hand downward against the iliac crest to prevent the lateral trunk muscles from elevating the pelvis and leg off the table. The patient is instructed to abduct the thigh and leg while the examiner places downward pressure with his other hand against the distal lateral thigh. The leg nearest the table is then tested for hip adduction. The primary adductor is the adductor longus (L3, L4). The examiner holds the upper leg in slight abduction while the patient adducts the lower leg off the table against the resistance of the examiner's other hand proximal to the knee.

An alternative method for testing abduction and adduction enables the examiner to compare the two legs simultaneously. The patient lies supine with the legs fully extended and the hips moderately abducted. To test abduction, the patient actively pushes out against the examiners resistance against the lateral malleoli. Adduction is tested by movement against resistance at the medial malleoli.

Knee. The knee is a compound condylar joint with three articulations, the patellofemoral and the lateral and medial tibial femoral condyles with their fibrocartilaginous menisci. The joint is stabilized by the articular capsule, the ligamentum patellae, the medial and lateral collateral and anterior and posterior cruciate ligaments. The collateral ligaments provide medial and lateral stability, while the cruciates provide anteroposterior support and rotatory stability. Normal knee motion is a combination of flexion or extension and rotation. With flexion the tibia internally rotates, and with extension it externally rotates on the femur. The surrounding synovial membrane is the largest of any of the body's joints; it extends up to 6 cm proximal to the joint as the suprapatellar pouch beneath the quadriceps femoris muscle. There are several clinically significant bursae about the knee, including the superficial prepatellar bursa, the superficial and deep infrapatellar bursae, the anserine bursa distal to the medial tibial plateau, and the posterior medial semimembranous and posterolateral gastrocnemius bursae (Fig. 24–11). Knee extension is provided for primarily by the quadriceps femoris muscle and flexion by the hamstrings. The biceps femoris externally rotates the lower leg on the femur, while the popliteus and semitendinous muscles supply internal rotation.

Examination of the knees should always include observation of the standing patient. Weight bearing will place deforming stress on the knees. *Genu varum* or lateral deviation of the knee joint (with medial deviation of the lower leg), *genu valgum* or medial deviation of the knee (and lateral deviation of the lower leg), and genu recurvatum or posterior bowing are often more easily appreciated in the standing patient. Limp, flexion contracture, locking, or giving away should be noted. Locking is the sudden loss of ability to extend the knee; it is painful and may be associated with an audible noise such as a click, pop, or snap.

Asymmetry from swelling or muscle atrophy may be noted on initial inspection. Patellar malalignment should be noted, including high-riding or laterally displaced patellas. The examiner should inspect the knee from the rear to identify popliteal swelling due to a popliteal or Baker's cyst, which is most commonly a medial semimembranous bursal swelling. If the calves appear asymmetric, measurement of calf circumference should be performed when the patient is lying on the examination table. Popliteal cysts may dissect down into the calf muscles, producing enlargement and palpable fullness. Edema may be present if the cyst causes secondary venous or lymphatic obstruction. Acute dissection or rupture of a popliteal cyst can mimic thrombophlebitis, the so-called pseudothrombophlebitis syndrome, with local pain, heat, redness, and swelling.

The patient is next examined in the supine position. Inability to fully extend the knee may be related to a flexion contracture or a large synovial effusion. Suprapatellar swelling with fullness of the distal anterior thigh that obliterates the normal depressed contours along the side of the patella usually indicates a knee joint effusion or synovitis. Localized swelling over the surface of the patella is generally secondary to prepatellar bursitis, while localized anterolateral or medial swelling along the joint line may represent cystic swelling of menisci.

Figure 24–11. Medial and posterior aspects of the knee with important muscle attachments and bursae illustrated. (From Polley, H.F., and Hunder, G.G.: Rheumatologic Interviewing and Physical Examination of the Joints. Philadelphia, W.B. Saunders Company, 1978.)

Quadriceps femoris muscle atrophy usually develops in chronic arthritis of the knee. Atrophy of the vastus medalis is the earliest change and may be appreciated by comparing the two thighs for medial asymmetry and circumference. Usually measurement of the thigh circumference is performed at approximately 15 cm above the joint to avoid spurious results due to suprapatellar effusions.

To adequately palpate the knee, the joint must be relaxed. This is usually best accomplished with the patient supine, and the knees fully extended as possible and not touching. Palpation should begin over the anterior thigh approximately 10 cm above the patella. In order to identify the superior margin of the suprapatellar pouch, which is an extension of the knee joint cavity, the examiner should palpate the tissues moving distally towards the knee. Swelling, warmth, thickness, nodules, loose bodies, tenderness, should be noted. A thickened synovial membrane has a "boggy," doughy consistency different from the surrounding soft tissue and muscle. It is usually palpated earlier over the medial aspect of the suprapatellar pouch and medial tibiofemoral joint. To enhance detection of knee fluid, any fluid in the suprapatellar pouch is compressed with the palm of one hand placed just proximal to the patella. The synovial fluid forced into the inferior distal articular cavity is then palpated with the opposite thumb and index finger laterally and medially to the patella. If the examiner alternates compression and release of the suprapatellar pouch, the synovial thickening can be differentiated from a synovial effusion, since the effusion will intermittently distend the joint capsule under the thumb and index finger of the opposite hand, while the synovial thickening will not. The examiner should be cautious not to compress the suprapatellar pouch too firmly or push the tissues distally because the patella or normal soft tissue, including the fat pads, will fill the palpated space and be misinterpreted as synovitis or joint swelling. With a large effusion, the patella can be ballotted by pushing it posteriorly against the femur with the right forefinger while maintaining suprapatellar compression with the left hand.

At the other extreme, effusions as small as 4 to 8 ml can be detected by eliciting the bulge sign. This test is performed with the knee extended and relaxed. The examiner strokes or compresses the medial aspect of the knee proximally and laterally with the palm of one hand to move the fluid from the area. The lateral aspect of the knee is then tapped or stroked, and a fluid wave or bulge is noted to appear medially (Fig. 24–12A and B). If not positive with the first attempt, the maneuver should be repeated with the pressure applied to the other areas of the lateral side of the knee.

The medial and lateral tibiofemoral joint margins are palpated for tenderness and bony lipping or exostosis as seen in osteoarthritis. Palpating the joint margins can be done easily with the hip flexed to 45 degrees, the knee flexed to 90 degrees, and the foot resting on the examining table. Tenderness over joint margins may represent articular cartilage disease, involvement of the

Figure 24–12. Demonstration of the bulge sign for a small synovial knee effusion. The medial aspect of the knee has been shaded to move the synovial fluid from this area (shaded depressed area in *A*). *B* shows bulge in previously shaded area after lateral aspect of the knee has been tapped. (From Polley, H.F., and Hunder, G.G.: Rheumatologic Interviewing and Physical Examination of the Joints. Philadelphia, W.B. Saunders Company, 1978.)

medial meniscus or anterior cruciate ligament, or lateral involvement of the collateral ligament, iliotibial band, or fibial head.

Bursitis can be differentiated from articular synovitis by palpation of localized tenderness and swelling. The anserine bursa is located at the medial tibial plateau between the medial collateral ligament and the tendons of the sartorius, gracilis, and semitendinous muscles. The prepatellar bursa, if quite swollen, can be mistakenly interpreted as knee joint synovitis unless the bursal margins are carefully outlined by palpation. Infrapatellar bursitis is palpated either overlying the infrapatellar tendon at the level of the tibia (superficial) or lying beneath the tendon (deep). The infrapatellar fat pad beneath the tendon at the level of the joint line may also be tender.

Patellar palpation is best performed with the knee extended and relaxed. The patella is compressed and moved so that its entire articular surface will come into contact with the underlying femur. Slight crepitation may be observed in many normally functioning knees. Pain with crepitation may suggest patellofemoral degenerative arthritis or chondromalacia patellae. Retropatellar pain occurring with active knee flexion and extension and secondary to patellofemoral disease may be differentiated from tibiofemoral articular pain. To test this the examiner should attempt to lift the patella away from the knee while passively moving it through range of motion. Painless motion during this maneuver indicates that the patellofemoral joint is the source of the difficulty. In addition, the *patellar inhibition test* will also help to clarify the presence of patellofemoral arthritis. In this test the examiner compresses the patella distally away from the femoral condyles while instructing the patient to isometrically contract the quadriceps. Sudden patellar pain and quadriceps relaxation are interpreted as a positive test for chondromalacia, but frequency of false positives is very high.

The patella should be checked for stability in patients suspected of having recurrent patellar dislocation. The patella is pushed laterally with the patient supine and the knee extended and relaxed. A distressed reaction from the patient is considered a positive *apprehension test.* Subluxation of the patella can also be appreciated while moving the knee through range of motion from 0 to 90 degrees flexion or back to full extension.

Another cause of joint snapping and symptoms suggesting an internal derangement is the *plica syndrome* caused by bands of synovial tissue.[8] In cases of mediopatellar plica syndrome, a tender bandlike structure may be palpated parallel to the medial border of the patella. During flexion and extension, a palpable or audible snap is appreciated. Patellar crepitance may also be noted.

Ligamentous instability is tested by applying valgus and varus stress to the knee and by using the drawer test. The knee should be extended and relaxed. The *abduction* or *valgus test* is performed by stabilizing the lower femur while placing a valgus stress on the knee by abducting the lower leg with the other hand placed proximal to the ankle. A medial joint line separation with the knee fully extended indicates a tear of the medial compartment ligaments plus the posterior cruciate ligament. The test is then performed with the knee in 30 degrees of flexion. If the test is negative at 0 degrees but positive at 30 degrees, the instability represents a tear of the medial compartment ligaments with the posterior cruciate ligament remaining intact. The adduction or varus test is then performed at 0 degrees. Separation of the lateral joint line indicates a lateral compartment ligament tear with an associated tear of the posterior cruciate ligament. Rotatory instability of the knee may also exist. The *jerk test* measures anterolateral instability.[9] With the hip flexed to 45 degrees and the knee to 90 degrees, the tibia is internally rotated while valgus stress is applied to the knee. The leg is extended and at approximately 30 degrees of flexion subluxation of the lateral femorotibial articulation is appreciated. With further extension, the articulation relocates. The change in acceleration rate of the two joint surfaces (during the maneuver) is felt as a sudden jerk.

The degree of ligamentous laxity observed during testing should be graded on a scale of 1 to 3.[9] A mild grade 1 instability indicates that the joint surfaces separate 5

mm or less; moderate grade 2 represents a separation of 5 to 10 mm. A severe instability, grade 3, is a separation greater than 10 mm. In cases of trauma, opening of the joint space indicates ligamentous instability secondary to rupture or stretching of the ligaments. However, in cases of chronic arthritis of the tibiofemoral compartment, there may be apparent medial or lateral separation due to the "pseudolaxity" created by loss of cartilage and bone. If the ligaments are intact, the resulting degree of valgus or varus displacement with stressing will not be any greater than in the normal knee.

The *drawer test* is performed with the hip flexed to 45 degrees and the knee to 90 degrees. To stabilize the knee, the examiner either sits on the foot while grasping the posterior calf with both hands or supports the lower leg between his lateral chest wall and forearm. The anterior drawer test is performed by pulling the tibia forward. This maneuver has been said to test whether the anterior cruciate ligament is intact. However, anterior subluxation may actually represent more complex instability.[9] With the tibia in neutral, a positive anterior drawer test in which the lateral tibial plateau subluxes forward while the medial stays in normal position represent anterolateral rotatory instability. If both plateaus sublux, tears of the middle one third of the medial and lateral capsular ligaments are present. If the subluxation is not present with the tibia internally rotated, the posterior cruciate ligament is intact. A positive anterior drawer test with the leg in external rotation represents a tear of the medial capsular ligament. A posterior drawer test in a chronically unstable knee suggests that damage has occurred to the posterior cruciate ligament.

Meniscal injury should also be tested for during the survey for joint instability. Symptoms that suggest a meniscal tear include locking during extension, joint clicking or popping during motion, and localized line tenderness along the joint. To examine the medial meniscus, the medial tibiofemoral joint line should be palpated with the lower leg internally rotated and the knee flexed to 90 degrees. Localized tenderness suggests involvement of the medial meniscus. With the knee flexed to 90 degrees, the lateral joint line is palpated for localized tenderness that would indicate lateral meniscal injury. The *McMurray test* is performed to elicit evidence of a posterior meniscal tear. In this, the patient's knee is placed in full extension and the examiner places one hand over the knee with the fingers along the side of the knee along one joint line and the thumb along the other side. The other hand holds the leg at the ankle and is used to flex, extend, and rotate the lower leg. With the knee flexed and the lower leg externally rotated 15 degrees, a palpable or audible snap occurring when the knee is extended from full to 90 degrees of flexion is a positive test and suggests a tear of the medial meniscus. A lateral snap or click occurring with the knee internally rotated 30 degrees and moved into extension suggests a lateral meniscal tear. In addition, a positive lateral test may represent a tear of the popliteus tendon, which can accompany a lateral meniscal tear. The *Apley maneuver* also tests for a torn meniscus. With the patient lying prone and the knee flexed to 90 degrees, the examiner places downward compression on the foot while rotating the tibia on the femur. Pain elicited during this maneuver suggests a meniscal tear. The *distraction test* is then performed by the examiner placing his knee on the patient's posterior thigh to stabilize the leg while applying an upward distractive force on the foot. Pain from rotating the tibia suggests ligament damage.

Range of motion of the knee in flexion and extension should be from full extension (zero degrees), to full flexion of 120 to 150 degrees. Some normal persons may be able to hyperextend to up to 15 degrees. Loss of full extension due to a flexion contracture is a common finding that accompanies chronic arthritis of the knee. In advanced arthritis, such as seen in some cases of rheumatoid arthritis, a posterior subluxation of the tibia on the femur may be observed.

Muscle strength testing includes testing flexion supplied by the hamstrings, i.e., the biceps femoris, semitendinosus, and semimembranosus (L5-S3) and extension supplied by the quadriceps femoris (L2-4). The hamstrings are tested best with the patient prone and attempting to flex the knee from 90 degrees to beyond. The ankle should be kept in neutral position or dorsiflexed to remove gastrocnemius action. With the leg externally rotated, the biceps femoris, which inserts on the fibula and lateral tibia, is primarily tested, while flexion with internal rotation tests the semitendinosus and semimembranosus muscles, which insert on the medial side of the tibia. Extension is tested with the patient sitting upright with the knee fully extended. The examiner stabilizes the thigh with downward pressure just proximal to the knee and places downward pressure at the ankle to test the knee extensors.

Ankle and Foot. The ankle is a hinged joint, and movement is limited to plantar flexion and dorsiflexion. It is formed by the distal ends of the tibia and fibula and proximal aspect of the body of the talus. The tibia forms the weight-bearing portion of the ankle joint; the fibula articulates on the side of the tibia. The malleoli of the tibia and fibula extend downward beyond the weight-bearing part of the joint and articulate with the sides of the talus. Malleoli provide lateral stability by enveloping the talus in a mortise-like fashion.

The articular capsule of the ankle is lax on the anterior and posterior aspects of the joint, allowing extension and flexion, but is tightly bound bilaterally by ligaments. The synovial membrane of the ankle on the inside of the capsule usually does not communicate with any other joints, bursae, or tendon sheaths in the region of the ankle or foot.

Strong medial and lateral ligaments of the ankle contribute to the lateral stability of the joint. The medial or deltoid ligament, the only ligament on the medial side of the ankle, is a triangle-shaped fibrous band that tends to resist eversion of the foot. It may be torn in eversion sprains of the ankles. The lateral ligaments of the foot consist of three distinct bands forming the posterior talofibular, the calcaneofibular, and the anterior talofibular ligaments. These ligaments may be torn in inversion sprains of the ankle. All tendons crossing the ankle joint lie superficial to the articular capsule and are enclosed in synovial sheaths ($\sim$ 8 cm in length) for part of their course across the ankle. On the anterior aspect of the ankle the tendons and synovial tendon sheaths of the tibialis anterior, extensor digitorum longus, peroneus tertius, and extensor hallucis longus overlie the articular capsule and synovial membrane. On the medial side of the ankle posteriorly and inferiorly to the medial malleolus lie the flexor tendons and tendon sheaths of the tibialis posterior, flexor digitorum longus, and flexor hallucis longus (Fig. 24–13). All three of these muscles plantar flex and supinate the foot. The tendon of the flexor hallucis longus is located more posteriorly than the other flexor tendons and lies beneath the Achilles' tendon for part of its course. The tendo calcaneus (Achilles' tendon) is a common tendon of the gastrocnemius and soleus muscles and inserts into the posterior surface of the calcaneus, where it is subject to external trauma, various inflammatory reactions, and irritations from bony spurs beneath it. On the lateral aspect of the ankle, posteriorly and inferiorly to the lateral malleolus, a synovial sheath encloses the tendons of the peroneus longus and peroneus brevis. These muscles extend the ankle (plantar flex) and evert (pronate) the foot. Each of the tendons adjacent to the ankle may be involved separately in traumatic or disease processes.

There are three sets of fibrous bands or retinacula that hold down the tendons that cross the ankle in their passage to the foot. The extensor retinaculum consists of a superior part (transverse crural ligament) in the anterior and inferior portions of the leg and an inferior part in the proximal portion of the dorsum of the foot. The flexor retinaculum is a thickened fibrous band on the medial side of the ankle. On the lateral side of the ankle the peroneal retinaculum forms a superior and an inferior fibrous band. These bands bind down tendons of the peroneus longus and peroneus brevis as they cross the lateral aspect of the ankle.

The intertarsal joints provide additional mobility to the foot. The intertarsal joints allow the foot to be everted and abducted (pronated) or inverted and adducted (supinated) to maintain the arch of the foot during weight bearing. Intertarsal ligaments on the undersurface of the foot are particularly strong. The arch is supported also by the plantar aponeurosis, the short muscles of the foot, and the long tendons that cross the ankle in their course into the sole of the foot. The subtalar (talocalcaneal) joint permits inversion and eversion of the foot. No muscles insert on the talus.

The plantar aponeurosis or fascia is a fibrous structure of great strength that extends from the calcaneus forward as a single band, which then divides at about the middle of the foot into portions for each of the five toes. The plantar aponeurosis becomes thinner as it extends distally in a fashion similar to that of the palmar aponeurosis in the hands and fingers. The area of the plantar aponeurosis near the attachment to the calcaneus is particularly subject to the effects of trauma and inflam-

Tibialis anterior
muscle

Tibialis posterior
muscle

Tibia

Inferior extensor
retinaculum

Deltoid ligament

Extensor hallucis longus
tendon sheath

Abductor hallucis
brevis muscle
(cut)

Flexor digitorum
longus muscle

Soleus muscle
Flexor hallucis
longus muscle

Posterior tibial
artery
Posterior tibial
nerve

Tendo calcaneus

Flexor retinaculum

Tibialis posterior tendon

Flexor digitorum
longus tendon

Tibialis anterior
tendon

Flexor hallucis
longus tendon

MAYO
©1978

Figure 24–13. Medial aspect of the ankle demonstrating the relationships between the tendons, ligaments, and posterior tibial artery and nerve. (From Polley, H.F., and Hunder, G.G.: Rheumatologic Interviewing and Physical Examination of the Joints. Philadelphia, W.B. Saunders Company, 1978.)

matory reactions. Bony spurs are likely to form at this area.

Each of the metatarsophalangeal and interphalangeal joints has an articular capsule lined with synovial membrane. The extensor tendon completes the capsule dorsally, and the collateral ligaments strengthen the capsule on its sides and the plantar ligaments support the plantar portion of the capsule. The metatarsophalangeal joints normally undergo less flexion than the metacarpophalangeal joints.

Bursae in the foot are commonly located on the sides of the first and fifth metatarsophalangeal joints and about the heel, especially between the skin and Achilles' tendon, between the Achilles' tendon and calcaneus, and between the skin on the sole and plantar surface of both the calcaneous and metatarsal heads. Subcutaneous bursae are likely to develop in areas that are subject to abnormal weight bearing or friction. Thus, a bursal reaction may form between the thickened skin (callus) and the underlying bony prominence of the first metatarsal head in a hallux valgus deformity of the great toe.

The foot and ankle should be inspected while the patient is standing, walking, and in a non-weight-bearing position. The feet can be compared with each other for evidence of localized or diffuse swelling or atrophy, the position of nodules, cutaneous changes, and appearance of the nails (Fig. 24–14). The location of calluses and subcutaneous bursae should be noted because they indicate areas of pressure or friction due to alterations in foot structure.

Synovial swelling of the ankle joint is most likely to cause fullness over the anterior or anterolateral aspect of the joint, since the capsule is more lax in this area.

Mild swelling of the joint may not be apparent on inspection because of the many structures that cross the joint superficially to the synovial membrane. Efforts should be made to differentiate between superficial linear swelling localized to the distribution of the tendon sheaths from more diffuse fullness and swelling due to involvement of the ankle joint. Similarly, it is difficult to observe synovitis of the intertarsal joints. Intertarsal joint synovitis may produce an erythematous puffiness or fullness over the dorsum of the foot. Chronic inflammation of structures around the ligaments that hold the

Figure 24–14. Inspection of standing feet in a rheumatoid patient demonstrates synovitis of the second and third metatarsophalangeal joints of the right foot. The involved toes are more spread apart, and the third toe is raised from the floor. Subtle swelling extends onto the dorsum of the right forefoot. (From Polley, H.F., and Hunder, G.G.: Rheumatologic Interviewing and Physical Examination of the Joints. Philadelphia, W.B. Saunders Company, 1978.)

forefoot together may result in weakening of these ligaments and spreading of the metatarsals, resulting in separation of the toes and widening of the forefoot. Swelling of the metatarsophalangeal joints produces thickening of the forefoot, which may keep some of the toes from touching the floor when the patient is sitting with the feet in a resting position.

There are several abnormal positions of the foot that should be recognized. Lowering of the longitudinal arch (pes valgoplanus or flat foot) or elevation of the longitudinal arch (pes cavus) may be seen. Talipes equinus is the position of the foot in plantar flexion and often results from contracture of the Achilles' tendon. This tends to occur in patients who are confined to bed. The presence of varus or valgus positions of the heel is determined by noting the deviation of the foot either medially or laterally, respectively. Inversion of the foot (supination) exists when the sole of the foot is turned inward, and eversion of the foot (pronation) exists when the sole of the foot is turned outward. Adduction of the foot is present when the forepart of the foot is displaced inward in relation to the midline of the leg. Abduction of the foot occurs when the forepart of the foot is displaced outward in relation to the midline of the limb. The various abnormal positions are often combined in deformities of the foot or may be associated with abnormalities of the knees.

The most common deformity of the great toe is *hallux valgus.* This is a lateral or outward deviation of the great toe resulting in an abnormal angulation and rotation of the first metatarsophalangeal joint. The first metatarsal bone deviates medially, which increases the width of the forefoot and produces a prominence of the first metatarsal head. The big toe may overlap, or underlie the second toe. A callus and bursal reaction are commonly found over the prominence of the medial aspect of the head of the first metatarsal bone. *Hallux rigidus* is the term used when motion at the first metatarsophalangeal joint is markedly reduced.

The typical "hammer toe" deformity consists of hyperextension at the metatarsophalangeal joint and flexion at the proximal interphalangeal joint. The distal interphalangeal joint may be straight or hyperextended. When the distal interphalangeal joint remains straight and the tip of the toe touches the floor, the deformity also is referred to as "mallet toe." A "cock-up toe" refers to a dorsal subluxation of the proximal phalanx on the metatarsal head (Fig. 24–15). The metatarsal head becomes depressed towards the sole of the foot, where it can be palpated readily. The tip of the toe is elevated above the surface on which the foot is resting. Cock-up toes occur in patients with arthritis at the metatarsophalangeal joint, whereas hammer toes may occur in patients with or without joint disease. Various combinations of these alterations may be found in arthritic patients. Severe articular damage of the toes also may produce hyperextension deformities of the phalanges of the toes.

A painful heel may be caused by a variety of condi-

Figure 24–15. Rheumatoid foot demonstrating cock-up toe deformities of the fourth and fifth toes as well as loss of the longitudinal arch and pronation of the left foot due to subtalar joint involvement. (From Polley, H.F., and Hunder, G.G.: Rheumatologic Interviewing and Physical Examination of the Joints. Philadelphia, W.B. Saunders Company, 1978.)

tions such as osseus spurs, Achilles' tendinitis, calcaneal bursitis, fractures, periostitis, osteomyelitis, or tumors. Careful localization of swelling and tenderness by palpation may help reveal the cause of the symptoms. The Achilles' tendon is subjected to local trauma because of its prominent location and also because of the magnitude of stress applied to it during walking and other activities. Palpable swelling and tenderness at the attachment of the Achilles' tendon to the calcaneus suggest Achilles' tendinitis. Attempts should be made to distinguish by palpation more superficial swelling about the tendon due to local irritation from a deep bursal reaction, since the latter often signifies inflammation due to a systemic disease such as rheumatoid arthritis or ankylosing spondylitis. Xanthomas, tophi, rheumatoid nodules, or fibrous calluses may be palpable in the Achilles' tendon.

Complete or partial rupture of the Achilles' tendon is usually a sudden event and generally occurs during a burst of unaccustomed physical activity. Pain, swelling, ecchymosis, and tenderness are present at the site of the tear, but the swelling may become more diffuse and include the region of the ankle joint. Tenderness over the Achilles' tendon and a visible or palpable depression in the tendon at the site of the separation help in recognition of this condition.

When the Achilles' tendon has been ruptured, a defect in the tendon may be palpable. Pain in the Achilles' tendon region with flexion of the foot against resistance is present in partial tears. When the tear is complete, squeezing the calf while the patient is lying prone with the feet over the edge of the examining table will fail to cause plantar flexion of the foot. Rupture of the Achilles' tendon may be confused with thrombophlebitis or with rupture of fibers of the gastrocnemius muscle or plantaris tendon.

Periostitis associated with pain and tenderness diffusely over the calcaneus or over a localized area may be seen in Reiter's disease or ankylosing spondylitis.

Pain and tenderness in the heel with weight bearing may be seen occasionally in adolescence. The syndrome is self-limited and has been attributed to calcaneal epiphysitis or tenosynovitis of the Achilles' tendon at the level of its insertion into the os calcis. There is no swelling, but the posterior superior portion of the os calcis is tender when palpated.

Plantar fasciitis is a condition in which the patient has pain under the calcaneus on weight bearing and tenderness under the anterior portion of the heel. It is commonly attributed to excessive standing or walking, especially when the patient has been unaccustomed to such activity. But often such a history cannot be elicited. Radiographs may or may not show a bony spur at the attachment of the plantar fascia to the calcaneus.

The metatarsophalangeal joints should be palpated between the examiner's thumb and forefinger. On the plantar surface the soft tissues consist of thick skin, superficial fascia, and adipose tissue. On the dorsal surface the normal soft tissues are not as thick, and the outline of the metatarsophalangeal joint can be determined more precisely. Changes from normal depend on the amount of atrophy of fat pads and other subcutaneous tissue that may be associated with metatarsalgia. Synovitis causes thickness of the soft tissues in the area of these joints, which is most readily detected by palpating the joint margins on their dorsal surfaces. Tenderness on lateral compression of the metatarsophalangeal joints may be noted with mild synovitis of these joints. Dorsal subluxation of the metatarsophalangeal joints may result from chronic synovitis in which the capsule is stretched and soft tissue forces elevate the base of the proximal phalanges on the metatarsal head. A step upward of the base of the proximal phalanx can be palpated in most instances and may be associated with a cock-up deformity. Chronic synovitis also may result in separation of the toes and widening of the forefoot.

The proximal and distal interphalangeal joints of the toes are palpated between the thumb and index finger in a manner similar to palpation of the corresponding joints in the fingers. Synovitis usually is detected best on the medial and lateral aspects of these joints while varying degrees of pressure are applied by the palpating fingers to determine the presence of swelling, tenderness, or warmth. Synovitis of the interphalangeal joints may cause diffuse swelling of the entire toe, a finding sometimes referred to as "sausage toe."

From the normal position of rest in which there is a right angle between the leg and foot, labeled 0 degrees, the ankle normally allows about 20 degrees of dorsiflexion and about 45 degrees of plantar flexion. Inversion and eversion of the foot occur mainly at the subtalar and other intertarsal joints. From the normal position of the foot the subtalar joint normally permits about 20 degrees of eversion and 30 degrees of inversion. To test

the subtalar joint the examiner grasps the calcaneus with one hand and attempts to invert and evert it, holding the ankle motionless. To move the mid-tarsal joints the examiner holds the calcaneus in one hand and the forefoot in the other and rotates the mid-foot in both directions in relation to the calcaneus. Both feet should be compared. The metatarsophalangeal joint of the great toe extends to about 80 degrees and flexes to about 35 degrees. The second through fifth toes move only about 45 degrees in either direction. Flexion of the interphalangeal joints varies among individuals, but generally the interphalangeal joints flex to 40 or 50 degrees.

A general assessment of muscular strength of the ankle can be obtained by asking the patient to lift the weight of the body on the toes and heels. If the patient can walk on toes and heels, the muscle strength of the flexors and extensors of the ankle can be considered normal. In many instances, however, joint pains may prevent the patient from walking, or it is desired to test muscles individually.

Prime movers in plantar flexion of the ankle are the gastrocnemius (S1,2) and the soleus (S1,2) muscles. The prime mover in dorsiflexion and inversion of the foot is the tibialis anterior muscle (L4,5, S1). The examiner applies graded resistance on the medial and dorsal aspect of the foot when testing the tibialis anterior muscle. The prime mover in inversion is the tibialis posterior muscle (L5, S1). To test the tibialis posterior muscle the foot should be in plantar flexion. The examiner applies graded resistance on the medial border of the forefoot while the patient attempts to invert the foot. The prime movers in eversion of the foot are the peroneus longus (L4, 5, S1) and peroneus brevis (L4, 5, S1) muscles.

The prime mover in flexion of the first metatarsophalangeal joint is the flexor hallucis brevis muscle (L4, 5, S1). The prime mover in flexion of the interphalangeal joint of this toe is the flexor hallucis longus muscle (L5, S1, 2). The prime mover in extension of the first metatarsophalangeal joint is the extensor digitorum brevis (L5, S1), and the prime mover in extension of the interphalangeal joint is the extensor hallucis longus (L4, 5, S1). Prime movers in flexion of the second through fifth metatarsophalangeal joints are the lumbrical muscles (L4, 5). The interosseus muscles and flexor digitiquinti muscles also function in flexion.

The prime mover in flexion of the proximal interphalangeal joints of the toes is the flexor digitorum brevis (L4, 5), and the prime mover in flexion of the distal interphalangeal joints of these toes is the flexor digitorum longus (L5, S1).

The prime movers in extension of the second through fifth metatarsophalangeal joints and interphalangeal joints are the extensor digitorum longus (L4, 5, S1) and extensor digitorum brevis (L5, S1) muscles. Because of the shortness of the toes and underdeveloped state of their muscles, it is often difficult to distinguish between function at the proximal and distal interphalangeal joints.

When the synovial tendon sheaths become inflamed

(tenosynovitis) as they cross the ankle, the superficial linear swelling and fullness of tenosynovitis should be differentiated from the more generalized swelling and tenderness found in synovitis of the ankle joint. At times the swelling of the tendon sheath is obscured by a more diffuse overlying edema, but when the edema is reduced by rest in bed and elevation of the extremity, careful palpation may show that the swelling and tenderness follow the line of a tendon. Tenosynovitis frequently causes pain on movement of the involved tendon. Thus, inversion or eversion of the foot against resistance may cause pain when there is a synovial reaction on the respective medial or lateral aspect of the foot or ankle. However, failure to produce pain with these maneuvers does not exclude a tenosynovial reaction.

Metatarsalgia, or pain and tenderness of the plantar surface of the heads of the metatarsal bones or metatarsophalangeal joints, is a common complaint, which occurs alone or in association with many local and systemic conditions. In youth, trauma and osteochondritis of the second metatarsal head are common causes. In the adult, any disturbance that can affect the feet can manifest itself in the metatarsophalangeal joint region of one or both feet. Patients with metatarsalgia may have atrophy of fat pads under these joints.

Interdigital neuroma, or *Morton's toe*, is a fusiform enlargement of an interdigital nerve. It must be differentiated from metatarsalgia. Interdigital neuroma is most commonly located between or distal to the heads of the third and fourth metatarsal bones. It is often bilateral and more common in women. Pain associated with interdigital neuroma is sharp or burning in quality and occurs initially with activity and later also at rest. Sharply localized tenderness is characteristic and is present in the soft fleshy tissues either between or distal to the heads of the third and fourth metatarsals, less often between the second and third toes. The location of tenderness helps differentiate it from metatarsophalangeal joint disease. Altered sensation or decreased 2-point discrimination may be found over the skin between the third and fourth toes. Occasionally large interdigital neuromas may be palpable and movable between the heads of the metatarsals.

"*March foot*" is caused by severe or prolonged use of the foot, such as during strenuous walking and usually is caused by a transverse fracture of the metatarsal shaft. The second metatarsal is affected most frequently and the third metatarsal next most frequently. However, any of the metatarsals can be involved. Localized pain develops over the dorsum of the forefoot, causing the patient to limp. The most common and significant findings on physical examination are palpable tenderness and swelling over the fracture. The diagnosis is confirmed by roentgenograms or bone scans of the foot. March

fracture may also occur in the calcaneus or the lower part of the tibia or fibula.

Reflex sympathetic dystrophy is an incompletely understood syndrome that involves the entire foot and ankle and easily can be mistaken for an atypical polyarthritis. It can be a sequel to, or complication of, trauma or synovitis, but frequently it has no obvious or detectable organic cause. Typically the foot is cyanotic or mottled, edematous, tender, cool, moist, and shiny. Hyperalgesia, although present, often does not conform to any definite nerve distribution.

When transient or regional osteoporosis involves the foot, it is similar to reflex dystrophy in some ways. Tenderness of the tarsal and metatarsal bones is present, and weight bearing is painful. In transient osteoporosis, however, the color of the skin is likely to be more normal, but occasionally some evidence of inflammation is present. In addition, in transient osteoporosis recurrences may be seen, and the knee and hip may also be involved. In this syndrome, the findings generally resolve in 4 to 8 months.

Tarsal tunnel syndrome is discussed in detail in Chapter 110. Excess accumulation of fat, tenosynovitis, fibrosis, or trauma may produce symptoms of the tarsal tunnel syndrome. Characteristic symptoms include burning pain, tingling, or numbness in the toes, forefoot, or heel in the distribution of the particular branch or branches entrapped.

Tinel's sign may be elicited by tapping over the posterior tibial nerve at the site of compression. Decreased sensation to pinprick or to 2-point discrimination is found earlier and more commonly than weakness or atrophy of the foot muscles. Electromyograms may show an increase in the nerve conduction time of the entrapped nerve.

References

1. Polley, H.F., and Hunder, G.G.: Rheumatological Interviewing and Physical Examination of the Joints. 2nd ed. Philadelphia, W.B. Saunders Company, 1978.
2. Hoppenfeld, S.: Physical Examination of the Spine and Extremities. Englewood Cliffs, New Jersey, Appleton-Century-Crofts, 1976.
3. Moll, J.M.H., and Wright, V.: Normal range of spinal mobility. An objective clinical study. Ann. Rheum. Dis. 30:381, 1971.
4. Nelson, M.A., Allen, P., Clamp, S.E., and DeDombal, F.T.: Reliability and reproducibility in low back pain. Spine 4:97, 1979.
5. Russell, A.S., Maksymowych, W., and LeClercq, S.: Clinical examination of the sacroiliac joints: A prospective study. Arthritis Rheum. 24:1575, 1981.
6. Waddell, G., McCulloch, J.A., Kummel, E., and Venner, R.M.: Nonorganic physical signs in low back pain. Spine 5:117, 1980.
7. Pace, J.B., and Nogle, D.: Piriform syndrome. West. J. Med. 124:435, 1976.
8. Hardaker, W.T., Whipple, T.L., and Bassett, F.H.: Diagnosis and treatment of the plica syndrome of the knee. J. Bone Joint Surg. 62A:221, 1980.
9. Hughston, J.C., Andrews, J.R., Cross, M.J., and Moschi, A.: Classification of knee ligament instabilities. Part I. The medial compartment and cruciate ligaments. J. Bone Joint Surg. 58A:159, 1976.

Chapter 25

Approach to Monarticular Arthritis

Frank R. Schmid

GENERAL CONSIDERATIONS

No other presentation for a rheumatic disease tests the physician's knowledge and skill as does monarticular arthritis. Often the onset is acute and the threat of infection real, so that urgency is required in decision making; sometimes the involved joint is the only apparent abnormality, so that every clue must be gleaned from the history, systemic and local examination, and the laboratory to make a diagnosis. While the challenge is demanding and, perhaps for that reason, exciting, solution of the problem can often be the most rewarding experience in rheumatology.

Definition of Monarticular Arthritis. Diarthrodial joints throughout the body have the same basic composition: synovium, capsule, articular cartilage, and bone. Periarticular structures such as tendons and bursae, although lacking bone and cartilage, have a similar synovial lining. Thus, they undergo many of the same pathologic processes as joints. Since they are anatomically adjacent to joints, their involvement may be mistakenly attributed to the joint itself unless a careful examination is performed. For these reasons, the approach to their management is included along with that of the joints under the overall chapter heading, monarticular arthritis.

By definition, monarticular means one joint or joint-related structure. In practice, involvement of as many as two or three separate joints still qualifies as a monarticular problem because of the frequency with which the classic monarticular syndromes are actually oligoarticular (Table 25–1). Involvement of more than this number of joint structures, however, even if the development is migratory and noncumulative, tends to suggest an entirely different set of causes.

Obviously every patient who ultimately has polyarthritis must at some point during the onset have a monarticular syndrome, if only for a short while. Therefore, awareness of subsequent polyarticular spread and the diagnostic possibilities that this raises must be kept in mind when the patient is first seen. Appropriate studies to test for their presence must be carried out. However, further discussion of such polyarthritic diseases as rheumatoid arthritis, rheumatic fever, and generalized osteoarthritis is not included in this chapter unless the duration of the monarticular phase is prolonged (Table 25-2). A related point to remember is that some patients present with a false monarticular history. Lesser degrees of involvement in other joints are ignored because attention becomes focused upon the major process in one or two joints. The true polyarthritic nature of the disease will be uncovered only by a careful and complete examination.

Broad Spectrum of Possible Diagnoses. Monarticular arthritis can be caused by many factors: genetic and biochemical abnormalities, as seen in the structural defects of the inherited connective tissue diseases as hy-

Table 25–1. Monarticular Diseases

Septic arthritis[1-4]
Gout[5]
Pseudogout[6]
Traumatic arthritis
Neuropathic arthropathy[7]
Mechanical derangement of joint
Localized syndromes (tendinitis, bursitis)
Arthritis with bleeding–clotting disorders (hemophilia, von Willebrand's disease, anticoagulant use)[8,9,10]
Familial Mediterranean fever[11]
Gaucher's disease[12]
Hyperlipoproteinemia (type II)[13]
Congenital dysplasia of hip
Juvenile osteochondroses
Avascular necrosis of bone[14]
Osteochondritis dissecans[15]
Loose joint body
Foreign body
Pigmented villonodular synovitis[16]
Synovioma[17]
Juxta-articular bone tumors[18-20]
Osteochondromatosis[21]
Fat necrosis in pancreatic disease[22]

Table 25–2. Polyarticular Diseases with Frequent Monarticular Component

Reiter's syndrome[23]
Juvenile rheumatoid arthritis (including ankylosing spondylitis)[24]
Psoriatic arthritis[25,26]
Colitic arthritis, Whipple's arthritis[27-29]
Sarcoid arthritis[30]
Pseudogout[6]
Arthritis with bleeding–clotting disorders (hemophilia, scurvy, von Willebrand's disease)[8,9,10]
Hemochromatosis[31]
Septic arthritis (especially due to *N. gonorrhoeae* and *meningitidis*)*[4]
Osteoarthritis (selected sites, as hip)[32]
Amyloid arthritis[33]
Relapsing polychondritis[34]
Hyperlipoproteinemia (Types II, IV)[35,36]

*Onset is frequently polyarticular before monarticular localization. Other syndromes usually have monarticular presentation initially.

permobility and in gout; trauma; infection; neoplasia; hormonal changes, as in parathyroid disease and pseudogout; immunologic mechanisms, as in amyloidosis; and finally, for the majority of patients, a nonspecific inflammatory process. The diagnostic net must be cast widely at the outset to ensure that the unusual cause for monarthritis is not overlooked.

Systemic diseases often include joint involvement in their spectrum of symptoms, in part because the connective tissue of joints is duplicated throughout the supporting structures of various parenchymal organs and also in part because a disorder in the mechanical function of joints is so readily perceived by the patient even if only minor. Therefore, a thorough general history and examination are mandatory. Focus upon the painful or swollen joint alone will not allow the correct diagnosis to be made in many cases. However, because so much of the severity of the illness falls upon one or just a few joint structures rather than multiple joint structures, the role of local factors in the causation of monarticular arthritis is usually more evident than in polyarticular arthritis. In fact, it may be helpful to analyze the patient's problem from the standpoint of the reason why one particular joint became involved and not another. For example, even though the bacteremia that precedes most cases of septic arthritis could potentially allow any joint in the body to become infected, only one or two, perhaps because of prior trauma, actually do become involved. Another example is the unusual instance in which a foreign body such as a plant thorn might have been introduced into the joint. This event may not be recalled by the patient unless all circumstances connected with the prior history of the involved part are reviewed.

The lesson in monarticular arthritis is that while no less a general history and examination are required than for any general medical problem, a more meticulous inspection of the local site adds insight into the pathogenesis and sometimes the specific cause.

Urgency for Diagnosis and Treatment. Among the prominent causes for monarthritis is infectious arthritis. Suspicion for this diagnosis must be raised upon initial examination even if the severity of joint pain and swelling is only minimal. Sometimes, as in the elderly or debilitated, systemic findings of sepsis may be absent. Since cure of this disease is possible and full restoration of joint function expected, confirmation or exclusion of this entity assumes major importance in the first few hours and days. In addition, other possible causes for monarticular arthritis, such as gout and pseudogout, are painful and disabling. Diagnosis of these diseases can be verified easily and quickly by examination of joint fluid, so that undue delay in making the diagnosis is not warranted. For these reasons, every patient with an undiagnosed monarticular arthritis should be considered a medical emergency.

Planning Ahead. Along with dispatch in handling the multiple aspects of examination and laboratory procedures, the physician must make both immediate and long-range decisions within the larger framework of a comprehensive approach to the problem. Less obvious diagnostic possibilities must be pursued as more likely ones are being investigated. Furthermore, no treatment carried out early should alter important clinical findings. Thus, use of anti-inflammatory drugs such as corticosteroids or even aspirin at the outset may mask some of the indicators of disease, e.g., fever and inflammation, that must be observed if one is monitoring the response of an infectious process to treatment. Drugs such as codeine should be given instead for pain relief.

In this chapter, the approach to diagnosis and management will be covered in a chronologic fashion in much the same manner as is seen in practice. Emphasis will be placed upon the use of a predetermined plan that can be followed for patients with monarthritis (Table 25–3).

INITIAL HISTORY AND EXAMINATION

The Involved Joint. Initial attention is directed to the patient's presenting complaint, the involved joint. Diagnostic clues can be obtained by analysis of events that may have precipitated the problem, by the type of onset, and by the nature of the findings both within and around the joint.

Precipitating Factors. When recognized, trauma to a limb may readily be shown to account for a painful or swollen joint. Occasionally, instances of trauma are more elusive, as for example when the patient is unable to provide an accurate history because of stupor from alcoholism, drug addiction, or an illness such as diabetic coma. In these cases, monarthritis may be the direct result of an unappreciated injury, although septic arthritis too is a well known complication of each of these situations. In other cases joint or bone disease caused by trauma may not show external evidence of soft tissue injury such as bruising or laceration, thus obscuring the diagnosis. A march fracture of a metatarsal may not be suspected on physical appearance or may not even be visible on the roentgenogram until callus appears weeks later. Meanwhile attention may be directed toward a presumed arthritis of an adjacent metatarsophalangeal or intertarsal joint as the cause of the problem. As noted earlier, a history of a penetrating injury that occurred days or weeks earlier may not be forthcoming unless a specific inquiry is made. Only then may it be obvious that a foreign body could have entered the joint. Trauma can also cause disease in more insidious ways. Forces applied for long periods of time to the arm of a cellist or violinist, to the forefoot of a ballet dancer, or to the shoulders of a gymnast can at one moment of time induce musculoskeletal symptoms in a joint or tendon. The patient who is hypermobile experiences long continued stress that can also produce an overt synovitis at some point, as in the metacarpophalangeal joint of the hand of a laboratory technician who had done extensive pipetting.

Other precipitating events for monarticular arthritis include the classic story of surgery or myocardial infarction 5 to 7 days before the abrupt onset of gout; the role of drugs such as corticosteroids in the development of aseptic necrosis; and the triggering effect of infection due to certain gram-negative bacilli such as *Salmonella* in causing the appearance of one or two swollen joints in Reiter's syndrome.

Further examples of precipitating factors for monarticular arthritis could be given, but these should suffice to underline the critical importance of their recognition in defining the cause of the disease. Caution is in order, however, in accepting each triggering event at face value. The arthritis presumed to have been induced by an identifiable precipitating factor must still be confirmed by more direct evidence, as discussed below. In some cases, the suspected precipitating factor may be largely irrelevant to the subsequent arthritis.

Type of Onset. Most patients with monarticular arthritis have an acute onset, with the peak intensity of symptoms reached in a few days' time. As such, a fairly exact time of onset can be given. In a few cases, the acuteness can be as dramatic as in gout. The patient may retire for the night perfectly well and be awakened before morning by exquisite pain in the joint. Less often, the onset is insidious, as might occur in some patients with psoriatic arthritis or sarcoidosis or with a more chronic presentation of chondrocalcinosis.

Age and Sex. Generally these characteristics afford some help in approaching the diagnosis. Male patients account for the largest fraction of cases of gouty arthritis, Reiter's syndrome, Whipple's disease, and the peripheral arthritis of juvenile ankylosing spondylitis. Female patients more often are candidates for a polyarthritic syndrome but are at greater risk for monarticular arthritis related to the gonococcus or hypermobility. Youngsters tend to be the victims of inherited and congenital disorders such as acetabular dysplasia of the hip or juvenile osteochondritis, and, with regard to septic arthritis, to be infected with *Hemophilus* species. Some diseases, such as chondrocalcinosis, are much more common in aged people. Gout when it occurs in women almost always appears postmenopausally.

Anatomic Localization of Joint Disease. Certain joints have the undeserved reputation of being so closely associated with certain types of arthritis that their involvement is tantamount to the diagnosis. Inflammation of the first metatarsal-phalangeal joint of the foot or podagra, although characteristic of gout, in fact can be found in other forms of arthritis. Similarly, heel pain, particularly at the weight-bearing portion of the calcaneus, is often found in Reiter's syndrome and in other spondyloarthropathies but again is not diagnostic. Distal interphalangeal joint involvement occurs in many diseases but is a more characteristic feature of osteoarthritis (Heberden's nodes), psoriatic arthritis, and, rarely, lupus erythematosus. The first carpometacarpal joint at the base of the thumb is often tender in patients with osteoarthritis who have Heberden's nodes. Thus, the specific site of the arthritis, while helpful, can only be suggestive in arriving at a diagnosis.

Inflammation of a single joint with rapid extension to an adjacent joint along with considerable overlying soft tissue swelling is a characteristic feature in gout, the so-called satellite phenomenon. Migratory polyarthritis of short duration followed by localization of the infection to but one of two joints is often seen in some forms of infectious arthritis such as gonococcal arthritis. However, by its very nature, monarticular or oligoarticular disease will be confined to but a few joints so that various anatomic or temporal patterns of involvement that could aid the diagnosis will not usually be seen.

Articular vs. Periarticular Involvement. A detailed history and examination will indicate whether the symptomatic musculoskeletal structure is actually within the joint and, if so, in which portion of the joint, or whether it is periarticular, involving the associated ligaments, tendons, or other supporting structures (Table 25-4). The physician, on examination, should gently pinpoint the exact source of pain with slight pressure over different parts of the joint. With confidence gained from the patient in this manner, motion of the part can be attempted. A primary intra-articular problem can be shown to encompass the entire circumference of a joint or to be localized within a portion of the joint, as, for example, a meniscal cartilage tear in the knee. Periarticular disease, in contrast, is confined to the unique region that conforms to the outline of the involved structures, as, for instance, the linear pattern of pain and swelling overlying the thumb extensor tendons near the wrist in de Quervain's disease.

Disease in other tissues of the extremity can mimic musculoskeletal symptoms. Neurologic pain has a burning or tingling quality and may follow the distribution of a dermatome or a peripheral nerve. As such it can occur as part of an unrelated disease or at times as a symptom resulting from a primary arthritic disease, as, for instance, compression of the median nerve in the carpal tunnel. Ischemic vascular disease is expressed as pallor or cyanosis, sometimes with but often without changes in the major pulses if vessels of small caliber are involved. Occasionally, the circulatory disturbance is the direct cause of both the musculoskeletal and vascular symptoms, as in polyarteritis nodosa. In gout and in the rarer disease of familial Mediterranean fever, a diffuse subcutaneous swelling and erythema can appear in an extremity and be confused with an infectious cellulitis. Therefore, in the approach to the patient who presents with symptoms in an extremity or the trunk, precision in interpretation of the clinical findings by a detailed history and a systemic examination of the affected part is required to define the problem accurately.

Symptoms of Joint Disease. Pain, whether severe or mild, is a cardinal feature of joint disease and can be felt directly at the site of involvement or referred to tissues at a distance from the joint. A well known example of referred pain is the pattern of pain felt in the anterior thigh or knee region caused by hip joint disease. Glenohumeral pain may be referred to the deltoid, and knee pain may be felt in the gastrocnemius muscle. In each case, careful examination will fail to reveal objective

Table 25–3. Algorithm for the Diagnosis of Monarticular Arthritis

(Continued on next page)

(Continued from previous page)

This algorithm may be used in the analysis of the problem presented by a patient with monarticular arthritis. The time frame development of these steps is several weeks. At each step the scope of diagnostic possibilities is named within the box; directions for further evaluation follow if the diagnosis has not been ascertained within the flow chart itself or by reference to tables in this chapter.

findings at the site of the referred pain, but pain, swelling, or limitation of motion can be detected in the involved joint. The relationship of pain to other factors can be a clue to the diagnosis. Pain at rest suggests inflammation of the joint structure; pain on use tends to speak for a mechanical defect such as cartilage damage in osteoarthritis or a meniscal injury to the knee. Pain beneath the patella that grows worse on descending stairs suggests chondromalacia or other injury to the patellar cartilage. Pain also may be expressed in unexpected ways, as in weakness or a feeling that a joint might give way on weight-bearing. The absence of pain in circumstances in which it might be expected suggests a diagnosis of a neuropathic joint or Charcot's arthritis. Some children with juvenile rheumatoid arthritis experience considerable joint inflammation but paradoxically have little or no pain.

Stiffness may be the term by which pain is expressed, but usually the finding expresses a difficulty with the easy or natural motion of the joint. This symptom is felt after prolonged inactivity, often after arising from sleep. Stiffness that persists for periods beyond 15 to 30 minutes usually is associated with inflammatory disease of the joint, and its duration affords a measure of the degree of such inflammation. However, other joint diseases such as degenerative arthritis may also have associated but briefer periods of stiffness.

Loss of joint motion occurs as a consequence of pain and/or stiffness as well as the result of a structural change in the joint. Motion may also be lost because of rupture of a tendon or a muscle attachment. Detection of this latter possibility requires meticulous examination of the joint structure for absence of tendon tightening on attempts at motion.

Swelling may be due to effusion within the joint capsule or to thickening of joint structures. A distinction between these two causes of swelling sometimes is difficult. The presence of fluid is revealed by its ability to be shifted from one compartment of the joint to another. Various maneuvers are applied for this purpose. In general, displacement of fluid by compression applied by one hand and detection of this by the fingers of the other hand indicates fluid. Swelling also may be due to bony proliferation, as is seen with Heberden's nodes or Bouchard's nodes in osteoarthritis or with a neuropathic joint. Bony swelling will characteristically be hard in contrast to the soft boggy reaction of soft tissue swelling. In addition, soft tissue swelling will tend to assume a fusiform shape conforming to the gross outline of the joint, whereas bony swelling tends to be asymmetrical.

Systemic Features of Monarticular Arthritis. While much information is gained by focusing attention on the involved joint, other systems of the body must also be examined, since either overt or minimal findings in these regions can shed light on the diagnosis of the musculoskeletal problem. Details concerning such a review are presented in other portions of this text; suggestions concerning the application of systemic findings to the interpretation of some of the causes of monarticular arthritis are presented in Table 25–5.

Table 25–4. Regional Articular and Periarticular Syndromes of Peripheral Joints

Region	Joint	Periarticular Syndrome	Nonarticular Syndrome
Jaw	Temporomandibular	Temporomandibular joint dysfunction	Temporal arteritis Molar dental problems Parotid swelling Preauricular lymphadenitis
Shoulder	Glenohumeral Acromioclavicular Sternoclavicular	Subacromial bursitis Long head bicipital tendinitis	
Elbow	Humeroulnar Proximal radioulnar	Olecranon bursitis Epicondylitis	Ulnar nerve entrapment
Wrist	Radiocarpal Intercarpal, second to fifth carpometacarpal First carpometacarpal	Extensor tendinitis (including de Quervain's tenosynovitis)	Carpal tunnel syndrome
Hand	Metacarpophalangeal Proximal interphalangeal Distal interphalangeal	Palmar fasciitis (Dupuytren's contracture)	
Hip	Acetabular-femoral	Greater trochanteric bursitis Adductor syndrome Ischial bursitis Fascia lata syndrome	Meralgia paresthetica
Knee	Condylar-tibial Patellar-condylar	Anserine bursitis Prepatellar bursitis Meniscal injury Ligamentous tear–laxity	
Ankle	Tibiotalar Subtalar (talonavicular, calcaneocuboid, talocalcaneal)	Peroneal tendinitis Subachilles bursitis Calcaneal fasciitis	Tarsal tunnel syndrome
Foot	Intertalar Metatarsophalangeal Interphalangeal	First metatarsophalangeal bursitis (bunion)	Morton's neuroma

Table 25–5. Systemic Features of Monarticular Arthritis

System	Mono- or Oligoarticular Arthritis
Skin	Juvenile chronic arthritis (Still's variety)
	Psoriatic arthritis
	Reiter's syndrome
	Colitic arthritis
	Sarcoid arthritis
	Familial Mediterranean fever
	Septic arthritis (esp. *N. gonorrhoeae* and *meningitidis*)
	Hyperlipoproteinemia
	Hemochromatosis
	Hemophilia, scurvy
	Fat necrosis due to pancreatic disease
	Amyloidosis
Nasopharynx and ear	Reiter's syndrome
	Gout
	Relapsing polychondritis
Eye	Juvenile rheumatoid arthritis
	Reiter's syndrome
	Relapsing polychondritis
	Sarcoid arthritis
Gastrointestinal tract	Colitic arthritis
	Whipple's disease
	Hemochromatosis
	Fat necrosis due to pancreatic disease
Heart and circulation	Amyloidosis
	Reiter's syndrome
	Relapsing polychondritis
Respiratory tract	Sarcoidosis
	Relapsing polychondritis
Nervous system	Neuropathic arthropathy
Renal system	Amyloidosis
	Gout
Hematologic system	Hemophilia
	Gaucher's disease
	Hemochromatosis

uable information that can direct the physician's attention toward the appropriate diagnosis (Table 25–7).

Roentgenograms and Radioisotopic Scans. Most often the roentgenogram of the involved site will reveal normal bone density and structure and a preserved cartilage space. Nevertheless, films should always be obtained at the outset, both of the affected and of the contralateral joint. Comparison of the films of paired joints is especially valuable in monarticular arthritis, since the normal joint acts as a control for the diseased joint and permits greater confidence in the interpretation of borderline abnormalities. Sometimes, as in chondrocalcinosis, the stippled line of calcific density on the articular surface can be seen in both the inflamed and the quiescent joint, thereby adding to the confidence of the diagnosis. Even totally normal films have value. They offer a baseline against which the efficacy of treatment can be measured. Findings that can be noted on roentgenograms are listed in Table 25–7.

In contrast, radioisotopic scans are often positive even in the early stages of disease and regardless of the type of process affecting the joint (Table 25–7). For this purpose, radioactive technetium is usually coupled to a polyphosphonate compound that has a preferential affinity for sites of active bone metabolism. Superficial joints can be more accurately appraised by clinical examination, but in deep-seated joints such as the hip or the shoulder as well as the spine, the scan can indicate that the site of pathology is confined within the joint or the bone rather than spread out into the surrounding soft tissues. Distinction between cellulitis and synovitis is possible by this method. The scan also can help identify areas of aseptic necrosis. Patients in whom uncertainty exists about the anatomic localization of disease should be checked by the radioisotopic scan; in others, this procedure may not be required.

IMMEDIATE LABORATORY STUDIES

Joint Fluid Examination. Patients with monarticular arthritis may demonstrate a joint effusion, and its possible presence should be carefully sought. Even a trace amount of excess joint fluid can be aspirated and used for microscopic examination or for culture. The selection of which tests should be run when only a small volume of sample is available must take into account the most likely diagnoses being considered, but as a general rule should include a wet-mount preparation for a semi-quantitative assessment of the number and type of cells and the demonstration of monosodium urate or calcium pyrophosphate dihydrate crystals; a gram-stained smear for rapid identification of the common bacterial invaders of the joint; and finally a standard culture preparation. All these critical procedures can be performed with as little as 2 or 3 drops of fluid. Given a larger amount of fluid, a more extended analysis can be performed (Table 25–6).

Urine, Blood, and Other Body Fluid Examinations. Conventional laboratory procedures may provide val-

IMMEDIATE MANAGEMENT

Apart from the urgency to begin treatment at once for a potential joint infection even before the diagnosis is confirmed or for a crystal-induced arthritis, the natural course of the disease can well be observed during the first few days. Drugs that might modify the inflammatory response, such as corticosteroids, and even non-steroidal anti-inflammatory drugs, such as aspirin, should be withheld. Comfort for the patient can be achieved by the use of splints or other supportive devices and an analgesic medication such as codeine or propoxyphene. Intra-articular injection of corticosteroids should be avoided, not only because of its dramatic effect on the reduction of inflammation but also because it can facilitate extension of an infectious process.

In monarticular arthritis, three common situations present during the first few days that require special mention. Foremost is consideration of septic arthritis. All patients with monarticular arthritis must be consid-

Table 25–6. Diagnostic Findings from Joint Fluid Examination in Monarticular Arthritis (After Harris)

Test	Finding	Possible Diagnosis
Appearance	Bloody	Traumatic arthritis
		Bleeding/clotting disorder
		Neuropathic arthropathy
		Pigmented villonodular synovitis
	Turbid	Septic arthritis
		Other inflammatory arthritides
	Clear	Degenerative joint disease
		Mechanical derangement of joint
White blood cell count	<2000/mm^3	Osteoarthritis
		Amyloidosis
		Osteochondromatosis
		Osteochondritis dissecans
		Gaucher's disease
		Hemochromatosis
		Arthritis with pancreatic disease
	2000–50,000/mm^3	Juvenile chronic arthritis
		Psoriatic arthritis
		Reiter's syndrome
		Colitic arthritis
		Familial Mediterranean fever
		Gout
		Pseudogout
		Septic arthritis
	>50,000/mm^3	Septic arthritis
		Gout
		Pseudogout
		Reiter's syndrome
Microscopy, wet mount	Sodium monourate crystals	Gout[37]
	Calcium pyrophosphate dihydrate crystals	Pseudogout[6]
	Lipid droplets	Traumatic arthritis, arthritis with pancreatic disease[22,38]
Glucose (simultaneous blood glucose normal)	<20 mg%	Septic arthritis
	>20 mg%	Septic arthritis
		Nonseptic inflammatory arthritides
Wright's stained smear	Mononuclear phagocytic cells	Reiter's disease (nonspecific)[39]
Gram-stained smear/culture	Gram-positive and gram-negative microorganisms	Septic arthritis[2]
Miscellaneous stained smear	Acid-fast microorganisms	Tuberculous, lepromatous arthritis[40]
	PAS-positive fungal bodies	Fungal arthritis[1,3]
	Congo red positive debris	Amyloid arthritis[41]
	PAS-positive intracellular inclusions	Whipple's disease[42]

ered candidates for this disease until it has been definitely excluded. Next is the approach that can be taken when a crystal-induced arthritis such as gout or pseudogout is thought to exist. Lastly, the most common situation is represented by those patients with an inflammatory disease not caused by either of these specific conditions. Further details concerning the diagnosis and management of each of these diseases, as well as the host of others that might present as a monarticular arthritis, are given elsewhere in this text.

Possible Septic Arthritis. Clues that an infection is a probable diagnosis may be found in the history and examination as well as in the joint fluid. Demonstration of microorganisms on smear of joint fluid is absolute evidence of infection; indirect evidence might be a markedly decreased synovial fluid glucose concentration in a turbid fluid containing large numbers of polymorphonuclear leukocytes. However, infection may still have to be considered in the absence of these findings. In gonococcal arthritis, the smear and indeed the culture may

be negative and the synovial fluid glucose only moderately decreased. Whenever the clinical findings suggest the possibility of infection, the proper course of action is to initiate antibiotic treatment, preferably intravenously or intramuscularly, and to monitor the response of the patient during the next several days. In gonococcal disease, the decrease in joint swelling and the return of the synovial fluid abnormalities toward normal usually occur in this time. Disease caused by other microorganisms may respond more slowly, but even if the response to antibiotic therapy directed at the presumed infectious agent is not completely convincing, results of the culture will be returned during this period. Based upon whether the culture is positive or negative, a more rational therapeutic decision can then be made.

Possible Crystal-Induced Arthritis. In almost every instance, the diagnosis of gout or pseudogout can be made with absolute certainty within the first several hours by careful examination of joint fluid for the appropriate crystal: a strongly negative needle-shaped

Table 25–7. Diagnostic Findings from Laboratory Tests and Procedure in Monarticular Arthritis*

Test	Finding	Possible Diagnosis
Urinalysis	Protein	Amyloidosis
	WBC/RBC	Gout
	Stones	Gout
Hematology	Leukocytosis	Septic arthritis
		Gout (mild elevation)
	Bleeding/clotting abnormality	Hemophilia, scurvy
Sedimentation rate	Elevated	Inflammatory arthritides
C-reactive protein		
Chemistry		
Urea nitrogen, creatinine	Elevated	Amyloidosis, gout
SGOT, LDH	Elevated	Hemochromatosis
Uric acid	Elevated	Gout
Globulin	Elevated	Sarcoidosis, amyloidosis
Calcium	Elevated	Pseudogout, sarcoidosis
Amylase	Elevated	Fat necrosis in pancreatic disease
Cholesterol	Elevated	Hyperlipoproteinemia
Radiology	Normal bone film	Inflammatory arthritides (early or mild)
	Bone erosion/cartilage loss	Neuropathic arthropathy
		Gout (tophi)
		Juvenile chronic arthritis (late)
		Septic arthritis
		Avascular necrosis
	Lytic lesions/cysts	Juxta-articular bone tumors
		Osteoarthritis
		Osteochondritis dissecans
	Calcification (articular and/or synovial)	Pseudogout
		Osteochondromatosis
Radioisotopic scan	Polyphosphonate localization	Most arthropathies

*Excluding synovial fluid analysis.

monosodium urate crystal or a weakly positive needle- or rhomboid-shaped calcium pyrophosphate dihydrate crystal. Once the diagnosis is made, specific therapy can be started. In most patients with gout, colchicine can be used, either orally or by intravenous injection. The latter technique reduces the likelihood of such gastrointestinal side effects as nausea, vomiting, and diarrhea. Colchicine remains one of the relatively few drugs that are effective in one or only a few diseases. The dramatic improvement in pain and the slower reduction of swelling within the first 24 hours of its use are strong evidence for a diagnosis of gout. Another situation in which it may be effective is familial Mediterranean fever, but this disease can be distinguished from gout on clinical grounds and by the absence of crystals in joint fluid. Alternative drugs would be the nonsteroidal anti-inflammatory compounds, but, as opposed to the selectivity of colchicine for gout, these drugs are wholly nonspecific in their ability to control inflammation. They are more reasonable for treatment of pseudogout, in which the action of colchicine is usually far less effective.

Nonspecific Inflammatory Monarthritis. The dilemma faced most often is the management of the patient with but one or two inflamed joints in whom no data that could establish a diagnosis are available within the first 24 to 72 hours. In some of these patients, infection may still be a consideration. Whenever this possibility cannot be definitely excluded, one might choose a course of antibiotics or perhaps just observation. Pain relief should be attempted by drugs or physical measures that will not modify the inflammatory process. Antipyretic drugs such as aspirin or acetaminophen and the nonsteroidal anti-inflammatory drugs should not be used. Fever and the possibility of extension of arthritis to other joints are helpful indicators of the nature of the underlying disease. Once sufficient evidence is at hand that infection is no longer a likely problem, then analgesic or anti-inflammatory treatment may be employed.

In the past, the striking effect of aspirin in rheumatic fever led to the notion that it could be used in a therapeutic trial in this disease. If an arthritic process rapidly abates, perhaps in 2 to 3 days, during the use of aspirin, rheumatic fever might well be considered; but, unfortunately from the standpoint of the selectivity of aspirin, other unrelated inflammatory arthritides do also. Thus, as indicated above, aspirin and other nonsteroidal anti-inflammatory drugs should only be prescribed in the initial phases of management, particularly in monarticular arthritis, after careful consideration has been given to the need to monitor the natural course of the illness, especially to response of more truly specific drugs as colchicine or an antibiotic drug.

Generally, early in the evaluation of the patient with monarticular arthritis, the physician will choose between colchicine, an antibiotic, aspirin, or observation for the reasons described above.

REASSESSMENT

Diagnosis Confirmed. During the first week, a diagnosis will have been established for most patients with an arthritis whose cause or pathogenesis is well understood. Some solutions will be direct, as is often the case with, among others, gout, pseudogout, septic arthritis, and traumatic arthritis. Other solutions will be reached upon completion of special diagnostic studies or after the appearance of additional clinical findings, as with the recognition of the bowel lesion of regional enteritis in a puzzling case of oligoarthritis or the detection of a *Salmonella* species in the stool culture of a HLA-B27 positive young adult with a similar arthritis.

Diagnosis Unconfirmed. Other patients, perhaps even a majority, with monarticular arthritis remain an enigma. With mixed emotions, the physician will observe that a large number undergo a spontaneous remission, leaving unanswered, at least for the moment, why the disease occurred and whether it will return. For most of these patients, optimism is in order. The frequency of unexplained types of monarthritis is much higher than is generally realized, with only a small portion likely to recur. In part this is due to the one-time nature of the illness: a viral disease or a traumatic event. Even for conditions that are thought to be progressive and persistent, such as rheumatoid arthritis, it is reasonable to assume that mild forms of disease occur that undergo a spontaneous cure.

In some patients, arthritis may persist, still lacking a definite diagnosis. In these, the dictum postulated above, that one should observe their natural history without modification by treatment, may now pay off. Some will slowly develop additional features of their illness. Although most patients with psoriatic arthritis show skin lesions before arthritis, a few develop psoriatic plaques later, thus providing an explanation for the previously unknown type of oligoarthritis. The rare syndrome of systemic fat necrosis seen with chronic pancreatitis or pancreatic carcinoma becomes obvious upon the radiologic demonstration of calcific deposits in the pancreas, a high serum amylase, or the necrotic lesion in a biopsy of the subcutaneous adipose tissue. In others, concern for a possible infection may remain, so that additional diagnostic tests will be required.

Among such procedures are those that provide more information about the diseased joint. A tomogram can reveal details of a juxta-articular bone tumor, osteomyelitis, osteochondromatosis, avascular necrosis, juvenile osteochondrosis, or osteochondritis dissecans. A dye and/or air-contrast arthrogram can define a meniscal tear or the filling defect of nonradiopaque osteochondromatosis. Computerized tomograms can define abnormalities of an internal structure with increasingly distinct precision, particularly if the structure has a density that contrasts with that of surrounding tissues. Metal, bone, or calcified tissues stand out, as does adipose tissue, against connective tissues and muscle, tendons, and capsule. This method can help identify foreign bodies such as plant thorns or tumors within the joint.

Synovial biopsy can provide direct information about the pathology of the disease.[43] In pigmented villonodular synovitis, the brownish, hemosiderin-laden tissue can be diagnostic. The electron-dense bodies of Whipple's disease have been found in synovium as well as in the small bowel mucosa. The granulomatous lesions of sarcoid and tuberculosis can be seen, with the further opportunity provided by the biopsy to inoculate tissue samples into appropriate culture media. In mycobacterial infections, including leprosy and atypical tuberculosis in addition to infection with *M. tuberculosis,* in fungal infections, and in infections caused by some common pyogenic invaders such as staphylococci and gonococci, culture of synovial tissue has proved to be positive when culture of joint fluid remained negative.

Direct inspection of the synovium can be accomplished by use of open biopsy rather than closed needle biopsy. Instances when this may be helpful are, for example, the diagnosis of a foreign body in synovium or the opportunity to exclude a mechanical defect such as a torn cartilage in a chronically inflamed joint. Some of these problems can now be more conveniently explored by arthroscopy.[44] This procedure allows inspection of the interior of large joints, especially the knee, and biopsy under direct vision of selected areas of synovium or cartilage.

THE UNDIAGNOSED MONARTICULAR ARTHRITIS

For those patients in whom a diagnosis of a persistent arthritis cannot be made despite all tests, therapy with intra-articular steroid may be useful. Negative cultures and tissue examination will have excluded all reasonable possibility of sepsis. Control of synovitis is sometimes dramatic by this approach, particularly when combined with a period of several weeks of either immobilization or absence of weight bearing. Injections can be repeated at intervals of at least 2 to 3 months; if after several injections, such maneuvers fail to control the disease, synovectomy should be considered, in the hope that this surgical approach will permit eradication of the process, or at least give information about the cause of the arthritis. Close cooperation among the various physicians involved in the care of the patient—the primary physician, the rheumatologist, the orthopedic surgeon, and others, including the team from rehabilitation medicine—is the best way to manage these difficult cases. Not only must all efforts to eliminate the disease be carried out before a state of chronic disability is accepted; appropriate planning for future activities at home or at work is also necessary.

Although most cases of monarticular arthritis yield a satisfactory answer, the temptation to apply a specific diagnostic label to the truly undiagnosed case should be scrupulously avoided even if it offends the physician's pride. Some problems are idiopathic. The main reason for use of a term as "nonspecific inflammatory monarthritis" is to encourage future studies to help clarify the diagnosis. Periodic reviews at appointed intervals offer both the patient and the physician the opportunity to observe new developments. The uncomfortable presence of these patients with a nonspecific arthritis has been a strong challenge to clinical investigators. Their efforts have led to renewed interest in synovial histopathology, to the acceptance of diagnostic arthroscopy, and to a detailed analysis of all circumstances surrounding the earliest stages of such cases. In the future, these approaches along with others will reduce still further the numbers of patients for whom no exact diagnosis can be made.

References

1. Schumacher, H.R.: Joint pathology in infectious arthritis. Clin. Rheum. Dis. 4:33, 1978.
2. Goldenberg, D.L., and Cohen, A.S.: Acute infectious arthritis. A review of patients with nongonococcal joint infections (with emphasis on therapy and prognosis). Am. J. Med. 60:369, 1976.
3. Goldenberg, D.L., and Cohen, A.S.: Arthritis due to tuberculous and fungal microorganisms. Clin. Rheum. Dis. 4:211, 1978.
4. Brogadir, S.P., Schimmer, B.M., and Myers, A.R.: Spectrum of the gonococcal arthritis-dermatitis syndrome. Semin. Arthritis Rheum. 8:177, 1979.
5. Grahame, R., and Scott, J.T.: Clinical survey of 354 patients with gout. Ann. Rheum. Dis. 29:461, 1970.
6. McCarty, D.J.: Calcium pyrophosphate dihydrate deposition disease—1975. Arthritis Rheum. 19:275, 1976.
7. Katz, I., Rainowitz, J.G., and Dziadiw, R.: Early changes in Charcot's joints. Am. J. Roentgenol. 86:965, 1961.
8. Hilgartner, M.W.: Hemophilic arthropathy. Adv. Pediatr. 21:139, 1975.
9. Ahlberg, A., and Silwer, J.: Arthropathy in von Willebrand's disease. Acta Orthop. Scand. 41:539, 1970.
10. Wild, J.H., and Zvaifler, N.J.: Hemarthrosis associated with sodium warfarin therapy. Arthritis Rheum. 19:98, 1976.
11. Heller, H., Gafni, J., Michaeli, D., Shahin, N., Sohar, E., Ehrlich, G., Karten, I., and Sokoloff, L.: Arthritis of familial Mediterranean fever (FMF). Arthritis Rheum. 9:1, 1966.
12. Silverstein, M.N., and Kelly, P.J.: Osteoarticular manifestations of Gaucher's disease. Am. J. Med. Sc. 253:569, 1967.
13. Glueck, C.J., Levy, R.I., and Fredrickson, D.S.: Acute tendinitis and arthritis. A presenting symptom of familial Type II hyperlipoproteinemia. JAMA 206:2895, 1968.
14. Martel, W., and Sitterly, B.H.: Roentgenologic manifestations of osteonecrosis. Am. J. Roentgenol. 106:509, 1969.
15. Bauer, G.C.H.: Osteonecrosis of the knee. Clin. Orthop. 130:210, 1978.
16. Byers, P.D., Cotton, R.E., Deacon, R.W., Lowy, M., Newman, P.H., Sissons, H.A., and Thomas, A.D.: The diagnosis and treatment of pigmented villonodular synovitis. J. Bone Joint Surg. 50B:290, 1968.
17. Cadman, N.L., Soule, E.H., and Kelly, P.J.: Synovial sarcoma: An analysis of 134 tumors. Cancer 18:613, 1965.
18. Calabro, J.J.: Cancer and arthritis. Arthritis Rheum. 10:553, 1967.
19. Goldenberg, D.L., Kelley, W., and Gibbons, R.B.: Metastatic adenocarcinoma of synovium presenting as an acute arthritis. Arthritis Rheum. 18:107, 1975.
20. Lagier, R.: Synovial reaction caused by adjacent malignant tumors: Anatomico-pathological study of three cases. J. Rheumatol. 4:65, 1977.
21. Milgram, J.W.: Synovial osteochondromatosis: A histologic study of 30 cases. J. Bone Joint Surg. 59A:792, 1977.
22. Gibson, T., Schumacher, H.R., Pascual, E., and Brighton, C.: Arthropathy, skin and bone lesions in pancreatic disease. J. Rheum. 2:7, 1975.
23. Calin, A.: Reiter's syndrome. Med. Clin. North Am. 61:365, 1977.
24. Cassidy, J.T., Brody, G.L., and Martel, W.: Monarticular juvenile rheumatoid arthritis. J. Pediatr. 70:867, 1967.
25. Sherman, M.: Psoriatic arthritis: Observations on the clinical, roentgenographic and pathological changes. J. Bone Joint Surg. 34A:831, 1952.
26. Wright, V.: Psoriasis and arthritis. Ann. Rheum. Dis. 15:348, 1956.
27. Haslock, I., and Wright, V.: The musculo-skeletal complications of Crohn's disease. Medicine 52:217, 1973.
28. Wright, V., and Watkinson, G.: The arthritis of ulcerative colitis. Br. Med. J. 2:670, 1965.
29. Kelly, J.J. III, and Weisiger, B.B.: The arthritis of Whipple's disease. Arthritis Rheum. 6:615, 1963.
30. Spilberg, I., Siltzbach, L.E., and McEwen, C.E.: The arthritis of sarcoidosis. Arthritis Rheum. 12:126, 1969.
31. Dymock, I.W., Hamilton, E.B.D., Laws, J.W., and Williams, R.: Arthropathy of haemochromatosis. Clinical and radiologic analysis of 63 patients with iron overload. Ann. Rheum. Dis. 29:469, 1970.
32. Solomon, L.: Patterns of osteoarthritis of the hip. J. Bone Joint Surg. 58B:176, 1976.
33. Cohen, A.S., and Canoso, J.J.: Rheumatological aspects of amyloid disease. Clin. Rheum. Dis. 1:149, 1975.
34. O'Hanlan, M., McAdam, L.P., Bluestone, R., and Pearson, C.M.: The arthropathy of relapsing polychondritis. Arthritis Rheum. 19:191, 1976.
35. Khachadurian, A.K.: Migratory polyarthritis in familial hypercholesterolemia (Type II hyperlipoproteinemia). Arthritis Rheum. 11:385, 1968.
36. Goldman, J.A., Abrams, N.R., Glueck, C.J., Steiner, P., and Herman, J.H.: Musculoskeletal disorders associated with Type IV hyperlipoproteinemia. Lancet 2:449, 1972.
37. McCarty, D.J., and Hollander, J.L.: Identification of urate crystals in gouty synovial fluid. Ann. Intern. Med. 54:452, 1961.
38. Graham, J., and Goldman, J.A.: Fat droplets and synovial fluid leukocytes in traumatic arthritis. Arthritis Rheum. 21:76, 1978.
39. Pekin, T.J. Jr., Malinin, T.I., Zvaifler, N.J.: Unusual synovial fluid findings in Reiter's syndrome. Ann. Intern. Med. 66:677, 1967.
40. Wallace, R., and Cohen, A.S.: Tuberculous arthritis. A report of two cases with a review of biopsy and synovial fluid findings. Am. J. Med. 61:277, 1976.
41. Gordon, D.A., Pruzanski, W., and Ogryzlo, M.A.: Synovial fluid examination for the diagnosis of amyloidosis. Ann. Rheum. Dis. 32:428, 1973.
42. Hawkins, C.F., Farr, M., Morris, C.J., Hoare, A.M., and Williamson, N.: Detection by electron microscope of rod-shaped organisms in synovial membrane from a patient with the arthritis of Whipple's disease. Ann. Rheum. Dis. 35:502, 1976.
43. Goldenberg, D.L., and Cohen, A.S.: Synovial membrane histopathology in the differential diagnosis of rheumatoid arthritis, gout, pseudogout, systemic lupus erythematosus, infectious arthritis and degenerative joint disease. Medicine 57:239, 1978.
44. Johnson, L.L.: Comprehensive Arthroscopic Examination of the Knee. St. Louis, C.V. Mosby Co., 1977.

Chapter 26
Polyarticular Arthritis

Ronald J. Anderson

THE DIFFERENTIAL DIAGNOSIS OF POLYARTICULAR SYMPTOMS

In evaluating a patient with polyarticular joint complaints the initial decision is to determine whether one is dealing with (1) polyarticular synovitis, (2) multiple structural lesions, or (3) diffuse myalgias. There are several features of the latter two conditions that permit one to make such a diagnosis based primarily on history and physical examination alone (Table 26–1).

MULTIPLE STRUCTURAL LESIONS

Although degenerative joint disease is most frequently a monarticular process, it may occur in either a symmetrical or a polyarticular fashion. The occurrence of premature polyarticular degenerative joint disease should alert one to the possibility of a primary defect in cartilage metabolism such as is seen in either hemachromatosis or ochronosis.

Features of Structural Lesions

Historical Features. *Progressive Increase in Symptoms.* Because of the irreversibility of cartilage loss, the symptoms tend to become progressively more severe. However, because of the gradual process of cartilage wear, the time course necessary for the development of these symptoms is prolonged and usually entails several years.

Absence of Symptoms at Rest. As the genesis of pain in structural lesions would appear to be due to the opposition of two imperfect surfaces against each other, the predominant early symptoms of structural lesions occur only with use. It is only late in the course of the degenerative process that pain at rest occurs.

Absence of Reversible "Flares." As the process is a gradual degenerative one, "flares" of increased symptoms are rare and should be attributed to some other cause (e.g., bursitis, pseudogout) rather than to an increase in cartilage degeneration itself.

Lack of Response to Anti-inflammatory Therapy. Because synovitis or other inflammatory conditions play little or no role in causing symptoms, the clinical response to the use of these agents is minimal. A frequent exception, however, is a beneficial symptomatic response to indomethacin seen in osteoarthritis of the hip.

Absence of Systemic Symptoms. Since the disease process is local and primarily degenerative, there is an absence of systemic malaise or other generalized symptoms.

Absence of Prolonged Morning Stiffness. Morning stiffness in structural lesions is a "gelling" phenomenon, with maximal relief occurring in 5 to 10 minutes. This is in contradistinction to the chronic rheumatic diseases, which have prolonged morning stiffness.

Objective Data. 1. Localization to weight-bearing joints. It is unusual for degenerative changes to occur in such non-weight-bearing joints as the shoulder, elbow, wrist, or metacarpal-phalangeal joints.

2. Radiographic evidence of cartilage loss in the involved joints.

3. Radiographic evidence of hypertrophic new bone formation. This feature is absent in the synovitic conditions because the erosive inflammatory process precludes new bone formation. Because significant synovitis is not seen in osteoarthritis, the reparative process is allowed to occur and hypertrophic spurs are frequently seen.

4. Noninflammatory characteristics of synovial fluid.

Diffuse Myalgia

This entity encompasses a large group of conditions, the primary features of which are benignity, nonprogressiveness, and generally an absence of physical findings. The symptoms seem to arise out of the muscles

Table 26–1. Cardinal Distinctions Between Structural and Synovial Lesions

Structural Lesions	Synovial Lesions
Subjective Features	
Symptoms only with use	Symptoms at rest
"Gelling" phenomenon	Morning stiffness common
Progressive worsening course	Variable course
Flares not seen	Flares common
Minimal response to medical treatment	Patient often benefits from medical treatment
Patient systematically well	Patient often systemically ill
Objective Features	
Crepitus and bony hypertrophy on physical examination	Soft tissue swelling on physical examination
Noninflammatory joint fluid	Inflammatory joint fluid
X-ray:	X-ray:
Usually positive	Negative early in course
Local cartilage loss	Diffuse cartilage loss
Often new bone growth	No new bone growth
Weight-bearing joints involved	Any joint involved (e.g., elbow)
Therapy	
Surgical	Medical

and periarticular structures. Patients with these complaints range from a group of patients best described as "achey" to another group who appear to use their symptoms for secondary gain. The "genuinely achey" group would seem to be analogous to patients with a spastic colon in that they are anatomically normal and do not develop any specific lesion. Laboratory examinations in the rheumatic diseases are relatively nonspecific. In the area of "false-positives" approximately 30 percent of "normals" will be latex positive, ANA positive, or hyperuricemic. It may also be stated, parenthetically, that no one over age 40 has a normal spinal radiograph. In regard to "false-negatives," skeletal radiographs are invariably normal in early synovitis, and the latex, ANA, and serum uric acid are frequently normal in those patients afflicted with the corresponding conditions. Therefore, as in most of rheumatology, it may be said regarding benign myalgias that if the physician does not know whether a patient is sick or not prior to laboratory evaluation, the laboratory and radiologic data will not answer this basic question.

FEATURES OF BENIGN MYALGIAS

Intermittent Pattern of Symptoms with Asymptomatic Intervals. This pattern is frequently abrupt in onset, with symptoms lasting only several minutes to hours, a distinguishing point from synovitis, in which the inflammatory process can seldom arise and subside in less than 3 days. The major value of this historical feature is in the differentiation from the generally irreversible structural lesions, which, with the exception of a deranged knee meniscus, are never intermittent. A corollary of this feature is that radiographic abnormalities of an intermittently asymptomatic joint are meaningless, as the radiograph shows irreversible changes that can never improve.

Lack of Functional Loss. There is no functional loss, or what functional loss exists is "illogical." Any condition with the ability to alter or destroy the anatomy of a joint will be associated with a dysfunction or loss of function of that particular joint. For example, patients with diseases affecting the hands will become unable to open jars or turn faucets. Hip or knee disease is associated with an inability to arise from a bathtub or a low chair. These specific dysfunctions are virtually universally found in disorders of these joints, and their absence implies that a significant disorder of these joints does not exist. Patients with benign myalgias, on the other hand, do not lose function over time, or whatever function they do lose is illogical (e.g., the patient no longer is employed but he still goes bowling). The usual history obtained is: "I've slowed down," but one cannot elicit a specific function that the patient cannot do.

Negative or Static Physical Examination. The physical examination is negative or static over an extended period of time. Occasionally a patient will be examined on a "good day" when he is asymptomatic and the physical examination is negative. If this is the situation

and the patient states, "You should have seen me 10 days ago when I was bad," the logical diagnostic approach is to have him return on a day when he is symptomatic and examine him at that time to determine if a change has occurred. If, on the other hand, the examination is negative in a patient with persistent symptoms, a logical approach is to record functions quantitatively (e.g., grip strengths, range of motion, timed walk of 50 feet) and then re-examine the patient several months later. If the measurements are unchanged, one can infer that no active destructive process, despite persistent symptoms, has occurred during the interim.

THE DIAGNOSIS OF SYNOVITIS

The ultimate requirement for the diagnosis of synovitis is the demonstration of inflammatory changes in a joint. The techniques used to perform this are as follows.

Evaluation of Historical Features. The author's experience has lead him to believe that patients are frequently unreliable in describing swelling within their own joints. More credence may be lent to a description by family members of the appearance of the joint, particularly when it is unilateral. The description by the patient of swelling in joints in which synovitis is never physically apparent (i.e., spine or hips) leads the physician to doubt the patient's reliability as an examiner of himself. However, several historical features are valuable.

The Significance of Morning Stiffness. Any musculoskeletal disorder, even a sprained ankle, has accentuated symptoms following prolonged immobility. However, in benign myalgias, most of the acute inflammatory disorders such as gout, and osteoarthritis, in general the stiffness tends to be short lived, and maximal alleviation of the symptoms is noted after 5 to 10 minutes of activity. In contrast, in the chronic inflammatory disorders (rheumatoid arthritis, spondylitis, psoriatic arthritis, and systemic lupus erythematosus), the morning stiffness tends to be prolonged for several hours' duration. This is not only a subjective phenomenon. Objective signs of synovitis may be detected on early-morning examinations but disappear as the day progresses. Measurements of joint function (i.e., grip strengths) also tend to improve in the same pattern.

It is advisable to quantitate the duration of morning stiffness in a standardized fashion. A phrase such as: "How long does it take, once you get up in the morning, until you're as good as you'll ever be?" usually will result in a reproducibly quantitative answer. The duration is a valuable bit of data for two reasons:

1. Significant (greater than one hour) morning stiffness tends to differentiate the chronic inflammatory processes from other disorders.

2. The duration of morning stiffness tends to parallel the severity of the synovitis. This is of particular value in assessing the effectiveness of anti-inflammatory therapy in patients whose symptoms represent a combina-

tion of potentially reversible synovitis and irreversible structural lesions. In such patients, a remission may be associated with a complete disappearance of morning stiffness but only minor or no improvement in the functional status. As medical therapy has the ability only to alter the reversible inflammatory aspects of these conditions, it becomes apparent that the duration of morning stiffness serves as a useful parameter in evaluating the effectiveness of such therapy.

Gradual Variability of Course. The inflammatory process of synovitis is potentially reversible, and periods of remission when the patient may be asymptomatic are seen in several conditions of this type. The minimal time required for a joint to become inflamed and then totally remit would seem to be in the range of 36 to 48 hours. Symptomatic flares in benign myalgias tend to be brief periods of symptoms lasting less than 24 hours.

It is more common for the synovitis to follow a course of gradual variability, with a rate of change measured in weeks and months. Specific dysfunctions occur during periods of synovitic activity, a distinguishing point in comparison with benign myalgias.

In contradistinction, the symptoms of structural lesions, with the exception of a deranged meniscus of the knee, are persistent and progressive in severity.

Symptoms at Rest. The presence of pain at rest is a feature of synovitis, neuropathies, and periarticular lesions (tendinitis, bursitis). Rest pain is seen in structural lesions only in the most far-advanced conditions in which a several-year history of increasing pain with activity is obtained.

Rapidity of Onset of Symptoms and Flares of Accentuated Activity. The degeneration of articular cartilage is a gradual process. Flares are rarely seen, and rapid improvement from accentuated symptoms is never seen. On the other hand, flares are common with synovitis.

Physical Examination. The appearance of an obviously inflamed, swollen joint makes the diagnosis easy. On the other hand, the hip and the spine will never appear swollen on physical examination, and one is forced to rely upon range of motion to elicit an objective abnormality. In addition, palpable effusions are rarely seen in the shoulder joint and are frequently subtle in the metacarpophalangeal and tarsal joints. In these latter two regions, one may employ examination techniques aimed at demonstrating spasm and shortening of muscles adjacent to inflamed joints. These techniques are as follows:

Bunnel's Sign. The intrinsic muscles of the hand, which consist of the lumbricales and the interossei, arise from the metacarpals, pass across the metacarpophalangeal joint, and serve to flex the metacarpophalangeal joint and extend the proximal interphalangeal joint. In the inflammation of the metacarpophalangeal joint, these muscles become tight and produce a situation in which proximal interphalangeal flexion is limited when the metacarpophalangeals are extended but normal when the metacarpophalangeals are flexed. Because the metacarpophalangeals are exclusively involved in synovitic processes and are not affected by osteoarthritis

or Bouchard's nodes, this sign is pathognomonic of synovitis of the metacarpophalangeal joint. In addition, in a patient with obvious synovitis it will distinguish between proximal interphalangeal and metacarpophalangeal disease as the cause of proximal interphalangeal dysfunction.

The principle of Bunnel's sign is also useful as a screening technique in evaluating generalized hand stiffness. A patient who can fully extend his fingers and also touch his fingertips to his palms with his metacarpophalangeals extended has normal metacarpophalangeals, proximal interphalangeals, and distal interphalangeals (Fig. 26-1; see Plate I, p. xxxv).

Peroneal Spasm. The peroneal muscles arise from the lateral calf, run across the tarsal bones, and serve to evert the foot. In tarsal inflammation, particularly of the talonavicular joint (the tarsal joint most commonly involved in rheumatoid arthritis), the peroneal musculature tightens up and everts the foot, and pain localized to the peroneal area is felt on forced inversion of the ankle. The associated tenderness localized to the talonavicular joint adds specificity to this maneuver (Fig. 26-2).

Laboratory Examination. The only direct technique of establishing the presence of synovitis in an inflamed joint is the determination of the white blood cell (WBC) count within the synovial fluids (Table 26-2).

The major diagnostic distinction that may be made based upon the synovial fluid WBC count is between an inflammatory condition and normal or osteoarthritic joint fluid. Although patients with septic arthritis may present with pus, they may also have a WBC count in the range found with sterile inflammatory conditions.

Figure 26-2. Peroneal spasm. Tenderness to palpation over the talonavicular-joint (cross-hatched area) in conjunction with painful spasm within the peroneal musculature (dotted area) upon passive inversion of the foot is indicative of talonavicular synovitis.

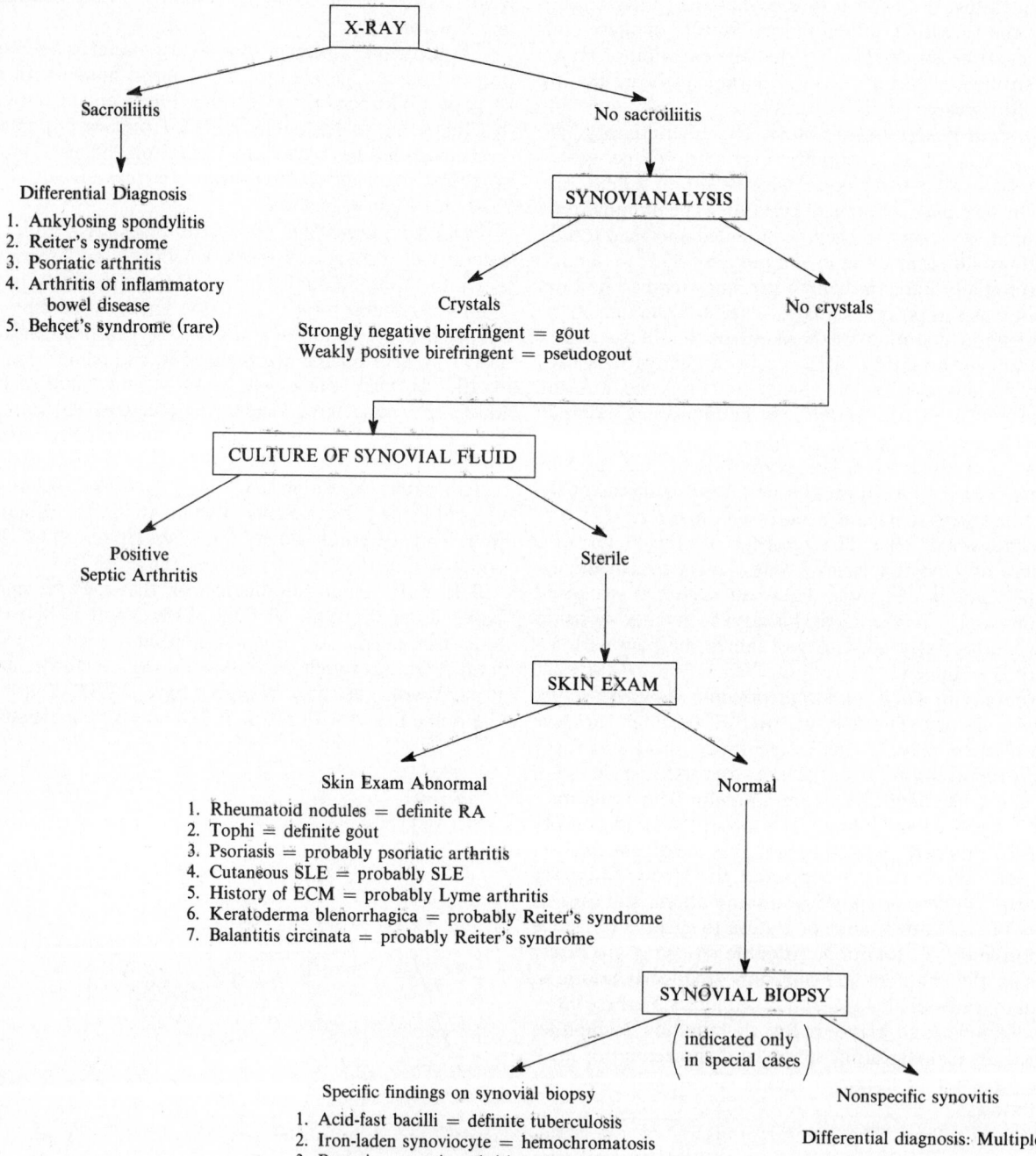

X-RAY

Sacroiliitis

No sacroiliitis

Differential Diagnosis

1. Ankylosing spondylitis
2. Reiter's syndrome
3. Psoriatic arthritis
4. Arthritis of inflammatory bowel disease
5. Behçet's syndrome (rare)

SYNOVIANALYSIS

Crystals

Strongly negative birefringent = gout
Weakly positive birefringent = pseudogout

No crystals

CULTURE OF SYNOVIAL FLUID

Positive
Septic Arthritis

Sterile

SKIN EXAM

Skin Exam Abnormal

1. Rheumatoid nodules = definite RA
2. Tophi = definite gout
3. Psoriasis = probably psoriatic arthritis
4. Cutaneous SLE = probably SLE
5. History of ECM = probably Lyme arthritis
6. Keratoderma blenorrhagica = probably Reiter's syndrome
7. Balantitis circinata = probably Reiter's syndrome

Normal

SYNOVIAL BIOPSY

(indicated only
in special cases)

Specific findings on synovial biopsy

1. Acid-fast bacilli = definite tuberculosis
2. Iron-laden synoviocyte = hemochromatosis
3. Bacteria = septic arthritis
4. Crystals = crystal-induced synovitis
5. Amyloid = amyloidosis
6. Plant thorn = plant thorn synovitis

Nonspecific synovitis

Differential diagnosis: Multiple

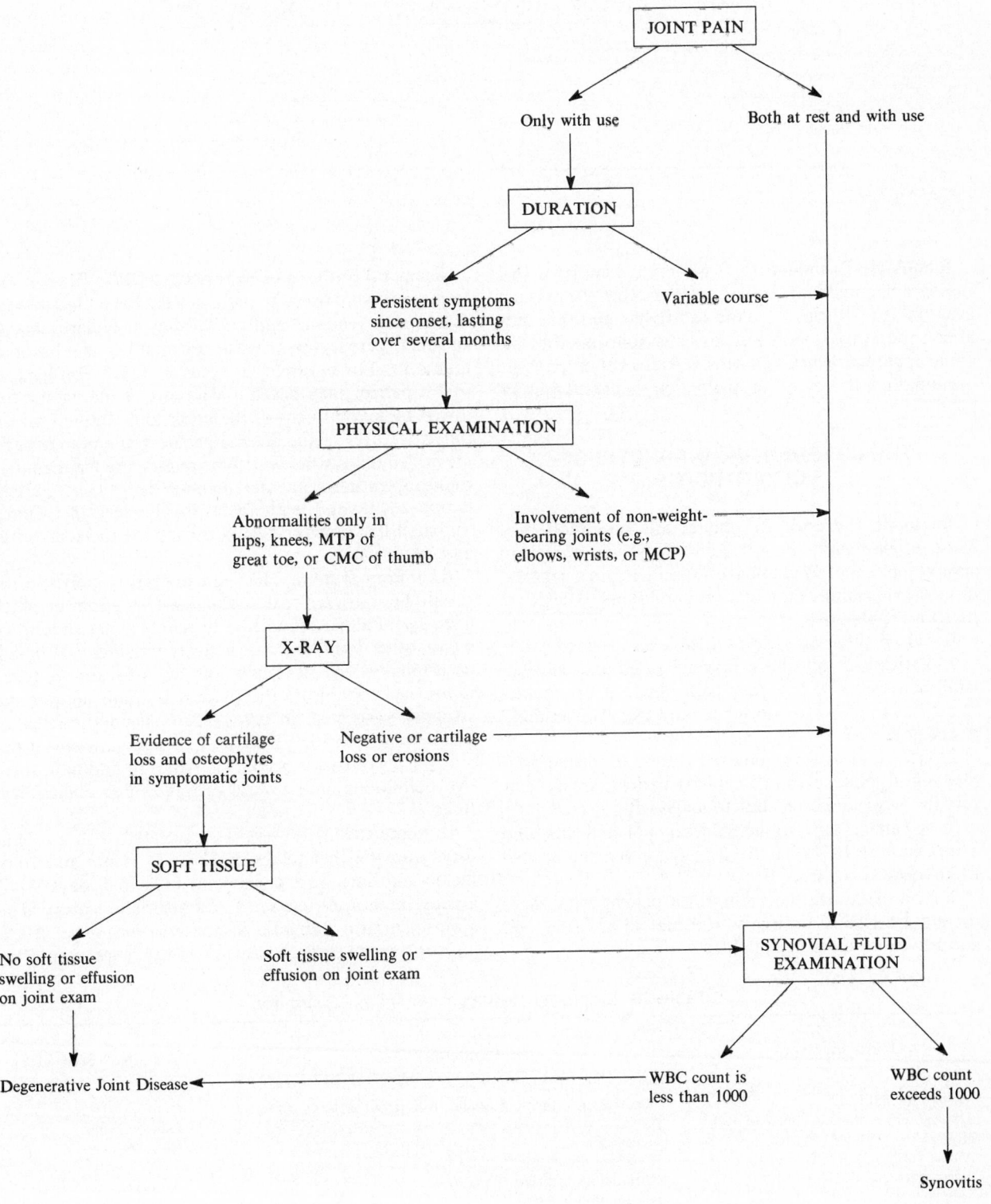

Table 26–2. White Blood Cell Count ($\times 10^3$)

Condition	0	1	2	4	8	16	32	64	128	Pus
Normal	—									
Osteoarthritis	————									
Rheumatoid arthritis			————————————————————							
Juvenile rheumatoid arthritis			————————————————————							
Gout						————————————				
Sepsis							————————————			

Radiologic Examination. It is well to remember that radiographs predominantly show bone, that the primary event in synovitis involves the soft tissue, and that only after a prolonged course do osseous abnormalities become apparent. When synovitis is equivocal on physical examination, it is even less distinct on roentgenography.

THE DIFFERENTIAL DIAGNOSIS OF POLYARTHRITIS

Anatomic Patterns. In general any condition may cause inflammation in any joint. However, there are several joints that seem to have a specificity, in a negative or positive manner, for certain conditions. These are listed in Table 26–3.

Based on these data, a few points can be made:

1. Patients complaining of generalized musculoskeletal pain who also have jaw pain usually have "something," as opposed to "nothing," and that "something" is not gout.

2. Deformities of the elbows, wrists, or metacarpophalangeal joints, even in an elderly patient, are due not just to "wear and tear" but to a synovitic process.

3. A patient with urethritis, fever, polyarthritis, and a *stiff neck* probably has Reiter's syndrome as opposed to gonococcal arthritis.

4. Low back pain occurring in a patient with rheumatoid arthritis is not due to rheumatoid arthritis, and another cause must be sought.

Temporal Patterns of Synovitis. *Additive Pattern.* The term additive pattern is used to describe a clinical syndrome that tends to add on features as it flares and to subtract these features in a similar manner as it becomes quiescent. For example, in systemic lupus erythematosus, a patient may develop synovitis of the wrists, followed by involvement of the knees and elbows. All the initial features of the disease persist while new features are added on. As the syndrome remits, the features tend to disappear in a sequential manner. This type of pattern is nonspecific and is characteristically seen in rheumatoid arthritis, lupus erythematosus, postrubella arthritis, and spondylitis.

Migratory Pattern. The term migratory polyarthritis should be restricted to describe those situations in which initially inflamed joints totally remit while, simultaneously, other joints become actively inflamed. Although occasionally seen in rheumatoid arthritis and systemic lupus erythematosus, the pattern is quite unique and strongly suggestive of either acute rheumatic fever or gonococcal arthritis. In each of these conditions, a migratory polyarthritis is characteristic. In addition, these two conditions have several distinguishing clinical features.

1. Acute rheumatic fever is associated with a migratory synovitis that peaks in 12 to 24 hours and completely subsides in a given joint in 2 to 5 days while arising in another region. A characteristic feature is an almost uniform dramatic response to full doses of salicylates, which seem capable of totally suppressing the

Table 26–3. Specific Joint Involvement in Polyarthritis

Joints Involved	Common With	Not Seen In
Temporomandibular	Rheumatoid arthritis, juvenile rheumatoid arthritis, psoriasis	Gout, myalgias
Elbows, wrists, metacarpophalangeals	Any synovitis	Osteoarthritis
Hips	Nonspecific	Gout
Ankles (only)	Erythema nodosum	
Cricoarytenoid	Rheumatoid arthritis	
Talonavicular	Rheumatoid arthritis	All other
Cervical spine	Rheumatoid arthritis, juvenile rheumatoid arthritis, psoriasis, osteoarthritis, spondylitis, myalgias	Gout, gonococcal arthritis

Thoracolumbar spine	Spondylitis:
	  Ankylosing spondylitis
	  Psoriasis
	  Reiter's syndrome
	  Inflammatory bowel disease
		Gout, rheumatoid arthritis

synovitis within 2 to 4 days after the initiation of therapy. If the salicylates are abruptly discontinued, the synovitis tends to reappear in a few days' time.

2. Gonococcal arthritis has two major patterns of joint involvement.[1,2] One pattern involves a migratory polyarthritis and tenosynovitis, predominantly of the small joints; bacteremia; petechial skin lesions, which progress to pustules; and sterile synovial fluid. Because of the difficulty of aspirating fluid from either the small joints or the inflamed tenosynovium, samples of synovial fluid are seldom obtainable for culture. The second pattern, which may be the initial presentation or may occur following an initial migratory polyarthritis, is the "septic joint" syndrome in which the presentation is of an acute septic, usually monarticular, arthritis. In these patients the blood cultures are often sterile and the synovial fluid cultures are often positive. Skin lesions are rarely reported in this presentation.

In 1974 Brandt and colleagues,[3] on the other hand, had surveyed 31 patients with acute arthritis and proved gonococcal infection. Although the presence of positive blood and synovial fluid cultures was mutually exclusive, they found no correlation between the source of the positive culture and the clinical picture. In addition, the clinical features were variable, and two distinct patterns were not seen.

Despite these conflicting reports, several points seem to be in agreement and of definite clinical value:

1. Positive cultures of either the synovial fluid or the blood seem to be mutually exclusive, and either may occur in any presentation. Therefore appropriate diagnosis requires bacteriologic examination from both sources.

2. Migratory polyarthritis should alert the physician to the possibility of gonococcal arthritis. This is particularly important also in evaluating a patient with acute, apparently septic monarticular arthritis. There is essentially no other condition except gonococcal arthritis in which an antecedent history of migratory polyarthritis will be obtained prior to the onset of acute monarticular arthritis. Therefore, one should always search for this history when evaluating a patient with a hot, inflamed joint.

Meningococcemia may have a presentation identical with that of gonococcal arthritis. With regard to patient screening, all patients with a migratory pattern of synovitis warrant immediate and complete evaluation, as the two predominant conditions associated with this pattern are both significantly treatable and ominous.

Palindromic or Intermittent Patterns. The term palindromic polyarthritis is used to describe those conditions associated with repetitive attacks of polyarticular synovitis that completely remit without sequelae or spread to other joints. Migratory conditions have already been discussed elsewhere. In evaluating patients with these complaints, two useful points should come to mind:

1. The definition of a palindromic state requires a period of observation to establish that the condition will spontaneously remit. Despite this, a prior history of palindromic flares makes it more likely that the current process will follow the same pattern.

2. At the time of initial examination the patient may be completely asymptomatic with a negative physical examination. Rather than obtaining laboratory data blindly and randomly, it is best to request that the patient return during a symptomatic interval when the true nature of the lesion may better be evaluated.

There is some value in separating palindromic conditions according to temporal patterns based upon the duration of inflammation. Short courses (2 to 3 days) are almost exclusively seen in rheumatoid arthritis, although they may also occur in sarcoidosis, familial Mediterranean fever, and sickle cell anemia.[4] Longer courses (7 to 100 days) occur in the peripheral synovitis of spondylitis, the arthropathy of inflammatory bowel disease,[5] Whipple's disease,[6] the polyarthritis associated with intestinal bypass,[7] Behçet's syndrome,[8] familial Mediterranean fever, and sickle cell anemia.[4] Acute polyarthritis has also been described in gout as an initial presentation. In 1974 Hadler and colleagues[9] reviewed the records of 1830 patients discharged from the Massachusetts General Hospital with the diagnosis of gout, gouty arthritis, or hyperuricemia. Of these patients 34 presented with acute polyarticular gout confirmed by the identification of sodium urate crystals in the synovial fluid. Twelve patients within this subgroup of 34 had polyarthritis as the initial manifestation of gout. The unique features of the presentation were asymmetry and preponderant involvement of the foot, ankle, and knee.

While polyarticular gout, particularly as an initial manifestation of the disease, would appear to be decidedly rare, "cluster attacks" of polyarthritis are not rare in pseudogout.[10]

Fever and Polyarticular Arthritis. The presence of fever may serve as an important clue in the diagnosis of polyarthritis. Septic arthritis is discussed elsewhere, and only the sterile processes will be discussed here. Any synovitic process may be associated with a fever, which tends to reflect the activity of the apparent synovitis. Gout would be a classic example of this situation, and temperatures in the 100 to 102° F range are not uncommon.[9] The examiner is usually able to examine the joint, assay the degree of inflammation, and make a relatively accurate guess as to what level of fever will be found.

On the other hand, there are several sterile processes that may present as polyarthritis in which the fever would appear to be in excess of the degree of inflammation observable in the joints. In this situation the cause of the excessive fever would seem to be an inflammatory process not readily apparent on physical examination. Conditions in which this is the case are as follows:

1. Rheumatoid arthritis. The excessive fever is often due to one of three situations: (a) vasculitis; (b) serositis affecting the pleura or pericardium; or (c) a recent abrupt decrease in the steroid dose in a patient maintained on chronic steroids (this may occur even though an adequate physiologic dose of steroids is administered).

2. Systemic lupus erythematosus.

3. Erythema nodosum. Fever can occur even in the absence of skin or joint lesions.

4. Familial Mediterranean fever.

5. Henoch-Schönlein purpura.

6. Behçet's syndrome.

7. Acute rheumatic fever.

8. Whipple's disease.

9. Lyme arthritis.

10. Sarcoidosis with or without erythema nodosum.

11. Juvenile rheumatoid arthritis. In the Still's disease variant of this disorder, fever without synovitis, or fever tremendously in excess of that expected from the apparent synovitis, is the rule. The characteristic truncal, evanescent skin rash is often the only observable lesion, and the true cause of the fever is not known. When the presentation occurs in adulthood, the diagnosis may be particularly obscure.[11]

12. Inflammatory bowel disease. The bowel lesion may be either inapparent or quiescent. Clubbing of the fingers is a distinctive and almost diagnostic feature of this condition if it is present and if subacute bacterial endocarditis has been excluded in a patient with febrile polyarthritis.

13. Reiter's syndrome and ankylosing spondylitis. The articulations of the spine are sufficiently "buried" so that inflammation is not apparent to palpation. This is a possible explanation for the fever's being often in excess of the apparent joint inflammation.

PATTERNS OF THERAPEUTIC RESPONSE

Therapeutic response to specific pharmacologic agents is highly variable in the rheumatic diseases, and few firm conclusions can be drawn. Even the classic specificity of colchicine for gout suffers from the sizable proportion of gouty attacks that do not respond, and the ability of colchicine to abort attacks of familial Mediterranean fever and occasionally erythema nodosum. Diagnostic decisions based on this type of evidence are usually not sound. However, a few points may be of diagnostic value:

1. The dramatic response of acute rheumatic fever to salicylates seems highly specific. Usually the findings and symptoms may be completely suppressed when therapeutic levels of the drug are obtained.

2. Indomethacin and phenylbutazone are usually equipotent to the other nonsteroidal anti-inflammatory agents in most polyarticular inflammatory diseases. However, in gout and the spondyloarthropathies they are usually dramatically more effective.

3. The institution of steroids in a prednisone dose of about 20 mg per day usually will initially almost completely suppress the synovitic features of rheumatoid arthritis and systemic lupus erythematosus but often will have little effect upon the synovitis of the spondyloarthropathies.

SYSTEMIC ASSOCIATIONS WITH POLYARTICULAR ARTHRITIS

Under this heading, associations will be recorded between polyarthritis and lesions or specific diseases of other organ systems. As pulmonary diseases are not covered separately in this text, they will be discussed here in somewhat greater depth.

Pulmonary Manifestations of Rheumatic Diseases. *Tracheolaryngeal Lesions.* Inflammation of the cricoarytenoid joint is a common manifestation of rheumatoid arthritis and is seen in virtually no other form of polyarthritis. Symptoms are chronic laryngeal pain and dysphonia, often accentuated with morning stiffness. A dysphagia of the globus hystericus type may also be seen. Tracheal pain is a common feature of relapsing polychondritis, and tracheal collapse is a fatal complication of this rare condition. The chronic mucous membrane dryness of Sjögren's syndrome may also provoke laryngeal symptoms.

Bronchial Lesions. An undocumented clinical suspicion exists that chronic bronchitis is more common in rheumatoid arthritis. The only documented lesion is atrophy of the glands of the respiratory tract in Sjögren's syndrome.

Pulmonary Fibrosis. Symptoms of dyspnea usually present only in the later stages of fibrosis owing to the tendency of patients to decrease their activity in accordance with their reduced pulmonary function. This is particularly significant in evaluating patients with crippling disorders who, because their primary musculoskeletal disease limits their exercise capacity, are seldom stressed to the limits of their pulmonary capacity. The exact incidence of parenchymal pulmonary dysfunction in the rheumatic diseases is unknown and varies with the sensitivity of the assay employed.

Pulmonary fibrosis is seen frequently in rheumatoid arthritis, systemic lupus erythematosus, polymyositis or dermatomyositis, and scleroderma. It appears to be much less common in the spondyloarthropathies. The current understanding implies that the disorder encompasses a spectrum that probably progresses from alveolitis to interstitial fibrosis. One cannot distinguish between the different arthropathies based on the pulmonary features; nor can the pulmonary lesion be distinguished from idiopathic pulmonary fibrosis.[12,13]

Pulmonary Infiltrates. Pulmonary infiltrates are relatively common as a transient event in systemic lupus erythematosus and may occur in any vasculitis, particularly in Wegener's granulomatosis, and rarely in Sjögren's syndrome.

Pulmonary Nodules. Among the rheumatic diseases, nodules occur almost exclusively in rheumatoid arthritis. They are usually multiple, do not calcify, and range from 0.5 to 5 cm in diameter. Rheumatoid pulmonary nodule formation is associated with peripheral nodules, a higher titer of rheumatoid factor, the male gender, and pneumoconiotic exposure. Their natural tendency to involute and their multiplicity tend to differentiate them from malignant nodules.

Lesions of the Pulmonary Vasculature. Pulmonary hypertension may develop secondary to the chronic hypoxia associated with pulmonary fibrosis or may arise de novo and not correlate with either arterial hypoxia or pulmonary fibrosis. In the latter situation Raynaud's phenomenon is usually present and the condition is seen in scleroderma, other rheumatic disorders with Raynaud's phenomenon, or Raynaud's syndrome alone.

Pleural Disorders. Inflammatory pleuritis is a common manifestation of rheumatoid arthritis, systemic lupus erythematosus, and the other vasculitides. It is not seen in noninflammatory rheumatic disorders and has not been described in psoriatic arthritis, Reiter's syndrome, or the spondyloarthropathies. The fluid characteristically will have a leukocytosis, elevation of the lactic dehydrogenase, and a protein content consistent with an exudate. In rheumatoid arthritis a low glucose content, usually less than 10 mg per 100 ml, is almost pathognomonic of the disease but is not universally seen in rheumatoid pleural effusions.

Dermatological Manifestations of Polyarticular Arthritis. This topic is covered in Chapter 36, and will be discussed here only briefly.

Nodules. These lesions are almost exclusively seen in rheumatoid arthritis and gout. There is a predilection in both conditions for them to form on the olecranon surfaces. Although the biopsy of each is distinctive, the appearance on physical examination may be identical. Several features tend to distinguish the two:

1. Rheumatoid nodules may occur simultaneously, soon after, or even prior to the onset of rheumatoid arthritis. Tophi occur later and are seldom evident within the first 2 years of the disease. Therefore, a patient with polyarthritis of less than 2 years' duration and olecranon nodules probably has rheumatoid arthritis.

2. Aspiration of tophi will reveal urate crystals.

3. Rheumatoid nodules usually arise abruptly, with a definite inflammatory reaction, and tend to regress in size with time. Tophi increase in size in a gradual manner and an inflammatory reaction is seldom seen, particularly early in their course.

Erythema. In Still's disease a transient, primarily truncal rash with the Koebner phenomenon is characteristic. It is usually seen in the late afternoon.

Squamous Eruptions. These are characteristic of Reiter's syndrome and psoriasis and are indistinguishable from each other by both physical and histological examination. Subungual hyperkeratoses are also seen in both diseases. Pitting of the nails seems to be limited to psoriasis.

Pustules. These are found in neisserial bacteremia and usually occur distally, progressing from papules to vesicles to pustules.

Urticaria. This may be seen in any vasculitis but is found most characteristically in the arthritis seen in the preicteric phase of infectious hepatitis.

Scarring. Any deep vasculitis may result in scarring. Paradoxically the relatively benign condition discoid lupus erythematosus tends to produce a scarring alopecia, which is rare in the more malignant condition, systemic lupus erythematosus. Behçet's syndrome produces scarring and has two associated unique features: the oral mucosal ulcerations usually heal to form a "pursed-lipped" appearance; and scars and phlebitis often occur at phlebotomy sites, a finding not seen in other conditions causing polyarticular disease.

Renal and Urological Manifestations of Polyarticular Disease. Nephritis is seen commonly in systemic lupus erythematosus, Wegener's granulomatosis, and the other vasculitides. It is virtually absent in rheumatoid arthritis. The resulting hematuria could also be associated with the nephrolithiasis seen in gout or hyperparathyroidism and its associated chondrocalcinosis. Phenacetin and cyclophosphamide are two commonly used drugs in arthritis which may also be associated with hematuria.

Proteinuria may be a feature of any nephritis or amyloidosis, or may be due to the toxicity of either gold or penicillamine.

Urethritis is essentially exclusively seen with gonococcal arthritis and Reiter's syndrome. Painless penile skin lesions often accompany Reiter's syndrome. Painful penile lesions are seen in Behçet's syndrome.

Cardiac Manifestations of Polyarticular Disease. Pericarditis is commonly seen in rheumatoid arthritis and systemic lupus erythematosus. It is also seen in scleroderma and may serve as an indicator of precipitant renal failure.[14]

Cardiomyopathies may be a clinical problem most commonly in amyloidosis, hemochromatosis, and scleroderma. Valvular heart disease is seen in subacute bacterial endocarditis and acute rheumatic fever. It has also been a rare clinical problem in rheumatoid arthritis, systemic lupus erythematosus, and ankylosing spondylitis—usually in the later stages of these diseases.

Hepatic Manifestations of Polyarticular Disease. Despite their tendency to involve almost all organs within the body, the systemic rheumatic diseases in general create little in the way of hepatic dysfunction, and most postmortem studies in these conditions describe only minimal abnormalities. Elevations of the hepatocellular enzymes (e.g., SGOT, SGPT) are found primarily in two situations: (1) in hepatitis-associated arthritis, and (2) in patients with either juvenile rheumatoid arthritis or systemic lupus erythematosus receiving salicylates.[15,16] The abnormally elevated enzymes will revert with the cessation of salicylates. Hepatomegaly or cirrhosis should alert the clinician to the possibility of amyloidosis, Wilson's disease, or hemochromatosis.

Gastrointestinal Manifestations of Polyarticular Disease. The vast majority of the anti-inflammatory medications are ulcerogenic, so it is difficult to define the specific effect of the drug or the disease upon this condition. Esophageal dysfunction is a common lesion in scleroderma, in any condition associated with Raynaud's phenomenon, or in Raynaud's phenomenon alone.

Diarrhea or the presence of malabsorption should alert one to the possibility of inflammatory bowel disease, scleroderma with small bowel atony, or Whipple's disease. Diarrhea may also frequently precede the onset of typical Reiter's syndrome, which may occur after *Salmonella, Shigella,* or *Yersinia* infections.

Neurologic Manifestations of Polyarticular Disease. Peripheral neuropathies may be found in all forms of vasculitis, usually as a result of an infarction of the *vasa nervorum* or secondary to entrapments as is discussed in Chapter 3. Vertebral instability can lead to the development of a myelopathy. This is most commonly seen in association with the later stages of rheumatoid arthritis. The *cauda equina* syndrome has been described in far-advanced ankylosing spondylitis.[17] Neither of these syndromes is seen early in the course of the disease, however, so they are not distinguishing features in the differential diagnosis of polyarthritis of recent onset. Seizures or diffuse abnormalities of cerebral functions are features usually associated with systemic lupus. However, Lyme arthritis, Behçet's syndrome, and the use of ibuprofen in patients with systemic lupus[18] may be associated with a picture of aseptic meningitis.

References

1. Holmes, K.K., Counts, G.W., and Beaty, H.N.: Disseminated gonococcal infection. Ann. Intern. Med. 74:979, 1971.
2. Keiser, H., Ruben, E.L., Wolinsky, E., and Kushner, I.: Clinical forms of gonococcal arthritis. N. Engl. J. Med. 279:234, 1968.
3. Brandt, K.D., Cathcart, E.S., and Cohen, A.S.: Gonococcal arthritis. Clinical features correlated with blood, synovial fluid, and genitourinary cultures. Arthritis Rheum. 17:503, 1974.
4. Schumacher, H.R., Andrews, R., and McLaughlin, G.: Arthropathy in sickle cell disease. Ann. Intern. Med. 78:203, 1973.
5. Haslock, I., and Wright, V.: The musculoskeletal complications of Crohn's disease. Medicine 52:217, 1973.
6. Caughey, D.E., and Bywaters, E.G.L.: The arthritis of Whipple's syndrome. Ann. Rheum. Dis. 22:327, 1963.
7. Shagrin, J.W., Frame, B., and Duncan, H.: Polyarthritis in obese patients with intestinal bypass. Ann. Intern. Med. 75:377, 1971.
8. O'Duffy, J.D., Carney, J.A., and Deodhar, S.: Behçet's disease: Report of 10 cases, 3 new manifestations. Ann. Intern. Med. 75:561, 1971.
9. Hadler, N.M., Franck, W.A., Bress, N.M., and Robinson, D.R.: Acute polyarticular gout. Am. J. Med. 56:715, 1974.
10. McCarty, D.J.: Diagnostic mimicry in arthritis—patterns of joint involvement associated with calcium pyrophosphate dihydrate crystal deposits. Bull. Rheum. Dis. 25:803, 1975.
11. Bujak, J.S., Aptekar, R.G., Decker, J.L., et al.: Juvenile rheumatoid arthritis presenting in the adult as fever of unknown origin. Medicine 52:431, 1973.
12. Crystal, R.G., Fulmer, J.D., Roberts, W.C., Moss, M.L., Line, B.R., and Reynolds, H.Y.: Idiopathic pulmonary fibrosis, Ann. Intern. Med. 85:769, 1976.
13. Walker, W.C., and Wright, V.: Pulmonary lesions and rheumatoid arthritis. Medicine 47:501, 1968.
14. McWhorter, J.E., IV, and LeRoy, E.C.: Pericardial disease in scleroderma (systemic sclerosis). Am. J. Med. 56:566, 1974.
15. Rich, R.R., and Johnson, J.S.: Salicylate hepatotoxicity in patients with JRA. Arthritis Rheum. 16:1, 1973.
16. Seaman, W.E., Ishak, K.G., and Plotz, P.H.: Aspirin-induced hepatotoxicity in patients with systemic lupus erythematosus. Ann. Intern. Med. 80:1, 1974.
17. Gordon, A.L., and Yudell, A.: Cauda equina lesion associated with ankylosing spondylitis. Ann. Intern. Med. 78:555, 1973.
18. Widener, H.L., and Littman, B.H.: Ibuprofen-induced meningitis in systemic lupus erythematosus. JAMA 239:1062, 1978.

Chapter 27
Muscle Weakness

Walter G. Bradley

INTRODUCTION

The techniques of history-taking and examination of patients are part of the basic tools of the trade of medicine. Nevertheless, it is always instructive to watch an expert in any specialty handling the interview and examination of a patient with a disease within his area. Speed, accuracy, and completeness come from years of experience.

The doctor who is asked to give a diagnostic opinion should approach the patient like a detective, albeit a sympathetic one, with every faculty attuned to the task. One of the key attributes of the great detective in fact or fiction is intuition—that is, the feeling that all is not as it should be. This is no sixth sense, but rather the ability to collect every piece of data, to make judgments on the reliability of the data, to match them against a vast experience of similar situations, and to see where the fault lies and where further investigation is required.

This is the era of science in medicine. No sooner is a symptom recorded than a list of investigations flashes into mind. It is important to reiterate the old teaching that the way to come to a diagnosis is through the history, examination, and formulation of a differential diagnosis, before it is possible to plan the investigations. The finding of a raised creatine kinase (CK) does not necessarily prove the presence of a diffuse muscle disease. Intramuscular injections, excessive exercise, focal muscle injury, and ischemic heart disease may all produce a raised serum CK. The findings in a muscle biopsy of necrosis and regeneration of muscle fibers may be due to a muscular dystrophy or polymyositis, and the diagnosis may depend on the clinical picture rather than the muscle pathology.

This chapter is aimed at providing a framework for searching out all relevant clues from patients complaining of muscle weakness. The various conditions that may cause muscle weakness are briefly considered in Chapter 79. The diagnostic tests of value in defining and separating conditions considered in the differential diagnosis are outlined in Chapter 47.

HISTORY OF THE PRESENT ILLNESS

It is curious how infrequently patients complain of the loss of a motor function when suffering from muscle weakness. They usually use terms like "tiredness" or "fatigue," rather than complaining of difficulty with performing a certain action, such as climbing stairs or doing their hair. This may be because the universal experience of muscle fatigue or tiredness on prolonged exercise, which is built into our linguistic framework, is equated with the symptoms of excessive exertion required to perform a standard task by a person with muscle weakness.

Sometimes the term "numbness" or "deadness" is used to indicate muscle weakness, though further questioning indicates the absence of true sensory loss. The patient is using the term to draw an analogy with the paralysis of an arm following sleeping on it at night, and of the loss of function following a dental anesthetic. It is thus important that the physician-detective try to find out exactly what the patient is experiencing. It is classic teaching that the patient should be allowed to tell his own story in his own words, but this should not be construed as preventing the questioning of the patient to clarify his words. Such *positive history-taking* should be directed to allow the physician to understand the symptoms just as well as if he had experienced them himself.

It is extremely difficult to quantify symptoms of weakness or fatigability. The only way in which this can be achieved is to relate it to functional capacity. If the patient complains of leg weakness, how far can he walk on the flat? Can he climb stairs with or without the bannisters? Can he get up out of a chair or off the floor? Is the weakness proximal or distal? For instance, is the main difficulty in getting up from a chair, or does the patient trip easily? If the complaints are of weakness of the arms, is it distal or proximal? Is there difficulty in opening bottles and holding tools, or is lifting objects above the head or doing the hair difficult?

The time-scale of the development of the symptoms is important. Was it sudden, gradual, or episodic? This is of diagnostic importance, since every disease has a different time course. If the weakness is variable, what are the modifying factors, such as diet, exercise, or environmental temperature?

SYSTEMATIC INQUIRY

As can be seen from the paragraphs above, the physician-detective is more than a passive recorder of the patient's words when taking the history of the illness. The physician will already have asked many questions by the time the patient has completed the story to his own satisfaction. At that time there will still be many other points of systematic inquiry which need to be checked.

Patients may not complain of extraocular, facial, bulbar, or neck weakness, particularly if these are mild.

Has anyone commented on a change in the facial appearance? Has there been any diplopia or difficulty in keeping the eyelids opened, as in myasthenia gravis? Are the muscles of mastication weak on chewing steak? Is there difficulty in swallowing (a symptom which is present in about a quarter of the patients with polymyositis, and about which patients rarely complain)? Do liquids go up the nose or into the larynx on swallowing, indicating bulbar involvement? Is there any difficulty in lifting the head off the pillow, suggesting weakness of neck flexion, or difficulty in holding up the head while working at the desk, suggesting weakness of neck extensors? Has there been any change in the posture, or wasting of muscles? Have the shoulders changed, or is there an alteration in the gait? Has there been any pain? If so, is it spontaneous pain, tenderness to palpation, or cramps after exercise or at rest? Pain and tenderness of the muscles after exercise are frequently present in normal individuals. If the patient is weak, increased exertion is required to perform the same tasks, with consequently greater postexertional pain. It is thus important to assess complaints of pain or tenderness carefully. Is it a prominent feature, or is it simply compatible with the degree of weakness? Pain and weakness are often symptoms of a local arthropathy, and separation of muscle pains from joint pains is often difficult despite detailed questioning.

Cramps are common in the general population, and some individuals are particularly susceptible. Cramps are particularly prominent in patients with upper motor neuron diseases, including multiple sclerosis and amyotrophic lateral sclerosis (ALS), but may also occur in the muscular dystrophies and polymyositis. This is the time to seek for clues about whether muscle weakness may be due to upper motor neuron conditions by inquiring about flexion spasms and sphincter control. Inquiries about sensory symptoms will help indicate the presence of a peripheral neuropathy or central nervous disease. Muscle fasciculations are an important symptom of lower motor neuron degeneration, as in ALS. Has the patient been aware of flickering of the muscles, and if so, in what distributions? Has there been any change in the urine suggestive of myoglobinuria? Myoglobinuria occurs if there is massive muscle breakdown in acute polymyositis, acute rhabdomyolysis, carnitine palmityl-transferase deficiency, and a number of other conditions.

A search for symptoms of systemic disease—endocrine, metabolic, dietary, respiratory, intestinal, immunologic, or inflammatory—is of major importance. Muscle weakness may be due to metabolic aberrations related to many primary diseases of other systems of the body. Weakness may also be due to peripheral nerve or skeletal muscle damage from toxic exposures in the patient's occupation or hobbies, or pharmaceutical or self-abusive drugs.

PAST HISTORY

Patients will often forget many past illnesses, even hospitalizations and surgical procedures. These illnesses may be of considerable significance, and it is important to spend time delving into the past. A previous cancer operation may be relevant in a man of 60 with dermatomyositis. A blind loop syndrome from gastric resection might be a cause of a painful proximal myopathy from malabsorption of vitamin D. There are great satisfactions for the physician-detective in the past history.

FAMILY HISTORY

Many of the neuromuscular diseases run in families. Some, such as facioscapulohumeral (FSH) muscular dystrophy, dystrophia myotonica, and peroneal muscular atrophy, are dominantly inherited, and the condition is passed on by an affected parent. Some, such as Duchenne muscular dystrophy, are X-linked recessive conditions, affecting only males but transmitted by females, so that a search of the maternal line for affected male relatives is needed. Some, for example, limb-girdle muscular dystrophy and infantile spinal muscular atrophy (Werdnig-Hoffmann disease), are inherited as recessive traits, and a history of consanguinity or affected sibs may be present.

In an overt disease such as peroneal muscular atrophy, patients often recognize their own condition and know which individuals in the family are also affected. However, formes frustes of the condition are frequent in such diseases. Knowledge of this allows search among relatives for the presence of such features as high arches, difficulty in obtaining shoes, and the development of calluses, which may indicate that the individual bears the gene for the disease. A vague history of a child who died with paralysis or a diagnosis of "polio" may be of relevance. Further information and search of medical records may be helpful when there are any pointers toward inherited disease.

Sometimes a patient will deny a family history in a disease that is frequently dominantly inherited. There are many possibilities: Inheritance may be through an individual who has a forme fruste of the disease. There may have been a spontaneous mutation or a rare autosomal recessive form of inheritance. The social parents may not be the biological parents. There may be poor family contact so that a child does not know about his parents. Sometimes patients will accept a feature as a family characteristic and not think it relates to a disease. The typical "fruity" transverse or pouting smile and drooped shoulders of FSH muscular dystrophy are examples in point. Sometimes there is a positive attempt to cover up a disease; this is particularly true in dystrophia myotonica, in which patients often refuse permission for contact to be made with relatives, and relatives may refuse to have anything to do with the inquiring physician.

Family photographs are useful for recognizing ocular myopathy, FSH dystrophy, and dystrophia myotonica. A careful search of the family history is important, since it may aid and confirm the diagnosis in the patient. Diagnosing the familial condition may avoid complex investigations. It may also lead to important genetic counseling for the patient and relatives.

EXAMINATION

The specialist in rheumatology, neurology, neuromuscular disease, or any other field must be a good general physician. The complete physical examination is an obligatory part of the examination of any patient complaining of muscle weakness. For instance, detection of an endocrine disturbance or carcinoma may reveal the cause of the muscle disease.

In examining the neuromuscular apparatus, as in any other part of the body, a systematic approach is essential. The neuromuscular examination includes inspection, palpation, assessment of contractures, assessment of muscle strength, and elicitation of tendon reflexes.

Inspection. *General.* The patient should be undressed to the underclothes or completely, and observed standing and walking. If standing or walking is impossible, that must be recorded. When standing is there any unusual postural change, such as hyperlordosis, kyphoscoliosis, or fixed flexion of a joint? Is there any wasting of muscles such as the "champagne bottle" or more severe "hock bottle" wasting of the distal legs seen in peroneal muscular atrophy? Are the shoulders forwardly ptosed as in limb-girdle dystrophy, or horizontally drooped as in FSH dystrophy? In the latter, outward rotation of the shoulder blades may cause the angle of the scapula to rise and bulge into the line of the shoulders, producing a spurious appearance of muscularity. Hypertrophy of calf and other muscles may be seen in X-linked and some other muscular dystrophies.

Regional. Is the face normal at rest, or is there abnormal posture of the eyes, eyelids, or lips? Is there any abnormal asymmetry, ptosis, or strabismus? The lips are abnormally pouting in FSH dystrophy, and may droop in the other facial myopathies. This is the stage at which to examine the facial muscles, as well as the cranial nerves, skull, and cranial vasculature. Is there eyelid ptosis from weakness of the levator palpebrae superioris? Is there difficulty on burying the eyelashes, indicating weakness of the orbicularis oculi? A horizontal smile is due to weakness of the levator anguli oris, and difficulty in puffing out the cheeks may be due to weakness of the orbicularis oris, preventing the air from being held anteriorly, or, less commonly, to palatal weakness, preventing the air from being held posteriorly. The bulk of the temporalis and masseter muscles should be checked. Is the tongue normal in size and movements, or is it wasted and fasciculating? Most normal individuals find it difficult to keep the tongue still, so that it is generally advisable to diagnose fasciculation from denervation only when wasting is present.

Is the neck normal in position? The head may be thrust forward due to neck extensor weakness, perhaps caused by polymyositis or some other proximal myopathy. Wasting of the sternomastoid muscles occurs in dystrophia myotonica. Are the shoulder or arm muscles wasted? For instance, wasting of the deltoid muscle, causing the shoulder to be sharply right-angled, is not common in a muscular dystrophy but may occur in polymyositis. Is there any wasting of the muscles of the arms or legs, and any abnormal posture such as the claw hand of an ulnar palsy or pes cavus? Keep watch for fasciculations, small spontaneous twitches of groups of muscle fibers causing dimpling of the skin. Tapping the muscle may sometimes bring these out, but they must be distinguished from the normal twitches seen in poorly relaxed muscles and after heavy exertion.

Inspection should always include examination of the gait. Is it waddling (Trendelenburg gait), indicating weakness of hip abduction? Or is the abdomen thrust forward (the aldermanic gait) as a result of weakness of hip extensors? Are the arms and hips used excessively in walking, indicating weakness of hip flexors? Is there a footdrop, indicated by high-stepping? Excessive wearing of the toes of the shoes may prove the presence of the footdrop. There are many techniques for recording gaits, including force plates, cinematographic means, and computerized facilities, but these are still in the realm of research into their clinical usefulness and will not be discussed here.

Palpation. Palpation is best done during the examination of each muscle when the object is to assess (1) *bulk*—the grade of atrophy in percentage of expected bulk for the sex, age, and body habitus; (2) *consistency*—normal, fibrotic, or abnormally soft; or (3) *strength,* which is detailed below. During examination of the consistency of the muscle, tenderness to pressure should also be assessed.

Determination of Contractures. In clinical terms, contracture indicates restriction of the normal range of movement of a joint. There are several causes of this, including alteration of the joint surfaces, excessive thickening of the joint capsule or ligaments, and alterations of the muscles and tendons. Contraction caused by the muscles and tendons may be recognized by variation in the range of restriction in relation to differing positions of intervening joints. Thus clawed fingers may be due to alterations of the ligaments and joints, or to contracture of the long flexor muscles of the fingers. In the latter case, the fingers may be straightened when the wrist is hyperflexed.

The exact basis of this type of contracture of skeletal muscle is not certain. It is seen in conditions in which muscle damage produces fibrosis, such as the muscular dystrophies and polymyositis, and may also be seen in muscles chronically denervated, for instance by poliomyelitis or by chronic spinal muscular atrophy. Probably the amount of collagen deposited around the muscle fibers in these conditions reduces the normal degree of stretch of each muscle fiber.

It is important to assess the degree of contracture prior to attempting to assess voluntary strength of a muscle. Strength can only be assessed over the range of free movement of the joint and muscle. The examiner tests the strength by pulling against a contracting muscle; if he is pulling against a fibrotic contracture, he may get a false impression of muscle strength. The degree of contracture of the muscle can be measured with a simple protractor.

Muscle Strength Testing. There are many different ways to assess the strength of a muscle: the maximum force on voluntary contraction of that muscle; that maximum force expressed as a percentage of the expected normal for the age, sex, and body habitus; the duration for which it is possible to maintain a given percentage of the maximum voluntary contraction; whether a certain action is possible, such as, for the deltoid muscle, lifting the extended arm to 90 degrees away from the body; or the time taken to perform a certain action, such as the biceps lifting 10 kg ten times at maximum speed. Consideration of the more important of these parameters is given below.

It is important that the examiner have a good knowledge of myology and neurology, particularly with regard to the action and range of each muscle. The body functions in terms of whole movements, often produced by several muscles. To isolate and test only one muscle is difficult. Patients with weakness of one muscle learn trick maneuvers involving various agonists. It is essential to have knowledge of such trick movements, and of the correct position for examining each muscle in as pure isolation as possible.

Several other factors must also be taken into account in assessing muscle strength. The degree of extension of a muscle governs its power output; it is weakest at the extremes of contraction or relaxation, and strongest in the mid-range of movement. The apparent contradiction to this rule provided by the quadriceps femoris muscle, which appears strongest in full extension, is due to the mechanical locking of the knee joint in that position. Thus the quadriceps muscle strength must be tested in midposition. The effect of gravity must not be forgotten; when tested with the patient supine, the hip flexors appear weaker than with the body vertical owing to the necessity of lifting the additional weight of the leg in the supine position.

It is also important to recognize that the maximum voluntary strength of a muscle is proportional to the amount of effort expended by the subject. In experimental terms the maximum strength of an animal muscle produced by nerve stimulation is several times that exerted by the animal in maximum voluntary contraction. Thus, because of central nervous phenomena, the maximum *voluntary* contraction is less than the *absolute* maximum. Similarly "fatigue," i.e., the loss of ability to sustain a maximum effort, is a central rather than a peripheral phenomenon. If the subject *does not want* to exert full effort, either consciously or unconsciously, then the muscle will appear weak. The examiner must be on the continuous lookout for such central phenomena related to muscle strength. Thus conscious malingering may produce inability to contract the quadriceps against gravity, although the patient gets up from a chair readily. Wavering or variability of effort with a sudden "give" may be due either to psychogenic causes or to local pain.

Clinical Assessment. The strength of each muscle group can be assessed by simply finding how much effort the examiner has to impose to overcome maximum contraction. Details of the techniques for estimation of the strength of each muscle are outside the scope of this chapter, and readers should consult Walton and Gardner-Medwin (1981),[1] the Medical Research Council War Memorandum (1943),[2] and the Mayo Clinic "Clinical Examinations in Neurology."[3]

Medical Research Council (MRC) Grading of Strength (1943). Muscle strength can be quantitated in a crude but reproducible fashion on the following grades: 5—normal power; 4—muscle contraction possible against gravity and resistance combined; 3—muscle contraction possible only against gravity; 2—movement of a joint possible with gravity eliminated but not possible against gravity; 1—flicker of contraction; 0—no contraction.

The grades are relatively absolute, and different observers are generally concordant in their observations. However, MRC grade 4 encompasses the vast majority of clinically weak muscles, and any attempt to subdivide this category into 4 minus, 4, and 4 plus returns subjectivity to the field.

Muscle Dynamometry. Numerous systems of measuring muscle strength have been devised. Among the simplest are the various pulley and weight or spring balance devices. Optimally the limb is placed in a frame so that the joint is in its midposition of movement, and only the muscle under test can move the joint. Consideration must be given to whether the contraction is to be isometric, i.e., in which no movement shall result from the contraction, or whether it is to be isotonic, in which case the range of movement must be defined. During repeated tests the power usually increases for a few times owing to a learning effect; it then reaches a plateau and eventually fades owing to fatigue. It is thus important to take measurements in a standardized fashion, frequently as the maximum of the first three contractions. Vigorous reinforcement and urging by the examiner are necessary to obtain the *maximum* voluntary contraction.

The apparatus required for such measurements as those outlined above is cumbersome, and a useful compromise between dynamometry and clinical examination is a hand-held dynamometer. Various models are available. The strictures already described above in relation to the clinical examination without additional apparatus apply equally to dynamometry, and the need for a rigorously standardized technique must be emphasized.

Functional Tests. Tests of the all-or-none ability to perform an action or of the time taken to perform such an action are of major help in muscle assessment, particularly in serial studies of a patient. The ability or inability to rise from the floor is one such test. Aberrations of the method of rising from the floor, including the Gower's maneuver, offer refinements of characterization.[4] The time that a patient takes to get from sitting on the floor to the vertical may be used for monitor of

muscle power when weakness of hip and knee extensors becomes significant. Similar tests include the time to get out of a chair, to walk a measured distance on the flat, to climb a standard flight of stairs, to hold the legs horizontally without support, or to hold the extended arms horizontally.

Tendon Reflexes. Elicitation of the tendon reflexes is a standard part of medical training and will not be described in detail here. The patient should be completely relaxed and the muscle in midposition. The tendon should be carefully struck a sharp blow. Reflexes should be categorized as 0 absent; ± present only with reinforcement maneuvers such as jaw or hand clenching; 1+ present but depressed; 2+ normal; 3+ exaggerated; 4+ sustained clonus.

It is important to know the changes in reflex patterns with age, including the loss of the ankle jerks in many patients over the age of 60. The pattern of reflex change is important in the diagnosis of the cause of muscle weakness. Thus upper motor neuron disease causes exaggeration of reflexes with spread of the reflex beyond the nerve and myotomal supply of the muscle which is struck. In addition, there are pathological reflexes indicative of upper motor neuron damage, such as extensor plantar responses. Lower motor neuron disease generally causes depressed or lost reflexes, particularly if this is due to a peripheral neuropathy affecting both the sensory and the motor fibers, and particularly in demyelinating rather than axonal diseases. Neuronal degenerations of either the anterior horn cell or the dorsal root ganglion tend to cause the reflexes to be lost rather later than in peripheral neuropathies. In amyotrophic lateral sclerosis, coexistent upper motor neuron motor disease causes increased reflexes in muscles that are atrophied owing to lower motor neuron damage, thus producing a characteristic clinical picture. Loss of tendon reflexes in primary muscle disease is probably due to involvement of muscle spindles, and possibly due to secondary involvement of intramuscular nerves. Only late in the disease is extrafusal muscle fiber damage sufficiently severe as to abolish reflexes. Thus, in primary muscle disease, the reflexes may be relatively spared compared with peripheral nerve disease until there is a greater degree of muscle weakness and wasting. In polymyositis, surprisingly, the tendon reflexes may occasionally be somewhat exaggerated. The explanation for this is not clear but may be related to membrane damage in muscle spindles causing hyperexcitability.

The distribution of reflex change may be characteristic. In muscular dystrophy such as that of Duchenne, the ankle jerks may be preserved though the knee and biceps reflexes are lost. In a distal polyneuropathy the peripheral reflexes such as the ankle jerk may be lost, while proximal reflexes such as those of the knee and elbow may remain.

The Examination of the Peripheral Nervous System. The recognition of whether weakness is due to skeletal muscle or nervous system damage relates to the distribution of the muscle weakness and the presence or absence of associated features. Distal muscle weakness is usually of peripheral nerve origin, while proximal muscle weakness is more likely to be due to a primary muscle problem. A specific distribution of muscle weakness may be diagnostic, as in the patterns seen in muscular dystrophy, in an upper motor neuron lesion, or in a peripheral nerve or root lesion. Thus in a muscular dystrophy such as that of Duchenne or Becker, the muscles earliest and most severely affected are the quadriceps, hip flexors, hip extensors, anterior tibialis, biceps, and brachioradialis, while others such as the gastrocnemius, triceps, deltoids, wrist flexors, and extensors are spared until later. This specific distribution cannot be explained on the basis of any root or peripheral nerve distribution.

In a chronic spinal muscular atrophy, the distribution of muscle involvement may be very variable. Commonly all muscles are very atrophic, but certain muscles or muscle groups are particularly weak. The distribution of muscle involvement, whatever its specific pattern, again cannot be explained on the basis of any nerve or root involvement. It may, in fact, imitate the distribution of a muscular dystrophy, when the term "pseudomyopathic spinal muscular atrophy" is applied. Further investigations are then required to separate the muscular dystrophy and spinal muscular atrophy.

In an upper motor neuron disease, the characteristic distribution of muscle weakness is concentrated in the extensors of the upper limbs, the deltoid, triceps, and wrist and finger extensors, and in the flexors of the lower limbs, the hip flexors, hamstrings, and anterior tibialis muscles. Here, the presence of the associated features of increased tendon jerks and pathologic reflexes confirms the anatomic diagnosis. In a lesion of one or more peripheral nerves or roots, the pattern of nerve and superficial sensory involvement is such that it can be explained solely and entirely from the known distribution of the nerve(s) or root(s). A knowledge of the myotonal and dermatomal map[5] is essential.

The presence of definite sensory loss proves that the nervous system is involved. Detailed individual examination of all modalities of sensation over the whole of the body is required.

As an aid to anatomic diagnosis it is best to tabulate the distribution of muscle weakness and sensory impairment, first listing the clearcut abnormalities and then listing more dubious abnormalities. It is important to develop a mental image of the dermatomes, myotomes, and peripheral nerve distribution in the body, having tables and figures[5] readily available for repeated comparison.

SUMMARY AND CONCLUSIONS

The diagnostic interview is a major part of the investigation of every patient, and this is particularly so in those with muscle weakness. It provides a guide to further investigation by laboratory and other procedures. These investigations are considered elsewhere; those dealing with the investigations of a patient with neuromuscular symptoms and signs are dealt with in Chapter 47. By the end of the interview and examination, the physician-detective should have a clear idea of the differential diagnosis, and thus the investigations required. Such investigations should always be directed; the shotgun approach is both expensive and sometimes misleading.

A final word is necessary concerning the diagnosis of neuromuscular involvement in the presence of rheumatologic conditions, for this is often difficult. Local joint pain makes it impossible for patients to exert their maximum voluntary effort, with resultant *apparent* weakness. Disuse of a limb from pain causes muscle atrophy, predominantly of type 2 muscle fibers. It is thus important to assess as well as possible the degree of joint involvement and consequent joint pain. At times it is clear that the degree of weakness and atrophy may simply be ascribable to the joint problems. At other times it is difficult to exclude some degree of neuromuscular involvement, and the investigations outlined in Chapter 47 are then required. The importance of recognizing the superimposition of a neuromuscular involvement upon the underlying rheumatologic condition is that the prognosis may be altered by such involvement, and the treatment may have to be altered to take account of this involvement. For instance, the development of polymyositis during the course of progressive systemic sclerosis may necessitate the addition of glucocorticoids or immunomodulation drugs to the treatment regimen; the development of a multiple mononeuropathy in rheumatoid arthritis may indicate the appearance of a diffuse vasculitis.

References

1. Gardner-Medwin, D.: The clinical examination of the neuromuscular system. *In* Walton, Sir John (ed.): Disorders of Voluntary Muscle. 4th ed. Edinburgh, Churchill Livingstone, 1981. p. 448.
2. Medical Research Council War Memorandum, No. 7. Revised 2nd ed. London, HMSO, 1943.
3. Mayo Clinic Staff: Clinical Examinations in Neurology. 4th ed. Philadelphia, W.B. Saunders Company, 1977.
4. Brooke, M.H.: A Clinician's View of Neuromuscular Diseases. Baltimore, Williams & Wilkins Company, 1977.
5. Bradley, W.G.: Disorders of Peripheral Nerves. Oxford, Blackwell Scientific Publications, 1974.

Chapter 28

Neck Pain

Kenneth K. Nakano

INTRODUCTION

When localized by a patient to the neck, pain can often produce a confusing diagnostic problem. Pain can originate from the involved tissues or may be so perceived but due to referral from another site (Table 28–1). Musculoskeletal conditions involve neurologic tissues, and the converse appears equally true.

Neck pain in clinical practice occurs slightly less frequently than low back pain; a major difference is that neck pain becomes far less disabling, seldom compromising work capacity. Neck stiffness exists as a common disorder; for the age group 25 to 29 years of age in our working population there is a 25 to 30 percent frequency of one or more attacks of stiff neck.[1] For the work population over 45 years of age this figure rises to 50 percent. Episodes of "simple" stiff neck last 1 to 4 days and seldom require medical care. Brachial neuralgia (pain radiating to the shoulder and arm) occurs later in life than stiff neck, with a frequency of 5 to 10 percent in the 25 to 29 year age group and subsequently rising to 25 to 40 percent after age 45. Overall, 45 percent of working men experience at least one attack of stiff neck, 23 percent report at least one attack of brachial neuralgia, and 51 percent suffer both these symptoms. The frequency of brachial neuralgia is approximately three times higher in those who complain of stiff neck, suggesting common factors in their pathogensis.

Pain in the neck exists in all occupational groups. Stiff neck appears first, followed by headache and shoulder-arm pain.[1] The pain-sensitive structures of the neck include the ligaments, the nerve roots, the articular facets and capsules, the muscles, and the dura. Pain in the

Table 28–1. Structures Causing Neck Pain

Acromioclavicular joint
Heart and coronary artery disease
Apex of lung, Pancoast's tumor, bronchogenic cancer (C3, C4, C5 nerve roots in common)
Diaphragm muscle (C3, C4, C5 innervation)
Gallbladder
Spinal cord tumor
Temporomandibular joint
Fibrositis and fibromyositis syndromes (upper thoracic spine, proximal arm and shoulder)
Aorta
Pancreas
Disorders of any somatic or visceral structure (produces cervical nerve root irritation)
Peripheral nerves
Central nervous system (posterior fossa lesions)
Hiatus hernia (C3, C4, C5)
Gastric ulcer

Table 28–2. Cervical Spine Syndromes

Localized Neck Disorders
Osteoarthritis (apophyseal joints, C1-C2-C3 levels most often)
Rheumatoid arthritis (atlantoaxial)
Juvenile rheumatoid arthritis
Sternocleidomastoid tendinitis
Acute posterior cervical strain
Pharyngeal infections
Cervical lymphadenitis
Osteomyelitis (staphylococcal, tuberculosis)
Meningitis
Ankylosing spondylitis
Paget's disease
Torticollis (congenital, spasmodic, drug-involved, hysterical)
Neoplasms (primary or metastatic)
Occipital neuralgia (greater and lesser occipital nerves)
Diffuse idiopathic skeletal hyperostosis
Rheumatic fever (infrequently)
Gout (infrequently)
Lesions Producing Neck and Shoulder Pain
Postural disorders
Rheumatoid arthritis
Fibrositis syndromes
Musculoligamentous injuries to neck and shoulder
Osteoarthritis (apophyseal and Luschka)
Cervical spondylosis
Intervertebral osteoarthritis
Thoracic outlet syndromes
Nerve injuries (serratus anterior, C3-C4 nerve root, long thoracic nerve)
Lesions Producing Predominantly Shoulder Pain
Rotator cuff tears and tendinitis
Calcareous tendinitis
Subacromial bursitis
Bicipital tendinitis
Adhesive capsulitis
Reflex sympathetic dystrophy
Frozen shoulder syndromes
Acromioclavicular secondary osteoarthritis
Glenohumeral arthritis
Septic arthritis
Tumors of the shoulder
Lesions Producing Neck and Head Pain with Radiation
Cervical spondylosis
Rheumatoid arthritis
Intervertebral disc protrusion
Osteoarthritis (apophyseal and Luschka joints; intervertebral disc; osteoarthritis)
Spinal cord tumors
Cervical Neurovascular syndromes
   Cervical rib
   Scalene muscle
   Hyperabduction
     syndrome
   Rib-clavicle compression

neck region can originate from many tissue sites and result from a number of mechanisms (Table 28–2).

Normal function of the cervical spine requires physiologic movements of the joints, bones, spinal cord, nerve roots through the intervertebral foramina, muscles, ligaments, tendons, fascia, sympathetic nervous system, and the vascular supply of all these structures. Since most structures in the neck potentially become pain sensitive, a knowledge of the dermatome pattern of pain distribution is necessary in clinical diagnosis.

ANATOMY AND BIOMECHANICS

The most mobile segment of the spine is the neck. Through a cylinder connecting the head to the thorax pass structures requiring the greatest protection and possessing the least: the carotid and vertebral arteries, the spinal cord, and the spinal nerve roots. The head, weighing 6 to 8 pounds, balances on the seven cervical vertebrae in a flexible chain held together by 14 apophyseal joints, 5 intervertebral discs, 12 joints of Luschka, and a system of ligaments (anterior longitudinal, posterior longitudinal, ligmentum flavum, interspinous and ligamentum nuchae) and muscles (14 paired anterior, lateral and posterior) (Figs. 28–1 and 28–2).

The shape and mode of articulation of the joints influence the axes and ranges of movement of the neck. Plates of avascular hyaline cartilage cover, and the intervertebral discs unite, the articular surfaces of the vertebral bodies. The intervertebral discs increase in area from below the axis (C2) downwards, and the cervical lordosis results from their wedge shape (Figs. 28–1 and 28–2). The thickness of the discs vary; the two deepest

lie below the sixth and fifth vertebra, respectively. Each intervertebral disc consists of fibrocartilage and contains a nucleus pulposus, which, in turn, changes in shape but cannot be compressed.

Anterior and posterior longitudinal ligaments extend up to the occipital bone and down into the sacrum, joining the vertebral bodies. The anterior longitudinal ligament attaches to the bodies and becomes tightly fixed at the discs (Fig. 28–2); a sudden extending force may rupture it and lead to severe hyperextension associated with damage to the spinal cord. The posterior ligament attaches to the discs and adjacent bones but not to the center.

The specialized atlanto-occipital and atlantoaxial joints are controlled by intersegmental muscles. The head and atlas move together around the odontoid peg and the upper articular facets of the axis (Fig. 28–1B), the long transverse processes of the atlas providing the levers used in rotation. The anterior surface of the odontoid process articulates with the posterior surface of the anterior arch of the atlas. The total excursion of the head can be measured in flexion, extension, rotation, and lateral flexion (Table 28–3). The overall range of movement in the sagittal plane (flexion and extension) approximates 90 degrees, about three quarters being due to extension.[2] Approximately 10 degrees of flexion and 25 degrees of extension occur at the atlanto-occipital joints.[3] In this range of movement, the ligaments help protect the spinal cord from damage by the normal,

Figure 28–1. *A,* Cervical spine: anterior view of articulated cervical vertebrae. *B,* Posterior view of the skull, seven cervical vertebrae and first thoracic vertebra.

Figure 28–2. Sagittal view of the lower head and neck to show the relationship of the spinal cord and brainstem to the bones, ligaments, and joints between the bodies of the cervical vertebrae. The cervical lordosis can be seen as can the relationship of the anterior and posterior longitudinal ligaments to intervertebral discs and the ligaments at the craniovertebral junction.

fractured, or dislocated odontoid process. The lower parts of the cervical spine contribute to the remainder of full range in this plane. The maximum range of movement between individual vertebrae occurs at the level of the joints between the fourth and fifth vertebrae in young children and between the fifth and sixth in teenagers and adults. The total range of rotation of the head and neck encompasses 80 to 90 degrees. Approximately 35 to 45 degrees occurs at the atlantoaxial joint and is associated with a screwing movement of the upper on the lower vertebra, a movement that reduces the cross-sectional area of the spinal canal. Lateral flexion does not occur in isolation but accompanies some rotation. Usually there exists about 30 degrees of lateral mobility on both sides in the lower cervical spine.[3] The spinal canal shortens on the side of the concavity of the spine and lengthens on the side of the convexity.

With age, the nucleus pulposus becomes vulnerable

Table 28–3. Age and the Normal Cervical Spine Motion

Age in Years	Flexion Extension (degrees)	Lateral Rotation (degrees)	Lateral Flexion (degrees)
< 30	90	90	45
31–50	70	90	45
> 50	60	90	30

to acute and chronic trauma.[4] With loss of disc substance the annulus fibrosus may bulge into the spinal canal, and on account of its eccentric position, the nucleus tends to prolapse backward if any tear develops in the annulus. The commonest sites for both types of herniation are the most mobile regions (viz., at C5-C6 and C6-C7). With degenerative changes, the disc space narrows and the spinal column shortens. The intervertebral foramina become narrowed, movements become restricted, and unusual mechanical strains on the synovial joints result. These changes may be confined to a localized area or may become widespread in generalized degenerative disease. The formation of osteophytes leads to encroachment on the spinal canal and intervertebral foramina. The canal may also be further narrowed by bulging of the ligamenta flava. Changes in the caliber of the vertebral arteries can result because of degenerative changes in the joints of the cervical spine. Arterial branches supplying joints and nervous tissue can be constricted at rest and further obstructed with movement. Occasionally, with severe vertebral artery stenosis, syncope results from rotation of the head.

Mere bony changes do not necessarily correspond to the segmental level of neurologic damage. Two reasons exist for this. The first relates to the disproportionate growth of the spinal cord and column. The first thoracic segment of the spinal cord lies opposite the seventh cervical vertebra (Fig. 28–2), and the upper rootlets of the lower cervical and first thoracic nerves cross over two intervertebral discs, while normally the lower rootlets of these two nerves cross only one disc (Fig. 28–3). Second, severe degeneration of the discs may shorten the vertebral canal to such an extent that the spinal cord, which remains unaltered in length, drops down relative to the bones. The spinal nerve roots may then become acutely folded as they travel toward the intervertebral foramina, the lowest roots becoming the most severely affected.

Familiarity with the distribution of sensory, motor, and autonomic components in segmental nerves becomes necessary for localization of neurologic segments in clinical examinations (Fig. 28–4 and Table 28–4). For practical purposes, the lower fibers of the cervical plexus supply the top of the shoulder; C5 and C6 nerve roots supply the lateral side of the arm and forearm; C6, C7, and C8 nerve roots innervate the hand; and C8 extends into the forearm. The T1 segment innervates the medial side of the arm and forearm. Visceral pain can be referred in some cases to well-defined segmental areas (Fig. 28–5); for example, pain of the point of the shoulder (C3-C4) may be associated with acute cholecystitis. The segmental supplies of individual muscles are listed in Table 28–4.

Nerve Root Compression. Normally a radicular nerve occupies 20 to 25 percent of the intervertebral foramen. There may be considerable variation in the anatomy of the lower cervical nerves and their root pouches, and as age advances, they become relatively fixed and vulnerable to damage.[5] Two types of disc lesions cause pressure on the radicular nerves or nerve roots: first, a dorsolat-

Figure 28–3. Brachial plexus and lower cervical spine. Note nerve roots, trunk, cords, and the peripheral nerves. The brachial plexus goes under the clavicle and over the first rib, accompanied by the subclavian artery and vein.

upper trunk
middle trunk
suprascapular n.
lateral cord
posterior cord
subscapular ns.
musculo-cutaneous n.
axillary n.
radial n.
median n.
ulnar n.
lower trunk
medial cord

Figure 28–4. Dermatome distribution of nerve fibers from C1 through T5 carrying senses of pain, heat, cold, vibration, and touch to the head, neck, arm, hand, and thoracic area. The sclerotomes and myotomes will be similar but with some overlap. Pain arising from structures deep to the deep fascia (myotome and sclerotome) do not precisely follow the dermatome distribution.

Table 28–4. Nerves and Tests of Principal Muscles

Nerve	Nerve Roots	Muscle	Test
Accessory	Spinal	Trapezius	Elevation of shoulders Abduction of scapula
	Spinal	Sternocleidomastoid	Tilting of head to same side with rotation to opposite side
Brachial Plexus		Pectoralis major	
	C5,C6	Clavicular part	Adduction of arm
	C7,C8,T1	Sternocostal part	Adduction, forward depression of arm
	C5,C6,C7	Serratus anterior	Fixation of scapula during forward thrusting of the arm
	C4,C5	Rhomboid	Elevation and fixation of scapula
	C4,C5,C6	Supraspinatus	Initiate abduction arm
	(C4),C5,C6	Infraspinatus	External rotation arm
	C6,C7,C8	Latissimus dorsi	Adduction of horizontal, externally rotated arm, coughing
Axillary	C5,C6	Deltoid	Lateral and forward elevation of arm to horizontal
Musculocutaneous	C5,C6	Biceps Brachialis	Flexion of supinated forearm
Radial	C6,C7,C8	Triceps	Extension of forearm
	C5,C6	Brachioradialis	Flexion of semiprone forearm
	C6,C7	Extensor carpi radialis longus	Extension of wrist to radial side
Posterior Interosseous	C5,C6	Supinator	Supination of extended forearm
	C7,C8	Extensor digitorum	Extension of proximal phalanges
	C7,C8	Extensor carpi ulnaris	Extension of wrist to ulnar side
	C7,C8	Extensor indicis	Extension of proximal phalanx of index finger
	C7,C8	Abductor pollicis longus	Abduction of first metacarpal in plane at right angle to palm
	C7,C8	Extensor pollicis longus	Extension of first interphalangeal joint
	C7,C8	Extensor pollicis brevis	Extension at first metacarpophalangeal joint
Median	C6,C7	Pronator teres	Pronation of extended forearm
	C6,C7	Flexor carpi radialis	Flexion of wrist to radial side
	C7,C8,T1	Flexor digitorum superficialis	Flexion of middle phalanges
	C8,T1	Flexor digitorum profundus (lateral part)	Flexion of terminal phalanges, index and middle fingers
	C8,T1	Flexor pollicis longus (anterior interosseous nerve)	Flexion of distal phalanx, thumb
	C8,T1	Abductor pollicis brevis	Abduction of first metacarpal in plane at right angle to palm
	C8,T1	Flexor pollicis brevis	Flexion of proximal phalanx, thumb
	C8,T1	Opponens pollicis	Opposition of thumb against 5th finger
	C8,T1	1st and 2nd lumbricals	Extension of middle phalanges while proximal phalanges are fixed in extension
Ulnar	C7,C8	Flexor carpi ulnaris	Observe tendons while testing abductor digiti minimi
	C8,T1	Flexor digitorum profundus (medial part)	Flexion of distal phalanges of ring and little fingers
	C8,T1	Hypothenar muscles	Abduction and opposition of little finger
	C8,T1	3rd and 4th lumbricals	Extension of middle phalanges while proximal-phalanges are fixed in extension
	C8,T1	Adductor pollicis	Adduction of thumb against palmar surface of index finger
	C8,T1	Flexor pollicis brevis	Flexion of proximal phalanx, thumb
	C8,T1	Interossei	Abduction and adduction of fingers

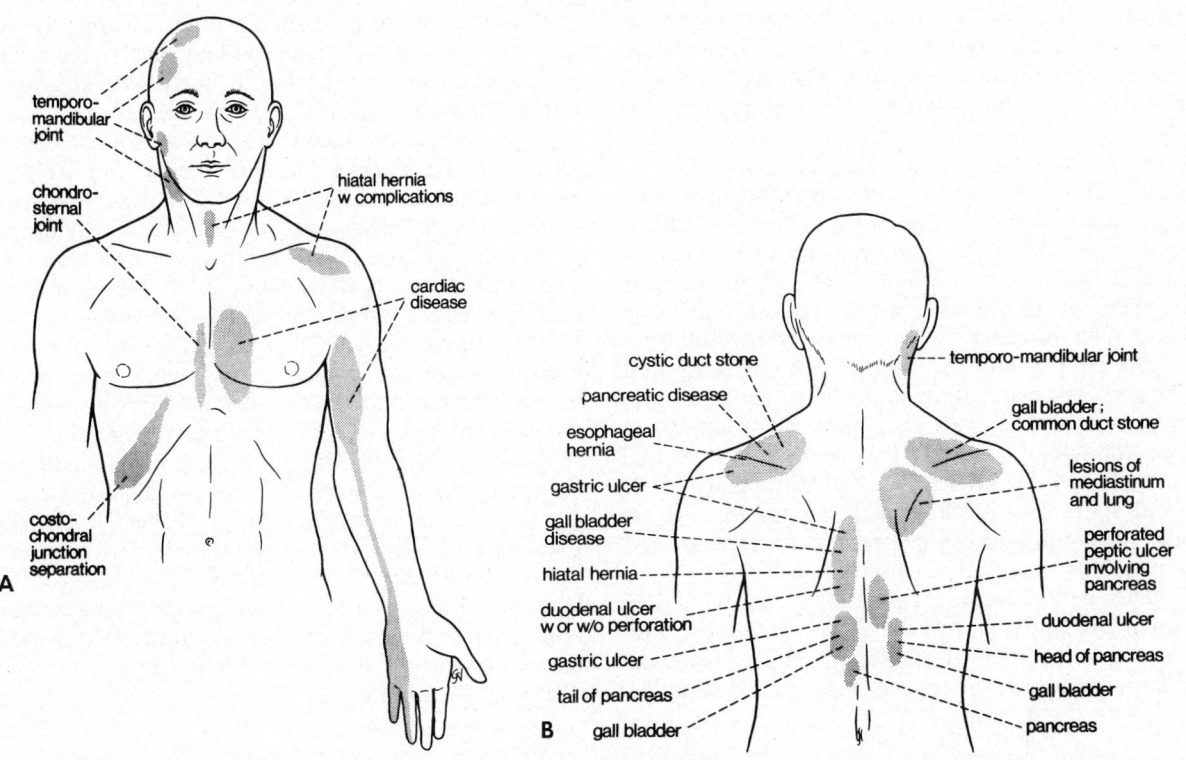

Figure 28-5. Patterns of reflexly referred pain from visceral and somatic st ructures. Anterior distribution (*A*); posterior distribution (*B*).

eral protrusion that does not invade the intervertebral foramen but compresses the intrameningeal nerve roots against the vertebral laminae; and second, an intraforaminal protrusion from the uncinate part of the disc that compresses the radicular nerve against the articular process. The extent of root compression depends on the angulation of the radicular nerve and its location in the foramen as well as on the size and position of the protrusion. Marginal lipping of the vertebrae and narrowing of the discs lead to secondary osteophyte formation of the articular processes and consequent posterolateral narrowing of the foramen.

Blood Supply. Variations in the pattern of blood vessels in the cervical spinal cord exist, but the main blood supply comes through a few major articular arteries.[6] The anterior and posterior spinal arteries act more as connecting links than as main channels of blood. The blood supply to the spinal cord can be impaired in patients with cervical spondylosis when one or more radicular arteries become compressed. The resultant ischemia may be either continuous or intermittent, and sometimes the maximum impairment occurs only when the head is in a certain position (usually extension).

The vertebral arteries vary in size, and one (usually the left) may be larger than the other. The vertebral arteries lie within the vertebral canal, on their medial aspect closely related to the neurocentral joint, and pass immediately anterior to the emerging cervical nerve roots. Each nerve root receives a small arterial branch. Spondylotic changes of the cervical vertebrae may displace the artery laterally and, in severe cases, posteriorly as well. The degree of displacement depends on the size

and position of the body prominence that arises as a result of spondylosis. Atheroma of the vertebral artery also may be important in the production of symptoms. Cerebellar infarction may result from a critical reduction of blood flow to the vertebral artery in the neck. When the block occurs in the cervical part of the vertebral artery, the cerebellar infarcts tend to be bilateral, approximately symmetrical, and in the territory of the superior cerebellar artery. Most often the obstruction will be incomplete, and blood flow may be reduced only when the patient turns or extends his head. Rotation and extension of the head to one side can obstruct the contralateral vertebral artery; and in patients with atherosclerosis, rotation and extension of the head can produce posterior circulation abnormalities such as nystagmus, vertigo, weakness, dysarthria, drop attacks, and a Babinski response. An anterior spinal-artery–spinal-cord syndrome results either from compromise of the anterior spinal artery or from compression of one of the main radicular arteries by osteophytes or adhesions associated with nerve root-sleeve fibrosis. In diseases involving the major blood vessels (e.g., arteriosclerosis, diabetes, syphilis) the blood supply of the spinal cord may be impaired, especially if the condition is associated with spondylosis.

CLINICAL EVALUATION

The essential means in the diagnosis and management of cervical pain include elicitation of the history and the physical examination. Radiologic and electrodiagnostic procedures assist in confirming the clinical formulation.

History and Symptoms. *Pain.* The most common symptom of cervical spine disorders will be pain (Fig. 28–6). Cervical nerve root irritation causes a well-localized area of pain (Fig. 28–4), while poorly defined areas of pain arise from deep connective tissue structures, muscle, joint, bone, or disc. The patient's ability to describe the pain provides the examiner with essential clues to diagnosis. Retro-orbital, temporal, and occipital pain reflects a referral pattern from the atlas, axis, and C3 and their surrounding structures. In cervical spine disorders pain may appear in the back, sides, or front of the neck and may radiate to the upper thoracic spine, shoulders, or scapular regions or into one or both upper limbs. Additionally, this pain may be produced, relieved, or exaggerated by various normal movements of the cervical spine. The areas of pain designation may be tender (e.g., transverse process, spinous process, apophyseal joints, anterior vertebral bodies).

Stiffness with consequent limitation of motion of neck, shoulder, elbow, wrist, and even fingers may occur subsequent to prior injury response, articular involvement, nerve root irritation, or reflex sympathetic dystrophy.

Tenosynovitis and tendinitis often accompany syndromes of the cervical spine and may involve the rotator cuff; tendons about the wrist or hand, with stenosis or fibrosis of tendon sheaths; and palmar fascia.

Paresthesias. Numbness and tingling follow the segmental distribution of the nerve roots (Fig. 28–4) in cervical spine disorders; however, this occurs frequently without demonstrable sensory change. The symptoms appear on one side or bilaterally upon awakening and frequently abate with a change in the position of the neck and upper limbs. Paresthesias involving the face, head, or tongue suggest involvement of the upper three nerve roots of the cervical plexus, while numbness of the neck, shoulders, arm, forearms, and fingers indicates, involvement of the C5-T1 nerve roots (Fig. 28–4).

Weakness. Muscular weakness, hypotonia, and fasciculation indicate a lower motor neuron disorder secondary to an anterior radiculopathy (Table 28–4). More than one root innervates a given muscle, and when muscle weakness and atrophy appear, they suggest dysfunction of several roots. Pain and guarding produce functional weakness. On the other hand, a motor deficit may elicit sensory symptoms, for example, a feeling of "heaviness" of the limbs.

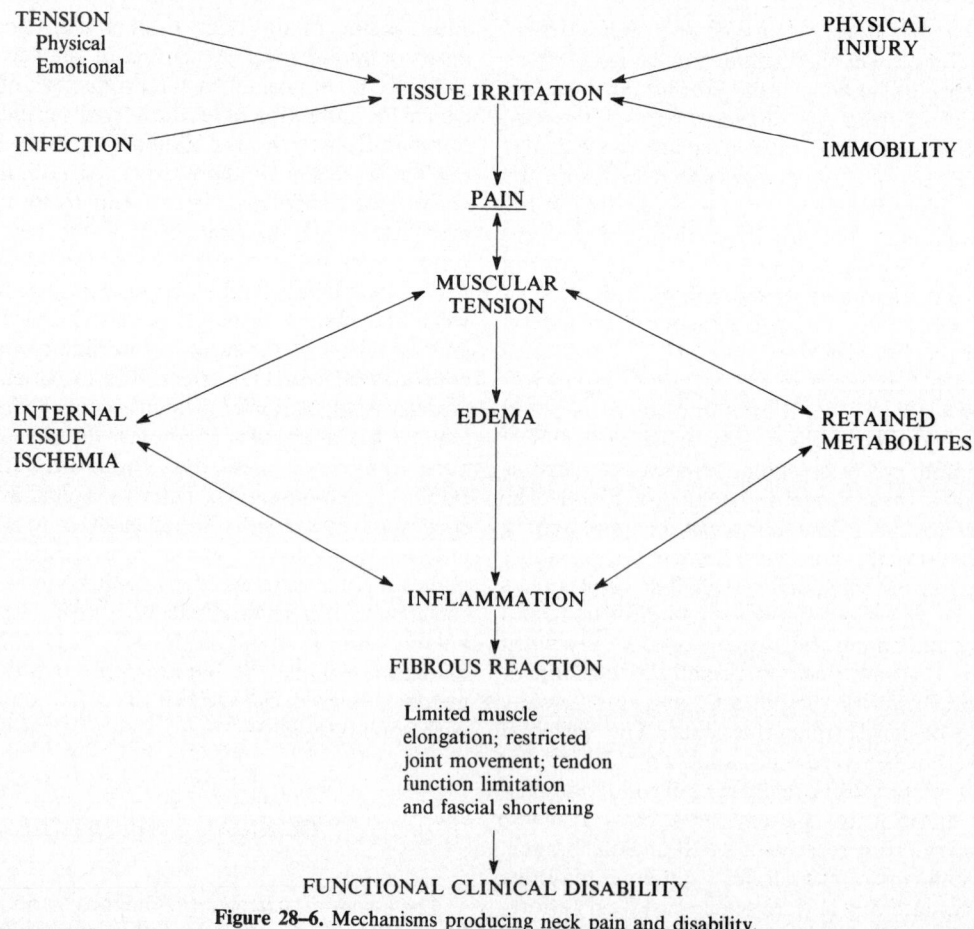

Figure 28–6. Mechanisms producing neck pain and disability.

Headache and Occipital Neuralgia. Head pain appears commonly and is characteristic of cervical spine disorders and results from nerve root compression, vertebral artery pressure, compression of sympathetic nerves, autonomic dysfunction, and posterior occipital muscle spasm as well as from osteoarthritic changes of the apophyseal joints of the upper three cervical vertebrae.[7] Occipital headache occurs commonly in the age group in which spondylosis appears, and becomes associated with pain in the neck and upper limbs. The pain may, in turn, spread to the eye region and may become dull rather than pulsating. It will be aggravated by strain, sneeze, and cough as well as by movements of the head and neck. Furthermore, the headache begins upon arising and worsens as the day progresses.

Pseudoangina Pectoris. A lesion at C6 and C7 may produce neurologic or myalgic pain with tenderness in the precordium or scapular region, raising confusion with angina pectoris. Pain from C6 and C7 may become compressive or may be increased with exercise, referred down the arm, aggravated by neck movement, or associated with torticollis or muscle spasm in the neck. Differentiation between heart disease and a radiculopathy can be made in the presence of other neurologic signs of C6-C7 dysfunction (e.g., muscle weakness, fasciculation, sensory changes). However, difficulty will arise in clinical situations in which true angina and pseudoangina coexist.

Eye Symptoms. "Blurring" of vision relieved by changing neck position, increased tearing, pain in one or both eyes, retro-orbital pain, and descriptions of the eyes being "pulled backward or pushed forward" may be reported by the patient with a cervical spine disorder. These symptoms result from irritation of the cervical sympathetic nerve supply to eye structures via the plexuses surrounding the vertebral and internal carotid arteries and their branches.

Ear Symptoms. Changes in equilibrium develop with irritation of sympathetic plexuses surrounding the vertebral arteries or with vascular insufficiency of these same arteries. Associated gait disturbances with or without tinnitus and altered auditory acuity result from vascular insufficiency secondary to vasospasm or compression of the vertebral arteries by cervical structures.

Throat Symptoms. Dysphagia results from muscle spasm, anterior osteophyte compression of the pharynx and esophagus, or abnormalities of cervical cranial nerve and sympathetic communications.

Miscellaneous Symptoms. Occasionally, bizarre symptoms appear in patients with cervical spine disorders. Dyspnea ("can't get a deep breath . . . or enough air") results from a C3-C4-C5 deficit (innervation of the respiratory muscles). Cardiac palpitations and tachycardia associated with unusual positions or hyperextension of the neck appear with irritation of the C4 nerve root, which innervates the diaphragm and pericardium, or with irritation of the cardiac sympathetic nerve supply. Nausea and emesis, ill-defined pain, and paresthesias may accompany spinal cord compression. Drop attacks, with abrupt loss of proprioception, and collapse without loss of consciousness may suggest posterior circulation insufficiency.

A complex variety of symptoms and signs result from cervical nerve root dysfunction, sympathetic nervous system involvement, cervical spinal cord compression, and posterior circulation insufficiency as well as diseases and injury of cervical bone, muscles, and joints. The clinician must consider all of these factors in evaluating patients with neck pain before diagnosing the symptoms as "functional" or psychoneurotic.

Clinical Examination. Systematic examination of patients with cervical spine syndromes includes head, neck, upper thoracic spine, shoulders, arms, forearms, wrists, and hands with the patient fully undressed. The clinician observes the patient's posture, movements, facial expression, gait, and various positions (e.g., sitting, standing, supine). As the patient walks into the office, the clinician observes the patient's head position and how naturally and rhythmically the head and neck move with body movement.

The neck should be inspected for normal anatomic position of the hyoid bone, thyroid cartilage, and thyroid gland and for normal cervical lordosis as well as scars or pigmentation. Palpation of bony structures in the neck should be performed with the patient supine in order to relax the overlying muscles. In palpating the anterior neck, the examiner stands at the patient's side and supports the neck from behind with one hand, palpating with the other, relaxing the spine as much as possible. The horseshoe-shaped hyoid bone lies above the thyroid cartilage and is at the level of the C3 vertebra. With the index finger and thumb (pincerlike) the examiner feels the stem of the horseshoe, and as the patient swallows, the hyoid bone moves up and then down. The thyroid cartilage possesses a superior notch and a flaring upper portion (sits at the C4 vertebra level); the lower border lies at the C5 level. Below the lower border of the thyroid cartilage the examiner palpates the first cricoid ring (opposite the C6 vertebra), and this will be the upper border of the trachea and just superior to the site of emergency tracheostomy. The cricoid ring moves with swallowing. About 2 to 3 cm lateral to the first cricoid ring, the carotid tubercle, the anterior tubercle of the transverse process of C6, can be felt. The carotid arteries lie adjacent to the tubercle, and their pulsation can be appreciated. Palpation of both carotid tubercles simultaneously results in restriction of carotid arterial flow, causing a carotid reflex. The carotid tubercle proves useful as a landmark in stellate sympathetic ganglion injections. The transverse process of C1 lies between the angle of the jaw and the styloid process of the skull. Since it will be the broadest transverse process of the cervical spine, palpation will be facilitated. Normal anatomic movements of the atlanto-occipital and atlantoaxial joints and bony structures can be appreciated by a lateral sliding movement, holding the atlas between the thumb and index finger by the transverse processes.

The posterior landmarks of the cervical spine include the occiput, inion, superior nuchal line, mastoid process, spinous processes of each vertebra, and apophyseal joints. Initially, the examiner palpates the occiput, then the inion, marking the center point of the superior nuchal line (the line will feel like a transverse ridge extending out on both sides of the inion). The round mastoid process sits at the lateral edge of the superior nuchal line (Fig. 28–1*B*). The spinous process of the axis (C2) can be palpated below the indented area immediately under the occiput. As each spinous process from C2 to T1 is palpated, the examiner notes the cervical lordosis. Occasionally the bifid spinous processes of C3 to C6 can be appreciated. The C7 (vertebra prominens) and T1 spinous processes will be larger than the others. Alignment of the spinous processes should be noted. The apophyseal joints can be felt as small rounded domes deep to the trapezius muscles about 1 inch lateral to the spinous processes. In order to palpate these joints the patient must be relaxed, as spasm and tension preclude access on examination. The joint involved can be determined by alignment with the hyoid bone at C3, the thyroid cartilage at C4 and C5, and the first cricoid ring at C6. These joints often become tender with osteoarthritis, especially in the upper cervical spine, whereas the C5-C6, C6-C7 level will be most often involved in cervical spondylosis.

Examination of soft tissues in the neck should be divided into two anatomic areas, anterior and posterior, the anterior being bordered laterally by the two sternocleidomastoid muscles, superiorly by the mandible, and inferiorly by the suprasternal notch (an upside-down triangle); the posterior aspect includes the whole area posterior to the lateral border of the sternocleidomastoid muscle. The supine position appears optimal in the examination. Anteriorly the sternocleidomastoid muscle can be examined by asking the patient to turn the head to the opposite side; the muscle then stands out and can be palpated from origin to insertion. The opposite muscle can be compared for any discrepancies in size, bulges, or strength. Hyperextension injuries overstretch the muscle, with resultant hemorrhage into the tissue. Localized swelling may be due to hematomas. In torticollis the sternocleidomastoid muscles will be involved. The lymph node chain resides along the medial border of the sternocleidomastoid muscle and in the normal situation cannot be palpated. Small tender lymph nodes can be palpated if they are enlarged secondary to infections (throat, ear), metastases, or primary tumor. Enlarged lymph nodes may, in turn, produce torticollis. The thyroid gland overlies the thyroid cartilage in an H pattern, the bar being the isthmus between the two laterally situated lobes. Normally, the thyroid gland will be smooth and palpable without enlargement. Diffuse enlargement of the thyroid gland, cysts, nodules, or tenderness from thyroiditis should be noted. The carotid arteries, best felt near the carotid tubercle on C6, should be examined separately, owing to the carotid reflex secondary to simultaneous palpation. Normally carotid pulsation should be symmetric.

The parotid gland overlies part of the sharp angle of the mandible, which is usually indistinct to palpation; but when the parotid gland is enlarged, the usually sharp and bony angle of the mandible feels soft and boggy owing to overlying glandular tissue (e.g., mumps, Sjögren's syndrome, and endocrine disorders). The supraclavicular fossa above the clavicle should be examined for lymph nodes, unusual excursion with respiration, swelling, fat accumulation, and asymmetry with the opposite side. The platysma muscle crosses the supraclavicular fossa but will be too thin to alter the contour of the fossa. Observation during voluntary platysma contracture may reveal lumps or asymmetry. The apex and dome of the lung extend up into the supraclavicular fossa. At times cervical ribs can be palpated.

Posteriorly, with the patient sitting, the clinician examines the trapezius muscle, lymph nodes, the greater occipital nerves, and the superior nuchal ligament. The trapezius muscle origin extends from the inion to the spinous process of T12 and inserts laterally in a continuous arc into the clavicle, the acromion, and the spine of the scapula. The trapezius should be felt from origin to insertion, beginning high up on the neck. Flexion injuries may traumatize the trapezius, and hematomas in the muscle occur frequently. Furthermore, the trapezius will be the site of focal points of pain and tenderness in fibrositis syndromes. Two trapezius muscles should be palpated bilaterally and simultaneously, while looking for tenderness, lumps and swelling, and asymmetry of the two muscles. Embryologically the trapezius and sternocleidomastoid muscles begin as one muscle and later split, but they retain a common attachment along the base of the skull to the mastoid process and their nerve supply remains the same, the spinal accessory nerve (ninth cranial nerve). The lymph node chain lies at the anterolateral border of the trapezius and normally cannot be palpated. The greater occipital nerves sit laterally to the inion, extending up in the scalp, and can be easily palpated when tender and inflamed. Commonly a flexion-extension injury of the spine produces traumatic inflammation and swelling of the occipital nerves with resultant painful occipital neuralgia, a frequent cause of headache. The superior nuchal ligament arises from the inion and extends to C7 and T1 spinous processes. It will be under the examining finger when the physician is feeling the spinous processes. It may become tender, irregular, and lumpy if overstretched or injured.

Range of Motion. There exists a large range of motion of the cervical spine (Table 28–3), which, in turn, provides a wide scope of vision and is essential to the sense of balance. The basic movements of the neck include flexion, extension, lateral flexion to the right and left, and rotation to the right and left. About half of the total flexion and extension of the neck occurs at the occiput-C1 level, the other half being equally distributed among the other six cervical vertebra, with a slight increase at the C5-C6 level. Approximately half of rotation occurs at the atlantoaxial joint (odontoid); the other half distributes equally among the other five vertebrae. All vertebrae share in lateral flexion. A decrease in specific motion may occur with blocking at a joint, pain, fibrous contractures, bony ankylosis, muscle spasm, mechanical alteration in joint and skeletal structures, or a tense and uncooperative patient. Other causes of muscle spasm include injury to muscles, involuntary splinting over painful joints or skeletal structures, and irritation or compression of cervical nerve roots of the spinal cord.

All range of cervical spine motion should be performed as follows: (1) actively and to the extreme of motion (to assess muscle function and strength), as observed by the examiner; (2) passively (to assess nonmobile structures, ligaments, capsules, and fascia), by which the examiner moves the relaxed cervical spine through all its motions; and (3) against resistance (to study origin and insertions of tendon and ligaments and assess motor strength), with each motion maximally attempted against force of the examiner's hand.

Flexion and Extension. The patient nods his head forward and touches chin to sternum. If one of the examiner's fingers can be placed between the patient's chin and sternum, there exists 10 degrees' limitation of flexion while 30 degrees of limitation exists if three fingers can be inserted within the above area. Observation of the curve of the cervical spine should be done as the examiner instructs the patient to look from floor to ceiling. The arc of neck motion normally remains smooth and not halting or irregular. In full hyperextension the base of the occiput normally touches the spinous process of T1.

Lateral Flexion. The patient attempts to touch his ear to his shoulder without rotation or shoulder shrugging. Normal people can laterally flex 45 degrees in either direction.

Rotation. The patient rotates the head maximally, usually being able to bring his chin into alignment with his shoulder. Normally, the motion remains smooth, while torticollis restricts motion.

Passive Range of Motion. The examiner asks for complete relaxation and takes the patient's head firmly in his hands, putting the spine through maximal flexion, extension, lateral flexion, and rotation. Passive motion may be more extensive than active motion if muscles remain stiff, painful, or possess involuntary spasm. In cases of head or cervical spine injury, passive range of motion should not be done because of the risk of neurologic trauma to an unstable spine.

Motion Against Resistance. All ranges of neck motion can be performed with the examiner offering firm resistance to each movement. The anchorage of muscle, tendon insertion and origin, muscle strength, and muscular function should be assessed. This phase of the examination should be performed with the patient seated. The primary (sternocleidomastoids) and secondary (three scalenes and small prevertebral muscles) flexors of the neck can be assessed by the examiner placing his left hand flat on the patient's upper sternum and his right (resisting) hand, with the palm cupped, on the patient's forehead; the patient then flexes his neck, slowly increasing the power to maximal pressure. The primary (paravertebral extensor mass, splenius and semispinalis capitis, and trapezius muscles) and secondary extensor muscles (small intrinsic neck muscles) should

be assessed by the examiner placing his left hand over the patient's upper posterior chest and scapular area, with his right palm cupped over the patient's occiput; the patient then gradually increases neck extension to his maximum. Lateral flexor muscles (three scalenes and the small intrinsic neck muscles) can be examined by placing the examiner's left hand on the patient's shoulder (for stability) and his right palm (fingers extended) against the side of the patient's head; the patient then laterally flexes against the examiner's resistance. The rotators of the neck (sternocleidomastoid and intrinsic neck muscles) can be tested to right lateral rotation by placing the stabilizing left hand of the examiner on the patient's left shoulder and his right hand along the right side of the patient's mandible while the patient rotates against resistance. Left rotation is tested in the reverse fashion. Either sternocleidomastoid muscle functioning alone provides the main pull to the side being tested.

Special Clinical Tests of the Cervical Spine. *Head Compression Test (Fig. 28–7).* With narrowing of the intervertebral foramina, pressure and shearing forces on the apophyseal joint surfaces, intervertebral disc compression, or pressure on stiff ligamentous and muscle structures there will be pain on compression of the head onto the cervical spine. If radicular pain or paresthesias with referral to the upper limb occur with the head compression test, it strongly suggests nerve root irritation. On the other hand, if the pain remains in the neck, soft connective tissues or joints appear as the pain-sensitive structures involved. The test should be performed with the patient sitting; the examiner places one hand across the other on the top of the patient's head with gradually increased downward pressure; the patient then reports any pain or paresthesias and its distribution. Application of pressure may also be down with the head tilted to either side, backward, or forward.

Head Distraction Test (Fig. 28–7). This test should be done with the patient seated; the open palm of the examiner's hand should be placed under the patient's chin.

NECK EXTENSION   NECK COMPRESSION

Figure 28–7. Neck compression and distraction tests in the examination of patients with cervical spine syndromes.

while the examiner's other hand goes under the patient's occiput; gradually the force of lifting the patient's head increases, removing the weight of the skull and distracting the foramina, discs, and joints. Nerve root compression may be relieved, with disappearance of symptoms with opening of the intervertebral foramina or extension of the disc spaces. Additionally, pressure on joint capsules of apophyseal joints diminishes with head distraction.

Valsalva Maneuver. Holding one's breath against a closed glottis raises intrathecal pressure. If an intraspinal tumor or a herniated disc exists in a person, then this test will produce pain, which radiates in a dermatome distribution. Vigorous cough or sneeze, likewise, will elicit pain in the above situations.

Dysphagia Test. Soft tissue swelling, hematoma, vertebral subluxation, or cervical osteophytic projections produce pain or restriction to swallowing.

Ophthalmologic Tests. Pupillary signs may differ from one side to the other or vary from one time to another in certain patients with cervical spine disorders, thereby indicating irritability of sympathetic nerve supply in the neck controlling the pupillary muscles. This should not be confused with Horner's syndrome, which follows complete interruption or paralysis of the sympathetic fibers, resulting in miosis, vasomotor and sweating changes, and ptosis on the affected side.

Adson Test. The Adson test examines the subclavian artery when it may be compressed by a cervical rib, the scalene muscles, or other thoracic outlet abnormalities. The examiner palpates the patient's radial pulse in abduction, extension, and external rotation of the arm. The patient then takes a deep inspiration while rotating his head maximally toward the side being tested. With subclavian artery compression there results a marked decrease in volume or absence of the radial pulse on the affected side.

Shoulder Depression Test. This test indirectly determines if there exists irritation on compression of nerve root, dural root sleeve fibrosis or adhesions, foraminal encroachment, or adjacent joint capsule thickening and adhesions. The examiner stands beside the patient who tilts the head to one side. With one of the examiner's hands on the patient's shoulder and the other hand on the patient's head, the examiner exerts downward pressure on the patient's shoulder and lateral flexion pressure on the patient's head in the opposite direction. This test places a tug on the nerve roots; with root sleeve fibrosis, foraminal osteophytes, or adhesions, radicular pain or paresthesias often result.

Muscle Weakness and Atrophy. Weakness of the muscles may be difficult to assess, as innervation of shoulder girdle, arm, forearm and muscles occurs by two or more roots (Table 28–4).

Muscular weakness has many possible causes; to narrow the choice down to one or a few, one must ascertain the anatomic localization of the patient's complaints. Tables 28–5 and 28–6 provide guidelines and offer differential clinical features separating upper and lower

Table 28–5. Clinical Features Differentiating Upper and Lower Motor Neuron Weakness

Clinical Feature	Upper Motor Neuron Weakness	Lower Motor Neuron Weakness
Weakness	Greater in extensors of upper limbs and in flexors of lower limbs (pyramidal distribution); usually involves one side of body but may also produce paraparesis, quadriparesis, or (rarely) monoparesis; usually does not produce weakness in one muscle group or bilateral cranial weakness	Nonpyramidal distribution; May be present in one muscle group; paraparesis, quadriparesis, and bilateral cranial nerve weakness also seen
Deep tendon reflexes	Usually increased, but acutely may be decreased; also may be decreased with parietal and cerebellar lesions	Decreased
Tone to passive motion	Increased; may be decreased with cerebellar and parietal lesions	Decreased
Pathologic reflexes associated	Babinski and others Defect of cortical association areas; frontal-release signs defect of sensation; cerebellar defects; cranial nerve defects	Absent Cranial nerve signs; sensory sign

motor neuron weakness. Atrophy may follow weakness owing to disuse or pain. Interossei hand muscle atrophy can appear with cervical spine disease (Fig. 28–8).

Reflexes. Reflexes indicate the state of the nervous system and its afferent pathways (Table 28–7). Certain abnormal reflexes appear only with spasticity and paralysis; these indicate injury to the corticospinal tract. The primary deep tendon reflexes (Table 28–8 and 28–9), abdominal reflexes, and plantar responses should be routinely examined; bulbocavernosus and anal reflexes should be tested in all suspected lower spinal cord (conus or cauda equina) lesions and in cases of sphincter disturbances.

In eliciting the deep-tendon reflexes, adequate relaxation of the patient and a mild degree of passive tension on the muscle becomes essential, especially in the radial (supinator) and ankle jerks. The examiner varies the tension on the muscle by manipulating the joint, and reinforcement procedures enable the patient to relax completely, as by pulling one of his hands with the other (Jendrassik maneuver). When the examiner elicits the triceps jerk, the small contraction of the triceps muscle should be disregarded, for most muscles will contract if directly percussed.

The tendon jerk normally occurs in only a part of each muscle, and in a myopathy, the reflex jerk may be

Table 28–6. Differentiating Symptoms of Lower Motor Neuron Weakness

Signs and Symptoms	Neuropathy	Myopathy*	Motor Neuron or Anterior Horn Cell Dysfunction	Neuromuscular Junction Dysfunction
Weakness	Mainly distal or nerve distribution	Proximal	May be distal or proximal and involve midline muscles (neck flexor weak)	Mainly bulbar respiratory, and proximal
Deep tendon reflexes	Decreased	Decreased	Increased	Normal
Myotatic reflexes	Increased	Decreased	Increased	Normal
Sensory loss paresthesias	Usually present	Absent	Absent	Absent
Fasciculations	May be present	Absent	Present	Absent
Atrophy	May be present	May be present	Present	Absent
Fatigue	Mild	Mild	Mild	Severe
Tenderness	May have dysesthesias	May be present	Cramps	Absent

*Myoglobinuria or myotonia may differentiate certain myopathies.

lost in the quadriceps through wasting in the vastus internus, though the power of contraction of the remainder persists to a fair degree. Some clinically normal people show reduced reflexes, and before the examiner decides, he should ascertain whether there exists other evidence of peripheral nerve (sensory loss, atrophy, etc.) or muscle disease.

Examination of Related Area. Shoulder lesions may closely mimic cervical spine disease, and a complete shoulder examination becomes necessary in these situations. The shoulder syndromes usually demonstrate little or no neurologic involvement. Rotator cuff tendinitis, calcareous deposits in tendons, and capsulitis often coexist with cervical spine disease. Reflex sympathetic dystrophy may occur, with the initial triggering pain mechanism arising in the spine. Similar changes may occur at the elbow, wrist, and fingers. Finger motion may be limited because of swelling secondary to circulatory reflex ischemic changes from sympathetic nerve irritation. Fibrous nodules and contracture of palmar fascia occur following cervical spine disease or injury.

Infections of the temporomandibular joint, teeth,

lower jaw, or scalp may refer pain to the temporomandibular joint area and to the neck. The jaw reflex (mediated by the fifth cranial nerve and involving the masseter and temporalis muscles) can be examined by placing the index finger on the mental area of the chin with the patient's mouth in the rest position (slightly open); a reflex hammer then taps the fingers and the jaw reflexly closes. An absent or decreased jaw jerk suggests abnormality in the course of the trigeminal nerve, while a brisk reflex suggests an upper motor neuron lesion. The jaw jerk proves useful in separating cervical spine disease from primary trigeminal nerve dysfunction.

Radiographic Examination. X-rays are essential in evaluation of the patient with a cervical spine disorder. The clinicians should assess both the clinical and the radiographic studies of his patient and not depend solely on the radiologist. Clinical correlation will be necessary, as gross radiologic signs and abnormalities may be associated with minimal or no clinical disturbance while the reverse situation (minimal radiographic change and neurolgic signs) may also occur.

Figure 28–8. Interossei hand muscle weakness in a patient with severe cervical spondylosis.

Table 28–7. Relation of Reflexes to Peripheral Nerves and Spinal Cord Segments

Reflex	Site and Mode of Elicitation	Response	Muscle(s)	Peripheral Nerve(s)	Cord Segment
Scapulohumeral reflex	Tap on lower end of medial border of scapula	Adduction and lateral rotation of dependent arm	Infraspinatus and teres minor	Suprascapular (axillary)	C4 to C6
Biceps jerk	Tap on tendon of biceps brachii	Flexion at elbow	Biceps brachii	Musculocutaneous	C5 and C6
Supinator jerk (also called radial reflex)	Tap on distal end of radius	Flexion at elbow	Brachioradialis (and biceps brachii and brachialis)	Radial (musculocutaneous)	C5 and C6
Triceps jerk	Tap on tendon of triceps brachii above olecranon, with elbow flexed	Extension at elbow	Triceps brachii	Radial	C7 and C8
Thumb reflex	Tap on tendon of flexor pollicis longus in distal third of forearm	Flexion of terminal phalanx of thumb	Flexor pollicis longus	Median	C6 to C8
Extensor finger and hand jerk	Tap on posterior aspect of wrist just proximal to radiocarpal joint	Extension of hand and fingers (inconstant)	Extensors of hand and fingers	Radial	C6 to C8
Flexor finger jerk	Tap on examiner's thumb placed on palm of hand; sharp tap on tips of flexed fingers (Tromner's sign)	Flexion of fingers	Flexor digitorum superficialis (and profundus)	Median	C7 and C8 (T1)
Epigastric reflex (exteroceptive)	Brisk stroking of skin downwards from nipple in mammillary line	Retraction of epigastrium	Transversus abdominis	Intercostal	T5 and T6
Abdominal skin reflex (exteroceptive)	Brisk stroking of skin of abdominal wall in lateromedial direction	Shift of skin of abdomen and displacement of umbilicus	Muscles of abdominal wall	Intercostal, hypogastric, and ilioinguinal	T6 and T12
Cremasteric reflex (exteroceptive)	Stroking skin on medial aspect of thigh (pinching adductor muscles)	Elevation of testis	Cremaster	Genital branch of genitofemoral	L2 and L3 (L1)
Adductor reflex	Tap on medial condyle of femur	Adduction of leg	Adductors of thigh	Obturator	L2, L3, and L4
Knee jerk	Tap on tendon of quadriceps femoris below patella	Extension at knee	Quadriceps femoris	Femoral	(L2), L3, and L4
Gluteal reflex (exteroceptive)	Stroking skin over gluteal region	Tightening of buttock (inconstant)	Gluteus medius and gluteus maximus	Superior and inferior gluteal	L4, L5, and S1
Posterior tibial reflex	Tap on tendon of tibialis posterior behind medial malleolus	Supination of foot (inconstant)	Tibialis posterior	Tibial	L5
Semimembranosus and semitendinosus reflex	Tap on medial hamstring tendons (patient prone and knee slightly flexed)	Contraction of semimembranosus and semitendinosus muscles	Semimembranosus and semitendinosus	Sciatic	S1
Biceps femoris reflex	Tap on lateral hamstring tendon (patient prone and knee slightly flexed)	Contraction of biceps femoris	Biceps femoris	Sciatic	S1 and S2
Ankle jerk	Tap on tendo calcaneus	Plantar flexion of foot	Triceps surae and other flexors of foot	Tibial	S1 and S2
Bulbocavernosus reflex (exteroceptive)	Gentle squeezing of glans penis or pinching of skin of dorsum of penis	Contraction of bulbocavernosus muscle, palpable at root of penis	Bulbocavernosus	Pudendal	S3 and S4
Anal reflex (exteroceptive)	Scratch or prick of perianal skin (patient lying on side)	Visible contraction of anus	Sphincter ani externus	Pudendal	S5

Table 28-8. The Six Primary Reflexes

Reflex	Nerve Roots Necessary for Reflex	Muscle Carrying Out the Reflex
Ankle jerk	S1	Gastrocnemius
Posterior tibial	L5	Posterior tibial
Knee	L2-L4	Quadriceps
Biceps	C5, C6	Biceps
Radial	C5, C6	Brachioradialis
Triceps	(C6) C7, C8	Triceps

Routine x-ray views include (1) anteroposterior views of the atlas and axis through the open mouth (Fig. 28-9); (2) anteroposterior views of the lower five vertebra; (3) lateral views in flexion, neutral, and extension (Fig. 28-10); and (4) both right and left oblique (Fig. 28-11) views.

Planograms and tomograms may be necessary in certain instances (e.g., trauma, tumors, infection). Nuclear bone scans can be used in patients suspected of having infection, tumor, certain metabolic diseases, and compression fractures. Computed tomography (CT) scan and myelography with iodinated contrast material will be necessary in cervical disc disease, tumors, and syringomyelia.

Electrodiagnostic Studies: Electromyography (EMG), Nerve Conduction Velocities (NCV), Somatosensory Evoked Responses (SER). Various EMG, NCV, and SER patterns help differentiate the normal from diffuse polyneuropathy, focal entrapment neuropathy, radiculopathy, myopathy, disorders of the neuromuscular junction (e.g., myasthenia gravis), and anterior horn cell disease (e.g., amyotrophic lateral sclerosis) (Table 28-10). No one feature of the EMG (except for true myotonia) gives a diagnosis; rather, it requires the summated information of needle EMG coupled with NCV and SER as well as the clinical examination as performed by a clinician.

Clinicians often face the problem of a patient with weakness. Weakness, in turn, may be secondary to disease within the muscle, nerve, neuromuscular junction, or upper motor neuron (spinal cord, brainstem, or cerebrum) (Tables 28-5 and 28-6). The specific need for definitive therapy, including surgery, can be established only when the physician becomes aware of the cause, extent, and prognosis of the weakness. Evaluation of the electrical activity of muscle tissue and of muscle response to nerve stimulation solves many of these problems.

Other Laboratory Tests. The clinical laboratory offers some help in diagnosis and management of neck pain

Table 28-9. Four Point Grading Scale for Reflexes

Grade	State of Reflexes
0	Absent despite full relaxation and reinforcement maneuvers
1	Reduced but not absent
2	Normal physiologic reflexes
3	Increased response but no reduplication or excessive spread
4	Marked increase with reduplication, clonus, and spread

in specific diseases (e.g., rheumatoid arthritis, hyperparathyroidism, multiple myeloma, ankylosing spondylitis, and metastatic malignant cancer). Cerebrospinal fluid (CSF) evaluation should be done in patients with neck pain suspected of having infection (meningitis, meningismus) or subarachnoid hemorrhage. In the latter conditions, the CSF will be diagnostic.

DIFFERENTIAL DIAGNOSIS

Many clinical conditions arising outside the cervical spine but perceived in or about the neck area (Fig. 28-5) mimic cervical nerve root irritation, muscle spasm, ligament strain, bone disease, and joint disorders. Although Table 28-1 lists multiple structures potentially causing neck pain, clinical evaluation usually differentiates between the entities.

Disorders of somatic or visceral structures having cervical nerve root innervation (same embryologic origin) cause pain felt in the neck. Since these areas constitute reflexly referred pain along the segmental distribution of the nerve roots, such areas of referral will not be tender on deep palpation. Areas of superficial peripheral tenderness develop owing to reflex or direct sympathetic irritation secondary to vasomotor changes. Referred painful areas do not have muscle spasm and often will be described as having a burning or cramping sensation. Nausea, emesis, and pallor may accompany this type of pain.

Peripheral neuropathy may produce pain both proximal as well as distal to the irritative site. However, muscle spasm will not be associated with peripheral neuropathy. Spinal cord tumor produces a poorly localized and ill-defined neck pain, hyper-reflexia, spasticity; immobilization will not relieve the pain, and deep tenderness and local muscle spasms will be absent. Furthermore, in spinal cord lesions there exists paralysis or weakness below the cord level (not dermatome) associated with sensory changes and Babinski signs. Cerebral or subarachnoid hemorrhage, meningitis, head and neck trauma, or a central tumor produces cervical spine pain, mimicking cervical spine syndromes producing nerve root irritation. In these instances the clinical examination, CT scan, CSF tests, and angiographic studies will differentiate between the various conditions.

An important point to remember in the differential diagnosis of neck pain is that compression or irritation of cervical nerve roots with radiation of pain is associated with deep tenderness at the site of pain. Segmental areas of deep tenderness that are not painful until palpated indicate nerve root involvement. A 1 percent injection of lidocaine in the painful area results in transient reproduction of the radicular pain followed by relief from pain for days or weeks in the patient with nerve root irritation. If local anesthetic injection fails to reproduce (and relieve) the pain, one then looks at potential visceral or somatic structures having the same segmental nerve supply.

Figure 28–9. Open mouth cervical spine x-ray showing the atlanto-occipital relationship, symmetry, joint space, and the bony configuration. The atlas-axis relationship and odontoid can also be seen. The arrow to the left shows the atlanto-axial joint; the middle arrow, the odontoid process; and the arrow to the right, the atlanto-occipital joint.

Figure 28–10. Lateral x-ray view showing the normal cervical lordosis with anterior convexity; spinous processes and the apophyseal joints are seen. The lower arrow marks the C6-C7 disc space. The upper right arrow shows the anterior arch of the atlas while the upper left arrow shows the posterior surface of the odontoid. In a C1-C2 subluxation, the space between the posterior surface of the arch of the atlas and the anterior surface of the odontoid opens up (normal will be up to 2.5 mm); this is seen best in flexion. The sagittal diameter may be measured from the middle of each vertebra to the point of union of the lamina; 10 mm or less will usually indicate pathologic narrowing and a myelopathy.

Figure 28–11. Oblique cervical x-rays display the intervertebral foramina, normally 10 mm vertical height and 5 mm transverse. Osteophyte projection from the uncovertebral joints, the vertebrae themselves, and the apophyseal joints can be seen (arrows).

Table 28–10. Summary of EMG, NCV, and SER Findings by Location in Disease in the Motor Unit

	Location						
	Spinal Cord		Nerve Root				Muscle
Study	Anterior Horn Cell	Anterior Motor	Dorsal Pre-	Ganglion Post-	Peripheral Nerve	Neuromuscular Junction	
Motor NCV	N	N	N	N	+	N	N
Sensory NCV	N	N	N	±	+	N	N
EMG	+	+	N	N	+	±	+
Repetitive stimulation	±	±	N	N	±	+	N
F wave	+	+	N	N	+	N	N
H reflex	+	+	+	+	+	N	N
SER	±	±	+	+	+	N	N

N = Normal
+ = Abnormal
± = Occasional Abnormality
SER = Somatosensory Evoked Response

Neck pain occurs in malingerers, depressed individuals, patients seeking compensation, hysterical and psychoneurotic patients, and automobile accident victims. If these patients possess no concomitant nerve root irritation, then they will derive no relief from local anesthesia injected in the painful area(s). Absence of muscle spasm, an antalgic position, and feigning of limitation of motion should arouse the examiner's suspicion.

Skilled clinical elicitation of historical data and the physical examination constitute the principal and most reproducible means of making a differential diagnosis[6,8,9] (Fig. 28–12). In evaluating the patient with neck pain the examiner soon realizes that there may be a syndrome of neck pain alone, head and neck pain, neck and shoulder pain, shoulder pain alone, shoulder and arm pain, or just arm, forearm, hand, or finger pain. Symptoms of altered sensation and vascular insufficiency often accompany the complaint of neck pain. Symptoms or signs arising in the head and upper cervical spine arise only from structures at the C1 to C4 level; symptoms in the lower neck, shoulder, and arm arise from structures at the C4 to T1 levels. When the examiner observes muscle weakness in the patient with neck pain, he must differentiate among nerve root compromise, myelopathy, pe-

Figure 28–12. Algorithm for the clinical evaluation of patients with neck pain.

ripheral neuropathy, and a primary muscle disease (Table 6).

TREATMENT

Medical Regimen. Opinions differ as to the best treatment of neck pain and the various cervical spine syndromes discussed in this chapter. Cautious clinical, electrodiagnostic, and x-ray assessment must precede the planning of treatment, and it becomes important to exclude other causes of pain in the neck and upper limbs before treatment commences. In any treatment regimen, the clinician must consider the following: (1) severity of the symptoms, (2) the presence or absence of neurologic findings, and (3) the severity of the condition as seen by electrodiagnostic evaluation and radiographic procedures (which may necessitate CT and myelography).

Bed Rest. Medical therapy aims at the relief of pain and stiffness in the neck and arms. Bed rest should be reserved for severe acute cases, for chronic cases with an acute exacerbation of symptoms, or for patients in whom ambulatory treatment fails. The patient lies flat in bed with one pillow and with the head in the most comfortable position. For the relief of pain, adequate analgesics should be prescribed. Salicylates and anti-inflammatory and analgesic medications usually suffice; however, if severe pain develops, codeine, meperidine, or morphine may become necessary. Muscle relaxant medications, hypnotics, or diazepam may be utilized concomitantly. With complete bed rest and sufficient analgesic, anti-inflammatory, and muscle relaxant medications, acute neck pain usually subsides within 7 to 10 days. When the acute pain subsides, the patient commences active exercises.

Cervical Collar. In cervical spondylosis and other musculoskeletal-type syndromes, limitation of neck movement benefits the patient, and cervical collars can be used to achieve this end. The several types of cervical collars range from those that immobilize the cervical spine to those intended merely to provide temporary support and limit excessive movement. Patients with nerve root pain often find relief of symptoms after wearing a collar. Generally, patients with generalized spondylosis do less well than those with focal spondylosis. Before prescribing a cervical collar, it is essential to assess the degree of disability, and the type of collar selected should depend on the degree of immobilization desired. Felt, foam, and rubber collars restrict gross movement, while plastic and plaster collars give more secure immobilization. Any collar must fit well and maintain the neck in the most comfortable position. Most people dislike wearing collars; however, some patients seem to become addicted to wearing collars, and it becomes difficult to persuade them to remove them. In general, the patient should leave his collar off after about 2 months to prevent weakness and wasting of the neck muscles. After the acute painful stage abates, active exercise in conjunction with collar use is encouraged.

Traction. Traction, either continuous or intermittent, should be considered when bed rest fails. Continuous traction should be reserved for more severe cases with symptoms of nerve root compression. Many patients cannot tolerate traction, and a few will become worse with it. Analgesics and muscle relaxants can be used in doses sufficient to prevent restlessness. Sometimes it becomes necessary to set up a traction apparatus utilizing only 5 pounds of weight; this keeps the patient immobile in bed and avoids the unpleasant effects of heavier traction. There exists some difference in opinion as to the correct direction of pull in traction. Some authors feel that the most comfortable position should be found and traction exerted in this direction; others recommend that the head be in extension, while other authorities consider slight flexion as the best postion. A weight of 10 pounds should be attached to a pulley at the head of the bed, and the bed raised to increase the pull and prevent the trunk from sliding up. The weight may be increased to 20 pounds according to muscular development or may be varied during the day: some authorities recommend 10 to 12 pounds by day and 5 to 8 pounds at night.[10] Intermittent traction may be applied manually or mechanically by pulley and weight with the head halter. The direction of pull should be in the most comfortable position. A weight between 15 and 25 pounds and traction applied for 15 to 20 minutes generally suffice. Treatment should be repeated daily if necessary. Occasionally, side effects of traction occur, and rarely, hemianopic visual field defects develop. Traction appears unsuitable for patients with visible gross x-ray changes of the cervical spine, because of danger of spinal cord compression or pressure on the vertebral arteries.

Exercises. Active exercises should be utilized in most regimens of treatment. The exercises can be grouped as follows: (1) anterior-neck-mobilizing exercises, (2) shoulder-raising exercises, and (3) muscle-strengthening exercises. Shoulder exercises, aimed at elevating the shoulder girdle and relieving drag on the nerve roots, can be combined with the use of a cervical collar.

Head positioning may be employed to relieve symptoms, as placing the head in certain positions relieves pain. The head should be carried at all times in its optimum position of slight flexion with the chin indrawn.

Other Measures. Massage may be useful in patients with painful muscle spasms; however, in most cases massage is not prescribed in cervical spine disorders. Injection of local anesthetic or steroids into painful areas may provide relief of pain and spasm with subsequent improvement in cervical movement. Ice applied to painful areas in the acute situations often helps, while heat in the form of ultrasound or infrared radiations helps subsequently to relieve muscle spasm.

Sometimes catastrophes, with severe neurologic complications and even death, have occurred with neck manipulation as a treatment of neck pain.[11] These complications usually result from vascular disturbances of the vertebral arteries, which appear to be particularly vulnerable at the first cervical vertebra where they enter the skull. Rotation and hyperextension can become dangerous movements.

Surgery. Two main groups of patients appear appropriate for surgical consideration.[12] In the first group, symptoms relate principally to the nerve roots emerging from the cervical spine, and the condition presents itself with either neck or arm pain. In the second situation, a slowly progressive spinal cord syndrome involves the legs first and then the arms.

Careful clinical investigation supplemented by EMG, NCV, and SER to exclude peripheral nerve disease becomes essential in patients with radicular symptoms.

Patient Education. Finally, an important aspect in the treatment of patients with neck pain entails "patient education." The clinician should define the problem, instruct the patient in the rationale of the treatment, and teach the patient how to care for his neck in standing, sitting, driving, and other activities of daily living.

SUMMARY

Many medical conditions produce neck pain both locally and in its referred aspect. Confirming the source of dysfunction in the neck, understanding the mechanism by which the symptoms occur, and recognizing the tissues capable of eliciting clinical signs assume importance. A careful, thorough history and complete physical examination usually reveal the problem clearly. When the clinician recognizes which symptoms can be reproduced and which movements and positions reproduce them, he will arrive at a diagnosis and direct effective therapy. Following the principals so established reaffirms the fact that a diagnosis need not be a diagnosis of exclusion.

References

1. Holt, L.: Frequency of symptoms for different age groups and professions. *In* Hirsch, C., and Zotterman, Y. (eds.): Cervical Pain. New York, Pergamon Press, 1971, pp. 17–20.
2. Waltz, T.A.: Physical factors in the production of the myelopathy of cervical spondylosis. Brain 90:395, 1967.
3. Penning, L.: Functional Pathology of the Cervical Spine. Amsterdam, Excerpta Medica, 1968.
4. Schmorl, G., and Junghans, H.: The Human Spine in Health and Disease. New York, Grune and Stratton, 1959.
5. Brain, W.R.: Some unsolved problems in cervical spondylosis. Br. Med. J. 1:771, 1963.
6. Nakano, K.K.: Neurology of Musculoskeletal and Rheumatic Disorders. Boston, Houghton-Mifflin, 1979.
7. Bull, J.W.D., Nixon, W.L.B., and Pratt, R.T.C.: The radiological criteria and familial occurrence of primary basilar impression. Brain 78:229, 1956.
8. Hoppenfeld, S.: Orthopaedic Neurology. Philadelphia, J.B. Lippincott Company, 1977.
9. Cailliet, R.: Neck and Arm Pain. Philadelphia, F.A. Davis Company, 1964.
10. Cyriax, J.: Textbook of Orthopedic Medicine. Volume 2. London, Cassell, 1965.
11. Miller, R.G., and Burton, R.: Stroke following chiropractic manipulation of the spine. JAMA 229:189, 1974.
12. Dunsker, S.B.: Cervical Spondylosis. Seminars in Neurological Surgery. New York, Raven Press, 1981.

Chapter 29

The Painful Shoulder

Thomas S. Thornhill

INTRODUCTION

Pain about the shoulder girdle is one of the more common patient problems seen in an outpatient setting. The clinician must differentiate between pain from a local musculoskeletal problem and that referred from another source. Owing to its role as the link between the thorax and the upper extremity and the close proximity of major neurovascular structures, shoulder pain is frequently an early manifestation of systemic disease. The purpose of this chapter is to provide the reader with practical guidelines for the diagnosis and treatment of painful shoulder disorders seen in a rheumatology practice. A detailed analysis of shoulder problems and the treatment of major trauma are beyond the scope of this chapter and have been covered by other authors.[1-5] The conditions to be discussed are divided, albeit artificially, into (1) disorders of the periarticular structures, (2) disorders of the glenohumeral joint, and (3) regional disorders (Table 29–1).

DIAGNOSTIC AIDS

Anatomy. An understanding of the structural and functional anatomy is a requisite for the clinician treating shoulder pain. One must visualize the three dimensional relationships, the muscular function, the ligamentous and tendinous attachments, and the routing of neurovascular structures. Figure 29–1 shows the musculoskeletal and topographic localization of pain in association with common shoulder disorders. By understanding the relationship between the rotator cuff and the subacromial region bounded inferiorly by the humeral head and superiorly by the undersurface of the acromion, the clinician not only can visualize the problems of an im-

Table 29–1. Common Causes of Shoulder Pain

I. **Periarticular Disorders**
   1. Rotator cuff tendinitis/impingement syndrome
   2. Calcific tendinitis
   3. Rotator cuff tear
   4. Bicipital tendinitis
   5. Acromioclavicular arthritis
II. **Glenohumeral Disorders**
   1. Inflammatory arthritis
   2. Osteoarthritis
   3. Osteonecrosis
   4. Cuff arthropathy
   5. Septic arthritis
   6. Glenoid labral tears
   7. Adhesive capsulitis
III. **Regional Disorders**
   1. Cervical radiculopathy
   2. Brachial neuritis
   3. Nerve entrapment syndromes
   4. Sternoclavicular arthritis
   5. Reflex sympathetic dystrophy
   6. Fibrositis
   7. Neoplasms
   8. Miscellaneous
      Gallbladder disease
      Splenic trauma
      Subphrenic abscess
      Myocardial infarction
      Thyroid disease
      Diabetes mellitus
      Renal osteodystrophy

pingement syndrome but can also accurately aspirate and inject this space. Knowledge of the route of the tendon of the long head of the biceps through the bicipital groove and onto the superior aspect of the glenoid helps in an understanding of bicipital tendinitis. Before attempting to diagnose and treat shoulder pain the reader should review in some detail one of the many sources describing the structural and functional relationships of the shoulder girdle.[2,3]

History. Most shoulder problems can be diagnosed by taking a detailed history. The association with trauma, the rapidity of onset, and the character and localization of the pain will frequently lead the clinician to the proper diagnosis. For instance, dislocations of the glenohumeral joint are usually associated with a force directed to the arm with the shoulder in an abducted and externally rotated position, while dislocations of the acromioclavicular joint are usually due to direct trauma to the shoulder. The gradual onset of pain in the subacromial region that is worse on forward elevation of the shoulder is characteristic of rotator cuff tendinitis with impingement. The presence of a snap or click on forward elevation frequently will indicate rotator cuff tear associated with impingement. The burning quality and characteristic radiation of pain are indicative of a neuropathic process.

Physical Examination. A detailed physical and neurologic examination with particular attention to the involved extremity is essential. Careful recording of range of motion should include both active and passive forward flexion, abduction, internal and external rotation

in a neutral position and at 90 degrees of abduction, and forward elevation. Forward elevation is defined as the arc between forward flexion and abduction and represents the most important arc in terms of placing the hand into a functional position. Abduction should be divided into that which occurs at the glenohumeral joint and that which occurs at the scapulothoracic joint. Careful recording of these values on serial examination will aid in judging response to therapy.

The localization of tenderness can help differentiate common entities such as glenoid labral tears, rotator cuff tendinitis, and bicipital tendinitis. While all three are associated with tenderness in the anterior aspect of the shoulder, the tenderness of rotator cuff tendinitis is generally subacromial and that of bicipital tendinitis migrates laterally and superiorly as the shoulder is abducted and externally rotated. Tenderness in the quadrilateral space or suprascapular notch is frequently associated with nerve entrapment syndromes. Neurologic examination should include sensory testing of the upper extremity with particular reference to the area innervated by the axillary nerve. All muscle systems should be graded and recorded, and the presence of atrophy or fasciculations noted.

Examination of the ipsilateral elbow, wrist, and hand is important not only in planning therapy but also in determining functional expectations.

Plain Radiographs. For most nontraumatic painful shoulder syndromes the use of an anteroposterior or glenohumeral view of the involved shoulder in internal and external rotation will suffice. In cases of trauma, a "trauma series," involving an anteroposterior view, scapular Y view, and axillary view, has become standard protocol. In cases of suspected acromioclavicular joint injury, an AP view of the shoulder with a weight held in the ipsilateral hand will frequently demonstrate subluxation at the AC joint.

Scintigraphy. ^{99}Technetium-MDP or gallium may be of diagnostic help in evaluating the painful shoulder. This benefit usually occurs when evaluating skeletal lesions about the shoulder joint. Bone scans are generally not helpful in the diagnosis of non-neoplastic or non-infectious shoulder disease.

Arthrography. Single-contrast arthrography, double-contrast arthrography, and double-contrast arthrotomography are valuable tools in evaluating problems of the rotator cuff, the glenoid labrum, the biceps tendon, and the shoulder capsule.[6-9] Figure 29–2 shows a normal double-contrast arthrogram of the shoulder. Rotator cuff tears can be demonstrated by both single- and double-contrast studies. The proponents of double-contrast arthrography feel that the extent of the tear, the preferred surgical approach, and the quality of the rotator cuff tissue are best determined by double-contrast studies.[7-9] Figure 29–3 demonstrates extravasation of contrast into the subacromial space from a rotator cuff tear. Arthrography can be misleading by underestimating the extent of a rotator cuff tear.

Tears of the glenoid labrum without shoulder dislocation are now being recognized as sources of anterior

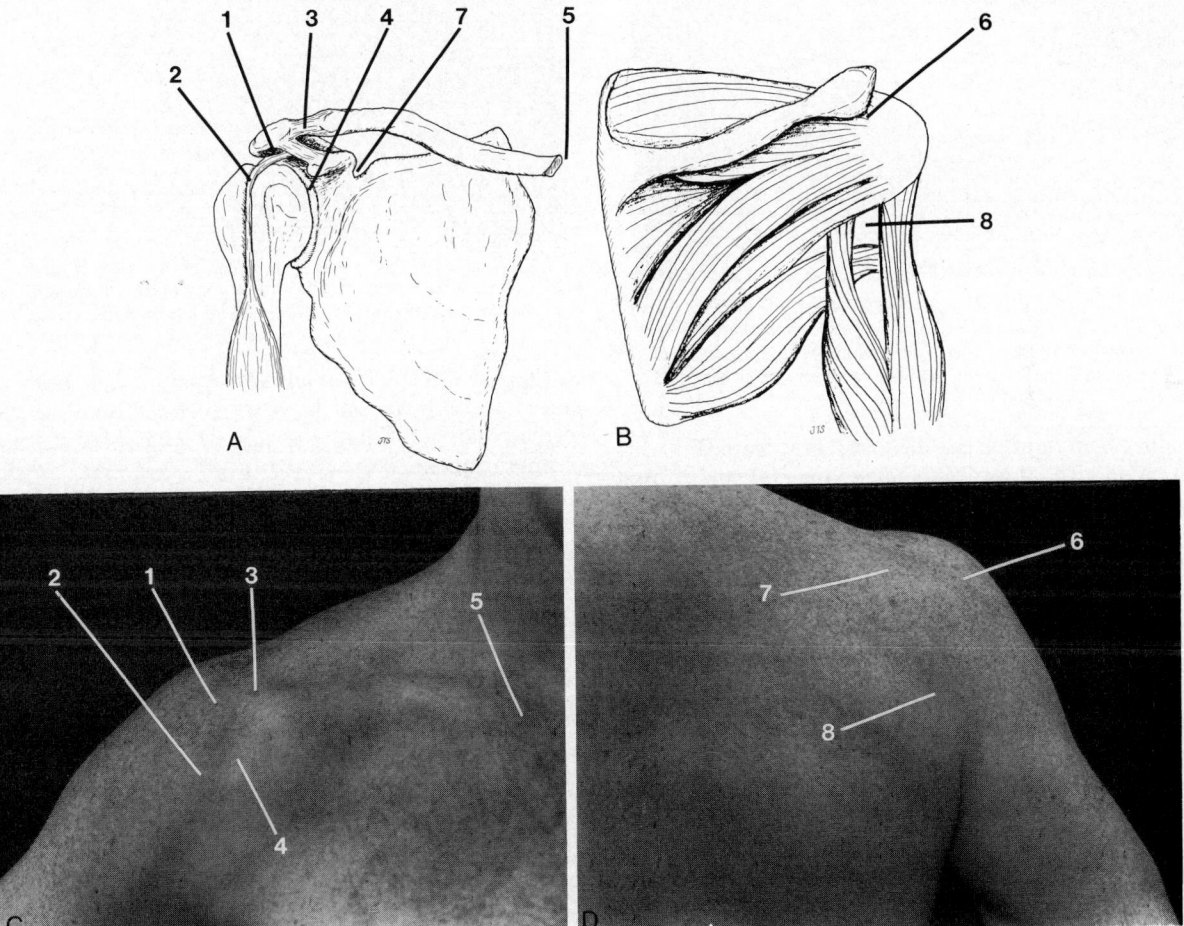

Figure 29–1. Musculoskeletal (*A* and *B*) and topographical (*C* and *D*) areas localizing pain and tenderness associated with specific shoulder problems. *1*, Subacromial space (rotator cuff tendinitis/impingement syndrome, calcific tendinitis, rotator cuff tear). *2*, Bicipital groove (bicipital tendinitis, biceps tendon subluxation and tear). *3*, Acromioclavicular joint. *4*, Anterior glenohumeral joint (glenohumeral arthritis, osteonecrosis, glenoid labral tears, adhesive capsulitis). *5*, Sternoclavicular joint. *6*, Posterior edge of acromion (rotator cuff tendinitis, calcific tendinitis, rotator cuff tear). *7*, Suprascapular notch (suprascapular nerve entrapment). *8*, Quadrilateral space (axillary nerve entrapment). These areas of pain and tenderness frequently overlap.

Figure 29–2. Normal double-contrast arthrogram showing the inferior edge of the rotator cuff (*RC*) as it courses through the subacromial space to the greater tuberosity; the tendon of the long head of the biceps (*BT*); and the articular cartilage of the humeral head (*AC*).

shoulder pain in athletes. Glenoid labral tears (Fig. 29–4) with or without associated glenohumeral subluxation can frequently be identified by double-contrast arthrotomography.[9] Shoulder arthrography can confirm a diagnosis of adhesive capsulitis by showing a contracted capsule with an obliterated axillary recess (Fig. 29–5).

Figure 29–3. Single-contrast arthrogram demonstrating a massive rotator cuff tear with extravasation of contrast into the subacromial space (see arrow).

Figure 29–4. A double-contrast arthrotomogram demonstrating a tear of the anteroinferior portion of the glenoid labrum (see arrow).

The use of subacromial bursography has been reported to be beneficial in visualizing the outer surface of the rotator cuff and the subacromial space in cases of impingement.[10,11]

Computed Tomography. CT has been shown to be helpful in evaluating the musculoskeletal system, but its use around the shoulder has been limited (see Chapter 40).

Electromyography and Nerve Conduction Velocity Studies. EMG and NCV studies can be helpful in differentiating shoulder pain from pain of neurogenic origin (see Chapter 47). They may also be beneficial in deter-

Figure 29–5. Double-contrast arthrogram in patient with calcific tendinitis (see arrow) and adhesive capsulitis. Note the contracted capsule with diminution of the synovial space and obliteration of the axillary recess.

mining the localization of neurogenic pain to a particular cervical root, the brachial plexus, or a peripheral nerve.[12,13]

Arthroscopy. Diagnostic arthroscopy and arthroscopic surgery have greatly aided in the diagnosis and treatment of knee injuries (see Chapter 41). Recent interest has focused on the use of arthroscopy for glenohumeral pain. It has been recommended for evaluating glenohumeral synovitis, articular cartilage damage, loose bodies and particularly for the diagnosis of labral tears. The added benefit of arthroscopy over arthrography remains to be shown. Arthroscopic surgery of the shoulder to date has been limited to removal of loose bodies and shaving of injuries of the glenoid labrum.

Injection. Injection of local anesthetics and corticosteroids is an extremely useful technique for both the diagnosis and treatment of shoulder pain (see Chapter 37). The physician must have a thorough knowledge of the anatomy of the shoulder girdle and a presumptive diagnosis in order to direct the injection properly. Injection of referred pain areas may be misleading. For example, in the patient with lateral arm pain due to deltoid bursal involvement from calcific tendinitis of the supraspinatus tendon, injection should be in the subacromial space and not the area of referred pain in the deltoid muscle.

It is often better to use a posterior subacromial approach when injecting a rotator cuff tendinitis in a patient with anterior impingement symptoms, as it is not only easier to enter the subacromial region posteriorly but also less traumatic to the contracted anterior structures.

The instillation of rapidly acting local anesthetics can be beneficial in determining the source of shoulder pain. Obliteration of pain, for instance, by injection of a local anesthetic along the bicipital groove can confirm a diagnosis of bicipital tendinitis. The use of local anesthetics is somewhat less helpful when injecting the subacromial space, owing to its extensive communications with the rest of the shoulder girdle, but relief of symptoms by such an injection can rule out pain from conditions such as cervical radiculopathy or an entrapment neuropathy.

PERIARTICULAR DISORDERS

Rotator Cuff Tendinitis/Impingement Syndrome. The majority of painful nontraumatic conditions about the shoulder joint are caused by tendinitis of the rotator cuff. E.A. Codman published his classic text reviewing the nature of these lesions and pointed out their importance in work-related disabilities.[1] Degenerative tendinitis has been labeled pericapsulitis, subacromial bursitis, subdeltoid bursitis, supraspinatus tendinitis, rotator cuff tear, and impingement syndrome. The variation in clinical description, method of treatment, and response to treatment perhaps is due to descriptions of the same condition at various points in time. Neer has clarified this condition by pointing out the various stages in which this disorder presents.[14] Though stratified into

three stages the process represents a continuum of inflammation, degeneration, and attrition of the rotator cuff by impingement on the anterior edge and undersurface of the anterior third of the acromion, the coracoacromial ligament, and occasionally the acromioclavicular joint.[15] The wear and attritional tears of the cuff occur in the supraspinatus tendon and may extend into the infraspinatus and the long head of the biceps.[16] The mechanical impingement of the rotator cuff may be influenced by variations in the shape and slope of the acromion.[16,17]

According to Neer,[14] the three stages of impingement are as follows: *Stage I, edema and hemorrhage,* usually occurs in active individuals younger than age 25 who engage in activities requiring excessive overhead arm usage. In stage I, treatment is conservative, and the patient generally responds to rest, nonsteroidal antiinflammatory agents, and occasional corticosteroid injection. *Stage II, fibrosis and tendinitis,* represents the biologic response of fibrosis and thickening due to repeated episodes of mechanical impingement. This stage is usually seen in active individuals between 25 and 40 years of age. They may respond to conservative treatment as in stage I but experience recurrent attacks. *Stage III, rotator cuff tears, biceps rupture, and bone changes,* rarely appears before the age of 40 years. Stage III represents the attritional wear of the supraspinatus tendon and occasionally the infraspinatus and long head of the biceps from repeated impingement. Patients with stage III disease present with varying weakness, crepitus, and supraspinatus atrophy, depending upon the extent of the tear and its chronicity.

The predominant feature of degenerative tendinitis is pain. The pain can be sudden and incapacitating or present as a dull ache. It can be focal and pinpointed as an area of tenderness along the anterior edge of the acromion (see Fig. 29–1). It also may present as a diffuse pain around the anterolateral or even posterior edge of the acromion or, at times, radiate to the subdeltoid bursa. This pain can be differentiated from other nontraumatic painful conditions about the shoulder by its position and response to treatment. For instance, the tenderness from bicipital tendinitis will follow the bicipital groove as the arm is externally rotated. Tenderness from a glenoid labral tear is generally beneath the coracoid and over the anterior edge of the glenoid. The impingement sign as elicited in Figure 29–6 is useful in the diagnosis of rotator cuff tendinitis. The patient with stage I and even stage II disease will frequently describe a catch as the arm is brought to an overhead position. They will frequently raise their arm by abduction and rotation to bypass the painful "spot." This observation underscores the Codman paradox, which states that the arm can be brought fully overhead from an anatomic position by either external rotation and abduction in the coronal plane or internal rotation and forward flexion in the sagittal plane.[1] In patients with focal tenderness of the supraspinatus the pain may disappear under the edge of the acromion as the arm is abducted (Dawbarn's sign).[3] Instillation of short-acting local anesthetics into

Figure 29–6. The "impingement sign" is elicited by forced forward elevation of the arm. Pain results as the greater tuberosity impinges on the acromion. The examiner's hand prevents scapular rotation. This maneuver may be positive in other periarticular disorders. (Reproduced with permission from Neer, C.S., II: Clin. Orthop. 173:70, 1983.)

the subacromial space can frequently obliterate the symptoms and confirm the diagnosis of degenerative tendinitis with impingement. It is important to remember that trigger point injection alone can be misleading and that injection of the subacromial space is necessary to assure validity of this diagnostic test.

Radiographs in the early stages of degenerative tendinitis with impingement are normal. As the disease progresses there may be some sclerosis, cyst formation, and eburnation of the anterior third of the acromion and the greater tuberosity. An anterior acromial traction spur may appear on the undersurface of the acromion lateral to the acromioclavicular joint and represent contracture of the coracoacromial ligament. The late radiographic findings include narrowing of the acromiohumeral gap, superior subluxation of the humeral head in relationship to the glenoid, and erosive changes of the anterior acromion.[18] Arthrography, as discussed earlier, can be helpful in diagnosing a full-thickness tear of the rotator cuff in association with stage III disease.

The choice of treatment, and frequently its result, is a function of the stage of the impingement. In stage I disease, in which there is little mechanical impingement, most patients will respond to rest. It is important not to immobilize the shoulder for any period of time, as contraction of the shoulder capsule and periarticular structures can produce an adhesive capsulitis. After a period of rest, a progressive program of stretching and strengthening exercises will generally restore the shoulder to normal function. Use of aspirin and other nonsteroidal antiinflammatory agents may shorten the symptomatic period. Modalities such as ultrasound, neuroprobe, and transcutaneous electrical nerve stimulation (TENS) are generally not necessary. Patients with stage I and stage II disease may have a dramatic response to

local injection of corticosteroids. In stage II disease, in which there is fibrosis and thickening anteriorly, it is frequently better to inject through a posterior approach. The author prefers a combination of 3 ml of 1 percent xylocaine, 3 ml of 0.5 percent bupivacaine and 20 mg of triamcinolone. This combines a short-acting anesthetic for diagnostic purposes, a longer-acting anesthetic for analgesic purposes, and a steroid preparation in a depot form. Neer has suggested that the patient with refractory stage II disease may respond to division of the coracoacromial ligament and bursectomy of the subacromial bursa. Division of the coracoacromial ligament alone has been performed under a local anesthetic.

Treatment of stage III disease depends upon the chronicity of the symptoms and the presence or absence of a rotator cuff tear. Neer recommends arthrography in those patients over 40 years of age who fail to respond to conservative treatment or experience sudden weakness of abduction and external rotation suggesting extension of a tear.[14] The surgical treatment of choice is an anterior acromioplasty.[15] Lateral acromionectomies and complete acromionectomies unnecessarily weaken the deltoid muscle.[18] Indications for anterior acromioplasty include (1) failure to respond to one year of conservative therapy and (2) chronic impingement and a rotator cuff tear shown on arthrography. The surgical technique and rehabilitation measures are beyond the scope of this discussion.[14,15]

Calcific Tendinitis. While most rotator cuff tendinitis probably represents one of the stages of mechanical impingement, there appears to be a subset of patients predisposed to inflammation in this area. These patients frequently have bilateral disease and give a history of other periarticular conditions such as trochanteric bursitis of the hip or symptoms of fibrositis. One particular subset within this group is made up of those individuals with calcific tendinitis.

Calcific tendinitis is a painful condition about the rotator cuff in association with deposition of calcium salts, primarily hydroxyapatite.[19,21,22] It is most common in patients over 30 years of age and shows a predilection for females.[19,20] While more common in the right shoulder, there is at least a 6 percent incidence of bilaterality.[19] Codman pointed out the localization of the calcification within the tendon of the supraspinatus.[1] He provided a detailed description of the symptoms and natural history of this condition. In describing the phases of pain, spasm, limitation of motion and atrophy, he pointed out the lack of correlation between symptoms and the size of the calcific deposit. According to Codman the natural history includes degeneration of the supraspinatus tendon, calcification, and eventual rupture into the subacromial bursa. During this latter phase, pain and decreased motion can lead to adhesive capsulitis (Fig. 29–5).

The pathogenesis of calcific tendinitis of the supraspinatus is recognized as a degenerative process with secondary calcification within the tendon fibers.[1,19,21,22] The localization of the calcium within the supraspinatus is most likely due to one of two reasons. Many of these patients have an early stage of impingement, and it is the supraspinatus that is compressed by the anterior portion of the acromion.[14,15] This longstanding impingement may lead to local degeneration of the tendon fibers. In patients without impingement the localization of the calcium within the supraspinatus may be related to the blood supply of the rotator cuff, which normally comes from an anastomatic network of vessels from either the greater tuberosity or the bellies of the short rotator muscles.[21] The watershed of these sources is just medial to the tendinous attachment of the supraspinatus.[23] Rathburn and MacNab referred to this watershed as the "critical zone" and pointed out that during adduction this area was rendered ischemic.[24]

The stimulation for calcification in calcific tendinitis has been the focus of considerable study.[4,21,22,25] Steinbrocker postulated that the process begins with necrosis and fraying of the tendon fibers, with secondary formation of a fibrinoid mass surrounded by leukocytes. This mass then serves as a template for calcification.[25] Others have suggested that the process of degeneration of the tendon causes formation of small particles consisting primarily of calcium salts.[4] The hyperemia associated with the acute episode would cause coalescence of the calcium with formation of a liquified calcium mass. As the increased vascularity subsides, this calcified mass would return to its "dry state."

It is also possible that the hypervascularity may, in fact, "wash out" an inhibitor substance and allow calcification to occur on the denuded fibers of the frayed tendon. It would be attractive to consider proteoglycans in this inhibitory role, as they are ubiquitous in tendons and articular cartilage, both of which do not calcify in the normal state.

Uhthoff has proposed that the pathogenesis of this process is not associated inflammation or scarring but suggests that the primary stimulus is hypoxia, which results in transformation of portions of the tendon into fibrocartilage.[21] The chondrocytes then would mediate calcification in a way similar to that occurring in the calcifying zone of the epiphyseal plate. In a subsequent study it was pointed out that the ultrastructure of calcifying tendinitis failed to demonstrate the arrangement or cell types seen in the epiphyseal plate.[22] The calcification occurred in extracellular matrix vesicles located in areas that had undergone fibrocartilagenous transformation. The authors pointed out the similarity to extracellular vesicles noted in other normal and pathologic conditions.[22] After calcification, the foci became surrounded by mononuclear and multinucleated cells, with phagocytized material within the cytoplasm.[21] Vascular invasion occurred as part of the reparative process. By restoring normal perfusion and oxygen tension to the tissue, the calcium could then be resorbed and the tendon returned to its normal state.[21]

Treatment of calcific tendinitis depends upon the clinical presentation and the presence of associated impingement. These patients can present with an acute inflammatory reaction that may resemble gout. They seem to be the most acutely painful patients with rotator cuff

tendinitis. The acute inflammation can be treated with local corticosteroid injection or the use of nonsteroidal agents or both. On occasion the use of ultrasound may be of some benefit. If there is associated impingement, treatment depends upon the stage of presentation, as discussed earlier. The radiographic appearance of the calcification can direct and perhaps predict the response to therapy. In the resorptive phase, the deposits appear floccular, suggesting that the process is in the phase of repair and that a conservative program is indicated. Those patients with discrete calcification and perhaps associated adhesive capsulitis (Fig. 29–5) may be at a stable phase at which the calcium produces a mechanical block and is unlikely to be resorbed. In patients who have failed to respond to conservative means, excision of the calcium salts and decompression of associated impingement is indicated.

Rotator Cuff Tear. Spontaneous tear of the rotator cuff in an otherwise normal individual is rare.[14] It can occur in patients with rheumatoid arthritis or lupus as part of the pathologic process with invasion from underlying pannus. Metabolic conditions such as renal osteodystrophy or agents such as corticosteroids are occasionally associated with spontaneous cuff tears.

Most patients will report a traumatic episode such as falling upon an outstretched arm of lifting a heavy object. The usual presenting symptoms are pain and weakness of abduction and external rotation. There may be associated crepitus and even a palpable defect. Longstanding tears are generally associated with atrophy of the supraspinatus and infraspinatus muscles.

It may be difficult to differentiate a partial thickness cuff tear from a painful tendinitis. Plain radiographs are helpful only during a later stage of the process when there may be narrowing of the acromiohumeral gap, proximal subluxation of the humeral head, and even erosion on the undersurface of the acromion.[27] Arthrography, as reported earlier, is helpful in diagnosing an acute tear but frequently underestimates its size.

Because of the overlap in diagnosis of complete tears and incomplete lesions, it is difficult to develop a rational form of treatment. DePalma reports that 90 percent of patients with rotator cuff tears respond to conservative measures such as rest, analgesics, anti-inflammatory agents, and physiotherapy.[28]

During the acute phase of pain the arm may be supported in a sling, but early restoration of motion is important to prevent adhesive capsulitis. Instillation of corticosteroids into the subacromial bursa may provide dramatic relief of symptoms.

Consideration of surgical treatment depends upon the patient's symptoms, the functional demand, and the etiology of the tear. Most acute tears represent extension of a tear associated with chronic impingement.[14] Patients in this group who fail to respond to conservative means should be treated by an anterior acromioplasty with rotator cuff repair.

In elderly patients whose pain and weakness do not create a functional problem, a conservative program is preferable. Wolfgang pointed out that surgical results were less satisfactory with advancing patient age.[29] Earnshaw reviewed 37 patients who had undergone rotator cuff repair and found an overall 65 percent with good results.[30] Patients in the fourth and fifth decades of life generally did well, while only 60 percent of patients in the sixth and seventh decades had a good result. In their study, the mechanism of injury, the extent of the tear, and the timing of repair had no influence on the outcome. The authors pointed out that most shoulders showed radiographic progression of proximal subluxation despite surgical repair. In this small series, good functional results were reported in two patients with irreparable tears and in some patients with postoperative arthrograms showing leakage of contrast. They concluded that relief of impingement and debridement of the edge of the tear were important determinants in the relief of symptoms.[30]

The surgical approach, technique of repair, and postoperative management are beyond the scope of this discussion and are well covered in other sources.[2,3,28,30,31]

Bicipital Tendinitis and Rupture. Bicipital tendinitis, subluxation of the biceps tendon within the bicipital groove, and rupture of the long head of the biceps are generally associated with anterior shoulder pain.

The long head of the biceps is an intracapsular and extrasynovial structure. It passes through the bicipital groove and over the head of the humerus and inserts on the superior rim of the glenoid (see Fig. 29–1A).[32] The biceps tendon aids in flexion of the forearm, supination of the pronated forearm if the elbow is flexed, and forward elevation of the shoulder.[3] As it crosses the humeral head, the biceps tendon is fixed within the bicipital groove. Meyer described a bony ridge on the lesser tuberosity and suggested this as a source of tendon wear and eventual rupture.[33] Shallowness of this groove has been reported as a cause of subluxation and dislocation of the bicipital tendon.[34]

Crenshaw and Kilgore reported that the early phases of bicipital tendinitis were associated with hypervascularity, edema of the tendon, and tenosynovitis.[35] Persistence of this process leads to adhesions between the tendon and its sheath, with impairment of the normal gliding mechanism in the groove. Stretching of these adhesions may be associated with chronic bicipital tendinitis.[34] The diagnosis of bicipital tendinitis is based upon the localization of tenderness (see Fig. 29–1). It is often confused with impingement symptoms and, in fact, is frequently seen in association with an impingement syndrome.[14] Isolated bicipital tendinitis can be differentiated by the fact that the tender area will migrate with the bicipital groove as the arm is abducted and externally rotated. There are many eponyms associated with tests to identify bicipital tendinitis.[3] Yergason's supination sign refers to pain in the bicipital groove when the examiner resists supination of the pronated forearm with the elbow at 90 degrees. Ludington's sign refers to pain in the bicipital groove when the patient interlocks his fingers on top of the head and actively abducts the arms.

Treatment is generally conservative and consists of rest, analgesics, nonsteroidal agents, and local injection of corticosteroids. The use of ultrasound and neuroprobe is more beneficial in this condition than in isolated rotator cuff tendinitis.

Patients with refractory bicipital tendinitis and recurrent symptoms of subluxation are treated by opening the bicipital groove and resecting the proximal portion of the tendon with either tenodesis of the distal portion into the groove or transfer to the coracoid process. The proponents of tenodesis believe that this prevents proximal migration of the humeral head, while those who advocate transfer to the coracoid feel that it maintains biceps power.

Rupture of the long head of the biceps is easily diagnosed by the appearance of the contracted belly of the biceps muscle ("Popeye sign"). The patient will frequently relate a snap and acute pain in association with lifting an object. In older patients, in whom rupture is due to attrition, presentation is frequently spontaneous and is associated with few or no symptoms. Acute ruptures in young active individuals are best treated surgically with either tenodesis of the distal stump into the bicipital groove or transfer to the coracoid. Patients with longstanding symptoms of impingement and acute biceps tendon rupture are treated with anterior acromioplasty and tenodesis of the distal stump into the bicipital groove. In older patients without symptoms of impingement, a conservative program is preferable, as these patients are generally asymptomatic and have sufficient strength and the contracted belly of the biceps muscle serves to impress their grandchildren.

Acromioclavicular Arthritis. The majority of painful conditions about the acromioclavicular joint are the result of trauma with resultant acromioclavicular joint instability, meniscal tears, and secondary degenerative change.[36] Most patients present with a history of direct trauma to the shoulder girdle. The pain may be generalized, but tenderness and, at times, crepitus can be palpated directly over the acromioclavicular joint. The pain is increased by abduction of the arm and particularly by adducting the arm across the chest and compressing the joint.[2]

Plain radiographs may be normal unless there is a true dislocation or degenerative change. It is important to differentiate the traction spur at the insertion of the coracoacromial ligament from an osteophyte associated with degenerative change of the joint. An anteroposterior radiograph with the patient holding a weight in the ipsilateral hand may demonstrate joint instability in acute cases.

Acute injuries are treated by rest, strapping, or surgical repair, depending upon the degree of instability and the functional demand of the patient. Acute injuries without subluxation (grade I) or partial subluxation (grade II) are best treated by conservative means. Complete dislocations (grade III) are treated by early mobilization, strapping to reduce the dislocation, or surgical repair according to the patient's functional demand and the surgeon's preference.[36-38]

Patients with degenerative change in the acromioclavicular joint and symptoms that cannot be controlled by conservative means are best treated by debridement of the joint and resection of the distal clavicle.[37,39] At no time should this joint be surgically fused.

GLENOHUMERAL DISORDERS

The various arthritides that affect the shoulder joint are discussed in detail in other chapters. They are presented here in order to discuss aspects that are unique to the glenohumeral joint.

The usual presentation of intra-articular disorders is pain with motion. The pain is generalized throughout the shoulder girdle and at times referred to the neck, back, and upper arm. The usual response to pain is to decrease glenohumeral motion and to substitute for it with increased scapulothoracic mobility. Patients with adequate elbow and scapulothoracic motion require little glenohumeral motion for activities of daily living; in fact, patients with glenohumeral arthrodesis can achieve adequate function.[40,41] The secondary response to pain, therefore, is diminution of motion and secondary soft tissue contractures with muscle atrophy. With increasing weakness and involvement of adjacent joints, the pain, limitation of motion, and weakness cause a substantial functional deficit.

Inflammatory Arthritis. While the most common inflammatory arthritis involving the shoulder joint is rheumatoid arthritis, other systemic disorders such as systemic lupus erythematosus, psoriatic arthritis, ankylosing spondylitis, Reiter's syndrome, and scleroderma may cause glenohumeral arthritis. The pathogenesis of the joint involvement in these conditions is discussed in detail in other chapters.

All patients with significant involvement present with pain. The limitation of motion is either secondary to splinting of the joint with secondary soft tissue contractures or primary soft tissue involvement with scarring or rupture. Plain radiographs will confirm glenohumeral involvement (Fig. 29–7A). There is narrowing of the glenohumeral joint space, with erosion and cyst formation without significant sclerosis or osteophytes. As the disease progresses, superior and posterior erosion of the glenoid with proximal subluxation of the humeral head may occur. Eventually, there may be secondary degenerative changes and even osteonecrosis of the humeral head.

Treatment is initially conservative and directed towards control of pain, inducing a systemic remission (see Chapter 63) and maintaining joint motion by physical therapy. The use of intra-articular corticosteroids may be beneficial in controlling local synovitis. In rheumatoid arthritis, the involvement of periarticular structures with subacromial bursitis and rupture of the rotator cuff magnifies the functional deficit.

Once the synovial cartilage interactions produce significant symptoms and radiographic changes that cannot be controlled by conventional therapy, glenohumeral resurfacing should be considered. The treatment of choice is an unconstrained shoulder arthroplasty of the type reported in detail in Chapter 115.[42,43] Total shoulder arthroplasty is best performed in patients with rheumatoid arthritis before end-stage bony erosion and soft tissue contractions have occurred.[44]

Acute inflammatory arthritis of the glenohumeral joint may also occur in association with gout, pseudogout, hydroxyapatite deposition of renal osteodystrophy, and recurrent hemophilic hemarthrosis.

Osteoarthritis. Osteoarthritis of the glenohumeral joint is less common than in the hip, its counterpart in the lower extremity. This is a result of both the nonweight-bearing characteristics of the shoulder joint and the distribution of forces throughout the shoulder girdle.

Figure 29–7. Plain radiographs demonstrating (*A*) rheumatoid arthritis with loss of joint space, cyst formation, glenohumeral erosion, and early proximal subluxation of the humerus indicating a rotator cuff tear. *B*, Osteoarthritis with narrowing of the glenohumeral joint space, sclerosis, and osteophyte formation. Note the preservation of the subacromial space, suggesting an intact rotator cuff.

Osteoarthritis is divided into those conditions associated with high unit loading of articular cartilage and those in which there is an intrinsic abnormality within the cartilage that causes abnormal wear at normal loads. Since the shoulder is normally a non-weight-bearing joint and less susceptible to repeated high loading, the presence of osteoarthritis of the glenohumeral joint should alert the physician to consider other associated factors. Has the patient engaged in unusual activities such as boxing, heavy construction, or chronic use of a pneumatic hammer? Is there some disorder such as epiphyseal dysplasia that has created joint incongruity with high unit loading of the articular cartilage? Is this a neuropathic process caused by diabetes, syringomyelia or leprosy? Is there associated hemachromatosis, hemophilia, or gout that may have altered the ability of articular cartilage to withstand normal loading? Is unrecognized chronic dislocation responsible?

Pain is the usual presentation, but it is generally not as acute or associated with the spasm seen in inflammatory conditions. Plain radiographs show narrowing of the glenohumeral joint, osteophyte formation, sclerosis, and some cyst formation (Fig. 29–7B). As the rotator cuff is generally intact there is less bony erosion of the glenoid and proximal subluxation of the humerus.

Patients with osteoarthritis of the glenohumeral joint frequently do well by functional adjustment and conservative therapy. Analgesics and nonsteroidal agents may provide symptomatic relief. The use of corticosteroid injections is less beneficial unless there is evidence of synovitis. Those patients with severe involvement who fail to respond are best treated by shoulder arthroplasty[42-44] (see Chapter 116).

Osteonecrosis. Osteonecrosis of the shoulder refers to necrosis of the humeral head seen in association with a variety of conditions. Symptoms are due to synovitis and joint incongruity secondary to resorption, repair, and remodeling. The pathogenesis and various etiologies are discussed in Chapter 107.

The most common cause of osteonecrosis of the shoulder is avascularity due to fractures through the anatomic neck of the humerus.[45] Fracture through this area disrupts the intramedullary and capsular blood supplies to the humeral head. Another common cause of osteonecrosis of the shoulder is steroid therapy in conjunction with organ transplantation, systemic lupus erythematosus, or asthma.

The mechanism by which steroids are associated with osteonecrosis is unknown. There appears to be a host susceptibility, which may be genetically predetermined. Patients will generally develop osteonecrosis shortly following steroid use, although symptoms may not present for a considerable period. At least in renal transplant patients, the association of osteonecrosis is independent of steroid dosage. The proposed pathogenesis of steroid-induced osteonecrosis includes increased free fatty acids with obliteration of intramedullary blood supply and steroid-induced vasculitis. This may elevate the intramedullary pressures within the humeral head and cause bone ischemia and death.[46] Other conditions associated with osteonecrosis of the humeral head include systemic lupus erythematosus, hemoglobinopathies, pancreatitis, and hyperbarism.

Early diagnosis is difficult, as there is frequently a considerable delay until symptoms are present. Bone scans may be helpful in early cases before radiographic changes are present. Plain radiographs demonstrate progressive phases of necrosis and repair and are discussed in detail in Chapter 107. In the early stages, the films may be normal or show either osteopenia or bony sclerosis. A crescent sign representing subchondral fracture or demarcation of the necrotic segment will appear during the reparative process. Patients who fail to remodel will show collapse of the humeral head with secondary degenerative changes.

There is often a considerable discrepancy between symptoms and radiographic involvement. Patients with extensive bony changes may be asymptomatic. Treatment should be directed by the patient's symptoms rather than the radiographs and is similar to that for osteoarthritis. Patients with severe symptoms that cannot be controlled by conservative means are best treated with an unconstrained shoulder arthroplasty or hemiarthroplasty.[42]

Cuff Arthropathy. Neer and colleagues have reported an unusual condition in which untreated massive tears of the rotator cuff with proximal migration of the humeral head are associated with erosion of the humeral surface.[17] The erosion of the humeral head is different from that seen in other arthritides and is presumed to be due to a combination of mechanical factors and nutritional factors. As the humeral head migrates superiorly, it is no longer contained and its cartilage cannot be nourished by the synovial fluid.

Patients with cuff tear arthropathies present a difficult therapeutic problem, as the bony erosion and disruption of the cuff jeopardizes the functional result from an unconstrained prosthesis.[44] In such patients a constrained total shoulder arthroplasty may be indicated.[47,48]

Septic Arthritis. Septic arthritis can masquerade as any of the conditions listed under periarticular or glenohumeral disorders. Sepsis must be included in any differential diagnosis of shoulder pain, as early recognition and prompt treatment are necessary to achieve a good functional result. The diagnosis is confirmed by joint aspiration with synovianalysis and culture. Cultures should include aerobic, anaerobic, mycobacterial, and fungal studies. Septic arthritis is extensively covered in Chapters 96, 97, and 98.

Glenoid Labral Tears. The increasing popularity of throwing sports and racket sports in 25- to 60-year-old individuals has led to the recognition of tears of the glenoid labrum as a cause of anterior shoulder pain (see Fig. 29–1).

This diagnosis is easily confused with rotator cuff tendinitis or bicipital tendinitis and can best be confirmed by double-contrast arthrotomography[9] or arthroscopy (see Fig. 29–4). Glenoid labral tears may be seen in association with anterior or even posterior instability. Surgical treatment is directed toward excision or repair of the torn labral portion and correction of any joint instability.

Adhesive Capsulitis. Adhesive capsulitis, or "frozen shoulder," is a condition characterized by limitation of motion of the shoulder joint with pain at the extremes of motion. It was first described by Putnam in 1882[49] and later by Codman.[1] The initial presentation is pain, which is generalized and referred to the upper arm, the back, and the neck. As the pain increases, loss of joint motion ensues. The process is generally self-limiting and in most cases resolves spontaneously within 10 months unless there is an underlying problem.

Adhesive capsulitis is slightly more common in females than in males.[50] There is usually an underlying condition producing pain and restricted motion of the glenohumeral joint. Adhesive capsulitis may be seen as an end result of rotator cuff tendinitis, calcific tendinitis (see Fig. 29–5), bicipital tendinitis, and glenohumeral arthritis.[51,52] It is also seen in a variety of conditions, including apical lung tumors, pulmonary tuberculosis, cervical radiculopathy, and postmyocardial infarction.[51-54]

DePalma reported that any condition that hindered scapulohumeral motion caused muscular inactivity and predisposed the patient to adhesive capsulitis.[52] Neviaser[55] found capsular adhesions to the underlying humeral head upon surgical exploration for adhesive capsulitis.

It is unclear whether the contracture of the shoulder capsule is a passive process related to lack of motion or an active process associated with capsular inflammation. Bulgen and colleagues reported an association between adhesive capsulitis and HLA-B27 antigen positivity.[56] He also reported decreased IgA levels in patients with the condition.[57] Lundberg and Neviaser failed to demonstrate synovitis or capsular inflammation when surgically exploring patients with adhesive capsulitis.[55,58]

Treatment of adhesive capsulitis is directed towards pain relief, restoration of function, and correction of the underlying cause. Many patients will have associated depression or emotional lability either as an underlying problem or secondary to their pain and functional limitation. The physician must direct a long-term therapy program and reassure the patient that this condition is usually self-limiting. As symptoms may last for a year, daily visits to the physical therapist become impractical and a home program should be outlined.

In patients with restriction of motion that prevents activities of daily living, a closed manipulation is indicated. This is best achieved at the time of arthrography (to confirm the diagnosis) and entails passive manipulation after the joint is inflated with a local anesthetic. The combination of inflating the joint and passive manipulation may free some adhesions and improve joint motion. On occasion, a general anesthetic is indicated for closed manipulation. Surgical intervention for adhesive capsulitis should be limited to treatment of an underlying problem such as calcific tendinitis or an impingement syndrome.

REGIONAL DISORDERS

Because the shoulder girdle connects the thorax with the upper extremity and the major neurovascular structures pass in close proximity to the joint, shoulder pain is a hallmark of many nonarticular conditions.

Cervical Radiculopathy. Cervical neck pain, with or without radiculopathy, may be associated with shoulder pain. When cervical radiculopathy presents as shoulder pain, it is frequently due to involvement of the upper cervical roots. It can be differentiated from shoulder pain on the basis of history, physical examination, electromyographs, cervical radiographs, and myelography when indicated. Since conditions causing cervical neck pain and those causing shoulder pain, such as calcific tendinitis and cervical radiculopathy, may co-exist, it is often difficult to distinguish which lesion is causing the symptoms. These conditions can often be distinguished by injection of local anesthetics to block certain components of the pain.

As cervical neck pain is reviewed extensively in Chapter 28 its diagnosis and treatment will not be discussed here.

Brachial Neuritis. In the 1940s, Spillane,[59] and Parsonage and Turner[60,61] described a painful condition of the shoulder associated with limitation of motion. As the pain subsided and motion improved, muscle weakness and atrophy became apparent.[62] The deltoid, supraspinatus, infraspinatus, biceps, and triceps are the most frequently involved muscles,[62] although diaphragmatic paralysis has also been reported.[61] The etiology remains unclear, but the clustering of cases suggests a viral or postviral syndrome.[60,61] Occasionally an associated influenza-like syndrome or previous vaccination has been reported.[62]

The prognosis for recovery is excellent, although full recovery may take two to three years. Tsiaris reported 80 percent recovery within two years and more than 90 percent by the end of three years.[63]

Nerve Entrapment Syndromes. Entrapment of peripheral nerves as either a primary or a secondary process may present with pain about the shoulder girdle. The clinical picture and neurophysiology of nerve entrapment syndromes are covered in Chapter 110 and in other detailed sources.[64-67] Two entrapment neuropathies, namely, axillary nerve entrapment and suprascapular nerve entrapment, are frequently overlooked and bear further discussion.

The axillary nerve arises from the posterior cord of the brachial plexus and exits posteriorly through the quadrilateral space. This space is bordered superiorly by the teres major, inferiorly by the teres minor, medially by the long head of the triceps, and laterally by the humeral shaft and lateral triceps heads. After sending a sensory branch to the upper lateral cutaneous surface and a motor branch to the teres minor, the nerve courses anteriorly to innervate the deltoid.[32]

Entrapment of the axillary nerve as it exits through the quadrilateral space is an infrequent cause of pain, weakness, and atrophy about the shoulder girdle. It is most commonly seen in the dominant shoulder of young athletic individuals such as pitchers, tennis players, and swimmers who function with excessive overhead activity. The pain may occur throughout the shoulder girdle and radiate down the arm in a nondermatomal pattern. It may be elicited by abduction and external rotation or by palpation of the quadrilateral space (see Fig. 29–1).

This condition represents entrapment of the axillary nerve as it leaves the posterior cord, penetrates the quadrilateral space, and moves anteriorly to innervate the deltoid. On surgical exploration the nerve has been found to be tethered upon the aponeurosis of the hypertrophied muscle or by fibrous bands encroaching upon the quadrilateral space.[68]

The suprascapular nerve is a branch of the upper trunk of the brachial plexus formed by the 5th and 6th cervical nerves. It passes obliquely beneath the trapezius and crosses the scapula through the suprascapular notch.[32] The suprascapular nerve has no cutaneous sensory branches, but supplies motor branches to the supraspinatus and infraspinatus muscles.

The suprascapular nerve entrapment syndrome is the result of compression and tethering of the nerve as it passes through the suprascapular notch. Rengachary and colleagues described variations in the size and shape of the fossa and the suprascapular ligament, which forms its superior border. The authors demonstrated variations in the fossa from a complete bony foramen to a smooth depression on the upper border of the scapula.[69] Patients with a true bony foramen or a deep notch should be more susceptible to the development of entrapment in this area.

The primary symptom is pain, which generally is described as a deep ache felt over the upper border and body of the scapula. The pain is well localized and does not radiate down the arm. Any activity that brings the scapula forward, such as reaching across the chest, may aggravate the pain.[70] Palpation of the suprascapular notch may elicit local tenderness (see Fig. 29–1).

Since the suprascapular nerve has no cutaneous innervation, there is no associated numbness, tingling, or paresthesias. With time, the patients will develop atrophy and weakness of the supraspinatus and infraspinatus muscles. This syndrome must be differentiated from rotator cuff tendinitis, which also could be associated with a similar pattern of pain and muscle atrophy.[71] It also must be differentiated from brachial neuritis and a cervical radiculopathy involving the 5th and 6th roots.[72] Selective EMG determinations of the supraspinatus and infraspinatus may reveal motor atrophy. Instillation of local anesthetics into the supraspinous notch may relieve the symptoms.

As with axillary nerve entrapment, this syndrome is often associated with athletic young individuals with excessive overhead activity. It has also been reported in relationship to trauma.[73,74] Once confirmed, the treatment of choice is surgical decompression of the suprascapular notch. If the entrapment is in association with

trauma, a substantial period of time should be given to rule out a neuropraxia, which is likely to resolve.

Sternoclavicular Arthritis. Occasionally, traumatic and nontraumatic conditions can cause pain about the sternoclavicular joint (see Fig. 29–1). The most common problem is ligamentous injury and painful subluxation or dislocation. This can be diagnosed by palpable instability and crepitus over the sternoclavicular joint. Sternoclavicular views may radiographically demonstrate dislocation.[37]

Inflammatory arthritis of the sternoclavicular joint has been seen in association with rheumatoid arthritis, ankylosing spondylitis, and septic arthritis. Two other conditions involving the sternoclavicular joint are Tietze's syndrome, a painful nonsuppurative swelling of the joint and adjacent sternochondral junctions, and Friedrich's disease, a painful osteonecrosis of the sternal end of the clavicle.[3]

Reflex Sympathetic Dystrophy. Since its original description by Weir Mitchell in 1864,[75] reflex sympathetic dystrophy (RSD) has remained a poorly understood and frequently overlooked condition. Its etiology is unknown but may be related to sympathetic overflow or short circuiting of impulses through the sympathetic system. Any clinician dealing with painful disorders must be familiar with the diagnosis and treatment of this condition. Bonica has provided an excellent review, which covers the clinical presentation, the various stages of the disease, and the importance of early intervention to ensure a successful outcome.[76]

Reflex sympathetic dystrophy has been confusingly called causalgia, shoulder-hand syndrome, and Sudeck's atrophy. It is generally associated with minor trauma and is to be differentiated from causalgia that involves trauma to major nerve trunks.[76] RSD is divided into three phases, which are important in the determination of the stage of involvement and the mode of treatment.[77] Phase one is characterized by sympathetic overflow with diffuse swelling, pain, increased vascularity, and radiographic evidence of demineralization. If left untreated for 3 to 6 months, this may progress to phase two, which is characterized by atrophy. The extremity may now be cold and shiny with atrophy of the skin and muscles. Phase three refers to progression of the trophic changes, with irreversible flexion contractures and a pale, cold, painful extremity. It has been speculated that phase one is related to a peripheral short circuiting of nerve impulses, phase two represents short circuiting through the internuncial pool in the spinal cord, and phase three is controlled by higher thalamic centers.[76,77]

Steinbocker reported that as long as there is evidence of vasomotor activity with swelling and hyperemia, there remains a chance for recovery.[78] Once the trophic phase two or three is established, the prognosis for recovery is poor. Prompt recognition of the syndrome is important, as early intervention to control pain is mandatory. Careful supervision and reassurance are critical, as many of these patients are emotionally labile, as a result of either their pain or an underlying problem. The syndrome may be remarkably reversed by a sympathetic block. Patients who receive transient relief from sympathetic blockade may be helped by surgical sympathectomy.

Fibrositis. Fibrositis and other diffuse musculoskeletal syndromes are characterized by multiple trigger points about the shoulder girdle. This subject is discussed in Chapter 32.

Neoplasms. Primary and metastatic neoplasms may cause shoulder pain by direct invasion of the musculoskeletal system or by compression with referred pain.[2,66] Primary tumors are more likely to occur in younger individuals. The more common lesions have a typical distribution, such as the predilection of a chondroblastoma for the proximal humeral epiphysis or of an osteogenic sarcoma for the metaphysis.[79] The differential diagnosis of spontaneous onset of shoulder pain in older individuals should include metastatic lesions and myeloma. Neoplasms are best identified by plain radiographs, ^{99}Tc-MDP scintigraphy, and computed tomography.

The Pancoast or apical lung tumor may present as shoulder pain owing to invasion of the brachial plexus.[52,80] With invasion of the cervical sympathetic chain the patient may also develop Horner's syndrome.

Miscellaneous. A variety of other conditions may present as shoulder pain and should be mentioned in this discussion. Acute abdominal disorders such as gallbladder disease, splenic injuries, and subphrenic abscess can refer pain to the shoulder. The pain of acute angina and myocardial infarction may be referred to the left shoulder and down the inner aspect of the left arm. Metabolic disorders such as hypo- and hyperthyroidism,[81] diabetes mellitus,[82] and secondary hyperparathyroidism in association with renal osteodystrophy are infrequently associated with pain about the shoulder girdle.

References

1. Codman, E.A.: The Shoulder-Rupture of the Supraspinatus Tendon and Other Lesions in or about the Subacromial Bursa. Boston, Thomas Todd Company, Printer, 1934.
2. Bateman, J.E.: The Shoulder and Neck. 2nd ed. Philadelphia, W. B. Saunders Company, 1978.
3. Post, M.: The Shoulder—Surgical and Nonsurgical Management. Philadelphia, Lea & Febiger, 1978.
4. Cailliet, R.: Shoulder Pain. 2nd ed. Philadelphia, F. A. Davis Company, 1981.
5. Greep, J.M., Lemmens, H.A.J., Roos, D.B., and Urschel, H.C.: Pain in Shoulder and Arm. An Integrated View. The Hague, Martinus Nijhoff, 1979.
6. Goldman, A.B.: Shoulder Arthrography. Boston, Little, Brown & Company, 1982.
7. Goldman, A.B., and Ghelman, B.: The double contrast shoulder arthrogram. A review of 158 studies. Radiology 127:655, 1978.
8. Mink, J., and Harris, E.: Double contrast shoulder arthrography: Its use in evaluation of rotator cuff tears. Ortho. Trans. 7:71, 1983.
9. Braunstein, E.M., and O'Connor, G.: Double-contrast arthrotomography of the shoulder. J. Bone Joint Surg. 64A:192, 1982.
10. Strizak, A.M., Danzig, L., Jackson, D.W., Greenway, D., Resnick, D., and Staple, T.: Subacromial bursography. J. Bone Joint Surg. 64A:196, 1982.
11. Lie, S.: Subacromial bursography. Radiology 144:626, 1982.
12. Nakano, K.K.: Neurology of Musculoskeletal and Rheumatic Disorders. Boston, Houghton Mifflin, 1979.
13. Leffert, R.D.: Brachial plexus injuries. N. Engl. J. Med. 291:1059, 1974.
14. Neer, C.S., II: Impingement lesions. Clin. Orthop. 173:70, 1983.
15. Neer, C.S., II: Anterior acromioplasty for the chronic impingement syndrome in the shoulder. A preliminary report. J. Bone Joint Surg. 54A:41, 1972.
16. Neer, C.S., II, Bigliani, L.U., and Hawkins, R.J.: Rupture of the long head of the biceps related to subacromial impingment. Ortho. Trans. 1:111, 1977.
17. Neer, C.S., II, Craig, E.V., Fukada, H., and Mendoza, F.X.: Cuff tear arthropathy. Exhibit at the annual meeting of the American Academy of Orthopedic Surgeons. Jan., 1982.
18. Neer, C.S., II, and Marberry, T.A.: On the disadvantages of radical acromionectomy. J. Bone Joint Surg. 63A:416, 1981.
19. McKendry, R.J.R., Uhthoff, H.K., Sarkar, K., and Hyslop, P.: Calcifying tendinitis of the shoulder: Prognostic value of clinical, histologic, and radiographic features in 57 surgically treated cases. J. Rheumatol. 9:75, 1982.
20. Vebostad, A.: Calcific tendinitis in the shoulder region. A review of 43 operated shoulders. Acta. Orthop. Scan. 46:205, 1975.
21. Uhthoff, H.K., Sarkar, K., and Maynard, J.A.: Calcifying tendinitis, a new concept of its pathogenesis. Clin. Orthop. 118:164, 1976.
22. Sarkar, K., and Uhthoff, H.K.: Ultrastructural localization of calcium in calcifying tendinitis. Arch. Pathol. Lab. Med. 102:266, 1978.
23. Moseley, H.F., and Goldie, I.: The arterial pattern of the rotator cuff of the shoulder. J. Bone Joint Surg. 45B:780, 1963.
24. Rathbun, J.B., and MacNab, I.: The microvascular pattern of the rotator cuff. J. Bone Joint Surg. 52B:540, 1970.
25. Steinbrocker, O.: The Painful Shoulder. In Hollander, J.E. (ed.): Arthritis and Allied Conditions. 8th ed. Philadelphia, Lea & Febiger, 1972.
26. Thompson, G.R., Ting, Y.M., Riggs, G.A., Fenn, M.E., and Denning, R.M.: Calcific tendinitis and soft tissue calcification resembling gout. JAMA 203:122, 1968.
27. Kotzen, L.M.: Roentgen diagnosis of rotator cuff tear. Am. J. Roentgenol. 112:507, 1971.
28. De Palma, A.F.: Surgery of the Shoulder, 2nd ed. Philadelphia, J. B. Lippincott Company, 1973.
29. Wolfgang, G.L.: Surgical repair of tears of the rotator cuff of the shoulder. Factors influencing the result. J. Bone Joint Surg. 56A:14, 1974.
30. Earnshaw, P., Desjardins, D., Sarkar, K., and Uhthoff, H.K.: Rotator cuff tears: The role of surgery. Can. J. Surg. 25:60, 1982.
31. Post, M., Silver, R., and Singh, M.: Rotator cuff tear, diagnosis and treatment. Clin. Orthop. 173:78, 1983.
32. Goss, C.M.: Gray's Anatomy of the Human Body. 28th ed. Philadelphia, Lea & Febiger, 1966.
33. Meyer, A.W.: Spontaneous dislocation and destruction of the tendon of the long head of the biceps brachii, fifty-nine instances. Arch. Surg. 17:493, 1928.
34. Hitchcock, H.H., and Bechtol, C.O.: Painful shoulder. Observations on the role of the tendon of the long head of the biceps brachii in its causation. J. Bone Joint Surg. 30A:263, 1948.
35. Crenshaw, A.H., and Kilgore, W.E.: Surgical treatment of bicipital tenosynovitis. J. Bone Joint Surg. 48A:1496, 1966.
36. Wright, P.E.: Dislocations. In Edmonson, A.S., and Crenshaw, A.H. (eds.): Campbell's Operative Orthopedics. St. Louis, C. V. Mosby Company, 1980.
37. Rockwood, C.A., Jr.: Fractures and dislocations of the shoulder. Part II. In Rockwood, C.A., Jr., and Green, D.P. (eds.) Fractures. Philadelphia, J. B. Lippincott Company, 1975.
38. Glick, J.: Acromioclavicular dislocations in athletes. Orthop. Rev. 1:31, 1972.
39. Taylor, G.M., and Tooke, M.: Degeneration of the acromioclavicular joint as a cause of shoulder pain. J. Bone Joint Surg. 59B:507, 1977.
40. Cofield, R.H., and Briggs, B.T.: Glenohumeral arthrodesis. J. Bone Joint Surg. 61A:668, 1979.
41. Rowe, C.R.: Arthrodesis of the shoulder used in treating painful conditions. Clin. Orthop. 173:92, 1983.
42. Neer, C.S., II, Watson, K.C., and Stanton, F.J.: Recent experience in total shoulder replacement. J. Bone Joint Surg. 64A:319, 1982.
43. Cofield, R.H.: Unconstrained total shoulder prosthesis. Clin. Orthop. 173:97, 1983.
44. Thornhill, T.S., Karr, M.J., Averill, R.M., Batte, N.J., Thomas, W.H., and Sledge, C.B.: Total shoulder arthroplasty, the Brigham Experience. 50th Annual Meeting of the American Academy of Orthopedic Surgeons, Anaheim, March, 1983.
45. Neer, C.S., II: Fracture and Dislocations of the Shoulder. Part I. In Rockwood, C.A., Jr., and Green, D.P. (eds.): Fractures. Philadelphia, J. B. Lippincott, Company, 1975.
46. Ficat, R.P., and Arlet, J.: Ischemia and Necrosis of the Bone. Baltimore, Williams & Wilkins Company, 1980.

47. Post, M., Haskell, S.S., and Jablon, M.: Total shoulder replacement with a constrained prosthesis. J. Bone Joint Surg. 62A:327, 1980.
48. Post, M., and Jablon, M.: Constrained total shoulder arthroplasty: Long-term follow-up observations. Clin. Orthop. 173:109, 1983.
49. Putnam, J.J.: The treatment of a form of painful periarthritis of the shoulder. Boston Med. Surg. J. 107:536, 1882.
50. Lippman, R.K.: Frozen shoulder; periarthritis; bicipital tenosynovitis. Arch. Surg. 47:283, 1943.
51. McLaughlin, H.L.: The "frozen shoulder." Clin. Orthop. 20:126, 1961.
52. DePalma, A.F.: Loss of scapulohumeral motion (frozen shoulder). Ann. Surg. 135:193, 1952.
53. Johnson, J.T.H.: Frozen shoulder syndrome in patients with pulmonary tuberculosis. J. Bone Joint Surg. 41A:877, 1959.
54. Dee, P.E., Smith, R.G., Gullickson, M.J., and Ballinger, C.S.: The orthopedist and apical lung carcinoma. J. Bone Joint Surg. 42A:605, 1960.
55. Neviaser, J.S.: Adhesive capsulitis of the shoulder. A study of the pathological findings in periarthritis of the shoulder. J. Bone Joint Surg. 27:211, 1945.
56. Bulgen, D.Y., Hazelman, B.L., and Voak, D.: HLA-B27 and frozen shoulder. Lancet 1:1042, 1976.
57. Bulgen, D.Y., Hazelman, B.L., Ward, M., and McCallum, M.: Immunological studies in frozen shoulder. Ann. Rheum. Dis. 37:135, 1978.
58. Lundberg, B.J.: The frozen shoulder. Acta Orthop. Scand. Suppl. 19, 1969.
59. Spillane, J.D.: Localized neuritis of the shoulder girdle. A report of 46 cases in the MEF. Lancet 2:532, 1943.
60. Parsonage, M.J., and Turner, J.W.A.: Neurologic amyotrophy. The shoulder-girdle syndrome. Lancet 1:973, 1948.
61. Turner, J.W.A., and Parsonage, M.J.: Neurologic amyotrophy (paralytic brachial neuritis). With special reference to prognosis. Lancet 2:209, 1957.
62. Bacevich, B.B.: Paralytic brachial neuritis. J. Bone Joint Surg. 58A:262, 1976.
63. Tsiaris, P., Dyck, P.J., and Mulder, D.W.: Natural history of brachial plexus neuropathy. Arch. Neurol. 27:109, 1972.
64. Omer, G.E., Jr., and Spinner, M.: Management of Peripheral Nerve Problems. Philadelphia, W. B. Saunders Company, 1980.

65. Kelly, T.R.: Thoracic outlet syndrome, current concepts and treatment. Ann. Surg. 190:657, 1979.
66. Brown, C.: Compressive invasive referred pain to the shoulder. Clin. Orthop. 173:55, 1983.
67. Bateman, J.E.: Neurologic painful conditions affecting the shoulder. Clin. Orthop. 173:44, 1983.
68. Cahill, B.R.: Quadrilateral space syndrome. In Omer, G.E., Jr., and Spinner, M.D. (eds.): Management of Peripheral Nerve Problems. Philadelphia, W. B. Saunders Company, 1980.
69. Rengachary, S.S., Neft, J.P., Singer, P.A., and Brackett, C.E.: Suprascapular entrapment neuropathy: A clinical, anatomical and comparative study. Neurosurgery 5:441, 1979.
70. Kopell, H.P., and Thompson, W.A.L.: Pain and the frozen shoulder. Surg. Gynecol. Obstet. 109:92, 1959.
71. Drez, D.: Suprascapular neuropathy in the differential diagnosis of rotator cuff injuries. Am. J. Sports Med. 4:43, 1976.
72. Khalili, A.A.: Neuromuscular electrodiagnostic studies in entrapment neuropathy of the suprascapular nerve. Orthop. Rev. 3:27, 1974.
73. Rask, M.R.: Suprascapular nerve entrapment. A report of two cases treated with suprascapular notch resection. Clin. Orthop. 123:73, 1977.
74. Solheim, L.F., and Roaas, A.: Compression of the suprascapular nerve after fracture of the scapula notch. Acta Orthop. Scand. 49:338, 1978.
75. Mitchell, S.W.: Phantom limbs. Lippincott's, Mag. 8:563, 1871.
76. Bonica, J.J.: Causalgia and other reflex dystrophies. In Bonica, J.J. (ed.): Management of Pain. Philadelphia, Lea & Febiger, 1979.
77. Evans, J.A.: Reflex sympathetic dystrophy. Surg. Gynecol. Obstet. 82:36, 1946.
78. Steinbocker, O.: The shoulder-hand syndrome: Present perspective. Arch. Phys. Med. 49:388, 1968.
79. Dahlin, D.C.: Bone Tumors. Springfield, Charles C Thomas, 1978.
80. Pancoast, H.K.: Importance of careful roentgen ray investigation of apical chest tumors. JAMA 83:1407, 1924.
81. Golding, D.N.: Hypothyroidism presenting with musculoskeletal syndromes. Ann. Rheum. Dis. 29:10, 1970.
82. Bridgman, J.F.: Periarthritis of the shoulder and diabetes mellitus. Ann. Rheum. Dis. 31:69, 1972.

Chapter 30

Low Back Pain

Stephen J. Lipson

INCIDENCE AND DISABILITY

Low back pain is extremely common, is estimated to affect about 65 to 80 percent of populations sampled,[1-3] and accounts for one third of rheumatic complaints.[4] Particular groups, notably those doing heavy industrial labor, have a higher incidence.[5] Back pain has accounted for a 63 percent rate of sick leave among manual laborers,[6] about 500 work days lost per 1000 workers per year,[7] prolonged disability with pain of up to 3 months' duration in 87 percent of those afflicted,[8] and a 60 percent incidence of recurrent bouts of pain in the first year of an attack. Back pain accounts for 4.2 percent of all consultations in general practice in Great Britain[4,9] where 1.1 million persons see general practitioners for a total of 3.1 million consultations per year[10] and where it creates an annual cost of over 500 million dollars in medical care, disability benefits, and lost work. In the United States, a family practice study over a 3-year period showed that 11 percent of men and 9.5 percent of women reported low back pain.[11] Associated risk factors are considered to be occupation, anxiety, depression, pregnancy, and cigarette smoking.[11] Over 5 billion dollars are spent annually for diagnosis and treatment, while lost productivity, compensation payments, and litigation costs add up to more than 14 billion dollars per year.[12]

OVERALL ADVANCES

The understanding of back disorders has tended to be overshadowed by the syndrome of the herniated nucleus pulposus as delineated by Mixter and Barr.[13] Disc herniations, however, account for only 5 percent of back disorders[14] and do not increase in incidence with a heavy lifting population,[15] as does low back pain. More recent progress in back pain has been directed away from this limited condition. Improvement in the understanding and management of low back pain has come from the recognition of the multiple factors involved in disability secondary to low back pain, methods to elucidate better the source of the pain and therefore attempt more specific therapy, definition of the syndromes, which encompass types of spinal disorders and their pathology, advances in radiologic imaging techniques, subsequent refinements of operative indications, and, finally, improved operative techniques. It is the goal of this chapter to review these advances, except for operative techniques, in terms of patient evaluation and disease states with consideration of any known underlying pathophysiology. An intended emphasis is placed on disc degeneration. Tumors, traumatic fractures, and metabolic bone disease are not discussed.

BACK PAIN AND CLINICAL EVALUATION

Relevant Anatomy and Pain Sources. Adjacent vertebrae are connected by an articular triad composed of the intervertebral disc anteriorly and two zygoapophyseal facet joints lined with synovium posteriorly. The unit is further stabilized by the anterior longitudinal ligament on the ventral side of the intervertebral disc and the posterior longitudinal ligament on the dorsal side. The latter is thinner and consists of bands fanning out over the posterior surface of the disc and loosely attached to it. In the vertebral arches the ligamentum flavum acts as a ligament and blends into the medial superior aspect of the facet joint capsule; it may prevent the synovium from being pinched in the joint during motion and protect the spinal nerves from protrusion of the capsule into the spinal nerve foramen. The interspinous ligament runs between the posterior spinous processes and is a true ligament. The supraspinous ligament connects the spinous processes.

The muscles of the lumbar region are the sacrospinalis and multifidus muscles. The sacrospinalis attaches to the posterior surface of the sacrum and iliac crest, inserts at the lateral angulus of the ribs, and acts as the posterior longitudinal support. The multifidus covers the intervertebral facet joints while running from the mamillary and transverse processes to insert on the spinous process one or two vertebrae above. These act as rotator muscles of the spine. The abdominal muscles via the abdomen provide anterior support to the spine.

The innervation of the lumbar spine has been well reviewed.[16] It consists of the sinuvertebral nerve and the posterior primary ramus (Fig. 30–1). The sinuvertebral nerve, first described by Luschka,[17] arises from the anterior aspect of the spinal nerve just distal to the spinal ganglion. After turning medially it is joined by a sympathetic branch from the ramus communicans, and the composite nerve passes through the intervertebral foramen into the spinal canal where it branches. Adjacent to the posterior longitudinal ligament it divides into ascending, descending, and transverse branches anastomosing with branches from the contralateral side and adjacent levels above and below. The branches are felt

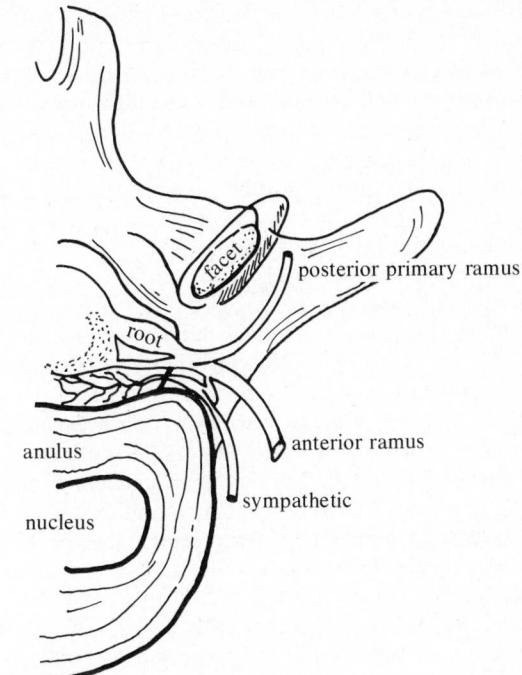

Figure 30–1. The innervation of the spine showing the relationships of the posterior primary ramus and the sinuvertebral nerve.

to innervate the vertebral body, laminae, intervertebral discs at the same level and one above and below, the posterior longitudinal ligament, the internal vertebral plexus, the epidural tissues, and the dura. The normal intervertebral disc is believed to be innervated only to the extent of the outer layers of the anulus fibrosus.

The posterior primary ramus arises from the spinal nerve just lateral to the intervertebral foramen in association with the major branch, the anterior ramus. It then divides into medial and lateral branches. The medial branch descends in a notch posterior to the transverse process and is covered by the medial part of the intertransverse ligament. It immediately gives off a small branch to the inferior part of the capsule of the facet joint. The medial branch then continues caudally, innervating the dorsal musculature, anastomosing with nerves from adjacent levels, and then innervating the superior part of the capsule of the facet joint below. The lateral branches of the upper three lumbar levels have cutaneous nerves reaching as far as the greater trochanter, and the two lower lumbar posterior primary rami have no skin supply.

There have been a number of clinical experimental studies to demonstrate pain sources in the low back. Smyth and Wright[18] used nylon thread loops to stimulate structures. The dura, ligamentum flavum, and interspinous ligaments were insensitive. The anulus gave back pain, and the nerve root caused sciatic pain when stimulated. Kellgren[19] injected hypertonic saline into spinal muscles and interspinous ligaments and produced back pain with sclerotomal referral. Hirsch[20] also injected hypertonic saline into the facet joint, which gave back pain with sclerotomal referral. Injection of the disc gave severe back pain resembling patients' attacks, whereas injection of the ligamentum flavum gave mild discomfort. Mooney and Robertson[21] demonstrated that facet irritation gave not only back pain but also marked patterns of referred pain into the thigh and leg, depending upon level. Hamstring muscle activity was enhanced, as evidenced by electromyographic findings and diminished straight leg raising. There was return of depressed reflexes when the facet was anesthetized.

Pain sources in the back, then, appear to originate from the disc and the facet joint. The root may contribute to the pain of sciatica, but it is clear that the pain pattern seen clinically can also be produced by facet joint irritation. It is because of the overlap of contributing pain sources that evaluation must be done carefully to sort out the pathologically significant anatomy; otherwise, surgical measures in particular may be aimed at noncontributing structures and fail.

Presenting Complaints. Low back pain is age related. Back pain begins in the second decade, and the incidence increases through the fifth decade of life[1] and then decreases.[3,22] Sciatica is rarely seen before the second decade and peaks in the third.[23] Back pain is increased in heavy lifting laborers,[5] and therefore a work history is necessary both for documentation and for purposes of certifying disability. Pain presents with a number of patterns, and the history will facilitate an accurate assessment of what is or is not its cause. Traditional analysis of low back pain demonstrates that the pain is usefully categorized as local, radicular, referred, or spasmodic.[24]

Local pain, presumably from a pathologic process stimulating sensory nerve endings, is usually steady, is occasionally intermittent, changes with position, is sharp or dull, and is felt in the affected part. It most often gives reflex paravertebral spasm.

Referred pain from pelvic and abdominal viscera is referred to dermatomal areas and takes on a deep and aching characteristic. Referred pain from spinal sources is noted in the sacroiliac area, buttocks, and posterior thigh and is noted as sclerotomal pain, since the referral area has the same embryonic origin as the mesodermal tissue involved.

Radicular pain relates to a spinal nerve root distribution, worsens with root stretching maneuvers such as

bending, and usually improves with rest. If pain is worsened by rest, particularly at night, a spinal cord tumor may be suspected. The pain has neurologic characteristics of paresthesias and numbness, and there may be associated motor weakness. The characteristic of walking giving rise to the spinal claudication symptom of spinal stenosis should be noted, as well as the effect of sitting, which will improve spinal stenosis symptoms but worsen those of disc herniation. Bladder, bowel, and sexual function should be determined, since they are involved in central midline herniations of the disc, conus tumors, and occasionally spinal stenosis. Pain from muscular spasm will have cramping, achy characteristics, usually in the sacrospinalis and gluteus maximus. A summary of the characteristics of back pain of various origins is given in Table 30–1.

A useful analysis of back pain arises out of an evaluation of further mechanical relationships of the pain. These mechanical relationships reflect the pathophysiologic origins of the pain. Low back pain and the pain of disc herniation tend to worsen with postural positions of prolonged duration. Positions that increase intradiscal pressure exacerbate pain; those that decrease pressure improve the pain, as outlined by the intradiscal pressure measurements done by Nachemson.[71] However, it is not established that intradiscal pressure causes pain, only that this relationship exists. Another pattern of pain, commonly seen in degenerative spinal stenosis, is that of neurogenic claudication, pain produced in the back or leg by walking or by assuming an erect position. This pain tends to be more diffuse than the pain caused during root entrapment by a herniated lumbar disc. In neurogenic claudication, when the spine is in flexion, room in the lumbar canal enlarges and the pain lessens. A summary of mechanical relationships is given in Table 30–2.

A past medical history of medications, other medical conditions, and a family history, especially of arthritic diseases, is necessary. It is useful at the initial encounter to ascertain work status, compensation, litigation, disability at work and home, and the patient's own assessment of how well he is coping with his affliction, as these factors can markedly alter the assessment, management, and outcome of treatment.[25-28]

Physical Examination. Examination should be done

Table 30–1. Summary of the Characteristics of Low Back Pain of Various Origins

Source of Pain	Distribution	Nature	Aggravating Factors	Neurologic Changes
Spinal pain	Sclerotomal Local	Sharp Dull	Motion	None
Discogenic pain	Sclerotomal	Deep, aching	Increased intradiscal pressure, e.g., bending, sitting, Valsalva maneuver	None
Nerve root pain	Radicular	Paresthesias Numbness	Root stretching	Present
Multiple lumbar spinal stenosis pain	Radicular Sclerotomal	Paresthesias Spinal claudication pattern	Lumbar extension Walking	Present
Referred visceral pain	Dermatomal	Deep, aching	Related to affected organ	None

Table 30–2. Mechanical Relationships Noted in Discogenic Low Back Pain and Herniated Nucleus Pulposus as Compared with Spinal Stenosis

	Herniated Nucleus Pulposus/Discogenic Low Back Pain	Spinal Stenosis
Standing/walking	▼	▲
Sitting	▲	▼
Valsalva maneuver	▲	—
Bending	▲	—
Lifting	▲	—
Bed rest	▼	▼

with the patient undressed. The spine and stance are inspected while the patient is standing to note lumbar lordosis, thoracic kyphos, scoliosis, tilt from "sciatic scoliosis," flexed lower extremities to relieve root tension, muscle spasm, and skin nevi over the spine. Gait and motion are noted, including toe and heel gait, to determine muscular weakness and to observe any inconsistent or exaggerated posturing.

Forward bending is measured and can be crudely quantitated by an estimate of flexion or the distance of the fingers from the floor. Lateral bending may be asymmetric with unilateral root entrapment. Hyperextension will elicit pain from inflamed facet joints. The spine is palpated to determine local tenderness, the stepoff of spondylolisthesis, or the defect of spina bifida, and percussed to produce local pain or sciatica and in the costovertebral angle to elicit pain of renal origin. The iliac crests are palpated and may be tender, particularly over the posterior iliac spine where local injection may give symptomatic relief. The sciatic nerve is palpated in its notch and along its course to determine hyperesthesia and tenderness. Calf tenderness may be found, reflecting sciatic hyperesthesia.

A thorough neurologic examination is done for objective signs of lumbar root involvement. In disc herniations, L5-S1 and L4-5 are most common, followed by L3-4. Disc herniations at L5-S1 usually involve the S1 root, L4-5 the L5 root, and L3-4 the L4 root. L4-5 herniation may involve both the L5 and S1 roots, and there is a 10 percent incidence of two-level herniations.[29] The neurologic findings are summarized in Table 30–3.

The findings according to level should be regarded as guidelines since, although these patterns are generally accurate as to level of entrapment, they can be misleading. The distribution of paresis in the lower extremity in herniated discs at the L4-5 and L5-S1 levels was studied by Weber,[30] who noted that although there is localization of paresis according to nerve root, in 30 to 40 percent of other muscle groups in the lower extremity are also affected. Impairment of the knee jerk has been shown to be affected more often by L4-5 herniations than by those at L3-4.[31] Neurologic assessment must be done carefully, since often only subtle motor weakness is present and must be elicited by repetitive testing. This is particularly true for the gastrosoleus, which is so powerful that manual testing may not demonstrate weakness. Repetitive toe lifts while standing on one foot are useful in this respect, as is examining a toe-toe and heel-heel gait. Reflexes can be enhanced by an isometric maneuver with the hands or, in the case of the ankle jerk, having the patient kneel on a chair. Sensory findings are often confusing and must be mapped carefully. It is of value to perform both pin and vibration tests to ascertain that all columns of the cord are intact.

The patient can then be placed supine and thigh and leg girths measured for atrophy. Leg lengths are measured, since leg length inequality may be associated with back pain that can be helped symptomatically with a shoe lift. Maneuvers are then done to stretch the sciatic nerve and elicit pain. Straight leg raising is done by lifting the leg by the heel with the knee extended until the patient expresses pain and the hamstrings tighten. The site of the pain is asked, since only radicular pain, not back pain, is indicative of a herniated disc. The test is of value only with distal roots and is therefore most accurate with lesions involving the L5 and S1 roots. Young patients have a marked tendency toward a positive straight leg raising test with disc herniations. Its absence fairly accurately excludes a disc herniation up to the age of 30, when it no longer excludes the diagnosis.[32] Variations of the straight leg raising test include dorsiflexion of the foot at the end point of straight leg raising to further stretch the sciatic nerve. Lasègue's test is done by having the hip and knee flexed and then

Table 30–3. Nerve Root Findings

Nerve Root	Pain and Dysesthesia	Weakness and Atrophy	Decreased Reflexes
L4	Posterolateral thigh across knee Anteromedial leg	Quadriceps	Knee jerk
L5	Posterior thigh Anterolateral leg Medial foot and hallux	Tibialis anterior Extensor hallucis longus Atrophied anterior compartment of the leg	None or decreased tibialis posterior
S1	Posterior thigh Posterior leg Posterolateral foot Lateral toes	Gastrosoleus	Ankle jerk
Sacral roots S2-4	Buttocks and perineum Posterior thigh Posterior leg Plantar foot	Gluteus maximus Hamstrings Gastrosoleus Foot intrinsics and long flexors Anal and bladder sphincters	Ankle jerk Absent plantar toe responses

slowly extending the knee. It can also be done with the patient seated over the side of the examining table. The crossed straight leg raising test is done by elevating the leg contralateral to the symptomatic side. Reproduction of radicular pain by this maneuver is considered the most indicative sign of disc herniation.[31]

To stretch the more proximal roots to the femoral nerve, the patient is turned prone and the Ely test for rectus femoris contracture done. The knee is flexed and the hip is hyperextended. This motion will be limited by irritation of the L3 and L4 roots. The Patrick or fabere test, to implicate the sacroiliac rather than the hip joint, is done by flexing, abducting, externally rotating, and extending the hip (giving rise to the mnemonic "fabere").[33] A painful response points to the sacroiliac joint as the source of the complaint.

If it is felt that the patient has too much emotional overlay, is too coached in examination by multiple previous consultations, or is guilty of outright malingering, there are some tests to help reveal this. In straight leg raising, the foot is both dorsiflexed and plantar flexed to ascertain the correct anatomical result. When the patient is sitting on the table, the knees are casually extended to note the presence of Lasègue's sign and to see if the patient sits back to relax sciatic tension. With the patient supine, he is asked to do an active straight leg raising maneuver while the examiner's hand is under the contralateral heel. A true effort will give a downward push on the opposite heel, while a feigned attempt will not produce it. A true list will persist while bending forward in a chair. These and other useful tests are reviewed elsewhere.[34,35]

An assessment of peripheral circulation should be performed as well as abdominal, rectal, and pelvic examination, since the source of some back pain may be found here. Chest expansion is measured with a tape measure as a screen for ankylosing spondylitis; it is highly significant when chest excursion is reduced to 1 inch.

Laboratory Examination. It is useful to perform a simple battery of tests as a screen for metabolic and specific diseases early on in the assessment and management of back pain. These, like the initial radiograph of the spine, provide a baseline for the exclusion of some diseases as the underlying cause of the pain. They can be tailored when appropriate. The tests include a complete blood count, sedimentation rate, rheumatoid factor, antinuclear antibodies, serum calcium, phosphorus, alkaline phosphatase, acid phosphatase when appropriate, uric acid, blood sugar, immunoelectrophoresis, protein electrophoresis, and urinalysis.

Psychologic Evaluation. For better or worse, back pain involves a significant number of emotional factors, and it is necessary to recognize them early in assessing pain. When personality factors are unfavorable, management will be unsuccessful no matter how skillfully performed.[27] Fortunately, emotional factors can be made more objective by psychological testing. The Minnesota Multiphasic Personality Inventory (MMPI) has become the most accurate guideline for detecting personality

traits that will predict poor results.[28,36] The hysteria (Hy) and hypochondriasis (Hs) scales of the MMPI have been shown to be the best predictors of a symptomatic result of surgery and chemonucleolysis for disc disease. A simple pain diagram has been correlated with the MMPI.[37] This makes it possible to have a quick, simple office assessment of personality traits that may confuse pain assessment. These tests cannot be used in an absolute sense to rule in or out functional versus organic pain,[38] but help in deciding whether to pursue invasive therapy, to seek psychologic and psychiatric consultation, or, in the case of chronic pain, to enter into behavior modification by operant conditioning.[39,40]

Anatomically based aid is given by the Pentothal interview,[41] utilizing the straight leg raising test. The patient's straight leg raising endpoint is established, and he is then given intravenous Pentothal anesthesia until a noxious stimulus such as toe squeeze or heel cord pinching no longer produces a response. The anesthetic is allowed to wear off, and at intervals the noxious stimulus, given in the limb examined, is tested. Upon return of a response such as a grimace, deep sigh, or withdrawal, the straight leg raising is repeated. If there is organic disease and lumbar root irritation, an appropriate response to this noxious stimulus will be registered. In this manner, further information as to the severity and organic nature of the pain described is gained.

Radiologic Evaluation. *Plain Radiographs and Common Anomalies of the Low Back.* The lumbosacral spine film is a necessary part of early evaluation. A lateral lumbosacral radiograph delivers a 2 rem skin dose, which is 15 times the exposure delivered by a chest radiograph.[42] Although the yield of causes of low back pain by radiography is low and the radiation dose relatively high, it serves to rule out serious conditions such as tumor and infection. It should be obtained with some discretion. One study has shown that the risks and costs of obtaining a lumbar radiograph at the initial visit does not justify the small associated benefit.[43] The standard anteroposterior, lateral, coned-down lateral, and 45-degree oblique views comprise the standard series. Early signs of disc degeneration are decreased height of the anterior disc space and anteroposterior intervertebral shift on flexion-extension lateral views.[44] The so-called vacuum sign of intranuclear gas also reflects disc degeneration.[45] Later radiographic signs of disc degeneration are further collapse of the disc space, sclerosis, and osteophyte formation. Osteophytes also occur in Reiter's syndrome, ankylosing spondylitis, and psoriatic arthritis. The presence of disc degeneration radiographically does not imply that a disc is the cause of pain. Lawrence[46] surveyed lumbosacral spine films in persons 35 years of age and older. Sixty-five percent of the males and 52 percent of the females showed disc degeneration, but in only 13 percent were there symptoms of pain. Nerve root involvement occurred in only 10 percent of those with signs of moderate to severe degeneration. In a large series of disc herniations proved at operation, the plain radiograph predicted a correct diagnosis in only 34 percent of cases.[47] Epstein[48] found 46 percent narrowing at L5-S1 and only 25 percent narrowing at L4-5 in 300 proved herniations. Therefore a disc can often appear radiographically normal when it is symptomatic, and when a disc is symptomatic, radiography is not an accurate predictor of the symptomatic level.

Various structural anomalies, definable on plain radiographs and associated with back pain and disc degeneration, have been reviewed.[49] A defect in the pars interarticularis (spondylolysis) increases the likelihood of symptomatic back pain by about 25 percent. Disc herniation, however, is unusual. The incidence of disc degeneration defined by discogram is increased by bilateral pars defects, and the degeneration is felt to be more rapidly progressive. Wiltse[49] believes that unilateral pars defects increase the rate of disc degeneration. Tropism, or a rotational asymmetry of the lumbosacral facets from a sagittal to a coronal direction, produces accelerated disc degeneration. Farfan and Sullivan[50] found a 23 percent incidence of asymmetry in asymptomatic backs. In symptomatic backs they found a very high incidence of asymmetry and disc herniations on the side of the more coronal facet.

Scoliosis in the thoracolumbar region does not increase the incidence of low back pain up to the age of 56.[4,5,51] There is progressive disc degeneration at the apex of the curve in progressive scoliotic curves. Lumbar lordosis does not increase the incidence of back pain.[1,5] Lumbosacral tilt from a unilateral anomalous lumbosacral facet or unilateral hypoplasia of the sacrum and pelvis is not known to produce rapid disc degeneration, although it might be expected to.[49] Leg length discrepancy producing tilt is known not to produce symptoms with up to 1 to 2 cm of discrepancy.[1,5] With greater than 4.5 cm of discrepancy, the incidence of back pain increases.[49]

Spina bifida occulta does not produce back pain.[1,5] Transitional vertebrae are either a sacralized lumbar vertebra or a lumbarized sacral vertebra, and neither produces increased back pain.[1,5] Five percent of people have six lumbar vertebrae, 2.5 percent have four, and the rest have the usual five.[52] Wiltse[49] advances a guideline that the more sacralized a vertebra, the more vestigial its disc and the less likely it is to herniate. If there is disc herniation, it is usually at the level above the transitional vertebra.

Bone Scan. Bone scanning with ^{99}Tc diphosphonate can be of use in defining the origin of back pain in some situations. It can demonstrate bony infections or tumors, and is useful in detecting early evidence of ankylosing spondylitis with increased activity in the sacroiliac, facet, and costovertebral joints. A developing pars interarticularis defect, not visible on plain radiography, can be demonstrated by bone scan. Advanced degenerative disc and facet disease produces increased uptake, and bone scan yields little useful information.[53] Ga-citrate scanning offers the possibility of early diagnosis of infections.[54]

Discography. Discography, the injection of radiologic water-soluble contrast material into the intervertebral disc, is felt to be a safe procedure and has been used since 1948.[55] Some large series have revealed no complications,[56,57] although there are reports of occasional infections, ranging from 1 in 622[58] to 1 in 2500.[59] The effect of puncture of the disc has been examined. Discography in dogs with followup at 6 to 12 months did not reveal significant radiologic or histologic changes.[60] Nuclear herniation with protruded disc has been caused with a 20-gauge needle in dogs,[61] and in clinical studies changes have varied from none at 1 to 3 months[58,62] to loss of disc height in about one fourth of patients 12 months after discography.[63]

Disc degeneration evidenced by discography increases with age and progression down the lumbar spine.[58] In cadavers, 90 percent of lumbar discs are normal in the age group 14 to 34 years, but only 5 percent are normal at 60 years.[64] Holt[65] found 34 percent degenerative changes in normal volunteers. Because of the marked prevalence of age-related disc degeneration, discography has been felt to be of little use in correctly diagnosing a herniated disc and was a reliable diagnostic method in only 30 percent of cases of surgically proved disc herniation.[47]

In normal discs it is difficult to inject more than 1 ml of contrast material into the nucleus. There is marked resistance to the injection but no pain. A degenerative disc is usually easy to inject, although firm resistance is reported in 15 percent of a large series.[59] The injection may be painful in up to two thirds of degenerative discs,[59] but pain may also be produced by injection of the anulus and by an irritant in the contrast medium. The radiologic appearance of degeneration is that of diffusion of contrast material through the disc and occasional extravasation through anular cracks into the epidural space. The appearance is variable and of no significance in diagnosing symptomatic herniation. Pain can be of diagnostic value, but only if it reproduces the symptomatic pain.[41] Discography produces back pain in 15 percent of normal males,[65] so that the simple production of pain is not diagnostic.

Discography in the lumbar spine, then, has certain indications.[41] It is useful in assessing the state of degeneration in a disc above the level of a proposed fusion, since that disc will be subject to progressive degeneration and will fail if unrecognized degeneration already exists. If myelography is negative but disc herniation is still suspected, discography can help define the disc degeneration. In patients in whom there is intractable low back pain without evidence of disc degeneration on the plain radiograph, discography can demonstrate the degeneration. The source of usual pain patterns may be confirmed by its reproduction on discography. Discography is routinely used in chemonucleolysis prior to the injection of chymopapain to ensure that a normal disc is not injected. Macnab[41] assesses a symptomatic pseudarthrosis, following fusion, by discography. Disc injection at the level of pseudarthrosis is painful, but it is painless if the fusion is solid. He feels that this technique is 80 percent reliable.

Myelography. Myelography is used as a preoperative

investigation, not as a diagnostic technique.[29,41] It is recommended preoperatively for two reasons: (1) it will reveal a tumor presenting as a disc herniation which might be missed if it is not at the level examined at surgery; and (2) it more precisely localizes the site of disc herniation and root entrapment. Lateral bony root entrapments may present with a negative myelogram. Diffuse anular bulges will give a waisted, hourglass appearance. Multiple disc herniations occur with a 5 to 10 percent incidence.[42] Myelographic information will thus allow the surgeon to modify his approach so that excessive exposure will be avoided, minimizing postoperative perineural scarring. As has been previously noted, neurologic examination is not completely accurate in localizing the level of involvement. In disc herniations, neurologic symptoms associated with the last two lowest spaces point to the correct level only about 60 percent of the time.[31] Neurologic signs are more accurate, reaching 75 to 80 percent.[31] Myelography is accurate 80 to 90 percent of the time,[47,66,67] but it is not foolproof in that lateral disc herniations are detected in only 70 to 80 percent of myelograms[42] and 11 percent of cases of sciatica have a negative myelogram as well as a negative neurologic exam.[68] Over two thirds of disc herniations with false-negative myelography are in the L5-S1 space,[31] because the dural sac may be short or may lie away from the disc by 3 to 4 mm.

Traditional myelography has been done with Pantopaque (iodophenylundelic acid), which is an oil-soluble contrast medium. The complications are numerous and include fever, headache, nausea, meningismus, backache, urinary changes, paresthesias, ileus, and acute and chronic arachnoiditis. Complications related to technique include extradural injections, epidural hematomas, contrast retention, venous intravasation, pulmonary embolism, epidermoid cyst formation, chronic dural leaks, chemical arachnoiditis secondary to the mixing of blood with Pantopaque, and others that are well reviewed.[69,70] Complications are infrequent, but the most common are the acute, transient systemic reactions secondary to inflammation caused by the Pantopaque, the extradural or mixed injection, and retention of contrast caused by faulty technique.[69]

Water-soluble myelography has replaced oil-soluble myelography and has been used extensively in Europe. Oil-soluble contrasts are now banned in Scandinavia.[71] Meglumine[70] and more recently metrizamide[71] are the agents used. These water-soluble contrast media are found to fill the root sleeves more completely because of their solubility in cerebrospinal fluid and their low viscosity. Therefore lateral disc herniations are more readily detected. These agents are less inflammatory and they are resorbed, leaving no retained contrast. The major complications are those of meningeal irritation, increased radicular symptoms, transient hypotension, and seizures.[70] Metrizamide is the most improved of the contrasts, but is still regarded as epileptogenic. It is reported to have 95 percent accuracy in disc herniations.[71]

The abnormalities noted on myelography vary with the size and location of the lesion. Lateral disc herniations usually cause incomplete filling of the root sleeve, lateral dural sac indentation, and a double density of the sac (Fig. 30–2). Central midline herniations often give a complete block with ventral indentation. Sequestered free fragments may migrate and will be seen as circumscribed masses. Chronic degeneration with a diffuse anular bulge will give a waisted, hourglass appearance at the level of the disc space and osteophytes (Fig. 30–3). Artifacts encountered are from the needle, hematomas, and scarring from previous surgery.

Lumbar Epidural Venography. Lumbar epidural venography is of particular use in demonstrating lumbar disc herniation and has achieved success by selective catheterization of the ascending lumbar veins.[72] The ascending lumbar veins off the external iliac veins and ascending sacral veins off the internal iliac veins are catheterized, and defects in filling of the anterior internal vertebral and radicular veins are noted (Fig. 30–4). In Macnab's series,[72] the diagnostic accuracy of venography was 98 percent, compared with 90 percent for myelography, in patients with lumbar disc herniation and no prior surgery. It cannot distinguish postoperative scarring from recurrent disc herniation. Epidural venography is indicated in patients who have not had a previous operation and in those patients in whom the myelogram is normal or equivocal but in whom there is a strong clinical suspicion of disc herniation.

Computed Tomography. Computed tomography (CT) has replaced many of the alternative methods of radiologic imaging described above. With fourth-generation scanners, the need for myelography has decreased and therefore the morbidity of investigation has decreased. CT scanning has the disadvantage of not being useful as a screening procedure, as myelography is, and may not visualize intradural lesions unless contrast is present intrathecally. The reliability of CT scanning in detecting herniated disc appears to be well over 95 percent. Herniated disc can be easily visualized on thin-cut CT scan, as seen in Figure 30–5. Spinal stenosis can be visualized as in Figure 30–6, with bulging of the disc, thickening of the ligamentum flavum, osteophytic entrapment from the facets, and the obliteration of epidural fat.

These techniques should be reserved for cases in which there is clinical suspicion of an anatomic lesion. Imaging techniques should not be used to find a lesion and thereby provide a presumptive diagnosis of the cause of pain. If one uses this latter approach, false positives from asymptomatic degeneration will confuse the evaluation. Such degeneration in the cervical and lumbar region was found following myelography in 28 percent of patients who had no spinal symptoms and were being studied for other reasons.[73]

Other Techniques. Epidurography is a technique of injecting epidural water-soluble contrast medium to outline the dural sac and root sleeves.[74] It is placed via the sacral hiatus, but in one series 7.5 percent of patients could not be injected successfully.[67] Subarachnoid injections carry a risk of seizure and death.

Nerve root infiltration is of value in localizing the

Figure 30–2. A metrizamide myelogram with L5-S1 herniated nucleus pulposus and root sleeve cutoff (arrows).

Figure 30–3. A metrizamide myelogram of a patient with degenerative spinal stenosis demonstrating central exclusion of the contrast with the hourglass configuration at the level of the discs (arrows). Tomography was used to enhance visualization.

Figure 30–4. Normal lumbar epidural venogram demonstrating the radicular vein (*RV*), ascending lumbar vein (*ALV*), and anterior internal vertebral vein (*AIVV*).

Figure 30–5. Computerized tomographic scan of a herniated intervertebral disc with unilateral obliteration of the root by disc material.

level of root involvement.[41] It is done under image intensification with oil-soluble contrast medium injected into the sleeve for definition and Xylocaine injected to determine if clinical relief of pain occurs.

Facet blocks offer both a diagnostic and therapeutic measure for relief of back pain.[21,53] Under image intensification a needle is placed into the facet joint. Water-soluble contrast can be used to outline the facet and a local anesthetic and/or a deposteroid injected for prolonged relief of symptoms. The relief of pain is the only endpoint of significance.

Figure 30–6. Computerized tomographic scan of spinal stenosis with bulging of the anulus, osteophytic overgrowth of the facet joints, and thickening of the ligamentum flavum.

DISEASE STATES

Degenerative Disc Disease. *Spinal Stenosis and Lumbar Root Entrapment.* Intervertebral disc degeneration is the central factor in many of the conditions of age-related degenerative disease of the lumbar spine. As already noted under Radiologic Evaluation, disc degeneration progresses with age and as one progresses down the lumbar spine. Mixter and Barr[13] first emphasized the role of herniation of the nucleus pulposus in producing lumbar root entrapment. In more recent years, much work has focused on disc degeneration itself and lumbar root entrapment as a result of anatomical changes secondary to disc degeneration. Clinically, lumbar root entrapment is now encompassed in the broad classification of spinal stenosis,[75] which includes narrowing of the spinal canal, nerve root canals, and intervertebral foramina. The process may be local, segmental, or generalized. It may be secondary to soft tissue or bone and may involve the canal, dural sac, or both. This definition includes classical disc herniation and a variety of entrapment syndromes described by Macnab.[76] The classification of spinal stenosis is outlined in Table 30–4.[75]

Historically, spinal stenosis was originally used to describe root entrapment caused by a congenital narrowing of the spinal canal produced by thickening of the neural arches, interpedicular narrowing, and a trefoil configuration of the canal.[77,78] The term was subsequently extended[79,80] to include degenerative and other changes causing root entrapment (illustrated in Fig. 30–7). Prior to their inclusion in the definition of spinal stenosis, it was already known that degenerative changes caused root entrapment,[81] and it had been shown that in an already compromised canal, small changes causing further root entrapment can have marked neurologic consequences.[82] Iatrogenic spinal stenosis has been shown to produce symptomatic narrowing of the canal by thickening of the laminae after decortication—particularly after posterior fusion. Scar tissue from laminectomy may cause compression. Epidural fat involved

Table 30–4. Classification of Spinal Stenosis

Congenital
  Idiopathic
  Achondroplastic
Acquired stenosis
  Degenerative
    Central portion of the spinal canal
    Lateral portion of the spinal canal
    Degenerative spondylolisthesis
  Combined—any combination of congenital, degenerative, and disc herniations
  Spondylolytic, spondylolisthetic
  Iatrogenic
    Postlaminectomy
    Postfusion
    Postchemonucleolysis
  Post-traumatic
  Miscellaneous
    Paget's disease
    Fluorosis

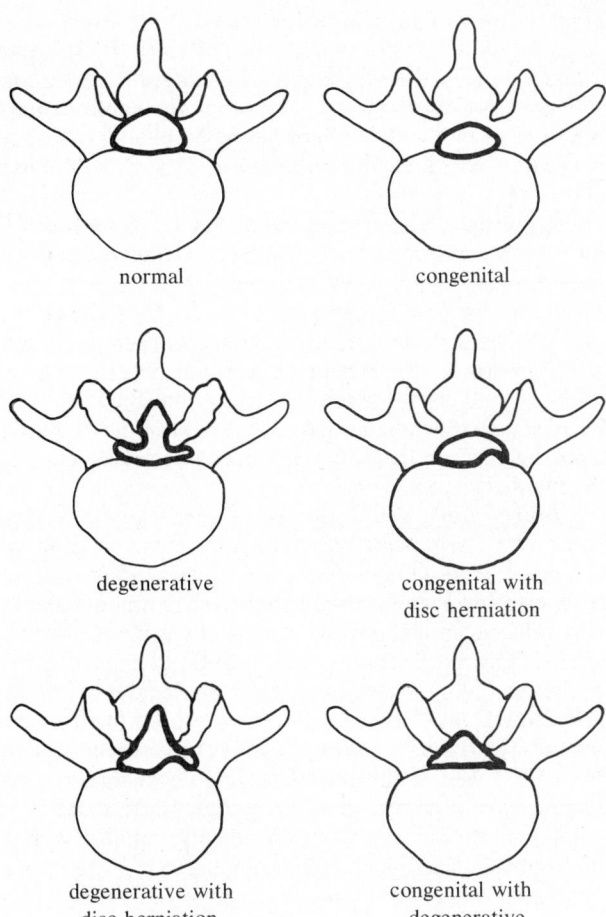

normal   congenital

degenerative   congenital with
                        disc herniation

degenerative with   congenital with
disc herniation   degenerative

Figure 30–7. Outlines of the cross section of the spinal canal in different types of spinal stenosis.

The anulus is well developed by 6 months of life, and in the first decade it fills with ground substance and attaches to the anterior and posterior longitudinal ligaments. The fibers are distinct, but by the end of the second decade the tissue is more hyalinized and less cellular. It then becomes coarse with fissuring, signs of cell death, deposition of pigment, and vascularization. In the fifth decade the anulus loses its lamellar distinction, the fibrils shorten and thicken, and there is hypocellularity. Degeneration is progressive with fissuring, nuclear herniation, and vascular invasion.

The nucleus pulposus starts as a cellular structure with a gelatinous matrix. In the first decade the notochordal cells disappear and fibroblasts distribute toward the periphery. Vacuoles are present in the nucleus pulposus. This arrangement is preserved into the second decade when it gradually loses its mucoid appearance and a fibrillar network appears. The nucleus-anulus border becomes less distinct in the third decade, and by the fourth decade it is obscured by a proliferation of fibrous tissue and cartilage cells. The fibrous change continues with pigment formation, desiccation, cleft formation, and calcium salt deposition. The pathology of symptomatic discs is the same, except that the changes appear more advanced than one might expect on an age basis.[87] Work over recent years has sought to delineate the causes of these changes and has focused on the biochemistry, immunology, nutrition, and biomechanics of the disc.

Biochemical Changes. Investigations on the biochemical changes with age and degeneration have been reviewed,[88-90] and work has focused on the changes in the collagen and proteoglycans of the intervertebral disc. The collagen of the disc is known to exhibit polymorphism and to change with age. Eyre and Muir[91] demonstrated types I and II collagen in the anulus fibrosus of young pigs, but only type II in the nucleus. They later demonstrated a smooth transition of types I and II with respect to outer versus inner parts of the anulus.[92] Other workers[93,94] have found evidence of type I collagen in degenerated nuclei, implying new collagen synthesis, but of an inappropriate type. The collagen crosslinks in aging discs change,[95] and interactions with proteoglycans are altered.[96] Noncollagenous proteins change in disc degeneration with the appearance and progressive accumulation of β-proteins,[97] but the significance of these changes is unclear.[90]

The proteoglycans of the disc are known to change with age.[98] With age and progression down the lumbar spine the composition of the proteoglycans in the anulus and the nucleus changes in that in both regions the size of the proteoglycans decreases, the keratan sulfate content increases, and they become less extractable.[99] Hyaluronate content parallels the distribution of proteoglycans in the disc, increases with age, and is present in adequate amounts to permit complete aggregation of available proteoglycans.[100] Proteoglycan structure in the human disc is similar to proteoglycans from cartilage except for a shorter core protein region. Anular proteoglycans have higher aggregation properties than do nu-

in lipomatosis can cause spinal stenosis.[83] Degenerative stenosis is the most common kind of spinal stenosis encountered.[84]

In the following paragraphs we will review what is known about degenerative disc disease and then consider the clinical states of lumbar root entrapment which result from these changes.

Pathologic Changes. The changes in the intervertebral disc with age have been well documented[85-87] and involve the central nucleus pulposus, the surrounding anulus fibrosus, and the cartilaginous endplates on the adjacent vertebral bodies. By the third decade the incidence of progressive degenerative change in the lumbar intervertebral disc shows a marked increase. In the cartilaginous endplate, early changes of fibrillation occur without evidence of repair. Some fissures and fibrous invasion occur, and breaks in the endplate with nuclear extrusion are seen. In the fourth and fifth decades the endplate is thinned and sometimes absent, and nuclear extrusion with Schmorl's node formation is more frequent. Calcium salts are deposited and progress from this stage on. The chondrocytes of the endplate show signs of senescence and frank necrosis. At older ages the changes are more progressive, with gradual loss of the endplate.

clear proteoglycans.[101] The water content of the disc decreases with age but may be due not so much to simple changes in the osmotic properties of the proteoglycans as to alterations in matrix interactions.[102]

Role of Immunity. Bobechko and Hirsch[103] postulated an autoimmune mechanism of disc degeneration after autologous nucleus pulposus implanted in rabbit ears caused lymph node stimulation. Humoral antibodies have not been found in patients with disc disease,[104,105] but leukocyte migration inhibition[105,106] and lymphocyte transformation[107,108] have been demonstrated in disc material. A proteoglycan fraction may be the antigenic stimulus.[108] Previous work on uncomplicated disc degeneration and nuclear herniation in the human[86,88,109] and experimental animal herniation[110] have not shown inflammatory infiltrates, although they have been observed in nerve roots involved in disc herniations.[111] The nucleus implants of Bobechko and Hirsch[103] also did not show cellular infiltrates. There is no evidence, therefore, that the target tissue is involved in a cell-mediated immune response, although it may contain something that exhibits lymphokine activity. Further work is needed to clarify the possible involvement of the immune mechanism in disc degeneration.

Disc Nutrition. Intradiscal pH measurements show that the pH is low in degenerated discs.[112] This was found to be due to increased lactate levels.[113] Since lactate is a product of anaerobic metabolism and the disc in young adults is avascular, disc nutrition was investigated to determine a possible contributing factor. Solute diffusion occurs through the anulus and central portion of the endplate[114] where vascular contacts are made. These contacts are reduced in degeneration. The cellularity of the disc is greatest in the anulus,[115] and by calculating energy requirements it was found that the center of the disc was unable to support much cellular activity. Glucose and oxygen enter the disc via the endplate and anulus,[115] but sulfate, an anion, is partially excluded by the polyanionic glycosaminoglycans of the nucleus and enters primarily by the anulus.[115] It is postulated that changes in the endplate with a consequence of nutritional deprivation may have a role in disc degeneration.

Biomechanical Factors. Mechanical factors are of importance in disc degeneration, and not just those due to an upright position, since dogs and other animals have disc degeneration.[117,118] The area of the spine subjected to the most mechanical stress appears to fail. Extensive intradiscal pressure studies have been performed and reviewed by Nachemson[71] and have shown that the nucleus acts as a liquid contained by the anular fibers. When the disc is loaded, intradiscal pressure exceeds the applied axial force with particularly high tensile stresses in the posterior anulus where herniations are most common. Axial loads per se produce failure first in the vertebral body with fracture of the subchondral endplate.[119] Schmorl's nodes can result, representing nuclear herniations through an endplate fracture.[120] Farfan[121] believes that rotational forces are the most important forces involved, producing early outer anular cracks with progression of the cracks until a radial fissure forms, allowing nuclear herniation. Progressive damage occurs with degenerative changes occurring in the posterior facet joints. A complete biomechanical description of the disc is not yet available, and there is a need to correlate the mechanical data with biologic status.[122]

Intradiscal pressure measurements by Nachemson[71] have given invaluable insight into measures used in the management of low back pain and its prevention. Postural and dynamic lifting measurements have shown the optimal positions to minimize intradiscal pressure. Lumbar supports are of benefit, and isometric exercises reduce the load delivered to the lumbar spine by traditional exercises. In this manner patients can be guided to better back hygiene and particularly stressful maneuvers can be avoided.

Clinical States and Treatment. Degenerative disc disease can present with backache and no nerve root entrapment or with nerve root involvement with or without backache. As the disc degenerates, segmental instability is produced and abnormal degrees of motion are permitted. This produces excessive motion and subluxation in the facet joints which undergo small degrees of trauma and can fracture.[43] As the disc loses height, further subluxation of the facets occurs, and degenerative arthritis in these joints is the sequela. Disc degeneration may remain asymptomatic, may be symptomatic because of changes in the disc itself, or may be symptomatic because of trauma in the facet joints and ligaments. Root entrapment occurs when roots are involved in disc herniations or entrapment by settling structures or osteophytic processes, yielding pain with discogenic or neurogenic claudication mechanics. The differences are presumably on the basis of different pathophysiologic mechanisms involving nociception to a radicular irritation or inflammatory phenomenon versus radicular ischemia.

Backache without nerve involvement is managed conservatively. Pain can be prolonged, lasting up to 3 months in 87 percent of those affected,[8] and has a 60 percent incidence of recurrent bouts within the first year of an attack. It is managed with bedrest, analgesics, muscle relaxants, corsets, weight loss, and exercises that emphasize back stretching and abdominal strengthening. Bed rest can decrease discomfort and hasten recovery, but analgesics do not speed recovery and nonsteroidal anti-inflammatories are ineffective.[123] Outlines of treatment programs vary with the treating physician but usually follow these measures.[34,124] Spinal fusion may be warranted in cases of chronic backache, but thorough investigation of the patient, including a psychological assessment,[124,125] is required to give some preoperative estimate of the likelihood of success.

Lumbar nerve root entrapment in disc degeneration was classically ascribed to disc herniation.[13] With anular radial fissures, the nucleus, as long as it is mobile, can herniate. The nomenclature describing disc herniations has been confusing, but certain patterns are established (Fig. 30-8). If the nucleus is confined by a few outer

Concealed

localized bulge   diffuse bulge

Prolapsed

sequestered

Figure 30–8. A classification of disc herniations.

anular fibers so that it does not enter the epidural space, it may present as a concealed disc with a localized or diffuse anular bulge. If the anular fibers are disrupted so that the nucleus leaves the confines of the anulus and enters the epidural space, it is prolapsed. If a piece of herniated material breaks off and is free in the epidural space, it is a sequestered disc or free fragment. The mechanism of root pain is not clear. Originally it was thought to be compression, but root compression is not necessarily found at surgery. All observers agree that involved roots exhibit stages of inflammation and that these inflamed roots will reproduce sciatic symptoms when stimulated. There is biopsy substantiation of intraneural inflammation.[111] Possible mechanisms of neural damage have been reviewed by Murphy.[126]

Symptoms of disc herniation may include backache, backache and sciatica, sciatica, and those of cauda equina compression. The onset is usually sudden and severe. Sciatic symptoms are radicular in nature and are exacerbated by activities such as Valsalva maneuvers and bending, which increase intradiscal pressure. Signs present are those reflecting root tension; these have been outlined previously. The phenomenon of sciatic scoliosis may suggest the relation of the herniation to the root. If the herniation is lateral to the root, the patient leans away from the symptomatic side. He leans toward the symptomatic side if the herniation is medial to the root. The clinical examination is directed toward establishing the diagnosis as accurately as possible. Neurologic symptoms give the correct level only 46 percent of the time,[47] whereas signs raise the accuracy to about 75 percent. Complete loss of a reflex is much more reliable as a diagnostic sign than simple depression.[31] A positive straight leg raising test is 75 to 80 percent diagnostically accurate, with crossed straight leg raising almost pathognomonic for disc herniation. Electromyography raises diagnostic accuracy to 80 percent.[127] Plain radiographs are essentially nondiagnostic. Water-soluble myelography raises accuracy to 90 to 95 percent.

Conservative therapy for disc herniation centers on bed rest, analgesics, muscle relaxants, and anti-inflammatory medications. Pelvic traction may be of benefit in some patients. The degree of bed rest is dependent on the severity of symptoms. Once they abate, a program of exercises and back protection is started. For severe symptoms more enforced bed rest over a 2-week period is used. Most disc herniations respond to conservative therapy, but in those that are unresponsive further measures may be needed.

Chemonucleolysis, the injection of chymopapain into the disc space, is now available in the United States. When previously in use it had about a 75 percent rate of good results, about the same as laminectomy and discectomy.[128] More recent studies indicate an 89 percent good result.[129] It is indicated in patients with a proven disc herniation who would otherwise be surgical candidates. Other techniques available for symptomatic relief are facet blocks[21] and radiofrequency facet denervation.[53] Intrathecal and epidural steroids have had some success in the symptomatic relief of discogenic pain,[130] although some authors find it no better than placebo.[131] Nerve root sleeve infiltrations with steroid may give relief.[124] Intradiscal steroids have been used.[132]

The one indisputable indication for surgery for removal of a disc is the cauda equina syndrome, in which a central midline herniation causes paralysis of the sacral roots, with bladder and bowel dysfunction and inability to walk (see Table 30–2). It occurs in about 2.4 percent of operative disc herniations.[133] The loss of bladder and bowel function is disastrous and return is limited, so that this entity is a true surgical emergency. Perineal anesthesia seldom recovers, and bladder paralysis may have a worse rate of recovery than somatic sensory deficits.[134]

Other indications for laminectomy are marked muscular weakness and progressive neurologic deficit in spite of bed rest.[124,125] There have been studies to dispute these indications as absolute. Andersson and Carlsson[135] found that the time since onset, duration of symptoms, and operative findings have no relationship to the return of motor activity in foot drop secondary to disc herniation. Estimates of motor return after loss from disc herniation are 50[23] to 80[136] percent and are not different in operative compared with nonoperative patients. After 1 year of followup the prognosis of motor return is no better after delayed surgery than with conservative therapy. Immediate surgical treatment is regarded as adequate therapy for the pain of disc herniation, but there is some doubt as to the use of paresis as an indication.[30]

Relative indications for laminectomy are intolerable

pain unrelieved by bed rest and recurrent episodes of incapacitating pain. Laminectomy for definite disc herniation remains a highly successful procedure.[2,68,133] Hirsch and Nachemson[68] reported that if disc herniation is a prolapse, 96 percent of operative patients have improvement. If concealed disc herniation is found with scarring and inflammation the predominant findings, 70 percent of patients have relief regardless of whether or not the disc is removed. Improvement in these patients is a matter of degree, and only 15 percent have complete and permanent relief. The remainder are improved but have recurrent symptoms. About one third will have persistent backache after discectomy.[133] The relationship between complete prolapse and a high degree of relief after surgery has been substantiated in other series.[133] Negative explorations prolong disability.[23] The overall long-term relief of sciatica has been shown to be the same in operative versus nonoperative patients, although the operative patients achieve their degree of relief more rapidly.[23] These studies imply that a relative indication for surgery offering optimal results is the emotionally stable patient with unequivocal disc herniation who for personal and socioeconomic reasons cannot sustain prolonged or repeated bouts of incapacitating pain. The most common cause for surgical failure is poor initial patient selection.[137]

Adhesive radiculitis is a condition in which the nerve root is found to be extensively involved in fibrous tissue in proximity to a disc space. It is presumably the result of chronic inflammation and clinically presents with persistent sciatic pain. Neurolysis is the only treatment, but the results are variable.

The remainder of the lumbar root entrapment syndromes fall into the broad definition of degenerative spinal stenosis. They are predominantly bony entrapments. As these are changes resulting from more advanced disc degeneration, they usually occur in patients over age 50. Prior to this, disc herniation is the common cause of radicular pain, but over age 50 bony entrapment predominates. The entrapment may be more lateral, giving only root symptoms, or more central, giving cauda equina symptoms. Unlike those with disc herniations, patients with these spinal stenosis syndromes have a long history of back pain and more recent sciatica. There is often a claudicating character to the pain, with pain in the back or in the legs with walking. The pain is not relieved by standing still but rather by flexing the back, as in sitting. Therefore these patients can walk up hills more easily than down and can bicycle, but cannot tolerate lumbar extension. These changes are usually progressive. There may be bowel and bladder symptoms, with the latter mimicking prostatic bladder outlet obstruction. These patients do not give marked root tension signs such as straight leg raising and may have multiple levels of root involvement. Radiographs reveal changes of degenerative disc disease with disc height narrowing, facet subluxation and degeneration, retrolisthesis, and pseudospondylolisthesis. The cross section of the spinal canal is difficult to visualize, but can be done with trans-

verse axial tomography,[138] and computed axial tomography[139] has dramatically lessened the difficulty. Myelography[84] reveals the canal diameter. In the anteroposterior dimension it is normally a minimum of 14 to 15 mm.[140,141] Degenerative stenotic changes are noted centrally at the discs, producing hourglass waisting of the contrast column by a thickened ligamentum flavum and bulging degenerative discs (Fig. 30–3). Peripherally the facets produce "cut-off" root sleeves produced by subluxation and osteophyte formation, leading to canal and foraminal encroachment. Water-soluble contrast media will give better definition of lateral entrapment by filling the root sleeve more fully. CT scan (Fig. 30–6) easily demonstrates the entrapment via disc, bone, and ligamentum flavum.

Macnab has described a variety of root entrapment syndromes resulting from degenerative change.[41,76,124] Central stenosis can occur with the bulging degenerative disc and posteriorly with a "shingling" overlap of the laminae, thickening of the ligamentum flavum, and subluxation and osteophyte formation in the facet joints. Subarticular entrapment occurs when the superior articular facet enlarges and compresses the root against a bulging disc or against the dorsum of a vertebral body. Foraminal encroachment occurs in the foramen where the superior facet lies in close relationship to the root. With subluxation and osteophytic outgrowths from the facet and the vertebral body, the root may be entrapped. Pedicular kinking occurs when there is loss of disc height, particularly asymmetrically whereby the root is kinked by the descending pedicle and commonly is entrapped between a bulging disc and a pedicle about it. Extraforaminal entrapment occurs after the root has left the foramen where it may be involved in diffuse or discrete anular bulge and, in the case of L5, trapped by the corporotransverse ligament against the sacral ala.

The treatment of all these spinal stenosis syndromes with severe symptoms is surgical, with emphasis placed on adequate decompression of the entrapped roots.[76,142] Once the symptoms are severe, they tend not to improve. If symptoms are not severe, regimens of back protection, isometric exercises, back supports, and anti-inflammatory medications are used. Operation is withheld until symptoms are no longer tolerable. Neurologic changes are not usually severe enough to warrant surgery. The symptomatic relief offered by adequate surgical decompression is considered particularly good.[142]

Systemic Inflammatory Disease of the Low Back. Rheumatoid arthritis is known to involve the lumbar spine. An increased incidence of subluxation and disc narrowing, apophyseal destruction, and osteoporosis was found in rheumatoid patients.[143] Rheumatoid erosions in facet joints have been demonstrated by stereoscopic radiographic examination.[144]

The inflammatory spondyloarthropathies, of which ankylosing spondylitis is the prototype, produce back pain of a diffuse and often severe nature.[145-149] They are discussed in detail in Section VI.

Hyperostotic spondylosis, described by Forestier and

Rotes-Querol,[150] is a disease of new bone formation in the thoracic and thoracolumbar spine. The spine stiffens and spurs form at multiple levels, often forming a bony ankylosis more marked on the right side of the spine. The disc spaces remain intact.[151] There may be subperiosteal new bone formation in the pelvis.[152] The cause is unknown, but there is associated glucose intolerance, diabetes, and obesity.[153]

Infections. *Pyogenic Vertebral Osteomyelitis.* Hematogenous osteomyelitis has a predilection for the vertebral column,[154,155] and pyogenic vertebral osteomyelitis has a predilection for older adults.[156] This is felt to be secondary to the marked vascularity of adult vertebrae[154] with seeding of the capillary beds at the endplate while the disc has no vascular channels in the adult.[157] An associated causative factor is that the incidence of urinary tract infections rises in adults, and these organisms may be seeded to the vertebrae by Batson's plexus, the vertebral, ascending lumbar, and sacral veins, freely communicating with the external vertebral, internal vertebral, and intraosseous vertebral veins.[158,159] Pyogenic infection then starts in the vertebral body and frequently involves the next body by spread to the epidural space and formation of an abscess, with compression, fracture, and collapse of the involved vertebra and spinal cord vascular compromise. These complications, plus bacteremia, accounted for most of the deaths in the older literature. Mortality now is expected to be less than 10 percent.[160]

Staphylococcus aureus traditionally has been the responsible organism, but gram-negative bacilli, especially related to genitourinary manipulations, are increasingly common.[156,161-163]

Patients present with backache of slow onset with or without radicular symptoms, low-grade fever, night sweats, and weight loss.[164] Paravertebral and hamstring spasms are present. Diabetes is frequently associated and should be sought.[155,165] The sedimentation rate is elevated, but the white blood cell count may be normal. Early radiographic signs are an eroded subchondral endplate, followed by involvement of the adjacent vertebra and loss of disc height. There is progressive loss of disc height over 6 to 8 weeks, progressive bony destruction, and reactive bone formation. Serial radiographs help to confirm the diagnosis.[166] Bone scan is useful in early detection. Multiple blood cultures and urine cultures should be obtained to determine the responsible organism. A biopsy for culture, either by closed Craig needle biopsy or open biopsy, is strongly advised, especially if blood cultures are negative. Antibiotics are recommended for 6 weeks[156] with monitoring of blood levels of the appropriate antibiotic to achieve bactericidal levels. The sedimentation rate can be used to follow the disease.[165,167] Bed rest is used during the treatment period, and a plaster jacket is used for 3 months. Fusion occurs in half the patients within 1 year, and most patients obliterate the disc space over 2 years.

Disc Space Infections. Disc space infections can result from any procedure inoculating the disc space. The most common is disc excision, the incidence of which is estimated to be 1 to 2.8 percent.[168,169] The hallmark of the disease is severe, excruciating pain, which may have an onset as late as 3 months postoperatively; in some cases, however, postoperative pain may not disappear but increase. There is marked muscle spasm. Laboratory evidence is not present or is obscured by the recent operation, although an elevated sedimentation rate after operation will normally fall over 3 months. Aspiration biopsy of the disc space is needed to determine the specific organism and its antibiotic sensitivity. Radiographic signs include dissolution of the subchondral bone but lag behind clinical signs by 2 to 3 weeks. There is a progression of loss of disc space height and sclerotic bony reaction.[170] Bone scan is of no diagnostic value because of postoperative changes. The disc space often goes on to fusion when infected.[171] Treatment is with antibiotics and cast immobilization.

Disc space infections in children are different from pyogenic vertebral osteomyelitis and offer a different prognosis.[172] They also differ from adult postoperative disc space infections. An irritable child will have progressive backache or limp, or refuse to walk. Night pain is common. There is paravertebral spasm. Early radiographic findings are absent. Later, progressive loss of disc space height with irregularity of the vertebral endplates is seen. The sedimentation rate is elevated. *Staphylococcus aureus* is the most common organism. Gallium bone scan may be useful for early detection.[54] Treatment is aimed toward 6 to 12 weeks of immobilization in a body jacket or spica cast. Antibiotics are not necessarily indicated and may not affect prognosis. They should be used when pain is not relieved by immobilization, when paravertebral spasm does not subside, or if the sedimentation rate remains elevated and the child is systemically ill. Aspiration biopsy is recommended if there are progressive and prolonged symptoms despite prolonged immobilization.

Other Infections of the Spine. Nontubercular granulomatous infections of the spine are widely reported and have been reviewed by Pritchard.[173] Blastomycosis in the vertebrae infects the disc space, adjacent bodies, and frequently the adjacent ribs. Cryptococcosis of the spine is uncommon and is thought to be hematogenous in origin. It produces little periosteal reaction and has lucent lesions. Actinomycosis may involve the anterior and posterior elements and has a tendency toward paravertebral abscesses. The vertebral body produces a "soap bubble" radiographic appearance, and the disc is spared. Coccidioidomycosis usually causes multiple vertebral lesions with relative sparing of the disc space. Brucellosis has a spondylitic form with involvement of the disc and adjacent vertebra.

Tuberculosis of the spine is now found primarily in third world countries. The spine accounts for about half the cases of bone and joint tuberculosis. There is a predilection for L1 to be the most commonly involved vertebra, and this is thought to be due to invasion by bacteria transported from the urinary tract via Batson's plexus.[174] The vertebral body is invaded and the disc is spared. The symptoms are insidious backache, increasing over many months. Constitutional symptoms can usually be elicited and paravertebral spasm with an acute kyphosis is found on examination. The sedimentation rate is elevated. Radiographs initially reveal osteopenia, followed by erosion on each side of the disc. Collapse follows, producing a variety of radiographic signs described by Hodgson[174] as concertina collapse, aneurysmal syndrome, lateral deviation, bony bridging, reversal of height-width ratio of the body, and wedging of the intervertebral disc. Paraplegia is a relatively frequent complication. Management is with multiple drug therapy; there is debate about the role of surgery and immobilization.[173]

Syphilitic spondylitis is rare,[120] and occurs secondary to gummatous destruction with collapse and a great deal of reactive bone. The more common manifestation is that of destructive change with excessive bony reaction from a Charcot neuropathic arthropathy, usually at the thoracolumbar junction.

Hydatid disease of bone is known but rare. The midthoracic spine is usually involved and the vertebral body is permeated by cysts, which often progress into the spinal canal. Vertebral collapse is common because of pathologic fractures. The incidence of paraplegia is high, as is the mortality.[175]

Spondylolysis and Spondylolisthesis. Spondylolisthesis designates a slipping of one vertebra forward on the one below. Spondylolysis indicates a separation at the pars interarticularis, permitting the slipping or "olisthesis." A classification of spondylolysis and spondylolisthesis has been proposed (Table 30–5).[176] Spondylolysis and, more frequently, spondylolisthesis can be involved with back pain. As previously noted, a pars interarticularis defect increases the incidence of back pain.[49] A vertebra may slip forward on the one below as a whole, or it may separate at the isthmus and slip. The entire unit may slip with subluxated posterior facets in degenerative or pseudospondylolisthesis. The slippage is graded either as a percent subluxation or I to IV by quarterly increments of slipping.

In the dysplastic type there is congenital dysplasia of the upper sacrum or the neural arch of L5 and the lowest free lumbar vertebra slips forward, usually in adolescence. The pars may remain unchanged, and the slippage will not exceed 25 percent, preventing cauda equina

Table 30–5. Classification of Spondylolysis and Spondylolisthesis

Dysplastic—congenital abnormalities of the upper sacrum or the arch of L5 allow the olisthesis
Isthmic—a pars interarticularis lesion of one of three types:
  Lytic—fatigue fracture of the pars
  Elongated, but intact pars
  Acute fracture
Degenerative—secondary to longstanding intervertebral instability
Traumatic—secondary to bony fractures in areas other than the pars
Pathological—secondary to generalized or local bone disease

paralysis. Usually the pars elongates or separates. Dysplastic changes of the upper sacrum with inadequate development of the L5 to S1 facets most commonly produce the instability.[177] The pars is often dysplastic, and the sacrum and L5 may have a wide spina bifida, giving rise to a high-grade slippage. It appears to be twice as common in girls as in boys.[176]

Isthmic spondylolisthesis involves a lesion in the pars interarticularis. The lytic lesion is a separation of the pars and is a fatigue fracture.[178] It is the most common type in patients less than 50 years old and is rarely seen in those less than 5 years old. The incidence in white children is 5 percent at 7 years and increases to 5.8 percent by 18 years old, mostly during the 11- to 15-year-old period.[176] There is a hereditary component,[179] the incidence increasing to 35 percent in families in which one member has spondylolysis or spondylolisthesis. Female gymnasts have been noted to have a fourfold increase in pars defects and spondylolisthesis,[180] and football interior linemen have an even higher incidence over the normal population.[181] Of the mechanical forces involved—flexion overload, unbalanced shear forces, and forced rotation—it is not yet known[182,183] which is primarily responsible for the slippage.

Elongation of the pars without separation is the same disease as the lytic lesion, but with repeated microfractures healing in an elongated position. The pars may taper out and then separate, in which case the defect is reclassified as lytic. Acute pars fractures are secondary to trauma and usually have only spondylolysis without slippage.

Degenerative spondylolisthesis is secondary to degenerative disc disease, with intersegmental instability[81,120] producing a local spinal stenosis. It is seldom seen before the age of 50, is ten times more frequent at L4 than at L5 or L3, is six times more frequent in women, and is three times more frequent in blacks. Sacralization is four times more frequent in degenerative spondylolisthesis as in the general population. It does not occur with spina bifida or isthmic spondylolisthesis, and the slippage is never more than 30 percent. Predisposing factors are a straight, stable lumbosacral joint putting more stress on the L4-5 facets. The disc and ligaments degenerate and allow hypermobility and facet degeneration, permitting forward slipping.[184]

Traumatic spondylolisthesis is secondary to a fracture in the posterior elements other than the pars such as a facet or pedicle.[176]

Pathological spondylolisthesis is due to a local or generalized bone disease in the pedicle, pars, or facets, where the forward forces are inadequately opposed and forward slippage results. It is known in osteopetrosis with pars fractures giving spondylolysis, arthrogryposis in Eskimos,[185] Paget's disease with pars elongation, syphilis secondary to gummas,[186] neurogenic arthropathies, tuberculous spondylitis, giant cell tumors of the posterior elements, and metastatic tumors.[177] Spondylolysis and spondylolisthesis aquisita are known to occur at the upper end of lumbar spine fusions[187-192] and are reported below a thoracolumbar scoliosis fusion.[193]

These are complications and are not seen with lateral fusions.[176]

Management of spondylolisthesis is age and lesion dependent. Wiltse and Jackson[194] have provided guidelines for the management of children with spondylolisthesis. A child, especially if less than 10 years old, who is found to have an isthmic spondylolisthesis is examined, and radiographs obtained, every 4 months for a year, then every 6 months up to the age of 15, then annually until growth is completed. This is especially important in girls, who have twice the incidence of high-grade olisthesis (slippage). In cases with up to 25 percent slippage and without symptoms, the child is followed and advised to avoid a career of heavy labor. In those with up to 50 percent slippage without symptoms, avoidance of traumatic sports is recommended. Those children with symptoms but recovery by conservative measures are followed. In a child with greater than 50 percent slippage, fusion is recommended regardless of symptoms. A child with persistent symptoms regardless of degree of slippage is advised to undergo fusion. A child less than 10 years old with a 50 percent slippage is often fused. Slippage will usually occur before 18 years of age if it is going to occur and rarely past 25 years of age. The most rapid slippage is between 9 and 15 years of age.[195] The onset of pain may be sudden and produce a "listhetic crisis" with the sudden onset of backache. On examination, a rigid lumbar spine, spastic scoliosis, flattened sacrum, and often hamstring spasm are found. There is usually no nerve root involvement; but if such involvement is present, laminectomy and possibly decompression will be required in addition to lumbosacral fusion.[124]

The presence of a pars defect does not mean that it is always the cause of back pain. Macnab[124] examined a large series of patients with backache and found a 7.6 percent incidence of pars defects, similar to the overall incidence in asymptomatic individuals. Dividing these patients by age, he showed that for those over 40 years of age the incidence is the same as in the general population. Under 26, however, about 19 percent of symptomatic individuals had a defect. Therefore if the patient is younger than 26, the defect is probably the cause of the back pain. Between ages 26 and 40 it is possibly the cause. Over age 40 it is rarely the cause.

Root irritation can occur with lytic spondylolisthesis by a variety of mechanisms. The neural arch of L5 may rotate forward on the sacrum and encroach on the foramen. Small ossicles and traction spurs make foraminal encroachment worse. Bony entrapment, described by Macnab,[124] occurs with forward and downward descent. The pedicles may kink the roots. Disc degeneration with bulging may cause entrapment lateral to the foramen. The corporotransverse ligament of L5 may compress the L5 root against the sacral ala with descent of L5. Disc herniation of L4-5 may involve the L5 root. Disc degeneration itself may be painful, and in patients over 35 lumbodorsal disc degeneration may be symptomatic.[124] Therefore clinical evaluation with myelography and root sleeve injection is necessary in the older patient with

back pain and spondylolisthesis. Foramenotomy may be necessary with fusion if there is a long history of backache. In this case discography is used to determine the upper extent of the fusion. If there is L4-5 degeneration or the slip is greater than 50 percent, an L4-S1 fusion is indicated.

In adults older than 40 with painful spondylolisthesis, the Gill procedure of removal of the loose posterior elements has been successful.[196] In adults without evidence of root entrapment and minimal slip, Newman[197] recommends direct repair of the defect.

Degenerative spondylolisthesis is a form of local spinal stenosis and a result of disc degeneration. It produces root entrapment and cauda equina symptoms with back pain, sciatic symptoms, and occasionally spinal claudication symptoms. Ten percent of Rosenberg's series[184] came to decompression. The question of fusion is unresolved. Guidelines of management are essentially those for degenerative disc disease and spinal stenosis.

Nonspinal Sources of Back Pain. Back pain can occur from disorders of the abdominal, retroperitoneal, and pelvic viscera, but it is rarely the only symptom. Pain is referred in a dermatomal distribution from viscera and is not aggravated by activity or relieved by rest, as is most pain of spinal origin. Peptic ulcer disease, gastric, duodenal, and pancreatic tumors, retroperitoneal lymphoma, sarcoma, and colonic tumors can all give rise to back pain. Retroperitoneal bleeding in anticoagulated patients can give back pain. In the pelvis, endometriosis and uterine, cervical, and bladder invasive carcinoma may give back pain, and tumors invading the lumbosacral plexus give rise to radicular pain. Sacral menstrual pain occurs, and uterine malposition and prolapse can give rise to sacral pain with standing. Fibroids may cause back pain. Chronic prostatitis can give sacral pain. Renal pain is located in the costovertebral angle and frequently radiates to the groin and testis.

Abdominal aortic aneurysm may give rise to back pain, which is particularly acute during dissection. Intermittent claudication of peripheral vascular disease may mimic sciatic pain and can be confused with spinal stenosis, but can be differentiated by the relief of vascular claudication pain on standing still.

References

1. Horal, J.: The clinical appearance of low back disorders in the city of Gothenburg, Sweden. Acta Orthop. Scand. Suppl. 118, 1969.
2. Hirsch, C.: Efficiency of surgery in low-back disorders. J. Bone Joint Surg. 47A:991, 1965.
3. Kelsey, J.L., and White, A.A.: Epidemiology and impact of low back pain. Spine 5:133, 1980.
4. Wood, P.H.N., and MacLeish, C.L.: Digest of data on the rheumatic diseases. 5. Morbidity in industry and rheumatism in general practice. Ann. Rheum. Dis. 33:93, 1974.
5. Hult, L.: The Munk Fors investigation. Acta Orthop. Scand. Suppl. 16, 1954.
6. Anderson, J.A.D.: Back pain in industry. In Jayson, M. (ed.): The Lumbar Spine and Back Pain. London, Sector Publishing, Ltd., 1976.
7. Glover, J.R.: Prevention of back pain. In Jayson, M. (ed.): The Lumbar Spine and Back Pain. London, Sector Publishing, Ltd., 1976.
8. Berquist-Ullman, M., and Larsson, U.: Acute low back pain in industry. Acta Orthop. Scand. Suppl. 170, 1977.
9. Wood, P.H.N.: Epidemiology of back pain. In Jayson, M. (ed.): The Lumbar Spine and Back Pain. London, Sector Publishing, Ltd., 1976.

466 General Approach to the Patient

10. Benn, R.T., and Wood, P.H.N.: Pain in the back: An attempt to estimate the size of the problem. Rheum. Rehab. 14:121, 1975.
11. Frymoyer, J.W., Pope, M.H., Cogtanza, M.C., Rosa, J.C., Goggin, J.E., and Wilder, D.G.: Epidemiologic studies of low back pain. Spine 5:419, 1980.
12. Akeson, W.H., and Murphy, R.W.: Low back pain. Clin. Orthop. 129:2, 1977.
13. Mixter, W.J., and Barr, J.S.: Rupture of the intervertebral disc with involvement of the spinal canal. N. Engl. J. Med. 211:210, 1934.
14. Hirsch, C.: Etiology and pathogenesis of low back pain. Israel J. Med. Sci. 2:362, 1966.
15. Kelsey, J.L.: An epidemiological study of acutely herniated lumbar intervertebral discs. Rheum. Rehab. 14:144, 1975.
16. Edgar, M.A., and Ghadially, J.A.: Innervation of the lumbar spine. Clin. Orthop. 115:35, 1976.
17. Luschka, H.: Die Nerven des menschlichen Wibelkanales. Verlag der H. Lappschen Buchhandelung P. V. 4850:8:1, 1850.
18. Smyth, M.J., and Wright, V.J.: Sciatica and the intervertebral disk. An experimental study. J. Bone Joint Surg. 40A:1401, 1958.
19. Kellgren, J.H.: Observations on referred pain arising from muscle. Clin. Sci. 3:175, 1938.
20. Hirsch, C., Ingelmark, B., and Miller, M.: The anatomical basis for low back pain. Acta Orthop. Scand. 33:1, 1963.
21. Mooney, V., and Robertson, J.: The facet syndrome. Clin. Orthop. 115:149, 1976.
22. Nachemson, A.L.: The natural course of low back pain. In White, A.A. and Gordon, S.L. (eds.): A.A.O.S. Symposium on Idiopathic Low Back Pain. St. Louis, C. V. Mosby Company, 1982, p. 46.
23. Hakelius, A.: Long term follow-up in sciatica. Acta Orthop. Scand. Suppl. 129, 1972.
24. Mankin, H.J., and Adams, R.D.: Pain in the back and neck. In Thorn, G.W., Adams, R.D., Braunwald, E., Isselbacher, K.J., and Petersdorf, R.G. (eds.): Harrison's Principles of Internal Medicine. 8th ed. New York, McGraw-Hill Book Company, 1977.
25. Macnab, I.: The "whiplash syndrome." Orthop. Clin. North Am. 2:389, 1971.
26. Wilfling, F.J., Klonoff, H., and Kokan, P.: Psychological, demographic and orthopaedic factors associated with prediction of outcome of spinal fusion. Clin. Orthop. 90:153, 1973.
27. White, A.W.M.: The compensation back. Applied Therap. 8:871, 1966.
28. Wiltse, L.L., and Rocchio, P.D.: Preoperative psychologic tests as predictors of success of chemonucleolysis in the treatment of low-back syndrome. J. Bone Joint Surg. 57A:478, 1975.
29. Rothman, R.H., and Simeone, F.A.: Lumbar disc disease. In Rothman, R.H., and Simeone, F.A. (eds.): The Spine. Philadelphia, W. B. Saunders Company, 1975.
30. Weber, H.: The effect of delayed disc surgery on muscular paresis. Acta Orthop. Scand. 46:631, 1975.
31. Hakelius, A., and Hindmarsh, J.: The significance of neurologic signs and myelographic findings in the diagnosis of lumbar root compression. Acta Orthop. Scand. 43:239, 1972.
32. Sprangfort, E.: Lasegue's sign in patients with lumbar disc herniation. Acta Orthop. Scand. 42:459, 1971.
33. Hoppenfeld, S.: Physical Examination of the Spine and Extremities. New York, Appleton-Century Crofts, 1976.
34. Finneson, B.E.: Low Back Pain. Philadelphia, J. B. Lippincott Company, 1973.
35. Wiltse, L.L.: Lumbosacral strain and instability. In American Academy of Orthopedic Surgeons: Symposium on the Spine. St. Louis, C. V. Mosby Company, 1969.
36. Caldwell, A.B., and Chase, C.: Diagnosis and treatment of personality factors in low back pain. Clin. Orthop. 129:141, 1977.
37. Ransford, A.O., Cairns, D., and Mooney, V.: The pain drawing as an aid to the psychologic evaluation of patients with low back pain. Spine 1:127, 1976.
38. Sternbach, R.A.: Psychologic aspects of chronic pain. Clin. Orthop. 129:150, 1977.
39. Fordyce, W.E., Fowler, R.S., Lehman, J.F., DeLateur, B.J., Sand, P.L., and Trieschmann, R.B.: Operant conditioning in the treatment of chronic pain. Arch. Phys. Med. Rehab. 54:399, 1973.
40. Anderson, T.P., Cole, T.M., Gullickson, G., Hudgens, A., and Roberts, A.H.: Behavior modification of chronic pain: A treatment program by a multidisciplinary team. Clin. Orthop. 129:97, 1977.
41. Macnab, I.: Surgical treatment of degenerative disc disease of the lumbar spine. In McKibbin, B. (ed.): Recent Advances in Orthopaedics. Edinburgh, Churchill Livingstone, 1975.
42. Park, W.: Radiological investigation of the intervertebral disc. In Jayson, M. (ed.): The Lumbar Spine and Back Pain. London, Sector Publishing, Ltd., 1976.
43. Liang, M., and Komaroff, A.L.: Roentgenograms in primary care patients with acute low back pain. A cost-effective analysis. Arch. Intern. Med. 142:1108, 1982.

44. Harris, R.I., and Macnab, I.: Structural changes in the lumbar intervertebral discs. Their relationship to low back pain and sciatica. J. Bone Joint Surg. 36B:304, 1954.
45. Edeiken, J., and Pitt, M.J.: The radiologic diagnosis of disc disease. Orthop. Clin. North Am. 2:405, 1971.
46. Lawrence, J.S.: Disc degeneration. Its frequency and relationship to symptoms. Ann. Rheum. Dis. 28:121, 1969.
47. Hakelius, A., and Hindmarsh, J.: The comparative reliability of preoperative diagnostic methods in lumbar disc surgery. Acta Orthop. Scand. 43:234, 1972.
48. Epstein, B.: The Spine. A Radiological Text and Atlas. 3rd ed. Philadelphia, Lea & Febiger, 1969.
49. Wiltse, L.L.: The effect of common anomalies of the lumbar spine upon disc degeneration and low back pain. Orthop. Clin. North Am. 2:569, 1971.
50. Farfan, H.F., and Sullivan, J.D.: The relation of facet orientation to intervertebral disc failure. Can. J. Surg. 10:179, 1967.
51. Collis, D.K., and Ponseti, I.V.: Long term followup of patients with idiopathic scoliosis not treated surgically. J. Bone Joint Surg. 51A:425, 1969.
52. Roche, M.B., and Rowe, G.G.: The incidence of separate neural arch and coincident bone variations. Anat. Rec. 109:233, 1951.
53. Shealy, C.N.: Facet denervation in the management of back and sciatic pain. Clin. Orthop. 115:157, 1976.
54. Norris, S.H., Ehrlich, M.G., McKusick, K., and Provine, H.: The radioisotope study of an experimental model of disc space infection. J. Bone Joint Surg. 60B:281, 1978.
55. Lindblom, K.: Diagnostic puncture of intervertebral discs in sciatica. Acta Orthop. Scand. 7:321, 1948.
56. Cloward, R.B., and Buzaid, L.L.: Discography technique—indications and evaluation of normal and abnormal intervertebral disc. Am. J. Roentgenol. 68:552, 1952.
57. Collis, J.S., and Gardner, W.J.: Lumbar discography—an analysis of 1000 cases. J. Neurosurg. 19:452, 1962.
58. Massie, W.K., and Stevens, D.B.: A critical evaluation of discography. J. Bone Joint Surg. 49A:1243, 1967.
59. Wiley, J.J., Macnab, I., and Wortzman, G.: Lumbar discography and its applications. Can. J. Surg. 11:280, 1968.
60. Garrick, J.G., and Sullivan, C.R.: Long-term effects of diskography in dogs. Minn. Med. 53:81, 1970.
61. Key, J.A., and Ford, L.T.: Experimental intervertebral disc lesions. J. Bone Joint Surg. 30A:621, 1948.
62. Goldie, I.: Intervertebral disc changes after discography. Acta Chir. Scand. 113:438, 1957.
63. DeSeze, S., and Levernieux, J.: Accidents in discography. Rev. Rheum. 19:1027, 1952.
64. Gresham, J.L., and Miller, R.: Evaluation of the lumbar spine by diskography and its use in selection of proper treatment of the herniated disk syndrome. Clin. Orthop. 67:29, 1969.
65. Holt, E.P.: The question of lumbar discography. J. Bone Joint Surg. 50A:720, 1968.
66. Friberg, S., and Hult, L.: Comparative study of Abrodil myelogram and operative findings in low back pain and sciatica. Acta Orthop. Scand. 20:303, 1951.
67. Luyendijk, W., and Van Voorthuisen, A.E.: Contrast examination of the spinal epidural space. Acta Radiol. Scand. 5:1051, 1966.
68. Hirsch, C., and Nachemson, A.: The reliability of lumbar disc surgery. Clin. Orthop. 29:189, 1963.
69. Post, M.J.D., Brown, M.D., and Gargano, F.P.: The technique and interpretation of lumbar myelograms. Spine 2:214, 1977.
70. McNeill, T.W., Huncke, B., Kornblatt, I., Stiehl, J., and Kahn, H.A.:A new advance in water-soluble myelography. Spine 1:72, 1976.
71. Nachemson, A.: The lumbar spine. An orthopaedic challenge. Spine 1:59, 1976.
72. Macnab, I., St. Louis, E.L., Grabias, S.L., and Jacob, R.: Selective ascending lumbosacral venography in the assessment of lumbar-disc herniation. J. Bone Joint Surg. 58A:1093, 1976.
73. Hitselberger, W.A., and Witten, R.M.: Abnormal myelograms in asymptomatic patients. J. Neurosurg. 32:132, 1970.
74. Mathews, J.A.: Epidurography—a technique for diagnosis and research. In Jayson, M. (ed.): The Lumbar Spine and Back Pain. London, Sector Publishing, Ltd., 1976.
75. Arnoldi, C.C., Brodsky, A.E., Cauchoix, J., Crock, H.V., Dommisse, G.F., Edgar, M.A., Gargano, F.P., Jacobson, R.E., Kirkaldy-Willis, W.H., Kurihara, A., Langerskjold, A., Macnab, I., McIvor, G.W.D., Newman, P.H., Paine, K.W.E., Russin, L.A., Sheldon, J., Tile, M., Urist, M.R., Wilson, W.E., and Wiltse, L.L.: Lumbar spinal stenosis and nerve root entrapment syndrome. Definition and classification. Clin. Orthop. 115:4, 1976.
76. Macnab, I.: Negative disc exploration. An analysis of causes of nerve-root involvement in sixty-eight patients. J. Bone Joint Surg. 53A:891, 1971.

77. Verbeist, H.: A radicular syndrome from developmental narrowing of the lumbar vertebral canal. J. Bone Joint Surg. 36B:230, 1954.
78. Verbeist, H.: Further experiences on the pathological influence on the developmental narrowness of the lumbar vertebral canal. J. Bone Joint Surg. 37B:576, 1955.
79. Kirkaldy-Willis, W.H., Paine, K.W.E., Cauchoix, J., and McIvor, G.W.D.: Lumbar spinal stenosis. Clin. Orthop. 99:30, 1974.
80. Schatzker, J., and Pennal, G.F.: Spinal stenosis. A cause of cauda equina compression. J. Bone Joint Surg. 50B:606, 1968.
81. Macnab, I.: Spondylolisthesis with an intact neural arch. The so-called pseudospondylolisthesis. J. Bone Joint Surg. 32B:325, 1950.
82. Schlesinger, E.B., and Taveres, J.M.: Factors in the production of "cauda equina" syndromes in lumbar discs. Trans. Am. Neurol. Assoc. 78:263, 1953.
83. Lipson, S.J., Naheedy, M.H., Kaplan, M.M., and Bienfang, D.C.: Spinal stenosis caused by epidural lipomatosis in Cushing's syndrome. N. Engl. J. Med. 302:36, 1980.
84. McIvor, G.W.D., and Kirkaldy-Willis, W.H.: Pathologic and myelographic changes in the major types of lumbar spinal stenosis. Clin. Orthop. 115:72, 1976.
85. Coventry, M.B., Ghormley, R.K., and Kernohan, J.W.: The intervertebral disc: Its microscopic anatomy and pathology. Part II. Changes in the intervertebral disc concomitant with age. J. Bone Joint Surg. 27A:233, 1945.
86. Coventry, M.B., Ghormley, R.I., and Kernohan, J.W.: The intervertebral disc: Its microscopic anatomy and pathology. Part III. Pathological changes in the intervertebral disc. J. Bone Joint Surg. 27A:460, 1945.
87. Eckert, C., and Decker, A.: Pathological studies of intervertebral discs. J. Bone Joint Surg. 29A:447, 1947.
88. Naylor, A.: Intervertebral disc prolapse and degeneration. The biochemical and biophysical approach. Spine 1:108, 1976.
89. Bushell, G.R., Ghosh, P., Taylor, T.K.F., and Akeson, W.H.: Proteoglycan chemistry of the intervertebral disks. Clin. Orthop. 129:115, 1977.
90. Ghosh, P., Bushell, G.R., Taylor, T.K.F., and Akeson, W.H.: Collagens, elastin and noncollagenous protein of the intervertebral disk. Clin. Orthop. 129:124, 1977.
91. Eyre, D.R., and Muir, H.: Collagen polymorphism: Two molecular species in pig intervertebral disc. FEBS Letters 42:192, 1974.
92. Eyre, D.R., and Muir, H.: Types I and II collagens in intervertebral disc. Interchanging radial distributions in annulus fibrosus. Biochem. J. 157:267, 1976.
93. Herbert, C.M., Lindberg, K.A., Jayson, M.I.V., and Bailey, A.J.: Intervertebral disc collagen in degenerative disc disease. Ann. Rheum. Dis. 34:467, 1975.
94. Naylor, A., Shentall, R.D., and Micklethwaite, B.: An electron microscopic study of segment long spacing collagen from the intervertebral disc. Orthop. Clin. North Am. 8:217, 1977.
95. Herbert, C.M., Lindberg, K.A., Jayson, M.I.V., and Bailey, A.J.: Changes in collagen of human intervertebral disks during aging and degenerative disk disease. J. Molec. Med. 1:79, 1975.
96. Pearson, C.H., Happey, F., Naylor, A., and Turner, R.L.: Collagens and associated glycoproteins in the human intervertebral disk. Variations in sugar and amino acid composition in relation to location and age. Ann. Rheum. Dis. 31:45, 1972.
97. Blakely, P.R., Happey, F., Naylor, A., and Turner, R.L.: Protein in the nucleus pulposus of the intervertebral disk. Nature 195:73, 1962.
98. Gower, W.E., and Pedrini, V.: Age-related variations in proteinpolysaccharides from human nucleus pulposus, annulus fibrosus and costal cartilage. J. Bone Joint Surg. 51A:1154, 1969.
99. Adams, P., and Muir, H.: Qualitative changes with age of proteoglycans of human lumbar discs. Ann. Rheum. Dis. 35:289, 1976.
100. Hardingham, T.E., and Adams, P.: A method for the determination of hyaluronate in the presence of other glycosaminoglycans and its application to human intervertebral disc. Biochem. J. 159:143, 1976.
101. Stevens, R.L., Ewins, R.J.F., and Muir, H.: Proteoglycans of the intervertebral disc: Homology of structure with laryngeal proteoglycans. Biochem. J. 179:561, 1979.
102. Comper, W.D., and Preston, B.N.: Model connective tissue systems. A study of polyion-mobile ion and of excluded volume interactions of proteoglycans. Biochem. J. 143:1, 1974.
103. Bobechko, W.P., and Hirsch, C.: Autoimmune response to nucleus pulposus in the rabbit. J. Bone Joint Surg. 47B:574, 1965.
104. Naylor, A., Happey, F., Turner, R.L., Shentall, R.D., West, D.C., and Richardson, C.: Enzymic and immunological activity in the intervertebral disc. Orthop. Clin. North Am. 6:51, 1975.
105. Gertzbein, S.D., Tile, M., Gross, A., and Falk, R.: Autoimmunity in degenerative disc disease of the lumbar spine. Orthop. Clin. North Am. 6:67, 1975.
106. Elves, M.W., Bucknill, T., and Sullivan, M.F.: In vitro inhibition of leucocyte migration in patients with intervertebral disc lesions. Orthop. Clin. North Am. 6:59, 1975.
107. Gertzbein, S.D., Tait, J.H., and Devlin, S.R.: The stimulation of lymphocytes by nucleus pulposus in patients with degenerative disc disease of the lumbar spine. Clin. Orthop. 123:149, 1977.
108. Bisla, R.S., Marchisello, P.J., Lockshin, M.D., Hart D.M., Marcus, R.E., and Granda, J.: Autoimmunological basis of disk degeneration. Clin. Orthop. 121:206, 1976.
109. Lindblom, K., and Hultqvist, G.: Absorption of protruded disc tissue. J. Bone Joint Surg. 32A:557, 1950.
110. Smith, J.W., and Walmsley, R.: Experimental incision of the intervertebral disc. J. Bone Joint Surg. 33B:612, 1951.
111. Lindahl, O., and Rexed, G.: Histologic changes in spinal nerve roots of operated cases of sciatica. Acta Orthop. Scand. 20:215, 1951.
112. Nachemson, A.: Intradiscal measurements of pH in patients with lumbar rhizopathies. Acta Orthop. Scand. 40:23, 1969.
113. Diamant, B., Karlsson, J., and Nachemson, A.: Correlation between lactate levels and pH in discs of patients with lumbar rhizopathies. Experientia 24:1195, 1968.
114. Nachemson, A., Lewin, T., Maroudas, A., and Freeman, M.A.R.: In vitro diffusion of dye through endplates in the annulus fibrosus of human lumbar intervertebral disks. Acta Orthop. Scand. 41:589, 1970.
115. Maroudas, A., Stockwell, R.A., Nachemson, A., and Urban, J.: Factors involved in the nutrition of human lumbar intervertebral disk: Cellularity and diffusion of glucose in vitro. J. Anat. 120:113, 1975.
116. Urban, J.P.G., Holm, S., Maroudas, A., and Nachemson, A.: Nutrition of the intervertebral disk. An in vivo study of solute transport. Clin. Orthop. 129:101, 1977.
117. Olsson, S.E.: On disc protrusion in dog. Acta Orthop. Scand. Suppl. 8, 1951.
118. Hansen, H.J.: Comparative views on the pathology of disk degeneration in animals. Lab. Invest. 8:1242, 1959.
119. Rolander, S.D., and Blair, W.E.: Deformation and fracture of the lumbar vertebral endplate. Orthop. Clin. North Am. 6:75, 1975.
120. Junghanns, H., and Schmorl, G.: The Human Spine in Health and Disease. New York, Grune & Stratton, 1959.
121. Farfan, H.E.: A reorientation in the surgical approach to degenerative lumbar intervertebral joint disease. Orthop. Clin. North Am. 8:9, 1977.
122. Akeson, W.H., Woo, S.L.Y., Taylor, T.K.F., Ghosh, P., and Bushell, G.R.: Biomechanics and biochemistry of the intervertebral disks: The need for correlation studies. Clin. Orthop. 129:133, 1977.
123. Wiesel, J.W., Cuckler, J.M., DeLuca, F., James, F., Zeide, M.S., and Rothman, R.H.: Acute low back pain. An objective analysis of conservative therapy. Spine 5:324, 1980.
124. Macnab, I.: Backache. Baltimore, Williams & Wilkins Company, 1977.
125. Wiltse, L.L.: Surgery for intervertebral disk disease of the lumbar spine. Clin. Orthop. 129:22, 1977.
126. Murphy, R.W.: Nerve roots and spinal nerves in degenerative disk disease. Clin. Orthop. 129:47, 1977.
127. Knuttson, B.: Comparative value of electromyographic, myelographic and clinical neurological examination in diagnosis of lumbar root compression syndrome. Acta Orthop. Scand. Suppl. 49, 1961.
128. Nordby, E.J., and Brown, M.D.: Present status of chymopapain and chemonucleolysis. Clin. Orthop. 129:79, 1977.
129. McCulloch, J.A.: Chemonucleolysis: Experience with 2000 cases. Clin. Orthop. 146:128, 1980.
130. Brown, F.W.: Management of diskogenic pain using epidural and intrathecal steroids. Clin. Orthop. 129:72, 1977.
131. Snoek, W., Weber, H., and Jorgensen, B.: Double blind evaluation of extradural methylprednisolone for herniated lumbar discs. Acta Orthop. Scand. 48:635, 1977.
132. Feffer, H.L.: Therapeutic intradiscal hydrocortisone. A long term study. Clin. Orthop. 67:100, 1969.
133. Spangfort, E.V.: The lumbar disc herniation. A computer aided analysis of 2,504 operations. Acta Orthop. Scand. Suppl. 142, 1972.
134. Scott, R.J.: Bladder paralysis in cauda equina lesions from disc prolapse. J. Bone Joint Surg. 47B:224, 1965.
135. Andersson, H., and Carlsson, C.A.: Prognosis of operatively treated lumbar disc herniation causing foot extensor paralysis. Acta Chir. Scand. 132:501, 1966.
136. Weber, H.: An evaluation of conservative and surgical treatment of lumbar disc protrusion. J. Oslo City Hosp. 20:81, 1970.
137. Spengler, D.M., Freeman, C., Westbrook, R., and Miller, J.W.: Low back pain following multiple spine procedures. Failure of initial selection? Spine 5:356, 1980.
138. Sheldon, J.J., Russin, L.A., and Gargano, F.P.: Lumbar spinal stenosis. Radiographic diagnosis with special reference to transverse axial tomography. Clin. Orthop. 115:53, 1976.
139. Hammerschlag, S.B., Wolpert, S.M., and Carter, B.L.: Computed tomography of the spinal canal. Radiology 121:361, 1976.
140. Eisenstein, S.: Measurements of the lumbar spinal canal in 2 racial groups. Clin. Orthop. 115:53, 1976.
141. Paine, K.W.E., and Huang, P.W.H.: Lumbar disc syndrome. J. Neurosurg. 37:75, 1972.

142. Wiltse, L.L., Kirkaldy-Willis, W.H., and McIvor, G.W.D.: The treatment of spinal stenosis. Clin. Orthop. 115:83, 1976.

143. Lawrence, J.S., Sharp, J., Ball, J., and Bier, F.: Rheumatoid arthritis of the lumbar spine. Ann. Rheum. Dis. 23:205, 1964.

144. Sims-Williams, H., Jayson, M.I.V., and Baddeley, H.: Rheumatoid involvement of the lumbar spine. Ann. Rheum. Dis. 36:524, 1977.

145. West, H.F.: The aetiology of ankylosing spondylitis. Ann. Rheum. Dis. 8:143, 1949.

146. Lawrence, J.S.: The prevalence of arthritis. Br. J. Clin. Pract. 17:699, 1963.

147. deBlecourt, J.J., and deBlecourt-Meindersma, T.: Hereditary factors in rheumatoid arthritis and ankylosing spondylitis. Ann. Rheum. Dis. 20:215, 1961.

148. Schlosstein, L., Terasaki, P.I., Bluestone, R., and Pearson, C.M.: High association of HL-A antigen W27 with ankylosing spondylitis. N. Engl. J. Med. 288:704, 1973.

149. Brewerton, D.A., Caffrey, M., Hart, F.D., James, D.C.O., Nicholls, A., and Sturrock, R.D.: Ankylosing spondylitis and HL-A-27. Lancet 1:904, 1973.

150. Forestier, J., and Rotes-Querol, J.: Senile ankylosing hyperostosis of the spine. Ann. Rheum. Dis. 9:321, 1950.

151. Vernon-Roberts, B., Pirie, C.J., and Trenwith, V.: Pathology of the dorsal spine in ankylosing hyperostosis. Ann. Rheum. Dis. 33:281, 1974.

152. Harris, J., Carter, A.R., Glick, R.N., and Storey, G.O.: Ankylosing hyperostosis: Clinical and radiological features. Ann. Rheum. Dis. 33:210, 1974.

153. Julkunen, H., Heinonen, O.P., and Pyorala, K.: Hyperostosis of the spine in an adult population. Its relation to hyperglycemia and obesity. Ann. Rheum. Dis. 30:605, 1971.

154. Wiley, A.M., and Trueta, J.: The vascular anatomy of the spine and its relation to pyogenic vertebral osteomyelitis. J. Bone Joint Surg. 41B:796, 1959.

155. Stone, D.B., and Bonfiglio, M.: Pyogenic vertebral osteomyelitis: A diagnostic pitfall for the internist. Arch. Intern. Med. 112:491, 1963.

156. Waldvogel, F.A., Medoff, G., and Swartz, M.N.: Osteomyelitis: A review of clinical features, therapeutic considerations and unusual aspects (third of three parts). N. Engl. J. Med. 282:316, 1970.

157. Crock, H.V., Yoshzava, H., and Kame, S.K.: Observations on the venous drainage of the human vertebral body. J. Bone Joint Surg. 55B:528, 1973.

158. Batson, O.V.: The function of the vertebral veins and their role in the spread of metastasis. Ann. Surg. 112:138, 1940.

159. Batson, O.V.: The vertebral vein system. Am. J. Roentgenol. 78:195, 1957.

160. Musher, D.M., Thorsteinsson, S.B., Minuth, J.N., and Luchi, R.J.: Vertebral osteomyelitis: Still a diagnostic pitfall. Arch. Intern. Med. 136:105, 1976.

161. Stauffer, R.N.: Pyogenic vertebral osteomyelitis. Orthop. Clin. North Am. 6:1015, 1975.

162. Wedge, J.H., Onyschak, A.F., Robertson, D.E., and Kirkaldy-Willis, W.H.: Atypical manifestations of spinal infections. Clin. Orthop. 123:155, 1977.

163. Ross, P.M., and Fleming J.L.: Vertebral body osteomyelitis: Spectrum and natural history. Clin. Orthop. 118:190, 1976.

164. Bonfiglio, M., Lange, T.A., and Kim, Y.M.: Pyogenic vertebral osteomyelitis. Clin. Orthop. 96:234, 1973.

165. Garcia, A., and Grantham, S.A.: Hematogenous pyogenic vertebral osteomyelitis. J. Bone Joint Surg. 42A:429, 1960.

166. Guri, J.P.: Pyogenic osteomyelitis of the spine. Differential diagnosis through clinical and roentgenographic observations. J. Bone Joint Surg. 28A:29, 1946.

167. Griffiths, H.E.D., and Jones, D.M.: Pyogenic infection of the spine. J. Bone Joint Surg. 53B:383, 1971.

168. Ford, L.T., and Key, J.A.: Postoperative infection of the intervertebral disc space. South. Med. J. 48:1295, 1955.

169. Pilgaard, S.: Discitis (closed space infection) following removal of lumbar intervertebral disc. J. Bone Joint Surg. 51A: 713, 1969.

170. Thibodeau, A.A.: Closed space infection following removal of lumbar intervertebral disc. J. Bone Joint Surg. 50A:400, 1968.

171. Sullivan, C.R., Bickel, W.H., and Svien, H.J.: Infections of vertebral interspaces after operations on the intervertebral disks. JAMA 166:1973, 1958.

172. Boston, H.C., Bianco, A.J., and Rhodes, K.H.: Disk space infections in children. Orthop. Clin. North Am. 6:953, 1975.

173. Pritchard, D.J.: Granulomatous infections of bones and joints. Orthop. Clin. North Am. 6:1029, 1975.

174. Hodgson, A.R.: Infectious disease of the spine. In Rothman, R H., and Simeone, F. A. (eds.): The Spine. Philadelphia, W. B. Saunders Company, 1975.

175. Alldred, A.J., and Nisket, N.W.: Hydatid disease of bone in Australasia. J. Bone Joint Surg. 46B:260, 1964.

176. Wiltse, L.L., Newman, P.H., and Macnab, I.: Classification of spondylolysis and spondylolisthesis. Clin. Orthop. 117:30, 1976.

177. Taillard, W.F.: Etiology of spondylolisthesis. Clin. Orthop. 117:30, 1976.

178. Wiltse, L.L., Widell, E.H., and Jackson, D.W.: Fatigue fracture: The basic lesion in isthmic spondylolisthesis. J. Bone Joint Surg. 57A:17, 1975.

179. Wiltse, L.L.: Etiology of spondylolisthesis. Clin. Orthop. 10:45, 1957.

180. Jackson, D.W., Wiltse, L.L., and Cirincione, R.J.: Spondylolysis in the female gymnast. Clin. Orthop. 117:68, 1976.

181. Ferguson, R.J.: Low-back pain in college football lineman. J. Bone Joint Surg. 56A:1300, 1974.

182. Farfan, H.F., Osteria, V., and Lamy, C.: The mechanical etiology of spondylolysis and spondylolisthesis. Clin. Orthop. 117:40, 1976.

183. Troup, J.D.G.: Mechanical factors in spondylolisthesis and spondylolysis. Clin. Orthop. 117:59, 1976.

184. Rosenberg, N.J.: Degenerative spondylolisthesis. J. Bone Joint Surg. 57A:4, 1975.

185. Petajan, J., Momberger, G., Aase, J., and Wright, D.G.: Arthrogryposis syndrome (Kusokwim disease) in the Eskimo. JAMA 209:1481, 1969.

186. Karaharjii, E., and Hummuksela, M.: Possible syphilitic spondylitis. Acta Orthop. Scand. 44:289, 1973.

187. Anderson, C.E.: Spondyloschisis following spine fusion. J. Bone Joint Surg. 38A:1142, 1956.

188. Harris, R.I., and Wiley, J.J.: Acquired spondylolisthesis as a sequel to spine fusion. J. Bone Joint Surg. 45A:1159, 1963.

189. Unander-Scharin, L.: A case of spondylolisthesis lumbalis aquisita. Acta Orthop. Scand. 19:536, 1950.

190. DePalma, A.F., and Marme, P.J.: Spondylolysis following spine fusion. Clin. Orthop. 15:208, 1959.

191. Harrington, P.R., and Tullos, H.S.: Spondylolisthesis in children. Clin. Orthop. 79:75, 1971.

192. Strayer, L.M., Risser, J.C., and Waugh, T.R.: Results of spine fusion for scoliosis twenty-five years or more after surgery. J. Bone Joint Surg. 51A:205, 1969.

193. Tietjen, R., and Morgenstern, J.M.: Spondylolisthesis following surgical fusion for scoliosis. Clin. Orthop. 117:176, 1976.

194. Wiltse, L.L., and Jackson, D.W.: Treatment of spondylolisthesis and spondylolysis in children. Clin. Orthop. 117:92, 1976.

195. Laurent, L.E., and Einola, S.: Spondylolischisis in children and adolescents. Acta Orthop. Scand. 82:45, 1961.
Osterman, K., Lindholm, T.S., and Laurent, L.E.: Late results of removal of the loose posterior element (Gill's operation) in the treatment of lytic lumbar spondylolisthesis. Clin. Orthop. 117:121, 1976.

197. Newman, P.H.: Surgical treatment for spondylolisthesis in the adult. Clin. Orthop. 117:106, 1976.

Chapter 31
The Painful Foot

Bruce Wood

THE NORMAL FOOT

Normal feet should perhaps be defined as feet capable of providing pain-free function throughout a wide range of reasonable physical activities. More rigid definitions of normal structure and function become difficult as one encounters numerous structural variations which offer little or no impediment to function. Obversely, feet that could by other criteria be defined as "normal" may present severe functional limitations and challenge the most astute clinician.

The foot is an extremely adaptive organ, capable of functioning under extreme conditions imposed by both environmental and activity demands. Numerous small joints provide flexibility and adaptability; and yet when needed for walking or running propulsion, these same joints under the combined forces of gravity and muscle action transform the foot into an efficient rigid propulsive lever.[1]

The skin on the weight-bearing plantar surface is thick and, together with the dense fat pads under the calcaneus and metatarsal heads, provides protection against shear and impact stress.

The transition from normality to presentation of symptoms is often a gradual process clinically, except in the presence of acute traumatic, inflammatory, or infectious processes.

Symptoms presenting in the foot may be the first indication of numerous systemic disorders, such as diabetes mellitus, rheumatoid arthritis, gout, and occlusive vascular diseases. It is important when evaluating foot symptoms to consider the systemic ramifications that may be a factor in foot pain or dysfunction. The occurrence of swelling, sensory changes, skin changes, and deformity, while often found as local problems, may be associated with systemic disorders as well.

OSTEOARTHRITIS—DEGENERATIVE JOINT DISEASE

A National Health survey conducted between 1960 and 1962 showed a prevalance of osteoarthritis in feet to be nearly 20 percent in a population between 18 and 79 years of age. As would be expected, the incidence rose sharply in the fifth and sixth decades. At ages 75 to 79 the incidence was 48.6 percent for males and 53.1 percent for females. In this same age group moderate to severe arthritis was three times more prevalent in women, with 14.6 percent of women and 4.8 percent of men being reported with foot involvement.[2]

From a biomechanical standpoint, any change in the functional mechanisms of the foot may produce pain and dysfunction. Continued use or overuse of biomechanically deficient feet, together with trauma, is probably the most common precipating factor in secondary degenerative joint disease in the foot. The first metatarsophalangeal joint is a frequent site for a variety of degenerative changes ranging from cartilage erosion and bursitis to joint rigidity secondary to osteophyte formation with or without the presence of bunions and hallux valgus.

The Hallux and Lesser Toes. Among the most common and easily identified deformities are bunions, hallux valgus, and hammer toes. Hallux valgus refers to an abnormal position of the great or first toe in which the toe is deviated laterally or in a fibular direction. In relation to the sagittal plane of the body, this change may be defined as a position of abduction. Occasionally the toe will also rotate or evert about its long axis. The deformity occurs principally at the first metatarsophalangeal joint, where positional changes ranging from slight deviation to frank dislocation are found. In addition to the deviation of the first toe, the first metatarsal usually deviates medially or to a position of adduction in relation to the sagittal plane. In the presence of this deformity, the head of the first metatarsal becomes prominent medially. This bony prominence, or bunion, may be normal in size or may be significantly enlarged. As static deformities, symptoms may be less severe than suggested by the deformity; but under the stress of function, particularly in a shoe incapable of accommodating the deformity, pain and secondary lesions occur frequently. In the absence of inflammatory or other connective tissue disorders, these deformities are probably related to inherited structural factors. Persons, particularly between the ages of 30 and 50, with such predisposing factors are likely to develop these deformities, especially in the presence of obesity, inappropriate shoes, and prolonged periods of overuse of their feet.[1,31] These deformities do not usually occur as single entities but rather are seen in combination. The lateral displacement of the hallux interferes with the lesser toes and may lead to contracture deformities and overlapping toes. The hammer toe is the most common lesser toe deformity and may occur singly or multiply. The deformity is characterized by hyperextension at the metatarsophalangeal joint and marked flexion at the proximal interphalangeal joint.

Dorsally contracted digits, particularly the second toe, may exert retrograde and plantar forces on the metatarsal heads, causing pain and perhaps skin lesions under the metatarsal heads. Frequently corns may develop secondary to shoe pressure over the prominent proximal interphalangeal joints. As these deformities develop, muscle imbalances occur, which encourage further progressions of the deformity.[4,5]

Gout. The classic picture of gout at the first metatarsophalangeal joint, podagra, is usually quite evident with a history of sudden onset and rather extreme pain to both touch and motion. The adjacent soft tissues and skin are moderately inflamed and swollen. The necessary differential diagnosis from infection in some cases is made by the absence of streaks and node hypertrophy as well as by the response to medication. Often the acute attack has subsided before the laboratory has confirmed the presence of synovial fluid crystals or determined serum uric acid levels. (See Chapter 86.) Tophaceous gout often leaves residual foot deformities requiring special shoe modifications to prevent excess weight bearing and subsequent tissue breakdown over prominent tophaceous lesions. Occasionally surgical reconstruction of deformities is necessary.

Osteophytes over the dorsal area of the first metatarsophalangeal joint may initially cause an extensor tendinitis resulting from the irritation of tendon and sheath as the tendon glides over or is pressed against the bony prominence. Further growth of osteophytes results in painful impingement (hallux limitus, Fig. 31–1), reducing the capability of dorsiflexion, a motion essential in each normal gait cycle. The end result is hallux rigidus when no motion is possible. Although interfering with gait and shoe fit, the rigid toe is much less painful than hallux limitus. Local inflammation of the tendon, synovium, or bursa may be treated with moist heat and steroid injections. An extended shank, sole stiffener, and rocker bar are shoe modifications that may decrease the need for full range of motion and therefore reduce pain. The eventual treatment often involves an arthroplasty to remove the osteophytes or, with cartilage damage, either a fusion or joint replacement procedure.

The patient with chronic pronation, particularly when the foot is subjected to excessive occupational or athletic stress and obesity, exerts high stresses upon improperly aligned midtarsal joints, leading to the formation of osteophytes dorsally at the talonavicular, navicular-cuneiform, and cuneiform-metatarsal joints. Although conclusive studies are not available, the talonavicular joint may well be the most commonly involved foot joint in osteoarthritis.[6] As with the first metatarsophalangeal joint, the extensor tendons lying over these prominences frequently develop tendinitis, especially when shoe pressures are excessive. Arthritis in this area is initially treated with appropriately fitted shoes and an orthosis to control pronation. Occasionally arthroplasty or fusion is indicated.

On a theoretical if not practical basis, degenerative joint disease secondary to chronic excessive pronation could be prevented if proper control of pronation is initiated early and maintained on a continuous basis.

Heel Pain. Chronic pronation results in attempts to stretch the medial and plantar connective tissue structures, especially the plantar calcaneonavicular or Spring

Figure 31–1. Hallux limitus showing degenerative joint changes with osteophytes.

ligament, the capsule of the calcaneotalonavicular joint, and the plantar fascia, an extensive and complex band of fibers binding the joints of the foot together plantarly.[7] The fascia is subjected to considerable tension, particularly at the area of its medial and plantar attachments to the tuberosity of the calcaneus. Continued tension of this inelastic tissue may result in periostitis at the calcaneal attachment, with eventual proliferative changes producing a plantar calcaneal spur. As with the calcaneal valgus and pronation seen in rheumatoid arthritis, the first concern is the mechanical control of the deformity and its causes. This may be done initially with a supportive dressing of adhesive tape and felt, followed with an orthosis. Following initial mechanical support, heat, ultrasound, anti-inflammatory agents, and injection may be used.

The etiology of heel pain includes numerous other medical and orthopedic diseases, ranging from ischemia and nerve entrapment to bursitis and fat pad atrophy. Identifying and managing the underlying disease or deformity is the obvious direction to follow, while local treatment is often less obvious.

There are three principal bursae and six major medial, lateral, and posterior tendons subject to inflammation in the heel area.[8,9] The Achilles, peroneus longus, and posterior tibial tendons are most frequently involved with tendinitis. The anatomic bursae are located as follows: (1) retrocalcaneal, located between the Achilles tendon and the posterior surface of the calcaneus just above the Achilles insertion; (2) superficial, located between the tendon and the overlying fascia; and (3) plantar calcaneal, located between the plantar aponeurosis (fascia) and the calcaneus. Inflammation of the posterior bursae may be in conjunction with or confused with Achilles tendinitis and is frequently caused and certainly aggravated by a rigid shoe counter, particularly in high heeled shoes or pumps. Occasionally a bony prominence is present at the posterior lateral aspect of the calcaneus, which, when subjected to shoe irritation, may develop a periostitis or adventitious bursitis. Rest, heat, protective padding, and occasionally steroid injection may help.

Caution must be exercised when considering a steroid injection in the region of the Achilles insertion, as tendon rupture and soft tissue necrosis have been reported in this area following such injections. In some instances these "pump bumps" may require surgical removal. Achilles tendinitis will have pain, swelling, and possibly heat and crepitus along its course just proximal to its insertion, while bursitis is more localized to the anatomic location of the bursae. Plantar bursitis may not be distinguishable from fasciitis or periostitis. Each is appropriately treated with rest, heat, anti-inflammatory drugs, or injection. A heel lift may be a helpful adjunct inasmuch as it reduces stress slightly in the region of the Achilles insertion. Short-term use of a short leg cast is sometimes necessary for this and other inflammatory conditions of foot and ankle structures. Chronic inflammation in the area of the retrocalcaneal bursa may cause erosive changes of the posterior aspect of the calcaneus. The quality and quantity of the plantar calcaneal fat pad can be readily palpated. On weight bearing it will occasionally bulge both medially and laterally owing to weakness or herniation of its fascial covering. This can sometimes be helped with a plastic heel cup and/or a $1/2$ inch thickness of Plastazote or similar cushioning substance. Rheumatoid nodules directly under the calcaneus, as in other weight-bearing areas, may be protected with a suitable cushion or aperture pad but may ultimately require excision. Sudden onset of pain in the heel area during activity of a strenuous nature may indicate rupture of the plantaris tendon, a small but lengthy tendon which inserts laterally either into the calcaneus or Achilles tendon.

NEUROPATHIC ARTHROPATHY— CHARCOT'S JOINT

While most inflammatory and degenerative connective tissue diseases of the foot are pain producing and disabling, Charcot joint disease or neuropathic arthropathy is unique for developing only in the presence of neuropathy. The loss of pain and proprioceptive responses allows joints and their soft tissues to exceed normal ranges of motion and develop significant joint instability. Ultimately, dislocation and deformity occur. Associated with the destructive process are swelling and hyperemia. Trauma, often only normal weight bearing on insensitive joints, is always a factor in this process. Diabetes mellitus is the most commonly associated disease, but neuropathic arthropathy may occur in a variety of neurologic diseases which are accompanied by diminished sensation and position sense such as tertiary syphilis, leprosy, and syringomyelia.

Typically, on initial presentation, Charcot feet are warm, swollen, and relatively nonpainful in proportion to clinical appearances. A common deformity is a broadening of the midtarsal region and a rocker bottom foot caused by collapse and destruction of the midtarsal structures. In the diabetic a strong pulse may be present. Charcot's joint should be suspected in the presence of long-term diabetes mellitus, swelling, and pain-free joint destruction out of proportion to the patient's complaint. Neuropathic ulcers may also be present, particularly on the sole of the foot. These may lead to osteomyelitis of the underlying weight-bearing bone, producing a very confusing radiographic picture. Initial treatment of non-weight-bearing rest in a nondependent position should be continued until swelling and erythema subside. This is followed by non-weight-bearing cast immobilization until complete bone repair is demonstrated radiographically. Ultimately the patient will require shoes which accurately accommodate and support the foot and therefore prevent further trauma and destruction.[1,10]

RHEUMATOID ARTHRITIS

The management and prevention of pain, deformity, and dysfunction in the rheumatoid arthritic foot have become increasingly important as total knee and hip joint replacement procedures provide significant and predictable improvement in lower extremity function. The goal of management, as with other joints, is to prevent or reduce deformity and pain and maintain or increase function.

It is important to differentiate between dysfunction resulting from an active inflammatory process and that resulting from structural or mechanical changes and certain pre-existing biomechanical defects. Within a large cross section of persons foot problems and minor disabilities are common, and when rheumatoid arthritis is superimposed, it is too easy to ascribe all foot pain to the rheumatoid arthritis.[11] This consideration is particularly important in the patient who has a preexisting peripheral vascular disease, neuropathy, diabetes mellitus, or structural abnormality.[12,13]

The foot presents no exception to the desirability of providing a team approach to management of rheumatoid arthritis, with rheumatologists, orthopedists, podiatrists, physical therapists, and orthotists working closely together. The treatment and management approach will vary, depending on the stage of the disease and the extent of functional loss, with prevention of pain and deformity being indicated in the early stages and surgical correction of deformity in the later stages.[14] In stages I and II early foot symptoms result from the inflammation, swelling, and thickening of synovial tissues and the accompanying inability to achieve free moving joint and muscle function both at rest and on weight bearing. In stages III and IV, following structural damage to the bones and joints, pain may be related to attempts to bear weight on mechanically altered structures, and frequently both inflammatory and structural changes will be responsible concurrently for pain.

History. Initial symptoms of rheumatoid arthritis are reported to appear in the feet in 17 to 20 percent of patients, while throughout the course of the disease foot involvement may reach 90 percent. Patients with early foot involvement will often report aching, pain, swelling, and change in their manner of walking. Less commonly encountered is pain of a sharp or shooting nature. The early symptoms are most frequent in the forefoot.[1,15,16] Initial swelling is often noted with the need, particularly by women, to change to a larger size shoe but without improvement of symptoms. Pain and dysfunction usually increase following periods of rest, particularly in early morning. Because of the diffuse nature of pain in the arthritic foot, patients are often unable to identify, locate, and quantify specific areas of pain; therefore close manual examination is needed. A careful foot history should determine any pre-existing congenital, familial, or acquired deformities as well as functional disabilities and limitations and the need for prior foot care.[17] Answers to this line of questioning will help differentiate present symptoms and may also be of assistance in treatment. As an example, calcaneal valgus and flat feet may occur with or without symptoms in the nonarthritic patient. Such a pre-existing situation could increase the severity of both deformity and pain if rheumatoid arthritis were to involve the rear foot[18-21] and should be treated early in the attempt to correct and prevent deformities. It is important to inquire about a person's prearthritic abilities. The patient with a pre-existing pronated foot or calcaneal valgus invariably reports, for example, poor ice skating ability because of "weak ankles," or in other sports a tendency to "sprain" or turn the ankles. Inquiry about relative pain and comfort associated with various shoe styles, materials, and walking surfaces can be helpful in selecting changes which will benefit the patient. The person whose forefoot pain is lessened while walking on a thick, well-padded carpet can be expected to do well with properly fitted compliant footwear or Plastazote* inner soles. Forefoot pain, particularly in patients with depressed metatarsal heads and displaced or absent fat pads, will often be likened to walking on marbles or a bed of coals.[3] A history of ankle pain or weakness often cannot be accepted as stated, for frequently the source of pain or instability is in the subtalar and talonavicular joints.[22] Associated with tal-

onavicular disease, peroneal muscle spasm can be a frequent source of leg pain.

Evaluation. Early diagnostic and evaluative processes should include recording baseline data to include neurological, vascular, and integumentary systems as well as assessments of gait function, deformity, range of motion, and relative muscle strengths. This baseline information is an essential reference point for measuring both progress and future treatment requirements. Note that the posterior tibial pulse may often be obscured by swelling and thickening in the tarsal tunnel area and that occasionally the posterior tibial nerve may be compressed in this same area.[23,24]

It is helpful to observe walking gait both with and without shoes, but pain may limit this examination to stance only. Normal heel-to-toe gait is a complicated mechanical function in which the posterior-lateral aspect of the heel strikes the walking surface and weight is rapidly transmitted along the lateral margin of the foot and across the ball of the foot, where a compliant fat pad absorbs some of the shear and impact force. During the gait cycle, the foot briefly pronates and then supinates just before push-off.[25,26] Any mechanical or disease process interfering with this function may produce pain.

Such mechanical shortcomings are of particular importance when the foot attempts to accommodate to the surface incongruities or otherwise uneven and inclined terrain. Pain and functional limitations of the knee and hip joints will also affect gait and foot function and must be considered in evaluation.[27] The rheumatoid patient with forefoot involvement often fails to push off from the ball of the foot and toes but rather will slide, shuffle, or lift the foot and place it forward. With rearfoot deformity, the foot may remain pronated (flattened) throughout the gait cycle. Biomechanically, long-term weight bearing on a pronated foot may encourage the development of further forefoot deformity and pain, especially hallux valgus, splaying, and metatarsalgia. Excessive pronations may also increase the internal rotary motion of the entire lower extremity, with resulting torsional stresses having an effect at both the knee and hip joints.[25]

Observe the standing and walking foot from all angles. At normal stance, the foot presents an upright calcaneus and straight Achilles tendon when viewed from behind. The rheumatoid foot, particularly with subtalar or talonavicular joint involvement, often presents a valgus attitude of the calcaneus and a flattening of the medial longitudinal arch (Fig. 31–2). In addition, the navicular becomes prominent medially and small skin creases may appear lateral to the heel. Typical forefoot deformities are easily recognized and consist of dorsally contracted digits or the so-called cockup toe deformity with dorsiflexion at the metatarsophalangeal joint and flexion of one or both of the interphalangeal joints.[1] Occasionally the interphalangeal joints will resemble swan neck or boutonnière deformities as seen in fingers. Hallux valgus, or hallux abductus, in which the great toe deviates laterally, is frequently seen, as in the prominent medial bunion whose apparent size is often accentuated by a

---

*Smith and Nephew, Ltd., Hertfordshire, England.

Figure 31–2. Rheumatoid foot showing calcaneal valgue, hallux abductus, bunions, and cockup toes.

splaying of the forefoot in the region of the metatarsal heads. The lesser toes, in addition to dorsal contraction, may also deviate laterally (fibular deviation) and often overlap one another or the great toe[28,29] (Fig. 31–3).

Range of Motion. Normal gait function requires an adequate joint excursion but with defined limits at each extreme, and it is necessary for all lower extremity joints to work in close harmony with each other. The range of motion may be decreased by fibrous ankylosis and bony impingement, soft tissue contractures, and pain, as well as by other extra-articular changes occurring in response to the disease. Similarly, joint excursions can be increased following destruction of the joint or its related supportive structures. Additionally, whether excursion is altered or not, the formal relation of one joint to another can be altered and thus affect function. An example of this is found with marked valgus deformity of the knee in the presence of normal ankle and foot joints. The valgus deformity at the knee is compensated for by a marked varus position in the subtalar joint.

The active and passive range of motion of the ankle, subtalar, midtarsal, and metatarsophalangeal joints should be recorded, and the strength of the muscles

Figure 31–4. *Left,* Non–weight-bearing foot depicting forefoot varus. *Right,* Compensatory rearfoot valgus as foot bears weight.

controlling these joints should be evaluated. The relationship of the forefoot to the rearfoot and of the rearfoot to the leg both on weight bearing and at rest should be noted, as well as the sites of pain with both active and passive motion. One will frequently note that the forefoot is in a varus position relative to the rearfoot, that is, the forefoot is in an inverted position relative to the heel. This may represent a compensatory adaptation to a rearfoot valgus[25] (Fig. 31–4); however, it is also seen in the nonarthritic foot in a large population cross section and often precedes and causes the compensatory rearfoot valgus. Deformity at the metatarsophalangeal joint may advance to the point of subluxation or dislocation with the base of one or more proximal phalanges displaced over the metatarsal head. This may be appreciated by palpation and is readily seen on radiographs.

Palpation. On examination note the presence of thickening or swelling and heat, particularly in the region of the ankle, at the Achilles tendon, and both dorsally and plantarly at the metatarsophalangeal joints. Note the locations of tenderness of both articular and nonarticular structures. Associated with cockup toes, the anatomical plantar fat pad which protects the ball of the foot from

Figure 31–3. Hallux abductus, overlapping toes, splaying of forefoot, and bunion.

Figure 31–5. Prominent metatarsal heads and atrophic fat pads.

shearing and impact stress is displaced anteriorly to a position where it is ineffective (Fig. 31–5). The plantar surface should be palpated to evaluate both the quality and quantity of the fat pad, the prominence of the metatarsal heads, and the presence of keratoses, bursae, and rheumatoid nodules. In addition, the fat pads under the heel may become atrophic. The plantar surface of the heel is a common site for the occurrence of symptomatic rheumatoid nodules. A Harris Mat imprint may be used to provide a graphic representation of those areas, particularly in the forefoot, which are subject to the greatest amounts of weight-bearing stress. Its principal value is in documentation and confirmation of clinical findings noted on careful manual examination (Fig. 31–6).

Examination of shoe wear on both the sole and inner sole provides further evidence of weight-bearing stress areas, while the heel and shoe counter provide graphic evidence of rearfoot deformity.

Tenderness. Inflammation can cause pain, swelling, or thickening of the joints of the ankle or foot; pain that is not significantly changed by rest is most likely secondary to inflammation. Common sites include the Achilles tendon along its distal portion and at its insertion. Localized tenderness anterior to the tendon just proximal to its insertion may represent a bursitis as well as tendinitis of the Achilles and its sheath.[8,9] Compression of the heel and palpation of the plantar surface of the os calcis may elicit pain, especially with Reiter's syndrome and psoriatic arthritis. Palpation medially and laterally at the talocalcaneal joint yields confusing results. Thickening of the joint synovium may cause pain, but along the medial aspect other sources of pain could be tendinitis or nerve entrapment in the tarsal tunnel. The metatarsal compression test, performed by compressing the metatarsal bones together, elicits pain be-

tween metatarsal heads in the presence of synovitis (Fig. 31–7). When compressing or squeezing this area, it is important that the pressure be exerted on the shafts of the first and fifth metatarsals rather than over the metatarsophalangeal joint. Further confirmation is made by palpating in the intermetatarsal head space. A more selective procedure to localize inflammatory pain con-

Figure 31–6. Harris Mat imprint showing areas of increased weight-bearing pressure under first and third metatarsal heads.

Figure 31-7. Metatarsal compression test exerts pressure on tissues in the intermetatarsal head spaces.

occlusive vascular disease, rheumatoid vasculitis, and the locations and effects of weight bearing and shoe pressure stresses.[30,31] Note especially the presence and locations of pressure-induced lesions such as corns and calluses, and particularly note if these lesions have ulcerated or become infected. It is not unusual to find a hematoma or extravasated blood under or within these keratotic lesions, particularly under the metatarsal heads and over the proximal interphalangeal joints of cockup toes. This is not only an indication of the degree of trauma inflicted upon the area, but more importantly represents a high risk area where continued trauma could be expected to produce an ulceration or abscess. Ulceration may be of a low grade, slowly evolving nature and is easily over-looked.

Careful debridement of plantar and digital lesions is essential both to aid in relief of pain and also to locate and treat ulcerations. Proprietary medications should never be used by patients to treat corns and calluses. Ulcerations are especially prevalent in those patients on long-term steroid therapy, as well as in patients with diabetes mellitus, large and small vessel disease, peripheral neuropathy, vasculitis, plantarly located nodules, and absent or atrophic plantar fat pads.[32] Ulcerative lesions and abscesses take on an even greater significance when joint replacement surgery of the hip and lower extremity has been performed or is contemplated, for these lesions may seed infection to the operated joint. Patients with vasculitis or on steroid therapy may develop small hemorrhagic lesions, and when located in the subungual or periungual areas these may become a focus for infection.

Verrucous lesions are not common in the adult population but when present are usually painful. These lesions can be distinguished from corns and calluses by

sists of dorsiflexing the toes, if not already in a cockup position, and applying direct digital pressure plantarly and distally at the point where the base of the toe joins the metatarsal head (Fig. 31-8A). This test can be used to distinguish between synovial joint pain and metatarsal head pain secondary to mechanical problems, which is noted by applying pressure directly on the plantar weight-bearing surface of the metatarsal head (Fig. 31-8B). Extensor tendinitis can be appreciated by applying gentle pressure over each extensor tendon while putting the digit through a full range of motion. Pain may be elicited, and additionally a fine crepitus may be felt. Plantar metatarsal head pain secondary to mechanical forces occurs most often under the second and third heads and somewhat less frequently under the fourth head. The fifth head and first, under which glide the sesamoid bones, are less frequently involved. The previously mentioned pronated foot with a varus forefoot exerts considerable stress on the second metatarsal and relatively less on the first, and it will be commonly noted in this circumstance that the second metatarsal head will be the most tender.[25] Radiography of the chronically pronated foot may demonstrate a relative hypertrophy of the second metatarsal shaft.

Skin Changes. The skin and its lesions are a good barometer of foot health and may indicate the extent of

Figure 31-8. *A*, Pressure applied at the joint space and capsule may differentiate pain secondary to synovitis. *B*, Pain in response to pressure directly on the metatarsal head is more likely to be of mechanical origin.

the presence of multiple papillae with dark-colored blood clots of pinpoint size which bleed freely when the surface callus is removed. Rheumatoid nodules are frequently noted in the foot, appearing usually adjacent to bony prominences in both the forefoot and heel areas. They may be a source of pain from shoe and weight-bearing pressure, and may also occasionally ulcerate or become abscessed.

The arthritic patient often has difficulty caring for nails, and family members and nurses are often fearful or unwilling to perform this task. The periungual and subungual tissue offer a fertile medium for both bacterial and mycotic infection. Neglected nails, particularly in the presence of digital deformity, will frequently abrade or lacerate adjacent soft tissues, causing both pain and infection. Repetitive pressure of as little as 5 pounds per square inch, a quantity easily achieved with shoe pressure upon thickened nails, will cause development of subungual abscesses, especially in the diabetic, vascular diseased, neuropathic, or debilitated patient.[12] Such subungual abscesses may readily initiate an osteomyelitis of the distal phalanx. Appropriate attention to and care of the nails constitute a small but essential element in the management of the rheumatoid foot. Intertriginous areas of skin must be protected from maceration, abrasion, and infection.

The periodic care of even minor lesions could be essential to the health of the arthritic patient, particularly in the presence of lower extremity joint replacements.

Radiography. Radiography is essential to proper evaluation to assess both the extent of bone and joint destruction and the functional and mechanical alterations, as well as the approaches to be taken to deal with these problems. The standard views, anteroposterior, lateral, and lateral oblique, will be adequate in most instances; however, the medial oblique may occasionally be helpful. Less frequently required but of great value when taken properly are the Harris view, which displays the subtalar joints, and the axial metatarsal view, which profiles the weight-bearing condylar sufaces and sesamoids in the ball of the foot. When evaluating structural relationships and changes, the three standard views should be taken with the patient standing. With some radiographic equipment this is a difficult task, but relatively inexpensive equipment is available which is specially designed for weight-bearing foot films. The significance of a weight-bearing film can be appreciated by comparing weight-bearing and non-weight-bearing views of the same foot. It will be noted that most deformities become much more apparent or actually increase under the force of gravity and weight bearing. This is particularly true with valgus rearfoot deformities, hallux valgus, and splaying of the metatarsal heads. The location of the metatarsal head lesions is usually quite obvious in rheumatoid feet; when questions arise, a small lead marker on the lesion will clearly identify the metatarsal head associated with the lesion.

Less conventional radiological techniques may be of value in selected cases. Fine detail radiography with optical magnification has the capability of identifying erosive changes in small joints earlier and in a detail not appreciated with standard views.[33] This technique may also aid in clarifying the early presence of osteomyelitis, although a bone scan is more sensitive in this important determination. Xerography, as well as fine detail and magnification, can be of value in more clearly defining soft tissue changes and masses. Persistent pain and an elusive diagnosis, especially in the rear- and midfoot, may be indications for CT scanning. The talocaneal joints and the angular relationships of the tarsal joints can be evaluated effectively with this technique.[34] (See Chapter 39.)

Rearfoot and Midfoot. Patients will frequently attribute symptoms of pain, swelling, stiffness, and weakness to the ankle when in fact their disease is more likely to be in the subtalar or midtarsal joints.[20] In one clinical study, rearfoot pain interfered with walking in 16 percent of patients, while 42 percent reported some rearfoot disability.[20] Normal ankles move in one plane only, that being flexion and extension (dorsiflexion) in the sagittal plane. Motion of the foot from side to side (inversion and eversion) occurs primarily in the subtalar joint. Normal subtalar motion is about 30 degrees; when measured from a neutral position, inversion is greater than eversion in a 2:1 ratio. Reports of physical examination of these joints are often confusing, and clinicians should be encouraged to distinguish clearly between the motions of the true ankle joint and the subtalar joint. Occasionally following ankle sprains or fracture, a small amount of inversion or eversion will occur in the unstable ankle joint.

Calcaneal valgus is the most common rearfoot deformity, and it may involve any or all of the talocalcaneal (subtalar), talonavicular, and calcaneocuboid joints. These joints may be severely involved with joint loss, decreased motion, and severe pain and yet show no valgus deformity. At the other extreme the rearfoot valgus may be great enough to cause bone and soft tissue impingement of the calcaneus against the fibula.[20]

The talonavicular joint margins can be palpated medially and plantarly just behind the navicular tuberosity. The talonavicular joint with its associated soft tissue structures is a vitally essential component in the normal foot and is often the site of early symptoms and clinical findings in conditions ranging from functional overuse syndromes to the rheumatoid foot with rearfoot involvement. Tenderness at this location could be fascial, ligamentous, muscular, or synovial in origin. Often associated with advanced disease and deformity in this region is peroneal muscle spasm, which can be a source of significant lateral leg pain.[21] Confirmation of peroneal spasm can be determined by the following test. With the patient at rest, apply enough force to the lateral side of the fifth metatarsal head to push the forefoot into a position of adduction. Repeat this motion several times rapidly, and peroneal spasm and involuntary forefoot abduction will occur.

When ankle dorsiflexion is limited to 0 or less, pronation and forefoot abduction may occur to compensate for loss of this essential ankle motion.[22,25] The limitation of dorsiflexion may be caused by articular changes in the ankle or by a tight or shortened gastrocnemius-soleus group or Achilles tendon. When examining ankle joint motion, the ranges should be evaluated with the knee in full extension as well as in 90 degrees of flexion. If ankle dorsiflexion increases beyond neutral with the knee in flexion, the limiting factor is the gastrocnemius, which arises from the femoral condyles. Calcaneal varus deformity (inversion) occurs rarely in adult rheumatoid arthritis but is more frequently seen in juvenile rheumatoid arthritis.[20] When present in adults, it is more likely to be a deformity occurring in the ankle, where owing to bone and cartilage erosions the talus becomes inverted within the ankle mortise.

Conservative Management. *General Principles.* During stages I and II when secondary deformity is less likely to be a problem, pre-existing mechanically induced lesions and deformities should be dealt with, especially chronic pronation and calcaneovalgus, for in the presence of rheumatoid arthritis these deformities are likely to increase. While inflammatory processes are active, particularly if multiple foot joints are involved, local mechanical therapy is of limited value; however, this is an appropriate time to outline changes in both foot use and foot wear. A change to shoes designed for function and comfort is helpful, especially for female patients whose shoes are often uncomfortable for even a normal foot. Appropriate exercise and activity programs should be encouraged as tolerated. Inappropriate activity would include contact sports and activities involving high foot-to-ground impact and shearing forces such as tennis and racquet ball; more suitable activities include bicycling, either stationary or two- or three-wheeled, swimming, and certainly walking on a compliant yet smooth surface such as a golf course or well groomed park. Rough and uneven surfaces requiring compensatory inversion and eversion may be difficult, especially with later stages of disease. Static active, passive, and isometric exercise of all joints, but especially the ankle, subtalar, and metatarsophalangeal joints, is encouraged within reasonable limits for maintaining both muscle tone and strength and joint mobility. The use of moist heat applications may be helpful for temporary relief of pain and stiffness. Polypropylene ankle-foot orthoses may be used as a night or resting splint. Generally when used as a night splint, these devices do not require custom fabrication, although stock splints may require the addition or modification of Velcro strapping for both comfort of fit and maintenance of position.

Footwear. Comfort is the essential quality for footwear in rheumatoid arthritis. A comfortable shoe should be lightweight and flexible with room to accommodate forefoot deformity; it should have a low heel of 3/16 to 1/2 inch of height, and a sole thick enough to protect the foot from mechanical surface trauma and compliant to cushion impact. The upper leather should be soft and pliable with a minimum of stitching and decoration, and should have a laced closure. The ideal shoe would have a natural crepe sole 1/2 inch thick with a totally plain glove leather upper and a combination last to ensure adequate fit for both rear- and forefoot. The problem of closure in the presence of limited hand function is solved either with a Velcro strap or by using elastic shoelaces, which eliminate the task of tying. The traditional so-called "orthopedic shoe" is of limited value except in the presence of minimal deformity and discomfort. With more severe deformity this shoe is often uncomfortable until the supporting counter has broken down, at which point the initial supportive value of the shoe is lost. Custom-fabricated stabilizing or supportive devices can be added to the comfortable shoe when needed without compromising comfort and fit. Adding inserts or orthoses to deal with forefoot problems usually increases the difficulty of shoe fitting. The Extra Depth Shoe* has a removable innersole which when removed increases the depth of the shoe by 1/4 inch, which is usually ample to accept both deformed toes and an effective plantar insert (Fig. 31–9). Molded or "space" shoes, although good conceptually, have definite limitations with rheumatoid feet as they are usually too stiff and noncompliant. Any increase of deformity or swelling results in an uncomfortably poor fit. Some manufacturers are now using removable molded Plastazote or Aliplast inserts, which are an improvement. This shoe is most suitable for the fixed rigid deformity or for some osteoarthritic feet. The Plastazote sandal introduced by Paul Brand, M.D., has been successfully adapted as either a shoe or sandal for many patients other than those with the neuropathic lesions of Hansen's disease for whom it was originally designed (Fig. 31–10). The experience at the Robert B. Brigham Hospital has demonstrated a 25 percent reduction in surgery on the rheumatoid foot since the introduction of this material. Some manufacturers have developed a nonmolded shoe and sandal utilizing Plastazote (Fig. 31–11).†

The Forefoot. Treatment of plantar forefoot pain involves two principles, the first being provision of a compliant stress absorbing surface for weight bearing, and the second, redistribution of weight-bearing forces. The placement of compliant accommodative weight dispersive devices within a shoe is subject to obvious space limitations, and for this reason the extra depth shoe is often used. Microcellular rubber, closed cell neoprene, and closed cell foamed polyethylenes are representative of compliant materials available. In addition to these, materials such as adhesive-backed felt, cork, rubber, or leather can be used to fabricate accommodative weight distributing padding. Plastazote and Aliplast may be heated and molded to the contour of the foot or may be inserted without heating as an inner sole. Molded orthoses from these materials are capable of not only providing stress and impact absorbing qualities under metatarsal heads but also allowing the entire plantar surface of the foot to bear weight, thereby shifting some weight bearing away from metatarsal heads. Using a combination of materials, including the more firm varieties of Plastazote and Aliplast, these devices can also

---

*P.W. Minor & Son, Inc., Batavia, New York 14020.
†AliMed, Inc., Boston, Massachusetts 02111.

Figure 31–9. Extra Depth Shoes showing removable innersoles in variations of style and closure (manufactured by P.W. Minor & Son, Inc., Batavia, New York 14020).

be used for long arch support in the less severe cases of pronation of mid- and rearfoot disease. The same concept of distributing weight over the entire sole can be effective for both the treatment and prevention of plantar skin lesions, including ulcers, corns, and calluses. The addition of forefoot accommodative apertures either directly to the inside of the shoe itself or to the shoe insert is effective in unloading a specific head or heads. When multiple heads, usually more than two, are involved, a metatarsal bar can be added to the orthoses just behind the metatarsal head area. This has the effect of shifting the weight to an area proximal to the heads (Fig. 31–9).

Figure 31–10. Plastazote sandal with polypropylene rearfoot stabilizer (by Barry Bent, Robert B. Brigham Division, Brigham and Women's Hospital).

Orthoses. Custom-made orthoses can also be ordered for accommodating or cushioning forefoot lesions. As with rearfoot devices, they are best made from plaster foot molds in preference to using paper tracings. Skilled technical help for the fabrication of these devices is often difficult to locate. Most large urban areas will have laboratories with some experience in this area. As an alternative there are numerous laboratories having nationwide service via mail. Generally these laboratories provide clear instructions for selecting and ordering their devices.

Splinting and exercise may be of value in retarding the development of deformity but are of limited value once significant joint destruction and deformity have occurred. Splinting and protective padding or shielding of the toes are helpful in reducing irritation of the soft tissues caused by pressure from shoes. An effective device for both splinting and protection can be molded from MPC.* Polyurethane foam impregnated with liquid latex rubber can also be fabricated as a protective shield or splint. MPC splints can also be used to maintain digital alignments during forefoot postoperative periods. The use of splints and wedges to correct hallux valgus deformity is of no value; because of the great forces acting on this deformity, a wedge between the great and second toes may increase the fibular displacement of the lesser toes. Occasionally hyperextension will occur at the interphalangeal joint of the great toe with or without hallux valgus or rigidus. This is a painful deformity, and the site is subject to chronic ulceration. Although surgical intervention is often required, an accommodative orthotic or MPC protective splint may be of value.

*Siebe Norton Inc., Cranston, Rhode Island 02920.

Figure 31–11. AliMed Plastazote Shoe showing removable innersole and Velcro closure (manufactured by AliMed, Inc., Boston, Massachusetts 02111).

Shoe Modifications. The same principles of redistribution of weight can be applied directly to the sole of the shoe. Plantation crepe soles can be added to almost any shoe to cushion impact. Metatarsal bars likewise provide a quick and simple modification. The major drawback to bars is that when improperly placed, an unfortunately frequent occurrence, they will increase pain. To be effective the front edge of the bar must be located proximal to the metatarsal heads. This location can be determined by noting the location of wear of both the inner and outer soles. Transferable marks placed on the metatarsal heads with ball-point pen, lipstick, or marker pens will be imprinted within the shoe after a few steps and will provide an accurate placement. Many orthopedic shoe repair shops and orthotics laboratories have shoe-stretching apparatus (such as a Eupedus device) which can selectively stretch a shoe to accommodate a digital deformity.

For patients able to play golf, the removal of cleats, particularly from the forefoot area, will reduce some of the shearing and torsional stresses induced by golf shoes; however, in general, the more flexible crepe sole shoe is probably more appropriate.

The molded Plastazote shoe provides the ultimate in forefoot protection. When the need to protect the forefoot maximally is combined with rearfoot deformity requiring stabilization, a shoe utilizing a polypropylene rearfoot stabilizer in addition to the Plastazote forefoot can be made. The use of thin-soled elevated heel shoes with narrow toes should be discouraged both from a comfort standpoint and from the fact that they will increase forefoot deformity. As a practical matter this rule can be broken for occasional social functions.

Injections. Polyarticular inflammatory foot pain is best managed with rest, heat, and systemic treatment; how-

ever, recalcitrant pain, particularly when located within a specific joint or joints, may be selectively treated with an injection of steroids, as can bursae and tendon sheaths.[8,9] The foot, particularly its plantar and interdigital spaces, is a potentially dirty area surgically, and careful skin preparation is essential. Sterile technique, including gloving, is advised. Steroid injections into deep areas, particularly the plantar heel area, are easier when preceded by injection of anesthetic. With the exception of the ankle and subtalar joints, the foot joints should be treated as small joints in terms of the quantity and strength of steroid to be injected. Reference to anatomic diagrams is helpful unless one is familiar with foot joints. Tuberculin syringes provide excellent control with both insertion and introduction of fluids when dealing with small joints and superficial bursae and tendon sheaths. Aspiration from bursae and the ankle joint for purposes of fluid examination and volume reduction can be readily accomplished; the smaller joints, except in the presence of significant effusion, can be most difficult to enter for either aspiration or injection. The metatarsophalangeal and talonavicular joints are most readily entered by attempting to follow the natural joint contours rather than through a vertical approach to the joint space. Care must be taken when injecting in the region of the Achilles tendon and its adjacent bursae, as rupture of the Achilles tendon has been reported following steroid injection.

The subtalar joint can be entered with a 1½-inch needle inserted at a point anterior to the fibula approximately 1 cm from its tip, directing the needle in a posterior, plantar, and medial direction. This provides entrance into the sinus tarsi. From this point, redirecting to a medial direction permits entrance into the extensive capsular complex, which includes the middle and anterior facets of the talocalcaneal as well as the talo-navicular joints. Redirecting to a more posterior angle from the original insertion will locate the posterior joint.

Other midfoot joints are very difficult to locate and inject. Intermetatarsal head synovitis or bursitis does not require direct joint penetration, but a deposit along the sides of the joint may be helpful. Plantar heel injections, whether for bursitis, fasciitis, or heel spurs, are simplest when approached medially. Entrance is made just above the junction of the thick tough plantar skin and the much more delicate skin of the upper foot and at a point medial to the attachment of the plantar fascia. Skin in this area is much more readily prepped, and the injection is far less painful. In addition, since spurs, fasciitis, or bursae are rarely limited to the pencil point of bone spur seen on x-ray, medial injection allows a broader deposition of steroid in the region of pain and inflammation. When properly located, this injection site is a safe distance away from the posterior tibial nerve and vessels. Deep injections are often made easier by detaching the syringe from the well placed needle and reloading with steroid. This is likely to be less traumatic and probably is more accurate.

Rearfoot. Moderate deformity occurring on weight bearing in a foot capable of resupinating before toe off can be treated with an orthosis designed to control or minimize pronation.[26] In the presence of more severe deformities with joint destruction but with the capability for passive motion, the aim of an orthosis is to restore normal structural and functional alignment, reduce pain, and prevent further deformity.

Following total knee replacement procedures in which a significant valgus or varus deformity has been reduced, the foot frequently requires modification of shoes or orthotic appliances. With an adequate supple subtalar range of motion, the foot may easily accommodate to the correct functional planes. With limited subtalar motion the stabilizing orthoses can be used in an attempt to make a gradual realignment. When this fails or in the presence of a rigid joint, shoes and orthoses must be constructed that will provide adequate distribution of weight-bearing forces without increasing stress to the midtarsal and subtalar joints. The use of orthoses to realign these rearfoot joints may be a long-term treatment requiring periodic modifications of the device or fabication of new devices as changes in structural relationship occur. If bony ankylosis occurs with the subtalar and midtarsal joints in an adequate functional position, the use of a stabilizing orthosis may be discontinued. This procedure is followed also in candidates for talonavicular fusion or triple arthrodesis and may also be used postoperatively following cast immobilization.

Stabilizing orthoses may be constructed from a variety of materials, including Fiberglas, Rohadur, nylon, polypropylene, Celastic, and Cutter Cast. Such devices are fabricated over a plaster model of the foot. The cast for the model or mold is made with the foot held in the position which the orthosis is intended to maintain. The surface in contact with the foot is contoured to conform to the weight-bearing surfaces, while the surface in contact with the shoe is flattened. Modifying the angle of the flattened surface allows adjustment of the valgus and varus attitude. In some instances in which both ankle and rearfoot joints are involved, a polypropylene drop foot orthosis can be fabricated to support and stabilize both joint complexes. When a stabilizing orthosis fails to achieve relief of pain, a plaster cast may be used for 3 to 4 weeks, to be followed again with an orthosis and physical therapy. These conservative measures deserve trial before resorting to rear foot surgery. (See Chapter 118.) In addition to rheumatoid arthritis, Reiter's disease and psoriasis may present painful inflammatory periosteal changes, particularly in the rearfoot area. Reiter's disease especially presents a frustrating problem as one attempts to resolve or reduce heel pain. Psoriatic and Reiter's periostitis of the heel are usually not mechanical in origin and therefore do not respond well to orthotics designed to reduce traction on the plantar fascia. The use of Plastazote inserts, heel cups, and cushion-soled shoes is helpful. Rest, application of moist heat, and occasionally the timely injection of steroids may be of benefit.

JUVENILE RHEUMATOID ARTHRITIS

The juvenile rheumatoid arthritic presents difficult challenges from the standpoint of both preventing and correcting or accommodating foot deformities. Early detection of structural changes and institution of appropriate shoes, orthoses, splints, and physical therapy are necessary.[35,36] The physically active child should be watched for any tendency toward deformity, particularly in the rear- and midfoot, where, in contrast to the adult calcaneal valgus deformity, equinovarus deformity is more frequently encountered. Appropriate shoes and/or orthoses should be utilized to minimize or prevent this deformity. Night splints and foot boards may also be needed. The juvenile rheumatoid arthritic is often an unreliable historian and reporter, and treatment requirements and decisions must be based largely on clinical judgment. Correction of deformities before the occurrence of fibrous ankylosis is essential if proper functional alignments are to be achieved and maintained. Active and passive range of motion and muscle strengthening exercises should be encouraged at an early stage as pain tolerance permits. Once fibrous or bony ankylosis has occurred, correction is difficult at best and surgical revision may ultimately be required.

SUMMARY

Early detection and treatment of deformity and pain with proper shoes, exercise, orthoses, and splints when needed may prevent, delay, or minimize disability. Soft, compliant, nonrestrictive footwear with low heels and crepe soles together with supportive, stabilizing, compliant, or accommodative orthoses and shoe modifications will often increase levels of function and comfort. For purposes other than splinting and rest, or treatment of pre-existing deformity, other local medical and surgical techniques are most useful following effective systemic management of the inflammatory disease. The management of the rheumatoid arthritic foot requires that patients be informed of the nature and course of treatment and that realistic goals and limitations be set. The criteria for lower extremity surgical intervention are such that major foot surgical procedures and joint replacements are often of low priority and in most instances are best performed late. The presence of deformity is not by itself justification for intervention, and indeed surgical intervention usually should follow failure of conservative measures.[4,5,37]

References

1. Inman, V.T., and DuVries, H.: DuVries' Surgery of the Foot. 3rd ed. St. Louis, C. V. Mosby Company, 1973.
2. National Health Survey Vital and Health Statistics: Data. United States DHEW Publication, No. 1000, Series 11,20:9, 1966.
3. Stott, J.R.P., Hutton, W.C., and Stokes, I.A.F.: Forces under the foot. J. Bone Joint Surg. 55B:335, 1973.
4. Giannestras, N.: Foot Disorders, Medical and Surgical Management. 2nd ed. Philadelphia, Lea & Febiger, 1973.
5. Kelikian, H.: Hallux Valgus and Allied Deformities of the Forefoot. Philadelphia, W. B. Saunders Company, 1965.
6. Roth, D.R.: Talonavicular joint osteoarthritis (osteoarthrisis). JAPA 72:237, 1982.
7. Furey, J.G.F.: Plantar fasciitis, J. Bone Joint Surg. 57A:672, 1975.
8. Kech, S.W., and Kelly, P.J.: Bursitis of the posterior part of the heel. J. Bone Joint Surg. 47A:267, 1965.
9. Cozen, L.: Bursitis of the heel. Am. J. Orthop. 3:372, 1961.
10. Frykeberg, R.G., and Kozak, G.P.: Neuropathic arthropathy in the diabetic foot. Fam. Phys. 17:105, 1978.
11. Clark, M.: Trouble with Feet. London, G. Bell, 1969. p. 13.
12. Brand, P.W.: Repetitive Stress on Insensitive Feet—The Pathology and Management of Plantar Ulceration in Neurotrophic Feet. SRSG No. RC-75, MPO, U.S. Public Health Service, 1975.
13. Hall, O.C., and Brand, P.W.: The etiology of the neuropathic ulcer. JAPA 69:173, 1979.
14. Steinbrocker, O., Traeger, C.H., and Batterman, R.C.: Therapeutic criteria in rheumatoid arthritis. JAMA 140:659, 1949.
15. Vainio, S.: The rheumatoid foot: A clinical study with pathological roentgenological comments. Ann. Chir. Gynaec. Fenn. 45:Suppl. 1, 1956.
16. Black, J.R., Cahalin, C., and Germain, B.F.: Pedal morbidity in rheumatic diseases. JAPA 72:360, 1982.
17. Taylor, P.M.: A review of changes of the hands and feet in rheumatoid arthritis. JAPA 68:817, 1978.
18. D'Amico, J.C.: The pathomechanics of adult rheumatoid arthritis affecting the foot. JAPA 66:227, 1976.
19. Harris, R.L.: Rigid valgus foot. J. Bone Joint Surg. 37A:169, 1955.
20. King, J., Burke, D., and Freeman, M.A.R.: The incidence of pain in the rheumatoid hind foot and the significance of calcaneo-fibular impingement. Int. Orthop. 2:255, 1978.
21. Harris, R.I., and Beath, T.: Etiology of peroneal spastic flatfoot. J. Bone Joint Surg. 30B:624, 1948.
22. Inman, V.T.: The Joints of the Ankle. Baltimore, Williams & Wilkins Company, 1976.
23. Chater, E.H.: Tarsal tunnel syndrome in rheumatoid arthritis. Br. Med. J. 3:406, 1970.
24. Kopell, H.P., and Thompson, W.A.L.: Peripheral Entrapment Neuropathies. Baltimore, Williams & Wilkins Company, 1963.
25. Sgarlato, T.E.: A Compendium of Podiatric Biomechanics. San Francisco, California College of Podiatric Medicine, 1971.
26. Root, M., Orien, W., and Weed, J.: Abnormal Function of the foot. Los Angeles, Clinical Biomechanics Inc., 1978.
27. Close, J.R.: Functional Anatomy of the Extremities. Springfield, Ill., Charles C Thomas, 1973.
28. Benson, G.M., and Johnson, E.W.: Management of the foot in the rheumatoid arthritic. Orthop. Clin. North Am. 2:733, 1971.
29. Kuhns, J.G.: The foot in chronic arthritis. Clin. Orthop. 16:141, 1960.
30. Wilkinson, M., and Torrance, W.N.: Clinical background of rheumatoid vascular disease. Ann. Rheum. Dis. 26:475, 1967.
31. Soter, N.A., Austen, K.F., and Gigli, I.: Urticaria and arthralgias as manifestation of necrotizing angiitis (vasculitis). J. Invest. Dermatol. 63:485, 1974.
32. Scott, J.T.: Digital arteritis in rheumatoid disease. Ann. Rheum. Dis. 20:224, 1961.
33. Mall, J.C., Genant, H.K., Silcox, D.C., and McCarty, D.J.: The efficacy of fine-detailed radiography in the evaluation of patients with rheumatoid arthritis. Radiology 112:37, 1974.
34. Seltzer, S.: Unpublished data, Department of Radiology, Brigham and Womens Hospital, 1983.
35. Donovan, W.: Proceedings of the First ARA Conference on the Rheumatic Diseases of Childhood, March 1974.
36. Calabro, J.J., Katz, R.M., and Maltz, B.A.: A critical appraisal of juvenile rheumatoid arthritis. Clin. Orthop. 74:100, 1971.
37. Clayton, M.L.: Surgery of the forefoot in rheumatoid arthritis. Clin. Orthop.16:136, 1960.

Chapter 32
"Fibrositis" and Other Diffuse Musculoskeletal Syndromes

Hugh Smythe

INTRODUCTION

Patients often describe trunk or limb pain unaccompanied by new findings on physical or radiologic examination. In these circumstances, approaches to diagnosis may reflect several levels of clinical skill. Most commonly and superficially, this symptom is attributed to "arthritis," "bursitis," "nerve compression," or "fibrositis," on the basis of evidence that is trivial or irrelevant. A more skilled examiner may recognize that the joints, bursae, and nervous system are essentially normal, leaving the patient and physician incompletely reassured and leaving also a natural suspicion that either the patient or the diagnostic effort is inadequate. With still more care, previously unsuspected points of tenderness may be found; but there has been so little definition and discussion of the significance of these tender points that confident and accurate diagnosis is by no means assured. To the beginner, problems in diagnosis emerge from the diffuse and vague localization of much pain of deep origin and the absence of obvious findings in the area of complaint. At the more advanced level, a wealth of physical findings exist, and the problem lies in assessment of the significance of newly discovered sites of deep tenderness.

Often deep tenderness indicates subtle local pathology—an enthesopathy, a bursitis, or a soft tissue injury. More often, however, there is no histologically definable local pathology. Recent controlled studies have confirmed and extended our knowledge of the clinical associations of these findings.[1-3] The concept of pain amplification syndromes (Table 32–1) has been introduced to group these conditions. The term amplification implies that the increase in pain or tenderness has resulted from altered physiological mechanisms, independent of psychological influences. The effect is selective, not diffuse. Some sites become tender, but background pain threshold is unaltered.[2]

Referred Pain and Associated Phenomena. *Body Image.*[4] When a pin is stuck into a finger, the patient can accurately localize the site of the injury and identify the nature of the stimulus. With eyes closed, he can summon up an image of the finger—extended or flexed, accurately located in space—and draw a picture of the part and the site of injury. This kind of detailed knowledge of the position and environment of the hand is essential to function, and a considerable area of cerebral cortex is assigned to processing this information.

However, we have no comparable need for information about deeply lying structures, and no comparable cortical mechanism exists. We have no "body image" of these deeply lying structures, and pain arising in them cannot therefore be accurately located. The pain must be referred; it is misinterpreted as arising from other areas that are within the body image. This spread of pain is not dependent on nerve root compression, and the dysesthesia in the fourth and fifth fingers produced by trauma to the ulnar nerve is not a good general illustration of the nature of referred pain.

Quality of Referred Pain. The quality of referred pain is determined more by the site to which it is referred than by the nature of the original pain stimulus. Anginal pain is of course not localized to the myocardium, as we have no body image of the heart muscle. It may be felt in the precordial region, where it is appreciated as a heaviness or a crushing pressure. It may be referred to the shoulder region, where it is felt as a deep ache, perhaps exacerbated by a draft. It may be referred to the forearm or hand, which may be described as dead, numb, woody, or swollen. The same pain, arising in the same area of heart muscle, and traveling by the same pathways to association areas in the cerebral cortex, may simultaneously give three very different kinds of sensory impression to the patient struggling to find words to accurately describe the nature of his distress. The qualities of deadness, numbness, and swelling associated with distal referral should be particularly noted, as they are common to many pains referred distally in the limbs, and commonly are misinterpreted as evidence of neural involvement.

Referred Tenderness. The development of tenderness ("hyperalgesia") in areas to which pain is referred is part of all the classic descriptions of referred pain.[4-7] In these accounts, however, an inordinate emphasis has been placed on the development of exagerated skin tenderness, "cutaneous hyperalgesia." Deep referred tenderness is much more common than skin tenderness.

Associated Features. Two separate kinds of phenomena are commonly associated with referred pain; together they can give rise to the bizarre association of pain and numbness. Tenderness, involuntary muscle spasm, inhibition of voluntary motion, and increased blood flow belong to the first category and can be thought of as protective in nature, though often mislocated. Referred muscle spasm, interfering with some function, may give rise to deep "clicks" or "clunks" in otherwise normal structures, such as the temporomandibular joints (from cervical spine), scapulae (from neck or shoulder), or greater trochanter (from low back).

A provisional diagnosis is made on the basis of the carefully gathered initial clinical evidence, and then alternative diagnoses are considered. This process raises reasonable doubts, which must be resolved by review of specific features in history or examination, by special investigations, by a therapeutic trial, or not at all. With nonarticular rheumatic disease, the special investigations are mostly not helpful. They are useful only in the diagnosis of degeneration, fracture, tumor, abscess, or systemic disease. Most nonarticular pain is not due to these

Table 32–1. Pain Amplification Syndromes

Group One: Tenderness at "Fibrositic" Sites
1. Referred pain syndromes
2. "Fibrositis" syndrome
3. Experimental sleep deprivation
4. Narcotic withdrawal
5. Others

Group Two: Tenderness of Different Distribution
1. Reflex dystrophies
2. Tender shins of steroid therapy

Table 32–2. Special Features of Referred Tenderness

1. Usually distal to primary lesion
2. Often not in region of maximum pain
3. Deep more than cutaneous
4. Often unknown to patient
5. Most at predictable sites*
6. Often relieved by local anesthesia or counterirritant therapy

*See Table 32–4 and Figure 32–1.

Table 32–3. Local Causes of Soft Tissue Pain

1. Bursitis, tendinitis, tenosynovitis
2. Phlebitis, vasculitis, panniculitis
3. Bone-tendon junction syndromes, muscle-tendon junction syndromes, hematoma in muscle, postexercise myalgia
4. Referred pain syndromes
   Reflex dystophies
   Nerve entrapment syndromes
   Pain with central nervous system disease
   Traumatic neuromas
5. Writer's cramp, other habit spasms

conditions, and in most situations the correct diagnosis comes from a specifically directed review of the history and physical findings.

THE POINT COUNT

In order to review the findings on physical examination while assessing alternative diagnoses, the clinician must have a systemic and effective approach to the examination of the peripheral joints, of the spine, and of the nonarticular regions. There must be a practiced familiarity with the sites in which tenderness is likely to occur and a technique that measures the quantity of tenderness, allowing for differences among individuals in general responses to pain stimulus. One approach is to do a "point count," analogous to the "joint count" inevitably used in assessing changes in the severity of peripheral joint inflammation. The basic idea is simple enough, and to the novice examiner there are only two methodologic problems: where to press and how hard to press.

A list of 14 sites at which tenderness may be found has been published,[13] and is reviewed in Table 32–4 and Figure 32–1. This list is not all-inclusive and certainly need not be carved in stone, but it remains a useful start. The firmness of pressure is determined by using as reference sites clinically "silent" areas—the lower ribs, the forearm or thigh muscles, and the fat pad lateral to the knee. For humanity as well as precision, one works at the threshold of tenderness, reducing the stimulus for generally tender individuals. Pressure over the target site

Figure 32–1. Characteristic sites of referred tenderness.

should be somewhat less firm, about 80 percent of the pressure over adjacent nontender areas, and the site scored positive only if very distinct tenderness is reported. This comparison of two sites, target and reference, may have to be done with some care, as the patient often assumes that the exquisite tenderness is due to unnecessary roughness and must be assured that the pressure on the "target" site is in fact less than on the "reference" area. The quantity of tenderness may then be scored in terms of the number of tender points and the distribution of these points examined for clues as to the underlying mechanisms. A small number of points, clustered in a single region, unassociated with diffuse aching stiffness and fatigue, suggests a referred pain syndrome. A large number of tender sites, spread widely and symmetrically, with systemic symptoms, suggests the "fibrositis" syndrome.

THE "FIBROSITIS" SYNDROME

The "fibrositis" syndrome is a pain amplification syndrome, the essential clinical feature of which is the presence of a large number of specifically tender sites. While there are complex interactions between personality and pathogenesis in these patients, the evidence to be discussed below indicates that the magnification is not purely psychogenic, i.e., at the interpretive level, but physiogenic, predominantly a quantitative change in physiologically normal pain mechanisms. Four lines of evidence support this belief: the predictability of the tender sites, the reactive hyperemia, the strong association with a specific sleep disturbance, and the temporary reproduction of the syndrome in normal subjects.

Clinical Picture. The pain or aching is widespread, poorly circumscribed and deep, and is referred to mus-

Table 32–4. The Point Count: 14 Tender Sites

Trapezius, midpoint of upper fold	R	1
	L	2
Costochondral junctions, second; maximum just	R	3
lateral to junctions on upper surface	L	4
Lateral epicondyles, tennis elbow sites, 2 cm	R	5
distal to epicondyles, within muscle that tenses when long finger is actually extended	L	6
Supraspinatus, at origins, above scapular spine	R	7
near the medial border	L	8
Low cervical, anterior aspects of intertransverse C4-6		9
Low lumbar, interspinous ligaments L4-S1		10
Gluteus medius, upper outer quadrants of	R	11
buttocks, in anterior fold of muscle	L	12
Medial fat pad, overlying medial collateral	R	13
ligament of the knee, proximal to the joint line	L	14

Table 32–5. Cardinal Features of "Fibrositis"

1. Diffuse aching pain, stiffness, weakness
2. High point count, diffuse distribution
3. High sensitivity to internal and external stimuli
4. Nonrestorative sleep
5. Perfectionistic personality

cles or bony prominences. When central, it has an aching character; when peripheral, it may feel like a swelling, stiffness, or numbness. The stiffness is an increase of a sense of tissue tension or of muscular effort required toward the extremes of range. These symptoms are concentrated in the broad areas of reference of the cervical and lumbar segments and tend to shift with time, so that the patients recurrently present with "new" sites of complaints. The stiffness is noted at rest, is worse in the morning, and is increased by weather changes, cold, fatigue, or excess use. Simple analgesics are disappointing, but heat, massage, or a holiday may give relief.

The exhaustion may be most disabling and not clearly related to lack of rest. It is often marked in the morning and paralyzes as well as punishes initiative.

The patients emphasize their exhaustion but many minimize their sleep disturbance. They may have been light sleepers for years and relate their frequent and prolonged wakefulness to pain. Virtually all arise feeling unrefreshed (this is the key question to ask), more exhausted than at bedtime the night before. After stress, they may spend whole nights without sleep (see Table 32–6).

They are sensitive to cold, noise, and environmental irritants. Visceral sensations may be equally amplified. An example is urinary frequency, particularly nocturnal, due to a sense of bladder fullness despite small urinary volume. There is usually no pain on urination, and cultures are sterile, but recurrent cystitis is frequently misdiagnosed and inappropriately treated. The association of the irritable bowel syndrome with "fibrositis" has been well documented.[1]

These patients are apprehensive and relax poorly during examination, with spasmodic, inappropriate muscle contractions interrupting active and passive motion; a full range is achieved only after gentle persistence. Grip strength and other muscle power as measured by a modified blood pressure cuff is half normal or less and is

Table 32–6. Symptoms of Sleep Disturbance*

Symptom	"Fibrositis" Group (n = 22)	Control Group (n = 22)
Waking with aching, stiffness	100 percent	23 percent
Tired during the day	100	41
Waking tired	95	32
Waking frequently	68	59
Difficulty falling asleep	36	23
Waking early	36	36

*After Campbell, S.M., Clark, S., Findall, E.A., et al.: Clinical characteristics of fibrositis. Arthritis Rheum. 26:817, 983.

inconstant and poorly sustained. Yet the muscles show the conditioning effect of isometric exercise; they tend to be well preserved, in striking contrast to the weakness described and displayed. Tenderness is not simply reported; it may be demonstrated by sudden dramatic twisting leaps, the highly characteristic "jump sign." The interview is exhausting for the examiner as well as the patient, a significant sign given the professional experience of the physician, indicative of the stresses between the patient and the environment.

The Tender Points. Most of the multiple other points are unknown to the patient and are often not central to the areas of pain. They can be readily found because of their remarkably constant location. The published list (see Table 32–4 and Fig. 32–1) is by no means exclusive. Tenderness at the medial epicondyle, the lower pole of the coracoid process, the other costochondral junctions, and the margins of the greater trochanters and patellae is almost equally common. The cervical tenderness is most often missed or underestimated. The anterior aspects of the lower intertransverse spaces are strikingly more tender than lateral or posterior aspects of transverse processes or interspinous ligaments. The carefully controlled dolorimeter study of Campbell and associates[2] has shown the efficiency of specific point tenderness in differentiating between normal and "fibrositic" subjects (Fig. 32–2).

The tenderness involves a variety of tissues, including muscle, bone, fibrous tissue, and subcutaneous fat, and extensive histologic and electromyographic studies have not identified any concentration of neural structures or other consistent histologic bases.[14-16] They tend to be firmer than surrounding tissues.

Skinfold tenderness and reactive hyperemia are important witnesses to diagnosis and to underlying mechanisms. Both are most marked in the upper scapular region. Hyperesthesia to pinprick is much less marked. Both occur in the general regions of sites of deep tenderness and so are found at the tennis elbow and costochondral sites. The erythema is uncommon distally in the limbs or in the lower half of the body. Absence of laboratory evidence of inflammatory or muscle damage is a defined requirement for the diagnosis of "primary" fibrositis; but it must be re-emphasized that fibrositic mechanisms ("secondary fibrositis") commonly complicate the assessment and therapy of rheumatoid arthritis and other diseases.

The "Fibrositic" Personality.

. . . In the morning she was asked how she slept. "Oh, terribly badly!" said the Princess. "I have scarcely shut my eyes the whole night. Heaven only knows what was in the bed, but I was lying on something hard, so that I am black and blue all over. . . ." Nobody but a real princess could be as sensitive as that. So the prince took her for his wife, for now he knew he had a real princess. (From "The Princess and the Pea," *Arthur Rackham Fairy Book.*)

These patients set high standards and are as demanding of themselves as of others. They are caring, honest, tidy, committed, moral, industrious—virtuous

Figure 32–2. *A*, Frequency spectra and raw EEG from NREM (stage 4) sleep in a healthy 25-year-old subject. The spectrum shows that most amplitude is concentrated at 1 cps (delta). *B*, NREM sleep in a 42-year-old "fibrositis" patient. The spectrum shows amplitude at both 1 cps (delta) and 8–10 cps (alpha). *C*, NREM sleep of a healthy 21-year-old subject during stage 4 sleep deprivation. In the EEG there is a clear association between external arousal (auditory stimulation) and alpha onset. Again the frequency spectrum (obtained by 10-second analysis from stimulus onset) shows amplitude concentrated in the delta and alpha bands. (From Moldofsky, H., et al.: Psychosomat. Med. *37*:341, 1975.)

to a fault. Their perfectionism can be trying, but they are often very effective in their chosen field of activity and have unusual loyalty from employers and family. They are not abnormal, just characteristic. They deeply resent any suggestion that they are using their illness as a crutch, as they drive themselves harder than most, and dislike other crutches, such as alcohol and prescribed medication. They are not depressed,[17] and the concept of "masked depression" may have arisen because of the response of "fibrositic" symptoms to tricyclic medication.

The Sleep Disturbance. As yet unconfirmed key studies have provided evidence of a specific disturbance in sleep physiology. In the first study,[18] 10 "fibrositic" subjects showed a decrease in stages 3 and 4 slow-wave sleep, with intrusion of a rapid alpha rhythm, as determined by computer analysis of the energy frequency spectra (Fig. 32–3), and all showed an overnight increase in tenderness measured by dolorimeter. These observations have since been confirmed and extended in studies of a large number of other patients.[19,20] High-energy bursts of alpha waves intruding into slow-wave sleep

was described by Hauri and Hawkins as alpha-delta sleep,[21] and its association with aching, fatigue, and stiffness described.[22] This more florid pattern can be read by eye, and was recognized in 8 of 26 "chronic pain" patients.[23] Other studies on this point have been done,[2] but they have not been published in detail.

In another study, experimental reproduction of aspects of the "fibrositis" syndrome was achieved in healthy university students.[24] After control nights, for three nights they were deprived of rapid eye movement (REM), or stage 4 non-REM, sleep, by a buzzer, supplemented when necessary by hand arousal. The buzzer caused a rapid alpha rhythm to appear in the EEG superimposed on the slow-wave pattern, to mimic the pattern seen in the "fibrositis" patients. No increase in tenderness was associated with REM deprivation, but disturbance of slow-wave non-REM sleep was associated with a marked overnight increase in tenderness scores and symptoms of anorexia, overwhelming physical tiredness, and heaviness (Fig. 32–3).

"Fibrositic" Features and Other Rheumatic Diseases. Therapy is often determined by the urgency of the pa-

Figure 32–3. Tenderness at selected sites in patients with "fibrositis" and in controls. A low value indicates a more tender site. (After Campbell, S.M., Clark, S., Tindall, E. A., et al.: Clinical characteristics of fibrositis. Arthritis Rheum. 26:817, 1983.)

tient's complaints and not by the severity of the underlying disease. Patients with rheumatoid arthritis, cervical or lumbar disc disease, or a whole host of other conditions may have amplification of their symptoms by "fibrositic" mechanisms. The point count allows rapid recognition of this complication and avoidance of the excess of therapy that might otherwise follow.

Moldofsky and Chester identified a subgroup of "paradoxical responders" among hospitalized rheumatoid patients, identified by worsening mood with improving disease.[25] When first admitted, these patients seemed cheerful and cooperative; but they became depressed, complaining, and agitated as treatment progressed. They were more likely to receive prolonged hospitalization, extensive investigation, and hazardous medical and surgical therapies, with increased morbidity and even mortality. "The squeaky wheel gets the grease." Almost half the hospitalized rheumatoid patients showed this pattern, and on examination the "fibrositic" sites were characteristically more tender than their swollen joints.

Prevalence, Criteria, and Nomenclature. Figure 32–4 shows the number of tender points recorded in an

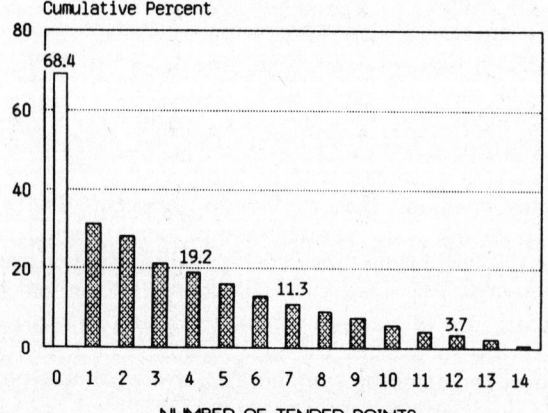

Figure 32–4. Prevalence of "fibrositic" tender points in 980 mixed rheumatic patients. (Data from Wolfe, F.: 1983.)

unselected group of rheumatic disease patients.[3] Clearly the prevalence of "fibrositis" in this population will be intolerably dependent on the point count criterion chosen. In published studies, the criteria have varied from 4 of 53 points[1] to 12 of 14.[16] The 20 percent with 4 or more points will include a majority with simple referred pain syndromes and without the other features listed in Table 32–2, characteristic of the disabling syndrome associated with large numbers of points. The pathogenesis, prognosis, and therapy are all different, and it seems inappropriate to apply the same name, be it "fibromyalgia"[1] or "fibrositis," to these very different groups. It would seem best to imbed "trigger points" and "localized fibrositis" within the primary diagnosis of which these are a manifestation, and develop a new name stressing the altered pain physiology of the more generalized syndrome. Moldofsky has suggested the "rheumatic pain modulation syndrome,"[26] a title that shares the disadvantages of other current names, that they are archaic and nonphysiologic, and therefore unsaleable to internists, neurologists, and other colleagues. The criteria are better than the names. Choosing subjects with a sufficient number of tender points leads to a group of patients with aching, fatigue, and irritable everything,[1] and selecting for aching and fatigue leads to patients with large numbers of tender points.[2]

Other Polymyalgic Syndromes. Widespread muscle aching and stiffness are seen acutely in association with viral and other infections or following unaccustomed exercise, and more chronically in association with a large variety of rheumatic, infectious, myopathic, endocrine, or malignant disorders. These manifestations have not been closely observed and warrant disciplined study. In acute illness the symptoms and tenderness are usually diffusely spread throughout the muscles, especially proximal muscles. About half the patients with the chronic syndromes show concentration of tenderness at "fibrositic" sites; but in others the tenderness is more diffuse, often with restriction of shoulder or other joint movement. In summary, almost any systemic disease, whether infectious, autoimmune, neoplastic, or metabolic in origin, may cause diffuse aching. In addition, the anxieties and frustrations of undiagnosed illness may unmask "fibrositic" elements in predisposed individuals.

PSYCHOGENIC MUSCULOSKELETAL PAIN SYNDROMES

For psychological reasons, symptoms may be invented or magnified, willfully or unconsciously. These classic varieties of psychiatric illness are relatively easy to suspect and to understand because of the obvious inconsistencies, exaggerations, emotional manipulations, and secondary gains. There remain two very difficult questions that frequently arise: (1) Does this obviously disturbed patient have an underlying organic disease? (2) By what mechanisms do psychological storms produce physiological changes?

Neither of these questions has received the attention

it deserves. The individual patient will require close and often repeated study with objective clinical and laboratory techniques; with such study, the number of symptoms resulting from purely cortical invention becomes very small. Magnification and modification of symptoms are common, and the interaction of personality and physical disability is so strong that psychogenic enhancement of tissue change is a distinct possibility. These questions require restatement in terms of phenomena that can be studied quantitatively. Many of the instruments used in these studies are inappropriate for rheumatology patients, scoring symptoms of disease and normal reactions to them as attributes of psychogenic origin.

PSYCHOGENIC REGIONAL PAIN OR HYSTERIA

Regional or generalized pain may be an important symptom in patients with hysteria of the classic type described by Charcot, Freud, and others, or it may be seen in patients with depression, schizophrenia, other neuroses, or even organic brain syndromes.[27]

The pain is regional rather than segmental and affects areas with large cortical or emotional representation, such as the face, anterior chest, or limbs. The boundary of the region affected is often sharply defined, at the root of a limb or the midline, but can be shifted dramatically by suggestion. There is often an extraordinary mixture of skin hyperesthesia plus numbness—marked distress when a hair is twitched but total inability to feel a pin. These features do not of course rule out the possibility of coexistent organic disease. Limitation of joint movement in these patients may stubbornly persist despite gently persistent persuasion, and re-examination after intravenous diazepam or Pentothal may be necessary. This examination should be carried out only with informed consent and detailed descriptive notes and in the presence of a qualified anesthetist and other witnesses.

OTHER SOFT TISSUE PAIN SYNDROMES

Diffuse Idiopathic Skeletal Hyperostosis (DISH, Ankylosing Hyperostosis, Forestier's Disease). The criteria for diagnosis of this syndrome are radiologic and spinal. Extraspinal involvement was described by Forestier and colleagues[28,29] and emphasized by Resnick and colleagues[30,31] with ossification of ligamentous attachments to bone at multiple sites. The diagnosis cannot now be made in the absence of extensive ossification, obviously a late event. Many of these patients describe widespread trunk and limb aching for decades prior to diagnosis, with points of tenderness where fibrous tissues attach to bone—a distribution quite different from the "fibrositic" points. This condition develops in heavy-boned, thick-limbed individuals, and must be considered, along with trauma and the B27-associated anthro-

pathies, in the differential diagnosis in patients presenting with pain under the heel or at other bone-tendon junction syndromes.

Tender Shins with Steroid Therapy. Slocumb[32] described "myalgias" associated with cortisone therapy, and later Rotstein and Good[33] described the occurrence of striking tenderness of the "muscles of the extremities" in five patients receiving high doses of oral steroids, coining the term "steroid pseudo-rheumatism." The tenderness is maximal in the lower legs, and affects bone, skin, tendon, and muscle but spares the feet. It is commonly associated with a waxlike shiny atrophy of the skin but not with edema, evidence of neuropathy, or tenderness at "fibrositic" sites. It is overwhelmingly associated with steroid therapy and may lessen if steroids are withdrawn but may also occasionally be seen in patients with maturity-onset diabetes. Its pathogenesis is unknown.

Malignant Hyperthermia Syndrome. Chronic widespread aching and stiffness have recently been emphasized as being characteristic and suggestive of the malignant hyperthermia syndrome,[34] a warning that general anesthesia may precipitate a catastrophe. The condition is fortunately rare, and the diagnosis is virtually impossible to confirm prior to the occurrence of a near-fatal event. Symptom analysis has therefore been retrospective in badly frightened patients and has not been sufficiently detailed to separate those caused by interaction of events and personality.

PROBLEMS IN THERAPY

The explanations are the most important and a difficult part of the treatment program. Multiple factors often combine to produce symptoms in patients with nonarticular rheumatism, and the therapeutic discussion may involve one or all of the following topics: (1) referred pain, tenderness, and reflex responses; (2) mechanical stress in neck and lower back; (3) the sleep disturbance; (4) measures for pain relief; and (5) attitudes and expectations.

One cannot cover all the areas in one interview, and the most urgent should be selected for explanations in depth. There may be varying emphasis on mechanical or "fibrositic" amplifying factors, but the same patterns occur so commonly that a printed handout covering this ground briefly may be of more value in this than in any other field of rheumatology. All explanations begin with the reassurance that the pain is real, not imaginary or neurotic in origin, a reassurance needed because of the absence of anatomic changes in the areas of pain.

Referred Pain, Tenderness, and Reflex Responses. The patient is given a brief but specific account of referred pain. All pain of deep origin is necessarily referred. The mental equipment to permit us to visualize our pancreas, apophyseal joints, or acetabulum does not exist, and pain arising in these structures is necessarily misinterpreted as arising in other structures sharing the same nerve supply and familiar enough to be included in the body image. The areas to which pain is referred often develop secondary reflex changes, misguided but protective in intent, including deep tenderness, circulatory changes, and strange mixtures of increased muscle tone and inhibition of voluntary action, and of pain and subjective numbness.

Mechanical Stresses in Neck and Low Back. For very good mechanical reasons, two regions of the spine account for the vast majority of complaints. No treatment program is adequate that fails to identify and correct these underlying mechanical problems, which are very often overlooked or neglected.

The cervical spine is particularly subjected to stresses during sleep. The skull and thorax are supported, but the neck forms an unsupported bridge, subjected to the compressive forces that give stability to the arch in architecture. Furthermore, the thoracic vertebrae are lifted by the support of the ribs, and the cervical vertebrae sag, inducing shear stresses. Slight exaggeration of these forces during examination with the patient in the sleeping position will reproduce the pain, which can be relieved nicely by using the examiner's forearm to provide support under the arch of the neck. The cause and the cure have been demonstrated, and it remains necessary only to find a similarly pleasant and effective support. A pair of cervical ruffs may be made by enclosing two 8-inch by 24-inch dressing pads within tubes of 3-inch stockinette; these should be loosely tied in front and worn during sleep as a pillow, not a splint. Neck-support pillows may give cooler long-term comfort, or a regular pillow can be doubled over and used with the fold under the neck. A variety of physical therapies can also be useful if gently applied; but 15 minutes of therapy three times weekly will not solve the problem if 8 hours per night is spent making it worse.

The lower lumbar spine is at the extreme limit of hyperextension in virtually all patients with low back problems, and many have such weak abdominal muscles they can neither improve their posture nor develop a positive intra-abdominal pressure during lifting to spare their back. The investigation and therapy are similar, using sit-ups with neck, trunk, hips, and knees flexed (for safety) and feet held. The test or exercise progresses through levels of difficulty, beginning with arms outstretched; then hands to opposite shoulders; hands behind neck; and finally arms behind head, with fingers touching opposite ears. Five repetitions faithfully performed once daily will restore abdominal power to level 3 or 4 within weeks, even for the aged. Postural training is designed to avoid lumbar hyperextension. The ideal is that of the athlete, with knees bent and spine slightly flexed. To be avoided is the military posture: chest out, shoulders back, and swaybacked.

The sleep disturbance is little helped by barbiturates, which do not restore the normal sleep pattern. Chlorpromazine is effective[20] in restoring deep sleep and relieving pain but leaves such unpleasant morning lethargy that it is unsuitable for long-term use. The benzodiazepines, such as diazepam, 5 to 20 mg at night, are occasionally helpful symptomatically. They do not abolish alpha intrusion into slow-wave sleep and are often in-

effective. Tricyclic antidepressants, such as amitriptyline or imipramine, can reduce alpha intrusion, and with an effect better sustained over prolonged periods.[22] In modest doses there is little effect for several hours after ingestion, but the quality of late morning sleep is improved. Some patients report frightening dreams, and others are sensitive to morning lethargy, so that appropriate evening dosage of amitriptyline may vary widely from 10 to 75 mg.

Counterirritant Therapies. A wide variety of popular or unusual therapies, including massage, heat, liniments, steroid injections, ethyl chloride spray, and acupuncture, are helpful in relieving pain. The "gate" theory of Melzack and Wall[8] has provided theoretical respectability, and recent studies have provided evidence for involvement of endorphins in the analgesic effect.[9] Factors influencing choice of counterirritant technique will include simplicity, safety, and availability and economy on one hand and maximal placebo effect on the other.

Compliance and Noncompliance. Among the most common reasons for failure to respond to conservative therapy is the failure to use it. The term noncompliance suggests that the fault lies with the patient. A better term might be faulty doctor-patient interaction, as noncompliant patients may have inadequate understanding of the program proposed and may have such apprehension of the doctor's anger that they will not reveal to the doctor their omissions and their reasons. Faced with failure, the patient and the doctor tend to try something new; this is ineffective strategy if the new remedy is similar to the old, and a dangerous decision if a hazardous course is taken unnecessarily. A certain decisiveness on the part of the therapist is obviously essential, but anger and ultimatums usually lead to evasions or countermanipulations. It is better to reduce the opportunities for personality conflicts, and to reinforce the continuing direction of therapy by sharing when possible clinical and laboratory evidence of improvement and compliance. The diary system can be very helpful, with the patient recording such variables as weight, abdominal muscle power, sedimentation rate, and salicylate level, with clearly defined target levels. Then the battle is between the patient and the chart, with the physician standing by as a helpful friend.

Attitudes and Expectations. Patients who are sensitive and perfectionistic set too high standards for themselves and may have to be specifically advised to take a holiday totally away from continuing responsibilities and cares. Such holidays should be consciously scheduled to take place once a year, once a month, once a week, and once a day. These patients are very sensitive to any implications that they are "quitters" or "fakers"—they are more characteristically unusually loyal and effective but at too high a cost.

Tension normally and necessarily accompanies major effort. It is normal for an athlete preparing for a major event to develop sweaty palms, a rapid heart rate, and the other physical responses to anticipated challenge. The body responds similarly to intellectual or emotional challenges, and this build-up of tension is essential to optimal performance. When the challenge is undramatic, is repeated daily, and arises from normal job and family duties, the relationship between tension and response to challenge may be inapparent or devalued. The defect does not lie in the exposure to tension but in the failure to get out from under self-imposed loads. Any variety of recreational release may be considered, but preference should be given to activities that give pleasure, are social, and involve physical activity. These patients are not helped by narrowing the scope of their life, and it is extremely important that their work patterns not be interrupted.

References

1. Yunus, M., Masi, A.T., Calabro, J.J., Miller, K.A., and Feigenbaum, S.L.: Primary fibromyalgia (fibrositis): Clinical study of 50 patients with matched normal controls. Semin. Arthritis Rheum. 11:151, 1981.
2. Campbell, S.M., Clark, S., Tindall, E.A., Forehand, M.E., and Bennett, R.H.O.: Clinical characteristics of fibrositis. Arthritis Rheum. 26:817, 1983.
3. Wolfe, F., and Cathey, M.A.: Prevalence of primary and secondary fibrositis. J. Rheumatol. 10:965, 1983.
4. Kellgren, J.H.: Deep pain sensibility. Lancet 1:943, 1949.
5. Kellgren, J.H.: Observations on referred pain arising from muscle. Clin. Sci. 3:174, 1938.
6. Kellgren, J.H.: On distribution of pain arising from deep somatic structures with charts of segmental pain areas. Clin. Sci. 4:35, 1939.
7. Lewis, T., and Kellgren, J.H.: Observations relating to referred pain, visceromotor reflexes and other associated phenomena. Clin. Sci. 4:47, 1939.
8. Melzack, R., and Wall, P.D.: Pain mechanisms: A new theory. Science 150:971.
9. Pomeranz, B.: Do endorphins mediate acupuncture analgesia? In Costa, E., and Trabucchi, M. (eds.): The Endorphins. Advances in Biochemical Psychopharmacology. Vol. 18. New York, Raven Press, 1977, p. 351.
10. Hinoki, M., and Niki, H.: Role of the sympathetic nervous system in the formation of the traumatic vertigo of cervical origin. Acta. Otolaryngol. 330(Suppl.):185, 1975.
11. Toglia, J.V.: Acute flexion-extension injury of the neck. Electronystagmographic study of 309 cases. Neurology 25:808, 1976.
12. Moldofsky, H.: Occupational cramp. J. Psychosomat. Res. 15:439, 1971.
13. Smythe, H.A., and Moldofsky, H.: Two contributions to understanding of the "fibrositis" syndrome. Bull. Rheum. Dis. 28:298, 1977.
14. Simons, D.G.: Muscle pain syndromes. Part 1. Am. J. Phys. Med. 54:289, 1975.
15. Simons, D.G.: Muscle pain syndromes. Part 2. Am. J. Phys. Med. 55:15, 1976.
16. Smythe, H.A.: Nonarticular rheumatism and the "fibrositis" syndrome. In Hollander, J.L., and McCarty, D.J., Jr. (eds.): Arthritis and Allied Conditions. 8th ed. Philadelphia, Lea & Febiger, 1972.
17. Payne, T.C., Leavitt, F., Garron, D.C., Katz, R.S., Golden, H.E., Glickman, P.B., and Vanderplate, C.: Fibrositis and psychogenic disturbance. Arthritis Rheum. 25:213–217, 1982.
18. Moldofsky, H., Scarisbrick, P., England, R., and Smythe, H.: Musculoskeletal symptoms and non-REM sleep disturbance in patients with "fibrositis syndrome" and healthy subjects. Psychosomat. Med. 37:341, 1975.
19. Moldofsky, H., and Scarisbrick, P.: Induction of neurasthenic musculoskeletal pain syndrome by selective sleep stage deprivation. Psychosomat. Med. 38:35, 1976.
20. Moldofsky, H., and Lue, F.: Alpha and delta EEG frequencies, pain and mood in "fibrositic" patients treated with chlorpromazine and L-tryptophan. EEG Clin. Neurophysiol. 50:71, 1980.
21. Hauri, P., and Hawkins, D.R.: Alpha-delta sleep. Electroencephalogr. Clin. Neurophysiol. 34:233, 1973.
22. Hauri, P.: The Sleep Disorders. Kalamazoo, The Upjohn Co., 1977, p. 51.
23. Wittig, R.M., Zorick, F.J., Blumer, D., Heilbronn, M., and Roth, T.: Disturbed sleep in patients complaining of chronic pain. J. Nerv. Ment. Dis. 170:429, 1982.
24. Moldofsky, H., and Scarisbrick, P.: Induction of neuresthenic musculoskeletal pain syndrome by selective stage sleep deprivation. Psychosomat. Med. 38:35, 1976.
25. Moldofsky, H., and Chester, W.J.: Pain and mood patterns in patients with rheumatoid arthritis. Psychosomat. Med. 32:309, 1970.
26. Moldofsky, H.: Rheumatic pain modulation syndrome: The interrelationships between sleep, central nervous system serotonin, and pain. In Critchley, M., Friedman, A.P., Sicuteri, F. (eds.): Advances in Neurology. Vol. 33. New York, Raven Press, 1982, p. 51.
27. Walters, A.: Psychogenic regional pain alias hysterical pain. Brain 84:1, 1961.
28. Forestier, J., and Rotes-Querol, J.: Senile ankylosing hyperostosis of the spine. Ann. Rheum. Dis. 9:321, 1950.
29. Forestier, J., and Lagier, R.: Vertebral ankylosing hyperostosis: Morphological basis, clinical manifestations, situation and diagnosis. In Hill, A. (ed.): Modern Trends in Rheumatology. Vol. 2. London, Butterworths, 1971, p. 323.
30. Resnick, D., Shall, S.R., and Robins, J.M.: Diffuse idiopathic skeletal hyperostosis (DISH): Forestier's disease with extraspinal manifestations. Radiology 115:513, 1975.
31. Utsinger, P.D., Resnick, D., and Shapiro, R.: Diffuse skeletal abnormalities in Forestier's disease. Arch. Intern. Med. 136:763, 1976.
32. Slocumb, C.H.: Symposium on certain problems are arising from clinical use of cortisone. Mayo Clin. Proc. 28:655, 1973.
33. Rotstein, J., and Good, B.A.: Steroid pseudorheumatism. Arch. Intern. Med. 99:545, 1957.
34. Henschel, E.O. (ed.): Malignant Hyperthermia: Current Concepts. New York, Appleton-Century-Crofts, 1977.

Chapter 33

Approach to the Patient with Hyperuricemia

William N. Kelley

Evaluation of the patient with hyperuricemia is directed toward answering the following questions: (1) Does the patient really have hyperuricemia? (2) Has damage to tissues or organs occurred as a result? (3) Are associated findings present? (4) What is the cause? (5) What, if anything, should be done? From a practical standpoint these inquiries are pursued simultaneously, since decisions about the significance of hyperuricemia and about therapy depend on the answers to all of them.

WHAT IS HYPERURICEMIA AND DOES THE PATIENT HAVE IT?

The serum urate value is elevated in an absolute sense when it exceeds the limit of solubility of monosodium urate in serum. At 37° C the saturation value of urate in plasma is about 7.0 mg per 100 ml; a value above this concentration represents supersaturation in a physicochemical sense. The serum urate concentration is elevated in a relative sense when it exceeds the upper limit of an arbitrary normal range, which is usually defined as the mean serum urate value plus two standard deviations in a sex- and age-matched healthy population. In most epidemiological studies, the upper limit has been rounded off at 7.0 mg per 100 ml in men and 6.0 mg per 100 ml in women. Finally, a serum urate value in excess of 7.0 mg per 100 ml begins to carry an increased risk of gouty arthritis or renal stones.

Many factors, including sex and age, have an important influence on the serum urate concentration. The serum urate concentration before puberty in both boys and girls averages approximately 3.6 mg per 100 ml. After the onset of puberty, the levels rise in males more than in females. Values in males reach a plateau in the early 20's and are essentially stable thereafter. Values in females are constant at a lower level than those found in males from age 20 through 40. With menopause the values in women rise and approach or equal those in men. Differences in the serum urate levels with sex and age are thought to be related to differences in the renal clearance of urate, perhaps determined, in turn, by the endogenous levels of estrogens and androgens. In addition to age and sex, other factors, including obesity, muscle mass, warm ambient temperature, higher social status, achievement, and intelligence, appear to correlate with a higher serum urate concentration.

Interpretation of the serum urate level must also take into account the laboratory method employed. Fluorimetric methods and most automated techniques will measure materials other than urate and may give higher values than the more specific uricase method. In addition, there may be substantial variation over a period of time in any single individual, an observation attributable to many causes, including some of the variables described above. Accordingly, a single serum urate value is of considerably less value than several determinations over time.

Hyperuricemia by one or more of the aforementioned definitions has been described in 2.3 to 17.6 percent of the populations studied. In one hospitalized population in the United States, 13.2 percent of all adult men exhibited a serum urate concentration in excess of 7.0 mg per 100 ml.[1]

HAS TISSUE OR ORGAN DAMAGE OCCURRED OWING TO THE HYPERURICEMIA?

Assessment of tissue damage that might be attributed to hyperuricemia is of major importance in the patient with arthritis, subcutaneous nodules, erosions or other changes on radiographs, aseptic necrosis, nephrolithiasis, or renal insufficiency. Any other clinical signs and symptoms that might result from sustained hyperuricemia would be rare in the absence of at least one of the above.

Arthritis. In the hyperuricemic patient with active joint disease, the most useful diagnostic test is direct examination of the synovial fluid. According to current dogma, the demonstration of intracellular monosodium urate crystals establishes the diagnosis of gout; it does not, of course, exclude other diseases that may occur simultaneously, e.g., septic arthritis, pseudogout, osteoarthritis, fractures, or torn ligaments or tendons, and these possibilities may have to be excluded. Intracellular monosodium urate crystals can be demonstrated in virtually all patients with gout if synovial fluid from the appropriate joint is carefully examined using compensated polarized light microscopy within the first 24 to 48 hours after onset of the attack. Thus, failure to demonstrate intracellular urate crystals in synovial fluid obtained from an acutely inflamed joint makes the diagnosis of gout highly unlikely as the cause of an acute episode of synovitis. However, when patients are examined several days after the onset of acute synovitis, the likelihood of finding urate crystals declines and the urate crystals observed may not be located in polymorphonuclear leukocytes. Extracellular urate crystals can be found in synovial fluid of 70 percent of gouty patients even during the intercritical period when they are asymptomatic.[2] The finding of extracellular urate crystals in synovial fluid does not carry the same degree of specificity for diagnosing gout as does the demonstration of intracellular urate crystals. This conclusion is based on the following observations. Although the patient with uncomplicated asymptomatic hyperuricemia rarely (<5 percent) exhibits extracellular urate crystals in synovial fluid, as many as 20 percent of patients with hyperuricemia secondary to renal failure may have extracellular urate crystals in the absence of any history of arthritis.[2]

When synovial fluid cannot be obtained or active joint disease is not present at the time of examination, the relationship of hyperuricemia to the clinical symptoms may be more difficult to evaluate. If there is a history of classic podagra or of an acute monoarticular arthritis strongly suggestive of gouty arthritis and dramatically responsive to colchicine, a working assumption that the patient has gout is justified. The diagnosis should be documented with demonstration of urate crystals at the first opportunity.

Nodules. The finding of subcutaneous nodules in the hyperuricemic subject raises the possibility that these are tophaceous deposits. The history is important in this connection, since tophi rarely occur without preceding gouty arthritis. However, if a question exists as to the nature of the nodule or deposit, material should be obtained for microscopic examination. This may be done most easily by closed aspiration of the nodule under aseptic conditions, using a sterile 22-gauge needle. Injection of a small amount of sterile saline may enhance the recovery of urate crystals if no material is obtained with aspiration alone. Suspected tophi in the helix of the ear can be confirmed by gentle abrasion of the skin and blotting the denuded surface with a sterile slide. If urate crystals are demonstrated, the nodule represents a tophus. If crystals are not demonstrated with this procedure, open surgical biopsy of the lesion may be performed. The tissue obtained at that time should be fixed in absolute alcohol in order to avoid dissolution of crystals if present.

Serologic tests for rheumatoid factor are also helpful in evaluating the patient with subcutaneous nodules. If the lesion is a rheumatoid nodule, over 90 percent of patients will have a positive screening test for rheumatoid factor and the test will usually remain positive at serum dilutions of 1:80 or greater. Only 30 percent of patients with gout exhibit positive screening tests for rheumatoid factor, and these are usually of low titer.

Radiographic Findings. Bony erosions seen on roentgenograms in a patient with hyperuricemia can present a difficult diagnostic problem. From a practical standpoint, erosions resulting from gout represent tophi, and consequently, they are usually preceded by a history of gouty arthritis. Tophi are not always evident in subcutaneous tissues on physical examination, however, at the time bony erosions are noted on roentgenograms. The radiographic appearance of the erosions may be of some help in determining the etiology of this lesion. Should this history be inconsistent with gout and the radiologic features atypical for gout, one would ordinarily assume that the erosions were not due to deposition of monosodium urate crystals. Biopsy may be indicated, particularly if a neoplastic lesion or infection is possible.

Tophi in the subcutaneous tissues are usually radiolucent, but they can become radiopaque if calcium is deposited in these lesions. In the latter circumstances radiographic examination may reveal the presence of tophaceous deposits, but physical examination will usually detect tophi in subcutaneous tissues before they are evident on roentenograms.

A possible relationship between hyperuricemia and aseptic necrosis of the femoral heads is suggested by the observation that aseptic necrosis may occur with an increased incidence in patients without gout and by the finding of monosodium urate crystals in synovium obtained from the hip at the time of surgery, even in some patients who give no history of gouty arthritis. Even though this relationship is not firmly established, it may be reasonable to consider treating the hyperuricemia if the necrosis is unilateral, or in an early stage if bilateral.

Nephrolithiasis. A history or laboratory finding indicative of a renal calculus provides information important to the future management of the patient. In contrast to the situation observed with tophi, renal calculi may antedate the onset of gouty arthritis. The typical uric acid stone is radiolucent and therefore is not visible on routine radiologic examination of the abdomen. It will appear as a filling defect with the use of radiopaque contrast material. As such it may be confused with other radiolucent stones, such as those composed of xanthine and adenine (which are very rare), as well as with tumors or blood clots. If a stone is passed or retrieved at surgery, it is important that it be subjected to chemical analysis.

The importance of hyperuricemia in patients with radiopaque stones deserves emphasis. First, radiopaque stones occur more commonly in patients with gout than in a nongouty population. In addition, reduction of uric acid production (and hence concentration in the urine) with allopurinol is associated with a striking decrease in the frequency of radiopaque stones containing calcium in both hyperuricemic and nonhyperuricemic subjects (Chapter 86). It is possible that the initial nidus for opaque stones in this setting is crystals of urate or uric acid. Whether or not this hypothesis accounts for the observation, the therapeutic implications are clear. Hyperuricemic subjects with calcium stones, but not other radiopaque stones such as magnesium ammonium phosphate or cystine, may benefit from a trial with allopurinol. In nonhyperuricemic subjects with hyperuricosuria (> 800 and > 750 mg of uric acid excreted per 24 hrs for men and women, respectively) who repetitively form calcium-containing stones a trial of allopurinol may also be indicated.[3]

Renal Insufficiency. One of the most difficult problems facing the clinician lies in his attempt to determine the relationship of hyperuricemia and renal insufficiency in the patient presenting with both abnormalities. In assessing the relationship between hyperuricemia and renal insufficiency it is important to consider the mechanisms by which uric acid and/or urate may injure the kidney. Urate can precipitate in the interstitium of the kidney, leading to slowly progressive renal insufficiency referred to as *urate nephropathy*; uric acid can precipitate in the collecting tubules, leading to acute renal failure, which is referred to as *uric acid nephropathy*; or uric acid crystals can grow into *calculi*, which leads to obstruction and/or infection of the kidney. If the patient has a history of gout preceding renal insufficiency and there is no evidence to suggest another cause of renal disease, such as hypertension or lead exposure, one may assume that urate nephropathy is the etiology of the renal failure. Attempts to reduce uric acid production are justified in that setting, in order to prevent further progress of the putative urate nephropathy. The patient with hyperuricemia and renal disease without a previous history of gout presents a more difficult problem. Since an understanding of the relationship of asymptomatic hyperuricemia to chronic renal disease is an important element in directing management of the former, this issue is discussed extensively later in this chapter. In the patient with acute renal failure, uric acid nephropathy should be considered. This entity is more likely to be encountered in patients with malignancies undergoing chemotherapy or radiation treatment than in gouty patients, with the exception of those individuals with inherited enzyme abnormalities leading to marked purine overproduction. The uric acid:creatinine ratio in a random urine sample from such a patient may help in his evaluation. The finding of a ratio in excess of 1.0 in a patient with acute renal insufficiency is indicative of a substantial increase in uric acid production and raises the possibility that uric acid deposition in the nephron or collecting system may be contributing to the renal insufficiency.[4] In this situation vigorous therapy is indicated. The more common finding in acute renal failure is a ratio of less than 1.0. In this situation the hyperuricemia may be due entirely to the renal disease and associated factors such as acidosis and dehydration. A history of renal calculi, especially if the stone is demonstrated to contain uric acid and/or calcium, may be another indication for antihyperuricemic therapy in the patient with renal insufficiency.

A general approach to the hyperuricemic patient is summarized in Figure 33–1. Most hyperuricemic patients will have no evidence of end-organ damage and thus have asymptomatic hyperuricemia. Management of asymptomatic hyperuricemia will depend on the associated findings and the cause of the hyperuricemia, as discussed in the following paragraphs.

ARE ASSOCIATED FINDINGS PRESENT?

Hyperuricemia and gout may be associated with obesity, ethanol consumption, and hypertension in a significant percentage of individuals. As a consequence it is not uncommon to also find glucose intolerance, hypertriglyceridemia, atherosclerosis, and renal, hepatic, and ischemic heart disease in hyperuricemic individuals. In evaluating hyperuricemic subjects it is important to keep these associated problems in mind. It may be justified to include a complete blood count, urinalysis, 2-hour postprandial blood sugar, fasting triglycerides, creatinine, liver panel, electrocardiogram, and chest x-ray in the evaluation of the hyperuricemic patient who is overweight or hypertensive or consumes significant amounts of ethanol. In the normotensive hyperuricemic patient who is not overweight and does not drink, a search for these associated findings would probably not be cost effective.

WHAT IS THE CAUSE OF HYPERURICEMIA?

Hyperuricemia may be defined as primary, first in order of time or development, or secondary, second in order of time or development (see Chapter 86).[5] In the latter setting, the hyperuricemia develops in the course of another disease or as a consequence of its therapy. Hyperuricemia, whether primary or secondary, may be due to overproduction of purines, reduced renal clearance of uric acid, or a combination of the two processes.

In 70 percent of hyperuricemic patients an underlying cause of hyperuricemia can be readily defined by history and physical examination.[1] Hyperuricemia may be the initial clue to the presence of a previously unsuspected disorder. In addition, the nature of the underlying cause may be useful in predicting the potential consequence, if any, of the chemical abnormality. Thus the possibility of an underlying cause should be explored in every hyperuricemic patient.

A scheme for investigating the cause of hyperuricemia, including the secondary causes, is summarized in Figure 33–2. It would seem most reasonable that one be guided by the initial history and physical examination. If an acquired cause commonly associated with normal uric acid excretion is present in the patient with asymptomatic hyperuricemia, further evaluation is probably unnecessary. If the patient has an underlying disorder usually associated with an overproduction of uric acid, determination of 24-hour urinary uric acid may be useful. The higher the urinary uric acid in this group of patients, the higher the incidence of renal calculi[6] and acute uric acid nephropathy,[7] and thus the more likely that treatment will be indicated. If no findings suggestive of a secondary cause are forthcoming, then 24-hour urinary uric acid should be measured in those with a serum urate in excess of 11 mg per 100 ml. Further rationale underlying this approach is described later in this chapter under Management of Hyperuricemia.

THE GENERAL WORKUP

At this point the general workup of the patient with hyperuricemia may be reviewed.

History. In beginning to sort out clues that will help in directing the physician toward a correct understanding of the problem, it is useful to formulate questions that will decide the following:

1. Is the hyperuricemia primary or secondary? (a) Is the patient obese? If so, for how long? (b) Does the patient consume alcohol regularly and liberally? (c) Has the patient consumed unbonded alcohol? (d) Is the patient taking thiazide diuretics, salicylates, or other drugs? (e) Is there evidence of volume depletion? (f) Is there a history suggestive of renal disease? (g) Is there a history suggestive of a myeloproliferative syndrome, chronic hemolytic anemia, or solid tumor malignancy?

2. Is there a history of acute arthritic attacks? If so, what was their character? Was there a response to colchicine? Has the patient noted any tophi?

3. Is there a history of kidney stones?

4. Has there been hypertension or any history of cardiovascular disease?

5. Is there a family history of hyperuricemia, gout, kidney stones, or renal disease?

Physical Examination. Special attention should be directed toward the following:

1. Habitus should be noted, and height and weight recorded.

2. Is there plethora or pallor? Is there lymphadenopathy, splenomegaly, or hepatomegaly?

3. What is the status of the vascular system? Is there evidence of present or previous hypertension?

4. Are there tophi present in the ears, tendons, joints, digits, or fingertips? Is joint disease present?

Laboratory Data. The need for laboratory studies will depend on the severity of the hyperuricemia and findings elicited from history and physical examination. In general, the laboratory studies will be those that would be

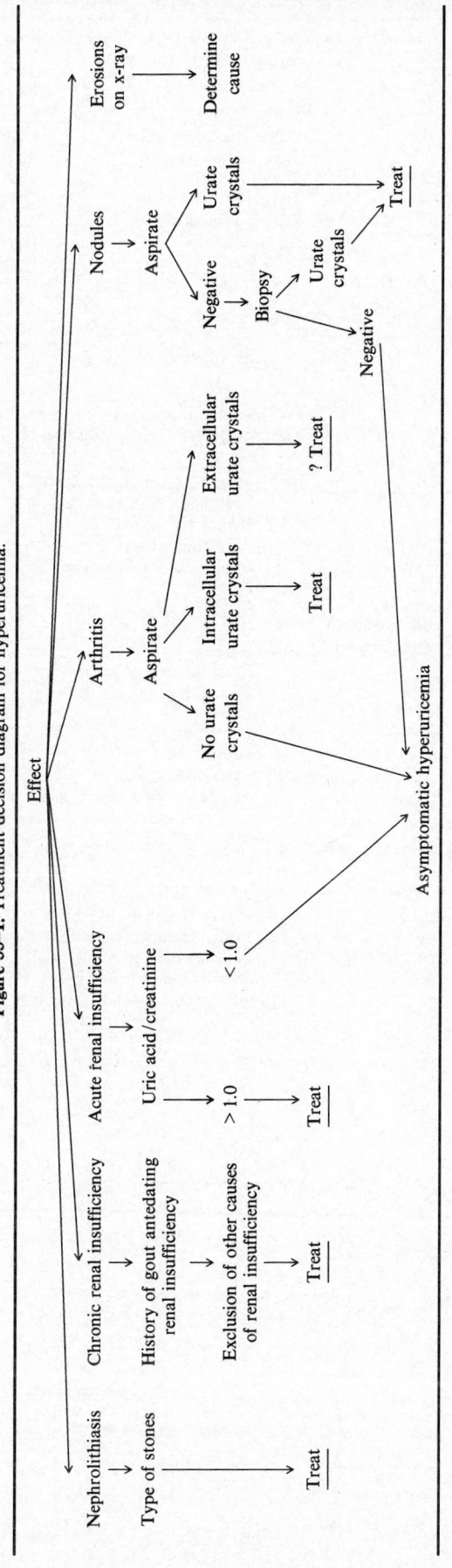

Figure 33–1. Treatment decision diagram for hyperuricemia.

Figure 33–2. Evaluation of the patient with hyperuricemia.

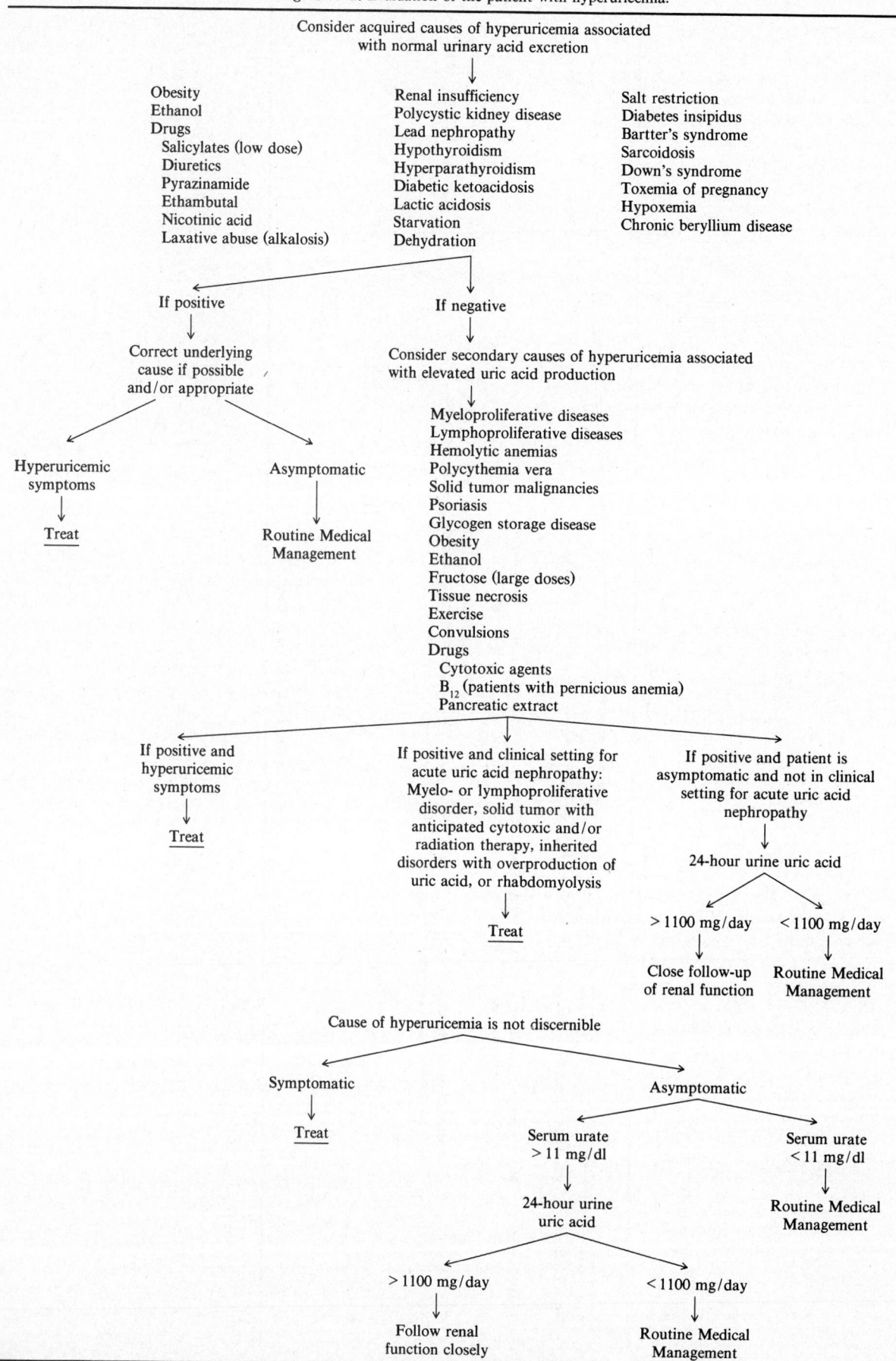

Consider acquired causes of hyperuricemia associated
with normal urinary acid excretion

Obesity
Ethanol
Drugs
   Salicylates (low dose)
   Diuretics
   Pyrazinamide
   Ethambutal
   Nicotinic acid
   Laxative abuse (alkalosis)

Renal insufficiency
Polycystic kidney disease
Lead nephropathy
Hypothyroidism
Hyperparathyroidism
Diabetic ketoacidosis
Lactic acidosis
Starvation
Dehydration

Salt restriction
Diabetes insipidus
Bartter's syndrome
Sarcoidosis
Down's syndrome
Toxemia of pregnancy
Hypoxemia
Chronic beryllium disease

If positive

Correct underlying
cause if possible
and/or appropriate

Hyperuricemic
symptoms

Treat

Asymptomatic

Routine Medical
Management

If negative

Consider secondary causes of hyperuricemia associated
with elevated uric acid production

Myeloproliferative diseases
Lymphoproliferative diseases
Hemolytic anemias
Polycythemia vera
Solid tumor malignancies
Psoriasis
Glycogen storage disease
Obesity
Ethanol
Fructose (large doses)
Tissue necrosis
Exercise
Convulsions
Drugs
   Cytotoxic agents
   B_{12} (patients with pernicious anemia)
   Pancreatic extract

If positive and
hyperuricemic
symptoms

Treat

If positive and clinical setting for
acute uric acid nephropathy:
Myelo- or lymphoproliferative
disorder, solid tumor with
anticipated cytotoxic and/or
radiation therapy, inherited
disorders with overproduction of
uric acid, or rhabdomyolysis

Treat

If positive and patient is
asymptomatic and not in clinical
setting for acute uric acid
nephropathy

24-hour urine uric acid

> 1100 mg/day

Close follow-up
of renal function

< 1100 mg/day

Routine Medical
Management

Cause of hyperuricemia is not discernible

Symptomatic

Treat

Asymptomatic

Serum urate
> 11 mg/dl

24-hour urine
uric acid

> 1100 mg/day

Follow renal
function closely

< 1100 mg/day

Routine Medical
Management

Serum urate
< 11 mg/dl

Routine Medical
Management

indicated because of the basic disease process whether or not the patient had hyperuricemia or gout. Some of these have been reviewed earlier in the chapter. Several special tests, however, are worthy of emphasis.

1. The most useful of special tests in determining whether the hyperuricemic patient has gout are those that may disclose urate crystals: (a) Synovial fluid analysis. Note should be made of gross appearance, total and differential cell count, bacteria if present, quality of the mucin clot, and crystals if present. The fluid should be examined with standard light, as well as with polarized light microscopy (see Chapter 38). (b) Needle aspiration or biopsy of suspected superficial or bony tophus with search for urate crystals.

2. If a renal stone is recovered, it should be analyzed for uric acid and other constituents by the most definitive methods available. If there is a history of renal colic, IVP may be required to visualize radiolucent stones.

3. If there is a suspicion of lead-induced hyperuricemia or gout, one should perform a calcium EDTA-infusion test with measurement of urinary lead, or analyze erythrocyte δ-aminolevulinic acid dehydratase activity.

MANAGEMENT OF HYPERURICEMIA

The management of patients with symptoms related to hyperuricemia is discussed in detail in Chapter 86. In general, such patients should be treated with antihyperuricemic agents. The decision of whether or not to treat hyperuricemia uncomplicated by articular gout, urolithiasis, or nephropathy is an exercise in clinical judgment on which there is less than universal agreement among physicians. The lack of unanimity reflects the paucity of firm data on hyperuricemia as an independent risk factor for hypertension, atherosclerosis, and renal disease. The weight of evidence favors the view that hyperuricemia is directly important only as it may predispose to articular tophi, gout, urate nephropathy, uric acid stones, and acute uric acid nephropathy. Accordingly, the risks engendered by asymptomatic hyperuricemia can be reduced to the statistical risks of development of these manifestations and their consequences.

The magnitude of the risk of articular gout or tophi is related to the degree and duration of hyperuricemia and the sex and age of the patient. Gouty arthritis and tophi are treatable and reversible whenever they occur and by themselves are not life threatening. It would be reasonable to withhold antihyperuricemic therapy in patients with hyperuricemia if the only goal of such therapy was to prevent the development of gout. Clearly, such therapy could be instituted when these manifestations occurred.

Urate nephropathy is an entity that may not be reversible. This manifestation is difficult to document, is probably a very late event, and is very rarely reported to occur in the absence of previous episodes of gouty arthritis.

Several studies relevant to the relationship between hyperuricemia and urate nephropathy deserve comment in this regard. In one study, no examples of renal disease were found in 15 patients at the time of their initial gouty attack.[8] Another group of investigators has evaluated renal function in asymptomatic hyperuricemic subjects.[9] Studies performed included the examination of urinary sediment, urine culture, Pitressin concentration test, PSP excretion, intravenous pyelogram, glomerular filtration rate, 24-hour urinary protein, and an acid load test. Abnormality in one or more of these tests was found in 63 percent of the hyperuricemic individuals. The Pitressin concentration test, PSP excretion, and acid load tests were the studies most frequently found to be abnormal. From these data, however, one cannot tell (1) if these abnormalities were due to an adverse effect of an increased filtered load of urate, (2) if hyperuricemia is simply a very sensitive marker for intrinsic renal disease, or (3) if hyperuricemia is a reflection of a fundamental metabolic disturbance that also affects renal tubular function. In a subsequent study renal function was monitored prospectively with serum creatinine determination for 8 years in 113 asymptomatic hyperuricemic subjects and 193 normouricemic patients.[10] During this extended follow-up the development of azotemia, as reflected by an increase in serum creatinine concentration, was not different in the hyperuricemic and control subjects. To the extent that an increase in serum creatinine concentration can be used to detect urate nephropathy, we conclude from this study that this particular abnormality is not a major contributor to renal dysfunction in hyperuricemic subjects who do not have articular manifestations of gout.

Urate nephropathy may not be a very common cause of renal dysfunction even in the patient with gout. In one study of 524 gouty patients followed for up to 12 years, hyperuricemia alone appeared to have no deleterious effect on renal function.[11] Renal functional deterioration was mainly associated with aging, renal vascular disease, renal calculi, and pyelonephritis, and the correlation with hypertension and resultant nephrosclerosis was much stronger than with hyperuricemia. In another study of 168 gouty patients followed for 10 years, the development of azotemia appeared to be unrelated to control of the hyperuricemia and was mild when it occurred.[10] Thus, although an association appears to exist between gout and renal disease, a causal role of the hyperuricemia per se in the production of urate nephropathy has yet to be established.

The lack of proof of a direct causal role of hyperuricemia in the genesis of urate nephropathy serves to emphasize the importance of a study designed to determine if control of hyperuricemia has an effect on renal function; one such short-term study exists. A study of 116 patients followed for a mean of 2.5 years compared the effects of allopurinol and placebo therapy in nongouty patients matched for serum urate concentration, mean creatinine clearance, blood pressure, and body weight.[12] No statistically significant differences were consistently found between the placebo-treated and allopurinol-treated groups, and it was concluded that normalization of the plasma urate concentration did not significantly alter renal function.

At present, therefore, the available data, which are admittedly incomplete, suggest that (1) renal function is not necessarily affected in an adverse manner by an elevated serum urate concentration; (2) the renal disease that accompanies hyperuricemia may often be related to inadequately controlled hypertension; and (3) correction of hyperuricemia has no apparent effect on renal function. When these observations are coupled with the side effects of the antihyperuricemic drugs, our current recommendation is that asymptomatic hyperuricemia per se is not an indication for antihyperuricemic agents if the goal is to prevent urate nephropathy.

Uric acid nephrolithiasis and calcium oxalate nephrolithiasis occur more commonly in the patient with hyperuricemia or hyperuricaciduria. Fessel[10] found an incidence of one stone per 114 patients per year in gouty patients, one stone per 295 patients per year in subjects with asymptomatic hyperuricemia, and one stone per 852 patients per year in normouricemic control subjects. In a careful long-term follow-up of gouty patients by Yu and Gutman,[13] the risk of uric acid nephrolithiasis was related to the height of the serum urate level and, to a greater degree, to the magnitude of urinary uric acid excretion. For example, risk of stone formation was less than 20 percent if the serum urate level was 7.1 to 9.0 mg per 100 ml, and reached 50 percent if it was over 13 mg per 100 ml. In similar patients the risk of nephrolithiasis was less than 21 percent if urinary uric acid excretion was less than 700 mg per day and increased substantially with uric acid excretion over 700 mg per day, reaching 50 percent if the excretion was over 1100 mg per day.

The most common type of stone in patients with gout is a uric acid calculus, but gouty subjects also have an increased prevalence of calcium-containing stones. From 1 to 3 percent of the gouty population have a history of calcium stone formation as compared with an overall prevalence of calcium stones in the population of about 0.1 percent. In addition, patients selected because of calcium oxalate or calcium phosphate stones have a high prevalence of hyperuricemia. In one series the mean serum urate in 67 patients with calcium oxalate stones was 7.2 mg per 100 ml compared with the mean serum urate in 10 patients with uric acid stones of 7.8 mg per 100 ml.[14] Perhaps more importantly, Coe and Kavalach[15] noted that 46 of 105 male patients and 9 of 41 female patients with idiopathic recurrent calcium stone disease had a urinary uric acid value over 750 (females) or 800 (males) mg per day while on an unrestricted diet. Hyperuricemia occurred in only 26 of the 55 hyperuricosuric patients. These studies have clearly identified a relationship between hyperuricemia, hyperuricaciduria, and idiopathic calcium oxalate nephrolithiasis. The incidence of calcium oxalate stone disease in a group of patients with asymptomatic hyperuricemia, however, has not been determined.

While both uric acid and calcium nephrolithiasis are often responsive to appropriate therapeutic regimens, including allopurinol, several observations militate against routine antihyperuricemic prophylaxis in asymptomatic patients at putative risk for developing renal stone disease: (1) The actual prevalence of stone disease in the asymptomatic patient with hyperuricemia is only twice as high as it is in the normouricemic population. (2) When a stone is formed, it rarely produces a life-threatening or irreversible series of events. In fact, stone disease related to hyperuricemia and/or hyperuricaciduria is often reversible with appropriate therapy. At this point, in the author's opinion, antihyperuricemic therapy should not be instituted as prophylaxis against the development of stone disease but should be started promptly with discovery of a stone in the hyperuricemic or hyperuricaciduric patient. Identification of the patient with a substantial risk of developing a stone in the future may be valuable to the physician in counseling the patient and in recommending frequency of follow-up visits (see below).

Uric acid nephropathy is a severe form of acute renal failure that may occur in hyperuricemic subjects as a result of the precipitation of uric acid crystals in collecting ducts and ureters. This condition occurs most commonly (1) in patients with profound overproduction of uric acid, particularly those with leukemia or lymphoma subjected to aggressive chemotherapy, (2) in patients with gout and marked hyperuricaciduria, and possibly (3) in patients after severe exercise or convulsions. Postmortem studies in patients with acute uric acid nephropathy reveal intraluminal precipitates of uric acid with dilatation of proximal tubules. Therapy designed to decrease the formation of uric acid and to increase the fraction of uric acid present as the more soluble ionized form, monosodium urate, is highly effective in the prevention or reversal of this process. Indeed, it is in this small group of patients that prophylactic antihyperuricemic therapy may be useful.

Based on the considerations discussed above the author has developed an approach to the hyperuricemic patient, and it is summarized in Figure 33–2. Determine, if possible, whether the patient has one of the conditions listed in this figure which might account for the hyperuricemia. If the underlying cause cannot be corrected, a decision regarding therapy and future management is required. When a symptom such as articular gout, tophi, bone lesions, or renal calculi is documented, antihyperuricemic therapy is justified. In the absence of symptoms, the following guidelines are helpful: (1) If the hyperuricemia is associated with one of the conditions that leads to a decrease in renal clearance of urate, the patient can be observed, without instituting hypouricemic therapy, at intervals dictated by his other medical problems. (2) If the hyperuricemia is related to one of the conditions associated with increased uric acid production, these patients may be at greater risk of developing renal calculi or acute uric acid nephropathy. In clinical settings in which acute uric acid nephropathy is likely, prophylactic treatment is probably justified. In other situations, although immediate antihyperuricemic therapy may not be indicated, quantitation of 24-hour urine uric acid excretion may be helpful in directing future management of the hyperuricemic subject. Based on studies of gouty patients and subject with malignancies, we have selected 1100 mg of uric acid excreted per day as a cut-off for potentially identifying those patients at higher risk for developing renal calculi and acute uric acid nephropathy. In our opinion those individuals who excrete > 1100 mg of uric acid per day warrant close follow-up of their renal function and immediate therapy at the first onset of symptoms or evidence of renal dysfunction. (3) If the probable cause of hyperuricemia cannot be determined to identify those patients with increased uric acid production and excretion, the serum urate concentration may be indicative of the amount of uric acid excreted in the urine. Studies in nongouty subjects with normal renal function have demonstrated that there is an abrupt increase in the rate of excretion of urinary uric acid when the serum urate concentration is increased to $\simeq 11$ mg per 100 ml, and the amount of uric acid excreted at these rates exceeds 1000 mg per day.[16] In our opinion those patients with serum urate concentrations of > 11 mg per 100 ml in whom a secondary cause of hyperuricemia cannot be determined deserve further evaluation with quantitation of 24-hour urine uric acid excretion. This level of serum urate concentration should not lead to the unnecessary evaluation of large numbers of asymptomatic hyperuricemic subjects, but should identify those patients who need further evaluation and close follow-up of their renal function.

References

1. Paulus, H.E., Coutts, A., Calabro, J.J., et al.: Clinical significance of hyperuricemia in routinely screened hospitalized men. JAMA 211:277, 1970.
2. Rouault, T., Caldwell, D.S., and Holmes, E.W.: Aspiration of the asymptomatic metatarsophalangeal joint in gouty patients and hyperuricemic controls. Arth. Rheum. 25:209, 1982.
3. Coe, F.L.: Hyperuricosuric calcium oxalate nephrolithiasis. Contemporary Issues in Nephrology 5:116, 1980.
4. Kelton, J., Kelley, W.N., and Holmes, E.W.: A rapid method for the diagnosis of acute uric acid nephropathy. Arch. Intern. Med. 138:612, 1978.
5. Wyngaarden, J.B., and Kelley, W.N.: Gout and Hyperuricemia. New York, Grune & Stratton, 1976.
6. Boyce, W.H., Garvey, F.K., and Strawcutter, H.E.: Incidence of urinary calculi among patients in general hospitals, 1948 to 1952. JAMA 161:1437, 1956.
7. Rieselbach, R.E., Bentzel, C.J., Cotlove, E., et al.: Uric acid excretion and renal function in the acute hyperuricemia of leukemia: Pathogenesis and therapy of uric acid nephropathy. Am. J. Med. 37:872, 1964.
8. Colton, R.S., Ward, L.E., Maher, F.I., et al.: Occult renal impairment in gouty and hyperuricemic individuals. Am. J. Med. Sci. 252:575, 1966.
9. Klinenberg, J.R., Dornfield, L.P., and Gonick, H.C.: Renal function in patients with asymptomatic hyperuricemia (abstr.). Arthritis Rheum. 12:307, 1969.
10. Fessel, W.J.: Renal outcomes of gout and hyperuricemia. Am. J. Med. 67:74, 1979.
11. Berger, L., and Yu, T-F.: Renal function in gout. IV. An analysis of 524 gouty subjects including long-term follow-up studies. Am. J. Med. 59:605, 1975.
12. Rosenfeld, J.B.: Effect of long-term allopurinol administration on serial GFR in normotensive and hypertensive hyperuricemic subjects. In Sperling, O., de Vries, A., and Wyngaarden, J.B. (eds.): Purine Metabolism in Man. New York, Plenum Press, 1974, p. 581.
13. Yu, T-F., and Gutman, A.B.: Uric acid nephrolithiasis in gout. Predisposing factors. Ann. Intern. Med. 67:1133, 1967.
14. Smith, M.J.V., Hunt, L.D., King, J.S., Jr., et al.: Uricemia and urolithiasis. J. Urol. 101:637, 1969.
15. Coe, F.L., and Kavalach, A.G.: Hypercalcemia and hyperuricosuria in patients with calcium nephrolithiasis. N. Engl. J. Med. 291:1344, 1974.
16. Wyngaarden, J.B.: Gout. Adv. Metab. Dis. 2:1, 1965.

Chapter 34

Psychological and Sexual Health in Rheumatic Diseases

Barbara Figley Banwell and Beth Ziebell

INTRODUCTION

Patients with rheumatic diseases are among those who need comprehensive health care. The types of care that physiatrists, physical therapists, and occupational therapists can offer are described in Chapter 111, and the help that can be gained by close collaboration with orthopedists is discussed in Chapters 112 through 121.

It is not a paradox that the rheumatologist, a subspecialist within the specialty of internal medicine, must be concerned with providing comprehensive care to patients, since he or she is often the co-ordinator of treatment activities. Comprehensive care includes a commitment to understanding emotional responses to chronic disease and knowledge sufficient to treat normal, exaggerated, and pathologic psychological reactions to chronic diseases or to refer the patient to qualified mental health professionals. The most compelling reason for such an approach is that most patients and health care professionals would agree that comprehensive care with sensitive and knowledgeable appreciation of psychosocial-sexual issues has a positive effect on outcome and attitude. There is a growing body of information in the literature that describes psychosocial and biologic variables as they shape and are shaped by the pattern of chronic recurring illness. A number of studies can be cited that trace physiologic responses to emotional states and the behaviors that accompany or result from those states.[1-3] Knowledge of these psychological factors influences the success of management and treatment programs in rheumatic disease.[4-11]

This chapter will discuss the following points: (1) specific features of rheumatic disease that are likely to evoke a psychological response, (2) common emotional responses to rheumatic disease, (3) a framework, for management of psychosocial problems in rheumatology, including the behavioral aspects of pain, (4) a framework for recognition and management of sexual problems in rheumatic disease, (5) methods and data pertinent to psychobiosocial research in rheumatic diseases, and (6) the psychosocial factors in juvenile arthritis.

FEATURES OF RHEUMATIC DISEASES THAT EVOKE PSYCHOLOGICAL RESPONSES

Psychological reaction to rheumatic disease is an interaction between the disease, its treatment, and the patients' perception of their illness. Some features of the disease are more likely than others to have psychological effects. However, one should not assume that all patients have similar reactions, since people perceive and experience symptoms differently.[12] Illness and disability represent catastrophic events to some people; to others they are an expected part of the human experience.[13]

The first psychological reactions are evoked by the symptoms or diagnosis of arthritis. The prior state of good health is disrupted. Some people consider good health a principal goal in life and pride themselves on its achievement and maintenance. Others have taken good health for granted. Good health is intimately related in some to self-respect, and even temporary change in health status may carry with it a sense of loss or vulnerability. The diagnosis of arthritis, so often associated with "wearing out" or old age, may carry a special negative meaning. Terms such as "chronic disease," "rheumatism," or "crippling" carry strong connotations in many subcultures of our society.

Change in physical appearance that results in disrupted body image can occur as a result of disease or treatment and is difficult to handle for the average patient. An attractive body image is particularly important for the patient whose self-esteem is already eroded by pain, loss of function, and decreased activity. An obvious disability can be a barrier to satisfactory social interaction.[14,15] The malar rash and alopecia of systematic lupus erythematosus, the swollen joints of rheumatoid arthritis, and the drawn appearance of those with scleroderma are sometimes the most disturbing symptoms of the disease. When drug treatment causes changes in physical appearance, the patient may be reluctant to take the medication and compliance with medication schedules may be threatened. For example, many patients fear rejection because of a changed physical appearance produced by corticosteroids. Each person considers his appearance a part of his identity and self-image; a change in this self-perception may have a greater or lesser impact than might be predicted. It is the physician's responsibility to be aware of how patients react to physical changes.

Pain exerts a powerful influence upon the personality and emotions. Whether intermittent or persistent, it dulls the environment and interrupts well-established patterns of behavior. Pain interferes with intellectual and emotional functioning.[16,17] The "chronic pain syndrome," in which pain becomes interwoven with a series of behavioral responses and patterns, is frequently seen in rheumatic diseases. Family interactions, particularly intimate ones involving broad and deep emotion, undergo stress when one member is in pain. In addition to the reaction to pain, many patients are affected by the anticipation of pain, a phenomenon that affects even the pain-free segments of their lives. This reaction to anticipated pain may change activity patterns more than pain itself. Pain is the most disconcerting problem encountered by the patient with a rheumatic disease. Chronic pain in the patient with arthritis will be discussed in a later section.

Weakness, fatigue, and loss of energy are discouraging concomitants of rheumatic disease. "If I just didn't get so tired" is a frequent complaint in almost every diagnostic category. Those who value accomplishment and achievement seem particularly dismayed by lack of energy. "Strength" is often defined culturally as a personality characteristic rather than a measure of the ability to do physical work. Thus, physical weakness may represent to the patient a character or personality flaw. This is complicated by the fact that persons with rheumatic diseases are often advised to rest and avoid hard physical tasks as a part of treatment. This contrasts with cultural advice to "fight the disease" or "conquer the symptoms."

The loss of functional ability is the result of pain, weakness, or other physiological impairment. The significance of the patient's functional loss is by no means correlated with the number of joints or muscles involved. The patient's perception of disability is subjective.[18] Those who do not easily adapt to change may experience prolonged depression or anger. Many adults are socially defined primarily by the name of their occupation—e.g., cooks, teachers, truck drivers, painters, or surgeons. Loss of the ability to carry out these tasks and function in these roles may cause loss of social identity and diminished self-esteem, even though function in another role would be quite possible.

When loss of function causes *dependence on others*, the effect may be even more devastating. Independence has great cultural significance, particularly for men. However, women forced to be dependent may be no less depressed than men. Dependence means seeking and requesting assistance, and asking for help is a difficult task. It involves timing (neither too soon nor too late), judgment (asking the right person), and humility. Each request presents the risk of rejection for the patient needing help. The helper is also at risk, and must be skilled in offering assistance without exerting control. Being helpful without being patronizing is a difficult skill. This tenuous interaction is repeated many times daily for those who are not independent. Independence is a quality achieved throughout life by accomplishing a series of tasks that began in childhood. For most people, losing independence symbolizes a return to previous states of immaturity. This reaches its ultimate expression in those patients who are unable to perform tasks of personal hygiene. Many patients express the view that the ongoing negotiation of assistance is one of the most difficult challenges of arthritis.

One last feature that has considerable psychological impact is the *financial cost of chronic illness.* Even with excellent comprehensive health insurance plans, many patients must still pay for drugs or laboratory tests. Common aspirin can become expensive when taken in large quantities over a period of years. In long-term illnesses, the costs of treatment, travel for medical care, special equipment, and child and home care can strain resources.

Although discussion to this point has centered upon the patient, the family and others who interact closely with the patient can also be expected to react to their perceptions of the disease. Their interactions with the patient will be tempered by their own experiences with illness. Medical personnel do not encounter all family members and are thus often unaware of their concerns. As the disease interferes with the patient's ability to fulfill his or her role within the family, conflicts and misunderstandings can develop. Family members are often confused about the fluctuating symptoms and function of the patient. When good communication does not exist between family members, problems and feelings often go unrecognized and unresolved. Resentment, anger, and depression have been described within many families. Patterns of reaction will be influenced by previous family patterns and structure. It is heartening to note in some families that adjustment has improved after participation in therapeutic programs.[19,20]

PSYCHOLOGICAL RESPONSES COMMON TO RHEUMATIC DISEASES

As the individual notices symptoms of disease, the initial response is *anxiety.* Fear and uneasiness grow as symptoms persist. Anxiety can precipitate positive action: the patient may seek medical advice. In contrast, it may also engender *denial* as the patient ignores symptoms or insists they have no meaning. Another component of denial may involve rejection of assistance. A form of denial is manifest in those who wander from specialist to specialist in search of assurance that they will "get well." When pain becomes constant or when a diagnosis of arthritis is made, most patients begin to accept or reach equilibrium with their disease. Seeking medical evaluation, diagnosis, and treatment represents a reasonable attempt to deal with circumstances.

Anger is a frequent response to disease or disability. Anger may be generated about the injustice of illness,

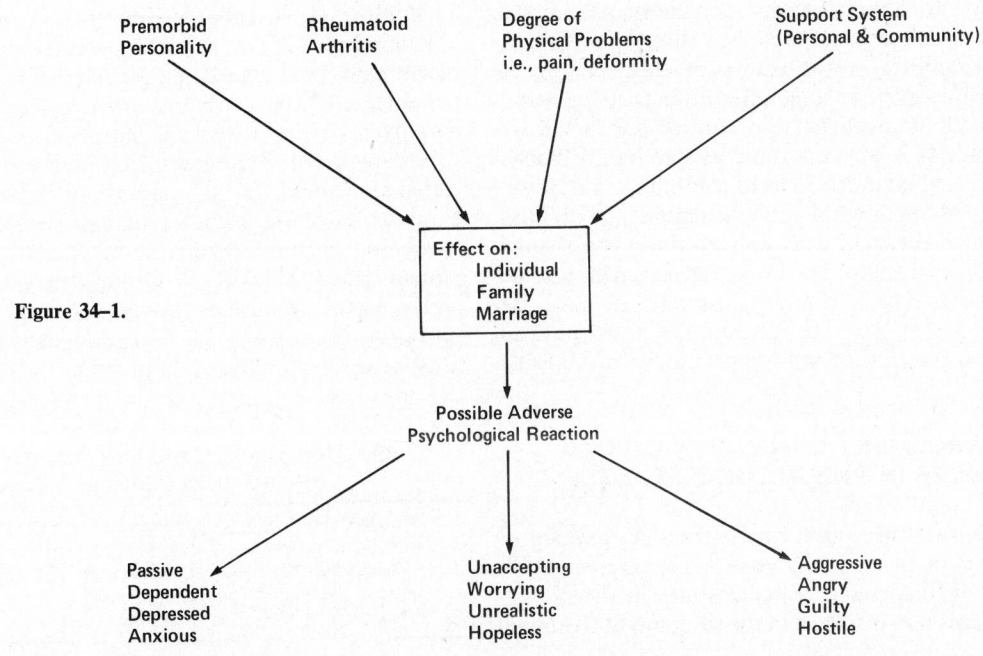

POSSIBLE ADVERSE PSYCHOLOGICAL REACTIONS ASSOCIATED WITH RHEUMATOID ARTHRITIS

Figure 34–1.

dependency, pain, the interruption of life patterns, or the moratorium on opportunity induced by functional handicap. Anger may be poorly focused and expressed in the most convenient way at the time, frequently being directed inappropriately at family or friends. Patients who refuse medication or resist educational programs may be expressing anger in the only way available to them. Persons with physical disabilities may have lost access to the usual means by which anger is diffused. They cannot easily "get away from things," engage in vigorous physical activity, or risk expressing emotions spontaneously. Unexpressed or unrecognized anger often leads to adverse reactions, among them depression.

Depression is one of the most commonly noted emotions in people with arthritis. A study of 50 psychiatric consultations for hospitalized arthritis patients revealed depression to be the most common psychological diagnosis.[21] It is a natural reaction to actual or perceived loss, and may be a useful temporary defense, allowing one to rest and reorder life's priorities. However, prolonged depression results in loss of energy and motivation. In rheumatic diseases it appears to accentuate pain and to be counterproductive to the therapy designed to strengthen muscles and restore function.

The reactions described above can be experienced at varied times throughout the course of one chronic illness. Each new symptom, frustration, or exacerbation of disease activity stimulates responses, which usually are consistent in the same patient. It is important for patient, family, and health professionals to recognize that experiencing these emotions again and again is not regression.

Ideally, as the patient experiences emotional responses to a disease activity, a decision is made to deal with the circumstances based on a realistic appraisal of the situation. The coping resources include the patient's previously established ways of dealing with personal problems, external help, and the influence of the environment. The decision to come to terms is made many times in the course of disease, in each new situation. Patients differ considerably in the extent of their coping resources. Adjustment is sometimes influenced by others who facilitate its occurrence or create barriers to its development. It is an important psychological mechanism which enables individuals to continue a satisfactory life in spite of impaired health and diminished abilities. Adjustment is easier to achieve from the stage of anger and resentment resulting from the development and activity of the disease, and is progressively less easily attained from the stages of depression, decreased physical activity, and diminished self-image and/or invalidism.

MANAGEMENT OF PSYCHOLOGICAL ISSUES IN RHEUMATIC DISEASES

There are two purposes for understanding psychological concepts in rheumatic disease: (1) to appreciate the role of personality and emotional states in the physiologic mechanism of disease and the response to treatment and (2) to facilitate successful psychologic adaptation to disease and its consequences. The physician should develop a conceptual framework that incorporates these concepts into a philosophy of treatment. A longitudinal approach, including assessment and appropriate intervention in psychosocial events, is ideal both as a treatment and as a research model.[20] A comprehensive model will include preventive, therapeutic, and rehabilitative components.

Discussion of health issues, including psychological components, occurs best in an atmosphere of trust and acceptance. Time must be provided for thorough assessment and understanding of the psychodynamics of specific situations. Time should be allotted for communication with other health professionals who contribute to the care of the patient.

Effective use of health professionals knowledgeable about arthritis is often the solution to providing comprehensive care with minimal cost of physician's time. During their longer treatment contacts therapists and nurses often make observations about a patient's emotional status that the physicians may miss.

Consideration of psychosocial issues and concerns must be based upon effective assessment of the patient's personal and social adjustment. This evaluation may be accomplished by psychometric testing,[22] interview, observation, or other clinical data collection methods. Each professional who participates in the treatment activities should develop a knowledge of the psychological status of the patient and the family. Included in the health interview must be a series of questions about psychological issues. Such questions might include the following: (1) How have your symptoms affected your life? (2) How have those around you been affected? (3) What are some of the feelings or emotions you have experienced lately? (4) What has been the biggest change in your life since your illness or symptoms began? (5) How have you adjusted to situations like this in the past? This information, enhanced by observations and available history, should provide a sense of the patient's recent emotional state, the effect of the disease upon the patient's life style, and the previous coping strategies employed by the patient (Table 34–1).

A network of resources, including lay support groups (often sponsored by such organizations as the Arthritis Foundation or the Lupus Foundation), social workers, psychologists, and others, is invaluable for complete patient care (Table 34–2). Group interaction is particularly useful because it provides the members an opportunity to test new patterns and behavior in an atmosphere of familiarity and trust. Groups can be

Table 34–1. Questions to Elicit Information About Psychological Issues in Arthritis

1. How have your symptoms affected your life?
2. How have those around you been affected?
3. What feelings have you experienced lately?
4. What is the biggest change in your life in the past year?
5. What has helped you cope with arthritis?

Table 34–2. Some Resources for Psychological Support

Arthritis health professionals
   physicians
   psychologists
   social workers
   nurses
   therapists
Mutual support groups (e.g., Arthritis Foundation, Lupus Foundation)
Community mental health agencies
Clergy
Family and friends
Self-help literature

structured to include opportunities for education about disease and treatment, mutual support, expression of concerns, and skill training for dealing with these concerns. The leaders of groups concerned with persons affected by rheumatic disease should have knowledge of the specific disease and its effects. In one of the few controlled studies of the effects of group counseling, Kaplan and Kozin note its value in improving knowledge and self-concept.[23]

When considering the best treatment for emotional problems, Achterberg-Lawlis[24] has found, "The traditional mental health models for therapy simply appear unacceptable for people who are brought together with a common diagnosis of arthritis." A stress management approach for dealing with psychosocial issues is often more acceptable for people who are hesitant to discuss feelings and emotions and for those who believe their problems are entirely physical. Some people even consider a suggestion for psychological help to be a strong criticism, whereas nearly everyone today accepts the logic of the importance of managing stress well.

A good stress management program includes better communication skills; assertiveness training; dealing with the negative emotions of anger, depression, worry, and guilt; relaxation techniques; pain management, and development of a less stressful lifestyle. All of these stress management concepts contribute to emotional health.

Following initial assessment, the physician should continue to both observe the patient's psychological health and be closely in touch with members of the patient care team who are directly involved with the patient's emotional health. Some indicators to be aware of include behavior changes, sleep patterns, sexual interest, personal appearance, work difficulties, and personal interactions with family and friends. Subsequent interviews should assess the patient's physical and emotional reactions to the treatment program. The patient and family should be given an opportunity to express opinions regarding the effect of medication and therapy. Faithfulness to treatment regimens should be monitored both for the sake of successful treatment and as an indicator of psychologic status.

In addition to the best possible medical and psychological management of the patient with arthritis, patients benefit from being involved in a "wellness" approach to their care. In such a wellness[25] approach, the patient will learn that everyone can be healthier than they are, in spite of having arthritis or any other chronic disease or disability. The patients discover that there are many aspects of their lives that only they can control, such as diet, exercise, personal growth and development, maintaining satisfying relationships, personal habits such as smoking, stress management, attitudes, lifestyle, and nonpharmaceutical pain management. The awareness of the many factors that contribute to a total health picture for each person can be taught in groups or on an individual basis by the physician or other health care providers. Psychological health can be improved when people give up a helpless, passive attitude and become more active in their own health care.

Until this point, the information presented has emphasized the patient and family as recipients of services and attention. It is also worthwhile to consider influencing the social and physical environment in which these persons live. Social and personal attitudes are in many instances the cause of depression, loss, and hopelessness among persons affected by chronic disease or disability.[26] Support is needed to provide barrier-free physical environments, accessible transportation, and nondiscriminatory employment for the handicapped. Equitable Social Security, medical care programs, and educational opportunities for the physically exceptional can provide wide-reaching impact on the consequences of disease.

In a study examining the relative contributions of selected disease, social, and work-related factors to disability status in a population of 180 people with rheumatoid arthritis, it was determined that social and work factors combined have a far larger effect on work disability than all disease factors.[27] The work factors of "control over the pace" and "activities of the job" had the greatest effect on continued employment, and "self-employment" was the favored work status. It was suggested that work disability is not strongly associated with the physical requirements of the job among persons with rheumatoid arthritis. These findings imply that the probability of work disability could be reduced by more flexible roles and pace in work settings. The responsibility of educating employers and other labor-management personnel lies with the physician or other health professional, and a climate of social responsibility makes the success of such efforts more likely.

The trauma of rheumatic disease might not be as overwhelming if the opportunity to fulfill roles and responsibilities within society were better protected.

BEHAVIORAL ASPECTS OF PAIN

Pain is perhaps the most potent stimulus of adverse psychological reactions for people experiencing arthritis. Although recent developments in the scientific study of pain have produced a greater understanding of some of its mechanisms and characteristics,[28,29] many misconceptions prevail about the experience and management of pain. These misconceptions and misunderstandings contribute to inadequate pain management techniques by health professionals. Many physicians who encounter patients with primary pain problems are frustrated both by the patient and by the failure of traditionally prescribed treatments.[30] Because patients with primary pain problems are so difficult to treat, and the impact of their disability so significant, multidisciplinary pain management programs have been developed.[31] These programs attempt to treat the complex psychological components of the experience in addition to the physical symptoms. These units are established on the premise that every pain patient who truly wants to get better can be helped at least to some degree. This basic premise has yet to be refuted.

In all pain programs, an individual management program is developed for each patient. A broad range of available techniques could include biofeedback, group and individual psychotherapy, heat or cold modalities, electrotherapy, hypnosis, therapeutic massage, exercise, and relaxation techniques. Various drug therapies and nerve blocks might be included, but the emphasis is on patient participation and the utilization of the person's inner resources. Every effort is made to eliminate feelings of helplessness and hopelessness. Numerous studies have been done to assess the effectiveness of behavorial pain management programs. Gottlieb and colleagues[32] reported 50 of 72 patients to have attained a preset level of satisfactory functioning. A significant level of improvement was retained on a 1-month follow-up. Thirty-six chronic pain patients with histories of treatment failure in other modalities were enrolled in the behavioral program summarized by Fordyce and colleagues.[33] On follow-up 22 months post-treatment, the patients reported a stable and significant decrease in pain intensity as well as a significant decrease in the degree to which pain interfered with activities. Pain management programs continue to develop with emphasis on rehabilitation principles and careful evaluation.

There are several characteristics of arthritis pain that set this condition apart from other pain management problems. First, arthritis pain is not one pain, but many pains, ranging in nature from acute to chronic. People with arthritis must learn to live and function with chronic pain while still attending to the signals of acute pain. Patient education materials for people with arthritis emphasize the need to "respect pain"[34] and "alter activities which cause pain lasting more than 1–2 hours,"[35] thus clearly implying the control that pain is to have over the patient's life. While it is relatively easy to cope with acute pain of short duration, facing a lifetime with pain as a constant companion can be an overwhelming experience. Even when arthritis is well managed or in remission, serious pain often still exists because of remaining joint damage. Guidelines for dealing with this type of pain may be very different from those for dealing with acute inflammatory pain. Another factor that makes arthritis pain difficult to manage is the unpredictable course and nature of the disease. Unexpected pain and flare-ups make long-range planning virtually an impossibility for the patient and family. And finally, patients who experience pain from arthritis are frequently told by health professionals and other advisors that because there is no cure for arthritis, they must "learn to live with it," thus reinforcing their hopelessness and diminishing their belief in the ability to alleviate the distress.

Therefore, the first challenge in developing a pain management program for arthritis patients is to help them to become less passive and begin to accept some personal responsibility for their own comfort level. This initial phase is primarily educational, teaching the relationship between stress, muscle tension, and feelings of pain. This framework of personal responsibility and control over the physical experience is the basis for positive management of pain in arthritis.

Once a stress management program is underway, the specific problem of dealing with pain can be addressed. Patients with arthritis react quite differently both to pain and to pain management techniques, so a many faceted approach is generally best. Because pain is a personal and subjective experience, every person with an ongoing, chronic pain problem will benefit from developing his own personal "bag of tricks" containing tried and proven ideas and techniques that are effective in reducing the pain experience for that individual.

The three major categories of useful techniques for nonmedicinal management of pain are physical measures, distraction, and relaxation. These measures, used individually or in combination, are central in the long-term management of arthritis pain (Fig. 34–2).

Physical measures often originate in a medical environment even though the patient will then have the responsibility for carrying them out at home. The patient may receive information from the physician, physical therapist, or occupational therapist about such things as paraffin dips for hands, warm showers and baths, hot or cold packs, exercises, splinting, and so on. In this category also belongs appropriate shoes and clothing, self-help devices, and joint protection.

COMPONENTS OF NON-MEDICINAL PAIN MANAGEMENT

Personal Responsibility for Comfort

Stress Management

Non-Modicinal Techniques

Physical Techniques   **Relaxation**

Distraction

Figure 34–2.

A VARIETY OF AVAILABLE RELAXATION METHODS

AUTOGENICS

BIOFEEDBACK

HYPNOSIS

FANTASY

PSYCHOCYBERNETICS

RELAXATION RESPONSE

VISUALIZATION IMAGERY

TRANSCENDENTAL MEDICATION

JACOBSEN'S PROGRESSIVE RELAXATION

YOGA

SELF HYPNOSIS

Figure 34–3.

Distraction techniques are useful because nearly everyone is capable of forgetting pain when their attention becomes focused on something else. What takes the person's mind off himself? Because of the personal nature of this activity, each person will need to find his own list of items that divert attention from the pain, at least for short periods of time. Chronic pain is easier to live with if one is able to achieve periods of relief. For one person, listening to music might be effective; for another, playing with a puppy or grandchild or both. The list of possibilities is endless and includes such diverse activities as working puzzles, singing, or doing crafts.

The third category of pain relief measures is relaxation. Tension always intensifies pain, so that decreased tension, both physical and emotional, provides comfort and relief. Being deeply relaxed in mind and body can profoundly diminish the experience of pain. There are many different kinds of relaxation methods, including Jacobson's Progressive Relaxation,[36] Yoga,[37] Autogenic Training,[38] and Transcendental Meditation[39] (Fig. 34–3). Benson simplifies the matter of choice by explaining that the outcome is more important than the specific technique used.[40]

One more adjunct to pain management is counseling or psychotherapy. If a patient's personal life is unsettled and unhappy, the resulting stress and tension cannot help but worsen existing pain problems. When emotions can be maintained on a relatively even level, people seem to be better able to manage the pain caused by arthritis.

As each person accumulates his own personal "bag of tricks," he can continue to add ideas as he learns and tries new things. Of course, gathering this collection of helpful pain management tools and skills is only the beginning, since they must be used and practiced in order to be effective. Patients can make a valuable contribution to their pain management when they are taught the necessary skills.

In summary, only the rare patient with arthritis will be in need of a formal comprehensive chronic pain management program. On the other hand, certain components of these programs such as stress management and relaxation are appropriate for almost any arthritis patient with pain. No health professional should ever advise a person with arthritis to simply "learn to live with pain." Patients have a right to learn about the rich repertoire of creative alternatives for dealing with pain rather than hearing a statement of helplessness.

SEXUAL HEALTH AND RHEUMATIC DISEASE

Sexual health is vulnerable to the effects of rheumatic disease. Sexuality is a concept that should be viewed from several perspectives. In the broad sense, it embodies all those aspects of personality relating to masculinity and femininity, including factors such as gender identity and behavior, self-perception, societal and personal roles, and interpersonal skills. In contrast, the narrow definition focuses on genital behavior and expressions. To the individual, sexuality is a construct of life experiences framed by values and attitudes. It is probably impossible for one person to define sexuality for another; yet it is useful to strive for mutual understanding.

One's perception of self as a sexual person is likely to be influenced by the physical changes caused by chronic disease. In rheumatic disease, whether acute or chronic, the characteristics of pain, loss of function, and physical change may disrupt many components of the life pattern, including sexual health. A seldom recognized consideration is that some drugs used in the treatment of rheumatic disease affect sexuality. They may also alter physical appearance and thus affect sexual interest or energy. Cytotoxic agents may be toxic to sperm and öocytes and/or may induce fetal wastage or sterility.

Although sexuality is gaining wider acceptance as a legitimate concern for health care professionals, adequate resources of skill, knowledge, and attitudes within the medical community remain to be developed to provide needed and appropriate services. A significant body of information now exists regarding sexuality in neuromuscular disabilities such as quadriplegia or paraplegia.[41,42] Although some aspects of this knowledge are relevant to rheumatic disease, there are some differences. It must be recognized that achieving satisfactory adjustments regarding sexuality may be particularly complicated by the fluctuating nature of the physical and emotional states that occur in rheumatic diseases.

The health practitioner who seeks to develop an approach that considers the sexual health of patients must first possess three requisite qualities: (1) recognition of the sexual aspects of his or her own personality ("comfort" with sexuality), (2) a commitment to respect the personal attitudes and values of others, and (3) a commitment and adherence to ethical professional standards regarding sex education, counseling, and therapy. Knowledge of anatomy, sexual physiology, and the manner in which sexual functioning might be affected by disease or disability is essential.

Approaches to sexuality should be sensitive and non-sexist. Perhaps because of the predominance of rheumatic disease in females, an inordinate portion of existing literature about sexuality and arthritis deals with women's sexual concerns. The sexual role of women is often described as the more passive and their societal role as that of traditional feminine homemaker. Men are usually described by their professional or work roles. If family and societal roles are to be considered as an aspect of sexuality, then consideration should be given to the woman whose work or professional career is interrupted by arthritis, and to the man whose domestic interests and roles are rendered difficult to fulfill.

Lief[43] has described the following as the effective physician's tasks in dealing with the sexual problems of patients, but these are certainly applicable to all health practitioners: (1) Be comfortable with sexual topics. (2) Listen well and know how to take a sexual history. (3) Show concern for the patient's feelings. (4) Judge whether the sexual problems identified are within the practitioner's competence, and, if the patient is in agreement, set up a plan of treatment with the patient's full knowledge and consent. (5) For problems not within the practitioner's competence, refer the patient to another professional person who has the required knowledge and skills. The physician may choose also not to deal with dysfunction that predated the disease or disability. Appropriate referral may be effective in this situation. The goal of intervention is to provide the recipient with information and assistance so that ultimately he or she can make decisions about sexuality within his or her own value system.

Creating an atmosphere in which discussion of sexual issues can occur is the first and most important step in any program. It has often been observed that patients rarely initiate discussion of sexual concerns, and yet this does not indicate a lack of importance of such concerns. Gathering information as part of a total health assessment provides a comfortable avenue for discussion for both health professionals and patients with sexual concerns. A few carefully worded questions about sexual function can show that the subject is open for discussion and is viewed as a health concern. The initial interview need not be a detailed sex history but will serve to identify areas of change or difficulty. If concerns are expressed, the subsequent information obtained should detail (1) the duration of the problem, (2) how it affects the patient at this time, (3) what, if anything, helps, (4) what the patient believes is the cause, and (5) how the patient feels about dealing with the problem. With this information, professionals can make a decision about their competence to work with the patient and whether the patient desires assistance at this time. Asking all patients about sexual concerns provides an opportunity to learn from patients who have made satisfactory adjustment. Interviews at this level also provide the opportunity to introduce ideas and concepts which can reduce vulnerability to sexual dysfunction.

In one study a comprehensive plan to consider sexuality in rheumatic disease not only resulted in greater attention to patient concerns; it also provided an opportunity to document problems and interventions.[44] In this study, half the patients indicated that they had concerns about sexual function, and some identified multiple problems. Table 34–3 depicts ten potential problems, the specific information needed for assessment,

Table 34–3. Sexual Counseling Protocol*

Problem	Assessment	Intervention
Pain or weakness	Specify cause, location, and nature	Recommend measures to relieve or minimize, i.e., position, warm bath, medication
Fatigue	Time of day, cause, nature	Pacing, scheduling, establishing priorities
Lack of interest	Determine influencing factors, i.e., medication, disease activity, depression	Educate to promote understanding of the effect of pain, fatigue, and disease activity on interest
Limited range of motion	Define functional limitations	Suggestions about positioning, alternative forms of expression
Lack of lubrication	Determine cause	Suggest psychological or physical measures as indicated
Erectile difficulties	Determine contributing factors, i.e., medical or psychological	Consider altering medications if possible; appropriate counseling measures
Fear of pregnancy, interfering medical problems (e.g., vaginal or penile ulcers, urinary tract infection)	Refer to physican or nurse to determine appropriate medical intervention; assess implications for individual and/or partner	Recommend appropriate medical measures; provide counseling regarding impact of decisions
Feelings of unattractiveness	Determine if perception is by self, partner, and/or others	Promote positive body image and acceptance of body, enhance feelings of self-worth
Problems with partner	Assess cause, e.g., fear of causing pain, partner's disinterest, responsibility for satisfaction, sexual roles, general relationship problems	Education and counseling as appropriate
Lack of partner	Evaluate possibilities for meeting other people, individual's own response	Discuss self-pleasuring, affirmation of self, encourage social contacts

*From Ferguson, K., and Figley, B.: Sexuality Disability 2:130,1979.

and examples of interventions. It demonstrates that concerns range from physical to psychological and require a variety of strategies. In an interdisciplinary approach, the physical therapist may be the most appropriate person to work with problems of sexual functioning that are due to limited range of motion or weakness; the social worker may best address issues of emotions, personality, or interpersonal relationships; the occupational therapist may offer principles of pacing and energy conservation which enable the patient to deal with fatigue and function; education by the nurse about the disease and medications may prepare the patient and family to cope with aspects of the disease that have implications for sexual function. The physician will view concerns in the context of the total health picture. Issues of birth control, fertility, or contraindication to pregnancy can be best addressed by the physician. By expressing interest, the physician who acts as coordinator of services also sanctions sexuality as a health concern. It should be noted that none of these people require highly trained or developed skills in sex therapy in order to contribute to a positive approach to sexual health.

It is important to plan a system for documentation of sexual issues in the patient's medical record. The record must accurately convey information to other medical staff without violating sensitivities or confidentiality. Documentation will avoid duplication of professional efforts and improve communication.

One conceptual model of a structured approach to sexual health is known as the PLISSIT model.[45] It describes the need for varying levels and types of education or intervention regarding sexuality. The model demonstrates that by offering permission to talk about sexual issues, providing limited information to those with questions and specific suggestions for specific concerns, there will be only a few people who require intensive therapy.

PSYCHOSOCIAL RESEARCH IN RHEUMATIC DISEASES; METHODOLOGY AND RESULTS

Many investigators have attempted to define psychologic concepts in rheumatic disease.[46] Their methods ranged from personal viewpoints based upon clinical observation[47,48] to intricate designs evaluating dependent and independent variables in controlled settings on multiple population samples.[2,11,20] Most populations studied have been patients with rheumatoid arthritis. Although early case studies were impressionistic and descriptive, they did generate interest and energy for future studies. More recent work has produced a wealth of descriptive data enticing to many. Nevertheless one must make careful assessment and interpretation of each study.

Studies of psychological factors in arthritis have been carried out by researchers in various disciplines and orientations, including rheumatology, psychiatry, sociology, and psychology. The scope and focus of a particular study may be influenced by the professional or philosophical orientation of the researcher; the social scientist may be unfamiliar with the subtleties of rheumatic disease, a rheumatologist not aware of the intricacies of psychological testing. These differences should be recognized and appreciated by the reader.

An assumption persists through much of the literature that persons of one diagnostic category represent a homogeneous group. However, clinical experience reveals that people with rheumatoid arthritis or lupus erythematosus, for instance, are heterogeneous. They are different in terms of severity and activity of disease, physical function or disability, sex, age, serology, and length of symptoms. These differences should be stated and defined as completely as possible. Experimental and control groups should be utilized with dependent and independent variables stated.

Several techniques have been used to observe or measure psychologic variables. Many early studies which produced "personality profiles" were based on case studies and interviews in therapy settings.[48,49] The case study approach represents a subjective and minimally controlled research strategy. Some later designs have included a combination of interview and testing in attempts to gain more objective information. Interpretive tests such as the Rorschach, Thematic Apperception Test (TAT), and Draw-a-Person (DAP) were at times utilized in attempts to construct personality descriptions unique to persons with arthritis.[50,51] It must be recognized that these tests and the validity of interpretation may be particularly affected by the method of administration, scoring, and circumstances of testing.

Self-report questionnaires are another method designed to obtain information without the intervening influence of the interviewer.[52] These seem to provide relevant information regarding perception and knowledge of disease or physical and functional status, but more extensive interpretation may lead to subjective decision on the part of the interpreter. Fries has confirmed the usefulness of one self-report scale.[53]

The Minnesota Multiphasic Personality Inventory is a long and complex psychometric instrument,[54] used in some of the studies which sought quantitative and objective descriptors.[55-57] The personality profiles have been standardized with nonclinical, psychiatric, and other criterion groups in the interest of extending usefulness. Moos and Solomon[56] point out that the demonstrated differences between arthritis and nonarthritis populations may be due to variables other than diagnosis such as physical disability or pain. Some test items have content only indirectly related to or influenced by arthritis. The implications of these on the validity of this instrument have been pointed out by Nalven and O'Brien.[58]

These issues in methodology are not presented in skepticism of earlier research, but rather to encourage caution in interpretation of biopsychosocial research and to provide guidelines for assessment. A systemized evaluation will include consideration of (1) orientation of the researcher, (2) description of experimental and control samples, (3) inclusion of control groups, (4) variables measured, (5) instruments of evaluation, and (6) whether the hypothesis was answered by the methods employed.

Much of the existing literature about psychologic concepts in rheumatoid arthritis addresses two questions: (1) Do common personality patterns and characteristics exist among those with rheumatoid disease—i.e., is there a rheumatoid personality? (2) What relationship exists between biological and psychosocial variables in rheumatoid arthritis?

A number of investigators have assessed patients with arthritis for common premorbid personality patterns.[46-48] They argue that some patterns predisposed a person to develop the disease. Most of the characteristics cited were described with negative words like "self-punitive," "rigid," "depressed," and "angry." It was suggested[50,58,59] that persons with rheumatoid arthritis repress hostility and direct rage against themselves. Other authors believe that patients with rheumatoid arthritis had often endured negative life experiences such as poor parental relationships, stressful marriage, or separation. However, the methodological problems inherent in these studies have been emphasized in recent reviews.[60-62] It is now concluded by these recent reviewers that many but not all patients with rheumatoid arthritis demonstrate certain common personality characteristics, but that these patterns are probably a result of the disease process rather than factors related to the development of rheumatoid arthritis.

There is a striking lack of research describing the presence or development of positive emotional states even though practitioners recognize that some people do manage to adjust to disease. Characteristics such as flexibility, confidence, and sense of humor are seldom measured or discussed. An urgent need exists for longitudinal studies tracing the course of adjustment and coping. As suggested by Crown and Crown,[12] such research would document the experiences of people with arthritis as they learn to live in spite of diminished resources of energy, mobility, skill, and strength. Studies with this perspective have great instructive and therapeutic value.

Another category of research has examined the relationship between psychological and physiological variables. It has been suggested that psychological and biological variables interact to influence the onset, pattern, and course of rheumatoid arthritis.[63] In a group of adult monozygotic twins, all of whom were discordant for rheumatoid arthritis, evidence was found for stress as the initiating factor in those who developed rheumatoid arthritis.[64] Solomon and colleagues reviewed the literature about the relationship of immunity, emotions, and stress.[65] They hypothesized a central mechanism which controls the immune system and links the physical and emotional affective systems with physiological responses, but the data to support this are tentative. Many more studies are in progress about these relationships; and this promises to be a major focus of research, particularly since it has preventive and therapeutic meaning.

There is growing interest in the relationship of psychosocial factors to other rheumatic diseases such as SLE, primary gout, and juvenile rheumatoid arthritis. In gout, Katz and Weiner[2] have developed a model demonstrating that some gouty attacks are precipitated by definite and predictable factors (see also Chapter 86). These precipitants include alcohol, dietary indiscretion, and/or noncompliance in taking medications. In some instances these factors lead to other, more direct precipitating causes. For example, stress in the job setting may lead to consumption of alcohol and noncompliance with medication, leading to an attack of gout. In systemic lupus erythematosus the neurologic involvement of the central nervous system complicates assessment. Psychological change may be due to disease pathology (organic) or emotional reaction to the symptoms (functional). Existing research in SLE has been reviewed by Gurland et al.[66] Compared with the psychological literature in rheumatoid arthritis, research in other rheumatic diseases is sparse.

Several important factors have emerged in recent years that contribute to a better understanding of psychological issues in rheumatic disease through expanded research. Among these factors are the following:

1. The overall increased interest and support for comprehensive multidisciplinary arthritis management programs such as the Multipurpose Arthritis Centers created by the National Institutes of Health in 1976. These Centers and others have provided a focus for the innovation, implementation, and evaluation of creative arthritis management strategies. The emphasis on program evaluation has served to foster more critical thinking among arthritis health professionals.

2. The growth of behavioral medicine, which seeks to link the biology and pathophysiology of disease and its treatment to associated psychological factors. Many new approaches to psychological assessment and intervention have thus taken into account the physical as well as the emotional or affective aspect of the individual patient, yielding a more unified and cohesive body of information. Behavioral medicine is experiencing particular growth in the field of rehabilitation, where function is usually more important than cure. Behavioral research in such areas as compliance with exercise[67,68] and control of Raynaud's phenomenon[69] is especially applicable to rheumatic disease. Achterberg has demonstrated the positive affect of relaxation training on functional indices in patients with rheumatoid arthritis.[70] While admittedly in early stages, such research does attempt to measure the outcomes of particular behavioral techniques in treatment.

3. The development of standardized, computer systems of patient classification and description such as ARAMIS (American Rheumatism Association Medical Information System). These systems facilitate the aggregation of large sample populations and information resources. In such systems, information about patients from all parts of the country and world can be assimilated and analyzed.

4. The creation of new multidimensional health status indices either appropriate for or specific to the rheumatic diseases. These instruments, such as the Arthritis Impact Measurement Scale,[71,72] the Sickness Impact Profile,[73] and the Stanford Health Assessment Questionnaire,[74]

measure discrete physical, emotional, and social factors and produce as well a summative score of the particular construct of items. These instruments are, as a rule, convenient and practical to administer, thus encouraging more widespread utilization. The instruments have provided a better method of defining the problems encountered by the person with arthritis and recognizing the inter-relationship of these problems. As validation of these instruments continues, more information will be obtained about their utility in detecting change along health status levels.

The expanding field of research in psychological issues in rheumatic disease seeks both to describe the current status of the individual with arthritis and to evaluate the effects of intervention. More emphasis now is placed on the therapeutic value of understanding these issues, rather than simply describing an existing personality construct.

PSYCHOLOGICAL FACTORS IN JUVENILE ARTHRITIS

Children with arthritis have been studied extensively for psychological variables. However, these investigations have suffered from the same problems as the work that has been reported in adults. The investigations are made following the development of the disease process so that the psychological factors noted in the patients are colored by the disability itself.

Even though there is a variability in the types and activity of juvenile arthritis (JA)—changed from the former term of juvenile rheumatoid arthritis JRA to include all forms of childhood arthritis—data obtained from these children are usually pooled and reported for JA as a single disease entity. In one exception McAnarney and her colleagues did a detailed investigation of 42 children from a pediatric rheumatology clinic.[75] As would be expected, they found that children with arthritis had more psychological problems than the normal controls. Surprisingly, children who were in Functional Class 1 (without evidence of disability) had more psychosocial problems than children who had moderate to severe functional disability. During the childhood years the children with mono- or pauciarticular disease appeared to have more problems in coping with their illness than did those who had polyarthritis with obvious disability. The authors felt that the latter group were more recognizable as handicapped and thus had more allowances made for them by parents and teachers, whereas the children with minimal disease, such as an involved knee or ankle concealed by trousers, were not thought to be sick or disabled. However, such children still might have joint involvement and pain, take medication, and be seen at regular intervals by a physician, indicating at least, to the children themselves, that they have an active and chronic disease. The expectations by parents, teachers, and peers that these children should behave and perform normally is probably the unsettling feature in their lives.

In psychological studies of a number of children, a Paris group found that before the age of 7 the defense mechanisms in children with juvenile rheumatoid arthritis were poor.[76,77] Beyond age 8, boys appeared to show more rigidity and obsessional features, whereas the girls were able to show variety in their responses and more compensation for depression. It was also noted that these children did well intellectually but performed poorly in social settings.[77]

It has also been found that arthritic children are unusually expressive in physical and motor actions.[78] They also show significantly higher activity in tasks emphasizing motor skills compared to verbal tests. The investigators also looked at the responses of the parents to the disease; as might be expected, there were feelings of guilt in the mothers, who thought that they might have contributed to the appearance of the disease.

Recently studies have emphasized life stresses as precipitating factors in the onset of juvenile arthritis. In one, 50 patients with JA were studied in Finland.[79] The investigators found a depressive reaction in 17 of the children, and in 13 of this group depression occurred after the onset of JA. Disturbed father-child relationships were observed in 46 percent of the families. Problems in sibling interrelationships were uncommon. Evidence of an increased intensity of overprotection in the mother-child relationship was not found. The two most frequent family problems were divorce or marital separation (18.5 percent) and death or hospitalization of a parent because of serious illness (11 percent). The investigators could not find a typical personality profile in the children. The life stress factors were present during the year before the onset of the JA in 37 percent of the patients.

In the Pediatric Arthritis Clinic in Rochester, New York, 88 patients with JA and their families were surveyed.[80] There was a high frequency of broken homes (Table 34–4), as defined by a home in which there had been divorce, separation, or death of a parent.

Statistical analysis showed this population of JA to be consonant with a sample of about 3000 children in this region. In the large control group the frequency of single-parent homes was 10.6 percent. This was significantly different from the data obtained with JRA (28.4 percent). It is obvious that although divorce, separation, and death are discrete events, situations may persist over a period of time within the household which could be

Table 34–4. Frequency of Broken Homes Among Children With JA*

Population	Parents (%) Married	Unmarried†	Single Parent(%)
JA	69.3	28.4	2.3
Control	87.6	10.6	1.8
Welfare	21.0	35.8	43.2

*From Henoch, M., Batson, J., and Baum, J.: Psychosocial factors in juvenile rheumatoid arthritis. Arthritis Rheum. 21:229, 1978.
†Divorce, separation, death.

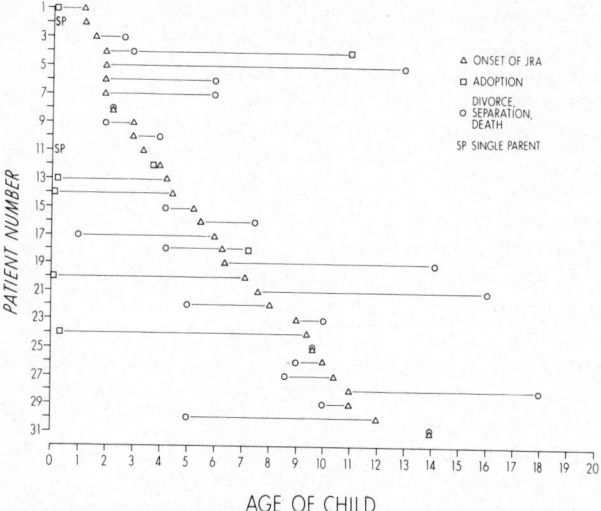

Figure 34–4. The time span of events in the lives of the children with JRA who have been adopted, or who come from broken or single parent homes, is presented. Each set of points connected by a line represents the time period between the event and the onset of disease for the individual patients. (From Henoch, M.J., Batson, J.W., and Baum, J.: Arthritis Rheum. 21:229, 1978.)

viewed as more traumatic than the actual separation or divorce. A more precise relationship is shown in Figure 34–4, which depicts the occurrence of the family trauma in relation to the onset of the arthritis in the child. Even with the noted variability, it was found that 48 percent of the events took place within the 2-year period preceding or following the development of arthritis in the child.

On the basis of these and Rimon's studies, a strong correlation has been found between stressful family life events and the development of juvenile rheumatoid arthritis.[79,80]

Others have noted that children with JA had problems achieving emotional separation from their mothers, a tendency to depression, and an impairment in their ability to show anger.[81] Again, these findings are consistent with the reactions of any patient with a chronic disease who is forced to become dependent. In some children it is particularly striking, because at the age when children are expected to show more independence from their parents, they often have the frustration of becoming more and more dependent.

Because of the potentially serious impact that childhood illness can have on personality development, intervention strategies have been developed that can help families as well as children with arthritis.

Parent support groups have been formed in many communities. These groups offer emotional support, understanding, and education to parents who have been previously quite isolated because of the relatively small number of children with arthritis. Parents are often given the advice that their child with arthritis should lead as normal a life as possible without clear information about how to incorporate this concept into everyday life.[82] In conjunction with studies of the child's perception of the

disease and experience of pain in juvenile chronic arthritis, Beales and colleagues point out that the child may have inaccurate interpretations of joint sensations and changes. Formal education and counseling sessions for the child and family are recommended to improve understanding and prevent unnecessary fears and fantasies.[83]

Parents and teachers usually need help in understanding that too much overprotection and pity rob the child of the chance to be strong and feel good about himself. The experiences the young child has as a child strongly influence the personality traits he will have as an adult.

Teen groups or rap sessions can be of great value for helping young people in this age group understand and cope with the many personal problems of adjustment that are a part of having arthritis. Often previously isolated, these teens appreciate the support and problem-solving advice from other kids their age who also have arthritis. They often feel better understood by their peers than by family or medical care providers.

Now that Public Law 94-142 (The Education for All Handicapped Children Act) has been in place for some time, support services should be provided in schools for all children. However, in reality one cannot expect even necessary services to be provided automatically because of the budget problems within school districts. Often it is necessary for parents and sometimes physicians to fight hard to obtain essential programs for individual children.

With the present emphasis on "mainstreaming," some children with quite severe handicaps may find themselves in a regular classroom for the first time. If there are any significant adjustment problems, the child might need the support of a psychologist or social worker trained to deal with school problems.

Many school districts now have a program called "adapted physical education" that allows all youngsters to participate in physical education according to their abilities. Unfortunately, one cannot assume that the physical education teacher has any expertise in childhood arthritis. It is more and more apparent that even when services are mandated by public law, there is not a guarantee of appropriate or adequate treatment. Thus, all of these activities need to be closely monitored by the rheumatology team, extending their scope of interest from the medical setting into the community itself.

A VIEW TO THE FUTURE

In looking to the future with regard to psychological issues in rheumatic disease, several intriguing questions can be considered. What is the impact of "holistic" philosophy on the care of arthritis? Who should be primarily responsible for the emotional and mental health care of the patient with arthritis? To what extent does this care belong in the medical as opposed to community mental health or lay volunteer organizations? How does one measure the outcome of attention to psychological health, and if such outcome measures do not indicate

Death   Sickness   Average Wellness   High Level Wellness

TRADITIONAL MEDICINE

all resources directed toward
taking care of illness

MANPOWER TRAINING
RESEARCH
INSTITUTIONS
PATIENT CARE

HOLISTIC HEALTH CARE

includes resources of TRADITIONAL MEDICINE *plus*
emotional and spiritual aspects of life and personal responsibility for health

PREVENTION
SPIRITUAL AND EMOTIONAL RESOLUTION
EDUCATION ABOUT NUTRITION, EXERCISE
HABIT CONTROL (Smoking, Weight, Stress)

Figure 34–5. A model of holistic health care.

an improved physical condition, how much effort and therapy ought to be afforded them?

First, the question of "holistic" approaches to arthritis. Such approaches are based on the philosophy that the patient is a whole person, and that any disease affects all aspects of being, not simply the physical being. "Holistic" approaches include emphasis on health as well as illness and tend to be more positive in nature (Fig. 34–5) with significant attention to psychological issues. Yet they also include activities which, while not in the category of "quackery," are sometimes unproven or untested by traditional measures. The previously discussed "wellness" approaches may be considered in the category of "holistic" medicine. Holistic medicine has appeal for many people and should be at least understood by the more traditional medical community. Evaluation of the various approaches as they relate to arthritis care should be supported and vigorously pursued.

Who is primarily responsible for mental and emotional health of the patient with arthritis? In multidisciplinary settings where physicians, social workers, nurses, and therapists—and sometimes clerical staff and maintenance personnel—have been trained in listening skills and supportive counseling, the primary responsibility must be assigned by some method in order to avoid conflict of advice and wasted effort. When is referral to psychiatry indicated? Does every patient with significant depression warrant psychiatric evaluation, or can this become the function of a highly trained nurse or social worker? What is the place of the psychologist or psychometrician, and how are their skills best used? To what extent does psychological care belong in the

medical system, where costs are high and continuing to rise? Recently, more attention has been given to programs of Arthritis Self Management skills, including many strategies to cope with psychological concerns.[84] The question of how much medical supervision is needed for such lay or volunteer programs has not yet been answered. What is the role of the community health program, and how much information about the medical aspects of arthritis is necessary for effective psychotherapy?

Finally, how are the outcomes of attention to psychological needs measured, and if a positive effect is not documented, how is the value of such attention justified to the medical community? In previous times the focus was to ascertain and describe various psychological health issues associated with arthritis. Now that a body of knowledge about those issues has been accumulated, the focus shifts to dealing with the concerns raised by them.

CONCLUSION

The symptoms and consequences of rheumatic disease can cause a variety of emotional reactions in patients and their families. These reactions are not specific to the diagnosis of the disease, but rather to the nature of the changes brought about by disease. Most people initially experience negative emotional reactions such as anxiety, fear, denial, and depression. These psychological states and altered sexual function need not and usually do not remain unchanged throughout the course of disease. It is possible for those affected by rheumatic disease to evolve psychologically to more positive states of adjustment. One strategy for helping people with arthritis achieve better psychological health is through stress and pain management techniques. Children with arthritis and their families require particular support and understanding so that the label of "sick child" does not preclude experiences for growth and development. Responsibility for psychological health and quality of life should be shared by health care professionals and the person with arthritis.

References

1. Moos, R.H., and Solomon, G.F.: Personality correlates of the rapidity of progression of rheumatoid arthritis. Ann. Rheum. Dis. 23:145, 1964.
2. Katz, J.L., and Weiner, H.: Psychobiological variables in the onset and recurrence of gouty arthritis: A chronic disease model. J. Chron. Dis. 28:51, 1975.
3. Solomon, G.F., Amkraut, A.A., and Kasper, P.: Immunity, emotions, and stress. Ann. Clin. Res. 6:313, 1974.
4. Carpenter, J.O., and Davis, L.J.: Medical recommendations—followed or ignored? Factors influencing compliance in arthritis. Arch. Phys. Med. Rehabil. 57:241, 1976.
5. Ferguson, K., and Bole, G.G.: Family support, health beliefs, and therapeutic compliance in patients with rheumatoid arthritis. Pat. Counsel. Health Ed. 2:101, 1979.
6. Moldofsky, H., and Rothman, A.I.: Personality, disease parameters and medication in rheumatoid arthritis. J. Chron. Dis. 24:363, 1971.
7. Rosillo, R.H., and Vogel, M.L.: Correlation of psychological variables and progress in physical rehabilitation. I. Degree of disability and denial of illness. Arch. Phys. Med. 51:227, 1970.
8. Vogel, M.L., and Rosillo, R.H.: Correlation of psychological variables and progress in physical rehabilitation. II. Motivation, attitude and flexibility of goals. Dis. Nerv. Syst. 30:593, 1969.
9. Vogel, M.L., and Rosillo, R.H.: Correlation of psychological variables and progress in physical rehabilitation. III. Ego functions and defensive and adaptive mechanism. Arch. Phys. Med. 52:15, 1971.
10. Rosillo, R.H., and Vogel, M.L.: Correlation of psychological variables and progress in physical rehabilitation. IV. The relation of body image to success of physical rehabilitation. Arch. Phys. Med. 52:182, 1971.
11. Earle, J.R., et al.: Psycho-social adjustment of rheumatoid arthritis patients from two alternative treatment settings. J. Rheumatol. 6:80, 1979.
12. Crown, S., and Crown, J.M.: Personality in early rheumatoid arthritis. J. Psychosomat. Res. 17:189, 1973.
13. Edwards, M.H.: The relationship of the arthritis patient to the community. In Lamont-Havers, R.W., and Hislop, H.J. (eds.): Arthritis and Related Disorders. New York, American Physical Therapy Association, 1965.
14. Comer, R.J., and Piliavin, J.A.: The effects of physical deviation on face-to-face interaction. J. Pers. Soc. Psychol. 23:33, 1972.
15. Goffman, E.: Stigma: Notes on the Management of Spoiled Identity. Englewood Cliffs, N.J., Prentice-Hall, 1969.
16. Moldofsky, H., and Chester, W.J.: Pain and mood patterns in patients with rheumatoid arthritis. Psychosomat. Med. 32:309, 1970.
17. Petrie, A.: Individuality in Pain and Suffering. Chicago, University of Chicago Press, 1969.
18. Moos, R.H., and Solomon, G.F.: Personality correlates of the degree of functional incapacity of patients with physical disease. J. Chron. Dis. 18:1019, 1965.
19. Katz, S. Vignos, P.J., Moskowitz, R.W., Thompson, H.M., and Svec, K.H.: Comprehensive outpatient care in rheumatoid arthritis: A controlled study. JAMA 206:1244, 1968.
20. Vignos, P.J., Thompson, H.M., Katz, S., Moskowitz, R.W., Fink, S., and Svec, K.H.: Comprehensive care and psycho-social factors in rehabilitation in chronic rheumatoid arthritis: A controlled study. J. Chron. Dis. 25:388, 1972.
21. Rogers, M.P., Reich, P., Kelly, M.J., and Liang, M.H.: Psychiatric consultation among hospitalized arthritis patients. Gen. Hosp. Psychiatry 2:89, 1980.
22. Shontz, F.C., and Fink, S.L.: A method for evaluating psychosocial adjustment of the chronically ill. Am. J. Phys. Med. 40:63, 1962.
23. Kaplan, S., and Kozin, F.: A controlled study of group counseling in rheumatoid arthritis. J. Rheumatol. 8:91, 1981.
24. Achterberg-Lawlis, J.: The psychological dimensions of arthritis. J. Consult. Clin. Psychol. 50:984, 1982.
25. Zeibell, B.: Wellness: An Arthritis Reality. Dubuque, Kendall Hunt, 1981.
26. Comer, R.J., and Piliavin, J.A.: As others see us: Attitudes of physically handicapped and normals toward own and other groups. Rehabil. Lit. 36:206, 1975.
27. Yelin, E., Meenan, R., Nevitt, M., and Epstein, W.: Work disability in rheumatoid arthritis: effects of disease, social, and work factors. Ann. Intern. Med. 93:551, 1980.
28. Melzack, R., and Wall, P.N.: Pain mechanisms: A new theory. Science 150:971, 1975.
29. Lim, R.K.S.: Neuropharmacology of pain and analgesia. In Pharmacology of Pain. Elmsford, New York, Pergamon, 1968.
30. Reuler, J.B., Girard, D.E., Nardone, D.A.: The chronic pain syndrome: Misconceptions and management. Ann. Intern. Med. 93:588, 1980.
31. Bonica, J.J.: Organization and function of a pain clinic. Adv. Neurol. 4:563, 1974.
32. Gottlieb, H., Strite, L.C., Koller, R., Madorsky, A., Hockersmith, V., Kleeman, M., and Wagner, T.: Comprehensive rehabilitation of patients having chronic low back pain. Arch. Phys. Med. Rehabil. 58:101, 1977.
33. Fordyce, W.E., Fowler, R., Lehmann, J., DeLateur, R., Sand, P., and Trieschmann, R.: Operant conditioning in the treatment of chronic clinical pain. Arch. Phys. Med. Rehabil. 54:399, 1973.
34. Melvin, J.: Rheumatic Disease. Occupational Therapy and Rehabilitation. Philadelphia, F.A. Davis Company, 1982, p. 353.
35. Haviland, N., Kamil-Miller, L., and Sliwa, J.: A Workbook for Consumers with Arthritis. Rockville, Maryland, AOTA, 1978.
36. Jacobson, E.: You Must Relax. New York, McGraw-Hill, 1976.
37. Hrena, S.F.: Yoga and Medicine: The Merging of Yogic Concepts with Modern Medicine Knowledge. New York, Penguin, 1973.
38. Shealy, C.N.: 90 Days to Self-health. New York, Bantam Books, 1978.
39. Bloomfield, H.H., Cain, M.P., Jaffe, D.T., and Kory, R.B.: TM*: Discovering Inner Energy and Overcoming Stress. New York, Dell, 1975.
40. Benson, H.: The Relaxation Response. 1st ed. New York, Avon, 1975.
41. Griffith, E.B., et al.: Sexual functioning in spinal cord injured patients: A review. Arch. Phys. Med. Rehabil. 56:18, 1975.
42. Cole, T.M.: Sexuality and the Spinal Cord Injured. In Green, R. (ed.): Human Sexuality: A Health Practitioner's Text. Baltimore, Williams & Wilkins Company, 1975, Chapter 12.
43. Lief, H.: Sexual knowledge, attitudes and behavior of medical students; implications for medical practice. In Abse, D.W., Nash, E.M., and London, L.M. (eds.): Marital and Sexual Counseling in Medical Practice. Hagerstown, Md., Harper & Row, 1974.
44. Ferguson, K., and Figley, B.: Sexuality and rheumatic disease: A prospective study. Sexuality Disability 2:130, 1979.
45. Annon, J.: The Behavioral Treatment of Sexual Problems. Honolulu, Kapiolani Health Services, 1974.
46. Ludwig, A.: Rheumatoid arthritis. In Wittkower, E.D., and Cleghorn, R.A. (eds.): Recent Developments in Psychosomatic Medicine. Philadelphia, J.B. Lippincott Company, 1954, pp. 232–244.
47. Dunbar, H.F.: Psychosomatic Diagnosis. New York, Paul Hoeber, 1943.
48. Robinson, C.E.: Emotional factors and rheumatoid arthritis. Can. Med. Assoc. J. 77:344, 1957.
49. Alexander, F.: Psychosomatic Medicine. New York, W.W. Norton, 1950.
50. Cleveland, S.E., and Fisher, S.: Behavior and unconscious fantasies of patients with rheumatoid arthritis. Psychosomat. Med. 16:327, 1954.
51. Cormier, B.M., and Wittkower, E.D.: Psychological aspects of rheumatoid arthritis. Can. Med. Assoc. J. 77:533, 1957.
52. Edwards, M.H., et al.: Patient's attitudes and knowledge concerning arthritis. Arthritis Rheum. 7:425, 1964.
53. Fries, J.F., Spitz, P.W., and Kraine, R.G.: Measurement of patient outcome in arthritis. Arthritis Rheum. 23:137, 1980.
54. Dahlstrom, W.G., et al.: An MMPI Handbook. Revised ed. Minneapolis, University of Minnesota Press, 1972.
55. Nalven, F.B., and O'Brien, J.F.: Personality patterns of rheumatoid arthritis patients. Arthritis Rheum. 7:18, 1964.
56. Moos, R.H., and Solomon, G.F.: Minnesota Multiphasic Personality Inventory response patterns in patients with rheumatoid arthritis. J. Psychosomat. Res. 8:17, 1964.
57. Bourestom, N.C., and Howard, M.T.: Personality characteristics of three disability groups. Arch. Phys. Med. Rehabil. 46:626, 1965.
58. Cobb, S.: Contained hostility in rheumatoid arthritis. Arthritis Rheum. 2:419, 1959.
59. Geist, H.: The Psychological Aspects of Rheumatoid Arthritis. Springfield, Ill., Charles C Thomas, 1966.
60. Scotch, N.A., and Geiger, H.J.: The epidemiology of rheumatoid arthritis: A review with special attention to social factors. J. Chron. Dis. 15:1037, 1962.
61. Hoffman, A.: Psychological factors associated with rheumatoid arthritis. Nurs. Res. 23:218, 1974.

62. Wolff, B.B.: Current psychosocial concepts in rheumatoid arthritis. Bull. Rheum. Dis. 22:656a, 1971–72.
63. Robinson, H., Kirk, R., Frye, R., and Robertson, J.T.: A psychological study of patients with rheumatoid arthritis and other painful diseases. J. Psychosomat. Res. 16:53, 1972.
64. Meyerowitz, S., Jacox, R.F., and Hess, D.W.: Monozygotic twins discordant from rheumatoid arthritis. Arthritis Rheum. 11:1, 1968.
65. Solomon, G.F., Amkraut, A.A., and Kasper, P.: Immunity, emotions and stress. Ann. Clin. Res. 6:313, 1974.
66. Gurland, B.J., Ganz, V.H., Fleiss, J.L., and Zubin, J.: The study of the psychiatric symptoms of systemic lupus erythematosus: A critical review. Psychosomat. Med. 34:199, 1972.
67. Waggoner, C.D., and Le Lieuvre, R.B.: A method to increase compliance to exercise regimens in rheumatoid arthritis patients. J. Behav. Med. 4:191, 1981.
68. Martin, J.E., and Dubbert, P.M.: Exercise applications and promotion in behavioral medicine: Current status and future directions. J. Consult. Clin. Psychol. 50:1004, 1982.
69. Surwit, R.S.: Behavioral treatment of Raynaud's syndrome in peripheral vascular disease. J. Consult. Clin. Psychol. 50:922, 1982.
70. Achterberg, J., Mc Graw, P., and Lawlis, G.F.: Rheumatoid arthritis: A study of relaxation and temperature biofeedback training as adjunctive therapy. Biofeedback Self Regul. 6:207, 223, 1981.
71. Meenan, R.F., Gertman, P.M., and Mason, J.H.: Measuring health status in arthritis. The Arthritis Impact Measurement Scales. Arthritis Rheum. 23:145, 1980.
72. Meenan, R.F., Gertman, P.M., and Mason, J.H.: The Arthritis Impact Measurement Scales: Further investigation of a health status measure. Arthritis Rheum. 25:1048, 1982.
73. Fries, J.F., Spitz, P.W., and Young, D.Y.: The dimensions of health outcomes; The Health Assessment Questionnaire, Disability and Pain Scales. J. Rheum. 9:789, 1982.
74. Deyo, R.A.: Physical and psychosocial function in rheumatoid arthritis. Clinical use of a self-administered health status instrument. Arch. Intern. Med. 142, 879, 1982.
75. McAnarney, E.R., Pless, I.B., Satterwhite, B., and Friedman, S.B.: Psychological problems in children with chronic juvenile arthritis. Pediatrics 53:523, 1974.
76. Rapoport, D., Hatt, A., Weil-Halpern, F., Hayem, F., and Mozziconacci, P.: La polyarthrite chronique juvenile dans la structure hospitaliere. IV. Étude psychologique des enfants atteints. Ann. Pédiat. 23:437, 1976.
77. Tursz, A.: La polyarthrite chronique juvenile dans la structure hospitaliere. V. Scolarité, vie sociale et familiale. Ann. Pédiat. 23:442, 1976.
78. Cleveland, S.E., Reitman, E.E., and Brewer, E.J., Jr.: Psychological factors in juvenile rheumatoid arthritis. Arthritis Rheum. 8:1152, 1965.
79. Rimon, R., Belmaker, R.H., and Ebstein, R.: Psychosomatic aspects of juvenile rheumatoid arthritis. Scand. J. Rheumatol. 6:1, 1977.
80. Henoch, M.J., Batson, J.W., and Baum, J.: Psychosocial factors in juvenile rheumatoid arthritis. Arthritis Rheum. 21:229, 1978.
81. Blom, G.E., and Nicholls, G.: Emotional factors in children with rheumatoid arthritis. Am. J. Orthopsychiat. 24:588, 1954.
82. Ziebell, B.A.: As Normal as Possible. 1st ed. Tucson, Arizona, Arthritis Foundation, Southern Arizona Chapter, 1976.
83. Beales, J.C., Keen, J.H., and Holt, P.J.: The child's perception of the disease and the experience of pain in juvenile chronic arthritis. J. Rheumatol. 10:61, 1983.
84. Lorig, K., and Fries, J.F.: The Arthritis Helpbook. Reading, Massachusetts, Addison Wesley, 1982.

Chapter 35

Ocular Manifestations of Rheumatic Diseases

Andrew P. Ferry

INTRODUCTION

Not many of the detailed clinical studies of rheumatic diseases reported in the literature include a detailed ocular examination by an ophthalmologist as an integral part of the study. Although most rheumatologists are aware of eye involvement in rheumatic disease, they are not necessarily well informed about how often the eyes are involved in patients with rheumatic diseases, which ocular abnormalities are most likely to be present in each of these conditions, and what the management should entail. Many of the associated ocular lesions are potentially blinding. In some instances (e.g., rheumatoid scleritis) the presence of an ocular abnormality may be obvious on casual examination, but in other cases the presence of an ocular abnormality may be overlooked on careful rheumatologic examination. For example, it is well known that the uveitis that leads to cataract formation in juvenile rheumatoid arthritis is usually asymptomatic. This *demands* ocular examination as part of the management protocol for children with this disease. Furthermore, even when ocular symptoms are present, the patient may not report them to the rheumatologist. Patients seldom relate their ocular symptoms to their nonocular disorders.

Detailed ophthalmic examination should be included in the protocol for future prospective studies of the rheumatic diseases. This will benefit the individual patients involved and will help fill some of the many gaps that remain in our understanding of the various types of ocular lesions that develop in patients afflicted with rheumatic disease.

In some of the diseases within the purview of the rheumatologist (e.g., the mucopolysaccharidoses, ochronosis, and Marfan's syndrome) ocular involvement is an integral part of the disorder. These ocular abnormalities are described in the chapters of this book devoted to these particular rheumatic diseases. Ocular involvement may also occur in certain other diseases (e.g., hemochromatosis) which I have not included in this chapter because of their rarity.

The entities discussed in this chapter are rheumatic fever, rheumatoid arthritis, juvenile rheumatoid arthritis, ankylosing spondylitis, systemic lupus erythematosus, connective tissue diseases other than rheumatoid arthritis and lupus erythematosus (scleroderma, periarteritis nodosa, and polymyositis), giant cell arteritis and polymyalgia rheumatica, Wegener's granulomatosis, relapsing polychondritis, enteropathic arthropathy, sarcoidosis, amyloidosis, and gout.

RHEUMATIC FEVER

Ocular complications are very uncommon in rheum atic fever. In a retrospective study of 200 patients with rheumatic fever examined at the Johns Hopkins Hospital, Smith found ocular manifestations in 12.[1] Most of these ocular lesions were inconsequential, and some probably were nonspecific responses to fever. Duke-Elder lists the following as ocular complications of rheumatic fever: palpebral edema, characteristic arborizations of the conjunctival vessels, subconjunctival hemorrhages, episcleritis and scleritis, and, more rarely, uveitis or embolic phenomena.[2]

RHEUMATOID ARTHRITIS

The eyes are affected considerably more often and more seriously in patients with rheumatoid arthritis than in patients with rheumatic fever. Keratoconjunctivitis sicca is the most common ocular complication of rheumatoid arthritis in adults.[3] But the most dramatic complications occur in the sclera, episclera, and corneal periphery. Anterior uveitis, band keratopathy, secondary cataract, palpebral edema, orbital myositis, and transitory palsies of the oculomotor nerves are all uncommon complications (although anterior uveitis and band keratopathy do occur with increased frequency in juvenile rheumatoid arthritis).

Keratoconjunctivitis Sicca. The normal precorneal tear film has a rather complex structure. It consists of three layers: (1) the outermost, oily layer derived from the palpebral sebaceous glands; (2) the innermost, mucoid layer derived from conjunctival goblet cell secretions; and (3) a watery, middle layer interposed between the oily and mucoid layers. The watery layer is formed by the secretions of the main and accessory lacrimal glands.

Keratoconjunctivitis sicca results from a decreased amount of tear elaboration by the main and accessory lacrimal glands. This failure of lacrimal secretion is caused by atrophic and cirrhotic changes in the lacrimal glands and leads to reduction of the middle layer of the precorneal tear film, the latter becoming attenuated and more viscous. Patients with keratoconjunctivitis sicca have tear lysozyme levels that are below normal.

Dryness of the mouth and oropharynx consequent to salivary gland atrophy is a frequent associated finding. This combination of xerostomia and keratoconjunctivitis sicca is commonly referred to as the *sicca syndrome.*[4] When associated with rheumatoid arthritis the resultant triad is known as *Sjögren's syndrome.* Components of the sicca syndrome have been found in up to one third of patients with rheumatoid arthritis, the incidence being particularly high in those patients with advanced joint disease. Sjögren's syndrome also has been described in patients with other connective tissue diseases, including systemic lupus erythematosus, polyarteritis nodosa, and scleroderma.

Keratoconjunctivitis sicca is usually of insidious onset and bilateral, occurs far more commonly in women than in men (about 90 percent of cases occur in women), and is extremely uncommon in those below age 40. Affected patients usually complain of itching or burning of the eyes. Photophobia is another common symptom. When first seen by the ophthalmologist, only a minority of these patients complain of ocular dryness. Because itching and burning of the eyes are such common symptoms among the general population, the presence of keratoconjunctivitis sicca often goes unsuspected by the ophthalmologist for months or years. Treatment of the supposed infection or allergy with various types of ointment only worsens the condition.

The eyes often appear slightly to moderately red and irritated (Fig. 35–1, Plate II, p. xxxvi). On slit-lamp biomicroscopic examination tiny, punctate gray opacities are seen that stain prominently with fluorescein solution. This epithelial keratopathy is usually most prominent in that portion of the cornea located in the interpalpebral fissure. Because this area is not covered by the lids during most of the waking hours it is particularly subject to drying. Rose bengal solution (1 percent) causes bright red staining of the abnormal corneal and conjunctival epithelium in the interpalpebral fissure. (Although much written about, rose bengal staining is used only infrequently by American ophthalmologists as a practical aid in diagnosis.)

In keratoconjunctivitis sicca the conjunctival goblet cells are stimulated to secrete an overabundance of mucus. A common finding is the presence of ropelike strands of mucus, often 1 cm or more long, arrayed over the eye or resting in the inferior fornix. Less often a so-called filamentary keratitis may develop. Plaques of diseased epithelium desquamate but remain attached to the adjacent epithelium at one end, forming epithelial filaments that may reach several millimeters in length and which simulate strands of mucus on clinical examination. A relatively rare complication of keratoconjunctivitis sicca is severe corneal opacification resulting from an infectious ulcer developing in the dry cornea.

When keratoconjunctivitis sicca is suspected, the Schirmer test of tear secretion often helps establish the diagnosis. This procedure can be carried out by the internist as well as by the ophthalmologist. A strip of filter paper that has been cut to size 5 × 35 mm is folded at one end, and the small, folded end is placed in the unanesthetized conjunctival sac (Fig. 35–2). At the end of 5 minutes the amount of wetting of the strip by tears is measured. Although there are many variables, such as the patient's age, 5 mm or less of wetting in 5 minutes is regarded as strongly indicating abnormally low tear secretion.

Patients with Sjögren's syndrome show a wide variety of organ-specific and non-organ-specific antibodies.[4] Rheumatoid factor tests are positive in 75 to 90 percent of the patients.

Treatment of keratoconjunctivitis sicca is unsatisfactory. Chronic replacement of tears by artificial substances is required. A variety of such agents are available. Some of the most popular ones at present are

Figure 35–2. The Schirmer test. *A,* The paper strips are supplied in a packet bearing a scale in millimeters. *B,* Each test strip has been folded partially at its indented area, and the shorter end has been placed in the conjunctival sac. After remaining there for 5 minutes the strips will be removed and the extent of wetting will be measured against the millimeter scale.

Adsorbotear (Burton, Parsons), Tears Naturale (Alcon), and Liquifilm Tears (Allergan). These are helpful in mild to moderate cases and typically must be instilled at least four times daily. Slowly dissolving hydroxypropyl cellulose pellets (Lacriserts) that are placed in the lower conjunctival fornix once daily have recently become available and have allowed many patients to circumvent the need for frequent instillation of drops. Many patients with keratoconjunctivitis sicca go through periods in which their symptoms lessen markedly, or even disappear. During these asymptomatic periods the ophthalmologist may advise reducing the frequency with which the artificial tears are instilled. In unusually severe cases conservation of any tears available may be accomplished by occluding the lacrimal drainage apparatus. This is done by applying diathermy to the superior and inferior puncta and canaliculi. In extreme cases tarsorrhaphy is required to protect the cornea.

Scleritis and Episcleritis. *Anatomy of Sclera and Episclera.* The sclera is composed of three layers which, from without inward, are (1) the episcleral tissue, (2) the sclera proper, and (3) the lamina fusca (Fig. 35–3). The episclera is a loose structure of delicate fibrous and elastic tissue that is continuous superficially with the loose trabeculae of Tenon's space. (Tenon's capsule

is covered, in turn, by the bulbar conjunctiva.) The loose structure of the episclera gradually gives way to a denser arrangement as the episclera merges with the sclera proper. The peculiar feature of the episclera is the large number of small vessels that it possesses in contradistinction to the sclera proper, which is almost avascular. The episcleral vessels are not seen easily in the uninflamed eye. But as soon as the eye becomes congested, three quite separate vascular plexuses become readily visible.[5]

The sclera proper is made up of a dense mass of fibrous tissue arranged in compact bundles. Each bundle consists of parallel collagenous fibers, interspersed among which are numerous elastic fibers. Between the bundles are the fixed cells of the scleral tissue (Fig. 35–3*B*). They are fibroblasts with small nuclei and long, branching processes.

Incidence of Scleritis and Episcleritis in Rheumatoid Arthritis. It has been known for many years that the incidence of scleritis and episcleritis is higher in patients with rheumatoid arthritis than it is in the general population. In an attempt to determine the incidence of these inflammatory lesions in patients with rheumatoid arthritis, and to differentiate rheumatoid scleritis and episcleritis from nonrheumatoid scleritis and episcleritis, a cooperative study was undertaken by the Center for Rheumatic Diseases in Glasgow and the Tennent Institute of Ophthalmology in that city.[6]

Between 1965 and 1973, 4210 patients with rheumatoid arthritis were examined at the Center for Rheumatic Diseases. Twenty-eight (0.67 percent) had scleritis, and seven (0.17 percent) had episcleritis.[6] (One assumes that some patients in this cohort with rheumatoid arthritis who did not have episcleritis or scleritis at the time of initial examination will develop one of these lesions in the future, thereby increasing the overall incidence of scleritis and episcleritis in the group of 4210 patients.)

Correspondingly, in 1971 and 1972 a total of 27 patients with scleritis and 35 patients with episcleritis were seen at the Tennent Institute of Ophthalmology. Of the 27 patients with scleritis, nine (33 percent) had clinical and radiological evidence of rheumatoid arthritis. Of the 35 patients with episcleritis, two (6 percent) had rheumatoid arthritis.[6] Of the 159 patients with episcleritis reported from London by Watson and Hayreh, seven (4 percent) had rheumatoid arthritis, as did 21 (10 percent) of their 207 patients with scleritis.[5]

Combining their patients, investigators at the two cooperating institutions in Glasgow found that all nine of their patients with rheumatoid episcleritis, and 25 of their 37 patients with rheumatoid scleritis, were women.[6] Among nonrheumatoid patients with episcleritis, men and women were affected equally. But among nonrheumatoid patients with scleritis, women were affected about five times as often as were men.[6]

The mean age of all patients with rheumatoid scleritis, rheumatoid episcleritis, and nonrheumatoid scleritis was in the sixth decade. Patients with nonrheumatoid episcleritis were younger, having a mean age of 45 years.

Figure 35–3. Normal eye. *A,* Anterior portion of a normal eye. The clear cornea (*C*) joins the opaque sclera (*S*) at the limbus (*L*). The bulbar conjunctiva (double arrows) is artifactitiously separated from the underlying Tenon's capsule (single arrow) and sclera at the left hand side of the field. Farther anteriorly the conjunctival epithelium merges with the corneal epithelium. The iris (*I*) merges posteriorly with the ciliary body (*CB*), the latter being separated artifactitiously from the overlying sclera. The periphery of the lens is visible behind the iris. Much of the lenticular substance has been lost in sectioning. Hematoxylin and eosin; magnification × 13. *B,* Wall of posterior portion of eye. The retina occupies the upper half of the field and the sclera fills the lower one fourth of the field. The choroid is interposed between the retina and sclera. The retinal layers are as follows: internal limiting membrane (top of the field), the nerve fiber layer (containing two prominent blood vessels), the ganglion cell layer (*G*), the inner plexiform layer, the inner nuclear layer, the outer plexiform layer, the outer nuclear layer, and the photoreceptors (rods and cones; *P*). The retinal pigment epithelium traverses the field below the photoreceptors. The choroid lines the outer surface of the retinal pigment epithelium and merges with the sclera at S. Only the inner half of the sclera is included in this field. Hematoxylin and eosin; magnification × 150.

With regard to bilaterality, among patients with rheumatoid scleritis both eyes were involved in 25 of 37 cases (68 percent). Among patients with rheumatoid episcleritis, both eyes were affected in about half the cases.[6]

Rheumatoid scleritis and rheumatoid episcleritis generally occur in patients whose arthritis is of longer duration than that of rheumatoid control patients. Also, patients with rheumatoid scleritis and episcleritis usually have more widespread systemic disease—particularly of the cardiovascular and respiratory systems—and have radiological evidence of more advanced joint disease than do rheumatoid control patients. Subcutaneous granulomatous nodules and atrophy of the skin are much more common in patients with rheumatoid scleritis and episcleritis than in rheumatoid control patients.[6]

The erythrocyte sedimentation rate is significantly higher in patients with rheumatoid scleritis and episcleritis than in rheumatoid control patients. Autoantibody studies in patients with rheumatoid scleritis and episcleritis show little variation from results expected in rheumatoid arthritis.[6]

Signs and Symptoms of Scleritis and Episcleritis. Inflammatory lesions of the sclera and episclera have been subjected to a variety of classifications. For a traditional view the reader is referred to Duke-Elder's System of Ophthalmology.[7]

Scleritis and episcleritis are clinically distinct, with different symptoms, signs, and prognoses. They require different forms of management. From a series involving many years of experience in treating patients with scleral

Table 35–1. Classification of Episcleritis and Scleritis*

Episcleritis		217 eyes
Simple episcleritis	170	
Nodular episcleritis	47	
Scleritis		301 eyes
Anterior scleritis	295	
Diffuse scleritis	119	
Nodular scleritis	134	
Necrotizing scleritis	42	
With inflammation	29	
Without inflammation	13	
(scleromalacia perforans)		
Posterior scleritis	6	

*From Watson, P. G., and Hayreh, S. S.: Br. J. Ophthalmol. *60*:163, 1976.

inflammatory disease, Watson and Hayreh have put forth a simplified classification which is useful clinically and which has gained wide acceptance[5] (Table 35–1).

Visual Status. Episcleritis rarely or never causes loss of vision. Scleritis may cause loss of vision by leading to one or more of a variety of complications such as uveitis, keratitis, or secondary cataract formation. In the series of Watson and Hayreh, 14 percent of patients with scleritis lost a significant amount of vision after the disease had been present for 1 year.[5]

Pain. Scleritis is one of the very few diseases that cause severe ocular pain. Some 60 percent of patients with scleritis have severe ocular pain. Although about half the patients with episcleritis will complain of ocular discomfort, severe pain is not a clinical feature of episcleritis.

Redness. In simple episcleritis the onset is often extremely rapid, the eye becoming flushed within several minutes of the beginning of symptoms. In nodular episcleritis and in scleritis the onset is much more gradual. In scleromalacia perforans there often is little or no redness of the eye at all.

It is of great importance to examine these patients in daylight, for this often is the only way to distinguish episcleritis from the much more serious scleral disease. In episcleritis the color is salmon-pink to bright red (Fig. 35–4, Plate II, p. xxxvi); in scleritis the redness has a deeper, purple hue (Fig. 35–5*B*, Plate II, p. xxxvi).

Conjunctival Discharge. This is not a feature of either scleritis or episcleritis. Indeed, if there is a discharge, and if it is anything but watery, the patient probably has neither of these disorders.

Location of the Inflammatory Focus. In episcleritis the areas in the interpalpebral fissures, both nasally and temporally, are most commonly affected (Fig. 35–4, Plate II, p. xxxvi). In scleritis there is no marked predilection for one meridian to be involved more often than the others, but scleritis does occur somewhat more often in the upper quadrants than in the lower quadrants of the sclera.

Scleral Edema. In scleritis there is scleral edema and involvement of the scleral vessels. With the slit-lamp biomicroscope scleral edema can be detected by observ-

ing the outward displacement of the deep vascular network of the episclera. Avascular zones of episclera may be identified overlying or adjacent to the site of severe necrotizing scleritis.

In episcleritis the sclera is not edematous. The episcleral vessels will be congested (Fig. 35–4, Plate II, p. xxxvi), and the episcleral tissues are infiltrated by inflammatory cells. (In scleritis, the overlying episclera will also be secondarily inflamed in many cases. But instillation of 1:1000 epinephrine or 2.5 percent phenylephrine in the conjunctival sac will constrict these secondarily affected superficial vessels, thereby revealing any underlying scleral disease.)

Scleral Thinning. In eyes that have been subjected to previous bouts of scleritis the sclera in the affected area often appears blue when viewed in daylight. (In daylight it is often possible to see areas of scleral thinning that are not recognizable with the slit-lamp biomicroscope or in rooms illuminated by tungsten or fluorescent lights.)

The blue color is imparted by the underlying ciliary body or choroid. In the past it had been assumed that the reason the uveal tract was more visible in these eyes was that the sclera had become thinned by the previous bout of inflammation. But more recently, it has become recognized that this increased visibility of the underlying uveal tract often is on the basis of increased scleral translucency, rather than scleral thinning. In the series of patients reported by Watson and Hayreh, scleral thinning occurred only in patients who had necrotizing scleritis.[5] Early in the pathogenesis of scleral thinning an avascular zone appears in the center of an area of scleritis. This avascular zone then breaks down to form a slough, the end result of which is an area of thinned sclera.

Scleral Defects. Scleral defects, as opposed to scleral thinning or increased scleral translucency, occur only in the severest forms of necrotizing disease.

Sir William Read, who was Royal Ophthalmologist in the reign of Queen Anne and who was unable to read or write, has been credited with the following description of the danger of perforation in deep scleritis: "For it is most certain that this horny membrane . . . by how much deeper the blister is hidden in the membrane . . . in danger to make an ulceration by breaking through the membrane, whereupon may ensue an utter loss and decay of all the humours."[6] But a different view of this worthy is provided by Garrison.[8] Sir William was a quack who started out as a tailor but set up as an oculist in London in 1694, having hired someone to write a book on ocular diseases in his name and having hired a poet to praise him in verse. His success attracted the attention of Queen Anne, whose bad eyesight made her an easy victim. After gaining her good graces Read was actually knighted and subsequently became oculist to George I.

In *necrotizing scleritis with adjacent inflammation* (see Table 35–1) the disease begins as a localized area of scleritis associated with severe congestion. About one fourth of these patients will also exhibit avascularity of a patch of episcleral tissue overlying or adjacent to the

A

Figure 35–5. Necrotizing scleritis. *A*, The lesion is located in the temporal aspect of the right eye of a 77-year-old woman whose antinuclear antibody titer was markedly elevated. (The eye is adducted, the temporal periphery of the cornea and iris being just visible in the far right hand side of the field.) Arrows delineate the borders of the scleral ulceration. An oblong avascular patch of episclera extends across the center of the scleral defect, reaching the rim of the ulcer inferonasally. *B*, Same patient as shown in *A*, 2 weeks later (see Plate II, p. xxxvi).

area of scleral edema (Fig. 35–5*A*). The inflammation may remain localized or may spread in both directions around the globe. In those areas where necrosis has occurred there will be scleral thinning or even absence of the sclera, with exposure of the underlying uvea (Fig. 35–5*B*; Plate II, p. xxxvi).

In *necrotizing scleritis without adjacent inflammation* ("*scleromalacia perforans*"; see Table 35–1), the patient initially has no ocular symptoms in many cases. Either she or an acquaintance may notice a grayish or yellow scleral patch which already may have progressed to a complete loss of scleral tissue in a localized area. Any clinical evidence of inflammatory change is minimal. After a variable period the yellowish-gray area separates as a sequestrum together with the overlying episclera. The resulting defect is covered by a thin layer of conjunctiva. Although unsupported by sclera, the underlying uvea tends not to bulge through the defect unless the intraocular pressure becomes elevated (Fig. 35–6).

About half the patients with scleromalacia perforans have rheumatoid arthritis, usually of long standing. Virtually all these patients are women.

Uveitis. In episcleritis severe uveitis is rare. But careful examination of the anterior chamber with the slit-lamp biomicroscope will reveal evidence (cells and flare) of a mild anterior uveitis in a small minority of cases.

In scleritis, about one third of the patients will have an anterior uveitis (iridocyclitis) and a smaller number will have posterior uveitis (choroiditis). The uveitis is believed to be caused by inflamed sclera overlying the uveal tract. (But in patients with Wegener's granulomatosis and necrotizing scleritis I have found well-developed foci of granulomatous inflammation in the uveal tract, apparently unrelated to scleral disease, on histopathological examination of several eyes.) In adult rheumatoid arthritis, when scleritis is not present, the incidence of uveitis is believed to be no greater than it is in the nonrheumatoid population.

Figure 35–6. Scleromalacia perforans (necrotizing scleritis without adjacent inflammation) in a 54-year-old woman with severe rheumatoid arthritis. The left upper and lower eyelids are separated by a speculum and the eye is directed inferotemporally. The sclera has perforated supranasally, and the underlying uveal tissue bulges through the scleral defect. (Courtesy of Milton Boniuk, M.D.)

Figure 35–7. Nodular scleritis and sclerosing keratitis. Prominent scleral nodules are present just behind the limbus of the left eye superiorly and supratemporally. The nodules were immobile and were separate from the overlying, inflamed episcleral tissues. An area of sclerosing keratitis appears as the limbus-parallel grayish infiltrate in the corneal periphery, extending from the site of the reflex of the photographic flash to the point where the cornea is covered by the lower eyelid temporally. Slit-lamp biomicroscopic examination revealed that the corneal edema and vessels were located in the deepest layers of the corneal stroma.

Keratitis. Mild corneal changes occur in a small minority of patients with episcleritis, but these are never severe.

In patients with scleritis, corneal changes of a type characteristically seen in scleritis occur in about 30 percent of cases.[5] Two of the most important of these are sclerosing keratitis and marginal corneal ulcer ("ring ulcer"; "limbal guttering").

In sclerosing keratitis the cornea adjacent to the swollen sclera becomes edematous and blood vessels grow into this edematous zone. The patient shown in Figure 35–7 has both nodular scleritis (see Table 35–1) and sclerosing keratitis.

Marginal corneal ulcers (see Fig. 35–15, Plate II, p. xxxvi) are potentially devastating because of the risk of perforation. They occur in about 5 percent of all patients with scleritis. Marginal corneal ulcers are more common in patients whose scleritis is associated with rheumatoid arthritis and other connective tissue diseases than in nonrheumatoid patients with scleritis.

Pathology of Scleritis and Episcleritis. The characteristic histologic picture in rheumatoid scleritis is a zonal type of granulomatous inflammatory reaction (Fig. 35–8). A central area of necrotic scleral collagen is surrounded by a palisade of epithelioid cells and giant cells. These epithelioid and giant cells are in turn surrounded by a mantle of chronic inflammatory cells, chiefly plasma cells and lymphocytes, which often involve the overlying episclera and the underlying uvea. In eyes with scleromalacia perforans the nongranulomatous component of the inflammatory reaction is often inconspicuous.

In simple episcleritis and in most cases of nodular episcleritis the usual histologic changes consist of hyperemia, edema, and infiltration by lymphocytes and plasma cells. But some rheumatoid episcleral nodules have exhibited all the features of subcutaneous rheumatoid nodules on pathologic examination (Fig. 35–9).[9]

Treatment. Episcleritis is a benign, self-limiting disorder for which no treatment is necessary in most patients. There is a tendency for recurrence in many cases.

Should it seem desirable to treat a particular patient, topical corticosteroids may be used.

Scleritis is a much more serious condition and requires skilled management. Topical corticosteroids alone are seldom effective in arresting the disease. Topical therapy with corticosteroids (e.g., prednisolone or dexamethasone) must be supplemented in most cases with systemic anti-inflammatory agents such as oxyphenbutazone, indomethacin, or prednisone. Complications of the scleritis (e.g., uveitis and secondary glaucoma) will require appropriate treatment by the ophthalmologist.

Some authorities believe that subconjunctival injection of corticosteroids, which is beneficial in various other types of ocular inflammation, is contraindicated in treating scleritis. In several cases patients have developed scleral thinning at the site of steroid injection. The relationship, if any, of the scleral thinning to the preceding subconjunctival injection of corticosteroids has not been established.

In extreme cases more heroic forms of medical and surgical treatment have been used. A variety of antimetabolites and alkylating compounds, including methotrexate, 5-fluorouracil, azathioprine, chlorambucil, nitrogen mustard, duazomycin, and cyclophosphamide, have been used with favorable results. Among these drugs, the one now believed to be most effective is cyclophosphamide (Cytoxan). Scleral grafting has been done to bridge over gaps that have developed at the site of necrotizing scleritis. Donor sclera, fascia lata, and periosteum are some of the substances that have been used for this purpose.

JUVENILE RHEUMATOID ARTHRITIS (STILL'S DISEASE)

Juvenile rheumatoid arthritis differs from adult rheumatoid arthritis in many ways that are well known to the rheumatologist. These differences include both clin-

Figure 35–8. Granulomatous scleritis. A 64-year-old woman who had rheumatoid arthritis with crippling deformities for several years consulted an ophthalmologist because of gradual diminution of vision over a 6-month period. He observed a lesion that "... perforated and destroyed the sclera at about three o'clock." The ophthalmologist did not suspect the possibility of rheumatoid scleritis with perforation and exposure of the uvea. Rather, he made a diagnosis of malignant melanoma of the ciliary body with perforation of the overlying sclera, and enucleated the eye. *A,* The sclera has been destroyed by an inflammatory process from the limbus (*L*) to the equatorial region of the eye at the bottom of the field. It is completely absent in the zone between the arrows, thereby exposing the underlying ciliary body. Hematoxylin and eosin; magnification × 6; Armed Forces Institute of Pathology Negative Number 57-1167. (Courtesy of Lorenz E. Zimmerman, M.D.) *B,* In this field only a small island of necrotic sclera (*S*) remains. It is being attacked and surmounted by polymorphonuclear neutrophils and a mantle of epithelioid cells. Several well-developed giant cells are present at the left hand side of the field, directly opposite the scleral fragment. The granulomatous inflammatory reaction is surrounded, in turn, by an outpouring of inflammatory cells consisting chiefly of plasma cells and lymphocytes. These are seen best in the lower portion of the field. Hematoxylin and eosin; magnification × 115; Armed Forces Institute of Pathology Negative Number 57-1163. (Courtesy of Lorenz E. Zimmerman, M.D.)

Figure 35–9. Rheumatoid episcleral nodule. The patient was a 63-year-old woman with a history of recurrent attacks of rheumatoid arthritis during a 20-year period. *A*, Slightly elevated, yellowish-white episcleral lesion (arrows) is surrounded by dilated blood vessels. *B*, Section of the episcleral nodule shown in *A*. A central zone of fibrinoid necrosis of the episcleral collagen is surrounded by a mantle of epithelioid cells, which are seen better in *C*. Hematoxylin and eosin; magnification × 45. *C*, From the upper right hand portion of the episcleral nodule shown in *B*. Fibrinoid necrosis of episcleral collagen fibers is present in the lower and central portions of the field. Epithelioid cells are palisaded in planes perpendicular to the central zone of necrosis and are sharply demarcated from the surrounding episcleral connective tissue, which contains a light scattering of lymphocytes and plasma cells. Hematoxylin and eosin; magnification × 90.

ical and laboratory features. For example, in juvenile rheumatoid arthritis no more than 10 percent of sera are positive in the commonly employed tests for rheumatoid factor. The frequency of antinuclear antibody is higher in children with rheumatoid arthritis than in adults with rheumatoid arthritis. These two disorders also differ in the nature of associated ocular involvement. In juvenile rheumatoid arthritis the classic triad of ocular lesions consists of anterior uveitis, band keratopathy, and secondary cataract. In adults with rheumatoid arthritis, uveitis (except as a complication of scleritis) probably occurs no more often than it does in the general population. And, except for individuals who have scleritis or who have drug-induced lenticular opacities, cataract is no more common in these adults than in normal controls. Nor is band keratopathy a feature of adult rheumatoid arthritis. Conversely, scleritis and keratitis, both of which are major problems in adult rheumatoid arthritis, are seldom seen in patients with juvenile rheumatoid arthritis. Keratitis sicca, which is so common in adults with rheumatoid arthritis, occurs only rarely in children with rheumatoid arthritis.

In virtually all cases the *uveitis* is an anterior uveitis (iridocyclitis). It is of nongranulomatous type (epithelioid cells and giant cells are not components of the inflammatory exudate) and is bilateral in about 50 to 70 percent of cases. Iridocyclitis occurred in 17 percent of 210 patients with juvenile rheumatoid arthritis reported by Chylack and co-workers in Boston.[10] Girls are affected more often than are boys, the ratio of involvement being 2:1 in the aforementioned series of patients.[10] Uveitis is far more likely to occur in children with the mono-pauciarticular form of the disease than in those with polyarticular involvement, and it is particularly likely to occur in children who develop rheu-

matoid arthritis before 4 years of age. Kanski studied 160 patients (102 girls and 58 boys) with anterior uveitis and seronegative juvenile arthritis.[11] *Chronic* uveitis occurred in 131 patients, 76 percent of whom were girls. (This is only slightly higher than would be expected from the proportion of girls in the study: 64 percent.) The remaining 29 patients with anterior uveitis had an *acute* form of uveitis, and 27 of them were boys. The acute form of iridocyclitis is bilateral in only about 15 percent of cases.

Band keratopathy occurs as a complication of iridocyclitis in many children whose uveitis is of a *chronic* nature. The incidence often has been put at about 50 percent. Band keratopathy occurred in 41 percent of the eyes that had a chronic anterior uveitis in Kanski's series. But Chylack and co-workers found band keratopathy in only 13 percent of the eyes with anterior uveitis in their study.[10]

Band keratopathy is not pathognomonic of juvenile rheumatoid arthritis. It occurs in a variety of other disorders and results from deposition of calcium in Bowman's layer (Fig. 35–10). Typically, the first areas of the cornea to be involved are located just inside the limbus nasally and temporally. Calcification of Bowman's layer then progresses across the cornea, eventually connecting the two original sites of involvement. The result is a band-like opacity located in the interpalpebral fissure. Although a slit-lamp biomicroscope is required to detect the incipient stage of the lesion, the opacity soon becomes visible to the naked eye.

The cause and pathogenesis of band keratopathy are unknown. Calcium and phosphorus metabolism are no different in the affected children than in those who do not develop band keratopathy. The fact that the calcification is usually confined to the zone of the interpal-

Figure 35–10. *A*, Band keratopathy in a 12-year-old girl with severe juvenile rheumatoid arthritis. (Courtesy of Torrence A. Makley, M.D.) *B*, Normal cornea. Bowman's layer (B, upper left), a modified portion of the stroma, is the clear zone traversing the cornea beneath the epithelium. In band keratopathy calcium is deposited in Bowman's layer. Beneath Bowman's layer lies the stroma proper, consisting of collagenous lamellae, keratocytes, and ground substance. Descemet's membrane (arrow) is elaborated by the single layered corneal endothelium, behind which lies the anterior chamber. Hematoxylin and eosin; magnification × 120.

pebral fissure suggests that drying of the cornea may play a role in deposition of calcium in this region.

Cataract is said to occur as a complication in about half of the children who have *chronic* uveitis,[12] and developed in 42 percent of the eyes with chronic iridocyclitis in Kanski's study.[11] But Chylack and co-workers found cataract in only 22 percent of eyes with uveitis.[10] The lower incidence of band keratopathy and secondary cataract in the patients reported by these investigators may reflect their diligent search for early, and often asymptomatic, uveitis, thereby enabling institution of appropriate therapy.

Treatment of eyes affected with the *acute* form of anterior uveitis is usually relatively simple, the inflammation responding well to topical medications. Because these eyes usually exhibit pain and redness that is obvious to the parents and to the rheumatologist, there seldom is any delay in beginning treatment. Serious ocular complications (e.g., cataract and band keratopathy) seldom occur.[11] In Kanski's study of 29 patients with the acute type of anterior uveitis, the mean age at onset of arthritis was 11.5 years. On followup, 21 of the 29 patients had developed typical ankylosing spondylitis, and five patients had sacroiliitis.

Treatment of the *chronic* form of uveitis is often difficult, but about 40 percent of cases can be brought under control in 3 months or less.[10] The mainstays of therapy are topical corticosteroids and atropine. Systemic corticosteroids may be required to treat those eyes that fail to respond to topical medications. Immunosuppressive drugs other than corticosteroids have seldom been used in treating iridocyclitis occurring in patients with juvenile rheumatoid arthritis.[11] This is attributable both to the lack of convincing evidence for their effectiveness and to the rheumatologist's reluctance to subject these young individuals to the major toxic effects of chemotherapy.

Chelation of the calcium in Bowman's layer with topically applied sodium versenate solution will result in clearing of band keratopathy and improvement of vision in many cases. In those children who eventually require ocular surgery (e.g., for a cataract dense enough to cause major visual loss or for glaucoma consequent to synechia formation) the results are often discouraging.

Many observers have commented on the lack of symptoms reported by children with the *chronic* form of uveitis when the ocular inflammation begins. Only a minority report symptoms of iridocyclitis or exhibit evidence of ocular inflammation that is apparent to their parents or to the rheumatologist. In view of this often asymptomatic onset of ocular inflammation, and because treatment of the uveitis at an early stage will often forestall development of complications such as band keratopathy and cataract, it is of great importance that children with rheumatoid arthritis be subjected to periodic examination by an ophthalmologist in a search for anterior uveitis. A 6-month interval between ophthalmic examinations would be appropriate in most cases. The children who are at greatest risk are those with the pauciarticular form of the disease, and they should be seen, at least initially, at even more frequent intervals.

ANKYLOSING SPONDYLITIS

Because one third to one half of the patients with ankylosing spondylitis exhibit synovitis in peripheral joints, the disease was formerly viewed as a variant of rheumatoid arthritis. But ankylosing spondylitis differs from rheumatoid arthritis in several ways: (1) Preponderance of involvement in men (male:female ratio 8:1). (2) Evidence of genetic transmission in related kindreds. (The disease is 30 times more prevalent among the relatives of spondylitis patients than in relatives of controls. The striking association of ankylosing spondylitis with the histocompatibility antigen HLA-B27 provides further insight into the genetic aspect of this disorder.) (3) The absence of rheumatoid factor and rheumatoid nodules. (4) Prominent calcification of the longitudinal ligaments of the peripheral portions of the intervertebral discs. (5) A tendency to bony ankylosis. (An ophthalmologic aphorism is that a young man with anterior uveitis who has difficulty in placing his chin in the slit-lamp apparatus should be suspected of having ankylosing spondylitis.) (6) The association of certain extra-articular manifestations, such as iridocyclitis and aortitis. (7) Symptomatic benefit with medications that are only minimally effective in rheumatoid arthritis (e.g., phenylbutazone and indomethacin).[13]

In various series, from 4 to 50 percent of patients with ankylosing spondylitis have had an anterior uveitis, with 25 percent being, perhaps, the most commonly accepted figure. Recent studies suggest that among patients with ankylosing spondylitis, uveitis occurs far more commonly in those who are HLA-B27 positive than it does in those who are HLA-B27 negative. Although uveitis may be the presenting sign of the disease, characteristically the ocular inflammation develops in a patient already known to have spondylitis. Typically the inflammation is an acute, nongranulomatous anterior uveitis. The signs and symptoms include photophobia, some decrease in visual acuity, a variable degree of ocular pain, congestion of the episcleral vessels, fine cellular precipitates on the corneal endothelium, cells and flare in the anterior chamber, and miosis. A severe plastic iritis, with formation of dense synechiae, is decidedly uncommon.[14]

Treatment of the iridocyclitis consists of the usual topical corticosteroids, cycloplegics (e.g., atropine), and mydriatics. The iritis generally runs a favorable course and tends to clear in 3 to 6 weeks, with few sequelae. Relapses are typical of the disease and may occur repeatedly over the course of many years.[13]

SYSTEMIC LUPUS ERYTHEMATOSUS

In the realm of the ophthalmologist the most common manifestation of this disease is the *butterfly eruption*,[15] which occurs in some 40 percent of cases and which is discussed in Chapter 36. Signs and symptoms of *central nervous system* involvement occur in some 30 percent of patients with systemic lupus erythematosus, and some of these individuals will be seen by the ophthalmologist because of ptosis, diplopia, or nystagmus.[16]

With regard to the *eye* itself, "cotton wool patches" in the retina often have been cited as being the most common lesion, followed in frequency by corneal and conjunctival involvement, with only a very occasional patient exhibiting uveitis or scleritis. But one encounters difficulty in attempting to determine the incidence of ocular involvement in systemic lupus erythematosus. For example, many observers have remarked that the retinal lesions occur much more often in acutely ill patients than they do in those who are in remission or who have only a relatively mild form of the disease. The investigation of Gold and co-workers, in which they reported the ocular findings in their 61 patients with systemic lupus erythematosus and reviewed ten similar series reported in the literature by other workers, is of interest in this regard.[17] They found retinal hemorrhages reported in from 5 to 28 percent of cases (not one of their 61 patients had a retinal hemorrhage) and cotton wool spots described in from 6 to 28 percent of cases (only 3 percent of their patients had cotton wool spots). Gold and associates remarked that all 61 of their patients had been referred to them for ocular examination from the systemic lupus erythematosus clinic at Bellevue Hospital. Most of these patients had been treated already with systemic antimalarials and/or corticosteroids, and were no longer acutely ill.

Another consideration in determining the incidence of ocular involvement in systemic lupus erythematosus is the fact that greater clinical awareness and better laboratory diagnostic aids in recent years have led to the detection of many mild cases of lupus. These patients are the very ones who are least likely to exhibit ocular complications.

Retinopathy. Retinal damage from antimalarials used in treating systemic lupus erythematosus is a greater cause of visual loss than is retinal involvement occurring in the natural course of the disease.

Cotton wool spots occur in lupus and in a variety of other disorders, most notably the "connective tissue" diseases, vascular hypertension, central retinal vein occlusion, diabetic retinopathy, papilledema, the dysproteinemias, leukemia, and severe anemia.[18] On ophthalmoscopic examination one or more (but usually less than ten) cotton wool spots are seen. They occur preferentially in the posterior part of the retina, rendering them detectable by casual examination. The optic nerve head is often involved. Each cotton wool spot appears as a grayish-white, soft, fluffy exudate, usually situated more closely to the arterioles than to the veins, lying in the inner layers of the retina and bulging slightly toward the vitreous body (Fig. 35–11). They are small, averaging about one third of a disc diameter in width. (The normal diameter of the optic nerve head is from 1.5 to 2.0 mm.) Cotton wool spots usually clear within 1 to 3 months of their appearance.

Pathologic examination of tissue from a cotton wool spot confirms the clinical impression that the lesion in-

Figure 35–11. A typical cotton wool spot in a young woman with systemic lupus erythematosus. The lesion is situated along the upper border of a retinal arteriole, about midway between the optic nerve head and the macula.

volves chiefly the inner retinal layers (Fig. 35–12). The ganglion cell nerve fiber layer is greatly thickened in a disciform, sharply circumscribed fashion. In this region some of the nerve fibers have been interrupted, and in many cases "*cytoid bodies*" are seen. The latter are globular bodies, 10 to 20 microns in diameter. Each bears a superficial resemblance to a cell because of a centrally located structure simulating a nucleus. (Thus, "cotton wool spot" is an ophthalmoscopic term, and "cytoid body" is a histologic feature of the cotton wool spot.)

The nature of cytoid bodies has been argued since their discovery in 1856. In recent years Wolter has shown conclusively that cytoid bodies arise from the axons of retinal ganglion cells. The axons of the retinal ganglion cells have their synapses in the lateral geniculate body. In a patient with a cotton wool spot these nerve fibers become interrupted as they course through the lesion which is located between the ganglion cell and the optic nerve head. Prominent terminal swelling of the axonal stump on the side remaining in contact with the retinal ganglion cell occurs. This bulbous terminal swelling of the interrupted nerve fiber, together with aggregation of the lipid debris of the degenerating axonal structures to form a pseudonucleus, constitutes a cytoid body.[18]

It is generally agreed that focal ischemia is the cause of cotton wool spots and the cotton wool spot is, therefore, a microinfarct of the retina. The precise nature of the vascular insufficiency is unsettled. Recent work suggests that the white material seen in a cotton wool spot may consist at least partially of accumulated axoplasmic debris at the site of an obstruction in the normal orthograde axoplasmic transportation system in axons of retinal ganglion cells.

Hemorrhages in the inner retinal layers are another feature of the retinopathy occurring in systemic lupus erythematosus. And, as is true of cotton wool spots,

Figure 35–12. A cotton wool spot in the retina of a 26-year-old woman who died of systemic lupus erythematosus. *A* (compare with Fig. 35-3*B*). The ganglion cell nerve fiber layer is greatly thickened in a disciform, sharply circumscribed fashion (arrows). It bulges internally toward the vitreous body (*V*), and also externally, distorting the inner nuclear layer of the retina. The rods and cones are separated artifactitiously from the underlying layer of retinal pigment epithelium. *S* = Sclera. Hematoxylin and eosin; magnification × 75. *B*, Same lesion shown in *A*. Nerve fibers (*NF*) are interrupted as they enter the area of the cotton wool spot. Many "cytoid bodies" are visible in the lesion. *G* = Ganglion cell layer of retina. Hematoxylin and eosin; magnification × 120. *C*, From near the center of the field shown in *B*. Many "cytoid bodies" (arrows) are present. *NF* = Nerve fiber layer of retina. *G* = Retinal ganglion cell. Hematoxylin and eosin; magnification × 480.

they are not necessarily mere reflections of a concomitant vascular hypertension. They can result from an independent effect of the disease on the retinal tissues and they are found in the absence of hypertension.[17] Other retinal lesions that may occur with or without concomitant hypertension are retinal *microaneurysms, arteriovenous crossing changes,* and *arteriolar narrowing.*[17]

Corneal and Conjunctival Lesions. A variety of these have been described.[19] The most common are *conjunctivitis* (3 to 20 percent of cases) and mild *epithelial degeneration,* rendering the affected cells stainable with topical fluorescein.[17] *Sjögren's syndrome* has been documented in association with various connective tissue diseases, including systemic lupus erythematosus, and any of these may replace rheumatoid arthritis in the classic triad of Sjögren's syndrome.[4]

CONNECTIVE TISSUE DISEASES OTHER THAN RHEUMATOID ARTHRITIS AND LUPUS ERYTHEMATOSUS

Scleroderma (systemic sclerosis) is a rare disease. Some three to five new cases per million population appear each year in the United States. In this disorder the ocular adnexa and the outer coats of the eye are affected relatively often, but involvement of the inner eye, particularly the retina, is unusual.[20] The most common finding is tightness of the eyelids. Keratoconjunctivitis sicca and Sjögren's syndrome occur less often.

Ocular involvement is uncommon in *periarteritis nodosa* (polyarteritis nodosa.) Reported abnormalities of the outer coats of the eye include chemosis (conjunctival edema), subconjunctival hemorrhages, conjunctivitis, keratitis, scleritis, marginal corneal ulceration, and Sjögren's syndrome. Choroidal angiitis has been found in many eyes examined post mortem, but clinical signs of choroidal involvement are seen only seldom. Retinal lesions are rarer than choroidal involvement, and the majority of these result from the effects of vascular hypertension upon the retinal vessels.[21]

Involvement of the eye is rare in *polymyositis* and in *dermatomyositis.* Conjunctivitis, episcleritis, iritis, and retinal cotton wool spots have been reported. The eyelids are involved more often. A peculiar bluish to violaceous ("heliotrope") erythematous suffusion develops in the eyelids in many cases and is often associated with closely set telangiectasias of the palpebral skin and with marked palpebral edema. The orbicularis oculi muscles and the extraocular muscles may participate in the widespread myositis, leading to pain, tenderness, oculomotor palsies, and nystagmus.[22]

GIANT CELL ARTERITIS (TEMPORAL ARTERITIS, CRANIAL ARTERITIS) AND POLYMYALGIA RHEUMATICA

The association of giant cell arteritis with polymyalgia rheumatica is discussed in Chapter 73. Henkind and Gold have emphasized that the incidence of giant cell arteritis in patients with polymyalgia rheumatica is much higher than the often cited 20 percent.[23] For those patients with polymyalgia rheumatica who do *not* have clinical evidence of giant cell arteritis and whose symptoms are controllable with small amounts of corticosteroids (10 mg or less of prednisone daily), the risk of visual complications is far lower than it is for patients with polymyalgia rheumatica who have clinical evidence of giant cell arteritis. Spiera and Davison followed for a minimum of 4 years 56 patients with polymyalgia rheumatica who had no clinical evidence of giant cell arteritis. None became blind or developed any other visual disturbance.[24] The outlook is much grimmer for patients with giant cell arteritis. Ocular involvement formerly occurred in 40 to 50 percent of patients, with unilateral blindness developing in 10 to 15 percent, and both eyes becoming blind in 12 to 15 percent.[25] Blindness in these patients is particularly unfortunate because it is usually preventable if the disease is diagnosed promptly and corticosteroids are administered immediately. In a recently reported series of cases, 15 of 126 patients with giant cell arteritis (12 percent) suffered ocular complications.[26] Earlier diagnosis and awareness of the need for immediate treatment probably account for the decreased frequency with which visual catastrophes currently occur in patients with giant cell arteritis.

The systemic disorder known today as "giant cell arteritis" was described first by the British ophthalmologist Jonathan Hutchinson in 1890. Subsequently it was studied in detail by others and was given the name "temporal arteritis" because involvement of the temporal arteries is a dominating feature. But because many patients also have evidence of involvement of other arteries in the cranial region (e.g., the cerebral and lingual arteries), there has been a more recent tendency to supplant the term "temporal arteritis" with the designation "cranial arteritis." Other authors prefer the term "giant cell arteritis" because, although the brunt of the disease is borne by the carotid arteries and their branches, other vessels (e.g., the aorta, innominate, subclavian, and coronary arteries) have been involved in many cases. Furthermore, this designation emphasizes one of the salient histologic features of the lesion. HLA tissue typing for A, B, and C antigens has been unremarkable in patients with giant cell arteritis, as have serum levels of IgA, IgG, IgM, antinuclear antibodies, and complement components C3 and C4.

A frequent characteristic feature is the presence of a prominent, thickened, tortuous, tender temporal artery that often shows no pulsation. An affected artery exhibits patchy areas of necrosis in the tunica media with fragmentation of the internal elastic lamina. A prominent granulomatous inflammatory reaction, with many giant cells, is found in the necrotic areas, particularly along the outer aspect of the internal elastic lamina, while marked fibrosis occurs on the intimal side. This diffuse, chronic, granulomatous inflammatory reaction produces such a severe amount of intimal reaction that the vascular lumen may be occluded (Fig. 35–13).

Only the ocular symptoms and signs occurring in this systemic disease will be considered here. The ocular complications of giant cell arteritis appear within several weeks or months of the onset of systemic manifestations. Typically the visual loss is abrupt and progresses rapidly to blindness. Less often the blindness is preceded by episodes of unilateral visual loss (amaurosis fugax). Both eyes often are affected, the second eye becoming involved from 1 day to 3 weeks after the first. Visual loss may be complete or may be limited to a sector of the visual field. When only part of the visual field is lost, an inferior altitudinal defect is the most common finding.

The visual loss results from ischemic infarction of the optic nerve (ischemic optic neuropathy) caused by giant cell arteritis involving branches of the ophthalmic artery supplying the optic nerve. Much less often the central retinal artery is occluded. The site of predilection for optic nerve involvement is just behind the lamina cribrosa. Low-grade papilledema results and the swollen optic nerve head tends to be more pallid than is the disc in cases of inflammatory optic neuritis (Fig. 35–14).

The presence of giant cell arteritis should be suspected in any patient above age 50 years with abrupt visual loss and ischemic optic neuropathy. The erythrocyte sedimentation rate should be determined immediately. It usually is elevated markedly in giant cell arteritis; but if the patient has been taking corticosteroids, it may be only slightly increased or even normal. If the sedimentation rate is found to be elevated, or if the patient has other evidence of giant cell arteritis, systemic corticosteroids should be administered immediately in large doses (60 to 120 mg of prednisone or its equivalent daily), and the temporal artery should be biopsied. Institution of corticosteroid therapy should not await the biopsy report. A negative temporal artery biopsy does not rule out the presence of giant cell arteritis. Skip areas of involvement occur. As the erythrocyte sedimentation rate falls, the dose of corticosteroids may be decreased to the lowest level sufficient to maintain the sedimentation rate at a normal level for at least 4 to 6 months, after which the steroids may be cautiously discontinued. If the temporal artery biopsy was negative, but the trial of corticosteroids has lowered a high sedimentation rate to normal, continued treatment is probably warranted. A patient with a normal sedimentation rate and a negative temporal artery biopsy is unlikely to have the disease and should not be subjected to the hazards of long-term, high-dose corticosteroid therapy.

Corticosteroid therapy usually will prevent involvement of the second eye, but only seldom will it improve vision in the first eye to be affected in patients with giant cell arteritis.

Figure 35–13. Giant cell arteritis. *A*, The temporal artery's lumen has been reduced profoundly in diameter by the inflammatory process in its wall and by subintimal proliferation. Hematoxylin and eosin; magnification × 30. *B*, In many areas epithelioid cells have fused to form giant cells. A prominent giant cell is located just to the left of the center of this field. Many lymphocytes and plasma cells also are present. Hematoxylin and eosin; magnification × 150.

Figure 35–14. Giant cell arteritis. (Same patient whose temporal artery biopsy is shown in Fig 35–13.) The optic nerve head is edematous. Retinal arteriolar narrowing is present. The retinal veins are slightly dilated, and the venous blood column is darker than normal. (A nuclear cataract was present, rendering the fundus details slightly indistinct.)

WEGENER'S GRANULOMATOSIS

The classic triad of Wegener's granulomatosis consists of granulomas of the upper or lower respiratory tract, focal necrotizing glomerulonephritis, and arteritis. But, as Wegener has emphasized, the condition should not be considered primarily an angiitis.[27] Angiitis is a prominent feature in the lungs in some patients, but it is not responsible for the extravascular granulomatous lesions. In some cases it is difficult or impossible to demonstrate angiitis.

Ocular involvement is common in Wegener's granulomatosis and may be the first sign of the disease.[28] Haynes and colleagues reported the ocular findings in 29 patients with Wegener's granulomatosis seen at the National Institutes of Health during a 15-year span and reviewed ocular involvement in cases reported in the English language literature since 1957.[29] Among the overall total of 342 patients, 39 percent had ocular disease. In 286 of the 342 patients the nature of the ocular involvement had been recorded. The most common abnormalities among these 286 patients were proptosis (18 percent); conjunctivitis, scleritis, episcleritis, or corneoscleral ulcer (16 percent); vasculitis of retina or optic nerve (8 percent); dacryocystitis (inflammation of the tear sac; 3 percent); and uveitis (2 percent).

I have seen several patients in whom ring ulcers of the corneal periphery were the initial sign of Wegener's granulomatosis.[28] The woman whose eye is shown in Figure 35–15, Plate II, p. xxxvi, had been treated initially for conjunctivitis. When I first examined her, 3 weeks after the onset of her ocular symptoms, she had a deep ring ulcer in the superotemporal periphery of her cornea. She also gave a history of recent weight loss and had several areas of cutaneous ulceration over her lower legs. Examination of her urine disclosed the presence of albuminuria and erythrocyte casts. Pulmonary cavities were demonstrated on roentgenography. The corneal lesion progressed and she soon developed a necrotizing scleritis of the type seen in rheumatoid arthritis. Death occurred from a cerebral hemorrhage 14 months after the onset of her symptoms. On pathological examination of the affected eye a granulomatous reaction to collagen fibers was found in the corneal ring ulcer and in the broad area of necrotizing scleritis (Fig. 35–16). There was no evidence of vasculitis in serial sections of the entire eye.

Although topical and systemic corticosteroids often are helpful in controlling some of the ocular lesions that occur in Wegener's granulomatosis, cyclophosphamide (Cytoxan) is regarded currently as the drug of choice in treating this disorder.[29]

RELAPSING POLYCHONDRITIS

Relapsing polychondritis is a rare disorder characterized by inflammation and destruction of cartilage. The condition has some features of rheumatoid arthritis, Wegener's granulomatosis, and midline lethal granuloma. The cause and pathogenesis are unknown.

Although the human eye does not contain cartilage, ocular involvement in relapsing polychondritis is common, occurring in about 65 percent of cases. Hyaline cartilage, such as articular cartilage, contains exclusively type II collagen. Fibrocartilages are composed of type II as well as type I collagen. With regard to the eye, corneal collagen is type I. Type II collagen is found in the retina and the vitreous body, but neither of these two tissues is an ocular site of predilection for involvement in relapsing polychrondritis. The most common ocular abnormalities associated with this disorder are episcleritis, iritis, and conjunctivitis.[23,30]

ENTEROPATHIC ARTHROPATHY

The disorders of main interest in this group are ulcerative colitis, Crohn's disease, and Whipple's disease.

The reported incidence of arthritis complicating *ulcerative colitis* and *Crohn's disease* is generally in the range of 10 percent, although Greenstein and associates reported involvement in 53 of 202 patients (26 percent) with ulcerative colitis and in 111 of 498 patients with Crohn's disease (22 percent).[31] The most common rheumatic pattern is an asymmetric polyarthritis involving a few joints. The reported incidence of spondylitis, which is indistinguishable from ankylosing spondylitis, in patients with ulcerative colitis and Crohn's disease varies from 2 to 6 percent. In contrast to Crohn's disease, the

Figure 35–16. Wegener's granulomatosis. (From the same patient whose eye is shown in Fig. 35–15.) *A*, In this plane of section the corneal ring ulcer (U) has become re-epithelialized. Epithelioid cells and giant cells attack the interrupted corneal collagen fibers. The limbal tissues (*L*) and the anterior portion of the sclera (left hand side of field) are severely necrotic. Hematoxylin and eosin; magnification × 30. *B*, Higher magnification of superficial portion of corneal ulcer shown in *A*. Two large giant cells are present. One of them is apposed to the interrupted collagen fibers (arrow) in the wall of the ulcer. Corneal collagen is type 1. Hematoxylin and eosin; magnification × 480. *C*, Most of the sclera (*S*) has been destroyed. Giant cells (the most prominent ones are located near the center of the field) attack the remaining scleral collagen fibers. The undulating structure traversing the upper portion of the field is the retina. Hematoxylin and eosin; magnification × 75. *D*, Epithelioid cells and giant cells form a granulomatous lesion (arrows) in ciliary body. *V* = Vitreous body. Hematoxylin and eosin; magnification × 95.

Figure 35–17. Whipple's disease. The patient was a 52-year-old man with vitreous body opacities thought to be on the basis of a uveitis. He had a 25-year history of intermittent polyarthritis and was regarded as having rheumatoid arthritis. The presence of Whipple's disease was diagnosed only on postmortem examination. *A*, The inner retinal layers are infiltrated by macrophages (*M*) with pale-blue cytoplasm and eccentric or paracentral small nuclei. Several macrophages (arrow) have migrated across the internal limiting membrane (*I*) into the vitreous body. Hematoxylin and eosin; magnification × 400. Armed Forces Institute of Pathology Negative Number 77-7146. (Courtesy of Ramon L. Font, M.D.) *B*, The retinal nerve fiber layer contains myriads of macrophages with intensely PAS-positive cytoplasm. Many macrophages have traversed the wrinkled internal limiting membrane (arrow) and are interposed between it and a fine preretinal membrane. The choroid and the inner layers of the sclera are present at the bottom of the field. (Compare with Fig. 35-3*B*.) PAS-hematoxylin; magnification × 170. Armed Forces Institute of Pathology Negative Number 77-7147. (Courtesy of Ramon L. Font, M.D.)

extraintestinal manifestations of ulcerative colitis (involvement of joints, eyes, and skin) seldom precede the intestinal symptoms.

There is an increased incidence of uveitis, particularly iritis, in patients with ulcerative colitis. Episcleritis and (rarely) marginal ring ulceration of the cornea are other types of ocular abnormalities that occur in these individuals. Patients with ulcerative colitis and spondylitis are much more likely to have iritis than are those without such joint involvement.[23] For example, Wright and colleagues found that 12 percent of 144 patients with ulcerative colitis had iritis and 17 percent had spondylitis.[32] There was a close association of uveitis with sacroiliac involvement. Of their 25 patients with spondylitis and ulcerative colitis, 13 (52 percent) had uveitis. But among the patients with colitis who did not have spondylitis, only 3 percent had uveitis.

Ocular involvement was found in 41 of 820 patients with Crohn's disease (5 percent).[31,33] (But because not all of the 820 individuals had undergone ophthalmologic examination, the prevalence of ocular involvement was undoubtedly higher than the reported 5 percent.) The most common ocular disorders were conjunctivitis, episcleritis, uveitis (especially iridocyclitis), and peripheral corneal ulceration.[31,33] Ocular lesions were much more common in those patients whose disease affected the colon than in those whose disease was in the small intestine.[31] (Similarly, joint involvement was also much more prevalent in patients whose Crohn's disease occurred in the colon than in those whose disease was limited to the small bowel.[31]) And there was a striking association of ocular involvement with joint involvement: Those patients with Crohn's disease who had joint lesions were far more likely to also have ocular lesions than were those patients with Crohn's disease whose joints were unaffected.[33]

In patients with *Whipple's disease* there is heavy infiltration of the intestinal wall and lymphatics by macrophages filled with glycoprotein. Steatorrhea and diarrhea are frequent signs. Nondeforming migratory arthritis is common and is often the initial complaint. Fever occurs in about one third of patients with Whipple's disease. Many of these individuals have been regarded erroneously as having rheumatoid arthritis.

Opacities in the vitreous body are the most common ocular abnormality in patients with Whipple's disease. They consist of macrophages that have migrated from the inner layers of the retina into the vitreous body. Thus, the basic abnormality is a retinitis (Fig. 35–17). The strong PAS-positivity of the macrophages' cytoplasm is attributed to the high content of polysaccharides present in bacterial wall remnants that are located within the cytoplasmic granules.[34] Electron microscopic examination of these macrophages in the retina and vitreous body has displayed intracytoplasmic, degenerating, rod-shaped bacteria and membranous structures identical with those seen in the intestine, brain, heart, and other tissues of patients with Whipple's disease.[34]

SARCOIDOSIS

The eyes and ocular adnexa are involved in many patients with sarcoidosis. The precise incidence varies widely in different studies and depends upon several factors. Involvement of the eyes in about 25 percent of patients with sarcoidosis is a widely accepted approximation. Considerable suffering and visual loss often occur.

Uveitis is the most common type of ocular involvement.[35] It is granulomatous in nature, is usually bilateral, and characteristically affects the anterior uvea (iris and ciliary body) more often and more severely than it does the posterior uvea (choroid). The severe inflammation leads to cataract formation and, by adhesion of the iris to the corneal periphery (anterior synechia formation) or by adhesion of the iris to the lens (posterior synechia formation), may result in chronic secondary glaucoma (Fig. 35–18). Much less often inflammation of the posterior portion of the uveal tract (choroid) predominates. A relatively common event is the development of *retinal perivasculitis*. The inflammatory cells aggregated about the retinal vessels account for the ophthalmoscopic picture known as "candle wax drippings." *Optic neuritis* and central nervous system sarcoidosis occur more often in patients with retinal perivasculitis than in those who do not have retinal lesions. Corticosteroids, topically and systemically, and topical atropine are the mainstays in treating sarcoid uveitis.

Involvement of the *outer coats* of the eye occurs much less often than do uveitis and retinitis. Major scleral

Figure 35–18. Iridocyclitis in sarcoidosis. The peripheral and mid-zones of the iris are massively infiltrated by discrete, noncaseating epithelioid cell tubercles. The pupillary zone of the iris is uninvolved and, in this plane of section, only the most anterior aspect of the ciliary body participates in the inflammatory reaction. Peripheral anterior synechia formation (adhesion of the iris to the anterior chamber angle structures and to the corneal periphery) has caused obstruction of the major outflow channels of the aqueous humor, resulting in intractable secondary glaucoma. Hematoxylin and eosin; magnification × 20. (Courtesy of Lorenz E. Zimmerman, M.D.)

Figure 35–19. Sarcoidosis of eyelids. The inflammatory infiltrate has caused plaque-like thickening of the skin of the left upper lid and the left inner canthus. Smaller lesions are present in the right lower lid, the right inner canthus, and near the tip of the nose.

lesions are great rarities. But particularly in patients with erythema nodosum small granulomatous lesions may develop in the episclera or in the outer scleral layers. In patients with hypercalcemia calcium deposition in Bowman's layer may cause band keratopathy.

Involvement of the *ocular adnexa* is common. The eyelids often are affected (Fig. 35–19). The lacrimal glands and fornical conjunctiva also are involved frequently. Although sarcoidosis of the main and accessory lacrimal glands may lead to diminished tear formation and thereby to keratoconjunctivitis sicca in a small minority of patients, in most cases involvement of the lacrimal gland and conjunctiva is asymptomatic. But simple clinical inspection of the conjunctiva, especially

the conjunctiva in the inferior fornix, and the lacrimal gland often will reveal abnormalities in the form of conjunctival nodules and lacrimal gland enlargement (Fig. 35–20).

The lacrimal gland and conjunctiva are located superficially and are readily available for *biopsy*. In an unpublished series of patients at The Mount Sinai Hospital in New York with "proved" systemic sarcoidosis, biopsy of the lacrimal gland exhibited noncaseating epithelioid cell tubercles in 25 percent of patients in whom the lacrimal glands were of normal size, and in 75 percent of those in whom the lacrimal glands were enlarged. At the University of Pennsylvania, biopsy of conjunctiva that appeared normal clinically was performed in 146 patients who were being evaluated for sarcoidosis. In 55 patients the diagnosis of systemic sarcoidosis was established by transbronchial biopsy, mediastinoscopy with biopsy, liver biopsy, or biopsy of another nonocular site. Thirty of these 55 patients (55 percent) with sarcoidosis documented by biopsy of a nonocular site also had positive conjunctival biopsies.[36]

Biopsy of the conjunctiva or lacrimal gland has many advantages over such invasive procedures as biopsy of a scalene lymph node, mediastinoscopy, or the recently introduced transbronchial biopsy of the lung. These latter procedures require hospitalization and, in the case of mediastinoscopy, subjection of the patient to general anesthesia. Because the cutaneous tuberculin test is positive in 20 to 40 percent of patients with sarcoidosis, the significance and specificity of granulomas found in mediastinal and scalene lymph nodes are open to question and require the most careful professional judgment. (But tuberculosis of the conjunctiva is rare—so rare that I have never seen a case. Thus, upon detecting a conjunctival granuloma with the histologic features of sarcoidosis the ophthalmic pathologist, unlike the general surgical pathologist examining a mediastinal or scalene

Figure 35–20. Sarcoidosis of lacrimal gland. *A,* The right upper lid is partially everted for photographic purposes, and the patient is directing her gaze inferonasally. The palpebral lobe of the lacrimal gland is moderately to markedly enlarged. *B,* Biopsy of the lacrimal gland revealed many discrete, noncaseating epithelioid cell tubercles of the type seen near the center of the field. Hematoxylin and eosin; magnification ×150.

lymph node, seldom is concerned about the possibility that the lesion might really be of tuberculous origin.)

The yield of positive biopsies is higher with the invasive procedures noted above, wherein positive results are obtained in 70 to 90 percent of cases, than it is in biopsies of the conjunctiva or lacrimal gland. But the yield of positive results in patients with proved sarcoidosis whose conjunctiva and lacrimal glands appear normal on clinical examination ranges from 25 to 55 percent.[36] And the yield is even higher in patients with obvious conjunctival nodules or with frank lacrimal gland enlargement. Biopsy of the conjunctiva or lacrimal gland is accomplished in a matter of a few minutes on an outpatient basis, using a local anesthetic. Conjunctival biopsy is well known to be a safe procedure, and none of the 115 patients who have undergone lacrimal gland biopsy on my service have developed any complication. Thus, when attempting to establish histologic confirmation in a patient suspected of having sarcoidosis, it seems prudent to offer her biopsy of the lacrimal gland or conjunctiva. Should these simple procedures prove negative (the results will be available within a day or two), the patient can then be subjected to the more formidable invasive procedures involving thoracic surgery.

Although the Kveim-Siltzbach test is a satisfactory and noninvasive way of establishing a tissue diagnosis, it entails a number of disadvantages: (1) the antigen is not widely available; (2) the clinician must wait a month to 6 weeks before obtaining the result; (3) biopsy of the skin is required eventually; and (4) the test is often negative in the later stages of sarcoidosis.

Thus, instead of merely referring the patient with suspected sarcoidosis to the ophthalmologist for ocular examination, I believe the internist should suggest that biopsy of the lacrimal gland and/or conjunctiva be done if a histologic diagnosis has not been established already.

Detection of altered levels of serum angiotensin converting enzyme (ACE) may also be helpful in establishing the diagnosis of sarcoidosis. In a series of patients with sarcoid uveitis studied at the Medical College of Virginia, both serum lysozyme and serum ACE were elevated in 90 percent. We have also been studying tear enzymes in patients with sarcoid uveitis. Dr. Robert S. Weinberg found a remarkably high correlation between levels of ACE in the serum and in the tears of patients with sarcoid uveitis. In the normal population, tear lysozyme levels usually are very high, but this does not appear to be the case with tear ACE levels. Thus, based on these preliminary observations, it appears that studying tear ACE levels in patients suspected of having sarcoid uveitis may be of great help in establishing the diagnosis.

AMYLOIDOSIS

Secondary systemic amyloidosis (pattern II type, perireticulin type) is a well-known complication of chronic inflammatory diseases, including rheumatoid arthritis and other connective tissue disorders. In secondary amyloidosis small, clinically unimportant deposits of ocular amyloid have been described only rarely, and ophthalmic signs attributable to the presence of amyloid are virtually unknown.[37]

But in *primary systemic amyloidosis* (pattern I type, pericollagenous type) ocular involvement occurs often.[37,38] Amyloid depositions in the collagenous sheaths of the retinal vessels are visible ophthalmoscopically as "vascular sheathing." From this pericollagenous location the amyloid passes into the vitreous body, resulting in opacities of a peculiar type that often reduce vision severely (Fig. 35–21, Plate II, p. xxxvi). Involvement of the uvea, particularly the choroid, is common but usually causes no clinical symptoms. Amyloid deposition in the trabecular meshwork drainage apparatus of the anterior chamber is often a cause of intractable open angle glaucoma. Lattice dystrophy of the cornea results from amyloid deposition in the corneal stroma. (The amyloid is arranged in a network configuration; hence the descriptive clinical term "lattice dystrophy.")

In primary systemic amyloidosis conjunctival involvement is very rare, but the skin of the eyelids is a site of predilection, the palpebral skin being affected more often in this disease than is any other cutaneous site in the body. Amyloid deposition in the soft tissues of the orbit may cause proptosis, and involvement of the orbital nerves produces a variety of abnormalities such as ophthalmoplegia and pupillary disturbances.[37]

GOUT

In the latter part of the nineteenth century and the first part of the twentieth century gout was accorded a major role in the causation of a broad variety of ocular disease. "Gouty iritis" was a frequently used term, and as many as 3.5 percent of all cases of iritis were attributed to gout. Today gout is seldom listed in tabulations of the causes of uveitis. Although gout is now less common than in the days when overindulgence in food and drink was the necessary attribute of a gentleman, it is obvious that the term "gouty iritis" was in many cases merely a convenient label assigned on most unconvincing evidence to many cases of ocular inflammation. Features of gouty iritis were as follows: (1) the onset was abrupt, and the iritis was preceded by inflammation of the outer coats of the eye (conjunctiva, episclera, and sclera); (2) the eye was intensely congested and very painful; (3) the attack preceded or accompanied an attack of acute gouty arthritis; (4) the attack was of short duration—a matter of only several days; and (5) relatively complete resolution, with few postinflammatory sequelae, was the rule.

A variety of other ocular abnormalities were also attributed to gout: (1) "the gouty hot eye" of Jonathan Hutchinson, wherein the eyes appeared chronically red and irritated, this persistent state being subject to periodic exacerbations; (2) gouty episcleritis and scleritis; and (3) tophi in the eyelids.

In the 1960s, when allopurinol was being evaluated

for its potential in treating patients with gout, I had the opportunity to perform complete eye examinations on 70 patients being cared for by Drs. Alexander Gutman and Tsai-Fan Yü. Most of these patients had severe gouty arthritis and had been selected for inclusion in this study because their disease was not controllable with conventional medications. Not one of these patients with severe gouty arthritis had uveitis, a history of uveitis, or residual evidence of past uveitis on ocular examination. But almost all of them exhibited congestion of the conjunctival and episcleral vessels, and in nearly half of the patients redness of the eyes was a source of cosmetic concern. There were no other noteworthy ocular findings in these 70 patients with severe gouty arthritis.

Acknowledgment

Supported in part by a grant from the National Society Southern Dames of America.

References

1. Smith, J.L.: Ocular complications of rheumatic fever and rheumatoid arthritis. Am. J. Ophthalmol. 43:575, 1957.
2. Duke-Elder, S., and Soley, R.E.: Summary of Systemic Ophthalmology. Vol. XV in System of Ophthalmology (Duke-Elder, S., ed.). St. Louis, C. V. Mosby Company, 1976, p. 139.
3. Ibid., p. 15.
4. Duke-Elder, S., and MacFaul, P.A.: The Ocular Adnexa. Vol. XIII in System of Ophthalmology (Duke-Elder, S., ed.). St. Louis, C. V. Mosby Company, 1974, pp. 625–635.
5. Watson, P.G., and Hayreh, S.S.: Scleritis and episcleritis. Br. J. Ophthalmol. 60:163, 1976.
6. McGavin, D.D., Williamson, J., Forrester, J.V., Foulds, W.S., Buchanan, W.W., Dick, W.C., Lee, P., Macsween, R.N., and Whaley, K.: Episcleritis and scleritis. A study of their clinical manifestations and association with rheumatoid arthritis. Br. J. Ophthalmol. 60:192, 1976.
7. Duke-Elder, S., and Leigh, A.G.: Diseases of the Outer Eye. Vol. VIII in System of Ophthalmology (Duke-Elder, S., ed.). St. Louis, C. V. Mosby Company, 1965, pp. 1003–1049.
8. Garrison, F.H.: An Introduction to the History of Medicine. 4th ed. Philadelphia, W. B. Saunders Company, 1929, p. 385.
9. Ferry, A.P.: The histopathology of rheumatoid episcleral nodules. An extra-articular manifestation of rheumatoid arthritis. Arch. Ophthalmol. 82:77, 1969.
10. Chylack, L.T., Bienfang, D.C., Bellows, A.R., and Stillman, J.S.: Ocular manifestations of juvenile rheumatoid arthritis. Am. J. Ophthalmol. 79:1026, 1975.
11. Kanski, J.J.: Anterior uveitis in juvenile rheumatoid arthritis. Arch. Ophthalmol. 95:1794–1797, 1977.
12. Duke-Elder, S., and Perkins, E.S.: Diseases of the Uveal Tract. Vol. IX in System of Ophthalmology (Duke-Elder, S., ed.). St. Louis, C. V. Mosby Company, 1966, pp. 533–553.
13. Christian, C.L.: Ankylosing spondylitis. In Wyngaarden, J.B., Smith, L.H.

(eds.): Cecil Textbook of Medicine. 16th ed. Philadelphia, W. B. Saunders Company, 1982, pp. 878–1879.
14. Duke-Elder, S., and Perkins, E.S.: Diseases of the Uveal Tract. Vol. IX in System of Ophthalmology (Duke-Elder, S., ed.). St. Louis, C. V. Mosby Company, 1966, pp. 542–544.
15. Duke-Elder, S., and MacFaul, P.A.: The Ocular Adnexa. Vol. XIII in System of Ophthalmology (Duke-Elder, S., ed.). St. Louis, C. V. Mosby Company, 1974, pp. 321–327.
16. Lessell, S.: The neuro-ophthalmology of systemic lupus erythematosus. Doc. Ophthalmol. 47:13, 1979.
17. Gold, D.H., Morris, D.A., and Henkind, P.: Ocular findings in systemic lupus erythematosus. Br. J. Ophthalmol. 56:800, 1972.
18. Ferry, A.P.: Retinal cotton wool spots and cytoid bodies. Mt. Sinai J. Med. 39:604, 1972.
19. Duke-Elder, S., and Leigh, A.G.: Diseases of the Outer Eye. Vol. VIII in System of Ophthalmology (Duke-Elder, S., ed.). St. Louis, C. V. Mosby Company, 1965, pp. 1098–1100.
20. Duke-Elder, S., and Soley, R.E.: Summary of Systemic Ophthalmology. Vol. XV in System of Ophthalmology (Duke-Elder, S., ed.). St. Louis, C. V. Mosby Company, 1976, p. 145.
21. Ibid., p. 129.
22. Ibid, p. 43.
23. Henkind, P., and Gold, D.H.: Ocular manifestations of rheumatic disorders. Rheumatology 4:13, 1973.
24. Spiera, H., and Davison, S.: Long-term follow-up of polymyalgia rheumatica. Mt. Sinai J. Med. 45:225, 1978.
25. Duke-Elder, S., and Scott, G.I.: Neuro-Ophthalmology. Vol. XII in System of Ophthalmology (Duke-Elder, S., ed.). St. Louis, C. V. Mosby Company, 1971, pp. 116–122.
26. Bengtsson, B.-A., and Malmvall, B.-E.: The epidemiology of giant cell arteritis, including temporal arteritis and polymyalgia rheumatica. Incidences of different clinical presentations and eye complications. Arthritis Rheum. 24:899, 1981.
27. Wegener, F.: About the so-called Wegener's granulomatosis with special reference to the generalized vascular lesions. Morgagni 1:5, 1968.
28. Ferry, A.P., and Leopold, I.H.: Marginal (ring) corneal ulcer as presenting manifestation of Wegener's granuloma. A clinicopathologic study. Trans. Am. Acad. Ophthalmol. Otolaryngol. 74:1276, 1970.
29. Haynes, B.F., Fishman, M.L., Fauci, A.S., and Wolff, S.M.: The ocular manifestations of Wegener's granulomatosis. Fifteen years (sic) experience and review of the literature. Am. J. Med. 63:131, 1977.
30. Anderson, W.B.: Ocular lesions in relapsing polychondritis and other rheumatoid syndromes. Am. J. Ophthalmol. 64:35, 1967.
31. Greenstein, A.J., Janowitz, H.D., and Sachar, D.B.: The extra-intestinal complications of Crohn's disease and ulcerative colitis: A study of 700 patients. Medicine 55:401, 1976.
32. Wright, R., Lumsden, K., Luntz, M.H., Sevel, D., and Truelove, S.C.: Abnormalities of the sacro-iliac joints and uveitis in ulcerative colitis. Quart. J. Med. 34:229, 1965.
33. Hopkins, D.J., Horan, E., Burton, I.L., Clamp, S.E., de Dombal, F.T., and Goligher, J.C.: Ocular disorders in a series of 332 patients with Crohn's disease. Br. J. Ophthalmol. 58:732, 1974.
34. Font, R.L., Rao, N.A., Issarescu, S., and McEntee, W.J.: Ocular involvement in Whipple's disease. Light and electron microscopic observations. Arch. Ophthalmol. 96:1431, 1978.
35. Duke-Elder, S., and Soley, R.E.: Summary of Systemic Ophthalmology. Vol. XV in System of Ophthalmology (Duke-Elder, S., ed.). St. Louis, C. V. Mosby Company, 1976, p. 143.
36. Nichols, C.W., Eagle, R.C., Yanoff, M., and Menocal, N.G.: Conjunctival biopsy as an aid in the evaluation of the patient with suspected sarcoidosis. Ophthalmology 87:287, 1980.
37. Ferry, A.P., and Lieberman, T.W.: Bilateral amyloidosis of the vitreous body. Arch. Ophthalmol. 94:982, 1976.
38. Duke-Elder, S., and Soley, R.E.: Summary of Systemic Ophthalmology. Vol. XV in System of Ophthalmology (Duke-Elder, S., ed.). St. Louis, C. V. Mosby Company, 1976, p. 9.

Chapter 36
Cutaneous Manifestations of Rheumatic Disorders

Nicholas A. Soter

INTRODUCTION

Dermatologic lesions may indicate associated disorders of organ systems other than the skin. The presence of skin lesions is especially noteworthy in patients with rheumatic diseases. Thus, the integument should be assessed with the same precision that is devoted to an examination of the joints and musculoskeletal system. In addition, it is important to ascertain whether topical medicaments have been applied to the skin inasmuch as these therapeutic agents can modify the gross and histopathologic features of the dermatologic lesions.

INTERPRETATION OF ALTERATIONS IN THE SKIN

Visual Examination of the Skin. Skin lesions may be the presenting complaint of the patient, may occur in association with other symptoms and signs, such as fever or arthralgia, or may be incidental findings observed during the routine physical examination. When examining the skin, one should consider the specific type of lesion and its configuration or shape as well as distribution. Eruptions may be localized or generalized. When the eruption occurs in bilateral and symmetrical distribution, the pathologic stimulus is usually endogenous or is hematogenously disseminated.

Aids in Examination of the Skin. Certain signs are recognized more easily by magnification of the skin lesions. Sidelighting of the skin lesions, which is preferably done in a darkened room, is often required to detect slight degrees of elevation or depression. The technique known as diascopy is performed by firmly pressing a piece of glass, such as a microscope slide, over a skin lesion; in the examination of erythematous lesions, blanching reflects capillary dilatation and lack of blanching reflects extravasated blood. Diascopy thus permits the differentiation of purpura from the erythema of vasodilatation. Diascopy performed on dermal papules may show a yellow-brown appearance that is characteristic of granulomas, which occur in such disorders as sarcoid of the skin.

Wood's lamp, which emits long-wave ultraviolet light (360 nm), is useful in the assessment of variations in skin pigmentation. When hyperpigmentation occurs in the epidermis, the pigmented areas show an increased intensity under Wood's lamp, which is not seen when the pigmentation occurs in the dermis. Areas of depigmentation appear more prominent when the melanocyte has been destroyed; in contrast, the hypopigmentation of impaired melanogenesis with intact melanocytes is not enhanced with Wood's lamp examination.

All lesions consisting of crusts and purulent exudates should be examined with Gram's stain and bacterial cultures.

The application of 10 percent potassium hydroxide to a portion of scale, which is then gently heated and examined with a light microscope, is used to search for fungi.

The microscopic examination of cells obtained from the base of vesicles, known as the Tzanck test, may allow the detection of isolated epithelial cells that occur in the pemphigus group of disorders or the giant cells with multiple nuclei that are present in herpes simplex or varicella-zoster viruses. Material obtained from the base of a vesicle is applied to a glass slide and stained with Giemsa's or Wright's reagent for examination.

Microscopic examination of skin lesions is particularly useful, since biopsy specimens are easily obtained for diagnosis by the use of a skin trephine or punch. A tubular blade is rotated between the thumb and index finger to cut through the entire thickness of the abnormal skin; the resulting cylinder of skin is secured with forceps and is cut at its base with a scissors. This simple operation is performed after local anesthesia, preferably with a solution without epinephrine which could theoretically alter blood vessels. Specimens from nodular lesions are best obtained by incision with a scalpel.

Classification of Skin Lesions. A macule is a circumscribed area of alteration in normal skin color without elevation or depression of its surface relative to the surrounding skin. Macules may be of any size and are the result of pigmentary or vascular abnormalities of the skin.

A papule is a solid lesion, most of which is elevated above, rather than deep within, the plane of the surrounding skin. The elevation may be caused by localized hyperplasia of cellular elements in the dermis or epidermis, by metabolic deposits in the dermis, or by dermal edema.

A nodule is a solid, round, or ellipsoidal lesion usually located in the dermis or subcutaneous tissue; however, it may occur in the epidermis. The depth of involvement rather than the diameter primarily differentiates a nodule from a papule. Nodules result from infiltrates, neoplasms, or metabolic deposits in the dermis or subcutaneous tissue and often indicate systemic disease.

A plaque is an elevation above the skin surface that occupies a relatively large surface area in comparison with its height above the skin. Frequently, it is formed by the confluence of papules.

A wheal is an edematous, flat-topped, erythematous elevation of the skin that is evanescent. Wheals reflect edema in the superficial layer of the dermis; when the edema occurs in the deep dermis or subcutaneous tissue, the term angioedema is used.

Vesicles and bullae are circumscribed elevated lesions containing fluid. They arise either from separation within the epidermis (intraepidermal vesiculation) or from separation at the dermoepidermal junction (subepidermal vesiculation).

A pustule is a circumscribed elevation of the skin that contains a neutrophilic polymorphonuclear cell infiltrate that may be white, yellow, or greenish yellow. These lesions may be sterile, as in psoriasis, or may reflect a purulent exudate. All pustules should be examined with Gram's stain and culture.

Erosions are superficial lesions in which there is destruction of the epidermis; when there is extension into the dermis, the lesion becomes an ulcer.

Figure 36–1. Rheumatoid nodule. Subcutaneous nodule over the ulnar aspect of the forearm in a patient with rheumatoid arthritis.

CUTANEOUS MANIFESTATIONS OF CERTAIN RHEUMATOLOGIC DISORDERS

Rheumatoid Arthritis. A variety of skin alterations occur in patients with rheumatoid arthritis; the most frequently recognized lesion is the rheumatoid nodule (Fig. 36–1).[1,2] These lesions occur over areas subjected to trauma or pressure, especially the ulnar aspect of the forearm and the lumbosacral area. They vary in size up to several centimeters in diameter, are firm in consistency, and may ulcerate after trauma. These subcutaneous nodules occur in approximately 20 percent of patients with rheumatoid arthritis, especially in those individuals with severe forms of the disease and rheumatoid factor.

The skin is often pale, translucent, and atrophic, especially over the hands, fingers, and toes. The presence of swelling of the proximal interphalangeal joints in addition to the atrophic skin may mimic the appearance of sclerodactyly. Palmar erythema is a frequent feature; however, its presence does not imply underlying liver disease. A few patients manifest telangiectases of the nail folds. Raynaud's phenomenon may occur, as well as a bluish coloration over the distal portions of the toes. Although longitudinal ridges with beading of the nail plate are claimed to be present more frequently in patients with rheumatoid arthritis,[3] the fact that this change also occurs in a high proportion of normal people casts doubt on this association.[4] Pyoderma gangrenosum occasionally may occur in individuals with severe rheumatoid arthritis.[5]

Vasculitis in patients with rheumatoid arthritis appears as a variety of syndromes; the clinical and path-

ologic features reflect involvement of vessels of different sizes.[6] Rheumatoid vasculitis is frequently described as an arteritis that involves the small arteries, such as the vasa nervorum and the digital arteries (Fig. 36–2). The clinical features in these patients with severe rheumatoid arthritis include a peripheral neuropathy, digital gangrene, nailfold infarcts, cutaneous ulcers, and, in some instances, pericarditis as well as coronary or mesenteric arteritis.[7,8] Patients with nodular and erosive disease and high titers of rheumatoid factor are particularly prone to develop arteritis.[9]

Figure 36–2. Necrotizing arteritis. Necrosis of the fingers in a patient with rheumatoid arthritis. Note bulla at top right.

Figure 36–3. Necrotizing venulitis. *A*, Palpable purpura over the dorsum of the fingers in a patient with rheumatoid arthritis. *B*, Necrosis in a reticulate array over the thigh.
batch 36 p. 535

Occasional patients experience involvement of medium rather than small arteries. The segmental pathologic lesions in these instances resemble those of polyarteritis nodosa.[10] These individuals manifest a form of arteritis with clinical features similar to those of patients with vasculitis of small arteries.

A common form of necrotizing vasculitis in patients with rheumatoid arthritis involves the venules, especially of the skin. *Cutaneous necrotizing venulitis* is recognized as erythematous papules (palpable purpura), in which the erythema does not blanch when pressed (Fig. 36–3). These vascular lesions may occur over any portion of the body; however, they most often appear on the lower extremities or over dependent areas in recumbent patients. The venular lesions are not related to the duration of the arthritis but rather are associated with severe articular disease, which is generally but not invariably seropositive. The duration and evolution of the venulitis do seem to correlate with the levels of rheumatoid factor and involvement of the complement system.[11] In one study, when the palpable purpura was present less than 1 month, rheumatoid factor levels tended to be low or absent, and the complement system was normal. When the skin lesions were present longer than 1 month, the rheumatoid factor titer was high, and hypocomplementemia was present. Arteritic, arteriolar, and venular lesions may coexist in the same patient.[11]

Sjögren's Syndrome. The dermatologic manifestations in patients with Sjögren's syndrome usually reflect glandular dysfunction with desiccation of the skin and mucous membranes and less frequently are a manifestation of involvement of blood vessels. Approximately 50 percent of individuals manifest dry skin (xerosis); however, the ability to sweat is normal as assessed by pilocarpine iontophoresis, and the sweat contains normal amounts of sodium and chloride.[12] The mucous membranes of the eyes, oral cavity (including the tongue), and vagina are usually involved in the sicca complex. A burning sensation of the eyes may occur with erythema, pruritus, a decreased ability to form tears, and the accumulation of inspissated rope-like material at the inner canthus. The lack of tears is confirmed by decreased wetting of a measured distance of filter paper strips placed under the eyelids (Schirmer test); however, this test should be used only for screening patients inasmuch as false-positive tests may be obtained in elderly persons. The oral cavity and tongue may be red and dry with oral erosions and decreased amounts of saliva. Scaling of the lips and fissures at the angles of the mouth may be noted; the teeth readily decay. Desiccation of the vagina is manifested as burning, pruritus, and dyspareunia. Enlargement of parotid glands is frequently noted; Raynaud's phenomenon may occur.

Cutaneous necrotizing venulitis[11] occurs in patients with Sjögren's syndrome[13] with or without underlying cryoglobulinemia. The venular lesions are present predominantly over the lower extremities, appear after exercise, and are associated with hyperpigmentation and cutaneous ulcers. Autoantibodies to small-molecular-weight ribonucleoprotein Ro(SS-A) are noted in individuals with Sjögren's syndrome and systemic or cutaneous necrotizing vasculitis with hematologic and serologic abnormalities.[14] Sjögren's syndrome occurs in association with other disorders such as hypergammaglobulinemic purpura, systemic lupus erythematosus, scleroderma, biliary cirrhosis, and lymphoproliferative disorders;[15] certain dermatologic features may thus reflect the coexistent disorder.

Spondyloarthropathies. *Reiter's Syndrome.* Reiter's syndrome[16] is recognized as a clinical symptom complex which consists of conjunctivitis, urethritis, arthritis, and skin lesions and usually occurs in men. The conjunctitis and urethritis tend to be transient in contrast to the arthritis and skin manifestations. Approximately 50 to 80 percent of patients experience mucocutaneous alterations[17] with involvement of the acral regions, especially soles, toes, and fingers. The most characteristic skin lesions, which are rare, begin as vesicles on erythematous bases, become sterile pustules, evolve to manifest keratotic scale, and are known as *keratoderma blennorrhagica* (Fig. 36–4). In addition, keratotic papules and plaques occur on the scalp and elsewhere on the skin. These psoriasiform plaques are reminiscent of psoriasis. Indeed, there have been patients reported with both Reiter's syndrome and psoriasis, yet the skin lesions in these two disorders are often difficult or impossible to distinguish clinically and histologically.[18] This relation between Reiter's syndrome and psoriasis takes on even greater importance, owing to the association of the histocompatibility antigen HLA-B27 with each disorder.[19,20] Sterile pustules develop beneath the nail plate; onychodystrophy frequently is noted.

Conjunctivitis, which occurs in 50 percent of patients,[21,22] is usually bilateral; a sterile purulent exudate frequently is noted. Balanitis occurs in 25 percent of individuals; it appears as papules and plaques with scale over the glans. Mouth erosions have been noted.

Psoriatic Arthritis. Psoriasis occurs in a variety of patterns and may be associated with several forms of arthritis. Classic psoriasis appears as papules and plaques with layers of scales; the individual lesion (Fig. 36–5) is erythematous, covered with layers of silver-white scale, and rather sharply demarcated from adjacent uninvolved skin. Removing the scale results in punctate bleeding that reflects rupture of the superficial blood vessels in the tips of the dermal papillae (Auspitz sign). Individual lesions heal with transient hyperpigmentation or hypopigmentation.

Psoriasis may occur over any portion of the integument, especially the elbows, knees, lumbosacral area,

Figure 36–4. Keratoderma blennorrhagica. Keratotic plaques and nodules in a patient with Reiter's syndrome.

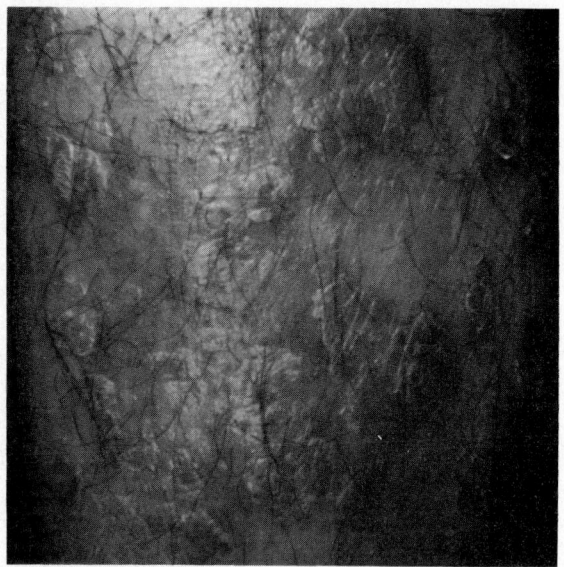

Figure 36–5. Psoriasis. Erythematous plaques with layers of scale.

scalp, gluteal cleft, and genitalia. The glans penis is frequently affected; the oral mucosa is infrequently involved, and the tongue is rarely affected.[23] The extent of involvement is quite variable and may range from minimal lesions of the elbows and knees to extensive numbers of lesions scattered over the skin. Uncommonly, there are considerable numbers of small, drop-like plaques designated as guttate psoriasis. Rarely fissures and scale of the distal portions of the fingers may be a predominant manifestation.[24] The skin lesions often appear at sites of trauma (Koebner reaction or isomorphic phenomenon).[25,26] Although the stimulus is usually mechanical, excess exposure to sunlight and the administration of drugs have been implicated.

The nails[27] are frequently affected; the extent of involvement varies in severity and may include one or several nails. The nail plate manifests a translucent quality with a yellow or brown coloration. There may be subungual accumulations of keratotic material, which frequently contains *Candida* species or *Pseudomonas* species; however, dermatophyte infections are rare.[28] The most widely recognized alteration of the nail plate is the presence of discrete pits (Fig. 36–6).

Generalized erythroderma or exfoliative dermatitis has been reported to occur in 20 percent of patients with psoriasis.[29-32] This reaction may develop spontaneously or occur after systemic illness, the administration of medications, or excessive exposure to the sun. Associated abnormalities include abnormal thermoregulation, increased transepidermal water loss, enhanced absorption of topically applied medicaments, loss of protein and iron,[33] and the possibility of high-output cardiac failure in persons with heart disorders.[34]

Pustular types of psoriasis are uncommon and occur in two forms: one is generalized[35,36] and the other is localized to the palms and soles.[37] Patients with generalized pustular psoriasis manifest an extensive sterile

Figure 36–6. Psoriasis. Onychodystrophy of the proximal portion of the nail plate with pits.

pustular eruption that may involve the mucous membranes. The onset is sudden with pyrexia and other signs of systemic toxicity, such as myalgia and arthralgia. The skin lesions consist of superficial pustules that may evolve into large purulent areas; existing psoriatic plaques may also contain sterile pustules. The episodes of pustules may continue over intervals of days to weeks. It has been suggested that patients with psoriatic arthritis are more likely to develop generalized pustular psoriasis than are patients without arthritis.[38,39]

Localized pustular psoriasis of the palms and soles is bilateral and recalcitrant without systemic manifestations. Onychodystrophy is common, and the plaques of ordinary psoriasis may be found elsewhere.

There are increased numbers of *Staphylococcus aureus* on lesional skin of patients with psoriasis.[40] Shedding of scale has been suggested as a source of hospital infection.[41]

Psoriasis may occur in association with various forms of inflammatory arthritis[42,43] (see Chapters 58 to 67), which include asymmetric oligoarthritis, symmetric arthritis, spondyloarthritis, and arthritis mutilans. The presence of psoriasis in patients with rheumatoid arthritis is considered to be the coincidental association of two common disorders. Onychodystrophy in patients with symmetric psoriatic arthritis may help to differentiate them from patients with rheumatoid arthritis.

Lupus Erythematosus. Lupus erythematosus may occur as a systemic disease or as a disorder, in which the lesions are restricted to the skin. The term *discoid lupus erythematosus*[44,45] has been used to refer to disease restricted to the skin as well as to refer to the gross appearance of the atrophic skin lesions irrespective of whether there is systemic disease. The term *subacute cutaneous lupus erythematosus* defines a mild systemic form with symmetrical, nonscarring skin lesions.[46] When lupus erythematosus is restricted to the skin, available data suggest that fewer than 5 percent of individuals are at risk to develop systemic disease. These data, however, are influenced by definition, vary in studies from different centers, and need re-examination.

The skin is involved at some time during the course of disease in approximately 80 percent of patients with lupus erythematosus.[47] The most widely recognized manifestation is an erythematous eruption (butterfly rash) over the malar areas of the face (Fig. 36–7), which occurs in patients with acute exacerbations of systemic lupus erythematosus. Rarely, bullous skin lesions occur that contain aggregates of neutrophilic leukocytes in the superficial dermis.[48]

The discoid skin lesion in patients with lupus erythematosus is a circumscribed, slightly indurated, red-purple plaque which manifests scaling, follicular plugs, telangiectases, atrophy, and hyperpigmentation or hypopigmentation (Fig. 36–8). The pigmentary alterations are especially prominent in black patients, in whom the cosmetic alteration may be disfiguring. The cutaneous lesions may be single but are usually multiple and occur over any portion of the body, including the scalp. In some individuals there is a predilection for sun-exposed areas. The skin lesions are usually asymptomatic.

Skin lesions in subacute cutaneous lupus erythematosus are symmetrical and affect the neck, extensor surfaces of the arms, and the upper portions of the trunk. The early lesions are edematous and erythematous papules and plaques that evolve into lesions with scales, producing a psoriasiform picture, or into annular polycyclic or figurate configurations.[46,49] These individuals have a mild systemic illness with fever, arthralgia, and malaise and without central nervous system and pro-

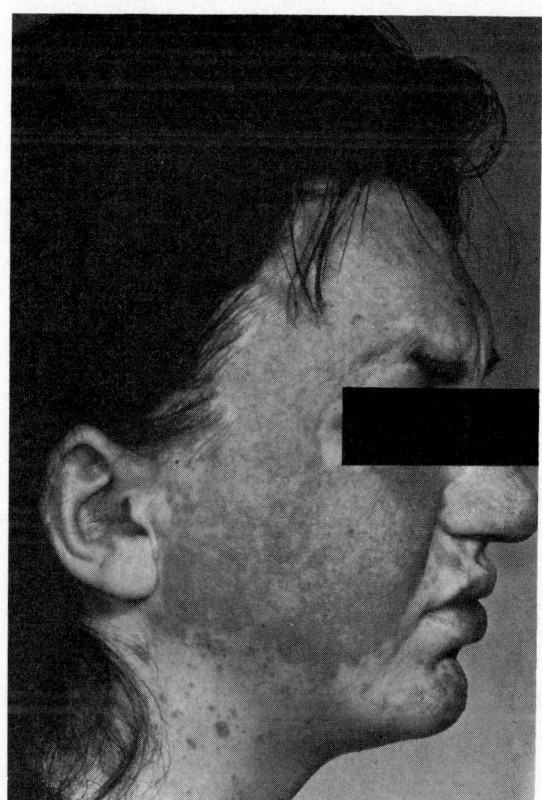

Figure 36–7. Systemic lupus erythematosus. Erythema with slight scale over the malar areas and forehead. Note that the distribution is determined by exposure to sunlight.

Figure 36–8. Cutaneous lupus erythematosus. Circumscribed atrophic patches with hypopigmentation and hyperpigmentation on the face.

gressive renal disease. There is an association with HLA-B8 and DR3 as well as anti-Ro and anti-La antibodies.[50,51]

Alopecia is common in patients with lupus erythematosus; it occurs in both scarring and nonscarring forms. Atrophic patches are present as solitary or multiple areas with the characteristic features of erythema, scale, follicular plugs, and pigmentary alterations. Diffuse hair loss without scarring may occur, especially in individuals with subacute cutaneous lupus erythematosus or with systemic lupus erythematosus.

Although many patients with subacute or systemic lupus erythematosus develop telangiectases over the nail folds, this sign also occurs in patients with rheumatoid arthritis, dermatomyositis, and scleroderma.[52]

A variety of other skin lesions occur in patients with lupus erythematosus. Raynaud's phenomenon is reported to occur in 10 to 30 percent, and episodes of urticaria or angioedema may be a manifestation.[53] The urticarial lesions in some instances have been shown to be a manifestation of underlying necrotizing venulitis.[54] Another manifestation of cutaneous necrotizing venulitis is palpable purpura, which appears to occur during exacerbations of the systemic disease.[11] Involvement of larger arterial blood vessels is present as peripheral gangrene.[55] In addition, flat purpura and petechiae may occur as manifestations of thrombocytopenia or the administration of corticosteroid preparations. Livedo reticularis may be present as a reticulate, erythematous mottling of the skin.

Photosensitivity[56,57] occurs in at least one third of patients with systemic lupus erythematosus and may be associated with flares of both the cutaneous and the systemic manifestations of the disease. The skin lesions have been experimentally induced by exposure to discrete wavelengths of light from an artificial light source.[58]

The oral and lingual lesions are more common in patients with systemic lupus erythematosus and consist of erythematous patches, dilated blood vessels, and erosions, which are frequently painful. Ulcers of the nasal septum may occur.

A rare skin manifestation is panniculitis (lupus profundus),[59] which appears as firm, deep nodules that have a predilection for the face, buttocks, and upper arms. The overlying skin may be erythematous, atrophic, or ulcerated. Healing results in a depressed scar.

Direct immunofluorescence techniques have been applied to the study of the skin of patients with lupus erythematosus as an aid in diagnosis and prognosis.[60-64] This procedure is known as the *lupus band test* (Fig. 36–9). In the skin lesions of both systemic and cutaneous lupus erythematosus, immunoglobulins and complement proteins are deposited in a granular pattern along the dermoepidermal junction in 90 to 95 percent of patients, whereas these immunoreactants are detected in uninvolved non-sun-exposed skin of approximately 50 percent of patients with systemic but not cutaneous lupus erythematosus—an important distinguishing feature. When uninvolved sun-exposed skin is examined, the lupus band test is usually negative in cutaneous lupus erythematosus and is positive in about 80 percent of individuals with systemic lupus erythematosus.[65]

The types of immunoglobulins detected in the deposited materials include mainly IgG and IgM. Complement factors from both the classic activating and amplification pathways are deposited at the same site,[66-68] notably Clq, C4, C3, properdin, and B as well as those

Figure 36–9. Positive lupus band test. Note bright intensity of granular deposits of IgM along basement membrane zone. Vascular staining is likewise present. × 25. (Courtesy of Terrence J. Harrist, M.D.)

of the terminal membrane attack complex, C5b, C6-C9.[69]

It has been suggested that the deposition of immunoreactants in uninvolved non-sun-exposed skin of patients with systemic lupus erythematosus can be correlated with renal disease.[70-72] This observation at present remains speculative inasmuch as there are reports unable to confirm it.[73,74] The suggestion has been offered that direct immunofluorescence techniques may have value as an indicator of the efficacy of therapy, especially with immunosuppressive agents;[75] however, long-term data in humans are unavailable.

Mixed Connective Tissue Disease. Mixed connective tissue disease is a disorder with clinical features of systemic lupus erythematosus, scleroderma, and/or polymyositis in association with circulating antibody to a saline-soluble nuclear antigen.[76] The dermatologic manifestations include a diffuse nonscarring alopecia, areas of hyperpigmentation and hypopigmentation, sclerodactyly, sclerosis reminiscent of the alterations observed in patients with scleroderma, and a variety of skin changes similar to those observed in patients with lupus erythematosus.[77] Raynaud's phenomenon is frequently present.

Necrotizing Vasculitides. *Necrotizing angiitis* or *vasculitis* is a term applied to disorders in which there is segmental inflammation with fibrinoid necrosis of the blood vessels. Clinical syndromes are based on criteria that include the gross and histologic appearance of the vascular lesions, the caliber of the affected blood vessels,[78-80] the frequency of involvement of specific organs, and the absence or presence of hematological and serological abnormalities. Although all sizes of blood vessels may be affected, necrotizing vasculitis of the skin in the majority of instances involves venules.[81-83] Cutaneous necrotizing venulitis may occur in association with coexistent chronic diseases, may be precipitated by infections or drugs, or may develop for unknown reasons.[84]

Although the manifestations of cutaneous necrotizing venulitis are polymorphous, the most characteristic lesion is an erythematous papule, in which the erythema does not blanch when the skin is pressed (*palpable purpura*) (Fig. 36–10; for color of part *B* see Plate III, p. xxxvii),[11,85] Transient areas of urticaria or angioedema are less frequent manifestations;[86-90] rarely, punctate petechiae are noted in the edematous lesions. Nodules, pustules,[91] vesicles, ulcers, necrosis, and a netlike mottling of the skin (livedo reticularis) may occur. Occasionally there is subcutaneous edema in the area of the vascular lesions.

The vascular eruption most often appears on the lower extremities and frequently over dependent portions of the body or areas under local pressure. The lesions may occur anywhere on the skin, but are uncommon on the face, palms, soles, and mucous membranes. The skin lesions occur in episodes that may recur for various periods of time ranging from weeks to years. Palpable purpuric lesions persist from 1 to 4 weeks and then resolve, leaving hyperpigmentation and/or atrophic scars. The urticarial lesions, which may last fewer than

Figure 36–10. *A*, Necrotizing venulitis. Palpable purpura distributed over the lower extremities. *B*, Close-up view of the lesions (see Plate III, p. xxxvii).

24 hours and at times up to 72 hours, resolve without residua except for occasional hyperpigmentation. Lesional symptoms include pruritus or burning and, less commonly, pain. Rarely, there are no symptoms. An episode of cutaneous vascular lesions may be attended by pyrexia, malaise, arthralgias, or myalgias. When present, associated systemic involvement of the small blood vessels most commonly occurs in kidneys, muscles, peripheral nerves, gastrointestinal tract, and joints.

Involvement of large blood vessels occurs in periarteritis nodosa, which is recognized in the skin as nodular lesions over an artery,[92-94] and giant cell (temporal) arteritis, which is present as erythema overlying the affected vessel.[95] Both Wegener's granulomatosis[96] and granulomatous angiitis (Churg-Strauss)[97,98] affect large and small vessels; the skin lesions in both disorders are present as erythematous nodules with or without necrosis and a variety of less specific erythematous, edematous, purpuric, papular, and pustular lesions.

Cutaneous necrotizing venulitis has been associated with collagen-vascular diseases, notably rheumatoid arthritis, Sjögren's syndrome, and systemic lupus erythematosus, as previously mentioned.

Hypergammaglobulinemic purpura, defined by the presence of circulating intermediate-sized complexes of immunoglobulin with sedimentation rates between 9S and 17S,[99] occurs predominantly in older women and may be associated with Sjögren's syndrome, systemic lupus erythematosus, and chronic lymphocytic lymphoma.[100] The recurrent purpuric skin lesions are a manifestation of necrotizing venulitis.

Cutaneous necrotizing venulitis also has been reported in association with lymphoproliferative disorders, especially Hodgkin's disease and lymphosarcoma.[101]

Cryoglobulins may occur in patients with cutaneous necrotizing venulitis with and without concomitant collagen-vascular and lymphoproliferative disorders,[11,102] in patients with hepatitis B virus,[103,104] and idiopathically.[105]

Infections and drugs are known to precipitate cutaneous necrotizing venulitis. The most commonly recognized infectious agents are hepatitis B virus[103,104,106] Group A streptococci.[107] *Staphylococcus aureus*,[107] and *Mycobacterium leprae*.[107-109] In hepatitis B virus disease, transient urticaria may be present early in the course and represents immune complex–induced vasculitis.[104] Episodes of palpable purpura may occur in patients with chronic active hepatitis.[110]

The most commonly incriminated medications are sulfonamides, thiazides, penicillin, and serum. Inasmuch as this is an infrequent form of drug-induced reaction, the literature consists of case reports rather than prospective or retrospective studies.

Genetic C2 deficiency has been noted in patients with cutaneous necrotizing venulitis[111,112] that was labeled anaphylactoid purpura.

In perhaps 50 percent of instances the cause of cutaneous necrotizing venulitis remains unknown. The Henoch-Schönlein syndrome or anaphylactoid purpura is the most widely recognized subgroup. A history of upper respiratory tract symptoms and signs is occasionally obtained. The syndrome, which occurs predominantly in children[113] and less frequently in adults,[114] includes involvement of the skin, joints, gastrointestinal tract, and kidneys.

The urticarial form of cutaneous necrotizing venulitis[86-90] (Fig. 36–11, Plate III, p. xxxvii) affects mainly women and is associated with arthralgias that tend to be episodic and are related in time to the appearance of the skin lesions. Abdominal pain, lymphadenopathy, and diffuse glomerulonephritis[86,90,115,116] have also been reported. Additional skin manifestations include occasional macular erythema, angioedema, and foci of purpura. This array of cutaneous lesions may have led to the description of similar patients with hypocomplementemia and Clq precipitins under the terms systemic lupus erythematosus–like syndrome and erythema multiforme.[117-121]

Erythema elevatum diutinum[122,123] consists of erythematous papules, plaques, and nodules predominantly disposed over the buttocks and extensor surfaces and is often accompanied by arthralgias of the associated joint. Other systemic manifestations are lacking.

Dermatomyositis-Polymyositis. A variety of cutaneous lesions, which develop insidiously or abruptly, occur in patients with dermatomyositis-polymyositis. Inasmuch as the clinical features and histopathologic alterations in involved muscles are similar in the absence or presence of skin lesions, dermatomyositis and polymyositis are considered as manifestations of a single disease. Dermatomyositis occurs in approximately 25 percent of patients with polymyositis. The most characteristic skin changes are periorbital edema and a purple-red color of the eyelids, which is frequently described as heliotrope.[124] Erythematous macules with scale occur on the face, scalp, neck, and upper portion of the trunk. Especially characteristic are purple-red papules that

evolve into atrophic plaques with telangiectases and pigmentary alterations (Fig. 36–12); these lesions, known as Gottron's sign, occur over the dorsal aspects of the interphalangeal joints. Ulcers of the oral mucous membranes may occur;[125] less frequently the conjunctivae and genitalia are affected. Various degrees of alopecia may be present; telangiectases are noted frequently over the nail folds.

Calcification has been noted in both muscle and subcutaneous tissues; this change is more frequent when the disease begins in childhood.[126] Calcification occurs especially over the shoulders, elbows, and buttocks, and is rare over the fingers in contrast to scleroderma.[128] Cutaneous ulcers and sinuses may develop after the extrusion of deposited calcium. Raynaud's phenomenon may be present in adults but is rare in children. Children often manifest facial erythema[127] and involvement of blood vessels of the gastrointestinal tract leading to intestinal perforation.[128]

The skin manifestations[129] in patients with dermatomyositis are at times reminiscent of those occurring in individuals with systemic lupus erythematosus and scleroderma. Occasionally a reticulated erythema known as poikiloderma is noted with telangiectases, atrophy, and pigmentary alterations.

Although the emergence of dermatomyositis in persons past middle age has been associated with the presence of internal malignant disorders, the reported frequency is undoubtedly too high.

Figure 36–12. Dermatomyositis. Atrophic plaques with telangiectases and pigmentary alterations over the interphalangeal joints of the fingers. Note telangiectases of the nail folds.

Scleroderma. Scleroderma may occur as a systemic disorder or as various localized forms that primarily affect the skin (see Chapters 76 and 77). The most common type is *morphea,* in which the skin lesions are present as circumscribed areas of atrophy with an ivory color in the center and a violet hue at the periphery. The lesions of morphea commonly persist for years; however, they may disappear spontaneously, healing with or without residual pigmentary alterations. Rarely, morphea may progress to systemic scleroderma.[130,131]

Linear scleroderma appears in a bandlike distribution. The lower extremities are most frequently affected.[132] In addition to the skin, underlying muscles and bones may be involved with deformities. Linear scleroderma begins most frequently during the first two decades of life. It has been associated with abnormalities of the axial skeleton, especially occult spina bifida.[133] Other variants of scleroderma include frontal or frontoparietal involvement of the head known as *coup de sabre,* which is characterized by an atrophic furrow that extends below the plane of the skin, and progressive facial hemiatrophy (Parry-Romberg syndrome).

In systemic scleroderma[134] or progressive systemic sclerosis the cutaneous alterations especially affect the face and hands. Features include a masklike expressionless face with a fixed stare, inability to wrinkle the forehead, tightening of the skin over the nose with a beaklike appearance, and restriction of the mouth with radial folds and a loss of tissue such that the teeth are prominent. An early sign is indolent nonpitting edema over the dorsum of the fingers, hands, and forearms. Sclerodactyly is noted with tapered fingers over which the skin is atrophic; flexion contractures may be present. Raynaud's phenomenon is common; recurrent painful ulcers occur over the fingers and toes (Fig. 36–13). Cutaneous calcification may be present, especially about the fingers, elbows, and knees; when calcification occurs in association with Raynaud's phenomenon, sclerodactyly, and telangiectases, the clinical symptom complex is known as the CRST syndrome. Although this form of scleroderma is alleged to pursue a more benign

Figure 36–14. Scleroderma. Telangiectases and telangiectatic macules over the palms.

course,[135] pulmonary hypertension[136] and esophageal abnormalities have been reported.

Telangiectases occur commonly, especially on the nail folds; telangiectatic macules, which are square, may involve the face, lips, tongue, and hands (Fig. 36–14). Other features may include generalized hyperpigmentation and alopecia.

Disorders with cutaneous sclerosis that should be considered in the differential diagnosis of scleroderma include eosinophilic fasciitis,[137] porphyria cutanea tarda, papular mucinosis (scleromyxedema),[138] lichen sclerosus et atrophicus, melorheostosis,[139,140] and the chronic form of graft-versus-host disease.[141]

Juvenile Rheumatoid Arthritis. The cutaneous eruptions that occur in association with juvenile rheumatoid arthritis are not adequately characterized. The most frequently recognized form is an evanescent, erythematous eruption that accompanies the late afternoon temperature rise in 25 to 40 percent of patients.[142,143] The skin lesions appear as small erythematous or salmon-colored macules and papules distributed over the face, trunk, and extremities. They are usually not pruritic and once formed do not move or enlarge. They occur when the disease is active, subside with remission, and heal without residua. Subcutaneous nodules may be noted and must be differentiated from the subcutaneous form of granuloma annulare.[144]

Rheumatic Fever. A variety of erythematous eruptions have been noted in patients with rheumatic fever.[145] The most specific eruption is *erythema marginatum.*[146,147] It appears as erythematous rings, usually with raised margins, that rapidly spread peripherally to form polycyclic or geographic outlines, leaving a pale or pigmented center. The essential feature is the rapid spread, which may be 2 to 10 mm in 12 hours.[148] The lesions occur on the trunk and extremities; they are rarely pruritic. The flat or macular form is known as *erythema circinatum.* Both erythema marginatum and circinatum are usually associated with carditis and are unaffected

Figure 36–13. Scleroderma. Ulcers and scars of the tips of the digits in an individual with Raynaud's phenomenon.

by treatment of the underlying disease. Small, multiple subcutaneous nodules may be noted over the hands, elbows, and occiput.[149]

A rare manifestation is *erythema papulatum*, which appears as indolent papules, especially over the elbows and knees.[150]

Infiltrative Systemic Diseases. *Amyloid.* Amyloid may be present as a primary cutaneous disease, may occur with genetic disorders, or may be associated in a secondary fashion with chronic inflammatory conditions.[151,152] Skin lesions occur in primary amyloid; secondary amyloid rarely has skin lesions. It is of note, however, that clinically uninvolved skin may contain amyloid deposits in both primary and secondary types, suggesting that a skin biopsy of such uninvolved skin can have a high diagnostic yield.[153]

The skin lesions appear as firm papules that are translucent and occur on the face (especially about the eyes), neck, intertriginous areas, and extremities. They vary in color from rose to yellow to brown; pruritus is absent. A conspicuous feature is hemorrhage; in fact the tendency to develop purpura is the basis for a diagnostic maneuver, in which purpura develops after a blunt instrument is used to traumatize the lesions.[154] Ecchymoses may occur in the absence of papules. Macroglossia is present in 25 to 40 percent of patients and appears with papules of the tongue; it is occasionally accompanied by ulcers and purpura.

Other clinical disorders associated with amyloid include familial Mediterranean fever, in which erythema and lesions resembling those of erysipelas occur; the syndrome of amyloid, urticaria, and deafness,[155,156] in which papules are present over the trunk; the Portuguese form, in which hyperkeratosis and ulcers of the feet occur;[157] and the carpal tunnel syndrome.

Sarcoid. A variety of cutaneous manifestations have been noted in patients with sarcoid.[158] Skin lesions occur in 25 percent of patients, and erythema nodosum occurs in 30 percent.[159-161] The most characteristic lesions observed in the United States are yellow-brown to violaceous papules and plaques with a predilection for the face, especially the alae nasi and the periocular areas (Fig. 36–15). Similar lesions may be widely distributed over the trunk and extremities. The papules may arise in a scar,[160] a valuable diagnostic sign. Especially in Europe, livid purple plaques have been described on the nose, cheeks, and lobes of the ear; these lesions are known as *lupus pernio*.[158] Other skin manifestations include an ichthyosiform dermatosis over the lower legs, subcutaneous calcification,[162] and areas of hypopigmentation.[163] The relation of the cutaneous lesions with specific internal manifestations and with prognosis is not adequately documented.

References

1. Collins, D.H.: The subcutaneous nodule of rheumatoid arthritis. J. Pathol. Bacteriol. 45:97, 1937.
2. Bennett, G.A., Zeller, J.W., and Bauer, W.: Subcutaneous nodules of rheumatoid arthritis and rheumatic fever: A pathologic study. Arch. Pathol. 30:70, 1940.
3. Hamilton, E.B.D.: Nail studies in rheumatoid arthritis. Ann. Rheum. Dis. 19:167, 1960.
4. Samman, P.D.: The Nails in Disease. London, Heinemann Medical Books, Ltd., 1965, p. 67.
5. Stolman, C.P., Rosenthal, D., Yaworsky, R., and Horan, F.: Pyoderma gangrenosum and rheumatoid arthritis. Arch. Dermatol. 111:1020, 1975.
6. Glass, D.N., Soter, N.A., and Schur, P.H.: Rheumatoid vasculitis. Arthritis Rheum. 19:950, 1976.
7. Sokoloff, L., Wilens, S.L., and Bunim, J.J.: Arteritis of striated muscle in rheumatoid arthritis. Am. J. Pathol. 27:157, 1951.
8. Schmid, F.R., Cooper, N.S., Ziff, M., and McEwen, C.: Arteritis in rheumatoid arthritis. Am. J. Med. 30:56, 1961.
9. Mongan, E.S., Cass, R.M., Jacox, R.F., and Vaughan, J.H.: A study of the relation of seronegative and seropositive rheumatoid arthritis to each other and to necrotizing vasculitis. Am. J. Med. 47:23, 1969.
10. Sokoloff, L., and Bunim, J.J.: Vascular lesions in rheumatoid arthritis. J. Chronic Dis. 5:668, 1957.
11. Soter, N.A., Austen, K.F., and Gigli, I.: The complement system in necrotizing angiitis of the skin. Analysis of complement component activities in serum of patients with concomitant collagen-vascular diseases. J. Invest. Dermatol. 63:219, 1974.
12. Bloch, K.J., Buchanan, W.W., Wohl, M.J., and Bunim, J.J.: Sjögren's syndrome: A clinical, pathological, and serological study of sixty-two cases. Medicine 44:187, 1965.
13. Shearn, M.A.: Sjögren's syndrome. Semin. Arthritis Rheum. 2:165, 1972.
14. Alexander, E.L., Arnett, F.C., Provost, T.T., and Stevens, M.B.: Sjögren's syndrome: association of anti-Ro (SS-A) antibodies with vasculitis, hematologic abnormalities, and serologic hyperreactivity. Ann. Intern. Med. 98:155, 1983.
15. Bloch, K.J., and Bunim, J.J.: Sjögren's syndrome and its relation to connective tissue diseases. J. Chronic Dis. 16:915, 1963.
16. Weinberger, H.W., Ropes, M.W., Kulka, J.P., and Bauer, W.: Reiter's syndrome, clinical and pathologic observations. A long term study of 16 cases. Medicine 41:35, 1962.
17. Montgomery, M.M., Poske, R.M., Barton, E.M., Foxworthy, D.T., and Baker, L.A.: The mucocutaneous lesions of Reiter's syndrome. Ann. Intern. Med. 51:99, 1959.
18. Wright, V., and Reed, W.B.: The link between Reiter's syndrome and psoriatic arthritis. Ann. Rheum. Dis. 23:12, 1964.
19. Brewerton, D.A., Caffrey, M., Nicholls, A., Walters, D., and James, D.C.O.: Acute anterior uveitis and HL-A 27. Lancet 2:994, 1973.
20. Lambert, J.R., Wright, V., Farjah, S.M., and Moll, J.M.H.: Histocompatibility antigens in psoriatic arthritis. Ann. Rheum. Dis. 35:526, 1976.
21. Csonka, G.W.: The course of Reiter's syndrome, Br. Med. J. 1:1088, 1958.
22. Hancock, J.: Surface manifestations of Reiter's disease in the male. Br. J. Vener. Dis. 36:36, 1960.
23. Schuppner, H.J.: Das klinische Bild der Schleimhautbeteiligung bei Psoriasis pustulosa. Arch. Klin. Exp. Dermatol. 209:600, 1960.
24. Baer, R.L., and Witten, V.H.: Psoriasis: A discussion of selected aspects.

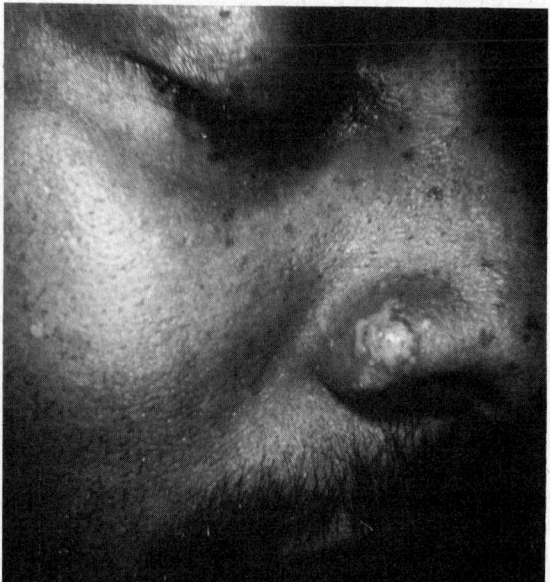

Figure 36–15. Sarcoid. Firm papules and plaques of the face.

In Baer, R.L., and Witten, V.H. (eds.): Yearbook of Dermatology, 1961–1962 Series. Chicago, Year Book Medical Publishers, 1962, p. 9.

25. Farber, E.M., Roth, R.J., Aschheim, E., Eddy, D.D., and Epinette, W.W.: Role of trauma in isomorphic response in psoriasis. Arch. Dermatol. 91:246, 1965.

26. Reinertson, R.P.: Vascular trauma and pathogenesis of the Koebner reaction in psoriasis. J. Invest. Dermatol. 30:283, 1958.

27. Zaias, N.: Psoriasis of the nail: A clinical-pathologic study. Arch. Dermatol. 99:567, 1969.

28. White, C.J., and Laipply, T.C.: Histopathology of nail diseases. J. Invest. Dermatol. 19:121, 1952.

29. Montgomery, H.: Exfoliative dermatitis and malignant erythroderma: The value and limitations of histopathologic studies. Arch. Dermatol. Syphilol. 27:253, 1933.

30. Wilson, H.T.H.: Exfoliative dermatitis: Its etiology and prognosis. Arch. Dermatol. Syphilol. 69:577, 1954.

31. Gentele, H., Lodin, A., and Skog, E.: Dermatitis exfoliativa. Acta Dermatol. Venereol. 38:296, 1958.

32. Abrahams, I., McCarthy, J.T., and Sanders, S.L.: 101 cases of exfoliative dermatitis. Arch. Dermatol. 87:96, 1963.

33. Marks, J., and Shuster, S.: Iron metabolism in skin disease. Arch. Dermatol. 98:469, 1968.

34. Fox, R.H., Shuster, S., Williams, R., Marks, J., Goldsmith, R., and Condon, R.E.: Cardiovascular, metabolic, and thermoregulatory disturbances with patients with erythrodermic skin diseases. Br. Med. J. 1:619, 1965.

35. von Zumbusch, L.R.: Psoriasis und pustulöses exanthem. Arch Dermatol. Syphilis 99:335, 1909–1910.

36. Tolman, M.M., and Moschella, S.L.: Pustular psoriasis (von Zumbusch). Arch. Dermatol. 81:400, 1960.

37. Barber, H.W.: Acrodermatitis continua vel perstans (dermatitis repens) and psoriasis pustulosa. Br. J. Dermatol. Syphilol. 42:500, 1930.

38. Ingram, J.T.: Pustular psoriasis. Arch. Dermatol. 77:314, 1958.

39. Champion, R.H.: Generalized pustular psoriasis. Br. J. Dermatol. 71:384, 1959.

40. Marples, R.R., Heaton, C.L., and Kligman, A.M.: *Staphylococcus aureus* in psoriasis. Arch. Dermatol. 107:568, 1973.

41. Payne, R.W.: Severe outbreak of surgical sepsis due to *Staphylococcus aureus* of unusual type and origin. Br. Med. J. 4:17, 1967.

42. Moll, J.M.H., and Wright, V.: Psoriatic arthritis. Semin. Arthritis Rheum. 3:55, 1963.

43. Kammer, G.M., Soter, N.A., Gibson, D.J., and Schur, P.H.: Psoriatic arthritis: a clinical, immunologic and HLA study of 100 patients. Semin. Arthritis Rheum. 9:75, 1979.

44. Rothfield, N.F., March, C.H., Miescher, P., and McEwen, C.: Chronic discoid lupus erythematosus: Study of 65 patients and 65 controls. N. Engl. J. Med. 269:1155, 1963.

45. Beck, J.S., and Rowell, N.R.: Discoid lupus erythematosus: A study of clinical features and biochemical and serological abnormalities in 120 patients with observation on relationship of this disease to systemic lupus erythematosus. Quart. J. Med. 35:119, 1966.

46. Sontheimer, R.D., Thomas, J.R., and Gilliam J.N.: Subacute cutaneous lupus erythematosus—a cutaneous marker for a distinct LE subset. Arch. Dermatol. 115:1409, 1979.

47. Tuffanelli, D.L., and Dubois, E.L.: Cutaneous manifestation of systemic lupus erythematosus. Arch. Dermatol. 90:377, 1964.

48. Hall, R.P., Lawley, T.J., Smith, H.R., and Katz, S.I.: Bullous eruption of systemic lupus erythematosus. Dramatic response to dapsone therapy. Ann. Intern. Med. 97:165, 1982.

49. Gilliam, J.N., and Sontheimer, R.D.: Distinctive cutaneous subsets in the spectrum of lupus erythematosus. J. Am. Acad. Dermatol. 4:471, 1981.

50. Sontheimer, R.D., Stastny, P., and Gilliam, J.N.: HLA associations in subacute cutaneous lupus erythematosus. J. Clin. Invest. 67:312, 1981.

51. Sontheimer, R.D., Stastny, P., Maddison, P., Reichlin, M., and Gilliam, J.N.: Anti-Ro and La antibodies and further HLA associations in subacute cutaneous lupus erythematosus (SCLE). Arthritis Rheum. 23:750, 1980.

52. Ross, J.P.: Nail fold capillaroscopy—a useful aid in the diagnosis of collagen vascular diseases. J. Invest. Dermatol. 47:282, 1966.

53. Harvey, A.M., Shulman, L.E., Tumulty, P.A., Conley, C.L., and Schoenrich, E.H.: Systemic lupus erythematosus: Review of the literature and clinical analysis of 138 cases. Medicine 33:291, 1954.

54. O'Loughlin, S., Schroeter, A.L., and Jordon, R.E.: Chronic urticaria-like lesions in systemic lupus erythematosus: A review of 12 cases. Arch. Dermatol. 114:879, 1978.

55. Dubois, E.L., and Arterberry, J.D.: Gangrene as a manifestation of systemic lupus erythematosus. JAMA 181:366, 1962.

56. Epstein, J.H., Tuffanelli, D.L., and Dubois, E.L.: Light sensitivity and lupus erythematosus. Arch. Dermatol. 91:483, 1965.

57. Baer, R.L. and Harber, L.C.: Photobiology of lupus erythematosus. Arch. Dermatol. 92:124, 1965.

58. Freeman, R.G., Knox, J.M., and Owens, D.W.: Cutaneous lesions of lupus erythematosus induced by monochromatic light. Arch. Dermatol. 100:677, 1969.

59. Tuffanelli, D.L.: Lupus erythematosus panniculitis (profundus): Clinical and immunologic studies. Arch. Dermatol. 103:231, 1971.

60. Burnham, T.K., Neblett, T.R., and Fine, G.: The application of the fluorescent antibody technique to the investigation of lupus erythematosus and various dermatoses. J. Invest. Dermatol. 41:451, 1963.

61. Cormane, R.H.: "Bound" globulin in the skin of patients with chronic discoid lupus erythematosus and systemic lupus erythematosus. Lancet 1:534, 1964.

62. Tan, E.M., and Kunkel, H.G.: An immunofluorescent study of the skin lesions in systemic lupus erythematosus. Arthritis Rheum. 9:37, 1966.

63. Tuffanelli, D.L., Kay, D., and Fukuyama, K.: Dermal-epidermal junction in lupus erythematosus. Arch. Dermatol. 99:652, 1969.

64. Harrist, T.J., and Mihm, M.C. Jr.: The specificity and clinical usefulness of the lupus band test. Arthritis Rheum. 23:479, 1980.

65. Provost, T.T., Andres, G., Maddison, P.J., and Reichlin, M.: Lupus band test in untreated SLE patients. Correlation of immunoglobulin deposition in the skin of the extensor forearm with clinical renal disease and serological abnormalities. J. Invest. Dermatol. 74:407, 1980.

66. Jordon, R.E., Schroeter, A.L., and Winkelmann, R.K.: Dermoepidermal deposition of complement components and properdin in systemic lupus erythematosus. Br. J. Dermatol. 92:263, 1975.

67. Schrager, M.A., and Rothfield, N.F.: Clinical significance of serum properdin levels and properdin deposition in the dermo-epidermal junction in systemic lupus erythematosus. J. Clin. Invest. 57:212, 1976.

68. Provost, T.T., and Tomasi, T.B.: Evidence for complement activation via the alternate pathway in skin diseases. I. Herpes gestationis, systemic lupus erythematosus, and bullous pemphigoid. J. Clin. Invest. 52:1779, 1973.

69. Biesecker, G., Lavin, L., Ziskind, M., and Koffler, D.: Cutaneous localization of the membrane attack complex in discoid and systemic lupus erythematosus. N. Engl. J. Med. 306:264, 1982.

70. Pohle, E.L., and Tuffanelli, D.L.: Study of cutaneous lupus by immunohistochemical methods. Arch. Dermatol. 97:520, 1968.

71. Gilliam, N.J., Cheatum, D.E., Hurd, E.R., Stastny, P., and Ziff, M.: Immunoglobulin in clinically uninvolved skin in systemic lupus erythematosus: Association with renal disease. J. Clin. Invest. 53:1434, 1974.

72. Dantzig, P.I., Mauro, J., Rayhanzadeh, S., and Rudofsky, U.H.: The significance of a positive cutaneous immunofluorescence test in systemic lupus erythematosus. Br. J. Dermatol. 93:531, 1975.

73. Caperton, E.M. Jr., Bean, S.F., and Dick, F.R.: Immunofluorescent skin test in systemic lupus erythematosus: Lack of relationship with renal disease. JAMA 222:935, 1972.

74. Grossman, J., Callerame, M.L., and Condemi, J.J.: Skin immunofluorescence studies on lupus erythematosus and other antinuclear-antibody-positive diseases. Ann. Intern. Med. 80:496, 1974.

75. Gilliam, J.N.: The significance of cutaneous immunoglobulin deposits in lupus erythematosus and NZB/NZW F$_1$ hybrid mice. J. Invest. Dermatol. 65:154, 1975.

76. Sharp, G.C., Irvin, W.S., LaRoque, R.L., Velez, C., Daly, V., Kaiser, A.D., and Holman, H.R.: Association of antibodies to different nuclear antigens with clinical patterns of rheumatic disease and responsiveness to therapy. J. Clin. Invest. 50:350, 1971.

77. Gilliam, J.N., and Prystowsky, S.D.: Mixed connective tissue disease syndrome: Cutaneous manifestations of patients with epidermal nuclear staining and high titer serum antibody to ribonuclease-sensitive extractable nuclear antigen. Arch. Dermatol. 113:583, 1977.

78. Zeek, P.M.: Periarteritis nodosa: A critical review. Am. J. Clin. Pathol. 22:777, 1952.

79. Zeek, P.M.: Periarteritis nodosa and other forms of necrotizing angitis. N. Engl. J. Med. 248:764, 1953.

80. Fauci, A.S., Haynes, B.F., and Katz, P.: The spectrum of vasculitis: Clinical, pathologic, immunologic, and therapeutic considerations. Ann. Intern. Med. 89:660, 1978.

81. Copeman, P.W.M., and Ryan, T.J.: The problem of classification of cutaneous angiitis with reference to histopathology and pathogenesis. Br. J. Dermatol. 82(Suppl. 5):2, 1970.

82. Soter, N.A., Mihm, M.C., Jr., Gigli, I., Dvorak, H.F., and Austen, K.F.: Two distinct cellular patterns in cutaneous necrotizing angiitis. J. Invest. Dermatol. 66:344, 1976.

83. Braverman, I.M., and Yen, A.: Demonstration of immune complexes in spontaneous and histamine-induced lesions and in normal skin of patients with leukocytoclastic angiitis. J. Invest. Dermatol. 64:105, 1975.

84. Soter, N.A., and Austen, K.F.: Cutaneous necrotizing angiitis. *In* Samter, M., et al. (eds.): Immunological Diseases. Boston, Little, Brown & Company, 1978, pp. 993–1001.

85. Braverman, I.M.: The angiitides, *In* Skin Signs of Systemic Disease. Philadelphia, W.B. Saunders Company, 1970, p. 199.

86. McDuffee, F.D., Sams, W.M., Jr., Maldonado, J.E., Andreini, P.H.,

Conn, D.L., and Samayoa, E.A.: Hypocomplementemia with cutaneous vasculitis and arthritis: Possible immune complex syndrome. Mayo Clin. Proc. 48:340, 1973.

87. Soter, N.A., Austen, K.F., and Gigli, I.: Urticaria and arthralgias as manifestations of necrotizing angiitis (vasculitis). J. Invest. Dermatol. 63:485, 1974.

88. Soter, N.A.: Chronic urticaria as a manifestation of necrotizing venulitis. N. Engl. J. Med. 296:1440, 1977.

89. Monroe, E.W.: Urticarial vasculitis: an updated review. J. Am. Acad. Dermatol. 5:88, 1981.

90. Sanchez, N.P., Winkelmann, R.K., Schroeter, A.L., and Dicken, C.H.: The clinical and histopathologic spectrums of urticarial vasculitis: Study of 40 cases. J. Am. Acad. Dermatol. 7:599,. 1982.

91. Diaz, L.A., Provost, T.T., and Tomasi, T.B., Jr.; Pustular necrotizing angiitis. Arch. Dermatol. 108:114, 1973.

92. Borrie, P.: Cutaneous polyarteritis nodosa. Br. J. Dermatol. 87:87, 1972.

93. Diaz-Perez, J.L., and Winkelmann, R.K.: Cutaneous periarteritis nodosa. Arch. Dermatol. 110:407, 1974.

94. Kussmaul, A., and Maier, R.: Über eine bisher nicht beschriebene ei-genthumliche Arterienerkrankung (Periarteritis nodosa), die mit Mor-bus brightii und rapid fortschreitender allgemeiner Muskellahmung einhergeht. Dtsch. Arch. Klin. Med. 1:484, 1866.

95. Hamilton, C.R., Jr., Shelley, W.M., and Tumulty, P.A.: Giant cell ar-teritis: Including temporal arteritis and polymyalgia rheumatica. Med-icine 50:1, 1971.

96. Fauci, A.S., and Wolff, S.M.: Wegener's granulomatosis: Studies in eight-een patients and a review of the literature. Medicine 52:535, 1973.

97. Churg, J., and Strauss, L.: Allergic granulomatosis, allergic angiitis and periarteritis nodosa. Am. J. Pathol. 27:277, 1951.

98. Chumbley, L.C., Harrison, E.G., and DeRemee, R.A.: Allergic granu-lomatosis and angiitis (Churg-Strauss Syndrome): Report and analysis of 30 cases. Mayo Clin. Proc. 52:447, 1977.

99. Capra, J.D., Winchester, R.J., and Kunkel, H.G.: Hypergammaglobuli nemic purpura: Studies on the unusual anti-γ-globulins characteristic of the sera of these patients. Medicine 50:125, 1971.

100. Kyle, R.A., Gleich, G.J., Bayrd, E.D., and Vaughan, J.H.: Benign hy-pergammaglobulinemic purpura of Waldenström. Medicine 50:113, 1971.

101. Sams, W.M., Jr., Harville, D.D., and Winkelmann, R.K.: Necrotising vasculitis associated with lethal reticuloendothelial diseases. Br. J. Der-matol. 80:555, 1968.

102. Brouet, J.-C., Claurel, J.-P., Danon, F., Klein, M., and Seligmann, M.: Biologic and clinical significance of cryoglobulins: A report of 86 cases. Am. J. Med. 57:775, 1974.

103. Levo, Y., Gorevic, P.D., Kassab, H., Zucker-Franklin, D., Gigli, I., and Franklin, E.C.: Mixed cryoglobulinemia—an immune complex disease often associated with hepatitis B virus infection. Trans. Assoc. Am. Physicians 90:167, 1977.

104. Dienstag, J.L., Rhodes, A.R., Bhan, A.K., Dvorak, A.M., Mihm, M.C. Jr., and Wands, J.R.: Urticaria associated with acute viral hepatitis type B. Ann. Intern. Med. 89:34, 1978.

105. Meltzer, M., and Franklin, E.C.: Cryoglobulinemia—a study of twenty-nine patients. I. IgG and IgM cryoglobulins and factors affecting cryo-precipitability. Am. J. Med. 40:828, 1966.

106. Gower, R.G., Sausker, W.F., Kohler, P.F., Thorne, G.E., and McIntosh, R.M.: Small vessel vasculitis caused by hepatitis B virus immune com-plexes. Small vessel vasculitis and HBsAg. J. Allergy Clin. Immunol. 62:222, 1978.

107. Parish, W.E.: Cutaneous vasculitis: The occurrence of complexes of bac-terial antigens with antibody, and of abnormalities associated with chronic inflammation. In Beutner, E.H., Chorzelski, T.P., Bean, S.F., and Jordon, R.E.: Immunopathology of the Skin; Labelled Antibody Studies. Chicago, Year Book Medical Publishers, Inc., 1974, p. 153.

108. Moschella, S.L.: The lepra reaction with necrotizing skin lesions: A report of six cases. Arch. Dermatol. 95:565, 1967.

109. Quismorio, F.P., Jr., Rea, T., Chandor, S., Levan, N., and Friou, G.J.: Lucio's phenomenon: An immune complex deposition syndrome in lepromatous leprosy. Clin. Immunol. Immunopathol. 9:184, 1978.

110. Duffy, J., Lidsky, M.D., Sharp, J.T., Davis, J.S., Person, D.A., Hollinger, F.B., and Min, K.-W.: Polyarthritis, polyarteritis, and hepatitis B. Medicine 55:19, 1976.

111. Sussman, M., Jones, J.H., Almeida, J.D., and Lachmann, P.J.: Deficiency of the second component of complement associated with anaphylactoid purpura and presence of mycoplasma in the serum. Clin. Exp. Immunol. 14:531, 1973.

112. Gelfand, E.W., Clarkson, J.E., and Minta, J.O.: Selective deficiency of the second component of complement in a patient with anaphylactoid purpura. Clin. Immunol. Immunopathol. 4:269, 1975.

113. Gairdner, D.: The Schönlein-Henoch syndrome (anaphylactoid purpura). Quart. J. Med. 66:95, 1948.

114. Cream, J.J., Gumpel, J.H., and Peachey, R.D.G.: Schönlein-Henoch pur-

pura in the adult: A study of 77 adults with anaphylactoid or Schönlein-Henoch purpura. Quart. J. Med. 34:461, 1970.

115. Sissons, J.G.P., Williams, D.G., Peters, D.K., Boulton-Jones, J.M., and Goldsmith, H.J.: Skin lesions, angio-oedema, and hypocomplementae-mia. Lancet 2:1350, 1974.

116. Feig, P.U., Soter, N.A., Yager, H.M., Caplan, L., and Rosen, S.: Vas-culitis with urticaria, hypocomplementemia, and multiple system in-volvement. JAMA 236:2065, 1976.

117. Agnello, V., Winchester, R.J., and Kunkel, H.G.: Precipitin reactions of the C1q component of complement with aggregated γ-globulin and immune complexes in gel diffusion. Immunology 19:909, 1970.

118. Agnello, V., Koffler, D., Eisenberg, J.W., Winchester, R.J., and Kunkel, H.G.: C1q precipitins in the sera of patients with systemic lupus er-ythematosus and other hypocomplementemic states: Characterization of high and low molecular weight types. J. Exp. Med. 134:228s, 1971.

119. Agnello, V., Ruddy, S., Winchester, R.J., Christian, C.L., and Kunkel, H.G.: Hereditary C2 deficiency in systemic lupus erythematosus and acquired complement abnormalities in an unusual SLE-related syn-drome. Birth Defects 11:312, 1975.

120. Agnello, V.: Association of systemic lupus erythematosus and SLE-like syndromes with hereditary and acquired complement deficiency states. Arthritis Rheum. 21(Suppl.5):S146, 1978.

121. Marder, F.J., Burch F.X., Schmid, F.R., Zeiss, C.R., and Gewurz, H.: Low molecular weight C1q-precipitins in hypocomplementemic vas-culitis-urticaria syndrome: Partial purification and characterization as immunoglobulin. J. Immunol. 121:613, 1978.

122. Mraz, J.P., and Newcomer, V.D.: Erythema elevatum diutinum: Pres-entation of a case and evaluation of laboratory and immunological status. Arch. Dermatol. 96:235, 1967.

123. Katz, S.I., Gallin, J.I., Hertz, K.C., Fauci, A.S., and Lawley, T.J.: Ery-thema elevatum diutinum: Skin and systemic manifestations, immu-nologic studies, and successful treatment with dapsone. Medicine 56:443, 1977.

124. Keil, H.: The manifestations in the skin and mucous membranes in dermatomyositis, with special reference to the differential diagnosis from systemic lupus erythematosus. Ann. Intern. Med. 16:828, 1942.

125. O'Leary, P.A., and Waisman, M.: Dermatomyositis: A study of 40 cases. Arch. Dermatol. Syphilol. 41:1001, 1940.

126. Muller, S.A., Winkelmann, R.K., and Brunsting, L.A.: Calcinosis in dermatomyositis: Observations on course of disease in children and adults. Arch. Dermatol. 79:669, 1959.

127. Everett, M.A., and Curtis, A.D.: Dermatomyositis: A review of nineteen cases in adolescents and children. Arch. Intern. Med. 100:70, 1957.

128. Banker, B.Q., and Victor, M.: Dermatomyositis (systemic angiopathy) of childhood. Medicine 45:261, 1966.

129. Christianson, H.B., Brunsting, L.A., and Perry, H.O.: Dermatomyositis: Unusual features, complications, and treatment. Arch. Dermatol. 74:581, 1956.

130. Curtis, A.C., and Jansen, T.G.: The prognosis of localized scleroderma. Arch. Dermatol. 78:749, 1958.

131. Jabłońska, S., Bubnow, B., and Szczepański, A.: Morphea: Is it a separate entity or a variety of scleroderma? Dermatologica 125:140, 1962.

132. Christianson, H.B., Dorsey, C.S., O'Leary, P.A., and Kierland, R.R.: Localized scleroderma: A clinical study of two hundred thirty-five cases. Arch. Dermatol. 74:629, 1956.

133. Rubin, L.: Linear scleroderma: Association with abnormalities of spine and nervous system. Arch. Dermatol. Syphilol. 58:1, 1948.

134. Tuffanelli, D.L., and Winkelmann, R.K.: Systemic scleroderma: Clinical study of 727 cases. Arch. Dermatol. 84:359, 1961.

135. Carr, R.D., Heisel, E.B., and Stevenson, T.D.: CRST syndrome: Benign variant of scleroderma. Arch. Dermatol. 92:519, 1965.

136. Salerni, R., Rodnan, G.P., Leon, D.F., and Shaver, J.A.: Pulmonary hypertension in the CREST syndrome variant of progressive systemic sclerosis (scleroderma). Ann. Intern. Med. 86:394, 1977.

137. Schumacher, H.R.: A scleroderma-like syndrome with fasciitis, myositis, and eosinophilia. Ann. Intern. Med. 84:49, 1976.

138. Rudner, E.J., Mehregan, A., and Pinkus, H.: Scleromyxedema: A variant of lichen myxedematosus. Arch. Dermatol. 93:3, 1966.

139. Morris, J.M., Samilson, R.L., and Corley, C.L.: Melorheostosis: Review of the literature and report of an interesting case with a nineteen-year follow-up. J. Bone Joint Surg. 45:1191, 1963.

140. Wagers, L.T., Young, A.W., Jr., and Ryan, S.F.: Linear melorheostotic scleroderma. Br. J. Derm. 86:297, 1972.

141. Hood, A.F., Soter, N.A., Rappeport, J., and Gigli I.: Graft-versus-host reaction: cutaneous manifestations following bone marrow transplan-tation. Arch. Dermatol. 113:1087, 1977.

142. Isdale, I.C., and Bywaters, E.G.L.: The rash of rheumatoid arthritis and Still's disease. Quart. J. Med. 25:377, 1956.

143. Calabro, J.J., and Marchesano, J.M.: Rash associated with juvenile rheu-matoid arthritis. J. Pediatr. 72:611, 1968.

144. Taranta, A.: Occurrence of rheumatic-like subcutaneous nodules without

evidence of joint or heart disease: Report of a case. N. Engl. J. Med. 266:13, 1962.

145. Canizares, O.: Cutaneous lesions of rheumatic fever: A clinical study in young adults. Arch. Dermatol. 76:702, 1957.

146. Perry, C.B.: Erythema marginatum (rheumaticum). Arch. Dis. Child. 12:233, 1937.

147. Keil, H.: The rheumatic erythemas: A critical survey. Ann. Intern. Med. 11:2223, 1938.

148. Bywaters, E.G.L.: Skin manifestations of rheumatic diseases. In Fitzpatrick, T.B., et al. (eds.): Dermatology in General Medicine. New York, McGraw-Hill Book Company, 1971, p. 1534.

149. Bywaters, E.G.L., and Thomas, G.T.: Bed rest, salicylates and steroid in rheumatic fever. Br. Med. J. 1:1628, 1961.

150. Bass, M.H.: The cutaneous manifestations of acute rheumatic fever in childhood. Med. Clin. North Am. 2:201, 1918.

151. Goltz, R.W.: Systematized amyloidosis: A review of the skin and mucous membrane lesions and a report of two cases. Medicine 31:381, 1952.

152. Rukavina, J.G., Block, W.D., Jackson, C.E., Falls, H.F., Carey, J.H., and Curtis A.C.: Primary systemic amyloidosis: A review and an experimental, genetic, and clinical study of 29 cases with particular emphasis on the familial form. Medicine 35:239, 1956.

153. Rubinow, A., and Cohen, A.S.: Skin involvement in generalized amyloidosis: A study of clinically involved and uninvolved skin in 50 patients with primary and secondary amyloidosis. Ann. Intern. Med. 88:781, 1978.

154. Hurley, H.J., and Weinberg, R.: Induced intralesional hemorrhage in primary systemic amyloidosis. Arch. Dermatol. 89:678, 1964.

155. Muckle, T.J., and Wells, M.: Urticaria, deafness and amyloidosis: A new heredo-familial syndrome. Quart. J. Med. 31:235, 1962.
Black, J.T.: Amyloidosis, deafness, urticaria, and limb pains: A hereditary syndrome. Ann. Intern. Med. 70:989, 1969.

157. Andrade, C.: A peculiar form of peripheral neuropathy: Familiar atypical generalized amyloidosis with special involvement of peripheral nerves. Brain 75:408, 1952.

158. James, D.G.: Dermatological aspects of sarcoidosis. Quart. J. Med. 28:109, 1959.

159. James, D.G., Thomson, A.D., and Willcox, A.: Erythema nodosum as a manifestation of sarcoidosis. Lancet 2:218, 1956.

160. Löfgren, S.: Erythema nodosum: Studies on etiology and pathogenesis in 185 adult cases. Acta Med. Scand. Suppl. 174, 1946.

161. Wood, B.T., Behlen, C.H., and Weary, P.E.: The association of sarcoidosis, erythema nodosum, and arthritis. Arch. Dermatol. 94:406, 1966.

162. Kroll, J.J., Shapiro, L., Koplon, B.S., and Feldman, F.: Subcutaneous sarcoidosis with calcification. Arch. Dermatol. 106:894, 1972.

163. Cornelius, C.E., Stein, K.M., Hanshaw, W.J., and Spolt, D.A.: Hypopigmentation and sarcoidosis. Arch. Dermatol. 108:249, 1973.

Section III
Diagnostic Tests

Chapter 37
Aspiration and Injection of Joints and Soft Tissues

Duncan S. Owen, Jr.

INTRODUCTION

Shortly after systemic cortisone and hydrocortisone were first used in the management of rheumatoid arthritis, Dr. George Thorn[1] injected 10 mg of hydrocortisone into the knee joint of a patient with rheumatoid arthritis. The knee improved locally, but the patient also improved generally; it was concluded that the improvement resulted from systemic absorption of the intra-articularly injected material. No further studies of intra-articular corticosteroid injections were carried out until 1951, when Dr. Joseph Hollander and his associates[2] reported a study from their clinic at the University of Pennsylvania. In an early study from the Mayo Clinic[3] short-lived improvement of 2 to 8 days was reported in patients with rheumatoid arthritis or osteoarthritis following intra-articular injections of hydrocortisone. Ten years later a series of over 100,000 injections of joints, bursae, and tendon sheaths in 4000 patients was reported by Hollander and colleagues.[4] They called attention to the usefulness of intra-articular corticosteroids as temporary, palliative, repeatable, local adjunct treatments of a variety of rheumatic conditions[5] and to the more prolonged benefits afforded by preparations less rapidly hydrolyzed than hydrocortisone.

MECHANISM(S) OF ACTION OF INTRASYNOVIAL CORTICOSTEROIDS

The anti-inflammatory mechanisms of corticosteroids are still not fully understood.[6] Early clinical studies demonstrated a decrease in erythema, swelling, heat, and tenderness to palpation of the inflamed joints.[3] An increase in viscosity and hyaluronate concentration of the synovial fluid was observed.[7] Studies with liver lysosomes indicated stabilization of the lysosomal membrane and prevention of release of lysosomal enzymes, which can induce further inflammation.[8-10] Experiments using phagocytic leukocytes and bacterial systems failed to document stabilization by hydrocortisone of the lyso-

somes in these cells.[11-13] Measurement of the action of hydrocortisone, dexamethasone, and prednisone on intact lysosomes isolated from human peripheral blood polymorphonuclear leukocytes demonstrated protection of these organelle membranes from either detergent lysis or heat incubation as assessed by the release of the lysosomal marker β-glucuronidase. Polymorphonuclear leukocyte lysosomes isolated from human volunteers treated with prednisolone were no more stable than those from untreated normals, and the serum from these treated volunteers did not protect intact lysosomes from detergent lysis.[14] The investigators felt the anti-inflammatory activity of corticosteroids was best explained by inhibitory effects on cellular metabolism rather than by their direct interaction with lysosomal membranes.

There is evidence of an anti-inflammatory effect mediated by a peptide hormone that inhibits polymorphonuclear microtubular assembly.[15] Many peptide hormones are believed to act by increasing the action of adenosine monophosphate within target cells, and this mechanism could explain the inhibitory effect of corticosteroids on phagocytic cells.

Corticosteroids are potent inhibitors of prostaglandin synthesis by several types of cells and tissues, including rheumatoid synovial tissue.[16-20] One of the effects is a decreased release of arachidonic acid from phospholipids.[19-21] Since only unesterified fatty acids are used by cyclooxygenase, this decreased release of arachidonic acid depresses all cyclooxygenase-derived products.[22]

Corticosteroids decrease levels of serum immunoglobulins and complement.[23,24] One study of intra-articular corticosteroids demonstrated a transient decrease in synovial fluid complement.[25] In another study, 12 patients received intra-articular methylprednisolone. Six showed no alteration of synovial fluid total hemolytic complement, C4 protein level, or rheumatoid factor titer. The other 6 showed a 50 percent or greater change in only one of the synovial fluid values. Most had reductions in total leukocyte counts, polymorphonuclear leukocyte counts, and acid phosphatase levels.[26]

Dick and co-workers in 1970[27] reported the results of

studies using intra-articular radioactive xenon (^{133}Xe). They demonstrated a fall in the rate of disappearance of ^{133}Xe after an intra-articular injection of hydrocortisone hemisuccinate. They felt corticosteroids diminish synovial permeability. A 1979 study of patients with rheumatoid arthritis from this same laboratory,[28] using intra-articular ^{133}Xe and triamcinolone hexacetonide in one group of patients and ^{133}Xe and lidocaine in a second group, revealed no difference in the rate of clearance of ^{133}Xe after 40 minutes in the triamcinolone-treated group. Therefore, they felt triamcinolone had no immediate effect on synovial blood vessels. However, the lidocaine-treated group showed a decrease in the rate of ^{133}Xe clearance.

In 1982, Eymontt and colleagues[29] reported the effects of intra-articular triamcinolone hexacetonide, prednisolone tebutate, and saline administration on both synovial permeability and synovial fluid leukocyte counts in patients with symptomatic osteoarthritis. In their study, they employed a radioactive blood-pool tracer, ^{99m}Tc human serum albumin. Their results indicated that corticosteroids decrease synovial permeability but produce an increase in synovial fluid leukocytes.

POTENTIAL SEQUELAE (TABLE 37–1)

In the late 1950s, there first appeared a few reports of Charcot-like arthropathy attributed to intra-articular corticosteroid therapy.[30,31] One study by Mankin and Conger, in 1966, reported that intra-articularly administered hydrocortisone acetate reduced the incorporation of glycine-^{3}H into rabbit articular cartilage to approximately one-third of control values within 6 hours. They interpreted the decrease in utilization to a decrease in matrix protein synthesis caused by hydrocortisone.[32]

In 1969, Bentley and Goodfellow[33] advised strongly against recurrent intra-articular injections because of potential severe arthropathy.

In 1970, Moskowitz and associates showed that intra-articular triamcinolone acetonide produced nuclear degeneration of chondrocytes and prominent cyst formation.[34]

In 1972, Mankin, Zarins, and Jaffe reported that intramuscular cortisone reduced the incorporation of glycine-^{3}H, $^{35}SO_4$, and was associated with a progressive decline in the concentration of hexosamine.[35]

Table 37–1. Potential Sequelae from Intra-Articular and Soft Tissue Corticosteroid Injections

1. Radiologic deterioration of joints—"steroid arthropathy"; Charcot-like arthropathy; osteonecrosis
2. Iatrogenic infection—very low incidence
3. Rupture of tendon
4. Tissue atrophy and fat necrosis
5. Nerve damage, e.g., inadvertent injection of median nerve in carpal tunnel syndrome
6. "Postinjection flare"
7. Uterine bleeding
8. Pancreatitis
9. Cushing's syndrome

In 1975, Behrens and associates found an increased number of fissures in rabbit cartilage after intra-articular injections of hydrocortisone. Hexosamine incorporation decreased, as did synthesis of proteoglycans; collagen production was reduced to one-fifth. They hypothesized that the anti-anabolic effects of the corticosteroids cause a massive decrease in the synthesis of all major matrix components. The loss of proteoglycan content led to a decrease in cartilage stiffness such that the impact of cyclic loading with weight-bearing caused death of cells, cystic degeneration of matrix, and fissuring in the midzonal areas of weight-bearing surfaces.

Completely different data were reported in 1976 by Gibson and associates.[37] They repeatedly injected the knee joints of 10 *Macaca irus* monkeys with either methylprednisolone or a control solution. Minor degenerative changes of femoral condyles were shown by India ink staining and by a system of histochemical grading, but changes in the joints injected with corticosteroids were *not* significantly different from those seen in control joints.

In 1981, Tenenbaum and colleagues[38] reported on a continuing study of the long-term effects of intra-articular dexamethasone TBA on rabbit knee cartilage. There was an acceleration of the calcific degenerative arthropathy that occurs in mature New Zealand rabbits. Under these experimental conditions, the cartilage injury seems limited and did not progress with repeated injections.

In 1969, Sweetnam[39] cautioned against steroid injection of inflamed tendons in athletes because of the possibility of tendon rupture. Wrenn and associates[40] in 1954 demonstrated a 40 per cent reduction in tensile strength of a tendon after the use of corticosteroids. (We have rarely observed a rupture of the long head of the biceps tendon or Achilles tendon following the injection of the tendon sheath for tendinitis.) Other complications include soft-tissue atrophy, especially noted when the small joints such as finger proximal interphalangeal joints are injected. Periarticular calcifications and ecchymoses around the atrophied areas have been reported.[41]

The intra-articular injection of corticosteroids occasionally produces what has been called a "postinjection flare."[42] This increase in local inflammation may develop a few hours after injection and last up to 48 hours. The difficulty of distinguishing this reaction from an iatrogenic infection may be worrisome. The flare is noted more frequently with the needle-shaped corticosteroid crystals and may be a form of crystal-induced arthritis produced by synovial fluid leukocytes phagocytosing the crystals and subsequently releasing lysosomal enzymes.

Systemic absorption of intra-articular corticosteroid, or from other soft tissue injections, occurs in almost all patients. Usually, this is clinically manifested, for example, in a patient with rheumatoid arthritis, by subjective and objective improvement of inflamed joints other than the one(s) injected. There may be other effects, such as eosinopenia, lymphopenia, and, depending upon the corticosteroid injected, changes in serum and urine cortisol levels. There may be suppression of the hypothalamic-pituitary-adrenal axis.[43] Patients with diabetes mellitus may note a severalfold rise in their blood glucose levels.

Prominent erythema, warmth, and diaphoresis of the face and torso may occur within minutes to hours after an intra-articular corticosteroid injection.[44] This reaction is noted mainly with triamcinolone acetonide. Some feel it is an uncommon reaction, but we note it in greater than 10 percent of patients injected with this medication. Some of these patients note headache. In this regard, it resembles the nitratoid reaction occasionally observed with the injection of gold salts, especially gold sodium thiomalate. These corticosteroid reactions may last a few minutes to a few days. However, some patients are so frightened by these reactions they refuse further injections.

Abnormal uterine bleeding may occur from injection of corticosteroids, especially triamcinolone acetonide. The exact mechanisms are unknown, but ovulation may be inhibited.[45,46] Also, corticosteroids may produce uterine bleeding in a postmenopausal patient. This alarms both patient and physician.

Pancreatitis, apparently induced by injectable corticosteroids, is rarely noted.

PRECAUTIONS

When performing arthrocenteses or soft-tissue injections, strict adherence to aseptic procedures is required. The physician should use the same precautions as for a lumbar spinal puncture. Iatrogenic infections may be disastrous but are rare if these precautions are taken. At the Medical College of Virginia we have observed one, or possibly two, infections in over 35,000 injections.

In theory, arthrocentesis may provide a focus for septic arthritis in a patient with bacteremia, such as staphylococcal endocarditis.[47] It is well known that a patient with damaged joints from, for example, rheumatoid arthritis, is more susceptible to developing spontaneous septic arthritis from blood-borne bacteria. Arthrocentesis in such instances has enabled rapid diagnosis and prevented the patient's joint from being destroyed. "Routine" therapeutic arthrocenteses should be avoided, however, if the patient is being treated for a condition associated with bacteremia.

Because of tissue atrophy with corticosteroids, one should use extreme caution when injecting near peripheral nerves. For example, carpal tunnel syndrome, either idiopathic or induced by rheumatoid arthritis, may be benefited by corticosteroid injection in the carpal tunnel. An injection directly into the median nerve could result in nerve necrosis or atrophy.

Gottlieb reported two cases of hypodermic needle separations during arthrocenteses.[48] It was recommended that the needles be inspected after arthrocentesis to ascertain that they are intact, and he advised keeping a hemostat within easy access to enable the operator to remove a separated needle from the soft tissues.

EFFICACY OF INJECTIONS

Intra-articular Injections. Despite the fact thousands of intra-articular corticosteroid preparations have been injected in thousands of patients, there are few good studies of their efficacy.[49] The length of symptomatic improvement appears related to the particular preparation used. Most patients with rheumatoid arthritis will benefit from an injection, but the effect may last only days. Hydrocortisone acetate may give improvement for a few days to a week or more; and prednisolone tebutate, for two weeks or more. Triamcinolone hexacetonide, which is poorly water soluble and one of the longest-acting agents, has been shown to provide reversal of inflammation in some patients for longer periods.[41] As with oral nonsteroidal anti-inflammatory drugs, responses among different patients are extremely varied. If one or two injections prove ineffective or give only short-lived benefit, there is no logic in persistently injecting the same joint.

Results of injections in osteoarthritic joints conflict. The data range from no benefit to outstanding benefit.[1,50-52] The differences may relate in part to the joint injected. For example, degenerative arthritis of the first carpometacarpal joint is a fairly common and painful condition in which there is little synovial thickening or increase in synovial fluid. The injection of corticosteroid is often painful, probably because of the moderate to marked decrease in joint space, but dramatic symptomatic improvement usually occurs within 12 hours, and may last many months. This contrasts with injection for osteoarthritis of the hip, in which it is very difficult to know if the hip joint space has been entered, even with use of the fluoroscope as a guide. Improvement of hip symptoms within 12 to 24 hours after injection probably indicates the corticosteroid was injected intra-articularly, but benefit often lasts only 2 days to a week. The mechanical problem of bone rubbing against bone in a weight-bearing joint may be the reason for the short-lived benefit, and repeated injections may be expected to be of little value.

Osteoarthritis of the knee may be very painful and may be associated with large volumes of synovial fluid. Even though it is the usual practice to remove as much synovial fluid as possible, the efficacy of this procedure in osteoarthritis is questionable. Usually the corticosteroid injection is associated with dramatic symptomatic relief, which lasts days to weeks or more. If the injections give short-lived benefit, repeated injections are probably contraindicated because the primary problem is in the cartilage, and repeated injections could hasten cartilage deterioration for reasons previously outlined.

A weight-bearing joint probably should be rested as much as possible for 24 to 48 hours after injection. Additionally, some recommend resting all corticosteroid-injected joints for a prolonged period of time.[53] There is no consensus about this, however.

Non-Articular Injections. In contrast to intra-articular injections that are used adjunctively, certain soft-tissue inflammatory conditions may be more or less permanently eradicated by judicious injections of corticosteroids with or without local anesthetics.[54-57] The conditions having the longest benefits from injections are those precipitated by trauma, especially when the activity causing the inflammation is avoided. For example, a patient troubled by recurrent lateral epicondylitis who derives short-lived benefit from a corticosteroid injection into the inflamed area may improve more permanently by discontinuing golf or tennis.

Many cases of apparent tendinitis and bursitis may be secondary manifestations of rheumatoid arthritis, in which injections may give an outstanding initial benefit that, unfortunately, is temporary. In such patients appropriate treatment of the underlying disease should be instituted, and the injections must be considered as adjunctive management.

The poorly understood but apparently quite common "fibrositis syndrome"[58,59] is associated with various "trigger points" and is discussed in detail in Chapter 32. These exaggerated tender areas may respond dramatically to the injection of a local anesthetic directly into the most tender area, but the addition of a corticosteroid in the same syringe may give more lasting relief.

TYPES OF PREPARATIONS

The original intra-articular corticosteroid, hydrocortisone acetate, is still available, is widely used, and is inexpensive. Other preparations of various potency and solubility are now available, and these are listed in Table 37-2. Few comparative studies of the efficacy or duration of action of the various agents have been reported. As previously mentioned, McCarty[41] has noted longterm benefits with triamcinolone hexacetonide, and thinks this is the least soluble and produces the most

prolonged effect of the agents commercially available. Such "longer-acting and more potent" suspensions are much more expensive than hydrocortisone. Some investigators are of the opinion that the more potent preparations are also more efficacious,[49] but the evidence for this is not strong.

Many clinicians, over months or years of practice, have settled on a preparation that seems to have, in their opinion, good benefit and few side effects. Some prefer, for example, a preparation of a "short-acting" solution and a "long-acting" suspension of betamethasone (Celestone Soluspan). They feel the solution works rapidly and prevents the possibility of a postinjection flare. For the same reason, others prefer to inject a "short-acting" solution, such as dexamethasone sodium phosphate, together with a more long-acting suspension.

Mixing the corticosteroid suspension with a local anesthetic, particularly procaine or lidocaine, may be helpful when injecting small joints and tendons, thereby preventing the injection in a single area of a very concentrated suspension, which could produce soft-tissue atrophy. However, one must be concerned over the compatibility of the two preparations. In the Aristospan package brochure dated February, 1978, the following is written:

Aristospan suspension may be mixed with 1% or 2% lidocaine hydrochloride, using the formulations which do not contain parabens. Similar local anesthetics may also be used. Diluents containing methylparaben, propylparaben, phenol, etc., should be avoided since these compounds may cause flocculation of the steroid.

A review of package inserts of intra-articular corticosteroids from the larger pharmaceutical companies revealed that most do not recommend the use of a mixture of corticosteroids and local anesthetics containing preservatives.

Local anesthetics usually contain preservatives. Ones without them are usually more expensive and are usually not available in the average arthrocentesis tray. Lidocaine for intravenous use does not contain preservatives. A brief survey of several rheumatologists and orthopedic surgeons throughout the country revealed that approximately one half used a corticosteroid and local anesthetic mixture, and only one was aware of the potential problem of flocculation. A few orthopedists, however, reported finding "steroid chalk" in joints, especially wrists, that had been injected with the "older steroids." There is no way of knowing if these joints had been injected with corticosteroid and local anesthetic combinations.

There is no consensus concerning the amount of material that should be injected into the various sized joints. Some clinicians tend to inject a smaller amount in volume of the "more potent" corticosteroids, but many, probably the majority, tend to inject 1 ml in the large joints and a lesser amount in the medium and small joints. Table 37-3 is a rough guide of the amount to be injected.

Table 37-2. Corticosteroids and Prednisone Equivalents*

Intra-articular Preparations (generic name, strength, and trade names)	Prednisone Equivalents
Betamethasone sodium phosphate and acetate suspension 6 mg/ml (Celestone Soluspan)	10
Dexamethasone sodium phosphate 4 mg/ml (Decadron and Hexadrol)	8
Dexamethasone acetate 8 mg/ml (Decadron-LA)	16
Hydrocortisone acetate 25 mg/ml (Hydrocortone)	1
Methylprednisolone acetate 20, 40, and 80 mg/ml (Depo-Medrol)	5, 10 and 20
Prednisolone tebutate 20 mg/ml (Hydeltra-T.B.A.)	4
Triamcinolone acetonide 10 and 40 mg/ml (Kenalog-10 and Kenalog-40)	2.5 and 10
Triamcinolone hexacetonide 20 mg/ml (Aristospan)	5

*One equivalent = 5 mg prednisone.

Table 37–3. Amount of Intra-Articular Corticosteroid for Injection

Size of Joint	Examples	Range of Dosage
Large	Knees Ankles Shoulders	1–2 ml
Medium	Elbows Wrists	0.5–1.0 ml
Small	Interphalangeal Metacarpophalangeal	0.1–0.5 ml

INDICATIONS

Intra-articular and soft-tissue corticosteroid injections are considered adjunctive therapy. Rarely are they considered primary therapy. Exceptions, as previously noted, include bursitis, tendinitis, or documented gout in a single joint. Table 37–4 lists the indications for intra-articular corticosteroid injections. This therapeutic list is not arranged in any particular order of preference or likelihood of response.

Articular. *Rheumatoid Arthritis.* Rheumatoid arthritis (with the possible exception of tendinitis and bursitis) is probably the one illness for which the most injections are given. The efficacy of injections in this illness is the most controversial, for reasons previously discussed. If systemic regimens were uniformly efficacious in patients with rheumatoid arthritis, there would be no need to inject corticosteroids in the joints. Since this is not the case, the judicious use of intra-articular corticosteroids may enable a patient to lead a more productive life and one of better quality. Injections may especially be indicated when the patient has failed to respond or when there are contraindications to nonsteroidal anti-inflammatory drugs, hydroxychloroquine, gold salts, or other systemic agents. Usually the injections will enable the patient to better participate in physical therapeutic procedures. The number of injections on a single day should be limited to two, but other joints may be injected on other days. There are no data as to how often the same joint may safely be re-injected. Not more than three times a year seems prudent.

Gout. Acute gouty arthritis (monosodium urate monohydrate crystal deposition disease) on occasion is refractory to so-called conventional regimens, that is, colchicine, phenylbutazone, or other nonsteroidal anti-

Table 37–4. Indications for Intra-articular Corticosteroid Injections

1. Rheumatoid arthritis
2. Gout
3. Pseudogout
4. Acute traumatic "arthritis"
5. Osteoarthritis
6. Synovitis of ipsilateral knee following total hip arthroplasty
7. Juvenile rheumatoid arthritis
8. Inflammatory bowel disease with peripheral joint involvement
9. Miscellaneous conditions with peripheral joint manifestations: ankylosing spondylitis, psoriatic arthritis, and Reiter's disease

inflammatory drugs. If this is the case, and if phagocytized sodium urate crystals continue to be present in the synovial fluid, complete aspiration of the inflamed joint followed by corticosteroid injection may be helpful. One has to be very sure that an infectious process is not the reason for the persistent inflammation.

Pseudogout. The diagnosis of pseudogout (calcium pyrophosphate dihydrate crystal deposition disease) requires the identification of the calcium pyrosphosphate crystals in synovial fluid. Aspirating as much fluid as possible may alleviate not only pain but also inflammation. That is, aspiration may remove a sufficient number of crystals to reduce the inflammatory process. On occasion, however, the inflammatory response does not respond to this and/or the usual nonsteroidal anti-inflammatory drugs, and intra-articular corticosteroids prove efficacious.

Acute Traumatic "Arthritis." Acute trauma to joints is usually treated with a conservative regimen of cold packs, rest, and, after an appropriate time, an increase in activity. Many feel that injuries to the soft tissues of the shoulder and ankle will cause serious sequelae if range of motion is not instituted after a short period of rest. Intra-articular corticosteroids may help in these situations by allowing early movement.

Osteoarthritis. Osteoarthritic joints, as previously discussed, can be extremely painful. The efficacy of intra-articular corticosteroids is debated; however, on occasion injections give outstanding and prolonged benefit. This is especially true if inflammation is present and there is little cartilage loss. If one or two injections do not give benefit, there is no good reason to keep injecting the joint.

Synovitis of Knee after Hip Arthroplasty. Synovitis of the ipsilateral knee after total hip arthroplasty is noted on occasion and may resolve spontaneously after a few days. It may persist, however, and injection of the knee with a corticosteroid usually is quite beneficial.

Juvenile Rheumatoid Arthritis. In children with rheumatoid arthritis, the number of systemic drugs that can be administered is limited. The judicious use of intra-articular corticosteroids may prove quite helpful. This is especially true when only a few joints are involved; for example, in the pauci (oligo) articular type.

Synovitis of Inflammatory Bowel Disease. Inflammatory gastrointestinal diseases may be associated with peripheral or axial arthritis. Sometimes, depending upon the type of intestinal disorder, an exacerbation of the intestinal problem is associated with an exacerbation of the joint symptoms. In certain situations, control of the intestinal disease also controls the joint disease. If, however, the arthropathy is not helped, injections of intra-articular corticosteroids may give rapid and prolonged relief.

Miscellaneous. Peripheral joint manifestations of other inflammatory arthritides such as ankylosing spondylitis, psoriatic arthritis, and Reiter's disease may be benefited by intra-articular corticosteroids.

Nonarticular. Nonarticular inflammatory conditions may be greatly benefited by the injection of a corticosteroid with or without a local anesthetic. Table 37–5 lists various soft tissue conditions which may benefit from the injections.

Shoulder. The main shoulder problems are bicipital tendinitis, subacromial bursitis, and supraspinatus tendinitis. As previously mentioned, these problems can be primary or part of a systemic problem, for example, rheumatoid arthritis. Injection of the specifically inflamed tendon or bursa usually gives relief within a few hours. However, when mixed with a local anesthetic, relief is usually immediate if the physician injected the correct area.

The possible sequelae of intratendinous injections have previously been mentioned. If the inflammatory problems involve the bicipital tendon or subacromial bursa, some physicians prefer to inject the shoulder joint directly. This seems especially true in patients with rheumatoid arthritis because arthrographic studies in these patients have frequently shown a communication between the subacromial bursa, the bicipital tendon sheath, and the shoulder joint. Thus, the drug can have a local effect in all these areas.

Elbow. Inflammation of the elbow epicondylar areas is frequently noted in patients who are quite active in sports, especially tennis and golf. Lateral epicondylitis is frequently a sequela of these activities, and it can be very painful. Injecting the inflamed region can give good to excellent benefit. Mixing the corticosteroid with local anesthetic can give immediate benefit; however, when the effect of the local anesthetic subsides, there is frequently an exacerbation of pain, apparently as a result

Table 37–5. Indications for Non-articular Corticosteroid Injections

1. Shoulder
   a. Bicipital tendinitis
   b. Subacromial bursitis
   c. Supraspinatus tendinitis
2. Elbow
   a. Lateral epicondylitis—"tennis elbow"
   b. Medial epicondylitis—"golfer's elbow"
   c. Olecranon bursitis
   d. Cubital tunnel syndrome
3. Wrist and Hand
   a. Ganglion
   b. de Quervain's disease—stenosing tenosynovitis of extensor pollicis brevis and abductor pollicis longus
   c. Trigger (snapping) fingers
   d. Carpal tunnel syndrome
4. Hip
   a. Trochanteric bursitis
5. Knee
   a. Anserine bursitis
   b. Prepatella bursitis
6. Pelvis
   a. Ischial bursitis
   b. Iliopectineal bursitis
7. Back
   a. "Fibrositic" trigger points
8. Foot
   a. Achilles tendinitis
   b. Achilles bursitis
   c. Calcaneal bursitis
   d. Tarsal tunnel syndrome

of a crystal-induced postinjection flare. Medial epicondylitis also can be very painful and usually responds well to an injection. However, one should be careful not to inject the nearby ulnar nerve.

Olecranon bursitis may be a primary condition, usually from trauma, but may be secondary to conditions such as gout, infection, and rheumatoid arthritis. Therefore, aspiration of the fluid and synovianalysis are essential before corticosteroids are injected.

Cubital tunnel syndrome, an entrapment of the ulnar nerve at the elbow, may be caused by tenosynovitis. The symptoms are usually more motor related than sensory. Injections can be administered by experienced operators; however, surgical decompression is usually necessary.[60]

Wrist and Hand. A ganglion on the dorsal aspect of the wrist can be treated by aspiration and injection. Again, there may be considerable discomfort several hours after injection. Between two thirds and three fourths of patients have their ganglia "cured" by this conservative approach.[42,61]

Stenosing tenosynovitis of the extensor pollicis brevis and abductor pollicis longus (de Quervain's disease) may cause considerable discomfort over the distal aspect of the radius. Conservative management with corticosteroid and local anesthetic injection may be quite helpful.[57,62] If immediate benefit is noted, this usually indicates the injection was in the proper area. Recurrence is common, however.

Trigger and snapping fingers may be caused by a primary nonspecific hand flexor tenosynovitis or tenosynovitis of rheumatoid arthritis. The tendinous sheath injection of corticosteroid and local anesthetic has been shown to be efficacious in over 90 percent of the cases, and median length of relief has been two years.[55]

Carpal tunnel syndrome has multiple etiologies, but the rheumatoid and idiopathic types may be helped by corticosteroid injections. Extreme care is necessary to prevent median nerve damage.[62] One should receive personal instruction in this technique before attempting it.

Hip. Trochanteric bursitis can give considerable discomfort and may be relieved by injections. There are one or more bursae about the femoral trochanter at the gluteal insertion. The tender region is easily palpated unless there is obesity.

Knee. The anserine bursa is present on the medial aspect of the knee where the tendons of the sartorius, semitendinosus, and gracilus muscles insert on the tibia. When it is inflamed, there is pain, palpable swelling, and tenderness over the medial anterior aspect of the tibia just below the knee. There may be associated degenerative arthritis of the knee, obesity, or a history of physical activity such as jogging, frequent knee bending, or frequent going up and down stairs. Some authors do not consider the condition a true bursitis and classify it as Dercum's disease (painful adiposity) or place it in the "fibrositis syndrome" category.[58] Whatever one wishes to call it, most cases are greatly benefited by injection of corticosteroid and local anesthetic. If the material is injected in the proper place, immediate relief is usually experienced.

Prepatellar bursitis may be secondary to trauma, for example, "housemaid's knee," or could be secondary to systemic illnesses such as rheumatoid arthritis or gout. It may be asymptomatic or quite painful. Some patients request treatment for cosmetic reasons. If clinically indicated, the bursal fluid can be examined by techniques similar to those used for synovial fluid. Injections are usually effective.[63]

Pelvis. Ischial or ischiogluteal bursitis may be more common than is generally thought and may be misdiagnosed as herniated nucleus pulposus, lumbosacral strain, or thrombophlebitis.[64] The ischiogluteal bursa overlies the sciatic nerve and the posterior femoral cutaneous nerve. Therefore, the pain may radiate and the wrong diagnosis may be made. Palpation over the ischial tuberosity should cause significant pain. Injections are helpful but are not recommended for the inexperienced operator.

Iliopectineal (iliopsoas) bursitis is an inflammation of the bursa that is located between the iliopsoas muscle and the iliopectineal eminence. It may communicate with the hip joint. There is tenderness over the anterior aspect of the hip in the region of the middle portion of the inguinal ligament. Hyperextension, adduction, or internal rotation of the hip elicits pain. Differential diagnoses include femoral hernia, psoas abscess, and septic arthritis of the hip. When these other diagnoses have been excluded, and if more conservative regimens have failed or are not practical, an injection of corticosteroid with or without local anesthetic can be tried.[65]

Back. Painful subjective and objective areas of the back may be noted and may be difficult to explain anatomically. Tender areas to moderate deep palpation, the so-called "trigger points," may be noted especially around the upper medial border of the trapezius, various periscapular areas, inferior posterior cervical area, and presacral regions. The latter may represent herniated presacral fatpads. These painful areas may be part of the "fibrositis syndrome."[58] An injection of corticosteroid, local anesthetic, or a combination of the two, into the "trigger points" frequently gives relief.

Foot. Achilles tendinitis may be secondary to trauma or to systemic illnesses such as rheumatoid arthritis or gout. The former may be associated with rheumatoid nodules in the tendon and the latter with tophi. Rest, analgesics, and anti-inflammatory medications are preferable to injections. If little benefit is obtained from these conservative measures, a small amount of a mixture of corticosteroid and local anesthetic may be injected.

Achilles bursitis may represent inflammation of the retrocalcaneal bursa between the calcaneus and Achilles tendon, or a subcutaneous bursitis between the skin and tendon. One should not forget the possibility of gout being the cause, and if the bursae are punctured, an attempt at aspiration is a good idea. The contents should then be examined. Conservative management of nonspecific bursitis is similar to that of Achilles tendinitis; but if this is ineffective, an injection may prove beneficial.

Calcaneal bursitis is an inflammation of the bursa at the attachment of the plantar fascia to the os calcis.

Pain is present in the center of the plantar aspect of the heel. Conservative management such as a rubber doughnut may help. If not, an intrabursal injection of corticosteroid mixed with local anesthetic usually gives good relief, but the injection frequently causes considerable pain.

Tarsal tunnel syndrome is an entrapment neuropathy of all or part of the posterior tibial nerve as it passes under the flexor retinaculum of the ankle. Burning pain and paresthesias in the affected foot are the symptoms. Injections by an experienced operator may help, but relief is usually temporary.[66]

CONTRAINDICATIONS TO INTRA-ARTICULAR CORTICOSTEROID INJECTIONS

The main contraindications to intra-articular corticosteroid injections are listed in Table 37–6. As previously stated, even though rare, iatrogenic infections occur. Therefore, it is essential to adhere to strict aseptic procedures, and certainly the physician must avoid inserting a needle through any area of cellulitis.

The previously mentioned bacteremia, as would be noted in certain cases of pneumonia, endocarditis, and pyelonephritis, is considered a contraindication by some. Therefore, if a patient is hospitalized for a condition that may be associated with bacteremia, and the patient concomitantly has active rheumatoid arthritis, it is probably wise not to institute therapeutic arthrocenteses and corticosteroid injections because of the possibility of an iatrogenic infection. (If one is concerned that bacteremia may have produced septic arthritis, arthrocentesis and special studies on the synovial fluid are mandatory.)

Instability of joints may be part of the Charcot-like arthropathy from intra-articular corticosteroids. Theoretically, further injections could make the instability worse. In general, joints of the spine are considered inaccessible, and injections are contraindicated because of potential sequelae. One should keep in mind that articular pain following trauma could represent an intra-articular fracture. Corticosteroid injection is contrain-

Table 37–6. Contraindications to Intra-Articular Corticosteroid Injections

1. Periarticular sepsis
2. Bacteremia
3. Unstable joints
4. Essentially inaccessible joints, e.g., spinal
5. Intra-articular fracture
6. Septic joint; do *not* forget possibility of tuberculosis
7. Possibly the nondiathrodial joints, e.g., symphysis pubis; however, sternomanubrial injections may prove very helpful on occasion
8. Marked juxta-articular osteoporosis
9. Failure to respond to prior injections
10. Blood clotting disorders
11. Probably total joint arthroplasty

dicated because of its potential for retarding the healing of a fracture.

Injection of a septic joint with a corticosteroid could greatly increase the morbidity of the infection. Purulent appearance of synovial fluid should alert the physician to this possibility, but tuberculous synovitis may produce a synovial fluid with minimal inflammatory findings, and the physician may thus be misled. The possibility should always be kept in mind and further studies of synovial fluid and even percutaneous synovial biopsy considered.

Nondiarthrodial joints, such as the symphysis pubis, are involved with certain arthritides, but these joints are difficult to inject. If they are accessible, injections are helpful on occasion, but several punctures may be necessary.

Juxta-articular osteoporosis of a marked degree may be worsened by intra-articular corticosteroid. This type of osteoporosis is more commonly seen in the patient with rheumatoid arthritis, and the arthritis itself plus lack of motion in the joint may be the main cause of the osteoporosis. Therefore, theoretically one or two corticosteroid injections may improve the problem. If one or two corticosteroid injections in the same joint provide no benefit, there is no sound reason to keep injecting it. Blood clotting disorders, such as factor VIII deficiency, may produce a destructive type of arthritis. Arthrocentesis could produce both intra-articular and external hemmorrhage. This problem should definitely be considered when undiagnosed synovitis is noted in a child.

There is an increased incidence of infections in the operated joints of patients who have total joint arthroplasties. These patients are seriously jeopardized by these injections. Even if these patients have an excerbation of their primary disease—for example, rheumatoid arthritis—in their operated joints, it is probably unwise to inject these joints with corticosteroids.

ANESTHESIA

As previously discussed, some physicians prefer mixing the corticosteroid with a local anesthetic, usually procaine or lidocaine, for two reasons. First, when injecting a bursa, tendon sheath, or periarticular region, this combination usually would give immediate subjective relief if the materials were injected in the proper space. This immediate benefit, of course, would be from the local anesthetic, not the corticosteroid, and the patients should be told they may experience further pain in an hour or two but should improve a few hours later, when the anti-inflammatory actions of the corticosteroids begin. Second, a mixture may be preferable because the corticosteroid would be diluted and there should be less soft tissue atrophy at the sites of injection.

A physician experienced in arthrocenteses may elect not to use any anesthesia when injecting large joints. If the patient is cooperative and relaxed, and if disposal needles are used, there should be very little pain associated with the arthrocenteses. If the physician is inexperienced or the patient is anxious and tense, a short burst of ethyl chloride spray on the skin over the joint to be injected is helpful.

The injection of a local anesthetic is the other option. First, a skin wheal should be made, followed by infiltration of the subcutaneous tissue and joint capsule. After a few minutes arthrocentesis can be performed and should be painless.

TECHNIQUES

To perform an arthrocentesis, the specific area of the joint to be aspirated is palpated and is then marked with firm pressure with a ballpoint pen that has the writing portion retracted. This will leave an impression that will last 10 to 30 minutes. (The ballpoint pen technique can also be used with soft tissue injection.) Strict asepsis is important and deserves re-emphasis. The area to be aspirated or injected should be carefully cleansed with a good antiseptic, such as the iodinated compounds. Then the needle can be inserted through the ballpoint pen impression. This method does not require the use of rubber gloves.

A tray for arthrocentesis can be prepared and kept available for use. This includes the following items: alcohol sponges; iodine or merthiolate; pHisoHex; sterile gauze dressings (2×2); sterile disposable 2-, 10-, and 20-ml syringes; 18- and 20-gauge 1½ inch needles; 20-gauge spinal needles; 25-gauge ½ inch needles; plain test tubes; heparinized tubes; vial of normal saline solution; clean microscope slides and coverslips; heparin to add to heparinized tubes if a large amount of inflammatory fluid is to be placed in the tube; fingernail polish to seal wet preparation; chocolate agar plates or Thayer-Martin medium; tryptic soy broth for most bacteria; anaerobic transport medium (replace periodically to keep culture media from becoming outdated); tubes with fluoride for glucose; plastic adhesive bandages; ethyl chloride; hemostat; tourniquet for drawing of simultaneous blood samples; and 1 percent lidocaine.

Articular. *Knee.* The knee is the easiest joint to inject. If fluid is to be aspirated, the patient should be in a supine position with the knee fully extended. The puncture mark is made just posterior to the medial portion of the patella, and an 18 to 20 g, 1½ inch needle directed slightly posteriorly and slightly inferiorly. The joint space should be entered readily and synovial fluid easily aspirated. On occasion thickened synovium or villous projections may occlude the opening of the needle, and it may be necessary to rotate the needle to facilitate aspiration of fluid. An infrapatellar plica, a vestigial structure that is also called the ligamentum mucosum, may prevent adequate aspiration of the knee when using the medial approach.[67] However, the plica should not adversely affect aspiration from the lateral aspect. If corticosteroid is injected, one should not have any feeling of obstruction as it is being injected. The supine technique is illustrated in Figure 37–1. The patient

Figure 37–1. Diagram of knee arthrocentesis. The needle is inserted just posterior to the medial portion of the patella and is directed slightly posteriorly and slightly inferiorly.

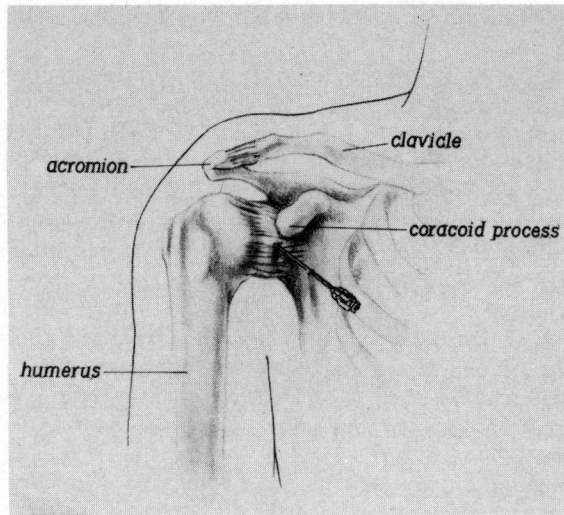

Figure 37–2. Diagram of shoulder arthrocentesis. With the shoulder externally rotated, the needle is inserted at a point just medial to the head of the humerus and slightly inferiorly and laterally to the coracoid process. The needle is then directed posteriorly and slightly superiorly and laterally.

should be relaxed if this technique is used. An anxious patient may tighten the patella to the point of making arthrocentesis very difficult. If this is the case or if fusion or osteophytes make the medial or lateral approaches to the knee joint very difficult, an easy technique, which usually avoids these problems, is to inject the knee with the patient sitting with the knee flexed. The mark is made at the medial aspect of the distal border of the patella, and the needle directed slightly superiorly towards the joint cavity. It is usually difficult to obtain fluid with this technique.

The suprapatellar "bursa" may be distended if a large amount of synovial fluid is present. In this instance, the "bursa" may be aspirated in a very easy and essential asymptomatic fashion.

Shoulder. The shoulder arthrocentesis is most easily accomplished with the patient sitting and the shoulder externally rotated. A mark is made just medial to the head of the humerus and slightly inferiorly and laterally to the coracoid process. A 20 to 22 g, 1½ inch needle is directed posteriorly and slightly superiorly and laterally. One should be able to feel the needle enter the joint space. If bone is hit, the operator should pull back and redirect the needle at a slightly different angle. This technique is illustrated in Figure 37–2.

The acromioclavicular joint may be palpated as a groove at the lateral end of the clavicle just medial to the shoulder. A mark is made and a 22 to 26 g, ⅝ to 1 inch needle is carefully directed inferiorly. Rarely is synovial fluid obtained.

The sternoclavicular joint is most easily entered from a point directly anterior to the joint. Caution is necessary to avoid a pneumothorax. The space is fibrocartilaginous and rarely can fluid be aspirated.

Ankle Joint. The patient should be supine and the leg-foot angle should be at 90 degrees. A mark is made just medial to the tibialis anterior tendon and lateral to the medial malleolus. A 20 to 22 g, 1½ inch needle is directed posteriorly and should enter the joint space easily without striking bone. Figure 37–3 illustrates injection of the ankle joint.

Subtalar Ankle Joint. Again, the patient is supine and the leg-foot angle is at 90 degrees. A mark is made just

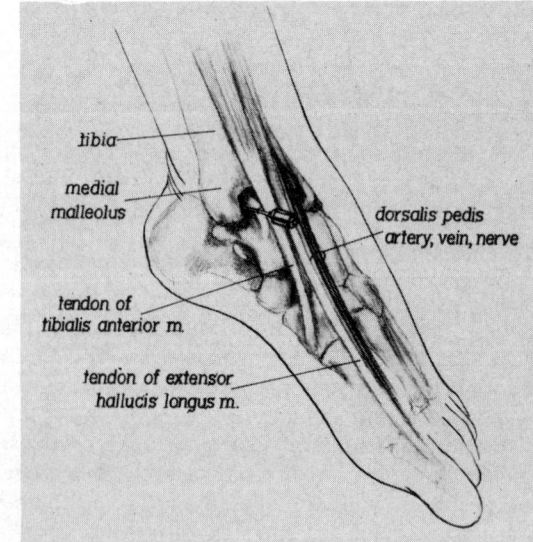

Figure 37–3. Diagram of ankle arthrocentesis. With the leg-foot angle at 90 degrees, the needle is inserted at a point just medial to the tibialis anterior tendon and just lateral to the medial malleolus. The needle is then directed posteriorly.

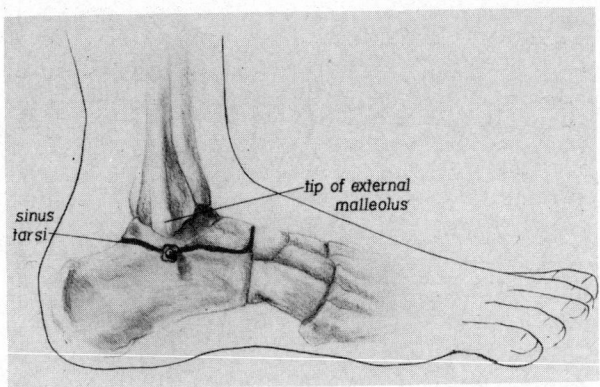

Figure 37–4. Diagram of ankle subtalar arthrocentesis. With the leg-foot angle at 90 degrees, the needle is inserted at a point just inferior to the tip of the lateral (external) malleolus and is directed perpendicularly.

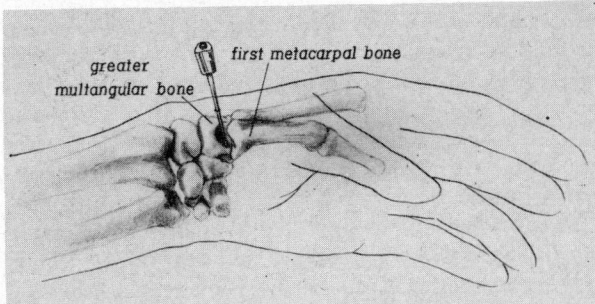

Figure 37–6. Diagram of first carpometacarpal arthrocentesis. The thumb is flexed across the palm toward the tip of the fifth finger. The needle is inserted at the base of the metacarpal bone away from the border of the snuffbox. It is then directed toward the proximal end of the fourth metacarpal.

inferior to the tip of the lateral malleolus. A 20 to 22 g, 1½ inch needle is directed perpendicular to the mark. With this joint, the needle may not enter the first time and another attempt or two may be necessary. Because of this and the associated pain, local anesthesia may be helpful. Figure 37–4 illustrates injection of this joint.

Wrist. This is a complex joint, but fortunately most of the intercarpal spaces communicate. A mark is made just distal to the radius and just ulnar to the so-called anatomic snuff box. Usually a 24 to 26 g, ⅝ to 1 inch needle is adequate, and the injection is made perpendicular to the mark. If bone is hit, the needle should be pulled back and slightly redirected toward the thumb. This type of injection is illustrated in Figure 37–5.

First Carpometacarpal Joint. Degenerative arthritis frequently involves this joint. Frequently the joint space

is quite narrowed, and arthrocenteses may be difficult and painful. A few simple maneuvers may make the injection fairly easy. The thumb is flexed across the palm toward the tip of the fifth finger. A mark is made at the base of the first metacarpal bone away from the border of the snuff box. A 22 to 26 g, ⅝ to 1 inch needle is inserted at the mark and directed towards the proximal end of the fourth metacarpal. This approach avoids hitting the radial artery. Figure 37–6 illustrates injection of this joint.

Metacarpophalangeal Joints and Finger Interphalangeal Joints. Synovitis in these joints usually causes the synovium to bulge dorsally, and a 24 to 26 g, ½ to ⅝ inch needle can be inserted on either side just under the extensor tendon mechanism. It is not necessary for the needle to be interposed between the articular surfaces. Some prefer having the fingers slightly flexed when injecting the metacarpophalangeal joints. It is unusual to obtain synovial fluid. When injecting corticosteroids, consider mixing them with a small amount of local anesthetic using the precautions previously discussed. This will distend the joint on all sides and possibly help prevent soft tissue atrophy. These injections are illustrated in Figure 37–7.

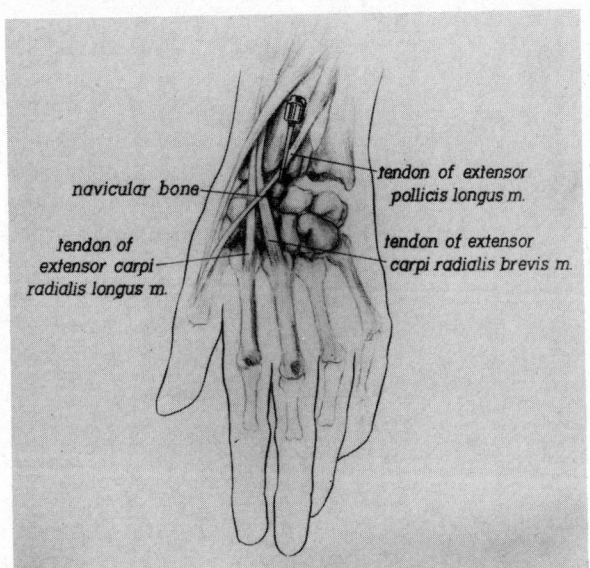

Figure 37–5. Diagram of wrist arthrocentesis. The needle is inserted at a point just distal to the radius and just ulnar to the anatomic snuffbox. It is then directed perpendicularly. If bone is hit, the needle should be pulled back and slightly redirected towards the thumb.

Figure 37–7. Diagram of metacarpophalangeal and interphalangeal arthrocenteses. With the digit straight or slightly flexed a small and short needle is inserted on either side just under the extensor tendon mechanism. It is not necessary for the needle to be interposed between the articular surfaces.

Metatarsophalangeal Joints and Toe Interphalangeal Joints. The techniques are quite similar to those of the metacarpophalangeal and finger interphalangeal joints, but many prefer to inject more dorsally and laterally to the extensor tendons. Marking the area(s) to be injected is helpful, as is gentle traction on the toe of each joint that is injected.

Elbow. A technique preferred by many is to have the elbow flexed at 90 degrees. The joint capsule will bulge if there is inflammation. A mark is made just below the lateral epicondyle of the humerus. A 22 g, 1 to 1½ inch needle is inserted at the mark and directed parallel to the shaft of the radius or can be directed perpendicular to the skin. Figure 37–8 illustrates these two approaches.

Hip. This is a very difficult joint to inject, even when using a fluoroscope as a guide. Rarely is the physician quite sure the joint has been entered; synovial fluid is rarely obtained. Two approaches can be used, anterior or lateral. A 20 g, 3½ inch spinal needle should be used for both approaches.

For the anterior approach, the patient is supine and the extremity fully extended and externally rotated. A mark should be made about 2 to 3 cms below the anterior superior iliac spine and 2 to 3 cms lateral to the femoral pulse. The needle is inserted at a 60-degree angle to the skin and directed posteriorly and medially until bone is hit. The needle is slightly withdrawn, and possibly a drop or two of synovial fluid can be obtained, indicating entry into the joint space.

Many prefer the lateral approach because the needle can "follow" the femoral neck into the joint. The patient is supine and the hips should be internally rotated—the knees apart and toes touching. A mark is made just anterior to the greater trochanter, and the needle is inserted and directed medially and slightly cephalad toward a point slightly below the middle of the inguinal ligament. One may feel the tip of the needle slide into the joint. Figure 37–9 illustrates the lateral approach to the hip joint.

Temporomandibular Joint. The temporomandibular joint is palpated as a depression just below the zygo-

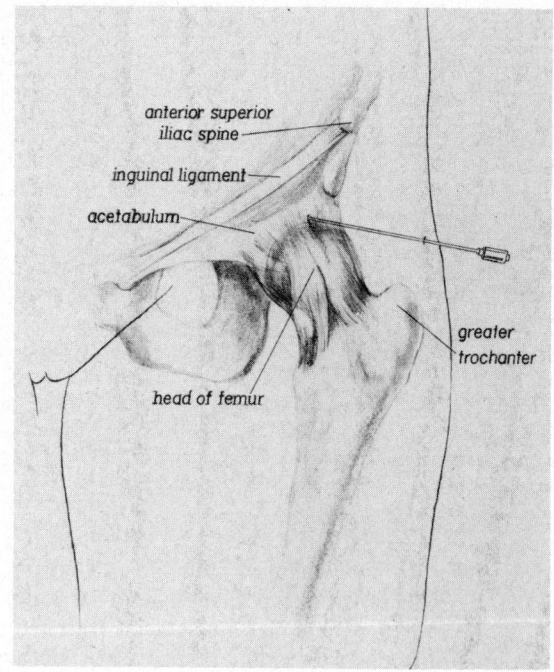

Figure 37–9. Diagram of hip arthrocentesis illustrating lateral technique. Using this technique, the patient is supine with the hips internally rotated—knees apart and toes touching. The needle is inserted just anterior to the greater trochanter and is directed medially and slightly cephalad toward a point slightly below the middle of the inguinal ligament. One may feel the needle slip into the joint. For the *anterior approach,* the patient is supine and the extremity fully extended and externally rotated. A mark is made 2 to 3 cm below the anterior superior iliac spine and 2 to 3 cm lateral to the femoral pulse. The needle is inserted at a 60-degree angle to the mark and directed posteriorly and medially until bone is hit.

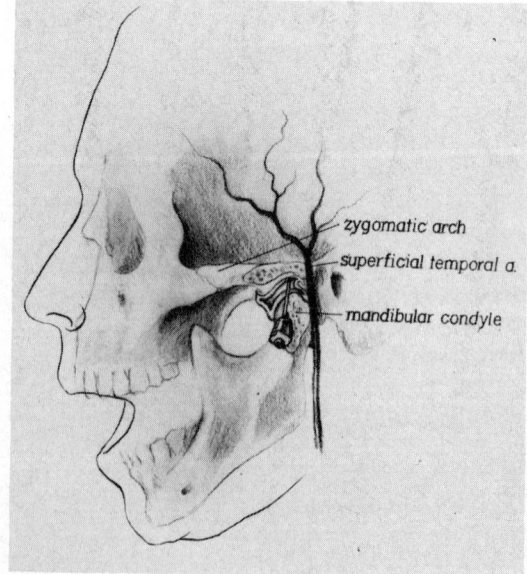

Figure 37–10. Diagram of temporomandibular arthrocentesis. With the mouth open, the joint space is palpated as a depression just below the zygomatic arch and 1 to 2 cm anterior to the tragus. The needle is inserted just perpendicular to the skin and directed slightly posteriorly and superiorly.

Figure 37–8. Diagram of elbow arthrocenteses illustrating parallel and perpendicular techniques. With the elbow flexed at 90 degrees, the needle is inserted just below the lateral epicondyle of the humerus and is directed parallel to the shaft of the radius, or it can be directed perpendicularly to the skin.

matic arch and 1 to 2 cms anterior to the tragus. The depression is more easily palpated by having the patient open and close the mouth. A mark is made and with the mouth open, a 22 g, ½ to 1 inch needle is inserted perpendicular to the skin and directed slightly posteriorly and superiorly. Figure 37–10 illustrates injection of the temporomandibular joint.

Nonarticular. *Shoulder.* Bicipital tendinitis can be treated by injecting the shoulder joint or by injecting the tendon sheath. The tendon is tender, is easily palpated in the bicipital groove of the humerus, and can be rolled from side to side. If it is elected to inject the sheath, the point of maximal tenderness is marked. A 22 g, 1½ inch needle is inserted in the sheath at the mark, and a portion of 0.5 ml of corticosteroid, with or without local anesthetic, is injected at this site. Then the needle is directed superiorly along the tendon, in the sheath, for about 2 to 3 cm, and more material is injected. The needle is then partially withdrawn and redirected inferiorly along the tendon for about 2 to 3 cm, and the remainder of the material injected. Figure 37–11 illustrates the bicipital tendon sheath injection.

Subacromial bursitis can be treated by injecting the shoulder joint or the bursa. The bursitis is frequently secondary to supraspinatus tendinitis. If only the subacromial bursa is to be injected, the most tender area is marked, and using a 20 to 22 g, 1 to 1½ inch needle, 0.5 ml corticosteroid with or without local anesthetic is injected. Calcification of the supraspinatus tendon may be present, and there may be an acute and severe pain. In this circumstance, one should consider aspirating and irrigating the bursa using a 16 to 18 g, 1½ inch needle.

Then 0.5 to 1.0 ml of corticosteroid with or without local anesthetic can be injected. Figure 37–12 illustrates the injection of the subacromial bursa.

The supraspinatus tendon can be directly injected by palpating the groove between the acromium and the humerus on the lateral aspect of the shoulder and marking this spot. Then a 20 to 22 g, 1 to 1½ inch needle is directed medially on a horizontal plane for about 2.5 cm and 0.5 ml of corticosteroid and 2.5 to 4.0 ml of local anesthetic injected. The technique of injecting the supraspinatus tendon is also illustrated in Figure 37–12.

Elbow. Lateral epicondylitis, or "tennis elbow," can be very painful, disabling, and chronic. With the elbow flexed and pronated, there is usually marked tenderness to palpation of a small area on the anterolateral surface of the external condyle of the humerus. This spot should be marked. A 20 to 22 g, 1 to 1½ inch needle is inserted about 2 cm distal to the mark, and 0.5 ml of corticosteroid mixed with 4 to 4.5 ml local anesthetic is injected in several small doses by injecting, withdrawing, redirecting the needle, and reinjecting the mixture. The injection of a "tennis elbow" is shown in Figure 37–13.

"Nodule." A nodule—for example, in the olecranon region or on the proximal aspect of the extensor surface of the ulna—may be a diagnostic dilemma: is it a tophus or a rheumatoid nodule? A simple punch needle biopsy should answer the question. Figure 37–14 illustrates the technique. Prepare the nodule with an antiseptic solution. Then insert a disposable 18 to 20 g, 1 to 1½ inch needle at a 90-degree angle and rotate it. The needle is then retracted almost completely and is inserted at a

Figure 37–11. Diagram of bicipital tendon sheath injections. At the point of maximal tenderness, the needle is inserted just under the sheath, and corticosteroid, with or without local anesthetic, is injected. The needle can then be directed superiorly and then inferiorly, with further injections at each site.

Figure 37–12. Diagram of subcromial bursa and supraspinatus tendon injections. For the subacromial bursa, the most tender area is palpated, and the needle is inserted directly into this area. To inject the supraspinatus tendon, the groove between the acromium and the humerus on the lateral aspect of the shoulder is palpated. The needle is inserted at this point and directed medially on a horizontal plane for 2.5 cm, and the materials are injected at this point.

Figure 37–13. Diagram of "tennis elbow" injection(s). With the elbow flexed and pronated, the needle is inserted at the most tender area on the anterolateral aspect of the external condyle of the humerus. A combination of corticosteroid and local anesthetic is injected in several areas.

45-degree angle and again rotated (Fig. 37–14A). Repeat this in three other quadrants of the nodule. Remove the needle from the nodule and slightly loosen it. Pull back on the syringe plunger to the 2 to 3 ml level, tighten the needle, and expel the contents onto a microscopic slide. In addition, use a 25 g needle to pick out collected material from the biopsy needle (Fig. 37–14B). Examine the specimen under the microscope for sodium urate crystals, preferably using polarizing filters. With a little

Figure 37–14. Diagram of punch needle biopsy of forearm nodule. The needle is inserted at a 90-degree angle and is rotated. The needle is then retraced almost completely, and is inserted at a 45-degree angle. Repeat this in three other quadrants (A). The contents of the needle are placed on a microscopic slide (B) and examined.

experience, you can virtually exclude the possibility of a tophus if no crystals are observed.

Wrists and Hands. Aspiration of a ganglion on the dorsal aspect of the wrist is done by using an 18 g, 1½ inch needle. After as much material as possible is aspirated, 0.5 to 1.0 ml of an intra-articular corticosteroid is injected.

De Quervain's disease (stenosing tenosynovitis of the extensor pollicis brevis and abductor pollicis longus) may be helped by injection. The most tender area in the region of the radial styloid is located by performing a modified Finkelstein's test, clasping the fingers over the thumb and gradually flexing the wrist in ulnar deviation. The most tender point is marked. Then a 22 g, 1½ inch needle is inserted about 1 cm proximal to the most tender spot and directed almost parallel to the skin toward the styloid process. As the needle is being advanced in the tendon sheath, 0.5 ml of corticosteroid and 2.5 ml of local anesthetic can be injected.

Trigger fingers are usually associated with chronic stenosing tenosynovitis of the finger flexor tendons. The main pathology usually lies over the head of the metacarpal bones in the palm, and a localized swelling may be palpated in this area. A mark is made over the palmar aspect of the metacarpal head, a 22 g, 1½ inch needle is inserted at a 45-degree angle and then directed proximally, almost parallel to the skin, and a mixture of 0.5 ml of both corticosteroid and local anesthetic is injected. Lack of resistance during injection should indicate proper needle placement.

Carpal tunnel syndrome injections should not be performed by an inexperienced operator. Theoretically, an injection of a long-acting corticosteroid directly into the medial nerve will damage it. If one elects to perform the procedure, a mark is made over the carpal tunnel just on the ulnar side of the long palmar tendon. A 25 g, ⅝ inch needle is directed perpendicular to the mark and inserted its full length. If the needle meets obstruction, or if the patient experiences paresthesias, the needle should be withdrawn and redirected in a more ulnar fashion. An injection of 0.5 ml corticosteroid may give benefit. The carpal tunnel may be injected again, but if relief is short-lived, surgery should be considered.

Hip. With trochanteric bursitis, there is an area that is tender to palpation in the region of the greater trochanter of the femur. After marking this area, a 20 to 22 g, 1½ to 3½ inch needle is inserted perpendicular to the skin directly into the tender area(s). Since several bursae may be inflamed, it is usually more effective to inject several areas superior and inferior to the mark with a mixture of 0.5 to 1.0 ml corticosteroid and 4.5 to 9.0 ml local anesthetic.

Knee. Anserine bursitis produces pain on the medial aspect of the tibia. In this same region may be noted pain from a fat pad, from another bursa, or from medial collateral ligament strain. All may benefit from injection. The point of maximal tenderness is marked. A 20 to 22 g, 1½ inch needle is inserted perpendicular to the skin and continued until bone is hit. It is then withdrawn slightly

Aspiration and Injection of Joints and Soft Tissues

and 0.25 to 0.50 ml corticosteroid and 2.5 to 4.5 ml local anesthetic injected.

The prepatellar bursa is easily aspirated. An 18 g, 1½ inch needle is recommended because sometimes the fluid is very gelatinous and difficult to obtain through a small-bore needle. After aspirating as much fluid as possible, 0.5 to 1.0 ml corticosteroid is injected. On occasion very little fluid is obtained during the initial aspiration, but reaspiration 24 hours after corticosteroid injection may yield a large amount of fluid.

Pelvis. When inflamed, the ischial (ischiogluteal) bursa is usually easily palpated as a tender area when the patient is lying on his side with the knees flexed. Theoretically this position will cause the ischium to be more exposed and the gluteal muscles and sciatic nerve to be pulled away. The point of maximal tenderness is marked, and 0.5 to 1.0 ml corticosteroid and 2.5 to 4.0 ml of local anesthetic are mixed in a syringe with a 20 g, 3½ inch needle attached. It is helpful to "fix" the skin over the mark. Then the needle is inserted into the mark until bone is hit. The needle is withdrawn slightly and all the mixture injected; alternatively, the needle is redirected in one or two other directions and portions of the mixture injected.

Iliopectineal (iliopsoas) bursitis, as previously mentioned, must be differentiated from psoas abscess, femoral hernia, and septic arthritis of the hip. If one elects to inject the bursa, a 20 to 22 g, 3½ inch spinal needle is used. Many use the technique of hip arthrocentesis. A dose of 0.5 to 1.0 ml of corticosteroid is injected with or without 4 to 4.5 ml local anesthetic.

Back. The "fibrositis syndrome" and the "trigger points" of the back have been briefly discussed. These "trigger points" can be marked and each injected with 0.25 ml corticosteroid or 1 ml or more of local anesthetic, or as many physicians prefer, a combination of the two. The shorter-acting corticosteroids, in contrast to the repository forms, have been recommended.[59] The physician must be careful to avoid injury to the underlying structures.

Foot. Achilles tendinitis may respond to injection. If this is done, a 22 g, 1½ inch needle is inserted just under the tendon sheath and a mixture of 0.25 ml corticosteroid and 2.5 ml local anesthetic injected. Direct injection of the tendon should be avoided.

An inflammation of the subcutaneous Achilles bursa between the skin and tendon is usually readily palpable, can be marked, and should be easily aspirated with a 20 g, 1 inch needle. The retrocalcaneal bursa is located between the Achilles tendon and the posterior facet of the calcaneus. A lateral or medial approach is probably better. Careful injection of either location with 0.25 to 0.50 ml corticosteroid with or without local anesthetic is usually beneficial.

Calcaneal bursitis can be treated by inserting a 20 g, 1½ inch needle perpendicular to the plantar surface of the midcalcaneal region, pushing the needle in until bone is hit, withdrawing slightly, and injecting 0.5 ml corticosteroid and 3.5 ml local anesthetic.

References

1. Hollander, J.L.: Arthrocentesis and intrasynovial therapy. *In* McCarty, D.J. (ed.): Arthritis and Allied Conditions. Philadelphia. Lea and Febiger, 1979.
2. Hollander, J.L.: The local effects of compound F(hydrocortisone) injected into joints. Bull. Rheum. Dis. 2:3, 1951.
3. Young, H.H., Ward, L.E., and Henderson, E.D.: The use of hydrocortisone acetate (compound F acetate) in the treatment of some common orthopaedic conditions. J. Bone Joint Surg. 36A:602, 1954.
4. Hollander, J.L., Jessar, R.A., and Brown, E.M., Jr.: Intrasynovial corticosteroid therapy: A decade of use. Bull. Rheum. Dis. 11:239, 1961.
5. Hollander, J.L.: Intrasynovial corticosteroid therapy in arthritis. Maryland State Med. J. 19:62, 1970.
6. Ragan, C., Howes, E.L., Plotz, C.M., Meyer, K., Blunt, J.W., and Lattes, R.: The effect of ACTH and cortisone on connective tissue. Bull. N.Y. Acad. Med. 26:251, 1950.
7. Jessar, R.A., Ganzell, M.A., and Ragan, C.: The action of hydrocortisone in synovial inflammation. J. Clin. Invest. 32:480, 1954.
8. de Duve, C., Wattiaux, R., and Wibo, M.: Effects of fat-soluble compounds on lysosomes in vitro. Biochem. Pharmacol. 9:97, 1962.
9. Weissman, G., and Thomas, L.: Studies on lysosomes: II. The effect of cortisone on the release of acid hydrolases from a large granule fraction of rabbit liver induced by an excess of vitamin A. J. Clin. Invest. 42:661, 1963.
10. Weissmann, G.: The role of lysosomes in inflammation and disease. Ann. Rev. Med. 18:97, 1967.
11. Wright, D.G., and Malawista, S.E.: Mobilization and extracellular release of granular enzymes from human leukocytes during phagocytosis: Inhibition by colchicine and cortisol but not by salicylate. Arthritis Rheum. 16:749, 1973.
12. Mandell, G.L., Rubin, W., and Hook, E.W.: The effect of an NADH oxidase inhibitor (hydrocortisone) on polymorphonuclear leukocyte bacterial activity. J. Clin. Invest. 49:1381, 1970.
13. Wiener, E., Marmary, Y., and Curelaru, Z.: The in vitro effect of hydrocortisone on the uptake and intracellular digestion of particulate matter by macrophages in culture. Lab. Invest. 26:220, 1972.
14. Persellin, R.H., and Ku, L.C.: Effects of steroid hormones on human polymorphonuclear leukocyte lysosomes. J. Clin. Invest. 54:919, 1974.
15. Stevenson, R.D.: Mechanism of anti-inflammatory action of glucocorticosteroids. Lancet. 1:225, 1977.
16. Lewis, G.P., and Piper, P.J.: Inhibition of release of prostaglandins as an explanation of some of the actions of anti-inflammatory corticosteroids. Nature 254:308, 1975.
17. Kantrowitz, F., Robinson, D.R., McGuire, M.B. and Levine, L.: Corticosteroids inhibit prostaglandin production by rheumatoid synovia. Nature 258:737, 1975.
18. Tashjian, A.H., Jr., Voelkel, E.F., McDonough, J., and Levine, L.: Hydrocortisone inhibits prostaglandin production by mouse fibrosarcoma cells. Nature 258:739, 1975.
19. Gryglewski, R.J.: Steroid hormones, anti-inflammatory steroids, and prostaglandins. Pharmacol. Res. Commun. 8:337, 1976.
20. Hong, S.-C.L., and Levine, L.: Inhibition of arachidonic acid release from cells as the biochemical action of anti-inflammatory corticosteroids. Proc. Natl. Acad. Sci. 73:1730, 1976.
21. Gryglewski, R.J., Panczenko, B., Korbut, R., Grodzinska, L., and Ocetkiewicz, A.: Corticosteroids inhibit prostaglandin release from perfused mesenteric blood vessels of rabbit and from perfused lungs of sensitized guinea pig. Prostaglandins 10:343, 1975.
22. Kuehl, F.A., Jr., and Egan, R.W.: Prostaglandins, arachidonic acid, and inflammation. Science 210:978, 1980.
23. Butler, W.T., and Rossen, R.D.: Effect of corticosteroids on immunity in man. I. Decreased serum IgG concentration caused by 3 or 5 days of high doses of methylprednisolone. J. Clin. Invest. 52:2629, 1973.
24. Atkinson, J.P., and Frank, M.M.: Effect of cortisone therapy on serum complement components. J. Immunol. 111:1061, 1973.
25. Hunder, G.G., and McDuffie, F.C.: Effect of intra-articular hydrocortisone on complement in synovial fluid. J. Lab. Clin. Med. 79:62, 1972.
26. Goetzl, E.J., Bianco, N.E., Alpert, J.S., Sledge, C.B., and Schur, P.H.: Effects of intra-articular corticosteroids in vivo on synovial fluid variables in rheumatoid synovitis. Ann. Rheum. Dis. 33:62, 1974.
27. Dick, W.C., Whaley, K., St. Onge, R.A., Downie, W.W., Doyle, J.A., Nuki, G., Gillespie, F.C., and Buchanan, W.W.: Clinical studies on inflammation in human knee joints: Xenon (Xe133) clearances correlated with clinical assessment in various arthritides and studies on the effect of intra-articular administered hydrocortisone in rheumatoid arthritis. Clin. Sci. 38:123, 1970.
28. DeCeulaer, K., Balint, G., El-Ghobarey, A., and Dick, W.C.: Effects of corticosteroids and local anaesthetics applied directly to the synovial vascular bed. Ann. Rheum. Dis. 38:440, 1979.
29. Eymontt, M.J., Gordon, G.V., Schumacher, H.R., and Hansell, J.R.: The

effects on synovial permeability and synovial fluid leukocyte counts in symptomatic osteoarthritis after intra-articular corticosteroid administration. J. Rheumatol. 9:198, 1982.

30. Chandler, G.N., and Wright, V.: Deleterious effect of intra-articular hydrocortisone. Lancet 2:661, 1958.

31. Chandler, G.N., Wright, V., and Hartfall, S.J.: Intra-articular therapy in rheumatoid arthritis. Comparison of hydrocortisone tertiary butyl acetate and hydrocortisone acetate. Lancet 2:659, 1968.

32. Mankin, H.J., and Conger, K.A.: The acute effects of intra-articular hydrocortisone on articular cartilage in rabbits. J. Bone Joint Surg. 48A:1383, 1966.

33. Bentley, G., and Goodfellow, J.W.: Disorganization of the knees following intra-articular hydrocortisone injections. J. Bone Joint Surg. 51B:498, 1969.

34. Moskowitz, R.W., Davis, W., Sammarco, J., Mast, W., and Chase, S.W.: Experimentally induced corticosteroid arthropathy. Arthritis Rheum. 13:236, 1970.

35. Mankin, H.J., Zarins, A., and Jaffe, W.L.: The effect of systemic corticosteroids on rabbit articular cartilage. Arthritis Rheum. 15:593, 1972.

36. Behrens, F., Shepard, N., and Mitchell, N.: Alteration of rabbit articular cartilage by intra-articular injections of glucocorticosteroids. J. Bone Joint Surg. 57A:70, 1975.

37. Gibson, T., Barry, H.C., Poswillo, D., and Glass, J.: Effect of intra-articular corticosteroid injections on primate cartilage. Ann. Rheum. Dis. 36:74, 1976.

38. Tenenbaum, J., Pritzker, K.P.H., Gross, A.E., Cheng, P-T, Renlund, R.C., and Tenenbaum, H.: The effects of intraarticular corticosteroids on articular cartilage. Sem. Arthritis Rheum. 11:140, Suppl. 1, 1981.

39. Sweetnam, R.: Corticosteroid arthropathy and tendon rupture (editorial) J. Bone Joint Surg. 51B:397, 1969.

40. Wrenn, R.N., Goldner, J.L., and Markee, J.L.: An experimental study of the effect of cortisone on the healing process and tensile stength of tendons. J. Bone Joint Surg. 36A:588, 1954.

41. McCarty, D.J.: Treatment of rheumatoid joint inflammation with triamcinolone hexacetonide. Arthritis Rheum. 15:157, 1972.

42. McCarty, D.J., Jr., and Hogan, J.M.: Inflammatory reaction after intrasynovial injection of microcrystalline adrenocorticosteroid esters. Arthritis Rheum. 7:359, 1964.

43. Koehler, B.F., Urowitz, M.B., and Killinger, D.W.: The systemic effects of intra-articular corticosteroid. J. Rheum. 1:117, 1974.

44. Gottlieb, N.L., and Riskin, W.G.: Complications of local corticosteroid injections. JAMA 243:1547, 1980.

45. Carson, T.E., Daane, T.A., Lee, P.A., Tredway, D.R., and Wallin, J.D.: Effect of intramuscular triamcinolone acetonide on the human ovulatory cycle. Cutis 19:633, 1977.

46. Cunningham, G.R., Goldzieher, J.W., de la Pena, A., and Oliver, M.: The mechanism of ovulation inhibition by triamcinolone acetonide. J. Clin. Endocrinol. Metab. 46:8, 1978.

47. McCarty, D.J., Jr.. A basic guide to arthrocentesis. Hosp. Med. (Nov.) 4:77, 1968.

48. Gottlieb, N.L.: Hypodermic needle separation during arthrocentesis. Arthritis Rheum. 24:1593, 1981.

49. Fitzgerald, R.F., Jr.: Intrasynovial injection of steroids. Mayo Clin. Proc. 51:655, 1976.

50. Miller, J.H., White, J., and Norton, T.H.: The value of intra-articular injections in osteoarthritis of the knee. J. Bone Joint Surg. 40B:636, 1958.

51. Friedman, D.M., and Moore, M.F.: The efficacy of intra-articular corticosteroid for osteoarthritis of the knee. Arthritis Rheum. 21:556, 1978.

52. Utsinger, P.D., Resnick, D., Shapiro, R.F., and Wiesner, K.B.: Roentgenologic, immunologic, and therapeutic study of erosive (Inflammatory) osteoarthritis. Arch. Intern. Med. 138:693, 1978.

53. McCarty, D.J.: Intrasynovial therapy with adreno-corticosteroid esters. Wis. Med. J. 77:875, 1978.

54. Henderson, E.D., and Henderson, C.C.: The use of hydrocortisone acetate (compound F acetate) in the treatment of post-traumatic bursitis of the knee and elbow. Minn. Med. 36:142, 1953.

55. Gray, R.G., Kiem, I.M., and Gottlieb, N.L.: Intratendon sheath corticosteroid treatment of rheumatoid arthritis-associated and idiopathic hand flexor tenosynovitis. Arthritis Rheum. 21:92, 1978.

56. Steinbrocker, O.: Management of some non-articular rheumatic disorders. Mod. Treatment 1:1254, 1964.

57. Steinbrocker, O., and Neustadt, D.H.: Aspiration and injection therapy in arthritis and musculoskeletal disorders. Hagerstown, Md., Harper and Row, 1972.

58. Smythe, H.A., and Moldofsky, H.: Two contributions to understanding of the "fibrositis" syndrome. Bull. Rheum. Dis. 28:928, 1977.

59. Brown, B.B., Jr.: Diagnosis and therapy of common myofascial syndromes. JAMA 239:646, 1978.

60. Clark, C.B.: Cubital tunnel syndrome. JAMA 241:801, 1979.

61. Lapidus, P.W., and Guidotti, F.P.: Report on the treatment of one hundred and two ganglions. Bull. Hosp. Joint Dis. 28:50, 1967.

62. Phalen, G.S.: Soft tissue affection of the hand and wrist. Hosp. Med. 7:47, 1971.

63. Blau, S.P.: All those joint pains may not be arthritis. Drug Therapy (Nov.) 1976, p. 144.

64. Swartout, R., and Compere, E.L.: Ischiogluteal bursitis. JAMA 227:551, 1974.

65. Hucherson, D.C., and Freeman, G.E., Jr.: Iliopectineal bursitis: A cause of hip pain frequently unrecognized. Am. J. Orthop. 4:220, 1962.

66. Kaplan, P.E., and Kernahan, W.T.: Tarsal tunnel syndrome. J. Bone Joint Surg. 63A:96, 1981.

67. Hardaker, W.T., Whipple, T.L., and Bassett, F.H.: Diagnosis and treatment of the plica syndrome of the knee. J. Bone Joint Surg. 62A:221, 1980.

Chapter 38
Synovial Fluid Analysis

H. Ralph Schumacher

INTRODUCTION

Joint fluid examination is to evaluation of joint disease as urinalysis is to renal disease. Analysis of joint fluid should be performed as part of the diagnostic evaluation in any patient with joint disease. Even small amounts of joint fluid can be aspirated and systematically examined. One to three drops of synovial fluid can be obtained from virtually any first MTP joint, for example.[1]

Some common diseases such as gout, pseudogout, septic arthritis, and systemic lupus erythematosus, as well as other less common diseases, can be quickly and definitively diagnosed by examination of joint fluid. Even if joint fluid examination is not diagnostic in other patients, it can be one of the most useful of a battery of clinical and laboratory tests used in differential diagnosis. Gross examination and leukocyte count as described later allow narrowing of diagnostic possibilities to the diseases causing "noninflammatory" effusions; "inflammatory" fluids, including septic effusions; and hemarthroses (Tables 38–1 to 38–3).

Even in patients in whom the diagnosis has been established, synovianalysis can show clues to new developments such as low-grade infection in a joint of a patient with lupus erythematosus or rheumatoid disease,

superimposition of calcium pyrophosphate crystal deposition in osteoarthritis, or crystals of intra-articularly injected steroids causing a transient crystal-induced synovitis.

TABLE 38–1. "NONINFLAMMATORY" JOINT EFFUSIONS (LEUKOCYTE COUNT LESS THAN 2000 PER CUBIC MILLIMETER)

Osteoarthritis
Traumatic arthritis
Acromegaly
Gaucher's disease
Hemochromatosis
Hyperparathyroidism
Ochronosis
Paget's disease
Mechanical derangement
Erythema nodosum
Villonodular synovitis, tumors
Aseptic necrosis
Ehlers-Danlos syndrome
Sickle cell disease
Amyloidosis
Hypertrophic pulmonary osteoarthropathy
Pancreatitis
Osteochondritis dissecans
Charcot's joints
Wilson's disease
Epiphyseal dysplasias

TABLE 38–2. INFLAMMATORY JOINT EFFUSIONS (LEUKOCYTE COUNT GREATER THAN 2000 PER CUBIC MILLIMETER)

Rheumatoid arthritis
Psoriatic arthritis
Reiter's syndrome
Ulcerative colitis
Regional enteritis
Postileal bypass arthritis
Ankylosing spondylitis
Juvenile rheumatoid arthritis
Rheumatic fever
Collagen-vascular disease
   Systemic lupus erythematosus
   Scleroderma
   Polymyositis
   Polychondritis
   Polyarteritis
Polymyalgia rheumatica
Giant cell arteritis
Sjögren's syndrome
Wegener's granulomatosis
Goodpasture's syndrome
Henoch-Schönlein purpura
Familial Mediterranean fever
Whipple's disease
Behçet's syndrome
Erythema nodosum
Sarcoidosis
Multicentric reticulohistiocytosis
Erythema multiforme (Stevens-Johnson)
Postsalmonella, shigella, yersinia arthritis
Infectious arthritis
   Parasitic
   Viral (hepatitis, mumps, rubella, others)
   Fungal
   Mycoplasmal
   Bacterial (staphylococcal, gonococcal, tuberculous, others)
   Treponemal
Carcinoid
Subacute bacterial endocarditis
Crystal-induced arthritis
   Gout
   Pseudogout
   Post-intra-articular steroid injection
   Hydroxyapatite arthritis
Hyperlipoproteinemias
Serum sickness
Agammaglobulinemia
Leukemia
Hypersensitivity angiitis
Palindromic rheumatism

TABLE 38–3. HEMARTHROSIS

Trauma with or without fractures
Pigmented villonodular synovitis
Synovioma, other tumors
Hemangioma
Charcot joint or other severe joint destruction
Hemophilia or other bleeding disorders
Von Willebrand's disease
Anticoagulant therapy
Myeloproliferative disease with thrombocytosis
Thrombocytopenia
Scurvy
Ruptured aneurysm
Arteriovenous fistula
Idiopathic

Only by examining the joint fluid can one be best informed about what is occurring in that joint. Abnormal blood tests such as rheumatoid factor, antinuclear antibodies, and elevated uric acid can be misleading and do not establish the nature of disease in the joint.

Normal joint fluid is described in detail in Chapter 16. Briefly, normal synovial fluid is an ultrafiltrate of plasma, with only small amounts of larger molecular weight proteins such as fibrinogen, beta 1C globulin, and other globulins, to which has been added hyaluronate-protein produced in the synovial membrane. Normal fluid is compared with that seen in various diseases in Table 38–4.

TECHNIQUE FOR ARTHROCENTESIS

The techniques used, appropriate precautions, and routes for arthrocentesis are described in Chapter 37.

If no fluid is identified in the syringe after attempted aspiration, try to express a drop of blood or tissue fluid from the needle. One can use such a single drop for examination for crystals, Gram stain, or culture. If no fluid is obtained and infection is suspected, irrigate the joint with a small amount of normal saline and culture this irrigating fluid. The patient should be fasting if synovial fluid and serum glucose are to be compared.

Consider the studies most likely to be helpful in each case before arthrocentesis and prepare a list of priorities for the fluid obtained. Not all tests by any means need be performed on each specimen.

GROSS EXAMINATION

This can partly be done at the bedside to help plan which of the other studies are most pertinent and should be done on small volume effusions.

Volume. The amount of effusion can help serve as one measure of the severity of arthritis and can be used for comparison with previous arthrocenteses. Low volume does not mean absence of an important intra-articular process. Effusions may be difficult to aspirate because of thick fibrin, rice bodies, and other debris. Fluid may be loculated and not accessible by the route chosen.

Viscosity. This is estimated by watching the synovial fluid as it is slowly expressed from the syringe and by manipulating several drops of fluid between the thumb and index finger. Fluid of normal viscosity holds together and stretches to a string of 1 to 2 inches before separating. Low-viscosity fluid drips from a syringe like water. Recent studies show that viscosity is less reliable than previously thought in classification of effusions.[3] Very viscous fluid is seen in hypothyroid effusions and in ganglia. Viscosity is generally decreased in inflammation but also is low in edema fluid. Greater degrees of quantitation are generally not needed; but if they are desired, a simple technique using a white blood cell diluting pipette has been described.[3] Viscosity tends to parallel the concentration of hyaluronate, which is measured as uronic acid as a research tool.[2] In purulent effusions the massive numbers of leukocytes may make the fluid seem more viscous. The usual patterns of viscosity and many of the other examination findings are given in Table 38–4. Hyaluronidase can be used to de-

Table 38–4. Classification of Synovial Effusions*

Gross Examination	Normal	"Noninflammatory" (Group I)	Inflammatory (Group II)	Septic (Group III)
Volume (ml) (knee)	< 3.5	Often > 3.5	Often > 3.5	Often > 3.5
Viscosity	High	High	Low	Variable
Color	Colorless to straw	Straw to yellow	Yellow	Variable
Clarity	Transparent	Transparent	Translucent	Opaque
Routine laboratory examination				
WBC (mm³)	< 200	200 to 2000	2000 to 75,000	Often > 100,000†
PMN leukocytes (%)	< 25	< 25	> 50 often	> 75†
Culture	Negative	Negative	Negative	Often positive
Mucin clot	Firm	Firm	Friable	Friable
Glucose (AM fasting)	Nearly equal to blood	Nearly equal to blood	< 50 mg% lower than blood	> 50 mg% lower than blood

*See Tables 38–1 and 38–2 for diseases in the noninflammatory and inflammatory groups.
†WBC and % PMN leukocytes will be less if organism is less virulent or partially treated.

crease synovial fluid viscosity before performing other tests, provided that the normal values using this enzyme have been standardized in the laboratory. Hyaluronidase use reportedly gives slightly higher synovial fluid leukocyte counts.[4]

Color and Clarity (Fig. 38–1). If print cannot be read easily through the fluid, the effusion is cloudy and this should suggest an inflammatory process. The plastic of some syringes makes fluids appear falsely cloudy, so fluids should be examined in glass. The value of gross examination in classifying effusions is summarized in Table 38–4. Generally, the more cloudy fluids have more cells, but not all very cloudy or opaque fluids are inflammatory. Microscopic examination is still needed to be certain that the opacity is not due to massive numbers of crystals, triglycerides, fibrin, amyloid, or cartilage fragments. Sometimes chronically inflamed joints have effusions containing rice bodies, which might also be confused grossly with pus. Rice bodies are end results of synovial proliferation and degeneration; they contain collagen, cell debris, and fibrin (Fig. 38–2, Plate IV, p. xxxviii).

Ochronotic fluid may be speckled with dark particles ("ground pepper" sign).[5] Black or gray debris from metal or plastic fragments after prosthetic arthroplasty can also discolor the fluid.[6]

Rheumatoid and other chronic effusions occasionally have a greenish hue; pigmented villonodular synovitis can be grossly bloody or may produce an orange-brown color. Gouty fluid tends to be unusually white when it contains massive amounts of crystals. Streaks of blood are the result of injury to a small vessel during the procedure. Causes of diffusely bloody fluid are listed in Table 38–3. Partially treated or low-grade infection can make the synovial fluid look like any other moderately inflammatory but not purulent fluid. Very slightly inflammatory or clear fluids are common in systemic lupus erythematosus, rheumatic fever, polymyositis, and scleroderma and can be seen in the interim between attacks of gout and pseudogout.

LEUKOCYTE COUNT

Quantitation of the synovial fluid leukocyte count is a very important part of synovial fluid analysis, especially as it is the major basis for classification of an effusion as "septic," "inflammatory," or "noninflammatory" (Table 38–4). Note the many important systemic diseases such as hypertrophic pulmonary osteoarthropathy and sickle cell disease that can be associated with noninflammatory effusions. Synovial fluid leukocyte counts along with volumes can be used as a rough measure of the intensity of inflammation in sequential samples.

The standard white blood cell (WBC) counting chamber and techniques are used, except that ordinary WBC counting fluid should be replaced with normal or 0.3 percent saline. The 0.3 percent saline will lyse erythrocytes. The acid of ordinary WBC counting fluid clots synovial fluid and gives inaccurate leukocyte counts. The fluid should be placed in a heparinized tube and shaken to mix it thoroughly. The count must be done promptly, as there may be some spontaneous clotting and clumping of leukocytes. A small amount of methylene blue can be added for easier identification of leukocytes. Rheumatoid arthritis fluid usually has leukocyte counts from 2000 to 75,000. Counts over 60,000 should raise a suspicion of infection. However, it should be noted that partially treated infections or "low-grade" infections with gonococci, mycobacteria, and fungi often have lower leukocyte counts. Patients with rheumatoid disease, Reiter's syndrome, and crystal-induced arthritis may have counts over 100,000 WBC per cubic millimeter.

Figure 38–1. Synovial effusions. *A,* Normal or edema fluid is clear, pale yellow, or colorless. Print is easily read through the tube. *B,* Fluid from noninflammatory joint disease is yellow and clear. *C,* An inflammmatory effusion is cloudy and yellow. Print may be blurred or completely obliterated, depending on the number of leukocytes. The effusion is translucent. *D,* A purulent effusion from septic arthritis contains a dense clump that does not even allow light through the many leukocytes. *E,* Hemorrhagic fluid is red. The supernatant may be darker yellow-brown (xanthochromic). A traumatic tap is less uniform and often has blood streaks.

Leukocyte counts of 200 to 2000 per cubic millimeter have generally been termed noninflammatory. Actually, truly normal joint fluid usually has only up to 50 WBC per cubic millimeter, so that counts over 200 clearly represent at least a low-grade inflammatory response, which is seen, for example, in some patients with osteoarthritis. Patients who have predominantly degenerative arthritis, as in hemochromatosis, can have "inflammatory" effusions with high WBCs if associated chondrocalcinosis leads to crystal-induced arthritis. The significance of occasional erythrocytes has not been evaluated. Noncrenated red cells may have been introduced by the arthrocentesis.

Figure 38–3. Synovial fluid leukocytes with cytoplasmic inclusions, "ragocytes," that have been felt to represent phagocytic vacuoles. Inclusions can appear pale or dark depending on focus.

MICROSCOPIC STUDIES

Wet Preparation. Probably the single most important step in synovial fluid analysis is prompt microscopic examination of a fresh drop of synovial fluid as a wet preparation. Even if only a single drop of fluid is obtained with aspiration, this can be examined for crystals and other constituents as a wet preparation and then the same fluid allowed to dry for staining with Gram's stain if required. Express 1 to 3 drops of unadulterated synovial fluid from the syringe or transfer the fluid with a flamed loop onto a clean glass slide. We usually examine uncentrifuged fluids, but examination of a button after centrifugation can help concentrate rare crystals or cells in a clear-appearing fluid. Dirty slides can be washed in acetone and air dried. Lens paper used to clean slides can introduce birefringent paper fibrils.

Cover the drops of synovial fluid with a glass cover slip. If any delay is expected before examination, the cover slip margins may be sealed with nail polish. This allows several hours of delay, but slides may still dry out and produce birefringent drying artifacts if left overnight. Remember that the nail polish at the margins is birefringent with polarized light.

Regular Light Microscopy. First examine each joint fluid with regular light microscopy. Red and white cells can be noted and their numbers estimated. Fragments of cartilage can be seen and, if numerous enough, concentrated by centrifugation and fixed for staining as a biopsy. Some leukocytes will be seen to contain cytoplasmic inclusions (Fig. 38–3) that have been felt to represent distended phagosomes and/or lipid droplets. Such cytoplasmic inclusion-containing cells[7] or "ragocytes" were first detected in rheumatoid arthritis but are also seen in other inflammatory arthropathies. Staining with fluorescein-conjugated antibodies to immunoglobulins and complement has shown these materials in vacuoles of some synovial fluid cells in rheumatoid arthritis and other diseases.

Erythrocytes may be noted to be sickled in patients with sickle cell disease or trait, but this does not establish that their current effusion is due to the sickle cell disease.

A variety of fibrillar materials can be seen in joint fluids. Some of these fibrils are fibrin, whereas others can be shown to be collagen from synovium or cartilage fragments.[8,9] Such fibrils (and crystals) can often be seen better by lowering the condenser or closing the diaphragm to produce a partial phase effect. Both collagen and fibrin are faintly birefringent. Ferrography has also been used to concentrate and analyze cartilage wear fragments.[10] Dark, irregularly shaped metal fragments can be seen in effusions of patients with implant arthroplasties.[6] Polymer fragments might also be seen.[11] The rare shards of ochronotic cartilage are yellow or ochre fragments with regular transmitted light microscopy[12] (Fig. 38–4, Plate IV, p. xxxviii).

Large numbers of lipid droplets may be noted in traumatic arthritis,[13,14] in inflammatory effusions of various types, including some otherwise unexplained effusions,[15] and in pancreatic fat necrosis,[16] or a few droplets can simply result from the arthrocentesis. Fat droplets should rise to the top of a spun specimen. Oil red O will stain lipid red. The origin and full significance of lipid droplets is not yet clear. In trauma some lipid presumably comes from marrow and synovium. Marrow spicules may be found if fracture into the joint has occurred. Such spicules tend to adhere to glass and must be sought carefully.[17]

Amorphous globular and irregular material, usually without birefringence, can be seen and can be due to amyloid masses[18] in patients with primary amyloid, multiple myeloma, and Waldenström's macroglobulinemia. Congo red will stain this pink or red on the wet preparation. Other globular or "coinlike" clumps can be seen from hydroxyapatite aggregates in joint and bursa fluids.[19] Apatite often appears to be phlogistic in bursae and joints.

Crystals can be noted with regular light microscopy and may be especially well seen with the illumination low or with the help of phase microscopy. Urate crystals are often acicular but may be blunt rods. Calcium pyrophosphate crystals can be rods or rhomboids. Other crystals also occasionally occur in joint fluids. All these crystals can be further differentiated with compensated polarized light.

Compensated Polarized Light Microscopy.[20,21] In a polarized light microscope, ordinary incandescent light is oriented in a single plane by a polarizer over the light source. When a second polarizer is added and rotated

90 degrees to the first, all light is blocked and the microscope field viewed through the ocular appears totally dark. If crystalline (birefringent) material is placed in the light path between the polarizers, light is deflected and split into fast and slow rays vibrating at different angles from the incident light. The vibration planes of these two new rays are mutually perpendicular, but neither is parallel to the original ray of plane polarized light. Some of these rays now pass through the second polarizer (also termed the analyzer) and are brightly visible on the dark field. This brightness is common to all birefringent material.

In clinical use different birefringent materials such as crystals can be distinguished in part by the altered behavior of light that passes through another birefringent structure (the compensator) placed between the first polarizer and the specimen. The compensator generally used is a "first order red plate," which eliminates green from the background and produces a rose-colored, instead of black, background field. The first order red compensator quality and thickness can be expressed numerically as 540 nm. If the slow ray of a birefringent crystal is parallel to the slow ray from the compensator, the additive effect of a urate or pyrophosphate crystal creates a value of about 700 nm and a blue color. If the same crystal is now rotated 90 degrees so that its fast ray is parallel to the compensator's slow ray, a color subtraction of the same number of nanometers will give a yellow color.

Monosodium urate crystals can be differentiated from calcium pyrophosphate dihydrate (CPPD) because with urate crystals the fast ray is in the long axis of the crystal, giving a yellow color when the crystal axis is parallel to the slow ray of the compensator. This is termed a negative optical sign or negative birefringence. CPPD crystals have their slow ray in the long axis of the crystal, and thus when parallel to the axis of slow vibration of the compensator they appear blue.

Monosodium urate crystals of gout tend to be 3 to 20μ long, rod or needle shaped, and very brightly negatively birefringent (Fig. 38–5, Plate IV, p. xxxviii). Crystals are generally identifiable within cells during active gouty arthritis. Crystals obtained from puncturing a tophus in a joint or elsewhere are often longer needles that are predominantly extracellular. Calcium pyrophosphate crystals have a weaker birefringence, are rarely as long as urates, are often rhomboid, and normally exhibit a blue color when the crystal axis is parallel to the slow ray of the compensator (i.e., positive optical sign or positive birefringence) (Fig. 38–6, Plate IV, p. xxxviii).

A variety of other birefringent materials will be seen on polarized light examinations of joint fluids. Depot corticosteroid preparations are crystalline[22] and can remain in joints or adjacent connective tissue for long periods after local injections. These crystals can be phagocytized and occasionally induce a transient inflammation several hours after intra-articular injections (Fig. 38–7), Plate V, p. xxxix). Corticosteroid crystals can appear as positively or negatively birefringent rods similar in size to urates or CPPD, as granules, or as irregular debris. Most other irregular birefringent material is artifact, such as dust from the slide or cover slip. Powder from rubber gloves is birefringent and generally shows a Maltese cross appearance.

Erroneous use of an oxalate[23] or lithium heparin[24] anticoagulant can introduce anticoagulant-derived crystals. Such crystals can be phagocytized by leukocytes in vitro and can thus be seen intracellulary. Oxalate and lithium heparin crystals are positively birefringent.

Cholesterol crystals can be seen in chronic joint effusions, especially in rheumatoid arthritis.[25] Crystals are usually platelike with a notch in one corner (Fig. 38–8, Plate V, p. xxxix) and larger than a cell, but crystals in cholesterol-laden effusions can occasionally also be negatively birefringent needles. Oxalate crystals recently described in joint effusions of patients with chronic renal failure may be pleomorphic but typically include some large bipyramidal forms.[26]

Calcium hydrogen phosphate dihydrate crystals are brightly positively birefringent and have been identified in joint fluids and tissues.[27,28] These crystals might be confused with CPPD and can only be definitely differentiated by x-ray diffraction. Apatite crystal clumps occasionally have some birefringence.

Commercial polarizing microscopes are readily available and should generally be used.[20] One can also obtain polarizing filters to be inserted in a regular light microscope. One filter is placed between the light source and condenser; another is placed above the objective or in the eyepiece. Filters are rotated until a black field is obtained. This produces the white birefringence that shows crystals more easily than ordinary light but cannot separate positive and negative birefringence. An effect similar to that obtained with a commercial compensated polarizing microscope can be achieved by applying two layers of cellophane tape to the top of a clean glass slide and placing this over the polarizing filter above the light source.[29,30] The long axis of the slide then is substituted for the axis of slow vibration of the first order red compensator. Some variation has been noted with different tapes; newer tapes that appear semiopaque before use do not appear to work. Before using such a set-up, findings should be clinically compared on several crystals with the findings using a commercial compensator.

Absolutely definitive diagnosis of crystals is made only by x-ray diffraction, but sufficient numbers of crystals are needed for this. Uricase digestion may be helpful in that urates but not other crystals will be digested with uricase.[31] Fortunately this is rarely required. Occasionally crystals of urate or CPPD are so few or so small that they are detected only by electron microscopy.(EM)[32,33] Urate crystals are dissolved out in usual electron microscopic preparations, but CPPD crystals are not. Individual apatite crystals can only be seen by EM. Electron diffraction or electron probe analysis can be done on such crystals, but techniques for this are less well standardized than those for x-ray diffraction.[19] Infrared spectroscopy using Fourier transformation or electron microscopy can identify small amounts of crystals mixed with other predominant crystals.

Dried Smears for Staining. Synovial smears are made using 1 to 2 drops of heparinized fluid on slides or coverslips in the same manner as with peripheral blood smears. If the leukocyte count is greater than approximately 5000, a good smear can generally be made from the whole fluid. Fluids with lower counts often produce better smears if the fluid is centrifuged and the button is resuspended in a few drops of the supernatant before smearing. It should be allowed to air dry.

Wright's Stain. For this single most useful stain, cover the smear with Wright's stain and let it stand for 2 minutes. Add distilled water to the stain on the slide until a metallic sheen appears. Let this stand 4 to 5 minutes, wash with distilled water, air dry, and examine.

Smears should be examined briefly under low magnifications to look for such findings as LE cells. LE cells have so far been reported frequently in systemic lupus erythematosus and only very rarely in rheumatoid arthritis, but they need not be present in typical systemic lupus erythematosus. Round, homogeneous hematoxylin bodies might also suggest lupus erythematosus, although their specificity has not been evaluated in synovial fluids. Cartilage and synovial fragments may be seen and should be examined for any characteristic changes. Iron-laden chondrocytes have been seen in a cartilage fragment in hemochromatosis. Blue to brown pigmented debris or brown cytoplasmic granules can be seen in ochronosis. Bone marrow spicules with fat cells or other marrow elements may also be seen.

The smear is next examined carefully under oil immersion. Cells can be separated into polymorphonuclear leukocytes, monocytes, small lymphocytes, and large mononuclear cells. The latter probably include some transformed lymphocytes, monocytes, and synovial lining cells. Although classification of individual large mononuclear cells may be difficult, it may be worth attempting, since transformed lymphocytes are seen in rheumatoid arthritis and not in acute gout or pseudogout.[34] Other diseases have received insufficient study. Synovial lining cells (Fig. 38–9, Plate V, p. xxxix) typically are 20 to 40 μ in diameter, with an eccentric nucleus that occupies less than 50 percent of the cytoplasm. Some large monocyte-derived cells are similar in size, although they often have larger nuclei. These two large mononuclear cells can best distinguished with nonspecific esterase or Sudan black stains,[35] since these stains are positive in monocytes but not in most lining cells. Other large cells (15 to 25 μ in diameter) that have nuclei filling the majority of the cytoplasm and are Sudan negative are the transformed lymphocytes or lymphoblasts (Fig. 38–10, Plate V, p. xxxix). Both the lining cells and lymphoblasts often have prominent nucleoli. Mononuclear cells in joint fluid can now also be classified by monoclonal antibodies.[36] The percentage of polymorphonuclear cells (PMN) is helpful in distinguishing some diseases (see Table 38–4). Among the inflammatory effusions, lower polymorphonuclear cell counts have been seen in early rheumatoid arthritis, systemic lupus erythematosus, rheumatic fever, scleroderma, and chronic infections such as tuberculosis. Lin-

ing cells or large monocytes can be seen to have phagocytized polymorphonuclear leukocytes in a variety of diseases in which there are both exudation of neutrophils and lining cell proliferation. Such cells are common in Reiter's syndrome but are by no means diagnostic (Fig. 38–11). A variety of unidentified cells are also seen. These require further study, as they may be clues to presently unrecognized processes or mechanisms occurring in some patients. Dark purple inclusions in phagocytic cells can be from cell debris but also can be clumps of apatite crystals. Bacteria can occasionally be seen in cells even with Wright's stain. Urate or calcium pyrophosphate crystals can often be seen in Wright's stained specimens, although the urates are dissolved out of some smears.

Eosinophils are uncommon in differential counts, having been reported after arthrography with just air or contrast medium,[37,38] but also occasionally in a variety of other effusions.[37] Malignant cells can occasionally be identified in synovial fluid with Wright's or the Papanicolaou stain.[39]

Gram's Stain. Smears for Gram's stain are made as for Wright's stain. Sometimes the addition of a single drop of serum to the slide prior to the drying stage allows better adherence of organisms. Flame the smear, specimen side down, three times through a blue flame. Let it cool and then flood the slide with crystal violet for 1 minute. Wash the slide with water, then flood with Gram's iodine and let it stand for 2 minutes. Pour off the iodine and wash the slide with 95 percent alcohol until it runs off clear. Flood the slide with Safranin for 30 seconds, wash it with water, and air dry. Bacteria can be quickly classified into broad groups, but mucin artifacts can be confusing. The absence of bacteria on Gram's stain is much too common in infection and does not rule out a septic joint.

Figure 38–11. "Reiter's cell." This is a phagocytic mononuclear cell with its nucleus marked (N) that has phagocytized a polymorpho nuclear leukocyte (arrow) with a pyknotic nucleus.

Other Stains. Ziehl-Neelsen stain may be helpful in evaluation of possible tuberculosis, although cultures and synovial biopsy are often needed. Fat stains and alcian blue–PAS stains for proteoglycans (mucopolysaccharide) may show deposition of these materials in synovial macrophages. Other stains that may be useful include a Prussian blue stain that may show iron in synovial lining cells in pigmented villonodular synovitis or in hemochromatosis.

Amyloid deposits stained with Congo red show an apple-green birefringence on polarized light examination of wet smears of synovial fluid or of paraffin-embedded specimens.

The Von Kossa stain or Alizarin red S[40] will stain calcium- and phosphate-containing CPPD crystals or clumps of apatite crystals.

SPECIAL TESTS

Mucin Clot Test.[41] Several drops of synovial fluid are added to about 20 ml of 5 percent acetic acid in a small beaker. Allow 1 minute for a "clot" to form and then shake the beaker. A good clot from normal or osteoarthritic fluid forms a firm mass that does not fragment on shaking. A poor clot, like those that result from many inflammatory effusions, fragments easily and forms flakes, shreds, and cloudiness in the surrounding fluid. Effusions from patients with systemic lupus erythematosus and rheumatic fever, although mildly inflammatory, often have good mucin clots.

Good mucin generally reflects the normal integrity of hyaluronate. Poor mucin indicates both dilution and destruction of hyaluronate protein (see Table 38–4). Unfortunately the mucin test and viscosity give only rough clues and are not as reliable as leukocyte counts in classification of effusions.

Glucose. Synovial fluid glucose can be measured by the standard Somogyi-Nelson true glucose method or the ortho-toluidine method and should be done simultaneously on fasting serum and synovial fluid for comparison[41] (see Table 38–4). Synovial fluid glucose concentration is normally very slightly less than that of blood glucose. Equilibration between blood and synovial fluid after a meal is slow and unpredictable, so that fasting levels are most reliable. Effusions for glucose should be placed in a fluoride tube to stop glucose metabolism in vitro by the synovial fluid leukocytes, which would further lower the glucose level. Glucose measurements should not have a high priority, but a very low level of glucose in the synovial fluid suggests joint infection. Most effusions in rheumatoid arthritis have a synovial fluid sugar level of less than half that of the blood, and some will be near zero.

Complement. Total hemolytic complement is determined by the technique of Kabat and Mayer.[42,43] Synovial fluid complement is predominantly of value when compared with serum levels and with serum and synovial fluid protein determinations. Fluid must be centrifuged promptly and the supernatant stored at $-70°$ C. In rheumatoid arthritis the serum complement is usually normal, while the synovial fluid level is often less than 30 percent of this.

In systemic lupus erythematosus and hepatitis both serum and synovial fluid levels may be low. Synovial fluid complement levels in infectious arthritis, gout, and Reiter's syndrome may be high, but this is largely due to elevated serum levels. Beta$_1$ globulin can also be measured by immunodiffusion in addition to or instead of hemolytic complement. Prompt storage at $-70°$ C is not as critical with this. It is useful to measure serum and synovial fluid protein[44] and globulin levels when evaluating complement, because synovial fluid complement may be very low in normal or noninflammatory fluids in which there is little escape of complement or other proteins into the joint space from the circulation.

Cultures. Prompt and careful culture of synovial fluid is very important if there is any suspicion of infection. Most bacteria will grow well in tryptic soy broth or sheep blood agar. Planting the cultures at the time of aspiration may be useful if prompt transport and handling in the laboratory cannot be assured. Try to obtain laboratory help in planning cultures needed. If certain organisms are a possibility, specific media are necessary. If anaerobic organisms are suspected, expel any air from the syringe and use anaerobic transport medium and/or take the fluid directly to the laboratory for planting on prereduced anaerobically sterile blood agar or a comparable culture medium.

Gonococci can be successfully cultured in only 25 to 30 percent of cases of apparent gonococcal arthritis. When this is suspected, plate the fluid immediately on chocolate agar or Thayer-Martin medium and have the culture continued in the laboratory under CO_2. There are CO_2 transport systems if delay is expected. If a mixed infection is possible, Thayer-Martin medium should retard the growth of organisms other than gonococci.

For suspected fungal infections the fluid should be transported in a sterile tube and processed in the laboratory for culture on Sabouraud's dextrose agar. Lowenstein-Jensen medium is used for mycobacterial infections.

Other Tests. Antinuclear factors, rheumatoid factor, immunoglobulins, and other substances involved in immune reactions can be measured in synovial fluid, but these assays have so far added little to the simple studies described here. Antinuclear factors, for example, are seen in synovial effusions in many conditions in which they are not identifiable in serum. Latex fixation tests for rheumatoid factor are occasionally positive in effusions when negative in the serum. However, the significance of such positive synovial fluids is not established. Several causes for false-positive tests for rheumatoid factor in synovial fluid have been described.[45] Immune complexes can be measured with a variety of techniques but are still largely investigational.

Other studies are not of much diagnostic value. The pH of normal fluid is 7.4, and this is slightly lower in inflammation.[46] Joint fluid pO_2 also falls in many inflammatory conditions. This tends to correlate with severity of leukocytosis and also with synovial fluid volume, which may lower pO_2 by affecting blood flow to the joint.[47] Total protein normally averages only 1.7 g per dl, but rises with inflammation. Uric acid, electrolytes, and urea nitrogen tend to reflect the serum values. Fibrinogen and its products are normally absent, so that normal fluid does not clot upon standing. Bence Jones kappa light chains have been demonstrated in amyloid arthropathy secondary to multiple myeloma. For research lymphokines, fibronectin, proteinases, and prostaglandins can be assayed in joint fluid.

Gas chromatography on synovial fluid has been suggested as an aid in identifying bacterial products in culture-negative infections.[48] Elevated synovial fluid lactic acid measurements have been found in untreated nongonococcal septic arthritis.[49] Succinic acid levels are also elevated in septic arthritis and tend to persist even after treatment.[50] Neither lactic nor succinic acid is specific for infection but may complement other tests for early diagnosis of infectious arthritis. Bacterial antigens can also be sought in synovial fluid by counter immunoelectrophoresis.

References

1. Agudelo, C.A., Weinberger, A., Schumacher, H.R., Turner, R., and Molina, J.: Definitive diagnosis of gout by identification of urate crystals in asymptomatic metatarsophalangeal joints. Arthritis Rheum. 22:559, 1979.
2. Bitter, T., and Muir, H.M.: A modified uronic acid carbazole reaction. Anal. Biochem. 4:330, 1962.
3. Hasselbacher, P.: Measuring synovial fluid viscosity with a white blood cell diluting pipette. Arthritis Rheum. 19:1358, 1978.
4. Palmer, D.G.: Total leukocyte enumeration in pathologic synovial fluids. Am. J. Clin. Pathol. 49:812, 1968.
5. Hunter, T., Gordon, D.A., and Ogryzlo, M.A.: The ground pepper sign of synovial fluid; a new diagnostic feature of ochronosis. J. Rheum. 1:45, 1974.
6. Kitridou, R., Schumacher, H.R., Sbarbaro, J.L., and Hollander, J.L.: Recurrent hemarthrosis after prosthetic knee arthroplasty: Identification of metal particles in the synovial fluid. Arthritis Rheum. 12:520, 1969.
7. Hollander, J.L., McCarty, D.J., and Rawson, A.J.: The "RA cell," "ragocyte," or "inclusion body cell." Bull. Rheum. Dis. 16:382, 1965.
8. Kitridou, R., McCarty, D.J., Prockop, D.J., and Hummeler, K.: Identification of collagen in synovial fluid. Arthritis Rheum. 12:580, 1969.
9. Cheung, H.S., Ryan, L.M., Kozin, F., and McCarty, D.J.: Identification of collagen subtypes in synovial fluid sediments from arthritic patients. Am. J. Med. 68:73, 1980.
10. Evans, C.H., Mears, D.C., and Stanitski, C.L.: Ferrographic analysis of wear in human joints. J. Bone Joint Surg. 64B:572, 1982.
11. Crugnola, A., Schillar, A., and Radin, E.: Polymeric debris in synovium after total joint replacement: Histological identification. J. Bone Joint Surg. 59A:860, 1977.
12. Schumacher, H.R., and Holdsworth, D.E.: Ochronotic arthropathy. I. Clinicopathologic studies. Semin. Arthritis Rheum. 6:207, 1977.
13. Graham, J., and Goldman, J.A.: Fat droplets and synovial fluid leukocytes in traumatic arthritis. Arthritis Rheum. 21:76, 1978.
14. Weinberger, A., Schumacher, H.R.: Experimental joint trauma: Synovial response to blunt trauma and inflammatory response to intra-articular injection of fat. J. Rheum. 8:380–389, 1981.
15. Reginato, A.J., Schumacher, H.R., Allan, D., and Rabinowitz, J.L.: Acute monoarthritis with lipid liquid crystals. Arthritis Rheum. 25:S35, 1982 (Abst).
16. Gibson, T., Schumacher, H.R., Pascual, E., and Brighton, C.: Arthropathy, skin and bone lesions in pancreatic disease. J. Rheum. 2:7, 1975.
17. Lawrence, C., and Seife, B.: Bone marrow in joint fluid: A clue to fracture. Ann. Intern. Med. 74:740, 1971.
18. Gordon, O.A., Pruzanski, W., and Ogryzlo, M.A.: Synovial fluid examination from the diagnosis of amyloidosis. Ann. Rheum. Dis. 32:428, 1973.
19. Schumacher, H.R., Somlyo, A.P., Tse, R.L., and Maurer, K.: Apatite crystal associated arthritis. Ann. Intern. Med. 87:411, 1977.
20. Phelps, P., Steele, A.D., and McCarty, D.J.: Compensated polarized light microscopy. JAMA 203:508, 1968.
21. Gatter, R.A.: Use of the compensated polarizing microscope. Clin. Rheum. Dis. 3:91, 1977.
22. Kahn, C.B., Hollander, J.L., and Schumacher, H.R.: Corticosteroid crystals in synovial fluid. JAMA 211:807, 1970.
23. Schumacher, H.R.: Intracellular crystals in synovial fluid anticoagulated with oxalate. N. Engl. J. Med. 274:1372, 1966.
24. Tanphaichitr, K., Spilberg, I., and Hahn, B.: Lithium heparin crystals simulating calcium pyrophosphate dihydrate crystals in synovial fluid. Arthritis Rheum. 19:966, 1976 (letter).
25. Zuckner, J., Uddin, J., Gantner, G.E., and Dorner, R.W.: Cholesterol crystals in synovial fluid. Ann. Intern. Med. 60:436, 1964.
26. Hoffman, G., Schumacher, H.R., Paul, H., Cherian, V., Reed, R., Ramsay, A., and Franck, W.: Calcium oxalate microcrystalline associated arthritis in end stage renal disease. Ann. Int. Med. 97:36–42, 1982.
27. Moskowitz, R.W., Harris, B.K., Schwartz, A., and Marshall, G.: Chronic synovitis as a manifestation of calcium crystal deposition disease. Arthritis Rheum. 14:109, 1971.
28. Gaucher, A., Faure, G., Netter, P., Pourel, J., and Duheille, J.: Identification des cristaux observés dans les arthropathies destructrices de la chondrocalcinose. Rev. Rheum. 44:407, 1977.
29. Owen, D.S.: A cheap and useful compensated polarizing microscope. N. Engl. J. Med. 285:115, 1971.
30. Fagan, T.J., and Lidsky, M.D.: Compensated polarized light microscopy using cellophane adhesive tape. Arthritis Rheum. 17:256, 1974.
31. McCarty, D.J., and Hollander, J.L.: Identification of urate crystals in gouty synovial fluid. Ann. Intern. Med. 54:452, 1961.
32. Schumacher, H.R., Jimenez, S.A., Gibson, T., Pascual, E., Traycoff, R.B., Dorwart, B.B., and Reginato, A.J.: Acute gouty arthritis without urate crystals identified on initial examination of synovial fluid. Arthritis Rheum. 18:603, 1975.
33. Honig, S., Gorevic, P., Hoffstein, S., and Weissmann, G.: Crystal deposition disease, diagnosis by electron microscopy. Am. J. Med. 63:161, 1977.
34. Traycoff, R.B., Pascual, E., and Schumacher, H.R.: Mononuclear cells in human synovial fluid. Identification of lymphoblasts in rheumatoid arthritis. Arthritis Rheum. 19:743, 1976.
35. Shehan, H., and Storey, G.: An improved method of staining leukocyte granules with Sudan black. Br. J. Pathol. Bacteriol. 59:336, 1947.
36. Duclos, M., Zeidler, H., Liman, W., Pichler, W.J., Rieber, P., and Peter, H.H.: Characterization of blood and synovial fluid lymphocytes from patients with rheumatoid arthritis and other joint diseases by monoclonal antibodies (OKT Series) and acid α-naphthyl esterase staining. Rheum. Internat. 2:75, 1982.
37. Hasselbacher, P., and Schumacher, H.R.: Synovial fluid eosinophilia following arthrography. J. Rheum. 5:173, 1978.
38. Murray, R.C., and Forrai, E.: Transitory eosinophilia localized in the knee joint after pneumarthrography. J. Bone Joint Surg. 32B:74, 1950.
39. Fam, A.G., Kolin, A., and Lewis, A.J.: Metastatic carcinomatous arthritis and carcinoma of the lung. J. Rheum. 7:98, 1980.
40. Paul, H., Reginato, A.J., and Schumacher, H.R.: Alizarin red S staining as a screening test to detect calcium compounds in synovial fluid. Arthritis Rheum. 26:191, 1983.
41. Ropes, M.M., and Bauer, W.: Synovial Fluid Changes in Joint Disease. Cambridge, Mass., Harvard University Press, 1953.
42. Pekin, I., and Zvaifler, N.J.: Hemolytic complement in synovial fluid. J. Clin. Invest. 43:1372, 1964.
43. Townes, A.S., and Sowa, J.M.: Complement in synovial fluid. Johns Hopkins Med. J. 125:23, 1970.
44. Bunch, T.W., Hunder, G.G., McDuffie, F.C., O'Brien, P.C., and Markowitz, H.: Synovial fluid complement determination as a diagnostic aid in inflammatory joint disease. Mayo Clin. Proc. 49:715, 1974.
45. Seward, C.W., and Osterland, C.K.: The pattern of anti-immunoglobulin activities in serum, pleural and synovial fluids. J. Lab. Clin. Med. 81:230, 1973.
46. Ward, T.T.: Acidosis of synovial fluid correlates with synovial fluid leukocytosis. Am. J. Med. 64:933, 1978.
47. Richman, A.I., Su, E.Y., and Ho, G.: Reciprocal relationship of synovial fluid volume and oxygen tension. Arthritis Rheum. 24:701, 1981.
48. Brooks, J.B., Kellogg, D.S., Alley, C.C., Short, H.B., Handsfield, H.H., and Huff, B.: Gas chromatography as a potential means of diagnosing arthritis. I. Differentiation between staphylococcal, streptococcal, gonococcal and traumatic arthritis. J. Infect. Dis. 129:660, 1974.
49. Brook, I.: Abnormalities in synovial fluid of patients with septic arthritis detected by gas-liquid chromatography. Ann. Rheum. Dis. 39:168, 1980.
50. Borenstein, D.G., Gibbs, C.A., and Jacobs, R.P.: Gas-liquid chromatographic analysis of synovial fluid. Arthritis Rheum. 25:947, 1982.

Chapter 39

Radiographic Evaluation of Articular Disorders

Robert O. Cone, III, and Donald Resnick

INTRODUCTION

The radiographic examination is a keystone in the diagnosis and management of the patient with articular disease. In some patients the diagnosis may initially be suggested by radiographic techniques, while in other patients with a known clinical diagnosis, the extent and the severity of the disease process may be documented by such techniques. Furthermore, serial radiographic examinations provide evidence of the therapeutic response of the disease process.

In this chapter we will discuss radiographic techniques and modalities and cardinal roentgen signs of articular disease as well as the radiographic findings at specific "target" areas of the major articular disorders.

RADIOGRAPHIC TECHNIQUES AND MODALITIES

Plain Film Examination. Appropriately selected plain films form the initial step in the radiologic evaluation of articular disease. The choice of radiographic projections for each anatomic area is a decision that deserves careful consideration. The need for a comprehensive examination to document the extent and configuration of the disease must be balanced with the consideration of expense, comfort, and radiation exposure to the patient, who may be expected to have numerous radiographic examinations over many years.

In most cases multiple radiographic projections of a number of joints are indicated. In Table 39–1, the suggested radiographic projections for the optimal evaluation of specific anatomic areas are listed. In the patient with monoarticular or pauciarticular disease, such a list may be closely followed. In the patient with polyarticular disease, however, obtaining the numerous radiographic views listed in Table 39–1 would be considered excessive in almost all cases. In these patients the initial radiographic examination should be individually tailored to as great an extent as is possible.

A "tailored" arthritis series is useful in those patients with polyarthritis who have either a known or a highly likely clinical diagnosis. In this setting, plain films are selected that most optimally visualize the major "target" areas of the disease as well as additional areas of clinical significance. For example, the patient with rheumatoid arthritis requires careful radiographic evaluation of the hands, wrists, feet, knees, shoulders, and cervical spine, whereas the patient with calcium pyrophosphate dihy-

drate (CPPD) crystal deposition disease usually requires analysis of only the hands, wrists, knees, and symphysis pubis.

The situation often arises in which a patient has polyarthritis without a specific clinical diagnosis. In this case, a "standard" arthritis series is useful. In this radiographic series, projections are selected to provide adequate visualization of a large number of major target areas with a minimum of radiation exposure. A suggested standard arthritis series, consisting of fifteen radiographs, is listed in Table 39–2.

The follow-up radiographic examination obtained during the course of treatment does not need to be as extensive as the initial survey. In many cases it can be limited to a few symptomatic areas or areas where unsuspected progression of disease may lead to catastrophic consequences, such as the cervical spine in patients with rheumatoid arthritis.

The intensifying screen in a radiographic film cassette combined with double emulsion radiographic film allows formation of a radiographic image with considerably less radiation exposure to the patient. A small decrease in radiographic resolution, however, is the price that is paid for this considerable diminution in radiation exposure. Occasionally, in evaluating diseases such as rheumatoid

Table 39–1. Radiographic Projections

Hand	Posteroanterior, oblique
Wrist	Posteroanterior, oblique, lateral
Elbow	Anteroposterior, lateral
Shoulder	Anteroposterior with internal rotation of the humerus; anteroposterior with external rotation of the humerus
Foot	Anteroposterior, oblique, lateral (including calcaneus)
Ankle	Anteroposterior, lateral
Knee	Anteroposterior, lateral, "tunnel" (anteroposterior in semiflexion), axial patellar ("sunrise")
Hip	Anteroposterior of pelvis, anteroposterior of hip with internal rotation of leg, anteroposterior of hip with external rotation of leg ("frog leg")
Sacroiliac Joint	Anteroposterior, anteroposterior with 30 degrees cephalic angulation of central ray
Lumbar Spine	Anteroposterior, obliques, lateral, lateral coned-down to L5-S1
Thoracic Spine	Anteroposterior, lateral
Cervical Spine	Anteroposterior, obliques, lateral with neck in flexion, lateral with neck in extension, "open-mouth" odontoid view

Table 39–2. Arthritis Survey

Hand and Wrist	Posteroanterior, obliques
Feet	Anteroposterior (2), obliques (2), lateral (2)
Knees	Anteroposterior (2), lateral (2)
Pelvis and Hips	Anteroposterior
Thorax and Shoulders	Anteroposterior
Cervical Spine	Lateral with neck in flexion

arthritis, osteomyelitis, septic arthritis, or hyperparathyroidism, increased resolution may be important in establishing a diagnosis at an early stage.[1-3] In these instances, increased radiation exposure to a relatively radioresistant area of the body, such as the hand, the wrist, or the foot, may be acceptable in order to obtain important diagnostic information. With virtually any radiographic unit, use of single emulsion film and a nonscreen vacuum-packed cassette will allow high-resolution images to be obtained. Furthermore, optical or radiographic magnification can be extremely helpful. In the latter case, these images may be obtained using microfocal spot radiographic tubes, such as are present on many angiographic units, or specially designed magnification units. It should be emphasized that these are specialized techniques and should be used only in selected clinical situations.

Radiographs of an articulation obtained during weight-bearing or the application of stress or traction may provide valuable supplemental information to the plain film radiographic examination. Weight-bearing views of the knees are especially useful in the evaluation of patients with osteoarthritis[4] and may allow a more exact delineation of cartilaginous loss as well as abnormal varus or valgus angulation of the joint. Stress radiographs may be utilized to assess soft tissue and bony stability following injury to the knee, ankle, acromioclavicular joint, or first metacarpophalangeal joint.[5] Upright lateral radiographs of the lumbar spine obtained after prolonged standing may accentuate bony neural arch defects (spondylolysis) or intervertebral slippage (spondylolisthesis). Radiographs of the pelvis obtained with the patient standing on one leg at a time may demonstrate instability of the sacroiliac joint or symphysis pubis.[6]

Radiographs obtained during application of traction across a joint may prove useful in selected circumstances. Subtle transchondral fractures in osteonecrosis of the femoral head may be accentuated with this technique.[7] Such traction may also stimulate the release of gas, primarily nitrogen, into the joint cavity, an occurrence that usually excludes the presence of a joint effusion and allows visualization of a portion of the cartilaginous surface.

Conventional Tomography. Conventional tomography can aid in the identification of subtle abnormalities as well as in the more precise delineation of previously identified lesions. In some anatomic areas, such as the temporomandibular, sternoclavicular, and costovertebral articulations, plain radiographs are rarely adequate and tomography is often indicated.

Arthrography and Bursography. Injection of radiopaque contrast material or air, or both, into a joint or bursa may be essential in evaluating a number of articular disorders.[8] Contrast arthrography is most often utilized in the knee and shoulder to identify surgically repairable soft tissue injuries such as meniscal or rotator cuff tears. Aspiration-arthrography allows confirmation of suspected joint sepsis; fluoroscopically guided intra-articular needle placement is particularly useful in recovering fluid from deep articulations such as the glenohumeral joint or the hip. Subsequent instillation of a small amount of radiographic contrast agent verifies that the joint space was indeed entered and may also yield important information concerning the extent of periarticular soft tissue destruction. Evaluation of the patient with a painful total hip prosthesis is an important indication for aspiration-arthrography to conclusively differentiate between chronic infection and aseptic loosening of the prosthesis.[9] Air arthrography, usually combined with conventional tomography, is often of great value in the identification of transchondral fractures as well as intra-articular osteocartilaginous bodies. Arthrography may also provide a firm diagnosis in cases of pigmented villonodular synovitis[10] or idiopathic synovial osteochondromatosis.[11]

Bursography has its greatest value in evaluating lesions of the subacromial bursa in the shoulder.[12,13] In this location, bursitis, intrabursal osteocartilaginous bodies, partial rotator cuff tears, and causes of shoulder impingement may be identified. At the same time, instillation of local anesthetic agents or anti-inflammatory medications directly into the bursa serves as both a diagnostic and a therapeutic procedure.

Computed Tomography. Computed axial tomography has only recently been applied to the evaluation of diseases of the musculoskeletal system. These diseases include sacroiliitis[14] and a number of vertebral disorders, such as spinal stenosis, apophyseal joint osteoarthritis, ossification of the posterior intraspinal ligaments, and intervertebral disc herniation.[15] Analysis of bone mineral content in the axial skeleton with computed tomography is now performed in many medical centers.[16]

RHEUMATOID ARTHRITIS

Rheumatoid arthritis is a common disease whose features are familiar to most physicians. For this reason it tends to be the clinical and radiographic standard against which other arthritides are evaluated. A thorough understanding of the roentgenographic features of this important disease provides a firm basis for evaluating articular disease in general.

General Distribution. Rheumatoid arthritis demonstrates a propensity toward symmetric involvement of synovial articulations. In the appendicular skeleton, the hands, wrists, feet, knees, hips, shoulders, and elbows are frequently affected. The small joints of the hands and feet are the earliest and most frequent sites of radiographic changes. In the axial skeleton, involvement of the cervical spine is common, while thoracolumbar and sacroiliac joint involvement is uncommon. Cartilaginous articulations, such as the symphysis pubis and manubriosternal joints, and entheses, where ligaments and tendons attach to bone, may be involved in rheumatoid arthritis, but such involvement is both less frequent and less severe than in the seronegative spondyloarthopathies.

General Radiographic Features. *Symmetry.* The symmetry of rheumatoid arthritis constitutes an important diagnostic criterion for this disease. Asymmetric involvement may be noted in male patients and in men and women with early disease or neurologic deficit.[17]

Osteoporosis. Osteoporosis is a characteristic feature of rheumatoid arthritis. Early in the course of the disease, it tends to be localized to the juxta-articular region of the small peripheral joints. Later, generalized osteoporosis may be present in the axial and appendicular skeleton, often exacerbated by medications (i.e., salicylates, corticosteroids) and disuse or immobilization. In a few patients with rheumatoid arthritis, osteomalacia may be observed.[18]

Soft Tissue Changes. Radiographic changes in the soft tissues can be of diagnostic importance in the patient with rheumatoid arthritis. Diffuse (fusiform) periarticular soft tissue swelling (Fig. 39–1) is an early finding about the small joints of the hands and feet. Intra-

Figure 39–1. Rheumatoid arthritis. Marginal erosions are present on both sides of the interphalangeal joint. Joint space narrowing and fusiform soft tissue swelling are also evident.

articular effusions are common radiographic findings in the knees, elbows, and ankles, producing characteristic displacements of adjacent fat planes. Occasionally, similar effusions in the small joints of the hand may lead to mild joint space widening. Bursal involvement can be identified as asymmetric soft tissue prominence, particularly in the knee (prepatellar bursa), elbow (olecranon bursa), heel (retrocalcaneal bursa), and shoulder (subacromial bursa). Tendinitis and tenosynovitis are most frequently identified in the wrist when involvement of the extensor carpi ulnaris tendon and its synovial sheath causes prominent soft tissue swelling adjacent to the ulnar styloid process. Rheumatoid nodules may occasionally be observed on radiographs as noncalcified, eccentric, lobular soft tissue masses, which may cause pressure erosion of adjacent bones.

Joint Space Narrowing. Progressive joint space narrowing due to destruction of articular cartilage by pannus is another hallmark of rheumatoid arthritis, which may allow its differentiation from gout, a disease in which preservation of joint width is typical. In rheumatoid arthritis, the diffuse cartilaginous loss and the tendency toward pancompartmental involvement of complex joints, such as the knee and the wrist, limit additional diagnostic possibilities. Bony ankylosis is common only in the wrist and in the midfoot; it is distinctly unusual at other sites.

Bony Erosions. Three types of bony erosions may be identified in rheumatoid arthritis. *Marginal erosions* occur at intra-articular sites that are not protected by overlying cartilage. Typically these "bare" areas are the initial points of attack by the proliferating synovial tissue (Fig. 39–1). *Compressive erosions* occur when collapse of osteoporotic subchondral bone leads to invagination of one bone into another. These changes occur at articulations exposed to strong muscular actions or significant weight-bearing forces. The most characteristic site of compressive erosion is the hip, where protrusio acetabuli may be identified (Fig. 39–2). Other important sites are at the metacarpophalangeal joints, where collapse of the base of a proximal phalanx by a metacarpal head produces a ball-in-socket-type articulation, and the radiocarpal joint of the wrist, where the scaphoid may appear to be "countersunk" into the distal radius. The third type of erosion seen in rheumatoid arthritis is *surface resorption*, usually related to inflammation of an adjacent tendon sheath (Fig. 39–3). This is an important finding in the wrist, where a characteristic erosion of the outer margin of the ulnar styloid process, due to extenor carpi ulnaris tenosynovitis, provides an early radiographic sign of rheumatoid arthritis.

Bony Cysts. Subchondral cystic lesions are frequent in rheumatoid arthritis and have been described as cysts, pseudocysts, geodes, and granulomas. Most commonly, multiple small, ill-defined subchondral radiolucencies are identified at any articulation involved in rheumatoid arthritis. The identification of larger cystic areas, especially in the hands and wrists of physically active men, has been termed rheumatoid arthritis of the robust reaction pattern.[19] Occasionally very large cystic lesions

Figure 39–2. Rheumatoid arthritis. Symmetric destruction of the cartilaginous surface has resulted in axial migration of the femoral head. The femoral head has become small and flattened. Sclerosis is apparent.

may be encountered in the elbow (olecranon process of ulna, distal humerus), femoral neck, or knee (distal femur, proximal tibia, patella) and have been described as pseudocystic rheumatoid arthritis (Fig. 39–4).[20] These large lesions may subsequently fracture.

Figure 39–3. Rheumatoid arthritis. An osseous erosion is present in the lateral margin of the ulnar styloid (surface erosion) (arrow) due to synovitis of the extensor carpi ulnaris tendon sheath. A second erosion is present at the point of insertion of the triangular fibrocartilage on the ulnar head (arrowhead). (From Resnick, D., and Niwayama, G.: Diagnosis of Bone and Joint Disorders. Philadelphia, W.B. Saunders Co., 1981.)

Figure 39–4. Pseudocystic rheumatoid arthritis. In this patient, large cystic erosions are present, giving the appearance of "hollow" carpal bones. Also note the narrowing of the radiocarpal joint with ulnar translocation of the carpus. (From Resnick, D., and Niwayama, G.: Diagnosis of Bone and Joint Disorders. Philadelphia, W.B. Saunders Co., 1981.)

Deformities and Instabilities. Many types of articular deformity and instability are observed in rheumatoid arthritis (Fig. 39–5). Most of these relate to tendinous or ligamentous laxity or disruption, with alteration of the normal muscle pull across one or more articulations (e.g., boutonnière or swan-neck deformity of the fingers, ulnar deviation at the metacarpophalangeal joints, fibular deviation at the metatarsophalangeal joints, or at-

Figure 39–5. Rheumatoid arthritis. In this patient note the prominent thumb deformity with flexion at the metacarpophalangeal joint and extension of the interphalangeal joint. This constitutes the boutonnière deformity.

lanto-axial subluxation). In some cases, however, the abnormality may relate directly to bone or cartilage destruction (e.g., protrusio acetabuli). These characteristic deformities and instabilities are summarized in Table 39–3.

Abnormalities at Specific Sites. *Hand.* The target areas of rheumatoid arthritis in the hands are the metacarpophalangeal and proximal interphalangeal joints. The earliest changes consist of fusiform soft tissue swelling, juxta-articular osteoporosis, diffuse joint space loss, and marginal bony erosions (Fig. 39–1). A particularly characteristic finding is indistinctness and focal loss of continuity of the dorsoradial subchondral bone plate (dot-dash pattern) of the metacarpal head.[21] In general, these radiographic findings appear initially at the second and third metacarpophalangeal joints and third proximal interphalangeal joint. The marginal osseous erosions tend to be more prominent on the proximal bone of the articulation, which tends to have a larger bare area. With progression of the disease, large erosions, complete joint space obliteration, and finger deformities appear. The end stage is usually fibrous ankylosis of the articular cavity; bony ankylosis is rare in the hand but, when present, almost exclusively involves the proximal interphalangeal joints.[17]

Wrist. The wrist is a complex articulation that should properly be viewed as a series of distinct synovial compartments: (1) radiocarpal, (2) inferior radioulnar, (3) midcarpal, (4) pisotriquetral, (5) common carpometacarpal, and (6) first carpometacarpal. Rheumatoid arthritis demonstrates distinctive pancompartmental involvement of the wrist, which helps to differentiate it from other arthropathies.[22] The least commonly involved area is the first carpometacarpal compartment, which may be spared even in the presence of advanced disease elsewhere in the wrist.

The distal ulna, being bounded by three important sites of synovial proliferation, occupies a prominent role as a target area in rheumatoid arthritis[23] (Fig. 39–3). Erosions along the outer margin of the ulnar styloid are related to tenosynovitis of the extensor carpi ulnaris tendon; erosions of the styloid tip are related to involvement of the prestyloid recess of the radiocarpal compartment; and erosions of the base and juxta-articular area of the distal ulna indicate inferior radioulnar compartment involvement.

Early erosions may involve any bone in the wrist; in addition to the distal ulna, some of the more characteristic sites[24,25] include the radial styloid, lateral scaphoid waist, triquetrum, and pisiform. These changes may be manifested as distinct erosions or as cystic lesions which give the radiographic appearance of hollow carpal bones. With time, the characteristic pancompartmental involvement becomes evident with loss of articular spaces. Bony ankylosis of the carpus is a relatively common end result of advanced rheumatoid arthritis. In some cases diffuse carpal destruction may occur, culminating in complete disintegration of the wrist.

Numerous deformities related to soft tissue destruction and muscular imbalances may be seen. The most characteristic wrist deformities consist of ulnar translocation of the proximal carpal row, related to destruc-

Table 39–3. Instabilities and Deformities in Rheumatoid Arthritis

Site	Name	Abnormality
Hand		
D.I.P. joint	Mallet finger	Flexion D.I.P.
P.I.P. and D.I.P. joints	Boutonnière deformity	Flexion P.I.P., extension D.I.P.
	Swan-neck deformity	Extension P.I.P., flexion D.I.P.
M.C.P. joint		Ulnar deviation
		Volar subluxation
Wrist		
Distal radioulnar joint	Caput ulna	Subluxation/dislocation D.R.U. joint
Radiocarpal joint		Radial deviation
		Ulnar translocation
Intercarpal joints	Scapholunate dissociation	Scapholunate space > 2 mm
	Dorsal intercalary segment instability	Dorsiflexion lunate, volar flexion caphoid
	Volar intercalary segment instability	Volarflexion lunate, dorsiflexion scaphoid
		Subluxation extensor carpi ulnaris tendon
Hip	Protrusio acetabuli	Acetabular wall medial to ilioischial line
		> 3 mm in male
		> 6 mm in female
Knee	Genu varus	Inward deviation of tibia
	Genu valgus	Outward deviation of tibia
Foot		
First M.T.P. joint	Hallux valgus (bunion)	Lateral deviation first M.T.P. joint
M.T.P. (all)		Fibular deviation M.T.P. joints (I–IV)
		Plantar subluxation M.T.P. joints
	Cock-up toe	Hyperextension and dorsal subluxation M.T.P.
P.I.P. and D.I.P.	Hammer toe	Hyperflexion P.I.P. or D.I.P.
Cervical spine		
Atlanto-axial joint	Atlanto-axial subluxation	Atlanto-odontoid space > 3 mm
	Vertical atlanto-axial subluxation	Superior displacement odontoid
All levels	Stair-step deformity	Subluxation apophyseal joints

tion of the triangular fibrocartilage-meniscus homologue complex, and radial deviation at the radiocarpal joint (Fig. 39–6).[26]

Elbow. The elbow is a frequent site of abnormality, particularly in patients with advanced disease. In this area a common radiographic finding consists of a positive "fat pad" sign, representing displacement of the fat pads anterior and posterior to the distal humerus owing to intra-articular effusion or synovial hypertrophy.[27,28] Soft tissue swelling over the ulnar olecranon, related to olecranon bursitis, and about the proximal ulna, related to rheumatoid nodules, is another frequent finding. Eventually, extensive osteolysis of the humerus, radius, and ulna may resemble the findings in neuroarthropathy. Large medullary cystic lesions of the distal humerus and ulnar olecranon may be the sites of pathologic fracture.[29]

Shoulder. Two main anatomic sites are frequently involved in rheumatoid arthritis of the shoulder, the glenohumeral and acromioclavicular joints. In the former location, changes of rheumatoid arthritis are prominent joint space narrowing, bony sclerosis, and cyst formation.[24] Osseous erosions are most prominent along the superolateral margin of the humerus, adjacent to the greater tuberosity, and may resemble the Hill-Sachs fracture associated with anterior shoulder dislocation. Erosions may be present at other sites on the proximal humerus and glenoid region of the scapula. Subacromial bursitis, bicipital tendinitis, and rotator cuff tears are frequent complications.

At the acromioclavicular joint, soft tissue swelling and erosions, which tend to be more prominent on the clavicular side of the joint, are early findings.[17] Later, destruction of a large portion of the distal clavicle may be seen.

Foot. Sites of foot involvement in rheumatoid arthritis may be divided into the forefoot, the midfoot, and the heel. The forefoot is very commonly affected (80 to 90 percent) in rheumatoid arthritis, especially the metatarsophalangeal joints.[30-32] The earliest changes involve the metatarsal heads at the first and fifth metatarsophalangeal articulations (Fig. 39–7).[17] At the fifth metatarsophalangeal joint, an early and characteristic erosion occurs on the dorsolateral aspect of the metatarsal head and may be visualized only on oblique radiographs. At the first metatarsophalangeal joint, the earliest involvement is along the medial aspect of the metatarsal head, with later erosions involving the adjacent sesamoid bones. With progression, diffuse joint space loss and larger erosions may be seen. Forefoot deformities in rheumatoid arthritis include hallux valgus, hammer toes, and "cock-up" toes, as well as fibular deviation of the digits and plantar subluxation of the metatarsal heads.

In the midfoot, rheumatoid arthritis is characterized by diffuse joint space loss, bony sclerosis, and osteophytosis, with osseous erosions being uncommon.[17] Osseous fusion in longstanding disease is relatively common. Differentiation of this disease from degenerative, post-traumatic, or neuropathic disorders may be difficult in this region.

In the heel, abnormalities of rheumatoid arthritis are related to involvement of the retrocalcaneal bursa, Achilles tendon, and plantar fascia. With the utilization of soft tissue–enhancing radiographic techniques, swelling of the Achilles tendon (> 1 cm in diameter at the level of the posterosuperior margin of the calcaneus) or soft tissue masses adjacent to the posterosuperior margin

Figure 39–6. Rheumatoid arthritis. Prominent juxta-articular osteoporosis is present with radial deviation of the radiocarpal joint and ulnar translocation of the carpus. Extensive erosive changes of the radial and ulnar styloid processes and multiple carpal bones are also present. (From Resnick, D., and Niwayama, G.: Diagnosis of Bone and Joint Disorders. Philadelphia, W.B. Saunders Co., 1981.)

Figure 39–7. Rheumatoid arthritis. The classical forefoot deformities are well illustrated in this patient. Note the subluxation and fibular deviation at the MTP joints and the prominent marginal erosions of the first metatarsal head (arrowhead). (From Resnick, D., and Niwayama, G.: Diagnosis of Bone and Joint Disorders. Philadelphia, W.B. Saunders, Co., 1981.)

of the calcaneus as the result of an engorged retrocalcaneal bursa may be early findings.[17,33,34] Osseous erosions at the posterosuperior margin of the calcaneus (Fig. 39–8) are subsequently noted. Well-defined plantar calcaneal spurs, which are identical to those seen in "normal" individuals, can be distinguished from the fluffy, proliferative calcaneal excrescences seen in the seronegative spondyloarthropathies.

Ankle. Although the ankle may be the site of radiographically identifiable joint effusions in the patient with rheumatoid arthritis, bony changes at this site are relatively uncommon. In some cases diffuse osteoporosis and joint space narrowing as well as marginal and central bony erosions may be seen.[35] Rarely, with severe disease, loss of integrity of the ankle mortice may occur.

Knee. The knee is commonly affected in rheumatoid arthritis. Engorgement of the suprapatellar space of the knee joint by effusion or synovial hypertrophy is noted on the lateral radiographic projection. Small erosions along the medial and lateral margins of the tibia and femur are the earliest bony changes and are followed by joint space loss involving the medial femorotibial, lateral femorotibial, and patellofemoral compartments.[17] Subchondral cysts may be seen in the femoral condyles or proximal tibia, and subchondral sclerosis due to bony collapse may be prominent.[36] Versus or valgus deformity of the knee joint or patellar instability may be present. Rupture of the quadriceps or patellar tendon may occur with corresponding abnormalities of the soft tissue shadows about the knee. The knee is also a common site of large synovial cysts, especially in the popliteal region.[37] These synovial cysts may extend along fascial planes for a considerable distance in a proximal or distal direction.

Hip. Hip involvement in rheumatoid arthritis is less common than knee involvement. A characteristic radiographic abnormality is diffuse concentric loss of articular space, with migration of the femoral head along the plane of the axis of the femoral neck.[38] Radiolucent zones at the bone cartilage junction of the femoral head are related to circumferential marginal erosions.[17] Central erosions of the femoral head and, less commonly, of the acetabulum may be seen. Occasionally large pseudocystic lesions of the femoral neck occur and are liable to pathologic fracture. Acetabular protrusion is present if the inner margin of the acetabulum is medial to the ilioischial line by 3 mm or more in men or 6 mm or more in women. Mild sclerosis and small osteophytes may be noted, related to secondary degenerative disease (osteoarthritis). Osteonecrosis of the femoral heads may be encountered in rheumatoid arthritis, usually in association with corticosteroid therapy.

Sacroiliac Joints. Asymptomatic sacroiliac joint changes are common in rheumatoid arthritis of long duration.[40] In general the findings consist of bilateral but asymmetric bony erosions that primarily involve the iliac side of the synovial articulation.

Spine. The cervical spine is one of the more common and important areas of involvement in rheumatoid arthritis. The apophyseal joints of the cervical spine are diffusely affected with bony erosion, joint space narrowing and, eventually, subluxation that leads to a "stair-step" type of deformity (Fig. 39–9), with contiguous vertebral bodies being offset like the steps of a staircase.[42] Erosions and destruction involving the uncovertebral joints (Luschka) as well as the discovertebral junctions are also common. Between the spinous processes, the formation of adventitious bursae and their subsequent inflammation lead to characteristic erosions and a "sharpened" appearance of these processes on lateral radiographs of the cervical spine.

The most important site of cervical spine abnormality is the craniocervical junction. Erosions involving the anterior or posterior margins of the odontoid process as well as joint space narrowing and marginal osseous erosions involving the lateral occipito-atlanto-axial articulations are early findings.[42] Subsequently, laxity or destruction of the transverse atlanto-axial ligament can lead to horizontal (in the sagittal plane) atlanto-axial subluxation with encroachment of the odontoid process on the vertebral canal during flexion of the neck.[42,43] The diagnosis of this complication is based upon the identification of an abnormally wide space (> 5 mm in the adult) between the posterior margin of the anterior arch of the atlas and the anterior surface of the odontoid process on lateral radiographs of the cervical spine exposed during flexion of the patient's neck. Large odontoid erosions may predispose to pathologic fracture. A second, less common but potentially fatal, pattern of cevical instability in rheumatoid arthritis is vertical atlanto-axial subluxation in which compression of the lateral masses of the atlas in association with disease of the lateral atlanto-axial and atlanto-occipital joints allows the odontoid process to be elevated vetically, becoming intimate with the brainstem.[44,45] Furthermore,

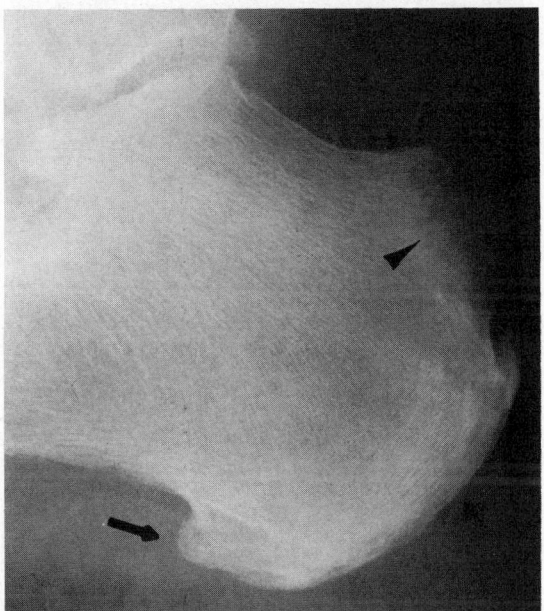

Figure 39–8. Rheumatoid arthritis. Erosions are present on the posterior (arrowhead) calcaneal surface. A plantar calcaneal spur is evident (arrow).

Figure 39–9. Rheumatoid arthritis. The "stair-step" deformity of the cervical spine is present with subluxation at multiple contiguous levels. Diffuse loss of intervertebral disc height and erosion of articular surfaces of the apophyseal joints are also present. (From Resnick, D., and Niwayama, G.: Diagnosis of Bone and Joint Disorders. Philadelphia, W.B. Saunders Co., 1981.)

occipito-atlanto-axial instability in the coronal plane can lead to lateral tilting of the head.

In contrast to the frequency of cervical spine involvement, changes in the thoracic and lumbar spine are uncommon in rheumatoid arthritis. However, erosive and destructive abnormalities about the lumbar apophyseal joints are well documented, as are irregularity, erosion, and loss of definition of the bony vertebral endplates.[17] Synovial cysts arising from the apophyseal joints are rare causes of neurologic symptoms and signs.[41]

Other Locations. Other synovial joints that may be involved in rheumatoid arthritis include the temporomandibular and sternoclavicular joints. Not infrequently, cartilaginous articulations, such as the sternomanubrial joint and symphysis pubis, may show erosive change and narrowing.

JUVENILE ARTHRITIS

General Radiographic Features. Juvenile arthritis (JA) is a generic term used to describe a group of childhood articular disorders that share, to a variable degree, certain clinical, laboratory, and radiologic features. Each specific subgroup of JA has its own distinctive radi-

ographic appearance. However, many of the changes are nonspecific and related to effects of the disorder on growth and development of the immature skeleton. It is useful to first consider these general features of childhood arthritis prior to considering abnormalities in specific subgroups of disease.

Growth Disturbances.[46-48] Epiphyseal enlargement is a common feature of JA and is related to growth stimulation associated with epiphyseal hyperemia. The changes occur diffusely but often are most marked at the femoral condyles, humeral condyles, and radial head. Epiphyseal overgrowth is combined with subnormal growth of the diaphyseal portion of the bone, resulting in a constricted appearance to the diaphysis with "ballooning" of the epiphysis (Fig. 39–10). The time of appearance and the size of individual bones in the wrist and midfoot may be increased. In some cases, overall bone length may be diminished owing to premature closure of the physis or, in other cases, increased owing to hyperemia.

Periostitis.[48] Periostitis is a common and nonspecific component of virtually all forms of JA. This is in contrast to the specificity of periostitis in the differential diagnosis of adult arthropathies. In childhood the periosteum is relatively loosely attached to the underlying bone, a situation that allows it to be easily lifted and stimulated to produce new bone in response to inflammation. Periostitis is most common in the phalanges, metacarpals, and metatarsals but may occasionally be

Figure 39–10. Juvenile chronic arthritis. Note the prominent juxta-articular osteoporosis with "ballooning" of the distal tibial and fibular epiphyses and a constricted appearance to the bone shafts.

seen in the metaphyses and diaphyses of long tubular bones. In the small bones of the hands and feet, exuberant periosteal new bone formation may result in a "squared" appearance.

Epiphyseal Compression Fractures.[48] Flattening and deformity of the epiphyseal centers in weight-bearing articulations are common in JA. Cupping of the epiphyseal centers of the proximal phalanges is also frequent. These changes are related to the abnormal stresses associated with joint contracture and subluxation acting on the osteoporotic epiphyses.

Osteopenia. Osteopenia, representing increased skeletal radiolucency, is generally most striking in the metaphyseal region of a bone, resulting in the formation of horizontally oriented radiolucent metaphyseal bands.[48] These lucent bands are commonly noted in the femur, tibia, fibula, and radius and are identical to those seen in childhood leukemia, metastatic neuroblastoma, and congenital infections. With time, diffuse osteoporosis can develop. Growth recovery lines (Fig. 39–11) are thin, horizontally oriented radiodense bands visualized in the diametaphyseal region of tubular bones in children with chronic illness. Presumably they are manifestations of accelerated bone growth in the intervals following exacerbations of disease. Occasionally, widespread metaphyseal sclerosis is seen (Fig. 39–11).

Juvenile-Onset Adult-Type (Seropositive) Rheumatoid Arthritis. Soft tissue swelling, juxta-articular osteoporosis, and marginal erosions are present, as in the typical adult case.[46] However, two features help differentiate this disorder from adult-onset rheumatoid arthritis: the presence of periostitis, especially of the small bones of the hands and feet, and the frequent occurrence of prominent marginal erosions without associated joint space narrowing.[50,51]

Seronegative Chronic Arthritis (Still's Disease).[49] Classic systemic Still's disease is an acute systemic illness that rarely manifests radiographic articular changes.

Polyarticular disease may occur in the presence or absence of classic Still's disease. Symmetric involvement of the hands, wrists, knees, ankles, feet, and cervical spine is common. In the hands and feet, osteoporosis is associated with joint space narrowing, and the small bones assume a "squared" shape as a result of new bone formation. Osseous erosions are unusual in this disorder and, when present, are usually of small size. Intra-articular bony ankylosis (Fig. 39–12) is a common late complication in the small joints, in contrast to its rarity in adult-onset rheumatoid arthritis. In the larger articulations such as the knee and the hip, osteoporosis and epiphyseal overgrowth are the most typical manifestations, often occurring without joint space narrowing or bony erosions. The cervical spine is frequently the only spinal level involved in this disorder (Fig. 39–13); abnormalities predominate in the upper cervical region. The growth disturbance results in a constriction of vertebral body width and depth with relatively normal height, resulting in a slender, gracile appearance. Apophyseal joint space narrowing, bony ankylosis, and osseous erosions occur with hypoplasia of the intervertebral discs and bony ankylosis of vertebral bodies. As in adults, atlanto-axial subluxation is a frequent complication in children.

Figure 39–11. Juvenile chronic arthritis. There is overgrowth of the epiphyses about the knee. Juxta-articular osteoporosis is evident, with several horizontally oriented growth recovery lines (arrowhead). Metaphyseal sclerosis (arrows) can be visualized in the proximal tibia.

Figure 39–12. Juvenile chronic arthritis. There are prominent finger deformities, osteoporosis, and bony ankylosis, especially in the carpus. Note the elongated, slender appearance of the tubular bones, which is related to growth disturbance.

Figure 39–13. Juvenile chronic arthritis. Intervertebral and apophyseal joint bony ankylosis is present at multiple levels. The overall appearance of the cervical spine is gracile, owing to the relatively normal height of the vertebral bodies and the diminished anteroposterior vertebral diameter. (From Resnick, D., and Niwayama, G.: Diagnosis of Bone and Joint Disorders. Philadelphia, W.B. Saunders Co., 1981.)

Pauciarticular and monoarticular forms of seronegative chronic arthritis are occasionally seen.[51,52] Changes are generally confined to the larger articulations such as the knee, hip, ankle, elbow, and wrist; the small joints of the hands and feet are spared. Radiographic abnormalities are the same as those in the polyarticular pattern of disease.

Juvenile-Onset Ankylosing Spondylitis. Juvenile-onset ankylosing spondylitis is generally first manifest in the articulations of the lower extremity, particularly the hips, knees, ankles, and small joints of the feet.[46] The joints of the upper extremities are relatively spared. Sacroiliitis and spondylitis occur but are usually identified later in the course of the disease, in contrast to adult-onset ankylosing spondylitis. In the spine, thoracic and lumbar involvement is common with involvement of the cervical spine being distinctly unusual.

Radiographic changes in the peripheral skeleton consist of joint space narrowing, bony erosions and proliferation, and intra-articular osseous fusion.[53] Osteoporosis is frequently not prominent. In the sacroiliac articulations and the thoracolumbar spine, the radiographic changes are identical to those of adult-onset ankylosing spondylitis.[54] Useful features in differentiating this disorder from other types of JA include the absence of diffuse osteoporosis, relative sparing of the articulations of the upper extremity and cervical spine, and sacroiliitis and spondylitis.

Juvenile-Onset Psoriatic Arthritis. Juvenile-onset psoriatic arthritis is occasionally encountered. Radiographic changes simulate those in adults. Hand in-

volvement is characterized by resorption of the terminal tufts of the distal phalanges and interphalangeal joint destruction.[49] Although sacroiliitis is common in this disorder, the normal indistinct appearance of the sacroiliac articulations in children and adolescents makes accurate radiographic diagnosis of sacroiliitis difficult.

Adult-Onset Still's Disease. Rarely, an adult patient may be encountered with a febrile illness identical to classic Still's disease.[55] When present, radiographic changes involve the wrists, knees, and fingers. Bony erosions are unusual. A peculiar tendency toward narrowing or ankylosis of the common carpometacarpal joint, especially that portion at the level of the second and third metacarpal bases, and the intercarpal joint in a pericapitate distribution has been reported.[97]

Others. Enteropathic arthropathy may be identified in childhood accompanying regional enteritis, ulcerative colitis, or bowel infections (*Salmonella, Shigella*). Its appearance is identical to that of juvenile-onset ankylosing spondylitis. Other rare causes of childhood arthropathy include systemic lupus erythematosus and familial Mediterranean fever.

THE SERONEGATIVE SPONDYLOARTHROPATHIES

Ankylosing Spondylitis. Synovial and cartilaginous joints as well as sites of tendon and ligament insertion (entheses) may be involved in ankylosing spondylitis and the other seronegative spondyloarthropathies.[57,58] Axial skeletal involvement is characteristic, with a predilection for the sacroiliac, apophyseal, discovertebral, and costovertebral articulations. The initial sites of involvement are the sacroiliac joints and lumbosacral and thoracolumbar vertebral junctions. Subsequently, ascending and descending spinal disease may be encountered.[59,60] Peripheral joint involvement, although frequent (50 percent), is usually mild.[54] The hips and glenohumeral joints are the most common extraspinal locations of disease.

Sacroiliac Joints. Involvement of the sacroiliac joint is the hallmark of ankylosing spondylitis. It is difficult to verify the diagnosis of this disease in the absence of such involvement. Rarely, spinal disease occurs in the absence of significant sacroiliac joint abnormality. Sacroiliitis occurs early in the course of ankylosing spondylitis and is characteristically bilateral and symmetric in its distribution.[59-62] On rare occasions, initial unilateral or asymmetric sacroiliac joint changes are observed. Changes occur both in the synovial and the ligamentous portions of the joint, with the abnormalities being more prominent on the iliac side of the articulation.[58] Osteoporosis, subchondral bony resorption with loss of definition of the articular margins, and superficial osseous erosions are interspersed with focal areas of bony sclerosis. Radiographically, in this stage, the articulation may appear widened. With progression of the disease, a wide, ill-defined band of sclerosis is seen on the iliac side of the joint with larger subchondral erosions (Fig. 39–14). In the late proliferative stage, bony bridges trav-

Figure 39–15. Ankylosing spondylitis. A specimen radiograph from a cadaver with the disease demonstrates complete intra-articular ankylosis of the ligamentous (arrowhead) and synovial (arrow) portions of the joint. (*SAC*, sacrum; *IL*, ilium).

Figure 39–14. Ankylosing spondylitis. Note the ill-defined band of sclerosis and prominent erosions of the subchondral bone plate (arrowheads), which are most conspicuous on the iliac side of the articulation.

erse the joint space, initially isolating islands of intact cartilage. Such segmental ankylosis may be followed by complete intra-articular bony fusion (Fig. 39–15) and disappearance of the periarticular sclerosis. The ligamentous (syndesmotic) portions of the sacroiliac joint may also be affected, leading to bony erosions and proliferation. In general, involvement of the ligamentous portion of the articulation is less prominent in ankylosing spondylitis than in psoriatic arthritis and Reiter's syndrome.

Spine. The initial sites of spinal involvement, especially in men, are the lumbosacral and thoracolumbar junctions. In women, the cervical spine may be affected at an early stage of disease. "Osteitis" is an initial finding, related to inflammation of the anterior portion of the discovertebral junction.[58] A focal erosive lesion at the anterosuperior and anteroinferior vertebral margins leads to loss of the normal concavity of the anterior aspect of the vertebral body, resulting in a "squared" configuration of the vertebral body in the lateral radiographic projection. This appearance is more easily identified in the lumbar spine as the thoracic vertebral bodies may normally have a squared appearance. In ankylosing spondylitis, bony sclerosis adjacent to the sites of erosion produces a "shiny corner" sign on radiographs.

Syndesmophytes are vertically oriented bony excrescences, which represent ossification of the outer fibers of the annulus fibrosus of the intervertebral disc.[63] They predominate on the anterior and lateral aspects of the spine and eventually bridge the intervertebral disc. (Fig. 39–16A). In the late stages of the disease, extensive syndesmophytic formation produces a smooth, undulating spinal contour, the "bamboo" spine.

It is of critical importance that the syndesmophytes that characterize ankylosing spondylitis (and enteropathic spondyloarthritis) be differentiated from other spinal and paraspinal bony excrescences (Figs. 39–16, 39–23, 39–38, and 39–39). Vertebral excrescences in spondylosis deformans arise several millimeters from the discovertebral junction, are triangular in shape, and demonstrate a horizontally oriented segment of variable length at their point of origin. In diffuse idiopathic skeletal hyperostosis (DISH), bone formation in the anterior longitudinal ligament results in a flowing pattern of ossification, thicker than that seen in ankylosing spondylitis. Such ossification is best demonstrated on lateral spine radiographs. Furthermore, in DISH, there is absence of erosion or bony ankylosis in the sacroiliac joints. The paravertebral ossifications that characterize psoriatic arthritis and Reiter's syndrome arise in an asymmetric fashion in the soft tissues adjacent to the outer layer of the annulus fibrosus. They are initially unattached to the vertebral body but, with time, they fuse with the margins of the vertebral body at a point several millimeters from the discovertebral junction.

Figure 39–16. Ankylosing spondylitis. Lateral (*A*) and frontal (*B*) radiographs of the spine demonstrate complete intervertebral ankylosis, which produces the characteristic "bamboo spine" appearance. Note the thin, vertically oriented syndesmophytes (arrowheads) arising from the discovertebral junction, owing to ossification in the outermost layer of the annulus fibrosus.

Erosions at one or more discovertebral junctions can be prominent radiographic findings in ankylosing spondylitis. These may be classified as focal or diffuse.[64] Focal lesions may relate to intraosseous herniation of disc material (cartilaginous or Schmorl's node) or enthesitis. Diffuse destruction of the discovertebral junction may be related to a pseudarthrosis following fracture. Discal calcification is common and usually seen in association with apophyseal joint ankylosis at the same spinal level.

Early alterations in the apophyseal joints in the lumbar, thoracic, and cervical segments consist of ill-defined erosions accompanied by reactive sclerosis. Capsular ossification or intra-articular bony ankylosis may subsequently occur. On frontal radiographs of the spine, such ossification produces vertically oriented, parallel, radiodense bands, which, when combined with a central radiodense band related to ossification of the interspinous and supraspinous ligaments, lead to the "trolley-track" sign (Fig. 39–16*B*).[58]

Erosions of the odontoid process and atlanto-axial subluxation may be observed in ankylosing spondylitis, although with less frequency than in rheumatoid arthritis.[44,59] Ankylosis of the atlanto-axial articulation, either in its normal position or in a position of subluxation, may occasionally be noted. At other levels in the cervical spine, the changes, when present, are identical to those in the thoracolumbar spine.

Extraspinal Locations. The hip is the most commonly involved peripheral articulation in ankylosing spondylitis, with the changes most frequently being bilateral and symmetrical in distribution.[65] Concentric joint space narrowing with axial migration of the femoral head and marginal osteophyte formation characterizes the hip disease of ankylosing spondylitis (Fig. 39–17). Osteophytes are first observed at the lateral margin of the femoral head-neck junction and, with progression, proliferate circumferentially to produce a characteristic "ring osteophyte."[65,66] Subchondral cysts and erosions as well as intra-articular bony ankylosis may be seen in some cases. Such hip disease can lead to significant clinical manifestations requiring surgical intervention. However, patients with ankylosing spondylitis who undergo hip surgery, including total joint replacement, are prone to develop exuberant deposits of juxta-articular heterotopic bone, which may severely restrict postoperative hip motion.[67]

The shoulder is the second most common peripheral site of involvement in ankylosing spondylitis.[54] Bilateral involvement is common; changes are osteoporosis, joint space narrowing, bony erosions, and rotator cuff disruption. A characteristic large destructive abnormality involving the superolateral aspect of the humeral head in this disease has been termed the "hatchet" sign[68] (Fig. 39–18).

Changes in other peripheral joints occur with variable frequency. In general, these changes, which are similar to but less extensive than those in the other seronegative spondyloarthropathies, include soft tissue swelling, mild osteoporosis, joint space narrowing, bony erosions, and osseous proliferation.[58] The erosions tend to be less prominent than in rheumatoid arthritis. The presence of bone proliferation (whiskering) and periostitis in an-

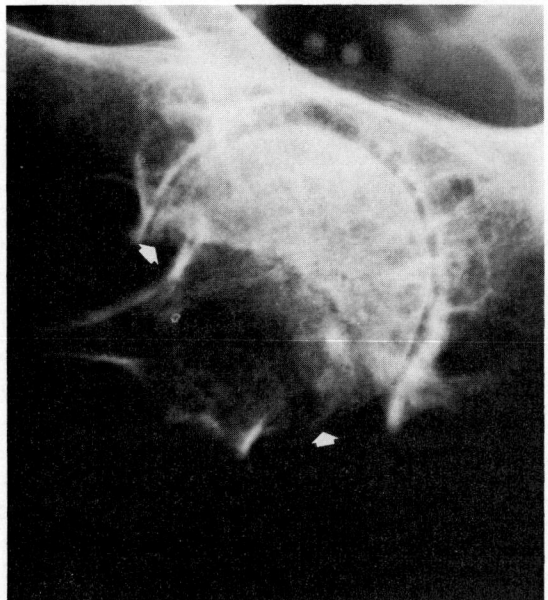

Figure 39–17. Ankylosing spondylitis. Concentric joint space narrowing with axial migration of the femoral head is present. Osteophytes (arrows) are present at the medial and lateral margins of the femoral head.

kylosing spondylitis (and the other seronegative spondyloarthropathies) is another helpful diagnostic feature.

Inflammation with bony proliferation at sites of tendon and ligament insertion (enthesopathy), especially those of the pelvis, patella, and calcaneus, is prominent in ankylosing spondylitis (as well as in the other seronegative spondyloarthropathies). Plantar and posterior calcaneal spurs are common and may be either well-defined or indistinct with feathery margins, representing the combination of erosive and proliferative change. Erosions of the posterior calcaneal margin due to inflammation in the retrocalcaneal bursa and thickening of the Achilles tendon may be present (Fig. 39–19).[34] The inflammatory enthesopathy of the seronegative spondyloarthropathies[58,69] differs from the degenerative enthesopathy seen in DISH (see Fig. 39–41). In the latter disease, bony outgrowths (enthesophytes) are sharply marginated and well-defined.

Other sites of involvement in ankylosing spondylitis[58] include the symphysis pubis and manubriosternal, temporomandibular, and sternoclavicular joints.

Psoriatic Arthritis. In general, psoriatic arthritis is asymmetric or unilateral with involvement of synovial and cartilaginous joints as well as entheses.[70] The most common sites of involvement are the interphalangeal joints of the hands and feet, metatarsophalangeal joints, metacarpophalangeal joints, sacroiliac joints, and spine. Changes in the knees, ankles, elbows, and wrists and manubriosternal, acromioclavicular, and sternoclavicular joints, as well as pelvic entheses, are not uncommon. Hip or glenohumeral joint involvement is rare.

The arthritis of psoriasis is associated with periarticular soft tissue swelling, which in some cases may be manifested by diffuse, sausage-like enlargement of an

Figure 39–19. Ankylosing spondylitis. Erosive change of the posterior calcaneal margin is present (arrowhead) as well as thickening of the Achilles tendon (between arrows).

Figure 39–18. Ankylosing spondylitis. There is disruption of the musculotendinous rotator cuff with superior migration of the humeral head. The large erosion (arrow) of the superolateral aspect of the humeral head ("hatchet deformity") is a characteristic radiographic sign of the disease.

entire digit. The absence of osteoporosis is remarkable in many cases of psoriatic arthritis and is an important consideration in the differential diagnosis. However, osteoporosis may occasionally be evident; thus, its presence does not exclude the diagnosis of psoriatic arthritis. Joint space narrowing or widening may be encountered, the latter being more common in the small joints of the hands and feet. Erosions progress from marginal areas in a central direction, often resulting in a "whittled" or "pencil-in-cup" deformity of the involved articulation.[72] In cases in which this severe destructive change is predominant, in combination with marked joint deformity, the term *arthritis mutilans* is frequently used. Bony proliferation is a striking feature of psoriatic arthritis and the other seronegative spondyloarthropathies (Fig. 39–20).[73] Proliferation around erosions produces a "whiskered" appearance. Diaphyseal and metaphyseal periostitis is also common.[74] In fact, osseous proliferation involving the distal phalanges may produce diffuse increased radiodensity, termed the "ivory phalanx."[75] Intra-articular bony fusion, especially involving the proximal and distal interphalangeal joints of the hands and feet, is a common finding. An inflammatory enthesopathy consisting of fine, feathery, bony proliferation at sites of tendon and ligament insertion is also prominent in many cases.

Hands. In the hands, involvement of the distal interphalangeal joints is frequent and may be unilateral or bilateral, symmetric or asymmetric in distribution (Fig. 39–20). Erosions occur at the joint margins and progress centrally, with irregular destructive changes. Protrusion

of one joint surface into its articular counterpart produces the pencil-in-cup deformity. Resorption of the terminal tufts of the distal phalanges may be seen. Psoriatic arthritis can lead to intra-articular bony ankylosis, a finding that is rare in rheumatoid arthritis.

Feet. Psoriatic arthritis involves two major areas in the foot: the forefoot and the calcaneus.[70] In the forefoot, changes are usually bilateral and asymmetric, predominating at the interphalangeal and metatarsophalangeal articulations. Marginal erosion, joint space narrowing (or widening), and bony proliferation are present, characteristically without significant osteoporosis. Severe destruction of the interphalangeal articulation of the great toe can be seen in psoriatic arthritis (and in Reiter's syndrome). Sesamoid involvement is also common in the foot as well as in the hand.

As in the other seronegative spondyloarthropathies, the combination of proliferative and erosive changes in the posterior and inferior surfaces of the calcaneus is an important radiographic finding of psoriatic arthritis. Erosions of the posterior surface of the calcaneus with surrounding proliferation adjacent to the retrocalcaneal bursa are common. Irregular and poorly defined spurs are typically present at the insertion of the plantar aponeurosis (Fig. 39–21), although in time, such spurs may become relatively well defined.

Sacroiliac Joints. A bilateral and symmetric distribution constitutes the most common radiographic pattern of sacroiliac joint abnormalities in psoriatic arthritis, although asymmetric involvement is not rare (Fig. 39–22).[70,76] Initially subchondral bony erosions and ill-defined sclerosis with apparent joint space widening are noted, abnormalities identical to those in ankylosing spondylitis. However, the frequency of intra-articular

Figure 39–20. Psoriatic arthritis. The distal interphalangeal joint is narrowed, with proliferative bony erosions (arrows). Also note the prominent soft tissue swelling and the abnormality of the fingernail.

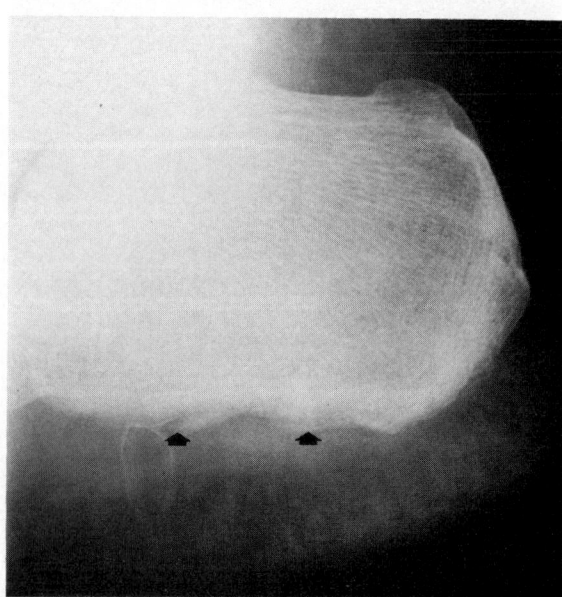

Figure 39–21. Psoriatic arthritis. The inferior surface of the calcaneus reveals the characteristic combination of erosive and proliferative changes (arrows) that form the hallmark of the seronegative spondyloarthropathies.

Figure 39–22. Psoriatic arthritis. Bilateral and asymmetric changes of the sacroiliac joints are present with erosions and sclerosis of the subchondral bone plate.

bony ankylosis in psoriatic arthritis is less than that in ankylosing spondylitis or the spondyloarthritis associated with inflammatory bowel diseases. Furthermore, in psoriatic arthritis (as in Reiter's syndrome), blurring and eburnation of apposing sacral and iliac surfaces within the ligamentous portion of the sacroiliac joint are more common than in ankylosing spondylitis.

Spine. The characteristic spinal lesion of psoriatic arthritis (as well as Reiter's syndrome) is paravertebral ossification.[77] These ossifications initially appear as either thick and irregular or thin and curvilinear densities, asymmetrically distributed parallel to the lateral surface of the intervertebral disc and vertebral body (Fig. 39–23). At this stage, the outgrowths are not attached to the vertebral body, although in later stages, the ossific densities merge with the lateral margins of the vertebral body several millimeters distal to the discovertebral junction. Occasionally, syndesmophytes identical to those in ankylosing spondylitis do occur in psoriatic arthritis[70] and Reiter's syndrome; however, in the great majority of cases, they are interspersed with the more characteristic paravertebral ossifications. "Corner osteitis," vertebral body "squaring," and apophyseal joint ankylosis are less common than in ankylosing spondylitis.

Cervical spine changes in psoriatic arthritis may be dramatic, even in patients with minimal thoracolumbar spinal involvement.[76,78] Discovertebral joint irregularity with extensive bony proliferation about the anterior aspect of the vertebra and extensive apophyseal joint erosion and narrowing may be seen. Atlanto-axial subluxation is common.[76]

Other Locations. In longstanding or severe disease, virtually any articulation may be involved. In most sites, the characteristic combination of erosive and proliferative change is present.

Reiter's Syndrome. Radiographic alterations occur in approximately 60 to 80 percent of patients with Reiter's syndrome.[79] These radiographic changes demonstrate morphologic characteristics that are virtually indistinguishable from those in the other seronegative spondyloarthropathies, especially psoriatic arthritis; differentiation is usually possible only by means of the distribution of abnormalities and the clinical history. Synovial joints, cartilaginous joints, and entheses may be affected. Characteristically these changes are bilateral and asymmetric, with a predilection for involvement of the lower extremity.[79]

The most common sites of involvement are the small joints of the foot and the posterior and inferior calcaneal surfaces, followed, in order of frequency, by the ankle and the knee. Involvement of the hip and upper extremity is considerably less common. In the axial skeleton the sacroiliac joints, spine, symphysis pubis, and manubriosternal joints are the most common sites of alteration.

The general radiographic features of Reiter's syndrome are soft tissue swelling, joint space narrowing, and bony erosion and proliferation. Osteoporosis is variable in frequency and extent but may be present during acute exacerbations of arthritis. Osseous proliferation at insertions of tendons and ligaments is a frequent finding, especially in the pelvis and the calcaneus.

Feet and Ankles. Asymmetric abnormalities of the metatarsophalangeal and interphalangeal joints of the forefoot are the most common manifestations of Reiter's syndrome (Fig. 39–24).[80] Frequently, effusions in the

Figure 39–23. Psoriatic arthritis. Note the thick asymmetric paravertebral ossifications (arrows) arising from the vertebral margins in this patient with psoriatic spondylitis. These lesions, which are best visualized in the anteroposterior projection of the spine, are characteristic of psoriatic arthritis and Reiter's syndrome.

Figure 39–24. Reiter's syndrome. There is destructive change of the second and third proximal interphalangeal joints with subtle periosteal proliferative reaction along the phalangeal shafts (arrow). Marginal erosions of the metatarsal heads and proximal phalanges are also evident.

retrocalcaneal bursa may be identified as radiodense shadows obliterating the normal fat plane between the posterosuperior aspect of the calcaneus and the Achilles tendon.[34] Thickening of this tendon may also be evident. Ill-defined plantar calcaneal spurs are characteristic but, as in the other seronegative spondyloarthropathies, the spurs may be relatively well-defined in the later stages of the disease. Marginal erosions are somewhat uncommon about the ankle, but joint space narrowing, with adjacent soft tissue swelling, and fluffy periostitis of the distal tibia and fibula are seen.[79]

Knee. The most common abnormality in the knee in Reiter's syndrome is the presence of a joint effusion, which in some instances becomes massive. Osteoporosis, joint space narrowing, and periostitis of the patella and distal femoral shaft also occur. Bony erosions in the femur or tibia are rare.

Sacroiliac Joints. Sacroiliac joint abnormalities are common and may be bilateral and asymmetric or unilateral in distribution. These abnormalities are identical to those of psoriatic arthritis.

Spine. Spinal involvement is less frequent in Reiter's syndrome than in ankylosing spondylitis and psoriatic arthritis. Although in some instances the changes may be identical to those of ankylosing spondylitis, a more characteristic finding consists of asymmetrically distributed paravertebral ossifications involving the thoraco-

lumbar spine.[81] Cervical spine involvement in unusual, and atlanto-axial subluxation is rare.

Other Locations. In the cartilaginous manubriosternal and pubic symphyseal articulations, the changes of Reiter's syndrome consist of erosions of the articular surfaces with adjacent bony proliferation and sclerosis.[79]

Severe and diffuse involvement of joints of the upper extremity is rare in Reiter's syndrome,[79] although scattered lesions, particularly in the proximal interphalangeal joints of the hands, may occasionally be seen. Distal interphalangeal or metacarpophalangeal joint alterations are less frequent. Fusiform or "sausage-like" soft tissue swelling, joint space narrowing, periarticular osteoporosis, and bony erosion and proliferation are observed.

Enteropathic Arthropathies and Related Conditions. The frequency of peripheral joint involvement in enteropathic arthritis is variable. Several types of involvement are seen:[82-86] a mild, inflammatory, self-limited peripheral arthritis in which the radiographic changes consist principally of soft tissue swelling and juxta-articular osteoporosis; a progressive, destructive peripheral arthropathy characterized by soft tissue swelling, variable osteoporosis, joint space narrowing, osseous erosions, bony proliferation; and sacroiliitis or spondylitis. In patients with spondyloarthritis the changes are identical to those in ankylosing spondylitis, although the male predominance of ankylosing spondylitis is less marked in this group of disorders and isolated sacroiliitis without spinal involvement is more common.

In primary biliary cirrhosis a severe destructive arthropathy of the hands has been described[87] characterized by the asymmetric distribution of well-defined marginal erosions primarily involving the proximal and distal interphalangeal joints with relative sparing of the metacarpophalangeal joints. Chondrocalcinosis may be present in some patients, and occasionally, severe involvement of the hips and shoulders resembling osteonecrosis has been noted.[88]

A number of pancreatic diseases, including carcinoma, inflammation, and pancreatic duct calculi, may be associated with a syndrome characterized by subcutaneous nodules, polyarthritis, and medullary fat necrosis.[89,90] The polyarthritis is radiographically nonspecific, with osteoporosis and soft tissue swelling being most commonly encountered. The radiographic appearance of medullary fat necrosis consists of diffuse osteolytic lesions with a "moth-eaten" appearance and periostitis. These changes closely resemble those of osteomyelitis and osteonecrosis.

CONNECTIVE TISSUE DISEASES

A number of connective tissue disorders, including systemic lupus erythematosus, progressive systemic sclerosis, dermatomyositis, polymyositis, periarteritis nodosa, and mixed connective tissue disease, may be associated with musculoskeletal radiographic abnormalities.

Systemic Lupus Erythematosus. The roentgenographic changes of systemic lupus erythematosus (SLE) include symmetric polyarthritis, deforming nonerosive arthropathy, spontaneous tendon rupture, osteonecrosis, soft tissue calcification, infection, acrosclerosis, and tuftal resorption.[91-100] With the polyarthritis the radiographic changes are nonspecific and consist of soft tissue swelling and periarticular osteoporosis.[91,92]

Joint space narrowing and bony erosions are unusual. Deforming nonerosive arthropathy is seen in 5 to 40 percent of patients with SLE.[92] Symmetric involvement of the hands is typical. The specific type of deformity is variable.[91-93] Swan-neck or boutonnière deformity can be evident. Other deformities include hyperextension of the interphalangeal joint of the thumb, ulnar drift at the metacarpophalangeal joints, and subluxation of the first carpometacarpal joint (Fig. 39–25). It is the prominent thumb deformity that is especially characteristic of lupus arthropathy. Although bony and cartilaginous abnormalities are generally not present, joint space narrowing, "hook-like" erosions of the radial and volar aspects of the metacarpal heads, and subchondral cyst formation are occasionally encountered (Fig. 39–26).[95] The radiographic findings of osteonecrosis in patients with SLE include transchondral fractures, subchondral sclerosis with cyst formation, and osseous collapse. Secondary osteoarthritis may eventually be prominent.

Linear or nodular calcific deposits in the subcutaneous tissues, particularly in the lower extremities, may occasionally be seen in SLE.[97] Sclerosis (acrosclerosis) or

Figure 39–26. Systemic lupus erythematosus. An unusual pattern of involvement is seen. Severe erosive changes are present in the first and second metacarpophalangeal joints and third PIP joint. Juxta-articular osteoporosis is prominent.

Figure 39–25. Systemic lupus erythematosus. This patient demonstrates juxta-articular osteoporosis with ulnar deviation at the metacarpophalangeal joints. No erosions are present.

resorption of the tufts of the terminal phalanges is occasionally evident in SLE.[100]

Progressive Systemic Sclerosis (PSS, Scleroderma). Soft tissue or bony involvement in PSS is common. The radiographic abnormalities can be divided into four main categories:[100] (1) soft tissue resorption, (2) soft tissue calcification, (3) osteolysis, and (4) erosive articular disease.

Soft tissue resorption is most commonly noted in the fingertips in association with Raynaud's phenomenon (Fig. 39–27). Early changes can be identified by noting a reduction in the normal distance between the phalangeal tips and the skin (normal $\geq$ 20 percent of the transverse diameter of the base of the same distal phalanx).[131] In time the fingertip assumes a conical shape and soft tissue calcification is often present.

Soft tissue calcification is most common in the hand but may occur at virtually any site.[102,103] Calcification may be present in subcutaneous tissue, joint capsule, tendons, or ligaments (Fig. 39–28). The calcification typically is composed of hydroxyapatite crystals and has a soft cloudlike radiographic appearance. Occasionally large tumoral collections may be present adjacent to a joint. Intra-articular or intra-osseous calcification may also be noted (Fig. 39–29).

Figure 39–27. Scleroderma. Juxta-articular osteoporosis, soft tissue calcification, and resorption of the terminal tufts of the distal phalanges are present. Also note the tapered appearance of the soft tissues of the second finger and a hooklike erosion in the radial aspect of the third metacarpal head.

Figure 39–29. Scleroderma. Prominent soft tissue calcification and intra-articular calcification are present as well as severe erosive change of the first carpometacarpal joint. This is a characteristic "target" area of scleroderma. (From Resnick, D., and Niwayama, G.: Diagnosis of Bone and Joint Disorders. Philadelphia, W.B. Saunders, 1981.)

Extra-articular osteolysis is a frequent manifestation of PSS. The most common site is the tuft of the distal phalanx of the hand or occasionally the foot, usually in association with Raynaud's phenomenon and soft tissue calcification. The earliest change is in the volar aspect of the tuft with continuing resorption leading to a "sharpened" appearance of the phalanx (Fig. 39–30).[100] Elsewhere, thickening of the periodontal membrane about the roots of the teeth[104] or localized mandibular osteolysis may be seen, the latter predisposing to pathologic fracture.[105] Localized osteolysis involving the ribs, acromion, clavicle, radius, ulna, and cervical spine has also been reported.[106-109]

A severe articular disease consisting of joint space narrowing, marginal and central osseous erosions, and deformity may occur.[109] There is a distinctive tendency toward involvement of the first carpometacarpal joint (Fig. 39–29).[100] Indeed, bilateral destructive changes of the first carpometacarpal articulation with joint subluxation should arouse suspicion of PSS. Other relatively common sites of joint involvement in PSS include the distal interphalangeal, proximal interphalangeal, inferior radioulnar, and metatarsophalangeal joints.

Dermatomyositis and Polymyositis. Articular abnormalities in dermatomyositis and polymyositis are usually without radiographic manifestations, although periarticular soft tissue swelling and osteoporosis may occasionally be noted.[112] More dramatic roentgenographic

Figure 39–28. Scleroderma. A large tumoral calcific collection is present adjacent to the hip.

Figure 39–30. Scleroderma. There is osteolysis of the volar aspect of the distal phalanges of the thumbs with adjacent soft tissue calcification. Also note the tapered appearance of the adjacent soft tissues.

changes occur in the skeletal musculature, especially the large proximal muscle groups of the thorax, arm, forearm, thigh, and calf. Initial inflammation produces increased bulk and radiodensity of muscles with loss of the normal intermuscular fat planes.[113] In later stages, muscle atrophy or contractures may be prominent. The most characteristic soft tissue abnormality is calcification[114] in subcutaneous tissue, intermuscular fascia, tendons, or fat (Fig. 39–31). Subcutaneous calcific deposits simulate those of progressive systemic sclerosis, but the presence of marked linear calcific collections favors the diagnosis of polymyositis or dermatomyositis.

Periarteritis Nodosa. Plain film radiographic findings are unusual in this disorder, although joint effusions or periostitis of the tubular bones identical to that of hypertrophic osteoarthropathy may occasionally be seen.[115] Angiography is an important diagnostic modality in evaluating the extent of vascular damage in this disease.

Mixed Connective Tissue Disease and "Overlap" Syndromes. A broad spectrum of radiographic abnormalities may be present in mixed connective tissue disease (MCTD),[116,117] including soft tissue swelling and calcification, osteoporosis, joint space narrowing, bony erosions, and joint deformity. Useful radiographic clues include (1) a radiographic pattern suggestive of more than one collagen vascular disease, (2) an erosive arthropathy with an asymmetric distribution or with prominent involvement of the distal interphalangeal joints, and (3) sausage-like soft tissue swelling of a digit. However, none of these changes is specific for MCTD.

There is a group of patients with clinical and radiographic features of more than one collagen vascular disease in whom serologic testing fails to document the presence of MCTD. Such patients are considered to have an "overlap" syndrome. Roentgenographic alterations generally indicate findings of rheumatoid arthritis, SLE, PSS, and dermatomyositis in various combinations.

Figure 39–31. Dermatomyositis. There is prominent calcification of the subcutaneous tissue and the muscle in the leg.

DEGENERATIVE JOINT DISEASE

The most characteristic sites of osteoarthritis (OA) include the proximal and distal interphalangeal joints of the hand, first carpometacarpal and trapezioscaphoid joints of the wrist, acromioclavicular and sacroiliac joints, hip, knee, and first metatarsophalangeal joint of the foot. Degenerative joint disease may also affect cartilaginous joints (such as the manubriosternal joint and symphysis pubis) and tendinous and ligamentous attachments to bone or entheses (such as in the pelvis, patella, and calcaneus). Degenerative disease of the spine is a separate subject and will be discussed later.

Osteoarthritis. In spite of a diversity of etiologies of OA, certain common radiographic characteristics allow a confident diagnosis in most cases. Joint space narrowing is a key diagnostic feature of the disease (Fig. 39–32).[118] In contrast to the inflammatory arthropathies, in which diffuse joint space narrowing of an involved articulation is expected, the joint space loss in OA tends to involve the portion of the joint exposed to the greatest stress (i.e., the lateral aspect of the hip, the medial compartment of the knee). Subchondral bone abnormalities are also characteristic of OA and include sclerosis (eburnation) and cyst formation, both of which predominate in the stressed area of the articulation. Subchondral

Figure 39–32. Osteoarthritis. There is narrowing of multiple interphalangeal joints with interdigitating osteophytes.

Figure 39–33. Osteoarthritis. Narrowing of the articular space and subchondral sclerosis about the first carpometacarpal joint are apparent.

eburnation results from cartilage denudation with subsequent bone-to-bone contact. The origin of subchondral cysts remains in debate.[119,120]

Osteophytes are the single most characteristic radiographic and pathologic abnormality in OA.[118] They tend to arise from endochondral ossification in areas of low stress where islands of cartilage are preserved, most commonly at joint margins. In some cases osteophytes may arise from the synovium or joint capsule.

Hand and Wrist. The interphalangeal joints of the hand are frequent target areas of OA. (Fig. 39–32). The appearance of articular space narrowing with closely apposed interdigitating bony surfaces and marginal osteophytes is characteristic. Metacarpophalangeal joint involvement may also occur but not as an isolated event; rather, such involvement is associated with alterations at interphalangeal articulations. At the metacarpophalangeal joints, it is interosseous space narrowing that is the predominant abnormality. Osseous erosions are not apparent. The first carpometacarpal (trapeziometacarpal) joint is the characteristic site of degenerative abnormalities in the wrist (Fig. 39–33). Joint space narrowing with bony eburnation, subchondral cysts, and osteophyte formation is typical. Radial subluxation of the first metacarpal base is common. The trapezioscaphoid space is the only other common site of OA in the wrist; involvement at this site is generally combined with that at the first carpometacarpal joint. Trapezioscaphoid joint disease in the absence of first carpometacarpal joint involvement should suggest another diagnosis, especially calcium pyrophosphate crystal deposition disease. Similarly, a degenerative disease-like arthropathy elsewhere in the wrist, especially at the radiocarpal joint, in the absence of significant occupational or accidental trauma, is generally related to a disease other than OA.

Sacroiliac Joint. OA of the sacroiliac joint is very common in the older age group. Joint space narrowing with a thin, well-defined band of subchondral sclerosis, especially in the ilium, is typically present. Osteophyte formation is most common at the superior and inferior margins of the synovium-lined portion of the joint. At the former location, these osteophytes may appear as localized radiodensities projected over the joint in the anteroposterior radiographic projection. Bony erosion and intra-articular osseous fusion are not features of OA of the sacroiliac joint.

Hip. OA of the hip is exceedingly frequent and may lead to significant patient disability. In the typical case, cartilage loss is focal, involves the superolateral aspect of the joint, and leads to upward migration of the femoral head (Fig. 39–34). Osteophyte formation is most prominent at the lateral acetabular and medial femoral margins, often in combination with thickening (buttressing) of the cortex in the medial aspect of the femoral neck. Subchondral sclerosis and cyst formation on both sides of the joint space may be marked. Focal loss of cartilage on the medial aspect of the articulation occurs in approximately 20 percent of patients with OA. Diffuse loss of cartilage with axial migration of the femoral head (along the axis of the femoral neck) is rare in OA. This latter feature is important in the differentiation of OA from inflammatory arthropathies such as rheumatoid arthritis.

Knee. The knee is a common site of OA. The most characteristic pattern of disease consists of involvement of the medial femorotibial compartment with joint space narrowing, osseous eburnation, subchondral cysts, and

Figure 39–34. Osteoarthritis. Moderately advanced osteoarthritic changes are present in *A* with asymmetric joint space narrowing and superior migration of the femoral head. Eburnation and cystic changes are seen in the subchondral region. In *B* advanced changes have occurred, with collapse of the superior articular surface and the formation of large marginal osteophytes.

marginal osteophytes.[122] Sharpening of the tibial spines or the presence of osteophytes arising from the intercondylar notch of the femur may also be observed. A true assessment of cartilage destruction may not be possible on standard anteroposterior radiographs (obtained with the patient supine) but is better provided by radiographs obtained either in the "tunnel" projection (Fig. 39–35) or with the patient in a weight-bearing

Figure 39–35. Osteoarthritis. Anteroposterior (*A*) and tunnel (*B*) projections reveal typical osteoarthritic changes of the knee. Note the asymmetric involvement with subchondral eburnation of the lateral articular surfaces. In this case the actual degree of joint space narrowing is much more apparent in the tunnel projection. An osteophyte arising from the intercondylar notch is identified (arrow).

position.[124] Varus angulation of the knee is the most common deformity in OA, reflecting the more severe involvement of the medial femorotibial compartment compared with the lateral one. Symmetric medial and lateral femorotibial compartment disease is unusual. Osteoarthritic changes in the patellofemoral compartment are also common, either in isolation or accompanying medial femorotibial compartment disease.

Osseous or cartilaginous debris may be present as intra-articular bodies ("joint mice") either free within the joint cavity or embedded in the synovial membrane. Degeneration of the fibrocartilaginous menisci is a typical feature of advanced OA.

Foot. OA in the foot typically affects the first metatarsophalangeal joint. Articular space narrowing, bony eburnation, osteophyte formation, and subchondral cysts are common. Hallux rigidus is a specific pattern of OA, which may be seen in adolescent or young adults; there is painful restriction of dorsiflexion at the first metatarsophalangeal joint.[124] Hallux valgus is another common pattern of OA about this joint, with lateral angulation of the first toe and prominent sclerosis, cyst formation, and osteophytosis on the medial aspect of the first metatarsal head.

Other Locations. Typical osteoarthritic changes in the elbows, acromioclavicular and glenohumeral joints, and ankles may be encountered, usually in patients with a history of trauma or pre-existing disease. In general, without such a history, a radiographic pattern consistent with OA[118] at an unusual site should suggest another disease process, including acromegaly, calcium pyrophosphate crystal deposition disease, ochronosis, and epiphyseal dysplasia.

Inflammatory Osteoarthritis. Inflammatory osteoarthritis is a disease most common in middle-aged women. It is characterized by acute episodic inflammation of the interphalangeal joints of the hand.[125] On roentgenograms, typical marginal osteophytes with or without bony erosions are seen. The erosions are first evident in the central portion of the subchondral bone, appearing as sharply marginated defects (Fig. 39–36).[118] Intra-articular ankylosis may subsequently result.[126] It must be emphasized that the clinical syndrome of inflammatory osteoarthritis can occur in the absence of radiographically demonstrable bony erosions; therefore, the term erosive osteoarthritis is not an ideal one for this disorder.

Degenerative Enthesopathy. Coarse bony proliferation at sites of ligamentous and tendinous attachment is a manifestation of a degenerative enthesopathy. This is most commonly observed in the pelvis, patella, ulnar olecranon, and calcaneus. The resulting bony excrescences are identical to those encountered in diffuse idiopathic skeletal hyperostosis. They are usually coarser and better defined than the outgrowths accompanying the inflammatory enthesopathy of the seronegative spondyloarthropathies.

Degenerative Disease of the Spine. The vertebral column is composed of a complex series of synovial, cartilaginous, and fibrous articulations. Degenerative diseases of the spine can involve any of these articulations

Figure 39–36. Inflammatory osteoarthritis. The combination of interphalangeal joint involvement, prominent marginal osteophytes, and central erosions of the articular surfaces (arrows) is characteristic of this disease. (From Resnick, D., and Niwayama, G.: Diagnosis of Bone and Joint Disorders. Philadelphia, W.B. Saunders Co., 1981.)

as well as ligamentous insertions (entheses).[128] Many distinct degenerative processes can be identified.

Intervertebral (Osteo)chondrosis. Primary degenerative disease of the nucleus pulposus of the intervertebral disc, termed intervertebral (osteo)chondrosis, is a common disorder, especially in the elderly, which may occur at any spinal level but is more commonly identified in the lumbar and cervical regions.[1]

The earliest radiographic change consists of linear or circular collections of gas ("vacuum phenomena") within the disc substance (Fig. 39–37).[129] These gas collections are more prominent on radiographs obtained with the spine in extension and may disappear in flexion. The presence of a vacuum phenomenon is a very useful observation, since it virtually excludes the possibility of infection.[130] Progressive narrowing of the intervertebral disc and sclerosis beneath the subchondral bone plate are additional manifestations of intervertebral (osteo)chondrosis. Herniation of portions of the intervertebral disc into the adjacent vertebral body (Schmorl's node, cartilaginous node) is a further radiographic sign. Small triangular osteophytes at the discovertebral junction are also seen (Fig. 39–37).

Spondylosis Deformans. Spondylosis deformans[127] refers to the formation of multiple large osteophytes predominantly along the anterior and lateral aspects of the vertebral bodies (Fig. 39–38).[131] These osteophytes may occur at any level; in the thoracic spine, they predom-

Figure 39–37. Intervertebral osteochondrosis. Lateral projections of the cervical spine (*A*) and lumbar spine (*B*) reveal typical abnormalities of intervertebral (osteo)chondrosis. Intervertebral disc space narrowing with sclerosis of the vertebral endplates and the formation of small triangular osteophytes from the anterior vertebral margins are evident. Prominent vacuum phenomena (arrows) are present in the lumbar spine. (From Resnick, D., and Niwayama, G.: Diagnosis of Bone and Joint Disorders. Philadelphia, W.B. Saunders Co., 1981.)

inate on the right side, presumably because their formation is inhibited on the left side by the constant pulsation of the descending thoracic aorta.[132] Narrowing of the intervertebral disc space, vacuum phenomena, and endplate bony sclerosis are not features of spondylosis deformans. The differentiation of the osteophytes of spondylosis deformans from the vertebral lesions of the seronegative spondyloarthropathies has been discussed previously.

Apophyseal Joint Osteoarthritis. The synovium-lined apophyseal joint is a frequent site of degenerative disease.[128] Changes are most common in the mid and lower cervical spine, the mid thoracic spine, and the lower lumbar spine. The radiographic changes are identical to those of OA in peripheral articulations,[133] with joint space narrowing, osseous eburnation, and marginal osteophyte formation. Capsular laxity may result in apophyseal joint malalignment. In this setting or with large osteophytes arising from the joint margins, impingement of a spinal nerve root within the neural foramen may occur.

Uncovertebral Arthrosis. Degenerative changes in the cervical uncovertebral articulations (Lushka) are often identified on the frontal radiograph of the cervical spine. The nature of this process is debated, since these articulations have been shown to represent intervertebral disc extensions in early life and to contain synovium-like

Figure 39–38. Spondylosis deformans. The frontal projection of the spine reveals multiple large interdigitating osteophytes arising from the lateral margins of the vertebral bodies. Note that the initial portion of the osteophytes has a horizontal orientation.

tissue in later life. Radiographic changes consist of osseous sclerosis, joint space loss, and osteophyte formation.

Costovertebral Osteoarthritis. Osteoarthritic changes of the synovium-lined costovertebral joints are very common, especially at the level of the eleventh and twelfth ribs.[128] Radiographic demonstration of these abnormalities (joint space narrowing, bony sclerosis, osteophytes) is frequently difficult, owing to the superimposition of ribs and vertebral bodies over the articulations on conventional radiographic studies.

Diffuse Idiopathic Skeletal Hyperostosis. Diffuse idiopathic skeletal hyperostosis (DISH) is a common degenerative enthesopathy and has been described under a variety of terms,[134-136] including Forestier's disease, spondylitis ossificans ligamentosa, spondylosis hyperostotica, and ankylosing hyperostosis of the spine. Although radiographic changes are evident in both the axial and the appendicular skeleton, the diagnosis of DISH is based on the presence of characteristic spinal alterations. In fact, the radiographic change in the vertebral column must fulfill three criteria before a diagnosis of DISH can be made: (1) the presence of flowing calcification or ossification along the anterolateral aspects of at least four contiguous vertebral levels, (2) relative preservation of intervertebral disc height in the involved vertebral segments without extensive changes of primary degenerative disc disease, and (3) the absence of apophyseal joint ankylosis or sacroiliac joint erosions, sclerosis, or intra-articular bony ankylosis.

The most characteristic radiographic abnormality of DISH is calcification and ossification of the anterior longitudinal ligament (ALL) of the spine.[137] This is most commonly identified in the mid thoracic spine but is also evident in the cervical and lumbar levels. Early in the disease, an undulating radiodense band forms along the anterolateral aspect of the spine separated from the anterior aspect of the vertebral body by a thin radiolucent line (Fig. 39–39); with progression of the disease, the lucency may disappear. These changes, which are best demonstrated in the lateral radiographic projection of the thoracic spine, may resemble the "bamboo spine" of ankylosing spondylitis but several important diagnostic features exist. Syndesmophytes arise from the anterosuperior and anteroinferior margins of the vertebral body, whereas the ossification in DISH attaches to the vertebral body several millimeters from these margins. In addition, syndesmophytes may be best seen in the frontal radiographic projection, in contrast to DISH, in which changes are most prominent on the lateral radiographic projection. The presence of sacroiliac joint erosions and intra-articular bony ankylosis of the sacroiliac or apophyseal joints in ankylosing spondylitis constitutes another important differential diagnostic point.

In the cervical spine, bony outgrowths characteristically appear at the anteroinferior margin of the vertebral body and extend inferiorly around the disc space. With progression, a thick, armorlike mass of bone bridges the intervertebral disc, leading to markedly diminished cer-

Figure 39–39. Diffuse idiopathic skeletal hyperostosis (DISH). The lateral view of the thoracic spine in this patient with DISH demonstrates ossification of the anterior longitudinal ligament (ALL). Note the characteristic lucencies between the ossified ALL and the anterior vertebral margin (arrowheads).

vical motion and, in some cases, dysphagia (Fig. 39–40).[138] Linear or Y-shaped radiolucencies in the bony mass may be noted at the level of the intervertebral disc space owing to herniation of disc material into the ossific mass. Ossification adjacent to the inferior margin of the anterior arch of the atlas is common and may be confused with traumatic changes. Ossification of the posterior longitudinal ligament may be seen as a distinct entity but occurs with increased frequency in patients with DISH (Fig. 39–40).[139] DISH may also be associated with a rare syndrome, sternocostoclavicular hyperostosis (SCCH),[139,140] in which extensive ossification of the soft tissues between the anterior ribs, medial clavicle, and sternum is evident.

In the lumbar spine, changes of DISH resemble those in the cervical region; osteophytes are present.

Extraspinal manifestations of DISH[142] are especially common in the pelvis. Bony proliferation at sites of ligamentous and tendinous attachment (enthesopathy) results in the formation of coarse, well-marginated bony excrescences, in contrast to the fine, spiculated, ill-defined bony proliferative changes of the seronegative spondyloarthropathies (Fig. 39–41). Calcification of the iliolumbar and sacrotuberous ligaments is an additional characteristic feature (Fig. 39–42). Para-articular osteophytes are commonly noted about the hip and along the inferior aspect of the sacroiliac joints.

Figure 39–40. Diffuse idiopathic skeletal hyperostosis (DISH). The lateral view of the cervical spine in this patient demonstrates thick, flowing ossification along the anterior margins of the vertebral bodies. Ossification of the posterior longitudinal ligament (OPLL) is also present (arrows).

Figure 39–41. Diffuse idiopathic skeletal hyperostosis (DISH). The degenerative enthesopathy of DISH is well demonstrated with coarse bony excrescences arising from sites of ligament and tendon insertion along the lateral aspect of the ilium, superior acetabular margin, and lesser trochanter (arrows). This appearance differs from that of the finely spiculated inflammatory enthesopathy of the seronegative spondyloarthropathies.

Figure 39–42. Diffuse idiopathic skeletal hyperostosis (DISH). Calcification of the sacrotuberous ligaments (arrows) has occurred.

Other extraspinal sites of prominent bony proliferation include the patellar poles, calcaneus, and olecranon process of the ulna. The "spurs" that form at these sites may be identical in appearance to localized degenerative changes in otherwise normal individuals, but they demonstrate a tendency toward increased size and multiplicity. In the hand, hyperostotic changes of the metacarpal and phalangeal heads, with proliferation in the terminal tufts, may be noted. Irregular excrescences may also be seen at the femoral trochanters, deltoid tuberosity of the humerus and anterior tibial tuberosity and about the interosseous membranes of the forearm and leg.

NEUROARTHROPATHY

Neuroarthropathy (Charcot joint) refers to destructive and productive articular abnormalities occurring in association with loss of pain or proprioceptive sensation, or both. Although debate exists as to the precise pathogenesis of neuroarthropathy, it is believed that the cumulative effect of trauma and joint laxity due to relaxation of periarticular supporting structures is contributory.

One of the early radiographic changes of neuroarthropathy is the presence of a joint effusion, which may become large. Mild joint subluxation may then appear.[142] Subsequently, fragmentation of the articular surface occurs with eburnation of bony surfaces, leading, in time, to complete joint disorganization. These radiographic abnormalities have been subdivided into hypertrophic and atrophic types. The hypertrophic reaction is more common in central lesions, as in tabes dorsalis and syringomyelia. There is prominent periosteal new bone formation as well as metaplasia of the synovium with the formation of bone and cartilage within its deeper layers. Large osteocartilaginous bodies of synovial origin in combination with fragments originating from the articular surfaces result in a fragmented, disorganized articulation with a great deal of osseous debris (Fig. 39–43). The atrophic reaction occurs more commonly with dis-

eases, such as diabetes mellitus, in which the abnormality involves the peripheral nerve (Fig. 39–44). Fragmentation occurs, but the osteocartilaginous debris is resorbed, resulting in disappearance of the articular surfaces. It should be emphasized that hypertrophic and atrophic patterns are not completely reliable in identifying the level of neurologic abnormality, since exceptions to these rules are common.

A great number of disorders lead to neuropathic changes. In general the morphologic aberrations produced by these disorders are similar; however, there are differences in articular distribution among these disorders, which provide clues to the specific diagnosis.

Tabes Dorsalis.[142-144] Five to 10 percent of patients with tabes dorsalis demonstrate neuroarthropathy. The articulations of the lower extremity are most commonly affected, with the knee and the hip being the most frequent target sites (Fig. 39–43A and B). Other sites include the ankle and the articulations in both the upper extremity and the spinal column. In peripheral joints, typic radiographic features are large effusions, bony eburnation, and fragmentation. Bilateral and symmetric changes are not uncommon. In the axial skeleton, intervertebral disc space narrowing, vertebral body sclerosis, and formation of large osteophytes may resemble the changes of unusually severe degenerative disease.

Syringomyelia.[145] Approximately 20 to 50 percent of patients with syringomyelia develop neuroarthropathy. There is a distinct predilection for upper extremity involvement, especially the glenohumeral joint, elbow, and wrist. Lower extremity or spinal alterations may occur in some cases. Bilateral and symmetric involvement is less frequent in syringomyelia than in tabes dorsalis.

Diabetes Mellitus.[146-148] Diabetes mellitus is probably the most common cause of neuroarthropathy, although less than 1 percent of patients with this disease develop such changes. The articulations of the foot are affected in the majority of cases, although the ankle, knee, spine, and joints of the upper extremity may occasionally be affected. Abnormalities predominate in the tarsal and tarsometatarsal articulations, consisting of bony ebur-

Figure 39–43. Tabes dorsalis with neuroarthropathy. Radiographs of the elbow (*A*) and knee (*B*) in patients with tabes dorsalis demonstrate changes of neuroarthropathy. Bony sclerosis, fragmentation, and instability of the joints are present with dramatic soft tissue swelling.

nation and fragmentation. Spontaneous fractures are common and a Lisfranc fracture-dislocation pattern may be seen (Fig. 39–44). In the forefoot a resorptive pattern is most typical, with tapering or "sharpening" of metatarsal and phalangeal shafts. Concurrent or superimposed infection is a common problem in the diabetic individual. There is great difficulty in differentiating the radiographic changes of neuroarthropathy from those of infection; however, the indistinctness of bony margins in infection compared with the sharp margins in neuroarthropathy aids in correct diagnosis.

Other Disorders. Although peripheral neuropathy is common in the alcoholic patient, neuroarthropathy is rare. It resembles that in diabetes mellitus with characteristic involvement of the articulations of the foot.[149] In amyloidosis, knee and ankle involvement is most typical.[150] Neuropathic changes in childhood should suggest the possibility of congenital indifference to pain or meningomyelocele.[142] In both of these disorders involvement of the ankle and tarsal articulations is seen, and changes may appear at the physis, or growth plate, with osseous irregularity, sclerosis, epiphyseal separation, and periostitis. An idiopathic form of neuroarthropathy of the elbow has been described, and neuroarthropathic changes have been observed following intra-articular administration of steroids.

CRYSTAL–RELATED ARTHROPATHIES

Several types of articular disease are related to abnormal deposition or accumulation of crystalline material in and about articulations. These include gout, calcium pyrophosphate dihydrate (CPPD) crystal deposition disease, hemochromatosis, and hydroxyapatite crystal deposition disease (HADD).[151] Two other entities that may be included in this group are Wilson's disease and ochronosis (alkaptonuria).

Figure 39–44. Diabetic neuroarthropathy. A Lisfranc's type of fracture-dislocation has occurred as a complication of neuroarthropathy in this diabetic patient. Note the lateral displacement of the second through fifth metatarsal bases with sclerosis and fragmentation of the adjacent tarsal bones.

Gout. The earliest radiographic change in gout consists of reversible soft tissue swelling about the involved articulation during an acute gouty attack. With chronicity of disease, tophi lead to nodular, lobulated soft tissue densities, especially in the feet, ankles, knees, elbows, and hands. Calcification within a tophus may be evident, particularly in individuals with gouty nephritis, whereas ossification of a tophus is rare.[151,152] Bony erosions are common in longstanding gout and may be intra-articular or extra-articular in location. Intra-articular erosions most commonly involve the joint margins and proceed centrally (Fig. 39–45). Extra-articular erosions involve the cortex of the bone, frequently in association with a soft tissue mass (tophus) (Fig. 39–46). These erosions are usually round or oval in shape, often with a sclerotic border and a "punched-out" appearance.[153] The presence of an "overhanging lip" of bone at the margin of an erosion is a characteristic feature of gout. Occasionally a more extensive proliferative bony reaction, presumably due to a reparative process, may be noted, typically at the first metatarsophalangeal joint, intertarsal joints, and knee.[155] The joint space is usually preserved in gouty arthritis until the late stages of the disease. In fact, the presence of prominent intra-articular osseous erosions with relative preservation of the joint space suggests the diagnosis of gout. Intra-articular bony ankylosis is occasionally seen, especially involving the interphalangeal joints of the hands and feet as well as the carpal region.[154] Although transient localized osteoporosis may be present during an acute gouty attack, extensive osteoporosis is not a feature of this disease.

Figure 39–46. Gout. A large extra-articular erosion of the lateral aspect of the fifth metatarsal shaft is bordered by reactive bony sclerosis (arrow). A smaller erosion is present more proximally (arrowhead) with an adjacent calcified soft tissue tophus. (From Resnick, D., and Niwayama, G.: Diagnosis of Bone and Joint Disorders. Philadelphia, W.B. Saunders Co., 1981.)

The general radiographic features of gout are similar at all sites; however, involvement at several specific areas may be of diagnostic importance.[151] The first metatarsophalangeal joint is the most characteristic site of involvement (Fig. 39–45). Erosions are most frequent on the dorsal and medial aspects of the metatarsal head, usually in association with a hallux valgus deformity. They are best demonstrated in the oblique radiographic projection. In the hand, proximal and distal interphalangeal joint involvement is more common than metacarpophalangeal joint involvement. Wrist abnormality is frequently pancompartmental, but extensive involvement of the common carpometacarpal articulation is important, since this area is relatively spared in most other arthropathies. Erosions of the olecranon process of the elbow and the dorsal surface of the patella strongly suggest gouty bursitis.

Chondrocalcinosis is occasionally seen in patients with gout. It is usually localized to a few articulations and predominates in fibrocartilage.

Secondary gout is associated with a wide variety of situations, including glycogen storage disease (type I),[156] Lesch-Nyhan syndrome,[157] myeloproliferative disorders,[158] endocrine diseases,[159] and the administration of certain drugs.[160] In general, secondary gout resembles primary gout radiographically, although unusual sites may be affected.[156-160]

Figure 39–45. Gout. Typical erosions of the metatarsal head and proximal phalangeal base (arrows) are present in this patient with gouty arthritis of the first metatarsophalangeal joint.

Calcium Pyrophosphate Dihydrate (CPPD) Crystal Deposition Disease. CPPD crystal deposition disease is characterized by the deposition of calcium pyrophosphate dihydrate crystals in hyaline cartilage and fibrocartilage as well as in synovium, capsule, tendons, and ligaments.[151] CPPD crystal deposition disease is a general term indicating the presence of CPPD crystal in or around joints. Chondrocalcinosis refers to calcification of hyaline cartilage or fibrocartilage, regardless of its etiology. Pyrophosphate arthropathy refers to a pattern of structural joint damage with or without radiographically demonstrable chondrocalcinosis. There are two main types of radiographic abnormalities in CPPD crystal deposition disease: (1) abnormal calcification and (2) destructive arthropathy. These changes may be present in combination or in isolation.

Abnormal calcification related to CPPD crystal deposition disease may be identified in articular or periarticular structures. The most comon intra-articular site of calcification is within cartilage, either hyaline cartilage or fibrocartilage (Fig. 39–47). Hyaline cartilage calcification may occur in any joint but is most common in the wrist, knee, elbow, and hip. It appears as thin curvilinear radiodensities parallel to, but distinct from, the subchondral bone plate.[151] Fibrocartilage calcification most commonly involves the menisci of the knee, triangular fibrocartilage of the wrist, symphysis pubis, annulus fibrosus of the intervertebral disc, or labra of the glenoid and acetabulum. (Fig. 39–48). It appears as thick, irregular radiodensities within the involved structure. Cloudlike or speckled radiodensities, representing calcific deposits within synovium, may be seen at many locations, including bursal cavities, but are most common about the wrist. Additional sites of calcification include joint capsule, tendons, bursae, and ligaments.[161] Calcification at these sites is less frequent than within cartilage.

Pyrophosphate arthropathy exhibits a degenerative disease–type pattern of structural joint disease. Its general radiographic features include a bilateral symmetric or asymmetric distribution and changes characterized by joint space narrowing, bony sclerosis, and prominent subchondral cysts.[161] The latter, representing an important diagnostic feature of the arthropathy, are frequently numerous and large and may simulate neoplasm. These cysts may progress rapidly in size, undermining the articular surface and resulting in collapse and deformity of the joint. At times, this progression may be so rapid as to resemble infection or neuroarthropathy (Fig. 39–49). In some patients, large osteophytes may be present about involved articulations.

Pyrophosphate arthropathy is most commonly seen in the knee, wrist, and metacarpophalangeal joints, although any joint may be involved. The relatively common involvement of the wrist, elbow, and shoulder contrast with the situation in degenerative joint disease in which these areas are usually spared. In the hand there is a tendency toward selective involvement of the second and third metacarpophalangeal joints. In the wrist, the radioscaphoid space is frequently involved, with collapse of the proximal pole of the scaphoid into the distal radial articular surface (Fig. 39–50). Narrowing of the capitolunate space is also frequent, as is involvement of the trapezioscaphoid articulation with or without involvement of the first carpometacarpal joint. Associated calcification of the triangular fibrocartilage, intercarpal ligaments, or articular cartilage may be encountered. In the knee, the distribution of abnormalities may mimic that of osteoarthritis with involvement of the medial femorotibial and patellofemoral compartments. At times, there is isolated involvement of the patellofemoral space. In the hip, superior joint space narrowing, mimicking osteoarthritis, or axial migration of the femoral head, simulating rheumatoid arthritis, can be seen.

Figure 39–48. Calcium pyrophosphate crystal deposition disease. A frontal radiograph of the wrist demonstrates calcification of the triangular fibrocartilage (open arrow) and several intercarpal ligaments (arrowheads). (From Resnick, D., and Niwayama, G.: Diagnosis of Bone and Joint Disorders. Philadelphia, W.B. Saunders Co., 1981.)

Figure 39–47. Calcium pyrophosphate crystal deposition disease. A frontal radiograph of the knee reveals calcification of hyaline articular cartilage (*H*) as well as fibrocartilaginous menisci (*F*). (From Resnick, D., and Niwayama, G.: Diagnosis of Bone and Joint Disorders. Philadelphia, W.B. Saunders Co., 1981.)

Figure 39–49. Calcium pyrophosphate crystal deposition disease. *A* and *B* are radiographs of the hip obtained 16 months apart. In *A*, there is preservation of the joint space with subtle cystic change within the femoral head (arrow). In *B*, there is collapse of the femoral head with large cystic lesions (arrows) and fragmentation of the acetabulum (arrowhead). This rapidly progressive arthropathy is characteristic of pyrophosphate arthropathy. (From Resnick, D., and Niwayama, G.: Diagnosis of Bone and Joint Disorders. Philadelphia, W.B. Saunders Co., 1981.)

Figure 39–50. Calcium pyrophosphate crystal deposition disease. In this patient, the changes of pyrophosphate arthropathy include narrowing of the radiocarpal joint with collapse of the scaphoid into the radial articular surface (arrow) as well as the presence of numerous subchondral cystic lesions. Calcification of the triangular fibrocartilage can also be noted.

Calcium Hydroxyapatite Crystal Deposition Disease (HADD). HADD may be a primary idiopathic disorder or secondary to other diseases and is characterized by the deposition of calcium hydroxyapatite crystals in periarticular or, rarely, intra-articular structures. In idiopathic disease, calcification is most commonly seen about the shoulder, although involvement of the hand, wrist, hip, foot, and paraspinal tissues may be seen. Hydroxyapatite deposits appear on radiographs as soft, cloudlike densities within tendons, ligaments, joint capsules, bursae, and periarticular soft tissues. These deposits may vary in size from small collections, 1 to 2 mm in diameter, to large lobulated masses, many centimeters in diameter. On serial radiographs, deposits may enlarge, remain unchanged, or diminish in size. They can even disappear completely.

In the shoulder, HADD is most commonly identified in the supraspinatus tendon of the fibromuscular rotator cuff. Here, it is frequently referred to as calcific tendinitis, peritendinitis calcarea, or hydroxyapatite rheumatism (Fig. 39–51).[151] Other sites of calcification in the shoulder include the infraspinatus, teres minor, subscapularis, and bicipital tendons.[162] It should be emphasized that in most cases these deposits are not symptomatic; the majority of patients with shoulder discomfort and periarticular calcific deposits will have another cause of

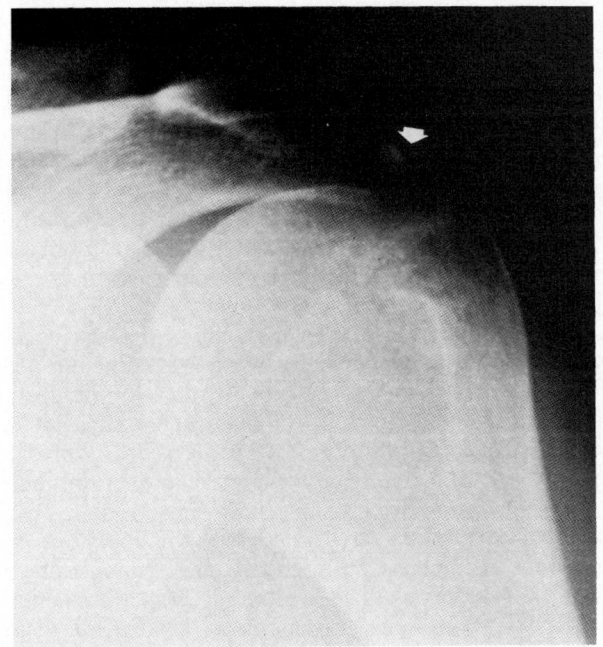

Figure 39–51. Hydroxyapatite crystal deposition disease. Calcification (arrow) of the supraspinatus tendon of the musculotendinous rotator cuff is present. This constitutes the single most common manifestation of this disorder. (From Resnick, D., and Niwayama, G.: Diagnosis of Bone and Joint Disease. Philadelphia, W.B. Saunders Co., 1981.)

pain, frequently subacromial bursitis or rotator cuff tendinitis.

Intra-articular HADD may be seen as an isolated event or in association with osteoarthritis or collagen vascular disease. Radiographically, cloudlike calcific collections within the joint are apparent. Rarely, severe articular destruction, especially in the glenohumeral joint, may be an associated feature.

Periarticular calcification, representing hydroxyapatite crystal deposition, is seen in a variety of disorders,[151] including hyperparathyroidism, renal osteodystrophy, collagen vascular diseases, hypoparathyroidism, milk-alkali syndrome, hypervitaminosis D, and sardoidosis.

Hemochromatosis. Radiographically the manifestations of hemochromatosis may be divided into three major categories: (1) osteoporosis, (2) articular calcification, and (3) structural joint damage.

Diffuse osteoporosis is an important feature of hemochromatosis,[163] in contrast to idiopathic CPPD crystal deposition disease, and may involve the axial and appendicular skeleton. In the spine, collapse of the vertebral endplates leads to biconcave deformities of the vertebral body ("fish" vertebra). Osteoporosis in the appendicular skeleton tends to be diffuse without a tendency toward a periarticular distribution.[165]

Articular calcification, related to CPPD crystal deposition (chondrocalcinosis), occurs in approximately 30 percent of patients with hemochromatosis.[151] In general this calcification is identical to that of idiopathic CPPD crystal deposition disease, but several characteristics may help to distinguish between these two disorders. In

hemochromatosis, hyaline cartilage calcification tends to be more prominent and the fibrocartilage of the symphysis pubis is more commonly involved than in idiopathic CPPD crystal deposition disease.[151]

Structural articular alterations in hemochromatosis occur in slightly less than half of the cases.[166,167] In general, the arthropathy of hemochromatosis is similar to that of idiopathic CPPD crystal deposition disease with joint space narrowing and subchondral cyst formation being prominent features. Although the two disorders cannot be absolutely separated on a radiographic basis, several features may be useful in differential diagnosis.[151] "Hook" osteophytes are distinctive bony excrescences, most commonly identified at the radial margins of the metacarpal heads, in patients with hemochromatosis. These osteophytes tend to be small, triangular, and sharply defined (Fig. 39–52). They are not prominent in osteoarthritis or idiopathic CPPD crystal deposition disease. The distribution of abnormalities may also be a useful diagnostic feature. In both CPPD crystal deposition disease and hemochromatosis, the second and third metacarpophalangeal joints are the most commonly involved sites in the hands, but additional alterations of the fourth and fifth metacarpophalangeal joints are more frequent in hemochromatosis. In addition, the radiocarpal joint may be spared in hemochromatosis, whereas it is almost always involved in idiopathic CPPD crystal deposition disease. The arthropathy of hemochromatosis is usually slowly progressive in contrast to idiopathic pyrophosphate arthropathy, in which a rapidly progressive arthropathy may be seen.

Wilson's Disease. Wilson's disease is a rare inherited disorder characterized by abnormal accumulation of copper in body tissues. The age of onset is typically the first through fourth decades of life. The general radi-

Figure 39–52. Hemochromatosis. There is joint space narrowing with erosive change about the second through fifth metacarpophalangeal joints. "Hook" osteophytes (arrowheads) occur at the radial margins of the metacarpal heads. (From Resnick, D., and Niwayama, G.: Diagnosis of Bone and Joint Disorders. Philadelphia, W.B. Saunders Co., 1981.)

ographic features consist of osteopenia and arthropathy.[151,168] Chondrocalcinosis has been considered an important feature of this disorder, but it appears to be very rare. Osteopenia, present in approximately 50 percent of patients, is most prominent in the hands, feet, and spine. It may relate to osteoporosis or osteomalacia, or both. Changes of rickets, with Looser's zones or "pseudofractures," are prominent in some cases.[169]

The arthropathy of Wilson's disease is most commonly identified in the wrist, hand, foot, hip, shoulder, elbow, and knee. Irregularity and indistinctness of the subchondral bone plate ("paintbrush" appearance) in combination with focal radiodense excrescences at the central and peripheral joint margins are characteristic. Subchondral cysts and focal areas of fragmentation of the articular surface may also be observed. An additional manifestation is the occurrence of small distinctly corticated ossicles about affected joints, especially prominent in the wrist. These structures resemble the accessory ossicles frequently seen in normal individuals but are more numerous and appear in unusual locations. Joint effusions are not prominent, but spiculated bony proliferative changes are frequently noted at entheses, resembling the inflammatory enthesopathy seen in the seronegative spondyloarthropathies.

Ochronosis (Alkaptonuria). The major radiographic features of ochronosis consist of osteoporosis, abnormal calcification and ossification, and arthropathy.[151] Osteoporosis, although generally diffuse in nature, is most prominent in the spine, where it may be associated with vertebral body collapse.[170]

Abnormal calcification and ossification are most prominent in the intervertebral discs, especially those in the lumbar spine. Additional sites of calcification and ossification include the symphysis pubis, costal cartilage, helix of the ear, and peripheral tendons and ligaments.[171] The crystals are composed of calcium hydroxyapatite and demonstrate a typical "cloudlike" appearance.

In the spine osteoporosis with waferlike calcification of the intervertebral disc is an early radiographic finding. Intervertebral disc narrowing with the formation of radiolucent discal collections (vacuum phenomena) are also common, often obscuring the calcification.[172] Progressive discal ossification and the formation of peripheral bony bridges in the outermost layer of the annulus fibrosus may lead to the appearance of a "bamboo spine," similar to that in ankylosing spondylitis. At some levels, osteophytes may also be prominent.

In the peripheral skeleton, the knees, hips, and shoulders are most commonly involved, with relative sparing of the small joints of the hands and feet.[172] In these locations, changes resemble those of degenerative joint disease; however, osteophytes and subchondral cysts are not prominent in ochronosis. In addition the location of abnormalities, such as the lateral femorotibial compartment of the knee, may help in differentiating ochronosis from OA. Occasionally, a rapidly progressing destructive peripheral arthropathy characterized by fragmentation of articular surfaces may be observed.

SEPTIC ARTHRITIS

Mechanisms. In general the radiographic features of joint sepsis consist of periarticular soft tissue swelling, intra-articular effusions, cartilage destruction with joint space narrowing, and irregular erosions of the subchondral bone plate.[173-175] In the initial stage of disease, the joint may appear widened, owing to the presence of a large effusion, but rapid cartilage destruction results in articular space narrowing with confluent irregular erosions of the subchondral bone plate (Fig. 39–53). In children, epiphyseal centers may completely disappear as a result of the hyperemia associated with the infected joint. Diabetic patients are prone to develop indolent, slowly progressive joint infections, usually adjacent to soft tissue ulcerations. In this setting the loss of distinctiveness of articular margins may be the only radiographic manifestation of infection (Fig. 39–54).

In contrast to bacterial infection, granulomatous infection (tuberculosis and fungal) may demonstrate a more slowly progressive pattern of joint destruction (Fig. 39–55). Osseous erosions first appear at the joint margins ("bare" areas) where synovial inflammatory tissue is in direct contact with bone. In fact, prominent juxta-articular osteoporosis and marginal bone erosions, in the absence of significant joint space loss, are characteristics of granulomatous infection. The late complications of joint sepsis include intra-articular fibrous or bony ankylosis as well as joint instability. In the spine the latter complication may result in spinal cord or nerve root compromise.

Figure 39–53. Septic arthritis. In this patient with a pyogenic arthritis of the ankle, note the soft tissue swelling, joint space loss, and large confluent subchondral erosions.

Figure 39–54. Septic arthritis. In this specimen radiograph of an infected foot in a diabetic patient, note the erosions of the lateral margins of the articular surfaces of the first metatarsal head and proximal phalanx (arrowheads).

Figure 39–55. Tuberculosis. Note the gradual progression of destructive changes in radiographs obtained 18 months apart. In *A* there is prominent soft tissue swelling and osteoporosis with marginal osseous erosions at multiple sites. In *B* the process has progressed to virtually complete destruction of the carpus. A large erosion of the distal radius is also present.

The role of various imaging modalities in the diagnosis of joint sepsis should be emphasized. Early detection is important in order to avoid irreversible joint destruction, or in the child, significant growth disturbance. Radionuclide studies are useful in this regard, both in detecting infection early in the course of the disease and in documenting the extent of involvement. However, adjacent soft tissue or bone infections, recent surgery, or post-traumatic changes may render this important tool useless in some cases. Recognition of articular effusions and periarticular soft tissue swelling on roentgenograms is of critical importance in the early diagnosis of joint infection. Magnification radiography may provide additional diagnostic information, especially in the diabetic patient with a foot infection. Fluoroscopically guided aspiration may play an important role in the evaluation of joint sepsis, especially in deep joints such as the hip or the shoulder or in sites such as the spine where surgical exploration may be required. Although the principal aim of this procedure is to procure a specimen for laboratory analysis, instillation of a small amount of radiopaque contrast agent may be helpful in ascertaining the extent of articular destruction and in detecting extra-articular spread of contaminated material.

MISCELLANEOUS ARTHROPATHIES

Osteonecrosis. Early in the course of epiphyseal osteonecrosis, radiographic changes are not evident. Subsequently a characteristic progression of radiographic changes will be seen. The earliest findings are a subtle, arclike radiolucent subchondral band (crescent sign) and the formation of patchy subchondral lucent and sclerotic foci (Fig. 39–56). Fragmentation and collapse of the articular surface follow. The joint space is usually preserved until late in the course of the disease when secondary osteoarthritis may supervene.

A peculiar form of spontaneous osteonecrosis is seen in the knee, most commonly involving the medial femoral condyle. It is manifested by the sudden appearance of pain and the radiographic changes of sclerosis, flattening, and irregularity of the femoral surface (Fig. 39–57).

Paget's Disease. Articular disease is a recognized complication of Paget's disease. Gout,[176] CPPD crystal deposition disease,[177] and rheumatoid arthritis[176] have each been observed in patients with Paget's disease. More importantly, individuals with this disease demonstrate an increased incidence of osteoarthritis in association with juxta-articular pagetic bony involvement.[121] This is most common in the hip and knee. Although radiographic features resemble those in idiopathic osteoarthritis (Fig. 39–58), more specific changes, such as acetabular protrusion, may be seen.

Acromegaly. Acromegalic arthropathy most closely resembles degenerative joint disease. Some features that aid in its recognition are (1) increased soft tissue thickness (e.g., heel pad > 21 mm) (Fig. 39–59), (2) promi-

Figure 39–56. Osteonecrosis. An early radiographic change of osteonecrosis is an arclike radiolucent band (arrowheads) parallel to the articular surface.

Figure 39–57. Spontaneous osteonecrosis. In this adult with the sudden onset of knee pain, the frontal radiograph demonstrates a defect in the articular surface of the medial femoral condyle (arrow). This is the characteristic location of this lesion. (From Resnick, D., and Niwayama, G.: Diagnosis of Bone and Joint Disorders. Philadelphia, W.B. Saunders Co., 1981.)

Figure 39–58. Paget's disease. Observe the prominent osteoarthritislike changes of the hip with asymmetric joint space loss and large marginal osteophytes. The juxta-articular bone is coarsened and enlarged.

Figure 39–60. Acromegaly. There is proliferation of the margins of the base and terminal tuft of the distal phalanx resulting in the classic "arrowhead" appearance.

Figure 39–59. Acromegaly. Note the soft tissue prominence of the heel pad with the formation of multiple osteophytes from the plantar and posterior surfaces of the calcaneus. (From Resnick, D., and Niwayama, G.: Diagnosis of Bone and Joint Disorders. Philadelphia, W.B. Saunders Co., 1981.)

Figure 39–61. Acromegaly. In this case, the most striking finding is the abnormally increased height of the intervertebral disc spaces (between arrowheads). Note posterior concavity of the vertebral bodies and degenerative changes.

Figure 39–62. Amyloidosis. Observe the diffuse soft tissue swelling and the presence of destructive lesions in the third and fourth metacarpal bases (arrows), radius, and ulna.

Figure 39–63. Hemophilia. There is overgrowth of the epiphyses, especially the radial head. Joint space narrowing and subchondral cysts are seen.

nent phalangeal tufts and bases ("arrowhead" phalanges) (Fig. 39–60), (3) "hooklike" osteophytes in the metacarpal heads, (4) joint space widening, (5) exuberant spinal osteophytosis with widened intervertebral discs (Fig. 39–61), and (6) prominent thoracic kyphosis.[178,179] In the later stages of the disease, loss of joint space becomes apparent. Acromegaly should be considered if a degenerative process occurs in an unusual articulation, such as the glenohumeral joint.

Hemoglobinopathies. Hemoglobinopathies may affect articular structures. The major changes in sickle cell anemia relate to vascular occlusion with osteonecrosis, which may involve epiphysis, metaphysis, or diaphysis of a tubular bone as well as flat bones. In sickle cell dactylitis (hand-foot syndrome), the changes of bone infarction are accompanied by prominent soft tissue swelling and exuberant periosteal reaction.[180] Osteomyelitis and, less commonly, septic arthritis can be seen in sickle cell anemia. Salmonella is frequently implicated.

Amyloidosis. Radiographically the diagnosis is suggested by the occurrence of a bilateral symmetric erosive arthropathy similar to rheumatoid arthritis but without joint space narrowing.[181,182] Large soft tissue masses and osteolytic defects in the diaphyses of tubular bones are other prominent findings in this disorder (Fig. 39–62).

Hemophilia. The arthropathy of hemophilia is related to destructive changes associated with repeated episodes of intra-articular hemorrhage (hemarthrosis).[183] Any joint may be involved, but changes in the knee, ankle, and elbow are most frequently identified. The earliest finding consists of juxta-articular soft tissue swelling with large intra-articular effusions. This is followed by prominent osteoporosis and, in the immature skeleton,

by epiphyseal overgrowth (Fig. 39–63). Subchondral cysts and bony erosions appear, initially with preservation of the cartilaginous coat, and subsequently with cartilage destruction and joint space narrowing. Late abnormalities include complete joint disorganization

Figure 39–64. Idiopathic synovial (osteo)chondromatosis. A radiograph of the elbow reveals multiple calcified bodies of varying sizes within the confines of an enlarged joint capsule.

Figure 39–65. Idiopathic synovial (osteo)chondromatosis. A plain film (*A*) and arthrogram (*B*) reveal typical changes. In *A*, observe intra-articular calcified bodies along the synovial sheath of the bicipital tendons. The arthrogram defines multiple radiolucent filling defects.

with obliteration of the articular space, large bony erosions, and joint instability. In the knee, radiographic features of hemophilia include widening of the intercondylar notch of the distal femur and squaring of the inferior patellar pole. The radiographic features of hemophilia may be difficult to differentiate from those of juvenile chronic arthritis.

Synovial (Osteo)chondromatosis and Pigmented Villonodular Synovitis. The typical radiographic picture of synovial (osteo)chondromatosis is that of numerous calcific densities confined to the articular cavity (Fig. 39–64). Pressure erosions of adjacent bony surfaces may be seen. Osteoporosis and joint space narrowing are generally not prominent. In cases where the bodies are not calcified, arthrography may confirm the diagnosis (Fig. 39–65).

Multiple erosions and cysts on both sides of the joint are seen in pigmented villonodular synovitis. Osteoporosis and joint space narrowing are usually not prominent.[184,186] During arthrography, nodular soft tissue masses may be demonstrated and aspiration of joint fluid will yield a characteristic "rusty" fluid.

Synovial Sarcoma. The typical roentgenographic finding of a synovial sarcoma is a soft tissue mass, which contains calcification in approximately 30 percent of cases. Erosion of neighboring bone is seen in 25 to 35 percent of lesions.

References

1. Mall, J.C., Genant, H.K., Silcox, D.C., and McCarty, D.J.: The efficacy of fine-detail radiography in the evaluation of patients with rheumatoid arthritis. Radiology 112:37, 1974.
2. Genant, H.K.: Magnification radiography. *In* Resnick, D., and Niwayama, G. (eds.) Diagnosis of Bone and Joint Disorders. Philadelphia, W. B. Saunders Company, 1981, p. 335.
3. Genant, H.K., Vardez Horst, J., Lanzl, L.H., Mall, J.C., and Doi, K.: Skeletal demineralization in primary hyperparathyroidism. *In* Mazesi, R.B. (ed.): Proceedings of the International Conference on Bone Min-

eral Measurement. Washington D.C., National Institute of Arthritis, Metabolism and Digestive Diseases, 1973, p. 177.
4. Leach, R.E., Grett, T., and Ferris, J.S.: Weight-bearing radiography in osteoarthritis of the knee. Radiology 97:265, 1970.
5. Resnick, D., and Danzig, L.: Arthrographic evaluation of injuries of the first metacarpophalangeal joint: Gamekeeper's Thumb. Am. J. Roentgenol. 126:1046, 1976.
6. Chamberlain, W.E.: The symphysis pubis in the roentgen examination of the sacroiliac joint. Am. J. Roentgenol. 24:621, 1930.
7. Martel, W., and Poznanski, A.K.: The value of traction during roentgenography of the hip. Radiology 94:497, 1970.
8. Resnick, D.: Arthrography, tenography and bursography. *In* Resnick, D., and Niwayama, G. (ed.): Diagnosis of Bone and Joint Disorders., Philadelphia, W. B. Saunders Company, 1981, p. 510.
9. Gelman, M., Coleman, R.E., Stevens, P.M., and Davey, B.W.: Radiography, radionuclide imaging, and arthrography in evaluation of painful total hip and knee replacements. Radiology 128:677, 1978.
10. Wolfe, R.D., and Giuliano, V.J.: Double-contrast arthrography in the diagnosis of pigmented villonodular synovitis of the knee. Am. J. Roentgenol. 110:793, 1970.
11. Prager, R.J., and Mall, J.C.: Arthrographic diagnosis of synovial chondromatosis. Am. J. Roentgenol. 127:344, 1976.
12. Strizak, A.M., Danzig, L.A., Jackson, D.W., Greenway, G., Resnick, D., and Staple, T.: Subacromial bursography: an anatomic and clinical study. J. Bone and Joint Surg. 64A:196, 1982.
13. Cone, R., Danzig, L., and Resnick, D.: The shoulder impingement syndrome. Radiology 150:29, 3, 10, 1984.
14. Carrera, G.F., Foley, W.D., Kozin, F., et al.: CT of sacroiliitis. Am. J. Roentgenol. 136:41, 1981.
15. Sheldon, J.J., Sersland, T., and Leboranc, J.: Computed tomography of the lower lumbar vertebral column. Radiology 124:183, 1977.
16. Genant, H.K.: Quantitative bone mineral analysis. *In* Resnick, D., and Niwayama, G. (eds.): Diagnosis of Bone and Joint Disorders. Philadelphia, W. B. Saunders Company, 1981, p. 686.
17. Resnick, D., and Niwayama, G.: Rheumatoid arthritis. *In* Resnick, D., and Niwayama, G. (eds.): Diagnosis of Bone and Joint Disorders. Philadelphia, W. B. Saunders Company, 1981, p. 906.
18. O'Driscoll, S., and O'Driscoll, M.: Osteomalacia in rheumatoid arthritis. Ann. Rheum. Dis. 39:1, 1980.
19. DeHaas, W.H.D., DeBoer, W., Griffin, F., and Oosten-Elst, P.: Rheumatoid arthritis of the robust reaction type. Ann. Rheum. Dis. 33:81, 1974.
20. Renneic, C., Mainzer, F., Multz, C.V., and Genant, H.K.: Subchondral pseudocysts in rheumatoid arthritis. Am. J. Roentgenol. 129:1069, 1977.
21. Norgaard, F.: Tidligste rontgenoligiske forandringer ved polyarthritis. Ugeskr. Laeger 125:1312, 1963.
22. Resnick, D.: Rheumatoid arthritis of the wrist. The compartmental approach. Med. Radiog. Photog. 52:50, 1976.
23. Resnick, D.: Rheumatoid arthritis of the wrist: Why the ulnar styloid? Radiolgy 112:29, 1974.

24. Berens, D.L., and Lin, R.K.: Roentgen Diagnosis of Rheumatoid Arthritis. Springfield, Ill., Charles C Thomas, 1969.

25. Resnick, D.: Early abnormalities of the pisiform and triquetrum in rheumatoid arthritis. Ann. Rheum. Dis. 35:46, 1976.

26. Linscheid, R.L.: The mechanical factors affecting deformity at the wrist in rheumatoid arthritis. In Proceedings of the twenty-fourth annual meeting of the American Society for Surgery of the Hand. New York, Jan. 17–18, 1969. J. Bone Joint Surg. 51A:790, 1969.

27. Jackman, R.J., and Pugh, D.G.: The positive elbow fat pad sign in rheumatoid arthritis. Am. J. Roentgenol. 108:812, 1970.

28. Weston, W.J.: The synovial changes at the elbow in rheumatoid arthritis. Australas. Radiog. 15:170, 1971.

29. Rappaport, A.S., Sosman, J.L., and Weissman, B.N.: Spontaneous fractures of the olecranon process in rheumatoid arthritis. Radiology 119:83, 1976.

30. Short, C.L. Bauer, W., and Reynolds, W.E.: Rheumatoid Arthritis. Cambridge, Massachusetts, Harvard University Press, 1957.

31. Thould, A.K., and Simon, G.: Assessment of the radiological changes in the hands and feet in rheumatoid arthritis. Ann. Rheum. Dis. 25:220, 1966.

32. Calabro, J.J.: The feet as an aid in the differential diagnosis of arthritis (abstr.). Arthritis Rheum. 3:435, 1960.

33. Bywaters, E.G.L.: Heel lesions in rheumatoid arthritis. Ann. Rheum. Dis. 13:42, 1954.

34. Resnick, D., Feingold, M.L., Curd, J., Niwayama, G., and Goergen, T.G.: Calcaneal abnormalities in articular disorders. Rheumatoid arthritis, ankylosing spondylitis, psoriatic arthritis, and Reiter's Syndrome. Radiology 125:355, 1977.

35. Kirkup, J.R.: Ankle and tarsal joints in rheumatoid arthritis. Scand. J. Rheumatol. 3:50, 1974.

36. Magayar, E., Talerman, A., Feher, M., and Wouters, H.W.: Giant bone cysts in rheumatoid arthritis. J. Bone Joint Surg. 56B:121, 1974.

37. Genovese, G.R., Jayson, M.I.J., and Dixon, A.S.: Protective value of synovial cysts in rheumatoid knees. Ann. Rheum. Dis. 31:179, 1972.

38. Resnick, D.: Patterns of migration of the femoral head in ostoearthritis of the hip: roentgenographic-pathologic correlation and comparison with rheumatoid arthritis. Am. J. Roentgenol. 124:62, 1975.

39. Armbuster, T., Guerra, J., Resnick, D., Georgen, J.G., Feingold, M.L., Niwayama, G., and Danzig, L.: The adult hip: An anatomic study. Part I. The bony landmarks. Radiology 128:1, 1978.

40. Sievers, K., and Caine, V.: The sacroiliac joint in rheumatoid arthritis in adult females. Acta Rheum. Scand. 9:222, 1963.

41. Linquist, P.R., and McDonnell, D.E.: Rheumatoid cyst causing extradural compression. J. Bone Joint Surg. 52A:1235, 1970.

42. Martel, W.: The occipito-atlanto-axial joints in rheumatoid arthritis. In Carter, M.E. (ed.): Radiological Aspects of Rheumatoid Disease. Proceedings of an international symposium, Amsterdam, 1963. Amsterdam, Excerpta Medica, 1964, p. 189.

43. Mathews, J.A.: Atlanto-axial subluxation in rheumatoid arthritis. A 5-year follow-up study. Ann. Rheum. Dis. 33:526, 1974.

44. Martel, W.: The occipito-atlanto-axial joints in rheumatoid arthritis and ankylosing spondylitis. Am. J. Roentgenol. 86:223, 1961.

45. Rana, N.A., Hancock, D.O., Taylor, A.R., and Hill, A.G.S.: Upward translocation of the dens in rheumatoid arthritis. J. Bone Joint Surg. 55B:471, 1973.

46. Ansell, B.M., and Kent, P.A.: Radiological changes in juvenile chronic polyarthritis. Skel. Radiol. 1:129, 1977.

47. Ansell, B.M., and Bywaters, E.G.L.: Growth in Still's Disease. Ann. Rheum. Dis. 15:295, 1956.

48. Martel, W., Holt, J.F., and Cassidy, J.T.: Roentgenologic manifestations of juvenile rheumatoid arthritis. Am. J. Roentgenol. 88:400, 1962.

49. Resnick, D., and Niwayama, G.: Juvenile chronic arthritis. In Resnick, D., and Niwayama, G. (ed.): Diagnosis of Bone and Joint Disease. Philadelphia, W. B. Saunders Company, 1981, p. 1008.

50. Ansell, B.M.: Chronic arthritis in childhood. Ann. Rheum. Dis. 37:107, 1978.

51. Schaller, J., and Wedgewood, R.J.: Juvenile rheumatoid arthritis: A review. Pediatrics 50:940, 1972.

52. Cassidy, J.T., Brody, G.L., and Martel, W.: Monoarticular juvenile rheumatoid arthritis. J. Pediatr. 70:867, 1967.

53. Kleinman, P., Rivelas, M., Schneider, R., and Kaye, J.J.: Juvenile ankylosing spondylitis. Radiology 125:775, 1977.

54. Resnick, D.: Patterns of peripheral joint disease in ankylosing spondylitis. Radiology 110:523, 1977.

55. Bywaters, E.G.L.: Still's disease in the adult. Ann. Rheum. Dis. 30:121, 1971.

56. Medsger, T.A. Jr., and Christy, W.C.: Carpal arthritis with ankylosis in late onset Still's disease. Arthritis Rheum. 19:232, 1976.

57. Bluestone, R.: Histocompatibility antigens and rheumatic disease. In Current Concepts. Kalamazoo, Michigan, Upjohn Company, 1978, p. 17.

58. Resnick, D., and Niwayama, G.: Ankylosing spondylitis. In Resnick, D., and Niwayama, G. (eds.): Diagnosis of Bone and Joint Disorders. Philadelphia, W. B. Saunders Company, 1981, p. 1040.

59. Wilkinson, M., and Bywaters, E.G.L.: Clinical features and course of ankylosing spondylitis as seen in a follow-up of 222 hospital referred cases. Ann. Rheum. Dis. 17:209, 1958.

60. Rosen, P.S., and Graham, D.C.: Ankylosing (Strumpell-Marie) Spondylitis (A clinical review of 128 cases). AIR 5:158, 1962.

61. Berens, D.L.: Roentgen features of ankylosing spondylitis. Clin. Orthop. Rel. Res. 74:20, 1971.

62. Resnick, D., Niwayama, G., and Goergen, T.G.: Comparison of radiographic abnormalities of the sacro-iliac joint in degenerative joint disease and ankylosing spondylitis. Am. J. Roentgenol. 128:189, 1977.

63. Forestier, J., Jacqueline, F., and Rotes-Querol, J.: Ankylosing Spondylitis. Springfield, Ill., Charles C Thomas, 1956.

64. Cawley, M.I.D., Chalmers, T.M., Kellgren, J.H., and Ball, J.: Destructive lesions of vertebral bodies in ankylosing spondylitis. Ann. Rheum. Dis. 31:345, 1972.

65. Dwosh, I.L., Resnick, D., and Becker, M.P.: Hip involvement in ankylosing spondylitis. Arthritis Rheum. 19:683, 1976.

66. Glick, E.N.: A radiological comparison of the hip joint in rheumatoid arthritis and ankylosing spondylitis. Proc. Roy. Soc. Med. 59:1229, 1976.

67. Resnick, D., Dwosh, I.L., Goergen, T.G., Shapiro, R.F., and D'Ambrosia, R.: Clinical and radiographic "reankylosis" following hip surgery in ankylosing spondylitis. Am. J. Roentgenol. 216:1181, 1976.

68. Rosen, P.S.: A unique shoulder lesion in ankylosing spondylitis. Clinical Comment. J. Rheum. 7:109, 1980.

69. Ball, J.: Enthesopathy of rheumatoid and ankylosing spondylitis. Ann. Rheum. Dis. 30:213, 1971.

70. Resnick, D., and Niwayama, G.: Psoriatic arthritis. In Resnick, D., and Niwayama, G. (eds.): Diagnosis of Bone and Joint Disorders. Philadelphia, W. B. Saunders Company, 1981, p. 1103.

71. Wright, V.: Psoriatic arthritis. In Scott, J.T. (ed.): Copeman's Textbook of the Rheumatic Diseases. 5th ed. Edinburgh, Churchill Livingstone, 1978, p. 537.

72. Zaias, N.: Psoriasis of the nail: A clinico-pathological study. Arch. Dermatol. 99:567, 1967.

73. Resnick, D., and Niwayama, G.: On the nature and significance of bony proliferation in "rheumatoid variant" disorders. Am. J. Roentgenol. 129:275, 1977.

74. Forrester, D.M., and Kirkpatrick, R.W.: Periostitis and pseudoperiostitis. Radiology 118:597, 1976.

75. Resnick, D., and Broderick, R.W.: Bony proliferation of terminal phalanges in psoriasis. The "Ivory" phalanx. J. Can. Assoc. Radiol. 28:187, 1977.

76. Killebrew, K., Gold, R.H., and Sholkoff, S.D.: Psoriatic spondylitis. Radiology 108:9, 1973.

77. Sundaram, M., and Patton, J.T.: Paravertebral ossification in psoriasis and Reiter's disease. Br. J. Radiol. 48:628, 1975.

78. Kaplan, D., Plotz, C.M., Nathanson, L., and Frank, L.: Cervical spine in psoriasis and psoriatic arthritis. Ann. Rheum. Dis. 23:50, 1964.

79. Resnick, D., and Niwayama, G.: Reiter's syndrome. In Resnick, D., and Niwayama, G. (eds.): Diagnosis of Bone and Joint Disorders, Philadelphia, W. B. Saunders Company, 1981, p. 1130.

80. Sholkoff, S.D., Glickman, M.G., and Steinbach, H.L.: Roentgenology of Reiter's syndrome. Radiology 97:497, 1970.

81. Cliff, J.M.: Spinal bony bridging and carditis in Reiter's disease. Ann. Rheum. Dis. 30:171, 1971.

82. Resnick, D., and Niwayama, G.: Enteropathic arthropathies. In Resnick, D., and Niwayama, G. (eds.): Diagnosis of Bone and Joint Disorders. Philadelphia, W. B. Saunders Company, 1981, p. 1149.

83. Jayson, M.I.V., Salmon, P.R., and Harrison, W.J.: Inflammatory bowel disease in ankylosing spondylitis. Gut 11:506, 1970.

84. McEwen, C., Ditata, D., Lingg, C., Porini, A., Good, A., and Rankin, T.: Ankylosing spondylitis and spondylitis accompanying ulcerative colitis, regional enteritis, psoriasis, and Reiter's disease. Arthritis Rheum. 14:291, 1971.

85. Haslock, I.: Enteropathic arthritis. In Scott, J.T. (ed.): Copeman's Textbook of the Rheumatic Diseases. 5th ed. Edinburgh, Churchill Livingstone, 1978, p. 567.

86. Ferguson, R.H.: Enteropathic arthritis. In Hollander, J.L., and McCarty, D.J. (eds.): Arthritis and Allied Conditions. 8th ed. Philadelphia, Lea & Febiger, 1972, p. 846.

87. O'Connell, D.J., and Marx, W.J.: Hand changes in primary biliary cirrhosis. Radiology 129:31, 1978.

88. Clarke, A.K., Galbraith, R.M., Hamilton, E.B.D., and Williams, R.: Rheumatic disorders in primary biliary cirrhosis. Ann. Rheum. Dis. 37:42, 1978.

89. Lucas, P.F., and Owen, T.K.: Subcutaneous fat necrosis, "polyarthritis", and pancreatic disease. Gut 3:146, 1962.

153. Vyhanek, L., Lavicka, J., and Blahos, J.: Roentgenological findings in gout. Radiol. Clin. 28:256, 1960.
154. Good, A.E., and Rapp, R.: Bony ankylosis: A rare manifestation of gout. J. Rheumatol. 5:335, 1978.
155. Kawenoki-Minc, E., Eyman, E., Leo, W., and Werynska-Przybylska, J.: Zwyrodnienie stawow i kregoslupa u chorych na dne. Analiza 262 przypadkowdny. Reumatoligia 12:267, 1974.
156. von Hoyningen-Huene, C.B.J.: Gout and glycogen storage disease in preadolescent brothers. Arch. Intern. Med. 118:471, 1966.
157. Riley, J.D.: Gout and cerebral palsy in a three-year-old boy. Arch. Dis. Child. 35:293, 1960.
158. Gutman, A.B.: Primary and secondary gout. Ann. Intern. Med. 39:1062, 1953.
159. Grahme, R., Sutor, D.J., and Mitchener, M.B.: Crystal deposition in hyperparathyroidism. Ann. Rheum. Dis. 30:597, 1971.
160. Dmartini, F.E.: Hyperuricemia induced by drugs. Arthritis Rheum. 8:823, 1965.
161. Resnick, D., Niwayama, G., Goergen, T.G., Utsinger, P.D., Shapiro, R.F., Hasselwood, D.H., and Wiesner, K.B.: Clinical, radiographic and pathologic abnormalities in calcium pyrophosphate dihydrate deposition disease (CPPD): Pseudogout. Radiology 122:1, 1977.
162. Vigario, D.G., and Keats, T.E.: Localization of calcific deposits in the shoulder. Am. J. Roentgenol. 108:806, 1970.
163. Schumacher, H.R. Jr.: Hemochromatosis and arthritis. Arthritis Rheum. 7:41, 1964.
164. Hamilton, E., Williams, R., Barlow, K.A., and Smith, P.M.: The arthropathy of hemochromatosis. Q. J. Med. 37:171, 1968.
165. Atkins, C.J., McIvor, J., Smith, P.M., Hamilton, E., and Williams, R.: Chondrocalcinosis and arthropathy: Studies in haemochromatosis and in idiopathic chondrocalcinosis. Q. J. Med. 39:71, 1970.
166. Seze, S. de, Solnica, J., Mitrovic, D., Miravet, L., and Dorfmann, H.: Joint and bone disorders and hypoparathyroidism in hemochromatosis. Semin. Arthritis Rheum. 2:71, 1972.
167. Hirsch, J.H., Killien, C., and Troupin, R.H.: The arthropathy of hemochromatosis. Radiology 118:591, 1976.
168. Feller, E.R., and Schumacher, H.R.: Osteoarticular changes in Wilson's disease. Arthritis Rheum. 15:259, 1972.
169. Finby, N., and Bearn, A.G.: Roentgenographic abnormalities of the skeletal system in Wilson's disease (hepatolenticular degeneration). Am. J. Roentgenol. 79:603, 1958.
170. Cervenansky, J., Sitaj, S., and Urbanek, T.: Alkaptonuria and ochronosis. J. Bone Joint Surg. 41A:1169, 1959.
171. Mueller, M.N., Sorenson, L.B., Strandjord, N., and Kappas, A.: Alkaptonuria and ochronotic arthropathy. Med. Clin. North Am. 49:101, 1965.
172. Martin, W.J., Underahl, L.O., Mathieson, D.R., and Pugh, D.G.: Alkaptonuria: Report of 12 cases. Ann. Intern. Med. 42:1052, 1955.
173. Resnick, D., and Niwayama, G.: Osteomyelitis, septic arthritis, and soft tissue infection: the mechanisms and situations. In Resnick, D., and Niwayama, G. (eds.): Diagnosis of Bone and Joint Disorders. Philadelphia, W. B. Saunders Company, 1981, p. 2042.
174. Chuinard, R.G., and D'Ambrosia, R.: Human bite infections of the hand. J. Bone Joint Surg. 59A:416, 1977.
175. Patterson, F.P., and Brown, C.S.: Complications of total hip replacement arthroplasty. Orthop. Clin. North Am. 4:503, 1973.
176. Franck, W.A., Bress, N.M., Singer, F.R., and Krane, S.M.: Rheumatic manifestation of Paget's disease of bone. Am. J. Med. 56:592, 1974.
177. McCarty, D.J. Jr.: Pseudogout: articular chondrocalcinsis. In Hollander, J.L., and McCarty, D.J., Jr. (eds.): Arthritis and Related Disorders. 8th ed. Philadelphia, Lea & Febiger, 1972, p. 410.
178. Steinbach, H.L., and Russell, W.: Measurements of the heel pad as an aid to diagnosis of acromegaly. Radiology 82:418, 1964.
179. Lang, E.K., and Bessler, W.T.: The roentgenologic features of acromegaly. Am. J. Roentgenol. 86:321, 1961.
180. Watson, R.J., Burko, H., Megas, H., and Robinson, M.: Hand-foot syndrome in sickle cell disease in young children. Pediatrics 31:975, 1963.
181. Grossman, R.E., and Hensley, G.T.: Bone lesions in primary amyloidosis. Am. J. Roentgenol. 101:872, 1967.
182. Weinfield, A., Stern, M.H., and Marx, L.H.: Amyloid lesions of bone. Am. J. Roentgenol. 108:799, 1970.
183. Pettersson, H., Ahlberg, A., and Nilsson, I.M.: A radiologic classification of hemophilic arthropathy. Clin. Orthop. Rel. Res. 149:153, 1980.
184. Resnick, D.: Tumors and tumor-like lesions in or about joints. In Resnick, D., and Niwayama, G. (eds.): Diagnosis of Bone and Joint Disorders. Philadelphia, W. B. Saunders Company, 1981, p. 2638.
185. Prager, R.J., and Mall, J.C.: Arthrographic diagnosis of synovial chondromatosis. Am. J. Roentgenol. 127:344, 1976.
186. Breimer, C.W., and Freiberger, R.H.: Bone lesions associated with villonodular synovitis. Am. J. Roentgenol. 79:618, 1958.

Chapter 40

Nuclear Medicine, and Special Radiologic Imaging and Technique in the Diagnosis of Rheumatic Diseases

Thomas C. Namey

INTRODUCTION

Prior to the advent of modern serologic studies, radiology was the physician's major ally in the diagnosis of rheumatic diseases. In recent years, electronic microcircuitry and information processing have re-expanded the radiologist's imaging armamentarium. Studies once available only at university centers are now commonplace in the community hospital: nuclear medicine, ultrasound, and computed tomography. Refinements and defined applications of existing studies in thermography, arthrography, and xeroradiography have increased their specific utilities. Cost effectiveness as well as outcome is a major concern and accentuates the need for a discussion of strategies in utilization of special imaging studies.

This chapter deals with this expanded technologic base, covering the uses of nuclear medicine, thermography, ultrasound, xeroradiography, arthrography, and computed tomography in the diagnosis of rheumatic diseases.

NUCLEAR IMAGING

The uses of the early bone-seeking radionuclides, strontium-85 (^{85}Sr), strontium-87m (^{87m}Sr), and fluorine-18(^{18}F), were generally restricted to the detection of metastatic or primary bone malignancies.[1-3] This was because of high cost or limited availability, excessive radiation per study (^{85}Sr), or a too short half-life (^{87m}Sr). In 1971, technetium-99m-phosphates were introduced. They had an optimal half-life (6 hours), low radiation dose to the patient, and low cost.[4,5] Early clinical trials verified the superior bone-imaging properties of the ^{99m}Tc phosphates, which were readily applicable to the evaluation of nonmalignant bone disease.[3,6] Gallium-67 (^{67}Ga), a radiolanthanide introduced in the search for alternative bone-seeking agents, was found to localize in lymphomas and other malignancies, but also in active pyogenic inflammatory sites to a greater degree than in bone.[7,8] ^{67}Ga scintiscanning has now proved to be a useful adjunct to ^{99m}Tc-phosphate imaging of bone and joints.[9-11] The important properties and utilities of the radiopharmaceuticals used in rheumatic imaging, ^{99m}Tc-pertechnetate, phosphate and sulfur colloid, and ^{67}Ga, are discussed in the following sections and are summarized in Table 40-1.

Radiotechnetium (^{99m})Tc-Pertechnetate. ^{99m}Tc-pertechnetate binds primarily to serum albumin, and the free TcO_4^- in equilibrium with albumin-bound TcO_4^- is taken up rapidly by organs that "trap" iodide, including the thyroid, gastric mucosa, salivary glands, choroid plexus, and kidneys. Organ uptake may be competitively inhibited by administration of pharmacologic amounts of perchlorate (ClO_4^-). Irrespective of ClO_4^- administration, sufficient pertechnetate is bound to albumin to serve as a "blood-pool" imaging agent if scin-

tigraphy is performed within 5 to 15 minutes after administration.

Synovial inflammation increases articular blood flow and juxta-articular venous capacitance, the principal determinants of "blood-pool" size.[12-14] The inflamed synovium binds no more pertechnetate than normal tissue on a weight basis.[15] Radiopertechnetate joint scintigraphy is analogous to "nuclear thermography." Many studies have confirmed that *quantitative* ^{99m}Tc-pertechnetate synovial scintigraphy provides a reliable, measurable, and reproducible index of acute articular inflammation.[14,16-19] Unfortunately the sensitivity for *qualitative* diagnostic imaging is too low relative to ^{99m}technetium-phosphate bone and joint studies, and the primary utility for joint study is quantitative, where it retains practical superiority.

Salivary gland imaging remains the most important clinical utility of radiopertechnetate. Both qualitative salivary gland imaging and quantitative computer studies can be performed, supplying complementary data for diagnostic purposes in Sjögren's syndrome, sarcoidosis, and salivary duct obstruction.[20-22] Functional uptake occurs because the iodide-trapping mechanism of the salivary acini cannot distinguish iodide from pertechnetate. Abnormalities are defined by abnormally low rates of accumulation, assymetric accumulation, overaccumulation (as in the case of duct calculi), and impaired excretion after standard stimuli to salivation (e.g., lemon juice or 500 mg. of ascorbic acid).[21,23-25]

Technetium-99m-Phosphates. The initial mechanism considered responsible for osseous uptake of the ^{99m}Tc-phosphates was ionic "adsorption" to the surface of microcrystalline hydroxyapatite by a phosphate–calcium ionic interaction.[26] Factors that would modify uptake by this mechanism include blood flow in tissues[27,28] and

Table 40–1. Commonly Used Radionuclide Imaging Agents

Radiopharmaceutical	Half-Life (hours)	Photon(s)	Clinical Study
^{99}Tc^m Pertechnetate	6.1	140	Quantitative synovial blood-pool imaging Salivary gland imaging
^{99}Tc^m Phosphates	6.1	140	Standard bone and joint scintigraphy Quantitative bone and joint studies (i.e., sacroiliac joints) Immediate blood-pool imaging
^{99}Tc^m Sulfur colloids	6.1	140	Liver-spleen imaging Bone marrow imaging—useful in avascular necrosis, bone infarcts
^{67}Gallium (citrate)	78	93(40%) 184(24%) 296(22%) 388(7%)	Infection Granulomatous disease, e.g., sarcoidosis Lymphoreticular diseases (lymphoma, Hodgkin's disease) Occult carcinoma

the rate of bone turnover or remodeling, factors that alter the available surface area of hydroxyapatite.[29,30] However, the original premise of ionic binding has been challenged by observation in vivo, in which uptake occurs in tissue with little or no histochemical evidence for salts of calcium.[26]

An alternative mechanism is that uptake of ^{99m}Tc-phosphates depends on binding to collagen, in the presence of normal blood flow.[31,32] There is a correlation between 5-hour bone–soft tissue uptake and urinary hydroxyproline excretion in renal osteodystrophy, Paget's disease, and hyperparathyroidism.[33] Hydroxyproline is found almost exclusively in collagen, the primary structural protein in bone. Because reutilization does not occur in vivo, urinary hydroxyproline reflects bone matrix degradation. In most circumstances, bone formation parallels bone destruction. Thus, an agent localized in areas of bone matrix synthesis will be paralleled by evidence for matrix breakdown. In three patient groups, including controls, patients with Paget's disease, and those with renal osteodystrophy, there was no difference in the early rate of accumulation in bone of ^{99m}Tc-pyrophosphate, despite the increased osseous blood flow in Paget's disease. After 5 hours, the highest bone–soft tissue ratios occurred in the patients with Paget's disease and renal osteodystrophy. Patients with hyperparathyroidism maintained their increased 5-hour bone–soft tissue ratios for several weeks after parathyroidectomy during the phase of reparative bone formation, despite a marked decrease in bone turnover.[33,34]

In vitro incubation studies on the rat tibia with ^{99m}Tc-pyrophosphate demonstrated a higher uptake in unmineralized osteoid than in bone (Fig. 40–1).[32] Using agents that inhibited crosslinking of collagen, data have been presented that indicate that immature, recently synthesized, incompletely crosslinked collagen is the substrate for ^{99m}Tc-phosphate uptake. Garcia and coworkers showed that after intramuscular implants of bone-forming demineralized matrix and "bone-resorbing" dead bone, only the bone-forming system accumulated ^{99m}Tc-pyrophosphate, whereas the lytic, bone-resorbing system accumulated less radiopharmaceutical than normal bone.[35] The "bone-seeking" technetium phosphates have a greater affinity for cartilage than for bone, and direct proof has been provided for nonmineral binding of technetium phosphates.[36]

In summary, factors associated with mineralization of bone appear to be responsible for the increased uptake of ^{99m}Tc-phosphates in vivo. Increased uptake may be expected to occur in areas of hyperemia (probably secondary to an increase in absolute metabolic activity of the cells as well as in delivery of the carrier) and in areas of osteogenesis irrespective of the net accumulation or loss of bone. Decreased activity is seen in areas of mature, quiescent bone and in areas where the vascular supply is deficient or absent.

Technetium Sulfur Colloid. Technetium-99m sulfur colloid is an established imaging agent for liver and spleen. The reticuloendothelial cells of these organs phagocytize the radiolabeled sulfur colloid, providing an

Figure 40–1. In vivo uptake ratios of treated bone to normal untreated bone with various radiopharmaceuticals. While ^{14}C-EHDP exhibits preferential binding for bone mineral, the technetium-99m-phosphates bind to demineralized bone (matrix) to a greater extent than to the mineral. (From Rosenthall, L., and Kaye, M.: Semin. Nucl. Med. 6:59, 1976. Reprinted by permission.)

estimation of size and macrophage phagocytic capacity. Uptake also occurs in bone marrow but to a lesser extent with the sulfur colloid preparations used in liver–spleen scintigraphy. However, this uptake is enhanced in states in which marrow activity is increased, such as megaloblastic anemias, hemolytic anemias, and hemoglobinopathies and when reticuloendothelial tissue of the liver and spleen is bypassed or replaced, as in portal hypertension or metastatic carcinoma. The preferential uptake by the phagocytic cells of the liver and spleen of the sulfur colloid versus the marrow cells is a function of the size distribution of the sulfur colloid in standard preparations (a mean of 100 microns). The reticuloendothelial cells in the marrow optimally phagocytize particles in the range of 10 microns.[37] However, adequate imaging of bone marrow tissues can be accomplished when the vascular clearance of the larger particles has occurred, which is after 15 to 20 minutes in normal individuals.[38] Alternatively, preparations of sulfur colloid particles with a smaller size distribution or other colloid aggregates of [99m]technetium, such as antimony colloid, will provide more efficient and selective marrow reticuloendothelial studies.[37] The clinical indications for bone-marrow imaging are avascular necrosis, bone infarction, viability of bone after fracture, and determination of erythropoietic marrow mass in disease states in which it is increased or decreased.

[67]**Gallium.** While bone binds some ionic gallium, much greater uptake occurs by microsomes in nonosseous cells, particularly polymorphonuclear (PMN) leukocytes and monocytes.[39-44] Gallium binds to serum and cellular transferrin and lactoferrin, suggesting that molecular

substrates for ferric ion are the principal determinants for tissue distribution of [67]gallium in vivo (Fig. 40–2).[45-49] Cellular uptake is mediated by a transferrin-specific ferric ion receptor, although this may not be the mechanism for uptake in tumor tissue.[50,51] PMN leukocytes bind greater amounts of gallium than do lymphocytes, probably because of the high concentration of lactoferrin in PMN leukocytes, and this rapid uptake establishes the means by which ^{67}Ga localizes at sites of infection and pus.[52] However, certain tumors take up gallium independent of leukocytes, enabling ^{67}Ga imaging to aid in the diagnosis of occult tumors as well as infection.[8,50] Deferoxamine mesylate, a potent iron-chelating agent, has been shown to effectively displace bound ^{67}Ga from tissues but increase target–nontarget tissue activity ratio.[53]

Because of different mechanisms for localization, ^{67}Ga imaging complements ^{99m}Tc-phosphate bone imaging in the detection of osteomyelitis and septic arthritis.[10,11,52] Imaging with ^{67}Ga should always *follow* rather than *precede* the studies using radiotechnetium, because of its long half-life (70 hours). Imaging should be performed at 8 to 24 hours and again at 72 hours using [67]Ga. Gallium is normally excreted in the terminal ileum, and normally some activity in the bowel may be seen. The multiple energies of emitted photons limit the resolution of radiogallium imaging and contribute to the substantially higher radiation dose used compared with radiotechnetium. The radiation exposure, while not excessive, should cause concern over the casual use of ^{67}Ga imaging, particularly in children or women of child-bearing age.

IMAGING METHODS AND DEVICES

The radioisotopes ^{99m}Tc and ^{67}Ga may be imaged with conventional rectilinear scanning devices or the Anger-type gamma scintillation camera, using several different collimators. Dual-probe scanners have shortened the time necessary to perform a skeletal or whole-body survey with any of the ^{99m}Tc or ^{67}Ga complexes. Nonethe-

less, the images obtained, although often sufficient for diagnostic purposes, do not contain the information density, resolution, or projections needed for complete studies.[3,11] The use of the Anger-type gamma camera is recommended for optimal visualization of abnormalities, since resolution is independent of the "focusing" effect seen in dual-crystal rectilinear scanning devices, and proximity of the lesion to the collimator surface leads to improved resolution.[1,11] For further definition, particularly of internal articulations that cannot closely approximate the collimator surface (e.g., hips and the axial skeleton), a pinhole collimator affords greater detail and magnification. This collimator is of particular value in pediatric imaging, since active epiphyseal growth plates often obscure early osseous inflammatory lesions.[11,54]

Survey scintigraphy with a rectilinear camera or gamma camera, followed by special views with a gamma camera employing a high-resolution parallel-hole or pinhole collimator, is the best approach in inflammatory bone or joint disease. Any abnormal or suspicious areas seen on the survey images and areas clinically suspect for osseous or articular involvement should be subjected to special study.[11] Finally, it is important to image the contralateral side for comparison, which increases accurate recognition of inflammatory lesions. Blood-pool imaging with immediate scanning after ^{99m}Tc-phosphate injection should be done if cellulitis or a soft tissue abscess is present and could obscure the diagnosis of an underlying bone lesion. Specialized or quantitative studies should be discussed in advance of imaging with the nuclear medicine specialist. Standard bone imaging is not optimal for assessment of inflammatory articular disease. Technicians and referring physicians acquaint themselves with the views constituting a "joint" scan.[55]

PERIPHERAL JOINT SCINTIGRAPHY IN INFLAMMATORY ARTHRITIS

The first agents used to assess joint inflammation were blood-pool markers, labled albumin, and [99]TcO$_4$[-].[56]

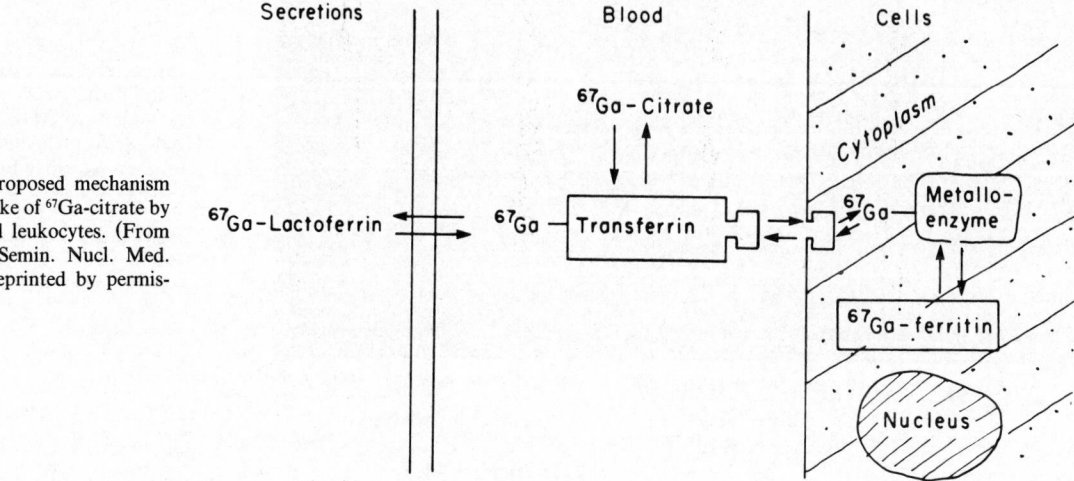

Figure 40–2. Proposed mechanism for cellular uptake of ^{67}Ga-citrate by tumor cells and leukocytes. (From Larson, S.M.: Semin. Nucl. Med. 8:200, 1978. Reprinted by permission.)

While the low sensitivity of pertechnetates precluded broader diagnostic use, use of this isotope presented a new and relatively simple approach to quantifying inflammation and was particularly applicable to research. Superiority of the newer ^{99m}Tc-phosphate bone-seeking radiotracers over blood-pool imaging with pertechnetate for diagnostic was demonstrated in 1975.[57] In some instances, articular "positivity" on ^{99m}Tc-PYP scanning predated the patient's awareness of joint inflammation, which was confirmed by the development of clinical synovitis weeks to months after the joint scan.[57] Numerous studies have since appeared and confirmed the efficacy of joint scanning with the bone-seeking radiotracers in documenting preradiographic articular involvement in rheumatoid arthritis, psoriatic arthritis, ankylosing spondylitis, gout, and other arthropathies.[58-69] Arguments for the use of joint imaging include the following:

1. Extreme sensitivity. The presence of articular or juxta-articular inflammation is virtually excluded by the presence of a normal joint scan. This was suggested by the long-term follow-up of 22 patients with "polyarthralgias" who had negative or noninflammatory scintigrams. None demonstrated inflammatory joint disease, although one had SLE and two had polymyalgia rheumatica (now considered as having an inflammatory articular component by author)[70].

2. Reduced radiation. Judicious use of joint and bone scanning can reduce the radiation exposure in diagnosing inflammatory rheumatic diseases, since multiple joints are frequently radiographed before disease becomes radiographically manifest.[71,74] For conventional imaging, radiographic exposure is "additive." This is not true for scintimaging. Only one radiation dose is accrued per study no matter how many images are made during the radioisotopic procedure. This concern varies for the age and sex of the patient and for the joint in question. It is most critical in lumbosacral studies in women of childbearing age, since gonads cannot be shielded. Since sacroiliac disease develops more slowly in women than men, this point cannot be overemphasized.[75-77] Gonadal exposure approximates 390 mREM in women during conventional lumbosacral radiography versus 140 mREM for [99]Tc[m]- phosphate scintigraphy using 15 mCi of [99]Tc[m]-EHDP.[78,79]

3. Cost. This is often inapparent to many clinicians. While the cost of bone and joint imaging is higher than one or two conventional radiographs, once survey studies are considered or the number of joints radiographed increases, economic considerations favor the radioisotopic study. Technetium phosphate bone and joint studies remain substantially less costly than computed tomography.

4. Early diagnosis. Documentation of the pattern of articular disease is the most important consideration in establishing a specific diagnosis. In rheumatoid arthritis, considered to be a symmetric polyarticular disease, patients may initially present with asymmetric oligo- or monoarticular synovitis. Alternatively, disease activity in one joint may obscure pain at another joint. In early disease, when standard radiographs are normal, joint imaging has the greatest value in documenting clinical and subclinical synovitis and establishing the pattern of articular activity crucial to diagnosis[80-82] (Figs. 40–3 and 40–4).

In summary, joint imaging offers the most sensitive documentation of the extent and pattern of early arthritis.[57,59,60,63,64,66-69,83] Normal studies are useful in ruling

R

L

Figure 40–3. Reiter's syndrome. This joint scan is virtually diagnostic for Reiter's syndrome. Readily apparent is the periostitis of the os calcanei, or "lover's heels." In addition the patient has plantar fasciitis on the right, synovitis of the right ankle, sacroiliitis, and abnormally increased uptake at the knees and shoulders. The patient's initial complaint was right ankle pain following an episode of "presumed" gonococcal urethritis. Within two weeks, both heels and sacroiliac joints were symptomatic.

22yoW ♂   REITER'S SYNDROME,   [99m]TcEDP 20miC 1/16/76
HLA— A(2,−)   Joint Scintograms
        B(27,−)

SIJ/Sacrum = 1.7

Figure 40–4. Technetium joint scan of a young male with acute reactive arthritis. Note the presence of tibial-fibular disease, which is occasionally seen in "enthesopathic" arthritis. This site of his knee pain was clinically "missed" by three different rheumatologists who examined the patient prior to imaging. Intense unilateral plantar fasciitis and asymmetric interphalangeal disease of the hands is also seen. QSS demonstrated unilateral (left) sacroiliitis (not shown).

out inflammatory arthropathy, as in the case of fibromyositis. The patient avoids multiple and expensive radiographs in preradiographic "early disease."

It is mandatory that joint imaging, when used, follow a specific protocol.[55] While it is true that no diagnosis is established by imaging one joint, the specificity for diagnosis comes from the composite pattern established by imaging multiple joints. Contralateral joints should be imaged for equal durations rather than by counts accumulated or activity. For some articulations, the subjective appreciation of inflammation is enhanced by a quantitative study, as is the case for the sacroiliac joints.[57,63,64,67]

Rheumatoid Arthritis and Seronegative Spondyloarthropathies. Scintimaging has been found to be a more sensitive indicator of disease activity compared with standard radiography, and the symmetric pattern of articular inflammation (particularly in the hands), which characterizes rheumatoid arthritis, can be distinguished from the rheumatoid variants, which tend toward asymmetry and greater axial involvement[68] (Fig. 40–5A, B, and C). Scintigraphic changes are, however, less specific than the radiographs in distinguishing between rheumatoid and seronegative diseases. Documentation of articular disease by scintimaging often antedates both clinical and radiographic abnormalities. Late abnormalities demonstrated by standard radiographic studies are more specific than are radioisotopic studies; early disease is more sensitively investigated by radionuclide joint imaging. This conclusion was confirmed in a comparison of ^{99m}Tc-EHDP imaging with both ^{99}TcO$_4^-$ imaging and fine-detail radiographs in hand studies in patients with rheumatoid arthritis.[58] It was concluded that the pattern of normal hand activity was maximal activity in the wrist, relative diminution in activity from the first to fifth MCPs, and a progressive decrease of activity from the proximal to more distal joints in each digit[58] (Fig. 40–5).

Lateral bone images of the ankle and heel are particularly important when imaging the feet in patients suspected of having Reiter's syndrome or psoriatic arthritis. Periostitis of the os calcis, plantar fasciitis, and Achilles tendonitis can and should be readily distinguished, since they are not typical in rheumatoid arthritis[67,68,84,85] (Figs. 40–3, 40–4, and 40–6). Asymmetric uptake in the metatarsal and interphalangeal joints of the feet or isolated distal interphalangeal uptake is also more characteristic of the rheumatoid variants.[67,68,84,85] Of unknown significance is the finding that patients with severe psoriasis demonstrate diffuse juxta-articular increased activity with ^{99m}Tc-phosphate imaging.[85-87] This finding has focused interest on abnormal juxta-articular connective tissue metabolism in psoriasis. Other peripheral features of the spondyloarthropathies suggest manifestations of "enthesitis" and include insertional tendonitis, patellar involvement, and asymmetric oligoarthritis.[61,67,68,84]

In spondyloarthropathies, increased uptake may be seen in the sacroiliac joints, the lumbar, thoracic, and cervical spine, and the sternoclavicular and costoclavicular joints.[61,63,64,67-69,88] Focal discitis can be noted, if present.[61,64,69,88] Intense sacroiliitis can often be identified, particularly if asymmetric or unilateral, without resorting to quantitative studies.[61,67-69,89] However, even though sacroiliac joint involvement may be noted visually, there is a great deal of observer error, since normal sacroiliac joints demonstrate a higher physiologic uptake than either adjacent iliac or sacral bone. Technical factors in imaging that affect contrast further impair visual estimation (Fig. 40–7), leading to attempts to quantify the uptake in the sacroiliac joints to aid in the documentation of inflammatory sacroiliitis.

Quantitative Sacroiliac Joint Imaging. Techniques have been developed that interface a computer with the gamma camera to both document and quantify the presence of inflammatory sacroiliitis. The uptake of bone-seeking radiotracer at the sacroiliac joints is compared

Figure 40–5. ^{99m}Tc-EHDP joint scintimages of hands. *A*, Normal hands. *B*, Rheumatoid arthritis. Increased articular uptake is essentially symmetric and greatest at the wrists and MCPs, with moderately increased PIP activity and near normal DIP activity. *C*, Psoriatic arthritis (HLA-B27+). Asymmetric involvement of the MCPs and PIPs is not characteristic of RA. Intense wrist and MCP disease would not occur in DJD. *D*, Erosive osteoarthritis. Sometimes intense activity is seen in osteoarthritis, usually when accompanied by clinical signs of inflammation. The abnormal joint uptake is localized to PIPs and DIPs. *E*, Reflex dystrophy syndrome. Diffuse increase in juxta-articular activity involving all articulations of the affected hand. Focal areas of increased activity represent osteoarthritic changes in right CMC and left wrist.

Figure 40–6. Acute right Achilles tendinitis (black arrowhead). Some uptake is also seen in the tendon itself (white arrow). Radiographs were normal.

2 hr post ^{99m}Tc EDP, 3/16/76

Figure 40–7. *A,* This 23-year-old male complained of right-sided low back pain, which he developed while working on an oil rig at sea. Because of "atypical" sciatica, a bone scan was performed and interpreted as normal. Closer inspection revealed relatively greater activity in the right sacroiliac joint, which was partially obscured by bladder activity (a technical mistake in bone imaging). Increased activity was also seen in the knees and right 1st MTP and DP of the foot. The patient underwent a myelogram, which was normal, but still had "exploratory" back surgery. *B,* Two months later, quantitative sacroiliac joint scintigraphy revealed definite, active, right-sided sacroiliitis. Patient was HLA-B27 positive.

with uptake at "normal" adjacent bone. The ratio of counts is expressed as an index. This procedure, quantitative sacroiliac scintigraphy (QSS), has become one of the more controversial areas of radioisotopic imaging in the diagnosis of rheumatic diseases. Historically, increased uptake of bone-seeking radiotracers, fluorine-18 and strontium-67, was seen in the sacroiliac joint of patients with sacroiliitis, often preceding radiographic change.[90-92] Early attempts to quantify sacroiliac joint uptake using the newer ^{99m}Tc-phosphates demonstrated significant differences between the sacroiliac indices of patients with active sacroiliitis and those of controls.[93] The highest values appeared in patients with ankylosing spondylitis with early sacroiliitis (radiographic grade 1 or 2) compared with patients with advanced disease (grade 3 or 4)[93,94] (Fig. 40–8). In one study of patients with Reiter's syndrome, 24 of 33 had sacroiliitis by QSS, suggesting that sacroiliitis is more common than previously thought in acute Reiter's and is possibly overshadowed by peripheral disease in some and transient in others, since fewer would have been expected to develop radiographic disease.[89]

Proposed technical modifications for QSS are fractional analysis of the sacroiliac joints (three horizontal activity profiles) and "background" subtraction to eliminate activity unrelated to bone due to overlying soft tissue and incomplete vascular clearance[63] (Fig. 40–9).

In another study, employing background subtraction to calculate a single sacroiliac index, QSS was found to be of value in the diagnosis of sacroiliitis.[95] Patients with active disease had significantly higher indices than patients with a similar grade of radiographic sacroiliitis but with clinically inactive disease. Overlap between patients with back pain of a "mechanical" etiology and those with sacroiliitis was found, however.[95] A more recent study concluded that QSS was useful in the diagnosis of early sacroiliitis and suggested that multilevel analysis, background subtraction, and drug washout techniques improved reliability of the study.[96] Using similar techniques for QSS, a good discrimination between patients with early sacroiliitis and controls has been observed.[97]

Other investigators, however, have reported results to the contrary.[98-103] Similar lack of correlation between increased sacroiliac joint uptake and the presence of radiographic disease or clinical disease has been reported.[98,99] Other investigators have reported some correlation of the sacroiliac index with QSS and the presence or absence of radiographic or clinical sacroiliitis, but they have noted poor specificity or too great an overlap with the broad range of normal values obtained for the quantitative sacroiliac study to be clinically useful.[100-102] Recently, a comparative study of the various techniques used for quantitative sacroiliac imaging was performed, with the conclusion that quantitative sacroiliac scintigraphy was useful as an objective tool for determination of sacroiliac joint inflammation, and that technical differences between the studies reported were the major reason for disparate results.[103]

Two long-term follow-up studies of patients identified as having sacroiliitis determined by QSS who had normal sacroiliac joint radiographs have been performed, concluding that QSS will identify patients with preradiographic sacroiliitis.[104,105] It is apparent, however, that not all patients with scintigraphic disease develop radiographic changes, and it is argued that clinical circumstances must be considered; an elevated sacroiliac index, while suggestive of sacroiliitis, is not specific.[104,105] Elevated sacroiliac indices have been demonstrated in sacroiliac ligament strain and metabolic bone disease and in those occasional patients with degenerative changes.[101,102]

Radiographic changes suggestive of "sacroiliitis" are not specific for inflammatory disease.[106] Likewise, inflammatory sacroiliitis is also known to occur in a number of inflammatory conditions not previously considered in the family of spondyloarthropathies; namely, gout, pseudogout, polymyalgia rheumatica, and familial Mediterranean fever.[106,107] Since "sacroiliitis" will eventually appear radiographically in many patients with paraplegia or hyperparathyroidism,[106] it seems reasonable to apply standards of specificity to quantitative sacroiliac scintigraphy when the accepted basis for diagnosis of "sacroiliitis" is itself fallible. It is probable that sacroiliitis is more common than previously thought, and this possibility is raised by the finding of "transient" sacroiliitis, present clinically and scintigraphically, in patients with Whipple's disease and acute sarcoid arthritis.[108,109] Both scintigraphic and radiographic sacroiliitis have recently been shown to be sequelae of both acute and chronic pelvic inflammatory

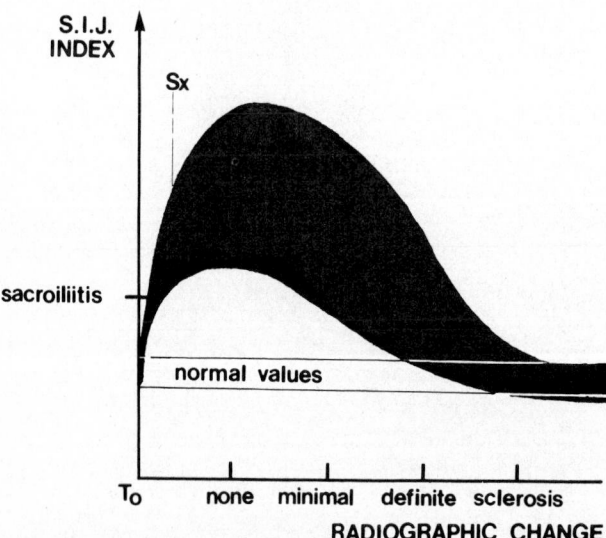

Figure 40–8. The relationships between sacroiliac joint indices by quantitative sacroiliac scintigraphy for *untreated* patients with various radiographic stages of sacroiliitis. In eary *active* sacroiliitis, quantitative sacroiliac joint scintigraphy is more helpful than conventional x-rays. Once radiographic disease develops, the sacroiliac indices fall and become normal with complete sclerosis. Normal indices may be seen for any stage of disease, if inactive or successfully treated. (From Namey, T. et al.: Arthritis Rheum. 20:1058, 1977. Reprinted with permission.)

Figure 40–9. Composite profiles of three regions (upper, middle and lower thirds) of each sacroiliac joint generated by a computer macrofunction performing quantitative sacroiliac joint scintigraphy. The central sacral region for each profile is assigned a value of 100 for ease of visual interpretation of the sacroiliac peak to sacral peak ratio. By looking at the curves, the sacroiliac indices and asymmetry of activity can be assessed. *A* is a normal study. *B* represents the profile of a patient with ankylosing spondylitis of two years' duration. Activity is symmetric and greatest in the upper third of each sacroiliac joint.

disease.[110-112] Differences in the laterality of unilateral sacroiliitis demonstrated by QSS has been offered as support for the etiologic role of Batson's vertebral venous plexus in triggering inflammatory sacroiliitis.[112]

In summary, QSS appears to be an independently useful marker for sacroiliitis that is clinically active, if the procedure is methodologically sound. It is not specific for "inflammatory" sacroiliac disease and must be clinically evaluated with other findings in the overall assessment of the patient. QSS is most logically employed during the performance of peripheral joint scintigraphic studies rather than as an isolated procedure.

Septic Arthritis. The diagnosis of septic arthritis, in contrast to osteomyelitis, is usually made without resort to radionuclide imaging. This statement specifically excludes pyarthrosis of the hip, sacroiliac joint, and intervertebral discs, where the problems of clinical assessment and difficulty with arthrocentesis increase the importance of radioisotopic studies.[11] A number of recent clinical reports have suggested that 99mTc-phosphate bone scintigraphy is an important indirect study in diagnosing septic sacroiliitis.[113-118] Also, several clinical situations generate a need to consider 99mTc-phosphate or

67Ga scintigraphy: (1) the evaluation of arthritis in the patient with known osteomyelitis or endocarditis; (2) the patient with underlying rheumatic disease; (3) acute arthritis and coexistant hemoglobinopathy; (4) persistent joint pain and fever following joint prosthesis insertion[11,119-121]; and (5) cellulitis overlying the questionably inflamed joint.[122,123]

Both negative and positive studies are clinically relevant. Because most inflammatory arthropathies involve more than one articulation, the presence of monoarticular disease on the bone or joint scan should always include septic arthritis in the differential diagnosis.[11] The bone scan becomes positive between 24 and 48 hours after pyarthrosis develops.[11,120,121] It remains positive for weeks to months after therapy, depending on when therapy was initiated. Septic arthritis always increases activity on both sides of the joint(s) affected, particularly in juxtasynovial bone within the joint capsule, and this is a general rule for synovitis.[1,125] Bone scan positivity represents attempted osteogenesis of repair. The negative joint scan presents a strong argument against the diagnosis of pyarthroses, especially when there is no known underlying arthropathy.[11,124] Radiographic changes take 10 to 14 days to become manifest in septic arthritis, in contrast to the changes seen within 2 days on the bone or joint scan. They, too, may be ambiguous if coexistent arthropathy is present.[120-122]

Cellulitis without pyarthrosis will generate a positive "blood-pool" study with the bone-seeking tracer, while delayed "osseous" imaging reveals only normal or slightly increased bone activity.[11,117-121] Several groups have recommended inclusion of an immediate postinjection radionuclide angiogram with the "blood-pool" and osseous phases of bone imaging (the "three-phase" study), but rarely is this essential in ruling out pyarthrosis.[11] The blood-pool study is necessary, particularly when superficial edema or erythema suggestive of cellulitis is present. One important observation has been made regarding the significance of focal photon-lucency, or photopenia, on blood-pool imaging. The presence of joint effusion, particularly in the hip, may cause an area of nonactivity, a possible result of capsular pressure diminishing the venous blood-pool or the mass of the nonvascular effusion itself.[127,128] When identified, especially in the presence of increased periarticular uptake, it most likely signals the presence of effusion. The blood-pool study should be routinely requested when ordering a $^{99}Tc^m$-phosphate bone and joint scan for possible joint infection.

Sequential imaging with ^{67}Ga should be considered when the ^{99m}Tc-phosphate scan is difficult to interpret, as in the case of children, whose active epiphyseal growth centers normally demonstrate greater uptake than adjacent bone, or in patients with underlying inflammatory disease.[11,119-121,124] The benefit of dual studies with ^{99m}Tc-phosphate/^{67}Ga in patients with rheumatoid arthritis and possible septic arthritis has been contested, however.[129] In the setting of a possible infected prosthesis, specifically in the hip, combined bone-gallium scanning does appear to enhance diagnostic accuracy.[130] ^{67}Ga scintigraphy should always follow ^{99m}Tc-phosphate imaging.[11,121,124] Early gallium scan positivity (increased activity seen on images obtained in the first 8 to 24 hours after administration of the ^{67}Ga) is a feature of acute pyogenic inflammation. Late positivity with minimally increased joint uptake seen at 8 to 12 hours is more typical of chronic infection, such as fungal or tuberculous arthritis. The gallium scan may also demonstrate nonosseous involvement, which is not demonstrable by the bone scan or radiograph (Fig. 40–10).

Osteomyelitis. The results of most clinical reports establish the bone scan as a primary diagnostic tool in evaluating osteomyelitis in children and adults.[131-136] An abnormal bone scan is usually seen within 1 or 2 days after the initial spread of infection to bone (not including fungal or tuberculous disease), which is days to weeks before radiographic changes occur.[1,3,11,54,120,121] In one series of patients with osteomyelitis, 20 of 33 cases had radiographic abnormalities prior to bone imaging.[132] This underscores the fact that many patients present to the physician "late" in the disease course or elude diagnosis on first contact, a fact that reinforces the need to recognize the earliest radiographic changes. The sensitivity and specificity of radionuclide bone studies in diagnosing osteomyelitis approach or exceed 90 percent

Figure 40–10. *A*, ^{99m}Tc-EHDP scan of patient with tuberculous osteomyelitis of the left patella and secondary tuberculous arthritis of the knee. *B*, ^{67}Ga scan at 24 hours also reveals extensive distal quadriceps involvement, later demonstrated pathologically after surgery.

in most series, if patients with sickle cell disease are excluded.[11,126,131,136] This is not true of neonates, in whom a much higher "false negativity" has been noted in "proven" osteomyelitis.[137-139]

The bone scan demonstrates an area of increased concentration of ^{99m}Tc-phosphate at the site of osteomyelitis, with a diffuse, less intense perimeter of activity occurring in adjacent uninvolved bone secondary to hyperemia and increased metabolic activity (Fig. 40–11). This pattern may be absent acutely if septic embolization, medullary vessel thrombosis, or compression of the osseous microcirculation by subperiosteal or interosseous pus has occurred.[127,140-143] In these cases a transient central area of photon-lucency, or nonuptake, surrounded by an area of increased activity, may be seen. Exclusion of bone infarction is impossible at this stage.

In acute osteomyelitis, hyperemia increases distal bone and periarticular activity, which develop as a consequence of the central focus of acute osteomyelitis acting as a low resistance "shunt" augmenting distal blood flow.[11] This is a valuable clue in discriminating most acute forms of osteomyelitis from the subacute variant (Brodie's abscess) or chronic and/or granulomatous osteomyelitis (Fig. 40–12). Blood-pool imaging and immediate radionuclide angiography, in conjunction with the delayed osseous phase of bone imaging in suspected cases of osteomyelitis, do not increase the sensitivity of the scan in diagnosing osteomyelitis, but markedly decrease the rate of false-positive diagnosis and increase diagnostic accuracy.[126,144] Hence, specificity of diagnosis is augmented by radionuclide angiography and blood-pool studies in cases of suspect osteomyelitis, particu-larly in children with normally "hot" epiphyseal growth centers. Combination blood-pool studies are also particularly valuable in a patient with superficial ulcers or cellulitis and should precede static bone imaging.[144] Both radionuclide angiography and blood-pool imaging are important parts of the "complete" bone scan when osteomyelitis is considered as a possible diagnosis.

Sequential imaging with ^{67}Ga citrate is helpful, particularly in children with possible hematogenous osteomyelitis, because of the proximity of metaphysis (the usual initial nidus of infection) to the epiphysis.[123,124] Gallium scanning may also better indicate disease activity if there is a question of recrudescence, since technetium bone scan positivity will lag behind relative clinical response, now reflecting osseous repair.[11,120,124] [67]Ga scintigraphy has been shown to be valuable in detecting osteomyelitis following total joint replacement, when increased activity around the prosthesis on bone scan, normally present, may be impossible to differentiate from an infected prosthesis.[130]

Bone Infarction and Avascular Necrosis. Avascular necrosis of bone is a common complication of sickle cell anemia, fractures of the femoral neck, steroid therapy, pancreatitis, and numerous systemic entities (see Chapter 107). Radiography cannot detect the acute phase of avascular necrosis because of the equivalent densities of acutely devitalized and normal bone.[37,38,145,146] Hence, the changes that become radiographically manifest with time are those of subsequent repair, sclerosis, and damage to the articulating surfaces, if localized to subchondral bone.

Early attempts to detect avascular necrosis by scin-

Figure 40–11. ^{99m}Tc-EHDP joint scans of acute and subacute osteomyelitis. The image on the left reveals increased distal uptake beyond the focus of osteomyelitis in the wrist and MCP joints of the same hand, compared with the contralateral extremity. The study on the right demonstrates the uptake seen in a patient with a Brodie abscess of the left radius, a subacute condition. In more chronic osteomyelitis or joint infection, an increase in distal osseous or articular uptake is not seen or is much less marked.

Figure 40–12. Acute ischemic necrosis of the right proximal humeral head seen in the bone scan of a 23-year-old female with acute sickle cell crisis. The entire area of infarction is seen as a region of nonuptake (large arrows) surrounded by an area of reactive, increased activity. The left shoulder is normal.

tigraphy were limited by the physical properties of the early bone-seeking tracers, [85]Sr and [18]F. Both were ineffective in delineating the acute necrosis phase, and late uptake was nonspecific, requiring radiographic, arthrographic, or surgical confirmation of diagnosis.[145,147,148]

Once available, the clear superiority of the newer ^{99m}Tc-phosphates in the diagnosis of avascular necrosis was readily demonstrated.[149-152] For the first time, the acute phase of injury, a region of nonuptake surrounded by an area of increased activity, could be routinely visualized, provided imaging was performed soon after the initial insult (Fig. 40–12). Once the reparative phase began, uptake nonspecifically increased without evidence for the once present avascular area, and differentiation of ischemic necrosis from inflammatory or severe degenerative arthritis would be impossible.

One recent study compared the ^{99m}Tc-phosphate bone scan with radiograph sensitivity in detecting steroid-induced avascular necrosis of bone in 36 patients. The sensitivity of the scan was 89 versus 41 percent for radiography when compared with interosseous pressure measurements.[153] While the bone scan specificity was only 50 percent, the predictive value of the scan was 92 percent. In children, epiphyseal growth center activity often obscures bone scan evidence for avascular necrosis, unless high-resolution studies with a pinhole collimator are obtained.[152]

To effectively diagnose avascular necrosis in bone, marrow imaging with ^{99m}Tc-sulfur colloid (SC) or antimony colloid may be necessary. ^{99m}Tc-SC, the agent used for conventional liver/spleen imaging, is phagocytized by the reticuloendothelial cells of both liver-spleen (85 percent) and the bone marrow (15 percent).

Because the large joints are anatomically far enough from the liver, imaging of bone is possible with the colloids, since some colloid is phagocytized by reticuloendothelial cells in bone marrow. Since both vascularity, necessary for delivery, and vital marrow, necessary for uptake, must be intact, ^{99m}Tc-SC imaging demonstrates avascular necrosis with greater specificity, both in the acute phase (vascular flow interrupted) and the late phase (vital marrow has been replaced by fibrous marrow)[11,37,38,150] (Fig. 40–13).

Ischemic necroses of bone and marrow are frequent complications of many hemoglobinopathies and storage diseases, but they are by far most common in sickle cell disease. The differential diagnosis between infarction and infection is exceedingly difficult, and both may be present simultaneously. Roentgenographic evaluation is invariably negative in the early stages of both. Most episodes of infarction during sickle crisis are polycentric, which often aids in distinguishing between infarction and osteomyelitis. Scintigraphic bone imaging frequently reveals periostitis in the long bones, a known and common feature of bone infarction. Bone scan abnormalities also frequently suggest skull and vertebral involvement. In a study of 30 patients with sickle cell anemia by bone marrow imaging using [99]Tc[m]-SC, one half had evidence for previous bone infarction, i.e., photopenic areas representing regions of marrow fibrosis.[150] Because there is normally extreme marrow expansion in patients with sickle disease, previous infarction even in more distal long bones, such as the tibia or fibula, can usually be seen[150,152] (Fig. 40–14). This contrasts with the absence of active marrow at these sites in normals but emphasizes the reason for the inherent clinical advantage of [99m]Tc-

Figure 40–13. Avascular necrosis of the right femoral head documented by ^{99m}Tc-SC scan. Note diminished uptake in the right femoral head compared with the left. Also note that in the normal individual, active marrow rarely extends below the knee. Compare with sickle cell patient in Figure 40–14.

SC imaging in sickle cell crisis. The bone scan will demonstrate a "mottled" pattern at these distal sites.[150]

Radiocolloid imaging for diagnosis of avascular necrosis is important in assessing viability of the femoral head after femoral neck fracture.[37,38] Colloid imaging has a 95 percent correlation with surgical findings in several reports.[37,38] The utility of sulfur colloid imaging is greatest in cases of unilateral avascular necrosis of the hip. This is because partial nonuptake in the femoral head is a normal finding in up to 40 percent of adults, but it is bilateral when present.[155,156] Unilateral nonuptake of ^{99m}Tc-SC is generally significant and much more specific for the scintigraphic diagnosis of avascular necrosis.[155,156]

Paget's Disease of Bone. Radionuclide bone imaging with the ^{99m}Tc-phosphates is the diagnostic procedure of choice in evaluating suspected or symptomatic Paget's disease.[157-167] The bone scan's sensitivity in detection and assessment of disease is superior to conventional radiography.[157-164,166,167] Scintigraphic changes will improve, but rarely revert to normal during or after treatment with mithramycin, calcitonin, or etidronate.[158,159,161,163,164,166-167] Bone scanning is more sensitive in detecting Paget's disease than measurement of serum alkaline phosphatase, which is frequently normal in mild or inactive disease.[158,160,165]

Paget's disease is most commonly polyostotic; multiple lesions are seen in 75 percent of patients[158-160] (Fig. 40–15). Diagnosis is rarely a problem in polyostotic disease, and differentiation between Paget's disease and osteomyelitis, tumor, or fracture is easily made. The difficulty lies in choosing between monostotic Paget's disease, when present, and metastatic disease in bone. Recent studies suggest that ^{67}Ga scanning may be even more sensitive than bone scanning agents in diagnosing

A   B

Figure 40–14. [99m]Technetium sulfur colloid liver/spleen scan and bone marrow scan in acute sickle cell crisis. *A,* Liver is slightly enlarged, but spleen is not visualized due to acute "functional asplenia," often noted in sickle crisis. *B,* The marrow scan is typical of the patient with active compensatory erythropoiesis, with extreme proximal marrow extension through both tibias. The patient had severe left tibial pain, shown to represent acute bone infarction of the left tibia. Note central absence of marrow uptake of the ^{99m}Tc-SC.

Figure 40–15. Paget's disease of bone. *A*, ^{99m}Tc-EHDP scintimages of cranial involvement typical of some patients with Paget's disease; few other entities will demonstrate such widespread cranial increased activity. *B* illustrates the polycentric nature of Paget's disease. Left scapular, "skip" vertebral, sacral, and left scapular disease are present by the abnormal uptake. Such patterns are virtually diagnostic of Paget's disease.

Paget's disease and evaluating therapy, but considerations of increased cost, patient inconvenience, and radiation dosimetry make routine use as yet impractical.[168]

Hypertrophic Osteoarthropathy and Periostitis. Hypertrophic osteoarthropathy is a osseous disease frequently associated with pulmonary, cardiac, or hepatic disorders, characterized by periosteal inflammation and reaction primarily of long bones, although all bones may be affected (Fig. 40–16) (see Chapter 103). The patient may be symptomatic with diffuse periosteal pain for months before radiologic periosteal thickening or elevation is seen.[169-173] In the early symptomatic phase, radionuclide bone scanning may suggest the diagnosis.[171,172] Findings include increased periosteal activity, which generates the "double stripe" sign at the ends of long bones (femur or humerus). Scintigraphic periostitis may also be found at the radius, ulna, tibia, and fibula. A patchy "skip" pattern to the periostitis is not uncommon. Increased patellar uptake is frequent. The terminal phalanges rarely demonstrate a significant increase in activity, even with marked "clubbing." Or importance to the scintigraphic diagnosis is the presence of "articular sparing," despite the reported infrequent synovitis. Resolution of scintigraphic abnormalities will accompany

resection of an etiologic pulmonary tumor or surgical correction of a cardiac left-to-right shunt, despite the persistence of radiographic findings.[172] "Spot" periostitis is sometimes seen following bone trauma and, when seen in children, should raise the possibility of the battered child syndrome and support such a diagnosis.[152]

Reflex Sympathetic Dystrophy. Reflex sympathetic dystrophy (RSD) is often post-traumatic and is considered to be an abnormal, excessive sympathetic nervous system response affecting distal extremities. Pain, swelling, and vasomotor disturbances are present with an initial increase in vascular flow and subsequent trophic dermal changes, radiographic osteoporosis, and juxta-articular erosions.[174,175] Unfortunately, early disease is frequently misdiagnosed when visible changes are minimal or absent, or is confused with local articular disease or nerve entrapment syndromes. Although 80 percent of patients with RSD develop eventual radiographic abnormalities that suggest the diagnosis, bone scintigraphy combined with early vascular studies presents a method of early diagnosis with objective findings that mirror abnormal physiology at a time when radiographs are normal.[174-181]

Scan findings include increased distal osseous uptake

Figure 40–16. Increased periosteal activity on bone scan characteristic of hypertrophic osteoarthropathy. Activity is greatest in the long bones (large arrows) with occasional "skipping." Note that activity is *decreased* over articulations (small arrows). The periosteum of small bones is also involved. These scintigraphic findings will precede radiographic changes.

in the affected extremity with mild juxta-articular accentuation[126,175,178-180] (Fig. 40–5*E*). Bone activity is usually increased from the forearm or calf, extending distally, although increased activity may extend to the elbow or knee. When unilateral, these findings are relatively specific, although they have also been described

in hemiplegia, following immobilization, or with diffuse cellulitis of the hand or foot.[181] The vascular flow studies demonstrate excessive arterial flow and the blood pool marked hyperemia on the affected side.[126,175,178-180] While RSD is clinically bilateral in one fourth of patients, scintigraphic studies have suggested a much higher frequency of bilaterality in clinically unilateral RSD. A few patients will develop changes of contralateral disease after bilaterality had been noted on the scan.[174,179,180] Carlson has verified the value of scanning for RSD of the lower limbs in patients whose disease followed a herniated lumbar disc.[177] It has also been seen in the lower extremities following sacroiliitis.[182] Abnormal scintigraphic changes revert with successful therapy and precede radiographic return to normalcy.[174,179,180]

Orthopedic and Sports Medicine Applications. Bone and joint scintigraphic examinations have been used by orthopedic surgeons to evaluate compartmental knee disease in planning arthrotomy and in interpreting pain after total hip or knee replacement.[183-185] In one study scintigraphy was compared with arthrography in confirming medial or lateral compartment degeneration and found to be as sensitive[183] (Fig. 40–17). The problem of possible loose prostheses is a major diagnostic dilemma in which ^{99m}Tc-phosphate bone imaging appears clinically useful. When compared with standard radiographs in 20 patients with total hip replacement, scintigraphy and arthrography were of equal, but complementary value in identifying prosthetic loosening.[184] In another study evaluating 94 total hip prostheses, the bone scan was found to best differentiate loosening from infection.[186] Bone scintigraphy for loosening was used to study 35 patients with 39 total knee prostheses. The authors concluded that there were highly correlated findings on the bone scans that suggested loosening, and that while the scan could not serve as the sole method of evaluation, it was a useful adjunct to clinical criteria and conventional radiography.[187]

Figure 40–17. Medial compartment osteoarthritis of the left knee demonstrated by scintimaging with ^{99m}Tc-EHDP in the left panel. The right panel reveals increased subchondral uptake increased across the entire tibial plateau, suggestive of severe osteoarthritis involving both medial and lateral compartments, much worse in the right knee.

Recently, nuclear arthrography using ^{99m}Tc-sulfur colloid has been used to study prosthetic loosening.[188-190] Its theoretical advantages include the fact that any radioactivity at the bone–prosthesis interface will *always* be abnormal and indicates communication with the joint space.

Because of the extreme sensitivity of bone and joint scintigraphy, these studies have been used, with a great deal of clinical success, to evaluate the athlete with unexplained pain and normal radiographs. The conditions diagnosed or suggested by bone scan include "shin splints,"[191,192] stress fractures, including those of the sesamoids of the feet, femur and femoral neck, tarsal, and wrist;[193-198] traumatic periostitis of the heel and plantar fasciitis;[191,199] insertional tendinitis;[191] damage to the pars interarticularis;[200] severe trauma following car, cycle, or other collisions that result in possibly severe musculoskeletal injury.[201]

^{67}Ga and ^{99m}Tc-pertechnetate Imaging in Sarcoidosis and Sjögren's Syndrome.

One of the first reports evaluating ^{67}Ga scanning included two patients with sarcoidosis, both of whom had positive scans.[9] One patient had marked perihilar uptake, and this has been subsequently demonstrated to be a significant finding in patients with sarcoidosis studied by ^{67}Ga imaging.[9,201,202] (Fig. 40–18). In another study, 9 of 27 patients had bilateral parotid uptake, a feature of sarcoid not typical for most other granulomatous or lymphomatous diseases.[203,204] Salivary uptake with ^{67}Ga is occasionally seen in Sjögren's syndrome but without coexistent hilar uptake.[205] Coupling the ^{67}Ga scan with the assay for angiontensin-converting enzyme (ACE) activity, Nosal and associates found that the combined studies increased the diagnostic specificity for sarcoidosis compared with either test alone by 98 versus 83 percent.[206] Because both tests are noninvasive, together they represent an alternative to surgical biopsy in the confirmation of the diagnosis of sarcoidosis. Increased uptake is also typically seen in the orbits, nasal mucosa, and smaller salivary glands, all of which are known sites of sarcoid activity (Fig. 40–18).

Recently, in one study of 12 patients with sarcoid and chronic hilar lymphadenopathy, the positivity of the ^{67}Ga scan or ACE-assay, while sensitive to the presence of disease, did not appear to discriminate between those patients remaining asymptomatic and those developing further pulmonary disease.[208] In a larger series of 54 patients, the ^{67}Ga scan was considered sensitive to the presence of disease (97 percent), but it did not correlate well with activity assessed clinically. However, the negative ^{67}Ga scan was considered to be an excellent predictor of clinical inactivity.[209]

The salivary gland uptake usually seen in sarcoid rarely progresses to functional abnormality demonstrable by ^{99m}Tc-pertechnetate imaging but is common in both primary and secondary Sjögren's syndrome.[20-23,25] There is a good correlation between labial biopsy abnormalities and pertechnetate scanning, which is therefore held useful in following disease progression.[21-25]

ARTHROGRAPHY

Technical and Clinical Considerations. Arthrography is the technique of radiographic visualization of intra-articular anatomy after arthrocentesis and instillation of

Figure 40–18. *A,* ^{67}Ga scan in acute sarcoidosis after 48 hours, demonstrating abnormally high parotid (large arrow), conjunctival (small arrow), and nasal mucosal activity, in addition to the perihilar uptake seen in the thorax (small arrowheads). *B,* ^{67}Ga imaging at 48 hours in this patient with primary Sjögren's syndrome reveals abnormal parotid uptake, but the hilar activity and uptake in the nasal and conjunctival mucosa are not seen.

a contrast agent, one of several radiopaque, iodinated, water-soluble compounds. The contrast medium may be used alone (single or positive contrast) or with injected air or CO_2 in a 1 to 5–10 ratio (double contrast). The amount injected is enough to mildly distend the joint capsule.[210-213] If joint effusion is present, the physician should send fluid for analysis prior to injection of contrast medium; if present in large amounts enough should be removed to prevent dilution of the contrast agent, particularly in double-contrast studies. Occasionally, air, CO_2, or other gas may be used above as a "contrast" agent if the patient is allergic to the iodinated contrast medium (negative contrast). The first arthrographic studies performed in Germany in 1905 used air for negative contrast.[214] Since then, extensive refinements have enhanced arthrographic studies: fluoroscopic guidance of the procedure and positioning; improved radiopaque media; stress devices for optimal opening of the joint space; spot filming of specific intra-articular structures; and finally the use of tomography or computed tomography in conjunction with standard imaging.[212,213,215-217]

Double-contrast studies are usually preferred because of superior detail and are most always indicated except for arthrography of the smaller joints, i.e., interphalangeal, or bursography, when the differences between the two methods are less significant. Although usually performed by a radiologist, simple studies may be performed by the rheumatologist or orthopedic surgeon in the outpatient setting if x-ray equipment is available and fluoroscopic guidance is unnecessary.[218]

Arthrography in adults (with the exception of certain hip arthrograms) does not require general anesthesia, although mild sedation may be of value, particularly in young children or infants. This contrasts with arthroscopy in which general or regional anesthesia is almost always required. The most common complication is increased articular pain in the first 24 hours after the completion of the study, which occurs in 25 percent of patients following knee arthrography and in up to 75 percent of patients undergoing shoulder study.[219,220] Mild synovitis secondary to the contrast agent is the most likely explanation rather than distention of the joint capsule.[212,213,218-222] The appearance of postprocedural pain is unrelated to sex, age of the patient, or arthrographic findings.[220] Double-contrast studies are usually better tolerated than positive-contrast arthrograms, but reaspiration of contrast agent (and air) after imaging does not lessen the likelihood of discomfort.[219] Reaspiration should be performed, nonetheless, in painful cases, in larger weight-bearing joints for psychic benefit, and to lessen mechanical discomfort. True allergic reactions to the contrast are uncommon. Pyogenic arthritis is rare, and the appearance of postprocedure pain is usually transient and benign and should not alarm either patient or clinician in the first 24 hours.[212,213,218-221]

Internal anatomic derangements are the single most common indication for arthrography. Usually the internal derangement is post-traumatic, but many arthrographically defined lesions develop as sequelae to underlying arthropathy, particularly in the shoulder and knee.[212,213,222] While virtually all articulations may be evaluated arthrographically, commonly studied joints include knee, shoulder, hip, ankle, wrist, elbow, and interphalangeal joints. Arthrographic technique is also frequently applied to juxta-articular structures, including bursa (bursography) and tendon sheaths.

Arthrography of the Knee. The most frequent indication for knee arthrography is confirmation of the presence or absence of clinically suspect meniscal injury[210-213] (Fig. 40–19). Medial meniscal tears predominate, since the medial meniscus is larger than the lateral meniscus and more vulnerable to trauma because of its firmer capsular attachment. Accuracy of arthrography in diagnosing medial meniscal lesions approaches 95 percent, when compared with findings at arthroscopy or surgery.[212,213] Lateral meniscal tears develop more frequently when knee stability is reduced by previous medial meniscal injury, ligamentous or capsular tears, adhesions, or osteoarthritis. Certain meniscal tears are common to specific settings. Vertical tears often follow acute trauma or athletic injury. Horizontal tears generally are seen in older individuals whose knees sustain continual stress, often occupational, without specific history of trauma. Osteonecrosis of the medial femoral condyle (most commonly developing in the sixth or seventh decade) was associated with medial meniscal tears in one report (21 of 27 patients), suggesting a causal relationship.[223]

Other indications for knee arthrography include the suspicion of loose bodies, abnormalities of articular cartilage, and ligamentous injury. Intra-articular loose bodies tend to migrate to synovial recesses or the intercondylar notch and are, hence, less accurately identified than meniscal lesions.[212,213] Cruciate ligamentous tears may be diagnosed, although the indications for arthrography in this instance are in question. Pathology of the posterior cruciate ligament poses more difficulty in delineation relative to the anterior.[224,225] Arthrography, although accurate in identifying anterior cruciate tear,

Figure 40–19. Medial meniscus "bucket handle" tear demonstrated by double-contrast arthrography. The tear is filled with air (arrows).

offers no diagnostic advantages over the simple "drawer" test.[226] Arthrographically demonstrable lesions of articular cartilage include osteochondritis dissecans, osteochondral fractures, and chondral fractures (which must be distinguished from each other), and chondromalacia patellae.[211-213,227,228]

Arthrography can usefully evaluate communicating cysts or bursae of the knee, particularly in patients with underlying inflammatory disease.[212,213,218,229,230] Fifty percent of all individuals have a posteromedial, synovia-lined bursa called the gastrocnemius-semimembranosus (G-S) bursa which communicates with the knee and is frequently bilateral. The G-S bursa may enlarge, causing pain with increased intra-articular pressure and chronic effusion (Fig. 40–20). The clinical term for the cyst in this clinical situation is Baker's cyst. While definition is possible with ultrasound or radioisotopic scanning, ultrasound cannot accurately delineate the ruptured cyst,

nor identify internal derangement when it is etiologic. Arthrography is therefore preferred in the context of a Baker's cyst occurring with possible meniscal lesion, or if the possibility of rupture is a diagnostic consideration, or when surgical removal of a Baker's cyst is contemplated.[212,218,231]

Arthrography is useful in the preoperative evaluation of juxta- or intra-articular masses of the knee, particularly when combined with tomography. In cases of malignant or locally aggressive lesions for which amputation is *not* planned, preoperative arthrography can determine if synovial or capsular invasion is present.[228] In selected benign osseous and synovial lesions, including both intra- and extra-articular chondromatosis and pigmented villonodular synovitis, arthrography can be helpful in deciding whether an arthrotomy is needed, and if so, how extensive the surgical exploration should be.[228,232-234] Certain lesions, such as synovial plicae, are

A   B

Figure 40–20. *A,* Large popliteal cyst extending into the calf. It was asymptomatic and detected in a patient studied for possible medial meniscal tear. *B,* This Baker's cyst was symptomatic, even though smaller than the one in *A.* This double-contrast study was performed in the office after simultaneous arthrocentesis for an effusion.

better dealt with by arthroscopy, since they are both diagnosed and treated with one procedure.[235]

Arthrography of the Shoulder. Arthrography to evaluate acute or chronic shoulder pain can demonstrate adhesive capsulitis, tears of the rotator cuff or joint capsule, lesions of the bicipital tendon, loose bodies, pigmented villonodular synovitis, and many other conditions.[212,222,236-238] It is also helpful in managing acute, recurrent, and chronic shoulder dislocation.[212,239,240] As with the knee, double-contrast studies are preferred for inherently greater anatomic detail (Fig. 40–21).

The rotator cuff is a musculotendinous aponeurosis of four muscles: the supraspinatus, infraspinatus, teres minor, and subscapularis. Damage occurs with acute or chronic dislocations or with chronic inflammation, as in patients with rheumatoid arthritis, calcific tendonitis, or pseudogout.[212,222,236,237] The usual presentation of rotator cuff tears is decreased range of motion with associated pain. The most common tear involves the supraspinatus tendon and separates the subacromial-subdeltoid bursa from the joint capsule. Diagnosis is made when contrast medium enters the subdeltoid bursa covering the greater tuberosity after instillation of the medium into the glenohumeral space[212,222,236,237] (Fig. 40–22). Tomography combined with double-contrast studies of the shoulder in rotator cuff tears has the ability to accurately demonstrate the size of the cuff tear and the thickness of remaining cuff tissue.[238] This information provides the surgeon with a better preoperative estimate of the difficulty of repair and prognosis for functional recovery.

Adhesive capsulitis (pericapsulitis), both a presentation or late complication of spondyloarthropathies, may also be post-traumatic or idiopathic. Exquisite pain, followed by progressively limited glenohumeral motion, with a concomitant decrease in external and internal rotation, is the characteristic clinical picture. During arthrography, much greater force than usual is required to instill both contrast medium and/or air, and the principal findings include a small capsular volume with (Fig. 40–23). Periarticular lymphatics are sometimes visualized because of the force required for injection.[218,222,236] Occasionally, the capsulitis appears treated as well as definitively diagnosed by the procedure, since large volumes of air and contrast medium can free capsular adhesions.[212,239] Since occult trauma to the rotator cuff is not uncommon, in instances of long-standing adhesive capsulitis arthrography may aid in the diagnosis of a coexistant rotator cuff tear.

The unstable, subluxing, or dislocating shoulder is probably better studied by arthrotomography, and in some instances by computed arthrotomography. Ten patients with unstable shoulders in which 3 had occult Hill-Sachs lesions were not successfully diagnosed by conventional studies.[240] Double-contrast arthrotomograms were also shown to be of value in lesions of the shoulder accompanied by known history of dislocation, since assessment of the integrity of the glenoid labrum has implications in the operative management of patients with shoulder trauma.[241] Subacromial bursography has been shown to be of value in differentiating "impinge-

Figure 40–21. Normal double-contrast arthrogram of the shoulder. Positive contrast and air outline the joint capsule (white arrows) and humeral articular cartilage (black arrowheads). Note that *no* air is found adjacent to either acromion or the greater tuberosity. (Courtesy of William A. Murphy, M.D.)

Figure 40–22. Rotator cuff tear. A double-contrast arthrogram demonstrates air in the subacromial and subdeltoid bursae (white arrows), which connects to the shoulder joint through the rotator cuff tear (black arrowheads). (Courtesy of William A. Murphy, M.D.)

ment syndrome" from subtle instability of the glenohumeral joint and/or rotator cuff disease. Strizak and associates suggested in their recent series that a normal bursogram literally rules out the diagnosis of chronic impingement syndrome.[243]

Arthrography of the Hip. Arthrography of the hip is technically much easier to perform than arthroscopy. Unexplained hip pain after total hip replacement with a differential diagnosis of loose hip prosthesis from hip infection and adhesive capsulitis represents a major indication in the adult.[212,221,243-245] Subtraction radiography is frequently necessary to differentiate contrast media

Figure 40–23. Frozen shoulder or adhesive capsulitis. A double-contrast shoulder arthrogram with needle in place reveals the small joint volume and obliteration of axial pouch recess.

surrounding the prosthesis, which has a similar radiopaque density. There is approximately a 20 to 50 percent error rate for arthrographic findings, compared with subsequent operative findings.[245,246] Errors are more likely to be false-positive for the acetabular component and false-negative for the femoral component in the diagnosis of loose prosthesis made on the basis of arthrography, although arthrography is more accurate than conventional radiography alone.[245] In one recent study, concomitant measuring of intracapsular pressure during arthrography was said to enhance the accuracy of the procedure.[246] A series has been reported of ten patients in whom intracapsular pressure recordings were made during arthrographic evaluation of loose hip prosthesis. A surprising finding was the evidence for postoperative adhesive capsulitis in five of the ten patients.[247] Hip arthrography has been used in infants to diagnose infection, congenital hip dislocation, and Legg-Calvé-Perthes disease.[212,221]

Arthrography of Other Articulations. The ankle may be safely studied for diagnosis of ligament and capsular tears.[212,218,248-251] Since treatment modalities for various types of ankle sprains differ greatly, it is held by several authors that ankle arthrography is grossly underutilized by clinicians.[248-252] Elbow studies provide aid in diagnosis and management of ligamentous tears, loose bodies, chondromatosis, villonodular synovitis, and osteochondritis.[212,216] Arthrographic examination of the wrist is useful in planning the extent of surgical synovectomy or in evaluating the site of median nerve compression prior to surgical release or for patients with chronic post-traumatic pain.[212,218,253-256] Finger arthrography combined with magnification radiography was of use in defining the pathology of chronic finger pain in a series of fifteen patients. Both single and double-contrast studies were used.[257] Rheumatologists should also be aware of the use of arthrography in the diagnosis and management of patients with temporomandibular joint pain and dysfunction, which are characteristic of many inflammatory arthropathies.[258,259]

ULTRASOUND

Ultrasonography, diagnostic imaging with high-frequency (1 to 5 megahertz) sound waves, represents a safe, noninvasive imaging technique for virtually all abdominal and pelvic organs, the heart (cardiac chambers, valves, and pericardium), and orbit of the eye. Applications have multiplied with the development of B-mode compound scanning and gray-scale imaging, which provide a two-dimensional echographic map based on the echoes arising from the boundaries of tissues with differential acoustic impedance, the product of the density of a substance multiplied by the speed of sound in the substance. The greater the difference in acoustic impedance, the larger the portion of sound reflected from the acoustic interface.[260,261] Bone presents a boundary with high reflectance (greater than 70 percent at the tissue-bone interface) too great for satisfactory echo imaging.[260,262] This has been the major drawback in musculoskeletal imaging. Collagen is responsible for the majority of internal echoes on gray-scale ultrasonography[262,263] and ultrasound has been described as a distribution and density map of the collagenous macrostructural support elements of human tissues.[264]

The general applications of ultrasound, mass delineation and determination of consistency, have proved valuable in delineating soft tissue lesions, such as tumors arising from the spine and bony pelvis.[260,265] The most specific musculoskeletal application has been the evaluation of the popliteal fossa and the noninvasive diagnosis of Baker's cyst.[266-271] Other uses particularly relevant to the rheumatologist include the echocardi-

ographic diagnosis of pericardial disease and effusions in rheumatoid arthritis,[272-276] systemic lupus erythematosus,[277] scleroderma,[278] and other collagen vascular diseases;[279] the accurate detection of dilated bile ducts in the differentiation of medical versus surgical jaundice; and the diagnostic and therapeutic percutaneous biopsy or aspiration of viscera, masses, and cysts. The percutaneous localization of biopsy site by ultrasonography has been reported to be more accurate than corresponding radiographic or radioisotopic methods.[260] A preliminary report has suggested the sonographic diagnosis of preradiographic myositis ossificans.[280] No doubt many other uses will be proposed, but their specific role in disease management will be unclear until large prospective studies are completed.

Ultrasonography of Baker's Cyst. Although the presence of a popliteal mass should suggest the diagnosis of a Baker's cyst in a patient with rheumatoid arthritis or in an individual with a history of knee effusion, clinical definition is usually uncertain and it is difficult to distinguish such a cyst from hematoma, popliteal artery aneurysm, or lipoma[212,218,266-271,281] (Fig. 40–24). Problems arise when posterior calf pain, often accompanied by distal edema and dilated veins, makes the clinical distinction between acute thrombophlebitis impossible (i.e., the so-called pseudothrombophlebitis syndrome or PTS). Only 25 percent of patients in one series of 34 patients with the clinical entity of PTS had rupture or rupture concurrent with acute dissection.[282] While most patients with PTS could be sorted out by ultrasound and spared more invasive diagnostic procedures, two pitfalls become apparent. First, patients may have both thrombophlebitis *and* Baker's cyst.[283,284] Thus, caution must be entertained, even when a Baker's cyst is documented. Second, ultrasound studies will frequently miss cyst rupture.[212,218,266,269,282] If cyst rupture is considered, then arthrography may be indicated, particularly if surgery is entertained.

Reports on ultrasound studies of articulations other than the knee are lacking. While able to diagnose effusion, ultrasound is more expensive than needle aspi-

Figure 40–24. Ultrasound of Baker's cyst of the right knee.

ration and does not provide synovial fluid, which may be diagnostic. Although the latter procedure is *invasive*, in the hands of a skilled rheumatologist or orthopedic surgeon the procedure is rapid, simple, safe, and relatively painless. One study did combine ultrasound with arthrography successfully in evaluation of elbow, hip, and shoulder joints,[285] but it is unclear what was gained by the two procedures other than cost.

THERMOGRAPHY

The development of modern thermography represents an interesting study in the application of technology. The existence of infrared emissions from the sun and other warm bodies was the observation of the royal astronomer to King George III of England, Sir William Herschel, in 1800. His son, John, took an interest in these studies and created the first primitive thermograph.[286] In 1880, Langley invented the bolometer, which was sensitive enough to detect a cow at 400 meters.[287] Hardy verified that human skin radiates infrared energy like the perfect "black body."[288] Interest in clinical applications waned until the use of thermography to detect night movements in World War II provided a technology for precise human measurements.

In 1949, Horvath and Hollander demonstrated the correlation between intra-articular temperature and clinical activity of the joint in patients with rheumatoid arthritis.[289] Skin temperature, lower than the tissue beneath it, is determined by the blood flow, the metabolic activity, and external temperature. This difference at the knee was shown by Hanson to be between 4 and 5 degrees Centigrade.[290] These facts form the basis for clinical assessment of inflammation by thermography.

Modern emission thermography utilizes equipment capable of 0.1°C temperature discrimination. This precision is available using modern electronic telethermography, which must be performed in a temperature-controlled room, whose technical features add to the cost of true quantitative thermography. Collins and associates have described a complicated "thermographic index" for normal joints, a basis for comparative thermographic assessment of inflammatory activity in joint disease,[291] but noted that there is a diurnal variation in the thermographic index. It has been used successfully in measuring the articular response to steroid injections, oral nonsteroidal drugs, penicillamine, and cytotoxic drugs.[292,293]

A second, less precise method of thermography more widely utilized employs a device for liquid crystal thermography (LCT). The "liquid" crystals are derivatives of cholesterol esters and polarize light in narrow wavebands. Phase transition with temperature is characterized by specific color-temperature response, allowing color thermography applications with color-temperature gradients of 0.2 to 0.4 degrees Centigrade in the most sensitive response zone.[294,295] Recently, these liquid crystals have been embedded in elastomeric sheets, which can be contoured to the torso, allowing for convenient

application of thermographic studies at lower cost.[296] The area of study is restricted to the area covered by the liquid crystal sheeting and similar controlled temperature environs must be maintained for accuracy.

Diagnosis of Low Back Pain. One of the first clinical uses for thermography was in the evaluation of lumbar disc disease by Albert and associates in 1964,[297] and by several other groups who demonstrated abnormal infrared emission patterns in lumbar spine disease.[298-304] Because of a high frequency of thermographic abnormalities in lumbar disc disease, it has been argued that lumbar thermography might rationally precede myelography for evaluating patients with possible disc herniation.[299-301] The procedure has not gained widespread acceptance because of a high rate of false negatives,[301] although a claim has been entered for both higher accuracy (91 versus 86 percent) and fewer false negatives (1 versus 6 of 42 patients) for LCT compared with myelography in patients who had undergone subsequent surgery.[302,303] However, the precise surgical diagnosis was not given, nor was it correlated with clinical information or electromyographic findings in this study. In another report, thermography compared favorably with myelography in the diagnosis of disc herniation but was ineffective in diagnosis of spinal stenosis.[301] There is also a high false positive rate in diagnosing herniated disc in patients with spondylitis, many of whom present with symptoms of sciatica suggestive of disc disease.[305]

Unfortunately, the litigious nature of low back pain and the need for more accurate diagnosis has led to the publication of articles emphasizing the specificity of thermographic diagnosis in legal journals.[306] Diagnostic thermography has much potential in neurologic disease of the spine, and more critical studies are needed. Raskin has suggested that lumbar thermography also be used to screen for muscular and ligamentous injuries, since lumbar and paraspinal spasm is probably responsible for the abnormal heat pattern in noninflammatory lumbar disease, to add to the clinical impression with a perfectly noninvasive procedure.[301] Lumbar thermography has been applied to the diagnosis of metastatic spine disease and spondylitis.[307,308] Thermographic assessment of sacroiliitis in a study by Scott and associates suggested value only in serial follow-up of the individual patient rather than in comparison between patients.[309]

Peripheral Disease. Thermography has not been used for the diagnosis of peripheral arthritis, possibly because of the greater ease in clinically documenting peripheral synovitis versus axial inflammation. Nonetheless a consistent series of observations has verified the value of thermographic measurement of inflammation of peripheral joints.[291-293] Thermography has also been of value in quantifying the inflammation of adjuvant or carrageenan-induced arthritis in the rat, thereby providing a tool for drug study.[292] While skin temperature differs from the articular temperature by a near constant for each joint, early studies with radiometers suggested that skin temperature varies with blood flow measured by xenon clearance or plethysmography. Recent studies employing peripheral thermography suggest that this skin

39yo BF with SHOULDER-HAND SYNDROME. Infrared Thermography performed at room temp. 72°F

Repeat Thermography after hand immersion in water at 58°F for 30 seconds.

Figure 40–25. Abnormal distal hyperemia in reflex dystrophy contributing to the positive telethermogram. Diminished relative vasoconstriction was seen after immersion in cold water, indicating aberrant sympathetic outflow.

temperature variation renders the thermographic assessment of the small peripheral joints of the phalanges unsatisfactory, but the effect is inconsequential for quantifying inflammation of the knee, ankle, elbow, and wrists.[310] Thermography has been found useful in the evaluation of the reflex dystrophy syndrome (Fig. 40–25).

COMPUTED TOMOGRAPHY

Donald Resnick, M.D.

In a little more than a decade since its introduction, computed tomography (CT) has already had a dramatic impact on the diagnosis of disease processes that affect virtually any organ system or tissue. In this brief time period, generations of CT scanners have appeared, each succeeding one striving for an increase in image resolution and a decrease in the time necessary for the examination.[311-314] Initially, CT scanners were found predominantly at a few large patient referral centers; subsequently, their numbers have increased at an incredible rate, and currently, they are found in even small and isolated hospitals as well as private medical offices.

The potential advantages of CT relative to conventional radiography are many, but foremost is an ability to display cross-sectional anatomy utilizing a series of images; these images, typically 2 to 13 mm in thickness, can be spaced at variable intervals, generally 2 to 10 mm apart. Specific x-ray attenuation values can be calculated for tissues within the slices and are expressed as CT numbers, usually on a scale of −1000 for air, 0 for water, and +1000 for dense bone.[311] The ability to differentiate among tissues with only subtle differences in radiodensity is, therefore, possible with CT and represents another significant advantage of this modality compared with routine radiography.

With regard to image format, a two-dimensional matrix of picture elements called pixels is displayed in a video monitor using, most commonly, shades of gray corresponding to the CT numbers. The range of such numbers can be adjusted by changing the window width and level in the monitor. Although cross-sectional image display is the classic format that is used, reconstruction of the image in a coronal or sagittal plane, or in any other plane, is possible.

The spatial resolution, a measure of image sharpness, is about 1.5 mm, slightly less than that for conventional radiography; the density resolution, a measure of the ability to differentiate subtle soft tissue densities, is about 0.5 percent greater than that for conventional radiography; and the radiation exposure for a series of images is in the acceptable range of 1 to 3 rads for the entire examination.[35]

In the last decade, the application of CT to the diagnosis of musculoskeletal disorders has been emphasized in hundreds of scientific articles. In general, CT is most valuable when utilized to evaluate regions such as the spine, pelvis, and hips, where anatomy is complex, and is less useful in the examination of the peripheral parts of the body. The following comments will serve as an overview of the more important clinical applications of this modality.

Low Back Pain. CT is quickly replacing myelography as the procedure of choice for the diagnosis of herniated intervertebral discs.[316,317] Methods of evaluation by CT vary with respect to slice interval and thickness as well as the utilization of either parallel cross-sectional images ("stacked coins") or images obtained along the axes of the intervertebral discs using angulation of the gantry. Furthermore, debate exists regarding the advantages of plain CT or that obtained following the introduction of intraspinal metrizamide,[318] and regarding the ability of reconstructed images in the sagittal or coronal plane to further increase the accuracy of CT in the diagnosis of discal herniation.[319] Although central herniation of the intervertebral disc is well evaluated with both myelography and CT, the latter modality is superior in the recognition of lateral lumbar disc herniation.[320]

With CT, a herniated disc appears as a soft tissue density located posterior to the normal intervertebral disc or vertebral body or both (Fig. 40–26). This density

Figure 40–26. Herniation of an intervertebral disc. On this cross-sectional image at the level of the intervertebral disc, observe a soft tissue density protruding into the spinal canal (arrow), obliterating the adjacent nerve root. The root on the opposite site (arrowhead) is visible.

is generally easy to recognize, although differentiation from a bulging anulus fibrosus[319,321] and conjoined nerve roots[322] can present diagnostic difficulty.

The evaluation of spinal stenosis related to congenital or acquired disorders is well accomplished with CT.[323] The cross-sectional display of CT provides information regarding the anteroposterior and transverse diameters of the spinal canal, and measurements of the diameter can be compared with available normal values.[324] In this fashion, stenosis of the central canal, the lateral recesses, and the neural foramina can be detected.[325,326] Alterations of the apophyseal joints are also well shown.

High-resolution CT can be indispensable in the evaluation of patients with persistent or recurrent symptoms and signs following lumbar spine surgery.[327] In these individuals, routine radiography generally provides little diagnostic information. With CT, extradural fibrosis or hematoma, postlaminectomy pseudomeningocele, recurrent discal herniation, and postoperative bony stenosis can be accurately defined, although in some cases administration of intraspinal or intravenous contrast material may be required.[328]

Sacroiliitis. The precise role of CT in the diagnosis of sacroiliitis is not clear. Although some reports have indicated an increased sensitivity of this modality compared with conventional radiography in the detection of early or minor abnormalities of the sacroiliac articulation,[329,330] others disagree with this assessment.[331] Carefully performed investigations comparing CT and conventional tomography[332] in detecting sacroiliitis have not yet been provided. However, CT can be useful in delineating the extent of disease in patients with infective sacroiliitis (Fig. 40–27) and in evaluating those with ankylosing spondylitis who have the cauda equina syn-

Figure 40–27. Tuberculosis of the sacroiliac joints. Observe the destruction of the left sacroiliac joint and a large cystic mass anterior to the articulation, representing soft tissue extension of the infection.

drome.[333,334] In these latter patients, multiple erosions of the posterior elements of the lumbar spine correlate with thecal diverticula demonstrated with myelography (Fig. 40–28). Furthermore, in individuals with ankylosing spondylitis, CT provides dramatic evidence of the degree of atrophy of posterior spinal muscles.[335]

Trauma. The value of CT in the assessment of the traumatized patient is not debated. This modality allows evaluation of such patients without the discomfort and the hazard required in their movement.[336] Identification of both bone and soft tissue injuries is facilitated.[337] CT is ideal for the delineation of injury to the axial skeleton. Trauma to the spine or spinal cord is one prime example of a situation in which evaluation by CT is advantageous. It allows identification of fractures of both the vertebral bodies and the posterior elements, of the extent of compromise to the adjacent spinal cord by displaced osseous fragments or hematoma formation, and of the degree of spinal instability.[323,338,339]

Figure 40–28. Ankylosing spondylitis and thecal diverticula. A CT image of a lumbar vertebra demonstrates scalloped erosions of the posterior elements, diagnostic of thecal diverticula.

Injuries to the hip or shoulder can also be well delineated with CT. In the former area, identification of complex fractures of the acetabulum and the proximal femur and of intra-articular bone fragments is possible.[340,341] In the shoulder, identification of similar fractures of the glenoid fossa and humerus is accomplished. In addition, compression fractures of the posterolateral surface of the humeral head (Hill-Sachs lesion) occurring in association with an anterior dislocation of the glenohumeral joint can be detected.[342] CT accomplished in conjunction with arthrography of this joint will allow diagnosis of subtle abnormalities of the glenoid labrum[343] (Fig. 40–29).

Further examples of injuries that are well defined by CT include fractures of the sacrum and sternum and dislocations of the sacroiliiac and sternoclavicular articulations (Fig. 40–30).

Tumors and Infections. Although in most cases CT does not significantly contribute to the histologic diagnosis of primary bone tumors (with the exception of simple cysts and lipomas), its cross-sectional display allows analysis of the degree of soft tissue extension and the compromise or violation of surrounding neurovascular structures.[344] This information can be vital to the surgeon in the management of the tumor and to the radiologist as an aid in the planning of percutaneous biopsy. CT can also be utilized as a diagnostic tool in the patient with suspected skeletal metastasis in whom plain films are unrewarding; although the spatial resolution of even the latest generation scanners is inferior to that of plain films, a cross-sectional image may occasionally delineate a lesion that was not evident with routine radiography. Furthermore, a potential exists for CT in differentiating benign and malignant pulmonary nodules in individuals who are suspected of having widespread metastatic disease.[345]

With regard to infections of bone, CT may reveal an increase in the density of the marrow (a phenomenon also evident with neoplasms) related to edema and vascular congestion at a time when plain films are negative,[346] although scintigraphy still appears to be the most

Figure 40–30. Posterior dislocation of the sternoclavicular joint. Note the posterior location of the medial end of the left clavicle and its intimate relationship with the adjacent trachea and vascular channels.

sensitive modality in the early diagnosis of osteomyelitis. CT can also demonstrate bone abscesses or cortical sequestration[347] and the extent of soft tissue involvement, the latter being particularly helpful in cases of spinal infection.

Articular Diseases. The role of CT in evaluating patients with articular disease is limited. This modality appears to have little or no advantage when compared with routine radiography or conventional tomography in delineating cartilaginous destruction or bony erosion with the exception of sites, such as the sternoclavicular, costovertebral, temporomandibular, and apophyseal articulations, that are difficult to visualize with usual imaging techniques.[348-350] Even in the latter locations, examination with CT frequently requires meticulous positioning of the patient and the utilization of re-for-

Figure 40–29. Abnormality of the glenoid labrum. A CT image following intra-articular administration of air reveals absence of the anterior portion of the glenoid labrum (arrow). A compression fracture of the humerus (arrowhead) is consistent with a Hill-Sachs lesion.

Figure 40–31. Pigmented villonodular synovitis. Multiple erosions of the right femoral head, well demonstrated with CT, are consistent with the diagnosis of pigmented villonodular synovitis.

Figure 40–32. Synovial cyst of the hip. In a patient with rheumatoid arthritis, observe erosion of the femoral head and femoral neck and a large cystic mass, located anterior to the hip (arrow).

Figure 40–34. Talocalcaneal tarsal coalition. A bony bridge extending between the sustentaculum tali of the calcaneus and the middle facet of the talus is indicative of a bony coalition. Compare the appearance to that of the opposite normal side.

matted images. CT, utilized with or without the introduction of intra-articular contrast agents, can be useful, however, in certain articular disorders, including osteochondritis dissecans, osteocartilaginous bodies, idiopathic synovial osteochondromatosis, and pigmented villonodular synovitis[351,352] (Fig. 40–31). Although not proven useful in detecting meniscal lesions in the knee, CT may be utilized in the diagnosis of tears of the cruciate ligaments.[353]

With respect to joint disease, CT is perhaps best suited to the evaluation of para-articular soft tissue masses. Synovial cysts arising adjacent to the glenohumeral joint, hip, and knee are well visualized in this fashion (Fig. 40–32), although the simultaneous administration of an arthrographic contrast agent is often required.

Osteoporosis. In recent years, CT has been applied to the diagnosis of generalized osteoporosis by allowing measurement of the degree of attenuation of the x-ray beam at a specific skeletal site. Although such quantitative techniques can be applied to the peripheral skel-

Figure 40–33. Ossification of the posterior longitudinal ligament. On a cross-sectional image in the upper cervical spine, a radiodensity seen posterior to the vertebral body (arrow) represents ossification of the posterior longitudinal ligament. Contrast around the spinal cord is related to the prior administration of metrizamide.

eton, it appears advantageous to investigate the vertebral spongiosa in this manner.[354-356] It has been suggested that CT can recognize a 1 percent change in the content of vertebral bone; however, errors occur owing to changes in patient position so that different sections of the bone are obtained.[357] It is expected that with refinement in and more widespread availability of this technique, quantitative CT analysis will become the noninvasive modality of choice in evaluating patients with osteoporosis and other metabolic disorders.

Miscellaneous Diseases. Diastomatomyelia, myelomeningocele, and ligamentous calcification and ossification (Fig. 40–33) are examples of spinal disorders that are well delineated with CT.[358] Tibial torsion and femoral or humeral anteversion can be evaluated with conventional radiography, but the technique is complex and time consuming; CT may be more advantageous in this evaluation. Coalition, or fusion, of tarsal bones, especially that between the talus and the calcaneus (Fig. 40–34), is best visualized in a coronal plane, which can be achieved with CT.[359] Although this modality has been applied to the diagnosis of ischemic necrosis, especially in the femoral head,[360] its precise role in this regard, particularly with respect to any advantage over scintigraphy, is not established.

A variety of soft tissue problems, in addition to tumors, can be defined with CT. Examples include entrapment neuropathies, especially in the carpal tunnel,[361] foot infections in the diabetic patient, foreign body localization,[362] and calcification or ossification. In the latter situation, the differentiation of myositis ossificans and osteosarcoma of the soft tissue is possible.[363]

References

1. Koenigsberg, M., and Freeman, L.: Radionuclide bone imaging. Curr. Prob. Diagn. Radiol. 6:1, 1976.
2. Lentle, B., Russell, A., Percy, J., Scott, J., and Jackson, F.: Bone scintiscanning updated. Ann. Intern. Med. 84:297, 1976.
3. Thrall, J.F.: Technetium-99m labelled agents for skeletal imaging. CRC Crit. Rev. Clin. Radiol. Nucl. Med. 8:1, 1976.
4. Subramanian, G., McAfee, J., Blair, R., Mehter, A., and Connor, T.: 99mTc-EHDP: A potential radiopharmaceutical for skeletal imaging. J. Nucl. Med. 13:947, 1972.
5. David, M., and Jones, A.: Comparison of 99Tc-labeled phosphate agents for skeletal imaging. Semin. Nucl. Med. 7:19, 1976.
6. Pendergrass, H., Potsaid, M., and Catronovo, F.: The clinical use of

^{99m}Tc-diphosphonate (HEDSPA): A new agent for skeletal imaging. Radiology 109:557, 1973.

7. Hayes, R.L.: The medical use of gallium radionuclides: A brief history with some comments. Semin. Nucl. Med. 8:183, 1978.

8. Turner, D., Fordham, E.W., Ali, A., and Slayton, R.E.: Gallium-67 imaging in the management of Hodgkin's disease and other malignant lymphomas. Semin. Nucl. Med. 8:205, 1978.

9. Higasi, T., Nakayama, Y., Murata, A., Nakamura, M., Sugiyama, M., and Suzuki, S.: Clinical evaluation of ^{67}Gacitrate scanning. J. Nucl. Med. 13:196, 1972.

10. Staab, E.V., and McCartney, W.: Role of gallium 67 in inflammatory disease. Semin. Nucl. Med. 8:219, 1978.

11. Namey, T.C., and Halla, J.: Radiographic and nucleographic techniques in the diagnosis of septic arthritis and osteomyelitis. Clin. Rheum. Dis. 4:95, 1978.

12. Hays, M., and Green, F.: The pertechnetate joint scan: I. Timing. Ann. Rheum. Dis. 31:272, 1972.

13. Hays, M., and Green, F.: The pertechnetate joint scan: II. Clinical correlations. Ann. Rheum. Dis. 31:278, 1972.

14. Weiss, T.E., and Shuler, S.E.: I. New techniques for identification of synovitis and evaluation of joint disease. II. Joint imaging as a clinical aid in diagnosis and therapy. Bull. Rheum. Dis. 25:786, 1974.

15. Hays, M.T., and Green, F.A.: In vitro studies of ^{99m}Tc-pertechnetate bending by human serum and tissues. J. Nucl. Med. 14:149, 1973.

16. Dick, W.C., and Grennan, D.: Radioisotopes in the study of normal and inflamed joint. Clin. Rheum. Dis. 2:67, 1976.

17. Huskisson, E., Scott, J., and Balme, H.: Objective measurement of rheumatoid arthritis using technetium index. Ann. Rheum. Dis. 35:81, 1976.

18. Boerbooms, A., and Buys, W.: Rapid assessment of ^{99m}Tc-pertechnetate uptake in the knee joint as a parameter of inflammatory activity. Arthritis Rheum. 20:348, 1978.

19. Szanto, E., and Lindvall, N.: Quantitative ^{99m}Tc pertechnetate scanning of the sacro-iliac joints. Scand. J. Rheumatol. 7:93, 1978.

20. Schaal, G., Anderson, L., Wolf, R., et al.: Xerostomia in Sjögren's syndrome: Evaluation by sequential salivary scintigraphy. JAMA 216:2109, 1971.

21. Parret, J., and Peyrin, J.: Radioisotopic investigations in salivary pathology. Clin. Nucl. Med. 4:250, 1979.

22. Daniels, T.E., Powell, M.R., Sylvester, R., and Talal, N.: An evaluation of salivary gland scintigraphy in Sjögren's syndrome. Arthritis Rheum. 22:809, 1979. (Please note minor change on salivary slides.)

23. Ohrt, H., and Shafer, R.B.: An atlas of salivary gland disorders. Clin. Nucl. Med. 7:370, 1982.

24. Janin-Mercier, A., Sauvezie, B., Ristori, M., Betail, G., Veyre, A., and Rampon, S.: Histological and immunological study in patients with rheumatoid arthritis showing isolated abnormalities of salivary scintigraphy. J. Clin. Immuno. 2:282, 1982.

25. Chaudiri, T.K., and Stadalnik, R.C.: Salivary gland imaging. Semin. Nucl. Med. 10:400, 1980.

26. Jones, A., Francis, M., and Davis, M.: Radionuclide reaction mechanisms. Semin. Nucl. Med. 7:3, 1976.

27. Siegel, B., Donovan, R., Alderson, P., and Mack, G.: Skeletal uptake of ^{99m}Tc-diphosphonate in relationship to local blood flow. Radiology 120:121, 1976.

28. Charkes, N.D.: Skeletal blood flow: Implications for bone-scan interpretation. J. Nucl. Med. 21:91, 1980.

29. Krishnamurthy, G.T., Brickman, A., and Blahd, W.: Technetium-99m-Sn-pyrophosphate pharmaco-kinetics and bone image changes in parathyroid disease. J. Nucl. Med. 18:236, 1977.

30. Christensen, S.B., and Krogsgaard, O.W.: Localization of Tc-99m MDP in epiphyseal growth plates of rats. J. Nucl. Med. 22:237, 1981.

31. Rosenthall, L., and Kaye, M.: Technetium-99m-pyrophosphate kinetics and imaging in metabolic bone disease. J. Nucl. Med. 16:33, 1975.

32. Kaye, M., Silverton, S., and Rosenthall, L.: Technetium-99m-pyrophosphate: Studies in vivo and in vitro. J. Nucl. Med. 16:40, 1975.

33. Rosenthall, L., and Kaye, M.: Observations on the mechanism of ^{99m}Tc-labeled phosphate complex uptake in metabolic bone disease. Semin. Nucl. Med. 6:59, 1976.

34. Wiegmann, T., Kirsh, J., Rosenthall, L., and Kaye, M.: Relationship between bone uptake of ^{99m}Tc-pyrophosphate and hydroxyproline in blood and urine. J. Nucl. Med. 17:711, 1976.

35. Garcia, D., Tow, D., and Kaperr, K.: Relative accretion of ^{99m}Tc-polyphosphate by forming and resorbing bone systems in rats. Significance in the pathologic basis of bone scanning. J. Nucl. Med. 17:93, 1976.

36. Evans, C.H., and Mears, D.C.: ^{99m}Tc-1-hydroxyethylidene-1, 1-diphosphonic acid to cartilage and collagen in vitro and its stimulation by Er^{3+} and low pH. Calcif. Tissue Int. 32:91, 1980.

37. Turner, J.H.: Post-traumatic avascular necrosis of the femoral head predicted by preoperative technetium-99m antimony-colloid scan. J. Bone Joint Surg. 65A:786–796, 1983.

38. Meyers, M.H., Telfer, N., and Moore, T.M.: Determination of the vascularity of the femoral head with technetium-99m-sulphur-colloid. J. Bone Joint Surg. 59A:568, 1977.

39. Brown, D., Byrd, B., Carlton, J., Sartzendruber, D., and Hayes, R.: A quantitative study of the subcellular localization of ^{67}Ga^{2+}. Cancer Res. 36:956, 1976.

40. Takeda, S., Uchida, T., and Matsuzawa, T.: A comparative study on lysosomal accumulation of gallium-67 and indium-III in Morris hepatoma 7316A. J. Nucl. Med. 18:835, 1977.

41. Tsan, M., Chen, W., Scheffel, U., and Wagner, H.N.: Studies on gallium accumulation in inflammatory lesions. I. Gallium uptake by human polymorphonuclear leukocytes. J. Nucl. Med. 19:36, 1978.

42. Menon, S., Wagner, H.N., and Tsan, M.: Studies on gallium accumulation in inflammatory lesions. II. Uptake by Staphylococcus aureus. J. Nucl. Med. 19:44, 1978.

43. Hayes, R.: The tissue distribution of gallium radionuclides. J. Nucl. Med. 18:740, 1977.

44. Larson, S.: Mechanisms of localization of gallium-67 in tumors. Semin. Nucl. Med. 8:193, 1978.

45. Hill, J., Merz, T., and Wagner, N., Jr.: Iron-induced enhancement of ^{67}Ga uptake in a model human leukocyte culture system in vitro. J. Nucl. Med. 8:193, 1978.

46. Hoffer, P., Huberty, J., and Khayam-Bashi, H.: The association of Ga-67 and lactoferrin. J. Nucl. Med. 18:713, 1977.

47. Bradley, W., Alderson, P., Eckelman, W., and Weiss, J.: Decreased tumor uptake in animals after whole body radiation. J. Nucl. Med. 19:204, 1978.

48. Larson, S., Rasey, J., Grunbaum, Z., and Allen, D.: Pharmacologic enhancement of gallium-67 tumor-to-blood ratios for EMT-6 sarcoma (BALB/c mice). Radiology 130:241, 1979.

49. Weiner, R., Hoffer, P.B., and Thakur, M.L.: Lactoferrin: Its role as a Ga-67 binding protein in polymorphonuclear leukocytes. J. Nucl. Med. 22:32, 1981.

50. Hayes, R.L., Rafter, J.J., Byrd, B.L., and Carlton, J.E.: Studies of the in vivo entry of Ga-67 into normal and malignant tissue. J. Nucl. Med. 22:325, 1981.

51. Emery, T., and Hoffer, P.B.: Siderophore-mediated mechanism of gallium uptake demonstrated in the microorganism Ustilago sphaerogena. J. Nucl. Med. 21:935, 1980.

52. Hoffer, P.: Gallium and infection. J. Nucl. Med. 21:484, 1980.

53. Oster, Z.H., Som, P., Sacker, D.F., and Atkins, L.: The effects of deferoxamine mesylate on gallium-67 distribution in normal and abscess-bearing animals: Concise communication. J. Nucl. Med. 21:421, 1980.

54. Handmaker, H., and Leonards, R.: Bone scan in inflammatory osseous disease. Semin. Nucl. Med. 6:95, 1976.

55. Kontzen, F., Namey, T., Tobin, M., Debovsky, E., and Tauxe, W.N.: Technical aspects of joint imaging. J. Nucl. Med. Tech. 6:110, 1978.

56. Weiss, T., Maxfield, W., Murison, P., and Hidalgo, J.: Iodinated human serum albumin (I^{131}) localization studies of rheumatoid arthritis joints by scintillation scanning. Arthritis Rheum. 8:979, 1965.

57. Desaulniers, M., Fuks, A., Hawkins, D., Lacourciere, Y., and Rosenthall, L.: Radiotechnetium polyphosphate joint imaging. J. Nucl. Med. 15:421, 1974.

58. Bekerman, C., Genant, H., Hoffer, P., Kozin, F., and Ginsberg, M.: Radionuclide imaging of the bones and joints of the hand. Radiology 118:653, 1975.

59. Mirtl, B., Leb, G., Klein, G., Goebel, R., and Eber, O.: Gelenksszintigraphie mit ^{99m}-Tc-pyrophosphat. Z. Rechtsmed. 34:149, 1975.

60. Hoffer, P.B., and Genant, H.K.: Radionuclide joint imaging. Semin. Nucl. Med. 6:121, 1976.

61. Barraclough, D., Russell, A., and Percy, J.: Psoriatic spondylitis: A clinical, radiological, and scintiscan survey. J. Rheumatol. 4:282, 1977.

62. Namey, T.C., McIntyre, J., LeRoy, E.C., and Bennett, J.C.: Early psoriatic arthritis: Nucleographic and HLA studies. Proceedings of the XIV International Congress of Rheumatology, 1977, p. 210.

63. Namey, T., McIntyre, J., Buse, M., and LeRoy, E.: Nucleographic studies of axial spondarthritides. I. Quantitative sacroiliac scintigraphy in early HLA-B27-associated sacroiliitis. Arthritis Rheum. 20:1058, 1977.

64. Lentle, B.C., Russell, A., Percy, J., and Jackson, F.: The scintigraphic findings in ankylosing spondylitis. J. Nucl. Med. 18:524, 1977.

65. Namey, T., and Rosenthall, L.: Generalized periarticular uptake of ^{99m}-Tc-pyrophosphate in progressive systemic sclerosis. Clin. Nucl. Med. 2:26, 1977.

66. Rosenthall, L., and Hawkins, D.: Radionuclide joint imaging in the diagnosis of synovial disease. Semin. Arthritis Rheum. 7:49, 1977.

67. Namey, T.: Joint and quantitative sacroiliac scintigraphy in the diagnosis of rheumatic diseases. In Tauxe, W. (ed.): Functional Studies in Nuclear Medicine, 1978. Southeastern Society of Nuclear Medicine (11) 1978, pp. 1–19.

68. Weissberg, D., Resnick, D., Taylor, A., Becker, M., and Alazraki, N.: Rheumatoid arthritis and its variants: Analysis of scintiphotographic, radiographic, and clinical examinations. AJR 131:665, 1978.

69. Esdaile, J., Hawkins, D., and Rosenthall, L.: Radionuclide joint imaging in the seronegative spondyloarthropathies. Clin. Orthop. 143:46, 1979.

70. Shearman, J., Esdaile, J., Hawkins, D., and Rosenthall, L.: Predictive value of radionuclide joint scintigrams. Arthritis Rheum. 24:83, 1982.

71. Abrams, H.: The "overutilization" of x-rays. N. Engl. J. Med. 300:1213, 1979.

72. Baldrusson, H., and Gustafsson, M.: Total radiation dosage from x-ray examinations in rheumatoid arthritis and other chronic skeletal diseases. Acta Orthop. Scand. 48:138, 1977.

73. Godderidge, C.: Female gonadal shielding. Appl. Radiol. (Mar./Apr.):65, 1979.

74. Manny, E., Brown, F., and Shaver, J.: Gonad shielding in diagnostic radiology. Postgrad. Med. 65:207, 1979.

75. Hill, H.F., Hill, A.G., and Bodner, J.G.: Clinical diagnosis of ankylosing spondylitis in women and relation to presence of HLA-B27. Ann. Rheum. Dis. 35:267, 1976.

76. Cheatum, D.: "Ankylosing spondylitis" without sacroiliitis in a woman without HLA-B27 antigen. J. Rheumatol. 3:420, 1976.

77. Nasrallah, N., Masi, A., Chandler, R., Feigenbaum, S., and Kaplan, S.: HLA-B27 antigen and rheumatoid factor negative (seronegative) peripheral arthritis. Am. J. Med. 63:379, 1977.

78. Ross, J.: Biomedical effects of ionizing radiation. In Blahd, W. (ed.): Nuclear Medicine. 2nd ed. New York, McGraw-Hill Book Company, 1971.

79. Physicians' Desk Reference for Radiology and Nuclear Medicine, 1978/79 Oradell, N.J., Medical Economics Company, p. 134.

80. Editorial: Ankylosing spondylitis and its early diagnosis. Lancet 2:591, 1977.

81. Hockberg, M., Borenstein, D., and Arnett, F.: The absence of back pain in classical ankylosing spondylitis. Johns Hopkins Med. J. 143:181, 1978.

82. Bernstein, B., and Singsen, B.: Juvenile ankylosing spondylitis: Are adult criteria appropriate? (abstract). Arthritis Rheum. 22:593, 1979.

83. Wahner, H., and O'Duffy, J.: Peripheral joint scanning with technetium pertechnetate. Mayo Clin. Proc. 51:525, 1976.

84. Khalkhali, I., Stadalnik, R., Wiesner, K., and Shapiro, R.: Bone imaging of the heel in Reiter's syndrome. AJR 132:110, 1979.

85. Holzmann, H., Hoede, N., Eibner, D., and Hahn, K.: Die psoriatische Osteoarthropathie. Hautarzt 30:343, 1979.

86. Namey, T., and Rosenthall, L.: Periarticular uptake of ^{99m}technetium diphosphonate in psoriatics. Arthritis Rheum. 19:607, 1976.

87. Hoede, N., Holzmann, H., Eissner, D., and Hahn, K.: Uber die Häufigkeit von Gelenkbeteiligungen bei Psoriasis. Verh. Dtsch. Ges. Rheumatol. 4:229, 1976.

88. Lin, M.S., Fawcett, H.D., and Goodwin, D.A.: Bone scintigraphy demonstrating arthropathy of central joints in ankylosing spondylitis. Clin. Nucl. Med. 8:364, 1980.

89. Russell, A., Davis, P., Percy, J., and Lentle, B.: The sacroiliitis of acute Reiter's syndrome. J. Rheumatol. 4:293, 1977.

90. Webb, J., Collins, L.T., and Southwell, P.B.: Fluorine-18 isotope scans in the early diagnosis of sacroiliitis. Med. J. Aust. 2:1270, 1971.

91. Lovgren, O., and Dowen, S.A.: Strontium (85SR) scintigrams of the sacro-iliacal joints. Acta Rheum. Scand. 15:327, 1969.

92. VanLaere, M., Veys, E.M., and Mielants, H.: Strontium 87m scanning of the sacroiliac joints in ankylosing spondylitis. Ann. Rheum. Dis. 31:201, 1972.

93. Russell, A., Lentle, B., and Percy, J.: Investigation of sacroiliac disease: Comparative evaluation of radiological and radionuclide techniques. J. Rheumatol. 2:45, 1975.

94. Lentle, B., Russell, A., Percy, J., and Jackson, F.: The scintigraphic investigation of sacroiliac disease. J. Nucl. Med. 18:529, 1977.

95. Lugon, M., Torode, A., Travers, R., Lavender, J.P., and Hughes, G.R.: Sacro-iliac joint scanning with technetium-99m-diphosphonate. Rheumatol. Rehabil. 18:131, 1979.

96. Dunn, E., Ebringer, R., and Ell, P.: Quantitative scintigraphy in the early diagnosis of sacro-iliitis. Rheum. Rehabil. 19:69, 1980.

97. Scott, D., Smith, A., Eastmond, C., Hayter, C., and Wright, V.: An evaluation of the techniques of sacro-iliac scintiscanning. Rheum Rehabil. 19:76, 1980.

98. Dequeker, J., Goddeeris, T., Walravens, M., and DeRoo, M.: Evaluation of sacroiliitis: Comparison of radiological and radionuclide techniques. Radiology 128:687, 1978.

99. Spencer, D.G., Adams, F.G., Horton, P.W., and Buchanan, W.W.: Scintiscanning in ankylosing spondylitis. J. Rheumatol. 6:426, 1979.

100. Berghs, H., Remans, J., Drieskens, L., Kiebooms, A., and Polderman, J.: Diagnostic value of sacroiliac joint scintigraphy with ^{99m}technetium pyrophosphate in sacroiliitis. Ann. Rheum. Dis. 37:190, 1978.

101. Goldberg, R., Genant, H., Shimshak, R., and Shames, D.: Applications and limitations of quantitative sacroiliac joint scintigraphy. Radiology 128:683, 1978.

102. Ho, G., Sadovinikoff, N., Malhotra, C.M., and Claumch, B.C.: Quantitative sacroiliac joint scintigraphy. Arthritis Rheum. 22:837, 1979.

103. Pfannenstiel, P., Semmler, U., Adam, W., Halbsguth, A., Bandilla, K., and Berg, D.: Comparative study of quantitating ^{99m}Tc-EHDP uptake in sacroiliac scintigraphy. Eur. J. Nucl. Med, 5:49, 1980.

104. Szanto, E., and Lindvall, N.: Quantitative ^{99m}Tc pertechnetate scanning of the sacro-iliac joints: A follow-up study of patients with suspected sacroiliitis. Scand. J. Rheumatol. 7:93, 1978.

105. Chalmers, I., Lentle, B., Percy, J., and Russell, A.: Sacroiliitis detected by bone scintiscanning: A clinical, radiological and scintigraphic follow-up study. Ann. Rheum. Dis. 38:112, 1979.

106. Bellamy, N., Park, W., and Rooney, P.J.: What do we know about the sacroiliac joint? Sem. Arthritis Rheum. 12(3), 1983.

107. O'Duffy, J., Hunder, G., and Wahner, H.: A follow-up study of polymyalgia rheumatica: Evidence of chronic axial synovitis. J. Rheumatol. 7:685, 1980.

108. Ho., G., Claunch, B.C., and Sadovnikoff, N.: Scintigraphic evidence of transient unilateral sacroiliitis in a case of Whipple's disease Clin. Nucl. Med. 12:548, 1980.

109. Namey, T., Horowitz, J., and Hardin, J.: Transient sacroiliitis in acute sarcoid arthropathy. 65th Meeting, Radiology Society of North America, Atlanta, 1979.

110. Szanto, E., and Hagenfeldt, K.: Sacro-iliitis and salpingitis. Scand. J. Rheumatol. 8:129, 1979.

111. Szanto, E., and Hagenfeldt, K.: Sacro-iliitis in women—a sequela to acute salpingitis. Scand. J. Rheumatol. 12;89, 1983.

112. Namey, T.C., and Biondo, J.J.: Scintigraphic patterns of early inflammatory sacroiliitis: The possible significance of unilateral sacroiliitis in Reiter's syndrome. Trans. Orthop. Res. Soc. 1980.

113. Gordon, G., and Kabins, S.A.: Pyogenic sacroiliitis. Am. J. Med. 69:50, 1980.

114. Lopez-Majano, V., and Miskew, D.: Sacro-iliac joint disease in drug abusers: The role of bone scintigraphy. Eur. J. Nucl. Med. 5:549, 1980.

115. Lewkonia, R., and Kinsella, T.: Pyogenic sacroiliitis: Diagnosis and significance. J. Rheumatol. 8:153, 1981.

116. Iczkovitz, J., Leek, J., and Robbins, D.: Pyogenic sacroiliitis. J. Rheumatol. 8:157, 1981.

117. Horgan, J.G., Walker, M., Newman, J.H., and Watt, I.: Scintigraphy in the diagnosis and management of septic sacro-iliitis. Clin. Radiol. 34:337, 1983.

118. Kumar, R., and Balachandran, S.: Unilateral septic sacro-iliitis: Importance of the anterior view of the bone scan. Clin. Nucl. Med. 8:413, 1983.

119. Murray, I.P.C.: Bone scanning in the child and young adult. Part I. Skeletal Radiol. 5;1, 1980.

120. Murray, I.P.C.: Bone scanning in the child and young adult. Part II. Skeletal Radiol. 5:65, 1980.

121. Kirchner, P.T., and Simon, M.A.: Current concepts review radioisotopic evaluation of skeletal disease. J. Bone Joint Surg. 63A:673, 1981.

122. Atcheson, S., Coleman, R., and Ward, J.: Septic arthritis mimicking cellulitis: Distinction using radionuclide bone imaging. Clin. Nucl. Med. 4:79, 1979.

123. Lisbona, R., and Rosenthall, L.: Radionuclide imaging of septic joints and their differentiation from periarticular osteomyelitis, and cellulitis in pediatrics. Clin. Nucl. Med. 2:337, 1977.

124. Lisbona, R., and Rosenthall, L.: Observations on the sequential use of ^{99m}Tc-phosphate complex and ^{67}Ga imaging in osteomyelitis, cellulitis, and septic arthritis. Radiology 123:123, 1977.

125. Gaucher, A., Colomb, J.N., Naoun, A., Pourel, J., Robert, J., Faure, G., and Netter, P.: Radionuclide imaging in hip abnormalities. Clin. Nucl. Med. 5:214, 1980.

126. Maurer, A.H., Chen, D.C.P., Camargo, E.E., Wong, D.F., Wagner, H.N., and Anderson, P.O.: Utility of three-phase skeletal scintigraphy in suspected osteomyelitis: Concise communication. J. Nucl. Med. 22:941, 1981.

127. Murray, I.P.C.: Photopenia in skeletal scintigraphy of suspected bone and joint infection. Clin. Nucl. Med. 7:14, 1982.

128. Kloiber, R., Pavlosky, W., Portner, O., and Gartke, K.: Bone scintigraphy of hip joint effusions in children. AJR 140:995, 1983.

129. Coleman, R.E., Samuelson, C.O., Balm, S., Christian, P.E., and Ward, J.R.: Imaging with Tc-99m MDP and Ga-67 citrate in patients with rheumatoid arthritis and suspected septic arthritis: Concise communication. J. Nucl. Med. 23:479, 1982.

130. Horoszowski, H., Ganel, A., Kamhin, M., Zaltzman, S., and Farine, L.: Sequential use of technetium 99m MDP and gallium 67 citrate imaing in the evaluation of painful total hip replacement. Br. J. Radiol. 53:1169, 1980.

131. Duszynski, D., Kuhn, J., Afshani, E., and Riddlesburger, M.: Early radionuclide diagnosis of acute osteomyelitis. Radiology 117:337, 1975.

132. Gilday, D., Paul, D., and Peterson, J.: Diagnosis of osteomyelitis in

children by combined blood pool and bone imaging. Radiology 117:331, 1975.

133. Letts, R., Afifi, A., and Sutherland, J.: Technetium bone scanning as an aid in the diagnosis of atypical acute osteomyelitis in children. Surg. Gynecol. Obstet. 140:89, 1975.

134. Majd, M., and Frankel, R.: Radionuclide imaging in skeletal inflammatory and ischemic disease in children. AJR 126:823, 1976.

135. Gelfand, M., and Silberstein, E.: Radionuclide imaging: Use in diagnosis of osteomyelitis in children. JAMA 237:245, 1977.

136. Nelson, H.T., and Taylor A.: Bone scanning in the diagnosis of osteomyelitis. J. Nucl. Med. 19:696, 1978.

137. Sullivan, J.A., Vasileff, T., and Leonard, J.C.: An evaluation of nuclear scanning in orthopaedic infections. J. Pediatr. Orthop. 1:73, 1981.

138. Sullivan, D.C., Rosenfield, N., Ogden, J., and Gottschalk, A.: Problems in the scintigraphic detection of osteomyelitis in children. Radiology 135:731, 1980.

139. Ash, J.M., and Gilday, D.L.: The futility of bone scanning in neo-natal osteomyelitis: Concise communication. J. Nucl. Med. 21:417, 1980.

140. Sy, W., Westring, D., and Weinberger, G.: "Cold" lesions on bone imaging. J. Nucl. Med. 16:1013, 1975.

141. Trackler, R., Miller, K., Sutherland, D., and Chadwick, D.: Childhood pelvic osteomyelitis presenting as a "cold" lesion on bone scan: Case report. J. Nucl. Med. 17:620, 1976.

142. Armbruster, T., Georgen, T., Resnick, D., and Catanzaro, A.: Utility of bone scanning in disseminated coccidiodomycosis: Case report. J. Nucl. Med. 18:450, 1977.

143. Garnett, E., Cockshott, W., and Jacobs, J.: Classical acute osteomyelitis with a negative bone scan. Br. J. Radiol. 50:757, 1977.

144. Park, H.M., Wheat, L.J., Siddiqui, A.R., Burt, R.W., Robb, J.A., Ransburg, R.C., and Kernek, C.B.: Scintigraphic evaluation of diabetic osteomyelitis: Concise communication. J. Nucl. Med. 23:569, 1982.

145. Shoju, H., Asnis, S., Bohne, W., Rovere, G., and Gristina, A.: Further observations on ^{85}Sr scintimetry in intracapsular fracture of the hip. South. Med. J. 68:1249, 1975.

146. Hungerford, D., and Zizic, T.: Alcoholism-associated ischemic necrosis of the femoral head: Early diagnosis and treatment. Clin. Orthop. 130:144, 1978.

147. D'Ambrosia, R., Riggins, R., Stadalnik, R., and DeNardo, G.: Scintigraphy in the avascular necrotic disorders of bone. Clin. Orthop. 121:146, 1975.

148. D'Ambrosia, R., Shoju, H., Riggins, R., Stadalnik, R., and DeNardo, G.: Scintigraphy in the diagnosis of osteonecrosis. Clin. Orthop. 130:139, 1978.

149. D'Ambrosia, R., Riggins, R., Stadalnik, R., and DeNardo, G.: Experience with ^{99m}Tc-diphosphonate in studying vascularity of the femoral head. Surg. Forum 26:521, 1975.

150. Lutzker, L.G., and Alavi, A.: Bone and marrow imaging in sickle cell disease: Diagnosis of infarction. Semin. Nucl. Med. 6:83, 1976.

151. D'Ambrosia, R., Riggins, R., Stadalnik, R., and DeNardo, G.: Vascularity of the femoral head: ^{99m}Tc-diphosphonate scintigraphy validated with tetracycline labeling. Clin. Orthop. 121:143, 1976.

152. Harcke, H.T.: Bone imaging in infants and children: A review. J. Nucl. Med. 18:231, 1977.

153. Conklin, J.J., Alderson, P.O., Zizic, T.M., Hungerford, D.S., Densereaux, J.Y., Gober, A., and Wagner, H.N.: Comparison of bone scan and radiograph sensitivity in the detection of steroid-indiced ischemic necrosis of bone. Radiology 147:221, 1983.

154. Gelfand, M., Ball, W., Oestreich, A., Crawford, A., Jolson, R., and Perlman, A.: Transient loss of femoral head Tc-99m diphosphonate uptake with prolonged maintenance of femoral head architecture. Clin. Nucl. Med. 8:347, 1983.

155. Spencer, R.P., Lee, Y.S., Sziklas, J.J., Rosenberg, R.J., and Karimeddinni, M.K.: Failure of uptake of radiocolloid by the femoral heads: A diagnostic problem: Concise communication. J. Nucl. Med. 24:116, 1983.

156. Williams, A.G., Mettler, F.A., and Christie, J.H.: Sulfur colloid distribution in normal hips. Clin. Nucl. Med. 8:490, 1983.

157. Khairi, M.R., Wellman, H., Robb, J., and Johnson, C.: Paget's disease of bone (osteitis deformans): Symptomatic lesions and bone scan. Ann. Intern. Med. 79:348, 1973.

158. Wellman, H., Sckauwecker, D., Robb, J., and Johnson, C.: Skeletal scintimaging and radiography in the diagnosis and management of Paget's disease. Clin. Orthop. 127:55, 1977.

159. Shirazi, P.H., Ryan, W.G., and Fordham, E.W.: Bone scanning in evaluation of Paget's disease of bone. CRC Crit. Rev. Clin. Radiol. Nucl. Med. 5:523, 1974.

160. Serafini, A.: Paget's disease of bone. Semin. Nucl. Med. 6:47, 1976.

161. Vellenga, C., Paurvels, E., Bjjvoet, O., and Hoshing, D.: Evaluation of scintigraphic and roentgenologic studies in Paget's disease under therapy. Radiol. Clin. (Basel) 45:292, 1976.

162. Lentle, B., Russell, A., Heslip, P., and Percy, J.S.: The scintigraphic findings in Paget's disease of bone. Clin. Radiol. 27:129, 1976.

163. Waxman, A., Ducker, S., McKee, D., Siemsen, J., and Singer, F.: Evaluation of ^{99m}TC diphosphonate kinetics and bone scans in patients with Paget's disease before and after calcitonin treatment. Radiology 125:761, 1977.

164. Lavender, J., Evans, I., Arnot, R., Bowring, S., Doyle, F., Joplin, G., and MacIntyre, I.: A comparison of radiography and radioisotope scanning in the detection of Paget's disease and in the assessment of response in human calcitonin. Br. J. Radiol. 50:243, 1977.

165. Frame, B., and Marel, G.M.: Paget's disease: A review of current knowledge. Radiology 141:21, 1981.

166. Vellenga, C.J.L.R., Pauwels, E.K.J., Bijvoet, O.L.M., and Frijink, W.B.: Scintigraphic aspects of the recurrence of treated Paget's disease of bone. J. Nucl. Med. 22:510, 1981.

167. Lee, J.Y.: Bone scintigraphy in evolution of didionel therapy for Paget's disease. Clin. Nucl. Med. 6:356, 1981.

168. Waxman, A.D., McKee, D., Siemsen, J.K., and Singer, F.R.: Gallium scanning in Paget's disease of bone: Effect of calcitonin, AJR 134:303, 1980.

169. Brower, A., and Teates, C.: Positive ^{99m}TC-polyphosphate scan in a case of metastatic osteogenic sarcoma with hypertrophic osteoarthropathy. J. Nucl. Med. 15:53, 1974.

170. Kay, C., and Rosenberg, M.: Positive Tc-99m polyphosphate scan in a case of secondary hypertrophic osteoarthropathy. J. Nucl. Med. 15:312, 1974.

171. Terry, D., Isitman, A., and Holmes, R.: Radionuclide bone images in hypertrophic pulmonary osteoarthropathy. AJR 124:571, 1975.

172. Rosenthall, L., and Kirsh, J.: Observations on radionuclide imaging in hypertrophic pulmonary osteoarthropathy. Radiology 120:359, 1977.

173. Sty, J.R., Sheth, K., and Starshak, J.: Bone scintigraphy in childhood idiopathic hypertrophic osteoarthropathy. Clin. Nucl. Med. 7:421, 1982.

174. Kozin, F., McCarty, D., Sims, J., and Genant, H.: The reflex sympathetic dystrophy syndrome. I. Clinical and histologic studies: Evidence for bilaterality, response to corticosteroids and articular involvement. Am. J. Med. 60:321, 1976.

175. Kozin, F., McCarty, D., Sims, J., and Genant, H.: The reflex sympathetic dystrophy syndrome. II. Roentgenographic and scintigraphic evidence of bilaterality, and of periarticular accentuation. Am. J. Med. 60:332, 1976.

176. Genant, H., Hozin, F., Bekerman, C., McCarty, D., and Sims, J.: the reflex sympathic dystrophy syndrome. Radiology 117:21, 1975.

177. Carlson, D., Simon, H., and Wegner, W.: Bone scanning and diagnosis of reflex sympathetic dystrophy secondary to herniated lumbar disks. Neurology 27:791, 1977.

178. Simon, H., and Carlson, D.H.: The use of bone scanning in the diagnosis of reflex sympathetic dystrophy. Clin. Nucl. Med. 5:116, 1980.

179. Kozin, F., Soin, J., Ryan, L., Carrera, G., and Wortmann, R.L.: Bone scintigraphy in the reflex sympathetic dystrophy syndrome. Radiology. 138:437, 1981.

180. Kozin, F., Ryan, L.M., Carerra, G.F., and Soin, J.S.: The reflex dystrophy syndrome (RSDS). III. Scintigraphic studies, further evidence for therapeutic efficacy of systemic corticosteroids and proposed diagnostic criteria. A.J. Med. 70:23, 1981.

181. Sy, W., Bay, R., and Camera, A.: Hand images: Normal and abnormal. J. Nucl. Med. 18:419, 1977.

182. Namey, T.: Unpublished data.

183. Thomas, R., Resnich, D., Daniel, D., and Greenfield, R.: Compartmental evaluation of osteoarthritis of the knee: A comparative study of available modalities. Radiology 116:585, 1975.

184. Gelman, M., Coleman, R., Stevens, P., and Davey, B.: Radiography, radionuclide imaging, and arthrography in evaluation of total hip and knee replacement. Radiology 128:677, 1978.

185. Williams, E., Tregonning, R., and Hurley, P.: 99Tcm-diphosphonate scanning as an aid to diagnosis of infection in total hip joint replacements. Br. J. Radiol. 50:562, 1977.

186. Tehranzadeh, J., Schneider, R., and Freiberger, R.H.: Radiological evaluation of painful total hip replacement. Radiology 141:355, 1981.

187. Hunter, J.C. Hattner, R.S., Murray, W.R., and Genant, H.K.: Loosening of the total knee arthroplasty: Detection by radionuclide bone scanning. AJR 135:131–136, 1980.

188. Abdel-Dayem, H.M., Barodawala, Y., and Papademetriou, T.: Scintigraphic arthrography: A new imaging procedure. Clin. Nucl. Med. 6:246, 1981.

189. Abdel-Dayem, H.M., Barodawala, Y.K., and Papademetriou, T: Scintigraphic arthrography: Comparison with contrast arthrography and future applications. Clin. Nucl. Med. 7:516, 1982.

190. Hussein, A., Barodawala, Y., and Papademetrious, T.: Loose knee prosthesis detection by scintigraphic arthrography. Clin. Nucl. Med. 8:355, 1983.

191. Brill, D.R.: Bone imaging for lower extremity pain in athletes. Sports Nucl. Med. 8:101, 1983.

192. Spencer, R.P., Levinson, E.D., Baldwin, R.D., Sziklas, J.J., Witek, J.T., and Rosenberg, R.: Diverse bone scan abnormalities in "shin splints." J. Nucl. Med. 20:1271, 1979.

193. Van Hal, M., Keene, J., Lange, T., and Clancy, W.: Stress fractures of the great toe sesamoids. Am. J. Sports Med. 10:122, 1982.

194. Lombardo, S., and Benson, D.: Stress fractures of the femur in runners. Am. J. Sports Med. 10:219, 1982.

195. Butler, J., Brown, S., and McConnell, B.: Subtrochanteric stress fractures in runners. Am. J. Sports Med. 10:228, 1982.

196. Hajek, M., and Nobel, B.: Stress fractures of the femoral neck in joggers. Am. J. Sports Med. 10:112. 1982.

197. Pavlov, H., Torg, J., and Freiberger, R.: Tarsal navicular stress fractures: Radiographic evaluation. Radiology 148:641, 1983.

198. Manzione, M., and Pizzutillo, P.: Stress fracture of the scaphoid waist. Am. J. Sports Med. 9:268, 1981.

199. Sewell, J.R., Black, C.M., Chapman, A.H., Statham, J., Hughes, G.R.V., and Lavender, J.P.: Quantitative scintigraphy in diagnosis and management of plantar fasciitis (calcaneal periostitis): Concise communication. J. Nucl. Med. 21:633, 1980.

200. Jackson, D., et al.: Stress reactions involving the pars interarticularis in young athletes. Am. J. Sports Med. 9:304, 1981.

201. Matin, P.: The appearance of bone scans following fractures, including immediate and long-term studies. J. Nucl. Med. 20:1227, 1979.

202. Isreal, H., Park, C., and Mansfield, C.: Gallium scanning in sarcoidosis. Ann. N. Y. Acad. Sci. 278:514, 1976.

203. Wiener, S., and Potal, B.: ^{67}Ga-citrate uptake by the parotid glands in sarcoidosis. Radiology 130:753, 1979.

204. Oren, V., Uszler, J., and White, J.: Diagnosis of uveo-parotid fever by 67-Ga citrate imaging. Clin. Nucl. Med. 3:127, 1978.

205. Ball, G., and Logic, J.: Unpublished data.

206. Nosal, A., Schleissner, L., Miskkin, F., and Lieberman, J.: Angiotensin-1-converting enzyme and gallium scan in non-invasive evaluation of sarcoidosis. Ann. Intern. Med. 90:3282, 1979.

207. Reginato, A., Schiappaccasse, V., Guzman, L., and Claure, H.: 99m Technetium-pyrophosphate scintophotography in bone sarcoidosis. J. Rheumatol. 3:426, 1976.

208. Gupta, B., Bekerman, C., Sicilian, L., Oparil, Z., Pinsky, S., and Szidon, J.: Gallium-67 citrate scanning and serum angiotensin converting enzyme levels in sarcoidosis. Radiology 144:895, 1982.

209. Israel, H.L., Sperber, M., and Steiner, R.M.: Course of chronic hilar sarcoidosis in relation to markers of granulomatous activity. Invest. Radiol. 18:1, 1983.

210. Butt, W., and McIntyre, J.: Double-contrast arthrography of the knee. Radiology 92:487, 1969.

211. Freiberger, R., Killoron, P., and Cardona, G.: Arthrography of the knee by double contrast method. AJR 197:736, 1966.

212. Pudlowski, R., Gilula, L., and Murphy, W.: Arthrography. In Taplick, G., and Haskin, M., (eds.): Surgical Radiology. Philadelphia, W. B. Saunders Company, 1980.

213. Dalinka, M., Coren, G., and Wershba, M.: Knee arthrography. CRC Crit. Rev. Clin. Radiol. Nucl. Med. 4:1, 1973.

214. Werndoff, K., and Robinsohn, L.: Kongressverhandlung. Deutsch. Gesellsch. Orthop. 1905.

215. Anderson, P., and Maslin, P.: Tomography applied to knee arthrography. Radiology 110:271, 1974.

216. Eto, R., Anderson, P., and Harley, J.: Elbow arthrography with the application of tomography. Radiology 115:283, 1975.

217. Gilula, L.: A simplified stress device for knee arthrography. Radiology 122:828, 1977.

218. Dixon, A., and Rasher, J.: Synoviography. Clin. Rheum. Dis. 2:129, 1976.

219. Hall, F.M., Rosenthall, D.I., Goldberg, R.P., and Wyshok, G.: Morbidity from shoulder arthrography. AJR 136:59, 1981.

220. Goldberg, R.P., Hall, F.M., and Wyshok, G.: Pain on knee arthrography: Comparison of air versus CO_2 and reaspiration versus no reaspiration. AJR 136:377, 1981.

221. Grech, P.: Hip Arthrography. Philadelphia. J.B. Lippincott Company, 1977.

222. Neviaser, J.: Arthrography of the Shoulder. Springfield, Ill., Charles C Thomas, 1975.

223. Norman, A., and Baker, N.: Spontaneous osteonecrosis of the knee and medial meniscal tears. Radiology 129:653, 1978.

224. Pavlov, H., and Torg, J.: Double contrast arthrographic evaluation of the anterior cruciate ligament. Radiology 126:661, 1978.

225. Dalinka, M., and Garofola, J.: Infrapatella synovial fold: Cause for confusion in the evaluation of the anterior cruciate ligament. Radiology 126:661, 1978.

226. Braunstein, E.M.: Anterior aiecrote ligament injuries: A comparison of arthrographic and physical diagnosis. AJR 138:423, 1982.

227. Gilley, J.S., Geiman, M.I., Edson, M., and Metcalf, R.W.: Chondral fractures of the knee. Radiology 138:51, 1981.

228. DeSmet, A., and Neff, J: Knee arthrography for the preoperative evaluation of juxta-articular masses. Radiology 143:663, 1982.

229. Hall, A., and Scott J.: Synovial cysts and rupture of the knee joint in rheumatoid arthritis: An arthrographic study. Ann. Rheum. Dis. 25:32, 1966.

230. Wolfe, R., and Colloff, B.: Popliteal cysts: An arthrographic study and review of the literature. J. Bone Joint Surg. 54A:1057, 1972.

231. Taylor, A., and Ansell, B.: Arthrography of the knee before and after synovectomy in rheumatoid patients. J. Bone Joint Surg. 54B:110, 1972.

232. Lowenstein, M.D., Smith, J.R.V., and Cole, S.: Infrapatellar pigmented villonodular synovitis: Arthrographic detection. AJR 135:279, 1980.

233. Wolfe, R., and Giuliano, V.: Double-contrast arthrography in the diagnosis of pigmented villonodular synovitis of the knee. Radiology 110:793, 1970.

234. Goergen, T., Resnick, D., and Niwayama, G.: Localized nodular synovitis of the knee: A report of two cases with abnormal arthrograms. AJR 126:641, 1976.

235. Boven, F., DeBoeck, M., and Potvliege, R.: Synovial plicae of the knee. Radiology 147:805, 1983.

236. Killoran, P., Morcove, R., and Frieberger, R.: Shoulder arthrography. AJR 103:658, 1968.

237. Desment, A., Ting, Y., and Weiss, J.: Shoulder arthrography in rheumatoid arthritis. Radiology 116:601, 1975.

238. Kilcoyne, R.F., and Matsen, F.A.: Rotator cuff tear measurement by arthropneumotomography. AJR 140:315, 1983.

239. Andren, L., and Lundberg, B.: Treatment of rigid shoulders by joint distension during arthrography. Acta Orthop. Scand. 36:45, 1965.

240. Kinnard, P., Tricoire, J., Levesque, R., and Bergeron, D.: Assessment of the unstable shoulder by computed arthrography. Am. J. Sports Med. 11:157, 1983.

241. Braunstein, E., and O'Connor, G.: Double-contrast arthrotomography of the shoulder. J. Bone Joint Surg. 64A:192, 1982.

242. Strizak, A., and Danzig, L., Jackson, D., Greenway, G., Resnick, D., and Staple, T.: Subacromial bursography. J. Bone Joint Surg. 64A:196, 1982.

243. Gelman, M.: Arthrography in total hip prosthesis complications. AJR 126:743, 1975.

244. Murphy, W., Siegel, M., and Gilula, L.: Arthrography in the diagnosis of unexplained chronic hip pain with regional osteopenia. AJR 129:283, 1977.

245. Phillips, W.C., and Kattapuram, S.V.: Prosthetic hip replacements: Plain films and arthrography for component loosening. AJR 138:677, 1982.

246. Hendrix, R., Wixson, R., Rana, N., and Rogers, L.: Arthrography after total hip arthroplasty: A modified technique used in the diagnosis of pain. Radiology 148:647, 1983.

247. Cone, R., Yaru, N., Resnick, D., Gershuni, D., and Guerra, J.: Intracapsular pressure monitoring during arthrographic evaluation of painful hip prostheses. AJR 141:885, 1983.

248. Brostrom, L., Liljedahl, S., and Lindvall, N.: Sprained ankles. II. Arthrographic diagnosis of recent ligament ruptures. Acta Chir. Scand. 130:560, 1965.

249. Brostrom, L.: Sprained ankles. III. Clinical observations in recent ligament ruptures. Acta Chir. Scand. 130:560, 1965.

250. Goldman, A., Katz, M., and Freiberger, R.: Post-traumatic adhesive capsulitis of the ankle: Arthrographic diagnosis. AJR 127:585, 1976.

251. Sanders, H.: Ankle arthrography and ankle distortion. Radiol. Clin. 46:1, 1977.

252. Brostrom, L.: Sprained ankles. I. Anatomic lesions in recent sprains. Acta Chir. Scand. 128:483, 1964.

253. Harrison, M., Freiberger, R., and Ranawat, C.: Arthrography of the rheumatoid wrist joint. AJR 112:480, 1971.

254. Resnick, D.: Arthrography in the evaluation of arthritic disorders of the wrist. Radiology 113:331, 1974.

255. Iveson, J., Hill, A., and Wrigert, V.: Wrist cysts and fistulae. Ann. Rheum. Dis. 34:388, 1975.

256. Levinsohn, E.M., and Palmer, A.K.: Arthrography of the traumatized wrist. Radiology 146:647, 1983.

257. Rosenthal, D., Murray, W., and Smith, R.J.: Finger arthrography. Radiology 137:647, 1980.

258. Lynch, T., and Chase, D.: Arthrography in the evaluation of the temporomandibular joint. Radiology 126:667, 1978.

259. Doyle, T.: Arthrography of the temporomandibular joint: A simple technique. Clin. Radiol. 34:147, 1983.

260. Ferrucci, J.: Body ultrasonography, I and II. N. Engl. J. Med. 300:358, 590, 1979.

261. Griffiths, H., and Sarno, R.: Contemporary radiology: An introduction to imaging. Philadelphia, W.B. Saunders Company, 1979.

262. Fields, S., and Dunn, F.: Correlation of echographic visualizability of tissue with biologic composition and physiologic state. J. Accout. Soc. Am. 54:809, 1973.

263. Lemons, R., and Quate, C.: Acoustic microscopy: Biomedical applications. Science 188:905, 1975.

264. Birnholtz, J.: On maps comparing cross-sectional imaging methods. AJR 129:1133, 1977.

265. DeSantos, L.A., and Goldstein, H.: Ultrasonography in tumors arising from the spine and bony pelvis. AJR 129:1061, 1977.

266. Meire, H., Lindsay, D., Swinson, D., and Hamilton, E.: Comparison of ultrasound and positive contrast arthrography in the diagnosis of popliteal and calf swellings. Ann. Rheum. Dis. 33:221, 1974.

267. Moore, C., Sarti, D., and Louie, J.: Ultrasonographic demonstration of popliteal cysts in rheumatoid arthritis. Arthritis Rheum. 18:577, 1975.

268. Ambanelli, U., Manganelli, A., and Nervetti, A.: Demonstration of articular effusions and popliteal cysts with ultrasound. J. Rheumatol. 3:134, 1976.

269. Carpenter, J., Hattery, R., Hunder, G., Bryan, R., and McLeod, R.: Ultrasound evaluation of the popliteal space: Comparison with arthrography and physical examination. Mayo Clin. Proc. 51:498, 1976.

270. Rudikoff, J., Lynch, J., and Phillips, E.: Ultrasound diagnosis of Baker's cyst. JAMA 235:1054, 1976.

271. Cooperberg, P., Tsang, L., Truelove, L., and Knickerbocker, J.: Gray scale ultrasound in the evaluation of rheumatoid arthritis of the knee. Radiology 126:759, 1978.

272. Nomeir, A., Turner, R., Watts, E., Smith, D., and Edmonds, J.: Cardiac involvement in rheumatoid arthritis. Ann. Intern. Med. 79:800, 1973.

273. Pakroski, R., Atassi, A., Poska, R., and Rosen, K.: Prevalence of pericardial effusion and mitral valve involvement in patients with rheumatoid arthritis without cardiac symptoms. N. Engl. J. Med. 289:593, 1973.

274. Davia, J., Cherthn, M., deCastro, C., and Nievu, L.: Absence of echocardiographic abnormalities of the anterior mitral valve leaflet in rheumatoid arthritis. Ann. Intern. Med. 83:500, 1975.

275. Schorn, D., Hough, I., and Anderson, I.: The heart in rheumatoid arthritis: An echocardiographic study. S. Afr. Med. J. 50:8, 1975.

276. John, J.T., Hough, A., and Sergent, J.S.: Pericardial disease in rheumatoid arthritis. Am. J. Med. 66:38, 1979.

277. Elkayam, U., Weiss, S., and Laniado, S.: Pericardial effusion and mitral valve involvement in systemic lupus erythematosus. Ann. Rheum. Dis. 36:349, 1977.

278. Smith, J., Clements, P., Furst, D., and Ross, M.: Echocardiographic features of progressive system sclerosis. Am. J. Med. 66:28, 1979.

279. Berstein, B., Takakashi, M., and Hanson, J.: Cardiac involvement in juvenile rheumatoid arthritis. J. Paediatr. 85:313, 1974.

280. Kramer, F., Kurtz, A., Rubin, C., and Goldberg, B.: Ultrasound appearance of myositis ossificans. Skeletal Radiol. 4:19, 1979.

281. McDonald, D., and Leopold, R.: Ultrasound B-scanning in the differentiation of Baker's cyst and thrombophlebitis. Br. J. Radiol. 45:829, 1972.

282. Katz, R.S., Zizic, T.M., Arnold, W.P., and Stevens, M.D.: The pseudothrombophlebitis syndrome. Medicine 56:151, 1977.

283. Khan, M.A.: Ruptured popliteal cyst and thrombophlebitis. Arthritis Rheum. 20:1560, 1977.

284. Gordon, G.V., Edell, S., Brogadir, S.P., Schumacher, H.R., Schimmer, B.M., and Dolinka, M.: Baker's cysts and true thrombophlebitis: Report of two cases and review of the literature. Arch Intern. Med. 139:40, 1979.

285. Seltzer, S.E., Finberg, H.J., and Weissman, B.N.: Arthrosonography: Technique, sonographic anatomy, and pathology. Invest. Radiol. 15:19, 1980.

286. Basel, S.K.: Medical thermography. Bibl. Radiol. 5:12, 1968.

287. Ryan, J.: Thermography. Australas. Radiol. 8:23, 1969.

288. Hardy, J.D.: The radiation from the human body. III. The human skin as a black body radiator. J. Clin. Invest. 13:615, 1934.

289. Horvath, S.M., and Holander, J.: Intra-articular temperature as a measure of joint reaction. J. Clin. Invest. 28:469, 1949.

290. Hanson, B., Linstroni, J., Ericson, E., Laine, V., and Honsson, I.: Intra-articular temperature in man under normal and pathologic conditions. Abstr. V. Eur. Cong. Rheum. Dis., 1963.

291. Collins, A., Ring, E., Cosh, J., and Bacon, P.: Quantification of thermography in arthritis using multithermal analysis. I. The thermographic index. Ann. Rheum. Dis. 33:113, 1974.

292. Collins, A., and Ring, E.: Measurement of the inflammation in man and animals by radiometry. Br. J. Pharmacol. 44:145, 1972.

293. Bacon, P., Collins, A., Ring, F., and Cosh, J.: Thermography in the assessment of inflammatory arthritis. Clin. Rheum. Dis. 2:51, 1976.

294. Logan, W.W., and Lind, B.: Improved liquid cholesterol ester crystal thermography of the breast. J. Surg. Oncol. 8:363, 1964.

295. Crissy, J.J., Gordy, E., Ferguson, J., and Lyman, R.B.: A new technique for demonstration of skin temperature patterns. J. Invest. Dermatol. 43:89, 1970.

296. Pochaczevsky, R., and Meyers, P.H.: The value of vacuum contoured liquid crystal dynamic breast thermography. Acta Thermgraphica 4:8, 1979.

297. Albert, S., Glickman, M., and Kallish, M.: Thermography in orthopaedics. Ann. N. Y. Acad. Sci. 121:157, 1964.

298. Heinz, E., Golberg, H., and Taveras, J.: Experience with thermography in neurologic patients. Ann. N. Y. Acad. Sci. 121:177, 1964.

299. Goldberg, H., Heinz, E., and Taveras, J.: Thermography in neurological patients. Acta Radiol. 5:786, 1966.

300. Edeiken, J., Wallace, J., and Curley, R.: Thermography and herniated lumbar discs. AJR 102:790, 1968.

301. Raskin, M., Martinez-Lopez, M., and Sheldon, J.: Lumbar thermography in discogenic disease. Radiology 119:149, 1976.

302. Pochaczevsky, R., Wexler, C.E., Meyers, P.H., Epstein, J.A., and Marc, J.A.: Liquid crystal thermography of the spine and extremities: Its value in the diagnosis of spinal root syndromes. J. Neurosurg. 56:386, 1982.

303. Pochaczevsky, R.: The value of liquid crystal thermography in the diagnosis of spinal root compression syndromes. Orthop. Clin. North Am. 14:271, 1983.

304. Pochaczevsky, R.: Assessment of back pain by contact thermography of extremity dermatomes. Orthop. Rev. 12:45, 1983.

305. Namey, T.: Scintigraphy, sacroiliitis, and sciatica. Presented to the 2nd annual meeting of the Academy of Neurological Orthopaedic Surgeons, Las Vegas, November 1978.

306. Meyer, D.A., and Meyers, P.H.: Would you like to know what pain looks like? Louisiana Bar. J. 27:77, 1979.

307. Raskin, M.: Thermography of the spine. Appl. Radiol. 118:123, 1976.

308. Agarwal, A., Lloyd, K.N., and Dovey, P.: Thermography of the spine and sacroiliac joint in spondylitis. Rheumatol. Phys. Med. 10:349, 1970.

309. Scott, D., Ring, E., and Bacon, P.: Problems in the assessment of disease activity in ankylosing spondylitis. Rheumatol. Rehabil. 20:74, 1981.

310. Rajapakse, C., Grennan, D., Jones, C., and Jayson, M.: Thermography in the assessment of peripheral joint inflammation: a re-evaluation. Rheumatol. Rehabil. 20:81, 1981.

311. Alfidi, R.J., MacIntyre, W.J., Meany, T.F., Chernack, E.S., Janicki, R., Tarar, R., and Levin, H.L.: Experimental studies to determine application of CAT scanning to the human body. AJR 124:199, 1973.

312. Ambrose, J.: Computerized transverse axial scanning (tomography) II. Clinical application. Br. J. Radiol. 46:1023, 1973.

313. Boyd, D.P., Korobkin, M.T., and Moss, A.: Engineering status of computerized tomographic scanning. Optical Eng. 16:37, 1977.

314. Hounsfield, G.N.: Computerized transverse axial scanning (tomography) I. Description of a system. Br. J. Radiol. 46:1016, 1973.

315. Genant, H.K.: Computed tomography. Resnick, D., and Niwayama, G. (eds.): In Diagnosis of Bone and Joint Disorders. Philadelphia. W.B. Saunders Company, 1981, p. 380.

316. Raskin, S.P., and Keating, J.W.: Recognition of lumbar disk disease: Comparison of myelography and computed tomography. Am. J. Neuroradiol. 3:215, 1982.

317. Williams, A.L., Haughton, V.M., and Syversten, A.: Computed tomography in the diagnosis of herniated nucleus pulposus. Radiology 135:95, 1980.

318. Anand, A.K., and Lee, B.C.P.: Plain and metrizamide CT of lumbar disk disease: comparison with myelography. Am. J. Neuroradiol. 3:567, 1982.

319. Williams, J.P., Joslyn, J.N., and Butler, T.W.: Differentiation of herniated lumbar disk from bulging annulus fibrosus. Use of reformatted images. J. Comp. Assist. Tomogr. 6:89, 1982.

320. Williams, A.L., Haughton, V.M., Daniels, D.L., and Thornton, R.S.: CT recognition of lateral lumbar disk herniation. Am. J. Neuroradiol. 3:211, 1982.

321. Williams, A.L., Haughton, V.M., Daniels, D.L., and Grogan, J.P.: Differential CT diagnosis of extruded nucleus pulposus. Radiology 148:141, 1983.

322. Helms, C.A., Dorwart, R.H., and Gray, M.: The CT appearance of conjoined nerve roots and differentiation from a herniated nucleus pulposus. Radiology 144:803, 1982.

323. Roub, L.W., and Drayer, B.: Spinal computed tomography: Limitations and applications. AJR 133:267, 1979.

324. Ullrich, C.G., Binet, E.F., Sanecki, M.G., and Kieffer, S.A.: Quantitative assessment of the lumbar spinal canal by computed tomography. Radiology 134:137, 1980.

325. Ciric, I.M., Mickhael, M.A., Tarkington, J.A., and Vick, N.A.: The lateral recess syndrome: A variant of spinal stenosis. J. Neurosurg. 53:433, 1980.

326. Chafetz, N., and Genant, H.K.: Computed tomography of the lumbar spine. Orthop. Clin. North Am. 14:147, 1983.

327. Teplick, J.G., and Haskin, M.E.: Computed tomography of the postoperative lumbar spine. A.J.R. 141:865, 1983.

328. Schulbiger, O., and Valavanis, A.: CT differentiation between recurrent disc herniation and postoperative scar formation: The value of contrast enhancement. Neuroradiology 22:251, 1982.

329. Kozin, F., Carrera, G.F., Ryan, L.M., Foley, D., and Lawson, T.: Computed tomography in the diagnosis of sacroiliitis. Arthritis Rheum. 24:1479, 1981.

330. Carrera, G.F., Foley, W.D., Kozin, F., Ryan, L., and Lawson, T.L.: CT of sacroiliitis. AJR 136:41, 1981.

331. Borlaza, G.S., Seigel, R., Kuhns, L.R., Good, A.E., Rapp, R., and Martel,

W.: Computed tomography in the evaluation of sacroiliiac arthritis. Radiology 139:437, 1981.

332. DeSmet, A.A., Gardner, J.D., Lindsley, H.B., Goin, J.E., and Fritz, S.L.: Tomography for evaluation of sacroiliitis. AJR 139:577, 1982.

333. Young, A., Dixon, A., Getty, J., Renton, P., and Vacher, H.: Cauda equina syndrome complicating ankylosing spondylitis: use of electromyography and computerised tomography in diagnosis. Ann. Rheum. Dis. 40:317, 1981.

334. Grosman, H., Gray, R., and St. Louis, E.L.: CT of long-standing ankylosing spondylitis with cauda equina syndrome. Am. J. Neuroradiol. 4:1077, 1983.

335. Sage, M.R., and Gordon, T.P.: Muscle atrophy in ankylosing spondylitis: CT demonstration. Radiology 149:780, 1983.

336. Tadmore, R., Davis, K.R., Roberson, G.H., New, P.F.J., and Taveras, J.M.: Computed tomographic evaluation of traumatic spinal injuries. Radiology 127:825, 1978.

337. Rosenthal, D.I., Mankin, H.J., and Bauman, R.A.: Musculoskeletal applications for computed tomography. Bull. Rheum. Dis. 33:1, 1983.

338. Faerber, E.N., Wolpert, S.M., Scott, R.M., Belkin, S.C., and Carter, B.L.: Computed tomography of spinal fractures. J. Comput. Assist. Tomogr. 3:657, 1979.

339. Handelberg, F., Bellemans, M.A., Opdecam, P., and Castelen, P.P.: The use of computerized tomography in the diagnosis of thoracolumbar injury. J. Bone Joint Surg. 63B:336, 1981.

340. Sauser, D.D., Billimoria, P.E., Roase, G.A., and Mudge, K.: CT evaluation of hip trauma. AJR 135:269, 1980.

341. Shirkoda, A., Brasheer, H.R., and Staab, E.V.: Computed tomography of acetabular fractures. Radiology 134:683, 1980.

342. Danzig, L.A., Resnick, D., and Greenway, G.: Evaluation of unstable shoulders by computed tomography. Am. J. Sports Med. 10:138, 1982.

343. Shuman, W.P., Kilcoyne, R.F., Matsen, F.A., Rogers, J.V., and Mack, L.A.: Double-contrast computed tomography of the glenoid labrum. AJR 141:581, 1983.

344. Griffiths, H.J., Hamlin, D.J., Kiss, S., and Lovelock, J.: Efficacy of CT scanning in a group of 174 patients with orthopedic and musculoskeletal problems. Skeletal Radiol. 7:87, 1981.

345. Siegelman, S.S., Zerhoun, E.A., Leo, F.P., Khouri, N.F., and Stitik, F.P.: CT of the solitary pulmonary nodule. AJR 135:1, 1980.

346. Khun, J.P., and Berger, P.E.: Computed tomographic diagnosis of osteomyelitis. Radiology 130:503, 1979.

347. Azouz, E.M.: Computed tomography in bone and joint infections. J. Can. Assoc. Radiol. 32:102, 1981.

348. Carrera, G.F., Haughton, V.M., Syversten, A., and Williams, A.L.: Computed tomography of the lumbar facet joints. Radiology 134:145, 1980.

349. Destouet, J.M., Gilula, L.A., Murphy, W.A., and Sagel, S.S.: Computed tomography of the sternoclavicular joint and sternum. Radiology 138:123, 1981.

350. Manzione, J.V., Katzberg, R.W., Brodsky, G.L., Seltzer, S.F., and Mellins, H.Z.: Internal derangement of the temporomandibular joint: diagnosis by direct sagittal computed tomography. Radiology 150:111, 1984.

351. Rosenthal, D.I., Aronow, S., and Murray, W.T.: Iron content of pigmented villonodular synovitis detected by computed tomography. Radiology 133:409, 1979.

352. Zinman, C., and Reis, N.D.: Osteochondritis dissecans of the talus: use of high resolution computed tomography scanner. Acta Orthop. Scand. 53:697, 1982.

353. Pavlov, H., Hirschy, J., and Torg, J.S.: Computed tomography of the cruciate ligaments. Radiology 132:389, 1979.

354. Genant, H.K., and Boyd, D.: Quantitative bone mineral analysis using dual energy computed tomography. Invest. Radiol. 12:545, 1977.

355. Cann, C.E., Genant, H.K., and Young, D.R.: Comparison of vertebral and peripheral mineral losses in disuse osteoporosis in monkeys. Radiology 134:525, 1980.

356. Cann, C.E., and Genant, H.K.: Precise measurement of vertebral mineral content using computed tomography. J. Comput. Asst. Tomogr. 4:493, 1980.

357. Breatnach, E., and Robinson, P.J.: Repositioning errors in measurement of vertebral attenuation values by computed tomography. Br. J. Radiol. 56:299, 1983.

358. Miyasaka, K., Kaneda, K., Ito, T., Takai, H., Sugimoto, S., and Tsuru, M.: Ossification of spinal ligaments causing thoracic radiculomyelopathy. Radiology 143:463, 1982.

359. Deutsch, A.L., Resnick, D., Campbell, B.: Computerized tomography and bone scintigraphy in the evaluation of tarsal coalition. Radiology 144:137, 1982.

360. Dihlmann, W.: CT analysis of the upper end of the femur: The asterisk sign and ischaemic bone necrosis of the femoral head. Skeletal Radiol. 8:251, 1982.

361. Cone, R.O., Szabo, R., Resnick, D., Gelberman, R., Taleisnik, J., and Gilula, L.A.: Computed tomography of the normal soft tissues of the wrist. Invest. Radiol. 18:546, 1983.

362. Bauer, A.R., and Yutani, D.: Computed tomographic localization of wooden foreign bodies in children's extremities. Arch. Surg. 118:1084, 1983.

363. Amendola, M.A., Glazer, G.M., Agha, F.P., Francis, I.R., Weatherbee, L., and Martel, W.: Myositis ossificans circumscripta: computed tomographic diagnosis. Radiology 149:775, 1983.

Chapter 41

Arthroscopy

John B. McGinty

INTRODUCTION

Arthroscopy is the endoscopic examination of the interior of a joint, and therefore can provide more direct diagnostic information than any other ancillary procedure. However, it must be emphasized that it cannot replace a good history, a thorough physical examination, laboratory studies, and appropriate roentgenograms. Only after a clinical impression based on these time-tested methods has been acquired should an arthroscopic examination be considered to provide additional or confirmatory information to arrive at a diagnosis.

Although the history of endoscopy goes back to Bozzini's Lichtleiter in 1805 and Nitze's[1] first cystoscope in 1876, it was not until after the development of the incandescent lamp by Edison in 1880 that other forms of endoscopy came into being. Professor Kenji Takagi[2] of Tokyo University first looked inside cadaver knees with a cystoscope in a gas medium. Between 1918 and 1931 he developed an arthroscope small enough to be practical and learned to take color photographs through his endoscopic system. In 1931 and 1934 the first papers on arthroscopy appeared in the American literature in the *Journal of Bone and Joint Surgery*.[3-5] Interest in arthroscopy faded in the western world while Masaki Watanabe was continuing Dr. Takagi's work in Tokyo, developing an array of instruments and his classic *Atlas of Arthroscopy*.[6,7] In the late 1960s, through the work of Jackson,[8-13] Casscells,[14] O'Connor,[15-18] and others, the Japanese experience was brought to the United States; fiberoptic instrumentation was developed,[1,19] techniques were established,[11, 20-26] and arthroscopy, as an accepted diagnostic procedure, flourished. Today, arthroscopy is being taught in most orthopedic and some rheumatology training programs, in seminars and workshops conducted by universities and by the American Academy of Orthopaedic Surgeons, and in fellowships and preceptorships with experts.

The techniques of arthroscopic surgery have changed the surgical approach to problems of the knee. At the present time many pathological situations can be solved utilizing arthroscopic techniques with consequent lower morbidity and fewer complications. These procedures include removal of loose bodies, synovectomy, partial meniscectomy, resection of synovial plicae, chondroplasty or shaving of articular cartilage for various types of chondromalacia, surgery for osteochondritis dissecans, and extensive debridement of the joint and lavage for osteoarthritis. Newer techniques of meniscal suture and repair of peripheral detachment, anterior cruciate ligament repair, and reconstruction are being developed. Techniques of arthroscopy are being utilized for surgical problems in other joints with increasing frequency.

Indications. There is no better way to establish a diagnosis of intrinsic joint pathology than to be able to see the lesion. The first indication for arthroscopy is the presence of a confusing diagnostic problem, when the specific diagnosis has not been made after history, physical examination, and laboratory and roentgenographic evaluation. The author no longer does an arthrotomy of the knee for mechanical problems without preceding it with an arthroscopy. With experience the inside of the knee can be examined better with an arthroscope than by an arthrotomy with limited exposure.

The need for tissue diagnosis is easily met arthroscopically. A tissue biopsy can be obtained blindly through the sheath of the arthroscope, or under direct vision through a single puncture by placing a smaller arthroscope and a biopsy forceps through a standard sheath.[27-29]

Planning surgical approaches is an important indication for arthroscopy. There is no better and efficient method for a surgeon to plan his approach to an intra-articular problem than to know exactly what the pathology is, and where it is located.

Finally, the need to document intra-articular pathology is an indication for arthroscopy. It is a simple matter to document lesions seen at arthroscopic examination with still photographs or television, as will be discussed later in this chapter.[30-31] Documentation is essential not only for teaching but also for medicolegal purposes, such as liability litigation and workmen's compensation arbitration.

Contraindications. Probably the only absolute contraindication to arthroscopy is sepsis. In the face of systemic sepsis with bacteremia, the possibility of seeding a joint contraindicates the use of arthroscopy. Overlying sepsis of the skin or subcutaneous tissue obviously must be brought completely under control before attempting an elective diagnostic procedure. On the other hand, the possibility of a septic joint is an indication for arthroscopy to inspect the synovium and articular cartilage, obtain material for culture, and irrigate the joint.

Limited joint motion may be a contraindication to arthroscopy. A certain range of motion is necessary to obtain a satisfactory examination, e.g., 30 to 75 degrees in the knee. Thorough examination requires manipulation of the joint as well as manipulation of the instrument (Fig. 41–1).

Figure 41–1. Examination of patellofemoral joint. The right hand of the operator is manipulating the patella while he is scanning the articular surface of the patella with the arthroscope.

Coagulation defects obviously must be identified and controlled before an arthroscopic examination is undertaken.

Anesthesia. Techniques for the reliable performance of arthroscopy on the ambulatory outpatient with local anesthesia have been established. The patient is brought directly to the operating room without premedication; arthroscopic examination is performed, using lidocaine and bupivacaine (Fig. 41–2); and the patient leaves the hospital immediately without external support. In this way the risk and morbidity of general anesthesia, the cost of an anesthesiologist, and time in the recovery room are eliminated.

There are certain situations in which general or spinal anesthesia is necessary. In the young child, arbitrarily, under 10 years of age, local anesthesia should probably not be used. With a very apprehensive patient or with a physician learning the procedure, local anesthesia is contraindicated. Finally, if a prolonged endoscopic procedure is contemplated, particularly if the prolonged use of a tourniquet is necessary, general or spinal anesthesia should be used.

General or spinal anesthesia is useful when doing arthroscopic surgical procedures. Local anesthesia frequently is inadequate, although it may be used in some situations. When one is performing arthroscopic surgical procedures, frequently the level of concentration and tension is such that the surgeon cannot give adequate attention to his patient who is awake and is under local anesthesia. Therefore, in this author's opinion general or spinal anesthesia is preferable in these situations.

The procedure of arthroscopy must be performed in the operating room with the same aseptic precautions as followed for arthrotomy. No infections have been reported.

Instruments. Many American arthroscopists learned the procedure with the Watanabe No. 21 arthroscope, an instrument illuminated with a tungsten bulb. The instrument had severe limitations: breakage of a bulb in the knee, short circuit of the fine wire filaments with consequent loss of illumination, and a hot light source requiring constant irrigation. The development of fiberoptics has made the use of tungsten illumination in endoscopy obsolete.

Today, virtually all arthroscopists use fiberoptic instrumentation. Fiberoptics allow a cool light source remote from the joint being examined. Fiberoptic arthroscopes come in different diameters, from the 1.7-mm Needlescope to a 6.0-mm operating arthroscope used for endoscopic surgery. The larger the diameter of the optical instrument, the larger the field of view, and the more light delivered for photographic exposure. There are a variety of angles of the objective lens of the arthroscope to provide different directions of orientation, from 0 to 120 degrees. The orientation for best general use, in the author's opinion, is the foreoblique (30-degree) lens, giving a larger field of view simply by rotating the instrument, but still providing enough of a direct, forward view to avoid confusion and disorientation. The 70-degree arthroscope should be part of the instrument table on the routine arthroscopic examination of the knee to provide sufficient visualization of the posterior compartments through the intercondylar notch. Biopsy forceps are available to biopsy under direct view through the same sheath, or through a second puncture.

The standard fiberoptic light source, located remote

Figure 41–2. Procedure under local anesthesia. Lidocaine can be injected directly into knee through the sheath at any time during the procedure.

from the operating field, contains a 150-watt tungsten bulb. Although still photographs can be taken with this light source using high-speed film, a high-intensity light source is necessary for adequate use of television.

TECHNIQUE OF ARTHROSCOPY

Arthroscopic examination can be performed on almost all joints. The knee will be used in this chapter to describe the basic technique.

The examination must be performed in the operating room with strict aseptic technique. The patient is placed in the supine position on the operating table, and the tourniquet is not used, unless endoscopic surgery or immediate subsequent surgery is anticipated. If local anesthesia is used, 4 ml of 0.5 per cent lidocaine (Xylocaine) is infiltrated into the skin, subcutaneous tissue, and capsule, followed by 5 ml intrasynovially. A 1-cm incision is made just lateral to the patellar tendon and just above the lateral joint line, and the sheath with a sharp trochar is inserted through the capsule, but not the synovium (Fig. 41–3). The sharp trochar is replaced with a blunt trochar, and the sheath is pushed into the knee, under the patella, into the suprapatellar pouch. The trochar is replaced with the arthroscope and 10 ml of 0.5 per cent bupivacaine (Marcain) is injected directly into the joint (see Fig. 41–2). Anesthesia has been adequate over an hour with these dosages, well within the margin of toxicity. If the examination is to be done with general or spinal anesthesia, 50 to 100 ml of normal saline is injected into the joint cavity before inserting the sheath.The examination is conducted using intermittent saline irrigation directly through the sheath.

The routine examination of the knee is divided into four parts. The *suprapatellar pouch and patellofemoral joint* (see Fig. 41–1) are first examined. This is an excellent location to study the character and vascularity of the synovium (Fig. 41–4; see Plate VI, p. xl). The entire undersurface of the patella can be seen by scanning with the instrument while the operator's opposite hand manipulates the patella. Similarly, the relationships of the patellofemoral joint can be observed in flexion and in extension. The arthroscope is then moved over the medial femoral condyle into the *medial compartment* (Fig. 41–5). The medial meniscus is examined anteriorly to posteriorly (Fig. 41–6; see Plate VI, p. xl). The peripheral 50 per cent of the posterior horn of the medial meniscus cannot be seen in most knees from an anterior approach. The medial femoral condyle can be seen by flexing and extending the knee. The arthroscope is then moved into the *intercondylar notch*. Again the character of the synovium is readily apparent in the notch. The anterior cruciate ligament is examined from its proximal to its distal attachment (Fig. 41–7; see Plate VI, p. xl). The posterior cruciate ligament cannot be seen from an anterior approach if the anterior cruciate ligament is intact. The extremity being examined is then crossed over the uninvolved extremity, allowing the knee to drop into varus. The arthroscope is moved into the fourth area, the *lateral compartment* (Fig. 41–8). The lateral meniscus is examined from its posterior attachment around to its anterior attachment. The popliteal tendon can be seen in the posterolateral corner. Femoral and tibial surfaces are evident by flexing and extending the knee. After conclusion of the routine examination the operator can return to areas of particular interest for further study, photographic documentation, or biopsy.

Figure 41–3. The index finger is used as a guard to prevent overpenetration when the sheath and trochar are inserted, thereby averting damage to the articular cartilage.

Figure 41–5. With the foot over the side of the table, the operator can open up the medial compartment simply by leaning on the lateral side of the knee.

It should be part of every examination of the knee to examine the posteromedial compartment. This is done most effectively through the intercondylar notch. The arthroscope is removed from the sheath, and the blunt trochar is reinserted into the sheath. The interval between the medial femoral condyle and the tibial plateau is palpated with the blunt trochar until the tip of the trochar falls into the interval between the anterior cruciate ligament and the lateral surface of the medial femoral condyle. The sheath with trochar is then maneuvered directly posteriorly and allowed to drop through that interval into the posteromedial compartment. The

Figure 41–8. With the extremity in 90 degrees of flexion, gravity allows the knee to drop into varus, thereby opening the lateral compartment for better visualization.

trochar is removed, and the 70-degree arthroscope is placed in the sheath to allow visualization across the medial femoral condyle and through the entire postero-medial compartment. The compartment can then be completely inspected by rotating the arthroscope. A similar approach can be used on the lateral side of the knee by inserting the sheath between the anterior cruciate ligament and the lateral femoral condyle through an anteromedial portal. This is not necessary as a routine maneuver, inasmuch as the entire posterior horn of the medial meniscus, including the popliteus, can be inspected from the anterior approach. The posterior cruciate ligament, on the other hand, can be visualized most easily by inserting the arthroscope behind the medial collateral ligament in the posteromedial approach.

Synovial Biopsy. The importance of synovial biopsy cannot be overestimated in the evaluation of synovial disease. With the arthroscope, biopsy can be accomplished in three ways. Blind biopsy can be done in the suprapatellar pouch at the conclusion of the examination by inserting a biopsy forceps through the sheath after removal of the arthroscope, feeling the tip of the forceps with the other hand through the skin, and then taking the biopsy without actually seeing the tissue to be biopsied. If a particular lesion is seen during arthroscopic examination, the arthroscope is removed from the sheath, a smaller arthroscope with a biopsy forceps is reinserted through the same sheath, and a biopsy is taken under direct vision. Finally, if a particular lesion is seen and the operator wishes to keep the lesion in view, a biopsy forceps can be inserted through a second puncture wound, and the biopsy taken under direct, uninterrupted visualization.

Arthroscopic examination can be performed on most peripheral joints. The *shoulder* is usually approached posteriorly just below the spine of the scapula where it becomes the acromion. The main internal landmark is the long head of the biceps. The undersurface of the rotator cuff and the entire glenoid can be seen. The head of the humerus is visualized by taking the shoulder through a range of motion.

The *elbow* must be approached both medially and laterally to adequately visualize the capitellum, the radial head, and the trochlea. Traction on the forearm and taking the joint through a range of motion help visualization.

The *wrist* and joints of the *hand* require a small-diameter arthroscope because of the many small compartments.[32] Multiple punctures are usually required in the examination of the wrist.

The *hip* presents a different problem to the arthroscopist because of its tight twisting capsule and because so much of the femoral head is covered by the acetabulum. The examination can be facilitated by placing the patient on the fracture table and applying traction to distract the joint. The hip is then approached anteriorly one fingerbreadth below the inguinal ligament and one fingerbreadth lateral to the femoral pulse.

The *ankle* is approached anterolaterally and antero-medially, and usually a good view of the dome of the talus and the undersurface of the tibia is possible when the joint is taken through a range of motion.

The *foot* with its many small joints must be examined like the hand, with a small-diameter arthroscope.

INTRA-ARTICULAR PATHOLOGY

Direct visualization of *synovial lesions* with an arthroscope can be quite dramatic. The arthroscope magnifies by a factor of ten at a distance of 1 mm. Therefore, detail can be seen that may not be visible to the naked eye. Color balance and vascular patterns may be very important, particularly in lesions such as rheumatoid arthritis and pigmented villonodular synovitis. Color differentiation and vascular engorgement may be obliterated if a tourniquet is used. Chondrocalcinosis and crystalline synovitis can also be observed. Proliferative synovitis, villous synovitis and synovial chondromatosis can be biopsied under direct vision[15, 33-38] (Fig. 41-9; see Plate VI, p. xl).

One author[15] has performed arthroscopic examinations with joint lavage with normal saline on 88 joints with crystalline synovitis. These joints had both urate and calcium pyrophosphate crystals. He noted marked improvement with only saline lavage in joints with and without involvement of articular cartilage compared with controls. In synovial disease arthroscopy may have therapeutic as well as diagnostic value (Fig. 41-10; see Plate VI, p. xl).

Lesions of the patellofemoral joint can be examined through various phases of flexion and extension, both passively and actively (under local anesthesia). Subluxation of the patella can be identified by the overhang of the lateral facet of the patella over the lateral femoral condyle. Chondromalacia can be localized, graded, followed, and in some instances treated. Osteochondral fractures can be identified and fragments replaced or removed (Fig. 41-11; see Plate VI, p. xl).

Lesions of the meniscus probably represent the most important pathology to be identified arthroscopically. Tears can be localized and quantitated. The recognition of a peripheral detachment, as opposed to a tear in the substance of the meniscus, is an important therapeutic differentiation, since some peripheral detachments heal and tears of the avascular fibrocartilage rarely do. The arthroscope has probably contributed to the reduction of unnecessary arthrotomies more than any other diagnostic tool. With increasing experience the arthroscopist will not remove menisci with small tears, particularly if they do not appear to be related to symptomatology. It is a simple matter to perform a second arthroscopy at a later date to see if the lesion has changed. Of even greater importance, evidence is accumulating that surgical absence of the meniscus appears to contribute to the ultimate development of degenerative arthritis of the knee.[39-46] It is becoming apparent that meniscal tears are not infrequently associated with various levels of anterior cruciate damage, resulting in some degree of rotary instability of the knee. This in all likelihood contributes to the development of degenerative change of articular cartilage and progression of osteoarthritis. Therefore, it is extremely important to preserve as much meniscal tissue as possible because of its cartilage-sparing effect in sharing the load and because of its role in stability of the knee by virtue of the meniscoligamentous complex. It has been shown that the blood supply to the meniscus itself is somewhat greater than we had previously believed. Microvascular studies have shown that vessels enter from the periphery at least one third of the way into the meniscal substance in humans. Efforts are being made at the present time to repair meniscal tears and to assess the results of such surgery (Fig. 41–12; see Plate VI, p. xl).

Lesions of articular cartilage can be identified and quantitated with the arthroscope and can be followed with relative ease. Osteochondritis dissecans in teenagers can be followed to the point of healing, so that if the fragment becomes loose, surgical management can be instituted. Roentgenograms show only the subchondral bone, not the overlying articular cartilage. Surgical decisions on osteotomy versus arthroplasty can be facilitated in unicompartmental degenerative arthritis by examining the "uninvolved" compartment with the arthroscope. The course of degenerative arthritis can be easily followed, leading to more rational therapeutic decisions. In rheumatoid arthritis the condition of articular cartilage can be determined prior to the surgical decision to undertake synovectomy.[40,47,48] Attempts are under way at resurfacing the articular cartilage utilizing techniques of "abrasion arthroplasty." This procedure abrades the subchondral exposed bone in osteoarthritis with the idea of revascularization and formation of a fibrocartilaginous surface. This technique is based on concepts that are in conflict with our knowledge of the healing of articular cartilage. Adequate long-term controlled follow-up studies are not yet available to document the efficacy of this procedure (Fig. 41–13; see Plate VI, p. xl).

Lesions of ligaments are usually the result of trauma. Arthroscopy is useful in acute trauma. Collateral ligaments, being extrasynovial, cannot be seen directly. However, damage to them may be inferred by subsynovial hemorrhage or synovial rupture. Tears of the anterior cruciate ligament are readily apparent both in the presence of acute injury and with chronic tears. The posterior cruciate ligament can also be examined anteriorly if the anterior cruciate ligament is gone, or posteromedially if the anterior cruciate ligament is intact.[16, 50-52] Procedures are being attempted to repair and reconstruct the anterior cruciate ligament by arthroscopic technique. Intra-articular arthroscopic stapling of the anterior cruciate ligament at its proximal attachment has been attempted. Most tears of the anterior cruciate ligament are interstitial and are not from one end to the other, which prevents an adequate tight repair by the utilization of surgical techniques, whether arthroscopic or open. Therefore, when one is considering the repair of anterior cruciate deficiencies, one has to also consider the possibilities of primary augmentation with some other structure. Arthroscopic attempts at

reconstructing the anterior cruciate ligament using other tendons, free fascia lata grafts, and synthetic ligaments are being researched. At the present time thorough, reliable methods and controlled long-term follow-up studies are not available.

Usually *loose bodies* can be located and removed with the arthroscope. The author has removed a loose body as large as 3 cm by bringing it to a subcutaneous position and then enlarging the skin incision. Once a loose body is identified endoscopically, a grasping forceps is inserted through a second incision and the object removed.

ACCURACY OF ARTHROSCOPY

As papers have accumulated in the literature in recent years, the reported accuracy of arthroscopy has steadily improved. In the first follow-up study in the American literature, Casscells[14] reviewed 150 cases using arthrotomy as an end point, with 80 percent accuracy. In 1972 Jackson and Abe[8] reported 90 percent accuracy in 200 cases. In 1975 Dandy and Jackson[12] reported 98.6 percent accuracy in 800 cases. DeHaven and Collins[41] did a prospective study of 100 cases comparing clinical evaluation, arthrography, and arthroscopy and reported an accuracy of 94 percent with arthroscopy. McGinty and Matza[53] reviewed 287 consecutive cases and found no difference in accuracy when arthroscopy was performed with local anesthesia compared to general or spinal anesthesia.

Most orthopedic surgeons will admit to about 80 to 85 percent accuracy in the diagnosis of abnormalities of the meniscus on clinical criteria alone. The addition of arthroscopy not only decreases the number of errors by 50 percent, it also allows the magnitude of pathology to be assessed before definitive management is undertaken. McGinty and Freedman[46] in a review of 221 consecutive arthroscopic examinations showed that one patient in three avoided arthrotomy by virtue of the arthroscopic examination.

DOCUMENTATION IN ARTHROSCOPY

One of the major benefits of arthroscopy is the ability to easily document intra-articular pathology. With the standard endoscopic light source and a 35-mm camera, using high-speed film, good quality slides or color prints can be made for the patient's record. Documentation of findings is important in planning future surgery, as evidence in liability litigation and workmen's compensation arbitration and in teaching, both in small conferences and large meetings. It is of considerable value when a surgeon opens a knee to be able to compare the findings with a photograph from a previous arthroscopy.

With the use of a high-intensity light source videotapes can be readily made during arthroscopic examinations. Color television cameras weighing only 2 ounces are easily attached to the arthroscope either directly or through a beam splitter (85 percent of the light to the camera and 15 percent to the eye of the arthroscopist). These cameras are becoming so small that the cuplet connecting the camera to the arthroscope is larger than the camera itself. This allows the camera to sit by itself on the end of the telescope, with much easier manipulation by the arthroscopist while he is doing other procedures. With these cameras the endoscopic image can be put on a monitor so more than one individual can observe the examination, an assistant can follow a procedure on the monitor, or an instant videotape can be made.[31]

FUTURE OF ARTHROSCOPY

The arthroscope as a diagnostic tool is well-established. Intra-articular surgery with 1-cm incisions, using the arthroscope and small instruments, is already a reality. Loose bodies are being removed; partial meniscectomies are accomplished; chondroplasties are being done for chondromalacia with small battery-powered tools; and lateral retinacular release is being performed with the arthroscope for subluxation of the patella. Arthroscopy is now carried out utilizing not only a saline medium but a gas medium of CO_2, which provides for a larger field of view and a somewhat more realistic appearance in comparison with that obtained with the techniques of open surgery. Newer, more efficient, and better controlled power tools are now available to tailor menisci, to remove synovium, and to trim articular cartilage. Electrosurgical and laser techniques are being utilized on humans. At the present time the use of laser techniques is extremely limited and dangerous, but refinements will undoubtedly occur. Techniques for suture of meniscal lesions are already a reality with their appropriate instrumentation.

Arthroscopy will find greater use as a research tool in following both intra-articular pathology and innovations in intra-articular surgery. Will there be a place for local chemical synovectomy under arthroscopic control? Injection of dyes to identify predegenerative lesions of articular cartilage is being tried.

The arthroscope in intra-articular surgery, like the operating microscope in neurosurgery, otolaryngology, and hand surgery, has opened up a whole new approach to intra-articular problems. The growth and potential of this approach are limited only by the imagination and zeal of its advocates.

References

1. Berci, G.: Endoscopy. New York, Appleton-Century-Crofts, 1976.
2. Takagi, K.: Practical experiences using Takagi's arthroscope. J. Japan Orthop. Assoc. 8:132, 1933.
3. Burman, M.S.: Arthroscopy or direct visualization of joints: An experimental cadaver study. J. Bone Joint Surg. 13A:669, 1931.
4. Burman, M.S., Finkelstein, H., and Mayer, L.: Arthroscopy of the knee joint. J. Bone Joint Surg. 16A:255, 1934.
5. Finkelstein, H., and Mayer, L.: The arthroscope. A new method of examining joints. J. Bone Joint Surg. 13A:583, 1931.
6. Watanabe, M., Takeda, S., and Ikeuchi, H.: Atlas of Arthroscopy. 2nd ed. Tokyo, Igaku Shoin Ltd., 1969.
7. Watanabe, M.: The development and present status of the arthroscope. J. Japan Med. Inst. 25:11, 1954.
8. Jackson, R.S., and Abe, I.: The role of arthroscopy in the management of disorders of the knee. J. Bone Joint Surg. 54B:310, 1972.
9. Jackson, R.W.: The role of arthroscopy in the management of the arthritic knee. Clin. Orthop. 101:28, 1974.
10. Jackson, R.W., and DeHaven, K.E.: Arthroscopy of the knee. Clin. Orthop. 107:87, 1975.
11. Jackson, R.W., and Dandy, D.J.: Arthroscopy of the Knee. New York, Grune & Stratton, 1976.
12. Dandy, D.J., and Jackson, R.W.: The impact of arthroscopy in the management of disorders of the knee joint. J. Bone Joint Surg. 57B:346, 1975.
13. Dandy, D.J., and Jackson, R.W.: The diagnosis of problems after meniscectomy. Bone Joint Surg. 57B:349, 1975.
14. Casscells, S.W.: Arthroscopy of the knee joint. J. Bone Joint Surg. 53A:287, 1971.
15. O'Connor, R.L.: The arthroscope in the management of crystal induced synovitis of the knee. J. Bone Joint Surg. 55A:1443, 1973.
16. O'Connor, R.L.: Arthroscopy in the diagnosis and treatment of acute ligament injuries of the knee. J. Bone Joint Surg. 56A:333, 1974.
17. O'Connor, R.L.: Arthroscopy of the knee. Surg. Ann. 9:265, 1977.
18. O'Connor, R.L.: Arthroscopy. Philadelphia, J. B. Lippincott Company, 1977.
19. Ohnsarge, J.: Arthroscopy of the knee joint by means of glass fibers. Z. Orthop. 106:759, 1969.
20. Dorfman, H., and Dreyfus, P.: Arthroscopy of the knee. Methods and results. Minerva Med. 62:2621, 1971.
21. Eikelaar, H.R.: Arthroscopy of the Knee. Thesis for doctorate in orthopaedic surgery at the University of Groningen. The Netherlands Royal United Printers, Hoitsema, B. V., 1975.
22. Eikelaar, H.R.: Looking inside, gaining insight. Aspects of arthroscopy of the knee joint. Ned. Tijdschr. Gneeskd. 119:1882, 1975.
23. Gilliquist, J., and Hagberg, G.: A new modification of the technique of arthroscopy of the knee joint. Acta Chir. Scand. 142:123, 1976.
24. Johnson, L.L., and Becker, H.L.: Arthroscopy technique and role of the assistant. Orthop. Rev. 5:31, 1976.
25. Johnson, L.L.: Comprehensive Arthroscopic Examination of the Knee. St. Louis, C. V. Mosby Company, 1977.
26. Johnson, L.L., Schneider, D., Goodman, F., Bullock, J.M., and DeBruin, J.A., Jr.: Cold sterilization method for arthroscopes using activated dialdehyde. Orthop. Rev. 6:75, 1977.
27. Mortya, H.: The use of arthroscopy and biopsy in the diagnosis of monarticular chronic arthritis of the knee joint. Ryumachi 16:12, 1976.
28. Robles, G.J., Katona, G., and Banoso, M.R.: Arthroscopy as an aid to diagnosis and investigation. Exerpta Medica, International Congress Series 143:6, 1968.
29. Takeda, S.: Relationship between arthroscopic findings and histological change of the synovial membrane. J. Japan Orthop. Assoc. 34:373, 1960.
30. Wruhs, O.: Arthroscopy and endophotography for diagnosis and documentation of knee joint injuries. Wien. Med. 120:126, 1970.
31. McGinty, J.B.: Closed-circuit television in arthroscopy. Int. Rev. Rheumatol. special edition, pp. 45–49, 1976.
32. Watanabe, M.: Arthroscopy of small joints. J. Japan Orthop. Assoc. 45:908, 1975.
33. Andersen, R.B., and Rosse, I.: Arthroscopy of the knee joint in rheumatic diseases. Ugeskr. Laeger 135:71, 1973.
34. Camerlain, M.: Arthroscopy and its rheumatologic perspective. Union Med. Con. 103:1262, 1974.
35. Delbarre, F., Aignan, T., and Ghozlan, R.: L'arthroscopie de Genou. Institute of Rheumatology, Faculty of Medicine, Paris, Cochin, 1976.
36. Dorfman, H., and Figuerda, M.: Value of arthroscopy in isolated monoarthritis of the knee. Sem. Hop. Paris 50:179, 1974.
37. Hertel, E.: Possibilities and limits of arthroscopy of rheumatic joints. A. Orthop. 113:798, 1975.
38. Jayson, M.I., and Dixon, A.S.: Arthroscopy of the knee in rheumatic diseases. Ann. Rheum. Dis. 27:503, 1968.
39. Alm, A., Gillquist, J., and Liljedahl, S.C.: The diagnostic value of arthroscopy of the knee joint. Injury 5:319, 1974.
40. Axer, A., Segal, D., Hendel, D., Shikias, S., Rabinowitz, J., Halperin, N., Rzetelny, V., and Gershwin, D.: Arthrography and arthroscopy in the diagnosis of internal derangement of the knee. Harefuah 91:61, 1976.
41. DeHaven, K.E., and Collins, H.R.: Diagnosis of internal derangement of the knee. The role of arthroscopy. J. Bone Joint Surg. 57A:802, 1975.
42. Gallannaugh, S.: Arthroscopy of the knee joint. Br. Med. J. 3:285, 1973.
43. Glintz, W.: Arthroscopy in meniscus injuries. Z. Unfallmed. Berufskr. 69:106, 1976.
44. Kreuscher, P.H.: Semilunar cartilage disease: A plea for early recognition by means of the arthroscope and early treatment of this condition. Ill. Med. J. 47:290, 1925.
45. Norwood, L.A. Jr., Shields, C.L. Jr., Russo, J., Kerland, R.K., Jobe, F.W., Carter, V.S., Blazina, M.E., Lombardo, S.J., and DelPizzo, W.: Ar-

throscopy of the lateral meniscus in knees with normal arthrograms. Am. J. Sports Med. 5:271, 1977.

46. McGinty, J.B., and Freedman, P.A.: Arthroscopy of the knee. Clin. Orthop. 121:171, 1976.
47. Glenby, W.: Diagnostic importance of arthroscopy in prearthrosis of the knee joint. Z. Ufallmed. Berufskr. 67:260, 1974.
48. Glintz, W.: Diagnosis of chondral injury in trauma of the knee joint. Langenbechs Arch. Clin. 345:423, 1977.
49. Glintz, W.: Arthroscopy diagnoses of the traumatic cartilage lesions of the knee joint. Hefte Unfallheilkd. 129:242, 1977.

50. Gilliquist, J., Hagbey, G., and Oretrop, N.: Arthroscopy in acute injuries of the knee joint. Acta Orthop. Scand. 48:190, 1977.
51. Okmura, T.: An arthroscopic study of the traumatic disorders of the knee joint. J. Japan Orthop. Assoc. 23:28, 1945.
52. Pochling, G.G., Bassett, F.H., and Goldner, J.L.: Arthroscopy: Its role in treating non-traumatic and traumatic lesions of the knee. South. Med. J. 70:465, 1977.
53. McGinty, J.G., and Matsa, R.: Arthroscopy of the knee. J. Bone Joint Surg. 60A:787, 1978.

Chapter 42
Synovial Biopsy and Pathology

H. Ralph Schumacher

INTRODUCTION

Biopsy of the synovial membrane should be considered in patients in whom diagnosis is not clear after clinical evaluation. Synovial fluid analysis as described in Chapter 38 should generally be performed before consideration of a biopsy if a synovial effusion can be aspirated. Examinations on synovial tissue may be the only way to make a definite diagnosis in some infectious, infiltrative, and deposition diseases of joints such as granulomatous infections, sarcoidosis, osteochondromatosis, the rare synovial leukemia or other malignancy, multicentric reticulohistiocytosis, pigmented villonodular arthritis, hemochromatosis, Whipple's disease, ochronosis, and amyloidosis. While the diagnosis of gout or pseudogout is best made by joint fluid analysis, occasionally the deposited materials or crystals are first found in synovial membrane when joint fluid is absent or not noted to contain crystals.[1]

Synovial membrane findings of villous proliferation, superficial fibrin, marked lining cell increase, focal necrosis, plasma cells, and lymphoid follicles may strongly suggest rheumatoid arthritis (RA), but are not specific. In RA as with several other systemic rheumatic diseases, diagnosis is often made by accumulation of criteria. Aid from a synovial biopsy showing a definite inflammatory process may help, as, for example, in the ARA diagnostic criteria.[2] Even if not giving a definite diagnosis, synovial biopsy by illustrating the presence or absence of inflammation may help guide symptomatic treatment. Synovial fluid findings can help in the same way, but both inflammatory and infiltrative synovial membrane lesions are not infrequently found with "noninflammatory" effusions.[3] Approximately 35 percent of needle biopsies performed in diagnostic problems are of clinical assistance.[3]

METHODS FOR OBTAINING SYNOVIUM

Needle Biopsy. Probably the most popular current technique for diagnostic synovial biopsy is use of the Polley-Bickel technique[4] or one of the newer, smaller Parker-Pearson needles[3, 5] (Fig. 42–1). Needle synovial biopsy can be performed in the hospital or in the clinic or office.

The knee is by far the most frequently biopsied joint, but successful biopsies can also be obtained from shoulders, elbows, wrists, ankles, olecranon bursae, and occasionally even smaller joints if they are sufficiently swollen. The route of entry is generally that described for arthrocentesis. The procedure can be performed by a single operator with one assistant. Meperidine is occasionally used for very anxious patients. Young children may even need general anesthesia. The biopsy area is widely prepared with soap and then iodine, and washed with alcohol. The operator then dons gloves and drapes a transparent plastic drape with a 2-inch hole over the biopsy site. The skin and subcutaneous tissue is infiltrated to the capsule with 1 percent lidocaine, using a 25-gauge needle. Caution is exercised to avoid instilling anesthetic into the joint space, which would distort the synovianalysis findings. Next, either the trochar or a 20- to 22-gauge needle is forcefully thrust through the anesthetized area into the joint space. We previously always inserted the smaller needle first but now often find it acceptable to most patients to use only the trochar and avoid the additional insertion. Fluid is aspirated for synovianalysis through the trochar or needle. It is not necessary to distend the joint with fluid. Two to 4 ml of 1 percent lidocaine can be instilled into the joint space, but biopsy can also be done without this if it is felt important to avoid any possible artifact that might be introduced by the local anesthetic. The biopsy needle is now inserted through the outer needle. The side with the hooked notch is approximated against the synovium, and suction is applied with a 20- to 50-ml Luer-lock syringe. The needle is always directed away from the site of initial lidocaine infiltration, to avoid possible artifacts in this area. Three to eight specimens (to minimize sampling error) from the various parts of the joint are taken by angling the needle without reinserting the outer needle. Suction is maintained with one hand on the syringe while the other retracts the inner crete localized lesions which can then be biopsied with a needle technique under direct visualization. The procedure is generally limited to larger joints.

Open Surgical Biopsy. If one is concerned about the possibility of focal granulomas, deeper lesions such as a vasculitis in larger capsular vessels, or other lesions that might have been missed on a needle biopsy, open surgical biopsy can be considered. Surgical biopsy is also very useful at small joints not suitable for needle biopsy. A small incision over a metacarpophalangeal joint is very effective and offers virtually no morbidity.

Open biopsy even of a knee can be done with a small incision; but if one wants the advantage of the full joint exploration, a large surgical incision and some postoperative immobilization are obviously needed.

Fragments of Synovial Membrane. Synovial membrane fragments can occasionally be found floating in joint fluid after arthrocentesis. These can be examined in a wet smear for crystals and can also be collected by centrifugation and fixed for processing as with any biopsy.

METHODS OF HANDLING TISSUE

The multiple small pieces of synovium from needle biopsy or the large specimens obtained at operation should be distributed among several methods of handling, depending on the questions being asked. Specimens for routine light microscopy are placed into neutral buffered formalin or Bouin's fixative. Some slides should be stained with hematoxylin and eosin and other tissue saved for consideration of special stains. If gout is a possibility, a portion of the biopsy should be placed in absolute alcohol, since urates are water soluble. Specimens thus should be processed without water and stained with the DeGolantha stain for urate or sections examined with compensated polarized light. Frozen sections of unfixed biopsies can also be used for polarized light examination for urates.

Immunofluorescent study of synovium has not been of any convincing clinical value but is of research interest. One study[9] suggested that demonstration of synovial IgM deposition favored the diagnosis of rheumatoid arthritis. Specimens for this study should be placed in saline until transferred to O.C.T. compound (Miles Laboratories) on a cryostat chuck which is then quick frozen by immersion in liquid nitrogen.

Electron microscopy (EM) of synovium is also largely of research interest. For example, it can show electron-dense deposits in vessel walls in early rheumatoid arthritis[10] and in palidromic rheumatism[11] and also in the syndrome of hypertrophic pulmonary osteoarthropathy[12] (Fig. 42–2). EM may be a major diagnostic aid in identifying apatite crystals (Fig. 42–3), viruses, small amounts of amyloid, bacilliform bodies of Whipple's disease, and Gaucher cell tubules. Any specimen for EM should be placed immediately in a fixative such as 3 percent glutaraldehyde or half-strength Karnovsky's fixative.[13] Specimens should be minced into 0.5 ×

Figure 42–1. Parker-Pearson synovial biopsy needle. The hooked biopsy needle on the left is inserted through the center 14-gauge needle, and tissue is drawn into the notch proximal to the hook by suction.

needle through the outer with a slight twist. The outer needle remains in place. One must become familiar with the appearance of the specimens, so as not to mistake fibrin or necrotic material (yellow-white) for synovial tissue (pink). Specimens may be transferred carefully from the needle by a 25-gauge needle to the fixative on a small piece of sterile paper.

Patients are instructed to rest biopsied joints until the following day, when they are permitted to resume usual activity, providing no increased pain or swelling has been noted. Hemarthrosis and infection are theoretical complications, but only two patients of more than 400 in our series have had hemarthrosis that required aspiration the next day for pain relief. There are reports of needle tips breaking off in the joint.[6] Care must be taken before biopsy to check that the needle fits easily through the trochar and that the tip is not bent or weakened.

Other needles that have been used for synovial biopsy are those of Cope, Williamson,[7] and Franklin and Silverman.[8]

Other Methods for Obtaining Synovial Biopsies. *Arthroscopy.* This allows the advantage of identifying dis-

Figure 42–2. Electron-dense deposit (arrows) in vessel wall of synovium of patient with rheumatoid arthritis of recent onset. E = vascular endothelium, L = lumen, P = pericyte. Electron micrograph × 16,000.

0.5 mm pieces, ideally fixed for up to 4 hours, and then switched into a buffer before further processing.

Culture of synovial membrane can on occasion be more useful than that of synovial fluid, especially with mycobacteria, fungi, and gonococci. Techniques for cultures are described in Chapter 38. Synovial membrane can also be grown in tissue culture for investigative purposes. Biopsies for this are placed promptly in tissue culture medium and taken to the laboratory.

Figure 42–3. Apatite crystals (arrow) in vacuole of a synovial lining cell in a patient with osteonecrosis of the knee. N = nucleus of cell. Electron micrograph × 17,000.

FINDINGS ON LIGHT MICROSCOPIC EXAMINATION OF SYNOVIAL BIOPSIES

Normal. Normal synovial membrane (Fig. 42–4; see Plate VII, p. xli) consists of one or two layers of synovial lining cells overlying a richly vascular areolar or fibrous connective tissue. A biopsy containing several pieces of normal synovium does not absolutely exclude intra-articular disease, but should direct the search toward very focal disease or extrasynovial processes. Failure to identify a characteristic lesion does not exclude the diagnosis of the diagnosable diseases listed in the Introduction. For example, gouty, tuberculous, or ochronotic synovium can show only mild proliferation or changes indistinguishable from rheumatoid arthritis in tissue adjacent to a tophus, granuloma, or typical pigmented shard.

Rheumatoid Arthritis and "Variants." In rheumatoid arthritis the combination of villous hypertrophy, lining cell proliferation, infiltration by lymphocytes and plasma cells (Fig. 42–5; see Plate VII, p. xli) with a tendency to form "lymphoid nodules," fibrin deposition, and focal necrosis is typical. This is not diagnostic with similar changes seen sometimes in systemic lupus erythematosus (SLE) and other diseases. Especially in RA of very recent onset all the aforementioned findings may not be present, and vascular occlusion or mild vasculitis may be prominent.[10]

Rheumatoid nodules are only very rarely seen in synovium. There may be multinucleated giant cells beneath the lining cells.

Psoriatic arthritis and ankylosing spondylitis can show synovial changes indistinguishable from RA. Early Reiter's syndrome[13] has a typical superficial congestion and polymorphonuclear leukocyte infiltration, which can, however, also be seen in some early RA, Behçet's disease,[14] and regional enteritis, as well as other conditions. Chronic Reiter's syndrome synovium is indistinguishable from that of RA.

Collagen-Vascular Diseases. The synovial membrane in SLE typically shows less intense lining cell hyperplasia and less leukocyte infiltration than in RA,[15,16] although, as noted above, inflammation may occasionally mimic RA. In polyarteritis synovial inflammation is usually mild and inflammatory cell infiltration of medium-sized vessel walls is only a rare finding.[17] Early scleroderma[18] shows sparse lining cells, superficial fibrin, and chronic inflammatory cell infiltration (Fig. 42–6; see Plate VII, p. xli). Similar findings with paucity of lining cells can be seen also in some SLE, polymyositis, rheumatic fever, and some infections. In later scleroderma synovial fibrin and fibrosis predominate.

Infectious Arthritis. Infection is one of the types of joint disease that can be definitively diagnosed by synovial biopsy.[19] In acute bacterial arthritis clusters or sheets of neutrophils can be seen (Fig. 42–7). Bacteria can sometimes be demonstrated in synovium with a tissue Gram's stain. Cultures may be positive on synovial biopsy specimens even when they have been negative on

Figure 42–7. Massive infiltration of synovium with neutrophils and some lymphocytes in untreated septic arthritis of 10 days' duration. × 100. Hematoxylin and eosin stain.

blood and synovial fluid.[20] In chronic or resolving infections there are often large numbers of lymphocytes and plasma cells.

Chronic infections such as tuberculosis and fungus disease can produce focal lesions that may be missed on limited biopsies. Mycobacterial granulomas in the superficial synovium do not always show caseation (Fig. 42–8; see Plate VII, p. xli). Ziehl-Neelsen and Kinyoun's stains can show acid-fast organisms. Staining for fungi should be attempted with Grocott and Gridley stains. Treponemes can be sought in secondary syphilis with fluorescent and silver stains. Only a mild nonspecific synovitis has been seen in three cases of secondary syphilis.

Sarcoidosis. Sarcoidosis can involve the synovium with typical granulomas,[21] but other patients, especially those with erythema nodosum, more often have predominantly periarthritis or only scattered lymphocytes in the synovium.

Infiltrative or Deposition Diseases. These diseases have specific findings that are amenable to diagnosis by synovial biopsy.

Crystal-Induced Arthritis. Both gout and pseudogout often have tophuslike deposits in synovial membrane (Fig. 42–9; see Plate VII, p. xli). Precautions for tissue handling to demonstrate urate tophi are described above.

Calcium pyrophosphate crystals are not as water soluble but can be dissolved by decalcification in specimens submitted along with bone. Thus pseudogout synovium occasionally can have lucent areas where crystals were lost, as in gout. Usually only a fibrous capsule, a few histiocytes, and giant cells surround the tophi. In acute crystal-induced arthritis there are areas of neutrophil infiltration, but in chronic disease large numbers of lymphocytes and plasma cells can be seen. Clumps of apatite crystals in synovium can appear as hematoxyphilic areas.[22] The tiny crystals forming these clumps are identifiable by EM. Oxalate crystals have also recently been found as pleomorphic birefringent bodies in synovium of one patient receiving chronic hemodialysis for chronic renal failure.[23]

Amyloidosis. In patients with primary amyloidosis, multiple myeloma, and Waldenström's disease amyloid can be deposited in the synovium. This appears pink on hematoxylin and eosin stain, and red with Congo red. The Congo red–stained material has an apple-green birefringence when viewed with plain polarized light.[24] In our experience most amyloid has been on the synovial surface (Fig. 42–10; see Plate VIII, p. xlii) and in the interstitium, but rarely in vessel walls.

Ochronosis. The synovial membrane in ochronosis is embedded with brownish-pigmented shards from the friable cartilage[25] (Fig. 42–11; see Plate VIII, p. xlii). Macrophages adjacent to the cartilage fragments often contain pigment granules. Clusters of lymphocytes can also be seen and can also be found in areas of synovium in other patients with cartilage degeneration, such as in primary or secondary osteoarthritis. It should be noted that cartilage and bone fragments without the ochronotic pigment can also be seen embedded in synovium in osteoarthritis, rheumatoid arthritis, and other destructive arthropathies.[26]

Hemochromatosis. Golden-brown hemosiderin pigment deposition in synovial lining cells and to a lesser degree in deeper phagocytes is characteristic of hemochromatosis[27] and other diseases with systemic iron overload. Iron in synovium from bleeding into the joint space or extravasation of erythrocytes into tissue produces hemosiderin mainly in deep macrophages. Iron stains blue with Prussian blue for confirmation (Fig. 42–12; see Plate VIII, p. xlii). Calcium pyrophosphate crystals can be seen in these synovia as well as in several other metabolic joint diseases.

Tumors. A variety of benign and malignant tumors or tumor-like conditions can involve the synovial membrane. Metastatic malignancies are occasionally identified in synovium.[28] Blast forms have been found infiltrating synovium in a few but by no means all patients with leukemia or lymphoma and arthritis.[29] Malignant synovioma is an extra-articular tumor that is very rarely seen in joint synovium. Osteochondromas developing in synovium can be seen as foci of osteo- and chondrometaplasia in the synovial connective tissue. Pigmented villonodular synovitis, generally involving a single joint or tendon sheath, is characterized by giant cells, foamy cells, and hemosiderin deposits predominantly in the

Figure 42–13. Giant cells, foam cells, and hemosiderin deposits are seen in pigmented villonodular synoistes. Some areas contain lymphocytes and plasma cells.

deep synovium (Fig. 42–13; see Plate VIII, p. xlii). There is villous or nodular proliferation with areas also showing some lymphocytes and plasma cells.

Other Diseases. *Multicentric Reticulohistiocytosis* [30] shows extensive infiltration of synovium with large foamy cells and/or multinucleated cells with eosinophilic "ground glass" cytoplasm.

Whipple's Disease. Whipple's disease synovial membrane often shows just mild lining cell hyperplasia and scattered lymphocytes and neutrophils, but PAS-positive macrophages can be seen in some cases to suggest the diagnosis.[31] EM can suggest the typical bacilliform bodies.[32]

Hypertrophic Osteoarthropathy (HPO). Despite large painful effusions, HPO tends to have virtually no inflammatory cell infiltration in synovium but marked vascular congestion in early disease.[12] Electron-dense deposits in vessel walls can be seen in some biopsies by EM. In chronic HPO lymphocytic infiltration is reported.

Scurvy. Scurvy of the synovium shows edema, extravasation of erythrocytes, and large fibrocytes that have been unable to release their collagen precursors because of the lack of vitamin C.[33]

Familial Arthropathy. A familial arthropathy with synovial coating with fibrin-like material and giant cells has been described in children.[34]

Sickle Cell Disease. Synovium in sickle cell disease can show obliterated vessels and occasionally some lymphocyte and plasma cell infiltration.[35]

Exogenous Particles. Thorns or animal spines can occasionally penetrate into joints and be visible in biopsies as well as producing a chronic synovitis.[36] Metallic or plastic particles in patients with joint arthroplasties can also occasionally be found in synovium.[37]

Pancreatic Disease. Synovial fat necrosis and lipid laden macrophages can be associated with pancreatic disease.[38] Rare, unexpected new findings will occasionally be encountered if undiagnosed cases are biopsied. For example, an eosinophilic infiltration with fibrin dep-

osition was found in a case later determined to have the hypereosinophilic syndrome.[39]

CONCLUSIONS

Synovial biopsy specimens obtainable by a variety of mechanisms can give specific diagnoses in some diseases or can provide additional criteria supporting diagnoses in other situations. Careful consideration of the questions to be asked before performing a diagnostic biopsy will allow optimal handling of the tissue.

References

1. Agudelo, C., and Schumacher, H.R.: The synovitis of acute gouty arthritis. Hum. Pathol. 4:265, 1973.
2. Ropes, M.W., Bennett, G.A., Cobbs, S., et al.: 1958 revision of diagnostic criteria for rheumatoid arthritis. Arthritis Rheum. 2:16, 1959.
3. Schumacher, H.R., and Kulka, J.P.: Needle biopsy of the synovial membrane. Experience with the Parker-Pearson technique. N. Engl. J. Med. 286:416, 1972.
4. Polley, H.F., and Bickel, W.H.: Punch biopsy of synovial membrane. Ann. Rheum. Dis. 10:277, 1951.
5. Parker, R.H., and Pearson, C.M.: A simplified synovial biopsy needle. Arthritis Rheum. 6:172, 1963.
6. Bocanegra, T.S., McClelland, J.J., Germain, B.F., et al.: Intraarticular fragmentation of a new Parker-Pearson synovial biopsy needle. J. Rheum. 7:248, 1980.
7. Williamson, N., and Holt, L.P.T.: A synovial biopsy needle. Lancet 1:799, 1966.
8. Moon, M-S., Kim, I., and Kim, J-M.: Synovial biopsy by Franklin-Silverman needle. Clin. Orthop. 150:224, 1980.
9. Bayliss, C.E., Dawkins, R.L., Cullity, G., et al.: Laboratory diagnosis of rheumatoid arthritis. Ann. Rheum. Dis. 34:395, 1975.
10. Schumacher, H.R.: Synovial membrane and fluid morphologic alterations in early rheumatoid arthritis: Microvascular injury and virus-like particles. Ann. N.Y. Acad. Sci. 256:39, 1975.
11. Schumacher, H.R.: Palindromic onset of rheumatoid arthritis. Clinical, synovial fluid and biopsy studies. Arthritis Rheum. 25:361, 1982.
12. Schumacher, H.R.: The articular manifestations of hypertrophic pulmonary osteoarthropathy in brochogenic carcinoma. Arthritis Rheum. 19:629, 1976.
13. Karnovsky, M.J.: A formaldehyde-glutaraldehyde fixative of high osmolality for use in electron microscopy (abstr.). J. Cell. Biol. 27:441A, 1965.
14. Abdou, N.I., Schumacher, H.R., Colman, R.W., et al.: Behçet's disease: Possible role of secretory component deficiency, synovial inclusions and fibrinolytic abnormality in the various manifestations of the disease. J. Lab. Clin. Med. 91:409, 1978.
15. Goldenberg, D.L., and Cohen, A.S.: Synovial membrane histopathology in the different diagnosis of rheumatoid arthritis, gout, pseudogout, systemic lupus erythematosus, infectious arthritis and degenerative joint disease. Medicine 57:239, 1978.
16. Labowitz, R., and Schumacher, H.R.: Articular manifestations of SLE. Ann. Intern. Med. 74:911, 1974.
17. Smukler, N.M., and Schumacher, H.R.: Chronic non-destructive arthritis associated with cutaneous polyarteritis. Arthritis Rheum. 20:1114, 1977.
18. Schumacher, H.R.: Joint involvement in progressive systemic sclerosis (scleroderma). Am. J. Clin. Pathol. 60:593, 1973.
19. Schumacher, H.R.: Joint pathology in infectious arthritis. Clin. Rheum. Dis. 4:33, 1978.
20. Wofsy, D.: Culture-negative septic arthritis and bacterial endocarditis. Diagnosis by synovial biopsy. Arthritis Rheum. 23:605, 1980.
21. Sokoloff, L., and Bunim, J.J.: Clinical and pathological studies of joint involvement in sarcoidosis. N. Engl. J. Med. 260:841, 1959.
22. Reginato, A.J., and Schumacher, H.R.: Synovial calcification in a patient with collagen-vascular disease. Light and electron microscopic studies. J. Rheumatol. 4:261, 1977.
23. Hoffman, G.S., Schumacher, H.R., Paul, H., et al.: Calcium oxalate microcrystalline-associated arthritis in end-stage renal disease. Ann. Intern. Med. 97:36–42, 1982.
24. Canoso, J.J., and Cohen, A.S.: Rheumatological aspects of amyloid disease. Clin. Rheum. Dis. I:149, 1975.
25. Schumacher, H.R., and Holdsworth, D.E.: Ochronotic arthropathy. Semin. Arthritis Rheum. 6:207, 1977.
26. Resnick, D., Weisman, M., Goergan, T.G., and Feldman, P.S.: Osteolysis with detritic synovitis. Arch. Intern. Med. 138:1003, 1978.

27. Schumacher, H.R.: Ultrastructural characteristics of the synovial membrane in idiopathic hemochromatosis. Ann. Rheum. Dis. 31:465, 1972.
28. Goldenberg, D.L., Kelley, W., and Gibbons, R.B.: Metastatic adenocarcinoma of synovium presenting as an acute arthritis. Arthritis Rheum. 18:107, 1975.
29. Spilberg, I., and Meyer, G.J.: The arthritis of leukemia. Arthritis Rheum. 15:630, 1972.
30. Krey, P.R., Comerford, F.R., and Cohen, A.S.: Multicentric reticulohistiocytosis. Arthritis Rheum. 17:615, 1974.
31. Delcambre, B., Luez, J., Leonardelli, J., et al.: Les manifestations articulaires de la maladie de Whipple. Semin. Hop. Paris 50:847, 1974.
32. Rubinow, A., Canoso, J.J., Goldenberg, D.L., and Cohen, A.S.: Synovial fluid and synovial membrane pathology in Whipple's disease. Arthritis Rheum. 19:820, 1976.
33. Bevilaqua, F.A., Hasselbacher, P., and Schumacher, H.R.: Scurvy and hemarthrosis. JAMA 235:1874, 1976.
34. Athreya, B., and Schumacher, H.R.: Pathologic features of a recently recognized form of familial arthropathy. Arthritis Rheum. 21:429, 1978.
35. Schumacher, H.R.: Rheumatological manifestations of sickle cell disease and other hereditary hemoglobinopathies. Clin. Rheum. Dis. 1:37, 1975.
36. Schumacher, H.R., and Majno, G.: Thorns in the skin and joints of monkeys. Arch. Pathol. 84:536, 1967.
37. Kitridou, R.C., Schumacher, H.R., Sbarbaro, J.L., and Hollander, J.L.: Recurrent hemarthrosis after knee arthroplasty. Arthritis Rheum. 12:520, 1969.
38. Smukler, N.M., Schumacher, H.R., Pascual, E., et al.: Synovial fat necrosis associated with ischemic pancreatic disease. Arthritis Rheum. 22:547, 553, 1979.
39. Brogadir, S.P., Goldwein, M.I., and Schumacher, H.R.: A hypereosinophilic syndrome mimicking rheumatoid arthritis. Am. J. Med. 69:799, 1980.

Chapter 43

The Acute Phase Reactants

Irving Kushner

THE ACUTE PHASE RESPONSE IN MAN

General Characteristics of Acute Phase Proteins. The concentration of a number of plasma constituents is substantially altered within the first few days following an inflammatory stimulus, as part of the general systemic and metabolic response to tissue injury and infection.[1] These alterations are referred to collectively as the *acute phase response*. Major increases are noted in the concentrations of a heterogeneous group of plasma proteins; these *acute phase proteins* will be the primary focus of this chapter.[2,3,3a] Very low density lipoproteins and triglyceride concentrations rise, while high density lipoprotein levels fall.[4,5] In addition, there are changes in concentration of the cations copper, zinc, and iron.[6,7,8] Finally, alterations are noted in concentration of fibronectin[9,10] and of a group of substances originally recognized because of their biologic activities, at times due to substances whose precise chemical nature is still poorly defined.[11,12,13] A number of functional activities have been found to be due to factors that have the characteristics of interleukin I and endogenous pyrogen.[14-17] If the inflammatory stimulus is self-limited, there is a return of acute phase proteins to normal levels within a matter of days or weeks, while persisting tissue alterations may often lead to similarly persisting "acute phase" plasma changes.

The best studied human acute phase proteins are listed in Table 43–1. With the exception of C-reactive protein (CRP) and SAA protein, neither of which is glycosylated, these proteins are glycoproteins with carbohydrate contents ranging between 2.7 and 42 percent. SAA is an apoprotein and circulates in plasma with the high density lipoproteins.[19]

Following appropriate stimuli the concentrations of acute phase proteins rise to levels at least 25 percent greater than normal. In the cases of SAA protein and C-reactive protein several hundredfold increases above concentrations seen in some normal individuals occur commonly and concentrations one-thousandfold or more above these levels may be seen with severe infections.[20,21] A number of other human plasma proteins, including several complement components, have been reported to display acute phase behavior; in general they have not been as well studied as the proteins tabulated.[1] There is great species variability in the acute phase response. The major acute phase reactants in man are CRP and SAA. These acute phase changes are of great interest, both because their measurement can be of clinical value and because of the questions they raise concerning the mechanisms governing their changes in concentration and the functions served by these proteins.

Varieties of Stimuli. The acute phase response has been noted following a large variety of inflammatory or injurious stimuli. These include surgical or other trauma, acute myocardial infarction, pulmonary embolism, dissecting aneurysm of the aorta, bone fracture, and injection of typhoid vaccine, among others. Many acute bacterial infections, including pneumococcal pneumonia, streptococcal pharyngitis, salpingitis, pyelonephritis, and peritonitis elicit the acute phase response. It has recently been emphasized that severe viral infections can similarly elicit an increase in C-reactive protein and SAA levels.[22,23,24] Increased concentrations of the acute phase proteins are seen in acute abdominal crises (such as cholecystitis and pancreatitis), in a number of connective tissue diseases, including rheumatic fever and rheumatoid arthritis, and in some patients with advanced malignancies. Marked physical exertion can also lead to the acute phase response.[24a]

Table 43-1. Best Studied Acute Phase Proteins in Humans*

	Electrophoretic Mobility on Paper	Molecular Weight (daltons)	Normal Plasma Concentration (mg/dl)
Group I			
Concentration may increase by about 50%			
Ceruloplasmin	α_2	151,000	15–60
C3 (complement component)	β	180,000	80–170
Group II			
Concentration may increase two- to four-fold			
α_1-Acid glycoprotein	α_1	40,000	55–140
α_1-Antitrypsin	α_1	54,000	200–400
α_1-Antichymotrypsin	α_1	68,000	30–60
Haptoglobin	α_2	100,000[†]	40–180
Fibrinogen	β	340,000	200–450
Group III			
Concentration may increase 100- to 1000-fold			
C-reactive protein	β–γ	105,000	< 1.0
Protein SAA (serum amyloid A)	A1b[18a]	12,000	< 0.5[‡]

*These values are derived, for the most part, from reference 18.
[†]MW for Hp 1-1.
[‡]Derived from studies in the mouse.[19]

Mechanisms, Teleology, and Clinical Usefulness. The increase in concentration of acute phase proteins following inflammatory stimulus has been shown, in each instance in which it has been studied, to result from an increase in synthesis by hepatocytes,[1,2] with occasional implication of other sites as well. It is presumed that this increased synthesis results from the action of a mediator system, which originates at the site of tissue injury and ultimately affects the hepatocytes. Plasma changes characteristic of the acute phase response can be produced in experimental animals by injection of preparations derived from leukocytes and indistinguishable from interleukin I (and endogenous pyrogen).[25,26] More recently, monokines, products of activated macrophages, have been reported to induce increases in synthesis of mouse SAA, rat fibrinogen, and other acute phase proteins in hepatocyte culture systems. The SAA-inducing activity co-purified with and may be identical to interleukin I,[27] while the fibrinogen-inducing activity was attributed to a molecule of greater molecular size.[28] It is possible that different mechanisms are responsible for induction of different acute phase proteins.[28a]

Teleologic speculations would suggest that the changes in concentration of these proteins lead to improved functional capacity to cope with the consequences of tissue injury or infection in one way or another. Thus, one might presume that increased amounts of haptoglobin would result in an improved capacity to bind the hemoglobin released by destroyed erythrocytes; in addition to leading to removal of this potentially toxic substance from the circulation, such binding might exert a bacteriostatic effect on certain pathogenic bacteria.[29] Similarly, increased amounts of fibrinogen could provide additional substrate for clotting as well as for forming complexes with intravascular fibrin; ceruloplasmin might be useful during the course of inflammation because it displays superoxide dismutase activity;[30] and α_1-antitrypsin and α_1-antichymotrypsin would provide increased inhibition of protease activity. While such speculation seems reasonable, the precise role played by each of the acute phase proteins in the response to tissue injury is difficult to establish, since demonstration of in vitro effects is not always relevant to in vivo phenomena.

The most widely employed indicators of the acute phase response in clinical medicine are measurements of the erythrocyte sedimentation rate and of C-reactive protein concentration. The bulk of this chapter will deal with these two tests and their significance. The erythrocyte sedimentation rate may reflect alterations in concentration of some acute phase proteins, while C-reactive protein may be regarded as the quintessential acute phase protein. Their measurement has been employed clinically for determining the presence and the degree of inflammation, both in initial evaluation and in monitoring the course of disease in a given patient, where they may serve as guides to management.

ERYTHROCYTE SEDIMENTATION RATE

Introduction. In this test anticoagulated blood is placed in a vertical cylindrical tube and the rate of sedimentation of the erythrocytes is measured. It has been known since the time of the ancient Greeks that the sedimentation rate may be altered in disease states, and this test has been widely employed in clinical medicine for about 60 years. The continued widespread use of the erythrocyte sedimentation rate (ESR) results from its relative simplicity, its familiarity, and the wealth of information about its clinical significance that has accumulated over this period.[31] As with all elements of the acute phase response, abnormal findings do not have diagnostic specificity but may accompany many abnormal states. The ESR should be viewed as an indirect way of screening for increased concentrations of fibrinogen, and to a lesser extent, of other acute phase proteins; such changes cause increased aggregation of erythrocytes suspended in plasma, causing them to fall more rapidly.[32]

Mechanisms Governing the Rate of Erythrocyte Sedimentation. The major influence on the rate of sedimentation of red cells suspended in plasma is the degree to which they aggregate with one another. Our understanding of erythrocyte aggregation stems, to a large extent, from studies of the physicochemical aspects of antibody-induced hemagglutination.[33, 34] There are three major factors that influence erythrocyte aggregation: (1) the surface *free energy* of the cells, (2) the charge on the cells, and (3) the dielectric constant (Fig. 43–1).

The *surface free energy* (interfacial tension) of red cells results from van der Waals' forces and exerts a *cohesive force,* tending to attract the cells to one another.

The *charge on erythrocytes* is similar on all cells, and acts as a *repulsive force.* This red cell charge is itself the sum of the negative potentials due to the sialic acid components of the erythrocyte membrane and the oppositely charged cloud of ions that surrounds each erythrocyte. The resultant of these two groups of charges, called the zeta potential, exists on the outer edge of this cloud of cations and determines the force of repulsion between red cells. In normal individuals the zeta potential is great enough to overcome the cohesive van der Waals' forces, and little aggregation occurs.

The *dielectric constant* is not a property of the red cells but rather of the medium, in this instance the plasma, in which the cells are suspended. The dielectric constant measures the *charge dissipation characteristics* of the medium. It is influenced by the concentration and degree of asymmetry of the molecules dissolved in plasma, particularly the plasma proteins. The dielectric constant is raised when the concentration of molecules that can become oriented or polarized by the electric field of the red cells is increased. The more asymmetric the molecule, the more likely it is to be polarized. Thus, with an increase in concentration of such molecules, the increase in dielectric constant tends to diminish the repulsive effect of the zeta potential; the cohesive effects of the surface free energy predominate, and aggregation ensues.

When erythrocytes align themselves in aggregates that resemble a stack of coins (rouleaux), there is an increase in mass of each stack of erythrocytes out of proportion to the increase in surface area. The increase in downward forces is significantly greater than any concomitant opposing increase in the upward forces exerted by plasma, which retard red cell fall. As a result, the cells fall rapidly. The greater the number of erythrocytes in each aggregate, the more rapid the rate of fall.

Effects of Plasma Protein Abnormalities. Rouleaux formation and consequent elevation in ESR may result from either a moderate increase in concentration of extremely asymmetric proteins (such as fibrinogen) or a major increase in concentration of only moderately asymmetric molecules (such as the immunoglobulins). There are thus two classes of change in plasma proteins that may result in an elevation in ESR.[35] One is the acute phase response. Fibrinogen is the most asymmetric of the acute phase proteins present in substantial concentration in plasma and has the greatest effect on the ESR. Other acute phase proteins, and the immunoglobulins present in increased concentrations in chronic inflammatory states, show lesser degrees of asymmetry, and less of an effect on erythrocyte aggregation. The other class of plasma protein abnormalities leading to elevation of ESR is seen in multiple myeloma and Waldenström's macroglobulinemia. In these instances, elevation in ESR is primarily due to a massive increase in concentration of a single molecular species of immunoglobulin. It is not clear that plasma lipids have any effect on ESR.[36]

Effects of Erythrocyte Abnormalities and Drugs. Alterations in the shape and size of red blood cells influence the ability of these cells to form rouleaux. Anisocytosis, poikilocytosis (such as that seen in sickle cell anemia), microcytosis, spherocytosis, and acanthocytosis all physically interfere with rouleaux formation.[31] These erythrocyte abnormalities may result in the finding of a paradoxically normal ESR when major acute phase plasma protein abnormalities are, in fact, present. In addition, alterations in the concentration of erythrocytes may affect the ESR. Anemia appears to result in a more rapid rate of fall of red cells, while polycythemia may cause a very low ESR.

The administration of certain drugs to patients or their addition to blood may alter the ESR. It has recently been found that ESR is spuriously elevated when de-

Figure 43–1. Factors influencing erythrocyte aggregation and sedimentation.

termined on heparinized specimens of blood or on blood from heparinized patients.[37] In contrast, patients receiving high doses of sodium valproate have been found to show significantly reduced ESR;[38] the mechanism responsible for this change is uncertain.[39] A diurnal variation in ESR has been found to be related to ingestion of food.[40]

Methods of ESR Determination. Arguments have persisted over the decades about which of the various methods of ESR determination is the most reliable, and if (and how) correction for anemia should be performed. The former argument seems to have been resolved for the moment by the decision of the International Committee for Standardization in Hematology that the Westergren technique be designated as the standardized selected method.[41] Correction for anemia has now generally been abandoned. Wintrobe's textbook has summarized the reasons for doing so: Correcting for anemia is only approximate, and it is an artificial ultrarefinement. It is misleading, particularly since no correction is made for alterations in size and shape of erythrocytes, which may be more important.[42]

In the standard Westergren method, 2 ml of venous blood is collected in 0.5 ml of sodium citrate solution. The blood is drawn up to a level of 200 mm in the cylindrical Westergren tube, which is then placed vertically in a rack. At the end of 1 hour the height of the zone of clear plasma above the sedimented column of red cells is measured; this distance is the rate of fall, expressed as millimeters in the first hour.[41]

The upper limits of normal originally suggested by Westergren, 3 mm per hour for males and 7 mm per hour for females, are undoubtedly too low. Commonly accepted values for screening purposes in young adults are 15 mm per hour for males and 20 mm per hour for females. With aging, even higher values seem to be the norm, although specific standards are uncertain.[43] In one study, the distribution of ESR values was found to be skewed in an apparently healthy elderly population; 12 percent of such individuals showed values over 40 mm per hour.[44]

As an alternative to the Westergren method, the Wintrobe method is used today primarily in small laboratories, often in physicians' offices. Its major virtue is its great simplicity. No diluent is used; anticoagulated blood is merely added to a mark in a graduated tube, and the cells are permitted to fall for 1 hour.[42] There are three major drawbacks to this method: (1) The Wintrobe tube, only 100 mm long, is half the length of the Westergren tube. Therefore ESR values greater than about 60 mm per hour can rarely be measured, since further fall is impeded by packing of red blood cells. As a result, degrees of increase in ESR, and hence of severity of inflammation, cannot be distinguished. (2) In contrast to the Westergren method, it is not as clear that correction for anemia can be safely ignored; the results may thus be difficult to interpret. (3) The narrow bore of the Wintrobe tube may lead to nonreproducible results at times.

A "zeta sedimentation ratio" has been proposed as a method of measuring the effect of altered plasma protein concentrations on erythrocyte aggregation, while avoiding the necessity of correcting for anemia.[45] Since the main virtues of the ESR are simplicity and familiarity, it seems unlikely that this method, which requires a specialized centrifuge, will be widely adopted.

Clinical Significance. Elevation in ESR has no diagnostic specificity but tends to reflect the presence either of tissue injury and inflammation on the one hand or of certain lymphoproliferative disorders on the other, as discussed above. High ESR values are usually seen in bacterial infections. Mild viral infections are usually accompanied by a normal ESR, while patients with severe manifestations of viral infections (such as mumps orchitis or poliomyelitis) usually have a high ESR. In general, mild elevations reflect mild tissue alterations, while marked elevations reflect major tissue injury. In a number of protracted or chronic illnesses, the course of the disease process is reflected by the rise and fall of the ESR.

The ESR is often employed as a rough screening test, in which a normal finding tends to be reassuring, while an elevated ESR may lead to a search for a source of inflammation or tissue injury. It must be emphasized that a normal ESR does *not* by any means rule out the presence of disease. Similarly, markedly elevated ESR values are occasionally seen in patients in whom no specific diagnoses can be made and whose ESR subsequently returns to normal.[46, 47]

Several specific cases deserve mention. The ESR normally rises in the latter portion of pregnancy and occasionally in women taking oral contraceptives.[48] Elevation in ESR has been reported in several diseases not clearly accompanied by tissue necrosis, e.g., hypothyroidism and hyperthyroidism. In one study, individuals participating in a vigil involving stressful days and sleepless nights demonstrated a moderate but significant increase in ESR.[36] Some intramuscular injections, particularly benzathine penicillin, may cause a rise in ESR and CRP levels.[49] At times high ESR values may be due to red blood cell agglutinins.

The Current Status of the ESR. The use of the ESR has been attacked as unsuitable, imprecise, and outmoded for a variety of reasons: (1) It is impossible to correct accurately for alterations in size, shape, or concentration of erythrocytes. (2) The ESR is abnormal in the presence of monoclonal immunoglobulins as well as of acute phase proteins; an elevation does not necessarily reflect inflammation or tissue injury. (3) The ESR is merely an indirect reflection of acute phase protein concentration. Direct measurement of a number of acute phase proteins themselves is now readily available and is more valuable than the indirect information provided by the ESR. (4) Plasma viscosity is highly correlated with ESR. Measurement of viscosity itself, without the need to correct for anemia or red cell abnormalities, can provide a simpler screening test for those abnormalities detected by the ESR.[50] (5) There is uncertainty about the effect of age and sex on the ESR; no one is quite sure what the range of normal is. (6) Serum C-reactive protein levels rise and fall faster than ESR and reflect the current status of a patient more accurately.[51] All these criticisms are true. Nonetheless, the ESR still manages to maintain an important place in medical practice. In the current era of sophisticated and automated laboratory testing, the fact that a practitioner can easily perform this familiar test himself in the simplest of laboratory settings probably assures a place for the ESR for some time to come.

C-REACTIVE PROTEIN

History, Structure, and Function. C-reactive protein (CRP) owes its name to the circumstances surrounding its discovery. It was originally detected in human serum because of its ability to precipitate with the somatic C-polysaccharide of the pneumococcus in the presence of calcium ion.[52,53] Although this method is no longer used to detect this protein, the name persists. CRP was felt for many years to be absent from normal sera, appearing only in response to inflammation. However, it has recently been shown to be present in trace amounts in all subjects,[54,55] the concentration rising dramatically after tissue injury. CRP has an electrophoretic mobility on paper in the rapid γ range. It is an aggregate of five apparently identical noncovalently linked subunits arranged in cyclic symmetry[56] (Fig. 43–2). Based on studies of its primary structure, a molecular weight of 105,000 daltons can be computed.[57] There is substantial homology of amino acid sequence between CRP and the plasma protein which appears to be the precursor of the amyloid P component, protein SAP.[58] Both CRP and SAP display a pentameric structure,[56] and both demonstrate calcium-dependent ligand-binding properties.[59] SAP is not a noteworthly acute phase protein in man;[60] even when acute phase behavior has been claimed, mean increases less than 25 percent have been found.[61]

The likelihood that CRP plays a significant biologic role is supported by the conservation of this protein over hundreds of millions of years of evolution; proteins demonstrating characteristics of CRP have been demonstrated in a variety of lower animals, including chickens, many species of fish, including some dogfish, and the horseshoe crab *Limulus polyphema*.[62,63] However, it is of interest that CRP does not demonstrate acute phase behavior in many of these species.[3a]

The magnitude and rapidity of the CRP response in man also suggest that an important physiologic role is played by this protein. While the precise functions of CRP during the acute phase are not known, this protein has been shown to exhibit a large number of in vitro recognition and activation functions with the potential for influencing inflammation and other defense mechanisms.[64] Among the recognition functions are binding to phosphocholine moieties, galactans, and polycations. The complexing of human CRP to its ligands leads to

Figure 43–2. Electron micrograph of CRP molecule. (Courtesy of Dr. Henry Gewurz).

activation of the complement system, initiating all of the major known complement-dependent reactivites.[65] Binding of CRP to phospholipase A–treated erythrocytes, rabbit erythrocyte ghosts and model membrane lipid systems has been shown.[66] In addition, binding of ligand-complexed CRP to subsets of peripheral blood monocytes has been reported; this interaction may promote complement-dependent phagocytosis by mononuclear phagocytes.[67] About 3 percent of peripheral blood lymphocytes bind such complexed CRP.[68] Thermally modified CRP is reported to cause platelet aggregation and secretion.[69] Evidence has been presented suggesting that some natural killer cells bear surface CRP,[70,71] that CRP can inhibit T lymphocyte-dependent antibody formation,[72] and that liposome-bound CRP can activate macrophages.[73]

In contrast to the large number of in vitro functional capabilities that have been reported for CRP, relatively few in vivo studies have been reported. CRP has been shown to deposit in areas of necrosis in inflammatory lesions but not in adjacent normal tissue.[74,75] Passively administered human CRP has been found to increase survival in mice infected with *S. pneumoniae*.[76,77] Liposome-bound CRP has been shown to inhibit tumor growth in mice.[78] The pattern of organ sequestration and clearance of injected erythrocytes in mice has been found to be altered if CRP is bound to these cells.[79]

This plethora of observations makes it unlikely that CRP serves only a single function and strongly suggests that CRP plays a broad range of physiologic roles in response to tissue injury and infection. However, precise delineation of the extent of its involvement in physiologic events in vivo is still not possible. Several of these observations, taken together, have led to the suggestion that *one* role of CRP might be to combine with phospholipid constituents of necrotic cell membranes at inflammatory sites; such binding would lead to adherence of phagocytic cells and to activation of the complement system, with consequent formation of mediators of inflammation and eventual phagocytosis and removal of damaged tissue.[64,65,80]

Role of CRP in Disease. Only a few reports have thus far suggested that CRP participates in the pathogenesis of human disease. Evidence has been presented indicating that CRP plays a role in causing hemolytic disease following envenomation by the brown recluse spider,[81] and in the formation of microemboli following administration of intravenous fat emulsions.[82] The demonstration that interaction of CRP with urate crystals may lead to complement activation suggests that this mechanism might contribute to the precipitation of acute gouty attacks following surgical and other stresses.[83]

Magnitude and Time Course of the CRP Response. The true range of normal for serum CRP levels has not been defined precisely, and may never be, since minor degrees of injury occurring in normal individuals in the course of everyday life probably cause slight degrees of CRP elevation. Concentrations less than 0.01 mg per deciliter are commonly found in umbilical cord sera, and many adults show levels less than 0.05 mg per dl.[55] While most apparently healthy individuals have CRP levels of less than 0.2 mg per dl, concentrations as high as 1 mg per dl are found frequently enough in such normal subjects[54,55,84,85] to justify regarding concentrations lower than this value as clinically insignificant.[20]

Following a variety of acute inflammatory stimuli, a sharp increase in serum concentration of CRP is noted, usually beginning within a few hours. In a group of patients with acute myocardial infarction, for example, a mean serum doubling time of about 8 hours was noted[86] (Fig. 43–3). The rise in serum concentration is caused by a progressive increase in the number of CRP-forming hepatocytes, with a resulting increase in rate of hepatic CRP synthesis.[87] The magnitude of the CRP rise reflects the extent of tissue injury; more extensive lesions cause longer periods of rising CRP levels and higher CRP concentrations.[86] As a useful approximation, concentrations of less than 1 mg per dl may be regarded as normal or as insignificant elevations; concentrations between 1 and 10 mg per dl, as *moderate* increases; and concentrations over 10 mg per dl, as *marked* increases.[20] Patients with severe acute inflammatory states may attain serum CRP levels of 20 mg per dl or greater; values greater than 30 mg per dl are occasionally seen. Such values are over 1000 times the concentrations found in many normal individuals. No other acute phase protein, with the exception of protein SAA, is known to increase its concentration this markedly.

Serum CRP levels generally reach a peak in 2 or 3 days following acute stimuli and then fall relatively rapidly. In a number of patients, CRP levels have been found to fall to half their peak concentrations within 24 hours, following effective control of the inflammatory stimulus,[88] and studies in rabbits indicate a serum half life of about 4 to 6 hours.[89] However, persistently elevated serum CRP concentrations are often seen in chronic inflammatory states such as pulmonary tuberculosis or active rheumatoid arthritis, or in the presence of extensive malignant disease.

Methods of CRP Detection. Early methods for detection of CRP made use of the relatively insensitive method of precipitation with C-polysaccharide or of the capacity of CRP to cause nonspecific capsular swelling of type 27 pneumococci.[90] Purification and crystallization of CRP in 1947, with subsequent raising of specific antisera, permitted immunochemical detection of this protein.[91] The first such method, and one still widely used, was the capillary precipitin technique, which represented a substantial improvement over previous methods.[92] However, this method is only semiquantitative and is relatively insensitive. Subsequently, the radial and electroimmunodiffusion techniques have permitted accurate quantitation of as little as 0.2 mg per dl.[93]

While sensitive radioimmunoassays have been developed,[55,84] their high degree of sensitivity is not necessary for clinical purposes; radial immunodiffusion and electroimmunodiffusion methods are sufficiently sensitive and provide quantitative data in the range of clinical significance. Newly developed nephelometric methods and enzyme immunoassays are likely to find widespread use as a result of the speed with which results are obtainable.[94-96] In light of the availability of quantitative methods, nonquantitative procedures such as the capillary precipitin test and latex agglutination methods must be regarded as of limited value; their replacement by quantitative techniques will greatly enhance the clinical value of CRP determination.[20]

Clinical Significance of Rise in CRP Levels. Unfor-

Figure 43–3. Serum CRP response in a representative patient with acute myocardial infarction. Note rapidity of rise and fall in this semilogarithmic plot. (From Kushner, I. et al.: J. Clin. Invest. *61*:235, 1978.)

tunately, most published studies of the clinical significance of serum CRP determinations were carried out before quantitative methods were available, and results were frequently expressed as the "presence" or "absence" of CRP. The precise clinical value of CRP determinations must be redefined using quantitative methods; such studies are increasingly being reported.[20, 97]

Generally speaking, CRP elevation occurs in the variety of infectious, traumatic, and inflammatory states enumerated in the introductory paragraphs of this chapter. Mildly elevated levels are found in sera of a small percentage of pregnant women at term. CRP is rarely elevated in cord blood. However, the majority of neonates will demonstrate elevated levels by the third postpartum day, presumably in response to umbilical cord necrosis.[98] The prevalence of significantly elevated CRP levels found in population surveys does not vary with age.[99] Serial determinations showing elevation in CRP above baseline levels are more likely to be significant than a single elevated reading, especially on a background of chronic inflammation. However, values greater than 10 mg per dl should raise the possibility of bacterial infection.[20] It is important that CRP levels be interpreted with caution in light of the rapid changes that occur from day to day and hour to hour.[86]

OTHER ACUTE PHASE REACTANTS

Early methods of assessing the acute phase response included a variety of measurements reflecting the concentrations of the large number of glycoproteins among the acute phase proteins: serum seromucoids, protein-bound hexose, hexosamine, sialic acid, and glucosamine. These determinations are rarely employed today. A frequently observed acute phase finding is elevation of the α_2- and, to a lesser extent, the α_1-globulin fractions on serum protein electrophoresis. Such changes usually reflect an increase in concentration of the many acute phase proteins with α-globulin electrophoretic mobilities.

Although an increase in concentration of any of the proteins listed in Table 43-1 might be expected to reflect inflammatory states, they are rarely studied with that end in mind. None of these offers an advantage over CRP determination; their concentrations rise more slowly, and the magnitude of rise is nowhere near as great, except for SAA.[21,100,101] SAA levels are said to be increased in apparently healthy elderly individuals,[102] although one report casts doubt on this claim.[103] Haptoglobin levels may be normal in the presence of inflammation if concomitant intravascular hemolysis is present. Similarly, serum ferritin levels, normally elevated in inflammatory states,[104] may be normal or may be depressed in the presence of concomitant iron deficiency. Consumption coagulopathies may lead to decreased fibrinogen levels, even in the presence of inflammation.

CLINICAL VALUE OF ASSESSMENT OF ACUTE PHASE REACTANTS

General Comments. While most studies of the clinical value of acute phase reactants have dealt with the ESR, critical quantitative studies of CRP have recently begun to be reported.[20,97] Studies of the relationship between ESR and CRP have uniformly suggested that CRP levels correlate better with degree of activity in rheumatoid arthritis and ankylosing spondylitis than does ESR.[105-107] Nonetheless, the continued use of the ESR in clinical medicine can be defended as long as its limitations and drawbacks are understood.[108,109] In general, assessment of the acute phase proteins is only occasionally of value in diagnosis. It is more often helpful in the management of rheumatic diseases by aiding in monitoring of disease activity during therapy.

The detection of elevated ESR or CRP levels in patients who do not present a clear-cut clinical picture suggests a significant inflammatory element to their illness, and renders diagnoses of psychogenic or trivial maladies less likely. On the other hand, relatively normal ESR or CRP levels may permit limited reassurance, if no alarming findings are noted on physical examination or other laboratory testing. Assessment of acute phase reactants is of limited value in management of conditions in which it is possible to monitor the target organ injury reasonably well, as in polymyositis, or in which there are serologic abnormalities highly correlated with activity of disease, as in systemic lupus erythematosus. In a number of illnesses, however, such ancillary clinical guides are lacking. In these patients, study of the acute phase reactants may be of value in allowing adjustment of drug dosage to the level of disease activity.

Importance of Quantitative CRP Determination. It is now apparent that description of serum CRP levels as simply "elevated" provides inadequate information and that differing degrees of CRP elevation have different implications.[20] To be clinically valuable, CRP levels should be expressed quantitatively. For example, while serum CRP levels are elevated in both Behçet's disease and Still's disease, CRP elevation in Behçet's disease is usually modest, levels rarely exceeding 2 mg/dl,[110] while CRP levels as high as 20 mg per dl may occur in Still's disease.[106]

Most chronic inflammatory diseases are accompanied by mild or moderate elevations in serum CRP concentrations. In general, CRP levels parallel disease severity as assessed clinically.[107,111,112] Thus, in juvenile arthritis, systemic (Still's) disease is generally accompanied by marked CRP elevation, polyarticular disease by a moderate increase, and pauciarticular disease by a very modest increase.[107] CRP levels average about 3 to 4 mg per dl in adult rheumatoid arthritis patients with moderate disease activity, but there is considerable variation: about 7 percent of such patients have values in the normal range, while a few patients with severe active disease show levels of 14 mg per dl or more.[107,113] In active ankylosing spondylitis CRP levels generally range between 2 and 3 mg per deciliter.[113]

Specific Diseases. In the following paragraphs several rheumatologic diseases have been chosen to illustrate some clinical situations in which evaluation of the acute phase response may be of value, or to illuminate areas of controversy.

Rheumatoid Arthritis. A time-honored method of distinguishing rheumatoid arthritis from other varieties of arthritis, particularly osteoarthritis, is the detection of an elevated ESR. Today this finding must be regarded as of limited value for a variety of reasons. Not all patients with rheumatoid arthritis have elevated ESR. Many of the diseases from which rheumatoid arthritis must frequently be differentiated are themselves often accompanied by an elevated ESR. Most patients with osteoarthritis are in an age group in which an elevated ESR is frequently found as a result of associated diseases, and aging itself is not infrequently associated with elevated ESR.[44] Finally, as a result of better and more widespread training in rheumatology, clinicians are frequently more perspicacious than was formerly the case; our experience is that careful physical examination and assessment of other laboratory findings usually permit the diagnosis of rheumatoid arthritis to be made without the need for determination of ESR, or in the presence of a normal ESR.

Several authors have reported that a relatively good prognosis is suggested by detection of low ESR values early in the course of rheumatoid arthritis, but there is controversy about this point.[114-116] In general, a high ESR at onset is correlated with a relatively poor prognosis.[117] Paradoxically, a very high ESR, in association with severe, acute onset of polyarthritis, has been correlated with a favorable prognosis.[114,115] This clinical presentation may possibly represent a subgroup within the spectrum of conditions currently regarded as seronegative rheumatoid arthritis.

The true value of determination of acute phase reactants such as ESR and CRP in the evaluation of new drugs for rheumatoid arthritis is uncertain. The major criteria employed in evaluation of such drugs have tended to be signs and symptoms, assessed as objectively as possible. However, in a number of studies, improvement in acute phase reactants has been accepted as reflecting the beneficial effect of a drug quite independent of changes in signs or symptoms. Thus, the ESR is the most important laboratory criterion in the American Rheumatism Association criteria for determining remission.[118] Such measurement has the virtue of being totally objective, in contrast to the symptoms and physical findings usually evaluated. In addition, a fall in acute phase reactants probably reflects greater degrees of improvement in elements of the local inflammatory process than does clinical improvement without an accompanying fall in acute phase reactants.

However, arguments have been advanced suggesting that improvement in acute phase reactants has more fundamental implications, and that a drug that lowers levels of acute phase reactants influences underlying pathogenic mechanisms rather than merely modifying the inflammatory process.[119] Viewed in this way, drugs that lower acute phase reactants can be felt to have induced remission. Support for the view that slow-acting, suppressive agents,[120] such as gold and penicillamine, actually are capable of modifying the natural history of disease is based at least in part on the observation that serum CRP levels frequently fall in patients manifesting clinical improvement on treatment with these drugs,[121] while they usually do not in those receiving nonsteroidal anti-inflammatory drugs.[122] In addition, higher CRP levels have been correlated with progressive erosive disease.[123,124]

Taken together, these considerations have suggested to some that erosive and destructive disease is less likely to occur if ESR or CRP are returned to normal,[123,124] that nonsteroidal anti-inflammatory drugs will not achieve this goal in most patients, and that in such instances drugs such as gold, which is capable of lowering acute phase protein levels, be employed.[125] This view presumes that improvement in acute phase reactants on treatment indicates that a remission has been induced[119] and that progressive joint destruction will be retarded or prevented. However, it is at least equally likely that improvement in acute phase reactants merely reflects the *degree* of suppression of inflammation rather than a basic, qualitative alteration of the fundamental disease process. At present, there is insufficient evidence to conclude with assurance that treatment that lowers acute phase reactants to normal will affect the chronic inflammatory mechanisms that lead to destruction of bone and cartilage. Only prospective drug studies and correlation with radiographic changes will permit such a conclusion.[126]

Polymyalgia Rheumatica and Giant Cell Arteritis. The diagnoses of polymyalgia rheumatica (PMR) and of the associated condition giant cell arteritis (GCA) are supported by finding an elevated ESR, often over 100 mm per hour.[127,128] Although ESR elevation is widely and falsely regarded as a sine qua non of these states, it should be pointed out that periodic reports continue to appear describing patients with PMR and GCA who have normal ESR.[128-130] The detection of extreme elevation of ESR in the absence of symptoms of PMR or GCA is not likely to be due to these states; the majority of such patients have underlying infection or malignancy.[46,47,131]

In patients with PMR or GCA, the return of the ESR to normal levels following initial treatment usually indicates that inflammation has been brought under control. In such patients, overt clinical manifestations of disease activity may be absent or subtle during subsequent attempts to decrease the dose of therapeutic agents, institute alternate-day corticosteroid therapy, or discontinue therapy. Disease activity may be monitored by following the ESR; elevation would suggest recurrence of activity and call for more aggressive therapy. Of course, clinical manifestations of disease, even in the presence of a normal ESR, should not be ignored.

Ankylosing Spondylitis. When the diagnosis of ankylosing spondylitis is considered, usually in young individuals with unexplained chronic backache and no history of trauma, the finding of an elevated ESR or CRP might support this diagnosis, being present in about 75 percent of patients with active spondylitis.[113] However, other studies would be required to confirm the diagnosis.[132]

Systemic Lupus Erythematosus. Determination of ESR has generally been felt to be of some value in the management of systemic lupus erythematosus (SLE).[132a] However, there is controversy about the value of CRP determination in patients with this disease. Two issues have been raised.[3a] (1) Are serum CRP levels sufficiently different in systemic lupus erythematosus and rheumatoid arthritis (RA) to play a diagnostically useful role in distinguishing between these diseases? (2) Is CRP elevation in lupus patients an indication of infection, or may it be due to lupus itself?

CRP levels are elevated above the normal range in most patients with active SLE and tend to fall and rise as the disease improves or becomes more active. However, a number of patients with active SLE do not show CRP elevation, and median CRP levels in series of patients with SLE have been found to be lower than in RA patients who are felt to have comparable degrees of disease, leading to the suggestion that CRP levels be employed as a diagnostic criterion.[133,134] However, comparing degree of severity in these two diseases is difficult, a bit like comparing apples and oranges, since they differ in their clinical manifestations, the major organs involved, and, undoubtedly, in their pathogenesis. Since the precise mechanisms linking the CRP response to tissue injury and inflammation are unknown, it is difficult to estimate what degree of CRP elevation ought to be expected in a given patient. Serum CRP levels may be quite elevated in some patients with SLE,[123,135-138] especially those with acute serositis and chronic synovitis, and may be normal in many rheumatoids.[113,124] The use of serum CRP levels as a diagnostic criterion does not seem to be a practical suggestion, in view of the considerable overlap in CRP concentrations observed between SLE and RA patients and the finding that CRP levels are only minimally elevated in many patients with mild to moderate RA.[107,113]

The second issue, the suggestion that CRP elevation in the course of SLE is more likely to be due to superimposed bacterial infection than to activation of lupus, can be confronted more clearly if CRP levels are expressed in quantitative terms; "elevated" has little precise meaning. It has now become clear that markedly elevated serum CRP levels are seen most frequently, but not exclusively, with bacterial infection.[20] Occurrence in the course of SLE of CRP levels in excess of 6 to 8 mg per dl should serve as a stimulus to rule out the possibility of infection. However, such values should not be regarded as proof of such infection; marked CRP elevation due to SLE is not infrequently seen.[133,135-139]

Acute Rheumatic Fever. Treatment of acute rheumatic fever with salicylates or corticosteroids results in a return of acute phase reactants toward normal. Elevations of ESR or CRP are often seen after cessation of a standard course of anti-inflammatory therapy. In the absence of clinical signs or symptoms of rheumatic activity these can be regarded as "laboratory rebounds," are usually transient, and can generally be left untreated. It should be noted that the ESR is frequently normal when Sydenham's chorea appears as a manifestation of rheumatic activity.

References

1. Kushner, I.: The phenomenon of the acute phase response. Ann. N.Y. Acad. Sci. 389:39, 1982.
2. Koj, A.: Acute phase reactants. *In* Allison, A.C. (ed.): Structure and Function of plasma proteins. Vol. 1. London and New York, Plenum Press, 1974, pp. 73–131.
3. Kushner, I., Volanakis, J., and Gewurz, H. (eds.): C-reactive protein and the plasma protein response to tissue injury. Ann. N.Y. Acad. Sci. 389:1, 1982.
3a. Pepys, M.B., and Baltz, M.L.: Acute phase proteins with special reference to C-reactive protein and related proteins (pentoxins) and serum amyloid A protein. Adv. Immunol. 34:141, 1983.
4. Coombes, F.J., Shakespeare, P.G., and Batstone, G.F.: Lipoprotein changes after burn injury in man. J. Trauma 20:971, 1980.
5. Cabana, V.G., Gewurz, H., and Siegel, J.N.: Inflammation-induced changes in rabbit CRP and plasma lipoproteins. J. Immunol. 130:1736, 1983.
6. Falchuk, K.H.: Effect of acute disease and ACTH on serum zinc proteins. N. Engl. J. Med. 296:1129, 1977.
7. Konijn, A.M., and Hershko, C.: Ferritin synthesis in inflammation. I. Pathogenesis of impaired iron release. Br. J. Haematol. 37:7, 1977.
8. Torrance, J.D., Charlton, R.W., Simon M.O., Lynch, S.R., and Bothwell, T.H.: The mechanism of endotoxin-induced hypoferremia. Scand. J. Haematol. 21:403, 1978.
9. Saba, T.M., and Jaffe, E.: Plasma fibronectin (opsonic glycoprotein); its synthesis by vascular endothelial cells and role in cardiopulmonary integrity after trauma as related to reticuloendothelial function. Am. J. Med. 68:577, 1980.
10. Deno, D.C., McCafferty, M.H., Saba, T.M., and Blumenstock, F.A.: Mechanism of depletion of plasma fibronectin after burn injury. Fed. Proc. 42:1035, 1983.
11. Constantian, M.B., Menzoian, J.O., Nimberg, R.B., Schmid, K., and Mannick, J.A.: Association of a circulating immunosuppressive polypeptide with operative and accidental trauma. Ann. Surg. 185:73, 1977.
12. Lentnek, A.L., Schreiber, A.D., and MacGregor, R.R.: The induction of augmented granulocyte adherence by inflammation: mediation by a plasma factor. J. Clin. Invest. 57:1098, 1976.
13. Clowes, G.H.A., Jr., George, B.C., Villee, C.A., Jr., and Saravis, C.A.: Muscle proteolysis induced by a circulating peptide in patients with sepsis or trauma. N. Engl. J. Med. 308:545, 1983.
14. George, B.C., Clowes, G.H.A., Jr., Saranis, C., Heideman, M., and Lane, B.: Plasma proteolysis inducing factor produced by human macrophages. Fed. Proc. 42:1039, 1983.
15. Oppenheim, J.J., and Gery, I.: Interleukin 1 is more than an interleukin. Immuno. Today 3:113, 1982.
16. Baracos, V., Rodemann, H.P., Dinarello, C.A., and Goldgerg, A.L.: Stimulation of muscle protein degradation and prostaglandin E_2 release by leukocytic pyrogen (interleukin-1): a mechanism for the increased degradation of muscle proteins during fever. N. Engl. J. Med. 308:553, 1983.
17. Biesel, W.R.: Mediators of fever and muscle proteolysis. N. Engl. J. Med. 308:586, 1983.
18. Putnam, F.W.: Alpha, beta, gamma, omega—the roster of the plasma proteins. *In* Putnam, F.W. (ed.): The Plasma proteins: Structure, function and genetic control. 2nd ed. Vol I. New York, Academic Press, 1975, pp. 58–131.
18a. Teppo, A.M., Maury, C.P., and Wegelius, O.: Characteristics of the amyloid A fibril-degrading activity of human serum. Scand. J. Immunol. 16:309, 1982.
19. Hoffman, J.S., and Benditt, E.P.: Changes in high density lipoprotein content following endotoxin administration in the mouse. J. Biol. Chem. 257:10510, 1982.
20. Morley, J.J., and Kushner, I.: Serum C-reactive protein levels in disease. Ann. N.Y. Acad. Sci. 389:406, 1982.
21. McAdam, K.P.W.J., Elin, R.J., Sipe, J.D., and Wolff, S.M.: Changes in human serum amyloid A and C-reactive protein after etiocholanolone-induced inflammation. J. Clin. Invest. 61:390, 1978.
22. Salonen, E-M., and Vaheri, A.: C-reactive protein in acute viral infections. J. Med. Virol. 8:161, 1981.
23. Shainkin-Kestenbaum, R., Zimlichman, S., Winikoff, Y., Pras, M., Chaimovitz, C., and Sarov, I.: Serum amyloid A (SAA) in viral infection:

rubella, measles and subacute sclerosing panencephalitis (SSPE). Clin. Exp. Immunol. 50:503, 1982.

24. Shainkin-Kestenbaum, R., Zimlichman, S., Winikoff, Y., and Chaimovitz, C.: Serum amyloid A levels in patients with infections due to cytomegalovirus, varicella-zoster virus, and herpes simplex virus. J. Infect. Dis. 146:443, 1982.

24a. Liesen, H., Dufaux, B., and Hollman, W.: Modifications of serum glycoproteins the day following a prolonged physical exercise and the influence of physical training. Europ. J. Appl. Physiol. 37:243, 41977.

25. Bornstein, D.L.: Leukocytic pyrogen: a major mediator of the acute phase reaction. Ann. N.Y. Acad. Sci. 389:323, 1982.

26. Kampschmidt, R.F., Upchurch, H.F., and Pulliam, L.A.: Characterization of a leukocyte-derived endogenous mediator responsible for increased plasma fibrinogen. Ann. N.Y. Acad. Sci. 389:338, 1982.

27. Sztein, M.B., Vogel, S.N., Sipe, J.D., Murphy, P.A., Mizel, S.B., Oppenheim, J.J., and Rosenstreich, D.L.: The role of macrophages in the acute-phase response: SAA inducer is closely related to lymphocyte activating factor and endogenous pyrogen. Cellular Immunol. 63:164, 1981.

28. Ritchie, D.G., and Fuller, G.M.: Hepatocyte stimulating factor: a monocyte-derived acute-phase regulatory protein. Ann. N.Y. Acad. Sci., 408:490, 1983.

28a. Baumann, H., Jahreis, G.P., and Gaines, K.C.: Synthesis and regulation of acute phase proteins in primary cultures of mouse hepatocytes. J. Cell. Biol. 97:866, 1983.

29. Eaton, J.W., Brandt, P., Mahoney, J.R., and Lee, J.T., Jr.: Haptoglobin: A natural bacteriostat. Science 215:691, 1982.

30. Goldstein, I.M., Kaplan, M.B., Edelson, H.S., and Weismann, G.: Ceruloplasmin: a scavenger of superoxide anion radicals. J. Biol. Chem. 254:4040, 1979.

31. Lascari, A.D.: The erythrocyte sedimentation rate. Pediatr. Clin. North Am. 19:1113, 1972.

32. Rovel, A., L'Huillier, J.F., and Vigneron, C.: Mechanisms of erythrocyte sedimentation. Biomedicine 28:248, 1978.

33. Pollack, W.: Some physicochemical aspects of hemagglutination. Ann. N.Y. Acad. Sci. 127:892, 1965.

34. Pollack, W., Hager, H.J., Reckel, R., Toren, D.A., and Singher, H.O.: A study of the forces involved in the second stage of hemagglutination. Transfusion 5:158, 1965.

35. Talstad, I., and Haugen, H.F.: The relationship between the erythrocyte sedimentation rate (ESR) and plasma proteins in clinical materials and models. Scand. J. Clin. Lab. Invest. 39:519, 1979.

36. Palmblad, J., Karlsson, C.-G., Levi, L., and Lidberg, L.: The erythrocyte sedimentation rate and stress. Acta. Med. Scand. 205:517, 1979.

37. Penchas, S., Stern, Z., and Bar-or, D.: Heparin and the ESR. Arch. Intern. Med. 138:1864, 1978.

38. Nutt, J.G., Neophytides, A.N., and Lodish, J.R.: Lowered erythrocyte-sedimentation rate with sodium valproate. Lancet 2:636, 1978.

39. Hutchinson, R.M., Clay, C.M., Simpson, M.R., and Wood, J.K.: Lowered erythrocyte-sedimentation rate with sodium valproate. Lancet 2:1309, 1978.

40. Mallya, R.K., Berry, H., Mace, B.E.W., deBeer, F.C., and Pepys, M.B.: Diurnal variation of erythrocyte sedimentation rate related to feeding. Lancet 1:389, 1982.

41. International Committee for Standardization in Hematology: Recommendation for measurement of erythrocyte sedimentation rate of human blood. Am. J. Clin. Pathol. 68:505, 1977.

42. Wintrobe, M.W., Lee, G.R., Boggs, D.R., Bithell, T.C., Athens, J.W., and Foerster, J.: Clinical Hematology. 7th ed. Philadelphia, Lea & Febiger, 1974.

43. Hayes, G.S., and Stinson, I.N.: Erythrocyte sedimentation rate and age. Arch. Ophthalmol. 94:939, 1976.

44. Sharland, D.E.: Erythrocyte sedimentation rate: the normal range in the elderly. J. Am. Geriatrics Soc. 28:346, 1980.

45. Editorial: E.S.R. or Z.S.R. Lancet 1:1394, 1976.

46. Zacharski, L.R., and Kyle, R.A.: Significance of extreme elevation of erythrocyte sedimentation rate. JAMA 202:264, 1967.

47. Ford, M.J., Innes, J.A., Parrish, F.M., Allan, N.C., Horn, D.B., and Munro, J.F.: The significance of gross elevations of the erythrocyte sedimentation rate in a general medical unit. Eur. J. Clin. Invest. 9:191, 1979.

48. Burton, J.L.: Effect of oral contraceptives on erythrocyte sedimentation rate in healthy young women. Br. Med. J. 3:214, 1967.

49. Haas, R.C., Taranta, A., and Wood, H.F.: Effect of intramuscular injections of benzathine penicillin G on some acute-phase reactants. N. Engl. J. Med. 256:152, 1957.

50. Hutchinson, R.M., and Eastham, R.D.: A comparison of the erythrocyte sedimentation rate and plasma viscosity in detecting changes in plasma proteins. J. Clin. Pathol. 30:345, 1977.

51. Editorial: C-reactive protein or E.S.R.? Lancet 2:1166, 1977.

52. Tillett, W.S., and Francis, T., Jr.: Serologic reactions in pneumonia with a non-protein somatic fraction of pneumococcus. J. Exp. Med. 52:561, 1930.

53. McCarty, M.: Historical perspective on C-reactive protein. Ann. N.Y. Acad. Sci. 389:1, 1982.

54. Kindmark, C.-O.: The concentration of C-reactive protein in sera from healthy individuals. Scand. J. Clin. Lab. Invest. 29:407, 1972.

55. Claus, D.R., Osmand, A.P., and Gewurz, H.: Radioimmunoassay of human C-reactive protein and levels in normal sera. J. Lab. Clin. Med. 87:120, 1976.

56. Osmand, A.P., Friedenson, B., Gewurz, H., Painter, R.H., Hoffman, T., and Shelton, E.: Characterization of C-reactive protein and the complement subcomponent Clt as homologous proteins displaying cyclic pentameric symmetry (pentraxins). Proc. Natl. Acad. Sci. USA 74:739, 1977.

57. Oliveira, E.B., Gotschlich, E.C., and Liu, T.Y.: Primary structure of human C-reactive protein. Proc. Natl. Acad. Sci. USA 74:3148, 1977.

58. Anderson, J.K., and Mole, J.E.: Large scale isolation and partial primary structure of human plasma amyloid P-component. Ann. N.Y. Acad. Sci. 389:216, 1982.

59. Pepys, M.B., Dash, A.C., Munn, E.A., Feinstein, A., Skinner, M., Cohen, A.S., Gewurz, H., Osmand, A.P., and Painter, R.H.: Isolation of amyloid P component (protein AP) from normal serum as a calcium-dependent binding protein. Lancet 1:1029, 1977.

60. Pepys, M.B., Dash, A.C., Markham, R.E., Thomas, H.C., Williams, B.D., and Petrie, A.: Comparative clinical study of protein SAP (amyloid P component) and C-reactive protein in serum. Clin. Exp. Immunol. 32:119, 1978.

61. Levo, Y., Ehrenfeld, M., and Wollner, S.: Serum amyloid P-component levels in rheumatoid arthritis. Isr. J. Med. Sci. 18:715, 1982.

62. Baltz, M.L., deBeer, F.C., Feinstein, A., Munn, E.A., Milstein, C.P., Fletcher, T.C., March, J.F., Taylor, J., Bruton, C., Clamp, J.R., Davies, A.J.S., and Pepys, M.B.: Phylogenetic aspects of C-reactive protein and related proteins. Ann. N.Y. Acad. Sci. 389:49, 1982.

63. Liu, T.-Y., Robey, F.A., and Wang, C.-M.: Structural studies on C-reactive protein. Ann. N.Y. Acad. Sci. 389:151, 1982.

64. Gewurz, H., Mold, C., Siegel, J., and Fiedel, B.: C-reactive protein and the acute phase response. Adv. Intern. Med. 27:345, 1982.

65. Volanakis, J.E.: Complement activation by C-reactive protein complexes. Ann. N.Y. Acad. Sci. 389:235, 1982.

66. Narkates, A.J., and Volanakis, J.E.: C-reactive protein binding specificities: artificial and natural phospholipid bilayers. Ann. N.Y. Acad. Sci. 389:172, 1982.

67. Mortensen, R.F., Osmand, A.P., Lint, T.F., and Gewurz, H.: Interaction of C-reactive protein with lymphocytes and monocytes: complement-dependent adherence and phagocytosis. J. Immunol. 117:774, 1976.

68. James, K., Baum, L.L., Vetter, M.L., and Gewurz, H.: Interactions of C-reactive protein with lymphoid cells. Ann. N.Y. Acad. Sci. 389:274, 1982.

69. Fiedel, B.A., Simpson, R.M., and Gewurz, H.: Effects of C-reactive protein (CRP) on platelet function. Ann. N.Y. Acad. Sci. 389:263, 1982.

70. Baum, L.L., James, K.K., Glaviano, R.R., and Gewurz, H.: Possible role for C-reactive protein in the human natural killer cell response. J. Exp. Med. 157:301, 1983.

71. James, K.K., Baum, L.L., Adamowski, C., and Gewurz, H.: C-reactive protein antigenicity on the surface of human lymphocytes. J. Immunol. 131:2930, 1983.

72. Mortensen, R.F.: Inhibition of the polyclonal antibody plaque-forming cell response of human B lymphocytes by C-reactive protein (CRP) and CRP complexes. Cell. Immunol. 66:99, 1982.

73. Barna, B.P., Deodhar, S.D., Gautam, S., Yen-Lieberman, B., and Roberts, D.: Macrophage activation and generation of tumoricidal activity by liposome-associated human C-reactive protein (CRP). Cancer Research, 44:305, 1984.

74. Kushner, I., and Kaplan, M.H.: Studies of acute phase protein: I. An immunohistochemical method for the localization of Cx-reactive protein in rabbits: association with necrosis in local inflammatory lesions. J. Exp. Med. 114:961, 1961.

75. DuClos, T.W., Mold, C., Paterson, P.Y., Alroy, J., and Gewurz, H.: Localization of C-reactive protein in inflammatory lesions of experimental allergic encephalomyelitis. Clin. Exp. Immunol. 43:565, 1981.

76. Mold, C., Nakayama, S., Holzer, T.J., Gewurz, H., and DuClos, T.W.: C-reactive protein is protective against Streptococcus pneumoniae infection in mice. J. Exp. Med. 154:1703, 1981.

77. Yother, J., Volanakis, J.E., and Briles, D.E.: Human C-reactive protein is protective against fatal Streptococcus pneumoniae infection in mice. J. Immunol. 128:2374, 1982.

78. Deodhar, S.D., James, K., Chiang, T., Edinger, M., and Barna, B.P.: Inhibition of lung metastases in mice bearing a malignant fibrosarcoma by treatment with liposomes containing human C-reactive protein. Cancer Research 42:5084, 1982.

79. Nakayama, S., Mold, C., and Gewurz, H.: Opsonic properties of C-reactive protein in vivo. J. Immunol. 128:2435, 1982.

80. Kaplan, M.H., and Volanakis, J.E.: Interaction of C-reactive protein complexes with the complement system. I. Consumption of human complement associated with the reaction of C-reactive protein with pneumococcal C-polysaccharide and with the choline phosphatides, lecithin and sphingomyelin. J. Immunol. 112:2135, 1974.

81. Hufford, D.C., and Morgan, P.N.: C-reactive protein as a mediator in the lysis of human erythrocytes sensitized by brown recluse spider venom. Proc. Soc. Exp. Biol. Med. 167:493, 1981.

82. Hulman, G., Pearson, H.J., Fraser, I., and Bell, P.R.F.: Agglutination of intralipid by sera of acutely ill patients. Lancet 2:1426, 1982.

83. Russell, I.J., Papaioannou, C., McDuffie, F.C., Macintyre, S., and Kushner, I.: Effect of IgG and C-reactive protein on complement depletion by monosodium urate crystals. J. Rheumatol. 10:425, 1983.

84. Shine, B., deBeer, F.C., and Pepys, M.B.: Solid phase radioimmunoassays for human C-reactive protein. Clinica Chemica Acta 117:13, 1981.

85. Drahovsky, D., Dunzendorfer, U., Ziegenhagen, G., Drahovsky, M., and Kellen, J.A.: Reevaluation of C-reactive protein in cancer sera by radioimmunoassay and radial immunodiffusion: I. Diagnostic value and use in battery of conventional tumor markers. Oncology 38:286, 1981.

86. Kushner, I., Broder, M.L., and Karp, D.: Control of the acute phase response: serum C-reactive protein kinetics after acute myocardial infarction. J. Clin. Invest. 61:235, 1978.

87. Kushner, I., and Feldmann, G.: Control of the acute phase response. Demonstration of C-reactive protein synthesis and secretion by hepatocytes during acute inflammation in the rabbit. J. Exp. Med. 178:466, 1978.

88. Kushner, I., Edgington, R.S., Trimble, C., Liem, H.H., and Muller-Eberhard, U.: Plasma hemopexin homeostasis during the acute phase response. J. Lab. Clin. Med. 80:18, 1972.

89. Chelladurai, M., Macintyre, S.S., and Kushner, I.: In vivo studies of serum C-reactive protein turnover in rabbits. J. Clin. Invest. 71:604, 1983.

90. Hedlund, P.: The appearance of acute phase protein in various diseases. Acta. Med. Scan. 128(Suppl. 196):579, 1947.

91. McCarty, M.: The occurrence during acute infections of a protein not normally present in the blood: IV. Crystallization of the C-reactive protein. J. Exp. Med. 85:491, 1947.

92. Anderson, H.C., and McCarty, M.: Determination of C-reactive protein in the blood as a measure of the activity of the disease process in acute rheumatic fever. Am. J. Med. 8:445, 1950.

93. Nilsson, L.-A.: Comparative testing of precipitation methods for quantitation of C-reactive protein in blood serum. Acta Pathol. Microbiol. Scand. 73:129, 1968.

94. Harmoinen, A., Hallstrom, O., and Gronroos, P.: Rapid quantitative determination of C-reactive protein using laser-nephelometer. Scand. J. Clin. Lab. Invest. 40:293, 1980.

95. Gill, C.W., Bush, W.S., Burleigh, W.M., and Fischer, C.L.: An evaluation of a C-reactive protein assay using a rate immunonephelometric procedure. Am. J. Clin. Pathol. 75:50, 1980.

96. Gushaw, J.B., Briscoe, R., Eimstad, W.M., Chang, C., Greenwood, H.M., and Allen, J.D.: A simple, rapid enzyme immunoassay for C-reactive protein. Ann. N.Y. Acad. Sci. 389:448, 1982.

97. Pepys, M.B.: C-reactive protein (CRP), serum amyloid P-component (SAP) and serum amyloid A protein (SAA) in autoimmune disease. In Holborow, E.J. (ed.): Autoimmunity. Clinics in Immunology and Allergy. Vol. 1. Eastbourne, W. B. Saunders Company, Ltd, 1981, pp. 7–101.

98. Hanson, L.A., and Nilsson, L.A.: Studies on C-reactive protein: 2. The presence of C-reactive protein during the pre- and neonatal period. Acta Pathol. Microbiol. Scand. 56:409, 1962.

99. Nilsson, L.-A.: C-reactive protein in apparently healthy individuals (blood donors) related to age. Acta Pathol. Microbiol. Scand. 73:619, 1968.

100. Ignaczak, T.F., Sipe, J.D., Linke, R.P., and Glenner, G.G.: Immunochemical studies on the nature of the serum component (SAA) related to secondary amyloidosis. J. Lab. Clin. Med. 89:1092, 1977.

101. Benson, M.D., Scheinberg, M.A., Shirahama, T., Cathcart, E.S., and Skinner, M.: Kinetics of serum amyloid protein A in casein-induced murine amyloidosis. J. Clin. Invest. 59:412, 1977.

102. Rosenthal, C.J., and Franklin, E.C.: Variation with age and disease of an amyloid A protein-related serum component. J. Clin. Invest. 55:746, 1975.

103. Hijmans, W., and Sipe, J.D.: Levels of the serum amyloid A protein (SAA) in normal persons of different age groups. Clin. Exp. Immunol. 35:96, 1979.

104. Birgegard, G., Hallgren, R., Killander, A., Stromberg, A., Venge, P., and Wide, L.: Serum ferritin during infection: A longitudinal study. Scand. J. Haematol. 21:333–340, 1978.

105. Walsh, L., Davies, P., and McConkey, B.: Relationship between erythrocyte sedimentation rates and serum C-reactive protein in rheumatoid arthritis. Ann. Rheum. Dis. 38:367, 1979.

106. Mallya, R.K., deBeer, F.C., Berry, H., Hamilton, E.D.B., Mace, B.E.W., and Pepys, M.B.: Correlation of clinical parameters of disease activity in rheumatoid arthritis with serum concentration of C-reactive protein and erythrocyte sedimentation rate. J. Rheumatol. 9:224, 1982.

107. Gwyther, M., Schwarz, H., Howard, A., and Ansell, B.M.: C-reactive protein in juvenile chronic arthritis: an indicator of disease activity and possibly amyloidosis. Ann. Rheum. Dis. 41:259, 1982.

108. Editorial: The ESR—an outdated test? Lancet 1:377, 1982.

109. Editorial: Is it time to abandon the ESR? Acta. Med. Scand. 212:353, 1982.

110. Adinolfi, M., and Lehner, T.: Acute phase proteins and C9 in patients with Behcet's syndrome and aphthous ulcers. Clin. Exp. Immunol. 25:36, 1976.

111. Farr, M., Kendall, M.J., Young, D.W., Meynell, M.J., and Hawkins, C.F.: Assessment of rheumatoid activity based on clinical features and blood and synovial fluid analysis. Ann. Rheum. Dis. 35:163, 1976.

112. Dixon, J.S., Bird, H.A., Pickup, M.E., and Wright, V.: A human model screening system for the detection of specific antirheumatic activity. Semin. Arthritis Rheum. 12:185, 1982.

113. Dixon, J.S., Bird, H.A., and Wright, V.: A Comparison of serum biochemistry in ankylosing spondylitis, seronegative and seropositive rheumatoid arthritis. Ann. Rheum. Dis. 40:404, 1981.

114. Duthie, J.J.R., Brown, P.E., Truelove, L.H., Baragar, F.D., and Lawrie, A.J.: Course and prognosis in rheumatoid arthritis. A further report. Ann. Rheum. Dis. 23:193, 1964.

115. Masi, A.T., Maldonado-Cocco, J.A., Kaplan, S.B., Feigenbaum, S.L., and Chandler, R.W.: Prospective study of the early course of rheumatoid arthritis in young adults: comparison of patients with and without rheumatoid factor positivity at entry and identification of variables correlating with outcome. Semin. Arthritis Rheum. 5:299, 1976.

116. McConkey, B., Crockson, R.A., and Crockson, A.P.: The assessment of rheumatoid arthritis: a study based on measurement of the serum acute phase reactants. Quart. J. Med. 162:115, 1972.

117. Fleming, A., Crown, J.M., and Corbett, M.: Prognostic value of early features in rheumatoid disease. Br. Med. J. 1:1243, 1976.

118. Roth, S.H.: Remission: the goal of rheumatic disease therapy. J. Rheumatol. 9(Suppl. 8):120, 1982.

119. Editorial: Inducing remission in rheumatoid arthritis. Lancet 1:193, 1981.

120. Huskisson, E.C.: The problems of studying disease-remittive agents in RA. J. Rheumatol. 9(Suppl. 8):201, 1982.

121. Dixon, J.S.: Biochemical and clinical changes in rheumatoid arthritis: their relation to the action of antirheumatoid drugs. Semin. Arthritis Rheum. 12:191, 1982.

122. McConkey, B., Crockson, R.A., Crockson, A.P., and Wilkinson, A.R.: The effects of some anti-inflammatory drugs on the acute-phase proteins in rheumatoid arthritis. Quart. J. Med. 42:785, 1973.

123. Amos, R.S., Constable, T.J., Crockson, R.A., Crockson, A.P., and McConkey, B.: Rheumatoid arthritis: relation of serum C-reactive protein and erythrocyte sedimentation rates to radiographic changes. Br. Med. J. 1:195, Jan. 22, 1977.

124. Nusinow, S., and Arnold, W.J.: Prognostic value of C-reactive protein (CRP) levels in rheumatoid arthritis. Clin. Res. 30:474A, 1982.

125. Amos, R.S., Crockson, R.A., Crockson, A.P., Walsh, L., and McConkey, B.: Rheumatoid arthritis: C-reactive protein and erythrocyte sedimentation rate during initial treatment. Br. Med. J. 1(612Y):1396, May 27, 1978.

126. Iannuzzi, L., Dawson, N., Zein, N., and Kushner, I.: Does drug therapy slow radiographic deterioration in rheumatoid arthritis? (Submitted to N. Engl. J. Med., 309:1023, 1983)

127. Hamilton, C.R., Jr., Shelley, W.M., and Tumulty, P.A.: Giant cell arteritis: including temporal arteritis and polymyalgia rheumatica. Medicine 50:1, 1971.

128. Bruk, M.I.: Articular and vascular manifestations of polymyalgia rheumatica. Ann. Rheum. Dis. 26:103, 1967.

129. Kansu, T., Corbett, J.J., Savino, P., and Schatz, N.J.: Giant cell arteritis with normal sedimentation rate. Arch. Neurol. 34:624, 1977.

130. Biller, J., Asconape, J., Weinblatt, M.E., and Toole, J.F.: Temporal arteritis associated with normal sedimentation rate. JAMA 247:486, 1982.

131. Schimmelpfennig, R.W., Jr., and Chusid, M.J.: Illnesses associated with extreme elevation of the erythrocyte sedimentation rate in children. Clin. Pediatr. 19:175, 1980.

132. Khan, M.A., and Kushner, I.: Diagnosis of ankylosing spondylitis: In Cohen, A.S. (ed.): Progress in Clinical Rheumatology. Vol. I. New York, Grune and Stratton (in press).

132a. DuBois, E.L.: Lupus erythematosis. Los Angeles, University of Southern California Press, 2nd edition, 1976.

133. Becker, G.J., Waldburger, M., Hughes, G.R.V., and Pepys, M.B.: Value

of serum C-reactive protein measurement in the investigation of fever in systemic lupus erythematosus. Ann. Rheum. Dis. 39:50, 1980.

134. Pereira Da Silva, J.A., Elkon, K.B., Hughes, G.R.V., Dyck, R.F., and Pepys, M.B.: C-reactive protein levels in systemic lupus erythematosus: a classification criterion? Arthritis Rheum. 23:770, 1980.

135. Zein, N., Ganuza, C., and Kushner, I.: Significance of serum C-reactive protein elevation in patients with systemic lupus erythematosus. Arthritis Rheum. 22:7, 1979.

136. Morrow, W.J.W., Isenberg, D.A., Parry, H.F., and Snaith, M.L.: C-reactive protein in sera from patients with systemic lupus erythematosus. J. Rheumatol. 8:599, 1981.

137. Rothschild, B.M., James, K.K., Jones, J.V., Thompson, L.D., Pifer, D.D., and Chesney, C.M.: Quantitation of C-reactive protein in SLE correlates with disease activity. Clin. Res. 30:476A, 1982.

138. Sturfelt, G., Sjoholm, A.G., and Svensson, B.: Complement components, Cl activation and disease activity in SLE. Int. Arch. Allergy Appl. Immun. 70:12, 1983.

139. Bertouch, J.V., Roberts-Thompson, P.J., Feng, P.H., and Bradley, J.: C-reactive protein and serological indices of disease activity in systemic lupus erythematosis. Ann. Rheum. Dis. 42:655, 1983.

Chapter 44

Rheumatoid Factor

Dennis A. Carson

INTRODUCTION

Rheumatoid factors are autoantibodies directed against antigenic determinants on the Fc fragment of immunoglobulin G (IgG) molecules (Fig. 44–1). Their importance was recognized in the 1940s when Waaler, and then Rose and co-workers, noted that the agglutination of sheep red blood cells by specific rabbit antibody was augmented by rheumatoid arthritis sera.[1,2] This was one of the first clues suggesting that rheumatoid arthritis was an autoimmune disease. However, it soon became clear that rheumatoid factors are not exclusively nor uniformly associated with rheumatoid arthritis. Investigations over several years have attempted to elucidate what the presence of rheumatoid factor signifies regarding the etiology of rheumatoid disease and how the autoantibody might contribute to the development of synovitis.

In this chapter we shall discuss (1) the nature of rheumatoid factors and how they are assayed; (2) the specificity and sensitivity of rheumatoid factors for rheumatoid arthritis; (3) genetic and environmental factors which influence rheumatoid factor production, structure, and specificity; (4) immunochemical properties of rheumatoid factors; (5) the probable physiologic role of IgM rheumatoid factors; and (6) the contribution of rheumatoid factors to the pathogenesis of chronic synovitis and extra-articular rheumatoid disease.

ASSAY METHODS

Rheumatoid factors have been found among the IgM, IgA, IgG and IgE classes of immunoglobulin.[3-7] Most methods developed for the measurement of antibodies against exogenous antigens have also been applied to the assay of rheumatoid factor. These include agglutination, precipitation, complement fixation, and immunofluorescence assays.[8-11] Technical problems have arisen because the IgG antigens with which rheumatoid factors react are present in high concentration in serum and may interfere with a particular detection system. The recent development of radioimunoassay and ELISA (enzyme-linked immunoabsorbent sandwich assay) methods has facilitated the more precise quantification of IgM, IgG, and IgA rheumatoid factors.[12-18]

IgM Rheumatoid Factors. IgM rheumatoid factors, like other IgM antibodies, are multivalent and hence are efficient agglutinators of antigen-coated particles. Commercially available sources of the latter include latex beads or bentonite particles that have been passively coated with human IgG. Cross-linking of the IgG-coupled latex or bentonite by IgM rheumatoid factor in serum produces a visible flocculus (Fig. 44–2). The quantity of IgM rheumatoid factor is then expressed as the highest dilution of serum yielding detectable agglutination. Nephelometry and particle counting techniques

Figure 44–1. Structure of an IgG molecule of the G1 subclass containing kappa light chains. The antigens reacting with rheumatoid factor are in the Fc region.

Figure 44–2. Latex fixation reaction. Multivalent IgM rheumatoid factor cross-links IgG-coated latex particles to produce a visible flocculus.

LATEX COATED WITH IgG   IgM RHEUMATOID FACTOR   AGGLUTINATION

permit a more exact expression of IgM rheumatoid factor levels.[19]

Red cells coated with human or rabbit IgG are likewise agglutinated by IgM rheumatoid factors. Human red cells sensitized with certain incomplete IgG anti-Rh antibodies are well suited for the detection of IgM rheumatoid factors, particularly those with anti-Gm specificities.[20-23] Sheep red blood cells coated with rabbit IgG antibody are cross-linked by rheumatoid factor in the classic Rose-Waaler reaction. This test can be modified for the detection of complement-fixing rheumatoid factors.[10]

A positive Rose-Waaler test may be more specific for rheumatoid arthritis than the bentonite or latex flocculation assays, since the latter detect antiallotypic antibodies resulting from transplacental immunization or transfusion, as well as true autoantibodies.[23] However, because only a minor proportion of the anti-IgG antibodies in rheumatoid sera cross-react with rabbit IgG, titers in the Rose-Waaler test are usually lower than in those systems that employ human IgG as antigen. Furthermore, anti-sheep heterophile antibodies may give a false positive reaction unless the sera are preabsorbed with sheep red blood cells. This problem can be avoided by using latex particles coated with rabbit IgG.[24]

IgM rheumatoid factors will precipitate aggregated IgG, in either solution or agar-containing gels.[9,25] In some instances precipitation is enhanced by decreasing the temperature and ionic strength of the incubation medium. The reaction of such cold reactive IgM rheumatoid factors with monomeric IgG or soluble immune complexes in poorly perfused areas may contribute to the pathogenesis of mixed cryoglobulinemic states.[26,27] More commonly, IgM rheumatoid factors combine with monomeric IgG to form soluble 22S complexes, which can be visualized in many rheumatoid sera by analytical ultracentrifugation (Fig. 44–3).[3]

Serum IgG will compete with IgG-coated particles for reaction with IgM rheumatoid factor. Through multivalent interactions, nonspecifically aggregated IgG in improperly treated sera or specific immune complexes will inhibit rheumatoid factor binding to a marked degree. Such "hidden rheumatoid factors" can be revealed by separation of the IgM and IgG fractions under dissociating conditions prior to performing the rheumatoid factor assays.[28] The Clq component of complement will agglutinate IgG-coated particles, particularly in plasma anticoagulated with calcium chelators.[29] Unlike IgM, however, the Clq molecule is denatured by heating serum at 56° C for 30 minutes.

Recently, sensitive radioimmunoassay and ELISA methods have been developed for the detection of IgM rheumatoid factors.[12-15,17,18] In a typical assay, plastic tubes or microtiter plates are coated with IgG (Fig. 44–4). IgM rheumatoid factors in serum or synovial fluid specifically bind to the IgG fixed to the plates. After washing, the amount of IgM rheumatoid factor bound is quantitatively determined with an anti-IgM antibody that has been radioiodinated or linked to an enzyme such as alkaline phosphatase. In the latter case, the amount of enzyme-linked antibody bound to the solid phase is determined by adding an appropriate substrate and then assaying product formation in a spectrophotometer.

Figure 44–3. Analytical ultracentrifugation of serum from a rheumatoid arthritis patient (bottom) and a normal subject (top). Pictures were taken 32, 48, and 64 minutes after reaching a speed of 52,000 rpm. The peak to the right in the rheumatoid serum represents 22S complexes formed by the reaction of IgM rheumatoid factor with IgG.

Figure 44–4. Radioimmunoassay of IgM rheumatoid factor.

One significant advantage of radioimmunoassay and ELISA methods is that they readily detect IgM rheumatoid factors in rheumatoid sera diluted 1000- to 100,000-fold. At such high dilutions, serum IgG and immune complexes infrequently compromise the accurate determination of IgM rheumatoid factor levels.

IgG and IgA Rheumatoid Factors. IgG rheumatoid factors are abundant in the sera, and particularly the synovial fluids, of many patients with severe rheumatoid arthritis.[13,14,17,30-32] Unfortunately, the routine assay of IgG rheumatoid factors presents several difficulties (Table 44–1). All assays for IgM rheumatoid factor take advantage of the markedly increased avidity of pentavalent IgM rheumatoid factors for aggregated IgG as compared to monomeric IgG. With IgG rheumatoid factor, this phenomenon is not nearly as marked. For the same reason IgG rheumatoid factors are inefficient agglutinators of IgG-coated particles or red blood cells. High concentrations of IgG in serum, and the tendency of IgG rheumatoid factors to self-associate rather than bind aggregated IgG, further make the assay of this antibody difficult. On occasion, IgG rheumatoid factor complexes precipitate in the cold or when serum is diluted 1:15 with water. This type of Ig rheumatoid factor

is frequently monoclonal and is more commonly found in hypergammaglobulinemic purpura, cryoglobulinemia, and Sjögren's syndrome than in typical rheumatoid arthritis.[33,34]

IgG rheumatoid factors in rheumatoid arthritis are most definitely detected by their characteristic sedimentation profile as intermediate complexes in the analytical ultracentrifuge (Fig. 44–5).[35,36] Other assays for IgG rheumatoid factor require the prior removal of multivalent IgM rheumatoid factor by gel filtration, ion exchange chromatography, or digestion with the proteolytic enzyme pepsin. The latter technique has the additional advantage of destroying the Fc portion of IgG, thereby releasing IgG rheumatoid factors trapped in self-associating complexes (Fig. 44–6).[37] Care must be taken, however, to prevent further proteolysis of the IgG molecule with subsequent loss of antigen binding activity.

If serum contains sufficient quantities of IgG rheumatoid factor, a positive latex or sensitized sheep cell reaction can be detected in an isolated IgG fraction, or in pepsin-digested IgG.[32-36] IgG rheumatoid factor will also precipitate with aggregated IgG. In some cases IgG

Table 44–1. Comparison of Rheumatoid Factors of the IgM and IgG Class

Property	IgM Rheumatoid Factor	IgG Rheumatoid Factor
Valence for IgG	5	2
Intrinsic affinity for antigen (liters/mole)	$1 \times 10^4 - 5 \times 10^5$	$1 \times 10^4 - 5 \times 10^5$
Agglutination of IgG-coated latex particles	Strong	Weak
Enhanced binding to aggregated IgG	Marked	Moderate
Usual sedimentation constants in ultracentrifuge	19S–22S	10S–18S
Self-association	No	Yes
Binding to IgG after treatment with:		
Reducing agents	Decreased	Unchanged
Pepsin	Decreased	Unchanged or increased

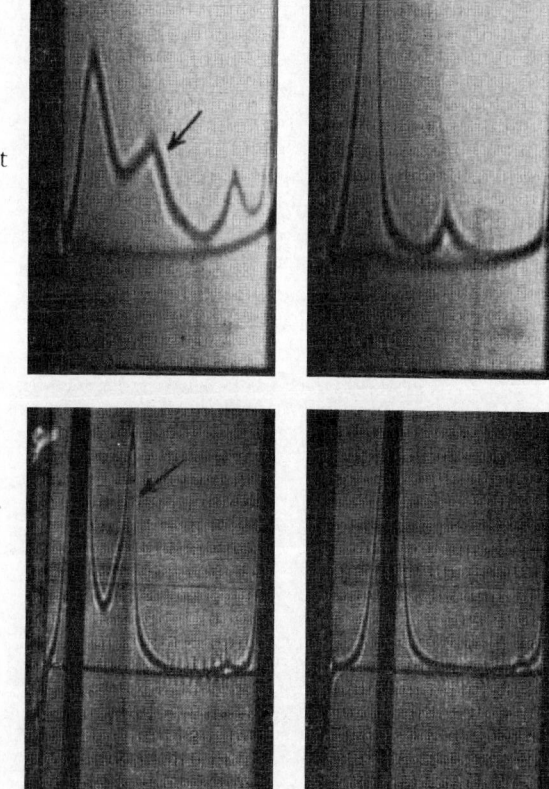

Figure 44–5. Analytical ultracentrifugation of IgG rheumatoid factor–containing sera in isotonic saline (*A*) and acetate buffer pH 4.5 (*B*). The arrows indicate the large intermediate complexes which disappear in the acetate buffer. (From Kunkel, H.G., et al.: J. Clin. Invest. 40:117, 1961.)

Figure 44–6. Effect of pepsin on IgG rheumatoid factor complexes. The pepsin destroys the Fc fragment of IgG, preventing IgG rheumatoid factor molecules from self-associating and releasing Fab'2 fragments with antibody activity. (Reprinted from Munthe, E., and Natvig. J.: Scand J. Immunol. 1:217, 1972.)

rheumatoid factors have been assayed as the quantity of serum IgG specifically adhering to IgG agarose immunoabsorbent columns, and eluting only under denaturing conditions.[38] This assay is not specific for IgG rheumatoid factor but may also detect normal IgG passively adhering to the immunoabsorbent via multivalent IgM rheumatoid factor.

Recently, both ELISA and radioimmunoassay methods have been developed for the detection of IgG rheumatoid factor.[13,14,17,39,40] They are performed analogously to the IgM rheumatoid factor assay described in Figure 44–4 except that anti-IgG antibody is substituted for anti-IgM in the final step. Nonetheless, IgM rheumatoid factor must still be removed or destroyed prior to the IgG rheumatoid factor assay to avoid false positive results.

The quantitative assay of IgG rheumatoid factor in serum is occasionally helpful in confirming a diagnosis of rheumatoid arthritis,[13,14,17,38] or hypergammaglobulinemic purpura.[34] In patients with rheumatoid vasculitis or the hyperviscosity syndrome, IgG rheumatoid factor levels may assist in monitoring the response to therapy.[40] However, indications for the routine clinical assay of IgG rheumatoid factor have not been well defined.

IgA and IgE Rheumatoid Factors. Rheumatoid factors of the IgA class have been measured in rheumatoid serum by immunoelectrophoresis, quantitative immunoabsorption, and radioimmunoassay and ELISA methods using class specific anti-immunoglobulin reagents to distinguish them from the more abundant IgM rheumatoid factors.[6,16,38,41]

IgA rheumatoid factors are also found in the saliva of patients with rheumatoid arthritis, and with the sicca syndrome. Most salivary IgA, and presumably IgA rheumatoid factor, is produced locally.[41] The role of IgA rheumatoid factors in chronic inflammation of the exocrine glands is not known.

With sensitive radioimmunoassays, IgE rheumatoid factors have been detected in the sera of most patients with rheumatoid arthritis, and a few with bronchial asthma.[7] They do not have any established diagnostic or prognostic significance.

INCIDENCE OF RHEUMATOID FACTOR

Rheumatoid factors are not specific for rheumatoid arthritis. Rather, they are found in the sera of a variable portion of patients with acute and chronic inflammatory diseases, and in some apparently normal individuals.[42-45] The exact incidence of rheumatoid factor in a population depends upon the assay system and the titer chosen to separate positive and negative reactors.

The titer of rheumatoid factor in a population, whether measured by the sensitized sheep cell agglutination test or by latex fixation, usually behaves as a continuous variable, but differs among various ethnic groups (e.g., Fig. 44–7).[45] With increasing age both the percentage of individuals with a particular titer and the mean titer of a population as a whole increase (Fig. 44–8).[46] In most populations, the distribution of titers among men and women is similar. Some studies have shown that the prevalence of rheumatoid factors and other autoantibodies in the general population tends to decline beyond the age of 70 to 80.[47] This decrease may be related to an increased mortality—particularly from hypertension and vascular disease—among autoantibody positive individuals.

Diseases other than rheumatoid arthritis in which positive rheumatoid factor tests are frequent include other rheumatic diseases, viral infections, chronic inflammatory diseases, and neoplasms after chemotherapy or radiotherapy.[42-45,48,49] Many of these conditions are also associated with either hypergammaglobulinemia, indicative of polyclonal B lymphocyte activation, or circulating immune complexes.[44,45,48,50] In one study, levels of circulating immune complexes, measured by both the solid phase and solution Clq binding assays, were strongly associated with the presence of IgM rheumatoid factor.[51] Table 44–2 is a partial list of diseases in which an increased incidence of rheumatoid factor has been reported.

In most but not all nonrheumatic conditions, titers of rheumatoid factor are lower than in rheumatoid arthritis. Thus the specificity of the rheumatoid factor reaction for rheumatoid arthritis increases with serum titer (Fig. 44–9).[52] At a dilution of serum that excludes 95 percent of the normal population, at least 70 percent or more patients with rheumatoid arthritis, as diagnosed by other criteria, will be positive by latex agglutination. The remaining patients are considered seronegative, i.e., having rheumatoid factor titers falling in the normal range. Some of the latter sera, particularly from patients with juvenile rheumatoid arthritis, may contain hidden IgM rheumatoid factors.[28,53,54] A few have IgG rheumatoid factors in the absence of IgM. Some seronegative patients, upon repeated testing, convert to seropositive.

A variable percentage of adult rheumatoid patients, which in the author's experience represent not more than 10 percent of the total, remain seronegative by the usual criteria. These patients usually have milder synovitis than the seropositive patients, and they seldom develop extra-articular rheumatoid disease.[55,56]

Figure 44–7. Titers of rheumatoid factor in the Pima and Blackfoot Indians as measured by bentonite flocculation (left panel) and sensitized sheep cell agglutination (right panel) assays. (From Bennett, P. H., and Burch, T. A., *In* Bennett, P. H., and Wood, P. H. N. (eds.): Population Studies in the Rheumatic Diseases. Amsterdam, Excerpta Medica, 1968.)

For uncertain reasons, the peripheral blood lymphocytes of the seronegative patients are relatively deficient in the B cells necessary for IgM rheumatoid factor synthesis.[57] Seropositive and seronegative rheumatoid ar-

thritis may actually represent different diseases with overlapping clinical manifestations.[56-59] In both adults and children, the histocompatibility antigen HLA-DR4 is associated significantly with seropositive rheumatoid arthritis, but not with seronegative arthritis, at least in most studies.[58,60-63]

Figure 44–8. Incidence of positive latex fixation tests in varying age groups in Tecumseh, Mich. (From Mikkelsen, W. M., et al.: J. Chronic Dis. 20:351, 1967.)

Figure 44–9. Relationship of latex fixation and sensitized sheep cell agglutination titers to rheumatoid arthritis. (From Valkenburg, H. A., et al.: Ann. Rheum. Dis. 25:497, 1966.)

Table 44-2. Diseases Commonly Associated with
Rheumatoid Factor

Table 44-2. Diseases Commonly Associated with
Rheumatoid Factor

Rheumatic diseases: rheumatoid arthritis, systemic lupus erythematosus, scleroderma, mixed connective tissue disease, Sjögren's syndrome

Acute viral infections: mononucleosis, hepatitis, influenza, and many others; after vaccination (may yield falsely elevated titers of antiviral antibodies)

Parasitic infections: trypanosomiasis, kala-azar, malaria, schistosomiasis, filariasis, etc.

Chronic inflammatory diseases: tuberculosis, leprosy, yaws, syphilis, brucellosis, subacute bacterial endocarditis, salmonellosis

Neoplasms: after irradiation or chemotherapy

Other hyperglobulinemic states: hypergammaglobulinemic purpura, cryoglobulinemia, chronic liver disease, sarcoid, other chronic pulmonary diseases

As noted previously, the sensitized sheep cell agglutination test is slightly more specific for rheumatoid arthritis than is the latex fixation test. Positivity by both latex fixation and sensitized sheep cell agglutination is more specific for rheumatoid arthritis than is positivity by either test alone.[48,52] In general, the specificity of rheumatoid factor for rheumatoid arthritis is increased by (1) positivity on two or more consecutive occasions, (2) high titer, (3) reactivity with both human and rabbit IgG, and (4) distribution among the IgM, IgG, and IgA classes.

Whether or not the presence of rheumatoid factor in the serum of a normal individual is a risk factor for the development of rheumatoid arthritis is controversial. In an English study, 8 of 22 individuals with strongly positive sensitized sheep cell agglutination tests for rheumatoid factor, but only 4 of 29 seronegative subjects, developed polyarthritis when followed over a 5-year period.[48] On the contrary, other prospective studies from Tecumseh and Framingham found no prognostic value for rheumatoid factor tests as measured by latex fixation, but suggested that serologic conversion usually occurred simultaneously with or subsequent to the development of clinical arthritis.[64,65]

ETIOLOGY OF RHEUMATOID FACTOR

Genetic Influences. Two types of immune response (Ir) genes have been described in animals, and recently in humans. The first are the histocompatibility-linked Ir genes. These encode the Ia antigens that restrict the interactions of certain T lymphocytes with antigen presenting macrophages and B lymphocytes. The second are the immunoglobulin variable region structural genes. These encode the diverse light and heavy polypeptide chain amino acid sequences responsible for antibody heterogeneity and specificity.

The histocompatibility-linked immune response genes play an undefined but important role in the etiology of seropositive rheumatoid arthritis. As mentioned previously, seropositive rheumatoid arthritis is associated with the HLA-DR4 antigen, located on the membrane of B lymphocytes, macrophages, and certain other cell types.[60-63] In animals, the Ia analogs of the HLA-DR antigens are the known products of genes that regulate the immune response to exogenous antigens and even some autoantigens.[66] Depending on the population studied, HLA-DR4–positive individuals have about a four- to eightfold increased risk of developing seropositive rheumatoid arthritis, as compared to HLA-DR4–negative subjects. Among normal blood donors, however, no significant correlation exists between IgM rheumatoid factor, as measured by the latex fixation test, and a particular HLA-DR type.[67]

Population studies among the Pima and Blackfoot Indians have failed to show a genetically determined familial aggregation of IgM rheumatoid factor positivity by either the latex fixation or sensitized sheep cell agglutination test.[68] In a family study in Leigh and Wensleydale, England, however, positivity by both assays showed a significant tendency toward familial aggregation, which was supported by twin studies.[48] As noted previously, such doubly reactive rheumatoid factors are the type most frequently associated with rheumatoid arthritis.

While genetic factors probably exert but a modest influence on the absolute ability to make IgM rheumatoid factor, they almost certainly influence the structure and specificity of the particular autoantibodies produced (Table 44-3). Insight concerning such possible genetic regulation of rheumatoid factor specificity came initially from structural studies of monoclonal proteins with rheumatoid factor activity. These monoclonal proteins, although arising in unrelated individuals, share common amino acid sequences and antigenic determinants (termed idiotypes) in the variable regions of the light and heavy chains.[69-71] Monoclonal IgG anti-gamma globulins also occur frequently in patients with cryoglobulinemia or hypergammaglobulinemia.[33,34] In one study the light chains isolated from two IgG rheumatoid factors had identical sequences through the first 42 amino acid residues, but differed from the light chains isolated from IgM rheumatoid factors.[72] The chance synthesis of nearly identical amino acid sequences in immunoglobulin molecules from unrelated individuals, even with similar antigenic reactivity, is distinctly unusual.

Recently, the IgM rheumatoid factors from some arthritis patients have been shown to share idiotypic antigens with monoclonal IgM rheumatoid factor cryoglobulins.[73-77] The rheumatoid factors from one instructive family with multiple seropositive members spanning three generations displayed a common idiotype

Table 44-3. Possible Role of Immunoglobulin Structural
Genes in Rheumatoid Factor Synthesis

1. Cross-reactive idiotypes among monoclonal and polyclonal rheumatoid factors from unrelated individuals
2. Familial clustering of private idiotypes on rheumatoid factors
3. Ability to make IgM rheumatoid factor present at birth
4. Linkage of rheumatoid factor synthesis to the heavy chain structural gene locus in mice

that was lacking on rheumatoid factors from unrelated individuals.[78] The common occurrence in the human population of antibody structural genes coding for rheumatoid factor light or heavy chains would explain all these results. In inbred mouse strains, breeding studies have definitively linked the synthesis of rheumatoid factors with defined specificities to the genetic locus for immunoglobulin heavy chains.[79]

Environmental Influences. If the ability to make rheumatoid factors is inherited, then (1) IgM rheumatoid factor precursors should be detectable among immature B lymphocytes and (2) IgM rheumatoid factor should function beneficially for the survival of the species. Recent evidence lends support to both these conclusions. IgM rheumatoid factor precursor B lymphocytes are present in human umbilical cord blood (Fig. 44–10) and are abundant in normal adult bone marrow.[59,80,81] Moreover, IgM rheumatoid factors comprise up to 10 percent of the Waldenström's macroglobulins that likely arise from neoplastic proliferation of immature lymphocytes.

Between birth and young adulthood, the frequency of IgM rheumatoid factor B lymphocytes in human blood rises severalfold, remaining fairly stable thereafter[59,80] (Fig. 44–10). Evidently the childhood infections and vaccinations that transiently induce low levels of IgM rheumatoid factor simultaneously increase the numbers of rheumatoid factor–bearing, long-lived memory B cells[81,82] (Fig. 44–11).

Experimental evidence has identified three types of environmental stimuli that potentially can trigger active rheumatoid factor synthesis in normal adults. They are (1) immunization with aggregated IgG in the form of immune complexes,[83-88] (2) polyclonal B cell activa-

Figure 44–11. Representative examples of changes in peripheral blood IgM rheumatoid factor B cell frequency after tetanus toxoid vaccination in two individuals. ■ = IgM rheumatoid factor B cell frequency; ● = plasma IgM rheumatoid factor; ○ = IgM. (From Welch, M. J., et al.: Clin. Exp. Immunol. 51:299, 1983.)

tion,[89-94] and (3) unexpected cross-reactions between IgG and exogenous antigens.[85,95-98] Other possible, but probably less likely, mechanisms include somatic mutations among antibody-producing cells, alloimmunization with maternal immunoglobulins, and acquired structural abnormalities of the IgG molecule which render it antigenic.[99-101]

In adult animals of several species, rheumatoid factors of both the IgM and IgG class have been produced experimentally by repeated immunization with aggregated or denatured IgG, with particulate bacterial antigens from streptococci and *E. coli,* and even with soluble protein antigens.[83,84] The significant results of these diverse experimental models can be summarized as follows. In most cases the experimentally produced rheumatoid factors were polyclonal; occasionally they were monoclonal.[85] Except when markedly denatured IgG was used for autoimmunization, the rheumatoid factors reacted to varying degrees with native immunoglobulin.[83,86] In some rabbits immunized with streptococci, the elicited IgG rheumatoid factors had double specificity, reacting with both streptococcal peptidoglycans and autologous IgG.[85] The sustained production of rheumatoid factor usually required continual antigenic or mitogenic stimulation. Neither a self-perpetuating sensitization to autologous IgG nor a chronic synovitis was successfully produced in most cases.

IgM and IgA rheumatoid factors are detectable in the sera of many adult mice, in the absence of overt arthritis or chronic inflammatory disease.[102] In the MRL/l mouse strain, a chronic synovitis of the lower extremities develops in 25 percent of adult animals and is associated with large amounts of circulating IgM and IgG rheumatoid factors.[103] Although the MRL/l has a widespread lupus erythematosus-like disease affecting many organs, it is the only autoimmune mouse strain with both spontaneously developing arthritis and rheumatoid factor.

Rheumatoid factors in human beings develop during the course of many acute and chronic inflammatory diseases. While IgM rheumatoid factors predominate in most of these conditions, IgG rheumatoid factors are occasionally produced. As in the experimental models,

Figure 44–10. Frequency of IgM rheumatoid factor precursor B cells in the peripheral blood of normal subjects, as a function of age. The relative frequency was estimated by stimulation with Epstein-Barr virus under limiting dilution conditions. (From Fong, S., et al.: Arthritis Rheum. 25:959, 1982.)

sustained rheumatoid factor production usually depends upon the continual presence of the immunologic stimuli. A well-studied example is subacute bacterial endocarditis, in which elimination of bacteria by antibiotics leads to the subsequent decline in rheumatoid factor titers (Fig. 44–12).[87,88]

With few exceptions, the nonrheumatic diseases and the animal models associated with rheumatoid factor induction are characterized by either elevated levels of nonrheumatoid factor containing immune complexes and/or a diffuse elevation of serum immunoglobulins, indicating polyclonal B lymphocyte activation.

There are several possible mechanisms through which circulating immune complexes could induce the formation of rheumatoid factor. These include (1) the creation of neoantigens on the Fc portion of IgG by the combination of antibody with antigen, immunoglobulin aggregation, or denaturation,[99-101] (2) the enhanced binding of aggregated IgG to low affinity receptors on potential rheumatoid factor forming cells,[104,105] (3) the ability of exogenous antigen trapped in an immune complex to stimulate helper T lymphocytes, and hence to break self-tolerance,[106] and (4) nonspecific activation of B lymphocytes by aggregated IgG.[107]

The potential importance of polyclonal B lymphocyte activation in inducing rheumatoid factor production in humans has recently been emphasized.[89-94] Polyclonal B lymphocyte activators are mitogens that nonspecifically stimulate lymphocytes to secrete immunoglobulins in the absence of antigenic stimulation. They are widespread in nature and include many bacteria,[108] mycoplasmas,[109] certain viruses such as the Epstein-Barr (EB) virus,[110] proteolytic enzymes, and various soluble macromolecules derived from plants or activated T lymphocytes.

In vitro experiments have shown that lymphocytes from many normal adult humans and mice secrete low-affinity IgM rheumatoid factors after mitogenic stimulation by polyclonal B lymphocyte activators, including pokeweed mitogen and Epstein-Barr virus[89-94] (Fig. 44–13). The latter is of particular interest in rheumatoid

Figure 44–13. In vitro secretion of rheumatoid factor by lymphocytes from patients with rheumatoid arthritis (R) and normal subject (N) after infection with Epstein-Barr virus (EBV). (From Slaughter, L., et al.: J. Exp. Med. 148:1427, 1977.)

arthritis, because it is a permanent but quiescent resident of the B lymphocytes of many normal adults which can be reactivated by certain immunologic stimuli.[111,112] In addition, the Epstein-Barr virus is the only well-described polyclonal activator of immature human B lymphocytes.[80,113] Most other polyclonal activators presumably exert their action via T lymphocyte-generated factors. The latter stimulate primarily mature B lymphocytes, which are already active in vivo.[114,115] In normal subjects, rheumatoid factor precursors are uncommon among the mature B lymphocyte subset, but abundant among the Epstein-Barr virus sensitive immature B lymphocyte subset.[71,80,114,115]

When compared with normal subjects, patients with rheumatoid arthritis have a distinctive cellular and humoral immune response to the Epstein-Barr virus.[90,116-120] The peripheral blood lymphocytes from rheumatoid arthritis patients frequently spontaneously transform in vitro to become permanent cell lines.[90,118,119] Patients with rheumatoid arthritis, when compared with normal subjects, have a fourfold increased titer of antibodies against Epstein-Barr virus–associated transformation antigens found in the nucleus of virally infected B lymphoblasts.[116,117] Whether these serologic and cellular abnormalities contribute in some way to the rheumatoid disease process is uncertain. In any event, they suggest that the differentiation and proliferation of B lymphocytes in rheumatoid arthritis patients might be improperly regulated.

The reasons for the common occurrence of rheumatoid factors after polyclonal activation of B lymphocytes may relate to the low affinity of the autoantibodies for IgG. Animal experiments have shown that the induction of either immunity or tolerance requires a minimum energy of interaction between antigen and antibody re-

Figure 44–12. Decline of rheumatoid factor levels after treatment of subacute bacterial endocarditis. Rheumatoid factor was measured by quantitative precipitation with aggregated gamma globulin as well as by latex and sheep cell agglutination. (From Williams, R. C., Jr., and Kunkel, H. G.: J. Clin. Invest. 41:666, 1962.)

ceptors on cells, which has been estimated to be in the order of 10^5 liters per mole.[121] Cells with receptors of lower affinity can be neither triggered nor tolerized by antigen under physiologic conditions. But most rheumatoid factors, either in the sera of patients or induced by polyclonal activators in vitro, are of low affinity. This implies that (1) there is no absolute tolerance for IgG in any normal person, and (2) rheumatoid factors probably are not specifically elicitable by autologous IgG antigen under normal circumstances.

In both experimental animals and human beings, some rheumatoid factors of the IgM and IgG classes have the unusual property of reacting with antigens apparently unrelated to IgG.[85,95-98] Thus certain rabbits hyperimmunized with streptococci develop high titers of IgG rheumatoid factors that react with both streptococcal cell walls and with IgG.[85] Similarly, in humans many polyclonal IgM and IgG factors bind to histones or other nuclear proteins.[95-98] These strange cross-reactions perhaps may be explained by the ontogeny of the B lymphocyte.[71] If genes coding for rheumatoid factor are indeed inherited, they likely give rise to somatic variants, through recombination and mutation. It would not be surprising if a somatically generated antibody occasionally retained evidence of its lineage by binding to the original germ line specificity, albeit with low affinity. There is no conclusive evidence for or against this hypothesis. Nevertheless it is consistent with the experimental data and does explain how a variety of antigens in the environment could unexpectedly give rise to rheumatoid factors during the course of normal immunization.

IMMUNOCHEMICAL PROPERTIES OF RHEUMATOID FACTOR

Antigenic Specificity. Polyclonal IgM rheumatoid factors from the sera of patients with rheumatoid arthritis react with a diverse array of antigenic determinants localized to the Fc portion of the IgG molecule in both the CH_2 and CH_3 domains[99] (Fig. 44–1). These determinants include (1) cross-reactive antigens shared by human and animal IgG;[122-124] (2) species-specific antigens found in human but not animal IgG;[28,123] (3) subclass-specific antigens found on one or more but not all of the four subclasses of human IgG;[125] (4) genetically defined alloantigens of the Gm type, which are autosomally inherited and differ from person to person, depending on their inheritance (each human IgG subclass has its own set of Gm antigens);[21-23] and (5) neoantigens better expressed on aggregated, denatured, or enzymatically digested IgG than on monomeric native IgG,[99-101] including the so-called "pepsin agglutinators," which react with antigenic determinants exposed in Fab'2 fragments of IgG but not in the native molecule.[126]

Recent experiments have also identified IgM and IgG antibodies in rheumatoid sera reactive with antigens on the Fab region of intact, native IgG.[93,127] Strictly speaking, such anti-Fab antibodies are not true rheumatoid factors. They may be representative of the anti-idiotypic antibodies that regulate interactions among lymphocytes in an "immune network."[128]

The many specificities of IgM rheumatoid factors have been utilized by immunologists to unravel the genetic control of human IgG synthesis. However, no one antigenic determinant on the IgG molecule, with the possible exception of the Ga antigen, has yet been shown to be of unique importance in rheumatoid arthritis.[129] The important point to remember is that IgM rheumatoid factors in rheumatoid sera react with multiple antigenic determinants on autologous IgG. While a proportion of rheumatoid factors do react better with Gm alloantigens, with animal IgG's or with denatured IgG than with native, autologous IgG, the difference is never absolute.

The varied array of antigenic determinants reacting with IgM rheumatoid factors reflects the polyclonality of the antibody molecules themselves. By means of quantitative immunoabsorptions with animal gamma globulins, the IgM rheumatoid factors from a single serum can be separated into multiple species with different antigen-binding profiles.[122,123] Each animal gamma globulin shares but a fraction of the antigenic determinants found on human IgG. Thus the chance of a particular serum reacting with an animal gamma globulin increases with the heterogeneity of the autoantibody response. Because rheumatoid factors in rheumatoid arthritis tend to be more heterogeneous and of higher titer than in nonrheumatic diseases, they more frequently react with animal IgG. This is one of the reasons for the slightly greater specificity of the Rose-Waaler test, as compared with the latex fixation test, for rheumatoid arthritis.

The specificity and polyclonality of IgG and IgA rheumatoid factors have been analyzed in only a few studies.[130] Isolated IgG rheumatoid factors contain both kappa and lambda light chains, although the kappa chains predominate.[34,95,131] They react with human IgG, as indicated by their ability to form immune complexes in autologous serum. A recent study reported that horse IgG was more sensitive, whereas rabbit IgG was more specific, for the detection of IgG rheumatoid factor by radioimmunoassay.[39] Some IgG rheumatoid factors have antinuclear antibody reactivity.[95]

In the future, rheumatoid factors may be divided according to their particular complement of idiotypic antigens. As discussed earlier, idiotypic antigens are serologic indicators of the three-dimensional structure of immunoglobulin variable regions. A series of monoclonal antibodies against human rheumatoid factors has been prepared by the hybridoma technique.[76,77] Eventually these homogeneous reagents should facilitate the systematic classification of rheumatoid factors, including the IgG and IgA rheumatoid factors that frequently escape detection in ordinary assays.

Kinetics of Interaction of Rheumatoid Factor with IgG. The affinity of rheumatoid factors for IgG has been determined by analytical ultracentrifugation and equilibrium molecular sieving.[105,132-134] Typical association constants for both IgM and IgG rheumatoid factors average from 1×10^4 to 5×10^5 liters per mole.[135] These values are from ten- to 100-fold less than the affinities of common heteroantibodies produced after exogenous immunization. A proportion of rheumatoid factors produced by plasma cells in vitro, or eluted from synovium, may have higher affinity.[28,136] These rheumatoid factors may not be detected in serum because of prior reaction with IgG and clearance by the reticuloendothelial system.

In spite of their intrinsically low affinity for antigen, rheumatoid factors can produce stable complexes with IgG under appropriate conditions. For multivalent IgM rheumatoid factor, this occurs when the IgG antigen is aggregated (Fig. 44–14). While each individual antigen-antibody bond in such an IgM-IgG aggregate probably is individually of insufficient energy to yield a long-lived complex, the sum total of multiple interactions produces a stable structure.[104] From a biologic standpoint, the potentiating effect of multivalency is probably greater for those IgM rheumatoid factors of low affinity, since high affinity antibodies, by definition, bind antigens securely even at low concentrations.

IgG rheumatoid factors have unique kinetic properties which distinguish them from all other autoantibodies and heteroantibodies, in that the antigens with which they react reside on the antibody molecule itself. Hence IgG rheumatoid factors can self-associate and form immune complexes in the absence of exogenous antigen.[130,137-139] This self-associating ability favors the formation of immune complexes by anti-Ig antibodies of lower affinity than would be required to produce a similar reaction in a heterologous antigen-antibody system. By analogy with other systems, the ability of IgG rheumatoid factor to form high molecular weight complexes probably depends upon (1) the concentration and affinity of the autoantibody and (2) the ratio of IgG rheumatoid factor to normal IgG. IgM rheumatoid factor may, in addition, enhance the formation of IgG rheumatoid factor containing complexes by cross-linking the reversibly aggregated IgG.[25]

Physiologic Role of Rheumatoid Factors. The regular

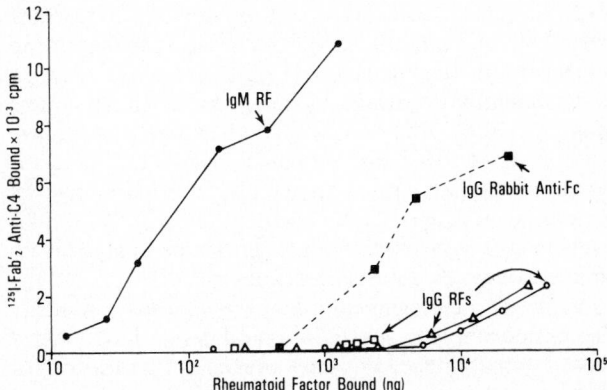

Figure 44–15. Comparison of the complement-fixing ability of IgM rheumatoid factor (RF), IgG rheumatoid factor, and rabbit IgG antibody against human Fc. The ordinate shows the amount of C4 fixed, as a function of the amount of antibody bound to antigen on a solid phase, as shown on the abscissa. (From Sabharwal, U.K., et al.: Arthritis Rheum. 25:1261, 1982.)

appearance of IgM rheumatoid factors during polyclonal B lymphocyte activation strongly suggests that the autoantibodies have an important physiologic function. Polyclonal B lymphocyte activation represents a primitive response of the humoral immune system to bacterial or parasitic exposure.[140] It leads to the production of diverse, low-affinity IgM and IgG antibodies. The IgM antibodies bind efficiently only to repeating antigenic determinants on the offending organism. The IgG antibodies typically interact only weakly with antigen. IgM rheumatoid factors have the ability to crosslink the low affinity IgG antibodies, aligned on a surface.[141] The net result is the formation of a relatively stable, multivalent and multispecific complex.

When bound to aggregated IgG, rheumatoid factors of the IgM class activate complement remarkably efficiently[142-144] (Fig. 44–15). If the IgG is bound to a bacteria or parasite, the end result probably is either the lysis of the invading organism or its clearance from the circulation via the abundant complement receptors of the reticuloendothelial system. For this reason, IgM rheumatoid factor synthesis may represent an essential component of an effective polyclonal antibody response.

Recent experiments in rats provide direct evidence for an important protective role of IgM rheumatoid factor in parasitic infections.[145] Lactating rats, and their suckling offspring, have a serum factor that renders them naturally resistant to infection with pathogenetic trypanosomes. The protective component has been identified as an IgM rheumatoid factor that amplifies a low level IgG response to the parasite.

ROLE OF RHEUMATOID FACTOR IN RHEUMATOID ARTHRITIS

The several mechanisms which have been proposed for the etiology of rheumatoid arthritis are discussed in detail in Chapters 58 and 59. Here, we wish to emphasize

Figure 44–14. Interaction of IgM rheumatoid factor with monomeric and aggregated IgG.

only the salient properties of rheumatoid factors which may contribute to the etiology, tissue specificity, and chronicity of rheumatic disease.

Rheumatoid arthritis is an extravascular immune complex disease predominantly affecting synovial tissues.[146] Thus the synovial fluid of rheumatoid arthritis patients, unlike serum, frequently has markedly depressed complement levels and contains high molecular weight IgG aggregates as detected in the analytical ultracentrifuge or by cryoprecipitation.[30,31,147,148] Partial isolation and characterization of the immune complexes from rheumatoid synovial fluids and tissues have yielded IgG rheumatoid factors, sometimes complexed with IgM rheumatoid factor, in the absence of other known antigens.[31] Thus rheumatoid factors are likely to be of prime importance in the pathogenesis of the extravascular immune complex disease which produces rheumatoid synovitis.

Because of the common occurrence of rheumatoid factor, as measured by latex fixation, in the sera of patients without rheumatic disease, the importance of rheumatoid factor has often been downgraded. In several respects, however, the rheumatoid factors in rheumatoid arthritis patients differ from those in the nonrheumatic diseases (Table 44-4). Rheumatoid factors in rheumatoid arthritis, when compared to those in nonrheumatic conditions, are of higher titer, react better with animal gamma globulins, are produced primarily in the synovium and other extravascular sites, and are enriched in self-associating IgG rheumatoid factor molecules. While no one of these differences is diagnostic of rheumatoid arthritis, the constellation of high titers of heterogeneous IgM and IgG rheumatoid factor produced in the synovium is highly characteristic of rheumatoid arthritis.

The immunochemical properties of rheumatoid factors may have implications important in understanding the pathogenesis of immune complex–mediated synovitis. Most of the immunoglobulin in rheumatoid synovium probably is produced in situ rather than being deposited from the circulation.[149,154] Moreover, many of the IgG-producing plasma cells in rheumatoid synovium contain IgG rheumatoid factor (Fig. 44-16).[138,152,155] At these sites of IgG rheumatoid factor production, the

local concentration of antibody is high while the concentration of normal IgG is low in comparison (Fig. 44-17). This imbalance permits the formation of large IgG rheumatoid factor containing complexes.[37,130,137,138] The ability of IgG rheumatoid factor in rheumatoid arthritis to react with multiple antigenic determinants on the Fc piece could further enhance large complex formation. When the IgG rheumatoid factor containing complexes escape into the circulation, however, where the concentration of normal IgG is high, they may be dissociated into immunoglobulin dimers and trimers. Through the formation of cyclical structures, self-associating IgG rheumatoid factor dimers are probably exceptionally stable.[130,137,138]

Soluble immune complexes with less than three IgG molecules are incapable of fixing complement and bind relatively poorly to IgM rheumatoid factors.[156] Hence the IgG-IgG dimers seen in the sera of patients with rheumatoid arthritis by analytical ultracentrifugation may not be of pathogenic import. The large IgG complexes in rheumatoid synovium, on the other hand, fix complement, bind to IgM rheumatoid factor, and perhaps have the capacity to stimulate other antigen sensitive cells.

In some patients with hypergammaglobulinemic purpura, hyperviscosity syndromes, and monoclonal gammopathies, as well as in some patients with widespread, severe rheumatoid arthritis, the IgG rheumatoid factor concentration in serum may achieve very high concentrations.[33,34,137,138] Under these unusual circumstances, large complement fixing complexes are formed just as they are in the synovium, leading to a diffuse and sometimes life-threatening vasculitis. Additionally, the unique cryoglobulinemic properties of some rheumatoid factors may facilitate precipitation even in the presence of excess normal IgG. In both cases, the IgG aggregates, besides fixing complement, may interfere with granulocyte and lymphocyte function, with a cascade of secondary abnormalities. Nevertheless the larger IgG-IgG complexes in the sera of patients with rheumatoid vasculitis can still be dissociated in vitro to typical IgG dimers by the addition of massive concentrations of normal IgG (Fig. 44-18).

Through the cross-linking of immunoglobulin Fc fragments, IgM rheumatoid factors stabilize and enhance the precipitation of antigen-antibody complexes.[31] On the other hand, IgM rheumatoid factors sterically hinder the binding of IgG molecules to complement and Fc receptor bearing macrophages and neutrophils.[157,158] Thus the effect of IgM rheumatoid factors on such biological consequences of immune complex formation as complement fixation, phagocytosis, and antibody dependent cellular toxicity depends upon the particular system studied. There is no doubt, however, that IgM rheumatoid factors themselves fix complement (Fig. 44-15).[9] Indeed, serum levels of hemolytic rheumatoid factor correlate significantly with in vivo complement turnover rates in patients with rheumatoid arthritis (Fig. 44-19).[159]

Table 44–4. Common Properties of Rheumatoid Factors in Rheumatoid Arthritis and Nonrheumatic Disease

	Rheumatoid Arthritis	Nonrheumatic Disease
Titer	High	Low
Double reactivity with human and animal gamma globulin	Frequent	Infrequent
Immunoglobulin class	IgM, IgG, IgA	Mainly IgM
Site of production	Synovium and other extravascular sites	Unknown, but no synovial localization

Figure 44–16. Demonstration of IgG rheumatoid factor containing plasma cells in rheumatoid synovium by immunofluorescence after digestion with pepsin. *A*, Stained with anti-IgG Fc before pepsin treatment (arrow indicates plasma cell with two nuclei). *B* and *C*, The effect of different pepsin concentrations on intracellular F(ab′)₂-fragments. Stained with anti-F(ab′)₂ after treatment with 0.15 M pepsin in *B* and 0.20 M pepsin in *C*. *D*, Stained with anti-IgG Fc after treatment with 0.15 M pepsin. No staining. *E*, Stained with heat-aggregated IgG before pepsin treatment. No staining. *F*, Stained with native IgG after pepsin treatment. *G*, Stained with heat-aggregated IgG after pepsin treatment. (From Munthe, E., and Natvig, J. B.: Clin. Exp. Immunol. 12:55, 1972.)

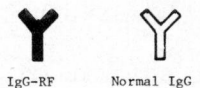

Figure 44–17. Possible mechanisms of immune complex formation by IgG rheumatoid factor in synovial tissues and serum.

Figure 44–18. *A* and *B*, Effect of adding monomeric IgG on the distribution of IgG rheumatoid factor containing intermediate complexes. Lower patterns with albumin added show no effects; upper patterns with γ-globulins added show a shift to smaller complexes. (From Kunkel, H. G., et al.: J. Clin. Invest. 40:117, 1961.)

SUMMARY

Rheumatoid factors are autoantibodies reacting with the Fc portion of autologous IgG. IgM rheumatoid factors are commonly measured by the agglutination of particles coated with human or rabbit IgG. The detection of poorly agglutinating IgG and IgA rheumatoid factors often requires special techniques such as analytical ultracentrifugation, immunofluorescence, or radioimmunoassay. IgM rheumatoid factors are not specific for rheumatoid arthritis but are found in a wide variety of acute and chronic inflammatory diseases and even in some normal individuals. The higher the titer of rheumatoid factor reacting with human and rabbit immunoglobulin, the greater the specificity of rheumatoid factor for rheumatoid arthritis. A variable percentage of rheumatoid patients are seronegative by conventional tests. Some may have hidden rheumatoid factor bound to serum IgG, or undetected IgG rheumatoid factor complexes. A certain percentage of rheumatoid arthritis patients, however, are true seronegatives. Some investigators believe that these patients actually have a different disease from seropositive rheumatoid arthritis.

Most human beings apparently have an inborn ability to make low-affinity rheumatoid factor after stimulation with polyclonal B cell activators, aggregated IgG, or cross-reacting antigens. Immunoglobulin variable region structure genes may influence the particular idiotypic antigens displayed on IgM rheumatoid factors. The role of histocompatibility antigens in rheumatoid factor production is still undefined. By analogy with animal systems, T lymphocytes may regulate the production of IgA and IgA rheumatoid factors.

IgM rheumatoid factors probably function normally in the defense against parasitic and bacterial infection. They substantially amplify the stability of interaction, and hence the biologic activity, of low-affinity IgG antibodies generated during polyclonal B lymphocyte activation.

The antigens on IgG with which rheumatoid factors react are heterogeneous. Most, but perhaps not all, are present on monomeric IgG. The increased reactivity of IgM rheumatoid factor with aggregated as opposed to monomeric IgG probably results from the enhanced stability of antigen-antibody complexes linked at multiple sites.

IgG rheumatoid factors have unique immunochemical properties. Even at low concentrations they form IgG-IgG dimers through preferential self-association. At higher rheumatoid factor concentrations, larger immune complexes are formed. Most of the immunoglobulin in rheumatoid synovium is produced locally. The synovial tissues and fluids of rheumatoid arthritis patients often

Figure 44–19. Relation between the in vivo fractional catabolic rate (FCR) of the C4 component of complement, and hemolytic IgM rheumatoid factor levels, in sixteen patients with rheumatoid arthritis. (From Kaplan, R. A., et al.: Arthritis Rheum. 23:911, 1980.)

contain many IgG rheumatoid factor–producing plasma cells and large complement fixing immune complexes. The restriction of complement-fixing immune complexes in rheumatoid arthritis to the extravascular space in most cases may result from a concentration-dependent aggregation of locally produced IgG rheumatoid factor. In the synovium and other extravascular sites where the concentration of antibody is high and antigen is low, the formation of complement-fixing complexes, with subsequent inflammation, is favored. In serum, where the concentration of normal IgG is high, complement-fixing immune complexes usually do not form. If serum rheumatoid factor levels are very high, however, or if their interaction with IgG results in cryoprecipitation, a systemic immune complex vasculitis may develop.

References

1. Waaler, E.: On the occurrence of a factor in human serum activating the specific agglutination of sheep blood corpuscles. Acta Path. Microbiol. Scand. 17:172, 1940.
2. Rose, H.M., Ragan, C., Pearce, E., and Lipman, M.O.: Differential agglutination of normal and sensitized sheep erythrocytes by sera of patients with rheumatoid arthritis. Proc. Soc. Exp. Biol. Med. 68:1, 1949.
3. Franklin, E.C., Holman, H.R., Muller-Eberhard, H.J., and Kunkel, H.G.: An unusual protein of high molecular weight in the serum of certain patients with rheumatoid arthritis. J. Exp. Med. 105:425, 1957.
4. Lospalluto, J., and Ziff, M.: Chromatographic studies of the rheumatoid factor. J. Exp. Med. 110:169, 1959.
5. Kunkel, H.G., Muller-Eberhard, H.J., Fudenberg, H.H., and Tomasi, T.B.: Gamma globulin complexes in rheumatoid arthritis and certain other conditions. J. Clin. Invest. 40:117, 1961.
6. Heimer, R., and Levin, F.M.: On the distribution of rheumatoid factors among the immunoglobulins. Immunochemistry 3:1, 1966.
7. Zuraw, B.L., O'Hair, C.H., Vaughan, J.H., Mathison, D.A., Curd, J.G., and Katz, D.H.: Immunoglobulin E-rheumatoid factor in the serum of patients with rheumatoid arthritis, asthma and other diseases. J. Clin. Invest. 68:1610, 1981.
8. Singer, J.M., and Plotz, C.M.: The latex fixation test. I. Application to the serologic diagnosis of rheumatoid arthritis. Am. J. Med. 21:888, 1956.
9. Epstein, W., Johnson, A., and Ragan, C.: Observations on a precipitin reaction between serum of patients with rheumatoid arthritis and a preparation (Cohn Fraction II) of human gamma globulin. Proc. Soc. Exp. Biol. Med. 91:235, 1956.
10. Tanimoto, K., Cooper, N.R., Johnson, J.S., and Vaughan, J.H.: Complement fixation by rheumatoid factor. J. Clin. Invest. 55:437, 1975.
11. McCormick, J.N.: An immunofluorescence study of rheumatoid factor. Ann. Rheum. Dis. 22:1, 1963.
12. Franchimont, P., and Suteneau, S.: Radioimmunoassay of rheumatoid factor. Arthritis Rheum. 12:483, 1969.
13. Carson, D.A., Lawrance, S., Catalano, M.A., Vaughan, J.H., and Abraham, G.: Radioimmunoassay of IgG and IgM rheumatoid factors reacting with human IgG. J. Immunol. 119:295, 1977.
14. Hay, C., Nineham, L.J., and Roitt, I.M.: Routine assay for detection of IgG and IgM anti globulins in seronegative and seropositive rheumatoid arthritis. Br. Med. J. 3:203, 1975.
15. Koopman, W.J., and Schrohenloher, R.E.: Sensitive radioimmunoassay for quantification of IgM rheumatoid factor. Arthritis Rheum. 34:302, 1980.
16. Dunne, J.V., Carson, D.A., Spiegelberg, H.L., Alspaugh, M.A., and Vaughan, J.H.: IgA rheumatoid factor in the sera and saliva of patients with rheumatoid arthritis and Sjögren's syndrome. Ann. Rheum. Dis. 38:161, 1979.
17. Pope, R.M., and McDuffy, S.J.: IgG rheumatoid factor. Relationship to seropositive rheumatoid arthritis and absence in seronegative disorders. Arthritis Rheum. 22:988, 1979.
18. Gripenberg, M., Wafis, F., Isomaki, H., and Lindes, E.: A simple enzyme immunoassay for the demonstration of rheumatoid factor. J. Immunol. Methol. 31:109, 1979.
19. Finley, P.R., Hicks, M.J., Williams, R.J., Hinlicky, J. and Lichti, D.A.: Rate nephrometric measurement of rheumatoid factor in serum. Clin. Chem. 25:1909, 1979.
20. Waller, M.V., and Vaughan, J.H.: Use of anti-Rh sera for demonstrating agglutination activating factors in rheumatoid arthritis. Proc. Soc. Exp. Biol. Med. 92:198, 1956.
21. Grubb, R., and Laurell, A.B.: Hereditary serological human serum groups. Acta Pathol. Microbiol. Scand. 39:390, 1956.
22. Natvig, J.B., and Kunkel, H.B.: Detection of genetic antigens utilizing gamma globulins coupled to red blood cells. Nature 215:68, 1967.
23. Steinberg, A.C., and Wilson, J.A.: Hereditary globulin factors and immune tolerance in man. Science 140:303, 1963.
24. Grieble, H.G., Bosh, G.L., Szarto, M., and Anderson, T.O.: Serologic diagnosis of RA. The latex gamma globulin fixation test. J. Chron. Dis. 21:667, 1967.
25. Winchester, R.J., Kunkel, H.G., and Agnello, V.: Occurrence of γ-globulin complexes in serum and joint fluid of rheumatoid arthritis patients. Use of monoclonal rheumatoid factors as reagents for their demonstration. J. Exp. Med. 134:2865, 1971.
26. Meltzer, M., Franklin, E.C., Elias, K., McCluskey, K.J., and Cooper, N.: Cryoglobulinemia—a clinical and laboratory study. II. Cryoglobulins with rheumatoid factor activity. Am. J. Med. 40:837, 1966.
27. Levo, Y., Gorevic, P.P., Kassab, H.J., Zucker-Franklin, D., and Franklin, E.C.: Association between hepatitis B virus and essential mixed cryoglobulinemia. N. Engl. J. Med. 296:501, 1977.
28. Allen, J.C., and Kunkel, H.G.: Hidden rheumatoid factors with specificity for native γ globulin. Arthritis Rheum. 9:758, 1966.
29. Ewald, R.W., and Schubart, A.F.: Agglutinating activity of the complement component C1q in the F-II latex fixation test. J. Immunol. 97:100, 1966.
30. Hannestad, K.: Presence of aggregated γ-globulin in certain rheumatoid synovial effusions. Clin. Exp. Immunol. 2:511, 1967.
31. Winchester, R.J., Agnello, V., and Kunkel, H.G.: Gamma globulin complexes in synovial fluids of patients with rheumatoid arthritis. Partial characterization and relationship to lowered complement levels. Clin. Exp. Immunol. 6:689, 1970.
32. Theofilopoulos, A.N., Burtonboy, G., LoSpalutto, J.J., and Ziff, M.: IgM rheumatoid factor and low molecular weight IgM. An association with vasculitis. Arthritis Rheum. 17:272, 1974.
33. Grey, H.M., Kohler, P.F., Terry, W.D., and Franklin, E.C.: Human monoclonal γ-G cryoglobulins with anti-γ-globulin activity. J. Clin. Invest. 47:1875, 1968.
34. Capra, J.D., Winchester, R.J., and Kunkel, H.G.: Hypergammaglobulinemic purpura. Studies on the unusual anti-γ-globulins characteristic of the sera of these patients. Medicine 50:125, 1971.
35. Chodirker, W.B., and Tomasi, T.B.: Low molecular weight rheumatoid factor. J. Clin. Invest. 42:876, 1963.
36. Schrohenloher, R.E.: Characterization of the γ-globulin complexes present in certain sera having high titers of anti-γ-globulin activity. J. Clin. Invest. 45:501, 1961.
37. Munthe, E., and Natvig, J.B.: Complement fixing intracellular complexes of IgG rheumatoid factor in rheumatoid plasma cells. Scand. J. Immunol. 1:217, 1972.
38. Torrigiani, G., and Roitt, I.M.: Antiglobulin factors in sera from patients with rheumatoid arthritis and normal subjects. Quantitative estimation in different immunoglobulin classes. Ann. Rheum. Dis. 26:334, 1967.
39. Pope, R.N., and McDuffy, S.J.: IgG rheumatoid factor: Analysis of various species of IgG for detection by radioimmunoassay. J. Lab. Clin. Med. 97:842, 1981.
40. Scott, D.G.I., Bacon, T.A., Allen, C., Elson, C.J., and Wallington, T.: IgG rheumatoid factor, complement and immune complexes in rheumatoid synovitis and vasculitis: Comparative and serial studies during cytotoxic therapy. Clin. Exp. Immunol. 43:54, 1981.
41. Elkow, K.B., Delacroix, D.L., Gharevi, A., Vauman, J.P., and Hughes, G.R.: Immunoglobulin A and polymeric IgA rheumatoid factors in systemic sicca syndrome: Partial characterization. J. Immunol. 129:577, 1982.
42. Dresner, E., and Trombly, P.: The latex-fixation reaction in nonrheumatic diseases. N. Engl. J. Med. 261:981, 1959.
43. Howell, D.S., Malcolm, J.M., and Pike, H.: The FII agglutinating factors in the serum of patients with nonrheumatic diseases. Am. J. Med. 29:662, 1960.
44. Kunkel, H.G., Simon, H.J., and Fudenberg, H.: Observations concerning positive serologic reactions for rheumatoid factor in certain patients with sarcoidosis and other hyperglobulinemic states. Arthritis Rheum. 1:289, 1958.
45. Bennett, P.H., and Wood, P.H.N. (eds.): Population Studies of the Rheumatic Diseases. Amsterdam, Excerpta Medica, 1968.
46. Mikkelson, W.M., Dodge, H.J., Duff, I.V., and Kato, H.: Estimates of the prevalence of rheumatic disease in the population of Tecumseh, Michigan, 1950–60. J. Chron. Dis. 20:351, 1967.
47. Hooper, B., Whittingham, S., Mathews, J.D., Mackay, I.R., and Curnow, D.H.: Autoimmunity in a rural community. Clin. Exp. Immunol. 12:79, 1972.

48. Lawrence, J.S.: Rheumatism in Populations. London, William Heinemann, Ltd., 1977.

49. Twomey, J.J., Rossen, R.D., Lewis, V.M., Laughter, A.H., and Douglass, C.C.: Rheumatoid factor and tumor-host interaction. Proc. Natl. Acad. Sci. USA 73:2106, 1976.

50. Theofilopoulos, A., and Dixon, F.J.: The biology and detection of immune complexes. Adv. Immunol. 28:89, 1979.

51. Pope, R.N., Yoshinoya, S., and McDuffy, J.J.: Detection of immune complexes and their relationships to rheumatoid factor in a variety of autoimmune disorders. Clin. Exp. Immunol. 46:259, 1981.

52. Valkenburg, H.A., Ball, J., Burch, T.A., Bennett, P.H., and Lawrence, J.S.: Rheumatoid factors in a rural population. Ann. Rheum. Dis. 25:497, 1966.

53. Moore, T.L., Donner, R.W., Weiss, T.D., Baldassare, A.R., and Zuckner, J.: Hidden 19S rheumatoid factor in juvenile rheumatoid arthritis. Pediatric Res. 14:1135, 1980.

54. Moore, T.L., Donner, R.W., Weiss, T.P., Baldassane, A.R., and Zuckner, J.: Specificity of hidden 19S 19M rheumatoid factor in patients with juvenile rheumatoid arthritis. Arthritis Rheum. 24:1283, 1981.

55. Masi, A.T., Maldonado-Cocco, J.A., Kaplan, S.B., Feigenbaum, S.L., and Chandler, R.W.: Prospective study of the early course of rheumatoid arthritis in young adults. Sem. Arthr. Rheum. 5:299, 1976.

56. Milzaao, S.C.: Seronegative peripheral arthritis. Clin. Rheum. Dis. 3:345, 1977.

57. Pasquali, J.-L., Fong, S., Tsoukas, C.D., Hench, P.K., Vaughan, J.H., and Carson, D.A.: Selective lymphocyte deficiency in seronegative rheumatoid arthritis. Arthritis Rheum. 24:770, 1981.

58. Alarcon, G., Koopman, W.J., Acton, R.T., and Barger, B.O.: Seronegative rheumatoid arthritis: A distinct immunogenetic disease? Arthritis Rheum. 25:502, 1982.

59. Fong, S., Miller, J.J., III, Moore, T.L., Tsoukas, C.D., Vaughan, J.H., and Carson, D.A.: Frequencies of Epstein-Barr virus inducible IgM anti-IgG B lymphocytes in normal children and in children with juvenile rheumatoid arthritis. Arthritis Rheum. 25:959, 1982.

60. Stastny, P.: Mixed lymphocyte cultures in rheumatoid arthritis. J. Clin. Invest. 57:1148, 1976.

61. McMichael, A.J., Sasayuki, T., McDevitt, H.O., and Payne, R.O.: Increased frequency of HLA-DW4 in rheumatoid arthritis. Arthritis Rheum. 20:1037, 1977.

62. Stastny, P.: Association of the B cell alloantigen DRw4 with rheumatoid arthritis. N. Engl. J. Med. 298:869, 1978.

63. Dobloug, J.H., Forre, O., Kass, E., and Thorsby, E.: HLA antigens and rheumatoid arthritis. Association between HLA-DRw4 positivity and IgM rheumatoid factor production. Arthritis Rheum. 23:309, 1980.

64. Mikkelson, W.M., and Dodge, H.: A 4-year follow-up of suspected rheumatoid arthritis. Arthritis Rheum. 12:87, 1967.

65. Hall, A.P.: Observations on subjects developing a positive test for rheumatoid factor. Arthritis Rheum. 12:301, 1969.

66. Ferrone, S., and David, C. (eds.): H-2, Ia and HLA-DR antigens. Hialeah, Florida, CRC Press, 1981.

67. Engleman, E.G., Sponzilli, E.E., Batey, M.E., Ramcharan, S., and McDevitt, H.O.: Mixed lymphocyte reaction in healthy women with rheumatoid factor. Lack of association with HLA-DW4. Arthritis Rheum. 21:690, 1978.

68. Bennett, P.H., and Burch, T.A.: The distribution of rheumatoid factor and rheumatoid arthritis in the families of Blackfeet and Pima Indians. Arthritis Rheum. 11:546, 1968.

69. Kunkel, H.G., Agnello, V., Joslin, F.G., Winchester, R.J., and Capra, J.D.: Cross idiotypic specificity among monoclonal IgM proteins with anti-γ-globulin activity. J. Exp. Med. 137:331, 1973.

70. Capra, J.D., and Kehoe, J.M.: Structure of antibodies with shared idiotypy: the complete sequence of the heavy chain variable regions of two immunoglobulin M anti-gamma globulins. Proc. Natl. Acad. Sci. USA 71:4032, 1974.

71. Carson, D.A., Pasquali, J.-L., Tsoukas, C.D., Fong, S., Slovin, S.F., Lawrance, S.K., Slaughter, L., and Vaughan, J.H.: Physiology and pathology of rheumatoid factors. Springer Semin. Immunopathol. 4:161, 1981.

72. Capra, J.D., Kehoe, J.M., Winchester, R.J., and Kunkel, H.G.: Structure function relationships among anti-gamma globulin antibodies. Ann. N.Y. Acad. Sci. 190:371, 1971.

73. Forre, O., Dobloug, J.H., Michaelsen, T.E., and Natvig, J.B.: Evidence for similar idiotypic determinants on different rheumatoid factor populations. Scand. J. Immunol. 9:281, 1979.

74. Bonagura, V.R., Kunkel, H.G., and Pernis, B.: Cellular localization of rheumatoid factor idiotypes. J. Clin. Invest. 69:1356, 1982.

75. Fong, S., Gilbertson, T., and Carson, D.A.: The internal image of IgG in anti-idiotypic antibodies against human rheumatoid factors. J. Immunol. 131:719, 1983.

76. Carson, D.A., and Fong, S.: A common idiotope on human rheumatoid factors identified by a hybridoma antibody. Molec. Immunol. 20:1081, 1983.

77. Pasquali, J.-L., Urlacher, A., and Storck, D.: A highly conserved determinant on human rheumatoid factor idiotypes defined by a monoclonal antibody. Eur. J. Immunol. 13:197, 1983.

78. Pasquali, J.-L., Fong, S., Tsoukas, C.D., Vaughan, J.H., and Carson, D.A.: Inheritance of IgM rheumatoid factor idiotypes. J. Clin. Invest. 66:863, 1980.

79. Van Snick, J.L.: A gene linked to the Igh-C locus controls the production of rheumatoid factors in the mouse. J. Exp. Med. 153:738, 1981.

80. Fong, S., Tsoukas, C.D., Frincke, L.A., Lawrance, S.K., Holbrook, T.L., Vaughan, J.H., and Carson, D.A.: Age associated changes in Epstein-Barr virus-induced human lymphocyte autoantibody responses. J. Immunol. 126:910, 1981.

81. Fong, S., Vaughan, J.H., Tsoukas, C.D., and Carson, D.A.: Selective induction of autoantibody secretion in human bone marrow by Epstein-Barr virus. J. Immunol. 129:1941, 1982.

82. Welch, M.J., Fong, S., Vaughan, J., and Carson, D.: Increased frequency of rheumatoid factor precursor B lymphocytes after immunization of normal adults with tetanus toxoid. Clin. Exp. Immunol. 51:299, 1983.

83. McCluskey, R.T., Miller, F., and Benacerraf, B.: Sensitization to denatured autologous gamma globulins. J. Exp. Med. 115:253, 1962.

84. Bokisch, V.A., Bernstein, D., and Krause, R.M.: Occurrence of 19S and 7S anti-IgG during hyperimmunization of rabbits with streptococci. J. Exp. Med. 136:799, 1972.

85. Bokisch, V.A., Chiao, J.W., Bernstein, D., and Krause, R.M.: Homogeneous rabbit 7S anti-IgG with antibody specificity for peptidoglycans. J. Exp. Med. 138:1184, 1973.

86. Abruzzo, J.L., and Christian, C.L.: The induction of a rheumatoid factor-like substance in rabbits. J. Exp. Med. 114:791, 1961.

87. Williams, R.C., and Kunkel, H.G.: Rheumatoid factor, complement and conglutinin aberrations in patients with subacute bacterial endocarditis. J. Clin. Invest. 41:666, 1962.

88. Carson, D.A., Bayer, A.S., Eisenberg, R.A., Lawrance, S., and Theofilopoulos, A.: IgG rheumatoid factor in subacute bacterial endocarditis: Relationship to IgM rheumatoid factor and circulating immune complexes. Clin. Exp. Immunol. 31:100, 1978.

89. Dresser, D.W.: Most IgM-producing cells in the mouse secrete autoantibodies (rheumatoid factor). Nature 274:480, 1978.

90. Slaughter, L., Carson, D.A., Jensen, F.C., Holbrook, T.L., and Vaughan, J.H.: In vitro effects of Epstein-Barr virus on peripheral blood mononuclear cells from patients with rheumatoid arthritis and normal subjects. J. Exp. Med. 148:1429, 1978.

91. Izui, S., Eisenberg, R.A., and Dixon, F.J.: IgM rheumatoid factors in mice injected with bacterial lipopolysaccharide. J. Immunol. 122:2096, 1979.

92. Dziarski, R.: Preferential induction of autoantibody secretion in polyclonal activation by peptidoglycan and lipopolysaccharide. II. In vivo studies. J. Immunol. 128:1026, 1982.

93. Van Snick, J.L., and Coulie, P.: Monoclonal anti-IgG antibodies derived from lipopolysaccharide-activated spleen cells of 129/S_v mice. J. Exp. Med. 155:219, 1982.

94. Birdsall, G.H.H., and Rossen, R.D.: Production of antibodies specific for Fc, Fab', and streptokinase-streptodornase in vitro by peripheral blood cells from patients with rheumatoid arthritis and normal donors. J. Clin. Invest. 69:75, 1982.

95. Hannestad, K., and Johannessen, A.: Polyclonal human antibodies to IgG (rheumatoid factors) which cross-react with cell nuclei. Scand. J. Immunol. 5:541, 1976.

96. Hannestad, K., Reckvig, O.P., and Husebekk, A.: Cross-reacting rheumatoid factors and lupus erythematosus (LE)-factors. Springer Semin. Immunopathol. 4:133, 1981.

97. Johnson, P.M.: IgM rheumatoid factors cross-reactive with IgG and a cell nuclear antigen: Immunopathological implications. Ann. Rheum. Dis. 39:586, 1980.

98. Agnello, V., Arbetter, A., DeKasep, G.I., Powell, R., Tan, E.M., and Joslin, F.: Evidence for a subset of rheumatoid factors that cross-react with DNA-histone and have a distinct cross-idiotype. J. Exp. Med. 151:1514, 1980.

99. Johnson, P.M., and Faulk, W.P.: Rheumatoid factor: Its nature, specificity, and production in rheumatoid arthritis. Clin. Immunol. Immunopathol. 6:414, 1976.

100. Dodon, N.D., and Quash, G.A.: The antigenicity of asialylated IgG: Its relationship to rheumatoid factor. Immunology 42:401, 1981.

101. Brown, C.S., and Brown, J.C.: Preferential reactivity of certain human and rabbit IgM and IgG rheumatoid factors with mildly reduced and amidoethylated IgG. J. Immunol. 126:2373, 1981.

102. Van Snick, J.L., and Masson, P.L.: Incidence and specificities of IgA and IgM anti-IgM anti-IgG autoantibodies in various mouse strains and colonies. J. Exp. Med. 151:45, 1980.

103. Andrews, B.S., Eisenberg, R.A., Theofilopoulos, A.N., Izui, S., Wilson, C.B., McConahey, P., Murphy, E.D., Roths, J.B., and Dixon, F.J.: Spontaneous murine lupus-like syndromes. Clinical and immunologic manifestations in several strains. J. Exp. Med. 148:1198, 1978.

104. Metzger, H.: Effect of antigen binding on the properties of antibody. Adv. Immunol. 18:169, 1974.

105. Eisenberg, R.: The specificity and polyvalency of binding of a monoclonal rheumatoid factor. Immunochemistry 13:355, 1976.

106. Weigle, W.O.: Immunological unresponsiveness. Adv. Immunol. 16:61, 1973.

107. Pisko, E.J., Turner, R.A., and Foster, S.L.: Induction of rheumatoid factor producing cells by aggregated IgG. Arthritis Rheum. 25:1108, 1982.

108. Banck, G., and Forsgren, A.: Many bacterial species are mitogenic for human blood B lymphocytes. Scand. J. Immunol. 8:347, 1978.

109. Biberfield, G.: Activation of human lymphocyte subpopulations by *Mycoplasma pneumoniae.* Scand. J. Immunol. 6:1145, 1977.

110. Rosen, A., Gergely, P., Jondal, M., Klein, G., and Britton, S.: Polyclonal Ig production after Epstein-Barr virus infection of human lymphocytes in vitro. Nature 267:52, 1977.

111. Nillson, K., Klein, G., Henle, W., and Henle, G.: The establishment of lymphoblastoid cell lines from adult and fetal human lymphoid tissue and its dependence on EBV. Int. J. Cancer 8:443, 1971.

112. Tovey, M., Lenoir, G., and Begon-Lours, J.: Activation of latent Epstein-Barr virus by antibody to human IgM. Nature 276:270, 1978.

113. Fu, S.M., and Harley, J.N.: Human cell lines containing Epstein-Barr virus but distinct from the common B lymphoblastoid cell lines. Proc. Natl. Acad. Sci. USA 76:6637, 1979.

114. Tsoukas, C.D., Carson, D.A., Fong, S., Pasquali, J.-L., and Vaughan, J.H.: Cellular requirements for pokeweed mitogen induced autoantibody production in rheumatoid arthritis. J. Immunol. 125:1125, 1980.

115. Pasquali, J.-L., Fong, S., Tsoukas, C.D., Slovin, S.F., Vaughan, J.H., and Carson, D.A.: Different populations of rheumatoid factor idiotypes induced by two polyclonal B cell activators, pokeweed mitogen and Epstein-Barr virus. Clin. Immunol. Immunopathol. 21:184, 1981.

116. Alspaugh, M.A., Jensen, F.C., Rabin, H., and Tan, E.M.: Lymphocytes transformed by Epstein-Barr virus. Induction of nuclear antigen reactive with antibody in rheumatoid arthritis. J. Exp. Med. 147:1018, 1978.

117. Catalano, M.A., Carson, D.A., Slovin, S.F., Richman, D.D., and Vaughan, J.H.: Antibodies to Epstein-Barr virus determined antigens in normal subjects and in patients with seropositive rheumatoid arthritis. Proc. Natl. Acad. Sci. USA 76:5825, 1979.

118. Depper, J.M., and Zvaifler, N.J.: Epstein-Barr virus—its relationship to the pathogenesis of rheumatoid arthritis. Arthritis Rheum. 24:755, 1981.

119. Tosato, G., Steinberg, A.D., and Blaese, R.M.: Defective EBV-specific suppressor T-cell function in rheumatoid arthritis. N. Engl. J. Med. 305:1238, 1981.

120. Vaughan, J.H.: Rheumatoid arthritis, rheumatoid factor and the Epstein-Barr virus. J. Rheumatol. 6:381, 1979.

121. Metcalf, E.S., and Klinman, N.R.: In vitro tolerance induction of neonatal murine B cells. J. Exp. Med. 143:1327, 1971.

122. Williams, R.C., and Kunkel, H.G.: Separation of rheumatoid factors of different specificities using columns conjugated with gamma-globulins. Arthritis Rheum. 6:665, 1963.

123. Butler, V.P., Jr., and Vaughan, J.H.: The reaction of rheumatoid factor with animal gamma globulins. Quantitative considerations. Immunology 8:144, 1965.

124. Gaardner, P.I., and Michaelsen, T.E.: Specificity of rheumatoid factors cross-reacting with human and rabbit IgG. Acta Path. Microbiol. Scand. 82:733, 1970.

125. Natvig, J.B., Gaardner, P.I., and Turner, M.W.: IgG antigens of the Cγ2 and Cγ3 homology regions interacting with rheumatoid factors. Clin. Exp. Immunol. 12:177, 1972.

126. Osterland, C.K., Harboe, M., and Kunkel, H.G.: Anti-γ-globulin factors in human sera revealed by enzymatic splitting of anti-Rh antibodies. Vox Sang. 8:133, 1963.

127. Nasu, H., Chia, D.S., Knutson, D.W., and Barrett E.V.: Naturally occurring human antibodies to the F(ab')₂ portion of IgG. Clin. Exp. Immunol. 42:378, 1980.

128. Jerne, N.K.: Towards a network theory of the immune system. Ann. Immunol. (Inst. Pasteur) 125c:374, 1974.

129. Gaardner, P.I., and Natvig, J.B.: Hidden rheumatoid factors reacting with "non a" and other antigens of native autologous IgG. J. Immunol. 105:928, 1970.

130. Nardella, F.A., Teller, D.C., and Mannik, M.: Studies on the antigenic determinants in the self-association of IgG rheumatoid factor. J. Exp. Med. 154:112, 1981.

131. Carson, D.A., and Lawrance, S.: Light chain heterogeneity of 19S and 7S anti-γ-globulins in rheumatoid arthritis and subacute bacterial endocarditis. Arthritis Rheum. 21:438, 1978.

132. Stone, M.J., and Metzger, H.: Binding properties of a Waldenström macroglobulin antibody. J. Biol. Chem. 243:5977, 1968.

133. Normansell, D.E.: Anti-γ-globulins in rheumatoid arthritis sera. II. The reactivity of anti-γ-globulin rheumatoid factors with altered γG-globulin. Immunochemistry 8:593, 1971.

134. Lyet, J.P., and Normansell, D.E.: Low molecular weight rheumatoid factors in rheumatoid arthritis sera. Immunochemistry 11:417, 1974.

135. Wager, O., and Teppo, A.-M.: Binding affinity of human autoantibodies: Studies of cryoglobulin IgM rheumatoid factors and IgG autoantibodies to albumin. Scand. J. Immunol. 7:503, 1978.

136. Robbins, D.L., Morre, T.L., Carson, D.A., and Vaughan, J.H.: Relative reactivities of rheumatoid factors in serum and cells. Arthritis Rheum. 21:820, 1978.

137. Gabriel, D.A., and Hadler, N.M.: The physical characterization of an aggregating IgG heteropolymer containing rheumatoid factor. J. Biol. Chem. 256:3240, 1981.

138. Pope, R.M., Teller, D.C., and Mannik, M.: The molecular basis of self-association of antibodies to IgG (rheumatoid factors) in rheumatoid arthritis. Proc. Natl. Acad. Sci. USA 71:517, 1974.

139. Pope, R.M., Mannik, M., Gilliland, B.C., and Teller, D.C.: The hyperviscosity syndrome in rheumatoid arthritis due to intermediate complexes formed by self-association of IgG-rheumatoid factors. Arthritis Rheum. 18:97, 1975.

140. Clagett, J.A., and Engel, D.: Polyclonal activation: a form of primitive immunity and its possible role in pathogenesis of inflammatory diseases. Dev. Comp. Immunol. 2:235, 1978.

141. Schmid, F.R., Roitt, I.M., and Rochas, M.J.: Complement fixation by a two component antibody system: Immunoglobulin G and immunoglobulin M antiglobulin (rheumatoid factor). J. Exp. Med. 132:673, 1970.

142. Zvaifler, N.J., and Schur, P.H.: Reaction of aggregated mercaptoethanol treated gamma globulin with rheumatoid factor-precipitin and complement fixation studies. Arthritis Rheum. 11:523, 1968.

143. Taylor-Upsahl, M.M., Johnson, P.M., Mellbye, O.J., and Natvig, J.B.: A study of complement fixation by rheumatoid factor using a hemolytic assay system. Clin. Exp. Immunol. 28:204, 1977.

144. Sabharwal, U.K., Vaughan, J.H., Fong, S., Bennett, P.H., Carson, D.A., and Curd, J.G.: Activation of the classical pathway of complement by rheumatoid factors. Arthritis Rheum. 25:161, 1982.

145. Clarkson, E.B., Jr., and Mellon, G.H.: Rheumatoid factor-like immunoglobulin M protects previously uninfected rat pups and dams from *Trypanosoma lewisi.* Science 214:186, 1981.

146. Zvaifler, N.J.: The immunopathology of joint inflammation in rheumatoid arthritis. Adv. Immunol. 13:265, 1973.

147. Hedberg, H.: Studies on the depressed hemolytic complement activity of synovial fluid in adult rheumatoid arthritis. Acta Rheumatol. Scand. 9:165, 1963.

148. Pekin, T.J., Jr., and Zvaifler, N.J.: Hemolytic complement in synovial fluid. J. Clin. Invest. 43:1372, 1964.

149. Sliwinski, A.J., and Zvaifler, N.J.: In vivo synthesis of IgG by the rheumatoid synovial membrane. J. Clin. Invest. 76:304, 1970.

150. Vaughan, J.H., Chihara, T., Moore, T.L., Robbins, D.L., Tanimoto, K., Johnson, J.S., and McMillan, R.: Rheumatoid factor-producing cells detected by direct hemolytic plaque assay. J. Clin. Invest. 58:933, 1976.

151. Taylor-Upsahl, M.M., Abrahamsen, T.G., and Natvig, J.B.: Rheumatoid factor plaque-forming cells in rheumatoid synovial tissue. Clin. Exp. Immunol. 28:197, 1977.

152. Munthe, E., and Natvig, J.B.: Immunoglobulin classes, subclasses and complexes of IgG rheumatoid factor in rheumatoid plasma cells. Clin. Exp. Immunol. 12:55, 1972.

153. Fehr, K., Valbart, M., Rauber, M., Knoppel, M., Baici, A., Salgam, T., and Boni, A.: Production of agglutinators and rheumatoid factors in plasma cells of rheumatoid and non-rheumatoid synovial tissue. Arthritis Rheum. 24:510, 1981.

154. Munthe, E., and Natvig, J.B.: Characterization of IgG complexes in eluates from rheumatoid tissue. Clin. Exp. Immunol. 8:249, 1971.

155. Petersen, J., Heilmann, C., Bjerium, O.J., Ingemann-Hansen, T., and Halkjair-Kristensen, J.: IgG rheumatoid factor secreting lymphocytes in rheumatoid arthritis. Evaluation of a haemolytic plaque forming cell technique. Scand. J. Immunol. 17:471, 1983.

156. Hyslop, N.E., Jr., Dourmashkin, R.R., Green, N.M., and Porter, R.R.: The fixation of complement and the activated first component (C1) of complement by complexes formed between antibody and divalent hapten. J. Exp. Med. 130:703, 1970.

157. McDuffie, F.C., and Brumfield, H.W.: Effect of rheumatoid factor on complement mediated phagocytosis. J. Clin. Invest. 57:3007, 1972.

158. Bolton, W.K., Schroek, J.H., and Davis, J.T.: IV. Rheumatoid factor inhibition of in vitro binding of IgG complexes to the human glomeruli. Arthritis Rheum. 25:297, 1982.

159. Kaplan, R.A., DeHeer, D.H., Carson, D.A., Pangburn, M.K., Muller-Eberhard, H.J., and Vaughan, J.H.: Metabolism of C4 and Factor B in rheumatoid arthritis: Relation to rheumatoid factor. Arthritis Rheum. 23:911, 1980.

Chapter 45
Immune Complexes

E. Dayer and P.H. Lambert

INTRODUCTION

Although the immunopathogenesis of most inflammatory rheumatic diseases is certainly multifactorial, antigen-antibody complexes can be involved in several of these diseases. They can often be detected in blood or in synovial space throughout the clinical course, with increased levels at the time of exacerbation.

The formation of immune complexes (ICs) by binding of antigens to their corresponding antibodies is a physiologic process usually of benefit to the host; IC formation allows the neutralization or the elimination of microbial antigens and of other exogenous antigens. Usually, ICs are eliminated rather efficiently by the fixed mononuclear phagocytic system, particularly by Kupffer cells in the liver.[1] Therefore, circulating ICs can be detected for only a short period of time after a specific antigenic challenge.

Immune complexes can play a role in the pathogenesis of autoimmune and immunological disorders. Indeed, in animals injected with bovine serum albumin,[2] the onset of glomerulonephritis, arthritis, or vasculitis coincided with the appearance of soluble ICs in the circulation and the deposition of ICs in renal glomeruli, synovial tissues, or vessel walls. In man, there is also evidence that ICs are directly involved in the pathogenesis of a variety of rheumatic diseases and that ICs formed during infections may participate in the development or the persistence of major inflammatory lesions.

The level of ICs in blood or in interstitial fluids reflects the balance between their generation and their clearance.

GENERATION OF IMMUNE COMPLEXES

The formation of circulating ICs in human diseases is a function of the availability of antigen molecules to react with the corresponding antibodies. Immune complexes primarily involve antigens from (a) exogenous sources (food, drugs, heterologous serum proteins); (b) microbial sources (viral, bacterial or parasitic); and (c) autologous sources (autoantigens, tumor antigens). For example, exogenous antigens are found in ICs from patients receiving antilymphocyte globulins or in those with food allergy.[1] Microbial antigens can be found in immune complexes associated with some infectious diseases. In hepatitis B, there is a transient phase during which a significant proportion of HB surface antigen is present in serum as a complex with anti-HBs antibodies.[3] Among autoantigens, the presence of DNA has been

suspected in ICs from patients with systemic lupus erythematosus, although it certainly does not represent a major antigen in the circulating immune complexes.[4]

Recently, advances have been made in the direct analysis of antigens present in ICs purified from human sera. Such purification can be done using columns filled with C1q or conglutinin-coated plastic beads.[5] The purified ICs have been shown, by SDS-polyacrylamide gel electrophoresis (SDS-PAGE), to contain complement components (C1q, C1r, C1s, and C3) and immunoglobulins (Fig. 45–1). In some instances (e.g., lepromatous leprosy), an antigen from the infectious agent has been identified as a component of the IC.[6] In most cases, however, the identification of specific antigens has proved to be difficult and only immunoglobulins and complement can be regularly demonstrated in purified immune complexes.

Antibodies directed toward the individual's own immunoglobulin may be important. A frequent feature of many IC diseases is hypergammaglobulinemia, which usually reflects a nonspecifically increased immunoglobulin synthesis.

Polyclonal activation produced in experimental animals by lipopolysaccharide or by protozoan parasites led to the production of a large variety of antibodies, including autoantibodies, and resulted in the formation and the persistence of ICs in circulation.[7] No heterologous antigen was detected within these circulating ICs; therefore, autoantibodies might be involved. There is evidence that anti-immunoglobulin autoantibodies may be of particular importance. Thus, the possibility that ICs may result from specific interactions between immunoglobulin molecules, without the involvement of exogenous antigen, should be considered in many clinical situations.

Autoantibodies against immunoglobulin can be directed against either the constant region or the antibody combining site. Antibodies produced against a constant portion of the IgG molecule (rheumatoid factors) occur frequently during polyclonal B-lymphocyte activation and in some rheumatic or infectious diseases. In rheumatoid arthritis, there is a close correlation between the production of such anti-IgG antibodies and the appearance of ICs.[8] The other antigenic site of immunoglobulins is located on the hypervariable region, or antibody combining site (idiotypic determinant). Each antibody has its own idiotype, which distinguishes it from antibody produced by other B-lymphocyte clones in the same individual. Cross-reactions can exist between idiotypes of immunoglobulin produced by different clones (cross-reacting idiotypes). It has been suggested

IgM

150 → ← IgG
136 → ← Prot.A-reactive
128 → ← C3(bi)
117 → ← Prot.A-reactive

92 → ← C1r̄
89 → ← C1s̄

68 → ← (C1s̄')
63 → ← C1q

49 → ← *

30.7 →
28.7 →
24.4 → ← *

MW(kD)   identification

Figure 45–1. Immune complexes from SLE patients are analyzed by sodium dodecylsulfate-polyacrylamide gel electrophoresis. Some components of IC have been identified after transfer to nitrocellulose sheets and reaction with appropriate antisera. Some bands (*) do not react with an antiserum against normal human serum proteins.

that the antibody repertoire of an individual consists of a network of idiotypes and anti-idiotypic antibodies. In this network each immunoglobulin would function both as an antibody directed toward the combining site of other immunoglobulins and as an immunogen for yet other immunoglobulins.[9]

Interactions between idiotype and anti-idiotype could play a role in the immunopathology of certain diseases. The frequent stimulation of antigen-specific antibodies and their corresponding anti-idiotypic antibodies could result in the formation of idiotype–anti-idiotype complexes. If many B lymphocytes were stimulated simultaneously and nonspecifically, as in polyclonal B-lymphocyte activation, many different idiotypic clones might produce immunoglobulin synchronously with their corresponding anti-idiotypic clones. Thus, some of the complexes appearing could consist of a wide variety of idiotype–anti-idiotype complexes. Such complexes have been shown to occur in animal models.[10] Recently idiotype–anti-idiotype complexes have been found in human patients with mixed cryoglobulinemia (type II).[11] The presence of anti-idiotypic antibodies (anti-anti DNA) has been suggested in systemic lupus erythematosus.[12] The idiotypic network provides, therefore, a large source of potential antigens and corresponding antibodies, and the formation of ICs may often represent

a perturbation of physiologic interactions in this network.

Mechanisms Leading to the Clearance of Immune Complexes. In vitro, immune complexes have been shown to bind to phagocytic cells through the Fc and C3 receptors found on their surface.[13] The adherence of immune complexes is usually enhanced after complement fixation[14] and is followed by the cellular uptake of ICs. In vivo, the clearance rate of immune complexes from the circulation depends on their removal by the mononuclear phagocytic system (MPS) (Fig. 45–2). In animals, the fate of preformed immune complexes depends on the lattice structure, on the nature of each component of the IC, and on the status of the mononuclear phagocytic system. Large latticed immune complexes are cleared much faster than small latticed ones.[15] Carbohydrate moieties on IgG[16] and IgM[17] may play a role in the hepatic uptake of ICs. The mononuclear phagocytic system can be saturated by large numbers of ICs, favoring the persistence of large latticed immune complexes in circulation.[18]

The role of the complement system in the clearance of immune complexes is still controversial. The persistence of ICs is not influenced by a depletion of circulating complement components,[19,20] but complexes that do not fix complement efficiently persist for a long time in the circulation.[21] In man, the capacity to clear circulating ICs has been estimated by measuring the clearance of IgG-sensitized red blood cells. However, such cells are preferentially removed by the spleen, rather than by the liver, as with soluble immune complexes.[22] Some patients with systemic lupus erythematosus (SLE) have an impaired clearance, which correlates with increased C1q binding activity.[23]

Immune complexes may be unequally distributed be-

IN VIVO FORMATION OF IMMUNE COMPLEXES

Figure 45–2 Possible sites of formation of immune complexes in vivo. IC may be formed in circulating blood or in extravascular spaces, according to the localization of the antigens at the time when antibodies appear; ag represents a source of antigen, e.g. a microorganism and ab the antibody MPS = mononuclear phagocytic system. The fate of the complexes is dependent on the site of their formation.

tween the intravascular and extravascular body fluid compartments. When immune complexes are formed in extravascular spaces, their clearance will depend (a) on the diffusion of ICs to the blood or to the lymphatic system and (b) on the accumulation of phagocytic cells, mostly polymorphonuclear leukocytes and monocytes, at the site of formation of ICs in tissues.

Interaction of Complement and Immune Complexes. Complement activation by ICs can, on the one hand, be responsible for changes of the IC structure and, on the other hand, can generate small peptides mediating the inflammatory response and favoring the elimination of ICs. The activation of the complement system by ICs brings C3b in close contact with the Fc part of the immunoglobulins in the ICs. Together with C3b, Factors B and P generate an alternative pathway convertase (C3b-Bb-P), which increases the cleavage of native C3 to C3b and leads to the intercalation of more C3b molecules in the IC lattice.[24] This results in a decrease of the size of the immune complexes, usually called *solubilization*. In vivo, the presence of C3b or C3bi on immunoglobulins facilitates the *binding to cells* expressing C3b or C3bi receptors. These have been found on erythrocytes, neutrophils, eosinophils, macrophages, and lymphocytes. Most complexes bound to nonphagocytic cells are released in the environment after the interaction of the IC with the complement regulatory proteins, Factors I and H.[25] Complexes bound to phagocytic cells can be eliminated by phagocytosis. In the course of complement activation, the release of peptides increases vascular permeability and attracts leukocytes.[26] This *inflammatory response* favors the accumulation of phagocytic cells at the site of complement activation and eliminates the immune complexes. In man, the interaction of ICs with the complement system seems of importance for their clearance from extravascular spaces. Indeed, in a study of synovial fluids from patients with rheumatoid arthritis (RA), the largest ICs were observed in those with the least capacity to solubilize ICs in vitro.[27] Factors that increase the size of ICs may also limit their diffusion from extravascular spaces and favor the persistence of the local inflammation.

Influence of the Structure of Immune Complexes on Their Pathogenicity. The properties of ICs may modify their clearance and binding to extravascular structures. Immune complexes usually result from the interaction of several different antigenic determinants on an antigen molecule with the corresponding *antibodies*. Therefore, they represent a heterogeneous material. Some particular properties of ICs depend on the affinity, class, and subclass of the antibodies involved (Table 45–1). For example, it has been shown that antibodies of low avidity do not form ICs with a stable lattice. Such ICs are not efficiently eliminated and would be preferentially deposited in renal glomeruli.[28] Properties of the *antigenic* component such as size, charge, and reactivity with tissue structures also influence the persistence of ICs and their potential pathogenicity. DNA, which is a negatively charged antigen, has a particular affinity for collagen structures[29] and presumably DNA-containing ICs

Table 45–1. Factors Influencing the Properties of Immune Complexes

1. Nature of antigen(s)	Size, charge, reactivity with biologic structures, antigenic determinants
2. Nature of antibodies	Class, subclass, affinity
3. Antigen-antibody ratio	
4. Secondary binding of IC-reactive molecule	Complement, rheumatoid factor, immunoconglutinin

are preferentially bound to such structures. The *relative concentration of the antigen and of the antibody* influences the size, and solubility, and the reactivity of the complexes. Small ICs may be trapped in small blood vessels or may be stuck in filtering membranes (glomerular basement membrane, choroid plexus). Such localization of ICs is favored by an increased vascular permeability and possibly by a decrease of the density of anionic sites in basement membranes.[30] Finally, the structure and properties of ICs are directly influenced by the *secondary binding of IC-reactive molecules,* particularly complement components and rheumatoid factors.

PRINCIPLES OF THE METHODS FOR DETECTION OF IMMUNE COMPLEXES IN SERUM AND SYNOVIAL FLUID

Immune complexes have been demonstrated in human disease[31] by the analysis of tissue specimens and by serologic testing of samples from various biologic fluids. Conventional histology or electron microscopy of pathologic specimens may reveal similarities with lesions induced experimentally by immune complexes. Immunohistochemical staining allows a more direct demonstration of immunoglobulin deposits, with or without associated complement components. Studies of biologic fluids provide evidence for the association of immune complexes with particular pathologic conditions, either by the direct detection of ICs or by demonstration of serologic changes, which are often associated with their presence. The initial assays for detecting soluble immune complexes in body fluids were based on their physicochemical properties, such as the size of the immune complexes, which is in turn dependent on the degree of aggregation of the complexed immunoglobulins. More recent methods have focused on the biologic properties of antibody and/or antigen molecules, detecting either the increased density of these molecules in complexes or the generation of immune mediators. Thus, aggregated antibodies bind more avidly than monomeric antibodies to C1q or to cellular receptors.

Differentiation of Immune Complexes From Monomeric IgG by Physical Properties. The new molecular structures generated after the antigen-antibody interactions are characterized by an increased molecular size and by changes of the surface properties, solubility, and electric charge as compared with the corresponding free antigens and antibodies. Molecular size and solubility of ICs are most widely used for their detection by physical methods.

Analytic ultracentrifugation allows the demonstration in various biologic fluids of an abnormal level of material sedimenting at a high velocity. The use of preparative methods for separation of macromolecular aggregates such as *sucrose gradient ultracentrifugation* or *gel filtration* permits the analysis of the various fractions and the study of their specific immunologic properties and concentrations. Additional evidence for the presence of ICs has been obtained by comparing the pattern at neutral pH with that at acid pH, which dissociates ICs. Ultracentrifugation and gel filtration are sometimes used in the purification of immune complexes, but are limited by contamination of the complexes with monomeric immunoglobulins. They can be combined with the use of labeled markers for ICs such as C1q[32,33] or antiglobulins[34] but are too time consuming for routine use.

Material with a decreased solubility in well-defined conditions (temperature, medium) occurs frequently in serum or other biologic fluids containing ICs. Abnormal precipitation of proteins in a serum sample under such defined conditions may therefore indicate the presence of ICs. The simplest procedure is precipitation at cold temperature. *Cryoglobulins* may frequently represent a particular type of IC, but monoclonal immunoglobulins or other proteins are often involved. Extensive immunochemical analysis of cryoprecipitates is required when considering cryoglobulins as possible immune complexes.[35] The extent of precipitation of serum proteins in *polyethylene glycol* (PEG, MW = 6000), an uncharged linear polymer, is generally proportional to the protein molecular size and to the concentration of PEG.[36] At low concentrations of PEG, high molecular weight proteins and ICs are preferentially precipitated before monomeric IgG. Although an increase in the amount of PEG precipitate often indicates ICs, such precipitation is influenced by other serum proteins and is a rather nonspecific screening test for ICs. More accurate informa-

tion may be obtained by analysis of the proteins (e.g., IgG, C1q, C4) precipitated at low PEG concentrations. Precipitation in PEG can be combined with the use of radiolabeled markers for immune complexes, such as C1q or staphylococcal protein A.[37]

Differentiation of Immune Complexes from Monomeric IgG by Interaction with Biologic Recognition Units. Soluble immune complexes can be detected by their reactivity with some plasma proteins or with biologic recognition units on cell membranes. (Fig. 45–3).

Interaction with Recognition Sites on Plasma Proteins. The reaction of immune complexes with complement components affords several methods for IC recognition. Complement-fixing immune complexes may be detected either by indirect measurement of complement consumption (e.g., anticomplementary activity, C1q deviation test)[38,39] or by direct evaluation of the binding of immune complexes to C1q, the first component of complement (C1q binding fluid phase[33] or solid phase assays[40]). In addition, because the reaction of immune complexes with complement leads to the persistence of some complement components on the immune complexes, such immune complexes coated with complement bind to molecules with an affinity for fixed activated complement components (e.g., conglutinin-binding assays,[41] anti-C3 assays[42]). The general feature of this group of methods is their dependence on the reactivity of the immune complex with complement. Although most circulating immune complexes may fulfill this requirement, those containing only IgG4, IgA, or IgE would not. The reactivity of substances other than immune complexes with complement components especially limits the specificity of inhibition assays (e.g., anticomplementary activity, C1q deviation test). A second group of assays that discriminate aggregated from monomeric immunoglobulins are based on the interaction of ICs with low-avidity anti-immunoglobulin antibodies.[43] Most of these methods are sensitive only for ICs containing IgG antibodies and are influenced to some extent

Figure 45–3. Assays for the detection of IC can be divided in 3 groups: solid phase, fluid phase, and cellular binding assays. In solid phase assays, the recognition unit is coated on a plastic tube, then interacted with the sample, and finally revealed with a radiolabeled anti-immunoglobulin reagent. In fluid phase assays, the radiolabeled recognition unit is incubated with the sample and the bound and free recognition units are separated by differential precipitation. In cellular assays, appropriate cells are incubated with the sample and immune complexes attached to cells are quantitated by a radiolabeled anti-immunoglobulin reagent.

by the concentration of monomeric IgG in the tested sample.

Interaction with Cell-Bound Receptors. The analysis of specific interactions of immune complexes with cells may provide information directly relevant to important biologic effects of such complexes. The use of living cells makes standardization difficult and is limited by the possible occurrence of factors interfering with the cell metabolism and by the occasional binding of antibodies directly to cell membranes. Many cells expressing a receptor for the Fc part of immunoglobulin can be used to detect ICs, since they usually bind more avidly aggregated immunoglobulins or ICs than monomeric immunoglobulins. All methods using this property for the detection of ICs are influenced to some extent by the concentration of immunoglobulins in the tested samples. The interaction of complement-coated ICs with complement receptors on cells may also be used. Various cells exhibit a high affinity for complement-coated ICs owing to the presence of receptors for complement components on the cell surface. Most of these receptors interact preferentially with C3b or its breakdown products, C3bi and C3d. One lymphoblastoid cell line, derived from a patient with Burkitt's lymphoma (the Raji cell line) is particularly suitable for the detection of ICs because it has a high density of complement receptors and lacks surface immunoglobulins.[44]

Methods Specific for Antigen. In particular clinical conditions it may be useful to know whether a specific antigen is contained in immune complexes and to distinguish between free antigen molecules and those bound specifically to immunoglobulins. In the case of particulate antigen, such as a virus, the detection of aggregated virus particles by electron microscopy suggests their involvement in immune complexes.[45] Free and complex-bound antigen can be further differentiated by measuring the amount of antigen removed from a serologic sample when the host immunoglobulins are specifically absorbed or precipitated. Thus, the virus titer of sera from mice infected with lactic dehydrogenase virus decreased strikingly after the specific precipitation of immunoglobulins.[46] The differential precipitation of the antigen bound to IC and free antigen was applied to HBs antigen using, in a first step, an incubation with radiolabeled anti-HBs Fab. In a second step the percentage of HBs antigen bound to immunoglobulins was determined by precipitation with an anti-Fc antibody and was compared with the precipitation of all HBs antigen using PEG 10 percent.[3] Further improvement of the method has been achieved by absorbing immune complexes on conglutinin-coated tubes and revealing free antigen-binding sites with labeled antibody to specific antigen (e.g., anti-HBs, anti-idiotype). This approach usually requires knowledge of the nature of the antigen in ICs. Antigen will be demonstrable only if free antigenic sites are exposed, and, therefore, this approach does not work when antibody is present in large excess.

Antigen-specific methods can be of clinical use for the diagnosis of some infectious diseases at the early stage of the immune response, when neither free antigen nor free antibody can be detected in the circulation. Considering the multiplicity of antigen-antibody systems possibly involved in the in vivo formation of ICs, it is unlikely that such antigen-specific methods would be routinely used in clinical situations. Their use would probably be restricted to the assessment of the immune status in well-defined conditions.

METHODS COMMONLY USED FOR THE DETECTION OF IMMUNE COMPLEXES

The sensitivity of each method for detecting immune complexes varies according to the nature of the ICs involved and the influence of various interfering factors. Difficulty in standardizing reagents and the complexity of the procedure may also impair applicability and reproducibility of some methods. Only a limited number of methods are suitable for routine laboratory investigation. A few operational principles of the most widely used methods will be described here.

Assays Involving Solid Phase Binding. Test samples are incubated in plastic tubes coated with an IC-recognition unit. Bound ICs are then quantitated using radiolabeled or enzyme-conjugated antibodies directed toward immunoglobulins. Such methodology has been successfully applied with various IC-recognition units: C1q, conglutinin, anti-C3 F(ab)2, and rheumatoid factor. Solid phase assays have many advantages over other methods of detection: they do not require any centrifugation, and results are quickly available when enzyme-conjugated reagents are used. They also allow for the quantitation of specific classes of immunoglobulin using labeled anti-immunoglobulin against IgG, IgM, IgA, or labeled staphylococcal protein A. However, the washing steps may favor the dissociation of low avidity antibodies from antigens and of ICs from the recognition unit. Such tests may also be influenced by the presence of rheumatoid factor in the sample.

C1q Solid Phase Binding Assay (C1q SP). The EDTA-treated sample is placed in a plastic tube previously coated with C1q, and the amount of ICs bound to the tube is determined, using the anti-Ig reagent.[40] The test (Fig. 45-4) may be influenced by the level of C1q in the tested sample, and only immune complexes reacting with C1q are detected.

Conglutinin Solid Phase Binding Assay (KgB). The test sample is incubated in the presence of calcium in a plastic tube coated with bovine conglutinin, which reacts with C3bi-bearing ICs. Bound ICs are determined after

Figure 45-4. Detection of IC by binding to solid phase conglutinin.

addition of labeled staphylococcal protein A or anti-immunoglobulin.[41] The test detects ICs that activate either the classical or the alternative complement pathway and bind C3. An excess of conglutinin should be used to coat the tubes in order to avoid inhibition by free C3 fragments generated either in vivo or during the in vitro manipulation of the sample.

Anti-C3 Solid Phase Binding Assay. Plastic tubes are coated with (Fab)'2 fragments of an antibody to C3 and then interacted with the serum samples. The amount of bound immune complex is measured with a radiolabeled anti-Ig reagent.[42]

Monoclonal Rheumatoid Factor Binding Inhibition Assay (mRF-I). This test (Fig. 45–5) is based on the inhibition by immune complexes of the binding of radiolabeled aggregated IgG to monoclonal RF, that has been coupled to microcrystalline cellulose.[43] Because monomeric IgG also binds to RF, although less avidly than aggregated IgG, serum samples must be diluted to a constant IgG content prior to analysis. Sample, labeled aggregates, and RF-cellulose are incubated together; the cellulose is then washed and the amount of bound IgG is measured. This assay is sensitive only for IC containing IgG.

Assays Involving Fluid Phase Binding. Fluid phase assays are based on the differential precipitation of free radiolabeled IC-recognition unit (C1q, conglutinin) from the same receptor bound to the IC.

C1q Binding Assay (C1q BA). Radiolabeled C1q is added to EDTA-treated serum in the presence of polyethylene glycol (PEG 2.5 percent, final concentration). After 1 hour, free C1q is separated from the precipitated bound C1q by centrifugation.[33] The percentage of radioactivity precipitated corresponds to the C1q binding activity of the sample and indicates the level of ICs. PEG favors the binding of C1q to ICs preventing their dissociation, and therefore, is suitable for the detection of low avidity ICs. Labeled C1q reacts as a tracer molecule and reflects the binding of endogenous C1q to IC during the test. Thus there is some competition between endogenous C1q and labeled C1q. This test is particularly sensitive for complexes containing IgM and this may explain the high level of positivity usually observed in RA. The binding of non–IC substances (e.g., polyanions) to C1q is not a major cause of false results at the ionic strength used except for heparin used to collect plasma.

Assays Involving Binding to Cells. Aggregates of Ig

Figure 45–6. Two kinds of immune complex tests involving C1q: Fluid phase binding and PEG precipitation or solid phase binding.

or immune complexes bind to Fc and complement receptors on the surfaces of various cell types, and the activities of the cell may change after binding ICs. Two approaches have been used to quantify the binding of immune complexes to cells: either direct quantitation with a labeled anti-immunoglobulin (e.g., Raji cell assay) or indirect quantitation by measurement of changes of cell function (e.g., platelet aggregation).

Raji Cell Binding Assay. This assay (Fig. 45–7) is based on the binding of IC to C3b and C3bi receptors on a continuous lymphoblastoid cell line (Raji cells). The Raji cell line is particularly suitable for detecting IC, since these cells lack surface Ig and have few or low affinity receptors for IgG Fc and a large number of receptors for complement. IC bound to cells are quantitated with a labeled anti-IgG antibody;[44] the level of IC is extrapolated from a standard curve prepared with increasing amounts of aggregated immunoglobulins mixed with human serum as a source of complement. The Raji cell assay is very sensitive for IC containing IgG. Detection of IgM-containing complexes is complicated in some diseases (e.g., SLE) by falsely high levels produced by antilymphocyte antibodies (IgM). The technique requires experience in continuous cell culture.

Platelet Aggregation Assay. Freshly collected platelets aggregate after the interaction of their surface Fc receptor with IC containing IgG. In the presence of immune complexes, the titer can be measured using microplates.[47] The test has also been done using serum that had been heat inactivated in order to prevent inhibition caused by high concentration of C1q. Some variation occurs with platelets from different donors. Antiplatelet antibodies, some myxoviruses, and some enzymes can also aggregate platelets. Recently, this test has been modified,

Figure 45–5. Detection of IC by inhibition of binding of aggregated IgG to solid phase monoclonal rheumatoid factor.

Figure 45–7. Detection of IC by binding to complement receptors on Raji cells.

using labeled anti-IgG reagents to measure platelet-bound immune complexes.

Interpretation of Results. The biologic activity and some of the physical characteristics of ICs may change after *collection of serum samples.* In order to obtain accurate results, one should take care in collecting and storing the samples. Blood should be allowed to clot for 2 hours without cooling (minimum temperature 25° C) in order to avoid the cryoprecipitation of some ICs. The serum samples should be kept frozen, if possible, at $-70°$ C and repeated freezing and thawing should be avoided. The use of plasma samples may lead to false results. For tests based on reactivity with complement, the presence of heparin, even at low concentrations, may interfere.

The *manipulation of the samples* at the time of testing is also of importance. Heat inactivation is not advisable, since it can aggregate IgG or alter the reactivity of IC with Fc or C3 receptors. Similarly, treating samples with reducing agents or with IgG immunoabsorbents in order to decrease RF activity before the test, may partially deplete ICs or change the IC structure. For all tests performed with living cells, toxic preservatives should be avoided.

The *expression of the results* may differ according to the test system used. Frequently, test levels are referred to standard curves with various concentrations of aggregated IgG. It should be pointed out that considerable variations exist between aggregated IgG preparations used in different laboratories. It is now possible to standardize the expression of the results, since reference preparations for IC measurement (tetanus toxoid–anti-tetanus toxoid IC and stabilized aggregated IgG) have been made available by a joint WHO/IUIS Committee.* The apparent level of IC in a serum sample may differ according to the test used. This reflects the heterogeneity of ICs in relation to their biologic activity or physical characteristics.

Because methods of detection of ICs are indirect, do not allow for a specific quantitation of the protein content, and are susceptible to interference by other substances, appropriate *control experiments* are required whenever ICs are demonstrated in a new clinical entity. These include (1) characterization of the size of the putative ICs, since immune complexes are larger than monomeric immunoglobulin; (2) fractionation in physicochemical conditions known to dissociate immune complexes and to decrease their size and biologic activities; and (3) confirmation that the test becomes negative after removal of immunoglobulins from the tested sample (e.g., by immunoabsorption) or after treatment known to alter the biologic properties of ICs (e.g., reduction and alkylation).

Factors interfering with the detection of ICs in biologic fluid should be considered for each test system. Tests based on the interaction with C1q may be influenced

by the presence in the sample of bacterial lipopolysaccharides or polyanions (e.g., heparin, DNA). Treatment of serum samples with DNAase can eliminate the interference by DNA. The recognition of activated C3 on the ICs may be inhibited by the presence of C3 fragments or non-IC C3 binding material (e.g., CRP complexes) in the tested sample. Conglutinin assays cannot be performed on EDTA or citrated samples because calcium is required. False positive results may be observed with cellular assays because of antilymphocyte antibodies. Other assays using living cells or platelets can also be influenced by a direct effect of various non-IC substances (e.g., bacterial lipopolysaccharides, mitogens, toxic agents) or by antibodies against cell membrane antigens (e.g., anti-HLA, anti-platelet).

EVALUATION OF IMMUNE COMPLEX DETECTION IN RHEUMATIC DISEASE

Critical Evaluation. The evaluation of methods for IC measurements in clinical investigation should be based on the sensitivity and specificity of each test. The *sensitivity* of a given method cannot be related only to the detection of aggregated immunoglobulins or of artificial complexes. Indeed, the sensitivity for IC detection will vary according to the type of ICs occurring in each disease considered. For example, using six techniques to measure IC levels in SLE and RA, it was found that some methods (fluid phase C1q binding, mRF-inhibition) are most sensitive for ICs from patients with RA; other methods (Raji cell assay, conglutinin solid phase assay, C1q solid phase assay) were more sensitive for ICs from patients with SLE. In most diseases studied, the *specificity* of the commonly used methods is generally sufficient to assert that the detected activity is due to ICs. Therefore, the selection of methods for the measurement of ICs in a given rheumatic disease should be influenced by the *sensitivity* of the method in this disease and by knowledge of the possible interfering factors in these patients. For example, although all three tests have a similar sensitivity, the C1q solid phase assay or the conglutinin solid phase assay would be preferable to the Raji cell assay in following patients with SLE, who may have circulating antibodies to lymphoblastic cells. In patients with RA, the C1q fluid phase assay would be preferable to the conglutinin solid phase assay in view of its higher sensitivity for the low avidity IgM-containing ICs encountered in this disease.

With all tests used, the *upper normal value* for ICs can only be based on a statistical analysis, since low amounts are formed in physiologic conditions. The distribution of normal values is asymmetrical, and therefore it is not advisable to use, as the upper limit, the value of the mean $\pm$ 2 SD. It is preferable to determine the limit of the 90th or 95th percentile in a normal population and to use it as the upper normal value.

Clinical Usefulness. The detection of ICs may be helpful in certain clinical conditions. The *diagnostic value* of a measurement by itself is limited, however, since the

---

*The preparations can be obtained on request from Dr. U. Nydegger, Central Laboratory of the Swiss Red Cross, Wankdorfstrasse 10, Bern, Switzerland.

presence of immune complexes is not specific to any particular disease. However, IC levels should be considered as an integral part of the laboratory diagnosis in a number of rheumatic diseases. For example, in a prospective study, Jones and associates[49] followed 53 patients with early arthritis for up to 3 years. During this time, 24 developed sufficient features for definite RA to be diagnosed and the others simply had arthralgias. Abnormal C1q-binding activity was found mainly in RA patients (79 percent) several months before the disease could be diagnosed. In suspected but not definite RA, the *absence* of detectable ICs may be of diagnostic value in ruling out this disease, provided the test used is of high sensitivity (e.g., C1qBA). Immune complex detection could be applicable to seronegative RA patients since positive tests have been reported for up to 70 percent of the cases.[50,53]

A *single* measurement in a given patient does not give a good indication of the clinical activity of the diseases in SLE[50] or in RA.[54] A better application is probably serial determination of IC levels during therapy. In individual patients with SLE or with rheumatoid arthritis, there is a good correlation between the clinical activity of the disease and serial measurement of IC levels. Lloyd and Shur[56] followed 37 patients with SLE before, during, and after clinical exacerbation. Patients developing active renal disease had marked increases in IC levels along with low levels of CH50 and C3. In a similar study, Hamburger[55] observed a good correlation between the IC level and clinical activity (Fig. 45–8). In RA patients,

serial studies of ICs in serum or in synovial fluids also suggest that in a given individual the IC level may be one biological indicator of clinical activity (Fig. 45–9).[67]

In a collaborative double-blind study for the evaluation of levamisole in the treatment of rheumatoid arthritis, a progressive decrease of IC levels was found in the treated groups, but not in the placebo group.[52] The measurement of IC levels has also been used to monitor therapeutic plasma exchange in SLE and in RA.

In RA patients, the presence of rheumatoid nodules is associated with higher levels of circulating IC (Fig. 45–10). However, the findings of a high IC level in a given patient does not have a predictive value for this type of complication.

Immune Complexes in Rheumatic Diseases and Their Relevance to Clinical Status.

Rheumatoid Arthritis. Anti-immunoglobulins of the IgG and IgM class have been shown to form ICs in serum and joint fluid either by IgG-IgG self-association or by reaction of IgM-RF with native IgG. These ICs react with C1q and IgM-RF and may be responsible for intravascular activation of the complement system.

Several techniques for detecting circulating ICs have been used to study sera and synovial fluids of patients

Figure 45–8. Changes in levels of immune complexes (C1q BA) and clinical status in SLE. Chronologic order from left to right (exception is M, whose chronologic order is right to left). Letters represent 13 individual patients with SLE. The disease activity was assessed by two physicians independently on a scale of 0 to 3+, according to all available clinical and laboratory findings. From Hamburger, M.I., et al.: A serial study of systemic reticuloendothelial system Fc receptor functional activity in systemic lupus erythematosus. Arthritis Rheum. 25:1, 1982.

Figure 45–9. Disease course of a patient with RA during 6 months. Periods with active disease were associated with high C3d and C1q BA levels in plasma or serum and synovial fluid, and remissions were followed by improvement of these parameters. Note inflammatory exacerbation on March 31. ESR = erythrocyte sedimentation rate. (From Nydegger U.E., et al.: Circulating complement breakdown products in patients with rheumatoid arthritis. Correlation between plasma C3d, circulating immune complexes and clinical activity. J. Clin. Invest. 59:862, 1977.)

Figure 45–10. Correlation of immune complex levels in serum (%[125]I-C1q binding activity, C1qBA) and the C3d concentrations in plasma with the occurrence of subcutaneous nodules in patients with rheumatoid arthritis. The means of the values (± 2 SD) from each group are indicated. The shadowed area represents the normal ranges (means ± 2 SD) of the value observed in healthy donors. ● = %; ○ = mg%.

with rheumatoid arthritis. Of the 18 techniques for the detection of ICs evaluated in a multicenter study, six were particularly effective.[48] The Raji cell binding test and the C1q binding test were positive in 71 and 83 percent, respectively. As previously detailed, the presence of vasculitis or other extra-articular features is generally associated with positive IC tests (C1q binding test, Raji cell binding test and conglutinin binding test). The level of circulating ICs is correlated with the presence of IgM-RF as well as the erythrocyte sedimentation rate.

Detecting immune complexes in serum may be *helpful for diagnosis* in the following situations: (a) in early arthritis, circulating immune complexes may be detected in serum several months prior to the definite diagnosis of RA;[49] (b) because circulating immune complexes are found in 70 percent of sera from patients with seronegative RA, their presence may help to distinguish seronegative RA from other arthropathies;[50] (c) the absence of circulating ICs has some exclusion value. For example, circulating ICs are usually absent in Reiter's disease, and this can be considered in the differential diagnosis of RA.[51] The detection of circulating ICs may be helpful for the *follow-up of individual RA patients* during therapy as one of the biologic indicators of clinical activity (see Clinical Usefulness).[52]

Systemic Lupus Erythematosus. The nature of circulating immune complexes and cryoprecipitates in sera from patients with SLE has not been well defined. Occasionally, ICs have been shown to contain anti-Ig and anti-DNA antibodies. Large amounts of circulating ICs generally correspond with active SLE, as well as with high levels of anti-double-strand DNA antibody and reduced complement levels. In a comparative study, the highest frequency of immune complexes in sera from SLE patients was observed using the Raji cell binding assay (91 percent), the fluid phase C1q binding test (78 percent), and platelet aggregation (74 percent).[48] In fol-

low-up studies, there was a close relationship between the immune complex levels and the changes in the disease activity.[54,55] Lloyd and Schar confirmed this correlation and found that patients with active renal disease showed higher C1qBA, as well as decreased CH50 and C3, in comparison with patients with only extrarenal manifestations.[56] The diagnostic value of circulating ICs is limited, but significant renal disease is unlikely when low complement levels are not associated with appreciably elevated C1q binding activity. The measurement of IC levels has been used to monitor therapeutic plasma exchange in SLE.[57]

Juvenile Rheumatoid Arthritis. In this heterogeneous group, circulating immune complexes have been observed, particularly in the clinical subsets marked by systemic onset or polyarticular disease. In a collaborative study of chronic juvenile arthritis, ICs were found more frequently in children with severe disease.[58]

Ankylosing Spondylitis. In most studies, no significant increase of circulating IC levels has been found.[51,59-61]

Scleroderma. Approximately half of the patients with scleroderma have circulating ICs.[62-64] In a recent study of 92 patients with progressive systemic sclerosis serum levels of ICs measured by the Raji cell assay were elevated in 72 percent.[65] In this study a positive result in the Raji cell binding test was most often associated with diffuse scleroderma, tendon friction rub, and positive antinuclear antibody. Individuals with immune complexes detected by the C1q binding test more frequently had evidence of pulmonary involvement and positive serum rheumatoid factor than patients with a negative C1q binding test.

Mixed Connective Tissue Disease (MCTD). Circulating ICs have been found by the C1q binding test, the Raji cell test and the mRF-I test. Approximately 81 to 90 percent of the sera were positive by one test and 65 percent were positive by two methods. Changes in IC levels seemed to parallel clinical activity.[66]

Degenerative Joint Diseases. Although ICs can be occasionally detected in synovial fluid from patients with osteoarthritis, circulating ICs are generally absent in these diseases.[27,50]

References

1. Nydegger, U.E., Kazatchkine, M.D., and Lambert, P.H.: Immune complexes. *In* Fougereau, M., and Dausset, J. (eds.): Progress in Immunology IV, Paris, New York, Academic Press, 1980.
2. Dixon, F.J.: The role of antigen-antibody complexes in disease. The Harvey Lectures 58:21, 1963.
3. Lambert, P.H., Tribollet, E., Celada, A., Madalinski, K., Frei, P.C., and Miescher, P.A.: Quantitation of immunoglobulin-associated HBs antigen in patients with acute and chronic hepatitis, in healthy carriers and in polyarteritis nodosa. J. Clin. Lab. Immunol. 3:1, 1980.
4. Harbeck, R.J., Bardana, E.J., Kohler, P.F., and Carr, R.I.: DNA-anti-DNA complexes: Their detection in systemic lupus erythematosus sera. J. Clin. Invest. 52:789, 1973.
5. Casali, P., and Lambert, P.H.: Purification of soluble immune complexes from serum using PMMA beads coated with conglutinin or C1q. Clin. Exp. Immunol. 37:295, 1979.
6. Maire, M., Barnet, M., and Lambert, P.H.: Identification of components of immune complexes purified from human sera. I. Immune complexes purified from sera of patients with systemic lupus erythematosus. Clin. Exp. Immunol. 51:215, 1983.

7. Louis, J., and Lambert, P.H.: Lipopolysaccharides: From immunostimulation to autoimmunity. Springer Sem. Immunopathol. 2:215, 979.

8. Winchester, R.J., Kunkel, H.G., and Agnello, V.: Occurrence of gammaglobulin complexes in serum and joint fluid of rheumatoid arthritis patients: Use of monoclonal rheumatoid factors as reagent for their demonstration. J. Exp. Med. 134:286s, 1971.

9. Jerne, N.K.: Towards a network theory of the immune system. Ann. Immunol. (Inst. Pasteur) 125C:373, 1974.

10. Rose, L.M., Goldman, M., and Lambert, P.H.: The production of anti-idiotype antibodies and of idiotype-anti-idiotype immune complexes following polyclonal B-cell activation by bacterial LPS. J. Immunol. 128:2126, 1982.

11. Geltner, D., Franklin, E.G., and Frangione, B.: Anti-idiotypic activity of the IgM fractions of mixed cryoglobulins. J. Immunol. 125:1530, 1980.

12. Agnello, V., Koffler, D., Eisenberg, J.W., Winchester, R.J., and Kunkel, H.: Clq precipitins in the sera of patients with systemic lupus erythematosus and other hypocomplementemic states: Characterization of high and low molecular weight types. J. Exp. Med. 144:428, 1971.

13. Munthe-Kaas, A.C., Kaplan, G., and Seljelid, R.: On the mechanism of internalization of opsonized particles by rat Kupffer cells in vitro. Exp. Cell. Res. 103:201, 1976.

14. Kijlstra, A., Van Es, L.A., and Daha, M.R.: Enhanced degradation of soluble immunoglobulin aggregates by macrophages in the presence of complement. Immunology 37:673, 1979.

15. Mannik, M., and Arend, W.P.: Fate of preformed immune complexes in rabbits and rhesus monkeys. J. Exp. Med. 134:19s, 1971.

16. Thornburg, R.W., Day, J.F., Thorpe, S.R., and Baynes, J.W.: Carbohydrate-mediated clearance of immune complexes from circulation. A role for galactose residues in hepatic uptake of IgG-antigen complexes. J. Biol. Chem. 255:6820, 1980.

17. Day, J.F., Thornburg, R.W., Thorpe, S.R., and Baynes, J.W.: Carbohydrate-mediated clearance of antibody-antigen complexes from the circulation. The role of high mannose oligosaccharides in the hepatic uptake of IgM-antigen complexes. J. Biol. Chem. 255:2360, 1980.

18. Haakenstad, A.O., and Mannik, M.: Saturation of the reticuloendothelial system with soluble immune complexes. J. Immunol. 112:1939, 1974.

19. Harkiss, G.D., and Brown, D.L.: Clearance kinetics of soluble preformed immune complexes containing IgM antibodies in normal and decomplemented rabbits. Immunology 42:217, 1981.

20. Bockow, B., and Mannik, M.: Clearance and tissue uptake of immune complexes in complement-depleted and control mice. Immunology 42:497, 1981.

21. Haakenstad, A.O., and Mannik, M.: The disappearance kinetics of soluble immune complexes prepared with reduced and alkylated antibodies in mice. Lab. Invest. 35:283, 1976.

22. Frank, M.M., Schreiber, A.D., Atkenson, J.P., and Jaffe, C.J.: Pathophysiology of immune hemolytic anemia. Ann. Intern. Med. 87:210, 1977.

23. Frank, M.M., Hamburger, M.I., Lawley, T.J., Kimberley, R.P., and Plotz, P.H.: Defective reticuloendothelial system Fc-receptor function in systemic lupus erythematosus. N. Engl. J. Med. 300:518, 1979.

24. Miller, G.W., and Nussenzweig, V.: A new complement function: Solubilization of antigen-antibody aggregates. Proc. Nat. Acad. Sci. 72:418, 1975.

25. Ehlenberger, A.G., and Nussenzweig, V.: The role of membrane receptors for C3b and C3d in phagocytosis. J. Exp. Med. 145:357, 1977.

26. Ward, P.A., and Zwaifler, N.J.: Complement-derived leukotactic factors in inflammatory synovial fluids of humans. J. Clin. Invest. 50:606, 971.

27. Dayer, E., Gerster, J.C., Aguado, M.T., and Lambert, P.H.: Capacity to solubilize immune complexes in sera and synovial fluids from patients with rheumatoid arthritis. Arthritis Rheum. 27:156, 1983.

28. Steward, M.W.: Chronic immune complex disease in mice: The role of antibody affinity. Clin. Exp. Immunol. 38:414, 1979.

29. Izui, S., Lambert, P.H., and Miescher, P.A.: In vitro demonstration of a particular affinity of glomerular basement membrane and collagen for DNA. A possible basis for a local formation of DNA-anti-DNA complexes in systemic lupus erythematosus. J. Exp. Med. 144:428, 1976.

30. Cavallo, T., Goldman, M., Graves, K., and Lambert, P.H.: Altered glomerular permeability in the early phase of immune complex nephritis. Kidney Int. 24:632, 1983.

31. Zubler, R.H., and Lambert, P.H.: Detection of immune complexes in human diseases. Prog. Allergy 24:1, 1978.

32. Bokisch, V.A., Muller-Eberhard, H.J., and Dixon, F.J.: Complement: A potential mediator of the hemorrhagic shock syndrome. Adv. Biosc. 12:417, 1974.

33. Zubler, R.H., Lange, G., Lambert, P.H., and Miescher, P.A.: Detection of immune complexes in unheated sera by a modified ^{125}I-Clq binding test. Effect of heating on the binding of Clq by immune complexes and application of the test to systemic lupus erythematosus. J. Immunol. 116:232, 1976.

34. Ludwig, F.J., and Cusumans, C.L.: Detection of immune complexes using ^{125}I-goat anti(human IgG) monovalent (Fab) antibody fragments. J. Natl. Can. Instit. 52:1529, 1974.

35. Brouet, J.C., Clauvel, J.P., Danon, F., Klein, M., and Seligmann, M.: Biological and clinical significance of cryoglobulins. Am. J. Med. 57:775, 1974.

36. Zubler, R.H., Perrin, L.H., Creighton, W.D., Lambert, P.H., and Miescher, P.A.: The use of polyethylene glycol (PEG) to concentrate immune complexes from serum or plasma samples. Ann. Rheum. Dis. 36(Suppl. 1)23, 1977.

37. Hällgren, R., and Wide, L.: Detection of circulating IgG aggregates and immune complexes using ^{125}I protein A from Staphylococcus aureus. Ann. Rheum. Dis. 35:306, 1976.

38. Nielsen, H., and Svehag, S.E.: Detection and differentiation of immune complexes and IgG aggregates by a complement consumption assay. Acta. Path. Microbiol. Scand. 84:261, 1976.

39. Sobel, A.T., Bokisch, V.A., and Muller-Eberhard, H.J.: Clq deviation test for the detection of immune complexes, aggregates of IgG and bacterial products in human sera. J. Exp. Med. 142:139, 1975.

40. Hay, F.C., Nineham, L.J., and Roitt, I.M.: Routine assay for the detection of immune complexes of known immunoglobulin class using solid phase Clq. Clin. Exp. Immunol. 24:396, 1976.

41. Casali, P., Bossus, A., Carpentier, A.N., Lambert, P.H., and Miescher, P.A.: Solid phase enzyme immunoassay or radioimmunoassay for the detection of immune complexes based on their recognition by conglutinin: Conglutinin binding test. Clin. Exp. Immunol. 29:342, 1977.

42. Pereira, A.B., Theofilopoulos, A.N., and Dixon, F.J.: Detection and partial characterization of circulating immune complexes with solid-phase anti-C3. J. Immunol. 125:763, 1980.

43. Luthra, H.S., McDuffie, F.C., Hunder, G.G., and Samayoa, E.A.: Immune complexes in sera and synovial fluids of patients with rheumatoid arthritis. Radioimmunoassay with monoclonal rheumatoid factor. J. Clin. Invest. 56:458, 1975.

44. Theofilopoulos, A.N., Wilson, C.B., and Dixon, F.J.: The Raji cell radioimmune assay for detecting immune complexes in human sera. J. Clin. Invest. 57:169, 1976.

45. Almeida, J.D., and Waterson, A.P.: The morphology of the virus-antibody interaction. Adv. Virus. Res. 15:307, 1969.

46. Notkins, A.L., Mahar, S., Scheele, C., and Goffman, J.: Infectious virus-antibody complex in the blood of chronically infected mice. J. Exp. Med. 124:81, 1966.

47. Penttinen, K.: The platelet aggregation test. Ann. Rheum. Dis. 36(Suppl. 1):55, 1977.

48. Lambert, P.H., Dixon, F.J., Zubler, R.H., Agnello, V., Cambiaso, C., Casali, P., Clark, J., Cowdery, J.S., McDuffie, F.C., Hay, F.C., McLennan, I.C., Masson, P., Muller-Eberhard, H.J., Penttinen, K., Smith, M., Tappeiner, G., Theofilopoulos, A.N., and Verroust, P.: A collaborative study for the evaluation of eighteen methods for detecting immune complexes in serum. J. Lab. Clin. Immunol. 1:1, 1978.

49. Jones, V.E., Jacoby, R.K., Wallington, T., and Holt, P.: Immune complexes in early arthritis. I. Detection of immune complexes before rheumatoid arthritis is definite. Clin. Exp. Immunol. 44:512, 1981.

50. Zubler, R.H., Nydegger, U.E., Perrin, L.H., Fehr, K., McCormick, J., Lambert, P.H., and Miescher, P.A.: Circulating and intraarticular immune complexes in patients with rheumatoid arthritis. J. Clin. Invest. 57:1308, 1976.

51. Gabay, R., Zubler, R.H., Nydegger, U.E., and Lambert, P.H.: Immune complexes and complement catabolism in ankylosing spondylitis. Arthritis Rheum. 20:913, 1977.

52. Vischer, T.L., Veys, E., Symoens, J., Rosenthal, M., and Huskisson, E.C.: Levamisole in rheumatoid arthritis. A randomized double-blind study comparing two dosage regimens of Levamisole with placebo. Lancet 2:1007, 1978.

53. McDougal, J.S., Hubbard, M., McDuffy, F.C., Strobel, P.L., Smith, S.J., Bass, N., Goldmann, J.A., Hartman, S., Myerson, G., Miller, S., Morales, R., and Wilson, C.H.: Comparison of five assays for immune complexes in the rheumatic diseases. An assessment of their validity in rheumatoid arthritis. Arthritis Rheum. 25:1156, 1982.

54. Abrass, C., Nies, K.M., Louie, J.S., Border, W.A., and Glassock, R.J.: Correlation and predictive accuracy of circulating immune complexes with disease activity in patients with systemic lupus erythematosus. Arthritis Rheum. 23:273, 1980.

55. Hamburger, M.I., Lawley, T.J., Kimberley, R.P., Plotz, P.H., and Frank, M.M.: A serial study of systemic reticuloendothelial system Fc receptor functional activity in systemic lupus erythematosus. Arthritis Rheum. 25:1, 1982.

56. Lloyd, W., and Schur, P.H.: Immune complexes, complement and anti-DNA in exacerbations of systemic lupus erythematosus (SLE). Medicine 60:208, 1981.

57. Wei, N., Klippel, J.H., Huston, D.P., Hall, R.P., Lawley, T.J., Balow, J.E., Steinberg, A., and Decker, J.L.: Randomised trial of plasma exchange in mild systemic lupus erythematosus. Lancet 1:17, 983.

58. Rossen, R.D., Brener, E.J., Person, D.A., Templeton, J.W., and Lipsky, M.D.: Circulating immune complexes and antinuclear antibodies in juvenile rheumatoid arthritis. Arthritis Rheum. 20:1485, 1977.
59. Rosenbaum, J.T., Theofilopoulos, A.N., Mc DeWitt, H.O., Pereira, A.B., Carson, D., and Calin, A.: Presence of circulating immune complexes in Reiter's syndrome and ankylosing spondylitis. Clin. Immunol. Immunopathol. 18:291, 1981.
60. Moksymowych, W., Dasgupta, M.K., Rothwell, R.S., Dossetor, J.B., and Russel, A.S.: The absence of circulating immune complexes in patients with ankylosing spondylitis. Rheumatol. Int. 1:107, 1981.
61. Duquesnoy, R., Santoro, F., Wattre, P., and Delcombre, B.: Failure to find C1q binding material and anti-IgG antibodies in ankylosing spondylitis. Ann. Rheum. Dis. 39:449, 1980.
62. Cunningham, P.H., Andrews, B.S., and Davis, J.S.: Immune complexes in patients with progressive systemic sclerosis (PSS) and mixed connective tissue disease (MCTD). Clin. Res. 26:374A, 1978.
63. Husson, J.M., Druet, P., Contet, A., Fiessinger, J.N., and Camillari, J.P.: Systemic sclerosis and cryoglobulinemia. Clin. Immunol. Immunopathol. 6:77, 1976.

64. Pisko, E., Gallup, K., Turner, R., Parker, M., Nomeir, A.M., Box, J., Davis, J., and Rothberger, H.: Cardiopulmonary manifestations of progressive systemic sclerosis: Associations with circulating immune complexes and fluorescent antinuclear antibodies. Arthritis Rheum. 22:518, 1979.
65. Seibold, J.R., Medsger, T.A., Winkelstein, A., Kelly, R.H., and Rodnan, G.P.: Immune complexes in progressive systemic sclerosis (scleroderma). Arthritis Rheum. 25:1167, 1982.
66. Halla, J.T., Volanakis, J.E., and Schrohenloher, R.E.: Circulating immune complexes in mixed connective tissue disease. Arthritis Rheum., 22:484, 1979.
67. Nydegger, U.E., Zubler, R.H., Gabay, R., Joliat, G., Karagevrekis, C.H., Lambert, P.H., and Miescher, P.A.: Circulating complement breakdown products in patients with rheumatoid arthritis. Correlation between plasma C3d, circulating immune complexes and clinical activity. J. Clin. Invest. 59:862, 1977.

Chapter 46

Antinuclear Antibodies

Morris Reichlin

INTRODUCTION

Antibodies to nuclear antigens (ANA) are found in the sera of patients with a variety of rheumatic diseases. This chapter will describe ANA determination as a screening test as well as a means of identifying antibodies to specific organelles. In some patients with systemic lupus erythematosus (SLE) and Sjögren's syndrome, antibodies to cytoplasmic antigens predominate, and these will also be discussed. Newly discovered ANA in progressive systemic sclerosis and the polymyositis syndromes will be described. Characterizing the ANA as to antigenic specificity will provide information about nosology, subset definition within diseases, clinical activity, specific organ involvement, and prognosis.

HISTORY

In 1948, Hargraves and colleagues initiated the study of antibodies to nuclei with the description of the LE phenomenon.[1] The demonstration of the ingestion of traumatized cells from SLE patients by polymorphonuclear leukocytes was readily confirmed[2] and is now known to be due to the reaction of antibodies against nucleoprotein (DNA-histone) with nuclei and the subsequent phagocytosis of such sensitized nuclei. The LE test, although still performed in many laboratories, is being replaced by tests that are more sensitive and specific. The next major advance was the indirect immunofluorescent assay (IFA) for the detection of ANA.[3-5] The assay detects antibodies with various antigenic specificities but is very useful as a screening test. It is the

method of choice in the initial search for autoantibodies relevant to the diagnosis of SLE.

Resolution of total ANA into individual antigen-antibody reactions required purified nucleic acid antigens and antigens solubilized from crude extracts detected by precipitation in agar utilizing the Ouchterlony method. Improved analytical methods for chemically defined autoantigens (e.g., DNA) have provided greater sensitivity and precision in antibody detection. Two recent approaches to antigenic analysis involve the use of human tissue culture lines as immunofluorescent substrates and a molecular biological analysis of autoantigens containing intrinsically labeled RNA.

ANA CLASSIFICATION

The antinuclear and anticytoplasmic antibodies that occur in the rheumatic diseases and have relevance for clinical diagnosis and disease classification are listed in Table 46-1. Each antibody specificity will be discussed in the context of its measurement, chemical nature, disease specificity, association with clinical subsets, and disease activity. Antibodies to DNA-histone, ds (double-stranded) and ss (single-stranded) DNA, RNA, histone, nRNP, and Sm* all occur in SLE, while antibodies to Ro*/SSA† and La*/SSB†/Ha* occur in SLE and Sjögren's syndrome. Antibodies to PM-Scl,‡ Mi₁,* Mi₂,* Jo₂,* and Ku* all occur in patients with polymyositis

---

*Represent the first two letters of the patient's name whose serum was used to identify the reaction in agar diffusion.
†Sjögren's syndrome A and B.
‡Polymyositis-scleroderma.

Table 46–1. Antibodies to Nuclear or Cytoplasmic Antigens (ANA and ACA)

Anti-DNA-histone
Anti-DNA
  Anti–single-stranded (ss) DNA (denatured)
  Anti–double-stranded (ds) DNA (native)
Anti-histone
Anti-nRNP*
Anti-Sm*
Anti-Ro/SSA*
Anti-La/SSB/Ha*
Anti-RNA, Poly IC, Poly GC, Poly ADP, Poly A
Anti-Ma
Anti-PM-Scl, PM_1
Anti-Mi_1, Mi_2
Anti-Ku
Anti-Jo_1, Jo_2
Anti-Scl_{70}
Anti-centromere
Anti-nucleosome (cross-reactive with Fc of human IgG)

*All shown to be RNA-protein conjugates.

(PM), while antibodies to Scl_{70} and centromere occur in patients with progressive systemic sclerosis (PSS). Finally antibodies to nucleosomes occur in patients with rheumatoid arthritis (RA).

DETECTION OF ANTINUCLEAR ANTIGENS

Immunofluorescence. The indirect immunofluorescent test is widely considered to be the most reliable screening test for ANA (Fig. 46–1). A dilution of human serum is placed on a cryostat section of mouse liver, which leads to attachment of Ig molecules with antinuclear specificity. After suitable washing, an antibody against human Ig is added, and after washing, the bound fluorescein-tagged antihuman Ig is visualized by fluorescence microscopy. Figure 46–2 illustrates the appearance of normal human serum and a human serum positive for ANA binding to the nuclei of mouse liver sections. Note the dark appearance of the nuclei in the upper part of the figure (negative ANA test) and the whitish nuclei in the lower part of the figure in a positive ANA test. When viewed through the microscope, the positive nuclei appear apple-green, reflecting the color of the bound fluorescein-tagged antihuman Ig.

Diagnosis of SLE. A positive ANA test by itself is not diagnostic of any disease, but a positive ANA in association with the characteristic clinical features of SLE supports the diagnosis. If the ANA test is performed on cryostat sections of mouse liver or kidney and standardized commercially available fluorescent conjugates of antihuman gamma globulin are employed, about 95 percent of active untreated SLE patients will have positive tests. The titers of positive ANA tests vary greatly, but at least 50 percent of the titers will exceed 1:100, and a small proportion (10 percent or less) will be positive only at the screening dilution (1:10 or 1:20 in most laboratories). If the screening test is performed on commercially available human tissue culture lines such as KB or Hep2 cells, the percentage of positive tests approaches 98 percent of active untreated SLE patients. The difference between the two substrates largely represents the relative absence of the Ro/SSA antigen in mouse or rat liver and kidney sections and its presence in the tissue culture lines.

There is great variation in ANA test results acquired from different laboratories. This variation includes whether the test is positive or negative, the titer determined, and the pattern reported. ANA titers tend to be higher on tissue culture lines. The factors that lead to variable results include not only the use of different substrates but also different fluoresceinated antibodies directed toward human immunoglobulin, varying skill of technicians, microscopes of differing power and sensitivity (transmission versus epiilluminated optics), as well as the age of the bulb in the microscope and failure to include positive control sera directed toward very soluble antigens such as Sm and La/SSB.

The clinician must then decide how to evaluate disparate results from different laboratories. The answer is not easy, but clinical laboratories differ in quality and the clinician must make a judgement based on performance. The clinician should be more persistent in pursuing a negative ANA test in the face of impressive clinical data for SLE than in being concerned about a positive test accompanying limited or nonspecific clinical findings. The latter situation should be viewed with circumspection. The first situation could be due to faulty ANA testing or to one of the uncommon serologic situations to be described below. The second situation requires continued observation of the patient until disease expression is more complete. Finally, there are numerous laboratories with a strong research interest in

Fluorescence Test for ANA

Place Frozen Mouse Liver on Slide

Apply Test Serum for ANA

ANA attach to Cell Nuclei

wash; then wash again

add Fluorescein-tagged Rabbit Anti-human Ig;

Positive Fluorescence Test for ANA

(excitation light source)

Figure 46–1. Stepwise diagram of the fluorescence test for anti-nuclear antibodies (ANA). The ANA bind to a variety of nuclear antigens; they are then identified by fluorescein-tagged antibodies to the human Ig.

Figure 46–2. The fluorescence ANA (FANA) test at low power ($\times 80$). *A* is a negative control of mouse liver substrate. *B* is the same substrate with a positive homogeneous ANA pattern.

ANA testing, and they can perform an ANA test when the clinician is faced with this problem.

A negative test for ANA occurs in about 5 percent of patients with otherwise typical SLE. Almost two thirds of these patients have serum antibodies to Ro/SSA or La/SSB or both, and of the remainder, the great majority have antibodies to ssDNA demonstrable by radioimmunoassay. Five recognized antibody specificities that are not measured by immunofluorescent assay on rodent liver or kidney sections have been described

(Table 46–2). Ro/SSA and ssDNA have already been mentioned, and the other three antigens that are germane to the clinical diagnosis of PM and PSS will be subsequently discussed. As is well known, antibodies to ssDNA when present alone do not bind to resting interphase nuclei.[161] Less than 1 percent of SLE patients have *none* of the autoantibodies characteristic of the disease; absence of a positive ANA on tissue culture lines and anti-ssDNA by radioimmunoassay therefore makes the diagnosis of SLE unlikely. The presence of

Table 46–2. Antigens Poorly Represented in Cryostat Sections of Rodent Epithelial Tissues

Antigen	Relevant Disease	Method of Detection
Ro/SSA	SLE Sjögren's syndrome	IFA* on human tissue culture lines Double diffusion†
ssDNA	SLE and wide spectrum of rheumatic diseases	Hemagglutination Radioimmunoassay ELISA‡
Jo₁	Polymyositis	Double diffusion
Ku	Polymyositis-scleroderma overlap	Double diffusion IFA on human or calf tissues
Centromere	Scleroderma CREST variant	IFA with human tissue culture lines, e.g., Hep2 or KB cells

*Immunofluorescence assay.
†Double diffusion or Ouchterlony method.
‡Enzyme-linked immunosorbent assay.

these antibodies tends to confirm the diagnosis but must be accompanied by clinical findings consistent with SLE in order to establish the diagnosis of SLE. For example, a patient with only Raynaud's phenomenon, polyarthritis (nonerosive, nondeforming), and a positive ANA test might have SLE, scleroderma, or polymyositis. The presence of typical skin or muscle findings would make the latter two diagnoses likely, but in their absence one could neither confidently exclude those two diagnoses nor make a diagnosis of SLE. On the other hand, the presence of a photosensitive malar rash or leukopenia or any of a number of other characteristic SLE findings not present in the other two diseases (mucous membrane ulceration, glomerulonephritis, thrombocytopenia, seizures, psychosis, discoid skin lesions, and alopecia) accompanying the limited clinical and serologic findings described would make the diagnosis of SLE virtually certain.

ANA Pattern. The ANA pattern is of some value but is a far less powerful criterion than the identification of a specific antigen-antibody reaction (e.g., anti-dsDNA, anti-Sm, anti-Ro/SSA, etc.). There are four major patterns recognized on cryostat sections of rodent liver or kidney. They are homogeneous or solid, peripheral or rim, speckled, and nucleolar. The homogeneous pattern is illustrated in Figure 46–2B while the peripheral, speckled, and nucleolar patterns of fluorescence are illustrated in Figure 46–3. The homogeneous pattern can be seen in all the connective tissue diseases as well as in drug-induced LE. Both the antibody associated with the

Figure 46–3. The fluorescence ANA (FANA) test at high power (×320). *A* is a negative control. *B* shows an example of the shaggy, rim or peripheral pattern which frequently correlates with antibodies to DNA. *C* is an example of the speckled pattern, frequently associated with antibodies to non–DNA-containing antigens. *D* shows the nucleolar pattern.

LE phenomenon and the histone-dependent antibodies arising in drug-induced SLE can produce this pattern of immunofluorescence. The speckled pattern is seen in sera from patients with SLE, RA, PSS, and Sjögren's syndrome. Sm, nRNP, La/SSB, Scl_{70}, and probably other antigens are targets for antibodies that give rise to the speckled patterns of fluorescence.

The peripheral pattern of fluorescence is seen most frequently in SLE sera and correlates with antibodies to dsDNA but is found in only a small proportion of sera containing these antibodies. Nucleolar fluorescence is seen most frequently in sera from scleroderma patients but also occurs to a lesser extent in sera from Sjögren's syndrome and SLE. The presence of multiple antibodies in SLE sera gives rise to patterns of fluorescence that vary with serum dilution. Often homogeneous fluorescence is observed at a low serum dilution and a speckled pattern at higher serum dilutions.

Positive ANA tests are found in 5 to 10 percent of patients with discoid lupus erythematosus without systemic involvement. A positive ANA test without clinical evidence of systemic involvement does portend the development of such involvement in some but not all patients. One cannot, therefore, confidently conclude that a patient with discoid LE and a positive ANA has SLE. Because the frequency of low-titer positive ANA tests increases with age in the normal population, a positive ANA test is much more significant in a young patient with discoid LE than in an older one.

ANA in Diseases Other Than SLE. A positive ANA test occurs to a variable extent in all the connective tissue diseases. Representative data are listed in Table 46–3. In arteritis, myositis, and RA the frequency of positive tests varies from 33 to 52 percent, and 70 to 90 percent of these positive tests occur at titers of 1/160 or less. On the other hand, high titers are quite common in SLE, mixed connective tissue disease, and PSS. Positive ANA tests are also seen in patients (5 to 20 percent) with juvenile RA, chronic active hepatitis, in-

fectious mononucleosis, and lepromatous leprosy. The titers are rarely impressive in these clinical settings.

ANAs are not usually specific for organ and species[7] but there are exceptions. Most notable is the presence of granulocyte-specific ANA, which are found in the sera of patients with RA.[8-11] As many as 50 percent of RA patients have such antibodies, which are not detectable with mouse liver nuclei. At least one antibody specificity, anti-Ku, is species specific, and does not bind to rodent tissue but does bind to bovine and human tissue.[12]

IDENTIFICATION OF INDIVIDUAL ANTIGEN–ANTIBODY REACTIONS

Immunodiffusion. Double diffusion in agar has been an important initial method for the identification and analysis of the specificities of autoantibodies. The antigen-antibody systems that were first characterized in this way include Sm, nRNP, Ro/SSA, La/SSB/Ha, Ma, Mi, Jo_1, Jo_2, Ku, PCNA, and PM_1 (PM-Scl). The nomenclature for these reactions rests on two conventions: (1) the first two letters of the name of the patient whose serum served as a monospecific prototype (e.g., Sm, Ro) and (2) a putative disease specificity of the antibody (e.g., SSA, PM_1). Such nomenclature is provisional and will give way to a chemical nomenclature when this information becomes available. Most of these antigens have now been well characterized biochemically, but their original antigenicity and clinical relevance were established with the double diffusion method. With an appropriate monospecific prototype serum and a crude extract of thymus or spleen tissue, definitive identification of a specific precipitin in an unknown serum can be made by the observation of line fusion as illustrated in Figure 46–4. The serum Da forms a thick precipitin line with an antigen in calf thymus extract (CTE), which fuses with a similar precipitin line formed by antibodies

Table 46–3. Fluorescent Antinuclear Antibody in Various Conditions*

	SLE (662)†	RA (201)	Scleroderma (91)	MCTD (57)	Myositis (30)	Arteritis (70)
Positive tests (%)	95	52	55	95	40	33
Titer of test Mean	298	142	338	508	173	50
Percent with titer ≤ 1:40	34	72	46	7	50	90
titer 1:80	17	8	9	5	10	10
titer 1:160	19	10	18	14	10	0
titer 1:320	20	6	13	48	17	0
titer ≥ 1:640	10	4	14	26	13	0
Pattern of fluorescence						
Diffuse (%)	64	73	29	10	27	51
Speckled (%)	30	22	58	86	17	33
Nucleolar (%)	3	5	13	4	56	16
Peripheral (%)	3	0	0	0	0	0

*From Fries, J.F.: Systemic Lupus Erythematosus: A Clinical Analysis. Philadelphia, W. B. Saunders Company, 1975.
†Number of observations in parentheses.

Figure 46–4. Precipitating antibodies to nRNA protein antigen. In the center well is calf thymus extract (CTE) and in the adjacent wells are serum specimens from patients Da and Mo. (Reprinted with permission from the New England Journal of Medicine 286:908, 1972).

in serum Mo with the antigen in CTE. The serum Mo forms a second line with CTE, which was identified as the Sm–anti-Sm system using a prototype anti-Sm serum in an adjacent well. The antigen forming the precipitin shared by sera Da and Mo proved to be of nuclear origin, and its antigenicity was completely destroyed by treatment with either RNAase or trypsin. This is the system now designated the nRNP system. Agar diffusion for the identification of specific antibodies is limited by insensitivity and the nonquantitative nature of the measurement. Precipitin reactions in agar require specific antibody concentrations of roughly 0.1 mg antibody protein per ml of serum if the precipitin is of the IgG class. Moreover, certain large macromolecules such as DNA diffuse poorly through agar gels, further reducing the sensitivity of this method for detection of the DNA–anti-DNA system by this technique. Several more sensitive and quantitative techniques are now available to measure anti-DNA. Indeed, it is anticipated that all precipitin reactions will be supplanted by more sensitive and quantitative techniques, the two most important being enzyme-linked immunosorbent assay (ELISA) and radioimmunoassay (RIA).

Counterimmunoelectrophoresis. Counterimmunoelectrophoresis is more sensitive than agar diffusion. Acidic antigens (e.g., DNA, RNA, and most of the precipitating antibodies described in the preceding section) are electrophoresed from a cathodal ($-$) well for a reaction with specific antibody, which has moved from an anodal well ($+$). This is illustrated in Figure 46–5, in which the technique is used for the measurement of antibodies to dsDNA in an SLE serum. The advantages of the method are improved sensitivity, certain identification of specific antigen-antibody reactions by line fusion even when crude extracts are used as the antigen source, and the potential resolution by electrophoresis of several antigens that differ in charge and may not resolve into independent lines in agar diffusion experiments.

The disadvantages of the method are that it will not detect basic antigens, and it will not measure antibodies that do not move cathodally by endosmosis (e.g., IgA, IgM); while it is more sensitive than double diffusion, it is still relatively insensitive, requiring 0.01 to 0.05 mg of antibody protein per ml for a positive test. Nonetheless, it has been successfully used for the detection of antibodies to the acidic antigens, dsDNA, ssDNA, nRNP, Sm, Ro/SSA, and La/SSB/Ha.[13-17] The technique is still far less sensitive and quantitative than hemagglutination, ELISA, or RIA methods and is being replaced by these methods as purified antigens become available.

Immunofluorescence. The use of the indirect immunofluorescence technique for the detection of antibodies to specific antigens has found its most intensive application in the measurement of antibodies to dsDNA. The Crithidia technique developed by Aarden, deGroot, and Feltkamp employs the hemoflagellate *Crithidia luciliae* as a substrate.[56] Binding of Ig to the kinetoplast, which contains exclusively circular double-stranded DNA, indicates antibody to dsDNA. The technique is also versatile, since Ig class can be determined by utilizing fluoreseinated antisera specific for heavy chains. Furthermore, the complement-fixing ability of the anti-DNA can be assessed by overlaying fresh normal human serum after binding of the anti-DNA and detection of fixed C3 with fluoreseinated anti-C3. This method has established itself as a standard technique for the measurement of anti-dsDNA.[18-20,56-58] No other immunofluorescent technique is known to identify antibodies directed toward a specific macromolecule, although antibodies to subcellular organelles have proved clinically useful. These include antibodies to the nucleolus,[21] the centromere,[22] and the mitotic spindle apparatus.[23] Measurement of antibodies to these organelles has clin-

undiluted $\ominus$

1:2

1:4 $\quad\oplus$

$\ominus\quad$ 1:8

1:16

1:32

Figure 46–5. Counterimmunoelectrophoresis (CIE) shows a "standard curve" of the method in which serial dilutions of an SLE serum are tested against a constant concentration of dsDNA (4 μg milliliter). DNA is negatively charged and thus migrates towards the positive pole while the antibody moves to the negative pole by endosmosis.

ical utility, as will be discussed in the context of individual diseases. It is already known from both biochemical and immunochemical studies that there are several distinct nucleolar antigens with potential clinical significance.[24-27,157,158]

Radioimmunoassay. The measurement of antibodies to DNA has preoccupied students of SLE since the first demonstration of these antibodies in 1957,[28,29] and the first radioimmunoassay for the detection of autoantibodies in SLE was developed for the measurement of anti-DNA. The Farr technique takes advantage of the ready solubility of radio-labeled DNA and the insolubility of labeled DNA–anti-DNA complexes in 50 percent saturated ammonium sulfate solutions.[30-33] The solubility differences of free and bound DNA permitted easy separation and measurement of the complexes by centrifugation and led to practical assays, which are still widely used today. Later modifications employing nitrocellulose filters for the separation of bound from free labeled DNA have also led to assays for anti-DNA that have found wide application.[34-36] Subsequently, RIAs were developed for numerous polynucleotides, including polydeoxy adenylate-thymidylate (dAT),[36] polyribo-inosinate-cytidylate (poly IC),[37] ribosomal RNA,[38] polyriboadenylate (poly riboA),[39] ultraviolet (UV) light–denatured DNA,[40] polyadenosine diphosphate ribose (poly ADP ribose),[41-43] and polyguanylate-cytidylate (poly GC).[44] While none of these assays has yet taken a clinically important place in the serological analysis of SLE patients, their detection and study raise many interesting questions. The utility of poly dAT is in its impeccably double-stranded character, so that antibodies to ssDNA do not bind to poly dAT. Binding of anti-ssDNA to the single-stranded regions of many putatively native DNA preparations commercially available created much confusion in the early literature on the specificity of antibodies to dsDNA in SLE.

Double-stranded RNA functions biologically as the replicative form of many RNA viruses, and such RNA is not a normal constituent of uninfected mammalian cells. The presence of antibodies to double-stranded RNA, poly IC, and poly GC in SLE has fueled much speculation about viral infection as an etiologic factor in SLE patients. Antibodies to ribosomal RNA, poly riboA, poly ADP ribose, and UV-denatured DNA have raised provocative questions about the nature of the immunogen and the immune dysregulation that regularly features antibodies to various polynucleotides in the rheumatic diseases in general and SLE in particular.

Enzyme-Linked Immunosorbent Assay (ELISA). Antibodies to DNA were first measured by the ELISA method in 1974[45] and a flurry of modifications followed which permitted the measurement of antibodies to either dsDNA or ssDNA.[46-52] As in all areas of medicine, the less expensive, safer, equally sensitive, and quantitative ELISA methods are rapidly replacing RIA techniques for the measurement of antigens and/or antibodies in the picogram to nanogram range. ELISA requires a purified antigen that will adhere to plastic, and as the various autoantigens are purified, it is expected that an

ELISA method will be developed for the detection and quantitation of the appropriate autoantibodies.

SPECIFIC AUTOANTIBODIES CHARACTERISTIC OF RHEUMATIC DISEASES

Antibodies to DNA. Antibodies to DNA have been of central interest in the immunology of SLE since their discovery in the late 1950s by several groups.[59,60,28,29] The development of serologic methods has led to increasing sensitivity and precision in the detection of these antibodies (Table 46–4). The earliest techniques were relatively insensitive precipitation methods. Complement fixation and passive hemagglutination methods for detecting anti-DNA were the first assays that detected antibody in more than half of the active untreated patients and were the standard techniques of the 1960s. These methods have now been largely supplanted by RIA, IFA on *Crithidia*, and ELISA methods for detecting and quantitating antibody to DNA. As can be seen, these techniques detect anti-DNA in 75 to 95 percent of active untreated patients. The lower figures seen in the table are from series in which no distinction is made between active and inactive disease. The crithidia technique measures only anti-dsDNA, while the RIA and ELISA methods are readily adapted to measure either anti-ssDNA or anti-dsDNA.

Antibodies to DNA have the widest clinical applicability and include those with the highest specificity for the diagnosis of SLE. There are two large categories of specificities that have clinical relevance: native (ds or double-stranded) and denatured (ss or single-stranded) DNA. Antibodies to dsDNA are directed to some aspect of the double-helical conformation of nDNA, the exact structure as yet being undetermined. Such antibodies do not bind to the free purine and pyrimidine bases but paradoxically can be absorbed out with ssDNA. In an investigation of this problem it has been shown that secondary structure in ssDNA is responsible for its reaction with anti-dsDNA antibodies in SLE sera.[63] Studies by the latter authors demonstrated that S_1 nuclease-resistant and heat-susceptible cores of double-helical structure in ssDNA were the source of reactivity for antibodies in SLE sera with specificity for dsDNA. In a related study it was determined that among antibodies

Table 46–4. Detection Methods for Antibodies to dsDNA

	Percent Positive Tests
Precipitation in agar gel[13,53]	7–33
Counterimmunoelectrophoresis[13,52]	37
Passive hemagglutination[54]	60
Complement fixation[28,29,53]	48–68
Radioimmunoassay[30-35,55]	50–75
IFA by the crithidia technique[18-20,52,56-58]	58–95
ELISA[45-52]	70–92

to dsDNA in SLE sera, great heterogeneity existed in binding specificity, which could be characterized by the pattern of reactivity exhibited by such antibodies with native DNA fragments varying in size from 20 to 1200 base pairs.[64] These studies support the long-held contention that specific antibodies to dsDNA exist, and they throw light on the previously puzzling observation that denatured DNA could absorb out antibodies to dsDNA.[65]

Antibodies to dsDNA are highly specific for the clinical diagnosis of SLE, although a rare report of the occurrence of such antibodies in patients with RA does exist. The ultimate diagnosis of such RA patients should be reserved, since some may develop other findings typical of SLE, including glomerulonephritis. Table 46–5 shows that anti-dsDNA is generally specific for SLE and that anti-ssDNA is found in a variety of diseases.

Since antibodies to dsDNA frequently fluctuate with disease activity and often disappear rapidly with immunosuppressive therapy, their occurrence is very rare in SLE patients who experience either a spontaneous or a steroid-induced remission. Demonstration of these antibodies requires impeccably native DNA in the assay procedure. The kinds of antigen preparations thought to be free of single-stranded regions include poly dAT, *Crithidia* kinetoplast DNA, PM_2 DNA, KB or *E. coli* nDNA treated with S_1 nuclease, and KB or *E. coli* dsDNA suitably purified on benzoylated DEAE columns. The requirement of dsDNA free of single-stranded regions for anti–native DNA detection was shown in a study in which apparent reactivity of human sera for dsDNA from patients with diseases other than SLE was due to antibody to single-stranded regions in the putative dsDNA preparations.[66]

Antibodies to dsDNA not only have considerable diagnostic specificity but have also been shown to be closely related to disease activity.[67,53] There is considerable evidence pointing to an important pathogenic role for dsDNA–anti-dsDNA immune complexes, particularly in lupus nephritis.[68-70]

As mentioned previously, the crithidia test has gained wide acceptance as a test for anti-dsDNA and when compared directly with a Farr assay has identical sensitivity.[62] In a recent large study,[52] the ELISA test for anti-dsDNA was positive in 80 percent of the samples, while the crithidia test was positive in only 58 percent of the samples. If these data are confirmed, the ELISA test may prevail as the most sensitive and quantitative test for anti-dsDNA. In that study, the sera that were positive by ELISA and negative by crithidia were the lowest positive samples, and the possibility of small amounts of single-stranded regions in the dsDNA bound to the plate is difficult to exclude.

Antibodies to ssDNA occur with even higher frequency in SLE patients than do antibodies to dsDNA, as illustrated in Table 46–5. The relevance of anti-ssDNA in SLE is emphasized not only by the observation that the specificity of antibodies to DNA is most commonly to ssDNA[71,72] but also by the identification of ssDNA in sera from lupus patients[73,74] and the demonstration of the alternating appearance of antigen and antibody in the circulation, in cryoprecipitates,[75] in renal lesions,[76] and in renal eluates.[77] In addition, in acid elution studies of nephritic kidneys from SLE patients such antibodies to ssDNA are invariably found in higher titers than antibodies to dsDNA and about 20 percent of the time are found when no antibodies are present that bind dsDNA.[77]

These antibodies are, therefore, at least as important as anti-dsDNA in immunopathogenesis and in some patients constitute the major demonstrable immune complex system. Thus, while antibodies to ssDNA are of both diagnostic and immunopathogenetic importance, their imperfect specificity must be recognized if their determination is to be useful without being misleading.

A question that has recently been reinvestigated is why some SLE patients with substantial antibody titers to dsDNA fail to develop nephritis. Two recent studies point to the absence of complement-fixing ability of the anti–native DNA in patients without clinical evidence

Table 46–5. Incidence of Antibodies to Native and Single-Stranded DNA*

Sera		Antibodies Positive (Percent)	
Source	Number Tested	Native DNA	Single-Stranded DNA
SLE	50	60.0(7.1)†	92.0(5.1)
Normal	280	0.3(5.0)	3.7(4.0)‡
Hospital§	65	0	16.8(4.3)
Procainamide	14	0	57.1(4.5)
Chronic active hepatitis	43	2.3(3.0)	58.2(5.1)
Infectious mononucleosis	20	0	40.0(5.7)
Rheumatoid arthritis	32	3.1(3.0)	59.5(5.5)
Chronic glomerulonephritis	40	2.5(4.0)	7.5(4.6)
Primary biliary cirrhosis	20	0	15.0(3.6)

*From Koffler, D., et al.: Science 166:1648, 1969. Copyright 1969 by the American Association for the Advancement of Science.
†Mean titer of group of sera expressed as log base 2, shown in parentheses.
‡Of 280 sera, 170 were tested for antibodies to single-stranded DNA.
§Random hospital sera obtained from patients with a variety of diseases.

of nephritis.[78,79] By inference it is reasoned that the complement-fixing properties of anti-DNA are necessary for the development of the inflammatory process in lupus nephritis.

The RNA-Protein Antigens. Anderson and associates[80] first described the presence of precipitating antibodies to antigens in tissue extracts in the sera of patients with Sjögren's syndrome, and since then, several such precipitating antibody systems have been characterized in the sera of SLE patients. Although some laboratories have used passive hemagglutination as a method to detect and quantitate antibodies to these antigens, immunodiffusion is the only technique that can confirm immunologic identity between different sera because of the heterogeneous nature of the commonly available antigen preparations. All of the antigens to be discussed behave as soluble materials and are prepared by ultracentrifugation of tissue extracts. There are four of these RNA-protein conjugate antigens, antibodies to which are made with substantial frequency in SLE patients. They include nRNP (40 to 45 percent), Sm (25 percent), Ro/SSA (25 to 40 percent), and La/SSB/Ha (10 to 15 percent).[61]

Antibodies to Sm and nRNP. The Sm and nRNP antigens are nuclear in origin, and recent work has shed much light on their structure. Early characterization of the Sm antigen showed it to be periodate-sensitive, but trypsin, RNAase, and DNAase did not affect its antigenicity in precipitin reactions.[81] The ability of the nRNP antigen to precipitate[82] or coat cells for a hemagglutination reaction[83,84] was ablated by either RNAase or trypsin. The frequent simultaneous occurrence of antibodies to Sm and nRNP was noted,[85] and their molecular association demonstrated by immunochemical methods.[86] These early studies[86] and later more elegant immunoaffinity studies have shown that Sm and nRNP antigenic determinants exist in a molecular complex and that there exists a molecular form of Sm free of nRNP.[87-89]

Two major advances have enhanced the understanding of the antigenic structure of these antigens. One is the work of Lerner and Steitz, who characterized the RNA components of RNA-protein particles that carry the Sm and nRNP epitopes.[90] The second development was the application of the "immunoblot" or Western blot technique as well as other quantitative analyses (elution from SDS polyacrylamide gels) of the antigenicity of the protein components of the Sm and nRNP particles.[87-89,91]

The particle bound by anti-nRNP is composed of an RNA component designated U_1 complexed to at least 7 proteins varying in molecular weight from 12 to 65K; the Sm particle is composed of the same 7 proteins as well as U_2, U_1, U_4, U_5, and U_6 RNAs containing 196, 171, 145, 120, and 95 nucleotides, respectively. As already mentioned, there is a smaller antigenic version of the Sm particle lacking RNA but having several small protein bands and a total molecular weight of 70K. Precipitation reactions of nRNP with its antibody require the whole particle, both RNA and protein. Protein alone is sufficient for the precipitation of Sm with anti-

Sm. Takano and colleagues[88] have shown direct binding of protein components of MW 65K and 30K with anti-nRNP and direct binding of protein components of 30K and 13K to anti-Sm. Douvas found nRNP antigenicity associated with a 30K-protein and Sm antigenicity related to a 13K-protein by the immunoblot technique.[90] Differences in elution conditions (3 M KSCN vs. 0.01 M HCl) may account for some of the differences in antigenicity noted by these two groups. There is no evidence for the direct binding of RNA to either antibody. The antigenic epitopes for both Sm and nRNP may be represented only on protein molecules, but more work is necessary to settle this issue. Moreover it is quite possible that individual patients may have antibodies that bind to different epitopes on the same protein or even different protein subunits within the same particle. Recently a hybridoma producing anti-Sm was formed by fusion of spleen cells from an autoimmune MRL/1 mouse with an appropriate myeloma cell line.[91] This mouse monoclonal antibody precipitates the same RNA-protein particle as does the human antibody, and the immunoblot technique indicates that the monoclonal antibody binds a 26K protein. The monoclonal antibodies of human-human hybridomas with activity against the Sm and nRNP antigens should provide powerful tools for the definitive analysis of these autoantigens.

The clinical significance of antibodies to nRNP and Sm has received much attention and only a brief summary of that information will be presented. There is agreement among workers in this area that antibodies to the Sm antigen are highly specific for SLE patients.[55] No characteristic clinical features are apparent for this group of patients, although there are reports that the nephritis of such patients is mild and follows a benign course.[92,93] It has also been reported that antibodies to Sm are associated with central nervous system involvement when it occurs as an isolated clinical manifestation of the disease.[94] A recent report provides evidence for fluctuation of anti-Sm levels with disease activity, suggesting participation in immune complex disease and use as a possible indicator of clinical activity in some patients.[101]

Patients who have antibodies only to nRNP have a low incidence of antibodies to DNA and a low incidence of clinically apparent renal disease.[83,84,95] These SLE patients with anti-nRNP in their sera develop nephritis only when antibodies of other specificities are present, notably anti-DNA.[96,97] Nephritis also occurs when anti-nRNP is associated with antibodies to Sm or Ro/SSA.

Much attention has centered on a group of patients with overlapping features of SLE, scleroderma, and polymyositis, who have been designated as having mixed connective tissue disease (MCTD) by Sharp and his associates.[83,84] These patients all possess antibodies to nRNP in their sera and, like other patients with anti-nRNP who lack overlapping features, have a low frequency of antibodies to DNA and a low frequency of nephritis.

Two reports of immune complex nephropathy in patients with MCTD and anti-nRNP have appeared,[98,99] but in neither report were antibodies to Ro/SSA[100] or ssDNA[77] sought in the sera of the nephritic patients. Both of these systems have been shown to participate in immune complex nephritis and to occur in 10 to 15 percent of patients with anti-nRNP. Special tests are required for their detection, and unless specifically sought, they are easily overlooked.

MCTD patients present with very heterogeneous clinical features, a point noted in the initial description and re-emphasized in the follow-up of the original 25 patients.[102] The only uniform finding in these patients is, by definition, the presence of antibodies to nRNP. No immunologic, clinical, genetic, or biochemical characteristic has yet been described that gives this syndrome definition. The finding(s) that will distinguish MCTD from its component connective tissue diseases (SLE, myositis, and PSS) awaits recognition.

Antibodies to Ro/SSA and La/SSB/Ha. Antibodies to the soluble antigens Ro and La were originally described in patients with SLE and Sjögren's syndrome.[103,104] Both antigens were thought to be cytoplasmic, since they were quantitatively recovered from the cytoplasmic fraction of cells prepared in strong sucrose solutions. Moreover, specifically purified antibodies to the Ro antigen predominantly stained the cytoplasm of KB* cells, thymocytes, and Wil$_2$ (a lymphoblastoid B-cell line) cells, while specifically purified antibodies to La stained both the nucleus and the cytoplasm of these cells (Maddison and Reichlin, unpublished data).

Alspaugh and Tan described two nuclear antigens extracted from Wil$_2$ cells, termed SSA and SSB, which precipitated with the sera of patients with Sjögren's syndrome.[105] Akizuki and colleagues described a soluble nuclear antigen, termed Ha, which precipitated with the sera of patients with SLE-Sjögren's syndrome overlap.[106] Interlaboratory exchange of sera and antigen extracts has clearly shown that Ro and SSA on the one hand, and La, SSB, and Ha on the other are antigenically identical. Problems still remain about the cellular localization of Ro/SSA and La/SSB/Ha, but these antigens are both RNA-protein conjugates.[107] While all RNA is synthesized in the nucleus, much RNA is eventually found in the cytoplasm. Some of the confusion about the cellular localization of these antigens might result from differences in the location of the antigen at different stages of the cell cycle. Examination of the cellular location of such antigens during different phases of the cell cycle employing monospecific specifically purified antibodies or monoclonal antibodies should provide definitive answers to these questions.

The antigenicity of La/SSB/Ha from all sources is trypsin sensitive and is RNAase sensitive only under certain circumstances.[104] Ro/SSA is trypsin sensitive only when derived from Wil$_2$ cells and is not RNAase sensitive. In neither case does isolated RNA have antigenic activity, and the consensus is that the antigenic epitopes in both instances are on protein subunits of the RNA protein conjugates. Venables and colleagues have shown with the immunoblot technique that antigenicity for La/SSB/Ha resides on polypeptides of molecular weight 40K and 29K.[108]

The clinical importance of antibodies to these antigens in North American populations is that they occur principally in two diseases: SLE and Sjögren's syndrome. Antibodies to Ro/SSA occur in 25 to 40 percent of unselected SLE patients when the assay utilized is the relatively insensitive agar diffusion method. Antibodies to La/SSB/Ha occur in 10 to 15 percent of SLE patients, all of whom also have antibodies to Ro/SSA in their sera.

Anti-Ro/SSA is found much more frequently in Japanese patients with connective tissue diseases than in North American patients. The frequency of occurrence in SLE is 58 percent, while the frequencies in RA, scleroderma, polymyositis, and undifferentiated connective tissue diseases are 24, 29, 15, and 45 percent, respectively. This difference is not explained by a more frequent occurrence of Sjögren's syndrome in the Japanese patients. Analysis of this difference in anti-Ro/SSA frequency in Japanese versus North American patients with connective tissue diseases should yield important clues to the genesis and regulation of this specific immune response.

Several clinical phenomena that are associated with the presence of anti-Ro/SSA in SLE patients are listed in Table 46-6. ANA-positive anti-Ro/SSA SLE patients are not clinically distinguishable from SLE patients without these antibodies except for a high frequency of rheumatoid factors that occur in 75 to 80 percent of these patients.[110] Antibodies to Ro/SSA occur in 62 percent of the patients with clinical SLE but negative ANA tests on cryostat sections of rodent liver or kidney sections. On the other hand, within the ANA-positive subset of SLE patients who have anti-Ro/SSA, important clinical and serologic differences distinguish patients who produce anti-Ro/SSA *alone* from those who produce *both* anti-Ro/SSA *and* anti-La/SSB.[111]

Table 46-6. Clinical and Serological Phenomena Associated with Anti-Ro/SSA in SLE Patients

1. Rheumatoid factor occurs in 80 percent of patients.
2. SLE patients with anti-Ro have a high frequency of nephritis, while those with both anti-Ro and anti-La have a low frequency of nephritis.
3. Anti-Ro/SSA found in 62 percent of "ANA-negative SLE" patients.
4. Anti-Ro/SSA occurs in 63 percent of instances of subacute cutaneous LE.
5. There is increased frequency of DR2 and DR3 antigens in SLE patients with anti-Ro/SSA.
6. Eighty-five percent of homozygous C2-deficient patients with SLE picture have anti-Ro/SSA. No other precipitins are demonstrable.
7. Anti-Ro/SSA and/or anti-La/SSB occur almost invariably in neonatal SLE. No other precipitin is found.

*A human tissue culture line.

There is a great similarity in nonrenal findings in these two groups of patients but a striking difference in the frequency and severity of renal disease. Thus, 16 of 30 (53 percent) anti-Ro/SSA patients had one or more of the following three findings: a serum creatinine greater than 3.0 mg per dl, proteinuria exceeding 1.5 g in 24 hours, and cellular casts in the urine. Only 2 of 23 (9 percent) of the anti-Ro/SSA *and* anti-La/SSB patients had such evidence for nephritis. The serologic correlation of this difference in renal disease was a 77 percent incidence of anti-DNA in the anti-Ro/SSA group and a 30 percent incidence of such antibodies in the anti-Ro/SSA and anti-La/SSB group. The titers of both anti-dsDNA and anti-ssDNA were higher in the patients with anti-Ro/SSA alone than in the patients who had both anti-Ro/SSA and anti-La/SSB in their sera.[111]

Recently, a subset of lupus patients with a characteristic nonscarring dermatitis designated subacute lupus erythematosus (SCLE) has been described.[112,113] The skin disease is intermediate in severity between the acute erythematous eruption of SLE and the chronic indolent scarring lesions of discoid LE. The patients exhibit a wide distribution of lesions, with the face, arms, and trunk being affected. Seventy percent of these patients are ANA-positive on KB cells, and they have a mild systemic illness very similar in character to that described in the so-called ANA-negative SLE patients.[6] The common factor shared by the ANA-negative SLE patients and the SCLE patients that may relate to their mild disease and the low frequency of nephritis is the low frequency of antibodies to dsDNA.

It has also been reported that 73 percent of these SCLE patients are DR3-positive, a great increase above the control frequency of 24 percent for this particular HLA antigen.[113] These patients' sera have recently been examined for the presence of antibodies to soluble cellular antigens, and it has been found that 63 percent have antibodies to Ro/SSA and/or La/SSB antigens.[113] As mentioned previously, 25 to 40 percent of SLE patients and only 3 percent of discoid LE patients have anti-Ro/SSA in their sera. In a recent report by Bell and Maddison, an even closer association of antibodies to Ro/SSA with the HLA antigen DR3 has been demonstrated.[114] In their SLE population, all the anti-Ro/SSA patients (10/10) were positive for the DR3 antigen. The frequency of DR3 in their control populations was 26 percent. These data suggest that a set of genetic determinants in the major histocompatibility complex (MHC) is associated with the production of anti-Ro/SSA.

Further data supporting a genetic influence on anti-Ro/SSA production comes from a study of homozygous C2 deficiency. The genes for C2 are known to reside in the MHC on chromosome 6. Antibodies to Ro/SSA were detected in 10 of 20 such C2-deficient sera and were the only precipitins detected. Of even greater interest is that of 11 of these patients with an SLE picture, 9 possessed anti-Ro/SSA, and the remaining anti-Ro/SSA patient had discoid LE. Therefore, 9 of the 10 homozygous C2-deficient, anti-Ro/SSA-positive pa-

tients were symptomatic.[115] As it is known that all homozygous C2-deficient patients studied thus far carry the DR2 antigen, it appears that antibodies to Ro/SSA can be associated with either the DR2 or DR3 antigen.

It has long been known that in children who develop neonatal SLE, the major clinical features are dermatitis and complete heart block. Recent studies show that antibodies to Ro/SSA or La/SSB or both have been found in every child and mother examined in this clinical setting.[116,117] The dermatitis and the anti-Ro/SSA disappear over the same time course, suggesting the possible participation of the anti-Ro/SSA in the pathogenesis of the dermal lesion. Some of the mothers have not been clinically ill, and the anti-Ro/SSA and anti-La/SSB have been demonstrated in their sera in the course of evaluating the clinical and serologic status of the children.

A final caveat of genetic interest derives from the study of a child with neonatal lupus in which mother and female child both had antibodies to Ro/SSA and La/SSB/Ha.[118] HLA typing of the mother and child revealed a dissociation of antibodies and DR antigens in that the mother was DR3 and the child was DR2. The child has had normal growth and development with no skin rash since four months of age, but the mother, initially asymptomatic, has developed some evidence of Sjögren's syndrome 17 months after delivery. Such data suggest that antibody production in the mother and clinical expression of disease in the neonate are controlled by independent factors.

Antibodies to PCNA and Ma. Two recently described antibodies that occur in small groups of SLE patients are of interest for various reasons. Antibodies to proliferating cell nuclear antigen (PCNA), described by Miyachi and colleagues,[119,120] occur in 2 percent of SLE sera.[120] This antigen is not only seen in interstitial cells in epithelial tissues like liver but is also seen in the majority of cells of actively proliferating tissues such as spleen. Antibodies may therefore exist in SLE sera which are directed to antigens poorly represented in tissues used as standard immunofluorescent substrates such as rodent liver and kidney. A similar situation exists for all the antigens listed in Table 46-2.

The Ma antigen is an acidic nuclear protein described by Winn and colleagues.[121] Antibodies to Ma occur in a subset (approximately 10 percent) of SLE patients with particularly severe disease. Of interest, if confirmed, is the association of this particular antibody with aggressive active disease and nephritis. Evidence was also presented demonstrating the alternating presence of antigen and antibody in the patients' sera, suggesting that immune complexes involving this system may be forming in the circulation of these patients.

Antibodies to Histones. Antibodies to histones were first measured by the complement fixation reaction of free histones with SLE sera.[122,123] More recently the reconstitution of acid-extracted nuclei with histones by the immunofluorescent technique has been utilized as an assay for antibodies to histone or histone-dependent antigens.[124,125] Antibodies to histone measured by immunofluorescence reconstitution were found in 30 percent of idiopathic SLE but in virtually all (22 of 23) patients with drug-induced SLE. An intriguing recent study utilizing free histone in an ELISA assay detects antihistone antibodies in 56 percent of idiopathic SLE and in all (9/9) active untreated SLE patients.[126] Contrary to the reports, by histone reconstitution of immunofluorescence, 0 of 9 patients with drug-induced SLE had antibodies to histone detected by the ELISA method.[126] These disparate results may only be apparent, since the histone reconstitution method always has DNA present and a likely candidate for the reactive antigen is DNA-histone, which requires both DNA and histone for antigenic activity.[127-130]

Because most of the reactions in the sera of patients with drug-induced SLE are histone-dependent, the restricted nature of this immune response in such patients is apparent. Four drugs are frequently implicated in drug-induced SLE with positive ANA tests: procainamide, isoniazid, hydralazine, and chlorpromazine. Occasional instances of drug-induced SLE with positive ANA have been reported with sulfonamides, diphenylhydantoin, trimethadione, penicillamine, and chlorthalidone.

Sjögren's Syndrome. In 1961 Anderson and colleagues reported two precipitin reactions designated SjD and SjT between concentrated tissue extracts and the sera of patients with Sjögren's syndrome.[80] Antigenicity of SjD was not affected by nucleolytic or proteolytic enzymes, while antigenicity of SjT was resistant to DNAase and RNAase but was destroyed by trypsin. In 1962 in a more extensive clinical survey they reported the occurrence of antibodies to SjD in 6 of 28 SLE patients, in 3 of 90 patients with RA, and in 3 of 10 patients with PSS.[132] Clinical studies indicated that antibodies to SjD and SjT occurred much more frequently in patients with keratoconjunctivitis sicca (KCS) alone (so-called primary Sjögren's syndrome) than in those with both KCS and RA (secondary Sjögren's syndrome)[133].

It is very likely if not certain that SjD is Ro (which is antigenically equivalent to SSA) and that SjT is La (which is antigenically equivalent to SSB and Ha). The frequency and mutuality of their occurrence, disease specificity, and physicochemical properties are similar. Indeed, like the reports in the early 1960s in which antibodies to SjD and SjT were reported to occur almost exclusively in KCS alone, the early studies of Alspaugh and Tan found anti-Ro/SSA and anti-La/SSB/Ha almost exclusively in primary Sjögren's syndrome.[134] Subsequent studies from Scotland[135] and Baltimore[136] have failed to exhibit this specificity, and an equal number of patients, amounting to 40 to 50 percent of the patients with both primary and secondary Sjögren's syndrome, have antibodies to these antigens. A unifying feature noted in the Baltimore patients is that the presence of anti-Ro/SSA is tightly linked to vasculitis and extraglandular disease whether these complications occur in the presence or absence of RA.

When KCS occurs with SLE[136] and scleroderma,[137] at least half of the patients with anti-Ro/SSA also have anti-La/SSB/Ha in their sera. In patients with primary biliary cirrhosis (PBC) who have Sjögren's syndrome, only anti-Ro/SSA is found in such sera. Sera from 12 such cases with anti-Ro/SSA were found in a series of 63 PBC patients.*

An association has been noted between vasculitis and antibodies to Ro/SSA or La/SSB or both, particularly in patients with Sjögren's syndrome but also in patients with Waldenström's benign hyperglobulinemic purpura or the hypocomplementemic urticaria vasculitis syndrome.[136] In a group of 75 patients with Sjögren's syndrome of whom 28 had biopsy-documented vasculitis, 24 (or 86 percent) had antibodies to Ro/SSA or La/SSB or both. Only 4 of the anti-Ro/SSA–negative Sjögren's syndrome patients (10 percent) had vasculitis, demonstrating the close association of the vasculitis and antibodies to Ro/SSA. The pathology exhibited was either a leukocytoclastic vasculitis or a mononuclear infiltrate in the vessel wall. The vasculitis was associated with central nervous system involvement in many patients, with peripheral vasculitis demonstrable in nerve and muscle[138] as well as skin.[139] Many of these patients, especially those with hypocomplementemia, have cryoglobulins in their sera, and preliminary studies suggest enrichment of antibodies to Ro/SSA in these cryoprecipitates.[140]

Progressive Systemic Sclerosis. Antinuclear antibodies in the sera of PSS patients have long been known to produce a variety of speckled and nucleolar patterns on frozen tissue sections and touch prints of tissue.[21,27,131,141] A maximum of 70 percent of the patients had positive tests on such substrates and no associations with any clinical features were established.

Employing tissue culture cells as substrate (Hep2) for immunofluorescence led to detection of ANA in almost all cases of PSS, the centromere pattern was described, and the relationship of anticentromere to the CREST (calcinosis, Raynaud's phenomenon, esophageal involvement, sclerodactyly, and telangietasia) syndrome was described.[22] Antibody to centromere occurs in about 50 percent of unselected cases of PSS but in 90 percent of PSS patients with the CREST variant.[22,24] This association has been confirmed.[142-143] Antibody to centromere seems to be associated with a very low (≤ 5 percent) frequency of renal, cardiac, pulmonary, and lower gastrointestinal involvement.[144]

A rich variety of staining patterns has been described which are produced by PSS sera on Hep2 cells, of which six are nuclear and three are nucleolar.[24] One precipitating antibody that occurs in 25 percent of PSS sera is directed to the Scl_{70} antigen, so designated because the MW of the reactive antigen is 70K. Thus far, this antibody appears highly specific for PSS patients. It is anticipated that identification of additional individual antigen-antibody reactions will lead to further serological and clinical correlations analogous to that described for the centromere antibody. Certainly the ability to

---

*Unpublished data of Penner, E., Maddison, P.J., Dickson, E.R., Weiser, M.M., Milgrom, F., and Reichlin, M.

detect ANA in virtually all cases of PSS has strengthened the view of this disorder as having an important immunologic component.

Polymyositis. Although it has long been known that 30 to 40 percent of patients with polymyositis (PM) have positive ANA tests (see Table 46–3), only recently have antigen-antibody reactions with specificity for this disorder been described. As in PSS, immunofluorescent studies on tissue culture cells (Hep2) detect antibodies in 86 percent of myositis patients (M. Reichlin, unpublished data).

The first antinuclear antibody characteristic for this disorder was detected by a complement-fixing antibody to a nuclear antigen Mi, which occurred in 60 percent of dermatomyositis (DM) patients and a smaller proportion of PM patients.[145] Soon thereafter, a precipitating antibody to a nuclear antigen designated PM$_1$ was described by Wolfe and associates and was said to be present in 60 percent of PM patients.[146] It is now recognized that no single precipitin reaction utilizing crude extracts and patient sera is present in more than 30 percent of PM sera and that the system originally designated PM$_1$ was a collection of precipitins, one of which (PM$_1$) occurred in a subset of PM patients, at least half of whom had an overlap of PSS and PM. This system has been renamed the PM-Scl system, is probably of nucleolar antigen, and occurs in 8 to 10 percent of unselected PM patients.[147]

Figure 46–6. The patterns depicted here are developed by the reaction of fluorescinated anti-Ig reacting with differing antigens in Hep2 cells. The antibodies detected are all from patients with polymyositis. (1) At the upper left is a relatively homogeneous nuclear pattern; (2) at the upper right is a fine speckled pattern with nucleolar sparing; (3) at the bottom left is a homogeneous cytoplasmic pattern; and (4) at the bottom right is a nucleolar pattern.

The most frequently found precipitating antibody in PM patients is designated Jo_1 and occurs in 30 percent of idiopathic PM and in less than 10 percent of DM patients. This antibody is not found in SLE, RA, or PSS patients' sera. The antigen is a nuclear acidic molecule of MW 150K, and no particular extramuscular features seem associated with such antibodies in North American patients.[148,149] There are genetic factors influencing production of these antibodies, since 67 percent of patients with anti-Jo_1 carry the DR3 antigen on their Ia-positive cells, while only 25 percent of non–anti-Jo_1 myositis patients possess the DR3 antigen.[149] Interestingly, while this antigen is nuclear and can be demonstrated on spleen cells, it is poorly represented in mouse liver and kidney sections, and negative ANA tests are the rule on these substrates as well as tissue culture cells. This antibody is best demonstrated by the agar diffusion method.

Several other precipitating antibodies are seen in myositis patients, often with features overlapping other rheumatic diseases. Thus anti-nRNP is seen in the majority of patients with SLE-myositis, the previously mentioned PM_1 or PM-Scl is seen in PSS-myositis patients in North America, and a system designated Ku, which is seen in PSS-myositis, has thus far only been found in Japanese patients.[12] Exchange of reagents has established the independent indentities of the nRNP, PM-Scl (PM_1), and Ku systems. Although the Ku antigen is nuclear, it is not present in mouse tissue, and ANA tests are positive only on bovine or human tissues.

There is clearly great heterogeneity in the antinuclear antibodies characteristic of PM and DM and an aggregate of antigens represented in crude extracts of tissue form precipitates with 60 percent of these sera. PM-Scl (PM_1), nRNP, and Jo_1 are major systems occurring in 10 to 30 percent of PM patients, but a number of other minor reactions constitute the total spectrum of antigens toward which antibodies are demonstrable.[150] Of the remaining 40 percent of sera that do not form precipitates with tissue extracts, fewer than 10 percent are ANA positive on cryostat sections of rodent liver or kidney. About 80 percent of such sera, however, do bind to Hep2 cells in a series of immunofluorescent patterns depicted in Figure 46–6. While none of these patterns is specific for the myositis syndromes, they illustrate the heterogeneity that exists among these antibodies. In addition, it is notable here as in PSS that almost all the patients exhibit some autoantibody. These findings also re-emphasize the capacity of the human tissue culture lines to detect autoantibodies not demonstrable on cryostat sections of rodent tissues.

Rheumatoid Arthritis. The nature of ANA in RA has recently received renewed attention. At least a portion of this ANA has been rigorously shown to have a dual specificity of great interest. Surprisingly, the reactive antigen(s) for this ANA is contained in the Fc of IgG, thus exhibiting rheumatoid factor activity, and is also contained in the core constituent of chromatin, the nucleosome, which is a DNA-histone complex.[151,152] This observation raises new questions about the nature of the antigenic stimulus for the production of rheumatoid factors as well as the possibility of the development of practical tests for the detection of this specificity.

MOLECULAR SPECIFICITIES OF ANA

Since the first report of Lerner and Steitz[90] defining the nRNP and Sm antigens as residing on small ribonucleoprotein particles, there has been an explosion of

Figure 46–7. Small RNAs from Ehrlich ascites cells precipitated by antibodies from patients with lupus erythematosus. Ehrlich ascites cells were labeled with $^{32}PO_4$, and total cell extracts were prepared: 10^8 cells in 5 ml of 50 mM tris-HCl and 150 mM NaCl p11 7.5, at 0° C were ruptured by sonication for 15 seconds with a Branson sonifier at setting 2; the homogenate was centrifuged at 15,000 g for 10 minutes to obtain a clear solution. RNAs were isolated from immune precipitates or extracts and were fractionated on a gel 400 mm long, 200 mm wide, and 0.5 mm thick, consisting of 10 percent polyacrylamide, 0.38 percent bisacrylamide, 7M urea, 1 mM EDTA, and 50 m Mtris borate, at pH 8.3. Lane 9 shows small RNAs from a total Ehrlich ascites cell extract. Lanes 1 to 8 show small RNAs precipitated by immunoglobulin G isolated from serums. Lane 6 shows normal serum; the other lanes show serums containing antibodies to (lane 1) Sm, (lane 2) RNP, (lane 3) Ro^b, (lane 4) Ro^a, (lane 5) La, (lane 7) Sm and Ro^a, and (lane 8) Sm, RNP, Ro^a and 1 a. (Reprinted from Lerner, M.R., Boyle, J.A., and Steitz, J.A.: Science. 211:398, 1981.)

activity, which promises to shed light on the nature of many autoantigens reactive with the sera of patients with connective tissue diseases. The Lerner-Steitz method for the characterization of small RNAs bound by antibodies from SLE patients is depicted in Figure 46–7.

U_1 RNA, which is an integral part of the nRNP antigen, has a base sequence that is complementary to the intron-exon junctions of eukaryotic DNA. The hypothesis was made therefore that U_1 RNA was the recognition unit for the RNA splicing reaction that is an integral part of RNA processing.[153] Evidence supporting the role of U_1 RNA in the splicing reaction has been published.[154]

Similar studies have been done on the nature of the Ro/SSA and La/SSB/Ha antigens.[107] AntiRo/SSA is directed against cytoplasmic particles containing protein and five small RNAs, designated Y_1-Y_5, containing 80 to 140 bases. Thus far, no biological or biochemical function has been associated with the Ro particles. Antibodies to La/SSB bind a particle containing a very heterogeneous set of small RNAs and protein from normal cells but also bind to an RNA particle containing RNA encoded by adenovirus and RNA particles that are encoded by EB virus.[155] Anti-La/SSB reacts predominantly with nuclear particles whose RNA components are all products of RNA polymerase III, including pre-tRNAs, pre-5S rRNA, and viral transcripts. It may be that the La/SSB protein plays a special role in the processing of RNAs that are products of RNA polymerase III.[156]

A recent report describes antibodies in scleroderma sera[157] (anti-To) that bind a 300-base nucleolar ribonucleoprotein (7-2) and a novel 350-base cytoplasmic ribonucleoprotein (8-2). Other scleroderma sera were found that specifically bound the U_3 ribonucleoprotein particle. Hashimoto and Steitz have described an SLE serum (anti-Th) that binds the nucleolar 7-2 ribonucleoprotein particle as well as the 8-2 ribonucleoprotein particle.[158] In this report evidence was presented that a precursor form of the 7-2 ribonucleoprotein was bound by anti-La/SSB, thus adding the 7-2 RNA protein particle as another for which the La/SSB protein plays a role in processing.[158]

Finally it has been shown that polymyositis sera containing anti-Jo_1 all bind an RNA-protein particle, the RNA component of which is histidyl transfer RNA.[159] Preliminary evidence suggests that the protein component of this particle is the histidyl-specific amino acid activating enzyme (R. Bernstein and M.B. Matthews, personal communication). This remarkable specificity is only shown by myositis sera containing anti-Jo_1 and not by myositis sera with other antibodies.

A survey of ANA-positive sera for their ability to bind RNA-protein particles and free RNA has emphasized the multiplicity of antigens that are targets for autoantibodies among patients with rheumatic diseases. Study of these reactions should shed light on the nature of these autoimmune responses as well as provide probes for the molecular biologists to explore the functions of these molecules in normal cells.[160]

SUMMARY

The intensive application of the agar diffusion method and tissue culture lines as substrates for immunofluorescence has led to the recognition of numerous new antibody specificities to nuclear and cytoplasmic antigens. Extensive biochemical and molecular biological study of these antigens has in many instances led to their molecular definition. The clinical applicability of all this new knowledge remains to be determined. It is, however, clear that the limit of the usefulness of ANA testing in the rheumatic diseases is yet to be reached.

References

1. Hargraves, M.M., Richmond, H., and Morton, R.: Presentation of two bone marrow elements: The "tart" cell and "L.E." cell. Proc. Staff Meet. Mayo Clin. 23:25, 1948.
2. Haserick, J.R., and Sunderberg, R.D.: The bone marrow as a diagnostic aid in acute disseminated lupus erythematosus. J. Invest. Dermatol. 11:209, 1948.
3. Friou, G.J.: Clinical application of lupus serum-nucleoprotein reaction using fluorescent antibody technique (abstract). J. Clin. Invest. 36:890, 1957.
4. Holman, H.R., and Kunkel, H.G.: Affinity between the lupus erythematosus serum factor and cell nuclei and nucleoprotein. Science 126:162, 1957.
5. Holborow, E.J., Weir, D.M., and Johnson, G.D.: A serum factor in lupus erythematosus with affinity for tissue nuclei. Br. Med. J. 2:732, 1957.
6. Maddison, P.J., Provost, T.T., and Reichlin, M.: ANA-negative systemic lupus erythematosus: Serological analysis. Medicine (Baltimore) 60:87, 1981.
7. Beck, J.: Antinuclear antibodies: Methods of detection and significance. Mayo Clin. Proc. 44:600, 1960.
8. Wiik, A., and Munthe, E.: Restrictions among heavy and light chain determinants of granulocyte-specific antinuclear factors. Immunology 23:53, 1972.
9. Elling, P., Grandal, H., and Faber, V.: Granulocyte-specific antinuclear factors in serum and synovial fluid in rheumatoid arthritis. Ann. Rheum. Dis. 27:225, 1968.
10. Rosenberg, J.N., Johnson, G.D., Holborow, E.J., and Bywaters, E.G.L.: Eosinophil-specific and other granulocyte-specific antinuclear antibodies in juvenile chronic polyarthritis and adult rheumatoid arthritis. Ann. Rheum. Dis. 24:350, 1975.
11. Hoyeraal, H.M.: Granulocyte-reactive antinuclear factors in juvenile rheumatoid arthritis. Scand. J. Rheumatol. 5:84, 1976.
12. Mimori, T., Akizuki, M., Yamagata, H., Inada, S., Yoshida, S., and Homma, M.: Characterization of a high molecular weight acidic nuclear protein recognized by autoantibodies in sera from patients with polymyositis-scleroderma overlap. J. Clin. Invest. 68:611, 1981.
13. Davis, J.S., and Winfield, J.B.: Serum antibodies to DNA by counterimmunoelectrophoresis (CIE). Clin. Immunol. Immunopathol. 2:510, 1974.
14. Davis, J.S.: Determination of DNA and anti-DNA by counterimmunoelectrophoresis: A rapid and sensitive assay. Arthritis Rheum. 14:377, 1971.
15. Schur, P.H., DeAngelis, D., and Jackson, J.M.: Immunological detection of nucleic acids and antibodies to nucleic acids and nuclear antigens by counterimmunoelectrophoresis. Clin. Exp. Immunol. 17:209, 1974.
16. Kurata, N., and Tan, E.M.: Identification of antibodies to nuclear acidic antigens by counterimmunoelectrophoresis. Arthritis Rheum. 19:574, 1976.
17. Keiser, H.D., and Weinstein, J.: The detection and identification of antibodies to saline extractable nuclear antigens by counterimmunoelectrophoresis. Arthritis Rheum. 23:1026, 1980.
18. Davis, P., Christian, B., and Russell, A.S.: Immunofluorescent technique for the detection of antibodies to nDNA: Comparison with radioimmunoassay. J. Rheumatol. 4:15, 1977.
19. Sontheimer, R.D., and Gilliam, J.N.: An immunofluorescence assay for double-stranded DNA antibodies using Crithidia luciliae kinetoplast as a double-stranded DNA substrate. J. Lab. Clin. Med. 91:550, 1978.
20. Ballou, S.P., and Kushner, I.: Antinative DNA detection by the Crithidia luciliae method: An improved guide to the diagnosis and clinical management of systemic lupus erythematosus. Arthritis Rheum. 22:321, 1979.

21. Ritchie, R.F.: Antinucleolar antibodies: Their frequency and diagnostic association. N. Engl. J. Med. 282:1174, 1970.

22. Tan, E.M., Rodnan, G.P., Garcia, I., Moroi, I., Fritzler, M.J., and Peebles, C.: Diversity of antinuclear antibodies in scleroderma: Anticentromere antibody and its relationship to CREST. Arthritis Rheum. 23:617, 1980.

23. McCarty, G.A., Barada, F.A., Fritzler, M.J., and Snyderman, R.: A new antinuclear antibody staining the mitotic spindle apparatus: Immunologic characteristics, clinical occurrence and cytoskeletal studies. Arthritis Rheum. 24:S109, 1981.

24. Bernstein, R.M., Steigerwald, J.C., and Tan, E.M.: Association of antinuclear and antinucleolar antibodies in progressive systemic sclerosis. Clin. Exp. Immunol. 48:43, 1982.

25. Pinnas, J.L., Northway, J.D., and Tan, E.M.: Antinucleolar antibodies in human sera. J. Immunol. 111:996, 1973.

26. Miyawaki, S., and Ritchie, R.F.: Nucleolar antigen specific for antinucleolar antibody in the sera of patients with systemic rheumatic disease. Arthritis Rheum. 16:726, 1973.

27. Beck, J.S.: Autoantibodies to cell nuclei. Scot. Med. J. 8:373, 1963.

28. Robbins, W.C., Holman, H.R., Deicher, H., and Kunkel, H.G.: Complement fixation with cell nuclei and DNA in lupus erythematosus. Proc. Soc. Exper. Biol. Med. 96:575, 1957.

29. Seligmann, M., and Milgrom, F.: Mise en évidence par la fixation du complement de la reaction entre acid desoxyribonucleique et serum de malades atteints de lupus erythemateux disséminé. C. R. Acad. Sci. 245:1472, 1957.

30. Wold, R.T., Young, F.E., Tan, E.M., and Farr, R.S.: Deoxyribonucleic acid antibody: A method to detect its primary interaction with deoxyribonucleic acid. Science 161:806, 1968.

31. Pincus, T., Schur, P.H., Rose, J.A., Decker, J.L., and Talal, N.: Measurements of serum DNA-binding activity in SLE. N. Engl. J. Med. 281:701, 1969.

32. Pincus, T.: Immunochemical conditions affecting the measurement of DNA antibodies using ammonium sulfate precipitation. Arthritis Rheum. 14:523, 1971.

33. Webb, J., and Whaley, K.: Evaluation of the native DNA-binding assay for DNA antibodies in systemic lupus erythematosus and other connective tissue diseases. Med. J. Aust. 2:324, 1974.

34. Kredich, N.M., Skyler, J.S., and Foote, L.J.: Antibodies to native DNA in systemic lupus erythematosus. A technique of rapid and quantitative determination. Arch. Intern. Med. 131:639, 1973.

35. Ginsberg, B., and Keiser, H.: A millipore filter assay for antibodies to native DNA in sera of patients with systemic lupus erythematosus. Arthritis Rheum. 16:199, 1973.

36. Lentz, K., Winfield, J.B., and Barland, P.: Antibodies to dAT detected by membrane filtration. Arthritis Rheum. 19:867, 1976.

37. Steinberg, A.D., Baron, S., and Talal, N.: The pathogenesis of autoimmunity in New Zealand mice. I. Induction of antinucleic acid antibodies by polyinosinic-polycytidylic acid. Proc. Natl. Acad. Sci. (USA) 63:1102, 1969.

38. Eilat, D., Steinberg, A.D., and Schechter, A.N.: The reaction of SLE antibodies with native single-stranded RNA: Radioassay and binding specificities, J. Immunol. 120:550, 1978.

39. Pillarisetty, R.J., and Talal, N.: Clinical studies of antibodies binding polyriboadenylic acid in SLE. Arthritis Rheum. 19:505, 1976.

40. Davis, P., Russell, A.S., and Percy, J.S.: Antibodies to UV light denatured DNA in systemic lupus erythematosus: Detection by filter radioimmunoassy and clinical correlations. J. Rheumatol. 3:375, 1976.

41. Kanai, Y., Kawaminami, Y., Miwa, M., Matsushima, T., and Sugimura, T.: Naturally occurring antibodies to poly (ADP-ribose) in patients with systemic lupus erythematosus. Nature 265:175, 1977.

42. Okobie, E.E., and Shall, S.: The significance of antibodies to poly (ADP-ribose) in patients with systemic lupus erythematosus. Clin. Exp. Immunol. 36:151, 1979.

43. Morrow, W.J.W., Isenkey, D.A., Parry, H.F., Shen, L., Okobie, E.E., Farzanek, F., Shall, S., and Snaith, M.L.: Studies on autoantibodies to poly (adenosine-diphosphate ribose) in SLE and other autoimmune diseases. Ann. Rheum. Dis. 41:396, 1982.

44. Nabon, E., Deffraissy, J.F., Kahn, M.F., Jeusset, J., Galanand, P., and Lacour, F.: Anti-poly (G)-poly (C) antibodies in the serum of patients with systemic lupus erythematosus. Clin. Immunol. Immunopathol. 22:349, 1982.

45. Pesce, A.J., Mendoza, N., Boreisha, I., Gaizutis, M.A., and Pollock, V.E.: Use of enzyme-linked antibodies to measure serum anti-DNA antibody in systemic lupus erythematosus. Clin. Chem. 20:353, 1974.

46. Gripenberg, M., Linder, E., Kurki, P., and Engvall, E.: A solid phase enzyme-linked immunoabsorbent assay (ELISA) for the demonstration of antibodies against denatured, single-stranded DNA in patient sera. Scand. J. Immunol. 7:151, 1978.

47. Klotz, J.L., Minami, R.M., and Teplitz, R.L.: An enzyme-linked immunosorbent assay for antibodies to native and denatured DNA. J. Immunol. Meth. 29:155, 1979.

48. Pisetsky, D.S., and Peters, D.V.: A simple enzyme-linked immunosorbent assay for antibodies to native DNA. J. Immunol. Meth. 41:187, 1981.

49. Miller, T.E., Lahita, R.G., Zario, V.J., MacWilliam, J., and Koffler, D.: Clinical significance of anti-double stranded DNA antibodies detected by a solid phase radioimmunoassay. Arthritis Rheum. 24:602, 1981.

50. Halbert, S.P., Karsh, J., and Anken, M.: Studies on antibodies to deoxyribonucleic acid and deoxyribonucleoprotein with enzyme immunoassay (ELISA). J. Lab. Clin. Med. 97:97, 1981.

51. Kavai, M., Banzai, A., Zsindely, A., Sonkoly, I., and Szegedi, G.: Enzyme-linked immunoabsorbent assay for antibodies to native DNA in sera of patients with SLE. J. Immunol. Meth. 48:169, 1982.

52. Eaton, R.B., Schneider, G., and Schur, P.H.: Enzyme immunoassay for antibodies to native DNA. Arthritis Rheum. 26:52, 1983.

53. Schur, P.H., and Sandson, J.: Immunological factors and clinical activity in systemic lupus erythematosus. N. Engl. J. Med. 278:533, 1968.

54. Koffler, D., Carr, R., Agnello, V., Feizi, T., and Kunkel, H.G.: Antibodies to polynucleotides: Distribution in human serum. Science 166:1648, 1969.

55. Notman, D.D., Kurata, N., and Tan, E.M.: Profiles of antinuclear antibodies in systemic rheumatic diseases. Ann. Intern. Med. 83:464, 1975.

56. Aarden, L.A., de Groot, E.R., and Feltkamp, T.E.W.: Immunology of DNA. III. *Crithidia lucilae*: A simple substrate for the detection of anti-dsDNA with the immunofluorescence technique. Ann. N. Y. Acad. Sci. 254:505, 1975.

57. Slater, W.G., Cameron, J.S., and Lessoff, M.H.: The *Crithidia luciliae* kinetoplast immunofluorescence test in systemic lupus erythematosus. Clin. Exp. Immunol. 25:480, 1976.

58. Chubick, A., Sontheimer, R.D., Gilliam, J.N., and Ziff, M.: An appraisal of tests for native DNA antibodies in connective tissue diseases: Clinical usefulness of *Crithidia luciliae* assay. Ann. Intern. Med. 89:186, 1978.

59. Ceppellini, R., Polli, E., and Celada, F.: A DNA-reacting factor in serum of a patient with lupus erythematosus diffusus. Proc. Soc. Exp. Biol. Med. 96:572, 1957.

60. Deicher, H.R.G., Holman, H.R., and Kunkel, H.G.: The precipitin reaction between DNA and a serum factor in systemic lupus erythematosus. J. Exp. Med. 109:97, 1959.

61. Reichlin, M.: Current perspectives on serological reactions in LE patients. Clin. Exp. Immunol. 44:1, 1981.

62. Aarden, L.L., Lakmeker, F., de Groot, E.F., Swaak, A.J.G., and Feltkamp, T.E.W.: Detection of antibodies to DNA by radioimmunoassay and immunofluorescence. Scand. J. Rheum. Suppl. 11:12, 1975.

63. Stollar, B.D., and Papalian, M.: Secondary structure in denatured DNA is responsible for its reaction with antinative DNA antibodies of systemic lupus erythematosus sera. J. Clin. Invest. 66:210, 1980.

64. Papalian, M., Lafer, E., Wong, R., and Stollar, B.D.: Reaction of systemic lupus erythematosus antinative DNA antibodies with native DNA fragments from 20-1200 base pairs. J. Clin. Invest. 65:469, 1980.

65. Stollar, B.D.: Nucleic acid antigens. *In* Sela, M. (ed.): The Antigens. Vol. 1. New York and London, Academic Press, 1973.

66. Locker, J.D., Medof, M.E., Burnett, R.M., and Sukhupunyaraska, S.: Characterization of DNA used to assay sera for anti-DNA antibodies: Determination of the specificities of anti-DNA antibodies in SLE and non-SLE rheumatic disease states. J. Immunol. 118:694, 1977.

67. Koffler, D., Agnello, V., Thoburn, R., and Kunkel, H.G.: Systemic lupus erythematosus: Prototype of immune complex nephritis in man. J. Exp. Med. 134:109, 1971.

68. Tan, E.M., Schur, P.H., and Carr, R.I.: Deoxyribonucleic acid (DNA) and antibodies to DNA in the serum of patients with systemic lupus erythematosus. J. Clin. Invest. 45:1732, 1966.

69. Koffler, D., Schur, P.H., and Kunkel, H.G.: Immunological studies concerning the nephritis of systemic lupus erythematosus. J. Exp. Med. 126:607, 1967.

70. Cochrane, C.G., and Koffler, D.: Immune complex disease in experimental animals and man. Adv. Immunol. 16:185, 1973.

71. Koffler, D., Carr, R.I., Agnello, V., Thoburn, R., and Kunkel, H.G.: Antibodies to polynucleotides in human sera: Antigenic specificity and relation to disease. J. Exp. Med. 134:294, 1971.

72. Samaha, R.J., and Irvin, W.S.: Deoxyribonucleic acid strandedness: Partial characterization of the antigenic region binding antibodies in lupus erythematosus serum. J. Clin. Invest. 56:446, 1975.

73. Barnett, E.V.: Detection of nuclear antigens (DNA) in normal and pathologic human fluids by quantitative complement fixation. Arthritis Rheum. 11:407, 1968.

74. Koffler, D., Agnello, V., Winchester, R.V., and Kunkel, H.G.: The occurrence of single-stranded DNA in the serum of patients with systemic lupus erythematosus and other diseases. J. Clin. Invest. 52:198, 1973.

75. Winfield, J.B., Koffler, D., and Kunkel, H.G.: Specific concentration of polynucleotide immune complexes in the cryoprecipitates of patients with systemic lupus erythematosus. J. Clin. Invest. 56:563, 1975.

76. Andres, G.A., Accini, G.A., Beiser, S.M., Christian, C.L., Cinotti, G.A., Erlanger, B.F., Hsu, K.C., and Seegal, B.C.: Localization of fluorescein-

labelled antinucleoside antibodies in glomeruli of patients with systemic lupus erythematosus nephritis. J. Clin. Invest. 49:2106, 1971.

77. Koffler, D., Agnello, V., and Kunkel, H.G.: Polynucleotide immune complexes in serum and glomeruli of patients with systemic lupus erythematosus. Am. J. Pathol. 74:109, 1974.

78. Miniter, M.F., Stollar, B.D., and Agnello, V.: Reassessment of the clinical significance of native DNA antibodies in systemic lupus erythematosus. Arthritis Rheum. 22:959, 1979.

79. Beaulieu, A., Ruismorio, F.P., Friou, G.J., Vayuvegula, B., and Mirick, B.: IgG antibodies to double-stranded DNA in systemic lupus erythematosus: Independent variation of complement-fixing activity and total antibody content. Arthritis Rheum. 22:565, 1979.

80. Anderson, J.R., Gray, K.G., Beck, J., and Kinnear, W.F.: Precipitating autoantibodies in Sjögren's disease. Lancet ii:456, 1961.

81. Tan, E.M., and Kunkel, H.G.: Characteristics of a soluble nuclear antigen precipitating with the sera of patients with systemic lupus erythematosus. J. Immunol. 96:464, 1966.

82. Mattioli, M., and Reichlin, M.: Characterization of a soluble nuclear ribonucleoprotein antigen reactive with LE sera. J. Immunol. 197:1281, 1971.

83. Sharp, G.C., Irvin, W.S., Laroque, R. L., Velez, C., Daly, V., Kaiser, A.D., and Holman, H.R.: Association of autoantibodies to different nuclear antigens with clinical patterns of rheumatic disease and responsiveness to therapy. J. Clin. Invest. 50:350, 1971.

84. Sharp, G.C., Irvin, W.S., Tan, E.M., Gould, R.G., and Holman, H.R.: Mixed connective tissue disease—an apparently distinct rheumatic disease syndrome associated with a specific antibody to an extractable nuclear antigen (ENA). Am. J. Med. 52:148, 1972.

85. Reichlin, M., and Mattioli, M.: Antigens and antibodies characteristic of systemic lupus erythematosus. Bull. Rheum. Dis. 24:756, 1974.

86. Mattioli, M., and Reichlin, M.: Physical association of two nuclear antigens and mutual occurrence of their antibodies: The relationship of the Sm and RNA protein (Mo) systems in SLE sera. J. Immunol. 110:1318, 1973.

87. Takano, M., Agris, P.F., and Sharp, G.C.: Purification and biochemical characterization of nuclear ribonucleoprotein antigen using purified antibody from serum of a patient with mixed connective tissue disease. J. Clin. Invest. 65:1449, 1980.

88. Takano, M., Golden, S.S., Sharp, G.C., and Agris, P.F.: Molecular relationship between two nuclear antigens, ribonucleoprotein and Sm: Purification of active antigens and their biochemical characterization. Biochemistry 21:5929, 1981.

89. Douvas, A.S.: Autoantibodies occurring in two different rheumatic diseases react with the same ribonucleoprotein particle. Proc. Natl. Acad. Sci. (USA) 79:5401, 1982.

90. Lerner, M.R., and Steitz, J.A.: Antibodies to small nuclear RNAs complexed with proteins are produced by patients with systemic lupus erythematosus. Proc. Natl. Acad. Sci. (USA) 76:5495, 1979.

91. Lerner, E.A., Lerner, M.R., Janeway, Jr., C.A., and Steitz, J.A.: Monoclonal antibodies to nucleic acid–containing cellular constituents: Probes for molecular biology and autoimmune disease. Proc. Natl. Acad. Sci. (USA) 78:2737, 1981.

92. Powers, R., Akizuki, M., Boehm-Truitt, M.J., Daly, V., and Holman, H.R.: Substantial purification of the Sm antigen and association of high titer antibody to Sm with a clinical subset of systemic lupus erythematosus. Arthritis Rheum. 20:131 (abstract), 1977.

93. Winn, D.M., Wolfe, J.R., Lindberg, D.A., Fristoe, F.A., Kingsland, L., and Sharp, G.C.: Identification of a clinical subset of systemic lupus erythematosus by antibodies to the Sm antigen. Arthritis Rheum. 22:1334, 1979.

94. Winfield, J.B., Brunner, C.M., and Koffler, D.: Serologic studies in patients with systemic lupus erythematosus and central nervous system dysfunction. Arthritis Rheum. 21:289, 1978.

95. Reichlin, M., and Mattioli, M.: Correlation of a precipitin reaction to an RNA protein antigen and a low prevalence of nephritis in patients with systemic lupus erythematosus. N. Engl. J. Med. 286:908, 1972.

96. Parker, M.D.: Ribonucleoprotein antibodies: Frequency and clinical significance in systemic lupus erythematosus, scleroderma, and mixed connective tissue disease. J. Lab. Clin. Med. 82:769, 1973.

97. Maddison, P.J., Mogavero, H., and Reichlin, M.: Patterns of clinical disease associated with antibodies to nuclear ribonucleoprotein. J. Rheumatol. 5:407, 1978.

98. Fuller, T.J., Richman, A.V., Auerbach, D., Alexander, R.W., Lottenberg, R., and Longley, S.: Immune complex glomerulonephritis in a patient with mixed connective tissue disease. Am. J. Med. 62:761, 1977.

99. Bennett, R.M., and Spongo, B.H.: Immune complex nephropathy in mixed connective tissue disease. Am. J. Med. 63:534, 1977.

100. Madison, P.J., and Reichlin, M.: Deposition of antibodies to a soluble cytoplasmic antigen in the kidneys of patients with systemic lupus erythematosus. Arthritis Rheum. 22:858, 1979.

101. Barada, F.A., Jr., Andrews, B.S., Davis, J.S., IV, and Taylor, R.P.: Antibodies to Sm in patients with systemic lupus erythematosus. Arthritis Rheum. 24:1236, 1981.

102. Nimelstein, S.H., Brody, S., McShane, D., and Holman, H.R.: Mixed connective tissue disease: A subsequent evaluation of the original 25 patients. Medicine (Baltimore) 59:239, 1980.

103. Clark, G., Reichlin, M., and Tomasi, T.B.: Characterization of a soluble cytoplasmic antigen reactive with sera from patients with systemic lupus erythematosus. J. Immunol. 102:117, 1968.

104. Mattioli, M., and Reichlin, M.: Heterogeneity of RNA protein antigens reactive with sera of patients with systemic lupus erythematosus. Arthritis Rheum. 17:421, 1974.

105. Alspaugh, M.A., and Tan, E.M.: Antibodies to cellular antigens in Sjögren's syndrome. J. Clin. Invest. 55:1067, 1975.

106. Akizuki, M., Powers, R., and Holman, H.R.: A soluble acidic protein of the cell nucleus which reacts with serum from patients with systemic lupus erythematosus and Sjögren's syndrome. J. Clin. Invest. 59:254, 1977.

107. Lerner, M.R., Boyle, J.A., Hardin, J.A., and Steitz, J.A.: Two novel classes of small RNA proteins detected by antibodies associated with lupus erythematosus. Science 211:400, 1981.

108. Venables, P.J.W., Charles, P.J., Buchanan, R.R.C., Yi, I., Mumford, P.A., Schreiber, L., Roon, G.R.W., and Maini, R.N.: Quantitation and detection of isotypes of antiSSB antibodies by ELISA and Farr assays using affinity purified antigens. Arthritis Rheum. 26:146, 1983.

109. Yamagata, H.: The antibodies to the SS-A antigen in patients with connective tissue diseases. Keio Igaku 58:381, 1981 (Japanese).

110. Maddison, P.J., Mogavero, H., Provost, T.T., and Reichlin, M.: The clinical significance of autoantibodies to a soluble cytoplasmic antigen in systemic lupus erythematosus and other connective tissue diseases. J. Rheumatol. 6:189, 1979.

111. Wasicek, C.A., and Reichlin, M.: Clinical and serological differences between systemic lupus erythematosus patients with antibodies to Ro versus patients with antibodies to Ro and La. J. Clin. Invest. 69:835, 1982.

112. Sontheimer, R.D., Thomas, J.R., and Gilliam, J.N.: Subacute cutaneous lupus erythematosus. A cutaneous marker for a distinct lupus erythematosus subset. Arch. Dermatol. 115:1409, 1979.

113. Sontheimer, R.D., Maddison, P.J., Reichlin, M., Jordan, R.E., Stastny, P., and Gilliam, J.N.: Serologic and HLA associations in subacute cutaneous lupus erythematosus, a clinical subset of lupus erythematosus. Ann. Intern. Med. 97:664, 1982.

114. Bell, D.A., and Maddison, P.J.: Serologic subsets in SLE: An examination of autoantibodies in relationship to clinical features of disease and HLA antigens. Arthritis Rheum. 23:1268, 1980.

115. Provost, T.T., Arnett, F.C., and Reichlin, M.: C_2 deficiency, lupus erythematosus and anticytoplasmic Ro (SSA) antibodies. Arthritis Rheum. 25:S41, 1982 (Abstract).

116. Franco, H.L., Weston, W.L., Peebles, C., Forstat, S.L., and Phanaphak, P.: Autoantibodies directed against sicca syndrome antigens in the neonatal lupus syndrome. Am. Acad. Dermatol. 4:67, 1981.

117. Kephart, D.C., Hood, A.F., and Provost, T.T.: Neonatal lupus erythematosus: New serological findings. J. Invest. Dermatol. 77:331, 1981.

118. Lockshin, M.D., Gibofsky, A., Peebles, C.L., Gigli, I., Fotino, M., and Hurwitz, S.: Neonatal lupus erythematosus with heart block: Family study of a patient with anti-SSA and SSB antibodies. Arthritis Rheum. 26:210, 1983.

119. Miyachi, I., Fritzler, M.J., and Tan, E.M.: Autoantibody to a nuclear antigen in proliferating cells. J. Immunol. 121:228, 1978.

120. Fritzler, M.J., McCarty, G.A., Ryan, J.P., and Kinsella, T.D.: Clinical features of patients with antibodies directed against proliferating cell nuclear antigen. Arthritis Rheum. 26:140, 1983.

121. Winn, D.M., Wolfe, J.F., Harmon, D., and Sharp, G.C.: Characterization of a distinct nuclear acidic protein antigen (MA) and clinical findings in systemic lupus erythematosus patients with MA antibodies. J. Clin. Invest. 64:820, 1979.

122. Kunkel, H.G., Holman, H.R., and Deicher, H.R.G.: Multiple autoantibodies to cell constituents in systemic lupus erythematosus. Ciba Found. Symp. 8:429, 1960.

123. Stollar, B.D.: Reactions of systemic lupus erythematosus sera with histone fractions and histone DNA complexes. Arthritis Rheum. 14:495, 1971.

124. Tan, E.M., Robinson, J., and Robitaille, P.: Studies on antibodies to histones by immunofluorescence. Scand. J. Immunol. 5:89, 1976.

125. Fritzler, M.J., and Tan, E.M.: Antibodies to histones in drug-induced and idiopathic lupus erythematosus. J. Clin. Invest. 62:560, 1978.

126. Gioud, M., Faci, M.A., and Monia, J.C.: Histone antibodies in systemic lupus erythematosus. Arthritis Rheum. 25:407, 1982.

127. Friou, G.J.: Identification of the nuclear component of the interaction of lupus erythematosus globulin and nuclei. J. Immunol. 80:476, 1958.

128. Holman, H.R., and Deicher, H.R.: The reaction of the lupus erythe-

matosus (LE) cell factor with deoxyribonucleoprotein of the cell nucleus. J. Clin. Invest. 38:2059, 1959.
129. Tan, E.M.: An immunologic precipitin system between soluble nucleoprotein and serum antibody in systemic lupus erythematosus. J. Clin. Invest. 46:735, 1967.
130. Stollar, B.D.: Studies on nucleoprotein determinants for systemic lupus erythematosus serum. J. Immunol. 99:959, 1967.
131. Burnham, T.K., Fine, G., and Neblett, T.R.: The immunofluorescent tumor imprint technique. II. The frequency of antinuclear factors in connective tissue diseases and dermatoses. Ann. Intern. Med. 65:9, 966.
132. Anderson, J.R., Gray, K.G., Beck, J.S., Buchanan, W.W., and McElhanney, A.J.: Precipitating autoantibodies in the connective tissue diseases. Ann. Rheum. Dis. 21:360, 1962.
133. Bunim, J.J.: Hypergammaglobulinemia and autoantibodies in Sjögren's syndrome. Ann. N. Y. Acad. Sci. 124: 852, 1965.
134. Alspaugh, M.A., Talal, N., and Tan, E.M.: Differentiation and characterization of autoantibodies and their antigens in Sjögren's syndrome. Arthritis Rheum. 19:216, 1976.
135. Alspaugh, M.A., Buchanan, W.W., and Whaley, K.: Precipitating antibodies to cellular antigens in Sjögren's syndrome, rheumatoid arthritis and other organ and non-organ-specific diseases. Ann. Rheum. Dis. 37:244, 1978.
136. Alexander, E.L., Hirsch, T.J., Arnett, F.C., Provost, T.T., and Stevens, M.B.: Ro (SSA) and La (SSB) antibodies in the clinical spectrum of Sjögren's syndrome. J. Rheum. 9:239, 1982.
137. Osial, T.A., Whiteside, T.L., Buckingham, R.B., Singh, G., Barnes, E.L., and Rodnan, G.P.: Antibodies to SS-A, SSB and RANA in progressive systemic sclerosis (PSS) with and without Sjögren's syndrome (SS) (abstract). Arthritis Rheum. 25:S34, 1982.
138. Alexander, E.C., and Alexander, G.E.: Central nervous system disease in primary Sjögren's syndrome association with vasculitis and antibodies to Ro/SSA. Arthritis Rheum. 25:15, 1982 (abstract).
139. Alexander, E.L., and Provost, T.T.: Cutaneous manifestations of Sjögren's syndrome (SS). Reflections of immune vasculitis. Arthritis Rheum. 25:S15, 1982 (abstract).
140. Reichlin, M.: Clinical and immunologic significance of antibodies to Ro and La in systemic lupus erythematosus. Arthritis Rheum. 25:767, 1982.
141. Rothfield, N.F., and Rodnan, G.P.: Serum antinuclear antibodies in progressive systemic sclerosis (scleroderma). Arthritis Rheum. 11:607, 1968.
142. Fritzler, M.J., Kinsella, T.D., and Garbutt, E.: The CREST syndrome: A distinct serologic entity with anticentromere antibodies. Am. J. Med. 69:520, 1980.
143. Kallenberg, C.G.M., Pastoor, G.W., Wouda, A.A., and The, T.H.: Antinuclear antibodies in patients with Raynaud's phenomenon: Clinical significance of anticentromere antibodies. Ann. Rheum. Dis. 41:382, 1982.
144. McCarty, G.A., Rice, J.R., Bembe, M.L., and Barada, F.A., Jr.: Anticentromere antibody. Clinical correlations and association with favorable prognosis in patients with scleroderma variants. Arthritis Rheum. 26:1, 1983.
145. Reichlin, M., and Mattioli, M.: Description of a serological reaction characteristic of polymyositis. Clin. Immunol. Immunopathol. 5:12, 1976.
146. Wolfe, J.F., Adelstein, E., and Sharp, G.C.: Antinuclear antibody with distinct specificity for polymyositis. J. Clin. Invest. 59:176, 1977.
147. Reichlin, M., Maddison, P.J., Targoff, I., Bunch, T., Arnett, F., Sharp, G.C., Treadwell, E., and Tan, E.M.: Antibodies to a nuclear/nucleolar antigen in patients with polymyositis-overlap syndromes. J. Clin. Immunol. 4:40, 1984.
148. Nishikai, M., and Reichlin, M.: Heterogeneity of precipitating antibodies in polymyositis and dermatomyositis. Characterization of the Jo₁ antibody system. Arthritis Rheum. 23:881, 1980.
149. Arnett, F.C., Hirsch, T.J., Nishikai, M., Bias, W., and Reichlin, M.: The Jo₁ antibody system. Clinical and immunogenetic associations in myositis. J. Rheumatol. 8:925, 1981.
150. Reichlin, M.: Marker antibodies for polymyositis syndromes. In Antibodies to Nuclear Antigens, Immunological Specificity and Clinical Implications. Excerpta-Medica 2, 1981.
151. Agnello, V., Ibanez de Kasip, G., Arbetter, A.E., and Spitz, J.J.R.: Significance of rheumatoid factors cross reactive with DNA-protein (DNP). Arthritis Rheum. 21:540, 1978.
152. Hannestad, K., and Stollar, B.D.: Certain rheumatoid factors react with nucleosomes. Nature 275:671, 1978.
153. Lerner, M.R., Boyle, J.A., Mount, S.M., Wolin, S.L., and Steitz, J.A.: Are snRNP's involved in splicing? Nature (London) 283:220, 1980.
154. Yang, V.W., Lerner, M.R., Steitz, J.A., and Flint, S.J.: A smaller nuclear ribonucleoprotein is required for splicing of adenoviral early RNA sequence. Proc. Natl. Acad. Sci. (USA) 78:1371, 1981.
155. Lerner, M.R., Andrews, N.C., Miller, G., and Steitz, J.A.: Two small RNA's encoded by Epstein Barr virus and complexed with protein are precipitated by antibodies from patients with systemic lupus erythematosus. Proc. Natl. Acad. Sci. (USA) 78:805, 1981.
156. Rinke, J., and Steitz, J.A.: Precursor molecules of both human 5S ribosomal RNA and transfer RNAs are bound by a cellular protein reactive with anti-La lupus antibodies. Cell 29:149, 1982.
157. Reddy, R., Tan, E.M., Henning, D., Nohga, K., and Busch, H.: Detection of a nucleolar 7-2 ribonucleoprotein and a cytoplasmic 8-2 ribonucleoprotein with autoantibodies from patients with scleroderma. J. Biol. Chem. 258:1383, 1983.
158. Hashimoto, C., and Steitz, J.A.: Sequential association of nucleolar 7-2 RNA with two different autoantigens. J. Biol. Chem. 258:1379, 1983.
159. Rosa, M.D., Hendrick, J.D., Lerner, M.R., Reichlin, M., and Steitz, J.A.: A mammalian tRNA His-containing antigen is recognized by the polymyositis specific antibody anti-Jo-1. Nucleic Acids Res. 11:853, 1983.
160. Hardin, J.A., Rahn, D.R., Shen, C., Lerner, M.R., Wolin, S.L., Rosa, M.D., and Steitz, J.A.: Antibodies from patients with connective tissue diseases bind specific subsets of cellular RNA-protein particles. J. Clin. Invest. 70:141, 1982.
161. Tan, E.M., and Vaughn, J.H.: Antinuclear antibodies. Significance of biochemical specificities. In Beutner, E.M., Chorezelski, T.P., Bean, S.F., and Jordon, R.E. (eds.): Immunopathology of the Skin. Wiley, New York, 1973, p. 369.

Chapter 47

Diagnostic Tests in Neuromuscular Diseases

Walter G. Bradley

INTRODUCTION

A wide range of rheumatologic immunologic conditions may be associated with neuromuscular disease. The most common of these are listed in Table 47–1. These may cause pain secondary to nerve entrapment or compression. Sensory symptoms such as paresthesia and sensory loss may occur in a number of the conditions, such as the sensorimotor polyneuropathy associated with rheumatoid arthritis. Muscle weakness may be due to muscle involvement in polymyositis, to motor nerve involvement in entrapments, or to the ischemic neuropathies of polyarteritis nodosa and other vasculitides.

The diagnosis of neuromuscular involvement in patients with rheumatologic conditions is not always easy, as indicated in Chapter 27. A debilitating systemic illness

Table 47–1. Neuromuscular Conditions Which May Be
Associated with Rheumatologic Diseases

Muscle

Polymyositis—pure or associated with rheumatoid arthritis,
  progressive systemic sclerosis, polyarteritis nodosa, systemic
  lupus erythematosus, etc.
Type 2 fiber atrophy—associated with painful local joints, or a
  systemic collagen-vascular disease
Sarcoid myopathy
Polymyalgia rheumatica
Myopathy associated with drugs—corticosteroid myopathy,
  penicillamine polymyositis

Nerve

Entrapment or compression neuropathy—secondary to joint
  capsule thickening or bony displacement, e.g., carpal tunnel
  syndrome
Mononeuropathy—nerve infarcts due to collagen-vascular disease,
  including polyarteritis nodosa, Wegener's granulomatosis,
  rheumatoid arthritis vasculitis, systemic lupus erythematosus,
  etc.
Polyneuropathy—in vasculitides, rheumatoid arthritis, etc.
Radiculopathy—associated with ankylosing spondylitis,
  rheumatoid arthritis
Polyneuropathy with dysproteinemias
Polyneuropathy associated with drugs—e.g., gold

Neuromuscular Junction

Myasthenia gravis—associated with autoimmune disease,
  including rheumatoid arthritis, scleroderma, systemic lupus
  erythematosus, thyroid disease, pernicious anemia, diabetes
  mellitus, etc.

such as progressive systemic sclerosis or rheumatoid arthritis may cause muscle atrophy. Local joint pain may produce restriction of movement and thereby apparent muscle weakness. If motor and sensory involvement are present, it is necessary to decide whether this is a secondary effect of the underlying rheumatologic condition or due to some unrelated cause. The presence of nerve and muscle involvement has considerable importance for both prognosis and therapy in rheumatologic diseases, and it is important to have a high index of suspicion for such involvement.

The diagnostic investigations of neuromuscular disease are relatively sophisticated and require some expertise for their interpretation. These investigations fall into three categories:

(1) *Screening*, such as the serum levels of enzymes released from the skeletal muscles.

(2) *Electrophysiology*, including electromyography and nerve conduction studies.

(3) *Morphology*, including muscle and nerve biopsies.

SCREENING TESTS FOR MUSCLE DAMAGE

A number of substances are highly concentrated in skeletal muscle and released into the bloodstream when muscle fibers undergo necrosis. From the blood they may eventually make their way to the urine. Determination of the level of such substances in the blood or urine may demonstrate the presence of muscle fiber ne-

crosis and indicate its severity. The general rule is that such substances are not released when muscle undergoes primary atrophy without loss of sarcolemmal integrity, as in disuse atrophy, denervation, thyrotoxicosis, and corticosteroid myopathy, but are released in such necrotizing conditions as muscle injury, polymyositis, and muscular dystrophy.

Urinary Creatine. Creatine phosphate provides the high-energy phosphate reserve of skeletal muscle. The average adult urinary excretion of creatine is about 60 to 150 mg in 24 hours in normal males and approximately twice that level in females. Muscle fiber atrophy from any cause produces an increased urinary excretion of creatine.

Urinary Myoglobin and 3-Methylhistidine. Necrosis of muscle fibers releases myoglobin into blood and thence into urine. Highly sensitive radioimmunoassays are now available for the detection and quantification of myoglobin. The substituted amino acid 3-methylhistidine is almost specifically localized to skeletal muscle. Thus the rate of excretion of the substance (providing that the patient is on a meat-free diet) is proportional to the total amount of muscle fiber breakdown occurring in unit time, whether this breakdown is the result of atrophy or of muscle fiber necrosis.

Serum Levels of Skeletal Muscle Enzymes. Aldolase, glutamic oxalacetic and glutamic pyruvic transaminases (SGOT and SGPT), lactic dehydrogenase (LDH), and creatine kinase* (CK) are all released into the plasma when muscle fibers undergo necrosis. Aldolase was the first enzyme in which this release was first recognized.[1] SGOT,[2] and CK[3] release were also reported to be important in muscle diseases. In most conditions causing muscle necrosis, the percentage rise of serum CK activity is higher than that of the other two enzymes, and thus serum CK levels provide the most sensitive index of muscle fiber breakdown. The role of serum levels of muscle enzymes in diagnosing neuromuscular disease has been extensively reviewed.[4-6]

A number of conditions causing muscle damage, including intramuscular injections, muscle needling during electromyography, and muscle biopsy, all cause a rise of serum enzymes, particularly CK. Thus it is important for blood to be drawn for the determination of the serum CK activity early in the investigations of patients, *before* any such manipulations are undertaken. The serum enzyme levels may not return to normal for several weeks following a muscle biopsy and electromyography. Because the serum CK is such a sensitive indicator of muscle damage, it is a useful screening test for muscle disease. However, the level may be raised in many different disorders, in heart disease, and in individuals performing heavy manual work.

Serum Isozymes. Many enzymes exist in several different molecular forms or isozymes. These are often dimers or tetramers of two or more subunits. The type

---

*Creatine kinase is frequently misdescribed as creatine phosphokinase. The kinases are a group of enzymes catalyzing phosphorylation of substances, and the term "phospho" is therefore redundant.

or proportion of the isozymes may vary from tissue to tissue. Different isozymes of CK are present in adult skeletal muscle (MM form), in brain (BB form), and in cardiac muscle (MB form). Thus skeletal and cardiac muscle damage and, rarely, cerebral damage may cause a rise in the plasma CK levels. The isozymes will often allow separation of these conditions. However, unfortunately this is not always so, since the skeletal muscle in the fetus and during extensive regeneration after injury contains a high proportion of the MB form. Thus the finding that the major proportion of the plasma CK is the MB form does not necessarily prove its cardiac origin.

LDH similarly exists as five different isozymes, the largest proportion normally being the slowest migrating LDH_5. Where extensive skeletal muscle necrosis and regeneration occur, there is a significant shift of isozymes toward the faster moving LDH_1 and LDH_2.[7] Such isozyme changes may help in the recognition of skeletal muscle damage when the total level of enzymes is relatively normal.

ELECTROPHYSIOLOGIC STUDIES OF NEUROMUSCULAR FUNCTION

Although extensively available in the United States and many other countries, electrophysiologic studies of neuromuscular function are frequently employed with insufficient knowledge of how the changes should be interpreted. These are investigations requiring considerable expertise and experience, and it is thus important that they should be undertaken by well-trained individuals.

These studies may be divided into electromyography, motor and sensory nerve conduction studies, and studies of neuromuscular junction function. It is important that the physician caring for the patient should understand the significance and limitation of these electrophysiological investigations. This chapter is intended to provide an outline of these tests and the alterations produced by diseases. For fuller descriptions the reader should consult Buchthal,[8] Bradley,[9] and Lenman and Ritchie.[10]

Motor Nerve Conduction Studies. The principle of these studies is illustrated in Figure 47–1, which deals with the median nerve. The supramaximal stimulus to the median nerve is first applied at the wrist (S_1), and the conduction time between the onset of the stimulus and the first deflection from the baseline of the evoked muscle action potential (MAP) is measured from the oscillograph record (T_1). The distance between the stimulating cathode and the proximal recording electrode (D_1) is also measured. The procedure is repeated with stimulation in the antecubital fossa (S_2) and the axilla (S_3), and the appropriate conduction time is measured (T_2 and T_3). The distance between the cathode-stimulating sites for S_1 and S_2 (D_2) and S_2 and S_3 (D_3) are also measured. The maximum motor conduction velocity (MMCV) for the segment elbow to wrist is given by the equation:

$$MMCV = \frac{D_2 \text{ (mm)}}{T_2 - T_1 \text{ (msec)}} m/\sec$$

T_1 is the terminal latency expressed as "x msec for y cm." The latency depends upon the distance from the stimulating to the recording electrodes, and comprises the time for the conduction of nervous impulses to the synapse, the synaptic delay, and the time for the conduction of the muscle action potential along the muscle fibers to the recording electrodes. The amplitude of the evoked MAP provides an index of the number of muscle fibers capable of activation. The duration of the MAP is prolonged in demyelinating neuropathies. *Late waves* (the F wave and the H reflex) result from conduction of the nerve impulse to the spinal cord and back to the muscle and are of use in studying conduction in the proximal parts of the nerve fibers. The F wave travels in a retrograde direction up the motor axons to the cord before returning to the muscle; the H reflex travels up the Ia afferent fibers and through the intraspinal monosynaptic reflex before returning down the motor axons.

Sensory Nerve Conduction Studies. A similar principle applies to sensory nerve conduction studies. Purely sensory nerves can be studied by stimulating digital (i.e., purely sensory nerves) and recording from the mixed nerves (orthodromic stimulation), or by stimulating mixed nerves and recording from the digital nerves (antidromic stimulation). The sensory nerve action potential (SNAP) is of much lower amplitude than the MAP, and averaging techniques are required to record them. Sensory nerve conduction may be expressed as a latency or as a conduction velocity.

It is important that each laboratory define its own *normal* values, since these depend upon observer and instrumentation. It is also important that the temperature of the electrophysiology room be carefully controlled at about 25° C and time allowed for equilibration, since nerve conduction is greatly influenced by limb temperature.

Figure 47–1. Diagram showing the techniques of measuring the maximum motor conduction velocity in the median nerve. (From Bradley, W.G.: Disorders of Peripheral Nerves. Oxford, Blackwell Scientific Publications, 1974.)

Nerve conduction is markedly slowed in segmental demyelinating neuropathies. This slowing is probably due to a combination of delayed activation of the widened nodes of Ranvier, which have paranodal demyelination; the slower continuous, rather than saltatory, conduction along totally demyelinated internodes; the current leakage through thin, partly remyelinated myelin sheaths; and the abnormally short intercalated internodes, causing an increased number of saltatory steps. The degree of reduction of nerve conduction velocity is related to the degree of segmental demyelination, and the conduction velocity is frequently slowed to less than 50 per cent of normal (less than 25 m per second), as in hypertrophic neuropathy. The terminal latency is greatly increased in such conditions; for instance, in the median nerve it may be greater than 6 msec, the normal being less than 3.0 msec.

In axonal degeneration, on the other hand, provided that some large myelinated fibers remain, the maximum nerve conduction velocity remains normal. Loss of axons is indicated by reduction of the amplitude of the evoked MAP, and sometimes by fragmentation of the MAP. The terminal latency is generally normal, although atrophy or regeneration of the distal axons, producing thin sprouts, may increase the terminal latency.

Electromyography. The principles of electromyography (EMG) are illustrated in Figures 47–2 and 47–3. The recording electrode is a needle, usually with a concentric insulated wire in the middle. Only the tip of the wire is free of insulation, potential differences being recorded between this bare tip and the outer part of the needle, which acts as the second electrode. This needle records the electrical events occurring in muscle fibers around its tip, and this activity is amplified and recorded by an oscilloscope.

The Normal Electromyogram. At rest, when the needle

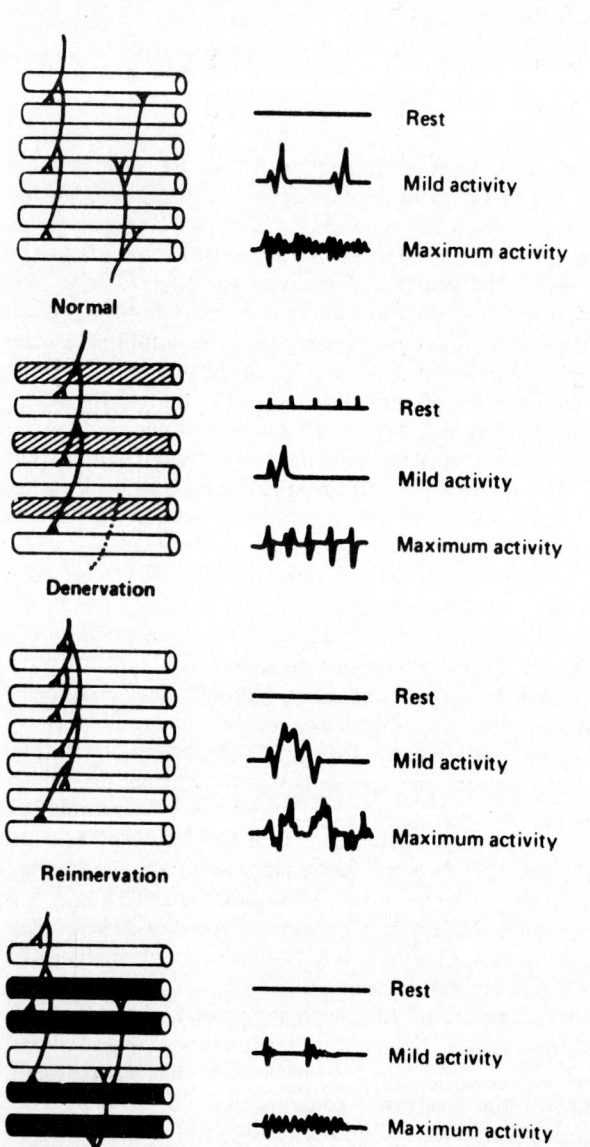

Figure 47–2. Classic interpretation of electromyography in the normal state, denervation, reinnervation, and myopathy, showing the electrical pattern at rest, on mild activity, and on maximum voluntary effort.

Figure 47–3. Diagram of the basis of the electromyogram during weak muscle contraction in normal muscle, and in denervation and myopathy. (From Bradley, W.G.: Disorders of Peripheral Nerves. Oxford, Blackwell Scientific Publications, 1974.)

is inserted there is a brief discharge from injured muscle fibers and then electrical silence. Weak contraction evokes isolated motor unit action potentials (MUAP) usually of 8 to 12 msec duration and 200 to 800 uV amplitude. The exact values depend on the muscle being studied. Each MUAP is the summation of the electrical events occurring in the muscle fibers of a single motor unit. It is irregular in outline because the electrical events in the individual muscle fibers do not reach the recording unit in a smoothly synchronized fashion. The normal MUAP has three or four phases. With maximum voluntary effort the superimposition of large number of MUAPs completely obliterates the baseline. This is called *a full interference pattern.*

Electromyogram in Neuropathic Disorders. Denervation and reinnervation produce atrophy of some muscle fibers and reinnervation of others by axonal sprouting from surviving motor neurons; the latter process produces enlarged motor units. At rest fibrillation potentials may be seen, which usually have two or three phases, and are about 2 to 3 msec in duration and 30 to 150 uV amplitude. They arise from spontaneous discharge of denervated muscle fibers. Weak contraction produces isolated MUAPs which are of large amplitude and longer duration than normal owing to the enlarged motor units. Also because of the sprouting of intramuscular nerves,

the MUAPs are even less synchronized than normal, with a resultant increase in the normal 5 to 10 percent of potentials with more than four phases (polyphasic potentials). Because of the fallout of motor units consequent upon the denervating condition, on maximum voluntary effort individual MUAPs may still be seen, and the baseline is not completely obliterated. This is termed *an incomplete* or *single unit interference pattern.*

Electromyogram in Myopathies. The patchy loss of whole or parts of individual muscle fibers with the retention of the normal numbers of motor nerves or motor units produces a characteristic picture. At rest the muscle is silent in most myopathies, although in polymyositis there is a marked increase in insertional activity presumably because of diffuse damage to the sarcolemma of the muscle fibers. Weak contraction elicits MUAPs which are of lower amplitude and shorter duration than normal owing to loss of muscle fibers. They are more polyphasic than normal since loss of muscle fibers prevents the smoothing effect of summation of large numbers of muscle fiber potentials. Mild contraction produces a full interference pattern, because all the motor units must be contracted to produce even a moderate force in the weakened muscle. Maximum voluntary effort produces a full interference pattern with a decreased maximum amplitude compared to normal.

Although the preceding description provides the classic changes recognized by electromyographers, the picture may not always be as simple. For instance, a muscle which is very severely damaged (end stage) by any process may produce aberrant results.

Single Fiber Electromyography. This recently developed technique uses an electrode with a recording surface that is capable of picking up the impulses of only two or three muscle fibers. In only a few instances will these be from the same motor unit because of the overlap of motor units in skeletal muscle. In denervated/reinnervated muscle, the density of fibers from the same unit in one area is increased, and synchronous discharges of two or three fibers is often seen. Failure of transmission in the nerve terminal can also be detected by this technique, which is therefore of help in diagnosing myasthenia gravis.

Repetitive Nerve Stimulation. Neuromuscular transmission in a normal individual will tolerate repetitive stimulation of up to 40 per second for 10 seconds with less than a 30 percent decrement of the amplitude of the evoked MAP. In patients with myasthenia gravis, if repetitive nerve stimulation at 2 to 10 per second is applied, there is a rapid decrement of the amplitude of the response which may fall to 50 percent of the initial response within a few seconds.[11] A maximum voluntary effort will similarly cause a decrement of the immediately succeeding evoked MAP. Unfortunately the response is not necessarily seen in every muscle in myasthenia gravis, the diagnosis of which may require advanced and sophisticated techniques such as single fiber EMG and the regional curare test.[12] In the myasthenic syndrome of Eaton and Lambert the electrophysiological findings are of an abnormally small first evoked muscle action potential, followed by an *incremental* response of more than 50 percent with stimuli applied at 10 to 30 per second.

PATHOLOGICAL STUDIES

Pathological studies of nerve and muscle aid considerably in the diagnosis of neuromuscular diseases, particularly when advanced techniques are applied. The following paragraphs provide a brief outline of these techniques, and of the pathological changes and their interpretation.

Muscle Biopsy. The following is a brief outline of the techniques of muscle biopsy. For further descriptions the reader should consult Dubowitz and Brooke[13] and Bradley.[9] The procedure is performed under local or general anesthesia. If the former, infiltration of the muscle with local anesthesia must be avoided. A 3-inch incision is made in line with the muscle fibers, the deep fascia is opened, and the muscle fascicles are separated by sharp dissection. A small fascicle about 3 mm in diameter and 2 to 3 cm long is removed in a biopsy clamp. Several models of such clamps are available to keep the muscle at the in vivo length during fixation. It is important to avoid direct handling of the tissue to be studied histologically, since this produces gross histological artifacts. Three specimens are usually removed: (1) Histology—fixation with formalin and embedding in paraffin wax. Stained sections allow examination of large amounts of transverse and longitudinally sectioned muscle. (2) Electron microscopy—fixation in glutaraldehyde and embedding in epoxy resins allowing ultrastructural investigation. (3) Histochemistry—the specimen is usually taken without clamps and rapidly frozen in liquid nitrogen; transverse sections are cut in a cryostat and stained for histochemical reactions.

Histochemistry has provided very important advances in the understanding of muscle diseases, and thus some details must be provided here. A battery of stains are available to show different metabolic systems; mitochondrial oxidative enzymes are revealed by NADH or SDH stains; phosphorylase required for initiating glycolysis may be stained; periodic acid-Schiff (PAS) stains glycogen; the enzyme of myosin responsible for the transduction of high energy phosphate bonds into contraction, myofibrillary ATPase, may also be demonstrated histochemically. Other histochemical reactions often used include acid phosphatase and nonspecific esterase which stain lysosomes and macrophages. Hematoxylin and eosin and the Gomori trichrome stains are also performed on cryostat sections. The latter will reveal increased numbers of mitochondria in mitochondrial myopathies, nemaline rods in patients with nemaline myopathy, and other structural changes.

Histochemical stains of normal human muscle show two classes of fiber, one stained darkly and the other lightly, and there is reciprocity between the oxidative and glycolytic enzyme stains in the same muscle fiber seen in serial sections. In some animals certain muscles are almost entirely made up of either oxidative or glycolytic fibers, and this histochemical separation of the muscles correlates well with the physiological twitch characteristics which are respectively slow and fast. In normal muscle in man, however, both oxidative and glycolytic fibers are randomly distributed throughout every muscle.

The separation of fiber types is sometimes less than absolute, and histochemistry has had its "lumpers" and "splitters," some wishing to differentiate only two types of fibers[14] while others have recognized up to nine fiber types.[15] Much confusion has arisen because of the lack of agreement between different workers over the terminology of these different fiber types. Not only have oxidative and glycolytic stains been used to separate the fibers, but staining techniques for myosin ATPase carried out after preincubation at various pHs have also been widely used. Myosin ATPase of fast-twitch muscle is more alkaline stable, acid labile and formaldehyde stable than that of slow muscle,[16] and by varying the pH and other parameters the density of staining can be varied to separate fiber subtypes. The glycine-formaldehyde calcium technique of Tunell and Hart[17] is a useful single technique, type 1 fibers being light, type 2A being

Table 47–2. Outline of the Criteria for Typing of Muscle Fibers on Histochemical and Physiologic Grounds (0, 1+, 2+, 3+ Indicate the Relative Intensity of Histochemical Staining)

Criteria	1	2A	2B	2C
Twitch speed	Slow	Fast	Fast	?
Susceptibility to fatigue	Resistant	Resistant	Susceptible	?
Myosin ATPase pH 9.4	1+	3+	3+	3+
Myosin ATPase pH 4.6	3+	0	3+	3+
Myosin ATPase pH 4.3	3+	0	0	2+
Myosin ATPase formaldehyde-glycine	0	1+	2+	?
NADH-TR	3+	2+	1+	2+
SDH	3+	2+	1+	2+
α-GPDH-ML	0	2+	2+	1+
PAS	1+	3+	2+	2+
Phosphorylase	1+	3+	3+	3+
Oxidative/glycolytic	Oxid.	Oxid./glyc.	Glyc.	Glyc.
Electron microscopy				
Proportion of mitochondria and lipid droplets	3+	2+	1+	2+
Z-line thickness (nm)	~120	~8	~8	?

ATPase = Myosin ATPase.
NADH-TR = NADH-tetrazolium reductase.
SDH = Succinic dehydrogenase.
α-GPDH-ML = Menadione-linked α-glycerophosphate dehydrogenase.
PAS = Periodic acid–Schiff.

intermediate, and type 2B being darkly stained. The fiber type can probably be recognized in electron micrographs.[18-20]

Some authors have combined physiological, histochemical, and biochemical criteria to define the individual muscle fiber types.[21] Such a nomenclature based upon several criteria has many advantages, but is impractical for everyday discussion. The following enumeration of fiber types is now generally accepted:

Type 1 = slow twitch, oxidative, fatigue-resistant.

Type 2A = fast twitch, glycolytic-oxidative, fatigue-resistant.

Type 2B = fast twitch, glycolytic, fast-fatiguing.

Type 2C = (perhaps) undifferentiated fibers.

Table 47–2 shows the physiological and various histochemical characteristics of these fiber types, and Table 47–3 gives a comparison of this terminology with several of the previously proposed nomenclatures. As seen in Figure 47–4, the histochemical typing of fiber is usually but not always reliable. Transposition of this terminology of fiber types to pathological muscle is not always easy, since both altered innervation and altered use may change the fiber type. Loss of clear differentiation of fiber types is a frequent finding in chronically diseased muscle.

For detailed descriptions of the pathological changes of skeletal muscle the reader should consult Dubowitz and Brooke.[13] *Denervation* tends to be associated with angulated atrophic fibers which are often very dark with the oxidative enzyme stains. *Reinnervation* produces aggregation of fibers all of the same type, i.e., fiber type grouping. *Denervation of such reinnervated groups* pro-

Table 47–3. Comparison of Fiber Type Terminology

Authors	Fiber Type			
	1	2A	2B	2C
Dubowitz and Pearse, 1960[24]	I	II	II	—
Stein and Padykula, 1962[25]	B	C	A	—
Romanul, 1964[15]	III	II	I	—
Padykula and Gauthier, 1966[26]	Intermediate	Red	White	—
Yellin and Guth, 1970[27]	β	β	α	—
Ashmore and Doerr, 1971[28]	β-red	α-red	α-white	—
Burke et al., 1971[29]	S	FR	FF	—
Close, 1972[30]	Slow twitch—fatigue resisting	Fast twitch—fatigue resisting	Fast twitch—fast fatiguing	—
Peter et al., 1972[21]	Slow twitch—oxidative	Fast twitch—oxidative-glycolytic	Fast twitch—glycolytic	

a) NADH - TR

b) Myosin ATPase pH 9.5

c) Myosin ATPase pH 4.6

d) Myosin ATPase pH 4.3

e) EM of Type I fiber

f) EM of Type 2 fiber

Bar for (a) - (d) 100 μm
Bar for (e), (f) 1 μm

Figure 47–4. *Above,* Serial sections of a normal muscle stained for *(a)* NADH-TR, *(b)* myosin ATPase at pH 9.5, *(c)* myosin ATPase at pH 4.6, and *(d)* myosin ATPase at pH 4.3. The fiber type is marked on each fiber. Although the staining characteristics of each fiber correspond in most cases to those shown in Table 46–2, this is not true of all fibers. *Below,* Electron micrographs of longitudinal sections of *(e)* Type 1 fiber and *(f)* Type 2 muscle fiber. The Type 1 muscle fiber has more mitochondria and a thicker Z-line than the Type 2 fiber, which has more glycogen between the myofibrils.

duces grouped fiber atrophy. A *necrotizing myopathy* causes muscle fiber necrosis, phagocytosis, and later regeneration, and this is typically seen in Duchenne muscular dystrophy. Rounding and increased random variation of fiber size are typical *myopathic* changes, as are the presence of internal nuclei, fibrosis, and fat cell replacement. However, all the latter changes may also be seen in chronic denervation.[22] Histochemistry has allowed the recognition and separation of a considerable number of specific neuromuscular diseases, such as the congenital myopathies. These include nemaline myopathy (see above); mitochondrial myopathies (see above); central core disease (with the central part of each fiber being devoid of mitochondrial enzyme activity); centronuclear myopathy with type 1 fiber hypotrophy (with abnormally small type 1 fibers, which all have central nuclei); and congenital fiber-type disproportion (with type 1 fibers being abnormally small). Type 2 fiber atrophy is a common finding in many conditions, including muscle atrophy of disuse, cachexia, and painful conditions of local joints and nerve roots. Corticosteroid myopathy tends to produce type 2 fiber atrophy with mitochondrial changes in type 1 fibers, although these changes are nonspecific.

Nerve Biopsies. Only a brief description of this procedure will be given here. For further descriptions the reader should consult Bradley[9] and Dyck and colleagues.[23] Usually a sensory nerve is biopsied, and this may be done under either local or general anesthesia. The most commonly approached are the sural nerve in the calf or the superficial branch of the radial nerve at the wrist. It is possible to biopsy the whole nerve or to take only a fascicular biopsy of a small portion of the nerve. The latter may cause no sensory loss, and is preferable unless total sensory loss is already present or one is looking for a vasculitis or a similarly "patchy" process. It is possible to take a fascicular biopsy of a mixed motor nerve, provided that only about one twentieth of the total transverse area is taken and considerable care is applied, but this should not be viewed as a routine investigation.

The nerve is exposed and carefully removed, touching only the ends where it is necessary to cut the fibers. Any pressure or other manipulation of the main portion of the nerve which is to be taken for histological examination will cause marked crush artifact changes in the nerve fibers.

It is a difficult decision whether any benefit is to be obtained from nerve biopsy. This decision is greatly aided by consultation with a person experienced in the clinical and pathological studies of patients with peripheral nerve disease. Nerve biopsy may be diagnostic in a few conditions like a vasculitis, leprosy, or amyloidosis. Apart from these conditions, unless a laboratory with a specific interest in peripheral nerve pathology is available, little useful information is likely to be gained from nerve biopsy.

It is particularly important that the nerve be prepared in the appropriate fashion. It is generally recommended that frozen sections be prepared for enzyme and lipid stains; that a portion of the nerve be fixed under tension in glutaraldehyde for embedding in epoxy resin for light and electron microscopic studies, and for the microdissection of single nerve fibers; and that a portion be fixed under tension in Susa fixative for paraffin embedding for hematoxylin and eosin, Bodian, or other silver stains for axons, and for PTAH or solochrome cyanin staining for myelin sheaths.

Details of the techniques and of the changes in various diseases are given in Bradley.[9] *Axonal degeneration* causes loss of axonal continuity and secondary degeneration of the myelin sheath into a string of myelin ovoids. *Segmental demyelination* is a process in which myelin breaks down, leaving the axon intact. These processes tend to occur in different diseases. For instance, toxic neuropathies are usually associated with axonal degeneration, whereas diphtheritic neuropathy causes segmental demyelination. Extensive segmental demyelination may give rise to onion bulb hypertrophy of the nerves with a characteristic pathological picture. A vasculitis may cause both axonal degeneration and segmental demyelination, with patchy loss of myelinated nerve fibers in some fasciculi and preservation in others;

the nerve biopsy may show an involved blood vessel. In most diseases causing peripheral neuropathy, such as diabetes mellitus, both segmental demyelination and axonal degeneration are present. The proportion of these two changes may aid in the recognition of the cause of the neuropathy, but this is rarely diagnostic.

SUMMARY AND CONCLUSIONS

The detailed biochemical, electrophysiological, and pathological studies described in this chapter are of great importance in the recognition and elucidation of neuromuscular disorders associated with rheumatologic diseases. The collaboration of several different experts is required to undertake these investigations, and the physician who is caring for the patient must have sufficient knowledge of these techniques to be able to integrate their results and interpret them in terms of the overall clinical picture.

References

1. Sibley, J.A., and Lehringer, A.L.: Aldolases in the serum and tissues of tumor bearing animals. Natl. Cancer. Inst. Monogr. 9:303, 1949.
2. Pearson, C.M.: Serum enzymes in muscular dystrophy and certain other muscular and neuromuscular diseases. I. Serum glutamic oxaloacetic transaminase. N. Engl. J. Med. 256:1069, 1075, 1957.
3. Ebashi, S., Toyokum, Y., Momoi, H., and Sugita, H.: Creatine phophokinase activity of sera of progressive muscular dystrophy patients. J. Biochem. (Tokyo) 46:103, 1959.
4. Zellweger, H., Durnin, R., and Simpson, J.: The diagnostic significance of serum enzymes and electrocardiogram in various muscular dystrophies. Acta Neurol. Scand. 48:87, 1972.
5. Munsat, T.L., Baloh, R., Pearson, C.M., and Fowler, W.: Serum enzyme alterations in neuromuscular disorders. JAMA 226:1536, 1973.
6. Munsat, T.L.: Creatine phosphokinase alterations in neuromuscular diseases. Isr. J. Med. Sci. 13:93, 1977.
7. Hooshmand, H., Dove, J., and Suter, C.: The use of serum lactate dehydrogenase isoenzymes in the diagnosis of muscle diseases. Neurology 19:26, 1969.
8. Buchthal, F.: An Introduction to Electromyography. Copenhagen, Scandinavian University Books, 1957.
9. Bradley, W.G.: Disorders of Peripheral Nerves. Oxford, Blackwell Scientific Publications, 1974.
10. Lenman, J.A., and Ritchie, E.: Clinical Electromyography. 2nd ed. Philadelphia, J. B. Lippincott Company, 1977.
11. Desmedt, J.E., and Borenstein, S.: The testing of neuromuscular transmission. In Vinken, P.J., and Bruyn, G.W. (eds.): Handbook of Clinical Neurology. Amsterdam, North Holland, 1970, pp. 104–115.
12. Brown, J.C., and Charlton, J.E.: Study of sensitivity to curare in myasthenic disorders using a regional technique. J. Neurol. Neurosurg. Psychiat. 38:27, 1975.
13. Dubowitz, V., and Brooke, M.H.: Muscle Biopsy: A Modern Approach. London, W. B. Saunders, 1973.
14. Engel, W.K.: Fiber-type nomenclature of human skeletal muscle for histochemical purposes. Neurology 24:344, 1974.
15. Romanul, F.C.A.: Enzymes in muscle. I. Histochemical studies of enzymes in individual muscle fibers. Arch. Neurol. 11:355, 1964.
16. Guth, L., and Samaha, F.J.: Qualitative differences between actomyosin ATPase of slow and fast mammalian muscle. Exp. Neurol. 25:138, 1969.
17. Tunell, G.L., and Hart, M.N.: Simultaneous determination of skeletal muscle fiber, types I, IIA, and IIB by histochemistry. Arch. Neurol. 34:171, 1977.
18. Fardeau, M.: Caractéristiques cytochimiques et ultrastructurales des différents types de fibres musculaires squelettiques extra-fusales (chez l'homme et quelques mammifères). Ann. Anat. Pathol. 18:7, 1973.
19. Eisenberg, B.R., and Kuda, A.M.: Retrieval of cryostat sections for comparison of histochemistry and quantitative electron microscopy in a muscle fiber. J. Histochem. Cytochem. 25:1169, 1977.

20. Saltis, L.M., and Mendell, J.R.: The fine structural differences in human muscle fiber types based on peroxidatic activity. J. Neuropath. Exp. Neurol. 33:632, 1974.
21. Peter, J.B., Barnard, R.J., Edgerton, V.R., Gillespie, C.A., and Stemple, K.E.: Metabolic profiles of three fiber types of skeletal muscle in guinea-pigs and rabbits. Biochemistry 11:2627, 1972.
22. Fewings, J.D., Harris, J.B., Johnson, M.A., and Bradley, W.G.: Progressive denervation of skeletal muscle induced by spinal irradiation in rats. Brain 100:157, 1977.
23. Dyck, P.J., Thomas, P.K., and Lambert, E.H. (eds.): Peripheral Neuropathy. Philadelphia, W. B. Saunders Company, 1975.
24. Dubowitz, V., and Pearse, A.G.E.: A comparative histochemical study of oxidative enzyme and phosphorylase activity in skeletal muscle. Histochemie 2:105, 1960.
25. Stein, J.M., and Padykula, H.A.: Histochemical classification of individual skeletal muscle fibers of the rat. Am. J. Anat. 110:103, 1962.
26. Padykula, H.A., and Gauthier, G.F. (1966). Quoted by Peter et al., Reference 21.
27. Yellin, H., and Guth, L.: The histochemical classification of muscle fibres. Exp. Neurol. 26:424, 1970.
28. Ashmore, C.R., and Doerr, L.: Comparative aspects of muscle fibre types in different species. Exp. Neurol. 31:408, 1971.
29. Burke, R.E. Levine, D.M., Zajac, F.E., Tsairis, P., and Engel, W.K.: Mammalian motor units: Physiological-histochemical correlation in three types in cat gastrocnemius. Science 174:709, 1971.
30. Close, R.I.: Dynamic properties of mammalian skeletal muscles. Physiol. Rev. 52:129, 1972.

Section IV
Clinical Pharmacology

Chapter 48
Principles of Pharmacodynamics and Pharmacokinetics

Donald S. Robinson

FACTORS INFLUENCING DRUG PHARMACODYNAMICS AND CLINICAL EFFECTS

Importance of Individualizing Drug Dosage. The need for individualizing drug dosage for patients in order to achieve optimal therapeutic effect is being increasingly recognized and accepted. The clinician can be aided in this by the clinical laboratory in the case of certain drugs for which therapeutic ranges of blood levels have been defined. The adjustment of dosage according to plasma level allows careful monitoring of treatment with such drugs. Unfortunately, there are only a few drugs for which plasma levels are of demonstrated clinical value and a therapeutic range has been defined. In the field of rheumatology, only salicylate and acetaminophen levels are routinely measured, although it is likely with the advent of sensitive modern methods of assaying drugs that additional drugs will be monitored using the laboratory in the near future.

For most drugs, dosage is still regulated by the process of prescribing the "usual dose," with subsequent adjustments, if any, based on observation of clinical effects. An understanding of certain basic principles governing pharmacodynamics and pharmacokinetics common to most drugs can aid physicians in this important matter of selecting and individualizing drug dose. The primary goal is to maximize therapeutic benefit and to minimize toxicity, side effects, and drug interaction.

The intensities of therapeutic and toxic effects are proportional to drug concentration at receptor sites in target tissues. Factors affecting distribution of a drug to these various receptor sites can significantly influence its clinical effects. The single most important determinant of drug concentration at receptor sites is *drug dosage*. Furthermore, it has been conclusively established that the majority of adverse drug reactions are dose related rather than idiosyncratic.[1] Therefore, more precise individualization of dosage can serve to avoid or reduce toxic and side effects for most drugs. Only for the minority of drugs with a high therapeutic ratio (ben-

efit-risk) is careful attention to dosage unimportant. The practice of increasing drug dosage until toxic manifestations appear and then decreasing the dose slightly is feasible for some drugs but it can be uncomfortable or occasionally hazardous.[2]

Pharmacokinetic and Pharmacodynamic Principles Important in Adjusting Dose. Since most drugs have a narrow therapeutic ratio (and since drug levels are usually not available), it is important for the clinician to adjust the "standard" dosage for each individual patient according to his assessment of several *pharmacokinetic processes*, which may be operative to either increase or decrease drug concentrations at receptor sites, and other *pharmacodynamic processes*, which can modify receptor response for a given drug concentration at the site of action (Fig. 48–1). *Concentration* of drug at the target site is primarily governed by the *pharmacokinetic* processes of absorption, distribution, metabolism, and excretion. Both genetic and environmental factors can alter these pharmacokinetic processes, but one can usually anticipate significant deviations from the norm in an individual patient and modify the "standard" dosage accordingly. These pharmacokinetic processes and the factors that influence them are discussed in more detail below.

For a given drug concentration at the receptor site, the *intensity* of the pharmacologic effects can further show additional variability owing to other influences on drug *pharmacodynamics* (Fig. 48–1). These include the less easily quantifiable factors such as functional changes in receptor activity, disease-induced changes in end-organ physiology, development of tolerance with chronic drug exposure, competition for binding at receptors by interacting drugs, and so forth. Thus, the pharmacodynamic effects of a drug are influenced both by pharmacokinetic processes (absorption, distribution, metabolism, and excretion) and by changes in target organs and receptor sites, all of which summate in the individual patient and determine his optimal dose. The following discussion examines these various processes in more detail with specific applications to rheumatologic drugs cited.

717

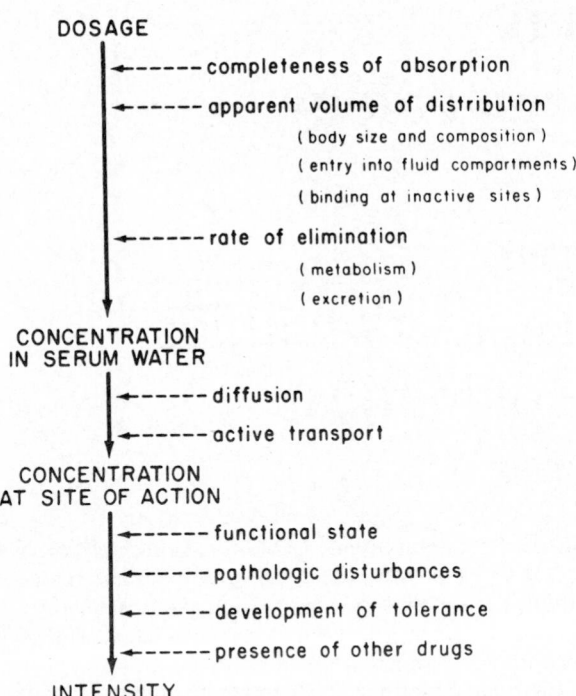

Figure 48–1. Factors that influence pharmacologic response to a drug. (Reprinted, with permission, from Koch-Weser, J.: N. Engl. J. Med. 287:227, 1972.)

EFFECTS OF IONIZATION ON DRUG BEHAVIOR

Most drugs used in clinical practice are either weak acids or weak bases.[3] They exist in an equilibrium of ionized and un-ionized forms, varying according to the pH of the biological fluid or tissue (Fig. 48–2). Small fluctuations in intracellular or plasma pH can produce significant shifts in the proportion of polar (ionized) or nonpolar (nonionized) drug. Since the polar and non-polar forms of a drug have different pharmacokinetic properties, some understanding of how ionization influences drug behavior is essential to enlightened therapeutics. Ionized (polar) drug passively diffuses across

STATE OF IONIZATION

	Acid (low pH) Medium	Alkaline (high pH) Medium
Weak acid drug	R–COOH	R–COO^{-} + H
Weak basic drug	R–NH$_3^{+}$	R–NH$_2$

Figure 48–2. Influence of pH on ionization (polarity) of drugs that are either weak acids or bases. (From Robinson, D.S.: J. Urol. 113:300, 1975. Copyright 1975, The Williams & Wilkins Company, Baltimore.)

Table 48–1. Commonly Prescribed Acidic and Basic Drugs and Drug Classes

Acidic Drugs	Basic Drugs
Salicylates, indomethacin, phenylbutazone, oxyphenbutazone, and the other nonsteroidal anti-inflammatory agents	Opiates (e.g., codeine)
	Major and minor tranquilizers
	Antidepressants
	Anti-arrhythmics:
Probenecid	Lidocaine
Anticoagulants	Procainamide
Sulfonamides and their derivatives:	Quinidine
Thiazide and loop diuretics	Amphetamines
Sulfonylurea hypoglycemic agents	Antihistamines
	Guanethidine
Phenytoin (Dilantin)	Reserpine
Penicillins and cephalosporins	Erythromycin
Barbiturates	Beta-adrenergic blocking agents
Clofibrate	
Methotrexate	Anticholinergic agents

lipid-rich cell membranes poorly, if at all, while nonpolar drug crosses such barriers relatively easily. Thus, drug in the ionized state is absorbed slowly, while nonionized drug is more readily absorbed from the gastrointestinal tract. Similarly, following glomerular filtration, drug in ionized form is less readily reabsorbed in the renal tubule with more rapid excretion.

Drug ionization also predisposes to certain drug interactions. For example, the ionic species of acidic drugs may compete for shared plasma protein–binding sites or for active transport processes in the kidney or central nervous system, resulting in clinically significant drug interactions.

Clinicians should be familiar with the acidic or basic nature of the drugs they use in practice, since such knowledge permits prediction of drug behavior and drug interactions (and therefore avoidance of many troublesome drug effects). Table 48–1 lists the more common drugs and drug classes as to their acidic or basic properties. It is readily apparent that many of the therapeutic agents employed in rheumatology are acidic with similar, and often competing, actions. Examples of the clinical significance of drug ionization in therapeutics are discussed subsequently.

DRUG ABSORPTION

A number of variables can influence either the rate of absorption or the amount of a dose that is absorbed after oral administration. Drug bioavailability can vary among manufacturers and among lots of the same manufacturer, depending on factors such as size of drug crystals, amount of compression, and hardness of coating substances used in a tablet. The *rate* of absorption of drug products can be quite variable, since the process of absorption must be preceded by the drug going into *solution* (in the stomach or small bowel), not just the tablet or capsule disintegrating. While much is made of this issue in advertising of analgesics, the absorption *rate* usually has little relevance in long-term drug treatment, in which steady state levels rather than intermittent peak levels of drug are important.

Because of the acidic nature of aspirin and the nonsteroidal anti-inflammatory agents, drugs of this class tend to be nonionized in the stomach (Fig. 48–2), so that some drug absorption can take place at the low pH present in the stomach, once it goes into solution. Salicylates tend to be less soluble at low pH so that the buffered forms of aspirin solubilize more readily in the stomach and may be absorbed more rapidly. Salicylate is often prescribed in an enteric-coated form to reduce the local gastric irritation caused by slowly dissolving tablets. Since rate of absorption is much less a consideration in the anti-inflammatory use of salicylate, many clinicians prescribe enteric-coated aspirin. In this instance, the remnants of enteric coatings may be detected in the stool, but most of the salicylate contents have usually been absorbed. Other studies have shown twice-a-day dosage forms of salicylate to be therapeutically equivalent to plain aspirin and other anti-inflammatory agents, with resultant improved compliance and lower incidence of side effects.[4-6]

DRUG DISTRIBUTION, PLASMA LEVELS, AND DRUG BINDING INTERACTIONS

Concurrent with absorption and entry into the plasma, drugs also undergo distribution, metabolism, and excretion. For most drugs, the absorption and distribution phases are short in comparison with metabolism and excretion. The clinical relevance of absorption, distribution, and elimination half-lives ($T^{1}/_{2}$) and their implications in regulating drug treatment is further discussed under Pharmacokinetics and Drug Dosing Strategies.

Plasma Protein Binding and Competition of Acidic Drugs for Binding Sites. Many drugs are bound in plasma to proteins, and this bound fraction serves as an inactive "reservoir" of drug. Many of the acidic drugs listed in Table 48–1 are significantly ionized in the slightly alkaline environment (pH 7.4) of plasma; i.e., they will exist largely in their anionic form. This accounts for the general tendency of acidic drugs to bind to sites on plasma albumin. Only the free (unbound) fraction of drug is in equilibrium with drug in other tissue compartments. Therefore, conditions that favor an increase in free drug fraction may be expected to potentiate drug effect. The concurrent administration of two acidic drugs (whose negatively charged anionic forms are both present in plasma) can result in competition for protein binding sites. This can increase the free fraction of one or both drugs, thereby potentiating their pharmacologic effects. Although the clinical importance of this type of interaction may be minor for many acidic drugs, including the nonsteroidal anti-inflammatory agents, it can be very significant in the case of certain drugs with very narrow therapeutic ratios.

Thus, phenylbutazone and oxyphenbutazone and salicylates markedly potentiate the anticoagulant effect when they are administered to a patient receiving warfarin. Similarly they enhance the hypoglycemic effects of the sulfonylurea antidiabetic agents (e.g., tolbutamide, chlorpropamide). As shown in Table 48–1, many anti-inflammatory drugs are acidic and are thus theoretically prone to this type of interaction.

Since phenylbutazone and oxyphenbutazone are highly bound to plasma protein (99 percent), they are especially susceptible to the drug displacement type of interaction. The high affinity of these two drugs for protein-binding sites also accounts for their long half-lives in plasma (around 3 days).

In a classic example of this particular interaction with the anticoagulant warfarin, a patient received phenylbutazone therapy for 1 day for relief of gouty symptoms, and the following day was started on warfarin therapy. Despite the use of a "standard" dose of warfarin, the patient manifested an excessive anticoagulant response, because the major part of the phenylbutazone administered the preceding day remained in the body bound to plasma and tissue proteins, competing with warfarin. The marked increase in the free fraction of warfarin produced an excessive anticoagulant response to an ordinarily usual dose of anticoagulant.[3]

Although it has been estimated that up to 30 percent of rheumatoid patients receive more than one nonsteroidal anti-inflammatory agent concurrently, documented pharmacokinetic interactions of clinical significance are few.[7] Protein binding of anionic drugs is complex, with nine affinity sites shown for indomethacin binding to serum albumin.[8] Furthermore, salicylates failed to affect this high degree of indomethacin binding.

Protein Binding and Drug Plasma Levels. Interacting drugs displacing one another from protein binding sites also can complicate the proper interpretation of plasma drug levels. The drug concentrations reported by clinical laboratories represent total drug content (both free and bound drug) in plasma. When the normal degree of drug binding is altered for any reason (e.g., interacting drug, renal disease, hypoalbuminemia), the reporting of total drug concentration in plasma can be misleading. Many chronic diseases are associated with lowered plasma albumin, and chronic renal insufficiency can result in both hypoalbuminemia and altered drug binding properties of albumin. Since drug levels reported by the laboratory do not distinguish between free and bound drug, care must be taken in interpreting such data in these settings (Fig. 48–3). A patient may be toxic at a "normal" dose and with a "normal" blood level because the percentage of unbound drug is increased even though the *total* drug content in plasma is within the normal range (frequent examples are salicylate or diphenylhydantoin toxicity encountered in renal failure or pregnancy). Anti-inflammatory doses of aspirin have been shown to produce a 25 percent decline in phenytoin levels.[9] Thus, proper interpretation of blood levels requires a knowledge of the total clinical picture, including associated drugs and disease-induced changes in pharmacokinetics.

Figure 48–3. Effect of drug displacement interaction on plasma drug level. The unbound drug fraction (cross-hatched column) is initially increased by a second competing drug. After equilibration occurs, the unbound drug fraction returns to the original concentration and the level of total drug (free and bound) is decreased due to a decline in the bound fraction (open column).

DRUG BIOTRANSFORMATION

Drug metabolism is largely a function of the liver, although for certain drugs there may be significant extrahepatic metabolism by intestinal mucosa (phenothiazines) or kidney (several drugs). Hepatic drug metabolism can be characterized as the general process of converting less polar compounds to more polar drug metabolites. These drug metabolites may be pharmacologically active or inactive. Because of their increased tendency to ionize, the increased polarity of metabolites usually promotes more rapid excretion in urine or bile and resultant shorter $T_{1/2}$'s than the parent drug. There are a few glaring exceptions to this general rule. For example, active metabolites of diazepam, chlordiazepoxide, and most other benzodiazepines, which are nonpolar and highly lipid soluble, accumulate in brain and other lipid-rich tissues to a greater extent than the parent compounds, and, being pharmacologically active, account for the gradually cumulative and prolonged clinical effects of these drugs.

First Order vs. Zero Order Kinetics. The major metabolic pathways of drug biotransformation are not generally saturated at usual clinical doses. Therefore, most drugs follow so-called *first order* kinetics, which signifies that a constant *percentage* of drug is metabolized per unit time independent of dosage. As will be discussed under Pharmacokinetics and Drug Dosing Strategies, first order kinetics implies that drug plasma and tissue levels will be linearly related to drug dose. However, for certain drugs (particularly those administered daily in gram quantities, such as the salicylates), the primary metabolic pathway may become saturated so that secondary and less efficient biotransformation pathways may become operative with advancing dosage. This results in so-called *zero order* kinetics, in which a constant *amount* rather than percentage of drug is metabolized

per unit of time. The implication of zero order kinetics is that the relationship between dosage and drug level is nonlinear, so that disproportionately high drug concentrations are produced by small increases in drug dose. Commonly used drugs that exhibit zero order kinetics include the salicylates, heparin, and diphenylhydantoin. In the case of all three of these drugs, it is fortunate that laboratory monitoring of drug concentration or effect allows the drugs to be administered in adequate therapeutic dosage, often approaching toxic levels, with reasonable precision and safety.

Drug Interactions that Inhibit Hepatic Drug Metabolism. Drug interactions involving hepatic metabolism may either inhibit or enhance the biotransformation of a second drug. Inhibition may produce unexpected toxicity when a second drug inhibiting metabolism is added to a patient's therapeutic regimen. For example, the potent xanthine oxidase inhibitor allopurinol is now known to weakly inhibit other drug oxidation metabolic pathways. Thus, mercaptopurine, azathioprine, and allopurinol should be used with caution in patients receiving warfarin because it can nonspecifically inhibit liver microsomal enzymes, the major pathway for warfarin degradation. The concurrent administration of allopurinol and warfarin is not recommended unless special precautions are taken for intensive monitoring of prothrombin times. It is possible, although not conclusively established at present, that allopurinol may inhibit the liver metabolism of other drugs such as the sulfonylurea hypoglycemic agents.

As mentioned previously, salicylates in the doses used for anti-inflammatory effect can saturate primary pathways of drug metabolism. Although the full clinical significance of this problem has not yet been established, there is compelling evidence that highdose salicylate therapy may inhibit not only its own metabolism but also that of a number of other anti-inflammatory agents and analgesics. Salicyluric acid (the glycine conjugate of salicylic acid) formation is inhibited when salicylate and salicylamide are co-administered.[10] Salicylamide also decreases the formation of acetaminophen sulfate and, to a lesser extent, acetaminophen glucuronide.

The first indication that saturation effects may be encountered with even relatively small doses of drugs was the observation that the rate of formation of salicyluric acid does not increase proportionally with dose when the daily amount of salicylate exceeds 300 to 500 mg in healthy adults. The elimination $T_{1/2}$ of salicylate increases from 3 to more than 20 hours as dosage increases; the elimination of the larger doses are not according to first order kinetics, and the *fraction* eliminated as salicylurate *decreases* with increasing dose. The rate of salicylurate formation becomes essentially independent of the amount of salicylate in the body when that amount exceeds about 15 mg per kilogram.[10] Secondary pathways of salicylate metabolism then come into play at higher doses.

These examples of potential drug interactions are of interest because often these drugs are unwittingly taken in combination as nonprescription over-the-counter products. Further investigation is required to establish the true clinical significance of these potentially troublesome interactions resulting in salicylism or, in the case of acetaminophen, possible low-grade liver toxicity.

Another example of drug interaction of this type is the effect of hydrocortisone in competitively inhibiting oxidation of such drugs as ethylmorphine and hexabarbital and in prolonging the $T^{1/2}$ of nortriptyline.[11] Conversely, it has also been established that drugs such as phenobarbital and diphenylhydantoin can accelerate the metabolism of cortisol and dexamethasone (see below), thereby decreasing steroid effect.[11]

The antiulcer drug cimetidine significantly impairs the metabolism of many other drugs, including warfarin, theophylline, phenytoin, diazepam, and propranolol.[12] The mechanism of h_2-blocker inhibition of hepatic drug metabolism may involve both direct microsomal enzyme impairment and altered liver blood flow. The possibility of significant interaction with salicylates and other antiinflammatory agents that can cause gastrointestinal ulceration should be kept in mind and requires further investigation.

Liver Microsomal Enzyme Induction. Phenylbutazone, like phenobarbital and diphenylhydantoin, is a potent inducer of liver microsomal enzymes and over a few days of administration can thereby stimulate the metabolism of a second drug that is primarily metabolized by microsomal enzymes. While the acute effect of phenylbutazone may be to enhance the action of other acidic drugs (by competition for plasma protein binding), its long-term administration may result in significant induction of metabolism of other drugs. Thus, it is obvious that the potential drug interactions of phenylbutazone are complex, encompassing the pharmacokinetic processes of distribution, metabolism and, as we will see later, excretion. Phenylbutazone stimulates steroid metabolism, shortening the $T^{1/2}$ of prednisolone and cortisol, but potentiates the acute toxicity of the anticoagulant warfarin and the oral hypoglycemic agents (probably by both displacing drugs from protein-binding sites and perhaps acutely inhibiting their liver metabolism). The best policy to adopt for phenylbutazone is to reserve it for short-term episodic use and to anticipate significant interactions with a large number of drugs. It should never be prescribed with warfarin or the sulfonylurea hypoglycemic agents.

RENAL FUNCTION AND DRUG PHARMACOKINETICS

Drug Excretion. Renal excretion constitutes a major elimination pathway for many drugs and their metabolites. The mechanism can be either by passive glomerular filtration (with varying amounts of tubular reabsorption) or by active secretion by the proximal tubule. Irrespective of the method of drug excretion, some fraction of drug may be reabsorbed as it traverses the nephron, depending on the degree of drug polarity in the tubular fluid. Thus, small shifts in urine pH may sig-

Figure 48–4. Renal mechanisms for glomerular filtration (passive), proximal tubular secretion (active), and tubular reabsorption (passive or active) of drugs. (From Robinson, D.S.: J. Urol. 113:100, 1975. Copyright 1975, The Williams & Wilkins Company, Baltimore.)

nificantly enhance or retard passive drug reabsortion of the nonpolar drug fraction in the nephron (Fig. 48–4).

The factors that influence the amount of drug appearing passively in the glomerular filtrate are the fraction of free (unbound) drug for plasma protein–bound drugs, and the size of the drug molecule. As shown in Fig. 48–4, there are two active transport processes for drug secretion in the proximal tubule, one shared by organic acids and one by organic bases. Acidic or basic drugs may be actively secreted by one of these routes and, as in the example of penicillin and probenecid, can compete with each other for this active transport secretory process. By so doing, probenecid markedly prolongs the elimination $T^{1/2}$ of penicillin, an acidic drug which is predominantly excreted via this route rather than metabolized. Other acidic drugs also share this property. Therapeutic doses of phenylbutazone also markedly prolong penicillin $T^{1/2}$, and even modest doses of aspirin increase the elimination time of penicillin through completion for the anionic transport pathway.[13] Salicylate and other acidic drugs can also slow the rate of elimination of another weak acid drug, methotrexate, thereby potentiating its toxic effects on bone marrow and tissues.[14] Another clinically significant example of drug interaction involving that old culprit phenylbutazone is its competition for proximal tubular secretion with hydroxyhexamide, the active metabolite of acetohexamide. This interaction with phenylbutazone has produced marked potentiation of this potent hypoglycemic agent, resulting in dangerous hypoglycemic episodes.[15] The hyperuricemia produced by chronic thiazide diuretic therapy similarly involves, in part, this mechanism of competition for secretory process.

Influence of Urine pH on Drug Excretion. Regardless of whether a drug is filtered or secreted by the kidney, it undergoes varying degrees of reabsorption from the filtrate by nonionic diffusion. The ratio of nonionized to ionized form of the drug will depend on the pH of the urine filtrate and the pKa of the weak acid. The renal tubule cell behaves as a membrane that permits nonionized drug to diffuse across it but prevents ionic species of the drug from undergoing reabsorption (Fig. 48–4). As urine traverses the tubule, it tends to become more concentrated and more acidified and the extent of drug ionization changes. Thus, salicylates, for example, tend to be present in urine mainly in nonionized form, while basic drugs like quinidine and procainamide are largely ionized in this milieu. The nonionic diffusion of salicylate in the renal tubule is obviously greater than for these basic drugs since it is predominantly nonionized at a pH less than 7. It has been shown that the coadministration of therapeutic doses of "nonabsorbable" antacids (e.g., Maalox) can alter the urine acidification process by a small but significant amount. This produces changes in steady state levels of salicylates as a result of the altered urine pH and excretory rate. Thus, salicylate levels in patients receiving chronic aspirin therapy are decreased by magnesium-containing and other antacids.[16] In a crossover study in a normal population, antacid administration decreased steady state salicylate levels from 16.6 to 13.7 mg per dl while raising urine pH only 0.3 units from 5.7 to 6.0[17] The profound effects of urine pH on salicylate elimination is illustrated by the fact that subjects with very acid urine excrete only 2 to 3 percent of a dose of aspirin as the unchanged drug (with the balance metabolized), while subjects with alkaline urine excrete approximately 25 percent of a dose and metabolize 75 percent.[18]

Impaired Renal Function and Anti-inflammatory Drugs. The contribution of renal mechanisms to the elimination of salicylates has been emphasized. However, other agents important in the practice of rheumatology which are also eliminated primarily by renal excretion include oxipurinol, colchicine, corticosteroids, and probably the gold salts.[19,20] In patients with end-stage renal disease, these drugs require extensive reduction in dose when treating coexisting gout or arthritis.[21] The use of drugs such as ibuprofen and probenecid in severe renal failure has not been as extensively studied, so guidelines regarding dosage adjustments are not well established.

PHARMACOKINETICS AND DRUG DOSING STRATEGIES

Most drugs are administered at intervals shorter than their elimination T½, so that with chronic administration accumulation in plasma and tissue occurs until equilibrium is reached. Steady-state plateau levels of drug are achieved when the amount of drug administered in one dose equals the amount of drug eliminated (by either metabolism or excretion) during that dosing interval.

First Order Elimination Kinetics and Steady-State Drug Levels. Most drugs are eliminated according to exponential kinetics, such that a *constant fraction of drug present* is eliminated per unit time (first order kinetics). This means that the elimination kinetics of drug is independent of dose, and therefore the elimination T½ remains constant irrespective of dosage. A simple calculation shows that any drug following first order kinetics is virtually completely eliminated (greater than 95 percent) from the body in 4 to 5 T½'s.[22,23]

Also, when a drug is given over a long term, it *accumulates* according to an exponential curve and achieves a plateau concentration with an "accumulation" half-time equal to its elimination T½ (Fig. 48–5). Thus for most drugs (those which follow first order kinetics), plateau values are achieved independent of the administered dose within 4 to 5 T½'s after initiating therapy. The *time* to reach steady-state levels depends solely on the elimination T½ and is constant for a given individual. The *concentration* of drug achieved at plateau, however, depends on both the size of the dose and the elimination T½ for that individual.

When the dose of a drug is changed in a patient receiving long-term therapy, the time to achieve a new

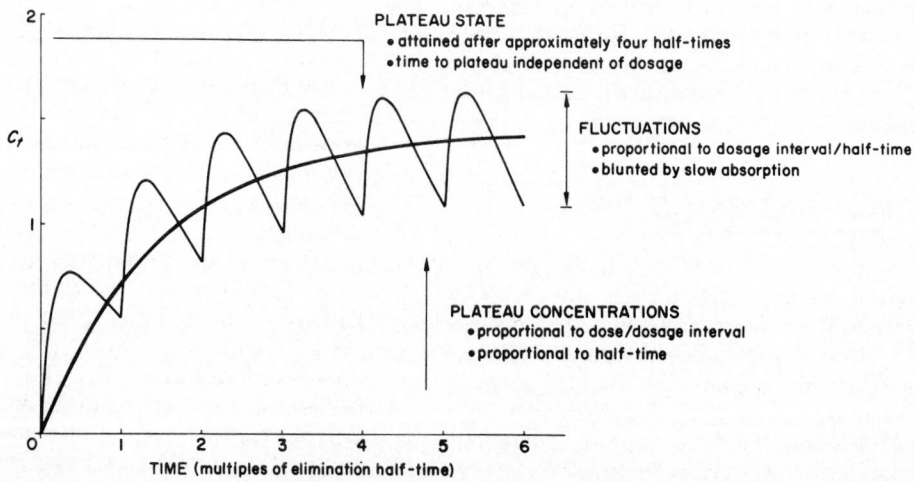

Figure 48–5. Drug accumulation during repeated administration of a drug at intervals equal to its elimination half-time (T½). (From Mayer, S.E., Melmon, K.L., and Gilman, A.G.: *In* Goodman, L.S., and Gilman, A. (eds.): The Pharmacological Basis of Therapeutics, 6th ed. New York, Macmillan, 1980.)

steady-state drug level is also 4 to 5 T½'s from the time of the change.[22,24] It is important for the physician to have a general understanding of the pharmacokinetics of drugs he prescribes, particularly their modes of elimination and elimination T½'s, since a rational plan for initiating therapy and for monitoring the patient until steady state is achieved depends on knowledge of such drug properties.[22]

Thus, anti-inflammatory drugs with long T½'s, such as phenylbutazone, oxyphenbutazone, probenecid, and high dose salicylate may require days to weeks of drug accumulation before plateau levels are achieved in many patients. This has obvious implications regarding development of toxicity or likelihood of drug interactions, and patients treated with these agents should be carefully monitored until this process of drug accumulation is complete.

Zero Order Elimination Kinetics and Steady-State Drug Levels. As previously mentioned, certain drugs (the notable examples being salicylates, heparin, and diphenylhydantoin) undergo elimination via saturable metabolic processes so that at higher doses given chronically a constant *amount* of drug is eliminated per unit of time rather than a constant *fraction* of drug. The resulting zero order kinetics produces a highly dose-dependent elimination T½. In this situation, the time taken to achieve plateau levels of drug becomes increasingly longer with each increment in dosage because of the longer elimination T½, and disproportionately higher final concentrations of drug in plasma and tissue result. As human pharmacology is better studied and understood, we can identify more and more drugs whose metabolism converts from first order to zero order at high doses. Such drugs, especially those with low therapeutic ratios, must be carefully monitored both during initiation of therapy and following any dosage increase. Obviously, plasma levels of a drug, if they are available, can be helpful in this situation. Since salicylates are the only anti-inflammatory agents for which routine plasma levels are of proved value, careful *clinical* observation of the patient for therapeutic and toxic effects is crucial for most drugs during the induction of therapy and until the response to drug is stabilized.

Zero Order Absorption Kinetics and Steady-State Drug Levels. One of the primary goals of effective therapy with anti-inflammatory agents is to reduce fluctuations in blood and tissue drug levels associated with absorption peaks and valleys. Many nonsteroidal anti-inflammatory agents have elimination half-lives of less than 8 hours, so that steady-state levels with chronic administration tend to vary excessively during each dosing interval. This is a factor in the case of several drugs, including aspirin, indomethacin, ibuprofen, and tolmetin, resulting in fluctuating efficacy, side effects, and erratic pain relief.

Recent innovations in drug delivery design have corrected this "sawtooth" effect by making the absorption half-life of a drug much longer than its elimination half-life. The latter ordinarily is the controlling factor governing steady-state levels and duration of drug effect. The recent introduction of a new precision-release oral dosage form of indomethacin has remedied many of the drawbacks of fluctuating drug levels with this agent.[25] Osmotically driven, controlled-release dosage forms of indomethacin can deliver a constant rate of 7 mg per hour and maintain a therapeutic level over a release time of 10 to 12 hours after oral administration.[26] The plasma drug levels achieved with this constant delivery oral dosage form are predictable, since the release of drug into the gut can be precisely controlled.[27] Thus, steady-state levels become dependent on rate of drug delivery rather than rate of drug biotransformation. This has proved to be a unique and useful advance in the area of pharmaceutics for short half-life drugs that do not undergo extensive first-pass metabolism.

How to Use Plasma Drug Levels. Plasma levels are helpful and of established value for such commonly used drugs as digitalis, anticonvulsants, antiarrhythmics, salicylate, theophylline, and lithium. Of these, the anticonvulsant drug diphenylhydantoin, like salicylate, also follows zero order kinetics, underscoring the value of drug level monitoring during therapy and when potential interacting drugs such as the sulfonylureas, diphenylhydantoin, phenylbutazone, or high-dose salicylates are coadministered.

Once the decision has been made to use drug levels in dosing strategy, the following guidelines are important:

1. Choose a target serum level, keeping in mind the factors that can modify individual response to a particular level (protein binding, hypoalbuminemia, development of tolerance, metabolic derangements such as uremia or acidosis [Fig. 48–1]).

2. In selecting an initial dose for rheumatologic agents, loading doses are usually not employed, since this is generally reserved for therapeutic emergencies in which full therapeutic effects without waiting are essential. For most situations, a maintenance dose is selected, taking care to make adjustments in the dose based on suspected impairment of the drug's major mode of elimination. For example, downward adjustment would be indicated in the presence of significant renal insufficiency for allopurinol in renal insufficiency.[11]

3. Ordinarily, wait until steady state levels have been reached (4 to 5 half-lives) before drawing a plasma level. If intervening toxicity is suspected before plateau is reached, a drug level is indicated at that time.

4. If necessary, adjust the next dose according to the following formula: New dose/old dose = desired level/measured level. This formula would *not* apply to drugs with zero order kinetics. For these drugs, smaller dose increments should be used.

Problems in the Correct Interpretation of Drug Levels. Drug levels should never be a substitute for careful observation and sound clinical judgment, which always take precedence when conflicting data are obtained. Several factors must be considered in the interpretation of blood levels. The ultimate effect at the receptor site of a given drug concentration may be altered by both pharmacokinetic and pharmacodynamic factors (Fig. 48–1). Obviously, a digoxin level in the "therapeutic range" can be a toxic level for a particular patient with altered receptor response resulting from hypokalemia, hypercalcemia, hypomagnesemia, acidosis, or hypoxia. The time elapsed since the last administered dose must be precisely known, especially to avoid absorption and redistribution artifacts in plasma levels, and to properly interpret rapidly fluctuating levels in the case of drugs with relatively short $T\frac{1}{2}$'s (e.g., procainamide, quinidine, propranolol).

For drugs that are highly protein bound, it is important to know the serum albumin level and state of renal function. For example, a patient with an albumin of 1.3 and a salicylate level of 25 mg per 100 ml (therapeutic range 25 to 30 mg percent) would probably be in the toxic range, since salicylate is normally 70 to 90 percent protein bound. In this setting, the free (unbound) fraction of salicylate may be excessively high, and toxicity might intervene in spite of a "normal" plasma level. Increased free drug fractions (percent) have been observed in renal disease for several drugs, including salicylates, diphenylhydantoin, and a number of cardiac agents. The mechanism for this may involve either plasma accumulation of acidic substances or altered plasma protein binding characteristics secondary to uremia.[21] Patients with chronic illnesses (associated with hypoalbuminemia) usually require redefinition of therapeutic ranges for these drugs as well.

Finally, some drugs have active metabolites with $T\frac{1}{2}$'s significantly different from the parent compound, and an unmeasured metabolite may exhibit more accumulation than the parent drug (benzodiazepines, allopurinol, procainamide, tricyclic antidepressants). A drug level (if available) would underestimate the combined therapeutic or toxic effects of the parent compound and its active metabolite(s). This predicament does not presently apply to any rheumatologic agents for which routine blood levels are available (salicylates, acetaminophen) as far as is known. However, as mentioned above, the active metabolite of allopurinol, oxipurinol, has a significantly longer $T\frac{1}{2}$ (mean 28 hours) compared to the parent drug (mean 2 to 4 hours). The net pharmacologic and therapeutic effects of long-term allopurinol administration are largely due to the metabolite oxipurinol, because it reaches high steady state levels in comparison to the parent drug, especially in the patient with renal insufficiency in whom the $T\frac{1}{2}$ is apt to be markedly prolonged.

References

1. Koch-Weser, J., Sidel, V.W., Sweet, R.H., Kanarek, P., and Eaton, A.E.: Factors determining physician reporting of adverse drug reactions: Comparison of 2000 spontaneous reports with surveillance studies at the Massachusetts General Hospital. N. Engl. J. Med. 280:20, 1969.
2. Koch-Weser, J.: Serum drug concentrations as therapeutic guides. N. Engl. J. Med. 287:227, 1972.
3. Robinson, D.S.: The application of basic principles of drug interaction to clinical practice. J. Urol. 113:100, 1975.
4. Biechman, W.J., and Lechner, B.L.: Clinical comparative evaluation of choline magnesium trisalicylate and acetylsalicylic acid in rheumatoid arthritis. Rheumatology and Rehabilitation 18:119, 1979.
5. Ehrlich, G.E., Miller, S.B., and Zeiders, R.S.: Choline magnesium trisalicylate versus ibuprofen in rheumatoid arthritis. Rheumatology and Rehabilitation 19:30, 1980.
6. Guliano, V., and Scharff, E.V.: Clinical comparison of two salicylates in rheumatoid arthritis patients on maintenance gold therapy. Curr. Therap. Res. 28:61, 1980.
7. Miller, D.R.: Combination use of nonsteroidal anti-inflammatory drugs. Drug Intelligence and Clin. Pharmacy 15:3, 1981.
8. Zini, R., D'Athis, P., Barre, J., and Tillement, J.P.: Binding of indomethacin to human serum albumen. Its displacement by various agents, influence of free fatty acids and the unexpected effect of indomethacin on warfarin binding. Biochem. Pharmacol. 28:2661, 1979.
9. Leonard, R.F., Knott, P.J., Rankin, G.O., Robinson, D.S., and Melnick, D.E.: Phenytoin-salicylate interaction. Clin. Pharmacol. Therap. 29:56, 1981.
10. Levy, G.: Drug biotransformation interactions in man: Nonnarcotic analgesics. In Vesell, E.S. (ed.): Drug Metabolism in Man. New York, New York Academy of Science, Vol. 179, 1971.
11. Dujovne, C.A., and Azarnoff, D.L.: Clinical complications of corticosteroid therapy: A selected review. In Azarnoff, D.L. (ed.): Steroid Therapy. Philadelphia, W. B. Saunders Company, 1975.
12. Sriwatanakul, K., and Mehta, G.: Clinically significant drug interactions. Rational Drug Therapy 17:1, 1983.
13. Kampmann, J., Hansen, J.M., Siersboek-Nielsen, K., and Laursen, H.: Effect of some drugs on penicillin half-life in blood. Clin. Pharmacol. Ther. 13:516, 1972.
14. Liegler, D.G., Henderson, E.S., Hahn, M.A., and Oliverio, V.T.: The effect of organic acids on renal clearance of methotrexate in man. Clin. Pharmacol. Ther. 10:849, 1969.
15. Field, J.B., Ohta, M., Boyle, C., and Remer, A.: Potentiation of acetohexamide hypoglycemia by phenylbutazone. N. Engl. J. Med. 277:889, 1967.
16. Levy, G., Lampman, T., Kamath, B.L., and Garrettson, L.K.: Decreased serum salicylate concentrations in children with rheumatic fever treated with antacid. N. Engl. J. Med. 293:323, 1975.
17. Hansten, P.D., and Hayton, W.L.: Effect of antacid and ascorbic acid on serum salicylate concentrations. J. Clin. Pharmacol. 20:326, 1980.
18. Hollister, L., and Levy, G.: Some aspects of salicylate distribution and metabolism in man. J. Pharm. Sci. 54:1126, 1965.
19. Bennett, W.M., Singer, I., Golpher, T., Feig, P., and Coggins, C.J.: Guidelines for drug therapy in renal failure. Ann. Intern. Med. 86:754, 1977.
20. Hansten, P.D. (ed.): Drug Interactions. 3rd ed. Philadelphia, Lea & Febiger, 1976.
21. Reidenberg, M.M. (ed.): Renal Function and Drug Action. Philadelphia, W. B. Saunders Company, 1971.
22. Robinson, D.S.: Pharmacokinetic mechanisms of drug interaction. Postgrad. Med. 57:55, 1975.
23. Fengl, E., and Woodbury, D.M.: General principles. In Goodman, L.S., and Gilman, A. (ed.): The Pharmacological Basis of Therapeutics. 5th ed. New York, Macmillan, 1975.
24. Rowland, M.: Drug administration and regimens. In Melmon, K.L., and Morrelli, H.F. (eds.): Clinical Pharmacology: Basic Principles in Therapeutics. 2nd ed. New York, Macmillan, 1978.
25. Robinson, D.S.: Pharmacokinetics and pharmacodynamics of drug delivery. Curr. Med. Res. Opinion 8(suppl. 2):10, 1983.
26. Bayne, W., Place, V., Theeuwes, F., Rogers, J.D., Lee, R.B., Davies, R.O., and Kwan, K.C.: Kinetics of osmotically controlled indomethacin delivery systems after repeated dosing. Clin. Pharmacol. Therap. 32:270, 1982.
27. Heimlich, K.R.: The evolution of precision drug delivery. Curr. Med. Res. Opinion 8(suppl. 2):28, 1983.

Chapter 49

Aspirin and Salicylate

Paul H. Plotz

INTRODUCTION

The salicylates have a recorded history of over two millennia of continuous medicinal use[1] in treating fever, and over a century in treating rheumatism. Only when they were synthesized commercially in 1874, however, did their modern pharmacologic history begin. Aspirin was introduced widely in 1899 and first used in the United States in that year,[2] but the salicylates were only slowly accepted as efficacious therapy in rheumatoid arthritis.[3] Today salicylates are available in hundreds of forms,[4] and the annual consumption of pills is measured in the billions. Never more than today, there is vigorous research on the action and toxicity of the salicylates, stimulated by the seminal discovery that they inhibit prostaglandin synthetase,[5] and by a desire to rescue them from threatened oblivion by perfecting them.

STRUCTURE, ABSORPTION, AND METABOLISM*

Salicylic acid is the common name for 2-hydroxybenzoic acid, and aspirin was originally a trade name but is now the common name for the salicylate ester of acetic acid (Fig. 49–1). Both are white powders relatively insoluble in aqueous solutions. Their sodium salts are more soluble, particularly in a slightly alkaline solution. The ionization constant, pKa, for the carboxyl hydrogen is

---

*This subject is well reviewed in Reference 6.

Figure 49–1. The chemical structure of the principal salicylates.

3.5 for aspirin and 3.0 for salicylic acid. Consequently, in the highly acid stomach both will be un-ionized, and in the body fluids, both will be largely ionized, though aspirin slightly less so. Because it is probable that the un-ionized rather than the ionized form of both drugs diffuses across cell membranes, it is worth remembering that, even far from the pKa, changes in pH can have marked changes in the proportion of drug that is ionized.[6]

When uncoated aspirin or salicylate tablets are placed in an aqueous solution, they visibly disintegrate with a speed that depends largely on various factors in their manufacture but in all events faster than the active drug goes into solution. The dissolution rate, too, is controlled by factors in tablet manufacture and plays a role in the subsequent fate of both aspirin and salicylate, since once dissolved, the drug is absorbed very rapidly.[6] Generally aspirin or salicylate taken as a solution (for example, effervescent buffered aspirin) or in an easily soluble form such as sodium aspirin is more rapidly absorbed than standard aspirin.[7-9] Buffering may also accelerate dissolution.[10,11] The drugs are available in many guises, none demonstrably better than the others for treating connective tissue diseases.

Acid in the stomach may cause the un-ionized form of the drug to form and precipitate, or the drug may remain in supersaturated solution,[7] but relatively little is known of the physical state of aspirin or salicylate in either the secreting or the nonsecreting stomach. Studies on the state of the drug in the overnight fasted stomach from which secretions have been aspirated may bear little relation to its state in a subject who eats and drinks and takes drug in irregular relation to food. Early observations of particles of aspirin in the stomach wall of patients who ingested drug just prior to gastrectomy have so many possibilities for artifact that they cannot be taken as having generality.[12] When awake subjects are gastroscoped after taking aspirin, such particles are not usually visible.

Aspirin and salicylate are absorbed to a certain extent by the gastric mucosa,[13-15] and it is likely that the low pH of the stomach contents, by causing the drugs to be un-ionized, facilitates absorption.[16,17] Nevertheless, they can be absorbed from the neutralized stomach at a considerable rate.[18] Both drugs become ionized as they pass into the small intestine, because the pH is near neutrality. While this enhances solubility, it obviously diminishes the amount of un-ionized drug. Since the drugs are well absorbed from the intestine, either the ionized form is absorbed or the effective pH in the unstirred layer near the wall is much lower, thus allowing the proportion of un-ionized drug to rise,[16] or the enormous surface allows the rapid absorption of any un-ionized drug so that the drugs are continually pushed toward the un-ionized form. Although aspirin can spontaneously hydrolyze to acetate and salicylate in aqueous solution, the rate of spontaneous hydrolysis is low enough so that little or no free salicylate is found in the intestine; it is absorbed as aspirin, not as salicylate.[7] The current enteric coating of cellulose acetate phthalate is stable to acid but dissolves readily above pH 6 in the small intestine.

Aspirin is the dominant form of the drug in plasma within the first 10 to 20 minutes after ingestion;[7,20,21] it can be detected for several minutes before there is any measurable salicylate,[22] and it even appears in joint fluid before salicylate. But it disappears very fast (T½ 15 minutes), and consequently the blood level of aspirin is quite sensitive to the rate of absorption.[6] Consequently, serum aspirin levels are lower with a sustained-release form than with plain or heavily buffered aspirins.[23]

Aspirin disappears by deacetylating to salicylate by one of three routes. It spontaneously deacetylates in plasma as it will in vitro in aqueous solution. It acetylates proteins, of which prostaglandin synthetase is the most notable example[24] but by no means the only one. Both hemoglobin[25] and albumin[26] have been shown to be acetylated, and doubtless other proteins and macromolecules are, too, including perhaps some cell surface macromolecules. And it is hydrolyzed enzymatically to salicylate, although it is by no means clear that this enzymatic activity is specific in any way for aspirin.[27] Probably several enzymes in the circulation are involved, including cholinesterase, an esterase that moves electrophoretically with albumin, and an esterase in red blood cells.[28,29] Furthermore, since hepatic venous salicylate exceeds portal venous salicylate after an oral dose of aspirin, the enzymatic hydrolysis probably takes place in the liver, but it has not been localized to a well-characterized enzyme.[7,30]

Aspirin and salicylate are partially bound to serum proteins, mainly albumin.[31] They diffuse into cells and across various membranes into body fluids such as the cerebrospinal fluid[33] and synovial fluid,[22] and they freely cross the placenta[31] and are secreted into breast milk.[32] The diffusion is fairly rapid, and joint fluid levels, although never so high as serum levels, do reach 60 to 75 percent of serum levels in acute experiments, and drug can be detected there within 20 minutes of ingestion.[22] With increasing dose, the proportion of drug in plasma that is not protein bound increases. Likewise, when plasma albumin is low, as in severe rheumatoid arthritis, less drug is protein bound. Since it is the free drug that diffuses to the site of its action, the pharmacologic and toxic effects of an increment in dose are greater when the dose is already high and when the plasma albumin is low. It is likely that many other factors influence the rates of passage of the drugs across biologic membranes, for example, the proportion of un-ionized drug, which is sensitive to pH, and local protein binding.[34]

Salicylate appears to be metabolized principally if not exclusively by the liver, although formal proof of this is lacking. There are three major and several minor metabolites of the drug, which together satisfactorily account for its fate. They are all excreted into the urine, and drug recovery in the urine after an acute ingestion approaches 100 percent of the ingested drug. The major metabolite is the glycine conjugate, called salicyluric acid, and there are two glucuronide conjugates, one on the phenolic hydroxyl and one on the carboxyl group. At no time do these principal metabolites reach any significant proportion of the circulating salicylate.[35] The metabolites appear to be excreted quantitatively as soon as they reach the kidneys and can be found in the plasma only by sensitive chemical techniques. Their excretion depends on glomerular filtration and tubular secretion, is independent of urine flow or urine pH, and approaches but does not exceed renal plasma flow.[35] The quantitatively minor metabolite, gentisic acid, is important only because it has occasionally been shown to have prostaglandin synthetase-inhibiting properties,[36] but it is highly unlikely that it contributes to the clinical effects of aspirin.

It has long been known that serum levels of salicylate (it is impractical to measure serum levels of aspirin in a clinical setting) bear only the crudest relationship to the dose ingested even when corrected for body size, and that the full effect on serum level of an increase in dose may be reflected only after several days. Most strikingly, a small increment in dose may lead to a profound increment in serum level (for example, in one study the mean serum level was three-fold higher when the dose was 100 mg per kilogram per day than when it was 65 mg per kilogram per day),[37] and marked fluctuations in serum level may be observed without a change in dose. Furthermore, in contrast to aspirin, the plasma half-life of salicylate is many hours and is directly proportional to the serum levels; *the higher the serum level, the slower the disappearance.* The mystery of this erratic behavior has been solved by a number of excellent studies which have shown that the two major determinants of the serum level of salicylate are the urinary pH[38-40] and the activity of the enzyme that synthesizes salicylurate by conjugating glycine to salicylate.[41-44]

Urinary pH variations over the normal range profoundly affect clearance of salicylate by the kidneys. Salicylate is filtered at the glomerulus, and is both reabsorbed and secreted by the tubules. Below pH 6, salicylate clearance is about one tenth of creatinine clearance.[35] Above neutrality, salicylate clearance rises steeply and may reach almost twice the creatinine clearance in a slightly alkaline urine. Consequently, salicylate excretion may change from hour to hour, depending on the quantity and composition of ingested food, exercise, the normal diurnal fluctuations of urinary pH, pulmonary events, and the ingestion of antacids.[45] Because of these factors, and because below pH 6 there is no significant variation of salicylate clearance, metabolic studies are often carried out with concomitant urinary acidification.

The ingestion of antacid not only facilitates absorption by solubilizing drug in the intestines and accelerating gastric emptying; it also facilitates excretion by the kidneys. This property is found with both absorbable and the "nonabsorbable" antacids, which can lower steady-state serum salicylate levels despite a constant salicylate dose by their effect on urinary pH.[40] Likewise, withdrawal of antacids can cause a sudden rise in salicylate levels.

The other major determinant of serum salicylate is the rate of conjugation to glycine. Since the glycine conjugate salicylurate is the major metabolite when salicylate excretion is suppressed by acidification, the serum level is determined principally by the rate of production of salicylurate. In acute metabolic studies it has been found that above a serum level of about 6 mg per deciliter the rate of fall of serum salicylate is constant because there is a constant rate of production of salicylurate independent of the serum level.[37,43] It appears that the extraordinary variation in serum levels among different individuals on a similar dose (serum levels ranged from 4 to 33 mg per deciliter in a group of patients with rheumatoid arthritis who took 50 mg per kilogram per day)[43] reflects variation in the level of the conjugating enzyme rather than in the kinetic parameters of the enzyme. The level of enzyme seems to be at least partially under genetic control; identical twins have very closely matched rates of salicylurate formation, while fraternal twins do not.[44] But the matter is not so simple, since with the continued ingestion of salicylate or aspirin, at least over several days, the level of enzyme rises somewhat.[44] With the chronic ingestion of a sustained release aspirin, the serum salicylate level may drift down after a few days before reaching a steady state. This adjustment may be due to increased salicylate formation, but it is not completely understood, since overall urinary recovery of salicylate metabolites also declines.[46] There may be other determinants of the level of this enzyme too, for example, the ingestion of other drugs. The production of salicylate phenolic glucuronide is also saturable within the clinical dose range,[41] but since it accounts for only about a fifth of excreted metabolites when salicylate excretion is suppressed, variation in its metabolism will have little effect on serum levels. It should be noted that because of the limited capacity of the two major metabolic pathways of salicylate, as the serum level rises the proportion of unconjugated salicylate will rise, and hence the effect of urinary pH on excretion will be more profound.

Although aspirin and salicylate are rapidly absorbed and metabolized, under steady-state chronic ingestion with as many variables as possible removed, the serum salicylate level fluctuates little between doses. With a 4-hour dosing interval, the mean fluctuation is only 1 mg per deciliter, and with an 8-hour interval, 2.5 mg per deciliter, although individual patients may vary by as much as 3 and 6.3 mg per deciliter, respectively.[32] With enteric-coated aspirin, a large dose taken twice a day can lead to a sustained serum salicylate level in the therapeutic range about as efficiently as the same amount taken four times a day, and with as little fluctuation in serum level.[47] The overall kinetic model for the metabolism of single doses of aspirin developed by Levy, Tsuchiya, and Amsel[41] is well substantiated by experimental results.[42]

Aspirin or salicylate can be given topically, intra-articularly, or intravenously, but these routes are either ineffective[48,49] or offer no real advantage.[50] Two new salicylates, salicylsalicylate[51] and diflunisal, a fluorobenzene derivate of salicylate,[52] have been introduced recently. Both may be as efficacious as plain aspirin, may have better gastrointestinal tolerance, and have a longer therapeutic interval than plain aspirin. They share many of the extratherapeutic effects of other salicylates; diflunisal adds several of its own.[53-55] They have no apparent advantages over enteric-coated aspirin, and are substantially more expensive. Formulations of salicylate with salts other than sodium are available[56,57] or under study[58] and may be useful alternatives upon occasion.

What is the clinical importance to the rheumatologist of the studies on the absorption and metabolism of salicylates? It can be safely said that some patients are symptomatically sensitive to the dosing interval, that if the drugs are stopped for a day or so disease will measurably flare, and that the symptoms and signs of most inflammatory arthritides fluctuate more in response to physical activity and emotional state than in response to fluctuations in the serum salicylate level.

MAJOR THERAPEUTIC ACTIONS

Antipyresis. The antipyretic property of the salicylates was known by the middle of the eighteenth century, and today antipyresis is a prime indication for salicylates. By the 1940s, it appeared likely that the antipyretic action was central, not peripheral, and the details have unfolded beautifully over the past decade. Jackson established in 1967 that endotoxin caused fever only after a considerable latency but that a substance liberated from leukocytes did so rapidly.[61] In the same year Cooper and associates showed that the leukocyte pyrogen but not endotoxin was 100-fold more potent when given into the brain than intravenously and established that a neurotransmitter other than epinephrine or norepinephrine was involved.[62] Circulating monocytes and fixed mononuclear phagocytes are the source of the pyrogen, which is probably identical to the lymphocyte-activating protein known as interleukin I.[63] When Milton and Wendlandt showed that prostaglandin E$_1$ injected into the third ventricle of a cat caused an immediate fever that acetaminophen could not affect,[64] the broad outlines of the story were evident. Over the next 2 years it was shown that aspirin injected into the anterior hypothalamus was more potent than aspirin injected into the third ventricle and that injections into the carotid artery and intravenously were progressively less potent.[65,66] Soon after Flower and Vane[19] discovered the prostaglandin details, they showed not only that rabbit brain prostaglandin synthetase was blocked by aspirin, indomethacin, and acetaminophen, but also that their relative potencies were far different from their potencies

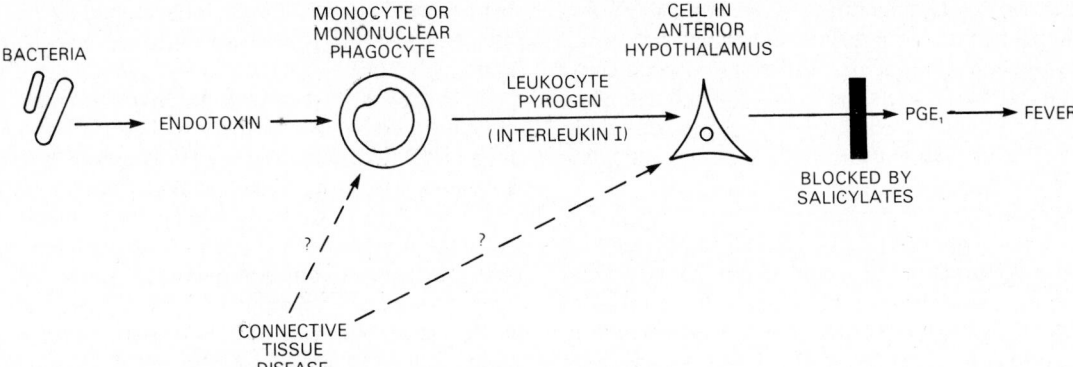

Figure 49–2. Leukocyte pyrogen liberated by monocytes and mononuclear phagocytes in response to bacteria stimulates the synthesis of prostaglandins in the anterior hypothalamus. The antipyretic action of salicylates is to block this synthesis.

in other enzyme systems.[67] In particular, acetaminophen and aspirin were almost equipotent and only about 10-fold less potent than indomethacin against the brain enzyme, whereas they were spread over a greater than 5000-fold potency range for dog spleen enzyme. Furthermore, it had long been known that sodium salicylate was almost as potent as aspirin in lowering fever despite doubts about their equivalence in other respects.[68]

It is now evident that PGE_1-like material appears in the third ventricle when fever is produced by an endotoxin,[69] that antipyretics of the PG-synthetase inhibiting class block that appearance,[69] that aspirin can block leukocyte pyrogen-induced but not PGE_1-induced fever,[69-71] that in vitro leukocyte pyrogen production is unaffected by high levels of salicylate,[72] that leukocyte pyrogen and aspirin do not compete for a common binding site, that in the brain as elsewhere PGE may mediate its effects through cyclic nucleotides,[73] and that the anterior hypothalamus is the principal site of action of this class of antipyretics.[74-76] (Fig. 49–2).

Although the mechanism of fever in the connective tissue diseases is unknown and may or may not depend upon the release of leukocyte pyrogen from sites of inflammation, the efficacy of salicylates and other prostaglandin synthetase-inhibiting drugs does suggest that prostaglandins serve as mediators of fever. Because of the sensitivity of fever to aspirin (inhibition of fever is maximal with about 600 mg every 4 hours), the antipyretic effects in many inflammatory conditions are achieved at doses below those necessary to suppress other measures of inflammation.

In adult rheumatoid arthritis, fever is unusual, and hypothermia is not a consequence of aspirin therapy. In rheumatic fever and in juvenile rheumatoid arthritis, in which fever may be the most prominent feature early in the illness, aspirin and other salicylates are powerful antipyretics and do not usually cause hypothermia. The antipyretic action is a principal indication for salicylates in lupus and often succeeds in lowering a fever in lupus when steroids fail. In fact, fever in lupus should preferentially be treated with nonsteroidal drugs.

Analgesia.* In general, aspirin and salicylate are properly classified as mild analgesics, equivalent to moderate doses of codeine, and less potent than full doses of narcotic analgesics[78,79] but more effective than narcotics against inflammatory pain.[80] It is likely that a maximum response is reached with 600 or 625 mg in an adult; with this dose, the serum salicylate level will not usually exceed 5 mg per dl. It has been asserted, though without published proof, that aspirin is a more effective analgesic than sodium salicylate in man.[81] Aspirin is clearly four times more potent than salicylate in blocking the painful response to intraperitoneal or intrasplenic bradykinin in dogs (see below),[82,83] and the period of analgesia in man does correspond roughly with the period when unhydrolyzed acetylsalicylic acid is still present in the blood after oral ingestion.[77] Nevertheless, as the long and successful history of salicylates prior to the synthesis of aspirin establishes, salicylate itself is analgesic in man.

Aspirin can act as an analgesic peripherally to reduce the inflow to the central nervous system of nerve impulses from a painful stimulus.[84,85] This has been shown in an elegant series of cross-circulation experiments in dogs.[82,83] The spleen of a recipient dog, with its nerve supply intact, received its arterial blood supply from a donor dog (Fig. 49–3). An injection of bradykinin into that splenic artery caused pain in the recipient as manifested by barking. An injection of aspirin into the donor dog blocked the pain, whereas an injection into the recipient (but not into the spleen) was ineffective. With narcotic analgesics, the reverse was true. If aspirin was injected directly into the splenic artery, the effective dose was 3.8 mg per kg, whereas it was 50 mg per kg if it was injected intravenously into the donor. Drug administered into the recipient's carotid artery was not analgesic. Again, with morphine the opposite was true. Propoxyphene was active by both routes. Furthermore, aspirin but not morphine blocked nerve impulses evoked in the splenic nerve by the bradykinin injection. In these

---

*This subject is well reviewed in Reference 77.

ANALGESIA FOLLOWING BRADYKININ-INDUCED PAIN

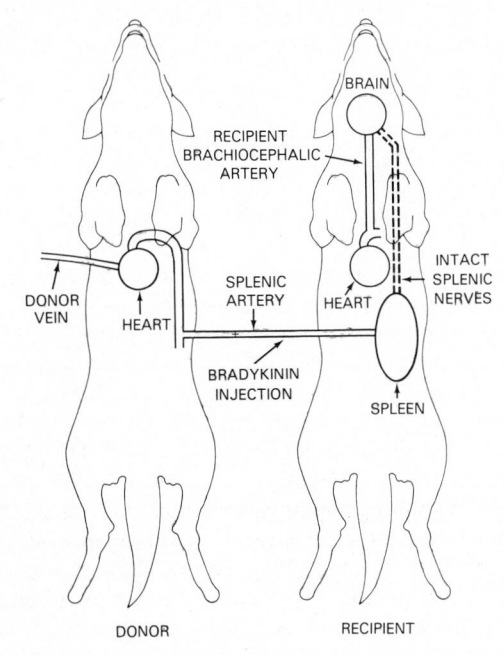

	SPLENIC ARTERY	DONOR VEIN	BRACHIOCEPHALIC ARTERY
SALICYLATES	+++	+	0
MORPHINE	0	0	+++

Figure 49–3. Bradykinin injected into the splenic blood supply of a vascularly isolated spleen causes the recipient dog to bark if the nervous connections of the spleen are left intact. Aspirin injected with the bradykinin blocks the pain response, but is without effect if injected into the brachiocephalic artery. With morphine, the opposite is true. (See Reference 83.)

experiments, sodium salicylate was an effective analgesic in doses fourfold higher than aspirin. In analogous experiments, in which a leg was supplied with arterial blood from a donor dog, intra-arterial sodium salicylate blocked the bradykinin-evoked pressor response in the recipient.[86] In an assay in which rats writhe in response to a bradykinin injection, aspirin was the most potent of a number of salicylate derivatives and analogues.[87] None of aspirin's metabolites beyond salicylate has analgesic action.[77]

What is known of the mechanism of the analgesic action? In response to an intra-arterial injection of bradykinin into the dog spleen, the splenic venous circulation had an increased output of prostaglandin-like material, and there was a rise in systemic blood pressure.[88] If PGE_1 or PGE_2 was given along with the bradykinin, the hypertension was augmented, although alone these prostaglandins lower the blood pressure. Indomethacin, a powerful inhibitor of prostaglandin synthesis, blocked the hypertension induced by bradykinin. Thus, prostaglandins appear to mediate some bradykinin effects. Experiments in rats showed that prostaglandins lowered

the threshold to pain from a mechanical stimulus,[89] and in humans that intradermal PGE_1 lowered the threshold to pain from a subsequent injection of bradykinin or histamine.[90] Aspirin cannot interfere with the pain induced by an intraarterial injection of either PGE_1 or PGE_2 in the dog.[91] Salicylates are generally ineffective against nonpathologic pain: that is, they appear to work only on some painful process already under way. For example, they raise the pain threshold to mechanical pressure in a rat's paw inflamed by an injection of yeast without altering the pain threshold in a normal paw.[89] A plausible case can thus be made for the view that part of the pain of inflammation is due to the stimulation by mediators such as bradykinin of the synthesis of prostaglandins which sensitize nerves to painful stimuli, and that salicylates are effective analgesics because they block that synthesis. Their analgesic property, however, is not identical to their anti-inflammatory property, since in both animal experiments and human experience analgesia occurs in doses below those that reduce heat and edema.

However plausible and satisfying the case may be for a unitary hypothesis of action of these drugs, the experiments are so far from providing the details necessary for verisimilitude that skepticism is unavoidable. One cannot yet dismiss theories concerning the direct effect of salicylates on nerve cell membranes,[92] or a central action under certain circumstances. For example, aspirin given to the rat so alters histamine metabolism that there is an increase in the production of indoleacetic acid, which has narcotic properties in that species.[93,94] Furthermore, many individuals, particularly the elderly, experience apparently central effects of aspirin such as dizziness, somnolence, and slurred speech, not to mention that hyperpnea and antipyresis are clearly central effects of the drugs. Any unitary hypothesis of aspirin and salicylate analgesic action must account for their ability to counteract pain of diverse sorts: headache, both vascular and muscular, and deep visceral or skeletal pain, whether neoplastic or mechanical, as well as pain related to inflammation. It seems likely that the proof of such a hypothesis will have to rest on a deeper understanding of the mechanism of pain than presently exists.

Anti-inflammation. In favoring aspirin and its pharmacologic relatives (and steroids) over propoxyphene, pentazocine, codeine, morphine, or even acetaminophen in the treatment of connective tissue diseases, especially arthritis, rheumatologists lean upon the belief that they provide not only freedom from addiction but the positive property of suppressing inflammation. Since one can obtain analgesia without measurably affecting other aspects of inflammation, the optimal use of these drugs in inflammatory disease depends on using them so as to obtain the anti-inflammatory effects.

What is the reason for believing that aspirin and salicylates have anti-inflammatory effects over and above analgesia? Inflammation is a term used to describe a global reaction that involves vascular events leading to the translocation of blood cells, protein, electrolytes, and fluid to the extracellular space; stimulation, proliferation, and transformation of cells; the production, diffusion, and destruction of mediators of great variety; the stimulation of nerve endings; the destruction of tissues; and ultimately a return to the uninflamed state. The inciting cause, the location, the species, the chronicity, and many other factors determine the course of inflammation and doubtless the response to intervention. Measuring the effects of intervention might therefore appear to be despairingly difficult, but in fact a good deal of useful information has been gathered on the global response and its less subtle manifestations, edema, erythema, and pain (see Analgesia).

The evidence for a reduction of edema and effusion in human arthritis is relatively limited. The clearest effect was in a study with patients with rheumatoid arthritis in which it was shown that aspirin at 5.3 grams per day reduced both joint pain and joint swelling as measured by jeweler's rings, whereas aspirin at 2.6 grams per day and acetaminophen affected only pain.[95] In other studies, some unpublished, aspirin has been shown to reduce swelling or increase joint motion, presumably measures of inflammation. There is evidence, too, that prostaglandins are elevated in the active synovial effusion of rheumatoid arthritis and even that therapy with aspirin can reduce that level, but the story is distinctly incomplete.[96] There is no useful, independent evidence on the mechanism or anti-inflammatory effects of aspirin or salicylate in any nonarthritic condition, although any clinician who has treated the serositis of lupus erythematosus with them will attest to their efficacy.

Animal models have provided substantial evidence for anti-inflammatory effects of aspirin and salicylate. Aspirin or salicylate reduced edema in rat paws injected with the algal polysaccharide carrageenan as a subacute irritant.[97-100] Furthermore they reduced the accumulation of effusion and cells when carrageenan was injected intrapleurally.[101] They reduced edema and warmth as well as the hyperesthesis of yeast-induced inflammation in the rat paw.[102,103] Urate-induced edema and ellagic acid-induced edema in both the rat paws and the dog stifle joint were reduced by aspirin.[104] Chemical- or ultraviolet-induced skin erythema was reduced only by very large doses.[105] Among chronic models of inflammation, aspirin effectively inhibited and also treated established adjuvant arthritis in the rat.[106-108] It did not have a beneficial effect on the inflammation of a traumatized joint,[109] and it had a variable effect in an antigen-induced arthritis.[110] Although it is likely that prostaglandins are important in the inflammation in some of these models, and that the interaction between bradykinin and prostaglandins is important in edema as well as pain, it is premature to suggest that aspirin works in them solely because of its effects of prostaglandin synthesis, or, conversely, that prostaglandin synthesis does or does not have a role in inflammation because inhibition of synthesis affects the process. Aspirin is not effective against inflammation caused by histamine or by injected or previously synthesized prostaglandins.

Recent tissue culture experiments have shed new light on the role of prostaglandin in rheumatoid inflammation. Human rheumatoid synovial fragments produced PGE_2 and a collagenase and can accelerate the release of calcium from mouse fetal bones; furthermore, mitogen-activated lymphocytes produce a substance or substances which stimulate these fragments to produce more prostaglandin.[111,112] It might seem possible, then, that adequate long-term suppression of prostaglandin synthesis would inhibit the bone destruction process in rheumatoid joints. Unfortunately, although such a possibility has not been formally ruled out, there is no clinical evidence on which to build such a hope.

In mechanistic terms, the influence of aspirin and salicylate upon the migration of neutrophils and monocytes seems to be important, particularly since prostaglandins can influence migration.[113,114] The complex effects of various prostaglandins on vascular permeability offer another point of intervention. There appears to be a direct effect of aspirin on the surface of granulocytes which might influence their ability to enter the extravascular space.[115] Aspirin and other prostaglandin-synthetase inhibitors may affect the many points in the immune response in which prostaglandins participate in complex or contradictory ways.[116]

Inflammation doubtless has an important beneficial role, so that interference with it might be hazardous as well as helpful. Such is the case with corticosteroids. With aspirin, salicylate, and other prostaglandin synthesis-inhibiting drugs, however, the course of infection, both chronic and acute, is unaffected, demonstrating the limitations of those drugs in the face of a powerful stimulus.[117]

Aspirin and sodium salicylate have rarely been compared for potency in animal models of inflammation; investigators tend to prefer to use aspirin, but sodium salicylate has been effective in some studies. In humans with arthritis, only the undocumented assertion by several investigators can be cited to support a greater anti-inflammatory potency for aspirin, although many clinicians favor it.[81] Even if the unitary hypothesis for the action of these drugs on prostaglandin synthesis is correct, it is unlikely that the inhibition of a single enzyme is solely responsible for anti-inflammatory effects.

Probably some effects of prostaglandin synthetase inhibition are the result of increased synthesis in the other wing of arachidonic acid metabolism, the leukotriene pathway, rather than just decreased prostaglandins, prostacyclins, and thromboxanes. In view of the great range of tissue sensitivities to inhibition, one should not a priori expect that the overall inhibition by salicylate will be appreciably less than that by aspirin.

However unproved and uncertain the unitary prostaglandin theory,[118,119] none of the other proposed theories of aspirin's anti-inflammatory action has plausible evidence in support of it. The possibility that aspirin works by inhibiting phosphodiesterase is remote, since only high levels are inhibitory.[120] Some of the older theories on the interactions of aspirin with various parts of the inflammatory system have been well reviewed.[105]

THE CLINICAL USE OF ASPIRIN AND SALICYLATES IN THE RHEUMATIC DISEASES

The major indications for aspirin and salicylate in the rheumatic diseases are fever, pain, and inflammation. They are useful for the fevers that commonly accompany rheumatic fever, systemic lupus erythematosus, and juvenile polyarthritis and, less commonly, rheumatoid arthritis, the spondyloarthritides, and other connective tissue diseases. They are useful for the pain of arthritis of any origin, including osteoarthritis and mechanical joint pain even when inflammation is not evident, and they are useful for the inflammatory arthritis, pleurisy, and pericarditis that accompany rheumatoid arthritis, lupus erythematosus, and occasionally other connective tissue diseases. They are not in general useful for the treatment of myositis, rash, nodules, renal disease, or serologic tests. It should be noted, however, that the anti-inflammatory effect in systemic lupus erythematosus, juvenile arthritis, and rheumatic fever may be accompanied by the fading of rash, and the sedimentation rate, too, responds as inflammation recedes in many diseases.

The antipyretic action and simple analgesia require relatively small doses of either aspirin or salicylate. One or two 300 mg tablets four to six times a day suffice for all but the largest adults. When the drugs are used to combat inflammation, higher doses are necessary, and although salicylate itself may not be so powerful and anti-inflammatory as aspirin, the serum level of salicylate is best used to guide therapy.

Plain aspirin is the cheapest place to start. Provided it is kept dry, it will remain as aspirin; otherwise it will slowly decay to salicylic acid and acetic acid and acquire a vinegary smell. Such preparations are not unsafe to use and are no less efficacious than the salicylate they contain. Today, however, enteric-coated aspirin is the best form of the drug. Indeed, since the gastrointestinal side effects, the principal drawback of plain aspirin, are so much reduced and since the drug is so well-absorbed, enteric-coated aspirin is a close to perfect nonsteroidal anti-inflammatory drug. It is available in several sizes and can even be given twice a day with adequate serum levels. The starting dose should be about 2.4 to 3.6 g per day in adults. The abrupt introduction of higher doses of plain aspirin often leads to patient resistance because of gastrointestinal side effects. Recalling the unusual metabolism of salicylates, in which the serum half-life gets longer as the serum level goes higher, the dose should be raised by one tablet per day no more often than once per week until tinnitus occurs or until the salicylate level is between 20 and 30 mg per dl. A slow-release form used at bedtime sometimes reduces early morning stiffness and pain. Since the drugs are most often introduced outside the hospital, and since frequent determinations of serum salicylate are impractical or impossible, older patients should raise the dose even more slowly, and all patients should be told about tinnitus, diminished hearing, and hyperpnea that accompany high serum salicylate levels. Patients know about

the gastrointestinal side effects well enough, but if a physician is committed to the use of salicylates, he can help a patient avoid them by a variety of maneuvers which may not make pharmacologic sense or be supported by controlled trials, but work. Plain aspirin can be given with meals, with antacids, crushed in milk, dissolved in water, or even crushed with Jell-O. The hour can be varied and the brand can be varied; a buffered preparation, sodium salicylate, timed-release aspirin, choline salicylate, and even various magnesium and calcium salts are available substitutes and will overcome gastrointestinal side effects in some patients. Enteric-coated aspirin is, I believe, the drug of choice except in the rare patient with gastric outlet obstruction in whom salicylism from retained undigested pills may occur.[121] Table 49–1 lists many of the common nonprescription and prescription forms in which aspirin and other salicylates are marketed.

It has often been observed that for some reason, pharmacological or psychological, individual patients may respond differently to different formulations. There are many variations in the formation of aspirin and salicylate designed to reduce the symptoms of gastrointestinal upset, to accelerate the absorption of the drug, or to reduce the microbleeding (see below). There is good evidence that sufficient buffering with either bicarbonate, citrate, or nonabsorbable alkali to bring the intragastric pH to neutrality will reduce microbleeding and accelerate absorption. The price, however, is a level of sodium intake unacceptable for long-term therapy (521 mg of sodium per 322 mg of aspirin in the most popular effervescent form, Alka-Seltzer) and/or accelerated excretion of the drug so that serum levels with long-term therapy are lower. Although the small amounts of buffering in commonly sold buffered aspirin may marginally accelerate absorption, they do not alter microbleeding. No formulation has proved dependably better at reducing gastric upset in blinded trials. In practical terms, if a patient has good symptomatic relief of arthritis with aspirin or salicylate but complains of gastrointestinal side effects, it is sensible to switch preparations; it is not necessary to abandon salicylates.

If the patient also takes corticosteroids or drinks any alcohol, nonabsorbable antacids should be used, bearing in mind that higher doses of the salicylate may then be necessary to maintain an adequate serum salicylate level.

Although it may be irrational, other nonsteroidal drugs can be added to aspirin with psychological if not pharmacological therapeutic benefit and no clear evidence for harm.

In rheumatoid arthritis, aspirin should be used in full anti-inflammatory doses, which means until a salicylate level of at least 20 mg per dl is reached or until tinnitus or diminished hearing occurs. Indeed, aspirin or another nonsteroidal anti-inflammatory drug should be given in anti-inflammatory doses along with all other classes of antirheumatic drug if inflammation is present.

Generally a reduction in dose suffices to reverse most symptomatic toxicities, although some require that the drug be stopped. The elderly patient is particularly sus-

Table 49–1. Some Commonly Used Nonprescription and Prescription Drugs Containing Salicylates*

Drug	Salicylate Concentration	Drug	Salicylate Concentration
Nonprescription			
Analgesics†			
		Momentum	162.5 mg aspirin,
Alka-Seltzer	324 mg aspirin		325 mg salsalate
Anacin products	400 mg and 500 mg aspirin	P-A-C Compound	227 mg aspirin
Arthralgen	250 mg salicylamide	Persistin	160 mg aspirin,
Arthritis Pain Formula	487.5 mg aspirin		485 mg salsalate
A.S.A.	325 mg aspirin	Trigesic	230 mg aspirin
A.S.A. Compound	227 mg aspirin	Vanquish caplets	227 mg aspirin
Ascriptin products	325 mg aspirin	**Cold remedies**	
Aspergum	210 mg aspirin	Alka-Seltzer Plus	324 mg aspirin
Bancap products	200 mg salicylamide	Codimal products	150 mg salicylamide
Bayer	325 mg aspirin	Coricidin products	325 mg aspirin
BC Tablets	325 mg aspirin,	Dristan tablets	325 mg aspirin
	95 mg salicylamide	Hista-Compound No. 5	227.5 mg salicylamide
BC Powder	650 mg aspirin,	Pyrroxate	200 mg aspirin
	195 mg salicylamide	Rhinocaps	162 mg aspirin
Bufferin	324 mg aspirin	Rid-A-Col	390 mg aspirin
Cama Inlay-Tabs	600 mg aspirin	Saleto-D	120 mg salicylamide
Capron	227 mg aspirin	Sine-Off tablets	325 mg aspirin
Cope	421.2 mg aspirin	Sinulin tablets	250 mg salicylamide
Doan's pills	325 mg magnesium	Triaminicin	450 mg aspirin
	salicylate	Viro-Med	325 mg aspirin
Duragesic	325 mg aspirin,	4-Way Cold Tablets	324 mg aspirin
	162 mg salsalate	**Miscellaneous**	
Ecotrin	325 mg aspirin	Midol	454 mg aspirin
Empirin	325 mg aspirin	Quiet World	227 mg aspirin
Excedrin capsules	250 mg aspirin		
Excedrin tablets	194.4 mg aspirin,		
	129.6 mg salicylamide		
Measurin	650 mg aspirin		
Prescription			
Analgesics†			
		Trilisate products	500 mg and 750 mg
Darvon Compound	227 mg and 325 mg aspirin		total salicylate
products		Zactirin tablets	325 mg aspirin
Disalcid	500 mg salicylic acid	Zactirin Compound-100	227 mg aspirin
Equagesic	250 mg aspirin	**Cold remedies**	
Fiorinal products	200 mg aspirin	Emprazil	200 mg aspirin
Meprogesic	250 mg aspirin	Omnicol	227 mg salicylamide
Percodan products	325 mg aspirin	Partuss T.D.	300 mg salicylamide
Synalgos products	356.4 mg aspirin	**Muscle relaxants**	
Talwin Compound	325 mg aspirin	Norgesic	385 mg aspirin
		Robaxisal	325 mg aspirin

*From Andrea S. Vivian, PharmD, and Ira B. Goldberg, PharmD: Facts and Comparisons, April 1982; The Redbook, 1982; The Handbook of Nonprescription Drugs, 6th ed, 1979.
†Analgesics labeled "compound" usually contain aspirin.

ceptible to salicylism.[122,123] The hepatic and renal side effects of the drug can be safely ignored in rheumatoid arthritis unless frank symptoms of hepatitis develop. It is unnecessary to monitor transaminase levels, creatinine, or urea in the patient on long-term therapy unless, especially in the elderly patient, there is a change that sharply alters fluid and electrolyte balance.

In juvenile arthritis and in rheumatic fever, aspirin is usually used in doses of 80 to 100 mg per kg per day, although sometimes doses up to 130 mg per kilogram per day are used. Children seem to tolerate high serum levels of salicylates better than adults, and therapeutic levels of over 30 mg percent are considered tolerable. The mild hepatitis that can be detected by blood tests is not a contraindication to continuing the drug, but any signs of bleeding or jaundice are.[124] The principles of aspirin administration in children have been clearly explained in pediatric literature.[125,126]

dren have been clearly explained in pediatric literature.[125,126]

In osteoarthritis and fibrositis, doses well short of supposed anti-inflammatory doses are usually adequate for analgesia, and there is no reason to push higher in the absence of overt inflammation.

In systemic lupus erythematosus, aspirin is often as good as or even better than corticosteroids for fever, arthritis, pleurisy, and pericarditis, and it is the drug of first choice in many clinics.[127] The starting dose should not exceed 2.4 g per day, but it can be raised to anti-inflammatory levels for arthritis and serositis. It is uncertain (see Side Effects and Toxicities) whether chronic liver damage occurs as a very rare sequel to salicylate-induced hepatitis, and it is true that the hepatitis may fade away as disease activity recedes, but it is safest to reduce the dose or stop temporarily if the serum transaminase rises rapidly in a hospitalized patient or is found to exceed about ten times normal in an ambulatory patient. If a random elevation of less than that is found in an otherwise reasonably well patient, the drug can be safely continued if the observation will be close. Minor alterations in renal function can occur with almost all the prostaglandin synthetase-inhibiting anti-inflammatory drugs and are not an indication for stopping therapy unless the change is marked or is accompanied by proteinuria, edema, or oliguria. Measurements of renal function to be used in therapeutic decisions, however, should not be made while a patient is taking those drugs.[128]

In ankylosing spondylitis, some patients will respond to anti-inflammatory doses of aspirin, and it may be worth trying. The same is true for the other spondyloarthritides and psoriatic arthritis.

Aspirin and salicylates no longer have a place in the treatment of crystal-induced disease. Not only are they not as effective as other drugs, but the peculiar effect of salicylates on the serum uric acid and urinary urate excretion can complicate evaluation and management.

Aspirin or salicylate can be tried for symptomatic relief in a variety of other connective tissue diseases, but is likely to be ineffective for the major manifestations of scleroderma, dermatopolymyositis, polyarteritis, polymyalgia rheumatica, and temporal arteritis.

INTERACTIONS WITH OTHER DRUGS*

Of the many drugs likely to be given with aspirin or salicylates, with few are there significant interactions. Much of the writing on the subject deals with the interactions of aspirin with acetaminophen, with indomethacin, and with the newer nonsteroidal anti-inflammatory drugs, and is concerned with the influence of one drug on the absorption or half-life of the other, not with their clinical interactions. These writings generally teach that there is little pharmacologic reason to give these drugs in combination but even less to forbid them. There are other interactions that are occasionally important: with coumarin anticoagulants, with uricosurics, with corticosteroids, with methotrexate, and with oral hypoglycemics (Table 49–2).

Salicylate displaces indomethacin from a plasma protein binding site, raising the unbound drug level, and thereby accelerating its clearance and metabolism.[130] Thus, aspirin at a dose of 3 to 6 g per day slightly lowers the peak serum indomethacin level when the two drugs are given simultaneously and has an inconstant effect on the serum disappearance.[131-134] This is altogether a small effect of no clinical significance. Indomethacin does not alter serum salicylate levels.[135] Both drugs are potent inhibitors of prostaglandin synthetase, and they may act at the same site on the enzyme, since indomethacin inhibits acetylation of the platelet enzyme by

aspirin.[136] Since this enzyme inhibition is responsible for some or perhaps all the pharmacologic action of both drugs, and since at full doses of either roughly the same effects are achieved, they would be expected neither to be additive nor significantly to interfere with one another. Such is the case in the few human and animal studies in which their clinical interaction has been measured. The long-lasting effects of both drugs in an animal model are probably irrelevant.[107] Despite some common side effects, there is no evidence that toxicities are additive. Of great theoretical and probably practical interest are the observations on interactions between salicylates and aspirin. Salicylate, like indomethacin, can prevent aspirin's irreversible inactivation of platelet prostaglandin synthetase by acetylation, and it can blunt some of aspirin's effects on the stomach (see Side Effects and Toxicities).

Aspirin has minor effects on the metabolism of acetaminophen,[137,138] including a reduction in acetaminophen-induced hepatotoxicity in mice.[139] Of greater interest is the finding in man that when a single dose of acetaminophen (650 mg) is given simultaneously with a single dose of aspirin (650 mg), total serum acetylsalicylic acid levels are higher and remain high much longer than when aspirin is given alone, but total salicylate levels are unchanged. At 1 hour, the serum level of aspirin was 3.32 μg per milliliter when the drug was given alone and 9.33 μg per milliliter when given with acetaminophen.[140] The mechanism for this effect on deacetylation is unknown and its clinical value unexplored. Although it would be useful to prolong the pharmacologic effects of aspirin, possible adverse effects on the liver of such combination therapy suggest caution.

What is true of the similarity in pharmacologic effects between aspirin and indomethacin is true also of the similarities among all the newer nonsteroidal anti-inflammatory drugs that can inhibit prostaglandin synthesis, although doubtless there will be subtle differences that are due to different sensitivities of the enzymes in various tissues. Consequently there is little interest in details of their interaction. From the few clinical studies, it was learned that ibuprofen can increase the level of free as opposed to protein-bound salicylate as measured in vitro by equilibrium dialysis;[141] a single dose of aspirin could slightly lower peak naproxen levels, probably by displacement from protein, leading to further excretion, but there was no effect on salicylate levels,[142] and aspirin lowered fenoprofen levels both acutely and chronically, possibly by increasing hydroxylation of the drug, but fenoprofen did not affect salicylate levels.[143] None of these interactions appear to be of any clinical significance. There is no indication that toxicities of drugs in this class are additive.

The interaction with the coumarin family of anticoagulants is variable and often not significant in an individual patient. Aspirin alone may have minor effects on prothrombin time and may reduce the amount of anticoagulant necessary to maintain a given prothrombin time.[129,144,145] Of far greater importance is the fact that they are inhibitors of different steps in the coagu-

---

*This subject is well reviewed in Reference 129.

Table 49–2. Interactions of Aspirin (A) and Salicylates (S) with Other Drugs

Drugs or Class of Drugs	Interaction	Clinical Implications
Nonsteroidal anti-inflammatory		
Indomethacin	A lowers serum levels slightly; not vice versa	None
Ibuprofen	Protein-bound S level reduced	None
Naproxen	A lowers serum levels slightly	None
Fenoprofen	A lowers serum levels slightly; not vice versa	None
Salicylate	Blocks A's irreversible inactivation of platelet prostaglandin synthetase	Uncertain
Acetaminophen	Raises serum A level but leaves total S level unchanged	None
Coumarin anticoagulants	A variably reduces prothrombin time further when added	Reduction of anticoagulant dose
Uricosuric agents	A/S blocks uricosuric effect	A/S should not be used with them
Sulfonylurea oral hypoglycemics	A/S variably potentiates hypoglycemic action	Reduction of sulfonylurea dose
Corticosteroids	Lower serum S levels	Observe S level when steroids reduced
Diuretics		
Furosemide	S blunts diuresis	Observe for this effect
Spironolactone	S blunts diuresis	
Antacids	Accelerate both absorption and excretion of A/S	Overall tendency to lower serum S levels when added
Methotrexate	A displaces methotrexate from protein-binding sites and enhances marrow depression	Caution, especially when using large doses of methotrexate
Ethanol	Synergistic effect with aspirin on gastrointestinal bleeding and bleeding time	Do not mix

lation scheme and consequently may increase the tendency for bleeding as a side effect of oral anticoagulant therapy. It is for this reason that these drugs should be given together only when necessary and that aspirin should be avoided when any other defect in the coagulation system, inherited or acquired, is present.

Salicylate has complicated dose-dependent effects on both uric acid reabsorption and secretion, probably in part through its competition as an organic anion. In low doses, these actions raise serum uric acid, and in high doses they may lower it. Any dose of aspirin or salicylate can block the uricosuric action of both probenecid and sulfinpyrazone and consequently should not be used together with them.[146] The newer uricosuric, benzbromarone, is less affected.[147] Aspirin, in common with other prostaglandin-synthetase inhibitors, can blunt a furosemide- or spironolactone-induced diuresis, especially under circumstances in which prostaglandins are contributing to the maintenance of renal blood flow (see Side Effects and Toxicities).[148,149]

Although aspirin and salicylates do not lower blood sugar in normal subjects, they may potentiate the hypoglycemic effects of the sulfonylurea drugs by unknown mechanisms, perhaps stimulating insulin secretion,[150] and doses may have to be modified accordingly.[129]

Any drugs that markedly alter urine pH can have an effect on salicylate levels, since salicylate excretion is markedly accelerated at high urine pH. Theoretically, ascorbate or other urine acidifiers could raise serum salicylate levels, but this does not appear to be a problem. A problem with ascorbate potentially related to

aspirin is that it can make the routine tests for stool occult blood falsely negative, thus obscuring a gastrointestinal blood loss.[151] Nonabsorbable as well as absorbable antacids can influence both the absorption and excretion of salicylates (see above).

Corticosteroids can lower the level of serum salicylate so that, when they are withdrawn, the serum level at a constant dose may rise substantially, even into the toxic range.[152] It is the impression of many clinicians that adverse effects of the two drugs on the gastrointestinal tract are additive or even synergistic.

Ethanol in the form of alcoholic beverages and aspirin probably are synergistic in their tendency to cause gastrointestinal bleeding from gastritis and gastric ulcer, and ethanol prolongs and potentiates aspirin's effect on bleeding time.[153]

Aspirin, probably by displacing methotrexate from protein-binding sites, enhances the bone marrow depressing effects of the antimetabolite. This has been shown clinically in studies with patients given large intra-arterial doses of methotrexate for malignancies.[154] Bone marrow depression, usually on the day after the injection, occurred almost exclusively in those patients who also received aspirin during the infusion. Studies in mice have confirmed this interaction experimentally.[155] It does not appear to potentiate the toxicity of the small doses of methotrexate used in current rheumatologic practice.

An interaction between phenytoin (Dilantin) and salicylate involving protein binding is not clinically important.[156]

ASPIRIN AND SALICYLATES IN PREGNANCY

In this day it is unnecessary to caution against the use in pregnancy of a drug even so apparently benign as aspirin.[157] The issue is how to assess the risk to the pregnant woman whose own illness demands anti-inflammatory therapy. The risk of congenital malformation that can be attributed to aspirin is negligible,[158] and neither hypoglycemia nor bleeding problems are more common in babies born of mothers taking salicylates.[159] The clinical significance of the altered hemostasis found in newborns of mothers taking aspirin in the last 10 days of pregnancy is doubtful.[160,161] In a large study of women taking aspirin at least twice a week, no increased incidence of stillbirth or perinatal mortality was found, and mean birth weight was unaffected.[162] That study, however, did not focus on women who took aspirin daily. In a smaller study of women in Australia who took salicylate-containing powders daily more for social than for genuine medical indications, mean birth weight, even corrected for the high incidence of smoking in this population, was significantly lower (3283 grams vs. 3502 grams in controls), and there were four stillbirths near term compared with none in a control group.[159] Pregnancy was an average of a week longer, ante-partum and post-partum hemorrhage was more common, and anemia in the mother was more frequent (uncorrected for other factors such as smoking), but labor was not significantly prolonged.[163]

The only study to focus on women who took aspirin for rheumatologic disease during pregnancy was a retrospective chart survey covering a 20-year period, so its findings must be accepted cautiously.[164] Gestation was prolonged by about a week, labor prolonged by about 5 hours, and estimated blood loss increased by about 100 ml in aspirin-takers with rheumatologic disease compared with normal women or with women with rheumatologic disease not taking aspirin. Reduced birth weight was common to the children of women with rheumatologic disease whether or not the women took aspirin. In both studies of women who took aspirin daily, there was an increased incidence of pregnancies lasting more than 42 weeks. Although the prostaglandin synthetase–inhibiting drugs have the useful property of promoting closure of a patent ductus arteriosus in the newborn, the same effect may occur prematurely in the fetus, leading to persistent pulmonary hypertension of the newborn.[165]

For the woman who must take an anti-inflammatory agent during pregnancy, aspirin can be relied on not to increase the risk of congenital malformation but does add some risk of prolonged gestation and labor and an increase of perinatal maternal bleeding. Since these risks are probably related to the prostaglandin synthetase-inhibiting properties of the drug, they are likely to depend on continued use of the drug. For the same reason, other drugs that inhibit prostaglandin synthetase are likely to share those effects. A sensible course would seem to be to stop anti-inflammatory medication if possible in the last month.

The infants born to women taking salicylates until term pose no special medical problems, although it is interesting to note that they have higher serum salicylate levels than their mothers.[31]

SIDE EFFECTS AND TOXICITIES

Under this heading I will discuss those effects of aspirin that are extratherapeutic. They are not all toxicities, and they are not all unwanted. Aside from the relation to major gastrointestinal hemorrhage and a controversial and doubtful relation to analgesic nephropathy, the toxicities of aspirin and salicylate are neither chronic nor cumulative. Furthermore, they are rapidly and completely reversible with a reduction of dose or cessation of therapy.

Allergy. For the many rheumatologists who have never or only rarely seen an allergic response to aspirin, the problem may seem remote, but a patient with a tale of an allergic response to aspirin is not rare in the office of the allergist. The incidence is well below 1 percent in a normal population but considerably higher in an allergy practice.[166] The earliest good description is of four cases of severe asthma, one fatal, induced, ironically, by "M. Matte's German Asthma Powder," which contained aspirin and caffeine.[167] By the early 1950s the essential immunologic facts of aspirin "allergy" were clear:[168] skin tests are negative for aspirin,[169,170] sodium salicylate does not provoke the allergy;[169] and there is no antibody detectable by passive cutaneous anaphylaxis (and presumably, therefore, no IgE or homocytotropic IgG antibody).[170,171] Later studies have confirmed these findings more elegantly. By the end of the preprostaglandin era, a nonimmune mechanism already seemed likely. It is now apparent that the "allergy"-inducing potential of the class of drugs is related to their ability to affect prostaglandin synthesis; not only aspirin (as little as 30 mg)[172] but other prostaglandin synthetase inhibitors, indomethacin (as little as 5 mg), mefenamic acid, flufenamic acid, fenoprofen, ibuprofen, and phenylbutazone, reduce air flow in aspirin-sensitive patients, whereas salicylate, salicylamide, acetaminophen, and propoxyphene do not.[173,174] What remains unknown is the site of the affected enzyme, and the exact way in which prostaglandins and leukotrienes affect the airways.

Clinically, the patients fall roughly into two categories: those who react to aspirin with bronchospasm and those who react with urticaria and angioedema. About half of those who have the bronchospastic reaction also have nasal polyps, in contrast to fewer than 15 percent of those with the urticaria-angioedema reaction.[175] Of those with the asthmatic response, at least half can be classified as having "intrinsic" asthma (normal IgE, normal skin tests, no recognizable environmental provocation or seasonal variation).[176] It seems likely that these patients have a metabolic defect either making them unusually sensitive to inhibition of prostaglandin synthetase because of a property of the enzyme itself or causing their airflow regulation to be abnormally dependent on prostaglandins to remain adequate.

In a large series of patients attending an allergy clinic, 3.8 percent of the asthmatics had aspirin allergy, the rate being higher for those with intrinsic (4.7 percent) than extrinsic (3.5 percent) asthma.[176] Most asthmatics who react to aspirin have the bronchospastic response, whereas among the 1.4 percent of rhinitis patients with aspirin allergy, the angioedema response predominated. Tartrazine sensitivity occurred in fewer than 20 percent of aspirin-allergic patients. The reported rate of 0.9 percent of "allergic" aspirin intolerance among normals seems to me inordinately high.[176]

Because aspirin is used so widely and because the "allergic" response requires only small, not full, rheumatologic doses to provoke it, aspirin allergy is virtually never discovered by the rheumatologist. If a patient gives a convincing history of bronchospasm, urticaria, or angioedema in relation to taking aspirin, however, it is likely that indomethacin, ibuprofen, fenoprofen, naproxen, tolectin, and probably phenylbutazone will provoke a similar response and ought to be avoided. Nonacetyl salicylate preparations can be used in this setting.

Tinnitus and Hearing Loss. Patients treated with salicylates will often note a high-pitched ringing in the ear and diminished hearing. Occasionally, they will also have vertigo, dizziness, and loss of balance. These toxicities are dose related and are probably all due to effects on the inner ear rather than on the central nervous system.

A raised threshold for all sound frequencies can be demonstrated by audiometry.[177] The change is roughly proportional to the serum salicylate level and is rapidly and completely reversible within 24 to 72 hours even if the drug has been taken for many years. The loss amounts to 20 to 40 decibels and occurs preferentially in the frequency range in which hearing is normal in those with pre-existing high tone deafness, thus leading to a flatter audiogram. Salicylates have little or no effect on presbycusis in which there is already a flat depressed acuity. The hearing loss is sensorineural, can be produced in several animal species,[178-182] and is unassociated with any recognizable morphologic changes in either animals or man, even if the drugs have been taken for many years with a known effect on hearing.[183] Salicylate-intoxicated cats show some biochemical changes in enzymes of the endolymph and perilymph, but what relationship this has to the ototoxicity is unknown.[178] Vestibular changes can be measured in humans as changes in the nystagmus induced by caloric stimulation and presumably account for the dizziness, vertigo, and imbalance.[183]

Tinnitus occurs universally in patients with normal hearing who take sufficient salicylate or aspirin. It comes on only when the serum salicylate exceeds 20 mg per dl, occurring on the average at about 30 mg per dl.[184] In these patients it is a useful guide to dosage, since it appears when the serum level is in the supposed anti-inflammatory range; the dose can be raised gradually until the appearance of tinnitus and then held steady at a slightly lower dose. Patients who have a high-tone hearing loss prior to salicylates often do not experience tinnitus even with very high salicylate levels. If there is any suspicion of a hearing deficit, or in any older patient, serum salicylate ought to be measured rather than waiting for tinnitus to occur.

Gastrointestinal Effects. The effects of aspirin and salicylate on the gastrointestinal tract have played a large role in their history. Aspirin itself was first popularized as a salicylate with less tendency to irritate the gastrointestinal tract; then attempts were made to reduce the gastric irritancy of aspirin; and now the newer nonsteroidal anti-inflammatory drugs claim to be no better than aspirin, merely less irritating to the gastrointestinal tract.

Because of the confusion concerning the gastrointestinal effects of aspirin and salicylate, it is helpful to examine separately the three major effects: symptomatic gastrointestinal distress, microbleeding, and frank gastritis or ulcer.

Gastrointestinal Symptoms. Gastrointestinal symptoms following use of aspirin occur occasionally and range from a very mild discomfort elicited only by direct or repeated questioning to heartburn, nausea, or severe discomfort occurring after a single tablet. Many patients with rheumatoid arthritis will tolerate a minor gastrointestinal discomfort as they will tolerate tinnitus in order to keep the beneficial effects of aspirin or salicylate. In various surveys the incidence of complaint has ranged from less than 2 percent to almost 40 percent, reflecting many factors related to the study design: whether or not the subjects knew they were getting aspirin, how a history of side effects was elicited, what condition the drug was given for, the age of the subjects, the dose of the drug, and doubtless sometimes the expectation or prejudice of the investigator.[185-189] Toxicities as well as benefit are subject to a placebo effect.

The form of aspirin does not appear to influence the incidence of gastrointestinal distress; in several controlled studies, aspirin and buffered aspirin have been found equally guilty.[186,187,190] Nor do symptoms correlate with the presence or amount of microbleeding or gastroscopic abnormalities.[191-194] It is my impression, however, that currently available enteric-coated aspirins are better tolerated as well as objectively less irritating (see below).

The mechanisms responsible for gastrointestinal symptoms are largely unknown, but probably a direct irritation to the mucosa, psychological expectations, and a central nervous system effect of salicylate all contribute. A dose of sodium salicylate given intravenously caused nausea at the same serum salicylate level as when the drug was given by mouth.[195] Since it is known that salicylate does not diffuse from the serum into the gastrointestinal tract, an extraluminal, probably extraintestinal central nervous system effect must have been responsible.

In practical terms, if gastrointestinal intolerance occurs when aspirin or salicylate is begun or when the dose is raised, and if the drug is otherwise having a therapeutic benefit, it is wisest to switch preparations to buffered, to enteric-coated, or to a liquid form, or to use one of the maneuvers suggested above (see Clinical Use). A substantial proportion of patients will be able to continue the drug with such switches from time to time. It has been repeatedly observed that some people who claim gastric intolerance to aspirin are able to tolerate it if they are unaware that it is being given or if it is given in another form. Of course switching to another nonsteroidal drug is sensible if intolerance persists. Combining two nonsteroidals (including aspirin) in submaximal doses sometimes works, too.

Microbleeding and Gastroscopic Changes. The ingestion of aspirin causes the loss of small amounts of blood (about 2.5 ml per day above a background loss of about 0.5 ml per day) into the stool in about 70 percent of people.[191,193,196-202] Although a sensitive qualitative test may sometimes detect losses this small,[203] most patients taking aspirin will not have occult blood on routine testing, and investigation of the circumstances of this loss has required the measurement of fecal radioactivity after the injection of ^{51}Cr-labeled autologous red blood cells. There is a large literature devoted to studies of this sort, most predicated upon the view that this blood loss is somehow related to other gastrointestinal effects of aspirin and salicylates, a view that is open to serious doubt.

Aspirin, soluble aspirin, calcium aspirin, aspirin in solution, aspirin in suspension, aspirin given with milk, and over-the-counter buffered aspirins are roughly equivalent in their ability to cause blood loss.[196,204] Sodium salicylate, choline salicylate, effervescent aspirin, or aspirin given with enough sodium bicarbonate or nonabsorbable, nonsodium-containing buffers causes little or no blood loss,[8,193,203,205-209] and the presence of achlorhydria markedly diminishes the loss.[201,202] No minimum dose for this toxicity has been found, but the loss does increase with increasing dose in the clinical range.[196] Furthermore, some subjects lose a great deal more than the average and are probably those few whose chronic iron deficiency anemia may be due to aspirin.[193,210] Ethanol, which itself does not cause this sort of microbleeding, does potentiate aspirin's effect.[199,211] There does not appear to be any adaptation, since microbleeding at 4 weeks or even as long as a year after starting therapy continues at about the same rate.[212,213] Intravenous aspirin in doses leading to the same serum salicylate level and the same effect on bleeding time causes a negligibly small increment blood loss in subjects with a normal gastrointestinal tract.[204,214] Nor does the ingestion of coumarin anticoagulants increase the rate of blood loss.[215]

Normal volunteers and patients with rheumatoid arthritis have the same frequency of microbleeding (about 70 percent) and the same range of blood loss.[193] Even patients who have recently had a major gastrointestinal hemorrhage from peptic ulcer disease have a similar frequency and degree of microbleeding.[210] Most patients with rheumatoid arthritis do not develop a chronic anemia that can be attributed to aspirin. On the contrary, patients who take aspirin over the course of a year for arthritis are likely to have a slightly higher hemoglobin than before they began the drug, probably because their disease activity has been diminished.[216]

Gastroscopic abnormalities after aspirin have been known for over 40 years, although much has been made of them recently with the advent of easier endoscopy.[137] There has been controversy over their actual incidence, location, nature, and even their relation to drug ingestion, but there is no doubt that aspirin given to a fasting subject with an empty stomach can lead to visible abnormalities ranging from hyperemia, petechiae, and submucosal hemorrhage to superficial erosion or even frank ulceration with visible intraluminal blood.[137,217-222,237,238] This is not a placebo effect, although occasionally placebo-treated subjects show some abnormalities. It occurs more frequently with aspirin than with other nonsteroidal prostaglandin synthetase inhibitors, although like microbleeding, it is by no means absent with them,[237,238] and tolerance does not develop over several weeks. The reported incidence has varied considerably, even to as high as 100 percent,[221] but all observers do not use equivalent language to describe their findings; one observer's hyperemia may well be another's superficial erosion. From both animal and human studies, the microscopic damage that accompanies the visible abnormalities is extremely quick to reverse, being largely gone within an hour of the dose of drug and completely gone by 6 hours.[222]

In view of their similar frequency, the fact that tolerance develops to neither, and the fact that adequate buffering can prevent both of them, it is reasonable to conclude that the microscopic blood loss originates in the visible lesions. *Most important, however, from a practical point of view, is that these abnormalities are markedly reduced if aspirin is given in an enteric-coated form, both in normals and in patients with rheumatologic diseases.*[223-226]

Prostaglandin synthesis inhibition is probably a necessary but insufficient cause for aspirin's gastric effects. Oral aspirin does inhibit gastric prostaglandin synthesis in man,[227,228] and, strikingly, the administration of some prostaglandins along with aspirin largely inhibits fecal blood loss,[229-231] reduces endoscopic damage,[232] and prevents the changes in gastric wall potential and ion fluxes that are associated with gastric damage (see below).[233,234] Intravenous aspirin does not affect the gastric mucosa or ion fluxes,[235] but its effect on gastric prostaglandin synthesis is not known. It seems likely that the peculiar propensity for plain aspirin to produce gastric damage is related to a powerful direct local effect on gastric prostaglandin synthesis aided by either high local concentration of the drug due to its insolubility or a second irritative effect, perhaps on gastric mucous[229] or local blood flow.[236]

The mechanism of microbleeding and gastroscopic changes is mysterious. They are clearly not due to platelet effects or other effects on the measurable coagulation factors. Despite earlier evidence that particles of undissolved drug might be involved in mucosal damage, soluble aspirin can cause microbleeding (although it may be argued that, in the acid environment of the stomach, aspirin might be precipitated from sodium aspirin solutions). Acid does seem necessary, since adequate buffering prevents it.[219] The fact that achlorhydria is also protective may reflect not only the absence of acid but also the more rapid cell turnover of the gastric mucosa characteristic of that condition, thus allowing more rapid repair.[239] The Davenport model (see below) postulates that the back-diffusion of acid into the gastric wall caused by an effect of aspirin on the gastric mucosal barrier liberates histamine locally, which dilates capillaries, presumably leading to diapedesis of red cells, some of which make their way to the gastric lumen through ruptured intercellular bridges.[240]

Do they relate to major blood loss, either chronic or acute? They are probably responsible, in the rare person with a large asymptomatic daily loss, for a chronic iron deficiency anemia. If the visible lesions are the precursor of the rare gastric ulcer or gastritis leading to major blood loss, it is easy to imagine that any condition that impedes the repair process, such as uremia, stress, ingestion of ethanol or corticosteroids, or an intercurrent illness, could potentiate the danger of aspirin.[239,241] There is no direct evidence, however, to link them to acute gastrointestinal bleeding caused by gastritis or peptic ulcer. Major hemorrhage retrospectively related to aspirin ingestion is as likely to have occurred with buffered or even effervescent aspirin,[242-244] which does not cause microbleeding, as with plain aspirin, and while the visible mucosal changes and the microbleeding are very common, major gastrointestinal hemorrhage is uncommon or even rare. The relation among them remains uncertain.

Does microbleeding or the visible gastroscopic changes relate in any way to complaints of gastrointestinal distress? In every series in which microbleeding or mucosal changes and symptoms have been recorded there has been a dissociation; some have distress without microbleeding or changes, and most have microbleeding or changes without distress.[191-194]

Both microbleeding and visible gastroscopic changes can be prevented by adequate buffering with sodium-containing buffers as in effervescent aspirin, but only at a cost of a prohibitive sodium intake for the chronic aspirin taker, and it is difficult to incorporate sufficient nonabsorbable buffer into an oral tablet. Sodium salicylate is thought by many to be pharmacologically inferior to aspirin. With sufficient ingenuity, an uncoated preparation of aspirin that caused little microbleeding or visible mucosal changes could probably be developed.[208] The availability of well-absorbed enteric-coated aspirin with markedly diminished effects on the stomach probably renders further efforts to do so unnecessary.

Neither microbleeding nor visible mucosal changes are the more dangerous for our being able to measure them or see them. If the gastrointestinal effects of aspirin and salicylate are to influence the way we use them,

then it must, in my opinion, be those that relate to patient comfort, for which appropriate individual adjustments are made, or those that relate to clear-cut morbidity or mortality, such as ulcer or major hemorrhage, for which there is yet no evidence that aspirin is a worse offender than any of the alternatives.

Ulcer, Gastritis, and Gastrointestinal Bleeding. Does aspirin cause major gastrointestinal bleeding? Ulcer? How often? Who is particularly susceptible? Can anything prevent it? What should be done if it occurs? Does anything potentiate the risk? What is safer than aspirin?

The evidence that aspirin causes major gastrointestinal bleeding is roughly as follows: In a large number of surveys of patients admitted to the hospital or studied as outpatients for major gastrointestinal bleeding and/or ulcer, the patients have been from two to five times more likely to have taken aspirin in the few days prior to admission than a group of control patients.[185,242-249] The choice of controls has varied in the studies and has been the focal point for much criticism. It may be, for example, that patients with any gastrointestinal problem more readily remember taking aspirin because of its publicized gastrointestinal effects; or that they have taken aspirin (usually effervescent) to treat the early symptoms of their bleed; or that controls are more likely to have diseases which, like stroke, impair their ability to take part in a survey. Even more remarkable is the extraordinary range of frequency of aspirin ingestion in the various populations—from 25 percent to over 90 percent.[250] Despite the imperfections of such studies, the qualitative conclusion is inescapable: a proportion of major gastrointestinal bleeding or ulcer is related to the recent ingestion of aspirin.[251] Such surveys also have established that buffered aspirin and effervescent aspirins are often the culprits, probably no less often than plain aspirin,[242-244,252] and that alcohol ingestion increases the risk of aspirin.[242,246,247] The episodes have been gastrointestinal bleeding without a visible source and therefore attributed to gastritis, gastric ulcer with bleeding, or gastric ulcer without bleeding.[252] Duodenal ulcer does not appear related.

In another type of survey, chronic gastric ulcer in young women in Australia was found to be quite common and highly likely to be associated with the chronic ingestion of headache powders; the incidence of gastric ulcer in women rose markedly as these powders came into vogue.[253] Furthermore, ulcer disease leading to gastrectomy is very common in analgesic abusers who have developed analgesic nephropathy, although it is difficult in that population to point a finger with any assurance at any particular drug or to ignore psychological factors.[254]

In a survey of hospitalized patients, habitual aspirin ingestion (four or more times per week) contributed to uncomplicated benign gastric ulcer and to new episodes of gastrointestinal bleeding not due to duodenal ulcer.[252] In that study, it was estimated, based on the known populations from which the patients were drawn, that the drug added a total of 25 cases per 100,000 users of aspirin per year. This is a very small risk indeed. Aspirin also increased the risk of bleeding in heparinized patients, which reinforces the stricture against using aspirin when another coagulation deficit exists.[255]

While aspirin does not appear to cause duodenal ulcer, patients with duodenal ulcer are not immune from its effects on the stomach. No formal survey proves that such patients are unusually susceptible to aspirin, but most physicians are properly cautious about using it. The hypersecretion of acid and pylorospasm characteristic of duodenal ulcer disease might be expected to contribute to a gastric toxicity of aspirin. In the absence of a strong indication (see below), it should be avoided.

Factors such as stress, alcohol ingestion, concurrent illness, other medications, diet, age, sex, and season as well as others probably contribute to the tendency of aspirin to cause gastric ulcer and gastritis with or without bleeding. Increased acid secretion may be a factor; however, ulcer and bleeding may occur, although rarely, in the patient with achlorhydria, too.[256,257]

There is no evidence that regular antacid ingestion or a switch to salicylate or even enteric-coated aspirin can prevent a risk of major gastrointestinal bleeding, but establishing a change in the frequency of a rare event is extremely difficult. *Most importantly, there is no evidence whatever that the incidence of ulcer or major gastrointestinal bleeding is any different with any other nonsteroidal anti-inflammatory drug from what it is with aspirin.*

Are rheumatologic patients or any subgroup of them particularly susceptible to the gastrointestinal effects of aspirin? There is no evidence that this is so. The incidence of ulcer disease in patients with rheumatic diseases may be higher than in the general population, but not all studies are in agreement on this point, and in particular they have not adequately assessed the role of drugs. Patients with rheumatoid arthritis are not more susceptible to aspirin-related gastrointestinal discomfort or microbleeding.

Clinically, gastric ulcer and gastritis in the patient with arthritis and in the normal individual are no different. It is my impression that gastric ulcer is more common than symptomatic gastritis with bleeding or silent gastrointestinal hemorrhage among rheumatologic patients. Major gastrointestinal bleeding related to aspirin is probably very rare in children, although a report of 12 children with melena, hematemesis, or anemia,[258] with frank ulceration in two children,[259] following therapeutic doses of aspirin suggests that it does occur.

What should be done when ulcer or gastrointestinal bleeding occurs in the rheumatologic patient taking aspirin? Although we used to continue aspirin when peptic ulcer occurred if it appeared necessary to manage rheumatoid arthritis, and found that ulcers usually healed,[260] a more sensible course is to add cimetidine.[261-265] When the ulcer is healed, there is no contraindication to a return to aspirin with antacid.

Potential Difference. When unbuffered aspirin is instilled into the stomach of man or experimental animals, the electrical potential difference between the gastric mucosa and the skin or a peripheral vein is reduced from its normal of -40 mv to about -30 mv.[266,267] It is likely that this change in potential reflects a change in the mucosal barrier that protects the stomach from the high acid concentrations of gastric secretion. In experimental animals, particularly the dog with an isolated gastric pouch, the potential changes induced by aspirin parallel a back-diffusion of hydrogen ions into the stomach wall and leakage of sodium and chloride into the lumen.[268,269] Davenport's theory of the gastric damaging effects of aspirin postulates that this back-diffusion leads to the release of histamine, capillary dilatation, increased acid production, and, if there is a sufficient concentration of acid in the lumen initially, gastric erosion and bleeding. Because of the difficulty of measuring ion fluxes in man, measurement of changes in the potential difference has been used as a surrogate for changes in the gastric mucosal barrier.

Aspirin causes a reduction in potential, but not if accompanied by adequate buffer (effervescent aspirin, nonabsorbable antacids, or sodium bicarbonate).[270,271] Ethanol alone reduces the potential and potentiates the reduction induced by aspirin.[270,272] Indomethacin, prednisone, and phenylbutazone do not alter the potential.[272] Bile acids, which cause gastric damage in animals and exacerbate aspirin's tendency to do so, also reduce the potential difference.[270] Glucagon, PGE_2, and cimetidine all increase the potential difference and, in the proper dose, block the potential reduction induced by aspirin.[261,263,273] In the case of glucagon, the intragastric pH is unaltered (i.e., it remains low), but gastric damage is prevented. In the case of cimetidine, the pH is raised to 7 and cell damage is blocked.

Animal Studies. Gastrointestinal effects of aspirin and salicylate have been studied in dogs, cats, rabbits, guinea pigs, rats, and even frogs. There are pronounced differences among different species in their susceptibility, so that extrapolation to man is hazardous.

The most useful studies have been by Davenport, using the dog with a Heidenhain pouch, an exteriorized isolated gastric pouch with intact blood supplied that can easily be filled and emptied. In his experiments, he instilled drugs with or without acid at various concentrations and measured the changes in ion concentration and the appearance of blood in the gastric fluid over time. He showed that aspirin or sodium salicylate in a weak acid solution (0.001 M HCl) breaks the mucosal barrier to ion fluxes, allowing hydrogen ions to back-diffuse into the gastric mucosa and sodium to leak into the lumen, but only with strong acid (0.1 M HCl) does bleeding occur.[274] Ethanol potentiates the effect of aspirin by lowering the concentration of acid at which bleeding appears. Davenport has summarized his findings and his model in an excellent review.[240]

Studies in rats, which develop ulcers easily with aspirin, have shown that stress,[275,276] starvation,[277] and bile acids[278,279] potentiate its effect, while bicarbonate,[280] vagotomy, atropine,[280,281] metiamide,[262] and cimetidine[275] ameliorate it. Giving very large quantities of glutamine[282] or cupric sulfate[283] or giving aspirin methyl ester[284] prevents the ulcers without inhibiting the beneficial pharmacologic effects.

Although it has been established in animals that aspirin does reduce both gastric venous[285] and gastric juice prostaglandin levels,[286] what relation this has to changes in the mucosal barrier, to ion fluxes, and to cell damage remains unknown. Gastric blood flow may increase,[287] decrease[288] or remain unchanged after aspirin, depending on the animal model;[241] likewise acid production is inconstantly affected.[241,288] Most attention has focused on the stomach, but permeability changes also occur in the small intestine.[289-291]

Platelet and Coagulation Effects. Aspirin's effects on platelets and coagulation have commanded attention because they were discovered early, have been easy to study, and have raised the hope of safe and effective prophylaxis against venous and arterial thrombosis. The principal effects are on platelets and bleeding time; there is a minor effect on synthesis of the vitamin K-dependent clotting factors.

Aspirin prolongs the bleeding time as tested by any of the standard assays. Most subjects, normal or rheumatoid, can be shown to respond, although the final bleeding time may remain within the normal range.[292-297] Curiously, women may be less affected than men.[298] On the average, the bleeding time is prolonged 1.5- to 2-fold. Sodium salicylate is without effect.[295] Ethanol can both potentiate and prolong this effect.[153] A minimal effective dose of aspirin has not been defined, although less than 1 gram a day can do it, and 0.44 gram is as effective as 4 grams.[297,299] The crudeness of the assay has limited the information that can be extracted from these studies, and it is, in fact, not certain that the effects on platelet cyclooxygenase described below rather than other effects on platelets, capillaries, arterioles, or local tissues are responsible for the altered bleeding time.

Soon after the discovery of the effects on bleeding time, several laboratories discovered that aspirin in vitro entirely blocked the aggregation of platelets by collagen or connective tissue fragments, and blocked a second wave of aggregation when platelets were exposed to ADP or epinephrine, while not blocking the initial aggregation these substances caused.[300-303] Later it was shown that aspirin blocked the release from platelets of serotonin and ADP from the dense granules,[304,305] that the initial adherence of aspirin-treated platelets to an injured vascular endothelium was unaffected but subsequent build-up of larger aggregates was blocked,[305-308] and that all these effects occurred with doses or levels of aspirin well below what are achieved in vivo after aspirin ingestion.[309-311] Although details in the picture of platelet aggregation remain to be worked out, the broad outline is roughly as follows. Various mechanical and chemical stimuli, including exposure to collagen, to damaged vascular endothelium, to excessive agitation, and to thrombin, ADP, and epinephrine, cause platelets to adhere to surfaces and to each other. During that process, arachidonate is mobilized and is metabolized by the enzyme platelet cyclooxygenase to the cyclic endoperoxide PGG_2, which is converted successively to thromboxane A_2 and PGE_2 and PGF_2, as well as to a number of other substances whose functions are not known. Thromboxane A_2 and probably also PGG_2 are released from the platelet into the surrounding fluid, where they cause the release of ADP and serotonin from the dense granules of other platelets.[312-314] The released ADP in turn aggregates these other platelets, causing them to adhere to the nearby initial aggregate.[315] The mechanism of dense granule release probably involves both GMP and calcium but is not presently well understood.[316,317] Aspirin, by blocking the initial step of synthesis in the prostaglandin pathway, blocks the release of PGG_2 and thromboxane A_2, thereby preventing the so-called release reaction and secondary aggregation. Platelets exposed to aspirin in vivo or in vitro demonstrate this lesion, and it is irreversible. If PGG_2 or additional ADP is provided, however, secondary aggregation can take place.

It is now clear that the acetyl group of the aspirin specifically acetylates a single platelet microsomal protein of molecular weight 85,000, the cyclooxygenase, and that the acetylation stoichiometrically irreversibly inactivates the enzyme.[24,318,319] The human platelet cyclooxygenase is peculiarly sensitive to this inactivation, at least 30 times as sensitive as the only other cyclooxygenase studied in detail.[314]

One 300 mg tablet of aspirin by mouth has a demonstrable effect on human platelets within 5 minutes and is maximally effective soon thereafter.[309] As expected, the more slowly absorbed enteric-coated aspirin reaches a maximal effect later, but inhibition is as great and lasts as long as with plain aspirin.[320] Although the platelets and megakaryocytes whose enzyme has been inhibited do not recover, as few as one third of normal platelets partially restore aggregation so that continued suppression may require daily ingestion.[314,321] With prolonged ingestion of somewhat higher doses, however, platelet aggregation returns despite continued complete inhibition of platelet cyclooxygenase, so no single mechanism offers a complete explanation.[322]

One of the complications is that salicylate itself, as well as indomethacin and diflunisal, though not acetaminophen, can block the acetylation of platelet oxygenase by aspirin.[323-325] In the case of salicylate, there is no inhibition of the enzyme; in the case of indomethacin, there is powerful reversible inhibition. These effects may depend upon the existence of more than one inhibitory site on the platelet enzyme, but details are lacking.[326-328]

The recently recognized ability of aspirin to inhibit vascular prostacyclin synthesis has also added complexity, since prostacyclins synthesized by vessel walls inhibit coagulation. Thus aspirin might promote coagulation by inhibiting vascular tissues while blocking coagulation by inhibiting platelets. With a *single* dose of aspirin as low as 30 mg, the platelet enzyme is inhibited far more than the vascular enzyme, either arterial or venous, but a *single* 300- or 325-mg tablet has profound effects on both enzymes.[329,330] With repeated doses, however, the situation that more closely approximates the rheumatologic use of aspirin, both enzymes are about equally affected.[322,331]

Several investigators have described effects of aspirin on other platelet functions, particularly in activating platelet factors 3 and 4.[303,332] Although they are of rapid onset, they may require somewhat larger doses. The consequences of this aspect of aspirin's action are not known.

Aspirin has a small inconsistent effect on the synthesis of the vitamin K–dependent clotting factors.[144,294] Some investigators have not found it at all. Rarely a patient will demonstrate bleeding and prolonged prothrombin time as a manifestation of aspirin toxicity.[124] Several of the reported cases occurred in people with a probable nutritional deficiency which may have contributed to the prothrombin problem.[333]

Of what clinical importance are the effects on coagulation, particularly on platelet function? Under ordinary conditions of aspirin use in the rheumatic diseases, none. The effect on prothrombin time is so weak and variable that it need be considered only when coumarin anticoagulants are administered simultaneously because the dose of anticoagulant sometimes but not always needs to be reduced (see above). The effect on platelets cannot be wholly responsible for the anti-inflammatory action of aspirin, since it occurs at doses at least 10-fold below anti-inflammatory doses. It might be argued that the antiplatelet effect contributes to the gastrointestinal microbleeding. That is exceedingly unlikely, since aspirin administered by other routes or so that it can be absorbed only beyond the stomach has just as much platelet effect but does not cause gastric microbleeding. Finally, there is no evidence, clinical or epidemiologic, that patients with rheumatic disease who are taking aspirin, even at the time of operation or even if another coagulation problem is present simultaneously, are disposed to bleed excessively. In a rare exception, aspirin appears to have been responsible for well-documented intravascular coagulation and aspirin-induced hepatitis in a young boy with Still's disease[334] and in a 17-year-old girl with "adult onset" juvenile rheumatoid arthritis.[335]

It is interesting to note that there exist patients whose platelets closely mimic aspirin-treated platelets.[305] In fact, a patient with deficient or absent platelet cyclooxygenase had no significant clinical illness.[312] This reflects, I believe, the happy natural redundancy of the coagulation system; under normal circumstances and sometimes in fact under any circumstances, deficits in the coagulation scheme can go unnoticed throughout a lifetime unless special tests uncover them.

Aspirin and other drugs that depress platelet function, such as dipyridamole and sulfinpyrazone, have been explored for their ability to prevent arterial and venous thrombosis, especially in patients with coronary and cerebral circulatory insufficiency and in bedridden patients after major surgery. It is beyond the scope of this chapter to review the evidence of these studies except to say that they show some modest promise in several clinical circumstances but almost surely will not prove to prevent major arteriosclerotic and thrombotic arterial disease, which occur all too often in patients who have taken aspirin for decades.

Hematologic and Immunologic Effects. *White Cell Effects.* Some investigators have found that aspirin or salicylate inhibits various in vitro functions of human or animal lymphocytes, including transformation in response to mitogens,[336] the allogeneic mixed lymphocyte reaction,[336] transformation in response to antigens,[337] and the production of migration inhibitory factor.[338,339] In some but not all experiments, the lymphocytes isolated from subjects taking aspirin have been found to respond subnormally.[340,341] The inhibition was sometimes related to serum level. The in vitro effects do occur in the range of drug levels found in the serum of patients, but it should be noted that when drug is added in vitro to a culture containing 20 percent plasma, the proportion of unbound drug is higher since the albumin concentration is lower. Data on the reversibility of the effect are inconsistent. These effects may be in some way related to the depressed levels of cyclic AMP found in the lymphocytes of subjects taking aspirin.[342]

In the only experiments in which lymphocyte responses to mitogen and antigens and corresponding skin tests were performed in a double-blind trial of aspirin and placebo administration to normals, aspirin showed no effect despite substantial serum levels.[343] Thus a healthy skepticism for claims that aspirin's anti-inflammatory effects are mediated by direct effects on lymphocytes is warranted, but indirect effects are still possible.

There have been a number of early studies of other immunologic effects of aspirin, which have been well reviewed.[116,344] These studies do not support a primary action on antibody synthesis; effects that have been reported, such as protection against the Schwartzman phenomenon in the rabbit, are more reasonably attributable to other actions of this class of drugs or occur at doses far from the clinical range.

Aspirin ingested by normal volunteers modestly decreased the ability of their granulocytes to adhere to nylon fibers in vitro for several hours after a 1.2-g dose, although sodium salicylate added in vitro had no effect.[345] The mechanism is unknown, but the changes in migration of leukocytes into inflammatory lesions in several animal models may be related to the adherence and movement of leukocytes.

Aspirin in Genetic Hemolytic Anemias. In a large careful study, 22 patients with glucose-6-phosphate dehydrogenase did not show signs of hemolysis when given a 4-day course of aspirin at 50 mg per kilogram per day.[346] Glutathione levels in deficient red cells were not altered in vitro by exposure to aspirin or the metabolite gentisic acid, and Heinz bodies did not form. Neither chemical altered the hexose monophosphate shunt activity of normal red cells. There is a single case report alleging that a large dose of aspirin (6 grams per day) shortened the half-life of red cells to 16 days in an enzyme-deficient subject.[347] Because of the heterogeneity of the enzyme-deficiency state, caution is necessary in applying the results of observations to all patients.[348] It is likely that aspirin can be safely administered when clinically indicated to most deficient individuals.

A much rarer genetic defect, the severe anemia form of pyruvate kinase deficiency, may cause the red cells of affected individuals to be unusually susceptible to salicylates.[349] When exposed in vitro to aspirin, intracellular ATP falls and the cells have altered permeability and a decreased hexose monophosphate shunt, thereby diminishing their ability to manufacture glutathione. Consequently detoxification of other drugs may be impaired. The clinical importance of this is unknown.

Cytopenia. Aspirin and salicylate have almost never been convincingly implicated as a cause of anemia, leukopenia, or thrombocytopenia resulting from peripheral destruction of cells or marrow depression.[350]

Pulmonary and Cardiovascular Effects. *Pulmonary Edema.* The rare complication of pulmonary edema caused by salicylates was first recognized in patients being treated with full doses of salicylates for rheumatic fever, with or without carditis. It was described as "rheumatoid pneumonia," with the typical roentgenographic appearance of pulmonary edema.[351] The patients in whom it was originally described had an increased plasma volume, which was thought to account for the pulmonary edema. The presence of actual or possible carditis resulting from rheumatic fever clouded the early description,[352,353] although it was noted that a patient taking salicylates who had a roentgenographic picture of pulmonary edema might have no other signs of heart failure.[354,355] With the description of cases in otherwise healthy individuals, it became apparent that underlying heart disease was not a requirement.[356,357] In addition, there have been autopsies of two patients with fatal pulmonary edema which showed only congested lungs; the hearts were normal.[358] In one previously normal patient with pulmonary edema, catheterization showed a normal pulmonary artery pressure, normal pulmonary capillary wedge pressure, and normal pulmonary atrioventricular oxygen difference. The pathophysiology is most reminiscent of noncardiogenic pulmonary edema of the sort caused by morphine, heroin, and propoxyphene.[359] The only experimental evidence of a similar lesion was in awake sheep infused with aspirin.[360] They developed increased pulmonary lymph flow and leakage of serum proteins into pulmonary lymph but had normal cardiac function and pulmonary artery pressure. Thus, by a mechanism unknown, there is an outpouring of fluid into the pulmonary air spaces at a time when cardiac function is unimpaired. The physiologic consequences are dyspnea and cyanosis, and the radiologic consequence is pulmonary edema.

The syndrome is particularly likely to occur in elderly patients, often smokers, who have been taking salicylates chronically. The clinical presentation may be of lethargy, confusion, and metabolic acidosis.[122,123] The serum salicylate level is usually greater than 40 mg percent. The lesion is rare, but it may be the presenting manifestation of occult salicylism in the elderly and must therefore be kept in mind.[361] Although the mechanism of the hyperpnea regularly seen with high therapeutic doses of salicylates is central stimulation,[362] the clinical appearance may also be that of marked dyspnea. This effect is probably not due to the inhibition of prostaglandin synthesis, since neither indomethacin nor ibuprofen causes it in experimental animals.[363]

Cardiovascular Effects. Aspirin and salicylate are free of cardiac effects except as related to the anoxia of the drug-related pulmonary edema and acid-base disturbances. From the discovery that prostaglandin infusion could keep open a patent ductus in the newborn when that shunt was necessary for survival,[364,365] it was but a short step to the use of the prostaglandin synthetase inhibitors aspirin and indomethacin to close the duct in newborns in whom surgery might otherwise be necessary.[366,367] This simple and apparently benign therapy is now in wide use. In these infants, marked transient renal effects occur, probably the reflection of an unusual dependence on prostaglandins to maintain renal perfusion. In levels larger than those encountered even in severe intoxication there is a direct suppression of cardiac conduction tissue.[368] Some other vascular effects are probably of no clinical relevance.[369]

Hepatic Effects. The hepatitis caused by aspirin is in a sense a disease of advancing medical science; it was discovered when the serum transaminase test became available[370,371] and usually is discovered today only because that test is ordered routinely, not because symptomatic liver disease develops. It first was thought to be a chemical manifestation of liver disease in children with active rheumatic fever with carditis, and only later was it realized that the common factor was aspirin or salicylate therapy rather than the disease. Subsequently, children with rheumatoid arthritis,[372,373] especially females and those with the systemic type,[124] patients with active systemic lupus erythematosus,[374] and patients with any underlying liver disease have been found particularly but not exclusively susceptible.[375] Those with other forms of connective tissue disease and even otherwise healthy individuals may show hepatic injury, although often of but a trivial degree.[375,378]

Usually, abnormal transaminase occurs in the second or third week of therapy or after an increase of dose. A high proportion of patients who have active lupus erythematosus and some patients with juvenile rheumatoid arthritis will develop abnormalities, sometimes within a week of an increase in dose, and often rising to levels in the hundreds or even thousands. Most often the bilirubin remains normal even if transaminase is high for extended periods; the alkaline phosphatase may rise just into the abnormal range. Except in a few patients, usually children, prothrombin time is unaffected.[124] In those few, ecchymoses and frank bleeding may occur quite rapidly and drug should be immediately stopped and vitamin K and/or plasma given.

Although most patients with this hepatitis are asymptomatic, some develop nausea, anorexia, a loss of taste for cigarettes, and even an enlarging or tender liver.[374,378] Biopsies in cases of acute aspirin-related injury have generally shown a nonspecific toxic hepatitis with single cell necrosis, anisocytosis and aniso-nucleosis, and a mononuclear cell infiltrate in the lobule and in the portal areas.[376,379,380] Several patients have been seen in whom the lesion developed in the face of a recent normal liver biopsy, thereby establishing that underlying liver disease is not a precondition. There have been two patients reported in whom histologic chronic hepatitis has been found to be the probable result of long-term aspirin therapy.[375,379] Although this is probably a rare event, aspirin should be added to the list of potential inciting agents of idiopathic chronic hepatitis, especially if immunologic phenomena are a prominent feature, since systemic lupus erythematosus with aspirin-induced hepatitis may closely resemble chronic active hepatitis with immunologic features.

Early papers stressed the relationship to high serum salicylate levels, often over 30 mg per dl, but the hepatitis clearly can occur with a serum level below the therapeutic range, as low as 10 mg per dl. If abnormalities occur, they will disappear within a week or rarely 2 weeks when the drug is stopped or the dose is lowered. In addition, however, they will often disappear if the drug is continued in children with arthritis.[124,381] If aspirin is continued in a patient with active lupus who develops hepatitis, the abnormalities will occasionally disappear if the disease becomes less active. There are apparently spontaneous fluctuations, particularly in children with arthritis; if children are tested often enough, abnormal liver function tests will appear at some time or other in more than half of those on aspirin.[382]

The mechanism of this lesion is unknown. Eosinophilia and rash are not regularly associated with the hepatitis, and the toxicity is dose related. Together, these observations make a hypersensitivity type reaction very unlikely. Animal studies have not shed any light on this area. It is possible to show only trivial hepatic changes in rabbits despite long-term high-dose therapy with salicylate.[383] It is true that patients with liver disease are more susceptible and that such patients have a reduced level of aspirin esterase,[384] but it is unlikely that those observations are related, since hepatitis is caused as readily by salicylate as by aspirin.[373] It is possible that a metabolite, perhaps an otherwise minor metabolite, achieves toxic levels in certain disease states, but there is no evidence of this yet. Salicylate does appear to be directly toxic to rat hepatocytes in short-term tissue culture, causing the liberation of a cytoplasmic enzyme, LDH; this system may provide a window on the mechanism of the toxicity.[385]

In clinical practice, the best way to avoid aspirin hepatitis in adult rheumatoid arthritis is to avoid measuring transaminase levels unless frank symptoms related to the liver or upper abdomen are present. In children, the drug can be continued safely if there is no evidence of bleeding or ecchymosis and if any transaminase abnormalities do not suddenly worsen or reach levels above several hundred. Lowering the dose or temporarily stopping and then resuming the drug at a lower dose is usually adequate therapy. When transaminase levels rise sharply in lupus, we tend to stop and switch temporarily to another drug, although some patients do improve without lowering the dose. It should be borne in mind that the administration of two hepatotoxic drugs can be unusually dangerous and ought in general to be avoided.

Reye's syndrome, the catastrophic illness of children in which an apparently metabolic encephalopathy is coupled to hepatocellular failure and fatty degeneration, has been attributed to salicylates[386] and has even been described in a girl being treated in hospital with aspirin for polyarthritis.[387] Although in an individual case it is impossible to incriminate aspirin, there is good epidemiologic evidence gathered in case-control studies that aspirin ingestion contributes to the Reye's syndrome which may follow outbreaks of influenza and chicken pox.[388,389] There is a move to have the label of aspirin bottles carry a warning to that effect.[390] The liver pathology of Reye's syndrome is quite different from that found in aspirin-induced hepatotoxicity.

Renal Effects. There are five renal effects of aspirin or salicylates that may, under certain circumstances, be clinically significant: a transient shedding of tubular cells when therapy is begun; a possible relation to analgesic nephropathy; reduced glomerular filtration and renal blood flow, probably related to prostaglandin synthetase inhibition; interaction with furosemide and spironolactone; and alteration of urate excretion (see above).

When aspirin or salicylate administration is begun, there is an outpouring of cells into the urine which is due to the shedding of tubular cells.[391,392] The effect lasts several days and disappears. Its mechanism is obscure. In fact it defies easy speculation because none of the actions of salicylates or aspirin is known to attenuate so quickly. Perhaps it is caused by effects on prostaglandin biosynthesis for which compensatory mechanisms exist. While hematuria may also occur in association with salicylate therapy, the mechanism remains unclear.

Although analgesic nephropathy, by which I mean both papillary necrosis and its supposed late consequence, end-stage renal disease due to interstitial nephritis, has been recognized for over 20 years, it continues to arouse heated debate. It has been studied mainly in those countries where social patterns of drug use have encouraged many young women to ingest large quantities of proprietary analgesic powders or pills.[393]

The controversy surrounds the issue of which drug or drugs are responsible. Without trying to unravel its entirety, the following considerations are relevant to aspirin: (1) It is possible in animals to produce a lesion with aspirin and/or phenacetin that more or less resembles analgesic nephropathy, but the circumstances of drug administration are remote from the clinical setting of analgesic nephropathy.[394,395] (2) Although aspirin taken alone has been blamed in some cases of analgesic nephropathy, it is phenacetin, alone or in combination, that seems most culpable.[396,397] (3) Several older autopsy studies of rheumatoid arthritis patients have shown an alarming incidence of papillary necrosis or even end-stage renal disease,[398-400] but renal dysfunction has *not* been found in a number of carefully observed groups of arthritis patients who have taken large quantities of aspirin over many years under medical observation.[401-405] (4) Finally, and most important, in the only controlled observations on the subject, analgesic ingestion could not be shown to be a risk factor for developing end-stage renal disease among a large population of patients on renal dialysis compared with matched hospitalized patients.[406] Although caution is appropriate in extending these last observations beyond the population in which they were made, they seem to me to have wider implications.[407] In summary, the virtually hypothetical relationship of aspirin to analgesic nephropathy suggests that a physician should not consider it in selecting long-term therapy for rheumatologic diseases, and, indeed, most rheumatologists wisely do not.

Effects on renal function were first discovered in a series of dramatic experiments performed by Hanzlick and Scott and their colleagues over 60 years ago.[408,409] They described mild albuminuria, edema, and a rising blood nitrogen after giving 1 g of sodium salicylate hourly until intolerance, usually about 12 g. Recent experiments showed that aspirin or salicylate could alter creatinine clearance acutely in humans, and that patients with renal disease are more susceptible to these effects.[128,374,410-413] These effects may arouse clinical concern in patients with systemic lupus erythematosus even in the absence of detectable renal disease.[128] In patients with active lupus with or without renal disease, the administration of anti-inflammatory doses of aspirin regularly raises the BUN and serum creatinine and sometimes raises the serum $K+$ and reduces the serum $Na+$.[414] The effect can be dramatic and misleading in the patient with lupus; if aspirin or indeed any of the other prostaglandin synthetase–inhibiting anti-inflammatory agents are administered to a patient with lupus for the management of arthritis, fever, or serositis, any changes in BUN, creatinine, and creatinine clearance must be recognized as possibly due to the drugs in order to avoid unnecessary renal biopsies and therapy. When the drugs are stopped, the changes rapidly recede. Sometimes the changes recede while the drugs are continued, and much clinical experience in lupus suggests that chronic renal changes are not a consequence of continued aspirin therapy. Nevertheless, it is important to recognize that advancing renal disease may sensitize the kidney to the renal effects of this class of drug.

The mechanism probably involves the inhibition of intrarenal prostaglandin synthesis.[415] Urinary prostaglandins fall before creatinine clearance does; the fall in creatinine clearance correlates with a fall in renal blood flow and a fall in inulin clearance; plasma renin falls; and a number of drugs that inhibit prostaglandin synthesis, including indomethacin, ibuprofen, fenoprofen, and naproxen, have the same effect.[414] Although it is possible to demonstrate aspirin-induced changes in creatinine clearance in patients with rheumatoid arthritis and indeed in normals, they are smaller than the changes in lupus and clinically insignificant.[128] Such a difference in susceptibility supports the view that under certain conditions of renal function, renal blood flow is maintained to a greater than normal extent by mechanisms involving prostaglandin synthesis.[416] The prostaglandin synthetase–inhibiting properties of aspirin and indomethacin have been used to advantage to probe the mechanism of and successfully treat the rare Bartter's syndrome.[417]

The relationship between aspirin and the mineralocorticoids is probably complicated and fortunately rarely of clinical interest. Aspirin can compete with al-dosterone receptors in some experimental models,[418] and it can inhibit the action of spironolactone administered to man.[419] The latter action is worth noting for those situations in which the drugs are given together.

The relation to urate excretion is discussed under Interactions with Other Drugs.

In summary, with the exception of the reversible but occasionally dramatic effects of aspirin (and other prostaglandin synthetase-inhibiting drugs) on BUN, creatinine, and creatinine clearance in active lupus, the renal effects of aspirin, although interesting and controversial, are clinically rarely important.

Aspirin or Salicylate Overdose or Accidental Intoxication. The problem of salicylate toxicity caused by accidental overdosage in infants and in children lies beyond the scope of this book and beyond the experience of most rheumatologists. Aspirin or salicylate overdosage in adults occurs in a different setting and presents different metabolic problems. Overdose with suicidal intent is met in the emergency ward. Although the complicating late acidosis of children is not usually a problem in managing adults, and although with modern techniques of rapid laboratory determinations and dialysis fatality is uncommon, death may occur with blood levels less than twice therapeutic levels.[34,420] When it is recognized that the therapeutic serum level of salicylate is in the range of $10^{-3}M$, far higher than almost any other drug, it is not difficult to understand that an organic anion at $4 \times 10^{-3}M$ (the mean serum level in a group of fatal cases)[421] might have many effects beyond its sometimes subtle therapeutic effects.

Salicylate intoxication in adults, however, is by no means limited to the suicidal. On a medical or rheumatology ward, the new appearance of dyspnea, confusion, ataxia, oliguria, or a rising BUN or creatinine in a hospitalized patient who is taking aspirin ought to suggest the possibility of salicylism.[361] After recognition, temporary withdrawal of the drug is usually adequate therapy. In the emergency ward, salicylism should be considered in the differential diagnosis of cardiopulmonary disease presenting dyspnea, tachypnea, or pulmonary edema, or of almost any central nervous system problem, including seizures. Asterixis may be present.[422] Older individuals taking salicylates or aspirin, often for a good reason, are the usual victims of this syndrome.[122,123] It probably arises when a supervening event alters the already peculiar metabolism of salicylate to cause a sudden rise in serum level. Among the events that may do so are acidosis, e.g., from fasting, dehydration, and the ingestion of drugs which displace salicylate from protein-binding sites. In a series of 20 patients with an average age of 53 in whom diagnosis had not been made until 6 or more hours after admission, six died, a far higher mortality than among 53 patients who took the drug with suicide in mind. Therapy consists of a forced diuresis, maintaining the urinary pH in the alkaline range, hemodialysis if diuresis is unsatisfactory, and any other appropriate supportive measures, including removing residual drug from the gastrointestinal tract by emesis, a large-bore stomach tube, or the administration of activated charcoal if that seems indicated by the history. Keeping the urine alkaline abets the excretion of salicylate. Vitamin K has also been recommended because large doses of salicylate may interfere with the synthesis of the vitamin K-dependent clotting factors.

The near-universal tachypnea of salicylism is due not to a metabolic acidosis but to a direct effect on the central nervous system in the medullary respiratory center.[362] Salicylate given intravenously will cause tachypnea, an increase in oxygen consumption and pH, and a decrease in pCO_2 within 1 or 2 minutes, well before any measurable blood acidosis. It has even been proposed that this action of salicylates be harnessed to increased pO_2 and lower pCO_2 in patients with emphysema,[423] but it is doubtless too variable and hazardous, particularly since an effect of salicylate of less rapid onset is increased oxygen consumption and CO_2 production.

There are probably many causes of the diverse central effects of salicylate intoxication. Local brain hypoglycemia may occur, as it does in experimental animals, because high doses of salicylate uncouple oxidative phosphorylation, forcing the brain to maintain its energy supply by markedly increasing glycolysis.[424,425] Indeed, glucose prevents death from salicylate intoxication of experimental animals.

Miscellaneous Effects. Aspirin has been shown to inhibit RNA synthesis of the mouse oocyte,[426] to reduce the growth rate of several mouse tumors,[427] and to alter tumor induction by a mouse tumor virus.[428] These effects have not been shown to depend on those features of the aspirin molecule known to be related to its pharmacology in man. It is likely that they are irrelevant to the clinical action of the salicylates.

There are curious effects of aspirin on experimental traumatic osteoarthritis in dogs,[429,430] which ought not impinge upon the clinical use of aspirin or other prostaglandin synthetase inhibitors at our current state of knowledge.

CONCLUSION

The recent pharmacologic history of the drugs whose action in man depends on inhibition of the synthesis of prostaglandin strongly suggests that no new drug in this class will exceed in clinical efficacy those already in use, although a new drug might show a different spectrum of side effects and toxicities. What appears to limit efficacy is not the power of the drug but the extent to which the prostaglandin system is involved in the inflammation of the connective tissue diseases.

The durability of the salicylates is no accident. Just as the survival of buildings of earlier civilizations is most often rooted in strong materials and sound structure, so is the survival of salicylates rooted in their clear and powerful action and their safety. If they become obsolete in this century, it will be not an indictment of them, but a tribute to the ingenuity of chemists and pharmacologists.

References

1. Gross, M., and Greenberg, L.A.: The Salicylates. A Critical Bibliographic Review. New Haven, Hillhouse Press, 1948.
2. Floeckinger, E.C.: An experimental study of aspirin, a new salicylic-acid preparation. Med. News (N.Y.) 75:645, 1899.
3. Goodwin, J.S., and Goodwin, J.M.: Failure to recognize efficacious treatments: a history of salicylate therapy in rheumatoid arthritis. Perspectives Biol. Med. 25:78, 1981.
4. Leist, E.R., and Banwell, J.G.: Products containing aspirin. N. Engl. J. Med. 291:710, 1974.
5. Vane, J.R.: Inhibition of prostaglandin synthesis as a mechanism of action for aspirin-like drugs. Nature New Biol. 231:232, 1971.
6. Martin, B.K.: The formulation of aspirin. Adv. Pharm. Sci. 3:107, 1971.
7. Leonards, J.R.: Presence of acetylsalicylic acid in plasma following oral ingestion of aspirin. Proc. Soc. Exp. Biol. Med. 110:304, 1962.
8. Leonards, J.R.: The influence of solubility on the rate of gastrointestinal absorption of aspirin. Clin. Pharmacol. Ther. 4:476, 1963.
9. Levy, G., and Yacobi, A.: Assessment of aspirin absorption rate from urinary excretion rate measurements. J. Clin. Pharmacol. 15:525, 1975.
10. Davison, C., Smith, B.W., and Smith, P.K.: Effects of buffered and unbuffered acetylsalicylic acid upon the gastric acidity of normal human subjects. J. Pharm. Sci. 51:759, 1962.
11. Nayak, R.K., Smyth, R.D., Polk, A., Herczeg, T., Carter, V., Visalli, A.J., and Reavey-Cantwell, N.H.: Effect of antacids on aspirin dissolution and bioavailability. J. Pharmacokinet. Biopharm. 5:597, 1977.
12. Douthwaite, A.H., and Lintott, G.A.M.: Gastroscopic observation of the effect of aspirin and certain other substances on the stomach. Br. Med. J. 2:1222, 1938.
13. Hogben, C.A.M., Schanker, L.S., Tocco, D.J., and Brodie, B.B.: Absorption of drugs from the stomach. II. The human. J. Pharmacol. Exp. Ther. 120:540, 1957.
14. Truitt, E.B., and Morgan, A.M.: Absorption of aspirin from the stomach in man. Toxicol. Appl. Pharmacol. 2:237, 1960.
15. Dotevall, G., and Ekenved, G.: The absorption of acetylsalicylic acid from the stomach in relation to intragastric pH. Scand. J. Gastroenterol. 11:801, 1976.
16. Hogben, C.A.M., Tocco, D.J., Brodie, B.B., and Schanker, L.S.: On the mechanism of intestinal absorption of drugs. J. Pharmacol. Exp. Ther. 125:275, 1959.
17. Nogami, H., and Matsuzawa, T.: Studies on absorption and excretion of drugs. I. Kinetics of penetration of acidic drug, salicylic acid, through the intestinal barrier in vitro. Chem. Pharm. Bull. 9:532, 1961.
18. Davenport, H.W.: Damage to the gastric mucosa: Effects of salicylates and stimulation. Gastroenterology 49:189, 1965.
19. Flower, R.J., and Vane, J.R.: Some pharmacologic and biochemical aspects of prostaglandin biosynthesis and its inhibition. In Robinson, H.J., and Vane, J.R. (eds.): Prostaglandin Synthesis Inhibitors. New York, Raven Press, 1974.
20. Lester, D., Lolli, G., and Greenberg, L.A.: The fate of acetylsalicylic acid. J. Pharmacol. Exp. Ther. 87:329, 1946.
21. Mandel, H.G., Cambosos, N.M., and Smith P.K.: The presence of aspirin in human plasma after oral administration. J. Pharmacol. Exp. Ther. 112:495, 1954.
22. Soren, A.: Dissociation of acetylsalicylic acid in blood and joint fluid. Scand. J. Rheumatol. 6:17, 1977.
23. Petersen, T., Husted, S.E., Pedersen, A.K., and Gedary, E.: Systemic availability of acetylsalicylic acid in human subjects after oral ingestion of three different formulations. Acta Pharmacol. Toxicol. 51:285, 1982.
24. Roth, G.J., and Majerus, P.W.: The mechanism of the effect of aspirin on human platelets. I. Acetylation of a particulate fraction protein. J. Clin. Invest. 56:624, 1975.
25. Bridges, K.R., Schmidt, G.J., Jensen, M., Cerami, M., and Bunn, H.F.: The acetylation of hemoglobin by aspirin. In vitro and in vivo. J. Clin. Invest. 56:201, 1975.
26. Walker, J.E.: Lysine residue 199 of human serum albumin is modified by acetylsalicylic acid. FEBS Letters 66:173, 1976.
27. Mulinos, M.G., and Ardam, I.: An aspirin splitting enzyme in blood (abstract). J. Pharmacol. Exp. Ther. 98:23, 1950.
28. Rainsford, K.D., Ford, N.L.V., Brooks, P.M., and Watson, H.M.: Plasma aspirin esterases in normal individuals, patients with alcoholic liver disease and rheumatoid arthritis: characterization and the importance of the enzymic components. Eur. J. Clin. Invest. 10:413, 1980.
29. Costello, P.B., and Green, F.A.: Aspirin survival in human blood modulated by the concentration of erythrocytes. Arthritis Rheum. 25:550, 1982.
30. Lowenthal, D.T., Briggs, W.A., and Levy, G.: Kinetics of salicylate elimination by anephric patients. J. Clin. Invest. 54:1221, 1974.
31. Levy, G., Procknal, J.A., and Garrettson, L.K.: Distribution of salicylate between neonatal and maternal serum at diffusion equilibrium. Clin. Pharmacol. Ther. 18:210, 1975.

746

Clinical Pharmacology

32. Clark, J.H., and Wilson, W.G.: A 16-day-old breast-fed infant with metabolic acidosis caused by salicylate. Clin. Pediatr. 20:53, 1981.

33. Reed, J.R., and Palmisano, P.A.: Central nervous system salicylate. Clin. Toxicol. 8:623, 1975.

34. Hill, J.B.: Salicylate intoxication. N. Engl. J. Med. 288:1110, 1973.

35. Schachter, D., and Manis, J.G.: Salicylate and salicyl conjugates: Fluorimetric estimation, biosynthesis and renal excretion in man. J. Clin. Invest. 37:800, 1958.

36. Flower, R.J., and Vane, J.R.: Some pharmacologic and biochemical aspects of prostaglandin biosynthesis and its inhibition. In Robinson, H.J., and Vane, J.R. (eds.): Prostaglandin Synthesis Inhibitors. New York, Raven Press, 1974.

37. Paulus, H.E., Siegel, M., Mongan, E., Okun, R., and Calabro, J.J.: Variations of serum concentrations and half-life of salicylates in patients with rheumatoid arthritis. Arthritis Rheum. 14:527, 1971.

38. Smith, P.K., Gleason, H.L., Stoll, C.G., and Ogorzalek, S.: Studies on the pharmacology of salicylates. J. Pharmacol. Exp. Ther. 87:237, 1946.

39. Levy, G., and Leonards, J.R.: Urine pH and salicylate therapy (letter). JAMA 217:81, 1971.

40. Levy, G., Lampman, T., Kamath, B.L., and Garrettson, L.K.: Decreased serum salicylate concentration in children with rheumatic fever treated with antacid. N. Engl. J. Med. 293:323, 1975.

41. Levy, G., Tsuchiya, T., and Amsel, L.P.: Limited capacity for salicyl phenolic glucuronide formation and its effect on the kinetics of salicylate elimination in man. Clin. Pharmacol. Ther. 13:258, 1972.

42. Tsuchiya, T., and Levy, G.: Biotransformation of salicylic acid to its acyl and phenolic glucuronides in man. J. Pharm. Sci. 61:800, 1972.

43. Gupta, N., Sarkissian, E., and Paulus, H.E.: Correlation of plateau serum salicylate level with rate of salicylate metabolism. Clin. Pharmacol. Ther. 18:350, 1975.

44. Furst, D.E., Gupta, N., and Paulus, H.E.: Salicylate metabolism in twins. Evidence suggesting a genetic influence and induction of salicylurate formation. J. Clin. Invest. 60:32, 1977.

45. Ayres, J.W., Weidler, D.J., Mackichan, J., and Wagner, J.G.: Circadian rhythm of urinary pH in man with and without chronic antacid administration. Eur. J. Cin. Pharmacol. 12:415, 1977.

46. Rumble, R.H., Brooks, P.M., and Roberts, M.S.: Metabolism of salicylate during chronic aspirin therapy. Br. J. Clin. Pharmac. 9:41, 1980.

47. Keystone, E.C., Paton, T.W., Littlejohn, G., Verdejo, A., Piper, S., Wright, L.A., and Goldsmith, C.H.: Steady-state plasma levels of salicylate in patients with rheumatoid arthritis: effects of dosing interval and tablet strength. Canad. Med. Assoc. J. 127:283, 1982.

48. Algozzine, G.J., Stein, G.H., Doering, P.L., and Araujo, O.E.: Trolamine salicylate cream in osteoarthritis of the knee. JAMA 247:1311, 1982.

49. Rylance, H.J., Chalmers, T.M., and Elton, R.A.: Clinical trials of intra-articular aspirin in rheumatoid arthritis. Lancet 2:1099, 1980.

50. McAteer, E., and Dundee, J.W.: Injectable aspirin as a postoperative analgesic. Br. J. Anaesth. 53:1069, 1981.

51. Harrison, L.I., Funk, M.L., Ré, O.N., and Ober, R.E.: Absorption, biotransformation, and pharmacokinetics of salicylsalicylic acid in humans. J. Clin. Pharmacol. 21:401, 1981.

52. Verbeeck, R.K., Boel, A., Buntinx, A., and DeSchepper, P.J.: Plasma protein binding and interaction studies with diflunisal, a new salicylate analgesic. Biochem. Pharmacol. 29:571, 1980.

53. Chan, L.K., Winearls, C.G., Oliver, D.O., and Dunnill, M.S.: Acute interstitial nephritis and erythroderma associated with diflunisal. Br. Med. J. 280:84, 1980.

54. Wharton, J.G., Oliver, D.O., and Dunnill, M.S.: Acute renal failure associated with diflunisal. Postgrad. Med. J. 58:104, 1982.

55. Diflunisal. Medical Letter 24:76, 1982.

56. Mason, W.D.: Comparative plasma salicylate and urine salicylate levels following administration of aspirin, magnesium salicylate, and choline magnesium trisalicylate. J. Pharm. Sci. 69:1355, 1980.

57. Binus, M.H., Lyon, J.A., and Nicholas, J.L.: Comparable serum salicylate concentrations from choline magnesium trisalicylate, aspirin, and buffered aspirin in rheumatoid arthritis. Arthritis Rheum. 25:464, 1982.

58. Rainsford, K.D., and Whitehouse, M.W.: Biochemical gastroprotection from acute ulceration induced by aspirin and related drugs. Biochem. Pharmacol. 29:1281, 1980.

59. Aarons, L.J., Bochner, F., and Rowland, M.: A chronic dose-ranging kinetic study of salicylate in man (abstract). Br. J. Pharmacol. 61:456P, 1977.

60. Bernheim, H.A., and Kluger, M.J.: Fever: Effect of drug-induced antipyresis on survival. Science 193:237, 1976.

61. Jackson, D.L.: A hypothalamic region responsive to localized injection of pyrogens. J. Neurophysiol. 30:586, 1967.

62. Cooper, K.E., Cranston, W.I., and Honour, A.J.: Observations on the site and mode of action of pyrogens in the rabbit brain. J. Physiol. 191:325, 1967.

63. Dinarello, C.A., and Wolff, S.M.: Molecular basis of fever in humans. Am. J. Med. 72:799, 1982.

64. Milton, A.S., and Wendlandt, S.: A possible role for prostaglandin E₁

65. Chai, C.Y., Lin, M.T., Chen, H.I., and Wang, S.C.: The site of action of leukocytic pyrogen and antipyresis of sodium acetylsalicylate in monkeys. Neuropharmacology 10:715, 1971.

66. Lin, M.T., and Chai, C.Y.: The antipyretic effect of sodium acetylsalicylate on pyrogen-induced fever in rabbits. J. Pharmacol. Exp. Ther. 180:603, 1972.

67. Flower, R.J., and Vane, J.R.: Inhibition of prostaglandin synthetase in brain explains the antipyretic activity of paracetamol (4-acetamidophenol). Nature 240:410, 1972.

68. Seed, J.C.: A clinical comparison of the antipyretic potency of aspirin and sodium salicylate. Clin. Pharmacol. Ther. 6:354, 1965.

69. Feldberg, W., and Gupta, K.P.: Pyrogen fever and prostaglandin-like activity in cerebrospinal fluid. J. Physiol. 228:41, 1973.

70. Schoener, E.P., and Wang, S.C.: Sodium acetylsalicylate effectiveness against fever induced by leukocyte pyrogen and prostaglandin E₁ in the cat. Experientia 30:383, 1974.

71. Woolf, C.J., Willies, G.H., Laburn, H., and Rosendorff, C.: Pyrogen and prostaglandin fever in the rabbit. I. Effects of salicylate and the role of cyclic AMP. Neuropharmacology 14:397, 1975.

72. Bodel, P., Reynolds, C.F., and Atkins, E.: Lack of effect of salicylate on pyrogen release from human blood leucocytes in vitro. Yale J. Biol. Med. 46:190, 1973.

73. Schoener, E.P., and Wang, S.C.: Observations on the central mechanism of acetylsalicylate antipyresis. Life Sci. 17:1063, 1975.

74. Avery, D.D., and Penn, P.E.: Blockade of pyrogen induced fever by intrahypothalamic injections of salicylate in the rat. Neuropharmacology 13:1179, 1974.

75. Satinoff, E.: Salicylate: Action on normal body temperature in rats. Science 176:532, 1972.

76. Pittman, Q.J., Veale, W.L., and Cooper, K.E.: Observations on the effect of salicylate in fever and the regulation of body temperature against cold. Can. J. Physiol. Pharmacol. 54:101, 1976.

77. Lim, R.K.S.: Salicylate analgesia. In Smith, M.J.H., and Smith, P.K. (eds.): The Salicylates. A Critical Bibliographic Review. New York, Wiley, 1966.

78. Wallenstein, S.L., and Houde, R.W.: Clinical comparison of analgetic effectiveness of N-acetyl-p-aminophenol, salicylamide and aspirin (abstract). Fed. Proc. 13:414, 1954.

79. Houde, R.W., Wallenstein, S.L., and Rogers, A.: Clinical pharmacology of analgesics. I. A method of assaying analgesic effect. Clin. Pharmacol. Ther. 1:163, 1960.

80. Fremont-Smith, K., and Bayles, T.B.: Salicylate therapy in rheumatoid arthritis. A scientific exhibit. JAMA 190:383, 1964. (Cited in Reference 77.)

81. Lasagna, L.: Analgesic drugs. Am. J. Med. Sci. 242:620, 1960.

82. Guzman, F., Braun, C., Lim, R.K.S., Potter, G.D., and Rodgers, D.W.: Narcotic and non-narcotic analgesics which block visceral pain evoked by intra-arterial injection of bradykinin and other algesic agents. Arch. Int. Pharmacodyn. Ther. 149:571, 1964.

83. Lim, R.K.S., Guzman, F., Rodgers, D.W., Goto, K., Braun, C., Dickerson, G.D., and Engle, R.J.: Site of action of narcotic and non-narcotic analgesics determined by blocking bradykinin-evoked visceral pain. Arch. Int. Pharmacodyn. Ther. 152:25, 1964.

84. Winder, C.V.: Aspirin and algesimetry. Nature 184:494, 1959.

85. Guilbaud, G., Benoist, J.M., Gautron, M., and Kayser, V.: Aspirin clearly depresses responses of ventrobasal thalamus neurons to joint stimuli in arthritic rats. Pain 13:153, 1982.

86. Hashimoto, K., Kumakura, S., and Taira, N.: Vascular reflex responses induced by an intra-arterial injection of azaazepinophenothiazine, andromedotoxin, veratridine, bradykinin and kallikrein and blocking action of sodium salicylate. Jap. J. Physiol. 14:299, 1964.

87. Thompkins, L., and Lee, K.H.: Comparison of analgesic effects of isosteric variations of salicylic acid and aspirin (acetylsalicylic acid). J. Pharm. Sci. 64:760, 1975.

88. Ferreira, S.H., Moncada, S., and Vane J.R.: Further experiments to establish that the analgesic action of aspirin-like drugs depends on the inhibition of prostaglandin biosynthesis (abstract). Br. J. Pharmacol. 47:629P, 1973.

89. Willis, A.L., and Cornelsen, M.: Repeated injection of prostaglandin E₂ in rat paws induces chronic swelling and a marked decrease in pain threshold. Prostaglandins 3:353, 1973.

90. Ferreira, S.H.: Prostaglandins, aspirin-like drugs and analgesia. Nature New Biol. 240:200, 1972.

91. Rosenthale, M.E., Dervinis, A., Kassarich, J., and Singer, S.: Prostaglandins and anti-inflammatory drugs in the dog knee joint. J. Pharm. Pharmacol. 24:149, 1972.

92. Levitan, H., and Barker, J.L.: Effect of non-narcotic analgesics on membrane permeability of molluscan neurones. Nature New Biol. 239:55, 1972.

93. Beaven, M.A., Horakova, Z., and Keiser, H.R.: Interference with histamine and imidazole acetic acid metabolism by salicylates: A possible

contribution to salicylate analgesic activity? Experientia 32:1180, 1976.

94. Moss, J., De Mello, M.C., Vaughn, M., and Beaven, M.A.: Effect of salicylates on histamine and L-histidine metabolism. Inhibition of imidazoleacetate phosphoribosyl transferase. J. Clin. Invest. 58:137, 1976.

95. Boardman, P.L., and Hart, F.D.: Clinical measurement of the anti-inflammatory effects of salicylates in rheumatoid arthritis. Br. Med. J. 2:264, 1967.

96. Robinson, D.R., and Levine, L.: Prostaglandin concentrations in synovial fluid in rheumatic diseases: Action of indomethacin and aspirin. In Robinson, H.J., and Vane, J.R. (eds.): Prostaglandin Synthetase Inhibitors. New York, Raven Press, 1974.

97. Winter, C.A., Risley, E.A., and Nuss, G.W.: Carrageenan-induced edema in hind paw of the rat as an assay for anti-inflammatory drugs. Proc. Soc. Exp. Biol. Med. 111:544, 1962.

98. Mielens, Z.E., Drobeck, H.P., Rozitis, J., and Sansone, V.J.: Interaction of aspirin with non-steroidal anti-inflammatory drugs in rats (letter). J. Pharm. Pharmacol. 20:567, 1968.

99. Swingle, K.F., Grant, T.J., Jaques, L.W., and Kvam, D.C.: Interactions of anti-inflammatory drugs in carrageenan-induced foot edema of the rat. J. Pharmacol. Exp. Ther. 172:423, 1970.

100. Willis, A.L., Davison, P., Ramwell, P.W., Brocklehurst, W.E., and Smith, B.: Release and actions of prostaglandins in inflammation and fever: Inhibition by anti-inflammatory and antipyretic drugs. In Ramwell, P.W., and Pharriss, B.B. (eds.): Prostaglandins in Cellular Biology. New York, Plenum Press, 1972.

101. Vinegar, R., Truax, J.F., and Selph, J.L.: Some quantitative temporal characteristics of carrageenan-induced pleurisy in the rat. Proc. Soc. Exp. Biol. Med. 143:711, 1973.

102. Randall, L.O., Selitto, J.J., and Valdes, J.: Anti-inflammatory effects of xylopropamine. Arch. Int. Pharmacodyn. Ther. 113:233, 1957.

103. Gilfoil, T.M., Klavins, I., and Grumbach, L.: Effects of acetylsalicylic acid on the edema and hyperesthesia of the experimentally inflamed rat's paw. J. Pharmacol. Exp. Ther. 142:1, 1963.

104. Van Arman, C.G., Carlson, R.P., Risley, E.A., Thomas, R.H., and Nuss, G.W.: Inhibitory effects of indomethacin, aspirin and certain other drugs on inflammations induced in rat and dog by carrageenan, sodium urate and ellagic acid. J. Pharmacol. Exp. Ther. 175:459, 1970.

105. Smith, M.J.H.: Anti-inflammatory activity of salicylates. In Smith, M.J.H., and Smith, P.K. (eds.): The Salicylates. A Critical Bibliographic Review. New York, Wiley, 1966.

106. Winter, C.A., and Nuss, G.W.: Treatment of adjuvant arthritis in rats with anti-inflammatory drugs. Arthritis Rheum. 9:394, 1966.

107. Van Arman, C.G., Nuss, G.W., and Risley, E.A.: Interactions of aspirin, indomethacin and other drugs in adjuvant-induced arthritis in the rat. J. Pharmacol. Exp. Ther. 187:400, 1973.

108. Sofia, R.D., Knobloch, L.C., and Douglas, J.F.: Effect of concurrent administration of aspirin, indomethacin or hydrocortisone with gold sodium thiomalate against adjuvant-induced arthritis in the rat. Agents Actions 6:728, 1976.

109. Gold, E.W., Anderson, L.B., Schwartz, E.R., and Miller, C.W.: The effect of salicylate on prostaglandin levels in rabbit knees following inducement of osteoarthritic changes. Prostaglandins 12:837, 1976.

110. Goldlust, M.B., Rich, L.C., and Harrity, T.W.: Effects of anti-inflammatory agents on the acute response of immune synovitis in rabbits. Arthritis Rheum. 20:937, 1977.

111. Robinson, D.R., Tashjian, A.H., and Levine, L.: Prostaglandin-induced bone resorption by rheumatoid synovia. Trans. Assoc. Am. Physicians 88:146, 1975.

112. Dayer, J-M., Robinson, D.R., and Krane, S.M.: Prostaglandin production by rheumatoid synovial cells. J. Exp. Med. 145:1399, 1977.

113. Kaley, G., and Weiner, R.: Prostaglandin E_1: A potential mediator of the inflammatory response. Ann. N.Y. Acad. Sci. 180:338, 1971.

114. Higgs, G.A., McCall, E., and Youlten, L.J.F.: A chemotactic role for prostaglandins released from polymorphonuclear leukocytes during phagocytosis. Br. J. Pharmacol. 53:539, 1975.

115. MacGregor, R.R., Spagnuolo, P.J., and Lentnek, A.L.: Inhibition of granulocyte adherence by ethanol, prednisone, and aspirin, measured with an assay system. N. Engl. J. Med. 291:642, 1974.

116. Zurier, R.B.: Prostaglandins, immune responses, and murine lupus. Arthritis Rheum. 25:804, 1982.

117. Robinson, H.J., Phares, H.F., and Graessle, O.E.: Prostaglandin synthetase inhibitors and infection. In Robinson, H.J., and Vane, J.R. (eds.): Prostaglandin Synthetase Inhibitors. New York, Raven Press, 1974.

118. Stone, C.A., Van Arman, C.G., Peck, H.M., Minsker, D.H., and Ham, E.A.: Pharmacologic and toxicologic action of prostaglandin synthetase inhibitors: Potential role of prostaglandin synthesis blockade. In Robinson, H.J., and Vane, J.R. (eds.): Prostaglandin Synthetase Inhibitors, New York, Raven Press, 1974.

119. Ferreira, S.H., Moncada, S., and Vane, J.R.: Prostaglandins and signs and symptoms of inflammation. In Robinson, H.J., and Vane, J.R. (eds.): Prostaglandin Synthetase Inhibitors. New York, Raven Press, 1974.

120. Stefanovich, V.: Inhibition of 3', 5'-cyclic AMP phosphodiesterase with anti-inflammatory agents. Res. Commun. Chem. Pathol. Pharmacol. 7:573, 1974.

121. Halla, J.T., Fallahi, S., and Hardin, J.G.: Acute and chronic salicylate intoxication in a patient with gastric outlet obstruction. Arthritis Rheum. 24:1205, 1981.

122. Heffner, J.E., and Sahn, S.A.: Salicylate-induced pulmonary edema. Ann. Intern. Med. 95:404, 1981.

123. Walters, J.S., Woodring, J.H., Stelling, C.B., and Rosenbaum, H.D.: Salicylate-induced pulmonary edema. Radiology 146:289, 1983.

124. Athreya, B.H., Moser, G., Cecil, H.S., and Myers, A.R.: Aspirin-induced hepatotoxicity in juvenile rheumatoid arthritis. Arthritis Rheum. 18:347, 1975.

125. Doughty, R.A., Giesecke, L., and Athreya, B.H.: Salicylate therapy in juvenile rheumatoid arthritis. Am. J. Dis. Child. 134:461, 1980.

126. Baum, J.: New thoughts on aspirin. Am. J. Dis. Child. 134:455, 1980.

127. Ropes, M.W.: Systemic Lupus Erythematosus. Cambridge, Mass., Harvard University Press, 1976.

128. Kimberly, R.P., and Plotz, P.H.: Aspirin-induced depression of renal function. N. Engl. J. Med. 296:418, 1977.

129. Buckingham, R.B.: Interactions involving anti-rheumatic drugs, I and II. Bull. Rheum. Dis. 28:960, 1978.

130. Mason, R.W., and McQueen, E.G.: Protein binding of indomethacin: Binding of indomethacin to human plasma albumin and its displacement from binding by ibuprofen, phenylbutazone and salicylate, in vitro. Pharmacology 12:12, 1974.

131. Jeremy, R., and Towson, J.: Interaction between aspirin and indomethacin in the treatment of rheumatoid arthritis. Med. J. Aust. 2:127, 1970.

132. Champion, G.D., Paulus, H.E., Mongan, E., Okun, R., and Pearson, C.M.: The effect of aspirin on serum indomethacin. Clin. Pharmacol. Ther. 13:239, 1972.

133. Garnham, J.C., Raymond, K., Shotton, E., and Turner, P.: The effect of buffered aspirin on plasma indomethacin. Eur. J. Clin. Pharmacol. 8:107, 1975.

134. Kaldestad, E., Hansen, T., and Brath, H.K.: Interaction of indomethacin and acetylsalicylic acid as shown by the serum concentrations of indomethacin and salicylate. Eur. J. Clin. Pharmacol. 9:199, 975.

135. Barraclough, D.R., Muirden, K.D., and Laby, B.: Salicylate therapy and drug interaction in rheumatoid arthritis. Aust. N.Z. J. Med. 5:518, 1975.

136. Rome, L.H., Lands, W.E., Roth, G.J., and Majerus, P.W.: Aspirin as a quantitative acetylating reagent for the fatty acid oxygenase that forms prostaglandins. Prostaglandins 11:23, 1976.

137. Thomas, B.H., Zeitz, W., and Coldwell, B.B.: Effect of aspirin on biotransformation of 14C-acetaminophen in rats. J. Pharm. Sci. 63:1367, 1974.

138. Whitehouse, L.W., Paul, C.J., and Thomas, B.H.: Effect of aspirin on fate of 14C-acetaminophen in guinea pigs. J. Pharm. Sci. 64:819, 1975.

139. Whitehouse, L.W., Paul, C.J., and Thomas, B.H.: Effect of acetylsalicylic acid on a toxic dose of acetaminophen in the mouse. Toxicol. Appl. Pharmacol. 38:571, 1976.

140. Cotty, V.F., Sterbenz, F.J., Mueller, F., Melman, K., Ederma, H., Skerpac, J., Hunter, D., and Lehr, M.: Augmentation of human blood acetylsalicylate concentration by the simultaneous administration of acetaminophen with aspirin. Toxicol. Appl. Pharmacol. 41:7, 1977.

141. Muirden, K.D., Deutschman, P., and Phillips, M.: Competition between salicylate and other drugs in binding to human serum protein in vitro. Aust. N.Z. J. Med. 4:149, 1974.

142. Segre, E., Chaplin, M., Forchelli, E., Runkel, R., and Sevelius, H.: Naproxen-aspirin interactions in man. Clin. Pharmacol. Ther. 15:374, 1974.

143. Rubin, A., Rodda, B.E., Warrick, P., Gruber, C.M., and Ridolfo, A.S.: Interactions of aspirin with non-steroidal anti-inflammatory drugs in man. Arthritis Rheum. 16:635, 1973.

144. Quick, A.J., and Clesceri, L.: Influence of acetylsalicylic acid and salicylamide on the coagulation of blood. J. Pharmacol. Exp. Ther. 128:95, 1960.

145. Loew, D., and Vinazzer, H.: Dose dependent influence of acetylsalicylic acid on platelet functions and plasmatic coagulation factors. Haemostasis 5:239, 1976.

146. Kelley, W.N.: Effects of drugs on uric acid in man. Ann. Rev. Pharmacol. Toxicol. 15:327, 1975.

147. Sorensen, L.B., and Levinson, D.J.: Clinical evaluation of benzbromarone. A new uricosuric drug. Arthritis Rheum. 19:183, 1976.

148. Berg, K.J.: Acute effects of acetylsalicylic acid in patients with chronic renal insufficiency. Europ. J. Clin. Pharm. 11:111, 1977.

149. Mirouze, D., Zipser, R.D., and Reynolds, T.B.: Effect of inhibitors of prostaglandin synthesis on induced diuresis in cirrhosis. Hepatology 3:50, 1983.

150. Seino, Y., Usami, M., Nakahara, H., Takemura, J., Nishi, S., Ishida, H., Ikeda, M., and Imura, H.: Effect of acetylsalicylic acid on blood glucose and glucose regulatory hormones in mild diabetes. Prostaglandins Leukotrienes Med. 8:49, 1982.

151. Jaffe, R.M., Kasten, B., Young, D.S., and MacLowry, J.D.: False-negative stool occult blood tests caused by ingestion of ascorbic acid (vitamin C). Ann. Intern. Med. 83:824, 1975.

152. Klinenberg, J.R., and Miller, F.: Effect of corticosteroids on blood salicylate concentration. JAMA 194:601, 1965.

153. Deykin, D., Janson, P., and McMahon, L.: Ethanol potentiation of aspirin-induced prolongation of the bleeding time. N. Engl. J. Med. 306:852, 1982.

154. Mandel, M.A.: The synergistic effect of salicylate on methotrexate toxicity. Plast. Reconstr. Surg. 57:733, 1976.

155. Zuik, M., and Mandel, M.A.: Methotrexate-salicylate interaction: A clinical and experimental study. Surg. Forum 26:567, 1975.

156. Leonard, R.F., Knott, P.J., Rankin, G.O., Robinson, D.S., and Melnick, D.E.: Phenytoin-salicylate interaction. Clin. Pharmacol. Ther. 29:56, 1981.

157. Collins, E.: Maternal and fetal effects of acetaminophen and salicylates in pregnancy. Obstet. Gynecol. 58 (Suppl.):57S, 1981.

158. Slone, D., Siskind, V., Heinonen, O.P., Monson, R.P., Kaufman, D.W., and Shapiro, S.: Aspirin and congenital malformations. Lancet 1:1373, 1976.

159. Turner, G., and Collins, E.: Fetal effects of regular salicylate ingestion in pregnancy. Lancet 2:338, 1975.

160. Rumack, C.M., Guggenheim, M.A., Rumack, B.H., Peterson, R.G., Johnson, M.L., and Braithwaite, W.R.: Neonatal intracranial hemorrhage and maternal use of aspirin. Obstet. Gynecol. 58(Suppl):52S, 1981.

161. Stuart, M.J., Gross, S.J., Elrad, H., and Graeber, J.E.: Effects of acetylsalicylic-acid ingestion on maternal and neonatal hemostasis. N. Engl. J. Med. 307:909, 1982.

162. Shapiro, S., Siskind, V., Monson, R.P., Heinonen, O.P., Kaufman, D.W., and Slone, D.: Perinatal mortality and birth-weight in relation to aspirin taken during pregnancy. Lancet 1:1375, 1976.

163. Collins, E., and Turner, G.: Maternal effects of regular salicylate ingestion in pregnancy. Lancet 2:335, 1975.

164. Lewis, R.B., and Schulman, J.D.: Influence of acetylsalicylic acid, an inhibitor of prostaglandin synthesis, on the duration of human gestation and labor. Lancet 2:1159, 1973.

165. Levin, D.L.: Effect of inhibition of prostaglandin synthesis on fetal development, oxygenation, and the fetal circulation. Sem. Perinatol. 4:35, 1980.

166. Settipane, R.A., Constantine, H.P., and Settipane, G.A.: Aspirin intolerance and recurrent urticaria in normal adults and children. Allergy 35:149, 1980.

167. Lamson, R.W., and Thomas, R.: Some untoward effects of acetylsalicylic acid. JAMA 99:107, 1932.

168. Samter, M., and Beers, R.F.: Concerning the nature of intolerance to aspirin. J. Allergy 40:281, 1967.

169. Friedlaender, S., and Feinberg, S.M.: Aspirin allergy: Its relationship to chronic intractable asthma. Ann. Intern. Med. 26:734, 1947.

170. Feinberg, A.R., and Malkiel, S.: Aspirin sensitivity—experimental studies. J. Allergy 22:74, 1951.

171. Schlumberger, H.D., Lobbecke, E.A., and Kallos, P.: Acetylsalicylic acid intolerance. Acta Med. Scand. 196:451, 1974.

172. Delaney, J.C.: The diagnosis of aspirin idiosyncrasy by analgesic challenge. Clin. Allergy 6:177, 1976.

173. Szczeklik, A., Gryglewski, R.J., and Czerniawska-Mysik, G.: Relationship of inhibition of prostaglandin biosynthesis by analgesics to asthma attacks in aspirin-sensitive patients. Br. Med. J. 1:67, 1975.

174. Szczeklik, A., Gryglewski, R.J., Czerniawska-Mysik, G., and Zmuda, A.: Aspirin-induced asthma. Hypersensitivity to fenoprofen and ibuprofen in relation to their inhibitory action on prostaglandin generation by different microsomal enzymic preparations. J. Allergy Clin. Immunol. 58:10, 1976.

175. Settipane, G.A., and Pudupakkam, R.K.: Aspirin intolerance. III. Subtypes, familial occurrence, and cross-reactivity with tartrazine. J. Allergy Clin. Immunol. 56:215, 1975.

176. Settipane, G.A., Chafee, F.H., and Klein, D.E.: Aspirin intolerance. II. A prospective study in an atopic and normal population. J. Allergy Clin. Immunol. 53:200, 1974.

177. Myers, E.N., and Bernstein, J.M.: Salicylate ototoxicity. A clinical and experimental study. Arch. Otolaryngol. 82:483, 1965.

178. Silverstein, H., Bernstein, J.M., and Davies, D.G.: Salicylate ototoxicity. A biochemical and electrophysiological study. Ann. Otol. 76:118, 1967.

179. Aly, S., Mousa, S., el-Kahky, M., Saleh, A., and el-Mofty, A.: Toxic deafness. I. J. Egypt. Med. Assoc. 58:144, 1975.

180. Aly, S., el-Kahky, M., Eid, S., Mousa, S., Ramandan, M., Saleh, A., and el-Mofty, A.: Toxic deafness. II. J. Egypt. Med. Assoc. 58:158, 1975.

181. Crifo, S.: Aspirin ototoxicity in the guinea pig. ORL 37:27, 1975.

182. Krzanowski, J.J., Jr., and Matschinsky, F.M.: Adenosine triphosphate and phosphocreatinine levels in cochlear structures. Use rate and effect of salicylates. J. Histochem. Cytochem. 23:766, 1975.

183. Bernstein, J.M., and Weiss, A.D.: Further observations on salicylate ototoxicity. J. Laryngol. Otol. 81:915, 1967.

184. Mongan, E., Kelly, P., Nies, K., Porter, W.W., and Paulus, H.E.: Tinnitus as an indication of therapeutic serum salicylate levels. JAMA 226:142, 1973.

185. Muir, A., and Cossar, I.A.: Aspirin and ulcer. Br. Med. J. 2:7, 1955.

186. Batterman, R.C.: Comparison of buffered and unbuffered acetylsalicylic acid. N. Engl. J. Med. 258:213, 1958.

187. Cronk, G.A.: Laboratory and clinical studies with buffered and non-buffered acetylsalicylic acid. N. Engl. J. Med. 258:219, 1958.

188. Sadove, M.S., and Schwartz, L.: An evaluation of buffered versus non-buffered acetylsalicylic acid. Postgrad. Med. 24:183, 1958.

189. Miller, R.R.: Analgesics. In Miller, R.R., and Greenblatt, D.J. (eds.): Drug Effects in Hospitalized Patients. New York, Wiley, 1976.

190. Linnoila, M., and Lehtola, J.: Absorption, and effect on gastric mucosa, of buffered and non-buffered tablets of acetylsalicylic acid. Int. J. Clin. Pharmacol. Biopharm. 15:61, 1977.

191. Stubbe, L.: Occult blood in faeces after administration of aspirin. Br. Med. J. 2:1061, 1958.

192. Weiss, A., Pitman, E.R., and Graham, E.C.: Aspirin and gastric bleeding. Am. J. Med. 31:266, 1961.

193. Wood, P.H.N., Harvey-Smith, E.A., and Dixon, A. St.J.: Salicylates and gastrointestinal bleeding. Acetylsalicylic acid and aspirin derivatives. Br. Med. J. 1:669, 1962.

194. Metzger, W.H., McAdam, L., Bluestone, R., and Guth, P.H.: Acute gastric mucosal injury during continuous or interrupted aspirin ingestion in humans. Am J. Dig. Dis. 21:963, 1976.

195. Caravati, C.M., and Cosgrove, E.F.: Salicylate toxicity: The probable mechanism of its action. Ann. Intern. Med. 24:638, 1946.

196. Pierson, R.N., Holt, P.R., Watson, R.M., and Keating, R.P.: Aspirin and gastrointestinal bleeding. Am J. Med. 31:259, 1961.

197. Leonards, J.R.: Aspirin and gastrointestinal blood loss. Gastroenterology 44:617, 1963.

198. Croft, D.N., and Wood, P.H.N.: Gastric mucosa and susceptibility to occult gastrointestinal bleeding caused by aspirin. Br. Med. J. 1:137, 1967.

199. Goulston, K., and Cooke, A.R.: Alcohol, aspirin, and gastrointestinal bleeding. Br. Med. J. 4:664, 1968.

200. Leonards, J.R., and Levy, G.: Aspirin-induced occult gastrointestinal blood loss: Local versus systemic effects. J. Pharm. Sci. 59:1511, 1970.

201. Jabbari, M., and Valberg, L.S.: Role of acid secretion in aspirin-induced gastric mucosal injury. Can. Med. Assoc. J. 102:178, 1970.

202. St. John, D.J.B., and McDermott, F.T.: Influence of achlorhydria on aspirin-induced occult gastrointestinal blood loss: Studies in Addisonian pernicious anemia. Br. Med. J. 2:450, 1970.

203. Scott, J.T., Porter, I.H., Lewis, S.M., and Dixon, A. St.J.: Study of gastrointestinal bleeding caused by corticosteroids, salicylates and other analgesics. Quart. J. Med. 30:167, 1961.

204. Grossman, M.I., Matsumoto, K.K., and Lichter, R.J.: Fecal blood loss produced by oral and intravenous administration of various salicylates. Gastroenterology 40:383, 1961.

205. Stubbe, L., Pietersen, J.H., and van Heulen, C.: Aspirin preparations and their noxious effect on the gastrointestinal tract. Br. Med. J. 1:675, 1962.

206. Beeken, W.L.: Effect of five salicylate-containing compounds upon loss of ^{51}chromium-labeled erythrocytes from the gastrointestinal tract of normal man. Gut 9:475, 1968.

207. Leonards, J.R., and Levy, G.: Reduction or prevention of aspirin-induced occult gastrointestinal blood loss in man. Clin. Pharmacol. Ther. 10:571, 1969.

208. Leonards, J.R., and Levy, G.: Effect of pharmaceutical formulation on gastrointestinal bleeding from aspirin tablets. Arch. Intern. Med. 129:457, 1972.

209. Leonards, J.R., and Levy, G.: Gastrointestinal blood loss from aspirin and sodium salicylate tablets in man. Clin. Pharmacol. Ther. 14:62, 1973.

210. Parry, D.J., and Wood, P.H.N.: Relationship between aspirin taking and gastroduodenal hemorrhage. Gut 8:301, 1967.

211. Bouchier, I.A.D., and Williams, H.S.: Determination of faecal blood loss after combined alcohol and sodium acetylsalicylate. Lancet 1:178, 1969.

212. Leonards, J.R., Levy, G., and Niemczura, R.: Gastrointestinal blood loss during prolonged aspirin administration. N. Engl. J. Med. 289:1020, 1973.

213. Schmid, F.R., and Culic, D.D.: Anti-inflammatory drugs and gastrointestinal bleeding: A comparison of aspirin and ibuprofen. J. Clin. Pharmacol. 16:418, 1976.

214. Cooke, A.R., and Goulston, K.: Failure of intravenous aspirin to increase gastrointestinal blood loss. Br. Med. J. 3:330, 1969.

215. Watson, R.M., and Pierson, R.N.: Effect of anticoagulant therapy upon aspirin-induced gastrointestinal bleeding. Circulation 24:613, 1961.

216. Baragar, F.D., and Duthie, J.J.R.: Importance of aspirin as a cause of anaemia and peptic ulcer in rheumatoid arthritis. Br. Med. J. 1:1106, 1960.

217. Muir, A., and Cossar, I.A.: Aspirin and gastric bleeding: Further studies of calcium aspirin. Am. J. Dig. Dis. 6:1115, 1961.

218. Paul, W.D.: The effect of acetylsalicylic acid (aspirin) on the gastric mucosa, a gastroscopic study. J. Iowa Med. Soc. 33:155, 1943.
219. Thorsen, W.B., Western, D., Tanaka, Y., and Morrissey, J.F.: Aspirin injury to gastric mucosa. Gastrocamera observations of the effect of pH. Arch. Intern. Med. 121:499, 1968.
220. Kuiper, D.H., Fall, D.S., Overholt, B.F., and Pollard, H.M.: The effect of aspirin on fecal blood loss with gastroscopic correlation in healthy volunteers (abstract). Ann Intern. Med. 70:1069, 1969.
221. Edmar, D.: The effects of acetylsalicylic acid on the human gastric mucosa as revealed by gastrocamera. Scand. J. Gastroenterol. 10:495, 1975.
222. Baskin, W.N., Ivey, K.J., Krause, W.J., Jeffrey, G.E., and Gemmell, R.T.: Aspirin-induced ultrastructural changes in human gastric mucosa: Correlation with potential difference. Ann. Intern. Med. 85:299, 1976.
223. Silvoso, G.R., Ivey, K.J., Butt, J.H., Lockard, O.O., Holt, S.D., Sisk, G., Baskin, W.N., Mackercher, P.A., and Hewett, J.: Incidence of gastric lesions in patients with rheumatic disease on chronic aspirin therapy. Ann. Intern. Med. 91:517, 1979.
224. Lanza, F.L., Royer, G.L., and Nelson, R.S.: Endoscopic evaluation of the effects of aspirin, buffered aspirin, and enteric-coated aspirin on gastric and duodenal mucosa. N. Engl. J. Med. 303:136, 1980.
225. Hoftiezer, J.W., Silvoso, G.R., Burks, M., and Ivey, K.J.: Comparison of the effects of regular and enteric-coated aspirin on gastroduodenal mucosa of man. Lancet 2:609, 1980.
226. Morris, A.D., Holt, S.D., Silvoso, G.R., Hewitt, J., Tatum, W., Grandione, J., Butt, J.H., and Ivey, K.J.: Effect of anti-inflammatory drug administration in patients with rheumatoid arthritis. Scand. J. Gastroenterol. 67(Suppl.):131, 1981.
227. Konturek, S.J., Obtulowicz, W., Sito, E., Olesky, J., Wilkon, S., and Kiec-Dembinska, A.: Distribution of prostaglandins in gastric and duodenal mucosa of healthy subjects and duodenal ulcer patients: effects of aspirin and paracetamol. Gut 22:283, 1981.
228. Cohen, M.M., and MacDonald, W.C.: Mechanism of aspirin injury to human gastroduodenal mucosa. Prostaglandins Leukotrienes Med. 9:241, 1982.
229. Hunt, J.N., and Franz, D.R.: Effect of prostaglandin E₂ on gastric mucosal bleeding caused by aspirin Dig. Dis. Sci. 26:301, 1981.
230. Cohen, M.M.: Prevention of aspirin-induced fecal blood loss with oral prostaglandin E₂: Dose-response studies in man. Prostaglandins 21(Suppl.):155, 1981.
231. Cohen, M.M. Cheung, G., and Lyster, D.M.: Prevention of aspirin-induced faecal blood loss by prostaglandin E₂. Gut 21:602, 1982.
232. Simmons, T.C., Weinstein, W.M., Shapira, M., and Grossman, M.I.: A therapeutic trial of 15(R)-15-methyl prostaglandin E₂ in rheumatoid arthritis patients with gastroduodenal lesions. Prostaglandins 21(Suppl.):165, 1981.
233. Müller, P., Fischer, N., Kather, H., and Simon, B.: Prevention of aspirin-induced drop in gastric potential with 16,16-dimethyl-prostaglandin E₂. Lancet 1:333, 1981 (letter).
234. Cohen, M.M.: Prevention of aspirin-induced fall in gastric potential difference with prostaglandins. Lancet 1:785, 1981 (letter).
235. Ivey, K.J., Paone, D.B., and Krause, W.J.: Acute effects of systemic aspirin on gastric mucosa in man. Dig. Dis. Sci. 25:97, 1980.
236. Kauffman, G.L., Aures, D., and Grossman, M.I.: Intravenous indomethacin and aspirin reduce basal gastric mucosal blood flow in dogs. Am. J. Physiol. 238G:131, 1980.
237. Rahbek, I.: Gastroscopic evaluation of the effect of a new anti-rheumatic compound Ketoprofen (19:583 R.P.) on the human gastric mucosa. A double-blind cross-over trial against acetylsalicylic acid. Scand. J. Rheumatol. (Suppl.) 63, 1976.
238. Loebl, D.H., Craig, R.M., Culic, D.D., Ridolfo, A.S., Falk, J., and Schmid, F.R.: Gastrointestinal blood loss. Effect of aspirin, fenoprofen, and acetaminophen in rheumatoid arthritis as determined by sequential gastroscopy and radioactive fecal markers. JAMA 237:976, 1977.
239. Croft, D.N.: Cell turnover and loss and the gastric mucosal barrier. Am. J. Dig. Dis. 22:383, 1977.
240. Davenport, H.W.: Salicylate damage to the gastric mucosal barrier. N. Engl. J. Med. 276:1307, 1967.
241. Silen, W.: New concepts of the gastric mucosal barrier. Am. J. Surg. 133:8, 1977.
242. Brown, R.K., and Mitchell, N.: The influence of some of the salicyl compounds (and alcoholic beverages) on the natural history of peptic ulcer. Gastroenterology 31:198, 1956.
243. Alvarez, A., and Summerskill, W.H.J.: Gastrointestinal haemorrhage and salicylates. Lancet 2:920, 1958.
244. Jennings, G.H.: Causal influences in haematemesis and melena. Gut 6:1, 1965.
245. Muir, A., and Cossar, I.A.: Aspirin and gastric haemorrhage. Lancet 1:539, 1959.
246. Needham, C.D., Kyle, J., Jones, P.F., Johnston, S.J., and Kerridge, D.F.: Aspirin and alcohol in gastrointestinal haemorrhage. Gut 12:819, 1971.
247. Dagradi, A.E., Lee, E.R., Bosco, D.L., and Stempien, S.J.: The clinical spectrum of hemorrhagic erosive gastritis. Am. J. Gastroenterol. 60:30, 1973.
248. Cameron, A.J.: Aspirin and gastric ulcer. Mayo Clin. Proc. 50:565, 1975.
249. Jorgensen, T.G.: Drug consumption before perforation of peptic ulcer. Br. J. Surg. 64:247, 1977.
250. Langman, M.J.S.: Aspirin is not a major cause of acute gastrointestinal bleeding. In Inglefinger, F.J., Ebert, R.V., Finland, M., and Relman, A.S. (eds.): Controversy in Internal Medicine II. Philadelphia, W. B. Saunders Company, 1974.
251. Spiro, H.M.: Aspirin is dangerous for the peptic ulcer patient. In Inglefinger, F.J., Ebert, R.V., Finland, M., and Relman, A.S. (eds.): Controversy in Internal Medicine II. Philadelphia, W. B. Saunders Company, 1974.
252. Levy, M.: Aspirin use in patients with major upper gastrointestinal bleeding and peptic ulcer disease. N. Engl. J. Med. 290:1158, 1974.
253. Duggan, J.M.: Progress report. Aspirin in chronic gastric ulcer: An Australian experience. Gut 17:378, 1976.
254. Gault, M.H., Rudwal, T.C., Engles, W.D., and Dossetor, J.B.: Syndrome associated with the abuse of analgesics. Ann. Intern. Med. 68:906, 1968.
255. Walker, A.M., and Jick, H.: Prediction of bleeding during heparin therapy. JAMA 244:1209, 1980.
256. Winawer, S.J., Bejar, J., and Zamcheck, N.: Recurrent massive hemorrhage in patients with achlorhydria and atrophic gastritis. Arch. Intern. Med. 120:327, 1967.
257. Rafoth, R.J., and Silvis, S.E.: Gastric ulceration associated with aspirin ingestion in an achlorhydric patient: A case report. Am. J. Dig. Dis. 21:279, 1976.
258. Bergman, G.E., Philippidis, P., and Naiman, J.L.: Severe gastrointestinal hemorrhage and anemia after therapeutic doses of aspirin in normal children. J. Pediatr. 88:501, 1976.
259. Newman, L.J., Yu, W.-Y., Halata, M., and Wasserman, E.: Peptic ulcer disease in children. Aspirin induced. NY State J. Med. 81:1099, 1981.
260. Gerber, L.H., Rooney, P.J., and McCarthy, D.M.: Healing of peptic ulcers during continuing anti-inflammatory drug therapy in rheumatoid arthritis. J. Clin. Gastroenterol. 3:7, 1981.
261. MacKercher, P.A., Ivey, K.J., Baskin, W.N., and Krause, W.J.: Protective effect of cimetidine on aspirin-induced gastric mucosal damage. Ann. Intern. Med. 87:676, 1977.
262. Okabe, S., Takeuchi, K., Urushidani, T., and Takagi, K.: Effects of cimetidine, a histamine H2-receptor antagonist, on various experimental gastric and duodenal ulcers. Am. J. Dig. Dis. 22:677, 1977.
263. Tarnawski, A., Krause, W.J., and Ivey, K.J.: Effect of glucagon on aspirin-induced gastric mucosal damage in man. Gastroenterology 74:240, 1978.
264. Welch, R.W., Bentch, H.L., and Harris, S.C.: Reduction of aspirin-induced gastrointestinal bleeding with cimetidine. Gastroenterology 74:459, 1978.
265. O'Laughlin, J.C., Silvoso, G.R., and Ivey, K.J.: Healing of aspirin-associated peptic ulcer disease despite continued salicylate ingestion. Arch. Intern. Med. 141:781, 1981.
266. Geall, M.G., Phillips, S.F., and Summerskill, W.H.J.: Profile of gastric potential difference in man. Effects of aspirin, alcohol, bile, and endogenous acid. Gastroenterology 58:437, 1970.
267. Ivey, K.J., Morrison, S., and Gray, C.: Effect of salicylates on the gastric mucosal barrier in man. J. Appl. Physiol. 33:81, 1972.
268. Davenport, H.W., Warner, H.A., and Code, C.F.: Functional significance of gastric mucosal barrier to sodium. Gastroenterology 47:142, 1964.
269. Chvasta, T.E., and Cooke, A.R.: The effect of several ulcerogenic drugs on the canine gastric mucosal barrier. J. Lab. Clin. Med. 79:302, 1972.
270. Caspary, W.F.: The effect of aspirin, antacids, alcohol and bile acids on transmural potential difference of the human stomach. Dtsch. Med. Wochenschr. 100:1263, 1975.
271. Bowen, B.K., Krause, W.J., and Ivey, K.J.: Effect of sodium bicarbonate on aspirin-induced damage and potential difference changes in human gastric mucosa. Br. Med. J. 2:1052, 1977.
272. Murray, H.S., Strottman, M.P., and Cooke, A.R.: Effect of several drugs on gastric potential difference in man. Br. Med. J. 1:19, 1974.
273. Cohen, M.M., and Pollett, J.M.: Prostaglandin E₂ prevents aspirin and indomethacin damage to human gastric mucosa. Surg. Forum 27:400, 1976.
274. Davenport, H.W.: Gastric mucosal hemorrhage in dogs. Effects of acid, aspirin, and alcohol. Gastroenterology 56:439, 1969.
275. Brown, P.A., Sawrey, J.M., and Vernikos-Danillis, J.: Attenuation of salicylate and stress-produced gastric ulceration by metiamide. Proc. West. Pharmacol. Soc. 18:123, 1975.
276. Rainsford, K.D.: Aspirin and gastric ulceration: Light and electron microscopic observations in a model of aspirin plus stress-induced ulcerogenesis. Br. J. Exp. Pathol. 58:215, 1977.
277. MacDonald, A., Dekanski, J.B., Gottfried, S., Parke, D.V., and Sacra, P.: Effects of blood glucose levels on aspirin-induced gastric mucosal damage. Am. J. Dig. Dis. 22:909, 1977.

278. Semple, P.F., and Russell, R.I.: Role of bile acids in the pathogenesis of aspirin-induced mucosal hemorrhage in rats. Gastroenterology 68:67, 1975.

279. Guth, P.H., Paulsen, G., Lynn, D., and Aures, D.: Mechanism of prevention of aspirin-induced gastric lesions by bile duct ligation in the rat. Gastroenterology 71:750, 1976.

280. Brodie, D.A., and Chase, B.J.: Role of gastric acid in aspirin-induced gastric irritation in the rat. Gastroenterology 53:604, 1967.

281. Dagle, G.E., Brodie, D.A., and Bauer, B.G.: Comparison of gross and microscopic gastric lesions produced in rats after single doses of aspirin and 2-deoxyglucose. Toxicol. Appl. Pharmacol. 16:638, 1970.

282. Okabe, S., Honda, K., Takeuchi, K., and Takagi, K.: Inhibitory effect of L-glutamine on gastric irritation and back diffusion of gastric acid in response to aspirin in the rat. Am. J. Dig. Dis. 20:626, 1975.

283. Boyle, E., Freeman, P.C., Goudie, A.C., Mangan, F.R., and Thomson, M.: The role of copper in preventing gastrointestinal damage by acidic anti-inflammatory drugs. J. Pharm. Pharmacol. 28:865, 1976.

284. Rainsford, K.D., and Whitehouse, M.W.: Gastric irritancy of aspirin and its congeners: Anti-inflammatory activity without this side-effect. J. Pharm. Pharmacol. 28:599, 1976.

285. Cheung, L.Y., Jubiz, W., Torma, M.J., and Frailey, J.: Effects of aspirin on canine gastric prostaglandin output and mucosal permeability. Surg. Forum 25:407, 1974.

286. Child, C., Jubiz, W., and Moore, J.G.: Effects of aspirin on gastric prostaglandin E (PGE) and acid output in normal subjects. Gut 17:54, 1976.

287. Cheung, L.Y., Moody, F.G., and Reese, R.S.: Effect of aspirin, bile salt, and ethanol on canine gastric mucosal blood flow. Surgery 77:786, 1975.

288. Gerkens, J.F., Shand, D.G., Flexner, C., Nies, A.S., Oates, J.A., and Data, J.L.: Effect of indomethacin and aspirin on gastric blood flow and acid secretion. J. Pharmacol. Exp. Ther. 203:646, 1977.

289. Farris, R.K., Tapper, E.J., Powell, D.W., and Morris, S.M.: Effect of aspirin on normal and cholera toxin-stimulated intestinal electrolyte transport. J. Clin. Invest. 57:916, 1976.

290. Kingham, J.G., Whorwell, P.J., and Loehry, C.A.: Small intestinal permeability I. Effects of ischaemia and exposure to acetyl salicylate. Gut 17:354, 1976.

291. Arvanitakis, C., Chen, G-H., Folscroft, J., and Greenberger, N.J.: Effect of aspirin on intestinal absorption of glucose, sodium, and water in man. Gut 18:187, 1977.

292. Beaumont, J.L., and Willie, A.: Influence sur l'hémostase, de l'hypertension artérielle, des antivitamines K, de l'héparine et de l'acide acétyl salicylique. Sang 26:880, 1955.

293. Beaumont, J.L., Caen, J., and Bernard, J.: Influence de l'acide acétyl salicylique dans les maladies hémorragiques. Sang 27:243, 1956.

294. Gast, L.F.: Influence of aspirin on hemostatic parameters. Ann. Rheum. Dis. 23:500, 1964.

295. Weiss, H.J., Aledort, L.M., and Kochwa, S.: The effect of salicylates on the hemostatic properties of platelets in man. J. Clin. Invest. 47:2169, 1968.

296. Mielke, C.H., Kaneshiro, M.M., Maher, I.A., Weiner, J.M., and Rapaport, S.I.: The standardized normal Ivy bleeding time and its prolongation by aspirin. Blood 34:204, 1969.

297. Bick, R.L., Adams, T., and Schmalhorst, W.R.: Bleeding times, platelet adhesion, and aspirin. Am. J. Clin. Pathol. 65:69, 1976.

298. Young, V.P., Giles, A.R., Pater, J., and Corbett, W.E.N.: Sex differences in bleeding time and blood loss in normal subjects following aspirin ingestion. Thromb. Res. 20:705, 1980.

299. Dybdahl, J.H., Daae, L.N.W., Erika, C., Godal, H.D., and Larsen, S.: Acetylsalicylic acid-induced prolongation of bleeding time in healthy men. Scand. J. Haematol. 26:50, 1981.

300. Evans, G., Mustard, J.F., and Packham, M.A.: Spontaneous bruising (letter). Lancet 2:724, 1967.

301. Weiss, H.J., and Aledort, L.M.: Impaired platelet/connective tissue reaction in man after aspirin ingestion. Lancet 2:495, 1967.

302. O'Brien, J.R.: Effects of salicylates on human platelets. Lancet 1:779, 1968.

303. Zucker, M.B., and Peterson, J.: Inhibition of adenosine diphosphate-induced secondary aggregation and other platelet functions by acetylsalicylic acid ingestion. Proc. Soc. Exp. Biol. Med. 127:547, 1968.

304. Zucker, M.B., and Peterson, J.: Effect of acetylsalicylic acid, other nonsteroidal anti-inflammatory agents, and dipyridamole on human blood platelets. J. Lab. Clin. Med. 76:66, 1970.

305. Weiss, H.J., Tschopp, T.B., and Baumgartner, H.R.: Impaired interaction (adhesion-aggregation) of platelets with the subendothelium in storage-pool disease and after aspirin ingestion. A comparison with von Willebrand's disease. N. Engl. J. Med. 293:619, 1975.

306. Cazenave, J.P., Packham, M.A., Guccione, M.A., and Mustard, J.F.: Inhibition of platelet adherence to damaged surface of rabbit aorta. J. Lab. Clin. Med. 86:551, 1975.

307. Tschopp, T.B.: Aspirin inhibits platelet aggregation on, but not adhesion to, collagen fibrils: An assessment of platelet adhesion and deposited platelet mass by morphometry and ^{51}Cr-labeling. Thromb. Res. 11:619, 1977.

308. Baumgartner, H.R., Tschopp, T.B., and Weiss, H.J.: Platelet interaction with collagen fibrils in flowing blood. II. Impaired adhesion-aggregation in bleeding disorders. A comparison with subendothelium. Thromb. Haemostas. 37:17, 1977.

309. Stuart, R.K.: Platelet function studies in human beings receiving 300 mg of aspirin per day. J. Lab. Clin. Med. 75:463, 1970.

310. Rowan, R.M., McDonald, G.A., Renton, R.L., Corne, S.J., and Brown, D.F.: Inhibition of platelet release reaction by acetylsalicylic acid. Postgrad. Med. J. 52:71, 1976.

311. Seuter, F.: Inhibition of platelet aggregation by acetylsalicylic acid and other inhibitors. Haemostasis 5:85, 1976.

312. Malmsten, C., Hamberg, M., Svensson, J., and Samuelsson, B.: Physiological role of an endoperoxide in human platelets: Hemostatic defect due to platelet cyclo-oxygenase deficiency. Proc. Natl. Acad. Sci. 72:1446, 1975.

313. Weiss, H.J., Willis, A.L., Kuhn, D., and Brand, H.: Prostaglandin E$_2$ potentiation of platelet aggregation induced by LASS endoperoxide: Absent in storage pool disease, normal after aspirin ingestion. Br. J. Haematol. 32:257, 1976.

314. Burch, J.W., Stanford, N., and Majerus, P.W.: Inhibition of platelet prostaglandin synthetase by oral aspirin. J. Clin. Invest. 61:314, 1978.

315. Gerrard, J.M., White, J.G., Rao, G.H.R., Krivit, W., and Witkop, C.J.: Labile aggregation stimulating substance (LASS): The factor from storage pool deficient platelets correcting defective aggregation and release of aspirin treated normal platelets. Br. J. Haematol. 29:657, 1975.

316. Gerrard, J.M., and White, J.G.: The influence of aspirin and indomethacin on the platelet contractile wave. Am. J. Pathol. 82:513, 1976.

317. Glass, D.B., Gerrard, J.M., Townsend, D., Carr, D.W., White, J.G., and Goldberg, N.D.: The involvement of prostaglandin endoperoxide formation in the elevation of cyclic GMP levels during platelet aggregation. J. Cyclic Nucleotide Res. 3:37, 1977.

318. Smith, J.B., and Willis, A.L.: Aspirin selectivity inhibits prostaglandin production in human platelets. Nature New Biol. 231:235, 1971.

319. Roth, G.J., Stanford, N., and Majerus, P.W.: Acetylation of prostaglandin synthetase by aspirin. Proc. Natl. Acad. Sci. 72:3073, 1975.

320. Ali, M., McDonald, J.W.D., Thiessen, J.J., and Coates, P.E.: Plasma acetylsalicylate and salicylate and platelet cyclooxygenase activity following plain and enteric-coated aspirin. Stroke 11:9, 1980.

321. Bradlow, B.A., and Chetty, N.: Dosage frequency for suppression of platelet function by low dose aspirin therapy. Thromb. Res. 27:99, 1982.

322. FitzGerald, G.A., Oates, J.A., Hawiger, J., Maas, R.L., Roberts, L.J., Lawson, J.A., and Brash, A.R.: Endogenous biosynthesis of prostacyclin and thromboxane and platelet function during chronic administration of aspirin in man. J. Clin. Invest. 71:676, 1983.

323. Brantmark, B., Hender, U., Melander, A., and Wåhlin-Boll, E.: Salicylate inhibition of antiplatelet effect of aspirin. Lancet 2:1348, 1981 (letter).

324. Livio, M., Del Maschio, A., Cerletti, C., and de Gaetano, G.: Indomethacin prevents the long-lasting inhibitory effect of aspirin on human platelet cyclo-oxygenase activity. Prostaglandins 23:787, 1982.

325. Rao, G.H.R., Reddy, K.R., and White, J.G.: Effect of acetaminophen and salicylate on aspirin-induced inhibition of human platelet cyclo-oxygenase. Prostaglandins Leukotrienes Med. 9:109, 1982.

326. Cerletti, C., Livio, M., and de Gaetano, G.: Non-steroidal anti-inflammatory drugs react with two sites on platelet cyclo-oxygenase. Evidence from 'in vivo' drug interaction studies in rats. Biochim. Biophys. Acta 714:122, 1981.

327. Dejana, E., Cerletti, C., de Castellarnau, C., Livio, M., Galletti, F., Latini, R., and de Gaetano, G.: Salicylate-aspirin interaction in the rat. Evidence that salicylate accumulating during aspirin administration may protect vascular prostacyclin from aspirin-induced inhibition. J. Clin. Invest. 68:1108, 1981.

328. Humes, J.L., Winter, C.A., Sadowski, S.J., and Kuehl, F.A.: Multiple sites on prostaglandin cyclooxygenase are determinants in the action of nonsteroidal antiinflammatory agents. PNAS 78:2053, 1981.

329. Preston, F.E., Whipps, S., Jackson, C.A., French, A.J., Wyld, P.J., and Stoddard, C.J.: Inhibition of prostacyclin and platelet thromboxane A$_2$ after low dose aspirin. N. Engl. J. Med. 304:76, 1981.

330. Weksler, B.B., Pett, S.B., Alonso, D., Richter, R.C., Stelzer, P., Subramanian, V., Tack-Goldman, K., and Gay, W.A.: Differential inhibition by aspirin of vascular and platelet prostaglandin synthesis in atherosclerotic patients. N. Engl. J. Med. 308:800, 1983.

331. Preston, F.E., Greaves, M., Jackson, C.A., and Stoddard, C.J.: Low-dose aspirin inhibits platelet and venous cyclo-oxygenase in man. Thromb. Res. 27:477, 484, 1982.

332. Loew, D., and Vinazzer, H.: Dose-dependent influence of acetylsalicylic acid on platelet function and plasmatic coagulation factors. Haemostasis 5:239, 1976.

333. Goldsweig, H.G., Kapusta, M., and Schwartz, J.: Bleeding, salicylates, and prolonged prothrombin time: Three case reports and a review of the literature. J. Rheumatol. 3:37, 1976.

334. Pinedo, H.M., van de Putte, L.B.A., and Loeliger, E.A.: Salicylate-induced consumption coagulopathy. Ann. Rheum. Dis. 32:66, 1973.

335. Sbarbaro, J.A., and Bennett, R.M.: Aspirin hepatotoxicity and disseminated intravascular coagulation. Ann. Intern. Med. 86:183, 1977.

336. Opelz, G., Terasaki, P.I., and Hirata, A.A.: Suppression of lymphocyte transformation by aspirin. Lancet 2:478, 1973.

337. Panush, R.S., and Anthony, C.R.: Effects of acetylsalicylic acid on normal human peripheral blood lymphocytes. Inhibition of mitogen- and antigen-stimulated incorporation of tritiated thymidine. Clin. Exp. Immunol. 23:114, 1976.

338. Coeugniet, E., Bendtzen, K., and Bendixen, G.: Leukocyte migration inhibitory activity of concanavalin-A-stimulated human lymphocytes. Modification by dipyridamole, lysine-acetylsalicylate and heparin. Acta Med. Scand. 199:99, 1976.

339. Brown, K.A., and Collins, A.J.: Action of non-steroidal anti-inflammatory drugs on human and rat peripheral leucocyte migration in vitro. Ann. Rheum. Dis. 36:239, 1977.

340. Crout, J.E., Hepburn, B., and Ritts, R.E., Jr.: Suppression of lymphocyte transformation after aspirin ingestion. N. Engl. J. Med. 292:221, 1975.

341. Smith, M.J., Hoth, M., and Davis, K.: Aspirin and lymphocyte transformation. Ann. Intern. Med. 83:509, 1975.

342. Snider, D.E., and Parker, C.W.: Aspirin effects on lymphocyte cyclic AMP levels in normal human subjects. J. Clin. Invest. 58:524, 1976.

343. Duncan, M.W., Person, D.A., Rich, A.A., and Sharp, J.T.: Aspirin and delayed type hypersensitivity. Arthritis Rheum. 20:1174, 1977.

344. Austen, K.F.: Immunologic aspects of salicylate action. In Dixon, A. St.J., Martin, B.K., Smith, M.J.H., and Wood, P.N.H. (eds.): Salicylates. Boston, Little, Brown & Company, 1963.

345. MacGregor, R.R., Spagnuolo, P.J., and Lentnek, A.L.: Inhibition of granulocyte adherence by ethanol, prednisone, and aspirin measured with an assay system. N. Engl. J. Med. 291:642, 1974.

346. Glader, B.E.: Evaluation of the hemolytic role of aspirin in glucose-6-phosphate dehydrogenase deficiency. J. Pediat. 89:1027, 1976.

347. Chan, T.K., Todd, D., and Tso, S.C.: Drug-induced hemolysis in glucose-6-phosphate dehydrogenase deficiency. Br. Med. J. 2:1227, 1976.

348. Colonna, P.: Aspirin and glucose-6-phosphate dehydrogenase deficiency. Br. Med. J. 283:1189, 1981 (letter).

349. Glader, B.E.: Salicylate-induced injury of pyruvate-kinase deficient erythrocytes. N. Engl. J. Med. 294:916, 1976.

350. Wijnja, L., Snijder, J.A.M., and Nieweg, H.O.: Acetylsalicylic acid as a cause of pancytopenia from bone marrow damage. Lancet 2:768, 1966.

351. Reid, J., Watson, R.D., and Sproull, D.H.: The mode of action of salicylate in acute rheumatic fever. Quart. J. Med. 19:1, 1950.

352. Bywaters, E.G.L., and Thomas, G.T.: Bed rest, salicylates, and steroid in rheumatic fever. Br. Med. J. 1:1628, 1961.

353. Alexander, W.D., and Smith, G.: Disadvantageous circulating effects of salicylate in rheumatic fever. Lancer 1:768, 1962.

354. Sutcliffe, J.: Pulmonary oedema due to salicylates with report of a case. Br. J. Radiol. 28:314, 1955.

355. Granville-Grossman, K.L., and Sergeant, H.G.S.: Pulmonary oedema due to salicylate intoxication. Lancet 1:575, 1960.

356. Hrnicek, G., Skelton, J., and Miller, W.C.: Pulmonary edema and salicylate intoxication. JAMA 230:866, 1974.

357. Tashima, C.K., and Rose, M.: Pulmonary edema and salicylates. Ann. Intern. Med. 81:274, 1974.

358. Davis, P.R., and Burch, R.E.: Pulmonary edema and salicylate intoxication (letter). Ann. Intern. Med. 80:553, 1974.

359. Karliner, J.S.: Noncardiogenic forms of pulmonary edema. Circulation 46:212, 1972.

360. Bowers, R.E., Brigham, K.L., and Owen, P.J.: Salicylate pulmonary edema: The mechanism in sheep and review of the clinical literature. Am. Rev. Respir. Dis. 115:261, 1977.

361. Anderson, R.J., Potts, D.E., Gabow, P.A., Rumack, B.H., and Schrier, R.W.: Unrecognized adult salicylate intoxication. Ann. Intern. Med. 85:745, 1976.

362. Tenney, S.M., and Miller, R.M.: The respiratory and circulating actions of salicylate. Am. J. Med. 19:498, 1955.

363. Kuna, S.T., and Levine, S.: Relationship between cyclooxygenase activity (COA) inhibition and stimulation of ventilation by salicylate. J. Pharm. Exp. Therap. 219:721, 1981.

364. Starling, M.B., and Elliott, R.B.: The effects of prostaglandins, prostaglandin inhibition, and oxygen on the closure of the ductus arteriosus, pulmonary arteries and umbilical vessels in vitro. Prostaglandins 8:187, 1974.

365. Elliott, R.B., Starling, M.B., and Neutze, J.M.: Medical manipulation of the ductus arteriosus. Lancet 1:140, 1975.

366. Friedman, W.F., Hirschklau, M.J., Printz, M.P., Pitlick, P.T., and Kirkpatrick, S.E.: Pharmacologic closure of patent ductus arteriosus in the premature infant. N. Engl. J. Med. 295:526, 1976.

367. Heymann, M.A., Rudolph, A.M., and Silverman, N.H.: Closure of ductus arteriosus in premature infants by inhibition of prostaglandin synthesis. N. Engl. J. Med. 295:530, 1976.

368. Eisner, D.A., Ohba, M., and Ojeda, C.: The effect of salicylate in Purkinje fibre pace-maker activity. J. Physiol. 269:84P, 1977.

369. Jackson, H.R., Johnson, S.M., Ng, K.H., Pye, W., and Hall, R.C.: The effect of acetylsalicylic acid on the response of the cardiovascular system to catecholamines. Eur. J. Pharmacol. 28:119, 1974.

370. Nydick, I., Tang, J., Stollerman, G.H., Wroblewski, F., and LaDue, J.S.: The influence of rheumatic fever on serum concentrations of the enzyme, glutamic oxalacetic transaminase. Circulation 12:795, 1955.

371. Manso, C., Taranta, A., and Nydick, I.: Effect of aspirin administration of serum glutamic oxalacetic and glutamic pyruvic transaminases in children. Proc. Soc. Exp. Biol. Med. 93:84, 1956.

372. Russell, A.S., Sturge, R.A., and Smith, M.A.: Serum transaminases during salicylate therapy. Br. Med. J. 2:428, 1971.

373. Rich, R.R., and Johnson, J.S.: Salicylate hepatotoxicity in patients with juvenile rheumatoid arthritis. Arthritis Rheum. 16:1, 1973.

374. Scaman, W.E., and Plotz, P.H.: Effect of aspirin on liver tests in patients with RA or SLE and in normal volunteers. Arthritis Rheum. 19:155, 1976.

375. Okumura, H., Ichikawa, T., Aramaki, T., and Oobayaski, K.: Liver disorder caused by aspirin. Naika 17:749, 1966.

376. Saltzman, D.A., Gall, E.P., and Robinson, S.F.: Aspirin-induced hepatic dysfunction in a patient with adult rheumatoid arthritis. Am. J. Dig. Dis. 21:815, 1976.

377. Wilson, J.R.: Aspirin hepatotoxicity in adults with rheumatoid arthritis. Ohio State Med. J. 72:577, 1976.

378. O'Gorman, T., and Koff, R.S.: Salicylate hepatitis. Gastroenterology 72:726, 1977.

379. Seaman, W.E., Ishak, K.G., and Plotz, P.H.: Aspirin-induced hepatotoxicity in patients with systemic lupus erythematosus. Ann. Intern. Med. 80:1, 1974.

380. Wolfe, J.D., Metzger, A.L., and Goldstein, R.C.: Aspirin hepatitis. Ann. Intern. Med. 80:74, 1974.

381. Bernstein, B.H., Singsen, B.H., King, K.K., and Hanson, V.: Aspirin-induced hepatotoxicity and its effect on juvenile rheumatoid arthritis. Am. J. Dis. Child. 131:659, 1977.

382. Miller, J.J., and Weissman, D.B.: Correlations between transaminase concentrations and serum salicylate concentration in juvenile rheumatoid arthritis. Arthritis Rheum. 19:115, 1976.

383. Kalczak, M., Gutowska-Grzegorczyk, G., and Maldyk, E.: The effect of chronic administration of acetylsalicylic acid on the rabbit's liver. Polish Med. J. IX:128, 1970.

384. Menguy, R., Desbaillets, L., Okabe, S., and Masters, Y.F.: Abnormal aspirin metabolism in patients with cirrhosis and its possible relationship to bleeding in cirrhotics. Ann. Surg. 176:412, 1972.

385. Tolman, K.G., Peterson, P., Gray, P., and Hammar, S.P.: Hepatotoxicity of salicylates in monolayer cell cultures. Gastroenterology 74:205, 1978.

386. Rosenfeld, R.G., and Liebhaber, M.I.: Acute encephalopathy in siblings. Reye syndrome vs salicylate intoxication. Am. J. Dis. Child. 130:295, 1976.

387. Sillanpaan, M., Makela, A.L., and Koivikko, A.: Acute liver failure and encephalopathy (Reye's syndrome?) during salicylate therapy. Acta Paediat. Scand. 64:877, 1975.

388. Waldman, R.J., Hall, W.N., McGee, H., and Van Amburg, G.: Aspirin as a risk factor in Reye's syndrome. JAMA 247:3089, 1982.

389. Halpin, T.J., Holtzhauer, F.J., Campbell, R.J., Hall, L.J., Correa-Villasenor, A., Lanese, R., Rice, J., and Hurwitz, E.S.: Reye's syndrome and medication use. JAMA 248:687, 1982.

390. Fulginiti, V.A., Brunnel, P.A., Cherry, J.D., Ector, W.L., Gershon, A.A., Gotoff, S.P., Hughes, W.T., Mortimer, E.A., and Peter, G.: Aspirin and Reye syndrome. Pediatrics 69:810, 1982.

391. Clausen, E., and Harvald, B.: Nephrotoxicity of different analgesics. Acta Med. Scand. 170:469, 1961.

392. Scott, J.T.: Renal irritation caused by salicylates. In Dixon, A. St.J., Martin, B.K., Smith, M.J.H., and Wood, P.H.N. (eds.): Salicylates. Boston, Little, Brown and Company, 1963.

393. Stewart, J.H., and Gallery, E.D.M.: Analgesic abuse and kidney disease. Aust. N.Z. J. Med. 6:498, 1976.

394. Murray, T., and Goldberg, M.: Analgesic abuse and renal disease. Ann. Rev. Med. 26:537, 1975.

395. Robinson, M.J., Nichols, E.A., and Taitz, L.: Nephrotoxic effect of acute sodium salicylate intoxication in the rat. Arch. Pathol. 84:224, 1967.

396. Axelsen, R.A.: Analgesic-induced renal papillary necrosis in the Gunn rat: The comparative nephrotoxicity of aspirin and phenacetin. J. Pathol. 120:145, 1976.

397. Duggin, G.G.: Mechanisms in the development of analgesic nephropathy. Kid. Int. 18:553, 1980.

398. Clausen, E., and Pedersen, J.: Necrosis of the renal papillae in rheumatoid arthritis. Acta Med. Scand. 170:631, 1961.

399. Lawson, A.A.H., and Maclean, N.: Renal disease and drug therapy in rheumatoid arthritis. Ann. Rheum. Dis. 25:441, 1966.

400. Nanra, R.S., and Kincaid-Smith, P.: Renal papillary necrosis in rheumatoid arthritis. Med. J. Australia 1:194, 1975.

401. Salomon, M.I., Gallo, G., Poon, T.P., Goldblat, M.V., and Tchertkoff, V.: The kidney in rheumatoid arthritis. Nephron 12:297, 1974.
402. New Zealand Rheumatism Association: Aspirin and the kidney. Br. Med. J. 1:593, 1974.
403. Macklon, A.F., Craft, A.W., Thompson, M., and Kerr, D.N.S.: Aspirin and analgesic nephropathy. Br. Med. J. 1:597, 1974.
404. Akyol, S.M., Thompson, M., and Kerr, D.N.S.: Renal function after prolonged consumption of aspirin. Br. Med. J. 284:631, 1982.
405. Emkey, R.D., and Mills, J.A.: Aspirin and analgesic nephropathy: JAMA 247:55, 1982.
406. Murray, T.G., Stolley, P.D., Anthony, J.C., Schinnar, R., Helper-Smith, E., and Davies, J.: Epidemiologic study of regular analgesic use and end-stage renal disease. Arch. Intern. Med., 143:1687, 1983.
407. Plotz, P.H.: Analgesic nephropathy. For this time and this place. Arch. Intern. Med., 143:1676, 1983.
408. Hanzlik, P.J., Scott, R.W., and Thoburn, T.W.: The salicylates. VII. Further observations on albuminuria and renal functional changes following the administration of full therapeutic doses of salicylate. Arch. Intern. Med. 19:1029, 1917.
409. Hanzlik, P.J., Scott, R.W., and Reycraft, J.L.: The salicylates. VIII. Salicyl edema. Arch. Intern. Med. 20:329, 1917.
410. Beeley, L., and Kendall, M.J.: Effect of aspirin on renal clearance of ^{125}I-diatrizoate. Br. Med. J. 1:707, 1971.
411. Robert, M., Fillastre, J.P., Berger, H., and Malandain, H.: Effect of intravenous infusion of acetylsalicylic acid on renal function. Br. Med. J. 2:466, 1972.
412. Berg, K.J.: Acute effects of acetylsalicylic acid in patients with chronic renal disease. Eur. J. Clin. Pharmacol. 11:111, 1977.
413. Berg, K.J.: Acute effects of acetylsalicylic acid on renal function in normal man. Eur. J. Clin. Pharmacol. 11:117, 1977.
414. Kimberly, R.P., Bowden, R.E., Keiser, H.R., and Plotz, P.H.: Reduction of renal function by newer non-steroidal anti-inflammatory drugs. Am. J. Med. 64:804, 1978.
415. Kimberly, R.P., Gill, J.R., Bowden, R.E., Keiser, H.R., and Plotz, P.H.: Elevated urinary prostaglandins and the effects of aspirin on renal function in lupus erythematosus. Ann. Intern. Med. 89:336, 1978.
416. Plotz, P.H., and Kimberly, R.P.: Acute effects of aspirin and acetaminophen on renal function. Arch. Intern. Med. 141:343, 1981.
417. Norby, L., Flamenbaum, W., Lentz, R., and Ramwell, P.: Prostaglandins and aspirin therapy in Bartter's syndrome. Lancet 2:604, 1976.
418. Feldman, D., and Couropmitree, C.: Intrinsic mineralocorticoid agonist activity of some non-steroidal anti-inflammatory drugs. J. Clin. Invest. 57:1, 1976.
419. Tweedale, M.H., and Ogilvie, R.I.: Antagonism of spironolactone-induced natriuresis by aspirin in man. N. Engl. J. Med. 289:198, 1973.
420. Done, A.K.: Treatment of salicylate poisoning: Review of personal and published experiences. Clin. Toxicol. 1:451, 1968.
421. Irey, N.S.: Blood and tissue concentrations of drugs associated with fatalities. Med. Clin. North Am. 58:1093, 1974.
422. Anderson, R.J.: Asterixis as a manifestation of salicylate toxicity. Ann. Intern. Med. 95:188, 1981.
423. Wegria, R., Capeci, N., Kiss, G., Glaviano, V.V., Keating, J.H., and Hilton, J.G.: Effect of salicylate on the acid-base equilibrium of patients with chronic CO_2 retention due to pulmonary emphysema. Am. J. Med. 19:509, 1955.
424. Smith, M.J.H.: Metabolic effects of salicylates. In Smith, M.J.H., and Smith, P.K. (eds.): The Salicylates. A Critical Bibliographic Review. New York, Wiley, 1966.
425. Thurston, J.H., Pollock, P.G., Warren, S.K., and Jones, E.M.: Reduced brain glucose with normal plasma glucose in salicylate poisoning. J. Clin. Invest. 49:2139, 1970.
426. Mukherjee, A.B., Chan, M., Waite, R., Metzger, M.I., and Yaffee, S.J.: Inhibition of RNA synthesis by acetyl salicylate and actinomycin D during early development in the mouse. Pediat. Res. 9:652, 1975.
427. Hial, V., Horakova, Z., Shaff, F.E., and Beaven, M.A.: Alteration of tumor growth by aspirin and indomethacin: Studies with two transplantable tumors in mouse. Eur. J. Pharmacol. 37:367, 1976.
428. Seifter, E., Rettura, G., Levenson, S.M., Appleman, M., and Seifter, J.: Aspirin inhibits a murine viral infection. Life Sci. 16:629, 1975.
429. Palmoski, M.J., Colyer, R.A., and Brandt, K.D.: Marked suppression by salicylate of the augmented proteoglycan synthesis in osteoarthritic cartilage. Arthritis Rheum. 23:83, 1980.
430. Palmoski, M.J., and Brandt, K.D.: Aspirin aggravates the degeneration of canine joint cartilage caused by immobilization. Arthritis Rheum. 25:1333, 1982.

Chapter 50
Nonsteroidal Anti-inflammatory Drugs

Alfred Jay Bollet

INTRODUCTION

New drugs with anti-inflammatory and analgesic action have been introduced into the therapy of rheumatic diseases in the recent past; more are under study and development. Aspirin and other forms of salicylate could eventually be replaced as the first-line anti-inflammatory drugs by these newer agents.

A single mechanism of action, inhibition of prostaglandin synthesis, has been advocated as the primary basis for the clinical effects of these drugs; however, differences in effectiveness in different diseases and a variety of basic studies suggest that they do not all act in exactly the same fashion. These agents vary significantly in pharmacologic properties and toxicity, and individual patients vary in their responsiveness to different nonsteroidal anti-inflammatory agents. It is valuable to have a variety of drugs available to allow individualization of therapy, seeking the most effective

regimen for a given patient. The potential toxicity of these drugs must be kept in mind, however, and careful thought given to safety and long-term benefit in each patient.

There are several families of chemical agents with clinically useful anti-inflammatory and analgesic properties. The salicylates are the oldest group, and are covered extensively in another chapter; only important comparisons in the effects or toxicity of salicylates will be mentioned here. The nonsteroidal anti-inflammatory agents discussed in this chapter are listed in Table 50–1.

MECHANISMS OF ACTION

ANTI-INFLAMMATORY EFFECTS

A long list of mechanisms of action has been suggested, especially for the salicylates,[1] including effects

Table 50–1. The Nonsteroidal Anti-inflammatory Agents

Drugs by Chemical Group	Example of Trade Name in the United States
*Salicylates**	
Aspirin	
Sodium salicylate and other salts of salicylic acid	Trilisate
Salicylsalicylic acid	Disalcid
Diflunisal	Dolobid
Indole Derivatives and Related Compounds	
Indomethacin	Indocin
Sulindac	Clinoril
Tolectin	Tolmetin
Zomepirac	Zomax
Pyrazolones	
Phenylbutazone	Butazolidine
Oxyphenbutazone	Tandearil
Azopropazone[†]	
Feprazone[†]	
Phenylacetic Acids	
Alclonfenac[‡]	
Diclofenac[†]	
Fenclofenac[†]	
Phenylpropionic Acids	
Ibuprofen	Motrin
Naproxen	Naprosyn
Fenoprofen	Nalfon
Flurbiprofen[†]	Ansaid
Ketoprofen[†]	
Fenbufen[†]	Cincopal
Benoxaprofen[‡]	Oraflex
Carprofen[†]	
Fenamates	
Mefenamic acid	Ponstel
Meclofenamate	Meclomen
Flufenamic acid[†]	
Oxicams	
Piroxicam	Feldene
Isoxicam[†]	

*See chapter on salicylates for further details.
[†]Not marketed in the United States at present.
[‡]Withdrawn from the market because of toxicity.

on virtually all the known phenomena that occur in the process of inflammation. Effects occur on synovial cells, vessel walls, and infiltrating leukocytes. There is inhibition of the synthesis of products of arachidonic acid metabolism (prostaglandins and leukotrienes), and generation of toxic oxygen radicals; there are also effects on leukocyte mobility, chemotactic responsiveness, phagocytic activity, and release of lysosomal enzymes during phagocytosis. Inhibition of the activity of these enzymes, as well as effects on the generation of chemotactic and toxic factors from the complement, fibrinolytic, and kinin pathways are other possible modes of action. It is clearly unlikely that all effective drugs are acting on a single enzyme (the cyclooxygenase) in only one of these pathways.

Differences in Effectiveness in Different Diseases. Among the reasons for suggesting that these drugs do not all work through the same mechanism is the difference in their effectiveness in different rheumatic diseases. Crystal synovitis due to urate deposition is well suppressed by colchicine, which is ineffective in other rheu-

matic diseases, while aspirin, which works well in rheumatoid arthritis, is relatively ineffective in gout; other nonsteroidal anti-inflammatory agents work well in both diseases. Similarly, in some cases of juvenile arthritis with fever (Still's disease) aspirin may be ineffective in controlling the fever, but indomethacin or other nonsteroidal agents may be more effective, or corticosteroids may be needed. In rheumatic fever, aspirin was extremely effective in controlling the joint inflammation, but the carditis was often uncontrolled; newer drugs have not been tested systematically in rheumatic fever, since the disease became rare in this country before they were available; however, in other forms of pericarditis (e.g., uremia and postcardiotomy syndrome), aspirin may be ineffective, but other nonsteroidal anti-inflammatory agents, such as indomethacin, are quite useful. Ankylosing spondylitis is better controlled by several of the newer agents than by aspirin.

There are forms of inflammation, such as immediate hypersensitivity, that are unaffected by nonsteroidal anti-inflammatory agents but controlled by antihistaminics or corticosteroids. Clearly a variety of mechanisms of inflammation are operative in different diseases, and the differences in effectiveness of specific agents in specific diseases point to variations in mechanisms of action.

Inhibition of Prostaglandin Synthesis. In the early 1970s Vane[2] introduced the concept that the nonsteroidal anti-inflammatory agents suppress inflammation through inhibition of synthesis of prostaglandins. Effects on prostaglandin synthesis have been demonstrated both in vitro and in vivo for the agents now in use. Cells do not store prostaglandins; release as a result of an injurious stimulus requires fresh biosynthesis; anti-inflammatory drugs affect both steps. Their relative potency as inhibitors of prostaglandin synthesis by rheumatoid synovial tissue in vitro resembles their relative clinical potency in suppressing inflammation.[3]

Much of the toxicity of the nonsteroidal anti-inflammatory agents can also be explained by their action on prostaglandin synthesis. For example, prostaglandins play a key role in protection of the gastric mucosa from autodigestion, through inhibition of acid production and stimulation of production of protective mucus.[4,5] Most of these drugs inhibit prostaglandin synthesis by gastric mucosal cells, contributing to the tendency to erosions and ulcer formation.[5,6] Gastric toxicity occurs with parenteral as well as oral administration of these drugs, since both routes of administration affect prostaglandin synthesis.[7] Inhibition of the cyclooxygenase in platelets blocks thromboxane formation and the ability of platelets to aggregate and initiate clotting. Aspirin, because of its very reactive acetyl group, acetylates amino acids (primarily the e-amino group of lysine) in the enzyme protein. The acetylation is irreversible, and the platelets cannot restore enzyme function, since they have no nucleus and thus no protein synthesizing capacity. New platelets must be released from the bone marrow in sufficient quantities to restore platelet function, a phenomenon for which one must allow one week.

On the other hand, nonsteroidal anti-inflammatory agents other than aspirin inhibit the catalytic activity of the cyclooxygenase competitively, a reversible effect, and enzyme function is restored when the drug is cleared from the blood. The duration of this effect is thus related to the half-life of clearance of the specific drug.[8-10] A similar lasting effect of aspirin occurs in patients with rheumatoid arthritis; prior administration of aspirin caused a lasting effect on prostaglandin synthesis by synovial tissue removed surgically and cultured in vitro, whereas the effect of prior administration of other agents, while demonstrable in vivo, was no longer present in the cultured tissue. All these agents inhibited prostaglandin synthesis when added to the cultures in vitro.[11]

The nonsteroidal anti-inflammatory agents react with several sites on the enzyme protein. The reaction with the catalytic site is competitive with the substrate for the enzyme, arachidonic acid. Reactions with a supplementary site are more characteristic of weak inhibitors and can interfere with inhibition of the catalytic site by stronger inhibitors such as indomethacin.[12]

There are both species and tissue differences in the effects of the various nonsteroidal anti-inflammatory agents on prostaglandin synthesis.[9,13-17] The seminal vesicle is the richest source of the enzyme and is thus used in many in vitro studies, but aspirin is a very poor inhibitor of this enzyme.[9,12,18-21] Another example of the tissue and species specificity of effects on prostaglandin synthesis is the anti-inflammatory effectiveness of acetoaminophen in rats, in suppressing carrageenan pleurisy and other forms of experimental inflammation,[22,23] but acetaminophen lacks such anti-inflammatory effectiveness in humans. On the other hand, acetaminophen does inhibit prostaglandin synthesis in nervous tissue,[24] at least in the hypothalamus, and this accounts for its antipyretic effects and probably contributes to its analgesic effects in humans. Salicylic acid decreases the amount of prostaglandin excreted in the urine each day in normal individuals and clearly inhibits the cyclooxygenase in some tissues in vitro, including the pancreas, where prostaglandins inhibit insulin release.[25] As a result, insulin production is augmented; this may account for the hypoglycemic reactions occasionally seen in diabetics, receiving oral hypoglycemics, who are given aspirin or other salicylates.[25-27]

Salicylic acid, however, is a weak inhibitor of the cyclooxygenase in most tissues, including the platelet and the stomach. In rats it does not cause the gastric erosions seen with aspirin or indomethacin, and when given concomitantly with indomethacin decreases the number of gastric erosions.[28] Salicylic acid has a weak effect on platelet function, which allows its use in patients with bleeding problems with greater safety than other nonsteroidal anti-inflammatory agents. In rats the reaction with platelets does not inhibit their function but blocks the inhibitory effect of other nonsteroidal anti-inflammatory agents on platelets.[28] This interference phenomenon has not been tested in humans, to my knowledge, in part because of concern that the salicylate will interfere with the therapeutic effect of the indomethacin by inhibiting the effect on the cyclooxygenase in synovial and other tissues.

An experimental example of the differences in the effect on prostaglandin synthesis is the demonstration in some animals of a fatal effect of intravenous injection of large amounts of arachidonic acid, because of the mass action effect resulting in the synthesis of large quantities of thromboxane causing extensive intravascular platelet aggregation. Aspirin and indomethacin prevent the fatal outcome, but salicylic acid does not.[29] On the other hand, arachidonic acid given to rats causes diarrhea because of prostaglandin synthesis in the gut; indomethacin prevents this effect, but salicylate does not. If the salicylate is given beforehand, it blocks the effect of the indomethacin, suggesting binding to the enzyme in a fashion which blocks access of the second drug.[28]

Another difference between the effect of salicylic acid and other nonsteroidal anti-inflammatory agents, including aspirin, is the effect on the respiratory tract. Inhibition of the cyclooxygenase by blocking synthesis of prostaglandins augments conversion of arachidonic acid to leukotrienes. Prostaglandins of the E series are bronchodilators, but several leukotrienes are bronchoconstrictors. People who are sensitive to this effect develop asthma, rhinitis, and sometimes nasal polyps when given aspirin; the other nonsteroidal anti-inflammatory agents usually have the same effect in these patients, but generally the nonaspirin salicylate preparations are well tolerated.

Additional evidence that an effect on prostaglandin synthesis is not the entire mechanism of action of the nonsteroidal anti-inflammatory agents comes from the observation that arachidonic acid–deficient animals have much less inflammation than animals with normal nutrition, but the inflammatory reaction that does develop is still inhibited by a variety of drugs.[1]

Evidence for Other Mechanisms of Action. Many other mechanisms of action have been postulated. The ones with the most supporting experimental evidence include effects on the generation of toxic oxygen radicals; on the intracellular concentration of cyclic AMP; on cellular responses, including chemotaxis, phagocytosis, and lysosomal enzyme activity; on interference with complement generation or action; and on bradykinin and the fibrinolytic and coagulation systems.

Neutrophils, which generate small quantities of prostaglandins, consume a great deal of oxygen, converting it to superoxide; this process contributes to the inflammatory process. Oxygen radicals are also generated in the synthesis of prostaglandins, as a product of the reaction that converts prostaglandin G_2 to prostaglandin H_2, and these radicals are toxic to proteins, including the cyclooxygenase, causing a decrease in enzymatic activity in vitro unless the toxic oxygen radicals are constantly removed.[7]

Salicylates act directly as scavengers of hydroxyl radicals,[30] and there is evidence that sulindac is a scavenger of free radicals.[7] The active form of this drug, the sulfide, formed by reduction of the prodrug in the liver, inhibits the enzyme cyclooxygenase, decreasing prostaglandin synthesis, but it also consumes free oxygen radicals. In the process it is reversibly converted back to the parent sulindac. The drug is thus partially inactivated in the tissues, but the process may contribute to its anti-inflammatory effectiveness.[7]

Complement components, especially C5a, when added to plasma, stimulate neutrophils to generate oxygen radicals; nonsteroidal anti-inflammatory agents also block this response.[31]

Effect on Leukocytes. Migration of leukocytes into sites of inflammation is affected by various nonsteroidal anti-inflammatory agents. Some of the leukotrienes, products of the lipoxygenase pathway of arachidonic acid metabolism, are chemotactic for neutrophils. Since inhibition of prostaglandin synthesis increases the amount of arachidonic acid converted to leukotrienes, the nonsteroidal anti-inflammatory drugs can increase the number of neutrophils that accumulate in experimental inflammation.[32,33] A similar effect occurs in human synovial fluid.[34]

Observations made on benoxaprofen, although it has been removed from the market, are illustrative of the possible actions of nonsteroidal anti-inflammatory drugs. Benoxaprofen, which inhibited the lipoxygenase as well as the cyclooxygenase,[35] decreased the migration of leukocytes into sites of experimental inflammation, with a greater effect on monocytes than on neutrophils.[19] Higher doses were required to affect migration of neutrophils. These phenomena were demonstrated in a study of human peritoneal macrophages, as well as in guinea pigs and rats.[36] Benoxaprofen was also shown to affect migration of human leukocytes into the synovial fluid in patients with rheumatoid arthritis and spondyloarthropathy.[34]

Benoxaprofen had a direct effect on migration of mononuclear cells, inhibiting their response to chemotactic stimuli in vitro; an effect on the generation of chemotactic stimuli could not account for this action. A decreased binding of chemoattractant to plasma membrane receptors was demonstrated with decreased cytoskeletal rearrangement.[37]

Other nonsteroidal anti-inflammatory agents, including indomethacin, ibuprofen, ketoprofen, naproxen and aspirin, had similar effects on leukocyte responses to chemotactic stimuli following in vivo administration.[19,30,38-40] Sulindac is reported to have a moderate effect on the lipoxygenase pathway.[17]

In a study of pleurisy induced with carrageenan in rats, only phenylbutazone and indomethacin suppressed migration of mononuclear cells in vitro, while a battery of nonsteroidal anti-inflammatory agents suppressed migration of mononuclear cells in vivo; none suppressed migration of neutrophils into the pleural exudate. Steroids suppressed migration of both neutrophils and mononuclear cells. All the drugs tested suppressed inflammation in rats rendered leukopenic beforehand. Thus, there is evidence for differences in the mechanisms of action of various anti-inflammatory drugs, and it is an oversimplification to focus only on inhibition of prostaglandin synthesis, although that mechanism certainly is important.[41-44]

Nonsteroidal anti-inflammatory drugs counteract membrane permeability in a variety of cells and subcellular organelles. Stabilization of lysosomal membranes of migrating leukocytes, inhibition of lysosomal enzyme function, and inhibition of lymphocyte function all have been suggested as possible mechanisms of action of these agents. Indomethacin and some other nonsteroidal agents inhibit phosphodiesterase, resulting in elevated intracellular levels of cyclic AMP.[45] Since cAMP stabilizes cell membranes, including those of lysosomes in neutrophiles, and decreases generation of superoxide, this could explain such an effect of these drugs. In addition, piroxicam inhibits phagocytosis and release of lysosomal enzymes from neutrophils in experimental synovitis in dogs,[46] and ketoprofen stabilizes lysosomal membranes against osmotic shock.[47] In rheumatoid arthritis, inhibition of release of activity of lysosomal enzymes could decrease the rate of cartilage degradation, which occurs as a result of phagocytosis by neutrophils of immune complexes trapped in articular cartilage.

Complement components, especially C5a, cause granulocytes to become sticky, leading to clumping of cells and vaso-occlusion. This mechanism causes extension of infarction in experimental myocardial infarction. Nonsteroidal anti-inflammatory drugs inhibit the adhesiveness of the neutrophils to each other and to vascular endothelium; ibuprofen (but not aspirin) decreased the volume of myocardial infarcts in cats.[31]

Neutrophils produce small amounts of prostaglandins when stimulated, but an in vitro stimulus such as the peptide FMLP causes aggregation. Indomethacin, aspirin, piroxicam, and ibuprofen prevent this response by the neutrophils in concentrations in vitro similar to those achieved after in vivo administration.[48]

Oxidative phosphorylation is strongly inhibited by aspirin, other salicylates, phenylbutazone, and indomethacin and to a lesser extent by ibuprofen,[49] but numerous agents that are not anti-inflammatory also inhibit this pathway. Ibuprofen partially suppresses leukocyte mobility and phagocytosis, and it, along with other nonsteroidal anti-inflammatory agents, inhibits sulfate uptake by cartilage in vitro.[49] This effect may be relevant to the cartilage breakdown that occurs in osteoarthritis as a result of increased degradation of cartilage matrix components. Interestingly, one nonsteroidal anti-inflammatory agent, benoxaprofen, was shown to cause an increase in sulfate uptake in articular cartilage,[50] an effect that would be beneficial in osteoarthritis; other agents have not been as carefully studied in this system.

Immunologic Effects. The variety of effects of nonsteroidal anti-inflammatory agents on immune functions suggests an effect of these drugs beyond that of suppressing the obvious clinical manifestations of inflammation. For example, aspirin inhibits DNA synthesis by guinea pig lymphocytes stimulated by phytohemagglutinin in vitro.[51] The abnormal T-lymphocyte function described in patients with rheumatoid arthritis and progressive systemic sclerosis, a decreased responsiveness to in vitro stimulation by phytohemagglutinin compared with controls, is reversed toward normal by addition of tolectin in vitro. Oral administration of tolectin to patients with rheumatoid arthritis in a dose of 1200 mg for 7 weeks[52] increased T-lymphocyte responsiveness, an effect similar to that observed with levamisole.

In vitro, formation of prostaglandin E_2 inhibits proliferation of T-lymphocytes, lymphokine production, and other T-lymphocyte functions; incorporation of nonsteroidal anti-inflammatory agents in these systems removes this inhibitory effect. As a result immunostimulation occurs. In guinea pigs, indomethacin causes an increase in skin test reactivity, resulting in an increased area of induration. In a study of 20 anergic patients with chronic combined immunodeficiency syndrome, most developed positive skin test reactivity when given indomethacin; skin test reactivity was lost when the drug was stopped and reappeared on repeat administration.[53]

In vitro cultures of lymphocytes and monocytes from patients with rheumatoid arthritis synthesize rheumatoid factor; incorporation of indomethacin in the culture medium results in decreased production of rheumatoid factor. Apparently the prostaglandins formed in vitro inhibit the action of suppressor (OKT8) cells; nonsteroidal anti-inflammatory agents, by blocking synthesis of prostaglandins, release these cells from inhibition and rheumatoid factor production decreases. A similar effect can be demonstrated in vivo; piroxicam given to patients with rheumatoid arthritis caused a decrease in rheumatoid factor concentration in plasma, which was detectable using a sensitive radioimmunoassay for rheumatoid factor.[54]

Analgesic Effects

The analgesic effects of the nonsteroidal anti-inflammatory drugs have been assumed to be due to an inhibitory effect on the sensitivity of peripheral pain receptors, but a simple direct mechanism of action has not been established. Evidence points to more complex actions, including diminution of prostaglandin synthesis peripherally, which decreases the sensitivity of peripheral nerve receptors, and effects on both spinal cord and brain function, perhaps also mediated through inhibition of prostaglandin synthesis.

Prostaglandins cause a long-lasting sensitization of peripheral nerve endings, resulting in the perception of pain from stimuli, such as pressure, that are not ordinarily painful.[14] This phenomenon would account for the occurrence of tenderness at sites of inflammation, and inhibitors of prostaglandin synthesis decrease tenderness experimentally. Most of the nonsteroidal anti-inflammatory drugs relieve pain due to experimental inflammation, but not other types of pain.[55]

Prostaglandin E_2 infused intradermally or intramuscularly does not cause pain unless high concentrations are used; low concentrations sensitize nerve endings to low amounts of histamine (which causes itching) or bradykinin (which causes pain) in concentrations that do not themselves give symptoms. Aspirin and other nonsteroidal agents do not prevent this direct effect of prostaglandin infusion.[56] Leukopenia in rats diminishes edema due to carrageenan injection but does not prevent the development of a hyperalgesic state. Histamine, bradykinin, or acetylcholine intradermally produces short-lived pain, but when accompanied by prostaglandins, strong pain results.[14]

The nonsteroidal anti-inflammatory drugs affect transmission of pain at dorsal root ganglia and in the spinal cord, as well as at higher levels. One drug extensively studied in this fashion, zomepirac, penetrates the blood-brain barrier and decreases prostaglandin levels that occur in the cerebrospinal fluid after peripheral nerve stimulation. Zomepirac also decreases the background electrical activity of spinothalamic tract nuclei, as well as antagonizing the increase in activity of these nuclei that occurs after painful peripheral stimuli.[57] The levels of prostaglandins in the cerebrospinal fluid correlate with the background activity of the spinothalamic tract cells in the thalamus. Acetaminophen also decreases hyperalgesia in a dose-related manner when injected intraventricularly in rats.[14] The actions of nonnarcotic analgesics such as zomepirac are not reversed by naloxone, indicating that opiate receptors are not involved in its action, but narcotic drugs also decrease prostaglandin synthesis in the brain after a peripheral nerve stimulus.

The observation that morphine, given intrathecally, has potent analgesic effects without central depression, and that the nonsteroidal anti-inflammatory drugs have central effects, has eliminated the older distinction that the narcotics are centrally acting and the nonsteroidal anti-inflammatory drugs peripherally acting analgesics.

The analgesic effect of the nonsteroidal anti-inflammatory drugs is increased by increasing doses in several studies,[58] and it is not clear if a plateau level of effect occurs at a certain dose. In the case of aspirin, increased effect occurs with increasing single doses ranging from 300 mg to about 1300 mgm.[58] It is difficult to extend these studies to test higher doses, since only patients with moderately severe pain can be used for the studies, and most such patients achieve complete relief at moderate doses, precluding testing at higher doses. The slope of the dose-response curve is relatively flat compared with strong analgesics such as the narcotics; nevertheless, large doses of these agents are useful when necessary, unless there are side effects. Further, the narcotic analgesics work through an entirely different mechanism, and thus the effects of the two types of drugs can be additive; combination therapy with a narcotic and a non-narcotic analgesic, in relatively large dosage, is useful in difficult or prolonged painful states.

Suppression of Fever

Suppression of prostaglandin synthesis is probably responsible for the antipyretic effects of these agents.[51,59]

An increase in prostaglandin E–like activity can be demonstrated in the cerebrospinal fluid following injection of pyrogen into animals; prostaglandin E_1 injected into the anterior hypothalamus or cerebral ventricles is the most powerful pyrogen known. The various nonsteroidal anti-inflammatory agents, including aspirin and indomethacin, prevent the increase in prostaglandins following a pyrogenic stimulus; acetaminophen has a similar effect. The nonsteroidal anti-inflammatory agents do not prevent the febrile response to direct injection of prostaglandin into the third ventricle of cats.[59,60] Sodium injected into ventricles also produces fever; these drugs do not prevent this form of fever.[59]

Acetaminophen inhibits prostaglandin synthesis in vitro by brain tissue but not by spleen.[61] A similar tissue specificity of inhibitors of prostaglandin synthesis presumably occurs in humans, accounting for the antipyretic activity of this drug without an anti-inflammatory effect.

PHARMACOKINETICS OF THE NONSTEROIDAL ANTI-INFLAMMATORY DRUGS

Absorption and Bioavailability. All of the nonsteroidal anti-inflammatory drugs currently on the market are relatively rapidly and reliably absorbed. All are extensively bound to plasma protein, primarily albumin, and have a small apparent volume of distribution, generally about 0.1 to 0.2 liter per kg of body weight.[62] Disposition generally follows a two-compartment model, with rapid equilibration into the central compartment, primarily the plasma and remainder of the extracellular fluid, then slow diffusion into a peripheral compartment. Similarly, blood levels generally show a biphasic decline, an initial rapid phase and then a slower terminal phase, presumably modified by diffusion out of the peripheral compartment.

Bioavailability of all the formulations being marketed is good. Food impairs absorption of only one of the nonsteroidal anti-inflammatory agents, fenoprofen, although ibuprofen administered with a meal is absorbed slower, with a lower peak serum concentration.[63,64] Neutralization of gastric acidity by food decreases the gastric irritation caused by these drugs, and the effects on absorption are too small to outweigh the advantage of administering them with meals. In one instance, isoxicam, there is evidence that food increases absorption.[64]

All the nonsteroidal anti-inflammatory agents are relatively acidic molecules, with pK values between 4 and 5. Thus, in the presence of normal gastric acidity, they are un-ionized and are more soluble in lipids, entering gastric mucosal cells relatively well. Gastric toxicity is increased by local absorption in the stomach, where these drugs are directly toxic to mucosal cells. Neutralization of gastric acid raises the pH of the gastric juice above the pK of these drugs, making them more water soluble and less lipid soluble. Less is absorbed into gastric mucosal cells, and thus there is less gastric

Table 50–2. Some Pharmacologic Characteristics of the Nonsteroidal Anti-inflammatory Drugs

Drug	Volume of Distribution (L/kg)	Protein Binding (Percent)	Renal Excretion (Percent Unchanged)
Alclofenac	0.1–0.4	> 99	*†
Aspirin§	0.16	40–70	< 2
Azapropazone	—	> 95	40–60
Benoxaprofen	—	—	0
Carprofen	0.4	> 98	< 5
Diclofenac	1.2	99.7	< 2
Diflunisal	10–12	high	< 20
Fenbufen	—	> 99	42
Fenoprofen	0.07–0.1	> 95	< 5
Flufenamic acid	—	> 90	< 10
Flurbiprofen	0.1	> 99	< 10
Ibuprofen	0.1 (est.)	99	< 2
Indomethacin	0.8	90–99	< 15
Isoxicam	0.17	95–98	1–2
Ketoprofen	0.1		—†
Mefenamic acid	—	> 90	< 10‡
Naproxen	0.09	99.5	10
Phenylbutazone	0.09	98–99	< 2
Piroxicam	0.14	99	2–5
Salicylate	0.1–0.24	85–95	2–30 (pH dependent)
Sulindac	—	93–98	< 20
Tolmetin	0.1	> 99	< 10
Zomepirac	—	—	5

*Possible nonlinear kinetics with accumulation disproportionate to dose.
†Slower terminal phase of clearance known or likely.
‡Slow elimination of metabolites with enterohepatic recirculation.
§See chapter on aspirin and salicylates for details.

toxicity. The nonsteroidal anti-inflammatory agents enter the gastric mucosa from the plasma as well, and thus systemic administration causes gastric toxicity.[7]

As the drugs are highly protein bound, only the small amount of free drug may be available to enter tissues (Table 50–2). The free, unbound drug may be the effective form; free drug levels are extremely low, but they are in constant equilibrium with the bound form. There is no information on the effect of low serum albumin levels on the disposition or effect of these drugs. Concomitant administration of aspirin with indomethacin or fenoprofen results in competition for protein-binding sites, resulting in displacement and decreased plasma levels of the drug, with increased clearance by either the kidney, liver, or both. A similar phenomenon occurs for most but not all the nonsteroidal anti-inflammatory agents. Although displacement from protein usually decreases the half-life of clearance of the drug, it is possible that tissue penetration of the drug is increased; thus the effect of competition for protein binding on tissue levels is not clear.

Inflammation, by inducing exudation and thus increasing the concentration of serum proteins in extracellular fluids, may increase the concentration of drug in the areas where the effect is needed. Acidity at sites of inflammation causes dissociation from plasma proteins and enhances penetration of cell membranes locally. Thus, experimentally, nonsteroidal anti-inflammatory agents are concentrated at sites of inflammation.[30,65]

In general, synovial fluid levels lag several hours behind serum levels of these drugs, rising more slowly and declining in parallel to plasma levels. In some studies synovial fluid levels declined more slowly than plasma levels and thus were higher for a few hours during single-dose studies. The levels in synovial fluid are determined more by the rate of the terminal clearance phase than the initial phase which determines early plasma levels.[62] In general, synovial fluid levels at steady-state plasma concentration average about 40 percent of plasma levels,[34,62,66-70] probably reflecting the lower protein concentration in the synovial fluid.[62] Similar observations on salicylate levels averaged 44 percent of peak levels in serum, but there was a wide range (16 to 90 percent).[69]

Blood Levels. The few studies of plasma levels obtained with the nonsteroidal anti-inflammatory agents show considerable interindividual variation in the peak blood levels achieved after single doses, as well as in the plateau levels found after multiple doses. A fourfold or greater range of levels occurs on a single dosage,[71] although there is an increase in mean blood levels with increased dosage.[72,73] No detailed analysis has been made of the factors that affect these blood levels or of the therapeutic significance of the observed variation.

Optimum therapeutic blood levels have not been determined for the newer agents; studies of phenylbutazone have suggested that 50 to 100 μg per ml is optimum, with little additional therapeutic benefit and increased toxicity above 100 μg per ml.[62] Trough levels of free and total naproxen showed a good correlation with clinical responses.[74] The usefulness of these agents will be substantially enhanced when the maximum effectiveness of each of these drugs has been correlated with blood levels and blood levels have become readily available to the clinician.

Metabolic Clearance. In general, there is little renal clearance of unchanged drug; the nonsteroidal anti-inflammatory drugs are extensively metabolized in the liver, and most of the altered or conjugated metabolites are excreted by the kidney.[62] Hepatic clearance is much lower than blood flow to the liver; thus, there is no problem of extensive first-pass metabolism (except for aspirin, which is deacetylated rapidly by the liver). Biliary excretion is variable, ranging from 2 to 50 percent, with enterohepatic recirculation occurring for a few drugs. A significant proportion of sulindac and meclofenamate is excreted in the bile and appears in the feces. This may account for the relatively high incidence of side effects in the lower intestine with these agents. One of the drugs under development, isoxicam, is excreted into the bile in dogs and humans to the extent of 60 percent, but no clinical implications of this phenomenon have been reported yet.[75]

Some nonsteroidal anti-inflammatory agents, notably sulindac and fenbufen, are administered as relatively inactive "prodrugs," which have to be metabolized to more active compounds in the liver to be clinically effective. Since the prodrug does not inhibit the gastric cyclooxygenase directly in the stomach, there is less gastric irritation, but it does not eliminate the problem, since the circulating active form of the drug can still affect the gastric mucosa.[7,76]

Any drug that is metabolized extensively can show considerable variability in clearance. A genetic basis for differences in rates of clearance was suggested based on studies of identical and fraternal twins.[62] An age effect on rates of clearance occurs with phenylbutazone[62] and also benoxaprofen, for which a T½ of 29 hours was found in younger patients (average age 41 years) and a T½ of 111 hours was found in much older patients (average age 82 years).[77] Males and patients on steroids metabolize salicylate faster; there is no information on the effect of gender or steroids on rates of clearance of the newer nonsteroidal anti-inflammatory drugs. Disease can alter metabolism of drugs; for example, the clearance of salicylates varies in normals as compared with patients with rheumatoid arthritis.[78] Similar data are not yet available regarding the newer nonsteroidal anti-inflammatory agents. Plasma levels of these drugs are affected by displacement from protein-binding sites,[79] a phenomenon that occurs when a variety of agents are administered concomitantly.

In general, lipophilicity influences both the rate of absorption of these drugs and their rate of metabolism by the liver. A low pKa gives low lipophilicity, and slower absorption, but also a slower rate of metabolism or excretion. Drugs with a high pKa have higher lipophilicity and thus more rapid absorption, but more rapid renal excretion and a short half-life of clearance.[66] Lipophilicity may affect penetration of drug into the cerebrospinal fluid; for example, zomepirac, which has an oil/water solubility coefficient twice that of tolmetin, enters the cerebrospinal fluid better.[31] The sulfoxide group of the relatively inactive sulindac is reduced to a sulfide, increasing affinity for the lipid layer about 1000-fold, approximately the same magnitude as the increase in activity as a cyclooxygenase inhibitor. In addition, the increased lipid solubility results in the accumulation of the sulfide form in tissues, while the prodrug sulindac tends to have higher concentrations in body fluids.[7]

Rates of Clearance. The rates of clearance (see Table 50–2) of the various nonsteroidal anti-inflammatory agents from the plasma significantly influence the clinical properties of these agents. Reports of the half-life of clearance of these agents all give average figures, which are useful guides, but it must be kept in mind that all these studies showed considerable interindividual variation in the rate of clearance, often over more than a twofold range. In addition, there are few useful studies of the effect of age, sex, disease, and concomitant administration of other types of drugs, such as anticoagulants, diuretics, and so on, on the rates of clearance of these agents. Most of the data reported are based on studies of young, healthy adult males. Undoubtedly considerable variation exists in different patients, and this phenomenon may account in part for the variability in responsiveness to these drugs.

Accordingly, in Table 50–3 the drugs are grouped

Table 50–3. Duration of Action of the Nonsteroidal Anti-inflammatory Drugs

	Clearance t½ (Hours)	Recommended Daily Dosage

Agents with Relatively Short Duration of Action
Average half-life is 1 to 8 hours. Time to steady-state concentration ranges from 4 to 16 hours. These drugs have rapid initial effect but frequent doses are necessary.

Tolemetin	1*	600–2000 mg
Indomethacin	1.5–2	75–200 mg
Ibuprofen	1–3	1.2–2.4 g
Fenoprofen	2–3	2.4–3 g
Salicylate (low dose)	2–3	(under 2.5 g)
Alclofenac	<3	none
Mefenamic acid	4 (estimate)	1.5–2.0 g
Flufenamic acid	4 (estimate)	600–800 mg
Meclofenamate	2–4	200–400 mg
Flurbiprofen	6	150–400 mg
Zomepirac	7–8†	none

Agents with Medium Duration of Action (t½ = 10–20 Hours)
Once-daily dosage is usually satisfactory. Time to steady state concentration 2 to 4 days.

Fenbufen	10‡	600–1000 mg
Azapropazone	12	900–1800 mg
Naproxen	12–15	500–1000 mg
Diflunisal	10–15	500–1000 mg
Sulindac	18‡	200–400 mg
Salicylate (high doses)	20	3.0–6.0 g

Agents with Moderately Long Duration of Action (t½ = 24–36 Hours)
Once-daily dosage is usually satisfactory. Time to steady-state concentration 4 to 7 days.

Piroxicam	24–36	20 g
Isoxicam	31 (range 21–70)	200 mg§
Benoxaprofen	25–32	none

Agents with Very Long Duration of Action in Maintenance Doses (t½ over 48 Hours)
Once-daily dosage is satisfactory. Time to steady-state concentration 2 to 3 weeks; thus, prolonged monitoring for initial toxicity is important.

Phenylbutazone	72 (range 29–176)	300–400 mg
Oxyphenbutazone	72 (range 29–176)	300–400 mg

*Longer periods (4 to 6 hours) reported based on study of terminal phase of half-life.
†Half-life of zomepirac goes up to 9 to 10 hours after multiple doses.
‡Half-life figures given are those for the principal, active metabolites in the case of sulindac and fenbufen.
§Since drug is not yet on the market, recommended daily dosage is not fully established. The dosage listed was used in studies of clinical effectiveness of the drug.

based on duration of action, which correlates better with clinical experience than with the actual half-life of clearance figures reported for each individual agent.

Steady-State Concentrations. In general, with repeated dosage, it takes 4 to 5 half-lives of clearance for steady-state plasma levels of a drug to be reached. As a result, short-acting nonsteroidal anti-inflammatory drugs reach plateau levels after the first day of therapy; drugs that have a half-life of about 12 hours require two full days,

while those with half-lives of 24 to 36 hours require about a week to achieve full effect. In an urgent clinical situation, such as acute gouty arthritis, a loading dose is advisable if a larger amount of drug on the first day would not be too toxic. Phenylbutazone is often used in this manner.

Since the mechanism of inhibition of platelet function is based on competitive inhibition of the cyclooxygenase by all the nonsteroidal anti-inflammatory drugs except aspirin, this side effect of these drugs clears as the drug is cleared from the plasma. Bleeding from impairment of platelet function may not cease until the drug is cleared sufficiently; the time needed to achieve plateau blood levels is a reasonable guide to the time needed for restoration of platelet function after discontinuing the drug. Therefore, with very long-acting agents, such as phenylbutazone, it may take three weeks or more for bleeding to stop. On the other hand, with rapidly cleared drugs, such as tolectin, indomethacin, fenoprofen, or diclofenac, platelet function is restored rapidly, and it is possible to give these drugs close to the time of surgery.

Other Clinical Implications of Clearance Data. With the rapidly cleared drugs, if a dose is missed for any reason, symptoms may return quickly. Similarly, these drugs may lose their effectiveness overnight, resulting in pain, loss of sleep and severe morning stiffness. To compensate, a large bedtime dose of indomethacin may be given; the drug enters adipose and nervous tissue and is released slowly, prolonging its action. Central nervous system toxicity is usually minimal, since the patient sleeps through it.[80] Alternatively, a longer-acting drug at bedtime can be combined with a shorter-acting agent during the day, to give a sustained overnight effect.

CLINICAL EFFECTS OF NONSTEROIDAL ANTI-INFLAMMATORY AGENTS

The nonsteroidal anti-inflammatory agents that have reached the market are all effective in the treatment of various rheumatic diseases. Tests of effectiveness have established that the drugs are more effective than placebo in patients with rheumatoid arthritis, osteoarthritis, and painful musculoskeletal injuries and, in some instances, in other rheumatic diseases, including gout. These drugs are generally effective in the treatment of rheumatic diseases; but, in each instance, not all of the studies necessary have been performed to gain approval for labeling for every possible indication. Some of the drugs in this category, such as zomepirac, have been tested and marketed as analgesics but are inhibitors of prostaglandin synthesis and are anti-inflammatory.

Tests comparing the relative effectiveness of the newer drugs to aspirin, or to each other, have generally shown small, statistically insignificant differences, although differences in frequency of side effects may be found. It is important to keep in mind that it is difficult to demonstrate a statistically significant difference in effectiveness of two drugs in such studies. Most trials purposely exclude unresponsive patients who have failed to benefit from similar agents, concentrating on patients with mild to moderately severe disease. As a result, relatively complete suppression of symptoms and objective findings occurs with each drug and no difference in effectiveness is demonstrated. Differences that may occur in the few severe cases are lost in the overall statistics, which are dominated by the abundance of mild cases. These studies are often misinterpreted as having established that there is no difference in effectiveness between two drugs, whereas in fact a proper interpretation is that the study failed to refute the null hypothesis that no difference exists, or more simply, failed to establish that a difference exists.

Other problems with the interpretation of reported comparisons of these drugs arise from changes in recommended dosages with time. Most of these agents were first marketed in relatively low doses, just high enough to show a difference from placebo, with minimal risk of toxicity. As experience showed a need for more effect in many cases, and that higher doses were safe, the recommended doses were progressively increased; meanwhile large, multicenter trials were initiated using the earlier dosage schedule. By the time the study was completed, analyzed and published, the dosage tested was no longer being used.[81] Thus, the data in many reports are of limited value. Finally, it is well established that the maximum anti-inflammatory effect of aspirin is only achieved at relatively high plasma levels, which requires pushing the drug to tolerance in most patients; a similar phenomenon may also be apparent with the other nonsteroidal agents when this approach has been effectively tested.

In all studies comparing several drugs, groups of patients preferred each; this variation in preferences of individuals for specific drugs has been a general phenomenon for unclear reasons, and the possibility of greater effectiveness of one agent in an individual patient makes it wise to try several of the drugs in sequence if the first does not give a satisfactory response.[30,82]

There are many excellent reviews of the clinical effectiveness, mechanisms of action, and pharmacology of these drugs.[30,49,76,83-90]

Effects on Specific Clinical Problems

Rheumatoid Arthritis. Subjective, objective, and laboratory parameters of disease activity of rheumatoid arthritis show improvement, and most patients gain significant benefit from the nonsteroidal anti-inflammatory drugs. In many patients, however, control of the manifestations of the disease may be incomplete, and other forms of therapy may need to be added to the regimen. Some rheumatologists have replaced aspirin with one of these drugs as the first-line agent in the treatment of rheumatoid arthritis[82] despite their increased cost. In one noncontrolled study, patients showed about the same frequency of preference for aspirin as for each of several of the newer nonsteroidal anti-inflammatory agents;[91] thus, only a minority of the patients preferred

aspirin. In addition, repeated studies have shown more gastrointestinal side effects and more occult blood loss with plain but not coated aspirin than with the newer agents.[92,93] It is not clear, however, if the use of any of these drugs in full anti-inflammatory doses would have changed the results appreciably.

Increasing attention is being given to the possibility that these drugs have a suppressive effect on disease in rheumatoid arthritis. Since, in general, damage to rheumatoid joints is proportional to the severity of the inflammatory process, suppression of inflammation could retard damage to articular tissues.[30] The newer agents have a more complete suppressive effect on disease in many patients, and some can give smooth 24-hour suppression of the inflammation. A preliminary report suggests slowing of the rate of development of erosions in patients given benoxaprofen.[94] A progressive decrease occurred in the number of abnormal joints over a 2-year period in patients receiving tolectin,[52] and, as described above, improvement in immunologic abnormalities has been reported, including normalization of T-lymphocyte function in patients receiving tolectin or piroxicam treatment,[54,95] and a decrease in rheumatoid factor levels in those on piroxicam.[54] There is no clear-cut evidence of a relationship between the severity of the inflammation or the immunologic abnormalities with the extent of the joint destruction in rheumatoid arthritis, but these changes certainly seem to be in the right direction. More carefully designed, extensive studies, similar to those that demonstrated a disease-suppressive effect for gold and penicillamine, are being conducted with several of these agents.

Juvenile Arthritis. Only tolectin has received approval by the Food and Drug Administration (FDA) for use in children, perhaps reflecting the cost of studies needed to obtain such approval. Other drugs have been used in children, and there are reports of effectiveness of ibuprofen (using doses in the range of 40 to 50 mg per kg per day and a maximum dose of 2 g per day), and naproxen (in doses of 10 mg per kg per day, up to 750 mg per day).[96,97] Doses given to children on a weight basis should never exceed the maximum given adults.

Indomethacin is especially useful in boys with ankylosing spondylitis, in juvenile-onset pauciarticular arthritis with positive HLA B-27, and occasionally in patients with systemic onset with higher fever (Still's syndrome) unresponsive to other nonsteroidal anti-inflammatory agents. In addition, indomethacin may be useful in boys with hip pain due to benign synovitis unrelieved by other drugs. Indomethacin is used in doses of 1.5 to 3 mg per kg per day up to a maximum of 200 mg per day but reportedly is not well tolerated as chronic therapy and had to be stopped in 43 percent of patients in one series.[96] The main side effects with indomethacin were headache, dizziness, nausea, and severe gastrointestinal distress. The use of indomethacin in children has been inhibited by a report in 1967 of impaired response to infection.[98] There have been no subsequent similar reports,[30] but FDA approval for the use of indomethacin in children was withdrawn after reports of deaths due to hepatitis associated with larger doses in young children.[96]

Osteoarthritis. The analgesic effects of the nonsteroidal anti-inflammatory drugs are particularly useful in the management of osteoarthritis, and all the drugs currently on the market are effective in this disease, relieving pain and increasing functional capacity. Doses lower than those needed to suppress the inflammation in rheumatoid arthritis may be adequate, thus decreasing the frequency of side effects.[49] In addition it is possible to take advantage of the lack of a plateau in analgesic effect with increasing doses of these drugs, combining an agent such as acetaminophen, which does not cause gastric irritation, to gain more analgesia.

The effect of the nonsteroidal anti-inflammatory drugs on chondrocyte metabolism in osteoarthritis has not been thoroughly studied. Early reports showed inhibition of the uptake of radiosulfate by articular cartilage by phenylbutazone and salicylate in vitro.[99,100] One agent, benoxaprofen, stimulates proteoglycan synthesis by cartilage in vitro,[50] an effect that could slow progression of the basic process occurring in the cartilage in this disease.

Ankylosing Spondylitis. Aspirin is clearly less effective than most of the newer nonsteroidal anti-inflammatory agents in the treatment of ankylosing spondylitis. Indomethacin, naproxen, and fenoprofen were shown to be more effective than tolectin and aspirin in one study of ankylosing spondylitis in which the same drugs found about equal preference in the management of patients with rheumatoid arthritis.[91] Phenylbutazone also is useful in the treatment of ankylosing spondylitis.[101,102]

Other Diseases. The nonsteroidal anti-inflammatory agents are useful in the treatment of minor musculoskeletal problems and a variety of nonrheumatic diseases as well. Their effect on uterine function is particularly useful in treatment of *dysmenorrhea* as well as threatened abortion. Women who have dysmenorrhea have higher resting uterine pressure ("tonus') and higher active pressure ("amplitude") as well as a higher frequency of contractions; these changes are attributed to the effects of prostaglandins.[103] Ibuprofen reduces the intrauterine pressure and the frequency of cyclic activity of the uterus, apparently by inhibition of prostaglandin synthesis. Sodium naproxen also reduces intrauterine pressure and uterine pain in women with dysmenorrhea;[103] zomepirac is also effective,[104] as is flufenamic acid.[105] Several nonsteroidal anti-inflammatory agents, including aspirin, indomethacin, and fenoprofen, affect the motility of the pregnant rat uterus and can delay parturition; the dosage necessary for inhibition of uterine contractions is considerably higher for aspirin than other nonsteroidal anti-inflammatory agents studied,[106] which correlates with the greater effectiveness of the newer agents compared with aspirin in the treatment of dysmenorrhea.

Because of the role of prostaglandins in causing vascular dilatation, infants with *patent ductus arteriosus* have been treated with indomethacin. The drug is given in 2 doses, 12 hours apart, and if levels above 250 ng per ml are achieved, the ductus usually closes. But the high frequency of spontaneous closure of the ductus in prematures, and the side effects, including kidney damage, hemorrhage into a ventricle, and necrotizing enterocolitis, has led to caution in suggesting its use for this purpose, since surgery is effective and may be safer.[107]

The effects of aspirin and the nonsteroidal anti-inflammatory drugs on *platelet function* are described earlier in this chapter. Aspirin, because of its prolonged effect, is useful in the management of patients who have had transient ischemic attacks in the central nervous system; newer agents have not been tested in this syndrome. An unexplained potentiating effect of alcohol on bleeding time of patients who have taken aspirin or other nonsteroidal anti-inflammatory agents may be clinically significant.[108]

The vascular effects of the nonsteroidal anti-inflammatory drugs could be a problem in patients with *ischemic heart disease,* since a decrease in coronary blood flow has been reported in patients given indomethacin, along with an increase in systemic blood pressure due to generalized vasoconstriction. The resulting increase in cardiac work, with increased oxygen demand, combined with decreased coronary blood flow can lead to impaired myocardial performance.[109]

Nonsteroidal anti-inflammatory agents are effective in *ocular disease,* since several can inhibit prostaglandin synthesis in uveal and conjunctival tissues; aspirin does not have such an effect in these tissues, but indomethacin, phenylbutazone, and oxyphenbutazone do.[33]

Toxicity

Effect on the Gastrointestinal Tract. The main toxicity of these drugs occurs in the gastrointestinal tract. In almost all studies of these drugs, epigastric distress, nausea, vomiting, and occasionally more serious side effects such as upper gastrointestinal bleeding lead the list of undesirable effects. Occult blood in the stool is almost a universal finding, but in considerably smaller quantities than occurs in patients receiving aspirin. Activation of peptic ulcer can occur with any of these drugs.

The most important reason for the gastrointestinal side effects is the inhibition of gastric prostaglandin synthesis. Prostaglandins increase gastric blood flow, tighten the mucosal barrier, increase mucus production, and decrease acid secretion;[49] prostaglandin E_2 has 2000 times the potency of cimetidine as an inhibitor of gastric acid secretion. These effects protect against gastric erosions or ulcer formation.

Drugs that are administered in inactive form but are activated by metabolism in the liver generally cause less inhibition of prostaglandin synthesis in the stomach, and therefore usually are somewhat less toxic. However, in each instance studied, including that of aspirin, the drug given parenterally inhibits gastric mucosal cyclooxygenase and can cause gastric erosions.[7]

Most clinicians recommend administration of these drugs with food or antacids to minimize gastrointestinal toxicity. If the drugs are given with liquid, they may be left behind in the stomach, since liquid is emptied from the stomach faster than solids, resulting in severe local irritation. Therefore, instructing patients to take the medicine in the middle of a meal could minimize the gastric irritation, whereas the ambiguous instructions "take with meals" usually means that the patient will take the drug after the meal, with coffee or tea, which can add to the local irritation.

Cimetidine is said to be protective against the upper gastrointestinal toxicity caused by the nonsteroidal anti-inflammatory drug[110,111] and may be useful in particularly difficult patients, such as those with a history of peptic ulcer disease or gastrointestinal bleeding. The expense and the potential for added toxicity make it unwise to use cimetidine routinely.

Prostaglandins also influence the function of the lower gastrointestinal tract, the specific effect apparently varying with the functional state of the gut at the time. As a consequence, ibuprofen reportedly causes diarrhea in some patients and constipation in others; it has been used successfully in the treatment of idiopathic diarrhea.[49] Serious lower gastrointestinal toxicity occasionally occurs with these drugs. Crampy lower abdominal pain and colonic bleeding, often from pre-existing diverticular disease, has been reported with several of them.[112] A salicylate combined with a sulfonamide, sulfasalazine, is reportedly useful in the management of ulcerative colitis, probably because of an effect on prostaglandin synthesis in the gut,[113] but there are no reports of the use of newer nonsteroidal anti-inflammatory drugs in inflammatory bowel disease.

Secretion into the bile and enterohepatic recirculation occurs to a varying extent with these drugs. When it occurs, increased local concentration in the gastrointestinal tract results. This phenomenon may account for the higher frequency of lower gastrointestinal toxicity with some of them. For example, mefenamic acid (Ponstel), which is approved for short-term analgesic use in the United States but is marketed abroad as an anti-inflammatory drug, causes a higher frequency of diarrhea, sometimes associated with hemorrhage and inflammation of the bowel; hemolytic anemia was reported with this drug. Meclofenamate (Meclomen), a related substance, also causes a dose-related diarrhea more often than do the other nonsteroidal anti-inflammatory agents.[114] Some clinicians have the impression that sulindac, which also undergoes considerable enterohepatic recirculation, causes a higher incidence of crampy abdominal pain than do most other nonsteroidal antiinflammatory agents. The serious reactions to benoxaprofen appear to be attributable to the extensive enterohepatic circulation of the drug.

Pancreatitis. Pancreatitis has also been reported with these drugs; in one instance the patient received sulindac, plus aspirin, for severe osteoarthritis of the hip.[115,116]

Salicylates have been known to cause a decrease in blood sugar in some individuals, particularly in diabetics who are receiving oral sulfonylureas.[27] A possible mechanism of this effect is the inhibition of prostaglandin synthesis in the pancreas, where the prostaglandins locally inhibit insulin release.[25] The effect of other nonsteroidal anti-inflammatory drugs on islet cell function has not been studied, but hypoglycemic reactions are not reported.

Esophageal stricture was suggested as a side effect of nonsteroidal anti-inflammatory drugs, because of a report that patients with this problem had a higher frequency of ingestion of these drugs than did a control group without dysphagia. The recommendation that patients drink a lot of water after ingesting the drug and not go to bed immediately afterward seems a reasonable precaution.[117]

Hepatotoxicity. The side effect of hepatotoxicity has been reported with several of the newer nonsteroidal anti-inflammatory drugs as well as with aspirin and acetaminophen. Ibuprofen reportedly causes liver toxicity in children but has mild effects on liver function tests in adults.[49] Serious liver toxicity, especially in older people, with several deaths, led to the removal of benoxaprofen from the market in the United States and the United Kingdom.[77] Diclofenac has been reported to cause a hypersensitivity type of hepatitis,[118] and hepatotoxicity has been reported with sulindac,[116] including a report of cholestatic jaundice.[119]

Because of the compensatory effect of prostaglandins synthesized in the kidney on renal blood flow in patients with hypovolemia, patients with cirrhosis who have hypoalbuminemia, ascites, and edema may develop the hepatorenal syndrome if given nonsteroidal anti-inflammatory drugs.

Renal Effects. Local prostaglandin synthesis in the kidney regulates intrarenal blood flow, particularly under circumstances of decreased glomerular filtration and moderate impairment of renal function. Increased amounts of prostaglandins are usually found in the urine in such instances. Aspirin and most other nonsteroidal anti-inflammatory agents, by inhibiting synthesis of the prostaglandins in the kidney, affect this compensatory mechanism; a rise in BUN and serum creatinine results. Among patients with rheumatic diseases, this effect is most frequently seen in those with systemic lupus with renal involvement but can occur in any patient with hypovolemia or intrinsic renal disease. The effect of these drugs is reversible when the drug is stopped and only occasionally requires discontinuation of effective antirheumatic therapy.[120]

Inhibition of renal prostaglandin synthesis causes salt and water retention, occasionally resulting in frank edema. Prostaglandins also affect water handling by the kidney, probably by an effect on cAMP concentration in renal tubular cells. Inhibition of prostaglandin synthesis by indomethacin or meclofenamate enhanced the antidiuretic effect of antidiuretic hormone in rats undergoing water diuresis.[121]

The nonsteroidal anti-inflammatory drugs can block the action of diuretics, including furosemide.[122] This effect can complicate the management of hypertension or congestive heart failure. The combination of triamterine and indomethacin causes serious renal toxicity, with azotemia. Normal medical students given 200 mg per day of triamterene and 150 mg per day of indomethacin showed reversible acute renal failure.[123] No similar effect was found when indomethacin was given with furosemide, hydrochlorothiazide, or spironolactone, perhaps because they work at different sites in the renal tubule. The mechanism suggested was that the toxicity of triamterene is ordinarily prevented by a compensatory increase in prostaglandin synthesis, and this protective mechanism is blocked by indomethacin. The presence of high levels of prostaglandins in the urine may be an indicator of susceptibility to the azotemic effect of aspirin or other nonsteroidal anti-inflammatory agents.[123] Indomethacin has no influence on the half-life of clearance of hydrochlorothiazide.[124]

The inhibition of intrarenal prostaglandin synthesis also affects production of renin. Large doses of aspirin (3.9 g per day) cause a decrease in plasma renin concentration, with a rebound above control values after cessation of the drug.[125] An inhibitory effect of these drugs on renin and angiotensin II genesis may be clinically important in patients who develop hypovolemia as a result of gastrointestinal bleeding; the ability to adjust to blood loss could be impaired, resulting in earlier vasomotor collapse.

Inhibition of renal prostaglandin synthesis is clinically useful in the management of Bartter's syndrome. Increased renal prostaglandin synthesis is a key step in the pathogenesis of this syndrome, leading to increased urinary excretion of prostaglandins and increased formation of renin and aldosterone. Indomethacin and other inhibitors of renal prostaglandin synthesis correct the elevated plasma renin concentration, hyperaldosteronism, and decreased sensitivity to angiotensin infusion characteristic of Bartter's syndrome.[126,127]

Sulindac reportedly has less effect on renal prostaglandin synthesis and thus causes less salt and water retention, inhibition of the effect of diuretics, and azotemia than do the other nonsteroidal anti-inflammatory agents.[128,129]

Acute Allergic Interstitial Nephritis. This side effect has been reported with several of the nonsteroidal anti-inflammatory agents, most often with fenoprofen, but also with ibuprofen,[130] naprosyn, tolmetin, indomethacin, and zomepirac.[129-131] Characteristically such patients have eosinophils in the urine sediment and avid uptake of gallium by the kidney on nuclear scanning. Renal biopsy shows normal-appearing glomeruli on light microscopy, with fusion of glomerular foot processes on electron microscopy. There are interstitial infiltrates consisting of plasma cells and lymphocytes (which are mostly T-lymphocytes) and eosinophils as well as focal deposition of IgG on interstitial and tubular basement membranes. These observations are similar to those made with other instances of drug-induced allergic interstitial nephritis. All instances reversed after the drug was discontinued, with return of BUN to normal, although steroid therapy was given to some of these patients.[132]

Lipid Nephrosis. Lipid nephrosis has been reported with fenoprofen, and there are single case reports with naprosyn and indomethacin.[132,133]

Analgesic Nephropathy. Ingestion of enormous quantities of analgesic medications (averaging 11 kg of aspirin, 8 kg of phenacetin, or 50,000 tablets, usually of combinations of aspirin, phenacetin, and caffeine or codeine) has been associated with abdominal or flank pain, pyuria without evidence of infection, hematuria, acidosis, passage of renal papillae in the urine, hypertension, and azotemia, with many deaths.[134] Phenacetin was most frequently implicated; aspirin is thought to be safe, and a study of renal function in patients who took large amounts of aspirin for rheumatoid arthritis for 10 or more years showed no evidence of impairment of renal function.[135] With the availability of its active metabolite, acetaminophen, phenacetin was replaced and analgesic nephropathy seems to have decreased in frequency, but some investigators feel that any analgesic can cause this syndrome.[136]

All the newer nonsteroidal anti-inflammatory agents cause nephrotoxicity in high doses in a variety of laboratory animals, especially dogs and rats.[137] It is not yet certain whether analgesic nephropathy will turn out to be a problem when sufficient quantities of these drugs have been ingested. Clinicians should remain alert to the possibility that long-term therapy may be associated with serious renal toxicity.

Use of Nonsteroidal Anti-inflammatory Drugs in Renal Failure. Since little direct renal excretion of the nonsteroidal anti-inflammatory drugs occurs, there is no known problem of accumulation of these drugs in patients with lowered glomerular filtration rates. The metabolites of most of these agents are normally cleared by the kidney, and the danger of accumulation of them is unclear. The effect of hemodialysis on blood levels of the drugs and their metabolites is unknown.[138] Several of these agents, most notably indomethacin, have been used in chronic uremic patients in usual dosage without any apparent problem. Diclofenac is also safe in chronic renal failure (see below).

Pseudoallergic Reactions. After ingesting aspirin, some patients develop asthmatic wheezes, rhinitis, and nasal polyps; urticaria and angioedema can also occur. This reaction apparently results from inhibition of the cyclooxygenase, shifting the metabolism of the arachidonic acid into the lipoxygenase pathway, increasing the production of leukotrienes. This reaction to aspirin occurs more often in patients with chronic urticaria and asthmatics but in only about 0.3 percent of normal people.[139,140]

Repeated administration of aspirin usually causes the same reaction in a sensitive patient. Other nonsteroidal anti-inflammatory agents that inhibit the cyclooxygenase cause a similar reaction in these patients. Drugs that are poor inhibitors of the enzyme usually do not cross-react; thus, nonaspirin salicylate and acetaminophen usually can be given to such patients.[139]

Pregnancy. None of the nonsteroidal anti-inflammatory agents are approved for use in pregnancy, since careful studies of safety in pregnancy are impossible.

The effect of these agents on the pulmonary vasculature of the fetus is a concern; inhibition of prostacycline synthesis in arterial walls can cause vasoconstriction; experimentally, closure of the ductus arteriosus in utero can be induced by inhibitors of prostaglandin synthesis, leading to ischemia of the lower parts of the body and developmental abnormalities. Widespread narrowing of the pulmonary vasculature can occur, causing pulmonary hypertension. Instances of persistent pulmonary hypertension have been observed in infants following the use of aspirin or indomethacin by the mother during pregnancy, and a similar syndrome was induced in lambs.[141]

If use of a nonsteroidal anti-inflammatory agent is considered during pregnancy, the indication should be quite strong and informed consent obtained. If possible, use should be limited to the third trimester and discontinued several days to a few weeks before term because during labor the nonsteroidal anti-inflammatory agents can decrease uterine contractions and delay parturition; blood loss at the time of delivery can be increased because of the effect on platelet function.[63]

Other Side Effects. Stevens-Johnson syndrome was reported with several of these agents, including sulindac,[142,143] diflunisal, and diclofenac.[144] Other serious reactions to sulindac reported include toxic epidermal necrolysis, granulocytopenia, aplastic anemia, and thrombocytopenia;[116] aplastic anemia was also reported with fenoprofen.[145] A sterile meningitis has occurred in patients with systemic lupus erythematosus given ibuprofen or sulindac.[116]

Visual blurring occurs with all the nonsteroidal anti-inflammatory agents, but no actual retinopathy has been reported, and the visual effects are reversible when the drug is stopped. *Morbilliform rashes* occur with high doses of these agents; they clear promptly when the drug is discontinued and do not recur at lower doses; clearly these are not allergic rashes. They are probably related to an effect on arachidonic acid metabolism.[146] One of the nonsteroidal anti-inflammatory agents, alclofenac, caused a high incidence of rashes. It was withdrawn from the market because of toxicity, including the occurrence of vasculitis.[147] This drug was a phenylacetic acid derivative that contained a chlorine atom on the main ring. *Anaphylactic reactions* have been reported to occur with higher frequency with tolectin and with zomepirac than with other agents.[148,149]

Interaction with Anticoagulants. The possibility of significant interaction with anticoagulants such as warfarin is great, because of the high degree of protein binding by both types of agents, as well as the possibility of alterations in hepatic metabolism. Apparently, no significant interaction occurs with ibuprofen, tolectin, naproxen, diflunisal, or diclofenac,[27,144] but it is necessary to reduce the dose of warfarin when isoxicam is used concomitantly.[150] An increase in unbound warfarin occurs with concomitant administration of fenoprofen, and some additional prolongation of prothrombin time occurs.[84] Because of their effect on platelet function, extreme caution is necessary when any of these drugs is used in combination with anticoagulants.

COMMENTS ABOUT INDIVIDUAL AGENTS

Points made elsewhere in this chapter will not be repeated in this section, and thus comments are not thorough reviews of each drug.

Indomethacin. Indomethacin (Fig. 50–1) was one of the earliest of the nonsteroidal anti-inflammatory agents to be introduced, and it is the standard agent used in vitro for inhibition of prostaglandin synthesis. Clinically it is very useful and is particularly effective in ankylosing spondylitis and in acute gout; there is also a report of special effectiveness in osteoarthritis of the hip compared with other agents.[151] Although indomethacin may cause less gastric irritation and occult blood loss than aspirin,[93] gastrointestinal side effects are the main limitation to its clinical usefulness.[30,152,153]

Indomethacin has an indole nucleus, resembling serotonin, which may account for its unusual incidence of central nervous system side effects, of which headache is the most common. Dizziness, "light-headedness," depersonalization, loss of concentrating ability, and actual confusion can occur, requiring discontinuation of the drug.

Indomethacin is favored by many clinicians for control of fever in difficult cases, such as lymphomas, but careful comparisons with newer agents have not been performed. Indomethacin has been used to treat Bartter's syndrome because of its effect on renal prostaglandin synthesis, decreasing production of renin and thus of aldosterone;[154] however, in some patients, pseudotumor cerebri has developed.[155]

Because of the relatively rapid clearance of indomethacin, symptoms may return during the night, with bothersome morning stiffness. To achieve smoother control of symptoms, a bedtime dose of 100 mg, coupled with 25 mg three or four times during the day can minimize side effects (patients sleep through the headache) and achieve more prolonged effect, but gastrointestinal side effects are still a problem.[80] The bedtime dose can be added to another short-acting agent with less gastrointestinal toxicity given during the day. A sustained release form of indomethacin (Indocin-SR[R]), which is absorbed more slowly, can achieve smoother blood levels with the drug on a daily dosage of 75 mg twice daily.[156]

Metabolism of indomethacin involves demethylation and deacetylation in the liver, with subsequent excretion of the inactive metabolites in the bile and urine; thus caution is wise in patients with impaired liver function.

Figure 50–1. Chemical structure of indomethacin. (The figures in this chapter are taken from The Merck Index, An Encyclopedia of Chemicals and Drugs. 9th ed. Rahway, New Jersey, Merck Co., Inc., 1976.)

Only small amounts of indomethacin or other nonsteroidal anti-inflammatory agents are excreted unchanged by the kidney. Metabolites are excreted by both the kidney and the liver, but there are no careful studies of the clearance of the metabolites in chronic renal failure. Indomethacin is the nonsteroidal anti-inflammatory drug most frequently used in patients with chronic renal failure, particularly to control the manifestations of uremic pericarditis. No special adjustment of dosage is recommended, but extreme caution should be exercised, particularly in view of the gastrointestinal and central nervous system side effects of the drug, which can resemble manifestations of uremia.

Blood levels of indomethacin are increased by concomitant administration of probenecid.[157] This interaction has the potential of increasing the therapeutic effect of a moderate dose of the drug, with less direct gastric irritation; the systemic effect of indomethacin on the stomach remains, however, and the clinical value of the use of probenecid in this fashion had not been evaluated.

Sulindac. Sulindac (Fig. 50–2) is a chemical relative of indomethacin and is given as a relatively inactive prodrug; the methyl sulfinyl group is converted by the cytochrome system in the liver to a variety of oxidized forms which have increased anti-inflammatory activity.[158] These metabolites are more potent inhibitors of prostaglandin synthesis and are cleared from the plasma more slowly, making twice-a-day dosage satisfactory; 150 to 200 mg of sulindac twice a day is recommended and should rarely, if ever, be exceeded.

The effectiveness of sulindac has been established for rheumatoid arthritis, osetoarthritis, and acute gout,[86] but the relatively long period needed to achieve plateau blood levels (4 to 5 days) and the lack of established safety of a loading dose make it a little less satisfactory for the latter condition. It is less effective than indomethacin and phenylbutazone in the treatment of ankylosing spondylitis.[159] Upper gastrointestinal irritation and bleeding are much less common with sulindac than with aspirin,[30,159] and the drug is much better tolerated than either aspirin or indomethacin; although chemically similar to indomethacin, central nervous system side effects have not been reported with sulindac. However, about 25 percent of patients have other gastrointestinal problems, including constipation and abdominal pain, perhaps because of excretion of active metabolites in the bile affecting prostaglandin synthesis in the gut.

Rare instances of a variety of other types of toxicity have been reported with sulindac, including Stevens-Johnson syndrome; blood dyscrasias, including fatal aplastic anemia;[116] pancreatitis;[160] hepatotoxicity; and aseptic meningitis in patients with systemic lupus.[116] Sulindac does not inhibit diuresis induced by furosemide apparently because of less effect on renal cyclooxygenase activity. Sulindac therefore does not interfere with drugs used for the treatment of hypertension or congestive heart failure, and it does not cause increased azotemia in patients with mild renal failure, as do the other nonsteroidal anti-inflammatory drugs.[128,129] This organ specificity of the effect of the drug makes it particularly useful in many patients.

Sulindac is capable of trapping toxic oxygen radicals, and in the process, in vitro, the active metabolites are converted back to the less active parent sulindac. Thus, this drug has an anti-inflammatory action beyond that of inhibition of prostaglandin synthesis, which could account for its extra effectiveness in some patients.[7]

Tolmetin. A pyrrole acetic acid derivative, chemically related to indomethacin but lacking an indole nucleus, tolmetin (Fig. 50–3) is rapidly cleared from the blood, either unchanged or as a dicarboxylic acid metabolite or a conjugate. Tolmetin is easily displaced from protein-binding sites; for example, aspirin displaces tolmetin competitively and accelerates its already very rapid clearance from the blood.[30] Concomitant use with aspirin had no better effect than aspirin alone.[161] Tolmetin causes fewer gastrointestinal and central nervous system side effects than indomethacin, despite its chemical similarity; 75 percent of patients who could not tolerate indomethacin did tolerate tolectin.[30] Tolmetin is reported to be effective in a variety of rheumatic diseases and is approved for use in juvenile arthritis.

Ibuprofen. The first phenylpropionic acid derivative to be marketed in the United States, ibuprofen is relatively well tolerated and has a particularly low incidence of gastrointestinal side effects.[49] Ibuprofen (Fig. 50–4) is rapidly metabolized, primarily in the liver; less than 10 percent is excreted unchanged in the bile and urine. At the dosage initially recommended, ibuprofen was effective as an analgesic, but it was weakly anti-inflammatory; since then, considerably higher doses have been shown to be well tolerated, and its anti-inflammatory effectiveness has been established. Currently doses of up to 2.4 g per day are approved, but there are reports of the use of 3.2 g per day.[49] The relatively greater analgesic effectiveness makes the drug clinically useful in a variety of problems. It has achieved great favor in the treatment of dysmenorrhea[162] and is effective in osteoarthritis of

Figure 50–3. Chemical structure of tolmetin.

Figure 50–2. Chemical structure of sulindac.

Figure 50–4. Chemical structure of ibuprofen.

Figure 50–5. Chemical structure of fenoprofen.

the hip, in psoriatic arthritis,[163] and, in large doses, in the treatment of gout.[82,164]

Ibuprofen does not induce hepatic microsomal enzymes and reports show absence of interference with the protein binding of warfarin, thus making it safe to use in combination with anticoagulant therapy, although the effect on platelet function has to be kept in mind.[30,49]

There are reports of the occurrence of a meningitis-like syndrome[165] and of a nonspecific febrile reaction[166] in patients with systemic lupus erythematosus given ibuprofen but these are clearly rare events.[49]

Fenoprofen. Fenoprofen (Fig. 50–5) is also a propionic acid derivative with a relatively short half-life. Absorption of fenoprofen is decreased by concomitant food or aspirin, but it is questionable whether this effect is clinically significant.[63] Available in 300-mg capsules, the recommended dose is 2.4 g per day. The drug is effective in a variety of rheumatic diseases, and, as is true of each of these drugs, there are patients who prefer it over aspirin or other anti-inflammatory agents;[30] it is relatively well tolerated, but dyspepsia is its chief side effect. Fenoprofen may cause serious renal toxicity more frequently than the other nonsteroidal anti-inflammatory agents, but this phenomenon is statistically rare.

Naproxen. Naproxen (Fig. 50–6) is a phenylpropionic acid derivative with a relatively long half-life, making twice-a-day dosage satisfactory. It is also relatively well tolerated. Although excreted primarily as a glucuronide conjugate, unbound, free drug is excreted by the kidney. Early studies suggested that doses above 500 mg per day result in increased unbound drug, which is rapidly cleared, suggesting that higher doses would be of no added value; however, clinical trials have established progressively increasing effectiveness with increasing doses, although with a shallow dose response curve.[167] The approved dosage has been increased to 1 g per day, and 1.5 g per day is being tested.

Since the sodium salt of naproxen is more rapidly absorbed than the acid, pain relief occurs sooner, and it is marketed as an analgesic. This advantage applies only to the first dose of the drug, however; the acid form of naproxen is as effective as an analgesic, since it is the active moiety. Naproxen is effective in the treatment of dysmenorrhea,[168] postoperative pain,[169] and dental pain and in sports injuries[170] as well as in the treatment of various rheumatic diseases, including rheu-

Figure 50–6. Chemical structure of naproxen.

matoid arthritis, osteoarthritis,[171] and gout;[172] it was reported to be as effective as phenylbutazone in ankylosing spondylitis.[173]

Concomitant administration of aspirin caused a 16 percent decrease in blood levels of naproxen,[73] a change that was felt not to be clinically important, and a subsequent trial of moderate doses of both agents showed additive effect without additional toxicity.[174]

Probenecid increases the blood levels of naproxen, a surprising effect, since renal tubular secretion of the parent drug is negligible; apparently this effect results from competition for hepatic glucuronyl transferase.[73] There is no significant interaction between naproxen and the sulfonylureas, nor does it change the activity of warfarin, despite interference with protein binding of the warfarin, increasing the free serum fraction of that drug by 13 percent.[73]

Naproxen crosses the placenta, and thus its use in pregnancy is unwise. It may potentiate the toxicity of bilirubin in neonatal jaundice by competing for binding sites on albumin.[83]

As is the case with the other nonsteroidal anti-inflammatory agents, there are reports of severe gastrointestinal bleeding with naproxen,[175,176] but overall the drug is relatively well tolerated, and one study concluded that it can be given safely to patients with a history of peptic ulcer or hiatal hernia, although the patients should be closely followed.[177]

Judging by sales in the United States, the two most popular nonsteroidal anti-inflammatory agents are naproxen and ibuprofen.

Phenylbutazone. The first drug in this group to be introduced, phenylbutazone has been widely used despite initial reports of serious gastrointestinal and bone marrow toxicity. Use of lower doses has decreased the frequency of toxicity markedly. Oxyphenbutazone, a metabolite of phenylbutazone, is also active and is available as a drug; kinetics, efficacy, and side effects are the same for the two agents.

The half-life of phenylbutazone is about 20 hours for high doses, but clearance is much slower with lower doses. At the currently recommended maintenance dose of 300 mg per day, a half-life of over 100 hours occurs. It can take 2 to 3 weeks for plateau steady-state blood levels to be reached, and a similar amount of time for toxicity to clear. An even longer half-life of phenylbutazone is seen in some elderly subjects,[62] and its use in patients over age 60 should be restricted to periods of one week. Phenylbutazone causes salt and water retention, and its use can complicate the management of hypertension or congestive heart failure.

Despite the very slow clearance of phenylbutazone, a dosage of three or four times per day is recommended. Once a day is, in fact, adequate, but dividing the dosage may minimize direct gastric toxicity.

Phenylbutazone and indomethacin are superior to aspirin in the treatment of ankylosing spondylitis[102] and gout. It is also useful for musculoskeletal injuries, but because of potential toxicity it is usually used only when other agents are not satisfactory; however, in such instances it can be a very valuable drug and is widely used by veterinarians for this purpose. In the treatment of acute gout, the use of a loading dose of about 600 mg is recommended to achieve therapeutic levels rapidly. The recommended maintenance dose of 300 mg per day should not be exceeded. Both phenylbutazone and oxyphenbutazone are uricosuric, in contrast to most of the other nonsteroidal anti-inflammatory agents, which are useful in the management of gout without causing uricosuria. This difference in effect may be important in patients with a history of uric acid calculi.

There are patients who receive more benefit from phenylbutazone than any other nonsteroidal anti-inflammatory agent, a phenomenon that occurs with all these drugs. Reports of some differences in the mechanisms of action of phenylbutazone suggest a possible basis for this benefit. For example, in vitro, both chemotaxis and spontaneous motility of neutrophils are inhibited by corticosteroids and phenylbutazone, whereas the other nonsteroidal anti-inflammatory drugs inhibit only chemotaxis.[178]

Azopropazone. Azopropazone is also a pyrazolone derivative, chemically related to phenylbutazone. It has a half-life of about 12 hours, and a biologic half-life of about 20 hours.[179] Although three or four doses a day are recommended, twice-daily dosage should be satisfactory. It takes 4 days to a week for a full steady-state plasma level to be reached. The drug and its inactive metabolites are excreted by the kidneys. Azapropazone is well tolerated but does cause fluid retention and thus problems of hypertension and congestive heart failure may be aggravated; caution is therefore recommended in the use of the drug in the elderly, as with phenylbutazone. In view of the extremely tight protein-binding characteristic of this drug, the possibility of interactions with concurrent anticoagulant and antidiabetic drugs exists; a considerable reduction in dosage of anticoagulant, up to 50 to 75 percent of previous levels, is recommended.[179] Careful monitoring is also recommended when sulfonamides or oral hypoglycemic agents are used concomitantly.[179]

Azapropazone, like the other pyrazolone derivatives, is markedly uricosuric. Because of the hematologic toxicity of other pyrazolones, careful monitoring of bone marrow function is wise; marrow suppression is found in animal studies but not reported in humans; however, the recommended maximum dose of 1800 mg per day should not be exceeded.[179]

Diclofenac. A phenylacetic acid derivative, diclofenac is rapidly absorbed, with peak plasma levels in 1 to 2 hours; the drug is tightly bound to protein and eliminated by the liver, where it is metabolized mainly by hydroxylation, with extensive enterohepatic recirculation.[180] Elimination is biphasic, but it is 90 percent complete 1.5 to 2 hours after the peak plasma level is reached; thus, it is very difficult to obtain smooth, steady-state plasma levels with diclofenac, even with a dosage of three times a day.[144] Interestingly, the drug appears rapidly in the synovial fluid, where, as a result of protein binding, levels persist much longer than in plasma.[144]

Despite its tight binding to protein, diclofenac does not interact with oral hypoglycemic or anticoagulant drugs, and no adjustment in dosage of these agents has been found to be necessary with concomitant administration.[144]

Careful studies of the effect of chronic renal failure on the pharmacokinetics of diclofenac have been performed. In such patients, the drug and its metabolites reach higher plasma levels, but calculations of elimination half-lives are the same as in normal subjects. Excretion of diclofenac and its metabolites in the urine is decreased in proportion to the reduction in glomerular filtration rate, but a compensatory increase in elimination via the bile occurs, preventing accumulation. Thus, patients with renal insufficiency may be given the same dosage schedule as is used for patients with normal renal function.[144,181]

The main side effects of diclofenac are gastrointestinal, but a fatal case of Stevens-Johnson syndrome has been reported; other serious reactions, including fatal aplastic anemia, have occurred, but the patients were taking other drugs in much closer temporal relationship to the onset of symptoms of the marrow dyscrasia. Single instances of deaths from pancreatitis and other serious gastrointestinal reactions are also reported.[144]

Because of lowered plasma levels of diclofenac with concomitant aspirin administration, combined therapy is not recommended.[144]

Diflunisal. A salicylate derivative, diflunisal has a phenyl group containing two fluorines added to the parent salicylate molecule. Conjugated in the liver, the entire parent molecule, containing the fluorine atoms, is excreted in the urine. Excretion is impaired by chronic renal failure, and the drug is not removed by hemodialysis;[182] thus, it should be avoided in patients with chronic renal failure.

The elimination half-life of diflunisal is dose dependent, increasing from 7 to 8 hours at 125 mg to 8 to 10 hours at 250 mg, and at 15 hours to 500 mg, in single doses. The recommended dosage is 500 mg followed by 250 to 500 mg twice a day. At this dosage, steady-state plasma levels may not be reached for 7 to 9 days,[89] and a loading dose of 1 g may be useful.[183]

Diflunisal is marketed primarily as an analgesic. It has a long enough half-life to permit twice-daily dosage, accounting for its trade name in the United States, Dolobid. Although diflunisal has less effect on the platelet cyclooxygenase than aspirin, it is inhibitory, and platelet function is impaired. Since it lacks the acetyl group of aspirin, it does not acetylate the platelet enzyme, and its inhibitory effect is reversed as the drug is cleared from the blood.

Diflunisal causes an increase in the plasma concentration of hydrochlorothiazide and a decrease in its renal excretion, but the clinical significance of this interaction is unknown. Diflunisal does block the uric acid retention caused by hydrochlorothiazide, however,[89] and when given alone, causes uricosuria.

Diflunisal causes less upper gastrointestinal toxicity than aspirin preparations, and it is useful in osteoarthritis and other painful rheumatic syndromes, but full trials of its effect in inflammatory rheumatic diseases are not yet available. Concomitant administration of aluminum hydroxide gel decreased absorption of diflunisal, but food does not affect its bioavailability. Aspirin in doses of 300 mg four times a day did not affect plasma levels of diflunisal, but 600 mg four times daily did decrease trough steady-state plasma levels. Several cases of Stevens-Johnson syndrome have been reported with diflunisal.[89]

Piroxicam. Piroxicam (Fig. 50–7) is slowly cleared (T½ averaging 24 hours), permitting once-a-day dosage, thus enhancing patient compliance and round-the-clock suppression of inflammation. The drug is very potent, and only 20 mg a day is recommended; higher doses result in an increased incidence of toxicity, primarily gastric irritation. Double-blind studies have demonstrated effectiveness of piroxicam in rheumatoid arthritis,[184] osteoarthritis,[185] gout,[186] and ankylosing spondylitis.[187]

Since small quantities of piroxicam are given, the drug occupies few binding sites on the plasma protein, and there is no apparent interaction with other drugs on this basis. Coadministration of aspirin does not cause clinically significant alteration in the plasma concentration of either agent,[71,188] but a combination of 40 mg per day of piroxicam and aspirin caused a high incidence of peptic ulcer formation.[189]

Benoxaprofen. A phenylpropionic acid derivative like other "profens," benoxaprofen (Fig. 50–8) was withdrawn from the market because of hepatotoxicity. Nevertheless, it is worth keeping the drug in mind because it has several unusual properties. The long half-life (averaging 29 hours) allowed once-a-day dosage but also led to the problems of toxicity; like all drugs metabolized extensively in the liver, there was considerable variation in the rate of clearance. In the elderly, a particularly long half-life was observed,[123] reaching 111 hours in one study.[77] As a result of a single recommended dose schedule, 600 mg a day, and no convenient method of monitoring blood levels, toxicity developed, with cholestasis, jaundice, and liver failure, particularly in elderly patients.

Figure 50–7. Chemical structure of piroxicam.

Figure 50–8. Chemical structure of benoxaprofen.

Benoxaprofen had the apparently unusual property of inhibition of the lipoxygenase pathway as well as the cyclooxygenase pathway of arachidonic acid metabolism. As a result, it caused an inhibition of cell migration and chemotactic responsiveness, particularly in monocytes. Although similar effects occur with other nonsteroidal anti-inflammatory agents, they were particularly well studied with benoxaprofen and may be relevant to its clinical effects.

Benoxaprofen caused stimulation of cartilage proteoglycan synthesis,[50] an effect that could slow cartilage degradation, particularly in osteoarthritis and other destructive arthropathies. Slowing of the radiologic evidence for cartilage destruction in rheumatoid arthritis was reported with benoxaprofen,[94] suggesting a suppressive effect on disease.

Among the unusual toxic manifestations of benoxaprofen reported were a painful photosensitivity on exposure to ultraviolet light[190] and increased hair growth in areas of male-pattern baldness[191] (which made several physicians want to take the drug despite reports of its toxicity).

Zomepirac. Zomepirac is chemically related to indomethacin and tolectin but has a longer half-life (average 7.6 hours).[192] An inhibitor of prostaglandin synthesis, it was useful in the treatment of rheumatoid arthritis and other inflammatory diseases, but was marketed primarily for short-term use as an analgesic. A study of its value in osteoarthritis over a 2-year period was reported, with its effect comparing favorably with aspirin, with fewer side effects.[193] In general, its toxicity and safety are comparable to those of other agents in this group, but a higher incidence of anaphylactic reactions, particularly in patients who had stopped taking the drug and then restarted it, led to the withdrawal of zomepirac from the market in the United States.

Other interesting new drugs are under development. One, *fenbufen,* is given as a prodrug that is converted to an active metabolite in the liver.[194] The active metabolite has a half-life of clearance of 10 hours, which is not increased in elderly patients,[195] but it is prolonged in chronic renal failure to an average of 17 hours.[196]

CLINICAL USEFULNESS OF THE NONSTEROIDAL ANTI-INFLAMMATORY AGENTS

In the view of many rheumatologists, the newer nonsteroidal anti-inflammatory agents have the potential of replacing aspirin as the first-line, premier antirheumatic drug because of increased effectiveness at full doses in many diseases, lower toxicity (especially gastrointestinal), and greater patient compliance. One tablet a day instead of 12 to 16 is clearly preferable for many patients. On the other hand, the greater cost, the lack of availability of plasma levels with concomitant lack of experience in how to use them, and uncertainty regarding long-term safety have resulted in the continued, use of large amounts of aspirin, and few rheumatologists would switch patients who are doing well on aspirin to one of the newer agents.

A major potential advantage of these drugs over aspirin is the reduced incidence of gastric irritation and occult blood loss; however, serious upper gastrointestinal bleeding can occasionally occur with any of these agents. They have been shown to be clearly superior to aspirin in several diseases, both rheumatic (e.g., gout, ankylosing spondylitis) and nonrheumatic (e.g., dysmenorrhea). As analgesics, several are as good as large amounts of aspirin, and again the lower gastrointestinal toxicity gives them a clear advantage.

Many clinicians use newer agents in combination with aspirin. This practice began when phenylbutazone was found to be too toxic in large doses and often too weak as the sole agent in safe maintenance doses. The literature abounds in confusing statements and observations on this subject, and package inserts distributed with these drugs advise against concomitant use of aspirin. Since the gastric irritation may be additive, this is probably good routine advice, but should it be a general proscription? Although displacement from protein-binding sites occurs when these drugs are given in combination,[79] studies of the effects of combinations of these drugs on blood levels have yielded data too variable for definitive conclusions; no consistent pattern exists, and no guide to therapy can be found in such studies.

A bizarre interaction between these drugs occurs in the treatment of adjuvant arthritis in rats. Prior administration of any of them interferes with the effect of indomethacin in this model; even prior use of indomethacin interferes.[197] The effect of isoxicam, on the other hand, is not blocked by prior aspirin or other nonsteroidal anti-inflammatory drugs.[198]

Many authoritative statements have proscribed combined use as irrational, since all drugs act in the same fashion; but there are abundant data to point to subtle, perhaps important, differences in mechanisms of action, in tissue penetration, and in capacity to inhibit prostaglandin synthesis in specific organs. The variation in pharmacokinetics is clinically important. Certainly there are differences in the effectiveness of these drugs in different diseases, especially when compared with aspirin, suggesting there are differences in mechanisms of action.

It seems unwise to base clinical decisions on dogmatic statements about mechanisms of action that are not well supported by the little laboratory data available. Clearly empirical observation must establish whether combinations are helpful or deleterious.

Thus far, studies of clinical effectiveness of combinations are inconclusive; additive benefit is as difficult to establish as is an advantage of one effective drug over another. Interference with effectiveness or additive toxicity is easier to establish and has not been observed, except for one report of a 33 percent incidence of peptic ulcer disease with a combination of piroxicam and aspirin.[189] Additive benefit in rheumatoid arthritis was shown for naproxen plus aspirin using moderate doses of each drug.[174] Additive benefit of combinations of analgesic medications occurs in a variety of types of pain.

In my view combinations of aspirin or other salicylates and other nonsteroidal anti-inflammatory agents or combinations of the newer agents are worthy of careful trial in patients who do not respond satisfactorily to maximum safe doses of single drugs. Care should be taken to observe for increased toxicity and for a satisfactory effect; in the absence of additive benefit, the combination should be discontinued. Another indication for combination therapy is the additive benefit of drugs with differing pharmacokinetics. For example, if a patient is responding to a short-acting agent, such as tolmetin or ibuprofen, but still has morning stiffness because of loss of therapeutic blood levels overnight, a nighttime dose of a longer-acting agent may be useful. Either a drug such as naproxen in the evening or a large dose of indomethacin at bedtime can be useful. Similarly, if a patient is well controlled on a long-acting agent, such as naproxen twice a day or piroxicam daily, but has a flare-up due to overuse of a joint or trauma, it may be useful to add intermittent doses of a short-acting agent temporarily.

Are These Drugs Interchangeable? In my view there are significant, but subtle, differences in mechanisms of action, effectiveness in different diseases, and other properties of these drugs. The unpredictable differences in effectiveness in different patients make it worth while to try a series of agents if the first drug does not work satisfactorily in a particular patient. Although the reason for the differences in effectiveness in individual patients is unknown, there is clearly a clinical advantage to having so many drugs available, making it possible to try a series of them sequentially in a given patient.

Unfortunately blood level determinations are not available for any of the nonsteroidal anti-inflammatory agents except the salicylates; it is reasonable to assume that such determinations would be clinically useful, as are salicylate levels, and would minimize the occurrence of toxicity. Without determinations of blood levels, we are unaware of differences in metabolism of these drugs in different patients. Variations in plateau blood levels seem a likely basis for individual differences in effectiveness. In the studies reported there are wide variations in plateau levels achieved in normal individuals on a single-dose regimen of a specific drug; age, sex, disease, and effect of other drugs are variables that have not been studied at all.

Do These Drugs Have a Disease-Modifying Effect in Rheumatoid Arthritis? It took more than 30 years to establish a disease-modifying effect for gold in rheumatoid arthritis. Conventional wisdom says that the nonsteroidal anti-inflammatory agents do not have such an effect, but no data exist in this regard, even for aspirin, since there are no controls available who have not received aspirin. The newer agents have a more complete disease-suppressive effect in many patients. If the severity of the inflammation bears a relationship to the degree of joint destruction, complete suppression of the inflammation should minimize disease progression.

Suppression of the model for immunologically induced chronic inflammatory arthritis, adjuvant disease in rats, occurs with these agents, preventing cartilage and bone erosion. The relationship of this observation to human rheumatoid arthritis is, of course, questionable.

Several studies are under way to try to establish a disease-suppressive effect for a variety of the nonsteroidal anti-inflammatory agents. The meager data that support the hypothesis that these agents have a suppressive effect in rheumatoid arthritis are described earlier in this chapter. No conclusion regarding a disease-suppressive effect is warranted on the basis of present evidence. While definitive evidence is being sought, what is the most rational course of action for the prudent clinician to follow? My recommendation is to assume that a modest disease-suppressive effect will be demonstrated, and to try to achieve maximal, continuous suppression of the inflammation rather than simply symptomatic relief, if this can be achieved without toxicity.

References

1. Smith, M.J.H.: Aspirin and prostaglandins: Some recent developments. Agents Actions 8:427, 1978.
2. Vane, J.R.: Mode of action of aspirin and similar compounds. *In* Robinson, H.J., and Vane, J.R. (eds.): Prostaglandin Synthetase Inhibitors. New York, Raven Press, 1974.
3. Robinson, D.R., McGuire, M.B., Bastian, D., Kantrowitz, F., and Levine, L.: The effects of anti-inflammatory drugs on prostaglandin production by rheumatoid synovial tissue. Prostaglandins Med. 1:461, 1978.
4. Harvey, I., Main, M. and Whittle, B.J.R.: Prostaglandins and prostaglandin synthetase inhibitors in gastrointestinal function and disease. *In* Robinson, H.J., and Vane, J.R. (eds.): Prostaglandin Synthetase Inhibitors. New York, Raven Press, 1974.
5. Johansson, C., Kollberg, B., Nordemar, R., Samuelson, K., and Bergstrom, S.: Protective effect of prostaglandin E_2 in the gastrointestinal tract during indomethacin treatment of rheumatic diseases. Gastroenterology 78:479, 1980.
6. Whittle, B.J.R.: Temporal relationship between cyclooxygenase inhibition as measured by prostacyclin biosynthesis, and the gastrointestinal damage induced by indomethacin in rat. Gastroenterology 80:94, 1981.
7. Kuehl, F.A., Dougherty, H.W., Ham, E.A., Humes, J.L., Egan, R.W., and Winter, C.A.: Biochemical aspects of the mechanism of action of sulindac. *In* Miehlke, K., Otte, P., and Platz, C.M. (eds.): Current Concepts of Anti-Inflammatory Drugs. New York, Biomedical Information, 1980, p. 17.
8. Metz, S.A.: Anti-inflammatory agents as inhibitors of prostaglandin synthesis in man. Med. Clin. North Am. 65:759, 1981.
9. Flower, R.J., and Vane, J.R.: Some pharmacologic and biochemical aspects of prostaglandin biosynthesis and its inhibition. *In* Robinson, H.J., and Vane, J.R. (eds.): Prostaglandin Synthetase Inhibitors. New York, Raven Press, 1974.
10. Kocsis, J.J., Hernandovich, J., Silver, M.T., Smith, J.B., and Ingerman,

C.: Duration of inhibition of platelet prostaglandin formation and aggregation by ingested aspirin or indomethacin. Prostaglandins 3:141, 1973.
11. Crook, D., Collins, A.J., Bacon, P.A., and Chan, R.: Prostaglandin synthetase activity from human rheumatoid synovial microsomes. Ann. Rheum. Dis. 35:327, 1976.
12. Humes, J.L., Winter, C.A., Sadowski, S.J., and Kuehl, F.A.: Multiple sites on prostaglandin cyclooxygenase are determinants in the action of nonsteroidal antiinflammatory agents. Proc. Natl. Acad. Sci. USA 78:2053, 1981.
13. Dembinska-Kiec, A., Zmuda, A., and Krupinska, J.: Inhibition of prostaglandin synthetase by aspirin-like drugs in different microsomal preparations. *In* Samuelsson, B., and Paoletti, R. (eds.): Advances in Prostaglandin and Thromboxane Research. Vol. 1. New York, Raven Press, 1976.
14. Ferreira, S.H., Lorenzetti, B.B., Salete, M., Castro, A., and Correa, F.M.A.: Antialgic effect of aspirin-like drugs and the inhibitor of prostaglandin synthesis. *In* DuMonde, D.C., and Jasare, M.K. (eds.): Recognition of Anti-Rheumatic Drugs. Baltimore, University Park Press, 1977.
15. Vane, J.R.: The mode of action of aspirin-like drugs. Agents Actions 8:430, 1978.
16. Wiseman, E.H.: Preclinical studies with piroxicam. *In* O'Brien, W.M., and Wiseman, E.H. (eds.): *In* Piroxicam. The Royal Society of Medicine International Congress and Symposium Series, No. 1. London, Academic Press, 1977.
17. Shen, T.Y.: The discovery of indomethacin and the proliferation of NSAIDs. Semin. Arthritis Rheum. XII, 2 (Suppl. 1):89, 1982.
18. Gryglewski, R.J.: Structure-activity relationship of some prostaglandin synthetase inhibitors. *In* Robinson, H.J., and Vane, J.R. (eds.): Prostaglandin Inhibitors. New York, Raven Press, 1974.
19. Moncada, M.D., and Vane, J.R.: Mode of action of aspirin-like drugs. *In* Stollerman, G.H. (ed.): Advances in Internal Medicine. Chicago, Year Book Medical Publishers, 1979.
20. Kuehl, F.A., Humes, J.L., Egan, R.W., Ham, E.A., Beveridge, G.C., and Van Arman, C.G.: Role of prostaglandin endoperoxide PGG_2 in inflammatory processes. Nature 265:170, 1977.
21. Egan R.W., Humes, J.L., and Kuehl, F.A.: Differential effects of prostaglandin synthetase stimulators on inhibition of cyclooxygenase. Biochemistry 17:2230, 1978.
22. Glenn, E.M., Bowman, B.J., and Rohloff, N.A.: Anti-inflammatory and PG inhibitory effects of phenacetin and acetaminophen. Agents Actions 7:513, 1977.
23. Glenn, E.M., Bowman, B.J., and Rohloff, N.A.: Anti-inflammatory and PG inhibitory effects of phenacetin and acetaminophen. Agents Actions 7:513, 1977.
24. Fitzpatrick, F.A., and Wynalda, M.A.: In vivo suppression of prostaglandin biosynthesis by non-steroidal anti-inflammatory agents. Prostaglandins 12:1037, 1976.
25. Metz, S.A., Robertson, R.P., Fujimoto, W.Y.: Inhibition of prostaglandin E synthesis augments glucose-induced insulin secretion in cultured pancreas. Diabetes 30:551, 1981.
26. Cherner, R., Groppe, C.W., and Rupp, J.J.: Prolonged tolbutamide-induced hypoglycemia. JAMA 185:883, 1963.
27. Buckingham, R.B.: Interactions involving antirheumatic agents. Bull. Rheum. Dis. 28:960 and 966, 1977–78.
28. Sherwood, J., and Kreutner, W.: Salicylic acid prevents the inhibition of platelet prostaglandin synthetase by indomethacin-like anti-inflammatory agents. Fed. Proc. 37:605A, 1978.
29. DiPasquale, G., and Mellace, D.: Inhibition of arachidonic acid induced mortality in rabbits with several non-steroidal anti-inflammatory agents. Agents Actions 7:481, 1977.
30. Simon, S., and Mills, J.A.: Drug therapy. N. Engl. J. Med. 302:1179 and 1237, 1980.
31. Jacob, H.: Neutrophil activation as a mechanism of tissue injury. Presentation at the VIII Pan-American Congress of Rheumatology, Washington, D.C., June, 1982.
32. Higgs, G.A., and Flower, R.J.: Anti-inflammatory drugs and the inhibition of arachidonate lipoxygenase. *In* Piper, P.J. (ed.): SRS-A and Leukotrienes. New York, John Wiley and Sons, 1981.
33. Higgs, G.A., Eakins, K.E., Mugridge, K.G., Moncada, S., Vane, J.R.: The effects of non-steroid anti-inflammatory drugs on leukocyte migration in carrageenin-induced inflammation. Eur. J. Pharmacol. 66:81, 1980.
34. Klickstein, L.B., Shapleigh, C., and Goetzl, E.J.: Lipoxygenation of arachidonic acid as a source of polymorphonuclear leukocyte chemotactic factors in synovial fluid tissue in rheumatoid arthritis and spondyloarthritis. J. Clin. Invest. 66:1166, 1980.
35. Dawson, W., Boot, J.R., Harvey, J., and Walker, J.R.: The pharmacology of benoxaprofen with particular reference to effects of lipoxygenase product formation. Eur. J. Rheumatol. Inflamm. 5:61, 1982.
36. Walker, J.R., and Dawson, W.: Inhibition of rabbit PMN lipoxygenase activity by benoxaprofen. J. Pharm. Pharmacol. 31:778, 1979.

37. Snyderman, R., and Goetzl, E.J.: Molecular and cellular mechanisms of leukocyte chemotaxis. Science 213:830, 1981.

38. Kuehl, F.A.: Prostaglandin research: Clinical implications. Semin. Arthritis Rheum. 12 (Suppl. 1):119, 1982.

39. Stecher, V.J.: The chemotaxis of selected cell types to connective tissue degradation products. Ann. N.Y. Acad. Sci. 256:177, 1975.

40. Brown, K.A., and Collins, A.J.: In vitro effects of non-steroidal anti-inflammatory drugs on human polymorphonuclear cells and lymphocyte migration. Br. J. Pharmacol. 64:347, 1978.

41. Meacock, S.C.R., and Kitchen, E.A.: Effects of the non-steroidal anti-inflammatory drug benoxaprofen on leucocyte migration. J. Pharm. Pharmacol. 31:366, 1979.

42. Walker, J.R., Smith, M.J.H., and Ford-Hutchinson, A.W.: Anti-inflammatory drugs, prostaglandins and leucocyte migration. Agents Actions 6:602, 1976.

43. Dawson, W.: Mechanisms of action of antiinflammatory drugs. In Samuelsson, B., Ramwell, P.W., and Paoletti, R. (eds.): Advances in Prostaglandin and Thromboxane Research. New York, Raven Press, 1980.

44. Meacock, S.C.R., and Kitchen, E.A.: Effects of the non-steroidal anti-inflammatory drug benoxaprofen on leucocyte migration. J. Pharm. Pharmacol. 31:366, 1979.

45. Weiss, B., and Hait, W.N.: Selective cyclic nucleotidephosphodiesterase inhibitors as potential therapeutic agents. Annu. Rev. Pharmacol. Toxicol. 17:441, 1977.

46. Carty, T.J., Stevens, J.S., Lombardino, J.G., Parry, M.J., and Randall, M.J.: Piroxicam, a structurally novel anti-inflammatory compound, mode of prostaglandin synthesis inhibition. Prostaglandins 19:671, 1980.

47. Tamisier, J.N.: Ketoprofen. Clin. Rheum. Dis. 5:381, 1979.

48. Abramson, S.: Effects of nonsteroidal anti-inflammatory drugs on neutrophil activation in vitro and in vivo. Presentation at the VIII Pan-American Congress of Rheumatology, Washington, D.C., June, 1982.

49. Kantor, T.G.: Ibuprofen. Ann. Intern. Med. 91:877, 1979.

50. Palmoski, M.J., and Brandt, K.D.: Benoxaprofen (Benx) stimulates proteoglycan (GG) synthesis in normal articular cartilage. Arthritis Rheum. 25 (Suppl.):S29, 1982.

51. Mobarok Ali, A.T.M., and Morley, J.: Actions of aspirin on lymphocytes. Aspirin Symposium 1980. Proceedings of an International Symposium held by the Aspirin Foundation. London: Royal College of Surgeons, June 5, 1980.

52. Ehrlich, G.E.: Three years' clinical experience with tolmetin in rheumatoid arthritis. Presentation on Zomepirac and Tolmetin: Advances in Clinical and Pharmacologic Research. VIII Pan-American Congress of Rheumatology, Washington, D.C., June, 1982.

53. Goodwin, J.S., and Webb, D.R.: Regulation of the immune response by prostaglandins. Clin. Immunol. Immunopathol. 15:106, 1980.

54. Goodwin, J.: Effects of nonsteroidal anti-inflammatory drugs on cellular and humoral immunity in vitro and in vivo. Presentation at the VIII Pan-American Congress of Rheumatology, Washington, D.C., June, 1982.

55. Cashin, C.H., Dawson, W., and Kitchen, E.A.: The pharmacology of benoxaprofen (2-lf-chlorophenyl-a-methyl-5-benzoxazole acetic acid), LRCL 3794, a new compound with anti-inflammatory activity apparently unrelated to inhibition of prostaglandin synthesis. J. Pharm. Pharmacol. 29:330, 1977.

56. Moncada, S., and Vane, J.R.: Interaction between anti-inflammatory drugs and inflammatory mediators. A reference to products of arachidonic acid metabolism. In Bonta, L.I., Thompson, J., and Brune, K. (eds.): Inflammation: Mechanisms and Their Impact on Therapy. Birkhauser Verlag, Basel, 1977.

57. Muschek, L.D.: Zomepirac: Recent pharmacologic developments. Presentation on Zomepirac and Tolmetin: Advances in Clinical and Pharmacologic Research. VIII Pan-American Congress of Rheumatology, Washington, D.C., June, 1982.

58. Kantor, T.G., Streem, A., and Laska, E.: Estimates of doses of antiinflammatory drugs in man by testing for analgesic potency. Arthritis Rheum. 20:1381, 1977.

59. Feldberg, W.: Prostaglandins and prostaglandin synthetase inhibitors. Action on physiological function. In Robinson, H.J., and Vane, J.R. (eds.): Prostaglandin Synthetase Inhibitors. New York, Raven Press, 1974.

60. Moncada, S., Ferreira, S.H., and Vane, J.R.: Sensitization of pain receptors of dog knee joint by prostaglandins. In Robinson, H.J., and Vane, J.R. (eds.): Prostaglandin Synthetase Inhibitors. New York, Raven Press, 1974.

61. Ferreira, S.H., and Vane, J.R.: New aspects of the mode of action of nonsteroid anti-inflammatory drugs. Annu. Rev. Pharmacol. 14:57, 1974.

62. Champion, G.D., and Graham, G.G.: Pharmacokinetics of non-steroidal anti-inflammatory agents. Aust. N.Z.J. Med. 8 (Suppl. I):94, 1978.

63. Ridolfo, A.S., Nickander, R., and Mikulaschek, W.M.: Fenoprofen and benoxaprofen. Clin. Rheum. Dis. 5:393, 1979.

64. Chernish, S.M., Rubin, A., Rodda, B.E., Ridolfo, A.S., and Gruber,

C.M. Jr.: The physiological disposition of fenoprofen in man, IV. The effects of position of subject, food ingestion on the plasma levels of orally administered fenoprofen. J. Med. (Exp. Clin.) 3:249, 1972.

65. Brune, K., Graf, P., and Glatt, M.: Inhibition of prostaglandin synthesis in vivo by nonsteroid anti-inflammatory drugs: Evidence for the importance of pharmacokinetics. Agents Actions 6:159, 1976.

66. Wiseman, E.H., and Hobbs, D.C.: Review of pharmacokinetic studies with piroxicam. Am. J. Med. 72:19, 1982.

67. Robinson, D.R., and Levine, L.: Prostaglandin concentrations in synovial fluid in rheumatic diseases: Action of indomethacin and aspirin. In Robinson, H.J., and Vane, J.R. (eds.): Prostaglandin Synthetase Inhibitors. New York: Raven Press, 1974.

68. Furst, D.E.: Tolmetin kinetics in synovial fluid. Presentation on Zomepirac and Tolmetin: Advances in Clinical and Pharmacologic Research. VIII Pan-American Congress of Rheumatology, Washington, D.C., June, 1982.

69. Soren, A.: Transport of salicylates from blood to joint fluid. Arch. Intern. Med. 132:668, 1973.

70. Adams, S.S., and Buckler, J.W.: Ibuprofen and flurbiprofen. Clin. Rheum. Dis. 5:359, 1979.

71. Hobbs, D.C., and Twomey, T.M.: Piroxicam pharmacokinetics in man: Aspirin and antacid interaction studies. J. Clin. Pharmacol. 19:270, 1979.

72. Nuotio, P., and Makisara, P.: Pharmacokinetic and clinical study of piroxicam. In O'Brien, W.M., and Wiseman, E.H. (eds.): Piroxicam. The Royal Society of Medicine International Congress and Symposium Series, No. 1. London: Academic Press, 1977.

73. Segre, E.J.: Naproxen. Clin. Rheum. Dis. 5:411, 1979.

74. Day, R.O., Furst, D.E., Dromgole, S.H., Kamm, B., Roe, R., and Paulus, H.E.: Relationship of serum naproxen concentration to efficacy in rheumatoid arthritis. Clin. Pharmacol. Ther. 31:733, 1982.

75. Yakatan, G.J.: Pharmacology and pharmacokinetics of isoxicam. Semin. Arthritis Rheum. XII (Suppl. 2):154, 1982.

76. Brogden, R.N., Heel, R.C., Speight, T.M., and Avery, G.S.: Fenbufen: A review of its pharmacological properties and therapeutic use in rheumatic diseases and acute pain. Drugs 21:1, 1981.

77. Taggart, H.M., and Alderdice, J.M.: Fatal cholestatic jaundice in elderly patients taking benoxaprofen. Br. Med. J. 284:1372, 1982.

78. Graham, G.G., Champion, G.D., Day, R.O., and Paull, P.D.: Patterns of plasma concentrations and urinary excretion of salicylate in rheumatoid arthritis. Clin. Pharmacol. Ther. 22:410, 1977.

79. Mason, R.W., and McQueen, E.G.: Protein binding of indomethacin: binding of indomethacin to human plasma albumin and its displacement from binding by ibuprofen, phenylbutazone and salicylate, in vitro. Pharmacology 12:12, 1974.

80. Huskisson, E.C., Taylor, R.T., Burston, D., Chuter, P.J., and Hart, F.D.: Evening indomethacin in the treatment of rheumatoid arthritis. Ann. Rheum. Dis. 29:393, 1970.

81. Turner, R.A., April, P.A., and Robbins, D.L.: Double-blind multicenter study comparing piroxicam and ibuprofen in the treatment of rheumatoid arthritis. Am. J. Med. 72:34, 1982.

82. Huskisson, E.C., Woolf, D.L., Balme, H.W., Scott, J., and Franklyn, S.: Four new anti-inflammatory drugs: Responses and variations. Br. Med. J. 1:1048, 1976.

83. Brogden, R.N., Pinder, R.M., Sawyer, P.R., Speight, T.M., and Avery, G.s.: Naproxen: A review of its pharmacological properties and therapeutic efficacy and use. Drugs 9:326, 1975.

84. Brogden, R.N., Pinder, R.M., Speight, T.M., and Avery, G.S.: Fenoprofen: A review of its pharmacological properties and therapeutic efficacy in rheumatic disease. Drugs 13:241, 1977.

85. Brogen, R.N., Heel, R.C., Speight, T.M., and Avery, C.S.: Tolmetin: A review of its pharmacological properties and therapeutic efficacy in rheumatic diseases. Drugs 15:429, 1978.

86. Brogden, R.N., Heel, R.C., Speight, T.M., and Avery, G.S.: Sulindac: A review of its pharmacological properties and therapeutic efficacy in rheumatic diseases. Drugs 16:97, 1978.

87. Famaey, J.P.: Recent developments about non-steroidal anti-inflammatory drugs and their mode of action. Gen. Pharmac. 9:155, 1978.

88. Nickander, R., McMahon, F.G., and Ridolfo, A.S.: Nonsteroidal anti-inflammatory agents. Ann. Rev. Pharmacol. Toxicol. 19:469, 1979.

89. Brogden, R.N., Heel, R.C., Pakes, G.E., Speight, T.M., and Avery, G.S.: Diflunisal: A review of its pharmacological properties and therapeutic use in pain and musculoskeletal strains and sprains and pain in osteoarthritis. Drugs 19:84, 1980.

90. Brock, P.G., and Jackson, D.: UK general practitioners' experience of fenbufen in elderly patients. Eur. J. Rheum. Inflam. 5:326, 1982.

91. Wasner, C., Britton, M.D., Kraines, G., Kaye, R.L., Bobrove, A.M., and Fries, J.F.: Nonsteroidal anti-inflammatory agents in rheumatoid arthritis and ankylosing spondylitis. JAMA 246:2168, 1981.

92. Beirne, J.A., Bianchine, J.R., Johnson, P.C., and Wartham, G.P.: Gastrointestinal blood loss caused by tolmetin, aspirin and indomethacin. Clin. Pharmacol. Ther. 16:821, 1974.

93. Ridolfo, A.S., Crabtree, R.E., Johnson, D.W., and Rockhold, F.W.:

Gastrointestinal microbleeding: Comparisons between benoxaprofen and other nonsteroidal antiinflammatory agents. J. Rheumatol. 6(Suppl.):36, 1980.

94. Bluhm, G.B., Smith, D.W., and Mikulaschek, W.M.: Radiologic assessment of benoxaprofen therapy in rheumatoid arthritis. Eur. J. Rheum. Inflamm. 3:186, 1981.

95. Levy, J.: Immunological aspects of tolmetin. Presentation on Zomepirac and Tolmetin: Advances in Clinical and Pharmacologic Research. VIII Pan-American Congress of Rheumatology, Washington, D.C., June 11, 1982.

96. Lindsley, C.B.: Pharmacotherapy of juvenile rheumatoid arthritis. Pediatr. Clin. North Am. 28:161, 1981.

97. Moran, H. Hanna, D.B. Ansell, B.M., Hall, M., and Engler, C.: Naproxen in juvenile chronic polyarthritis. Ann. Rheum. Dis. 38:152, 1979.

98. Jacobs, J.C.: Sudden death in arthritic children receiving large doses of indomethacin. JAMA 199:932, 1967.

99. Bostrom, H., Berntsen, K., and Whitehouse, M.W.: Biochemical properties of anti-inflammatory drugs-II. Biochem. Pharmacol. 13:413, 1964.

100. Bollet, A.J.: Inhibition of glucosamine-6-PO4 synthesis by salicylate and other anti-inflammatory agents in vitro. Arthritis Rheum. 4:624, 1961.

101. Fowler, P.D.: Indomethacin and phenylbutazone. Clin. Rheum. Dis. 1:267, 1975.

102. Godfrey, R.G., Calabro, J.J., Mills, D., and Maltz, B.: A double-blind crossover trial of aspirin, indomethacin and phenylbutazone in ankylosing spondylitis. Arthritis Rheum. 15:110, 1972.

103. Pulkkinen, M.O., and Csapo, A.I.: The effect of ibuprofen on the intrauterine pressure and menstrual pain of dysmenorrheic patients. Prostaglandins 15:1055, 1978.

104. Budoff, P.W.: Zomepirac sodium in the treatment of primary dysmenorrhea syndrome. N. Engl. J. Med. 307:714, 1982.

105. Schwartz, A., Zor, U., Lindner, H.R., and Naor, S.: Primary dysmenorrhea. Obstet. Gynecol. 44:709, 1974.

106. Aiken, J.W.: Prostaglandins and prostaglandin synthetase inhibitors: Studies on uterine motility and function. In Robinson, H.J., and Vane, J.R. (eds.): Prostaglandin Synthetase Inhibitors, New York, Raven Press, 1974.

107. Nadas, A.S.: Indomethacin and the patent ductus arteriosus. N. Engl. J. Med. 305:97, 1981.

108. Deykin, D., and Janson, P.: The Ponte Vedre syndrome. An unexpected interaction between alcohol and aspirin. Trans. Am. Clin. Climatol. Assoc. 93:121, 1982.

109. Friedman, P.L., Brown, E.J., Gunther, S., Alexander, R.W., Barry, W.H., Mudge, G.H., and Grossman, W.: Coronary vasoconstrictor effect of indomethacin in patients with coronary-artery disease. N. Engl. J. Med. 305:1171, 1981.

110. Mann, N.S., and Sachdev, A.J.: Acute erosive gastritis induced by aspirin, ketoprofen, ibuprofen, and naproxen: Its prevention by metiamide and cimetidine. South. Med. J. 70:526, 1977.

111. O'Laughlin, J.C., Silvoso, G.R., and Ivey, K.J.: Healing of aspirin-associated peptic ulcer disease despite continued salicylate ingestion. Arch. Intern. Med. 141:781, 1981.

112. Schwartz, H.A.: Lower gastrointestinal side effects of nonsteroidal antiinflammatory drugs. J. Rheumatol. 8:952, 1981.

113. Sharon, P., Ligumsky, M., Rachmilewitz, D., and Zor, U.: Role of prostaglandins in ulcerative colitis: Enhanced production during active disease and inhibition by sulfasalazine. Gastroenterology 75:638, 1978.

114. Abruzzo, J.L.: Anti-inflammatory and antirheumatic drugs. Ann. Intern. Med. 94:270, 1981.

115. Lilly, E.L.: Pancreatitis after administration of sulindac. JAMA 246:2680, 1981.

116. Park, G.D., Spector, R., Headstream, T., and Goldberg, M.: Serious adverse reactions associated with sulindac. Arch. Intern. Med. 142:1292, 1982.

117. Heller, S., Fellows, I.W., Ogilvie, A.L., and Atkinson, M.: Nonsteroidal and anti-inflammatory drugs and benign esophageal stricture. Br. Med. J. 285:167, 1982.

118. Dunk, A.A., Walt, R.P., Jenkins, W.J., and Sherlock, S.S.: Diclofenac hepatitis. Br. Med. J. 284:1605, 1982.

119. Giroux, Y., Moreau, M., and Kass, T.G.: Cholestatic jaundice caused by sulindac. Canad. J. Surg. 25:334, 1982.

120. Dunn, M.J., and Zambraski, E.J.: Renal effects of drugs that inhibit prostaglandin synthesis. Kidney Int. 18:609, 1980.

121. Lum, G.M., Aisenbrey, G.A., Dunn, M.J., Berl, T., Schrier, R.W., and McDonald, K.M.: In vivo effect of indomethacin to potentiate the renal medullary cyclic AMP response to vasopressin. J. Clin. Invest. 59:8, 1977.

122. Laiwah, A.C., and Mactier, R.A.: Non-steroidal anti-inflammatory agents may impair furosemide induced diuresis in cardiac failure. Br. Med. J. 283:714, 1981.

123. Favre, L., Glasson, P., and Vallotton, M.B.: Reversible acute renal failure from combined triamterene and indomethacin. Ann. Intern. Med. 96:317, 1982.

124. Williams, R.L., Davies, R.O., Berman, R.S., Holmes, G.I., Huber, P., Gee, W.L., Lin, E.T., and Benet, L.Z.: Hydrochlorothiazide pharmacokinetics and pharmacologic effect: The influence of indomethacin. J. Clin. Pharmacol. 22:32, 1982.

125. Brooks, P.M., and Cossum, P.A.: Rebound rise in renin concentrations after cessation of salicylates. N. Engl. J. Med. 303:562, 1980.

126. Gill, J.R., Frolich, J.C., Bowden, R.E., Taylor, A.A., Keiser, H.R., Seyberth, H.W., Oates, J.A., and Bartter, F.C.: Bartter's syndrome: A disorder characterized by high urinary prostaglandins and a dependence of hyperreninemia on prostaglandin synthesis. Am. J. Med. 61:43, 1976.

127. Fichman, M.P., Telfer, N., Zia, P., Speckart, P., Golub, M., and Rude, R.: Role of prostaglandins in the pathogenesis of Bartter's syndrome. Am. J. Med. 60:785, 1976.

128. Calin, A.: Non-steroidal anti-inflammatory drugs and furosemide-induced diuresis. Br. Med. J. 283:1399, 1981.

129. Bunning, R.D., and Barth, W.F.: Sulindac. JAMA 248:2864, 1982.

130. Linton, A.L., Clark, W.F., Driedger, A.A., Turnbull, D.I., and Lindsay, R.M.: Acute interstitial nephritis due to drugs. Ann. Intern. Med. 93:735, 1980.

131. Mease, P.J., Ellsworth, A.J., Killen, P.D., and Wilkens, R.F.: Zomepirac, interstitial nephritis and renal failure. Ann. Intern. Med. 97:454, 1982.

132. Brezin, J.H., Katz, S.M., Schwartz, A.B., and Chinitz, J.L.: Reversible renal failure and nephrotic syndrome associated with nonsteroidal anti-inflammatory drugs. N. Engl. J. Med. 301:1271, 1979.

133. Finkelstein, A., Fraley, D.S., Stachura, I., Feldman, H.A., Gandy, D.R., and Bourke, E.: Fenoprofen nephropathy: Lipoid nephrosis and interstitial nephritis. Am. J. Med. 72:81, 1982.

134. Gault, M.H., Rudwal, T.C., Engles, W.D., and Dossetor, J.B.: Syndrome associated with the abuse of analgesics. Ann. Intern. Med. 68:906, 1968.

135. Emkey, R.D., and Mills, J.A.: Aspirin and analgesic nephropathy. JAMA 247:55, 1982.

136. Knapp, M., and Avioli, L.V.: Analgesic nephropathy. Arch. Intern. Med. 142:1197, 1982.

137. Wiseman, E.H., and Reinert, H.: Anti-inflammatory drugs and renal papillary necrosis. Agents Actions 54:322, 1975.

138. Bennett, W.M., Muther, R.S., Parker, R.A., Feig, P., Morrison, G., Golper, T.A., and Singer, I.: Drug Therapy in renal failure: Dosing guidelines for adults. Ann. Intern. Med. 93:286, 1980.

139. Settipane, G.A.: Adverse reactions to aspirin and related drugs. Arch. Intern. Med. 141:328, 1981.

140. Stevenson, D.D.: Aspirin and rhinosinusitis/asthma: Desensitization. N. Engl. Soc. Allergy Proc. 2:88, 1981.

141. Rudolph, A.M.: Effects of aspirin and acetaminophen in pregnancy and in the newborn. Arch. Intern. Med. 141:358, 1981.

142. Miller, J.L.: Marrow aplasia and sulindac. Ann. Intern. Med. 92:129, 1980.

143. F.D.A. Drug Bulletin: Clinoril adverse reactions. 9:29, 1979.

144. Fowler, P.: Phenylbutazone and indomethacin. Clin. Rheum. Dis. 5:427, 1975.

145. Ashraf, M., Pearson, R.M., and Winfield, D.A.: Aplastic anaemia associated with fenoprofen. Br. Med. J. 284:1301, 1982.

146. O'Brien, W.M.: Piroxicam treatment of inflammatory disease. In the Royal Society of Medicine, International Congress and Symposium Series, Number 1. The Royal Society of Medicine, London, Academic Press, 1977.

147. Brogden, R.N., Heel, R.C., Speight, T.M., and Avery, G.S.: Alclofenac: A review of its pharmacological properties and therapeutic efficacy in rheumatoid arthritis and allied rheumatic disorders. Drugs 14:241, 1977.

148. Corre, K.A., and Rothstein, R.J.: Anaphylactic reaction to zomepirac. Ann. Allergy 48:299, 1982.

149. Rossi, A.C., and Knapp, D.E.: Tolmetin-induced anaphylactoid reactions. N. Engl. J. Med. 307:499, 1982.

150. Farnham, J.: Studies of isoxicam in combination with aspirin, warfarin, sodium and cimetidine. Semin. Arthritis Rheum. XII(Suppl. 2):179, 1982.

151. Barnes, C.G., Goodman, H.V., Eade, A.W.T., Misra, H.N., Cochrane, G.M., Clarke, A.K., and Stoppard, M.: A double-blind comparison of naproxen with indomethacin in osteoarthrosis. J. Clin. Pharm. 15:347, 1975.

152. Boardman, P.L., and Hart, F.D.: Side effects of indomethacin. Ann. Rheum. Dis. 26:127, 1967.

153. Taylor, R.T., Huskisson, E.C., Whitehouse, G.H., Hart, F.D., and Trapnell, D.H.: Gastric ulceration occurring during indomethacin therapy. Br. Med. J. 4:734, 1968.

154. Littlewood, J.M., Lee, M.R., and Meadow, S.R.: Treatment of Bartter's syndrome in early childhood with prostaglandin synthetase inhibitors. Arch. Dis. Child. 53:43, 1978.

155. Konomi, H., Imai, M., Nihei, K., and Kamoshitas, T.H.: Indomethacin causing pseudotumor cerebri in Bartter's syndrome. N. Engl. J. Med. 298:855, 1978.

156. Rhymer, A.R., Hart, C.B., and Daurio, C.: A double-blind trial comparing indomethacin sustained release capsules (indocid-R) with indomethacin capsules in patients with rheumatoid arthritis. Rheumatol. Rehabil. 21:101, 1982.

157. Brooks, P.M., Bell, M.A., Sturrock, R.D., Famaey, J.P., and Dick, W.C.: The clinical significance of indomethacin-probenecid interaction. Br. J. Clin. Pharmacol. 1:287, 1974.

158. Van Arman, C.G., Risley, E.A., Nuss, G.W., Hucker, H.B., and Duggan, D.E.: Pharmacology of sulindac. In Huskisson, E.C., and Franchimont, P. (eds.): Clinoril in the Treatment of Rheumatic Disorders: A New Nonsteroidal Anti-Inflammatory/Analgesic Agent. Proceedings of a Symposium VIII European Rheumatology Congress, Helsinki, June 1–7, 1975 (New York, Raven Press, 1976).

159. Huskisson, E.C., and Franchimont, P.: Clinoril in the treatment of rheumatic disorders. In Huskisson, E.C., and Franchimont, P. (eds.): Clinoril in the Treatment of Rheumatic Disorders: A New Nonsteroidal Anti-Inflammatory/Analgesic Agent. Proceedings of a Symposium VIII European Rheumatology Congress, Helsinki, June 1–7, 1975 (New York: Raven Press, 1976).

160. Memon, A.N.: Pancreatitis and sulindac. Arch. Intern. Med. 97:139, 1982.

161. Robinson, H., Abruzzo, J.L., Miyara, A., and Ward, J.R.: Concomitant tolmetin and aspirin therapy for rheumatoid arthritis. In Ward, J.R. (ed.): Tolmetin. Amsterdam, Excerpta Medica, 1975.

162. Chan, W.Y., Dawood, N.Y., and Fuchs, F.: Relief of dysmenorrhea with the prostaglandin synthetase inhibitor ibuprofen: Effect on prostaglandin levels in menstrual fluid. Am. J. Obstet. Gynecol. 135:102, 1979.

163. Smith, D.L., and Regan, M.G.: Ibuprofen in psoriatic arthritis. Arthritis Rheum. 8:961, 1980.

164. Boss, G.R., and Seegmiller, J.E.: Hyperuricemia and gout: Classification, complications and management. N. Engl. J. Med. 300:1459, 1979.

165. Widener, H.L., and Littman, B.H.: Ibuprofen-induced meningitis in systemic lupus erythematosus. JAMA 239:1062, 1978.

166. Mandell, B., Shen, H.S., and Hepburn, B.: Fever from ibuprofen in a patient with lupus erythematosus. Arch. Intern. Med. 85:209, 1976.

167. Segre, E.J.: Naproxen metabolism in man. J. Clin. Pharmacol. 15:316, 1975.

168. Pulkkinen, M.O., Henzl, M.R., and Csapo, A.I.: The effect of naproxensodium on the prostaglandin concentrations of the menstrual blood and uterine "jet washings" in dysmenorrheic women. Prostaglandins 15:543, 1978.

169. Filtzer, H.S.: A double-blind randomized comparison of naproxen sodium, acetaminophen and pentazocine in postoperative pain. Current Therapeutic Research 27:293, 1980.

170. Williams, J.G.P., and Engler, C.: A double-blind comparative trial of naproxen and indomethacin in sports injuries. Rheumatol. Rehabil. 16:265, 1977.

171. Merton, J.W., III, Lussier, A., Ward, J.R., Neustadt, D., and Multz, C.: Naproxen vs. aspirin in osteoarthritis of the hip and knee. J. Rheumatol. 5:338, 1978.

172. Sturge, R.A., Scott, J.T., Hamilton, E.B.D., Liyanage, S.P., Dixon, A., Davies, J., and Engler, E.: Multicenter trial of naproxen and phenylbutazone in acute gout. Ann. Rheum. Dis. 36:80, 1977.

173. Van Gerwen, F., Vander Kost, J.K., and Gribnan, F.W.: Double blind trial of naproxen and phenylbutazone in alkylosing spondylitis. Ann. Rheum. Dis. 37:85, 1978.

174. Wilkens, R.F., and Segre, E.J.: Combination therapy with naproxen and aspirin in rheumatoid arthritis. Arthritis Rheum. 19:677, 1976.

175. Matts, S.P.F.: Naproxen (Naprosyn) and gastrointestinal haemorrhage. Br. Med. J. 2:52, 1974.

176. Hart, F.D.: Naproxen (Naprosyn) and gastrointestinal haemorrhage. Br. Med. J. 2:51, 1974.

177. Roth, S.H., and Boost, G.: An open trial of naproxen in rheumatoid arthritis patients with significant esophageal, gastric and duodenal lesions. J. Clin. Pharmacol. 15:378, 1975.

178. Rivkin, I., Foschi, C.V., and Rosen, C.H.: Inhibition of in vitro neutrophile chemotaxis and spontaneous motility by anti-inflammatory agents. Proc. Soc. Exp. Biol. Med. 153:236, 1976.

179. Sondervorst, M.: Azapropazone. Clin. Rheum. Dis. 5:465, 1979.

180. Riess, W., Stierlin, H., Degen, P., Faigle, J.W., Gerardin, A., Moppert, J., Sallmann, A., Schmid, K., Schweizer, A., Sule, M., Theobald, W., and Wagner, J.: Pharmacokinetics and metabolism of the anti-inflammatory agent Voltaren. Scand. J. Rheumatol. Suppl. 22:17, 1978.

181. Stierlin, H., Faigle, J.W., and Columbia, A.: Pharmacokinetics of diclofenac sodium (Voltaren) and metabolites in patients with impaired renal function. Scand. J. Rheumatol. Suppl. 22:30, 1978.

182. Verbeeck, R., Tjandramaga, T.B., Mullie, A., Berbesselt, R., Verberekmoes, R., and De Schepper, P.J.: Biotransformation of diflunisal and renal excretion of its glucronides in renal insufficiency. Br. J. Clin. Pharmacol. 7:273, 1979a.

183. Forbes, J.A., Beaver, W.T., White, E.H., White, R.W., Neilson, G.B., and Shackleford, R.W.: A new oral analgesic with an unusually long duration of action. JAMA 248:2139, 1982.

184. Wilkens, R.F., Ward, J.R., Louis, J.S., and McAdam, L.P.: Double-blind study comparing piroxicam and aspirin in the treatment of rheumatoid arthritis. Am. J. Med. 72:23, 1982.

185. Abruzzo, J.L., Gordon, G.V., and Meyers, A.R.: Double-blind study comparing piroxicam and aspirin in the treatment of osteoarthritis. Am. J. Med. 72:45, 1982.

186. Widmark, P.H.: Piroxicam: Its safety and efficacy in the treatment of acute gout. Am. J. Med. 72:63, 1982.

187. Romberg, O.: Comparison of piroxicam with indomethacin in ankylosing spondylitis. A double-blind crossover trial. Am. J. Med. 72:58, 1982.

188. Wiseman, E.H., and Hobbs, D.C.: Review of pharmacokinetic studies with piroxicam. Am. J. Med. 72:9, 1982.

189. Semble, E., Metcalf, D., Turner, R., Agudelo, C., Pisko, E., Johnson, A.M., and Heise, E.: Genetic predictors of patient response and side effects in the treatment of rheumatoid arthritis with a high dose of nonsteroidal antiinflammatory drug regimen. Arthritis Rheum. 25:370, 1982.

190. Kligman, A.M., and Kaidbey, K.H.: Phototoxicity to benoxaprofen. Eur. J. Rheumatol. Inflamm. 5:124, 1982.

191. Fenton, D.A., English, J.S., and Wilkinson, J.D.: Reversal of male-pattern baldness, hypertrichosis, and accelerated hair and nail growth in patients receiving benoxaprofen. Br. Med. J. 284:1228, 1982.

192. O'Neill, P.M., Yorgey, K.A., Renzi, N.L., Williams, R.L., and Benet, L.Z.: Disposition of zomepirac sodium in man. J. Clin. Pharmacol. 22:470, 1982.

193. Honig, S.: Long-term therapy with zomepirac: Two years of safety and efficacy data. Presentation on Zomepirac and Tolmetin: Advances in Clinical Pharmacologic Research. VIII Pan-American Congress of Rheumatology, June, 1982.

194. Mawdsley, P.: Fenbufen. Clin. Rheum. Dis. 6:615, 1980.

195. Braverman, A.M.: Single-dose pharmacokinetic study of 900 mg fenbufen in the elderly. Eur. J. Rheumatol. Inflamm. 5:304, 1982.

196. Armstrong, R., Bradbrook, I., Gibson, T.J., Morrison, P., Rogers, H.J., and Spector, R.G.: A study of repeated administration of fenbufen in patients with chronic rheumatic disorders and renal impairment. Eur. J. Rheumatol. Inflamm. 5:294, 1982.

197. Van Arman, C.G., Nuss, G.W., and Risle, E.A.: Interactions of aspirin, indomethacin and other drugs in adjuvant-induced arthritis in the rat. J. Pharmacol. Exp. Ther. 187:400, 1973.

198. DiPasquale, G., Rassaert, C., Welaj, P. and Tripp, L.: Anti-inflammatory activity of isoxicam in combination with aspirin or D-propoxyphene. Agents Actions 6:748, 1976.

199. Ackerman, N.R., Rooks, W.H., Shott, H.L., Genant, H., Maloney, P., and West, E.: Effects of naproxen on connective tissue changes in the adjuvant arthritic rat. Arthritis Rheum. 22:1365, 1979.

Chapter 51
Antimalarials

Richard I. Rynes

HISTORICAL PERSPECTIVE

The establishment of antimalarial medications as useful antirheumatic agents has been steeped in controversy. This group of drugs is derived from the bark of the Peruvian cinchona tree, which Jesuit missionaries brought to Spain in the early seventeenth century as a remedy for certain fevers. For a number of years, Jesuit bark, as it was often called in the European countries, was not widely accepted by the medical establishment, in part because it was used by the Jesuits, but more importantly because it did not conform to Galen's teachings.[1] Charlatans often dispensed the medicine in secret remedies.

Cinchona bark's active principles, quinine and cinchonine, were isolated by Pelletier and Caventau in 1820 at about the same time that salicylin, the progenitor of aspirin, was being isolated from the bark of the willow tree. It was not until 1894 that J. P. Payne,[2] physician to St. Thomas' Hospital in London, delivered a postgraduate lecture on lupus erythematosus in which he first described the successful use of quinine for a rheumatic disease. Four factors, later to become points of contention, were mentioned in his report. These were effectiveness, dose, toxicity, and mechanism of action.

Payne's study was uncontrolled, as were almost all subsequent studies. The benefits appeared conclusive, however, and he commented: "I can not say that quinine treatment is an absolute success, but has succeeded in a considerable number of cases. I also think, therefore, that the best thing to do is to begin with this." The optimum dosage was not known but "decidedly large doses should be given." Side effects were not recognized and "people with this complaint seem to bear quinine unusually well." Payne was not sure of the mechanism by which quinine worked but believed that there was a "circulatory disturbance very much influenced by quinine."

In light of current knowledge, Payne's assessment of antimalarial effectiveness has been confirmed, as has its low toxicity. His use of high dosage is decidedly out of favor, since it is only low-dose administration that is safe on a long-term basis. The mechanism of drug action has not yet been established, but there is some evidence supporting Payne's hypothesis.[3]

Despite Payne's optimistic report, the beneficial effects of quinine were not confirmed until 1938 when Davidson and Birt[4] reported improvement of discoid lupus in 19 of 29 patients.

During the first half of the 20th century extensive efforts were undertaken to synthesize antimalarial compounds with improved therapeutic/toxicity ratios. These new compounds were also successfully applied to the treatment of patients with lupus erythematosus. In 1928, Martenstein[5] reported that pamaquine was beneficial in 22 of 28 patients with discoid or subacute systemic lupus erythematosus. Another compound, quinacrine, was first shown to be effective against lupus erythematosus by the Russian Prokoptchouk,[6] who obtained good results in all 35 patients treated. Because this report was published in Russia in 1940, it remained generally unknown until after Page's independent observation.[7]

The seminal publication in Lancet by Page[8] in 1951 provided much of the impetus for use of antimalarials in patients with connective tissue diseases. He treated patients with lupus erythematosus with quinacrine in doses varying from 100 to 300 mg per day. Skin lesions improved in 17 of 18 patients. Associated "rheumatoid arthritis" remitted in two patients, and systemic symptoms including arthritis cleared in a third. The importance of dosage was noted. Some patients responded to an initial 100 mg per day, while others needed at least 300 mg per day. Side effects were mild except in one patient who developed a lichenoid skin reaction, which necessitated discontinuation of the drug.

The response of Page's patients with lupus and "rheumatoid arthritis" influenced several groups to treat rheumatoid arthritis with antimalarials.[9-11] Bagnall's[10] favorable report of the efficacy of chloroquine in patients with rheumatoid arthritis, published in 1957, stimulated the more widespread use of this compound in treating patients with rheumatoid arthritis. Of 108 patients, 36 percent went into remission and major improvement was found in another 35 percent. He used chloroquine, a compound that had been synthesized in 1934, in hopes that toxicity would be minimized. Ironically, chloroquine was not used extensively until after World War II because it had been judged to be too toxic for practical use in humans. This conclusion was based on studies of treatment of blood-induced vivax malaria in four paretics at the psychiatric clinic in Dusseldorf, Germany.[12] At the time of Bagnall's report others were finding that hydroxychloroquine, a compound structurally similar to chloroquine, might be equally effective and even less toxic.[13-15]

In distinction to these favorable reports, some studies dampened the enthusiasm for antimalarials. Double-blinded studies[16,17] failed to confirm Bagnall's impressive remission rate, although they did show effectiveness. More disturbing was the recognition by Hobbs and associates[18] in 1959 that long-term treatment of rheumatic diseases might result in serious drug-induced retinal toxicity. By 1964 editorials in four major journals[19-22] warned of this problem and questioned whether benefits justified the potential loss of vision. Even as late as as the period between 1976 and 1978 the British National Formulary[23] stated that "chloroquine is rarely effective and toxic effects are frequent and serious, including irreversible retinal damage; it is now regarded as obsolete." This assessment has not been substantiated by a careful analysis of studies describing drug efficacy and toxicity. Based on a more accurate appraisal, antimalarials continue to be widely used for rheumatic diseases.

DEFINITION AND STRUCTURE

The term "antimalarials" is somewhat misleading when applied to drugs used to treat rheumatic diseases. For these conditions the term is limited to the quinoline derivatives and the structurally similar acridine compound quinacrine (Fig. 51–1). Other drugs used to treat malaria, such as pyrimethamine, an inhibitor of dihy-

drofolate reductase, and sulfadoxine, a sulfonamide, are not employed as antirheumatic medications. Dapsone, a sulfone used in the treatment of malaria, has been reported to be effective in rheumatoid arthritis[24] but is not considered one of the "antimalarials."

Figure 51–1 illustrates the structure of the compounds that have been used to treat rheumatic diseases. Their corresponding proprietary names are listed in Table 51–1. Quinine is the parent compound. Pamaquine and primaquine are 8-aminoquinoline derivatives. Four drugs, amiodiaquin, amopyroquin, chloroquine, and hydroxychloroquine, are 4-aminoquinoline derivatives. The latter two differ only by the substitution of a hydroxyethyl group for an ethyl group on the tertiary amino-nitrogen of the side chain of chloroquine. Although quinacrine is a 9-aminoacridine compound, its structure does contain the chloroquine moiety.

Only two compounds are generally prescribed in current practice. Hydroxychloroquine is used almost exclusively in the United States, while chloroquine is also

Figure 51–1. Structural formulas of antirheumatic antimalarials.

Table 51–1. Antirheumatic Antimalarial Drugs and Their Proprietary Names

Generic Name	Proprietary Name
hydroxychloroquine	Plaquenil
chloroquine	Aralen
	Resochin
	Nivaquine
	Sanoquin
quinacrine	Atabrine
	Mepacrine
	Acriquin
amodiaquin	Camoquin
amopyroquin	Propoquin
primaquine	
pamaquine	Plasmochin

used in Europe. Occasionally quinacrine is added to achieve maximum effect[25] or used to treat patients unable to tolerate the other two.

PHARMACOKINETICS

The absorption of quinine and the synthetic antimalarials is rapid and essentially complete when given orally. There is less accumulation of quinine in the body and less localization in the tissues in comparison with the synthetic drugs. It is primarily eliminated by being altered metabolically.[26]

Quinacrine is widely distributed in tissues and is very slowly liberated. Significant amounts are detected in the urine for at least two months after therapy is discontinued.[27] Both pamaquine and primaquine reach the maximum level in the plasma about 2 hours after a single oral dose, but at the end of 8 hours little remains. Compared with other synthetic antimalarials, the drugs are concentrated to a smaller extent in the tissues.[28]

Chloroquine and hydroxychloroquine are also rapidly absorbed.[1,15] About 8 percent of the ingested dose is found in the feces, but this may not all represent unabsorbed drug, since fecal excretion of parenterally administered drugs occurs.[29] The drugs are quickly cleared from the plasma and localized largely unchanged in tissue to a degree intermediate between that of quinine and quinacrine.[30]

Plateau plasma levels are achieved in 8 to 14 days.[31,32] Frisk-Holmberg and associates[33] studied 100 patients receiving 250 mg of chloroquine phosphate daily for more than 2 months and found a fivefold variation in plasma levels, but most patients had levels between 200 and 400 μg per liter. Others, studying patients taking 500 mg of chloroquine per day, found similar plasma levels of 200 to 400 μg per liter and a plateau urinary excretion of 75 mg per day.[34] Corresponding values for daily doses of 400 mg of hydroxychloroquine are 500 to 700 μg per liter for plasma and 55 mg per day urinary excretion.[34] Zvaifler and associates[31] found somewhat higher plateau plasma chloroquine levels of 600 to 800 μg per liter but noted no differences in patients receiving dosages ranging from 125 mg to 750 mg per day.

The half-life of chloroquine in man has been reported to vary widely. In patients receiving either a single or a weekly dose, the half-life is about 3.5 days.[35] When patients received 500 mg of chloroquine phosphate daily for four weeks, the half-life increased to 6 to 7 days.[32] Others have found dose-dependent kinetics with a half-life as long as 12 days after receiving a single 1-gram dose of chloroquine.[33] Some of these differences may result from different methodologies of measurement.[33] By the 77th day after drug administration is discontinued, urinary daily output falls to about 1 mg.[32] At this time about 55 percent of the total ingested dose may be accounted for by urinary excretion.[32] However, small amounts of chloroquine may be found in plasma, red blood cells, and urine as long as 5 years after the last dose.[36] The rate of urinary excretion depends on pH and is increased when the urine is acidified.

The major metabolic conversion product of either chloroquine or hydroxychloroquine, accounting for about one-third of the total urinary excretory product, is the desethyl derivative formed by *N*-alkyl degradation of the terminal desethyl amino-ethyl group in the side chain.[29,37] Minor metabolic conversion products account for about 3 percent of excreted drug. They include compounds formed by ring hydroxylation and side chain degradation.[29,37]

Tissue concentrations of chloroquine and hydroxychloroquine are much greater than plasma levels.[38,39] Most studies have been conducted in animals, especially rats, but a few studies have been performed in military personnel[39,40] committing suicide by chloroquine ingestion[39] or dying from other causes.[40] In rats the lowest tissue concentrations are found in brain, followed by muscle, kidney, liver, lung, spleen, and the adrenal glands.[38] Studies in humans show rather similar tissue distribution.[39] Localization of the 4-aminoquinolines in the eye assumes great importance because of retinal toxicity. In albino rats drug concentration in the eye ranks between muscle and heart. In pigmented rats eye concentration is 10 to 20 times greater than any other tissue.[38] Bernstein and associates[41] found that this could be accounted for by deposition in the iris and choroid.

Despite the markedly increased deposition of chloroquine in pigmented ocular tissue, subcellular localization is not well established. McChesney and associates have found similar excretion rates in blacks and whites, suggesting that binding to skin melanin may not be substantial.[32] In vitro chloroquine binds to nucleic acids, but Vargo[42] has shown that only 10 percent of tissue levels are localized in the nucleus of rat liver or kidney cells. High concentrations have been measured in the lysosomal fraction of rat liver.[43]

POSSIBLE MECHANISMS OF THERAPEUTIC ACTION

Since Payne[2] first suggested that quinine corrected a circulatory disturbance in lupus erythematosus, much speculation and investigation have centered upon the mechanisms by which antimalarials act. Conclusions have not been definitive because the pathogenesis of the two major diseases responding to antimalarials, lupus erythematouss and rheumatoid arthritis, is complicated and incompletely understood (see Chapters 58, 59 and 68), and also because the antimalarials have multiple actions. A number of interacting pathways (described in Section I) have been implicated in disease pathogenesis, but the primary factors responsible for disease initiation, development, and severity have not been determined. Antimalarial drugs may inhibit several of these pathways. However, investigation of drug actions has generally been conducted in vitro, and it is not known if the drugs produce similar effects in vivo. Furthermore, concentrations of the drug in these experiments vary greatly and may not be obtained in the crucial in vivo sites.

The varied actions of antimalarials may be considered under several headings. They may impair several basic physiologic processes. These actions, possibly interacting with others, may moderate inflammatory or immunologic pathways. There are also a number of miscellaneous actions that may contribute to modulation of disease pathogenesis.

Primary Actions. Three basic processes affected by antimalarials are sulfhydryl-disulfide interchange, enzymatic reactions, and nucleoprotein interaction.

Sulfhydryl-disulfide interchange reactions participate in numerous biologic processes.[44] These include certain enzymatic reactions, proliferation of immunologically competent cells,[45] denaturation of some proteins, the Arthus reaction, cell wall integrity, and the formation of the mitochondrial network. Gerber[44] has shown that chloroquine binds to certain sulfhydryl groups of human serum protein. This occurs using concentrations of chloroquine obtainable in the serum of patients undergoing treatment. He also established that chloroquine can block sulfhydryl-disulfide interchange reactions during the denaturation of bovine serum albumin by heat or urea and can inhibit the reduction of ferricyanide by cysteine.

Enzymatic reactions participate in almost all biologic events. Chloroquine reduces the activity of many enzymes,[46] including phospholipase,[47] NADH-cytochrome C reductase, and cholinesterase. More specifically related to the pathogenesis of arthritis, Whitehouse and Coewy[48] demonstrated that chloroquine inhibits the protease-induced release of peptides from incubating cartilage slices and the hydrolysis of rat skin gelatin by bacterial collagenase. Chloroquine may also interfere with hyaluronidase actions, as shown indirectly by Whitehead and Hager.[49]

Antimalarials have been shown to form complexes with DNA by binding of the quinoline ring to the phosphate groups and nucleotide bases.[50] This appears to stabilize the DNA, block depolymerization by desoxyribonuclease,[51] inhibit the actions of DNA and RNA polymerases,[52] and interfere with DNA replication.[53] By binding to the DNA substrate, antimalarials block reactions between DNA and anti-DNA antibodies.[54] This is probably the explanation for the inhibition of the LE cell phenomenon observed by Dubois.[55] DNA binding might be expected to be an important modulator of DNA/anti-DNA antibody complex formation in lupus, but an in vivo effect has not been demonstrated.

Anti-inflammatory Actions. A number of antimalarial actions may inhibit inflammatory reactions. In addition to blocking sulfhydryl-disulfide interchange and a direct effect on enzymes, chloroquine also stablizes lysosomal membranes, thereby inhibiting the release of lysosomal enzymes.[56] Protection was observed against several different mechanisms of membrane destablization, including ultraviolet light. Prostaglandins, another set of mediators of inflammation, are elevated in rheumatoid synovial fluid. Chloroquine decreases total prostaglandin production.[57] It has a direct effect on phospholipase A, the enzyme initiating prostaglandin synthesis.[47] Prostaglandin F2 formation is inhibited to a greater extent than prostaglandin E2.[57]

Other inflammatory processes blocked by chloroquine include polymorphonuclear cell chemotaxis and phagocytosis.[58] This action may be one of the mechanisms causing the suppression of polymorphonuclear infiltration into implants of polyurethane foam impregnated with dead tubercle bacilli.[59] Chloroquine also appears to suppress the growth of fibroblasts, as shown by the inhibition of the development of connective tissue capsules about implants.[60]

Experimental evidence supports Payne's concept[2] that antimalarials may affect "circulatory disturbances." The activity of histamine,[61] which increases vasopermeability, is diminished. Another vascular abnormality inhibited by chloroquine is blood sludging, the intravascular aggregation of erythrocytes. Sludging has been observed in patients with rheumatoid arthritis[3] and was found to disappear when monitored in the retinal veins of 22 patients treated with chloroquine. Clinical improvement followed "desludging" in 51 percent of patients and a lowered erythrocyte sedimentation rate in 41 percent.

Immunologic Action. Abnormal immunologic reactivity is believed to play an important role in rheumatic disease pathogenesis. Experimental evidence concerning antimalarial action on immune reactivity is inconsistent. Animal studies suggest that chloroquine has no inhibitory effect on antibody production. Thompson and Bartholomew[62] found no difference between treated and control rabbits in the production of circulating antibodies to typhoid O and H antigens or to bovine serum albumin. Kalmonson and Gage[63] showed that hydroxychloroquine-treated rabbits produced a normal primary or secondary response to diphtheroid toxoid. They did note an enhanced tuberculin reaction in the hydroxychloroquine-treated rabbits infected with bacillus Calmette-Guérin.

Other studies demonstrated inhibition of immune reactions. Hurvitz and Hirschhorn[64] showed that chloroquine inhibited the proliferative response of cultured human lymphocytes induced by phytohemagglutinin, steptolysin O antigen, or foreign lymphocytes. Panaji and co-workers[65] extended these results by demonstrating decreased responsiveness to phytohemagglutinin by lymphocytes from patients treated with chloroquine and aspirin compared with those from patients treated with aspirin alone.

More recently Salmeron and Lipsky[66] observed that proliferation of lymphocytes suppressed by chloroquine was restored by purified monocytes. They showed that the generation of immunoglobulin-secreting cells could also be suppressed by concentrations of chloroquine as low as 1 μg per ml. Adding supernatants from cultures of purified monocytes reversed this action. Purified interleukin 1 could be substituted for monocyte supernatant with similar effect, suggesting that chloroquine interferes with the secretion of interleukin 1 by monocytes.[66a]

It has not been shown that antibody production in patients with rheumatic diseases is directly inhibited by antimalarials, but in vitro complex formation between antigens and antibodies is inhibited.[67,68] The fall in titers of rheumatoid factors observed in patients with rheumatoid arthritis[69-71] may merely be a nonspecific reflection of disease improvement.

Miscellaneous Action. Among the miscellaneous actions of antimalarials that may explain their improvement of lupus erythematosus is a photoprotective effect. McChesney and associates[72] showed that these drugs are present in the skin in high concentrations and can absorb ultraviolet radiation. Lester and co-workers[73] showed that hydroxychloroquine raises the minimal erythema-inducing dose of ultraviolet light between five- and tenfold in patients with photosensitive rashes or lupus erythematosus. Others have not found a sunscreening action.[74,75] They postulated that the photoprotective effect was mediated by "modifying the reaction pattern of the patient with polymorphous light eruption in a manner which supresses the abnormal but not the normal responses to ultraviolet light in the sunburn spectrum."[74]

Infectious agents may participate in the development of systemic lupus erythematosus or rheumatoid arthritis.[76] Chloroquine inhibits the replication of some bacteria[52] and protects tissue culture cells from viral infections.[77] Replication of the Maloney leukemia virus may be prevented even in the absence of an apparent effect on DNA or RNA synthesis.[78]

There is evidence that the Epstein-Barr virus may be a pathogenetic agent for rheumatoid arthritis.[79] While exposure to this agent is similar to that of nonrheumatoid individuals, patients develop an unusual host response that includes the production of rheumatoid arthritis precipitin (RAP), presumed to be an antibody to a nuclear antigen of Epstein-Barr-infected B lymphocytes. Chloroquine enhances the expression of the Epstein-Barr virus antigen, EA, in superinfected cells.[80] This could promote the immunologic inactivation of such cells in treated patients.

THERAPEUTIC EFFECTIVENESS

The effectiveness of antimalarial medications in the treatment of systemic lupus erythematosus and rheu-

matoid arthritis is generally accepted. They are probably helpful in treating other inflammatory arthritides, such as psoriatic arthritis, ankylosing spondylitis, and juvenile rheumatoid arthritis, although hard data supporting this are lacking.

Because antimalarials were synthesized to treat malaria and not connective tissue diseases, clinical trials to determine efficacy and toxicity and animal experiments elucidating mechanisms of action were not initially conducted for rheumatic diseases. Later studies have rectified some omissions, but there is a paucity of studies directly comparing different antimalarials or varying doses of a single drug.

Lupus Erythematosus. The variability of lupus erythematosus and the unevenness of its response to medication increase the difficulty of evaluating its response to antimalarials. Untreated lupus erythematosus is characterized by excerbations and remissions. The discoid variety undergoes spontaneous remission in 10 to 15 percent,[25] while the systemic form may have spontaneous remission in 40[81] to 70 percent.[82] This occurrence of spontaneous remissions, as well as the finding that various manifestations of systemic lupus erythematosus do not respond equally well to antimalarials, may lead to an overestimation of effectiveness in uncontrolled studies. It is particularly important not to attribute generalized benefit to treatment when only one manifestation is actually improved. Corticosteroids are generally more effective than antimalarials. When both are taken, the steroids may obscure benefits accruing from antimalarial treatment. On the other hand, improvement due to steroids may be incorrectly attributed to antimalarials.

Discoid Lupus Erythematosus. Even after considering these factors, the conclusion that discoid lupus erythematosus responds to antimalarials is inescapable. Compared with the spontaneous remission rate of 15 percent, remissions or major improvements have been noted in 60 to 90 percent of treated patients. Furthermore, all antimalarial compounds have been beneficial. However, daily dosages were often much larger than those currently acceptable.

Quinine was the first antimalarial used to treat discoid lupus erythematosus. Payne[2] did not report the percentage of responders and used doses as high as 1800 mg per day. Nineteen of 29 patients treated by Davidson and Birt[4] responded to doses half as large, while five were unimproved, and five were lost to follow-up. Erythematous lesions improved, but scaly ones did not.

The development of synthetic antimalarials provided other therapeutic agents. Martenstein[5] in 1928 used pamaquine, an 8-aminoquinoline, with good results in 79 percent of 28 patients. He too noted greater improvement of acutely inflamed lesions than of hyperkeratotic changes. Quinacrine was the first antimalarial agent for which responses of a large number of patients were described. Prokoptchouk[6] treated 35 patients with a series of 10-day courses interspersed with rest periods. Two to five courses were generally needed, but even chronic, scarred lesions improved. Page's report[8] of its effectiveness in 17 of 18 patients treated with doses of 100 to 300 mg per day stimulated further trials. In the next 10 years five of the papers published[83-87] reported good results in 215 of 276 patients with discoid lupus erythematosus, a 78 percent response rate. The 4-aminoquinoline compound amodiaquin was also found to be effective by several investigators.[25,88,89]

Goldman and associates[90] first treated discoid lupus erythematosus with chloroquine because it was less toxic than quinacrine and did not impart the yellowish skin staining found with quinacrine. Eleven of 18 patients showed great improvement with doses of 500 or 750 mg per day for 1 to 2 weeks followed by 250 mg per day for 4 to 6 weeks. Others noted similar or slightly better results.[25,91,92] Rogers and Finn[91] found chloroquine in doses of 250 mg per day as effective as quinacrine, beginning with 300 mg per day and tapering to 100 mg per day. Lesions cleared in 35 percent of 45 patients in each group, while another 15 percent of the quinacrine-treated and 30 percent of the chloroquine-treated patients were much improved.

Hydroxychloroquine was also initially used to diminish the toxicity seen with other antimalarials. In the study of Mullins and associates[13] localized edematous lesions cleared within two weeks in seven of eight patients, and excellent results were achieved over a somewhat longer time in five of eight patients with chronic discoid changes. Initial doses were quite high, averaging about 1000 mg per day, and maintenance doses were generally 400 to 600 mg per day. Seventeen of 22 patients treated with this drug by Lewis and Frumess[14] were more than 50 percent improved, with nine in remission after eight weeks.

A few controlled studies have substantiated antimalarial benefit. Dubois[25] substituted placebo for amodiaquin in seven patients. Five, who were initially controlled by amodiaquin alone, flared one to three months after placebo was substituted and then improved within several days after readministration of the drug.

Prakken reviewed the published results of the various treatments of discoid lupus erythematosus and found that 74 percent of those treated with metals (As, Au, Bi), 69 percent of those receiving antimalarials, and 72 percent of those given a miscellany of drugs were cured or much improved. As a result he participated in a double-blind trial with Kraak and co-workers.[93] There were 49 patients assigned to one of two groups. One was given hydroxychloroquine for one year, starting with two 200-mg tablets per day. If there was no improvement, the patient had his pills increased to four and then six, a maximum daily dose of 1200 mg. If a cure was obtained, the dose was reduced to a maintenance level. At the end of a year the patient was put on a placebo for three months. The other group reversed the procedure. Statistical analysis of the data showed that hydroxychloroquine was significantly more effective than the placebo.

The effectiveness of antimalarials in the treatment of skin lesions is often apparent within the first week when erythematous changes start to regress. Follicular plugging may then disappear, and after several months thickening and induration diminish or clear. Most patients responding to antimalarial medication suffer relapse after the drug is discontinued. Winkelmann and associates[85] found that only seven of 67 patients who took quinacrine or chloroquine for 10 weeks to 4 years maintained remission for 3 years after stopping treatment. Forty-eight patients who responded favorably to treatment had subsequent relapses after discontinuing medication. Most responded to additional courses of treatment.

Systemic Lupus Erythematosus. In distinction to the marked benefits of treatment of discoid lupus erythematosus with antimalarials, improvement of systemic lupus erythematosus is not nearly as well-documented. Much of the evidence suggesting that antimalarials are effective for the systemic variety comes from the inclusion of a few patients with "subacute" lupus in larger series of patients with only discoid skin lesions.[8,13,85,90] These patients have had findings such as arthritis, fever, fatigue, malaise, mildly depressed white blood cell counts, mild albuminuria, and a positive LE cell phenomenon. Quinacrine,[8] chloroquine even in low dosage,[90] and hydroxychloroquine[13] were each effective in such patients.

Dubois[94] treated 20 patients with systemic lupus erythematosus using rather high doses of quinacrine. Seven of nine patients with arthralgias and fever remitted on treatment, while only three of 11 patients with more severe acute systemic lupus erythematosus were benefited. In general, the less active the disease, the more rapid and better was the improvement.

Rudnicki and colleagues[95] provided some additional evidence that antimalarial treatment is effective for some systemic symptoms. They studied 43 patients who had been treated with antimalarials for at least two years and then had medication discontinued because of toxicity. Significantly fewer flare-ups occurred during the years on treatment, but no improvement in individual manifestations could be demonstrated for the entire group. When specific drugs and doses were studied, paired-t test analysis showed less fever, fatigue, and weight loss during the years on drug ($p < 0.05$) for the group who had received 500 mg of chloroquine daily. No significant corticosteroid-sparing effect was found. Others suggest that antimalarial treatment may have a steroid-sparing effect.[96]

Antimalarials are not appropriate treatment for the more severe manifestations of systemic lupus erythematosus according to Dubois[25] or Lanham and Hughes.[97] However, there is one study suggesting that antimalarials may be useful in treating lupus glomerulonephritis. Conte and associates[98] treated 12 patients with a combination of indomethacin (3 mg per kg per day) and hydroxychloroquine (800 mg per day). All patients had active diffuse proliferative glomerulonephritis, and four had more than 50 percent crescent formation on biopsy. Serum creatinine was initially elevated in all but two patients (median of 2.0 mg per dl) and all had 24-hour proteinuria of greater than 1 g (median 3.6 g). Duration of treatment ranged from 22 to 76 months in all but one patient. Follow-up evaluation demonstrated lasting remissions in 8 patients, including one with crescent formation and improvement in three others. Only one patient died. At the same time 16 patients treated with high-dose corticosteroids by this group did poorly, with nine deaths.

Rheumatoid Arthritis. Medications used for rheumatoid arthritis may be divided into several groups on the basis of their onset of action and their effect on the underlying disease process. The antimalarials belong to the class termed slow-acting antirheumatic drugs (SAARDs). Little or no improvement may be apparent for weeks or months after antimalarials are started. Benefits ensue gradually and may not be maximal for many months.[10,15] This contrasts with the more immediate effects of steroids or nonsteroidal anti-inflammatory agents that appear within one or two weeks. Analogously, when antimalarial treatment is discontinued, the disease will not flare within days but gradually worsen over weeks or months. It is this gradual action that suggests that SAARDs act indirectly. SAARDs may modify the disease process in such a manner that some patients enter a sustained remission.

Different types of studies have been helpful in determining the effectiveness of antimalarials. Factors considered are the drug used, dosage schedule employed, length of study, and whether the study is controlled. Double-blind controlled studies are most definitive, but prolonged placebo-controlled studies are often not feasible in patients with rheumatoid arthritis. Long-term open evaluation provides additional information, particularly in assessing late responses,[15] relapses on treatment,[10] and the effects of dosage. The response to different dosages may not be readily appreciated unless specifically studied.

Several of the antimalarials no longer employed have been shown to be effective. Encouraged by Page's[8] description of improvement of arthritis in two patients with lupus erythematosus treated with quinacrine, Freedman and Bach[9] used this medication to treat 23 patients with rheumatoid arthritis. All but one improved both subjectively and objectively. Primaquine was effective in each of 21 patients treated by Steck and associates,[99] 2 entering complete remission and 8 partial remission. Two 4-aminoquinoline drugs, amodiaquin and amopyroquin, have also been used with some benefit.[11,100-102] A 5-month double-blind cross-over study of amopyroquin was conducted on 15 patients by Bartholomew and Duff.[102] Even with this small number of patients, significant improvement in Lansbury's systemic index, grip strength, and erythrocyte sedimentation rate was found for drug but not placebo.

In 1953, Haydu[103] described chloroquine treatment of rheumatoid arthritis. Patients were treated for 6 months using the rather low dosage of 0.5 g three times a week. Considerable improvement was noted in 21 of 28 patients. Although only one patient went into complete remission, only one failed to show any improvement. Haydu believed that his data were not sufficient to judge the true efficacy of chloroquine but that the medication should be regarded as one additional antirheumatic substance.

Subsequent studies confirmed the efficacy of chloroquine and demonstrated that hydroxychloroquine was equally beneficial. One of the most influential[19] was that of Bagnall.[10] He treated 125 patients with 250 mg of chloroquine per day. Twenty-one of the 90 patients with rheumatoid arthritis were initially entered in a double-blind placebo-controlled study. The results so favored the chloroquine-treated group that Bagnall had no difficulty in determining which was the active compound. The controlled study was stopped because he believed he could not ethically enter seriously affected patients in a long-term placebo-controlled study. In the open study major improvement was noted in 71 percent, and half of those entered remission. Long duration of disease or gross articular damage was more prevalent in those failing to respond. Relapses during treatment were noted in 18 patients. They occurred most frequently in the second and third year of treatment, especially in patients unable to tolerate the standard dose. Sixteen of these 18 patients improved with continued treatment. Seven patients relapsed three to twelve months after treatment was stopped and again remitted when chloroquine was restarted. Bagnall emphasized that maximum benefit might not be apparent until after a year of treatment.

Results achieved by Scherbel and associates[15] supported Bagnall's findings. One hundred and six patients were treated with a 4-aminoquinoline compound and 60 percent obtained major benefit. Forty-six patients received chloroquine in an initial dose of 500 mg per day, which was later reduced to 250 mg, and 60 received hydroxychloroquine, 600 mg per day, which was later reduced to 400 mg. Equal improvement was noted for patients on each medication. Scherbel's group found that for the same dose of each medication hydroxychloroquine was one-half to two-thirds as effective as chloroquine and one-half as toxic. In distinction to Bagnall's[10] findings, Scherbel did not observe any correlation between response of rheumatoid arthritis to medication and American Rheumatism Association stage of disease, duration of disease, or functional capacity of patient. They too noted that maximum response might not be evident for one year or longer and that disease activity fluctuated during treatment.

Adams and co-workers[104] reported a response rate using hydroxychloroquine that was comparable to that noted by Bagnall[10] for chloroquine. One hundred and eight patients treated with 400 mg per day of hydroxychloroquine for a minimum of 6 months were analyzed. Sixty-three percent had at least 30 percent improvement in active joint count and morning stiffness. Thirteen patients went into remission, and another 15 had greater than 75 percent improvement. Kersley and Palen[11] found that dosage may affect response rate by demonstrating that a daily dose of 800 mg was more effective than 400 mg.

Controlled studies have consistently demonstrated that these two medications are effective. Dosage of the active drug and duration of these trials have varied. The first study, conducted by Freedman,[105] compared daily doses of 200 mg of chloroquine phosphate to placebo in 66 patients over a 16-week interval. Clinical improvement was greater on chloroquine, but erythrocyte sedimentation rate and hemoglobin did not change. Rinehart and co-workers[106] studied chloroquine in both placebo-controlled parallel fashion and a cross-over manner after recognizing its benefit in open studies. Observing 33 patients over 4 months, they found that the active drug group, who received 250 mg of chloroquine per day, did significantly better than controls. Cohen and Calkins[16] studied 22 patients in a cross-over trial of only 18 weeks' duration. Morning stiffness and pain were significantly improved during active treatment. Grip strength and erythrocyte sedimentation rate were little affected.

Two double-blind studies have been conducted using hydroxychloroquine. Hamilton and Scott[17] in a cross-over study of 41 patients compared 600 mg daily with a 3-mg placebo dose. Each was taken for a 3-month period. Patient estimation of fitness, number of aspirin tablets taken daily, joint tenderness and swelling, grip strength, and erythrocyte sedimentation rate all improved when patients received the active drug, but only a decrease in ingested aspirin tablets reached statistical significance ($p < 0.001$). The authors concluded that the drug had slight but definite antirheumatic activity.

The Cooperating Clinics of the American Rheumatism Association[71] conducted a 6-month placebo-controlled study in which 53 patients received 800 mg per day of hydroxychloroquine and 60 received placebo. Results are shown in Table 51–2. Changes in individual indexes (listed in the footnote) all favored the drug-treated group, but none reached statistical significance. More impressive were the changes in the overall assessments listed in Table 51–2, which were associated with hydroxychloroquine treatment. Furthermore, serum gamma globulin levels returned toward normal for only the drug-treated group. Latex agglutination tests became normal in seven of 36 drug-treated patients, but only in two of 44 patients receiving placebo. The authors concluded that the differences in response were a result of drug effectiveness.

Even more favorable results have been obtained in two 1-year studies. One hundred and seven patients entered the trial conducted by Freedman and Steinberg.[107] Forty-two patients treated with 400 mg of chloroquine sulfate daily and 40 placebo-treated patients completed the trial. The authors noted definite general improvement in 80 percent of the patients completing 1 year of chloroquine treatment compared with 30 percent of the placebo group. Deterioration was seen in only 5 percent of chloroquine-treated patients but in 25 percent of controls. All clinical parameters, including joint tenderness, walking time, and the erythrocyte sedimentation rate, improved in the drug-treated group. Only manual dexterity improved in the placebo group. Radiographic evaluation showed improvement in erosion score for two treated patients, with worsening in three. Twelve placebo patients had greater erosions, and none had improvement.

Popert and associates[69] conducted a similar trial in which 134 patients were entered. Dosage of chloroquine was 250 mg a day, although some patients received 500 mg per day during initiation of treatment. Disease activity, functional capacity, grip strength, and erythrocyte sedimentation rate were significantly better in the treated group. Improvement was more marked in those with shorter duration of disease. The sheep cell agglutination titer fell in 16 of 18 chloroquine-treated patients but in only three of 15 controls. Increased titers were noted in one treated patient and six controls. The only parameter not improved by treatment was radiologically assessed erosions. Each group showed slight progression.

Comparison with Other Slow-acting Antirheumatic Drugs (SAARDs). A few studies have compared various SAARDs in treating rheumatoid arthritis. Dwosh and colleagues[108] compared chloroquine (250 mg per day), gold thiomalate (50 mg weekly), and azothiaprine (1 to 2 mg per kg per day) in an open study of 33 patients with class II disease using American Rheumatism Association criteria. The five variables assessed were articular index, joint count, grip strength, morning stiffness, and erythrocyte sedimentation rate. At 24 weeks, each group was significantly better than at baseline. Analysis of variance showed no significant difference in improvement among the three groups except that the erythrocyte blood sedimentation rate was only decreased in the group receiving gold. Toxicity was minimal for all groups. On follow-up examination, most patients had maintained their improvement, although disease flares occurred in four of 10 patients treated with chloroquine. The authors concluded from their study that chloroquine is "a moderately effective anti-rheumatic drug and should be considered early in the management of rheumatoid arthritis."

Two studies analyzed termination of treatment using life table analysis.[109,110] In the first[109] gold was compared with hydroxychloroquine. Fifty percent of patients stopped hydroxychloroquine treatment at 13 months, with 36 percent discontinuing medication for lack of benefit and 7 percent because of side effects. Of patients receiving gold therapy, 60 months elapsed before 50 percent terminated treatment primarily because of toxicity. A subsequent report[110] from the same institution compared treatment terminations with those for patients taking gold, D-penicillamine, and levamisole. In this study hydroxychloroquine treatment resulted in fewer terminations than the other drugs, with only 30 percent

Table 51–2. Controlled Study of Hydroxychloroquine in Rheumatoid Arthritis:[71] Comparison by Overall Assessment

Parameter	Placebo (Percent Improved)	Hydroxychloroquine (Percent Improved)
Class II or I	9	50
Five-point scores*	54	75
Observer's assessment	35	64
Patient's assessment	60	75

*Five-point score is summation of five indices: duration of morning stiffness, number of active joints, time of 50-foot walk, erythrocyte sedimentation rate, and grip strength.

stopping treatment at 15 months. A 6 percent lack of effectiveness was found for hydroxychloroquine, a frequency similar to that for gold or penicillamine and less than that for levamisole. Commenting on the differences between the studies, the authors suggested that they may have discontinued hydroxychloroquine before full benefit was received or demanded a more complete remission in the first study. Patients treated with hydroxychloroquine in the second study may have had less active disease prior to treatment than those treated with the other drugs.

Combination with Other Medications. Combination treatment utilizing antimalarials and other antirheumatic drugs has not been extensively evaluated. Because the antimalarials appear to act differently from nonsteroidal anti-inflammatory drugs, these two groups of medications are used concomitantly. One report[111] suggests that chloroquine may decrease the need for steroids. Sievers and Hurri[112] found that antimalarials could be used in combination with gold to therapeutic advantage. Side effects appeared additive and in general could be attributed to only one medication.[113] On the other hand, Bunch and associates[114] found that hydroxychloroquine combined with D-penicillamine was less effective than either used alone.

Other Arthropathies. The response of other rheumatic diseases to antimalarials is mainly anecdotal. Bagnall[10] treated 17 patients with ankylosing spondylitis, 10 with rheumatoid arthritis and concomitant psoriasis, and eight with juvenile rheumatoid arthritis with chloroquine. Although the numbers were too small for statistical consideration, he found the results to be similar to those for classic rheumatoid arthritis. Scherbel[115] found moderate to great improvement in 84 percent of 73 patients with juvenile rheumatoid arthritis. Sixteen of 23 of his patients with psoriasis and rheumatoid arthritis improved satisfactorily.[15]

Some authors consider antimalarials to be contraindicated in patients with psoriatic arthritis because exacerbation of skin lesions may occur. Kammer and co-workers[116] employed hydroxychloroquine in doses of 200 to 400 mg per day for 50 courses of treatment in their series of 100 patients with psoriatic arthritis. Sixty-eight percent had beneficial responses. Twenty-four of the 34 patients who responded went into remission. No exacerbation of skin lesions was noted. Results of the study being conducted by the Pediatric Rheumatology Collaborative Study Group of the American Rheumatism Association of hydroxychloroquine treatment of juvenile rheumatoid arthritis[117] should help clarify its role in this disease.

SIDE EFFECTS AND TOXICITY

The decision to use a medication must be based on a comparison of therapeutic benefit with toxicity. After it was established that antimalarials could cause loss of vision, safety became the paramount issue and the major factor limiting antimalarial use. During the past two

decades more articles have appeared discussing retinal toxicity than commenting on effectiveness.

Much of the impetus for the development of chloroquine and hydroxychloroquine was the toxicity of the earlier synthetic antimalarials. These compounds frequently produced skin lesions, gastrointestinal problems, and neurologic symptoms. Thrombocytopenia, leukopenia, and aplastic anemia also occurred.[83-86,105,118] Yellowish staining of the skin, which could simulate jaundice, was a particularly distressing problem with quinacrine treatment.[8,25,90] 8-Aminoquinoline compounds may cause hemolysis and methemoglobinemia in patients with a genetically transmitted deficiency of glucose-6-phosphate dehydrogenase.[119] Amodiaquin was shown by Kersley and Palin[11] to produce severe side effects, including aplastic anemia, with daily doses of 400 mg. Even in the usually acceptable dosage of 200 mg per day, it was less well tolerated than 800 mg per day of hydroxychloroquine. Elevations of SGOT were reported in four of 15 patients treated with 150 mg per day of amopyroquin.[102]

Although hydroxychloroquine and chloroquine are relatively safe, the list of reported side effects is extensive (Table 51–3). Toxicity may be somewhat arbitrarily divided into five major types (headings in Table 51–3). Gastrointestinal reactions are most frequent, followed by lesions of the skin and hair. Neuromuscular side effects comprise a variety of findings. Eye toxicity and a small number of miscellaneous reactions complete the groups.

The incidence of untoward effects varies widely, depending on daily dosage. In man, hydroxychloroquine has been found to be half as toxic as chloroquine on a weight basis.[15] Scherbel and colleagues noted reactions in 440 of 805 (55 percent) patients treated with daily doses of 250 to 500 mg of chloroquine or 400 to 600 mg of hydroxychloroquine. Sixty-seven percent were transient reactions and disappeared spontaneously. Another 26 percent responded to reductions in dosage. Only 7 percent of reactions precluded further treatment. Bagnall reported similar findings.[10] Analysis of toxicity reported in double-blind studies suggests that open studies overestimate the incidence of side effects. Freedman and Steinberg[105] reported side effects in 33 of 53 chloroquine-treated patients and similar problems in 22 of 54 placebo-treated patients during a 1-year period. Withdrawals were necessitated in five treated and four control patients. The placebo-controlled study conducted by the Cooperating Clinics Committee of the American Rheumatism Association[71] revealed more side effects in the patients treated with 800 mg of hydroxychloroquine daily. However, the placebo-treated patients showed a considerable frequency of reactions, which might have been attributed to hydroxychloroquine in an uncontrolled study. No patient in either group had reactions necessitating drug withdrawal. Hydroxychloroquine has been found to be less toxic than gold, penicillamine, or levamisole.[110]

Gastrointestinal side effects may mimic those of nonsteroidal anti-inflammatory drugs, with epigastric burn-

Table 51–3. Toxic Effects of Chloroquine and Hydroxychloroquine

Gastrointestinal
  Anorexia*[15]
  Abdominal bloating[15]
  Abdominal cramps[15]
  Diarrhea[15]
  Heartburn[15]
  Nausea[15]
  Vomiting[15]
  Weight loss[15,20]
Skin and Hair
  Alopecia[15,33]
  Bleaching of hair[15,25]
  Dryness of skin[15]
  Exacerbation of psoriasis[121,122]
  Increased pigmentation of skin and hair[25]
  Pruritus[15]
  Rashes[15,120-122]
    Exfoliative
    Lichenoid
    Maculopapular
    Morbilliform
    Urticarial
Neuromuscular
  Convulsive seizures[154]
  Difficulty in visual accommodation[129]
  Headache[15]
  Insomnia[15]
  Involuntary movements[155]
  Lassitude[15]
  Myasthenic reaction[25]
  Mental confusion[15]
  Nervousness or irritability[15]
  Neuromyopathy[123,124]
  Ototoxicity
    Nerve deafness[15,156,157]
    Tinnitus[15,156]
  Polyneuropathy[33]
  Toxic psychosis[158,159]
  Vestibular dysfunction[15,158]
  Weakness[30]
Miscellaneous
  Birth defects†[160]
  Blood dyscrasias
    Leukopenia[10,85]
    Agranulocytosis[127,128]
    Aplastic anemia[161]
    Leukemia†[161]
  Chromosome changes[162]
  Death from overdosage[39,153]
    Peripheral circulatory collapse
  Heart
    Electrocardiogram changes[120]
    Cardiomyopathy[33,163]
  Precipitation of porphyria[164]
Ocular
  Corneal deposits[11,131]
    Halos around lights
  Diplopia[130]
  Defects in accommodation and convergence‡[129]
    Various mild visual difficulties[25,30,120]
  Loss of corneal reflex[145,165]
  Retinopathy[18,137,141,143,147]
    Loss of vision
    Pigment abnormalities
    Scotomata
    Visual field abnormalities

*References for toxic effects are selected.
†Effect not conclusively related to medication.
‡May be a neuromuscular toxic effect.

ing, nausea, and vomiting. However, gastrointestinal blood loss is not caused by antimalarials. Nausea and anorexia may begin shortly after medication is started, and weight loss may be significant.[120] Abdominal cramps, bloating, and diarrhea[15,90] are more unique to antimalarials. Scherbel and associates[15] found significantly fewer gastrointestinal reactions with hydroxychloroquine (11 percent) than with chloroquine (19 percent).

Cutaneous lesions occur with equal frequency in patients receiving hydroxychloroquine or chloroquine.[15] Rashes may be lichenoid, urticarial, morbilliform, or maculopapular. Patients with psoriatic arthritis may experience an exacerbation of psoriatic skin lesions. Occasionally this has progressed to exfoliative dermatitis.[120,121] Kammer's group[116] did not observe any worsening of psoriasis or exfoliative lesions in 50 patients treated with 200 to 400 mg of hydroxychloroquine daily, although generalized erythematous, pruritic macular and papular eruptions occurred in four.

Reversible changes in the skin pigment have been noted in 10 to 25 percent of patients on long-term treatment, particularly when high daily dosages are taken.[25] Grayness or bleaching may appear at the roots of scalp hair, eyebrows, or eye lashes. Bluish-black oval macules occur on the shins, and the lesions may coalesce. Initially they have been mistaken for ecchymoses. Less commonly, alopecia develops[15,33] and must be differentiated from that which is a sign of the disease, lupus erythematosus, and not its treatment.

The more frequently noted neurologic manifestations are often of little significance because of their mildness and reversibility on lower daily doses.[10] These include frontal or unilateral headaches, giddiness, blurring of vision, insomnia, and nervousness.[10,30,120] A myasthenic syndrome has been reported by Dubois[25] to develop several weeks after beginning chloroquine and to disappear within days after discontinuing the drug. More important is a neuromuscular syndrome[123,124] that may be confused with corticosteroid-induced muscle weakness or attributed to the disease treated. Weakness starts in the proximal lower extremity but may be delayed a year or more after starting medication. It progresses slowly and may involve the arms. Complete reversibility is noted after discontinuing the antimalarials. A neurogenic component is suggested by decreased deep tendon reflexes and some of the electromyographic changes.[123] Muscle biopsy reveals vacuolar changes, but serum enzyme levels are not elevated.[124] This same histologic lesion may be present in patients with systemic lupus erythematosus who have not been treated with antimalarials.[125,126]

Among the miscellaneous side effects attributed to chloroquine or hydroxychloroquine is agranulocytosis or aplastic anemia.[127,128] This complication occurs very infrequently but has proved fatal.[128] Fatal overdosage has also been documented.[39]

Recent studies have provided a much better understanding of the occurrence of various ocular toxicities. Chloroquine and hydroxychloroquine may cause three main reactions. Two, defects in accommodation or convergence and corneal deposits, are relatively frequent, especially with higher doses. Symptoms are variable but not severe. They are completely reversible and, therefore, benign. The third, retinal toxicity, has great significance, since it may cause permanent loss of vision.

Blurred vision, difficulty changing focus quickly from a near to a far object, and poorly defined visual difficulties were frequent findings in the first systematic analysis of chloroquine administration to human volunteers reported shortly after World War II.[30,120] These symptoms were reversible within days of discontinuing the medication. It is likely that these problems are mediated by a direct effect on neural centers controlling convergence and accommodation, although a peripheral effect on ocular muscles has not been excluded.[129] Occasionally diplopia may result from extraocular muscle palsy.[130] Corneal deposits were described by Hobbs and Colnan[131] in 1958 and may be associated with halos around lights. Similar symptoms can be caused by glaucoma, and steroid-induced glaucoma must be differentiated.

Retinal lesions were not found with the lower doses of chloroquine used for the prophylaxis or treatment of malaria. In 1957, Cabiaggi[132] reported a patient with systemic lupus erythematosus treated with chloroquine and later hydroxychloroquine who developed atrophic retinal lesions surrounded by a pigmented border, tiny pigmented granules, constricted visual fields, and decreased visual acuity. Lesions of this patient and of two others[133] with severe fundal changes and visual field constriction were attributed to the disease rather than the treatment. Hobbs and associates[18] first attributed retinopathy to chloroquine treatment in 1959. Three patients developed abnormalities approximately three years after starting treatment. Symptoms consisted of misty vision and inability to see entire words when reading. Examination revealed decreased visual acuity, field defects, paracentral scotomata, and narrowed vessels. Fundus pigment was irregular and mottled or clumped in one patient, and an atrophic area was noted in another. After Hobbs' publication appeared, multiple cases of chloroquine retinopathy were reported.[130,134-145] Hydroxychloroquine may cause similar lesions,[146-148] although only a handful of patients with visual loss on this medication have been described.

Classic chloroquine retinopathy shows pigmentary mottling or clumping, progressing to a "bull's eye" lesion (Fig. 51–2). Visual acuity may be decreased and associated with central scotomata, peripheral field constriction, and later more dense field loss. Histologic examination shows loss of rods and cones and migration of clumps of pigment.[149] Speculation about the etiology of retinopathy centers upon the binding of 4-aminoquinolines to melanin of the retinal pigment epithelium, with subsequent loss of its putative protective function.[149]

Following the reports of retinal toxicity, investigations were undertaken to find more specific factors related to toxicity. A search for early predictors of retinal toxicity revealed that many ophthalmologic parameters became abnormal in patients taking antimalarials. Some,[141,142]

Figure 51–2. Bull's eye lesion: a classic, but not specific, lesion of chloroquine or hydroxychloroquine retinopathy. (Courtesy of Dr. R. Reinecke.)

such as the photostress test[142] or time to recover visual acuity after the macula is "dazzled" by a bright light, became abnormal in almost all patients unrelated to the visual loss and are, therefore, not predictive of visual loss. Others, such as loss of color vision or abnormal electrooculograms,[135] were not sensitive enough to be routinely employed as predictors of visual loss.[130,145,147]

It was noted, however, that retinal pigment abnormalities were almost invariably present in patients with visual loss. Mild changes, such as increased granularity or mottling, were believed to be an early indication of toxicity.[135,145] Percival and Meanock[130] found that visual field abnormalities to red test objects appeared in certain patients who did not have loss of vision detected by visual acuity changes, or scotomata, or field lesions to a white test object. Rynes and associates[147] prospectively studied 99 patients on long-term hydroxychloroquine treatment with daily doses of 400 mg to determine if visual loss could be prevented by regular ophthalmologic evaluation of retinal pigment changes and visual fields using a red test object. Although four patients[147,148] had either pigmentary changes, scotomata, or field constriction using a red test object, none had visual loss or field changes using a white test object.

The question of whether large *cumulative* dosage or high *daily* dosage contributes to retinal toxicity is extremely important because rheumatic diseases require long-term treatment. If cumulative dosage is a major factor, the medication should not be used for long-term treatment. Several lines of evidence suggest that it is daily dosage that determines toxicity.

First, visual loss almost always occurred in patients receiving daily doses greater than 400 mg of hydroxychloroquine or 250 mg of chloroquine.[135,138,143,150] Second, Mackenzie[151] has calculated the daily dose received by patients developing toxicity and compared this with the daily dose of those treated with cumulative doses greater than 1 kilogram. He found that all patients who developed toxicity took over 4 mg per kg per day of chloroquine or 6.5 mg per kg per day of hydroxychloroquine.

Furthermore, toxicity developed at relatively low cumulative doses, with means of 375 g for chloroquine and 525 g for hydroxychloroquine. Third, in the study by Tobin and associates[148] of patients who were followed for up to 7 years (mean of 57 months), toxicity was manifest within 3.5 years of starting the medication and did not increase as higher cumulative doses were achieved. Frisk-Holberg's group[33] related toxicity to serum drug levels, which should not change with increased cumulative doses once metabolic equilibrium is reached.

Because visual loss has been reported to progress[136,137] or even start[140] after treatment is discontinued, it was important to determine if early lesions are reversible. Retinal lesions may be divided into two groups. Those that have been termed "premaculopathy"[145] are generally reversible when the medication is discontinued. They include loss of foveal reflex, abnormal recovery times following "macular dazzle" with a bright light, mild pigmentary stippling, and visual field loss to a red test object. The other group, termed "true retinopathy," is much more serious. The characteristic ophthalmologic findings are severe pigmentary changes, especially a "bull's eye" lesion (Fig. 51–2), and visual field loss to a white test object. Loss of vision is almost always present, rarely improves, and may even progress after the medication is discontinued.

GUIDELINES FOR USE OF ANTIMALARIALS

Antimalarial medications are now established as important drugs in the treatment of rheumatic diseases. The controversy over whether long-term use will result in retinal lesions with loss of vision has been resolved by the recognition that such toxicity is related to daily dose.[147,150,151] Recent studies have demonstrated that the two antimalarials currently used, hydroxychloroquine and chloroquine, are among the least toxic slow-acting antirheumatic medications.[109,110]

The absence of retinal toxicity is dependent upon strict adherence to the guidelines listed in Table 51–4; these are low daily dose and regular ophthalmologic monitoring. The maximum daily dose for hydroxychloroquine should be 400 mg and for chloroquine 250 mg. The ophthalmologic safety of these schedules has been es-

Table 51–4. Safety Guidelines for Antimalarial Drugs

Maximum Daily Dose	
Hydroxyhloroquine	400 mg
Chloroquine	250 mg

Ophthalmologic Monitoring

Frequency
    Baseline, then every 6 months
Protocol
    Question patient about visual disturbance.
    Determine best-corrected visual acuity.
    Examine fundus for pigmentary abnormalities.
    Assess visual fields with a red test object; use white test object at baseline and if red test object fields are abnormal.

tablished.[23,147] Mackenzie's[151] method of determining dose on the basis of the patient's lean body weight may provide an additional margin of safety. He recommends a maximum of 6.5 mg per kg per day for hydroxychloroquine and 4 mg per kg per day for chloroquine.

Ophthalmologic examinations should be conducted regularly and frequently in order to detect the mild changes that are reversible. It may be helpful to discuss the reasons for routine monitoring and the methods to be used with the ophthalmologist chosen to conduct eye examinations. Some ophthalmologists, not familiar with recent studies documenting antimalarial safety, still believe these medications should never be used. The examination protocol is not complicated, but visual field testing is tedious and often difficult to reproduce. It is important to use both a 5-mm red test object and a 3-mm white test object at baseline. The examination should look for field constriction as well as paracentral scotomata. Because testing with a red test object is more sensitive, the white test object need not be used in follow-up examinations if red test object fields remain unchanged. A 5-degree constriction compared with baseline fields should be considered abnormal.[147]

If funduscopic examination shows pigmentary changes or visual field examination demonstrates constriction or paracentral scotomata, the medication is discontinued. Even though this conservative ophthalmologic protocol may occasionally deny antimalarial treatment to some patients who have changes unrelated to medication, strict adherence has prevented loss of vision in all patients so monitored.[148]

Daily dosage also may be related to drug effectiveness as well as to toxicity,[11] and it is important to keep in mind that current dosage has been determined by toxicity studies rather than trials of efficacy. However, the lower dosages have been shown to be effective.[10,15,104]

Hydroxychloroquine sulfate, 200 mg twice a day, or chloroquine phosphate, 250 mg per day, may be used as the initial slow-acting antirheumatic drug in patients with rheumatoid arthritis who respond insufficiently to nonsteroidal anti-inflammatory medications.[110] Because their activity and toxicity differ substantially, the nonsteroidal anti-inflammatory drugs may be continued. Although antimalarials may be slightly less effective than gold salts, D-penicillamine or azathioprine, this difference has not been shown to be significant.[108] Furthermore, any difference in effectiveness is counterbalanced by decreased side effects with fewer drop-outs for toxicity.[110] Another advantage is the lower cost of monitoring toxicity. Although an ophthalmologic examination should be performed every 6 months, routine hematologic and urinary monitoring are not necessary. After the drug has been found to be well tolerated, the patient need not visit his physician more frequently than indicated by disease severity. If successful, treatment should be maintained until the patient is in complete remission. The dose of hydroxychloroquine may then be decreased to 200 mg once a day for 6 months before discontinuing the medication. Even with this protocol, some patients will have a relapse after discontinuing the drug. A treatment course should not be considered to have failed until tried for at least 6 months.

Antimalarials may be used with benefit in patients with other inflammatory arthritides, including psoriatic arthritis, peripheral joint disease of ankylosing spondylitis, and juvenile rheumatoid arthritis. Patients with psoriatic arthritis should be warned that their skin lesions may flare, and they should be monitored carefully for the first month on treatment. However, the potential exacerbation of skin lesions should not be considered a contraindication in such patients.[116] Dosage schedules in adults should be the same as for rheumatoid arthritis. Modification of dosage depending on the patient's weight is mandatory in treating children with juvenile rheumatoid arthritis. Laakenson and associates[152] believe the maximum safe dose of chloroquine diphosphate is 4 mg per kg per day and that of hydroxychloroquine sulfate is 7 mg per kg per day. It is important to remember that children are quite sensitive to chloroquine overdose. Death has resulted from ingestion of as little as 1 gram[153] (four tablets).

Antimalarials have an important role in the treatment of skin lesions in patients with lupus erythematosus and appear to be effective for articular disease and some systemic manifestations such as fever or malaise. There are several ways to use antimalarials in the treatment of lupus erythematosus. Hydroxychloroquine may be started in most patients when the diagnosis is established, using a dosage schedule similar to that for rheumatoid arthritis, and continued as long as the disease remains active. Alternatively, antimalarials may be used only in patients with those manifestations definitely shown to respond. Some physicians use intermittent rather than sustained courses of treatment.

Although much of the controversy surrounding antimalarial use has been resolved, additional studies documenting the effectiveness of low doses would be helpful. Studies elucidating the mechanism of antimalarial drug action would provide a more rational basis for therapy and might enable a more appropriate selection of patients to be treated.

References

1. Rollo, I.M.: Drugs used in the chemotherapy of malaria. *In* Goodman, A.G., Goodman, L.S., and Gilman, A. (eds.): The Pharmacological Basis of Therapeutics. 6th ed. New York, MacMillan Publishing Co., 1980, pp. 1038–1060.
2. Payne, J.F.: A post-graduate lecture on lupus erythematosus. Clin. J. IV:223, 1894.
3. Cecchi, E., and Ferraris, F.: Desludging action of hydroxychloroquine in rheumatoid arthritis. Acta Rheum. Scand. 8:214, 1961.
4. Davidson, A.M., and Birt, A.R.: Quinine bisulfate as a desensitizing agent in treatment of lupus erythematosus. Arch. Dermatol. 37:247, 1938.
5. Martenstein, H.: Subactue lupus erythematosus and tubercular cervical adenopathy. Treatment with plasmochin. Z. Haut. Geschlectkrankheit. 27:248, 1928.
6. Prokoptchouk, A.J.: Treatment of lupus erythematosus with acriquine. Vestn. Vencrol. Dermatol. No. 2–3, 1940, p. 23.
7. Zakon, S.J., and Gershenson, J.: Introduction of quinacrine in treatment of lupus erythematosus. (Includes a translation of the paper by Prokoptchouk.) Arch. Dermatol. Syph. 71:520, 1955.
8. Page, F.: Treatment of lupus erythematosus with mepacrine. Lancet 2:755, 1951.
9. Freedman, A., and Bach, F.: Mepacrine and rheumatoid arthritis. Lancet 2:231, 1952.
10. Bagnall, A.W.: The value of chloroquine in rheumatoid disease—a four year study of continuous therapy. Can. Med. Assoc. J. 77:182, 1957.
11. Kersley, G.D., and Palin, A.G.: Amodiaquine and hydroxychloroquine in rheumatoid arthritis. Lancet 2:886, 1959.
12. Coatney, G.R.: Pitfalls in a discovery: The chronicle of chloroquine. Am. J. Trop. Med. Hyg. 12:121, 1963.
13. Mullins, J.F., Watts, F.L., and Wilson, C.J.: Plaquenil in the treatment of lupus erythematosus. JAMA 161:879, 1956.
14. Lewis, H.M., and Frumess, G.M.: Plaquenil in the treatment of discoid lupus erythematosus. AMA Arch. Dermatol. 73:576, 1956.
15. Scherbel, A.L., Harrison, J.W., and Atdjian, M.: Further observations on the use of 4-aminoquinoline compounds in patients with rheumatoid arthritis or related diseases. Cleveland Clin. Quart. 25:95, 1958.
16. Cohen, A.S., and Calkins, E.: A controlled study of chloroquine as an antirheumatic agent. Arthritis Rheum. 1:297, 1958.
17. Hamilton, E.B.D., and Scott, J.T.: Hydroxychloroquine sulfate (Plaquenil) in treatment of rheumatoid arthritis. Arthritis Rheum. 5:502, 1962.
18. Hobbs, H.E., Sorsby, A., and Freedman, A.: Retinopathy following chloroquine therapy. Lancet 2:478, 1959.
19. Rothermich, N.O.: Editorial. Coming catastrophes with chloroquine? Ann. Intern. Med. 61:1203, 1964.
20. Editorial. Chloroquine retinopathy. JAMA 184:775, 1963.
21. Editorial. Ocular complications of treatment with chloroquine and related antimalarial drugs. Can. Med. Assoc. J. 88:530, 1963.
22. Editorial. Retinal damage from drugs. Br. Med. J. Vol. 1:929, 1962.
23. Marks, J.S.: Is chloroquine obsolete in treatment of rheumatic diseases? Lancet 1:371, 1979.
24. Swinson, D.R., Losnick, J., and Jackson, L.: Double-blind trial of dapsone against placebo in the treatment of rheumatoid arthritis. Ann. Rheum. Dis. 40:235, 1981.
25. Dubois, E.: Antimalarials in the management of discoid and systemic lupus erythematosus. Sem. Arthritis Rheum. 8:33, 1978.
26. Taggert, J.V., Earl, D.P., Berliner, R.W., Zubrod, C.G., Welch, W.J., Wise, N.B., Schroeder, E.F., London, I.M., and Shannon, J.A.: Studies on the chemotherapy of the human malarials. III. The physiological disposition and antimalarial activity of the cinchona alkaloids. J. Clin. Invest. (Suppl.) 27:80, 1948.
27. Rollo, I.M.: Miscellaneous drugs used in the treatment of protozoal infections. *In* Goodman, A.G., Goodman, L.S., and Gilman, A. (eds.): The Pharmacological Basis of Therapeutics. 6th ed. New York, MacMillan Publishing Co., 1980, pp. 1078–1079.
28. DiPalma, J.R. (ed.): Drill's Pharmacology in Medicine. 4th ed. New York, McGraw-Hill Book Company, 1971, pp. 1779.
29. McChesney, E.W., Conway, W.D., Banks, W.F., Jr., Rogers, J.E., and Shekosky, J.M.: Studies on the metabolism of some compounds of the 4-amino-7-chloroquinoline series. J. Pharmcol. Exp. Ther. 151:482, 1966.
30. Berliner, R.W., Earle, D.P., Jr., Taggert, J.V., ZuBrod, C.G., Welch, W.J., Conan, N.J., Bauman, E., Scuddar, S.T., and Shannon, J.A.: Studies on the chemotherapy of human malarias. VI. The Physiological deposition, antimalarial activity and toxicity of several derivatives of 4-aminoquinolines. J. Clin. Invest. 27(Suppl.):98, 1948.
31. Zvaifler, N.J., and Rubin, M.: The metabolism of chloroquine (abstract). Arthritis Rheum. 5:330, 1962.
32. McChesney, E.W., Fasco, M.J., and Banks, W.F., Jr.: The metabolism of chloroquine in man during and after repeated oral dosage. J. Pharmacol. Exp. Ther. 158:323, 1967.
33. Frisk-Holmberg, M., Bergkvist, Y., Domeij-Nyberg, B., Hellstrom, L., and Jansson, F.: Chloroquine serum concentration and side effects: Evidence for dose-dependent kinetics. Clin. Pharmcol. Ther. 25:345, 1979.
34. McChesney, E.W., and Rothfield, N.F.: Comparative metabolic studies of chloroquine and hydroxychloroquine (abstract). Arthritis Rheum. 7:328, 1964.
35. McChesney, E.W., Banks, W.F., Jr., and McAuliff, J.P.: Laboratory studies of the 4-aminoquinoline antimalarials. II. Plasma levels of chloroquine and hydroxychloroquine after various oral dosage regimens. Antibiot. Chemother. 12:583, 1962.
36. Rubin, M., Bernstein, H.N., and Zvaifler, N.J.: Studies on the pharmacology of chloroquine. Arch. Ophthalmol. 70:474, 1962.
37. Rubin, M.: The antimalarials and tranquilizers. Dis. Nerv. Syst. (Suppl.) 29:67, 1968.
38. McChesney, E.W., Banks, W.F., Jr., and Fabian, R.J.: Tissue distribution of chloroquine, hydroxychloroquine and desethylchloroquine in the rat. Toxicol. Appl. Pharmacol. 10:501, 1967.
39. Kiel, F.W.: Chloroquine suicide. JAMA 190:398, 1964.
40. Prouty, R.W., and Kuroda, K.: Spectrophotometric determination and distribution of chloroquine in human tissues. J. Lab. Clin. Med. 52:477, 1958.
41. Bernstein, H., Zvaifler, N., Rubin, M., and Mansour, A.M.: The ocular deposition of chloroquine. Invest. Ophthal. 2:384, 1963.

42. Varga, F.: Intracellular localization of chloroquine in the liver and kidney of the rat. Acat. Physiol. Acad. Sci. Hung. 34:327, 1968.

43. Matsuzawa, Y., and Hostetler, K.Y.: Studies on drug-induced lipidosis: Subcellular localization of phospholipid and cholesterol in the liver of rats treated with chloroquine or 4,4′-bis(diethylaminoethoxy) α,β-diethyldiphenylethane. J. Lipid Res. 21:202, 1980.

44. Gerber, D.H.: Effect of chloroquine on the sulfhydryl group and the denaturation of bovine serum albumin. Arthritis Rheum. 7:193, 1964.

45. Noelle, R.J., and Lawrence, D.A.: Modulation of T-cell function. II. Chemical basis for the involvement of cell surface thiol-reactive sites in control of T-cell proliferation. Immunology 60:453, 1981.

46. Sams, W.M.: Chloroquine: Mechanism of action. Mayo Clin. Proc. 42:300, 1967.

47. Matsuzawa, Y., and Hostetler, K.Y.: Inhibition of lysosomal phospholipase A and phospholipase C by chloroquine and 4,4′-bis-(diethylaminoethyoxy) α,β-diethyldiphenylethane. J. Biol. Chem. 255:5190, 1980.

48. Whitehouse, M.W., and Cowey, F.K.: Inhibition of connective tissue by proteases by antimalarial, antirheumatic drugs. Biochem. J. 98:118, 1966.

49. Whitehead, R.W., and Hager, J.P.: The anti-inflammatory and antihyaluronidase effect of chloroquine diphosphate. J. Pharmacol. Exp. Ther. 110:52, 1954.

50. Cohen, S.N., and Yielding, K.L.: Spectrophotometric studies of the interaction of chloroquine and deoxyribonucleic acid. J. Biol. Chem. 240:3123, 1965.

51. Kurnick, N.B., and Radcliffe, I.E.: Reactions between DNA and quinacrine and other antimalarials. J. Lab. Clin. Med. 60:669, 1962.

52. Cohen, S.N., and Yielding, K.L.: Inhibition of DNA and RNA polymerase reactions by chloroquine. Proc. Nat. Acad. Sci. USA 54:521, 1965.

53. Ciak, J., and Hahn, F.E.: Chloroquine: Mode of action. Science 151:347, 1966.

54. Stoller, D., and Levine, L.: Antibodies to denatured DNA in lupus erythematosus serum. V. Mechanism of DNA-anti-DNA inhibition by chloroquine. Arch. Biochem. 101:335, 1963.

55. Dubois, E.L.: Effect of quinacrine (Atabrine) upon lupus erythematosus phenomenon. Arch. Dermatol. 71:570, 1955.

56. Weissman, G.: Labilization and stabilization of lysosomes. Fed. Proc. 23:1038, 1964.

57. Greaves, M.W., and McDonald-Gibson, W.: Effect of non-steroidal antiinflammatory drugs and antipyretic drugs on prostaglandin biosynthesis by human skin. J. Invest. Dermatol. 61:127, 1973.

58. Ward, P.A.: The chemosuppression of chemotaxis. J. Exp. Med. 24:209, 1966.

59. Clarke, A.K., Vernon-Roberts, B., and Aurey, H.L.F.: Assessment of anti-inflammatory drugs in the rat using subcutaneous implants of polyurethane foam impregnated with dead tubercle bacilli. Ann. Rheum. Dis. 34:326, 1975.

60. Greiling, H., and Dother, G.: Biochemical studies on the mechanism of action of resorcin. Z. Rheumaforsch. 21:316, 1962.

61. Desphande, V.R., Sharma, M.L., and Dashputra, P.G.: Antihistaminic action of antimalarials. Indian J. Physiol. Pharmacol. 7:259, 1963.

62. Thompson, G.R., and Bartholomew, L.E.: The effect of chloroquine on antibody formation. Univ. Mich. Med. Cent. J. 30:227, 1964.

63. Kalmonson, G.M., and Gage, I.G.: Effects of hydroxychloroquine on immune mechanisms. Clin. Res. 11:106, 1963.

64. Hurvitz, D., and Hirschhorn, K.: Suppression of "in vitro" lymphocyte responses by chloroquine. N. Engl. J. Med. 273:23, 1965.

65. Panayi, G.S., Neill, W.A., Duthie, J.J.R., and McCormick, J.N.: Action of chloroquine phosphate in rheumatoid arthritis. I. Immunosuppressive effect. Ann. Rheum. Dis. 32:316, 1973.

66. Salmeron, G., and Lipsky, P.E.: Immunosuppressive activity of chloroquine: Inhibition of human monocyte function. Arthritis Rheum. 25:S132, 1982.

66a. Salmeron, G., and Lipsky, P.E.: Immunosuppressive potential of antimalarials. (Suppl.). Am. J. Med. 18:19, 1983.

67. Szilagyi, T., and Kavai, M.: The effect of chloroquine on the antigen-antibody reaction. Acta Physiol. Acad. Sci. Hung. 38:411, 1970.

68. Holtz, G., Mantel, W., and Buck, W.: The inhibition of antigen-antibody reactions by chloroquine and its mechanism of action. Z. Immunitaetsforsch. 146:145, 1973.

69. Popert, A.J., Meijers, K.A.E., Sharp, J., and Bier, F.: Chloroquine diphosphate in rheumatoid arthritis. A controlled study. Ann. Rheum. Dis. 20:18, 1961.

70. Klinefelter, H.F., and Achurra, A.: Effect of gold salts and antimalarials on the rheumatoid factor in rheumatoid arthritis. Scand. J. Rheumatol. 2:177, 1973.

71. Mainland, D., and Sutcliffe, M.I.: Hydroxychloroquine sulfate in rheumatoid arthritis, a six month, double-blind trial. Bull. Rheum. Dis. 13:287, 1962.

72. McChesney, E.W., Nachod, F.C., and Tainter, M.L.: Rationale for treatment of lupus erythematosus with antimalarials. J. Invest. Dermatol. 29:97, 1957.

73. Lester, R.S., Burnham, T.K., Fine, G., and Murray K.: Immunologic concepts of light reactions in lupus erythematosus and polymorphous light eruptions. Arch. Dermatol. 96:1, 1967.

74. Cahn, M.M., Levy, E.J., and Shaffer, B.: Polymorphous light eruption: Effect of chloroquine phosphate in modifying reactions to ultraviolet light. J. Invest. Dermatol. 26:201, 1956.

75. Shaffer, B., Cahn, M.M., and Levy, E.J.: Absorption of antimalarial drugs in human skin: Spectroscopic and chemical analysis in epidermis and corium. J. Invest. Dermatol. 30:341, 1958.

76. Bartholomew, L.E., and Bartholomew, F.N.: Antigenic bacterial polysaccharide in rheumatoid synovial effusions. Arthritis Rheum. 22:969, 1979.

77. Watson, D.E.: Chloroquine protection against virus induced cell damage without inhibition of virus growth. J. Gen. Virol. 14:100, 1972.

78. Pazmino, N.H., Yuhas, J.M., and Tennant, R.W.: Inhibition of murine RNA tumor virus replication and oncogenesis by chloroquine. Int. J. Cancer 14:379, 1974.

79. Depper, J.M., and Zvaifler, N.J.: Epstein-Barr virus. Its relationship to the pathogenesis of rheumatoid arthritis. Arthritis Rheum. 24:755, 1981.

80. Karmali, R.A., Horrobin, D.F., Menezes, J., Patel, P., and Musto, J.: Chloroquine enchances Epstein-Barr virus expression. Nature 275:4444, 1978.

81. Dubois, E.L.: Systemic lupus erythematosus: Recent advances in its diagnosis and treatment. Ann. Intern. Med. 45:163, 1956.

82. Ropes, M.W.: Observations on the natural course of disseminated lupus erythematosus. Medicine 43:387, 1964.

83. O'Leary, P.A., Brunsting, L.A., and Kierland, R.R.: Quinacrine (Atabrine) hydrochloride in treatment of discoid lupus erythematosus. Arch. Dermatol. Syph. 67:633, 1953.

84. Kierland, R.R., Brunsting, L.A., and O'Leary, P.A.: Quinacrine hydrochloride in the treatment of lupus erythematosus. Mayo Clin. Proc. 28:22, 1953.

85. Winkelman, R.K., Merwin, C.F., and Brunsting, L.A.: Antimalarial therapy of lupus erythematosus. Ann. Intern. Med. 55:772, 1961.

86. Christiansen, J.V., and Nielsen, J.P.: Treatment of lupus erythematosus with mepacrine. Br. J. Dermatol. 68:73, 1956.

87. Buchanan, R.N.: Quinacrine in the treatment of discoid lupus erythematosus: A five-year follow-up survey-results and evaluation. South. Med. J. 52:978, 1959.

88. Pappenfort, R.B., and Lockwood, J.H.: Amodiaquine (Camoquin) in the treatment of chronic discoid lupus erythematosus. AMA Arch. Dermatol. 74:384, 1956.

89. Leeper, R.W., and Allende, M.F.: Antimalarials in the treatment of discoid lupus erythematosus. AMA Arch. Dermatol. 73:50, 1956.

90. Goldman, L., Cole, D.P., and Preston, R.H.: Chloroquine diphosphate in the treatment of discoid lupus erythematosus. JAMA 152:1428, 1953.

91. Rogers, J., and Finn, O.A.: Synthetic antimalarial drugs in chronic discoid lupus erythematosus and light eruptions. Arch. Dermatol. Syph. 70:61, 1954.

92. Crissey, J.T., and Murray, P.F.: A comparison of chloroquine and gold in the treatment of lupus erythematosus. Arch. Dermatol. 74:69, 1956.

93. Kraak, J.H., van Ketel, W.G., Prakken, J.R., and van Zwet, W.R.: The value of hydroxychloroquine (Plaquenil) for the treatment of chronic discoid lupus erythematosus: A double-blind trial. Dermatologica 130:293, 1965.

94. Dubois, E.L.: Quinacrine (Atabrine) in treatment of systemic and discoid lupus erythematosus. Arch. Intern. Med. 94:131, 1954.

95. Rudnicki, R.D., Gresham, G.E., and Rothfield, N.F.: The efficacy of antimalarials in systemic lupus erythematosus. J. Rheumatol. 2:323, 1975.

96. Ziff, M., Esserman, P., and McEwen, C.: Observations on the course and treatment of systemic lupus erythematosus. Arthritis Rheum. 1:332, 1956.

97. Lanham, J.G., and Hughes, G.R.V.: Antimalarial therapy in SLE. Clin. Rheum. Dis. 8:279, 1982.

98. Conte, J.J., Mignon-Conte, M.A., and Fournie, G.J.: Lupus nephritis: Treatment with indomethacin-hydroxychloroquine combination and comparison with corticosteroid treatment. Nouv. Presse Med. 4:91, 1975.

99. Steck, I.E., Zivin, S., Joseph, N., and Montgomery, M.M.: Influence of primaquine on the clinical findings and joint potentials in rheumatoid arthritis (abstract). Ann. Rheum. Dis. 11:310, 1952.

100. Bepler, C.R., Baier, H.N., McCracken, S., Rentschler, C.L., Rogers, F.B., and Lansbury, J.: A 15 month controlled study of the effects of amodiaquin (Camoquin) in rheumatoid arthritis. Arthritis Rheum. 2:403, 1959.

101. Pomeroy, H., Warren, C., Mills, D., and Clark, G.M.: The effect of amodiaquin (Camoquin) on the course of rheumatoid arthritis. Arthritis Rheum. 2:396, 1959.

102. Bartholomew, L.E., and Duff, I.F.: Amopyroquin (Propoquin) in rheumatoid arthritis. Arthritis Rheum. 6:356, 1963.

103. Haydu, G.G.: Rheumatoid arthritis therapy: Rationale and use of chloroquine diphosphate. Am. J. Med. Sci. 225:71, 1953.

104. Adams, E.M., Yocum, D.E., and Bell, C.L.: Hydroxychloroquine in the treatment of rheumatoid arthritis. Am. J. Med. 75:321, 1983.

105. Freedman, A.: Chloroquine and rheumatoid arthritis. Short-term controlled trial. Ann. Rheum. Dis. 15:251, 1956.

106. Rinehart, R.E., Rosenbaum, E.E., and Hopkins, C.E.: Chloroquine therapy in rheumatoid arthritis. Northwest Med. 56:703, 1957.

107. Freedman, A., and Steinberg, V.L.: Chloroquine in rheumatoid arthritis, a double blindfold trial of treatment for one year. Ann. Rheum. Dis. 19:243, 1960.

108. Dwosh, I.L., Stein, H.B., Urowitz, M.B., Smythe, H.A., Hunter, T., and Ogryzlo, M.A.: Azathioprine in early rheumatoid arthritis: Comparison with gold and chloroquine. Arthritis Rheum. 20:685, 1977.

109. Richter, J.A., Runge, L.A., Pinals, R.S., and Oates, R.P.: Analysis of treatment terminations with gold and antimalarial compounds in rheumatoid arthritis. J. Rheum. 7:153, 1980.

110. Husain, Z., and Runge, L.A.: Treatment complications of rheumatoid arthritis with gold, hydroxychloroquine, D-penicillamine and levamisole. J. Rheum. 7:825, 1980.

111. Scull, E.: Chloroquine and hydroxychloroquine therapy of rheumatoid arthritis. Arthritis Rheum. 5:30, 1962.

112. Sievers, K., and Hurri, L.: Combined therapy of rheumatoid arthritis with gold and chloroquine. 1. Evaluation of therapeutic effect. Acta Rheum. Scand. 9:48, 1963.

113. Sievers, K., Hurri, L., and Sievers, U.M.: Combined therapy of rheumatoid arthritis with gold and chloroquine. II. Evaluation of side effects. Acta Rheum. Scand. 9:56, 1963.

114. Bunch, T.W., O'Duffy, J.D., Tompkins, R.B., and O'Fallon, W.M.: Controlled study of hydroxychloroquine and penicillamine singly and in combination in the treatment of rheumatoid arthritis (abstract). Arthritis Rheum. 23:659, 1980.

115. Scherbel, A.L.: Long-term maintenance therapy with 4-amino-quinoline compounds in rheumatoid arthritis. In Mills, L.C., and Moyer, J.H. (eds.): Inflammation and Diseases of Connective Tissue. Philadelphia, W. B. Saunders Company, 1961, p. 555.

116. Kammer, G.M., Soter, N.A., Gibson, D.J., Schur, P.H.: Psoriatic arthritis: A clinical, immunologic and HLA study of 100 patients. Sem. Arthritis Rheum. 9:75, 1979.

117. Fink, C.W.: Treatment of juvenile arthritis. Bull. Rheum. Dis. 32:21, 1982.

118. Dubois, E.L.: Lupus Erythematosus. 2nd ed. Los Angeles, University of Southern California Press, 1974, pp. 548–554.

119. Beutler, E.: The hemolytic effect of primaquine and related compounds. A review. Blood 14:102, 1959.

120. Alving, A.S., Eichelberger, C.B., Jr., Jones, J.R., Wharton, C.M., and Pullman, T.N.: Studies on the chronic toxicity of chloroquine (SN-7618). J. Clin. Invest. (Suppl.) 27:60, 1948.

121. Cornbleet, T.: Action of synthetic antimalarial drugs on psoriasis. J. Invest. Dermatol. 26:435, 1956.

122. Reed, W.B.: Psoriatic arthritis. A complete study of 86 patients. Acta Dermatol. Venereol. 41:396, 1961.

123. Whisnant, J.P., Espinosa, R.E., Kierland, R.R., and Lambert, E.H.: Chloroquine neuropathy. Proc. Mayo Clin. 38:501, 1963.

124. Hicklin, J.A.: Chloroquine neuromyopathy. Ann. Phys. Med. 9:189, 1968.

125. Pearson, C.M., and Yamazaki, J.N.: Vacuolar myopathy in systemic lupus erythematosus. Am. J. Clin. Pathol. 29:455, 1958.

126. Sibrans, D.F., and Holley, H.L.: Vacuolar myopathy in a patient with positive LE cell populations. Arthritis Rheum. 10:141, 1967.

127. Polano, M.K., Cats, A., and van Older, G.A.J.: Agranulocytosis following treatment with hydroxychloroquine sulphate. Lancet 1:1275, 1965.

128. Propp, R.P., and Stillman, J.S.: Correspondence: Report of a non-fatal case of agranulocytosis on hydroxychloroquine therapy. N. Engl. J. Med. 277:492, 1967.

129. Rubin, M.L., and Thomas, W.C., Jr.: Diplopia and loss of accommodation due to chloroquine. Arthritis Rheum. 13:75, 1970.

130. Percival, S.P.B., and Meanock, I.: Chloroquine: Ophthalmological safety and clinical assessment in rheumatoid arthritis. Br. Med. J. 3:579, 1968.

131. Hobbs, H.E., and Calnan, C.D.: The ocular complications of chloroquine therapy. Lancet I:1207, 1958.

132. Cambiaggi, A.: Unusual ocular lesions in a case of systemic lupus erythematosus. Arch. Ophthalmol. 57:451, 1957.

133. Goldman, L., and Preston, R.H.: Reactions to chloroquine observed during treatment of various dermatologic disorders. Am. J. Trop. Med. Hyg. 6:654, 1957.

134. Voipio, H.: Incidence of chloroquine retinopathy. Acta Ophthalmol. 44:349, 1966.

135. Arden, G.B., and Kolb, H.: Antimalarial therapy and early retinal changes in patients with rheumatoid arthritis. Br. Med. J. 1:270, 966.

136. Nylander, U.: Ocular damage in chloroquine therapy. Acta Ophthalmol. 44:335, 1966.

137. Okun, G., Gouras, P., Bernstein, H., and VonSallmann, L.: Chloroquine retinopathy. Arch. Ophthalmol. 69:59, 1963.

138. Nozik, R.A., Weinstock, F.J., and Vignos, P.J.: Ocular complications of chloroquine. Ann. J. Ophthalmol. 58:774, 1964.

139. Crews, S.J.: Chloroquine retinopathy with recovery in early stages. Lancet 2:436, 1964.

140. Burns, R.P.: Delayed onset of chloroquine retinopathy. N. Engl. J. Med. 275:693, 1966.

141. Carr, R.E., Henkind, P., Rothfield, N., and Siegel I.M.: Ocular toxicity of antimalarial drugs: Long-term follow-up. Am. J. Ophthalmol. 66:738, 1968.

142. Carr, R.E., Gouras, P., and Gunkel, O.D.: Chloroquine retinopathy. Arch. Ophthalmol. 75:171, 1966.

143. Shearer, R.V., and Dubois, E.L.: Ocular changes induced by long-term hydroxychloroquine (plaquenil) therapy. Am. J. Ophthalmol. 64:245, 1967.

144. Henkind, P., Carr, R.E., and Siegel, I.: Early chloroquine retinopathy: Clinical and functional findings. Arch. Ophthalmol. 71:157, 1964.

145. Percival, S.P.B., and Behrman, J.: Ophthalmological safety of chloroquine. Br. J. Ophthalmol. 53:101, 1969.

146. Shearer, R.V., and Dubois, E.L.: Ocular changes induced by long-term hydroxychloroquine (plaquenil) therapy. Am. J. Ophthalmol. 64:245, 1967.

147. Rynes, R.I., Krohel, G., Falbo, A., Reinecke, R.D., Wolfe, B., and Bartholomew, L.E.: Ophthalmologic safety of long-term hydroxychloroquine treatment. Arthritis Rheum. 22:832, 1979.

148. Tobin, D.R., Krohel, G.B., and Rynes, R.I.: Hydroxychloroquine. A seven-year experience. Arch. Ophthalmol. 100:81, 1982.

149. Bernstein, H.N., and Ginsberg, J.: The pathology of chloroquine retinopathy. Arch. Ophthalmol. 71:238, 1964.

150. Scherbel, A.L., Mackenzie, A.H., Nousek, J.E., and Atdjian, M.: Ocular lesions in rheumatoid arthritis and related disorders with particular reference to retinopathy. A study of 741 patients treated with and without chloroquine drugs. N. Engl. J. Med. 273:360, 1965.

151. Mackenzie, A.H.: Ocular safety of huge cumulative antimalarial dosage (abstract). Arthritis Rheum. 24:70, 1981.

152. Laaksonen, A.L., Koskiahde, V., and Juva, K.: Dosage of antimalarial drugs for children with juvenile rheumatoid arthritis and systemic lupus erythematosus. Scand. J. Rheumatol. 3:103, 1974.

153. Cann, H.M., and Verhulst, H.L.: Fatal acute chloroquine poisoning in children. Pediatrics 27:95, 1961.

154. Torrey, E.F.: Chloroquine seizures. JAMA 204:867, 1968.

155. Umez-Eronimi, E.M., and Eronimi, E.A.: Chloroquine-induced involuntary movements. Br. Med. J. 1:945, 1977.

156. Dewar, W.A., and Mann, H.M.: Chloroquine in lupus erythematosus (letter). Lancet 1:780, 1954.

157. Mukherjee, D.K.: Chloroquine ototoxicity—a reversible phenomenon? J. Laryngol. Otol. 93:809, 1979.

158. Burrell, Z.L., and Marinez, A.C.: Chloroquine and hydroxychloroquine in the treatment of arrhythmias. N. Engl. J. Med. 258:798, 1958.

159. Rab, S.M.: Two cases of chloroquine psychoses. Br. Med. J. 1:1275, 1963.

160. Hart, C.W., and Naunton, R.F.: The ototoxicity of chloroquine phosphate. Arch. Otolaryngol. 80:407, 1964.

161. Nagaratnam, N., Chetiyawardana, A.N., and Rajiyah, S.: Aplasia and leukemia following chloroquine therapy. Postgrad. Med. J. 54:108, 1978.

162. Neill, W.A., Panayi, G.S., Duthie, J.J.R., and Prescott, R.J.: Action of chloroquine phosphate in rheumatoid arthritis. II. Chromosome-damaging effect. Ann. Rheum. Dis. 32:547, 1973.

163. Magnussen, I., and deFine Olivamus, B.: Cardiomyopathy after chloroquine treatment. Acta Med. Scand. 202:429, 1977.

164. Baler, C.R.: Porphyria precipitated by hydroxychloroquine treatment of systemic lupus erythematosus. Cutis 17:96, 1976.

165. Henkind, P., and Rothfield, N.F.: Ocular abnormalities in patients treated with synthetic antimalarial drugs. N. Engl. J. Med. 269:433, 1963.

Chapter 52

Gold Compounds

Norman L. Gottlieb

HISTORY OF GOLD TREATMENT

Gold has been advocated for the treatment of numerous diseases of man, animals, and plants since the eighth century. A combination of gold and mercury was called an elixir of life by Paracelsus in the early sixteenth century.[1] It was not until 1890, when Koch[2] reported the in vitro inhibition of tubercle bacilli by gold cyanide, that gold compounds were used for specific medical disorders. A mixture of gold and magnesium was used to treat tuberculosis in 1894; gold salts alone were recommended for the treatment of lupus vulgaris in 1913 and pulmonary tuberculosis in 1924.[3]

The beneficial effects of aurothioglucose (Solganal) in patients with bacterial endocarditis, rheumatic fever, and other poorly defined disorders, based on the hypothesis that gold had nonspecific antiseptic effects, was reported by Landé in 1927.[4] Shortly after their introduction, gold compounds were used for luetic infection, ankylosing spondylitis (especially with prominent peripheral joint involvement), and degenerative and gonococcal arthritis with less impressive results.[5] Chrysotherapy is not presently recommended for these conditions.

Believing that tuberculosis and rheumatoid arthritis (RA) had a common (infectious) etiology, Forestier[6] applied gold–thiopropanol sodium sulfanate (Allochrysine) for the treatment of RA. His favorable experience with more than 550 cases, in which improvement was noted in 70 to 80 percent, was published in 1935. Subsequently, numerous authors have confirmed these observations, including Hartfall and associates,[7] who noted "apparent cure or striking improvement" in 80 percent of 900 RA cases. Two double-blind studies, reported in 1945[8] and in the early 1960s,[9,10] reaffirmed the value of parenteral gold in RA. More recent work has documented the efficacy of gold compounds in reducing joint pain and inflammation, and maintaining articular function;[11,12] one long-term blinded study found that gold altered the natural history of RA by protecting articular cartilage and subchondral bone.[12]

In addition to RA, gold treatment is advocated for selected cases of juvenile rheumatoid arthritis (JRA) and psoriatic arthritis affecting the peripheral joints. Exceptionally, it is prescribed for severe palindromic rheumatism, an infrequent arthropathy.[13] In addition, gold currently is offered as a therapeutic alternative for certain nonrheumatic disorders such as pemphigus,[14] a serious bullous skin disorder, and is used in the Far East for bronchial asthma.[15]

An orally administered gold compound, auranofin (Ridaura), is the first slow-acting antirheumatic drug developed specifically for RA.[16]

INDICATIONS AND PATIENT SELECTION

Gold treatment is used primarily for progressively severe polyarticular RA that is not controlled by measures such as rest, physical therapy, nonsteroidal anti-inflammatory agents, mild to moderately potent analgesics, and occasional intra-articular injections of microcrystalline corticosteroids. Most rheumatologists practicing in the United States advocate an initial trial of chrysotherapy in preference to other disease-modifying drugs. Whether or not the risk-to-benefit ratio warrants the use of chrysotherapy in early or mild RA, to prevent or delay irreversible joint damage, is unresolved. Some studies have shown that gold therapy is most effective in early, nonerosive RA,[17,18] whereas others have demonstrated its value in active disease of long duration despite the presence of joint deformity and destruction.[7,19] Gold is not indicated for advanced RA without evidence of active synovitis, and is generally not advised for mono- or pauciarticular arthritis.[17]

Factors that do not significantly influence the response to chrysotherapy include patient age, sex, and race, magnitude of serum immunoglobulin and erythrocyte sedimentation rate (ESR) elevation, presence or absence of serum rheumatoid factor (RF),[11,13,20] or subcutaneous nodules (personal experience). In one recent report gold-treated ANA-negative RA patients improved more than ANA-positive subjects (but the opposite was true for levamisole).[21] Although not conclusively tested, therapeutic benefit does not seem related to histocompatibility antigens on the A, B, and D loci.[22] Concomitant systemic medications, other than chelating agents, which enhance gold excretion, also do not alter the efficacy of gold. Systemic corticosteroids and gold compounds may be administered concurrently. When chrysotherapy is initiated in corticosteroid-treated RA patients, steroids may be tapered gradually after several months of uninterrupted gold treatment, if clinical improvement is evident.

Gold compounds may be employed in RA patients with Felty's or Sjögren's syndrome or in RA accompanied by pre-existing neutropenia or eosinophilia.[23-28] Available evidence suggests the drug is efficacious in these circumstances, and the prevalence, type, and severity of toxicity are not greater than anticipated. Importantly, neutropenia and splenomegaly that has been documented by clinical examinations and liver-spleen scan, have improved during chrysotherapy.[23,24] Despite earlier admonitions against gold in RA-associated Sjögren's syndrome, recent studies indicate it is generally well tolerated.[25] Similarly, nonprogressive proteinuria unaccompanied by renal insufficiency, or the presence of a single normally functioning kidney does not interdict gold treatment.[13,29]

EFFICACY

The favorable influence of chrysotherapy on RA has been documented in numerous studies and in several double-blind controlled trials in which gold was compared with placebo. (Table 52–1).[8,10-12,18,30-38] More recently, gold compounds have been compared with other potent antirheumatic agents, including penicillamine, cyclophosphamide, azathioprine, and antimalarials.[39-41]

The first double-blind study involved 110 RA patients treated with 100 mg weekly of gold sodium thiomalate (Myochrysine) or with an inactive control substance.[8] Sixty-three percent of gold-treated patients but only 21 percent of controls experienced great or moderate improvement after 12 months. "Toxicity" occurred in 75 percent and 37 percent of gold-treated and control subjects, respectively.

The second double-blind study, conducted under the auspices of the Empire Rheumatism Council, provided strong impetus for the use of chrysotherapy in RA.[9,10] This multicenter effort involved nearly 200 patients, half of whom received a cumulative dose of 1000 mg of gold sodium thiomalate and the remainder (controls) a total dose of 0.01 mg over a 6-month period; a maintenance gold schedule was not provided. After 3 months of therapy the gold-treated group improved to a greater degree than the controls as assessed by functional capacity, subjective fitness, joint involvement, grip strength, num-

ber of analgesic tablets required, hemoglobin level, serum RF titer, and ESR. The reduction in number of involved joints is illustrated in Figure 52–1. Radiologic progression, as measured by joint space narrowing, the number of new bone erosions, or the extension of existing erosions, was statistically similar in both groups, although less marked in those receiving gold. The beneficial effects still were discernible 12 months after cessation of therapy, but were not evident 24 months after treatment was discontinued.

A trial similar to the British effort was undertaken in the United States, but only 68 RA patients were recruited, and after withdrawals because of toxicity, change of residence, and lack of benefit, just 43 were available for re-evaluation at 6 months.[11] In part a consequence of the small number of patients studied, the only parameter that changed significantly was the ESR.

The efficacy of auranofin has been examined in numerous protocols involving more than 3000 RA patients worldwide.[16,42-52] Oral gold has been compared with placebo,[43,44] aurothioglucose,[48] gold sodium thiomalate,[43,45-47] gold sodium thiopropanolsulphonate,[49] penicillamine,[47,52] hydroxychloroquine,[50] and levamisole.[51] While some were well-designed double-blind controlled trials, others were open-label or suffered from various methodologic deficiencies. Reliable data come from a 21-week trial completed by the Cooperative Systematic Studies of Rheumatic Diseases group, a multicenter effort involving 209 RA patients who received either gold sodium thiomalate (n = 82), auranofin (n = 77), or placebo (n = 50).[43] There were no statistically significant differences in benefit between intramuscular and oral gold for any clinical parameter measured (joint pain/tenderness, joint swelling, patient assessment, morning

Table 52–1. Results of Intramuscular Chrysotherapy in Selected Controlled and Uncontrolled Studies

Investigator	Year	Number of Patients	Greatly Improved (%)*	Partially Improved (%)*	Treatment Failure (%)*
Controlled Trials					
Ellman et al.[30]	1940	60 (30)†	37 (3)	57 (73)	6 (23)
Fraser[8]	1945	57 (46)	63 (21)	19 (24)	18 (55)
Waine et al.[31]	1947	58 (62)	57 (29)	24 (27)	19 (43)
ERC[10]	1961	90 (95)	41 (22)‡		
CCC[11]	1973	22 (21)		77 (38)*	
Uncontrolled Trials					
Forestier[32]	1934	500+		75*	
Hartfall and Garland[33]	1935	100	70	20	10
Cecil et al.[18]	1942	245	66	20	14
Adams and Cecil[34]	1950	106 (83)§	89 (57)	8 (25)	3 (18)
Snorrason[35]	1952	295 (169)§	72 (23)		
Lockie et al.[36]	1958	369 (566)§	57 (38)	35 (48)	7 (11)
Rothermich et al.[37]	1976	73	73		27
Sharp et al.[38]	1982	73	37	27	36

*Greatly improved includes disease categorized as "in remission, arrested, marked-moderate improvement, and excellent response"; partially improved includes "some and slight improvement"; treatment failure includes "limited or no improvement and worse." The degree of improvement could not be ascertained in the CCC study or Forestier's report.

†Figures in parentheses are control group data.

‡Patient's estimate of fitness at 6 months.

§Results in non-gold-treated patients but not controlled studies.

Figure 52–1. Mean number of involved joints declines significantly in gold-treated RA patients, but not in controls. (Adapted from the Empire Rheumatism Council Study, Ann. Rheum. Dis. 19:95, 1960.)

stiffness, and ARA functional class). Certain laboratory tests (hemoglobin and platelet count) improved more with gold sodium thiomalate, but serum rheumatoid factor titer and erythrocyte sedimentation rate declined similarly. Both compounds fared better than placebo, reaffirming the value of chrysotherapy for RA. In another trial of 340 RA patients followed for six months, auranofin was superior to placebo, 67 and 43 percent of patients evincing moderate or marked improvement, and 9 and 29 percent being withdrawn for lack of efficacy, respectively.[44] Other reports support these findings and further suggest that auranofin is equal to or superior to all the other disease-modifying drugs enumerated above.

Two 6-month controlled, blinded studies examined the effects of changing from intramuscular to oral gold treatment.[53,54] Only patients who were clinically stable and responded adequately to parenteral treatment were enrolled. Disease activity, erythrocyte sedimentation rate, and serum immunoglobulin levels followed similar patterns, whether patients remained on the injectable preparation or received auranofin.

In 1974, a 30-month double-blind study compared a standard course of gold sodium thiomalate followed by a maintenance gold schedule with placebo.[12] Serial radiograms of the hands and wrists revealed fewer bone erosions and less joint space narrowing in the gold-treated group. These findings document for the first time that gold compounds favorably alter the natural history of RA by reducing bone and cartilage destruction, a consequence presumably of its suppressive action on synovial inflammation.

Roentgenographic progression was correlated with clinical disease activity in a 2-year gold sodium thiomalate trial involving 73 RA patients.[38] As anticipated, given our understanding of the pathophysiology of rheumatoid joint destruction, patients whose synovitis was suppressed the most developed fewest hand and wrist erosions and least joint space narrowing.

A longitudinal roentgenographic study of hand and

wrist erosions in auranofin-treated RA patients,[55] used as controls radiographs from the Cooperating Clinics Committee trial comparing gold sodium thiomalate with placebo.[11] Both gold compounds were superior to placebo in reducing the rate of osseous erosions, auranofin having the more profound effect. These conclusions would be more convincing if concomitant rather than historical controls were used for this assessment.

As mentioned above, chrysotherapy may partially correct or restore to normal certain laboratory tests. Hemoglobin, hematocrit, and serum albumin levels increase, while serum RF-titer, ESR, C-reactive protein, plasma glycoproteins, fibrinogen, gamma and total globulins, immune complexes, and IgG, IgA, and IgM decrease significantly during gold treatment.[56,57] Figure 52–2 shows mean changes in immunoglobulins, gamma globulin, and albumin levels in a group of RA patients reported previously.[56] Serum complement (C3) levels fall initially but return to pretreatment concentrations with time; antinuclear antibody titers rise during chrysotherapy.[58] As with clinical manifestations, significant serologic changes generally do not develop until 3 to 6 months of treatment.

Gold sodium thiomalate and D-penicillamine were compared in a 6-month controlled study of 89 RA patients.[39] Both agents were similarly effective in reducing joint pain and swelling, articular index, morning stiffness, the number of subcutaneous nodules and ESR and RF titer, and in increasing grip strength. The gold group was probably at a disadvantage; an inflexible schedule (50 mg weekly until a cumulative dose of 1 gram) was given to all gold-treated patients, whereas variable doses (1 to 1.8 grams daily) were administered to penicillamine-treated patients, according to the clinical response. These doses of penicillamine are higher than recommended currently (see Chapter 53).

Gold sodium thiomalate, azathioprine (Imuran; 2.5 mg per kilogram per day), and cyclophosphamide (Cytoxan; 1.5 mg per kilogram per day) were compared in an 18-month double-blind trial of 121 patients with early RA (mean duration of disease, 5 years).[40] Improvement

Figure 52–2. Mean serum immunoglobulin (IgG, IgA, and IgM) concentrations decline during chrysotherapy. (Adapted from Gottlieb, N.L., et al.: J. Lab. Clin. Med. 86:962, 1975.)

in morning stiffness, grip strength, subjective assessment, joint size, and walking time and reduction in ESR and RF titer were comparable in all patient groups. Roentgenographic joint deterioration was least, and steroid sparing effect greatest, with cyclophosphamide at occasional assessment points, although differences among agents were not pronounced.

Gold sodium thiomalate (50 mg per week intramuscularly), azathioprine (1.0 to 2.0 mg per kilogram per day orally), or chloroquine (250 mg per day orally) was given to 33 patients with early RA (mean disease duration, approximately 2 years) in a nonblinded, randomly assigned 24-week study.[41] Articular index, total active joint count, synovial effusion count, grip strength, duration of morning stiffness, functional class, ESR, and RF titer were assessed serially. All drugs were beneficial, the gold and azathioprine groups faring marginally better than the chloroquine group at the final evaluation.

The value of chrysotherapy in psoriatic arthritis has not been studied extensively.[59,60] Double-blind, controlled reports comparing the efficacy of gold with placebo, nonsteroidal anti-inflammatory agents, or cytotoxic drugs are not available. The influence of gold treatment on a limited number of patients with psoriatic arthritis involving the peripheral joints has been contrasted with its effect on RA patients.[59] The psoriatic arthritis patients experienced a greater reduction in Lansbury index, greater improvement in functional activity, and lesser frequency of severe toxic reactions. These findings should be interpreted cautiously because the natural histories of the two disorders differ, the population surveyed was small, and few clinical (and no laboratory or roentgenographic) parameters were measured.

Certain additional aspects of chrysotherapy are worthy of comment. Some clinicians believe that gold compounds are capable of inducing a protracted or permanent remission in a minority of RA patients.[6,7,37] Reliable information on the frequency of gold (and other disease-modifying antirheumatic drugs)-induced remissions in RA is not available. Differences in study populations, definitions of RA and remissions, and spontaneous variations in disease activity are partly responsible for this void in our knowledge. At the extremes, Adams and Cecil[34] reported that 79 percent of 61 gold-treated patients with RA of less than 6 months' had remissions, while the Cooperative Systematic Studies of Rheumatic Disease group observed no remissions (applying the ARA Preliminary Criteria for Clinical Remission in RA[61]) in 159 patients treated with either parenteral or oral gold.[43] In a recent retrospective review of protracted chrysotherapy,[62] 73 percent of 39 patients who received gold for 3 or more years entered a remission in contrast to only 6 percent of 36 patients who discontinued treatment during the first 18 months. An example of such a response is shown in Figure 52–3. Others have documented healing of bone erosions in an occasional patient during gold treatment (Fig. 52–4).[41] On the other hand, a considerable proportion (15 to 60 percent) of RA patients are unresponsive to gold therapy, experience limited symptomatic relief, eventually

EFFECT OF GOLD ON JOINT INFLAMMATION

Figure 52–3. Schematic graph of the clinical course of a 76-year-old male with seropositive, nodular, progressive RA of 3 years' duration. The clinical remission he experienced at the fourth month of gold treatment persisted until his demise from other causes more than 1 year later.

escape its beneficial effects despite continued treatment, or must be withdrawn from treatment because of adverse side effects. In fact, only 16 percent of patients continued to receive gold injections 4 years after initiation of treatment in one recent trial,[63] while 50 percent remained on drug at 5 years in another study.[64] Also, it has been observed that patients unresponsive to an initial course of gold uncommonly respond to subsequent courses, and that a majority of patients who escape its favorable effects will not regain them despite ardent efforts by the physician.[10,37] But, other workers[65] recently reported that patients whose disease exacerbates while receiving monthly maintenance gold injections frequently benefit from a return to weekly treatment. The efficacy of gold treatment does not correlate positively with the development of gold toxicity,[66,67] as suggested by earlier reports.[68,69] Some data suggest that 6 months is insufficient time to accrue maximum benefit from chrysotherapy; treatment should be extended to 18 or more months before being discontinued for lack of improvement.[62] However, another report showed loss of efficacy after 2 to 4 years of maintenance therapy.[70] Lastly, the beneficial effects of gold compounds may persist several months or even years after treatment has been abandoned, presumably reflecting tissue gold stores.[9,10,13]

GOLD PREPARATIONS

The chemistry of gold-containing compounds is reviewed elsewhere.[71] Briefly, of the several oxidation states for gold compounds (viz., I, O, I, II, III, V), only complex gold I compounds are used therapeutically; gold (O), known as colloidal or metallic gold, is not biologically active; simple gold (I) salts (e.g., gold chloride) are unstable; gold (III) complexes are too toxic and, the biologic activities of the others have not been studied.

Numerous gold-containing compounds have been used to treat RA in the past 50 years. Gold sodium

Figure 52–4. Serial life-size contact-print radiographs of a middle-aged female with active RA of several years' duration. Note the articular erosions (*F* and *G*) and periarticular demineralization (*H*) in *A*, which developed during treatment with antimalarial agents. *B* shows the same hand after the patient has received continuous chrysotherapy for 5 years; most of the osseous lesions have healed. (Supplied through the courtesy of Paul Young, M.D.)

thiomalate, aurothioglucose, and gold thioglycoanilid (Lauron) are administered by intramuscular injection only; gold sodium thiosulfate (Sanocrysine) also may be given intravenously.[29] Until recently, gold has not been given orally because the commercially available preparations are insufficiently absorbed.

Gold sodium thiomalate and aurothioglucose are the two most widely used compounds in the United States; their structural formulas are shown in Figure 52–5. These preparations are water soluble, and contain a sulfur moiety attached to the gold.[29] Gold sodium thiomalate also has been given intra-articularly on an inves-

Figure 52–5. Gold sodium thiomalate and aurothioglucose, the two intramuscular gold preparations most widely used in the United States, are aurous salts, contain 50 percent gold by weight, and are attached to a sulfur moiety. Auranofin, a conjugated gold compound with two ligands, contains sulfur and is 29 percent gold by weight.

GOLD SODIUM THIOMALATE
(MYOCHRYSINE)

AUROTHIOGLUCOSE
(SOLGANAL)

(2,3,4,6-TETRA-O-ACETYL-1-THIO-β-D-GLUCOPYRANOSATO-S)
(TRIETHYLPHOSPINE) GOLD
AURANOFIN

tigational basis.[72] Gold sodium thiomalate, aurothioglucose, and gold thioglycoanilid are approximately 50 percent gold by weight; gold sodium thiosulfate is 37 percent gold.

While it is generally acknowledged that gold sodium thiomalate and aurothioglucose are similarly efficacious, mounting evidence suggests that aurothioglucose may be preferred because of lesser toxicity. Gold sodium thiomalate is associated with vasomotor (nitritoid) reactions[58,73] and with nonvasomotor reactions,[74] which rarely occur with aurothioglucose. Moreover, one prospective study found a significantly higher incidence of adverse reactions with gold sodium thiomalate (30 percent) than with aurothioglucose (9 percent).[37] This observation requires verification. On the other hand, aurothioglucose has the disadvantage of poor miscibility because of the sesame oil vehicle; if the vial is not thoroughly shaken, dosing may be inexact. Aurothioglucose may be associated with the development of firm intramuscular lumps at injection sites, presumably representing nonabsorbed sesame oil or a tissue response to the injectable. The long large-bore needle (1.5 inch, 20 gauge) required for injection of the viscous material increases patient discomfort. There are also pharmacokinetic differences in the compounds, absorption and peak serum levels being diminished with aurothioglucose (see Pharmacokinetics, below).

One study utilizing gold sodium thiomalate and aurothioglucose in oily suspensions and in aqueous solutions showed significantly more toxicity with the aqueous preparations of both compounds than with the oil suspensions.[75] This finding suggests that adverse effects in part may be a consequence of the vehicle, or of resultant altered gold kinetics, rather than differences in compounds.

Auranofin, a triethylphosphine gold compound that contains 29 percent gold by weight, is distinctly different physicochemically from the parenteral compounds.[71,76] Some of its unique characteristics include absorption after oral administration (approximately 25 percent of the administered dose), a monomeric form, lipid solubility, nonconductivity, and weak reactivity with sulfhydryl groups.

DOSAGE SCHEDULES

The currently recommended intramuscular gold dosage schedule was derived empirically following years of clinical experience; only recently has it been subject to rigidly controlled study and modification. In the early history of chrysotherapy, doses of 100 to 200 mg or more of gold compound were administered once weekly or more often.[6,33] The frequency of toxicity coupled with a 4 percent mortality rate led to a reduction in the sanctioned dose.[13]

Presently the conventional (standard) gold schedule for adults with RA consists of test doses of 10 mg and 25 mg given 1 week apart, followed by 50 mg weekly, until the cumulative dose totals 1 gram or toxicity or major clinical improvement supervenes. Injections of aurothioglucose and gold sodium thiomalate preferably are given deep into the gluteal musculature, alternating right and left sides, following skin cleansing with an alcohol swab or other antiseptic. Gold sodium thiomalate may also be given into the deltoid or other less bulky muscle groups, injection sites not recommended for aurothioglucose.

Numerous variations in the aforementioned schedule have been used by clinicians. Some prefer weekly injections of 25 rather than 50 mg of gold compound; others recommend 50 mg until 500 to 700 mg is attained, at which time the dose is reduced to 25 mg weekly, or increased by increments of 10 mg or more at fixed intervals in unresponsive cases. Alternative schedules include 100 to 150 mg or more weekly, until 1500 to 2500 mg is achieved, or adjusting the dose to maintain the serum concentration above 300 μg per deciliter or some other arbitrary figure.

One multicenter study compared the clinical results of administering 1000 mg or 2500 mg of aurothioglucose in 21 weeks, followed by maintenance therapy, to more than 200 RA patients.[77] The "low" dose group received 25 mg twice weekly for 11 weeks followed by 50 mg once weekly, while the "high" dose group received 100 mg twice weekly for 11 weeks and then 50 mg weekly for 10 weeks. The efficacy of both dosage regimens was similar; joint count, grip strength, morning stiffness, functional capacity, and ESR improved comparably. However, the frequency of toxicity was significantly greater in the "high" dose (58 percent) than with the "low" dose (24 percent) group (Table 52-2). A double-blind prospective trial in the United States, published in 1977, compared the efficacy of 50 mg and 150 mg of gold sodium thiomalate given weekly for 20 weeks.[78] Therapeutic effects were similar in the two patient groups. Toxicity of such severity as to require discontinuation of therapy occurred in 16 of 24 (67 percent) high dose patients and 3 of 23 (13 percent) low dose patients. Other investigators reported that 25 mg of gold sodium thiomalate was as efficacious as more than twice that amount using a flexible dose schedule.[58] There were no significant differences in joint pain score, ring size, grip strength, radiologic change, deformity, or laboratory tests when high and low dose groups were compared. The number of adverse reactions was similar in the two groups. The possible benefits of daily or alternate day, semimonthly or monthly injection, or other variations in frequency of gold administration have not been explored.

Patients failing to respond to 50 mg per week may benefit from higher gold doses, given in additive weekly to monthly increments of 10 to 25 mg, but rarely exceeding 100 mg. One report showed that 5-mg increases in gold dose each week until a maximum of 100 mg was reached caused improvement in the majority (82 percent) of patients without increasing the risk of toxicity.[68] Another showed that 43 percent of patients who failed to benefit from 50 mg of gold improved significantly when higher doses (1.5 to 2 times the initial dose) were em-

Table 52–2. Relationship of Intramuscular Gold Dose to Prevalence of Toxicity

Investigator	Conventional Gold Dose (50 mg per Week)		Alternative Gold Dose*		No Gold	
	Number of Patients: Toxic/Treated	Percent Toxic	Number of Patients: Toxic/Treated	Percent Toxic	Number of Patients: Toxic/Treated	Percent Toxic
ERC[9]	35/99	35	—		16/100	16
Cats[77]	29/119	24	64/111	58*a	—	
CCC[11]	12/36	33	—		2/32	6
Gordon et al.[25]	25/101	25	—		—	
Rothermich et al.[37]	10/55	18	9/42	21*b	—	
Sharp et al.[58]†	5/38	13	4/37	11*c	—	
Furst et al.[78]†	3/23	13	16/24	67*d	—	

*Alternative dosage schedules: *a = 200 mg per week; *b = 1 mg per kilogram per week; *c = 25 mg per week; *d = 150 mg per week.
†Only toxicity severe enough to withhold gold for 6 or more weeks, or to discontinue treatment, is included.

ployed, and that less than 10 percent developed untoward side effects.[37] However, some clinicians prefer to discontinue therapy after 1000 mg in unresponsive cases, whereas others administer an additional 10 to 20 injections of 50 mg, hoping that higher cumulative doses will prove beneficial. The best available evidence suggests that if no beneficial effect (and no toxicity) is noted after 1000 mg of gold (given in doses of 50 mg per week), then a gradual increase in weekly dose may be warranted.

Maintenance gold therapy, which generally consists of 25 to 50 mg of compound every 2 to 4 weeks, is advocated by many authorities upon completion of the initial course. Unfortunately, few studies have examined the efficacy of this commonly used protracted treatment schedule. In 1946, Ragan and Tyson commented that in their opinion, maintenance gold could prevent severe and disabling relapse of RA.[79] Freyberg and associates described the results of an uncontrolled study showing that maintenance chrysotherapy was of decided value in improving and maintaining functional capacity.[13] The value of maintenance gold therapy is indirectly substantiated by the data of Sigler and co-workers,[12] which shows roentgenographic protection of cartilage and bone; such benefit was absent in the Empire Rheumatism Council study, which provided the same initial course but no maintenance treatment.[10] The Dutch study found no significant benefit from maintenance gold treatment.[77] The data of Rothermich and associates suggest that maintenance therapy administered semimonthly rather than monthly more effectively prevents disease relapse,[37] findings refuted by a recent British study.[80]

Several gold schedules have been recommended for children with JRA. Doses of 1 mg per kilogram weekly of gold sodium thiomalate seemed more beneficial than similar doses given at 3- or 4-week intervals.[81] Some clinicians recommend lower doses (0.5 mg per kilogram),[82] whereas others have adopted a single dose schedule of 25 mg per week after test doses,[83] or have related dosage to age.[84]

Gold sodium thiomalate (100 mg) has been instilled periodically into the knee joints of a small number of patients with RA, experimentally.[72] Pharmacokinetic studies of radiolabeled([195]Au) gold sodium thiomalate indicate rapid clearance from the joint cavity with appearance in blood and urine.[85] The initial clinical results of intra-articular gold injection appeared promising, but this mode of administration has attracted little recent attention. It should not be confused with intra-articular radioactive *colloidal* gold ([198]Au) injection, whose short-term benefits derive from the effects of radiation on the synovium. This therapeutic modality is primarily used outside the United States.[86]

The proposed auranofin schedule derives from several studies of dosage range.[87-90] While 3 mg twice daily appears optimal for the majority of adults with RA, some improve with 1 mg daily, and others require 9 mg daily. Diarrhea and abdominal cramps are the commonest limiting factors to achieving high daily dosage. For JRA, 0.1 to 0.2 mg per kg per day was well tolerated and effective for some children in one small open-label trial.[91]

GOLD DISTRIBUTION

Gold concentrations have been measured in animal and human tissues using colorimetric methods, atomic absorption spectroscopy, neutron activation analysis, radionuclide, and other techniques. The tissue distribution of gold in animals is reviewed in detail elsewhere.[92-95] In general, the kidneys, adrenals, and reticuloendothelial system organs achieve highest gold concentrations.[92,93] Intracellularly, gold localizes predominantly in the nuclear, mitochondrial, and lysosomal fractions, attached to organelle membranes.[96]

In RA patients, gold is widely distributed throughout the tissues, but in markedly varying concentrations. At autopsy, one patient who received 5 grams of aurothioglucose during a 4-year period had higher gold levels in the reticuloendothelial system (lymph nodes, bone marrow, liver, and spleen) than in the joint structure (synovial membrane, articular cartilage, cortical bone, muscle, and synovial fluid).[97] The concentrations of gold found in these and other organs are shown in Figure 52–6. These findings generally have been confirmed by others.[98,99] However, one study found higher synovial gold levels during active chrysotherapy.[100] Only minuscule quantities of gold are found in the crystalline *lens*

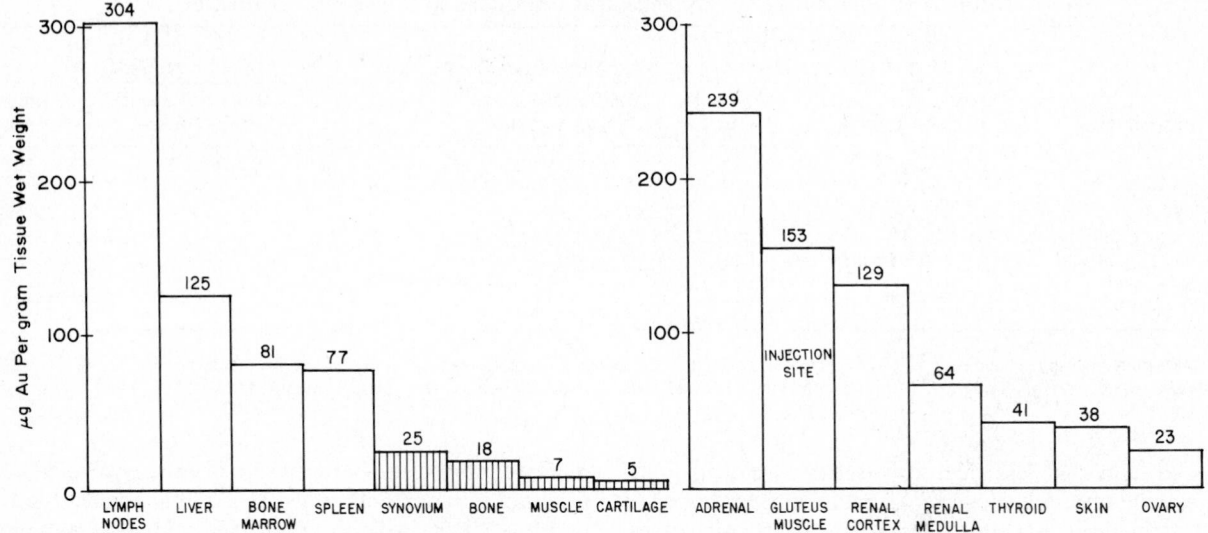

Figure 52–6. Gold concentrations in reticuloendothelial, articular, and other tissues from a deceased RA patient who received 5 grams of aurothioglucose during 4 years of chrysotherapy. Higher levels were found in lymph nodes and liver than in tissues composing the joint structure. (Adapted from Gottlieb, N.L., et al.: Arthritis Rheum. 15:16, 1972.)

of the eye, despite cumulative gold doses exceeding 10 grams.[101] The greatest quantities of gold are stored in the bone marrow, liver, skin, and bone, a function in part of their large mass (Table 52–3).[97]

Gold concentrations in *body fluids* are much lower than in most tissues. During a standard course of chrysotherapy, blood and urine gold levels generally average 300 to 400 μg per deciliter and 30 to 60 μg per deciliter, respectively, when measured 1 week after administration.[67,102,103] Synovial fluid gold levels generally are about 50 percent of serum concentrations;[104] other fluids (pericardial, bile, milk of lactating women) also contain small quantities of gold.[97,105,106]

Studies of diarthrodial joints indicate that gold preferentially localizes in the synovial membrane during active chrysotherapy;[97] gold levels in *synovium, cartilage, bone, and striated muscle* are similar after treatment is abandoned.[98] Electron probe roentgenographic analysis has shown that gold is present in synovial lining cells and in subsynovial mononuclear cells, enters lysosomes in synovial lining cells, and alters the lysosomal structure

seen electron microscopically.[107,108] Sulfur also is present in gold-containing lysosomes, but the sulfur to gold ratio is not identical to that found in gold sodium thiomalate.

In the *skin,* gold is confined largely to the dermis; 3 percent is present in the epidermis.[109] Electron dense particles, thought to represent gold, have been identified in the lysosomes of dermal histiocytes.[110]

Higher gold levels are found in the *renal cortex* than in the *renal medulla* of RA patients.[97] Gold has been identified in the proximal tubules, but not in glomerular subepithelial deposits, in patients with gold-induced proteinuria.[111]

Knowledge of the tissue distribution of gold during auranofin treatment is incomplete. In rats and guinea pigs, gold concentrations in kidney, spleen, and liver are 35 to 70 times higher with gold sodium thiomalate than with comparable or larger doses of oral gold.[112,113] During protracted auranofin treatment of RA patients, synovial fluid and skin gold levels are a fraction of those attained with gold sodium thiomalate, and corneal chrysiasis is observed rarely.[114]

PHARMACOKINETICS

Pharmacokinetic studies have provided important insights into the metabolism, excretion, and distribution of gold within the intravascular, serum protein, synovial fluid, tissue, and intracellular compartments. The metabolism of gold sodium thiomalate has been investigated most thoroughly, because it may be dosed precisely and consistently, and because radiolabeled compounds with long ([195]Au-gold sodium thiomalate; 183 days) and short ([198]Au-gold sodium thiomalate; 3 days) half-lives are available commercially.

Blood Gold. Serum contains less than 0.5 ng per deciliter of gold prior to initiation of therapy. Gold levels

Table 52–3. Distribution of Gold in Body Tissues*

Tissue	Gold Content (mg Gold)	Percent Total Gold Retained
Bone marrow	159	26
Liver	148	24
Skin	117	19
Bone	110	18
Muscle	33	5
Spleen	19	3
Other	33	5
Total	619	100

*Adapted from Gottlieb, N., et al.: Arthritis Rheum. 15:16, 1972. Based on tissues assayed; some organ weights used in determining gold content were estimated.

Figure 52–7. Higher blood gold concentrations are achieved with conventional doses of gold sodium thiomalate than with auranofin (triethylphosphine gold). Gold levels reach a plateau after 6 to 8 weeks of injectable treatment, and after 12 weeks of auranofin, reflecting the longer half-life of the oral compound. (Adapted from Gottlieb, N.L.: J. Rheumatol. 9 (Suppl. 8):99, 1982, and Finkelstein, A.E., et al.: J. Rheumatol. 7:160, 1980.)

rise gradually in the early phase of conventional treatment, and plateau after 6 to 8 weeks (Fig. 52–7). During chrysotherapy, and following intramuscular injection of gold sodium thiomalate (50 mg), a mean peak serum level of about 700 μg per deciliter is reached within 2 hours and maintained for several hours.[102,103] Levels decline on each successive day, reaching about 300 μg per deciliter at the end of 1 week[103] (Fig. 52–8). Gold concentrations are relatively constant, regardless of the duration of treatment, if the dose is unaltered. One-half the dose of *intravenous* radiogold is cleared from the serum in 5.5 days.[115] Aurothioglucose has a slower absorption rate and lower peak serum level, but values are similar after 7 days.[17,116]

Serum gold concentrations correlate directly with the administered gold dose. When 25 mg per week is given, levels approximate 165 μg per deciliter 1 week after injection;[58] with higher doses (150 mg per week) levels

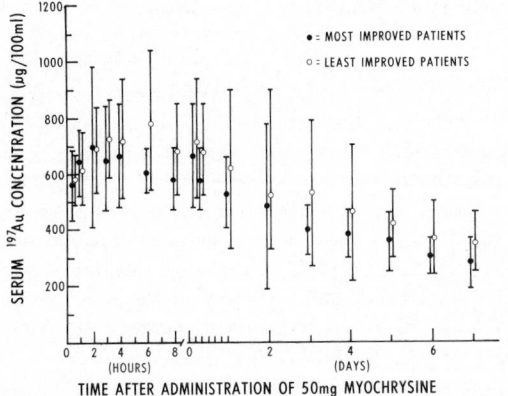

Figure 52–8. Mean hourly and daily serum gold concentrations in a group of RA patients receiving conventional chrysotherapy. Within several hours of intramuscular gold sodium thiomalate (50 mg), peak levels (700 μg per deciliter) are attained, which gradually fall to 300 μg per deciliter after 7 days. Gold concentrations in "most" and "least" improved patients are similar. (Adapted from Gottlieb, N.L., et al.: Arthritis Rheum. 17:161, 1974.)

of nearly 1000 μg per deciliter are achieved.[78] During maintenance therapy serum concentrations vary according to the dose and frequency of administration, generally ranging from 75 to 125 μg per deciliter when 50 mg of gold is given every 3 to 4 weeks.[102,103] Upon termination of treatment, levels of 10 to 30 μg per deciliter persist for many months, and gold is detectable as long as 1 year later.[17]

Studies of orally administered gold (auranofin, 6 mg per day) show gradually increasing serum levels during 3 months of therapy which then plateau.[87-89] At 1, 2, and 3 months, *whole blood* gold levels were 40, 60, and 70 μg per deciliter, respectively. A variation of 1 mg per day in auranofin dosage alters blood levels by approximately 10 μg per dl,[87] as shown in Figure 52–7. Serum gold concentrations are slightly lower than whole blood levels.[113,117] The blood gold half-life with auranofin is longer than with gold sodium thiomalate, increasing from 17 days prior to treatment to 26 days after 6 months of therapy with 6 mg per day.[118]

Ninety-two percent of gold in the intravascular compartment is protein bound and 8 percent is present as free gold, using 50 mg per week of an intramuscular compound.[102,119] Higher dosage programs increase the non-protein-bound gold fraction threefold.[119] The great majority of protein-bound gold is in the albumin fraction (95 percent); the remainder is in higher molecular weight fractions.[102] Enhanced binding to immunoglobulins, complement, and circulating lymphocytes is observed with serum gold levels in the range of 300 to 500 μg per deciliter.[120]

Gold is in the red cell fraction of one third of treated patients, averaging 16 percent of the total circulating gold 7 days after administration of an intramuscular compound, but is not detectable in leukocytes or platelets.[121] Serum levels are similar in patients with and without red blood cell gold, but total and fecal gold excretion are greater in those with red cell gold. Other investigators found minuscule quantities of gold in circulating lymphocytes.[122] Two recent reports demonstrate that cigarette smoking increases erythrocyte gold uptake during parenteral treatment.[123,124] During auranofin treatment, approximately 50 percent of intravascular gold is in the cellular fraction, the majority either attached to erythrocyte membranes or present intracellularly.[113] This finding may have some undefined therapeutic importance.

Gold diffuses from serum to synovial fluid rapidly, reaching a state of equilibrium several hours after intramuscular injection.[104] Disappearance of radiogold from synovial fluid conforms to first-order kinetics during the first week, clearance half-time approximating 6 days.

Gold Excretion. Approximately 40 percent of the administered dose of intramuscular gold is eliminated, 70 percent in the urine and 30 percent in the feces.[67,102] Considerable variation in excretory pattern exists, occasional individuals eliminating greater quantities of gold in stool than in urine.[67] On the day of injection, urinary gold content is highest, reflecting renal filtration of elevated serum gold levels, and declines progressively on successive days.[19,102] In contrast, daily fecal gold content is irregular, is not influenced by day-to-day variation in serum gold levels, and in part is a function of bowel habit and stool mass.[67] Forty percent of excreted gold derives from the current dose and 60 percent from previous doses.[67] The second, third, and fourth weeks following injection, 16, 12, and 10 percent of the administered dose are eliminated, respectively, if no additional gold is given. Keratinous tissues (skin, hair, and nail) have little avidity for gold, in contrast to certain other heavy metals (e.g., lead and arsenic); no meaningful quantity of gold is eliminated from the body via these excretory routes.[125]

The percentage of gold recovered in excreta during auranofin treatment is dose related, ranging from 76 to 100 percent of the administered dose, with 6 and 2 mg per day, respectively.[114] Approximately 95 percent of recoverable gold is in feces and only 5 percent is in urine.[114,118] Fecal gold content represents a combination of excreted and nonabsorbed gold, and gold adsorbed on mucosal cells that are subsequently sloughed.[126] The contribution from the biliary track is negligible.[126]

Gold Retention. Body gold retention has been measured following *intravenous* [195]Au-gold sodium thiomalate, using a whole body radiation counting chamber, and by classic metabolic methods. Applying the former technique, which monitors the kinetics of a *single* (the current) gold dose, RA patients retain 43 percent of the radionuclide 60 days after injection and approximately 25 percent after 250 days.[115] Fifteen percent of orally administered radiolabeled gold is retained after 10 days, while 1 percent remains 6 months later.[118] Utilizing the latter method, which reflects the kinetics of total body gold, approximately 60 percent of a 50 mg dose is retained each week during conventional intramuscular chrysotherapy.[67] Body retention approximates 45 and 30 percent of the injected dose, respectively, when 50 mg of compound is given every second or third week. After 20 weekly injections of 50 mg, approximately 300 mg of elemental gold is retained (20 weeks × 50 mg compound × 50 percent gold by weight × 60 percent retention = 300 mg). Lesser quantities of oral gold (auranofin) are retained; retention is dose dependent, varying from 30 percent with 6 mg per day to zero percent with 2 mg per day.[114] Following 20 weeks of therapy at 6 mg per day it is estimated that 73 mg of gold will be retained (140 days × 6 mg compound per day × 29 percent gold by weight × 30 percent retention = 73 mg), and considerably less when smaller doses are prescribed. The reduced body burden of gold with auranofin therapy may be therapeutically advantageous, although the form and biologic activity of the stored element or compound is unknown.

The existence of superficial and deep gold compartments, composed of tissues having varying avidity for gold, has been proposed.[58] The kinetics of gold interchange between compartments (tissues that store large quantities of the element such as bone marrow and liver, with the intravascular and intra- and extracellular fluids and synovial membrane) has not been defined.

CLINICAL-PHARMACOLOGIC CORRELATES

Investigators have sought to correlate the response to chrysotherapy with the pharmacokinetics of gold, to enhance efficacy and reduce the frequency and severity of toxicity. Blood gold concentrations have been examined most intensively, but urinary, fecal, and total gold excretion, skin, hair, and nail gold content, and body gold retention and distribution also have been studied. Unfortunately, meaningful correlates generally have not been identified.

More than 10 reports failed to define a relationship between serum gold concentration and efficacy, when measured at weekly intervals immediately prior to injection, during the course of therapy.[26,102,103] Peak, hourly, and daily serum blood gold levels also are comparable in gold responders and nonresponders, as shown in Figure 52–8.[103] Furthermore, serum radiogold disappearance curves do not correlate with response to treatment, and are similar in individual patients at different periods of chrysotherapy, independent of disease activity. Patients achieving mean concentrations of nearly 1000 μg per deciliter during high-dose therapy (150 mg per week) fared no better than those whose levels were 450 μg per deciliter during conventional treatment;[78] patients with gold levels of 167 μg per deciliter during low-dose treatment (25 mg per week) improved as much as patients receiving 50 mg per week (332 μg per deciliter).[58]

Serum gold levels are not helpful in monitoring adverse reactions; peak, hourly, daily, and weekly concentrations are similar in gold-toxic and nontoxic patients.[103] Serum radiogold disappearance curves also are comparable in both patient groups and in individuals studied twice, whether or not toxicity is present. However, as shown in Table 52–2, the frequency of severe toxicity is increased two- to fivefold when high-dose treatment schedules (150 to 200 mg per week) are employed.[77,78]

Recent trials indicate no relationship between urinary gold content and response to treatment of toxicity.[102,103,127] Body gold retention is not related to clinical outcome.[67,115] One small study observed a positive correlation between low fecal gold excretion and favorable clinical course, which may relate to organ (e.g., liver) gold distribution.[67]

Serial hair and nail gold concentrations are identical in gold-toxic and nontoxic patients during chrysotherapy.[125] Skin gold concentrations are similar in patients with and without gold dermatitis, and generally are comparable in skin lesions and in unaffected skin from patients with gold dermatitis.[125]

MECHANISMS OF ACTION

A myriad of in vitro and in vivo properties of gold compounds involving inflammatory cycles, the immune system, cellular biochemistry, and so forth have been elucidated in the past decades. But the mechanisms responsible for the favorable action of gold in RA remain enigmatic, and the information accrued has not substantially improved the results of chrysotherapy.

Gold compounds inhibit the growth of tubercle and other bacilli in vitro. Further support for the antimicrobial actions of gold derives from its protective effect on hamsters experimentally infected with Eaton's primary atypical pneumonia agent,[128] and from its purported beneficial effect in gonococcal arthritis.[5] More recently, gold sodium thiomalate was shown to inhibit the growth of *E. coli* when added to agar medium, but the addition of gold to human sera did not alter bacteriolytic activity.[129]

Gold sodium thiomalate inhibits acid phosphatase, beta glucuronidase, and malic dehydrogenase in guinea pig peritoneal macrophages,[130] acid phosphatase, beta glucuronidase, and cathepsin in human synovial fluid cells,[131] and several human epidermal enzymes.[132] These findings suggest that gold may ameliorate rheumatoid inflammation by inhibiting lysosomal enzymes. However, the release of hydrolases from lysosomes is unaffected by gold compounds, indicating that gold does not stabilize lysosomal membranes.[133]

The phagocytic activity of certain inflammatory cells is enhanced in patients with RA. Intramuscular gold compounds inhibit macrophage and polymorphonuclear leukocyte phagocytic activity at inflammatory sites in vivo, using a "skin-window" technique and measuring colloidal carbon particle uptake.[134] This action may alter cellular release of lysosomal enzymes, the initial handling of antigens in some immune responses, and several aspects of cell-mediated immunity. Chrysotherapy reduces the serum concentration of several trace metals (tin, molybdenum, manganese, barium, and cesium) that are elevated in RA patients; perhaps gold displaces other metal ions from biologically active compounds, successfully modifying a series of disease-producing biochemical interactions.[135] The effects of gold on serum protein, complement, and immunoglobulin concentrations, and on RF titer, have been discussed under Efficacy.

Gold sodium thiomalate inhibits the copper-catalyzed thermal aggregation of human gamma globulin in vitro; aggregated protein of this type is thought to be inflammatory, antigenic, and a stimulus to RF formation.[136] Gold compounds affect the classic and alternative complement systems in vitro.[137,138] Gold sodium thiomalate and thiosulfate and gold chloride partially inactivate the first component (C1) of the complement system in serum and synovial fluid, in concentrations achieved during conventional chrysotherapy.[137] An example of the effect of gold sodium thiomalate on C1, C4, and C2 in rheumatoid synovial fluid is shown in Figure 52–9. Highly purified human C1 and C1$_s$ were also irreversibly destroyed by gold. Thiomalic acid produced no such effects. The prostaglandin system, another important mediator of inflammation, is also affected by gold in vitro. Gold sodium thiomalate, in therapeutic serum concentrations, inhibits PGE_2 synthesis in a time- and concentration-dependent manner.[132] At a cellular level, gold acts directly on free sulfhydryl groups of proteins (e.g.,

Figure 52–9. Gold sodium thiomalate (GST) (3.1 μg per milliliter) partially inactivates the functional hemolytic activity of C1, and protects against C4 and C2 destruction, the natural substrates of C1, in vitro. Thiomalic acid (TA) has no effect on C1. (Supplied through the courtesy of Duane Schultz, Ph.D.)

cysteine), rendering them biologically inactive.[139] In contrast to certain antirheumatic agents, gold compounds do not inhibit connective tissue activation (CTAP).[140]

Most recently, the effects of gold on lymphocytes and monocytes have been reported. Gold sodium thiomalate inhibits antigen- and mitogen-triggered human lymphocyte DNA synthesis in vitro, an action that is increased by partially depleting the cell culture of monocytes, and that is reversed by culture supplementation with purified monocytes.[141] Preincubation of purified monocytes with gold renders them deficient in their ability to support mitogen-induced T-lymphocyte proliferation on subsequent culture. These and other observations suggest that gold blocks thymus-derived lymphocyte activation by interfering with monocyte function. Gold sodium thiomalate and thiosulfate inhibit transformation of human lymphocytes stimulated by other lymphocytes in the mixed lymphocyte culture, purified protein derivative, phytohemagglutinin, concanavalin A, and pokeweed mitogen in vitro.[142] Other investigators reported that gold sodium thiosulfate does not inhibit the incorporation of (³H) thymidine (a measure of DNA synthesis) and (¹⁴C) amino acids (a measure of protein synthesis) in human lymphocytes. Micromolar concentrations of gold sodium thiomalate and aurothioglucose also inhibit peptide-stimulated chemotactic responsiveness of human blood monocytes, but not of polymorphonuclear leukocytes.[143] However, others have shown that gold sodium thiomalate inhibits neutrophil chemotaxis and random migration in vitro, in normal subjects, and in gold-responsive RA patients but not in gold-resistant patients.[144]

Aurothioglucose and gold sodium thiomalate influence the immune response of mice, resulting in immunoenhancement or immunosuppression, depending upon gold concentration, as measured by direct and indirect plaque-forming cells, rosette-forming cells, and serum antibody assays.[145] Chrysotherapy interferes with the cytotoxic activity of macrophages from *Corynebacterium parvum*–treated mice.[146] But gold does not alter certain immunologic responses in other animal models. Delayed hypersensitivity to diphtheria toxoid and dinitrochlorobenzene in guinea pigs and antibody production to bovine serum albumin, typhoid-paratyphoid vaccine, and *E. coli* in rabbits are not influenced by 4 to 10 times the human equivalent dose of gold sodium thiomalate.[147] In the rat, gold suppresses the infiltration of inflammatory cells into subcutaneous implants of polyurethane foam impregnated with dead tubercle bacilli, but does not affect the fluid phase of the phlogistic response.[148] Gold sodium thiosulfate stains intravital collagen in rat tails, increases cross-linkages and shrinkage temperature, decreases swelling ability, and prolongs the contraction-relaxation period.[149] Gold is beneficial in treating adjuvant arthritis of rats.[150]

The pharmacologic and biologic actions of auranofin differ in many respects from those of the intramuscular gold compounds (Table 52–4). Oral gold exhibits anti-inflammatory activity in several animal models, suppresses humoral immune mechanisms, alters cell-mediated immunity, depresses polymorphonuclear and mononuclear leucocyte activity in vitro, and inhibits DNA synthesis in vitro and human cellular activity in vivo.[151] In many of these test systems the effect of auranofin is stronger than comparable or larger doses of the injectable gold compounds. One or more of these functions may explain the efficacy of auranofin in RA despite the low blood and tissue gold levels.

PRECAUTIONS, CONTRAINDICATIONS, AND COSTS

Efforts to predict gold toxicity and to reduce the frequency and severity of untoward gold reactions have had a modicum of success. Most strikingly, the mortality rate has fallen from an estimated 4 percent in the early years of chrysotherapy to less than 0.5 percent at present. Reasons for the reduced death rate are complex and speculative and are discussed more fully under Gold Toxicity. I believe that improved general medical care, the availability of life support systems, and lower gold doses largely account for the declining mortality rate. Because the prevalence of untoward reactions correlates directly with gold dose, especially when 50 mg per week is exceeded, the use of a conventional schedule should reduce the frequency of toxicity; however, wide variation in the prevalence of complications in recent and past reports prohibits accurate comparison. The presently available precautionary measures, described below, do not predict or prevent gold complications; they merely permit prompt recognition of early toxicity. Therefore, continued efforts should be directed toward defining the optimal gold schedule; new techniques, predictive of impending toxicity, must be developed. Immediate cessation of gold, coupled with appropriate therapeutic

Table 52–4. Pharmacologic and Biologic Actions of Gold Sodium Thiomalate and Auranofin

Action	Gold Sodium Thiomalate	Auranofin
Inflammation		
Carrageenan edema (rat)	↑/↓	↓
Kaolin edema (rat)	0	↓
Passive cutaneous anaphylaxis (rat)	↓ (weak)	↓
Ultraviolet erythema (guinea pig)	↓	↓
Adjuvant arthritis (rat)	↓	↓
Humoral Immunity		
IgG hemagglutinin (adjuvant arthritis; rat)	0	↓
Antibody-dependent cellular cytotoxicity (ADCC, rat)	0	↓
Antibody-dependent complement lysis (rat)	↑	↓
Hemagglutinin (mouse)	0	0
Hemolysin plaque-forming cells (rat)	0	↓
Hemolysin plaque-forming cells (mouse)	↑	↓/0
Cell-mediated Immunity (CMI)		
Sub-optimal CMI (mouse)*	↑	↑
Immunosuppressed CMI (mouse)*	0	↑
Experimental allergic encephalomyelitis (rat)	↓ (delay)	↓ (delay)
Polymorphonuclear Leukocyte Activity (in vitro)		
Chemotaxis (human)	–	↓
Aggregation (human)	↓ (weak)	↓
Superoxide production (human)	0/↓	↓
Phagocytosis (rat/human)	–/0	↓/↓
Lysosomal enzyme release (rat/human)	0/↓ (weak)	↓/↓
ADCC	0	↓
Mononuclear Leukocyte Activity (in vitro)		
Mononuclear (target cell destruction, rat)	–	↑
Monocyte (ADCC/chemotaxis, human)	0/↓	↓/↓
Lymphocyte (mitogen stimulation, human; antibody secretion, mouse; ADCC, human)	↓ (weak), ↓ (weak), 0	↓, ↓, ↓ (weak)
NK cell (target cell destruction, human)	–	↑/↓
DNA Synthesis (in vitro)		
Mitogen stimulated lymphocytes	↓ weak/0	↓
EBV-transformed lymphocytes	0	↓
HeLa carcinoma	–	↓
RAJI lymphoma	–	↓
Human Cellular Activity (in vivo)		
DNA synthesis (mitogen-stimulated lymphocytes)	↑/↓ (weak), (10–20 weeks)	↓ (2 weeks)
Delayed hypersensitivity (dinitrochlorobenzene skin test)	0	↓

*Using oxazolone-induced contact sensitivity and delayed hypersensitivity to sheep red blood cells.

measures, avoids severe or protracted target-organ damage in some cases.

My recommendations for monitoring chrysotherapy are as follows. Baseline history, physical, and laboratory examinations are mandatory. The physician inquires in detail for a past history of allergic drug reaction, pruritus, rash, oral lesions, renal disease, and proteinuria. The skin and oral mucosa are carefully examined for lesions such as psoriasis, fungal infection, leukoplakia, palatal or buccal mucosal ulceration, or inflammation from dental appliances. A complete blood count with differential, thrombocyte estimate from peripheral blood smear or platelet count, urinalysis, and biochemical profile are obtained.

During chrysotherapy, the patient is queried, preferably by the physician or by specially trained medical personnel under his direct supervision, about pruritus, dermatitis, stomatitis, and metallic taste and is examined prior to each injection. Most authorities recommend a complete blood count, thrombocyte count or estimate, and urinalysis every 1 to 3 weeks. I dip-stick test a urine specimen for proteinuria, using Uristix or other commercially available product, before each injection.

Chrysotherapy is terminated promptly should any of the aforementioned symptoms or significant eosinophilia, leukopenia, anemia, thrombocytopenia, microscopic hematuria, or proteinuria develop. Causes of such abnormality, other than gold toxicity, such as laboratory error, incidental skin or mucous membrane lesions, side effects from other medications, and so forth, are sought. If no alternative explanation is found, presumably the reaction is gold related, and treatment is temporarily or permanently abandoned, depending on the type and severity of reaction and the activity of the rheumatic process.

Gold compounds should not be administered to patients with a past history of severe gold toxicity (e.g., generalized dermatitis, significant depression of any blood cell type, or heavy proteinuria; see Gold Toxicity for additional discussion). Other heavy metal toxicity that has resulted in organ impairment (e.g., renal insufficiency from chronic plumbism) also interdicts the use of chrysotherapy.

Vasomotor responses (nitritoid reactions) are associated with gold sodium thiomalate treatment and may include dizziness and syncope as part of their symptom complex (see Gold Toxicity for further discussion). Because they occur within several minutes of administration, probably as a result of vasodilation with ensuing transient hypotension, it is advisable to give gold sodium thiomalate while the patient is recumbent. Furthermore, I recommend that the patient remain in the examining room or elsewhere in the doctor's office for 10 to 15 minutes after injection.

The concomitant use of certain other antirheumatic agents generally is interdicted during chrysotherapy. The pyrazolon-derived compounds (phenylbutazone, oxyphenbutazone), antimalarials, cytotoxic agents, and penicillamine are beneficial in RA, but they may cause side effects similar to those of gold, such as bone marrow depression, proteinuria, and dermatitis. Should an un-

toward reaction occur, the offending drug could not be readily identified, demanding discontinuation of both agents. Drug interactions and potentiation of toxicity have not been explored adequately, but they are additional considerations for avoiding conjunctive therapy. Some authorities believe that the concurrent use of systemic corticosteroids may reduce the efficacy of gold treatment, an opinion not substantiated by critical testing. Excessive sun exposure may contribute to the development of gold dermatitis and is discouraged; this admonition is based on anecdotal experience.

Gold compounds and penicillamine are commonly prescribed sequentially, usually in that order, for patients requiring slow-acting antirheumatic drugs who are unresponsive or intolerant to the initial choice.[152-154] The therapeutic response to the first agent does not predict the value of the second.[152] And, with the possible exceptions of proteinuria[152] and dermatitis,[154] patients who experience complications from the initial drug are not more likely to develop similar reactions from the next.

Gold therapy is not recommended for pregnant or lactating women because the safety for the fetus or newborn infant has not been established. What little evidence is available, however, anecdotal and otherwise, suggests a low magnitude of risk.[15] Women of childbearing age in whom chrysotherapy is contemplated are advised to use accepted contraceptive measures; treatment is terminated if pregnancy develops. The milk of gold-treated lactating women and the blood of their nursing infants contain small quantities of gold, the clinical significance of which has not been determined. Therefore, in the present state of knowledge, gold treatment is best avoided in nursing mothers.

Chrysotherapy may be used in conjunction with analgesics, salicylate compounds and other systemic nonsteroidal anti-inflammatory agents, and intraarticular corticosteroids without amelioration of benefit. Sjögren's syndrome, which develops in 10 to 15 percent of RA patients, is not a deterrent to gold therapy.[25] Similarly, ocular chrysiasis does not interdict chrysotherapy.[101] This incidental finding is not associated with visual disturbance or a higher prevalence of gold toxicity. Inasmuch as ocular complications from gold treatment occur rarely, periodic ophthalmologic examinations are not necessary.

The cost of administering and monitoring the initial phase (20 weeks) of intramuscular gold treatment is considerable. A survey conducted in 1976 indicated that the expense varies from $300 to $800, depending on the frequency and number of laboratory tests and physician (versus nurse or physician's assistant) visits, and on the established charges for these procedures.[155] The price of the injectable is approximately $50.00 for a 10 cc vial (50 mg per cubic centimeter) of aurothioglucose or gold sodium thiomalate. Transportation expenses, loss of income as a result of travel and waiting in the physician's office, and monies expended in evaluating and treating gold complications were not determined, raising the real cost of chrysotherapy well beyond the survey's estimates. Strategies to reduce costs include fewer and less frequent laboratory tests and administration of gold at home by a family member or nurse. The extent to which these cost-cutting measures jeopardize the patient's health (increase the frequency or severity of gold toxicity) or reduce the beneficial effects of treatment is speculative.

The cost of oral gold treatment is not fully established, and will be partly dependent upon (a) the retail price of auranofin capsules, (b) final guidelines for the number, type, and frequency of laboratory tests advised, and (c) recommended frequency of physician visits to monitor drug effects. Oral chrysotherapy will probably be less expensive than parenteral treatment during the first 6 months, when weekly visits to the physician's office and frequent blood and urine tests are required, but thereafter costs may be comparable.

GOLD TOXICITY

Adverse reactions develop in approximately one third of RA patients treated with intramuscular gold, varying from 5 to 80 percent in several reported series.[13] Most complications are inconsequential, consisting primarily of localized dermatitis, stomatitis, or transient mild proteinuria. More serious reactions involve the hematopoietic system, kidneys, liver, or other vital organs. Table 52–5 lists many of the toxic reactions associated with gold therapy.

Dermatitis and stomatitis account for 60 to 80 percent of all adverse gold reactions. The clinical and histologic appearance of gold rash is highly variable and may mimic other skin conditions such as lichen planus, idiopathic pityriasis rosea, psoriasis, and dermatophytosis. Erythema nodosum, exfoliative dermatitis, and bullous lesions develop rarely. One report indicated that 50 percent of lesions defied clinical classification into known dermatologic entities.[156]

The severity, distribution, and duration of gold rash varies from mild, localized, evanescent eruptions to those that are intensely pruritic or painful, generalized, and persistent for 1 year or longer. Most gold rashes last 1 to 2 months, are discrete, and are confined to the extremities or, less frequently, the trunk. Approximately 85 percent of eruptions are pruritic; other manifestations of gold toxicity such as eosinophilia, metallic taste, or proteinuria often accompany dermatitis.[13,156]

Skin punch biopsy may aid the clinician in defining gold dermatitis and in excluding incidental disorders that arise during chrysotherapy.[156] Immunofluorescent studies are of little value in differentiating gold rash from other conditions; immunoglobulins and complement components are found in a minority of gold eruptions but also are present in diverse dermatitides of other causes.[157]

The appearance of a rash during chrysotherapy in a patient without a pre-existing history of similar eruption, and especially if accompanied by pruritus or other manifestations of gold toxicity, is strongly suggestive of gold dermatitis. Chrysotherapy should be interrupted temporarily, pending evaluation and complete resolution of

Table 52–5. Adverse Reactions from Intramuscular Gold Compounds

Dermatologic
  Dermatitis—common
  Stomatitis—common
  Pruritus—common
  Alopecia—rare
  Chrysiasis—rare
  Photosensitivity—rare
Renal
  Proteinuria—common
  Hematuria—rare
  Nephrotic syndrome—rare
  Renal insufficiency or failure—rare
Hematologic
  Eosinophilia—common
  Thrombocytopenia—rare
  Granulocytopenia—rare
  Aplastic anemia—rare
Ophthalmic
  Corneal or lens chrysiasis—common
  Conjunctivitis, iritis, corneal ulcer—rare
Cardiopulmonary
  Vasomotor (nitritoid) reactions—common*
  Anaphylaxis—rare
  Syncope—rare
  Diffuse pulmonary infiltrates—rare
Musculoskeletal
  Myalgias—common*
  Joint pain, swelling, stiffness—common*
Gastrointestinal
  Enterocolitis—rare
  Cholestatic jaundice—rare
Miscellaneous
  Metallic taste—common
  Peripheral neuritis—rare
  Headaches—rare

*With gold sodium thiomalate (Myochrysine).

dermal pathology plus several additional weeks of observation. In some circumstances, treatment then may be reinstituted, using a reduced dosage schedule of 5 to 10 mg of gold compound weekly, with 5 to 10 mg increments every 1 to 4 weeks if toxicity does not recur. A lower dosage schedule, consisting of 1 to 2 mg initially with increments of similar magnitude, has also been advocated, and reportedly reduces the frequency of recurrent dermatitis.[158] Reinstitution of chrysotherapy in patients with a history of proved mild to moderately severe localized gold dermatitis that has resolved rarely results in exfoliative dermatitis or other generalized skin rash. The majority of patients tolerate a reduced dosage schedule without adverse reaction, but those with recurrent dermatitis tend to have eruptions similar to those manifest initially.[159]

Rarely, gray or blue discoloration of the skin develops with protracted intramuscular chrysotherapy.[160] This condition, known as chrysiasis, is asymptomatic, difficult to document objectively, does not influence the response to treatment, and is not associated with other side effects. Although gold is detectable in the skin of these patients, it is universally present during protracted injectable treatment, a critical gold concentration necessary to develop chrysiasis has not been defined, and the mechanisms responsible for this pigmentary change are not known.[125,161]

Transient proteinuria, microscopic hematuria, and nephrotic syndrome are well-described complications of gold therapy. The prevalence of transient proteinuria varies from 0 to 26 percent of patients receiving 50 mg of gold-compound weekly, as shown in Table 52–6. The frequency of proteinuria increases when higher gold doses are administered.[77,78] However, proteinuria has also been described in approximately 3 percent of non-gold-treated RA patients;[9,11] hypertension, diverse urinary tract disorders, and various medications used to treat RA are other conditions which may cause proteinuria. At times, urinary protein resolves spontaneously despite continuation of chrysotherapy in the absence of any identifiable cause.

Nephrotic syndrome is the most frequent serious renal abnormality associated with gold therapy, encountered in 0.2 to 2.6 percent of patients.[162-164] Histologically, the predominant lesion is membranous glomerulonephritis. IgG, IgM, and complement (C3) have been found in glomerular lesions. Particulate matter consistent with gold has been found in proximal and distal renal tubules, interstitium, and glomerular tufts.[162,163] Gold has been identified within proximal convoluted tubule cells, suggesting that gold may injure tubular epithelial cells, with subsequent release of antigen, antibody formation, and resultant immune complex deposition in glomerular tufts.[111] The prognosis with gold-associated nephrotic syndrome is generally favorable, 70 percent of patients recovering fully within months to years. The remainder have varying degrees of persistent proteinuria; renal insufficiency is observed rarely.[162]

Hematologic disorders resulting from chrysotherapy include eosinophilia, leukopenia or agranulocytosis, thrombocytopenia, anemia, pancytopenia, and aplastic anemia. Eosinophilia occurs in approximately 5 percent of gold-treated patients but, depending upon such factors as definition and patient population, varies from 0 to 40 percent in several published series.[13,165] Generally, eosinophilia is transient and of no significance; however, it may be a harbinger of impending toxicity affecting any organ system. Eosinophilia has been correlated positively with serum IgE levels and gold toxicity,[165] although others have not confirmed this finding.[157]

Thrombocytopenia is an infrequently (1 to 3 percent) recognized complication of gold treatment that is potentially serious and occasionally life threatening. It may develop shortly after gold is begun or as late as 18 months after cessation of therapy.[166,167] The initial manifestations of platelet reduction may be easy bruisability or spontaneous petechiae or purpura affecting the skin, mucous membranes of the mouth, and tongue. Less commonly, epistaxis or gingival, gastrointestinal, or genitourinary hemorrhage leads to the diagnosis of thrombocytopenia. Platelet counts above 25,000 per cubic millimeter uncommonly are associated with bleeding difficulties unless other hematologic abnormalities coexist.

Leukopenia may develop during gold therapy owing to granulocytopenia or agranulocytosis. The prevalence of leukopenia is low but not precisely established, and the extent and duration of white cell reduction are highly variable. Granulocytopenia may be asymptomatic or may be associated with clinical manifestations.

The most feared complication of chrysotherapy is severe pancytopenia or bone marrow aplasia. The incidence of the latter is low, existing evidence pointing to a prevalence of less than 0.5 percent.[168] However, the mortality rate is high, more than 60 percent of affected individuals succumbing to infection, bleeding, or other complications despite supportive and aggressive therapy.

Vasomotor (nitritoid) reactions, characterized by weakness, dizziness, nausea, vomiting, sweating, and facial flushing, may follow gold sodium thiomalate. The prevalence of this reaction has varied from not being cited to as high as 34 percent in several series.[78] Peripheral vasodilatation may ensue, causing hypotension from the action on arteriolar smooth muscle. Rarely, this results in myocardial infarction[73] or central nervous system injury, especially in the elderly population with arteriosclerotic or other forms of cardiovascular disease.[169] Nonvasomotor symptoms, including transient stiffness, arthralgias, myalgias, joint swelling, fatigability, and malaise, developed in 15 percent of patients treated with gold sodium thiomalate in one reported study.[74] Aurothioglucose exceptionally causes either symptom complex.

Organ systems rarely affected by gold treatment in-

Table 52–6. Prevalence of Proteinuria During Intramuscular Chrysotherapy

Investigator	Conventional Gold Dose (50 mg per Week)		Alternative Gold Dose*		No Gold	
	Number of Patients: Toxic/Treated	*Percent Toxic*	*Number of Patients: Toxic/Treated*	*Percent Toxic*	*Number of Patients: Toxic/Treated*	*Percent Toxic*
ERC[9]	4/99	4	–		3/100	3
Cats[77]	4/119	3	10/111	9	–	
CCC[11]	0/36	0	–		1/32	3
Gordon et al.[25]	7/101	7	–		–	
Rothermich et al.[37]	2/55	4	0/42	0	–	
Sharp et al.[58]	6/38	16	9/37	24	–	
Furst et al.[78]	6/23	26	9/24	38	–	

*Alternative gold schedules are given in Table 52–2.

clude the lungs, liver, and lower intestinal tract. Acute respiratory distress associated with diffuse pulmonary infiltration characteristically causes malaise, cough productive of small amounts of sputum, shortness of breath, pleuritic chest pain, and pulmonary rales.[170,171] Patchy areas of pulmonary consolidation without hilar adenopathy, but with alteration of respiratory function tests consistent with restrictive lung disease, are observed. Dramatic improvement follows withdrawal of chrysotherapy and administration of systemic corticosteroids.

Cholestatic jaundice, with hyperbilirubinemia, elevated serum glutamic oxaloacetic transaminase and other enzymes, and high alkaline phosphatase levels, has been ascribed to gold treatment in a few patients.[172,173] Findings generally include fatigability, pruritus, anorexia, painless icterus, dark urine, light-colored stool, and hepatomegaly. Liver biopsy may show bile stasis and thrombi in the biliary tree, or ballooning hepatocytes with sinusoidal compression and minimal cholestasis. Hepatotoxicity usually develops early in the course of treatment (less than 200 mg of compound), is often associated with peripheral blood eosinophilia, and recedes rapidly with cessation of gold therapy.

Enterocolitis is another uncommon complication of chrysotherapy, occurring primarily in middle-aged females who have received small total doses of gold.[174,175] Symptoms may include abdominal pain, bloody or nonbloody diarrhea, nausea, vomiting, and fever. Despite treatment with antibiotics, dimercaprol (BAL), corticosteroids, and life-support measures, the mortality rate approaches 50 percent.

Corneal chrysiasis, defined by slit-lamp microscopy, is directly related to cumulative dose, occurring in 75 percent of patients who receive greater than 1500 mg of intramuscular gold.[176,177] Lens chrysiasis occasionally develops despite minuscule lens gold levels.[101] Neither condition leads to the development of ocular disease. Conjunctivitis, iritis, and corneal ulcers have been rarely attributed to gold treatment.

Evolving information shows an association between certain untoward side effects from gold and antigens on the histocompatibility D locus. Specifically, gold-induced proteinuria and thrombocytopenia, which likely represent immune-mediated reactions, occur many times more frequently than anticipated (increased relative risk is 32 times for proteinuria and nine times for thrombocytopenia) in RA patients possessing HLA-DR3 and DRw3.[178-180] Interestingly, the more common forms of gold toxicity, such as dermatitis and stomatitis, are not related to this genetic background.[178,179] Given the prevalence of these antigens in the general population (31 percent),[179] the limited number of slow-acting antirheumatic drugs currently available, and the expense of HLA-D typing, routine HLA typing before initiating gold treatment is not warranted.

Extensive premarketing experience reveals that the type, severity, and time of complication developing from auranofin differ importantly from characteristics of complications of the injectable gold compounds (Table 52–7). Most side effects are mild and transient, affect the lower gastrointestinal tract, and are dose related. Changes in stool consistency and frequency, diarrhea, and abdominal cramps are the commonest untoward effects of oral gold.[16,42] These reactions generally occur within the first few weeks to months of treatment, improve spontaneously or remand with dose reduction, or very uncommonly require permanent drug abandonment.[16] The mechanisms of gastrointestinal irritation are unknown, but barium enema, sigmoidoscopy, and mucosal biopsy on a limited number of patients have not revealed significant pathologic change.[16] Gold colitis or persistent diarrhea after drug cessation has not been encountered. Mucocutaneous lesions and serious complications affecting the hematopoietic system, kidneys, and so forth occur less commonly with auranofin than with the intramuscular preparations.[16,42] Approximately four times as many patients were withdrawn from intramuscular gold treatment (20 percent) because of drug

Table 52–7. Adverse On-Therapy Experiences: Gold Sodium Thiomalate and Auranofin Compared

Complication	CSSRD Study*			Combined Data from Seven Studies Comparing Gold Sodium Thiomalate and Auranofin†	
	Gold Sodium Thiomalate (n = 81)	Auranofin (n = 78)	Placebo (n = 50)	Gold Sodium Thiomalate (n = 244)	Auranofin (n = 243)
Mucocutaneous	7 (%)	1 (%)	4 (%)	48 (%)	23 (%)
Vasomotor reactions	6	0	0	NR‡	NR
Proteinuria	0	0	0	6	2
Diarrhea	2	6	0	8	25
Other GI symptoms	2	1	0	6	12
Hematologic	0	0	0	7	1
Miscellaneous	15	5	0	31	22
Withdrawals due to adverse reactions	27	7	2	22	7

*Adapted from the Cooperative Systemic Studies of Rheumatic Diseases Report[43]; excludes adverse reactions leading to withdrawal.
†Adapted from Blodgett.[16]
‡NR = Not reported.

intolerance as from oral gold (5 percent) in the Cooperative Systematic Studies of Rheumatic Diseases 21-week controlled trial[43] and in cumulative data from seven protocols.[16] With more prolonged therapy, the drop-out rates rise, but the 4:1 withdrawal ratio between parenteral and oral gold remains.[16]

TREATMENT OF GOLD TOXICITY

The great majority of adverse gold reactions resolve spontaneously within weeks to months following cessation of chrysotherapy or require only symptomatic measures. Treatment of serious complications affecting the skin, kidneys, lungs and gastrointestinal and hematopoietic systems has been the subject of numerous reports but not of controlled studies.[13,29,156,159,162,164,166-168,170-174,181,182] Appraisal of the efficacy of corticosteroids, dimercaprol, penicillamine, ACTH, and other agents is further complicated by the variable natural history of gold reactions, and by the rare mortality from bone marrow aplasia, thrombocytopenia, or enterocolitis despite aggressive treatment.

Most patients with gold dermatitis of such severity as to require treatment benefit from oral antihistamines, topical corticosteroids, or emollients such as petrolatum, Crisco, Aquaphor, or Lubriderm. Colloidal baths, tranquilizers, sedatives, and the application of ice or cold compresses may relieve pruritus.[156] Prolonged sun exposure and contact with soap should be avoided. Symptoms resulting from severe or generalized pruritic eruptions may improve with systemic corticosteroids, although the literature fails to provide convincing evidence that the natural history of the eruption is altered favorably.

Stomatitis, glossitis, cheilitis, and gingivitis may be minimally symptomatic, demanding no treatment or only avoidance of spices and sour substances, or of such severity as to necessitate stronger measures. Frequent alkaline mouth washes or the application of Xylocaine Viscous or Kenalog in Orabase may afford relief of oral soreness, burning, or pain in severe or protracted cases.[159] Resultant anorexia and weight loss occasionally require nutritional supplementation with a liquid diet, baby food or blenderized soft foods, or, rarely, intravenous fluids or other forms of alimentation.

Moderate to high dose corticosteroid therapy (20 to 60 mg daily in divided doses of prednisone or its equivalent) reportedly is beneficial in some cases of gold-induced nephrotic syndrome, thrombocytopenia, and, less often, other hematologic disorders, enterocolitis, and pulmonary infiltrates. Higher doses of steroids may be justified in unresponsive cases. Treatment generally must be given for several weeks to months, and then tapered gradually. It is currently believed that corticosteroids act by reducing inflammation in the affected target organ, by altering the immunologic response, or by some other undefined mechanism. Gold metabolism is not affected.

Dimercaprol, penicillamine, N-acetylcysteine, and other chelating agents have been employed primarily in severe reactions unresponsive to corticosteroid therapy or in conjunction with steroids.[13,29,183-185] With the exception of penicillamine,[186,187] these drugs enhance urinary gold excretion and are thought to compete with gold for essential cellular enzymes. Dimercaprol is given intramuscularly in doses of 2.5 to 3.0 mg per kilogram every 6 hours for 3 or 4 days. Reduced doses may then be administered for an additional time period, depending on the therapeutic response. Some clinicians base the amount of BAL prescribed on the cumulative gold dose, applying greater quantities of BAL for patients with higher total gold doses.[188] Perhaps some drug failures result from inadequate courses of BAL. Penicillamine (Cuprimine) is given orally in divided doses of 1 to 2 grams daily for variable time periods. The use of these agents is attended by potentially serious side effects. Bone marrow depression, sterile abscesses, vomiting, carpopedal spasm, paresthesias, and severe headaches may develop from BAL. Complications associated with penicillamine are reviewed in Chapter 53.

In addition to these measures, patients with severe thrombocytopenia associated with hemorrhage may require volume repletion, whole blood or platelet transfusions, and life support measures. Vincristine,[189] other potent chemotherapeutic agents, and splenectomy[190] have also been used successfully. Those suffering from significant granulocytopenia or agranulocytosis often improved spontaneously within two weeks.[191] In unresponsive cases, and in those with bone marrow aplasia, reverse isolation techniques, systemic antibiotics, bed rest, blood or platelet transfusions, and extensive general medical and nursing care may be beneficial. Androgenic hormones, bone marrow transplantation,[192] and peritoneal dialysis[193] also have been recommended in recalcitrant cases.

SELECTION OF GOLD COMPOUND: ORAL OR INTRAMUSCULAR?

The advantageous safety profile of auranofin compared with the injectable gold compounds, coupled with similar efficacy profiles, provides an improved benefit-to-risk ratio. In addition, auranofin is easier to administer, may require less laboratory and clinical monitoring, and hopefully will be less expensive. On the other hand, this oral gold compound may not be fully as potent as the intramuscular agents, may be prescribed improperly by physicians unfamiliar with rheumatic disease treatment and used inappropriately by patients who self-administer medication, and may present compliance problems. Experience with the parenteral compounds spans 55 years, ample time for physicians to become familiar with these products, and for the identification of common and rare adverse reactions. For these and other reasons, the ultimate place of auranofin vis-à-vis the intramuscular compounds in the therapeutic hierarchy of RA is speculative. I believe auranofin will replace the injectables as the initial agent of choice, and may encourage the modification of criteria for instituting slow-acting drug treatment, so that it is used in milder forms and earlier phases of RA.

REFERENCES

1. Slot, G., and Deville, P.M.: Treatment of arthritis and rheumatism with gold. Lancet 226:73, 1934
2. Koch, R.: Reported at the 10th International Medical Congress, Berlin, August 4, 1890. Dtsch. Med. Wochenschr. 16:756, 1890.
3. Rodnan, G.P., and Benedek, T.G.: The early history of antirheumatic drugs. Arthritis Rheum. 13:145, 1970.
4. Landé, K.: Die gunstige beeinflussung schleichender Dauerinfekte durch Solganal. Munch. Med. Wochenschr. 74:1132, 1927.
5. Oren, J.: Arthritis and its treatment with gold salts. J. Med. Soc. N.J. 33:591, 1936.
6. Forestier, J.: Rheumatoid arthritis and its treatment by gold salts. J. Lab. Clin. Med. 20:827, 1935.
7. Hartfall, S.J., Garland, H.G., and Goldie, W.: Gold treatment of arthritis: A review of 900 cases. Lancet 233:838, 1937.
8. Fraser, T.N.: Gold treatment in rheumatoid arthritis. Ann. Rheum. Dis. 4:71, 1945.
9. Empire Rheumatism Council: Gold therapy in rheumatoid arthritis. Ann. Rheum. Dis. 19:95, 1960.
10. Empire Rheumatism Council: Gold therapy in rheumatoid arthritis: Final report of a multicentre controlled trial. Ann. Rheum. Dis. 20:315, 1961.
11. The Cooperative Clinics Committee of the ARA: A controlled trial of gold salt therapy in rheumatoid arthritis. Arthritis Rheum. 16:353, 1973.
12. Sigler, J.W., Bluhm, G.B., Duncan, H., et al.: Gold salts in the treatment of rheumatoid arthritis: A double-blind study. Ann. Intern. Med. 80:21, 1974.
13. Freyberg, R.H., Ziff, M., and Baum, J.: Gold therapy for rheumatoid arthritis. In Hollander, J.L., and McCarty, D.J. (eds.): Arthritis and Allied Conditions. 8th ed. Philadelphia, Lea & Febiger, 1972, pp. 455–482.
14. Penneys, N.S., Eaglstein, W.H., and Frost, P.: Management of pemphigus with gold compounds. Arch. Dermatol. 112:185, 1976.
15. Miyamoto, T., Miyaji, S., Horiuchi, Y., et al.: Gold therapy in bronchial asthma with special emphasis upon blood level of gold and its teratogenicity. J. Jap. Soc. Intern. Med. 63:1190, 1974.
16. Blodgett, R.C., Heuer, M.A., and Pietrusko, R.G.: Auranofin: A unique oral chrysotherapeutic agent. Semin. Arthritis Rheum. 13:255, 1984.
17. Freyberg, R.H., Block, W.D., and Wells, G.S.: Gold therapy for rheumatoid arthritis. Clinics 1:537, 1942.
18. Cecil, R.L., Kammerer, W.H., and DePrume, F.J.: Gold salts in the treatment of rheumatoid arthritis. Ann. Intern. Med. 16:811, 1942.
19. Gottlieb, N.L., and Bjelle, A.: Gold compounds in rheumatoid arthritis. Scand. J. Rheumatol. 6:225, 1977.
20. Mouridsen, H.T., Baerentsen, O., Rossin, N., et al.: Lack of effect of gold therapy on abnormal IgG and IgM metabolism in rheumatoid arthritis. Arthritis Rheum. 17:391, 1974.
21. Menard, H.A., Mathieu, J.T., de Medicis, R., and Lussier, A.: Slow-onset antirheumatic drugs in rheumatoid arthritis: Could the presence of antinuclear antibody influence the therapeutic results? J. Rheumatol. 6:156, 1979.
22. Vischer, T.L.: Pharmacogenetics in therapy with gold and other slow-acting anti-rheumatic drugs. International Gold Workshop, Munich, Germany, January 14, 1982.
23. Gowans, J.D.C., and Salami, M.: Response of rheumatoid arthritis with leukopenia to gold salts. N. Engl. J. Med. 288:1007, 1973.
24. Hurd, E.R., and Cheatum, D.E.: Decreased spleen size and increased neutrophils in patients with Felty's syndrome. JAMA 235:2215, 1976.
25. Gordon, M.H., Tiger, L.H., and Ehrlich, G.E.: Gold reactions are not more common in Sjögren's syndrome. Ann. Intern. Med. 82:47, 1975.
26. Gottlieb, N.L.: Chrysotherapy. Bull. Rheum. Dis. 27:912, 1976-77.
27. Luthra, H.S., Conn, D.L., and Ferguson, R.H.: Felty's syndrome: Response to parenteral gold. J. Rheumatol. 8:902, 1981.
28. Mastaglia, G.L., and Owen, E.T.: A study of the response of the leukopenia of rheumatoid arthritis to gold salt therapy. J. Rheumatol. 8:658, 1981.
29. Harvey, S.C.: Heavy metals. In Goodman, L.S., and Gilman, A.: The Pharmacologic Basis of Therapeutics. 3rd ed. New York, Macmillan Publishing Co., 1965, pp. 943-975.
30. Ellman, P., Lawrence, J.S., and Thorold, G.P.: Gold therapy in rheumatoid arthritis. Br. Med. J. 2:314, 1940.
31. Waine, H., Baker, F., and Mettier, S.R.: Controlled evaluation of gold treatment in rheumatoid arthritis. Calif. Med. J. 66:295, 1947.
32. Forestier, J.: Rheumatoid arthritis and its treatment by gold salts. Lancet 227:646, 1934.
33. Hartfall, S.J., and Garland, H.G.: Gold treatment of rheumatoid arthritis. Lancet 229:8, 1935.
34. Adams, C.H., and Cecil, R.L.: Gold therapy in early rheumatoid arthritis. Ann. Intern. Med. 33:163, 1950.
35. Snorrason, E.: Rheumatoid arthritis, sanocrysin treatment and prognosis. Acta Med. Scand. 142:249, 1952.
36. Lockie, L.M., Norcross, B.M., and Riordan, D.J.: Gold treatment in rheumatoid arthritis. JAMA 167:1204, 1958.
37. Rothermich, N.O., Philips, V.K., and Bergen, W.: Chrysotherapy: A prospective study. Arthritis Rheum. 19:1321, 1976.
38. Sharp, J.T., Lidsky, M.D., and Duffy, J.: Clinical responses during gold therapy for rheumatoid arthritis: Changes in synovitis, radiologically detectable erosive lesions, serum proteins, and serologic abnormalities. Arthritis Rheum. 25:540, 1982.
39. Huskisson, E.C., Gibson, T.J., and Balme, H.W.: Trial comparing D-penicillamine and gold in rheumatoid arthritis. Ann. Rheum. Dis. 33:532, 1974.
40. Currey, H.L.F., Harris, J., and Mason, R.M.: Comparison of azathioprine, cyclophosphamide, and gold in treatment of rheumatoid arthritis. Br. Med. J. 3:763, 1974.
41. Dwosh, I.L., Stein, H.B., Urowitz, M.B., et al.: Azathioprine in early rheumatoid arthritis. Comparison with gold and chloroquine. Arthritis Rheum. 20:685, 1977.
42. Heuer, M.A., and Morris, R.W.: Smith, Kline & French World-Wide Clinical Experience With Auranofin: A Review. Auranofin (Ridaura) International Symposium, Amsterdam, November, 1982.
43. Ward, J.R., Williams, H.J., Egger, M.J., et al.: Comparison of auranofin, gold sodium thiomalate, and placebo in the treatment of rheumatoid arthritis. Arthritis Rheum.26:1303, 1983.
44. Katz, W.A., Alexander, S., Bland, J.H., Blechman, W., Bluhm, G.B., Bonebreak, R.A., Falbo, A., Greenwald, R.A., Hartman, S., Hobbs, T., Indenbaum, S., Lergier, J.E., Lanier, B.G., Lightfoot, R.W., Phelps, P., Sheon, R.P., Torretti, D., Wenger, M.E., and Wilske, K.: The efficacy and safety of auranofin compared to placebo in rheumatoid arthritis. J. Rheumatol. 9 (Suppl. 8):173, 1982.
45. Menard, H.A., Beaudet, F., Davis, P., Harth, M., Percy, J.S., Russell, A.S., and Thompson, J.M.: Gold therapy in rheumatoid arthritis: An interim report of the Canadian multicenter prospective trial comparing sodium aurothiomalate and auranofin. J. Rheumatol. 9 (Suppl. 8):179, 1982.
46. Schattenkirschner, M., Kaik, B., Muller-Fassbender, H., Rau, R., and Zeidler, H.: Auranofin and sodium aurothiomalate in the treatment of rheumatoid arthritis: A double-blind, comparative multicenter study. J. Rheumatol. 9 (Suppl. 8):184, 1982.
47. Barraclough, D., Brook, A., Brooks, P., Boyden, K., and Thomas, K.: A comparative study of auranofin, gold sodium thiomalate, and D-penicillamine in rheumatoid arthritis: A progress report. J. Rheumatol. 9 (Suppl. 8):197, 1982.
48. van Riel, P.L.C.M., van de Putte, L.B.A., Gribnau, F.W.J., and MacRae, K.D.: A single-blind comparative study of auranofin and gold thioglucose in patients with rheumatoid arthritis. Auranofin International Symposium, Amsterdam, November, 1982.
49. DeQueiter, J., Franckx, L., and Deckers, Y.: Comparison of oral gold (auranofin) and injectable gold (gold sodium thiopropanol-sulphonate; Allochrysine) treatment in patients with rheumatoid arthritis: A double-blind study. Auranofin International Symposium, Amsterdam, November, 1982.
50. Bird, H.A., Gallez, P.L., Dixon, J.S., Sitton, N.G., and Wright, V.: A comparison of auranofin and hydroxychloroquine in rheumatoid arthritis. Auranofin International Symposium, Amsterdam, November, 1982.
51. Huskisson, E.C., and Scott, J.: Comparative study of auranofin in rheumatoid arthritis. 15th International Congress of Rheumatology, Paris, June, 1981.
52. Felix-Davies, D.D., Bateman, J.R.M., Delamere, J.P., and Wilkinson, B.R.: A comparative trial of auranofin and D-penicillamine in rheumatoid arthritis. 15th International Congress of Rheumatology, Paris, June, 1981.
53. Wenger, M.E., Weiss, T.E., Rosenthal, S.H., O'Brien, W.M., Bernhard, G.C., Heller, M.D., and Reese, R.W.: Rheumatoid arthritis patients treated with auranofin maintain clinical benefits when switched from Myocrisin. Auranofin International Symposium, Amsterdam, November, 1982.
54. Berry, H., Gibson, T.J., Crisp, A.J., Pitt, P., Irani, M., Clarke, B., Bloom, B., and Paney, G.S.: Double-blind comparison of auranofin and Myocrisin in patients stabilised on Myocrisin. Auranofin International Symposium, Amsterdam, November, 1982.
55. Gofton, J.P., and O'Brien, W.: Roentgenographic findings during auranofin treatment. Am. J. Med. 75 (Suppl.): 142, 1983.
56. Gottlieb, N.L., Kiem, I.M., Penneys, N.S. et al.: The influence of chrysotherapy on serum protein and immunoglobulin levels, rheumatoid factor, and antiepithelial antibody titers. J. Lab. Clin. Med. 86:962, 1975.

57. Highton, J., Panayi, G.S., Shephard, P., Faith, A., Griffin, J., and Gibson, T.: Fall in immune complex levels during gold treatment of rheumatoid arthritis. Ann. Rheum. Dis. 40:575, 1981.

58. Sharp, J.T., Lidsky, M.D., Duffy, J., et al.: Comparison of two dosage schedules of gold salts in the treatment of rheumatoid arthritis. Arthritis Rheum. 20:1179, 1977.

59. Dorwart, B.B., Gall, E.P., Schumacher, H.R., et al.: Chrysotherapy in psoriatic arthritis. Arthritis Rheum. 21:513, 1978.

60. Richter, M.B., Kinsella, P., and Corbett, M.: Gold in psoriatic arthropathy. Ann. Rheum. Dis. 39:279, 1980.

61. Pinals, R.S., Masi, A.T., and Larsen, R.A.: Preliminary criteria for clinical remission in rheumatoid arthritis. Arthritis Rheum. 24:1308, 1981.

62. Srinivasa, N.R., Miller, B.L., and Paulus, H.E.: Long-term chrysotherapy in rheumatoid arthritis. Arthritis Rheum. 22:105, 1979.

63. Sambrook, T.N., Browne, C.D., Champion, G.D., Day, R.O., Vallance, J.B., and Warwick, N.: Terminations of treatment with gold sodium thiomalate in rheumatoid arthritis. J. Rheumatol. 9:932, 1982.

64. Richter, J.A., Runge, L.A., Pinals, R.S., and Oates, R.P.: Analysis of treatment terminations with gold and anti-malarial compounds in rheumatoid arthritis. J. Rheumatol. 7:153, 1980.

65. Sagransky, D.M., and Greenwald, R.A.: Efficacy and toxicity of retreatment with gold salts: A retrospective review of 25 cases. J. Rheumatol. 7:474, 1980.

66. Empire Rheumatism Council: Relation of toxic reactions in gold therapy to improvement in rheumatoid arthritis. Ann. Rheum. Dis. 20:335, 1961.

67. Gottlieb, N.L., Smith, P.M., and Smith, E.M.: Gold excretion correlated with clinical course during chrysotherapy in rheumatoid arthritis. Arthritis Rheum. 15:582, 1972.

68. Smith, R.T., Peak, W.P., and Kron, K.M.: Increasing the effectiveness of gold therapy in rheumatoid arthritis. JAMA 167:1197, 1958.

69. Bayles, T.B., and Fremont-Smith, P.: Significant clinical remissions in rheumatoid arthritis resulting from "sensitivity" produced by gold salt therapy. Ann. Rheum. Dis. 15:394, 1956.

70. Rosenthal, M.: Loss of efficacy of antirheumatic drugs in rheumatoid arthritis. J. Rheumatol. 7:586, 1980.

71. Sadler, P.J.: The comparative evaluation of the physical and chemical properties of gold compounds. J. Rheumatol. 9 (Suppl. 8): 71, 1982.

72. Lewis, D.C., and Ziff, M.: Intra-articular administration of gold salts. Arthritis Rheum. 9:682, 1966.

73. Gottlieb, N.L., and Brown, H.E., Jr.: Acute myocardial infarction following gold sodium thiomalate induced vasomotor (nitritoid) reaction. Arthritis Rheum. 20:1026, 1977.

74. Halla, J.T., Hardin, J.G., and Linn, J.E.: Postinjection nonvasomotor reactions during chrysotherapy. Arthritis Rheum. 20:1188, 1977.

75. Lawrence, J.S.: Comparative toxicity of gold preparations in treatment of rheumatoid arthritis. Ann. Rheum. Dis. 35:171, 1976.

76. Walz, D.T., DiMartino, M.J., Griswold, D.E., Intoccia, A.P., and Flanagan, T.L.: Biological actions of auranofin. Am. J. Med. 75 (Suppl.): 90, 1983.

77. Cats, A.: A multicentre controlled trial of the effects of different dosage of gold therapy, followed by maintenance dosage. Agents Actions 6:355, 1976.

78. Furst, D., Levine, S., Srinivasan, R., et al.: A double-blind trial of high versus conventional dosages of gold salts for rheumatoid arthritis. Arthritis Rheum. 20:1473, 1977.

79. Ragan, C., and Tyson, T.L.: Chrysotherapy in rheumatoid arthritis. Am. J. Med. 1:252, 1946.

80. Griffin, A.J., Givson, T., Huston, G., and Taylor, A.: Maintenance chrysotherapy in rheumatoid arthritis: A comparison of two dose schedules. Ann. Rheum. Dis. 40:250, 1981.

81. Hanson, V.: Dosage of gold salts in treatment of juvenile rheumatoid arthritis. Arthritis Rheum. 20 (Supplement No. 2): 548, 1977.

82. Ansell, B.M.: The management of juvenile chronic polyarthritis (Still's disease). Practitioner 208 (1243): 91, 1972.

83. Brewer, E.J., Jr.: Juvenile Rheumatoid Arthritis. Philadelphia, W. B. Saunders Company, 1970, pp. 205-213.

84. Sairanen, E., and Laaksonen, A.L.: The results of gold therapy in juvenile rheumatoid arthritis. Ann. Paediat. Fenn. 10:274, 1964.

85. Gottlieb, N.L., and Smith, E.M.: Pharmacology of intraarticularly injected ^{195}Au-labeled Myochrysine (sodium aurothiomalate) used as a diagnostic and therapeutic aid in rheumatoid arthritis (abstract). J. Nucl. Med. 9:319, 1968.

86. Makin, M., and Robin, G.C.: Chronic synovial effusions treated with intra-articular radioactive gold. JAMA 188:725, 1964.

87. Finkelstein, A.E., Roisman, F.R., and Batista, V.: Oral chrysotherapy in rheumatoid arthritis: Minimum effective dose. J. Rheumatol. 7:160, 1980.

88. Champion, G.D., Bieri, D., Browne, C.D., Day, R.O., Graham, G.G., Haavisto, T.M., Sambrook, P.N., and Vallance, J.B.: Auranofin in rheumatoid arthritis. J. Rheumatol. 9 (Suppl. 8): 137, 1982.

89. Calin, A., Saunders, D., Bennett, R., Jacox, R., Kaplan, D., O'Brien, W., Paulus, H.E., Roth, S., and Weiss, T.: Auranofin: One mg or 9 mg? The search for the appropriate dose. J. Rheumatol. 9 (Suppl. 8): 146, 1982.

90. Bernhard, G.C.: Auranofin treatment for adult rheumatoid arthritis: Comparison of 2 mg and 6 mg daily dose. J. Rheumatol. 9 (Suppl. 8): 149, 1982.

91. Giannini, H., Brewer, E.J., Jr., and Person, P.A.: Auranofin in the treatment of juvenile rheumatoid arthritis. J. Pediatr. 102:138, 1983.

92. Block, W.D., Buchanan, O.H., and Freyberg, R.H.: Metabolism, toxicity, and manner of action of gold compounds used in the treatment of arthritis. J. Pharmacol. Exp. Ther. 82:391, 1944.

93. Bertrand, J.J., Waine, H., and Tobias, C.A.: Distribution of gold in the animal body in relation to arthritis. J. Lab. Clin. Med. 33:1133, 1948.

94. Jeffrey, M.R., Freundlich, H.F., and Bailey, D.F.: Distribution and excretion of radiogold in animals. Ann. Rheum. Dis. 17:52, 1958.

95. Stuve, J., and Galle, P.: Role of mitochondria in the handling of gold by the kidney. J. Cell. Biol. 44:667, 1970.

96. Penneys, N.S., McCreary, S., and Gottlieb, N.L.: Intracellular distribution of radiogold: Localization to large granule membranes. Arthritis Rheum. 19:927, 1976.

97. Gottlieb, N.L., Smith, P.M., and Smith, E.M.: Tissue gold concentration in a rheumatoid arthritic receiving chrysotherapy. Arthritis Rheum. 15:16, 1972.

98. Grahame, R., Billings, R., and Laurence, M.: Tissue gold levels after chrysotherapy. Ann. Rheum. Dis. 33:536, 1974.

99. Kamel, H., Brown, D.H., Ottoway, J.M., et al.: Gold levels in kidney, liver, and spleen (letter to editor). Arthritis Rheum. 19:1368, 1976.

100. Veron-Roberts, B., Dore, J.L., Jessop, J.D., et al.: Selective concentration and localization of gold in macrophages of synovial and other tissues during and after chrysotherapy in rheumatoid patients. Ann. Rheum. Dis. 35:477, 1976.

101. Gottlieb, N.L., and Major, J.C.: Ocular chrysiasis correlated with gold concentrations in the crystalline lens during chrysotherapy. Arthritis Rheum. 21:704, 1978.

102. Mascarhenas, B.R., Granda, J.L., and Freyberg, R.H.: Gold metabolism in patients with rheumatoid arthritis treated with gold compounds—reinvestigated. Arthritis Rheum. 15:391, 1972.

103. Gottlieb, N.L., Smith, P.M., and Smith, E.M.: Pharmacodynamics of ^{195}Au labeled auriothiomalate in blood. Correlation with course of rheumatoid arthritis, gold toxicity and gold excretion. Arthritis Rheum. 17:161, 1974.

104. Gerber, R.C., Paulus, H.E., and Bluestone, R.: Kinetics of aurothiomalate in serum and synovial fluid. Arthritis Rheum. 15:625, 1972.

105. Kapelowitz, R.H., Help, W.M., Headly, L.A., et al.: Urinary and fecal excretion of Au^{198} in gold-treated patients with rheumatoid arthritis (abstract). Arthritis Rheum. 7:319, 1964.

106. Gottlieb, N.L.: Gold metabolism (letter to the editor). Arthritis Rheum. 17:1057, 1974.

107. Ghadially, F.N., Oryschak, A.F., and Mitchell, D.M.: Ultrastructural changes produced in rheumatoid synovial membrane by chrysotherapy. Ann. Rheum. Dis. 35:67, 1976.

108. Nakamura, H., and Igarashi, M.: Localization of gold in synovial membrane of rheumatoid arthritis treated with sodium aurothiomalate. Ann. Rheum. Dis. 36:209, 1977.

109. Penneys, N.S., Kramer, K., and Gottlieb, N.L.: The quantitative distribution of gold in skin during chrysotherapy. J. Invest. Dermatol. 65:331, 1975.

110. Cox, A.J.: Gold in the dermis following gold therapy for rheumatoid arthritis. Arch. Dermatol. 108:655, 1973.

111. Viol, G.F., Minielly, J.A., and Bistricki, T.: Gold nephropathy: Tissue analysis by x-ray fluorescent spectroscopy. Arch. Pathol. Lab. Med. 101:635, 1977.

112. Kamel, H., Brown, D.G., Ottaway, J.M., Smith, W.E., Cottney, J., and Lewis, A.J.: A comparison of tissue gold levels in guinea pigs after treatment with Myochrysine intramuscularly and triethylphosphine gold chloride and Myochrysine administered orally. Agents Action 8:546, 1978.

113. Walz, D.T., Griswold, D.E., DiMartino, J., and Bumbier, E.E.: Distribution of gold in blood following administration of auranofin. J. Rheumatol. 6 (Suppl. 5): 56, 1979.

114. Gottlieb, N.L.: Comparative pharmacokinetics of parenteral and oral gold compounds. J. Rheumatol. 9 (Suppl. 8): 99, 1982.

115. Gerber, R.C., Paulus, H.E., and Jennrich, R.I.: Gold kinetics following aurothiomalate therapy: Use of a whole-body radiation counter. J. Lab. Clin. Med. 83:778, 1974.

116. Rubinstein, H.M., and Dietz, A.A.: Serum gold-levels in rheumatoid arthritis. Ann. Rheum. Dis. 32:128, 1973.

117. van Riel, P.L.C.M., Gribnau, F.W.J., and van de Putte, L.B.A.: Cell-bound gold in patients treated with aurothioglucose and with auranofin. A comparison of different methods of determination. J. Rheumatol. 10:574, 1983.

118. Blocka, K., Furst, D.E., Landaw, E., Dromgoole, S., Blomberg, A., and Paulus, H.E.: Single-dose pharmacokinetics of auranofin in rheumatoid arthritis. J. Rheumatol. 9 (Suppl. 8): 110, 1982.

119. Campion, D.S., Olsen, R., and Bohan, A.: Interaction of gold sodium thiomalate with serum albumin (abstract). J. Rheumatol. 1 (Suppl.): 112, 1974.

120. Lorber, A., Bovy, R.A., and Chang, C.C.: Relationship between serum gold content and distribution to serum immunoglobulins and complement. Nature New Biol. 236:250, 1972.

121. Smith, P.M., Smith, E.M., and Gottlieb, N.L.: Gold distribution in whole blood during chrysotherapy. J. Lab. Clin. Med. 82:930, 1973.

122. Lorber, A., Simon, T., and Wilcox, S.: In vivo gold kinetics—lymphocyte binding and effect on lymphocyte responsiveness (abstract). Arthritis Rheum. 20:126, 1977.

123. Graham, G.G., Haavisto, T.M., McNaught, P.J., Browne, C.D., and Champion, G.D.: The effect of smoking on the distribution of gold in blood. J. Rheumatol. 9:527, 1982.

124. James, D.W., Ludvigsen, N.W., Cleland, L.G., and Milazzo, S.C.: The influence of cigarette smoking on blood gold distribution during chrysotherapy. J. Rheumatol. 9:532, 1982.

125. Gottlieb, N.L., Smith, P.M., and Penneys, N.S.: Gold concentrations in hair, nail and skin during chrysotherapy. Arthritis Rheum. 17:56, 1974.

126. Weisman, M.H., Hardison, G.M., and Walz, D.: Studies of the intestinal metabolism of oral gold. J. Rheumatol. 7:633, 1980.

127. Lawrence, J.S.: Studies with radioactive gold. Ann. Rheum. Dis. 20:341, 1961.

128. Marmon, B.P., and Goodburn, G.M.: Effect of an organic gold salt on Eaton's primary atypical pneumonia agent and other observations. Nature 189:247, 1961.

129. Pruzanski, W., Leers, W.D., and Wardlaw, A.C.: Bacteriolytic and bactericidal activity of sera and synovial fluids in rheumatoid arthritis and in osteoarthritis. Arthritis Rheum. 17:207, 1974.

130. Persellin, R.H., and Ziff, M.: The effect of gold salt on lysosomal enzymes of the peritoneal macrophage. Arthritis Rheum. 9:57, 1966.

131. Paltemaa, S.: The inhibition of lysosomal enzymes by gold salts in human synovial fluid cells. Acta Rheum. Scand. 14:161, 1968.

132. Penneys, N.S., Ziboh, V., Gottlieb, N.L., and Simon, E.: Inhibition of prostaglandin synthesis and human epidermal enzymes by aurothiomalate in vitro: Possible actions of gold in pemphigus. J. Invest. Dermatol. 63:356, 1974.

133. Ennis, R.S., Granda, J.L., and Posner, A.S.: Effect of gold salts and other drugs on the release and activity of lysosomal hydrolases. Arthritis Rheum. 11:756, 1968.

134. Jessop, J.D., Vernon-Roberts, B., and Harris, J.: Effects of gold salts and prednisolone on inflammatory cells. Ann. Rheum. Dis. 32:294, 1973.

135. Niedermeier, W., Prillaman, W.W., and Griggs, J.H.: The effect of chrysotherapy on trace metals in patients with rheumatoid arthritis. Arthritis Rheum. 14:533, 1971.

136. Gerber, D.A.: Copper-catalyzed thermal aggregation of human gamma-globulin: inhibition by histidine, gold thiomalate, and penicillamine. Arthritis Rheum. 17:85, 1974.

137. Schultz, D.R., Volanakis, J.E., Arnold, P.I., et al.: Inactivation of C1 in rheumatoid synovial fluid, purified C1 and C1 esterase, by gold compounds. Clin. Exp. Immunol. 17:395, 1974.

138. Burge, J.J., Fearson, D.T., and Austen, K.F.: Inhibition of the alternative pathway of complement by gold sodium thiomalate in vitro. J. Immunol. 120:1625, 1978.

139. Libensen, L.: Toxicity and mode of action of the gold salts. Exp. Med. Surg. 3:146, 1945.

140. Castor, C.W.: Connective tissue activation. Arthritis Rheum. 15:504, 1972.

141. Lipsky, P.E., and Ziff, M.: Inhibition of antigen- and mitogen-induced human lymphocyte proliferation by gold compounds. J. Clin. Invest. 59:455, 1977.

142. Lies, R.B., Cardin, C., and Paulus, H.E.: Inhibition by gold of human lymphocyte stimulation. Ann. Rheum. Dis. 36:216, 1977.

143. Ho, P.P.K., Young, A.L., and Southard, G.L.: Methyl ester of N-formylmethionyl-leucyl-phenylalanine. Chemotactic responses of human blood monocytes and inhibition of gold compounds. Arthritis Rheum. 21:133, 1978.

144. Mowat, A.G.: Neutrophil chemotaxis in rheumatoid arthritis. Ann. Rheum. Dis. 37:1, 1978.

145. Measel, J.W., Jr.: Effect of gold on the immune response of mice. Infect. Immun. 11:350, 1975.

146. Ghaffar, A., McBride, W.H., and Cullen, R.T.: Interaction of tumor cells and activated macrophages in vitro: Modulation by Corynebacterium parvum and gold salt. J. Reticuloendothel. Soc. 20:283, 1976.

147. Persellin, R.H., Hess, E.V., and Ziff, M.: Effect of gold salt on the immune response. Arthritis Rheum. 10:99, 1967.

148. Clarke, A.K., Vernon-Roberts, B., and Currey, H.L.F.: Assessment of anti-inflammatory drugs in the rat using subcutaneous implants of polyurethane foam impregnated with dead tubercle bacilli. Ann. Rheum. Dis. 34:326, 1975.

149. Adam, M., Bartl, P., Deyl, Z., et al.: Uptake of gold by collagen in gold therapy. Ann. Rheum. Dis. 24:378, 1965.

150. Walz, D.T., DiMartino, M.J., and Misher, A.: Suppression of adjuvant-induced arthritis in the rat by gold sodium thiomalate. Ann. Rheum. Dis. 30:303, 1971.

151. Lewis, A.J., and Walz, D.T.: Immunopharmacology of gold. In Ellis, J.P., and West, G.B. (eds.): Progress in Medicinal Chemistry. Vol. 19. New York, Elsevier Biomedical Press, 1982, pp. 1–58.

152. Halla, J.T., Cassady, J., and Hardin, J.G.: Sequential gold and penicillamine therapy in rheumatoid arthritis: Comparative study of effectiveness and review of the literature. Am. J. Med. 72:423, 1982.

153. Kean, F.W., Lock, C.J.L., Howard-Lock, H.E., and Buchanan, W.W.: Prior gold therapy does not influence the adverse effects of D-penicillamine in rheumatoid arthritis. Arthritis Rheum. 25:917, 1982.

154. Webley, M., and Coomes, E.N.: An assessment of penicillamine therapy in rheumatoid arthritis and the influence of previous gold therapy. J. Rheumatol. 6:20, 1979.

155. Liang, M.H., and Fries, J.F.: Containing costs in chronic disease: Monitoring strategies in the gold therapy of rheumatoid arthritis. J. Rheumatol. 5:241, 1978.

156. Penneys, N.S., Ackerman, A.B., and Gottlieb, N.L.: Gold dermatitis. Arch. Dermatol. 109:372, 1974.

157. Iveson, J.M., Scott, D.G., Perera, W.D.H., et al.: Immunofluorescence of the skin in gold rashes—with particular reference to IgE. Ann. Rheum. Dis. 36:520, 1977.

158. Klinefelter, H.F.: Reinstitution of gold therapy in rheumatoid arthritis after mucocutaneous reactions. J. Rheumatol. 2:21, 1975.

159. Gottlieb, N.L., and Gray, R.G.: Diagnosis and management of adverse reactions from gold compounds. J. Anal. Tox. 2:173, 1978.

160. Beckett, V.L., Doyle, J.A., Hadley, G.A., and Spear, K.L.: Chrysiasis resulting from gold therapy in rheumatoid arthritis: Identification of gold by x-ray microanalysis. Mayo Clin. Proc. 57:773, 1982.

161. Jeffery, D.A., Biggs, D.F., Percy, J.S., and Russell, A.S.: Quantitation of gold in skin in chrysiasis. J. Rheumatol. 2:28, 1975.

162. Silverberg, D.S., Kidd, E.G., and Shnitka, T.K.: Gold nephropathy. A clinical and pathologic study. Arthritis Rheum. 13:812, 1970.

163. Törnroth, T., and Skrifvars, B.: Gold nephropathy prototype of membranous glomerulonephritis. Am. J. Pathol. 75:573, 1974.

164. Vaamonde, C.A., and Hunt, F.R.: The nephrotic syndrome as a complication of gold therapy. Arthritis Rheum. 13:826, 1970.

165. Davis, P., and Hughes, G.R.V.: Significance of eosinophilia during gold therapy. Arthritis Rheum. 17:964, 1974.

166. Deren, B., Masi, R., and Weksler, M.: Gold-associated thrombocytopenia. Arch. Intern. Med. 134:1012, 1974.

167. Stafford, B.T., and Crosby, W.H.: Late onset of gold-induced thrombocytopenia. JAMA 239:50, 1978.

168. McCarty, D.J., Brill, J.M., and Harrop, D.: Aplastic anemia secondary to gold-salt therapy: Report of a fatal case and a review of the literature. JAMA 179:655, 1962.

169. Harris, B.K.: Myocardial infarction after a gold-induced nitritoid reaction (letter to editor). Arthritis Rheum. 20:1561, 1977.

170. Winterbauer, R.H., Wilske, K.R., and Wheelis, R.F.: Diffuse pulmonary injury associated with gold treatment. N. Engl. J. Med. 294:919, 1976.

171. Gould, P.W., McCormack, P.L., and Palmer, D.G.: Pulmonary damage associated with sodium aurothiomalate therapy. J. Rheumatol. 4:252, 1977.

172. Favreau, M., Tannenbaum, H., and Lough, J.: Hepatic toxicity associated with gold therapy. Ann. Intern. Med. 87:717, 1977.

173. Howrie, D.L., and Gartner, Jr. J.C.: Gold-induced hepatotoxicity: Case report and review of the literature. J. Rheumatol. 9:727, 1982.

174. Stein, H.B., and Urowitz, M.B.: Gold-induced enterocolitis. J. Rheumatol. 3:21, 1976.

175. Fam, A.G., Paton, T.W., Shamess, C.J., and Lewis, A.J.: Fulminant colitis complicating gold therapy. J. Rheumatol. 7:479, 1980.

176. Hashimoto, A., Maeda, Y., Ito, H., et al.: Corneal chrysiasis—a clinical study in rheumatoid arthritis patients receiving gold therapy. Arthritis Rheum. 15:309, 1972.

177. Prouse, P.J., Kanski, J.J., and Gumpel, J.M.: Corneal Chrysiasis and clinical improvement with chrysotherapy in rheumatoid arthritis. Ann. Rheum. Dis. 40:564, 1981.

178. Wooley, P.H., Griffin, J., Panayi, G.S., Batchelor, J.R., Welsh, K.I., and Gibson, T.J.: HLA-DR antigens and toxic reaction to sodium thiomalate and D-penicillamine in patients with rheumatoid arthritis. N. Engl. J. Med. 303:300, 1980.

179. Coblyn, J.S., Weinblatt, M., Holdsworth, D., and Glass, D.: Gold-induced thrombocytopenia: A clinical and immunogenetic study of 23 patients. Ann. Intern. Med. 95:178, 1981.

180. Gran, J.T., Husby, G., and Thorsby, E.: HLA-DR antigens and gold toxicity. Ann. Rheum. Dis. 42:63, 1983.

181. Levinson, M.L., Lynch, J.P., III, and Bower, J.S.: Reversal of progressive, life-threatening gold hypersensitivity pneumonitis by corticosteroids. Am. J. Med. 71:908, 1981.

182. Gerber, R.C., and Paulus, H.E.: Gold therapy. Clin. Rheum. Dis. 1:307, 1975.

183. Lorber, A., Baumgartner, W.A., Bovy, R.A., et al.: Clinical application for heavy metal-complexing potential of acetylcysteine. J. Clin. Pharmacol. 13:332, 1973.

184. Bunch, T.W.: Gold overdose treated with BAL (letter editor). Arthritis Rheum. 19:123, 1976.

185. Godfrey, N.F., Peter, A., Simon, T.M., and Lorber, A.: IV. N-Acetylcysteine treatment of hematologic reaction to chrysotherapy. J. Rheumatol. 9:519, 1982.

186. Davis, P., and Barraclough, D.: Interaction of D-penicillamine with gold salts. Arthritis Rheum. 20:1413, 1977.

187. Schaeffer, N., Shaw, C.F., Thompson, H.O., and Satre, R.W.: Competition for protein-bound gold (1). Arthritis Rheum. 23:165, 1980.

188. Saphir, J.R., and Ney, R.G.: Delayed thrombocytopenic purpura after diminutive gold therapy. JAMA 195:7, 1966.

189. Ball, G.V.: Gold-induced thrombocytopenia: Response to vincristine? (letter to editor). Arthritis Rheum. 20:1288, 1977.

190. Marriott, H.J.L., and Peters, H.R.: Blood dyscrasias secondary to gold: With a case of hypoplastic anemia cured by splenectomy. Ann. Intern. Med. 32:864, 1950.

191. Gottlieb, N.L., Buchoff, H.S., Vidal, A.F., Germain, B.F., Gray, R.G., and Goldberg, E.S.: The course of severe gold-associated granulocytopenia. Clin. Res. 30:659-A, 1982 (Abstr.).

192. Baldwin, J.L., Storb, R., Thomas, E.D., et al.: Bone marrow transplantation in patients with gold-induced marrow aplasia. Arthritis Rheum. 20:1043, 1977.

193. Combs, R.J., Dentino, M.M., Lehrman, L., et al.: Gold toxicity and peritoneal dialysis. Arthritis Rheum. 19:936, 1976.

Chapter 53

D-Penicillamine

Israeli A. Jaffe

Penicillamine is a component of the penicillin molecule[1] which was identified in the urine of patients with chronic liver disease who were receiving penicillin for the treatment of intercurrent infections.[2] Walshe demonstrated its effectiveness as a copper chelating agent and introduced it into the treatment of Wilson's disease.[3] In addition, it has been shown to be effective in treatment of cystinuria,[4] heavy metal poisoning,[5] and rheumatoid arthritis (RA).[6] It has possible but as yet unproved efficacy in the management of biliary cirrhosis[7] and chronic active hepatitis.[8] It appears to have a role in the treatment of scleroderma,[9,10] but this has not been confirmed by controlled clinical trials.

CHEMISTRY

The structural formula of penicillamine (Fig. 53–1) shows that it is a sulfhydryl amino acid differing from cysteine by the presence of two methyl groups in the β-carbon position (β,β-dimethylcysteine, or 3-mercaptovaline). It may be prepared from natural penicillin by a semisynthetic process, or it may be made entirely synthetically. Regardless of the mode of preparation, all the penicillamine currently employed in clinical medicine is the pure D-form, and penicillamine will denote only the D-isomer unless otherwise specified.

METABOLISM

Penicillamine is well absorbed from the gastrointestinal tract but may react with certain constituents of the

Figure 53–1. The chemical structure of penicillamine. The drug is an analogue of the naturally occurring amino acid cysteine, with CH_3 groups replacing H^+ at the B carbon position.

diet, particularly metals,[11] and may also interact directly with other drugs in the upper gastrointestinal tract (see Dosage). Approximately 50 percent of an orally administered dose can be accounted for by analysis of urine and feces.[12] Using ^{14}C-D-penicillamine, recovery of radioactivity was 85 percent. The discrepancy between the results obtained by the chemical and radioactive measurements is believed to be due to bacterial degradation of the drug in the colon, which yields chemically nonidentifiable products.[12] Very little free penicillamine is found in the urine; most of it is present in the oxidized form, as either the internal disulfide (penicillamine-penicillamine) or the mixed disulfide (penicillamine-cysteine).[12] A third major metabolite has recently been identified, S-methyl penicillamine.[13] In animal studies using radioactive penicillamine, it was found that the drug had its greatest affinity and highest accumulation in collagen-containing organs such as skin and tendon, in contrast to liver and kidney.[14] There was also a high uptake in organs rich in protein content such as pancreas and testicle.[14] In the plasma, binding was greatest to albumin, α-globulin, and ceruloplasmin.[14] In dogs, it was found that following discontinuance of penicillamine the drug very rapidly disappeared from the urine; however, the mixed disulfide and internal disulfide were demonstrable for more than 3 months after the agent had been stopped.[15] This might explain the persistence of drug effect as well as certain of the toxicities for long periods after treatment has been discontinued.

CLINICAL PHARMACOLOGY

Penicillamine is prepared as a 250 mg or 125 mg capsule or scored tablet of 250 mg, and a 50 mg tablet is also available in England. The pharmacologic properties of the compound that have been demonstrated to occur in man are chelation of divalent cations,[3] SH-SS interchange,[16] and thiazolidine formation, which gives rise to dermolathyrism[17] and vitamin B_6 antagonism.[18] It is not known whether any of these actions are responsible for the antirheumatoid properties of the drug. The chelating properties form the basis for its use in the treatment of Wilson's disease and heavy metal poisoning. When administered to patients with RA or cystinuria, a minimal depletion of copper and zinc has been reported,[19] but this is generally well compensated for in a normal diet.[20] Depletion of these metals may, however, be partially responsible for the development of taste abnormalities (see below). The SH-SS interchange reaction between penicillamine and cystine gives rise to the mixed disulfide, penicillamine-cysteine.[16] This is considerably more soluble than cystine and results in a decrease in size of cystine calculi, and their ultimate dissolution.[4] The anti-vitamin B_6 effect of penicillamine is due to the formation of a thiazolidine between penicillamine and pyridoxal phosphate.[18] The anti-vitamin B_6 effect does not appear to be clinically significant, since concomitant administration of the vitamin does not influence either the efficacy of the drug or the incidence of side effects.[21] Vitamin B_6 supplements are recommended, however, for growing children and adult patients whose nutrition is marginal.

The dermolathyrogenic effect of penicillamine is also due to thiazolidine formation—in this reaction, between penicillamine and the aldehyde cross-links of collagen[22] (see Chapters 14 and 76). This may be demonstrated in skin biopsies from patients receiving penicillamine, particularly when given in large doses.[23] Wound healing is not impaired in patients receiving penicillamine.[24] The collagen formed in wound healing is the type III or embryonal form, whose keto crosslinks do not react with penicillamine, in contrast to the aldehyde crosslinks of type I collagen.[25]

INDICATIONS

Penicillamine is effective in treatment of active RA, seropositive or seronegative, and in patients with juvenile rheumatoid arthritis.[26] Its efficacy was first established by the United Kingdom Multi-Center trial,[27] and subsequent controlled clinical trials showed that it was as effective as gold[28] and azathioprine.[29] It was found that a 600-mg daily dose gave a therapeutic result comparable (statistically) to that produced by 1200 mg, with considerably fewer side effects and withdrawals.[30] It has been of particular value in RA associated with certain extra-articular manifestations, such as vasculitis,[31] rheumatoid lung disease,[32] Felty's syndrome,[33] rheumatoid nodulosis,[34] and amyloidosis.[35] A recent report demonstrated radiographic evidence of healing of osseous lesions in a child with juvenile rheumatoid arthritis (JRA) treated with penicillamine.[36]

Penicillamine is not effective in ankylosing spondylitis,[37] psoriatic arthritis, or other B-27 associated diseases for which it has been tried.[38] There have been further reports of the usefulness of penicillamine in the treatment of progressive systemic sclerosis[9,10] (see Chapter 76). These studies are anecdotal and retrospective, and a controlled clinical trial of penicillamine in this disease now seems warranted.

DOSAGE

Because of the high incidence of toxic and untoward reactions to the drug (see below), there have been continuous modifications in the dosage regimens employed for its use in RA.[39-41] The basic principle underlying all these schedules is that the drug is introduced gradually, with slow increments, until a clinical response is achieved. Usually, that dose may have to be adjusted according to the changing pattern of disease activity.

From the time that therapy is initiated to the earliest evidence of clinical response, a period of 8 to 12 weeks may be required. A similar latency is noted after increase or decrease in dosage. As a result, it is currently recommended that increments in the maintenance dose of penicillamine be made at 8- to 12-week intervals, particularly since the *rate of dosage increment* appears to be a more significant determinant for the development of certain untoward effects than the absolute magnitude of the maintenance dose.[41] Typically, a patient will be started at a single daily dosage of 250 mg, given approximately 1½ hours before a meal, and not together with any other medication.[42,43] If there is no clinical or laboratory evidence of response after approximately 2 months, the dosage is raised to 500 mg, which may also be given once daily. Alternatively, some workers include a treatment period at 375 mg per day after 8 weeks, rather than directly doubling the starting dose. At the end of 6 months, most patients who will benefit from the drug will have shown some evidence of clinical improvement. If required, the dose may be raised to 750 mg for the next 12 weeks and, in a limited number of cases, to 1000 mg a day, preferably given in a single dose. As indicated earlier, the maintenance dose of penicillamine is highly variable not only from patient to patient but in the evolution of the individual patient's own treatment program, and the aforementioned outline serves only as a guide. The availability of the 125-mg dosage form permits somewhat greater flexibility and better adjustments of the maintenance dose. In some patients who have shown an incomplete response, an increase in the daily dose by 125 mg may provide greater suppression of the disease without added toxicity. In addition, as will be indicated below, certain side effects are dose related, and a reduction in the maintenance level by as little as 125 mg per day may result in disappearance of an untoward reaction without significantly compromising the quality of the response. The 125-mg dosage is also useful in children with JRA, for whom the average daily dose is 500 to 625 mg.[44] Some patients report an increase in articular discomfort when therapy is begun. This usually subsides with time, but may be dose limiting and require discontinuance of therapy in some cases.

RESPONSE PATTERN

The pattern of improvement in a penicillamine-responsive patient is similar to that observed with a remission induced by gold salts. There is a gradual decrease in the *duration* of morning stiffness and in the severity and intensity of pain. This is often followed by a diminution in swelling, effusion, and the size of nodules. Often, patients will report an increased sense of well-being and a decrease in easy fatigability. Later in the course of treatment, laboratory studies will often reveal a fall in the RF titer, decrease in the ESR, and a rise in hemoglobin.[21]

When penicillamine therapy is begun, analgesics and anti-inflammatory drugs, including steroids, must be continued. As the clinical response evolves, these agents may be gradually decreased, although steroid withdrawal often requires several years to be completed. Exacerbations in rheumatoid disease activity may be seen during the first 1 to 2 years of therapy; however, these are often self-limited and usually subside within a 2- to 3-month period without the necessity of an increase in dosage. Late in the course of treatment, true secondary failures have been observed. In some patients, discontinuance of the drug for 6 to 12 months followed by gradual reintroduction may again give a good therapeutic response.

SIDE EFFECTS AND TOXICITY

The toxicities and untoward effects that may be produced by penicillamine are many and diverse and have limited its clinical usefulness. As indicated previously, experience with the newer dosage regimens has shown that certain of these side effects can be reduced in frequency and severity by the practice of "go low—go very slow." These reactions have been reported in patients given penicillamine regardless of their underlying disease, but most published reports of toxicity are in RA patients, since they comprise the largest number exposed to the drug. It has been observed that most of the side effects will be encountered during the first 18 months of therapy (Fig. 53–2), and it is less likely for a major toxic reaction to appear for the first time after that period.[45]

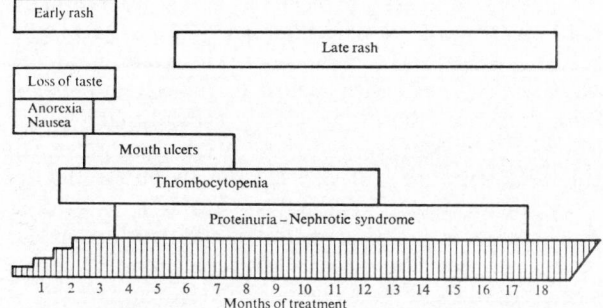

Figure 53–2. The chronopharmacology of penicillamine. (After Balme, H.W., and Huskisson, E.C.: J. Rheumatol. 4:Suppl. 8, 21-07, 1975.) This depicts the peak incidence of some of the more common side effects of penicillamine during a course of therapy with a maintenance dose of 1 gram per day. Most of the serious reactions will have developed during the first 18 months of treatment. Aplastic anemia was not included in this illustration, but it may occur at any time, particularly after an increment in dosage.

Hematologic toxicity is certainly the most serious of the untoward effects that may be produced by penicillamine. *Leukopenia, thrombocytopenia,* and *aplastic anemia* have all been observed. Thrombocytopenia may occur as an isolated event, when it may respond to a reduction in dosage, or it may herald the development of more widespread bone marrow failure. The presence of normal numbers of megakaryocytes in the bone marrow will resolve this question. A white blood cell count below 3000 per cubic millimeter or a platelet count below 100,000 per cubic millimeter mandates a temporary discontinuance of the drug until the severity of the reaction can be assessed. Complete blood counts, including platelet counts, must be done every 2 weeks for the first 6 months and monthly thereafter. Prescriptions for penicillamine should *never be labeled refillable.* If aplastic anemia develops, the patient should be hospitalized and placed in reverse isolation. Immediately after cultures have been obtained, a parenteral antibiotic regimen is instituted consisting of carbenicillin, 10 grams every 8 hours, oxacillin, 2 grams every 6 hours, and gentamicin, 80 mg every 8 hours. Mycostatin oral suspension, 15 ml by mouth every 4 hours, is given in an oral lavage, which is swirled and then swallowed. If the patient has been on corticosteroids, these must be maintained, but they should not be *added* to the regimen for the management of aplastic anemia. In some patients with thrombocytopenia only, steroids may be required to control bleeding. Weeks and rarely months may elapse before marrow function commences to return. During this time, the patient remains in constant risk of sepsis, and continued vigilance is mandatory. Granulocyte transfusions have not been effective, but fresh platelets have sometimes helped in an acute hemorrhagic crisis due to thrombocytopenia. Patients who have had major hematologic toxicity to penicillamine should never be rechallenged with the drug. In some patients who had thrombocytopenia only, retreatment has been accomplished without recurrence of the toxicity.

Proteinuria is secondary to an immune-complex, membranous glomerulopathy (Fig. 53–3) and has been encountered in up to 20 percent of patients receiving the drug.[46] Although the peak incidence for development of this side effect is usually between 6 and 9 months after commencement of treatment, proteinuria may clear with a slight reduction in daily dosage such as 125 to 250 mg. A complete urinalysis should be performed according to the same schedule as the hematologic studies. If urinary protein excretion exceeds 2 grams per 24 hours or if there is evidence of *nephrotic syndrome* or *gross hematuria,* the treatment should be terminated and the patient not rechallenged. After discontinuance of the drug, a period of up to 1 year may be required for urinary abnormalities to disappear completely. In patients who have been studied with renal biopsy following withdrawal of the drug, there was healing of the lesions and disappearance of the immune complexes.[47] Microscopic hematuria during the course of penicillamine treatment has been found to be a benign occurrence and does not mandate discontinuance of therapy provided that it remains stable.[48]

Figure 53–3. Renal biopsy from a patient with nephrotic syndrome secondary to penicillamine. The basement membrane of the glomerulus stains in an intense granular pattern with fluorescinated anti-human IgG and fluorescinated anti-human complement. Staining gradually disappears after treatment has been discontinued.

Dermatological reactions include skin rash, which is probably the most common of the side effects encountered with the drug. Simple pruritus can often be controlled by the addition of an antihistamine such as hydroxyzine (Atarax) or cyproheptadine (Periactin). Often pruritus and mild rash will be transitory and will clear despite continuance of the medication. Late rashes tend to be unresponsive to antihistamine therapy or to reduction in dosage, and generally require discontinuance of the drug. The occurrence of the skin rash and oral lesions simultaneously should alert the clinician to the possibility of a pemphigoid type reaction, which mandates discontinuance of the drug[49] (see below).

Mucous membrane lesions similar to those seen in aphthous stomatitis have been observed. Oral (or genital) ulcers may clear on reduction of the maintenance dose, but often therapy must be discontinued and the patient not rechallenged.

Autoimmune syndromes also occur. Penicillamine administration has been reported to be responsible for the development of Goodpasture's syndrome,[50] myasthenia gravis,[51] polymyositis,[52] pemphigus,[49] lupus erythematosus,[53] and Sjögren's syndrome.[54] While the number of individual case reports of each of these entities has been few, a high index of suspicion is warranted should a patient receiving penicillamine develop features of any of these syndromes. In such an instance, the drug must be discontinued and the patient not rechallenged. As noted previously with other toxicities, these entities have been encountered in patients receiving penicillam-

ine regardless of their underlying disease. It is not the rheumatoid diathesis per se that predisposes to their development, and the mechanism by which penicillamine produces these autoimmune phenomena is not understood (see below).

Hypogeusia or blunting or loss of taste perception is very commonly encountered and may persist for up to 3 months following its onset. It gradually clears even though therapy is continued, and patients should be urged not to discontinue the drug because of this particular reaction. Some investigators report an accelerated return to normal taste if supplements of copper or zinc are given,[55] but it has been shown that with the lower dosages of penicillamine currently employed, such supplementation may abrogate the therapeutic response.[56] No instances of permanent taste impairment have been reported.

In addition, certain miscellaneous side effects may infrequently be encountered. Drug fever has been described. It occurs usually during the third week of therapy, and is often associated with a morbilliform eruption. When the drug is stopped, fever and rash quickly subside, but these patients should not be rechallenged. Other side effects which have been infrequently observed have been a benign enlargement of the breasts (mammary gigantism)[57] and hepatotoxicity.[58]

INDICATIONS, CONTRAINDICATIONS, AND PRECAUTIONS

As indicated previously, penicillamine is employed in the treatment of patients with RA, seropositive or seronegative, whose disease has not responded to general, conservative measures. It usually will be considered after a trial of chrysotherapy has been abandoned, because of either toxicity or failure of response. Some workers will employ penicillamine before gold salts, particularly if there are present certain of the extra-articular manifestations which have been shown to be favorably influenced by penicillamine therapy.

Penicillamine is contraindicated in pregnancy, although the literature is in some conflict on this point.[59,60]

A history of allergy to penicillin is *not* a contraindication to the use of penicillamine.[61] There have been multiple studies on the relation of prior gold therapy to penicillamine, both with regard to toxicity and therapeutic response. There is general agreement that a failure to respond to either one of these drugs does not mean that the alternative will also fail. Furthermore, the development of a particular adverse reaction to gold or penicillamine is not a predictor of the development of the same or any other toxicity with the alternative drug. It is acknowledged that patients who develop a serious toxicity to gold, particularly proteinuria, are more likely to have proteinuria during penicillamine, but this is far from absolute.[62-65]

As indicated above, prescriptions for penicillamine should *never be made refillable.* Since hematologic toxicity may be precipitate in onset and develop in the

Figure 53–4. The effect of penicillamine therapy on complexes as measured by precipitation with a purified IgM rheumatoid factor. (Courtesy of Dr. Robert Winchester.) Well No. 1 contains synovial fluid, and well No. 2 contains serum from the same patient prior to treatment. Well No. 3 shows a decrease in the amount of complexes after 6 weeks on the drug. Wells No. 4 and No. 5 show the absence of serum complexes at 3 and 6 months, respectively. Well C is normal serum. A serial examination of synovial fluid was not possible as the effusion had reabsorbed.

interval between routine blood studies, patients should be alerted to report to the physician if they develop any evidence of mucocutaneous bleeding or unexplained fever. Bone marrow toxicity is particularly likely to occur *after a dosage increment*; hence careful surveillance is especially needed at these times. Patients over the age of 60 are at greater risk for development of hematologic toxicity and hence require more close supervision.

In summary, penicillamine therapy must be discontinued in the event that any of the following untoward reactions develop: aplastic anemia, leukopenia below 3000 per cubic millimeter, thrombocytopenia below 100,000 per cubic millimeter, nephrotic syndrome, increasing hematuria persistent for more than 30 days, or any of the autoimmune syndromes described above.

MECHANISM OF ACTION

The mechanism of action of penicillamine in RA, like that for gold salts, is not known. The drug is neither cytotoxic[66] nor anti-inflammatory,[67] and it is virtually without effect in animal models of experimental arthritis.[68] It has been shown that the prolonged administration of penicillamine to RA patients is associated with a reduction in or disappearance of immune complexes, in both the serum and synovial fluid (Figs. 53–4 and 53–5).[69] Whether this reduction in complexes is the mechanism by which penicillamine exerts its therapeutic effect or is simply a reflection of a more basic action, analogous to the fall in RF titer, is not clear at this time.

The effect of penicillamine on lymphocyte transformation in vitro has been the subject of study by several investigators. Some workers have shown an inhibition of transformation in the presence of the drug,[70,71] while others found that it enhanced responsiveness to mitogen.[72] This apparent discrepancy may be due to differences in experimental design, especially variation in timing of the addition of the penicillamine with respect to the mitogen. In vitro, the addition of copper in minute amounts to cell cultures with penicillamine greatly augments the suppression of lymphocyte responsiveness.[73] In a subsequent study, this synergistic inhibition by penicillamine and copper salts was found to be restricted solely to human helper T lymphocytes; suppressor T lymphocytes and B lymphocytes were not affected.[74]

Figure 53–5. The ultracentrifugal pattern of serum proteins before treatment (top) and after 3 months on the drug (bottom). (Kindly performed by Dr. Henry Kunkel.) Serum was diluted 1:1 with saline. Centrifugation was at 52,640 rpm and proceeds from left to right. Pictures were taken at 16, 32, 48, 64, 80, and 90 minutes. The post-treatment pattern shows a reduction in the 22S complex, 19S macroglobulin, and the intermediate gamma globulin complexes.

Peripheral blood lymphocytes obtained from patients receiving penicillamine, show a normal response to mitogenic stimulation.[75] Other possible explanations for the mode of action that have been suggested are the copper chelating properties,[76] the anti-vitamin B_6 effect,[77] the effect on collagen, and the inhibition by penicillamine in vitro of the denaturation of human gamma globulin.[78]

The effect of penicillamine on lymphocyte subpopulations is currently under investigation in several laboratories. The autoimmune syndromes produced by the drug have generated considerable interest with respect to the possibility that they might represent a clue as to the primary locus of action of the agent in RA. Simple haptene formation could explain certain of the autoimmune phenomena. A haptene between penicillamine and the interepithelial cement substance in skin, for example, could explain the development of pemphigus. Similar haptene formation between penicillamine and acetylcholine receptor might be expected to elicit antibody, resulting in development of clinical myasthenia gravis.[79] There is, however, an alternative explanation which has been suggested for these phenomena. An effect of penicillamine on a subpopulation of T lymphocytes might result in enhancement of certain components of the immune system, resulting in a partial loss of tolerance to self antigens. Such a perturbation of the immunoregulatory mechanism might be of therapeutic value in RA. The report of a patient who experienced both penicillamine-induced nephrotic syndrome and pemphigus[80] and the increased association of spontaneous myasthenia and pemphigus[81,82] indirectly support this hypothesis. Immunomodulation and immune enhancement are currently subjects of increasing interest with respect to their possible therapeutic implications in RA[83,84] (Chapter 55). It is perhaps relevant in this regard that thymic and lymph node hyperplasia was consistently found in rhesus monkeys during chronic penicillamine administration,[85] and thymic hyperplasia was recently reported in a penicillamine-treated RA patient who was subjected to thymectomy after development of drug-induced myasthenia gravis.[86]

References

1. Abraham, E.P., Chain, E., Baker, W., and Robinson, R.: Penicillamine: A characteristic degradation product of penicillin. Nature 151:107, 1943.
2. Walshe, J.M.: Disturbances of amino acid metabolism following liver injury. Quart. J. Med. 22:483, 1953.
3. Walshe, J.M.: Wilson's disease. New oral therapy. Lancet 1:25, 1956.
4. Crawhall, J.C., Scowen, E.F., and Watts, R.W.E.: Effects of penicillamine on cystinuria. Br. Med. J. 1:588, 1963.
5. Boulding, J.E., and Baker, R.A.: The treatment of metal poisoning with penicillamine. Lancet 2:985, 1957.
6. Jaffe, I.A.: Comparison of the effect of plasmapheresis and penicillamine on the level of circulating rheumatoid factor. Ann. Rheum. Dis. 22:71, 1963.
7. Jain, S., Scheuer, P.J., Samourian, S., McGee, J. O'D., and Sherlock, S.: A controlled trial of D-penicillamine in primary biliary cirrhosis. Lancet 1:831, 1977.
8. Stern, R.B., Wilkinson, S.P., Howorth, P.J.N., and Williams, R.: Controlled trial of synthetic D-penicillamine in maintenance therapy for active chronic hepatitis. Gut 18:19, 1977.
9. Kang, B., Veres-Thorner, C., Hereida, R., Cha, E., Bose, S., and Schwatrz, M.: Successful treatment of far-advanced progressive systemic sclerosis by D-penicillamine. J. Allergy Clin. Immunol. 69:297, 1982.
10. Steen, V.D., Medsger, T.A. Jr., and Rodnan, G.P.: D-Penicillamine therapy in progressive systemic sclerosis (scleroderma) a retrospective analysis. Ann. Intern Med. 97:652, 1982.
11. Lyle, W.H., and Pearcey, D.F.: Inhibition of penicillamine-induced cupruresis by oral iron. Proc. R. Soc. Med. 70(Suppl. 3):48, 1977.
12. Perett, D.: An outline of D-penicillamine metabolism. Proc. R. Soc. Med. 70 (Suppl. 3):61, 1977.
13. Perett, D., Sneddon, W., and Stephens, A.D.: Studies on D-penicillamine metabolism in cystinuria and rheumatoid arthritis: Isolation of S-methyl-D-penicillamine. Biochem. Pharmacol. 25:259, 1976.
14. Ruiz-Torres, A.: Zur Pharmakokinetik und zum Stoffwechsel von D- und L-Penicillamin, 2. Mitteilung: Verteilung von D- und L-Penicillamin-^{14}C im Organismus der Ratte nach peroraler Verabfolgung. Arzneim. Forsch. (Drug Res.) 24:1043, 1974.
15. Wei, P., and Sass-Kortsak, A.: Urinary excretion and renal clearances of D-penicillamine in humans and the dog. Gastroenterology 58:288, 970.
16. Tabachnik, M., Eisen, H.N., and Levine, B.: New mixed disulfide: Penicillamine-cysteine. Nature 174:701, 1954.
17. Nimni, M.E., and Bavetta, L.A.: Collagen defect induced by penicillamine. Science 150:905, 1965.
18. Kuchinskas, E.J., and du Vigneaud, V.: An increased vitamin B_6 requirement in the rat on a diet containing L-penicillamine. Arch. Biochem. 66:1, 1957.
19. Bostrom, H., and Wester, P.O.: Excretion of trace elements in two penicillamine-treated cases of cystinuria. Acta Med. Scand. 181:475, 1967.
20. Lyle, W.H.: Penicillamine and zinc. Lancet 2:1140, 1974.
21. Jaffe, I.A.: The effect of penicillamine on the laboratory parameters in rheumatoid arthritis. Arthritis Rheum. 8:1064, 1965.
22. Nimni, M.E., Deshmukh, K., Gerth, N., and Bavetta, L.A.: Changes in collagen metabolism associated with the administration of penicillamine and various amino and thiol compounds. Biochem. Pharmacol. 18:707, 1969.
23. Harris, E.D., and Sjoerdsma, A.: Effect of penicillamine on human collagen and its possible application to treatment of scleroderma. Lancet 2:996, 1966.
24. Ansell, B.M., Moran, H., and Arden, G.P.: Penicillamine and wound healing in rheumatoid arthritis. Proc. R. Soc. Med. 70(Suppl. 3):75, 1977.
25. Bailey, A.J., Bazin, S., Sims, T.J., Le Louis, M., Nicoletis, C., and Delaunay, A.: Characterization of the collagen of human hypertrophic and normal scars. Biochem. Biophys. Acta 405:412, 1975.
26. Hill, H.F.H.: Treatment of rheumatoid arthritis with penicillamine. Sem. Arthritis Rheum. 6:361, 1977.
27. Multi-Center Trial Group: Controlled trial of D(-) penicillamine in severe rheumatoid arthritis. Lancet 1:275, 1973.
28. Huskisson, E.C., Gibson, T.J., Balme, H.W., Berry, H., Burry, H.C., Grahame, R., Dudley Hart, F., Henderson, D.R.F., and Wojtulewski, J.A.: Trial comparing D-penicillamine and gold in rheumatoid arthritis. Preliminary report. Ann. Rheum. Dis. 33:532, 1974.
29. Berry, H., Liyange, R., Durance, C.G., and Berger, L.: Trial comparing azathioprine and penicillamine in treatment of rheumatoid arthritis. Ann. Rheum. Dis. 35:542, 1976.
30. Dixon, A. St. J., Davies, J., Dormandy, T.L., Hamilton, E.B.D., Holt, P.J.L., Mason, R.M., Thompson, M., Weber, J.C.P., and Zutshi, D.W.: Synthetic D(-) penicillamine in rheumatoid arthritis. Double-blind controlled study of a high and a low dosage regimen. Ann. Rheum. Dis. 34:416, 1975.
31. Jaffe, I.A.: Rheumatoid vasculitis report of a second case treated with penicillamine. Arthritis Rheum. 11:585, 1968.
32. Lorber, A.: Penicillamine therapy for rheumatoid lung disease: Effects of protein sulfhydryl groups. Nature 210:1235, 1966.
33. Blau, S., and Meiselas, L.: Regression of splenomegaly with hematologic recovery in Felty's syndrome due to D-penicillamine. A case report. Meadowbrook Hosp. J. 5:16, 1971–1972.
34. Ginsberg, M.H., Genant, H.K., Yü, T.S.F., and McCarty, D.J.: Rheumatoid nodulosis: An unusual variant of rheumatoid disease. Arthritis Rheum. 18:49, 1975.
35. Lake., B., and Andrews, G.: Rheumatoid arthritis with amyloidosis and malabsorption syndrome. Effect of D-penicillamine. Am. J. Med. 44:105, 1968.
36. Ansell, B.M.: Chronic arthritis in childhood. Ann. Rheum. Dis. 37:107, 1978.
37. Leca, A.P., and Camus, J.P.: Ankylosing spondylitis: Treatment failures with D-penicillamine. Nouv. Presse Med. 4:112, 1975.
38. Bird, H.A., and Dixon, A. St. J.: Failure of D-penicillamine to affect peripheral joint involvement in ankylosing spondylitis or HLA B-27 associated arthropathy. Ann. Rheum. Dis. 36:289, 1977.
39. Day, A.T., Golding, J.R., Lee, P.N., and Butterworth, A.D.: Penicillamine in rheumatoid disease: A long-term study. Br. Med. J. 1:180, 1974.
40. Jaffe, I.A.: The technique of penicillamine administration in rheumatoid arthritis. Arthritis Rheum. 18:513, 1975.
41. Jaffe, I.A.: D-Penicillamine. Bull. Rheum. Dis. 28:948, 1978.
42. Schnua, A., Osman, M.A., Patel, R.B., Welling, P.G., and Sundstrom,

W.R.: Influence of food on the bio-availability of penicillamine. J. Rheumatol. 10:95, 1983.

43. Harkness, J.A.L., and Blake, D.R.: Penicillamine nephropathy and iron. Lancet 2:1368, 1982.

44. Ansell, B., and Hall, M.: Penicillamine. Arthritis Rheum. 20(Suppl):536, 1977.

45. Balme, H.W., and Huskisson, E.C.: Chronopharmacology of penicillamine and gold. Scand. J. Rheumatol. 4(Suppl. 8):21, 1975.

46. Bacon, P.A., Tribe, C.R., Mackenzie, J.C., Verrier-Jones J., Cumming, R.H., and Amer, B.: Penicillamine nephropathy in rheumatoid arthritis. A clinical pathological and immunological study. Quart. J. Med. 45:661, 1976.

47. Jaffe, I.A., Treser, G., Suzuki, Y., and Ehrenreich, T.: Nephropathy induced by D-penicillamine. Ann. Intern. Med. 69:549, 1968.

48. Barraclough, D., Cunningham, T.J., and Muirden, K.D.: Microscopic haematuria in patients with rheumatoid arthritis on D-penicillamine. Aust. N. Z. J. Med. 11:706, 1981.

49. Benveniste, M., Crouzet, J., Homberg, J.C., Lessana, M., Camus, J.P., and Hewitt, J.: Pemphigus induced by D-penicillamine in rheumatoid arthritis. Nouv. Presse Med. 4:3125, 1975.

50. Sternlieb, I., Bennett, B., and Scheinberg, I.H.: D-Penicillamine induced Goodpasture's syndrome in Wilson's disease. Ann. Intern. Med. 82:673, 1975.

51. Bucknall, R.C., Dixon, A. St. J., and Glieb, E.N.: Myasthenia gravis associated with penicillamine treatment for rheumatoid arthritis. Br. Med. J. 1:600, 1975.

52. Schrader, P.L., Peters, H.A., and Dahl, D.S.: Polymyositis and penicillamine. Arch. Neurol. 27:456, 1972.

53. Crouzet, J., Camus, J.P., Leca, A.P., Guillien, P., and Lievre, J.A.: Lupus induced by D-penicillamine during the treatment of rheumatoid arthritis. Ann. Med. Interne 125:71, 1974.

54. May, V., Aristoff, H., and Lecoq, G.: Syndrome de Gougerot-Sjögren induit par la D-penicillamine. A propos d'un cas. Revue Rheumat. 44:497, 1977.

55. Henkin, R.I., Keiser, H.R., Jaffe, I.A., Sternlieb, I., and I.H.: Decreased taste sensitivity after D-penicillamine reversed by cooper administration. Lancet 2:1268, 1967.

56. Mery, C., Delrieu, F., Ghozlan, R., Saporta, F., Simon, B., Amor, C., Menkes, J., and Delbarre, F.: Controlled trial of D-penicillamine in rheumatoid arthritis. Dose effect and the role of zinc. Scand. J. Rheumatol. 5:241, 1976.

57. Desai, S.N.: Sudden gigantism of breasts: Drug induced? Br. J. Plast. Surg. 26:371, 1973.

58. Rosenbaum, J., Katz, W.A., and Schumacher, H.R.: Hepatotoxicity associated with use of D-penicillamine in rheumatoid arthritis. Ann. Rheum. Dis. 39:152, 1980.

59. Scheinberg, I.H., and Sternlieb, I.: Pregnancy in penicillamine treated patients with Wilson's disease. N. Engl. J. Med. 293:1300, 1975.

60. Mjolnerod, O.K., Rasmussen, K., Dommerud, S.A., and Gjeruldsen, S.T.: Congenital connective-tissue defect probably due to D-penicillamine. Lancet 1:673, 1971.

61. Bell, C.L., and Graziano, F.M.: The safety of administration of penicillamine to penicillin-sensitive individuals. Abstract, A.R.A. Ann. Meeting, Boston, Mass., 1981.

62. Webley, M., and Coomes, E.: An assessment of penicillamine therapy in rheumatoid arthritis and the influence of previous gold therapy. J. Rheumatol. 6:20, 1979.

63. Steven, M.M., Hunter, J.A., Murdoch, R.M., and Capell, H.A.: Does the order of second-line treatment in rheumatoid arthritis matter? Br. Med. J. 1:79, 1982.

64. Kean, W.F., Lock, C.J.L., Howard-Lock, H.E., and Buchanan, W.W.: Prior gold therapy does not influence the adverse effects of D-penicillamine in rheumatoid arthritis. Arthritis Rheum. 25:917, 1982.

65. Halla, J.T., Cassasy, J., and Hardin, J.G.: Sequential gold and penicillamine therapy in rheumatoid arthritis. Am. J. Med. 72:423, 1982.

66. Merryman, P., Jaffe, I.A., and Ehrenfeld, E.: Effect of D-penicillamine on poliovirus replication in HeLa cells. J. Virol. 13:881, 1974.

67. Friedrich, L., and Zimmerman, F.: Zur Pharmakologie von D-Penicillamin. Arzneim. Forsch. (Drug Res.) 25:162, 1975.

68. Liyange, S.P., and Currey, H.L.: Failure of oral D-penicillamine to modify adjuvant arthritis or immune response in the rat. Ann. Rheum. Dis. 31:521, 1972.

69. Jaffe, I.A.: Penicillamine treatment of rheumatoid arthritis: Effect on immune complexes. Ann. N.Y. Acad. Sci. 256:330, 1975.

70. Schumacher, K., Maerker-Alzer, G., and Preuss, R.: Effect of D-penicillamine on lymphocyte function. Arzneim. Forsch. (Drug Res.) 25:603, 1975.

71. Merryman, P., and Jaffe, I.A.: Effect of penicillamine on the proliferative response of human lymphocytes. Proc. Soc. Exp. Biol. Med. 157:155, 1978.

72. Maini, R.N., and Roffe, L.: D-Penicillamine and lymphocyte function in rheumatoid arthritis: The inhibitory and augmenting effects of D-penicillamine in vitro on phytohemagglutinin-induced lymphocyte transformation. In Munthe, E. (ed.): Penicillamine Research in Rheumatoid Disease. Oslo, Fabritius and Sonner, 1976, p. 172.

73. Lipsky, P.E., and Ziff, M.: The effect of D-penicillamine on mitogen-induced human lymphocyte proliferation: Synergistic inhibition by D-penicillamine and copper salts. J. Immunol. 120:1006, 1978.

74. Lipsky, P.E., and Ziff, M.: Inhibition of human helper T cell function in vitro by D-penicillamine and CuSO₄. J. Clin. Invest. 65:1069, 1980.

75. Zuckner, J., Ramsey, R.H., Dorner, R.W., and Gantner, G.E.: D-Penicillamine in rheumatoid arthritis. Arthritis Rheum. 13:131, 1970.

76. Whitehouse, M.W., Field, L., Denko, C.W., and Ryall, R.: Is penicillamine a precursor drug? Scand. J. Rheumatol. 4(Suppl. 8):183, 1975.

77. Axelrod, A.E., and Trakatellis, A.C.: Relationship of pyridoxine to immunological phenomena. Vitam. Horm. 22:591, 1964.

78. Gerber, D.A.: Inhibition of the denaturation of human gamma globulin by a mixture of D-Penicillamine disulfide and cooper. Biochem. Pharm. 27:469, 1978.

79. Masters, C.L., Dawkins, R.L., Zilco, P.L., Simpson, J.A., and Leedman, R.J.: Penicillamine-associated myasthenia gravis, antiacetylcholine receptor and antistriational antibodies. Am. J. Med. 63:689, 1977.

80. Sparrow, G.P.: Penicillamine pemphigus and the nephrotic syndrome occurring simultaneously. Br. J. Dermatol. 98:103, 1978.

81. Maize, J.C., Dobson, R.L., and Provost, T.T.: Pemphigus and myasthenia gravis. Arch. Dermatol. 111:1334, 1975.

82. Noguchi, S., and Nishitani, H.: Immunologic studies of a case of myasthenia gravis associated with pemphigus vulgaris after thymectomy. Neurology 26:1075, 1976.

83. Maini, R.N., and Berry, H. (eds): Modulation of Autoimmunity and Disease. Clinical Pharmacology and Therapeutics Series. Vol. 1. New York, Praeger Scientific, 1981.

84. Dawkins, R.L., Christiansen, F.T., and Zilko, P.J. (eds.): Immunogenetics in Rheumatology: Musculoskeletal Disease and D-Penicillamine. New York, Excerpta Medica, 1982.

85. Jacobus, D.P., Bokelman, D.L., and Majka, J.A.: D-Penicillamine in the monkey. In Munthe, E. (ed.): Penicillamine Research in Rheumatoid Disease. Oslo, Fabritius and —Sonner, 1976, p. 25.

86. Vincent, A., and Newsom-Davis, J.: Anti-acetylcholine receptor antibodies in D-penicillamine-associated myasthenia gravis. Lancet 1:1254, 1978.

Chapter 54
Glucocorticoids
Lloyd Axelrod

INTRODUCTION

The history of glucocorticoid therapy and the history of rheumatology are inseparable. From the beginning, during the initial studies of the effects of cortisone on patients with rheumatoid arthritis, it was apparent that the dramatic anti-inflammatory effects of glucocorticoids are frequently accompanied by the unwelcome manifestations of Cushing's syndrome.[1] The purpose of this chapter is to examine the risks associated with the use of glucocorticoids as anti-inflammatory and immunosuppressive agents and to provide guidelines for the long-term systemic use of these commonly prescribed substances. The indications for the use of glucocorticoids in the rheumatic disorders are discussed in the chapters of this book that consider the several rheumatic diseases for which these agents are sometimes indicated. This chapter is concerned primarily with the general principles of glucocorticoid therapy.

STRUCTURE OF COMMONLY USED GLUCOCORTICOIDS

Glucocorticoids are 21-carbon steroid molecules with numerous metabolic and physiologic effects. Figure 54–1 reveals the structures of several commonly employed glucocorticoids.[2] Cortisol (hydrocortisone) is the principal circulating glucocorticoid in man.

The existence of glucocorticoid activity depends on the presence of a hydroxyl group at carbon number 11 of the steroid molecule. Thus, cortisone and prednisone, which are 11-keto compounds, lack glucocorticoid activity until converted in vivo to cortisol and prednisolone, the corresponding 11-beta-hydroxyl compounds.[3,4] This transformation occurs predominantly in the liver.[5,6] The direct application of cortisone to the skin is ineffective in the treatment of dermatologic diseases that respond to topical application of cortisol.[4] Similarly, the anti-inflammatory action of cortisone is minimal compared with the effect of intra-articular administration of cortisol.[3] Cortisone and prednisone are available only for systemic therapy. All glucocorticoid preparations marketed for topical or local use are 11-beta-hydroxyl compounds, thus eliminating the need for biotransformation.

PHYSIOLOGY: THE REGULATION OF CORTISOL SECRETION

The production of cortisol by the adrenal cortex is regulated directly by the anterior pituitary gland and indirectly by the hypothalamus. Under normal circumstances, ACTH is released from the anterior pituitary gland in pulsatile fashion.[7] Although plasma ACTH levels are thus subject to minute-to-minute variation, these levels are higher on the average in the early morning hours than later in the day, i.e., there is a diurnal rhythm of ACTH release. ACTH is itself subject to release by corticotropin-releasing hormone, a substance synthesized in the hypothalamus and carried directly to the anterior pituitary gland by a local circulation, the hypophyseal-portal system. Stressful stimuli originating at a suprahypothalamic level lead to an augmented release of corticotropin-releasing hormone from the hypothalamus. This substance in turn provokes the discharge of ACTH from the anterior pituitary gland.

This sequence is subject to negative feedback inhibition. Increasing levels of cortisol or a synthetic glucocorticoid result in decreasing secretion of ACTH. It is not known whether this feedback control occurs predominantly at the hypothalamic level or the pituitary level.[8,9] In normal persons, stressful stimuli can overcome the effect of this feedback inhibition.[10]

PHARMACODYNAMICS

Half-Life, Potency, and Duration of Action. The important differences among the available glucocorticoid compounds are in duration of action, relative glucocor-

Figure 54–1. Commonly used glucocorticoids. In the representation of cortisol, the 21 carbon atoms of the glucocorticoid skeleton are designated by numbers, and the four rings are designated by letters. The arrows indicate the structural differences between cortisol and each of the other molecules. (From Axelrod, L.: Medicine 55:39, 1976.)

Table 54–1. Commonly Used Glucocorticoids*

Duration of Action[†]	Glucocorticoid Potency[‡]	Equivalent Glucocorticoid Dose (mg)	Mineralocorticoid Activity
Short-acting			
Cortisol (hydrocortisone)	1	20	Yes§
Cortisone	0.8	25	Yes§
Prednisone	4	5	No
Prednisolone	4	5	No
Methylprednisolone	5	4	No
Intermediate-acting			
Triamcinolone	5	4	No
Long-acting			
Betamethasone	25	0.60	No
Dexamethasone	30	0.75	No

*From Axelrod, L.: Medicine 55:39, 1976; and Axelrod, L.: *In* Miller, R. R., and Greenblatt, D. J. (eds.): Handbook of Drug Therapy. New York, Elsevier North Holland, 1979, p. 809.

†The classification by duration of action is based on the work of Harter (see text).[11]

‡The values given for glucocorticoid potency are relative. Cortisol is arbitrarily assigned a value of one. These values are approximations derived from several sources.[12-21]

§Mineralocorticoid effects are dose related. At doses close to or within the basal physiologic range for glucocorticoid activity, no such effect may be detectable.

ticoid potency, and relative mineralocorticoid potency (Table 54–1).[2] Commonly used glucocorticoids are categorized as short-, intermediate-, and long-acting on the basis of the duration of ACTH suppression following a single dose, equivalent in anti-inflammatory activity to 50 mg of prednisone (Table 54–1).[11] The values provided for relative glucocorticoid potency are approximations derived from several sources.[12-21] The relative potencies of the glucocorticoids correlate with their affinity for the cytoplasmic glucocorticoid receptor.[22,23] However, the observed potency of a glucocorticoid is a measure not only of the intrinsic biologic potency but also of the duration of action.[21,22] Consequently, the relative potency of two glucocorticoids will vary as a function of the time interval between the administration of the two steroids and the determination of the potency. In particular, failure to account for the duration of action may lead to a marked underestimation of the potency of dexamethasone.[21]

The half-life of cortisol in the circulation is in the range of 80 to 115 minutes.[2] Values for other commonly used agents are as follows: cortisone, 0.5 hours; prednisone, 3.4 to 3.8 hours; prednisolone, 2.1 to 3.5 hours; methylprednisolone, 1.3 to 3.1 hours; and dexamethasone, 1.8 to 4.7 hours.[2,21,24] The variability in the reported values for the half-life of an individual glucocorticoid may be a consequence in part of the fact that the pharmacokinetic characteristics of the glucocorticoids are dose dependent. With increasing intravenous doses of prednisolone, there is an increase in the volume of distribution and an increase in the clearance of this steroid.[24-26] The dose-dependent kinetic behavior of prednisolone may be due to the fact that the binding of prednisolone to plasma proteins is nonlinear; with an increase in dose, there is an increase in the percentage of the steroid that is unbound.[24-26]

The relationship between the circulating half-life of a glucocorticoid and its potency is not strict. Prednisolone and dexamethasone have comparable circulating half-lives, but dexamethasone is clearly more potent. Similarly, the correlation between the circulating half-life of a glucocorticoid and its duration of action is imprecise. The many actions of glucocorticoids do not have an equal duration, and the duration of action may be a function of the dose.[11,27-29]

For example, the duration of an elevation of the serum glucose of fasting subjects increases with increasing glucocorticoid dosage. It is 10 to 12 hours with 15 mg of methylprednisolone, 12 to 16 hours with 45 mg, and 18 to 22 hours with 90 mg.[27] In adult patients with stable chronic bronchial asthma, the duration of the response to a single oral dose of 40 mg of prednisolone depends on the aspect of pulmonary function that one observes.[28] Improvement in the peak expiratory flow rate, the forced expiratory volume in 1 second, and the maximum expiratory flow rate is still detectable 24 hours after administration of the dose, but not at 36 hours. However, improvement in forced vital capacity, residual volume/total lung capacity, and flow rate at 50 percent of vital capacity is still detectable at 12 hours, but not 24 hours. The differences in the duration of these effects may depend on the actual duration of the effects or on the variable sensitivity of the techniques utilized to measure the effects, or both.

Harter studied the duration of one effect of glucocorticoids, the length of time following a single dose during which ACTH remains suppressed.[11] He did this by administering metyrapone to a normal subject and measuring the urinary 17-ketogenic steroids during 6-hour periods as an index of ACTH secretion. He divided glucocorticoids into three groups based on the duration of ACTH suppression following a single dose of a glucocorticoid, equivalent in anti-inflammatory activity to 50 mg of prednisone. The first group, the short-acting steroids, is characterized by a return of ACTH activity within 24 to 36 hours. This group includes cortisone, hydrocortisone, prednisone, prednisolone, and methyl-prednisolone. The second group, the intermediate-acting steroids, consists of compounds that suppress ACTH for 48 hours. This group includes triamcinolone and paramethasone. The third group, the long-acting glucocorticoids, consists of substances that supress ACTH for well over 48 hours. This class includes dexamethasone and betamethasone. This formulation is based on studies in a single patient. It does not provide information about variations from individual to individual, about prolonged therapy, or about subjects who have not received metyrapone.

Since these variations in the duration of ACTH suppression are achieved by doses of glucocorticoids with comparable anti-inflammatory activity, the duration of ACTH suppression is not simply a function of the level of anti-inflammatory activity. However, the duration of ACTH suppression produced by an individual glucocorticoid is probably dose related. Harter found that as he increased the dose of prednisone from 25 mg to 100 mg, the duration of ACTH suppression was prolonged.[11] In another study, daily morning doses of 8 mg of triamcinolone taken for 1-week did not produce suppression of the 8 A.M. level of plasma 17-hydroxycorticosteroids, but daily morning doses of 12 mg produced suppression in some subjects and 16 mg produced suppression in all subjects.[29] Long-acting conjugates of the glucocorticoids given as intramuscular injections may be released slowly and exert an effect for much more prolonged periods, often several weeks.

The slight differences in the circulating half-lives of the glucocorticoids contrast with the marked differences between them in potency and in the duration of ACTH suppression. Also, the duration of ACTH suppression exceeds the half-life by more than the fivefold factor that would be expected if the duration of effect were a function of the circulating level of the steroid. Such data suggest that the duration of action of a glucocorticoid is not determined by its presence in the circulation. This is consistent with our understanding of the mechanism of action of steroid hormones. A steroid molecule passes through the cell membrane and enters the cytoplasm, where it binds to a specific cytoplasmic receptor protein.[30-32] This complex enters the nucleus, where it modifies the process of transcription, whereby RNA is synthesized (or transcribed) from the DNA template. The consequence is an alteration in the rate of synthesis of specific proteins. In this manner, the steroid modifies the phenotypic expression of the genetic information. Thus, the glucocorticoid continues to act within the cell after it has disappeared from the circulation. In addition, the series of events initiated by the glucocorticoid may continue to occur, or a product of this sequence (such as a specific protein) may be present after the disappearance of the glucocorticoid.

Bioavailability, Absorption, and Biotransformation. In normal subjects, plasma cortisol levels after oral administration of cortisone are much lower than after equal doses of cortisol.[33] This suggests that while oral cortisone may be adequate replacement therapy in chronic adrenal insufficiency, it is unwise to use this agent orally when pharmacologic effects are sought. In contrast, comparable plasma prednisolone levels are achieved in normal subjects following equivalent oral doses of prednisone and prednisolone.[24,26] There is wide variation in the prednisolone concentration after both drugs, which may reflect variability in absorption.[24]

In several instances in the past, therapeutic failure was attributed to diminished bioavailability of prednisone tablets; this has not been reported in recent years.[34] The serum prednisolone levels achieved following a single 50-mg tablet of prednisone and ten 5-mg tablets of prednisone given as a single oral dose of 50 mg are comparable.[35] Problems with in vivo bioavailability of prednisolone tablets have not been reported.[36] A comparison of the plasma prednisolone levels achieved after a single oral dose of prednisolone made by eight different American manufacturers indicates that the tablets tested were equivalent.[37] The bioavailability of dexamethasone does not vary when this agent is given intravenously, as an elixir, or in tablet form.[38]

Plasma cortisol levels after an intramuscular injection of cortisone acetate rise little or not at all, in contrast to the marked rises that follow the intramuscular injection of hydrocortisone.[39-45] Although intramuscular cortisone acetate has long been used for perioperative management, it may not provide adequate plasma cortisol levels and offers no advantage over hydrocortisone by the same route.

Plasma Transport Proteins. Under normal physiologic conditions, cortisol and, to a lesser extent, its synthetic derivatives are primarily bound to corticosteroid-binding globulin (CBG, transcortin), an alpha-globulin, in the plasma. CBG is a vehicle for the transportation of the steroid; the bound steroid is not active. Albumin binds most of the remaining glucocorticoid (10 to 15 percent) not complexed with CBG, leaving only a small portion of the steroid unbound and free to exert its physiologic and pharmacologic actions. Circadian fluctuations occur in the capacity of CBG to bind cortisol and prednisolone in normal subjects.[46] In contrast, patients who have been given prolonged treatment with prednisone have no diurnal variation in the binding capacity of CBG for cortisol of prednisolone, and both capacities are reduced in comparison with normal subjects.[46] Thus, long-term glucocorticoid therapy alters not only the endogenous secretion of steroids but also the transport of some glucocorticoids in the circulation. Possibly, this explains the observation that the disappearance of prednisolone is more rapid in those who have previously received glucocorticoids than in those who have not.[47,48]

Glucocorticoid Therapy in the Presence of Liver Disease. Plasma cortisol levels are normal in patients with liver disease.[49] Although cortisol clearance is reduced in cirrhotics, the hypothalamic-pituitary-adrenal homeostatic mechanism appears to be intact. Thus, a decreased rate of metabolism is accompanied by decreased synthesis of cortisol.[49]

In patients with active liver disease, the conversion of

prednisone to prednisolone is impaired.[48,50,51] This is offset in good measure by a decreased rate of elimination of prednisolone from the plasma in patients with active liver disease or cirrhosis.[51,52] In patients with liver disease, the plasma availability of prednisolone may be quite variable after oral doses of either prednisone or prednisolone.[51] The conversion of cortisone to cortisol has been studied in only one patient with hepatic disease and was normal.[33] The situation is further complicated by the fact that a lower percentage of circulating prednisolone is bound to protein in patients with active liver disease than in normal subjects;[48,50] the unbound fraction is inversely related to the serum albumin concentration.[50] An increased frequency of prednisone side effects is observed at low serum albumin levels;[53] possibly both findings reflect impaired hepatic function. Because the impairment of conversion of prednisone to prednisolone in the presence of liver disease is quantitatively small and is offset by a decreased rate of clearance of prednisolone, and because of the marked variability in plasma prednisolone levels after administration of either steroid, there is no clear mandate to use prednisolone rather than prednisone in the patient with active liver disease or cirrhosis.[24] Whichever agent is used, a somewhat lower dose than would otherwise be used should be employed if the serum albumin level is low.[24]

Glucocorticoids During Pregnancy. Glucocorticoid therapy appears to be well tolerated in pregnancy.[54] Although glucocorticoids cross the placenta, at present there is no convincing evidence that this produces clinically significant hypothalamic-pituitary-adrenal suppression or Cushing's syndrome in the neonate,[54] although subnormal responsiveness to exogenous ACTH may occur.[55,56] Nor is there evidence that glucocorticoids increase the incidence of congenital defects in humans.[54] Glucocorticoids appear to decrease the birthweight of full-term infants;[57] the long-term consequences of this effect are unknown. Owing to low concentrations of prednisone and prednisolone in breast milk, the administration of these drugs to the mother of a nursing infant is unlikely to produce deleterious effects.[58,59]

Drug Interactions. The concomitant use of other drugs can alter the effectiveness of the glucocorticoids.[60]

The metabolism of glucocorticoids is accelerated by compounds that induce hepatic microsomal enzyme activity, such as phenytoin,[61-64] barbiturates,[63,65,66] and rifampin.[67,68] Administration of these compounds can increase the steroid requirement of a patient with adrenal insufficiency[67] or lead to deterioration in the condition of a patient whose underlying disorder is well controlled by glucocorticoid therapy.[65,66,68] These substances should be avoided if possible in patients receiving steroids. Diazepam does not alter the metabolism of glucocorticoids[63] and is preferable to barbiturates. If an inducer of hepatic microsomal enzyme activity must be used in a patient on steroids, an increase in the required dosage of the steroid should be anticipated.

The bioavailability of prednisone is decreased by antacid doses comparable to those used clinically.[69]

The concurrent administration of a glucocorticoid and a salicylate may reduce serum salicylate levels; conversely, reduction of the steroid dose during administration of a fixed dose of salicylate may lead to higher and possibly toxic serum salicylate levels.[70-72] This interaction may reflect the induction of salicylate metabolism by glucocorticoids.[71]

Glucocorticoids may increase requirements for insulin or oral hypoglycemic agents, antihypertensive drugs, or glaucoma medications. They may also alter the requirement for sedative-hypnotic or antidepressant therapy. Digitalis toxicity can result from hypokalemia induced by glucocorticoids, as from hypokalemia of any cause. Glucocorticoids may reverse the neuromuscular blockade induced by pancuronium.[73,74] The mechanism is not known. The bioavailability of prednisolone is not impaired by the simultaneous use of cholestyramine.[75]

CONSIDERATIONS PRIOR TO THE USE OF GLUCOCORTICOIDS AS PHARMACOLOGIC AGENTS

Cushing's syndrome is a serious disorder. The 5-year mortality rate was over 50 percent in a series of patients studied at the beginning of the era of glucocorticoid and ACTH therapy.[76] Infection and cardiovascular complications are frequent causes of death in this disorder. High-dose exogenous glucocorticoid therapy is similarly hazardous.

Table 54–2 summarizes the important questions to consider prior to the initiation of glucocorticoid therapy.[77] These enable the physician to assess the potential risks that must be weighed against the potential benefits of treatment. The more severe the underlying disorder, the more readily glucocorticoid therapy can be justified. Thus, steroid therapy is usually employed in patients with some severe forms of systemic lupus erythematosus, active vasculitis, status asthmaticus, severe chronic active hepatitis, transplantation rejection, severe pemphigus, or diseases of comparable severity. Steroids gen-

Table 54–2. Considerations Prior to the Use of Glucocorticoids as Pharmacologic Agents*

1. How serious is the underlying disorder?
2. How long will therapy be required?
3. What is the anticipated effective steroid dose?
4. Is the patient predisposed to any of the known hazards of glucocorticoid therapy?
     Diabetes mellitus
     Osteoporosis
     Peptic ulcer, gastritis, or esophagitis
     Tuberculosis or other chronic infections
     Hypertension and cardiovascular disease
     Psychological difficulties
5. Which glucocorticoid preparation should be employed?
6. Have other modes of therapy been utilized to minimize the glucocorticoid dosage and to minimize the side effects of glucocorticoid therapy?
7. Is an alternate-day regimen indicated?

*Modified from Thorn, G.W.: N. Engl. J. Med. 274:775, 1966.

erally should not be administered to patients with rheumatoid arthritis or mild bronchial asthma, who should receive more conservative therapy first. Although they may experience symptomatic relief from glucocorticoids, it may prove difficult to withdraw steroids for this very reason. As a result, these patients may unnecessarily experience Cushing's syndrome and hypothalamic-pituitary-adrenal suppression.

The anticipated duration of glucocorticoid therapy is another critical variable. The use of glucocorticoids for 1 to 2 weeks for a condition such as poison ivy or allergic rhinitis is unlikely to be associated with serious side effects if there is no contraindication to their use. An exception to this rule is a steroid-induced psychosis, which may occur after only a few days of high-dose glucocorticoid therapy, even in patients with no previous history of psychiatric disease.[78,79] Because so many complications are dose and time related, the smallest possible dose should be prescribed for the shortest possible period.[78,80,81] If hypoalbuminemia is present, the dose should be appropriately reduced.[24,50,53] If long-term treatment is indicated, consideration should be given to the use of an alternate-day schedule.

Whenever possible, a local steroid preparation should be used, since systemic effects are minimal when these substances are properly administered. Examples are topical therapy in dermatologic disorders, steroid enemas in ulcerative proctitis, steroid aerosols in bronchial asthma and allergic rhinitis, and intra-articular steroids.[82,83]

Agents with minimal or no mineralocorticoid activity should be used when a glucocorticoid is prescribed for pharmacologic purposes. If the dose is to be tapered over a few days, a long-acting agent may be undesirable. For alternate-day therapy, a short-acting agent that generally does not cause sodium retention (e.g., prednisone, prednisolone, or methylprednisolone) should be used. There is no indication for the systemic administration of glucocorticoid conjugates that are designed to achieve a prolonged duration of action (several days or several weeks) following a single intramuscular injection. The absorption and bioavailability of such agents cannot be regulated precisely, the duration of action cannot be estimated reliably, and it is not possible to taper the dose rapidly in the event of an adverse reaction such as a steroid-induced psychosis. The use of such preparations may produce hypothalamic-pituitary-adrenal suppression more often than comparable doses of the same glucocorticoid given orally.[84] The use of supplementary agents to minimize the steroid dose and to minimize the side effects of systemic glucocorticoids should always be considered.

EFFECTS OF EXOGENOUS GLUCOCORTICOIDS

Anti-inflammatory and Immunosuppressive Effects. The effects of glucocorticoids on inflammatory and immune responses are exceedingly complex; this complexity derives from the complexity of the inflammatory and immune processes themselves and from the fact that glucocorticoids modify these processes in numerous ways.[85-90] Studies performed in steroid-sensitive species, such as the mouse, rat, and rabbit, may not apply to steroid-resistant species such as the guinea pig, monkey, and man.[85,86] In addition many studies in in vitro systems employ concentrations of glucocorticoids that are not attainable in man.[89,90]

It is not yet possible to identify a single mechanism of action underlying the numerous effects of glucocorticoids on inflammatory and immune responses. As noted above, glucocorticoid hormones (like other steroid hormones) act by binding to a specific cytoplasmic receptor protein. The steroid-receptor complex then enters the nucleus, where it modifies the transcription of RNA from the DNA template. This results in an alteration of the rate of synthesis of specific proteins. It is tempting to try to relate this receptor-mediated mechanism of action to the numerous effects of glucocorticoids on inflammation and immunity. In fact, glucocorticoid receptors have been demonstrated in normal human lymphocytes, monocytes, neutrophils, and eosinophils and in human neoplastic cells.[90] Although the number of cytoplasmic glucocorticoid receptors correlates with a clinical response to glucocorticoid therapy in some patients with lymphoid tumors, the presence of receptors in malignant tissue does not guarantee responsiveness.[90] Variations in corticosteroid receptor density, affinity, or binding constants do not correlate with the range of responses of immunoreactive cells to glucocorticoids.[90]

Glucocorticoid effects on inflammatory and immune phenomena include effects on leukocyte movement, leukocyte function, and humoral factors (Table 54–3). In general, glucocorticoids have a greater effect on leukocyte traffic than on function and more effect on cellular than humoral processes.[89] Probably the most important anti-inflammatory effect of glucocorticoids is their ability to inhibit recruitment of neutrophils and monocyte-macrophages to an inflammatory site.[89]

Glucocorticoids alter the traffic of all the major leukocyte populations within the circulation. The administration of a single dose of a glucocorticoid produces a neutrophilic leukocytosis; peak levels occur 4 to 6 hours after the steroid is given.[87,91] This leukocytosis is the consequence of an accelerated release of mature neutrophils from the bone marrow,[92] an increase in the circulating half-life of the neutrophils,[93] and decreased egress of neutrophils from the circulation to an inflammatory site.[92,94] The administration of a single dose of a glucocorticoid to normal human subjects produces a marked but transient lymphocytopenia; the nadir is reached 4 to 6 hours after administration (Fig. 54–2).[87,95-99] This lymphocytopenia involves all lymphocyte subpopulations. It is also selective, since thymus-derived lymphocytes are decreased to a greater degree than bone marrow-derived lymphocytes,[87,95,96,99] and within the total T lymphocyte population certain subsets are decreased to a greater extent than others.[90] The mechanism of the lymphocytopenia in humans involves the redistribution of lymphocytes out of the circulation.

Table 54–3. Effects of Glucocorticoids on Inflammatory and Immune Responses in Humans*

Effects on Leukocyte Movement

Lymphocytes
  Circulating lymphocytopenia 4 to 6 hours following drug administration, secondary to redistribution of cells to other lymphoid compartments
  Depletion of recirculating lymphocytes
  Selective depletion of T lymphocytes more than B lymphocytes
Monocyte-Macrophages
  Circulating monocytopenia 4 to 6 hours following drug administration, probably secondary to redistribution
  Inhibition of accumulation of monocyte-macrophages at inflammatory sites
Neutrophils
  Circulating neutrophilia
  Accelerated release of neutrophils from the bone marrow
  Blockade of accumulation of neutrophils at inflammatory sites
Eosinophils
  Circulating eosinopenia, probably secondary to redistribution
  Decreased migration of eosinophils into immediate hypersensitivity skin test sites

Effects on Leukocyte Function

Lymphocytes
  Suppression of delayed hypersensitivity skin testing by inhibition of recruitment of monocyte-macrophages
  Suppression of lymphocyte proliferation to antigens more easily than proliferation to mitogens
  Suppression of mixed leukocyte reaction proliferation
  Suppression of T lymphocyte–mediated cytotoxicity (at high concentrations in vitro)
  No effect on antibody dependent cell-mediated cytotoxicity
  Suppression of spontaneous (natural) cytotoxicity
  Regulatory effects on helper and suppressor cell populations
Monocyte-Macrophages
  Suppression of cutaneous delayed hypersensitivity by inhibition of lymphokine effect on the macrophage
  Blockade of Fc receptor binding and function
  Depression of bactericidal activity
  Possible decrease in monocyte chemotaxis
Neutrophils
  Possibly no effect on phagocytic and bactericidal capability (controversial)
  Increase in antibody-dependent cellular cytotoxicity
  Probable decrease in lysosomal release but little effect on lysosomal membrane stabilization at pharmacologic concentrations
  Inhibition of chemotaxis only by suprapharmacologic concentrations

Effects on Humoral Factors

Mild decrease in immunoglobulin levels but no decrease in specific antibody production
Probably no effect on complement metabolism
Decreased reticuloendothelial clearance of antibody-coated cells
Decreased synthesis of prostaglandins, and leukotrienes
Effects on kinins controversial
Inhibition of plasminogen activator release
Potentiation of the actions of catecholamines
Antagonism of histamine-induced vasodilatation

*Adapted from Parrillo, J. E., and Fauci, A.S.: Ann. Rev. Pharmacol. Toxicol. 19:179, 1979.

In general, there are two distinct populations of lymphocytes in the circulation.[87,89] The first population, the recirculating lymphocytes, freely migrates into and out of the intravascular space in equilibrium with the much larger total body pool of recirculating lymphocytes. The

second population, the nonrecirculating lymphocytes, remains in the intravascular space. Glucocorticoids cause the recirculating lymphocyte to leave the intravascular space, but they do not affect the nonrecirculating lymphocyte.[100] This alteration of the normal lymphocyte traffic may be due to suppression of entry of lymphocytes into the circulation.[101] Glucocorticoids also cause a profound monocytopenia and eosinopenia; the time courses after a single steroid dose are similar to that of the lymphocytopenia.

The mechanism of the decrease in the accumulation of inflammatory cells at an inflammatory site caused by glucocorticoids is not fully understood. Corticosteroids modify the increased capillary and membrane permeability that occurs at an inflammatory site.[102] By decreasing the dilatation of the microvasculature and the increased capillary permeability that occur during the inflammatory response, exudation of fluid and the formation of edema may be reduced, and the migration of

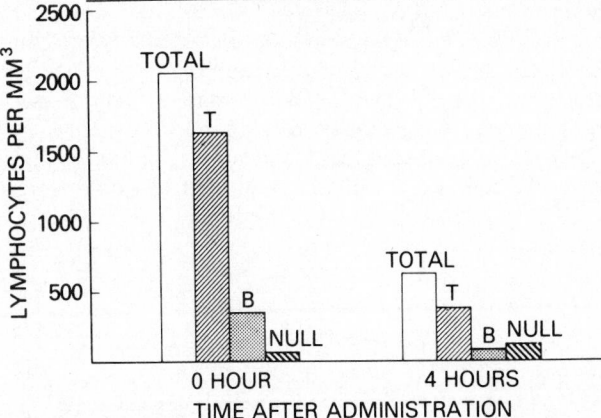

Figure 54–2. The effect of hydrocortisone administration on circulating lymphocytes and monocytes. Hydrocortisone, 400 mg, was administered intravenously in a single dose to a normal volunteer. The upper panel shows the effect on the total lymphocyte and monocyte counts. The lower panel shows the effect on circulating thymus-derived (T) and bone-marrow derived (B) lymphocytes, as well as lymphocytes without detectable surface markers (null cells), 4 hours after drug administration. T lymphocytes were measured by the sheep erythrocyte rosette assay, and B lymphocytes were measured by the complement receptor assay. (From Fauci, A.S., Dale, D.C., and Balow, J.E.: Ann. Intern. Med. 84:304, 1976.)

leukocytes may be impaired.[88,89,102,103] The decrease in accumulation of inflammatory cells may be due also to decreased adherence of the inflammatory cells to the vascular endothelium.[104-106] It is not presently possible to determine the relative contributions of a direct vascular effect, of an effect on inflammatory cell adherence to the vascular wall, and of an effect on chemotaxis to the reduction in the inflammatory response caused by glucocorticoids.

Glucocorticoids have numerous effects on leukocyte function. Steroid therapy suppresses cutaneous delayed hypersensitivity responses. This occurs after approximately 14 days of glucocorticoid therapy and disappears approximately 6 days after treatment is withdrawn; these rates vary considerably from patient to patient.[107] This suppression is a consequence of decreased recruitment of macrophages necessary for the expression of hypersensitivity and is not due to suppression of the sensitized lymphocyte.[107-110] Steroids antagonize the effects of migration inhibition factor (MIF) on the macrophage (Fig. 54–3).[111] Glucocorticoids do not suppress the production of lymphokines by lymphocytes, but they do inhibit the ability of these soluble mediators to recruit cells necessary for the expression of cellular immunity.[87,89,111] Although human lymphoid tissue is generally resistant to the lytic effect of glucocorticoids, certain activated lymphocyte subsets may be sensitive to the lytic effect of steroids. Other effects of glucocorticoids on lymphocyte function are summarized in Table 54–3.

Monocyte-macrophage traffic and function are relatively sensitive to glucocorticoids (Table 54–3). Glucocorticoids in divided daily doses depress the bactericidal activity of monocytes.[112,113] Because the monocyte is thought to be the principal cell involved in granuloma formation, the sensitivity of monocytes to glucocorticoids may explain the effectiveness of glucocorticoids in many granulomatous diseases.[89]

Although neutrophil traffic is quite sensitive to glucocorticoids, neutrophil function appears to be relatively resistant to these agents.[89] While most in vivo studies of neutrophil phagocytosis have found no evidence for impairment of phagocytosis or bacterial killing,[89] other data are consistent with the view that glucocorticoids

induce a generalized phagocytic defect, affecting granulocytes as well as monocytes.[114]

Glucocorticoid therapy retards the disappearance of sensitized erythrocytes, platelets, and artificial particles from the circulation.[89,114,115] This may explain the efficacy of glucocorticoids in the treatment of idiopathic thrombocytopenic purpura and autoimmune hemolytic anemia.

Glucocorticoids are potent inhibitors of prostaglandin synthesis.[116-120] This is of particular interest in view of the evidence for synthesis of prostaglandin E_2 by rheumatoid synovia[121] and the possibility that the bone resorption-stimulating activity of this prostaglandin accounts for the bone destruction in rheumatoid arthritis.[121] Corticosteroids inhibit prostaglandin synthesis by inhibition of arachidonic acid release from phospholipids.[119,120] This is distinct from the mechanism of action of the nonsteroidal anti-inflammatory agents, such as salicylates and indomethacin, which inhibit the cyclooxygenase that converts arachidonic acid to the cyclic endoperoxide intermediates in the prostaglandin synthetic pathway. Thus, the glucocorticoids and the nonsteroidal anti-inflammatory agents exert their anti-inflammatory effects at two distinct but adjacent loci in the synthetic pathway of a substance with known bone resorption-stimulating activity that is synthesized by rheumatoid synovia.

Glucocorticoids and nonsteroidal anti-inflammatory agents have a different spectrum of anti-inflammatory effects. Some of the therapeutic effects of steroids that are not produced by the nonsteroidal agents may be due to inhibition of leukotriene formation.[122] Leukotrienes are a class of substances originally found in leukocytes, which share a conjugated triene as a common structural feature.[122] Leukotriene B4 causes adhesion and chemotactic movement of leukocytes.[122] Leukotrienes C4, D4, and E4 (the constituents of the slow-reacting substance of anaphylaxis) increase vascular permeability.[122] These leukotrienes (B4, C4, D4, and E4) may act synergistically with the vasodilator prostaglandins PGE_2 and PGI_2 to mediate inflammation.[122] The glucocorticoid-mediated inhibition of arachidonic acid release prevents formation not only of prostaglandins and thromboxanes (as do the nonsteroidal anti-inflammatory agents) but also of leukotrienes and other oxygenated derivatives. Consequently, some of the therapeutic effects of steroids that are not shared by the nonsteroidal agents may be due to inhibition of leukotriene formation.[122]

Side Effects. Adverse reactions to glucocorticoids include the diverse manifestations of Cushing's syndrome and hypothalamic-pituitary-adrenal (HPA) suppression (Table 54–4).[16,80,81,123] Iatrogenic Cushing's syndrome differs from spontaneous Cushing's syndrome in several respects (Table 54–5).[124,125] These differences may be explained in part by the fact that in iatrogenic Cushing's syndrome caused by exogenous glucocorticoids, ACTH is suppressed, whereas in spontaneous, ACTH-dependent Cushing's syndrome, the elevated ACTH output results in bilateral adrenal hyperplasia. In the former circumstance, the secretion of adrenocortical androgens

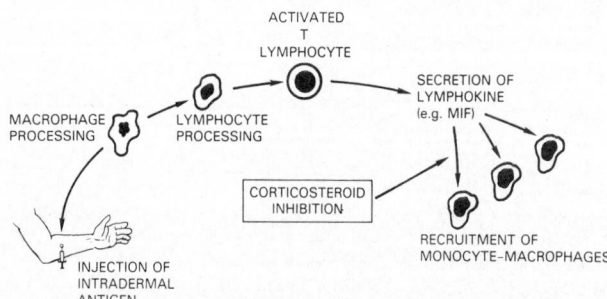

Figure 54–3. Schematic representation of the probable site of inhibition of the delayed hypersensitivity skin test response. Glucocorticoids inhibit the recruitment of the monocyte-macrophage, but do not affect the activated T lymphocyte. (From Parrillo, J.E., and Fauci, A.S.: Ann. Rev. Pharmacol. Toxicol. 19:179, 1979.)

Table 54–4. Adverse Reactions to Glucocorticoids*

Ophthalmic
  Posterior subcapsular cataracts, increased intraocular pressure and glaucoma, exophthalmos
Cardiovascular
  Hypertension
  Congestive heart failure in predisposed patients
Gastrointestinal
  Peptic ulcer disease, pancreatitis
Endocrine-metabolic
  Truncal obesity, moon facies, supraclavicular fat deposition, posterior cervical fat deposition (buffalo hump), mediastinal widening (lipomatosis), hepatomegaly due to fatty liver (rare)
  Acne, hirsutism or virilism, impotence, menstrual irregularities
  Suppression of growth in children
  Hyperglycemia; diabetic ketoacidosis; hyperosmolar, nonketotic diabetic coma; hyperlipoproteinemia
  Negative balance of nitrogen, potassium, and calcium
  Sodium retention, hypokalemia, metabolic alkalosis
  Secondary adrenal insufficiency
Musculoskeletal
  Myopathy
  Osteoporosis, vertebral compression fractures, spontaneous fractures
  Aseptic necrosis of femoral and humeral heads and other bones
Neuropsychiatric
  Convulsions
  Benign intracranial hypertension (pseudotumor cerebri)
  Alterations in mood or personality
  Psychosis
Dermatologic
  Facial erythema, thin fragile skin, petechiae and ecchymoses, violaceous striae, impaired wound healing
  Panniculitis (following withdrawal)
Immune, infectious
  Suppression of delayed hypersensitivity
  Neutrophilia, monocytopenia, lymphocytopenia, decreased inflammatory responses
  Susceptibility to infections

*From Axelrod, L.: *In* Miller, R. R., and Greenblatt, D. J. (eds.): Handbook of Drug Therapy. New York, Elsevier North Holland, 1979, p. 809.

and mineralocorticoids is not increased. When ACTH output is elevated, the secretion of adrenal androgens and mineralocorticoids may be increased.[2] The augmented secretion of adrenal androgens may account for the higher incidence of virilism, acne, and menstrual irregularities reported in the spontaneous form of Cushing's syndrome, and the enhanced production of mineralocorticoids may explain the higher incidence of hypertension.[2]

The complications that are virtually unique to iatrogenic Cushing's syndrome arise following prolonged use or large doses of glucocorticoids. This is the case with benign intracranial hypertension,[126,127] posterior subcapsular cataract,[128-130] and aseptic necrosis of bone.[131-137]

Although the association of glucocorticoid therapy and peptic ulcer disease is controversial,[138-143] it appears that glucocorticoids increase the risk of peptic ulcer disease and gastrointestinal hemorrhage.[142,143] The magnitude of the association between glucocorticoid therapy and these complications is small and is related to the total dose and duration of therapy.[139,142]

Glucocorticoid therapy, especially daily therapy, may

suppress the immune response to skin tests for tuberculosis.[107] When possible, tuberculin skin testing is advisable prior to the initiation of glucocorticoid therapy. Routine isoniazid prophylaxis for corticosteroid-treated patients, even those with positive tuberculin skin tests, is probably not indicated.[144]

Some patients respond to and develop side effects to glucocorticoids more readily than others at equivalent doses. Of course, variations in responsiveness to glucocorticoids may result from drug interactions (see above) or from variations in the severity of the underlying disease. Alterations in the bioavailability of administered glucocorticoids probably do not account for the variations in therapeutic response in most patients.[23] In patients who develop side effects, the metabolic clearance rate of prednisolone and the volume of distribution are lower[26,47] and the circulating half-life is longer[47] than in those who do not. Patients who develop a cushingoid habitus on prednisone have higher endogenous plasma cortisol levels than those who do not, perhaps owing to a resistance of the HPA axis to suppression by exogenous glucocorticoids.[145]

Variations in the effectiveness of steroids may be due to altered cellular responsiveness to steroids.[23,146-149] In patients with primary open-angle glaucoma, glucocorticoids produce a greater rise of intraocular pressure,[146] greater suppression of the 8 A.M. plasma cortisol level (when dexamethasone, 0.25 mg, is administered the previous evening at 11 P.M.),[148] and greater suppression of phytohemagglutinin-induced transformation of lymphocytes than in normal subjects.[147,149] Since primary open-angle glaucoma is not uncommon, these findings suggest that a distinct subpopulation of patients is hyper-re-

Table 54–5. Natural Versus Iatrogenic Cushing's Syndrome*

More common in natural Cushing's syndrome:
  Hypertension
  Acne
  Menstrual disturbances
  Impotence in males
  Hirsutism or virilism
  Striae
  Purpura
  Plethora
Virtually unique to iatrogenic Cushing's syndrome:
  Benign intracranial hypertension
  Glaucoma
  Posterior subcapsular cataract
  Pancreatitis
  Aseptic necrosis of bone
  Panniculitis
Nearly equal frequency in both syndromes:
  Obesity
  Psychiatric symptoms
  Edema†
  Poor wound healing

*Adapted from Ragan, C.: Bull. N.Y. Acad. Med. 29:355, 1953; and Christy, N.P.: The Human Adrenal Cortex. New York, Harper & Row, 1971, p. 395.

†The incidence of edema in iatrogenic Cushing's syndrome may depend on the glucocorticoid employed. Ragan utilized cortisone.[125]

sponsive to glucocorticoids and that this sensitivity is genetically determined.

Withdrawal from Glucocorticoids. The symptoms associated with glucocorticoid withdrawal include arthralgia, myalgia, anorexia, nausea, emesis, lethargy, headache, fever, desquamation, weight loss, and postural hypotension. Many of these symptoms can occur with normal plasma levels of glucocorticoids[150] and in patients with normal responsiveness of the HPA system.[151,152] Thus, the "steroid withdrawal syndrome" does not depend on the absence of glucocorticoids from the circulation or the impairment of HPA responsiveness. There is no satisfactory explanation for these observations. The "steroid withdrawal syndrome" may contribute to psychologic dependence on glucocorticoid treatment and to one's difficulties in withdrawing such therapy.[124]

SUPPRESSION OF THE HYPOTHALAMIC-PITUITARY-ADRENAL (HPA) SYSTEM

The Development of HPA Suppression. There are few well-documented cases of acute adrenocortical insufficiency following chronic glucocorticoid therapy and no such cases following ACTH therapy.[2] Therefore, the minimal duration of glucocorticoid therapy that can produce HPA suppression must be ascertained from studies of adrenocortical weight and adrenocortical responsiveness to provocative tests.[2,124,153] Adrenocortical atrophy is detectable 5 days after the onset of glucocorticoid therapy.[154] Abnormalities in responsiveness to ACTH and to metyrapone are observed in some but not all patients within 3 days of initiation of treatment with glucocorticoids.[2,124,153] Abnormalities in responsiveness to ACTH and to insulin-induced hypoglycemia occur following the administration of prednisone 25 mg twice daily for 5 days.[155] It must be emphasized that there is considerable variation from patient to patient[156] and from study to study.[124] These figures define the earliest time at which abnormalities are observed in some but not all patients. Because assessment of the onset of HPA suppression currently depends upon anatomic and biochemical (but not clinical) evidence, and because the biochemical abnormalities observed are sometimes mild, it is not possible to identify definitively the shortest interval or the smallest dose at which suppression may occur. On the basis of the available evidence, any patient who has received a glucocorticoid in doses equivalent to 20 to 30 mg of prednisone per day for more than 5 days should be suspected of having HPA suppression.[2] If the doses are closer to but above the physiologic range, 1 month is probably the minimal interval.[2] Once such suspicions are entertained, the physician has two alternatives. One may perform an ACTH test, or one may treat the patient as though adrenocortical insufficiency were present.

The adrenocortical response to an ACTH test is a useful guide to the presence or absence of suppression in glucocorticoid-treated patients (Table 54–6). The

Table 54–6. Assessment of Hypothalamic-Pituitary-Adrenal Function in Patients Treated with Glucocorticoids

Method

Withhold exogenous steroids for 24 hours

Give cosyntropin (synthetic alpha 1-24 ACTH) 250 μg (25 units) as IV bolus or IM injection

Obtain plasma cortisol level before administration of ACTH and 30 or 60 minutes afterward

Performance of the test in the morning is customary but not essential

Interpretation

Normal response: plasma cortisol level above 18 μg/dl at 30 *or* 60 minutes after ACTH administration

Note: Traditional recommendations also specify an increment above baseline of 7 μg/dl at 30 minutes or 11 μg/dl at 60 minutes and a doubling of the baseline value at 60 minutes. These parameters are valid in normal, unstressed subjects but are frequently misleading in ill patients with a normal hypothalamic-pituitary-adrenal axis, in whom stress may raise the baseline plasma level via an increase in *endogenous* ACTH levels.

maximal response of the plasma cortisol level to ACTH corresponds to the maximal plasma cortisol level observed during the induction of general anesthesia and surgery in patients who have received glucocorticoid therapy.[157-160] This is so when one uses a 6-hour infusion of ACTH[159,160] or a rapid intravenous injection of synthetic ACTH with measurement of the plasma cortisol level just before and then 30 minutes[158] or 60 minutes[157] after the injection. A normal response to ACTH preoperatively is unlikely to be followed by markedly impaired secretion of cortisol during anesthesia and surgery in steroid-treated patients. In general, other tests of the HPA system, such as insulin-induced hypoglycemia and the metyrapone test, are not indicated in the evaluation of the steroid-treated patient for possible HPA axis suppression.

The stress of general anesthesia and surgery is not hazardous to patients who have received only replacement doses (no more than 25 mg hydrocortisone, 5 mg prednisone, 4 mg triamcinolone, or 0.75 mg dexamethasone),[161] if the steroid is given early in the day.[162] If doses of this size are given late in the day, suppression may occur as a result of inhibition of the diurnal release of ACTH.[162,163]

ACTH and the HPA System. Pharmacologic doses of ACTH produce supranormal cortisol secretory rates and elevated plasma cortisol levels. One might expect such elevated levels to suppress ACTH release. In fact, there is no evidence of clinically significant hypothalamic-pituitary suppression in patients who have received ACTH therapy.[2] The failure of ACTH to cause suppression of HPA function is not explained by the dose of ACTH employed, the frequency of injections, the time of administration, or the plasma cortisol pattern following ACTH administration.[164] Another possible explanation is that the hyperplastic and overactive adrenal cortex that results from ACTH therapy might compensate for hypothalamic or pituitary suppression.[165] Although threshold adrenocortical sensitivity to ACTH is not changed in patients who have received daily ACTH therapy,[164] the possibility remains that there is altered adrenocortical responsiveness to ACTH in the physiologic range. In addition, evidence exists that the preservation of the normal response of the plasma cortisol level in patients treated with ACTH is due, at least in part, to the fact that ACTH treatment reduces the rate of ACTH secretion but not the total amount secreted, while glucocorticoids reduce both the rate of secretion and the total amount secreted.[166]

Recovery from HPA Suppression. During recovery from HPA suppression, hypothalamic-pituitary function returns before adrenocortical function.[167] Twelve months must elapse following withdrawal of large doses of glucocorticoids given for a prolonged period before homeostatic function, including responsiveness to stress, returns to normal.[2,167,168] In contrast, recovery from HPA suppression induced by a brief course of steroids (i.e., prednisone 25 mg twice daily for 5 days or prednisone 20 mg twice daily for 3 weeks) occurs within 5 days.[155,169] As a group, patients with mild suppression of the HPA axis (i.e., normal basal plasma and urine steroid levels but diminished responses to ACTH and insulin-induced hypoglycemia) resume normal functional capacity more rapidly than those with severe depression of the HPA axis (i.e., low basal plasma and urine steroid levels and diminished responses to ACTH and insulin-induced hypoglycemia).[170] The time course of recovery correlates with the total duration of previous glucocorticoid therapy and the total previous steroid dose.[170,172] Nevertheless, it is not possible in an individual patient to predict the time course of recovery from a course of glucocorticoid therapy at supraphysiologic doses lasting more than a few weeks, so persistence of HPA suppression should be suspected for 12 months after such a course of treatment. The course of recovery from suppression of the contralateral adrenal cortex by the products of an adrenocortical tumor may exceed 12 months.[162,173] Recovery from suppression induced by exogenous glucocorticoids may be more rapid in children than adults.[174]

WITHDRAWAL OF PATIENTS FROM GLUCOCORTICOIDS

Risks of Withdrawal. The decision to discontinue glucocorticoid therapy provokes apprehension among physicians. The untoward consequences of such an action include precipitation of adrenocortical insufficiency, the steroid withdrawal syndrome, or an exacerbation of the underlying disease. Rarely, the syndrome of nodular panniculitis may occur.[175-178] This syndrome is characterized by painful pruritic nodules involving the flexor surfaces of the extremities, the cheeks, and the trunk.[175-178] These lesions, which appear 1 to 35 days after withdrawal of glucocorticoids, have been noted almost exclusively in children with acute rheumatic fever. The lesions may be ameliorated by reinstitution of glucocorticoids.

Adrenocortical insufficiency following the withdrawal of glucocorticoids is justly feared. The likelihood of precipitating the underlying disease almost certainly depends upon the activity and natural history of the illness in question. When there is any possibility that the underlying illness may flare up, the glucocorticoid should be withdrawn gradually, over an interval of weeks to months, with frequent reassessment of the patient.

Management of the Patient with HPA Suppression. There is no proved means of hastening a return to normal HPA function once inhibition has resulted from glucocorticoid therapy. The use of ACTH does not appear to prevent or reverse the development of glucocorticoid-induced adrenal insufficiency.[152,179-181] Conversion to an alternate-day schedule permits but does not accelerate recovery.[182,183] In children, alternate-day glucocorticoid therapy may delay recovery.[184]

Recovery from steroid-induced adrenal insufficiency is time dependent and spontaneous. During this interval, small doses of hydrocortisone (10 to 20 mg) or prednisone (2.5 to 5 mg) in the morning may alleviate withdrawal symptoms. Recovery of HPA function does occur during the administration of small doses of glucocorticoids in the morning; the rate of recovery is determined not only by the doses given when the steroids are being tapered but also by the dose administered during the initial phase of treatment, before tapering is commenced.[170-172] The available studies do not exclude the possibility that small doses of glucocorticoids in the morning retard the rate of recovery from HPA suppression, even though they do not prevent recovery. This requires further investigation.

ALTERNATE-DAY GLUCOCORTICOID THERAPY

Alternate-day glucocorticoid therapy is defined as the administration of a short-acting glucocorticoid with no appreciable mineralocorticoid effect (such as prednisone, prednisolone, or methylprednisolone) once every 48 hours in the morning, at about 8:00 A.M. The objective is to minimize the adverse effects of glucocorticoids while retaining therapeutic effectiveness. The original basis for this approach was the hypothesis that the anti-inflammatory effects of glucocorticoids persist longer than the undesirable metabolic effects.[185-189] If so, it should be possible to find a schedule that allows rest periods between doses during which the patient is not exposed to the side effects of glucocorticoids while the desired anti-inflammatory action persists.[186,187] This hypothesis is not supported by observations of the duration of steroid effects (see above).

A second hypothesis emphasizes that intermittent rather than continuous administration produces a cyclic, though not diurnal, pattern of glucocorticoid levels in the circulation and within the target cells that simulates the normal diurnal cycle. This might prevent the development of Cushing's syndrome and HPA suppression but provide therapeutic benefit. Since the full expression of a disease frequently occurs only when the level of inflammatory activity increases over a protracted period of time, the intermittent administration of a glucocorticoid may be sufficient to shorten the interval during which the disorder develops without interruption, thereby preventing the level of disease activity from becoming clinically apparent (Fig. 54–4).[87] The duration of action of the glucocorticoids is important in this context. The selection of prednisone, prednisolone, and methylprednisolone as the agents of choice for alternate-day therapy and of 48 hours as the appropriate interval between doses has an empirical basis. Harter and associates found that intervals of 36, 24, and 12 hours were accompanied by adrenal suppression, and that an interval of 72 hours was therapeutically ineffective when prednisone (and, in some cases, triamcinolone) was employed. An interval of 48 hours was found to be optimal.[187]

Alternate-Day Glucocorticoids and Cushing's Syndrome. An alternate-day regimen can prevent or ameliorate the manifestations of Cushing's syndrome,[2,27,99,186,187,189-208] including not only the somatic and psychological manifestations but also quantifiable end-points such as high blood pressure,[191,194,195,200,206] retarded linear growth rate in children,[193,204-206] altered leukocyte kinetics,[99,197,202,203] impaired responsiveness to skin testing for delayed hypersensitivity,[192,203] impaired monocyte cellular function,[208] elevated urinary excretion rates of nitrogen and potassium,[27] impaired intestinal absorption of calcium,[207] reduced serum 25-hydroxyvitamin D levels,[207] and elevated serum cholesterol and triglyceride levels.[209]

The susceptibility to infections that characterizes Cushing's syndrome[76,210-212] may be alleviated by an alternate-day program. Cases in which refractory infections appeared to clear after conversion from daily to alternate-day therapy have been described.[194,195] Several studies report a low incidence of infections in patients on alternate-day therapy.[191,194,195,202,213] Children treated with alternate-day steroids regain or retain tonsillar and peripheral lymphoid tissue.[191] These reports strongly suggest that alternate-day therapy is associated with a lower incidence of infections than daily medication but do not firmly establish this point.

Host defense mechanisms have been studied in patients on alternate-day therapy. Patients maintained on such a program and studied on the day off the drug have normal blood neutrophil and monocyte counts, normal cutaneous inflammatory responses, and no abnormality of the neutrophil half-life; in contrast, patients on daily therapy demonstrate neutrophilia, monocytopenia, decreased cutaneous neutrophil and monocyte inflammatory responses, and prolongation of the neutrophil half-life.[99,202] Patients studied on the day off therapy do not have the lymphocytopenia observed in patients receiving daily treatment.[99,197,203] Monocyte cellular function is normal in patients on alternate-day therapy when studied 4 hours and 24 hours after a dose,[208] although daily therapy in divided doses depresses the bactericidal activity of monocytes.[113] Intermittently normal leukocyte kinetics,[99,197,202,203] preservation of delayed hypersensitivity,[192,203] and preservation of monocyte cellular function[208] may explain the apparently reduced susceptibility to infections of patients on alternate-day therapy.

Effects of Alternate-Day Steroid Therapy on HPA Responsiveness. Patients on alternate-day glucocorticoid therapy may have some suppression of basal steroid levels, but they have normal to nearly normal responsiveness to provocative tests such as ACTH stimulation tests,[187,214,215] insulin-induced hypoglycemia,[193,216] and the metyrapone test.[190,217] They also have less suppression of HPA function than patients on daily therapy.[184,187,218,219]

Effects of Alternate-Day Therapy on the Underlying Disease. Alternate-day glucocorticoid therapy is as effective or nearly as effective in controlling a diverse group of diseases as daily therapy in divided doses. This approach has been utilized with apparent benefit in patients with the following disorders: childhood nephrotic syndrome,[191] adult nephrotic syndrome,[198,220] membranous nephropathy,[221,222] renal transplantation,[194,195,199,200,204,206,223-226] mesangiocapillary glomerulonephritis,[227] lupus nephritis,[228] ulcerative colitis,[229,230] rheumatoid arthritis,[182,231] acute rheumatic fever,[232] myasthenia gravis,[233-239] Duchenne muscular dystrophy,[240] dermatomyositis,[241] idiopathic polyneuropathy,[242,243] asthma,[183,205,215,218,244] sarcoidosis,[196,201] alopecia areata and other chronic dermatoses,[186] and pemphigus vulgaris.[232,245] In one study, alternate-day therapy was not as effective as daily therapy in reducing the sedimentation rate in giant cell arteritis.[246] However, patients were transferred abruptly from daily therapy with divided doses to alternate-day therapy.[246] In addition, there were few adverse effects of steroids and no evidence of progression of the arteritis on the alternate-day regimen, so there may be a role for this approach in giant cell arteritis.[247] In another study, 18 of 27 patients with giant cell arteritis were treated successfully with an al-

Figure 54–4. The effect of glucocorticoid administration on the activity of the underlying disease. Full-blown disease activity may require the use of a divided daily dose schedule. When the disease is controlled, or from the start of therapy in certain diseases, alternate-day therapy may be effective. (From Fauci, A.S., Dale, D.C., and Balow, J.E.: Ann. Intern. Med. 84:304, 1976.)

ternate-day regimen after a gradual transition from daily single dose therapy.[248] Prospective controlled studies demonstrate the efficacy of alternate-day therapy in membranous nephropathy[221] and renal transplantation.[224,226]

Use of Alternate-Day Therapy. Since alternate-day therapy can prevent or ameliorate the manifestations of Cushing's syndrome, can avert or permit recovery from HPA suppression, and is as effective (or nearly as effective) as continuous therapy, whenever possible a patient for whom chronic glucocorticoid administration is indicated should be placed on such a program. Yet some physicians are reluctant to utilize alternate-day schedules, often because of an unsuccessful experience. Many efforts fail because of lack of familiarity with the indications for, and use of, such therapy.

The benefits of alternate-day glucocorticoid therapy are demonstrable only when steroids are used for a prolonged period. There is no reason to use an alternate-day schedule when the anticipated duration of therapy is no longer than several weeks.

Alternate-day therapy may not be necessary or appropriate during the initial stages of therapy or during exacerbation of the underlying disease. Nevertheless, patients with childhood and adult nephrotic syndrome,[191,193,198,220] membranous nephropathy,[221,222] lupus nephritis,[228] rheumatoid arthritis,[182,231] myasthenia gravis,[233-236] dermatomyositis,[241] asthma,[214,215,244] sarcoidosis,[196,201] rheumatic fever,[232] pemphigus vulgaris,[245] a variety of ocular diseases,[213] and several other disorders have been treated with an alternate-day regimen as initial therapy with apparent benefit. It appears to be easier to establish treatment with alternate-day steroids than to convert from daily therapy in patients with rheumatoid arthritis.[182,231] Studies in recipients of renal transplants have initially used daily therapy and then converted to an alternate-day schedule. Thus, an alternate-day schedule as initial therapy may be beneficial in some disorders but ineffective in others.

Alternate-day therapy may be hazardous in the presence of adrenocortical insufficiency of any cause because the patient is unprotected against glucocorticoid insufficiency during the last 12 hours of the 48-hour cycle.[182,187,194] In a patient who has been on glucocorticoids for more than a brief period, or who may have adrenal insufficiency on another basis, adequacy of HPA function should be determined before the initiation of an alternate-day program. It may be possible to surmount this obstacle by giving a small dose of a short-acting glucocorticoid (i.e., 10 mg of hydrocortisone) in the afternoon of the second day; this approach has not been studied.

Alternate-day glucocorticoid therapy may fail to prevent or ameliorate the manifestations of Cushing's syndrome or HPA suppression if a short-acting glucocorticoid is not used, or if it is used incorrectly.[11,214,249,250] For example, the use of prednisone four times per day on alternate-days may be less successful than use of the same total dose once every 48 hours.

An abrupt alteration from daily to alternate-day therapy should be avoided because the prolonged use of daily-dose glucocorticoids may have resulted in HPA suppression. In addition, patients with normal function of the HPA axis may experience withdrawal symptoms in these circumstances and have an exacerbation of the underlying disease.[204]

No program of conversion from continuous therapy to alternate-day therapy has been proved to be optimal. One approach is to reduce the frequency of drug administration each day, until the total dose for each day is given in the morning, and then gradually to increase the dose on the first day of each 2-day period and to decrease the dose on the second day. Another approach is to double the dose on the first day of each 2-day cycle, and to give this as a single morning dose, if possible, and then to taper gradually the dose on the second day.[251] It is not clear how often such changes should be made with any approach. This probably depends on the underlying disease involved, the duration of previous glucocorticoid therapy, the personality of the patient, and the physician's ability to utilize adjunctive therapy. In any event, the conversion should be made as quickly as the patient will tolerate it. If the patient develops evidence of adrenal insufficiency, of the steroid withdrawal syndrome, or of an exacerbation of the underlying disease, the previously effective regimen should be reinstituted and then tapered more gradually. Occasionally, it will be necessary to resume full daily doses temporarily. Changes in the dose should be approximately 10 mg of prednisone (or equivalent) at total daily doses of more than 40 mg, 5 mg at total doses of more than 20 mg, and 2.5 mg at lower doses. At small total daily doses, an absolute change of dose represents a larger percentage change in dose than at large total daily doses. The interval between changes in dose may be as short as one day or as long as many weeks.

Also, optimal results from alternate-day glucocorticoid therapy may not be achieved because of failure to utilize supplemental therapy for the underlying disorder. Conservative (nonglucocorticoid) therapy is often used until a glucocorticoid is initiated, at which time these less toxic therapeutic measures are ignored. Utilization of adjunctive therapy may facilitate the use of the lowest possible dose of glucocorticoids. On alternate-day therapy, these measures should be used especially during the end of the second day, when symptoms may be prominent. The potential benefits of nonsteroidal anti-inflammatory agents in the rheumatic diseases should not be neglected. Supplemental therapy may be especially helpful in disorders in which the patient is likely to experience symptoms of the disease on the day off therapy, such as asthma and rheumatoid arthritis. In illnesses in which disabling symptoms are less likely to appear on the alternate day, such as the childhood nephrotic syndrome, less difficulty may be encountered.

Alternate-day therapy may fail because of failure to inform the patient about the purposes of this regimen. Because glucocorticoids may induce euphoria, a patient may be reluctant to accept modification of a schedule of frequent doses. Careful explanation about the risks of glucocorticoid excess, attuned to the patient's intellectual and emotional ability to comprehend, will maximize the likelihood of success. Close communication between patient and physician is indispensable.

DAILY SINGLE–DOSE GLUCOCORTICOID THERAPY

In some situations, alternate-day therapy fails because the patient experiences symptoms of the underlying disease during the last few hours of the second day. In these cases, single-dose glucocorticoid therapy may be of value. This regimen appears to be as effective as divided daily doses in controlling such underlying diseases as rheumatoid arthritis, systemic lupus erythematosus, polyarteritis, and proctocolitis.[252-255] In giant cell arteritis, a daily dose in the morning is nearly as effective as daily therapy in divided doses.[246] Daily single-dose therapy appears to reduce the likelihood that a patient will develop HPA suppression.[29,254,256,257] On the other hand, the manifestations of Cushing's syndrome are probably not prevented or ameliorated by a daily single-dose regimen.[252,253]

GLUCOCORTICOIDS OR ACTH?

Disorders that respond to glucocorticoid therapy also respond to ACTH therapy if the adrenal cortex is normal. However, there is no evidence that ACTH is superior to glucocorticoids for the treatment of any disorder when comparable doses are used.[2,16,258] In fact, hydrocortisone and ACTH, when given intravenously in pharmacologically equivalent dosage (determined by plasma cortisol levels and urinary steroid excretion rates) are equally effective in the treatment of inflammatory bowel disease.[259] Since ACTH does not appear to offer any therapeutic advantage, glucocorticoids are preferable for therapeutic purposes;[2] they can be administered orally, the dose can be regulated precisely, the effectiveness does not depend on adrenocortical responsiveness (an important consideration in patients who have been treated with glucocorticoids), and they produce a lower incidence of certain side effects, such as acne, hypertension, and increased pigmentation.[260] When one is unable to use alternate-day therapy, ACTH might appear to be preferable because it does not suppress the HPA axis. This benefit is usually outweighed by the advantages of glucocorticoids enumerated above and by the fact that daily injections of ACTH are not superior to single daily doses of short-acting glucocorticoids; in both cases, HPA suppression is unlikely to result, but Cushing's syndrome is not prevented. In life-threatening situations, glucocorticoids are indicated because maximal blood levels are obtained immediately after intravenous administration, while with ACTH infusion the plasma cortisol level rises to a plateau over several hours.

The principal indication for ACTH continues to be the assessment of adrenocortical reserve.

References

1. Polley, H.F., and Slocumb, C.H.: Behind the scenes with cortisone and ACTH. Mayo Clin. Proc. 51:471, 1976.
2. Axelrod, L.: Glucocorticoid therapy. Medicine 55:39, 1976.
3. Hollander, J.L., Brown, E.M., Jr., Jessar, R.A., and Brown, C.Y.: Hydrocortisone and cortisone injected into arthritic joints. JAMA 147:1629, 1951.
4. Robinson, R.C.V., and Robinson, H.M., Jr.: Topical treatment of dermatoses with steroids. South. Med. J. 49:260, 1956.
5. Jenkins, J.S.: The metabolism of cortisol by human extrahepatic tissues. J. Endocrinol. 34:51, 1966.
6. Schalm, S.W., Summerskill, W.H.J., and Go, V.L.W.: Development of radioimmunoassays for prednisone and prednisolone: Application to studies of hepatic metabolism of prednisone. Mayo Clin. Proc. 51:761, 1976.
7. Krieger, D.T., Allen, W., Rizzo, F., and Krieger, H.P.: Characterization of the normal temporal pattern of plasma corticosteroid levels. J. Clin. Endocrinol. Metab. 32:266, 1971.
8. Gann, D.S., Dallman, M.F., and Engeland, W.C.: Reflex control and modulation of ACTH and corticosteroids. In McCann, S.M. (ed.): Endocrine Physiology III. Int. Rev. Physiol. Vol. 24. Baltimore, University Park Press, 1981, p. 157.
9. Giguère, V., Labrie, F., Côté, J., Coy, D.H., Sueiras-Diaz, J., and Schally, A.V.: Stimulation of cyclic AMP accumulation and corticotropin release by synthetic ovine corticotropin-releasing factor in rat anterior pituitary cells: Site of glucocorticoid action. Proc. Natl. Acad. Sci. USA 79:3466, 1982.
10. Estep, H.L., Island, D.P., Ney, R.L., and Liddle, G.W.: Pituitary adrenal dynamics during surgical stress. J. Clin. Endocrinol. Metab. 23:419, 1963.
11. Harter, J.G.: Corticosteroids: Their physiologic use in allergic diseases. N.Y. State J. Med. 66:827, 1966.
12. Boland, E.W.: 16-α-Methyl corticosteroids. Calif. Med. 88:417, 1958.
13. Boland, E.W., and Liddle, G.W.: Metabolic and antirheumatic activities of 6-methylprednisolone (Medrol). Ann. Rheum. Dis. 16:297, 1957.
14. Bondy, P.K.: The adrenal cortex. In Bondy, P.K., and Rosenberg, L.E. (eds.): Duncan's Diseases of Metabolism. 7th ed. Philadelphia, W. B. Saunders Company, 1974, p. 1105.
15. Bunim, J.J., Black, R.L., Lutwak, L., Peterson, R.E., and Whedon, G.D.: Studies on dexamethasone, a new synthetic steroid, in rheumatoid arthritis—a preliminary report. Arthritis Rheum. 1:313, 1958.
16. Cope, C.L.: Adrenal Steroids and Disease. 2nd ed. London, Pitman Medical, 1972.
17. Kleeman, C.R., Koplowitz, J., and Maxwell, M.H.: Metabolic effects of two newer adrenal analogs, 6-methylprednisolone (Medrol) and 6-methyl-9α-fluoro-21-desoxyprednisolone (9α-fluoro-21-desoxymedrol). Metabolism 7:425, 1958.
18. Liddle, G.W.: Studies of structure-function relationships of steroids. II. The 6α-methylcorticosteroids. Metabolism 7:405, 1958.
19. Liddle, G.W.: Clinical pharmacology of the anti-inflammatory agents. Clin. Pharmacol. Ther. 2:615, 1961.
20. Liddle, G.W.: The adrenal cortex. In Williams, R.H. (ed.): Textbook of Endocrinology. 5th ed. Philadelphia, W. B. Saunders Company, 1974, p. 233.
21. Meikle, A.W., and Tyler, F.H.: Potency and duration of action of glucocorticoids. Effects of hydrocortisone, prednisone and dexamethasone on human pituitary-adrenal function. Am. J. Med. 63:200, 1977.
22. Ballard, P.L., Carter, J.P., Graham, B.S., and Baxter, J.D.: A radioreceptor assay for evaluation of the plasma glucocorticoid activity of natural and synthetic steroids in man. J. Clin. Endocrinol. Metab. 41:290, 1975.
23. Morris, H.G.: Factors that influence clinical responses to administered corticosteroids. J. Allergy Clin. Immunol. 66:343, 1980.
24. Pickup, M.E.: Clinical pharmacokinetics of prednisone and prednisolone. Clin. Pharmacokinetics 4:111, 1979.
25. Pickup, M.E., Lowe, J.R., Leatham, P.A., Rhind, V.M., Wright, V., and Downie, W.W.: Dose dependent pharmacokinetics of prednisolone. Eur. J. Clin. Pharmacol. 12:213, 1977.
26. Gambertoglio, J.G., Amend, W.J.C., Jr., and Benet, L.Z.: Pharmacokinetics and bioavailability of prednisone and prednisolone in healthy volunteers and patients: A review. J. Pharmacokinet. Biopharm. 8:1, 1980.
27. Walton, J., Watson, B.S., and Ney, R.L.: Alternate-day vs. shorter interval steroid administration. Arch. Intern. Med. 126:601, 1970.
28. Ellul-Micallef, R., Borthwick, R.C., and McHardy, G.J.R.: The timecourse of response to prednisolone in chronic bronchial asthma. Clin. Sci. 47:105, 1974.
29. Grant, S.D., Forsham, P.H., and DiRaimondo, V.C.: Suppression of 17-

hydroxycorticosteroids in plasma and urine by single and divided doses of triamcinolone. N. Engl. J. Med. 273:1115, 1965.

30. Thompson, E.B., and Lippmann, M.E.: Mechanism of action of gluco-corticoids. Metabolism 23:159, 1974.

31. Baxter, J.D.: Glucocorticoid hormone action. Pharmacol. Ther. B 2:605, 1976.

32. Chan, L., and O'Malley, B.W.: Steroid hormone action: Recent advances. Ann. Intern. Med. 89:694, 1978.

33. Jenkins, J.S., and Sampson, P.A.: Conversion of cortisone to cortisol and prednisone to prednisolone. Br. Med. J. 2:205, 1967.

34. Sugita, E.T., and Niebergall, P.J.: Prednisone. J. Am. Pharm. Assoc. 15:529, 1975.

35. DiSanto, A.R., and DeSante, K.A.: Bioavailability and pharmacokinetics of prednisone in humans. J. Pharm. Sci. 64:109, 1975.

36. Thiessen, J.J.: Prednisolone. J. Am. Pharm. Assoc. 16:143, 1976.

37. Tembo, A.V., Hallmark, M.R., Sakmar, E., Bachmann, H.G., Weidler, D.J., and Wagner, J.G.: Bioavailability of prednisolone tablets. J. Pharmacokinet. Biopharm. 5:257, 1977.

38. Duggan, D.E., Yeh, K.C., Matalia, N., Ditzler, C.A., and McMahon, F.G.: Bioavailability of oral dexamethasone. Clin. Pharmacol. Ther. 18:205, 1975.

39. Nelson, D.H., Sandberg, A.A., Palmer, J.G., and Tyler, F.H.: Blood levels of 17-hydroxycorticosteroids following the administration of adrenal steroids and their relation to levels of circulating leukocytes. J. Clin. Invest. 31:843, 1952.

40. Gemzell, C.A., and Franksson, C.: Blood levels of 17-hydroxycorticosteroids in normal and adrenalectomized men following administration of cortisone acetate. Acta Endocrinol. 12:218, 1953.

41. Plumpton, F.S., Besser, G.M., and Cole, P.V.: Corticosteroid treatment and surgery. 2. The management of steroid cover. Anaesthesia 24:12, 1969.

42. Banks, P.: The adreno-cortical response to oral surgery. Br. J. Oral Surg. 8:32, 1970.

43. Kehlet, H., Nistrup Madsen, S., and Binder, C.: Cortisol and cortisone acetate in parenteral glucocorticoid therapy? Acta Med. Scand. 195:421, 1974.

44. Kehlet, H.: A rational approach to dosage and preparation of parenteral glucocorticoid substitution therapy during surgical procedures. A short review. Acta Anaesth. Scand. 19:260, 1975.

45. Fariss, B.L., Hane, S., Shinsako, J., and Forsham, P.H.: Comparison of absorption of cortisone acetate and hydrocortisone hemisuccinate. J. Clin. Endocrinol. Metab. 47:1137, 1978.

46. Angeli, A., Frajria, R., DePaoli, R., Fonzo, D., and Ceresa, F.: Diurnal variation of prednisolone binding to serum corticosteroid-binding globulin in man. Clin. Pharmacol. Ther. 23:47, 1978.

47. Kozower, M., Veatch, L., and Kaplan, M.M.: Decreased clearance of prednisolone, a factor in the development of corticosteroid side effects. J. Clin. Endocrinol. Metab. 38:407, 1974.

48. Schalm, S.W., Summerskill, W.H.J., and Go, V.L.W.: Prednisone for chronic active liver disease: Pharmacokinetics, including conversion to prednisolone. Gastroenterology 72:910, 1977.

49. Peterson, R.E.: Adrenocortical steroid metabolism and adrenal cortical function in liver disease. J. Clin. Invest. 39:320, 1960.

50. Powell, L.W., and Axelsen, E.: Corticosteroids in liver disease: Studies on the biological conversion of prednisone to prednisolone and plasma protein binding. Gut 13:690, 1972.

51. Davis, M., Williams, R., Chakraborty, J., English, J., Marks, V., Ideo, G., and Tempini, S.: Prednisone or prednisolone for the treatment of chronic active hepatitis? A comparison of plasma availability. Br. J. Clin. Pharmacol. 5:501, 1978.

52. Araki, Y., Yokota, O., Tatsuo, K., Kashima, M., and Miyazaki, T.: Dynamics of synthetic corticosteroids in man. In Pincus, G., Nakao, T., and Tait, J.F. (eds.): Steroid Dynamics. New York, Academic Press, 1966, p. 463.

53. Lewis, G.P., Jusko, W.J., Burke, C.W., Graves, L., and the Boston Collaborative Drug Surveillance Program: Prednisone side-effects and serum-protein levels, a collaborative study. Lancet 2:778, 1971.

54. Schatz, M., Patterson, R., Zeitz, S., O'Rourke, J., and Melam, H.: Corticosteroid therapy for the pregnant asthmatic patient. JAMA 233:804, 1975.

55. Ohrlander, S., Gennser, G., Nilsson, K.O., and Eneroth, P.: ACTH test to neonates after administration of corticosteroids during gestation. Obstet. Gynecol. 49:691, 1977.

56. Grajwer, L.A., Lilien, L.D., and Pildes, R.S.: Neonatal subclinical adrenal insufficiency: Result of maternal steroid therapy. JAMA 238:1279, 1977.

57. Reinisch, J.M., Simon, N.G., Karow, W.G., and Gandelman, R.: Prenatal exposure to prednisone in humans and animals retards intrauterine growth. Science 202:436, 1978.

58. Katz, F.H., and Duncan, B.R.: Entry of prednisone into human milk (letter). N. Engl. J. Med. 293:1154, 1975.

59. McKenzie, S.A., Selley, J.A., and Agnew, J.E.: Secretion of prednisolone into breast milk. Arch. Dis. Child. 50:894, 1975.

60. Jubiz, W., and Meikle, A.W.: Alterations of glucocorticoid actions by other drugs and disease states. Drugs 18:113, 1979.

61. Choi, Y., Thrasher, K., Werk, E.E., Jr., Sholiton, L.J., and Olinger, C.: Effect of diphenylhydantoin on cortisol kinetics in humans. J. Pharmacol. Exp. Ther. 176:27, 1971.

62. Haque, N., Thrasher, K., Werk, E.E., Jr., Knowles, H.C., Jr., and Sholiton, L.J.: Studies on dexamethasone metabolism in man: Effect of diphenylhydantoin. J. Clin. Endocrinol. Metab. 34:44, 1972.

63. Stjernholm, M.R., and Katz, F.H.: Effects of diphenylhydantoin, phenobarbital, and diazepam on the metabolism of methylprednisolone and its sodium succinate. J. Clin. Endocrinol. Metab. 41:887, 1975.

64. Petereit, L.B., and Meikle, A.W.: Effectiveness of prednisolone during phenytoin therapy. Clin. Pharmacol. Ther. 22:912, 1977.

65. Brooks, S.M., Werk, E.E., Ackerman, S.J., Sullivan, I., and Thrasher, K.: Adverse effects of phenobarbital on corticosteroid metabolism in patients with bronchial asthma. N. Engl. J. Med. 286:1125, 1972.

66. Brooks, P.M., Buchanan, W.W., Grove, M., and Downie, W.W.: Effects of enzyme induction on metabolism of prednisolone. Clinical and laboratory study. Ann. Rheum. Dis. 35:339, 1976.

67. Edwards, O.M., Courtenay-Evans, R.J., Galley, J.M., Hunter, J., and Tait, A.D.: Changes in cortisol metabolism following rifampicin therapy. Lancet 2:549, 1974.

68. Buffington, G.A., Dominguez, J.H., Piering, W.F., Hebert, L.A., Kauffman, H.M., Jr., and Lemann, J., Jr.: Interaction of rifampin and glucocorticoids. Adverse effect on renal allograft function. JAMA 236:1958, 1976.

69. Uribe, M., Casian, C., Rojas, S., Sierra, J.G., and Go, V.L.W.: Decreased bioavailability of prednisone due to antacids in patients with chronic active liver disease and in healthy volunteers. Gastroenterology 80:661, 1981.

70. Klinenberg, J.R., and Miller, F.: Effect of corticosteroids on blood salicylate concentration. JAMA 194:131, 1965.

71. Graham, G.G., Champion, G.D., Day, R.O., and Paull, P.D.: Patterns of plasma concentrations and urinary excretion of salicylate in rheumatoid arthritis. Clin. Pharmacol. Ther. 22:410, 1977.

72. Bardare, M., Cislaghi, G.U., Mandelli, M., and Sereni, F.: Value of monitoring plasma salicylate levels in treating juvenile rheumatoid arthritis. Arch. Dis. Childh. 53:381, 1978.

73. Meyers, E.F.: Partial recovery from pancuronium neuromuscular blockade following hydrocortisone administration. Anesthesiology 46:148, 1977.

74. Laflin, M.J.: Interaction of pancuronium and corticosteroids. Anesthesiology 47:471, 1977.

75. Audétat, V., and Bircher, J.: Bioavailability of prednisolone during simultaneous treatment with cholestyramine. Gastroenterology 71:1110, 1976.

76. Plotz, C.M., Knowlton, A.I., and Ragan, C.: The natural history of Cushing's syndrome. Am. J. Med. 13:597, 1952.

77. Thorn, G.W.: Clinical considerations in the use of corticosteroids. N. Engl. J. Med. 274:775, 1966.

78. Boston Collaborative Drug Surveillance Program: Acute adverse reactions to prednisone in relation to dosage. Clin. Pharmacol. Ther. 13:694, 1972.

79. Hall, R.C.W., Popkin, M.K., Stickney, S.K., and Gardner, E.R.: Presentation of the steroid psychoses. J. Nervous Mental Dis. 167:229, 1979.

80. deLange, W.E., and Doorenbos, H.: Corticotrophins and corticosteroids. In Meyler, L., and Herxheimer, A. (eds.): Side Effects of Drugs, Vol. 7. Amsterdam, Excerpta Medica, 1972, p. 516.

81. Newman, S.: Hormone-induced diseases. In Moser, R.H. (ed.): Diseases of Medical Progress: A Study of Iatrogenic Disease. Springfield, Ill., Charles C Thomas, 1969, p. 361.

82. Fitzgerald, R.H., Jr.: Intrasynovial injection of steroids. Uses and abuses. Mayo Clin. Proc. 51:655, 1976.

83. Balch, H.W., Gibson, J.M.C., El-Ghobarey, A.F., Bain, L.S., and Lynch, M.P.: Repeated corticosteroid injections into knee joints. Rheumatol. Rehab. 16:137, 1977.

84. Carson, T.E., Daane, T.A., and Weinstein, R.L.: Long-term intramuscular administration of triamcinolone acetonide. Effect on the hypothalamic-pituitary-adrenal axis. Arch. Dermatol. 111:1585, 1975.

85. Claman, H.N.: Corticosteroids and lymphoid cells. N. Engl. J. Med. 287:388, 1972.

86. Claman, H.N.: How corticosteroids work. J. Allergy Clin. Immunol. 55:145, 1975.

87. Fauci, A.S., Dale, D.C., and Balow, J.E.: Glucocorticosteroid therapy: Mechanisms of action and clinical considerations. Ann. Intern. Med. 84:304, 1976.

88. Schreiber, A.D.: Clinical immunology of the corticosteroids. Prog. Clin. Immunol. 3:103, 1977.

89. Parrillo, J.E., and Fauci, A.S.: Mechanisms of glucocorticoid action on immune processes. Ann. Rev. Pharmacol. Toxicol. 19:179, 1979.

90. Cupps, T.R., and Fauci, A.S.: Corticosteroid-mediated immunoregulation in man. Immunological Rev. 65:133, 1982.

91. Dale, D.C., Fauci, A.S., Guerry, D., IV, and Wolff, S.M.: Comparison of agents producing neutrophilic leukocytosis in man: Hydrocortisone, prednisone, endotoxin, and etiocholanolone. J. Clin. Invest. 56:808, 1975.

92. Bishop, C.R., Athens, J.W., Boggs, D.R., Warner, H.R., Cartwright, G.E., and Wintrobe, M.M.: Leukokinetic studies. XIII. A non-steady-state kinetic evaluation of the mechanism of cortisone-induced granulocytosis. J. Clin. Invest. 47:249, 1968.

93. Athens, J.W., Haab, O.P., Raab, S.O., Mauer, A.M., Ashenbrucker, H., Cartwright, G.E., and Wintrobe, M.M.: Leukokinetic studies. IV. The total blood, circulating and marginal granulocyte pools and the granulocyte turnover rate in normal subjects. J. Clin. Invest. 40:989, 1961.

94. Boggs, D.R., Athens, J.W., Cartwright, G.E., and Wintrobe, M.M.: The effect of adrenal glucocorticosteroids upon the cellular composition of inflammatory exudates. Am. J. Pathol. 44:763, 1964.

95. Fauci, A.S., and Dale, D.C.: The effect of in vivo hydrocortisone on subpopulations of human lymphocytes. J. Clin. Invest. 53:240, 1974.

96. Yu, D.T.Y., Clements, P.J., Paulus, H.E., Peter, J.B., Levy, J., and Barnett, E.V.: Human lymphocyte subpopulations: Effect of corticosteroids. J. Clin. Invest. 53:565, 1974.

97. Clarke, J.R., Gagnon, R.F., Gotch, F.M., Heyworth, M.R., MacLennan, I.C.M., Truelove, S.C., and Waller, C.A.: The effect of prednisolone on leucocyte function in man: A double blind controlled study. Clin. Exp. Immunol. 28:292, 1977.

98. Cooper, D.A., Petts, V., Luckhurst, E., and Penny, R.: The effect of acute and prolonged administration of prednisolone and ACTH on lymphocyte subpopulations. Clin. Exp. Immunol. 28:467, 1977.

99. Cook, J.D., Trotter, J.L., Engel, W.K., and Sciabbarrasi, J.S.: The effects of single-dose alternate-day prednisone therapy on the immunological status of patients with neuromuscular diseases. Ann. Neurol. 3:166, 1978.

100. Fauci, A.S., and Dale, D.C.: The effect of hydrocortisone on the kinetics of normal human lymphocytes. Blood 46:235, 1975.

101. Yu, D.T.Y., Clements, P.J., and Pearson, C.M.: Effect of corticosteroids on exercise-induced lymphocytosis. Clin. Exp. Immunol. 28:326, 1977.

102. Ebert, R.H., and Barclay, W.R.: Changes in connective tissue reaction induced by cortisone. Ann. Intern. Med. 37:506, 1952.

103. Zweifach, B.W., Shorr, E., and Black, M.M.: The influence of the adrenal cortex on behavior of terminal vascular bed. Ann. N.Y. Acad. Sci. 56:626, 1953.

104. MacGregor, R.R., Spagnuolo, P.J., and Lentnek, A.L.: Inhibition of granulocyte adherence by ethanol, prednisone, and aspirin, measured with an assay system. N. Engl. J. Med. 291:642, 1974.

105. MacGregor, R.R.: The effect of anti-inflammatory agents and inflammation on granulocyte adherence: Evidence for regulation by plasma factors. Am. J. Med. 61:597, 1976.

106. MacGregor, R.R.: Granulocyte adherence changes induced by hemodialysis, endotoxin, epinephrine, and glucocorticoids. Ann. Intern. Med. 86:35, 1977.

107. Bovornkitti, S., Kangsadal, P., Sathirapat, P., and Oonsombatti, P.: Reversion and reconversion rate of tuberculin skin reactions in correlation with the use of prednisone. Dis. Chest 38:51, 1960.

108. Cummings, M.M., and Hudgins, P.C.: The influence of cortisone on the passive transfer of tuberculin hypersensitivity in the guinea pig. J. Immunol. 69:331, 1952.

109. Seebohm, P.M., Tremaine, M.M., and Jeter, W.S.: The effect of cortisone and adrenocorticotropic hormone on passively transferred delayed hypersensitivity to 2,4-dinitrochlorobenzene in guinea pigs. J. Immunol. 73:44, 1954.

110. Weston, W.L., Mandel, M.J., Yeckley, J.A., Krueger, G.G., and Claman, H.N.: Mechanism of cortisol inhibition of adoptive transfer of tuberculin sensitivity. J. Lab. Clin. Med. 82:366, 1973.

111. Balow, J.E., and Rosenthal, A.S.: Glucocorticoid suppression of macrophage migration inhibitory factor. J. Exp. Med. 137:1031, 1973.

112. Rinehart, J.J., Balcerzak, S.P., Sagone, A.L., and LoBuglio, A.F.: Effects of corticosteroids on human monocyte function. J. Clin. Invest. 54:1337, 1974.

113. Rinehart, J.J., Sagone, A.L., Balcerzak, S.P., Ackerman, G.A., and LoBuglio, A.F.: Effects of corticosteroid therapy on human monocyte function. N. Engl. J. Med. 292:236, 1975.

114. Handin, R.I., and Stossel, T.P.: Effect of corticosteroid therapy on the phagocytosis of antibody-coated platelets by human leukocytes. Blood 51:771, 1978.

115. Frank, M.M., Schreiber, A.D., Atkinson, J.P., and Jaffe, C.J.: Pathophysiology of immune hemolytic anemia. Ann. Intern. Med. 87:210, 1977.

116. Lewis, G.P., and Piper, P.J.: Inhibition of release of prostaglandins as an explanation of some of the actions of anti-inflammatory corticosteroids. Nature 254:308, 1975.

117. Kantrowitz, F., Robinson, D.R., McGuire, M.B., and Levine, L.: Corticosteroids inhibit prostaglandin production by rheumatoid synovia. Nature 258:737, 1975.

118. Tashjian, A.H., Jr., Voelkel, E.F., McDonough, J., and Levine, L.: Hydrocortisone inhibits prostaglandin production by mouse fibrosarcoma cells. Nature 258:739, 1975.

119. Gryglewski, R.J.: Steroid hormones, anti-inflammatory steroids and prostaglandins. Pharmacol. Res. Commun. 8:337, 1976.

120. Hong, S.-C.L., and Levine, L.: Inhibition of arachidonic acid release from cells as the biochemical action of anti-inflammatory corticosteroids. Proc. Natl. Acad. Sci. 73:1730, 1976.

121. Robinson, D.R., Tashjian, A.H., Jr., and Levine, L.: Prostaglandin-stimulated bone resorption by rheumatoid synovia: A possible mechanism for bone destruction in rheumatoid arthritis. J. Clin. Invest. 56:1181, 1975.

122. Samuelsson, B.: Leukotrienes: Mediators of immediate hypersensitivity reactions and inflammation. Science 220:568, 1983.

123. Janoski, A.H., Shaver, J.C., Christy, N.P., and Rosner, W.: On the pharmacologic actions of 21-carbon hormonal steroids ('glucocorticoids') of the adrenal cortex in mammals. In Deane, H.W., and Rubin, B.L. (eds.): Handbuch der Experimentellen Pharmakologie. Vol. XIV, Part 3 (The Adrenocortical Hormones). Berlin, Springer-Verlag, 1968, p. 256.

124. Christy, N.P.: Iatrogenic Cushing's syndrome. In Christy, N.P. (ed.): The Human Adrenal Cortex. New York, Harper & Row, 1971, p. 395.

125. Ragan, C.: Corticotropin, cortisone and related steroids in clinical medicine: Practical considerations. Bull. N.Y. Acad. Med. 29:355, 1953.

126. Intracranial hypertension and steroids (leading article.) Lancet 2:1052, 1964.

127. Walker, A.E., and Adamkiewicz, J.J.: Pseudotumor cerebri associated with prolonged corticosteroid therapy. JAMA 188:779, 1964.

128. David, D.S., and Berkowitz, J.S.: Ocular effects of topical and systemic corticosteroids. Lancet 2:149, 1969.

129. Lubkin, V.L.: Steroid cataract—a review and a conclusion. J. Asthma Res. 14:55, 1977.

130. Pavlin, C.R., DeVeber, G.A., Cook, G.T., and Chisholm, L.D.J.: Ocular complications in renal transplant recipients. Can. Med. Assoc. J. 117:360, 1977.

131. Heimann, W.G., and Freiberger, R.H.: Avascular necrosis of the femoral and humeral heads after high-dosage corticosteroid therapy. N. Engl. J. Med. 263:672, 1960.

132. Velayos, E.E., Leidholt, J.D., Smyth, C.J., and Priest, R.: Arthropathy associated with steroid therapy. Ann. Intern. Med. 64:759, 1966.

133. Harrington, K.D., Murray, W.R., Kountz, S.L., and Belzer, F.O.: Avascular necrosis of bone after renal transplantation. J. Bone Joint Surg. 53A:203, 1971.

134. Fisher, D.E., and Bickel, W.H.: Corticosteroid-induced aseptic necrosis: A clinical study of seventy-seven patients. J. Bone Joint Surg. 53A:859, 1971.

135. Park, W.M.: Spontaneous and drug-induced aseptic necrosis. In Davidson, J.K. (ed.): Aseptic Necrosis of Bone. Amsterdam, Excerpta Medica, 1976, p. 213.

136. Cruess, R.L.: Cortisone-induced avascular necrosis of the femoral head. J. Bone Joint Surg. 59B:308, 1977.

137. Abeles, M., Urman, J.D., and Rothfield, N.F.: Aseptic necrosis of bone in systemic lupus erythematosus. Arch. Intern. Med. 138:750, 1978.

138. Fenster, L.F.: The ulcerogenic potential of glucocorticoids and possible prophylactic measures. In Azarnoff, D.L. (ed.): Steroid Therapy. Philadelphia, W. B. Saunders Company, 1975, p. 42.

139. Conn, H.O., and Blitzer, B.L.: Nonassociation of adrenocorticosteroid therapy and peptic ulcer. N. Engl. J. Med. 294:473, 1976.

140. Langman, M.J.S., and Cooke, A.R.: Gastric and duodenal ulcer and their associated diseases. Lancet 1:680, 1976.

141. Jick, H., and Porter, J.: Drug-induced gastrointestinal bleeding. Lancet 2:87, 1978.

142. Messer, J., Reitman, D., Sacks, H.S., Smith, H., Jr., and Chalmers, T.C.: Association of adrenocorticosteroid therapy and peptic-ulcer disease. N. Engl. J. Med. 309:21, 1983.

143. Spiro, H.M.: Is the steroid ulcer a myth? N. Engl. J. Med. 309:45, 1983.

144. Schatz, M., Patterson, R., Kloner, R., and Falk, J.: The prevalence of tuberculosis and positive tuberculin skin tests in a steroid-treated asthmatic population. Ann. Intern. Med. 84:261, 1976.

145. Frey, F.J., Amend, W.J.C., Jr., Lozada, F., Frey, B.M., and Benet, L.Z.: Endogenous hydrocortisone, a possible factor contributing to the genesis of cushingoid habitus in patients on prednisone. J. Clin. Endocrinol. Metab. 53:1076, 1981.

146. Becker, B.: Intraocular pressure response to topical corticosteroids. Invest. Ophthalmol. 4:198, 1965.

147. Bigger, J.F., Palmberg, P.F., and Becker, B.: Increased cellular sensitivity to glucocorticoids in primary open angle glaucoma. Invest. Ophthalmol. 11:832, 1972.

148. Becker, B., Podos, S.M., Asseff, C.F., and Cooper, D.G.: Plasma cortisol suppression in glaucoma. Am. J. Ophthalmol. 75:73, 1973.
149. Becker, B., Shin, D.H., Palmberg, P.F., and Waltman, S.R.: HLA antigens and corticosteroid response. Science 194:1427, 1976.
150. Good, T.A., Benton, J.W., and Kelley, V.C.: Symptomatology resulting from withdrawal of steroid hormone therapy. Arthritis Rheum. 2:299, 1959.
151. Amatruda, T.T., Jr., Hollingsworth, D.R., D'Esopo, N.D., Upton, G.V., and Bondy, P.K.: A study of the mechanism of the steroid withdrawal syndrome. Evidence for integrity of the hypothalamic-pituitary-adrenal system. J. Clin. Endocrinol. Metab. 20:339, 1960.
152. Amatruda, T.T., Jr., Hurst, M.M., and D'Esopo, N.D.: Certain endocrine and metabolic facets of the steroid withdrawal syndrome. J. Clin. Endocrinol. Metab. 25:1207, 1965.
153. Paris, J.: Pituitary-adrenal suppression after protracted administration of adrenal cortical hormones. Proc. Mayo Clin. 36:305, 1961.
154. Salassa, R.M., Bennett, W.A., Keating, F.R., and Sprague, R.G.: Postoperative adrenal cortical insufficiency: Occurrence in patients previously treated with cortisone. JAMA 152:1509, 1953.
155. Streck, W.F., and Lockwood, D.H.: Pituitary adrenal recovery following short-term suppression with corticosteroids. Am. J. Med. 66:910, 1979.
156. Christy, N.P., Wallace, E.Z., and Jailer, J.W.: Comparative effects of prednisone and of cortisone in suppressing the response of the adrenal cortex to exogenous adrenocorticotropin. J. Clin. Endocrinol. Metab. 16:1059, 1956.
157. Jasani, M.K., Freeman, P.A., Boyle, J.A., Reid, A.M., Diver, M.J., and Buchanan, W.W.: Studies of the rise in plasma 11-hydroxycorticosteroids (11-OHCS) in corticosteroid-treated patients with rheumatoid arthritis during surgery: Correlations with the functional integrity of the hypothalamic-pituitary-adrenal axis. Quart. J. Med. 37:407, 1968.
158. Kehlet, H., and Binder, C.: Value of an ACTH test in assessing hypothalamic-pituitary-adrenocortical function in glucocorticoid-treated patients. Br. Med. J. 2:147, 1973.
159. Marks, L.J., Donovan, M.J., Duncan, F.J., and Karger, R.: Adrenocortical response to surgical operations in patients treated with corticosteroids or corticotropin prior to surgery. J. Clin. Endocrinol. Metab. 19:1458, 1959.
160. Sampson, P.A., Winstone, N.F., and Brooke, B.N.: Adrenal function in surgical patients after steroid therapy. Lancet 2:322, 1962.
161. Danowski, T.S., Bonessi, J.V., Sabeh, G., Sutton, R.D., Webster, M.W., Jr., and Sarver, M.E.: Probabilities of pituitary-adrenal responsiveness after steroid therapy. Ann. Intern. Med. 61:11, 1964.
162. Nichols, T., Nugent, C.A., and Tyler, F.H.: Diurnal variation in suppression of adrenal function by glucocorticoids. J. Clin. Endocrinol. Metab. 25:343, 1965.
163. Chamberlain, M.A., and Keenan, J.: The effect of low doses of prednisolone compared with placebo on function and on the hypothalamic pituitary adrenal axis in patients with rheumatoid arthritis. Rheumatol. Rehab. 15:17, 1976.
164. Carter, M.E., and James, V.H.T.: Comparison of effects of corticotrophin and corticosteroids on pituitary-adrenal function. Ann. Rheum. Dis. 30:91, 1971.
165. Daly, J.R., and Glass, D.: Corticosteroid and growth hormone response to hypoglycaemia in patients on long-term treatment with corticotrophin. Lancet 1:476, 1971.
166. Daly, J.R., Fletcher, M.R., Glass, D., Chambers, D.J., Bitensky, L., and Chayen, J.: Comparison of effects of long-term corticotrophin and corticosteroid treatment on responses of plasma growth hormone, ACTH, and corticosteroid to hypoglycaemia. Br. Med. J. 2:521, 1974.
167. Graber, A.L., Ney, R.L., Nicholson, W.E., Island, D.P., and Liddle, G.W.: Natural history of pituitary-adrenal recovery following long-term suppression with corticosteroids. J. Clin. Endocrinol. Metab. 25:11, 1965.
168. Livanou, T., Ferriman, D., and James, V.H.T.: Recovery of hypothalamo-pituitary-adrenal function after corticosteroid therapy. Lancet 2:856, 1967.
169. Webb, J., and Clark, T.J.H. Recovery of plasma corticotrophin and cortisol levels after a three-week course of prednisolone. Thorax 36:22, 1981.
170. Spitzer, S.A., Kaufman, H., Koplovitz, A., Topilsky, M., and Blum, I.: Beclomethasone dipropionate and chronic asthma: The effect of long-term aerosol administration on the hypothalamic-pituitary-adrenal axis after substitution for oral therapy with corticosteroids. Chest 70:38, 1976.
171. Westerhof, L., Van Ditmars, M.J., DerKinderen, P.J., Thijssen, J.H.H., and Schwarz, F.: Recovery of adrenocortical function during long-term treatment with corticosteroids. Br. Med. J. 4:534, 1970.
172. Westerhof, L., Van Ditmars, M.J., DerKinderen, P.J., Thijssen, J.H.H., and Schwarz, F.: Recovery of adrenocortical function during long-term treatment with corticosteroids. Br. Med. J. 2:195, 1972.

173. Kyle, L.H., Meyer, R.J., and Canary, J.J.: Mechanism of adrenal atrophy in Cushing's syndrome due to adrenal tumor. N. Eng. J. Med. 257:57, 1957.
174. Morris, H.G., and Jorgensen, J.R.: Recovery of endogenous pituitary-adrenal function in corticosteroid-treated children. J. Pediat. 79:480, 1971.
175. Smith, R.T., and Good, R.A.: Sequelae of prednisone treatment of acute rheumatic fever. Clin. Res. Proc. 4:156, 1956.
176. Taranta, A., Mark, H., Haas, R.C., and Cooper, N.S.: Nodular panniculitis after massive prednisone therapy. Am. J. Med. 25:52, 1958.
177. Vince, D.J.: Nodular panniculitis after massive prednisone therapy. Can. Med. Assoc. J. 79:840, 1958.
178. Spagnuolo, M., and Taranta, A.: Post-steroid panniculitis. Ann. Intern. Med. 54:1181, 1963.
179. Young, I.I., DeFilippis, V., Meyer, F.L., and Wolfson, W.Q.: Maintenance of adrenal cortical responsiveness during prolonged corticoid therapy. Arch. Intern. Med. 100:1, 1957.
180. Fleischer, N., Abe, K., Liddle, G.W., Orth, D.N., and Nicholson, W.E.: ACTH antibodies in patients receiving depot porcine ACTH to hasten recovery from pituitary-adrenal suppression. J. Clin. Invest. 46:196, 1967.
181. Carter, M.E., and James, V.H.T.: An attempt at combining corticotrophin with long-term corticotrophin therapy: With a view to preserving hypothalamic-pituitary-adrenal function. Ann. Rheum. Dis. 29:409, 1970.
182. Carter, M.E., and James, V.H.T.: Effect of alternate-day, single-dose corticosteroid therapy on pituitary-adrenal function. Ann. Rheum. Dis. 31:379, 1972.
183. Portner, M.M., Thayer, K.H., Harter, J.G., Rayyis, S., Liang, T.C., and Kent, J.R.: Successful initiation of alternate-day prednisone in chronic steroid-dependent asthmatic patients. J. Allergy Clin. Immunol. 49:16, 1972.
184. Morris, H.G., Neuman, I., and Ellis, E.F.: Plasma steroid concentrations during alternate-day treatment with prednisone. J. Allergy Clin. Immunol. 54:350, 1974.
185. Haugen, H.N., Reddy, W.J., and Harter, J.G.: Intermittent steroid therapy in bronchial asthma. Nord. Med. 63:15, 1960.
186. Reichling, G.H., and Kligman, A.M.: Alternate-day corticosteroid therapy. Arch. Dermatol. 83:980, 1961.
187. Harter, J.G., Reddy, W.J., and Thorn, G.W.: Studies on an intermittent corticosteroid dosage regimen. N. Engl. J. Med. 269:591, 1963.
188. Jacobson, M.E.: The rationale of alternate-day corticosteroid therapy. Postgrad. Med. 49:181, 1971.
189. Soyka, L.F.: Alternate-day corticosteroid therapy. Adv. Pediat. 19:47, 1972.
190. Fleisher, D.S.: Pituitary-adrenal responsiveness after corticosteroid therapy in children with nephrosis. J. Pediat. 70:54, 1967.
191. Soyka, L.F.: Treatment of the nephrotic syndrome in childhood: Use of an alternate-day prednisone regimen. Am. J. Dis. Child. 113:693, 1967.
192. MacGregor, R.R., Sheagren, J.N., Lipsett, M.B., and Wolff, S.M.: Alternate-day prednisone therapy: Evaluation of delayed hypersensitivity responses, control of disease and steroid side effects. N. Engl. J. Med. 280:1427, 1969.
193. Sadeghi-Nejad, A., and Senior, B.: Adrenal function, growth, and insulin in patients treated with corticoids on alternate days. Pediatrics 43:277, 1969.
194. Reed, W.P., Lucas, Z.J., and Cohn, R.: Alternate-day prednisone therapy after renal transplantation. Lancet 1:747, 1970.
195. Siegel, R.R., Luke, R.G., and Hellebusch, A.A.: Reduction of toxicity of corticosteroid therapy after renal transplantation. Am. J. Med. 53:159, 1972.
196. Block, A.J., and Light, R.W.: Alternate day steroid therapy in diffuse pulmonary sarcoidosis. Chest 63:495, 1973.
197. Chai, H., and Gilbert, A.: The effect of alternate-day prednisone on the white blood count in children with chronic asthma. J. Allergy Clin. Immunol. 51:65, 1973.
198. Gulati, P.D., Malik, G.B., and Vaishnava, H.: Alternate-day steroid therapy in adult nephrotics. J. Med. 4:266, 1973.
199. McEnery, P.T., Gonzalez, L.L., Martin, L.W., and West, C.D.: Growth and development of children with renal transplants. Use of alternate-day steroid therapy. J. Pediatr. 83:806, 1973.
200. Sampson, D., and Albert, D.J.: Alternate day therapy with methylprednisolone after renal transplantation. J. Urol. 109:345, 1973.
201. Sheagren, J.N., Simon, H.B., and Rich, R.R.: Therapy of sarcoidosis initiated with alternate-day prednisone. J. Natl. Med. Assoc. 65:391, 1973.
202. Dale, D.C., Fauci, A.S., and Wolff, S.M.: Alternate-day prednisone: Leukocyte kinetics and susceptibility to infections. N. Engl. J. Med. 291:1154, 1974.
203. Fauci, A.S., and Dale, D.C.: Alternate-day therapy and human lymphocyte subpopulations. J. Clin. Invest. 55:22, 1975.

204. Potter, D.E., Holliday, M.A., Wilson, C.J., Salvatierra, O., Jr., and Belzer, F.O.: Alternate-day steroids in children after renal transplantation. Transplant. Proc. 7:79, 1975.
205. Reimer, L.G., Morris, H.G., and Ellis, E.F.: Growth of asthmatic children during treatment with alternate-day steroids. J. Allergy Clin. Immunol. 55:224, 1975.
206. Diethelm, A.G., Sterling, W.A, Hartley, M.W., and Morgan, J.M.: Alternate-day prednisone therapy in recipients of renal allografts: Risks and benefits. Arch. Surg. 111:867, 1976.
207. Klein, R.G., Arnaud, S.B., Gallagher, J.C., DeLuca, H.F., and Riggs, B.L.: Intestinal calcium absorption in exogenous hypercortisonism: Role of 25-hydroxyvitamin D and corticosteroid dose. J. Clin. Invest. 60:253, 1977.
208. Norris, D.A., Fine, R., Weston, W.L., and Spector, S.: Monocyte cellular function in asthmatic patients on alternate-day steroid therapy. J. Allergy Clin. Immunol. 61:255, 1978.
209. Curtis, J.J., Galla, J.H., Woodford, S.Y., Lucas, B.A., and Luke, R.G.: Effect of alternate-day prednisone on plasma lipids in renal transplant recipients. Kidney Int. 22:42, 1982.
210. Kass, E.H., and Finland, M.: Adrenocortical hormones in infection and immunity. Ann. Rev. Microbiol. 7:361, 1953.
211. Thomas, L.: Cortisone and infection. Ann. N.Y. Acad. Sci. 56:799, 1953.
212. Dale, D.C., and Petersdorf, R.G.: Corticosteroids and infectious diseases. In Azarnoff, D.L. (ed.): Steroid Therapy. Philadelphia, W. B. Saunders Company, 1975, p. 209.
213. Schutz, S., Newhouse, R., and Dello Russo, J.: Alternate-day steroid regimen in the treatment of ocular disease. Br. J. Ophthalmol. 52:461, 1968.
214. Easton, J.G., Busser, R.J., and Heimlich, E.M.: Effect of alternate-day steroid administration on adrenal function in allergic children. J. Allergy Clin. Immunol. 48:355, 1971.
215. Kuzemko, J.A., and Lines, J.G.: Adrenal cortical function in asthmatic children on alternate-day steroids. Arch. Dis. Child. 46:366, 1971.
216. Ackerman, G.L., and Nolan, C.M.: Adrenocortical responsiveness after alternate-day corticosteroid therapy. N. Engl. J. Med. 278:405, 1968.
217. Wyatt, R., Waschek, J., Weinberger, M., and Sherman, B.: Effects of inhaled beclomethasone dipropionate and alternate-day prednisone on pituitary-adrenal function in children with chronic asthma. N. Engl. J. Med. 299:1387, 1978.
218. Falliers, C.J., Chai, H., Molk, L., Bane, H., and Cardoso, R.R. de A.: Pulmonary and adrenal effects of alternate-day corticosteroid therapy. J. Allergy Clin. Immunol. 49:156, 1972.
219. Bakran, I., Jr., Korsic, M., Durakovic, Z., Vrhovac, B., and Tajic, M.: The effect of alternate-day prednisone therapy on cortisol secretion rate in corticosteroid-dependent asthmatics. Int. J. Clin. Pharmacol. 15:57, 1977.
220. Bolton, W.K., Atuk, N.O., Sturgill, B.C., and Westervelt, F.B., Jr.: Therapy of the idiopathic nephrotic syndrome with alternate day steroids. Am. J. Med. 62:60, 1977.
221. Collaborative Study of the Adult Idiopathic Nephrotic Syndrome: A controlled study of short-term prednisone treatment in adults with membranous nephropathy. N. Engl. J. Med. 301:1301, 1979.
222. Hopper, J., Jr., Biava, C.G., and Tu, W.-H.: Membranous nephropathy: High-dose alternate-day therapy with prednisone. West. J. Med. 135:1, 1981.
223. Bell, M.J., Martin, L.W., Gonzales, L.L., McEnery, P.T., and West, C.D.: Alternate-day single-dose prednisone therapy: A method of reducing steroid toxicity. J. Pediat. Surg. 7:223, 1972.
224. McDonald, F.D., Horensten, M.L., Mayor, G.B., Turcotte, J.G., Selezinka, W., and Schork, M.A.: Effect of alternate-day steroids on renal transplant function: A controlled study. Nephron 17:415, 1976.
225. Reimold, E.W.: Intermittent prednisone therapy in children and adolescents after renal transplantation. Pediatrics 52:235, 1973.
226. Curtis, J.J., Galla, J.H., Woodford, S.Y., Saykaly, R.J., and Luke, R.G.: Comparison of daily and alternate-day prednisone during chronic maintenance therapy: A controlled crossover study. Am. J. Kidney Dis. 1:166, 1981.
227. McAdams, A.J., McEnery, P.T., and West, C.D.: Mesangiocapillary glomerulonephritis: Changes in glomerular morphology with long-term alternate-day prednisone therapy. J. Pediatr. 86:23, 1975.
228. Ackerman, G.L.: Alternate-day steroid therapy in lupus nephritis. Ann. Intern. Med. 72:511, 1970.
229. Cocco, A.E., and Mendeloff, A.L.: An evaluation of intermittent corticosteroid therapy in the management of ulcerative colitis. Johns Hopkins Med. J. 120:162, 1967.
230. Powell-Tuck, J., Bown, R.L., Chambers, T.J., and Lennard-Jones, J.E.: A controlled trial of alternate-day prednisolone as a maintenance treatment for ulcerative colitis in remission. Digestion 22:263, 1981.
231. Ansell, B.M., and Bywaters, E.G.L.: Alternate-day corticosteroid therapy in juvenile chronic polyarthritis. J. Rheumatol. 1:176, 1974.
232. Haim, S., Benderly, A., Shafrir, A., and Levy, J.: Alternate-day corticosteroid regimen. Dermatologica 142:171, 1971.
233. Jenkins, R.B.: Treatment of myasthenia gravis with prednisone. Lancet 1:765, 1972.
234. Engel, W.K., Festoff, B.W., Patten, B.M., Swerdlow, M.L., Newball, H.H., and Thompson, M.D.: Myasthenia gravis. Ann. Intern. Med. 81:225, 1974.
235. Seybold, M.E., and Drachman, D.B.: Gradually increasing doses of prednisone in myasthenia gravis: Reducing the hazards of treatment. N. Engl. J. Med. 290:81, 1974.
236. Brunner, N.G., Berger, C.L., Namba, T., and Grob, D.: Corticotropin or corticosteroids in generalized myasthenia gravis: Comparative studies and role in management. Ann. N.Y. Acad. Sci. 274:577, 1976.
237. Mann, J.D., Johns, T.R., and Campa, J.F.: Long-term administration of corticosteroids in myasthenia gravis. Neurology 26:729, 1976.
238. Newball, H.H., and Brahim, S.A.: Effects of alternate-day prednisone therapy on respiratory function in myasthenia gravis. Thorax 31:410, 1976.
239. Johns, T.R.: Treatment of myasthenia gravis: Long-term administration of corticosteroids with remarks on thymectomy. Adv. Neurol. 17:99, 1977.
240. Drachman, D.B., Toyka, K.V., and Myer, E.: Prednisone in Duchenne muscular dystrophy. Lancet 2:1409, 1974.
241. Engel, W.K., Borenstein, A., DeVivo, D.C., Schwartzman, R.J., and Warmolts, J.R.: High-single-dose alternate-day prednisone (HSDAD-PRED) in treatment of the dermatomyositis/polymyositis complex. Trans. Am. Neurol. Assoc. 97:272, 1972.
242. DeVivo, D.C., and Engel, W.K.: Remarkable recovery of a steroid-responsive recurrent polyneuropathy. J. Neurol. Neurosurg. Psychiat. 33:62, 1970.
243. Schwartzman, R.J., Engel, W.K., and Rapoport, A.: Criteria for the prednisone treatment of idiopathic polyneuropathy (abstract). Neurology 27:364, 1977.
244. Walsh, S.D., and Grant, I.W.B.: Corticosteroids in treatment of chronic asthma. Br. Med. J. 2:796, 1966.
245. Rabhan, N.B., and Kopf, A.W.: Alternate-day prednisone therapy for pemphigus vulgaris. Arch. Dermatol. 103:615, 1971.
246. Hunder, G.G., Sheps, S.G., Allen, G.L., and Joyce, J.W.: Daily and alternate day corticosteroid regimens in treatment of giant cell arteritis: Comparison in a prospective study. Ann. Intern. Med. 82:613, 1975.
247. Abruzzo, J.L.: Alternate-day prednisone therapy. Ann. Intern. Med. 82:714, 1975.
248. Bengtsson, B.-A., and Malmvall, B.-E. An alternate-day corticosteroid regimen in maintenance therapy of giant cell arteritis. Acta Med. Scand. 209:347, 1981.
249. Jasani, M.K., Boyle, J.A., Dick, W.C., Williamson, J., Taylor, A.K., and Buchanan, W.W.: Corticosteroid-induced hypothalamo-pituitary-adrenal axis suppression: Prospective study using two regimens of corticosteroid therapy. Ann. Rheum. Dis. 27:352, 1968.
250. Rabhan, N.B.: Pituitary-adrenal suppression and Cushing's syndrome after intermittent dexamethasone therapy. Ann. Intern. Med. 69:1141, 1968.
251. Fauci, A.S.: Alternate-day corticosteroid therapy. Am. J. Med. 64:729, 1978.
252. Dubois, E.L., and Adler, D.C.: Single-daily dose oral administration of corticosteroids in rheumatic disorders: An analysis of its advantages, efficacy and side effects. Curr. Ther. Res. 5:43, 1963.
253. Nugent, C.A., Ward, J., MacDiarmid, W.D., McCall, J.C., Baukol, J., and Tyler, F.H.: Glucocorticoid toxicity: Single contrasted with divided daily doses of prednisolone. J. Chronic Dis. 18:323, 1965.
254. Myles, A.B., Schiller, L.G.F., Glass, D., and Daly, J.R.: Single daily dose corticosteroid treatment. Ann. Rheum. Dis. 35:73, 1976.
255. Powell-Tuck, J., Bown, R.L., and Lennard-Jones, J.E.: A comparison of oral prednisone given as single or multiple daily doses for active proctocolitis. Br. J. Gastroenterol. 13:833, 1978.
256. DiRaimondo, V.C., and Forsham, P.H.: Pharmacophysiologic principles in the use of corticoids and adrenocorticotropin. Metabolism 7:5, 1958.
257. Myles, A.B., Bacon, P.A., and Daly, J.R.: Single daily dose corticosteroid treatment: Effect on adrenal function and therapeutic efficacy in various diseases. Ann. Rheum. Dis. 30:149, 1971.
258. Allander, E.: ACTH or corticosteroids? A critical review of results and possibilities in the treatment of severe chronic disease. Acta Rheum. Scand. 15:277, 1969.
259. Kaplan, H.P., Portnoy, B., Binder, H.J., Amatruda, T., and Spiro, H.: A controlled evaluation of intravenous adrenocorticotropic hormone and hydrocortisone in the treatment of acute colitis. Gastroenterology 69:91, 1975.
260. Savage, O., Copeman, W.S.C., Chapman, L., Wells, M.V., and Treadwell, B.L.J.: Pituitary and adrenal hormones in rheumatoid arthritis. Lancet 1:232, 1962.
260. Savage, O., Copeman, W.S.C., Chapman, L., Wells, N.V., and Treadwell, B.L.J.: Pituitary and adrenal hormones in rheumatoid arthritis. Lancet 1:232, 1962.

Chapter 55

Cytotoxic and Other Immunoregulatory Agents

Anthony S. Fauci

INTRODUCTION

Immunoregulation can be broadly defined as the complex process whereby immunologic reactivity, either cellular or humoral, is constantly modulated to result in the net expression of an appropriate or, in certain circumstances, inappropriate immune response.[1] Recent intensive interest and investigation in immunology, which has led to certain rather striking advances in our understanding of the complexities of immune function and regulation in animal models as well as in man, together with the observations that many rheumatic diseases are at least associated with aberrancies of immune function, including immunoregulation,[1-5] form the intellectual basis for the use of immunoregulatory agents in the treatment of certain rheumatic diseases. It should be pointed out, however, that the use of cytotoxic and other immunoregulatory agents in these diseases antedated the most recent advances in our understanding of many of the subtle complexities of immune regulation. This is particularly true of the use of corticosteroids and cytotoxic agents in diseases whose clinicopathologic manifestations were strongly suggestive of aberrant inflammatory or immune-mediated phenomena. Since the use of these agents generally resulted in suppression of inflammation and immune function, it is not surprising that they have been extensively used in certain rheumatic, connective tissue, and autoimmune diseases.[7-10]

Unfortunately, despite the fact that recent advances in our understanding of immune function and regulation have allowed a greater intellectual understanding of the potential mechanisms of aberrant immune function in the diseases in question, the extraordinary complexity of the immune system, with its various inductive, regulatory, effector, and feedback mechanisms, has made it clear to clinical investigators that perturbation of the system by agents used for therapeutic purposes may have multifaceted effects on the system, some of which might be unpredictable, if not unrecognized. Indeed, this very complexity of the system in the face of the relatively crude and usually nonspecific modulation effected by most of the therapeutic agents in question may result in only a minor or temporary dampening of the expression of the disease process. On the other hand, the adverse side effects associated with perturbation of the immune system in this manner may place the therapeutic efficacy that results beyond the limits of the price that one is willing to pay for such an effect. Indeed, certain immunoregulatory agents have been used and are being used inappropriately in diseases whose severity or projected clinical course clearly do not warrant such an aggressive approach. Nonetheless, despite these general caveats, certain cytotoxic and other immunoregulatory agents have been successfully and appropriately employed in the treatment of a number of rheumatic diseases, and in certain situations with rather impressive results.[6,8-10]

It is the aim of this chapter to consider some of the real and potential mechanisms whereby one can feasibly and successfully modify the expression of aberrant inflammatory and immune responses and to discuss the mechanisms of action of the various categories of immunoregulatory agents as well as their proven and potential usefulness in the treatment of rheumatic diseases in order to better appreciate the positive and negative aspects of such a therapeutic approach.

THE IMMUNE SYSTEM AND ITS REGULATION

A number of models of the immune system and its regulation have been proposed, and each almost invariably has the common denominator of a cellular and humoral network of immune reactivity reflected by different cell types. The dual limbs of the immune response introduced several years ago[11-14] and now clearly substantiated are the thymus-derived (T) lymphocyte limb and the bone marrow–derived or bursa-equivalent (B) lymphocyte limb, both of which derive from a common stem cell. Other cell types, such as the monocyte-macrophage, play a major role in the inductive, regulatory, and effector phases of the immune response.[15]

A somewhat simplified scheme of the immune system is illustrated in Figure 55–1. As has been previously and extensively described, the expression of immune function can be conveniently looked upon as a series of phases. Both T and B lymphocytes mediate a number of critical immune functions, and each of these cell types, when given the appropriate signal, pass through phases, from activation or induction through proliferation, differentiation, and ultimately effector function.[3,5] The effector function that is expressed may be at the end point of a response, such as secretion of antibody by a differentiated B lymphocyte or plasma cell, or it might serve a regulatory function that modulates other end-stage functions, as is seen with inducer or suppressor T lymphocytes, which modulate the function of B lymphocytes,

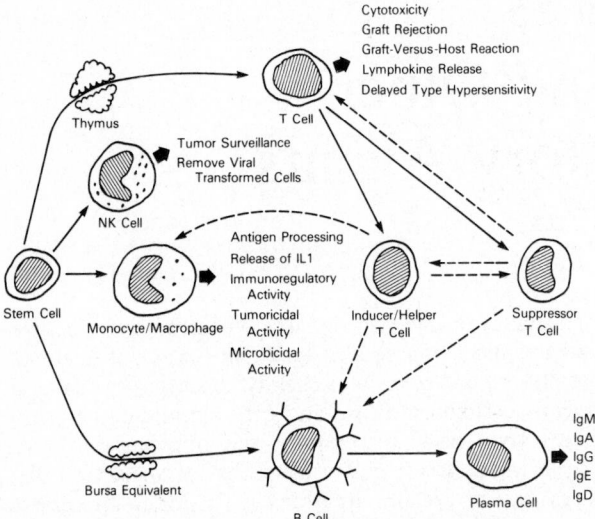

Figure 55–1. Schematic diagram of the human immune system. Virtually all of the components of the immune system derive from a common stem cell, which then gives rise to the various components of the system. Cells that come under the influence of the thymus evolve into thymus-derived (T) cells and are further subdivided into various subsets of immunoregulatory populations. In addition to the regulation of B lymphocyte function by induction and suppression, the T lymphocyte limb also manifests effector functions such as are indicated by the bold arrow stemming from the T cell. Lymphocytes that evolve through the bursa-equivalent differentiate into B lymphocytes, which upon appropriate stimuli further differentiate into antibody-secreting plasma cells, which are the ultimate effector cells of this limb of the immune response. Monocyte/macrophages and natural killer cells also evolve from the common stem cell, and these also have ultimate effector functions. Monocytes may be immunoregulated by T lymphocytes and their products, and they may also be involved in the immunoregulation of B and T lymphocyte function. The extraordinarily complex cellular and humoral interactions in this scheme, which are simplified here, particularly with regard to the delicate balance among positive and negative influences, ultimately result in the net expression of an appropriate immune response. Even the slightest imbalance in this immunoregulatory circuit may lead to the expression of aberrancies of immune function leading to clinically apparent immune-mediated disease.

T lymphocytes, other lymphoid cells, or even certain nonlymphoid cell types. Very briefly, in addition to induction and suppression, T lymphocytes mediate a number of other important immune functions, such as specific cell-mediated cytotoxicity, certain types of graft rejection, graft-versus-host phenomena, delayed-type hypersensitivity, and the production and release of a broad range of soluble mediators termed lymphokines, which have profound effects on virtually all phases of the immune response.

On the other hand, B lymphocytes subserve a much more uniform function. They are the precursors of antibody-forming cells, and when appropriately stimulated, they proliferate and differentiate into cells that secrete antibody of the various classes and subclasses. Natural killer cells are lymphoid cells. They are not of B lymphocyte lineage and may well not be of T lymphocyte lineage, although they share some, but not all, phenotypic characteristics of T lymphocytes.[16] These cells are felt to be involved in immune surveillance

against neoplastically transformed cells as well as in the elimination of virally transformed target cells.[17]

The monocyte-macrophage system, which is represented by monocytes in the peripheral blood and by macrophages in various tissues, plays a major role in the expression of immune reactivity by mediating a number of important functions, such as the presentation of antigen to lymphocytes and the secretion of factors such as interleukin 1 (IL 1) that are involved in the activation of lymphocytes. In addition, they directly mediate certain effector functions, such as the destruction of antibody-coated bacteria, tumor cells, or even normal cells such as hematologic elements in certain types of autoimmune cytopenias.[16,18] Furthermore, activated macrophages can directly eliminate various cell types even in the absence of antibody.

Finally, nonlymphoid cells such as neutrophils, eosinophils, and basophils play a major role in the inflammation that results from certain immune-mediated reactions and as such must be considered in the scheme of immune function despite the fact that they are not classically viewed as part of the immune system.

The net expression of immune function, be it a specific or nonspecific effector function, is the result of a balance between positive and negative influences mediated by the inducer or suppressor populations of cells alluded to above.[1,3,5] They may exert their influence either directly or via the release of soluble immunoregulatory molecules. In addition to the classic cellular regulation of immune reactivity, the idiotypic network has been proposed as a potentially important mechanism of immunoregulation.[19] Elaborate and complex schemes have been proposed for the mechanisms of such immunoregulation, with secreted idiotype and anti-idiotype antibodies as well as idiotype- and anti-idiotype–bearing cells having been demonstrated as playing a major role in the regulation of immune function in the murine system.[20] The demonstration of regulation of human immune function by idiotype–anti-idiotype reactions has been reported recently[21] and awaits further delineation before its role in the regulation of normal and abnormal lymphocyte physiology can be appreciated fully. In this regard, recent evidence suggests that the idiotype network may play a role in the regulation of autoimmune states such as systemic lupus erythematosus (SLE).[22]

ABERRANCIES OF IMMUNE REACTIVITY

The established and potential mechanisms of disease activity in the broad range of rheumatic diseases are discussed in the individual chapters dealing with these disorders. However, if one considers Figure 55–1 and the preceding discussion, it is clear that there are a number of potential mechanisms for the expression of aberrant immune reactivity related to the occurrence of even slight perturbations of the delicate balance in the cellular or humoral immunoregulatory network. This may take the form of a selective deficiency in suppressor cell function or an abnormal heightening of inducer cell activity. In addition to imbalances in immunoregulation, one can have primary hyper-reactivity of certain effector functions such as B-lymphocyte reactivity.[1] Under these circumstances, it is conceivable that even a normally functioning helper and/or suppressor cell network might not successfully dampen the aberrant B-lymphocyte hyper-reactivity. Even more likely, there may be a combination of hyperactive effector cell function such as hyper-reactivity at the B-lymphocyte level together with abnormalities of immunoregulatory T-lymphocyte function. In fact, this is precisely the situation that has been noted in SLE. It is still disputed whether the B-lymphocyte hyper-reactivity is a primary state independent of the deficiency of suppressor T-lymphocyte function, whether the B-lymphocyte hyper-reactivity is secondary to the suppressor cell defect, or whether the abnormalities of immune reactivity actually result from a combination of both of these phenomena together with a number of other recognized as well as ill-defined factors.[1]

In this regard, the net expression of immune function in most of the rheumatic diseases appears to be one of aberrant hyper-reactivity. As such, we generally distinguish these disorders from immunodeficiency diseases in which the net expression of immune function is generally that of hyporeactivity. However, given the balance between positive and negative influences in the immune network, one can easily appreciate that a deficiency of immune function such as suppressor cell activity (hence, strictly speaking a immunodeficiency state) can actually result in hyperactive effector immune function.[1,23] This point is not trivial and has important implications in appreciating the basis of certain of the therapeutic strategies that will be described below. Thus, although we commonly refer to the therapeutic strategy of immunosuppression for diseases of inflammation and/or immunologic hyper-reactivity, we would more correctly think in terms of therapeutic immunoregulation either by dampening hyperactive responses or by directly or indirectly enhancing defective negative immunoregulatory influences.

POTENTIAL AREAS OF MODIFICATION OF IMMUNE RESPONSES BY THERAPEUTIC AGENTS

Suppression. Abnormally hyperactive immune responses at either the T- or B-lymphocyte level can be theoretically as well as practically eliminated or at least dampened by nonspecifically suppressing the entire immune system. Clearly, sufficient amounts of cytotoxic agents, irradiation, antilymphocyte sera, and other immunosuppressive agents can be administered to eliminate virtually any immune response. These therapeutic modalities are truly nonspecific in that they do not selectively eliminate abnormally active lymphoid cells, nor do they spare normal lymphoid cells. Thus, although the desired effect can ultimately be obtained, the inevitable toxic side effects render such an approach non-

feasible in the treatment of non-neoplastic diseases. Thus, within the realm of nonspecific suppression of immune function, therapeutic strategies are employed that strike a balance between the desired effect of suppression of aberrant immune reactivity and maintenance of sufficient immune function as well as phagocytic, particularly neutrophil, cell number and function to maintain the integrity of the host defense system as well as the level of inflammatory and immune function required to maintain immunologic homeostasis.

This approach usually takes the form of administration of cytotoxic drugs in dose regimens which, while still nonspecific, would relatively more selectively dampen the ongoing aberrant immune response. An example is the use of chronically administered cyclophosphamide in doses of 2 mg per kg per day in certain of the severe systemic vasculitic syndromes.[24,25] These disorders are characterized by hyper-reactivity of B-lymphocyte responses with hypergammaglobulinemia, immune complex deposition, and spontaneous secretion of polyclonal immunoglobulin (Ig) by activated B lymphocytes.[26] Administration of cyclophosphamide in the above regimen results in a selective suppression of B-lymphocyte reactivity with relative sparing of T-lymphocyte responses despite the fact that a total lymphocytopenia inevitably results from such chronic therapy.[27] Thus, although all B-lymphocyte function is suppressed, rendering such an approach nonspecific, there appears to be a selective suppression of the hyperactive B lymphocytes more than other lymphoid cell function.[27]

Other nonspecific but less globally immunosuppressive modalities include thoracic duct drainage, plasmapheresis, leukopheresis, the use of antilymphocyte globulin or monoclonal antibodies directed against lymphocyte subsets, irradiation of groups of regional lymph nodes, and the use of agents such as cyclosporin A, which relatively selectively suppresses T-lymphocyte function while sparing other lymphoid and nonlymphoid cells. Each of these approaches represents an attempt within the realm of a fundamentally nonspecific immunosuppressive regimen to render the approach somewhat more selective.

Despite these attempts at introducing varying degrees of selectivity into nonspecific immunosuppressive regimens, the extraordinary complexity of the immune system, with its multiple levels of regulation and feedback mechanisms, adds a considerable degree of uncertainty to such approachs. This stems from the fact that the desired effect may not be realized, since perturbation of the on-going activity of the system may introduce feedback mechanisms that obviate the desired effect. Furthermore, the actual effect may be different from the desired effect and de facto undesirable in itself. One can view the situation as an attempt to employ extremely crude tools to fine tune an extraordinarily complex and delicate machine. Nonetheless, despite the limitations of such an approach, nonspecific immunosuppression has resulted in favorable therapeutic results in a number of rheumatic diseases.[6,8,9] However, given the state of the art at present, realization of these limitations is essential for proper application of such regimens as well as for providing an impetus to continuing the search for more specific and less toxic forms of immunosuppression.

Unfortunately, modalities of truly specific suppression are more theoretical than practical when one considers their use in rheumatic diseases in man. For example, classic experiments with cyclophosphamide have demonstrated that administration of an antigen together with the drug results in a selective suppression of the immune response to the antigen in question as opposed to the immune response in general.[28] However, since the actual responsible antigens in most, if not all, rheumatic diseases remain unclear, such an approach is at present not clinically feasible.

A number of suppressor systems in the mouse have proved to be specific, and antigen-specific suppressor cells and suppressor factors have been identified.[29] In the human system, virtually all of the suppressor systems are nonspecific,[23,30] and those that reflect a degree of specificity are almost invariably specific in their induction and nonspecific in their expression. Furthermore, although various systems of specific immunologic tolerance have been described in a number of animal models,[31] these cannot yet be extrapolated to an approach to the treatment of human disease for a variety of reasons, not the least important of which is our failure to recognize the putative antigen in most diseases.

Enhancement. As mentioned above, even disorders that express a net hyperactive immune response may have components that are hypoactive. In this regard, immune enhancement should theoretically be beneficial provided the defective element can be selectively enhanced. Since virtually all of the immune-enhancing drugs or agents that will be discussed below are indeed nonspecific, they suffer from the same limitations as immunosuppressive agents in the modulation of aberrant immune reactivity in disease states. Nonetheless, certain drugs that enhance immune responses have been used with limited success in certain immunologically mediated diseases and will be mentioned below.

The ultimate enhancement of the immune response would be complete replacement, as with ablation and bone marrow transplantation. However, given the nature of the diseases in question together with the logistic constraints on bone marrow transplants, such an approach is not feasible at present for rheumatic diseases. Transfer of mature immune competent lymphoid cells has the theoretical potential of reversing the imbalance of immunoregulatory lymphocyte subsets. Again, logistic constraints, with regard to histocompatibility requirements and restrictions, make such an approach untenable. However, of particular interest over the past few years has been the availability of purified preparations of lymphokines such as interleukin II (IL II) and the various interferons. These factors, particularly IL II, are capable of exerting profound enhancing effects on the immune response in vitro,[32] and the therapeutic use of such factors holds at least theoretical potential for the future.

CYTOTOXIC AGENTS

General Considerations

Of all the immunoregulatory agents that are used in the treatment of rheumatic diseases, the cytotoxic drugs pose perhaps the greatest difficulty for the clinician from both a theoretical and a practical standpoint. This stems largely from the fine line between risk and benefit, which exists for virtually all such agents used in the treatment of these diseases. Unfortunately, the terminology that is frequently employed with regard to the cytotoxic agents is somewhat misleading in that the term "cytotoxic" agent is used synonymously with the term "immunosuppressive" agent. Indeed, cytotoxic agents can be and are frequently immunosuppressive; however, a number of other drugs discussed in this chapter as well as the corticosteroids (see Chapter 54) can be potent immunosuppressive agents. The cytotoxic agents differ from many of these other agents in that the common denominator of their effect is that they destroy cells, hence the derivation of the term "cytotoxic," which means simply that the drugs are directly toxic or damaging to cells. It is this ability to kill cells that distinguishes the cytotoxic immunosuppressive agents from the other categories of immunosuppressive drugs and explains their extensive use in the treatment of a variety of neoplastic diseases. Indeed, their use as antineoplastic agents long antedates their use as immunosuppressive agents in non-neoplastic inflammatory and immune-mediated diseases. Only when the profound immunosuppressive effects of these agents as used in the treatment of neoplastic diseases became apparent did clinical investigators conceive of their use in diseases that manifested marked inflammatory responses and apparent immune-mediated mechanisms.[10] Certain of the mechanisms of action of cytotoxic agents on inflammatory and immunologic responses are listed in Table 55–1.[33]

It cannot be emphasized too strongly that the rationale for the use of cytotoxic agents as well as the goals that one wishes to achieve by therapy are for the most part quite different depending on whether one uses these agents in the treatment of non-neoplastic immune-mediated diseases or neoplastic diseases. The rationale and goal for the use of cytotoxic agents in the treatment of neoplastic diseases is simply to eliminate where possible every last tumor cell. This approach is almost invariably associated with significant destruction of the normal

Table 55–1. Principal Mechanisms of Action of Cytotoxic Agents on Inflammatory and Immunologic Reactions

1. Elimination of sensitized and immunologically committed lymphoid cells
2. Elimination of nonsensitized lymphoid cells secondarily engaged in aberrant immunologic reactivity
3. Elimination of nonlymphoid cells engaged in nonspecific inflammatory responses to aberrant immunologic reactions
4. Suppression of functional capabilities of surviving lymphoid cells

elements of host defense mechanisms, such that a life-threatening or near life-threatening state exists for variable periods of time during and following chemotherapy until the normal cellular elements can recover. If the tumor is sensitive to the chemotherapeutic agents used, such that a reasonable chance of remission and/or cure exists, then the attendant risks are clearly justifiable, since the malignant neoplasm will otherwise inevitably result in the death of the patient. Under such circumstances, the goals are rather clear-cut, and the options are few.

The situation is quite different when using these agents to treat non-neoplastic diseases. Since there are no recognizable malignant clones in the immune-mediated diseases, the rationale and goal are usually to suppress the aberrant inflammatory and immune-mediated reactions that are responsible for the tissue damage without markedly suppressing the normal host defense mechanisms, which would put the patient at significant risk for either an infection or a neoplasm resulting from the suppression of normal immune surveillance mechanisms.[24,25,33] Unfortunately, maintaining this balance between risk and benefit is not an easy task, since, as mentioned previously, the agents employed are almost always nonspecific in their suppressive effects, and suppression of normal immune mechanisms will invariably accompany suppression of the aberrant reactions. It is hoped that suppression of these abnormal immune responses will be effected prior to the point at which such a degree of suppression of normal immune mechanisms occurs, so that the patient would not be at a significant risk.

Of equal, if not greater, importance than the suppression of normal immunologic mechanisms is the suppression of normal nonspecific mechanisms of host defenses in the form of the circulating polymorphonuclear neutrophils. Due to the relatively rapid turnover of the neutrophil series in the bone marrow, cytotoxic agents are particularly effective in causing a neutropenia, which becomes one of the major limiting factors in the use of these agents. In this regard, another important difference in the use of these agents in neoplastic versus non-neoplastic diseases is the fact that in non-neoplastic diseases, the drugs are usually administered chronically over extended periods of time, ranging from months to years, and so the risk of a host defense defect is a relatively persistent problem as opposed to the relatively brief (albeit usually more severe) periods of defect seen following the intermittent courses of chemotherapy usually administered for neoplastic diseases.

Finally, the major difference in the use of these agents in the treatment of neoplastic versus non-neoplastic diseases lies in the area of exercising of clinical judgment as to when to employ such an aggressive chemotherapeutic approach in a non-neoplastic disease that might not be invariably fatal. The clinical course of most neoplastic diseases that are left untreated or that are not aggressively treated is usually rather clear, which makes the decision to initiate aggressive therapy relatively easy. In contrast, many of the rheumatic diseases, such as SLE, rheumatoid arthritis, the systemic vasculitides, scleroderma, and dermatomyositis/polymyositis, as well as several of the organ-specific autoimmune diseases in which cytotoxic agents have been used have variable clinical courses. Only when the disease seems to be progressing with irreversible organ system dysfunction that is not responsive to more conventional therapy, such as nonsteroidal anti-inflammatory agents or corticosteroids, does one consider employing a cytotoxic agent. This is often a difficult decision, since the efficacy of these agents in many of these diseases has not been conclusively proved by appropriately controlled studies. Furthermore, the chronicity of most of these diseases dictates that even though a cytotoxic agent may be effective in suppressing disease activity, the agent cannot be used indefinitely. Thus, it is essential to set reasonable goals for the use of cytotoxic agents in the treatment of rheumatic diseases.

Therapeutic Goals

Very few situations exist in which the use of cytotoxic agents can be expected to effect a true and long-term "cure" of a non-neoplastic disease. One such situation is the use of these agents, particularly cyclophosphamide, in the treatment of certain of the vasculitic syndromes. Paramount among these syndromes is Wegener's granulomatosis in which long-term remissions, which can indeed be called "cures," have been effected in as high as 90 percent of patients treated with cyclophosphamide, 2 mg per kg per day, together with prednisone, 1 mg per kg per day, administered first daily and then on an alternate-day schedule.[24,25] Similar results have been obtained with other of the vasculitic syndromes, particularly the polyarteritis nodosa group of the systemic necrotizing vasculitides.[34] Prior to the institution of this therapy, virtually all patients with Wegener's granulomatosis died of their disease, as did most patients with the polyarteritis nodosa type of systemic necrotizing vasculitis.[24,25] It is conceivable that the drug does not in fact "cure" the disease but merely suppresses the inflammatory and aberrant immune-mediated mechanisms long enough for the disease to spontaneously run its course and permanently remit. Therefore, given these reported therapeutic results, a reasonable goal for the use of cytotoxic agents (in this case cyclophosphamide) in these vasculitic syndromes is a true permanent remission or cure. One can hope that a single course of therapy, which is usually administered for over a year, will result in a situation in which the drug would not have to be used again in the patient. At worst, it may be necessary to treat a minor relapse with an additional brief course of therapy.

The goals for the use of cytotoxic agents in most of the other immune-mediated rheumatic diseases, particularly the classic connective tissue diseases, are somewhat different from those of the vasculitic syndromes. Since the connective tissue diseases usually run waxing and waning courses, which are characterized by exacerbations and remissions, the use of cytotoxic agents should be reserved for treatment of flares of disease in which there is a clear-cut danger of irreversible organ system dysfunction. Despite the fact that cytotoxic agents have been used for several years in the treatment of the severe manifestations of the connective tissue and other rheumatic diseases, there are unfortunately very few controlled studies that definitively document the efficacy of such an approach.[6,8,9] A few controlled trials of cytotoxic agents have been carried out, and they have documented short-term benefits in flares of disease activity. There is, however, still very little information available regarding long-term effects of these agents on the ultimate course of the disease.[6,8,9] Thus, given the present state of knowledge in this area, a reasonable goal for the use of cytotoxic agents in the connective tissue diseases would be to suppress flares of disease activity that are serious enough to be organ system- or life-threatening until such a point that the disease goes into remission and the drug can be withdrawn. Under such circumstances, the drug can be used again for a limited course should another relapse occur.

If it is necessary to continue the cytotoxic agent indefinitely in order to effect a sustained remission or even a partial remission, then one must carefully examine the risks of such long-term treatment with a drug whose potential adverse side effects are so substantial.[10,35,36] A classic example of this latter point would be the use of chronic cytotoxic therapy in a patient with rheumatoid arthritis. Given the normal life expectancy in patients with rheumatoid arthritis (see Chapter 60), it may be inappropriate to risk a serious and even fatal complication of therapy to suppress disease activity that is rarely life-threatening. On the other hand, the patient's life situation may be such that he or she feels that the risk is worth the benefit of suppressing certain unacceptable manifestations of disease activity. Thus, the goals may differ depending on the individual patient.

Individual Cytotoxic Agents

Although a wide variety of cytotoxic agents of various classes have been used in the chemotherapy of neoplastic diseases,[37] only a limited number of these have been regularly employed in the treatment of non-neoplastic, inflammatory, and immune-mediated diseases. The three major categories of cytotoxic drugs employed in the latter diseases are the alkylating agents and two groups of antimetabolites, the purine analogues and the folic acid antagonists. The mechanisms of action of these cytotoxic agents are outlined in Table 55–2, and their structures are illustrated in Figure 55–2. Other cytotoxic agents that are used almost exclusively in the treatment of neoplastic diseases are covered in detail elsewhere[37] and include other antimetabolites such as the pyrimidine analogues in the form of 5-fluorouracil, cytosine arabinoside, and triacetyl-6-azauridine. In addition, natural products used in the treatment of neoplastic diseases include the vinca alkaloids (vinblastine and vincristine) and antibiotics (actinomycin D, daunomycin, rubido-

mycin, adrioblastina, bleomycin, mithramycin, and mitomycin C). Finally, miscellaneous cytotoxic agents include cisplatin, hydroxyurea, procarbazine, and mitotane. The list is surely not complete, as newer agents are constantly being developed. Indeed, within this group of agents used predominantly in neoplastic processes are some that have also been used in certain non-neoplastic diseases. For example, as will be discussed below, vincristine has been successfully employed as a therapeutic modality in idiopathic thrombocytopenic purpura,[38] and hydroxyurea has been employed in the treatment of the idiopathic hypereosinophilic syndrome.[39]

Alkylating Agents. Alkylating agents are chemicals that can substitute alkyl radicals into other molecules. Biologically effective alkylating agents are usually bifunctional or polyfunctional in that each molecule has two or more alkylating groups.[10] Thus, each molecule

Table 55–2. Mechanisms of Action of Classes of Cytotoxic Agents Commonly Employed in the Treatment of Inflammatory and Immune-Mediated Non-Neoplastic Diseases

Class	Typical Agent	Mechanisms of Action
Alkylating agents	Nitrogen mustard Cyclophosphamide Chlorambucil	Under physiological conditions the drug reacts chemically with biologically vital macromolecules such as DNA by contributing alkyl groups to the molecule, resulting in crosslinkage
Purine analogues	6-Mercaptopurine Thioguanine Azathioprine	Although incorporation of the analogue into cellular DNA with subsequent inhibition of nucleic acid synthesis is generally considered the basic mechanism of action of these agents, they likely exert their cytotoxic effects by one or more of multiple mechanisms, including effects on purine nucleotide synthesis and metabolism as well as alterations in the synthesis and function of RNA and DNA.
Folic acid antagonists	Methotrexate	Binds with high affinity to dihydrofolate reductase, preventing the formation of tetrahydrofolate and thus causing an acute intracellular deficiency of folate coenzymes. Consequently, one-carbon transfer reactions critical for de novo synthesis of purine nucleotides and thymidylate cease, with resulting interruption of the synthesis of DNA and RNA.

of the alkylating agent can covalently bind with two or more molecules of other substances. In this manner, two or more molecules may be linked to each other, i.e., in crosslinkage. By virtue of the induction of these structural changes at the molecular level, alkylating agents can potentially alter the function of proteins and nucleic acids. For example, when the DNA of a cell such as a lymphocyte is crosslinked by the agent, replication of its strands is blocked, and the cell cannot divide properly, leading ultimately to cell death.[40]

Nitrogen Mustard. Mechlorethamine was the first of the nitrogen mustards to be used clinically. The drug is administered intravenously, and its clearance from the blood is extremely rapid. Following administration, the drug rapidly undergoes chemical transformation and combines with either water or reactive compounds of cells such that the drug is no longer present in its active form after only a few minutes.[10] Following detoxification, the drug is ultimately cleared via the urine. Because of this rapid clearance of the active component, it is theoretically possible to protect certain tissues from the effects of the agent by merely interrupting the blood supply to the area for a few minutes during and after injection of the drug. The usual dosage is 0.4 mg per kg intravenously every 3 to 4 weeks. Toxic side effects include severe local reactions if the drug comes into contact with surrounding tissues as well as phlebitis and thrombosis if the drug comes into direct contact with the intima of the injected vein. Nausea and vomiting occur quite commonly following drug administration and can usually be prevented or lessened by premedication. Leukopenia and thrombocytopenia constitute the major limitations in the amount of drug that can be given in a single dose; the onset is usually within a few days of drug administration and may last for as long as two to three weeks.

Nitrogen mustard has been virtually replaced by cyclophosphamide as the alkylating agent of choice in the treatment of non-neoplastic diseases. The former has the disadvantage of requiring intravenous administration, it has significant potential toxic side effects, and its therapeutic index in experimental animals has been shown to be much lower than cyclophosphamide with respect to immunosuppressive effects. However, historically nitrogen mustard is an important agent, which led the way for the use of cyclophosphamide in the treatment of immune-mediated diseases. For example, the early success in treatment of a patient with Wegener's granulomatosis with nitrogen mustard in 1954[41] laid the rational basis for the use of cyclophosphamide in the successful induction of remission in large numbers of patients with that disease.[25]

Cyclophosphamide. Cyclophosphamide is well absorbed orally and so has the advantage of administration by either the oral or intravenous route. The drug is inert and is activated by metabolism in the liver by the mixed-function oxidase system of the smooth endoplasmic reticulum.[42] The plasma half-life of cyclophosphamide is 6 to 7 hours; this may be significantly prolonged by prior treatment with allopurinol.[43] Maximal concentrations are reached in plasma 1 hour after administration and urinary recovery of unmetabolized drug is approximately 14 percent with negligible fecal recovery after intravenous administration.[10] Since approximately 60 percent of the drug is excreted through the kidney in the form of active metabolites, renal failure may result in impaired excretion of these active metabolites, with a resulting relative increase in immunosuppressive effect as well as in toxicity of a given dose of drug. Since certain enzymes of the mixed-function oxidase system can be induced by drugs such as barbiturates and corticosteroids, these agents can influence the metabolism of cyclophosphamide from its inert to its active form.[44] However, the biologic actions of cyclophosphamide seem to be more substantially affected by alterations in the rates of detoxification and elimination than by changes in the rate of generation of the active metabolites.[10] Indeed, the antitumor and therapeutic index of cyclophosphamide was shown not to be significantly modified by pretreatment of animals with phenobarbital.[45]

Although cyclophosphamide acts primarily during the S phase of the cell cycle and so has a profound effect on rapidly dividing cells, it also affects cells at all phases

Figure 55–2. Structure of cytotoxic agents used in the treatment of certain rheumatic diseases.

of the cell cycle, including resting (G_0) cells.[8] A large amount of literature has accumulated, particularly in the mouse and other animal models, demonstrating the effects of cyclophosphamide on virtually all components of the cellular and humoral immune responses.[46,47] Of particular note is the ability of cyclophosphamide to inhibit antibody production. Although this has been shown to occur most dramatically when the drug is administered before the antigen,[47,48] for practical purposes, cyclophosphamide inhibits antibody production when given at the same time or even after the antigen. Cyclophosphamide has been shown to selectively inhibit suppressor T lymphocytes as opposed to inducer or helper T lymphocytes.[49,50] However, in the therapeutic protocols in which cyclophosphamide is administered to patients with rheumatic diseases (see below), a more global rather than a selective suppression of T-lymphocyte function is seen. The immunosuppressive effects of chronically administered cyclophosphamide therapy in man are summarized in Table 55–3.[27,51-54] The most consistent finding in cyclophosphamide-treated patients is a lymphocytopenia of both T and B lymphocytes. B-lymphocyte function is clearly more profoundly suppressed than T-lymphocyte function,[27] and this is reflected at the cellular level as well as in the suppression of Ig production and serum levels of Ig in patients treated chronically with cyclophosphamide.

Cyclophosphamide is generally administered to patients with non-neoplastic diseases in a dosage regimen of 2 mg per kg per day orally. Immunosuppressive and clinical effects are usually seen within 2 to 3 weeks after initiation of therapy. An alternative regimen is the administration of single large intravenous bolus doses of 750 to 1000 mg per m². This latter regimen is usually reserved for patients with neoplastic diseases but is currently being evaluated in certain protocols for the treatment of rheumatic diseases such as SLE. As with the use of any cytotoxic and potentially myelosuppressive agent, the dosage must be modified throughout the therapeutic course in accordance with the degree of myelosuppression that occurs (see below).

Although cyclophosphamide has proved to be an extremely effective immunosuppressive agent in the treatment of non-neoplastic diseases,[33] its potential toxic side effects are considerable, and the physician must be aware of them whenever he or she undertakes the treatment of a patient with this agent (Table 55–4).[35,36] Although suppression of all marrow elements is seen with cyclophosphamide therapy, neutropenia is clearly the most important hematologic effect of the drug with regard to factors limiting its use. It should be appreciated that chronically administered cyclophosphamide will have a cumulative effect on the bone marrow reserve such that a dose that is well tolerated at one point in time may produce significant neutropenia after one or more years of therapy. This will necessitate frequent monitoring of the white blood cell count (WBC) and appropriate adjustment of dosage. Gonadal suppression is an almost invariable effect of chronic administration of cyclophosphamide and is due to the damaging effects of the drug on the germinal epithelium.[55,56] The oligo- and azospermia in males[57] and oligo- and amenorrhea in premenopausal women[55] may be permanent if treatment is continued for a year or longer. Although prepubertal testes are damaged, return of spermatogenesis after drug withdrawal occurs more frequently in this younger age bracket.[58]

Although significant alopecia occurs quite frequently after high doses of cyclophosphamide, only minor degrees occur during chronic low-dose therapy; in both cases, it is reversible upon cessation of the drug. Gastrointestinal intolerance is unpredictable and can be quite severe in certain patients. Although nausea and vomiting can usually be successfully treated with antiemetics, gastric discomfort may be refractory to the usual therapeutic modalities. The latter complication not infrequently disappears upon continuation of the drug.

Hemorrhagic cystitis is seen in from 15 to 30 percent of patients and can be a most difficult complication.[25,29] Although the cystitis usually clears upon cessation of the drug, bladder fibrosis, intractable hemorrhage, and bladder carcinoma have been reported.[59] Under most circumstances, the onset of hemorrhagic cystitis is an absolute indication for discontinuation of the drug. If the cystitis is severe, the drug must be stopped regardless of the circumstances. However, if it is necessary to continue the drug in a patient with only mild cystitis because of no adequate therapeutic substitute, the dosage should be decreased and the patient followed with urinary cytology and intermittent cystoscopies. If the cystitis per-

Table 55–4. Toxic Side Effects of Chronically Administered Low-Dose (2 mg per kg per day) Cyclophosphamide Therapy

1. Marrow suppression—predominantly neutropenia
2. Gonadal suppression—oligospermia, ovarian dysfunction
3. Alopecia
4. Gastrointestinal intolerance
5. Hemorrhagic cystitis
6. Hypogammaglobulinemia after extended use
7. Pulmonary interstitial fibrosis
8. Oncogenesis

Table 55–3. Immunosuppressive Effects of Chronically Administered Cyclophosphamide Therapy in Man

1. Absolute lymphocytopenia of both T and B lymphocytes, with early preferential depletion of B lymphotocytes
2. Significant suppression of in vitro lymphocyte blastogenic responses to specific antigenic stimuli, with only mild suppression of responses to mitogenic stimuli
3. Suppression of antibody response and cutaneous delayed hypersensitivity to a new antigen, with relative sparing of established cutaneous delayed hypersensitivity
4. Reduction of elevated serum immunoglobulin levels as well as occurrence of hypogammaglobulinemia in patients treated for extended periods of time (years)
5. Selective suppression on in vitro B-lymphocyte function, with diminution of increased spontaneous immunoglobulin production of individual B lymphocytes as well as suppression of mitogen-induced immunoglobulin production

sists or worsens on the lower dose, then the drug must be discontinued even though the alternative drug for the disease in question is inferior to cyclophosphamide.

We have noted a few patients who have developed hypogammaglobulinemia during chronically administered cyclophosphamide therapy. This is of potential importance because of the synergistic host defense defects created by neutropenia and hypogammaglobulinemia. Although pulmonary and cardiac toxicity are generally seen only at high doses of the drug,[60,61] interstitial pulmonary fibrosis can occur with chronically administered low-dose cyclophosphamide, and the physician should be alert to this possibility. In addition, an antidiuretic hormone effect has been reported with large doses of cyclophosphamide but not with lower doses.[62] Finally, neoplastic diseases, particularly lymphomas and leukemias, may occur as a result of cyclophosphamide therapy.[63]

Chlorambucil. Chlorambucil is available for oral administration, and absorption is adequate and reliable. The drug is related to nitrogen mustard in that the methyl group of the mustard is replaced by phenylbutyric acid. The drug is metabolized by beta oxidation of the butyric acid.[64] The drug is almost completely metabolized and has a plasma half-life of approximately 90 minutes. At recommended doses, chlorambucil is the slowest acting nitrogen mustard in clinical use.[10]

As chlorambucil is an alkylating agent, its mechanism of action is similar to the other alkylating agents. At high doses, it suppresses all myeloid elements, and the therapeutic strategy is to suppress immune function in the form of lymphocytes prior to the suppression of other bone marrow elements. In this regard, it has been reported that at lower doses, chlorambucil exerts a more selective effect on lymphopoiesis than on granulopoiesis.[65] Clearly, chlorambucil has not been as extensively studied as cyclophosphamide with regard to its immunosuppressive effects. However, it is generally felt that it is not as potent an immunosuppressive agent as cyclophosphamide, and although its toxic side effects may be somewhat less than cyclophosphamide, its efficacy in suppressing disease activity in the non-neoplastic diseases is probably less than that of cyclophosphamide. An example of this is the greater efficacy of cyclophosphamide than chlorambucil in suppressing disease activity in generalized Wegener's granulomatosis.[66] Nonetheless, chlorambucil has been used with some success in certain of the connective tissue diseases.[8]

Chlorambucil is generally administered to patients with non-neoplastic diseases in a dosage regimen of 0.1 and 0.2 mg per kg per day orally. The dose is adjusted according to the degree of nonlymphocytic myelosuppression that is encountered, i.e., neutropenia and thrombocytopenia. When severe myelosuppression occurs, the drug should be discontinued. Marrow function usually recovers rapidly; however, irreversible marrow failure has been reported in a number of patients treated with chlorambucil for non-neoplastic diseases.[67] Such complications highlight the inherent danger in the treatment of non-neoplastic diseases with cytotoxic agents

of any class. Other side effects include gastrointestinal discomfort with nausea and vomiting, hepatotoxicity, dermatitis, and infertility.[10] Oncogenesis is a particularly disturbing potential complication of chlorambucil therapy, and a marked increase in the incidence of leukemia and other tumors has been associated with the use of this agent.[68,69]

Purine Analogues. The two major purine analogues that have been used clinically are 6-mercaptopurine (6MP) and azathioprine, which is the purine analogue currently used almost exclusively. 6MP is an analogue of hypoxanthine in which the 6-OH radical is replaced by a thiol group. When an imidazole group is attached to the S of 6MP, azathioprine is formed. In vivo, azathioprine is metabolized to 6MP, which is the active drug. The ultimate mechanism of action of 6MP is the inhibition of nucleic acid synthesis. However, despite extensive studies in this area, the precise mechanism of action whereby these purine analogues cause cell death or cytotoxicity remain unclear. Certain potential mechanisms of action have been proposed, including the conversion of 6MP to its ribonucleotide, which inhibits the enzymes necessary for the conversion of inosinic acid to xanthylic and adenylosuccinic acids as well as the conversion of adenylosuccinic acid to adenylic acid, leading to the inhibition of DNA synthesis.[70] In addition, feedback inhibition of 5-phosphoribosylamine occurs with reduction of de novo purine biosynthesis and resulting inhibition of DNA synthesis and cell death.

Azathioprine and 6MP. Azathioprine and 6MP are available for oral administration, and absorption is quite good. Since azathioprine is converted in vivo to 6MP, which is the active drug, their pharmacokinetics can be considered together. About one half of an oral dose of drug is found excreted in the urine within the first 24 hours.[10] After an intravenous dose, the half-life of the drug is 60 to 90 minutes, with clearance from the blood resulting from uptake by cells, renal excretion, and metabolic degradation. There are two major pathways for the metabolism of 6MP. The first is the methylation of the sulfhydryl group and oxidation of the methylated derivatives. The second is the oxidation of 6MP to 6-thiouric acid by the enzyme xanthine oxidase.[10] Since allopurinol inhibits xanthine oxidase, this drug decreases the metabolism of 6MP and so accounts for the increase in toxicity of azathioprine and 6MP when allopurinol is simultaneously administered.

Azathioprine and 6MP inhibit both cell-mediated and humoral immunity. Because of the diversity of studies that have been carried out in animal models and humans, there have been certain disagreements with regard to the type and extent of immunosuppression that occurs during azathioprine and 6MP therapy.[46,70] Despite this, there have been some rather consistent findings with regard to the effects of azathioprine and 6MP on immune and inflammatory responses. Azathioprine and 6MP cause a total lymphocytopenia of both T and B lymphocytes.[71] Gammaglobulin synthesis is suppressed by azathioprine therapy,[72] as is the antibody response (particularly the secondary response) to vaccination.[73] In addition, B-lymphocyte proliferation is suppressed by azathioprine.[74] There has been some controversy with regard to the effects of these agents on T lymphocytes. Certain studies report a selective effect on T lymphocytes, including inhibition of sheep red blood cell rosette formation.[75] However, other studies claim no selective effect on T lymphocytes[71,74] and in fact demonstrate that treatment with azathioprine has very little suppressive effect on mitogen-induced blastogenesis of human T lymphocytes.[76,77] In this regard, there seems to be little question that azathioprine is not as effective as cyclophosphamide in the suppression of lymphocyte function. Azathioprine and 6MP can suppress the induction of de novo delayed hypersensitivity; however, it is generally agreed that established delayed hypersensitivity remains intact during drug therapy.[73,77] Azathioprine has potent anti-inflammatory effects, which are probably related to its ability to reduce the number of monocytes in an inflammatory site by inhibition of monocyte production.[78] This suppression of monocyte function may also explain the effects of these drugs on delayed hypersensitivity.[79]

Azathioprine and 6MP are generally administered in doses of approximately 2 mg per kg per day. As with the other cytotoxic agents, the dosage must be adjusted according to the degree of resulting myelosuppression. Immunosuppressive and clinical effects are usually seen within 3 or 4 weeks after initiation of therapy. Patients with impaired renal function may have reduced clearance of the drug and its metabolites, with a resulting cumulative effect and increased toxicity unless the dosage is appropriately adjusted downward.

The major toxicity of both 6MP and azathioprine is bone marrow suppression, with leukopenia rather than thrombocytopenia and anemia being the major manifestation. The major toxic side effects of chronically administered azathioprine or 6MP therapy are listed in Table 55–5.[80] Of note with regard to the neutropenia associated with these agents is the fact that a rapid fall in WBC within a week of starting therapy has been reported and resembles an idiosyncratic reaction. In addition, the peripheral WBC cannot always be an accurate measure of the host defense defect, since infections may occur in individuals with normal neutrophil counts, suggesting a functional impairment of immune-competent cells involved in host defense, most likely at the T lymphocyte-monocyte axis. The suppression of delayed hypersensitivity by these agents[78,79] as well as the fact that neutrophil function is generally normal in individuals

Table 55–5. Toxic Side Effects of Chronically Administered Azathioprine and 6-Mercaptopurine Therapy

1. Marrow suppression—predominantly neutropenia
2. Hepatotoxicity—probably on an allergic basis
3. Infectious disease complications—not necessarily correlated with neutropenia
4. Gastrointestinal intolerance
5. Oncogenesis—particularly lymphoid malignancies

receiving azathioprine[81] adds credence to this hypothesis. This point should be fully appreciated, since infectious disease complications cannot be totally predicted regardless of the level of the WBC. Finally, although the effects on gonadal function have not been fully evaluated with regard to azathioprine, it is clear that sterility is not the invariable rule, since several normal pregnancies have been reported in patients who had been receiving azathioprine. Fetal abnormalities do not appear to be a problem.[36]

Folic Acid Antagonists. The folic acid antagonists such as methotrexate bind competitively to dihydrofolate reductase with a much higher affinity than does the natural substrate dihydrofolic acid. This prevents the conversion by dihydrofolate reductase of hydrofolic acid to tetrahydrofolic acid, thus interfering with the transport of one-carbon fragments required for thymidine synthesis. In this manner, DNA synthesis, and ultimately cellular proliferation, is inhibited.[10] Folic acid antagonists kill cells predominantly in the S phase of the cell cycle, particularly during the logarithmic phase of growth rather than at the plateau phase; they have little effect on resting cells. This selective killing of rapidly proliferating cells forms the rational basis for the successful use of methotrexate in the treatment of psoriasis, which is characterized by an abnormally rapid proliferation of epidermal cells. Leucovorin (folinic acid) is a fully reduced, metabolically functional folate coenzyme that functions directly without the need of reduction by dihydrofolate reductase. Hence, it has been used to "rescue" normal cells from the toxicity of folic acid antagonists.[10]

Methotrexate. Methotrexate may be administered orally or parenterally. It is readily absorbed from the gastrointestinal tract when administered in doses of 0.1 mg per kg, but larger doses are less completely absorbed (approximately 60 percent absorption).[10] The plasma half-life of methotrexate is approximately 2 hours,[82] although it disappears from the plasma in a triphasic fashion following intravenous administration.[10] The drug has very poor penetration through the blood-brain barrier. Approximately 50 percent of the drug is bound to plasma proteins and may be displaced by certain drugs, such as sulfonamides, salicylates, tetracycline, and chloramphenicol. Most of the drug is excreted unchanged in the urine within the first 24 hours, predominantly during the first 8 hours, with very little fecal excretion.

Methotrexate exerts profound suppression on both primary and secondary antibody responses in man.[83-85] Although the drug has been demonstrated to markedly suppress the delayed hypersensitivity reaction in animals,[70] little if any effect on established delayed cutaneous hypersensitivity was noted in man during treatment with methotrexate.[85]

Methotrexate is administered orally or intravenously, usually in an intermittent fashion, and the dosages are usually determined on a weekly basis. The standard adult dose ranges from 5 to 50 mg per week. This total weekly dose may be given as a single intravenous dose once a week or orally as 3 divided doses, each separated by 12 hours, or orally daily for 5 days of the week. The drug dosage should be reduced in patients with renal failure, as increased toxicity has been noted.

Toxic side effects of methotrexate include marrow suppression, particularly leukopenia and thrombocytopenia, oral mucositis, nausea, vomiting, diarrhea, and occasional hepatotoxicity. Although an increased risk of malignancy has not been documented in patients receiving methotrexate, there is a significant risk to the fetus if the drug is administered during the first trimester of pregnancy.[10]

Other Agents

Vinca Alkaloids. The commonly used vinca alkaloids, vincristine and vinblastine, are cell cycle–specific agents that block mitosis by interfering with protein assembly of the mitotic spindle, leading to metaphase arrest.[10] Vincristine is administered intravenously in doses of 2 mg per m² of body surface weekly. After intravenous injection, vincristine is cleared almost entirely from the blood in approximately 30 minutes. The drug is excreted primarily by the liver into the bile, with less than 5 percent of the drug appearing in the urine.

Immunosuppression with these compounds has been negligible, and antibody formation in rabbits was shown not to be significantly affected by administration of vinca alkaloids.[46] Vinblastine has been employed in a unique immunosuppression protocol in the treatment of idiopathic thrombocytopenia in which the drug was bound to platelets for the purposes of delivering the toxic drug directly and selectively to the cells that were removing and killing the platelets.[86]

The major toxic side effect of the vinca alkaloids is neurotoxicity. This is usually manifested by peripheral neuropathy in the form of paresthesias, loss of deep tendon reflexes, neuritic pain, muscle weakness, and wasting. In addition, hoarseness due to vocal cord paralysis may be seen together with other cranial nerve palsies leading to ptosis and diplopia. Severe constipation, sometimes resulting in paralytic ileus, is commonly seen and may mimic an acute surgical abdomen. In this regard, adequate hydration as well as a program of prophylactic laxatives and stool softeners is recommended for all patients receiving these agents. Bladder atony may lead to urinary retention or incontinence. Other side effects of the vinca alkaloids include alopecia in about 20 percent of patients, leukopenia, thrombocytopenia (only at very high doses or after prolonged administration of the drug), pyuria, dysuria, fever, gastrointestinal symptoms, mutagenicity, and inappropriate secretion of antidiuretic hormone, leading to hyponatremia with high urinary sodium.[10] Finally, extravasation of the drug at the site of injection can lead to severe local inflammatory reactions.

5-Fluorouracil. 5-Fluorouracil is a pyrimidine analogue that competes with uracil in various metabolic pathways but cannot be converted to thymidine. Thus, it ultimately blocks DNA synthesis. In addition, it inhibits enzymes such as thymidylate synthetase required for the synthesis of ribonucleotides and deoxyribonucleotides. The drug has been used predominantly in the treatment of neoplastic diseases, and its precise immunosuppressive properties are not well studied in man.[10] The drug works throughout the cell cycle and is metabolized almost exclusively in the liver. It is usually administered intravenously, since absorption after oral ingestion is unpredictable and incomplete. The major toxic side effects result from the inevitable myelosuppression, particularly leukopenia. Other side effects include nausea and vomiting, alopecia, dermatitis, nail changes, atrophy of the skin, ulcerative stomatitis and gastroenteritis, and neurologic manifestations such as cerebellar ataxia.[10]

Hydroxyurea. Hydroxyurea inhibits the enzyme ribonucleotide diphosphate reductase, which catalyzes the reductive conversion of ribonucleotides to deoxyribonucleotides and which is a crucial step in the synthesis of DNA. The drug is specific for the S phase of the cell cycle.[10] It is readily absorbed from the gastrointestinal tract, and peak plasma concentrations are reached within two hours of administration of an oral dose. Within 24 hours, it is undetectable in the blood with approximately 80 percent of the drug recovered in the urine within 12 hours of oral or intravenous administration.[10] The drug is administered orally in doses of 20 to 30 mg per kg per day as a single dose. Although the drug has been used predominantly in the management of chronic granulocytic leukemia, it has recently been used in the treatment of the idiopathic hypereosinophilic syndrome.[87] Toxic side effects include myelosuppression, nausea and vomiting, gastrointestinal ulcerations, and mild skin rashes.

THEORETICAL AND PRACTICAL CONSIDERATIONS IN THE USE OF CYTOTOXIC AGENTS FOR THE TREATMENT OF NON–NEOPLASTIC DISEASES

As mentioned above, one of the major goals in the use of cytotoxic agents for the treatment of non-neoplastic diseases is to achieve a degree of immunosuppression that results in suppression of the aberrant inflammatory and immune reactivity in a disease state without seriously compromising host defense mechanisms, which would lead to an increased incidence of infectious disease complications. For reasons that are not entirely clear, in those inflammatory and immune-mediated diseases for which cytotoxic agents have proved to be beneficial, it appears that disease activity can indeed be suppressed without the invariable occurrence of a serious defect in clinically relevant host defense mechanisms.

Although the cytotoxic agents have a number of immediate and long-term toxic side effects that must be considered in the decision to employ such agents in a given patient, once the decision has been made to use a cytotoxic agent, awareness and recognition of these side effects become of paramount importance in the successful management of the patient. In this regard, although the different classes of cytotoxic agents used in the treatment of non-neoplastic diseases differ somewhat in their mechanisms of action, the major immediate limiting side effect common to virtually all of them is myelosuppression, particularly neutropenia and to a lesser extent thrombocytopenia and anemia.

When the physician undertakes the treatment of non-neoplastic diseases with these agents, it is essential to appreciate the necessity for careful and continuous monitoring of the WBC, with appropriate modification of the dosage regimen to maintain the WBC above the neutropenic range. It has been consistently observed that if the WBC is maintained above 3000 to 3500 cells per mm^3, which usually results in a neutrophil count of 1000 to 1500 per mm^3, there is very little chance of opportunistic infections as a result of drug-induced host defense defects, particularly when the agent employed is an alkylating agent such as cyclophosphamide or chlorambucil. For example, this has clearly been shown to be the case with the use of cyclophosphamide in the treatment of Wegener's granulomatosis[25] and other of the severe systemic vasculitic syndromes.[24,26] This observation holds true provided there is not a concomitant and synergistic cause of host defense defects, such as daily corticosteroid therapy. For this reason, it is suggested that corticosteroids be administered on an alternate-day basis, when possible, in patients receiving cytotoxic agents together with corticosteroids for the treatment of non-neoplastic diseases.[24-26] Using such a regimen of chronically administered cyclophosphamide at a dose of 2 mg per kg per day with frequent adjustments of dosage to maintain the WBC above 3000 per mm^3 together with prednisone 60 mg per day or less with conversion to alternate-day prednisone within 1 to 2 months of initiating therapy and maintenance of alternate-day prednisone together with the cyclophosphamide, there has been virtually no increased incidence of opportunistic infections in a large series of patients recently reported.[25] The exception to this was an increased incidence of herpes zoster infections in patients receiving chronic cyclophosphamide therapy.[88] The zoster did not disseminate viscerally in any patient, and there were no serious sequelae of the infection.

Maintaining the WBC above the neutropenic level while effecting remission of disease activity requires continuous monitoring of the WBC as well as appreciation that as patients receive a cytotoxic agent for extended periods of time, their tolerance for a given dose will decrease, necessitating adjustment downward of the dose. It should also be pointed out that an appreciation of the "slope of the curve" of the WBC is important, in that the effect of a given dose of drug on one day may be reflected several days later (Fig. 55–3). Therefore, one should not wait until the patient is already seriously neutropenic before decreasing the dose of cytotoxic agent but should decrease the dose based on the projection of the downward slope of the WBC curve. In this way, a smooth plateauing of the WBC can be

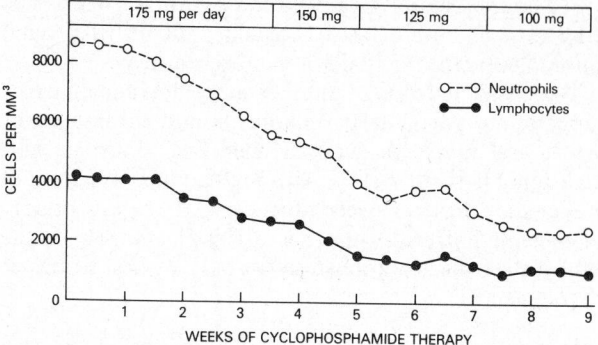

Figure 55–3. Schematic diagram of the use and modification of cyclophosphamide therapy according to the white blood cell count in a patient with Wegener's granulomatosis. The major goal in the treatment of non-neoplastic diseases with cytotoxic agents such as cyclophosphamide is the suppression of disease activity and avoidance of toxic side effects such as significant neutropenia. As shown with the patient indicated in this figure, the dose of drug must be continually modified in accordance with the white blood cell count so as to allow the total white blood cell count to remain above 3000 to 3500 per mm^3, which generally results in a neutrophil count above 1000 to 1500 per mm^3. It is essential to realize that the dosage must be decreased as the slope of the white blood cell count declines, since a given dose of drug will be reflected by the white blood cell count several days later. One must anticipate this and modify the dosage so as to arrive smoothly at a maintenance dose of cyclophosphamide, which is almost always lower than the initial induction dose. Once the maintenance dose is reached, the patient will usually be able to tolerate it for several months. However, usually even this dose must ultimately be decreased, as the bone marrow is less able to tolerate the drug over a period of time. Again, this requires frequent and consistent monitoring of the counts throughout the period of drug administration.

maintained and infectious disease complications largely avoided.

The preceding principles of the relationship between neutropenia and infection generally hold true except under certain circumstances, such as the concomitant use of other agents, which cause a host defense defect but do not cause neutropenia. As mentioned, this is the case with the use of daily corticosteroids, which negates our ability to use the WBC as an accurate gauge of the degree of host defense defect. Furthermore, agents such as azathioprine (see above) can result in an increased incidence of infectious disease complications even without neutropenia. When using such agents, it is still important to monitor the WBC; however, the danger of the occurrence of unpredicted infectious disease complications must be appreciated. In addition, the gradual dropping of the WBC on a constant dose of cytotoxic agent is the rule, but certain drugs such as azathioprine can give an idiosyncratic, precipitous drop in WBC. All of these possibilities must be taken into consideration in the use of these agents.

It should be pointed out that under certain circumstances the bone marrow reserve of a given patient may be suppressed to a point at which the dosage of cyclophosphamide must be reduced despite the fact that the disease is still active. In these situations, the addition of or increase in the dose of alternate-day prednisone may allow one to administer higher doses of cyclophosphamide with a lesser degree of leukopenia. It is felt that the mechanism of this marrow-sparing effect of corticosteroid in patients treated with cyclophosphamide is the result of a beneficial effect on marrow regeneration, due most likely to an altering of cell cycle characteristics of granulocyte progenitor cells.[25]

Once disease remission has been achieved and maintained for an adequate period of time with the use of cytotoxic agents, it is important to continually attempt to taper the dose of drug with the ultimate goal of discontinuation. The time for maintenance of remission on cytotoxic agents varies with each disease. However, the general principle stands that the physician should always have the ultimate discontinuation of the cytotoxic agent as a goal of the regimen.

Finally, a thorough familiarization with all of the other immediate as well as long-term potential side effects of these agents should be undertaken by the physician who prescribes them, and careful following of the patient during and after use of these agents is essential in order to detect the onset of these complications as early as possible.

THERAPEUTIC APHERESIS

The word apheresis is a Greek derivative meaning withdrawal. Therapeutic apheresis implies withdrawal of a substance from a patient, ultimately leading to clinical improvement in a disease state. Although the original aphereses were solely confined to the removal of plasma for hyperviscosity states such as Waldenström's macroglobulinemia, the recent development of sophisticated equipment for removal of plasma as well as selected cellular components has led to an acceleration of the use of apheresis in a number of different disease states, including hematologic, connective tissue, neurologic, and even neoplastic disorders.[89] Plasmapheresis is the removal of plasma without significant removal of cellular elements. Cytapheresis is the removal of cells without significant removal of noncellular elements such as plasma. For example, lymphocytapheresis is the selective removal of mononuclear cells, especially lymphocytes, without significant removal of either plasma or nonlymphoid cellular elements. Selective lymphocyte removal can be accomplished either by thoracic duct drainage (which strictly speaking is lymphocytapheresis) or by continuous flow cell separators via venous access. Lymphoplasmapheresis is the removal of both plasma and lymphocytes with sparing of nonlymphoid cellular elements.

In addition to the removal of the hyperviscous macroglobulin in Waldenström's macroglobulinemia, plasmapheresis has the theoretical and practical effect of removing pathogenic autoantibodies in diseases such as Goodpasture's syndrome, immune thrombocytopenia, autoimmune hemolytic anemia, myasthenia gravis, and severe Rh disease.[89,90-93] Most recently, plasmapheresis

has been used in the treatment of connective tissue diseases, particularly rheumatoid arthritis and SLE, and to a lesser degree in the treatment of certain of the vasculitic syndromes.[93-97] Given the evidence that lymphocytes appear to be involved in both the initiation and propagation of the inflammatory responses in rheumatoid arthritis, lymphocytapheresis and lymphoplasmapheresis have been performed in the treatment of this disease.[98,99] Finally, recent evidence has indicated that a form of plasmapheresis in which plasma is perfused over immobilized protein-A may be effective in inducing tumor rejection in patients with malignant neoplasms by removing serum factors that inhibit rejection.[100] In this regard, the area of selective removal of potentially harmful components of plasma by extracorporeal modification of plasma either by selective absorption, cryogelation, and membrane filtration or by chemical and physical precipitation is currently under intensive study.[101,102]

The major rationale for the use of plasmapheresis in the treatment of immune complex–mediated diseases such as SLE is the physical removal of the immune complexes from the circulation, making them unavailable for deposition in tissue. However, a further rationale may relate to abnormalities in reticuloendothelial system (RES) function seen in certain immune complex–mediated diseases such as SLE.[103] A recent study has demonstrated that plasmapheresis re-established previously abnormal splenic RES function, and this did not necessarily correlate with complete normalization of autoantibodies or immune complex levels.[96] In addition, recent studies have demonstrated that defective monocyte function improved following plasmapheresis.[104] Hence, the therapeutic efficacy of plasmapheresis may well extend beyond the mere removal of a substance that is directly toxic to tissues.

Plasmapheresis carries with it the potential problem of a rebound in production of antibodies to higher levels than pretreatment by removal of either feedback inhibitory mechanisms or actual suppressor factors.[90] However, this difficulty is generally obviated by the fact that most protocols employing plasmapheresis also call for the simultaneous administration of immunosuppressive agents, which not only synergize with the effects of the plasmapheresis but also blunt any potential rebound phenomena that might occur.[105]

Plasmapheresis protocols vary considerably in the specific details of the procedure. However, current uses of plasmapheresis are usually true plasma exchanges in that large amounts of plasma are removed and replaced by various types of replacement fluids. A commonly used protocol is the performance of plasma exchanges three times per week over a 2- to 6-week period. Each procedure usually lasts from 2 to 4 hours. At each procedure, variable amounts of plasma may be removed, but a relatively standard amount is 40 ml of plasma per kg of body weight or up to 3 liters per exchange. Plasma volume is usually replaced by a combination of albumin and normal saline with or without other fluids such as acid citrate dextrose.[94] Replacement of plasma volume and oncotic pressure are accomplished by these materials.

Theoretically, however, one must at least consider the replacement of other factors, such as Ig, clotting factors, and other proteins. It has been reported that a prolongation of prothrombin, partial thromboplastin, and thrombin times as well as a reduction in fibrinogen, clotting factors, and platelet counts occurred 4 hours after plasmapheresis; however, these all recovered by 24 hours.[106] The effect of plasmapheresis with albumin replacement on normal plasma constituents was also studied.[107] All plasma constituents were shown to have recovered within 48 hours except fibrinogen, C3, cholesterol, IgG, and IgM. Although fresh frozen plasma is the most physiologic replacement fluid available, as it supplies Ig, coagulation factors, complement, and possbily other factors that might be beneficial to and lacking in the patient, it does carry the risk of transmission of viral hepatitis. Thus, albumin and normal saline remain the standard replacement fluids.

Lymphapheresis, like plasmapheresis, has been carried out under a variety of protocols. In one study, lymphapheresis was carried out in a group of patients with rheumatoid arthritis, and each procedure was repeated 2 to 3 times per week for a total of 13 to 16 procedures over a 5-week period.[98] A mean of 13.7×10^{10} lymphocytes were removed per patient during the study, and every patient became lymphopenic. Although short periods of lymphapheresis resulted in equal losses of T and B lymphocytes, this extended 5-week course resulted in a disproportionate fall in circulating T lymphocytes by 26 to 58 percent. In addition, serum IgM fell by 30 percent.[98] Clearly significant lymphodepletion with resulting immunosuppression can be achieved with repeated lymphocytapheresis using continuous flow centrifugation.[108] In a double-blind controlled trial of lymphoplasmapheresis versus sham apheresis in patients with rheumatoid arthritis, by the ninth treatment, treated patients had significant reductions in absolute lymphocyte counts; total serum protein; alpha, beta, and gammaglobulins; IgG, IgM, IgA; C3; and circulating immune complexes; with no significant changes in WBC, serum sodium, potassium, or albumin.[99] Of note is the fact that Westergren sedimentation rates fell significantly, as did rheumatoid factor titers.

Lymphapheresis has for the most part replaced thoracic duct drainage as a modality for removing lymphocytes largely because of the ease, convenience, and relative lack of complications of the former. However, significantly favorable and sometimes dramatic clinical responses have been reported in a study of the effects of long-term thoracic duct drainage in a group of patients with autoimmune diseases.[109] Significant degrees of immunosuppression, particularly of T lymphocyte–mediated responses, was noted in the treated patients[109,110] and disease was transiently exacerbated in three patients in whom autologous lymphocytes were reinfused.[110]

Detrimental side effects and complications of apheresis include depletion of platelets as well as important components of plasma, such as clotting factors, with resulting bleeding diatheses, hypotension, fluid and electrolyte imbalance, and complications relating to access sites. The potential long-term complications of these procedures are unclear at present.

The long-term therapeutic benefits from apheresis are uncertain, and a number of controlled and uncontrolled studies are currently being conducted to determine the precise immediate and long-term benefits of this approach in several rheumatic diseases. Several studies have indicated at least a significant short-term clinical improvement in patients with rheumatoid arthritis treated with various apheresis protocols.[89,98,99] The situation is less clear in SLE, and a recent review of the currently available data indicates no significant benefit of plasmapheresis in the treatment of SLE.[95]

IONIZING RADIATION

Ionizing radiation exerts its effects on tissues by inducing the ionization of atoms. X-rays and gamma rays cause ejection of electrons from the atoms with which they interact, and thus ionize them. When the irradiation is of high enough energy, the ejected electrons themselves have considerable kinetic energy and in turn ionize other atoms. Ionization of atoms within a cell leads to the formation of highly reactive free radicals. These free radicals interact with biologically relevant macromolecules such as DNA. In fact, the lesion responsible for the most important biologic effects of radiation is scission of the DNA chain.[111] Such effects on nuclear DNA lead to the major cellular consequence of irradiation, which is impairment of cellular reproduction. It is for this reason that rapidly dividing cells such as bone marrow, intestinal epithelium, and certain types of lymphocytes appear to be selectively affected by irradiation. However, irradiation may also impair cell function and viability by mechanisms unrelated to the mitotic event.[111]

Ionizing radiation can have profound effects on lymphoid cells, including those involved in the initiation and propagation of immune-mediated connective tissue diseases. The ultimate effect of irradiation on the immune system of the host is highly dependent on the dose delivered. Although this may vary according to the protocol employed, there is generally a gradation of sensitivity of lymphoid subsets as well as lymphoid cells at various stages of differentiation to increasing doses of irradiation.[112] Precursor cells are usually exquisitely sensitive to irradiation. Low doses of irradiation may selectively kill certain subpopulations of T and B lymphocytes while sparing others. Resting or undifferentiated B lymphocytes are quite sensitive to irradiation, while fully differentiated plasma cells are rather resistant to the effects of radiation.[113] Among immunoregulatory T-lymphocyte subsets, suppressor T lymphocytes are generally more sensitive to irradiation than are helper T lymphocytes.[113] It should be pointed out that the net effect of irradiation on lymphocyte subpopulations in particular and immune function in general is usually highly dependent on the total dosage and the dosage schedule employed. For example, total body irradiation is profoundly immunosuppressive and is designed to eliminate as extensively as possible the immune competence of the host. The side effects of this modality are extreme and may be fatal. Therefore, this type of radiation protocol is reserved for special clinical circumstances such as preparation for bone marrow transplantation. For this reason, we will not discuss this modality in the present setting.

TOTAL LYMPH NODE IRRADIATION

A potentially important advance in the use of radiation therapy for non-neoplastic diseases has been made with the recent introduction of the use of fractionated total lymph node irradiation in the treatment of rheumatoid arthritis. The rationale for this approach is similar to that described for the use of lymphapheresis in that recent evidence indicates that lymphocytes, particularly T lymphocytes, appear to be involved in the immunopathogenic expression of rheumatoid arthritis. Total lymph node irradiation has been used for the past 20 years in the treatment of Hodgkin's disease and non-Hodgkin's lymphoma.[114,115] Of note is the fact that there have been no serious long-term sequelae of leukemia, second tumors, or serious host defense defects leading to infectious disease complications. Nonetheless, cell-mediated immunity was shown to be suppressed for several years following treatment.[116] Thus, this approach has recently been employed in the treatment of intractable rheumatoid arthritis as an alternative to the use of cytotoxic agents such as cyclophosphamide and azathioprine.

The results of at least two feasibility studies have been impressive.[117,118] Twenty-one patients were treated with 2000 to 3000 rad over 5 to 14 weeks with a follow-up of 12 to 18 months. Seventeen of 21 patients experienced significant clinical improvement. Virtually all patients experienced a lymphocytopenia with suppression of in vitro lymphocyte responses. In one study,[117] there was an increase in the ratio of suppressor to helper T lymphocytes. This reappearance of suppressor cell capability is analogous to the development of suppressor T lymphocytes accompanying long-lasting immunosuppression in mice treated with total lymph node irradiation.[119] It should be pointed out that abnormal antibody activities characteristic of rheumatoid arthritis as well as normal components of humoral immunity were not suppressed by the treatment protocol.[118] There were some partial recrudescences within a year in one study[118] and sustained remissions over an 18-month period in another study.[117] Thus, effective suppression of manifestations of severe rheumatoid arthritis can be accomplished for significant periods of time with total lymph node irradiation, and this is associated with substantial suppression of T lymphocyte function. In addition, immediate toxic side effects are few. Although it is uncertain whether the natural history of the disease will be altered by this approach, it clearly deserves further study and attention as a promising modality of therapy for severe connective tissue diseases mediated by lymphoid cells.

ANTILYMPHOCYTE ANTIBODIES

Standard Antisera. Heterologous antilymphocyte serum (ALS) refers to antiserum raised in one species against lymphocytes of another species. Since such antisera generally contain antibodies directed against cell types other than lymphoid cells, absorption of the serum with nonlymphoid cells is required to make the serum relatively specific for lymphocyte antigens. The serum may then be fractionated to obtain the IgG fraction with antilymphocyte activity; this is referred to as antilymphocyte globulin (ALG). This latter manipulation removes a number of serum factors that might be immunogenic and cause hypersensitivity reactions such as serum sickness.

Since the ultimate target of the ALS is usually T lymphocytes, it would be preferable to have the antiserum react only with T lymphocytes while sparing B lymphocytes. In this regard, further absorptions of the ALS with B lymphocytes may yield an antiserum that is relatively specific for T lymphocytes, i.e., anti–T lymphocyte serum (ATS).

The common denominator of the mechanism of immunosuppression of ALS is a lymphocytopenia. Although ALS bound to lymphocytes in the presence of complement in vitro can cause cytotoxicity[120] and ultimately cell death, the major mechanism of lymphocytopenia in vivo is the selective depletion of circulating T lymphocytes by opsonization and clearance via the RES, predominantly of the liver.[121] It should be pointed out that in the absence of complement, ALS may bind to the lymphocyte and induce blast transformation,[120] and so modulation of lymphocyte function can potentially occur, although the net effect is almost invariably the removal of cells from the recirculating pool. The potency of the immunosuppressive effects of a given batch of ALS depends on the relative ability of the antiserum to bind to and induce the clearance of lymphocytes.

ALS has been used extensively in man as an immunosuppressive agent in renal allograft recipients with rather impressive results.[122,123] With regard to the use of ALS in immune-mediated diseases, a number of investigators have employed this agent in uncontrolled trials of the treatment of diseases such as autoimmune hemolytic anemia, myasthenia gravis, multiple sclerosis, and a variety of connective tissue diseases.[120] Although several reports indicated favorable results, the use of ALS in connective tissue diseases has not been extensive, owing to the lack of convincing controlled trials demonstrating its efficacy.

Most recently, the toxic side effects of ALS preparations have been markedly decreased by the use of meticulous absorption procedures that remove non-Ig proteins, which might increase the incidence of serum sickness as well as antibodies to a variety of nonlymphoid cells, particularly platelets and erythrocytes. Nonetheless, one must be aware of the considerable potential toxic side effects of the use of ALS.[120] These include fever, chills, arthralgias, and back pain, usually occurring 3 to 12 hours after the first and second injection. Subsequently, fever may be minimal. With intramuscular injections, there may be pain at the site of injection, and with intravenous injections, there may be mild phlebitis as well as occasional episodes of bradycardia and hypotension. Infectious complications of the immunosuppression include herpes zoster; nephrotoxic nephritis caused by antiglomerular antibodies in the ALS preparation has been reported.[120] Furthermore, the long-range toxic side effects of ALS are unclear at this point, which adds to the reluctance to use these agents widely in the treatment of connective tissue diseases.

Monoclonal Antibodies. Immunologic research was virtually revolutionized by the demonstration by Köhler and Milstein in 1975 that somatic cell hybridization could be employed in the immortalization of B lymphocyte lines, producing monoclonal antibody.[124] This new dimension in immunobiologic analysis witnessed immediate application in immunodiagnosis.[125] However, the potential for the therapeutic use of monoclonal antibodies is clear, and already a number of studies are being conducted for the use of these agents in the treatment of certain neoplastic diseases. Preliminary studies have already demonstrated their potential efficacy in the treatment of certain lymphoid malignancies.[126,127] In addition, monoclonal antibodies directed against lymphoid tumor antigens have been used to deplete bone marrow of residual leukemia cells prior to autologous marrow transplantation.[128] Monoclonal antibodies directed against mature alloreactive T lymphocytes have been used to pretreat allogeneic bone marrow prior to transplantation for the purpose of preventing acute graft-versus-host disease with variable results.[129,130] However, of particular interest is the recent report of the use of a monoclonal antibody (T12) to treat an HLA haplotype–mismatched allogenic bone marrow prior to transplantation for severe combined immunodeficiency as well as to treat the recipient in vivo to terminate ongoing severe graft-versus-host disease.[131]

With regard to the use of monoclonal antibodies in the treatment of autoimmune diseases, experimental data have indicated at least the feasibility of employing this approach in diseases such as experimental allergic encephalitis[132] and myasthenia gravis.[133] Although it is tempting to envision the manipulation of immunoregulatory lymphocyte subsets in autoimmune diseases by the in vivo use of monoclonal antibodies directed against specific lymphocyte subsets, it should be pointed out that the complexity of the immune system with its intricate feedback mechanisms renders such an approach only speculative at present.

STEROID HORMONES

Glucocorticosteroids. Glucocorticosteroids are used extensively in the treatment of rheumatic diseases. These agents manifest both anti-inflammatory and immunosuppressive effects.[7] Although virtually any function of an inflammatory or immune competent cell can be suppressed by a high enough concentration of corticosteroid in vitro, in the dosages of drug that are generally employed in the treatment of rheumatic diseases, the effects of the drug are somewhat selective for one or another of the components of the inflammatory or immune response.[7,134] For example, the inductive phase of the immune response is clearly more sensitive to the immunosuppressive effects of corticosteroids than is the effector phase.[7] Furthermore, the T-lymphocyte or cell-mediated limb of immunity is clearly more sensitive to corticosteroids than is the B-lymphocyte or humoral limb.[135] In addition, within the T-lymphocyte fraction, certain subsets are selectively more sensitive to the drug than are others.[136]

Of particular importance in the understanding of the effects of corticosteroids on inflammatory and immune competent cells is an appreciation of the fact that the drugs can affect the inflammatory and immune response by a number of mechanisms. For example, administration of corticosteroids may affect the circulatory kinetics of a given cell type such as a neutrophil, monocyte, or lymphocyte subset and thus block the availability of these cells to the inflammatory site without directly suppressing the functional capability of the cell. On the other hand, the drug may directly affect the functional capability of a cell in a situation in which circulatory kinetics are not relevant.[7] In general, lower concentrations of the drug are required in order to affect circulatory kinetics, whereas higher concentrations are needed in order to directly suppress a functional capability of a cell.[7] Finally, the effects of corticosteroids on a given cell type may vary, depending on the state of activation of the cell in question. Understanding these concepts is important in the proper design of therapeutic protocols for the use of corticosteroids in the treatment of non-neoplastic diseases. A detailed discussion of the use of corticosteroid therapy is contained in Chapter 54.

Sex Hormones. The sex hormones, particularly the androgens, may have significant immunoregulatory effects. Indeed, male sex hormones have been shown to suppress a variety of immune responses in experimental animals.[137,138] Furthermore, in vitro testosterone has been shown to cause a mild decrease in blastogenic responses of phytohemagglutinin-stimulated human lymphocytes at hormone concentrations of 0.1 μg per ml and to completely ablate the response at 80 mg per ml.[139] Of potential clinical relevance is the observation that the administration of male sex hormones can decrease the degree of autoimmune phenomena and even prolong survival in the murine models of SLE.[140,141] Furthermore, a lack of male sex hormones may lead to a marked acceleration of autoimmunity.[142] These observations may not only provide insight into the pathophysiologic mechanisms of disease but also may provide the rational basis for the therapeutic use of these agents in certain autoimmune diseases. Although the male sex hormones have been shown to be immunosuppressive,[137,138] the precise mechanisms whereby these agents prevent or ameliorate autoimmune phenomena are unclear at present. It should be pointed out that male sex hormones have proved to be highly effective in the treatment of hereditary angioedema.[143,144] The mechanisms whereby these agents are effective in this latter disease include the reversal of the biochemical abnormality by inducing the synthesis of the deficient C1 esterase inhibitor.[144]

Other Hormones. A number of other hormones have been shown to have in vitro and in vivo effects on immune function. The clinical relevance of these effects with regard to rheumatic diseases is unclear at present, particularly with regard to therapeutic efficacy. However, an understanding of the potential immunologic effects of various hormonal imbalances is important for an appreciation of the scope of hormonal influences on the immune responses in general and on immune-mediated diseases in particular. A brief summary of certain representative effects of various nonglucocorticosteroid hormones on the immune responses is contained on Table 55–6.[145]

OTHER AGENTS

Levamisole. Levamisole is a three-ring molecule with the extremely low molecular weight of 241. It was introduced into veterinary practice in 1966 as a nematocidal agent and was subsequently used in man. It is highly active against a wide range of nematodes and is particularly effective in ascariasis. It has, however, received recent attention as an immunoenhancing agent in man. Levamisole is absorbed rapidly from the gastrointestinal tract. Following administration of a 150-mg dose in man, peak blood levels of 5 micrograms per ml are reached at 2 hours.[146] The plasma half-life is approximately 4 hours, and the drug is metabolized predominantly in the liver, with excretion of the breakdown products via the kidney and to a lesser extent in the feces.

Levamisole has been shown to augment the effector phase of the nonspecific inflammatory response as well as to truly potentiate the immune response by enhancing lymphoid cell function. The drug has been shown to be effective in correcting the chemotactic defect of monocytes[147] and neutrophils[148] in patients with viral infections. In addition, levamisole has been shown to be effective both in vitro and in vivo in correcting the chemotactic defect in neutrophils from patients with the syndrome of hyperimmunoglobulin E and recurrent infections.[149,150] However, a recent double-blind study demonstrated that despite restoration of normal chemotactic responsiveness in patients with the hyperimmunoglobulin E syndrome by treatment with levamisole, patients who received the drug tended to have more serious infectious complications than those patients given a placebo.[151]

A variety of lymphocyte functions have been shown to be enhanced in vivo by treatment with levamisole as well as in vitro by the addition of the drug to lymphocyte cultures. The drug appears to be most effective in immunopotentiation in individuals with abnormally low responses, with little effect under conditions of optimal responses. Delayed hypersensitivity skin tests have been shown to be enhanced in patients receiving levamisole therapy, particularly in those individuals with significant impairment of delayed cutaneous hypersensitivity.[152] The function of specific subpopulations of T lymphocytes are also augmented by levamisole. This includes enhancement of inducer or helper T-lymphocyte function and cytotoxic T-lymphocyte function as well as suppressor T-lymphocyte function.[153] Patients treated with levamisole generally do not manifest an increase in the absolute numbers or percentages of lymphocytes. However, reduced numbers of T lymphocytes are restored together with a reduction in the percentage of null cells (non-T, non-B cells).[154] Since null cells have been postulated to be precursors or immature forms of T and/or B lymphocytes, the increased numbers of T lymphocytes may represent an induction of differentiation or maturity from null cell to normally functioning T lymphocyte.[155] Although B lymphocytes are generally felt not to be directly stimulated by levamisole, a recent study described a booster response in antibody titers to recall antigens in patients treated with levamisole.[155] The mechanisms responsible for the phenomenon are unclear but could include a direct action on B lymphocytes or an

Table 55–6. Effects of the Nonglucocortoid Hormones on the Immune Response*

Growth Hormone	Appears essential for the maturation and function of thymic-dependent immune responses in the dwarf mouse
Thyroxine	Stimulatory to phytohemagglutinin blastogenic responses and antisheep erythrocyte plaque-forming cell production in mature mice; also appears to affect the maturation of thymic-dependent immune functions in immature mice
Insulin	In physiologic doses, stimulatory to thymic-derived immune responses in rats
Androgens	Prolong allograft survival in mice and decrease the phytohemagglutinin blastogenic responses in human lymphocytes *in vitro*
Estrogens and Oral Contraceptives	*In vitro* and *in vivo* administration inhibit human lymphocyte phytohemagglutinin blastogenic responses; also, decrease natural killer-cell activity and prolong allograft survival in animals *in vivo*

* From Stevenson, H.C., and Fauci, A.S.: The effect of glucocorticoids and other hormones on inflammatory and immune responses. *In* Oppenheim, J.J., Rosenstreich, D.L., and Potter, M. (eds.): Cellular Functions in Immunity and Inflammation. New York, Elsevier/North Holland, 1981.

indirect effect by enhancing inducer T lymphocytes or impeding suppressor cell function.

Levamisole has been used in malignant diseases as an adjuvant agent; it has also been used in a number of nonmalignant diseases. Of particular interest has been its use in the treatment of rheumatoid arthritis in which rather favorable clinical responses have been reported.[155,156] The drug is generally administered in doses of 150 mg orally on a daily basis for periods up to 16 weeks.[155] The major constraint of its use clinically is the incidence and severity of the toxic side effects. Side effects of the drug have included gastrointestinal disturbances, fatigue, fever, and skin rash. However, the most severe and limiting toxic side effect is granulocytopenia, which seems to be disproportionately more frequent in patients with rheumatic diseases. Of particular interest is the fact that agranulocytosis due to levamisole is particularly common in patients with HLA-B27.[157,158] In a recent study of the treatment of 20 rheumatoid arthritis patients with levamisole, agranulocytosis or neutropenia occurred at some time in 4 patients.[155] Despite the favorable clinical results with regard to the activity of the rheumatoid arthritis in that study, the toxicity clearly renders the drug unacceptable for routine use in rheumatoid arthritis.

Other Immune Enhancers and Adjuvants. Clearly, the most extensively employed adjuvant in experimental animals is complete Freund's adjuvant (CFA), which is composed of paraffin oil and an emulsifying agent to which killed mycobacteria have been added. Injection of emulsions of antigens in CFA into experimental animals results in markedly augmented antibody responses as well as delayed hypersensitivity.[159] Unfortunately, the severe local and systemic toxic side effects of CFA render it unacceptable for use in humans. Recently, preparations of adjuvants such as the synthetic N-acetylmuramyl-L-alanyl-D-isoglutamine have been shown to be effective enhancers of antibody production without appreciable toxic side effects.[160] Such studies may prove extremely fruitful in the ultimate development of a clinically acceptable adjuvant, which could be used in the enhancement of immune function in the absence of significant toxic side effects.

Cyclosporin A. Cyclosporin A was discovered in 1972 during a search for biologically produced antifungal agents. It is a 1200-dalton fungal metabolite, which proved to be only mildly active as an antifungal agent but did manifest certain profound effects on the immune response. Cyclosporin A is a cyclic endecapeptide of original chemical structure in which some amino acids are unconventional or modified (N-methylated.)[161] This latter property is responsible for the fact that the drug is effective by oral administration in that pH and enzymes of the gastrointestinal tract do not seem to inactivate it. It can be administered by both the parenteral and oral routes, it exhibits poor water solubility, and it does not need to be activated in vivo, as witnessed by the fact that it is directly active in vitro. The drug has been recently employed extensively as an immunosuppressive agent for organ (particularly renal) transplantation.[162] It is administered either as the sole immunosuppressive agent[163] or together with corticosteroids.[164] The optimal dose with regard to efficacy balanced against toxic side effects has not been precisely determined. However, recent studies in patients receiving cadaveric renal transplants have arrived at a dosage of 17 mg per kg per day with gradual tapering by about 2 mg per kg per day decrements at monthly intervals until a maintenance dose of 6 to 8 mg per kg per day is reached.[163]

Cyclosporin A differs from other known cytotoxic immunosuppressive agents in its mechanism of action and particularly by the fact that it manifests a low degree of myelotoxicity. It appears that the effect of the agent is selective for the immune system, particularly T lymphocytes. There is general agreement that cyclosporin A acts preferentially on proliferating T lymphocytes.[162] It has also been shown that the agent exerts its effects at an early stage in the triggering of T lymphocytes, since addition of cyclosporin A to lymphocyte cultures late after antigenic stimulation results in diminution of the inhibitory effect.[162]

It is currently debated exactly where in the mechanism of cell triggering cyclosporin A acts. Certain investigators have shown evidence that the drug acts by inhibiting the production of receptors for IL II or T lymphocyte growth factor.[165] Others claim that receptors for IL II are present despite the presence of the drug in culture and claim that IL II is missing from cultures.[162] In this regard, it is unclear whether cyclosporin A exerts this effect by blocking the synthesis of IL II or its secretion. In any event, cyclosporin A blocks a number of T lymphocyte functions, particularly those dependent on helper or inducer T lymphocyte activity.

In vitro studies have demonstrated suppressive effects of cyclosporin A on T helper lymphocytes for antibody production to T lymphocyte–dependent antigens,[166] inhibition of the generation[167] but not expression of the function[168] of cytotoxic T lymphocytes induced in the mixed lymphocyte reaction, and abrogation of concanavalin A–induced suppressor cell function.[169] It is unclear at this time whether the selective effects on helper T-lymphocyte function provide a balance in favor of T-lymphocyte suppression as being responsible for the initiation and maintenance of the immunosuppressed state. It has generally been felt that cyclosporin A affects B lymphocytes only insofar as it inhibits helper T lymphocyte function. However, recent studies suggest that the drug may have selective direct effects of enhancement or inhibition on certain subsets of B lymphocytes.[170] Of interest is the finding that in patients treated with cyclosporin A alone, IgG levels increased to become significantly elevated compared with those found in normal healthy controls.[162]

Cyclosporin A has received considerable attention as an extremely effective immunosuppressive agent for renal transplant rejection. Recently, favorable reports have appeared describing successes in transplantation of heart, lungs, pancreas, and liver in both experimental animals and certain small human studies.[162] The implications of these studies are extraordinary for the use of organ transplantation in a wide variety of clinical situations. In this regard, recent studies have demonstrated the efficacy of cyclosporin A in suppressing graft-versus-host reactions in bone marrow transplants.[171]

The major constraint in the use of cyclosporin A, as with other immunosuppressive agents, lies in its toxicity. Although it has few myelotoxic effects, use of the agent is not without risks. By far the most serious toxic side effect of the drug is its nephrotoxicity. This toxic side effect is particularly serious in a renal transplantation program, since it is often unclear whether the deterioration in renal function is due to insufficient drug, allowing for rejection to occur, or to too much cyclosporin A, causing nephrotoxicity.[162] Other toxic side effects include abnormalities of liver function tests, transient hirsutism, and gum hypertrophy. Bacterial infection has not been a problem with the use of this drug. However, reactivation of certain viral infections, particularly Epstein-Barr virus, have occurred sporadically. Of note is the fact that lymphomas have occurred in patients treated with cyclosporin A and were felt to result from the immunosuppressive effects rather than from any carcinogenicity of the drug.[162]

Of particular interest for the present discussion is the potential for the use of cyclosporin A in the treatment of rheumatic diseases characterized by hyper-reactivity or aberrant immune function at the T-lymphocyte level. Although no clinical trials have been performed with the use of cyclosporin A in rheumatic diseases, it is clear that the impressive immunosuppressive effects of this agent in the relative absence of myelosuppressive effects warrants at least consideration of the trial of this agent in certain selected immune-mediated connective tissue diseases.

Dapsone. Dapsone is a sulfone (4,4′-diaminodiphenyl sulfone) and first gained notoriety as an agent effective in the treatment of *Mycobacterium leprae*. Most recently it has been recognized as an effective agent in the treatment of dermatitis herpetiformis[172] and erythema elevatum diutinum[173] as well as the bullous eruptions of SLE.[174] Dapsone is available for oral administration and is slowly and nearly completely absorbed from the gastrointestinal tract. Peak concentrations of dapsone are reached in plasma 1 to 3 hours after oral administration, and its half-life ranges from 10 to 50 hours, with a mean of 28 hours.[175] Twenty-four hours after an oral dose of 100 mg, plasma concentrations range from 0.4 to 1.2 μg per ml. The sulfones are distributed throughout the total body water and are present in all tissues. They tend to be retained in skin, muscle, liver, and kidney, with traces of the drug present in these organs up to 3 weeks following cessation of administration. Dapsone is acetylated in the liver, and about 70 to 80 percent of a dose is excreted in the urine.

The mechanism of the bactericidal activity of dapsone is probably similar to the sulfonamides. However, the mechanisms whereby dapsone is effective in dermatitis herpetiformis and erythema elevatum diutinum and the bullous skin lesions of SLE are unclear at present. The common denominator of dermatitis herpetiformis and erythema elevatum diutinum is the infiltration of the lesions with neutrophils.[173] This has led investigators to put forth a number of hypotheses for mechanisms of effect, including blocking of complement deposition, which removes the chemotactic stimulus to neutrophils. However, other studies[176] have not substantiated these theories, and the mechanisms of action remain unknown in these diseases despite the dramatic clinical responses.

Given the fact that the underlying lesion in erythema elevatum diutinum is a leukocytoclastic vasculitis involving the postcapillary venules, it is conceivable that dapsone might be effective in other cutaneous vasculitis syndromes. However, there have been no prospective studies of the use of dapsone in other vasculitic syndromes, and anecdotal reports exist, but they are inconclusive.

The drug is administered orally in doses of 50 to 100 mg per day. The effect is seen within days, and particularly with erythema elevatum diutinum, relapses occur almost immediately after cessation of the drug,[173] which is somewhat paradoxical given the fact that the drug is present in organs for weeks after cessation of therapy. The sudden relapses following cessation might be explained by a need for a critical concentration of drug in plasma below which a dramatic deterioration in clinical condition is seen.

The limiting factor in the use of dapsone is its toxic side effects, which include hemolysis and methemoglobinemia and which occur relatively frequently. Other side effects include anorexia, nausea, and vomiting. Rarely, headache, nervousness, insomnia, and peripheral neuropathy have been reported.

Interferons. The interferons are relatively small glycoproteins that inhibit the multiplication of certain viruses. They first attracted significant attention because of their potential antiviral activities. They are elaborated from viral-infected cells and protect noninfected cells from viral infection.[177] They induce a transient state of refractoriness to viral infection by altering nucleotide metabolism and cytoplasmic enzyme induction.[177] However, it soon became clear that in addition to their antiviral properties, interferons had significant effects on cell differentiation, cell growth, the expression of surface antigens, cellular morphology, and most importantly for the purposes of this discussion, immunoregulation.[177,178]

The interferon nomenclature has recently been refined[179] and now includes the following three major types: (1) interferon alpha, which was previously known as classic interferon or leukocyte interferon, is pH 2 stable; (2) interferon beta, which was previously known as fibroblast interferon, is pH stable; and (3) interferon gamma, which was previously known as Type II or immune interferon, is produced by antigen-induced or mitogen-induced lymphocytes and is pH 2 labile.

In general, interferon gamma is much more potent in

Table 55–7. Effects of Interferon on Immune Function*

Humoral Immunity		Cellular Immunity	
Decreased	Increased	Decreased	Increased
IgE synthesis	Primary antibody response T-dependent and independent antigens	Antigenic, mitogenic, and allogeneic-stimulated proliferation	Allograft survival
Antibody response to T-dependent and independent antigens; affects both primary and secondary responses		Bone marrow cell growth Monocyte maturation in culture Delayed-type hypersensitivity Graft-versus-host disease in mice	Macrophage phagocytosis IgE-mediated histamine release in vitro Expression of surface antigens and Fc receptors T-cell mediated cytotoxicity Natural killer activity

*From Kotzin, B.L., Stroker, S., Engleman, E.G., et al.: Treatment of intractable rheumatoid arthritis with total lymphoid irradiation. N. Engl. J. Med. 305:969, 1981.

its immunoregulatory effects than are the other interferons. It should be pointed out that in the evaluation of the effects of interferon on the immune system, one must be aware of the fact that the type and degree of effect may be heavily dependent on the time and dose of interferon used in both in vivo and in vitro studies. A summary of the immunoregulatory effects of interferon is given in Table 55–7.[177]

Table 55–8. Pharmacologic Properties of Immunoregulatory Agents

Agent	Administration	Dosage	Gastrointestinal Absorption	Plasma Half Life	Major Side Effects
Cytotoxic Agents Nitrogen mustard	IV	0.4 mg/kg q. 3–4 weeks	—	Few minutes	Leukopenia, thrombocytopenia, nausea, vomiting, local reactions at injection site
Cyclophosphamide	IV or oral	2 mg/kg/day orally or IV; 750 mg/m² IV bolus	Excellent	6–7 hours	Neutropenia, gonadal suppression, cystitis, alopecia, oncogenesis, pulmonary fibrosis, gastrointestinal intolerance
Chlorambucil	IV or oral	0.1–0.2 mg/kg/day orally	Good	90 minutes	Leukopenia, thrombocytopenia, oncogenesis, gonadal suppression, gastrointestinal intolerance, hepatotoxicity, dermatitis
Azathioprine and 6-mercaptopurine	IV or oral	2 mg/kd/day orally	Excellent	60–90 minutes	Leukopenia, hepatotoxicity, gastrointestinal intolerance, oncogenesis, host defense defect
Methotrexate	IV or oral	5–50 mg per week as single IV dose or orally in 3 divided doses (q. 12 hours) or orally daily for 5 days of the week	Intermittent to Good	2 hours	Leukopenia, thrombocytopenia, oral mucositis, gastrointestinal intolerance, hepatotoxicity, fetal intolerance in first trimester of pregnancy
Vinca alkaloids (vincristine and vinblastine)	IV	2 mg/m²	—	Less than 30 minutes	Neurotoxicity

Table 55–8. Pharmacologic Properties of Immunoregulatory Agents *(continued)*

Agent	Administration	Dosage	Gastrointestinal Absorption	Plasma HalfLife	Major Side Effects
5-Fluorouracil	IV	12 mg/kg/day for 4 days followed by 6 mg/kg on alternate days for 2–4 doses; repeat monthly with adjustment of dose according to response	Unpredictable	10–20 minutes	Leukopenia, gastrointestinal intolerance, alopecia, dermatitis, mucositis
Hydroxyurea	IV or oral	20–30 mg/kg/day orally	Good	6–8 hours	Myelosuppression, gastrointestinal intolerance and ulcerations, mild skin rashes
Other Agents Levamisole	Oral	Up to 150 mg/day	Excellent	4 hours	Granulocytopenia, gastrointestinal intolerance, fever, skin rash, fatigue
Cyclosporin A	IV or oral	17 mg/kg/day with monthly tapering until maintenance dose of 6–8 mg/kg/day is reached	Fair to good	2–24 hours	Nephrotoxicity, hepatotoxicity, reactivation of viral infections, oncogenesis, transient hirsutism, gum hypertrophy
Dapsone	Oral	50–100 mg/day	Good	10–50 hours	Hemolysis, methemoglobinemia, gastrointestinal intolerance
Interferons (predominantly alpha)		Phase I trials in effect	—	Uncertain	Fever, nausea, vomiting, diarrhea, transient leukopenia, myocardial infarction, others to be determined

Administration of interferon alpha has been shown to be of some therapeutic value in herpes zoster infections, in patients with certain neoplasms, and in patients with hepatitis B infections.[177] Although there are no published controlled trials of the use of interferons in the treatment of non-neoplastic diseases such as the connective tissue diseases, their potent immunoregulatory capabilities may prove useful in attempts at manipulating the immune response in these diseases. However, it should be pointed out that the multifaceted effects of the interferons on the immune response renders the net effect unpredictable, and at this time, the use of these agents in the treatment of rheumatic diseases remains more hypothetical than practical. Perhaps when more purified preparations of interferons become available through gene cloning techniques, their effects will be more precisely delineated and trials can be undertaken. At this point, we can only say that the interferons, particularly interferon gamma, have potent immunoregulatory properties that may prove useful in the future

treatment of diseases characterized by abnormalities of immune function.

A summary of certain of the pharmacologic properties of several of the immunoregulatory agents discussed in this chapter is given in Table 55–8.

CONCLUSIONS

The use of cytotoxic and immunoregulatory agents has played a major role in the treatment of non-neoplastic, immune-mediated diseases. However, most of these agents are nonspecific and are invariably associated with a variety of toxic side effects. Since most of the rheumatic diseases in which these agents are used are chronic in nature and are rarely curable, the physician must establish the clear-cut goals of a given therapeutic regimen and must be aware of the actual as well as the potential and the immediate as well as the long-term toxic side effects of these agents. Insightful use of these agents under appropriate clinical circumstances can often lead to dramatic improvements in the clinical course as well as gratifying improvements in life style. Under other circumstances, the effects may even be life saving. However, use of these agents should be avoided in circumstances in which a less aggressive approach would be more appropriate given the nature of the illness and the projected balance between clinical results and toxic side effects. The treating physician should be acquainted as best as possible with the established results of controlled trials as they appear in the literature and should critically evaluate uncontrolled trials, which may indeed represent a true advance in therapy but which may also give a false sense of security that a particular agent will be beneficial. All things considered, sound clinical judgment applied to each individual patient with regard to the choice and actual usage of an immunoregulatory agent is indispensable.

References

1. Fauci, A.S.: Immunoregulation in autoimmunity. J. Allergy Clin. Immunol. 66:5, 1980.
2. NIAID Group: New Initiatives in Immunology. Report. Bethesda, Maryland, National Institute of Allergy and Infectious Diseases. DHHS Publication No. (NIH) 81-2215:1, 1981.
3. Paul, W.E.: Lymphocyte biology. In Parker, C.W. (ed.): Clinical Immunology. Vol. 1. Philadelphia, W. B. Saunders Company, 1980.
4. Fauci, A.S.: The revolution in clinical immunology. JAMA 246:2567, 1981.
5. Fauci, A.S., Lane, H.C., and Volkman, D.J.: Activation and regulation of human immune responses: Implications in normal and disease states. Ann. Intern. Med., 98:76, 1983.
6. Steinberg, A.D., Plotz, P.H., Wolff, S.M., Wong, V.G., Agus, S.G., and Decker, J.L.: Cytotoxic drugs in treatment of nonmalignant diseases. Ann. Intern. Med. 76:619, 1972.
7. Fauci, A.S., Dale, D.C., and Balow, J.E.: Glucocorticosteroid therapy: mechanisms of action and clinical considerations. Ann. Intern. Med. 84:304, 1976.
8. Gerber, N.L., and Steinberg, A.D.: Clinical use of immunosuppressive drugs. Part I. Drugs 11:36, 1976.
9. Gerber, N.L., and Steinberg, A.D.: Clinical use of immunosuppressive drugs. Part II. Drugs 11:90, 1976.
10. Calabresi, P., and Parks, R.E.: Antiproliferative agents and drugs used for immunosuppression. In Goodman, L.S., and Gilman A. (eds.): The Pharmacologic Basis of Therapeutics. 6th ed. New York, Macmillan, 1980.
11. Cooper, M.D., Peterson, R.D.A., and Good, R.A.: Delineation of the thymic and bursal lymphoid system in the chicken. Nature 205:143, 1965.
12. Cooper, M.D., Peterson, R.D.A., South, M.A., and Good, R.A.: The functions of the thymus system and the bursa system in the chicken. J. Exp. Med. 123:75, 1966.
13. Claman, H.N., Chaperon, E.A., and Triplett, R.F.: Thymus-marrow cell combinations. Synergism in antibody production. Proc. Soc. Exp. Biol. Med. 12:1167, 1966.
14. Miller, J.F.A.P., and Mitchell, G.F.: Cell-cell interactions in immune response. I. Hemolysin-forming cells in neonatally thymectomized mice reconstituted with thymus or thoracic duct lymphocytes. J. Exp. Med. 128:801, 1968.
15. Möller, G. (ed.): Role of macrophages in the immune response. Immunol. Rev. 40:1, 1978.
16. Möller, G. (ed.): Natural killer cells. Immunol. Rev. 44:1, 1979.
17. Herberman, R.B., and Ortaldo, J.R.: Natural killer cells: Their role in defenses against disease. Science 214:24 1981.
18. Gallin, J.I., and Fauci, A.S. (eds.): Advances in Host Defense Mechanisms. Vol. 1. New York, Raven Press, 1982.
19. Jerne, N.K.: Towards a network theory of the immune system. Ann. Immunol. (Inst. Pasteur) 125:373, 1974.
20. Möller, G. (ed.): Idiotypes on T and B cells. Immunol. Rev. 34:1, Copenhagen, Munksgaard, 1977.
21. Geha, R.S.: Presence of auto-anti-idiotypic antibody during the normal human immune response to tetanus toxoid antigen. J. Immunol. 129:139, 1982.
22. Abdou, N.I., Wall, H., Lindsley, H.B., Halsey, J.F., and Suzuki, T.: Network theory in autoimmunity. In vitro suppression of serum anti-DNA antibody binding to DNA by anti-idiotypic antibody in systemic lupus erythematosus. J. Clin. Invest. 67:1297, 1981.
23. Waldmann, T.A., and Broder, S.: Suppressor cells in the regulation of the immune response. In Schwartz, R.S. (ed.): Progress in Clinical Immunology. Vol. 3. New York, Grune and Stratton, 1977.
24. Fauci, A.S., Haynes, B.F., and Katz, P.: The spectrum of vasculitis: clinical, pathologic, immunologic, and therapeutic considerations. Ann. Intern. Med. 89:660, 1978.
25. Fauci, A.S., Haynes, B.F., Katz, P., and Wolff, S.M.: Wegener's granulomatosis: prospective clinical and therapeutic experience with 85 patients over 21 years. Ann. Intern. Med. 98:76, 1983.
26. Cupps, T.R., and Fauci, A.S.: The Vasculitides. In Smith, L.H. (ed.): Major Problems in Internal Medicine. Vol. XXL. Philadelphia, W. B. Saunders Company, 1981.
27. Cupps, T.R., Edgar, L.C., and Fauci, A.S.: Suppression of human B lymphocyte function by cyclophosphamide. J. Immunol. 128:2453, 1982.
28. Maguire, H.C., and Maibach, H.I.: Specific immune tolerance to anaphylactic sensitization (egg albumin) in the guinea pig by cyclophosphamide (cytoxan). J. Allergy 32:406, 1961.
29. Möller, G. (ed.): Suppressor T lymphocytes. Immunol. Rev. 26:1, 1975.
30. Fauci, A.S.: Assays for suppressor cells. In Rose, N.R., and Friedman, H. (eds.): Manual of Clinical Immunology. 2nd ed. Washington, D.C., Society for Microbiology, 1980.
31. Talal, N.: Tolerance and autoimmunity. In Parker, C.W. (ed.): Clinical Immunology. Vol. I. Philadelphia, W. B. Saunders Company, 1980.
32. Farrar, J.J., Benjamin, W.R., Hilfiker, M.L., Howard, M., Farrar, W.L., and Fuller-Farrar, J.: The biochemistry, biology, and role of interleukin 2 in the induction of cytotoxic T cell and antibody-forming B cell responses. Immunol. Rev. 63:129, 1982.
33. Fauci, A.S.: Clinical aspects of immunosuppression: use of cytotoxic agents and corticosteroids. In Bellanti, J.A. (ed.): Immunology II. Philadelphia, W. B. Saunders Company, 1978.
34. Fauci, A.S., Katz, P., Haynes, B.F., and Wolff, S.M.: Cyclophosphamide therapy of severe necrotizing vasculitis. N. Engl. J. Med. 301:235, 1979.
35. Decker, J.L.: Toxicity of immunosuppressive drugs in man. Arthritis Rheum. 16:89, 1973.
36. Schein, P.S., and Winokur, S.T.: Immunosuppressive and cytotoxic chemotherapy: long-term complications. Ann. Intern. Med. 82:84, 1975.
37. Calabresi, P., and Parks, R.E.: Chemotherapy of neoplastic diseases. In Goodman, L.S., and Gilman, A. (eds.): The Pharmacologic Basis of Therapeutics. 6th ed. New York, Macmillan, 1980.
38. Ahn, Y.S., Harrington, W.J., Seelman, R.C., and Eytel, C.S.: Vincristine therapy of idiopathic and secondary thrombocytopenias. N. Engl. J. Med. 291:376, 1974.
39. Fauci, A.S., Harley, J.B., Roberts, W.C., Ferrans, V.J., Gralnick, H.R., and Bjornson, B.J.: The idiopathic hypereosinophilic syndrome: clinical, pathologic and therapeutic considerations. Ann. Intern. Med. 97:78, 1982.
40. Roberts, J.J., Brent, T.P., and Crathorn, A.R.: Evidence for the inactivation and repair of the mammalian DNA template after alkylation by mustard gas and half mustard gas. Eur. J. Cancer 7:515, 1971.
41. Fahey, J.L., Leonard, E., Churg, J., and Godman, G.: Wegener's granulomatosis. Am. J. Med. 17:168, 1954.
42. Brock, N.: Pharmacologic characterization of cyclophosphamide (NSC-26271) and cyclophosphamide metabolites. Cancer Chemother. Rep. 51:315, 1967.
43. Bagley, C.M., Bostick, F.W., and DeVita, V.T., Jr.: Clinical pharmacology of cyclophosphamide. Cancer Res. 33:226, 1973.
44. Gershwin, M.E., Goetzel, E.J., and Steinberg, A.D.: Cyclophosphamide: use in practice. Ann. Intern. Med. 80:531, 1974.
45. Sladek, N.E.: Therapeutic efficacy of cyclophosphamide as a function of its metabolism. Cancer Res. 32:535, 1972.
46. Makinodan, T., Santos, G.W., and Quinn, R.P.: Immunosuppressive drugs. Pharmacological Rev. 22:189, 1970.
47. Shand, F.L.: The immunopharmacology of cyclophosphamide. Int. J. Pharmacol. 1:165, 1979.
48. Berenbaum, M.C., and Brown, I.N.: Dose-response relationships for agents inhibiting the immune response. Immunology 7:65, 1964.
49. Askenase, P.W., Hayden, B.J., and Gershon, R.K.: Augmentation of delayed-type hypersensitivity of doses of cyclophosphamide which do not effect antibody responses. J. Exp. Med. 141:697, 1975.
50. Sy, M.S., Miller, S.D., and Claman, H.N.: Immune suppression with supraoptimal doses of antigen in contact sensitivity. I. Demonstration of suppressor cells and their sensitivity to cyclophosphamide. J. Immunol. 119:240, 1977.
51. Fauci, A.S., Wolff, S.M., and Johnson, J.S.: Effect of cyclophosphamide

upon the immune response in Wegener's granulomatosis. N. Engl. J. Med. 285:1493, 1971.

52. Fauci, A.S., Dale, D.C., and Wolff, S.M.: Cyclophosphamide and lymphocyte subpopulations in Wegener's granulomatosis. Arthritis Rheum. 17:355, 1974.

53. Hurd, E.R., and Giuliano, V.J.: The effect of cyclophosphamide on B and T lymphocytes in patients with connective tissue diseases. Arthritis Rheum. 18:67, 1975.

54. Dale, D.C., Fauci, A.S., and Wolff, S.M.: The effect of cyclophosphamide on leukocyte kinetics and susceptibility to infection in patients with Wegener's granulomatosis. Arthritis Rheum. 16:657, 1973.

55. Warne, G.L., Fairley, K.F., Hobbs, J.B., and Martin, F.I.R.: Cyclophosphamide-induced ovarian failure. N. Engl. J. Med. 289:1159, 1973.

56. Schilsky, R.L., Lewis, B.J., Sherins, R.J., and Young, R.C.: Gonadal dysfunction in patients receiving chemotherapy for cancer. Ann. Intern. Med. 93:109, 1980.

57. Trompeter, R.S., Evans, P.R., and Barratt, T.M.: Gonadal function in boys with steroid-responsive nephrotic syndrome treated with cyclophosphamide for short periods. Lancet 1:1177, 1981.

58. Fairley, K.F., Barrie, J.U., and Johnson, W.: Sterility and testicular atrophy related to cyclophosphamide therapy. Lancet 1:568, 1972.

59. Plotz, P.H., Klippel, J.H., Decker, J.L., et al.: Bladder complications in patients receiving cyclophosphamide for systemic lupus erythematosus or rheumatoid arthritis. Ann. Intern. Med. 91:221, 1979.

60. Weiss, R.B., and Maggia, F.M.: Cytotoxic drug-induced pulmonary disease: update 1980. Am. J. Med. 68:259, 1980.

61. Appelbaum, F.R., Strauchen, J.A., Graw, R.G., Jr., et al.: Acute lethal carditis caused by high-dose combination chemotherapy. A unique clinical and pathological entity. Lancet 1:58, 1976.

62. De Fronzo, R.A., Braine, H., Colvin, O.M., and Davis, P.J.: Water intoxication in man after cyclophosphamide therapy. Time course and relation to drug activation. Ann. Intern. Med. 78:861, 1973.

63. Penn, I.: Depressed immunity and the development of cancer. Clin. Exp. Immunol. 46:459, 1981.

64. McLean, A., Newell, D., and Baker, G.: The metabolism of chlorambucil. Biochem. Pharmacol. 25:2331, 1976.

65. Stukov, A.N.: Experimental study of the combined effect of leukoran, degranol, and prednisolone. Neoplasma 22:181, 1976.

66. Israel, H., and Patchefsky, A.S.: Treatment of Wegener's granulomatosis of lung. Am. J. Med. 58:671, 1975.

67. Rudd, P., Fried, J.F., and Epstein, W.V.: Irreversible bone marrow failure with chlorambucil. J. Rheumatol. 2:421, 1975.

68. Cameron, S.: Chlorambucil and leukemia. N. Engl. J. Med. 296:1065, 1977.

69. Lerner, H.J.: Acute myelogenous leukemia in patients receiving chlorambucil as long-term adjuvant chemotherapy for Stage II breast cancer. Cancer Treat. Rep. 60:1431, 1978.

70. Gabrielsen, A.E., and Good, R.A.: Chemical suppression of adaptive immunity. Adv. Immunol. 6:91, 1967.

71. Yu, D.T., Clements, P.J., Peter, J.B., Levy, J., Paulus, H.E., and Barnett, E.V.: Lymphocyte characteristics in rheumatic patients and the effect of azathioprine therapy. Arthritis Rheum. 17:37, 1974.

72. Levy, J., Barnett, E.V., MacDonald, N.S., Klinenberg, J.R., and Pearson, C.M.: The effect of azathioprine on gammaglobulin synthesis in man. J. Clin. Invest. 51:2233, 1972.

73. Maibach, H.I., and Epstein, W.L.: Immunologic responses of healthy volunteers receiving azathioprine (Imuran). Int. Arch. Allergy 27:102, 1965.

74. Abdou, N.I., Zweiman, B., and Casella, S.R.: Effects of azathioprine therapy on bone marrow-dependent and thymus-dependent cells in man. Clin. Exp. Immunol. 13:55, 1973.

75. Fournier, C., Bach, M.A., Dardenne, M., and Bach, J.F.: Selective action of azathioprine on T cells. Transplantation Proc. 5:523, 1973.

76. Campbell, A.C., Skinner, J.M., Hersey, P., Roberts-Thompson, P., MacLennan, I.C.M., and Truelove, S.C.: Immunosuppression in the treatment of inflammatory bowel disease. I. Changes in lymphoid subpopulations in the blood and rectal mucosa following cessation of treatment with azathioprine. Clin. Exp. Immunol. 16:521, 1974.

77. Sharbaugh, R.J., Ainsworth, S.K., and Fitts, C.T.: Lack of effect of azathioprine on phytohemagglutinin-induced lymphocyte transformation and established delayed cutaneous hypersensitivity. Int. Arch. Allergy Applied Immunol. 51:681, 1976.

78. Gassman, A.E., and van Furth, R.: The effect of azathioprine (Imuran) on the kinetics of monocytes and macrophages during the normal steady state and an acute inflammatory reaction. Blood 46:51, 1975.

79. Phillips, S.M., and Zweiman, B.: Mechanisms in the suppression of delayed hypersensitivity in the guinea pig by 6-mercaptopurine. J. Exp. Med. 137:1494, 1973.

80. Rosman, M., and Bertino, J.R.: Azathioprine. Ann. Intern. Med. 79:694, 1973.

81. Losito, A., Williams, D.G., and Harris, L.: The effects on polymorphonuclear leukocyte function of prednisolone and azathioprine in vivo and prednisolone, azathioprine and 6-mercaptopurine in vitro. Clin. Exp. Immunol. 32:423, 1978.

82. Henderson, F.S., Adamson, R.H., and Oliverio, V.T.: The metabolic rate of tritiated methotrexate. II. Absorption and excretion in man. Cancer Res. 25:1018, 1965.

83. Hersh, E.M., Carbone, P.P., Wong, V.G., and Freireich, E.J.: Inhibition of the primary immune response in man by antimetabolites. Cancer Res. 25:997, 1965.

84. Hersh, E.M., Carbone, P.P., and Freireich, E.J.: Recovery of immune responsiveness after drug suppression in man. J. Lab. Clin. Med. 67:566, 1965.

85. Mitchell, M.S., Wade, M.E., DeConti, R.C., Bertino, J.R., and Calabresi, P.: Immunosuppressive effects of cytosine arabinoside and methotrexate in man. Ann. Intern. Med. 70:535, 1969.

86. Ahn, Y.S., Byrnes, J.J., Harrington, W.J., et al.: The treatment of idiopathic thrombocytopenia with vinblastine-loaded platelets. N. Engl. J. Med. 298:1101, 1978.

87. Fauci, A.S., Harley, J.B., Roberts, W.C., Ferrans, V.J., Gralnick, H.R., and Bjornson, B.H.: The idiopathic hypereosinophilic syndrome. Clinical, pathophysiologic, and therapeutic considerations. Ann. Intern. Med. 97:78, 1982.

88. Cupps, T.R., Silverman, G.J., and Fauci, A.S.: Herpes zoster in patients with treated Wegener's granulomatosis. A possible role for cyclophosphamide. Am. J. Med. 69:881, 1980.

89. Tindall, R.S.A. (ed.): Therapeutic Apheresis and Plasma Perfusion. New York, A. R. Liss, Inc., 1980.

90. Branda, R.F., Molodow, C.F., McCollough, J.J., and Jacob, H.S.: Plasma exchange in the treatment of immune disease. Transfusion 5:570, 1975.

91. Lockwood, C.M., Pearson, T.A., Rees, A.J., Evans, D.J., Peters, D.K., and Wilson, C.B.: Immunosuppression and plasma exchange in the treatment of Goodpasture's syndrome. Lancet 1:711, 1976.

92. Pinching, A.J., Peters, D.K., and Newsom Davis, J.: Remission of myasthenia gravis following plasma-exchange. Lancet 2:1373, 1976.

93. Vogler, W.R.: Therapeutic apheresis: Where we've been and where we are going. In Tindall, R.S.A. (ed.): Therapeutic Apheresis and Plasma Perfusion. New York, A. R. Liss, Inc., 1980.

94. Wallace, D.J., Goldfinger, D., Gatti, et al.: Plasmapheresis and lymphoplasmapheresis in the management of rheumatoid arthritis. Arthritis Rheum. 22:703, 1979.

95. Balow, J.E., and Tsokos, G.C.: Plasmapheresis in systemis lupus erythematosus: facts and perspectives. Int. J. Artif. Organs 5:286, 1982.

96. Lockwood, C.M., Worlledge, S., Nicholas, A., Cotton, D., and Peters, D.K.: Reversal of impaired splenic function in patients with nephritis or vasculitis (or both) by plasma exchange. N. Engl. J. Med. 300:524, 1979.

97. Kauffmann, R.H., and Houwert, D.A.: Plasmapheresis in rapidly progressive Henoch-Schoenlein glomerulonephritis and the effect on circulating IgA immune complexes. Clin. Nephrol. 16:155, 1981.

98. Karsh, J., Klippel, J.H., Plotz, P.H., Decker, J.L., Wright, D.G., and Flye, M.W.: Lymphapheresis in rheumatoid arthritis. A randomized trial. Arthritis Rheum. 24:867, 1981.

99. Wallace, D., Goldfinger, D., Lowe, C., et al.: A double-blind controlled study of lymphoplasmapheresis versus sham apheresis in rheumatoid arthritis. N. Engl. J. Med. 306:1406, 1982.

100. Terman, D.S., Young, J.B., Shearer, W.T., et al.: Preliminary observations of the effects on breast adenocarcinoma of plasma perfused over immobilized protein A. N. Engl. J. Med. 305:1195, 1981.

101. Saal, S.D., and Gordon, B.R.: Extracorporeal modification of plasma and whole blood. In Tindall, R.S.A. (ed.): Therapeutic Apheresis and Plasma Perfusion. New York, A. R. Liss, Inc., 1980.

102. Pineda, A.A.: Methods for selective removal of plasma constituents. In Tindall, R.S.A. (ed.): Therapeutic Apheresis and Plasma Perfusion. New York, A. R. Liss, Inc., 1980.

103. Hamburger, M.I., Lawley, T.J., Kimberly, R.P., Plotz, P.H., and Frank, M.M.: A serial study of splenic reticuloendothelial system Fc receptor functional activity in systemic lupus erythematosus. Arthritis Rheum. 25:48, 1982.

104. Steven, M.M., Tanner, A.R., Holdstock, T.J., and Wright, R.: Effect of plasma exchange on the in vitro monocyte function of patients with immune complex diseases. Clin. Exp. Immunol. 45:240, 1981.

105. Lockwood, C.M., Rees, A.J., Pearson, T.A., Evans, D.J., Peters, D.K., and Wilson, C.B.: Immunosuppression and plasma exchange in the treatment of Goodpasture's syndrome. Lancet 1:711, 1976.

106. Flaum, M.A., Cuneo, R.A., Appelbaum, F.A., Deisseroth, A.B., Engel, W.K., and Gralnick, H.R.: The hemostatic imbalance of plasma-exchange transfusion. Blood 54:694, 1979.

107. Orlin, J.B., and Berkman, E.M.: Partial plasma exchange using albumin replacement: removal and recovery of normal constituents. Blood 56:1055, 1980.

108. Wright, D.G., Karsh, J., Fauci, A.S., et al.: Lymphocyte depletion and immunosuppression with repeated leukapheresis by continuous flow centrifugation. Blood 58:451, 1981.

109. Machleder, H.I., and Paulus, H.: Clinical and immunological alterations observed in patients undergoing long-term thoracic duct drainage. Surgery 84:157, 1978.

110. Paulus, H.E., Machleder, H.I., Levine, S., Yu, D.T.Y., and Macdonald, N.S.: Lymphocyte involvement in rheumatoid arthritis. Studies during thoracic duct drainage. Arthritis Rheum. 20:1249, 1977.

111. Hutchinson, F.: The molecular basis for radiation effects on cells. Cancer Res. 26:2045, 1966.

112. Anderson, R.E., and Warner, N.L.: Ionizing radiation and the immune response. Adv. Immunol. 24:215, 1976.

113. Fauci, A.S., Pratt, K.R., and Whalen, G.: Activation of human B lymphocytes. VIII. Differential radiosensitivity of subpopulations of lymphoid cells involved in the polyclonally induced PFC responses of peripheral blood B lymphocytes. Immunology 35:715, 1978.

114. Kaplan, H.S.: Hodgkin's Disease. 2nd ed. Cambridge, Harvard University Press, 1980.

115. Hellman, S., Mauch, P., Goodman, R.L., Rosenthal, D.S., and Moloney, W.C.: The place of radiation therapy in the treatment of Hodgkin's disease. Cancer 42:971, 1978.

116. Fuks, Z., Strober, S., Bobrove, A.M., Sasazuki, T., McMichael, A., and Kaplan, H.S.: Long-term effects of radiation on T and B lymphocytes in peripheral blood of patients with Hodgkin's disease. J. Clin. Invest. 58:803, 1976.

117. Kotzin, B.L., Strober, S., Engleman, E.G., et al.: Treatment of intractable rheumatoid arthritis with total lymphoid irradiation. N. Engl. J. Med. 305:969, 1981.

118. Trentham, D.E., Belli, J.A., Anderson, R.J., et al.: Clinical and immunologic effects of fractionated total lymphoid irradiation in refractory rheumatoid arthritis. N. Engl. J. Med. 305:976, 1981.

119. Strober, S., Slavin, S., Gottlieb, M., et al.: Allograft tolerance after total lymphoid irradiation (TLI). Immunol. Rev. 46:87, 1979.

120. Taub, R.N., and Deutsch, V.: Antilymphocytic serum. Pharmacol. Ther. 2:89, 1977.

121. Harris, N.S., Merino, G., and Najarian, J.S.: Mode of action of antilymphocyte sera (ALS). Transplant. Proc. 3:797, 1971.

122. Starzl, T.E., Marchioro, T.L., Hutchinson, D.E., Porter, K.A., Cerilli, G.J., and Brettschneider, L.: The clinical use of antilymphocyte globulin in renal homotransplantation. Transplant. Suppl. 5:1100, 1967.

123. Sheil, A.G.R., Mears, D., Kelly, G.E., et al.: Controlled clinical trial of antilymphocyte globulin in patients with renal allografts from cadaver donors. Lancet 1:359, 1971.

124. Köhler, G., and Milstein, C.: Continuous cultures of fused cells secreting antibody of predefined specificity. Nature 256:495, 1975.

125. Kennett, R.H., McKearn, T.J., and Bechtol, K.B. (eds.): Monoclonal Antibodies. Hybridomas: A New Dimension in Biological Analyses. New York, Plenum Press, 1980.

126. Miller, R.A., and Levy, R.: Response of cutaneous T cell lymphoma to therapy with hybridoma monoclonal antibody. Lancet 2:226, 1981.

127. Miller, R.A., Malone, D.G., Warnke, R., and Levy, R.: Treatment of B-cell lymphoma with monoclonal anti-idiotype antibody. N. Engl. J. Med. 306:517, 1982.

128. Ritz, J., Sallan, S.E., Bast, R.C., Jr., et al.: Autologous bone-marrow transplantation in CALLA-positive acute lymphoblastic leukaemia after in vitro treatment with J5 monoclonal antibody and complement. Lancet 2:60, 1982.

129. Prentice, H.G., Blacklock, H.A., Janossy, G., et al.: Use of anti-T cell monoclonal antibody OKT3 to prevent acute graft-versus-host disease in allogeneic bone-marrow transplantation for acute leukemia. Lancet 1:700, 1982.

130. Filipovich, A.H., McGlave, P.B., Ramsay, N.K.C., Goldstein, G., Warkentin, P.I., and Kersey, J.H.: Pretreatment of donor bone marrow with monoclonal antibody OKT3 for prevention of acute graft-versus-host disease in allogeneic histocompatible bone marrow transplantation. Lancet 1:1266, 1982.

131. Reinherz, E., Geha, R., Rappeport, J.M., et al.: Reconstitution after transplantation with T-lymphocyte-depleted HLA haplotype-mismatched bone marrow for severe combined immunodeficiency. Proc. Natl. Acad. Sci. USA 79:6047, 1982.

132. Steinman, L., Rosenbaum, J.T., Sriram, S., and McDevitt, H.O.: In vivo effects of antibodies to immune response gene products: prevention of experimental allergic encephalitis. Proc. Natl. Acad. Sci. USA 78:7111, 1981.

133. Barkas, T., and Simpson, J.A.: Lack of inter-animal cross-reaction of anti-acetylcholine receptor antibodies at the receptor-binding site as demonstrated by heterologous anti-idiotype antisera: implications for immunotherapy of myasthenia gravis. Clin. Exp. Immunol. 47:119, 1982.

134. Cupps, T.R., and Fauci, A.S.: Corticosteroid-mediated immunoregulation in man. Immunol. Rev. 65:133, 1982.

135. Fauci, A.S., and Dale, D.C.: The effect of in vivo hydrocortisone on subpopulations of human lymphocytes. J. Clin. Invest. 53:240, 1974.

136. Haynes, B.F., and Fauci, A.S.: The differential effect of in vivo hydro-cortisone on kinetics of subpopulations of human peripheral blood thymus-derived lymphocytes. J. Clin. Invest. 61:703, 1978.

137. Eidenger, D., and Garrett, T.J.: Studies of the regulatory effects of sex hormones on antibody formation and stem cell differentiation. J. Exp. Med. 136:1098, 1972.

138. Steinberg, A.D., Klassen, L.W., Raveche, E.S., et al.: Study of the multiple factors in the pathogenesis of autoimmunity in New Zealand mice. Arthritis Rheum. 21:2190, 1978.

139. Wyle, F.A., and Kent, J.R.: Immunosuppression by sex steroid hormones. I. The effect upon PHA and PPD stimulated lymphocytes. Clin. Exp. Immunol. 27:407, 1976.

140. Roubinian, J.R., Papoian, R., and Talal, N.: Androgenic hormones modulate autoantibody responses and improve survival in murine lupus. J. Clin. Invest. 59:1066, 1977.

141. Melez, K., Reeves, P., and Steinberg, A.D.: Modification of NZB/NZW disease by sex hormones. J. Immunopharmacol. 1:27, 1978.

142. Roubinian, J.R., Talal, N., Greenspan, J.S., Goodman, J.R., and Sitteri, P.K.: Effect of castration and sex hormone treatment on survival, antinucleic acid antibodies and glomerulonephritis in NZB/NZW F¹ mice. J. Exp. Med. 147:1568, 1978.

143. Sheffer, A.L., Fearon, D.T., and Austen, K.F.: Methyltestosterone therapy in hereditary angioedema. Ann. Intern. Med. 53:199, 1977.

144. Gelfand, J.A., Sherrins, R.J., Alling, D.W., and Frank, M.M.: Treatment of hereditary angioedema with Danazole. Reversal of clinical and biochemical abnormalities. N. Engl. J. Med. 295:1444, 1976.

145. Stevenson, H.C., and Fauci, A.S.: The effect of glucocorticosteroids and other hormones on inflammatory and immune responses. In Oppenhiem, J.J., Rosenstreich, D.L., and Potter, M. (eds.): Cellular Functions in Immunity and Inflammation. New York, Elsevier/North Holland, 1981.

146. Symoens, J., and Rosenthal, M.: Levamisole in the modulation of the immune response: the current experimental and clinical state. J. Reticuloendothel. Soc. 21:175, 1977.

147. Snyderman, R., and Pike, M.C.: Pathophysiologic aspects of leukocyte chemotaxis: identification of a specific chemotactic factor binding site on human granulocytes and defects of macrophage function associated with neoplasia. In Gallin, J.I., and Quie, P.G. (eds.): Leukocyte Chemotaxis: Methods, Physiology, and Clinical Implications. New York, Raven Press, 1978.

148. Rabson, A.R., Whiting, D.A., Anderson, R., Glover, A., Koornhof, H.J.: Depressed neutrophil motility in patients with recurrent herpes simplex virus infections: In vitro restoration with levamisole. J. Infect. Dis. 135:113, 1977.

149. Wright, D.G., Kirkpatrick, C.H., and Gallin, J.I.: Effects of levamisole on normal and abnormal leukocyte locomotion. J. Clin. Invest. 59:941, 1977.

150. Hogan, N.A., and Hill, H.R.: Enhancement of neutrophil chemotaxis and alteration of levels of cellular cyclic nucleotides by levamisole. J. Infect. Dis. 138:437, 1978.

151. Donabedian, H., Alling, D.W., and Gallin, J.I.: Levamisole is inferior to placebo in the hyperimmunoglobulin E recurrent-infection (Job's) syndrome. N. Engl. J. Med. 307:290, 1982.

152. Tripodi, D., Parks, L.C., and Brugmans, J.: Drug-induced restoration of cutaneous delayed hypersensitivity in anergic patients with cancer. N. Engl. J. Med. 289:354, 1973.

153. Sampson, D., and Lui, A.: The effect of levamisole on cell-mediated immunity and suppressor cell function. Cancer Res. 36:952, 1976.

154. Rosenthal, M., Trabert, U., and Mueller, W.: The effect of levamisole on peripheral blood lymphocyte subpopulations in patients with rheumatoid arthritis and ankylosing spondylitis. Clin. Exp. Immunol. 25:493, 1976.

155. Miller, B., DeMerieux, P., Srinivasan, R., et al.: Double-blind placebo controlled crossover evaluation of levamisole in rheumatoid arthritis. Arthritis Rheum. 23:172, 1980.

156. Runge, L.A., Pinals, R.S., Lourie, S.H., and Tomar, R.H.: Treatment of rheumatoid arthritis with levamisole. A controlled trial. Arthritis Rheum. 20:1445, 1977.

157. Schmidt, K.L., and Mueller-Eckhardt, C.: Agranulocytosis, levamisole, and HLA-B 27. Lancet 2:85, 1977.

158. Veys, E.M., Mielants, H., and Verbruggen, G.: Levamisole-induced adverse reactions in HLA-B27-positive rheumatoid arthritis. Lancet 1:148, 1978.

159. Freund, J.: Some aspects of active immunization. Ann. Rev. Microbiol. 1:291, 1947.

160. Chedid, L., Audibert, F., LeFrancier, P., Chory, J., and Lederer, E.: Modulation of the immune response by a synthetic adjuvant and analogs. Proc. Natl. Acad. Sci. USA 73:2472, 1976.

161. Borel, J.F., Feurer, C., Gubler, H.U., and Stahelin, H.: Biological effects of cyclosporin A: A new antilymphocytic agent. Agents Actions 6:468, 1976.

162. White, D.J.G., and Calne, R.Y.: The use of cyclosporin A immunosuppression in organ grafting. Immunol. Rev. 65:115, 1982.

163. Preliminary results of a European trial: Cyclosporin A as a sole immunosuppressive agent in recipients of kidney allografts from cadaver donors. Lancet 2:57, 1982.

164. Starzl, T.E., Klintmalm, G.B.G., Weil, R., III, et al.: Cyclosporin A and steroid therapy in sixty-six cadaver kidney recipients. Surg. Gynecol. Obstet. 153:486, 1981.

165. Larsson, E.L.: Cyclosporin A and dexamethasone suppress T cell responses by selectively acting at distant sites of the triggering process. J. Immunol. 124:2828, 1980.

166. Cammisuli, S.: Inhibition of a secondary humoral immune response by cyclosporin A. Transplant. Clin. Immunol. 13:15, 1981.

167. Horsburgh, T., Wood, P., and Brent, L.: Suppression of in vitro lymphocyte reactivity by cyclosporin A. Existence of a population of drug-resistant cytotoxic lymphocytes. Nature 286:609, 1980.

168. Palacios, R.: Cyclosporin A inhibits the proliferative response and the generation of helper, suppressor and cytotoxic T cell functions in the autologous mixed lymphocyte reaction. Cell. Immunol. 61:453, 1981.

169. Palacios, R., and Möller, G.: T-cell growth factor abrogates concanavalin A induced suppressor cell function. J. Exp. Med. 153:1360, 1981.

170. Kunkel, A., and Klaus, G.G.B.: Selective effects of cyclosporin A on functional B cell subsets in the mouse. J. Immunol. 125:2526, 1980.

171. Powles, R.L., Clink, H.M., Spence, D., et al.: Cyclosporin A to prevent graft-versus-host disease in man after allogenic bone-marrow transplantation. Lancet 1:327, 1980.

172. Katz, S.I., Hall, R.P., Lawley, T.J., and Strober, W.: Dermatitis herpetiformis: The skin and the gut. Ann. Intern. Med. 93:857, 1980.

173. Katz, S.I., Gallin, J.I., Hertz, K.C., Fauci, A.S., and Lawley, T.J.: Erythema elevatum diutinum: skin and systemic manifestations, immunologic studies and successful treatment with dapsone. Medicine 56:443, 1977.

174. Hall, R.P., Lawley, T.J., Smith, H.R., and Katz, S.I.: Bullous eruption of systemic lupus erythematosus. Ann. Intern. Med. 97:165, 1982.

175. Mandell, G.L., and Sande, M.A.: Antimicrobial agents. Drugs used in the chemotherapy of tuberculosis and leprosy. *In* Goodman Gilman, A., Goodman, L.S., and Giulman, A. (eds.): The Pharmacologic Basis of Therapeutics. 6th ed. New York. Macmillan, 1980.

176. Katz, S.I., Hertz, K.C., Crawford, P.S., Gazze, L.A., Frank, M.M., and Lawley, T.J.: Effect of sulfones on complement deposition in dermatitis herpetiformis and on complement-mediated guinea pig reactions. J. Invest. Dermatol. 67:688, 1976.

177. Stiehm, E.R., Kronenberg, L.H., Rosenblatt, H.M., Bryson, Y., and Merigan, T.C.: Interferon: immunobiology and clinical significance. Ann. Intern. Med. 96:80, 1982.

178. Bloom, B.R.: Interferons and the immune system. Nature 284:593, 1980.

179. Steward, W.E. II, Blalock, J.E., Burke, D.C., et al.: Interferon nomenclature. J. Immunol. 125:2353, 1980.

Chapter 56

Antihyperuricemic Drugs

William N. Kelley and Edward W. Holmes

A large number of drugs are capable of reducing the serum urate concentration in hyperuricemic subjects. These antihyperuricemic agents may be classified into one of several general categories: those that enhance uric acid excretion and those that inhibit xanthine oxidase and thus uric acid synthesis.

URICOSURIC DRUGS

Many drugs with diverse chemical structures and pharmacologic properties decrease the serum urate concentration in man by enhancing the renal excretion of uric acid.[1-43] These compounds are listed in Table 56–1. At present, probenecid (Fig. 56–1) and sulfinpyrazone (Fig. 56–2) are most widely employed for this purpose in the United States. In Europe benzbromarone and zoxazolamine are used as well; the former agent may be available in the United States in the future.

Mechanism of Action. The uricosuric effect of a drug could be due to an increase in the quantity of urate filtered at the glomerulus, an inhibition of reabsorption of urate in the tubule, or an enhancement of its secretion by the tubule (see Chapter 21).

Effect on Urate Filtration. Drugs could increase the quantity of urate filtered by raising the glomerular filtration rate, the plasma concentration of free urate, or both. The former mechanism has not been demonstrated, but the latter may apply in some situations.[44-46] Several agents with uricosuric effects in man,

including sulfinpyrazone, probenecid, salicylates, phenylbutazone, sulfaethylthiadiazole, diflumidone, W 2354, and halofenate, have been shown to reduce the binding of urate to albumin in vitro.[18,44,45] Displacement of urate from plasma proteins in vivo could theoretically increase the filtered load of free urate and thus could account for at least part of the uricosuric effect of these drugs.

Table 56–1. Drugs Shown to Be Uricosuric in Man

Acetoheximide[1]*	Halofenate (MK 185)[25]
ACTH[2]	Iodopyracet[26,27]
Ascorbic acid[3]	Iopanoic acid[11,12]
Azapropazone[4]	Meclofenamic acid[28]
Azauridine[5]	Meglumine iodipamide[11]
Benzbromarone[6,7]	Mersalyl[29]
Benziodarone[8,9]	Metiazininic acid[30]
Calcitonin[10]	Niridazole[31,32]
Calcium ipodate[11,12]	Orotic acid[5]
Carinamide[13]	Outdated tetracyclines[33]
Chlorprothixene[14]	Phenolsulfonphthalein[26]
Cinchophen[15]	Phenylbutazone[34]
Citrate[16]	Phenylindandione[20]
Dicumarol[17]	Phenoxyisobutyric acid[35]
Diflumidone[18]	Probenecid and metabolites[36,37]
Estrogens[19]	Salicylates[38]
Ethyl biscoumacetate[20]	Sodium diatrizoate[12]
Ethyl p-chlorophenoxyiso- butyric acid[21]	Sulfaethylthiadiazole[18]
Glyceryl guaiacholate[22]	Sulfinpyrazone[39]
Glycine[23]	Ticrynafen[24,40,41]
Glycopyrrolate[24]	W 2354 (5-chlorosalicylic acid)[18]
	Zoxazolamine[43]

*Superscript numbers indicate references.

Figure 56–1. Structure of probenecid.

While there is indirect evidence that salicylates could displace bound urate in vivo,[47] the amount of urate actually bound to plasma proteins in vivo appears to be negligible.[48] Thus, any effect of drugs on the quantity of urate filtered, based on displacement from plasma proteins, must also probably be small.

Effect on Uric Acid Reabsorption. The uricosuric effect of most agents studied, including probenecid[49] and sulfinpyrazone,[49] has been attributed to inhibition of the tubular reabsorption of filtered urate. With several exceptions, drugs with a significant uricosuric effect in man[49] are, like uric acid itself, weak organic acids. Since tubular reabsorption of uric acid is thought to occur by a process common to many organic acids, it has been assumed that these drugs inhibit this process in a competitive manner. Steele and Rieselbach[50] have postulated two types of urate reabsorptive sites in the proximal tubule, only one of which is sensitive to inhibition by probenecid.[51] Probenecid secretion is required for its uricosuric effect.[52] This and other evidence[53] have suggested that probenecid and probably most other uricosuric agents inhibit reabsorption at a site in the nephron distal to the site responsible for secretion of organic acids such as uric acid and probenecid. The suggestion is that of the two reabsorptive sites that exist for uric acid, one is proximal to and the other is distal to uric acid secretion; only the latter is inhibited by probenecid.

Five drugs that are not organic acids have been shown to have uricosuric effects in man. Studies with two of these agents, outdated tetracycline[33] and chlorprothix-

Figure 56–2. Structure of sulfinpyrazone.

ene,[54] suggest that they may inhibit the reabsorption of uric acid in the proximal tubule in a nonspecific manner that also affects the reabsorption of other compounds in this segment of the nephron. Glycopyrrolate may exert its uricosuric effect by virtue of its anticholinergic properties.[24] The mechanisms of action of zoxazolamine and niridazole, the final agents in this group, have not been established.

Effect on Uric Acid Secretion. The uricosuric effects of several drugs, including glycine,[23] benziodarone,[55] azapropazone,[3] and the radiographic contrast agents,[12] have been attributed to enhanced tubular secretion of urate. This hypothesis was based on the finding that prior administration of pyrazinamide (PZA) partially or completely blocked the uricosuric effects of these drugs. At the time these studies were done, urate secretion was thought to occur beyond all urate reabsorptive sites in the proximal renal tubules. With the recognition that substantial reabsorption of uric acid also occurs at a postsecretory site,[53] it became clear that the effect of PZA had been misinterpreted and that the uricosuric action of these drugs, as with most others, could also be assigned to inhibition of uric acid reabsorption at a postsecretory site.[53] In fact, animal studies indicate that a number of uricosuric drugs, including probenecid, actually inhibit uric acid secretion as well as uric acid reabsorption. The predominance of evidence at this time favors the conclusion that uricosuric agents increase the renal clearance of uric acid by decreasing uric acid reabsorption in the proximal nephron.

Probenecid. *Biological Effects.* Probenecid, p-(di-n-propylsulfamyl) benzoic acid (Fig. 56–1), was originally developed as a drug more potent than carinamide in sustaining high blood levels of penicillin by interfering with the renal tubular secretion of the antibiotic. Both carinamide and probenecid were found to increase uric acid excretion in man and to lower serum urate levels.[13,36,37] The value of probenecid in the control of hyperuricemia was demonstrated in 1950 by Talbott and associates[37] and by Gutman.[36] Probenecid soon came to enjoy wide acceptance in the treatment of gout. As the first well-tolerated agent found to be consistently effective in lowering the serum urate concentration in gout, probenecid inaugurated the modern era in therapy that has made control of tophaceous disease an achievable goal.

The increase in uric acid clearance brought about by probenecid may be substantial, but rejection of filtered urate is never complete. Even with large doses and high plasma levels of probenecid the clearance of uric acid does not exceed 50 percent of filtered urate.[48,56]

Uricosuria in response to administration of probenecid is effectively countermanded by salicylates in low doses.[57] The physiologic mechanism of this effect is not established but may involve inhibition of secretion of urate at sites proximal to the probenecid-sensitive reabsorption sites. Curiously, salicylates do not block the probenecid-mediated renal retention of penicillin.[58]

Pharmacokinetics. Probenecid is readily absorbed in the gastrointestinal tract. The half-life of probenecid in plasma is dose dependent,[56] and ranges from 6 to 12 hours. This is prolonged by the concomitant administration of allopurinol.[59] Probenecid is extensively bound to plasma proteins (89 to 94 percent of drug) and is largely confined to the extracellular fluid. The maintenance dose of probenecid ranges from 500 mg per day to 3 grams per day given in three or four divided doses.[60]

Metabolism. Probenecid is rapidly metabolized in vivo as shown by recovery in the urine of less than 5 percent of the administered dose within 24 hours. The major urinary metabolite, probenecid acyl monoglucuronide, accounts for 41 percent of the administered compound within 48 hours. The remainder of the metabolites result from oxidative attack on the n-propyl side chain;[56,61,62] these side chain metabolites possess uricosuric activity in animals.[63]

Other Effects. Probenecid has a number of other effects that could be of physiologic significance. Probenecid blocks the transport of serotonin and dopamine out of the cerebrospinal fluid. An increase in the concentration of 5-hydroxyindoleacetic acid and homovanillic acid is observed in cerebrospinal fluid obtained from patients being treated with probenecid,[64-66] but this increase is less marked in patients with Down's syndrome.[67] In addition, probenecid reduces the renal excretion of pantothenic acid,[68,69] androsterone,[70] ACTH,[71] and diiodotyrosine[72] and may produce a modest salt and water diuresis in some persons.[73] Although probenecid may reduce the elevated serum phosphorus concentration in patients with hypoparathyroidism,[74-76] it appears to have no effect on serum phosphorus, amino acid excretion,[61,77] or glucose excretion[61] in normal subjects. This drug also inhibits the conjugation of benzoic acid derivatives with glycine by an unknown mechanism.[78] Finally, probenecid reduces the uptake and degradation of cAMP in kidney cortex and liver of the rat.[79]

Interaction with Other Drugs. Probenecid influences the renal excretion, volume of distribution, and hepatic uptake of a number of drugs.[61] These effects are summarized in Table 56–2. Because of these interactions certain drugs should be used with caution in patients receiving probenecid. Dapsone[91] and indomethacin,[92] for example, should be used at a lower dose in patients receiving probenecid. Not only does probenecid delay the renal excretion of salicylic acid and many of its glucuronide derivatives, but acetylsalicylate completely blocks the uricosuric effect of probenecid and most other uricosuric agents. Diuretics on the other hand do not abrogate the uricosuric effect of probenecid. Subtherapeutic doses of heparin may have a profound anticoagulant effect in patients receiving probenecid.[101]

The effect of probenecid on the metabolism of some drugs has been used to good advantage. Probenecid has been used, for example, to enhance the blood levels of ampicillin and penicillin.[94,95] In addition, the prolonged half-life of rifampin[100] and cephradine[97] in the presence of probenecid may be therapeutically useful. Probenecid reduces the volume of distribution of several antibiotics, including ampicillin, ancillin, nafcillin, and cephaloridine;[97] should the concentration of these antibiotics be

Table 56–2. Effects of Probenecid on Metabolism of Other Drugs

Decreased renal excretion
 p-Aminohippuric acid[60]
 Phenolsulfonphthalein[80-85]
 Salicylic acid and its acyl and phenolic glucuronides[86-89]
 Phlorizin and its glucuronide[90]
 Acetazolamide[88]
 Dapsone and its metabolites[91]
 Sulfinpyrazone and its parahydroxyl metabolite[92]
 Indomethacin[93]
 Ampicillin[94]
 Penicillin[95]
 Cephradine[96]
Reduced volume of distribution
 Ampicillin[97]
 Ancillin[97]
 Nafcillin[97]
 Cephaloridine[97]
Impairment of hepatic uptake
 Bromsulfonphthalein[98]
 Indocyanin green[99]
 Rifampcin[100]
Delayed metabolism
 Heparin[101]

significantly reduced in certain body fluids or spaces in the presence of probenecid, the net effect could be detrimental. Probenecid has no effect on the elimination of blood levels of gentamicin,[103] sulfonamides, streptomycin, chloramphenicol, or tetracyclines.[83]

Clinical Use. Probenecid should be given in two or three evenly spaced doses. The initial dose should be low, 0.25 gram (half a tablet) every 12 hours, so as to avoid sudden diuresis of large quantities of uric acid, and thus the risk of crystalluria and ureteral blockade. Fluids should be forced in order to prevent formation of concentrated urine, especially during the late hours of the night. After 3 or 4 days the dose of probenecid is increased to 0.5 gram every 12 hours. The serum urate concentration is checked at weekly intervals, and adjustments in dosage are made every 1 to 2 weeks, increasing the daily dose by 0.5 gram each time, until satisfactory control is achieved.

The largest critical experience in the use of probenecid is that of Gutman and Yu.[60,104,105] They found a dose of 1.0 gram per day to be most appropriate in about 50 percent of cases; 0.5 gram per day elicited the desired response in 10 percent of cases; 1.5 to 2.0 grams was required in 25 percent; and 2.5 to 3.0 grams in 15 percent.

In spite of careful management a significant percentage of patients are not brought under satisfactory control with probenecid. In one large clinic[60] 27 percent of patients receiving probenecid failed to achieve serum urate levels of less than 7 mg per 100 ml. In another series of patients[106] only half achieved serum urate levels of 6 mg per 100 ml. Leading causes of failure were poor patient compliance, drug intolerance, salicylate ingestion, and renal impairment. As a general rule, patients with glomerular filtration rates of 80 ml per minute or less are not likely to have an adequate response to a uricosuric drug, and patients with this degree of renal impairment are probably candidates for allopurinol therapy.

Complications. *Acute Gout.* A potential complication of all forms of antihyperuricemic drug therapy is the precipitation of an attack of acute gouty arthritis during the initial days or weeks of therapy, at a time when serum urate levels are being lowered. This complication occurs in 10[60,107] to 20[108] percent of patients started on probenecid alone. The incidence can be greatly reduced by concomitant administration of colchicine or indomethacin.

Nephrolithiasis. A complication of uricosuric drug therapy that is largely preventable is urinary uric acid crystal or stone formation. Initiation of uricosuric drug therapy leads to a transient increase in uric acid excretion. In some patients, particularly those with normal renal function who are overproducers of uric acid, who are given a full therapeutic dose of probenecid, there may be a very brisk and pronounced uricosuria. Since uric acid is relatively insoluble, especially in acid urine, this sudden increase in uric acid excretion can lead to the precipitation of uric acid crystals in the collecting ducts of the kidney or ureters. A more common complication is the development of uric acid stones. This complication was recorded in 9 percent of the patients treated by Gutman and Yu.[60] Uric acid precipitation with initiation of uricosuric therapy is unusual in the normal producer of uric acid.

In some patients at especially high risk of developing nephrolithiasis it may be advisable to alkalinize the urine, in addition to forcing fluids, in order to reduce the likelihood of uric acid stone formation. In these patients the pH of the urine should be raised 6.5 or above by ingestion of 2 to 6 grams per day of sodium bicarbonate or 20 to 60 ml per day of Shohl's solution (citric acid-sodium citrate) during the first days or weeks of therapy. These values may be difficult to achieve, as gouty subjects tend to produce acid urines. Alkalinization during the night may be achieved with a single 250-mg tablet of acetazolamide taken at bedtime. When hyperuricemia has been controlled and the urinary uric acid has returned toward normal, the special precautions regarding urinary uric acid stones are rarely necessary.

Toxicity. The frequency of side effects of probenecid in 2502 patients receiving the drug for periods ranging from 1 day to 4 years was tabulated by Boger and Strickland[109] in 1955. Most of the patients had been on probenecid for only a few days to a few months. The series represented reports compiled from many sources and included patients given probenecid in order to enhance penicillin blood levels. They reported hypersensitivity reactions in 0.3 percent, drug fever in 0.4 percent, skin rash in 1.35 percent, and gastrointestinal disturbances in 3.1 percent. In two longer-term studies involving direct observations of gouty patients, Gutman and Yu[60] found an 8 percent incidence of gastrointestinal complaints, and a 5 percent incidence of hypersensitivity and rash among 169 patients, whereas de Seze and associates[108] noted an 18 percent incidence of gastrointestinal complaints among 156 patients.

Serious toxicity of probenecid is rare. Hepatic necrosis has been reported in one patient[110] and the nephrotic syndrome in at least two.[111,112] One patient who took a massive overdose of probenecid (42.5 grams) in a suicide attempt developed seizures but had no apparent long-term sequelae.

In Talbott's[113] experience, only 2 percent of patients permanently discontinued probenecid because of side effects. In the clinic of Gutman and Yu[104,114] about 12 percent did so. However, in the experience of de Seze and colleagues[108,115] and Kuzell and colleagues[116] about one third of patients eventually became intolerant of probenecid and discontinued its use.

Sulfinpyrazone. *Biological Effects.* The uricosuric properties of phenylbutazone are attributable to one of its metabolites. Sulfinpyrazone is a derivative of that metabolite, and is one of the most potent uricosuric agents known (Fig. 56–2). It has no antiinflammatory properties.

Pharmacokinetics. Sulfinpyrazone is rapidly and completely adsorbed from the gastrointestinal tract with a peak concentration in the serum 1 hour after its oral administration. The half-life in serum is 1 to 3 hours.[39,117] At a serum concentration of 10 mg per 100 ml, 98 percent of the drug is bound to plasma proteins. As a result, sulfinpyrazone, like probenecid, is largely confined to the extracellular fluid.[117,118] Some 20 to 45 percent of the drug is excreted unchanged in 24 hours, predominantly during the first 6 hours.[39,118] Most of the drug is excreted in the urine as the parahydroxyl metabolite, which is also uricosuric in man.

A dose of sulfinpyrazone of 35 mg has a uricosuric effect comparable to 100 mg of probenecid,[39] and 400 mg per day has an effect similar to that observed with 1.5 to 2.0 grams of probenecid per day.[119] Hence, sulfinpyrazone is three to six times more potent than probenecid on a weight basis.[56]

Other Effects. It is not known whether sulfinpyrazone has all the effects on transport, excretion, or metabolism of endogenous substances as described for probenecid. Sulfinpyrazone does suppress the excretion of PAH[39] and phenolsulfonphthalein.[120]

One action of sulfinpyrazone of potential therapeutic significance is the reduction in platelet function observed following its administration. As a result, sulfinpyrazone decreases thrombosis in arteriovenous shunts[121] and prolongs platelet survival in patients with prosthetic heart valves, rheumatic heart disease, and recurrent venous thrombosis.[122,123] This effect of sulfinpyrazone on platelet function can be demonstrated in vitro and appears to be unrelated to its antihyperuricemic effect. This antiplatelet effect of sulfinpyrazone has been attributed to inhibition of prostaglandin synthesis in the platelet.[124]

Clinical Use. Sulfinpyrazone is given in initial doses of 50 mg (half a tablet) twice daily for 3 or 4 days, and then in doses of 100 mg twice daily, increasing the daily dose by 100-mg increments each week, until the serum urate concentration is in the desired range. The precautions of high fluid intake and alkalinization of urine discussed with use of probenecid apply even more critically in the case of sulfinpyrazone because of its potency and prompt action.

The usual maintenance dose ranges from 300 to 400 mg per day in three or four equally divided doses, although a maximal effect is frequently not reached until a dose of 800 mg per day is administered. Sulfinpyrazone has an additional uricosuric effect in subjects receiving the maximal effective dose of probenecid,[125] apparently because probenecid inhibits the tubular secretion of sulfinpyrazone and thus prolongs its uricosuric action.[92]

An extensive clinical experience[76,92,118,126,127] attests to the usefulness of sulfinpyrazone. Tolerance for sulfinpyrazone is somewhat better than for probenecid.[76,126] Nevertheless, according to Kuzell and associates[116] almost one quarter of patients stop the drug for one reason or another. Leading causes of failure of control, as with probenecid, are concomitant salicylate ingestion and renal insufficiency.

Toxicity. The incidence of gastrointestinal symptoms (10 to 15 percent) is roughly the same as that observed with probenecid.[115,116,119,126] In addition, the potential occurrence of uric acid stones after initiation of therapy with sulfinpyrazone represents a significant complication for the reasons discussed earlier with probenecid. Sulfinpyrazone appears to produce a higher incidence of bone marrow changes than probenecid.[76,119,127]

Benziodarone and Benzbromarone. Benziodarone[8,9,128,129] and benzbromarone[6,130-132] are potent uricosuric agents in man. Both agents inhibit the tubular reabsorption of uric acid.[133] The drugs differ in that benziodarone contains iodine whereas benzbromarone contains bromide (Fig. 56–3). The former compound has found limited clinical use, in part because of its effect on thyroid function.[134] The latter drug has been well tolerated for periods up to 6 years.[135]

In 50 gouty patients treated by de Gery and colleagues[135] the mean serum urate level fell from 9.2 to 4.8 mg per 100 ml, while the mean urinary uric acid excretion rose from 520 to 746 mg per day. In eight patients the serum creatinine concentration was greater than 2 mg per 100 ml. Zöllner and colleagues[136] have reported that benzbromarone is more effective than other uricosuric agents in patients with renal insufficiency.

Benzbromarone is a weak inhibitor of xanthine oxidase in vitro, but its action in vivo appears to be exclusively uricosuric. In full therapeutic doses there is no increase in urinary xanthine or hypoxanthine excretion.[130,135]

XANTHINE OXIDASE INHIBITORS

A second general approach toward controlling serum urate levels is that of regulating production of uric acid. At present, the only therapeutically effective method for decreasing uric acid formation is the inhibition of xanthine oxidase by allopurinol or its derivative oxipurinol.

The final steps in the synthesis of uric acid involve conversion of hypoxanthine to xanthine and xanthine to uric acid catalyzed by a single enzyme, xanthine oxidase. Many inhibitors of xanthine oxidase are known, including several pteridines,[137] certain substituted quinazolines,[138] and various purine analogues such as adenine and 2,6-diaminopurine,[139] 6-thiopurine,[140] symmetrical triazines,[141] and 4-diazoimidazole-5-carboxamide.[142] The pyrazolo (3,4-d) pyrimidines have also proved to be important members of this group. Pyrazolo (3,4-d) pyrimidines are purine analogues in which the positions of nitrogen-7 and carbon-8 of the purine ring are reversed (Fig. 56–4).

Allopurinol. Allopurinol was first synthesized for trial as a chemotherapeutic agent, but by itself had little or no effect on experimental tumors.[143,144] It was found to be an inhibitor of xanthine oxidase[145] and to block the conversion of 6-thiopurine to 6-thiouric acid in mouse and man.[146] It was first used clinically as adjunct therapy in patients receiving 6-thiopurine for leukemia.[147] Patients given allopurinol showed a pronounced reduction in both serum and urinary uric acid values.[147,148] These observations suggested a trial of the agent in gout. Allopurinol is now established as a standard form of therapy of hyperuricemia and uric acid stones.

Allopurinol [4-hydroxypyrazolo(3,4-d)pyrimidine] and its major metabolic product, oxipurinol [4,6-dihydroxypyrazolo(3,4-d)pyrimidine] are analogues of hypoxanthine and xanthine, respectively. Both are potent inhibitors of xanthine oxidase.[145,149-151] The Michaelis constant of allopurinol is some 15 to 20 times lower than that of xanthine, whereas that of oxipurinol is comparable to that of xanthine.[150] Allopurinol shows substrate-competitive kinetics. Both allopurinol and oxipurinol produce pseudoirreversible inactivation of xanthine oxidase; inactivation occurs when allopurinol and enzyme are incubated in the absence of substrate, but

Benziodarone

Benzbromarone

Figure 56–3. Structures of benziodarone and benzbromarone.

Figure 56–4. Comparison of structure of 4-hydroxypyrazolo(3,4-d) pyrimidine (allopurinol) with structure of hypoxanthine.

enzyme activity can be restored by prolonged dialysis. Oxipurinol has no effect on the enzyme alone, but inactivates it in the presence of xanthine when molecular oxygen is the hydrogen acceptor.[149]

Pharmacokinetics and Metabolism. Allopurinol is completely absorbed in the gastrointestinal tract. It has a half-life in vivo of 39 minutes to 3 hours.[150,152,153] Since allopurinol and oxipurinol both inhibit the oxidation of allopurinol, the half-life of allopurinol increases as the level of xanthine oxidase inhibition increases. Most of the allopurinol (45 to 65 percent) is rapidly oxidized to oxipurinol in vivo with a smaller portion being converted to allopurinol-1-N-ribonucleotide[154] and allopurinol-1-N-ribonucleoside[155] (Fig. 56–5). Most of the oxipurinol formed is excreted unchanged by the kidney with a half-life of 14[153] to 28 hours.[152] Small portions are metabolized to oxipurinol-7-N-ribonucleoside and oxipurinol-1-N-ribonucleoside[156] and to the corresponding 5'-phosphoribosyl derivatives.[157,158] The pathways involved in

the metabolism of allopurinol are summarized in Figure 56–5.

The renal clearance of allopurinol and oxipurinol ranges from 14 to 20 ml per minute and 23 to 31 ml per minute, respectively.[153] Factors that affect uric acid excretion generally alter oxipurinol excretion in a similar manner.[156] For example, uricosuric agents increase the renal excretion of oxipurinol and uric acid, and renal insufficiency reduces the excretion of both compounds.

Because of its prolonged half-life oxipurinol may be primarily responsible for xanthine oxidase inhibition in vivo when allopurinol is administered.[150] Although allopurinol is the more effective of the two agents when the two are compared daily, this reflects the relatively poor absorption of oxipurinol in the gastrointestinal tract.[159]

Biological Effects (Table 56–3). The administration of allopurinol in man is followed by a decrease in levels of serum and urinary uric acid[160,161] and by increases in

Figure 56–5. Metabolism of allopurinol.

Table 56–3. Metabolic Effects of Allopurinol

Clinical Effect	Mechanism	Effector
Antihyperuricemia	Xanthine oxidase inhibition	Allopurinol Oxipurinol
Decreased total purine production	Inhibition of amidophosphoribosyl-transferase	Allopurinol-1-N-ribosylphosphate; IMP
	PP-ribose-P depletion	Allopurinol
Orotidinuria	Inhibition of orotidine-5'-phosphate decarboxylase	Oxipurinol-7-N-ribosylphosphate Oxipurinol-1-N-ribosylphosphate Allopurinol-1-N-ribosylphosphate
Orotic aciduria	Inhibition of orotate phosphoribosyltransferase	?Orotidine-5'-phosphate
	PP-ribose-P depletion	Allopurinol
Prolongation of half-life of drugs metabolized by the microsomal-oxidizing system	Inhibition of hepatic microsomal drug-metabolizing enzymes	Unknown
Apparent increased activity of orotate phosphoribosyltransferase and orotidine-5'-P decarboxylase	?Stabilization of enzymes to extraction	Unknown

plasma and urinary concentrations of hypoxanthine and xanthine. Plasma levels reach only 0.5 to 1.0[147,162] or, rarely, 2.0 mg per 100 ml[163] because of the relatively high renal clearance of oxypurines. These oxypurine levels are well below the solubility limits of hypoxanthine or xanthine in serum.[162] Urinary increases of hypoxanthine and xanthine may reach several hundred milligrams a day, and are related to the degree of inhibition of xanthine oxidase and the level of HPRT activity.

In most patients the replacement of urinary uric acid by the oxypurines, hypoxanthine and xanthine, is less than stoichiometric.[147,161-164] The deficit ranges from 10 to 60 percent and in patients with normal HPRT activity is roughly proportional to the pretreatment level of uric acid excretion.[161-165] The total deficit may amount to several hundred milligrams of total purines (uric acid plus oxypurines) a day.[147,161,163] In addition, the reduction in total purine excretion is associated with a decreased incorporation of isotopic glycine into urinary uric acid.[166] This effect of allopurinol requires normal HPRT activity[165,167] and could be due to a combination of factors, including (1) reduction of purine biosynthesis de novo by the inhibitory effect of allopurinol ribonucleotide on amidophosphoribosyltransferase;[154] (2) reduction in purine biosynthesis de novo owing to the inhibitory action of purine ribonucleotides derived from IMP on PP-ribose-P synthetase and amidophosphoribosyltransferase;[168] and (3) depletion of PP-ribose-P,[169] an essential and limiting substrate of purine biosynthesis de novo, as a result of its enhanced consumption in the conversion of hypoxanthine and allopurinol[154] to their respective ribonucleotide derivatives.

Studies by Elion and Nelson[170] suggest that the first alternative is not important. The K_i for allopurinol ribonucleotide of the pigeon liver amidophosphoribosyltransferase of 0.6 mM[154] may be taken as a first approximation of concentration required to produce significant inhibition of the human enzyme. Tissue levels of allopurinol ribonucleotide in human liver are probably less than 10^{-7} M, and concentrations of di- or triphosphates of allopurinol or oxipurinol are not present at the 10^{-9} M level. Thus, the levels of allopurinol ribonucleotide in liver are far below the concentrations needed to inhibit amidophosphoribosyltransferase effectively.

The levels of natural purine ribonucleotides[157] lie much closer to the K_i values of pigeon liver[168] or human placental[171] or lymphoblast[172] enzymes. Reutilization of hypoxanthine[173] and xanthine[174] for nucleotide and nucleic acid synthesis is markedly enhanced in the intact rat when their oxidation is inhibited by allopurinol. Studies in patients are also consistent with the conclusion that there is enhanced purine salvage during allopurinol therapy.[175] The temporary increases in levels of IMP and XMP, and subsequently AMP and GMP, could increase feedback inhibition of purine biosynthesis de novo. This would be enhanced by the cooperative effect of AMP and GMP in the inhibition of amidophosphoribosyltransferase[168,171] and by a fall in PP-ribose-P levels.[169]

The administration of allopurinol leads to a substantial reduction of erythrocyte PP-ribose-P content, which occurs 3 to 5 hours after administration of the drug.[169] This effect in erythrocytes is most likely due to consumption of PP-ribose-P by the conversion of allopurinol to its ribonucleotide. It is not attributable to increased reutilization of hypoxanthine and xanthine, since PP-ribose-P levels do not fall after oxipurinol administration[169] and erythrocytes do not contain xanthine oxidase activity. This effect of allopurinol on PP-ribose-P content would be significant for purine biosynthesis only if it also occurs in tissues such as liver that actively synthesize purines de novo. This has not yet been demonstrated.

The administration of either allopurinol or oxipurinol in man is accompanied by a substantial increase in the excretion of orotidine and orotic acid.[176,177] Studies in vivo and in cell culture show that this results from inhibition of orotidine-5'-phosphate decarboxylase, which catalyzes a step in the conversion of orotic acid to uridine 5'-monophosphate (UMP). Inhibition of orotidine-5'-phosphate decarboxylase in vivo is not de-

Clinical Pharmacology

pendent on the presence of HPRT activity and therefore cannot be completely attributed to the formation of allopurinol-1-N-ribonucleotide, oxipurinol-1-N-ribonucleotide, or xanthosine-5'-monophosphate, each of which is a potent inhibitor of orotidine-5'-phosphate decarboxylase in vitro.[177,178] In HPRT-deficient cells, the inhibitory effect of these compounds on pyrimidine biosynthesis appears to involve formation of derivatives that are analogues of orotidine-5'-phosphate,[179,180] whose formation is catalyzed by orotate phosphoribosyltransferase.[158] In HPRT-competent cells it seems likely that the inhibition of orotidine-5'-phosphate decarboxylase is due primarily to both 1- and 7-N-ribonucleotide derivatives of oxipurinol.

The consequence of this allopurinol-mediated inhibition of pyrimidine biosynthesis remains to be defined in man. The administration of allopurinol to rats is associated with a transient decrease in UMP and UDP pools in the liver, whereas UTP levels are elevated; no change is observed in the level of uridine nucleotides in the kidney.[157] These studies suggest that, at least in the rat, any reduction of intracellular pyrimidine nucleotides resulting from the inhibition of pyrimidine biosynthesis de novo is rapidly corrected, presumably by an enhanced salvage of uridine resulting from nucleotide catabolism, through its reconversion to UMP.

The administration of allopurinol also leads to an apparent eightfold increase in the activity of orotate phosphoribosyltransferase and orotidine-5'-phosphate decarboxylase in circulating erythrocytes.[181-183] The increase can usually be demonstrated within 1 week of allopurinol therapy, and the activity appears to level off after 3 to 6 weeks. The mechanism responsible for this is complicated and poorly understood. The ribonucleotide derivatives of both allopurinol and oxipurinol are capable of shifting the configuration of the complex of orotate phosphoribosyltransferase and orotidine-5'-phosphate decarboxylase to a larger, more stable molecular species.[182] Most of the data currently available are consistent with the hypothesis that the apparent increase in enzyme activity is due to stabilization of the enzyme complex to the extraction procedure. Irrespective of mechanism, this change in enzyme activity during allopurinol therapy appears to be of little clinical consequence. These metabolic effects of allopurinol are summarized in Table 56–3.

Allopurinol also has a number of other metabolic effects that have been demonstrated in vitro or in lower animals. Through its action on xanthine oxidase it inhibits tryptophan pyrrolase,[184,185] probably by limiting the availability of H_2O_2 to the latter enzyme.[186,187] Allopurinol also inhibits purine nucleoside phosphorylase[155,188] and pyrimidine deoxyribosyltransferase[189] in vitro. It activates, and at higher concentration inhibits, urate oxidase.[190] Allopurinol does not inhibit liver aldehyde oxidase, an enzyme with substrates very similar to those of xanthine oxidase.[191]

Allopurinol and oxipurinol administration are not associated with visible changes in chromosome structure.[192]

Interaction with Other Drugs. There are potentially important drug-drug interactions involving allopurinol that deserve comment. The biological activities of purine analogues such as 6-mercaptopurine, azathioprine and hypoxanthine arabinoside, the major metabolic product of adenine arabinoside, which are inactivated by xanthine oxidase, are potentiated by the xanthine oxidase inhibition associated with allopurinol administration.[146,193] The toxicity of other cytotoxic agents such as cyclophosphamide also appears to be enhanced by the concomitant administration of allopurinol, although the mechanism is unclear. In addition, allopurinol has an inhibitory effect on the hepatic microsomal drug-metabolizing enzymes.[195] Thus, drugs such as antipyrine and bishydroxycoumarin, which are metabolized by this system, should be used with caution and at a lower dose in patients receiving allopurinol. The half-life of probenecid is prolonged by about 50 percent in the presence of allopurinol.[59] This has been attributed to the inhibitory effect of allopurinol on the microsomal drug-metabolizing system. The administration of allopurinol is associated with a threefold higher incidence of ampicillin-related skin rash.[196] However, it is not clear whether this potentiation is due to allopurinol or to the presence of hyperuricemia.[196] The toxic effects of allopurinol seem to be enhanced with the concomitant administration of a thiazide diuretic.[197,198]

Clinical Use. The administration of allopurinol to subjects with normal renal function is followed, within 24 to 48 hours, by a decrease in serum and urinary acid values. Maximum reductions are achieved in 4 days to 2 weeks, after which values remain relatively constant over prolonged periods of time.[160,161,197] (Fig. 56–6). With the inhibition of urate production by allopurinol, increased amounts of hypoxanthine and xanthine appear in urine, usually within 4 to 6 hours. Only trivial changes occur in the excretion of other urinary purine bases.[200]

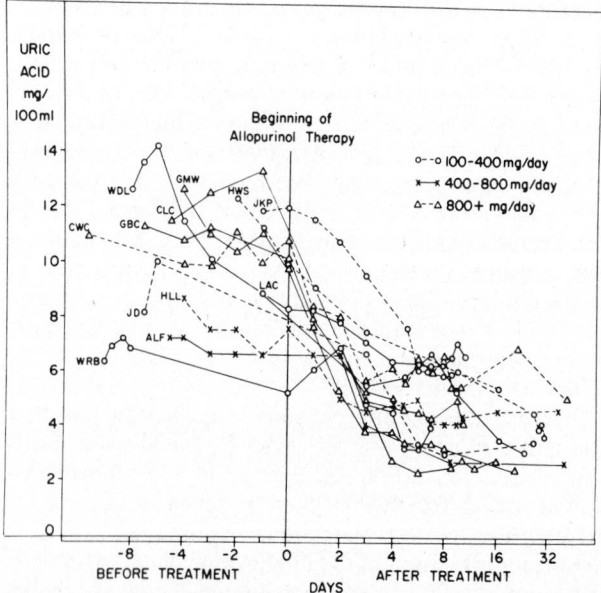

Figure 56–6. Effect of allopurinol on serum uric acid in 12 patients with gout.

Withdrawal of allopurinol results in a return to pretreatment serum urate levels within a few days. Occasional, more prolonged effects are associated with delayed excretion of oxipurinol.[151]

Normal serum urate values can be achieved in all but a few patients. The doses required to reduce the elevated levels to normal average 200 to 300 mg per day for patients with mild disease and 400 to 600 mg per day for those with moderately severe tophaceous disease; rarely, doses of 700 to 1000 mg per day have been required.[160] The average dose required to maintain the serum urate level between 6.0 and 6.9 mg per 100 ml in patients with normal renal function is 300 mg per day.[201] In individuals with reduced glomerular filtration rates it may be advisable to reduce the maintenance dose of allopurinol because of the prolonged half-life of oxipurinol in patients with renal failure. Table 56–4 lists suggested doses for allopurinol in patients with different glomerular filtration rates. In most patients with normal renal function allopurinol need not be initiated at a low dose. In some patients with frequent episodes of gout, however, beginning with a low dose will lessen the probability of precipitating a series of incapacitating attacks. Because of the long biological half-life of the active metabolite, oxipurinol, it is not necessary to divide the doses or to space them throughout the day. A single 300-mg tablet has been shown to be as effective as three divided doses of 100 mg each.[202] In all patients being treated with allopurinol, or any antihyperuricemic agent for that matter, the drug dosage should be adjusted to the individual's need through monitoring the serum urate concentration. The optimal end-point of antihyperuricemic therapy is to reduce the serum urate concentration to a level at which the urate concentration is no longer saturating, i.e., 7 mg per 100 ml or less.

An extensive clinical experience attests to the usefulness of allopurinol in gout. Resolution of tophi occurs gradually with maintenance of normal serum urate levels and is frequently extensive by 6 to 12 months. Destructive arthritis improves in most patients; in an occasional patient with rapid resolution of tophi, however, bony lesions will not heal, leading to telescoped digits.[203] Slower improvement can be anticipated in patients with renal insufficiency.[204] The progression of gouty nephropathy appears to halt in most patients.[163,195,202-206]

Loebl and Scott[207] noted a low incidence of recurrent gouty arthritis in 33 patients in whom allopurinol was discontinued after therapy for a mean of 2 years even though the serum urate rapidly returned to pretreatment levels. These observations suggest that after a few years of control of hyperuricemia the patient may re-enter an asymptomatic phase. Nevertheless, the current recommendation is that once antihyperuricemic therapy is instituted for firm medical indications it should be continued indefinitely if possible.

By selection of the appropriate dose of allopurinol, it is possible to reduce the serum urate level to normal or, if desired, to hold it as low as 2 or 3 mg per 100 ml indefinitely, unless renal function is markedly limited. Even then appreciable reduction of serum urate values can be achieved with allopurinol.[208-213] In patients with extensive tophaceous deposits it may not be possible to reduce the serum urate level to as low as 2 to 3 mg per 100 ml because of the ongoing resorption of preformed urate from the tophi, but the serum urate concentration can usually be lowered to nonsaturating levels, with a resultant decrease in the frequency of gouty attacks and eventual resorption of the tophi.

Uricosuric agents may be used concurrently with allopurinol to hasten mobilization of urate deposits.[161,199] Combined therapy may be particularly effective in the patient with extensive tophaceous deposits (and good renal function), in whom substantial amounts of preformed urate must be eliminated. The administration of a uricosuric agent to a patient receiving allopurinol usually results in appreciable increases of urinary uric acid excretion and a further decline in serum urate level.[161,199] Allopurinol lengthens the biologic half-life of probenecid and thus potentiates its uricosuric effect.[59] On the other hand, uricosuric drugs increase the clearance of oxipurinol in man[150,156] and thus diminish the degree of xanthine oxidase inhibition. They cause either no change or a decrease in excretion of oxypurines in patients receiving allopurinol.[156] Goldfinger and associates[214] cite evidence that hypoxanthine and xanthine are excreted by the renal tubules in man and that this process is inhibited by uricosuric agents. One would anticipate that plasma oxypurine levels would be further elevated upon addition of a uricosuric agent, but they have not been measured in this situation. The net effect of these drug interactions suggests that lower than usual doses of probenecid and greater than usual doses of allopurinol would be indicated when the drugs are used concurrently. Clinically, however, the drugs are tolerated so well that both can be used together without altering the usual dosages of either.

Complications. Acute Attacks of Gout. Most investigators have found the frequency of gouty attacks relatively high on initiation of therapy.[163] Typical attacks have occurred with serum urate levels as low as 2 mg per 100 ml and comparably low urinary urate excretions. Daily colchicine should be given during at least the first 6 to 12 months of therapy of gout with allopurinol in order to minimize the likelihood of recurrent acute attacks.

Xanthine Renal Stones. More than half of the urinary oxypurine increase observed with allopurinol consists of xanthine,[200] a sparingly soluble compound.[162] The levels

Table 56–4. Recommended Maintenance Dose of Allopurinol Based on the Glomerular Filtration Rate

GFR (ml/min)	Dose (mg)
100	300
80	250
60	200
40	150
20	100
10	100 every 2 days
0	100 every 3 days

attained with full doses of allopurinol equal those that in xanthinuric subjects (who lack xanthine oxidase activity as an inborn error of metabolism) have caused formation of urinary calculi composed of xanthine. Thus far, development of xanthine crystalluria or lithiasis as a complication of allopurinol therapy has been observed in only one patient given the drug for treatment of gout or uric acid stones.[215] This patient had a partial deficiency of HPRT.

Four instances of xanthine stone formation induced by allopurinol therapy have been reported in other circumstances. Two occurred in children with the Lesch-Nyhan syndrome[216,217] and a third in an adult patient with lymphosarcoma.[218] These three patients excreted approximately 1500 mg of uric acid a day prior to allopurinol therapy; one child, who received allopurinol at a dose of 9 mg per kilogram, excreted as much as 800 mg of xanthine a day while on therapy.[216,219] The fourth case occurred in a 9-year-old American boy with Burkitt's lymphoma, who was given 600 mg of allopurinol a day. He excreted 1976 mg of oxypurines, 240 to 950 mg of orotic acid, and 640 to 1530 mg of orotidine daily in the urine, and passed many crystals identified as xanthine.[220] Allopurinol should be given cautiously and in minimal doses to patients with extraordinarily great uric acid excretion values, particularly those with an inability to reutilize hypoxanthine and xanthine because of HPRT deficiency.

Oxipurinol Crystal Deposition. Watts and associates[221] have demonstrated microcrystalline deposits of oxipurinol as well as of hypoxanthine and xanthine in muscle biopsy specimens of patients receiving allopurinol for treatment of gout. There are no recognizable clinical consequences of this phenomenon. The concentration of hypoxanthine and xanthine in muscle is considerably less than observed in patients congenitally deficient in xanthine oxidase.[222]

Formation of oxipurinol sludge and stones in the urinary tract has been reported in an 8-year-old boy given both allopurinol and oxipurinol orally in doses of 15 and 37.5 mg per kilogram, respectively.[223] Surgical intervention was required because of urinary tract obstruction. Both sludge and stones showed infrared spectra virtually the same as authentic oxipurinol, and unlike the spectra of allopurinol and uric acid. In addition, a 33-year-old woman with regional enteritis and recurrent uric acid nephrolithiasis who was treated with 600 mg per day of allopurinol developed many small, soft, yellow stones, which were identified as oxipurinol by liquid and gas chromatograph/mass spectrophotometric techniques.[224]

Toxicity. Serious toxicity of allopurinol therapy appears to have been unusual during its initial decade of use. A small percentage of patients (perhaps 5 percent) find it necessary to discontinue the drug.[59] Allopurinol may lead to the development of gastrointestinal intolerance,[206] skin rashes, sometimes with fever,[204] occasionally toxic epidermal necrolysis,[225,226] alopecia,[227] bone marrow suppression with leukopenia and thrombocytopenia,[227] agranulocytosis,[228,229] granulomatous hepati-

tis,[230,231] severe jaundice,[232] sarcoidlike reaction,[233] and vasculitis.[234,235] The incidence of side effects of all kinds may be about 20 percent.

Toxic effects tend to occur more often in the presence of renal insufficiency and with thiazide therapy. A series of reports over the last 12 years have described a constellation of findings, including fever, skin rash, progressive renal insufficiency, eosinophilia, and hepatitis, in patients experiencing toxic reactions to allopurinol, and some authors have referred to this as an allopurinol hypersensitivity syndrome. In a group of 78 patients with this putative syndrome the following abnormalities were noted: skin rash, 92 percent; fever, 87 percent; worsening renal function, 85 percent; eosinophilia, 73 percent; hepatitis, 68 percent; and leukocytosis, 39 percent.[236] Twenty-one percent of these patients died. Diffuse vasculitis involving multiple organ systems was noted in a number of cases at post-mortem examination. The median dose of allopurinol was 300 mg per day, and the mean duration of therapy was 3 weeks (range of 1 to 30 weeks). Prior renal insufficiency was recorded in 81 percent of these patients, and 49 percent received concomitant diuretic therapy, leading some authors to postulate that pre-existing renal disease and thiazides might be predisposing factors to this syndrome.[236] While the incidence of this type of severe allergic reaction is not known, it is probably quite rare. However, the potential severity of this disorder emphasizes the need for restricting allopurinol therapy to those hyperuricemic patients who have specific indications for antihyperuricemic therapy as well as the need to reduce the dose of allopurinol in patients with renal insufficiency (Table 56–4) (see Chapter 86).

Skin rashes are more frequent and serious in patients receiving allopurinol and ampicillin. In the Boston Collaborative Drug Surveillance Program,[196] 2.1 percent of 283 patients receiving allopurinol without ampicillin, 7.5 percent of 1257 patients receiving only ampicillin, and 22.4 percent of 67 hospitalized patients receiving allopurinol and ampicillin experienced drug rashes. Although it could not be determined whether the threefold greater risk of drug rash in patients taking ampicillin plus allopurinol was associated with allopurinol or hyperuricemia, it would be prudent not to prescribe these two drugs together.

The occurrence of skin rash in a patient receiving allopurinol does not necessarily require that the drug be discontinued. The rash of allopurinol often involves the hands and feet alone, or at least chiefly. There may be swelling and intense itching, and the body and face may be involved. Provided there is no laryngeal edema, it may suffice to administer large doses of Benadryl or other antihistaminic agent to control the itching. A minimal amount of swelling of the hands and feet is often then well tolerated. After a few weeks, it may be possible to stop the antihistamine without recurrence of the rash. Reduction of the dose of allopurinol may also be helpful in reducing the severity of the skin lesions, especially in patients with renal insufficiency. Desensitization has apparently been effected in two patients allergic to allopurinol by initiating therapy with a very low dose of allopurinol (0.05 mg per day) and gradually increasing the amount given over a period of 30 days.[237,238]

Oxipurinol. Although the therapeutic effects of allopurinol are mediated at least in part by its metabolic product oxipurinol, whose half-life is about eightfold longer than that of allopurinol,[161] a direct comparison of the two agents given orally indicates that allopurinol is the more effective because of the relatively poor absorption of oxipurinol from the gastrointestinal tract.[164] Nevertheless, oxipurinol can be used therapeutically, and has been effectively employed in some patients who have been sensitive to allopurinol. In a study of 13 patients allergic to allopurinol, 70 percent had their hyperuricemia controlled with oxipurinol without evidence of toxicity.[239] Toxic reactions identical to those observed with allopurinol were observed in 30 percent of the patients treated with oxipurinol. Cross-sensitivity to the two drugs might be expected on the basis of their structural similarities. Oxipurinol is not marketed in the United States but is available in Europe and Japan.

OTHER THERAPEUTIC AGENTS

Thiopurinol. Thiopurinol[4-thiopyrazolo(3,4-d)pyrimidine], although developed for use as a xanthine oxidase inhibitor, reduces plasma urate concentrations and uric acid excretion values without a concomitant increase in plasma oxypurine levels or in oxypurine excretion.[240,241] These effects occur in gouty patients with normal renal function and normal HGPRT activity, but thiopurinol has no effect on plasma or urinary uric acid values in patients with nearly complete deficiency of erythrocyte HGPRT activity.[242] Effects of thiopurinol have been postulated to reflect inhibition of purine biosynthesis de novo by thiopurinol ribonucleotide, although this hypothesis has not yet been documented.

Orotic Acid. Orotic acid in doses ranging from 2 to 6 grams per day produces a modest reduction in serum urate concentration.[243,244] This is related both to its uricosuric effect[245] and to inhibition of purine biosynthesis de novo.[243,245] Orotic acid is a normal intermediate of pyrimidine biosynthesis and reacts with PP-ribose-P to form orotidine-5'-monophosphate (OMP), a precursor of uridine and cytidine nucleotides.[246] Several studies suggest that orotic acid inhibits purine biosynthesis by competing with L-glutamine for available PP-ribose-P.[247] Following the administration of orotic acid, erythrocyte PP-ribose-P levels fall and the incorporation of isotopic glycine into urinary uric acid is reduced.[244] Although short-term therapy with orotic acid in man was not associated with the development of a fatty liver,[244] as it is in the rat,[248,249] this agent does not appear to offer any therapeutic advantage over other antihyperuricemic drugs currently in use.

Uricase. The infusion of highly purified uricase has been shown to bring about a transient reduction in the serum urate level.[250-253] An increased clearance of uric acid appears to contribute to the response.[251] Use of uricase has been advocated in patients with hyperuricemia of renal origin.[254-255] Rapid development of antibodies to the enzyme is associated with diminished effectiveness.

References

1. Yu, T-F., Berger, L., and Gutman, A.B.: Hypoglycemic and uricosuric properties of acetohexamide and hydroxyhexamide. Metabolism 17:309, 1968.
2. Friedman, M., and Byers, S.O.: Mechanism by which ACTH increases the excretion of urate. Am. J. Physiol. 163:684, 1950.
3. Stein, H.B., Hasan, A., and Fox, I.H.: Ascorbic acid-induced uricosuria: A consequence of megavitamin therapy. Ann. Intern. Med. 84:385, 1976.
4. Frank, O.: Untersuchungen zur urikosurischen Wirkung von Azapropazon. Z. Rheumaforsch. 30:368, 1971.
5. Fallon, H.D., Frei, E., Block, J., et al.: The uricosuria and orotic aciduria induced by 6-azauridine. J. Clin. Invest. 40:1906, 1961.
6. Sternon, J., Kocheleff, P., Courturier, E., et al.: Effet hypouricémiant de la benzbromarone. Étude de 24 cas. Acta Clin. Belg. 22:285, 1967.
7. Podevin, R., Paillard, F., Amiel, C., et al.: Action de la benziodarone sur l'excrétion rénale de l'acide urique. Rev. Fr. Étud. Clin. Biol. 12:361, 1967.
8. Nivet, M., Marcovici, J., Laruelle, P., et al.: Note préliminaire sur l'action d'un benzofuranne sur l'uricémie. Bull. Soc. Med. Hôp. Paris 116:118, 1965.
9. Delbarre, F., Auscher, C., and Amor, B.: Action uricosurique et antigoutteuse de certains dérivés du benzofuranne. Presse Méd. 73:2725, 1965.
10. Blahos, J., Osten, L., Mertl, J., Kotas, O., Gregor, O., and Reisenauer, R.: The uricosuric effect of calcitonin. Horm. Metab. Res. 7:445, 1975.
11. Mudge, G.H.: Uricosuric action of cholecystographic agents. N. Engl. J. Med. 284:929, 1971.
12. Postlethwaite, A.E., and Kelley, W.N.: Uricosuric effect of radiocontrast agents: A study in man of four commonly used preparations. Ann. Intern. Med. 74:845, 1971.
13. Wolfson, S.Q., Cohn, C., Levine, R., et al.: Transport and excretion of uric acid in man. III. Physiologic significance of the uricosuric effect of caronamide (abstract). Am. J. Med. 4:774, 1948.
14. Healey, L.A., Harrison, M., and Decker, J.L.: Uricosuric effect of chlorprothixene. N. Engl. J. Med. 272:526, 1965.
15. Nicolaier, A., and Dohrn, M.: Über die Wirkung von Chinolicarbonsauren und ihrer Derivate auf die Ausscheidung der Harnsäure. Dtsch. Arch. Klin. Med. 43:331, 1908.
16. Koden, W.: Citric acid therapy in uraturia. Z. Arztl. Fortbild. 58:392, 1964.
17. Hansen, O.E., and Holten, C.: Uricosuric effect of dicoumarol. Lancet 1:1047, 1958.
18. Schlosstein, L.H., Kippen, I., Whitehouse, M.W., et al.: Studies with some novel uricosuric agents and their metabolites: Correlation between clinical activity and drug-induced displacement of urate from its albumin-binding sites. J. Lab. Clin. Med. 82:412, 1973.
19. Nicholls, A., Snaith, M.L., and Scott, J.T.: Effect of estrogen therapy on plasma and urinary levels of uric acid. Br. Med. J. 1:449, 1973.
20. Sougin-Mibashan, R., and Horwitz, M.: The uricosuric action of ethyl biscoumacetate. Lancet 1:1191, 1955.
21. Oliver, M.F.: Reduction of serum-lipid and uric acid levels by an orally active androsterone. Lancet 1:1321, 1962.
22. Ramsdell, C.M., Postlethwaite, A.E., and Kelley, W.N.: Uricosuric effect of glyceryl guaiacolate. J. Rheumatol. 1:114, 1974.
23. Yu, T-F., Kaung, C., and Gutman, A.: Effect of glycine loading on plasma and urinary uric acid and amino acids in normal and gouty subjects. Am. J. Med. 49:352, 1970.
24. Postlethwaite, A.D., Ramsdell, C.M., and Kelley, W.N.: Uricosuric effect of an anticholinergic agent in hyperuricemic subjects. Arch. Intern. Med. 134:270, 1974.
25. Jain, A., Ryan, J.R., Hague, D., et al.: The effect of MK-185 on some aspects of uric acid metabolism. Clin. Pharmacol. Ther. 11:551, 1970.
26. Talbott, J.H.: Gout. London and New York, Oxford University Press, 1943.
27. Bonsnes, R.W., Dill, L., and Dana, E.: The effect of Diodrast on the normal uric acid clearance. J. Clin. Invest. 23:776, 1944.
28. Robinson, R.G., and Radcliff, E.J.: The effect of meclofenamic acid on plasma uric acid levels. Med. J. Aust. 1:1079, 1972.
29. Coombs, F.S., Pecora, L.J., Thorogood, E., et al.: Renal function in patients with gout. J. Clin. Invest. 12:525, 1940.

30. Mochtey, I.: Serum uric acid levels following administration of metiazinic acid (Soripal). Clin. Chim. Acta 47:317, 1973.
31. Podevin, R., Paillard R., Voudiclari, S., and Richet, G.: Action of niridazole (CIBA 32,644 BA) on the metabolism of uric acid in man. Rev. Franc. Étud. Clin. Biol. 13:624, 1968.
32. Weintraub, M., Nash, T.E., Ottesen, E., and Becker, M.A.: Uricosuric effects of niridazole. Clin. Pharmacol. Ther. 22:568, 1977.
33. Fulop, M., and Drapkin, A.: Potassium depletion syndrome secondary to nephropathy apparently caused by "outdated tetracycline." N. Engl. J. Med. 272:986, 1965.
34. Kuzell, W.C., Schaffarzick, R.W., Brown, B., et al.: Phenylbutazone (Butazolidin) in rheumatoid arthritis and gout. JAMA 149:729, 1952.
35. Trevaks, G., and Lovell, R.R.H.: Effect of Atromid and its components on uric acid excretion and on gout. Ann. Rheum. Dis. 24:572, 1965.
36. Gutman, A.B.: Uric acid metabolism and gout. Combined staff clinic. Am. J. Med. 9:799, 1950.
37. Talbott, J.H., Bishop, C., Norcross, M., et al.: The clinical and metabolic effects of Benemid in patients with gout. Trans. Assoc. Am. Physicians 64:372, 1951.
38. See, G.: Études sur l'acid salicylique et le salicylates: Traitement du rheumatisme aigu et chronique, de la goutte, et de diverses affections du systeme nerveux sensitif par les salicylates. Bull. Acad. Med. Paris 6:689, 717, 926, 937, 1024, 1877.
39. Burns, J.J., Yu, T-F., Ritterband, A., et al.: A potent new uricosuric agent, the sulfoxide metabolite of the phenylbutazone analogue, G-25671. J. Pharmacol. Exp. Ther. 119:418, 1957.
40. Nemati, M., Kyle, M.C., and Freis, E.D.: Clinical study of ticrynafen, a new diuretic, antihypertensive, and uricosuric agent. JAMA 237:652, 1977.
41. Friedman, A., and Steele, T.H.: Supersaturation of urine with uric acid and urate: Response to a uricosuric diuretic. J. Lab. Clin. Med. 92:447, 1978.
42. de Carvalho, J.G.R., Dunn, F.G., Chrysant, S.G., and Frohlich, E.D.: Ticrynafen: A novel uricosuric antihypertensive natriuretic agent. Arch. Intern. Med. 138:53, 1978.
43. Burns, J.J., Yu, T-F., Berger, L., et al.: Zoxazolamine. Physiological deposition, uricosuric properties. Am. J. Med. 25:401, 1958.
44. Bluestone, R., Kippen, I., Klinenberg, J.R., et al.: Effect of some uricosuric and anti-inflammatory drugs on the binding of uric acid to human serum albumin in vitro. J. Lab. Clin. Med. 76:85, 1970.
45. Klinenberg, J.R., and Kippen, I.: The binding of urate to plasma proteins determined by means of equilibrium dialysis. J. Lab. Clin. Med. 75:503, 1970.
46. Kippen, I., Whitehouse, M.W., and Klinenberg, J.R.: Pharmacology of uricosuric agents. Ann. Rheum. Dis. 33:391, 1974.
47. Postlethwaite, A.E., Gutman, R.A., and Kelley, W.N.: Salicylate-mediated increase in uric acid removal during hemodialysis: Evidence for urate binding in vivo. Metabolism 23:771, 1974.
48. Kovarsky, J., Holmes, E.W., and Kelley, W.N.: Absence of significant urate binding to human serum proteins. J. Lab. Clin. Med. 93:85, 1979.
49. Gutman, A.B.: Uricosuric drugs, with special reference to probenecid and sulfinpyrazone. Adv. Pharmacol. 4:91, 1966.
50. Steele, T.H., and Rieselbach, R.E.: Renal urate excretion in normal man. Nephron 14:21, 1975.
51. Steele, T.H., and Bonar, G.: Origins of the uricosuric response. J. Clin. Invest. 52:1368, 1973.
52. Meisel, A.D., and Diamond, H.S.: Inhibition of probenecid uricosuria by pyrazinamide and para-aminohippurate. Am. J. Physiol. 232:F222, 1977.
53. Steele, T.H.: Urate secretion in man: The pyrazinamide suppression test. Ann. Intern. Med. 79:734, 1973.
54. Weinshilboum, R.M., Goldstein, J.L., and Kelley, W.N.: Prolonged hypouricemia associated with acute chlorprothixene ingestion. Arthritis Rheum. 18:739, 1975.
55. Lemierix, G., Vinay, P., Gougoux, A., et al.: Nature of the uricosuric action of benziodarone. Am. J. Physiol. 224:1440, 1973.
56. Dayton, P.G., Yu, T-F., Chen, W., et al.: The physiological disposition of probenecid, including renal clearance in man, studied by an improved method for its estimation in biological material. J. Pharmacol. Exp. Ther. 140:278, 1963.
57. Gutman, A.B., and Yu, T-F.: Benemid (p-[di-n-prophylsulfamyl]benzoic acid) as uricosuric agent in chronic gouty arthritis. Trans. Assoc. Am. Physicians 64:279, 1951.
58. Boger, W., Strickland, S.C., Bayne, G.M., et al.: Probenecid and salicylates: The question of interaction in terms of penicillin excretion. J. Lab. Clin. Med. 45:478, 1955.
59. Tjandramaga, T.B., Cucinell, S.A., Israeli, Z.H., et al.: Observations on the disposition of probenecid on patients receiving allopurinol. Pharmacology 8:259, 1972.
60. Gutman, A.B., and Yu, T-F.: Protracted uricosuric therapy in tophaceous gout. Lancet 2:1258, 1957.

61. Beyer, K.H., Russo, H.F., Tillson, E.K., et al.: "Benemid," p-(di-n-propylsulfamyl)benzoic acid. Its renal affinity and its elimination. Am. J. Physiol. 166:625, 1951.
62. Dayton, P.G., Perel, J.M., Cunningham, R.F., et al.: Studies of the fate of metabolites and analogs of probenecid. The significance of metabolic sites, especially lack of ring hydroxylation. Drug Metab. Dispos. 1:742, 1973.
63. Israeli, Z.H., Perel, J.M., Cunningham, R.F., et al.: Metabolites of probenecid. Chemical, physical and pharmacological studies. J. Med. Chem. 15:709, 1972.
64. Bowers, M.J., Jr.: CSF homovanillic acid: Effects of probenecid and alpha-methyltyrosine. Life Sci. [I] 9:691, 1970.
65. Tamarkin, N.R., Goodwin, F.K., and Axelrod, J.: Rapid elevation of biogenic amine metabolites in human CSF following probenecid. Life Sci. 9:1397, 1970.
66. Van Praag, H.M., Korf, J., and Puite, J.: 5-Hydroxyindoleacetic acid levels in the cerebrospinal fluid of depressive patients treated with probenecid. Nature 225:1259, 1970.
67. Airaksinen, E.M., and Kanko, K.: Effect of probenecid on 5-hydroxyindoles in cerebrospinal fluid in Down's syndrome. Ann. Clin. Res. 5:392, 1973.
68. Boger, W.P., Bayne, G.M., Gylfe, J., et al.: Renal clearance of pantothenic acid in man: Inhibition by probenecid ("Benemid"). Proc. Soc. Exp. Biol. Med. 82:604, 1953.
69. Markkanen, T., Toivanen, P., Toivanen, A., et al.: The effect of probenecid (p-(di-n-propylsulfamyl)-benzoic acid) on the spontaneous renal excretion of biologically active metabolites of thiamine, riboflavin and pantothenic acid. Scand. J. Clin. Lab. Invest. 15:511, 1963.
70. Gardner, L.I., Crigler, J.R., Jr., and Migeon, C.J.: Inhibition of urinary 17-ketosteroid excretion produced by "Benemid." Proc. Soc. Exp. Biol. Med. 78:460, 1951.
71. Bonar, J.A., and Perkins, W.H.: Inhibition of urinary excretion of iodine[131]-labeled corticotropin by probenecid. J. Clin. Endocrinol. 22:38, 1962.
72. Huang, K.C.: Renal excretion of L-tyrosine and its derivatives. J. Pharmacol. Exp. Ther. 134:257, 1961.
73. Sirota, J.H., Yu, T-F., and Gutman, A.B.: Effect of Benemid (p-[di-n-propylsulfamyl]benzoic acid) on urate clearance and other discrete renal functions in gouty subjects. J. Clin. Invest. 31:692, 1952.
74. Dubin, A., Kushner, D.S., Bronsky, D., et al.: Hyperuricemia in hypoparathyroidism. Metabolism 5:703, 1956.
75. Kolb, F.O., and Rukes, J.M.: Effects of Benemid (probenecid) in the treatment of hypoparathyroidism and pseudohypoparathyroidism (abstract). J. Clin. Endocrinol. 14:785, 1954.
76. Persellin, R.H., and Schmid, F.R.: The use of sulfinpyrazone in the treatment of gout reduces serum uric acid levels and diminishes severity of arthritis attacks, with freedom from significant toxicity. JAMA 175:971, 1961.
77. Bearn, A.G., and Kunkel, H.G.: Abnormalities of copper metabolism in Wilson's disease and their relationship to the aminoaciduria. J. Clin. Invest. 33:400, 1954.
78. Beyer, K.H., Wiebelhaus, V.D., Tillson, E.K., et al.: "Benemid," p-(di-n-propylsulfamyl)benzoid acid: Inhibition of glycine conjugative reactions. Proc. Soc. Exp. Biol. Med. 74:772, 1950.
79. Coulson, R., Bowman, R.H., and Roch-Ramel, F.: The effects of nephrectomy and probenecid on in vivo clearance of adenosine 3'5'-monophosphate from rat plasma. Life Sci. 15:877, 1974.
80. Benedek, T.G.: The effect of probenecid and of liver disease on the excretion of phenolsulfonphthalein. Am. J. Med. Sci. 242:448, 1961.
81. Beyer, K.H.: Functional characteristics of renal transport mechanisms. Pharmacol. Rev. 2:227, 1950.
82. Blondheim, S.H.: Effect of probenecid on excretion of bromosulphthalein. J. Appl. Physiol. 7:529, 1955.
83. Boger, W.P., Matteucci, W.V., and Schimmel, N.H.: Renal clearances of penicillin, phenolsulphonphthalein, and paraaminohippurate (PAH) modified by "Benemid" (abstract). Am. J. Med. 11:517, 1951.
84. Newcombe, D.S., and Cohen, A.S.: Uricosuric agents and phenolsulfonphthalein excretion. Arch. Intern. Med. 112:738, 1963.
85. Peck, H.M., and Beyer, K.H.: Renal function: Excretion of phenolsulfonphthalein by the amphibian (Rana pipiens) kidney (abstract). Fed. Proc. 13:393, 1954.
86. Gutman, A.B., Yu, T-F., and Sirota, J.H.: A study, by simultaneous clearance techniques, of salicylate excretion in man. Effect of alkalinization of the urine by bicarbonate administration; effect of probenecid. J. Clin. Invest. 34:711, 1955.
87. Schacter, D., and Manis, J.F.: Salicylate and salicyl conjugates: Fluorimetric estimation, biosynthesis and renal excretion in man. J. Clin. Invest. 37:800, 1958.
88. Weiner, I.M., Washington, J.A., II, and Mudge, G.H.: Studies on the renal excretion of salicylate in the dog. Bull. Johns Hopkins Hosp. 105:284, 1959.

89. Yu, T-F., and Gutman, A.B.: Study of the paradoxical effects of salicylate in low, intermediate and high dosage on the renal mechanisms for excretion of urate in man. J. Clin. Invest. 38:1298, 1959.

90. Braun, W., Whittaker, V.P., and Lotspeich, W.F.: Renal excretion of phlorizin and phlorizin glucuronide. Am. J. Physiol. 190:563, 1957.

91. Goodwin, C.S., and Sparell, G.: Inhibition of dapsone excretion by probenecid. Lancet 2:884, 1969.

92. Perel, J.M., Dayton, P.G., Snell, M.M., et al.: Studies of interactions among drugs in man at the renal level: Probenecid and sulfinpyrazone. Clin. Pharmacol. Ther. 10:834, 1969.

93. Skeith, M.D., Simkin, P.A., and Healey, L.A.: Renal excretion of indomethacin and its inhibition by probenecid. Clin. Pharmacol. Ther. 9:89, 1968.

94. Klein, J.O., and Finland, M.: Ampicillin activity in vitro and absorption and excretion in normal young men. Am. J. Med. Sci. 243:544, 1963.

95. Beyer, K.H.: Factors basic to the development of useful inhibitors of renal transport mechanisms. Arch. Int. Pharmacodyn. 98:97, 1954.

96. Mischler, T.W., Sugerman, A.A., Willard, D.A., et al.: Influence of probenecid and food on the bioavailability of cephradine in normal male subjects. J. Clin. Pharmacol. 14:604, 1974.

97. Gibaldi, M., and Schwartz, M.A.: Apparent effect of probenecid on distribution of penicillin in man. Clin. Pharmacol. Ther. 9:345, 1968.

98. Goetzee, A.E., Richards, T.G., and Tindall, V.R.: Experimental changes in liver function induced by probenecid. Clin. Sci. 19:63, 1960.

99. Vogin, E.E., Scott, W., Boyd, J., et al.: Effect of probenecid on indocyanine green clearance. J. Pharmacol. Exp. Ther. 152:509, 1966.

100. Kenwright, S., and Levi, A.J.: Impairment of hepatic uptake of rifamycin antibiotics by probenecid, and its therapeutic implications. Lancet 2:1401, 1973.

101. Sanchez, G.: Enhancement of heparin effect by probenecid. N. Engl. J. Med. 292:48, 1975.

102. Palmer, D.G., and T.C., Highton: A short trial assessment of uricosuric therapy in gout. Aust. Ann. Med. 17:242, 1968.

103. Bergan, T., Westlie, L., and Brodwall, E.K.: Influence of probenecid on gentamycin pharmacokinetics. Acta Med. Scand. 191:221, 1974.

104. Gutman, A.B.: Medical management of gout. Postgrad. Med. 51:61, 1972.

105. Yu, T-F.: Milestones in the treatment of gout. Am. J. Med. 56:676, 1974.

106. Thompson, C.R., Duff, I.F., Robinson, W.D., et al.: Long-term uricosuric therapy in gout. Arthritis Rheum. 5:384, 1962.

107. Gutman, A.B.: Treatment of primary gout: The present status. Arthritis Rheum. 8:911, 1965.

108. de Seze, S., Ryckewaert, A., and d'Anglejan, G.: The treatment of gout by probenecid. (A study based on 156 cases, 68 of which were treated from 1 to 9 years.) Rev. Rhum. Mal. Osteoartic. 30:93, 1963.

109. Boger, W.P., and Strickland, S.C.: Probenecid (Benemid). Its use and side-effects in 2502 patients. Arch Intern. Med. 95:83, 1955.

110. Reynolds, E.S., Schlant, R.C., Gonick, H.C., et al.: Fatal massive necrosis of the liver as a manifestation of hypersensitivity to probenecid. N. Engl. J. Med. 256:592, 1957.

111. Ferris, T.F., Morgan, W.S., and Levitin, H.: Nephrotic syndrome caused by probenecid. N. Engl. J. Med. 265:381, 1961.

112. Hertz, P., Yager, H., and Richardson, J.A.: Probenecid-induced nephrotic syndrome. Arch. Pathol. 94:241, 1972.

113. Talbott, J.H.: Gout. 2nd ed. New York, Grune & Stratton, 1964, p. 206.

114. Gutman, A.B., and Yu, T-F.: Prevention and treatment of chronic gouty arthritis. JAMA 157:1096, 1955.

115. de Seze, S., Ryckewaert, A., Caroit, M., et al.: Le traitement uricosurique de la goutte. Congres International de la goutte et de la lithiase urique, Sept. 4-6, Evian, 1964, p. 297.

116. Kuzell, W., Glover, R., Gibbs, J., et al.: Effect of Anturane on serum uric acid and cholesterol in gout. A long-term study. Acta Rheumatol. Scand. Suppl. 8:31, 1964.

117. Dayton, P.G., Sicam, L.E., Landrau, M., et al.: Metabolism of sulfinpyrazone (Anturane) and other thio analogues of phenylbutazone in man. J. Pharmacol. Exp. Ther. 132:287, 1961.

118. Gutman, A.B., Dayton, P.G., Yu, T-F., et al.: A study of the inverse relationship between pKa and rate of renal excretion of phenylbutazone analogs in man and dog. Am. J. Med. 29:1017, 1960.

119. Yu, T-F., Burns, J.J., and Gutman, A.B.: Results of a clinical trial of G-28315, a sulfoxide analog of phenylbutazone, as a uricosuric agent in gouty subjects. Arthritis Rheum. 1:532, 1958.

120. Domenjoz, R.: The pharmacology of the phenylbutazone analogues. Ann. N.Y. Acad. Sci. 86:263, 1960.

121. Kaegi, A., Pineo, G.F., Shimizu, A., et al.: Arteriovenous shunt thrombosis: Prevention by sulfinpyrazone. N. Engl. J. Med. 290:304, 1974.

122. Weily, H.S., and Genton, E.: Altered platelet function in patients with prosthetic mitral valves: Effects of sulfinpyrazone therapy. Circulation 42:967, 1970.

123. Steele, P.O., Weily, H.S., and Genton, E.: Platelet survival and adhesiveness in recurrent venous thrombosis. N. Engl. J. Med. 288:1148, 1973.

124. Ali, M., and McDonald, W.D.: Effects of sulfinpyrazone on platelet prostaglandin synthesis and platelet release of serotonin. J. Lab. Clin. Med. 89:868, 1977.

125. Seegmiller, J.E., and Grayzel, A.I.: Use of the newer uricosuric agents in the management of gout. JAMA 173:1076, 1960.

126. Emmerson, B.T.: A comparison of uricosuric agents in gout, with special reference to sulphinpyrazone. Med. J. Aust. 1:839, 1963.

127. Glick, E.N.: Sulphinpyrazone in the treatment of arthritis associated with hyperuricaemia. Proc. R. Soc. Med. 54:423, 1961.

128. Richet, G., Cottet, J., Amiel, C., et al.: Traitement de l'hyperuricémie des goutteux et des insuffisants rénaux par la Benziodarone. Presse Méd. 74:1247, 1966.

129. Delbarre, F., Auscher, C., Olivier, J.L., et al.: Traitement des hyperuricémies et de la goutte par des dérivés du benzofuranne. Semin. Hôp. Paris 24:1127, 1967.

130. Jain, A.K., Ryan, J.R., McMahon, F.G., et al.: Effect of single oral doses of benzbromarone on serum and urinary uric acid. Arthritis Rheum. 17:149, 1974.

131. Sinclair, D.S., and Fox, I.H.: The pharmacology of hypouricemic effect of benzbromarone. J. Rheum. 2:437, 1975.

132. Yu, T-F.: Pharmacokinetic and clinical studies of a new uricosuric agent—benzbromarone. J. Rheum. 3:305, 1976.

133. Kramp, R.A.: Effects of benzofuran derivatives on tubular permeability to 6-urate-2¹⁴C in the rat nephron. In Sperling, O., De Vries, A., and Wyngaarden, J.B. (eds.): Purine Metabolism in Man. New York, Plenum Press, 1974, p. 777.

134. Camus, J.P., Prier, A., Kartun, P., et al.: Thyréotoxicose et benziodarone. Rev. Rhum. Mal. Osteoartic. 40:148, 1973.

135. de Gery, A., Auscher, C., Saporta, L., et al.: Treatment of gout and hyperuricemia by benzbromarone, ethyl 2(dibromo-3,5-hydroxy-4-benzoyl)-3 benzofuran. In Sperling, O., De Vries, A., and Wyngaarden, J.B., (eds.): Purine Metabolism in Man. New York, Plenum Press, 1974, p. 683.

136. Zöllner, N., Griebsch, A., and Fink, J.K.: Über die Wirkung von Benzbromaron auf den Serumharnsäurespiegel und die Harnsäureausscheidung des Gichtkranken. Dtsch. Med. Wochenschr. 98:2405, 1970.

137. Petering, H.G., and Schmitt, J.A.: Studies in enzyme inhibition. I. Action of some simple pterines on xanthine oxidase. J. Am. Chem. Soc. 72:2995, 1950.

138. Priest, D.G., Hynes, J.B., Jones, C.W., et al.: Quinazolines as inhibitors of xanthine oxidase. J. Pharmacol. Sci. 63:1158, 1974.

139. Wyngaarden, J.B.: 2,6-Diaminopurine as substrate and inhibitor of xanthine oxidase. J. Biol. Chem. 224:453, 1957.

140. Silberman, H.R., and Wyngaarden, J.B.: 6-Mercaptopurine as substrate and inhibitor of xanthine oxidase. Biochim. Biophys. Acta 47:178, 1961.

141. Fridovich, I.: A new class of xanthine oxidase inhibitors isolated from guanidinium salts. Biochemistry 4:1098, 1965.

142. Baker, B.R., Wood, W.F., and Kozma, J.A.: Irreversible enzyme inhibitors. CXXVI. Hydrocarbon interaction with xanthine oxidase by phenyl substituents on purines and pyrazolo(3,4-d)pyrimidines. J. Med. Chem. 11:611, 1968.

143. White, F.R.: 4-Aminopyrazolo(3,4-d)pyrimidine and three derivatives. Cancer Chemother. Rep. 3:26, 1959.

144. Shaw, R.K., Shulman, R.N., Davidson, J.K., et al.: Studies with the experimental antitumor agent 4-aminopyrazolo(3,4-d)pyrimidine. Cancer 13:482, 1960.

145. Feigelson, P., Davidson, J.K., and Robins, P.K.: Pyrazolopyrimidines as inhibitors and substrates of xanthine oxidase. J. Biol. Chem. 226:993, 1957.

146. Elion, G.B., Callahan, S., Nathan, H., et al.: Potentiation by inhibition of drug degradation: 6-Substituted purine and xanthine oxidase. Biochem. Pharmacol. 12:85, 1963.

147. Rundles, R.W., Wyngaarden, J.B., Hitchings, G.H., et al.: Effects of a xanthine oxidase inhibitor on thiopurine metabolism, hyperuricemia and gout. Trans. Assoc. Am. Physicians 76:126, 1963.

148. Wyngaarden, J.B., Rundles, R.W., Silberman, H.R., et al.: Control of hyperuricemia with hydroxypyrazolopyrimidine, a purine analogue which inhibits uric acid synthesis. Arthritis Rheum. 6:306, 1963.

149. Massey, V., Komai, H., Palmer, G., et al.: On the mechanism of inactivation of xanthine oxidase by allopurinol and other pyrazolo(3,4-d)pyrimidines. J. Biol. Chem. 245:2837, 1970.

150. Elion, G.B.: Enzymatic and metabolic studies with allopurinol. Ann. Rheum. Dis. 25:608, 1966.

151. Rundles, R.W., Wyngaarden, J.B., Hitchings, G.H., et al.: Drugs and uric acid. Ann. Rev. Pharmacol. 9:345, 1969.

152. Elion, G.B., Kovensky, A., Hitchings, G.H., et al.: Metabolic studies of allopurinol, an inhibitor of xanthine oxidase. Biochem. Pharmacol. 15:863, 1966.

153. Hande, K., Reed, E., and Chabner, B.: Allopurinol kinetics. Clin. Pharmacol. Ther. 23:598, 1978.

154. McCollister, R.J., Gilbert, W.R., Jr., Ashton, D.M., et al.: Pseudo-feed-back inhibition of purine synthesis by 6-mercaptopurine ribonucleotide and other purine analogues. J. Biol. Chem. 239:1560, 1964.

155. Krenitsky, T.A., Elion, G.B., Strelitz, R.A., et al.: Ribonucleosides of allopurinol and oxoallopurinol. J. Biol. Chem. 242:2675, 1967.

156. Elion, G.B., Yu, T-F., Gutman, A.B., et al.: Renal clearance of oxipurinol, the chief metabolite of allopurinol. Am. J. Med. 45:69, 1968.

157. Nelson, D.J., Bugge, C.J.L., Krasny, H.C., et al.: Formation of nucleo-tides of 6-¹⁴C allopurinol and 6-¹⁴C oxipurinol in rat tissues and effects on uridine nucleotide pools. Biochem. Pharmacol. 22:2003, 1973.

158. Beardmore, T.D., and Kelley, W.N.: Mechanism of allopurinol-mediated inhibition of pyrimidine biosynthesis. J. Lab. Clin. Med. 78:696, 1971.

159. Chalmers, R.A., Kromer, H., Scott, J.T., et al.: A comparative study of the xanthine oxidase inhibitors, allopurinol and oxipurinol in man. Clin. Sci. 35:353, 1968.

160. Wyngaarden, J.B., Rundles, R.W., and Metz, E.N.: Allopurinol in the treatment of gout. Ann. Intern. Med. 62:842, 1965.

161. Rundles, R.W., Metz, E.N., and Silberman, H.R.: Allopurinol in the treatment of gout. Ann. Intern. Med. 64:229, 1966.

162. Klinenberg, J.R., Goldfinger, S.E., and Seegmiller, J.E.: The effectiveness of the xanthine oxidase inhibitor allopurinol in the treatment of gout. Ann. Intern. Med. 62:639, 1965.

163. Yu, T-F., and Gutman, A.B.: Effects of allopurinol (4-hydroxypyra-zolo(3,4-d)pyrimidine) on serum and urinary uric acid in primary and secondary gout. Am. J. Med. 37:885, 1964.

164. Dayton, P.G., Amor, B., Auscher, C., et al.: Treatment of gout with allopurinol, a study of 106 cases. Ann. Rheum. Dis. 25:627, 1966.

165. Kelley, W.N., Greene, M.L., Rosenbloom, F.M., et al.: Hypoxanthine-guanine phosphoribosyltransferase deficiency in gout. Ann. Intern. Med. 70:155, 1969.

166. Emmerson, B.T.: Discussion, symposium on allopurinol. Ann. Rheum. Dis. 25:621, 1966.

167. Kelley, W.N., Rosenbloom, F.M., Miller, J., et al.: An enzymatic basis for variation in response to allopurinol. N. Engl. J. Med. 278:287, 1968.

168. Caskey, C.T., Ashton, D.M., and Wyngaarden, J.B.: The enzymology of feedback inhibition of glutamine phosphoribosylpyrophosphate ami-dotransferase by purine ribonucleotides. J. Biol. Chem. 239:2570, 1964.

169. Fox, I.H., Wyngaarden, J.B., and Kelley, W.N.: Depletion of erythrocyte phosphoribosylpyrophosphate in man, a newly observed effect of al-lopurinol. N. Engl. J. Med. 283:1177, 1970.

170. Elion, G.B., and Nelson, D.J.: Ribonucleotides of allopurinol and oxi-purinol in rat tissues and their significance in purine metabolism. In Sperling, O., De Vries, A., and Wyngaarden, J.B. (eds.): Purine Me-tabolism in Man. New York, Plenum Press, 1974, p. 639.

171. Holmes, E.W., McDonald, J.A., McCord, J.M., et al.: Human glutamine phosphoribosylpyrophosphate amidotransferase: Kinetic and regula-tory properties. J. Biol. Chem. 248:144, 1973.

172. Wood, A.W., and Seegmiller, J.E.: Properties of 5-phosphoribosyl-1-pyrophosphate amidotransferase from human lymphoblasts. J. Biol. Chem. 248:138, 1973.

173. Pomales, R., Bieber, S., Friedman, R., et al.: Augmentation of the in-corporation of hypoxanthine into nucleic acids by the administration of an inhibitor of xanthine oxidase. Biochim. Biophys. Acta 72:119, 1963.

174. Pomales, R., Elion, G.B., and Hitchings, G.H.: Xanthine as a precursor of nucleic acid purines in the mouse. Biochim. Biophys. Acta 95:505, 1965.

175. Edwards, N.L., Recker, D., Airozo, D., et al.: Enhanced purine salvage during allopurinol therapy: An important pharmacologic property in humans. J. Lab. Clin. Med. 98:673, 1981.

176. Fox, R.M., Royse-Smith, D., and O'Sullivan, W.J.: Orotidinuria induced by allopurinol. Science 168:861, 1970.

177. Kelley, W.N., and Beardmore, T.D.: Allopurinol: Alteration in pyrimi-dine metabolism in man. Science 169:388, 1970.

178. Beardmore, T.D., Fox, I.H., and Kelley, W.N.: Effect of allopurinol on ɒyrimidine metabolism in the Lesch-Nyhan syndrome. Lancet 2:830, 1970.

179. Hatfield, D., and Wyngaarden, J.B.: 3-Ribosylpurines. I. Synthesis of (3-ribosyluric acid) 5'-phosphate and (3-ribosylxanthine) 5'-phosphate by a pyrimidine ribonucleotide pyrophosphorylase of beef erythrocytes. J. Biol. Chem. 239:2580, 1964.

180. Hatfield, D., and Wyngaarden, J.B.: 3-Ribosylpurines. II. Studies on (3-ribosylxanthine) 5'-phosphate and on ribonucleotide derivatives of cer-tain uracil analogues. J. Biol. Chem. 239:2587, 1964.

181. Beardmore, T.D., Cashman, J., and Kelley, W.N.: Mechanism of allo-purinol-mediated increase in enzyme activity in man. J. Clin. Invest. 51:1823, 1972.

182. Grobner, W., and Kelley, W.N.: Effect of allopurinol and its metabolic derivatives on the configuration of human orotate phosphoribosyl-transferase and orotidine 5'-phosphate decarboxylase. Biochem. Phar-macol. 24:379, 1975.

183. Fox, R.M., Wood, M.H., and O'Sullivan, W.J.: Studies on the coordinate activity and lability of orotidylate phosphoribosyltransferase and de-carboxylase in human erythrocytes and the effects of allopurinol admin-istration. J. Clin. Invest. 50:1050, 1971.

184. Becking, G.C., and Johnson, W.J.: The inhibition of tryptophan pyrrolase by allopurinol, an inhibitor of xanthine oxidase. Can. J. Biochem. 45:1667, 1967.

185. Chytil, F.: Activation of liver tryptophan oxygenase by adenosine 3',5'-phosphate and by other purine derivatives. J. Biol. Chem. 243:893, 1968.

186. Ghosh, D., and Forrest, H.S.: Inhibition of tryptophan pyrrolase by some naturally occurring pteridines. Arch. Biochem. 120:578, 1967.

187. Julian, J., and Chytil, F.: Participation of xanthine oxidase in the acti-vation of liver tryptophan pyrrolase. J. Biol. Chem. 245:1161, 1970.

188. Krenitsky, T.A., Elion, G.B., Henderson, A.M., et al.: Inhibition of human purine nucleoside phosphorylase. Studies with intact erythro-cytes and the purified enzyme. J. Biol. Chem. 243:2876, 1968.

189. Gallo, R.C., Parry, S., and Breitman, T.R.: Inhibition of human leukocyte pyrimidine deoxynucleoside synthesis by allopurinol and 6-mercapto-purine. Biochem. Pharmacol. 17:2185, 1968.

190. Truseve, R., and Williams, V.: The effect of allopurinol on urate oxidase activity. Biochem. Pharmacol. 17:165, 1968.

191. Johns, D.G.: Human liver aldehyde oxidase: Differential inhibition of oxidation of charged and uncharged substrates. J. Clin. Invest. 46:1492, 1967.

192. Stevenson, A.C., Silcock, S.R., and Scott, J.T.: Absence of chromosome damage in human lymphocytes exposed to allopurinol and oxipurinol. Ann. Rheum. Dis. 35:143, 1976.

193. Friedman, H.M., and T. Grasela: Adenine arabinoside and allopurinol: Possible adverse drug interaction. N. Engl. J. Med. 304:423, 1981.

194. Boston Collaborative Drug Surveillance Program: Allopurinol and cy-totoxic drugs. Interaction in relation to bone marrow depression. JAMA 227:1036, 1974.

195. Vesell, E.S., Passananti, G.T., and Greene, F.E.: Impairment of drug metabolism in man by allopurinol and nortriptyline. N. Engl. J. Med. 283:1484, 1970.

196. Boston Collaborative Drug Surveillance Program: Excess of ampicillin rashes associated with allopurinol or hyperuricemia. N. Engl. J. Med. 286:505, 1972.

197. Young, J.L., Jr., Boswell, R.B., and Nies, A.S.: Severe allopurinol hy-persensitivity: Association with thiazides and prior renal compromise. Arch. Intern. Med. 134:553, 1974.

198. Wood, M.H., O'Sullivan, W.J., Wilson, M., and Tiller, D.J.: Potentiation of an effect of allopurinol on pyrimidine metabolism by chlorothiazide in man. Clin. Exp. Pharmacol. Physiol. 1:53, 1974.

199. Goldfarb, E., and Smyth, C.J.: Effects of allopurinol, a xanthine oxidase inhibitor, and sulfinpyrazone upon the urinary and serum urate con-centrations in eight patients with tophaceous gout. Arthritis Rheum. 9:414, 1966.

200. Kelley, W.N., and Wyngaarden, J.B.: The effect of dietary purine re-striction, allopurinol and oxipurinol on the urinary excretion of ultra-violet absorbing compounds. Clin. Chem. 16:707, 713, 1970.

201. Yu, T-F.: The effect of allopurinol in primary and secondary gout. Ar-thritis Rheum. 8:907, 1965.

202. Rodnan, G., Robin, J.A., and Tolchin, S.F.: Efficacy of a single daily dose of allopurinol in gouty hyperuricemia. In Sperling, O., De Vries, A., and Wyngaarden, J.B. (eds.): Purine Metabolism in Man. New York, Plenum Press, 1974, p. 571.

203. Gottlieb, N.L., and Gray, R.G.: Allopurinol-associated hand and foot deformities in chronic tophaceous gout. JAMA 238:1663, 1977.

204. Delbarre, F., Lagrue, G., Frugier, J-C., et al.: Le traitement, par L-allopurinol, de la goutte avec insuffisance rénale. Semin. Hop. Paris 43:644, 1967.

205. Rundles, R.W., Silberman, H.R., Hitchings, G.H., et al.: Effects of xan-thine oxidase inhibitor on clinical manifestations and purine metabolism in gout. Ann. Intern. Med. 60:717, 1964.

206. Delbarre, F., Amor, B., Auscher, C., et al.: Treatment of gout with allopurinol, a study of 106 cases. Ann. Rheum. Dis. 25:627, 1966.

207. Loebl, W.Y., and Scott, J.T.: Withdrawal of allopurinol in patients with gout. Ann. Rheum. Dis. 33:304, 1974.

208. Emmerson, B.T.: The use of the xanthine oxidase inhibitor, allopurinol, in the control of hyperuricemia, gout and uric acid calculi. Aust. Ann. Med. 16:205, 1967.

209. Levin, N.W., and Abrahams, O.L.: Allopurinol in patients with impaired renal function. Ann. Rheum. Dis. 25:681, 1966.

210. Ogryzlo, M.A., Urowitz, M., and Weber, H.M.: Effects of allopurinol on gouty and nongouty uric acid nephropathy. Ann. Rheum. Dis. 25:673, 1966.

211. Stoberg, K-H.: Allopurinol therapy of gout with renal complications. Ann. Rheum. Dis. 25:688, 1966.

212. Rundles, R.W.: Allopurinol in gouty nephropathy and renal dialysis. Ann. Rheum. Dis. 25:694, 1966.

213. Wilson, J.D., Simmonds, H.A., and North, J.D.K.: Allopurinol in the treatment of uremic patients with gout. Ann. Rheum. Dis. 26:136, 1967.

214. Goldfinger, S., Klinenberg, J.R., and Seegmiller, J.E.: The renal excretion of oxypurine. J. Clin. Invest. 44:623, 1965.

215. Sperling, O., Brosh, S., Boer, P., Liberman, U.A., and De Vries, A.: Urinary xanthine stones in an allopurinol-treated gouty with partial deficiency of hypoxanthine-guanine phosphoribosyltransferase. Israel J. Med. Sci. 14:288, 1978.

216. Sorensen, L., and Seegmiller, J.E.: Seminars on the Lesch-Nyhan syndrome: Management and treatment, discussion. Fed. Proc. 27:1097, 1968.

217. Greene, M.L., Fujimoto, W.Y., and Seegmiller, J.E.: Urinary xanthine stones—a rare complication of allopurinol therapy. N. Engl. J. Med. 280:426, 1969.

218. Band, P.R., Silverberg, D.S., and Henderson, J.F.: Xanthine nephropathy in a patient with lymphosarcoma treated with allopurinol. N. Engl. J. Med. 283:354, 1970.

219. Wyngaarden, J.B.: Allopurinol and xanthine nephropathy. N. Engl. J. Med. 283:371, 1970.

220. Ablin, A., Stephens, B.G., Hirata, T., et al.: Nephropathy, xanthinuria, and orotic aciduria complicating Burkitt's lymphoma treated with chemotherapy and allopurinol. Metabolism 21:771, 1972.

221. Watts, R.W.E., Scott, J.T., Chalmers, R.T., et al.: Microscopic studies on skeletal muscle in gout patients treated with allopurinol. Quart. J. Med. 40:1, 1971.

222. Watts, R.E.W., Sneeden, W., and Parker, R.A.: A quantitative study of skeletal muscle purines and pyrazolo(3,4-d)pyrimidines in gout patients treated with allopurinol. Clin. Sci. 41:153, 1971.

223. Landgrebe, A.R., Nyhan, W.L., and Coleman, M.: Urinary tract stones resulting from excretion of oxypurinol. N. Engl. J. Med. 292:626, 1975.

224. Stote, R.M., Smith, L.H., Dubb, J.W., et al.: Oxypurinol nephrolithiasis in regional enteritis secondary to allopurinol therapy. Ann. Int. Med. 92:384, 1980.

225. Straitigos, J.D., Bartsokas, S.K., and Capetanakis, J.: Further experiences with toxic epidermal necrolysis incriminating allopurinol, pyrazolone and derivatives. Br. J. Dermatol. 86:564, 1972.

226. Kantor, G.I.: Toxic epidermal necrolysis, azotemia, and death after allopurinol therapy. JAMA 212:478, 1970.

227. Auerbach, R., and Orentrich, N.: Alopecia and ichthyosis secondary to allopurinol. Arch. Dermatol. 98:104, 1968.

228. Irby, R., Toone, E., and Owen, D., Jr.: Bone marrow depression associated with allopurinol therapy (abstract). Arthritis Rheum. 9:860, 1966.

229. Greenberg, M.D., and Zambrano, S.S.: Aplastic agranulocytosis after allopurinol therapy. Arthritis Rheum. 15:413, 1972.

230. Lidsky, M.D., and Sharp, J.T.: Jaundice with the use of 4-hydroxypyrazolo(3,4-d)pyrimidine (4-HPP) (abstract). Arthritis Rheum. 10:294, 1967.

231. Chawla, S.K., Patel, H.D., Parrino, G.R., Soterakis, J., Lopresti, P.A., and D'Angelo, W.A.: Allopurinol hepatotoxicity. Arthritis Rheum. 20:1546, 1977.

232. Simons, F., Feldman, B., and Gerety, D.: Granulomatous hepatitis in a patient receiving allopurinol. Gastroenterology 62:101, 1972.

233. Swank, L.E., Chejfec, G., and Nemchausky, B.: Allopurinol-induced granulomatous hepatitis with cholangitis and a sarcoid-like reaction. Arch. Intern. Med. 138:997, 1978.

234. Jarzobski, J., Ferry, J., Wombolt, D., et al.: Vasculitis with allopurinol therapy. Am. Heart J. 79:116, 1970.

235. Mills, R.M., Jr.: Severe hypersensitivity reactions associated with allopurinol. JAMA 216:799, 1971.

236. Hande, K.R., Noone, R.M., and Stone, W.J.: Severe allopurinol toxicity: Description and guidelines for prevention in patients with renal insufficiency. Am. J. Med., in press, 1984.

237. Fam, A.G., Paton, T.W., and Chaiton, A.: Reinstitution of allopurinol therapy for gouty arthritis after cutaneous reactions. Can. Med. Assoc. J. 123:128, 1980.

238. Meyrier, A.: Desensitization in a patient with chronic renal disease and severe allergy to allopurinol. Br. Med. J. 1:458, 1976.

239. Griffing, W.L., and O'Duffy, J.D.: Oxipurinol in allopurinol-allergic patients. Clin. Res. 31:803A, 1983.

240. Delbarre, F., Auscher, C., DeGery, A., et al.: Le traitement de la dyspurinie goutteuse par la mercaptopyrazolopyrimidine (MPP: thiopurinol). Presse Med. 76:2329, 1968.

241. Sarre, H., Simon, L., and Claustre, G.: Les urico-frenateurs dans le traitement de la goutte. A propos de 126 cas. Semin. Hop. Paris 46:3295, 1970.

242. Auscher, C., Mercier, N., Pasquier, C., et al.: Allopurinol and thiopurinol: Effect in vivo on urinary oxypurine excretion and rate of synthesis of their ribonucleotides in different enzymatic deficiences. In Sperling, O., De Vries, A., and Wyngaarden, J.B. (eds.): Purine Metabolism in Man. New York, Plenum Press, 1974, p. 657.

243. Delbarre, F., and Auscher, C.: Traitement de la goutte par l'acide uracil-6-carboxylique et ses dérivés. Presse Méd. 71:1765, 1963.

244. Kelley, W.N., Greene, M.L., Fox, I.H., et al.: Effects of orotic acid on purine and lipoprotein metabolism in man. Metabolism 19:1025, 1970.

245. Kelley, W.N., Fox, I.H., and Wyngaarden, J.B.: Regulation of purine biosynthesis in cultured human cells. I. Effects of orotic acid. Biochim. Biophys. Acta 216:512, 1970.

246. Lieberman, I., Kornberg, A., and Simms, E.S.: Enzymatic synthesis of uridine 5'-phosphate. J. Biol. Chem. 215:403, 1955.

247. Higgins, J.R., Ashton, D.M., Speas, M., et al.: An evaluation of relative roles of substrate diversion and feedback inhibition in the control of purine synthesis. Clin. Res. 9:181, 1961.

248. Standerfer, S.B., and Handler, P.: Fatty liver induced by orotic acid feeding. Proc. Soc. Exp. Biol. Med. 90:270, 1955.

249. Creasey, W.A., Hankin, L., and Handschumacher, R.E.: Fatty livers induced by orotic acid. I. Accumulation and metabolism of lipids. J. Biol. Chem. 236:2064, 1961.

250. Altman, K.I., Smull, K., and Guzman-Barron, E.S.: A new method for the preparation of uricase and the effect of uricase on the blood uric acid levels of the chicken. Arch. Biochem. 21:158, 1949.

251. London, M., and Hudson, P.B.: Uricolytic activity of purified uricase in two human beings. Science 125:937, 1957.

252. Royer, R., Vindel, J., Lamarche, M., et al.: Modalités d'élimination des purines au cours du traitement enzymatique de la goutte et des états hyperuricémiques par une urateoxydase. Presse Méd. 76:2325, 1968.

253. Kissel, P., Lamarche, M., and Royer, R.: Modification of uricemia and the excretion of uric acid nitrogen by an enzyme of fungal origin. Nature 217:72, 1968.

254. Brogard, J.M., Frankhauser, J.I., and Stahl, A.: Application de l'uricolyse enzymatique au traitement des hyperuricémies d'origine rénale. Schweiz. Med. Wochenschr. 103:404, 1973.

255. Brogard, J.M., Stahl, A., and Stahl, J.: Enzymatic uricolysis and its use in therapy. In Kelley, W.N., and Weiner, I.M. (eds.): Uric Acid. Berlin, Springer-Verlag, 1978, pp. 515–524.

Chapter 57

Colchicine

Stanley L. Wallace

INTRODUCTION

Colchicine is an ancient and traditional drug in the treatment of acute gout. Extracts of the plant *Colchicum autumnale,* also called the meadow saffron or the autumn crocus, have been utilized for this purpose at least since the sixth century A.D., when Alexander of Tralles first described such use.[1] However, undoubtedly because of the strong purgative effect, colchicine had lost its place in therapy by the seventeenth century.[2] Nicholas Husson, a French Army officer, reintroduced colchicum as a secret ingredient of L'eau Medicinale, a patent medicine panacea first offered in 1780.[3] L'eau Medicinale was shown to be particularly effective in acute gout. Want, in 1814, demonstrated that the active ingredient in this nostrum was colchicum.[4] Pelletier and Caventou[5] determined in 1820 that the active ingredient of colchicum was the alkaloid colchicine. The pure preparation has been in constant use for the treatment of gout for the past 160 years.

STRUCTURE-FUNCTION RELATIONSHIPS

The structure of the colchicine molecule was established in 1945 by Dewar.[6] The molecule has three rings; the first is benzenoid and the second and third are 7 carbon rings (Fig. 57–1). The first ring has three methoxyl groups attached. The second has an acetylamino side chain, while ring C is an analogue of tropolone methyl ether, with a ketone group and a methoxyl group attached to adjacent carbons (Fig. 57–2). The tropolonoid nature of the side chains of the third ring implies a resonating hydrogen shared by both side chains.

In a three-dimensional crystallographic study of desacetylmethylcolchicine, the benzenoid ring (ring A) and the ring with tropolonoid configuration (ring C) were planar, forming a dihedral angle of 54 degrees.[7] The other seven carbon ring was folded into a boatlike conformation. The two necessary structures for colchicine's activity on tubulin (see below) are the first and third rings and their side chains; the second ring plays little or no role.

Tropolone methyl ether is a precise analogue of ring C of colchicine. Andreu and Timasheff found that this simple molecule was capable of binding to a single site on the tubulin molecule.[8] The binding of tropolone methyl ether or of colchicine to tubulin inhibited the binding of the other, indicating that the two substances bound to the same site. Both tropolone and tropolone methyl ether inhibited tubulin polymerization into microtubules in vitro.[8]

Figure 57–2. Tropolone methyl ether and tropolone.

Mescaline is an analogue of the trimethoxyphenyl structure of the first colchicine ring. N-Acetylmescaline also binds to tubulin, and the binding is inhibited by colchicine. N-Acetylmescaline partly inhibits microtubular assembly. Studies by Andreu and Timasheff and others[8,9] indicated that colchicine was a bifunctional ligand that interacted with tubulin at two sites, presumably at the tropolone (ring C) and trimethoxyphenyl (ring A) locations. The evidence suggested that the tropolone endbound first, and that this binding induced in the tubulin a conformational change, bringing the trimethoxyphenyl binding site into proper position for this ring to fall into place on the protein.[8]

Garland reported that for each tubulin dimer, there was only one tight binding site for colchicine,[10] and the rate of binding was slow. It was again concluded that colchicine induced a conformational change in the tubulin dimer. The optical activity of a portion of the colchicine molecule, related to the tropolonoid configuration of the third ring, disappeared when colchicine was bound to tubulin. These results implied a conformational change in colchicine itself during binding, separate from a change in tubulin.[11]

The role of ring B in colchicine-tubulin binding was studied.[12] A wide variation in structure of the B-ring moiety was tolerated by the colchicine-binding site of tubulin. Even an analogue combining an A ring and a C ring, without significant representation of a B-ring-like structure, was able to inhibit colchicine-tubulin binding considerably.[12]

	R¹	R²	R³	R⁴
Colchicine	CH_3	$COCH_3$	O	OCH_3
Desacetylmethylcolchicine	CH_3	CH_3	O	OCH_3
Desacetylthiocolchicine	CH_3	H	O	SCH_3
Colchicoside	$C_6H_{11}O_5$	$COCH_3$	O	OCH_3
Trimethylcolchicinic acid	CH_3	H	O	OH
Colchiceine	CH_3	$COCH_3$	OH	O

Figure 57–1. Central colchicine nucleus.

Possible correlations between the structure of colchicine and of selected analogues, and their effects in the treatment of acute gout in man have been studied.[13,14] The colchicine analogues tested were desacetylmethylcolchicine, desacetylthiocolchicine, colchicoside, trimethylcolchicinic acid and colchiceine. The differences between each of these analogues and colchicine are shown in Figure 57–1. The conclusion of these early studies was that the tropolonoid configuration of the third ring was necessary for colchicine's antigout effect.[13,14] Animal data are less clear.[15-17] There is a significant degree of species variability and much less animal responsiveness to concentrations of colchicine that are effective in the human.[18]

Colchicine is highly sensitive to light. Exposure to sunlight or to ultraviolet light leads to the formation of three photoisomers, α, β, and γ lumicolchicine.[19,20] The photoisomers do not retain the tropolonoid structure of colchicine, although the trimethoxyl side chains of ring A persist. The lumicolchicines have not been tested in clinical acute gout, but they did not bind to tubulin[21] and were ineffective in arresting mitosis in metaphase in a variety of tissues.[21-23]

MECHANISM OF ACTION

Borisy and Taylor first demonstrated that colchicine bound to tubulin, the microtubule subunit protein.[24] This binding interfered with the aggregation of these subunits into microtubules. The formation of a colchicine-tubulin dimer was a prerequisite for the prevention of tubulin aggregation, since free colchicine did not itself detectably inhibit microtubule assembly.[25] A single colchicine-tubulin dimer complex bound to the microtubule assembly end, decreasing the rate of addition of free tubulin dimer. The colchicine-bound tubulin dimers dissociated significantly more slowly than the normal dissociation of tubulin dimers, in effect producing a tight "cap" at the assembly-end of the microtubule.[26] The colchicine binding stabilized a conformational isomer of tubulin. This change in tubulin conformation, after binding to colchicine, may lead both to increased affinity of the colchicine-tubulin complexes for microtubule assembly ends and to decreased affinity of free tubulin for the same assembly ends once the colchicine-tubulin complex is already there.[27]

Malawista[28,29] has presented strong arguments for the position that colchicine's mechanism of action in the treatment of acute gouty inflammation depends upon the effect on microtubules. Polymorphonuclear leukocytes are necessary for the propagation of urate crystal–induced inflammation,[30,31] and they have been shown to contain microtubules, which disappear or diminish on exposure to colchicine.[32] Phagocytosis in human polymorphonuclear cells is accompanied by a rapid assembly of microtubules, followed by disassembly.[33] Colchicine-induced microtubule disassembly is associated with cell membrane alterations in leukocytes and macrophages. The topography of cell membranes in general, as well

as membrane receptor mobility, is controlled by the cell cytoskeleton, including microtubules.[33,34] Membrane receptors for phagocytic particles are distributed topographically in a different manner after colchicine therapy than under normal cell circumstances. The precise relation of colchicine-induced membrane alterations to changes in polymorphonuclear leukocyte function is not completely clear. There is little doubt that in polymorphonuclear leukocytes, colchicine's membrane effect is mediated by microtubules.[35-37] The membrane-dependent processes of chemotaxis, phagocytosis, and lysosomal degranulation in neutrophils are all influenced by the cytoskeleton. Microtubules have been assigned the roles of directing molecular reorganization of neutrophil membranes and of providing orientation to gross membrane activities.[37]

There has been some suggestion of a direct colchicine effect on membranes, an effect not involving microtubules.[38,39] Colchicine affected the shape and surface ultrastructure of both human leukocytes and red blood cells in a similar fashion.[40] Since red blood cells do not contain microtubules, the inference was that this membrane effect, even in the leukocyte, did not require microtubules. Other evidence includes the lack of correlation between the inhibitory effect of colchicine on mast cell secretion of histamine and its action on mast cell microtubules,[41] and the differences between colchicine binding by mammalian liver cell nuclear membranes[42] and by their microtubules.[43]

Many leukocyte functions are sensitive to colchicine in vitro,[29] although most of these studies have been carried out at concentrations higher than those achievable in vivo with doses of therapeutic size.[18,44,45] Colchicine has been shown to inhibit lysosomal enzyme release from human polymorphonuclear leukocytes in a dose-related fashion.[46] In patients treated with 0.6 to 1.8 mg per day of colchicine to prevent recurrences of familial Mediterranean fever, neutrophils were capable of normal phagocytosis, produced normal amounts of pyrogen, and migrated normally, both randomly and in response to chemotactic stimuli.[47] Skin window responses were normal for the first 9 hours of study, but at 24 hours the mean number of neutrophils and monocytes was significantly reduced in colchicine-treated patients compared with controls.[47]

Thirteen patients with acute gout were treated with colchicine by mouth, until toxicity, in doses up to 6 mg in 24 hours. Then daily oral doses of 1.8 mg were given for one week. A statistically significant drop in phagocytic capacity and in phagocytic rate was found in comparison to pretreatment values.[48] The disparity in results may represent methodologic differences in these studies.

A variety of studies have demonstrated colchicine effects on polymorphonuclear leukocyte adherence and locomotion.[49-54] In one in vivo human experiment, 5 mg of colchicine given orally over 24 hours induced a reduction in the percentage of neutrophils adherent to nylon fiber columns, and a less marked change in random migration.[49] The daily administration for 8 days of

1 mg of colchicine to volunteers caused reductions in neutrophil chemotaxis within 24 hours of ingestion.[50]

Phagocytosis of urate crystals by human polymorphonuclear leukocytes induced the synthesis and release of an 8400 molecular weight glycoprotein by the cell. The glycoprotein had strong chemotactic activity that was not associated with complement.[51] This chemotactic factor was not a major mediator in other rheumatic diseases. Colchicine decreased both the production and the release by white cells of this urate crystal–associated chemotactic factor. The purified factor itself induced marked joint inflammation, which was not prevented by colchicine. It was suggested that preventing the production and release of the crystal-associated chemotactic factor, after phagocytosis of urate crystals, might explain the quasi-specificity of colchicine in the treatment of acute gout.[51]

Functional studies of migration of leukocytes in a millipore filter system showed that colchicine markedly inhibited directed migration (chemotaxis), had no effect on random migration, and minimally decreased activated random migration.[52] However, studies of leukocyte migration in filters involve a number of cell functions in addition to chemotaxis, including locomotion, orientation, and deformability of the cell. The last factor, deformability, was indirectly evaluated by measuring the effect of colchicine on leukocyte chemotaxis in an agarose system.[53] Deformability played a minor role in agarose, since the leukocytes were not required to squeeze through tortuous spaces as in the filter system. Colchicine in agarose had no effect on polymorphonuclear leukocyte locomotion or chemotaxis,[53] although presumably microtubules were affected. These findings suggested a dissociation between microtubule assembly and polymorphonuclear cell orientation.

In another study, colchicine was found to inhibit chemokinesis rather than chemotaxis;[54] again it was concluded that the integrity of microtubule function was not necessary for cells to discern a concentration gradient or to react with directional motion. Evidence has previously been adduced suggesting a separation between colchicine's effect on tubulin and its ability to interfere with urate crystal-induced inflammation. An analogue, trimethylcolchicinic acid, was effective in the therapy of acute gout in man,[55,56] inhibited the release of lysosomal enzymes on phagocytosis of urate crystals,[57] and interfered with the leukocyte response to a chemotactic stimulus, at least in a filter system,[58] but had no effect on tubulin[59] and was not antimitotic. Desacetamido-colchicine, on the other hand, had greater antimitotic potency than colchicine, but had very little antiinflammatory effect against urate crystal–induced inflammation.[15]

The phagocytic synoviocyte is involved in the mechanisms of acute inflammation induced in the joint by the urate crystal, as well as the polymorphonuclear leukocyte.[60,61] Colchicine at a concentration of 10^{-7} M induced the release of large amounts of prostaglandin E in rat peritoneal macrophages.[62] Colchicine also enhanced prostaglandin synthesis in human synovium,[63] although no direct studies of the effect of colchicine specifically on the phagocytic synovial cell have been reported. Colchicine did not affect phagocytosis in monocytes but did inhibit the release of monocytic lysosomal enzymes during phagocytosis.[64]

COLCHICINE–cAMP

It was initially suggested that cyclic AMP inhibited and cyclic GMP promoted the assembly of microtubules in leukocytes.[65] Subsequent studies demonstrated that the increased cyclic AMP levels developed as a consequence of microtubule assembly rather than as a cause.[66] Colchicine and other agents that interfere with microtubule assembly caused an increase in human leukocyte cyclic AMP levels.[67] They also potentiated beta-adrenergic and PGE stimulation of cyclic AMP levels. The effect of colchicine was mediated through cytoplasmic microtubules, rather than occurring as a direct effect on cell membranes or on the hormone receptor or on adenylate cyclase activity.[68] It was suggested that the mechanism for the cAMP effects of colchicine might be through a cytoplasmic microtubule influence on the mobility of membrane proteins, enabling an increased frequency of interaction between a hormone-hormone receptor-GTP-binding protein complex and the catalytic moiety of adenylate cyclase. Other observers denied an influence on cell membrane fluidity[69] but invoked a colchicine effect on GTP and GTPase as a possible mechanism for stimulating cAMP production.

There are two GTP-binding sites for each dimer of tubulin. One site is easily exchangeable with free GTP; the second is nonexchangeable, and GTP hydrolysis occurs at the exchangeable site only. Microtubule assembly is followed by the hydrolysis of exchangeable site GTP to GDP.[70] This facilitates depolymerization of the microtubule and permits the tubulin to cycle between dimer and microtubule. The hydrolysis of GTP accompanying microtubular assembly occurred in a kinetic first-order process following assembly, but kinetically uncoupled from it.[71] Colchicine, although it inhibited tubulin polymerization, stimulated GTPase activity of the protein.[71-73] The GTPase activity occurred with the formation of tubulin-colchicine complexes.[73] Tropolone, however, had no effect on GTP hydrolysis; most likely the trimethoxyl-benzene first ring moiety of the colchicine molecule was chiefly responsible for its effect on GTP hydrolysis.[72]

Colchicine also both stimulated the release of prostaglandin E by a variety of cells (see above)[62,63,74] and in turn increased tissue sensitivity and responsiveness to prostaglandin E stimulation.[67,74,75] In the rat jejunum, colchicine caused a marked increase in mucosal PGE_2 content, adenylate cyclase activity, and mucosal cAMP.[76] Pretreatment with indomethacin reduced the degree of change in adenylate cyclase.

COLCHICINE METABOLISM

Two general approaches for measuring colchicine in body fluids and cells have been reported in recent years. Colchicine labeled with ^{14}C on the methoxyl group of the third ring was used as a tracer in the first method;[18] the label was therefore within the tropolonoid structure shown to be necessary for colchicine's effect on microtubules[21-23] and for its action in the treatment in acute gout.[13,14] Thin-layer chromatography was used for separation.

The second approach involved radioimmunoassay.[44] Initially colchicine itself was conjugated to bovine serum albumin; the site of conjugation was in the tropolone structure of the third ring. Subsequent radioimmunoassay methods used colchicine analogues;[45,77-79] the binding site for several of these studies was on the amino group side chain of ring B.[45,77,78] The antisera therefore could be expected to have 100 percent cross-reactivity with lumicolchicine.[77] Three derivatives of colchicine have been synthesized and characterized to serve as haptens for the development of radioimmunoassay procedures.[79] The haptens were linked to bovine serum albumin through ring A, ring B, and ring C side chains.

With the use of the ^{14}C label,[18] after intravenous administration of 2 mg, the calculated zero-time concentration of colchicine was 1.8 ± 0.7 μg per dl. The apparent volume of distribution for colchicine was much larger than the extracellular volume, averaging 2.19 ± 0.80 liters per kg of body weight. The plasma half-time was only 19.3 ± 7.5 minutes. Excretion did not explain the rapid disappearance or large volume of distribution; clearly colchicine rapidly entered cells.

Radioimmunoassay as a method for measuring colchicine levels was more sensitive than the ^{14}C label, thin-layer chromatography approach. Following an intravenous dose of 1 mg, the colchicine levels declined biexponentially, fitting a two-compartment open body model, both in normal humans and in patients with familial Mediterranean fever.[45] A short distribution phase, with a 3- to 5-minute half-time, was followed by a longer elimination phase, with a 65 ± 15 minute half-time.[45] Central and peripheral compartment volumes were 10 to 14 liters and 49.5 to 76 liters. A study by radioimmunoassay after an intravenous dose of 2 mg, and using a single compartment model, found a mean half-time of 58 ± 10 minutes.[44] The calculated zero-time concentration with this method was 2.9 ± 1.5 μg per dl.

Studies of the plasma levels of colchicine after oral administration of 1 mg have also been accomplished.[45,77,80] Peak plasma concentrations, using the ^{14}C label, were achieved from 0.5 to 2 hours after oral administration.[80] The mean maximal plasma levels were around 0.2 μg per dl, approximately one-tenth the calculated zero-time concentration achieved after intravenous administration of twice the dose.[18] Similar concentrations, of 0.1 to 0.25 μg per dl,[45] after oral administration of 1 mg were measured in one radioimmunoassay study.

Another radioimmunoassay method, however, reported larger peak levels of 0.6 μg per dl.[77]

Circulating leukocytes represent an excellent tissue for measurement of colchicine entry into and concentration within cells. Leukocytes are easily accessible and are necessary for urate crystal–induced inflammation.[30,31] The first study of leukocyte concentrations of colchicine, after intravenous administration of the drug, using measurement by ^{14}C label, demonstrated a peak concentration at 10 minutes; stable levels of approximately ten times plasma concentration were maintained for 24 hours.[81] The drop in levels was slow; significant white cell concentrations of colchicine were measurable as late as 10 days after the single dose. White cell concentrations were also studied by radioimmunoassay after intravenous administration of colchicine.[82] The results differed from those obtained with ^{14}C; white cell concentrations reached plasma levels only at 24 hours but remained higher thereafter. At 96 hours after intravenous administration, the mean white cell concentration was 1.4 μg per dl.

The location of the colchicine gastrointestinal absorption site or sites is not specifically known. The administration of large doses of colchicine orally induces jejunal[83] and ileal dysfunction;[84] absorption therefore most likely occurs in the jejunum and ileum. After absorption, colchicine is carried to the liver. Biliary excretion of colchicine in animals, involving active transport against concentration gradients, has been demonstrated after intravenous administration.[85] Hepatic transport of colchicine is also evidenced by the fact that plasma colchicine levels in patients with severe liver disease were higher than in normals.[18] Enterohepatic recirculation is probable.

Maximal urinary excretion occurred within two hours after intravenous administration of colchicine.[44] Significant measurable amounts of colchicine were found in the urine for periods up to 10 days after a single intravenous dose.[44,81] Late urinary excretion presumably arose from previously cell-bound colchicine. As noted above, leukocyte concentrations of colchicine were still measurable 10 days after a single intravenous dose.[81] Colchicine excretion occurs in the feces as well as in urine but has not yet been quantitated there in humans.

With the use of either ^{14}C or radioimmunoassay methods, studies of colchicine metabolism have failed to demonstrate metabolites in plasma, urine, or cells.[18,44,80,81] In an in vitro system simulating the oxidative reactions of liver microsomes, colchicine was converted to four metabolic products, primarily involving oxidative monodemethylation.[86] In vitro metabolism of colchicine by mammalian liver microsomes has been shown, again by monodemethylation.[87] It is not clear why metabolites, if they do occur in vivo, have not been identified.

TOXICOLOGY

Approximately 80 percent of patients receiving a full therapeutic course of colchicine by mouth in the treatment of acute gout develop hyperperistalsis, abdominal cramping pain, diarrhea, and nausea or vomiting. In the process of transport across the jejunal and ileal mucosal cell membrane, enough colchicine must bind to microtubules in these cells to alter function and produce symptoms. In human volunteers receiving colchicine by mouth in doses ranging from 1.9 to 3.6 mg per day, for periods ranging from 4 days to 3 weeks,[83,84,88-90] all developed jejunal and ileal dysfunction. Jejunal effects included decreased absorption of D-xylose[83] and a fall in serum carotene levels.[90] Reduced jejunal mucosal lactase and sucrase activity was noted.[83] Histologic studies on jejunal mucosa during colchicine therapy revealed edema and round cell infiltration in 3 of 5 patients.[83] In the rat, colchicine stimulated jejunal adenylate cyclase activity, and significantly increased mucosal cAMP content.[76] Colchicine also induced increases in prostaglandin E_2, which in turn mediated increases in intestinal fluid volume.[76]

Ileal effects in human volunteers were manifested by decreased vitamin B_{12} absorption, increased excretion of fecal bile acids and sterols, most likely due to impaired reabsorption of acidic and neutral sterols in the distal ileum, and a consequent drop in serum cholesterol.[88-90] There were marked and consistent increases in fecal sodium and potassium and less marked increases in fecal nitrogen.

A single report of azoospermia in a patient on colchicine prophylactic therapy has been recorded.[91] A number of other studies, however, have revealed no effects on sperm counts, luteinizing hormone, follicle-stimulating hormone, testosterone, or prolactin levels induced in patients receiving prophylactic doses of colchicine.[92-94]

Colchicine overdoses, whether therapeutic[95] or suicidal,[96] can lead to more severe and more general toxic manifestations. The gastrointestinal side effects described above, when more profound, can cause severe dehydration, hypokalemia, hyponatremia, metabolic acidosis, renal shutdown, and death. Shock can be due to profound dehydration or to septicemia secondary to severe intestinal wall damage. Death has occurred after doses as small as 7 mg[97] or 10 mg[98] given in 4 or 5 days. Death is invariable after fairly rapid ingestion of more than 40 mg.[96] The risks of toxicity are greater in patients with chronic liver or kidney disease, because both organs are excretory pathways for colchicine.[18]

In colchicine overdose, the earliest hematologic manifestation of colchicine toxicity is disseminated intravascular coagulation;[99] the most severe changes occur at about 25 hours after the ingestion of a single, large suicidal dose. Marrow failure, characterized by leukopenia, thrombocytopenia, and bleeding, reaches its peak at about the fifth day.[99] Other toxic manifestations of colchicine overdose include hepatocellular failure and late central nervous system dysfunction, with seizures and loss of deep tendon reflexes.[96]

In a review of the use of colchicine as a suicidal drug, 28 of 36 patients were female.[100] When the ages were known, two thirds were under 20; the mean age was 23

$\pm$ 8. Taking of colchicine was generally impulsive and not designed to result in death. The choice of drug was considered a blatant gesture of getting even with the male parent.

Treatment of colchicine overdose is symptomatic, including gastric lavage if the patient is seen early enough after ingestion. Subsequent therapy is directed at the various manifestations of toxicity. Dehydration, electrolyte imbalance, metabolic acidosis, and shock must be corrected, infection eliminated, and seizures controlled. The patient must be supported during disseminated intravascular coagulation and marrow failure.

Attempts at hemodialysis and exchange transfusion have failed.[101] Since so little colchicine is present in blood,[18,44] dialysis and exchange transfusions would not be expected to be useful procedures. Some method for accelerating colchicine release from microtubules and from cells would be necessary first, without cell death, before approaches for removing colchicine from the blood could be of value.

References

1. Hartung, E.F.: History of the use of colchicum and related medicaments in gout. Ann. Rheum. Dis. 13:190, 1954.
2. Culpeper, N.: Pharmacopoiea Londonensis or the London Dispensatory. 6th Ed. London, Peter Cole, 1654, p. 4.
3. Wallace, S.L.: Colchicum, the panacea. Bull. N.Y. Acad. Med. 40:130, 1973.
4. Copeman, W.S.C.: A Short History of the Gout and the Rheumatic Diseases. Berkeley-Los Angeles, University of California Press, 1964.
5. Pelletier, P.S., and Caventou, J.B.: Examen chimique de plusiers végétaux de la famille des colchicées et du principe actif qu'ils renferment. Ann. Chim. Phys. 14:69, 1820.
6. Dewar, M.J.S.: Structure of colchicine. Nature 155:141, 1945.
7. Margulies, T.N.: Structure of the mitotic spindle inhibitor Colcemid. N-desacetyl-N-methylcolchicine. J. Am. Chem. Soc. 96:899, 1974.
8. Andreu, J.M. and Timasheff, S.N. Interaction of tubulin with single ring analogues of colchicine. Biochemistry 21:534, 1982.
9. Cortese, F., Bhattacharayya, B., and Wolff, J.: Podophyllotoxin as a probe for the colchicine-binding site of tubulin. J. Biol. Chem. 252:1134, 1977.
10. Garland, D.L.: Kinetics and mechanism of colchicine binding to tubulin: Evidence for ligand-induced conformational change. Biochemistry 17:4266, 1978.
11. Detrich, H.W., Williams, R.C., MacDonald, T.L., Wilson, L., and Puett, D.: Changes in the circular dichroic spectrum of colchicine associated with its binding to tubulin. Biochemistry 20:5999, 1981.
12. Ray, K., Bhattacharayya, B., and Biswas, B.B.: Role of B-ring of colchicine in its binding to tubulin. J. Biol. Chem. 256:6241, 1981.
13. Wallace, S.L.: Colchicine analogues in the treatment of acute gout. Arthritis. Rheum. 2:389, 1959.
14. Wallace, S.L.: Colchicine: Clinical pharmacology in acute gouty arthritis. Am. J. Med. 30:439, 1961.
15. Fitzgerald, T.J., Williams, B., and Uyeki, E.: Colchicine on sodium urate-induced paw swelling in mice: Structure-activity relationships of colchicine derivatives. Proc. Soc. Exp. Biol. Med. 136:115, 1971.
16. Zweig, M.H., Maling, H.M., and Webster, M.E.: Inhibition of sodium urate rat hind paw edema by colchicine derivatives. Correlation with antimitotic activity. J. Pharmacol. Exp. Ther. 182:344, 1972.
17. Chang, Y.H., and Malawista, S.E.: Mechanisms of action of colchicine IV. Failure of non-leukopenic doses of colchicine to suppress urate crystal-induced canine joint inflammation. Inflammation 1:143, 1976.
18. Wallace, S.L., Omokoku, B., and Ertel, N.H.: Colchicine plasma levels: Implications as to pharmacology and mechanisms of action. Am. J. Med. 48:443, 1970.
19. Grewe, L., and Wolfe, W.: Unwandlung des Colchizins durch Sonnenlicht. Chem. Ber. 84:621, 1951.
20. Wilson, L., and Friedkin, M.: The biochemical events of mitosis. I. Synthesis and properties of colchicine labelled with tritium in its acetyl moiety. Biochemistry 5:2463, 1966.
21. Wilson, L., and Friedkin, M.: The biochemical events of mitosis. II. The in vivo and in vitro binding of colchicine in grasshopper embryos and its possible relation to the inhibition of mitosis. Biochemistry 6:3126, 1967.

22. Sagorin, C., Ertel, N.H., and Wallace, S.L.: Photoisomerization of colchicine. Loss of significant antimitotic activity in tissue culture. Arthritis. Rheum. 15:213, 1972.

23. Linskens, H.F., and Wulf, W.: Uber die Trennung und Mitosewirkung der Lumicolchicine. Naturwissenschaften 40:487, 1953.

24. Borisy, G.G., and Taylor, E.W.: The mechanism of action of colchicine. Binding of colchicine-H^3 to cellular protein. J. Cell Biol. 34:525, 1967.

25. Farrell, K.W., and Wilson, L.: Proposed mechanism for colchicine poisoning of microtubules reassembled in vitro from Strongylocentrotus purpuratus sperm tail outer doublet tubulin. Biochemistry 19:3048, 1980.

26. Margolis, R.L., Rauch, C.T., and Wilson, L.: Mechanism of colchicine-dimer addition to microtubule ends: Implications for the microtubule polymerization mechanism. Biochemistry 19:5550, 1980.

27. Detrich, H.W., Williams, R.C., and Wilson, K.: Effect of colchicine binding on the reversible dissociation of the tubulin dimer. Biochemistry 21:2392, 1982.

28. Malawista, S.E.: Colchicine: A common mechanism for its anti-inflammatory and antimitotic effect. Arthritis Rheum. 11:191, 1968.

29. Malawista, S.E.: The action of colchicine in acute gouty arthritis. Arthritis Rheum. 18:835, 1975.

30. Phelps, P., and McCarty, D.J.: Crystal induced inflammation in canine joints. II. Importance of the polymorphonuclear leukocytes. J. Exp. Med. 124:115, 1966.

31. Chang, Y.H., and Gralla, E.J.: Suppression of urate crystal–induced canine joint inflammation by heterologous anti-polymorphonuclear leukocyte serum. Arthritis Rheum. 11:145, 1968.

32. Malawista, S.E., and Bensch, K.G.: Human polymorphonuclear leukocytes: Demonstration of microtubules and effect of colchicine. Science 156:521, 1967.

33. Walter, R.J., Berlin, R.D., Pfeiffer, J.R., and Oliver, J.M.: Polarization of endocytosis and receptor topography in cultured macrophages. J. Cell Biol. 86:199, 1980.

34. Devirgilius, L.C., Dini, L., Stefanini, S., and Autori, F.: Cytoskeletal control of concavalin A receptor mobility in isolated rat hepatocytes. Cell. Mol. Biol. 26:533, 1980.

35. Becker, J.S., Oliver, J.M, and Berlin, R.D.: Fluorescence techniques for following interactions of microtubules and membranes. Nature 254:152, 1975.

36. Berlin, R.D., and Fera, J.P.: Changes in membrane microviscosity associated with phagocytosis: Effects of colchicine. Proc. Soc. Natl. Acad. Sci. 74:1072, 1977.

37. Oliver, J.M.: Cell biology of leukocyte abnormalities—membrane and cystoskeletal function in normal and defective cells. Am. J. Pathol. 93:221, 1978.

38. Alstiel, L.D., and Landsberger, F.R.: Interaction of colchicine with phosphatidylcholine membranes. Nature 269:70, 1977.

39. Wunderlich, F., Muller, R., and Speth, V.: Direct evidence for a colchicine-induced impairment in the mobility of membrane component. Science 182:1136, 1973.

40. Lichtman, M.A., Santillo, P.A., Kearney, E.A., Roberts, G.W., and Weed, R.I.: The shape and surface morphology of human leukocytes in vitro. Effects of temperature, metabolic inhibitors and agents that influence membrane structure. Blood Cells 2:507, 1976.

41. Lagunoff, D., and Chi, E.Y.: Effect of colchicine on rat mast cells. J. Cell. Biol. 71:182, 1976.

42. Stadler, J., and Franke, W.W.: Characterization of colchicine binding of membrane fractions from rat and mouse liver. J. Cell. Biol. 60:297, 1974.

43. Stadler, J., and Franke, W.W.: Colchicine binding proteins in chromatin and membranes. Nature New Biol. 237:237, 1972.

44. Ertel, N.H., Mittler, J.C., Akgun, S., and Wallace, S.L.: A radioimmunoassay for colchicine in plasma and urine. Science 193:233, 1976.

45. Halkin, H., Dany, S., Greenwald, M., Shnaps, Y., and Tirosh, M.: Colchicine kinetics in patients with familial Mediterranean fever. Clin. Pharm. Ther. 28:82, 1980.

46. Hoffstein, S., Goldstein, I.M., and Weissmann, G.: Role of microtubule assembly in lysosomal enzyme secretion from human polymorphonuclear leukocytes. J. Cell. Biol. 73:242, 1977.

47. Dinarello, C.A., Chusid M.J., Fauci, A.S., Gallin, J.I., Dale, D.C., and Wolff, S.M. Effect of prophylactic colchicine on leukocyte function in patients with familial Mediterranean fever. Arthritis Rheum. 19:618, 1976.

48. Dalleverde, E., Fan, P.T., and Chang, Y-H.: Mechanism of action of colchicine V. Neutrophil adherence and phagocytosis in patients with acute gout treated with colchicine. J. Pharmacol. Exp. Ther. 223:197, 1982.

49. Fordham, J.N., Kirwan, J., Cason, J., and Currey, H.L.F.: Prolonged reduction in polymorphonuclear adhesion following oral colchicine. Ann. Rheum. Dis. 40:605, 1981.

50. Ehrenfeld, M., Levy, M., Bar Eli, M., Gallily, R., and Eliakim, M.: Effect of colchicine on polymorphonuclear leukocyte chemotaxis in human volunteers. Br. J. Clin. Pharmacol. 10:297, 1980.

51. Spilberg, I., Mandell, B., Mehta, J., Simchowitz, L., and Rosenberg, D.: Mechanism of action of colchicine in acute crystal-induced arthritis. J. Clin. Invest. 64:775, 1979.

52. Malech, H.L., Root, R.K., and Gallin, J.I.: Structural analysis of human neutrophil migration. J. Cell. Biol. 75:666, 1977.

53. Daughaday, C.C., Bohrer, A.N., and Spilberg, I.: Lack of effect of colchicine on human neutrophil chemotaxis under agarose. Experientia 137:199, 1981.

54. Valerius, N.H.: In vitro effect of colchicine on neutrophil granulocyte locomotion. Acta Path. Microbiol. Scand. 86B:149, 1978.

55. Wallace, S.L.: Trimethylcolchicinic acid in the treatment of acute gout. Ann. Intern. Med. 54:274, 1961.

56. Smyth, C.J., and Frank, L.S.: Treatment of acute gouty arthritis. Rheumatism 18:2, 1962.

57. Mikulikova, D., and Trnavsky, K.: Influence of colchicine derivatives on lysosomal enzyme release from polymorphonuclear leukocytes. Biochem. Pharmacol. 29:2146, 1980.

58. Phelps, P., and McCarty, D.J.: Crystal-induced arthritis. Postgrad. Med. 45:87, 1969.

59. Mizel, S.B., and Wilson, L.: Nucleoside transport in mammalian cells: inhibition by colchicine. Biochemistry 11:2573, 1972.

60. Agudelo, C.A., and Schumacher, H.R.: The synovitis of acute gouty arthritis: a light and electron microscopic study. Hum. Pathol. 4:265, 1973.

61. Ortel, R.W., and Newcombe, D.S.: Acute gouty arthritis and response to colchicine in the virtual absence of synovial fluid leukocytes. N. Engl. J. Med. 290:1363, 1974.

62. Gemsa, D., Kramer, W., Brenner, M., Tell, G., and Resch, K.: Induction of prostaglandin E. release from macrophages by colchicine. J. Immunol. 124:376, 1980.

63. Robinson, D.R., Smith, H., and Levine, L.: Prostaglandin synthesis by human synovial cultures and its stimulation by colchicine. Arthritis Rheum. 16:129, 1973.

64. Fleer, A., van Schark, M.L.J., Kr, A.E.G., and Engelfriet, C.P.: Destruction of sensitized erythrocytes by human monocytes in vitro: Effects of cytochalasin B., hydrocortisone and colchicine. Scand. J. Immunol. 8:515, 1978.

65. Weissmann, G., Goldstein, I., Hoffstein, S., and Tsung, P.K.: Reciprocal effects of cAMP and cGMP on microtubule-dependent release of lysosomal enzymes. Ann. N.Y. Acad. Sci. 253:750, 1975.

66. Malawista, S.E., Oliver, J.M., and Rudolph, S.A.: Microtubules and cyclic AMP in human leukocytes: on the order of things. J. Cell. Biol. 77:881, 1978.

67. Rudolph, S.A., Greengard, P., and Malawista, S.E.: Effects of colchicine on cyclic AMP levels in human leukocytes. Proc. Nat'l Acad. Sci. 74:3404, 1977.

68. Rudolph, S.A., Hegstrand, L.R., Greengard, P., and Malawista, S.E.: The interaction of colchicine with hormone sensitive adenylate cyclase in human leukocytes. Mol. Pharmacol. 16:805, 1979.

69. Hagmann, J., and Fishman, P.H.: Modulation of adenylate cyclase in intact macrophages by microtubules. J. Biol. Chem. 255:2659, 1980.

70. Timasheff, S.N., and Grisham, L.M.: In vitro assembly of cytoplasmic microtubules. Ann. Rev. Biochem. 49:565, 1980.

71. Hensel, C., and Carlier, M.F.: GTPase activity of the tubulin-colchicine in relation with tubulin-tubulin interactions. Biochem. Biophys. Res. Comm. 103:332, 1981.

72. Lin, C.M., and Hamel, E.: Effects of inhibitors of tubulin polymerization on GTP hydrolysis. J. Biol. Chem. 256:9242, 1981.

73. David-Pfeuty, T., Simon, C., and Pantaloni, D.: Effect of antimitotic drugs on tubulin GTPase activity and self-assembly. J. Biol. Chem. 254:11696, 1979.

74. Burch, R.M., and Halushka, P.V.: Inhibition of prostaglandin synthesis antagonizes the colchicine-induced reduction of vasopressin-stimulated water flow in the toad urinary bladder. Mol. Pharmacol. 21:142, 1982.

75. Gemsa, D., Steggemann, L., Till, G., and Resch, K.: Enhancement of PGE response of macrophages by colchicine. J. Immunol. 119:524, 1977.

76. Rachmilewitz, D., and Karmeli, F.: Effect of colchicine on jejunal adenylate cyclase activity, PGE_2 and cAMP contents. Eur. J. Pharmacol. 67:235, 1980.

77. Scherrmann, J.M., Boudet, L., Pontikis, R., Nguyen-Hong-Nam, and Fournier, E.: A sensitive radioimmunoassay for colchicine. J. Pharm. Pharmacol. 32:800, 1980.

78. Wolff, J., Capraro, H.G., Brossi, A., and Cook, G.H.: Colchicine binding to antibodies. J. Biol. Chem. 255:7144, 1980.

79. Pontikis, R., Scherrmann, J.M., Nguyen-Hong-Nam, Boudet, L., and Pichat, L.: Radioimmunoassay for colchicine: Synthesis and properties of three haptens. J. Immunoassay 1:449, 1980.

80. Wallace, S.L., and Ertel, N.H.: Plasma levels of colchicine after oral administration of a single dose. Metabolism 22:749, 1973.

81. Ertel, N.H., and Wallace, S.L.: Measurement of colchicine in urine and peripheral leukocytes. Clin. Res. 19:348, 1971.
82. Ertel, N.H.: Unpublished data.
83. Race, T.F., Paes, I.C., and Faloon, W.W.: Intestinal malabsorption induced by colchicine. Am. J. Med. Sci. 259:32, 1970.
84. Webb, D.I., Chodos, R.B., Maher, C.Q., and Faloon, W.W.: Mechanism of Vitamin B-12 malabsorption in patients receiving colchicine. N. Engl. J. Med. 279:845, 1968.
85. Hunter, A.L., and Klassen, C.D.: Biliary excretion of colchicine. J. Pharmacol. Exp. Ther. 192:605, 1975.
86. Schoenharting, M., Pfaender, P., Ricker, A., and Siebert, G. The metabolic transformation of colchicine. I. The oxidative formation of products from colchicine in the Udenfriend system. Hoppe-Seyler's Z. Physiol. Chem. 354:421, 1973.
87. Schoenharting, M., Mende, G., and Siebert, G.: The metabolic transformation of colchicine. II. The metabolism of colchicine by mammalian liver microsomes. Hoppe-Seyler's Z. Physiol. Chem. 355:1391, 1974.
88. Faloon, W.W., Webb, D.I., and Race, T.F.: Cholesterol-lowering effect of colchicine. Ann. Intern. Med. 66:1058, 1966.
89. Faloon, W.W.: Drug production of intestinal malabsorption. N.Y. State J. Med. 70:2189, 1970.
90. Rubulis, A., Rubert, M., and Faloon, W.W.: Cholesterol lowering, fecal bile and sterol changes during neomycin and colchicine. J. Clin. Nutr. 23:125, 1970.
91. Merlin, H.E.: Azoospermia caused by colchicine. Fertil. Steril. 23:180, 1972.
92. Bremmer, W.J., and Paulsen, C.A.: Colchicine and testicular function in man. New Engl. J. Med. 294:1384, 1976.
93. Levy, M., and Yaffe, C.: Testicular function in patients with familial Mediterranean fever on long term colchicine therapy. Fertil. Steril. 29:667, 1978.
94. Fukutani, K., Ishida, H., Shinohara, M., Minowada, S., Niijima, T., Hijkata, K., and Izowa, Y.: Suppression of spermatogenesis in patients with Behçet's disease treated with cyclophosphamide and colchicine. Fertil. Steril. 36:76, 1981.
95. Stennerman, G.N., and Hayashi, T.: Colchicine intoxication: A reappraisal of its pathology based on a study of three fatal cases. Hum. Pathol. 2:321, 1971.
96. Gaultier, M., Kaufer, A., Bismuth, C., Crabie, P., and Fregaville, J.-P.: Données actuelles sur l'intoxication aiguë par la colchicine. Ann Med. Interne. 12:605, 1969.
97. McLeod, J.G., and Phillips, L.: Hypersensitivity to colchicine. Ann. Rheum. Dis. 6:224, 1947.
98. Liu, Y.K., Hymovitz, R., and Carroll, M.G.: Marrow aplasia induced by colchicine. Arthritis Rheum. 21:731, 1978.
99. Crabie, P., Pollet, J., and Pebay-Peysoula, F.: Étude de l'hémostase au cours des intoxications aiguës par la colchicine. Eur. J. Toxicol. 3:373, 1970.
100. Baum, J., and Meyerowitz, S.: Colchicine: Its use as a suicidal drug by females. J. Rheumatol. 7:124, 1980.
101. Ellwood, M.G., and Robb, G.H.: Self-poisoning with colchicine. Postgrad. Med. J. 47:129, 1971.

Section V
Rheumatoid Arthritis

Chapter 58
The Etiology of Rheumatoid Arthritis

J. Claude Bennett

INTRODUCTION

Over the past two and a half decades much information has accrued regarding the nature of the inflammatory process and its interface with the immune system. Our views of how the immune response is activated, the nature of its molecular genetic regulation, and how it becomes expressed at the level of effector events have provided better insights into the nature of the rheumatic diseases. Even though there are indications that rheumatoid arthritis is an autoimmune disorder, in the sense that it involves antibodies against autologous immunoglobulin G, there are no solid data from which to infer that this has occurred de novo. On the contrary, there is much data indicating that some initiating event, such as a specific external etiologic agent, is responsible for setting the disease process in motion.

In considering disease phenomena associated with autoimmunity it is important to distinguish between states that are directly mediated by this process and those in which autoantibodies can be demonstrated but whose pathologic effects are unproved. Thrombocytopenic purpura and hemolytic anemia are situations in which there seems to be a true autoimmunity, with antibodies directed at the target cells,[1] leading to their destruction in the peripheral blood. In contrast, occurrence of rheumatoid factors in rheumatoid arthritis, antinuclear antibodies in a variety of connective tissue diseases, and antithyroid antibodies in many patients with diverse conditions are all associated with no obvious specific target pathology. In most of these situations it remains uncertain as to whether the apparent autoimmunity results from the acquisition of some new antigen from an external stimulus or from some primary abnormality in the regulation of the cells that mediate these reactions.[2]

Although the concept of "forbidden clones," as originally expounded by Burnet,[3] dominated our thinking for a while relative to autoimmunity, we came to believe that some kind of alteration of the immunoregulatory system must be at fault in certain of these autoimmune processes. This may be viewed as involving, for example, alteration of the control mechanisms in such a way that

the appropriate balance between immunologic "help" and "suppression" is disrupted.[4] Other levels of immunoregulation apparently are influenced by such things as anti-idiotypic antibodies, as was proposed by Jerne in his "network hypothesis."[5] In this latter concept, antibody itself acts in a manner of continuing regulation so that anti-antibodies from one clone act on the preceding clone to regulate its response. Such intricate regulatory mechanisms are of primary importance for keeping the immune system in smooth operating order. Absence of such regulation conceivably could allow an imbalance, permitting the initiation of an autoimmune process with clinical consequences.

Recently it has been suggested[6] that certain individuals are genetically predisposed to particular autoimmune diseases because they have "preforbidden" clones which may diversify into "forbidden" clones by somatic modification events of the immunoglobulin genome. The obvious prerequisite for such a sequence of events would be that preforbidden clones must have paratopes (receptors for antigen) that are within a few mutational changes of self-reactivity. Observations that certain people and particular animal strains are genetically predisposed to particular autoimmune disorders are compatible with this concept.[7]

On the other hand, examples can be found in which specific external agents seem to initiate an inflammatory arthritis that in many respects parallels true rheumatoid disease. It, therefore, seems logical to assume that an initiating agent activates an immune response in a host of appropriate genetic makeup and that the resultant inflammation leads to continual disease activity. It will be the purpose of this chapter to discuss those etiologic agents that have been studied, or for which model systems exist, in relation to rheumatoid arthritis. Although investigations in the general areas of bacteriology, virology, and immunology have contributed enormously to our understanding of inflammatory disease and host responses, the specific documentation of the etiologic agent in rheumatoid arthritis has proved disappointing. Even though the issue of the events responsible for the initiation of a chronic unrelenting arthritis of the rheumatoid type will be the emphasis of this chapter, other diseases will be discussed occasionally for illustrative purposes.

Perspective on this problem of etiology of rheumatoid arthritis is aided by categorization of the various infectious agents that can be involved in the pathogenesis of arthritis. Pyogenic bacteria, mycobacteria, certain fungi, and certain viruses, such as smallpox, are classic examples of multiplication of the agent directly within the joint space. The second situation is one in which the infectious agent localizes in the joint space and initiates the immune response. Examples of this include Lyme disease,[8] *Mycoplasma hyorhinis* in swine,[8] rubella in man,[10] herpes simplex in rabbits and guinea pigs, and certain organisms that might exist within immune complexes, such as hepatitis B virus[11] or the meningococcus.[12] Among those infections in which the agent is at a distant site but there is an associated immune response that causes arthritis is rheumatic fever, in which cross-reacting streptococcal antigens initiate an autoimmune response. Certain other disorders in which there may be an antecedent infection include those in which we find a Reiter-like syndrome[13] following *Shigella, Salmonella, Yersinia enterocolitica,* or other infections of the gastrointestinal tract. The fourth category represents those arthritides in which there is a toxicogenic process. These are best exemplified by certain of the arbovirus infections, in which there is a direct virus effect on the synovial tissue. Examples of these are chikungunya, O'-nyong-nyong, Mayaro, and Ross River.[14]

The important concept to recognize is that a whole variety of organisms and/or their products may be responsible for initiating an arthritis, if even through multiple and differing mechanisms. When the scope of processes that can be associated with infection and arthritis is realized, one becomes aware of the extraordinary difficulties involved in evaluating the possible etiology of rheumatoid arthritis from this standpoint. It may be that the way in which the host responds to an external agent is of the greatest importance in deciphering *which* events initiate the pathogenic process in *which* individuals.

THE LINK TO GENETICALLY CONTROLLED HOST RESPONSE FACTORS

No relationship is more basic to medicine than that which exists between the inciting agent of disease and the disease susceptibility of the host. Recent discoveries of the relationship of histocompatibility markers to the epidemiology of certain diseases have indicated a strong genetic relationship of these cell-surface molecules to apparent disease susceptibility. The associated molecules include those that are coded for by the major histocompatibility complex (MHC) located on the sixth chromosome.[15] They are specific glycoprotein molecules[16] whose presence as alloantigens has come to be associated strongly with certain rheumatic diseases. These associations are quite striking between HLA-B27 and ankylosing spondylitis, as well as with certain related diseases, including Reiter's syndrome and reactive arthritides.

Studies of the association of specific clinical subsets with the genetic markers coded for by genes within the MHC region have contributed to our knowledge of rheumatoid disease in general. Recent reports suggest that patient response to specific forms of therapy may be related to an individual's genetic make-up, such as the observation that patients with rheumatoid arthritis manifesting toxic responses to chrysotherapy exhibit a significant increase in the HLA-DR3 phenotype.[17] There is also evidence that DR4-positive individuals with seropositive arthritis have a more aggressive form of disease than patients who are DR4 negative. Other studies serve to clarify the relationship of clinical subsets common to different ethnic groups and may provide clues to the level of homogeneity that may exist between these various disease categories and the ethnic groups from which they are derived. Examples for this can be found in recent reports suggesting that blacks with seropositive RA exhibit the same associations with DR4 as are found in whites with seropositive RA.[18] It should be noted that the recent description of new MHC genetic loci, such as the SB locus, which codes for 5 polymorphisms,[19] adds to our repertoire of genetic probes.

The current notion is that the genes coding for the HLA-D or HLA-DR are in fact analogous to the immune response (Ir) genes in the murine major histocompatibility complex and code for some immune response antigens.[20] These relationships are of importance in that all patients who have ankylosing spondylitis are not B27 positive; it is also obvious that all patients who are B27 positive do not have ankylosing spondylitis. It follows then that the B27 marker itself does not cause disease, but rather alerts us to those factors or MHC determinants, such as Ir gene products on the cell surface, that might be more specifically related to the direct disease response and, hence, be a more faithful indication of disease susceptibility.

These observations encourage extensive studies at the epidemiologic level in order to better define host populations at risk and to evaluate familial associations in terms of specific genetic markers relative to expression of disease. Certainly, a combination of appropriate clinical, epidemiologic, and immunogenetic studies is necessary in order to define all these relationships at a population level.

IMMUNE COMPLEXES AND INDUCTION OF THE INFLAMMATORY PROCESS

Although the concept of immune complexes and the inflammatory process in general are the subject of other chapters, it is essential that certain correlations be made here in order that the implications for microbial agents in the etiology of rheumatoid arthritis might be apparent. It seems clear that immune complexes, whether produced in vivo or produced in vitro and injected into animals, can initiate an inflammatory process.[21] Several models exist to document this phenomenon in arthritis.[22] Immune complexes of various sizes and differing immunochemical properties can exist at different times in a given immune response, owing to simple relationships in the molecular parameters of the antigen (its size and valency) and antibody (its amount relative to antigen present in vivo at any time). Inflammation also depends upon the ability of these complexes to fix the first component of complement in order to initiate the complement cascade. It is important in this regard to recognize that our various techniques for detecting immune complexes, including the Raji cell assay, C1q-binding, and rheumatoid factor binding, may measure different kinds of complexes, as judged by the fact that results are not always parallel in all these systems.

In rheumatoid arthritis one cannot overemphasize the extraordinary correlation of antiglobulins (rheumatoid factors) with the presence of the disease.[23] What makes these antiglobulins form? Are they genuine antibodies against autologous 7S IgG? How are rheumatoid factors formed in relation to altered autologous immunoglobulins, and what is the alteration process? These kinds of relationships and questions must be accounted for within any etiologic mechanism that emerges for rheumatoid arthritis.

ORGANISMS IMPLICATED IN THE INITIATION OF THE RHEUMATOID PROCESS

Bacteria. Consideration of the potential infectious etiology of rheumatoid arthritis from the standpoint of modern bacteriology poses some difficulty in the strict application of Koch's postulates. The confusion results from the multiplicity of organisms that have been implicated from time to time in the rheumatic disorders. Although much evidence can be brought to bear to indicate that known microbial infections may be followed by polyarthritis and multisystem rheumatic disease in both animals and man, it is difficult to analyze such a course of events when dealing with human rheumatoid disease. Clearly, what is needed more than anything else in this area of investigation is the application of the tools of molecular microbiology to the problem of how host cells interact with microbes and their components. Such an approach could provide an understanding of how these agents give rise to an unrelenting, yet waxing and waning, course of inflammation.

Although the history of research in the human rheumatic diseases is interlaced with the development of streptococcal microbiology, data confirming that this organism actually initiates inflammatory arthritis as the sole etiologic agent exist only in the case of rheumatic fever.[24] It was this distinction that separated rheumatoid arthritis from "infectious arthritis."[25] The magnificent investigations on rheumatic fever and its relationship to the *Streptococcus* and streptococcal antigens represent

landmark achievements in the history of medicine. At present there is no evidence that human rheumatoid disease is initiated by *Streptococcus*.

Clostridia have been implicated from the studies of Mansson and Olhagen.[26] These researchers have observed that cultivation of feces reveals a high frequency of atypical *Clostridium perfringens* in rheumatoid arthritis and certain other chronic inflammatory rheumatic diseases. The abnormalities that they have noticed include a high count of *Clostridium perfringens,* i.e., more than 100,000 bacteria per gram of feces, and/or a potent alpha toxin production. Clostridia in normal individuals are present in very small numbers in the colon, but in conjunction with certain arthritides they become numerous and they have been observed even extending into the upper jejunum. In these studies, for example, 67 percent of patients with rheumatoid arthritis have abnormal intestinal flora, as indicated by the aforementioned assays. This compares with only 0.9 percent in healthy controls. It is of some significance that these studies have led them to carry out certain experiments involving dietary changes in pigs,[27] so that a change in bacterial flora resulted. This had the secondary effect of producing arthritis in these animals. The postulated mechanism is that a protein-rich diet produced a disturbance in secretory functions of the digestive tract so that clostridial overgrowth could take place. They suggest that this contributes to the development of a rheumatoid-like arthritis in these animals.

Stewart and his colleagues have drawn attention to the possible role that diphtheroid organisms might play in rheumatoid arthritis. They have found that approximately 28 percent of synovial membranes and 10 percent of synovial fluids from patients with rheumatoid arthritis yield diphtheroids.[28] These studies were performed using careful bacteriologic cultural techniques and appropriate controls; the observed differences between the patients with rheumatoid arthritis and the controls seem real. Further, there seems to be a serologic response in terms of agglutination titers to corynebacteria in the rheumatoid patients as compared to normals. These studies face many problems of interpretation in that diphtheroids are widely distributed in nature; they are notoriously difficult to isolate and identify by conventional methods; and they are frequently present as "contaminants" in many microbial cultures. Further, the serologic responses by no means parallel infectivity. Nevertheless, the data are indicative of some association, and it may be that diphtheroids do play a role in rheumatoid arthritis,[29] if only in some way to modify the immune mechanisms of the host. It could be that even if they do not cause rheumatoid arthritis, they might perhaps play some role in modulating its course.

Mycoplasmas have been the target of considerable discussion and investigative pursuit as related to the pathogenesis of rheumatoid arthritis and other arthritides.[30] Several groups of investigators reported the isolation of mycoplasma from both joint fluid and synovial tissues of patients with rheumatoid arthritis. In general, these reports have not been substantiated by results from other laboratories,[31] but interest in the agents continues, in view of the very striking association of animal mycoplasmal diseases with arthritis. Sometimes a close similarity is found between mycoplasma-caused arthritis in animals and rheumatoid arthritis in man. Although clinical evidence for the isolation of a mycoplasma organism in rheumatoid arthritis is very slim, this may be due to difficulties in the cultivation procedures and technical reproducibility. Perhaps these obstacles will be overcome in the future with new approaches to antigen detection and new techniques that will involve a search for the presence of mycoplasma genomes using the probes of molecular biology.[32,33]

Of particular interest to the field of mycoplasmology are investigations into the mode of pathogenicity of chronic infections. Recent work in this area would suggest that these organisms have the ability to associate very closely with the cells of the host organism. The intimate relationship developed by mycoplasma for the host cells is revealed by electron microscopy, and shows a bridging between the organism and the surface of the host lymphoid cells.[34] It has now been shown that mycoplasma adsorbs onto its own surface antigens from mammalian host cells.[35] These include histocompatibility markers of the mammalian cell, as well as certain unique T-lymphocyte antigens. This phenomenon may have its explanation in the fact that the mycoplasma has no real cell wall but only a membrane similar in nature to the external lipid bilayer of the eukaryotic cell.[34] Hence, the organism has the capability of functioning in a manner analogous to a synthetic liposome, and as such is able to take up solubilized molecules shed from cell surfaces.[36] This interaction presumably takes place through hydrophobic molecular interactions. It could be that the ability of the mycoplasma to escape the immune system of the host and to persist chronically is due to alteration of its own cell surface so that it mimics the host cell. It is hoped that at the molecular level the studies of this intimate mycoplasma–host cell association, the immune response of the host and the way in which mycoplasmal evasion of the immune defenses takes place will be fertile areas for investigation.

Viruses. Viruses can cause disease in any of several ways, ranging from acute short-lived infections to those that progress with age and last perhaps a lifetime. The ability of slow viruses to produce tissue pathology and the demonstration of this in the case of human disease may foretell a complete revolution in our understanding of chronic viral infections. Only recently are methods beginning to be developed that will allow us to study many of the diseases that have in the past been considered to have their origin in degenerative processes or in metabolic alterations.[37]

A number of investigators have studied the possible viral etiology of rheumatoid arthritis using both direct culture techniques and several indirect methodologies. Although no single virus has been repeatedly demonstrated in a consistent fashion from one laboratory to the other, some hints of a possible viral involvement in rheumatoid disease have occurred. For example, virus-like particles have been found in the synovium in patients with rheumatoid arthritis.[38] It appears, however, that these same particles are found in a number of different tissues in different disease states and they may represent no more than some sort of organized debris rather than virus or viral products.[39] Interest in the viral etiology of rheumatoid arthritis accelerated when it was found that the rubella virus was unable to infect and replicate in rheumatoid synovial cells.[40] This suggested that there might be a preformed virus already present in the synovial cell which produced the interference. This was of considerable importance, since the technique of interference by latent viruses had been used for some time to study rubella viruses. Unfortunately these original striking observations were not confirmed, and it seems now that rheumatoid synovial cells are able to support the replication of many viruses in the same way as do synovial cells from nonrheumatoid sources.[41]

The experience with kuru[37,42] and the realization of the role of slow viruses in the long-term production of disease have alerted us to the fact that viral infection can involve many patterns of disease and makes the search for filterable agents in rheumatoid tissues a continuing challenge. From time to time, reports of transmissible agents in rheumatoid tissues have appeared.[43] Unfortunately, these are generally not reproduced in other laboratories. It would be presumptive to dismiss all these experiments at this time, but taken in perspective the evidence is slim for a viral infection as a cause of rheumatoid arthritis. The work of Gajdusek and colleagues[37,42] and others in discovering the role of slow viruses in certain chronic diseases of the central nervous system may have a parallel in rheumatoid arthritis, and this possibility is likely to remain as a stimulus to research.

Of specific interest relative to the possible viral etiology of rheumatoid arthritis is the observation of Alspaugh and Tan that the serum of patients with rheumatoid arthritis reacts with an antigen extracted from the Epstein-Barr virus (EBV)–carrying cell line, Wil-2.[44] This rheumatoid arthritis precipitin (RAP) reacts with a nuclear antigen (RANA) extracted exclusively from EBV-infected cells. This antigen (RANA) is related to the Epstein-Barr nuclear antigen (EBNA), yet is distinct from it. Antibody to each develops over the same time course after primary EBV infection.

EBV can modulate the immune system as evidenced by its ability to cause lymphoid proliferation, B-cell activation, and increased immunoglobulin secretion. The data indicate that rheumatoid arthritis patients, as compared with normals, do not regulate in vitro EBV infection as efficiently. Even though one must keep in mind that EBV is not arthrotropic, it could exert special influence on the immune system of rheumatoid arthritis patients. It has been found, for example, that EBV-induced B-cell lines proliferate more rapidly from peripheral blood lymphocytes from patients with rheumatoid arthritis than from normals. This seems to be due to a defective regulation by rheumatoid arthritis T cells. Recently it has been shown that this defect is due to diminished generation of gamma interferon by the T cells.[45] Although we are learning much about the special effects of EBV on immune regulation, it is difficult to implicate the virus as the primary event in rheumatoid arthritis.

Several additional experimental approaches of sound molecular rationale have been pursued in studies of the viral etiology of rheumatoid arthritis. These include (1) serologic surveys of patients with rheumatoid arthritis to obtain clues to a specific antiviral antibody that might be present,[46] (2) an examination of synovial cell cultures for virally induced enzymes, particularly DNA-dependent DNA polymerase and RNA-dependent DNA polymerase,[47] (3) an examination of newly synthesized RNA and DNA by rheumatoid synovial cells to see if molecular parameters compatible with virus molecules were present,[48] and (4) examination of sera from patients with rheumatoid arthritis to test for cytotoxic antibodies that are reactive against lymphoid cell surface antigens, perhaps produced by virus modification.[49] Although these approaches produced interesting information relative to the molecular cell biology of rheumatoid cells, they have not clarified the question of a virus etiology of the disease. On balance the data must be summarized as negative. Clearly, some of the newer tools available for looking for viruses and viral genomes in host tissues, including hybridization methodologies and techniques of electron microscopy, should be applied to examine further the possibility that virus products are present.

Recent data on the type C oncornaviruses are particularly intriguing relative to the way in which viral genomes may be incorporated into a host cell and produce virally related proteins which may be expressed on the surface, thereby modifying the host cell surface antigenic expression.[50] These events have been studied from the standpoint of relevance to human disease, particularly in SLE, by Strand and August.[51] For example, the G_{IX} marker, found on the surface of certain murine lymphoblastoid cells, was described initially as a distinct genetically determined antigen.[52] Although this marker is present on certain cell lines in the absence of virus production, there is an unambiguous demonstration that in the mouse this molecule (G_{IX}) is identical to the gp69/70 viral coat protein of the type C oncornavirus.[53] That this molecule may be expressed on the surface of cells in which the viral genome is present, even though no virion production takes place, encourages further searches for possible new antigenic expression on surfaces of rheumatoid cells. Special note should be made for future studies of RA cells similar to those that have been done to define oncogenes in certain tumor cell lines.[54] Recent evidence for translocation of some oncogenes into the immunoglobulin gene region[55] may be of great importance.

There are several common viral diseases that are associated with inflammatory rheumatic syndromes. The most striking of these is synovitis following rubella infection[10] and the arthritis that may precede the onset of jaundice in infectious hepatitis.[11] Also, the occurrence of hepatitis B antigen–associated polyarteritis[56] should

be mentioned. In view of these situations it must be presumed that rheumatoid arthritis could result from a host immune response to antigens of a yet unknown virus, persisting either in the joint tissues with only localized inflammation or in the form of circulating immune complexes, which results in both systemic and local pathology. These possibilities again emphasize that the syndrome recognized as rheumatoid arthritis could have its origin in diverse etiologies.

ANIMAL MODELS

Mycoplasma Infections. As indicated previously, one of the major factors for considering mycoplasma in a discussion of the etiology of rheumatoid arthritis in man is its striking incrimination as a cause of arthritis in several animal species. Most of these organisms, however, can also be recovered from the respiratory tract, and in some instances, such as the *M. arthritidis* arthritis of rats, the condition is acute and purulent. The mycoplasma-induced arthritides that occur in pigs, mice, and turkeys, however, can often be of long duration and produce a chronic course.[57] In these situations, it is often possible to isolate the organisms from the infected joints only in the early phase of disease. These observations relate to *M. pulmonis* in the mouse and *M. hyorhinis* in pigs. In the latter situation, Barden and Decker[9,58] found it increasingly difficult to isolate the organism from the arthritic joints in the later stages of disease, but they found high titers of antibody in both the serum and joint fluids of these animals. A similar situation exists in the case of *M. gallisepticum* in the turkey arthritis model, but its exact correlation with antibody production is not yet defined. It seems clear from the animal models that mycoplasmas can initiate an arthritic process, and they may provide us with some new experimental tools for studies in man. For example, the strain, the dose, and the route of administration seem particularly important in defining whether or not an arthritis can be associated with a given mycoplasma infection. Furthermore, the newer serologic approaches for looking at mycoplasma antigens should provide some very interesting serologic reagents for analysis of rheumatoid tissues.[34,59] Conversely, the utilization of sera from patients with rheumatoid arthritis to screen for antibodies against known antigens of the mycoplasma may be a useful approach.

Erysipelothrix Arthritis in Pigs. *Erysipelothrix rhusiopathiae,* since its initial description by Löffler in 1885, has become recognized as an important cause of chronic arthritis in pigs, and is the organism most commonly isolated from arthritic joints in this species.[60] It also has marked similarities to rheumatoid arthritis in man and, in fact, in much of the veterinary literature is referred to as "rheumatoid arthritis in pigs." The organism is a small gram-positive nonmotile coccobacillus and will grow on blood agar under aerobic conditions.[61] It will also produce natural infections in a wide variety of domesticated and wild animals and will cause an erysipelas-like disease in man.

The disease caused by *E. rhusiopathiae* in pigs may take one of the following three possible courses: (1) an acute form with a high mortality in untreated cases, (2) a less acute form associated with urticaria and erythematous plaques over the entire body surface, or (3) no clinical evidence of infection but the pig becomes a carrier, with the organism being found in the spleen, tonsils, gut, or bone marrow.

It is in the chronic stages of the disease that arthritis and sometimes endocarditis may occur. Arthritis may also occur following apparent recovery from acute forms of the disease. Interestingly, the onset of arthritis may even be the first indication that the disease is present. This arthritis may be chronic; it may wax and wane and may be unrelenting. It produces a synovial pathology in which the membrane is thickened, villus formation occurs, and the cellular infiltrate is composed of lymphocytes and plasma cells. There is also a tendency to follicle formation.[62] Some investigators have also reported the presence of rheumatoid factor–like molecules in the sera of pigs with erysipelothrix arthritis, but this finding has been inconsistent.[63] Since the data indicate that the arthritis can be present and progress in the absence of living erysipelothrix organisms, much effort is underway at present to see if persistent bacterial debris is responsible for perpetuation of the inflammatory process.

Adjuvant Arthritis. Arthritis is produced[64] following the injection into rats of Freund's adjuvant, a mixture of whole heat-treated acid-fast bacilli, mineral oil, and an emulsifying agent. This occurs without any added tissue homogenate or other bacteria and is given by intradermal injection. Following a latent period of about 2 weeks there develops arthritis and periarthritis, which involves most of the joints and extremities. It is especially severe in the distant small joints of the paws, and also in the tail, presenting as intense red swellings of variable size and painfulness. The intensity of the arthritis waxes and wanes over several weeks, may completely remit, or may be followed by spontaneous recurrences. The general incidence of the disease is reproducible at about the 85 percent level in various strains. A striking aspect of the pathology is extensive extra-articular calcification, resulting finally in tissue destruction and ankylosis.

Current evidence suggests that the arthritogenic properties of bacterial adjuvants reside within the peptidoglycan dimer[65] (see Fig. 58–1). The possible role of peptidoglycans in producing chronic inflammation is a point of great current interest. These molecules are found internal to the capsule and the outer membrane of bacteria, and there is an extraordinary degree of similarity among the peptidoglycans found across the entire spectrum of bacteria. Such similarity of structure is not found among surface antigenic components—for example, those that are used for serologic identification of various types of bacteria. The chemical structure of the peptidoglycan is important for an appreciation of the role that it might have in initiating a chronic inflammatory response (Fig. 58–1). This molecule is an alternating chain of *N*-ace-

Figure 58–1. Structural representation of the peptidoglycan molecule. The basic unit consists of an alternating *N*-acetyl glucosamine and *N*-acetyl muramic acid, to which the peptide side-chain is attached. Polymerization occurs at the time of incorporation into the cell wall. In some bacteria, spacer linkages, such as (Gly)$_5$ or (Ala)$_{2-3}$, are inserted between polymeric units. (From Bennett, J.C.: Arthritis Rheum. 21:531, 1978, by permission.)

tylglucosamine and *N*-acetylmuramic acid. Attached to the lactic acid ether side chain of the muramic acid is a tetrapeptide L-Ala-D-Glu-L-Lys-D-Ala. A fifth residue, D-Ala is present on the precursor molecule before the monomers are polymerized and assembled to form the cell wall.[66] In some cases, the units are coupled directly during polymerization through the L-Ala to one of the L-Lys residues of an adjacent unit. In other cases, there may be a spacer linkage such as (Gly)$_5$ or (Ala)$_{2-3}$.

Cell Wall Antigens: A Streptococcal Model in Rats. Cromartie and associates[67] have shown that a chronic arthritis can be produced in rats by a single intraperitoneal injection of a sterile aqueous suspension of cell wall fragments of bacteria, particularly the *Streptococcus*. The arthritis that results within a week is striking. It is a proliferative, inflammatory, erosive pansynovitis that waxes and wanes but recurs in an unrelenting fashion until total joint destruction results. Evidence again indicates that it is the peptidoglycan-polysaccharide fragment of the cell wall that is responsible for the inflammatory process, just as in the adjuvant model. The differences, however, are that the bacterial constituents are given in aqueous solution, the arthritis is chronic, it is erosive from the very beginning, its pattern of recurrence is even more striking, and there is less extra-articular calcification. In short, it more directly relates to a true model for rheumatoid arthritis.

These studies are reinforced by previous investigations,[68] which examined the development of antibodies to streptococcal antigens in rabbits. These workers reported that occasionally animals immunized with streptococci developed rheumatoid factors that are capable of recognizing both peptidoglycan and the Fc component of IgG. Hence, these observations emphasize the possibility of a relationship between the peptidoglycan and the Fc region. Additional clinical observations reveal that patients with rheumatic fever, juvenile rheumatoid arthritis,[69] and rheumatoid arthritis[70] have antibodies that cross-react with peptidoglycans. These findings may have parallels in studies of patients with bacterial endocarditis, in which bacterial antigens are clearly present as the initiating factors of the inflammatory process.

Some limited studies of chronic rheumatoid arthritis synovial tissue, utilizing very sensitive (10^{-15} M) gas chromatographic and mass spectrographic techniques, have failed to detect bacterial muramic acid.[71] This is strong evidence against the bacterial debris concept for human rheumatoid disease, but studies in the early, more acute stages have not been carried out.

SUMMARY

Available information requires the interlocking of several concepts when considering the etiology of rheumatoid arthritis.[72] These include (1) genetics of the host, (2) the host-immune response, and (3) an inciting agent. The extraordinary achievements of cell biology and molecular genetics provide hope that we will soon be able to understand how these factors work together in the pathogenesis of rheumatoid disease.

References

1. Miescher, P.A., and Muller-Eberhard, H.J.: Textbook of Immunopathology. 2nd ed. New York, Grune & Stratton, 1976.
2. Stites, D.P., Stobo, J.D., Fudenberg, H.H., and Wells, J.V.: Basic and Clinical Immunology. 4th ed. Los Altos, Calif., Lange Medical Publications, 1982.
3. Burnet, F.M.: The Clonal Selection Theory of Acquired Immunity. Nashville and Cambridge, Vanderbilt and Cambridge University Presses, 1959.
4. Gershon, R.K., Eardley, D.D., Durum, S., Green, D.R., Shen, F.W., Yamauchi, K., Cantor, H., and Murphy, D.B.: Contrasuppression: A novel immunoregulatory activity. J. Exp. Med. 153:1533, 1981.
5. Jerne, N.K.: Towards a network theory of the immune system. Ann. Immunol. (Inst. Pasteur) 125c:373, 1974.
6. Knight, J.G.: Autoimmune diseases: Defects in immune specificity rather than a loss of suppressor cells. Immunology Today 3:326, 1982.
7. Knight, J.G., and Adams, D.D: In Receptors, Antibodies and Disease. Ciba Fnd. Sym. 90:35, 1982.
8. Steele, A.C., Bartenhagen, N.M., Craft, J.E., Huchinson, G.J., Newman, J.H., Rahn, D.W., Sigal, L.H., Spieler, P.N., Stenn, K.S., and Malawista, S.E.: The early clinical manifestations of Lyme arthritis. Ann. Intern. Med. 99:76–82, 1983.
9. Barden, J.A., and Decker, J.L.: *Mycoplasma hyorhinis* swine arthritis. I. Clinical and microbiological features. Arthritis Rheum. 14:193, 1971.
10. Ogra, P.L., and Herd, J.K.: Arthritis with induced rubella infection. J. Immunol. 107:810, 1971.
11. Alpert, A., Isselbacher, K.J., and Schur, P.H.: The pathogenesis of arthritis associated with viral hepatitis. N. Engl. J. Med. 285:185, 1971.
12. Whittle, H.C., Abdullahi, M.T., Fakunle, F.A., Greenwood, B.M., Bryceson, A.D.M., Parry, E.H.O., and Turk, J.L.: Allergic complications of meningococcal diseases. I. Clinical aspects. Br. Med. J. 2:733, 1973.
13. Catterall, R.D.: The role of microbial infection in Reiter's syndrome. In Dumonde, D.C. (ed.): Infection and Immunology in the Rheumatic Diseases. Oxford, Blackwell Scientific Publications, 1976.
14. Tesh, R.B. Arthritides caused by mosquito-borne viruses. Ann. Rev. Med. 33:31, 1982.
15. Sasazuki, T., McDevitt, H.O., and Grumet, F.C.: The association between genes in the major histocompatibility complex and disease susceptibility. Ann. Rev. Med. 28:425, 1977.
16. Terhorst, C., Robb, R., Jones, C., and Strominger, J.L.: Further structural studies on the heavy chain of HLA antigens and its similarity to immunoglobulins. Proc. Natl. Acad. Sci. USA 74:4002, 1977.
17. Coblyn, J.S., Weinblatt, M., Holdsworth, D., and Glass, D.: Gold-induced thrombocytopenia; a clinical and immunogenetic study of twenty-three patients. Ann. Intern. Med. 95:178, 1981.
18. Karr, R.W., Rodey, G.E., Lee, T., and Schwartz, B.: Association of HLA DR$_{w4}$ with rheumatoid arthritis in black and white patients. Arthritis Rheum. 23:1241, 1980.
19. Awdeh, Z.L., and Alper, C.A.: Inherited structural polymorphism of the fourth component of human complement. Proc. Natl. Acad. Sci. 77:3576, 1980.
20. Albert, E.D., and Gotze, D.: The major histocompatibility system in man. In Gotze, D. (ed.): The Major Histocompatibility System in Man and Animals. Berlin, Springer-Verlag, 1977.
21. Barnett, E.V.: Circulating immune complexes: Their immunochemistry, detection and importance. Ann. Intern. Med. 91:430, 1979.
22. Jones, J.V.: Autoimmunity and multi-system disease. In Holborow, E.J., and Reeves, W.G. (eds.): Immunology in Medicine. New York and London, Academic Press and Grune & Stratton, 1977.
23. Maini, R.N.: Immunology of Rheumatic Diseases: Aspects of Autoimmunity. London, Edward Arnold, Ltd. 1977.
24. Green, C.A.: Hemolytic streptococcal infections and acute rheumatism. Ann. Rheum. Dis. 3:4, 1942.
25. Copeman, W.S.C.: A Short History of the Gout and the Rheumatic Diseases. Berkeley, University of California Press, 1964.
26. Mansson, I., and Olhagen, B.: Fecal *Clostridium perfringens* and rheumatoid arthritis. J. Infect. Dis. 130:444, 1974.
27. Mansson, I., Norberg, R., Olhagen, B., and Bjorklund, N.E.: Arthritis in pigs induced by dietary factors. Clin. Exp. Immunol. 9:677, 1971.
28. Stewart, S.M., Alexander, W.R.M., and Duthie, J.J.R.: Isolation of diphtheroid bacilli from synovial membrane and fluid in rheumatoid arthritis. Ann. Rheum. Dis. 28:477, 1969.
29. Bartholomew, L.E., and Bartholomew, F.N.: Antigenic bacterial polysaccharide in rheumatoid synovial effusions. Arthritis Rheum. 22:969, 1979.
30. Taylor-Robinson, D., and Taylor, G.: Do mycoplasmas cause rheumatic disease? In Dumonde, D.C. (ed.): Infection and Immunology in the Rheumatic Diseases. Oxford, Blackwell Scientific Publications, 1976.
31. Cassell, G.H. and Cole, B.C.: Mycoplasmas as agents of human disease. New Engl. J. Med. 304:80, 1981.
32. Cole, B.C., Griffiths, M.M., Eichwald, E.J., and Ward, J.R.: New models of chronic synovitis in rabbits induced by mycoplasmas: Microbiological, histopathological, and immunological observation in rabbits injected with *Mycoplasma arthritidis* and *Mycoplasma pulmonis*. Infect. Immun. 16:383, 1977.
33. Cohen, S.N.: The manipulation of genes. Sci. Am. 233:24, 1975.
34. Cassell, G.H., Davies, J.K., Wilburn, W., and Wise, K.S.: Pathobiology of mycoplasmas. In Schlessinger, D. (ed.): Microbiology 1978. Washington, D.C., American Society of Microbiology, 1978.
35. Wise, K.S., Acton, R.T., and Cassell, G.H.: Selective association of murine T-lymphoblastoid cell surface alloantigens with *Mycoplasma hyorhinis*. Proc. Natl. Acad. Sci. USA 75:4479, 1978.
36. Bouma, S.R., Drislane, F.W., and Huestis, W.H.: Selective extraction of membrane-bound proteins by phospholipid vesicles. J. Biol. Chem. 252:6759, 1977.
37. Gajdusek, D.C.: Unconventional viruses and the origin and disappearance of kuru. Science 197:943, 1977.
38. Schumacher, H.R.: Synovial membrane and fluid morphologic alterations in early rheumatoid arthritis: Microvascular injury and virus-like particles. Ann. N.Y. Acad. Sci. 256:39, 1975.
39. Baringer, J.R.: Tubular aggregates in endoplasmic reticulum in herpes simplex encephalitis. N. Engl. J. Med. 285:943, 1971.
40. Grayzel, A.I., and Beck, C.: Rubella infection of synovial cells and the resistance of cells derived from patients with rheumatoid arthritis. J. Exp. Med. 131:367, 1970.
41. Person, D.A., Rawls, W.E., and Sharp, J.T.: Replication of rubella, Newcastle disease and vesicular stomatitis viruses in cultured rheumatoid synovial cells. Proc. Soc. Exp. Biol. Med. 138:748, 1971.
42. Gajdusek, D.C., and Gibbs, C.J.: Transmission of kuru from man to rhesus monkey (*Macaca mulata*) 8¼ years from inoculation. Nature 240:351, 1972.
43. Warren, S.L., Marmor, M.D., Leonard, M.D., Liebes, D.M., and Hollins, R.: An active agent from human rheumatoid arthritis which is transmissible in mice. Arch. Intern. Med. 124:629, 1969.
44. Alspaugh, M.A. and Tan, E.M.: Serum antibody in rheumatoid arthritis reactive with a cell-associated antigen: Demonstration by precipitation and immunofluorescence. Arthritis Rheum. 19:711, 1976.
45. Hasler, F., Bluestein, H.G., Zvaifler, N.J. and Epstein, L.B.: Analysis of the defects responsible for the impaired regulation of Epstein-Barr virus-induced B cell proliferation by rheumatoid arthritis lymphocytes. J. Exp. Med. 157:173, 1983.

46. Chandler, R.W., Robinson, H., and Masi, A.T.: Serological investigations for evidence of an infectious etiology of rheumatoid arthritis. Ann. Rheum. Dis. 30:274, 1971.

47. Spruance, S.L., Richards, O.C., Smith, C.B., and Ward, J.R.: DNA polymerase activity of cultured rheumatoid synovial cells. Arthritis Rheum. 18:229, 1975.

48. Person, D.A., Sharp, J.T., and Rawls, W.E.: A search for viruses and mycoplasmas in connective tissue diseases. Arthritis Rheum. 16:677, 1973.

49. Person, D.A., Sharp. J.T., and Lidsky, M.D.: The cytotoxicity of leukocytes and lymphocytes from patients with rheumatoid arthritis for synovial cells. J. Clin. Invest. 58:690, 1976.

50. August, J.T., and Strand, M.: Type-C oncornaviruses and autoimmunity. Arthritis Rheum. 20:S64, 1977.

51. Strand, M., and August, J.T.: Type-C RNA virus gene expression in human tissue. J. Virol. 14:1584, 1974.

52. Boyse, E.A.: The G_{IX} system in relation to C-type viruses and heredity. Immunol. Rev. 33:125, 1977.

53. Lerner, R.A., Wilson, C.B., Del Vilano, B.C., McConahey, P.J., and Dixon, F.J.: Endogenous oncornaviral gene expression in adult and fetal mice: Quantitative histologic and physiologic studies of the major viral glycoprotein, gp70. J. Exp. Med. 143:151, 1976.

54. Reshani, G., Givol, D. and Canaani, E.: Activation of a cellular oncogene by DNA rearrangement: possible involvement of an IS-like element. Nature 300:607, 1982.

55. Marcu, K.B., Harris, L.J., Stanton, L.W., Erickson, J., Watt, R., and Croce, C.M.: Transcriptionally active c-myc oncogene is contained within NIARD, a DNA sequence associated with chromosome translocation in B cell neoplasia. Proc. Natl. Acad. Sci. 80:519, 1983.

56. Gocke, D.J., Hsu, K., Morgan, C., Bombardieri, S., Lockshin, M., and Christian, C.L.: Association between polyarteritis and Australia antigen. Lancet 2:1149, 1970.

57. Ross, R.F.: Pathogenicity of swine mycoplasmas. Ann. N.Y. Acad. Sci. 225:347, 1973.

58. Decker, J.L., and Barden, J.A.: Mycoplasma arthritis in the pig. *In* Dumonde, D.C. (ed.): Infection and Immunology in the Rheumatic Diseases. Oxford, Blackwell Scientific Publications, 1976.

59. Brown, T.McP., Bailey, J.S., Felts, W.R., and Clark, H.W.: Mycoplasma antibodies in synovia. Arthritis Rheum. 9:495, 1966.

60. Ward, A.R.: The etiology of polyarthritis in swine. J. Am. Vet. Med. Assoc. 61:155, 1922.

61. Packer, R.A.: The use of sodium azide and crystal violet in a selective medium for streptococci and *Erysipelothrix rhusiopathiae.* J. Bacteriol. 46:343, 1943.

62. Drew, R.A.: Erysipelothrix arthritis in pigs as a comparative model for rheumatoid arthritis. Proc. R. Soc. Med. 65:994, 1972.

63. Timoney, J.: Antibody and rheumatoid factor in synovia of pigs with erysipelothrix arthritis. J. Comp. Pathol. 81:243, 1971.

64. Pearson, C.M.: Development of arthritis, periarthritis and periostitis in rats given adjuvants. Proc. Soc. Exp. Biol. Med. 91:95, 1956.

65. Kohashi, O., Pearson, C.M., Watanabe, Y., Kotani, S., and Koga, T.: Structural requirements for arthritogenicity of peptidoglycans from *Staphylococcus aureus* and *Lactobacillus plantarum* analogous synthetic compounds. J. Immunol. 116:1635, 1976.

66. Schleifer, K.H., and Seidl, H.P.: Structure and immunological aspects of peptidoglycans. *In* Schlessinger, D. (ed.): Microbiology 1977. Washington, D.C., American Society for Microbiology, 1977.

67. Cromartie, W.J., Craddock, J.G., Schwab, J.H., Anderle, S.K., and Yang, C.H.: Arthritis in rats after systemic injection of streptococcal cells or cell walls. J. Exp. Med. 146:1585, 1977.

68. Bokisch, V.A., Chiao, J.W., Bernstein, D., and Krause, R.M.: Homogeneous rabbit 7S anti-IgG with antibody specificity for peptidoglycan. J. Exp. Med. 138:1184, 1973.

69. Heymer, B., Schleifer, K.H., Read, S., Zabriske, J.B., and Krause, R.M.: Detection of antibodies to bacterial cell wall peptidoglycan in human sera. J. Immunol. 117:23, 1976.

70. Braun, D.G., and Holm, S.E.: Streptococcal anti-group A precipitins in sera from patients with rheumatic arthritis and acute glomerulonephritis. Int. Arch. Allergy 37:216, 1970.

71. Prtichard, D.G., Settine, R.L. and Bennett, J.C.: Sensitive mass spectrometric procedure for the detection of bacterial cell wall components in rheumatoid joints. Arthritis Rheum. 23:608, 1980.

72. Bennett. J.C.: The infectious etiology of rheumatoid arthritis: New considerations. Arthritis Rheum. 21:531, 1978.

Chapter 59

Pathogenesis of Rheumatoid Arthritis

Edward D. Harris, Jr.

INTRODUCTION

In order to treat rheumatoid arthritis effectively, a physician must understand the sequence that occurs within the joints and extra-articular tissues. After the initial inflammatory events, multiple systems of inflammation, cellular proliferation, and autacoid production are activated. Each activated system affects and amplifies others. Many different biologic responses are generated simultaneously.

The Stages of Rheumatoid Arthritis. Although beginning as nonspecific inflammation within the joint, rheumatoid arthritis (RA) progresses to a proliferative lesion within the synovium that can lead to joint destruction. The inflammatory lesion generates and drives the proliferative one. The rate of progression of the disease within an individual patient depends upon both the intensity and the chronicity of the disease. The disease of a patient who has intermittent flares of synovitis

will not progress as rapidly to joint destruction as that of one who has virtually continuous manifestations of synovitis. Similarly, the patient with a high grade of inflammation will progress to loss of joint function much more rapidly than the individual with a low-grade inflammatory response.

The stages in the pathogenesis of RA, chosen arbitrarily but of interest for discussion, are outlined in Table 59–1.

A WORKING SCHEME FOR THE PATHOGENESIS OF RHEUMATOID ARTHRITIS

The scheme outlined here and in Table 59–1 is based on data that will be discussed subsequently.

1. An immune response of the host is triggered and is sufficiently strong to perturb the host systems, which

Table 59-1. The Pathophysiology of Rheumatoid Arthritis

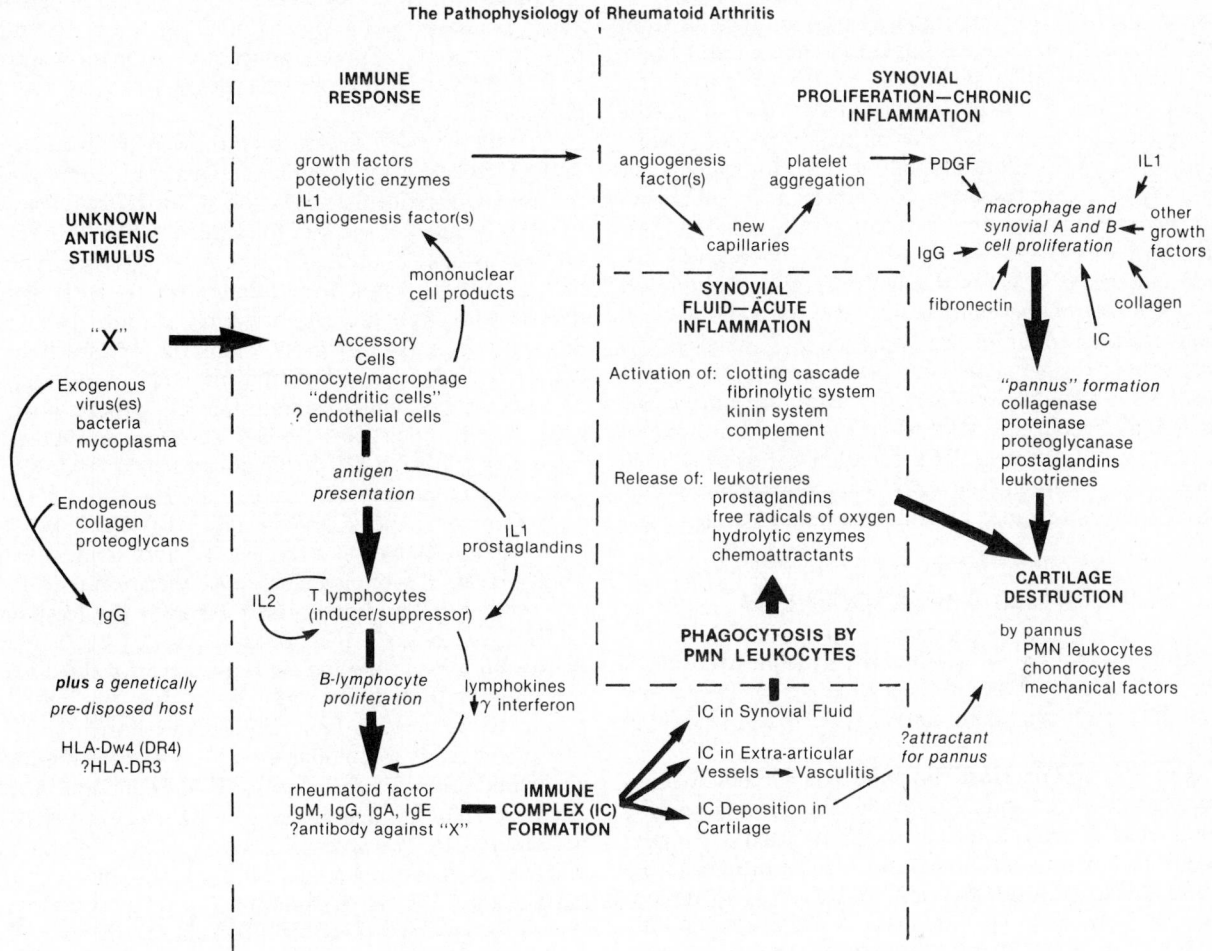

The Pathophysiology of Rheumatoid Arthritis

produce an inflammatory response directed against the self or nonself antigen(s). A major determinant in this process is the genetically controlled immune response, which programs the mode and intensity with which the antigen is recognized and the degree to which the immune response is amplified and the antigen localized.

2. In the synovial fluid the immune response catalyzes activation of many processes which interact to produce a self-sustaining active inflammation within the joint space. These systems include complement, kinins, clotting and fibrinolysis, phagocytosis by leukocytes, and lysosomal enzyme release by the same cells. Polymorphonuclear (PMN) leukocytes are attracted to the joint space by C5a and by leukotriene B_4 formed during the inflammatory response. During phagocytosis of debris and/or immune complexes the PMN leukocytes release proteolytic enzymes (elastase and collagenase), prostaglandins, and free radicals of oxygen.

3. In the synovium large numbers of helper T lymphocytes cluster about HLA-DR$^+$ (Ia$^+$) macrophage/dendritic cells. These cells are probably involved in the presentation of antigen to T lymphocytes. Induction of antibody formation by B lymphocytes follows. Rheumatoid patients may not be able to regulate polyclonal

B-lymphocyte proliferation (in response to the putative infectious agent and/or Epstein-Barr virus infection) which results from these inductive stimuli. At present it is believed that there are subsets among HLA-DR$^+$ cells, some of which can present antigen to T lymphocytes and others which cannot.

4. Antigen-antibody complexes form within the joint cavity and in avascular hyaline and fibrocartilage. This trapping may be mediated primarily by charge differences among matrix macromolecules and the immunoglobulins.

5. Mediators produced by interaction of mononuclear cells (and, perhaps, mast cells) stimulate target cells (i.e., synovial cells) to proliferate and to produce proteinases and prostaglandins. Deeper in the subsynovial layers, fibroblasts are activated to produce more connective tissue matrix.

6. In response to soluble products of activated mononuclear cells as well as other factors (see Chapter 13), endothelial cells begin to sprout and angiogenesis of capillaries begins. Without this development of new vessels the hypertrophied synovium could not be sustained.

7. The lesion becomes polarized. There is inflammation generated by phagocytosis of antigen-antibody com-

plexes in the synovial fluid and a marked proliferative response in the synovium. Beginning at the periphery of the joint, the synovium organizes into an invasive front and begins to replace cartilage and subchondral bone, utilizing several different enzyme systems. Neutral proteinases released by the synovial (pannus) cells and by recruited chondrocytes break up aggregates of proteoglycans. This, in effect, solubilizes them for pinocytosis and continued degradation by cathepsin D, sulfatases, and enzymes specific for the carbohydrate moieties. Elastase cleaves crosslinked regions among collagen fibrils, and collagenase cleaves the helical region. Solubilized collagen fragments spontaneously denature and are further catabolized by neutral proteinases, cathepsin B1, and other collagenolytic cathepsins. Fragments of collagen have strong chemotactic attraction for monocytes as well as fibroblasts. Mineral is resorbed from bone as osteoclasts are activated by prostaglandins or by soluble products of mononuclear cells. The demineralized substrate is then degraded by collagenases and proteinases.

DETAILS OF PATHOGENESIS

The remainder of this chapter will attempt to correlate the pathology with events occurring within the synovium, in the synovial fluid, and at the cell-cartilage junction.

The Susceptible Host: Immunogenetics and RA. As emphasized in Chapter 58, the likelihood of a specific single virus or infective agent being isolated as a cause of all rheumatoid arthritis is small. The difference between those who develop RA and those who do not may relate more to individual variations in the immune response than to selective contact with a specific etiologic agent (Table 59–1).

The most compelling of recent data linking genetic control of the immune response to RA is that demonstrating the association of the HLA-D4 locus to this disease. In two studies, 51 percent[1] and 36 percent[2] of patients with RA possessed the Dw4 haplotype compared with 13 percent and 7 percent of controls, respectively. D-related (DR) alloantigens of B lymphocytes (as well as macrophages, sperm, and vascular endothelium) are more easily assayed because, as with HLA-A, HLA-B, and HLA-C loci, serologic testing can be performed. HLA-DR4 has been reported in 70 percent of rheumatoid patients but in only 28 percent of controls.[3] It is of interest that HLA-DR typing of 59 individuals revealed a highly significant relationship (p < 0.0001) between HLA-DR4 and responsiveness of peripheral blood mononuclear cells to denatured collagen.[4] These studies are strong support for the hypothesis that genes linked to coding for HLA-DR4 constitute true immune response (Ir) genes for T lymphocyte-dependent reactivity to collagen.

Although HLA-DR4 has been convincingly associated with RA (a relative risk of 8.02) and positive tests for rheumatoid factor, data regarding "seronegative RA" have been inconsistent. In one recent study in which rigid diagnostic criteria were used, no statistically significant difference between seronegative RA patients and 123 control subjects was noted in the distribution of DR antigens.[5] Those seronegative patients who did have DR4 had a more rapidly progressive, destructive disease.

There are some exceptions to the general association of the DR4 locus and rheumatoid arthritis. For example, no increased frequency of HLA-Dw4 or HLA-DR4 was found in women of the Yakima Indian nation with rheumatoid arthritis,[6] although RA is a slightly atypical disease in these people (e.g., primary erosive wrist/MCP disease with high titers of antinuclear antibody in addition to rheumatoid factor). Similarly, 49 Israeli Jews with RA had no association with DR4;[7] seronegative patients were not included in this group. Other nonwhite rheumatoid populations studied have had an increased frequency of HLA-DR4, including blacks and Mexicans[8] and Japanese.[9]

In summary, the HLA-D4 and HLA-DR4 loci are probably associated with the genes determining susceptibility to an immunologic response that results in RA.

"Agent X": The Factor That Initiates the Response in RA. As noted in the previous chapter by Bennett, the search for one specific causative agent of the disease continues, although the promise of ever finding that "agent X" is perhaps less secure than before.

Proteoglycans and collagen are examples of endogenous candidates for the cause of RA. Induction in rats of an arthritis that may become chronic and erosive can be achieved by systemic injection of basic components of bacterial or mycobacterial cell walls that include peptidoglycans.[10,11] It is possible that bacterial peptidoglycans or oligosaccharides could become associated with proteoglycans being produced in connective tissue, and that these altered matrix components would become immunogenic and arthritogenic.[12]

Similarly, both humoral and cellular immunity to collagen and its denatured form (gelatin) have been demonstrated in RA. Circulating antibodies to collagen in RA have been noted, although these are not specific to certain types of collagen and do not correlate with the activity of the disease.[13] Forty percent of patients with serum antibodies to collagen (type I, native and denatured) have them in synovial fluid as well.[14] Most patients with active RA have some evidence for cellular sensitivity to type II and type III collagens.[15] Indeed, injection of purified type II collagen into a certain strain of rats at a certain age produces a chronic arthritis not unlike rheumatoid arthritis[16,17] that can be passively transferred by mononuclear cells or by immunoglobulins from one rat to another (see Chapter 14). It is of interest that although IgM antibody production in man is usually short-lived after an antigenic stimulus, in patients with RA, IgM as well as IgG antibody production to native type II collagen appears to persist at high levels.[18] Does this imply a persistence of antigenic stimulation?

The work generated recently concerning the role of Epstein-Barr virus (EBV) in RA is another example of the inability to determine whether an agent associated with RA has an etiologic relationship to the disease. Rheumatoid patients have a higher frequency than control populations of antibodies to EBV-associated nuclear antigens.[19-21] Rheumatoid patients have defective EBV-specific suppressor T-lymphocyte function; the RA T lymphocytes do not suppress the polyclonal B-lymphocyte stimulation induced by EBV infection.[22-25] RA T lymphocytes are specifically deficient in their ability to generate gamma interferon (which suppresses EBV-induced B lymphoblast transformation), although this deficiency is restored to normal if monocyte/macrophages are removed from the cell system or if cyclooxygenase inhibitors are added to it.[25] Perhaps the defect is an excessive sensitivity of T lymphocytes to factors such as prostaglandins produced by monocyte/macrophages.

There are data demonstrating that antibodies to EBV antigens in RA patients are *not* different from controls in patients with recent onset (< 6 weeks) of rheumatoid arthritis,[26] and that unlike patients with acute infectious mononucleosis, rheumatoid patients do *not* have an increased excretion from the oropharynx of infectious viral particles.[27] On the basis of these observations, the role of EBV appears to be that of a facilitator (not unlike a co-factor in an enzymatic process) of the chronic immune response in this disease.

No firm data exist implicating other exogenous (e.g., mycoplasma) agents or endogenous antigens as the cause, although as will be discussed below, many investigators believe that altered IgG is, in and of itself, sufficient to cause RA.

THE EARLY LESION IN RHEUMATOID ARTHRITIS: IMMUNE PROCESSING AND NEW BLOOD VESSEL FORMATION

If we assume that RA is generated by an immune response to an as yet unknown antigen, why does the inflammation begin and persist in the joint? There are three qualities that stand out as being peculiar to joints: (1) they are designed for movement; (2) they contain a potential space lined not by epithelial tissue but by mesenchyme with no basement membrane (see Chapter 16); and (3) within joints there are large areas of avascular connective tissue, the articular and meniscal cartilages.

The observation that arthritis is less severe in paralyzed limbs in patients has been supported by many observations, including quantitative ones demonstrating more cells in the synovial fluid of freely moving joints (after injection of phlogistic crystals) compared with joints that are immobilized. The quality of being developed for motion appears to confer upon joints a susceptibility to inflammation.

Another unusual quality of joints—the lack of limiting membrane between the joint space and synovial blood vessels—contributes to the rapidity with which alterations in blood flow are reflected in cell content and volume of synovial fluid. In addition, the redundant tissue of synovium necessary to allow full motion of the

joint makes the joint space a low pressure cavity, which offers minimal (sometimes negative) pressure resistance to inflow of low molecular weight solutes and biologically active precursors or products of inflammation into the joint. During inflammation, high molecular weight substances (e.g., α_2-macroglobulin and fibrinogen), which selectively are prevented from entering normal joints, pass readily through synovial capillaries with fenestrations between endothelial cells into the joint space.[28] Once within the joint space it is difficult for molecules of Mr greater than 100,000 to be cleared. The synovial fluid thus serves as a sink into which are spilled components of inflammation, including proteinases[29] and components of the complement system.[30]

The absence of blood vessels in cartilage makes it possible for antigen-antibody complexes to be sequestered without being cleared from the tissue. That this happens in experimental models as well as in human RA has been demonstrated in a number of studies.[31-33] The requirements for development of this phenomenon may be as follows[34]: (1) antibody must be present in the extravascular space, joint space, or synovium; (2) diffusion of antigen or or soluble complexes into the cartilage must occur; (3) antigen and antibody must combine to form larger, more insoluble complexes; and (4) these aggregates must then be trapped within the meshwork of collagen in cartilage, tendon, or menisci. Immunofluorescent studies have revealed intense staining for IgG, IgM, IgA, and C3 in hyaline cartilage from rheumatoid joints, while very little was present in cartilage from degenerative joint disease.[35] However, the deposition of immune complexes in cartilage is not the sole initiating factor in synovitis; this has been proved by demonstration of the persistence of antigen in nonarthritic joints.[36]

The *absence* of immune complexes in superficial areas of cartilage underlying invasive pannus tissue in RA[37] suggests that these complexes were phagocytized or otherwise freed by the cells of the pannus. It is intriguing to hypothesize that the immune complexes could serve both as a chemoattractant for pannus and, during the process of being phagocytized, as a stimulus to release by the pannus cells of enzymes capable of destroying cartilage.[38,39] Fibronectin binds to the Clq component of complement,[40] and since fibronectin stimulates endocytosis as well as being a chemoattractant in several systems, it is possible that fibronectin could function in facilitating clearance of Clq-coated material such as immune complexes.

These data reviewed here do not provide us with a definite answer to the question of why this early inflammatory response localizes within joints, but do help in understanding the unique setting that the joint offers for an inflammatory and proliferative reaction.

Once within the extracellular synovial tissues the antigen "X" is probably processed by HLA-DR–positive (Ia+) cells. (An alternative is that "X" is brought to the synovium by Ia+ nonresident cells.) In immunofluorescent studies of rheumatoid synovium, interdigitating reticular cells (D cells or "dendritic" cells) staining powerfully for HLA-DR(Ia+) antigens are found in close contact with inducer (helper) T lymphocytes.[41] The appearance of Ia+ on mononuclear cells appears to be induced by antigen presentation. Anatomically, this action occurs in what has been described as "transitional" areas[42] containing some lymphocytes (more suppressor [OK T8] than inducer [OK T4] cells), plasma cells, blast cells, macrophages and fibroblasts. This area is distinct from "lymphocyte-rich" areas around postcapillary venules (where more inducer [OK T4] than suppressor [OK T8] lymphocytes were found) and from the "proliferative" areas containing primarily fibroblasts and macrophages destined to become the effector components of synovium for joint destruction. Close cell-to-cell contact in these areas assures transfer of information among them (Fig. 59–1).

The synovial macrophage or "dendritic" cell-dependent T-lymphocyte activation is not dissimilar from delayed-type hypersensitivity reactions[43] seen in the skin. The synovial HLA-DR+ cells may be functionally similar to epidermal Langerhans cells in their role in antigen presentation. There appear to be different subsets of macrophages when they are characterized by their expression of Ia (HLA-DR); some bear Ia antigens only after activation,[44] whereas the so-called "dendritic cells" (assuming that data in mice can be extrapolated to humans) continuously express Ia antigen.[45]

Without proliferation of new blood vessels, synovitis could not be sustained. As noted in Chapter 13, the endothelial cell is programmed with all the genetic information needed to develop an entire capillary network in vitro so long as the cells are driven by a stimulus such as the angiogenic factors purified from rat tumors[46] or activated macrophages. For capillary growth to occur in vivo, three separate processes must occur: endothelial cell migration, endothelial cell replication, and extracellular matrix modification. Do macrophages in synovium activated during processing of antigen provide the signals to initiate these processes? Or can the endothelial cell itself provide these stimuli? Data suggesting that endothelial cells express Ia antigens on the cell surface and thus have the potential to restore mitogen responsiveness to monocyte-depleted human T lymphocytes[47] raise the possibility of an affirmative answer to the latter question.

ACUTE INFLAMMATION: A PHENOMENON IN RHEUMATOID SYNOVIAL FLUID BUT NOT SYNOVIUM

Early in rheumatoid synovitis in some patients mononuclear cells may predominate in synovial fluid,[48] but once synovitis is established, the PMN leukocyte is the predominant cell.

Polymorphonuclear Leukocytes. Although PMN leukocytes must come from blood vessels and traverse the endothelium to appear in subsynovial tissue, they are rarely found there. The rule is that they migrate almost immediately into the synovial fluid, to which they are drawn by chemotactic factors. Once in the joint space they contribute to the sometimes intense inflammatory response characteristic of RA. It is inevitable that products of this inflammatory activity diffuse back into the

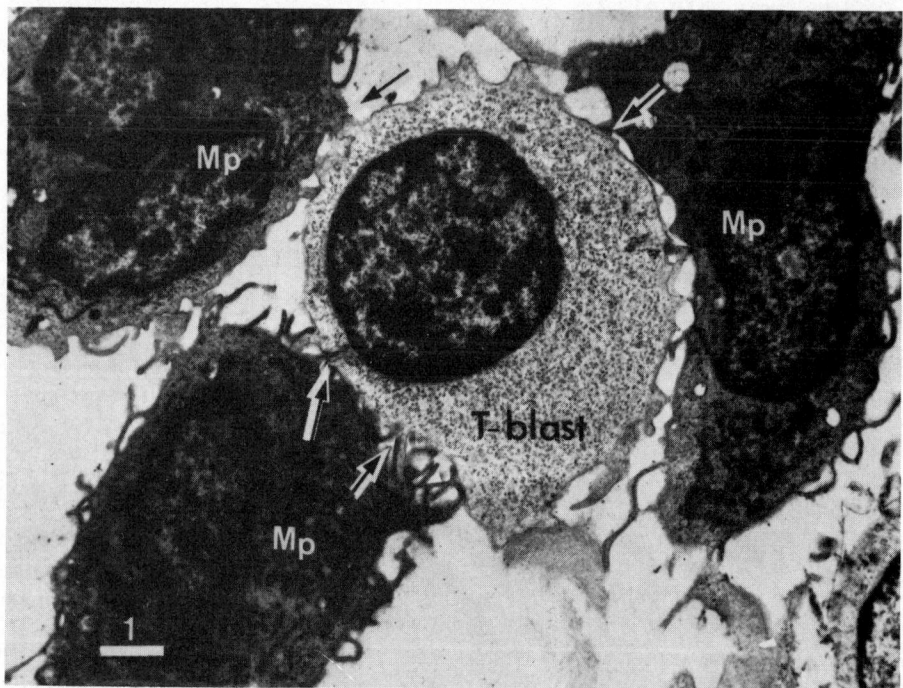

Figure 59–1. T lymphoblast surrounded by three macrophages (*Mp*). The arrow points to probable intercellular bridging. (Photograph provided by Hitoshi Ishikawa and Morris Ziff, University of Texas Southwestern Medical Center, Dallas, Texas.)

Figure 59–2. This sequence of scanning electron photomicrographs shows polymorphonuclear (PMN) leukocytes as they migrate through a capillary or venule wall into extravascular connective tissue. *A,* A PMN leukocyte is about to emigrate from a venule through the opening subjacent to it. The cell and vessel wall are viewed from the luminal side. × 6400. *C,* PMN leukocytes present in the extracellular tissue after emigration from vessels. The copious strands may be fibrin. × 1280. (Photographs courtesy of Morris J. Karnovsky and Graeme B. Ryan, Harvard Medical School.)

synovium and contribute to the proliferative disease seen there.

Figure 59–2 is a sequence showing the migration of PMN leukocytes through a capillary or venule wall into the extracellular matrix. Little damage to the blood vessels results from this emigration of cells, although changes varying in degree from swelling to fibroblastic transformation are seen.[49] Although PMN leukocytes are rarely found in the synovial membrane itself, with the use of histochemical methods for demonstrating PMN neutrophil granules it is estimated that in occasional samples PMN leukocytes may be found at the cartilage-pannus junction.[50] There is no evidence that PMN leukocytes return to the circulation. Rather, they

are trapped within the joint. The influx of new cells is quite rapid and it has been estimated by studies of DFP-labeled PMN leukocytes that in a rheumatoid effusion containing 25,000 granulocytes per cubic millimeter, the breakdown in the synovial cavity may exceed one billion cells per day.[51] The mechanism of this postulated destruction is unknown, and the PMN leukocyte degradation has not been measured or observed directly. In addition to cell death, there are several mechanisms that result in release of lysosomal enzymes from PMN leukocytes into synovial fluid (these have been reviewed in detail in Chapter 9).

The direct result of lysosomal enzyme release into the synovial fluid "sink" is generation of a significant potential for tissue damage. Enzymes accumulate more rapidly than they can be cleared from the fluid through exit by synovial capillaries. Eventually the large quantity of proteinases saturate the capacity of proteinase inhibitors present in synovial fluid, and enzyme activity (e.g., collagenase) is expressed unopposed.[29] In addition, it is likely (see Chapters 9 and 10) that lysosomal contents have a direct capability for provoking tissue injury and potentiating a proliferative response in synovial tissue.[52-54]

In order for PMN leukocytes to accumulate within the joint space, chemotactic factors (CF) must be elaborated (Table 59–2). Chemotactic substances (as detailed in Chapter 9) react with specific receptors on the PMN leukocyte cell surface, resulting in a polarized appearance of the cell as ion flux occurs and phospholipase, methyltransferase, and adenylate cyclase are activated. One of the substances listed in Table 59–2, leukotriene B_4 (LTB_4),[57] is a product of the 5-lipoxygenase pathway of arachidonate metabolism (see Chapters 6 and 9). PMN leukocytes metabolize LTB_4 quickly, and for this reason it is not known how important a role LTB_4 plays in chemotoxis in vivo. Elevated LTB_4 has been measured in rheumatoid synovial effusions, and these levels are acutely lowered by glucocorticoids.[58]

The binding of chemotactic substances to the PMN leukocyte and "fluidizing" of the cell membrane appear to be sufficient in and of themselves to generate free radicals from oxygen metabolism, leading to an increased lysosomal enzyme release from the cells. PMN leukocytes in peripheral blood from patients with RA may be deficient in their capability for both phagocytosis and response to chemoattractants.[55,56] This may reflect a form of down-regulation by cells that have phagocytized immune complexes or have saturated the receptors for chemotactic stimuli.

Table 59–2. Endogenous Chemotactic Factors (CF) Found in Chronic Inflammation*

1. Complement-derived CF
   C5a
   C3 fragment
   C567
2. Lymphocyte-derived CF
   These are chemotactic for monocytes, fibroblasts, and eosinophils as well as PMN leukocytes.
3. PMN leukocyte-derived CF
4. Leukotriene B_4
   This substance also may be needed for PMN leukocyte responsiveness to other CF.
5. Platelet-derived growth factor
6. Platelet factor IV
7. Enzymes
   Kallikrein
   Plasminogen activator
8. Coagulation-related factors
   Fibrinopeptide B
   Fibrin degradation products
9. Fibronectin
10. Collagen fragments

*Derived from O'Flaherty, J.T., and Ward, P.A.: Chemotactic factors and neutrophil. Sem. Hematol. 16:163, 1979.

Free radicals associated with reduction of molecular oxygen by PMN leukocytes and by mononuclear phagocytes are generated within the joint in response to phagocytosis or by binding of chemotactic substances to cell membrane receptors.[59] The radicals—superoxide (O_2^-, hydroxyl ion (OH^+), and singlet oxygen ($^1O_2^*$)—have the potential to damage lipid membranes,[60] degrade hyaluronic acid,[61] inactivate proteinase inhibitors such as α_1-proteinase inhibitor[62] and catalyze production of chemotactic lipids from polyunsaturated fatty acids. Solid evidence for pathologic activity in vivo of these free radicals is sparse because they are scavenged quickly by numerous naturally occurring superoxide dismutases within mitochondria as well as in the cytosol of cells. The naturally occurring copper-binding protein ceruloplasmin[63] has superoxide dismutase activity. Orgotein, a substance with anti-inflammatory activity isolated from bovine liver, is in fact a superoxide dismutase and has demonstrated anti-inflammatory effects.[64] Copper-penicillamine complexes may generate H_2O_2 nonenzymatically, which in turn can damage cell membranes, inhibiting cellular functions such as the T-lymphocyte response to mitogens (the presumptive mechanism of action of this disease-modifying drug [Lipsky, unpublished observations]). PMN leukocytes also produce N-chloroamines,[64a] by chlorination of endogenous amines in the presence of H_2O_2 and myeloperoxidase. These chloroamines are potent oxidizers of sulfhydryl groups and/or thioether groups, which are crucial to the activity of certain proteins. Chloroamines have a longer T½ than do superoxide, hydroxyl radicals, etc.

Complex functions of granulocytes in RA such as rates of phagocytosis have been reported to be normal by some investigators[65] and impaired by others.[66,67] Similarly, response to chemoattractants of PMN leukocytes from patients with RA was reported to be depressed in some studies[68] but normal in others.[69] It must be stressed that factors other than the underlying disease affect integrated neutrophil functions, including drug therapy and nutritional status. For example, it has been demonstrated in a crossover study of 13 rheumatoid patients that a 7-day fast (i.e., no food; noncaloric liquids ad lib) produced a mean weight loss of 5.1 kg., an increased response to chemoattractants, and improved serum bactericidal activity.[69] An association was found between improvement in inflammatory activity of the joints and enhancement of neutrophil bactericidal capacity.

The full potential for tissue destruction and enhancement of inflammation by PMN leukocytes is treated completely in Chapters 9 and 12. It is probable that this cell is one of the most important amplification mechanisms in the inflammatory process of RA. Once responding to chemoattractants or being activated during phagocytosis, the broad range of powerful phlogistic effects is sufficient to generate painful symptoms in patients, particularly since the cells and their inflammatory constituents are trapped within the joint space.

Synovial Fluid Pathology in the Inflammatory Lesion of RA. It must be emphasized again that there is no membrane barrier isolating synovium from synovial fluid and that the interactions among systems within synovial fluid can effect change in the proliferative rate of synovial cells. Conversely, substances generated by lymphocytes, macrophages, and synovial cells may amplify inflammation through effects on cellular or extracellular substances in synovial fluid.

Complement. Just as data have indicated that immunoglobulins and anti-immunoglobulins are synthesized by rheumatoid synovial tissue,[71,72] radioisotope dilution studies have provided evidence that 50 percent of intra-articular C3 may be derived from local synthesis[73] and that biologically active C2, C4, C5, and properdin factor B are synthesized there as well.[77] Despite local production of complement components, the activities of C4, C2, and C3 and total hemolytic complement in rheumatoid (seropositive) synovial effusions are lower than in synovial fluids from patients with other joint diseases.[70,74,75]

Using a sensitive solid-phase radioimmunoassay to quantitate the activation of the classic pathway of complement by rheumatoid factor, it has been demonstrated[76] that IgM-rheumatoid factor is a much more important determinant of complement activation than is IgG-rheumatoid factor in both serum and synovial fluids. Combined with other data showing that there is an accelerated catabolism of C4 in RA[77] and that the presence of C4 fragments[78] in plasma of rheumatoid patients correlates with titers of rheumatoid factor, the weight of evidence indicates a role in vivo for IgM-rheumatoid factor in complement activation.

The biologically active products produced during complement activation are probably the most important consequence of intra-articular complement consumption. Like proteinases from PMN leukocytes, these inflammatory components may build up in synovial fluid during acute inflammation. The potential for interaction between PMN leukocytes and the complement system is substantial. Neutrophil lysosomal lysates contain enzymatic activity capable of generating chemotactic activity (probably C5a) from fresh serum,[79,80] and an enzyme acting at neutral pH found in rheumatoid synovial fluid produced chemotactic factor in significant quantity when incubated with purified C5.[81] C5a, in addition to being a principal chemotactic factor in inflammatory effusions, is capable of mediating lysosomal release from human PMN leukocytes.[79,80,82] This sets up one of many amplification loops in inflammatory synovial fluid.

Another amplification loop in synovial inflammation may involve complement activation by C-reactive protein (CRP). As reviewed in Chapter 43, CRP concentrations in plasma increased up to 1000 times the concentrations found in normal individuals following an inflammatory stimulus. CRP may combine with phospholipid constituents of necrotic cell membranes at inflammatory sites or with the first complement components.[83-85]

Kinin-Forming Systems. One of the primary mediators of acute inflammation generated in synovial fluid is bradykinin. Bradykinin is a nonapeptide (see Chapter 8). The increased vascular permeability and local vasodi-latation it produces could be principal factors in generating warm joints and synovial effusions.[86] As with the clotting system, activation of Hageman factor (factor XII) is the initial step in kinin formation.[87] Kinins and arthritis may be related at multiple steps in development of inflammation. Rheumatoid factor–IgG complexes have been reported to activate kininogens, although rheumatoid factor plus unaltered IgG did not.[88] Kallikrein activator and kininase are both present in human granulocytes. Kallikrein itself is a potent and versatile proteinase that can activate plasminogen to plasmin, and precursor to active Hageman factor, and latent to active collagenase.

Fibrin Formation and Fibrinolysis. The end point of activation of the clotting sequence is the formation of fibrin. The accumulation of fibrin is one of the most striking pathologic features of rheumatoid synovitis. Fibrin accumulates on the synovial surface, on cartilage surfaces, in areas of subsynovial hemorrhage or infarction, and as particulate aggregates in synovial fluid. At the final stages of fibrin formation, fibrinopeptides are formed (released from fibrinogen by the action of thrombin during clotting), which may have the capacity in and of themselves to increase vascular permeability. What initiates the clotting sequence? It has not been demonstrated that immune complexes of rheumatoid factor and IgG can activate this Hageman factor–dependent pathway,[89] but plasmin (activated by plasminogen activator from plasminogen) has this capability, as (possibly) does collagen. Production of a procoagulant by mononuclear cells in culture is stimulated by immune complexes.[90]

The presence of fibrin on synovium and cartilage may impede normal nutrition to these tissues and may amplify conditions that lead to hypoxia and acidosis in synovial fluid. In addition, homologous fibrin appears to generate a chronic immunologic response in experimental animals.[91] It is possible that in addition to being entrapped in collagen matrix, immune complexes may be caught up in fibrin clots within the joint space, a factor that would perpetuate the inflammatory and proliferative disease. Like the buildup of other components of the inflammatory reaction, the accumulation of fibrin in joints reflects an imbalance caused by the inadequacy of the joint lining to clear the large quantities of byproducts of inflammation. In some rheumatoid joints a strong inhibition of fibrinolysis by plasmin has been observed as well as diminished activity of plasminogen activator.[92]

Arachidonic Acid Metabolites. The prostaglandins produced from membrane phospholipids have been discussed extensively (see Chapter 6). Their presence and activity have been equated with the degree of inflammation in RA. However, their role has been diminished recently, in part because it is appreciated that although PGE_2 and PGI_2 cause vasodilatation and are synergistic with other substances (e.g., histamine, C5a, LTB_4) in increasing vasopermeability, the leukotrienes (especially LTB_4) may have more potent phlogistic effects than do the products of cyclooxygenase. In addition, it is appreciated that certain harmful effects of nonsteroidal anti-inflammatory drugs (e.g., renal insufficiency, toxic amblyopia, CNS effects, and hepatotoxicity) may be directly related to prostaglandin inhibition. Also, increasing data support a beneficial role for prostaglandins in synovial biology. As potential good effects within connective tissue, PGE_2 may suppress synovial cell proliferation, suppress production of plasminogen activator by certain cells, and inhibit formation of free radicals.[94,95] Underlying these facts is the principle that biologic effects of pluripotent substances such as prostaglandins are multiple, and while inhibition of one function in vivo may help suppress inflammation, inhibition of another may amplify it.

Synovial Fluid Oxygen. It has been calculated that glucose uptake in rheumatoid synovium may be five times greater than in normal tissue, and that anaerobic glycolysis increases fractionally more than aerobic glycolysis.[96,97] Despite the increase in blood flow and a shift toward anaerobic glycolysis, there exists a state of relative hypoxia in the synovial fluid and, presumably, the synovium as well. There is an inverse linear correlation between pH of rheumatoid synovial fluid on one hand and lactic acid and pCO_2 on the other.[98] The pH remains relatively constant until pO_2 falls to approximately 30 mm Hg, at which point it begins to fall precipitously as the pO_2 continues to fall.[98] Only those patients with severe active RA had a synovial fluid pO_2 of less than 27 mm Hg.[98] The severe rheumatoid patient, therefore, may have ischemic joint tissues. In the presence of large tense joint effusions the intra-articular pressure may be great enough to obliterate small vessel blood flow. In those without elevated intra-articular pressures, inflammation-associated increases in synovial blood supply may still be insufficient for adequate oxygenation of the proliferated, hypermetabolic synovial tissues. This may lead to focal infarction and necrosis and may be a factor in generating "rice bodies" in joints. Consistent with this concept of "metabolic-circulatory imbalance" is the fact that the temperature of joint effusions in the sickest rheumatoids is often low; it has been inferred that the decline in local temperature reflects a hypoperfused or ischemic synovium.[99]

Iron. Rupture of small vessels in RA must be relatively common, because iron deposits in the form of hemosiderin are observed frequently. The foci of iron granules are often not in just the lining cells, as in hemophilic arthritis, but in deep synovial cells as well[100] (Fig. 59–3). As illustrated by the proliferative synovitis seen in hemophilic arthritis,[101] red blood cell products (including iron) may supplement the other inflammatory and proliferative stimuli within the joint. Iron may have deleterious effects upon cells when it accumulates in tissues to the degree it does in rheumatoid synovium. In the presence of traces of free iron salts, superoxide and hydrogen peroxide can react together to produce the hydroxyl radical, the most toxic of the univalent reduction products derived from oxygen.[102] Deposition of iron within reticuloendothelial cells probably requires oxidation of ferrous iron, since it is stored in the more

Figure 59–3. In this section of rheumatoid synovium prepared with Prussian blue stain, large collections of iron, the product of many microhemorrhages, are found deep in the subsynovial tissue. × 315. (Courtesy of K. Muirden, M.D.)

stable ferric form; this oxidation may necessitate activation of molecular oxygen.[103] Iron, even in soluble complexes, can induce synovial cells to produce significant amounts of neutral proteinases.[104]

THE CHRONIC IMMUNOPROLIFERATIVE REACTION IN SYNOVIUM

The heterogeneity of cells found in rheumatoid synovium is a fact that has great implications for function of this diseased tissue. As more is learned about individual cell types in the chronic immunoproliferative response, it has become clear that cellular function in the synovium is dependent upon and determined by communication among different cell types.

The early stage of the immune response in synovium has been described above. It involves presentation of antigen by accessory cells such as endothelial cells and/or macrophages to T lymphocytes, which subsequently activate multiple clones of B lymphocytes. As Ziff[105] pointed out in 1974, the synovial tissues of patients with rheumatoid arthritis have many of the properties of a secondary lymphoid organ involved in an active immune response with the synthesis of immunoglobulin. Most of the small lymphocytes in the rheumatoid synovial membrane appear to be T lymphocytes. Immunofluorescent studies have revealed positive staining with anti–T-lymphocyte antisera, and the same cells do not demonstrate EAC receptors.[106,107] Even the aggregates of small lymphocytes adjacent to plasma cell–rich areas in rheumatoid synovial membranes are T lymphocytes.[108] B lymphocytes, on the other hand, may be rapidly transformed into plasma cells after arrival in the synovium. The T-lymphocyte predominance in synovial tissue does not apply to peripheral blood. Although some investigators have detected fewer B lymphocytes in rheumatoid patients,[109] others have reported finding increased numbers of B lymphocytes,[110] while still others report no differences in B- and T-lymphocyte ratios in normal and rheumatoid patients.[111]

The functional subsets of the T lymphocytes vary from one anatomic area to another within the synovium. In the "transitional" areas suppressor T lymphocytes are more numerous, while in the "lymphocyte-rich" areas inducer T lymphocytes predominate.[42] B lymphocytes in synovium are localized primarily within reactive lymphoid centers.[112]

Compared with cells found in peripheral blood of both rheumatoid and normal individuals, many more lymphocytes in rheumatoid synovium express Ia+ antigens on their surface. One study demonstrated a strong preferential expression on suppressor/cytotoxic subsets compared with helper/inducer cells.[113] Although variable among different studies, the $T_5:T_H$ lymphocyte ratio in synovial fluid is generally higher than in peripheral blood of rheumatoid patients,[114] a phenomenon possibly related to localization of T helper cells within synovium around accessory/antigen-presenting cells. This variability may reflect the expected variation in both intensity and focus of the immune response in different patients at different stages of their diseases. It is important to emphasize that it is only after activation that T lymphocytes express Ia antigen.[115,116]

In peripheral blood, as in synovium, the most striking change in lymphocyte surface antigens in rheumatoid arthritis is not fluctuations in lymphocyte subsets but an increase in Ia+ antigens found on lymphocytes.[117] This nonspecific phenomenon is seen also after immunization with tetanus toxoid or PPD and may serve as an index in any individual of immunologic stimulation.[117] Similarly, using methods that separate activated from resting lymphocytes by density gradient centrifugation,[118] a direct correlation between clinical disease activity and numbers of activated B lymphocytes (B-blasts) in peripheral blood lymphocyte populations has been observed.

One of the subsets of lymphoid cells that has received increased interest for its relevance to rheumatoid arthritis has been that of natural killer (NK) cells.[119] These are nonadherent, nonphagocytic cells that express surface receptors for the Fc portion of IgG and share a variety of T-lymphocyte markers. Morphologically, they appear as large granular lymphocytes. Functionally, they share features with both macrophages and PMN leukocytes, having spontaneous activity in normal individuals and augmented activity in response to interferon and other stimuli. Unlike macrophages and PMN leukocytes they proliferate in response to Interleukin 2 (T cell growth factor). Killing of other cells may be mediated by membrane-associated serine proteinases or phospholipases. There are very few studies of NK cells in rheumatoid arthritis. One study[120] has reported a decreased cytotoxicity of unfractionated synovial tissue lymphocytes from RA compared with peripheral blood lymphocytes from both rheumatoid and control populations.

No immunospecific response of lymphocytes from rheumatoid patients to rheumatoid synovium has been observed, although lymphocytes from some patients did show greater cytotoxic activity than did control lymphocytes when tested against young cultures of synovial cells.[121] These observations were not confirmed in another study.[122] Using the very sensitive antibody-dependent cell-mediated cytotoxicity (ADCC) assays, Griffiths and co-workers found no antibody to synovial cells in ten autologous rheumatoid sera.[123] However, since immunoglobulin is produced by plasma cells in rheumatoid synovium,[71] and peripheral blood mononuclear leukocytes from RA produce IgM rheumatoid factor in vitro (in contrast to controls),[124] and since there are Fc receptor–bearing lymphocytes in rheumatoid synovial tissues,[125] the effector mechanisms needed to mobilize ADCC are clearly present.

The histologic picture in rheumatoid synovium is one of extreme proliferation, and "cytotoxicity" is not obvious. One hypothesis designed to reconcile this apparent contradiction is that the normal mechanism of ADCC in RA may be inhibited by antigen present in excess (e.g., IgG) or by antigen-antibody complexes. Thus, the ADCC that normally would inhibit cell proliferation would be inhibited in the rheumatoid patient and proliferation could develop unopposed.

One other subset of lymphocytes should be considered in the context of rheumatoid synovitis. A prostaglandin-producing lymphocyte subpopulation has been defined.[126] There are more indomethacin-sensitive (i.e., prostaglandin-producing) peripheral blood mononuclear cells in rheumatoid than in normal patients.[127] Prostaglandin production by rheumatoid synovial cells is enormously increased in RA.[129]

Soluble mediators (lymphokines) are produced by active lymphocytes and have many biologic effects.[130] In RA there is evidence for activity in synovium of lymphokines, which have the effect (1) of increasing vascular permeability; (2) of being chemotactic for granulocytes and monocytes; (3) of activating monocyte-macrophages, osteoclasts, and synovial cells; and (4) of being mitogenic. The name "lymphokine" may be misleading. Certain soluble factors once thought to be produced by lymphocytes are now known to be released by monocyte-macrophages with some sort of assistance from lymphocytes. In addition, there is evidence that B lymphocytes can produce such soluble mediators. It may be most helpful to consider the soluble mediators of inflammation as being produced by the interaction of monocyte-macrophages and lymphocytes. Injection of partially purified preparations of lymphokines into rabbit knee joints has produced a chronic inflammatory reaction in the subsynovial tissue.[127] This may be another example of the cyclic augmentation found in chronic rheumatoid synovitis; in this case, inflammation produces activation of mediators, which in turn stimulate more inflammation.

Much current debate exists concerning transfer factor.[131,132] More studies are needed to determine whether or not this is a discrete factor or rather represents heterogeneous, nonspecific helper factors from lymphocyte cultures that stimulate immune responses directly or by inhibition of suppressor factors.

A primary role for lymphocytes as determinants of activity of RA is suggested indirectly by studies of their depletion in this disease.[133,134] Thoracic duct drainage and depletion of lymphocytes often ameliorate, although temporarily, the course of RA. Collagen-induced arthritis can be transferred from affected to nonaffected animals using lymphocytes from the sick animals.[135,136] That B lymphocytes capable of differentiating into antibody-secreting plasma cells are less crucial for development of arthritis than are T lymphocytes can be inferred from the fact that an illness like RA can develop in patients with congenital agammaglobulinemia.[137]

Antibody Production by Rheumatoid Synovial Lymphocytes: The Role of Rheumatoid Factor in Pathogenesis. B lymphocytes and plasma cells synthesize and release immunoglobulins from their sites in the synovium of RA,[71] and immunofluorescent studies reveal that significant amounts of rheumatoid factor are produced by these cells as well.[138,139] Most of the plasma cells contain IgG, but IgM-containing cells are also observed, particularly in seropositive patients. The lymphocytes in rheumatoid synovium appear to be committed to different antigens than are the peripheral blood lymphocytes of the same individual. IgG produced by synovial culture explants of numerous patients with RA contained an average of 41 percent IgG$_3$ compared with 12 percent IgG$_3$ in the serum IgG of the same patients.[140] However, IgG$_1$ is by far the predominant IgG type produced by synovial lymphocyte/plasma cells in RA.

Repeated immunizations with tetanus toxoid of rheumatoid patients before joint surgery have failed to induce antitetanus antibody production by synovial cells even though peripheral blood lymphocytes were producing specific antibody at a brisk rate.[142] Lymphocytes from nonarticular tissues (e.g., pericardium) involved in the inflammatory process also synthesize IgG and IgM and RF. Factors involved in "spread" of rheumatoid disease from articular to nonarticular tissues are not known.

Although there are no data clearly implicating rheumatoid factor as a principal causative agent in RA, the role of antiglobulins in the amplification and perpetuation of the process is well supported:

1. Despite the fact that some patients with virtually no circulating IgG develop RA,[137] it is known that patients with a positive test for rheumatoid factor in blood have more severe clinical disease and complications[141] than do seronegative patients.

2. Some data have indicated that rheumatoid factor is "hidden" or masked by other proteins in some seronegative patients.[143] However, recent studies that examined production in vitro by peripheral blood mononuclear leukocytes have indicated that (a) lymphocytes/monocyte populations from seropositive RA patients spontaneously elaborate IgM RF and (b) similar populations of cells from both normal and seronegative patients produced no IgM RF unless induced by lectins, and then produced significantly less than cells from seropositive patients.[144] These studies support with immunologic evidence the hypothesis that seronegative RA represents a disease distinct from seropositive RA.

3. Polyclonal IgM rheumatoid factor is able to fix and activate complement by the classic pathway.[145]

4. Using a cell assay for anti-IgG (rheumatoid factor) plaque-forming cells, Vaughan found that the appearance of these cells coincided with flares of clinical activity of the disease.[146] Anti-IgG plaque-forming cells were more concentrated in bone marrow and synovial fluid than in peripheral blood.

5. Most IgG-rheumatoid factors are directed against antigenic determinants on the Fc fragments of IgG and may self-associate to form dimers of larger polymers[147] (Fig. 59–4). These complexes stimulate their own formation and this, another example of cyclic amplification, continues long after any exogenous infective agent has been cleared from the system. Self-associating rheumatoid factors are almost impossible to detect unless the Fc region of the molecules bearing antigenic determinants is removed by prior pepsin digestion.[148] Isolated IgG that had self-associated to form RF was able to activate the human complement cascade in the fluid phase, even though its effectiveness was only 1/100th that of aggregated IgG or large-latticed immune complexes.[149] If one postulates that high concentrations or further polymerization of self-associating IgG-RF occurs in joints, perhaps bound to cartilage surfaces, a mechanism would be available for explaining depressed levels of complement in rheumatoid synovial effusions.[150]

6. Immune complexes containing rheumatoid factor have been localized within synovial tissues by immunofluorescent techniques[151,153] (Fig. 59–5). A hyperviscosity syndrome, which affects the central nervous system (producing headache, tinnitus, vertigo, and seizures)

Figure 59–4. Scheme for development of self-associating IgG, which may increase in size sufficient to fix complement or be phagocytized by PMN leukocytes, or both. The Fab positions of one molecule have affinity for the Fc portion of another, and the lattice begins to build. (After Pope, R.M., et al.: Proc. Natl. Acad. Sci. USA 71:517, 1974.)

Figure 59–5. Section of rheumatoid synovial tissue stained with fluorescein-labeled anti-IgG. A similar staining pattern was observed in the same sections with fluorescein-labeled anti-C3, indicating the presence of immune complexes. (From Natvig, J.B., et al.: Scand. J. Rheumatol. 5 [Suppl. 12]:77, 1975.)

and causes striking retinal pathology and diffuse hemorrhages, has been reported in a number of patients with RA,[154,155] and circulating intermediate-size immune complexes have been demonstrated. Another clinical association between severe disease and rheumatoid factor has been the finding of IgM rheumatoid factor in pulmonary lesions of patients with rheumatoid lung disease.[156]

7. Increased levels of IgG–anti-IgG have been associated with a high frequency of subcutaneous nodules, vasculitis,[157,158] elevated erythrocyte sedimentation rate, decreased complement levels, and increased number of involved joints. IgG-IgG complexes in joint fluids of rheumatoid patients have been shown after isolation and purification to be almost completely IgG rheumatoid factor.[158,159] IgG rheumatoid factor has been identified in plasma cells from rheumatoid synovial membranes.[160] In seropositive patients about 60 percent of plasma cells contained rheumatoid factor, while none of the cells from control tissue did.[161,162] Polymorphonuclear leukocytes from rheumatoid synovial effusions contain intracytoplasmic granules of immunoglobulins, including rheumatoid factor.[163-166] PMN leukocytes from synovial fluid which contain intracytoplasmic inclusions, called "ragocytes," are easily seen on wet preparations visu-

alized without staining, although they are seen more clearly using immunofluorescence. Such inclusions often contain rheumatoid factor. Recent data suggest that within rheumatoid synovial effusions IgG rheumatoid factor is preferentially reduced compared with serum, in contrast to IgA and IgM RF.[167] These data suggest that IgG RF may be specifically utilized in the pathogenesis of the proliferative, chronic synovitis.

8. In experiments performed in patients with RA, a marked inflammatory response was elicited when rheumatoid factor from the patient was injected into the joint, but not when normal IgG was given.[168] Rheumatoid factor becomes involved in pathogenesis when it forms immune complexes sufficiently large to activate complement[169] and/or be phagocytized by macrophages or polymorphonuclear leukocytes. Detection of the immune complexes independent of their antigenic specificity has given a new perspective to clinical studies.[170] Immune complex assays using binding to Clq are most frequently positive in RA (see Chapters 44 and 45).

Several hypotheses have been advanced to explain how IgG could become immunogenic.

i. New determinants on IgG may be exposed following polymerization as an aggregate or in antigen-antibody complexes.[171]

ii. A structural anomaly in the IgG of rheumatoid patients may render it immunogenic. Studies using circular dichroism spectropolarimetry have suggested that there may be a defect at the hinge region of rheumatoid IgG which could increase the binding affinity to membrane Fc receptors on B lymphocytes.[172]

iii. Depletion of suppressor T lymphocytes might allow B lymphocytes to produce autoantibodies against certain determinants on IgG.[173]

iv. Rheumatoid factor development could represent idiotype–anti-idiotype interaction. Jerne proposed[174] that in the course of an immune response, specific idiotypes present in higher concentration might stimulate anti-idiotypic antibody formation, which could modulate the immune response. Monoclonal antibodies have been developed against idiotypes on IgM rheumatoid factor. In one study the mouse antibody reacted with an identical or similar determinant located on (or close to) the binding site of all tested monoclonal or polyclonal IgM RF. The significance of these highly conserved determinants on rheumatoid factor idiotypes is not yet understood.[75]

Studies of lymphocyte antibody production in vitro have contributed to dissection of the immune response in RA. Using the hemolytic plaque-forming assay,[176] one can test for lymphocytes producing antibody against specific antigens as well as quantitate the number of cells with this specificity. Lymphocytes from rheumatoid patients in the plaque-forming assay have been observed to produce rheumatoid factor which is not present in peripheral blood and which has a much higher affinity for IgG than does rheumatoid factor in blood.[177] Were these high-affinity rheumatoid factors produced in vivo, they might never gain access to the circulation but rather be bound to autologous IgG in the immediate environment of the cell. These high-affinity complexes could aggregate and activate complement or be phagocytized, or both, initiating inflammation in the tissues (e.g., synovium) in which the antiglobulins were formed.

In addition to rheumatoid factors of the γ, α, and δ isotypes in RA, ϵ isotypes also have been demonstrated in certain patients.[178,179] Of 13 sera containing IgE immune complexes, 11 were from patients with extra-articular manifestations.[179] It was suggested that IgE-RF could complex with aggregated (self-associating) IgG in synovial tissue and that the IgG-IgE complexes could activate mast cells and basophils in the synovium, resulting in accentuation of the inflammatory response in this organ.[178] This has particular interest in light of recent reports that there are numerous mast cells in rheumatoid synovium and that these may release factors capable of stimulating collagenase production by synovial cells.[180]

Circulating Immune Complexes (CIC). The availability of multiple assays for CIC in serum has led to a proliferation of studies demonstrating correlation of the presence of CIC with certain articular and extra-articular manifestations of RA. In particular, vasculitis is frequently associated with high levels of immune complexes.[181,182] Interpretation of data on CIC in RA has been confused by a plethora of different assays for CIC as well as by interference with the test by rheumatoid factor. Different assays give different results using the same sera, and the differences are not due to different sensitivities of the assays. One recent study compared the following five different assay systems for CIC in rheumatoid sera: (1) bovine conglutinin assay; (2) ^{125}I-Clq binding assay; (3) monoclonal rheumatoid factor inhibition assay; (4) Raji cell assay; and (5) staphylococcal binding assay.[183] Different tests discriminated better for different parameters of disease activity (e.g., articular disease severity and extra-articular manifestations). None was of more use for measuring disease activity than the erythrocyte sedimentation rate or the IgG rheumatoid factor immunoassay.

THE SYNOVIAL CELLS IN RHEUMATOID ARTHRITIS

The synovial cells in rheumatoid arthritis are hyperplastic and usually become the dominant cell in the thickened, highly vascular synovium, which may weigh up to a thousandfold more than the normal membrane surrounding the joint cavity. As mentioned previously, many of the synovial cells become Ia antigen positive as synovitis develops.

Dissociated Adherent Rheumatoid Synovial Cells. In recent years the cells in rheumatoid synovium have been characterized by studying them in a freshly dissociated state. Thirty to 50 percent appear to be lymphocytes, some of which are partially adherent. The remaining cells are heterogeneous.[184,185] Most have been described as larger (15 to 60 μm) than lymphocytes with a high ratio of cytoplasm to nucleus. Many of these are mul-

tinucleate. In culture up to 40 percent of adherent cells may have a classic stellate or dendritic appearance (Fig. 59–6) and have knobby inclusions within a ribbed cytoplasm of the cell processes. Forty to 70 percent of the cells are phagocytic in early cultures. There does appear to be a subset of adherent synovial cells that have receptors for C3 and the Fc portion of IgG[186] and are similar in other respects to monocyte/macrophages. Most of the stellate cells do not have Fc receptors, nor do they produce lysozyme.[184] Cultures containing these mixtures of cells produce very large amounts of collagenase and prostaglandins.

In primary cultures the stellate cells begin to lose their striking appearance as monocytes/macrophages decrease or after cells are passaged. The stellate appearance is related to changes in biochemical parameters within cells. There are data[187] suggesting that mononuclear cell factor (Interleukin I) produced by monocytes/macrophages stimulates PGE_2 production, which in turn induces activity of adenylate cyclase, which produces increased cellular cAMP levels. As cAMP levels increase, the cells take on a stellate appearance. Despite the relationship of stellate cells and collagenase production, and the relationship of the stellate appearance with PGE_2 levels, there is no proven direct link in human synovial cells between PGE_2 and collagenase biosynthesis.

It is tempting to focus on the similarities among the collagenase/PGE_2-producing stellate cell of rheumatoid synovium, the DR-positive (Ia+) human epidermal Langerhans cells,[188] and the human dendritic (stellate) (Ia+) cells which circulate in peripheral blood and may be the principal accessory cell for antigen presentation to lymphocytes. It has not been demonstrated directly that the same cells expressing enhanced Ia+ positivity are those induced by Interleukin 1 to produce large amounts of collagenase; indeed, the latter cell type seems to be larger than the Ia+ accessory cell.

Rheumatoid Synovial Cells Grown from Explants. Most studies of rheumatoid synovial cells have been carried out using the cells that grow out from explants in organ culture. The advantage to this technique is that a morphologically homogeneous fibroblast-like population is produced. However, these cells have passed through several generations when functional characteristics are first studied; differentiated cells with a primary role in the rheumatoid process may not survive trypsinization or other routine methods of cell passage, and the original admixture of different cell types is lost. Nevertheless, the "synovial fibroblasts" that have been grown out from explants of rheumatoid synovium have a number of qualities different from cells obtained from normal tissue: (1) The rheumatoid cells in early cultures have higher growth rates than cells from noninflammatory synovitis and reach a higher final saturation density.[189] There are insignificant differences, however, in these parameters between rheumatoid cells and cells from nonrheumatoid but inflammatory synovitis. (2) The rheumatoid cells produce hyaluronic acid of lower molecular weight.[190] (3) The rheumatoid cells have a

Figure 59–6. Scanning electron photomicrographs of a classic dendritic cell from rheumatoid synovium. Cells were dissociated from matrix and grown in monolayer culture on a thin film of collagen. Individual collagen fibrils are seen, presenting a matte-like surface. Knobby inclusions within the cell processes are as yet undefined, although transmission electron microscopic studies show that they are not mitochondria. In *B*, a thin linear "ribbing" is seen below the plasma membrane and is stretched over the knobby inclusions. Magnification: *A*, × 2490; *B*, × 17,600. The bar in *A* is 20 μm; in *B* it is 2 μm.

markedly increased rate of glucose utilization and lactate production.[190] (4) The rheumatoid cells produce larger quantities of lysosomal enzymes.[191,192] (5) The rheumatoid cells are reported to be resistant to the effects produced in normal cells by corticosteroids, such as an

accelerated rate of cell growth, reduction in cell volumes, and reduction in the rate of hyaluronate and collagen synthesis.[190]

These differences between normal and rheumatoid cell lines persist through many passages (generations) of cells, implying a long-lasting alteration in cell function. Co-culture of normal human synovial cells with human blood lymphocytes, PMN leukocytes, or platelets results in the same profound changes in the synovial cells. Castor and his colleagues[193,194] have isolated polypeptides of molecular weight 10,000 to 15,000 from these cells which produce these effects. Called connective tissue activating peptides (CTAP), they initiate in cells the metabolic changes which can be considered "reparative" as opposed to phlogistic. CTAP derived from spleen increased glucose uptake and lactate formation as well as hyaluronate synthesis in human synovial cells, but produced lesser effects on cells derived from other connective tissues, and none at all upon fibroblasts from thyroid tissue. The data were different when CTAP derived from platelets was used. The data emphasize a cellular specificity for both target and effector cells and imply a deep complexity in these interactions. The CTAP polypeptides are mimicked in action by prostaglandin E_1, by dibutyryl cyclic AMP (but only at supraphysiologic concentrations),[193] and by fractions of serum containing nonsuppressible insulin-like activity.

It must be remembered that although one can estimate intensity and perhaps chronicity of inflammation using these in vitro systems, no qualitative differences have been described to suggest a defect intrinsic to rheumatoid cells not found in synovial cells from other types of chronic synovitis.

Macrophages. As discussed in Chapter 16, embryologic studies have provided data to indicate that histiocytes derived from blood-borne cells are found early in synovial tissue.[195] Experimental studies using guinea pigs have provided evidence that in an immunologically induced inflammatory lesion of synovium, most inflammatory cells appear to be derived from nonlymphocyte mononuclear cells of the blood.[196] Macrophages are the most versatile cells in the synovial lesion in RA. This is emphasized by the many receptors they possess on cell membranes and the many products that they secrete. Simple enumeration of factors secreted does not indicate the variation in expression of receptors and subsequently in secretion of products as functions of the activation of such cells. Chapter 10 gives listings of the many gene products secreted by monocytes in both the resting and activated state.

The activation of macrophages (referring to the marked change in metabolism and secretory and phagocytic function occurring over many hours after exposure to activating substances) could occur in rheumatoid synovial tissue through several mechanisms. Products of activated T lymphocytes activate macrophages to release a number of mediators, substances that have direct action upon other systems or else affect immune function and production of enzymes such as collagenase[197] and plasminogen activator.[198] Cellular immunity to many stimuli[199] and immune complexes stimulate selective release of lysosomal enzymes.[200] Evidence of the cyclic amplification mechanism within inflammatory states is found in the observation that cleavage of complement components may cause spreading and lysosomal release

by macrophages.[201,202] Proteinase(s) released by macrophages can cleave these complement proteins. Adding to the substrate supply for this enzyme activity is macrophage secretion of C3 and factor B, as well as agents that control this process, such as specific inhibitors Factor I (C3b-inactivator) and (B1H globulin), and general proteinase inhibitors such as α_2 macroglobulin.

Once activated in synovial tissue, the products of macrophages can have multiple roles in production and perpetuation of RA. One enzyme secreted by macrophages, plasminogen activator, may be of singular importance because it is secreted in an active state, not as a latent precursor or zymogen. In the presence of plasminogen, plasmin is formed. Plasmin has broad specificity and can initiate fibrinolysis and activate the clotting, kinin, complement, and collagenolytic systems[203] (see Chapter 8). Proteinases themselves may stimulate macrophage secretory activity by induction of plasma membrane spreading activity.[204] Similarly, proteinases can stimulate directly the secretion of collagenase from fibroblasts in culture.[205] Macrophages secrete an angiogenesis factor, potentially one of their most potent gene products.[206]

Cell-Cell Interactions in Rheumatoid Synovitis. The synovial cells proliferate enormously in rheumatoid arthritis. They must be considered stimulated cells, and their products (new connective tissue and proteinases) in this activated and proliferative state are responsible for altered appearance and function of joints. It is unlikely that these cells initiate a proliferative state sui generis, but rather that they are responding to stimuli from other cells. Stimulation of cells to proliferate involves interaction of ligands with at least two types of cell membrane receptors, the so-called "competency" and "progression" factors. In vitro, ligands for both receptors must be present if transformation or mitogenesis is to occur.

Proliferation of the number of cells in the synovium is the result of the inflammatory process. In experimental models of arthritis, synovial lining cells began to increase synthesis of DNA very soon after the inflammatory stimulus was injected and continued to manifest DNA synthetic activity for more than two months.[207] By inference, even short periods of inflammatory stimuli may be sufficient to sustain synovial proliferation in a rheumatoid joint.

Proliferation of growth of mesenchymal cells (including synovial cells) has been achieved in vitro with many different substances,[193] including: (1) connective tissue activating peptides (CTAP I-III), (2) human platelet–derived growth factor which has been purified into two homogeneous active fractions,[211] (3) somatomedin, (4) nonsuppressible insulin-like material in plasma, (5) fibroblast growth factor, (6) "low molecular weight constituents" (LMWC) from regenerating liver,[208] and (7) fibronectin. The monocyte/macrophage is perhaps the most influential cell upon activity and proliferation of the fibroblast. Mixtures of monocyte/macrophages and lymphocytes after antigen or mitogen stimulation produce in cell culture many different substances that affect fibroblast (and therefore, presumably, synovial cell) activity. Proteins that induce fibroblasts to proliferate in vitro can be separated biochemically from other factors produced by monocyte/lymphocyte cultures which are chemotactic for fibroblasts.[209] Highly purified Interleukin 1 itself appears to have two effects upon cultured fibroblasts which would amplify the proliferative and destructive potential of rheumatoid synovium; it induces fibroblast proliferation[210] and stimulates collagenase[212,215] and prostaglandin production[213,214] by the same populations of cells.

Work using passaged nonrheumatoid human synovial fibroblasts treated in vitro with conditioned medium from both concanavalin A–stimulated and streptococcal cell wall–stimulated human peripheral blood monocytes has identified a polypeptide that stimulates plasminogen activator biosynthesis by these cells. Named synovial activator, it is believed to be a different biochemical moiety from other mediators.[219] However, its action is similar to that of mononuclear cell factor or Interleukin 1.

Cells in rheumatoid synovium not only interact with other cells but also are influenced by contact with the extracellular matrix. Collagen, proteoglycans, fibronectin, and laminin are principal matrix constituents that have been shown to affect the growth and behavior of mesenchymal cells. Collagen, for example, appears both to directly stimulate synovial cells or other fibroblasts to synthesize collagenase[216] and to induce mononuclear cells to produce mononuclear cell factor (Interleukin 1), which in turn stimulates synovial cells to generate more collagenase and prostaglandins.[217] Fibronectin produced by macrophages has been shown to be a potent chemoattractant for fibroblasts in vitro.[218]

Complicating the study of substances produced by one cell that influence others is the profusion of "factors" isolated and named by many different laboratories. Helping to unify and consolidate "factor" proliferation has been the determination that Interleukin 1 is probably the same molecule (or a very similar molecule) as the one responsible for activities previously attributed endogenous leukocyte pyrogen, chondrocyte stimulating factor, fibroblast proliferation factor, B-cell activating factor, lymphocyte-activating factor, and mononuclear cell factor. It is likely that other "activities," such as human monocyte-derived growth factor for mesenchymal cells or the factor derived from activated cultures of peripheral blood mononuclear cells which stimulates production of plasminogen activator by synovial fibroblasts[219] may, in the future, be purified and shown to have structural homology with well-characterized molecules such as Interleukin 1.

THE BIOCHEMISTRY OF TISSUE DESTRUCTION IN RHEUMATOID ARTHRITIS

The aggressive invasion of cartilage, bone, and tendon by proliferative synovium is accomplished by destruction and replacement of the extracellular matrix proteo-glycans and collagen. Enzymes present in synovial fluid and released by the proliferative pannus are responsible for initiating this destruction.

Collagen Degradation. In cartilage, the type II collagen fibers have variable size (some up to 250 nm in diameter).[220] Cartilage collagen is characteristically very difficult to solubilize, indicating a high degree of intermolecular crosslinking (see discussion of crosslinks in collagen in Chapter 14). Figure 59–7 summarizes various pathways of collagen degradation applicable to replacement of cartilage by the invasive pannus. It is useful to think of cartilage as being exposed to destructive enzymes from two sources: the synovium and synovial fluid. In most cases, enzymes free in synovial fluid are regulated by proteinase inhibitors in synovial fluids, principally α_2 macroglobulin[222] and α_1-proteinase inhibitor (α_1-antitrypsin).[223,224]

As mentioned previously, PMN leukocytes are trapped in synovial fluid in large numbers. Proteinases and polysaccharidases are released as cells die and are lysed, or as they release lysosomal enzymes, including elastase and collagenase,[224] while phagocytosing debris or immune complexes. It has been demonstrated that in synovial fluid with particularly large numbers of PMN leukocytes ($> 50,000$ per mm[3]), free collagenase activity may be present, implying that proteinase inhibitors are saturated by enzymes[29] or else inactivated by substances such as N-chloroamines. Proteinases in synovial fluid are very likely responsible for damage to the superficial

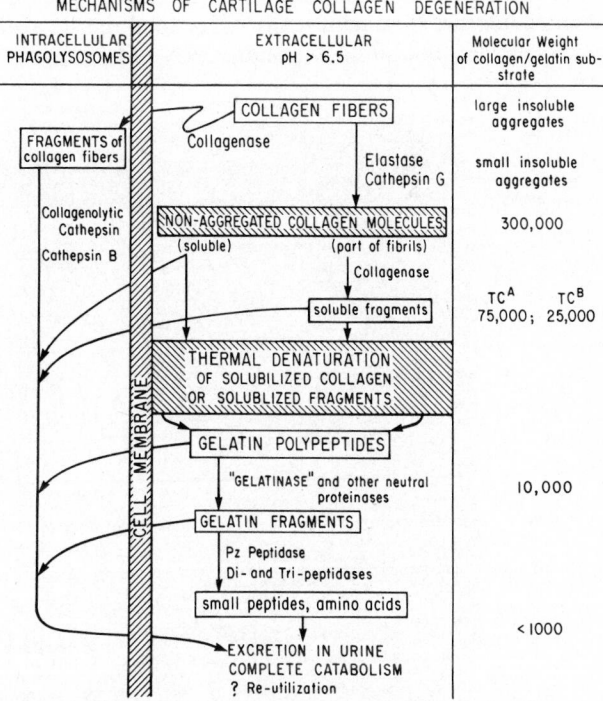

Figure 59–7. Mechanisms of cartilage collagen breakdown in rheumatoid arthritis. A schema. The left side describes intracellular (within phagolysosomes) events potentially involved in collagen breakdown. Extracellular events are depicted in the middle, and on the right are approximate molecular weights of collagen or gelatin fragments during sequential steps of degradation.

layers of cartilage demonstrated in RA,[225] and in experimental systems it has been shown that PMN leukocytes adhere to cartilage in greater numbers when there are immune complexes entrapped within the avascular cartilage.[226] Small foci or microabscesses of PMN leukocytes can be seen occassionally at the pannus-cartilage junction. Release of lysosomal enzymes occurs at the cartilage surface as viable PMN leukocytes are "frustrated" in phagocytosis of immune complexes bound superficially to substrate. Active proteinases, in addition to saturating proteinase inhibitors, may permanently inactivate inhibitors by limited proteolysis.[227]

As reviewed in Chapter 14, crosslinked collagen fibrils are relatively resistant to collagenases. PMN leukocyte serine proteinases have the ability to cleave the nonhelical crosslink region, which contains the intermolecular crosslinks.[228] Noncrosslinked molecules could remain in fibril conformation as insoluble aggregates or could become soluble. The individual molecules are readily cleaved by specific collagenases produced by synovial cells and macrophages.[229] The fragments produced are very susceptible to thermal denaturation and as gelatin polypeptides can be degraded by multiple enzymes, including relatively specific "gelatinases" (metalloproteinases active at neutral pH).[230]

There are two forms of inactive proteinases in extracellular tissues. One is proteinase complexed with α_2 macroglobulin[231] or α_1-proteinase inhibitor[232] or tissue proteinase inhibitors. There is little evidence that these forms are easily restored to active enzymes. The inactive complexes are eliminated from the circulation by the reticuloendothelial system.[233] Clearance must be slower from synovial fluid and the complexes could be disso-

ciated if α_2 macroglobulin molecules were gradually denatured or degraded, releasing active proteinases. There is increasing evidence that inhibitor-enzyme complexes are more avidly taken up by phagocytic cells than are either inhibitors or enzymes alone.

The second form of inactive enzymes are proenzymes, the precursor forms produced by the cells. Within the extracellular space it is probable that other proteinases activate proenzymes. For example, plasmin is an effective activator of latent rheumatoid synovial collagenase. Rheumatoid synovial cells also produce plasminogen activator.[203] Since plasminogen is among the high molecular weight proteins that are increased in concentration in synovial fluid in RA, it seems probable that sufficient plasmin is present in synovial tissue to activate latent forms of collagenase or latent activators essential for activation of procollagenase.

Molecule by molecule destruction of collagen in the extracellular space, as portrayed above, may be bypassed in the presence of a very aggressive synovitis in which entire pieces of fibrils are phagocytized and, presumably, degraded by lysosomal proteinases (cathepsin B and collagenolytic cathepsin) within phagolysosomes (Fig. 59–8).

Tissue inhibitors of metalloproteinases (TIMP) are present in all connective tissues. These proteins (Mr less than 30,000) inhibit collagenases and other tissue metalloproteinases.[234] In situations of active, aggressive synovitis, however, the TIMP probably are saturated and inactivated by proteinases released into the extracellular tissues in large quantities. TIMP from all tissues in a single species are immunologically identical.

Pharmacologic control of synovial collagenase bio-

Figure 59–8. The leading edge of a pannus cell extends diffusely into cartilage. Collagen fibers, characterized by 69 nm periodicity, can be seen about to be or actually engulfed by the cell. This very close contact of synovium and cartilage is found in < 10 percent of patients but is the type of process associated with phagocytosis of collagen by this leading edge of cells. × 30,000. (Electron photomicrograph by Andrey M. Glauert. From Harris, E.D., Jr., et al.: Arthritis Rheum. 20:657, 1977.)

synthesis is suggested by the data showing that gluco-corticoids and retinoid compounds inhibit production of the enzyme.[235] That different mechanisms regulate the production of both collagenase and plasminogen activator (both are neutral proteinases secreted by mesenchymal cells in response to polypeptide stimulating factors produced by monocytes) is emphasized by the evidence that while retinoids inhibit collagenase production they also stimulate plasminogen activator production by human synovial fibroblasts.[236]

Proteoglycan Degradation. Proteoglycans in cartilage are quickly depleted when synovitis develops.[237] As shown in Figure 59–9, although the cartilage has a normal thickness and gross appearance (using metachromatic stain), there is very little tinctorial evidence for proteoglycans. As with collagen, it is likely that enzymes active at neutral pH are essential for solubilization or mobilization of the components of the proteoglycan molecule. Neutral metalloproteinases found in cartilage are the leading candidates for this role,[238] although PMN leukocyte elastase and cathepsin G can bring about essentially complete release of proteoglycan from cartilage as well.[228] Once the aggregates are broken up, the soluble components of proteoglycans can be degraded intracellularly by lysosomal enzymes, especially cathepsins B and D.[239] There are increased amounts of enzymes with the potential to break down the polysaccharide side chains of chondroitin sulfate and keratan sulfate in rheumatoid synovium as well. Levels of N-acetylglucosaminidase, β-galactosidase, arylsulfatase A, and glucuronidase activity are all higher in rheumatoid synovium than in controls, although this increase of enzyme activity is seen in reactive synovitis of many varieties and is not specific for RA.[240]

It is probable that in response to inflammation in the joint, cartilage generates its own destruction. Cultures of synovium release a factor of low molecular weight that induces chondrocytes to generate proteinases, which degrade proteoglycans. This substance(s) has been named catabolin[241] and is similar to Interleukin 1 and mononuclear cell factor that mediates cartilage proteoglycan degradation through chondrocyte activation.[242] That this mechanism operates in vivo is suggested by the enhanced size of lacunae around chondrocytes near invasive fronds of the pannus cells (see Fig. 59–11).

Some of the proteinase activity in proliferating rheumatoid synovial cells in vitro is associated with the cell membrane surface rather than being secreted into the culture medium.[243] The pathophysiologic significance of surface-associated proteinases can only be speculated upon at this time.

Bone Resorption. Collagenase and elastase cannot degrade bone unless it has been demineralized. In vivo, then, either some component of the inflammatory lesion must be able to mobilize bone mineral or else osteoclasts (or cells with equivalent capabilities) must develop and create resorption. Both mechanisms are possible in the rheumatoid lesion. Multinucleate cells have been described at the resorbing interface of pannus and bone. Prostaglandins stimulate bone resorption by stimulating osteoclastic activity.[244,245] Prostaglandin endoperoxides (PGG_2 and PGH_2) cause a transient stimulation of calcium release that is quite different from the prolonged resorption resulting from PGE_2, suggesting that more needs to be learned about which of the arachidonic acid metabolites are principally responsible for the bone resorption induced by this system.[246] An immunologic mechanism is also applicable to bone resorption. Osteoclast-activating factor (OAF) is a soluble product of cultured human mononuclear leukocytes,[247] produced, it is believed, by the mononuclear cells found deep in rheumatoid synovium.

Both of these potential mechanisms can be synergistic in causing the resorption and replacement of bone at the bone-pannus junction as well as the juxta-articular osteopenia that develops as an early sign of proliferative synovitis.

PATHOLOGY OF RHEUMATOID ARTHRITIS

The pathology of RA is best understood in the context of cellular, immunologic, and biochemical mechanisms discussed in detail in the preceding sections.

The rheumatoid process has minimal destructive capability until it becomes chronic. The disease is such

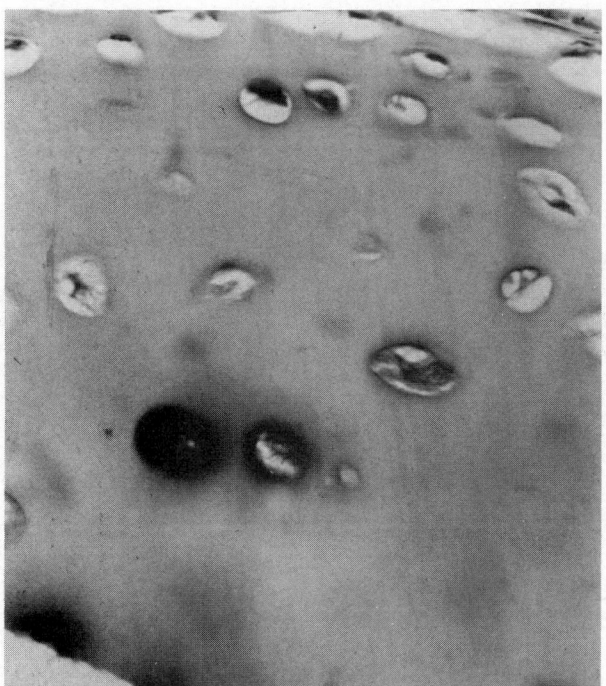

Figure 59–9. Human articular cartilage from active rheumatoid arthritis removed at joint arthroplasty and stained for metachromasia. The only metachromatic stain surrounds a few chondrocytes, which, presumably, are actively making proteoglycan only to have it broken down by proteinases derived from synovial fluid, chondrocytes, and/ or synovial tissue. The form of this depleted cartilage is normal; however, its functional capacity to rebound from a deforming load is seriously impaired.

that at any point in the development of the highly proliferative polarized and destructive lesion it may regress.
It is not known how long this "maturation" process
takes to occur, but extrapolation from clinical observations suggests that it is unlikely that significant erosive
disease can develop before 8 weeks after the first symptoms, even in the most aggressive lesions.

Synovium. Figure 59–10 is a photomicrograph of synovium from an inflamed knee obtained 3 days after the
onset of arthritis, which subsequently evolved into classic RA. The synovial lining cells have not proliferated
much, but the small blood vessels are very prominent
deep in the subsynovial tissue, not so much because they
are dilated but because of a large increase in numbers
of vascular cells and lymphocytes in the perivascular
areas. Accumulation of an increased amount of interstitial fluid is indicated by the low density of cells and
matrix. The lymphocytes of the synovial lesion have been
identified primarily as T lymphocytes[106,107] in other studies. No plasma cells are seen in the earliest lesions. As
the lesion matures, a striking heterogeneity of cell types
is found. Macrophages, lymphocytes, endothelial cells,
"synovial cells," and fibroblast-like cells are all present.

The first vascular change in rheumatoid synovitis is
one of venular dilatation.[93] Deposition of fibrin within
the vessel wall occurs, and there is proliferation of endothelium.[248] But as new tissue develops, an enlarged

Figure 59–11. Low power scanning electron microscopic view of the
surface of synovium early in rheumatoid arthritis. × 120. (Courtesy
of Dr. Gilbert Fauré. Assistant des Hôpitaux, Chief de Clinique,
Service de Rhumatologic Hospital de Nancy-Brabois.)

capillary network appears and sustains the proliferating
cells, invading the relatively avascular cartilage and subchondral bone. Factors responsible for generation of new
capillaries are discussed in Chapter 13. Extracellular
proteinases released by cells (?endothelial cells, ?mast
cells, ?tissue histiocytes) may include plasminogen ac-

Figure 59–10. Photomicrograph of synovium with three days of clinically identifiable inflammation, later evolving into definite rheumatoid
arthritis. Histologic details are described in the text. *SLC,* Synovial
lining cells. × 180. (From Schumacher, H.R., and Kitridou, R.D.:
Arthritis Rheum. 15:465, 1972.)

Figure 59–12. Scanning electron microscopic view of rheumatoid synovium. Villous fronds are beginning to appear. Fibrin debris coats the
surface. × 35. (Courtesy of Dr. G. Fauré.)

Figure 59–13. This scanning electron photomicrograph represents more chronic, established disease than Figure 59–12. × 35. The villi are more numerous; there is much more synovial surface area. (Courtesy of Dr. G. Fauré.)

tivator and collagenase. Proteinases may inactivate the inhibitors of angiogenesis normally found in cartilage, permitting the vascular pannus to erode into cartilage.

The early lesion in RA viewed by scanning electron microscopy of the synovial surface is shown in Figure 59–11. The folds are possible artifacts, but the finely pebbled appearance of individual cells on the surface is not unlike the normal synovium. As the synovial lesion progresses, it becomes more and more a heterogeneous mixture of cells.

Progression to chronicity is associated with an enormous increase in the synovial surface area. This is accomplished by formation of villi (compare Figs. 59–12 and 59–13 with 59–14). The development of villi is accompanied by deposition of fibrin on the synovial surface. In chronic progressive disease multiple long microvilli have developed and the fine pebbled appearance of individual cells is less distinct, perhaps because of a diffuse film of fibrin that coats the cell surface. The microvilli shown in Figure 59–13 are probably prone to infarction and autoamputation from the stalk, with subsequent existence in synovial fluid as "rice bodies."

High-power views of the surface of rheumatoid synovium reveal multiple cell processes and surface irregularities (Fig. 59–15). Seen in many such scanning election micrographs is the suggestion of intercellular bridging among cells. These conduits would certainly assure information transfer from cell to cell.

In the advanced process, then, there are four levels of cell surface area multiplication: (1) macrovillous formation, visible to the naked eye; (2) microvilli, visible by low-power microscopy; (3) the nodular surface of the villi caused by cells protruding from the surface; and (4) multiple processes from individual cells. When stained in such a way as to emphasize cell processes as well as extracellular matrix, the clear area surrounding synovial cells at the cartilage-pannus junction can be shown to contain thin cell processes, suggesting that these cells could be the stellate cells that are found in cultures of freshly dissociated rheumatoid synovial cells in vitro (Fig. 59–16, Plate III, p. xxxvii).

Ultrastructural studies of the synovial lining cells show a marked increase in the number of type B cells

Figures 59–14 and 59–15. High power scanning electron microscopic views of individual cells on the synovial villus surface. There is a suggestion of intercellular bridging via thin cell processes in both figures. Magnification: Figure 59–14, × 4800; Figure 59–15, × 10,000. (Courtesy of Dr. G. Fauré.)

(fibroblast-like; see Chapter 16), those containing moderate numbers of lysosomes as well as well-developed endoplasmic reticulum and Golgi bodies.[249]

The type A cells (macrophage-like) remaining in these tissues have a different appearance from normal cells. They have fewer cell processes and contain swollen, distorted mitochondria and numerous membrane-bound granular dense bodies, which have been interpreted to be phagolysosomes.[250] Breakdown products of erythrocytes (membrane fragments and hemosiderin), which are easily visible as granules in cells on routine stains of tissue, are prominent in electron photomicrographs. The red blood cells presumably originate from intra-articular microhemorrhages.[251]

Multinucleate cells are found often in rheumatoid tissues (Fig. 59–17)[252] and in adherent cell cultures that have been freshly dissociated from matrix. It is tempting to presume presence of a virus that could be implicated as a fusogen. Lysolecithinase produced by phospholipase from neutrophils may be present transiently, and it has the capacity to fuse cells. A heat-labile protein of Mr of about 60,000 is released from antigen- or mitogen-stimulated lymphocytes and promotes the formation of multinucleated giant cells from human monocyte precursors.[253] Multinucleate cells formed among synovial fibroblasts have been demonstrated in vitro to secrete more collagenase than cultures of unfused cells. Their presence in tissues may be associated with accelerated rates of matrix degradation. Indirect support for this hypothesis is found in the nonrheumatoid but very destructive arthropathy, multicentric reticulohistiocytosis, that is characterized by multinucleate, lipid-laden histiocytes, resembling foreign body–type giant cells[254] (see Chapter 95).

The functional results of pathologic change are apparent in the joint capsule, tendons, and articular cartilage.

Figure 59–17. Phase microscopy of a thin section of succulent rheumatoid synovium prepared for electron microscopy, emphasizing the heterogeneity of this tissue. A multinucleate cell, which probably is a hypersecretor of proteinases, is visible. × 100. (Courtesy of Dr. Donald D. DiBona.)

The Joint Capsule. Proliferation of new tissue (highly vascularized collagen bundles with moderate perivascular inflammation) leads to altered physiology. Compliance is decreased, and accompanying this are redundancy and instability as ligaments are stretched. Subluxation from stretched capsular ligaments can lead directly to cartilage damage from mechanical incongruity. Periodic fluctuations in the amount of extracellular fluid present in the thickened capsule and overlying soft tissues are responsible for the variations in stiffness felt by patients.

The thickening of the rheumatoid joint capsule and the large accumulations of synovial fluid produce very high pressures in joints. [255] Flexion pressures in the knee joint of as high as 1000 mm Hg have been recorded.[256] It follows that high pressures in joints may compromise synovial blood flow, decreasing further the already low oxygen tensions in synovial fluid.[257]

Tendons. Tendons are remarkably homogeneous bundles of collagen sparsely populated with fibroblasts, blood vessels, and nerves. Tendons are exposed to both proliferative and destructive stimuli. Proliferative stimuli result in the formation of tendon nodules, which histologically are the same as subcutaneous rheumatoid nodules. Tendon nodules interfere with normal gliding function. Destructive effects of proliferative synovium in the tendon sheaths, accompanied by altered use patterns and, occasionally, trauma from eroded bone edges can lead to tendon rupture.

Articular Cartilage. The initial response in cartilage is loss of proteoglycans. The functional result of this is loss of stiffness, loss of ability to rebound from a comprehensive force, and a diminished capacity to resist deformation.[258,259] Thus, while the erosive pannus replaces the cartilage at the periphery of the joints, the central cartilage on the weight-bearing surfaces is more susceptible to mechanical fibrillation and fragmentation.

The Cartilage-Synovial Interface. Histopathologic studies early in the erosive phase of RA have revealed that the initial focus of bone and cartilage destruction is the periphery of the joint. "Recruitment" of perichondral and periosteal cells (as well as the chondrocytes themselves) occurs in this destructive process (Fig. 59–18).[260] Often a cartilage "lip" appears as subchondral bone is eroded underneath cartilage. Perhaps this protection of cartilage is provided by proteinase inhibitors, so-called "anti-invasive factors" in cartilage.[261] Similar inhibitors, some specific for collagenase, are present in tendon as well.

Although the invasive tissue may not often appear similar to synovial villi by histologic examination, there is little reason to doubt that the invasive pannus is an extension of proliferative synovium. As shown in Figure 59–19, where cartilage has been completely replaced, the appearance of the proliferative tissue at the surface resembles synovium, with the same polarity apparent that is seen in synovial lining cells. PMN leukocytes are found rarely at the pannus-cartilage interface.[262]

Tongues of proliferative cells penetrate the cartilage (Fig. 59–20), and destruction takes place in a very nar-

Figure 59–18. The periphery of a joint near the insertion of synovium at the osseous-chondral junction in rheumatoid arthritis. This shows proliferation of general mesenchymal tissue, including chondrocytes (*Ch*), as the destructive process begins. *C* is cartilage; *B* is bone. The arrow points to either a reduplicating chondrocyte or a cross section through a tongue of the invasive lesion.

Figure 59–19. A section from a metacarpal head replaced at joint arthroplasty. The surface at the upper left is the joint space. Residual cartilage at the left is surrounded by fibrous tissue. The superficial layers of pannus have taken on the appearance of synovium. At the bottom center, an area where subchondral bone has been completely degraded is seen as the pannus extends down into marrow space.

Figure 59–20. High power light microscopy at the pannus-synovial junction. The space between them is shrinkage artifact. Tongues of proliferating tissue have invaded the residual cartilage shown at the upper left. Small blood vessels (*BV*) are seen just below the cartilage-pannus junction. Small, darkly staining cells, probably lymphocytes (*L*) are just below the invading surface.

Figure 59–21. High power electron microscopic view of the junction between articular cartilage and rheumatoid synovium. The process is moving from the lower right to the upper left. Cartilage collagen fibers (distinguished by their 64-mm banding patterns, left center) are only faintly visible in the amorphous zone (1 to 3 μm wide) between cells and cartilage. Both a macrophage-like cell (*A*) and a cell filled with dilated endoplasmic reticulum (*B*) are at this leading edge of invasion.

row zone between the cells and cartilage. Ultrastructural studies have revealed several different patterns at this interface. One common form (Fig. 59–21) is a narrow, amorphous zone (2 to 4 μm wide), which well separates structural cartilage components from the invading cells.[263,264] Penetrating this zone are long thin processes from the cellular edge. The amorphous zone appears to contain debris. Probably in this setting cartilage is being destroyed extracellulary by enzymes active at neutral pH released by the adjacent cells.

Specimens of the cartilage-synovial junction from other patients have shown small blood vessels penetrating close to the cartilage, carrying with them some lymphocytes and plasma cells as well as mesenchymal cells and macrophages.[265] Although blood vessels do not often penetrate closer than 100 μm from the junction, it must be re-emphasized that without the capillary network which is built within the proliferative lesion there could be no progressive erosive synovitis.

Yet another pattern of synovial-cartilage interface is one of intimate contact between cells and cartilage, with cell borders and processes penetrating deeply into the cartilage matrix (Fig. 59–8). Cells at the interface may include PMN leukocytes, mast cells, and dendritic cells as well as macrophages and fibroblast-like cells. In this pattern, perhaps associated with more aggressive and rapidly progressive disease, intracellular collagen fibrils have been observed within membrane-bound vesicles and in various stages of digestion. It appears that this synovial-cartilage junction has special qualitative differences from the remaining synovium. Immunoreactive collagenase (antibody formed against active, not latent, enzyme) has been demonstrated at this junction around cells in proximity to cartilage, but rarely in cells deep in the synovium or even in the lining cells of synovium. There is much to be learned about the microenvironment at the pannus-cartilage junction, including the pH, the type and activity of cellular metabolism, and the qualitative nature of enzymes released by cells.

Pressure-Induced Pathology in RA. Normal joint function involves operation under very large forces, often greater than body weight. The effect of these forces begins to potentiate enzymatic destruction of joints from the earliest stages of the disease. Another example of cyclic augmentation in this disease is the fact that movement itself potentiates inflammation, so that the two are closely related.

One example of the destructive effects of pressure is the formation of subchondral pseudocysts. These lesions are round or pear shaped and contain fibrotic granulation tissue, necrotic debris, and detached pieces of cartilage and bone.[266] Often they are found in patients who are bothered little by pain and inflammation and continue an active life despite much proliferative synovitis in many joints. A connection between the cysts and joint cavity can be demonstrated in virtually all cases studied carefully.[267] Rarely, such a cyst may lead to weakened bone structure and fracture (Fig. 59–22).

Rheumatoid Nodules: The Extra-Articular Proliferative Lesion of RA. Rheumatoid nodules have been well

Figure 59–22. This radiograph demonstrates a pathologic fracture through a very large subchondral cyst in the proximal tibia. This patient had severe proliferative arthritis and many subchondral cysts, but had never missed a day of work and suffered very little from his disease. Biopsy of the involved subcortical lucent area showed typical rheumatoid granulation tissue. (Courtesy of Dr. Ed Olson and the Radiology Department, White River Junction, Vt., Veterans Administration Hospital.)

characterized morphologically.[268,269] These nodules are most often found subcutaneously over pressure points and represent a proliferative diathesis of mesenchymal tissue. In response to minimal trauma there is an intriguing combination of tissue destruction following proliferation and vasculitis to give the final result. Anatomically there is a central necrotic zone surrounded at a fairly sharp border by a highly cellular area of radially arranged cells amid strands of collagen (Figure 59–23, Plate III, p. xxxvii). The intense cellularity gives way at the periphery to more densely packed connective tissue. Mononuclear cells infiltrate around blood vessels in this capsular zone. Electron microscopic studies of the central necrotic areas have shown a mixture of collagen fibers in varying stages of degradation, noncollagenous filamentous material, granular debris, cell membranes, and fat globules.[270]

Study of nodules shortly after they have developed has revealed a marked inflammation of venules with deposition of fibrin within vessel walls and in surrounding tissue. Intense proliferation of fibroblasts in these early lesions is often found. The intense exudation from small blood vessels accounts for the space-occupying qualities of these nodules and explains how they can appear in less than 24 hours. The cellular proliferation is induced, somehow, by the vascular inflammation and gives structure to the nodule. The necrosis is probably a result of two processes: the microinfarctions resulting from thrombosis of terminal vessels, and the enormous quantities of proteinases and collagenase produced by the cellular palisading area.[271] Rarely, rheumatoid nodules appear in patients with a clinical diagnosis of RA but in whom no circulating rheumatoid factor can be demonstrated.[271a]

End Stages of Rheumatoid Arthritis. Progression of the process defined above results in loss of cartilage. With subluxation, thinning of bone, muscle atrophy, and fibrosis, movement of the joint diminishes and this facilitates fibrous ankylosis across joints. Rarely is ankylosis accompanied by mineralization, so that a true arthrodesis does not occur. Accompanying ankylosis there is a marked decrease in the inflammatory process with loss of the cellularity and vascularity. Whether these signs of decreased disease activity reflect the loss of movement or loss of cartilage as a trophic factor is not known. It has been reported that there is less inflammation in joints after insertion of a prosthesis and removal of all cartilage whether or not synovium is left within the joint.[272]

Vasculitis. The most prominent of extra-articular pathology in RA is vasculitis. It may present clinically as a variety of syndromes and may be associated with involvement of medium-sized arteries, small arteries, and venules. All layers of the vessel wall are infiltrated by lymphocytes.[273] Intimal proliferation and thrombosis occasionally are found, particularly in digital arteries. Deposits of IgG, IgM, and C3 have been noted in the walls of involved arteries,[152,274] notably in those patients with severe disease, high titers of rheumatoid factor, low serum C3, and clinical features such as peripheral neuropathy, digital gangrene, nailfold infarcts, and cutaneous ulcers.

In some patients, involvement of medium sized rather than small arteries with necrosis, fibrinoid change, PMN leukocyte infiltration, and disruption of the internal elastic lamina may resemble closely the pathology of polyarteritis nodosa.[275]

Palpable purpura, reflecting involvement of venules in a leukocytoclastic vasculitis, is the third pattern of involvement. Immunofluorescense sometimes reveals the presence of immunoglobulins and complement in and around the venules,[276] although studies of cutaneous vessel immune deposits have been positive in more than 50 percent of seropositive RA patients whether or not they have clinical vasculitis.[277] The persistence of fibrin in chronic lesions of vasculitis involving small arteries has led to the speculation that fibrin may play an active role in the genesis of these chronic and occlusive arterial lesions.[278]

References

1. Stastny, P.: Mixed lymphocyte cultures in rheumatoid arthritis. J. Clin. Invest. 57:1148, 1976.
2. McMichael, A.J., Sasazubi, T., McDevitt, H.O., and Payne, R.O.: Increased frequency of HLA-3C and HLA-Dw4 in rheumatoid arthritis. Arthritis Rheum. 20:1037, 1977.
3. Stasny, P.: Association of the B-cell alloantigen DR4 with rheumatoid arthritis. N. Engl. J. Med. 298:869, 1978.
4. Solinger, A.M., Bhatnagar, R., and Stabo, J.D.: Cellular, molecular, and genetic characteristics of T cell reactivity to collagen in man. Proc. Natl. Acad. Sci. (USA) 78:3877, 1981.
5. Alarcon, G.S., Koopman, W.J., Acton, R.T., and Barger, B.O.: Seronegative rheumatoid arthritis. A distinct immunogenetic disease? Arthritis Rheum. 25:502, 1982.
6. Willikens, R.F., Hansen, J.A., Malmgren, J.A., Nisperos, B., Mickelson, E.M., and Watson, M.A.: HLA antigens in Yakima Indians with rheumatoid arthritis. Lack of association with HLA-Dw4 and HLA-DR4. Arthritis Rheum. 25:1435, 1982.
7. Schiff, B., Mizrachi, Y., Orgad, S., Yaron, M., and Gazit, E.: Association of HLA-Aw31 and HLA-DR1 with adult rheumatoid arthritis. Ann. Rheum. Dis. 41:403, 1982.
8. Ueno, Y., Iwaky, Y., Terasaki, P.I., Park, M.S., Barnett, E.V., Chia, D., and Nakata, S.: HLA-DR4 in Negro and Mexican rheumatoid arthritis patients. J. Rheumatol. 8:804, 1981.
9. Stastny, P.: Joint report: Rheumatoid arthritis. In Terasaki, P.I. (ed.): Histocompatibility Testing 1980. Los Angeles, UCLA Tissue Typing Laboratory, 1980, pp. 681–686.
10. Schwab, J.H., Anderle, S.K., and Yank, C.H.: Arthritis in rats after systemic injection of streptococcal cells or cell walls. J. Exp. Med. 146:1585, 1977.
11. Pearson, C.M., Wood, F.D, and Tavaka, A.: Adjuvant and arthritogenic effects of some fractions of wax D from mycobacteria. Arthritis Rheum. 7:746, 1964.
12. Hamerman, D.: New thoughts on the pathogenesis of rheumatoid arthritis Am. J. Med. 40:1, 1966.
13. Andriopoulos, N.A., Mostecky, J. Wright, G.P., et al.: Characterization of antibodies to the native human collagens and to their component α-chains in the sera and the joint fluids of patients with rheumatoid arthritis. Immunochemistry 13:709, 1976.
14. Menzel, J., Steffen, C., Kolarz, G., Kojer, M., and Smolen, J.: Demonstration of anti-collagen antibodies in rheumatoid arthritis synovial fluids by ^{14}C radioimmunoassay. Arthritis Rheum. 21:243, 1978.
15. Trentham, D.E., Dynesius, R.A., Rocklin, R.E., and David, J.R.: Cellular sensitivity to collagen in rheumatoid arthritis. N. Engl. J. Med. 299:327, 1978.
16. Trentham, D.E., Townes, A.S., Kang, A.H., et al.: Humoral and cellular sensitivity to collagen in Type II collagen-induced arthritis in rats. J. Clin. Invest. 61:89, 1978.
17. Trentham, D.E., Townes, A.S., and Kang, A.H.: Autoimmunity to type II collagen: An experimental model of arthritis. J. Exp. Med. 146:857, 1977.
18. Claque, R.B., Shaw, M.J., and Holt, P.J.L.: Incidence and correlation between serum IgG and IgM antibodies to native type II collagen in patients with chronic inflammatory arthritis. Ann. Rheum. Dis. 40:6, 1981.
19. Alspaugh, M.A., and Tan, E.M.: Serum antibody in rheumatoid arthritis reactive with a cell-associated antigen: Demonstration by precipitation and immunofluorescence. Arthritis Rheum. 19:711, 1976.
20. Catalano, M.A., Carson, D.A., Slovin, S.F., Richman, D.D., and Vaughn, J.H.: Antibodies to Epstein-Barr virus-determined antigens in normal subjects and in patients with seropositive rheumatoid arthritis. Proc. Natl. Acad. Sci. (USA) 76:5825, 1979.
21. Alspaugh, M.A., Henle, G., Lennette, E.T., and Henle, W.: Elevated

levels of antibodies to Epstein-Barr virus antigens in sera and synovial fluids of patients with rheumatoid arthritis. J. Clin. Invest. 67:1134, 1981.

22. Tosato, G., Steinberg, A.D., and Blaese, R.M.: Defective EBV-specific suppressor T-cell function in rheumatoid arthritis. N. Engl. J. Med. 305:1238, 1981.

23. Depper, J.M., Bluestein, H.G., and Zvaifler, N.J.: Impaired regulation of Epstein-Barr virus-induced lymphocyte proliferation in rheumatoid arthritis is due to a T cell defect. J. Immunol. 127:1899, 1981.

24. Hasler, F., Bluestein, H.G., Zvaifler, N.J., and Epstein, L.B.: Analysis of the defects responsible for the impaired regulation of Epstein-Barr virus-induced B cell proliferation by rheumatoid arthritis lymphocytes. I. Diminished gamma interferon production in response to antalogous stimulation. J. Exp. Med. 157:173, 1983.

25. Lai, P.K., Alpers, M.P., and MacKay-Scollary, E.M.: Epstein-Barr herpes virus infection: inhibition by immunologically-induced mediators with interferon-like properties. Int. J. Cancer 20:21, 1977.

26. Silverman, S.L., and Schumacher, H.R.: Antibodies to Epstein-Barr viral antigens in early rheumatoid arthritis. Arthritis Rheum. 24:1465, 1981.

27. Depper, J.M., Zvaifler, N.J., and Bluestein, H.G.: Oropharyngeal Epstein-Barr virus excretion in rheumatoid arthritis. Arthritis Rheum. 25:427, 1982.

28. Kushner, I., and Somerville, J.: Permeability of human synovial membrane to plasma proteins. Relationship to molecular size and inflammation. Arthritis Rheum. 14:560, 1971.

29. Harris, E.D., Jr., Faulkner, C.S., III, and Brown, F.E.: Collagenolytic systems in rheumatoid arthritis. Clin. Orthop. 110:303, 1975.

30. Ruddy, S., and Austen, K.F.: Activation of the complement system in rheumatoid synovitis. Fed. Proc. 32:134, 1973.

31. Cooke, T.D., Hurd, E.R., Ziff, M., and Jasin, H.E.: The pathogenesis of chronic inflammation in experimental antigen-induced arthritis. II. Preferential localization of antigen-antibody complexes to collagenous tissues. J. Exp. Med. 135:323, 1972.

32. Cooke, T.D., Hurd, E.R., and Jasin, H.E.: Identification of immunoglobulins and complement in rheumatoid articular collagenous tissues. Arthritis Rheum. 18:563, 1975.

33. Ohno, O., and Cooke, T.D.: Electromicroscopic morphology of immunoglobulin aggregates and their interactions in rheumatoid articular collagenous tissues. Arthritis Rheum. 21:516, 1978.

34. Jasin, H.E.: Mechanism of trapping of immune complexes in joint collagenous tissues. Clin. Exp. Immunol. 22:473, 1975.

35. Ohno, O., and Cooke, T.D.V.: Immunoelectron microscope investigation of complexed immunoglobulins in rheumatoid (RA) and osteoarthrosis (OA) articular collagenous tissue. J. Bone Joint Surg. 60A:923, 1978.

36. Fox, A., and Glynn, L.E.: Persistence of antigen in nonarthritic joints. Ann. Rheum. Dis. 34:431, 1975.

37. Shiozawa, S., Jasin, H.E., and Ziff, M.: Absence of immunoglobulins in rheumatoid cartilage-pannus junctions. Arthritis Rheum. 23:816, 1980.

38. Cardella, C.J., Davies, P., and Allison, A.C.: Immune complexes induce selective release of lysosomal hydrolases from macrophages. Nature (Lond.) 274:46, 1974.

39. Dayer, J-M, Parswell, J.H., Schnaeberger, E.E., and Krane, S.M.: Interactions among rheumatoid synovial cells and monocyte-macrophages: Production of collagenase-stimulating factor by human monocytes exposed to concanavalin A or immunoglobulin Fc fragments. J. Immunol. 124:1712, 1980.

40. Bing, D.H., Alrneda, S., Isliker, H., Lattav, J., and Hynes, R.O.: Fibronectin binds to the C1q component by complement. Proc Natl. Acad. Sci. (USA) 79:4198, 1982.

41. Janossy, G., Duke, O., Poulter, L.W., Panayi, G., Bafill, M., and Goldstein, G.: Rheumatoid arthritis: A disease of T-lymphocyte/macrophage immunoregulation. Lancet 2:839, 1981.

42. Kurosaka, M., and Ziff, M.: Immunoelectron microscopic study of distribution of T cell subsets and HLA-DR expressing cells in rheumatoid synovium. Arthritis Rheum. 26(Suppl. 4):553, 1983.

43. Klareskog, L., Forsum, U., Scheyniers, A., Kabelitz, D., and Wigzell, H.: Evidence in support of a self-perpetuating HLA-DR-dependent delayed-type cell reaction in rheumatoid arthritis. Proc. Natl. Acad. Sci. (USA) 29:3632, 1982.

44. Bellu, D.I., and Unanue, E.R.: Regulation of macrophage populations. II. Synthesis and expression of Ia antigens by peritoneal exudate macrophages is a transient event. J. Immunol. 126:263, 1981.

45. Steinman, R.M., Kaplan, G., Witmer, M.D., and Cohn, Z.A.: Identification of a novel cell type in peripheral lymphoid organs of mice. I. Purification of spleen dendritic cells, new surface markers and maintenance in vitro. J. Exp. Med. 149:1, 1979.

46. Fensclan, A., Watt, S., and Mello, R.J.: Tumor angiogenic factor. Purification from the Walker 256 rat tumor. J. Biol. Chem. 256:9605, 1981.

47. Ashida, E.R., Johnson, A.R., and Lipsky, P.E.: Human endothelial cell-lymphocyte interaction. J. Clin. Invest. 67:1490, 1981.

48. Schumacher, H.R., and Kitrodou, R.C.: Synovitis of recent onset. A clinicopathologic study during the first month of disease. Arthritis Rheum. 15:465, 1972.

49. Gerber, P., Whang-Peng, J., and Monroe, J.H.: Transformation and chromosomal changes induced by Epstein-Barr virus in normal human leukocyte cultures. Proc. Natl. Acad. Sci. USA 63:740, 1969.

50. Mohr, W., and Wessinghage, D.: The relationship between polymorphonuclear granulocytes and cartilage destruction in rheumatoid arthritis. Z. Reichtsmed. 37:81, 1978.

51. Hollingsworth, J.W., Siegel, E.R., and Creasey, W.A.: Granulocyte survival in synovial exudate of patients with rheumatoid arthritis and other inflammatory joint diseases. Yale J. Biol. Med. 39:289, 1967.

52. Weissman, G., Spilberg, I., and Krakauer, K.: Arthritis induced in rabbits by lysates of granulocyte lysosomes. Arthritis Rheum. 12:103, 1969.

53. Weissman, G., and Spilberg, I.: Breakdown of cartilage protein polysaccharide by lysosomes. Arthritis Rheum. 9:162, 1968.

54. Desmukh, K., and Hemrick, S.: Metabolic changes in rabbit articular cartilage due to inflammation. Arthritis Rheum. 19:199, 1976.

55. Mowat, A.G., and Baum, J.: Chemotaxis of polymorphonuclear leukocytes from patients with rheumatoid arthritis. J. Clin. Invest. 50:2541, 1971.

56. Turner, R.A., Schumacher, H.R., and Myers, A.R.: Phagocytic function of polymorphonuclear leukocytes in rheumatic diseases. J. Clin. Invest. 52:1632, 1973.

57. Goetzl, E.J., and Pickett, W.C.: Novel structural determinates of the human neutrophil chemotactic activity of leukotriene B. J. Exp. Med. 153:482, 1981.

58. Klickstein, L.B., Shapleigh, C., and Goetzl, E.J.: Lipoxygenation of arachidonic acid as a source of polymorphonuclear leukocyte chemotactic factors in synovial fluid and tissue in rheumatoid arthritis and spondyloarthritis. J. Clin. Invest. 66:1166, 1980.

59. Fridovich, I.: The biology of oxygen radicals. Science 201:875, 1978.

60. Goldberg, B., and Stern, A.: The generation of O_2 by the interaction of the hemolytic agent phenylhydrazine with human hemoglobin. J. Biol. Chem. 250:2401, 1975.

61. McCord, J.M.: Free radicals and inflammation: Protection of synovial fluid by superoxide. Science 185:529, 1974.

62. Carp, H., and Janoff, A.: Potential mediator of inflammation. Phagocyte-derived oxidants suppress the elastase-inhibitory capacity α_1-proteinase inhibitor in vitro. J. Clin. Invest. 66:987, 1980.

63. Goldstein, I., Edelson, H.S., Kaplan, M.B., and Weissman, G.: Ceruloplasmin: A scavenger of superoxide anion radicals. J Biol. Chem. 254:4040, 1979.

64. Oyanagui, Y.: Participation of superoxide anions in the prostaglandin phase of carrageenan foot-oedema. Biochem. Pharmacol. 25:1465, 1976.

64a. Weiss, S.J., Lampert, M.B., and Test, S.T.: Long-lived oxidants generated by human neutrophils: Characterization and bioactivity. Science 222:625, 1983.

65. Hallgren, R., Hukansson, L., and Venge, P.: Kinetic studies of phagocytosis. 1. The serum independent particle uptake by PMN from patients with rheumatoid arthritis and SLE. Arthritis Rheum. 21:107, 1978.

66. Corberand, J., Amigues, H., deLarrard, B., and Pradere, J.: Neutrophil functions in rheumatoid arthritis. Scand. J. Rheumatol. 6:49, 1977.

67. Wilton, J.M.A., Gibson, T., and Chuck, C.M.: Defective phagocytosis by synovial fluid and blood PMN leukocytes in patients with rheumatoid arthritis. I. The nature of the defect. Rheumatol. Rehabil. Supplement, 1978, pp. 25–35.

68. Mowat, A.G., and Baum, J.: Chemotaxis of PMN leukocytes from patients with rheumatoid arthritis. J. Clin. Invest. 50:2541, 1971.

69. Udein, A-M., Trang, L., Venizelos, N., and Palmblad, J.: Neutrophil functions and clinical performance after total fasting in patients with rheumatoid arthritis. Ann. Rheum. Dis. 42:45, 1983.

70. Ruddy, S., and Colten, H.R.: Biosynthesis of complement proteins by synovial tissues. N. Engl. J. Med. 290:1284, 1974.

71. Smiley, J.D., Sachs, C., and Ziff, M.: In vitro synthesis of immunoglobulin by rheumatoid synovial membrane. J. Clin. Invest. 47:624, 1968.

72. Slirvinski, A.H., and Zvaifler, N.H.: In vivo synthesis of IgG by rheumatoid synovium. J. Lab Clin. Med. 76:304, 1970.

73. Ruddy, S., Britton, M.C., Schur, P.H., and Austen, K.F.: Complement components in synovial fluid: Activation and fixation in seropositive rheumatoid arthritis. Ann. N.Y. Acad. Sci. 168:161, 1969.

74. Ruddy, S., and Austen, K.F.: The complement system in rheumatoid synovitis. I. An analysis of complement component activities in rheumatoid synovial fluids. Arthritis Rheum. 13:713, 1970.

75. Pekin, T.J., Jr., and Zvaifler, N.J.: Hemolytic complement in synovial fluid. J. Clin. Invest. 43:1372, 1964.

76. Sabharwal, U.K., Vaughan, J.H., Fong, S., Bennett, P.H., Carson, D.A., and Curd, J.G.: Activation of the classical pathway of complement by rheumatoid factors. Assessment by radioimmunoassay for C4. Arthritis Rheum. 25:161, 1982.

77. Kaplan, R.A., Curd, J.G., DeHeer, D.H., Carson, D.A., Pangburn, M.K., Muller-Eberhard, H.J., and Vaughan, J.H.: Metabolism of C4 and

factor B in rheumatoid arthritis: Relation to rheumatoid factor. Arthritis Rheum. 23:911, 1980.

78. Sabharwal, U.K., Vaughan, J.H., Fong, S., Bennett, P.H., Carson, D.A., and Curd, J.G.: Activation of the classical pathway of complement by rheumatoid factors: Assessment by radioimmunoassay for C4. Arthritis Rheum. 25:161, 1982.

79. Goldstein, I.M., and Weissmann, G.: Generation of C5-derived lysosomal enzyme-releasing activity (C5a) by lysates of leukocyte lysosomes. J. Immunol. 113:1583, 1974.

80. Borel, J.F., Keller, H.U., and Sorkin, E.: Studies on chemotaxis. XI. Effect on neutrophils of lysosomal and other subcellular fractions from leukocytes. Int. Arch. Allergy Appl. Immunol. 35:194, 1969.

81. Ward, P.A., and Zvaifler, N.J.: Complement-derived leucotactic factors in inflammatory synovial fluids of humans. J. Clin. Invest. 50:606, 1971.

82. Goldstein, I.M., Hoffman, S., Gallin, J., and Weissman, G.: Mechanisms of lysosomal enzyme release from human leucocytes. Microtubule assembly and membrane fusion induced by a component of complement. Proc. Natl. Acad. Sci. USA 70:2916, 1973.

83. Kaplan, M.H., and Volanakis, J.E.: Interaction of C-reactive protein complexes with the complement system. I. Consumption of human complement associated with the reaction of C-reactive protein with pneumococcal C-polysaccharide and with the choline phosphatides, lecithin and sphingomyelin. J. Immunol. 112:2135, 1974.

84. Kushner, I., Rakitu, L., and Kaplan, M.H.: Studies of acute phase protein. II. Localization of C-reactive protein in heart in induced myocardial infarction in rabbits. J. Clin. Invest. 42:286, 1963.

85. Wuepper, K.D.: Cutaneous responses to human C3a anaphylatoxin in man. Clin. Exp. Immunol. 11:13, 1972.

86. Pisano, J.J., and Austen, K.F.: Chemistry and Biology of the Kallikrein Kinin System in Health and Disease. Washington, D.C., U.S. Government Printing Office, 1976.

87. Epstein, W., Melmon, K.L., Tan, E.M., and Stoff, J.: Kinin generation by human IgG rheumatoid factor complex (abstract). J. Clin. Invest. 47:90, 1968.

88. Melmon, K.L., and Cline, M.J.: Kallikrein activator and kininase in human granulocytes: A model of inflammation. In Rocha, E., and Silva, M. (eds.): Symposium on Vasoactive Polypeptides: Bradykinin and Related Kinins. Oxford, Pergamon Press, 1967.

89. Cochrane, C.G., et al.: The interaction of Hageman factor and immune complexes. J. Clin. Invest. 51:2736, 1972.

90. Rothberger, H., Zimmerman, T.S., Spiegelberg, H.L., and Vaughan, J.H.: Leucocyte procoagulant activity: Enhancement of production in vitro by IgG and antigen-antibody complexes. J. Clin. Invest. 59:549, 1977.

91. Glynn, L.E.: Heberden Oration. The chronicity of inflammation and its significance in rheumatoid arthritis. Ann. Rheum. Dis. 27:105, 1968.

92. Van de Putte, L.B.A., Hegt, V.N., and Overbeek, T.E.: Activators and inhibitors of fibrinolysis in rheumatoid and non-rheumatoid synovial membranes. Arthritis Rheum. 20:671, 1977.

93. Kulka, P.J.: Microcirculation impairment as a factor in inflammatory tissue damage. Ann. N.Y. Acad. Sci. 116:1018, 1964.

94. Metzger, F., Haffeld, J.F., and Oppenheim, J.J.: Regulation by PGE_2 of the production of oxygen intermediates by LPS-activated macrophages. J. Immunol. 127:1109, 1981.

95. Vassalli, J-D, Hamilton, J., and Reich, E.: Macrophage plasminogen activator: Modulation of enzyme production by anti-inflammatory steroids, mitotic inhibitors, and cyclic nucleotides. Cell 8:281, 1976.

96. Roberts, J.E., McLees, B.D., and Kerby, G.P.: Pathways of glucose metabolism in rheumatoid and non-rheumatoid synovial membrane. J. Lab. Clin. Med. 70:503, 1967.

97. Thomas, P.P.L., and Dingle, J.T.M.: Studies on human synovial membrane in vitro. The metabolism of normal and rheumatoid synovia and the effect of hydrocortisone. Biochem. J. 68:231, 1958.

98. Falchuk, K.H., Goetzl, E.J., and Kulka, J.P.: Respiratory gases of synovial fluids. An approach to synovial tissue circulatory-metabolic imbalance in rheumatoid arthritis. Am. J. Med. 49:223, 1970.

99. Wallis, W.J., Simkin, P.A., Nelp, W.B., and Foster, D.M.: Synovial fluid temperature in rheumatoid synovitis. Arthritis Rheum. 26:517, 1983.

100. Muirden, K.D.: The anaemia of rheumatoid arthritis: The significance of iron deposits in the synovial membrane. Aust. Ann. Med. 19:97, 1970.

101. Mainardi, C.L., Levine, P.H., Werb, Z., and Harris, E.D., Jr.: Proliferative synovitis in hemophilia. Biochemical and morphologic observations. Arthritis Rheum. 21:137, 1978.

102. Blake, D.R., Hall, N.D., Bacon, P.A., Dieppe, P.A., Halliwell, B., and Gutteridge, J.M.C.: The importance of iron in rheumatoid disease. Lancet 2:1142, 1981.

103. Chichton, R.R.: Interreaction between iron metabolism and oxygen activation. In: Oxygen Free Radicals and Tissue Damage. Ciba Foundation Symposium 65 (new series). Amsterdam, Excerpta Medica, 1979, pp. 57–76.

104. Okazaki, I., Brinckeroff, C.E., Sinclair, J.F., Sinclair P.R., Bronkowsky, H.L. and Harris, E.D., Jr.: Iron increases collagenase production by rabbit synovial fibroblasts J. Lab. Clin. Med. 97:396–402, 1981.

105. Ziff, M.: Relation of cellular infiltration of rheumatoid synovial membrane to its immune response. Arthritis Rheum. 17:313, 1974.

106. VanBoxel, J.A., and Paget, S.A.: Predominantly T cell infiltrate in rheumatoid synovial membrane. N. Engl. J. Med. 293:517, 1975.

107. Bankhurst, A.D., Husky, G., and Williams, R.C., Jr.: Predominance of T cells in the lymphocytic infiltrates of synovial tissues in rheumatoid arthritis. Arthritis Rheum. 19:555, 1976.

108. Van de Putte, L.B.A., de Vries, E., Van Leuwen, A.W.F.M., and Meijer, C.J.L.M.: T-lymphocytes and rheumatoid inflammation. In Feltkamp, A., and Leiden, T.E.W. (eds.): Non-Articular Forms of Rheumatoid Arthritis. Amsterdam, Staflen's Scientific Publishing, 1977, pp. 103–110.

109. Mellbye, O.J., Messner, R.P., DeBord, J.R., and Williams, R.C.: Immunoglobulin and receptors for C3 on lymphocytes from patients with rheumatoid arthritis. Arthritis Rheum. 15:371, 1975.

110. Papamichael, M., Brown, J.C., and Holborow, E.J.: Immunoglobulins on the surface of human lymphocytes. Lancet 2:850, 1971.

111. Micheli, A., and Brom, J.: Studies on blood T and B lymphocytes in rheumatoid arthritis. Ann. Rheum. Dis. 33:435, 1974.

112. Konttinen, Y.T., Reitamo, S., Ranki, A., Hayry, P., Kankaanapaa, U., and Wegelius, O.: Characterization of the immunocompetent cells of rheumatoid synovium from tissue sections and eluates. Arthritis Rheum. 24:71, 1981.

113. Burmester, G.R., Yu, D.T.Y., Irani, A-M, Kunkel, H.G., and Winchester, R.J.: Ia+ T cells in synovial fluid and tissues of patients with rheumatoid arthritis. Arthritis Rheum. 24:1370, 1981.

114. Fox, R.I., Fong, S., Sabharwal, N., Carstens, S.A., Kung, P.C., and Vaughan, J.H.: Synovial fluid lymphocytes differ from peripheral blood lymphocytes in patients with rheumatoid arthritis. J. Immunol. 128:351–354, 1982.

115. Winchester, R.J., and Kunkel, H.G.: The human Ia system. Adv. Immunol. 28:221–292, 1979.

116. Reinberg, E.L., Kung, P.C., Pesando, J.M., Ritz, J., Goldstein, G., and Schlossman, S.F.: Ia determinants on human T-cell subsets defined by monoclonal antibody. Activation stimuli required for expression. J. Exp. Med. 150:1472, 1979.

117. Yu, D.T., Winchester, R.J., Fu, S.M., Givofsky, A., Ko, H.S., and Kunkel, H.G.: Peripheral blood Ia-positive T cells, increases in certain diseases and after immunization. J. Exp. Med. 151:91, 1980.

118. Carter, S.D., Bacon, P.A., and Hall, N.D.: Characterization of activated lymphocytes in the peripheral blood of patients with rheumatoid arthritis. Ann Rheum. Dis. 40:293, 1981.

119. Herberman, R.B., and Ortaldo, J.R.: Natural killer cells: Their role in defenses against disease. Science 214:24, 1981.

120. Dohlong, J.H., Førre, O., Kvien, T.K., Egeland, T., and Degre, M.: Natural killer (NK) cell activity of peripheral blood, synovial fluid, and synovial tissue lymphocytes from patients with rheumatoid arthritis and juvenile rheumatoid arthritis. Ann. Rheum. Dis. 41:490, 1982.

121. Griffiths, M.M., Smith, C.B., Ward, J.R., and Klauber, M.R.: Cytotoxic activity of rheumatoid and normal lymphocytes against allogeneic and autologous synovial cells in vitro. J. Clin. Invest. 58:613, 1976.

122. Ghose, T., Woodbury, J.F., and Hansell, M.M.: Interaction in vitro between synovial cells and autologous lymphocytes and sera from arthritis patients. J. Clin. Pathol. 28:550, 1975.

123. Griffiths, M.M., Smith, C.B., and Pepper, B.J.: Susceptibility of rheumatoid and non-rheumatoid synovial cells to antibody-dependent cell-mediated cytotoxicity. Arthritis Rheum. 21:97, 1978.

124. Koopman, W.J., and Schrohenloher, R.E.: Enhanced in vitro synthesis of IgM rheumatoid factor in rheumatoid arthritis. Arthritis Rheum. 23:985, 1980.

125. Abrahamsen, T.G., Froland, S.S., Natvig, J.B., and Pahle, J.: Elution and characterization of lymphocytes from rheumatoid inflammatory tissue. Scand. J. Immunol. 4:823, 1975.

126. Goodwin, J.S., Bankhurst, A.D., and Messner, R.P.: Suppression of human T-cell mitogenesis by prostaglandin. J. Exp. Med. 146:1719, 1977.

127. Panayi, G.S., and Corrigall, V.: Lymphocyte function in rheumatoid arthritis. In Panayi, G.S., and Johnson, P.M. (eds.): Immunopathogenesis of Rheumatoid Arthritis. Chertsey, Reedbooks, Ltd. 1979, p. 31.

128. Andreis, M., Stastny, P., and Ziff, M.: Experimental arthritis produced by injection of mediators of delayed hypersensitivity. Arthritis Rheum. 14:537, 1971.

129. Dayer, J.M., Robinson, D.R., and Krane, S.M.: Prostaglandin production by rheumatoid synovial cells. J. Exp. Med. 145:1399, 1977.

130. Waksman, B.H., and Namba, Y.: On soluble mediators of immunologic regulation. Cell Immunol. 21:161, 1976.

131. Lawrence, H.S., and Valentine, F.T.: Transfer factor and other mediators of cellular immunity. Am. J. Pathol. 60:437, 1970.

132. Lawrence, H.S.: Transfer factor and cellular immune deficiency disease. N. Eng. J. Med. 283:411, 1970.

133. Wegelius, O., Laire, W., Lindstrom, B., and Klockars, M.: Fistula of the thoracic duct as immunosuppressive treatment in rheumatoid arthritis. Acta Med. Scand. 187:539, 1970.

134. Paulus, H.E., Machleder, H.I., and Peter, J.B.: Clinical improvement of rheumatoid arthritis during prolonged thoracic duct lymphocyte drainage. Arthritis Rheum. 16:562, 1973.

135. Whitehouse, M.W., Whitehouse, D.J., and Pearson, C.M.: Passive transfer of adjuvant-induced arthritis and allergic encephalomyelitis in rats using thoracic duct lymphocytes. Nature 224:1322, 1969.

136. Pearson, C.M.: Transfer of adjuvant arthritis by means of lymph node or spleen cells. J. Belg. Rheumatol. Med. Phys. 24:150, 1969.

137. Good, R.A., Rotstein, J., and Mozzitello, W.F.: The simultaneous occurrence of rheumatoid arthritis and agammaglobulinemia. J. Lab. Clin. Med. 49:343, 1957.

138. Mellors, R., Heimer, R., Corcos, J., et al.: Cellular origin of rheumatoid factor. J. Exp. Med. 110:875, 1959.

139. Munthe, E., and Natvig, J.B.: Immunoglobulin classes, subclasses and complexes of IgG rheumatoid factor in rheumatoid plasma cells. Clin. Exp. Immunol. 12:55, 1972.

140. Hoffman, W.L., Goldberg, M.S., and Smiley, J.D.: Immunoglobulin G_3 subclass production by rheumatoid synovial tissue cultures. J. Clin. Invest. 69:136, 1982.

141. Cats, A., and Hazevoet, H.M.: Significance of positive tests for rheumatoid factor in the prognosis of rheumatoid arthritis. Ann. Rheum. Dis. 29:254, 1970.

142. Herman, J.H., Bradley, J., Ziff, M., and Smiley, J.D.: Response of the rheumatoid synovial membrane to exogenous immunization. J. Clin. Invest. 50:266, 1971.

143. Allen, J.C., and Kunkel, H.G.: Hidden rheumatoid factors with specificity for native gamma globulins. Arthritis Rheum. 9:758, 1966.

144. Cone, R.E., Feldmann, M., Marchalones, J.J., and Nossal, G.J.V.: Cytophilic properties of surface immunoglobulin of thymus-derived lymphocytes. Immunology 26:49, 1974.

145. Veys, E.M., Gabriel, P.A., and Goegne, E.: Rheumatoid factor and serum IgG, IgM and IgA levels in rheumatoid arthritis with vasculitis. Scand. J. Rheumatol. 5:1, 1976.

146. Vaughan, J.H.: Lymphocyte function in rheumatic disorders. Arch. Intern. Med. 135:1324, 1975.

147. Pope, R.M., Teller, D.C., and Mannik, M.: The molecular basis of self-association of antibodies to IgG (rheumatoid factor) in rheumatoid arthritis. Proc. Natl. Acad. Sci. USA 71:517, 1974.

148. Winchester, R.J.: Characterization of IgG complexes in patients with rheumatoid arthritis. Ann. N.Y. Acad. Sci. 256:73, 1975.

149. Brown, P.B., Nardella, F.A., and Mannik, M.: Human complement activation by self-associated IgG rheumatoid factors. Arthritis Rheum. 25:1101, 1982.

150. Pekin, T.J., Jr., and Zvaifler, N.J.: Hemolytic complement levels in synovial fluids. J. Clin. Invest. 43:1372, 1964.

151. Rodman, W.S., Williams, R.C., Jr., Bilka, P.J., and Muller-Eberhard, H.J.: Immunofluorescent localization of the third and fourth component of complement in synovial tissues from patients with rheumatoid arthritis. J. Lab. Clin. Med. 69:141, 1967.

152. Conn, D.L., McDuffie, F.C., and Dyck, P.J.: Immunopathologic study of sural nerves in rheumatoid arthritis. Arthritis Rheum. 15:135, 1972.

153. Zvaifler, N.J.: Immunopathology of joint inflammation in rheumatoid arthritis. Immunology 16:265, 1973.

154. Pope, R.M.: Rheumatoid arthritis associated with hyperviscosity syndrome and intermediate complex formation. Arch. Intern. Med. 135:281, 1975.

155. Jasin, H.E., LoSpalluto, J.J., and Ziff, M.: Rheumatoid hyperviscosity syndrome. Am. J. Med. 49:484, 1970.

156. DeHoratius, R.J., Abruzzo, J.L., and Williams, R.C., Jr.: Immunofluorescent and immunologic studies of rheumatoid lung. Arch. Intern. Med. 129:441, 1972.

157. Theofilopoulos, A.N., Burtonboy, G., LoSpalluto, J.J., and Ziff, M.: IgM rheumatoid factor and low molecular weight IgM: An association with vasculitis. Arthritis Rheum. 17:272, 1977.

158. Allen, C., Elson, C.J., Scott, D.G.I., Bacon, P.A., and Bucknall, R.C.: IgG antiglobulins in rheumatoid arthritis and other arthritides: relationship with clinical features and other parameters. Ann. Rheum. Dis. 40:127, 1981.

159. Winchester, R.J., Agnello, V., and Kunkel, H.G.: Gamma globulin complexes in synovial fluids of patients with rheumatoid arthritis. Partial characterization and relationship to lowered complement levels. Clin. Exp. Immunol. 6:689, 1970.

160. Munthe, E., and Natvig, J.B.: Characterization of IgG complexes in eluates from rheumatoid tissue. Clin. Exp. Immunol. 8:249, 1971.

161. Munthe, E., and Natvig, J.B.: Immunoglobulin classes, subclasses and complexes of IgG rheumatoid factor in rheumatoid plasma cells. Clin. Exp. Immunol. 12:55, 1972.

162. Munthe, E., and Natvig, J.B.: Complement-fixing intracellular complexes of IgG rheumatoid factor in rheumatoid plasma cells. Scand. J. Immunol. 1:217, 1972.

163. McCarty, D.J., and Hollander, J.L.: Identification of urate crystals in gouty synovial fluid. Ann. Intern. Med. 54:452, 1961.

164. Hollander, J.L., McCarty, D.J., Astorga, G., and Castro-Mirillo, E.: Studies on the pathogenesis of rheumatoid joint inflammation. I. The R.A. "cell" and a working hypothesis. Ann. Intern. Med. 62:271, 1965.

165. Britton, M.C., and Schur, P.H.: The complement system in rheumatoid synovitis. II. Intracytoplasmic inclusions of immunoglobulins and complement. Arthritis Rheum. 14:87, 1971.

166. Rodman, W.S., Williams, R.C., Jr., Bilka, P.J., and Muller-Eberhard, H.J.: Immunofluorescent localization of the third and the fourth component of complement in synovial tissue from patients with rheumatoid arthritis. J. Lab. Clin. Med. 69:141, 1967.

167. Cecere, F., Lessard, J., McDuffy, S., and Pope, R.M.: Evidence for the local production and utilization of immune reactions in rheumatoid arthritis. Arthritis Rheum. 25:1307, 1982.

168. Rawson, A.J., Hollander, J.L., Quismorio, F.P., and Abelson, N.M.: Experimental arthritis in man and rabbit dependent upon serum anti-immunoglobulin factors. Ann. N.Y. Acad. Sci. 168:188, 1969.

169. Tanimoto, K., Cooper, N.R., Johnson, J.S., and Vaughan, J.H.: Complement fixation by rheumatoid factor. J. Clin. Invest. 55:437, 1975.

170. Theofilopoulos, A.N., Dixon, F.J., and Bokish, V.A.: Binding of soluble immune complexes to human lymphoblastoid cells. I. Characterization of receptors for IgG, Fc and complement and description of the binding mechanism. J. Exp. Med. 140:877, 1974.

171. Henney, G.S., Stanworth, D.R., and Gell, P.G.H.: Demonstration of the exposure of new antigenic determinants following antigen-antibody combination. Nature 205:1079, 1965.

172. Johnson, P.M., Watkins, J., Scopes, P.M., and Tracey, B.M.: Differences in serum IgG structures in health and rheumatoid disease. Ann. Rheum. Dis. 33:366, 1974.

173. Allison, A.C.L.: Heberden Oration: Mechanism of tolerance and autoimmunity. Ann. Rheum. Dis. 32:283, 1973.

174. Jerne, N.K.: Towards a network theory of the immune system. Ann. Immunol. (Inst. Pasteur) 115C:373, 1974.

175. Pasquali, J.L., Urlacher, A., Storck, D.: A highly conserved determinant on human rheumatoid factor idiotypes defined by a mouse monoclonal antibody. Clin. J. Immunol. 13:197–201, 1983.

176. Jerne, N.K., Nordin, A.A., and Henry C.: The agar plaque technique for recognizing antibody-producing cells. In Amos, B., and Koprowski, H. (ed.): Cell Bound Antibodies. Philadelphia, Wistar Institute Press, 1963, p. 109.

177. Vaughan, J.H., Chihara, T., Moore, T.L., Robbins, D.L., Tanimoto, K., Johnson, J.S., and McMillan, R.: Rheumatoid factor–producing cells detected by direct hemolytic plaque assay. J. Clin. Invest. 58:933, 1976.

178. Zuran, B.L., O'Hair, C.H., Vaughan, J.H., Mathison, D.A., Curd, J.G., and Katz, D.H.: Immunoglobulin E–rheumatoid factor in the serum of patients with rheumatoid arthritis, asthma, and other diseases. J. Clin. Invest. 68:1610, 1981.

179. Meretey, K., Falus, A., Erhardt, C.C., and Maini, R.N.: IgE and IgE–rheumatoid factors in circulating immune complexes in rheumatoid arthritis. Ann. Rheum. Dis. 41:405, 1982.

180. Crisp, A.J., Chapman, C.M., Kirkham, S., Schiller, A.L., and Krane, S.M.: Synovial mastocytosis in adult rheumatoid arthritis. Arthritis Rheum. 26:552, 1983.

181. Abel, T., Andrews, B.S., Cunningham, P.H., Brunner, C.M., Davis, J.B., and Horwitz, D.A.: Rheumatoid vasculitis: Effect of cyclophosphamide on the clinical course and levels of circulating immune complexes. Ann. Intern. Med. 93:407, 1980.

182. Rapoport, R.J., Kozin, F., Macket, S.E., and Jordan, R.E.: Cutaneous vascular immunofluorescence in rheumatoid arthritis: correlation with circulating immune complexes and vasculitis. Am. J. Med. 68:325, 1980.

183. McDougal, J.S., Hubbard, M., McDuffie, F.C., Strobel, P.L., Smith, S.J., Bass, N., Goldman, J.A., Hartman, S., Myerson, G., Miller, S., Morales, R., and Wilson, C.H., Jr.: Comparison of five assays for immune complexes in the rheumatic diseases. An assessment of their validity for rheumatoid arthritis. Arthritis Rheum. 25:1156, 1982.

184. Dayer, J.M., Krane, S.M., Russell, R.G.G., and Robinson, D.F.: Production of collagenase and prostaglandins by isolated adherent rheumatoid synovial cells. Proc. Natl. Acad. Sci. USA 73:945, 1976.

185. Abrahamsen, T.G., Johnson, P.M., and Natvig, J.B.: Membrane characteristics of adherent cells dissociated from rheumatoid synovial tissue. Clin. Exp. Immunol. 28:474, 1977.

186. Theofilopoulos, A.N., Carson, D.A., Tovassoli, M., Slotrim, S.F., Speers, W.C., Jensen, F.B., and Vaughan, J.H.: Evidence for the presence of receptors for C3 and IgG Fc on human synovial cells. Arthritis Rheum. 23:1, 1980.

187. Baker, D.G., Dayer, J.M., Roelke, M., Schumacher, H.R., and Krane, S.M.: Rheumatoid synovial cell morphologic changes induced by a mononuclear cell factor in culture Arthritis Rheum. 26:8, 1983.

188. Pollack, M.S., Goldenhersch, M., Chin-Louie, J., and Safai, B.: The functional study of DR-positive human epidermal Langerhans cells in mixed cell cultures with allogeneic lymphocytes. Clin. Immunol. Immunopathol. 24:15, 1982.

189. Anastassiades, T.P., Ley, J., Wood, A., and Irwin, D.: The growth kinetics of synovial fibroblast cells from inflammatory and noninflammatory arthropathies. Arthritis Rheum. 21:461, 1978.

190. Castor, C.W.: Connective tissue activation II. Abnormalities of cultured rheumatoid synovial cells. Arthritis Rheum. 14:55, 1971.

191. Goldfischer, S., Smith, C., and Hamerman, D.: Altered acid hydrolase activities in rheumatoid synovial cells in culture. Am. J. Pathol. 52:569, 1968.

192. Henderson, B.: The contribution made by cytochemistry to the study of the metabolism of the normal and rheumatoid synovial lining cell (synoviocyte). Histochemical J. 14:527, 1982.

193. Castor, C.W., and Lewis, R.B.: Connective tissue activation. X. Current studies of mediators and the process. Scand. J. Rheumatol. 5:41, 1975.

194. Castor, C.W., Ritchie, J.C., Scott, M.E., and Whitney, S.L.: Connective tissue activation. XI. Stimulation of glycosaminoglycan and DNA formation by a platelet factor. Arthritis Rheum. 20:859, 1977.

195. Andersen, H.: Development, morphology and histochemistry of the early synovial tissue in human foetuses. Acta Anat. 58:90, 1964.

196. Loeuvi, G.: Experimental immune inflammation in the synovial membrane. Immunology 17:489, 1969.

197. Wahl, L.M., Wahl, S.M., Mergenhagen, S.E., and Martin, G.R.: Collagenase production by lymphokine-activated macrophages. Science 187:261, 1975.

198. Vasalli, J.D., and Reich, E.: Macrophage plasminogen activator: Induction by products of activated lymphoid cells. J. Exp. Med. 145:427, 1977.

199. David, J.R., and David, R.R.: Cellular hypersensitivity and immunity. Inhibition of macrophage migration and the lymphocyte mediators. Prog. Allergy 16:200, 1972.

200. Cardella, C.J., Davies, P., and Allison, A.C.: Immune complexes induce selective release of lysosomal enzymes. Nature 247:46, 1974.

201. Schorlemmer, H.U., and Allison, A.C.: Effects of activated complement components on enzyme secretion by macrophages. Immunology 31:781, 1976.

202. Gotze, D., and Bianco, C.: In van Furth, R. (ed.): Mononuclear Phagocytes: Functional Aspects. The Hague, Martinus Nijhoff, 1979.

203. Werb, Z., Mainardi, C.L., Vater, C.A., and Harris, E.D., Jr.: Endogenous activation of a latent collagenase by rheumatoid synovial cells. Evidence for a role of plasminogen activator. N. Engl. J. Med. 296:1017, 1977.

204. Bianco, C., Eden, A., and Cohn, Z.A.: The induction of macrophage spreading: Role of coagulation factors and the complement system. J. Exp. Med. 144:1531, 1976.

205. Werb, Z., and Aggler, J.: Proteases induce secretion of collagenase and plasminogen activator by fibroblasts. Proc. Natl. Acad. Sci. USA 75:1839, 1978.

206. Polvernie, P.J., Cottran, R.S., Gimbrone, M.A., Jr., and Unanue, E.R.: Activated macrophages induced vascular proliferation. Nature 269:804, 1977.

207. Henderson, B., Glynn, L.E., and Chayen, J.: Cell division in the synovial lining in experimental allergic arthritis: Proliferation of cells during the development of chronic arthritis. Ann. Rheum. Dis. 41:275, 1982.

208. Krane, S.M.: Heberden Oration, 1980. Aspects of the cell biology of the rheumatoid synovial lesion. Ann. Rheum. Dis. 40:433, 1981.

209. Postlethwaite, A.E., and Kang, A.H.: Characterization of fibroblast proliferation factors elaborated by antigen- and mitogen-stimulated guinea pig lymph node cells: Differentiation from lymphocyte-derived chemotactic factor for fibroblasts, lymphocyte mitogenic factor, and Interleukin 1. Cellular Immunol. 73:169, 1982.

210. Schmidt, J.A., Mizel, S.B., Cohen, D., and Green, I.: Interleukin 1, a potential regulator of fibroblast proliferation. J. Immunol. 128:2177, 1982.

211. Devel, T.F., Huang, J.S., Proffitt, R.T., Baenziger, J.U., Chang, D., and Kennedy, B.B.: Human platelet-derived growth factor. J. Biol. Chem. 256:8896, 1981.

212. Dayer, J.-M., Russell, R.G.G., and Krane, S.M.: Collagenase production by rheumatoid synovial cells: Stimulation by a human lymphocyte factor. Science 135:181, 1977.

213. Dayer, J.-M., Robinson, D.R., and Krane, S.M.: Prostaglandin production by rheumatoid synovial cells. Stimulation by a factor from human mononuclear cells. J. Exp. Med. 145:1393, 1977.

214. Mizel, S.B., Dayer, J.-M, Krane, S.M., and Mergenhagen, S.E.: Stimulation of rheumatoid synovial cell collagenase and prostaglandin production by partially purified lymphocyte-activating factor (Interleukin 1). Proc. Natl. Acad. Sci. (USA) 78:2474, 1980.

215. Postlethwaite, A.E., Lachman, L.B., Mainardi, C.L., and Kang, A.H.: Interleukin 1 stimulation of collagenase production by cultured fibroblasts. J. Exp. Med. 157:801, 1983.

216. Biswas, C., and Dayer, J.-M.: Stimulation of collagenase production by collagen in mammalian cell cultures. Cell 18:1035, 1979.

217. Dayer, J.-M., Trentham, D.E., David, J.R., and Krane, S.M.: Collagens stimulate the production of mononuclear cell factor (MCF) and prostaglandins (PGE$_2$) by human monocytes. Trans. Assoc. Am. Phys. 93:326, 1980.

218. Tsukamoto, Y., Helsel, W.E., and Wahl, S.M.: Macrophage production of fibronectin, a chemoattractant for fibroblasts. J. Immunol. 127:673, 1981.

219. Hamilton, J.A., and Slywka, J.: Stimulation of human synovial fibroblast plasminogen activator production by mononuclear cell supernatants. J. Immunol. 126:851, 1981.

220. Harris, E.D., Jr., and McCroskery, P.A.: The influence of temperature and fibril stability on degradation of cartilage collagen by rheumatoid synovial collagenase. N. Engl. J. Med. 290:1, 1974.

221. Werb, Z., Burleigh, M.C., Barrett, A.J., and Starkey, P.M.: Binding and inhibition of mammalian collagenases and other metal proteinases. Biochem. J. 139:359, 1974.

222. Starkey, P.M., and Barrett, A.J.: α_2-Macroglobulin, a physiological regulator of proteinase activity. In Barrett, A.J. (ed.): Proteinases in Mammalian Cells and Tissues. New York, North-Holland Publishing Company, 1977, pp. 663–696.

223. Ohlsson, K., and Delshammar, M.: Interactions between granulocyte elastase and the plasma proteinase inhibitors in vitro and in vivo. In Burleigh, P.M., and Poole, A.R. (eds.): Dynamics of Connective Tissue Macromolecules. New York, North-Holland Publishing Company, 1975, pp. 259–275.

224. Ohlsson, K.: Granulocyte collagenase and elastase and their interaction with α_1-antitrypsin and α_2-macroglobulin. In Reich E. et al.(eds.): Protease and Biological Control. Cold Springs Harbor Laboratories, 1975, pp. 591–602.

225. Kimura, H., Tateishi, H., and Ziff, M.: Surface ultrastructure of rheumatoid articular cartilage. Arthritis Rheum. 20:1085, 1977.

226. Jasin, H.E.: Deposition of immune complexes within articular connective tissues. In Panayi, G.S., and Johnson, P.M. (eds.): Immunopathogenesis of Rheumatoid Arthritis. Reedbooks, Ltd., 1979, p. 89.

227. Banda, M.J., Clark, E.J., and Werb, Z.: Limited proteolysis by macrophage elastase inactivates human α_1-proteinase inhibitor. J. Exp. Med. 152:1563, 1980.

228. Barrett, A.J.: The possible role of neutrophil proteinases in damage to articular cartilage. Agents Actions 8:3, 1978.

229. Harris, E.D., Jr., and Krane, S.M.: Collagenases. N. Engl. J. Med. 291:557, 605, 652, 1974.

230. Harris, E.D., Jr., and Krane, S.M.: An endopeptidase from rheumatoid synovial tissue culture. Biochim. Biophys. Acta 258:566, 1972.

231. Abe, S., and Nagai, Y.: Evidence for the presence of a complex of collagenase with α_2-macroglobulin in human rheumatoid synovial fluid. A possible regulatory mechanism of collagenase activity in vivo. J. Biochem. 73:897, 1973.

232. Delshammar, M., and Ohlsson, L.: Granulocyte collagenase and elastase and the plasma proteinase inhibitors in human plasma. Surgery 83:323, 1978.

233. Ohlsson, K., and Laurell, C.B.: The disappearance of enzyme inhibitor complexes from the circulation of man. Clin. Sci. Molec. Med. 51:87, 1976.

234. Reynolds, J.J., Murphy, G., Sellers, A., and Cartwright, E.: A new factor that may control collagen resorption. Lancet 2:333, 1977.

235. Brinckerhoff, C.E., McMillan, R.M., Dayer, J.-M., and Harris, E.D., Jr.: Inhibition by retinoic acid of collagenase production in rheumatoid synovial cells. N. Engl. J. Med. 303:432, 1980.

236. Hamilton, J.A.: Stimulation of the plasminogen activator activity of human synovial fibroblasts by retinoids. Arthritis Rheum. 25:432, 1982.

237. Hamerman, D.: Cartilage changes in the rheumatoid joint. Clin. Orthop. 64:91, 1969.

238. Sapolsky, A.I., Keiser, H.D., Howell, D.S., and Woessner, J.F., Jr.: Metalloproteases of human articular cartilage that digest cartilage proteoglycan at neutral and acid pH. J. Clin. Invest. 58:1030, 1976.

239. Sapolsky, A.I., Howell, D.S., and Woessner, J.F., Jr.: Neutral proteases and cathepsin D in human articular cartilage. J. Clin. Invest. 53:1044, 1974.

240. Kar, N.C., Cracchiolo, A., Mirra, J., and Pearson, C.M.: Acid, neutral and alkaline hydrolases in arthritic synovium. Am. J. Clin. Pathol. 65:220, 1976.

241. Dingle, J.T., Saklatvala, J., Hembry, R.M., Tyler, J., Fell, H.B., and Jabb, R.: A cartilage catabolic factor from synovium. Biochem. J. 184:177, 1979.

242. Jasin, H.E., and Dingle, J.T.: Human mononuclear cell factors mediate cartilage matrix degradation through chondrocyte activation. J. Clin. Invest. 68:571, 1981.

243. Hatcher, V.B., Borg, J.P., Levitt, M.A., and Smith, C.: Enhanced neutral protease activity in proliferating rheumatoid synovial cells. Arthritis Rheum. 24:919, 1981.

244. Klein, D.C., and Raisz, L.G.: Prostaglandins: Stimulation of bone resorption in tissue culture. Endocrinology 85:1436, 1970.

245. Robinson, D.R., Tashjian, A.H., Jr., and Levine, L.: Prostaglandin E$_2$-induced bone resorption by rheumatoid synovia. A model for bone

destruction in rheumatoid arthritis. J. Clin. Invest. 56:1181, 1975.

246. Raisz, L.G., Dietrich, J.W., Simmons, H.A., Seyberth, H.W., Hubbard, W., and Oates, J.A.: Effect of prostaglandin endoperoxides and metabolites on bone resorption in vitro. Nature 267:532, 1977.

247. Horton, J.F., Oppenheim, J.J., Mergenhagen, S.E., et al.: Macrophage lymphocyte synergy in the production of osteoclast-activating factor. J. Immunol. 113:1278, 1974.

248. Cruickshank, B.: The arteritis of rheumatoid arthritis. Ann. Rheum. Dis. 13:136, 1954.

249. Ghadially, F.N., and Roy, S.: Ultrastructure of synovial membrane in rheumatoid arthritis. Ann. Rheum. Dis. 26:426, 1967.

250. Barland, P., Novikoff, A.B., and Hamerman, D.: Fine structure and cytochemistry of the rheumatoid synovial membrane with special reference to lysosomes. Am. J. Pathol. 44:853, 1964.

251. Muirden, K.D.: Ferritin in synovial cells in patients with rheumatoid arthritis. Ann. Rheum. Dis. 25:387, 1966.

252. Grimley, P.M., and Sokoloff, L.: Synovial giant cells in rheumatoid arthritis. Am. J. Clin. Pathol. 49:931, 1966.

253. Postlethwaite, A.E., Jackson, B.K., Beachey, E.H., and Kang, A.H.: Formation of multinucleated giant cells from human monocyte precursors. J. Exp. Med. 155:168, 1982.

254. Gold, R.H., Metzger, A.L., Mirra, J.M., Weinberger, H.J., and Killebrew, K.: Multicentric reticulohistiocytosis (lipoid dermatoarthritis). Am. J. Roentgenol. 124:610, 1975.

255. Jayson, M.I.V., and Dixon, A. St. J.: Intra-articular pressure in rheumatoid arthritis of the knee. 1. Pressure changes during passive joint distention. Ann. Rheum. Dis. 29:261, 1970.

256. Dixon, A. St. J., and Grant, C.: Acute synovial rupture in rheumatoid arthritis. Clinical and experimental observation. Lancet 1:742, 1964.

257. Jayson, M.I.V., and Dixon, A. St. J.: Intra-articular pressure in rheumatoid arthritis of the knee. 2. Effect of intra-articular pressure on blood circulation to the synovium. Ann. Rheum. Dis. 29:266, 1970.

258. Harris, E.D., Jr., Parker, H.G., Radin, E.L., and Krane, S.M.: Effects of proteolytic enzymes on structural and mechanical properties of cartilage. Arthritis Rheum. 15:497, 1972.

259. Kempson, G.E., Muir, H., Swanson, S.A.V., et al.: Correlations between stiffness and the chemical constituents of cartilage of the human femoral head. Biochim. Biophys. Acta 215:70, 1970.

260. Mills, K.W.: Pathology of the knee joint in rheumatoid arthritis. J. Bone Joint Surg. 52B:746, 1970.

261. Kuettner, K.E., Harper, E.J., and Eisenstein, R.: Protease inhibitors in cartilage. Arthritis Rheum. 20:5124, 1977.

262. Mohr, W. and Wessinghage, D.: The relationship between polymorphonuclear granulocytes and cartilage destruction in rheumatoid arthritis. Z. Rheumatol. 37:81, 1978.

263. Harris, E.D., Jr., DiBona, D.R., and Krane, S.M.: A mechanism for cartilage destruction in rheumatoid arthritis. Trans. Assoc. Am. Phys. 83:267, 1970.

264. Harris, E.D., Jr., DiBona, D.R., and Krane, S.M.: Mechanisms of destruction of articular structures in rheumatoid arthritis. In Forscher, B. (ed.): Proceedings of the Third International Symposium on Inflammation. International Congress Series No. 229. Amsterdam, Excerpta Medica, 1971, pp. 243–253.

265. Kobayashi, I., and Ziff, M.: Electron microscope studies of the cartilage/pannus junction in rheumatoid arthritis. Arthritis Rheum. 18:475, 1975.

266. Freund, E.: The pathological significance of intra-articular pressure. Edinburgh Med. J. (NS) 47:192, 1970.

267. Maggar, E., Talerman, A., Fether, M., and Wouters, H.W.: The pathogenesis of the subchondral pseudocysts in rheumatoid arthritis. Clin. Orthop. 100:341, 1974.

268. Collins, D.H.: The subcutaneous nodule of rheumatoid arthritis. J. Pathol. Bacteriol. 45:97, 1937.

269. Bennett, G.A., Zeller, J.W., and Bauer, W.: Subcutaneous nodules of rheumatoid arthritis and rheumatic fever. A pathologic study. Arch. Pathol. 30:70, 1970.

270. Cochrane, W., Davies, D.V., Dorleng, J., and Bywaters, E.G.L.: Ultramicroscopic structures of the rheumatoid nodule. Ann. Rheum. Dis. 23:345, 1964.

271. Harris, E.D., Jr.: A collagenolytic system produced by primary cultures of rheumatoid nodule tissue. J. Clin. Invest. 51:2973, 1972.

271a. Kaye, B.R., Kaye, R.L., and Bobrove, A.: Rheumatoid nodules. Review of the spectrum of associated conditions and proposal of a new classification, with a report of four seronegative cases. Am. J. Med. 76:279, 1984.

272. Lance, E.M.: The effect of joint replacement on rheumatoid synovitis and its significance. Arthritis Rheum. 25 (Suppl.): 41, 1982.

273. Sokoloff, L., Wilikens, S.L., and Bunim, J.J.: Arteritis of striated muscle in rheumatoid arthritis. Am. J. Pathol. 27:157, 1951.

274. Conn, D.L., McDuffie, F.C., and Dyck, P.J.: Immunopathologic study of sural nerves in rheumatoid arthritis. Arthritis Rheum. 15:135, 1972.

275. Sokoloff, L., and Bunim, J.J.: Vascular lesions in rheumatoid arthritis. J. Chron. Dis. 5:668, 1957.

276. Glass, D., Soter, N.A., and Schur, P.H.: Rheumatoid vasculitis. Arthritis Rheum. 19:950, 1976.

277. Conn, D.L., Schroeter, A.L., and McDuffie, F.C. Cutaneous vessel immune deposits in rheumatoid arthritis. Arthritis Rheum. 19:15, 1976.

278. Conn, D.L., and McDuffie, F.C.: The pathogenesis of rheumatoid neuropathy. In Eberl, R., and Rosenthal, M. (eds.): Organic Manifestations and Complications in Rheumatoid Arthritis. New York, F.K. Schattaner Verlag, 1975, pp. 295–306.

Chapter 60

Rheumatoid Arthritis: The Clinical Spectrum

Edward D. Harris, Jr.

INTRODUCTION

Review of medical history has shown us how difficult it has been to precisely define clinical entities, and this problem is particularly evident when attempts are made to determine when rheumatoid arthritis (RA) was first described. Some have concluded that RA developed only recently as a clear-cut entity, and was not seen in Europe until the end of the eighteenth century.[1,2] Short has evaluated the data provided by human paleopathology and by medical writings that appeared before 1800.[3] Hip-

pocrates described a form of arthritis that developed in a man at about age 35, which first involved the hands and feet and next the elbows, knees, and hips.[4] Soranus, an Ephesian who lived in the second century A.D., wrote a treatise[5] describing a polyarthritis with morning stiffness in which the joints became twisted ". . . with the toes and fingers either turned sideways or bent over backwards, or resting immovable upon their neighbors." The problem with accepting this or other early descriptions as being the first case reports of RA is that each of them has clear references to what must have been tophaceous gout spread among references to what may have been RA or psoriatic arthritis.

In contrast, perhaps because of the sclerotic nature of the disease process, evidence for ankylosing spondylitis in antiquity is solid. Lumbar spines with bony ankylosis and fused sacroiliac joints have been demonstrated in specimens from men living before 1800 B.C.[6] Small bones of the hand have been examined less rigorously,[3] and the proliferative soft tissue characteristic of rheumatoid synovitis is poorly preserved. For these reasons, perhaps, there is no definite evidence for the existence of RA before relatively recent times.

In this chapter the epidemiology of RA will be discussed first, and then a detailed survey of its modes of presentation and criteria necessary for its diagnosis will be presented. Then, with diagnosis established, exploration of the natural history of the disease as it affects the joints and extra-articular tissues will be outlined.

EPIDEMIOLOGY AND DIAGNOSIS

RA is a diagnosis made primarily on clinical grounds. Despite the usefulness of rheumatoid factor in both di-

agnosis and understanding of the pathophysiology of the disease, the presence of anti-IgG is not specific for RA. No other test specific for diagnosis is available. A set of criteria for diagnosis designed by Ropes and committee for the American Rheumatism Association[7] has proved useful for both epidemiologic and demographic studies as well as for diagnosis of individual patients in physicians' offices (Table 60–1). The weakness of the ARA criteria is in application to the "probable" class of diagnosis. When only three criteria are necessary, the firmness of the diagnosis varies considerably, depending on which three are picked. For instance, a patient with morning stiffness and a single painful swollen joint would meet criteria for "probable" RA. This problem is mirrored in marked discrepancies between series in the ratios of "probable" to "definite" RA, of female to male cases,[8] and in the large number of patients who meet criteria for diagnosis of probable RA who evolve either to a healthy state or into another process.[9]

Mitchell and Fries have published a systematic analysis of the ARA criteria[10] using a population of 840 patients over age 16 in whom a clinical diagnosis of RA was made. These patients are believed to represent al-

Table 60–1. American Rheumatism Association Criteria for the Diagnosis of RA

Eleven criteria available. For three different degrees of certainty of diagnosis, different numbers of criteria must be met. Unlike the Jones criteria for rheumatic fever, there are no major and minor criteria.

Classic RA—7 criteria needed
Definite RA—5 criteria needed
Probable RA—3 criteria needed

To meet criteria 1 to 5, symptoms or signs must be present for at least 6 weeks.

Criteria	Comments
1. Morning stiffness	This symptom is very useful as an indicator of inflammation; the absence of morning stiffness in a chronically painful joint is good evidence that synovial inflammation is minimal or absent
2. Pain on motion or tenderness in at least one joint	Criteria 2 to 6 must be observed by a physician
3. Swelling of one joint, representing soft tissue or fluid	Bony overgrowth is usually representative of a degenerative process, not synovial inflammation
4. Swelling of at least one other joint (soft tissue or fluid) with an interval free of symptoms no longer than 3 months	
5. Symmetrical joint swelling (simultaneous involvement of the same joint, right and left)	Terminal interphalangeal joints are rarely involved in RA and therefore are not acceptable for this or other criteria
6. Subcutaneous nodules over bony prominences, extensor surfaces or near joints	See exclusions in second footnote below
7. Typical roentgenographic changes which must include dimineralization in periarticular bone as an index of inflammation; degenerative changes do not exclude diagnosis of RA	Demineralization may result from disease of muscles around inflamed joints as well as from release of prostaglandins (see Chapter 59) by inflamed synovial tissue
8. Positive test for rheumatoid factor in serum	Laboratory quality control is essential here; in general, positive tests should be in a titer of 1:64 or greater
9. Synovial fluid; a poor mucin clot formation on adding synovial fluid to dilute acetic acid	This is strictly a qualitative test and can be used only as a crude estimate of sustained joint inflammation

10. Synovial histopathology consistent with RA (see Chapter 59)
  a. Marked villous hypertrophy
  b. Proliferation of synovial cells
  c. Lymphocyte/plasma cell infiltration in subsynovium
  d. Fibrin deposition within or upon microvilli	

11. Characteristic histopathology of rheumatoid nodules biopsied from any site	These are nonspecific; granuloma annulare is indistinguishable on routine histological preparations from the rheumatoid nodule

A diagnosis of *possible* RA requires that morning stiffness, history of pain or swelling of joints, subcutaneous nodules, or an elevated ESR or C-reactive protein—any two of these criteria—be present for a least 3 weeks.

Exclusions are based principally on presence of evidence for other diseases that have criteria for their own diagnosis (e.g., systemic lupus erythematosus, scleroderma) or more specific diagnostic techniques (e.g., the crystal deposition diseases). Some may be inappropriate. For instance, it is known that gout and RA can be present in the same patient. Exclusions are covered under Differential Diagnosis of Rheumatoid Arthritis later in this chapter.

most all of the patients with RA in the northern half of Saskatchewan. Their analyses revealed the following interesting points.:

1. The fist 5 "clinical" criteria (see Table 60–1) were each present in two thirds of the patients at their initial visit to the rheumatologist.

2. Of these 5 criteria, joint pain/tenderness was the most frequent and morning stiffness was the least common.

3. Nodules were present at the initial visit in 19 percent, and rheumatoid factor in 47 percent.

4. Elimination of the last 3 criteria—"poor mucin" in synovial fluid and typical histopathology of synovium or nodules—would have resulted in reclassification of only 3 patients. These criteria are rarely (1 to 2 percent) met at time of diagnosis.

5. Patients who met ARA criteria at the first visit of "definite" or "classic" RA, when contrasted with those in the "probable" group, (a) were older (5 to 8 years); (b) had their disease longer; and (c) had more fatigue, weaker grip strength, more frequent elbow and ankle involvement, and a higher number of active joints.

Another set of criteria was proposed at the third International Symposium of Population Studies of the Rheumatic Diseases in New York City in 1966.[11] These are listed in Table 60–2. Meeting these criteria is more rigorous and clearly would exclude mono- or diarticular disease, seronegative arthritis, and mild, nondeforming disease.

An interesting comparison of the ARA and New York criteria was carried out by O'Sullivan and Cathcart in Sudbury, Massachusetts.[12] In 1964, of 4522 persons examined, 17 appeared to be affected by RA according to the New York criteria, and 118 had either probable or definite RA by the ARA criteria. Follow-up data are shown in Table 60–3. These data indicate that the New York criteria identify persons whose disease remains clinically meaningful and establish the prevalance of RA as 0.5 percent of women and 0.1 percent of men. The data do not define the nature of the disease manifested in the 88 patients who initially met criteria for RA and who failed to meet criteria on later examination. We can infer, however, that early RA (probable or definite by ARA criteria) is a relatively benign process with a high probability for remission within several years. Therefore,

Table 60–3. Follow-up of RA (3 to 5 Years), Diagnosed by ARA and NY Criteria*

1. Diagnosed originally by ARA criteria:

Initial ARA Class		Final ARA Class	
		Probable	Definite
Definite RA	40	7	12
Probable RA	78	7	4
Total	118	14	16	30

2. Diagnosed originally by NY Criteria:
Initial (by ARA Criteria)

		Final		
		NY Criteria		ARA Criteria
		RA Present	RA Absent	
17 {	2 probable	11	6	2 negative
	15 definite			10 definite
				2 probable
				3 negative

*Collated from O'Sullivan, J.B., and Cathcart, E.S.: Ann. Intern. Med. 76:573, 1972.

one of the most significant determinants of prognosis in RA may be which criteria (ARA versus New York) are used to establish the diagnosis!

Wolfe[13] summarized the results of 14 studies of population samples, including the National Health Examination survey,[14] the survey of Tecumeseh, Michigan,[15] studies of various Native American Groups,[16] and representative atomic bomb survivors from Hiroshima and Nagasaki.[17] Using criteria for "definite" RA, the prevalence rate varied from 0.3 to 1.5 percent. In 1984 it is reasonable to estimate that there are 4 to 6 million cases of RA in the United States. A conservative estimate would be that 100,000 to 200,000 new cases of definite or classic RA developed in the USA in 1984.

Variations from these prevalence data are very rare, indicating that specific genetic and environmental influences on the development of RA, if significant, are widespread in the world. A few populations with an apparent predisposition to RA exist. One study, using both the ARA and New York criteria, found a frequency of definite RA of 3.4 percent in Yakima Indian women, ages 18 to 79, compared with a prevalence of 1.4 percent in the general population.[18] In a geographically and socially isolated band of 227 Chippewa Indians, the minimum prevalence of RA was found to be 5.3 percent. Clinically, the RA in this group was typical: additive, symmetrical, and persistent. The prevalence of HLA-DR4 was 68 percent, significantly higher than in most general populations, and all of the 12 with RA expressed HLA-DR4.[19]

Subgroups within the total population with RA have been identified. There is a striking increase in prevalence of RA in urban South African blacks[20] (3.3 percent) compared with rural blacks (0.87 percent).[21] Definite RA is two to three times more common in females than in males, although if groups of early "probable" RA are considered, the male to female ratio may approach 1.0.

Table 60–2. New York Criteria for the Diagnosis of RA

RA is present if criteria 1 and 2 plus either 3 or 4 are met:

1. History of an episode of three painful limb joints. Each group of joints (e.g., proximal interphalangeal joint) is counted as one joint, scoring each side separately
2. Swelling, limitation of motion, subluxation and/or ankylosis of three limb joints. *Necessary inclusions*: (1) at least one hand, wrist or foot; (2) symmetry of one joint pair. *Exclusions*: (1) distal interphalangeal joints; (2) fifth proximal interphalangeal joints; (3) first metatarsophalangeal joints; (4) hips
3. Radiographic changes (erosions)
4. Serum positive for rheumatoid factors

In Rochester, Minnesota, there has been a decline in the incidence of RA in the female population since 1960.[22] However, a case-control study of this population showed no association between rheumatoid arthritis and the use of oral contraceptives, or the use of estrogens for menopause-related or postmenopausal symptoms. These data contradict those[23] from England, which reported that patients with rheumatoid arthritis were found to have used oral contraceptives only half as much as control subjects.

The disease has an increasing prevalence with advancing age up to the seventh decade. It is well described in children (see Chapter 80), and new cases appear in even the very aged.[14,15] The National Health Survey[14] data indicated a higher prevalence of RA in patients of either sex with less than 5 years of education and in those with lower yearly incomes.

Future epidemiologic studies will be based on new genetic information, which has identified specific polymorphic cell surface glycoprotein antigens associated with RA (see Chapters 4 and 59). RA has been shown to be associated with HLA-Dw4[24] and with the B-cell alloantigen HLA-DR4 related to HLA-Dw4.[25] The C locus antigen Cw3 is also present with an increased frequency.[26] Although only a small percentage of persons with HLA-Dw4 develop RA, probably because the disease is multifactorial, these data give insight into possible immune response genes in humans. In the future, immunogenetics must be a constant associate of clinical observations in epidemiologic studies of RA.

Since 1948, when the studies of Rose and colleagues[27] re-emphasized the studies of Waaler[28] linking a factor in serum of patients with RA to agglutination of normal and sensitized sheep red blood cells, the presence or absence of rheumatoid factor in serum has occupied attention of epidemiologists in this field. Rheumatoid factor is found more frequently in population studies (3 to 5 percent) than is RA, and in these individuals the prevalence of seropositivity is approximately equal in male and females.[15,29,30] A recent study set out to determine whether HLA-Dw4 (sometimes referred to as Dw4x7x10), the histocompatibility antigen associated with RA, was associated with the presence of rheumatoid factor.[31] The frequency of HLA-Dw4 was determined in 24 healthy women with a significant titer for rheumatoid factor (median titer 1:160). Only three carried the Dw4 antigen, suggesting that the genes linked to HLA-Dw4 mediate susceptibility to RA via mechanisms other than control of rheumatoid factor synthesis. Frequently patients present with definite RA and are seronegative.[32] However, these individuals probably have a distinct immunogenetic disease.[33] In one series, although HLA-DR3 was significantly less prevalent and HLA-DR4 more common in patients positive for rheumatoid factor, a clinically matched group (except for the absence of vasculitis or nodules in the seronegative patients) who were seronegative had no difference from controls in distribution of DR antigens. In this series the seronegative DR4+ patients had more erosive/destructive disease than seronegative DR4- patients.[33]

An increased prevalence of RA in first-degree relatives of patients with RA would indicate that some genetic or environmental factor influences appearance of the disease. Twin studies are a principal tool for dissecting out genetic influences in many diseases. The data in twin studies have varied, ranging from evidence for discordance[34] to, in one study, almost 50 percent concordance.[35] In another study,[36,37] the risk of erosive arthritis in monozygous co-twins was about 30 times the reference population, while in dizygous co-twins and in nontwin siblings the risk was about 6 times that of control groups. It also was determined that functionally incapacitating (Grade 3 or 4) RA was found in four times the expected rate in first-degree relatives of probands with seropositive disease; erosive radiographic changes were found at three times the expected rate. Study of serology in first-degree relatives of patients with RA has revealed no higher frequency of rheumatoid factor than in relatives of matched controls.[38]

A number of observations suggest that certain factors are or are not associated with RA. Some of these are listed below. None has been substantiated by independent studies: (1) RA was less common in schizophrenics than in a control population.[39] (2) In studies of identical twins discordant for RA, a history of psychologic stress was more common in the affected twin.[34] (3) Heavy outdoor occupations or work in health fields was associated with RA.[40] (4) Rheumatoid patients had an increased frequency of exposure to pets (e.g., dogs, cats, birds, or other sick animals) in the 5 years before developing their disease than did a control group.[41] All such epidemiologic studies are subject to scrutiny; they are difficult to compile without introducing bias.

EARLY RHEUMATOID ARTHRITIS

It has been said that duration of continuous symptoms and signs correlates better with more severe RA than does any other index of disease activity.[42] Although this is almost simplistic, there are many corollaries of it that can be useful for both diagnosis and therapy. Continuous synovitis implies activation of multiple pathogenetic mechanisms within the synovium and joint space (see Chapter 59), and virtually ensures sufficient proliferation and polarization to result in progressive joint destruction. Conversely, disease that has clinical remission is associated with regression of the proliferative inflammation.

Early diagnosis of RA is rarely important to the patient. RA presents with acute severe symptoms so infrequently that the best course is often to effectively rule out other diagnoses and resist making an early diagnosis in a new patient with synovitis. If criteria are met in the proper time, a diagnosis of RA can be given. As mentioned above, many patients (perhaps 80 percent) given a diagnosis of RA early in the course of their disease will go into a sustained remission. The implication of this is either that the course of early RA is benign or that most diagnoses of RA that are made early and with few criteria having been met are wrong. The patients who demand a diagnosis should be reassured that, unlike the situation with malignancies, there are no data to suggest that very early, forced diagnoses and prompt treatment are associated with a better prognosis. Fortunately, a forced wait for diagnosis (6 weeks) is built into ARA criteria for diagnosis.

In the Northern Hempisphere, the onset of RA is more frequent in winter than in summer. In several series, the onset of RA from October to March is twice as frequent as in the other 6 months,[43,44] and exacerbations of the disease are more common in winter.[45]

Although it is often impossible to identify a day in a patient's life when arthritis began, it is of interest to search for prodromal symptoms. Some patients speak of transient joint symptoms or a history of recurrent bursitis. Ganglion cysts at the wrists have been noted to precede development of RA, but their frequency in a control population is not known.

Much more diffuse, subjective, and difficult to study are precipitating factors of arthritis. There is no evidence that any have a direct cause-and-effect relationship. Trauma is one of the most common preludes to arthritis; this can include surgery. Other episodes, including infections, vaccine inoculations, and emotional trauma, have been implicated by many patients as the cause of their problems, but there is no proof of their association.

Patterns of Onset (Table 60–4)

Insidious Onset. RA usually has an insidious slow onset over weeks to months. Fifty-five to 70 percent of cases begin this way.[43,46] The initial symptoms may be systemic or articular. In some patients, fatigue, malaise, or diffuse musculoskeletal pain may be the first nonspecific complaint, with joints involved later. Although symmetrical involvement is common, asymmetric presentation (often becoming more symmetrical later in the course of disease) is not rare. The reasons for symmetry of joint involvement remain a complete mystery, but the fact of symmetry in RA stands as a useful criterion for

Table 60–4. Characteristics of Onset of RA in 300 Patients with Definite or Classic Disease*

		Percent
1. Mode of onset:	rapid† (days or weeks)	46
	insidious—54 percent	54
2. Site of onset:	small joints	32
	medium-sized joints	16
	large joints	29
	combined	26
3. Pattern of onset:	monoarticular	21
	oligoarticular	44
	polyarticular	35

*From Fallahi, S., Halla, J.T., and Hardin, J.G.: Clin. Res. 31:650A, 1983.

†This time frame includes patients described in other studies as having "intermediate" onset.

diagnosis. Morning stiffness may be the first symptom, noted even before pain. This phenomenon is probably related to accumulation of edema fluid within inflamed tissues during sleep. Morning stiffness disappears as edema and products of inflammation are absorbed by lymphatics and venules and returned to the circulation by motion accompanying use of muscles. Pain and stiffness may develop in other joints, but it is rare for symptoms to remit completely in one set of joints while developing in another. This lack of a migratory quality of arthritis sets RA somewhat apart from rheumatic fever, in which migratory arthritis is common.

A subtle, early change in RA is development of muscle atrophy around affected joints. This decreases efficiency and strength, and the patient develops weakness out of proportion to pain. Opening doors, climbing stairs, and doing repetitive work become more demanding. A low-grade fever without chills is often overlooked unless the patient is a very good observer of his or her body functions. Depression, anxiety, and fear of the future affect the patient and accentuate symptoms. Weight loss is common, and anorexia contributes to this.

Acute Onset. Eight to 15 percent of patients have an acute onset of symptoms. The term "acute" refers to the rate of build-up of symptoms. Very rarely, a patient can pinpoint onset of disease to an instant, such as opening a door or driving a golf ball. Symptoms mount, with pain developing in other joints, often in a less symmetrical pattern than in patients who have an insidious type of onset. Pain may be generated also by surrounding muscles, and muscle pain can be so severe as to mimic ischemic pain. The differential diagnosis here is extremely broad, ranging from septic arthritis to myositis or viral infections.

Intermediate Onset. Fifteen to 20 percent of patients have an intermediate type of onset. Symptoms develop over days or weeks. Systemic complaints are more noticeable than in the insidious type of onset.

Patterns of Joint Involvement in Early Rheumatoid Arthritis

By far the most commonly involved joints in RA are the metacarpophalangeal joints, proximal interphalangeal joints, and wrists.[47] The combined data from two series are listed in Table 60–5. Larger joints generally become symptomatic after small joints. This raises the question of whether early disease in large joints remains asymptomatic for a longer time. The answer was sought in one study by performing xenon clearances on clinically normal knees of patients with early RA.[48] Seven of 22 had abnormal (high) perfusion, supporting this hypothesis. Although rheumatoid factor eventually becomes positive in 80 to 90 percent of cases with definite RA, it is apparent that the development of seropositivity lags behind clinical manifestations (Table 60–6). There seems to be little indication for repeating the laboratory test for rheumatoid factor if a patient has had one positive test at significant titer.

Table 60–5. Joints Involved in RA*

	Percent Initially Involved[47]			Percent Ultimately Involved[43]
	Right	Left	Bilateral	
Metacarpophalangeal	65	58	52	87
Wrist	60	57	48	82
Proximal Interphalangeal	63	53	45	63
Metatarsophalangeal	48	47	43	48
Shoulder	37	42	30	47
Knee	35	30	24	56
Ankle	25	23	18	53
Elbow	20	15	14	21

*Other joints (e.g., distal interphalangeal joints) are not tabulated here.

Unusual Patterns of Onset of Disease

Adult Onset Still's Disease. This disease appears in adults, usually in the third or fourth decade, as a syndrome like that seen in children with the acute, febrile onset of juvenile arthritis. That it can occur in adults supports those who would say that Still's disease is distinct from RA, rather than a different presentation of the same process. It was first described by Bywaters, who presented 14 of his patients.[49] Females are more commonly affected by adult-onset Still's disease. Most patients present with fever. Serology (rheumatoid factor and antinuclear antibody) is negative, and patients have not developed subcutaneous nodules.[50] Fever patterns in these patients are usually quotidian (i.e., reaching normal levels at least once each day). Patients have a skin rash—salmon-colored or pink macules that are evanescent and become more prominent when patients are febrile. The arthritis in this process usually involves fewer joints than RA in most adults. Erosive disease is rare. The cervical spine is involved, and loss of neck motion may be striking. Pericarditis and pleural effusions and severe abdominal pain (mesenteric adenitis)[51] may be present and confound diagnostic attempts. Unlike systemic lupus erythematosus, serum complement is normal or high.[52] In a recent series, 11 patients (all of whom were white women), followed for a mean of 20.2 years after disease onset, had the following characteristics:[53]

(1) Ten had a polycyclic pattern (characterized by remissions and exacerbations).

(2) Patterns of exacerbations were similar to but less severe than the original presentations.

(3) Loss of wrist extension was the most common

Table 60–6. Interval from Onset of Disease to Development of a Positive Rheumatoid Factor Test in 100 Patients with RA*

	Positive Result (Time in Months)					Negative
	Within 3	4–6	7–12	After 12	Total	
Number of patients	33	22	21	12	88	12

*From Jacoby, R.K., et al.: Br. Med. J. 2:96, 1973.

clinical abnormality, and carpal ankylosis was present in 10.

(4) Five out of 11 patients developed DIPJ involvement.

(5) Biopsy of the characteristic skin rash of Still's and juvenile rheumatoid arthritis showed perivascular infiltrate of neutrophils in the superficial dermis.

Palindromic Pattern of Onset. Palindromic rheumatism was described by Hench and Rosenberg in 1941.[54] Like many other clinical complexes in rheumatology, it should be considered a syndrome that can be either the initial manifestation of many different organic processes or never evolve into anything more. The syndrome is more like gout than anything else. Pain usually begins in one joint; symptoms worsen for several hours and are associated with swelling and erythema. An intercritical period, as in gout, is asymptomatic. It is likely that 30 to 50 percent of patients with palindromic rheumatism develop RA. In these, multiple joints become involved, swelling does not subside completely between attacks, and tests become positive for rheumatoid factor. Neither the characteristics of joint fluid nor the pathology of synovial biopsies allows the prediction that palindromic rheumatism will develop into RA.[55]

Age- and Sex-Related Modes of Onset. Certain types of presentation of arthritis appear more often in certain age groups. In late adolescent females a chronic, rarely erosive synovitis of the knees often presents without involvement of other joints, and without systemic signs. The erythrocyte sedimentation rate is usually normal, and rheumatoid factor is absent. Stiffness and pain are directly proportional to joint swelling, and this, in turn, is a function of use. Rest or assiduous use of crutches results in fairly prompt resolution of joint swelling, but with even mild activity, swelling recurs. Synovial biopsy has revealed moderate synovial cell hyperplasia and variable infiltration with mononuclear cells. Synovial fluid leukocyte counts are usually less than 10,000 per cubic millimeter. The course is one of gradual improvement with occasional flares of activity, without relationship to menstrual cycles. The process is self-limited and rarely lasts longer than 5 to 6 years. It is not known whether this represents an oligoarticular form of juvenile rheumatoid arthritis in older girls, a variant of adult RA, or another entity.

RA developing in older men (60 years of age and older) is often dominated by stiffness and diffuse boggy swelling of the hands, wrists, and forearms. Onset is slow, but the stiffness is often incapacitating. In other respects, the disease is similar to other forms of adult RA, but the therapy is not the same. Nonsteroidal anti-inflammatory drugs are rarely effective, but low-dose corticosteroids (< 7.5 mg prednisone per day) may be helpful in reducing edema and increasing motion and function.

RA and Paralysis: Asymmetric Disease. Being relatively common, RA is likely to occur with many other types of chronic disease. A striking asymmetry or even unilateral involvement has been described in patients with poliomyelitis, meningioma, encephalitis, neurovascular syphilis, strokes, and cerebral palsy.[56,57] Joints are spared on the paralyzed side, and the degree of protection demonstrates a rough correlation with the extent of paralysis.[58] Protective effect is less if a neurologic deficit develops in a patient already suffering from RA.[59]

"Arthritis Robustus." This is not so much an unusual presentation of disease as it is an unusual reaction of patients to the disease.[60,61] Men usually form this group. Their disease is characterized by proliferative synovitis, which appears to cause little pain. Patients are athletic and invariably keep working (often at physical labor). Osteopenia is less, and new bone proliferation at joint margins is common. Bulky subcutaneous nodules develop. Subchondral cysts develop, presumably from the excessive pressure developed from synovial fluid within a thick joint capsule during muscular effort (see Chapter 59).

The Course of Rheumatoid Arthritis

Before studying the evolution of the disease from synovitis to destruction of normal tissues and the development of complications of this disease, it is important to emphasize that there are many forms of the disease. As noted in the studies by O'Sullivan and Cathcart,[12] a large number—perhaps 80 percent—of patients who early in the course of their disease meet the criteria for possible or probable RA go on to develop another disease, or, more likely, become completely better. Here we will outline the different courses of RA. Prognosis and methods available to assess progression and/or treatment will be discussed at the end of this chapter.

Intermittent Course of RA. This course is marked by partial to complete remissions without need for continuous therapy. This type of disease is usually mild. Initially, only a few joints are involved. Insidious return of disease is often marked by more joint involvement than at first. Twenty to 30 percent of patients with RA enjoy these periods of remission.[62,63] Within this group it is reported that approximately half had remissions lasting more than a year, and in the entire group remissions lasted longer than exacerbations.

Long Clinical Remissions of RA. In one group of 250 patients receiving only simple medical and orthopedic treatment[45] almost 10 percent were in clinical remission for 12 to 31 years (mean, 22 years). Although most of these patients had RA for less than 6 months at time of inclusion, 40 percent had remained in remission. The fact that many of these patients had an acute onset of symptoms with marked fever and severe joint pain and inflammation raises the question of whether they truly had RA. Nevertheless, some sign of disease activity (e.g., an elevated erythrocyte sedimentation rate) persisted in many throughout the "clinical remission," and occasional patients had brief but true flares of disease in one or a few joints.

Progressive Disease. This group may pursue a rapid or slow course, but the end point is the same: disabling, destructive disease. In modern times, this group should be divided into two subgroups: those who respond to aggressive therapy and those who do not. Fortunately, the latter group is small and probably represents less than 3 percent of patients with definite or classic rheumatoid arthritis.

Diagnosis of Rheumatoid Arthritis

Diagnosis of RA must be by established criteria that are based upon effective clinical history and examination, laboratory tests, and diagnoses that exclude it. The criteria are discussed above. Before discussion of the exclusions (i.e., the findings that point to the presence of another disease process), we will address diagnosis positively, listing factors typical of the disease.

The characteristic patient with RA complains of pain and stiffness in multiple joints. The joint swelling is boggy and includes both soft tissue and synovial fluid. These joints are slightly to moderately tender to touch, especially the small joints of the hands and feet. Often palmar erythema and prominent veins on the dorsum of the hand are found. Distal interphalangeal joints are involved rarely. Temperature over the involved joints (except the hip) is elevated, but the joints are not usually red. Range of motion is limited, and muscle strength and function around inflamed joints are diminished. Soft, poorly delineated subcutaneous nodules are often found on the extensor surface of the forearm. General physical examination is normal except for a possible low-grade fever (~38° C), pallor, and asthenia. Movement is guarded, and apprehension often dominates facial expressions. Initial laboratory tests often show[64] (1) a slight leukocytosis with normal differential white blood cell count (WBC); (2) thrombocytosis; (3) a slight anemia (~10 grams hemoglobin per deciliter), normochromic and either normocytic or microcytic; (4) normal urinalysis; (5) erythrocyte sedimentation rate (Westergren) of ~30 mm per hour and up, sometimes to over 100 mm per hour; (6) normal renal, hepatic, and metabolic function; (7) a normal serum uric acid (before initiation of salicylate therapy); (8) positive rheumatoid factor test and negative ANA; (9) elevated α_2-globulins and α_1-globulins; and (10) normal or elevated serum complement.

A "typical" arthrocentesis reveals the following: joint fluid is straw-colored and slightly cloudy and contains many flecks of fibrin. Within the fluid a clot forms on standing at room temperature. There are 5000 to 25,000 WBC per cubic millimeter, and 85 percent of these are PMN leukocytes. Occasional large PMN leukocytes with granules staining positively for IgG, IgM, and C3 are found. No crystals are present. The mucin clot is fair. C4 and C2 are slightly depressed, but C3 is normal. IgG in synovial fluid may approach serum concentrations. In contrast, synovial fluid glucose is depressed, occasionally to less than 25 mg percent. Cultures are negative. A full discussion of synovial fluid analysis is found in Chapter 38.

Differential Diagnosis of Rheumatoid Arthritis

It is important to exclude many other diseases before making a diagnosis of RA.[65] In the discussion of the many entities that follows, the relative frequency of the entities is recorded as common, uncommon, or rare; they are listed in alphabetical order.

Ankylosing Spondylitis, Seronegative Spondyloarthropathy, and Reactive Arthritis (Common). Short, Bauer, and Reynolds,[66] in their complete and well-referenced monograph on RA, felt that clinical evidence was strong enough to include ankylosing spondylitis as a variant of RA ("the spinal equivalent of rheumatoid arthritis"). Nevertheless, these authors established as an objective for future study the determination of whether or not rheumatoid spondylitis constituted a distinct disease entity. The question may have been clouded somewhat by the observation that in many children with RA, roentgenographic evidence of spondylitis was found.[67] This phenomenon is now recognized, of course, as spondylitis occurring in juveniles and related (as in the adult disease) to HLA-B27.

The problem in differentiating spondylitis arises with the patient (particularly a female) who presents with minimal back pain and peripheral joint involvement. Suspicion that this is not RA is generated when small joints are not involved, when joint disease is asymmetrical, and when the cervical spine is involved with limitation of motion.

In some cases, the conclusion is inescapable that RA and ankylosing spondylitis are present in the same patient. In one series[68] nine seropositive patients presented with spinal ankylosis and symmetrical erosive polyarthritis; eight of the nine carried HLA-B27. If one assumes that these two diseases occur completely independently of each other, simultaneous occurrence in the same patient should occur once in every 50,000 to 200,000 of the adult population.

In distinguishing patients with Reiter's syndrome from those with RA, a careful history and physical examination to look for heel pain or tenderness and ocular or urethral symptoms are of greatest importance. Polyarthritis persists chronically in over 80 percent of patients with Reiter's syndrome (see Chapter 65), and indeed Reiter's syndrome may have a worse prognosis than RA. The characteristics of enthesopathy in patients with Reiter's syndrome (e.g., sausage digits indicating juxta-articular disease), insertional tendinitis, periostitis, and peri-insertional osteoporosis or erosions may point to the diagnosis.

The differential diagnosis between "RA and psoriasis" and "psoriatic arthritis" may by artificial (see Chapter 66). Some patients with distal interphalangeal joint involvement and severe skin involvement obviously have a disease that is not RA. Others, however, have a seropositive symmetrical polyarthritis that appears to be RA; yet they also have psoriasis. A search in these patients for evidence of enthesopathy, distal interphalangeal joint disease, and/or spondylitis or sacroiliitis may reveal enough abnormalities to define a symptom complex different from RA.

Inflammatory bowel disease (IBD) (ulcerative colitis and Crohn's disease) is associated with arthritis in 20 percent of cases.[69] Peripheral arthritis is more common in many series[70] than spondylitis. Ankles, knees, and elbows are the most often involved of peripheral joints, with proximal interphalangeal joints and wrists next in frequency. Simultaneous attacks of arthritis and development of erythema nodosum are not uncommon. Attacks of joint pain begin more rapidly than do most attacks of RA, and usually only two to three joints are affected at once. Involvement is usually asymmetrical, and erosions are uncommon. The occurrence of peripheral arthritis in IBD is not related to HLA-B27.

Behçet's syndrome is marked by an asymmetric polyarthritis in 50 to 60 percent of cases.[71] Joint deformity is unusual. The painful oral and genital ulcers and CNS involvement are unusual in RA. Uveal tract involvement (Behçet's syndrome) must be differentiated from scleritis (RA) in patients with ocular and joint disease. Spondylitis, as in the other disorders classified here, is found in Behçet's syndrome, principally when HLA-B27 is present.

Enteric infections are complicated occasionally by inflammatory joint disease resembling RA. The joint disease associated with *Yersinia enterocolitica* infections occurs several weeks after the gastrointestinal illness.[72] Knees and ankles are the joints most commonly involved, and most patients (even those with peripheral arthritis and no spondylitis) have HLA-B27.[73]

Arthropathy may precede other findings of Wipple's disease (see Chapter 67). The pattern is that of a migratory poly- or oligoarthritis involving ankles, knees, shoulders, elbows, and fingers, as with IBD. Remission may occur when diarrhea begins. As with the arthritis of IBD, joint destruction is rare,[74] presumably because the synovitis lacks sustained chronicity.

Arthritis Associated with Oral Contraceptives (Uncommon). A syndrome of persistent arthralgias, myalgias, and morning stiffness with occasional development of polyarticular synovitis has been described in women in their third decade of life taking oral contraceptives (estrogens and progestins).[75] Positive tests for antinuclear antibodies are common, and several patients have had circulating rheumatoid factor. Symptoms resolve after the contraceptive is discontinued.

Arthritis of Thyroid Disease (Uncommon) (see Chapter 102). In hypothyroidism, synovial effusions and synovial thickening simulating RA have been described.[76] The sedimentation rate may be elevated because of hypergammaglobulinemia. Joint fluid is noninflammatory and may have an increased viscosity. Knees, wrists, hands, and feet are involved most often, and not infrequently coexisting calcium pyrophosphate deposition disease is found.

The syndrome of thyroid acropachy complicates less than 1 percent of hyperthyroid patients.[77] This represents periosteal new bone formation, which may be associated with a low-grade synovitis similar to hypertrophic osteoarthropathy. Although impossible to quantitate, it is said that patients with coexisting RA and hyperthyroidism have pain from their arthritis that appears to exceed that expected from the degree of inflammation.

Bacterial Endocarditis (Uncommon). Arthralgias, arthritis, and myalgias occur in approximately 30 percent of patients with subacute bacterial endocarditis.[78] The joint symptoms are usually in one or several joints, usually proximal large ones. It is possible that this synovitis could be caused by circulating immune complexes, which have been demonstrated, along with hypocomplementemia, in subacute bacterial endocarditis.[79] Fever out of proportion to joint findings in the setting of leukocytosis should lead to consideration of infective endocarditis as a diagnostic possibility, even in the absence of a significant heart murmur. It is wise to obtain blood cultures in all patients with a presentation of polyarthritis and significant fever. Embolic phenomena with constitutional symptoms, including arthralgias, can be presenting symptoms of *atrial myxoma,* but this process usually mimics systemic vasculitis or SBE more than it does RA.[80]

Calcium Pyrophosphate Deposition Disease (CPPD) (Common) (see Chapter 87). This crystal-induced synovitis presents in many different forms, ranging from a picture of indolent osteoarthrosis to that of an acute, hot joint. About 5 percent of patients have a chronic polyarthritis (sometimes referred to as pseudorheumatoid arthritis) which is associated with proliferative erosions at subchondral bone.[81] Although radiographs are of great help when chondrocalcinosis is present, CPPD may be present in the absence of calcification on radiographs.[82] Diagnosis then can be made only by arthrocentesis. One of the radiographic signs of CPPD that help differentiate it from RA is the presence of unicompartmental disease in the wrist.

Diffuse Connective Tissue Disease: Systemic Lupus Erythematosus, Scleroderma, Dermatomyositis-Polymyositis, Vasculitis, Mixed Connective Tissue Disease (MCTD) (Common). These entities, all discussed in depth elsewhere in the text, may begin with a syndrome of mild systemic symptoms and minimal polyarthritis involving the proximal interphalangeal and metacarpophalangeal joints. It is crucial to remember that at this point it may be appropriate not to make a definitive diagnosis. Also, it is not uncommon for one of these entities, diagnosed at one point in time, to evolve into another as years go by. Finally, it is not even agreed that MCTD is a distinct entity (see Chapters 71 and 76); argument exists that it is a common form of presentation of several rather specific entities. The following list contains rules of thumb for characterizing joint disease of the various entities:

1. In systemic lupus erythematosus, an organized synovitis that causes erosions is rare. Soft tissue and muscle inflammation may lead to dislocation of normal tendon alignment, resulting in ulnar deviation similar to Jaccoud's arthropathy.

2. Limitation of joint motion in scleroderma is almost always secondary to taut skin bound down to underlying fascia. The same considerations hold for dermatomyositis-polymyositis; proliferative synovitis is rarely sustained in these processes.

3. In reports of MCTD (patients having arthralgias, arthritis, hand swelling, sclerodactyly, Raynaud's phe-

nomenon, esophageal hypomotility, and myositis with circulating antibody to a ribonucleoprotein) 60 to 70 percent have arthritis. Many are given an initial diagnosis of RA. Numerous series have shown deforming, erosive arthritis. In one series, for example, 8 of 17 patients presented in a fashion like RA.[83] Articular osteopenia alone was found in 8. Six had loss of joint space, and 5 had erosions typical of RA. Despite the serologic specificity for MCTD (see Chapter 71), there is still debate as to whether all patients with apparent RA diagnosed by clinical patterns should be classified as having MCTD if serum antibody to nuclear ribonucleoprotein is found in his or her serum.

Familial Mediterranean Fever (Uncommon). The articular syndrome in this disease is an episodic monarthritis or oligoarthritis of the large joints that appears in childhood or adolescence, mimicking oligoarthritic forms of JRA.[84] Episodes of arthritis come on acutely with fever and all cardinal signs of inflammation and can precede other manifestations of the disease. Usually self-limited (days to weeks), attacks occasionally will last for months, associated with radiographic changes of periarticular osteopenia without erosions.

Gout (Common) (see Chapter 86). Before a diagnosis of chronic erosive RA is made, chronic tophaceous gout must be ruled out. The reverse applies as well. Features of gouty arthritis that mimic RA include polyarthritis, symmetrical involvement, fusiform swelling of joints, subcutaneous nodules, and subacute presentation of attacks. Conversely, certain presentations of RA that suggest gouty arthritis include hyperuricemia (after treatment with low doses of aspirin), periarticular nodules, and seronegative disease (particularly in the male).[85] Radiographic findings may be similar, with appearance of the subcortical erosions of RA being similar to small osseous tophi in gout.[86] Although large asymmetrical erosions with ballooning of the cortex are more likely to be gout than RA, this is not always the case.[87] Serologic tests may be misleading as well; positive tests for rheumatoid factor have been found in as many as 30 percent of patients with chronic tophaceous gout,[88] and these patients have had no clinical or radiographic signs of RA. The coexistence of RA and gout is rare, and curiously so. Only 10 cases of gout coexisting with RA have been reported in the medical literature since 1881. Wallace and associates[89] have calculated that considering the prevalence of the two diseases, 10,617 cases should be anticipated to coexist within the United States. It is possible that numerous coexistent cases either have not been reported or have been missed, with physicians assuming that acute joint pain in a rheumatoid patient represents a flare of this process. Arthrocentesis, even in established rheumatoid joints, may be indicated to rule out sepsis or gout.

Hemochromatosis (Uncommon) (see Chapter 94). The characteristic feature of hemochromatosis that is almost diagnostic is firm bony enlargement of the metacarpophalangeal joints, particularly the second and third, with associated cystic degenerative disease on radiographs and, not infrequently, chondrocalcinosis.[90] Marginal erosions, juxta-articular osteoporosis, synovial proliferation, and ulnar deviation are not seen in the arthropathy of hemochromatosis but are common in RA. Wrists, shoulders, elbows, hips, and knees are involved less often than the metacarpophalangeal joints. More than a third of patients with this iron overload syndrome have an arthropathy.[91]

Hemoglobinopathies (Uncommon) (see Chapter 101). In homozygous (S-S) sickle cell disease, the most common arthropathy is associated with crises and is believed to be a result of microvascular occlusion in articular tissues.[92] However, in some cases a destructive arthritis with loss of articular cartilage has been defined,[93] and this resembles severe RA. In most patients with sickle disease and joint complaints, periosteal elevation, bone infarcts, fish-mouth vertebrae, and aseptic necrosis can be found on radiographs.[92] Episodic polyarthritis and noninflammatory synovial effusions are also found in sickle cell–β-thalassemia.[94]

Hemophilic Arthropathy (Uncommon) (see Chapter 100). A deficiency of factor VIII and IX sufficient to produce clinical bleeding frequently results in hemarthroses. The clotting abnormality rarely is overlooked, however, and it is unlikely that a diagnosis of RA would be made in the setting of hemophilia A or B.

Hyperlipoproteinemia (Uncommon). Achilles tendinitis and tenosynovitis in familial type II hyperlipoproteinemia can be presenting symptoms in this affliction and may be accompanied by arthritis.[95] Synovial fluid findings may resemble those of mild RA, and the tendon xanthomas may be mistaken for rheumatoid nodules or gouty tophi. Similarly, bilateral pseudoxanthomatous rheumatoid nodules have been described.[96] Asymmetrical and oligoarticular synovitis has been described in type IV hyperlipoproteinemia.[97] The absence of morning stiffness and noninflammatory synovial effusions helps rule out RA. The treatment of hyperlipoproteinemia with clofibrate may cause an acute muscular syndrome,[98] but this resembles myositis or polymyalgia rheumatica more than it does RA.

Hypertrophic Osteoarthropathy (Uncommon) (see Chapter 103). This process may present as oligoarthritis involving knees, ankles, or wrists. The synovial inflammation accompanies periosteal new bone formation, which can be seen on radiographs. Correction of the inciting factor (e.g., cure of pneumonia in a child with cystic fibrosis) will very likely alleviate the synovitis. The synovium is characterized primarily by an increased blood supply and synovial cell proliferation. Very little infiltration by mononuclear cells is seen.[99] Pain, which increases when extremities are dependent, is characteristic, although not always present. If clubbing is not present or is not noticed, this entity is easily confused with RA.

Infectious Arthritis (Common) (see Chapters 96 to 98). Bacterial sepsis may present superimposed in the setting of RA, and will be discussed below. Viral infections, however, may present as arthritis with many characteristics of RA. Rubella arthritis occurs more often in adults than in children and often affects small joints of the hands.[100] Lymphocytes predominate in synovial effusions. Synovitis (pain greater than swelling) occurred following vaccination with rubella vaccine, particularly with the dog kidney preparations, which are no longer used.[101]

Arthritis often precedes viral hepatitis and is associated with the presence of circulating hepatitis B surface antigen (HB_sAg) and hypocomplementemia.[102] HB_sAg has been found in synovial tissues by direct immunofluorescence, supporting the concept that this synovitis is mediated by immune complexes.[103] A relatively acute onset of diffuse polyarthritis with small joint effusions and minimal synovial swelling should prompt the physician to obtain liver function tests in the patient with a history of exposure to hepatitis. With the onset of icterus, the arthritis usually resolves, leaving no trace.

Fever, sore throat, and cervical adenopathy followed by a symmetric polyarthritis are compatible with infection due to hepatitis B, rubella, adenovirus type 7, ECHO virus type 9, *Mycoplasma pneumoniae,* or Epstein-Barr virus as well as acute rheumatic fever or adult-onset Still's disease.[104]

Lyme Disease (see Chapter 99). This interesting disease is caused by infection with a spirochete classified as a *Borrelia* species. It can closely simulate RA in adults or children by having an intermittent course with development of chronic synovitis.[105] Erosive synovitis necessitating synovectomy has evolved in several cases. The proliferative synovium is not different from that of RA. The differentiating point from RA is history of a tick bite or an expanding erythematous skin lesion with central pallor preceding the arthritis. The disease is being recognized in many parts of the country. Clinical abnormalities affecting the central nervous system and heart in Lyme disease may produce a syndrome mimicking systemic lupus erythematosus or vasculitis.

Multicentric Reticulohistiocytosis (MR) (Rare) (see Chapter 95). This process is particularly interesting because it is one that causes severe arthritis mutilans with an "opera-glass hand" (*main en lorgnette*).[106] Other causes of arthritis mutilans are RA, psoriatic arthritis, erosive osteoarthritis treated with glucocorticoids, and gout (after treatment with allopurinol). The cell that appears to effect damage to tissues is the multinucleate lipid-laden histiocyte, which appears to release degradative enzymes sufficient to destroy connective tissue. Differential characteristics from RA include the following:[107]

1. Skin manifestations: In MR, nodules are often widely disseminated and the histology is entirely different.

2. Joint manifestations: In MR, distal interphalangeal joints are frequently and extensively involved.

3. Radiographic manifestations: In MR, joint spaces appear to widen as destruction of subchondral bone occurs faster than cartilage is lost.

4. Laboratory tests: In MR, the erythrocyte sedimentation rate is often normal in face of severe resorptive disease, and rheumatoid factor is not present in MR.

Osteoarthritis (Common) (see Chapter 89). Although

Table 60–7. Factors Useful for Differentiating Early RA from Osteoarthrosis (Osteoarthritis)

	RA	Osteoarthrosis
Age of onset	Childhood and adults; peak incidence in 50's	Increases with age
Predisposing factors	HLA-DR4	Trauma, congenital abnormalities (e.g., shallow acetabulum)
Symptoms, early	Morning stiffness	Pain increases through the day and with use
Joints involved	Metacarpophalangeal joints, wrists, proximal interphalangeal joints most often; distal interphalangeal joints almost never	Distal interphalangeal joints (Heberden's nodes), weight-bearing joints (hips, knees)
Physical findings	Soft tissue swelling, warmth	Bony osteophytes, minimal soft tissue swelling early
Radiologic findings	Periarticular osteopenia, marginal erosions	Subchondral sclerosis, osteophytes
Laboratory findings	Increased erythrocyte sedimentation rate; rheumatoid factor, anemia, leukocytosis	Normal

osteoarthritis begins as a degeneration of articular cartilage and RA begins as inflammation in the synovium, each process approaches the other pathologically, and therefore clinically, as the diseases progress. In osteoarthritis, as cartilage deteriorates and joint congruence is altered and stressed, a reactive synovitis often develops. Conversely, as the rheumatoid pannus erodes cartilage, secondary degenerative changes in bone and cartilage develop and in end stages of either degenerative joint disease or RA the involved joints appear the same. To differentiate clearly between the two, therefore, the physician must delve into the early history and functional abnormalities of the disease. Factors useful in separating the two processes are listed in Table 60–7.

One overlap condition exists: erosive osteoarthritis. This occurs in middle-aged women (more than men) and is characterized by inflammatory changes in proximal interphalangeal joints, with destruction and functional ankylosis of the joints. The proximal interphalangeal joints can appear red and hot, yet there is almost no synovial proliferation or effusion. The erythrocyte sedimentation rate may be slightly elevated, but rheumatoid factor is negative.[108]

Parkinson's Disease (Common). Although the tremor and/or rigidity of Parkinson's Disease is rarely confused with rheumatoid arthritis, Parkinson's patients have a predilection for developing swan-neck deformities of the hands (Fig. 60–1), which is generally unappreciated by rheumatologists. This abnormality, the pathogenesis of which still is unknown, was first described in 1864.[109]

Polychondritis (Uncommon) (see Chapter 91). This process can mimic infectious processes, vasculitis, granulomatous disease, or RA. Patients with RA and ocular inflammation (e.g., scleritis) usually have active joint disease before ocular problems develop. The reverse occurs in polychondritis. In addition, polychondritis is not associated with rheumatoid factor. The joint disease is usually episodic. Nevertheless, erosions can develop that are not unlike those of RA.

Polymyalgia Rheumatica (PR) (Common) (see Chapter 73). Although joint radionuclide imaging studies have indicated increased vascular flow in synovium of patients with classic polymyalgia rheumatica, it remains appropriate to exclude PR as a diagnosis if significant synovitis (soft tissue proliferation or effusions) can be

detected. Otherwise, many patients who actually have RA would be diagnosed as having PR and treated with potentially harmful doses of corticosteroids. A careful history will usually differentiate shoulder or hip girdle muscle pain from shoulder or hip joint pain. It is probable that RA and PR coexist in numerous patients, but careful descriptions of such patients are rare.

Rheumatic Fever (Uncommon) (see Chapter 81). Rheumatic fever is much less common now than it was previously, but still must be considered in adults with polyarthritis. In adults, the arthritis is the most prominent clinical finding of RF; carditis is less frequent than it is in children, while erythema marginatum, subcuta-

Figure 60–1. These swan neck deformities are a result of Parkinson's disease, not rheumatoid arthritis.[109]

neous nodules, and chorea are rare.[110,111] The presentation is often that of an additive, symmetrical, large joint polyarthritis (involving lower extremities in 85 percent of patients), developing within a week and associated with a severe tenosynovitis.[110] This extremely painful process is dramatically responsive to salicylates.[111,112] Unlike Still's disease in the adult, rheumatic fever generally has no remittent or quotidian fevers, has a less protracted course, and shows evidence for antecedent streptococcal infection. There are many similarities between the presentation of rheumatic fever in adults and "reactive" postinfectious synovitis developing after *Shigella, Salmonella, Brucella, Neisseria,* or *Yersinia* infections. These latter processes do not respond well to salicylates, however. As rheumatic fever becomes less frequent, and as penicillin prophylaxis effectively prevents recurrences of the disease, Jaccoud's arthritis (chronic postrheumatic fever arthritis) is becoming very rare. This entity, described first by Bywaters in 1950,[113] resulted from severe and repeated bouts of rheumatic fever and synovitis, which left stretched-out joint capsules and ulnar deformity of the hands without erosions due to ulnar displacement and shortening and fibrosis of extensor tendons.[114] The same deformity can develop in systemic lupus erythematosus characterized by recurrent synovitis and soft tissue inflammation, or in Parkinson's disease (Fig. 60–1). Differentiating rheumatic fever from RA is particularly difficult when subcutaneous nodules associated with rheumatic fever are found.[115]

Sarcoidosis (Uncommon) (see Chapter 93). The two most frequent forms of sarcoid arthritis are usually easily differentiated from RA. In the acute form with erythema nodosum and hilar adenopathy the articular complaints usually appear as periarthritis affecting large joints of the lower extremities. Differential diagnosis may be confused by the fact that many of these patients have rheumatoid factor present in serum.[116] Joint erosions and proliferative synovitis do not occur in this form of sarcoidosis.

In chronic sarcoidosis, cystlike areas of bone destruction, mottled rarefaction of bone, and a reticular pattern of bone destruction giving a lacelike appearance on radiographs may simulate destructive RA. This form of sarcoid is often polyarticular, and biopsy of bone or synovium for diagnosis may be essential, particular since there is often no correlation between joint disease and clinical evidence for sarcoid involvement of other organ systems.[117] It is very likely that Poncet's disease or tuberculous rheumatism[118] actually represents granulomatous "idiopathic" arthritis (i.e., sarcoidosis).

Miscellaneous Abnormalities That Can Be Mistaken for Rheumatoid Arthritis. *Sweet's syndrome* (rare) is called acute febrile neutrophilic dermatosis.[119,120] It has been described in adults, often following "flulike" illness. The three major features are an acute illness with fever, leukocytosis, and raised painful plaques on the skin that show neutrophilic infiltration of the dermis on biopsy. Joint disease occurs in 20 to 25 percent of cases and is characterized by acute, self-limited polyarthritis.

Because of the skin lesions, Sweet's syndrome is confused with systemic lupus erythematosus, erythema nodosum, and erythema elevatum diutinum more often than for RA. It has been treated effectively with indomethacin[120] and corticosteroids.

Thiemann's disease is a rare form of idiopathic vascular necrosis of the proximal interphalangeal joints of the hands with occasional involvement of other joints.[121,122] Bony enlargement begins relatively painlessly, and the digits (one or more may be involved) become fixed in flexion. The primary lesion is in the region of the epiphysis, and the lesion begins most often before puberty, distinguishing it from erosive osteoarthritis that it resembles radiographically. It is clearly a heritable disease, but the genetic factors have not been defined.

Calcific periarthritis can be easily confused with polyarthritis.[123] The skin is red over and around the affected joints; the tissues are boggy and tender, but no effusion is present. Passive motion is easier than active motion. Periarticular calcification is visible on radiographs. Unless the periarthritis can be differentiated from true arthritis (as in the periarthritis of sarcoid), the syndrome would seem like palindromic rheumatism or early RA.

The syndrome of *intermittent hydrarthrosis* describes periodic attacks of benign synovitis in one or few joints, usually the knee, beginning in adolescence.[124] The difference between this and oligoarticular JRA or RA is one of degree, not kind. In contrast to palindromic rheumatism, in which acute synovitis often may occur in different joints during successive attacks,[125] the same joint or joints are affected during each attack in intermittent hydrarthrosis.[126]

Although perhaps more appropriately classified with arthritis related to gastrointestinal disease (see Ankylosing Spondylitis, etc.) polyarthritis that occurs in obese patients after intestinal bypass surgery can present as RA.[127] Articular complaints occur in approximately 25 percent of these patients, but rarely are joint complaints persistent or severe. Circulating cryoproteins that may be immune complexes have been described. Bennett (see Chapter 58) has suggested that the shortened bowel may enable arthritogenic and immunogenic bacterial products to gain access to the host. Fortunately, this form of treatment for morbid obesity is rarely used.

The *fibrositis syndrome* (see Chapter 32) should not be confused with RA, because in fibrositis (syn., fibromyalgia) there is no evidence of synovitis. Although there are no specific diagnostic tests that define fibrositis, there are certain recurrent nonarticular locations for pain that are seen in different patients. These include[128] the midpoint of the upper border of the trapezius, forearm muscles distal to the lateral humeral epicondyle, the second costochondral junction, the fat pad medial to the knee, and intervertebral ligaments. Arousal syndromes of disordered sleep may be related to development of this syndrome. Evidence is accumulating that patients with RA may develop a superimposed fibromyalgia. This leads to very difficult therapeutic problems.

Although *glucocorticoids* suppress inflammation and pain, there is an arthropathy associated with their use[129] that resembles avascular necrosis. More likely confused with RA are the symptoms of corticosteroid withdrawal. These patients may suffer diffuse polyarticular pain, particularly in the hands, if the corticosteroid dose is tapered too rapidly.

The rheumatic syndromes associated with *malignancy* are outlined in detail in Chapter 104. Direct involvement by cancer of synovium usually presents as a monarthritic syndrome.[130] A more subtle association is represented by the patients who present with a slightly atypical RA at about the time a malignancy is developing. *Pigmented villonodular synovitis* is a nonmalignant but very proliferative disease of synovial tissue that has many functional characteristics similar to those of RA and usually involves only one joint. The histopathology is characterized by proliferation of histiocytes, multinucleate giant cells, and hemosiderin- and lipid-laden macrophages. Clinically, this presents as a relatively painless chronic synovitis (most often of the knee) with joint effusions and greatly thickened synovium.[131] Subchondral bone cysts and cartilage erosion may be associated with the bulky tissue. It is not clear whether this should be classified as an inflammation or neoplasm of synovium (see Chapter 108).

Multiple myeloma may present as a polyarthritis, mimicking RA. Amyloid deposits can be found in synovial and periarticular tissues[132] and are, presumably, responsible for the joint complaints. The synovial fluid in *amyloid arthropathy* is noninflammatory, and, on occasion, particulate material staining with apple green fluorescence after Congo red staining may be found in the fluid.

Idiopathic edema is a cause of nonarticular rheumatism that may be confused for RA with mild, early synovitis.[133]

ESTABLISHED RHEUMATOID ARTHRITIS: ITS COURSE AND COMPLICATIONS

The Involvement of Joints—Effects of Disease on Form and Function

Once rheumatoid synovitis is established by the sequence outlined in Chapter 59, the effects that the process has on joints are a complex function of the intensity of the underlying disease, its chronicity, and the stress put on individual involved joints by the patient. This is graphically illustrated by the radiographs of a patient's pelvis (Fig. 60–2). The patient was a 67-year-old female who developed arthritis in 1960 at the age of 49 years. Characterized by exacerbations and remissions initially, her disease became chronic and destructive, and in 1971 she was no longer able to bear weight on her right hip and was in a wheelchair or bed until 1978, when the second (lower) radiograph was taken. The changes in the 8-year interval are defined more by her being confined to inactivity in a wheelchair than by the activity

of her arthritis. In 1970, she had developed a significant protrusio acetabuli; the apparent joint space was almost completely obliterated, and significant sclerosis developed in both the acetabulum and femoral head. In contrast, after 8 years of non–weight bearing, there was a dramatic change in her radiographs: The protrusio was unchanged; however, the contour of the femoral head was smooth; the apparent joint space widened, suggesting the joint had been re-surfaced with fibrocartilage. Subchondral sclerosis diminished. While the hip was being remodeled, the lumbosacral spine was bearing her body weight in a wheelchair and impressive sclerosis and narrowing of the vertebral disc occurred.

Among other principles demonstrated by Figure 60–2 is the fact that there are reparative as well as destructive mechanisms in rheumatoid synovitis, and that expression of one or the other may be related more to motion and weight bearing than to other factors, including treatment.

Understanding the sequence of changes produced by arthritis in individual joints, therefore, is best achieved by attempting to define how the disease alters normal function of joints, bone, and muscle.

The Cervical Spine. Unlike other nonsynovial joints, such as the sternomanubrial joint or symphysis pubis, the discovertebral joints in the cervical spine often manifest osteochondral destruction in RA,[134,135] and on lateral radiographs may be found narrowed to less than 5 mm. Significant pain is the clinical presentation, and passive range of motion, in the absence of muscle spasm, may be normal. There are two possible mechanisms for this process: (1) extension of the inflammatory process from adjacent neurocentral joints, the joints of Luschka, which are lined by synovium, into the discovertebral area;[134,135] and (2) Chronic cervical instability initiated by apophyseal joint destruction leading to vertebral malalignment or subluxation.[136] This may produce microfractures of the vertebral endplates, disc herniation, and/or degeneration of disc cartilage.

The atlantoaxial joint is prone to subluxation in several directions: (1) The atlas moves *anteriorly* on the axis (most common). This results from laxity of the transverse cruciate ligament and the lateral alarodontoid ligaments induced by proliferative synovial tissue developing in adjacent synovial bursa, or from fracture or erosion of the odontoid process (Fig. 60–3). (2) The atlas moves *posteriorly* on the axis. This can occur only if the odontoid peg has been fractured off the axis or destroyed. (3) The vertical subluxation of the atlas in relation to the axis (least common). This results from destruction of the lateral atlantoaxial joints or of bone around the foramen magnum. One recently described patient with RA had superior, posterior, and lateral displacement of C1.[137]

The most common symptom of subluxation is pain radiating up into the occiput.[138] Two other less common clinical patterns include: (1) slowly progressive spastic quadriparesis, frequently with painless sensory loss of the hands, and (2) transient episodes of medullary or positive dysfunction associated with vertical penetration

Figure 60–2. Remodeling of the hip joint in a patient with rheumatoid arthritis during 7 years without weight-bearing (see text for details). In contrast, the lumbosacral spine, supporting the weight of the upper body and providing the only mobility while the patient was seated, has undergone progressive degeneration. (The radiographs are owned by the Radiology Section at the Dartmouth-Hitchcock Medical Center and were provided by Dr. Joshua Burnett.)

Figure 60–3. Anterior subluxation of C1 on C2 during flexion of the head. In this 21-year-old female there is a normal 3 mm distance between the atlas and the odontoid process while her head is held in extension (*right*). In flexion radiograph (*left*) subluxation to 7 mm has developed. (Courtesy of Gary S. Hoffman, M.D.)

of the dens and probable vertebral artery compression.[139] Paresthesias in the shoulders or arms may occur during movement of the head. Physical findings suggestive of atlantoaxial subluxation include (1) loss of occipitocervical lordosis, (2) resistance to passive spine motion, (3) abnormal protrusion of the axial arch, felt by the examining finger on the posterior pharyngeal wall, and (4) a "click" produced by anterior pressure on the spinous process of C2 when combined with posterior pressure on the forehead. The "click" indicates an intact odontoid process abutting the axial arch. Radiographic views (lateral, in flexion) should reveal more than a 3-mm separation between the odontoid peg and the axial arch.[140] In symptomatic patients, the films in flexion should be taken only after radiographs (including an open-mouth posteroanterior view) have ruled out an odontoid fracture or severe atlantoaxial subluxation. Recent studies have indicated that computerized tomography is useful for demonstrating spinal cord compression by loss of posterior subarachnoid space in patients with C1-2 subluxation.[141]

Neurologic symptoms often have little relationship to the degree of subluxation and may be related to individual variations in diameter of the spinal canal. Symptoms of spinal cord compression that demand intervention include[142] (1) a sensation of the head falling forward on flexion of the cervical spine; (2) changes in levels of consciousness; (3) "drop" attacks; (4) loss of sphincter control; (5) dysphagia, vertigo, convulsions, hemiplegia, dysarthria, or nystagmus; and (6) peripheral paresthesias without evidence for peripheral nerve disease or compression. Some of these symptoms may be related to compression of the vertebral arteries, which must wind through foramina in the transverse processes of C1 and C2, rather than to compression of the spinal cord.

Is mortality increased in patients with atlantoaxial subluxation? In one series of autopsies on 104 consecutive deaths in patients with RA,[143] 11 cases of severe dislocation were found. In all 11 cases the odontoid protruded posterosuperiorly and impinged upon the medulla within the foramen magnum. In five, spinal cord compression was determined to be the only cause of death. In only two cases was subluxation diagnosed before death. These patients must be at risk for even small falls and whiplash injuries and for general anesthesia with intubation. Cervical collars should be prescribed for stability. Operative stabilization may be considered if symptoms are progressive. In a series of 84 patients with some form of subluxation[144] but without cord or brainstem lesions, one fourth worsened and one fourth improved without surgery over 5 to 14 years of follow-up. Using survival tables, these authors concluded that cervical luxations per se do not significantly shorten life in patients with RA. In most series, less than 20 percent of patients with RA exhibited C1-2 disease. Glucocorticoid therapy appeared to have an adverse effect on forward luxations at C1-C2.

Vertical atlantoaxial subluxation is equally important, although less common, being present in 13 of 476 (3.7 percent) hospitalized patients with RA.[145] Symptoms associated with this collapse of the lateral support system of the atlas occur in patients with severe erosive disease. Neurologic findings have included decreased sensation in the distribution of cranial nerve 5 and sensory loss in the C2 area, nystagmus, and pyramidal lesions. Vertical subluxations are believed to have a worse prognosis than the other varieties.[146]

Bywaters has demonstrated bursal spaces between the cervical interspinous processes in autopsies of patients without joint disease, and in rheumatoid patients, bursal proliferation that led in several cases to radiographically demonstrated destruction of the spinous processes.[147]

Temporomandibular Joints (TMJ). TMJ are commonly involved in RA. In one series of 65 patients with classic or definite RA,[148] careful history revealed that 55 percent of patients had symptoms at some time during the course of their disease. Radiographic examination revealed structural alterations in 78 percent of the joints examined (86 percent of patients). An overbite may develop[149] as the mandibular condyle and the corresponding surface of the temporal bone, the eminentia articularis, are eroded. Physical examination of the rheumatoid patient should include palpation for tenderness and auscultation for crepitus. Occasional patients will present with acute pain and an inability to close the mouth, necessitating intra-articular glucocorticoids to suppress the acute process.

Cricoarytenoid Joints. The small diarthrodial joints have an important function, since they rotate with the vocal cords as they abduct and adduct to vary pitch and tone of the voice. Careful history may reveal hoarseness in up to 30 percent of rheumatoid patients.[150] This is not disabling in and of itself, but there is a danger that the cricoarytenoid joints may become inflamed and immobilized, with the vocal cords adducted to the midline, causing inspiratory stridor.[151] Autopsy examinations have demonstrated cricoarytenoid arthritis in almost half the patients with RA, suggesting that much significant disease of the larynx may be asymptomatic.[152] Symptomatic rheumatoid nodules within the vocal cord itself, mimicking laryngeal carcinoma, have been described. Asymptomatic cricoarytenoid synovitis may occasionally lead to aspiration of pharyngeal contents, particularly at night.

Ossicles of the Ear. Many rheumatoid patients suffer a decrease in hearing. In general this has been ascribed to salicylate toxicity, and it is believed to be reversible when the drug is discontinued (see Chapter 49). On the other hand, conductive hearing loss in patients not on salicylates was reported by Copeman.[153] Studies using otoadmittance measurements[154] have been carried out in patients with RA in an attempt to determine whether the interossicle joints were involved. The technique mea-

sured factors that impede the flow of sound through the ear: stiffness (tympanic membrane and ossicles), mass or inertia (the bulk of the ossicles), and resistance. The data showed that 38 percent of "rheumatoid ears" and 8 percent of controls demonstrated a pattern characteristic of an increase in the flaccidity of a clinically normal tympanic membrane. This is consistent with erosions and shortening of the ossicles produced by the erosive synovitis, not with ankylosis.

Sternoclavicular and Manubriosternal Joints. These joints, both possessing synovium and a large cartilaginous disc, are often involved in RA.[155] Because of the relative immobility there are a few symptoms. Patients occasionally complain of pain in sternoclavicular joints while lying on their sides in bed. When symptoms do occur, the physician must be concerned about superimposed sepsis. Computerized tomography may be a useful technique for careful delineation of the sternoclavicular joint. Manubriosternal involvement is almost never clinically important, although by tomographic criteria it is very common in RA.[156] Some patients develop manubriosternal joint subluxation. This deformity may be associated with cervical spine disease. In one study, of 10 patients with manubriosternal subluxation, 8 had radiographic evidence for significant atlanto-axial subluxation.[157]

The Shoulder. RA of the shoulder not only affects synovium within the glenohumeral joint, but also involves the distal third of the clavicle, various bursae and the rotator cuff, and multiple muscles around the neck and chest wall.

One of the most important principles of rehabilitation (see Chapter 111) is that joint pain causes decreased mobility of joints and that decreased mobility quickly leads to muscle weakness and atrophy. Often rheumatoid involvement of the shoulder can be detected by an examination that demands effort from various muscle groups. One of the first muscle groups to weaken in shoulder involvement in RA is the mid-thoracic group, which is responsible for normal scapular positioning on the chest wall. A common early change in RA is an anterolateral shift of the scapula, producing a "forward shoulder." Forward shifting of the scapula decreases stability of the glenohumeral joint. In a reaction to restore stability, the pectoralis major pulls the humerus into a position of adduction and internal rotation. Thus it is not unusual that limitation of rotation has been found to be the most consistent abnormality of shoulder function on physical examination.

In recent years it has been appreciated that involvement of the rotator cuff in RA is a principal cause of morbidity. The function of the rotator cuff is to stabilize the humeral head in the glenoid. Weakness of the cuff results in superior subluxation. Rotator cuff tears or insufficiency for other reasons can be demonstrated by shoulder arthrogram. In Ennevaara's series of 200 consecutive patients with RA, studied by arthrography, 21 percent had rotator cuff tears and an additional 24 percent had evidence for fraying of tendons.[158] One likely mechanism for tears is that the rotator cuff tendon insertion into the greater tuberosity is vulnerable to erosion by the proliferative synovitis that develops there[159] (Fig. 60–4). Previous injury and aging may predispose to the development of tears.[160] Sudden tears may present with pain and inflammation so great as to suggest sepsis.

Standard radiographic examinations[161] of the shoulder in RA reveal erosions (69 percent) and superior subluxation (31 percent). Arthrograms, in addition to showing tears of the rotator cuff, can demonstrate[162] (1) diffuse nodular filling defects, (2) irregular capsular attachment, (3) bursal filling defects, (4) adhesive capsulitis, and (5) dilatation of the biceps tendon sheath (perhaps unique to RA). Marked soft tissue swelling of the anterolateral aspect of the shoulders in RA may be secondary to chronic subacromial bursitis rather than to glenohumeral joint effusions.[163] In contrast to rotator cuff tears, bursal swelling is not necessarily associated with decreased range of motion or pain. Synovial proliferation within the subdeltoid bursa may explain resorption of the undersurface of the distal clavicle seen in this disease.[164]

The Elbow. Perhaps because it is a very stable hinge joint, severe pain in the elbow rarely is manifest in the disease. Nevertheless, involvement of the elbow is common, and if lateral stability at the elbow is lost as the disease progresses, disability can be severe.

The frequency of elbow involvement varies from 20 to 65 percent, depending on the severity of disease in the patient populations studied. The relatively low prevalence shown in Table 60–5 is in contrast with the 67 percent[165] involvement found in another study. One of the earliest findings—often unnoticed by the patient—is loss of full extension. Since the elbow is principally a connecting joint between the hand and trunk, the shoulder and wrists can compensate for loss of elbow motion.[166] For example, pronation at the wrists can be assisted 45 to 50 degrees by abducting the shoulder; and

shoulder elevation and wrist flexion can be substituted for flexion at the elbow.

The Hand and Wrist. These should be considered together because they form a functional unit. There are data,[167,168] for example, linking disease of the wrist to ulnar deviation of the metacarpophalangeal joints. The best hypothesis,[167] based on radiographic measurements, is that weakening of the extensor carpi ulnaris leads to radial deviation of the wrist as the carpal bones rotate (the proximal row in an ulnar direction, the distal ones in a radial one). Ulnar deviation of the fingers (a "zigzag" deformity) occurs in response to this, to keep the tendons to the phalanges in a normal line with the radius. A refinement of this hypothesis[168] is that the first anatomic abnormality may be volar subluxation of the ulnar side of the carpus. This may be caused by slippage of the movable insertion of the extensor carpi ulnaris in a lateral-volar direction, which results in a volar pull on the wrist bones only weakly opposed by residual extensors. This produces relative supination of the carpus, a prominent ulnar head, and in turn accentuates the weakness of the extensor carpi ulnaris, producing the same dominance of the radial carpi extensors and ulnar deviation of the metacarpophalangeal joints. Other factors, including the tendency for power grasp to pull the fingers into an ulnar attitude[169] and inappropriate intrinsic muscle action,[170] are undoubtedly involved as well (Table 60–8).[171-175] It is important to note that erosion of bone or articular cartilage is not essential for development of ulnar deviation. Significant although reducible ulnar deviation can result from repeated synovitis and myositis in the hands (e.g., systemic lupus erythematosus).

Dorsal swelling on the wrist within the tendon sheaths of the extensor muscles (fifth and sixth tendon compartments) is one of the earliest signs of disease. Rarely, cystic structures resembling ganglia will be early findings of RA.[176]

As the synovial proliferation develops within the wrist, pressure increases within the relatively nondistensible joint spaces. Proliferative synovium develops enzymatic machinery sufficient to destroy ligaments, tendons, and the articular disc distal to the ulnar head. Pressure and enzymes combine to produce communications between radiocarpal, radioulnar, and midcarpal joints in about 70 percent of patients with RA compared with 16 percent or less in controls.[177] Integrity of the distal radioulnar joint is lost; the ulnar collateral ligament, stretched by the proliferative synovium of the radioulnar joint, finally either ruptures or is destroyed and the ulnar head springs up into dorsal prominence, where it "floats" and can easily be depressed by the examiner's fingers.

On the volar side of the wrist, synovial protrusion cysts develop; they can be palpated, and their origins can be confirmed by arthrography.[178] The thick transverse carpal ligament prevents significant resistance to decompression, however, and the hyperplastic synovium compressing the median nerve can cause the carpal tunnel syndrome, which is described in detail in Chapter 110.

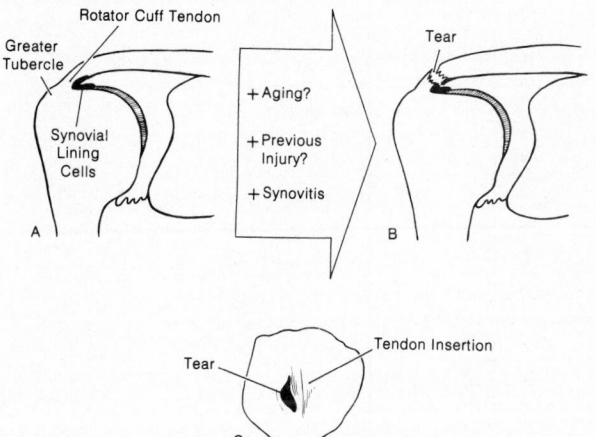

Figure 60–4. Pathogenesis of rotator cuff tears in rheumatoid arthritis. The small patch of synovium present at the reflection of insertion of the rotator cuff tendon can, in its proliferated state, produce enzymes sufficient to seriously weaken the tendon, predisposing it to rupture. (From Weiss, J.J., et al.: Arch. Intern. Med. 135:521, 1975.)

Table 60–8. A Sequence of Pathology in Development of Ulnar Deviation at Metacarpophalangeal Joints

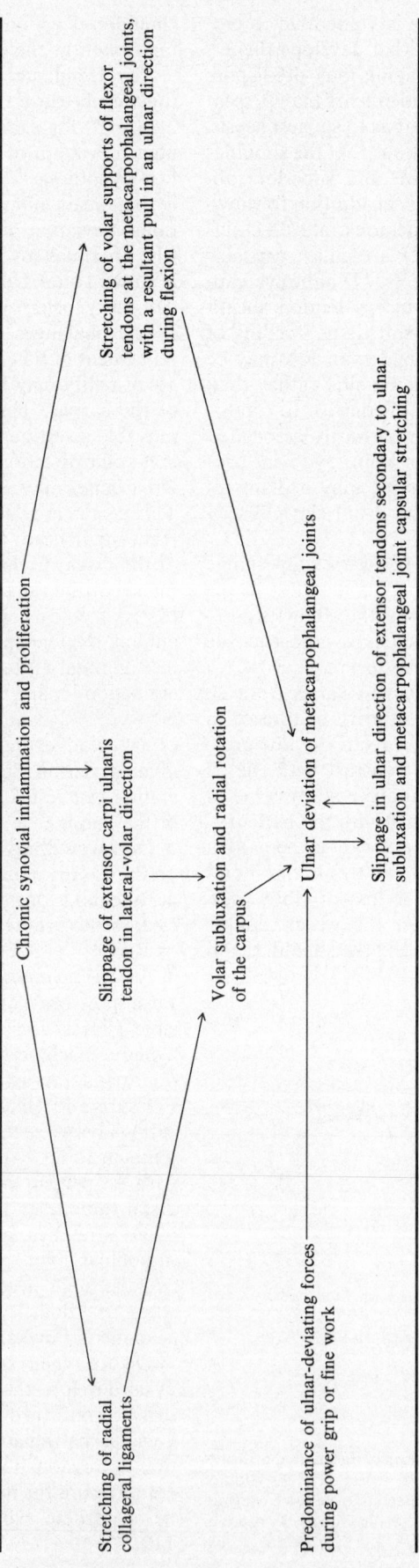

Common sites for bone erosion by proliferative synovitis in the wrist are at the periphery of the joint where no protective cartilage is found.[179] Enzymes and pressure may be synergistic in producing fracture, and osseous and cartilage debris may accumulate in the joint spaces.[180] Irregular bone edges from which fragments have been separated may serve as weapons to erode tendons already weakened and attenuated by action of proteinases.

Progression of disease in the wrist is characterized by loss of joint space and loss of bone. This foreshortening of the carpus has been quantitated as a carpal-metacarpal (c:mc) ratio (length of the carpus divided by that of the third metacarpal). Data showed a linear decrease in the c:mc ratio with progressive disease (Fig. 60–5).[181] This is caused by compaction of bone at the radiolunate, lunate-capitate, and capitate-third metacarpal joints, which usually accompanies severe disease.

The *hand* often has many joints involved in RA. One of the most sensitive indices of hand involvement is grip strength. The act of squeezing brings stress on all hand joints. As noted in Chapter 24, muscular contraction causes ligamentous tightening around joints, compressing inflamed synovium. The immediate result is weakness, with or without pain. Gerber (see Chapter 111) suggests that the reflex inhibition of muscular contraction secondary to pain may be a primary factor. Progression from early disease to severe deformity of the hands is shown in Figures 60–6 and 60–7.

Often before deformities demonstrable at rest in individual joints are discernible, there are two kinetic abnormalities that develop. (1) The normal arches of the hands may be increased or decreased. A transverse arch is formed by the carpal bones and lies at the base of the thenar and hypothenar eminences. A longitudinal arch runs from this carpal arch to each phalanx. Early edema and pain associated with spasm of the interosseous muscles lead to loss of these arches, with a "flat-handed" appearance. (2) Involuntary motion of one metacarpal on the next grasp is a normal phenomenon. This motion

Figure 60–5. The carpal-metacarpal ratio in relation to radiographic state of disease in 390 hand films of 73 female RA patients. (From Trentham, D.E., and Masi, A.J.: Arthritis Rheum. 19:939, 1976.) *B*, Radiograph of the right wrist of a 42-year-old woman with RA. The carpal-metacarpal index (see text) is 4.28, significantly below the lower limit of normal, consistent with destructive synovitis in the wrist, particularly in the radiocarpal joint. Despite severe disease this patient has developed no ulnar deviation at the metacarpophalangeal joints.

Figure 60–6. Subtle changes in RA developing in a 32-year-old woman. Fusiform swelling of proximal interphalangeal joints (the fourth in particular) is apparent. The hands are warm and slightly swollen (note the reflected light), and the veins are engorged.

is often lost as intrinsic muscles shorten during prolonged inflammation. Opposition of digits IV and V to the thumb is particularly hampered by loss of motion between the metacarpals. Thus, early loss of grip strength is often greatest in these digits.

The swan-neck deformity is one of flexion of the distal interphalangeal and metacarpophalangeal joints, with hyperextension of the proximal interphalangeal joint. The lesion probably begins with shortening of interosseous muscles and tendons, leading to a degree of metacarpophalangeal joint flexion during digital extension. Shortening of the intrinsic muscles exerts tension of the dorsal tendon sheath, leading to hyperextension of the proximal interphalangeal joint[182] (Fig. 60–8). Deep tendon contracture or, rarely, distal interphalangeal joint involvement with RA leads to the distal interphalangeal joint flexion.[183] Rupture of the sublimis tendon, which would reduce capacity to flex the proximal interphalangeal joint, could lead to the same sequence of events.[184]

If during chronic inflammation of a proximal interphalangeal joint, the extensor hood stretches or is avulsed, the proximal interphalangeal joint may pop up in flexion, producing a boutonnière deformity[172,183] (Fig. 60–9). The distal interphalangeal joint remains in hyperextension.

Without either of these deformities, limitation of movement develops at the proximal interphalangeal and distal interphalangeal joints. Limitation of full flexion of the distal interphalangeal joint is common in RA and represents incomplete profundus contraction. Similarly, tight intrinsic muscles may prevent full flexion of proximal interphalangeal joints when the metacarpophalangeal joints are in full extension.

Nalebuff's classification of thumb disease in RA gives a sequence of functional problems with this joint.[185] Three types of deformity have been described. In type I, metacarpophalangeal inflammation leads to stretching of the joint capsule and a boutonnière-like deformity. In type II, inflammation of the carpometacarpal joint

leads to volar subluxation during contracture of the adductor hallucis. In type III, after prolonged disease of both metacarpophalangeal joints, exaggerated adduction of the first metacarpus, flexion of the metacarpophalangeal joint, and hyperextension of the distal interphalangeal joint result from the patient's need to provide a means to pinch.

One of the most common manifestations of RA in hands is tenosynovitis in flexor tendon sheaths. Frequently overlooked during an examination that focuses on the dorsum of the hand, the tendon sheath lesion is manifested on the volar surface of the phalanges as diffuse swelling between joints or a palpable grating within flexor tendon sheaths in the palm.

In one series, hand flexor tenosynovitis was observed in 55 percent of 100 patients with RA,[186] a higher frequency than found in other studies and probably related more to careful examination than to any difference in population or disease. Although hand flexor tenosynovitis was not associated with more prolonged or severe disease, there was an association with a number of para-articular manifestations (distinct from extra-articular

Figure 60–7. A, Early ulnar deviation of the metacarpophalangeal joints without subluxation. Extensor tendons have slipped to the ulnar side. The fifth finger, in particular, is compromised with weak flexion, causing loss of power grip. B, Complete subluxation with marked ulnar deviation at the metacarpophalangeal joints of a 90-year-old woman with RA. Arrows mark the heads of the metacarpals, now in direct contact with the joint capsule instead of the proximal phalanges. (Courtesy of James L. McGuire, M.D.)

Table 60-9. Prevalence of Para-Articular Disorders Associated with RA*

Patients	Flexor Tenosynovitis	Without Flexor Tenosynovitis
Number of patients	55	45
Carpal tunnel syndrome	26	6
Extensor tenosynovitis	26	4
Epicondylitis	12	3
Dupuytren's contracture	6	0
De Quervain's tenosynovitis	5	0
Flexor carpi radialis tendinitis	7	0
Flexor carpi ulnaris tendinitis	2	0
Achilles tendinitis	5	0

*Adapted from Gray, R.C., and Gottlieb, N.L.: Arthritis Rheum. 20:1003, 1977.

manifestations) (Table 60–9).[187] De Quervain's tenosynovitis is particularly important to diagnose because it causes severe discomfort and yet is relatively easily treated. It represents extensor tenosynovitis in the thumb extensors. Pain originating from these sheaths can be demonstrated by Finklestein's test: ulnar flexion at the wrist after the thumb is maximally flexed and adducted. Pain on this maneuver is indicative of de Quervain's tenosynovitis. Many factors may lead to loss of hand strength in patients with RA (Table 60–10). Tenosynovitis rather than articular synovitis is probably the most significant of these factors.[188]

Figure 60–9. Early (A) and late (B) "boutonnière" deformity of the phalanges in RA. In B, moderate soft tissue swellings at the second and third metacarpophalangeal joints are visible.

Not infrequently, rheumatoid nodules will develop within the tendons, and they may "lock" the finger painfully into flexion, necessitating surgical excision or glucocorticoid injections when they become chronic and recurrent. If flexor tenosynovitis reduces active motion, peritendinous and pericapsular adhesions may develop secondarily and limit proximal interphalangeal joint motion.[188]

Table 60–10. Factors Diminishing Hand Grasp Strength in RA

1. Synovitis in joints
2. Reflex inhibition of muscular contraction secondary to pain
3. Altered kinesiology; distorted relation of joint, bones, and tendons during motion
4. Flexor tenosynovitis, with or without rheumatoid nodules on tendons
5. Vascular ischemia → pain; from altered sympathetic tone
6. Edema of all structures, from inflammation and perhaps altered lymphatic drainage
7. Intrinsic muscle atrophy and/or fibrosis

Figure 60–8. Multiple deformities of the hand in severe rheumatoid arthritis. This 60-year-old woman has had wrist surgery (dorsal synovectomy and resection of the ulnar head). The bones of the thumb have been destroyed and partially resorbed, producing redundant skin and a short digit ("main en lorgnette"). Hyperextension at the proximal interphalangeal joints with flexion of the distal interphalangeal joints, as in the third finger of her hand, are characteristic of the swan neck deformity. (Courtesy of James L. McGuire, M.D.).

Often hands are painful in RA without much evidence for inflammation. It has been suggested that ischemia secondary to vascular spasm from excess sympathetic tone may contribute to hand pain, particularly during grasp motion.[189] The improvement in peripheral hemodynamics following administration of propranolol has suggested that this claudication may be mediated primarily by beta-adrenergic receptors.[190]

Although classic teaching describes an absence of distal interphalangeal joint involvement in RA, some careful observations have found distal interphalangeal joint tenderness in the hands of up to 70 percent of patients with RA at some time during the course of their disease.

Hip. The hip is less frequently involved in adult forms of RA than in juvenile RA, and clinical involvement is difficult to evaluate if pain is not present. Pain on the lateral aspect of the hip is often a manifestation of trochanteric bursitis rather than synovitis, which usually produces pain or tenderness in the groin.

About half the patients with established RA will have radiographic evidence of hip disease.[191] The femoral head may collapse and be resorbed, while the acetabulum often remodels as it is pushed medially, leading to protrusio acetabuli. Significant protrusion occurs in about 5 percent of all patients with RA.[192] Loss of internal rotation on physical examination correlates best with radiographic findings. Similar to other weight-bearing joints, the femoral head may develop cystic lesions. Communication of these with the joint space can often be demonstrated on surgically resected femoral heads.[193] Radiography of the pelvis rarely shows localized erosions of the lower part of the sacroiliac joint in RA, a phenomenon probably associated with localized granuloma formation. Synovial cysts can develop around the hip joint. Communication between the iliopsoas bursa and the hip joint facilitates formation of a cyst that appears within the pelvis and can be large enough to obstruct venous return from the extremity.[194]

Knees. In contrast to the hips, synovial inflammation and proliferation are readily demonstrated. Synovial fluid in excess of 5 ml may be demonstrated by the "bulge" sign: milking fluid from the lateral superior recess of the joint across to the medial side, producing a fluid wave across the normally concave area inferomedial to the patella.[195] Very early in knee disease, often within a week after onset of symptoms, quadriceps atrophy is noticeable and may lead to the application of more force than usual through the patella to the femoral surface. Another early manifestation of knee disease in RA is loss of full extension, a functional loss that can become a fixed flexion contracture unless remedies are undertaken to correct it.[196]

Flexion of the knee markedly increases the intra-articular pressure (see Chapter 59) and may produce an outpouching of posterior components of the joint space, a popliteal or Baker's cyst. Jayson and Dixon have demonstrated that fluid from the anterior compartments of the knee may enter the popliteal portion but not readily return.[197] This one-way valve may produce pressures so high in the popliteal space that it may rupture down

into the calf or, rarely, superiorly into the posterior thigh. Rupture occurs posteriorly between the medial head of the gastrocnemius and the tendinous insertion of the biceps. Clinically, popliteal cysts and complications of them may present in several ways (Table 60–11). The intact popliteal cyst may compress superficial venous flow through to the upper part of the leg, producing dilation of superficial veins and/or edema. Rupture of the joint posteriorly with dissection of joint fluid into the calf may resemble acute thrombophlebitis with swelling and tenderness, as well as systemic signs of fever and leukocytosis. One helpful sign in joint rupture may be the appearance of a crescentic hematoma beneath one of the malleoli.[198] Part of the examination of rheumatoid patients should include observation from the rear while the patient stands. This often increases the observation of popliteal cysts. Ultrasound evaluation is a useful way to assess popliteal swelling and usually obviates the need for arthrography in these patients.[199]

Very often, radiographic evidence for destruction of the knee lags behind clinical evidence for it. It is important to assess the thickness of articular cartilage radiographically by taking films with the patient in a standing position. The proliferative destructive synovitis in RA may destroy meniscal cartilage and cruciate ligaments. Tests for lateral and anteroposterior stability will indicate the extent of damage to these structures before gross deformity or incongruity is visible.

Ankle and Foot. The ankle joint is involved less often than the knee in RA, but probably is a better measure of severe disease than is the knee; the ankle is rarely involved in mild or oligoarticular RA, but often is damaged in severe progressive forms of the disease. Clinical evidence for ankle involvement is soft, occasionally cystic, swelling anterior and posterior to the malleoli (Fig. 60–10). Much of the stability of the ankle depends upon integrity of ligaments holding the fibula to the tibia and these two bones to the talus. In RA, inflammatory and proliferative disease may loosen these connections by stretching and eroding the collagenous ligaments. The result is incongruity, which, once initiated, progresses to pronation deformities or eversion of the foot (Fig. 60–11).

The Achilles tendon is a major structural component and kinetic force in the foot and ankle. Rheumatoid nodules develop in this collagenous structure, and spontaneous rupture of the tendon has been reported when diffuse granulomatous inflammation is present.[203] The subtalar joint controls eversion and inversion of the foot on the talus, and is involved commonly in RA. Patients with RA invariably have more pain while walking on

Table 60–11. Differential Diagnosis of Popliteal Cysts[200-202]

Lipoma	Hemangioma
Xanthoma	Lymphadenopathy
Fibrosarcoma	Charcot joint
Vascular tumor	Thrombophlebitis
Varicose veins	

Figure 60–10. Marked synovial proliferation in the ankle joint of a 43-year-old woman with RA. (Courtesy of James L. McGuire, M.D.).

uneven ground, and this is related to the relatively common subtalar joint involvement in RA.[204]

More than one third of patients with RA have significant disease in the feet.[205] The foot in RA widens as the angle between metacarpals increases. Metatarsophalangeal joints are involved often, and gait is altered as pain develops during push-off in striding. It is of interest that the metatarsal heads sublux downward very soon after the metatarsophalangeal joints become involved, producing "cock-up" toe deformities (Fig. 60–12A). Hallux valgus and bunion-callus formation appear if disease continues (Fig. 60–12B). Cystic collections often develop under the metatarsophalangeal joints and occasionally represent outpouchings of flexor tendon sheaths.[206] Patients whose metatarsal heads sublux to the subcutaneous area may develop pressure necrosis. Alternatively, patients who have subluxed metatarsophalangeal joints often develop pressure necrosis over the proximal interphalangeal joints that protrude dorsally ("hammer toes") and are subject to irritation by shoes. An extensive discussion of RA and the foot is presented in Chapter 31.

The sequence of changes as disease progresses in the foot is as follows:[207,208] (1) intermetatarsal joint ligaments stretch; (2) spread of the forefoot occurs; (3) the fibrofatty cushion on the plantar surface migrates anteriorly; (4) toes sublux dorsally and extensor tendons shorten; (5) metatarsal heads sublux to a subcutaneous site on the plantar surface; and (6) development of hallux valgus often results in "stacking" of the second and third toes on top of the great toe. It is important to note that distal interphalangeal joints of the foot rarely are affected in rheumatoid arthritis.

Whereas Achilles tendinitis and plantar fasciitis are the principal causes of foot pain in patients with Reiter's syndrome or ankylosing spondylitis, patients with RA are more likely to develop plantar faciitis without Achilles tendinitis. Sub-Achilles bursitis is characterized by a tender mass bulging to the sides of the tendon and is found principally in women. A valgus deformity of the heel is the most characteristic change of the hindfoot in RA and develops along with instability of the mortise joint.

Another cause of foot pain in rheumatoid patients is the tarsal tunnel syndrome. In a group of 30 patients with RA, radiographically demonstrated erosions in the feet, and foot pain, 4 (13 percent) were shown by electrodiagnostic techniques to have slowing of medical

Figure o0–11. Valgus of ankle, pes planus, and forefoot varus deformity of the left foot related to painful synovitis of the ankle, forefoot, and metatarsophalangeal joint in a 24-year-old man with severe RA.

Figure 60–12. Foot problems in RA. *A*, Discrete cystic proliferation below subluxed metatarsal heads (2 and 3) in the foot of a patient with RA. *B*, Marked hallux valgus with proliferative tissue in the form of a "bunion" at the first metatarsophalangeal joint in a patient with RA. There is, in addition, diffuse cystic swelling below the metatarsal heads. (Courtesy of James L. McGuire, M.D.)

and/or lateral plantar nerve latency.[209] Clinically, these patients are difficult to distinguish from those with foot pain but without compression neuropathy.

Bone. Bones are involved in RA at more sites than the bone ends, where erosion by proliferative synovium occurs.

The para-articular osteopenia that accompanies persistent synovitis is an early sign that proliferative disease sufficient to result in significant destruction of joints is present. Long bones distant from joints also become involved in RA. Almost all patients with far-advanced long-standing RA develop diffuse demineralization of the entire skeleton.[210] Older age, the predominance of females in all groups of patients with RA, and the use of corticosteroids in treatment all potentiate the development of osteopenia.[211] Related to, and a possible cause of, this osteopenia are dietary deficiencies of both calcium and vitamin D.[212] All these factors combine to produce a much higher frequency of insufficiency (e.g., stress) fractures of long bones in this disease.[212,213,215] The

fibula is the most common site of fracture. The frequency of fracture has been increasing as the number of total joint prostheses are inserted and as patients formerly bedridden are now able to walk. Careful assays have shown an increased excretion of hydroxyproline by patients with active rheumatoid arthritis not treated with glucocorticoids.[214] Urinary hydroxyproline reflects bone matrix breakdown and correlates positively with the 24-hour whole-body retention of ^{99m}Tc methylene dephosphonate (an index of bone metabolism) and global index of disease activity.

Muscle. Clinical weakness is common in RA, but is it caused by muscle involvement by the rheumatoid process or is it a reflex weakness response to pain? Most rheumatoid patients have muscle weakness, but few have muscle tenderness. An exception to this is the occasional patient with a severe flare of active disease; such a patient may cry out in severe pain, unable to move either muscles or joints. These symptoms resemble vascular insufficiency (ischemic pain) in their intensity.

In an early autopsy series, focal accumulations of lymphocytes and plasma cells with some contiguous degeneration of muscle fibers were found in all rheumatoid patients and named "nodular myositis."[216] More recent and sophisticated studies[217] of patients with definite and classic RA revealed four groups of neuromuscular abnormalities: (1) chronic myopathy resembling a dystrophic process, probably the endstage of a myositis (8 cases); (2) diminution of muscle bulk, with atrophy of type II muscle fibers similar to that described in cachexia (13 cases); (3) peripheral neuropathy, possibly demyelinating (9 cases); and (4) steroid myopathy (4 cases). Each of these types of muscle pathology is overshadowed by serious joint disease when it is present. In most patients, muscle symptoms are not predominant.

Extra-Articular Complications of Rheumatoid Arthritis

Unlike joint disease per se, the complications of RA may be fatal. In general, the number and severity of extra-articular features vary with the duration and severity[218,219] of the disease. Some of these factors will be discussed under Prognosis.

Ocular and dermatologic complications will not be discussed in detail here; these are presented in the context of other manifestations in those organ systems in Chapters 35 and 36, respectively. Nerve compression syndromes commonly seen in RA are outlined in Chapter 110.

The interest in these extra-articular manifestations is enhanced by realization that RA is a systemic process, and that each organ and tissue reacts in a unique way to what is presumed to be the same inciting factor.

Rheumatoid Nodules. The pathology of rheumatoid nodules is well documented.[220,221] In the well-formed nodule there is a central area of necrosis rimmed by a corona of palisading fibroblasts that is surrounded by a collagenous capsule with perivascular collections of chronic inflammatory cells.

Careful histology of early lesions[222] has suggested that development of the nodule is mediated through affected small arterioles and the terminal vascular bed of tissues; small vessels proliferate, and this is associated with proliferation of resident histiocytes and fibroblasts, as well as an influx of monocytes and lymphocytes. The nodule tissue in organ culture has the capacity to produce collagenase and proteinase in large quantity, similar to synovial tissue.[223] It has been suggested that these enzymes released by the palisading layer of cells may be sufficient to result in destruction of the extracellular matrix collagen around the cells, leading to their death and a centrifugally expanding central necrosis commonly found in these nodules.

Occurring in 20 to 35 percent of patients with definite or classic RA, nodules are found most easily on extensor surfaces such as the olecranon process and the proximal ulna (Fig. 60–13A). They are subcutaneous and vary in consistency from a soft, amorphous, entirely mobile mass to firm rubber masses attached firmly to periosteum.

Rheumatoid factor is almost always found in the serum of patients with rheumatoid nodules. Rarely, such nodules are present without obvious arthritis.[224] Multiple

Figure 60–13. Manifestations of increased reactivity of mesenchymal tissue in rheumatoid arthritis appearing (*A*) as nodules on the elbow and (*B*) within the sclera of the eye. The eye lesion represents scleral perforation associated with a granulomatous scleral reaction. Treatment was placement of a scleral patch graft. Note the great increase in vascularity of the sclera. The dark areas represent scleral thinning with exposure of uveal pigment. (Patient of Drs. S. Arthur Bouchoff and G. N. Fouhls. Photograph courtesy of Marty Schener.)

nodules on the hands in the absence of clinical arthritis but with a positive test for rheumatoid factor has been called "rheumatoid nodulosis."[225,226] The differential diagnosis of rheumatoid nodules includes the five following types.

"Benign" Nodules. These usually are found in healthy children without rheumatoid factor or arthritis; they are nontender, appear often on the pretibial regions, feet, and scalp, increase rapidly in size, and are histologically identical to rheumatoid nodules.[227] They resolve spontaneously.

Granuloma Annulare. These nodules are intracutaneous but histologically identical to rheumatoid nodules. They slowly resolve, and are not associated with other disease.[228]

Xanthomatosis. These nodules usually have a yellow tinge, and patients have abnormally high plasma lipoproteins and cholesterol. There is no underlying bone involvement.

Tophi. These collections of monosodium urate crystals have small, punched-out bone lesions associated with them and are rarely found in patients with a normal serum urate. A search for crystals with a polarizing microscope will reveal the classic needle-shaped, negatively birefringent crystals.

Miscellaneous. The nodules of multicentric reticulohistiocytosis have been described (see the preceding Differential Diagnosis of Rheumatoid Arthritis). Numerous proliferative disorders affecting cutaneous tissue, including erythema elevatum diutinum, acrodermatitis chronica atrophicans, bejel, yaws, pinta, and leprosy, can resemble rheumatoid nodule.[229] A rheumatoid nodule, particularly when it occurs on the face, may simulate basal cell carcinoma.[230]

Appearance of nodules in unusual sites may lead to confusion in diagnosis. Sacral nodules may be mistaken for bedsores if the skin overlying them breaks down.[231] Occipital nodules also occur in bedridden patients. In the larynx, rheumatoid nodules on the vocal cords may cause progressive hoarseness.[232] Nodules found in the heart and lungs will be discussed below. A nodule in the eye is shown in Figure 60–13B.

Fistula Development. The rare development of cutaneous sinuses near joints occurs in seropositive patients with long-standing disease and positive tests for rheumatoid factor.[233] These fistulae can be either sterile or septic, and connect the skin surface either with a joint or with a para-articular cyst in bone or soft tissues.[234] The pathogenesis of fistulae without a septic origin is particularly difficult to understand because the rheumatoid process is usually so clearly centripetal in nature, that is, progressing toward the center of the joint, rather than centrifugal.

Infection. Infections have paralleled the use of corticosteroids and immunosuppressive agents as a complication of RA.[235] Pulmonary infections, skin sepsis, and pyarthrosis are most common.[236-238] In addition to the presence of drugs that suppress host resistance, the phagocytic capacity of leukocytes in RA may be less than normal.[239] Difficulty in diagnosis is accentuated by the similarity of aggressive RA to infection, particularly in joints. A full discussion of sepsis in RA is presented in Chapter 96.

Hematologic Abnormalities. The majority of patients with RA have a mild normocytic hypochromic anemia, which correlates with the erythrocyte sedimentation rate and with activity of the disease.[240-241] Hemoglobin rarely drops below 10 grams per dl in RA unless there is another contributing factor such as blood loss. Study of the dynamics in development of this anemia have confirmed early studies that this is an anemia of chronic disease related to ineffective erythropoiesis.[241-243] It is characterized by a low serum iron, a low total iron-binding capacity, and normal reticuloendothelial iron stores (except, for unknown reasons, in Felty's syndrome, in which iron stores may be absent). The mean red cell life is slightly shortened. Total erythroid heme turnover is slightly reduced, and ineffective erythropoiesis accounts for a much greater than normal percentage of total heme turnover. These patients also may demonstrate a diminished ability to absorb iron through the gastrointestinal tract, which is usually related to the irritative presence of one or another anti-inflammatory medications.[244] The presence or absence of stainable iron in the marrow of patients with RA may correlate approximately with serum ferritin levels alone.[245] By addition of the mean corpuscular volume and the erythrocyte sedimentation rate to the equation in a computer program, iron stores (presence or absence) can be predicted in 95 percent of patients. The remaining 5 percent identified by the computer will need bone marrow examination.[246] In contrast to anemia associated with blood loss, the ineffective erythropoiesis will return to normal if remission can be induced in RA. The ineffective erythropoesis is not related to "functional" iron deficiency (i.e., reduced availability of iron).[247]

Eosinophilia and thrombocytosis are often associated with RA. Eosinophilia (5 percent of total white blood cell count or greater) was observed in 40 percent of patients selected for having severe seropositive disease.[248] Similarly, a significant relationship has been shown to exist between thrombocytosis and extra-articular manifestations of rheumatoid disease.[249] This may be related in part to an increase in platelet production associated with active intravascular coagulation.

One of the most significant hematologic complications of RA, Felty's syndrome, is discussed in Chapter 61.

Vasculitis. In one sense, it is redundant to think of vasculitis as a complication of RA, since the initial pathology in RA is believed to rest in small blood vessels. However, it is useful to use the term vasculitis to group those extra-articular complications not related to proliferative granulomas but rather to inflammatory vascular disease.

Clinical vasculitis usually takes one or another of the following forms: (1) distal arteritis (ranging from splinter hemorrhages to gangrene); (2) cutaneous ulceration (including pyoderma gangrenosum); (3) peripheral neuropathy; (4) pericarditis; (5) arteritis of viscera, including heart, lungs, bowel, kidney, liver, spleen, pancreas,

lymph nodes, and testis; (6) acro-osteolysis; or (7) palpable purpura.

The pathology in rheumatoid vasculitis is that of a panarteritis. All layers of the vessel wall are infiltrated with mononuclear cells. Fibrinoid necrosis is seen in very active lesions. Intimal proliferation may predispose to thrombosis. When larger vessels are involved, the pathology resembles that of polyarteritis nodosa.[250] In addition, a venulitis associated with RA has been described.[251,252] In patients with hypocomplementemia the cellular infiltrate around the vessels contains neutrophils; in normocomplementemic patients, lymphocytes predominate.[252] Uninvolved skin from rheumatoid patients is positive for immunoglobulin and complement when sections for histopathology are stained with fluorescein-labeled antibodies to these components. The presence of IgG correlates directly with circulating immune complexes, vasculitic skin lesions, subcutaneous nodules and high titer rheumatoid factor.[253]

It is unusual for vasculitis to be active in any but the sickest patients, those with severe deforming arthritis and high titers of rheumatoid factor. Supporting the hypothesis that vascular injury is mediated by deposition of circulating immune complexes are the data indicating (1) depressed levels of C2 and C4;[254] (2) hypercatabolism of C3;[255] (3) deposition of IgG, IgM, and C3 in involved arteries;[256] and (4) the presence of large amounts of cryoimmunoglobulins in serum of patients with vasculitis.[257]

Neurovascular disease may be the only manifestation of vasculitis. The two common clinical patterns are a mild distal sensory neuropathy and a severe sensorimotor neuropathy (mononeuritis multiplex).[258] The latter form is characterized by severe arterial damage on nerve biopsy specimens. Symptoms of the milder form may be paresthesias or "burning feet" in association with decreased touch and pin sensation distally. Patients with mononeuritis multiplex have weakness (e.g., foot drop) in addition to sensory abnormalities. Symptoms and signs are identical to those found in polyarteritis. Rheumatoid pachymeningitis is a rare complication of RA. Confined to the dura and pia meter, this process may be limited to certain areas (e.g., lumbar cord and/or cisternae, etc).[259] Elevated IgG (including IgM and IgG rheumatoid factors allow molecular weight IgM) and immune complexes are found in the CSF.

Although there is a negative association between psychosis and RA, it is possible that organic brain syndromes may be related to RA in patients not taking corticosteroids or indomethacin,[263] and it is presumed that these manifestations are caused by small vessel disease.

Visceral lesions present generally as claudication or infarction of the organ supplied by the involved arteries. Intestinal involvement with vasculitis presents as abdominal pain, at first intermittent, progressing often to continuous pain and a tender, quiet belly on examination. If infarction develops, resection must be accomplished promptly.[260] Early studies of rheumatoid vasculitis implied that glucocorticoid therapy might be responsible for precipitating vasculitis in rheumatoid patients. A sudden reduction or cessation of glucocorticoid therapy also has been implicated as a precipitating cause of vasculitis.[261] A more recent large study, however, showed no relationship to steroid dose and vasculitis.[262]

Clinical features associated with a poor prognosis in rheumatoid vasculitis are renal impairment, intestinal vasculitis, neuropathy, weight loss, and histological evidence of vasculitis on rectal biopsy.[264]

The kidney is an example of an organ that is rarely involved directly in RA but often is compromised indirectly. Amyloidosis (see Chapter 92) is a complication of chronic RA. Another indirect cause of renal disease is toxicity from therapy. Phenacetin abuse causes renal papillary necrosis, and salicylates may cause abnormalities as well.[265] A membranous nephropathy is the pathologic lesion related to therapy with gold salts and D-penicillamine, but a long-term study has suggested that perhaps membranous nephropathy is related to the underlying disease and that gold treatment may exacerbate the underlying process.[266] This remains to be confirmed. Rarely, a focal necrotizing glomerulitis is seen in patients dying with disseminated vasculitis.[267]

Pulmonary Disease. There are five forms of lung disease in RA: (1) pleural disease, (2) interstitial fibrosis, (3) nodular lung disease, (4) pneumonitis, and (5) arteritis.

Pleural Disease. Pleuritis is very commonly found at autopsy of patients with RA, but clinical disease during life is seen less frequently.[268] Characteristics of the rheumatoid effusions are as follows: glucose = 10 to 50 mg per dL; protein = 4 g per dL; cells = 1000 to 3500 (mononuclear) per cu mm; lactic dehydrogenase = elevated; CH_{50} = depressed.

The low glucose concentrations are of interest. Sepsis (particularly tuberculosis) is the only other condition that commonly has such a low synovial fluid glucose. An impaired transport of glucose into the pleural space appears to be the cause.[269]

Interstitial Fibrosis. The increased reactivity of mesenchymal cells in RA is believed to be the cause of pulmonary fibrosis in this disease. Similar to findings in scleroderma, physical findings are of fine diffuse dry rales. Radiographs show a diffuse reticular or reticulonodular pattern in both lung fields,[270,271] which develop a "honeycomb" appearance. The pathologic findings are those of diffuse fibrosis in the midst of a mononuclear cell infiltrate.[272] The principal functional defect is impairment of alveolar-capillary gas exchange with decreased diffusion capacity, which is best measured utilizing single-breath carbon monoxide diffusion capacities.[273] In a prospective study of 155 rheumatoids and 95 control subjects, rheumatoids showed an increased frequency of chest crackles and abnormal chest radiographs and restrictive ventilatory defects. These abnormalities were associated with smoking.[274] It is likely that rheumatoids who smoke are at a higher risk for fibrotic complications in the lungs than are those in the general population.

Nodular Lung Disease. Pulmonary nodules may appear singly or in clusters that coalesce. Single ones appear as a coin lesion and, when significant peripheral arthritis and nodules are present, can be diagnosed by needle biopsy without thoracotomy. Caplan's syndrome,[275] in which pneumoconiosis and RA are synergistic and produce a violent fibroblastic reaction with obliterative granulomatous fibrosis, becomes a much less frequent occurrence as the respiratory environment in mining operations improves. Nodules may cavitate and create a bronchopleural fistula,[276] and may even precede arthritis.[277]

Pneumonitis. Very rare is an interstitial pneumonitis that progresses to alveolar involvement, respiratory insufficiency, and death. Pathologic studies show a very cellular loose fibrosis and proteinaceous exudate in alveoli (Fig. 60–14).

Arteritis. Pulmonary hypertension from arteritis of the pulmonary vasculature is very rare and is occasionally associated with digital arteritis.[278]

Cardiac Complications. Cardiac disease in RA can take many forms related to granulomatous proliferation or vasculitis. Involvement can be classified as follows: (1) pericarditis, (2) myocarditis (rheumatoid carditis), (3) endocardial (valve) inflammation, (4) conduction defects, (5) coronary arteritis, and (6) granulomatous aortitis.

Pericarditis. Infrequently diagnosed by history and physical examination in RA, pericarditis is present in up to 50 percent of patients at autopsy.[279,280] Use of echocardiography has enabled much more precise assessment of cardiac structure and function in patients with RA. In one study, 31 percent had echocardiographic evidence of pericardial effusion. The same study revealed only rare evidence for impaired left ventricular function in prospectively studied outpatients with RA.[281] Although unusual, cardiac tamponade with constrictive pericarditis develops in RA and may require pericardectomy.[282,283] This complication appears to be more frequent after sudden reduction of glucocorticoid treatment. Pericarditis usually develops after RA is established, but it may precede the arthritis. Most patients have a positive test for rheumatoid factor, and half will have nodules.

Myocarditis. This complication can take the form of either granulomatous disease or interstitial myocarditis. The granulomatous process resembles subcutaneous nodules[284] and could be considered specific for the disease. Diffuse infiltration of the myocardium by mononuclear cells, on the other hand, may involve the entire myocardium and yet have no clinical manifestations.[280]

Endocardial Inflammation. Echocardiographic studies have reported conflicting evidence for previously undiagnosed mitral valve disease diagnosed by a reduced E to F slope of the anterior leaflet of the mitral valve.[285,286] Although aortic valve disease and arthritis are generally associated through ankylosing spondylitis, a number of granulomatous nodules in the valve have been reported.[287] Aortic valve replacement has been successful in these cases.

Conduction defects such as atrioventricular block are

Figure 60–14. Severe, subacute inter-sitital pneumonitis in RA. This complication proved fatal in 5 weeks in this 66-year-old woman with severe, active seropositive RA. *A*, The gross photograph of the left lung shows dense interalveolar thickening by a fibrofibrinous exudate. Air sacs are becoming obliterated. Lungs were heavy and incompressible, but there was only a trace of excess fluid. *B*, Microscopic sections showed thickened alveolar septa with a rich fibrinous exudate present. (Courtesy of Charles Faulkner, III, M.D.)

rare in RA but are probably related to direct granulomatous involvement. The pathology may reveal proliferative lesions[284] or healed scars.[288]

Patients with severe RA and active vasculitis who develop a myocardial infarction are very likely to have coronary arteritis as a basis for the process.[289]

In severe rheumatoid heart disease, granulomatous disease can be found to spread to involve even the base of the aorta.[290]

PROGNOSIS IN RHEUMATOID ARTHRITIS

Natural History of RA. Epidemiologists have pointed out the multiple difficulties in attempting to establish change in patterns of RA in different time periods or different communities. The best data suggest that patients currently admitted to the hospital for RA are likely to have fewer joint contractures and less ankylosis of peripheral joints at admission than did patients admitted 20 years ago, whereas the prevalence of rheumatoid factor, subcutaneous nodules, and the mean number of affected joints has, if anything, increased slightly.[291] These and other data suggest that the disease is not changing, but that earlier, more effective treatment has perhaps diminished the morbidity.

As with other chronic diseases, both physicians and their patients are eager to know the chances for remission and anxious about the threat of severe morbidity or death.

There are now well-tested criteria for a clinical remission.[292] Six criteria have yielded optimal discrimination (Table 60–12). Very few patients achieve 5 of 6 of these criteria, and thus very few rheumatoids, whether or not they are being treated, ever achieve true remission. Thus, it would be more logical to refer to gold and D-penicillamine as "disease-modifying drugs" rather than "remission-inducing" substances. Most series of rheumatoid patients are weighted by those with more severe disease who have well-established disease.[293] In contrast, a large number of patients given a diagnosis of RA go into complete remission, and probably should not have been considered initially to have RA.[11]

Death associated with RA is generally associated with the complications—both articular and extra-articular—of RA. The probability of these deaths varies directly with the severity of complications. Such potentially morbid articular complications include the various forms of atlantoaxial subluxation, cricoarytenoid synovitis, and sepsis of involved joints. Extra-articular complications directly causing a higher mortality rate include Felty's syndrome (possible death from overwhelming infection), Sjögren's syndrome, cardiopulmonary complications, diffuse vasculitis, and amyloidosis. Infection has been one of the most common contributing factors to death in rheumatoid patients.[293-295]

Aside from the occurrence of death as an outcome in RA, there are a number of other variables in the disease that have been related to prognosis.

Presentation of Arthritis. *Good Prognosis.* Several investigators have observed that a clinical subgroup of patients with an acute, explosive onset of disease or early rapid progression of symptoms do better in the long run than do patients with an insidious onset of disease.[296-298]

Table 60–12. Preliminary Criteria for Complete Clinical Remission in Rheumatoid Arthritis

A minimum of five of the following requirements must be fulfilled for at least two consecutive months in a patient with definite or classic RA.
1. Morning stiffness not to exceed 15 minutes
2. No fatigue
3. No joint pain
4. No joint tenderness or pain on motion
5. No soft tissue swelling in joints or tendon sheaths
6. ESR (Westergren) less than 30 mm/hr (females) or 20 mm/hr (males)

Exclusions: Clinical manifestations of active vasculitis, pericarditis, pleuritis, or myositis and/or unexplained recent weight loss or fever secondary to RA prohibit a designation of complete clinical remission.[292]

Table 60–13. Comparative Mortality and Morbidity in Seronegative and Seropositive Patients*

	Seronegative (Percent)	Seropositive (Percent)
Deaths	15	27
Remissions†	70	38
Vasculitis	10	50

*From Kellgren, J.H., and O'Brien, W.M.: Arthritis Rheum. 5:115, 1962.
†In survivors.

Whether this is related to the patients coming earlier under good care or to other factors is unknown. However, a more recent study[299] of 235 patients in which an "acute" pattern of onset was present in 69 patients, intermediate in 55, and gradual in 111 revealed that radiologic destruction after 7 years from the beginning of the disease process was the same in each group, regardless of the rapidity of onset. Patients who evolve into RA from a palindromic type of presentation are reported to have a better prognosis.[300]

Poor Prognosis. Patients with a disease of insidious onset appear to do less well than others, but this may be due in part to their relatively late presentation for good care.[301] Factor analysis of one series by computer[302] has revealed poorer prognosis for patients who have at once the patterns of large proximal joint involvement (shoulder, elbow, wrist, and knee) and disease in the first and second metatarsophalangeal joints.

Rheumatoid Factor. Many studies have confirmed that seropositivity is associated with a poorer prognosis in RA. One series of 60 patients with active disease showed the associations seen in Table 60–13.[303] Patients with rheumatoid factor have more involved joints when they present to a physician for the first time, and develop more erosions and ligamentous instability.[304,305] As mentioned previously, more and more of those individuals who carry a diagnosis of seronegative rheumatoid arthritis[306] are being recognized as having other classifiable entities.

Rheumatoid Nodules. These occur almost always in patients with rheumatoid factor, although without correlation with titer of rheumatoid factor.[293,304,305] Therefore, similar to those patients with rheumatoid factor alone, patients with subcutaneous nodules have a poorer outcome and more frequent bone erosions.[293,297,307]

Sex. In young adults developing RA, females generally have a worse outcome with more swollen and tender joints and erosions than do males.[304]

Synovial Histopathology. Although it is generally agreed that persistence and intensity of synovial inflammation are related to joint destruction, no single feature or group of features demonstrable by routine histopathologic examination of synovium has been correlated with destructive lesions in RA.[308,309] In part, this may be related to the major variations in histology found from area to area within the synovium,[310] a factor that makes histopathologic prognostication from synovial needle biopsy practically useless. A finding of cartilage erosion associated with synovial lining cell proliferation and few subsynovial lymphocytes[311] has not been confirmed.[308,309]

Synovial Fluid Analysis (see Chapter 38). Chemotactic factors in synovial fluid in RA attract PMN leukocytes, which accumulate and are eventually lysed within the joint space. It has been demonstrated that when the joint fluid leukocyte count exceeds 50,000 to 60,000 cells per cubic millimeter, proteinase inhibitors in the fluid can be saturated or inhibitors damaged or rendered effete, so that proteinase activity is manifest.[312] Human neutrophils have been found to generate an unusual class of oxidants with a long half-life (about 18 hours), which appear to be N-chloroamines. These substances have oxidizing potential sufficient to inactivate thio ether-containing proteinase inhibitors such as α_1-proteinase inhibitor, and perhaps, α_2-macroglobulin.[313] It is probable that at times such as these, proteinases act unopposed upon cartilage components. Acidosis of synovial fluid correlates with leukocyte counts in synovial fluid;[314] severe acidosis may alter cellular metabolism in cartilage and synovium. Depression of glucose and complement components in synovial fluid can be roughly correlated with the intensity of inflammation in the fluid,[315] and levels of IgG with the degree of subsynovial lymphocyte accumulation.[315]

Other Laboratory Data. A number of laboratory tests in addition to those for rheumatoid factor have prognostic significance.

Eosinophilia. Patients with RA and an associated eosinophilia of 5 percent or greater have a higher incidence of vasculitis, pleuropericarditis, pulmonary fibrosis, and subcutaneous nodules.[248] The hypothesis has been put forth that immune complexes may induce the eosinophilia and that therefore the latter may correlate better with vasculitis than other simple tests in RA.

Thrombocytosis. A highly significant correlation between platelet count and disease severity, and platelet count and extra-articular manifestations of RA, has been described.[249] An inverse correlation between platelet count and hemoglobin was found as well.

Circulating Immune Complexes Each assay for immune complexes appears to detect different components of immune complexes. For example, the C1q binding assay, which detects complexes containing IgM rheumatoid factor, correlates poorly with indices of disease activity in RA.[216] The C1q solid phase assay may better parallel the articular index in RA[317] but does not correlate as well as the ESR or IgG rheumatoid factor.

C-Reactive Protein (CRP) (see Chapter 43). In a recent series of 56 patients with RA, the measurement of both the erythrocyte sedimentation rate (ESR) and CRP correlated directly with erosive disease better than did other tests, including the presence of rheumatoid factor.[318] In another group of 99 patients the serum C reactive protein concentration closely reflected the activity of RA as judged by a new multivariate analysis comprising morning stiffness, pain scale, grip strength, articular index, hemoglobin, and the erythrocyte sedimentation rate (ESR).[319] Changes in CRP level cover a much broader range than changes in ESR and appear to occur more rapidly (24 hours) in contrast to ESR (days or weeks).

Classification and Assessment in Rheumatoid Arthritis

The inflammatory lesion in RA is reflected reasonably well by heat, pain, swelling, and tenderness. Joint destruction can occur with minimal inflammation, however, and means to assess cartilage destruction are limited to radiographic determination of apparent joint space narrowing and erosions. A good noninvasive means to assess the erosive potential of synovitis does not exist, and until there are valid objective tests available to assess the proliferative lesion, clinical means of classification will be used. These are used frequently in drug studies and are reviewed in Chapter 48. The prototype for these has been Lansbury's systemic index, consisting of quick objective measurement of five features of activity in RA: morning stiffness, pain, fatigue, muscle weakness, and the ESR.[320,321]

Although easy to perform, the Lansbury indices and others like them have been difficult to standardize. One major difficulty is in the attempts to measure pain. As stated by Huskisson,[322] "The severity of pain is known only to the sufferer. . . . Pain is a personal psychological experience, and an observer can play no legitimate part in its direct measurement." For these reasons, direct (though subjective) measurement by a visual analogue scale is a good technique.

Classification of RA is best done by functional analysis. The criteria of Steinbrocker and associates[323] have long been used effectively (Table 60–14). It is appropriate to correlate functional class with an anatomic radiographic staging system[323] (Table 60–15). In evaluating the status of a particular patient, the physician can use, as a rough guide, the radiographic staging system as an index of whether the functional status of that individual is appropriate. For instance, if a functional Grade III patient has only Grade 2 radiographic

Table 60–14. Functional Capacity in RA*

Grade	Definition	Remarks
I	Capable of all activities	
II	Moderate restriction	Adequate for normal activities despite handicap of discomfort or limited motion at one or more joints
III	Marked restriction	Activity limited to self-care and few or no duties of a usual occupation
IV	Bed and/or chair	Capable of little or no self-care

*From Steinbrocker, O., et al.: JAMA 140:659, 1949.

Table 60–15. Radiographic Staging System for RA*

Grade	Definition
1	No destructive changes; periarticular osteopenia may be present
2	Osteoporosis is definite, with or without slight subchondral bone destruction; slight joint space narrowing may be present
3	Evidence for cartilage and bond destruction; joint deformity (e.g., subluxation, ulnar deviation); no bony or fibrous ankylosis
4	Stage 3 criteria plus fibrous or bony ankylosis

*From Steinbrocker, O., et al.: JAMA 140:659, 1949.

changes, it is likely that aggressive physical therapy and/or attention to care of nonarticular complications of the disease may improve functional status. Similarly, in treatment trials as well as with individual patients, it is essential to define when a remission has occurred. It is crucial to remember that if a patient with Grade 3 radiologic stages enters a complete remission, it still is unlikely that he or she would have a low Lansbury score or achieve Grade I functional status.

Care of the rheumatoid patient should include a careful record of the physical examination and functional and radiographic assessment. This permits care of patients in a prospective fashion and provides a systematic assessment of disease activity. With proper assessment, effective therapy, as outlined in Chapter 61, can be started, evaluated, and changed if necessary.

References

1. Snorrason, E.: Landre-Beauvais and his goutte asthenique primitive. Acta Med. Scand. 142(Suppl. 266):115, 1952.
2. Boyle, J.A., and Buchanan, W.W.: Clinical Rheumatology. Philadelphia, F.A. Davis Company, 1971, pp. 71–72.
3. Short, C.L.: The antiquity of rheumatoid arthritis. Arthritis Rheum. 17:193, 1974.
4. Copeman, W.S.C.: A Short History of the Gout and the Rheumatic Diseases. Berkeley, University of California Press, 1964.
5. Soranus of Ephesus: On Acute Diseases and on Chronic Diseases. Translated into Latin by Caelius Aurelianus (5th century A.D.). English translation by I.E. Drabkin. Chicago, University of Chicago Press, 1950, pp. 923–929.
6. Ruffer, M.A., and Rietti, A.: On osseous lesions in ancient Egyptians. J. Pathol. Bacteriol. 16:439, 1912.
7. Ropes, M.W., Bennett, E.A., Cobb, S., Jacox, R., and Jessar, R.: 1958 Revision of diagnostic criteria for rheumatoid arthritis. Bull. Rheum. Dis. 9:175, 1958.
8. Wood, P.H.N.: Epidemiology of rheumatic disorders: Problems in classification. Proc. R. Soc. Med. 63:189, 1970.
9. Schumacher, H.R., and Kitridou, R.C.: Synovitis of recent onset. A clinicopathologic study during the first month of disease. Arthritis Rheum. 15:465, 1972.
10. Mitchell, D.M., and Fries, J.F.: An analysis of the American Rheumatism Association criteria for rheumatoid arthritis. Arthritis Rheum. 25:481, 1982.
11. Bennett, P.H., and Burch, T.A.: New York symposium on population studies in the rheumatic diseases: New diagnostic criteria. Bull. Rheum. Dis. 17:453, 1967.
12. O'Sullivan, J.B., and Cathcart, E.S.: The prevalence of rheumatoid arthritis. Follow-up evaluation of the effect of criteria on rates in Sudbury, Massachusetts. Ann. Intern. Med. 76:573, 1972.
13. Wolfe, A.M.: The epidemiology of rheumatoid arthritis: A review. Bull. Rheum. Dis. 19:518, 1968.
14. Engel, A., Roberts, J., and Burch, T.A.: Rheumatoid arthritis in adults in the United States 1960–1962. In Vital and Health Statistics, Series 11, Data from the National Health Survery, Number 17. Washington, D.C., National Center for Health Statistics, 1966.
15. Mikkelsen, W.M., Dodge, H.J., Duff, I.F., and Kato, I.H.: Estimates of the prevalence of rheumatic disease in the population of Tecumseh, Michigan, 1959–60. J. Chronic Dis. 20:351, 1967.
16. O'Brien, W.M., Bennett, P.H., Burch, T.A., et al.: A genetic study of rheumatoid arthritis and rheumatoid factor in Blackfeet and Pima Indians. Arthritis Rheum. 10:163, 1967.
17. Wood, W.J., Kato, H., Johnson, K.G., et al.: Rheumatoid arthritis in Hiroshima and Nagasaki, Japan. Arthritis Rheum. 10:21, 1967.
18. Beasley, R.P., Willkens, R.F., and Bennett, P.H.: High prevalence of rheumatoid arthritis in Yakima Indians. Arthritis Rheum. 16:743, 1973.
19. Harvey, J., Lotze, M., Arnett, F.C., et al.: Rheumatoid arthritis in a Chippewa band. II. Field study with clinical serologic and HLA-D correlations. J. Rheum. 10:28, 1983.
20. Solomon, L., Robin, G., and Valkenburg, H.A.: Rheumatoid arthritis in an urban South African Negro population. Ann. Rheum. Dis. 34:128, 1975.
21. Beighton, P., Solomon, L., and Valkenburg, H.A.: Rheumatoid arthritis in a rural South African Negro population. Ann. Rheum. Dis. 34:136, 1975.
22. Linos, A., Worthington, J.W., O'Fallon, W.M., and Kurland, L.T.: The epidemiology of rheumatoid arthritis in Rochester, Minnesota. A study of incidence, prevalence and mortality. Am. J. Epidemiol. 11:87–98, 1980.
23. Wingrave, S., and Kay, C.R.: Reduction in incidence of rheumatoid arthritis associated with oral contaceptives. Lancet 1:569, 1978.
24. Stastny, P.: Mixed lymphocyte cultures in rheumatoid arthritis. J. Clin. Invest. 57:1148, 1976.
25. Stastny, P.: Association of the B-cell alloantigen DRw4 with rheumatoid arthritis. N. Engl. J. Med. 298:869, 1978.
26. McMichael, A.J., Sasazuki, T., McDevitt, H.O., and Payne, R.O.: Increased frequency of HLA-Cw3 and HLA-Dw4 in rheumatoid arthritis. Arthritis Rheum. 20:1037, 1977.
27. Rose, H.M., Ragan, C., Pearce, E., and Lipman, M.O.: Differential agglutination of normal and sensitized sheep erythrocyes by sera of patients with rheumatoid arthritis. Proc. Soc. Exp. Bio. Med. 68:1, 1948.
28. Waaler, E.: On the occurrence of a factor in human serum activating the specific agglutination of sheep blood corpuscles. Acta Pathol. Microbiol. Scand. 17:172, 1940.
29. Lawrence, J.S.: Prevalence of rheumatoid arthritis. Ann. Rheum. Dis. 20:11, 1961.
30. Lawrence, J.S., Laine, V.A.I., and DeGraaff, R.: The epidemiology of rheumatoid arthritis in northern Europe. Proc. R. Soc. Med. 54:454, 1961.
31. Engleman, E.G., Sponzilli, E.E., Batey, M.E., Rancharan, S., and McDevitt, H.O.: Mixed lymphocyte reaction in healthy women with rheumatoid factor. Arthritis Rheum. 21:690, 1978.
32. Plotz, C.M., and Singer, J.M.: The latex fixation test. II. Results in rheumatoid arthritis. Am. J. Med. 21:893, 1956.
33. Alarcon, G.S., Koopman, W.J., Acton, R.T., and Barger, B.O.: Seronegative rheumatoid arthritis. A distinct immunogenetic disease? Arthritis Rheum. 25:502, 1982.
34. Myerowitz, S., Jacox, R.F., and Hers, D.W.: Monozygotic twins discordant for rheumatoid arthritis. Arthritis Rheum. 11:1, 1968.
35. Harvald, B., and Hauge, M.: In Genetics and the Epidemiology of Chronic Diseases. Washington, D.C., U.S. Government Printing Office, 1965, p. 61.
36. Lawrence, J.S.: Genetics of rheumatoid factor and rheumatoid arthritis. Clin. Exp. Immunol. S2:769, 1967.
37. Lawrence, J.S.: Rheumatoid arthritis-nature or nurture. Ann. Rheum. Dis. 29:357, 1970.
38. Siegel, M., Lee, S.L., Widelock, D., Gwon, N.V., and Kravitz, H.: A comparative family study of rheumatoid arthritis and systemic lupus erythematosus. N. Engl. J. Med. 273:893, 1965.
39. Mellsop, G.W., Koadlow, L., Syme, J., et al.: Absence of rheumatoid arthritis in schizophrenia. Aust. N.Z. J. Med. 4:247, 1974.
40. Hellgren, L.: The prevalence of rheumatoid arthritis in occupational groups. Acta Rheumatol. Scand. 16:106, 1970.
41. Gottlieb, N.L., Dichek, N., Poiley, J., and Kiem, I.M.: Pets and rheumatoid arthritis: An epidemiologic survey. Arthritis Rheum. 17:229, 1974.
42. Beall, G., and Cobb, S.: The frequency distribution of episodes of rheumatoid arthritis as shown by periodic examination. J. Chronic Dis. 14:291, 1961.
43. Jacoby, R.K., Jayson, M.I.V., and Cosh, J.A.: Onset, early stages and prognosis of rheumatoid arthritis: A clinical study of 100 patients with 11 year follow-up. Br. Med. J. 2:96, 1973.
44. Lawrence, J.S.: Surveys of rheumatic complaints in the population. In Dixon, A.St.J. (ed.): Progress in Clinical Rheumatology. London, Churchill, 1965, p. 1.
45. Short, C.L., and Bauer, W.: The course of rheumatoid arthritis in patients receiving simple medical and orthopedic measures. N. Engl. J. Med. 238:142, 1948.

46. Fleming, A., Crown, J.M., and Corbett, M.: Early rheumatoid disease. I. Onset. Ann. Rheum. Dis. 35:357, 1976.
47. Fleming, A., Benn, R.T., Corbett, M., and Wood, P.H.N.: Early rheumatoid disease. II. Patterns of joint involvement. Ann. Rheum. Dis. 35:361, 1976.
48. Dick, W.C., Grayson, M.F., Woodburn, A., Nuki, G., and Buchanan, W.W.: Indices of inflammatory activity. Relationship between isotope studies and clinical methods. Ann. Rheum. Dis. 29:643, 1971.
49. Bywaters, E.G.L.: Still's disease in the adult. Ann. Rheum. Dis. 30:121, 1971.
50. Gupta, R.C., and Mills, D.M.: Still's disease in an adult: A link between juvenile and adult rheumatoid arthritis. Am. J. Med. Sci. 269:137, 1975.
51. Aptekar, R.G., Decker, J.L., Bujak, J.S., and Wolff, S.M.: Adult onset of juvenile rheumatoid arthritis. Arthritis Rheum. 16:715, 1973.
52. Strampl, I.J., and Lozar, J.D.: Adult-onset Still's disease. Variant of rheumatoid arthritis. Postgrad. Med. 58:175, 1975.
53. Elkon, K.B., Hughes, G.R.V., Bywaters, E.G.L., et al.: Adult-onset Still's disease. Twenty year follow-up and further studies of patients with active disease. Arthritis Rheum. 25:647, 1982.
54. Hench, P.S., and Rosenberg, E.F.: Palindromic rheumatism: New oft-recurring disease of joints (arthritis, periarthritis, para-arthritis) apparently producing no articular residues. Report of 34 cases. Proc. Mayo Clin. 16:808, 1942.
55. Schumacher, H.R.: Palindromic onset of rheumatoid arthritis. Arthritis Rheum. 25:361, 1982.
56. Yoghami, I., Rookolamini, S.M., and Faunce, H.F.: Unilateral rheumatoid arthritis: Protective effects of neurologic deficits. Am. J. Roentgenol. 128:299, 1977.
57. Bland, J., and Eddy, W.: Hemiplegia and rheumatoid hemiarthritis. Arthritis Rheum. 11:72, 1968.
58. Glick, E.N.: Asymmetrical rheumatoid arthritis after poliomyelitis. Br. Med. J. 3:26, 1967.
59. Thompson, M., and Bywaters, E.G.L.: Unilateral rheumatoid arthritis following hemiplegia. Ann. Rheum. Dis. 21:370, 1961.
60. Bywaters, E.G.L.: The hand. In Radiological Aspects of Rheumatoid Arthritis. International Congress Series. Amsterdam, Excerpta Medica Foundation, No. 64, 1964, p. 43.
61. de Haas, W.H.D., de Boer, W., Griftioen, F., and Oostenelst, P.: Rheumatoid arthritis of the robust reaction type. Ann. Rheum. Dis. 31:81, 1974.
62. Short, C.L., Bauer, W., and Reynolds, W.E.: Rheumatoid arthritis: A Definition of the Disease and a Clinical Description Based on a Numerical Study of 293 Patients and Controls. Cambridge, Harvard University Press, 1957.
63. Short, C.L.: Rheumatoid arthritis: Types of course and prognosis. Med. Clin. North Am. 52:549, 1968.
64. Cohen, A.S. (ed.): Laboratory Diagnostic Procedures in the Rheumatic Diseases. 2nd ed. Boston, Little, Brown & Company, 1975.
65. Hoffman, G.S.: Polyarthritis: The differential diagnosis of rheumatoid arthritis. Semin. Arthritis Rheum. 8:115, 1978.
66. Short, C.L., Bauer, W., and Reynolds, W.E.: Rheumatoid Arthritis. Cambridge, Harvard University Press, 1957.
67. Potter, T.A., Barkin, T., and Stillman, R.S.: Occurrence of spondylitis in juvenile rheumatoid arthritis. Ann. Rheum. Dis. 13:364, 1954.
68. Fallet, G.H., Mason, M., Berry, H., Mowat, A.G., Bonssina, I., and Gerster, J.-C.: Rheumatoid arthritis and ankylosing spondylitis occurring together. Br. Med. J. 1:604, 1976.
69. Morris, R.I., Metzger, A.L., Bluestone, R., et al.: HLA w27—a useful discriminator in arthropathies of inflammatory bowel disease. N. Engl. J. Med. 290:1117, 1974.
70. McEwen, C., Lingg, C., and Kirsner, J.B.: Arthritis accompanying ulcerative colitis. Am. J. Med. 33:923, 1962.
71. Zizic, T.M., and Stevens, M.B.: The arthropathy of Behçet's disease. Johns Hopkins Med. J. 136:243, 1975.
72. Ahvonen, P., Sievers, K., and Ano, K.: Arthritis associated with Yersinia enterocolitica infection. Acta Rheumatol. Scand. 15:232, 1969.
73. Ano, K., Ahvonen, P., Lassus, A., Sievers, K., and Tulisinen, A.: HL-A27 (sic) in reactive arthritis: A study of Yersinia arthritis and Reiter's disease. Arthritis Rheum. 17:521, 1974.
74. Hawkins, C.F., Farr, M., Morris, C.J., House, A.M., and Williamson, N.: Detection by electron microscope of rod-shaped organisms in synovial membrane from a patient with the arthritis of Whipple's disease. Ann. Rheum. Dis. 35:502, 1976.
75. Bole, G.G., Friedlaender, M.H., and Smith, C.K.: Rheumatic symptoms and serological abnormalities induced by oral contraceptives. Lancet 1:323, 1969.
76. Bland, J.H., and Frymoyer, J.W.: Rheumatic syndromes of myxedema. N. Engl. J. Med. 282:1171, 1970.
77. Gimlette, T.M.D.: Thyroid acropachy. Lancet 1:22, 1960.
78. Churchill, M.A., Geraci, J.E., and Hunder, G.G.: Musculoskeletal manifestations of bacterial endocarditis. Ann. Intern. Med. 87:754, 1977.

79. Bayer, A.S., Theofilopoulos, A.N., Eisenberg, R., Dixon, F.J., and Guze, L.B.: Circulating immune complexes in infective endocarditis. N. Engl. J. Med. 295:1500, 1976.
80. Bulkley, B.H., and Hutchins, G.M.: Atrial myxomas: A fifty year review. Am. Heart J. 97:639, 1979.
81. McCarty, D.J.: Diagnostic mimicry in arthritis—patterns of joint involvement associated with calcium pyrophosphate dihydrate crystal deposits. Bull. Rheum. Dis. 25:804, 1975.
82. Utsinger, P.D., Zvaifler, N.J., and Resnick, D.: Calcium pyrophosphate dihydrate deposition disease without chondrocalcinosis. J. Rheumatol. 2:258, 1975.
83. Halla, J.T., and Hardin, J.G.: Clinical features of the arthritis of mixed connective tissue disease. Arthritis Rheum. 21:497, 1978.
84. Heller, H., Gafni, J., Michaeli, D., et al.: Arthritis of familial Mediterranean fever (FMF). Arthritis Rheum. 9:1, 1966.
85. Talbott, J.H., Altman, R.D., and Yu, T-F.: Gouty arthritis masquerading as rheumatoid arthritis or vice versa. Semin. Arthritis Rheum. 8:77, 1978.
86. Resnick, D.: Gout-like lesions in rheumatoid arthritis. Am. J. Roentgenol. 127:1062, 1976.
87. Rappoport, A.S., Sosman, J.L., and Weissman, B.N.: Lesions resembling gout in patients with rheumatoid arthritis. Am. J. Roentgenol. 126:41, 1976.
88. Kozin, F., and McCarty, D.J.: Rheumatoid factor in the serum of gouty patients. Arthritis Rheum. 20:1559, 1977.
89. Wallace, D.J., Klinenberg, J.R., Morbaim, D., Berlanstein, B., Biren, P.C., and Callis, G.: Coexistent gout and rheumatoid arthritis: Case report and literature review. Arthritis Rheum. 22:81, 1979.
90. Hirsch, J.H., Killien, F.C., and Troupin, R.H.: The arthopathy of hemochromatosis. Diagn. Radiol. 118:591, 1976.
91. Dymock, I.W., Hamilton, E.B.D., Laws, J.W., and Williams, R.: Arthropathy of hemochromatosis. Ann. Rheum. Dis. 29:469, 1970.
92. Schumacher, H.R., Andrews, R., and McLaughlin, G.: Arthropathy in sickle cell disease. Ann. Intern. Med. 78:203, 1973.
93. Schumacher, H.R., Dorwart, B.B., Boud, J., Alavi, A., and Miller, W.: Chronic synovitis with early cartilage destruction in sickle cell disease. Ann. Rheum. Dis. 36:413, 1977.
94. Crout, J.E., McKenna, C.H., and Petitt, R.M.: Symptomatic joint effusions in sickle cell-β-thalassemia disease. JAMA 235:1878, 1976.
95. Glueck, C.J., Levy, R.I., and Fredickson, D.S.: Acute tendinitis and arthritis: A presenting symptom of familial type II hyperlipoproteinemia. JAMA 206:2895, 1968.
96. Watt, T.L., and Baumann, R.R.: Pseudoxanthomatous rheumatoid nodules. Arch. Dermatol. 95:156, 1967.
97. Buckingham, R.B., Bole, G.G., and Bassett, D.R.: Polyarthritis associated with Type IV hyperlipoproteinemia. Arch. Intern. Med. 135:286, 1975.
98. Langer, T., and Levy, R.I.: Acute muscular syndrome associated with administration of clofibrate. N. Engl. J. Med. 279:856, 1968.
99. Schumacher, H.R.: Articular manifestations of hypertropic pulmonary osteoarthropathy in bronchogenic carcinoma. Arthritis Rheum. 19:629, 1976.
100. Yanez, J.E., Thompson, G.R., Mikkelsen, W.M., and Bartholomew, L.E.: Rubella arthritis. Ann. Intern. Med. 64:772, 1966.
101. Spruance, S.L., and Smith, C.B.: Joint complications associated with derivatives of HPV-77 rubella virus vaccine. Am. J. Dis. Child. 122:105, 1971.
102. Alpert, E., Isselbacher, K.J., and Aschur, P.H.: The pathogenesis of arthritis associated with viral hepatitis. Complement component studies. N. Engl. J. Med. 285:185, 1971.
103. Schumacher, H.R., and Gall, E.P.: Arthritis in acute hepatitis and chronic active hepatitis. Pathology of the synovial membrane with evidence for the presence of Australia antigen in synovial membranes. Am. J. Med. 57:655, 1974.
104. Sigal, L.H., Steere, A.C., and Niederman, J.C.: Symmetric polyarthritis associated with heterophile-negative infectious mononucleosis. Arthritis Rheum. 26:553, 1983.
105. Steere, A.C., Malawista, S.E., Hardin, J.A., Ruddy, S., Askenasy, W., and Andiman, W.A.: Erythema chronicum migrans and Lyme arthritis. The enlarging clinical spectrum. Ann. Intern. Med. 86:685, 1977.
106. Gold, R.H., Metzger, A.L., Mina, J.M., Weinberger, H.J., and Killebrew, K.: Multicentric reticulohistiocytosis (lipoid dermato-arthritis). Am. J. Roentgenol. 124:610, 1975.
107. Orkin, M., Goltz, R.W., Good, R.A., Michael, A., and Fisher, I.: A study of multicentric reticulohistiocytosis. Arch. Dermatol. 89:641, 964.
108. Ehrlich, G.E.: Inflammatory osteoarthritis. I. The clinical syndrome. J. Chronic Dis. 25:317, 1972.
109. Ordenstein, L.: Sur la Paralysie Agitante et la Sclérose en Plaques Generalisée Paris. Imprimerie de E. Martinet, 1864 (original in Library of the New York Academy of Medicine)
110. McDanold, E.C., and Weissman, M.H.: Articular manifestations of rheumatic fever in adults. Ann. Intern. Med. 89:917, 1978.

111. Barnett, A.L., Terry, E.E., and Persellin, R.H.: Acute rheumatic fever in adults. JAMA 232:925, 1975.
112. Stollerman, G.H., Markowitz, M., Tarania, A., Wannamaker, L.W., and Whittemor, R.: Jones' criteria (revised) for guidance in the diagnosis of rheumatic fever. Circulation 32:664, 1965.
113. Bywaters, E.G.L.: Relation between heart and joint disease including "rheumatoid heart disease" and chronic post-rheumatic arthritis (type Jaccoud). Br. Heart J. 12:101, 1950.
114. Zvaifler, N.J.: Chronic postrheumatic-fever (Jaccoud's) arthritis. N. Engl. J. Med. 267:10, 1962.
115. Ruderman, J.E., and Abruzzo, J.L.: Chronic post rheumatic-fever arthritis (Jaccoud's): Report of a case with subcutaneous nodules. Arthritis Rheum. 9:640, 1966.
116. Spilberg, I., Siltzbach, L.E., and McEwen, C.E.: The arthritis of sarcoidosis. Arthritis Rheum. 12:126, 1969.
117. Kaplan, H.: Sarcoid arthritis. A review. Arch. Intern. Med. 112:162, 1963.
118. Poncet, A.: Address to the Congress Francais de Chirurgie, 1897. Bull. Acad. Med. Paris 46:194, 1901.
119. Krauser, R.E., and Schumacher, H.R.: The arthritis of Sweet's syndrome. Arthritis Rheum. 18:35, 1975.
120. Hoffman, G.S.: Treatment of Sweet's syndrome (acute febrile neutrophilic dermatosis) with indomethacin. J. Rheumatol. 4:201, 1977.
121. Thiemann, H.: Juvenile Epiphysenstorungen. Fortschr. Geb. Rontgenstr. Nuklearmed. 14:79, 1909–10.
122. Rubenstein, H.M.: Thiemann's disease. A brief reminder. Arthritis Rheum. 18:357, 1975.
123. Pinals, R.S., and Short, C.L.: Calcific periarthritis involving multiple sites. Arthritis Rheum. 9:566, 1966.
124. Weiner, A.D., and Ghormley, R.K.: Periodic benign synovitis. Idiopathic intermittent hydrarthrosis. J. Bone Joint Surg. 38A:1039, 1956.
125. Williams, M.H., Sheldon, P.J.H.S., Torrigiani, G., and Mattingly, S.: Palindromic rheumatism. Clinical and immunological studies. Ann. Rheum. Dis. 30:375, 1971.
126. Ehrlich, G.E.: Intermittent and periodic rheumatic syndromes. Bull. Rheum. Dis. 24:746, 1974.
127. Shagrin, J.W., Frame, B., and Duncan, H.: Polyarthritis in obese patients with intestinal bypass. Ann. Intern. Med. 75:377, 1971.
128. Smythe, H.A., and Moldofsky, H.: Two contributions to understanding of the "fibrositis syndrome." Bull. Rheum. Dis. 28:928, 1978.
129. Velayos, E.E., Leidholt, J.D., Smyth, C.J., and Priest, R.: Arthropathy associated wtih steroid therapy. Ann. Intern. Med. 64:759, 1966.
130. Moulsopoulos, H.M., Fye, K.H., Pugay, P.I., and Shearn, M.A.: Monoarthric arthritis caused by metastatic breast carcinoma. JAMA 234:75, 1975.
131. Granowitz, S.P., and Mankin, H.J.: Localized pigmented villonodular synovitis of knee. J. Bone Joint Surg. 49A:122, 1967.
132. Gordon, D.A., Pruzanski, W., Ogryzlo, M.A., and Little, H.A.: Amyloid arthritis simulating rheumatoid disease in five patients with multiple myeloma. Am. J. Med. 55:142, 1973.
133. Pinals, R.S., Dalakos, T.G., and Streeten, D.H.P.: Idiopathic edema as a cause of nonarticular rheumatism. Arthritis Rheum. 22:396, 1979.
134. Bland, J.: Rheumatoid arthritis of the cervical spine. J. Rheumatol. 1:319, 1974.
135. Ball, J.: Enthesopathy of rheumatoid and ankylosing spondylitis. Ann. Rheum. Dis. 30:213, 1971.
136. Martel, W.: Pathogenesis of cervical discovertebral destruction in rheumatoid arthritis. Arthritis Rheum. 20:1217, 1977.
137. Weiner, S., Bassett, L., and Speigel, T.: Superior, posterior, and lateral displacement of C1 in rheumatoid arthritis. Arthritis Rheum. 25:1378, 1982.
138. Stevens, J.C., Cartilage, N.E.F., Saunders, M., Appleby, A., Hall, M., and Shaw, D.A.: Atlantoaxial subluxation and cervical myelopathy in rheumatoid arthritis. Quart. J. Med. 40:391, 1971.
139. Nakano, K.K., Schoene, W.C., Baher, R.A., et al.: The cervical myelopathy associated with rheumatoid arthritis: Analysis of 32 patients with 2 postmortem cases. Am. Neuro. Assoc. 3:144, 1978.
140. Martel, W.: The occipito-atlanto-axial joints in rheumatoid arthritis and ankylosing spondylitis. Am. J. Roentgenol. 86:223, 1961.
141. Raskin, R.J., Schnapf, D.J., Wolf, C.R., Killian, P.J., and Lawless, O.J.: Computerized tomography in evaluation of athentoaxial subluxation in rheumatoid arthritis. J. Rheumatol. 10:32, 1983.
142. Mayer, J.W., Messner, R.P., and Kaplan, R.J.: Brain stem compression in rheumatoid arthritis. JAMA 236:2094, 1976.
143. Mikulowski, P., Wollheim, F.A., Rotmil, P., and Olsen, I.: Sudden death in rheumatoid arthritis with atlanto-axial dislocation. Acta Med. Scand. 198:445, 1975.
144. Smith, P.H., Benn, R.T., and Sharp, J.: Natural history of rheumatoid cervical luxations. Ann. Rheum. Dis. 31:431, 1972.
145. Henderson, D.R.F.: Vertical atlanto-axial subluxation in rheumatoid arthritis. Rheumatol. Rehab. 14:31, 1975.

146. Davidson, R.C., Horn, J.R., Herndon, J.H., and Oliver, G.D.: Brain stem compression in rheumatoid arthritis. JAMA 238:2633, 1977.
147. Bywaters, E.G.L.: Rheumatoid and other diseases of the cervical interspinous bursae, and changes in the spinous process. Am. Rheum. Dis. 41:360, 1982.
148. Ericson, S., and Lundberg, M.: Alterations in the temporomandibular joint at various stages of rheumatoid arthritis. Acta. Rheum. Scand. 13:257, 1967.
149. Marbach, J.J., and Spiera, H.: Rheumatoid arthritis of the temporomandibular joints. Ann. Rheum. Dis. 26:538, 1967.
150. Lofgren, R.H., and Montgomery, W.W.: Incidence of laryngeal involvement in rheumatoid arthritis. N. Engl. J. Med. 267:193, 1962.
151. Polisar, I.A., Burbank, B., Levitt, L.M., Katz, H.M., and Morrione, T.G.: Bilateral midline fixation of cricoarytenoid joints as a serious medical emergency. JAMA 172:901, 1960.
152. Bienenstock, H., Ehrich, G.E., and Freyberg, R.H.: Rheumatoid arthritis of the cricoarytenoid joint: A clinicopathologic study. Arthritis Rheum. 6:48, 1963.
153. Copeman, W.S.C.: Rheumatoid oto-arthritis. Br. Med. J. 2:1536, 1963.
154. Moffat, D.A., Ramsden, R.T., Rosenberg, J.N., Booth, J.B., and Gibson, W.P.R.: Otoadmittance measurements in patients with rheumatoid arthritis. J. Laryngol. Otol. 91:917, 1977.
155. Kalliomaki, J.L., Viitaneu, S-M., and Virtama, P.: Radiological findings of sternoclavicular joints in rheumatoid arthritis. Acta Rheumatol. Scand. 14:233, 1968.
156. Kormano, M.: A microradiographic and histological study of the manubriosternal joint in rheumatoid arthritis. Acta. Rheumatol. Scand. 16:47, 1970.
157. Khong, T.K., and Rooney, P.J.: Manubriosternal joint subluxation in rheumatoid arthritis. J. Rheumatol. 9:712, 1982.
158. Ennevaara, K.: Painful shoulder joint in rheumatoid arthritis. Acta Rheumatol. Scan. Suppl. 11, 1967, pp. 1–116.
159. Weiss, J.J., Thompson, G.R., Doust, V., and Burgener, F.: Rotator cuff tears in rheumatoid arthritis. Arch. Intern. Med. 135:521, 1975.
160. Mosley, H.F.: Ruptures of the Rotator Cuff-Shoulder Lesions. 3rd ed. Edinburgh, E & S Livingston Ltd., 1969, p. 73.
161. Edeiken, J., and Hodes, P.J.: Roentgen Diagnosis of Diseases of Bone. 2nd ed. Baltimore, Williams & Wilkins Company, 1978, pp. 690–709.
162. DeSmet, A.A., Ting, Y.M., and Weiss, J.J.: Shoulder arthrography in rheumatoid arthritis. Diagn. Radiol. 116:601, 1975.
163. Huston, K.A., Nelson, A.M., and Hunder, G.G.: Shoulder swelling in rheumatoid arthritis secondary to subacromial bursitis. Arthritis Rheum. 21:145, 1978.
164. Resnick, D., and Niwayama, G.: Resorption of the undersurface of the distal clavicle in rheumatoid arthritis. Diagn. Radiol. 120:75, 1976.
165. Laine, V., and Vainio, K.: The elbow in rheumatoid arthritis. In Hymans, W., Paul, W.D., and Herschel, H.: Early Synovectomy in Rheumatoid Arthritis. Amsterdam, Excerpta Medica, 1969, p. 112.
166. Peterson, L.F.A., and James, J.M.: Surgery of the rheumatoid elbow. Orthop. Clin. North Am. 2:667, 1971.
167. Shapiro, J.S.: A new factor in the etiology of ulnar drift. Clin. Orthop. 68:32, 1970.
168. Hastings, D.E., and Evans, J.A.: Rheumatoid wrist deformities and their relation to ulnar drift. J. Bone Joint Surg. 57A:930, 1975.
169. Inglis, A.E.: Rheumatoid arthritis in the hand. Am. J. Surg. 109:368, 1965.
170. Swezey, R.L., and Fiegenberg, D.S.: Inappropriate intrinsic muscle action in the rheumatoid hand. Ann. Rheum. Dis. 30:619, 1972.
171. Fearnley, G.R.: Ulnar deviation of the fingers. Ann. Rheum. Dis. 10:126, 1951.
172. Flatt, A.E.: Surgical rehabilitation of the arthritic hand. Arthritis Rheum. 11:278, 1959.
173. Hakstian, R.W., and Tubiana, R.: Ulnar deviation of the fingers. J. Bone Joint Surg. 49A:299, 1967.
174. Snorrason, E.: The problem of ulnar deviation of the fingers in rheumatoid arthritis. Acta. Med. Scand. 140:359, 1951.
175. Vainio, K., and Oka, M.: Ulnar deviation of the fingers. Ann. Rheum. Dis. 12:122, 1953.
176. Croft, J.D., and Jacox, R.F.: Rheumatoid "ganglion" as an unusual presenting sign of rheumatoid arthritis. JAMA 203:144, 1968.
177. Harrison, M.D., Freiberger, R.H., and Ranawat, C.S.: Arthrography of the rheumatoid wrist joint. Am. J. Roentgenol. 112:480, 1971.
178. Iveson, J.M.I., Hill, A.G.S., and Wright, V.: Wrist cysts and fistulae. An arthrographic study of the rheumatoid wrist. Ann. Rheum. Dis. 34:388, 1975.
179. Martel, W., Hayes, J.T., and Duff, I.F.: The pattern of bone erosion in the hand and wrist in rheumatoid arthritis. Radiology 84:204, 1965.
180. Resnick, D., and Gmelich, J.T.: Bone fragmentation in the rheumatoid wrist; radiographic and pathologic considerations. Diagn. Radiol. 114:315, 1975.
181. Trentham, D.E., and Masi, A.T.: Carpo: metacarpal ratio. A new quan-

titative measure of radiologic progression of wrist involvement in rheumatoid arthritis. Arthritis Rheum. 191:939, 1976.

182. Brewerton, D.A.: Hand deformities in rheumatoid disease. Ann. Rheum. Dis. 16:183, 1957.

183. McCarty, D.J., and Gatter, R.A.: A study of distal interphalangeal joint tenderness in rheumatoid arthritis. Arthritis Rheum. 9:325, 1966.

184. Vaughan-Jackson, O.J.: Rheumatoid hand deformities considered in the light of tendon imbalance. J. Bone Joint Surg. 44B:764, 1962.

185. Nalebuff, E.A.: Diagnosis, classification, and management of rheumatoid thumb deformities. Bull. Hosp. Joint Dis. 24:119, 1968.

186. Kellgren, J.H., and Ball, J.: Tendon lesions in rheumatoid arthritis: A clinicopathological study. Ann. Rheum. Dis. 9:48, 1950.

187. Gray, R.G., and Gottlieb, N.L.: Hand flexor tenosynovitis in rheumatoid arthritis. Arthritis Rheum. 20:1003, 1977.

188. Millis, M.B., Millender, L.H., and Nalebuff, E.A.: Stiffness of the proximal interphalangeal joints in rheumatoid arthritis. J. Bone Joint Surg. 58A:801, 1976.

189. Vyden, J.K., Callis, G., Groseth-Dittrich, M.F., Laks, M.M., and Weinberger, H.: Peripheral hemodynamics in rheumatoid arthritis (abstract). Arthritis Rheum. 14:419, 1971.

190. Vyden, J.K., Groseth, Dittrich, M.F., Callis, G., Laks, M.M., and Weinberger, H.: The effect of propranolol on peripheral hemodynamics in rheumatoid arthritis (abstract). Arthritis Rheum. 14:420, 1971.

191. Duthie, R., and Harris, C.: A radiographic and clinical survey of the hip joints in sero-positive rheumatoid arthritis. Acta Orthop. Scand. 40:346, 1969.

192. Hastings, D.E., and Parker, S.M.: Protrusio acetabuli in rheumatoid arthritis. Clin. Orthop. 108:76, 1975.

193. Colton, C., and Darby, A.: Giant granulomatous lesions of the femoral head and neck in rheumatoid arthritis. Ann. Rheum. Dis. 29:616, 1970.

194. Levy, R.N., Hermann, G., Haimov, M., et al.: Rheumatoid synovial cyst of the hip. Arthritis Rheum. 25:1382, 1982.

195. Cary, G.R.: Methods for determining the presence of subtle knee joint effusion. J. Louisiana St. Med. Soc. 118:147, 1966.

196. Gupta, P.J.: Physical examination of the arthritis patient. Bull. Rheum. Dis. 20:596, 1970.

197. Jayson, M.I.V., and Dixon, A.St.J.: Valvular mechanisms in juxta-articular cysts. Ann. Rheum. Dis. 29:415, 1970.

198. Kraag, G., Thevathasan, E.M., Gordon, D.A., and Walker, I.H.: The hemorrhage crescent sign of acute synovial rupture. Ann. Intern. Med. 85:477, 1976.

199. Gordon, G.V., and Edell, S.: Ultrasound evaluation of popliteal cyst. Arch. Intern. Med. 140:1453, 1980.

200. Hall, A.P., and Scott, J.T.: Synovial cysts and rupture of the knee joint in rheumatoid arthritis. Ann. Rheum. Dis. 25:32, 1966.

201. Hench, P.K., Reid, R.T., and Reames, P.M.: Dissecting popliteal cyst stimulating thrombophlebitis. Ann. Intern. Med. 64:1259, 1966.

202. Tait, G.B.W., Bach, F., and Dixon, A.St.J.: Acute synovial rupture. Ann. Rheum. Dis. 24:273, 1965.

203. Rask, M.R.: Achilles tendon rupture owing to rheumatoid disease. J. Amer. Med. Asso. 239:435, 1978.

204. Dixon, A.St.J.: The rheumatoid foot. In Hill, A.G.S. (ed.): Modern Trends in Rheumatology. Vol. 2. London, Butterworths, 1971, pp. 158–173.

205. Vidigal, E., Jacoby, R., Dixon, A.St.J., Rattiff, A.H., and Kirkup, J.: The foot in chronic rheumatoid arthritis. Ann. Rheum. Dis. 34:292, 1975.

206. Bienenstock, H.: Rheumatoid plantar synovial cysts. Ann. Rheum. Dis. 34:98, 1975.

207. Dixon, A.St.J.: The rheumatoid foot. Proc. R. Soc. Med. 63:677, 1970.

208. Calabro, J.J.: A critical evaluation of the diagnostic features of the feet in rheumatoid arthritis. Arthritis Rheum. 5:19, 1962.

209. McGuigan, L., Burke, D., and Fleming, A.: Tarsal tunnel syndrome and peripheral neuropathy in rheumatoid disease. Ann. Rheum. Dis. 42:128, 1983.

210. Vainio, K.: The rheumatoid foot: A clinical study with pathological and roentgenological comments. Ann. Clin. Gynaec. Fenn. 45(Suppl. 1):107, 1956.

211. Duncan, H., Frost, H.M., Villaneuva, A.R., et al.: The osteoporosis of rheumatoid arthritis. Arthritis Rheum. 8:943, 1965.

212. Saville, P.D., and Kharmosh, O.: Osteoporosis of rheumatoid arthritis: Influence of age, sex and corticosteroids. Arthritis Rheum. 10:423, 1967.

213. Maddison, P.J., and Bacon, P.A.: Vitamin D deficiency, spontaneous fractures and osteopenia in rheumatoid arthritis. Br. Med. J. 2:433, 1974.

214. Rajapakse, C., Thompson, R., Grennan, D.M., et al.: Increased bone metabolism in rheumatoid arthritis as measured by the whole-body retention of $^{99}Tc^m$ methylene diphosphonate. Ann. Rheum. 42:138, 1983.

215. Schneider, R., and Kaye, J.J.: Insufficiency and stress fractures of the long bones occurring in patients with rheumatoid arthritis. Diagn. Radiol. 116:595, 1975.

216. Steiner, G., Freund, H.A., Leichtentritt, B., and Maun, M.E.: Lesion of skeletal muscles in rheumatoid arthritis. Am. J. Pathol. 22:103, 1946.

217. Haslock, D.I., Wright, V., and Harriman, D.G.F.: Neuromuscular disorders in rheumatoid arthritis. A motor-point muscle biopsy study. Quart. J. Med. 39:335, 1970.

218. Hurd, E.R.: Extra-articular manifestations of rheumatoid arthritis. Semin. Rheum. Dis. 8:151, 1979.

219. Hart, F.D.: Rheumatoid arthritis: Extra-articular manifestations. Br. Med. J. 3:131, 1969.

220. Collins, D.H.: The subcutaneous nodule of rheumatoid arthritis. J. Pathol. Bacteriol. 45:97, 1937.

221. Bennett, G.A., Zeller, J.W., and Bauer, W.: Subcutaneous nodules of rheumatoid arthritis and rheumatic fever: A pathologic study. Arch. Pathol. 30:70, 1940.

222. Sokoloff, L.: The pathophysiology of peripheral blood vessels in collagen diseases. In Orbison, J.L., and Smith, D.E. (eds.): The Peripheral Blood Vessels. Baltimore, Williams & Wilkins Company, 1963, p. 297.

223. Harris, E.D., Jr.: A collagenolytic system produced by primary cultures of rheumatoid nodule tissue. J. Clin. Invest. 51:2973, 1972.

224. Ganda, O.P., and Caplan, H.I.: Rheumatoid disease without joint involvement. JAMA 228:338, 1974.

225. Ginsberg, M.H., Genant, H.K., Yu, T.F., and McCarty, D.J.: Rheumatoid nodulosis: An unusual variant of rheumatoid disease. Arthritis Rheum. 18:49, 1975.

226. Brower, A.C., NaPombejara, C., Stechschulte, D.J., Mantz, F., and Ketchum, L.: Rheumatoid nodulosis: Another cause of juxta-articular nodules. Diagn. Radiol. 118:669, 1977.

227. Simons, F.E.R., and Schaller, J.G.: Benign rheumatoid nodules. Pediatrics 56:29, 1975.

228. Wood, M.G., and Beerman, H.: Necrobiosis lipoidica, granuloma annulare. Report of a case with lesions in the galea aponeurotica of a child. Am. J. Dis. Child. 96:720, 1958.

229. Watt, T.L., and Baumann, R.R.: Pseudoxanthomatous rheumatoid nodules. Arch. Dermatol. 95:156, 1967.

230. Healey, L.A., Wilske, K.R., and Sagebiel, R.W.: Rheumatoid nodules simulating basal-cell carcinoma. N. Engl. J. Med. 277:7, 1967.

231. Sturrock, R.D., Cowden, E.A., Howie, E., Grennan, D.M., and Buchanan, W.W.: The forgotten nodule: Complications of sacral nodules in rheumatoid arthritis. Br. Med. J. 2:92, 1975.

232. Friedman, B.A., and Rice, D.H.: Rheumatoid nodules of the larynx. Arch. Otolaryngol. 101:361, 1975.

233. Bywaters, E.G.L.: Fistulous rheumatism: A manifestation of rheumatoid arthritis. Ann. Rheum. Dis. 12:114, 1953.

234. Shapiro, R.F., Resnick, D., Castles, J.J., D'Ambrosia, R., Lipscomb, P.R., and Niwayama, G.: Fistulization of rheumatoid joints: Spectrum of identifiable syndromes. Ann. Rheum. Dis. 34:489, 1975.

235. Baum, J.: Infection in rheumatoid arthritis. Arthritis Rheum. 14:135, 1971.

236. Gaulhofer de Klerch, E.H., and Van Dam, G.: Septic complications in rheumatoid arthritis. Acta Rheum. Scand. 9:254, 1963.

237. Huskisson, E.C., and Hart, F.D.: Severe, unusual and recurrent infections in rheumatoid arthritis. Ann. Rheum. Dis. 31:118, 1972.

238. Bodel, P.T., and Hollingsworth, J.W.: Comparative morphology, respiration, and phagocytic function of leukocytes from blood and joint fluid in rheumatoid arthritis. J. Clin. Invest. 45:580, 1966.

239. Mowat, A.G.: Hematologic abnormalities in RA. Semin. Arthritis Rheum. 1:195, 1971.

240. Engstedt, L., and Strandberg, O.: Haematological data and clinical activity of the rheumatoid diseases. Acta Med. Scand. 180:13, 1966.

241. Samson, D., Holliday, D., and Gumpel, J.M.: Role of ineffective erythropoiesis in the anaemia of rheumatoid arthritis. Ann. Rheum. Dis. 36:181, 1977.

242. Cartwright, G.E.: The anemia of chronic disorders. Semin. Hematol. 3:351, 1966.

243. Raymond, F.D., Bowie, M.A., and Dugan, A.: Iron metabolism in rheumatoid arthritis. Arthritis Rheum. 8:233, 1965.

244. Ridolfo, A.S., Rubin, A., Crabtree, R.E., and Gruber, C.M.: Effects of fenoprofen and aspirin on gastrointestinal microbleeding in man. Clin. Pharmacol. Ther. 14:226, 1973.

245. Smith, R.J., Davis, P., Thomson, A.B.R., Wadsworth, L.D., and Fackre, P.: Serum ferritin levels in the anemia of rheumatoid arthritis: J. Rheumatol. 4:389, 1977.

246. Beck, R.L., French, B., Brinck-Johnsen, T., Cornwell, G.G., and Rawnsley, H.M.: Multivariate approach to predictive diagnosis of bone-marrow iron stores. Am. J. Pathol. 70:665, 1978.

247. Williams, R.A., Samson, D., Tikerpae, J., Crowne, J., and Gumpel, J.M.: In-vitro studies of ineffective erythropoiesis in rheumatoid arthritis. Am. Rheum. Dis. 41:502, 1982.

248. Winchester, R.J., Litwin, S.D., Koffler, D., and Kunkel, H.G.: Observations on the eosinophilia of certain patients with rheumatoid arthritis. Arthritis Rheum. 14:650, 1971.

249. Hutchinson, R.M., Davis, P., and Jayson, M.I.V.: Thrombocytosis in rheumatoid arthritis. Ann. Rheum. Dis. 35:138, 1976.

250. Sokoloff, L., and Bunin, J.J.: Vascular lesions in rheumatoid arthritis. J. Chronic Dis. 5:668, 1957.

251. Kulka, J.P., Bocking, D., Ropes, M.W., and Bauer, W.: Early joint lesions of rheumatoid arthritis: Report of 8 cases with knee biopsies of less than one year's duration. Arch. Pathol. 59:129, 1955.

252. Soter, N.A., Mihm, M.C., Gigli, I., and Dvorak, H.F.: Two distinct cellular patterns in cutaneous necrotizing angiitis. J. Invest. Dermatol. 66:344, 1976.

253. Rapaport, R.J., Kozin, F., Mackel, S.E., and Jordon, R.E.: Cutaneous vascular immunofluorescence in rheumatoid arthritis. Am. J. Med. 68:325, 1980.

254. Mongam, E.S., Cass, R.M., Jacox, R.F., and Vaughan, J.H.: A study of the relation of seronegative and seropositive rheumatoid arthritis to each other and to necrotizing vasculitis. Am. J. Med. 47:23, 1969.

255. Weinstein, A., Peters, K., Brown, D., and Bluestone, R.: Metabolism of the third component of complement (C3) in patients with rheumatoid arthritis. Arthritis Rheum. 15:49, 1972.

256. Conn, D.L., McDuffie, F.C., and Dyck, P.J.: Immunopathologic study of sural nerves in rheumatoid arthritis. Arthritis Rheum. 15:135, 1972.

257. Weisman, M., and Zvaifler, N.: Cryoimmunoglobulinemia in rheumatoid arthritis. J. Clin. Invest. 56:725, 1975.

258. Schmid, F.R., Cooper, N.S., Ziff, M., and McEwen, C.: Arteritis in rheumatoid arthritis. Am. J. Med. 30:56, 1961.

259. Markenson, J.A., McDougal, J.S., Tsairis, P., et al.: Rheumatoid meningitis: a localized immune process. Ann. Intern. Med. 90:786, 1979.

260. Bienenstock, H., Minick, R., and Rogoff, B.: Mesenteric arteritis and intestinal infarction in rheumatoid disease. Arch. Intern. Med. 119:359, 1967.

261. Hart, F.D., Golding, J.R., and MacKenzie, D.H.: Neuropathy in rheumatoid disease. Ann. Rheum. Dis. 16:471, 1957.

262. Gordon, D.A., Stein, J.L., and Brody, I.: The extra-cellular features of rheumatoid arthritis. A systematic analysis of 127 cases. Am. J. Med. 54:455, 1973.

263. Siomopoulos, V., and Shah, N.: Acute organic brain syndrome associated with rheumatoid arthritis. J. Clin. Psych. 40:46, 1979.

264. Scott, D.G., Baron, P.A., Elliott, P.J., et al.: Systemic vasculitis in a district general hospital 1972–80. Quart. J. Med. 51:292, 1982.

265. Lawson, A.A.H., and MacLean, N.: Renal disease and drug therapy in rheumatoid arthritis. Ann. Rheum. Dis. 25:441, 1966.

266. Samuels, B., Lee, J.C., Engleman, E.P., and Hooper, J., Jr.: Membranous nephropathy in patients with rheumatoid arthritis: Relationship to gold therapy. Medicine 57:319, 1977.

267. Case Records of the Massachusetts General Hospital, Case 23-1965. N. Engl. J. Med. 272:1069, 1965.

268. Walker, W.C., and Wright, V.: Pulmonary lesions and rheumatoid arthritis. Medicine 47:501, 1968.

269. Dodson, W.H., and Hollingsworth, J.W.: Pleural effusion in rheumatoid arthritis: Impaired transport of glucose. N. Engl. J. Med. 275:1337, 1966.

270. Dixon, A.St.J., and Ball, J.: Honeycomb lung and chronic rheumatoid arthritis: A case report. Ann. Rheum. Dis. 16:241, 1957.

271. Stack, B.H.R., and Grant, I.W.B.: Rheumatoid interstitial lung disease. Br. J. Dis. Chest 59:202, 1965.

272. Walker, W.C., and Wright, V.: Diffuse interstitial pulmonary fibrosis and rheumatoid arthritis. Ann. Rheum. Dis. 28:252, 1969.

273. Frank, S.T., Weg, J.G., Harkleroad, L.E., and Fitch, R.F.: Pulmonary dysfunction in rheumatoid disease. Chest 63:27, 1973.

274. Hyland, R.H., Gordon, D.A., Broder, I., et al.: A systematic controlled study of pulmonary abnormalities in RA. J. Rheumatol. 10:395, 1983.

275. Caplan, A.: Certain unusual radiographic appearances in the chest of coal miners suffering from RA. Thorax 8:29, 1953.

276. Portner, M.M., and Gracie, W.A.: Rheumatoid lung disease with cavitary nodules, pneumothorax and eosinophilia. N. Engl. J. Med. 275:697, 1966.

277. Hull, S., and Mathews, J.A.: Pulmonary necrobiotic nodules as a presenting feature of rheumatoid arthritis. Ann. Rheum. Dis. 41:21, 1982.

278. Gardner, D.L., Duthie, J.J.R., MacLeod, J., and Allan, W.S.H.: Pulmonary hypertension in RA: Report of a case with intimal sclerosis of pulmonary and digital arteries. Scot. Med. J. 2:183, 1957.

279. Bonfiglio, T., and Atwater, E.: Heart disease in patients with sero-positive rheumatoid arthritis; a controlled autopsy study and review. Arch. Intern. Med. 124:714, 1969.

280. Lebowitz, W.B.: The heart in rheumatoid arthritis. A clinical and pathological study of 62 cases. Ann. Intern. Med. 58:102, 1963.

281. MacDonald, W.J., Jr., Crawford, M.H., Klippel, J.H., Zvaifler, N.J., and O'Rourke, R.A.: Echocardiographic assessment of cardiac structure and function in patients with rheumatoid arthritis. Am. J. Med. 63:890, 1977.

282. Lange, R.K., Weiss, T.E., and Ochsner, J.L.: Rheumatoid arthritis and constrictive pericarditis. A patient benefited by pericardectomy. Arthritis Rheum. 8:403, 1965.

283. Thadini, V., Iveson, J.M.I., and Wright, V.: Cardiac tamponade, constrictive pericarditis and pericardial resection in rheumatoid arthritis. Medicine 54:261, 1975.

284. Gowands, J.D.C.: Complete heart block with Stokes-Adams syndrome due to rheumatoid heart disease. N. Engl. J. Med. 262:1012, 1960.

285. Prakash, R., Atassi, A., Poske, R., and Rosen, K.M.: Prevalance of pericardial effusion and mitral-valve involvement in patients with rheumatoid arthritis without cardiac symptoms. N. Engl. J. Med. 289:597, 1973.

286. Weintraub, A.M., and Zvaifler, N.J.: The occurrence of valvular and myocardial disease in patients with chronic joint disease. Am. J. Med. 35:145, 1963.

287. Iveson, J.M.I., Thadani, V., Ionescu, M., and Wright, V.: Aortic valve incompetence and replacement in rheumatoid arthritis. Ann. Rheum. Dis. 34:312, 1975.

288. Lev, M., Bharati, S., Hoffman, F.G., and Leight, L.: The conduction system in rheumatoid arthritis with complete atrioventricular block. Am. Heart J. 90:78, 1975.

289. Swezey, R.L.: Myocardial infarction due to rheumatoid arteritis. JAMA 199:191, 1967.

290. Reimer, K.A., Rodgers, R.F., and Oyasu, R.: Rheumatoid arthritis with rheumatoid heart disease and granulomatous aortitis. JAMA 235:2510, 1976.

291. Valkenburg, H.A.: Pattern of rheumatoid disease in society: Change or disappearance? Scand. J. Rheumatol. 5(Suppl. 12):89, 1975.

292. Pinals, R.S., Masi, A.F., Larsen, R.A.: Special article: Preliminary criteria for clinical remission in RA. Arthritis Rheum. 24:1308,

293. Sharp, J.T., Calkins, E., Cohen, A.S., Schubart, A.F., and Calabro, J.J.: Observations on the clinical, chemical, and serological manifestations of rheumatoid arthritis, based on the course of 154 cases. Medicine 43:41, 1964.

294. Cobb, S., Anderson, F., and Baurer, W.: Length of life and cause of death in rheumatoid arthritis. N. Engl. J. Med. 249:553, 1953.

295. Baum, J.: Infection in rheumatoid arthritis. Arthritis Rheum. 14:135, 1971.

296. Short, C.L.: Long remissions in rheumatoid arthritis. Medicine 43:401, 1964.

297. Duthie, J.J.R., Brown, P.E., Truelove, L.H., Barago, E., and Lawrie, A.J.: Course and prognosis in rheumatoid arthritis. A further report. Ann. Rheum. Dis. 23:193, 1964.

298. Corrigan, A.B., Robinson, R.G., Terenty, T.R., Dick-Smith, J.B., and Walters, O.: Benign rheumatoid arthritis of the aged. Br. Med. J. 1:444, 1974.

299. Luukkainen, R., Isomaki, H., and Kajander, A.: Prognostic value of the type of onset of rheumatoid arthritis. Ann. Rheum. Dis. 42:274, 1983.

300. Mattingly, S.: Palindromic rheumatism. Ann. Rheum. Dis. 25:307, 1966.

301. Duthie, J.J.R., Thompson, M., Weir, M.M., and Fletcher, W.B.: Medical and social aspects of treatment of rheumatoid arthritis with special reference to the factors affecting prognosis. Ann. Rheum. Dis. 14:133, 1955.

302. Fleming, A., Benn, R.T., Corbett, M., and Wood, P.H.N.: Early rheumatoid disease. II. Patterns of joint involvement. Ann. Rheum. Dis. 35:361, 1976.

303. Kellgren, J.H., and O'Brien, W.M.: On the natural history of rheumatoid arthritis in relation to the sheep cell agglutination test (SCAT). Arthritis Rheum. 5:115, 1962.

304. Masi, A.T., Maldonado-Cocco, J.A., Kaplan, S.B., Feigenbaum, S.L., and Chandler, R.W.: Prospective study of the early course of rheumatoid arthritis in young adults: Comparison of patients with and without rheumatoid factor positivity at entry and identification of variables correlating with outcome. Semin. Arthritis Rheum. 5:299, 1976.

305. Jacoby, R.K., Jayson, M.I.V., and Cosh, J.A.: Onset, early stages and prognosis of rheumatoid arthritis: A clinical study of 100 patients with 11-year follow-up. Br. Med. J. 2:96, 1973.

306. Dixon, A.St.J.: "Rheumatoid arthritis" with negative serological reaction. Ann. Rheum. Dis. 19:209, 1960.

307. Ragan, C., and Farrington, E.: The clinical features of rheumatoid arthritis. JAMA 181:663, 1962.

308. Henderson, D.R.F., Jayson, M.I.V., and Tribe, C.B.: Lack of correlation of synovial histology with joint damage in rheumatoid arthritis. Ann. Rheum. Dis. 34:7, 1975.

309. Yates, D.B., and Scott, J.T.: Rheumatoid synovitis and joint disease. Relationship between arthroscopic and histological changes. Ann. Rheum. Dis. 34:1, 1975.

310. Cruickshank, B.: Interpretation of multiple biopsies of synovial tissue in rheumatic diseases. Ann. Rheum. Dis. 11:137, 1952.

311. Muirden, K.D., and Mills, K.W.: Do lymphocytes protect the rheumatoid joint? Br. Med. J. 4:219, 1971.

312. Harris, E.D., Jr., Faulkner, C.S., II, and Brown, F.E.: Collagenolytic systems in rheumatoid arthritis. Clin. Orthop. 110:303, 1975.

313. Weiss, S.J., Lampert, M.D., and Test, S.T.: Long-lived oxidants generated by human neutrophils: Characterization and bioactivity. Science 222:625, 1983.

314. Ward, T.T., and Steigbigel, R.T.: Acidosis of synovial fluid correlates with synovial fluid leukocytosis. Am. J. Med. 64:933, 1978.

315. Ruddy, S.: Synovial fluid: Mirror of the inflammatory lesion in rheumatoid arthritis. In Harris, E.D., Jr. (ed.): Rheumatoid Arthritis. New York, Medcom Press, 1974.

316. Hay, F.C., Nineham, L.J., Perumal, R., et al.: Intra-articular and circulating immune complexes and antiglobulins (IgG and IgM) in rheumatoid arthritis: correlation with clinical features. Ann. Rheum. Dis. 38:1, 1979.

317. Lessard, J., Nunnery, E., Cecere, F., et al.: Relationship between the articular manifestations of rheumatoid arthritis and circulating immune complexes detected by three methods and specific classes of rheumatoid factors. J. Rheumatol. 10:411, 1983.

318. Amos, R.S., Constable, T.J., Crockson, R.A., Crockson, A.P., and McConkery, B.: Rheumatoid arthritis: Relation of serum C-reactive protein and erythrocyte sedimentation rates to radiographic changes. Br. Med. J. 1:195, 1977.

319. Mallya, R.K., deBeer, F.C., Berry, H., et al.: Correlation of clinical parameters of disease activity in rheumatoid arthritis with serum concentration of C-reactive protein and erythrocyte sedimentation rate. J. Rheumatol. 9:224, 1982.

320. Lansbury, J.: Quantitation of activity of rheumatoid arthritis. Method for summation of systemic indices of rheumatoid activity. Am. J. Med. Sci. 232:300, 1956.

321. Lansbury, J.: Report of a three-year study on the systemic and articular indexes in rheumatoid arthritis: Theoretic and clinical considerations. Arthritis Rheum. 1:505, 1958.

322. Huskisson, E.C.: Measurement of pain. Lancet 2:1127, 1974.

323. Steinbrocker, O., Traeger, C.H., and Batterman, R.C.: Therapeutic criteria in rheumatoid arthritis. JAMA 140:659, 1949.

324. Fallahi, S., Halla, J.T., and Hardin, J.G.: The reassessment of the nature of onset of rheumatoid arthritis. Clin. Res. 31:650A, 1983.

Chapter 61
Felty's Syndrome

Robert Pinals

INTRODUCTION

In 1924 Felty[1] described five patients with chronic arthritis, splenomegaly, and leukopenia and proposed that this association represented a distinct clinical entity. The term *Felty's syndrome* was first used in 1932 by Hanrahan and Miller[2] in reporting a patient who responded to splenectomy but died 18 months later.[3] Most of the more recent literature has recognized that Felty's syndrome represents one of many systemic complications of seropositive rheumatoid arthritis occurring in a group of patients with unusually severe articular disease and immunologic abnormalities. The term "hypersplenism" was derived from the observation that splenectomy usually resulted in partial or complete resolution of the granulocytopenia, but the role of the spleen in pathogenesis has been an area of considerable controversy for many years. There is evidence for its participation both in the removal of granulocytes from the circulating pool and in the suppression of granulopoiesis. Thus an etiologic definition is still unavailable, and Felty's syndrome must be defined in descriptive terms as a variant of seropositive rheumatoid arthritis with splenomegaly and granulocytopenia (< 2000 per cubic millimeter). Although the complete triad is required for a diagnosis of Felty's syndrome, some patients may be encountered and considered for the diagnosis at a time when only two of the features are present, with appearance of the third only after a period of observation. Patients with rheumatoid arthritis may also develop superimposed illnesses which may result in splenomegaly or granulocytopenia; drug reactions, myeloproliferative disorders, reticuloendothelial malignancies, hepatic cirrhosis, amyloidosis, sarcoidosis, tuberculosis, and other chronic infections must be considered and excluded with reasonable clinical certainty before the diagnosis of Felty's syndrome is accepted.

The true prevalence of Felty's syndrome is unknown, but it is probably found in less than 1 percent of patients with rheumatoid arthritis.[4] Splenomegaly alone is more common, identified by palpation in 6.5 percent in one large series,[4] and even more frequently by radioactive scanning.[5]

CLINICAL FEATURES

About two thirds of patients with Felty's syndrome are women. HLA DRw4 was found in 95 percent of patients with Felty's syndrome, compared with 69 percent in other rheumatoid arthritis patients and 31 percent in controls.[6] This may account for the rarity of Felty's syndrome in blacks, who are known to have a low frequency of DRw4.[7] The condition is usually recognized in the fifth through the seventh decades of life in patients who have had rheumatoid arthritis for 10 years or more. However, since it is most often discovered by a routine blood count, the frequency of medical observation is an important factor in early recognition. Splenomegaly and granulocytopenia may be present before symptoms or signs of arthritis in rare instances.[8] The articular disease is usually more severe than in the average case of rheumatoid arthritis, with greater deformity and erosion,[9,10] but there are many examples of mild involvement.[11,12] About one third of the patients have relatively inactive synovitis, as judged by signs and symptoms, but even these patients continue to have an

Table 61–1. Frequency of Extra-Articular Manifestations in Felty's Syndrome*

Rheumatoid nodules	76%
Weight loss	68%
Sjögren's syndrome†	56%
Lymphadenopathy	34%
Leg ulcers	25%
Pleuritis	19%
Skin pigmentation	17%
Neuropathy	17%
Episcleritis	8%

*From a review of 10 reports since 1962.
†Determined by positive Schirmer test.

Figure 61–1. Ulceration of the leg developed 3 years previously in this patient with Felty's syndrome. The ulcer healed with local treatment but recurred on two occasions. The brown pigmentation proximal to the ulcer was also present on the other leg.

elevated erythrocyte sedimentation rate (ESR). In one large series the mean ESR was 85 mm per hour.[10]

The spleen size is variable. In 5 to 10 percent of patients it is not large enough to be palpable, but occasionally there is massive splenomegaly.[13] The median splenic weight in Felty's syndrome is about four times normal.[13] There is no correlation between spleen size and the degree of granulocytopenia.[9,10,14]

Patients with Felty's syndrome tend to have more extra-articular manifestations than others with rheumatoid arthritis (Table 61–1). Weight loss was mentioned by Felty and has been emphasized by later authors. It may be striking and unexplained, often occurring for several months before the diagnosis of Felty's syndrome is made. Felty also mentioned brown pigmentation over exposed surfaces of the extremities, especially over the tibia. Although noted by others,[9,15,16] it is not specific for Felty's syndrome, and may be related to stasis and to extravasation of red blood cells secondary to disease of small vessels. Leg ulcers are frequent but do not seem to differ from those in other rheumatoid arthritis patients in terms of chronicity, recurrence, and presumed relationship to vasculitis (Fig. 61–1).

Although about 60 percent of patients with Felty's syndrome are described as having one or more infections which may be attributable to the granulocytopenia, the literature is difficult to interpret because nonleukopenic rheumatoid arthritis patients may also be more susceptible to infection and because there is no suitable control group for comparison.[17] In addition, some reports of Felty's syndrome are limited to splenectomized patients, who may represent a more severely involved group. The degree of granulocytopenia correlates poorly with the number and severity of infections.[9,11] Most of the infec-

Table 61–2. Percentage of Felty's Syndrome Patients with Various Types of Infection*

Skin (abscess, cellulitis, furunculosis)	26%
Pneumonia	24%
Urinary tract	9%
Oral ulcers	4%
Sinusitis and otitis	4%
Septic arthritis	2%

*Taken from four reports[8,10,13,14] in which sufficient information was available on a total of 90 patients.

tions are caused by ordinary bacteria such as staphylococcus, streptococcus, and gram-negative bacilli,[10] and involve common sites, particularly the skin and respiratory tract (Table 61–2). In spite of the granulocytopenia, pus may accumulate in an appropriate fashion, suggesting that the site of infection is capable of competing successfully with the spleen for available granulocytes. The response to antibiotic therapy is usually adequate.[10]

Mild hepatomegaly is common in Felty's syndrome and liver function abnormalities, particularly elevations of alkaline phosphatase and the transaminases, which are described in about a quarter of the patients.[10] An unusual type of liver involvement may be associated with Felty's syndrome, but occurs rarely in other rheumatoid arthritis patients.[18] Histologically, the picture is described as nodular regenerative hyperplasia.[19] Although there is mild portal fibrosis or infiltration with lymphocytes and plasma cells, the appearance is not characteristic of cirrhosis. Obliteration of portal venules may compromise portal blood flow, leading to atrophy and regenerative nodule formation, portal hypertension, and gastrointestinal hemorrhage. It has been suggested that immune complex–mediated platelet activation may be the mechanism of venular injury and occlusion.[19] Other

primary disorders may be associated with nodular regenerative hyperplasia, but about a third of cases have
had Felty's syndrome.[18,19]

HEMATOLOGIC FEATURES

The leukopenia in Felty's syndrome is a relative and
absolute granulocytopenia, in contrast to systemic lupus
erythematosus (SLE), in which lymphopenia is a more
prominent feature. Few patients have blood counts often
enough to determine the rate at which granulocytopenia
develops at the onset of Felty's syndrome, but in some
cases only weeks have elapsed between normal and
grossly abnormal white blood cell counts. There is often
considerable spontaneous variation in the granulocyte
count. Patients with mild lowering may return to the
normal range, but this is rarely seen when depression is
severe. Thus, spontaneous remissions have been
observed[11,20] but are uncommon. During infections or
other stressful episodes the granulocyte count often returns to the normal range but is seldom elevated. This
may conceal the diagnosis temporarily, since blood
counts may be ordered in some patients mainly in the
setting of an infection or other acute illness.

The bone marrow may show no abnormality in some
cases, but in most there is a myeloid hyperplasia, with
a relative excess of immature forms, often described as
"maturation arrest." Although this might reflect an impaired myelopoietic response, early release of mature
forms would result in the same appearance.[9,10,11,14] Rarely
the marrow suggests a depression in myeloid activity.[11,14]
or shows an increased lymphocytic infiltration.[14]

A mild to moderate anemia is found in most patients,
representing the anemia of chronic disease with an additional component of shortened red blood cell survival,
which is corrected by splenectomy.[21] Reticulocyte count
elevations are common.[10] Thrombocytopenia (platelet
count < 150,000 per cubic millimeter) occurs in 38 percent but is seldom severe enough to cause purpura.

SEROLOGIC FEATURES

The alterations in immune response commonly found
in rheumatoid arthritis are amplified in patients with
Felty's syndrome, in keeping with the general picture of
unusually severe articular and systemic disease. Rheumatoid factor has been present in 98 percent of the
patients, generally in high titer.[10] Only a few seronegative
cases have been reported.[11,15,16,22] Positive LE cell tests
are found in one third and antinuclear antibodies (ANA)
in two thirds of the patients, with wide differences in
frequency (47 to 100 percent), probably reflecting the
variable sensitivity of the latter test. Patients with Felty's
syndrome also have granulocyte-specific ANA more
often than rheumatoid arthritis patients without neutropenia (85 percent vs 14 percent).[22,23] Anti-nDNA is
not elevated.[10] Immunoglobulin levels are higher than
in other rheumatoid arthritis patients;[9,10] complement

Table 61–3. Immune Complexes in Sera of Patients with
Rheumatoid Arthritis (RA) and Felty's Syndrome (FS)

Method	RA (% Positive)	FS (% Positive)
Intermediate complexes by ultracentrifugation[25]	27	100
Double diffusion against IgM rheumatoid factor[25]	27	75
Phagocytosed inclusions in normal granulocytes[25]	23	77
Cryoglobulins[24]	26	78
C1q binding[26]	12	60
Platelet aggregation[27]	8	68

levels are lower,[10,24] although most patients have levels
within the normal range. Immune complexes have been
detected by various techniques in the majority of Felty's
syndrome patients (Table 61–3). These complexes may
contain IgG, IgM, and complement.[25] A granulocyte-
reactive ANA is also selectively concentrated in the
cryoprecipitate in some sera,[24] suggesting the possibility
that this antibody might be available to act upon nuclear
antigen following ingestion of the immune complexes by
granulocytes.

PATHOGENESIS

Although the spleen certainly plays a key role in the
pathogenesis of granulocytopenia, little insight has been
gained by routine examinations of surgical specimens,
for they show only the predictable immune hyperactivity
(increased plasma cells, immunoblasts, and germinal
center hyperplasia) and inconstant evidence of phagocytic hyperfunction.[10,11,13] Amyloid is almost never
found, and the periarterial lamellar fibrosis, characteristic of SLE, described in one report[28] has not been
confirmed by others.

The hematologic improvement resulting from splenectomy led some to postulate that the spleen had been
producing a humoral inhibitor of granulocyte production[29] and others to support splenic sequestration
and destruction of granulocytes as the principal mechanism.[30] The debate appeared to be settled in favor of
the latter proposal when granulocyte counts were shown
to be lower in the splenic vein than in the artery.[31]
However, recent studies have suggested that the two
viewpoints are not mutually exclusive and that a number
of factors may contribute to the development of granulocytopenia (Fig 61–2).

Increased Removal of Granulocytes. Granulocyte sequestration and reduced survival might certainly result
from impaired motility of cells laden with immune complexes and difficulty in negotiating channels in the
splenic pulp. Many granulocytes with large cytoplasmic
inclusions containing immunoglobulins and complement
were identified in the spleens of patients with Felty's
syndrome.[32] Such phagolysosomal inclusions also form
when normal neutrophils are incubated with sera from
patients with Felty's syndrome.[33]

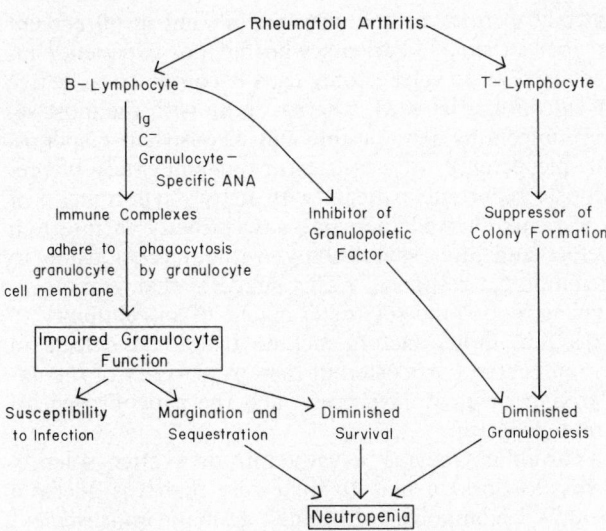

Figure 61–2. Pathogenesis of Felty's syndrome.

Neutrophil function and survival may also be compromised by the adherence of antibodies to cell surface receptors. The presence of granulocyte antibodies was suggested by early transfusion experiments in which plasma from a patient with Felty's syndrome produced transient granulocytopenia.[34] Granulocyte antibodies were demonstrated by fluorescent[24] and indirect antiglobulin consumption[35] techniques, and by inhibition of phagocytosis,[36] but antibodies could also be found in some non-neutropenic rheumatoid arthritis patients. In a direct antiglobulin consumption assay[37] there were high levels of surface immunoglobulin on the granulocytes in Felty's syndrome, not overlapping the levels found in rheumatoid arthritis without neutropenia and in other neutropenic controls with marrow failure. Curiously, the granulocyte surface immunoglobulins fell to the normal range after splenectomy, suggesting that most of these antibodies had been produced in the spleen. The surface immunoglobulins include granulocyte-specific ANA, which may be capable of fixing complement[23] and contributing to cell injury. A recent characterization of serum granulocyte binding activity in Felty's syndrome revealed that IgG was the principal immunoglobulin involved, and that both soluble immune complexes and specific antibodies to granulocytes participated.[38] Similar antibodies might also be directed against granulocyte precursors, leading to diminished production, but relevant studies have not yet been reported.

Granulocyte kinetic studies have been performed in Felty's syndrome, but technical problems and variations in these studies have led to disputed interpretations.[39] Early reports on small numbers of patients suggested that granulocyte survival was diminished,[40,41] but in a larger and more recent study excessive margination was demonstrated in all patients and was felt to represent the most significant defect.[42] The marginated pool consists of neutrophils adherent to the walls of venules in the spleen and elsewhere. Thus, neutrophils had shifted from the circulating to the marginated pool but had not been destroyed prematurely.

Impaired Production of Granulocytes. Evidence suggesting that suboptimal granulopoietic compensation might contribute to neutropenia was provided by the observation and the population of progenitor marrow cells in the synthetic phase was diminished in some patients with Felty's syndrome.[43] Bone marrow granulocyte precursor cells form colonies when grown in vitro in semi-solid agar; the number of colonies gives an indication of the proliferative state of the marrow. A glycoprotein colony-stimulating factor normally found in serum and urine is required for this growth. Colony-stimulating activity was found to be lower in Felty's syndrome than in other neutropenic disorders.[44,45] Retardation of mouse bone marrow colony counts was found after addition of sera from 87.5 percent of Felty's syndrome patients and only 12.5 percent of other rheumatoid arthritis sera, suggesting the possibility of an inhibitor. However, the effect of the sera on marrow cultures did not correlate with the degree of granulocytopenia, and no single serum fraction could be identified as the source of inhibition.[46] In a recent report, 8 of 19 Felty's syndrome patients were found to have a heat stable, nondialyzable serum factor capable of inhibiting colony formation by human marrow granulocyte precursors.[47]

Mononuclear cells were also shown to induce suppression of colony formation in normal human marrow cultures. This effect was found with peripheral blood mononuclear cells from Felty's syndrome patients, but not with their serum or with the cells of other patients with rheumatoid arthritis and neutropenia from other causes. The suppression correlated with granulocytopenia in Felty's syndrome.[48] The responsible cells are probably T lymphocytes.[49,50] The observation that occasional patients who have lymphocytic infiltration in the marrow respond poorly to splenectomy lends support to this mechanism.[14]

In summary, the granulocytopenia in Felty's syndrome appears to be multifactorial in origin. Ingestion and surface-coating of immune complexes leads to impaired granulocyte functions and facilitates their removal by the reticuloendothelial system. Specific antibodies directed against granulocyte cell surface antigens may also be involved. Sequestration of granulocytes in the spleen and venules results in a diminished circulating pool, either with or without actual premature destruction of granulocytes. Excessive utilization of leukocytes in the joints in patients with active synovitis places additional demands on granulopoiesis.[51] In some patients the marrow does not respond appropriately to granulocytopenia, apparently because of the presence of an unidentified humoral inhibitor and/or mononuclear cells which suppress myelopoiesis. There may be different subsets of Felty's syndrome, as illustrated by one report in which both humoral and cell-mediated mechanisms were investigated. About two thirds of the patients had high levels of neutrophil-bound IgG. In the remaining patients peripheral blood mononuclear cells inhibited colony growth in normal marrow.[52]

The increased susceptibility to infection is probably related to several factors in addition to granulocytopenia. Granulocyte reserves are diminished,[40,41,53,54] as determined by the increment in granulocyte counts after injection of epinephrine, endotoxin, or etiocholanolone, a steroid metabolite that mobilizes granulocytes, presumably from the marrow but possibly also from the marginal pool. Defective function of granulocytes in phagocytosis,[33] chemotaxis,[55,56] and bacterial killing[57] has been demonstrated. Hypocomplementemia may also play a role in some patients.[24,26]

SPLENECTOMY

Indications. Since splenectomy usually reverses the hematologic abnormalities in Felty's syndrome, it is indicated if the patient has experienced significant morbidity. The usual indication is recurrent or serious infection, but in rare instances splenectomy may be performed for thrombocytopenia, anemia, abdominal discomfort from splenomegaly, or esophageal varices. Amelioration of active synovitis after splenectomy occurs too inconsistently to justify surgery on those grounds alone. Dramatic healing of the leg ulcers has been reported often enough to indicate splenectomy if conservative measures have failed.[13,16] Some authors have advocated splenectomy in all cases of Felty's syndrome as a prophylaxis against infection,[58] and others only for those with severe granulocytopenia (< 500 per cubic millimeter) even in the absence of infection.[13] However, it must be noted that these patients often remain free of infection over periods of many years.[9,45]

Results. No prospective, randomized studies of splenectomy have been performed, and the value of the procedure in preventing serious infection and prolonging survival is not entirely clear. It is likely that the variable long-term success rate reflects patient selection factors in different centers. However, there is no dispute about the prompt hematologic response, which is observed within minutes or hours after splenectomy in most cases,[15] although a few may be leukopenic at the time of discharge but improve soon thereafter.[13] In five recent reports,[9,10,11,13,14] 88 percent of patients had a good short-term hematologic response to splenectomy. However, granulocytopenia recurred and persisted in 24 percent of patients available for follow-up examinations. The absolute granulocyte level in these cases was generally higher than it had been prior to splenectomy. Continuing immune-mediated granulocyte destruction may be responsible for these secondary failures. Persistently high levels of serum granulocyte-binding IgG may be associated with a poor response to splenectomy.[59] In another study antibody-dependent, lymphocyte-mediated granulocytotoxicity developed in three of six splenectomy failures. None of the patients with Felty's syndrome had evidence of such an immune response prior to splenectomy.[60] Recurrent or persistent infection was noted in

only 26 percent in one large series[13] but in 60 percent in four others.[9-11] Patients who did not experience infection prior to splenectomy usually continued to be free of infection afterward, whereas those with the most severe infections had variable and inconsistent responses to splenectomy. In a long-term outcome study of previously reported[10] patients with Felty's syndrome, 5 of 7 patients showed the same susceptibility to infection before and after splenectomy, without relationship to hematologic response.[61] This suggests that granulocytopenia is not the sole determinant of susceptibility to infection. Other factors include functional defects in granulocytes, corticosteroid therapy, severity of the underlying rheumatoid process, and the patient's general state of health.

Thrombocytopenia usually improves after splenectomy, as does anemia, to the extent that it is due to a hemolytic component. Although dramatic improvement in synovitis has been mentioned in several reports,[62,63] it is apparently not observed in most cases and is often temporary. Leg ulcers may also respond, even those which are not significantly infected,[13,15,16] but their variability in etiology and natural course makes these reports difficult to interpret.

OTHER TREATMENTS

The basic illness should be treated in the same manner as it would in the absence of Felty's syndrome. Frequently granulocytopenia may improve during treatment with gold[45,64] or penicillamine.[45] Low doses of corticosteroids do not produce consistent improvement in granulocytopenia and also predispose to infection.[9,11] High-dose parenteral testosterone may stimulate granulopoiesis and is also reported to reduce the infection rate in a small number of patients[65] but is not suitable for females. Lithium salts also stimulate granulopoiesis by augmenting colony-stimulating activity,[66] but long-term benefit has not yet been demonstrated, and the treatment has been unsuccessful in the experience of some investigators.[54]

References

1. Felty, A.R.: Chronic arthritis in the adult, associated with splenomegaly and leucopenia. Johns Hopkins Hosp. Bull. 35:16, 1924.
2. Hanrahan, E.M., Jr., and Miller, S.R.: Effect of splenectomy in Felty's syndrome. JAMA 99:1247, 1932.
3. Fitz, R.: Painful joints, splenomegaly, and anemia. Med. Clin. North Am. 18:1053, 1935.
4. Short, C.L., Bauer, W., and Reynolds, W.E.: Rheumatoid arthritis. Cambridge, Mass., Harvard University Press, 1957.
5. Isomäki, H., and Koivisto, O.: Splenomegaly in rheumatoid arthritis. Acta Rheum. Scand. 17:23, 1971.
6. Dinant, H.J., Muller, W.H., van den Berg-Loonen, E.M., Nijenhuis, L.E., and Engelfriet, C.P.: HLA DRw4 in Felty's syndrome. Arthritis Rheum. 23:1336, 1980.
7. Termini, T.E., Biundo, J.J., and Ziff, M.: The rarity of Felty's syndrome in blacks. Arthritis Rheum. 22:999, 1979.
8. Heyn, J.: Non-articular Felty's syndrome. Scand. J. Rheumatol. 11:47, 1982.
9. Ruderman, M., Miller L.M., and Pinals, R.S.: Clinical and serologic observations on 27 patients with Felty's syndrome. Arthritis Rheum. 11:377, 1968.

10. Sienknecht, C.W., Urowitz, M.B., Pruzanski, W., and Stein, H.B.: Felty's syndrome. Clinical and serological analysis of 34 cases. Ann. Rheum. Dis. 36:500, 1977.
11. Barnes, C.G., Turnbull, A.L., and Vernon-Roberts, B.: Felty's syndrome. Ann. Rheum. Dis. 30:359, 1971.
12. Cornwell, C.G., and Zacharski, L.R.: Neutropenia, elevated rheumatoid factor, splenomegaly and absence of rheumatoid arthritis. Ann. Inter. Med. 80:555, 1974.
13. Laszlo, J., Jones, R., Silberman, H.R., and Banks, P.M.: Splenectomy for Felty's syndrome: Clinicopathological study of 27 patients. Arch. Intern. Med. 138:597, 1978.
14. Moore, R.A., Brunner, C.M., Sandusky, W.R., and Leavell, B.S.: Felty's syndrome: Long-term follow-up after splenectomy. Ann. Intern. Med. 75:381, 1971.
15. DeGruchy, G.C., and Langley, G.R.: Felty's syndrome. Australas. Ann. Med. 10:292, 1961.
16. Williams, R.C., Jr.: Rheumatoid Arthritis as a Systemic Disease. Philadelphia, W.B. Saunders Company, 1974.
17. Baum, J.: Infection in rheumatoid arthritis. Arthritis Rheum. 14:135, 1971.
18. Thorne, C., Urowitz, M.B., Wanless, I., Roberts, E., and Blendis, L.M. Liver disease in Felty's syndrome. Am. J. Med. 73:35, 1982.
19. Wanless, I.R., Godwin, T.A., Allen, F., and Feder, A.: Nodular regenerative hyperplasia of the liver in hematologic disorders: A possible response to obliterative portal venopathy. Medicine 59:367, 1980.
20. Luthra, H.S., and Hunder, G.G.: Spontaneous remission of Felty's syndrome. Arthritis Rheum. 18:515, 1975.
21. Hume, R., Dagg, J.H., Fraser, T.N., and Goldberg, A.: Anaemia of Felty's syndrome. Ann. Rheum. Dis. 23:267, 1964.
22. Faber, V., and Elling, P.: Leucocyte-specific antinuclear factors in patients with Felty's syndrome, rheumatoid arthritis, systemic lupus erythematosus, and other diseases. Acta Med. Scand. 179:257, 1966.
23. Wiik, A., and Munthe, E.: Complement-fixing granulocyte-specific antinuclear factors in neutropenic cases of rheumatoid arthritis. Immunology 26:1127, 1974.
24. Weisman, M., and Zvaifler, N.J.: Cryoimmuno-globulinemia in Felty's syndrome. Arthritis Rheum. 19:103, 1976.
25. Andreis, M., Hurd, E.R., Lospalluto, J., and Ziff, M.: Comparison of the presence of immune complexes in Felty's syndrome and rheumatoid arthritis. Arthritis Rheum. 21:310, 1978.
26. Hurd, E.R., Chubick, A. Jasin, H.E., and Ziff, M.: Increased Clq binding immune complexes in Felty's syndrome. Arthritis Rheum. 22:697, 1979.
27. Bucknall, R.C., Davis, P., Bacon, P.A., and Verrier-Jones, J.: Neutropenia in rheumatoid arthritis: Studies on possible contributing factors. Ann. Rheum. Dis. 41:242, 1982.
28. Denko, C.W., and Zumpft, C.W.: Chronic arthritis with splenomegaly and leukopenia. Arthritis Rheum. 5:478, 1962.
29. Dameshek, W.: Hypersplenism. Bull. N.Y. Acad. Sci. 31:113, 1955.
30. Wiseman, B.K., and Doan, C.A.: Primary splenic neutropenia: A newly recognized syndrome, closely related to congenital hemolytic icterus and essential thrombocytopenic purpura. Ann. Intern. Med. 16:1097, 1942.
31. Wright, C.S., Doan, C.A., Bouroncle, B.A., and Zollinger, R.M.: Direct splenic arterial and venous blood studies in the hypersplenic syndromes before and after epinephrine. Blood 6:195, 1951.
32. Hurd, E.R.: Presence of leucocyte inclusions in spleen and bone marrow of patients with Felty's syndrome. J. Rheumatol. 5:26, 1978.
33. Hurd, E.R., Andreis, M., and Ziff, M.: Phagocytosis of immune complexes by polymorphonuclear leucocytes in patients with Felty's syndrome. Clin. Exp. Immunol. 28:413, 1977.
34. Calabresi, P., Edwards, E.A., and Schilling, R.F.: Fluorescent antiglobulin studies in leucopenic and related disorders. J. Clin. Invest. 38:2091, 1959.
35. Rosenthal, F.D., Beeley, J.M., Gelsthorpe, K., and Doughty, R.W.: White-cell antibodies and the aetiology of Felty's syndrome. Quart. J. Med. 43:187, 1974.
36. McIntyre, P.A., Laleli, Y.R., Hodkinson, B.A., and Wagner, H.N., Jr.: Evidence for anti-leukocyte antibodies as a mechanism for drug-induced agranulocytosis. Trans. Assoc. Am. Physicians 84:217, 1971.
37. Logue, G.: Felty's syndrome: Granulocyte-bound immunoglobulin G and splenectomy. Ann. Intern. Med. 85:437, 1976.
38. Starkebaum, G., Arend, W.P., Nardella, F.A., and Gavin, S.E.: Characterization of immune complexes and immunoglobulin G antibodies reactive with neutrophils in the sera of patients with Felty's syndrome. J. Lab. Clin. Med. 96:238, 1980.
39. Bishop, C.R.: The neutropenia of Felty's syndrome. Am. J. Hematol. 2:203, 1977.
40. Bishop, C.R., Rothstein, G., Ashenbrucker, H.E., and Athens, J.W.: Leukokinetic studies. XIV. Blood neutrophil kinetics in chronic steady-state neutropenia. J. Clin. Invest. 50:1678, 1971.
41. Greenberg, M.S., Zanger, B., and Wong, H.: Studies in granulocytopenic subjects. Blood 30:891, 1967.
42. Vincent, P.C., Levi, J.A., and MacQueen, A.: The mechanism of neutropenia in Felty's syndrome. Br. J. Haematol. 27:463, 1974.
43. Greenberg, P.L., and Schrier, S.L.: Granulopoiesis in neutropenic disorders. Blood 41:753, 1973.
44. Gupta, R., Robinson, W.A., and Albrecht, D.: Granulopoietic activity in Felty's syndrome. Ann. Rheum. Dis. 34:156, 1975.
45. Goldberg, J., and Pinals, R.S.: Felty's syndrome. Semin. Arthritis Rheum. 10:52, 1980.
46. Duckham, D.J., Rhyne, R.L., Smith, F.E., and Williams, R.C.: Retardation of colony growth of in vitro bone marrow culture using sera from patients with Felty's syndrome, disseminated lupus erythematosus (SLE), rheumatoid arthritis, and other disease states. Arthritis Rheum. 18:323, 1975.
47. Goldberg, L.S., Bacon, P.A., Bucknall, R.C., Fitchen, J., and Cline, M.J.: Inhibition of human bone marrow–granulocyte precursors by serum from patients with Felty's syndrome. J. Rheumatol. 7:275, 1980.
48. Abdou, N.I., NaPombejara, C., Balentine, L., and Abdou, N.L.: Suppressor cell–mediated neutropenia in Felty's syndrome. J. Clin. Invest. 61:738, 1978.
49. Bagby, G.C., Jr., and Gabourel, J.D.: Neutropenia in three patients with rheumatic disorders: Suppression of granulocytes by cortisol-sensitive thymus-dependent lymphocytes. J. Clin. Invest. 64:72, 1979.
50. Slavin, S., and Liang, M.H.: Cell-mediated autoimmune granulocytopenia in a case of Felty's syndrome. Ann. Rheum. Dis. 39:399, 1980.
51. Hollingsworth, J.W., Siegel, E.R., and Creasey, W.A.: Granulocyte survival in synovial exudate of patients with rheumatoid arthritis and other inflammatory joint diseases. Yale J. Biol. Med. 39:289, 1967.
52. Starkebaum, G., Singer, J.W., and Arend, W.P.: Humoral and cellular immune mechanisms of neutropenia in patients with Felty's syndrome. Clin. Exp. Immunol. 39:307, 1980.
53. Kimball, H.R., Wolff, S.M., Talal, N., Plotz, P.H., and Decker, J.L.: Marrow granulocyte reserves in the rheumatic diseases. Arthritis Rheum. 16:345, 1973.
54. Joyce, R.A., Boggs, D.R., Chervenick, P.A., and Lalezari, P.: Neutrophil kinetics in Felty's syndrome: Am. J. Med. 69:695, 1980.
55. Mowat, A.G., and Baum, J.: Chemotaxis of polymorphonuclear leukocytes from patients with rheumatoid arthritis. J. Clin. Invest. 50:2541, 1971.
56. Howe, G.B., Fordham, J.N., Brown, K.A., and Currey, H.L.F.: Polymorphonuclear cell function in rheumatoid arthritis and in Felty's syndrome. Ann. Rheum. Dis. 40:370, 1981.
57. Gupta, R.C., Laforce, F.M., and Mills, D.M.: Polymorphonuclear leukocyte inclusions and impaired bacterial killing in patients with Felty's syndrome. J. Lab. Clin. Med. 88:183, 1976.
58. Green, R.A., and Fromke, V.L.: Splenectomy in Felty's syndrome. Ann. Intern. Med. 64:1265, 1966.
59. Blumfelder, T.M., Logue, G.L., and Shimm, D.S.: Felty's syndrome: Effects of splenectomy upon granulocyte count and granulocyte-associated IgG. Ann. Intern. Med. 94:623, 1981.
60. Logue, G.L., Huang, A.T., and Shimm, D.S.: Failure of splenectomy in Felty's syndrome. The role of antibodies supporting granulocyte lysis by lymphocytes. N. Engl. J. Med. 304:580, 1981.
61. Thorne, C., and Urowitz, M.B.: Long-term outcome in Felty's syndrome. Ann. Rheum. Dis. 41:486, 1982.
62. Khan, M.A., and Kushner, I.: Improvement in rheumatoid arthritis following splenectomy for Felty's syndrome. JAMA 237:1116, 1977.
63. Gibberd, F.B., Gilbertson, C., and Jepson, E.M.: Felty's syndrome. Ann. Rheum. Dis. 24:46, 1965.
64. Luthra, H.S., Conn, D.L., and Ferguson, R.H.: Felty's syndrome: Response to parenteral gold. J. Rheumatol. 8:902, 1981.
65. Wimer, B.M., and Sloan, M.W.: Remission of Felty's syndrome with long-term testosterone therapy. JAMA 223:671, 1973.
66. Gupta, R.C., Robinson, W.A., and Kurnick, J.E.: Felty's syndrome. Effect of lithium on granulopoiesis. Am. J. Med. 61:29, 1976.

Chapter 62
Sjögren's Syndrome

Keith Whaley and Margaret A. Alspaugh

INTRODUCTION: DEFINITION AND HISTORICAL ASPECTS

There is no absolute definition of Sjögren's syndrome (SS); however, the diagnostic triad described by Bloch and colleagues[1] serves most clinical purposes. This triad includes keratoconjunctivitis sicca or dry eyes, with or without lacrimal gland enlargement; xerostomia (dry mouth), with or without salivary gland enlargement; and the presence of a connective tissue disease, usually rheumatoid arthritis.[2,3] More rarely systemic lupus erythematosus, scleroderma (systemic sclerosis), polyarteritis nodosa, or polymyositis may be present.[3] In order to establish the presence of SS, at least two of these three criteria should be present. Patients having only the ocular and oral components are said to have the sicca syndrome, whereas those having associated connective tissue diseases are categorized as SS with the specific diseases, e.g., SS with rheumatoid arthritis.

Historically, filamentary keratitis was described by Leber in 1888,[4] xerostomia by Hadden in 1888,[5] and lacrimal and salivary gland enlargement without keratoconjunctivitis sicca or xerostomia by Mikulicz.[6] Other components of SS were described between 1883 and 1933.[7] However, it was not until 1933 that a full de scription was given by Henrik Sjögren.[8] Histologically, SS and Mikulicz's disease are identical and thus are currently considered to be variants of the same disease.[9]

INCIDENCE AND PREVALENCE

As in most autoimmune diseases, there is a predilection for middle-aged and elderly females. However, in elderly persons in Scotland a high prevalence (16.7 percent) of keratoconjunctivitis sicca was found equally in males and females.[10] Xerostomia was also common in elderly females (18.2 percent), but less common in elderly males (2.8 percent). Definite sicca syndrome was found in 3.5 percent of females and 2.8 percent of males over the age of 80 years. It should be noted that there was no association between the prevalence of autoantibodies and keratoconjunctivitis sicca or xerostomia in these persons, suggesting that senile atrophy of the secretory apparatus rather than immunologic injury was the underlying etiology. The sicca syndrome, although not rare, is probably much less common than SS accompanied by a connective tissue disease. In the United Kingdom the incidence of keratoconjunctivitis sicca in rheumatoid arthritis is 11 percent,[11] whereas xerostomia occurs in only 1 percent of patients. It is likely that a

dry climate (e.g., Mexico) will accentuate symptoms of the sicca syndrome, whereas a cooler, moist climate (e.g., the United Kingdom) may help minimize them. As a result of the widespread clinical application of the newer and more sensitive techniques for the investigation of salivary gland disease, it is now becoming obvious that subclinical inflammation of the salivary glands is almost universal in patients with connective tissue diseases, although the extent of tissue destruction is insufficient to produce the overt signs of secretory insufficiency. Recent publications have shown extremely high incidences of salivary gland abnormalities in systemic lupus erythematosus,[12] scleroderma,[13,14] and mixed connective tissue disease.[15] Indeed, an autopsy examination of the submandibular glands of patients with rheumatoid arthritis has shown lymphocytic infiltrates in all cases.[16]

CLINICAL FEATURES

Ocular. The Schirmer tear test is a crude test for tear secretion[17] (Fig. 62–1). Normal individuals should wet 15 mm or more of the standard filter strip in 5 minutes. When subnormal wetting occurs, tear secretion should be stimulated by the inhalation of 10 percent ammonia held 6 inches below the nose.[3] Less than 15 mm of wetting during the forced Schirmer tear test demonstrates diminished secretion. However, the presence of diminished tear secretion alone is not diagnostic of keratoconjunctivitis sicca (Table 62–1). This may be confirmed by putting rose bengal dye (1 percent) into the conjunctival sac and using a slit lamp to find evidence of punctate or filamentary keratitis (Fig. 62–2). Keratitis alone is also not diagnostic of keratoconjunctivitis sicca and may occur in a number of other conditions (Table 62–2). When diminished tear secretion and a punctate or filamentary keratitis coexist, then keratoconjunctivitis sicca is considered present. Occasional patients may have SS with normal tear secretion, since patients may have only pronounced lacrimal gland enlargement (Table 62–3). Usually, however, lacrimal gland enlargement is associated with diminished tear secretion. In hot, dry atmospheres the standard Schirmer test gives false-positive results.[18] Hence, in certain geographical locations a

Table 62–1. Principal Causes of Diminished Tear Secretion

1. Senile atrophy of lacrimal glands
2. Inflammatory conditions, e.g., Sjögren's syndrome, sarcoidosis
3. Tumors, as listed in causes of lacrimal gland enlargement (Table 62-3)

Figure 62-1. Schirmer tear test. The filter paper strip is folded 5 mm from one end, and placed over the lower lid at the junction of the middle and outer thirds. The length of wetting after 5 minutes is measured; over 15 mm is normal.

Table 62-2. Etiology of Punctate or Filamentary Keratitis

1. Degenerative—e.g., keratoconjunctivitis sicca from any cause, keratoconus, neuropathic keratopathy, benign mucous membrane pemphigoid
2. Infective—e.g., punctate epithelial keratitis (adenovirus, herpes, or vaccinia) and bacterial keratitis (rare)
3. Edematous states—e.g., recurrent erosions, wearing of ill-fitting contact lenses
4. Traumatic—rare

falsely high prevalence of keratoconjunctivitis sicca can occur.

The symptoms and signs of keratoconjunctivitis sicca are shown in Table 62-4. No one symptom is specific, whereas some signs appear to be. Patients with connective tissue diseases rarely complain about keratoconjunctivitis sicca, and careful questioning is required. We have developed a statistical method for the diagnosis of keratoconjunctivitis sicca based on the frequency with which these symptoms and signs occur in patients and controls.[19] This method can save the ophthalmologist's time.[20]

Table 62-5 lists the ocular complications of keratoconjunctivitis sicca. These complications are secondary

Table 62-3. Causes of Lacrimal Gland Enlargement

1. Inflammation—unilateral or bilateral
   a. Acute dacryoadenitis, e.g., gonococcal, infectious mononucleosis
   b. Chronic dacryoadenitis, e.g., trachoma, tuberculosis, leprosy, actinomycosis
   c. Sarcoidosis
   d. Sjögren's syndrome
2. Tumors—usually unilateral
   a. Cysts
   b. Epithelial, e.g., adenoma, adenocarcinoma
   c. Lymphoreticular, e.g., Hodgkin's disease, leukemia, lymphosarcoma, Waldenström's macroglobulinemia
   d. Secondary tumors
   e. Miscellaneous, e.g., angioma, melanoma

to dryness of the cornea and conjunctiva rather than any direct immunological injury. The increased incidence of bacterial and viral infections of the eye in this condition is secondary to the breakdown of the local conjunctival defense mechanisms which depend on the antibacterial nature of tears and their physical flow properties.

Oral. Assessment of xerostomia is difficult. Mild xerostomia is occasionally found among healthy middle-aged people or patients with rheumatoid arthritis and other connective tissue diseases without evidence of SS. When salivary gland enlargement is present, the diagnosis is simple, as it is commonly found in association with xerostomia. Contrary to popular belief, gland enlargement is usually unilateral and episodic. In a study of 171 patients with SS, intermittent salivary gland enlargement was present in 37 patients (21.6 percent), of

Figure 62-2. Slit lamp appearance of punctate keratitis in a patient with keratoconjunctivitis sicca.

Table 62–4. Clinical Features of Keratoconjunctivitis Sicca*

Clinical Features	Normal (n=37)	With Kerato-conjunctivitis Sicca (n=40)
Symptoms:		
Foreign body sensation	2	32
Burning	2	30
Tiredness, with or without difficulty in opening the eyes	2	26
Dry feeling, with or without a poor response to physical or chemical irritants and emotions	1	28
Redness	2	19
Difficulty in seeing	1	10
Itchiness	10	16
Aches	1	15
Soreness or pain	2	9
Photosensitivity and excess of secretion which may appear to be watery, ropy, or as a film over the eye	2	15
Signs:		
Dilatation of the bulbar conjunctival vessels (usually interpalpebral)	2	11
Photophobia	7	31
Irregularity of the corneal image	3	21
White and frothy or yellow and tenacious on discharge	0	11
Dullness of the conjunctiva and/or cornea	0	11
Ptosis	0	6
Mild pericorneal injection	0	10

*Data from Anderson, J.R., et al.: Quart. J. Med. 41:175, 1972. Courtesy of the editor of the Quarterly Journal of Medicine.

whom only 13 had bilateral episodes of swelling. Persistent salivary gland enlargement was found in only seven patients (4.1 percent), and of these only five were bilateral.[3] One hundred and twenty-seven patients (74.3 percent) had no clinical salivary gland enlargement, and it is this group that provides the greatest diagnostic challenge. There are as yet no entirely satisfactory clinical or laboratory tests for the diagnosis of the oral component of SS. Probably the most reliable sign of xerostomia is the absence of pooling of saliva in the floor of the mouth. Severe xerostomia may cause lip cracking and chronic ulceration of the lip (Fig. 62–3), angular

Table 62–5. Ocular Complications of Keratoconjunctivitis Sicca

Infection, often asymptomatic
 Bacterial
 Fungal
 Viral
Symblepharon with secondary exposure keratitis
Pannus formation, causing essential shrinkage of the conjunctiva
Marginal gutter ulceration
Corneal ulceration with perforation, which may result in uveitis, cataract, and glaucoma

Figure 62–3. Patient with severe Sjögren's syndrome showing parotid gland enlargement and chronic ulceration of the lower lip.

stomatitis, oral soreness, fissuring and ulceration of the tongue, atrophy of the oral mucosa, and, rarely, secondary candidiasis. Severe dental caries may occur in xerostomia.

The differential diagnosis of xerostomia is often difficult; mild degrees are common in mouth breathers and heavy smokers, and extremely severe xerostomia may occur following drug therapy and extirpation or irradiation of the salivary glands as well as in SS. The xerostomia found in severe dehydration secondary to uremia and diabetic ketoacidosis is not a diagnostic problem.

Salivary gland enlargement is not pathognomonic of SS, as illustrated by the bewildering list of causes listed in Table 62–6. A good history and physical examination should discriminate between these possibilities. If there is any diagnostic doubt, biopsy is essential. The laboratory tests are aimed at demonstrating pathological changes within the gland or assessing the functional reserve. Sialography demonstrates dilations (sialectasia)

Table 62–6. Causes of Salivary Gland Enlargement

1. Neoplasms
 Primary salivary gland tumors (benign and malignant)
 Malignant lymphoma
 Waldenström's macroglobulinemia
2. Inflammation
 Sjögren's syndrome
 Sarcoidosis
 Acute bacterial and viral infections
 Chronic sialadenitis
 Tuberculosis
 Syphilis
 Actinomycosis
 Ancylostomiasis
 Histoplasmosis
3. Miscellaneous
 Iodide, lead, or copper hypersensitivity
 Hyperlipidemic states
 Cirrhosis of the liver
 Diabetes mellitus
 Malnutrition

and other changes (atrophy) occurring within the intrasalivary duct system[21,22] (Fig. 62–4). The technique of sialography is usually performed by injection of a predetermined volume of contrast media. This may lead to rupture of the duct system and aggravate the inflammatory process. It is our policy to use the hydrostatic technique, which virtually eliminates rupture of the duct system.[23] Sialectasia, with the retention of secretions, predisposes to staphylococcal parotitis with abscess formation.

Because of potential hazard, biopsy of the major salivary glands is recommended only when there is a suggestion of intraparotid malignancy or when serious diagnostic doubts are present. As changes in the minor glands mirror the changes in the major glands,[24] biopsy of the minor glands of the lip[25] or palate[26] is now a routine test. The technique is also useful in diagnosing sarcoidosis.[27] Histologically a positive biopsy of a major gland shows infiltration by lymphocytes, plasma cells, and occasional reticulum cells. These cells surround the

ducts and infiltrate the acinar tissue with consequent loss of secretory epithelium. The stroma of the salivary glands is usually still present; hence, the lobular architecture is preserved, which helps in the differentiation between SS and lymphoma of the salivary glands. The epithelial cells lining the ducts show degenerative changes, and the lumina of the ducts contain inspissated material. The ducts are frequently dilated, and basket cell hypertrophy leading to epimyoepithelial "islands" may occur (Fig. 62–5). These "islands" result from intense proliferation of the epimyoepithelial cells, with consequent occlusion of the ducts. Morgan and Castleman[9,28] considered these "islands" pathognomonic of SS, but they may also be seen in lymphoid tumors affecting the salivary glands. Polymorphonuclear and eosinophilic leukocyte infiltration may occur, the former usually being associated with secondary bacterial infection. Although the lymphoid infiltrates of SS do not have the general appearance of normal lymphatic tissue germinal centers, occasionally there are centers seen in

Figure 62–4. *A*, Normal sialogram. *B*, Dilatation of main parotid duct. *C*, Sialectasia. (Courtesy of Dr. Martin Ferguson.)

Figure 62–5. Epimyoepithelial cell island in the parotid gland. H&E. × 130. (Courtesy of Dr. G. MacDonald.)

the major glands,[1] indicating an ongoing immune response. Indeed, immunofluorescence studies have shown rheumatoid factor localized in and around the plasma cells in the infiltrate.[1] Although not conclusive, the evidence suggests that local synthesis of rheumatoid factor is occurring in the salivary gland in SS, as has been demonstrated in the synovial tissues in rheumatoid arthritis. Talal and his colleagues[29] have shown that rheumatoid factor is produced by minor salivary gland biopsy in tissue culture. As an end result of the chronic inflammatory process, complete atrophy of the acinar tissue may occur. The glands become completely replaced with fatty tissue, and little evidence of the original immune reaction remains (Fig. 62–6).

The histopathological changes that occur in the minor salivary glands are similar to those found in the major glands. For the purpose of diagnosis, diffuse lymphocytic infiltration must be ignored, as this is found in many other conditions.[30] However, focal lymphocytic infiltrates (Fig. 62–7) have a much higher degree of specificity for SS, and are seen in over 70 percent of patients.[3] Focal sialadenitis also occurs in other connective tissue diseases (Table 62–7),[3] an observation supporting the concept of subclinical SS.

Salivary gland flow rates, radionuclide scintiscanning, and iodide trapping capacity are all measures of function of salivary ducts. All are handicapped by the wide ranges found in normal individuals. Only salivary flow rates and scintiscanning are in regular clinical use; the iodide trapping capacity test is obsolete.[31] Salivary flow rates can only be properly assessed under conditions of maximal stimulation with lemon juice. Under these circumstances there is a marked age and sex difference in parotid salivary flow[3] (Table 62–8). There is no obvious change in salivary flow with age in males, whereas there is a pronounced fall in postmenopausal females. Inevitably, as with most tests of organ function in which the organ may be only partially destroyed, there is a marked overlap in salivary flow rates between patients with SS and healthy persons, which is markedly reduced when age and sex-matched controls are used.[3] Subnormal maximally stimulated salivary flow rates never occur in iatrogenic xerostomia, and stimulated levels of less than 0.5 ml per minute are virtually diagnostic of SS.

Figure 62–6. Late stages of inflammation in labial salivary glands. Lymphocytic infiltration associated with marked acinar atrophy, periductal fibrosis, and fatty infiltration. H&E. × 55. (Courtesy of Dr. G. MacDonald.)

Figure 62–7. *A,* Normal labial salivary gland biopsy. H&E. × 50. *B,* Biopsy from patient with Sjögren's syndrome showing focal and diffuse lymphocytic infiltration, predominantly periductal in distribution, and duct dilatation. H&E. × 50. (Courtesy of Dr. G. MacDonald.)

Radionuclide scanning of the salivary glands using radioactive technetium pertechnetate ($^{99m}TcO_4^-$) is of proved diagnostic value.[32–34] Serial scans on patients permit assessment of the progression of disease. Salivary gland pertechnetate scanning is currently the most promising procedure in terms of sensitivity and simplicity of performance.

Other isotopes such as [67]gallium, [111]indium and [113m]indium, and [75]selenium-labeled seleno-methionine appear to be selectively concentrated in sites of lymphoreticular neoplasia and may afford a simple means of screening for suspected lymphoid tumor involving the salivary gland.[34a,34b]

Involvement of Other Exocrine Glands. *Respiratory Tract.* Involvement of the nasal mucosa results in dryness and crusting of the nasal mucosa.[1,35] Abnormalities of taste and smell may occur.[36] Eustachian tube obstruction may result in conduction deafness secondary to serous otitis media.[1,35]

Involvement of the lower respiratory tract may be present as a chronic bronchitis, with cough and production of tenacious sputum. Histologically there is

Table 62–7. Grades of Lymphocytic Infiltration in the Labial Salivary Glands in Connective Tissue Diseases*

| Clinical Group | Number | Grade of Lymphocytic Infiltrate | | | | | Percent with Foci |
		0	1	2	3	4	
Sicca syndrome	21	1	3	4	5	8	61.9
Rheumatoid arthritis plus Sjögren's syndrome	50	1	10	4	15	20	70.0
Rheumatoid arthritis	73	30	20	9	12	2	19.2
Psoriatic arthritis	16	12	2	1	1	0	6.3
Ankylosing spondylitis	12	8	1	1	2	0	16.7
Reiter's syndrome	12	10	2	0	0	0	0
Systemic lupus erythematosus	5	1	1	1	0	2[†]	40.0
Scleroderma	4	1	2	0	0	1[†]	25.0
Dermatomyositis	1	1	0	0	0	0	0
Gout	2	2	0	0	0	0	0
Osteoarthritis	20	16	1	1	1	0	5.0

*From Whaley, K., et al.: Quart. J. Med. 42:279, 1973. Courtesy of the editor of the Quarterly Journal of Medicine.
†These patients also had Sjögren's syndrome.

chronic inflammatory cell infiltration around the bronchial glands. Recurrent pneumonitis and pleurisy, with or without effusion, may occasionally complicate SS, and during the acute episode pulmonary opacities may be seen on x-ray. Certain other patients develop chronic interstitial pulmonary fibrosis with varying degrees of severity. Many SS patients without overt evidence of respiratory disease have restrictive ventilatory defects and diminished gas transfer.[37] In addition to the lesion referred to as diffuse interstitial pulmonary fibrosis, a similar clinical syndrome can result from lymphoid cell infiltration of the pulmonary interstitium.[38] The type of infiltrate may range from the benign lymphocytic interstitial pneumonitis, through pseudolymphoma, to malignant lymphoma.[39] Bronchopneumonia may also occur. There is no evidence that chronic interstitial pulmonary fibrosis of SS is due to the intrapulmonary deposition of circulating immune complexes.[1,40]

Gastrointestinal Tract. In addition to the mouth, dryness of the pharynx and esophagus contributes to difficulty with the passage of food to the stomach. Mild dysphagia is therefore common in SS, and occasionally postcricoid webs, which are clinically, radiologically, and histologically indistinguishable from those found in the Plummer-Vinson syndrome, are seen.[35] These webs

occur in the absence of sideropenia and do not appear to undergo malignant transformation. Abnormal esophageal motility also occurs in the sicca syndrome.[41]

Although achlorhydria has been described in SS, its significance is uncertain as it occurs occasionally in patients with connective tissue disease or in the older age groups.[42] Gastric biopsies from patients with SS have shown chronic inflammatory cell infiltration of the mucosa.[43] In a series of 121 patients with SS, gastric parietal cell antibody was found in 35 (27.6 percent). As the presence of this antibody in the peripheral blood correlates with the histological changes of chronic atrophic gastritis,[44] it is reasonable to assume that SS of the gastric mucosa is relatively common. However, overt pernicious anemia occurs in only 3.5 percent of SS patients.[37] That SS involving the stomach differs from true pernicious anemia is suggested by the finding that there is no increased incidence of SS in pernicious anemia.[45]

Pancreas. Numerous case studies of pancreatic disease and SS have reported acute pancreatitis, chronic relapsing pancreatitis, and asymptomatic dense diffuse pancreatic calcification. Necropsy findings have included acute and chronic pancreatitis in a patient with hepatic cirrhosis,[47] parenchymatous disorganization and atrophy,[48] parenchymatous replacement by a heavy cel-

Table 62–8. Effect of Age on Lemon Juice–Stimulated Parotid Salivary Flow Rates* in Sjögren's Syndrome†

		<20 Years	21–40 Years	41–60 Years	≥61 Years
Controls	Male	1.49 ± 0.09	1.73 ± 0.09	1.69 ± 0.11	1.58 ± 0.16
	Female	1.99 ± 0.14	1.76 ± 0.09	1.36 ± 0.12	1.15 ± 0.08
Sicca syndrome	Male	—	—	—	0.65 ⎫ Only 3 0.45 ⎬ patients 0.50 ⎭ studied
	Female	—	—	0.24 ± 0.08	0.27 ± 0.05
Sjögren's syndrome plus rheumatoid arthritis	Male	—	—	0.93 ± 0.17	0.43[‡] (0.32–0.78)
	Female	—	0.56 ± 0.05	0.47 ± 0.077	0.41 ± 0.05

*Milliliters per minute (mean ± S.E.M.).
†From Whaley, K., et al.: Quart. J. Med. 42:279, 1973. Courtesy of the editor of the Quarterly Journal of Medicine.
‡Only four patients studied.

lular infiltrate and vascular connective tissue,[49] and "oncocytic" changes in several acini containing periodic acid–Schiff positive material in their lumina.[50] Systematic investigation of pancreatic functions in SS have shown impaired responses to secretin[1,51–53] and pancreozymin,[53] suggesting that widespread or subclinical pancreatic disease is a common feature of SS. A recent study has also shown evidence of associated gastric and gallbladder dysfunction.[54]

Liver. Hepatomegaly is found in 18 to 23 percent of SS patients, but until recently only sporadic case reports of significant pathology appeared.[1,37,55] Biochemical evidence of liver disease[56] and lymphocytic infiltration of the liver[57] have also been reported. Following the introduction of the mitochondrial antibody test as a marker of autoimmune liver disease,[58,59] it has become increasingly obvious that autoimmune liver disease is a feature of SS. The incidence of mitochondrial antibody in patients with the sicca syndrome is on the order of 10 percent, whereas it was found in the sera of 3 of 71 (4.2 percent) of patients with SS with rheumatoid arthritis.[60,61] The presence of antimitochondrial antibody in the serum is usually associated with the histological evidence of peripheral lymphocytic infiltration,[62] features indistinguishable from clinically obvious primary biliary cirrhosis. Thus, the involvement of the exocrine hepatic apparatus is clearly another manifestation of SS.

When patients with autoimmune liver disorders were screened, sicca syndrome was found in 35 percent of patients with chronic active hepatitis,[63] 24 percent with cryptogenic cirrhosis,[63,64] and 52 to 100 percent of patients with primary biliary cirrhosis.[64,65]

Renal Involvement. SS patients may develop renal tubular defects, usually nephrogenic diabetes insipidus or renal tubular acidosis (type I or II, but II is more common), but also more global defects of renal tubular function, including generalized aminoaciduria, diminished renal tubular reabsorption of uric acid, or glycosuria; phosphaturia[66–69] also occurs, in addition to overt tubular dysfunction. Patients with SS display an inability to concentrate urine and an inability to excrete an acid load.[37,68,70–72] Histological examination of renal biopsy material from these patients has revealed a variety of pathological changes, the most prominent being interstitial infiltration with lymphocytes and plasma cells associated with nephrocalcinosis and tubular atrophy.[68,71,72] It is more likely that the renal tubular defects are due to lymphocyte-mediated tubular injury rather than to hypersensitivity.[73] Evidence to support this hypothesis comes from the observation that patients in the early stages of renal homotransplant rejection may develop renal tubular acidosis associated with peritubular lymphocytic infiltration.[74] Granular deposits of IgG and C3 have been detected in the peritubular basement membrane of a patient with the sicca syndrome.[75] Electron microscopic studies showed the presence of electron-dense deposits in the same location, suggesting that these deposits were immune complexes.

Immune complex glomerulonephritis may occur in patients with primary SS who do not have systemic lupus erythematosus (SLE).[37,68,76] Immunofluorescence and electron microscopic examinations have revealed membranoproliferative and membranous glomerulonephritis.[76] In addition to acute glomerulonephritis, elevated blood urea levels are not infrequent in SS.[37] The reason for this finding is unclear but could represent subclinical glomerular injury. Occasionally patients with SS have elevated DNA binding capacities and may eventually develop systemic lupus erythematosus.[77]

Skin Manifestations. Dryness of the skin is a common complaint of SS patients.[1,37,49] The mechanism underlying the xeroderma of SS is still unclear; there is histological evidence of chronic inflammation of the sweat glands (Fig. 62–8),[37,48,49] but another study failed to find such evidence.[1] A case report of complete absence of sebaceous glands associated with severe sweat gland atrophy in a patient with SS[77] suggests that sebaceous gland function may be impaired.

Genital Dryness. It is now appreciated that the apocrine glands of the external genitalia are frequently involved in SS.[1] The skin of the vulva and vagina is dry and atrophic, and patients may complain of vaginal dryness, sometimes associated with a burning sensation

Figure 62–8. Inflammation of sweat glands in a patient with Sjögren's syndrome and xeroderma. (Courtesy of the late Professor J. Milne.)

or dyspareunia. Histologically nonspecific vaginitis may be present, but as the patients are frequently postmenopausal, such changes could be due to estrogen deficiency.

Disease of Nonexocrine Organs. *Thyroid Disease.* Serological evidence shows an increased incidence of autoimmune thyroiditis in SS,[37,79-82] and clinical thyroid disease occurs in 10 to 14 percent of patients.[1,37] There is no increased incidence of SS in patients with autoimmune thyroid disease.[83] Serum antithyroglobulin and antithyroid microsomal antibodies occur in about 40 percent of patients with SS, the incidence being the same in the sicca syndrome or in SS with associated connective tissue disease.[37]

Diabetes Mellitus. Diabetes mellitus occurred in 7 of 171 patients (4.1 percent), which approximates the predicted incidence in a population of similar age and sex distribution.

Neuropathy. Sjögren[8] noted bilateral facial neuritis in patients who also experienced transient sensory changes of the cornea and the facial skin, and Weber[84] reported a patient with bilateral ptosis and unequal irregular pupils. Since then, several reports of cranial neuropathy occurring in SS have appeared; isolated trigeminal neuropathy appears to be the most common presentation, but other isolated cranial nerves may be involved, and sometimes multiple cranial nerves are damaged.[85-87] Peripheral neuropathy may also complicate SS. The clinical picture is of either the sensory or the sensorimotor type.[37] Focal and diffuse involvement of the central nervous system, including the spinal cord, occurs uncommonly.[87] Vasculitis probably accounts for nervous system involvement.[48,87,88]

Myasthenia Gravis. Myasthenia gravis has been reported in patients with SS,[37,89-91] but only in those patients with associated rheumatoid arthritis. Three percent of myasthenics also have rheumatoid arthritis.

Muscle Disease. Polymyositis may be associated with SS.[1,92,93] In addition, focal myositis without muscle necrosis,[37] perivascular accumulations of lymphocytes, or a granulomatous myositis may occur.[1] Presumably the focal myositic lesions represent subclinical polymyositis.

Joint Disease. Approximately half to two thirds of patients with SS have it in association with a connective tissue disease, usually rheumatoid arthritis.[1] In addition to the association of SS and rheumatoid arthritis, there is accumulating evidence that a mild relapsing nonerosive polyarthritis affecting the knees and elbows may complicate the sicca syndrome.[1,94,95] This arthritis is apparently episodic and self-limiting, and causes no permanent joint damage. The pathogenesis of this arthropathy is obscure, but its clinical nature suggests an immune complex phenomenon. Although one patient with psoriatic arthropathy and SS has been reported, an extensive investigation of patients with various seronegative spondyloarthritides failed to show an increased incidence of even subclinical SS.[96] Surprisingly, the prevalence of mild incidences of asymptomatic keratoconjunctivitis sicca in 100 patients with rheumatoid arthritis of less than 1 year's duration was almost 40 percent.[97]

The generally accepted prevalence of keratoconjunctivitis sicca in rheumatoid arthritis is 15 to 25 percent, although very high incidences have been reported.[98]

Vasculitis. SS may rarely be a complication of polyarteritis nodosa.[59,99] Patients with severe sicca syndrome may develop a vasculitis of the medium and small vessels,[100] which gives rise to skin ulceration and peripheral neuropathy.[1] Hyperglobulinemic purpura gives rise to capillaritis[37,101-103] and is found in a minority of patients with SS. About 20 to 30 percent of patients with hyperglobulinemic purpura have or will subsequently develop SS.[103] The rash of hyperglobulinemic purpura occurs especially in the lower limbs when the patient is ambulatory. It appears as "crops" of purpura, which are hot and itchy. Rarely the rash may be confluent. As the name implies, the rash is always associated with hyperglobulinemia.

Raynaud's Phenomenon. Although Raynaud's phenomenon occurs frequently in patients with scleroderma and other connective tissue diseases associated with SS, it is also a frequent finding in patients with the sicca syndrome. The pathological basis of Raynaud's phenomenon is unclear, with the exception of scleroderma in which obliterative endarteritis of the digital vessels is present, or when cryoglobulinemia occurs. Cryoglobulinemia is an uncommon association of SS.

Cutaneous Manifestations. Apart from skin dryness, purpura, skin ulceration, lip ulceration, and angular stomatitis, all of which have been discussed earlier, vitiligo may rarely occur in the sicca syndrome.[37] Three patients with partial lipodystrophy and one with total lipodystrophy associated with SS have been reported.[104,105] One patient had associated diabetes mellitus, and two patients had hypocomplementemia.[104] Complement activation appeared to be by the alternative pathway, although the presence of nephritic factor was not sought.

Drug Allergy. Although Bloch and his colleagues[1] first drew attention to the undue frequency of drug hypersensitivity, in particular penicillin and gold, in patients with SS, it is still not generally appreciated that drug allergy may be a serious hazard in these patients.[106] A later study showed that penicillin allergy was increased in patients with rheumatoid arthritis, but this increase was wholly confined to those patients with coexistent SS. Thus, the occurrence of drug allergy in patients with rheumatoid arthritis should alert the physician to the possibility of coexistent SS. Gordon et al.[107] found no evidence of increased allergy to gold in patients with rheumatoid arthritis complicated by SS. We are unable to explain this discrepancy. In support of our earlier observations on penicillin and gold allergy, we have recently noted a very high incidence of allergic reactions to levamisole in patients with rheumatoid arthritis and coexistent SS.[108] Nine of ten patients with SS and rheumatoid arthritis developed allergy to this medication, whereas only five of 30 patients with rheumatoid arthritis alone developed allergic skin reactions. It has been suggested that SS may predispose to drug-induced systemic lupus erythematosus,[109] but the evidence for this is weak.[110]

LABORATORY FINDINGS

Hematology. Mild anemia is a common finding in patients with SS.[1-3,55,111] The anemia is usually normocytic and normochromic, or occasionally hypochromic, as in other chronic inflammatory diseases. Leukopenia has been reported in 19 to 33 percent of patients with SS,[1,2,55,80,111] but in our own series only 6 percent had leukopenia.[37] The pathogenesis of leukopenia is obscure; bone marrow biopsies have shown no evidence of depressed leukopoiesis,[2] although granulocyte kinetics and the occurrence of granulocyte autoantibodies have not been studied. Eosinophilia has been reported as a common abnormality in many series of patients with SS,[1,2,111] and occurred in 5 percent of our patients.[37] Thrombocytopenia was reported by Heaton[78] in most of his patients with SS, but other authors consider it infrequent.[1,2,55,111] In our own studies in Glasgow, thrombocytopenia was only present in three patients with associated systemic lupus erythematosus, and was probably associated with this disease.[37]

Serum Proteins. Diffuse elevation of serum immunoglobulins is a common finding in SS.[1,2,37] Extremely high levels may occur, and of course purpura hyperglobulinemia may complicate this development. In addition, a hyperviscosity syndrome may occur in SS, owing to the presence of either cryoglobulins or circulating IgG–anti-IgG complexes.[2,112-116]

All three major immunoglobulins may be elevated in the serum of patients with SS, compared to age- and sex-matched controls. This elevation is most marked for IgG and less for IgA.[37,117] However, the changes in IgM and IgA concentrations are relatively small.[29,72] Secretory IgA levels are also elevated in SS[37] but contribute a very small part of total IgA. However, serum secretory IgA levels are increased in many chronic diseases, even those not involving secretory surfaces.[118] Hypogammaglobulinemia has been seen in patients when malignant lymphoma supervenes in SS.[1,119-121] Circulating immune complexes are present in the sera of patients with SS.[122] Although a defect in Fc-receptor–mediated clearance by the cells of the reticuloendothelial system of patients with SS is not related to the presence of complexes, it occurs most commonly in patients with involvement of nonexocrine organ involvement.[123]

Cryoglobulinemia, as mentioned earlier, may complicate SS, and SS may be a complication of the Meltzer-Franklin syndrome.[124] A monoclonal IgG-K cryoglobulin from a patient with SS was shown to have an abnormal carbohydrate composition with a low fucose and hexose content, and abnormalities of the primary immunoglobulin structure also. The latter abnormalities included significant reductions in the isoleucine and arginine residues in the heavy chains. It is probable that the carbohydrate residue deficits are responsible for the incomplete solubility of this particular cryoglobulin.[125] It appears that mixed cryoglobulins frequently have reduced sialic acid content,[126-129] which is probably responsible for the cryoprecipitability of the complexes. In contrast, the solubility of monoclonal cryoglobulins is due to abnormalities of the amino acid composition and sequence.[130,131] Macroglobulinemia and cryomacroglobulinemia have been reported in patients with SS.[68,119,121,132,133]

Serum α-2 macroglobulin levels are normal in patients with SS.[37] Patients with SS have normal pancreatic amylase levels,[134] whereas 15 percent have elevated serum salivary amylase levels. The concentration of serum salivary amylase did not correlate with any clinical or laboratory features of SS. It is possible that patients with high levels probably had a different underlying pathological process from those with normal or reduced levels.

Proteins in Salivary Secretions. Salivary IgG and IgM levels are elevated in patients with SS,[135,136] and the concentrations of these two proteins are related to the severity of the gland destruction based on the sialography index.[136] Using a radioimmunoassay, elevated levels of IgA and IgM rheumatoid factor have been found in the saliva of SS patients.[137] It is probable that although local synthesis of immunoglobulins and rheumatoid factors occurs in the salivary glands,[29,138] the larger part of these salivary proteins are serum derived.[137]

Concentrations of β-2 microglobulin in the saliva of patients with SS are higher than serum levels,[139] suggesting that this low molecular weight cell membrane protein is secreted into saliva by tissue lymphocytes. Support for this hypothesis has been obtained by showing a correlation between the degree of inflammation seen on labial biopsy and the salivary concentration of β-2 microglobulins, especially in patients with lymphoproliferative complications. The observations that levels of serum concentrates rose during relapse and fell during remission suggested that serial measurements of serum β-2 microglobulin may be useful in monitoring disease activity, and measurement of salivary concentrations might permit the estimations of the degree of local inflammation.[140] Salivary lysozyme concentrations are frequently reduced in primary SS, especially in patients with parotid gland enlargement.[141]

Non–Organ-Specific Autoantibodies (Table 62–9). The most common autoantibody found in SS is rheumatoid factor reactive against both human and rabbit IgG. Rheumatoid factors in patients with SS and associated rheumatoid arthritis are directed to different antigenic determinants on the IgG molecule than are rheumatoid factors occurring in the sera of patients with the sicca syndrome.[142] In the former group, 51 percent of rheumatoid factors had anti-Gm specificity, a proportion similar to that found in uncomplicated rheumatoid arthritis, whereas only 20 percent of the SS patients had rheumatoid factors with anti-Gm specificity. However, the prevalence of auto- and isospecific anti-Gm rheumatoid factors was the same in both groups.[142]

Patients with SS not having rheumatoid factor demonstrable by conventional techniques have been shown to have IgG antiglobulin factors reacting with both horse and rabbit immunoglobulin fractions.[37] Previously such antiglobulin factors have been demonstrated in the sera of patients with seronegative rheumatoid arthritis,[143] ju-

Table 62–9. Prevalence of Autoantibodies in Sjögren's Syndrome

	Sicca Syndrome		Sjögren's Syndrome and Rheumatoid Arthritis	
	Glasgow*	Bethesda†	Glasgow	Bethesda
Rheumatoid factor				
Latex fixation	36/69 (52.1%)		93/94 (99%)	
Bentonitic flocculation		22/23 (96%)		30/30 (100%)
R3 agglutination titer	26/69 (39%)		79/94 (84%)	
SCA test		14/19 (74%)		21/29 (72%)
Antinuclear antibody	25/68 (37%)	14/16 (88%)%	50/91 (55%)	14/25 (56%)
Non–tissue-specific precipitins	12/62 (19%)	13/16 (81%)	15/73 (21%)	1/18 (6%)
Smooth muscle antibody	2/62 (3%)		7/70 (10%)	
Salivary duct antibody	7/69 (10%)‡		51/78 (65%)	
Thyroglobulin precipitating antibody	2/12 (17%)		2/16 (13%)	
Thyroglobulin tanned red cell test	17/50 (34%)		13/71 (18%)	
Thyroid microsomal antibody	22/51 (43%)		15/72 (21%)	
Gastric parietal cell antibody	15/51 (29%)		20/74 (27%)	
Coombs' test	0/19 (0%)		4/29 (14%)	
LE latex	2/61 (3%)		1/34 (3%)	
LE cells	1/12 (8%)	0/23 (0%)	0/11 (0%)	6/30 (20%)

*From Whaley, K., et al.: Quart. J. Med. 42:513, 1973.
†From Bloch, K. J., et al.: Medicine 44:187, 1965.
‡Salivary duct fluorescence in the sicca syndrome is probably due to mitochondrial antibody.

venile rheumatoid arthritis,[144] gout, psoriatic arthritis, and ankylosing spondylitis.[145] (The occurrence of these antiglobulin factors in such a wide variety of chronic arthritides suggests that they merely reflect the presence of chronic inflammatory disease.) Circulating intermediate rheumatoid factor IgG–anti-IgG immune complexes have been demonstrated in the sicca syndrome.[1]

The prevalence of antinuclear antibodies (ANA) in SS by immunofluorescence was 68 percent in one series.[1] The incidence in sicca syndrome as opposed to SS with rheumatoid arthritis in the United States and United Kingdom is shown in Table 62–9. More recently other investigators[146] have reported a higher incidence of ANA in sicca syndrome than in SS with rheumatoid arthritis.

ANA in SS are directed against a variety of nuclear antigens, and this is reflected in the different patterns of nuclear immunofluorescence.[37,147] Using rat liver as substrate, the most common pattern of nuclear fluorescence is the homogeneous type which is due to antibody to DNA-histone. This antibody lacks diagnostic specificity, as it is the most common type of ANA in systemic lupus erythematosus and rheumatoid arthritis.[148] LE cells are not found in the sicca syndrome but do occur in approximately 10 percent of patients with SS and accompanying rheumatoid arthritis. Using a modified clot test to detect LE cells, Baumer[149] found pseudo-LE cells in 22 patients with SS. These cells were monocytes or polymorphonuclear leukocytes containing numerous small or large intracytoplasmic inclusions with nuclear characteristics. It is possible that these cells are an immunocytological expression of an antinuclear factor other than the LE cell factor.

The morphological patterns of nuclear immunofluorescence that appear to have some degree of specificity for SS are the speckled and nucleolar varieties.[147,150] In sicca syndrome the speckled pattern is usually due to

the SS-B antibody, which will be discussed later.[150] The membranous (rim) pattern of nuclear fluorescence is usually not seen in SS unless it is associated with systemic lupus erythematosus. Antibodies to native DNA, almost diagnostic of systemic lupus erythematosus, occur infrequently in patients with the sicca syndrome.[36,37] It has been suggested that such patients will ultimately develop overt systemic lupus erythematosus,[77] but this has not been our experience.

Using an extract of a human lymphocyte cell line (WI-L2), Alspaugh and Tan[151] defined three precipitating antigen-antibody systems in the sera of patients with SS. These were denoted anti-SS-A, anti-SS-B, and anti-SS-C (Fig. 62–9). Anti-SS-A and anti-SS-B occurred more commonly in the sera of patients with the sicca syndrome (70 percent and 48 percent, respectively) than

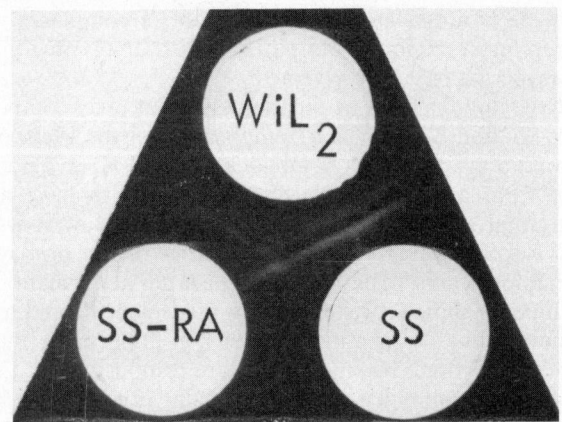

Figure 62–9. Immunodiffusion study showing nonidentity between precipitins of SS-RA (RAP) sera and the precipitins in SS-sicca (A and B). An extract of WI-L2 cells is shown in the upper wall. (From Alspaugh, M.A., and Tan, E.M.: J. Clin. Invest. 55:1067, 1975.)

in the sera of patients with SS and accompanying rheumatoid arthritis (9 percent and 3 percent, respectively) (Table 62–10). By contrast anti-SS-C has the same prevalence in SS with rheumatoid arthritis and in rheumatoid arthritis alone (68 percent), but is rare in the sicca syndrome.[57,150] These three antibodies were not found in certain other connective tissue diseases. The relationship of anti-SS-C to rheumatoid arthritis rather than SS led to its being referred to as rheumatoid arthritis precipitin (RAP).

Systemic lupus erythematosus appears to be the only other disease besides the sicca syndrome in which anti-SS-A is present. Approximately 33 percent of our lupus patients have this antibody.[152] While the incidence of SS in this group of patients has not been determined at this time, it should be noted that there is a very high incidence of SS in anti-SS-A positive patients. The relationship of anti SS-A and anti-Ro, and the characteristics of these antigen-antibody systems, is discussed fully in Chapter 46.

Serial studies have been performed on patients with SS. Titers of anti-SS-A antibody are generally stable but may increase with the onset of lymphoproliferation. In one patient with lymphoma and vasculitis, anti-SS-A antibody fell prior to death. In contrast, anti-SS-B titers fluctuate widely. Increased titers have occurred with the onset of myositis and lymphoproliferation. Treatment with corticosteroids apparently had little effect on anti-SS-A titers, but anti-SS-B levels fell dramatically.

Cryoprecipitates containing anti-SS-B—SS-B complexes have been found in two SS patients.[153] Ha, an acidic nuclear antigen, which reacts with antibodies in the sera of patients with SS or SLE,[154] has been shown to be immunologically identical with SS-B. In one patient, the appearance of anti-Ha (anti-SS-B) in the serum coincided with the onset of pseudolymphoma.[155]

Anti-insulin receptor antibodies have been demonstrated in one patient with SS and diabetes mellitus.[156] The hypocomplementemia of partial lipodystrophy is associated with circulating C3 nephritic factor. C3 nephritic factor is an oligoclonal immunoconglutinin, directed against the alternative pathway C3 convertase (C3bBb),[157-160] and it is therefore another non-organ specific autoantibody associated with SS.

Mitochondrial antibody is found in the sera of 10 percent of patients with the sicca syndrome and 4 percent of patients with rheumatoid arthritis and SS, and when present usually indicates clinical or subclinical evidence of liver disease.[37]

Smooth muscle antibody is an occasional feature of SS, but is not as good an index of hepatocellular disease.[37,161]

Antibodies to the Golgi complex have been found in the sera of a single patient with SS complicated by lymphoma. The antibody was not found in the sera of normal individuals, of individuals with uncomplicated SS (with or without RA), or of individuals with a wide variety of connective tissue diseases.[162] The significance of this antibody is unknown at present.

Organ-Specific Autoimmunity. Salivary duct antibody in sera from patients with SS was initially described by Bertram and Halberg.[163] Using an indirect immunofluorescent technique, sera stained the epithelial cytoplasm of the salivary duct. However, in a careful study of patients with various types of SS, MacSween and his colleagues[164] found a low prevalence in patients with sicca syndrome but a high prevalence in patients with SS accompanied by rheumatoid arthritis, and even in 20 to 25 percent of patients with rheumatoid arthritis alone. This result was confirmed in an extensive study by Whaley and his colleagues[37] (Table 62–9).

The small number of positive tests for salivary duct antibody in patients with the sicca syndrome is probably explained by the coexistence of mitochondrial antibody. All the patients in this group who had a positive salivary duct antibody test also had a positive mitochondrial antibody test. Mitochondrial antibody is a non–organ-specific antibody that reacts with the epithelial cytoplasms of many ductal systems, and therefore stains salivary duct epithelium. In contrast, salivary duct antibodies found in sera of patients with rheumatoid arthritis appear to be organ-specific, since they react only with the epithelial ducts of lacrimal and salivary glands.[164]

An antibody reacting with the cytoplasm of the epithelial cells of both intra- and interlobular pancreatic ducts has been detected by immunofluorescence. This antibody was found in the sera of 4 to 12 patients with

Table 62–10. Frequency of Precipitins SS-A and SS-B and RAP in Connective Tissue Diseases

Disease	Number Tested	Precipitins		
		SS-A	SS-B	RAP
SS–sicca complex	56	39 (70%)	27 (48%)	3 (5%)
SS–rheumatoid arthritis	33	3 (9%)	1 (3%)	25 (76%)
Systemic lupus erythematosus	85	28 (33%)*	0	2 (7%)
Discoid lupus erythematosus	22	0	0	0
Scleroderma	105	0	1	0
Mixed connective tissue disease	12	0	0	0
Rheumatoid arthritis (seropositive)	90	0	0	59 (67%)
Rheumatoid arthritis (seronegative)	51			9 18%)
Normal healthy subjects	70	0	0	1

*From Scopelitis, E., et al.: Arthritis Rheum. (in press).

SS, all of whom had an associated connective tissue disease, in eight of 31 (25.8 percent) patients with rheumatoid arthritis, but in none of 64 healthy controls.[165] The antibody cross-reacts with the duct cells of submandibular, parotid, and lacrimal glands, and thus appears to be salivary duct antibody. These data suggest that the duct cells of all the exocrine glands involved in SS contain common antigens against which the "autoimmune" response is directed.

Although clinical evidence of autoimmune thyroid disease is uncommon in SS, the prevalence of *thyroid autoantibodies* is significantly higher than in age- and sex-matched populations.[1,37] The presence of thyroid antibodies in the serum may indicate subclinical thyroiditis.[166]

Gastric parietal cell antibodies are found in approximately 30 percent of SS patients, the incidence being equally distributed between patients with sicca syndrome and patients with SS with accompanying rheumatoid arthritis.[37] In a similar study from Bethesda, it was found that American patients do not have an increased prevalence of parietal cell antibody.[167] Presumably, environmental factors are important in the pathogenesis of gastric parietal cell antibody in SS. This is in keeping with the results of a study of the prevalence of autoantibodies in monozygotic and dizygotic twins, from which it became clear that environmental factors exerted more control than genetic factors in the production of gastric parietal cell and other autoantibodies.[168,169]

Ten percent of SS patients have positive *Coombs' tests*, all of whom have connective tissue diseases.[1,37,51,55,170] Only two cases of patients with Coombs-positive autoimmune hemolytic anemia have been reported in patients with SS without systemic lupus erythematosus.[171]

Adrenal, parathyroid, pituitary, and ovarian antibodies are rare, and to date there is no evidence of their increased prevalence in patients with SS.

Humoral immune responses: Isohemagglutinin titers are significantly reduced in patients with the sicca syndrome whereas only levels of anti-A_1 and anti-A_2, but not anti-B levels, were reduced in patients with SS and rheumatoid arthritis.[172] Antibody responses to tetanus toxoid and pneumococcal polysaccharide vaccine are normal in patients with SS.[172,173] Neither immunogen precipitates disease exacerbation.

Complement: Patients with SS accompanied by rheumatoid arthritis have similar complement profiles to patients with rheumatoid arthritis alone. Raised levels of total hemolytic complement or individual complement proteins are the rule, but reduced levels occur when vasculitis is present. Patients with the sicca syndrome generally have normal serum complement levels with little evidence of complement activation.[174] However, when vasculitis occurs in the sicca syndrome, it is associated with profound hypocomplementemia, with reductions in the classic and also alternative pathway components. Genetic deficiencies of the complement system do not appear to be associated with the sicca syndrome.

Cellular immunity: Patients with sicca syndrome generally show normal delayed hypersensitivity responses to tuberculin and dinitrochlorobenzene (DNCB). However, patients with SS and rheumatoid arthritis, rheumatoid arthritis alone, or the sicca syndrome complicated by lymphoma have decreased response to these antigens.[172,175]

A number of abnormalities of T-lymphocyte numbers and functions have been recorded in SS. These include diminished numbers of T lymphocytes in the peripheral blood,[176,177] with reduction in the OKT8 (suppressor) cell population being most pronounced.[178] (The OKT4 [helper] population was normal.) The population of Ia-positive T lymphocytes is increased.[179] The autologous mixed lymphocyte reaction is reduced,[180] the mitogenic response to suboptimal concentrations of PHA is subnormal,[181] and the response of natural killer cells to immune interferon is reduced.[182] Serum levels of immune interferon are increased in SS.[183]

These findings could result from the disease process, or they could be the manifestations of an underlying abnormality that predisposes to SS. Alternatively, they could represent the result of both factors. Further work is required before their significance can be assessed.

In contrast, surface immunoglobulin positive lymphocytes (B lymphocytes) were not reduced in patients with the sicca syndrome of rheumatoid arthritis.[177] One communication reported a modest increase in circulating B lymphocytes in SS, which in itself is not remarkable. However, the authors showed a marked elevation in the number of B lymphocytes carrying multiple heavy chain determinants.[185] Similar findings have been reported in patients with chronic lymphocytic leukemia and other lymphoreticular neoplasms,[187-189] which is interesting in view of the predisposition of patients with SS to lymphoreticular neoplasms. Unlike SLE, patients with SS do not have increased numbers of B lymphocytes spontaneously secreting immunoglobulin in the blood or bone marrow.[186]

Antibody-dependent cell-mediated cytotoxicity is normal in SS and also in rheumatoid arthritis, showing that K cells, probably a subpopulation of T lymphocytes, are normal.[190]

Characterization of Lymphocytic Infiltrates. Immunofluorescent studies on frozen salivary gland sections from NZB/NZW mice demonstrated that the predominant cell types in the early lessions were immunoglobulin-bearing B lymphocytes and plasma cells. Later, as the lesions enlarged, the predominant cell type was the T lymphocyte, the B lymphocytes and plasma cells being smaller in number and situated more peripherally.[191] It has been shown in the minor salivary glands of human SS that small lymphocyte foci contain predominantly surface-immunoglobulin positive B lymphocytes and plasma cells, whereas larger lesions have a predominant T-lymphocyte infiltrate centrally situated, with B lymphocytes and plasma cells at the periphery.[177] It is not unreasonable to assume that the early lesion, which is predominantly periductal, is associated with B-lymphocyte infiltration and limited ductal damage, whereas with increasing T-lymphocyte infiltration considerable acinar destruction occurs. The predominant T-lymphocyte subset in the salivary gland infiltrates is OKT4 positive (i.e., of the helper-inducer population). The OKT4/OKT8 (helper:suppressor ratio) was greater than 3.0.[178]

Pseudolymphoma tissue showed primarily B-lymphocyte infiltration, while parotid tissue showed both B- and T-lymphocyte infiltration, i.e., B lymphocytes surrounded by larger numbers of T lymphocytes or null cells.

The early events in the evolution of such lesions could therefore be antigen recognition and/or early tissue damage by B lymphocytes and plasma cells migrating into the region. It is possible that the mechanism of tissue damage may be antibody-dependent cell-mediated lymphocytotoxicity or production of cytotoxic antibody. Recruitment of T lymphocytes could be by the production of lymphocyte chemotactic factors or other inflammatory factors which lack antigen specificity. Alternatively T lymphocytes might become specifically involved as part of a classic Type IV hypersensitivity reaction by becoming sensitized to tissue antigens released by B-lymphocyte–mediated tissue damage.

It is conceivable that the T-lymphocyte infiltration represents the early phase of human Sjögren's syndrome and that the smaller foci of B-lymphocyte and plasma cell infiltration represent a late lesion or, indeed, a different pathogenic process. Under these circumstances one could postulate that a cell-mediated immune response was the initial process and that the B lymphocytes and plasma cells were recruited later and increased tissue damage by antibody-dependent lymphocytotoxicity or the production of lymphocytotoxic antibody.[191]

Cell-mediated immunity to salivary gland extract has been demonstrated in patients with SS, using inhibition of polymorphonuclear leukocyte migration.[192] Despite these observations, Cremer and her colleagues were unable to demonstrate either lymphocyte- or antibody-mediated cytotoxicity for cultured autologous labial salivary gland tissue.[193]

Genetic Factors in Sjögren's Syndrome. The genes controlling the immune responses of mice map between the genes controlling the D and K determinants of the major histocompatibility complex,[194] and may not be separable from the genes coding for Ia surface antigens.[195] The Ia antigens, which are probably identical with the lymphocyte-defined antigens of mice,[196] appear to determine the intensity of the mixed lymphocyte reaction.[197] Although the immune-response genes in man have not yet been defined, by analogy with the mouse it is probable that they map within the HLA-D locus. Several organ-specific autoimmune diseases have been shown to be associated with HLA-B8, including celiac disease,[98] myasthenia gravis,[199] indiopathic Addison's disease,[200] Graves' disease,[201] chronic active hepatitis,[202] and juvenile diabetes mellitus.[203] A number of studies have shown the association of HLA-B8 with the sicca syndrome.[204-206] HLA-Dw3 is a lymphocyte-defined antigen in strong linkage dysequilibrium with HLA-B8,[207] and in both celiac disease[208] and sicca syndrome[209] the association of disease is primarily with HLA-Dw3 (69 percent association with sicca syndrome) and only secondarily with HLA-B8 (59 percent association) because of linkage dysequilibrium.[210] High levels of anti-SS-B antibodies were found in patients with the sicca syndrome and SS with SLE. In the sicca syndrome levels were higher in patients with HLA-Dw 2 or HLA-Dw3, or both than in patients with other HLA-DW types.[210a] This suggests that antigens or specific immune response genes close to the D region may be important for the development and antibodies to SS-B. All sicca patients have been shown to possess two immunologically distinct and genetically unrelated B-lymphocyte Ia antigens (AGS and #172).[211] Thus there is a strong argument in favor of the notion that immune-response genes located within the HLA-D locus are involved in the pathogenesis of SS and other organ-specific autoimmune diseases.

There are reports in the literature on the occurrence of SS in families. Table 62-11 presents the salient features of these reports. Although most of these cases had some symptoms and signs of SS, very few fulfilled the full diagnostic criteria. In addition some had associated con-

Table 62–11. Published Cases of Familial Sjögren's Syndrome

Reference	Cases	Comment
Lisch, 1937[247]	Twelve cases in 3 generations	—
Coverdale, 1948[248]	Father and daughter	—
	Mother and daughter	—
Pascucci, 1958[249]	Mother and daughter	Mother only had symptoms of xerophthalmia
Bloch et al., 1965[1]	Mother and daughter	—
	Mother and daughter	—
Doni et al., 1965[250]	Mother and son	
Camus et al., 1970[251]	Mother and daughter	Both had keratoconjunctivitis sicca and intermittent parotid gland enlargement; both had familial scleroderma
Shearn, 1971[2]	Two sisters	Both had systemic lupus erythematosus
Koivukangas et al., 1973[252]	Two sisters	Both had achalasia of the esophagus
Lichtenfield et al., 1976[253]	Four siblings—2 male, 2 female	One had an intraparotid lymphoma; most diagnoses did not fulfill diagnostic criteria
Frayha et al., 1977[254]	Mother and daughter	Both had CRST syndrome, mitochondrial antibody and Sjögren's syndrome
Vaillant et al., 1981[255]	Identical twin sisters	Both had sicca syndrome; no CTD

nective tissue disease, suggesting that the familial occurrence was of the connective tissue disease and not the SS.

A high incidence of abnormalities associated with SS has been described in the relatives of patients with SS.[1,212,213] In one study, relatives less than 45 years old had a higher incidence of probable rheumatoid arthritis, positive Schirmer test, serum autoantibodies, and increased gamma globulin levels than age- and sex-matched controls.[213] In another study relatives did not differ from age- and sex-matched controls, presumably because of the increased incidence of these abnormalities in older individuals.[10]

The other evidence for the genetic etiology of SS comes from the New Zealand black (NZB), and the NZB/NZW F1 hybrid mice. These mice have genetically determined autoimmune disease, very similar to systemic lupus erythematosus, and in addition have lymphocytic infiltrates in their lacrimal and salivary glands very similar to those seen in SS.[214] Although the genetics of serum autoantibodies, hemolytic anemia, and systemic lupus erythematosus are well documented,[215] the genetic control of the Sjögren's lesions has not yet been studied in depth. However, it is likely that they are strongly influenced by the murine genotype.

Infective Etiology. Serum levels of IgM antibody to cytomegalovirus (CMV) are increased in patients with SS.[216] This may be relevant, as the clinical features of CMV are similar to those of SS. This finding is made more striking by the observation that serum levels of antibodies to common respiratory viruses are not elevated (Whaley, unpublished observations).

There is an unconfirmed report on ultrastructural studies of the bronchial epithelium of a patient with SS associated with a lymphoid interstitial pneumonia which revealed the presence of round electron-dense virus-like particles, 70 to 120 Å in diameter. These particles are similar to the murine leukemia type A virus particles associated with tumors in laboratory and wild mice.[217]

Ultrastructural studies have shown tubuloreticular structures in the endothelium of renal glomeruli[218-220] and in the major and minor salivary glands.[221,222] These tubuloreticular structures are seen in vascular endothelium and in the lymphocytes in the minor salivary glands.[222] From studies of transplanted human lymphoid tumors, it has been suggested that tubuloreticular structures are associated with immunoglobulin synthesis, more particularly with gamma than with $m\mu$ heavy chain synthesis.[223] At present the exact nature of these particles is unknown, but current evidence suggests they are not viruses.

Lymphoproliferation. Lymphoproliferation, both benign and malignant, occurs in SS. Benign lymphoproliferation characteristically occurs in the major and minor salivary glands and the lacrimal glands. Initially it is periductal in distribution, but later becomes widespread with acinar destruction. There is considerable evidence that these lymphocytes are responding to an antigenic challenge; salivary duct antibody which has autoreactivity[224] occurs in the sera of patients with SS,[163,164] and circulating lymphocytes of patients may be sensitized to a salivary gland antigen.[192,225,226] These data suggest that some of the lymphocytes in the salivary and lacrimal glands are sensitized to a glandular antigen, possibly ductal, although many could be nonspecifically recruited by the sensitized lymphocytes. The local production of large quantities of IgG, IgM, and IgA by the lymphocyte cells in minor salivary gland tissue[29] may be in response to an antigenic challenge.

Lymphocytic infiltration of many exocrine organs is a feature of SS, and, although generally mild, it may on occasion be particularly intense. This progressive disease supervenes on what has previously been a rather stable disease process, and is termed pseudolymphoma. The clinical manifestations of pseudolymphoma depend upon organ involvement, but characteristically the lungs, kidneys, and salivary glands are involved, although occasionally generalized lymphoproliferation with lymphadenopathy, pulmonary infiltrates, fever, and weight loss suggest lymphoma.[227] Involvement of the lungs results in pulmonary infiltration, and renal infiltration results in renal tubular acidosis and nephrogenic diabetes insipidus.[69,121] Pseudolymphoma of the salivary glands presents with massive salivary gland enlargement and associated widespread cervical lymphadenopathy.[121] Histologically, two types of pseudolymphoma can be diagnosed: highly pleomorphic infiltrates which include small and large lymphocytes, or plasma cells and large reticulum cells. Occasionally histological evidence of distortion of normal lymph node architecture and infiltration beyond the capsule makes differentiation between malignant and benign lymphoproliferation very difficult.[121] Examination of biopsy tissue using immunohistochemistry may reveal areas of monoclonal proliferation,[228,229] and as a result, influence one's therapeutic approach. In addition to benign lymphoproliferation, the chances of developing a malignant lymphoreticular neoplasm are markedly increased in patients with SS. In our experience the chance of developing such a tumor is approximately 5 percent,[37] which is far higher than the expected incidence in the general population (1 in 10,000). Malignant lymphoproliferation may occur after many years of apparently benign disease, and pseudolymphoma itself has been shown to progress to malignancy in two patients.[119]

A report from the National Institutes of Health suggests that the risk rate for developing non-Hodgkins lymphoma in SS is 44 times normal and the risk rate for SS with rheumatoid arthritis is the same as for sicca syndrome.[230] Most authorities believe that malignant lymphoproliferation occurs almost exclusively in the sicca syndrome.

For the purposes of classification, lymphoreticular neoplasms complicating SS fall into two broad categories, those of intrasalivary and those of extrasalivary origin. The latter are probably more common and certainly have been reported more frequently. In addition to site of origin, the lymphoreticular neoplasms of SS can be divided into histological types. Although reticulum cell sarcoma and unclassified primitive stem cell lymphoma are the most commonly encountered lymphoid malignancies, lymphosarcoma, Hodgkin's disease, giant follicular lymphoma, thymoma, Waldenström's macroglobulinemia, and Franklin's heavy chain disease have all been reported (Table 62–12). There are several clinically important aspects of the association of malignant lymphoproliferation and SS. This complication generally occurs more commonly in patients with severe forms of the disease as shown by a high frequency of preceding vasculitis, neuropathy, splenomegaly, and lymphadenopathy.[119] It has been suggested that low-dose irradiation to salivary glands may predispose to malignant lymphoproliferation.[119,230] This could perhaps be the result of a degree of immunosuppression; such a conclusion is supported by the observation that the administration of azathioprine to a patient with SS was associated with the development of reticulum cell sarcoma.[231] Our experience argues against increased incidence after irradiation or immunosuppressive therapy; the incidence of lymphoma in our patients is probably no different from the incidence in the Bethesda series, yet none of our patients had ever received x-ray therapy or immunosuppressive medication. Another important point in the management of patients with SS with lymphoma is that serum immunoglobulin concentrations and autoantibody titers may fall as lymphoma develops. In fact, these falls may precede the clinical manifestations of the lymphoma, and should alert the clinician to this dramatic change in the patient's prognosis.[119,120] Intrasalivary lymphoid neoplasms are also a well-known

Table 62–12. Cases of Sjögren's Syndrome (SS) or Benign Lymphoepithelial Lesion (BLL) Associated with Lymphoreticular Neoplasia of Primarily Extrasalivary Origin*

References	Disorder	Number of Cases
Rothman et al., 1951[256]	SS—Stem cell lymphoma or reticulum cell sarcoma	1
Talal and Bunim, 1964[227]		3
Talal et al., 1967[119]		3
Hornbaker et al., 1966[257]		1
Miller, 1967[258]		1
Anderson and Talal, 1971[121]		1
Slater et al., 1976[231]		1
Present authors (unpublished)		1
Bark and Perzik, 1968[259]	BLL—	2
Pinkus and Dekker, 1970[133]		1
	Total:	15
Anderson and Talal, 1971[121]	SS—Malignant lymphocytic lymphoma	1
Bilder and Hornova, 1967[260]	SS—Lymphosarcoma	1
Thorpe, 1969[261]		1
Whaley et al., 1973[37]		1
Cited by Talal and Bunim, 1964[227]	SS—Hodgkin's disease	1
Whaley et al., 1973[37]		1
Senti-Parades et al., 1964[262]	SS—Giant follicular lymphoma	1
Yoshinaga, 1968[263]	SS—Lymphoma of vocal cords	1
Strimlan et al., 1976[39]	SS—Malignant lymphoma	6
Lattes, 1962[264]	SS—Thymoma	1
Dourov et al., 1968[265]		1
Alarcon-Segovia and Zavala-Mejia, 1971[266]		1
Pinkus and Dekker, 1970[133]	BLL—Thymoma	1
	Total:	18
Talal et al., 1967[119]	SS—Waldenström's macroglobulinemia	2
Whitehouse et al., 1967[132]		1
Maleville et al., 1967[267]		1
Pinkus and Dekker, 1970[133]		1
Anderson and Talal, 1971[121]		2
Wager et al., 1971[263]	SS—Franklin's heavy-chain disease	2
	Total:	9
	Overall total:	42

*More reports of extrasalivary lymphoreticular neoplasms have appeared since this table was originally prepared. They confirm the high incidence of such neoplasms in primary SS.

Figure 62–10. Intrasalivary primitive stem cell lymphoma (reticulum cell sarcoma) in a patient with the sicca syndrome. H&E. × 130. (Courtesy of Dr. G. MacDonald.)

complication of SS, but appear to be less frequent than their extrasalivary counterparts (Fig. 62–10). Malignant transformation may involve not only the lymphoreticular system, but also the epithelial elements of the salivary ducts[232] (Table 62–13). From the data of Hyman and Wolff,[233] it would appear that approximately 12 percent of cases of intraparotid lymphoreticular neoplasms are associated with SS or the benign lymphoepithelial lesion.

ANIMAL MODELS OF SJÖGREN'S SYNDROME

New Zealand black (NZB) and the hybrid NZB × NZW F1 mice develop lesions in the salivary[214] and lacrimal glands[234] that are similar to those seen in SS, although ductal proliferation and epimyoepithelial cell islands do not occur.[234a] The spontaneous development of these lesions has influenced ideas on the possible role of genetic and viral factors in the pathogenesis of human SS and lymphoma and has also helped elucidate the sequence in which various lymphocyte subpopulations infiltrate the target organs.[191]

Attempts to experimentally induce Sjögren-like lesions in animals have, until recently, met with little success. The use of saline extracts of salivary gland homogenates emulsified in complete Freund's adjuvant produces remarkably little sialadenitis; but when the newer adjuvants carbonyl iron and *Bordetella pertussis* vaccine are used, severe periductal infiltration of chronic inflammatory cell results. This is associated with marked acinar destruction.[235] This model has not yet been fully characterized.

Table 62–13. Intrasalivary Malignancies Complicating Sjögren's Syndrome (SS) and Benign Lymphoepithelial Lesion (BLL)

Reference	Disorder		Number of Cases
Bilder and Hornova, 1967[260]	SS—Lymphosarcoma		1
Lichtenfield et al., 1976[253]	SS—Lymphocytic lymphoma		1
Hyman and Wolff, 1976[233]	BLL—Lymphosarcoma		1
Whaley and Buchanan (unpublished)	BLL—Lymphocytic lymphosarcoma		1
		Total:	4
Azzopardi and Evans, 1972[269]	SS—Reticulum cell sarcoma		5
Whaley et al., 1973[37]			1
Strimlan et al., 1976[39]	SS—"Malignant lymphoma"		1
Hyman and Wolff, 1976[233]	BLL—Reticulum cell sarcoma		3
		Total:	10
Gravanis and Giansanti, 1970[232]	BLL—Carcinoma		3
Delaney and Balogh, 1966[270]	SS—Adenocarcinoma		1
		Total:	4
		Overall total:	18

TREATMENT

Treatment of SS can be divided into the treatment of the sicca components and treatment of the associated disorders. The most important aspect of patient management is regular outpatient supervision by a rheumatologist, ophthalmologist, and dentist, together with other specialist care as required. Regular physical examinations and serological testing may give early warning of intervening malignancy or other complications and should be mandatory. Patient education is valuable; explanation and reassurance at the time of diagnosis facilitate patient awareness of possible complications, especially common problems such as drug allergy. The use of unnecessary antibiotic, x-ray, or immunosuppressive therapy is to be avoided.

In approximately 50 percent of patients with keratoconjunctivitis sicca the instillation of 0.5 percent carboxymethyl cellulose eyedrops is sufficient to ameliorate symptoms and prevent any local complications.[236] Polyvinyl alcohol (5 percent) also improves eye symptoms.[237] Artificial tear preparations can also be obtained as slow-release tears and may be effective in resistant cases.[238] Ocular complications such as essential shrinkage of the conjunctiva, corneal ulceration, and perforation require intensive ophthalmologic supervision. Apart from their use as eyedrops, artificial tears can be applied using constant flow spectacles containing reservoirs of the tear substitute. Flow relies on gravity, on capillary attraction, or on battery driven pump mechanisms. We have no experience with these methods of application, and they seem unnecessary in view of the simplicity and effectiveness of the application of artificial teardrops.

Patients who have a limited residual tear flow benefit from occlusion of the nasolacrimal ducts by electrocoagulation. This maneuver permits the accumulation of residual tears whereby symptoms and complications may be avoided. Not only do patients with SS lack tears; they frequently suffer from the accumulation of large volumes of inspissated mucus. The use of artificial tears in some of these patients meets with failure, but treatment with the mucolytic agent in acetyl cysteine (5 to 10 percent solution) greatly improves the success rate. It is important to appreciate that the dry eye is susceptible to both bacterial and fungal infection.[239,240] Regular culture of swabs from the conjunctival sac is recommended. Infection must be treated energetically with the appropriate antibiotics; the possibility of allergy should always be considered. Oral bromhexine (48 mg per kg per day) increases tear secretion in patients with SS, clarifies mucoid eye discharge, and may improve xerostomia.[241,242]

Xerostomia is difficult to treat. Lubricants themselves tend to adhere to the mucous membranes, leaving the mouth feeling drier than before. In our experience simply increasing the oral fluids is the most effective way of alleviating symptoms. However, a number of studies have shown that saliva substitutes may ameliorate symptoms and possibly increase salivary flow.[243-245] The incorporation of fluoride into the substitute may help prevent caries.[245] Secondary oral infections lead to painful mouths. *Candida* infection is the most common problem and responds well to topical mycostatin. Regular dental supervision may prevent or delay the onset of the rapidly progressive caries that complicates SS. Careful brushing of the teeth and dental flossing are mandatory. The occasional occurrence of suppurative parotitis, already mentioned, requires early antibiotic therapy if surgical drainage is to be avoided.

Nasal dryness is best treated by the frequent application of saline soaks. The application of oil-based nasal lubricants may lead to lipoid pneumonia and is best avoided.

Skin dryness is rarely of sufficient severity to justify treatment, but vaginal dryness leading to dyspareunia usually responds to lubricants such as K-Y jelly.

Treatment of associated connective tissue diseases requires care, as allergy to gold and levamisole and perhaps other medications is common.[108] Usually the treatment of the complications of SS, such as primary biliary cirrhosis, does not differ from the treatment of primary biliary cirrhosis without SS. However, there is some evidence that renal tubular acidosis may be improved by cyclophosphamide.[69]

It has been suggested that slight improvement in lacrimal and salivary secretions may follow cyclophosphamide therapy.[138] There is also a report suggesting that lacrimal and salivary secretions increase after alkali therapy for renal tubular acidosis.[246]

The treatment of lymphoreticular neoplasia is difficult and is best performed in collaboration with an oncologist. Some patients with pseudolymphoma respond dramatically to corticosteroids and cyclophosphamide; others do not and may progress to overt lymphoma. Although the case for irradiation or immunosuppressive medication predisposing to lymphoid malignancy is not proved, it is prudent to avoid them.

References

1. Bloch, K.J., Buchanan, W.W., Wohl, M.J., and Bunin, J.J.: Sjögren's syndrome. A clinical, pathological and serological study of 62 cases. Medicine 44:187, 1965.
2. Shearn, M.A.: Sjögren's Syndrome. Philadelphia, W. B. Saunders Company, 1971.
3. Whaley, K., Williamson, J., Chisholm, D.M., Webb, J., Mason, D.K., and Buchanan, W.W.: Sjögren's syndrome. 1. Sicca components. Quart. J. Med. 42:279, 1973.
4. Leber, T.: Ueber die Entstehung der Netzhautablosung. Ber. Versamonl. Ophthal. Ges. Stuttg. 14:165, 1882.
5. Hadden, W.B.: On "dry mouth" or suppression of the salivary buccal secretions. Trans. Clin. Soc. Lond. 21:176, 1888.
6. Mikulicz, J.: Concerning peculiar symmetrical disease of lacrimal and salivary glands. Med. Classics 2:165, 1937-38.
7. Gougerot, H.: Insuffisance progressive et atrophie des glandes salivaires et muqueuses de la bouche, des conjunctives (et parfois des muqueuses nasale, laryngée, vulvaire): "Secheresse" de la bouche, des conjunctives, etc. Bull. Soc. Franc Derm. Syph. 32:376, 1925.
8. Sjögren, H.: Zur Kenntnis der Keratoconjunctivitis sicca (Keratitis filiformis bei Hypunfunktion der Tranendrusen). Acta Ophthalmol. 11:1, 1933.
9. Morgan, W.S., and Castleman, B.A.: Clinicopathologic study of Mikulicz's disease. Am. J. Pathol. 29:471, 1953.
10. Whaley, K., Williamson, J., Wilson, T., McGavin, D.D.M., Hughes, G.R.V., Hughes, H., Schmulian, L.R., MacSween, R.N.M., and Bu-

chanan, W.W.: Sjögren's syndrome and autoimmunity in a geriatric population. Age Ageing 1:197, 1972.

11. Williamson, J.: Personal communication, 1978.

12. Alarcón-Segovia, D., Ibanez, G., Velazquez-Forero, F., Hernandez-Ortiz, J., and Gomzalez-Jimenez, Y.: Sjögren's syndrome in systemic lupus erythematosus. Clinical and subclinical manifestations. Ann. Intern. Med. 81:577, 1974.

13. Alarcón-Segovia, D., Ibanez, G., Hernandez-Ortiz, J., Cetina, J.A., Gomzalez-Jimenez, Y., and Diaz-Jouanen, E.: Salivary gland involvement in diseases associated with Sjögren's syndrome. I. Radionuclide and roentgenographic studies. J. Rheumatol. 1:159, 1974.

14. Cipoletti, J.F., Buckingham, R.B., Barnes, E.L., Peel, R.L., Mahmood, K., Cignetti, F.E., Pierce, J.M., Rabin, B.S., and Rodman, G.P.: Sjögren's syndrome in progressive systemic sclerosis. Ann. Intern. Med. 87:535, 1977.

15. Alarcon-Segovia, D.: Symptomatic Sjögren's syndrome in mixed connective tissue disease. J. Rheumatol. 3:181, 1976.

16. Waterhouse, J.P., and Doniach, I.: Post-mortem prevalence of focal lymphocytic adenitis of the submandibular salivary gland. J. Pathol. Bact. 91:53, 1966.

17. Schirmer, O.: Studien zur Physiologie und Pathologie der Tranenabsorderung und Tranenabfulis. Arch Ophthalmol. 56:197, 1903.

18. Williamson, J., and Allison, M.: Effect of temperature and humidity in the Schirmer tear test. Br. J. Ophthalmol. 15:596, 1967.

19. Anderson, J.R., Whaley, K., Williamson, J., and Buchanan, W.W.: A statistical aid to the diagnosis of keratoconjunctivitis sicca. Quart. J. Med. 41:175, 1972.

20. Forrester, J.V., Anderson, J.A., Williamson, J., Jaczynowska, Z., and Buchanan, W.W.: Evaulation of a computer-assisted statistical diagnosis of keratoconjunctivitis sicca. Rheumatology 6:17, 1976.

21. Whaley, K., Blair, S., Low, P.S., Chisholm, D.M., Dick, W.C., and Buchanan, W.W.: Sialographic abnormalities in Sjögren's syndrome, rheumatoid arthritis and other arthritides and connective tissue diseases. A clinical and radiological investigation using hydrostatic sialography. Clin. Radiol. 23:474, 1972.

22. Blair, G.S.: Salivary gland radiology. Br. Dent. J. 140:15, 1976.

23. Park, W.M., and Mason, D.K.: Hydrostatic sialography. Radiology 86:116, 1966.

24. Chisholm, D.M., Waterhouse, J.P., and Mason, D.K.: Lymphocytic sialadenitis in major and minor glands: A correlation in post mortem studies. J. Clin. Pathol. 23:690, 1970.

25. Chisholm, D.M., and Mason, D.K.: Labial salivary gland biopsy in Sjögren's disease. J. Clin. Pathol. 21:656, 1968.

26. Bertram, U.: Xerostomia. Acta Adent. Scand. 25:Suppl. 49, 1967.

27. Hughes, G.R.V., and Gross, N.J.: Diagnosis of sarcoidosis by labial gland biopsy. Br. Med. J. 3:215, 1972.

28. Morgan, W.S.: The probable systemic nature of Mikulicz's disease and its relation to Sjögren's syndrome. N. Engl. J. Med. 251:5, 1954.

29. Talal, N., Asofsky, R., and Lightbody, P.: Immunoglobulin synthesis by salivary gland lymphoid cells in Sjögren's syndrome. J. Clin. Invest. 49:49, 1970.

30. Whaley, K., Chisholm, D.M., Downie, W.W., Dick, W.C., and Williamson, J.: Lymphocytic sialadenitis in the buccal mucosa in Sjögren's disease, rheumatoid arthritis and other arthritides. A clinical and laboratory study. Acta Rheum. Scand. 14:298, 1968.

31. Mason, D.K., Harden, R.McG., Boyle, J.A., Jasani, M.K., Williamson, J., and Buchanan, W.W.: Salivary flow rates and iodide trapping capacity in patients with Sjögren's syndrome. Ann. Rheum. Dis. 26:311, 1967.

32. Cummings, N.A., Schall, G.L., Asofsky, R., Anderson, L.G., and Talal, N.: Sjögren's syndrome—newer aspects of research, diagnosis and therapy. Ann. Intern. Med. 75:937, 1971.

33. Schall, G.L., Anderson, L.G., Buchignani, J.S., and Wolf, R.O.: Investigation of major salivary duct obstruction by sequential salivary scintigraphy; report of 3 cases. Am. J. Roentgenol. Radium Ther. Nuclear Med. 113:655, 1971.

34. Stephen, K.W., Chisholm, D.M., Harden, R.McG., Robertson, J.W. K., Whaley, K., and Stuart, A.: Diagnostic value of quantitative scintiscanning of the salivary glands in Sjögren's syndrome and rheumatoid arthritis. Clin. Sci. 41:555, 1971.

34a. Goode, R., Goodwin, D., Burgert, P., and Nelson, L.: Radioisotope scanning for tumours of the head and neck. Arch. Otolaryngol. 97:312, 1973.

34b. Garcia, R.R.: Differential diagnosis of tumors of the salivary glands with radioactive isotopes. Int. J. Oral Surg. 3:330, 1974.

35. Doig, J.A., Whaley, K., Dick, W.C., Nuki, G., Williamson, J., and Buchanan, W.W.: Otolaryngological aspects of Sjögren's syndrome. Br. Med. J. 4:460, 1971.

36. Henkin, R.I., Talal, N., Larson, A.L., and Mattern, C.F.T.: Abnormalities of taste and smell in Sjögren's syndrome. Ann. Intern. Med. 76:375, 1972.

37. Whaley, K., Webb, J., McAvoy, B.A., Hughes, G.R.C., Lee, P., Mac-

Sween, R.N.M., and Buchanan, W.W.: Sjögren's syndrome. 2. Clinical associations and immunological phenomena. Quart. J. Med. 42:513, 1973.

38. Weisbrot, I.M.: Lymphomatoid granulomatosis of the lung, associated with a long history of benign lymphoepithelial lesions of the salivary glands and lymphoid interstitial pneumonitis. Report of a case. Am. J. Clin. Pathol. 66:792, 1976.

39. Strimlan, C.V., Rosenow, E.C., Divertie, M.B., and Harrison, E.G.: Pulmonary manifestations of Sjögren's syndrome. Chest 70:354, 1976.

40. Tomasi, T.B., Fudenberg, H.H., and Finby, N.: Possible relationship of rheumatoid factors and pulmonary disease. Am. J. Med. 33:243, 1962.

41. Ramirez-Mata, M., Pena-Ancirez, F.F., and Alarcon-Segovia, D.: Abnormal oesophageal motility in primary Sjögren's syndrome. J. Rheumatol. 3:63, 1975.

42. Stenstam, T.: On the occurrence of keratoconjunctivitis sicca in cases of rheumatoid arthritis. Acta Med. Scand. 127:130, 1947.

43. Jebavy, M. von, Hradsky, M., and Herout, V.: Gastric biopsy in patients with Sjögren's syndrome. Zschr. Med. 16:930, 1961.

44. Adams, J.F., Glen, A.I., Kennedy, E.H., McKenzie, I.L., Morrow, J.M., Anderson, J.R., Gray, K.G., and Middleton, D.G.: The histological and secretory changes in the stomach in patients with autoimmunity to gastric parietal cells. Lancet 1:401, 1964.

45. Williamson, J., Paterson, R.W., McGavin, D.D., and Whaley, K.: Sjögren's syndrome in relation to pernicious anaemia and idiopathic Addison's disease. Br. J. Ophthalmol. 54:31, 1950.

46. Cardell, B.S., and Gurling, K.G.: Observations on pathology of Sjögren's syndrome. J. Pathol. Bact. 68:137, 1954.

47. Allington, H.V.: Dryness of the mouth. Arch. Dermatol. Syph. 62:829, 1950.

48. Szanto, L., Farkas, K., and Gyulae, E.: Sjögren's disease. Rheumatism 13:60, 1957.

49. Ellman, P., Weber, F.P., and Goodier, T.E.W.: Contribution to pathology of Sjögren's syndrome. Quart. J. Med. 20:33, 1951.

50. Bain, G.O.: The pathology of Mikulicz-Sjögren's disease in relation to disseminated lupus erythematosus. A review of the autopsy findings and presentation of a case. Can. Med. Assoc. J. 82:143, 1960.

51. Gordon, M.E., and Shanbrom, E.: The systemic manifestations of Sjögren's syndrome. Report of glandular function with histologic, bacterial and viral studies. Ann. Intern. Med. 48:1342, 1958.

52. Fenster, L.F., Buchanan, W.W., Laster, L., and Bunim, J.J.: Studies of pancreatic function in Sjögren's syndrome. Ann. Intern. Med. 61:498, 1964.

53. Hradsky, M., Bartos, V., and Keller, O.: Pancreatic function in Sjögren's syndrome. Gastroenterologia 108:252, 1967.

54. Dreiling, D.A., and Soto, J.M.: The pancreatic involvement in disseminated 'collagen' disorders. Studies of pancreatic secretion in patients with scleroderma and Sjögren's disease. Am. J. Gastroenterol. 1:546, 1976.

55. Vanselow, N.A., Dodson, V.N., Angell, D.D., and Duff, I.F.: A clinical study of Sjögren's syndrome. Ann. Intern. Med. 58:124, 1963.

56. Zawadzki, Z., and Edwards, G.A.: Dysimmunoglobulinemia associated with hepatobiliary disorders. Am. J. Med. 48:196, 1970.

57. Denko, C.W., and Bergenstal, D.M.: The sicca syndrome (Sjögren's syndrome). A study of sixteen cases. Arch. Intern. Med. 105:849, 1960.

58. Walker, J.G., Doniach, D., Roitt, J.M., and Sherlock, S.: Serological tests for the diagnosis of primary biliary circhosis. Lancet 1:827, 1965.

59. Goudie, R.B., MacSween, R.N.M., and Goldberg, D.M.: Serological and histological diagnosis of primary biliary cirrhosis. J. Clin. Pathol. 19:527, 1966.

60. Whaley, K., Goudie, R.B., Dick, W.C., Nuki, G., Williamson, J., and Buchanan, W.W.: Liver disease in Sjögren's syndrome and rheumatoid arthritis. Lancet 1:861, 1970.

61. Webb, J., Whaley, K., MacSween, R.N.M., Nuki, G., Dick, W.C., and Buchanan, W.W.: Liver disease in rheumatoid arthritis and Sjögren's syndrome: Prospective study using biochemical and serological markers of hepatic dysfunction. Ann. Rheum. Dis. 34:70, 1975.

62. Doniach, D., and Walker, J.G.: A limited concept of autoimmune hepatitis. Lancet 1:813, 1969.

63. Golding, P.L., Brown, R., Mason, A.M.S., and Taylor, E.: Sicca complex in liver disease. Br. Med. J. 4:340, 1970.

64. Golding, P.L., Smith, M., and Williams, R.: Multisystem involvement in chronic liver disease. Studies on the incidence and pathogenesis. Am. J. Med. 55:772, 1973.

65. Alarcon-Segovia, D., Diaz-Jouanen, F., and Fishbein, E.: Features of Sjögren's syndrome in primary biliary cirrhosis. Ann. Intern. Med. 79:31, 1973.

66. Kahn, M., Merritt, A.D., Wohl, M.J., and Orloff, J.: Renal concentrating defect in Sjögren's syndrome. Ann. Intern. Med. 56:883, 1962.

67. Shearn, M.A., and Tu, W.H.: Nephrogenic diabetes insipidus and other defects of renal tubular function in Sjögren's syndrome. Am. J. Med. 39:312, 1965.

68. Talal, N., Zisman, E., and Schur, P.H.: Renal tubular acidosis, glomer-

ulonephritis and immunologic factors in Sjögren's syndrome. Arthritis Rheum. 11:774, 1968.

69. Kaltreider, H.B., and Talal, N.: Impaired renal acidification in Sjögren's syndrome and related disorders. Arthritis Rheum. 12:538, 1969.

70. Shearn, M.A., and Tu, W.H.: Latent renal tubular acidosis in Sjögren's syndrome. Ann. Rheum. Dis. 27:27, 1968.

71. Tu, W.H., Shearn, M.A., Lee, J.C., and Hopper, J., Jr.: Interstitial nephritis in Sjögren's syndrome. Ann. Intern. Med. 69:1163, 1968.

72. Shioji, R., Furuyama, T., Onodera, S., Saito, H., Ito, H., and Sasaki, Y.: Sjögren's syndrome and renal tubular acidosis. Am. J. Med. 48:456, 1970.

73. Morris, R.C., and Fudenberg, H.H.: Impaired renal acidification in patients with hypergammaglobulinemia. Medicine 46:57, 1967.

74. Massry, S.G., Preuss, H.G., Maher, J.F., and Schreiner, G.E.: Renal tubular acidosis after cadaver kidney homotransplantation. Studies on mechanisms. Am. J. Med. 42:284, 1967.

75. Winer, R.L., Cohen, A.H., Sawhney, A.S., and Gorman, J.T.: Sjögren's syndrome with immune-complex tubulointerstitial renal disease. Clin. Immunol. Immunopathol. 8:494, 1977.

76. Moutsopoulos, H.M., Balow, J.E., Lawley, T.J., Stahl, N.I., Antonovych, T.T., and Chused, T.M.: Immune complex glomerulonephritis in sicca syndrome. Am. J. Med. 64:955, 1978.

77. Steinberg, A.D., and Talal, N.: The co-existence of Sjögren's syndrome and systemic lupus erythematosus. Ann. Intern. Med. 74:55, 1971.

78. Feuerman, E.J.: Sjögren's syndrome presenting as recalcitrant generalized pruritus. Some remarks about its relation to collagen diseases and the connection of rheumatoid arthritis with the sicca syndrome. Dermatologica 137:74, 1968.

79. Heaton, J.M.: Antimalarials in the treatment of Sjögren's syndrome. Br. Med. J. 1:1512, 1959.

80. Anderson, J.R., Goudie, R.B., Gray, K.G., and Buchanan, W.W.: Antibody to thyroglobulin in patients with collagen diseases. Scot. Med. J. 6:449, 1961.

81. Bunim, J.J.: Heberden Oration. A broader concept of Sjögren's syndrome and its pathogenic implications. Ann. Rheum. Dis. 20:1, 1961.

82. Bloch, K.J., and Bunim, J.J.: Sjögren's syndrome and its relationship to connective tissue diseases. J. Chron. Dis. 16:915, 1963.

83. Williamson, J., Cant, S., Mason, D.K., Greig, W.R., and Boyle, J.A.: Sjögren's syndrome and thyroid disease. Br. J. Ophthalmol. 51:721, 1967.

84. Weber, F.F.: Non-ocular features of Sjögren's syndrome. Med. Press 213:253, 1945.

85. Spillane, J.D., and Wells, C.E.C.: Isolated trigeminal neuropathy. A report of 16 cases. Brain 82:391, 1956.

86. Attwood, W., and Poser, C.M.: Neurologic complications of Sjögren's syndrome. Neurology 11:1034, 1961.

87. Kaltreider, H.B., and Talal, N.: The neuropathy of Sjögren's syndrome. Trigeminal nerve involvement. Ann. Intern. Med. 70:751, 1969.

88. Alexander, E.L., Provost, T.T., Stevens, M.B., and Alexander, G.E.: Neurologic complications of primary Sjögren's syndrome. Medicine (Baltimore) 61:247, 1982.

89. Downes, J.M., Greenwood, B.M., and Wray, S.H.: Autoimmune aspects of myasthenia gravis. Quart. J. Med. 35:85, 1966.

90. Brown, J.W., Nelson, J.R., and Hermann, C., Jr.: Sjögren's syndrome with myopathic and myasthenic features. Bull. Los Angeles Neurol. Soc. 33:9, 1968.

91. Osserman, K.E., and Genkins, G.: Studies in myasthenia gravis: Review of a twenty year experience in over 1200 patients. Mt. Sinai Med. J. 38:497, 1971.

92. Denko, C.W., and Old, J.W.: Myopathy in the sicca syndrome (Sjögren's syndrome). Am. J. Clin. Pathol. 51:631, 1969.

93. Fox, J.T.: Sjögren's syndrome and late-life myopathy. Arch. Neurol. 15:397, 1966.

94. Martinez-Lavin, M., Alspaugh, M.A., Taylor, D., Vaughan, J.H., and Tan, E.M.: Value of specific antibodies (SS-A and SS-B) in the diagnosis of Sjögren's syndrome (abstract No. 257). XIV International Congress of Rheumatology, June 26–July 1, 1977.

95. Ichikawa, Y., Komatsundo, M., Koriyama, K., and Arimori, M.: Co-operative clinical studies on Sjögren's syndrome between one with rheumatoid arthritis and one without rheumatoid arthritis. Arthritis Rheum. 25:137, 1976.

96. Whaley, K., Chisholm, D.M., Williamson, J., Dick, W.C., Nuki, G., and Buchanan, W.W.: Sjögren's syndrome in psoriatic arthritis, ankylosing spondylitis and Reiter's syndrome. Acta Rheum. Scand. 17:105, 1971.

97. Hernandez, L.A.: Unpublished data.

98. Sjögren, H.: Some problems concerning keratoconjunctivitis sicca and sicca syndrome. Acta Ophthalmol. 29:33, 1951.

99. Mason, A.M.S., Gumpel, J.M., and Golding, P.L.: Sjögren's syndrome—a clinical review. Semin. Arthritis Rheum. 2:301, 1973.

100. Soter, N.A.: Clinical presentations and mechanisms of necrotizing angiitis of the skin. J. Invest. Derm. 67:354, 1976.

101. Strauss, W.G.: Purpura hyperglobulinemia of Waldenström: Report of a case and review of the literature. N. Engl. J. Med. 260:857, 1959.

102. Waldenström, J.: Studies on conditions associated with disturbed gamma globulin formation. Harvey Lect. 56:211, 1961.

103. Talal, N.: Sjögren's syndrome. Bull. Rheum. Dis. 16:404, 1966.

104. Alarcon-Segovia, D., and Ramos-Niembro, F.: Association of partial lipodystrophy and Sjögren's syndrome (letter). Ann. Intern. Med. 85:474, 1976.

105. Ipp, M.M., Howard, N.J., Tervo, R.C., et al.: Sicca syndrome and total lipodystrophy: A case of a fifteen year old female patient. Ann. Intern. Med. 85:443, 1976.

106. Williams, B.O., St. Onge, R.A., Prentice, A., Dick, W.C., Nuki, G., and Whaley, K.: Penicillin allergy in rheumatoid arthritis with special reference to Sjögren's syndrome. Ann. Rheum. Dis. 28:607, 1969.

107. Gordon, M.H., Tiger, L.H., and Ehrlich, G.E.: Gold reactions are not more common in Sjögren's syndrome. Ann. Intern. Med. 82:47, 1975.

108. Balint, G., El-Ghobarey, A., Capell, H., Madkour, M., Dick, W.C., Ferguson, M.M., and Anwar-Ul-Haq, M.: Sjögren's syndrome: A contra-indication to levamisole treatment? Br. Med. J. 2:1386, 1977.

109. Grennan, D.M.: SLE precipitated by antibiotics in Sjögren's syndrome (letter). Br. Med. J. 1:460, 1976.

110. Sewell, J.R.: SLE precipitated by antibiotics in Sjögren's syndrome (letter). Br. Med. J. 1:385, 1976.

111. Stoltze, C.A., Hanlon, D.G., Pease, G.L., and Henderson, J.W.: Keratoconjunctivitis sicca and Sjögren's syndrome. Arch. Intern. Med. 106:513, 1960.

112. Bonner, H., Ennis, R.S., Geelhoed, G.W., and Tarpley, T.M.: Lymphoid infiltration and amyloidosis of lung in Sjögren's syndrome. Arch. Pathol. 95:42, 1973.

113. Alarcon-Segovia, D., Fishbein, E., Abruzzo, J.L., and Heimer, R.: Serum hyperviscosity in Sjögren's syndrome. Interaction between serum IgG and IgG rheumatoid factor. Ann. Intern. Med. 80:35, 1974.

114. Pruzanski, W.: Hyperviscosity and immunoglobulin complexes. Ann. Intern. Med. 80:107, 1974.

115. Blaylock, W.M., Waller, M., and Normansell, D.E.: Sjögren's syndrome: Hyperviscosity and intermediate complexes. Ann. Intern. Med. 80:27, 1974.

116. Waller, M., Edwards, W., Mullinax, F., Hymes, A.J., and Curry, N.: Hyperviscosity syndrome: Natural history in a patient with Sjögren's syndrome. Med. Coll. Va. Quart. 12:81, 1976.

117. Gumpel, J.M., and Hobbs, J.R.: Serum immune globulins in Sjögren's syndrome. Ann. Rheum. Dis. 29:681, 1970.

118. Waldman, R.H., Mach, J.P., Stella, M.M., and Rowe, D.S.: Secretory IgA in human serum. J. Immunol. 105:43, 1970.

119. Talal, N., Sokoloff, L., and Barth, W.F.: Extrasalivary lymphoid abnormalities in Sjögren's syndrome (reticulum cell sarcoma, "pseudolymphoma," macroglobulinemia). Am. J. Med. 43:50, 1967.

120. Whaley, K., and Buchanan, W.W.: Recent advances in Sjögren's syndrome. In Hill, A.G.S. (ed.): Modern Trends in Rheumatology, Vol. II. London, Butterworths, 1970, pp. 139–157.

121. Anderson, L.H., and Talal, N.: The spectrum of benign to malignant lymphoproliferation in Sjögren's syndrome. Clin. Exp. Immunol. 9:199, 1971.

122. Fischbach, M., Char, D., Christensen, M., Daniels, T., Whaley, K., Alspaugh, M., and Talal, N.: Immune complexes in Sjögren's syndrome. Arthritis Rheum. 23:791, 1980.

123. Hamburger, M.I., Moutsopoulos, H.M., Lawley, T.J., and Frank, M.M.: Sjögren's syndrome: A defect in reticuloendothelial system Fc-receptor-specific clearance. Ann. Intern. Med. 91:534, 1979.

124. Meltzer, M., Franklin, F.C., and Eilias, K.: Cryoglobulinemia—a clinical and laboratory study. II. Cryoglobulin with rheumatoid factor activity. Am. J. Med. 40:837, 1966.

125. Zinneman, H.H., and Caperton, E.: Cryoglobulinaemia in a patient with Sjögren's syndrome and factors of cryoprecipitation. J. Lab. Clin. Med. 89:483, 1977.

126. Zinneman, H.H., Levi, D., and Seal, U.S.: On the nature of cryoglobulins. J. Immunol. 100:594, 1968.

127. McIntosh, R.M., Kaufman, D.B., and Kulvinskas, C.: Cryoglobulins. I. Studies on the nature, incidence and clinical significance of serum cryoproteins in glomerulonephritis. J. Lab. Clin. Med. 75:566, 1970.

128. McIntosh, R.M., Kulvinskas, C., and Kaufman, D.B.: Cryoglobulins. II. The biological and chemical properties of cryoproteins in acute poststreptococcal glomerulonephritis. Int. Arch. Allergy 41:700, 1971.

129. Zlotnick, A., Salvin, S., and Eliakim, M.: Mixed cryoglobulinaemia, with a monoclonal IgM component, associated with chronic liver disease. Isr. J. Med. Sci. 8:1968, 1972.

130. Zinneman, H.H., Fromke, V.L., and Seal, U.S.: Some biochemical properties of a cryomacroglobulin. Clin. Chim. Acta 43:91, 1973.

131. Wang, A.C., Wells, J.V., and Fudenberg, H.H.: Chemical analyses of cryoglobulins. Immunochemistry 11:341, 1974.

132. Whitehouse, A.C., Buckley, C.E., Nagaya, H., and McCarter, J.: Mac-

roglobulinaemia and vasculitis in Sjögren's syndrome. Experimental observations relating to pathogenesis. Am. J. Med. 43:609, 1967.

133. Pinkus, G.S., and Dekker, A.: Benign lymphoepithelial lesion of the parotid glands associated with reticulum cell sarcoma. Report of a case and review of the literature. Cancer 25:121, 1970.

134. Wolf, R.O., Ross, M.E., and Rapley, T.M.: Changes in serum salivary isoamylases in Sjögren's syndrome. Am. J. Clin. Pathol. 65:1022, 1976.

135. Bluestone, R., Gumpel, J.M., Goldberg, L.S., and Holborrow, E.J.: Salivary immunoglobulins in Sjögren's syndrome. Int. Arch. Allergy Appl. Immunol. 42:686, 1972.

136. Mach, P.S., Amor, B., Messing, B., Chicault, P., Ghozlan, R., and Deltarre, F.: Salivary immunoglobulin determinations: Their diagnostic value in Sjögren's syndrome. Biomedicine 25:31, 1976.

137. Dunne, J.V., Carson, D.A., Speigelberg, H.L., Alspaugh, M.A., and Vaughn, J.H.: IgA rheumatoid factor in the sera and saliva of patient with rheumatoid arthritis and Sjögren's syndrome. Ann. Rheum. Dis. 38:161, 1979.

138. Anderson, L.G., Cummings, N.A., Asofsky, R., Hylton, M.B., Tarpley, T.M., Tomasi, T.B., Wolf, R.O., Schall, G.L., and Talal, N.: Salivary gland immunoglobulin and rheumatoid factor synthesis in Sjögren's syndrome. Natural history and response to treatment. Am. J. Med. 53:456, 1972.

139. Talal, N., Grey, H.M., and Zvaifler, N.: Elevated salivary and synovial fluid beta-2-microglobulin in Sjögren's syndrome and rheumatoid arthritis. Science 187:1196, 1975.

140. Michalski, J.P., Daniels, T.E., Talal, N., and Grey, H.M.: Beta$_2$ microglobulin and lymphocytic infiltration in Sjögren's syndrome. N. Engl. J. Med. 293:1228, 1975.

141. Moutsopoulos, H.M., Karsh, J., Wolf, R.O., Torpley, T.M., Tylenda, A., and Papadopoulos, N.M.: Lysozyme determination in parotid saliva from patients with Sjögren's syndrome. Am. J. Med. 69:39, 1980.

142. Bunim, J.J., Buchanan, W.W., Wertlake, P.T., Sokoloff, L., Bloch, K.J., Beck, J.S., and Alepa, F.P.: Clinical, pathologic, and serologic studies in Sjögren's syndrome. Combined clinical staff conferences at the National Institutes of Health. Ann. Intern. Med. 61:509, 1964.

143. Torrigiani, G., and Roitt, I.: Antiglobulin factors in sera from patients with rheumatoid arthritis and normal subjects. Quantitative estimation in different immunoglobulin classes. Ann. Rheum. Dis. 26:334, 1967.

144. Torrigiani, G., Ansell, B.M., Chown, E.E., and Roitt, I.M.: Raised IgG antiglobulin factors in Still's disease. Ann. Rheum. Dis. 28:424, 1969.

145. Howell, F.A., Chamberlain, M.A., Perry, R.A., Torrigiani, G., and Roitt, I.: IgG antiglobulin levels in patients with psoriatic arthropathy, ankylosing spondylitis and gout. Ann. Rheum. Dis. 31:129, 1972.

146. Ichikawa, Y.: Rheumatoid arthritis and Sjögren's syndrome. Reprinted from the Papers of the Institute for Thermal Spring Research. Okayama University, No. 42, 1973, pp. 25–29.

147. Beck, J.S., Anderson, J.R., Bloch, K.J., Buchanan, W.W., and Bunim, J.J.: Antinuclear and precipitating autoantibodies in Sjögren's syndrome. Ann. Rheum. Dis. 24:16, 1965.

148. Anderson, J.R., Buchanan, W.W., and Goudie, R.B.: Autoimmunity, Clinical and Experimental. Springfield, Ill., Charles C Thomas, 1967.

149. Baumer, A.: Immunozytologische, Phanomene bei verschidenen rheumatoischen Krankheiten. Z. Rheumaforsch.24:326, 1965.

150. Alspaugh, M.A., Talal, N., and Tan, E.M.: Differentiation and characterization of autoantibodies and their antigens in Sjögren's syndrome. Arthritis Rheum. 19:216, 1976.

151. Alspaugh, M.A., and Tan, E.M.: Antibodies to cellular antigens in Sjögren's syndrome. J. Clin. Invest. 55:1067, 1975.

152. Scopelitis, E., Biundo, J.J., and Alspaugh, M.A.: Anti-SS-A antibody and other nuclear antibodies in systemic lupus erythematosus. Clin. Res. 26:385A, 1978.

153. Wilson, M.R., Arroyave, C.M., Miles, L., and Tan, E.M.: Immune reactants in cryoproteins, relationship to complement activation. Ann. Rheum. Dis. 36:540, 1977.

154. Akizuki, M., Powers, R., and Holman, H.R.: A soluble acidic protein of the cell nucleus which reacts with serum from patients with systemic lupus erythematosus and Sjögren's syndrome. J. Clin. Invest. 59:264, 1977.

155. Kassan, S.S., Akizuki, M., Steinberg, A.D., Reddick, R.L., and Chused, T.M.: Antibody to a soluble acidic nuclear antigen in Sjögren's syndrome. Am. J. Med. 63:328, 1977.

156. Kawanishi, K., Kawamura, K., Nishina, Y., Goto, A., Okada, S., Ishida, T., Ofuji, T., Kahn, C.R., and Flier, J.S.: Successful immunosuppressive therapy in insulin resistant diabetes caused by anti-insulin reception autoantibodies. J. Clin. Endocrinol. Metab. 44:15, 1977.

157. Daha, M.R., Austen, K.F., and Fearon, D.T.: C3 nephritic factor (C3NeF): Heterogeneity, polypeptide chain structure and antigenic reactivity. J. Immunol. 120:1389, 1978.

158. Davis, A.E., III, Gelfand, E.W., Schur, P.H., Rosen, F.S., and Alper, C.A.: IgG subclass studies of C3 nephritic factor. Clin. Immunol. Immunopathol. 11:98, 1978.

159. Schrieber, R.D., and Muller-Eberhard, H.J.: Nephritis factor (T.A.): A

homogeneous immunoglobulin directed toward the complex of C3 and factor B of human complement. J. Immunol. 120: 1796, 1978.

160. Scott, D.M., Amos, N., Sissons, J.G.P., and Peters, D.K.: The immunoglobulin nature of the nephritic factor: NeF activity is found in Fab and Fab$_2$ as well as intact IgG. J. Immunol. 120:1797, 1978.

161. Feltkamp, T.E.W., and Rossum, A.L. van: Antibodies to salivary duct cells, and other autoantibodies, in patients with Sjögren's syndrome and other idiopathic autoimmune diseases. Clin. Exp. Immunol. 3:1, 1968.

162. Rodriguez, J.L., Gelpi, C., Thomson, T.M., Rial, F.J., and Fernandez, J.: Anti-golgi complex autoantibodies in a patient with Sjögren's syndrome and lymphoma. Clin. Exp. Immunol. 49:579, 1982.

163. Bertram, U., and Halberg, P.: A specific antibody against the epithelium of salivary ducts in sera from patients with Sjögren's syndrome. Acta Allerg. 19:458, 1965.

164. MacSween, R.N.M., Goudie, R.B., Anderson J.R., Armstrong, E., Murray, M.A., Mason, D.K., Janani, M.K., Boyle, J.A., Buchanan, W.W., and Williamson, J.: Occurrence of antibody to salivary duct epithelium in Sjögren's disease, rheumatic arthritis and other arthritides. A clinical and laboratory study. Ann. Rheum. Dis. 26:402, 1967.

165. Ludwig, H., Schernthaner, G., Scherak, O., and Kolarz, G.: Antibodies to pancreatic duct cells in Sjögren's syndrome and rheumatoid arthritis. Gut 18:311, 1977.

166. Buchanan, W.W., Harden, R.M., Koutras, D.A., and Gray, K.G.: Abnormalities of iodine metabolism in euthyroid nongoitrous woman with complement-fixing antimicrosomal thyroid autoantibodies. J. Clin. Endocrinol. Metab. 25:301, 1965.

167. Anderson, J.R., Beck, J.S., Buchanan, W.W., Bloch, K.J., and Bunim, J.J.: Sjögren's syndrome and autoimmunity. *In* Baldwin, R.W., and Humphrey, J.H. (eds.): Autoimmunity. A Symposium on the Fifth Congress of the International Academy of Pathology, Oxford, Blackwells, 1965, pp. 453–467.

168. Buchanan, W.W., Boyle, J.A., Greig, W.R., McAndrew, R., Barr, M., Gray, K.G., Anderson, J.R., and Goudie, R.B.: Distribution of certain autoantibodies on monozygotic and dizygotic twins. Ann. Rheum. Dis. 25:463, 1968.

169. Buchanan, W.W., Boyle, J.A., Greig, W.R., McAndrew, R., Barr, M., Gray, K.G., Anderson, J.R., and Goudie, R.B.: Occurrence of autoantibodies in healthy twins. Clin. Exp. Immunol. 2:(Suppl.) 803, 1967.

170. Pirofsky, B.: *In* Autoimmunization and the Autoimmune Hemolytic Anemias. Baltimore, Williams and Wilkins Company, 1969.

171. Sage, R.E., and Forbes, I.J.: A case of multiple autoimmune disease, lymphoid proliferation and hypogammaglobulinemia. Blood 31:536, 1968.

172. Whaley, K., Glen, A.C.A., MacSween, R.N.M., Deodhar, S., Dick, W.C., Nuki, G., Williamson, J., and Buchanan, W.W.: Immunological responses in Sjögren's syndrome and rheumatoid arthritis. Clin. Exp. Immunol. 9:721, 1971.

173. Karsh, J., Palvidis, N., Schiffman, G., and Moutsopoulos, H.M.: Immunization of patients with Sjögren's syndrome with pneumococcal polysaccharide vaccine: A randomized trial. Arthritis Rheum. 23:1294, 1981.

174. Whaley, K., Canesi, B., Moseley, A., Morrow, W., Sturrock, R., Mitchell, W., and Dick, W.C.: Complement metabolism in the sero-negative arthritides. Ann. Rheum. Dis. 33:495, 1974.

175. Leventhal, B.G., Waldorf, D.S., and Talal, N.: Impaired lymphocytic transformation and delayed hypersensitivity in Sjögren's syndrome. J. Clin. Invest. 46:1338, 1967.

176. Williams, R.C., Jr., DeBoard, J.K., Melbye, O.J., Messner, R.P., and Lindstrom, F.D.: Studies of T and B lymphocytes in patients with connective tissue diseases. J. Clin. Invest. 52:283, 1973.

177. Talal, N., Sylvester, R.A., Daniels, T.E., Greenspan, J.S., and Williams, R.C., Jr.: T and B lymphocytes in the peripheral blood and tissue lesions in Sjögren's syndrome. J. Clin. Invest. 53:180, 1974.

178. Fox, R.I., Carstens, S.A., Fong, S., Robinson, C.A., Howell, S.A., and Vaughan, J.H.: Use of monoclonal antibodies to analyze peripheral blood and salivary gland lymphocyte subsets in Sjören's syndrome. Arthritis Rheum. 25:419, 1982.

179. Sauvezie, B., Miyasaka, N., Charron, D., Kielich, C., Loeb, J., Daniels, T.E., and Talal, N.: An increase in peripheral blood Ia-positive T cells in Sjögren's syndrome correlates with a decrease in the autologous mixed lymphocyte response. Clin. Exp. Immunol. 49:50, 1982.

180. Miyasaka, N., Sauvezie, B., Pierce, D.A., Daniels, T.E., and Talal, N.: Decreased autologous mixed lymphocyte reaction in Sjögren's syndrome. J. Clin. Invest. 66:928, 1980.

181. Michalski, J.P., and McCombs, C.: Decreased lymphocyte reactivity to a suboptimal concentration of phytohemagglutinin in Sjögren's syndrome. Arthritis Rheum. 20:851, 1977.

182. Minato, N., Takedo, A., Kauo, S., and Takaku, F.: Studies of the function of natural killer-interferon system in patients with Sjögren's syndrome. J. Clin. Invest. 69:581, 1982.

183. Hooks, J.J., Moutsopoulos, H.M., Geis, S.A., Stahl, H.I., Decker, J.L.,

and Notkins, A.L.: Immune interferon in the circulation of patients with autoimmune disease. N. Engl. J. Med. 301:5, 1979.

184. Moutsopoulos, H., Fye, K.H., Sawada, S., Becker, M.J., Goldstein, A., and Talal, N.: In vitro effect of thymosin on T lymphocyte rosette formation in rheumatic diseases. Clin. Exp. Immunol. 26:563, 1976.

185. Van Boxel, J.A., Hardin, J.A., Green, I., and Paul, W.E.: Multiple heavy-chain determinants on individual B lymphocytes in the peripheral blood of patients with Sjögren's syndrome. N. Engl. J. Med. 289:823, 1973.

186. Fauci, A.S., and Moutsopoulos, H.M.: Polyclonally triggered B cells in the peripheral blood and bone marrow of normal individuals, and in patients with systemic lupus erythematosus and primary Sjögren's syndrome. Arthritis Rheum. 24:577, 1981.

187. Aisenberg, A.C., and Bloch, K.J.: Immunoglobulins in the surface of neoplastic lymphocytes. N. Engl. J. Med. 287:272, 1972.

188. Preud'Homme, J.L., and Seligmann, M.: Surface bound immunoglobulins as a cell marker in human lymphoproliferative diseases. Blood 40:777, 1972.

189. Piessens, W.F., Schur, P.H., and Moloney, W.C.: Lymphocyte surface immunoglobulins: Distribution and frequency in lymphoproliferative diseases. N. Engl. J. Med. 288:176, 1973.

190. Feldmann, J.L., Becker, M.J., Moutsopoulos, H., Fye, K., Blackman, M., Epstein, V., and Talal, N.: Antibody-dependent cell-mediated cytotoxicity in selected autoimmune diseases. J. Clin. Invest. 58:173, 1976.

191. Greenspan, J.S., Gutman, G.A., Weissman, I.L., and Talal, N.: Thymus-antigen and immunoglobulin-positive lymphocytes in tissue infiltrates of NZB/NZW mice. Clin. Immunol. Immunopathol. 3:16, 1974.

192. Berry, H., Bacon, P.A., and Savis, J.D.: Cell-mediated immunity in Sjögren's syndrome. Ann. Rheum. Dis. 31:298, 1972.

193. Cremer, N.E., Daniels, T.E., Oshiro, L.S., Marcus, F., Claypool, R., Sylvester, R.A., and Talal, N.: Immunological and virological studies of cultured labial biopsy cells from patients with Sjögren's syndrome. Clin. Exp. Immunol. 18:213, 1974.

194. McDevitt, H.O., Deak, B.D., Shreffer, D.C., Klein, J., Stimpeling, J.H., and Snell, D.D.: Genetic control of the immune response. Mapping the Ir1 locus. J. Exp. Med. 135:1259, 1972.

195. Cullen, S.E., David, C.S., Cone, J.L., and Sachs, D.H.: Evidence for more than one Ia antigenic speciality on molecules determined by the I-A subregion of the mouse major histocompatibility complex. J. Immunol. 116:549, 1976.

196. Bach, F.H., Widmer, M.B., Bach, M.L., and Klein, J.: Serologically defined and lymphocyte defined components of the major histocompatibility complex in the mouse. J. Exp. Med. 136:1430, 1972.

197. Lozner, E.C., Sachs, D.H., and Shearer, G.M.: B-cell alloantigens determined by the H-2 linked Ir region are associated with mixed lymphocyte culture stimulation. Science 183:757, 1974.

198. Falchuk, Z.M., Rogentine, G.N., and Strober, W.: Predominance of histocompatibility antigen HL-A8 in patients with gluten-sensitive enteropathy. J. Clin. Invest. 51:1602, 1972.

199. Fritze, D., Herrman, C., Jr., and Naeim, F.: HL-A antigens in myasthenia gravis. Lancet 1:240, 1974.

200. Platz, P., Ryder, L., Nielsen, L.S., Svejgaard, A., Thomsen, M., Nerup, J., and Christy, M.: HL-A and idiopathic Addison's disease (letter). Lancet 2:289, 1974.

201. Grumet, F.C., Payne, R.O., Konishi, J., and Kriss, J.: HLA antigens as markers for disease susceptibility and autoimmunity in Graves' disease. J. Clin. Endocrinol. Metab. 39:1115, 1974.

202. Mackay, I.R., and Morris, P.J.: Association of autoimmune active chronic hepatitis with HL-A1, 8. Lancet 2:793, 1972.

203. Nerup, J., Platz, P., Anderson, O.O., Christy, M., Lyngsoe, J., Poulsen, J.E., Ryder, L.P., Nielsen, L.S., Thomsen, W., and Sveygaard, A.: HL-A antigens and diabetes mellitus. Lancet 2:864, 1974.

204. Gershwin, M.E., Terasaki, P.I., and Graw, R.: Increased frequency of HL-A8 Sjögren's syndrome. Tissue Antigens 6:342, 1975.

205. Fye, K.H., Terasaki, P.I., Moutsopoulos, H., Daniels, T.E., Michalski, J.P., and Talal, N.: Association of Sjögren's syndrome with HLA-B8. Arthritis Rheum. 19:883, 1976.

206. Ivanyi, D., Drizhal, I., Erbenova, E., Horejs, J., Salavee, M., Macurova, H., Dostal, C., Balik, J., and Juran, J.: HLA in Sjögren's syndrome. Tissue Antigens 7:45, 1976.

207. Kissmeyer-Nielsen, F. (ed.): Histocompatibility Testing. Copenhagen, Munksgaard, 1972.

208. Keuning, J.J., Pena, A.S., Van Leeuwen, A., Hooff, J.P., and Rood, J.J. van: HLA-DW3 associated with coeliac disease. Lancet 1:506, 1976.

209. Chused, T.M., Kassan, S.S., Opelz, G., Moutsopoulos, H.M., and Terasaki, P.I.: Sjögren's syndrome associated with HLA-DW3. N. Engl. J. Med. 296:895, 1977.

210. Hirzova, E., Ivanyi, D., Sula, K., Horejs, J., Dostal, C., and Drizhal, I.: HLA-DW3 in Sjögren's syndrome. Tissue Antigens 9:8, 1977.

210a. Manthorpe, R., Teppo, A.M., Bendixen, G., and Wegelius, O.: Antibodies to SS-B in chronic inflammatory connective tissue diseases: Relationship with HLA-DW2 and HLA-DW3 in primary Sjögren's syndrome. Arthritis Rheum. 25:662, 1982.

211. Moutsopoulos, H.M., Chused, T.M., Johnson, A.H., Knudsin, B., and

Mann, D.C.: B lymphocyte antigens in sicca syndrome. Science 199:1441, 1978.

212. Burch, J.A., Bunim, J.J., and Bloch, K.T.: Clinical, radiological and serological studies on relatives of patients with Sjögren's syndrome and of patients' neighbours. Arthritis Rheum. 5:104, 1962.

213. Bloch, K.J., and Bunim, J.J.: Sjögren's syndrome and its relationship to connective tissue diseases. J. Chronic Dis. 16:915, 1963.

214. Kessler, H.S.: A laboratory model for Sjögren's syndrome. Am. J. Pathol. 52:671, 1968.

215. Whaley, K., Hughes, G.R.V., and Webb, T.: Systemic lupus erythematosus in animals and man. In Buchanan, W.W., and Dick, W.C. (eds.): Recent Advances in Rheumatology, Vol. 1. Edinburgh, Churchill Livingstone, 1975, pp. 67–136.

216. Shillitoe, E.J., Daniels, T.E., Whitcher, J.D., Vibeke-Strand, C., Talal, N., and Greenspan, J.S.: Antibody to cytomegalovirus in patients with Sjögren's syndrome, as determined by an enzyme-linked immunosorbent assay. Arthritis Rheum. 25:260, 1982.

217. Sutinen, S., Sutinen, S., and Huhti, E.: Ultrastructure of lymphoid interstitial pneumonia. Virus-like particles in bronchiolar epithelium of a patient with Sjögren's syndrome. Am. J. Clin. Pathol. 67:328, 1977.

218. Shearn, M.A., Tu, W.H., Stephens, B.G., and Lee, J.C.: Virus-like structures in Sjögren's syndrome. Lancet 1:568, 1970.

219. Talal, N.: Sjögren's syndrome, lymphoproliferation and renal tubular acidosis. Ann. Intern. Med. 74:633, 1971.

220. Gyorkey, F., Sinkovics, J.G., Min, K.W., and Gyorkey, P.: A morphologic study on the occurrence and distribution of structures resembling viral nucleocapsids in collagen diseases. Am. J. Med. 53:148, 1972.

221. Albegger, K.W., and Auböck, L.: The evidence of "virus-like" inclusions in myoepithelial sialadenitis of Sjögren's syndrome by electron microscopy. Arch. Klin. Exp. Ohren Nasen Kehlkopfheilkd. 203:153, 1972.

222. Daniels, T.E., Sylvester, R.A., Silverman, S., Dolando, V., and Talal, N.: Tubulo-reticular "virus-like" structures within labial salivary glands in patients with Sjögren's syndrome. Arthritis Rheum. 17:593, 1974.

223. Pothier, L., Uzman, B.G., Kasac, H., Saito, H., and Adams, R.A.: Immunoglobulin synthesis and tubular assays in the endoplasmic reticulum in transplanted human tumours of lymphoid origin. Lab. Invest. 259:607, 1973.

224. Whaley, K., Chisholm, D.M., Goudie, R.B., Downie, W.W., Dick, W.C., Boyle, J.A., and Williamson, J.: Salivary duct autoantibody in Sjögren's syndrome: Correlation with focal sialadenitis in the labial mucosa. Clin. Exp. Immunol. 4:273, 1969.

225. Soborg, M., and Bertram, U.: Cellular hypersensitivity in Sjögren's syndrome. Acta Med. Scand. 184:319, 1968.

226. Bertram, N., and Soborg, M.: Nye Immunologiske reaktioner ved Sjögren's syndrome. Tandlaegebladet 74:344, 1970.

227. Talal, N., and Bunim, J.J.: The development of malignant lymphoma in Sjögren's syndrome. Am. J. Med. 36:529, 1964.

228. Bender, B.L., and Jaffe, R.: Immunoglobulin production in lymphomatoid granulomatosis and relation to other "benign" lymphoproliferative disorders. Am. J. Clin. Pathol. 73:41, 1980.

229. Faquet, G.B., Webb, H.H., Agee, J.F., Ricks, W.B., and Sharbaugh, A.H.: Immunologically diagnosed malignancy in Sjögren's pseudolymphoma. Am. J. Med. 65:424, 1978.

230. Kassan, S.S., Hoover, R., and Kimberly, R.P.: Increased incidence of malignancy in Sjögren's syndrome (abstract). Arthritis Rheum. 20:123, 1977.

231. Slater, A., Whittaker, J.A., and Fisher, D.J.H.: Reticulum-cell sarcoma and Sjögren's syndrome in a patient treated with azathioprine (letter). N. Engl. J. Med. 296:51, 1976.

232. Gravanis, S.M.B., and Giansanti, J.S.: Malignant histopathologic counterpart of the benign lymphoepithelial lesion. Cancer 26:1332, 1970.

233. Hyman, G.A., and Wolff, M.: Malignant lymphomas of the salivary glands. Review of the literature and report of 33 new cases, including four cases associated with the lymphoepithelial lesion. Am. J. Clin. Pathol. 65:421, 1976.

234. Kessler, H.S., Cubberly, M., and Manski, W.: Eye changes in autoimmune NZB and NZB × NZW mice. Arch. Ophthalmol. 85:211, 1971.

234a. Carlson, B., and Ostberg, Y.: The autoimmune submandibular sialadenitis of the NZB/NZW hybrid mice. Arch. Otorhinolaryngol. 225:57, 1979.

235. Whaley, K., and MacSween, R.N.M.: Experimental induction of immune sialadenitis in guinea-pigs using different adjuvants. Clin. Exp. Immunol. 17:681, 1974.

236. Williamson, J., Doig, W.M., Forrester, J.V., Whaley, K., and Dick, W.C.: Management of the dry eye in Sjögren's syndrome. Br. J. Ophthalmol. 58:798, 1974.

237. Norn, M.S.: Treatment of keratoconjunctivitis sicca with liquid paraffin or polyvinyl alcohol in double-blind trial. Acta Ophthal. (Kbh) 55:945, 1977.

238. Werblin, T.P., Rheinstrom, S.D., and Kaufman, H.E.: The use of slow-release artificial tears in the longterm management of keratitis sicca. Ophthalmology (Rochester) 88:78, 1981.

239. Williamson, J., Wilson, T., Wallace, J., and Whaley, K.: Studies of the

bacterial flora in keratoconjunctivitis sicca. Eye Ear Nose Throat Monthly 50:257, 1971.

240. Williamson, J., Doig, W.M., Forrester, J.V., Whaley, K., and Dick, W.C.: Studies on the viral flora in keratoconjunctivitis sicca. Br. J. Ophthalmol. 59:45, 1975.

241. Avisar, R., Savir, H., Machtey, I., Ovaknin, L., Shaked, P., Menachie, R., and Allalouf, D.: Clinical trial of bromhexine in Sjögren's syndrome. Ann. Ophthalmol. 13:971, 1981.

242. Frost-Larsen, K., Isager, H., and Manthorpe, R.: Sjögren's syndrome treated with bromhexine: a randomised clinical study. Br. Med. J. 1:1579, 1978.

243. Shannon, I.L., and Edmonds, E.J. Effect of fluoride concentration on rehardening of enamel by a saliva substitute. Int. Dent. J. 28:421, 1978.

244. Klestov, A.C., Webb, J., Latt, D., Schiller, G., McNamara, L., Young, D.Y., Hobbes, J., and Fetherston, J. Treatment of xerostomia: A double-blind trial in 108 patients with Sjögren's syndrome. Oral Surg. 51:594, 1981.

245. Donatsky, O., Johnson, T., Holmstrup, P., and Bertram, U.: Effect of saliment on parotid salivary secretion and on xerostomia caused by Sjögren's syndrome. Scan. J. Dent. Res. 90:157, 1982.

246. Flynn, C.T., Negus, T.W., McHardy, and Rainford, D.J.: Improvement in lacrimal and salivary secretions after alkali therapy in Sjögren's syndrome with renal tubular acidosis. Ann. Rheum. Dis. 35:381, 1976.

247. Lisch, K.: Über hereditäres Vorkommen des mit Keratoconjunctivitis sicca verbundenen Sjögrenschen Symptomenkomplexes. Arch. Augenheilkd. 110:357, 1937.

248. Coverdale, H.: Some unusual cases of Sjögren's syndrome. Br. J. Ophthalmol. 32:669, 1948.

249. Pascucci, F.: La sindrome de Sjögren. Nota 1. Premesse metodo di esame. Contributo casistico. Riv. Crit. Clin. Med. 58:133, 1958.

250. Doni, N., Brancato, R., Bartoletti, L., and Berni, G.: La familiarita delta sindrome di Sjögren. Rev. Crit. Clin. Med. 65:750, 1965.

251. Camus, J.P., Emerit, I., Reinhart, P., Guillien, P., Crouzet, J., and Fourot, J.: Sclerodermie familiale avec syndrome de Sjögren et anomalies lymphocytaises et chromosomiques. Ann. Med. Interne 121:149, 1970.

252. Koivukangas, T., Similä, S., Heikkinen, E., Rasanen, O., and Wasz-Hockert, O.: Sjögren's syndrome and achalasia of the cardia in two siblings. Pediatrics 51:943, 1973.

253. Lichtenfield, J.L., Kirschner, R.H., and Wiernick, P.H.: Familial Sjögren's syndrome with associated primary salivary gland lymphoma. Am. J. Med. 60:286, 1976.

254. Frayha, R.A., Tabbara, K.F., and Geha, R.S.: Familial CRST syndrome with sicca complex. J. Rheumatol. 4:53, 1978.

255. Vaillant, J.M., Laudanbach, P., Schuller, E., Muller, J.Y., and Deboise, A.: Gougerot-Sjögren syndrome in two univitelline twin sisters. Ann. Med. Interne 132:408, 1981.

256. Rothman, S., Blocky, M., and Hauser, F.V.: Sjögren's syndrome associated with lymphoblastoma and hypersplenism. Arch. Derm. Syph. 63:642, 1951.

257. Hornbaker, J.H., Jr., Foster, E.A., Williams, G.S., and Davis, J.S.: Sjögren's syndrome and nodular reticulum cell sarcoma. Arch. Intern. Med. 118:449, 1966.

258. Miller, D.G.: The association of immune disease and malignant lymphoma. Ann. Intern. Med. 66:507, 1967.

259. Bark, C.J., and Perzik, S.L.: Mikulicz's disease, sialoangiectasis and autoimmunity based upon a study of parotid lesions. Am. J. Clin. Pathol. 49:683, 1968.

260. Bilder, J., and Hornova, J.: Lymfosarkom přiušní žlázy při Sjögrenově syndromu. Cesk. Stomat. 67:441, 1967.

261. Thorpe, P.: Polymyalgia rheumatica: A not so benign syndrome. Med. J. Aust. 2:678, 1969.

262. Senti-Parades, A., Canedo-Acea, R., Pulido-Ledesma, R., Borrajero, I., and Delgado, B.: Reporte de un caso de sindrome de Sjögren-Mikulicz. Rev. Cuba Med. 3:560, 1964.

263. Yoshinaga, T.: Two cases of Sjögren's syndrome with malignant tumour. Jap. J. Clin. Med. 26:2161, 1968.

264. Lattes, R.: Thymoma and other tumors of the thymus. Cancer 15:1224, 1962.

265. Dourov, N., Sternon, J., de Coster, A., and Chailly, P.: Thymome malin, myasthénie, thyröidite, syndrome de Gougerot-Sjögren bloc alvéolo-capillaire. A propos de in cas. Ann. Anat. Path. 13:201, 1968.

266. Alarcon-Segovia, D., and Zavala-Mejia, J.L.: Sindrome de Sjögren associado a timoma. Rev. Invest. Clin. 23:133, 1971.

267. Maleville, J., Heid, F., Rousselot, P., Bergoend, H., Grosshans, E., and Aroujo, A.: Purpura dysglobulinémique et syndrome de Gougerot-Sjögren. Révélation ultérieure d'une réticulose maligne à tendance plasmocytaire. Bull. Soc. Franc. Derm. Syph. 74:696, 1967.

268. Wager, O., Rasanen, J.A., and Lindenberg, L.: Cited by Shearn.[2]

269. Azzopardi, J.G., and Evans, D.J.: Malignant lymphoma of parotid associated with Mikulicz disease (benign lymphoepithelial lesion). J. Clin. Pathol. 24:744, 1971.

270. Delaney, W.E., and Balogh, K., Jr.: Carcinoma of the parotid gland associated with benign lymphoepithelial lesion (Mikulicz's disease) in Sjögren's syndrome. Cancer 19:853, 1966.

Chapter 63

The Management of Rheumatoid Arthritis

Shaun Ruddy

INTRODUCTION

Few diagnoses arouse more anxiety in both patient and physician than rheumatoid arthritis. Misapprehensions about the tractability and prognosis of this disease are common among both laity and medical professionals. The patient recalls a family member who, perhaps years ago, was afflicted with a severe crippling form of arthritis and wonders when she* will become similarly disabled. If she has been referred to a rheumatologist, she looks around the waiting room and sees patients with very active, progressive, and deforming disease who have been selected for referral precisely because of the extreme severity of their disease. As for the physician, very likely he or she was exposed to relatively little information about rheumatic diseases during medical school years; and, because most patients with rheumatoid arthritis are managed as outpatients, to relatively little training during hospital internship and residency. Like the patient, the physician also may selectively recall one or two patients with severe, active, and progressive disease who failed to respond to all of the treatment modalities available. And yet such pessimism is usually unwarranted. As illustrated in Chapter 60, rheumatoid arthritis is, in the majority of instances, a disease with a good prognosis. Most patients have gratifying responses to treatment, albeit not the immediate response measured in hours, or days seen with acute illnesses such as pneumococcal pneumonia. Even in the minority of patients whose response to treatment would be judged less than completely satisfactory, appropriate therapeutic measures usually allow them to continue to function harmoniously with their environment.

This chapter will outline the general approach for the prospective and aggressive management of rheumatoid arthritis. Detailed consideration of individual therapeutic modalities applicable to rheumatoid arthritis is given in 19 other chapters of this text. Table 63-1 provides a guide to the information contained in these chapters. Before proceeding to detailed considerations of the various aspects of the management of rheumatoid arthritis, a few general principles are worthy of emphasis.

1. *The time course of rheumatoid arthritis is measured in months and years.*[1] Although a few patients will experience brief, apparently self-limited episodes of ar-

thritis which do not recur, most will have had their disease for a prolonged period of time when initially seen by the physician, and most can be expected to have it, albeit in a moderate or reduced form, for months or even years to come.[2] One corollary of this extended time frame is that there need be no rush to make the diagnosis of rheumatoid arthritis, with all the attendant anxieties and fears it engenders. If the diagnosis is immediately obvious and inescapable from the history and physical examination, there is no sense in delaying and much to be gained in terms of patient trust and understanding by a forthright and honest exposition of the diagnosis. If, as is frequently the case, insufficient criteria are present for a firm diagnosis, it is perhaps wiser to institute conservative treatment and employ a label such as "polyarthritis of unknown etiology" until the disease declares itself or regresses.[3] Since treatment at this early stage would not likely be influenced by the use of a specific diagnostic category, little is to be gained by employing one which is uncertain and likely to be emotionally troublesome for the patient and her family.

A second corollary of the lengthy time course of rheumatoid arthritis involves the expectations of both patient and physician for the immediacy of response to therapy.

Table 63–1. Other Chapters in the Textbook of Rheumatology Relating to the Management of Rheumatoid Arthritis

Chapter Number	Topic
24	Examination of the joints
34	Psychological and sexual aspects
35	Ocular manifestations
36	Cutaneous manifestations
37	Aspiration and injection of joints
49	Salicylates
50	Nonsteroidal anti-inflammatory drugs
51	Antimalarials
52	Gold compounds
53	D-Penicillamine
54	Glucocorticoids
55	Immunoregulatory agents
111	Rehabilitation
113	Synovectomy
114	Hand surgery
115	Elbow surgery
116	Shoulder surgery
117	Knee surgery
118	Ankle and foot surgery
120	Hip surgery

---

*The feminine gender is used throughout this chapter to refer to patients because most patients with rheumatoid arthritis are women.

Rheumatologists, in particular, are often visited by patients with severe and progressive disease who believe that their multiple sore joints will forthwith be soothed and remedied, now that they have found a "specialist" in their disease. Even referring physicians find it difficult to accept the notion that it may be necessary to administer a potentially very toxic agent such as gold salts or penicillamine for up to 6 months before a decision about its effectiveness for a particular patient can be made with assurance. In both cases, it is helpful to point out that the patient has had months or even years to reach her present condition, and that it is reasonable to expect that it will take a long time to reverse the process. Fortunately, immediate institution of supportive measures often results in significant diminution of pain and improvement in function and sense of well-being, which convinces the patient that the course of her disease is at least going in the right direction.

2. *The extent and intensity of rheumatoid arthritis are highly variable.* As discussed in detail in Chapter 60, this variation applies both between different patients and between different times in the same patient. Notwithstanding the prognostic indicators mentioned in Chapter 60, which are most useful when large numbers of patients are involved, it is extremely difficult to prognosticate for an individual patient, particularly early in the disease.[3] As a rule, the best indication of how the disease will progress for an individual patient is the history of the disease in that patient previously. Most patients do not need to be told that their disease is one of remissions and exacerbations over time; they have learned this from experience. Surprisingly, however, not as many realize the implications of this variation in time for the assessment of therapy. It is often helpful to point out that, in a disease that gets better or worse on its own, it will sometimes be difficult for either doctor or patient to determine whether a particular form of treatment has been effective for her or whether the improvement may have been a coincidence. Reasoning from this, patients are usually able to understand how a particular remedy widely accepted as efficacious for the treatment of arthritis may not be of any real or lasting benefit. Conversely, patients may recognize the need for careful scientific evaluation of efficacy of new agents and be willing to participate in experiments designed for such evaluations.

3. *Optimal management of rheumatoid arthritis requires the combined efforts of multiple members of a health-care team.* The reverse of this statement is that no one individual is capable of meeting all the health-care needs of a patient with rheumatoid arthritis. While the administration of drugs has a central role in the treatment program, the prescription of one or more pharmaceutical agents by a physician represents only a fraction of the treatment modalities that can and should be involved. Depending upon the patient's individual problems, as many as a dozen different other health-care professionals may be required (Table 63–2).[4] Their function will be detailed later in this chapter. At any

Table 63–2. Members of the Arthritis Health-Care Team

Patient
Family physician
Rheumatologist
Orthopedist
Nurse specialist or nurse practitioner
Occupational therapist
Physical therapist
Rehabilitation or vocational counselor
Psychologist, sex therapist
Social worker
Pharmacist
Nutritionist
Clergy
Community agencies

one time a number of these individuals will be interacting with both the patient and those in her environment, including family, friends, social agencies, employers, and even the government. This web of interactions requires constant and close attention to communication between the participating individuals; like everyone else, patients have a way of filtering out that which they do not wish to hear and focusing on that which they do. Conflicting reports or advice, either real or imagined, may be received from different members of the team. One individual, therefore, needs to accept primary responsibility for relating to the patient and to function as the center of communications with the patient, avoiding the distortions or misinformation that may otherwise be introduced into the system. In many instances, this role may be filled by the patient's family physician; in others, a nurse practitioner or other allied health professional may serve this function. In all cases, it is incumbent upon the other members of the team to maintain close contact with this individual, preferably by direct verbal communication on a frequent basis. The ideal mechanism for fostering such communication is the case conference, where all members of the team involved in the care of an individual patient are able to meet and share their views of the patient's problems and progress.

GOALS OF MANAGEMENT

Proper management of rheumatoid arthritis results in the maintenance or restoration of the patient to a state of useful and harmonious function with her environment for the foreseeable future. Implicit is the relief of pain, the prevention of joint destruction, and the preservation or improvement of the patient's functioning. Since some remedies, e.g., systemic corticosteroids, may superficially accomplish the first of these goals, the provision of prolonged relief has been included.

Translation of these lofty and somewhat vague goals into specific ones for a particular patient defines the art of clinical rheumatology. Understanding by the patient, and members of the arthritis health care team of realistic therapeutic goals is the basis for a satisfactory outcome.[5]

In response to a few open-ended questions, usually the patient can outline appropriate solutions for her particular life problems. Even the most rudimentary inquiries into disability produced by rheumatoid arthritis often evince very definite responses from patients. After questioning the patient about her ability to function in her occupation, and establishing a rapport, the interviewer may focus on particular goals with such simple questions as: "What is one thing that you cannot do, that you would most like to do?" or "What is the major problem which led you to come here for medical care?" The tone of the question should not exclude multiple responses, but if these are offered, priorities need to be settled. Once such information has been elicited, definition of the patient's goals is greatly simplified; the realism of such goals is usually most fruitfully assessed by a conference among the health professionals who have met with the patient. In such a meeting, the relation between the patient's views of her needs and those that she can realistically be expected to accomplish can be weighed against the risks of various therapeutic options. Consider, for example, the 58-year-old concert cellist who develops rheumatoid arthritis at the height of her career and needs a few more years of active finger movement at the expense of aggressive corticosteroid and, possibly, immunosuppressive therapy. Against that, consider the 30-year-old heiress whose most important activity is communicating her judgment about investments to her employees; in this instance, a much more conservative approach might be warranted. Alternatively, the cellist may be grateful for an opportunity to retire, and the heiress may have been diligently perfecting her tennis serve in order to compete in the professional circuit. In such instances, goals of therapy would be entirely reversed and, with them, the acceptable risks of therapy.

SUPPORTIVE MEASURES

Patient Education. Once the diagnosis of rheumatoid arthritis has been made, the physician begins the process of informing the patient about her disease[6] (see Chapters 34 and 111). Education continues in time for the duration of active disease, and extends from the initial physician contact to involve many other members of the health care team. The form that the education takes usually involves a mixture of techniques. Certainly direct question and answer sessions between patient and physician, nurse practitioner, physical or occupational therapist, rehabilitation counselor, social worker, pharmacist, or even another patient with arthritis will be frequently employed. Some individuals are more at ease when acquiring their information by reading or watching a film or other instructional material, and for these, excellent literature is prepared and distributed by the Arthritis Foundation[7,8] and some hospitals provide appropriate audiovisual aids. Excellent monographs written for arthritis patients are also available.[9] Group in-

structional sessions, in which a particular topic of general interest to patients with arthritis is discussed, often prove to be extremely popular, perhaps because they afford an environment in which patients can share their embarrassment or anxiety about their disease.[10] Such group sessions may be conducted under the aegis of a hospital clinic, may be organized by a local chapter of the Arthritis Foundation or other social agency, or may even be structured as self-help classes completely independently by patients themselves.

The content of educational efforts should be designed to (1) provide basic information to the patient, (2) reinforce the physician's or other therapist's instructions to the patient, (3) help the patient in effecting appropriate behavioral changes, and (4) lend emotional support. Whenever possible an encouraging, active, aggressive approach toward the disease should be fostered in place of the "there's nothing that can be done and I'll just have to live with it" passive attitude into which patients sometimes are allowed to slip. A great deal can be done about rheumatoid arthritis, and, more often than not, the prognosis is for a favorable outcome. Once patients are informed of this, their ability to cooperate in treatment regimens is greatly enhanced. The listing of the patient as a primary member of the arthritis health-care team in Table 63-2 exemplifies this. Without making the patient feel guilty *for* her disease, it should be possible to make her responsible *about* it. Very early in the treatment program, the patient needs to understand that her disease has no known cause, and that in no way were errors of either commission or omission by her responsible for the development of the disease. Conversely, she needs to understand that her behavior and participation in the treatment program can very much influence the outcome.

Some of the areas that must be dealt with in any educational program are listed in Table 63-3. In most instances it will be obvious which member of the health care team will assume responsibility for a particular area. One of the most disquieting facts for the patient with rheumatoid arthritis to accept is that the cause of the disease remains unknown (see Chapter 58). Many patients infer from this that there is no effective treatment. A frontal approach to this issue is often helpful, citing examples of other diseases with unknown causes for which effective, even curative therapies exist. The patient should also be taught that maintenance of function when the disease is active will allow continued function for the years when it may become quiescent. When specifically discussed in advance, the concepts of intermittent activity and extended time frame may prevent dissatisfaction with the lack of immediate results or even a sudden worsening following the institution of a particular treatment. Knowledge that rheumatoid arthritis affects the entire body, not merely the joints, may allow the patient to accept the overwhelming fatigue, malaise, and weight loss, which she might otherwise attribute to some other cause.

The more the patient understands about treatment,

Table 63–3. Educational Topics for Patients with Rheumatoid Arthritis

I. Nature of basic disease process
    Joint anatomy and physiology
    Unknown cause
    Intermittent activity
    Extended time frame
    A systemic illness, not merely sore joints
II. Treatment
    Difficulty of assessing responses in intermittent disease
    Prevalence and avoidance of quack remedies
    Distinction between pain relief and reduction of inflammation
    Distinction between immediate anti-inflammatory effects and long-term remission
    Availability of multiple therapeutic agents (including surgery)
    Importance of follow-up
III. Behavior modification
    Importance of rest
    Exercise regimen to maintain function
    Usefulness of joint protection techniques and devices
    Proper nutrition and avoidance of weight gain
    Job modification or counseling
IV. Emotional support
    Alleviation of guilt; absence of precipitating factors or activity
    Absence of clinically important genetic factors
    Alterations in body image
    Diminished sexual libido or physical difficulties in performance
    Involvement of family

the more likely is she to cooperate to her fullest extent. Most patients will easily grasp the distinction between an analgesic, which merely relieves (or often only dulls) the pain of a sore joint, and an anti-inflammatory agent, which actually reduces the redness, heat, and swelling in conjunction with relieving the pain.[11] Similarly, most patients understand how foolish it is to purchase relatively expensive and widely advertised "special arthritis pills" when told that the major active ingredient in such nostrums is aspirin, which they might already be taking at a fraction of the cost. Even the more subtle difference between an anti-inflammatory agent, which takes effect in a few days or a week or two,[12] and a suppressive or remission-inducing agent, whose full effect may not be apparent for months,[13,14] can be made clear to the patient through iterative and graded instructional techniques. Most will quickly understand the difference between the apparently miraculous disappearance of symptoms afforded by systemic steroids and the relentless progression of joint destruction that occurs despite the feeling of well-being these drugs engender.[15]

With regard to particular drugs or other therapeutic regimens, careful and specific instructions about potential side effects or complications may make the difference between patient acceptance of the agent and refusal to take a drug at the first sign of unexpected nausea or lightheadedness. Because such effects may be multiple and complex and, therefore, difficult to remember when communicated verbally from physician to patient, reinforcement or relearning of these effects become very

important. Many clinics find printed take-home literature about side effects of a particular agent convenient. Review of the major untoward effects by the pharmacist when he provides the prescription is another useful mode of reinforcement, as is the use of a follow-up visit with an arthritis nurse specialist or nurse practitioner specifically for drug review. Ideally, the patient should be familiar with each of the drugs, its dosage, and possible side effects. Parenthetically, one side effect insufficiently discussed is the cost of the medicines. Compliance may be improved if the physician points out that $1.00 is a great deal of money to pay for a single tablet, and then explains why this expenditure is appropriate for the patient's particular circumstances.

Almost all patients with rheumatoid arthritis will find it necessary to modify their behavior to reach an equilibrium with their disease. The specific ways in which this may need to be accomplished will be detailed below.

To a large measure, supportive emotional therapy consists of sympathetic listening. The patient needs to be able to discuss her feelings of guilt—"What did I do to deserve this disease?"—her concerns about passing it on to other members of her family, and her inability to function completely satisfactorily in her role as employee, mother, or wife. In the area of altered body image or sexual function, a few open-ended questions may elicit the expression of great emotional concern which the patient might not otherwise have volunteered[16] (see Chapter 34). A conscious effort to raise such questions must be made by the therapist, since these areas are easily neglected, sometimes because of the therapist's own discomfort in discussing them. Depending upon the particular problem, referral to another member of the health care team who has a special interest in the area in question may be advisable.

Education of the immediate family in almost every area outlined in Table 63–3 is extremely important. If the family understands that the patient has a systemic disease, they will more readily accept the need for an enforced rest period in mid-afternoon, the need for help with the heavy housework, and other modifications in the patient's environment. Open communication between family and patient about ways in which the disease has impinged on family life is fostered by including the family in discussion groups or interviews with physicians or other members of the arthritis team whenever possible. The fine line between a supportive and helpful family attitude and an oversolicitous one in which the patient is made a self-conscious invalid requires constant monitoring. Every rheumatologist or orthopedist can relate stories about patients with rheumatoid arthritis who are brought to the hospital with severe flexion deformities and muscle atrophy, having been immobilized in bed some 5 years earlier by a well-meaning family.

Rest. In part the much debated question of the value of rest in the treatment of rheumatoid arthritis is moot, since most patients will adopt some form of rest irrespective of any advice from their physicians. In fact, the frequency of affirmative responses to the question, "Do you take a nap in the afternoon?" is sufficiently high as to be useful in the diagnosis of rheumatoid arthritis. Even though they may sleep well at night, patients with rheumatoid arthritis will often describe fatigue occurring abruptly and at a reproducible time during their daily activities.[17] Prescription of an hour's nap just prior to such a period may lead to significant improvement in symptoms for the remainder of the day. Despite its reliability as a symptom in rheumatoid arthritis and the advisability of preventing it, the mechanisms causing fatigue which accompanies active disease have eluded scientific understanding.

While most would agree about the virtues of modifying daily activities so as to include rest periods, and while there is strong evidence of the efficacy of rest or immobilization of individual joints in reducing inflammation (discussed below), the value of complete bed rest as a therapeutic adjunct in the treatment of rheumatoid arthritis remains controversial. In one study patients were randomly placed on a regimen of 18 to 22 hours of enforced bed rest per day or one of 8 hours per night with ad lib daytime activities; no significant difference after 10 weeks[18] was noted. Comparison of the effects of bed rest versus planned activity demonstrated only marginal advantage for bed rest.[18] When patients hospitalized for enforced rest were compared with outpatients, however, significant improvements in hospitalized groups were observed.[19] While acknowledging the absence of any rigidly controlled body of scientific evidence, most rheumatologists do favor enforced bed rest for patients with severe disease, prolonged morning stiffness, and involvement of many joints, particularly the weight-bearing ones. Further, most would recommend that such treatment be carried out in a hospital setting. The advantages of such an arrangement are multiple. It allows removal of the patient from the stressful setting in which she must attempt to cope with her daily activities as well as active disease, and it provides an environment in which rest is viewed as a goal rather than something to feel guilty about. Daily contact with the physician and other members of the arthritis team allows progressive patient education. Institution of physical therapy and other local measures usually unavailable at home often alleviates particular problems (e.g., the use of hot packs on arising often greatly reduces the symptoms of morning stiffness). The antiphogistic effect of enforced bed rest allows sufficient time for anti-inflammatory medications to begin to take effect, and the hospital environment ensures compliance with the prescribed medication routine. Sometimes the mere fact of hospitalization convinces an unconcerned family that the patient does indeed have a serious disease. The combined effect of all these benefits is often dramatic. Within a week or two, the patient is often feeling remarkably improved and is convinced that the physician and the arthritis team can exert some control over her disease, and her mental attitude often borders on the euphoric.[19] In fact, at this point, it may be wise to point out to the patient that the remarkable improvement is the result of being in an environment that greatly favors her well-being, and that maintenance of the complete extent of improvement should not be expected when she returns to her original environment, irrespective of how modified that may be. Without such a warning, the patient may be surprised and disappointed as some of her symptoms reappear when she returns home to re-enter a more active life.

One consequence of the rapidly rising costs of hospital care is the reticence of physicians to hospitalize patients for severe arthritis. With average costs now counted in hundreds of dollars daily, it becomes increasingly difficult to justify hospitalizing a patient with rheumatoid arthritis for assessment of the extent of the disease, enforced bed rest, institution of physical modalities, and drug therapy. Further, in today's acute care facility, the patient with rheumatoid arthritis who does not appear to have a life-threatening illness may be neglected by a busy hospital staff occupied in attempting the resuscitation of the patient in the adjacent bed from a fatal ventricular arrhythmia. Nonetheless, hospitalization in an acute-care facility may be of dramatic benefit, particularly when the physician or other members of the arthritis team take care to orient hospital staff to the specific needs of their patient. An optimal hospital program includes specially trained personnel and accommodations for dealing with the special problems presented by patients with disabling arthritis.

Exercise and Physical Therapy. Although it is difficult to demonstrate any long-term benefits from the use of physical modalities such as heat or hydrotherapy, such treatments definitely have a soothing effect on the patient's discomfort. Hot packs, warm baths, or showers on arising often dispel morning stiffness more rapidly. In a hospital setting, immersion in a Hubbard tank may be even more effective. The use of a paraffin bath for the relief of hand stiffness can be learned by the patient and employed at home. The rationale for these modalities is discussed in Chapter 111.

Apart from the improved sense of well-being for the patient, the purpose of the soothing, loosening, analgesic properties of heat and hydrotherapy is to allow sufficient relief of pain and spasm to permit each joint to go through a full range of motion and to permit muscle strengthening exercises.[20,21] In severely affected joints, especially those that may have been temporarily immobilized by casting, gentle passive range of motion by a skilled therapist may be required at least twice daily to maintain motion. The gentleness and skill with which such maneuvers must be performed deserves emphasis; vigorous passive range of motion may do more harm than good by overstretching ligamentous structures or, rarely, even by fracture through the shaft of an osteoporotic bone.

The most commonly employed form of physical therapy is active assisted exercise. In this instance, the patient initiates a particular motion and the therapist assists her in continuing it to its limit. Gradual increase in the limits of motion often results, and gradual reduction in the amount of assistance from the therapist eventually permits the patient to carry the joint through its range of motion unassisted. In this regard, assistance from devices such as pulleys or weights may be used by the patient to substitute for the therapist. A pulley attached to a door frame, which assists elevation and abduction of one shoulder by using the weight of the opposite limb as a controlled counterbalance, is a common example of such a device. Taking advantage of the buoyant effect of water to relieve weight, either in a specially designed hydrotherapy pool or in a plain swimming pool, is another means of assisting active exercise. In the case of the swimming pool, special devices may be required to allow convenient entry and exit by handicapped patients.

An active exercise program at home, in which all the patient's joints are put through a complete range of motion daily, is an integral part of the management of any patient with rheumatoid arthritis. The patient should be trained in this regimen, preferably using written instructions or diagrams, and its continuation should be reinforced periodically by follow-up visits with the therapist. The value of such a regimen in maintaining muscle tone and joint mobility, even in unaffected joints, requires emphasis by the physician or other member of the team who has primary contact with the patient. Specific inquiry as to whether the exercise program is continuing to be followed should be included frequently in routine follow-up visits.[22]

There is a contradiction inherent in recommending rest as a useful form of therapy and simultaneously insisting on exercise, and many patients will be confused by and call attention to this dichotomy. To a certain extent, judgments about rest and exercise will represent a compromise in which the patient should actively participate. Dependent patients will often demand specific prohibitions or encouragements of activity or rest from physicians. Most often it is wisest to let the patient judge for herself, using some common sense guides. Mechanical irritation of a joint already inflamed by rheumatoid arthritis only makes it more inflamed, and the patient whose knees are warm, grossly swollen, and much more painful on the morning after a night of dancing can appreciate this principle. No specific prohibition should be needed, merely an admonition to use common sense.

Although there may be controversy about the usefulness of complete bed rest in the treatment of rheumatoid arthritis, there is widespread agreement about the utility of local joint rest. Naturally enforced rest, such as paralysis of an extremity from a stroke,[23] poliomyelitis,[24] or a peripheral nerve lesion,[25] usually results in sparing of the paralyzed joints in patients who subsequently develop rheumatoid arthritis. In a study of 153 patients with rheumatoid arthritis, the degree of radiographically detectable erosions of the wrist was positively correlated with the degree of physical activity of the joint.[26] Physical therapists (and occupational therapists as well) play an important role in providing appliances to permit such rest and in instructing patients

in their use. By using bivalved or functional splints, a certain amount of mobility can be maintained, while at the same time providing partial rest to the involved joints.[27] A good example is the lightweight thermoplastic splint to the volar surface of the forearm, which allows motion at the metacarpophalangeal joints and distally but supports the wrist (see Chapter 111). Use of such splints nightly may make the difference between a good night's sleep and one of constant reawakening. Nocturnal splinting of the knees may also be used if on awakening the patient is troubled by marked stiffness and flexion contractures. Apart from the pain relief that the use of such splints may afford, actual diminution in the extent and severity of the synovitis may be observed.[28]

Occupational Therapy and Rehabilitation. A rudimentary assessment of the patient's functional capacity should be conducted by the physician in the initial evaluation of the patient. Consideration of the patient's relationship to those about her and the demands of her life will influence decisions about therapy, and the physician should have some knowledge of these factors. A much more detailed and meaningful analysis of the interaction between the patient and her environment can usually be accomplished by an occupational therapist, who has had special training in methods for such analysis. A verbal review of the activities of daily living will often reveal difficulties that can be remedied with readily available assistive devices. General principles of joint protection, e.g., sitting instead of standing, can be taught. Observation of the patient at work, either in a simulated environment, e.g., kitchen, carpentry shop, print shop, or directly in the home or on the job, may indicate unique problems requiring the construction of special appliances designed to deal with the problem. Attention to such details may make the difference between dependence and independence or between disability and keeping a job.[29,30]

Counseling about employment is a very important aspect of the management of rheumatoid arthritis. One of the major goals is the maintenance of useful vocational or domestic function; too often considerable loss of self-esteem accompanies the acceptance of disability. Interaction with a vocational or rehabilitation counselor needs to be begun early in the contact with the patient so that decisions regarding long-term outlook for continued employment can be arrived at gradually and realistically. While retraining of each patient into a position particularly adapted to her joint problems is an ideal goal, such a solution is the ideal rather than the norm. On the other hand, vocational counselors often prevent disability by identifying and removing impediments to work that are unrelated to the actual performance of the job itself, e.g., transportation to and from work. As an alternative, the patient can be helped to accept partial disability in a supportive yet realistic way. Time available from an early retirement may be focused on a useful avocation, for example. An imaginative approach to rehabilitation can prevent the loss of self-image, identity, and self-esteem and yet help the patient to accept realistically those functional impairments resulting from disease.

RELIEF OF PAIN

The choice of methods for reducing or relieving pain in joints of patients with rheumatoid arthritis requires a decision about the cause of the pain. The pain at rest in a joint with very active synovitis is caused by mechanisms very different from the pain with motion or weightbearing in a joint that has suffered severe structural damage from years of rheumatoid arthritis. Methods for the assessment of activity of disease have been discussed in Chapter 60. In addition to the commonly used indices such as length of morning stiffness, number of painful joints, number of swollen joints, grip strength, time for 50-foot walk, and erythrocyte sedimentation rate,[31] certain other symptoms or signs may provide useful clues to activity. Pain at rest, particularly at night, often indicates active synovitis. Systemic symptoms, including anorexia, weight loss, fever, or development of new nodules, are also quite reliable indices of activity.

If the pain is attributable to active synovitis, then the most effective agents for pain relief, in the long term, will be those designed to reduce the activity of the disease. If the pain is attributable to structural problems, then judicious use of analgesics, local measures such as immobilization, and, if necessary, surgery will be the most appropriate forms of pain relief.[32,33]

For the patient with severe and active synovitis, the advantages of hospitalization have already been discussed.[17-19] If the patient is already on an optimal anti-inflammatory regimen, further transient restriction of mobility may suffice. For the patient with a severe exacerbation, the proper course is usually a sympathetic and attentive interview followed by a thorough examination of the joints. The attempt is to identify one or two joints that are most inflamed and the major sources of complaints. If a single joint is extraordinarily hot, swollen, and very painful, the diagnosis of septic arthritis, which is more prevalent in rheumatoid joints, should be considered. Examination of fluid for crystals may reveal coincident gout or pseudogout. In the absence of such unusual circumstances, local measures directed at relieving the most severe joints, e.g., splints or local steroid injections, may be helpful.

Analgesics per se are not usually very effective in treating the pain of rheumatoid arthritis. The sympathetic physician will wish to do his utmost to relieve pain, but he must eventually realize and come to terms with the fact that, in the presence of active synovitis, his success will be limited.[34] Aspirin and the other nonsteroidal anti-inflammatory agents have analgesic effects in addition to their anti-inflammatory action, but the substitution of an agent with an equipotent analgesic effect but no anti-inflammatory effect usually results in much less satisfactory control of the arthritis and its accompanying pain. Occasional patients will experience

significant relief from propoxyphene or codeine, but most will either derive no benefit or complain of the dulled sensorium or other side effects these drugs induce. Much the same can be said for the stronger narcotic analgesics, whose use in a chronic disease such as rheumatoid arthritis is not recommended for obvious reasons. Such agents should not be withheld for the relief of other self-limited forms of pain, such as that associated with myocardial infarction, or, with a pathologic fracture of a long bone, but they should not be used for the pain of the arthritis in which an immediate improvement in the cause of the pain is not expected.

ANTI-INFLAMMATORY DRUGS

Aspirin. As indicated previously, patients readily understand the difference between drugs that simply reduce pain and those that reduce warmth, swelling, stiffness, and pain of inflammatory arthritis. Similarly, they are able to distinguish between the small amounts of aspirin all of us take for minor aches and pains and the very large amounts required for lessening the inflammation of rheumatoid arthritis. Emphasis on this distinction allows the patient to think of aspirin in a special way and prevents the "all he did was tell me to take some aspirin" reaction, which may otherwise occur. The appropriate drug for the initial treatment of rheumatoid arthritis is aspirin in sufficient dosage to achieve blood levels of greater than 20 mg per deciliter. Plain aspirin tablets are cheapest, and the best formulation with which to begin, though buffered, enteric-coated, or other salicylates may be used if necessary.[35] The only absolute contraindications are a history of severe gastrointestinal bleeding following previous aspirin administration or a history of asthma and nasal polyposis indicative of an idiosyncratic reaction to the drug.[36] Usually a dose of 0.9 g four times a day, with meal and at bedtime with a snack, is a useful starting dose. Patients are warned about tinnitus and are told that the optimal dose for them is going to be slightly less than that which causes tinnitus. From the initial dose of 12 tablets daily, the number is increased by one or two tablets a week until tinnitus is achieved, and then a dose slightly less than this is maintained after an appropriate halt in therapy to allow the cessation of tinnitus. In adjusting the dose, the physician must be aware that at high blood levels the pharmacokinetics of aspirin are those of a saturable enzyme system (see Chapters 48 and 49) so that the half-life is effectively quite prolonged and a week may be required to achieve a new steady-state blood level following a change in dosage.[37] In using tinnitus as a guide to dosage, the physician should also be aware that it is unreliable as a first sign of toxicity in children, in whom much more serious and potentially fatal metabolic disturbances may occur in the absence of tinnitus. In contrast, in the elderly gradual diminution in auditory acuity, reversible with cessation of therapy, may occur instead of tinnitus,[28] or tinnitus may occur at levels well below 20 mg per deciliter. In both instances, or in cases in which compliance is in question, measurement of the serum salicylate level is an inexpensive and reliable way to monitor dosage.

A certain firmness and persistence are required of the physician in order to be certain that aspirin has been given an adequate therapeutic trial. As a rule, in early rheumatoid arthritis, aspirin should be the only agent used initially. Often this has the salutary effect of convincing the patient of its efficacy. While small increases in gastrointestinal blood loss are common,[39] severe gastrointestinal hemorrhage fortunately is not. Further, there is no evidence relating dyspepsia following aspirin ingestion to the occurrence of severe hemorrhage. Thousands of patients have taken tons of aspirin over many years, and this agent remains the least expensive and perhaps the least toxic of any available for the treatment of rheumatoid arthritis. It is therefore worth tinkering with the dose form, timing of administration, and type of preparation used before giving up on aspirin and moving on to another agent which may be no more effective, possibly may be more toxic, and certainly will be more expensive. The prescribing physician should realize also that the decision to abandon aspirin (or any other therapeutic agent in rheumatoid arthritis) is likely to be an irrevocable one. It may require a rather brave and convincing therapist to reinstitute trial of a medicine in the face of statements such as: "I already tried that, and it upset my stomach terribly and didn't help my arthritis anyway!"

Nonsteroidal Anti-inflammatory Drugs (NSAIDs). Chapter 50 deals with the clinical pharmacology of the ever-lengthening list of agents which, like aspirin, interfere with prostaglandin metabolism and which, in clinical trials for the treatment of rheumatoid arthritis, appear to be as effective as aspirin and perhaps somewhat better tolerated.[12] If a patient is unable to tolerate sufficient aspirin to maintain therapeutic levels, it is appropriate to try one of the NSAIDs.

Most comparative studies have shown that NSAIDs are about as effective as aspirin in the treatment of rheumatoid arthritis[40] and usually they have caused less gastrointestinal irritation, although all of them may cause peptic ulceration. Increases in serum levels of hepatic enzymes sometimes occur during the first weeks of therapy, and serious hepatitis has been reported as well.[41] Inhibition of renal prostaglandin synthesis may impair renal blood flow and handling of fluid and electrolytes, especially in older patients with pre-existing renal or prerenal dysfunction.[42] Blood dyscrasias are rare but may be fatal; phenylbutazone and oxyphenbutazone have been associated with agranulocytosis, aplastic anemia, and leukemia, so that long-term use of these agents in treatment of rheumatoid arthritis is contraindicated.[43]

There are insufficient data comparing NSAIDs in the treatment of rheumatoid arthritis to permit a recommendation as to which is safer or more effective than the others. Physicians with long experience in using these

agents assert that they are unable to predict which patients will benefit most from or tolerate best which drugs. Some advocate sequential trials of 3 to 4 weeks until one that is effective in controlling the patient's disease is identified. Full beneficial effects may not be apparent for 10 to 14 days. Conversely, increased symptoms following withdrawal may not occur for a week or more, so that patients should be instructed not to conclude a drug was ineffective because they feel no worse after having missed a day or two of dosing. Irrespective of the number of tablets per day required to achieve full-dose therapy—six or more in the case of a short-acting agent versus one in the case of a long-acting one—the cost to the patient is of the order of $1.00 per day.

Systemic Corticosteroids. These agents, which may effect dramatic suppression of inflammation and relief of symptoms, are discussed under the heading Anti-inflammatory Drugs because available evidence indicates that, despite their dramatic effects, they have no effect on the underlying disease process.[15] Even patients who have excellent symptomatic responses will show radiographic evidence of progressive joint destruction over the years. The use of systemic steroids for the articular manifestations of rheumatoid arthritis is not ordinarily advisable. Taken in sufficient dose for such a chronic problem as rheumatoid arthritis, steroids predictably lead to a number of unpleasant side effects. For the patient with rheumatoid arthritis, the deleterious effects on bone are the most troublesome. Virtually every physician has been exposed to a patient with rheumatoid arthritis, treated with systemic corticosteroids, who now has severe osteopenia with multiple painful vertebral compression fractures added to her other musculoskeletal woes.

The use of systemic corticosteroids for articular rheumatoid arthritis is a drastic step, one to be taken only with full exposition of the potential side effects to the patient. The natural history of steroid administration is eventual failure of control of symptoms at one dose and a requirement for an increased dose. Attempts to reduce or withdraw these agents are usually attended by significant flares in disease activity and increases in symptoms, even when decrements of as little as 1 mg per day are involved. A firm control of dosage by the physician and agreement in advance about patient compliance with this control are mandatory. The patient who manipulates her own medicines as she sees fit is no candidate for systemic steroids: she will soon be taking 30 or 40 mg of prednisone or its equivalent daily.

Despite these warnings, there are some clinical situations in which the systemic administration of corticosteroids is warranted.[44] In patients with severe progressive active disease, administration of 5 or even 7.5 mg daily may allow continued functioning while other remission-inducing agents are administered simultaneously and allowed some time to begin working. Socioeconomic considerations often influence the decision to begin such therapy. If the patient is a wage-earner who is about to lose a job and has a dependent family, or if she is a mother of a young family and is about to be incapacitated by her disease, then the risks may be warranted. In each instance, the lowest possible dose should be used, and a maximum dose ever to be used should be agreed upon in advance. The steroid should be administered as a single daily dose in the morning and continual attempts made to reduce the dose or to convert to every-other-day dosage. In contrast to some of the other rheumatic diseases, the latter form of therapy is not often satisfactory for the control of the symptoms of rheumatoid arthritis.

Local Injections of Corticosteroids. Despite experimental evidence indicating that repeated intraarticular injection of steroids may have deleterious effects on cartilage, the judicious use of local corticosteroid injections is a valuable part of the therapeutic armamentarium in rheumatoid arthritis.[45] The pros and cons of and the techniques for their use are considered in detail in Chapter 37. Aspiration of a joint and instillation of corticosteroids are most useful when only a few joints are involved, particularly when these joints are interfering with the overall progress of the patient. Instillations of steroids into tendon sheaths or bursae are also effective local remedies; elimination of pain on pressure over a trochanteric or deltoid bursa may allow sound sleep for many nights. Injections of an area of nerve entrapment may elimate symptoms for a sufficiently long time as to permit slower-acting agents to control the synovitis, thereby eliminating the need for surgical release.

Duration of benefit following local injection is highly variable. Some patients will experience relief lasting several months, while other may benefit for only a few days. The length of time of relief seems to be reproducible for any given patient, so that one who has had only a few days of improvement is unlikely to derive months of relief following a second injection. Judgment is required in determining the number of joints to be injected and the frequency with which any particular joint can be injected. Some systemic absorption and systemic anti-inflammatory effects are observable following intra-articular injections, particularly of large joints where larger total amounts of steroids may be involved. The nature of this improvement and its cause should be explained to the patient, lest she develop unfounded optimism about the state of her disease.

REMISSION–INDUCING AGENTS

Most patients with rheumatoid arthritis report a lessening in symptoms after taking full-dose anti-inflammatory agents for a week or two, but very few experience a total disappearance of their disease. Most of these do so very early in their course, making the diagnosis suspect. Current criteria for a "clinical remission" include less than fifteen minutes of morning stiffness, no fatigue, no joint pain by history, no joint tenderness, no joint or tendon sheath swelling, and no elevation of erythrocyte sedimentation rate.[46] Although "outcome" is doubtless more significant for the patient than transient changes in the progress of her disease,[47] nearly all studies of efficacy have measured the latter. By these criteria, at least three agents—antimalarials (Chapter 51), gold salts (Chapter 52) and penicillamine (Chapter 53)—have been shown to induce remission. As knowledge about the dosage and toxicity of these agents has accumulated, the tendency has been to use them earlier in the course of the disease, before irreversible structural damage has occurred. Whereas formerly they were often considered measures of last resort, fraught with life-threatening complications, currently they are regularly prescribed for patients with aggressive disease, in the hope of preventing irreversible structural damage.[48] The decision to use such agents is influenced by the patient's age, the severity of disease, the distribution and number of joints affected, and the effect of the disease on the patient's functioning. Although remission-inducing agents tend to be prescribed earlier for young patients, there is no evidence that the results are better or the toxicity less in this age group.[49] In general, most rheumatologists would prescribe a remission-inducing agent after several months of progressive rheumatoid arthritis, irrespective of the intensity of disease or the patient's age. Since one agent may succeed where others have already failed, they are usually administered sequentially, beginning with those that are least toxic and progressing through increasingly more toxic ones, monitoring patient response at each step. Unfortunately, attempts to predict responses to individual agents by scrutinizing clinical or laboratory variables for individual patients have been unsuccessful.[50]

Antimalarials. Probably the least risky and most easily administered remission-inducing agent is the antimalarial. As discussed in Chapter 51, the efficacy of chloroquine or hydroxychloroquine in the treatment of rheumatoid arthritis has been repeatedly validated in controlled studies; the effects have not been dramatic, but they have been quite reproducible.[51-53] Ease of administration and relative freedom from minor nuisance-type side effects as well as from major life-threatening complications makes antimalarials the preferred initial remission-inducing agent in the opinion of many rheumatologists. These drugs have a slowly developing favorable effect of unknown nature, but they do not have immediate or dramatic anti-inflammatory influences. Patients who begin taking antimalarials need to understand that no beneficial effects may be apparent for several weeks, and that 3 or 4 months may be required before a decision about efficacy can be made in their particular case. As for any potentially toxic agent, full disclosure for possible complications is mandatory. The most important of these is pigmented macular degeneration of the retina. When this occurs, it may be catastrophic, since there is no effective treatment and it may progress even after the drug has been stopped. The patient must be informed that expert ophthalmologic consultation will be required periodically and will begin immediately (to detect patients with pre-existing retinal lesions such as senile macular degeneration, which may be difficult to differentiate from antimalarial retinopathy). As made clear in Chapter 51, however, the frequency of macular degeneration is probably overestimated, is dose related, and rarely occurs at doses currently recommended.[54] A trial of 6 to 12 weeks of an antimalarial is, therefore, often warranted early in the course of documented rheumatoid arthritis.

Gold. Of all the remission-inducing agents, gold has been used for the longest time and has been studied most extensively, and there is abundant evidence of efficacy.[13] Details of the use of gold salts are considered in Chapter 52. On the average, about one third of patients who are administered gold salts will experience dramatic and sustained improvement in their disease; depending upon definitions, as many as one quarter will have remissions.[13,31,55,56] Another third will experience some improvement, but it is often difficult to distinguish this improvement from that which might have occurred as part of the natural history of the disease. The remaining third will discontinue treatment either because of toxicity or failure to improve. During the first year or two, about two thirds of patients will improve either concomitantly with or because of gold salt therapy. With longer follow-up, however, the fraction of patients still taking gold continues to fall, due both to continuing development of toxic reactions and to recrudescence of disease in those who earlier had responded.[57,58] The usual treatment regime begins with a test dose of 10 mg the first week, 25 mg the second, and then 50 mg weekly for 20 weeks. When a clinical response is apparent, the frequency of injections can be reduced to every other week or eventually to once a month. Firm evidence supports the continued administration of gold salts in those who experience benefit; randomized and placebo-controlled cessation of therapy resulted in relapse for those who were not continued in treatment.[13] There is no specific limit to the length of time for which gold may be given, but complete discontinuation should be contemplated only after several symptom-free years and complete absence of laboratory evidence of active disease.

Most unwanted effects occur relatively early in the course of treatment, often between the fifth and fifteenth week of injections. The most common toxic reaction is a mild pruritic rash (which may not recur following cessation and reinstitution of therapy[59]), but more extensive skin eruptions, including exfoliative dermatitis, also occur. Oral or other mucocutaneous ulcers may be quite painful and occasionally persist for weeks following cessation of therapy. Renal toxicity is usually manifested by mild proteinuria, which may require adjustment of the dose. Moderate proteinuria is an indication for cessation of therapy, but subsequently treatment may be resumed.[60] Frank nephrotic syndrome or renal functional impairment is rare and usually reversible. Hematologic complications include thrombocytopenia, which is often reversible,[61] and agranulocytosis or aplas-

tic anemia, which is rarely so. These may occur late in the course of treatment, often without warning. Immediate cessation of gold therapy and institution of steroids is indicated, possibly with the addition of a gold-chelating agent. Use of a routine protocol, designed to inquire about symptoms of toxicity and to elicit signs or obtain laboratory data about toxicity, allows monitoring of untoward effects by members of the health-care team other than the physician, but the requirements for urine and blood screening make gold salt therapy quite costly.

A complex of gold with a trialkylphosphine, auranofin, has been shown to be well absorbed via the oral route.[62] In a number of controlled studies,[63,66] auranofin has been shown to be nearly as effective as the standard regimen of parenteral gold salts. Although gastrointestinal side effects such as diarrhea are more frequent with the oral preparation, cutaneous and renal toxicity is substantially less, so that discontinuation of therapy due to adverse reactions has generally been less frequent. Thrombocytopenia, proteinuria, elevated liver enzymes, "nitritoid" reactions, and "gold pneumonitis" are rarely observed in patients treated with auranofin. No correlation between mean blood levels of gold and clinical response has been noted, but the same absence of correlation has been observed following parenterally administered gold salts.[67]

Penicillamine. In the opinion of most rheumatologists, penicillamine is the next agent to be tried after antimalarials and gold have failed. As detailed in Chapter 53, this drug was chosen for the wrong reasons, namely its theoretical ability to reduce the disulfide bridges of IgM rheumatoid factor, which was believed to have a pathogenetic role in rheumatoid arthritis.[68] When it was reported that penicillamine not only led to a real fall in rheumatoid factor titers but also to clinical improvement in a patient with rheumatoid vasculitis, interest in the agent as treatment for the other manifestations of rheumatoid arthritis was generated.[69] Many years later its efficacy was documented by controlled studies of the Empire Rheumatism Council.[14] Today there is no issue about its efficacy, only about its rank among the remitting agents. Patient acceptance is probably lower than that observed with gold salts, owing to intolerable nausea, dyspepsia, and dysgeusia,[70] but such symptoms can often be avoided when the drug is begun at a very low dose (125 mg daily) and increased very slowly (125 mg each month). The side effects of penicillamine resemble those of gold and commonly include skin rash, proteinuria, and bone marrow suppression. Unique toxicities include the development of myasthenia gravis–like syndromes[71] and of pemphigus.[72] Like all remission-inducing agents, penicillamine has a delayed therapeutic response, so that full benefit may not appear for up to six months.

Azathioprine. The only other agent that may be disease modifying and is approved for use in rheumatoid arthritis is azathioprine.[73] Use of this anti-inflammatory and immunosuppressive drug is described in Chapter 55. Because it ordinarily affords only modest control of symptoms and has been associated with severe toxicity, including a potential for lymphoreticular malignancy, most rheumatologists employ azathioprine only after antimalarials, gold, and penicillamine have failed. Even relatively low doses, which would not usually be effective in the suppression of renal allograft rejection (for which the drug was first designed), appear to reduce the symptoms of rheumatoid arthritis.[74]

EXPERIMENTAL TREATMENTS

Although a minority of patients with rheumatoid arthritis experience a complete remission and the majority obtain a satisfactory result, a small fraction is afflicted with inexorable, progressive, and destructive disease despite the most careful and well-intentioned applications of currently approved therapy. Such patients often have life-threatening extra-articular manifestations which occur when the disease appears to "escape" the bounds of the joint capsule and involve vital organs (See Chapter 60). In such instances, use of drugs whose risk-benefit ratios are as yet imperfectly defined may be required in an attempt to preserve crucial joint function or even life. The wisest course of action in such circumstances is referral to a tertiary treatment center where the health-care team is familiar with the dosage and toxicity of the immunosuppressive or cytotoxic regimens to be employed, the means for monitoring toxicity and effects of therapy are immediately available, and the results of such experimental treatment are collected and analyzed in a systematic fashion.

Besides azathioprine, which has been approved in the United States for the treatment of rheumatoid arthritis, other drugs with potential beneficial effect include levamisole, cyclophosphamide, and methotrexate. As was true for many of the agents used for the treatment of rheumatoid arthritis, the discovery of *levamisole* was an accident. The original observation was made that animals dewormed with this antihelminthic appeared to have an enhanced antibody response.[75] Subsequent in vitro experiments demonstrated that levamisole potentiated a variety of T-lymphocyte responses, and even increased the severity of rat adjuvant arthritis. Several controlled trials in patients with rheumatoid arthritis have shown it to be efficacious in the treatment of this disease.[76–78] At doses of 150 mg three days weekly a response rate of 70 per cent was observed.[78] Unfortunately, frequent and severe toxicity had limited its use. In particular, granulocytopenia and agranulocytosis occur so frequently as to make levamisole unsatisfactory for routine use.

Double-blind controlled studies confirm the beneficial effects of *cyclophosphamide* in the short-term therapy of rheumatoid arthritis,[79,80] including reduction in the frequency of radiographic hand joint erosions. At a dose of 150 mg per day, most patients experience significant toxic effects, including bone marrow suppression (especially neutropenia), gonadal suppression, alopecia, and cystitis (with occasional bladder fibrosis and even carcinoma); an increased risk of lymphomas and leukemias also exists. A controlled trial of 150 mg versus 75 mg per day demonstrated significant improvement in both groups, but the frequency of side effects was also the same, with the exception of neutropenia, which was only 6 per cent in the low-dose group compared with 32 per cent in the high-dose group.[81] While short-term beneficial effects have consistently been demonstrated, the appropriate studies to determine the effect of cyclophosphamide on long-term outcome[47] have not been made.

The folic acid antagonist *methotrexate* has been used in low doses for the treatment of psoriasis and psoriatic arthritis for a number of years, but only recently has it been used to any extent in rheumatoid arthritis.[82] Typically three oral doses of 2.5 to 7.5 mg are administered at twelve-hour intervals once weekly. Experience with this regimen in the treatment of psoriasis indicates that it is not associated with the increased risk of malignancies seen with azathioprine or cyclophosphamide.[83] Hepatotoxicity, not necessarily heralded by changes in blood chemistries,[84] is the most serious side effect; marrow toxicity is not usually a problem with the low-dose schedule. There are no controlled prospective studies of the efficacy of methotrexate in the treatment of rheumatoid arthritis, but retrospective analyses have indicated definite improvement in approximately two thirds of patients, all of whom had been refractory to other remission-inducing agents.[85–87]

Cyclosporin A, a fungal metabolite that has had a major positive impact in the control of allograft rejection, appears to act specifically on T-lymphocyte function.[88] It might, therefore, be expected to have a beneficial effect in the control of rheumatoid arthritis. Partly because of nephrotoxicity, it has not been widely studied in any rheumatic diseases. In the one small uncontrolled series that has been published, only about one third of patients with rheumatoid arthritis showed any substantial improvement.[89]

Experience with *total lymphoid irradiation* in the treatment of Hodgkin's disease indicated that it was associated with few serious side effects and no increased risk of hematologic malignancy, but led to profound impairment of T-lymphocyte function, which often lasted for years.[90] Uncontrolled studies of small numbers of patients with rheumatoid arthritis refractory to the usual remission-inducing agents have demonstrated improvement in disease activity.[91,92] In one study,[92] partial recrudescence of disease was observed after about a year, but in another the beneficial effects and laboratory evidence of immunosuppression were observed to persist throughout a 13- to 28-month follow-up period.[93]

SURGERY

An integral part of the management of many patients with rheumatoid arthritis involves orthopedic or plastic surgery.[33] The technical aspects and details of procedures used in the surgical approach to rheumatoid arthritis are considered in Chapters 112 to 120. Here we will consider the influence of the disease on the fitness of the patient for surgery and the special attention required for such patients.

Influence of Rheumatoid Arthritis on Fitness and Response to Surgery. Despite the systemic nature of their disease and the multiplicity of medicines with which rheumatoid arthritis patients are often treated, their surgical morbidity and mortality are not extraordinary. While it is doubtless advantageous to postpone surgery until disease activity appears to have come under partial control, rarely is complete quiescence of the disease possible in a patient who requires surgery; moderate anemia or hypoalbuminemia is not in itself a contraindication.[95] The fact that many patients with rheumatoid arthritis are nearer to their ideal body weight than the general population or, especially, patients with osteoarthritis, may actually enhance their suitability as surgical candidates. When wound healing was studied in a matched group of patients with rheumatoid or osteoarthritis, no major differences were noted. Some problems peculiar to patients with rheumatoid arthritis require special attention by anesthesiologists or surgeons, however; and the primary therapist should be responsible for pointing out these problems.

Anesthesiologic Considerations. The possibility of cervical spine involvement, especially atlantoaxial subluxation, must always be kept in mind.[96] A careful history of symptoms of such involvement, together with preoperative radiographs in flexion and extension, if necessary, may prevent a catastrophe during endotracheal intubation. In patients with juvenile rheumatoid arthritis who may have extensive ankylosis of the cervical spine, intubation may present even more formidable problems. Rarely, temporomandibular joint involvement may make intubation difficult.

Continuation of Medical Therapy. Doubtless either the surgeon or the anesthesiologist will obtain a history of preceding therapy with systemic steroids and attend to appropriate adrenal steroid replacement during the perioperative period. On the other hand, the necessity for the patient to receive nothing by mouth for a day or two occasionally leads to prolonged cessation of anti-inflammatory or suppressive therapy, even when it could be given parenterally. The result may be a general increase in symptoms which progresses as the steroid coverage is reduced and finally removed. While it is true that aspirin and related anti-inflammatory drugs may have an effect on the coagulation process, significant postoperative hemorrhage attributable to these agents is uncommon. Similarly, the use of antimalarials, gold, penicillamine, or other agents is not contraindicated in the postoperative period. Often, however, their administration may simply be overlooked until either the patient complains of other joints or follow-up by other members of the arthritis health-care team calls attention to the omission.

References

1. Short, C.L., Bauer, W., and Reynolds, W.E.: Rheumatoid Arthritis. Cambridge, Mass., Harvard University Press, 1957.
2. Duthie, J.J.R., Brown, P.E., Truelove, L.H., Baraza, F., and Lawpie, H.: Course and prognosis in rheumatoid arthritis. Ann. Rheum. Dis. 23:193, 1974.
3. Feigenbaum, S.L., Masi, A.T., and Kaplan, S.B.: Prognosis in rheumatoid arthritis: A longitudinal study of newly diagnosed younger adult patients. Am. J. Med. 66:377, 1979.
4. Katz, S., Vignos, P.J., Moskowitz, R.W., Thompson, H.M., and Svec, K.H.: Comprehensive outpatient care in rheumatoid arthritis: A controlled study. JAMA 206:1244, 1968.
5. Decker, J.L.: The management of rheumatoid arthritis. Med. Times 105:28, 1977.
6. Kaye, R.L., and Hammond, A.H.: Understanding rheumatoid arthritis. Evaluation of a patient education program. JAMA 239:2466, 1978.
7. Arthritis Practical Information. Where to turn for help. Atlanta, The Arthritis Foundation, 1982.
8. Rheumatoid Arthritis. Medical Information Series. Atlanta, The Arthritis Foundation, 1983.
9. Fries, J.F.: Arthritis. A Comprehensive Guide. Reading, Mass., Addison-Wesley Publishing Company, 1979.
10. Valentine, L.R.: Self care through group learning. Am. J. Nursing 70:2110, 1976.
11. Boardman, P.L., and Hart, F.O.: Clinical measurements of the anti-inflammatory effects of salicylates in rheumatoid arthritis. Br. Med. J. 2:264, 1967.
12. Simon, L.S., and Mills, J.A.: Nonsteroidal anti-inflammatory drugs. New Engl. J. Med. 302:1179, 1237, 1980.
13. Empire Rheumatism Council: Gold therapy in rheumatoid arthritis: Final report of a multicentre controlled trial. Ann. Rheum. Dis. 20:315, 1961.
14. Multicentre Trial Group: Controlled trial of d (-) penicillamine in severe rheumatoid arthritis. Lancet 1:275, 1973.
15. Glass, D., Snaith, M.L., Russel, A.S., and Daly, J.R.: Possible unnecessary prolongation of corticosteroid therapy in rheumatoid arthritis. Lancet 2:234, 1971.
16. Ferguson, K., and Figley, B.: Sexuality and rheumatic disease: A prospective study. Sexuality Disability 2:130, 1979.
17. Mills, J.A., Pinals, R.S., Ropes, M.W., Short, C.L., and Sutcliffe, S.: Value of bedrest in patients with rheumatoid arthritis. N. Engl. J. Med. 284:453, 1971.
18. Alexander, G.J., Hortas, C., and Bacon, P.A.: Bed rest activity and the inflammation of rheumatoid arthritis. Br. J. Rheumatol. 22:134, 1983.
19. Lee, P., Kennedy, A.C., Anderson, J., and Buchanan, W.W.: Benefits of hospitalization in rheumatoid arthritis. Quart. J. Med. 43:205, 1974.
20. Nordemar, R.: Physical training in rheumatoid arthritis: A controlled long-term study. II. Functional capacity and general attitudes. Scan. J. Rheumatol. 10:25, 1981.
21. Wright, U., and Dawson, D.: Joint stiffness—its characterization and significance. Biomed. Engineering 4:8, 1969.
22. Wright, V., Hopkins, R., and Jackson, M.: Instructing patients in physiotherapy: An example using three methods. Rheumatol. Rehabil. 19:91, 1980.
23. Bland, J.H., and Eddy, W.M.: Hemiplegia and rheumatoid arthritis. Arthritis Rheum. 11:72, 1968.
24. Kammermann, J.S.: Protective effect of traumatic lesions on rheumatoid arthritis. Ann. Rheum. Dis. 25:361, 1966.
25. Glick, E.N.: Asymmetrical rheumatoid arthritis after poliomyelitis. Br. Med. J. 3:26, 1967.
26. Castillo, B.A., Sallab, R.A., and Scott, J.T.: Physical activity, cystic erosions, and osteoporosis in rheumatoid arthritis. Ann. Rheum. Dis. 24:522, 1965.
27. Gault, S.J., and Spyker, J.M.: Beneficial effect of immobilization of joints in rheumatoid and related arthritides: A splint study using sequential analysis. Arthritis Rheum. 12:34, 1969.
28. Harris, R., and Copp, E.P.: Immobilization of the knee joint in rheumatoid arthritis. Ann. Rheum. Dis. 21:353, 1962.
29. Brewerton, D.H., and Daniel, S.W.: Return to work: Experiences of a rehabilitation officer. Br. Med. J. 2:240, 1969.
30. Cochrane, G.M.: Rheumatoid arthritis: Vocational rehabilitation. Int. Rehabil. Med. 4:148, 1982.

31. The Cooperating Clinics Committee of the American Rheumatism Association: A controlled trial of gold salt therapy in rheumatoid arthritis. Arthritis Rheum. 16:353, 1973.

32. Ehrlich, G.E.: Total Management of the Arthritis Patient. Philadelphia, J. B. Lippincott Company, 1973.

33. Hall, A.P.: The decision to operate in rheumatoid arthritis. Orthoped. Clin. North Am. 6:675, 1975.

34. Hardin, J.G., and Kirk, K.A.: Comparative effectiveness of five analgesics for the pain of rheumatoid arthritis. Arthritis Rheum. 21:564, 1978.

35. Giuliano, V., and Scarff, E.V.: Clinical comparison of two salicylates in rheumatoid arthritis patients on maintenance gold therapy. Curr. Therap. Res. 28:61, 1980.

36. Samter, M., and Beers, R.F.: Concerning the nature of intolerance to aspirin. J. Allergy 40:281, 1967.

37. Cassel, S., Furst, D., Dromgoole, S., and Paulus, H.: Steady-state serum salicylate levels in hospitalized patients with rheumatoid arthritis. Arthritis Rheum. 22:384, 1979.

38. Mongan, E., Kelly, P., Nies, K., Porter, W.W., and Paulus, H.E.: Tinnitus as an indication of therapeutic serum salicylate levels. JAMA 226:142, 1973.

39. Leonards, J.R., Levy, G., and Niemczura, R.: Gastrointestinal blood loss during prolonged aspirin administration. N. Engl. J. Med. 289:1020, 1973.

40. Verbeeck, R.K., Blackburn, J.L., and Loewen, G.R.: Clinical pharmacokinetics of non-steroidal anti-inflammatory drugs. Clin. Pharmacokinet. 8:297, 1983.

41. Weinblatt, M.E., Tesser, J.R., and Gilliam, J.H., III: The liver in rheumatic diseases. Sem. Arth. Rheum. 11:399, 1982.

42. Zawada, E.T., Jr.: Renal consequences of nonsteroidal anti-inflammatory drugs. Postgrad. Med. 71:223, 1982.

43. Fowler, P.D.: Marrow toxicity of the pyrazoles. Ann. Rheum. Dis. 26:344, 1967.

44. Harris, E.D., Jr.: Glucocorticoid use in rheumatoid arthritis. Hosp. Pract. 18:137, 1983.

45. Gray, R.G., and Gottlieb, N.L.: Intra-articular corticosteroids: An updated assessment. Clin. Orthop. Rel. Res. 177:235, 1983.

46. Pinals, R.S., Masi, A.T., and Larsen, R.A.: Preliminary criteria for clinical remission in rheumatoid arthritis. Arthritis Rheum. 24:1308, 1981.

47. Fries, J.F.: The assessment of disability: From first to future principles. Br. J. Rheumatol. 22(Suppl. 3):48, 1983.

48. Pinals, R.S.: Approach to rheumatoid arthritis and osteoarthritis: An overview. Am. J. Med 75(Suppl. 4B):2, 1983.

49. Terkeltaub, R., Esdaile, J., Decary, F., and Tannenbaum, H.: A clinical study of older age rheumatoid arthritis with comparison to a younger onset group. J. Rheumatol. 10:418, 1983.

50. Christian, C.L.: Prognostic and therapeutic implications of immunologic test results in rheumatic disease. Hum. Pathol. 14:446, 1983.

51. Freedman, A., and Steinberg, V.L.: Chloroquine in rheumatoid arthritis—a double blindfold trial of treatment for one year. Ann. Rheum. Dis. 19:243, 1960.

52. Scherbel, A.L.: Use of synthetic antimalarial drugs and other agents for rheumatoid arthritis: Historic and therapeutic perspectives. Am. J. Med. 75:1, 1983.

53. Bell, C.L.: Hydroxychloroquine sulfate in rheumatoid arthritis: Long-term response rate and predictive parameters. Am. J. Med. 75:46, 1983.

54. Rynes, R.I., Krohel, G., Falbo, A., Reinecke, R.D., and Bartholomew, L.E.: Ophthalmologic safety of long-term hydroxychloroquine treatment. Arthritis Rheum. 21:588, 1978.

55. Sigler, J.W., Bluhm, G.B., Duncan, M.D., Sharp, J.T., Ensign, D.C., and McCrum, W.R.: Gold salts in the treatment of rheumatoid arthritis. Ann. Intern. Med. 80:21, 1974.

56. Sharp, J.T., Lidsky, M.D., and Duffy, J.: Clinical responses during gold therapy for rheumatoid arthritis. Changes in synovitis, radiologically detectable erosive lesions, serum proteins, and serologic abnormalities. Arthritis Rheum. 25:540, 1982.

57. Rothermich, N.O., Phillips, V.K., Bergen, W., and Thomas, M.H.: Follow-up study of chrysotherapy. Arthritis Rheum. 22:423, 1979.

58. Richter, J.A., Runge, L.A., Pinals, R.S., and Oates, R.P.: Analysis of treatment terminations with gold and antimalarial compounds in rheumatoid arthritis. J. Rheumatol. 7:153, 1980.

59. Klinefelter, H.F.: Reinstitution of gold therapy in rheumatoid arthritis after mucocutaneous reactions. J. Rheumatol. 2:21, 1975.

60. Newton, P., Swinburn, W.R., and Swinson, D.R.: Proteinuria with gold therapy: When should gold be permanently stopped? Br. J. Rheumatol. 22:11, 1983.

61. Coblyn, J.S., Weinblatt, M., Holdsworth, D., and Glass, D.: Gold-induced thrombocytopenia. A clinical and immunogenetic study of twenty-three patients. Ann. Intern. Med. 95:178, 1981.

62. Berglöf, F.E., Berglöf, K., and Walz, D.T.: Auranofin: An oral chrysoth-

erapeutic agent for the treatment of rheumatoid arthritis. J. Rheumatol. 5:68, 1978.

63. Menard, H.A., Beaudet, F., Davis, P., Harth, M., Percy, J.S., Russell, A.S., and Thompson, J.M.: Gold therapy in rheumatoid arthritis: Interim report of the Canadian multicenter prospective trial comparing sodium aurothiomalate and auranofin. J. Rheumatol. 9 (Suppl.):179, 1982.

64. Katz, W.A., Alexander, S., Bland, J.H., Blechman, W., Bluhm, G.B., Bonebrake, R.A., Falbo, A., Greenwald, R.A., Hartman, S., Hobbs, T., Indenbaum, S., Lergier, J.E., Lanier, B.G., Lightfoot, R.W., Phelps, P., Sheon, R.P., Torretti, D., Wenger, M.E., and Wilske, K.: The efficacy and safety of auranofin compared to placebo in rheumatoid arthritis. J. Rheumatol. 9 (suppl.):173, 1982.

65. Schattenkirchner, M., Kaik, B., Muller-Fassbender, H., Rau, R., and Zeidler, H.: Auranofin and sodium aurothiomalate in the treatment of rheumatoid arthritis, a double-blind, comparative, multicenter study. J. Rheumatol. 9 (Suppl.)184, 1982.

66. Ward, J.R., Williams, H.J., Egger, M.J., Reading, J.C., Boyce, E., Altz-Smith, M., Samuelson, C.O., Jr., Willkens, R.F., Solsky, M.A., Hayes, S.P., Blocka, K.L., Weinstein, A., Meenan, R.F., Guttadauria, M. Kaplan, S.B., and Klippel, J.: Comparison of. auranofin, gold sodium thiomalate and placebo in the treatment of rheumatoid arthritis. A controlled clinical trial. Arthritis Rheum. 26:1303, 1983.

67. Gottlieb, N.L., Smith, P.M., and Smith, E.M.: Pharmacodynamics of ¹⁹⁵Au labeled auriothiomalate in blood. Correlation with course of rheumatoid arthritis, gold toxicity and gold excretion. Arthritis Rheum. 17:161, 1974.

68. Griffin, S.W., Ulloa, A., Henry, M., Johnston, M.L., and Holley, H.L.: In vivo effect of pencillamine on circulating rheumatoid factor. Clin. Res. 8:87, 1960.

69. Jaffe, I.A.: Rheumatoid arthritis with arteritis. Report of a case treated with pencillamine. Ann. Intern. Med. 61:556,1964.

70. Tsang, I.K., Patterson, C.A., Stein, H.B., Robinson, H.S., and Ford, D.K.: D-Penicillamine in the treatment of rheumatoid arthritis. Arthritis Rheum. 20:666, 1977.

71. Bucknall, R.C., Dixon, A.S.J., Glick, E.N., Woodland, J., and Zutshi, D.W.: Myasthenia gravis associated with penicillamine treatment for rheumatoid arthritis. Br. Med. J. 1:600, 1975.

72. Marsden, R.A., Ryan, T.J., Van Hegan, R.I., Walshe, M., Hill, H., and Mowat, A.G.: Pemphigus foliaceus indicated by penicillamine. Br. Med. J. 2:1423, 1976.

73. Currey, H.L.F., Harris, J.R.M., Mason, R.M., Woodland, J., Beveridge, T., Roberts, C.J., Vere, D.W., Dixon, A.S.J., Davies, J., and Owen-Smith, B.: Comparison of azathioprine, cyclophosphamide and gold in treatment of rheumatoid arthritis. Br. Med. J. 3:763, 1974.

74. Abel, T., Urowitz, M.B., Smythe, H.A., Keystone, E.C., and Norman, C.B.: Long-term effects of azathioprine in rheumatoid arthritis. Arthritis Rheum. 21:539, 1978.

75. Symoens, J., and Schuermans, Y.: Levamisole. Clin. Rheum. Dis. 5:603, 1979.

76. Runge, L.A., Pinals, R.S., Lourie, S.H., and Tomas, R.H.: Treatment of rheumatoid arthritis with levamisole. A controlled trial. Arthritis Rheum. 20:1445, 1977.

77. Multicentre Study Group: Levamisole in rheumatoid arthritis. Final report on a randomised double-blind study comparing a single weekly dose of levamisole with placebo. Ann. Rheum. Dis. 41:159, 1982.

78. Miller, B., de Merieux, P., Ramachandran, S., Clements, P., Fan, P., Levy, J., and Paulus, H.: Double-blind placebo controlled crossover evaluation of levamisole in rheumatoid arthritis. Arthritis Rheum. 23:172, 1980.

79. Cooperating Clinics of the American Rheumatism Association: A controlled trial of cyclophosphamide in rheumatoid arthritis. N. Engl. J. Med. 283:883, 1970.

80. Steinberg, A.D., Plotz, P.H., Wolf, S., Wong, V.G., Agus, S.G., and Decker, J.L.: Cytotoxic drugs in the treatment of non-malignant disease. Ann. Intern. Med. 76:619, 1972.

81. Williams, H.J., Reading, J.C., Ward, J.R., and O'Brien, W.M.: Comparison of high and low dose cyclophosphamide therapy in rheumatoid arthritis. Arthritis Rheum. 23:521, 1980.

82. Willkens, R.F.: Reappraisal of the use of methotrexate in rheumatic disease. Am. J. Med. 75(Suppl. 4B):19, 1983.

83. Bailin, P.L., Tindall, J.P., Roenigk, H.H., Hogan, M.D.: Is methotrexate therapy for psoriasis carcinogenic? JAMA 232:359, 1975.

84. Weinstein, G.D., Roenigk, H.H., Maibach, H., et al.: Psoriasis-liver methotrexate interactions: Results of an international cooperative study. Arch. Dermatol. 108:36, 1973.

85. Groff, G.D., Shenberger, K.N., Wilke, W.S., and Taylor, T.H.: Low dose oral methotrexate in rheumatoid arthritis: An uncontrolled trial and review of the literature. Sem. Arthritis Rheum. 12:333, 1983.

86. Steinsson, K., Weinstein, A., Korn, J., and Abeles, M.: Low dose methotrexate in rheumatoid arthritis. J. Rheumatol. 9:860, 1982.

87. Michaels, R.M., Nashel, D.J., Leonard, A., Sliwinski, A.J., and Derbes,

S.J.: Weekly intravenous methotrexate in the treatment of rheumatoid arthritis. Arthritis Rheum. 25:339, 1982.

88. White, D.J.G., and Calne, R.Y.: The use of cyclosporin immunosuppression in organ grafting. Immunol. Rev. 65:115, 1982.

89. Graf, U., Marbet, U., Muller, W., and Thiel, G.: Cyclosporin A—Wirkungen und Nebenwirkungen bei der Behandlung der chronischen Polyarthritis und der Psoriasisarthritis. Immun. Infekt. 9:20, 1981.

90. Fuks, Z., Strober, S., Bobrove, A.M., Susazuki, T., McMichael, A., and Kaplan, H.S.: Long-term effects of radiation on T and B lymphocytes in peripheral blood of patients with Hodgkin's disease. J. Clin. Invest. 58:803, 1976.

91. Kotzin, B.L., Strober, S., Engelman, E.G., Calin, A., Hoppe, R.T., Kansas, G.S., Terrell, C.P., Kaplan, H.S.: Treatment of intractable rheumatoid arthritis with total lymphoid irradiation. N. Engl. J. Med. 305:969, 1981.

92. Trentham, D.E., Belli, J.A., Anderson, R.J., Buckley, J.A., Goetzl, E.J., David, J.R., and Austen, K.F.: Clinical and immunologic effects of fractionated total lymphoid irradiation in refractory rheumatoid arthritis. N. Engl. J. Med. 305:976, 1981.

93. Field, E.H., Strober, S., Hoppe, R.T., Calin, A., Engleman, E.G., Kotzin, B.L., Tanay, A.S., Calin, H.J., Terrell, C.P., and Kaplan, H.S.: Sustained improvement of intractable rheumatoid arthritis after total lymphoid irradiation. Arthritis Rheum. 26:934, 1983.

94. Mowat, A.G.: Surgical treatment of rheumatoid arthritis. In Scott, J.T. (ed.): Copeman's Textbook of the Rheumatic Diseases. 5th ed. New York, Churchill Livingstone, 1978, p. 459.

95. Garner, R.W., Mowat, A.G., and Hazleman, B.L.: Wound healing after operations on patients with rheumatoid arthritis. J. Bone Joint Surg. 55B:134, 1973.

96. Smith, P., Benn, R.T., and Sharp, J.: Natural history of rheumatoid cervical luxations. Ann. Rheum. Dis. 32:432, 1972.

Section VI
Spondylarthropathies

Chapter 64
Ankylosing Spondylitis

Andrei Calin

INTRODUCTION

Ankylosing spondylitis is not a new disease. However, during the last 10 years it has become a center of attention, intriguing clinicians, epidemiologists, pathologists, radiologists, and immunogeneticists. National societies, international workshops, numerous articles, and recent texts[1,2] attest to its new position in medicine. Once considered a rare disease, affecting primarily men and progressing relentlessly to total spinal fusion, it is now recognized as relatively common, affecting about 1 percent of the population, with a more equal sex distribution, although frequently more severe in males.

Nomenclature. The term ankylosing spondylitis derives from the Greek words *ankylos* (bent or crooked) and *spondylos* (vertebra). During its history, ankylosing spondylitis has been termed spondylitis ankylopoetica, spondylitis deformans, atrophic spondylitis, spondylitis atrophica ligamentosa, pelvospondylitis ossificans, spondylitis rhizomelica, von Bechterew's disease, Marie-Strümpell disease, and finally rheumatoid spondylitis. Because of its implication of a relation to rheumatoid arthritis, the last term, rheumatoid spondylitis, did more to harm the progress of our understanding than any of the other terms. Happily, the term "rheumatoid variants" has been replaced by the more appropriate "seronegative spondylarthritides."[2a] The latter term describes an interrelated group of disorders, the prototype of which is ankylosing spondylitis. The other conditions, Reiter's syndrome, psoriatic arthropathy, enteropathic spondylitis, and rarer disorders, are described in Chapters 65 to 67. The contrasting features between rheumatoid arthritis and ankylosing spondylitis are summarized in Tables 64–1 to 64–3. As will be seen, the conditions may be distinguished from each other on historic, geographic, epidemiologic, genetic, immunogenetic, clinical, immunologic, pathologic, radiologic, and therapeutic grounds.

Historic Review. Raymond,[3] in 1912, provided convincing illustrations of ankylosing spondylitis in mummies and graves of ancient Egypt. The paleopathologist Sir Mark Ruffer described a certain Nefermaat who lived about 2900 B.C. The mummified remains demonstrate a rigid block of bone from the mid-cervical region to the sacrum.[4] Likewise, there are impressive radiographic studies by Bourke.[5] Short[6] described 18 instances of ankylosing spondylitis extending over three millenia, 2900 B.C. to 200 A.D., derived from Egyptian sources. Other examples from the Danish and French neolithic periods exist, and there is a more recent account of a New Mexican Indian (1200 A.D.) with ankylosing spondylitis.[7] Although the occurrence of erosive digital arthritis in mummies from ancient Egypt has been suggested, the first accepted description of rheumatoid arthritis occurs no earlier than Sydenham's in 1676.[8] The separate descriptions of Bechterew, Strümpell, and Marie at the end of the nineteenth century promoted the general recognition of ankylosing spondylitis.

Table 64–1. Demographic Comparison Between Rheumatoid Arthritis and Ankylosing Spondylitis

	Rheumatoid Arthritis	Ankylosing Spondylitis
History	Data from 19th century; man only	Data from 3000 B.C.; crocodiles, monkeys, horses
Distribution	Worldwide	Racial
Prevalence	0.5–1%	0.5–1%
Etiology	Unknown	Unknown (?Klebsiella, etc.)
Family history	? slight increase	Increased familial prevalence
Sex distribution	2 ♂ > ♀	♂ ≥ ♀*
Age	All ages (peak 30–50)	Young (peak 20–30)

*Sacroiliitis per se has a male to female ratio of approximately 1–2:1. Classic ankylosing spondylitis is recognized in a ratio of 3–4:1.

Table 64–2. Contrasting Clinical Features Between Rheumatoid Arthritis and Ankylosing Spondylitis

	Rheumatoid Arthritis	Ankylosing Spondylitis
Joint distribution	Polyarthropathy Symmetrical Small and large Upper > lower limb	Oligoarthropathy Asymmetrical Large > small Lower > upper limb
Sacroiliacs	—	+
Spine involvement	Cervical	Total: ascending
Nodules	+	—
Eyes	Sicca syndrome Scleritis Scleromalacia perforans	Conjunctivitis Uveitis
Aortic regurgitation	—	+
Lungs	Caplan's syndrome Effusions	Upper lobe pulmonary fibrosis

DIAGNOSTIC CRITERIA

During recent years, criteria for the classification and diagnosis of different rheumatic diseases have been developed to help different clinicians in different locations to use the same diagnostic labels for similar groups of patients. In the case of ankylosing spondylitis, criteria were first formulated in Rome in 1961 (Table 64–4). A revised set of criteria was introduced at a subsequent symposium in New York in 1966.[9] (Table 64–5). The most frequent means of satisfying these criteria is an x-ray demonstration of Grade III or IV bilateral sacroiliitis, together with a history of pain. In fact, few clinicians rely on these criteria, and for the purpose of this discussion we can think of ankylosing spondylitis as "symptomatic sacroiliitis." As described below, the disease is considered "primary" if no other rheumatologic disorder is present, or "secondary" if the sacroiliitis is related to psoriatic arthropathy, inflammatory bowel disease, or Reiter's syndrome. Fortunately, the physician's subjective estimation of the clinical criteria usually correlates well with objective measurements.[10] Unfortunately, however, physicians and radiologists with little training in rheumatologic disease have difficulty in recognizing minimal sacroiliac change on the radiograph. Frequently, the radiologist is reluctant to describe sacroiliitis unless he sees totally obliterated joints on different views. In reality, a single anteroposterior pelvic view is sufficient.

A review of the Rome criteria reveals an obvious flaw. Limitation of movement is not defined. The New York criteria do define limitation of chest expansion as 1 inch (2.5 cm) or less. However, this figure is difficult to derive since some patients are reluctant to take a deep breath, and the measurement is difficult, for obvious reasons, in the female. More important, decreased chest expansion occurs late in the course of ankylosing spondylitis, at a time when the disease should be obvious. Pain, as such, is too sensitive and too nonspecific to be a useful criterion. An analysis of the nature of inflammatory spinal disease pain will be described below.

HLA-B27 histocompatibility antigen typing has led to immense strides in the understanding of ankylosing spondylitis. However, it should not be considered a diagnostic test or necessary for the diagnosis of ankylosing spondylitis. This condition is established by sacroiliac radiologic examination, a necessary but sufficient criterion for the diagnosis. The radiograph of the pelvis is readily available and is less expensive. A patient with symptomatic sacroiliitis, lacking the antigen HLA-B27, still has ankylosing spondylitis. The test may be negative in secondary forms of ankylosing spondylitis and in non-Caucasian patients. Occasionally, sacroiliitis is seen as a chance finding in the absence of pain. Presumably the precipitating trigger has been pulled in a susceptible individual. In epidemiologic and family studies, patients are sometimes found with unilateral sacroiliitis, dactylitis, syndesmophytes, and other stigmata of "undifferentiated spondylarthropathy."[11,12]

Table 64–3. Contrasting Laboratory, Pathologic, Radiologic, and Therapeutic Features Between Rheumatoid Arthritis and Ankylosing Spondylitis

	Rheumatoid Arthritis	ankylosing Spondylitis
Serology (rheumatoid factor)	+	—
HLA-B27 Association	No	Yes
HLA-DR4 Association	Yes	No
Pathology	Inflammatory synovitis	Enthesopathy
Radiology	Symmetrical erosive arthropathy	Asymmetrical erosive arthropathy with new bone formation, ankylosis, and sacroiliitis
Therapy	ASA, gold, penicillamine	Indomethacin, phenylbutazone

Table 64–4. Criteria for Diagnosing Ankylosing Spondylitis (Rome, 1961)

Clinical criteria:
1. Low back pain and stiffness for more than 3 months which is not relieved by rest
2. Pain and stiffness in the thoracic region
3. Limited motion in the lumbar spine
4. Limited chest expansion
5. History or evidence of iritis or its sequelae

Radiological criterion:
6. X-ray showing bilateral sacroiliac changes characteristic of ankylosing spondylitis (this would exclude bilateral osteoarthritis of the sacroiliac joints)

EPIDEMIOLOGY

During the 1950's it was recognized that ankylosing spondylitis occurred in twins, brothers, fathers, mothers, and other relatives.[13] Strecher and colleagues found the disease to be 30 times more prevalent among relatives of spondylitics than among controls.[14] These authors suggested that the disease was inherited by a single autosomal dominant factor with "70 percent penetrance in men and 10 percent penetrance in women." Elsewhere, de Blecourt and associates found the disease to be 23 times more common in relatives than in controls.[15] In 1964, Kellgren summarized the then available data and suggested a prevalence of ankylosing spondylitis of 0.1 percent in controls and 4 percent in relatives.[16] In 1967, Emery and Lawrence[17] studied 188 available first-degree relatives of 76 probands with ankylosing spondylitis and a similar number of age- and sex-matched controls. Among the first-degree relatives, 16 percent were found to have sacroiliitis. In retrospect, the striking aspect of their study was the relatively high frequency among female relatives (8 percent) compared to male relatives (20 percent), a ratio far higher than the often quoted one in ten.

The search for the explanation of this increased family prevalence took a dramatic step forward in 1973 when two reports defined the association of the genetic marker, HLA-B27, with ankylosing spondylitis.[18,19] Awareness

Table 64–5. Clinical Criteria for Ankylosing Spondylitis (New York, 1966)

Diagnosis:
1. Limitation of motion of the lumbar spine in all three planes— anterior flexion, lateral flexion, and extension
2. History or the presence of pain at the dorsolumbar junction or in the lumbar spine
3. Limitation of chest expansion to 1 inch (2.5 cm) or less, measured at the level of the fourth intercostal space

Grading:
Definite AS
1. Grade 3–4 bilateral sacroiliitis with at least one clinical criterion.
2. Grade 3–4 unilateral or Grade 2 bilateral sacroiliitis with clinical criterion 1 (limitation of back movement in all three planes) or with both clinical criteria 2 and 3 (back pain and limitation of chest expansion)

Probable AS
Grade 3–4 bilateral sacroiliitis with no clinical criteria

of the link between HLA-B27 and ankylosing spondylitis led to or explained several observations:

1. There is an increased prevalence of ankylosing spondylitis among relatives of patients. HLA-B27 is inherited as an autosomal codominant characteristic; 50 percent of first-degree relatives of probands with HLA-B27 possess this antigen.

2. Uveitis is a common accompaniment of ankylosing spondylitis. Brewerton and colleagues[20] studied 100 consecutive patients with uveitis. B27 was found not only in 29 of 33 patients with associated rheumatic disorders but also in 29 of 67 patients with no other rheumatologic disease.

3. Many patients with Reiter's syndrome develop sacroiliitis. Brewerton and others[21] showed that Reiter's syndrome, even in the absence of sacroiliitis, is HLA-B27 related. Whether the sacroiliitis in these patients should be considered a complication of Reiter's syndrome or a further manifestation of HLA-B27 associated disease remains unclear.

4. Juvenile chronic arthropathy, psoriatic arthropathy, and inflammatory bowel disease may all be "complicated" by sacroiliitis and ankylosing spondylitis. Repeated studies have shown an increased frequency of HLA-B27 in these disorders.[22] Even in patients *without* sacroiliitis, HLA-B27 may be present in up to 20 percent of those with psoriatic arthropathy or juvenile chronic arthropathy.

The shared genetic background partly explains these interrelationships. However, several observations remain unaccounted for:

1. Not all patients with HLA-B27 develop disease.

2. Some 5 percent of Caucasians with ankylosing spondylitis are not HLA-B27 positive.

3. Despite the increased frequency of HLA-B27 in patients with enteropathic sacroiliitis, some 50 percent of individuals with this condition do not possess the antigen.[23]

4. The association between ankylosing spondylitis and HLA-B27 in blacks[24] (40 to 50 percent) and Japanese[25] is not as striking as that in Caucasians.

5. The majority of patients with Reiter's syndrome are B27 positive but do not develop sacroiliitis.

6. Relatives of probands with both sacroiliitis and B27, even when carrying an identical HLA haplotype, frequently remain disease free.

7. The Pima[26] and Haida Indians, both with a high frequency of HLA-B27 and sacroiliitis, develop Reiter's syndrome only rarely.[27]

8. Ankylosing spondylitis and Reiter's syndrome tend to "breed-true" within families.[28,29]

9. We now know that B27-positive relatives of B27-positive patients are some R_n times more likely to develop ankylosing spondylitis than are B27-positive relatives of healthy B27-positive subjects.[29a]

These statements and others remind us that we still have only a limited understanding of the relationship between HLA-B27 and disease. Other genetic and environmental factors will be considered below.

The HLA-B27 rheumatic disease associations in var-

Table 64–6. Frequency of HLA-B27 in Different Healthy Populations

Population	%
Japan	< 1
Black (Africa)	< 1
Black (U.S.A.)	3–4
London (G.B.)	6
Geneva (Switzerland)	7
Los Angeles (U.S.A.)	8
Edmonton (Canada)	9
Zagreb (Yugoslavia)	14
Helsinki (Finland)	14
Pima Indians (U.S.A.)	18
Haida Indians (Canada)	50

ious ethnic groups are summarized in Tables 64–6 and 64–7.

Prevalence. With increased awareness and interest in the disease, many patients who previously were thought to have mechanical back problems, "seronegative rheumatoid arthritis," and other disorders are now recognized as having ankylosing spondylitis. It is to be hoped that the frequent occurrence of an ankylosing spondylitis patient undergoing a myelographic investigation followed by bedrest will be seen less frequently. The true prevalence of ankylosing spondylitis appears to be in the region of 1 percent. The figure contrasts sharply with the older data reporting a ratio of ankylosing spondylitis to rheumatoid arthritis ranging from a figure 1:11[30] to 1:19.[31] In 1949, West[32] estimated the prevalence to be 1 in 2000 of the general population, with a 10:1 male to female ratio.[32] Later, Lawrence[33] proposed a prevalence among males of 4 per 1000 and for females, 0.5 per 1000.

Table 64–7. HLA-B27 and Rheumatic Disease in Caucasians

Group	% Positive
Healthy Caucasians	5–14
Ankylosing spondylitis	90–100
Endemic Reiter's syndrome	70–90
Psoriasis	5–10
Psoriatic arthropathy without sacroiliitis	18–22
Psoriatic arthropathy with sacroiliitis	50–60
Seropositive "juvenile" rheumatoid arthritis	5–10
Juvenile chronic polyarthropathy without sacroiliitis	15–25
Juvenile chronic polyarthropathy with sacroiliitis	40–60
Inflammatory bowel disease	6
Inflammatory bowel disease with peripheral arthropathy	6
Inflammatory bowel disease with sacroiliitis	50–70
Yersiniosis	10
Yersinia-reactive arthropathy	80
Salmonellosis	10
Salmonella-reactive arthropathy	80–90
Shigellosis	10
Post-*Shigella* arthropathy (epidemic Reiter's syndrome)	80
Uveitis	40–50
Chronic balanitis	90
Rubella arthritis	6

With the availability of HLA-B27 as a genetic marker, a controlled study of HLA-B27 positive and negative supposedly healthy blood donors suggested that 20 percent of B27 positive individuals have symptomatic ankylosing spondylitis.[34] The majority of these patients had been inappropriately investigated and inappropriately treated. The sex distribution in this study was comparable. Since about 8 percent of Caucasians carry this antigen, extrapolating to the general population, the figures would suggest that 1 percent of Caucasians develop ankylosing spondylitis. This figure is comparable to the prevalence of rheumatoid arthritis. Data from other studies provide further evidence for this 20 percent risk factor, a figure that is in striking agreement with the number for Reiter's disease (see Chapter 65). Overall, the percentage ranges from a low of about 10 percent in western Australia[39] to a high of 50 percent in Pima males.[26]

Sex Distribution. That ankylosing spondylitis may occur almost as frequently in females as males (albeit with milder and more peripheral disease; see below) is suggested by several studies.[17,34,37,40] Distinguishing features between ankylosing spondylitis in male and female patients will be discussed later.[41]

Racial Distribution. It has long been recognized that ankylosing spondylitis occurs more rarely in non-Caucasian populations. The reason for this is now apparent. For example, HLA-B27 occurs in less than 1 percent of Japanese and black Africans. The disease is exceptionally rare in the former group and almost unknown in the latter. In the American Indian, B27 prevalence figures range from 18 to 50 percent, and ankylosing spondylitis is correspondingly frequent.[26,35] The American black has a B27 prevalence of 3 to 4 percent and a frequency of ankylosing spondylitis between the two extremes.[24]

Age Distribution. Sacroiliac and spinal disease usually develops about age 20 in patients with "primary" ankylosing spondylitis, but other ages are affected in the "secondary" forms. For example, individuals (mostly male, carrying the HLA-B27 antigen) with juvenile chronic arthropathy can develop spinal disease during their teens.[42] Individuals with spinal disease secondary to one of the other seronegative spondylarthropathies may develop ankylosing spondylitis as late as the fifth or sixth decade. A so-called seronegative enthesopathic arthropathy syndrome is recognized in children, often associated with HLA-B27 but with a normal pelvis.[43]

PATHOLOGY

The unique histopathology of ankylosing spondylitis and the seronegative spondylarthritides was clearly defined in 1971.[44] The primary pathologic site for rheumatoid disease is the synovium. In contrast, in ankylosing spondylitis, the primary site is the insertion of ligaments and capsules into bone (= the enthesis). Moreover, the latter disease is characterized by fibrosis and ossification rather than joint destruction and instability. An explanation for these clinical findings has been provided by the pathologist. Enthesopathic change explains the typical findings of ankylosing spondylitis: syndesmophyte formation, squaring of the vetebral bodies, vertebral end plate destruction, Achilles tendinitis, and other problems. The enthesis is a metabolically active site, at least during growth, a point of significance since ankylosing spondylitis begins at an early age. Further studies have enhanced our understanding of the pathological process in this disease.[45-47]

In summary, we now understand that ossification occurs in the region of discs, the apophyseal and sacroiliac joints, and extraspinal sites, initiated by lesions at the site of ligamentous insertions (= enthesopathy). The synovitis that occurs in patients with peripheral joint disease mimics that seen in rheumatoid diseases.[47]

CLINICAL FEATURES

Since we now know that the prevalence of ankylosing spondylitis is at least ten times greater in males than hitherto considered (and even a greater-fold in females),[34] it is clear that the majority of patients with ankylosing spondylitis remained undiagnosed. Unless the physician appreciates that ankylosing spondylitis is a common disease, his index of suspicion will remain low and the diagnosis missed.

Articular Disease

Spinal Symptoms. Although back pain affects some 30 percent of society at some stage in life, persistent back pain is much less common. The five characteristic features of back pain in inflammatory spinal disease such as ankylosing spondylitis are summarized in Table 64–8. These symptoms were derived from a controlled analysis of patients with mechanical spinal disease and ankylosing spondylitis.[48] Other features, useful in differentiating back pain of a mechanical and inflammatory nature, are summarized in Table 64–9. A typical patient with ankylosing spondylitis develops back pain or discomfort during the early 20's. Onset is insidious and tends to be persistent, having begun at least 3 months earlier than the first visit to a physician. In contrast to most mechanical back syndromes, the discomfort of ankylosing spondylitis improves with exercise. The morning stiffness usually lasts longer than that seen with mechanical spinal problems. Some patients present with a "pleuritic" chest pain that may cause sleep disturbance. This pain, worse on inspiration, is due to insertional tendinitis of the many costosternal and costovertebral

Table 64–8. Characteristic Features of Back Pain (or Discomfort) in Ankylosing Spondylitis

1. Age of onset below 40 years
2. Insidious onset
3. Duration greater than 3 months
4. Association with morning stiffness
5. Improvement with exercise

Table 64–9. Differential History in Back Symptoms of Mechanical and Inflammatory Type

	Mechanical	Inflammatory
Past history	±	+ +
Family history	−	+
Onset	Acute	Insidious
Age	15–90	< 40
Sleep disturbance	±	+ +
Morning stiffness	+	+ + +
Involvement of other systems	−	+
Effect of exercise	Worse	Better
Effect of rest	Better	Worse
Radiation of pain	Anatomical (S1, L5)	Diffuse (thoracic, buttock)
Sensory symptoms	+	−
Motor symptoms	+	−

muscle insertions. The back pain is not well localized by the patient. The pain may be centered on the low back but is often felt in the low dorsal area or buttocks with minimal radiation.

Late Spinal Complications. Relatively few patients progress relentlessly to the classic stage of bamboo spine. The fused spine may fracture following trivial or even unrecognized injury.[49] This event appears to be more common than once appreciated and may be evidenced by increased motion and/or pain. Fractures usually occur in the cervical region and may be multiple. Because of deformity, radiographic visualization of the fracture site may be difficult and special views required. In some patients the fracture site may be apparent only weeks after the injury. Conservative management with halo traction and body cast may be adequate, or surgical intervention may be required.

A sudden exacerbation of back pain may follow mild trauma. Radiologic evaluation reveals a localized defect in a vertebral end plate or destruction of the disc-bone border. Spondylodiscitis is the term given to this lesion.[50] Measures to reduce spinal mobility result in rapid symptomatic relief. This is in contrast to the more usual exercise regimen recommended for patients with ankylosing spondylitis.

Extraspinal Joint Disease. As many as 20 percent of patients may present with peripheral joint disease. Pain, swelling, and effusion of the peripheral joints are a frequent initial event. At some stage of the disease, up to 35 percent of patients exhibit peripheral joint involvement, often asymmetric in nature and more frequently affecting the lower limb joints. Hip ankylosis and shoulder disease may provide major disability. Any joint may be involved, and a recent study described temporomandibular joint disease in 10 percent of patients,[51] while another referred to peripheral arthropathy occurring after the spinal disease had become inactive.[52]

Published reports of "prevalence" figures for various complications of ankylosing spondylitis are mostly derived from university-based series of patients. Now that milder cases are being recognized, it is probable that these figures are an exaggeration. True figures will follow from new and detailed epidemiologic studies.

Enthesopathic Lesions. In view of the pathologic nature of the disorder, it is not surprising that patients may present with insertional tendinitis at any site, typified by lesions of the Achilles tendon, intercostal muscle insertions, plantar fasciitis, and dactylitis. These tendinitic episodes may be recurrent but leave little residual evidence of disease activity apart from new bone formation, as demonstrated by the plantar spur.

Extra-Articular Disease

Until recently, ankylosing spondylitis was thought to be a back disease with little or no constitutional or systemic involvement. During the last years it has become clear that the disorder may affect all body systems and indeed may not be the "immunologically silent" condition it was once considered. Direct questioning may reveal a history of conjunctivitis, uveitis, oligoarthritis (usually of the lower limbs), Achilles tendinitis, and other enthesopathic problems.

General Symptoms. Constitutional features include fatigue, weight loss, and low grade fever.[53] Hypochromic anemia and an increased erythrocyte sedimentation rate may occur.[54]

Certain features may be found early or at any time in the course of the disease. These include peripheral joint involvement and inflammation of the uveal tract.[55] Other manifestations occur only after years of active disease. Examples include aortic regurgitation,[56] cord compression,[57] upper lobe pulmonary fibrosis,[58] and amyloid deposition.[59]

Chronic Prostatitis. In 1958, Mason and others showed that chronic prostatitis, present in 30 percent of controls and patients with rheumatoid arthritis, occurred in 80 percent of patients with Reiter's syndrome and ankylosing spondylitis.[60] The significance of this possible chronic source of infection is not clear, and any etiological relationship remains speculative.

Eye Disease. Conjunctivitis and iritis may occur in up to 25 percent of patients during the course of their illness.[61] Hart stated that at presentation 13 percent of cases revealed past or present evidence of iridocyclitis and that more than 20 percent of patients develop this manifestation during a 10-year follow-up period.[53] Eye involvement seems to be unrelated to the severity of the spondylitis, but may be more frequent in subjects with peripheral joint involvement. That inflammation of the uveal tract may be a "forme fruste" of ankylosing spondylitis was suggested by the association of uveitis with B27 even in the absence of rheumatic disease.[20] Visual episodes are often self-limiting, but may require corticosteroid preparations given locally or even systemically.

Pulmonary Disease. In 1949, Hamilton described two patients with chronic infiltrative and fibrotic changes in the upper lobe of the lungs.[62] Many reports have appeared since that time, and upper lobe pulmonary fibrosis is now a well recognized late manifestation of ankylosing spondylitis.[58] Typically, the patient has severe spondylitis. Cough, sputum and dyspnea begin in the fifth decade, the sputum becoming profuse. Radio-graphic examination reveals diffuse bilateral upper lobe pulmonary fibrosis. Cyst formation and parenchymal destruction may occur, the lesions becoming invaded with *Aspergillus.* These changes mimic tuberculosis. Histology reveals patchy pneumonia with round cell and fibroblastic infiltration, progressing to interalveolar fibrosis with hyalinization. Dense pleural and pulmonary fibrosis may occur. Treatment is of no avail. Death may occur following massive hemoptysis.

Although a rigid chest wall may result from postinflammatory fusion of thoracic joints, pulmonary ventilation is usually well maintained by the diaphragm. In an analysis of deaths in patients with ankylosing spondylitis, Court-Brown and Doll noted 2.5 to 3 times excessive deaths from respiratory causes compared with expected individual rates. The influence of upper lobe pulmonary fibrosis and other infective etiologic factors was hinted at.[63]

Cardiovascular Disease. Cardiovascular involvement is now well recognized.[64,65,65a] The stated prevalence of this complication varies from 3.5 percent of cases with a 15-year history to 10 percent with up to 30 years of disease. Heart disease occurs more frequently in those with more severe spondylitis involvement, prominent systemic manifestations, and marked peripheral joint disease.

Aortic incompetence, cardiomegaly, and persistent defects in cardiac conduction are the most common findings. Complete atrioventricular block with the development of Stokes-Adams attacks may occur.[66] Pericarditis has also been described. Cardiac involvement may be clinically silent[65] or may dominate the picture.

Aortic incompetence is the best studied complication. Up to 20 percent of patients with ankylosing spondylitis may have anatomic disease of the aortic valve, but relatively few of these have clinically detectable valvular dysfunction. In a recent review[56] of the histology, the adventitial scar tissue and intimal fibrous proliferation affecting aortic valve cusps and aorta behind and above the sinuses of Valsalva were described. The scar tissue may extend below the base of the aortic valve, producing a subaortic fibrous ridge. This may involve the base of the anterior mitral leaflet, causing mitral regurgitation. Further extension may result in heart block. Aortitis may be apparent before definite changes of ankylosing spondylitis. Thus, the condition may be considered a forme fruste in a similar manner to that of uveitis. However, patients with "primary" aortic insufficiency do not appear to carry the antigen HLA-B27 more frequently than one would expect by chance alone.[67]

Amyloidosis. Amyloid is an occasional complication of ankylosing spondylitis.[68] In one study,[59] three of 35 patients with ankylosing spondylitis were found to have amyloid on routine rectal biopsy. Although relatively common, this event is rarely of clinical significance.

The Kidney in Ankylosing Spondylitis. In contrast to patients with rheumatoid arthritis, in whom impairment of renal function is an expression of the disease,[69] there appears to be no impairment of renal glomerular function in ankylosing spondylitis.[70] This is despite the recognized pathologic changes demonstrated by Pasternack and others.[71,72] In a study of 38 consecutive patients with severe ankylosing spondylitis, investigation of glomerular function failed to show any marked abnormality.[70] However, cases of IgA nephropathy have been described.[72a]

Neurological Syndromes. Involvement of the cauda equina may occur in the later stages of the disease.[73,74] The syndrome presents with insidious onset of leg or buttock pain with sensory and motor impairment, in association with bowel and bladder symptoms. Lumbar diverticulae are found on myelographic examination. Emergency neurosurgery may be required. One study[75] suggests that multiple sclerosis may occur in this disease more frequently than would be expected by chance alone.

PHYSICAL EXAMINATION

Spinal mobility is symmetrically decreased, in contrast to patients with mechanical spinal disease who may have limited anterior motion or lateral motion in one direction. Apart from spinal mobility, other physical findings include muscle spasm and loss of lumbar lordosis. Other measurements include the occiput to wall distance, a test of little use until late in the disease. Finger to floor measurements are likewise not helpful, the maneuver reflecting general flexibility, length of arms, and hip status rather than spinal mobility per se. A nonspecific but useful measurement is that of "intermalleolar straddle." The patient is asked to abduct the hips to the maximum, and the distance between the medial malleoli is measured. This distance seems to reflect overall pelvic mobility and decreases in patients with enthesopathic disease (for contrasting features with mechanical spinal disease, see Table 64–10).

Various techniques have been developed to measure spinal mobility.[76-78] The most useful single measurement is the modified Schober test.[77] A perpendicular line is drawn from the midpoint between the posterior iliac spines and an arbitrary point 10 cm above. The distraction of the line joining these two points is measured on anterior flexion. In a normal individual, this 10-cm line distracts to a total of between 16 and 22 cm. A

Table 64–10. Differential Findings on Examination Between Back Pain of Mechanical and Inflammatory Type

	Mechanical	**Inflammatory**
Scoliosis	+	—
Range of movement: Decreased	Asymmetrically	Symmetrically
Local tenderness	Local	Diffuse
Muscle spasm	Local	Diffuse
Straight leg raising	Decreased	Normal
Sciatic nerve stretch	Positive	Absent
Hip involvement	—	+
Neurodeficit	+	—
Other systems	—	+

Table 64–11. Sacroiliac Changes in Ankylosing Spondylitis*

Grade		
	0 Normal	
	I Suspicious	
	II Minimal sacroiliitis	Grade depends on degree of blurring of joint margins, juxta-articular sclerosis, erosive change, and narrowing
	III Moderate sacroiliitis	
	IV Ankylosis	

*According to New York criteria.

patient with severe disease may only have 1 or 2 cm of distraction. Lateral spinal flexion can be measured by noticing the distraction on contralateral flexion of a line drawn in the mid-axillary plane, 20 cm in length, with the upper point level to the xiphisternum. A "normal" individual distracts to a total of 26 to 32 cm, whereas a patient with inflammatory spinal disease may increase the distance by only 2 or 3 cm, or less.

RADIOLOGIC EVALUATION

The five grades of sacroiliitis, introduced by the New York criteria (Grades 0 through IV), are summarized in Table 64–11. Grade 0 refers to normal sacroiliac joints. The sacroiliac margin is clear, and there is a uniform joint space of normal width (Fig. 64–1). There is no bony sclerosis. Grade I signifies "suspicious" change but no specific abnormality. Grade II or "minimal sacroiliitis" refers to loss of definition at the edge of the sacroiliac joints (Fig. 64–2). There is some sclerosis and perhaps minimal erosions. There may be some joint space narrowing. Grade III or moderate sacroiliitis describes the situation in which there is definite sclerosis on both sides of the sacroiliac joint, blurring and indistinct margins, and erosive changes with loss of joint space (Fig. 64–3, left). Grade IV changes show complete fusion or ankylosis of the joint with or without some residual sclerosis (Fig. 64–3, right).

Sacroiliitis is frequently missed. Reliance on a single anteroposterior radiograph of the pelvis is sufficient to recognize sacroiliac disease. Sacroiliitis does not occur as an age-related phenomenon.[17] Other processes that may cause confusion with sacroiliitis include Paget's disease of bone and metastatic disease. Gout and infections such as brucellosis, staphylococcal disease, and other, rarer causes (e.g., *Serratia*) may lead to unilateral sacroiliitis.[79,80]

Osteitis condensans ilii is a sclerotic condition of unknown cause producing dense bone in one or both iliacs. The sclerosis is not on the sacral side of the joint. This radiologic change allows for an increased demarcation of the joint margin in contrast to sacroiliitis, in which a blurred margin and juxta-articular sclerosis on both sides of the joint occur. An example of a female patient with both conditions is shown in Figure 64–4.

One frequently sees patients with bilateral Grade IV

Figure 64–1. Normal pelvis. Note clearly defined sacroiliac joint margins and lack of sclerosis.

sacroiliitis and no extrapelvic spinal disease. Why some patients demonstrate this appearance while others have miminal (Grade II) sacroiliitis and marked spinal disease remains unknown. An example of an HLA-B27 positive patient with the latter configuration is given in Figure 64–5. The "end-stage" pelvis is shown in Figure 64–6.

In view of the enthesopathic nature of the disease (inflammation at the site of ligament insertion into bone), it is not surprising that radiologic changes occur at these sites. Thus, vertebral squaring, which may be an early *or* late change in spondylitis, results from destructive erosive disease at the upper and lower corners of the vertebrae at the site of insertion of the anulus fibrosus of the disc. Thus, the normal concavity of the

Figure 64–2. Minimal sacroiliitis (Grade II). Note juxta-articular sclerosis, blurring of joint margin, minimal erosions, and some joint space narrowing in this 35-year-old female.

Figure 64–3. Moderate sacroiliitis (Grade III) on left side; note juxta-articular sclerosis and further loss of joint space. Right side shows total ankylosis (Grade IV) in this 40-year-old female.

Figure 64–4. This 38-year-old HLA-B27-positive female has both osteitis condensans ilii (note ilial sclerosis) and sacroiliitis (note loss of joint space).

anterior border of the vertebral body is lost (Fig. 64–7). Ball has demonstrated that bony reaction to this destructive lesion results in syndesmophyte formation[43] (Fig. 64–8). At the later stage, progressive ossification occurs (Fig. 64–9). This new bone formation is in close juxtaposition to the spine, in contrast to the changes seen in hyperostosis.

Syndesmophytes must be differentiated from osteophytes (associated with disc space narrowing) and hyperostotic lesions. McEwen and colleagues studied the different radiologic spinal changes in primary ankylosing spondylitis and the other secondary spondyloarthropathies. As summarized in Table 64–12, primary ankylosing spondylitis and spondylitis secondary to inflammatory bowel disease mimic each other in contrast to the changes seen with Reiter's syndrome and psoriatic

Figure 64–5. Fifty-year-old HLA-B27–positive male with minimal sacroiliitis but marked spinal ankylosis. Note lumbar syndesmophytes.

Figure 64–6. Sixty-year-old HLA-B27–negative male with inflammatory bowel disease and total pelvic and spinal fusion. Note loss of joint space at symphysis pubis and sacroiliac joint, osteoporosis, and spinal ossification.

Figure 64–7. Ankylosing spondylitis. Note loss of concavity of lumbar vertebra due to enthesopathic disease.

arthropathy.[81] In essence, asymmetric sacroiliitis associated with skip lesions in the spine suggests Reiter's syndrome or psoriatic disease.

Radionuclide scanning may be more sensitive than radiography in detecting early sacroiliac disease.[82] However, this investigation is nonspecific and too sensitive and has no role to play. Computed tomography is expensive and unnecessary.

Extraspinal Radiologic Disease. Typical findings include an erosive destructive anthropathy of hip and, to a lesser extent, other joints and new bone formation at the site of enthesopathic lesions. Examples of the latter include plantar spurs and fluffy periostitis at the site of Achilles tendon insertion.

LABORATORY ABNORMALITIES

In rheumatoid arthritis abnormal chemical values are frequently found. Such abnormalities are less well rec-

ognized in ankylosing spondylitis. However, some 50 percent of patients with this disease have a rise in alkaline phosphatase.[83] Serum creatine phosphokinase is also frequently elevated.[84] The explanation for this elevated enzyme is not clear. The erythrocyte sedimentation rate may be high, but the rate bears little correlation to the disease activity. If searched for, circulating immune complexes may be found.[85]

As stressed, the diagnosis of ankylosing spondylitis depends on suspicion, history, clinical evaluation, and radiological confirmation. HLA-B27 plays little or no role in the diagnosis of this disease. The patient with symptoms suggesting ankylosing spondylitis but with normal radiographs does not have ankylosing spondylitis, regardless of HLA status. In contrast, a B27 negative individual with sacroiliitis does have the disease. This topic is explored elsewhere in more detail.[86,87]

ANKYLOSING SPONDYLITIS AND WOMEN

As mentioned, the prevalence of ankylosing spondylitis in women may approach the figure for men.[17,34,37,40]

The diagnosis is often missed in females because of a

Figure 64–8. Ankylosing spondylitis. Note syndesmophyte formation (ossification in anterior fibers of anulus fibrosus).

Figure 64–9. Ankylosing spondylitis. Late stage. Note paraspinal ossification and fused sacroiliac joint.

low degree of suspicion. Moreover, certain features of the disease in women make definition of ankylosing spondylitis more difficult. In Caucasians, Hill and others have shown that there is the same strong association between HLA-B27 and disease in the two sexes.[71]

The major differences between the disease in men and in women are summarized in Table 64–13. In women, the disease tends to present with peripheral joint involvement, to progress less rapidly, to be associated with less dramatic spinal changes, to have more cervical involvement, and to be relatively less severe.[41] These and other factors partly explain why the condition is diagnosed less frequently in women than in men. A typical delay in diagnosis of 10 years in women has been described.[88-90] Hitherto, many women with this disease carried the diagnostic label of "seronegative rheumatoid arthritis."[91] Pregnant women with the disease have few problems.[92]

The differential diagnosis between ankylosing spondylitis and rheumatoid disease is compounded by the fact that some patients with seropositive nodular erosive rheumatoid arthritis may fuse peripheral joints as well as the spine. The differentiation relies on the normal sacroiliac joints, strong seropositivity for rheumatoid factor, and absence of HLA-B27.[93]

ETIOLOGY

The cause of ankylosing spondylitis remains unknown despite an unsubstantiated claim that a specific Klebsiella serotype has an intimate relationship with B27-positive lymphocytes of patients.[94] A debate continues as to whether this organism is found more frequently in patients with AS than in controls or only in patients with extraspinal symptoms.[95] Our impression is that many different organisms could precipitate disease in susceptible individuals. The relationship among HLA-B27, other genes, and the environment is under intense study.[96] At this time, there are several intriguing pieces of information.

1. About 20 percent of B27-positive subjects develop disease.[29-31,97]

2. There may be a haplotypic influence conferring susceptibility greater than just that of B27 (e.g., B27/A28[98,99] and B27/A2[100]).

3. Relatives of healthy B27-positive subjects are less likely to develop disease than are relatives of B27 positive patients.[29a]

4. Both ankylosing spondylitis and Reiter's syndrome appear to breed-true within families.[28,29]

5. HLA-B27 may be heterogenic, there being at least two subpopulations of "B27" molecules as determined by monoclonal antibodies[102] and biochemical analysis with two-dimensional poly-acrylamide gel electrophoresis.[103]

Taken together these data suggest that there may be

Table 64–12. Radiologic Changes in Primary and Secondary Forms of Ankylosing Spondylitis

	Category I: Primary Ankylosing Spondylitis —and Ankylosing Spondylitis Associated with Inflammatory Bowel Disease	Category II: Ankylosing Spondylitis Associated —with Reiter's Syndrome and Psoriatic Arthropathy
Sacroiliac changes	Symmetrical	Asymmetrical
Osteitis pubis	++	+
Facetal joint involvement	+++	+
Squaring of vertebrae	++	+
Syndesmophytes	+++	+
Ossification	++	+
Spread	Ascending	Random

Table 64–13. Major Differences Between Ankylosing Spondylitis in Men and in Women

	Males	Females
HLA-B27	> 90 percent	> 90 percent
Delay in diagnosis	3 years	10 years
Progress	+ + +	+
Severity	+ + +	+
Peripheral joint disease:		
Initial	+	+ +
Subsequent	+	+ + +
Spinal ankylosis*	+ +	+
Cervical spine symptoms	+	+ +
Osteitis pubis	+	+ + +

*Skipping thoracic and lumbar spine in females.

genetic differences between healthy and diseased B27-positive subjects. Whether these differences relate to B27 epitopes, other genes on the 6th chromosome, or genes elsewhere remain unknown.

That ankylosing spondylitis is not an immunologically silent disorder is now well-recognized.[85,104–107] Nevertheless, the possibility that the disorder depends on a link between B27 and a putative immune response gene[108] is by no means certain, particularly since there is no HLA-DR association.[109] Recently, attention has been paid to two animal models that may clarify the situation.[110,111]

PROGNOSIS

The outcome for an individual patient is difficult to predict.[112] Some patients have disease limited to the pelvis while others have progressive spinal or extraskeletal disease. HLA-B27 homogeneity is not associated with more severe disease.[113] Long-term follow-up studies of groups of patients (followed, inevitably, in academic referral centers) have suggested decreased survival characteristics.[114–117] However, it is our impression that the individual patient may remain optimistic about the natural history, most leading a normal social, family, and professional life.

MANAGEMENT

General Considerations. The majority of patients with ankylosing spondylitis should expect a good prognosis for a successful life pattern, despite chronic discomfort over many years. The disease progresses to severe and total ankylosis in relatively few patients. Apart from inflammatory eye disease, systemic involvement is rare.

The patient should stop smoking. The combination of a fused chest and pulmonary disease is a tragic occurrence. Swimming is the best routine sport to pursue. For those few individuals with relentless disease, admission to an active rehabilitation unit is advisable. Hydrotherapy and aggressive remedial exercises may provide benefit.

Posture and Exercises. The patient must realize that the aim of therapy is to maintain normal posture and activity. Thus, a hard bed at night is more useful than a soft mattress. Extension exercises should remind the patient that the natural tendency of the disease is to produce loss of height and curvature. Thus, extension exercises must be performed at least twice daily. A hot shower provides decreased stiffness and allows the exercise regimen to be followed. During the day, adequate attention must be given to the position at work, the style of chairs, and the chance for mobility.

Nonsteroidal Anti-inflammatory Drug Therapy. There have been few adequately controlled studies comparing efficacy between different drugs and long-term outcome. One uncontrolled study suggests that continuous rather than intermittent phenylbutazone therapy is associated with less skeletal ossification.[118] Phenylbutazone appears to be the most efficacious agent, and aspirin has little place in the management of ankylosing spondylitis.[119]

Although phenylbutazone is probably the most efficacious agent, indomethacin is considered the drug of choice in view of the possible long-term toxicity of the former drug. This may be given in doses of 25 to 50 mg three times a day. For those patients who tolerate indomethacin in whom efficacy is lacking, phenylbutazone, 100 mg three to four times daily, is suitable for a few weeks. Thereafter, a safe drug can be given. If indomethacin is not tolerated, other, newer nonsteroidal agents may be useful[120,121] and are discussed in Chapter 50.

It is important for the patient to have adequate insight into the natural history of the disease, and the prognosis for almost normal function should be stressed. The patient must be aware that therapy should be continuous. The purpose of anti-inflammatory agent medication is to enable the patient to carry out an adequate exercise program, to maintain good posture, and to follow normal activities.

Other Modalities. Radiotherapy may be of limited value, but it has fallen into disrepute because of the risk of leukemia.[122] Surgical treatment is occasionally indicated. Vertebral wedge osteotomy may be useful for correcting deformity,[123] and hip arthroplasty performed for patients with inflammatory hip disease. Immunosuppressive agents have not been studied in this condition, and recent information suggests that penicillamine has little role to play.[124] Whether auranofin is efficacious remains to be seen.

Genetic Counseling. Debate continues as to whether family members of patients with ankylosing spondylitis and other HLA-B27 associated diseases should be routinely HLA typed. At present, we know that about 20 percent of B27 positive individuals will develop ankylosing spondylitis. However, as yet there is no cure for this disease, and considerations such as vaccination and other protective mechanisms are not yet viable possibilities. Moreover, with knowledge of the disease in the family, diagnosis can be reached early and adequate treatment introduced. At this stage, therefore, we would not advise routine HLA typing.

SUMMARY

Ankylosing spondylitis is a common disease. As the medical community becomes more aware of this fact, improved recognition, diagnosis, and therapy should follow.

There are still many aspects of the disease that remain poorly explained. For example, a recent epidemiologic study suggested that even in the absence of specific and recognized complications, the death rate in patients with ankylosing spondylitis is greater than in matched controls.[116] Despite this, the physician and patient should maintain an optimistic outlook, since few individuals with this chronic rheumatic syndrome are incapacitated.

In Britain, patients and physicians have combined to provide a national ankylosing spondylitis society, a group determined to enhance education, research, and care for this disease. Similar fora should be developed in the United States and elsewhere.

References

1. Calin, A., and Fries, J.F.: Ankylosing Spondylitis: Discussions in Patient Management. Garden City, N.Y., Medical Examination Publishing Company, Inc., 1978, pp. 1–117.
2. Moll, J.M.H. (ed.): Ankylosing Spondylitis. Edinburgh, Churchill Livingstone, 1980.
2a. Calin, A., (ed.): Spondylarthropathies. Stratton, Orlando, Florida, Grune & Stratton, 1984.
3. Raymond, P.: Les maladies de nosanc eancêtres à l'age de la piètre (The diseases of our ancestors in the stone age). Aeschlape, 2:121, 1912.
4. Ruffer, M.A., and Rietti, A.: On osseous lesions in ancient Egyptians. J. Pathol. Bacteriol. 16:439, 912.
5. Bourke, J.B.: A review of the Palaeopathology of Arthritic Diseases in Antiquity. Edited by D. Drothwell and A.T. Sardison. Springfield, Ill., Charles C Thomas, 1967, p. 352.
6. Short, C.L.: The antiquity of rheumatoid arthritis. Arthritis Rheum. 17:193, 1974.
7. Turner, C., and Bennett, P.H.: Personal communication.
8. Sydenham, T.: Medical Observations Concerning the History and Cure of Acute Diseases. Translated by R.G. Latham. London, The Sydenham Society, 1848, p. 254.
9. Bennett, P.H., and Burch, T.A.: Population Studies of the Rheumatic Diseases. Amsterdam, Excerpta Medica Foundation, 1968, p. 305.
10. Moll, J.M.H., and Wright, V.: New York criteria for ankylosing spondylitis: A statistical evaluation. Ann. Rheum. Dis. 32:354, 1973.
11. Burns, T., Marder, A., Becks, E., Sullivan, L. and Calin, A. "Undifferentiated Spondylarthritis: A Nosological Missing Link?" Arthritis Rheum., 25:S142, 1982.
12. Burns, T. and Calin, A.: Undifferentiated Spondylarthropathy. In Calin, A. (ed.): The Spondylarthropathies. New York, Grune & Stratton, 1984, pp. 253–264.
13. Graham, W., and Uchida, I.A.: Heredity in ankylosing spondylitis. Ann. Rheum. Dis. 16:334, 1957.
14. Strecher, R.M.: Heredity in joint diseases. Docum. Rheum. Geigy 12, 1957.
15. de Blecourt, J.J., Polman, A., and de Blecourt-Meindersma, T.: Hereditary factors in rheumatoid arthritis and ankylosing spondylitis. Ann. Rheum. Dis. 20:215, 961.
16. Kellgren, J.H.: The epidemiology of rheumatic diseases. Ann. Rheum. Dis. 23:109, 1964.
17. Emery, A.E., and Lawrence, J.S.: Genetics of ankylosing spondylitis. J. Med. Genet. 4:239, 1967.
18. Brewerton, D.A., Caffrey, M., Hart, F.D., et al: Ankylosing spondylitis and HL-A 27. Lancet 1:904, 1973.
19. Schlosstein, L., Terasaki, P.I., Bluestone, R., et al.: High association of an HL-A antigen, W27 with ankylosing spondylitis. N. Engl. J. Med. 288:704, 1973.
20. Brewerton, D.A., Caffrey, M., Nicholls, A., et al.: Acute anterior uveitis and HLA 27. Lancet 2:994, 1973.
21. Brewerton, D.A., Caffrey, M., Nicholls, A., et al.: Reiter's disease and HLA 27. Lancet 2:996, 1973.
22. Brewerton, D.A., and James, D.C.O.: The histocompatibility antigen (HL-A 27) and disease. Semin. Arthritis Rheum. 4:191, 1975.

23. Hyla, J.F., Franck, W.A., and Davis, J.S.: Lack of association of HLA B27 with radiographic sacroiliitis in inflammatory bowel disease. J. Rheumatol. 3:196, 1976.
24. Good, A.E., Kawanishi, H., and Schultz, J.S.: HLA B27 in blacks with ankylosing spondylitis or Reiter's disease. N. Engl. J. Med. 294:166, 1976.
25. Sonozaki, H., Seki, H., Chang, S., et al.: Human lymphocyte antigen, HLA 27 in Japanese patients with ankylosing spondylitis. Tissue Antigens 5:131, 1975.
26. Lisse, J.R., Bennett, P.H., Knowler, W.O., Gofton, J.P., Calin, A. and Mann, D.L.: High risk of sacroiliitis in HLA-B27 positive Pima Indian men. Arthritis Rheum. 25:236, 1982.
27. Gofton, J.P., and Bennett, P.: Personal communication, 1983.
28. Hochberg, M.C., Bias, W.B., and Arnett, F.C.: Family studies in HLA-B27 associated arthritis. Medicine 57:463, 1978.
29. Calin, A., Barnett, M., Marder, A., and Marks, S.: The nature and prevalence of spondylarthritis among relatives of probands with ankylosing spondylitis and Reiter's syndrome. J. Rheumatol. In press, 1984.
29a. Calin, A., Marder, A., Becks, E., et. al.: Genetic differences between B27 positive patients with ankylosing spondylitis and B27 positive healthy controls. Arthritis Rheum. 26:1460, 1983.
30. Dunham, C.L., and Kantz, F.G.: Spondylarthritis and ankylopoetica: Review and report of 20 cases. Am. J. Med. Sci. 201:232, 1941.
31. Hare, H.F.: Diagnosis of Marie-Strümpell arthritis with certain aspects of treatment. N. Engl. J. Med. 223:702, 1940.
32. West, H.F.: The aetiology of ankylosing spondylitis. Ann. Rheum. Dis. 8:143, 1949.
33. Lawrence, J.S.: The prevalence of arthritis. Br. J. Clin. Pract. 17:699, 1963.
34. Calin, A., and Fries, J.F.: The striking prevalence of ankylosing spondylitis in "healthy" W27 positive males and females. A controlled study. N. Engl. J. Med. 293:835, 1975.
35. Gofton, J.P., Chalmers, A., Price, G.E., et al.: HLA 27 and ankylosing spondylitis in B.C. Indians. J. Rheumatol. 2:318, 1975.
36. Cohen, L.M., Mittal, K.K., Schmid, F.R., et al.: Increased risk for spondylitis stigmata in apparently healthy HLA W27 men. Ann. Intern. Med. 84:1, 1976.
37. Kidd, K.K., Bernoco, D., Carbonara, A.O., et al.: Genetic analysis of HLA associated diseases: The "illness susceptible" gene frequency and sex ratio in ankylosing spondylitis. In Dausset, J., and Svegaard, A.: HLA and Disease. Copenhagen, Munksgaard, 1977.
38. Editorial. HLA-B27 and risk of ankylosing spondylitis. Br. Med. J. 2:650, 1978.
39. Dawkins, R.C., Owen, E.T., Cheah, P.S., Christiansen, F.T., Calin, A., et al.: Prevalence of ankylosing spondylitis and radiological abnormalities of the sacroiliac joints in HLA-B27 positive individuals. J. Rheumatol. 8:1025, 1981.
40. Dequeker, J., Decock, T., Walrarens, M., and van de Putte, I.: A systematic survey of the HLA-B27 prevalence in inflammatory rheumatic diseases. J. Rheumatol. 5:453, 1978.
41. Marks, S.H., Barnett, M., and Calin, A.: Ankylosing spondylitis in women and men: A case-control study. J. Rheumatol., 10:624, 1983.
42. Marks, S.H., Barnett, M., and Calin, A.: A case-control study of juvenile- and adult-onset ankylosing spondylitis. J. Rheumatol. 9:5, 1982.
43. Rosenberg, A.M. and Petty, R.E. "A Syndrome of Seronegative Enthesopathy and Arthropathy in Children." Arthritis Rheum. 25:1041–1047, 1982.
44. Ball, J.: Enthesopathy of rheumatoid and ankylosing spondylitis. Ann. Rheum. Dis. 30:213, 1971.
45. Cawley, M.I.D., Chalmers, T.M., Kellgren, J.H., et al.: Destructive lesions of the vertebral bodies in ankylosing spondylitis. Ann. Rheum. Dis. 31:345, 1972.
46. Sutherland, R.I.C., and Matheson, D.: Inflammatory involvement of vertebrae in ankylosing spondylitis. J. Rheumatol. 3:296, 1975.
47. Revell, P.A., and Mayston, V.: Histopathology of the synovial membrane of peripheral joints in ankylosing spondylitis. Ann. Rheum. Dis. 41:579, 1982.
48. Calin, A., Porta, J., and Fries, J.F.F.: The clinical history as a screening test for ankylosing spondylitis. JAMA 237:2613, 1977.
49. Hunter, T., and Dubo, H.: Spinal fractures complicating ankylosing spondylitis. Ann. Intern. Med. 88:546, 1978.
50. Sutherland, R.I.L., and Matheson, D.: Inflammatory involvement of vertebrae in ankylosing spondylitis. J. Rheumatol. 2:296, 1975.
51. Davidson C., Wojtulewski, J.A., Bacon, P.A., et al.: Temporomandibular joint disease in ankylosing spondylitis. Ann. Rheum. Dis. 34:87, 1975.
52. Cohen, M.D., and Ginsburg, W.W.: Late-onset peripheral joint disease in ankylosing spondylitis. Ann. Rheum. Dis. 41:574, 1982.
53. Hart, F.D.: The stiff aching back. The differential diagnosis of ankylosing spondylitis. Lancet 1:740, 1968.
54. Polley, H.F.: The diagnosis and treatment of rheumatoid spondylitis. Med. Clin. North Am. 39:509, 1955.

55. Birbeck, M.Q., Buckler, W.St.J., Mason, R.M., et al.: Iritis as the presenting symptom in ankylosing spondylitis. Lancet 2:802, 1951.

56. Bulkley, B.H., and Roberts, W.C.: Ankylosing spondylitis and aortic regurgitation. Description of the characteristic cardiovascular lesion from study of eight necropsy patients. Circulation 18:1014, 1973.

57. Sharp, J., and Purser, D.W.: Spontaneous atlanto-axial subluxation in ankylosing spondylitis and rheumatoid arthritis. Ann. Rheum. Dis. 20:47, 1961.

58. Editorial: The lungs in ankylosing spondylitis. Br. Med. J. 3:492, 1971.

59. Jayson, M.I.V., Salmon, P.R., and Harrison, W.: Amyloidosis in ankylosing spondylitis. Rheum. Phys. Med. 1:78, 1971.

60. Mason, R.M., Murray, R.S., Oates, J.K., et al.: Prostatitis and ankylosing spondylitis. Br. Med. J. 1:748, 1958.

61. Blumberg, B., and Ragan, C.: The natural history of rheumatoid spondylitis. Medicine 35:1, 1956.

62. Hamilton, K.A.: Pulmonary disease manifestations of ankylosing spondylarthritis. Ann. Intern. Med. 31:216, 1949.

63. Court-Brown, W.M., and Doll, R.: Mortality from cancer and other causes after radiotherapy for ankylosing spondylitis. Br. Med. J. 2:1327, 1965.

64. Graham, D.C., and Smythe, H.A.: The carditis and aortitis of ankylosing spondylitis. Bull. Rheum. Dis. 9:171, 1958.

65. Tucker, C.R., Fowles, R.E., Calin, A., et al.: Aortitis in ankylosing spondylitis: Early detection of aortic root abnormalities with two-dimensional echocardiography. Am. J. Cardiol. 9:680, 1982.

65a. Bergfeldt, L: HLA B27 associated rheumatic diseases with severe cardiac bradyarrhythmias: clinical features and prevalence in 223 men with permanent pacemakers. Am. J. Med. 75:210, 1983.

66. Julkunen, H., and Luomanmaki, M.: Complete heart-block in rheumatoid (ankylosing) spondylitis. Acta Med. Scand. 176:410, 1964.

67. Calin, A., Fries, J.F., Stinson, F.B., et al.: Normal frequency of HLA B27 in aortic insufficiency. N. Engl. J. Med. 294:397, 1976.

68. Cruickshank, B.: Pathology of ankylosing spondylitis. Bull. Rheum. Dis. 10:211, 1960.

69. Burry, H.C.: Reduced glomerular function in rheumatoid arthritis. Ann. Rheum. Dis. 31:65, 1972.

70. Calin, A.: Renal glomerular function in ankylosing spondylitis. Scand. J. Rheumatol. 4:241, 1975.

71. Pasternack, A., Tallquist, G., and Martio, J.: Renal vascular changes in ankylosing spondylitis. Acta Med. Scand. 187:519, 1970.

72. Pasternack, A., Tornroth, T., and Martio, J.: Ultrastructural studies of renal arteriolar changes in ankylosing spondylitis. Acta Pathol. Microbiol. Scand., Section A, 79:591, 1971.

72a. Jennette, J.C., Ferguson, A.L., Moore, M.A., et al.: IgA nephropathy associated with seronegative spondylarthropathies. Arthritis Rheum. 25:144, 1982.

73. Russell, M.L., Gordon, D.A., Ogryzlo, M.A., et al.: The cauda equina syndrome of ankylosing spondylitis. Ann. Intern. Med. 78:551, 1973.

74. Gordon, A.L., and Yudell, A.: Cauda equina lesion associated with rheumatoid spondylitis. Ann. Intern. Med. 78:555, 1973.

75. Thomas, D.J., Kendall, M.J., and Whitfield, A.G.W.: Nervous system involvement in ankylosing spondylitis. Br. Med. J. 1:148, 1974.

76. Moll, J.M.H., Liyanage, S.P., and Wright, V.: An objective clinical method to measure lateral spinal flexion. Rheum. Phys. Med. 11:225, 1972.

77. Moll, J.M.H., and Wright, V.: Normal range of spinal mobility: An objective clinical study. Ann. Rheum. Dis. 30:281, 1971.

78. Hart, F.D., Strickland, D., and Cliffe, P.: Measurement of spinal mobility. Ann. Rheum. Dis. 33:136, 1974.

79. Delbarre, F., et al.: Pyogenic infection of the sacro-iliac joint. J. Bone Joint Surg. 57A:819, 1975.

80. Donovan, T.L., Chapman, M.W., Harrington, K.D., et al.: Serratia arthritis. J. Bone Joint Surg. 58A:1009, 1976.

81. McEwen, C. DiTata, D., Lingg, C., et al.: Ankylosing spondylitis and spondylitis accompanying ulcerative colitis, regional enteritis, psoriasis, and Reiter's disease. Arthritis Rheum. 14:291, 1971.

82. Russel, A.S., Lentle, B.C., and Percy, J.S.: Investigation of sacroiliac disease: Comparative evaluation of radiological and radionuclide techniques. J. Rheumatol. 2:45, 1975.

83. Kendall, M.J., Lawrence, D.S., Shuttleworth, G.R., et al.: Haematology and biochemistry of ankylosing spondylitis. Br. Med. J. 2:235, 1973.

84. Calin, A.: Creatine phosphokinase in ankylosing spondylitis. Ann. Rheumatol. 34:244, 1975.

85. Rosenbaum, J.T., Theofilopoulos, A., McDevitt, H.O., Perreira, A., Carson, D., and Calin, A.: Presence of circulating immune complexes in Reiter's syndrome and ankylosing spondylitis. Clin. Immun. Immun. Pathol. 18:291, 1981.

86. Calin, A.: HLA-B27: To type or not to type? Ann. Intern. Med., 92:208, 1980.

87. Calin, A.: HLA-B27 in 1982. Reappraisal of a Clinical Test. Ann. Intern. Med. 96:114, 1982.

88. Hill, H.F.H., Hill, A.G.S., and Bodmer, J.G.: Clinical diagnosis of ankylosing spondylitis in women and relation to presence of HLA B27. Ann. Rheum. Dis. 35:267, 1976.

89. McBryde, A.M., and McCollum, D.E.: Ankylosing spondylitis in women. The disease and its prognosis. North Carolina Med. J. 34:34, 1973.

90. Resnick, D., Dwosh, I.L., Goergen, T.G., et al.: Clinical and radiographic abnormalities in ankylosing spondylitis: A comparison of men and women. Radiology 119:293, 1976.

91. Calin, A., and Marks, S.: The case against seronegative rheumatoid arthritis. Am. J. Med. 70:992, 1981.

92. Ostensen, M., Romberg, O., and Husby, G.: Ankylosing spondylitis in motherhood. Arthritis Rheum. 25:140, 1982.

93. Calin, A., Grahame, R., Tudor, M., et al.: Histocompatibility linked antigens in ankylosing rheumatoid arthritis and ankylosing spondylitis. Lancet 1:874, 1974.

94. Seager, K., Bashir, H.R., and Geczy, A.F.: Evidence for a specific B27-associated cell surface marker on lymphocytes of patients with ankylosing spondylitis. Nature 277:68, 1979.

95. Eastmond C.J., Calguneri, M., Shinebaum, R., et al.: A sequential study of the relationship between fecal Klebsiella aerogenes and the common clinical manifestations of ankylosing spondylitis. Ann. Rheum. Dis. 41:15, 1982.

96. Calin, A.: The relationship between genetics and environment in the pathogenesis of rheumatic diseases (medical progress). West. J. Med. 131:205, 1979.

97. Calin, A., and Fries, J.F.: An "experimental" epidemic of Reiter's syndrome revisited. Follow-up evidence on genetic and environmental factors. Ann. Intern. Med. 84:564, 1976.

98. Arnett, F., Schacter, B.Z., Hochberg, M.C., et al.: HLA-A28 in patients with B27 associated rheumatic diseases. Arthritis Rheum. 20:106, 1977.

99. Calin, A., Porta, J., and Payne, R.: HLA-A28 in B27 positive controls and patients with ankylosing spondylitis. Arthritis Rheum. 20:1428, 1977.

100. Terasaki, P.I., and Mickey, M.R.: HL-A haplotypes of 32 diseases. HLA and disease associations. Transplant. Rev. 22:105, 1975.

101. Calin, A., Marder, A., Sullivan, L., et al.: The prevalence of sacroiliitis among relatives of B27-positive spondylitics and relatives of healthy B27-positive blood donors: A controlled study. Arthritis Rheum. 25:S62, 1982.

102. Grumet, F.C., Fendly, B.M., Fish, L., Foung, S., and Engleman, E.G.: Monoclonal antibody (B27M2) subdividing HLA-B27. Human Immunology 5:61, 1982.

103. Kaneoka, H., Engleman, E.G., and Grumet, F.C.: Immunochemical variants of HLA-B27. J. Immunol., 130:1288, 1983.

104. Sturrock, R.D., Barrett, A.J., Versey, J., et al.: Raised levels of complement inactivation products in ankylosing spondylitis. J. Rheumatol. 14:428, 1974.

105. Veys, E.M., and Van Laere, M.: Serum IgG, IgM, and IgA levels in ankylosing spondylitis. Ann. Rheum. Dis. 32:493, 1973.

106. Kinsella, T.D., Espinoza, L., and Vasey, F.B.: Serum complement and immunoglobulin levels in sporadic and familial ankylosing spondylitis. J. Rheumatol. 2:308, 1975.

107. Corrigal, V., Panayi, G.S., Unger, A., et al.: Detection of immune complexes in serum of patients with ankylosing spondylitis. Ann. Rheum. Dis. 37:159, 1978.

108. McDevitt, H.D., and Bodmer, W.F.: HLA, immune response genes and disease. Lancet 1:1269, 1974.

109. Braun, W.E., Dejello, C.L., Clough, J.D., et al.: No association of known DR antigens with ankylosing spondylitis. N. Engl. J. Med. 298:744, 1978.

110. Rosenbaum, J.T.: Why HLA-B27?: An Analysis based on two animal models. Ann. Intern. Med. 94:261, 1981.

111. Rosenbaum, J.T., McDevitt, H.O., Guss, R.B., and Egbert, P.R.: Endotoxin-induced uveitis in rats as a model for human disease. Nature 286:611, 1980.

112. Calin, A.: Ankylosing spondylitis. In Fries, J.F., and Ehrlich, G.E. (eds.): Prognosis: Contemporary Outcomes of Disease. Bowie, Maryland, The Charles Press Publishers, 1981, pp. 357–359.

113. Albert, E.D., Schloz, S., and Christ, V.: Genetics of B27-associated disease. Ann. Rheum. Dis. 38S:142, 1979.

114. Carter, E.T., McKenna, C.H., Brian, D.D., et al.: Epidemiology of ankylosing spondylitis in Rochester, Minnesota, 1935–1978. Arthritis Rheum. 22:365, 1979.

115. Khan, M.A., Khan, M.K., and Kushner, I.: Evidence of decreased survival in ankylosing spondylitis by life-table analysis. Arthritis Rheum. 22:628, 1979.

116. Radford, E.P., Doll, R., and Smith, P.G.: Mortality among patients with ankylosing spondylitis not given x-ray therapy. N. Engl. J. Med. 297:572, 1977.

117. Smith, P.G., and Doll, R.: Mortality among patients with ankylosing spondylitis after a single treatment course with x-rays. Br. Med. J. 284:449, 1982.

118. Boersma, J.W.: Retardation of ossification of the lumbar vertebral column

in ankylosing spondylitis by means of phenylbutazone. Scand. J. Rheumatol. 5:60, 1976.

119. Godfrey, R.G., Calabro, J.J., Mills, D., et al.: A double-blind cross-over trial of aspirin, indomethacin and phenylbutazone in ankylosing spondylitis. Arthritis Rheum. 15:110, 1972.

120. Calin, A., and Grahame, R.: Double-blind cross-over trial of flurbiprofen and phenylbutazone in ankylosing spondylitis. Br. Med. J. 4:496, 1974.

121. Calin, A., and Britton, M.: Sulindac in ankylosing spondylitis. Double-blind evaluation of sulindac and indomethacin. JAMA 242:885, 1979.

122. Court-Brown, W.M., and Doll, R.: Leukaemia and aplastic anaemia in patients irradiated for ankylosing spondylitis. Spec. Rep. Ser. Med. Res. Coun. (London), No. 2950. London, Her Majesty's Stationers Office, 1965.

123. Scudese, V.A., and Calabro, J.J.: Vertebral wedge osteotomy—Correction of rheumatoid (ankylosing) spondylitis. JAMA 186:627, 1963.

124. Bird, H.A., and Dixon, A.St.J.: Failure of D-penicillamine to affect peripheral joint involvement in ankylosing spondylitis or HLA-B27 associated arthropathy. Ann. Rheum. Dis. 36:289, 1977.

Chapter 65
Reiter's Syndrome
Andrei Calin

INTRODUCTION

On August 21, 1916, a lieutenant in the Prussian army developed abdominal pain and diarrhea. This episode lasted 48 hours and was followed by a latent period of 7 days, at which time urethritis and conjunctivitis occurred. The following day he developed polyarthralgias and arthritis of the knees, ankles, elbows, wrists, and several interphalangeal joints. Within a few days the symptoms remitted and the patient remained well for 3 weeks. A relapse followed, with a recurrence of urethritis and uveitis. Unfortunately, we have no knowledge of the long-term course of this historic patient. These events were recorded by Professor Hans Reiter.[1] Apart from a few notable exceptions, few physicians paid much attention to this triad of urethritis, conjunctivitis, and arthritis. From a subject of relative obscurity, Reiter's syndrome has now become one of great fascination and major importance. This dramatic change has resulted from the recognition of the striking association between Reiter's syndrome, a chronic rheumatic disease, and the histocompatibility antigen, HLA-B27. This relationship highlights the link between the individual's genetic background and susceptibility to environmentally induced disease. Indeed, Reiter's syndrome may compare with systemic lupus erythematosus as the rheumatic disorder most likely to hold the answers to some of our many questions. The major developments during the last few years have been published as the proceedings of an international workshop on Reiter's disease.[2]

DEFINITION

Reiter's syndrome may be defined[3] as in Table 65–1, or it may be defined more simply as[11] an episode of arthritis lasting greater than one month in association with urethritis or cervicitis.[4] In the experience of the ARA Criteria Subcommittee, the sensitivity and specificity of these criteria were 84.3 and 98.2 percent, respectively.[4] Terminology often presents a problem in a rapidly developing field. The concept of Reiter's syndrome as a triad of features is being replaced by a more broadly based definition. Since many of the symptoms and signs of the syndrome are clinically silent and nonspecific, a requirement for *three* features is illogical. Patients with a "sexually acquired reactive arthritis"[5] may be considered to have Reiter's syndrome, but terms such as "incomplete Reiter's syndrome"[6] should be avoided. Reiter's syndrome, ankylosing spondylitis, and the other seronegative spondylarthritides are no longer classed as "rheumatoid variants." These conditions may be clearly differentiated from rheumatoid arthritis on historic, epidemiologic, genetic, immunologic, clinical, radiologic, pathologic, and therapeutic grounds (see Chapter 64).

Various formes frustes of Reiter's syndrome have been described, such as persistent balanitis[7] in the absence of other stigmata of the full syndrome, causing added difficulty with definition. There are no specific differential features between the reactive arthropathies associated with *Yersinia, Salmonella* and *Shigella* infections (post-dysenteric Reiter's disease). Reiter's syndrome may be used as a generic term for all these disorders. Alternatively, the eponym may be avoided and replaced by a nonspecific term such as "B27-associated reactive arthropathy." However, B27 is present in 80 percent or less of patients.

Table 65–1. Definition of Reiter's Syndrome

Seronegative asymmetric arthropathy (predominantly lower extremity)
Plus one or more of the following:
 Urethritis/cervicitis
 Dysentery
 Inflammatory eye disease
 Mucocutaneous disease: balanitis, oral ulceration, or keratodermia
Exclusions:
 Primary ankylosing spondylitis
 Psoriatic arthropathy
 Other rheumatic disease

HISTORICAL REVIEW

A search of the literature takes us from the Old Testament book of Leviticus (Chapter 15, verse 2) to 1983. No doubt, exciting developments will occur during the next few years. In Leviticus, we find a description of an individual with a urethral discharge but no clincial follow-up in regard to such sequelae as conjunctivitis or arthritis. More recently, in 1776, Stoll[8] demonstrated that the triad of urethritis, arthritis, and conjunctivitis may follow dysentery; in 1818, Sir Benjamin Brodie[9] found the same to be true following a venereal infection. In 1916, both Reiter on the Balkan front and the French physicians Fiessinger and Leroy[10] on the Somme described, respectively, "spirochaetosis arthritica" and "conjunctival-urethral-synovial syndrome," each syndrome following a dysenteric episode. In 1947, Harkness[11] reaffirmed that Reiter's syndrome may follow both dysenteric and venereal infections. Two major epidemics of Reiter's syndrome, one described by Paronen[12] in 1948 and the other by Noer[13] in 1966, and the subsequent follow-up studies[14,15] have enhanced our understanding of the disease. In the first, Paronen provides an exhaustive review of the Finnish *Shigella flexneri* epidemic in which over 150,000 succumbed to the enteric infection. Thereafter, 344 patients developed Reiter's syndrome. In the second, Noer relates the events leading up to his "experimental" epidemic in which nine cases of Reiter's syndrome developed among 602 crew members with *Shigella* dysentery, there being no cases among those crew members who remained free of the original infection. The significance of these long-term studies will be described later. Review articles describe the natural history and long-term sequelae.[16-18]

ETIOLOGY

The interrelationship between the environment and genetics is crucial in the pathogenesis of Reiter's syndrome.[19] Although the disease mechanism remains unknown, we now recognize several different relevant infective agents and a specific genetic background. How these two features interact in the pathogenesis of the disease remains unclear, but the problem forms the center of much research.

As discussed in the recent symposium on Reiter's syndrome,[2] several of the characteristic findings in Reiter's disease mimic those that occur in the adjuvant arthritis rat model. Originally, this model was thought to mimic rheumatoid arthritis, but it is now recognized that the clinical features in the rat mimic those found in the spondylarthropathies, particularly Reiter's disease. In adjuvant arthritis, the trigger can be mycobacterium in Freund's adjuvant. Both gram-positive and gram-negative peptidoglycans appear to be operative. The susceptibility is strain specific[20] and is controlled by an autosomal gene linked to the MHC. A delay in disease onset occurs in both conditions, with a primary focus on the sacroiliac joints and spine. Tendinitis, periostitis, urethritis, balanitis, keratodermia blennorrhag-

ica, diarrhea, and inflammatory eye disease occur in both disorders. Erythema nodosum is seen in the rat model, and this phenomenon also occurs in yersinia arthropathy, particularly in B27-negative women. Other animal models that may be relevant to our understanding of the B27-related arthropathies have recently been discussed.[21,22]

Environmental Considerations. Historically, Reiter's syndrome has been considered to occur in two forms: the epidemic or enteric form of the disease, and the endemic or postvenereal form. It may be that this artificial grouping is untenable, since, although many patients do fall into one of these two categories, some are not so readily classifiable. Moreover, some individuals develop recurrent exacerbations following neither definite infective diarrheal disease nor sexual indiscretion. Furthermore, the distinction between urethritis as a precipitating factor and urethritis as an integral manifestation of the postdysenteric syndrome remains unclear. Conceivably, *Shigella* and other organisms may not cause an obvious diarrhea but yet may precipitate a recurrence of Reiter's syndrome, since arthritogenic organisms may be carried silently.

The role of chronic persistent genitourinary infection also remains unclear. For example, there is a suggestion that individuals with Reiter's syndrome (and ankylosing spondylitis) are more likely to have prostatitis than age-matched patients with rheumatoid disease.[23] Streptococcal disease has also been incriminated, though without definite evidence, but it is important to realize that the list of arthritogenic agents continues to increase.[24] Reiter's original description of a spirochete on blood culture[1] has never been confirmed.

Epidemic Reiter's Syndrome. There have been several clearly defined postenteric epidemics of Reiter's syndrome.[12,13] Paronen's patients were known to have had *Shigella flexneri* dysentery. The specific *Shigella* serotypes associated with Reiter's syndrome have not been adequately defined. One report[25] described the isolation of *Shigella flexneri* 2a from a patient with Reiter's syndrome following an episode of traveler's diarrhea, and we have now confirmed this association.[26] Our further studies have determined that *Shigella flexneri* 1.g.[26] is also arthritogenic. Whether other *Shigella* infections are associated with a reactive arthropathy remains uncertain. In our controlled follow-up studies of post-*Shigella sonnei* epidemics, no cases of Reiter's syndrome occurred.[27] The disease is said to follow infection with *Shigella dysenteriae*[28], but there have been no recent reports of this occurrence.

Reactive arthritis, sometimes including other features of Reiter's syndrome, has followed infection with *Salmonella*[29,30] and *Yersinia enterocolitica.*[31] A recent study revealed an intriguing relationship between HLA-B27 molecules and *Yersinia* in patients with Reiter's syndrome.[32] These cases are of particular interest in view of the association with HLA-B27. Enteropathic *E. coli* have not, to date, been associated with a reactive arthropathy. It is not clear whether the term reactive arthritis should include the arthropathies associated with amebic dysentery,[33] Whipple's disease,[34] or rheumatic fever. These and other rarer syndromes will probably be more clearly demarcated in the future.

Postvenereal Reiter's Syndrome. Postvenereal or endemic Reiter's syndrome has often been considered the more common form of Reiter's syndrome, especially in the United States and Britain, in contrast to continental Europe, where the postdysenteric variety is allegedly more frequent. Certain cases of postvenereal disease appear to be associated with *Chlamydia*[5] or *Mycoplasma* infection.[35] However, there is no consensus as to the primary cause or causes of postnonspecific urethritis Reiter's syndrome. In a recent study, 531 men with nonspecific urethritis were followed prospectively.[5] Arthritis developed in 16 patients and only 5 of these 16 were positive for *Chlamydia trachomatis*, a similar frequency as in those men without reactive arthropathy. (Some 30 to 50 percent of men with nonspecific urethritis have *Chlamydia* isolated from the urethra.)

A recent study reveals that patients with Reiter's syndrome in the United States have a marked proliferative repose to Yersinia, although this organism is only rarely incriminated outside of Europe.[35a]

In summary, it is possible that a patient with a specific genetic background may react to a variety of different organisms and develop either a reactive arthropathy or the full picture of Reiter's syndrome, depending on other unknown genetic or environmental events.

Genetic Considerations. Since 1973, when Brewerton and colleagues[36] first defined the association between HLA-B27 and Reiter's disease, there have been numerous reports of this association. The original study was performed in individuals with nonspecific urethritis and thus no definite infective agent. More recently, two studies demonstrated that epidemic Reiter's syndrome is also HLA-B27 associated.[15,37] These studies were performed in Caucasian subjects. It has long been recognized that Reiter's syndrome is seen less frequently in non-Caucasians, a finding that may relate to the decreased prevalence of HLA-B27 among these populations. However, HLA-B27 is frequently found in both Haida[38] and Pima[39] Indians, two groups known to have a high prevalence of ankylosing spondylitis but few if any cases of Reiter's syndrome.[40,41] Since it is likely that the arthritogenic agents are ubiquitous, there are probably other relevant genetic determinants that explain this paradox. One possible explanation may relate to the finding that Reiter's syndrome and ankylosing spondylitis tend to breed true within families.[42-44] Moreover the use of monoclonal antibodies and biochemical analysis with two-dimensional polyacrylamide gel electrophoresis[45-47] has suggested that the B27 molecule may consist of at least two subpopulations.

Recently, it has been suggested that HLA-B27-negative individuals with Reiter's syndrome are likely to have one of the other cross-reacting antigens, HLA-B7, BW22, or BW42,[48] a finding that provides support for the theory that HLA-B27 itself (or cross-reacting antigen) is relevant in the disease's pathogenesis rather than a postulated immune-response linked gene.

INCIDENCE AND PREVALENCE

The incidence and prevalence of Reiter's syndrome are difficult to assess but are almost certainly underestimated for several reasons (Table 65-2):

1. There is no absolute diagnostic test.
2. The illness tends to affect young adults, members of a mobile community who are difficult to follow.
3. The early venereal features of the disease may be suppressed or forgotten, and the patient carries a diagnostic label of "undifferentiated chronic arthritis" or other nonspecific diagnosis.
4. The enteric features may have been minimal.
5. Several diagnostically significant features of the disease (including the often clinically inapparent mouth ulcers, balanitis, and urethritis) may be masked by the more severe arthritic component, resulting in failure to diagnose the disease appropriately.
6. Nonspecific but clinically significant features may be overlooked. These include eye disease and keratodermia (often misdiagnosed as fungal disease or psoriasis).
7. Urethritis, difficult to recognize in the male, is frequently impossible to establish in the female.
8. Cervicitis is nonspecific, usually asymptomatic, and rarely identified as a relevant feature in a female presenting with, for example, a swollen ankle.
9. Since the chronicity of the disorder has not been adequately recognized, many patients with persistent arthropathy and relatively minimal extra-articular disease are considered to have "seronegative rheumatoid arthritis."
10. There is overlap between the seronegative spondylarthritides. Thus, some patients considered to have ankylosing spondylitis as a primary event may in fact have sacroiliitis and spinal disease as a secondary manifestation of Reiter's syndrome. The earlier triad or tetrad of features may be long forgotten and the original diagnosis ignored. Likewise, some patients with ankylosing spondylitis may develop nonspecific urethritis and, in error, be considered to have Reiter's syndrome.
11. Because Reiter's syndrome is a multisystem disorder, care is often fragmented and the patient may be followed independently by the ophthalmologist, or-

Table 65–2. Explanation for Lack of Prognostic Data and Underestimated Prevalence of Reiter's Syndrome

1. No absolute diagnostic test
2. Young adults: mobile community
3. Venereal history suppressed
4. Enteric features forgotten
5. Clinically inapparent "diagnostic" features: silent mouth ulcers, silent balanitis, silent urethritis
6. Nonspecific but clinically significant eye disease or skin disease
7. Asymptomatic urethritis in females
8. Asymptomatic cervicitis
9. Misdiagnosis: "seronegative rheumatoid arthritis"
10. Overlap between seronegative spondylarthritides (e.g., Reiter's syndrome now considered ankylosing spondylitis)
11. Fragmented care (a multisystem disorder)

thopedic surgeon, rheumatologist, venereologist, or other subspecialty physician.

Nevertheless, a few studies have provided evidence that Reiter's syndrome is a relatively common rheumatic disease. Indeed, it may be claimed that the most common cause of an inflammatory arthropathy in a young male is Reiter's syndrome. Csonka[49,50] has stated that Reiter's syndrome develops in about 1 percent of subjects with nonspecific urethritis. More recent data[5] suggest that reactive arthritis develops in up to 3 percent of individuals with nonspecific urethritis. This latter study provides evidence that the risk to the HLA-B27 positive individual who contacts nonspecific urethritis is in the order of 20 percent, a figure remarkably similar to our own,[15] in which some 25 percent of B27 positive *Shigella* patients developed epidemic Reiter's syndrome. In that same group of patients, Noer[13] showed that the incidence of Reiter's syndrome among all *Shigella* patients (9 out of a total of 602) was 1.5 percent.

Several studies have provided evidence that some 20 percent of HLA-B27 positive individuals develop ankylosing spondylitis following an unknown event.[51-53] Why only 20 percent of B27 positive subjects are at risk following an unknown event (ankylosing spondylitis) or a specific infective episode (Reiter's syndrome) remains unknown. Detailed epidemiologic, family, genetic, and molecular studies should elucidate this problem.

GEOGRAPHIC DISTRIBUTION

It is possible that Reiter's syndrome has a worldwide distribution, the prevalence roughly following the frequency of HLA-B27, with certain exceptions as discussed above. A recent study from China described 22 cases.[54] Until detailed prospective studies have been performed, the worldwide distribution will not be clearly defined.

SEX DISTRIBUTION

The sex distribution is more difficult to assess, since the syndrome may be diagnosed only with difficulty in the female. The often quoted sex ratio of 20 males to 1 female is almost certainly an exaggeration. As discussed in Chapter 64, we now have evidence that ankylosing spondylitis occurs more frequently in females than was hitherto believed. Likewise, it is probable that Reiter's syndrome in females will be more clearly recognized in the future.[55] Balanitis and urethritis, two common diagnostic features in the male, cannot provide the same help in the female. In our own study, women represented 15 percent of the 131 patients.[3] Postdysenteric Reiter's disease does have an equal sex distribution.[26] That postvenereal Reiter's disease is more prevalent in men may relate to the fact that nonspecific urethritis itself occurs more often in men.

AGE DISTRIBUTION

Urethritis is difficult to recognize in children, and the diagnosis of Reiter's syndrome is only likely to be made during an epidemic of dysentery with Reiter's syndrome affecting many family members. Paronen[12] included four cases in children among his 344 epidemic cases.

Reiter's syndrome is most frequently recognized during the third decade. However, no age is exempt, and we have seen patients in their 50's and above with both postvenereal and postendemic Reiter's syndrome. The so-called seronegative enthesopathic arthropathy syndrome of children[56,57] has features that mimic those found in Reiter's disease and the other spondylarthropathies.

CLINICAL FEATURES

Almost every system in the body may be affected by Reiter's syndrome. The prevalence of the various features is difficult to ascertain, since different authors have used a different definition for Reiter's syndrome, some making the diagnosis only in the presence of the full triad. Since most published studies come from academic center patient populations, there is an inevitable bias toward more severe disease. In an attempt to overcome this problem, we have recently evaluated 131 patients seen both at a university clinic and in a community center.[3] The prevalence of the different features, at entry to the study, are summarized in Table 65–3. Polyarthritis and urethritis (or cervicitis) were seen in over 90 percent of patients. The third most common event was back pain, often due to insertional tendinitis, since many individuals had normal pelvic radiographs. Two thirds had eye disease. Balanitis and heel pain (including Achilles tendinitis) occurred in about half the patients. One quarter had oral lesions or keratodermia blennorrhagica. Nail involvement, aortitis, and other complications were rarely seen.

Every patient presenting with a mono- or oligoarthropathy, especially when involving lower limb joints,

Table 65–3. Characteristics of 131 Consecutive Patients with Reiter's Syndrome, at Initial Visit

Total (n = 131)	%
Arthritis:	100
Monoarthritis	4
Polyarthritis	96
Urethritis/cervicitis	90
Diarrhea	18
Eye disease	63
Back pain	72
Heel pain	56
Tendinitis	52
Balanitis	46
Stomatitis	27
Keratodermia	22
Nail lesions	6

must be questioned about possible urethritis, balanitis, eye disease, and mouth ulcers. The urethritis is frequently not apparent to the patient. Minimal stinging on passing urine or a small discharge, sometimes only noticed by the patient after being alerted by direct questioning, may be present. Likewise, the balanitis is frequently not evident unless the prepuce is retracted. Stomatitis is usually asymptomatic and will be apparent only on close inspection. A minimally inflamed eye is easily forgotten or passed off as a reaction to irritating fumes. The various skin lesions typified by keratodermia blennorrhagica may not be seen until later in the course of the disease and may then be considered nonspecific, fungal, or due to psoriasis. Questioning concerning bowel function may reveal a major diarrheal episode consisting of the frequent passage of bloody loose stools, a short episode of increased bowel activity lasting for 24 hours, or a hitherto forgotten event some weeks earlier. Because of the emotive nature of urethritis, the patient's confidence must be gained to ensure an adequate history in this respect.

Typically, there is a latent period between the onset of diarrhea or urethritis and the rheumatologic syndrome. Following an interval of 1 to 3 weeks, other features of the disease occur in varying order. Conjunctivitis (or uveitis) may be followed by tendinitis, arthralgias, or arthritis. When an episode of diarrhea is followed some days later by urethritis, it is difficult to be sure whether the Reiter's syndrome should be considered enteric or venereal in nature, since the urethritis may be a nonvenereal manifestation of the syndrome or either feature may be coincidental.

Arthritis. Until recently, the arthritis of Reiter's syndrome was said to be acute, short lived, and transient. Indeed, an occasional fortunate patient has a self-limiting process. However, more frequently patients are seen with a persistent or recurrent rather than transient arthropathy. Arthralgias, monoarthritis, polyarthritis, tendinitis, fasciitis, and spinal symptoms occur. Weight-bearing joints, particularly the knees and ankles, are most frequently involved. The arthritis may be florid with large effusions, knee involvement sometimes resulting in popliteal rupture early in the course of the disease.[58] A "sausage" toe (dactylitis) represents a typical lesion. The extrasynovial swelling is characteristic of the enthesopathic process (Fig. 65–1).

Although a persistent monarthropathy is rare, the patient frequently complains primarily of ankle and/or heel pain. It remains unknown why Reiter's syndrome preferentially involves the Achilles tendon, plantar fascia, ankle, and subtalar joints.

Ligament, Tendon, and Fascial Problems. Back pain, Achilles tendinitis, plantar fasciitis, chest wall pain, and other fleeting arthralgias are a frequent problem in Reiter's syndrome. The pathology is not always clear cut, but many of these symptoms may be due to insertional tendinitis or enthesopathic change as described by Ball[59] (see Chapter 64). Since intercostal muscle insertion tendinitis presents with a "pleuritic" type of chest pain, patients presenting with such pain and fever may be inappropriately investigated for thoracic disease.

Urogenital Lesions. Urethritis may be a postdysenteric phenomenon (a primary feature of the disease) or a precipitating event. In either case, it may be asymptomatic or a major component. Acute hemorrhagic cystitis has been described.[60] Prostatitis may occur in 80 percent of patients, a figure comparable to that seen in ankylosing spondylitis, but greater than the 30 percent figure for age-matched rheumatoid arthritis controls.[23] Since involvement of the urogenital tract may occur in the postdysenteric form of Reiter's syndrome, the inflammatory process must be due to mechanisms other than direct infection. Likewise, diarrhea may occur in venereally acquired Reiter's syndrome, according to some authors.[61,62] As discussed below, the urethral process may be considered an "allergic" phenomenon.

Ocular Lesions. Conjunctivitis is considered a part of the classic triad of Reiter's syndrome. However, it is not clear from the literature how many patients have conjunctivitis, a conjunctival reaction to uveitis, iritis alone, or a mixture. The symptoms are frequently mild and escape notice. The discharge, when present, is sterile and

Figure 65–1. Reiter's syndrome. Note two "sausage" digits (dactylitis) and typical nail change.

Figure 65–2. Reiter's syndrome. *A*, Keratodermia blennorrhagica on sole of foot. Note hyperkeratotic lesions. *B*, Same foot as shown in *A*, 6 weeks later. Note total healing of lesions.

Figure 65–3. Reiter's syndrome. Keratoderma blennorrhagica. Note hyperkeratotic lesions over lower limbs.

Figure 65–4. Reiter's syndrome. Keratodermia blennorrhagica. Note scaling lesions on palms.

body, resulting in exfoliation and even death.[69] Macroscopically, the skin lesions begin as discrete vesicles which become opaque as their wall thickens. Hyperkeratotic nodules result. Apart from a narrow erythematous base around the lesions, there is little evidence of local inflammation. The vesicles may coalesce, resulting in a hyperkeratotic crust lasting for days, weeks, or months. They may disappear without a trace and can frequently recur.

Microscopically, the lesions cannot be distinguished from those of psoriasis. Characteristic changes include hyper- and parakeratosis with elongation of the rete pegs. Spongiform pustules are found in the upper malpighian layer with varying degrees of polymorphonuclear leukocyte infiltration throughout the epidermis. Well-defined microabcesses may be found. These various changes have been reviewed by Hancock[70] and Csonka.[49,50] Prevalence figures derived from five separate studies are summarized in Table 65–4. Figures range from 1 to 31 percent. Representative lesions are shown in Figure 65–1 through 65–4.

The relationship between skin lesions and overall disease severity and prognosis has not been defined. In our study,[3] there appeared to be no correlation between the skin lesions and the course of the disease.

There is no specific treatment, although various keratolytic agents may be tried. Topical glucocorticoids should be avoided because of the risk of atrophy. The response to methotrexate and azathioprine appears favorable, but no formal double-blind control studies have been performed.

As shown in Table 65–4, the prevalence of mucosal lesions varies from 3 to 33 percent. These figures are probably an underestimate for the reasons mentioned above. The lesions occur on the palate, tongue, buccal mucosa, and lips. They appear as shallow ulcers, sometimes with an irregular erythematous base. The histopathology was described by Epstein in 1939.[71] Changes are similar to those found in the skin. Parakeratosis, elongation of the rete pegs, acanthosis, microabscesses, and mixed cellular infiltrate are found. The lesions require no therapy.

Circinate balanitis occurs as painless and superficial erosions on the glans penis (Fig. 65–5). Prevalence figures range from 23 to 50 percent (Table 65–4). Again, these figures may well be an underestimate. Balanitis may present with small vesicles which can rupture to form a painless superficial erosion with little surrounding erythema. Lesions may coalesce to form a circinate pat-

usually subsides in a few days. During the course of the disease, uveitis may become a more significant problem, causing serious debility.[14,15,63] Up to a third of all patients presenting to an ophthalmologist with uveitis may have underlying rheumatic disease.[64]

Mucocutaneous Manifestations. The association between keratodermia blennorrhagica and urethral infection has been known since 1893.[65] More recently, these lesions were recognized as part of Reiter's syndrome.[66] Stomatitis and balanitis were associated at the turn of the century.[67,68] As discussed above, the prevalence and natural history of these lesions remain unclear. The mouth ulcers are usually clinically inapparent and may disappear within a few days of their occurrence. Likewise, the skin lesions may go unnoticed by the patient and physician.

Keratodermia blennorrhagica occurs most frequently on the soles of the feet (Fig. 65–2), glans penis, and toes. Discrete lesions may be found elsewhere on the limbs (Fig. 65–3), scrotum, trunk, scalp, and palms (Fig. 65–4). In severe cases, keratodermia may affect the whole

Table 65–4. The Prevalence of Mucocutaneous Lesions in Reiter's Syndrome

Patients (No.)	Stomatitis (%)	Balanitis (%)	Keratodermia Blennorrhagica (%)	References
76	11	26	8	54
260	12	23	13	36, 37
16	33	50	31	45
344	3	33	1	11
131*	27	46	22	3
131†	22	29	17	3

*At initial visit.
†At mean follow-up, 6.4 years.

Figure 65–5. Reiter's syndrome. Circinate balanitis. Note superficial ulceration.

tern. The coronal margin of the prepuce and adjacent glans are most frequently affected. In circumcised individuals the lesions develop a hard crust, in contrast to uncircumcised patients in whom the lesions remain moist and may develop secondary infection.

Balanitis may predate other manifestations of Reiter's syndrome. Lassus[7] described a group of individuals with

Figure 65–6. Reiter's syndrome. Nail lesions. Note typical destructive nature of change with subungual hyperkeratotic accumulaltion of material.

persistent circinate erosive balanitis and no other stigmata of Reiter's syndrome, the majority of whom were HLA-B27 positive. Thus, balanitis may occur as a forme fruste of Reiter's syndrome. Four of our own 131 patients had balanitis for a mean of 4 years before the onset of urethritis, arthritis, and conjunctivitis.[3]

Nail involvement may be seen in association with keratodermia or may occur as a separate entity. Early change consists of a red rolled edge of a nail fold. Subungual corny material accumulates and may lift the nail plate, which becomes yellow and thickened (Fig. 65–6). The brittle nail may be shed. These changes may persist indefinitely or clear. Inflammatory areas in the skin adjacent to the subungual keratotic material may mimic paronychiae.

A striking aspect of the mucocutaneous phenomena seen in Reiter's syndrome is that ankylosing spondylitis, a closely related disease, does not have any of these lesions.

LATE SEQUELAE

In discussing Reiter's syndrome, it is conventional to describe the early symptoms and signs and then the late manifestations. Clearly, this artificial approach is not always justified. Some patients, seen early in their course, may already have an asymmetric sacroiliitis, a major ophthalmic problem that predated the other stigmata of Reiter's syndrome, or even an "idiopathic" aortic regurgitation.

Spinal Disease. It is recognized that some 20 percent of individuals with HLA-B27 develop sacroiliitis and ankylosing spondylitis.[51-53] It is also well recognized that a varying proportion of patients with Reiter's syndrome develop sacroiliitis or even the full picture of ankylosing spondylitis. It has been said that sacroiliac involvement is found particularly in patients with longstanding, recurrent disease, and figures as high as 80 percent have been quoted.[72] A reasonable figure is probably in the range of 20 to 30 percent. Whether the spinal disease should be considered a complication of Reiter's syndrome or rather a manifestation of HLA-B27 disease remains unclear. However, the fact that the spinal disease is said to occur more frequently in patients with severe Reiter's syndrome and that the involvement is often asymmetrical,[73,74] would suggest that the process is related to Reiter's syndrome itself, rather than to HLA-B27. Moreover, one occasionally sees patients with Reiter's syndrome who develop spondylitis at an older age than that of the usual onset of "primary" ankylosing spondylitis, analogous to the situation in which patients with inflammatory bowel disease may only develop sacroiliitis and spondylitis after the fifth or sixth decade. It remains unknown whether an HLA-B27 positive individual who develops Reiter's syndrome is more or less at risk of developing sacroiliitis and ankylosing spondylitis than an otherwise healthy HLA-B27 subject. Family studies, now in progress, may provide an answer to this intriguing question.

The patient with Reiter's syndrome should be directly questioned about back pain or stiffness and other symptoms suggestive of spondylitis. Typical features include insidious onset, predominant morning stiffness, discomfort after prolonged periods of rest, and improvement with exercise.[75] Physical examination may reveal a decreased range of spinal mobility. These symptoms and signs may be present before marked radiologic change.

Late Eye Disease. Progressive iridocyclitis with intraocular hemorrhage, optic neuritis, and other problems may occur.[76] Blindness may result. In contrast, uveitis may sometimes be considered a forme fruste of Reiter's syndrome, since even in the absence of rheumatologic symptoms or signs, patients presenting with uveitis may be found to have HLA-B27.[77]

Cardiovascular Disease. Involvement of the heart is well recognized. Electrocardiographic changes include prolongation of the PR interval, complete heart block, S-T segment changes, and abnormal Q waves.[62,78] Clinically, the patient may develop palpitations, transient murmurs, pericardial rub, and aortic regurgitation.[12,17] This last complication is clinically and histologically identical to that seen in ankylosing spondylitis.[79] Occasionally, one will see older patients with pulmonary or cardiac symptoms related to hitherto unrecognized or forgotten Reiter's syndrome. With sophisticated modern equipment, clinically unsuspected heart changes may be found.[80]

Central Nervous System Involvement. The prevalence of neurological complications is in the region of 1 percent. These include peripheral neuropathy, transient hemiplegia, cranial nerve lesions, and other nonspecific neurological findings.[76,78,81]

Pulmonary Complications. Pleurisy and pulmonary infiltrates have been described.[82] Since patients with Reiter's syndrome may have insertional tendinitis of the intercostal muscles and ligaments, "pleuritic" chest wall pain may occur.

Miscellaneous Complications. Rarely, purpura, thrombophlebitis,[83] and amyloidosis[84] may complicate Reiter's syndrome.

Nonspecific Features. Fatigue, malaise, weight loss, fever, and mental change are sometimes found in patients with Reiter's syndrome. These features may be a part of the disease process or may be related to drug therapy.

RADIOLOGIC EVALUATION

In the early stages no radiographic changes are found. With progression of disease juxta-articular osteoporosis, narrowing of the joint space, and erosive changes may be seen. Periostitis, as seen in juvenile chronic polyarthropathy, psoriatic arthropathy, and other seronegative spondyarthritides, occurs around the pelvis, metatarsals, tarsal bones, phalanges, and elsewhere. New bone reaction is also commonly found at the insertion of the plantar fascia. These plantar spurs may develop during a few weeks.

As mentioned above, sacroiliitis indistinguishable from that seen in ankylosing spondylitis may occur, or it may be asymmetric. Apophyseal joint erosions and ankylosis may be seen. The asymmetric spinal changes mirror those occurring in psoriatic arthropathy.[74] Lateral bony bridging between the vertebral bodies at the dorsolumbar junction has been described.[85] Skip lesions are also recognized, as seen with psoriatic arthropathy.

LABORATORY EVALUATION

The erythrocyte sedimentation rate may vary from 1 to 130 mm per hour. There appears to be little or no correlation between this and disease severity or prognosis. The abnormality may persist for weeks or return to normal despite progressive joint activity. Mild hypo- or normochromic anemia may be present. Serum proteins show minimal change. We have recently demonstrated immune complexes in about two thirds of patients with Reiter's disease.[86] Prostatic antibodies may be present, but this test is nonspecific.[87]

Synovial fluid analysis is rarely contributory in the differential diagnosis of inflammatory joint disease, unless crystals or infective agents are found. In the synovial fluid the white count may range from 500 to 50,000 cells per cubic millimeter. The glucose, protein, and other measurements are of no help. It is claimed[88] complement is normal or elevated in Reiter's syndrome synovial fluid, in contrast to the low titers seen in rheumatoid disease. However, this distinction should not be required to differentiate the two conditions. More recently, the synovial fluid-serum complement ratio has been shown to be reduced in Reiter's syndrome.[89]

HLA-B27

Although of great academic interest, the routine typing for the HLA-B27 antigen is an unnecessary and expensive "test." This topic is explored elsewhere in more detail.[90,91] Sometimes claimed to be of use in differentiating Reiter's syndrome from gonococcal disease, the B27 result would be too late to be of use. A detailed history and examination should suffice for the recognition of most cases of Reiter's syndrome. B27 typing may be helpful in the evaluation of mono- or oligoarthropathy in which no typical extra-articular features are present.

In 1973, the association between ankylosing spondylitis and HLA-B27 became apparent.[92,93] Thereafter, Brewerton reported a similar link between this antigen and Reiter's disease. The implications of this finding are manifold. The initial study[36] was performed with endemic (postvenereal) cases of Reiter's syndrome. The relevant infective agent in these cases may be *Mycoplasma, Chlamydia* or other agents.[35] More recently, studies have determined that postepidemic Reiter's syndrome and post-*Yersinia* and post-*Salmonella* reactive arthropathies are also HLA-B27 associated.[15,31,37]

In Caucasians, some 80 percent of Reiter's syndrome

patients are B27 positive.[3] In blacks, however, the link is less close.[94] The disparity between different races has been more clearly defined in ankylosing spondylitis in both blacks,[94] and Japanese.[95] The reason why some individuals without HLA-B27 still develop Reiter's syndrome is unclear. However, some B27-negative patients do carry cross-reacting antigens.[48]

As discussed above, the risk for the HLA-B27 positive individual of developing ankylosing spondylitis or a reactive arthropathy following infection appears to be about 20 percent.[5,15,51-53] Whether the same B27 positive individual is at risk for developing either ankylosing spondylitis or Reiter's syndrome remains unknown. However, recent family studies suggest that the two disorders run in families.[42-44] These and the evidence for molecular differences within the B27-positive lymphocytes[45-47] argue for a genetic explanation. There are two major theories: the first, that HLA-B27 is linked to a gene responsible for disease expression; and the second, that B27 itself may be directly related to disease pathogenesis by molecular mimicry or cross-reactivity.[96]

PATHOLOGY

Synovial biopsy in Reiter's syndrome is relatively unhelpful. The changes are nonspecific and show inflammatory change with edema, vascular congestion, and infiltration with neutrophils, lymphocytes, and occasional plasma cells. There is some proliferation of synoviocytes and fibroblasts. At a later stage, changes are indistinguishable from those seen in rheumatoid arthritis.[61]

Adequate biopsy material from extra-articular sites is not available. However, as discussed in Chapter 64, Ball[59] introduced the concept of enthesopathy (inflammatory change at the site of the enthesis: that area where ligaments insert into bone). Many of the clinical manifestations of Reiter's syndrome can be explained if one remembers the enthesopathic nature of the disease. Thus, whereas inflammation of the synovium is central to the disease process of rheumatoid arthritis, inflammation at the site of ligament and capsule insertion is the focus for disease activity in Reiter's syndrome. Typical examples of the enthesopathic process include insertional tendinitis of the Achilles tendon, the sausage digit with juxta-articular inflammation and radiologic evidence of periostitis, periinsertional osteoporotic change, erosions, and plantar spurs (Table 65–5). The explanation for these enthesopathic lesions remains unclear.

Table 65–5. Enthesopathic Features of Reiter's Syndrome

Sausage digits (juxta-articular disease)
Insertional tendinitis: Achilles tendon, intercostal muscles
Sacroiliitis
Periostitis, spurs
Peri-insertional osteoporosis, erosions

Table 65–6. Similarities Between Reiter's Syndrome and Gonococcal Arthropathy

	Reiter's Syndrome	Gonococcal Arthropathy
Oligoarthritis	+	+
Tenosynovitis	+	+
Conjunctivitis	+	+
Urethritis	+	+
Skin lesions	+	+
Fever	+	+
Urethral cultures for gonococcus	?+	?+
Sexual activity	+	+
Synovial fluid	Variable	Variable

REITER'S SYNDROME IN FEMALES AND CHILDREN

Reiter's syndrome is recognized only with difficulty in women. In our study,[3] 15 percent of 131 consecutive patients were women. Children with Reiter's syndrome are only likely to be recognized as such following an epidemic of *Shigella* dysentery when other adult family members are diagnosed as having Reiter's syndrome. The clinical course in women and children appears to be similar to that in men.[3,26,55,97] A report of Reiter's syndrome in a female, presenting as erythema nodosum, appeared recently.[98]

DIFFERENTIAL DIAGNOSIS

When Reiter's syndrome presents with a triad or tetrad of features, there should be no problems in reaching

Table 65–7. Differences Between Reiter's Syndrome and Gonococcal Arthritis

	Reiter's Syndrome	Gonococcal Arthritis
Sex distribution	Males > females	Males < females
Personal or family history of arthritis	+	−
Uveitis	+	−
Gonococcus culture:		
Joint	−	?+
Skin	−	?+
Pharynx	−	?+
Rectum	−	?+
Back pain	+	−
Migratory arthralgias	−	+
Joint distribution	Lower > upper	Lower < upper
Achilles tendinitis	+	−
Plantar fasciitis	+	−
Massive recurrent knee effusion	+	−
Stomatitis	+	−
Balanitis	+	−
Keratodermia blenorrhagica	+	−
Response to penicillin	−	+
HLA-B27 (%)	80	5
Course	Recurrent/chronic	Acute

Table 65–8. Similarities Between Reiter's Syndrome and Psoriatic Arthropathy

	Reiter's Syndrome	Psoriatic Arthropathy
Peripheral joint disease	+	+
Axial disease	25%	25%
Association with:		
Eye disease	+	+(rare)
Skin disease	+	+
Nail involvement	+	+
HLA-B27	+(80%)	+(20–50%)

a correct diagnosis. However, if only one or two features are present, the differential diagnosis will include infective arthritis, rheumatic fever, crystal synovitides, and other disorders. Since the disease is most commonly seen in young men, gonococcal disease provides a frequent diagnostic dilemma. The similarities and differences between these two disorders are summarized in Tables 65–6 and 65–7. Since both conditions may be venereally acquired, a coincidental positive culture for the gonococcus may be found in Reiter's syndrome. Gonococcal arthritis is more frequently encountered in women. HLA-B27 typing may be an academically useful test when the differential diagnosis between these two conditions remains in doubt, but is currently too slow for the result to be valuable in patient management.

Psoriatic arthropathy and Reiter's syndrome have many features in common. Indeed, there are times when the two cannot be differentiated. Some similarities and differences are summarized in Tables 65–8 and 65–9.[99]

Acute rheumatic fever is now rarely seen. Nevertheless, it is important to remember to include rheumatic fever in the differential diagnosis of Reiter's syndrome, especially in those cases in which the disease presents with fever and toxicity. Antistreptolysin 0 titer and other tests will help in the diagnosis.

THE RELATIONSHIP OF REITER'S SYNDROME TO ANKYLOSING SPONDYLITIS

The patient with progressive spinal disease may be followed for many years with a diagnosis of "ankylosing spondylitis," forgetting that the episode began with urethritis and conjunctivitis several decades earlier. In contrast, there are patients with ankylosing spondylitis who develop a coincidental urethritis. Eye lesions are common to both disorders, and so the differentiation sometimes remains difficult. Both conditions are associated with HLA-B27, and as yet there are few genetic differences, apart from a suggestion that there are HLA haplotype distinctions between the two conditions,[100] and both epidemiologic[42-44] and genetic[45-47] differences. Similarities and differences between these two conditions are summarized in Table 65–10.

NATURAL HISTORY AND PROGNOSIS

Such statements as "joint symptoms are characteristically acute, short lived, and transient"[101] may give the patient and physician a false expectation. For the occasional fortunate individual, Reiter's syndrome *may* be a self-limiting disease. In fact, the prognosis of Reiter's syndrome is notoriously difficult to assess. The reasons for this are protean (see Table 65–2). Long-term follow-up studies are few and suffer from the inherent problem that such studies are usually performed in academic centers where patients with more severe disease are followed.

In fact, a review of the literature suggests a relatively *poor* prognosis. The original Paronen epidemic,[12] in 1944, was reviewed 20 years later.[14] Three hundred and forty-four patients were originally affected. At follow-up, 100 patients were available for the study (no doubt including a bias toward those with more severe disease). Of these patients, 80 still had active disease. These included 32 with ankylosing spondylitis, 18 with recurrent acute arthropathy, 30 with chronic joint disease, 7 with recurrent uveitis, and 2 with aortic regurgitation. Some 40 (over 10 percent of the original Reiter's syndrome patients) were unable to work because of persistent Reiter's syndrome.

Csonka[49] followed 185 patients for a period of 2 to 15 years. Sixty-two percent had active disease, and he suggested a recurrence rate of 15 percent per patient per year. In another study, Good[102] followed 34 patients for 2 years and found that 24 had persistent disease at the

Table 65–9. Differences Between Reiter's Syndrome and Psoriatic Arthropathy

	Reiter's Syndrome	Psoriatic Arthropathy
Sex distribution	10 male: 1 female	3 female: 2 male
Age	20–30	Any age
Onset	Acute	Insidious
HLA	B27	B27, B13, BW17, BW38, DR4
Skin lesions	Plantar, palmar, penile	Widespread
Relationship of arthritis to severity of skin lesions	None	Fair
Mouth ulcers	Yes	No
Urethritis	Yes	No
Joint predilection	Lower limb	Upper limb
Distal interphalangeal joints	Rare	Frequent

Table 65–10. Similarities and Differences Between Ankylosing Spondylitis and Reiter's Syndrome

	Ankylosing Spondylitis	Reiter's Syndrome
Sex distribution		
Sacroiliitis	M = F	Postvenereal M > F
Sacroiliitis and spondylitis	M > F	Postdysenteric M = F
Sacroiliitis and peripheral joint disease	M < F	
Age at onset		
Primary	20–30	20–30 (Any age)
"Secondary"	20–60	
Sacroiliitis	100%	20%
Spine involvement	Symmetrical ascending	Asymmetrical patchy
Peripheral joint disease	25%	95%
Hip disease	15%	5%
Conjunctivitis/uveitis	20%	55%
Urethritis	0	95%
Skin/mucous membrane disease	0	60%
Aortic regurgitation	Rare	Rare
Onset	Gradual	Sudden
Course	Chronic	Remitting/relapsing
HLA-B27		
Caucasians	95%	80%
Blacks	40–60%	40–60%
Risk for B27-positive subjects	Approximately 20 %	Approximately 20% (if venereal or gut infection)

end of the period, including 13 with sacroiliitis. Our follow-up[15] of Noer's original study[13] revealed that four of the five patients contacted had active and severe disease, 13 years after the original epidemic. All four had persistent joint problems, two had deteriorating vision following iridocyclitis, and two had ankylosing spondylitis. Only one subject remained free from active disease. Of interest, this individual was the only one of the five who was HLA-B27 negative. In fact, he carried the cross-reacting antigen HLA-B7. McCluskey and others[103] have also suggested that individuals with HLA-B27 are more likely to develop severe disease than their HLA-B27 negative counterparts. However, a more recent study[3] throws some doubt on this concept.

In our recent investigation,[3] 131 patients were consecutively admitted to the study at both a university and a community medical center (in order to avoid selection bias). At a mean of 5.6 years, 122 patients (93 percent) were available for follow-up. In summary, there were no major differences between the two centers. Polyarthritis persisted in 83 percent of cases, urethritis and/or cervicitis in 42 percent, back pain and heel pain in about one half, eye disease in a third, and balanitis and mouth ulcers in a quarter. Of major importance, over one quarter of the patients were either unemployable or were forced to change occupation.

There was little difference in the disease between males and females or between B27-positive and B2-negative individuals.

Some patients have recurrent episodes with asymptomatic periods between exacerbations. However, in our experience, the majority of individuals have continuing but sometimes minimal background discomfort. These symptoms may include back pain, heel pain, or other problems. Many of our patients had a continuing chronic disease from the outset. Some recurrences were precipitated by sexual indiscretion, but many appeared following a diarrheal episode or de novo, with the urethritis

appearing as an "allergic" phenomenon rather than an infective event.

Thus, Reiter's syndrome *is* a major chronic rheumatic disease. The physician and patient must have a realistic concept of its natural history. Future works of reference should *not* include such statements as: "The disease is usually self-limited, subsiding in 6 weeks to 6 months, and complete remission with full recovery of peripheral joint function is the rule."

MANAGEMENT

There is no cure for Reiter's syndrome. Few rheumatic syndromes are more frustrating to treat. False expectations of the patient (and sometimes physician) frequently result in "doctor shopping." The plethora of new nonsteroidal anti-inflammatory drugs has not improved therapy.

A major role in management is one of explanation. The disease is frequently bewildering and disturbing for the patient and family. Feelings of guilt and anxiety about sexual misconduct should be allayed. Although anecdotal evidence suggests that certain patients with postvenereal Reiter's syndrome are more likely to develop relapse following sexual indiscretion, many individuals develop an exacerbation without obvious cause.

It may be useful to provide the patient with an "allergic" analogy; some individuals have a tendency to develop asthma or hay fever on exposure to known or unknown allergens, whereas others have a genetically determined susceptibility to develop Reiter's syndrome following contact with an unrecognized (or recognized) precipitating event. This allergic approach provides the patient with some insight into the recurrent nature of the condition and aids discussion about prognosis.

Although there are no control data, there is some suggestion that the use of a condom protects the patient from a postvenereal exacerbation. Apart from this maneuver and the recommended avoidance of multiple sexual partners, there is no way to avoid recurrent attacks or chronicity.

Symptomatic management of the acute episode includes the use of analgesics, nonsteroidal anti-inflammatory agents, and modalities of physical therapy. Use of antibiotic therapy is controversial. One uncontrolled study recommended the use of lincomycin,[105] but a more recent study[5] demonstrated that antibiotic therapy did not influence the development of Reiter's syndrome in patients with nonspecific urethritis.

The joint and soft tissue manifestations appear to respond better to indomethacin, phenylbutazone, and other newer nonsteroidal anti-inflammatory drugs than to aspirin, but there have been no controlled studies. Indomethacin, 25 to 50 mg three times a day, may decrease the inflammatory process. If this agent is not efficacious, phenylbutazone, 100 mg three or four times daily, may be given. If indomethacin is not tolerated, one of the newer nonsteroidal agents can be given. Whether long-term therapy decreases the chance of relapse or chronicity is unknown.

Patients with severe inflammation of the uveal tract may require steroid eye drops or subconjunctival preparation. However, apart from an anecdotal suggestion that systemic corticosteroids are useful,[106] they appear to have no role in management. Indeed, a failure to respond to steroids helps differentiate the enthesopathic disorders from the synovitides. For persistent monarthropathy, plantar fasciitis, or Achilles tendinitis, intralesional therapy with methylprednisolone, 40 to 80 mg, may be helpful.

For those patients with relentless progression of disease, more aggressive therapy must be given. Despite the recognized risks of cytotoxic therapy, experience with psoriatic arthropathy suggests that cytotoxic therapy may be useful. In a placebo-controlled study with azathioprine, we have shown that 1 to 2 mg per kg body weight daily may be helpful within 4 to 8 weeks.[107] Uncontrolled data suggest that methotrexate may also be suitable.[108,109] Therapy should be continued until improvement, usually within 2 to 12 weeks, and then the dosage tapered, as able. Support for the use of stilbestrol[110] has not been critically analyzed.

Reiter's syndrome is a major chronic rheumatic disease. Therapy is empirical and inadequate. Increased activity should be directed toward improving recognition, elucidating etiologic factors, and, ideally, providing a cure. Meanwhile, controlled studies of various therapies should be performed. At this time auranofin is under study.

References

1. Reiter, H.: "Ueber eine bisher unerkannte Spirochaeteninfektion (Spirochaetosis arthritica). Deut. Med. Wschr. 42:1435, 1916.
2. Symposium on Reiter's syndrome. Ann. Rheum. Dis. 38:Suppl. 1, 1979.
3. Fox, R., Calin, A., Gerber, R.C., and Gibson, D.: The chronicity of symptoms and disability in Reiter's syndrome: An analysis of 131 consecutive patients. Ann. Intern. Med. 91:190, 1979.
4. Willkens, R.F., Arnett, F.C., Bitter, T., Calin, A., et al.: Reiter's Syndrome: Evaluation of Preliminary Criteria for Definite Disease. Arthritis Rheum. 24:844–849, 1981.
5. Keat, A.C., Maini, R.N., Nkwazi, G.C., et al.: Role of Chlamydia trachomatis and HLA B27 in sexually acquired reactive arthritis. Br. Med. J. 1:605, 1978.
6. Arnett, F.C., McClusky, E., Schacter, B.Z., et al.: Incomplete Reiter's syndrome: Discriminating features and HLA-W27 in diagnosis. Ann. Intern. Med. 84:8, 1976.
7. Lassus, A.: Circinate erosive balanitis. Ann. Rheum. Dis. 34:(Suppl.) 55, 1975.
8. Stoll, M. (1776): Cited by Huette, in De l'arthrite dysenterique. Arch. Gen. Med. 14:29, 1869.
9. Brodie, B.C.: Pathologic and Surgical Observations on Diseases and Joints, London, Longman, 1818.
10. Fiessinger, N., and Leroy, E.: Contribution à l'étude d'une épidémie de dysenterie dans le somme. Bull. Soc. Med. Hôp. Paris 40:2030, 1916.
11. Harkness, A.H.: Reiter's disease. Br. Med. J. 1:72, 1947.
12. Paronen, I.: Reiter's disease; a study of 344 cases observed in Finland. Acta Med. Scand. (Suppl. 212) 131:1, 1948.
13. Noer, H.R.: An "experimental" epidemic of Reiter's syndrome. JAMA 198:693, 1966.
14. Sairanen, D., Paronen, I., and Mohonen, H.: Reiter's syndrome: A follow-up study. Acta Med. Scand. 185:57, 1969.
15. Calin, A., and Fries, J.F.: An "experimental" epidemic of Reiter's syndrome, revisited. Follow-up evidence on genetic and environmental factors. Ann. Intern. Med. 84:564, 1976.
16. Hawkes, J.G.: Clinical and diagnostic features of Reiter's disease: A follow-up study of 39 patients. New Zealand Med. J. 78:347, 1973.
17. Good, A.E.: Reiter's disease: A review with special attention to cardiovascular and neurologic sequelae. Semin. Arthritis Rheum. 3:253, 1974.
18. Calin, A.: Reiter's syndrome. In Calin, A. (ed.): The Spondylarthropathies. Orlando, Florida, Grune & Stratton, 1984, pp. 119–150.
19. Calin, A.: The relationship between genetics and environment in the pathogenesis of rheumatic diseases (medical progress). West. J. Med. 131:205, 1979.
20. Battisto, J.R., Smith, R.N., Beckman, K., et al.: Susceptibility to adjuvant arthritis in DA and F344 rats: A dominant trait controlled by an autosomal gene locus linked to the MHC. Arthritis Rheum. 25:1194, 1982.
21. Rosenbaum, J.T., McDevitt, H.O., Guss, R.B., and Eabert, P.R.: Endotoxin-induced uveitis in rats as a model for human disease. Nature 286:611, 1980.
22. Rosenbaum, J.T.: Why HLA-B27: An analysis based on two animal models. Ann. Intern. Med. 94:261, 1981.
23. Mason, R.M., Murray, R.S., Oates, J.K., and Young, A.C.: Prostatitis and ankylosing spondylitis. Br. Med. J. 1:748, 1958.
24. Iveson, J.M.I., Nanda, B.S., Hancock, J.A.H., et al.: Reiter's disease in three boys. Ann. Rheum. Dis. 34:364, 1975.
25. Good, A.E., and Schultz, J.S.: Reiter's syndrome following Shigella flexneri 2a. Arthritis Rheum. 20:100, 1977.
26. Kaslow, R., Simon, D., Calin, A., et al.: Reiter's disease following epidemic shigellosis. J. Rheumatol. 8:969, 1981.
27. Kaslow, R.A., Ryder, R.W., and Calin, A.: Search for Reiter's syndrome following an outbreak of Shigella sonnei dysentery. J. Rheum. 6:562, 1979.
28. Manson Bahr, P.H.: The Dysenteric Disorders. London, Cassel, 1939, p. 71.
29. Warren, C.P.W.: Arthritis associated with Salmonella infection. Ann. Rheum. Dis. 29:483, 1970.
30. Jones, R.A.K.: Reiter's disease after Salmonella typhimurium enteritis. Br. Med. J. 1:1391, 1977.
31. Aho, K., Ahronen, P., Lassus, A., et al.: HL-A27 in reactive arthritis. A study of Yersinia arthritis and Reiter's disease. Arthritis Rheum. 17:521, 1974.
32. Wiesenhutter, C.W., Brenner, M.B., Kobayashi, S., Huberman, A., and Yu, D.T.Y.: Participation of HLA molecules in the interaction between human lymphocytes and a Reiter's disease–causing bacterium. Arthritis Rheum. 24:S38, 1982.
33. Marche, J.: Spondylarthrite ankylosante et syndrome de N. Fiessinger-Leroy-Reiter. Deux aspects de la même maladie rhumatismale. France Med. 18:7, 1955.
34. Caughey, D.E., and Bywaters, E.G.L.: The arthritis of Whipples's syndrome. Ann. Rheum. Dis. 22:327, 1963.
35. Ford, D.K.: The etiology of non-gonococcal urethritis and Reiter's syndrome. Excerpta Medica International Congress Series 165:227, 1969.
35a. Brenner, M.B., Kobayashi, S., Weisenhutter, C.W., et al,: In-vitro T lymphocyte proliferative response to Yersinia enterocolitica in Reiter's syndrome. Arthritis Rheum. 27:250, 1984.
36. Brewerton, D.A., Caffrey, M., Nicholls, A., et al.: Reiter's disease and HLA 27. Lancet 2:996, 1973.
37. Aho, K., Ahvonen, P.I., Alkio, P., et al.: HLA 27 in reactive arthritis following infection. Ann. Rheum. Dis. 34:(Suppl.) 29, 1975.
38. Gofton, J.P., Chalmers, A., Price, G.E., et al.: HLA B27 and ankylosing spondylitis in British Columbia Indians. J. Rheumatol. 2:314, 1975.
39. Lisse, J.R., Bennett, P.H., Knowler, W.O., Gofton, J.P., Calin, A., and Mann, D.L.: High risk of sacroiliitis in HLA-B27 positive Pima Indian men. Arthritis Rheum. 25:236, 1982.

40. Gofton, J.P.: Personal communication, 1983.

41. Bennett, P.H., Personal communication, 1983.

42. Hochberg, M.C., Bias, W.B., and Arnett, F.C.: Family studies in HLA-B27-associated arthritis. Medicine 57:463, 1978.

43. Yunus, M., Calabro, J.J., Miller, K.A., and Masi, A.T.: Family studies with HLA typing in Reiter's syndrome. Am. J. Med. 70:1210, 1981.

44. Calin, A., Barnett, M., Marder, A., and Marks, S.: The nature and prevalence of spondylarthritis among relatives of probands with ankylosing spondylitis and Reiter's syndrome. Arthritis Rheum. 24:S78, 1981.

45. Grumet, F.C., Fendly, B.M., Fish, L., Foung, S., and Engleman, E.G.: Monoclonal antibody (B27M2) subdividing HLA-B27. Hum. Immun. 5:61, 1982.

46. Karr, R.W., Hahn, Y., and Schwartz, B.D.: Structural identity of human histocompatibility leukocyte antigen-B27 molecules from patients with ankylosing spondylitis and normal individuals. J. Clin. Invest. 69:443, 1982.

47. Kaneoka, H., Engleman, E.G., and Grumet, F.C.: Immunochemical variants of HLA-B27. J. Immun., 130:1288, 1983.

48. Arnett, F.C., Schacter, B.Z., Hochberg, M.C., et al.: HLA-B7 cross-reactive antigens in B27-negative Reiter's syndrome (abstract). Arthritis Rheum. 20:106, 1977.

49. Csonka, G.W.: Recurrent attacks in Reiter's disease. Arthritis Rheum. 3:164, 1960.

50. Csonka, G.W.: The course of Reiter's syndrome. Br. Med. J. 1:1088, 1958.

51. Calin, A., and Fries, J.F.: The striking prevalence of ankylosing spondylitis in "healthy" W27 positive males and females. A controlled study. N. Engl. J. Med. 293:835, 1975.

52. Cohen, L.M., Mittal, K.K., Schmid, F.R., et al.: Increased risk for spondylitis stigmata in apparently healthy HLA W27 men. Ann. Intern. Med. 84:1, 1976.

53. Kidd, K.K., Bernoco, D., Carbonera, A.O., et al.: Genetic analysis of HLA associated diseases: The "illness susceptible" gene frequency and sex ratio in ankylosing spondylitis. In Dausset, J., and Svegaard, A. (eds.): HLA and Disease. Copenhagen, Munksgaard, 1977.

54. Xing-hua, C., and Gui-ying, S.: Reiter's syndrome: Clinical analysis of 22 cases. Chinese Med. J. 95:533, 1982.

55. Smith, D.L., Bennett, R.M., and Regan, M.G.: Reiter's disease in women. Arthritis Rheum. 23:335, 1980.

56. Jacobs, J.C., Johnston, A.D., and Berdon, W.E.: HLA-B27 associated spondyloarthritis and enthesopathy in children. J. Pediatr. 100:521, 1982.

57. Rosenberg, A.M., and Petty, R.E.: A syndrome of seronegative enthesopathy and arthropathy in children. Arthritis Rheum. 25:1041, 1982.

58. Garner, R.W., and Mowat, A.G.: Joint rupture in Reiter's disease. Br. J. Surg. 59:657, 1972.

59. Ball, J.: Enthesopathy of rheumatoid and ankylosing spondylitis. Ann. Rheum. Dis. 30:213, 1971.

60. Berg, R.L., Weinberger, H., and Dienes, L.: Acute haemorrhagic cystitis. Am. J. Med. 22:848, 1957.

61. Weinberger, H.W., Ropes, M.W., Kulka, J.P., and Bauer, W.: Reiter's syndrome, clinical and pathological observations—a long term study of 16 cases. Medicine 41:35, 1962.

62. Hall, W.H., and Finegold, S.: A study of 23 cases of Reiter's syndrome. Ann. Intern. Med. 38:533, 1953.

63. Ford, D.K.: Arthritis and venereal disease. Br. J. Ven. Dis. 29:123, 1953.

64. Catterall, R.D.: Significance of non-specific genital infection in uveitis and arthritis. Lancet 2:739, 1961.

65. Vidal, E.: Eruption generalisée et symmetrique de croutes cornées, avec chute des ongles, d'origine blennorrhagique coincident avec une polyarthrite de même nature. Ann. Derm. Syph. 4:3, 1893.

66. Wiedmann, H.: Reitersche Erkrankung. Wien. Klin Wochenschr. 47:1245, 1934.

67. Stanislawski, W.: Über einen Fall von gonorrhoischer Urethritis mit Affection der Gelenke, symetrische hornartigen Hautausschlag und Ausfallen der Nagel. Krankh. Harn. Sex App. 5:643, 1900.

68. Chauffard, A.: Ann. Derm. Syph. Cited by Hauser (1958), 793, 1897.

69. Carr, J.L., and Friedman, M.: Keratodermia blennorrhagicum, report of a case with autopsy. Am. J. Pathol. 20:709, 1944.

70. Hancock, J.A.H.: Surface manifestations of Reiter's disease in the male. Br. J. Vener. Dis. 36:36, 1960.

71. Epstein, E.: Differential diagnosis of keratosis blenorrhagica and psoriasis arthropathica. Arch. Derm. Syph. 40:547, 1939.

72. Marche, J.: L'atteinte des articulations sacroiliaque dans le syndrome dit de Reiter. Rev. Rhumat. Malad. Osteoarticulaires 17:449, 1950.

73. Oates, J.K., and Young, A.C.: Sacroiliitis in Reiter's disease. Br. Med. J. 1:1013, 1959.

74. McEwen, C., DiTata, D., Lingg, C., et al.: Ankylosing spondylitis and spondylitis accompanying ulcerative colitis, regional enteritis, psoriasis, and Reiter's disease. Arthritis Rheum. 14:291, 1971.

75. Calin, A., Porta, J., and Fries, J.F.F.: The clinical history as a screening test for ankylosing spondylitis. JAMA 237:2613, 1977.

76. Oates, J.K., and Hancock, J.A.H.: Neurological symptoms and lesions occurring in the course of Reiter's disease. Am. J. Med. Sci. 238:79, 1959.

77. Brewerton, D.A., Caffrey, M., Nicholls, A., et al.: Acute anterior uveitis and HLA 27. Lancet 2:994, 1973.

78. Csonka, G.W., and Oates, J.K.: Pericarditis and electrocardiographic changes in Reiter's syndrome. Br. Med. J. 1:866, 1957.

79. Bulkley, B.H., and Roberts, W.C.: Ankylosing spondylitis and aortic regurgitation. Description of the characteristic cardio-vascular lesion from study of eight necropsy patients. Circulation 18:1014, 1973.

80. Tucker, C.R., Fowles, R.E., Calin, A., et al.: Aortitis in ankylosing spondylitis: Early detection of aortic root abnormalities with two-dimensional echocardiography. Am. J. Cardiol. 9:680, 1982.

81. Hancock, J.A.H.: In King, A. (ed.): Recent Advances in Venerology. London, Churchill, 1964, p. 395.

82. Thiers, H., and Pinet, A.: Syndrome de Reiter avec uretrite à inclusions, infiltrat pulmonaire labile et keratodermie. Lyons Med. 184:51, 1950.

83. Csonka, G.W.: Involvement of the nervous system in Reiter's syndrome. Ann. Rheum. Dis. 17:334, 1958.

84. Bleehen, S.S., Everall, J.D., and Tighe, J.R.: Amyloidosis complicating Reiter's syndrome. Br. J. Vener. Dis. 42:88, 1966.

85. Cliff, J.M.: Spinal bony bridging and carditis in Reiter's disease. Ann. Rheum. Dis. 30:171, 1971.

86. Rosenbaum, J.T., Theofilopoulos, A., McDevitt, H.O., et al.: Presence of circulating immune complexes in Reiter's syndrome and ankylosing spondylitis. Clin. Immun. Pathol. 18:291, 1981.

87. Grimble, A., and Lessof, M.H.: Anti-prostate antibodies in arthritis. Br. Med. J. 2:263, 1965.

88. Fostiropoulos, G., Austen, K.F., and Block, K.J.: Total haemolytic complement (CH50) and second component of complement (C2 hu) activity in serum and synovial fluid. Arthritis Rheum. 8:219, 1965.

89. Yates, D.B., Maini, R.N., Scott, J.T., and Sloper, J.C.: Complement activation in Reiter's syndrome. Ann. Rheum. Dis. 34:468, 1975.

90. Calin, A.: HLA-B27: To type or not to type? Ann. Intern. Med. 92:208, 980.

91. Calin, A.: HLA-B27 in 1982. Reappraisal of a clinical test. Ann. Intern. Med. 96:114, 1982.

92. Brewerton, D.A., Caffrey, M., Hart, F.D., et al.: Ankylosing spondylitis and HLA 27. Lancet 1:904, 1975.

93. Schlosstein, L., Terasaki, P.I., Bluestone, R., et al.: High association of an HLA antigen W27 with ankylosing spondylitis. N. Engl. J. Med. 288:704, 1973.

94. Good, A.E., Kawanish, H., and Schultz, J.S.: HLA B27 in blacks with ankylosing spondylitis or Reiter's disease. N. Engl. J. Med. 294:166, 1976.

95. Sonozaki, H., Seki, H., Chang, S., et al.: Human lymphocyte antigen HLA 27 in Japanese patients with ankylosing spondylitis. Tissue Antigens 5:131, 1975.

96. McDevitt, H.O., and Bodmer, W.F.: HLA, immune response genes and disease. Lancet 1:1269, 1974.

97. Lockie, N.G., and Hunder, G.G., Reiter's syndrome in children; a case report and review. Arthritis Rheum. 14:767, 1971.

98. McMillan, A.: Reiter's disease in a female, presenting as erythema nodosum. Br. J. Vener. Dis. 51:345, 1975.

99. Espinosa, L.R., Vasey, F.B., Oh, R., et al.: Association between HLA-BW38 and peripheral psoriatic arthropathy. Arthritis Rheum. 21:72, 1978.

100. Terasaki, P., and Mickey, M.R.: HLA haplotypes of 32 diseases. Transplant. Rev. 22:105, 1975.

101. Wright, V.: In Scott, J.T. (ed.): Copeman's Textbook of the Rheumatic Diseases. Churchill Livingstone, 1978, p. 553.

102. Good, A.E.: Involvement of the back in Reiter's syndrome. Ann. Intern. Med. 57:44, 1962.

103. McClusky, O.E., Lordon, R.E., and Arnett, F.C.: HLA 27 in Reiter's syndrome and psoriatic arthritis: A genetic factor in disease susceptibility and expression. J. Rheumatol. 1:263, 1974.

104. Primer on the rheumatic diseases. JAMA 224:(Suppl. 5) 71, 1973.

105. Mowat, A.G., Chalmers, T.M., Alexander, W.R.M., et al.: Case of Reiter's disease treated with lincomycin hydrochloride. Br. Med. J. 1:478, 1967.

106. Ogryzlo, M.A., and Graham, W.: "Reiter's syndrome: Effect of pituitary adrenocorticotrophic hormone (ACTH) and cortisone. JAMA 144:1239, 1950.

107. Burns, T.M., Marks, S.H., and Calin, A.: A double-blind, placebo-controlled, cross-over trial of azathioprine (AZA) in refractory Reiter's syndrome (RS). Abstract. ARA Annual Scientific Meeting, San Antonio, Texas, June, 1983.

108. Mullins, J.F., Maberry, J.D., and Stone, O.J.: Reiter's syndrome treated with folic acid antagonists. Arch. Dermatol. 94:335, 1966.

109. Farber, G.A., Forshner, J.G., and O'Quinn, S.E.: Reiter's syndrome treatment with methotrexate. JAMA 200:171, 1967.

110. Laird, S.M., Gill, A.J., and Pitkeathly, D.A.: Treatment of Reiter's disease with stilboestrol. Br. Med. J. 1:970, 1965.

Chapter 66
Psoriatic Arthritis

V. Wright

The French must be credited with initiating and developing the concept of psoriatic arthritis, and the name of Alibert is usually mentioned as the first to draw attention to the association, although there is some doubt about how clearly he was able to distinguish between leprosy and psoriasis. Bazin[1] first coined the name "psoriasis arthritique." Initially, there was resistance to regarding the disease as an entity distinct from rheumatoid arthritis.[2] However, several large well-conducted surveys were provided.[3-7] Increasing clinical, radiographic, serologic, and epidemiologic evidence supports the classification of psoriatic arthritis as a true entity.[8]

DEFINITION

Over the years different aspects of the disease have been singled out for emphasis, and often have been made the basis of a definition. A severely destructive form of arthritis associated with psoriasis has achieved quite undue prominence in the literature.[9,10] The appearances are striking, but the cases are rare. Because the distal interphalangeal joints may be involved in contrast to rheumatoid arthritis, there are some who have confined the definition to an arthritis affecting only the distal joints associated with psoriasis.[11,12] Hench[13] and later Carrier[14] required arthritis following longstanding, uncontrolled psoriasis. Some maintained that both the joint and skin changes must be atypical,[15] while others insisted on synchronous remissions and relapses of skin and joint changes.[16]

In fact all these patients would come within a global definition of psoriatic arthritis, a syndrome in which psoriasis is associated with inflammatory arthritis, usually having a negative sheep cell agglutination test.[17]

PREVALENCE

True figures for the frequency of psoriasis are difficult to obtain. Often psoriasis may be so minimal that even the patient is unaware of its presence, particularly when only the scalp or the navel is involved. It is all too easy to dismiss the scalp lesions as dandruff. The reported prevalence of psoriasis in inflammatory polyarthritis has ranged from 2.6 to 7.0 percent.[18] This compares with a population prevalence of 1.0 to 2.0 percent. Comparison of the available figures suggests that psoriasis occurs two or three times more often in patients with arthritis than in the population at large. Conversely, the prevalence of "arthritis" in psoriatic patients is reported as being 0.5 to 40.2 percent. These data are of little value, since in many studies the criteria for the diagnosis of arthritis are not given. A careful study by Leczinsky[19] demonstrated that 6.8 percent of 543 psoriatic inpatients had a rheumatoid type of polyarthritis (5.8 percent in men; 7.9 percent in women). This can be compared with a prevalence of 0.7 percent in 543 nonpsoriatic dermatologic patients. Another Scandinavian study[20] suggested a six- to ten-fold increase in arthritis among psoriatic patients compared with controls. In seropositive rheumatoid arthritis the frequency of psoriasis is similar to that of a control hospital population, but the prevalence in seronegative "rheumatoid arthritis" is over four times as great.[7] The prevalence of psoriatic arthritis in the population can only be estimated, but careful calculations suggest that it is 0.10 percent.[8,21] Lower estimates of the order of 0.02 percent have been made.[20,22] The lower figures may reflect more rigid criteria used for diagnosis. The sex ratio in psoriatic arthritis (male:female, 1:1.04) is not very different from that in uncomplicated psoriasis (1:1.4) or from that in rheumatoid arthritis (1:1.5). The male predominance in psoriatic arthritis reported by Bollet and Turner[23] and Reed[24] may well be explained by the fact that arthritis predominantly affecting distal joints occurs more frequently in men.[5]

ETIOLOGY

Heredity is the most prominent factor in the development of the cutaneous lesions of psoriasis. A family history is obtained in one third of patients, but the exact mode of inheritance is still not clear. Dominant transmission with incomplete penetrance[25,26] and a double recessive mechanism[27] have both been proposed. There is great variability in the pedigrees of psoriatic patients. This may be because there are different subgroups of psoriatic patients. Evidence of this is found in the study of HLA-B17, which seems to be a useful genetic marker for detecting a subgroup of psoriatic patients characterized by a high rate of affected relatives and a slightly earlier age of onset. HLA-B12, on the other hand, appears to characterize the subgroup with an infrequent family history of the disease.[28]

The increased frequency of HLA-B13 and HLA-B7 among patients with psoriasis has been noted by several authors.[28-34] There is a strong association between Cw6 and psoriasis.[33,35-38] Marcusson[38] in a careful family study showed that psoriasis often occurs in close relatives who share one disease-predisposing HLA haplotype with the proband. Some of the carriers of disease-associated HLA haplotypes have no signs of dermal involvement but have subjective or objective signs of arthritic lesions. He therefore suggested that psoriasis and/or arthritic lesions may be different clinical manifestations of disease in individuals carrying psoriasis-predisposing haplotypes. On the basis of these findings he favored a dominant inheritance pattern. Moreover, it was thought that at least two HLA-linked genes cooperated in the development of disease. These genes could occur in the cis-position on the same haplotype or in the trans-position on different haplotypes. In the former case, disease inheritance would seem to be dominant, whereas in the latter case disease would occur mainly in HLA-identical siblings of the proband.

The occurrence of psoriasis of guttate type following streptococcal infections in children is of some interest, as are exacerbations at sites of injury, the Koebner phenomenon.

In psoriatic arthritis heredity is likewise a significant factor. Evidence of this derives from individual pedigrees[39-42] and family surveys.[21,43-45] Our own studies showed that psoriatic arthritis was aggregated in first-degree relatives with psoriatic arthritis probands much more frequently than in the general population and in spouse controls.[17] There is a high concordance between HLA-B27 and sacroiliitis in patients with psoriatic arthritis.[30-32,65-86] The Guy's Hospital group [56] has confirmed the raised frequency of Cw6 in patients with psoriasis and has noted that those with arthritis had an increased frequency not only of B27 but also of DR7. DR3 in their series was associated with erosions. The genetic transmission appeared to be multifactorial. Environmental factors such as trauma, neurotrophic effect, capillary changes, and infection have all been suggested as etiologically important.[8]

PATHOLOGY

The microscopic appearance of the joints in psoriatic arthritis does not differ from that in rheumatoid arthritis. Moreover, arthroscopy has failed to differentiate the two diseases.[46] Histologic studies have failed to differentiate rheumatoid arthritis from psoriatic arthritis.[47,48] Some synovial biopsies from psoriatic arthritic patients showed pure round cell infiltration, more fibrosis, and many thick-walled small vessels. Characteristic rheumatoid granulomas have not been found.[23] The one possible differentiating feature has been the increased fibrosis in some joints, particularly the distal interphalangeal joints.[11] In a group of patients who died from other causes, marked articular destruction and reabsorption of bone producing shortening of the middle phalanges of the distal joints of the fingers and toes, was noted, with less marked resorption of the proximal end of the bone, so that a cup-like deformity was formed by a pronounced marginal overgrowth at the site of insertion of tendons.

CLINICAL FEATURES

A wide spectrum of clinical disease occurs, which has confused classification previously. Five broad clinical groups have been recognized:[17]

1. Patients in whom distal interphalangeal joints are predominantly, although rarely exclusively, involved.

2. A severely deforming type of arthritis, usually characterized by widespread ankylosis. Occasionally arthritis mutilans occurs because of dissolution of the bone, giving opera glass hands and a similar condition in the feet.

3. Patients who appear clinically indistinguishable from those with rheumatoid disease, apart from the absence of rheumatoid factor in the serum. However, the arthritis is less extensive and more benign in its course.

4. Patients with single or asymmetrical oligo- (or mono-) arthritis. In our original description these would have been included in group 3.

5. Patients in whom there is ankylosing spondylitis, accounting for about 5 percent of all types of psoriatic arthritis.

The fourth group of single or asymmetrical oligo- (or mono-) arthritis has received more attention in continental Europe.[49-51] Not all patients fall into these clear-cut categories, and some progress from one group to another. Patients who originally have distal joint involvement sometimes develop a polyarthritis in which the distal joint inflammation subsides, leaving features similar to Heberden's nodes. The distal joints are nearly always involved in arthritis mutilans. On the other hand, a single digit may show destructive mutilans changes of bone without the arthritis being widespread. Psoriasis and rheumatoid arthritis are both common, and the diseases may coincide. From population prevalences one might expect to find 1.4 cases per 10,000 women and 0.4 per 10,000 men. A group of patients we have reported with a positive sheep cell agglutination test appeared to be examples of coincidental psoriasis and rheumatoid arthritis, judging by their clinical course and the prevalence of subcutaneous nodules in 17 percent, which is a figure we found in our clinic population of rheumatoid patients. These nodules are strikingly absent from patients with true psoriatic arthritis.

Skin. In our 10-year follow-up of 227 patients the peak age of onset of skin lesions was 16 to 20 years, with a secondary peak around 45 to 55 years. The lesions commonly began on the elbows, followed by the legs, and then by the scalp and back. The psoriasis was usually mild in extent at the onset, although Leczinsky[19] has shown that arthritis is ten times more common in patients with severe involvement of the skin than in those with mild involvement. Molin[52] and Little and associates[53] also drew attention to this.

Skin lesions usually preceded the arthritis (Fig. 66–1). However, in 16 percent the arthritis preceded the skin lesions. On this basis we predicted that some patients with seronegative "rheumatoid arthritis" were destined to develop psoriasis. Dixon[54] followed 54 such patients and found that four indeed did so. In our follow-up study there were no particular precipitating factors

Figure 66–1. Relationship of onset of psoriatic arthritis to the onset of skin and nail changes. Simultaneous onset is indicated by the dark bars.

for the psoriasis. Synchronous exacerbations and remission of skin and joint changes have been reported,[16] but the dissociation of these manifestations is just as likely to occur. Most patients do not notice any relationship. The misapprehension may have been perpetuated by the fact that the arthritis of patients with skin disease sufficiently severe to require admission to hospital is likely to improve on bed rest: a common factor improves both without demonstrating a link between the two. Pustular psoriasis occurred in 25 percent of the severe group, compared with 4 percent of the other patients. These lesions occur on the palms and the soles.

Nails. The arthritis is more closely related to nail changes than to skin changes. Nail changes are much more frequent in psoriatic arthritis (85 percent) than in psoriatic patients without arthritis (31 percent), and the changes begin at the onset of the arthritis more frequently than skin changes (Fig. 66–1). Occasionally there is a topographical relationship between the involvement of the distal joints and affected nails. Since nail changes may occur without skin lesions, we have recently completed a study to ascertain the specificity of the nail lesions in this condition.[55] Although pitting is a characteristic feature, it is by no means specific. If more than 20 pits can be seen in all the fingernails, this is most likely due to psoriasis. Onycholysis is the most characteristic finding, and if it is associated with either ridging or pitting it is almost certainly due to psoriasis.

Arthritis. The peak age of onset is between 36 and 45 years, but in the deforming group the arthritis begins before the age of 20 three times as commonly as it does in the group indistinguishable from rheumatoid arthritis. The onset is acute in nearly half the patients. In the distal joint group the arthritis commonly begins in these joints. A synchronous onset of skin and joint changes is uncommon, but nail and joint changes often begin together.

Psoriatic arthritis may present with an acute gout-like onset,[15,47,57] and in some patients the big toe may be involved.

In a study of juvenile psoriatic arthritis 43 patients were examined.[58] There appeared to be two groups: one indistinguishable from patients with Still's disease, and one with the typical patterns of adult psoriatic arthritis. As in the adult, psoriasis can occur in seropositive juvenile rheumatoid arthritis. In some patients severe joint damage speedily occurs, the rate of destruction being greater than that observed in any other form of juvenile chronic arthritis. The arthritis may continue into adult life, although with an intermittent and frequently fairly mild course. These are major differences from Still's disease and suggest that initial assessment of prognosis should be guarded.

During the course of the arthritis disability tends to be less than in rheumatoid arthritis (Fig. 66–2), although one cannot ignore the selection factor in a university hospital with a particular interest in the condition. Involvement of the distal and proximal interphalangeal joints, together with flexor tenosynovitis, may give a sausage shape to the digit. The distal joint involvement is in sharp contrast to rheumatoid arthritis (Fig. 66–3). Asymmetry of joint involvement is seen more commonly than in rheumatoid disease. Spondylitic involvement in psoriatic patients is widely recognized.[3,4,47,59-61] Epidemiological studies have shown an increased prevalence of ankylosing spondylitis and of sacroiliitis in patients with psoriatic arthritis.[62-64] There is, moreover, a familial aggregation of sacroiliitis and of spondylitis in blood relatives of patients with psoriatic arthritis.[17]

In a review of 130 patients with psoriatic arthritis, spondylitis was noted in 40 percent and sacroiliitis in 21 percent.[65] Those with sacroiliitis and predominantly axial disease were usually men who had developed psoriasis later in life. Iritis, chronic back pain, and restriction of spinal mobility were common features. The disorder in this group resembled idiopathic ankylosing spondylitis. In those with sacroiliitis in association with peripheral polyarthritis, symptoms or signs of spondy-

Figure 66–2. Disability during the course of the disease in patients with psoriatic arthritis and with rheumatoid arthritis.

Figure 66–3. Hands of a patient with psoriatic arthritis showing pronounced distal joint involvement.

litis were frequently absent. Both groups, however, had a high incidence of HLA-B27.

Extra-articular Features. These are much less frequent in psoriatic arthritis than in rheumatoid arthritis. Subcutaneous nodules are characteristically absent and extensor tendon sheath effusions uncommon. Eye lesions may occur with conjunctivitis in 19.6 percent, uveitis in 10.1 percent, and scleritis in 1.8 percent.[66] Reed[24] has described spondylitic heart disease and suggested that in these patients skin lesions are usually pustular. In all our experience we have seen only one patient with fibrosing alveolitis, but it must be remembered that this is an unusual complication of rheumatoid arthritis, being present in only 1.5 percent of 512 patients with rheumatoid arthritis whom we studied.[67]

Prognosis. Psoriatic arthritis is not usually a severe disease, despite the undue prominence given in the literature to the rare destructive cases that occur. A 10-year follow-up suggests that it produces less pain and disability than rheumatoid arthritis.[68] Apart from the unusual deforming group, about one third lost no time from work at all, and 97 percent managed with less than 12 months off throughout the period of their arthritis (a minimum of 10 years). Over this period the patients showed little deterioration radiologically.

Of 32 deaths that we could trace, three patients had amyloidosis, and 15 died from conditions in which corticosteroid therapy may have been a contributory factor.[69] In our follow-up study in the United Kingdom, ischemic heart disease was the most common cause of death.

Ancillary Investigations. Rheumatoid factor is usually absent from the blood of polyarthritic patients in whom psoriasis is present. Over our 10-year follow-up period of 227 patients, the SCAT was positive in 16 percent in the group indistinguishable from rheumatoid arthritis and fluctuant in a further 10 percent. There may be some degree of anemia, and the erythrocyte sedimentation rate is raised in the active phase of the disease, although this may be moderate compared with rheumatoid arthritis.[70]

Antinuclear factor was positive in 7 percent of our patients, which is the same figure we obtained for controls, compared with 23 percent of our rheumatoid population. This is in keeping with the findings of Zachariae and Zachariae.[71]

The frequent biochemical abnormalities and evidence of hyperparathyroidism in patients with rheumatoid arthritis[72,73] prompted us to investigate this in 138 patients with psoriatic arthritis. These patients had less derangement of liver function tests and protein metabolism than patients with rheumatoid arthritis. There was no evidence of hyperparathyroidism or osteomalacia, although hypocalcemia was common. A low bilirubin level was often noted.

Hyperuricemia has been frequently cited as a feature of psoriasis.[27,74,75] It is said to be more common in patients with extensive involvement of skin.[76] However, a carefully controlled study of our patients, in which all drugs that might influence uric acid metabolism were withdrawn, failed to show any difference from a group of matched patients with rheumatoid arthritis (Fig. 66–4). Other abnormalities that have been reported are shown in Table 66–1.

Histocompatibility antigens have been studied extensively in this disease. HLA-B13 and -B17 are more fre-

Figure 66-4. Serum uric acid levels in patients not receiving drugs which would influence the levels. The vertical arrow indicates the upper limit of normal (mmol/l.). *A*, Uncomplicated psoriasis. *B*, Rheumatoid arthritis (off treatment one week). *C*, Psoriatic arthritis (off treatment one week).

Table 66–1. Investigations of the Blood of Patients with Psoriatic Arthritis

Author	Date	Investigation
Wright[77]	1956	Sheep cell agglutination test usually negative
Zachariae and Zachariae[71]	1969	Antinuclear factor usually absent
Lodin et al.[70]	1957	Anemia
Lodin et al.[70]	1957	Moderately raised erythrocyte sedimentation rate
Baker et al.[78]	1963	Transient leucocytosis
See Tables 66–2 and 66–3		HLA-B27 more frequent
Lambert and Wright[79]	1979	Liver function tests normal
Lambert and Wright[79]	1979	Bilirubin frequently low
Lambert and Wright[79]	1979	Hypoalbuminemia and hyperglobulinemia uncommon
Lambert and Wright[79]	1979	Calcium often low
Lambert and Wright[65]	1977	Uric acid normal (other authors differ)
Gaedicke et al.[80]	1970	Normal erythrocyte phosphoglucose isomerase
Robillard[81]	1968	Elevated gamma and alpha-2-globulin.
Petres and Majert[82]	1968	Decreased IgM in mild psoriatic arthritis; elevated in severe psoriatic arthritis
Danielsen[83]	1965	Elevated IgA levels
Heiskell et al.[84]	1962	Elevated beta globulins
Lambert et al.[85]	1978	Nitroblue tetrazolium scores often raised

quent in patients with psoriasis than in the general population. The frequencies of HLA-B27 in psoriatic arthritis with spinal involvement and with peripheral arthritis are shown in Tables 66–2 and 66–3. Taking all the series, it appears that even with spinal involvement B27 occurs less frequently than it does in uncomplicated ankylosing spondylitis. It is a good deal less in peripheral psoriatic arthritis, but still increased above the frequency in the general population. In a recent study of psoriatic spondylitis we found that 90 percent of patients with sacroiliitis and syndesmophytes had B27, and that when syndesmophytes occurred with normal sacroiliac joints B27 was present in 43 percent.[65] HLA-BW38 has been found more frequently in patients with peripheral psoriatic arthritis.[87]

RADIOLOGIC FEATURES

Many of the radiologic features of psoriatic arthritis are indistinguishable from those of rheumatoid arthritis,

Table 66–2. HLA-B27 in Psoriatic Arthritis (Peripheral)

Authors	Date	Number	Percent
Brewerton et al.[48a]	1974	47	24
Karnoven et al.[32]	1974	17	24
McClusky et al.[30]	1974	8	—
Metzger et al.[31]	1975	17	18
Lambert et al.[58]	1976	48	14.6

Table 66–3. HLA-B27 in Psoriatic Arthritis (Spinal)

Authors	Date	Number	Percent
Brewerton et al.[48a]	1974	22	64
Karnoven et al.[32]	1974	19	58
McClusky et al.[30]	1974	6	100
Medsger et al.[86]	1974	8	87.5
Metzger et al.[31]	1975	23	35
Lambert et al.[65]	1976	16	87.5

except that fewer joints tend to be involved. Table 66–4 summarizes features that are more specific to psoriatic arthritis. They are discussed by Resnik in Chapter 39. Marginal erosions[88] can produce an apparent widening of the joint space and expansion at the base of the terminal phalanx (Fig. 66-5 and 66-6). There may be erosion of the tuft of the terminal phalanx, especially of the big toe.

The rare arthritis mutilans shows a dissolution of bones, particularly of the metatarsal. A phalanx may virtually disappear, and it is easy to see why the opera glass effect is produced clinically (Fig. 66-7).

Our findings of sacroiliitis in 20 percent of patients[65] is similar to that reported by Baker and associates,[43] although higher than that reported by Dawson and Tyson,[15] Avila and associates,[88] and Bardnagni and Carlisimo.[89] Spinal involvement similar to that found in ankylosing spondylitis may develop, and this may effect the cervical spine.[61,90] It has been suggested that there is a specific cervical lesion associated with psoriasis (with or without arthritis) comprising apophyseal sclerosis, joint narrowing, and anterior ligamentous calcification.[91] Our specific study of psoriatic spondylitis[65] suggested that there is a chance association of psoriasis and ankylosing spondylitis, the prevalence being about 7 percent. However, psoriatic spondylitis is characterized radiologically by sacroiliitis and by syndesmophytes. This differs from ankylosing spondylitis clinically and radiologically. Sacroiliitis was more frequently associated with unilateral or asymmetrical syndesmophytes which occurred in small numbers and were more often nonmarginal (Fig. 66-8). HLA-B27 was associated with sacroiliitis and was present more often than normal in those with only syndesmophytes. A rare type of paravertebral ossification of the lumbar and thoracic areas may occur at some distance from the vertebral body.[48,92] On the basis of syndesmophyte morphology, McEwen and associates[93] placed the spondylitis associated with psoriasis in a group with Reiter's disease, and distinguished it from another group of patients with idiopathic ankylosing spondylitis and the spondylitis associated with

Table 66–4. Radiologic Features in Psoriatic Arthritis

1. Distal interphalangeal joint involvement with erosion and expansion of base of terminal phalanx
2. Terminal phalangeal osteolysis, especially of the hallux
3. Arthritis mutilans giving pencil-in-cup appearance
4. Oligoarthritis
5. Sacroiliitis
6. Spinal involvement—syndesmophytes may be present without sacroiliitis

Figure 66-7. Radiograph of dissolution of phalanges of second toe in psoriatic arthritis.

Figure 66-5. Erosion of a distal interphalangeal joint in psoriatic arthritis with expansion of base of terminal phalanx.

Figure 66-6. Negatives of radiographs showing (*A*) osteolysis resulting in "pencil-in-cup" appearance, and (*B*) osteolysis resulting in "fishtail" deformity of the proximal end of the distal phalanx. (After Wright and Moll.)

Figure 66-8. Radiograph of nonmarginal syndesmophytes of the lumbar spine in psoriatic arthritis.

ulcerative colitis. Recently it has been suggested that scintiscan studies are a more sensitive means of detecting sacroiliitis in those patients.[94]

DIFFERENTIAL DIAGNOSIS

Differentiating psoriatic arthritis from other diseases is best done by considering the skin lesions, the peripheral arthritis, and the spinal involvement.

The classic well-demarcated rash of psoriasis with silvery scales affecting the elbows, scalp, abdomen, or back (Fig. 66-9) poses no problems of diagnosis. Sometimes, however, the skin lesion may be so small that the patient may be unaware of it. This is particularly true of small lesions in the scalp, at the internatal cleft, on the perineum, around the umbilicus, under the breasts, or in the axillae and groins. Seborrheic dermatitis may be confusing, especially in postmenopausal women when psoriasis may occur in a seborrheic distribution. Seborrheic lesions are poorly demarcated and are usually not palpable.

Fungal infection is the most common cause of confusion with psoriatic nails, especially when only the toenails are involved. Scrapings must be examined for mycelia. Pitting is often regarded as characteristic of psoriasis, but it may occur with eczema or exfoliative dermatitis. In a study of this aspect we found that onycholysis in the absence of previous injury to the affected nail is suggestive of a psoriatic origin.[55] Two or all of onycholysis, horizontal ridging, and nail pitting in the same patient are likely to indicate psoriasis. Nail pitting

alone is a poor discriminator between psoriatic and other causes of nail dystrophy. However, more than 20 fingernail pits per person are suggestive of psoriasis, and more than 60 pits are unlikely to be found in the absence of psoriasis.

The skin and nail changes of Reiter's disease may be indistinguishable from those of psoriasis clinically and pathologically, especially the pustular variety. A well-defined link between these two diseases has been described in 11 patients who began with Reiter's syndrome and progressed to psoriatic arthritis.[95]

Clinically, acute Heberden's nodes and radiologically advanced distal joint osteoarthrosis may be confused with psoriatic arthritis. The involvement of the first carpometacarpal joints, the presence of Bouchard's nodes of the proximal interphalangeal joints, and a persistently normal ESR help to establish the diagnosis of primary generalized osteoarthrosis. Atypical forms of osteoarthrosis with erosion,[96-99] and with ankylosis,[100] may be even more confusing, but they are rare.

The clinical appearance of joints in psoriatic arthritis may simulate gout,[47] particularly in patients with distal joint arthritis.[77] A considerably raised level of serum uric acid makes the diagnosis of psoriatic arthritis unlikely. The detection of uric acid crystals in the synovial fluid will provide the diagnosis, and the response of the disease to colchicine may be a useful diagnostic aid.

Traumatic arthritis of the knee has been understandably but mistakenly diagnosed in a number of our patients with psoriasis.[101] Arthrotomy revealed synovial proliferation and not a torn meniscus. Any "traumatic" arthritis in patients with psoriasis which fails to settle in the usual way should be considered as monarticular psoriatic arthritis until proved otherwise.

Rheumatoid arthritis is distinguished by a positive SCAT; subcutaneous nodules are pathognomonic, although a colleague, Dr. John Moll, has treated a patient with erosive distal joint arthritis who also had nodules. Presumably this is an example of coincidental psoriatic arthritis and rheumatoid arthritis, which will rarely occur.

TREATMENT

In most patients treatment of psoriasis is no problem, and many require no therapy at all. Details of treatment of the skin manifestations of psoriasis are beyond the scope of this book. Most patients with mild to moderate arthritis respond to NSAIDS. Occasional patients will have more progressive joint disease and should be treated similarly to those with progressive rheumatoid arthritis.

Despite repeated claims, the evidence for the arthritis subsiding because of successful treatment of the skin is tenuous. The skin rash should be treated in its own right, and the type of treatment (e.g., inpatient therapy) will often benefit the arthritis concomitantly. Often the arthritis is sufficiently mild not to require treatment. Initially a regimen of nonsteroidal anti-inflammatory

Figure 66–9. Site of onset of skin lesions in three groups of patients with psoriatic arthritis. *Top,* Patients with distal disease, involving primarily the hands and/or feet. *Middle,* This group had a pattern of distribution similar to the one above but had a severe deforming process. *Bottom,* These patients had an arthritis that could not be distinguished from rheumatoid arthritis.

drugs suffices. A trial of indomethacin and diclofenac showed both to be effective.[110] Antimalarial drugs are avoided for fear of provoking exfoliation.[111,112] A review of 50 patients with psoriatic arthritis treated with hydroxychloroquine showed no exacerbation of skin lesions.[112] In reviewing the situation Luzar[114] reported a flare-up in one of three psoriatic patients whom he had so treated, and there appears to be a low incidence of such exacerbations, probably in the realm of 1 to 2 percent.[115] Clinicians have been reluctant to use gold for fear of producing a rash in a patient already suffering from one skin disease. There is no greater risk of this toxic reaction than in rheumatoid arthritis[62] (see Chapter 52). Uncontrolled studies have reported benefit for more resistant cases.[113,116,117] As a last resort cytotoxic agents may be used. In a small group of patients treated with 6-mercaptopurine the majority improved.[118] Low doses of 25 to 150 mg daily sufficed and produced little toxicity. After treatment was stopped, the remissions lasted for up to 10 months.

Feldges and Barnes[119] found the arthritis responded in nine of ten patients treated with azathioprine in a dose of 2.5 mg per kilogram per day. There was concomitant but fluctuating improvement of the skin lesions. In two patients treatment was stopped because of gut disturbances and in one because of mild thrombocytopenia. The antipyrimidine azaribine was used in 32 patients unresponsive to conventional therapy.[120] The spectrum of response varied from total remission of arthritis in five patients to no improvement in seven. Cyclosporin A brought about an impressive improvement in the psoriatic lesions of four patients, but the effect on the arthropathy was variable.[121] An enthusiastic report on the response of patients with psoriatic arthritis to the oral retinoid tigason was made on the basis of 24 patients treated, but the study was uncontrolled.[122] Systemic steroids are rarely used, since a high dose is often required and the condition usually relapses despite continued therapy. Moreover, a low dose can destabilize the disease. Methotrexate, a folic acid antagonist, has been used successfully in controlling the rash of psoriasis[102] and has been used systemically to control the arthropathy, but with serious side effects.[103] The major hazard of long-term treatment is the development of hepatic fibrosis. We do annual liver biopsies on our patients receiving this drug. Hall and associates[104] showed that intra-articular methotrexate had a short-term anti-inflammatory effect on patients with psoriatic arthritis, but not on those with rheumatoid arthritis. Azathioprine improved two thirds of a group of patients with psoriasis resistant to inpatient treatment and not responding to powerful drugs such as methotrexate and corticosteroids, or when the lesions were extensive and disabling.[105] In Leeds we have 25 patients with severe psoriasis under long-term treatment with such agents. Eighteen are receiving methotrexate. After a test dose of 5 mg the patients receive 25 mg intravenously weekly for 1 month, with blood checks 3 days after injection, and then every 2 weeks. The only examples of severe toxicity have been an ulcer at the injection site in one

patient and liver inflammation in another. Hydroxyurea is being given in three patients, 500 mg twice daily for 1 month and then 500 mg three times each day. A further four patients are receiving azathioprine, 50 mg twice daily for 1 month and then 50 mg three times each day.

The initial enthusiastic report on treating psoriasis by oral 8-methoxypsoralens followed 1 or 2 hours later by high-intensity long-wave ultraviolet radiation appeared in 1974, and the subject has been extensively reviewed.[106] A careful study at the National Institutes of Health suggests that the arthritis may improve concomitantly.[107]

The nails usually improve only with radiotherapy. Popp and Addington[108] suggested that this improved the distal joints as well. Triamcinolone acetonide, given with a needleless injector three times a week, improved 78 percent of patients.[109]

Orthopedic surgery is required in some of these patients. The tendency to fibrosis may hinder the mobilization of a joint postoperatively, but on the whole it does not jeopardize the results of surgery. Psoriatic scales are heavily infected and may produce cross-infection. It has been claimed that prosthetic replacement in these patients is hazardous because they are prone to infection.[123] We have not been able to confirm this. Even incisions through psoriatic plaques do not increase the frequency of wound infection.[79]

References

1. Bazin, P.: Théoriques et Cliniques sur les Affections Cutanées de Nature Arthritique et Arthreux. Paris, Delahaye, 1860, pp. 154–161.
2. Short, C.L., Bauer, W., and Reynolds, W.E.: Rheumatoid Arthritis. Cambridge, Harvard University Press, 1957, p. 38.
3. Vilanova, X., and Pinol, J.: Psoriasis arthropathica. Rheumatism 7:197, 1951.
4. Coste, F., Francon, J., Touraine, R., and Loyau, G.: Polyarthritis psoriasique. Rev. Rhum. Mal. Osteo-artic. 25:75, 1958.
5. Wright, V.: Psoriasis and arthritis. Arch. Dermatol. 80:27, 1959.
6. Wright, V.: Psoriasis and arthritis: A re-evaluation. Am. J. Med. 27:454, 1959.
7. Baker, H.: The Relationship Between Psoriasis, Psoriatic Arthritis and Rheumatoid Arthritis. An Epidemiological, Clinical and Serological Study. M.D. Thesis, University of Leeds, 1965.
8. Wright, V., and Moll, J.M.H.: Seronegative Polyarthritis. Amsterdam, North-Holland, 1976.
9. Fawcitt, J.: Bone and joint changes associated with psoriasis. Br. J. Radiol. 23:440, 1950.
10. Sterne, E.H., and Schneider, B.: Psoriatic arthritis. Ann. Intern. Med. 38:512, 1953.
11. Bauer, W., Bennett, G.A., and Zeller, J.W.: Pathology of joint lesion in patients with psoriasis and arthritis. Trans. Assoc. Am. Physicians 56:349, 1941.
12. Meany, T.F., and Hays, R.A.: Roentgen manifestations of psoriatic arthritis. Radiology 68:403, 1957.
13. Hench, P.S.: Arthropathia psoriatica. Proc. Mayo Clin. 2:89, 1927.
14. Carrier, J.W.: Psoriatic arthritis. Am. J. Roentgenol. 74:612, 1958.
15. Dawson, M.H., and Tyson, T.L.: Psoriasis arthropathica with observations on certain features common to psoriasis and rheumatoid arthritis. Trans. Assoc. Am. Physicians 53:303, 1938.
16. Jeghers, H., and Robinson, L.J.: Arthropathia psoriatica: Report of a case and discussion of the pathogenesis, diagnosis and treatment. JAMA 108:949, 1937.
17. Moll, J.M.H., and Wright, V.: Familial occurrence of psoriatic arthritis. Ann. Rheum. Dis. 32:181, 1973.
18. Baker, H.: Epidemiological aspects of psoriasis and arthritis. Br. J. Dermatol. 78:249, 1966.
19. Leczinsky, C.G.: The incidence of arthropathy in a ten-year series of psoriasis cases. Acta Derm.-Venereol. 28:483, 1948.
20. Hellgren, L.: Association between rheumatoid arthritis and psoriasis in total populations. Acta Rheum. Scand. 15:316, 1969.
21. Theiss, B., Schnyder, V.W., Boni, A., and Wagenhauser, F.: Intrafamiliare

Untersuchungen bei Psoriasis-Arthritis. Z. Rheumaforsch. 28:403, 1969.

22. Cats, A.: Psoriasis and arthritis. *In* Farber, E.M., and Cox, A.J. (eds.): Psoriasis. Proceedings of the International Symposium, Stanford University. Stanford University Press, 1971, pp. 127–135.

23. Bollet, A.J., and Turner, R.A.: Psoriatic arthritis. Ann. N.Y. Acad. Sci. 73:1013, 1958.

24. Reed, W.B.: Psoriatic arthritis. Acta Derm.-Venereol. 41:396, 1961.

25. Hoede, L.: Zur Frage Erblichkeit der Psoriasis. Hautarzt 8:433, 1957.

26. Lomholt, G.: Psoriasis: Prevalence, Spontaneous Course and Genetics. Copenhagen, Gad, 1963.

27. Steinberg, A.G., Becker, S.W., Fitzpatrick, T.B., and Kierland, R.R.: Genetic and statistical study of psoriasis. Am. J. Hum. Genet. 3:267, 1951.

28. Russell, T.J., Lorain, M.D., Schults, M., and Kuban, D.J.: Histocompatibility (H.L.A.) antigens associated with psoriasis. N. Engl. J. Med. 287:738, 1972.

29. White, S., Newcomer, V., Mickey, M., and Terasaki, P.: Disturbance of HLA antigen frequency in psoriasis. N. Engl. J. Med. 287:740, 1972.

30. McClusky, O.E., Cordon, R.E., and Arnett, F.C., Jr.: HL-A 27 in Reiter's syndrome and psoriatic arthritis; a genetic factor in disease susceptibility and expression. J. Rheumatol. 1:263, 1974.

31. Metzger, A.L., Morris, R.I., Bluestone, R., and Terasaki, R.I.: HL-A W27 in psoriatic arthropathy. Arthritis Rheum. 18:111, 1975.

32. Karnoven, J., Lassus, A., Sievers, V., and Tulikainen, A.: HL-A antigens in psoriatic arthritis. Ann. Clin. Res. 6:304, 1974.

33. Tsuji, K., Inouye, H., Nose, Y., Sasazuki, T., Ozawa, A., and Ohkido, M.: Further studies in HLA A B C D DR and haptotype antigen frequencies in psoriasis vulgaris. Acta Derm. Venereol. 59:107, 1979.

34. Green, L., Meyers, O.L., Gordon, W., and Briggs, B.: Arthritis in psoriasis. Ann. Rheum. Dis. 40:366, 1981.

35. Batchelor, J.R., and Morris, P.J.: HLA and disease—joint report. *In* Bodmer, W.F., Batchelor, J.R., Bodmer, J.G., Festenstein, H., and Morris, P.J. (eds.): Histocompatibility Testing 1977. Copenhagen, Munksgaard, 1978, p. 205.

36. Tiilikainen, A., Lassus, A., Karvonen, J., Vartainen, P., and Julin, M.: Psoriasis and HLA Cw6. Br. J. Dermatol., 102:179, 1980.

37. Hawkins, B.R., Tiwari, J.L., Lowe, N., Wolfish, P., Pollock, C.A., Cho, Y.W., and Terasaki, P.I. HLA and psoriasis. *In* Terasaki, P.I. (ed.): Histocompatibility Testing. Los Angeles, UCLA Tissue Typing Laboratory, 1981, p. 711.

38. Marcusson, J.: Psoriasis and arthritic lesions in relation to the inheritance of HLA genotypes. Acta Derm. Venereol. 59:Suppl. 82, 1979.

39. Bauer, J., and Vogl, A.: Psoriasis und Gelenkleiden, Klin. Wschr. 10:1700, 1931.

40. Tiedemann, G.: Symptomatologie und Aetiologie der Psoriasis arthropathica. Z. Menschl. Vererb. Konstit. Lehre 30:248, 1951.

41. Ward, J.H., and Stephens, F.E.: Inheritance of psoriasis in a Utah kindred. Arch. Dermatol. 84:589, 1961.

42. Wright, V.: Psoriatic arthritis. *In* Copeman, W.S.C. (ed.): Textbook of the Rheumatic Diseases. 4th ed. Edinburgh, Livingstone, 1969, p. 632.

43. Baker, H., Golding, D.N., and Thompson, M.: Psoriasis and arthritis. Ann. Intern. Med. 58:909, 1963.

44. Theiss, B., Schnyder, U.W., and Boni, A.: Intrafamiliare immunochemische Untersuchungen bei Psoriasis-Arthritis und Psoriasis-Spondylarthritis. Arch. Klin. Exp. Derm. 239:248, 1970.

45. Vilàghy, I., and Krebs, A.: Untersuchungen über die Vererblichkeit des Syndroms Psoriasis arthropathica. Dermatologica 140:209, 1970.

46. Jayson, M.I.V., and Henderson, D.R.F.: Arthroscopy in the diagnosis in inflammatory joint disease. Rheumatol. Rehabil. 12:195, 1973.

47. Sherman, M.: Psoriatic arthritis: Observations on the clinical, roentgenographic and pathological changes. J. Bone Joint Surg. 34A:831, 1952.

48. Coste, F., and Solnica, J.: Rev. Franc. Erud. Clin. Biol. 11:58, 1966.

48a Brewerton, D.A., Caffrey, M., Nicholls, A., Walters, D., and James, D.C.O.: HLA-B27 and arthropathies associated with ulcerative colitis and psoriasis. Lancet 1:956, 1974.

49. Serre, H., Simon, L., and Sany, J.: Le rhumatisme psoriasique. J. Med. Montpellier 4:3, 1969.

50. Schattenkirchner, M.: Zur Symptomatologie de Arthritis psoriatica. Med. Klin. 65:1360, 1970.

51. Nazzaro, P., and Gogante, D.: Observations on 100 cases of psoriatic arthritis. *In* Farber, E.M., and Cox, A.J. (eds.): Psoriasis. Proceedings of the International Symposium, Stanford University. Stanford University Press, 1971, p. 137.

52. Molin, L.: Psoriasis: A study of the course and degree of severity, joint involvement, socio-medical conditions, general morbidity, and influences of selection factors among previously hospitalized psoriatics. Acta Derm.-Venereol. 53:Suppl. 72, 1973, pp. 1–125.

53. Little, M., Harvie, J.N., and Lester, R.S.: Psoriatic arthritis in severe psoriasis. Can. Med. Assoc. J. 112:317, 1975.

54. Dixon, A.St.J.: Rheumatoid polyarthritis associated with a negative sheep cell agglutination test. A follow up study. Ann. Rheum. Dis. 17:252, 1958.

55. Eastmond, C.J., and Wright, V.: Nail dystrophy in psoriatic arthritis. Ann. Rheum. Dis. 38:226, 1979.

56. Armstrong, R.D., Panayi, G.S., Welsh, K.I.: Histocompatibility antigens in psoriasis, psoriatic arthropathy and ankylosing spondylitis. Ann. Rheum. Dis. In the press, 1983.

57. Barber, H.W.: Psoriasis. Br. Med. J. 1:219, 1950.

58. Lambert, J.R., Ansell, B.M., Stephenson, E., and Wright, V.: Psoriatic arthritis in childhood. Clin. Rheum. Dis. 2:339, 1976.

59. Fletcher, E., and Rose, F.C.: Psoriasis spondylitica. Lancet 1:695, 1955.

60. Graber-Duvernay, J.: À propos de la spondylarthrite psoriasique. Rev. Rhum. 24:288, 1957.

61. Wright, V.: Psoriasis and arthritis: A study of the radiographic appearances. Br. J. Radiol. 30:113, 1957.

62. Wright, V.: Psoriatic arthritis: A comparative study of rheumatoid arthritis and arthritis associated with psoriasis. Ann. Rheum. Dis. 20:123, 1961.

63. Jajic, I.: Radiological changes in the sacro-iliac joints and spine of patients with psoriatic arthritis and psoriasis. Ann. Rheum. Dis. 27:1, 1968.

64. Bruhl, W., and Maldykowa, H.: Analiza kliniczna 50 przypadkow artropatii tusczycowej. Pol. Tyg. Lek. 15:525, 1970.

65. Lambert, J.R., and Wright, V.: Psoriatic spondylitis: A clinical and radiological description of the spine in psoriatic arthritis. Quart. J. Med. 46:411, 1977.

66. Lambert, J.R., and Wright, V.: Eye inflammation in psoriatic arthritis. Ann. Rheum. Dis. 35:354, 1976.

67. Walker, W.C., and Wright, V.: Pulmonary lesions and rheumatoid arthritis. Medicine 47:501, 1968.

68. Roberts, M.E.T., Wright, V., Hill, A.G.S., and Mehra, A.C.: Psoriatic arthritis: A follow-up study. Ann. Rheum. Dis. 35:206, 1976.

69. Reed, W.B., and Wright, V.: Psoriatic arthritis. *In* Hill, A.G.S. (ed.): Modern Trends in Rheumatology. London, Butterworths, 1966, p. 375.

70. Lodin, A., Gentele, H., Lagerholm, B., and Karltorp, N.: Psoriatic arthritis and elevated E.S.R. Acta Derm.-Venereol. 37:459, 1957.

71. Zachariae, H., and Zachariae, E.: Antinuclear factors, the anti-human globulin consumption test, and Wassermann reaction in psoriatic arthritis. Acta Rheum. Scand. 15:62, 1969.

72. Cockel, R., Kendall, M.J., Becker, J.C., and Hawkins, C.F.: Serum biochemical values in rheumatoid disease. Ann. Rheum. Dis. 30:166, 1971.

73. Kennedy, A.C., Allam, B.F., Boyle, I.T., Nuki, C., Rooney, P.J., and Buchanan, W.W.: Abnormalities in mineral metabolism suggestive of parathyroid overactivity in rheumatoid arthritis. Curr. Med. Res. Opin. 3:345, 1975.

74. Barmann, R.R., and Jillson, O.F.: Hyperuricemia and psoriasis. J. Invest. Dermatol. 36:105, 1961.

75. Walton, R., Block, W.D., and Heyde, J.: A comparative study of uric acid values of whole blood in patients with psoriasis and other dermatoses. J. Invest. Dermatol. 36:125, 1961.

76. Eisen, A.Z., and Seegmiller, J.E.: Uric acid metabolism in psoriasis. J. Clin. Invest. 40:1486, 1961.

77. Wright, V.: Psoriasis and arthritis. Ann. Rheum. Dis. 15:348, 1956.

78. Baker, H., Golding, D.N., and Thompson, M.: Atypical polyarthritis in psoriatic families. Br. Med. J. 2:348, 1963.

79. Lambert, J.R., and Wright, V.: Surgery in patients with psoriasis and arthritis. Rheumatol. Rehabil. 18:35, 1979.

80. Gaedicke, H., Kaiser, W., and Mathies, H.: Die Bestimmung der Phosphoglucose-Isomerase-Aktivatat in den Erythrocyten und ihre Bedeutung als diagnostiches Kriterium der Arthritis psoriatica. Klin. Wschr. 48:1456, 1970.

81. Robillard, J.: Le Rheumatisme Psoriasique (à Propos de 53 Observations). Thesis. Lyon, 1968.

82. Petres, J., and Majert, P.: Immunelektrophorese bei psoriatischer Arthropathie. Arch. Klin. Exp. Dermtol. 233:398, 1968.

83. Danielsen, L.: Immuno-electrophoretic analysis of serum proteins in psoriasis and psoriatic arthritis. Acta Rheumatol. Scand. 11:112, 1965.

84. Heiskell, G.L., Reed, W.B., Weimer, H.E., Becker, S.W., and Carpenter, C.M.: Serum protein profiles in psoriasis and arthritis. Arch. Dermatol. 85:708, 1962.

85. Lambert, J.R., Roberts, M., and Wright, V.: Nitroblue tetrazolium test in psoriatic arthritis, rheumatoid arthritis and osteoarthrosis. Ann. Rheum. Dis. 37:363, 1978.

86. Medsger, T.A., Rodnan, G.P., Rabin, B., Birnbaum, N., and Porter, P.: HL-A 27 and psoriatic spondylitis. Arthritis Rheum. 7:323, 1974.

87. Espinoza, L.R., Vasey, F.B., Oh, J.H., Wilkinson, R., and Osterland, C.K.: Association between HLA-BW38 and peripheral psoriatic arthritis. Arthritis Rheum. 21:72, 1978.

88. Avila, R., Pugh, D.G., Slocumb, C.H., and Winkelmann, R.K.: Psoriatic arthritis: A roentgenological study. Radiology 75:691, 1960.

89. Bardagni, O., and Carlisimo, O.A.: Artropatia psoriatica. Policlinico Scz. Prat. 74:33, 1967.

90. Porrini, A., McEwen, C., Di Tata, C., Poppel, M., and Lingg, C.: A roentgenologic and clinical study of ankylosing spondylitis and spondylitis accompanying ulcerative colitis, psoriasis and Reiter's disease. Arthritis Rheum. 7:338, 1964.

91. Kaplan, D., Plotz, C.M., Nathanson, L., and Frank, L.: Cervical spine in psoriasis and in psoriatic arthritis. Ann. Rheum. Dis. 23:50, 1964.

92. Bywaters, E.G.L., and Dixon, A.St.J.: Paravertebral ossification in psoriatic arthritis. Ann. Rheum. Dis. 24:313, 1965.

93. McEwen, C., Di Tata, D., Lingg, C., Porrini, A., Good, A., and Rankin, T.: Ankylosing spondylitis accompanying ulcerative colitis, regional enteritis, psoriasis and Reiter's disease. Arthritis Rheum. 14:291, 1971.

94. Barraclough, D., Russell, A.S., and Percy, J.S.: Psoriatic spondylitis: A clinical radiological and scintiscan survey. J. Rheumatol. 4:282, 1977.

95. Wright, V., and Reed, W.B.: Reiter's syndrome and psoriatic arthritis. Ann. Rheum. Dis. 23:12, 1964.

96. Crain, D.C.: Interphalangeal osteoarthritis characterized by painful inflammatory episodes resulting in deformity of the proximal and distal articulations. JAMA 175:1049, 1961.

97. Peter, J.B., Pearson, C.M., and Marmor, L.: Erosive osteoarthritis of the hands. Arthritis Rheum. 9:365, 1966.

98. Kidd, K.L., and Peter, J.B.: Erosive osteoarthritis. Radiology 86:640, 1966.

99. Swezey, R.L., and Alexander, S.J.: Erosive osteoarthritis and the main en lorgnette deformity. Arch. Intern. Med. 128:269, 1971.

100. Smukler, N.M., Edeiken, J., and Giuliano, V.J.: Ankylosis in osteoarthritis of the finger joints. Radiology 100:525, 1977.

101. Wright, V.: Psoriatic arthritis. In Scott, J.T. (ed.): Textbook of Rheumatic Diseases. 5th ed. Edinburgh, Churchill-Livingstone, 1978, pp. 537–548.

102. Weinstein, G.D., and Frost, P.: Methotrexate for psoriasis. A new therapeutic schedule. Arch. Dermatol. 103:33, 1971.

103. Black, R.L., O'Brien, W.M., van Scott, E.J., Auerbach, R., Eisen, A.Z., and Bunim, J.J.: Methotrexate therapy in psoriatic arthritis. JAMA 189:743, 1964.

104. Hall, G.H., Jones, B.J.M., Head, A.C., and Jones, V.E.: Intra-articular methotrexate; clinical and laboratory studies in rheumatoid and psoriatic arthritis. Ann. Rheum. Dis. 37:351, 1978.

105. du Vivier, A., Munro, D.D., and Verbov, J.: Treatment of psoriasis with azathioprine. Br. Med. J. 1:49, 1974.

106. Leading article: PUVA. Br. Med. J. 3:2, 1978.

107. Perlman, S.G., Gerber, L.M., Roberts, R.M., Nigra, T.P., and Barth, W.F.: Photodermotherapy and psoriatic arthritis. Fourth Southeastern Regional Meeting of American Rheumatism Association, Atlanta, 1977.

108. Popp, W.C., and Addington, E.A.: Roentgen therapy for psoriasis of nails and psoriatic arthritis. Radiology 36:98, 1941.

109. Abell, E.: Treatment of psoriatic nail dystrophy. Br. J. Dermatol. 86:79, 1972.

110. Leatham, P.A., Bird, H.A., Wright, V., and Forbes, P.D.: The run-in period in trial design: A comparison of two nonsteroidal anti-inflammatory agents in psoriatic arthropathy. Agents Actions 12:221, 1982.

111. Cornbleet, T.: Action of synthetic antimalarial drugs on psoriasis. J. Invest. Dermatol. 26:435, 1956.

112. Reed, W.B., and Becker, S.W.: Psoriasis and arthritis. Arch. Dermatol. 11:577, 1960.

113. Kammer, G.M., Sotar, N.A., and Gibson, D.J.: Psoriatic arthritis: a clinical immunologic, and HLA study of 100 patients. Sem. Arthritis Rheum. 9:513, 1979.

114. Luzan, M.J.: Hydroxychloroquine in psoriatic arthropathy: Exacerbations of psoriatic skin lesions. J. Rheum. 9:462, 1982.

115. Mackenzie, A.H., and Scherbec, A.C.: Chloroquine and hydroxychloroquine. In Huskisson, E.C. (ed.): Clinics of Rheumatic Diseases. London, W. B. Saunders Co., 1980, p. 545.

116. Dorwart, B.B., Gall, E.P., and Schumacher, R.H.: Chrysotherapy in psoriatic arthritis: Efficacy and toxicity compared to rheumatoid arthritis. Arthritis Rheum. 21:513, 1978.

117. Richter, M.B., Kinsella, P., and Corbett, M.: Gold in psoriatic arthropathy. Ann. Rheum. Dis. 39:279, 1980.

118. Baum, J., Hurd, E., Lewis, D., Ferguson, J.L., and Ziff, M.: Treatment of psoriatic arthritis with 6-mercaptopurine. Arthritis Rheum. 16:139, 1973.

119. Feldges, D.H., and Barnes, C.G.: Treatment of psoriatic arthropathy with either azathioprine or methotrexate. Rheumatol. Rehabil. 13:120, 1974.

120. Levine, S., and Paulus, H.E.: Treatment of psoriatic arthritis with azaribine. Arthritis Rheum. 19:1, 1976.

121. Mueller, W., and Graf, U.: The use of cyclosporin A, a new immunosuppressant, in the treatment of psoriatic arthritis (German). Schweiz. Med. Wochenschr 111/12:408, 1981.

122. Stollenwerk, E., Fischer-Hoinkes, H., Komenda, K., and Schilling, F.: Clinical observations on oral retinoid therapy of psoriatic arthropathy (Ro 10-9359). In Orfanos, C.E. (ed.): Retinoids. Springer-Verlag, Berlin, Springer-Verlag, 1981, p. 205.

123. Kummerle, F., Weissinghage, D., and Schweikert, C-H.: Risks of alloplastic replacements in degenerative and inflammatory diseases of joints. Acta Orthop. Belg. 37:541, 1971.

Chapter 67

Enteropathic Arthritis

Armin E. Good and Peter D. Utsinger

INTRODUCTION

The term enteropathic arthritis refers to certain arthritides that are associated with intestinal disorders. While there are obvious limitations to the use of this generic term (just as there would be limitations to using neuropathic arthritis to refer to a group of diseases involving the central nervous system and associated with arthritis), there is usefulness in the term, at least in so far as it emphasizes the unusual association between diseases of both the peripheral and the axial skeleton and diseases of the gut. Until these diseases can be distinguished etiologically or pathogenetically, it seems worthwhile to group them together in this chapter with a brief review of the microbiology and immunology of the gut.

BACTERIOLOGY

The small intestine is not an important reservoir of bacteria, with the exception of the distal part of the ileum. In the jejunum, aerobic and facultative anaerobic organisms, including streptococci, lactobacilli, coliforms, and staphylococci, have been found in concentrations of less than 10^4 per ml of intestinal fluid.[1] Biopsies of the jejunum of normal humans show a tendency for intestinal bacteria to cling to the epithelial surface of the bowel, embedded in mucus.[2] In the ileum the microbial population increases in number and becomes more diverse. In the distal ileum, presumably because of its proximity to the colon, aerobes and facultative anaerobes (bacteroides, lactobacilli, and clostridia) are found, in concentrations up to 10^7 organisms per gram of feces. When the ileocecal valve is passed, the anaerobic population of the bowel exceeds aerobic organisms by several log titers. Anaerobic organisms within the lumen of the colon outnumber aerobic organisms by at least 5000 to 1, and the ratio may approach 10,000–12,000 to 1. The speciating of colonic organisms is most difficult because of problems in culturing strict anaerobes. However, biochemical analyses can also be helpful in defining the variety of colonic organisms.[3] As is the case with the small intestinal flora, colonic bacteria tend to adhere to the mucus on the lining epithelial cells.

IMMUNOLOGY

Organized Lymphoid Tissue. The most well-studied of the gut-associated lymphoid tissues (GALT) are those with highly organized structures—Peyer's patches (PP). PP are almost certainly not the mammalian equivalent of the chick bursa of Fabricius, a primary site of B lymphocyte development, since T lymphocytes are found in PP before B lymphocytes appear. Although PP are considered to be secondary lymphoid organs, the dome or the surface epithelium of the PP may be a primary lymphoid organ. While the dome is initially filled with T lymphocytes, later, with antigen stimulation from absorbed gut bacteria, the dome becomes packed with B-lymphocyte–rich follicles. In man, PP are distributed along the antimesenteric surface of the intestine as two hundred or more nodules and are most abundant in the distal ileum. The dome epithelium contains columnar cells, goblet cells, and unique cells called M cells.[4] The latter have a basal nucleus, prominent Golgi complexes, and numerous mitochondria and form intracellular bridges with adjacent M cells and tight contacts with lymphocytes and plasmablasts. Because M cells have pinocytotic vesicles, it is thought that they may be involved in antigen transport of gut luminal antigens to the intrafollicular cells. It is certain that inert particles and protein antigens traverse the dome epithelium, and also certain that the transport of some of these particles is assumed by the M cells.[5,7] Strong circumstantial evidence supports the concept that enteropathogenic bacteria also invade the host via the dome epithelium. PP also contain phagocytic cells, which are macrophage-like, and nonlymphocyte Ia-positive cells similar to the dendritic cells of the spleen.

Poorly Organized Lymphoid Tissue. Lymphoid cells and other cells of nonepithelial origin are scattered throughout the intestine, in the lamina propria and the intraepithelial compartment. The dominant lymphocyte in the intraepithelial compartment is a T cell with the OK T8 phenotype.[7,8] Still controversial is the suggestion that some of these T cells are transitional cells destined

to become mast cells, an idea based on the finding of some histamine-containing granules in some of the cells. The lamina propria contains T lymphocytes, a minority of which bear the OK T8 phenotype. The lamina propria is packed with IgA-secreting plasma cells, most probably migrating from the PP; others derive from in situ precursor B cells.

Macrophages are found near the apex of absorptive villi, shedding themselves and phagocytized debris from the lamina propria into the intestinal lumen, seemingly serving as intestinal scavengers.

IgA Structure and Function. The principal immunoglobulin in external secretions is IgA. It differs from serum IgA in that it is predominantly a dimer and contains two additional components—the secretory piece and J chain. Secretory IgA can neutralize viruses and is an effective barrier to transenteric mucosal bacterial invasion.

ARTHROPATHY WITH INFLAMMATORY BOWEL DISEASE

Ulcerative colitis is an inflammatory disease that involves the gastrointestinal mucosa in a diffuse manner. Crohn's disease is a focal granulomatous disease involving all layers of the gut wall. Features of both diseases, however, coexist in some cases, and multiple mucosal biopsies may be necessary for reasonably certain differentiation. In recent years granulomatous colitis has been split away from ulcerative colitis and joined to Crohn's disease, so that older studies contrasting the arthropathies of the two bowel diseases have been invalidated. The prevalence of arthritis appears to be related to the site of bowel involvement rather than to the specific diagnosis of ulcerative colitis or Crohn's disease. As far as possible, the discussion here will be unified under the noncommittal diagnosis of inflammatory bowel disease (IBD).

Peripheral Arthritis

Definition. The peripheral arthritides described with ulcerative colitis and Crohn's disease appear similar in every respect and have been defined according to four cardinal characteristics: (1) the articular manifestations usually begin after the onset of the intestinal disease; (2) attacks of arthritis are related temporally to flares of the bowel disease; (3) the attacks of arthritis are followed by complete remission of synovitis; and (4) rheumatoid factor is absent.[9] Musculoskeletal and other extraintestinal features of IBD are summarized in Figure 67–1.

Prevalence of Peripheral Joint Involvement. Using current diagnostic criteria, the frequency of peripheral arthritis among patients with Crohn's disease is 20 percent[10] and among those with ulcerative colitis, 9 to 11.5 percent.[11,12] Males and females are equally affected. The frequency is about the same in adults as among children with IBD;[13] with anemia and growth retarda-

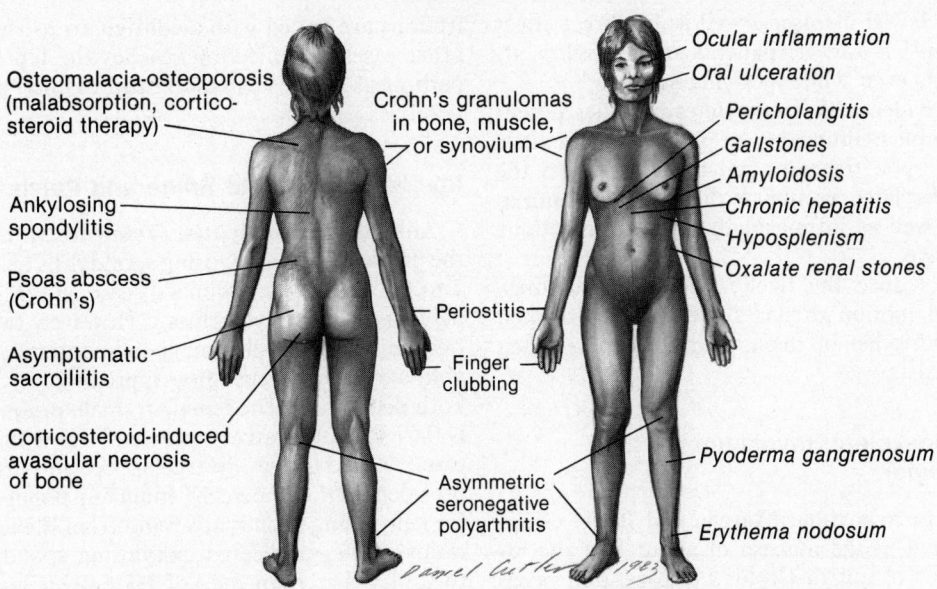

Figure 67–1. Diagramatic summary of musculoskeletal (left, center) and other extra-intestinal features (right, in italics) of inflammatory bowel disease.

tion, arthritis in the latter closely simulates juvenile rheumatoid arthritis.

Arthritis is more frequent in the face of complications of ulcerative colitis such as pseudomembranous polyposis, perianal disease, and massive hemorrhage[14] and is more common with extensive colitis than with distal proctocolitis only. The major complications of Crohn's disease, fistula formation and malabsorption, do not appear to increase the frequency of arthritis.[10] Crohn's disease limited to the colon is associated with the highest frequency of arthritis;[12,15] and Crohn's disease limited to the small bowel, the lowest.[12] Arthritis is more common in patients with extraintestinal manifestations such as erythema nodosum and aphthous stomatitis[12] as well as uveitis and pyoderma gangrenosum.[16]

Characterization. The peripheral arthritis has been characterized in detail by McEwen.[17] Attacks often appear abruptly, reaching a peak within 24 hours. While the pain may be more severe than that of rheumatoid arthritis, in 85 percent of attacks less than four joints are affected. As many as eight joints may be involved, frequently in a migratory fashion. In decreasing order of frequency, the knee, ankle, elbow, proximal interphalangeal joint of a finger, wrist, shoulder, and metacarpophalangeal joint are affected. The duration of attacks is less than a month in one half of cases, from 5 weeks to 2 months in a quarter, from 2 to 6 months in a tenth, and from 6 to 12 months in a tenth. The remaining patients have more or less continuous arthritis over periods of several years. The mean duration of the attacks in another series was 7 weeks (range of 1 to 16 weeks).[9]

The attacks predominate in the first few years of bowel disease. In patients followed for 5 years the average number of attacks was two, increasing only to 2.5 at the end of 15 years.[17] Most patients recover with no permanent articular damage. Only 25 percent of patients have clinical or radiographic evidence of residual damage, often without functional significance.

With ulcerative colitis a close association has been observed between exacerbations of the colitis and attacks of arthritis. The concurrence of flares of bowel disease with flares of arthritis is less clear-cut in Crohn's disease than in ulcerative colitis.

Laboratory and Radiographic Findings. The IBD itself may account for anemia, leukocytosis, and elevated erythrocyte sedimentation rate. Tests for serum rheumatoid factor and antinuclear antibodies are negative.

Synovial fluid analyses and synovial biopsies have been reported infrequently. Synovial fluid typically shows turbid sterile fluid with a fair mucin clot containing 5000 to 12,000 leukocytes, predominantly polymorphs. Synovial fluid protein and complement components are normal. Biopsies have revealed nonspecific features, namely, proliferation of synovial lining cells, increased vascularity, and infiltration of lymphocytes, plasma cells, and histiocytes.[17] Radiographs of involved joints are preponderantly negative; minimal destructive signs have been observed, such as cystic changes, erosion, and narrowing of the joint space.[18]

Therapy. Optimal therapy directed to the underlying bowel disease is also the most effective treatment for the peripheral arthritis. In one large series of patients with ulcerative colitis submitted to colectomy, there were no recurrences of joint symptoms postoperatively.[11,14] In Crohn's disease, bowel resections do not clearly induce remissions, probably because surgery can never remove all of the involved gut.

Corticosteroids prescribed for management of the colitis usually suppress the arthritis, possibly indirectly by controlling the bowel disease as well as by direct effect upon synovium.[17] However, patients may develop attacks of arthritis even while receiving steroids.[16,19]

There is no evidence that salicylates or other potent drugs such as phenylbutazone or indomethacin have adverse effects upon the intestinal disease beyond the duodenum. Salicylates or nonsteroidal anti-inflammatory agents as well as intra-articular steroid injections are often effective.

In order to reduce the likelihood of contractures, timely range of motion exercises are important when patients are bedridden or debilitated, especially when spondylitis coexists.

Other Musculoskeletal Involvement (Excluding Spine)

Granulomas in Synovium, Muscle, and Bone. Granulomas are found in the mucosa of about half the resected specimens of gut in Crohn's disease, and occasionally in the uveal tract, lymph nodes, and liver as well, and may also be involved in the musculoskeletal manifestations of Crohn's disease. These lesions are often difficult to find, even in large specimens of bowel. From experience with sequential surgical specimens, the granulomas appear to have a life history of about 3 months. In series of patients with Crohn's disease, there are isolated reports of persistent monarthritis contrasting with typically benign, transitory enteropathic arthritis.[20,21] Synovial biopsies in such cases have shown chronic granulomatous inflammation, including non-necrotizing, epitheloid cell granulomas with giant cells of the Langhans type.[22,23] In another case, biopsy of an indurated mass in the gastrocnemius muscle in a patient with myalgias and tenderness of both calves and multifocal electromyographic changes disclosed similar granulomas.[24]

Clubbing and Periostitis. Clubbing of digits is found in 12 percent of patients with Crohn's disease, particularly those with internal fistulas.[25] Periosteal proliferation, however, is unusual and generally asymptomatic. Massive periostosis with severe pain has been reported in a single exceptional case.[26]

Avascular Necrosis. When persistent articular involvement, particularly in the hip, occurs during or following treatment of IBD with corticosteroids, steroid-induced avascular necrosis should be considered. However, in spite of the widespread use of corticosteroid therapy in IBD, it is remarkable that this complication has been reported in only a single instance.[19]

Septic Arthritis of the Hip. Septic arthritis of the hip is an occasional febrile complication of Crohn's disease, the infection extending from the bowel via an internal fistula. The diagnosis may not be readily apparent, as fever and weight loss can be ascribed to the bowel disease, and anti-inflammatory drugs may blunt the signs of acute arthritis. Key findings may be a fluctuant mass near the inguinal ligament, a persistent flexion deformity at the hip, and a radiograph showing bulging of the psoas shadow or gas near the hip areas. Most hip infections are linked with a contiguous psoas abscess.[27] In other cases the infection reaches the hip from a retroperitoneal abscess extending through the greater sciatic notch.[28]

Involvement of the Spine and Pelvis

Ankylosing Spondylitis. *Prevalence.* In various studies the prevalence of ankylosing spondylitis has ranged from 2 to 6.9 percent in Crohn's disease and from 1.1 to 25.6 percent in ulcerative colitis.[17] However, two current series employing similar diagnostic criteria show remarkable agreement, reporting approximately 4 percent in both diseases.[4,21] The female to male ratio in spondylitis is 0.57 with ulcerative colitis and 1.0 with Crohn's disease.[25] These figures diverge appreciably from the mean prevalence of 0.1 percent found in population surveys for ankylosing spondylitis[30] and from the female to male ratios in uncomplicated ankylosing spondylitis of 0.25 to 0.11.[31] The frequency of HLA-B27 in patients with IBD and spondylitis is substantial but less than that encountered with ankylosing spondylitis alone and is reported as low as 53 percent in one study.[32] It has been suggested that the presence of putative genetic determinants for IBD predispose individuals to ankylosing spondylitis in the absence of B27.[33]

Relation to Bowel Disease. Any large series of spondylitis with IBD includes cases in which the spondylitis clearly precedes the onset of the bowel disease, sometimes by many years. In general, the activity of the spondylitic disease has not obviously paralleled that of the bowel. These observations have argued against a cause and effect relationship between the disease of the gut and spine and have supported the notion that the two diseases, though genetically linked in some manner, run separate and autonomous courses. Newer analyses, facilitated by histocompatibility data, have suggested that spondylitis with IBD is heterogeneous and, in some measure at least, is a response to disease in the gut. Three categories of spondylitis have been delineated by Dekker-Saeys and co-workers.[34] In category I, comprising one third of the total study group, are patients in whom spondylitis predominated and preceded the bowel disease. Seventy percent are positive for HLA-B27, 68 percent have radiographic involvement of the spine, and about 25 percent have had iritis.

In category II, one fourth of the group, are patients in whom spondylitis followed the bowel symptoms. These patients have severe disease of the gut, including internal fistulas, recurrent attacks, and multiple operations (Fig. 67–2). Thirteen percent are positive for HLA-B27, 36 percent have spinal radiographic changes, and none has had iritis. In category III, comprising the large remaining fraction, are patients with approximately simultaneous onset of disease in the spine and gut, with neither predominating.

These authors propose that the syndrome of spondylitis with IBD actually includes classic idiopathic ankylosing spondylitis, spondylitis "secondary" to the in-

Figure 67–2. Patient with spondylitis and Crohn's disease, who demonstrates loss of skeletal muscle and subcutaneous fat as well as the typical kyphotic posture of ankylosing spondylitis.

testinal inflammatory pathology, and an indeterminate group. Longitudinal studies correlating symptoms and radiologic progression with fluctuations in the bowel disease will be necessary to validate the attractive hypothesis that there is in fact "secondary" or enteropathic involvement of the spine.

Radiographic Findings. The radiographic features of spondylitis associated with inflammatory bowel disease are typical for those of spondylitis alone.[35] Compression fractures or pronounced demineralization should suggest superimposed osteomalacia-osteoporosis (Fig. 67–3).

Therapy. In patients who are free from gastric or duodenal ulcers, aspirin, phenylbutazone, or indomethacin can be used as in the management of ankylosing spondylitis alone. There is no evidence that these drugs exacerbate inflammatory bowel disease or promote infective complications. When corticosteroids are employed for the bowel disease, the spinal pain is also ameliorated.

Daily physical therapy is especially important in order to forestall irrevocable loss of mobility whenever these patients become bedridden or debilitated.

Asymptomatic Sacroiliac Disease. *Prevalence.* A finding that lends support to the notion of "secondary" spondylitis is the high prevalence of asymptomatic radiographic sacroiliitis (ARSI), which is consistently reported in series of patients with IBD. The prevalence rates, which are often double those for ankylosing spondylitis, range from 4 to 15 percent, clearly exceeding rates among population controls.[29] In contrast to classic ankylosing spondylitis, ARSI is not significantly associated with HLA-B27, and the female to male ratio is 1 or greater.[36]

Relation to Bowel Disease. A cause and effect association between bowel disease and ARSI cannot be ruled out. In ulcerative colitis, some studies have shown that greater duration[37,38] and extent[37] of disease favor the development of ARSI. Further evidence that ARSI may represent a response to an associated disease rather than to a genetic factor 'is derived from a family study of ulcerative colitis. Relatives of probands with asymptomatic sacroiliitis were not more likely to have sacroiliitis than relatives of probands without sacroiliitis, whereas relatives of probands with ankylosing spondylitis showed a significant excess of this disease compared with relatives of probands free from spondylitis.[39]

The meaning of ARSI is far from clear, but this sign may provide an important clue to the etiopathogenesis of various arthropathies discussed in this chapter. Longitudinal studies, perhaps using quantitative scintigraphy in patients encountered very early in their bowel disease, should establish whether this subtle, asymptomatic sacroiliac involvement is related to duration, chronicity, or complications; whether reversion to normal or progression to spondylitis occurs; and how asymptomatic, in fact, the process is.

From a practical standpoint, a presumptive diagnosis of early ankylosing spondylitis should not be made whenever ARSI is encountered with IBD. The odds are about 2 to 1 that the sacroiliac involvement will not surface symptomatically.

Osteoporosis-Osteomalacia. Compression fractures of the spine can occur in IBD from steroid-induced osteoporosis as well as osteomalacia, particularly when small bowel involvement is extensive. Malabsorption is found in 10 percent of cases of Crohn's disease.[12] Compression fracture may complicate coexistent ankylosing spondylitis (see Fig. 67–3) or produce kyphotic deformity, mimicking ankylosing spondylitis. The pain of pathologic fractures in the femora and tarsal bones can be misinterpreted as arthritis of peripheral joints.

Psoas Abscess. Crohn's disease may now be the single most common cause of psoas abscess. In a series of 185 patients with Crohn's disease seen from 1955 to 1969, five developed a psoas abscess.[27] The abdominal portion of the right psoas muscle lies behind the jejunum and sigmoid colon. Thus, infection can enter either psoas sheath via a penetrating posterior fistula. The patient usually presents with pain in the low back, hip, and anterolateral thigh. A flexion deformity of the hip and a limp are usually noted. Other frequent signs are a

Figure 67–3. Osteomalacia complicating ankylosing spondylitis with Crohn's disease. Compression fractures (arrows) of dorsal vertebral bodies appearing between August, 1972 (left), and January, 1973 (right), in patient with Crohn's disease, ankylosing spondylitis, and fecal wasting of calcium. Vitamin D and calcium supplements appeared to control pain and halt progression of the bone disease in this case.

tender mass in the groin or iliac fossa, weight loss, and fever. Near the insertion of the muscle on the lesser trochanter of the femur, the infection may penetrate the capsule of the hip joint.

REACTIVE ARTHRITIS FOLLOWING ENTERIC INFECTION

Reactive arthritis alone or with any or all of the other features of Reiter's syndrome is associated with a growing number of enteric bacterial pathogens: *Shigella flexneri*,[40] *Salmonella* species,[41] *Yersinia enterocolitica*,[42] *Campylobacter fetus* subspecies *jejuni*,[43] and possibly *Brucella* species.[44] These enteric syndromes contribute to the pool of patients diagnosed as having Reiter's syndrome (see Chapter 65) and, except for *Brucella*, demonstrate a HLA-B27–linked host susceptibility factor. Moreover, superinfections with any of these organisms may cause a flare-up of established IBD.[45] Reactive arthritis occurring in this setting could, in fact, account for some cases labeled as enteropathic arthritis

of IBD. Finally, except for *Shigella*, these organisms are capable of invading the bloodstream and producing septic arthritis.

The preceding considerations not only emphasize the role of infective disease in the differential diagnosis but also may provide insight into the mechanisms of the enteropathic arthritis of IBD. Current assessment of patients with arthritis linked to bowel disease thus may often require stool and synovial cultures as well as serum agglutinin tests for several enteric pathogens.

Prevalence. For many years dysentery has been recognized as a precipitating cause for arthritis that does not follow the "septic" pattern of destructive monarthritis but rather involves a few joints and clears completely. Oligo- or polyarthritis was described with dysentery in the eighteenth century and related to epidemic shigellosis by 1897. The incidence of arthritis in large epidemics of shigellosis in the late nineteenth and early twentieth centuries varied from 0 to 10 percent.[46] Military epidemics of shigellosis in World War I had 1 to 2 percent of cases with arthritis.[47] Similarly 2 percent of sailors involved in shipboard epidemic dysentery on an

American naval vessel during World War II had arthritis as well.[48] Subsequently *S. flexneri,* types *2a* or *1,* has been linked to virtually all cases of post-*Shigella* arthritis.[49] Arthritis is not associated with the more common *S. sonnei* enteritis.[50]

In the older literature, arthritis associated with *Salmonella* infection was considered first and foremost a manifestation of sepsis, usually by *Salmonella cholerae suis,* an organism also noted for septic arteritis.[51] Since 1943, however, reports have appeared of aseptic arthritis, usually polyarticular and invariably clearing completely. These cases of presumptive reactive arthritis have occurred preponderantly with *Salmonella typhimurium* and *Salmonella enteritidis.*[52] The incidence of the arthritis in *S. typhimurium* epidemics ranges from 1.6 percent to 9.5 percent.[53]

Yersinia enterocolitica is a gram-negative bacillus established only since 1964 as an enteric pathogen. Until recently the organism has not been routinely sought in bacteriologic laboratories and often has been misidentified. The organism is not a normal component of the intestinal flora. In acute infections, bacteria can be isolated from feces, lymph nodes, and, eventually, the bloodstream. In Scandinavia, serologic surveys indicate that 3 percent of the population have had recent or have current *Yersinia* infections.[54] Currently in Finland[42] and Denmark[54] reactive arthritis following *enterocolitica* infection is far more common than rheumatic fever. Estimates for the incidence of aseptic arthritis following enteritis range from 1.5[54] to 33 percent.[53]

Campylobacter subspecies *jejuni,* now recognized as the most common cause of acute bacterial diarrhea in North America, was linked to reactive arthritis in 1979.[43] In a rural outbreak that involved 88 persons with symptomatic gastroenteritis, one case of reactive arthritis occurred.[55] Elsewhere, arthritis was found in 24 percent of 33 patients hospitalized for *Campylobacter* enteritis, suggesting that severity of infection may have a bearing on subsequent development of arthritis.[56]

Evidence as yet scant and tentative suggests that an aseptic arthritis with brucellosis involving sacroiliac and other joints may belong within the group of reactive arthritides. A study of 16 such patients from a Peruvian mestizo population infected by *Brucella mellitensis* did not disclose an HLA-B27 association.[44] A previous study from Hungary noted an association between the B27 antigen and the spondylarthrosis of chronic brucellosis due to *B. abortus.*[57]

Characterization of the Arthritis. The onset of arthritis is predominantly in the second or third week after the onset of diarrhea; sometimes it is delayed as late as the eighth week. The joint disease with these reactive or aseptic arthritides is indeed virtually identical to that of venereally associated Reiter's disease. It is asymmetric, usually additive, and occasionally migratory; predominates in the lower extremity; and sometimes includes the sacroiliacs or low back. Fever is present in a large majority of cases.

Laboratory Features. Laboratory findings include mild anemia and elevated erythrocyte sedimentation rates. Synovial aspirates are mildly to markedly inflammatory in type, with polymorphonuclear leukocytes predominating. By definition synovial bacterial cultures are sterile but should be mandatory, to exclude septic arthritides following non-*Shigella* pathogens. Because of the latent period between the onset of diarrhea and the onset of arthritis, single stool cultures are often negative; the phenomenon of intermittent, and even prolonged, bacterial shedding, however, makes serial stool cultures worthwhile. Serum agglutination tests have a low sensitivity but are valuable when positive. The reactive arthritides with the above pathogens (excluding *Brucella*) demonstrate association with HLA-B27 in about 65 percent of cases.

Therapy. The treatment of aseptic arthritis has ranged from mild analgesics for lesser attacks to intra-articular steroids and low-dose steroids for severe prolonged attacks.

There is a reluctance to employ antimicrobials routinely in the uncomplicated acute bacterial diarrhea of the various organisms discussed above. Indications include bacteremia, coexistence of ulcerative colitis, immunocompromised patients, prolonged carrier state, and probably any patient whose illness is severe enough to warrant hospital admission.

Current first-choice agents are trimethoprim and sulfamethoxazole (Bactrim) for *Shigella,* ampicillin for *Salmonella,* tetracycline for *Yersinia,* and erythromycin for *Campylobacter* infections. With bacteremia or septic arthritis, final choice of the agent should depend upon antibiotic susceptibility studies.

BYPASS DISEASE

Bypass disease is a multisystem illness that follows intestinal bypass surgery for morbid obesity in about 15 percent of patients.[58-61]

Etiopathogenesis. The alteration or overgrowth of the bacterial flora in the colon, in the bypassed segment of the small bowel, and in the contiguous, normally nearly sterile jejunum may explain many of the extra-intestinal manifestations of bypass disease, as suggested by the occasional improvement in these symptoms following antibiotic treatment and the nearly uniform improvement following re-anastamosis or surgical procedures that prevent backwash of colonic or blind-loop contents. It is possible that bacteria themselves or bacterial products may be etiologic agents; it is almost certain that they contribute to the pathogenesis of the disease.[62] Patients with bypass disease often have serum cryoprecipitates that contain immunoglobulin classes and subclasses (including IgG_1, IgG_3, IgA, secretory IgA, and IgM), complement components (C1q, C3, C4, properdin factor B), and bacterial antigens (*E. coli. B. fragilis,* etc.). The precipitable cryoproteins are of the "mixed" types, presumably immune complexes, increasing in serum concentration temporally with the polyarthritis.[63] Dissociative techniques have shown that at least some of the immunoglobulin in these cryoproteins represents antibacterial antigen antibody.[64] In addition, bacteria have been identified in the cryoprotein by both stereochemical (immunologic) and biochemical (gas-liquid spectrophotometry) techniques.

Bacterial antigens such as peptidoglycans may pass through the hyperporous intestine, exceed the phagocytic capacity of the reticuloendothelial system, and become components of circulating immune complexes. These immune complexes have been found in skin, joints, kidney, and lung.[58-62] The fact that bacterial antigen, immunoglobulin, and complement have been identified in these numerous tissues suggests either in situ formation of complexes or deposition of complexes from the serum. Indeed, under certain exacting experimental conditions, ingested radiolabeled bacterial fragments can be identified in the serum of bypass disease patients, and subsequently in synovial fluid and skin.[62]

Exactly how the foregoing chain of events is effected is unknown, but contributing factors may include the genetic status of the host, the large bacterial pool in the bypassed gut, the effect of bile salts on the bacterial pool, the diseased liver and its altered function, changes in the bowel secretion of IgA, or altered secretory IgA, and changes in the patient's reticuloendothelial Fc receptor function.

Arthritis-Dermatitis Syndrome. Arthritis is a common complication of bowel bypass, occurring in 8 to 36 percent of cases.[65-71] The arthritis may develop at any time in the years after bypass[68] and may last for days or weeks in some and indefinitely in others.[72] The arthritis occurs more commonly in females and is more common with jejunocolic bypass than with jejunoileal bypass.[67-71] Any joint may be involved, but the most commonly affected include the metacarpophalangeal, proximal interphalangeal, wrist, knee, and ankle joints.[65-71] Frequently pain and tenderness are greater than expected, given the objective findings.[60] The synovitis is usually mild, but commonly the onset is abrupt, with intense inflammation. Usually the arthritis is periodic, remittent, and intermittent, and involves multiple joints for brief periods of time. However, there is extreme variability in the duration of arthritis: rare patients have episodes lasting more than years. Less frequent patterns of involvement include chronic arthritis with juxta-articular erosions, nodular seronegative polyarthritis, and intermittent monarthritis of the knee. Morning stiffness may be particularly marked, and when the arthritis is symmetrical, a rheumatoid arthritis–like picture emerges. Tenosynovitis is commonly seen. Myalgias and marked proximal muscle tenderness are not uncommon. The arthritis has no consistent histocompatibility associations and is but rarely associated with HLA-B27–positive spondylitis.

The rheumatoid factor is usually absent, as are antibodies to nuclear antigens, extractable nuclear antigens, DNA, and deoxyribonucleoprotein. The synovial fluid is often noninflammatory, with good mucin clot and few leukocytes, though white blood cell counts of from 500 to 27,000/mm^3, with 10 to 98 percent polymorphonuclear leukocytes, have been noted. Synovial biopsy demonstrates chronic synovitis with predominantly lymphocytes but no lymphoid follicles.

Skin lesions accompany the arthritis in over 80 percent of cases. The most common are vesiculopustular, papulovesicular, and urticarial. These most frequently evolve from a macular rash into discrete 2- to 13-mm lesions over arms, legs, trunk, and face. Patients are often seen with lesions at different stages of development; progression from a maculopapular to pustulovesicular rash may take from 24 to 72 hours. Other skin lesions include necrobiosis lipoidica, erythema nodosum, ecchymoses, and various forms of cutaneous vasculitis.

Recently it has been suggested that the "bowel bypass syndrome" may occur without bypass surgery in other chronic enteric diseases such as IBD and diverticulitis.[73]

Arthritis and associated conditions have apparently responded to antibiotics, especially tetracycline, in a minority of cases. Many cases may be treated with salicylates or nonsteroidal anti-inflammatory agents alone, particularly phenylbutazone. An excellent response is sometimes seen with relatively low doses of oral steroids. Partial surgical revision of the bypassed bowel results in an unsatisfactory therapeutic response, but complete bowel revision usually results in total remission.

WHIPPLE'S DISEASE

Whipple's disease or intestinal lipodystrophy is a rare multisystem disease associated with inflammatory lesions containing periodic acid Schiff (PAS)–staining macrophages packed with poorly characterized bacteria. Arthropathy, one of the most frequent manifestations, characteristically precedes the other cardinal signs of the disease (abdominal pain, diarrhea, and weight loss), sometimes by many years.

When confronted by any patient whose arthritis is resistant to diagnosis and treatment, the physician should consider Whipple's disease. In some cases when gastrointestinal symptoms are slight or in remission, the entity may masquerade as a collagen disease with protean manifestations over many years. Because effective therapy with antibiotics is at hand, it is important to establish the diagnosis as early as possible.

Prevalence. The disease is predominant among white patients aged 25 to 50 and has a male to female ratio of 10:1. Familial clustering of cases has been reported, most notably in a family with affected brothers whose grandmother also probably had the disease.[74]

Nonarticular Features. The nonarticular clinical features include the basic Whipple triad of malabsorption, diarrhea, and weight loss, but also may encompass many years of repeated inflammatory episodes in diverse organs, such as pneumonia, pleuritis, pericarditis, thyroiditis, and papilledema. Some patients have had progressive central nervous system involvement with minimal gastrointestinal symptoms.[75] Physical findings include hypotension, lymphadenopathy, hyperpigmentation, fever, edema, subcutaneous nodules, clubbing, hepatosplenomegaly, and signs of pleural effusion or a pleural friction rub.

Peripheral Arthritis. Arthritis in this disease can be regarded as the effect of bacterial colonization in synovium.

Prevalence. Arthralgia or arthritis occurs in 65 to 90 percent of patients. In 10 percent, this involvement precedes the diagnosis of Whipple's disease by more than 10 years. Indeed, arthritis may precede other features of Whipple's disease for as long as 35 years. The average age at onset of joint pain is 46.[76]

Characterization. The articular attacks are usually acute in onset and last from hours to a few days; more rarely a joint may be involved for several years. The characteristic pattern is that of a migratory poly- or oligoarthritis, involving ankles, knees, shoulders, elbows, and fingers. The attacks do not tend to coincide with diarrhea; to the contrary, they may remit spontaneously when diarrhea and abdominal pain appear. Prolonged remission may occur between attacks. Pain is not usually severe.

Physical examination may show swelling, effusion, and sometimes increased heat. Persistent inflammation of the knee with marked effusion and rupture of the synovium has occurred.[77] Residual deformity has not been reported and x-ray changes of the peripheral joints are limited to periarticular demineralization.

Synovial Fluid Analysis and Biopsy. Few reports of synovial fluid analyses have been published.[77-79] The mucin clot has been described as firm and the viscosity is relatively high.[79] Before antibiotic treatment was started, repeated aspirates in a single patient showed a range of 450 to 28,250 leukocytes per mm³ and 65 to 97 percent polymorphs. After treatment, the leukocyte counts ranged from 100 to 350 per mm³ (82 to 88 percent mononuclear cells).[79]

Synovial smears stained by PAS reagent have shown Schiff-positive material in polymorphonuclear and synovial cells; cultures are usually sterile.[77]

In contrast to the nonspecific synovial fluid findings, synovial biopsy may provide an early indication of the correct diagnosis, particularly if electron microscopy is included. Transmission electron micrographs have demonstrated microorganisms even in cases without PAS-staining granules in synovial macrophages by light microscopy.[77]

Axial Arthritis. Whipple's disease appears to have an association with sacroiliitis and spondylitis approaching that of inflammatory bowel disese. Back pain was present in 19 percent of a large series of patients reviewed in 1963. All patients with back pain also had peripheral joint involvement; only three had radiographic sacroiliac changes.[80] Five well-documented cases of ankylosing spondylitis have been reported.[81] It has been estimated that sacroiliitis alone and ankylosing spondylitis occur in 7 and 4 percent, respectively, of cases.[82]

Of 28 patients who have been HLA typed, 8 (29 percent) are B27 positive,[83] including one of two patients with ankylosing spondylitis who were tissue typed.[81,82]

Laboratory Diagnosis of Whipple's Disease. Laboratory features other than the synovial findings noted above include anemia in 90 percent, steatorrhea in 93 percent, and D-xylose malabsorption in 78 percent. Some patients show evidence of impaired delayed skin test and impaired lymphocyte responses to PHA. However, this immunologic dysfunction is probably merely secondary to the disease, because T-lymphocyte numbers and function return to normal after successful antibiotic treatment.[84]

X-rays of the gastrointestinal tract may show indentation of the barium column due to peritoneal lymphadenopathy.

Peroral jejunal biopsy is the key to the definitive diagnosis, which is established by PAS-positive inclusions in the macrophages of the small intestine. By electron microscopy, bacterial cells are identified within the inclusions. PAS-positive lesions have been encountered in many other sites: lymph nodes, pericardium, myocardium, peritoneum, liver, spleen, pancreas, brain, spinal cord, peripheral nerve plexuses, pleura, lung, kidney, urinary bladder, ovary, and bone marrow. Multiple biopsy sampling should be carried out in the small intestine, as skip areas of involvement have been encountered. In ruling out the disease, a negative jejunal biopsy carries more weight than a negative lymph node biopsy. Subcutaneous nodules have been noted in a few patients; biopsy in a recent case disclosed foamy histiocytes containing PAS granules and, by electron microscopy, remnants of bacilli within phagosomes.[85]

The discovery that bacterial cells account for the intracytoplasmic PAS-positive granules supports Whipple's hypothesis, put forth in 1907, that the disease is an infective process.[86] All organisms cultured to date are probably contaminants and the Whipple's bacillus, easily classified as a single bacillus on the basis of its uniform electron microscope and immunofluorescent staining characteristics, has yet to be convincingly cultured in vitro.[84]

Therapy. Antibiotic treatment has greatly improved the management of the disease. With a typical empirical regimen (a 10-day course of intramuscular penicillin, 1.2 million units per day, with streptomycin 1 gram per day, followed by one double-strength tablet of trimethoprim-sulfamethoxazole twice a day for 12 months) arthralgia ceases within 5 to 30 days and the patient promptly regains weight. However, some patients may relapse even while on tetracycline. In one case tetracycline controlled the bowel lesion but arthritis relapsed, responding in turn to erythromycin. More disturbing is a late relapse culminating as fatal central nervous system disease even while patients are on continuous antibiotic treatment.[75] Trimethoprim and sulfamethoxazole (Bactrim), which attains very high levels in cerebrospinal fluid, may be the best treatment for patients with central nervous involvement.[87] A recommended regimen is one double-strength tablet three times daily for two weeks followed by   tablet twice daily for one year.

All patients with Whipple's disease should be followed

for life. In the event of recrudescence, prompt and aggressive, albeit empiric, juggling of antibiotic regimens is indicated.

References

1. Gorbach, S.L.: Intestinal microflora. Gastroenterology 60:1110, 1971.
2. Gorbach, S.L., Nahas, J., and Weinstein, L.: Studies of intestinal microflora IX. The microflora of ileostomy effluent: A unique microbial ecology. Gastroenterology 53:874, 1967.
3. Moore, W.E.C., and Holdeman, L.V.: Identification of anaerobic bacteria. Am. J. Clin. Nutr. 25:1306, 1972.
4. Owens, R.L.: Epithelial cell specialization within human Peyer's patches: An ultrastructural study of intestinal lymphoid follicles. Gastroenterology 66:189, 1974.
5. Bockman, D.E., and Cooper, M.D.: Pinocytosis by epithelium associated with lymphoid follicles in the bursa of Fabricius, appendix, and Peyer's patches. An electron microscopic study. Am. J. Anat. 136:455, 1973.
6. Smith, M.W., and Peacock, M.A.: "M" cell distribution in follicle-associated epithelium of mouse Peyer's patch. Am. J. Anat. 159:167, 1980.
7. Joel, D.D., Laissue, J.A., and LeFevre, M.E.: Distribution and fate of ingested carbon particles in mice. J. Reticuloenothel. Soc. 24:477, 1978.
8. Selby, W.S., Janossy, G., Goldstein, G., and Jewell, D.P.: T lymphocyte subsets in human intestinal mucosa: The distribution and relationship to MHC-derived antigens. Clin. Exp. Immunol. 44:453, 1981.
9. Palumbo, P.J., Ward, L.E., Sauer, W.G., and Scudamore, H.H.: Musculoskeletal manifestations of inflammatory bowel disease: Ulcerative and granulomatous colitis and ulcerative proctitis. Mayo Clin. Proc. 48:411, 1973.
10. Haslock, I., and Wright, V.: The musculo-skeletal complications of Crohn's disease. Medicine 52:217, 1973.
11. Wright, V., and Watkinson, G.: The arthritis of ulcerative colitis. Br. Med. J. 2:670, 1965.
12. Greenstein, A.J., Janowitz, H.D., and Sachar, D.B.: The extra intestinal complications of Crohn's disease and ulcerative colitis: A study of 700 patients. Medicine 55:401, 1976.
13. Lindsley, C.B.: Arthritis in inflammatory bowel disease in children. Arthritis Rheum. 20:(Suppl.)411, 1977.
14. Wright, V., and Watkinson, G.: Articular complications of ulcerative colitis. Am. J. Proctol. 17:107, 1966.
15. Farmer, R.G., Hawk, W.A., and Turnbull, R.B., Jr.: Clinical patterns in Crohn's disease: A statistical study of 615 cases. Gastroenterology 68:627, 1975.
16. Wright, V., and Watkinson, G.: The arthritis of ulcerative colitis. Medicine 38:243, 1959.
17. McEwen, C.: Arthritis accompanying ulcerative colitis. Clin. Orthop. 57:9, 1968.
18. Clark, R.L., Muhletaler, C.A., and Margulies, S.I.: Colitic arthritis: Clinical and radiographic manifestations. Radiol. 101:585, 1971.
19. Brom, B., Bank, S., and Marks, N.: Periostitis, aseptic necrosis and arthritis occurring in a patient with Crohn's disease. Gastroenterology 60:1106, 1971.
20. Ansell, B.M., and Wigley, R.A.D.: Arthritis manifestations in regional enteritis. Ann. Rheum. 23:64, 1964.
21. Soren, A.: Joint affections in regional ileitis. Arch. Intern. Med. 117:78, 1966.
22. Lindstrom, C., Wramsby, H., and Ostberg, G.: Granulomatous arthritis in Crohn's disease. Gut 13:257, 1972.
23. Fraya, R., Stevens, M.B., and Bayless, T.M.: Destructive monarthritis and granulomatous synovitis as the presenting manifestations of of Crohn's disease. Johns Hopkins Med. J. 137:151, 1975.
24. Minard, D.B., Haddad, H., Blain, J.G., Beaudry, R., Devroede, G., and Masse, S.: Granulomatous myositis and myopathy associated with Crohn's colitis. N. Engl. J. Med. 295:818, 1976.
25. Wright, V., and Moll, J.M.H.: Seronegative polyarthritis. Amsterdam, North-Holland Publishing Company, 1976, pp. 271–328.
26. Arlat, I.P., Maier, W., Leupold, D., and Wolf, A.: Massive periosteal new bone formation in ulcerative colitis. Radiology 144:507, 1982.
27. Kyle, J.: Psoas abscess in Crohn's disease. Gastroenterology 61:149, 1971.
28. London, D., and Fitton, J.M.: Acute septic arthritis complicating Crohn's disease. Br. J. Surg. 57:536, 1970.
29. Dekker-Saeys, B.J., Meuwissen, S.G.M., van den Berg-Loonen, E.M., DeHaas, W.H.D., Agenant, D., and Tytgat, G.N.J.: II. Prevalence of peripheral arthritis, sacroiliitis, and ankylosing spondylitis in patients suffering from inflammatory bowel disease. Ann. Rheum. Dis. 37:33, 1978.
30. Kellgren, J.H.: The epidemiology of rheumatic diseases. Ann. Rheum. Dis. 23:109, 1964.
31. Wright, V., and Moll, J.M.H.: Seronegative polyarthritis. Amsterdam, North-Holland Publishing Company, 1976, p.87.
32. Nagant de Deuxchaisnes, C., Huaux, J.P., Fiasse, P., and DeBruyere, M.: Ankylosing spondylitis, sacroiliitis, regional enteritis and H1-A27. Lancet 1:1238, 1974.
33. Woodrow, J.C., and Eastmond, C.J.: HLA-B27 and the genetics of ankylosing spondylitis. Ann. Rheum. Dis. 37:504, 1978.
34. Dekker-Saeys, B.J., Meuwissen, S.G.M., van den Berg-Loonen, E.M., DeHaas, W.H.D., Meijers, K.A.F., and Tytgat, G.N.J.: III Clinical characteristics and results of histocompatibility typing (HLA-B27) in patients with both ankylosing spondylitis and inflammatory bowel disease. Ann. Rheum. Dis. 37:36, 1978.
35. McEwen, C.D., DiTata, D., Lingg, C., Porini, A., Good, A., and Rankin, T.: Ankylosing spondylitis accompanying ulcerative colitis, regional enteritis, psoriasis and Reiter's disease. Arthritis Rheum. 14:291, 1971.
36. Hyla, J.F., Frank, W.A., and Davis, J.S.: Lack of association of HLA-B27 with radiographic sacroiliitis in inflammatory bowel disease. J. Rheumatol. 3:196, 1976.
37. Wright, V., and Watkinson G.: Sacroiliitis and ulcerative colitis. Br. Med. J. 2:675, 1965.
38. Wright, R., Lumsden, K., Luntz, M.H., Sevel, D., and Truelove, S.C.: Abnormalities of the sacroiliac joints and uveitis in ulcerative colitis. Quart. J. Med. 34:229, 1965.
39. Macrae, I., and Wright, V.: A family study of ulcerative colitis with particular reference to ankylosing spondylitis and sacroiliitis. Ann. Rheum. Dis. 32:16, 1973.
40. Paronen, I.: Reiter's disease: A study of 344 cases observed in Finland. Acta. Med. Scand. 131(Suppl. 212):1, 1948.
41. Vartianen, J., and Hurri, L.: Arthritis due to Salmonella typhimurium: Report of 12 cases of migratory arthritis in association with Salmonellatyphimurium infection. Acta. Med. Scand. 175:771, 1964.
42. Sievers, K., Ahvonen, P., and Aho, K.: Epidemiological aspects of Yersinia arthritis. Int. J. Epidemiol. 1:45, 1972.
43. Berden, J.H.M., Muytjens, H.L., and van de Putte, L.B.A.: Reactive arthritis associated with Campylobacter jejuni enteritis. Br. Med. J. 1:380, 1979.
44. Alarcon, G.S., Bocanegra, T.S., Gotuzzo, E., Hinostroza, S., Carillo, C., Vasey, F.B., Germain, B.F., and Espinoza, L.R.: Reactive arthritis associated with brucellosis: HLA studies. J. Rheum. 8:621, 1981.
45. Newman, A., and Lambert J.R.: Campylobacter jejuni causing flare-up in inflammatory bowel disease (letter to the editor). Lancet 2:919, 1980.
46. Manson-Bahr, P.H.: The Dysenteric Disorders. London, Cassel, 1939, p. 71.
47. Schittenhelm, A., and Schlecht, H.: Uber polyarthritis enterica. Dtsch. Arch. Klin. Med. 126:329, 1918.
48. Noer, H.R.: An "experimental" epidemic of Reiter's syndrome. JAMA 198:693, 1966.
49. Simon, D.G., Kaslow, R.A., Rosenbaum, J., Kaye, R.L., and Calin, A.: Reiter's syndrome following epidemic shigellosis. J. Rheumatol. 8:969, 1981.
50. Lewis, R.B.: The absence of reactive arthritis after Shigella sonnei infection (letter to the editor). Arthritis Rheum. 25:1267, 1982.
51. David, J.R., and Black, R.L.: Salmonella arthritis. Medicine 39:385, 1960.
52. Warren, C.P.W.: Arthritis associated with Salmonella infections. Ann. Rheum. Dis. 29:483, 1970.
53. Masi, A.T.: Epidemiology of B27 associated diseases. Ann. Rheum. Dis. 1:131, 1979.
54. Larsen, J.H.: Yersinia enterocolitica infections and arthritis. In Dumonde, D.C. (ed.): Infection and Immunology in the Rheumatic Diseases. Oxford, Blackwell, 1976.
55. Eastmond, C.J., Rennie, J.A.N., and Reid, T.M.S.: An outbreak of Campylobacter enteritis—a rheumatological follow-up survey. J. Rheumatol. 10:107, 1983.
56. Gumpel, J.M., Martin, C., and Sanderson, P.J.: Reactive arthritis associated with Campylobacter enteritis. Ann. Rheum. Dis. 40:64, 1981.
57. Hodinka, L., Gomor, B., Meretey, K., Zahumenszky, Z., Geher, P., Telegdy, L., and Bozsoky, S.: HLA-B27 associated spondyloarthritis in chronic brucellosis. Lancet 1:499, 1978.
58. Utsinger, P.D.: Systemic immune complex disease after intestinal bypass surgery. Arthritis Rheum. 22:668, 1979.
59. Wands, J.R., LaMont, J.T., Mann, E., and Isselbacher, K.J.: Arthritis associated with intestinal bypass procedure for morbid obesity. N. Engl. J. Med. 294:121, 1976.
60. Utsinger, P.D., Farber, N., Shapiro, R.F., Ely, P.H., McLaughlin, G.E., and Wiesner, K.B.: Clinical and immunologic study of the post-intestinal bypass arthritis-dermatitis syndrome. Arthritis Rheum. 21:599, 1978.
61. Ginsberg, J., Quismorio, F.P., DeWind, L.T., and Mongan, E.S.: Musculoskeletal symptoms after jejunoileal shunt surgery for intractable obesity: Clinical and immunologic studies. Am. J. Med. 67:443, 1979.
62. Utsinger, P.D.: Absorption and articular depositions of ingested I¹³¹ E. coli cell wall in reactive arthritis. Arthritis Rheum. 24:56, 1981.
63. Utsinger, P.D.: Bypass arthritis: A bacterial antigen-antibody systemic immune complex disease. Arthritis Rheum. 27:758, 1980.

64. Utsinger, P.D.: Systemic immune complex disease following intestinal bypass surgery: Bypass disease. J. Am. Acad. Dermatol. 2:488, 1980.

65. Buchanan, W.W., Kean, W.F., and Rooney, P.J.: Some metabolic aspects of arthritis. S. Afr. Med. J. 61:467, 1982.

66. Buchanan, R.F., and Wilkens, R.F.: Arthritis after jejunoileostomy. Arthritis Rheum. 15:644, 1972.

67. Zapanta, M., Aldo-Benson, M., Biegel, A., and Madura, J.: Arthritis associated with jejunoileal bypass: Clinical and immunologic evaluation. Arthritis Rheum. 22:711, 1979.

68. Clegg, D.O., Samuelson, C.O., Williams, H.J., and Ward, J.R.: Articular complications of jejunoileal bypass surgery. J. Rheumatol. 7:65, 1980.

69. Shagrin, J.W., Frame, B., and Duncan, H.: Polyarthritis in obese patients following jejunocolonic bypass. Arthritis Rheum. 12:696, 1969.

70. Hess, R.J.: Polyarthritis after small bowel bypass. Okla. St. Med. J. 67:283, 1974.

71. Duncan, H.: Arthropathy and the intestinal bypass operation for obesity. J. Rheumatol. 4:115, 1977.

72. Ginsberg, J.H., Quismorio, F.P., Mongan, E.S., Friou, G.J., and DeWind, L.T.: Articular complications after jejuno-ileal shunt: Clinical and immunological studies. Arthritis Rheum. 19:797, 1976.

73. Jorizzo, J.L., Apisarnthanarax, P., Subrt, P., Hebert, A.A., Henry, J.C., Raimer, S.S., Dinehart, S.M., and Reinarz, J.A.: Bowel bypass syndrome without bowel bypass: Bowel-associated dermatosis syndrome. Arch. Intern. Med. 143:457, 1983.

74. Puite, R.H., and Tesluk, H.: Whipple's disease. Am. J. Med. 19:383, 1955.

75. Knox, D.L., Bayless, T.M., and Pittman, F.E.: Neurological disease in patients with treated Whipple's disease. Medicine 55:467, 1976.

76. LeVine, M.E., and Dobbins, W.O. III: Joint changes in Whipple's disease, Sem. Arthritis. Rheum. 3:79, 1973.

77. Hawkins, C.F., Farr, M., Morris, C.J., Hoare, A.M., and Williamson, N.: Detection by electron microscope of rod-shaped organisms in synovial membrane from a patient with the arthritis of Whipple's disease. Ann. Rheum. Dis. 35:502, 1976.

78. Rubinow, A., Canoso, J.J., Goldenberg, D.L., and Cohen, A.S.: Synovial fluid and synovial membrane pathology in Whipple's disease. Arthritis Rheum. 19:820, 1976.

79. Caughey, D.E., and Bywaters, E.G.L.: The arthritis of Whipple's disease. Ann. Rheum. Dis. 22:327, 1963.

80. Kelly, J.J. III, and Weisiger, B.B.: The arthritis of Whipple's disease. Arthritis Rheum. 6:615, 1963.

81. Canoso, J.J., Saini, M., and Hermos, J.A.: Whipple's disease and ankylosing spondylitis: Simultaneous occurrence in HLA-B27 positive male. J. Rheum. 5:79, 1978.

82. Robert d'Eshougues, J., Delcambre, B., and Defrance, D.: Les manifestations à articulariers de la maladie de Whipple. Rev. Rheum. Mal. Osteoartic. 43:565, 1976.

83. Dobbins, W.O. III: Personal communication, 1983.

84. Dobbins, W.O. III: Is there an immune deficit in Whipple's disease? Digest. Dis. Sci. 26:247, 1981.

85. Good, A.E., Beals, T.F., Simmons, J.L., and Ibrahim, M.A.H.: A subcutaneous nodule with Whipple's disease: Key to early diagnosis? Arthritis Rheum. 23:856, 1980.

86. Whipple, G.H.: A hitherto undescribed disease characterised anatomically by fat and fatty acids in the intestinal and mesenteric lymphatic tissues. Bull. Johns Hopk. Hosp. 18:382, 1907.

87. Ryser, R.J., Locksley, R.M., Eng, S.C., Dobbins W.O. III, Schoenknecht, F., and Rubin C.E.: Reversal of the dementia associated with Whipple's disease by antibiotics which penetrate the blood-brain barrier. Gastroenterology. 86:745, 1984.

Section VII
Systemic Lupus Erythematosus and Overlap Syndromes

Chapter 68
Etiology and Pathogenesis of Systemic Lupus Erythematosus

Nathan J. Zvaifler and Virgil L. Woods, Jr.

ETIOLOGY OF SYSTEMIC LUPUS ERYTHEMATOSUS

Introduction. Despite intensive efforts, no etiology has yet been found for systemic lupus erythematosus (SLE). Before ascribing this to a lack of insight or an insufficiency of current technology, it is important to consider other explanations. First, what we call SLE may be the expression of a common pathogenetic mechanism initiated by a variety of factors. A similar principle exists for immediate-type hypersensitivity reactions, such as urticaria or asthma, in which different insults produce an identical clinical picture. Second, the etiology may be multifactorial. For instance, the development of SLE may require contact with a specific pathogen plus a particular predisposition of the host. If the pathogen were a ubiquitous agent, then it would be difficult to demonstrate a difference in frequency of exposure between SLE patients and controls. Third, and perhaps most importantly, SLE may not be a single disease, but rather a constellation of signs and symptoms produced by a variety of etiologic agents. This latter possibility reflects both an appreciation of the protean manifestations of SLE and uncertainties about the extent of its boundaries.

In many textbooks SLE is described as a grave, multisystem disorder with a chronic, intermittent, unpredictable course. A revised operational definition was recently proposed by a committee of the American Rheumatism Association from a computer analysis of the most frequent manifestations of the disease and their ability to discriminate SLE from other closely related disorders.[1] Patients with 4 or more of the 11 criteria are said to have the disease with a 96 percent confidence. Adherence to these criteria, however, results in a definition of SLE that need not exclude the lupus-like illness induced by certain drugs or the related disease seen in patients with deficiencies of the complement system.

Lately, there has been an increasing effort to group SLE patients with features in common with the intention of identifying different outcomes. The usually benign course of discoid lupus can be contrasted with the dire prognosis of lupus nephritis, for example. Certain clusters of clinical, morphological and laboratory features are recognizable, usually associated with autoantibodies to cellular constituents (Table 68–1). Especially prominent are the antibodies to the nuclear antigens—native, double-stranded deoxyribonucleic acid (dsDNA), an acidic glycoprotein called Sm, and nuclear ribonucleoprotein (nRNP). Two other ribonucleoprotein antigens, SS-A (previously considered as cytoplasmic antigen Ro) and SS-B (previously La) are also important.[2,3] Some authors have ascribed a particular clinical picture or course to individuals whose serum contains antibodies against predominantly one or another of these antigens. For instance, antibody to dsDNA correlates with hypocomplementemia, glomerulonephritis, and a poorer prognosis.[4,5] High titers of anti-nRNP antibody usually accompany Raynaud's phenomenon, a characteristic swelling of the fingers, polyserositis, and a mild course.[6,7] Similarly, high titers of anti-Sm antibody are said to be found in patients with significant photosensitive skin rash and a mild, apparently nonprogressive arthritis. In other studies, Sm has been identified with SLE patients with milder CNS and renal disease.[8] Because of the unique association of antibodies with SLE, some would withhold the diagnosis unless there was antibody to dsDNA, thereby eliminating a third or more of the patients in most series. Most would require antinuclear antibody, as determined by immunofluorescence analysis, but there are a small number of patients who, although repeatedly negative for these antibodies in conventional assays, possess anti-SS-A or SS-B antibody, and have in common a classical photosensitivity dermatitis plus other features of SLE.[9,10] Many of those patients have detectable ANAs when cultured prolif-

Table 68–1. Autoantibodies to Intracellular Antigens*

Antigenic Specificity	Disease Association
Nuclear Antigens	
1. Antibodies to DNA	
a. Native (double-stranded) DNA	Usually restricted to systemic lupus erythematosus (SLE)
b. Antigenic determinant common to double- and single-stranded DNA	High antibody titers in SLE; lower titers in other rheumatic diseases
c. Single-stranded DNA (purine and pyrimidine determinants)	Rheumatic and nonrheumatic diseases
d. zDNA	SLE
2. Antibodies to histones:	
a. H2A-H2B	High prevalence in drug-induced LE; lower in SLE
b. H1, H3-H4	SLE
3. Antibodies to small nuclear ribonucleoproteins	
a. "Sm" antigen	Probably restricted to SLE
b. Nuclear ribonucleoprotein (n-RNP)	High antibody titers in mixed connective tissue disease; lower titers in other rheumatic diseases
c. "SS-A" antigen (Ro)	Sjögren's syndrome–sicca complex; SLE
d. "SS-B" antigen (La)	
4. Antibodies to other nuclear antigens:	
a. Proliferating cell nuclear antigens	SLE
b. Anticentromere antibody	CREST variant of scleroderma
c. RANA (rheumatoid arthritis–associated nuclear antigen)	Rheumatoid arthritis (RA) and Sjögren's syndrome with RA
Cytoplasmic Antigens	
1. Antibodies to "common" antigens:	
a. Ribosomal ribonucleoprotein (r-RNP)	SLE
b. Mitochondrial antigens	Primary biliary cirrhosis
c. Microsomal antigens	Chronic active hepatitis, malignancies
d. Single-stranded RNA, t-RNA, synthetic polynucleotides	SLE
2. Antibodies to tissue-specific antigens:	
a. Tissue-specific microsomes: gastric parietal cells, thyroid epithelial cells, adrenal cortical cells	Organ-specific autoimmunity: pernicious anemia, Hashimoto's disease, Addison's disease
Nucleolar Antigens	
1. Nucleolar 4s-6s RNA	Scleroderma and Raynaud's phenomenon
2. Other nucleolar antigens (demonstrated by immunofluorescence)	Scleroderma, SLE and Sjögren's syndrome

*Modified from Tan, E.M., Reyes, P., and Fritzler, M.J.: *In* Ruddon, E. (ed.): Biological Markers of Neoplasia: Basic and Applied Aspects. Amsterdam, Elsevier-North Holland, Inc., 1978.

erating cells are the substrate (see Chapter 46). The majority of patients with complement deficiencies who develop SLE also generally lack antinuclear antibodies and have a high incidence of photosensitivity skin rash.[11] It could be argued that these different clinical presentations and antibody profiles describe subsets of the disease resulting from different etiologies, but they might just as well indicate variable host responses.

So long as the etiology of SLE remains obscure it seems reasonable to use the broadest definition of the disease and consider the greatest range of possibilities. For the same reason, this review will consider animal models of the disease wherever appropriate, emphasizing differences between various strains rather than similarities. Animal models of SLE have been influential in shaping our concepts of the etiology and pathogenesis of the human disease. Studies in man often follow from results obtained in autoimmune mice. The major strains of interest are the New Zealand black (NZB) mouse; the F1 hybrid of the NZB strain and the New Zealand white mouse (NZW), called the NZB/NZW; and the MRL/1 and BXSB mice. Two forms of disease develop in each mouse strain. Early in life the animals show

multiple immunologic abnormalities; later each develops fatal immune complex nephritis and other features of human autoimmune diseases (Table 68–2). For instance, at an early age female NZB/NZW mice acquire antinuclear and antinative DNA antibodies (dsDNA) and routinely die during the first year of an immune complex nephritis.[12] In the MRL/1 strain, both sexes get a massive nonmalignant lymphadenopathy and permanent renal disease early (around the fourth month) in life. In the BXSB strain, only the males get a slowly progressive nephritis. The amount and type of antinuclear antibodies vary among the strains. For instance, most serum samples from MRL mice react with the Sm antigen and contain rheumatoid factor, while NZB/NZW hybrids and BXSB lack these antibodies. BXSB mice make little anti-dsDNA antibody in contrast to MRL and NZB/NZW mice.[13] Each mouse strain appears to have a genetic background that predisposes to autoimmune disease. Various superimposed factors then determine the time of appearance and severity of disease. Except for the BXSB, sex hormones function as accelerating factors. In the BXSB mouse, a gene linked to the Y chromosome exerts a major influence on the expression of disease,

Table 68–2. Immunological Abnormalities in Autoimmune Mouse Strains*

	NZB	NZB/NZW	BXSB	MRL/1
Numerical Abnormalities				
B cells	↓	↓	↑	N
T cells	↓	↓	N	↑
Lymphoid hyperplasia	+	+	++	+++
Functional Abnormalities				
B lymphocytes				
Decreased tolerance, polyclonal activation	+, early	+, early	+	+, late
Activated B-lymphocyte subpopulation	*xid* gene–sensitive, thymus-independent B lymphocyte	*xid* gene–sensitive, thymus-independent B lymphocyte	?	*xid* gene–insensitive, thymus-dependent B lymphocyte?
T lymphocytes				
Decreased tolerance	+	+	+	+
T helper,T suppressor	Lyt 23+ cells increased in aged animals, but decreased ability to generate new suppressors		?	increased T-cell help
Autoantibody production				
Anti-DNA	+	++	++	+++
Rheumatoid factor, anti-Sm	0	0	0	+
Sex Predilection Accelerating Factors	Female	Female	Male	Male = female
Sex hormone dependence	±	+	0	+
Genes	multiple autosomal	multiple autosomal	Y-chromosome–linked gene	lpr gene
Virus infection	+	+	+	+

Modified from Dixon, F.J.: Arthritis Rheum. 25:271, 1982; Steinberg, A.D., et al.: Arthritis Rheum. 25:734, 1982; and Theofilopoulos, A.N. et al.: Arthritis Rheum. 25:725, 1982. Symbols: ↑ = increased; ↓ = decreased; N = normal; 0 = absent; + = unclear; ? = not reported.

while in the MRL/1 strain, the *lpr* gene accelerates disease. Detailed genetic and virologic investigations have failed to demonstrate common denominators among the three strains, suggesting that murine lupus, perhaps like its human counterpart, is more a syndrome than a single disease.

Despite these reservations, enough is known about SLE to expect that any etiologic candidate must explain the persistence of the disorder, the associated abnormalities of immunologic regulation, and the immune complex–mediated tissue injury. Since chronic viral infections can meet all these requirements, they will be the first etiology considered. The reader should appreciate, however, that it is unlikely that any etiology to be discussed operates independently. Rather, the development of SLE probably requires a modification in the complex interrelationships between the host, the pathogen, and their environment.

Chronic Virus Infection. Enthusiasm for a viral etiology for SLE followed from electron microscopic obser-

vations of unusual inclusions in glomerular endothelial cells, skin, vascular endothelium, and lymphocytes, but these inclusions were not limited to material from patients with SLE.[14-18] Neither could they be demonstrated to be components of any known virus. Now the tubuloreticular structures are considered a nonspecific manifestation of cell injury.[18]

Antibodies to measles virus were investigated because of a superficial resemblance between the tubuloreticular structures and the internal nucleoprotein core of paramyxoviruses, of which measles is an example. They were higher in SLE compared with normal populations, but so were other serum virus antibody titers.[19] Although the results are somewhat conflicting, in most studies, antibodies to measles and rubella are usually high in serum samples from SLE patients, and parainfluenza, mumps, and Epstein-Barr virus titers are often elevated; whereas influenza, Newcastle disease, and respiratory syncytial virus antibody levels are no different than controls.[20] The increase in virus antibodies could merely reflect polyclonal B-lymphocyte activation and a general increase in antibodies characteristically found in SLE. Overall there is some correlation with IgG levels, but in any individual the total serum immunoglobulin is not a good predictor of viral antibody levels.[20,21] Interpretation of virus measurements is complicated by the observation that some SLE sera react with the uninfected human, monkey, and hamster cells used as antigen controls with titers equal to those found with the virus-infected cells.[22]

Direct virus isolation from SLE patients using either conventional or more sensitive co-cultivation techniques has been unrewarding.[23-25] The demonstration of viral antigens in tissues from SLE patients has been reported,[26-31] but human serum has low titers of natural antibody for mammalian type C and other retroviruses, thereby complicating investigation in this area.[32,33] Even if we accept these provocative findings, it remains to be shown that the virus expression is the cause rather than the result, of SLE. A similar situation exists with the observation of large amounts of interferon in serum from SLE patients with active disease. A portion is conventional alpha interferon; the remainder has unusual properties.[34] Although the interferon might reflect a response to viral infection, it is more likely an expression of immune hyperactivity.

The impetus for the study of type C oncornaviruses in human SLE derives from observations in New Zealand mice. Throughout life all New Zealand strains have large concentrations of type C virus-like particles and murine viral antigens in their tissues. Most endogenous mammalian type C viruses can only infect and replicate in the cells of the species in which they arise. Accordingly they are called ecotropic viruses. Murine species also harbor viruses that only grow to a limited extent in the natural host. These viruses cannot infect cells of their parent species, but they replicate well in heterologous cells; thus they are called xenotropic viruses.

Xenotropic viruses can be isolated from virtually all tissues of NZB mice. They appear to have a pathogenetic role in the nephritis of NZB/NZW hybrids because large amounts of antibody to virus-related antigens, especially viral envelope gp-70 antigen, can be identified in their glomerular deposits.[35] There is no clear demonstration, however, that the virus infection is responsible for the development of abnormalities of immunologic regulation or the perpetuation of the autoimmune process.

The role of oncornavirus infection in the induction of immunologic abnormalities has been analyzed in other murine strains. For instance, Swan mice develop an autoimmune disorder similar to NZB/NZW hybrids, with high titers of antinuclear and anti-dsDNA antibodies early in life and immunoglobulin deposits in the skin and kidneys. Other similarities include autoantibodies to T lymphocytes, functional alterations of the thymus, a poor response to thymus-dependent antigens, and a premature reduction of thymic hormone levels. But unlike the NZB/NZW, the tissues of Swan mice have no detectable xenotropic type C virus. Moreover, ecotropic

virus is only found long after the appearance of the immunologic abnormalities.[36]

Dixon and colleagues have identified the types of virus recovered from cultured cells of NZB/NZW, MRL/1, and BXSB mice and compared them to viruses from mice without recognizable autoimmune disease. As expected, NZB/NZW have easily recoverable xenotropic and ecotropic viruses. Isolates from MRL/1 mice were limited to ecotropic virus; the BXSB mice had no ecotropic virus and only an occasional xenotropic virus even after prolonged culturing. The cells of nonautoimmune strains—NZW, AKR, and BALB/c—all contained both ecotropic and xenotropic viruses.[37] Serum levels of viral antigens were measured using a radioimmunoassay for gp-70. In general, the strains with the most viral antigen had autoimmune disease, but there was no parallel between the severity of the disease and their level of serum gp-70.[37]

Finally, Datta and colleagues performed backcross experiments between virus-infected autoimmune NZB mice and virus-negative SWR mice. The development of autoimmunity in the offspring of the NZB mice was found to be independent of xenotropic virus expression.[38] Thus, while most mice carry one or more oncornaviruses, there is no consistent relationship between any one or combination of these and the development of autoimmune disease. Clearly viruses are one of several factors that can accelerate murine lupus, but they only induce disease in genetically susceptible hosts.[12] For this reason it is appropriate to consider the available information on the genetics of human SLE.

Genetics. Most diseases, including those with an infectious etiology, are multifactorial in their causation and have important genetic and environmental contributions. For instance, both the susceptibility to *Mycobacterium tuberculosis* and the severity of the disease are modified by the genetic constitution of the individual. McKusick has suggested that the genetic contribution to a multifactorial disorder can be elucidated by an analysis of the following: familial aggregation, twin studies, ethnic comparisons, immunogenetic analysis of blood groups and histocompatibility typing, and experimental breeding of animals with analogs of the human disease.[39] Information from all these areas supports the conclusion that genetic factors are important in the development of SLE.

Studies of familial aggregation are based on the rationale that more cases of a genetically determined disorder will appear in the relatives of persons with a given disease than among the relatives of appropriately selected control subjects. Epidemiologic investigations suggest that the prevalence of SLE is at least 10 affected persons per 100,000 of population.[40] In Rochester, Minnesota; San Francisco, California; Oahu, Hawaii; and Dunedin, New Zealand the number may be higher.[41-44] Regardless, SLE occurs in relatives of patients with the disease with a frequency between 0.4 and 5 percent, representing a several hundredfold increase over that of the general population.[45-47] Immunologic abnormalities are also found more often in family members of SLE patients than in controls.[45-49]

A comparison of the prevalance of a trait in monozygotic as compared to dizygotic twins is a classical method for distinguishing between genetic and environmental factors. Block and colleagues analyzed 12 twin pairs in which one or both of the twins had SLE; seven were definitely monozygotic and three definitely dizygotic. These were compared with 17 twin pairs (12 definitely monozygotic) described in the literature. More than 50 percent of monozygotic twin pairs appeared to be concordant for the disease. Moreover, there was a remarkable concordance of the presence of antinuclear antibodies (71 percent), hypergammaglobulinemia (87 percent) and disease expression between identical twins.[50,51] On the other hand, the frequency of SLE in dizygotic twins is probably no different than in other first-degree relatives.[46,50]

Certain ethnic groups have a high prevalence of SLE. Black people develop the disease three times more often than would be predicted by their representation in the general population,[40] but the feature of their disease are similar.[52] In one study SLE was diagnosed in 1 of every 245 black women between the ages of 15 and 54 years.[42] Certain Indian tribes have a much higher annual incidence of SLE than other tribes or control populations. Again, women make up a disproportionate number of those affected.[53] Women of Oriental and Polynesian ancestry appear to be at risk for more severe disease.[43]

Histocompatibility antigens (HLA) have been extensively studied in patients with SLE, in an attempt to discover differences in susceptibility, serology, and outcome. The results are conflicting.[49] The phenotypes HLA-A1, B8, B15, and B19 have all been reported increased.[47,55-58] Some of the discrepancies may represent differences in patient populations. For instance, in one well-controlled series, HLA-A1 was found more frequently in blacks with SLE, while HLA-B8 was increased in caucasians with SLE.[55] The HLA chromosomal complex in man is the equivalent of the major histocompatibility complex of rodents. Within this complex the HLA-D locus controls strong stimulation in the primary mixed lymphocyte culture (MLC) reaction. In addition, genes at this locus code for glycoproteins expressed principally on B lmphocytes, macrophages, activated T cells, and epithelial cells.These are similar to the immune response gene associated (Ia) antigens of mice. Like the murine Ia system, the human B-lymphocyte determinants are very polymorphic. Only a portion of the specificities are detected by MLC reactions; other specificities have been defined in population studies with appropriate alloantisera (see Chapter 4). It is not clear that identical specificities are being detected with these alloantisera, but HLA-DR2 and DR3 occur much more frequently in SLE patients than in controls.[59-62] Antinuclear antibodies are reported to correlate with HLA-A2, B7, and DR3.[63,64] An analysis of a small number of SLE families shows that one or another HLA haplotype is usually shared among the propositus and those members of the family with autoimmune abnormalities. But exceptions have been noted,[60] suggesting that there are probably multiple interacting genes within and outside of the MHC.[49]

Homozygous deficiencies of the early complement components, particularly C2, are frequently associated with SLE and discoid lupus erythematosus.[11,65] Genes controlling the production of several complement proteins map within the HLA region. There is a particularly strong association between C2 deficiency and the haplotypes A10 and B18.[66,67] An even closer linkage may exist with the HLA-D gene, D2.[68] Because of an association between immune response (Ir) genes and the HLA system, it has been proposed that the C2 deficiency gene is linked to an as yet unidentified Ir gene determining disease susceptibility. An argument against this notion is the observation that acquired deficiencies of C2 and C4, as seen in hereditary angioedema, also predispose to the development of SLE or DLE.[69,70] This suggests that alterations of the early complement components can alter host defenses, perhaps by allowing the proliferation of a pathogen (or pathogens) responsible for the symptom complex or impairing the clearance of immune complexes. Support for the latter comes from the observation that immune complexes are difficult to solubilize in the serum of SLE patients with hypocomplementemia.[71] Also, the erythrocytes of SLE patients have fewer receptors for the major cleavage fragment of the third component of complement (C3b). These receptors are important components of the mononuclear-phagocytic system. A pedigree analysis suggests that this defect is inherited in an autosomal codominant manner.[72]

Certain drugs, such as hydralazine and procainamide, induce an SLE-like disease, especially in those who metabolize the drug slowly.[73-76] The activity of the enzyme N-acetyltransferase, which acetylates these drugs, is genetically controlled.[77] The acetylator status of patients with idiopathic SLE has been determined. In five separate reports, two thirds or more of the subjects had the slow acetylator phenotype.[78-82] Three other investigations did not confirm these findings.[83-85] If this association is true, it could help explain genetically determined differential responses to environmental or infectious agents that precipitate the idiopathic form of SLE.

Analysis of murine lupus models cannot distinguish a single genetic basis for their disease. The H-2 genes of the various strains of mice that develop lupus are dissimilar.[12,37] Moreover, the H-2^d haplotype of NZB mice is shared by many strains that display no autoimmunity.[86] When F1 hybrids are made by crossing MRL mice with NZB, NZW, or BXSB, they do not develop an accelerated disease, unlike the offspring of the NZB by NZW matings.[87] To date, in a variety of breedings between lupus mice and normal strains, no particular phenotypic feature appears to segregate with disease.[86,88] For NZB/NZW mice, multiple unlinked genes appear to be responsible for disease manifestations, whereas in the MRL strains, a single gene has a major effect. [12,88] The congenic MRL/Mp−+/+ mouse is genetically identical to the MRL/Mp−lpr/lpr (MRL/1) except for the absence of *lpr* genes. This animal has mild autoimmune disease and lacks the marked lymphoproliferation seen in the mice with the *lpr* gene.[12] A single gene linked to the Y chromosome exerts a major effect on disease expression in the BXSB strain.[89] Analysis of canine SLE by backcross and outcross experiments does not support a genetic mechanism for the transmission of serologic abnormalities, but there is a suggestion of vertical passage of an infectious agent by nongenetic means.[90]

Environmental Factors. Epidemiologic studies provide a number of clues to the possible etiology of SLE. As noted above, certain populations seem to be at greater risk. This may reflect genetic factors, but environmental influences could also be important. Crowding, socioeconomic status, and migration do not appear to explain the increased susceptibility to SLE in the blacks in New York City,[40] but the effects of poverty, increased contact with animals, and environmental pathogens have not been analyzed in other populations.[91] Ultraviolet light, a recognized precipitant of dermal and systemic manifestations of SLE in those who already have the disease, is probably not an important risk factor for the development of SLE, because the ascertainment of the disease in Alabama and New York City is about the same.[40,91] Likewise, of the many Indian tribes studied, the three with the highest annual incidence of SLE reside in the northern half of the United States.[53]

The introduction of new pharmaceutical agents in the 1950s was followed by reports of a drug-induced disease similar to idiopathic SLE. Siegel and colleagues showed that the number of new cases of idiopathic SLE in New York City changed very little during the period 1957 through 1966, but there was a dramatic rise (four- to five-fold) in drug-induced SLE in 1965 and 1966, due primarily to procainamide.[92] The many other drugs with this potential were the subject of a recent conference.[73] No other environmental toxins or chemicals have a proven association with SLE, but a theoretical model for hydrazine-containing substances has been proposed.[93]

Several observations implicate contagious environmental factors. Some dogs in households that include patients with SLE show clinical or serologic features of the disease.[94,95] These findings suggested a common environmental exposure of family members and their pets, but subsequent reports have failed to confirm an association of canine SLE with human SLE.[96-98] Antibodies reactive with antigens on lymphocyte membranes are seen in a variety of acute and chronic viral infections. Similar cytotoxic antilymphocyte antibodies occur with great frequency (probably more than 80 percent) and in high titers in patients with SLE.[99,100] Messner and his associates found that more than a third of asymptomatic SLE relatives had lymphocytotoxic antibodies in their serum. The frequency was similar whether they were blood or nonblood relatives and significantly greater in

household contacts when compared with relatives who did not share the same abode.[100,101] Comparable results were obtained with families in New Mexico, Caracas, Venezuela, Mexico City, and Russia.[99,102,103] but no increase in lymphocytotoxic antibodies was found in SLE relatives studied in Boston or eastern Canada.[104,105] Differences in the assay could account for this discrepancy, but it is more likely due to variations in the patient populations, particularly the number with active versus inactive disease or the types of environmental exposures. A related observation is that physicians and laboratory personnel who handle SLE serum have a greater frequency and amount of antinuclear, anti-dsDNA and lymphocytotoxic antibodies than do controls.[99,106]

Hormonal Influences. The predilection for women in their child-bearing years to develop SLE has long been appreciated. This female prevalence is not as evident in children or in the aged.[107,108] Another unusual, and perhaps related, finding is the co-existence of SLE in males with the feminizing condition known as Klinefelters' syndrome (XXY karyotype). Eight such patients have been recorded, and in two there was evidence of chronic estrogen stimulation.[109] SLE patients excrete excessive amounts of material with high estrogenic activity. Several of the 16 hydroxylation metabolites of estrone are present in increased amounts in both men and women with SLE and in some of their first-degree relatives.[110] A French group reported that the activity of SLE was greater in women taking progestational but not estrogen-based oral contraceptives.[111]

Observations suggesting important hormonal influences on the evolution or expression of SLE are paralleled by findings in NZB/NZW mice. Female NZB/NZW mice have a worse disease than males. It is characterized by an earlier appearance of antibodies to dsDNA and polyadenylic acid, greater severity of immune complex nephritis, and a decreased life span. Artificial manipulation of the hormonal environment by castration or drug treatment modifies the expression of autoimmunity. An overall increase in male hormones supresses, while female hormones accelerate the disease.[12,112-115] Androgens favorably influence survival, with the immune complex nephritis being less severe in female animals treated with male sex hormones. Estrogens may exert their effects by increasing anti-DNA antibody production,[116] accelerating the switch from a benign (IgM) to a more nephrotoxic class (IgG) of anti-DNA antibody or by diminishing the clearance of circulating immune complexes.[112,113] Hormonal influences are not paramount, however, since in other murine strains, like the MRL/1 mice, males and females develop a lupus-like disease at approximately the same age, and in the BXSB mouse the disease is more severe in males, even though unrelated to sex hormones.[12,117]

Autoimmunity. The intricacies of the immune response are described in detail in Chapters 2 through 5. Immunity can be defined as a state of specific reactivity to a foreign substance resulting from prior exposure. Tolerance is a state of specific unresponsiveness to an antigen following initial exposure to that antigen. Initially, tolerance was thought to result from the elimination of clones of specific immunologically competent cells. Subsequently it was shown that unresponsiveness was not necessarily an all or none phenomenon. Administration of large amounts of antigen to adult animals over long periods or of minute amounts for a short time could induce nonresponsiveness, while intermediate amounts elicited antibody formation.[118] Thus, tolerance is a learned response determined in part by the nature, dose, and route of administration of the antigen and the state of maturity of the immune system when the antigen is introduced. In general, the more immature the host, the easier it is to induce tolerance to a particular antigen. The recognition that antibody responses depend on cooperation between helper T lymphocytes and B lymphocytes,[119,120] and that these can be paralyzed independently, increased the appreciation of the complexities of the problem.[121] Presently, the term tolerance does not cover a single state of immunologic nonreactivity brought about by a single mechanism, but rather self-tolerance exists and is maintained at a number of different levels in the immune system.

Ehrlich is credited with being the first to imagine the consequences of unrepressed immunologic reactivity against the body's own cells and tissues. He called this "horror autotoxicus" or, in modern parlance, autoimmunity. The initial theories designed to explain autoimmunity suggested a failure in ontogeny to eliminate clones of autoreactive cells.[122] Deletion or abortion of T-lymphocyte clones, especially those recognizing antigens of the major histocompatibility complex, likely occurs in the thymus, while B lymphocytes appear to be eliminated at an early phase in their development before they emerge from the fetal liver or bone marrow.[123] But this process is not complete, as evidenced by the fact that B lymphocytes reactive with autologous thyroglobulin or DNA can be detected in adult animals or man.[124,125] The existence of autoantibodies is by itself a cogent argument against the complete elimination of potentially responsive autoreactive immunocytes. Thus, other mechanisms must be involved in preventing autoimmunity.

In the humoral response the Ig-bearing B lymphocytes are the precursors of antibody-secreting plasma cells. T lymphocytes do not synthesize antibodies, but they play a crucial role in regulating the amount, class, and affinity of antibody produced by B lymphocytes.[126] The nature of the cooperation between T and B lymphocytes has been examined at the molecular level. When primed B lymphocytes are exposed to a hapten antigen bound to a protein carrier, they can only make a secondary antibody response if T lymphocytes primed to the carrier are also present. In other words, T lymphocytes recognize and respond to the carrier determinant of an antigen and help B lymphocytes specific for the hapten to develop into antibody-forming cells.[127,128] T lymphocytes can also suppress antibody formation through an interaction with T helper lymphocytes or by a direct effect on the B lymphocyte.[129] Finally, certain serum factors, including antibody alone or complexed with antigen, can block antibody production.[130,131] The factors responsible for upsetting this delicate immunologic homeostasis in SLE are not known, but a number of explanations have been proposed. These will be reviewed in light of the viral, genetic, and environmental factors outlined above.

An immunologic profile of typical patients with SLE would include multiple autoantibodies, impaired T-lymphocyte functions and generally normal antibody responses to exogenous antigens. If autoantibodies were produced by clones of autoreactive cells arising spontaneously by somatic mutation, as originally suggested by Burnett, then the emergence of such clones might result from a vertically transmitted viral infection. It is not altogether clear how a random phenomenon like somatic mutation can result in the rapid appearance late in life of autoantibodies specific for a given antigen, or the multiplicity of antinuclear autoantibodies. The "forbidden clone" hypothesis could be mimicked by the introduction of maternal lymphoid stem cells into the fetus at an early stage in its development,[132] before the fetal immune system develops the ability to discriminate self from non-self. Later in life, if these maternal cells were to become activated and recognize the host as foreign, they could induce autoantibody formation by mechanisms that will be discussed below with the chronic graft-versus-host reaction.

T lymphocytes only recognize antigens on cell surfaces when they are associated with membrane determinants coded by genes in the major histocompatibility complex (MHC).[133] Thus, in the instance of antibody formation, helper T lymphocytes can only respond to antigen if it is associated with Ia molecules. These determinants have a limited distribution in the body. They are found mainly on macrophages, some lymphocytes, including activated T lymphocytes, vascular endothelium and epidermal cells, but are absent from most differentiated cells. Mitchison uses this concept to explain autoimmunity.[134] He proposes that tolerance is preprogrammed because, although self macromolecules bear potentially immunogenic determinants, they cannot activate helper T lymphocytes owing to a nonassociation with Ia molecules. When cells (and probably other macromolecules) are injured or altered, they are processed by macrophages. If self antigens become associated with the Ia molecules on the macrophage surface in the course of processing, then autoantibodies could develop. Type C viruses which bud from cell membranes, or lipophilic membrane–reactive drugs such as procainamide or anticonvulsants would be ideal provocateurs of this type of self antigen processing.

Autoantibody formation can result from impaired B-lymphocyte regulation. An augmentation of T-lymphocyte help, or a failure to suppress B lymphocytes capable of making autoantibodies would have the same net effect. In situations in which tolerance to an antigen resides solely in T lymphocytes, tolerance can be broken by bypassing or removing the T-lymphocyte block. For instance, if a T lymphocyte can be induced to respond to a particular carrier moiety on an antigen, then a humoral response can be provoked to any hapten attached to that carrier provided that hapten-specific B lymphocytes are available. The host may lack T lymphocytes that recognize self antigens, but if these antigens are displayed to B lymphocytes on an immunogenic carrier, tolerance will be broached. For example, when a virus attaches to an erythrocyte membrane, it becomes an immunogenic unit. T lymphocytes can recognize the virus (as carrier) and collaborate with B lymphocytes that respond to red cell membranes (as hapten). The result would be antierythrocyte membrane antibodies (autoantibody). Similarly, if host determinants are incorporated into the capsid of a virus, as might occur with budding from a cell membrane, the virus would serve as the immunogenic carrier allowing successful T-B collaboration and the production of anti–cell membrane antibodies. This may be the mechanism responsible for antilymphocyte and other anti–surface membrane antibodies. Alternatively, tolerance might be abrogated if a portion of a self antigen were altered as a new immunogenic carrier (neoantigen) for the unaltered associated determinants. Incomplete enzymatic digestion of nucleoprotein or DNA, for instance, might result in antinuclear or anti-DNA antibodies. Finally, an exogenously administered carrier, such as a drug, binding to a host determinant could induce autoantibodies. Procainamide and hydralazine complex with nucleoprotein in vitro; this has been advanced as an explanation for their ability to induce antinuclear antibodies.[135]

An escape from tolerance accompanies nonspecific activation of T lymphocytes. In mice adjuvants, mitogens or allogeneic cells cause the release of soluble factors capable of activating large numbers of B lymphocytes.[136-138] One such material, termed allogeneic effect factor, is produced by T lymphocytes specifically activated by exposure to alloantigens on genetically unrelated cells.[139] An analogous situation develops in the chronic graft-versus-host (GVH) reaction in mice following the introduction of parental cells into an F1 hybrid. The donor's T lymphocytes respond to the host's transplantation antigens (i.e. the MHC structures on the F1 hybrid cells). Depending on the strain combinations and conditions, a variety of outcomes ensue, ranging from an acute, lethal runt disease to a chronic illness characterized by dermatitis, angiogenesis, extensive lymphadenopathy, and immune complex glomerulonephritis.[140,141] Red blood cell, nucleoprotein, and dsDNA antibodies are all observed.[141,142] T lymphocytes from the donor strain are required, but the autoantibodies are made by the B lymphocytes of the host, presumably stimulated by soluble products released by the activated T lymphocytes. In mice the strongest positive allogeneic effects result from reactions between parental T lymphocytes and incompatible structures of F1 cells that are coded by genes in the I region of the MHC.[141,143] Genetic factors, other than those residing in the histocompatibility complex, are also important.

Idiopathic SLE is probably not caused by an infusion of allogeneic cells, but T lymphocytes do react toward self MHC structures combined with foreign antigens in the same way that they react toward allogeneic MHC structures.[144] An alteration of self MHC by antigens binding to I region determinants on the surface of lymphocytes or epidermal cells could thus provoke a T-lymphocyte anti-MHC reaction between the cells of one individual analagous to a GVH reaction. This might be a common pathway by which multiple etiologic agents could produce an identical pathologic process.

Peripheral mononuclear cells respond vigorously when cultured with allogenic cells (mixed leukocyte reaction). They also contain a population of T lymphocytes that recognize and respond to determinants on autologous cells specified by genes of the major histocompatibility complex. The autoreactive responders are contained in a subset of T lymphocytes (a portion of those with the T4+ phenotype) that is distinct from those that proliferate to allo- and xeno-antigens. They function to induce suppressor and cytotoxic cells and produce growth factors (IL-2), which lead to proliferation of other T lymphocytes. The exact in vivo function of the autologous mixed leukocyte reaction is not known, but because it is so frequently abnormal in autoimmune disease, this reaction is considered to be important in the regulation of the normal immune response.[146,147]

A potential for autoimmunity likely exists in everyone. Under ordinary circumstances, however, this self reactivity is held in check. In mice, suppressor T lymphocytes control almost every phase of the immune response.[129] They can inhibit the development and/or expression of both T- and B-lymphocyte responses to antigen.[129,148] Sometimes the suppression is antigen specific; other times they block responses to a variety of unrelated antigens. Mitogens, such as concanavalin A, can induce the formation or differentiation of suppressor T lymphocytes.[149]

Immunologic Abnormalities in Autoimmune Mice. Abnormalities have been found in virtually every aspect of the immune system of autoimmune mice and vary from strain to strain. It remains unclear which of these defects are primary and responsible for the initiation of autoimmune disease and which are secondary immunologic disorders produced by autoimmune attack upon components of the immune system.

The immunologic defects differ in the various strains of autoimmune mice. Perhaps the best evidence for a primary B-lymphocyte defect is in the NZB/NZW mouse. B lymphocytes from these animals appear to be abnormally activated in that they produce exceptionally large amounts of IgM, are less readily rendered tolerant than normal B lymphocytes and have cell-surface immunoglobulin phenotypes indicative of accelerated maturation.[150-152] These abnormalities occur early in life, before the appearance of defects in other parts of the immune system and prior to the development of autoimmune disease.[153] NZB mice depleted of immunocompetent T lymphocytes continue to manifest hyperreactivity and autoimmune disease.[154-156] In NZB strains, B-lymphocyte hyperactivity appears to be limited to a subpopulation of B lymphocytes responsible for certain thymus-independent responses. The CBA/N mouse bears a gene (the *xid* gene) that renders this particular subpopulation of B lymphocytes inactive. Introducing this gene into NZB mice causes B-lymphocyte hyperactivity to disappear; autoantibodies are significantly reduced, and they do not develop immune complex disease.[157-159]

T-lymphocyte function is normal or increased early in the life of NZB animals.[160-162] This early T-lymphocyte hyperactivity appears to be independent of B-lymphocyte influences, since NZB animals bearing the *xid* gene, and therefore lacking B-lymphocyte hyperactivity or autoantibody continue to express the T-lymphocyte abnormalities.[161] With some assay systems there is evidence of reduced T suppressor lymphocyte function in adult NZB/NZW mice; it has been proposed that autoantibodies specific for suppressor T lymphocytes mediate the decrease.[163] This has not been confirmed with other assay systems.[164,165] Antiserum to murine lymphocyte membrane antigens can identify T-lymphocyte subsets that perform different functions. For instance, helper T lymphocytes display the Lyt 1+ phenotype whereas suppressor T lymphocytes are of the Lyt 23+ type.[166] The number of Lyt 23+ (suppressor phenotype) T lymphocytes is increased in aged NZB and NZB/NZW animals, even though these animals are deficient in their ability to express suppressor function.[167] It has been proposed that aged NZB mice are deficient in a Lyt 123+ precursor cell which under the influence of a Lyt 1+ helper cell normally differentiates into a mature T suppressor lymphocyte.[168] Perhaps early lymphocyte hyperactivity in these animals eventually exhausts the ability of the thymus to generate new suppressor T lymphocytes.

MRL/1 mice have little evidence of a primary B-lymphocyte defect, and B-lymphocyte hyperactivity only develops late in the course of their autoimmune disease. The B-lymphocyte subpopulation that produces anti-DNA antibody in this strain is different from the hyperactive subpopulation found in NZB mice. When the CBA/N *xid* gene is bred to MRL/1 mice, they continue to produce anti-DNA antibody.[169] Additionally, the MRL/1 anti-DNA antibody is of the IgG type, suggesting that the responsible B-lymphocytes are T-lymphocyte dependent, not T independent as in the NZB mouse.

T-lymphocyte defects probably account for the autoimmune disease in MRL/1 mice. MRL/1 mice develop massive lymphoid hyperplasia. The lymphocytes in these hyperplastic nodes are unusual in that each cell may express phenotypic markers of both T-suppressor and T-helper lymphocytes.[170,171] Functionally, however, they behave as helper T-lymphocytes, for both polyclonal immunoglobulin production by B in lymphocytes and spontaneous anti-DNA antibody production.[172] Neonatal thymectomy of MRL/1 mice decreases the expression of lymphoid hyperplasia and autoantibodies,[173] but when reconstituted with normal thymuses, these mice continue to express autoimmune disease, in-

dicating that the defect resides in the lymphoid stem cell and not the thymus.[174] MRL/1 T in lymphocytes spontaneously produce a B-lymphocyte differentiation factor that induces polyclonal IgG and IgM synthesis in lipopolysaccharide-activated B-lymphocytes.[175]

In the BXSB strain, polyclonally activated B-lymphocytes are found, associated with lymphoid proliferation and production of autoantibodies.[172] The male BXSB mouse early in life displays a resistance to tolerance induction similar to that seen in other autoimmune strains, whereas the female BXSB is easily tolerized. If male bone marrow cells are transferred to irradiated female recipients along with either male or female thymuses, the resulting animal displays the male pattern of tolerance resistance.[176] If female splenic T in lymphocytes are transferred into the recipient at the same time as male bone marrow cells, the animal displays the female pattern of autoimmune disease, indicating that the abnormalities induced by male bone marrow cells can be suppressed by female splenic T in lymphocytes.[177]

Immunologic Abnormalities in SLE. Practically every aspect of the immune system has been reported to be abnormal in patients with SLE. When considering the significance of individual defects, it is important to keep several points in mind. Just as the various strains of autoimmune mice can differ in their underlying immunologic abnormalities, subgroups of SLE patients may differ from one another in their immunologic abberations.[178] Generalization from studies involving limited numbers of patients or lack of appreciation of genetic influences is hazardous. Additionally, SLE is characterized by exacerbations and remissions over time, either spontaneous or induced by treatment; and in general, immunologic impairments are most pronounced when the disease is active, and diminished or absent when it is quiescent. Also, many of the drugs used to treat SLE can perturb the immune system, further complicating the interpretation of immunologic abnormalities.

It remains unclear which of the multiplicity of immunologic defects are fundamental to the cause of lupus and which are secondarily induced. For example, the production of antilymphocyte autoantibodies in SLE is likely secondary to an abrogation of normal mechanisms of tolerance. Once produced, these antibodies can interact in vivo with subpopulations of lymphocytes, impairing their function. There is abundant in vitro evidence that SLE antilymphocyte autoantibodies can produce a variety of cellular dysfunctions in normal lymphocytes. Some of these autoantibody-induced abnormalities may exacerbate the primary defect that initiated the autoantibody production. Under these circumstances, it is virtually impossible to discern which abnormality came first.

Humoral and Cellular Immunity. Studies of the in vivo humoral and cellular immune responses of patients with active SLE have produced conflicting results. Serum antibody responses to immunization are reported as either decreased or normal.[179,180] When decreased, primary responses are generally diminished to a greater extent than secondary responses, and IgM antibodies are more impaired than IgG. There is evidence of overall heightened immunoglobulin production by patients with SLE, in that patients with active disease often have hypergammaglobulinemia. Normal human serum contains a variety of antibodies reactive with environmental antigens, presumably generated by exposure to these antigens earlier in life. Though SLE patients have evidence of overall increased antibody production, their resting serum antibody levels to these environmental antigens may be normal, increased, or decreased when compared with control individuals.

Reports of the delayed hypersensitivity responses of SLE patients challenged with antigens such as *Candida,* trichophyton, and streptokinase-streptodornase are conflicting.[181,182] Some individuals with SLE are found to be anergic to all of these agents, whereas others have normal responses to some of them. A delayed hypersensitivity response requires a prior sensitization to the antigen. For most SLE patients, this immunization in all probability occurs years before the onset of clinical disease. Their response to challenge with these, or similar environmental antigens, will therefore depend on the state of the immune system, both prior to the onset of disease and at the time of challenge. When patients with active SLE are purposely immunized with "new" antigens such as dinitrochlorobenzene or keyhole-limpet hemocyanin, they consistently fail to become sensitized.[183,184] Taken together, these observations suggest that the sensitization phase of the immune response is much more intact before the onset of SLE, and that differences in preservation of premorbid immunologic memory may account for some of the variations seen to in vivo challenge with environmental antigens.

At the cellular level, abnormalities have been found in the manner in which lymphocytes from patients with active SLE interact with each other. The autologous mixed leukocyte reaction (MLR) has been proposed to be a model system for studying immunoregulatory events that normally occur between T in lymphocytes, B lymphocytes, and macrophages. In patients with active SLE, the autologous MLR is almost always deficient, while patients with inactive disease show near normal responses.[185] The defective response in active disease is due to an impairment of both the stimulator (B in lymphocytes, macrophages) and responder T in lymphocyte populations, including T-helper and T-suppressor lymphocytes.[186] There appears to be a selective deficiency in the T-lymphocyte population that is normally stimulated by autologous B-lymphocytes and a relatively normal response from T in lymphocytes stimulated by macrophages.[187] When SLE is inactive, only the T-suppressor subpopulation continues to demonstrate autologous MLR hyporeactivity, whereas the stimulatory activity of SLE B in lymphocytes and macrophages, and the proliferative responses of T-helper lymphocytes are normal. The marked abnormality of the autologous MLR in active SLE patients contrasts with the relatively

normal responses seen when SLE lymphocytes are cultured with allogeneic lymphocytes.[185] This difference in the perturbation of auto- versus allo-reactivity suggests that the cellular mechanisms responsible for these proliferative reactions may differ from each other.

Lymphocyte Enumeration. Lymphopenia is common in SLE, and the number of lymphocytes is related inversely to the activity of the disease. While B in lymphocytes are present in relatively normal numbers, peripheral blood T in lymphocytes are decreased in number, and the decrease is often most marked in the T-suppressor lymphocyte subpopulation, as defined by the presence of cell-surface receptors for aggregated IgG (T_γ), monoclonal antibodies (OKT5/8, anti-Leu 2a), or assays of suppressor cell function.[178,188] The number of circulating T-helper lymphocytes are less affected in active SLE. Additionally, there appears to be a preferential loss of those T in lymphocytes with the highest density of cell-surface markers.[189]

B-Lymphocyte Function. Although patients with SLE have a normal quantity of blood B lymphocytes, there is considerable evidence of B-lymphocyte hyperactivity. Increased numbers of peripheral blood lymphocytes have cell-surface phenotypes indicative of abnormal B in lymphocyte maturation and activation.[190,191] When cultured in vitro, SLE B in lymphocytes produce abnormally large amounts of immunoglobulin in the absence of an exogenous stimulus, and the percentage of B in lymphocytes spontaneously producing antibody is increased.[191-193] In contrast, when cultured SLE B in lymphocytes are challenged with mitogens, such as pokeweed, they are found to be markedly deficient in their ability to further proliferate or increase immunoglobulin synthesis, suggesting prior activation.[191,194] The antibodies spontaneously produced by SLE B in lymphocytes show a polyclonal pattern of activation, some of the antibodies being reactive with self constituents (autoantibodies) and others being reactive with nonself antigens.[192,195] It is still possible, however, that antibody production is not strictly polyclonal and that a disproportionate number of autoantibodies are generated toward particular self antigens, for example, components of the cell nucleus.

T-Lymphocyte Function. There is also evidence of T-lymphocyte hyperactivity. Patients with active SLE have increased numbers of circulating T-lymphocytes bearing Ia antigens, a phenotypic feature associated with T-lymphocyte activation.[196] Additionally, there is a tenfold increase in the number of circulating T in lymphocytes which are found to be secreting soluble factors.[197] Suppressor T-lymphocyte function in SLE has been extensively studied in vitro.[198-203] When the disease is active, the T in lymphocytes of SLE patients are almost always incapable of inhibiting mitogen-driven or spontaneous B-lymphocyte proliferation and differentiation, or the proliferative responses of other T in lymphocytes. It has been clearly demonstrated that the defect results from an inability of their T in lymphocytes to generate suppressive signals and not in the response of target cells to such signals. As the generation of normal suppressor T in lymphocytes is the result of a collaboration between several cell types, defects in any one of them could result in the apparent loss of suppressor function. Alternatively, the mechanism of production of T-suppressor lymphocytes may be intact, with normal generation of mature T-suppressor lymphocytes, but these are subsequently rendered inactive, or removed from the circulation, perhaps through the action of antilymphocyte autoantibodies.

Natural Killer Cell Function. Natural killer (NK) cell activity is diminished in most patients with SLE.[204,205] Interferon is normally an in vitro inducer of NK activity, and SLE NK cells appear to be hyporesponsive to the activating influences of interferon. SLE patients appear to have normal numbers of inactive NK cells but a deficiency of active, cytotoxic NK cells.[206] In this report, in vitro exposure of normal NK cells to SLE serum did not impair any phase of NK function, suggesting that this is an intrinsic defect in SLE, not induced by antilymphocyte antibodies. Other studies have suggested that autoantibodies in SLE serum can impair the function of NK cells from normal individuals.[207]

Antilymphocyte Antibodies. Autoantibodies to lymphocyte membrane antigens are assuming increasing importance in considerations of the pathogenesis of SLE[99,100] (Table 68–3). Some, primarily the cold-reactive IgM antibodies, are cytotoxic; whereas others, usually of the IgG class, interfere with in vitro lymphocyte functions.[208-212] Lymphocytotoxic antibodies are demonstrable in the serum of at least 80 percent of patients with SLE, and they react with lymphocytes from most normal donors as well as with autologous lymphocytes. Absorption studies reveal that most SLE sera contain a mixture of T-lymphocyte-specific, B-lymphocyte-spe-

cific, and antilymphocyte antibodies reactive with common determinants on T in and B in lymphocytes.

Antilymphocyte antibodies could perturb the immune system in a number of ways, either by effecting the removal of their target cells from the circulation into the reticuloendothelial system or by a variety of lytic mechanisms, including complement-mediated lysis or antibody-dependent cell cytotoxicity (ADCC).[213] Noncytotoxic lymphocyte membrane reactive antibodies might also be important. Cell-surface immunoglobulins, both IgM and IgD, are critical to antigen-specific triggering of B in lymphocytes, and antibodies to IgD produce an adjuvant-like effect in many experimental systems. Elevated concentrations of autoantibodies to IgD have been found in the sera of 45 percent of patients with SLE.[214] These autoantibodies may contribute to the B-lymphocyte hyperactivity seen in SLE.

Defects in T-suppressor function are one of the most constant findings in SLE; therefore it is of considerable interest that SLE antilymphocyte antibodies may show specific reactivity for, and an ability to inactivate or kill, suppressor T in lymphocytes.[215-217] Honda has shown that SLE serum contains certain autoantibodies specifically reactive with T in lymphocytes depleted of cell-surface sialic acid, but not normal T in lymphocytes.[218] These same antibodies appear to preferentially eliminate T-suppressor effector function. Other antilymphocyte antibodies can preferentially kill cell populations necessary for the generation of suppressor cells, but not mature suppressor cells. SLE serum can inhibit the autologous MLR by interfering with both the stimulator and responder populations. Recent work suggests that some SLE autoantibodies that can inhibit the autologous MLR do so by interacting with Ia antigens.[219,220]

Some antilymphocyte antibodies are specific for activated T in lymphocytes and their secreted products, introducing the possibility that some autoantibodies interfere with the immune system by their interaction with activated, proliferating lymphocytes.[222] It also indicates that our operational definition of an antilymphocyte autoantibody should not be restricted to antibodies primarily reactive with resting lymphocytes. One of the essential features of the immune system is rapid clonal proliferation of lymphocytes after an appropriate triggering event. Autoantibodies that are able to react with molecules needed for rapid proliferation, either soluble mediators or activation-dependent cell-surface molecules, could inhibit clonal expansion and thus markedly perturb both the immune response and immunoregulatory events.

To fully understand these mechanisms, it will be necessary to define the nature of the cell-surface antigens on lymphoid cells that are recognized by antilymphocyte antibodies. Reactivities with histocompatibility-associated antigens, such as the HLA-A, B, and C molecular complexes, β_2 microglobulin, and Ia antigens have all been described.[223-225] Additionally, cross reactivities have been reported between antilymphocyte cell-surface autoantibodies, constituents of the cell nucleus, and cell-

Table 68–3. Specificities of Antilymphocyte Antibodies in SLE*

A. Cell membrane antigens on populations of lymphoid cells
   1. T- and B-lymphocyte surface antigens
   2. Suppressor T cells
   3. Lymphoblasts including activated T lymphocytes
   4. Monocyte surface antigens
   5. Natural killer surface antigens
   6. Lymphoid cell lines
   7. Chronic lymphocyte leukemia cells
B. Crossreactive with other tissue antigens
   1. Nuclear antigens
   2. Neurons and glial cells
   3. Trophoblastic antigens
   4. Hematopoietic cells
C. Reactive with defined cell surface antigens
   1. Beta$_2$ microglobulin
   2. HLA heavy chain antigen
   3. Ia antigen
   4. Cord erythrocyte i antigen

*Modified from Searles, R.P., and Williams, R.C., Jr.: Lymphocyte-reactive antibodes in SLE. *In* Clin. Rheum. Dis., Vol. 8, No. 1, April, 1982.

surface antigens of CNS cell types.[226,227] These later auto-antibodies may be important in the pathogenesis of the CNS manifestations of SLE (discussed below).

In all probability, multiple immunologic defects, some inherited, are needed for the production of clinical disease, though just as in the autoimmune mice, particular lesions may be critical. The finding that otherwise normal family members of patients with SLE have abnormal suppressor T-lymphocyte function or serum antilymphocyte antibodies suggests that these isolated immunoregulatory abnormalities in themselves do not produce SLE, but when additional abnormalities are superimposed upon these immunologic lesions, recognizable disease results.

PATHOGENESIS OF SYSTEMIC LUPUS ERYTHEMATOSUS

Immune Complex Disease. While the etiology of SLE remains obscure, it is clear that much of the tissue damage, especially in blood vessels and kidney, is caused by the deposition of antigen-antibody complexes. Indeed, lupus is generally considered to be the prototype human immune complex disease. To better understand the pathogenesis of SLE, it will be useful to review the salient features of experimental immune complex diseases. More than 70 years ago, Von Pirquet postulated that injury to specific organs or tissues might result from immunologic reactions.[228] Subsequently, it was shown in animal experiments that the toxic compounds envisioned by Von Pirquet were the consequence of an interaction of antigen with antibody in the circulation to form a soluble macromolecular complex that induced acute or chronic inflammation.[229,230] Since these complexes localize in tissues for anatomic and physiologic reasons, and not because of any immunologic specificity, their physical properties are of great importance. Thus, the size and solubility of the complexes, their concentration, their ability to engage and activate the complement system, and the duration of their presence in the circulation are all significant determinants.[231]

The first form of immune complex disease studied experimentally was acute serum sickness in the rabbit. Rabbits given a single intravenous injection of a large quantity of foreign serum or a plasma protein will, after several days, produce antibodies against the injected protein. As these antibodies are released into the circulation they encounter an excess of antigen and form soluble complexes. With increasing antibody concentration more and larger complexes are formed. Most are quickly removed from the circulation by the reticuloendothelial system, but some are deposited in vascular endothelium and the renal glomerulus. Once deposited in tissue, the complexes interact with humoral and cellular elements of the host, causing characteristic biochemical, pharmacologic, and morphologic changes. Typical lesions can be found in the blood vessels, heart, and joints, but the best studied are in the glomerulus

Figure 68–1. Diagram of a glomerulus. The mesangial cells (M) are surrounded by capillaries which have a diameter slightly larger than a red blood cell (RBC). A basement membrane invests the capillaries and passes over the mesangium. The central portion of the endothelial cells (En) forms another mesangial boundary. The foot processes on the outer side of the basement membrane are frequently covered by processes from epithelial cells (Ep). (Adapted from Lotta, H.: *In* Gatta, S.R. (ed.): The Handbook of Physiology. Baltimore, Williams & Wilkins Company, 1973.)

(Fig. 68–1). With fluorescein-labeled antibodies the responsible antigen, host immunoglobulin, and complement components are detectable in a granular pattern along the glomerular basement membrane. This granular (lumpy-bumpy) appearance is the hallmark of immune complex disease in all species and tissues studied.[231] The remarkable phlogogenic capacity of such complexes can be appreciated by the fact that only about 20 micrograms of antigen are present in both kidneys of animals with acute serum sickness and severe glomerulonephritis.[232]

If instead of a single injection, foreign proteins are administered daily for a long time, certain animals respond by making amounts of antibody that lead to the formation of soluble complexes and the development of glomerulonephritis, but not arteritis. In other animals, those that make large amounts of antibody, the dose of antigen is usually insufficient to clear the circulating antibody and neither complexes nor nephritis develops. No disease is seen in animals that fail to respond to the antigen.[233] The level of antibody produced appears to be under genetic control. In the appropriate animals continual antigen administration leads to a progressive, fatal glomerulonephritis. Immunofluorescent staining reveals large granular deposits of antigen, host immunoglobulin, and C3 collecting along the outer edge of the basement membrane. These correspond to dense granular deposits seen by electron microscopy. Typically, in chronic serum sickness, the deposits are located on the epithelial side of the basement membrane, but they can also be seen along the endothelium or within the mesangium. Initially, only minute amounts (0.04 percent) of the daily dose of antigen is deposited in the glomeruli. Following weeks of exposure to complexes, some still unknown compensatory mechanism is overwhelmed, allowing larger amounts (about 0.5 percent) of the daily dose to be deposited in the glomerulus, with concomitant severe functional abnormalities.[234] Based on these findings, it has been suggested that the mechanisms of injury in acute and chronic immune complex glomerulonephritis are different. The evanescent lesion of acute serum sickness probably depends on the rapid release of inflammatory mediators, whereas the structural damage seen in the glomerulonephritis of chronic serum sickness is mediated by the complement system and polymorphonuclear leukocytes.[231]

A number of factors influence the deposition of immune complexes. Because the glomerulus is a high-volume ultrafilter and exposed to large amounts of plasma, any alteration of glomerular capillary permeability could enhance complex deposition. For instance, anything that releases vasoactive substances from mast cells and platelets or the administration of histamine or serotonin causes an increased endothelial deposition of colloidal carbon in mice and immune complexes in guinea pigs and rabbits.[235-238] Antihistamines and antagonists of serotonin reduce the severity of acute serum sickness in rabbits, may benefit the spontaneous glomerulonephritis of New Zealand mice, and protects against human serum sickness.[237,239-241] Hydrodynamic forces can also be influential. The arterial lesions in acute serum sickness of rabbits occur most often at the entrance to the coronary arteries and branches and bifurcations of the aorta. Endocarditis is a common finding. Superimposed arterial hypertension intensifies the lesions in serum sickness.[237,242]

A great deal has been learned about the toxic potential of immune complexes by following intravenously infused preformed complexes in experimental animals. Complexes of varying size and antigen-antibody ratio can be made and studied. Large complexes, formed near equivalence, are eliminated rapidly.[243] Smaller, soluble complexes formed in antigen excess disappear from the circulation more slowly.[244] Complexes smaller than 19S do not appear to be nephritogenic in rabbits with acute serum sickness, while larger complexes regularly deposit in the glomerulus and produce injury.[243]

The rate at which the reticuloendothelial system, especially the liver and spleen, clears complexes from the circulation is an important determinant of tissue injury.[245] Phagocytosis of antibody-coated materials or antigen-antibody complexes is preceded by binding to Fc and/or complement receptors on specialized mononuclear cells, such as the liver Kuppfer cells, alveolar mac-

rophages, cells lining the splenic sinusoids, and circulating and tissue-fixed macrophages. The function and expression of these receptors can be modulated by many agents, including lipopolysaccharide, lymphokines, interferons, corticosteroids, and even antigen-antibody complexes.[246] In the kidney, phagocytic functions are performed by the mesangium. Mesangial hypertrophy and localization of immune complexes in mesangial cells are the earliest findings in rabbits with chronic serum sickness.[234] Similar lesions, unaccompanied by renal dysfunction, are found in other animals with experimental or spontaneous immune complex disease. With continual exposure, the mesangial capacity appears to be compromised or exhausted, leading to immune complex deposition in the glomerulus and overt functional impairment.[231,234]

Exposure of bound immune complexes containing C3b to fresh serum generates a C3b convertase (from the alternate pathway) that can disrupt the primary bonds between antigen and antibody, eventually leading to disaggregation of the complexes. Such "solubilized" complexes can no longer bind to receptors or efficiently activate complement through the classical pathway.[247]

The strength of the bond between antigen and antibody is responsible for the stability of the complex. Low-affinity antibody binds less tightly or to a lesser number of sites on the antigen when compared with precipitating antibody. Antigens bound by low-affinity antibody are eliminated more slowly and theoretically have a greater opportunity to produce kidney damage.[248] In experimental chronic glomerulonephritis some rabbits develop renal lesions after many weeks of immunization during which time little precipitating antibody is observed.[249] Thus, the size, antigen-antibody ratio, and quality of the antibody are probably more important determinants of nephrotoxicity than the absolute quantity of circulating immune complex.

The renal disease of NZB/NZW mice bears an amazing resemblance to lupus nephritis. Its immune complex pathogenesis and the responsible antigens have been extensively investigated.[250,251] When examined by the electron microscope the glomerular basement membrane appears thickened, and there are dense deposits, initially in the mesangial region and then along the epithelial and to a lesser extent the endothelial margins. The characteristic immunofluorescence pattern includes granular deposits of mouse immunoglobulin and C3 in the mesangium and along the glomerular basement membrane.[250] Lambert and Dixon demonstrated DNA in an identical pattern to the mouse immunoglobulin deposits. Using acid buffers, they were able to elute antibody from the kidney. Approximately 50 percent of its activity was directed towards nuclear material, specifically nucleoprotein and DNA. The anti-DNA activity of the eluates was 80 times greater than the serum antibody.[251] Isoelectric focusing of the glomerular eluates from NZB/NZW and MRL/1 mice reveals a restricted population of anti-DNA antibodies (pI 8-9) in contrast to the more heterogeneous anti-DNA antibody in the serum.[252] Active immunization of young NZB/NZW mice with DNA-methylated albumin accelerates both the development of antinuclear antibodies and a more severe form of nephritis.

Complement is also important in murine lupus nephritis. The glomerular lesions regularly contain complement components and only complement-fixing antibodies (IgG2a) are present in the eluates.[251] Furthermore, when complement-deficient (C5) A/J mice that have anti-DNA antibodies are injected with DNA, they do not develop severe glomerular disease.[251]

Viral antigens are implicated in the nephritis of NZB and NZB/NZW hybrid mice. Mellors and his co-workers demonstrated that soluble Gross leukemia virus antigens appear in the eluates from the kidneys of the NZB mice at about six months of age. Antibody to Gross antigens can be detected several months earlier. Both antigen and antibody are present in the kidney prior to the development of proteinuria and well in advance of measurable free, circulating antibody.[35,253] A similar but more accelerated process is present in the NZB/NZW. Dixon and colleagues measured the concentration of IgG from acid eluates of washed renal homogenates before and after absorption with insoluble nuclear protein, Gross virus soluble antigen, and Gross virus. Thirty-five to 48 percent of the eluted IgG reacted with insoluble nuclear protein, whereas 5 to 21 percent was absorbed by viral antigens, suggesting that the Gross virus may be only one of several antigens contributing to the pathogenesis of the nephritis.[254] Although many mouse strains have gp-70 antigen-antibodyin their serum and proteinuria is correlated with the amount of antigen, only NZB/NZW mice have circulating gp-70 antigen-antibody immune complexes.[255,256]

Lupus Nephritis. Systemic lupus erythematosus resembles immune complex–mediated chronic experimental serum sickness. Antigen-antibody complexes are demonstrable in renal glomeruli, blood vessels, skin, and the choroid plexus of the brain. The evidence that these complexes mediate the renal injury in SLE rests on a number of observations, including studies of the complement system, serial observations of antibodies and antigens during the course of the disease, measurements of immune complexes and cryoprecipitable proteins in the serum, immunofluorescent and electron microscopic examination of renal biopsies and kidneys obtained at autopsy, and identification of the immunoreactants eluted from kidneys.

Complement. Total hemolytic complement activity is decreased in the serum of many patients with SLE at some time during their illness.[4,11,257,258] The degree of depression is often related to disease activity; the most marked hypocomplementemia occurs in patients with nephritis and less often in those with extensive skin or central nervous system disease. The reduction is most marked in the components that comprise the classical complement system, i.e., C1, C4 and C3, and the pattern suggests activation by immune complexes.[257,259-261] C2 levels are not usually depressed, except in association

with genetic defects.[257] Static measurements of hemolytic activity or protein concentrations of complement components give an incomplete picture of activation of the complement system. Hypercatabolism can be masked by an increase in synthesis. Turnover studies using radiolabeled components or measurements of the breakdown products of components released from the native molecule during the activation process provide a truer picture. SLE patients with hypocomplementemia, especially those with active nephritis, display a higher fractional catabolic rate,[262-265] an increased extravascular distribution of C3 and C5,[263,265] and a reduction of C3 synthesis when compared with normal subjects.[262,263] Breakdown products of C3 (C3d, C3c) and of factor B are detected in relatively high concentration in plasma from patients with SLE. The level of these fragments is inversely related to the serum C3 concentration.[266] Factor B and properidin concentrations are decreased.[267,268] This could reflect triggering of the C3b amplification loop or direct activation of the alternate complement pathway.[269] The plasma concentrations of beta 1 H globulin and the C3b inactivator, regulatory proteins of the alternate complement pathway, are also reduced.[270] The likelihood that the observed activation of the complement system in SLE is triggered by immune complexes is suggested both by the pattern of the complement profile and by a significant correlation between the increase of C3d plasma concentration and the serum levels of Clq binding activity.[271]

Serum Antigens and Antibodies. An enormous array of antibodies to cellular constituents is found in SLE serum (Table 68–1). Many crossreact with bacterial and viral polynucleotides, suggesting that the immunogens could be exogenous rather than due to native or altered tissue antigens. Antibodies to nucleohistone (the nucleoprotein complex formed between DNA and histone) were the first autoantibodies discovered in patients with SLE and were demonstrated to be responsible for the LE cell reaction.[272] Subsequently, a multiplicity of antinuclear and cytoplasmic antibodies were defined. The pathogenetic significance of many of them is questionable, but antibodies to DNA surely play an important role in immune complex–mediated lesions. Antibodies to native double-stranded DNA (dsDNA) are detected predominantly in SLE.[273-275] In contrast, antibodies reactive with single-stranded DNA (sDNA), while often found in SLE, are frequently demonstrated in other diseases. Only rarely do antibodies to dsDNA and sDNA have a unique specificity for either the denatured or single-stranded form; sDNA may be the major immunogen for both types of antibodies.[275] Recently, SLE autoantibodies specifically reactive with left-handed Z-DNA have been described.[276] A number of human monoclonal antibodies selected to react with denatured DNA were also found to bind to the phospholipid cardiolipin. The two compounds share appropriately spaced phosphodiester groups. The fact that some coagulation proteins, cardiolipin, and certain cell membranes share similar antigens might explain some of the serologic heterogeneity of SLE serum.[277] Antinucleoprotein antibody needs both the DNA and protein moieties present for its interaction.[272,278] Soluble nuclear antigens obtained by extraction of nuclei with saline also constitute important immunogens. Two immunogens, Sm and n-ribonucleoprotein (nRNP), have been well characterized and their relationship to SLE defined.[2,6,7,279] The nRNP and Sm determinants are each distinct antigenic sites present on small nuclear RNAs complexed to proteins that are critical to RNA splicing[280] and discussed further in Chapter 48. SS-A (Ro) and SS-B (La) antibodies may also react with small nuclear ribonucleoproteins.[281] Antibodies to single- and double-stranded RNA and RNA-DNA hybrids are found in the serum of some SLE patients. These antibodies are best detected using synthetic polyribonucleotides.[282]

Serial studies of some antinucleoprotein antibodies show a definite relationship between their concentration in serum and disease activity.[275] Titers of anti-dsDNA antibody correlate best with hypocomplementemia and active nephritis in SLE patients.[4,274,275] sDNA antibodies may occur intermittently during periods of disease exacerbation.[275,283,284] Antibodies reactive with double-stranded RNA may increase with peaks of disease activity, often concomitant with rises in anti-dsDNA and anti-sDNA antibodies, but on other occasions no direct relationship to disease activity has been observed.[275] Anti-nRNP antibodies show a different pattern. They remain at high titer throughout the patient's illness, showing little correlation with disease activity.[7,275] Often the appropriate immunogens, dsDNA, sDNA, dsRNA and nRNP, are found free in the circulation alternating with the presence of circulating antibody. This has led Koffler and his associates to implicate them as the important tissue-localizing antigen-antibody complexes.[231,274,275,284]

Both IgG and IgM antibodies to dsDNA are demonstrable in SLE serum, and there is some evidence that patients with IgM antibodies get nephritis less often.[285] There are other important qualitative differences among anti-DNA antibodies with respect to the development of nephritis. For instance, it has been claimed that patients whose antibodies both precipitate and bind to DNA have a greater incidence of nephritis, while those sera precipitate but do not form soluble complexes get nephritis only infrequently.[286,287] Differences in avidity of anti-DNA antibodies have been reported, and low avidity antibodies are claimed to be more nephrotoxic.[288-290] As will be discussed below, there are disagreements about the measurement of avidity, but it should be appreciated that serum antibodies may be the residua after more avid antibody has been deposited in the kidneys. It has been reported that the serum anti-DNA antibodies associated with nephritis are primarily of the complement-fixing subclasses.[291,292]

Reticuloendothelial System Dysfunction. In experimental animals defects in Fc receptors of mononuclear phagocytes can lead to a prolonged circulation and enhanced deposition of immune complexes. The reticuloendothelial septum (RES) has been less well studied in humans.[246,293] When IgG-sensitized autologous erythrocytes are administered intravenously, they are rapidly cleared by the spleen in normal individuals. Clearance rates are markedly prolonged in patients with active SLE, especially those with active renal disease.[293] Although these findings are interesting, it must be recognized that the disposal of most immune complexes occurs primarily in the liver, and there is currently no satisfactory system for measuring human hepatic Fc function. Moreover, when NZB/NZW mice were studied with artificial complexes that are preferentially removed by the liver, no defects were found.[294]

Membrane-associated C3b receptors probably participate in the clearance of complexes that have activated the complement system and become coated with C3b. Most human peripheral blood cells have C3b receptors, but because of the large numbers of red blood cells greater than 85 percent are erythrocyte associated. SLE red blood cells have a decrease in the number and function of C3b receptors, which is perhaps genetically determined.[72,295,296] A failure of these cells to bind circulating immune complexes could result in an enhanced delivery of complexes to the liver and spleen, causing overload and dysfunction of the RES.

Immune Complexes and Cryoglobulins. A number of methods are available for detecting immune complexes.[271] Some depend on the selective detection of a known antigen by discrimination between free and antibody-bound antigen in the complex. Others detect complexes independent of the nature of the antigen involved. These antigen-nonspecific methods are based on the distinct properties of complexed immunoglobulin molecules when compared with free immunoglobulin molecules. They take advantage of the physical changes induced by complex formation and biological activities of the immune complexes, such as complement fixation or binding to cell membranes. Cryoprecipitation and analytical ultracentrifugation are examples of the former; and C1q binding or reactions with Fc or C3 receptors on cultured lymphoblasts (Raji cells), mononuclear cells, or platelets, of the latter. In 1971 Agnello and associates reported that 23 of 30 hypocomplementemic SLE patients had a material in their serum that precipitated with C1q, whereas none of 53 normocomplementemic patients did.[297] Subsequently, immune complexes were demonstrated in the majority of patients with SLE by a variety of assay systems.[298,299] Levels of C1q binding activity often reflect disease activity or exacerbations but are not different in patients with renal manifestations as compared with those without nephritis.[271]

The nature of the antigens in SLE immune complexes is still a matter of disagreement, especially the important question of the relative involvement of the DNA-anti-DNA system. Several laboratories have reported isolation of DNA from SLE serum or plasma.[300-302] On the other hand, treatment of SLE serum with deoxyribonuclease did not decrease the activity of the immune complex material detected either by a C1q binding or a Raji cell assay, and Izui and collaborators failed to detect either DNA or anti-DNA in the complexes using radioimmunoassays specific for these constituents.[303,304] They have concluded, therefore, that although DNA–anti-DNA complexes are prominent in tissue lesions, they constitute only a minor part of the detectable immune complex activity in SLE sera.[303]

Cold precipitable proteins (cryoglobulins) can be isolated from the serum of patients with SLE, and their quantity is closely associated with disease activity and hypocomplementemia. There is much evidence that cryoglobulins are a manifestation of circulating immune complexes.[305] Early studies demonstrated that the SLE cryoglobulins contained IgG and IgM and the complement components C1q, C4, and C3. The IgM possessed anti-IgG reactivity.[306-308] Isolated cryoproteins were capable of fixing complement in vitro.[308] If cryoprecipitates represent circulating immune complexes of pathogenetic significance, they should contain antigens and specific antibodies in concentrations that are relatively enriched compared with their concentration in the serum. Several studies support this concept. A number of different polynucleotide antibodies are found in SLE cryoglobulins. Some, such as the antibodies to dsDNA, sDNA, and n-RNP are specifically concentrated, whereas antibodies to dsRNA are present in amounts proportional to their representation in serum. Ribosomal antibodies have not been found in cryoprecipitates even when detectable in accompanying serum.[309] There is an enrichment of both anti-immunoglobulin (rheumatoid factor) and antilymphocyte antibodies in the cryoprecipitates.[310,311] Each is a cold-reactive IgM antibody but can be distinguished from the other by appropriate absorptions. An anti-idiotype antibody was made to an IgM antiglobulin and fluoresceinated. It reacted with the IgM in the glomeruli of a renal biopsy from the patient's own kidney but not in other kidney specimens, indicating pathogenetic significance of the rheumatoid factor in that cryoglobulin.[312] Digestion of the precipitates with pronase to destroy immunoglobulin and other proteins allows DNA to be detected by counterimmunoelectrophoresis. The amount of DNA was shown to be enriched relative to the serum concentration.[300] SLE cryoglobulins appear to contain antigens from lymphocytes and neural tissues. Immunization of rabbits with cryoprecipitates results in the production of antibodies that react with distinctive determinants on both SLE and normal lymphocytes and cultured neuronal and glial cells.[313,314] Differential absorption studies provide evidence that these are separate antigens but cannot exclude the possibility that there are additional shared specificities.[314]

Identification of Immunoreactants in Renal Tissues. Immunofluorescent studies indicate that immunoglobulins, mainly IgG and IgM, are deposited in association

Figure 68–2. Schematic and immune fluorescent demonstration of immune complexes in various areas of the glomerulus. In *A*, the complexes are limited to the mesangial area. The specimen is a glomerulus from a patient with SLE showing minimal morphologic changes and mesangial deposits of IgG (upper left). The features demonstrated in *B* are seen in diffuse proliferative glomerulonephritis. Complexes are deposited in the mesangium and diffusely along the basement membrane, primarily in a subendothelial location. The glomerulus in the upper right is from a patient with diffuse proliferative lupus nephritis stained with a fluoresceinated antibody to IgG.

A

B

with complement in SLE nephritis.[315-318] Three major patterns of localization are recognized; namely, mesangial, subendothelial, and subepithelial (Fig. 68–2). The deposits are generally granular in appearance when located along the glomerular basement membrane. Mesangial immunofluorescence is characteristically irregular, with homogeneous strands lying between capillary loops, but may be granular.[318] Different immunoglobulin classes are observed in the glomeruli. IgG alone or in combination with IgM is most common. In some cases only IgM can be identified.[312,318] Certain IgG subclasses may be selectively deposited.[257,319]

Treatment of isolated glomeruli with acid buffers and deoxyribonuclease allows identification of some antigens and antibodies participating in lupus glomerulonephritis. Antinuclear antibodies and antibodies to sDNA and dsDNA are present in glomerular eluates from most kidneys.[283,320-322] Occasionally anti-RNP and Sm antibodies are detected, but anti-dsRNA antibodies are not found.[283,322] When the concentration of a particular antibody in the elute is compared with its concentration in serum (based on relative IgG concentrations), the antibodies to sDNA are dominant in both amount and frequency, occasionally being found in eluates when no antibody is present in the serum.[283,289] The avidity of the eluted antibody to dsDNA is significantly greater than the anti-dsDNA in the corresponding cryoprecipitates or serum.[289] Treatment of kidneys obtained at autopsy or by renal biopsy with high molarity salt solution or acid buffers releases antibody but retains the corresponding antigens. Using highly purified fluorescein-labeled antisera, both native and denatured DNA can be detected in extracellular locations, but nRNP antigen was not demonstrated.[321,323]

Immune complexes, identifiable by immunofluorescence or electron microscopy, are present in the tubular basement membrane and interstitium of 20 to 50 percent of patients with lupus nephritis.[324,325] They are associated with conspicuous interstitial fibrosis and mononuclear cell infiltration, as well as tubular cell damage, indicating their probable pathogenetic significance.

The complement components in SLE renal lesions have been analyzed. Evidence for classical complement pathway activation includes the finding of C1q, C4, and particularly C3 in kidney biopsies.[257,319,326,327] Deposits containing properidin and beta 1 H are seen, but rarely is factor B seen.[257,326,328] Indeed, even the complex of late-acting components (C5-C9) responsible for membrane injury can be demonstrated at glomerular and tubular sites.[329] Because of the association with immunoglobulin, it is presumed that complement resides in the renal tissues bound to antigen and antibody. What is not known is whether the complexes arrive in the kidney with complement bound to them, or if complement fixation occurs after their localization, or independent of immunoglobulin.

Although there is general agreement that lupus renal disease is mediated by immune complexes, other important questions remain unanswered. For instance, why do some patients get mild and others severe disease, and what accounts for the various types of SLE nephritis? The different patterns and locations of granular deposits and the variable immunoglobulin classes suggest a heterogeneity of complexes. Most studies fail to confirm that a particular immunoglobulin class or subclass relates to severity of disease, although in the instance of proliferative lesions the total amount of immunoglobulin deposited may be important.[330-332] There is a broad correlation between the amount of immunoglobulin found in mesangium and the degree of proliferation seen by light microscopy, suggesting that proliferation is a secondary response to these deposits. Subendothelial deposits are rarely seen in the absence of mesangial deposits.[330] The situation in membranous nephropathy is distinctively different; subepithelial deposits are unrelated to either subendothelial or mesangial deposits.

The reason for the localization of complexes in one area of the kidney or another is unknown. Impaired mesangial function could decrease the clearance of complexes from renal capillaries or lead to incomplete removal of deposited material from the subendothelial space. In either case, the net effect would be an increase in glomerular immunoglobulin deposits. Glomerular endothelial cells are separated by tiny fenestrations, which allow the passage of intact immune complexes and their subsequent localization against the basement membrane. But it is not clear how intact macromolecular complexes can penetrate the basement membrane to deposit in the subepithelial region. Indeed, we do not know if antigen and antibody pass individually and then combine or whether special characteristics of the immunoreactants are important.

In experimental models of autologous immune complex nephropathy in rats (Heymann nephritis) the subepithelial site where the complexes lodge corresponds to the localization of polyanionic glomerular sialoprotein on epithelial cells and in filtration slits. This negatively charged material is thought to regulate the permeability of the glomerular capillary wall to circulating macromolecules.[333,334] Manipulations that alter the charge of the sialoprotein or the antigen-antibody complex can enhance or decrease the localization of immune complexes.[333,335] The effect of DNA has not been studied in this system. However, DNA has been shown to have an affinity for the collagen component of the glomerular basement membrane (GBM) and under certain circumstances free DNA can bind in vivo to glomeruli.[336,337] Izui has suggested that a least some of the glomerular lesions in lupus nephritis result from a reaction of circulating anti-DNA antibodies to DNA bound to GBM acting like an immunoabsorbent (in situ immune complex formation). The antibody class may also be an important determinant. Patients with diffuse proliferative disease had a higher ratio of IgM to IgG anti-DNA antibody than those with focal changes, even though the total amount of anti-DNA antibody was the same in the two groups.[332]

An alternative explanation is provided by the studies of Winfield and colleagues, who found that SLE patients with the most severe forms of nephritis had the highest serum levels of anti-dsDNA antibodies, but the avidity of the antibody was low. This is in contrast to the almost tenfold higher avidity of the anti-dsDNA eluted from their glomeruli.[289] The most likely explanation is that the higher avidity anti-dsDNA antibodies are rapidly cleared from the circulation in the form of immune complexes and deposited in the Kidney. Estimations of antibody avidity are difficult and may account for the disagreement on this point.[288] Patients with membranous nephropathy appear to have less total anti-dsDNA antibody, and it is almost exclusively nonprecipitating. In diffuse proliferative glomerulonephritis, on the other hand, there are greater amounts of antibody and it is primarily precipitating in character.[338] Furthermore, using a C1q binding assay, Ooi and associates could not detect circulating immune complexes in the serum from patients with membranous nephropathy, while they were present in a high portion of patients with diffuse proliferative glomerulonephritis.[339]

Skin. The dermal manifestations of lupus erythematosus have been recognized since the 19th century.[340] In the early 1960s two groups of investigators independently reported the presence of immunoglobulins at the dermal-epidermal (D-E) junction in SLE skin lesions.[341,342] Subsequently, numerous others have identified immunoglobulins, primarily IgG and IgM, and components of the classical, alternate, and terminal complement pathways in this region of the skin.[343] The deposits are variously described as homogenous, granular, and thready. Characteristically the immunofluorescence appears as a band along the D-E junction, hence the name lupus band test. Most (80 to 100 percent) of the biopsies from lupus skin lesions show these changes.[344] Similar abnormalities are present in the uninvolved skin of some SLE patients, most often in sun-exposed areas.[345-350] Some disagreement exists concerning the relationship of the skin immunopathology to disease activity, involvement of other tissues, especially the kidney, and serologic abnormalities. The confusion stems in part from the use of different criteria for renal disease, varying sites of skin biopsy, and a tendency to compare biopsy findings from skin and kidney taken at different times. No correlations are obtained with biopsies from lesional skin or from sun-exposed, noninvolved areas. However, when the results are compared with the findings in uninvolved, non–sun-exposed skin, most studies indicate that a positive band test correlates with more severe disease, the presence of nephritis, hypocomplementemia, and raised anti-DNA antibody levels, but it cannot predict the morphology of the glomerular lesions.[345,347,348,351-355]

We do not understand why immunoglobulins and complement localize to the dermal-epidermal junction. Circulating complexes could be trapped in this region. Alternatively, there may be in situ formation of complexes. The dermal-epidermal junction has no phagocytic cells analagous to the mesangium, but it is a vascular area in which the circulation is sluggish in the long horizontal segments that run parallel to the basement membrane. Dense deposits are seen in the dermal vessels of normal and lesional SLE skin.[356] Immunofluorescent staining of blood vessel walls in the upper dermis is sometimes observed in combination with the subepidermal immunoglobulin deposits.[357,358] A correlation of serologic abnormalities and hypocomplementemia with the granular deposits in noninvolved skin is an argument in favor of the localization of circulating complexes. So is the finding of an identical immunofluorescent appearance in the skin of patients with other immune complex disorders such as leprosy and bacterial endocarditis.[359,360] On the other hand, it might be expected that the immunoglobulin makeup of trapped dermal and renal complexes would be similar, but that is often not the case.[352,354]

Acid eluates from normal skin of SLE patients contain antinuclear and antibasement membrane antibodies.[358,361-364] The latter react with dermal and esophageal basement membrane but not with glomerular basement membrane. On normal skin, it fixes complement and gives a linear pattern by immunofluorescence.[361,362,364] Antiglomerular basement membrane antibody injures the glomerulus in Goodpasture's syndrome, and it is possible that the antidermal basement membrane antibody behaves in a similar manner. The absence of linear fluorescence in samples from SLE skin suggests, however, that this is not the case.

An attractive explanation for the immune complexes found in SLE skin is a local reaction of nuclear antigens and antinuclear antibodies. During keratinization, epidermal nuclei are broken down, and nucleoprotein and DNA are thought to diffuse back into the dermis.[358] Normally, these substances would pass through the subepidermal region and be removed by the circulation, but in the presence of appropriate antibodies, precipitation occurs at the dermal-epidermal junction. This is consistent with the positive association of antinuclear and anti-dsDNA antibodies with D-E immunoglobulin deposits in normal skin, the presence of antinuclear antibodies in eluates from uninvolved SLE skin, and the occasional demonstration of immunoglobulins fixed to the nuclei of epidermal cells in biopsy specimens examined by the direct fluorescent antibody technique.[358,363,365-367] Support for this proposal comes from the experiments of Natali and Tan, who showed that immunoglobulin accumulates in a subepidermal band at sites of UV irradiation in mice that have circulating antibody to UV-altered DNA. Mice that were immunized to produce the antibody but were not irradiated did not develop similar lesions.[268]

A direct pathogenetic relationship between immune complex deposition in SLE skin and the development of typical dermal abnormalities is not likely. Early lupus skin lesions frequently lack immunofluorescence,[369] and those induced under controlled conditions of exposure to monochromatic light may not develop demonstrable immunoglobulin and complement complexes for several months.[370] Gilliam even suggests an inverse relationship between persistent, destructive SLE skin lesions and subepidermal immunoglobulin deposits in uninvolved skin.[358] Finally, it is difficult to imagine that dermatologic manifestations of SLE result from injury induced by immune complexes when identical immunofluorescent and electron-dense deposits are identified in normal, nonlesional skin from SLE patients. It is of interest, however, that although C1q and C3 are demonstrable in both lesional and nonlesional skin, only the abnormal skin shows the terminal (membrane attack complex) complement components in association with immunoglobulin.[343]

Antibodies to Cell Membranes. Until now the discussion of the pathogenesis of tissue lesions in SLE has focused primarily on antigen-antibody complexes. It is important, however, to emphasize the role played by antibodies to cell membrane antigens. Antibodies to circulating cellular elements are well known. Antierythrocyte autoantibody, which is similar to incomplete Rh antibody of the IgG class, is found in the serum of about 5 percent of SLE patients.[371] Many others have both gammaglobulin and complement on their red blood cells; some have only complement.[372,373] Positive Coombs' tests and occasionally hemolytic anemia can be a consequence of these antibodies.[372,374] Thrombocytopenia is common in SLE, and serum factors reactive with platelets are found in the majority of patients.[375-377] The antibodies are IgG and involve all four subclasses, in contrast to the predominance of IgG_3 antiplatelet antibodies found in idiopathic thrombocytopenic purpura.[378] It is not clear that all of the antibodies detected on platelets are directed to unique determinants on these cells. For instance, SLE autoantibodies reactive with β_2 microglobulin cause in vitro platelet aggregation, and platelet membranes have receptors for immune complexes.[379] Theoretically, antiplatelet antibodies could affect platelet survival by direct lysis or accelerated removal of the thrombocytes from the circulation.

Autoantibodies to lymphocyte membrane antigens are assuming increasing importance in considerations of the pathogenesis of SLE. As discussed earlier, they can have profound effects on lymphocyte numbers and functions both in vivo and in vitro. Patients with clinically active SLE have antilymphocyte antibodies more frequently and in higher titers than do patients with relatively inactive disease.[380-382] Besides an association with overall disease activity, certain clinical manifestations appear more often in patients with the IgM cold-reactive lymphocytotoxic antibody. Butler and associates reported an association with thrombocytopenia and central nervous system manifestations.[380] This has been confirmed in other studies.[383,384] Subsequently, Bluestein demonstrated neurocytotoxic antibodies in approximately 75 percent of serum samples from SLE patients.[385] The relationship of lymphocytotoxic and neurocytotoxic antibodies to one another and to the neuropsychiatric manifestations of systemic lupus will be detailed below.

Central Nervous System Manifestations of SLE. Neurologic and psychiatric illnesses are important features of SLE.[386,387] They occur commonly, perhaps in a third of the patients, and are responsible for a significant morbidity and mortality.[388] In contrast to lupus nephritis

there is little known about the pathogenesis of central nervous system disease. Post-mortem examination by light microscopy of the brains of patients dying with SLE have demonstrated degenerative and proliferative changes in small vessels similar to those of hypertensive encephalopathy and thrombotic thrombocytopenic purpura.[387,389] Scattered about the cerebral cortex are microinfarcts and gliosis around small blood vessels. Affected arterioles showed thickening of the intimal and medial coats and occasionally perivascular collections of mononuclear cells. The inflammatory cell infiltrates and fibrinoid necrosis of the walls of small and medium-sized arteries typically seen in other systemic lesions of SLE are only occasionally seen in the brain. While microvascular lesions can account for the clinical findings in some SLE patients, there is often a remarkable lack of correlations between clinical and pathologic findings. Patients with obvious lupus encephalopathy frequently show only minimal abnormalities at post-mortem examination. This has suggested that some features of CNS disease may be brought about by unique pathologic processes that do not appreciably perturb brain histology. SLE autoantibodies reactive with brain are potential mediators for such a process.

SLE-related neuropsychiatric problems are found signficantly more often in patients with increased serum lymphocytotoxic antibody titers.[380-383] A potential explanation of this association was suggested by the demonstration that more than 90 percent of the lymphocytotoxic activity in SLE sera is also reactive with antigenic determinants present in homogenized human brain and on cultured human neuronal and glial cells. In addition, SLE serum contains other CNS-reactive autoantibodies that are not crossreactive with antigenic determinants on lymphocytes; some of these anti-CNS autoantibodies may be specific for CNS cell subpopulations.[385,390]

The introduction of various brain constituent antibodies into the ventricles or cerebral cortex of experimental animals causes convulsions, meningitis, impaired memory, and motor dysfunction.[391-393] This suggests that brain-reactive autoantibodies might be responsible for certain forms of SLE CNS disease. If antibodies from the circulation are to be responsible for CNS disease, then they must escape the constraints of the blood-brain barrier, which normally prevents serum protein from coming into contact with cortical tissues. The best evidence for the exclusion of blood-borne autoantibodies is the finding that, though most SLE patients have neuron-reactive antibodies in their plasma, neither the amount nor specificity of these antibodies appears to be related to the neuropsychiatric manifestations of SLE patients.[394] Some investigators, however, have reported an association between the amount of IgG antineuronal antibody in serum and active CNS disease.[395,396]

Antineuronal antibodies can gain access to the nervous system. Approximately 75 percent of a group of patients investigated with active CNS lupus had increased IgG antineuronal activity in their cerebrospinal fluid (CSF) compared with less than 10 percent of other lupus patients.[394] Patients with more diffuse CNS manifestations, such as psychosis, organic brain syndrome, or generalized seizures, were more likely (90 percent) to have increased amounts of IgG antineuronal antibodies than were patients with anatomically localized lesions (25 percent). The manner by which antineuronal antibodies gain access to the central nervous system is still not clear. Local production of these autoantibodies seems unlikely, given the paucity of pathologic studies showing immunocopetent cells in the brain tissues of patients dying with active SLW-CNS disease. The finding in the CSF of immunoglobulins that are restricted in their electrophoretic mobility has been used as an indicator of local antibody production in the CNS, since it implies that most of the IgG is derived from a limited number of plasma cell clones. Such oligoclonal banding is typically found in patients with multiple sclerosis who have increased concentration of CSF IgG.[397] CSF proteins with restricted electrophoretic migration have been reported to be variously present or absent in CSF from SLE patients with active CNS disease and increased IgG concentration.[397a,397b]

Mechanisms that can alter the blood-brain barrier in SLE have been proposed. Atkins and colleagues observed immunoglobulins in the choroid plexi of two patients who had CNS manifestations of SLE during life.[398] They suggested that the patients' symptoms might be explained by alterations in choroidal function induced by immune complexes. Clinically there is an association of neuropsychiatric symptoms and other manifestations thought to be mediated by immune complexes, such as dermal vasculitis, arteritis, and hypocomplementemia.[384,399,400] This is not a universal experience, however.[401] It has been shown that choroidal deposits of immunoreactants are a regular feature of SLE—with or without a history of CNS disease—and are often found in other human diseases with immune complex–mediated vascular injury.[360,402,403] Subendothelial deposits in choroidal vessels are a feature of naturally occurring or experimental immune complex diseases of rodents and rabbits[404-407] (Fig. 68–3). These observations probably reflect the fact that the choroidal capillaries with their open fenestrations, reminiscent of the vessels of the glomerulus, allow the passage of immune complexes from the circulation into the interstitium of the choroid plexus where they are retained by cells bearing Fc receptors.[408] Serum antineuronal antibodies might gain access to the CNS through the choroid plexus after it has been damaged by immune complexes. Alternately, immune complex–mediated disease of the small blood vessels of the brain may allow plasma antineuronal antibodies to enter the central nervous system. If this is so, it remains to be explained how endothelial damage can occur in the absence of a typical inflammatory reaction. Evidence suggesting that antineuronal antibodies may pass through the CNS microvasculature and bind to neurons is shown in (Fig 68–4). Brain tissue was obtained immediately after death from a young woman with severe SLE organic psychosis. Tissue sections incubated with fluoresceinated rabbit antibodies to human proteins demonstrated that both human IgG and IgM, but not fibrinogen, were bound to neuronal cells. The intensity of the neuronal membrane immunofluorescence was pro-

Figure 68–3. Dense deposits in endothelial cells of the choroid plexus of a mouse with ferritin-antiferritin experimental immune complex disease (× 18,000). The vascular lumen is at the upper left and the epithelium facing the cerebrospinal fluid is on the lower right-hand side of the photomicrograph. (From Lambert, P., et al.: Acta Neuropathol. (Berlin) 38:83, 1977.)

Figure 68–4. Immunofluorescent staining of cerebral cortex of a young woman who died with active SLE-related organic brain syndrome. This photomicrograph of anti-IgM immunofluorescence shows a ring pattern of staining of the neuronal cells clustered about a cerebral blood vessel. IgG staining (not shown) showed a similar ring pattern on cells throughout the field. Control proteins such as albumin and fibrinogen gave no staining. (From Zvaifler, N.J., Bluestein, H.G.: The pathogenesis of central nervous system manifestations of systemic lupus erythematosus. Arthritis Rheum. 25:862, 1982.

portional to the distance of the cells from the cerebral vessels, suggesting that the vessel was the exit site for the autoantibody.

To fully understand the mechanisms by which anti-CNS autoantibodies produce disease it will be essential to define the molecular nature of the cell surface antigens that they recognize. Since a large percent of lymphocytotoxic autoantibody is reactive with neural tissues, it might be anticipated that some antineuronal antibodies will combine with antigenic structures known to be shared by these cell types. Candidates for crossreactive target antigens include the human Thy-1 equivalent and histocompatibility antigens of the A, B, and C series. Hirano and colleagues have reported that serum antibody to asialo GM_1 is associated with neurologic disorders in SLE patients.[409] Asialo GM_1, a neutral glycolipid, constitutes a relatively small proportion of the glycolipids in brain and has been identified on subpopulations of lymphoid cells.[410,411] Using rabbit antiserum to lupus serum cryoprecipitates, Klippel and co-workers have shown that lupus cryoglobulins contain antigens, presumably present as antigen-antibody complexes, that are crossreactive with cell surface structures of lymphoid and CNS cells.[412] These antisera are being employed to isolate and define the physiochemical characteristics of their target antigens.[413] A comparative analysis of the shared neuronal and lymphocyte antigenic determinants reactive with SLE anti-CNS autoantibodies may reveal the complex interrelationship between the altered immune regulation and neuropsychiatric problems that characterize SLE.

References

1. Tan, E.M., Cohen, A.S., Fries, J.F., Masi, A.T., McShane, D.J., Rothfield, N.T., Schaller, J.G., Talal, N., and Winchester, R.: The 1982 revised criteria for the classification of systemic lupus erythematosus. Arthritis Rheum. 25:1271, 1982.
2. Notman, D.D., Kurata, N., and Tan, E.M.: Profiles of antinuclear antibodies in systemic rheumatic diseases. Ann. Intern. Med. 83:464, 1975.
3. Reichlin, M.: Clinical and immunologic significance of antibodies to Ro and La in systemic lupus erythematosus. Arthritis Rheum. 25:767, 1982.
4. Schur, P.H., and Sandson, J.: Immunologic factors and clinical activity in systemic lupus erythematosus. N. Engl. J. Med. 278:533, 1968.
5. Pincus, T., Schur, P.H., Rose, J.A., Decker, J., and Talal, N.: Measurement of serum DNA–binding activity in systemic lupus erythematosus. N. Engl. J. Med. 281:701, 1969.
6. Reichlin, M., and Mattioli, M.: Correlation of a precipitation reaction to RNA-protein antigen and a low prevalence of nephritis in patients with systemic lupus erythematosus. N. Engl. J. Med. 286:908, 1972.
7. Sharp, G.C., Irvin, W.S., Tan, E.M., Gould, R.G., and Holman, H.R.: Mixed connective tissue disease—an apparently distinct rheumatic disease syndrome associated with a specific antibody to an extractable nuclear antigen (ENA). Am. J. Med. 52:148, 1972.
8. Winn, D.M., Wolfe, J.F., Lindberg, D.A., Firstoe, F.H., Kingsland, L., and Sharp, G.C.: Identification of a clinical subset of systemic lupus erythematosus by antibodies to the Sm antigen. Arthritis Rheum. 22:1334, 1979.
9. Fessel, W.J.: ANA-negative systemic lupus erythematosus. Am. J. Med. 64:80, 1978.
10. Gladman, D.D., Chalmers, A., and Urowitz, M.B.: Systemic lupus erythematosus with negative LE cells and antinuclear factor. J. Rheumatol. 5:142, 1978.
11. Agnello, V.: Complement deficiency states. Medicine 57:1, 1978.
12. Dixon, F.J.: Murine lupus—an overview. Arthritis Rheum. 25:721, 1982.
13. Eisenberg, R.A., Tan, E.M., and Dixon, F.J.: Presence of anti-Sm reactivity in autoimmune mouse strains. J. Exp. Med. 147:582, 1978.
14. Fresco, R.: Virus-like particles in SLE. N. Engl. J. Med. 283:1231, 1970.
15. Pincus, T., Blecklow, N.R., Grimley, P.M., and Bellanti, J.A.: Glomerular microtubules of SLE. Lancet 2:1058, 1970.
16. Gyorkey, F., Sinkovics, J.G., Min, K.W., and Gyorkey, P.: A morphologic study on the occurrence and distribution of structures resembling viral nucelocapsids in collagen disease. Am. J. Med. 53:148, 1972.
17. Dreyer, E.O., Muldiyarov, P.Y., Nassonova, V.A., and Alekberova, Z.S.: Endothelial inclusions in nuclear bodies in SLE. Ann. Rheum. Dis. 32:444, 1973.
18. Schaff, Z., Barry, D.W., and Grimley, P.M.: Cytochemistry of tubuloreticular structures in lymphocytes from patients with SLE and in cultured human lymphoid cells. Lab Invest. 29:577, 1973.
19. Phillips, P.E., and Christian, C.L.: Myxovirus antibody increases in human connective tissue disease. Science 168:982, 1970.
20. Phillips, P.E.: The role of viruses in systemic lupus erythematosus. Clin. Rheum. Dis. 1:505, 1975.
21. Rothfield, N.F., Evans, A.S., and Niederman, J.C.: Clinical and laboratory aspects of raised virus antibody titers in systemic lupus erythematosus. Ann. Rheum. Dis. 32:238, 1973.
22. Pincus, T.: Discussion. Virologic studies in murine human lupus. Arthritis Rheum. 21:S85, 1978.
23. Hicks, J.T., Aulakh, G.S., McGrath, P.P., Washington, G.C., Kim, E., and Alepa, F.P.: Search for Epstein-Barr and type C oncornaviruses in systemic lupus erythematosus. Arthritis Rheum. 22:845, 1979.
24. Phillips, P.E., and Hargrave-Granada, R.: Type C oncornavirus isolation studies in systemic lupus erythematosus. II. Attempted detection by viral RNA–dependent DNA polymerase assay. Ann. Rheum. Dis. 37:225, 1978.
25. Phillips, P.E., Sellers, S.A., and Contronei, S.L.: Type C oncornavirus isolation studies in systemic lupus erythematosus. III. Isolation of a putative retrovirus by triple cell fusion. Ann. Rheum. Dis. 37:234, 1978.
26. Lewis, R.M., Tannenberg, W., Smith, C., and Schwartz, R.S.: C-type viruses in SLE. Nature 252:78, 1974.
27. August, J.T., and Strand, M.: Type C oncornavirus in autoimmunity. Arthritis Rheum. 20:S64, 1977.
28. Panem, S., Ordonez, N.G., Kirstein, W.H., Katz, A.I., and Spargo, B.H.: C-type virus expression in SLE. N. Engl. J. Med. 295:470, 1976.
29. Mellors, R.C., and Mellors, J.W.: Antigen related to mammalian type-C RNA viral P30 proteins located in renal glomeruli in human SLE. Proc. Natl. Acad. Sci. USA 73:233, 1976.
30. Mellors, R.C., and Mellors, J.W.: Type C RNA viral genome expression in systemic lupus erythematosus (SLE). The New Zealand mouse model and the human disease. In Milgrom, F., and Albini, B. (eds.): Immunopathology. Sixth International Convocation on Immunology. Basel, S. Karger 1979, pp. 185–190.

31. Markenson, J.A., Phillips, P.E., Brinkmann, J.P., and Christian, C.L.: Type C virus related antigens on the surface of lymophocytes from normals and patients with SLE. Arthritis Rheum. 19:809, 1976.

32. Aoki, T., Walling, M.J., Bushar, G.S., Liu, M., and Hsu, K.C.: Natural antibodies in sera from healthy humans to antigens on surfaces of type C RNA viruses and cells from primates. Proc. Natl. Acad. Sci. USA 73:2491, 1976.

33. Kurth, R., Teich, N.M., Weiss, R., and Oliver, R.T.D.: Natural human antibodies reactive with primate type-C viral antigens. Proc. Natl. Acad. Sci. USA 74:1237, 1977.

34. Preble, O.T., Black, R.J., Friedman, R.M., Klippel, J.H., and Vilcek, J.: Systemic lupus erythematosus. Presence in human serum of an unusual acid labile leukocyte interferon. Science 23:429, 1982.

35. Yoshiki, T., Mellors, R.C., Strand, M., and August, J.T.: The viral envelope glycoprotein of murine leukemia virus and the pathogenesis of immune complex glomerulonephritis of New Zealand mice. J. Exp. Med. 140:1011, 1974.

36. Blaineau, C., Gisslebrecht, S., Piatier, D., Hurot, M.A., and Levy, J.P.: Swan mice: Autoimmune mice without xenotropic type C virus production*. Clin. Exp. Immunol. 31:276, 1978.

37. Dixon, F.J., Jenson, F.C., McConahey, P.J., and Croker, B.T.: Oncornavirus and immunologic disease. In Meischer, P. (ed.): Microbial Immunopathology. New York, Grune and Stratton, 1977, p. 131.

38. Datta, S.K., Manny, N., Andrzejewski, C., Andre-Schwartz, J., and Schwartz, R.S.: Genetic studies on autoimmunity and retrovirus expression in crosses of New Zealand black mice. I. Xenotropic virus. J. Exp. Med. 147:854, 1978.

39. McKusick, V.A.: Human Genetics, 2nd ed. Englewood Cliffs, N.J. Prentice-Hall Inc., 1969, p. 190.

40. Siegel, M., Holley, H.L., and Lee, S.L.: Epidemiologic studies on systemic lupus erythematosus. Comparative data for New York City and Jefferson County, Alabama, 1956:1965. Arthritis Rheum. 13:802, 1970.

41. Kurland, L.T., Hauser, W.A., Ferguson, R.H., and Holley, K.E.: Epidemiologic features of diffuse connective tissue disorders in Rochester, Minnesota 1951 through 1967 with special reference to systemic lupus erythematosus. Mayo Clin. Proc. 44:649, 1969.

42. Fessel, W.J.: Systemic lupus erythematosus in the community. Arch. Intern. Med. 134:1027, 1974.

43. Serdula, M.K., and Rhoads, G.G.: Frequency of systemic lupus erythematosus in different ethnic groups in Hawaii. Arthritis Rheum. 22:328, 1979.

44. Meddings, J., and Grennan, D.M.: The prevalence of systemic lupus erythematosus (SLE) in Dunedin. N.Z. Med. J. 91:205, 1980.

45. Leonhardt, T.: Family studies in systemic lupus erythematosus. Acta Med. Scand. 416:S1, 1964.

46. Arnett, F.C., and Shulman, L.E.: Studies in familial systemic lupus erythematosus. Medicine 55:313, 1976.

47. Lehman, T.J.A., Hamson, V., Singson, B.H., Kornreich, H.K., Bernstein, B., and King, K.K.: Serum complement abnormalities in the antinuclear antibody-positive relatives of children with systemic lupus erythematosus. Arthritis Rheum. 22:954, 1979.

48. Miller, K.B., and Schwartz, R.S.: Familial abnormalities of suppressor-cell function in systemic lupus erythematosus. N. Engl. J. Med. 301:803, 1979.

49. Winchester, R.J., and Nunez-Roldon, A.: Some genetic aspects of systemic lupus erythematosus. Arthritis Rheum. 25:833, 1982.

50. Block, S.R., Winfield, J.B., Lockshin, M., D'Angelo, W.A., and Christian, C.L.: Studies of twins with systemic lupus erythematosus. A review of the literature and presentation of 12 additional sets. Am. J. Med. 59:533, 1975.

51. Block, S.R., Lockshin, M.D., Winfield, J.B., Weksler, M.E., Masakatsu, I., Winchester, R.J., Mellors, R.C., and Christian, C.L.: Immunologic observations on 9 sets of twins either concordant or discordant for SLE. Arthritis Rheum. 19:545, 1976.

52. Ballou, S.P., Kahn, M., and Kusher, A.: Clinical features of systemic lupus erythematosus. Differences related to race and age of onset. Arthritis Rheum. 25:55, 1982.

53. Morton, R.O., Steinberg, A.D., Gershwin, M.E., and Brady, C.: The incidence of systemic lupus erythematosus in North American Indians. J. Rheum. 3:186, 1976.

54. Grumet, F.C., Coukell, A., Bodmer, J.G., Bodmer, W.F., and McDevitt, H.O.: Histocompatibility (HLA) antigens associated with systemic lupus erythematosus: A possible genetic predisposition to disease. N. Engl. J. Med. 285:193, 1971.

55. Goldberg, M.A., Arnett, F.C., Bias, W.B., and Shulman, L.E.: Histocompatibility antigens in systemic lupus erythematosus. Arthritis Rheum. 19:129, 1976.

56. Dostal, C., Ivanyi, D., Macurova, H., Hana, I., and Strejcek, J.: HLA antigens in systemic lupus erythematosus. Ann. Rheum. Dis. 36:83, 1977.

57. Nies, K.M., Brown, J.C., Dubois, E.L., Quismorio, F.P., Friou, G.J., and Terasaki, P.I.: Histocompatibility (HLA) antigens and lymphocyto-

58. Kampf, D., Malchus, R., Alexander, M., and Hoppe, I.: HLA-antigens in systematic lupus erythematosus (SLE). Arch. Dermatol. Res. 264:345, 1979.

59. Gibofsky, A., Winchester, R., Hansen, J., Patarroyo, M., DuPont, B., Paget, S., Lahita, R., Halper, J., Fotino, M., Yunis, E., and Kunkel, H.G.: Contrasting patterns of newer histocompatibility determinants in patients with rheumatoid arthritis and systemic lupus erythematosus. Arthritis Rheum. 21:S134, 1978.

60. Reinertsen, J.L., Klippel, J.H., Johnson, A.H., Steinberg, A.D., Decker, J.L., and Mann, D.L.: B-lymphocyte alloantigens associated with systemic lupus erythematosus. N. Engl. J. Med. 299:515, 1978.

61. Scherak, O., Smolen, J.S., and Mayr, W.R.: HLA-DRw3 and systemic lupus erythematosus. Arthritis Rheum. 23:954, 1980.

62. Celada, A., Barras, C., Benzonana, G., and Jeannet, M.: Increased frequency of HLA-DRw3 in systemic lupus erythematosus. Tissue Antigens 15:283, 1980.

63. Hawkins, B.R., and Dawkins, R.L.: Autoantibodies in an Australian population. II. Association with HLA antigens. J. Clin. Lab. Immunol. 2:217, 1979.

64. Griffing, W.L., Moore, S.B., Luthra, H.S., McKenna, C.H., and Fathman, C.G.: Associations of antibodies to native DNA and HLA-DRw3. A possible major histocompatibility complex-linked human immune response gene. J. Exp. Med. 152:319s, 1980.

65. Glass, D., Raum, D., Gibson, D., Stillman, J.S., and Schur, P.H.: Inherited deficiency of the second component of complement. Rheumatic diseases associations. J. Clin. Invest. 58:853, 1976.

66. Fu, S.M., Kunkel, H.G., Brusman, H.P., Allen, S.H., Jr., and Fotino, M.: Evidence for the linkage between HLA histocompatibility genes and those involved in the synthesis of the second component of complement. J. Exp. Med. 140:1108, 1974.

67. Berrens, L., Baart de la Faille, H., and Borst-Eilers, E.: HLA-linked C2 deficiency in a Dutch patient with systemic lupus erythematosus. J. Clin. Pathol. 32:528, 1979.

68. Fu, S.M., Stern, R., Kunkel, H.G., DuPont, B., Hansen, J.A., Day, N.K., Good, R.A., Jersild, C., and Fontino, M.: Mixed lymphocyte culture determinants and C2 deficiency: LD-7a associated with C2 deficiency in four families. J. Exp. Med. 142:495, 1975.

69. Kohler, P.F., Percy, J., Campion, W.M., and Smyth, C.J.: Hereditary angioedema and "familial" lupus erythematosus in identical twin boys. Am. J. Med. 56:406, 1974.

70. Donaldson, V.H., Hess, E.V., and McAdams, A.J.: Lupus-erythematosus-like disease in three unrelated women with hereditary angioneurotic edema. Ann. Intern. Med. 86:312, 1977.

71. Aquado, M.T., Perrin, L.H., Miescher, P.A., and Lambert, P.H.: Decreased capacity to solubilize immune complexes in sera from patients with systemic lupus erythematosus. Arthritis Rheum. 24:1225, 1982.

72. Wilson, J.G., Wong, W.W., Schur, P., and Fearon, D.T.: Mode of inheritance of decreased C3b receptors in erythrocytes of patients with systemic lupus erythematosus. N. Engl. J. Med. 307:981, 1982.

73. Hess, E.V.: Introduction to drug related lupus. Kroc Foundation Conference on Drug Induced Lupus. Arthritis Rheum. 24:979, 1981.

74. Perry, H.M., Jr., Tan, E.M., Carmody, S., and Sakamoto, A.: Relationship of acetyl transferase activity to antinuclear antibodies and toxic symptoms in hypertensive patients treated with hydralazine. J. Lab. Clin. Med. 76:114, 1970.

75. Woosely, R.L., Drayer, D.E., Reidenberg, M.M., Nies, A.S., Carr, K., and Oates, J.A.: Effects of acetylator phenotype on the rate at which procainamide induces antinuclear antibodies and the lupus syndrome. N. Engl. J. Med. 298:1157, 1978.

76. Sonnhag, C., Karlsson, E., and Hed, J.: Procainamide-induced lupus erythematosus-like syndrome in relation to acetylator phenotype and plasma levels of procainamide. Acta Med. Scand. 206:245, 1979.

77. Reidenberg, M.M., Drayer, D., DeMarco, A.L., and Bello, C.T.: Hydralazine elimination in man. Clin. Pharmacol. Ther. 14:970, 1973.

78. Johansson, E.A., Mustakallio, K.K., Mattila, M.M., and Tiilikainen, A.: Cutaneous reactions to drugs, acetylation phenotype and HLA antigens in patients with and without systemic lupus erythematosus (SLE). Ann. Clin. Res. 8:126, 1976.

79. Reidenberg, M.M., and Martin, J.H.: The acetylator phenotype of patients with systemic lupus erythematosus. Drug Metab. Dispos. 2:71, 1974.

80. Fishbein, E., and Alarcon-Segovia, D.: Phenotypically low acetyl transferase activity: A characteristic of systemic lupus erythematosus (SLE). Arthritis Rheum. 19:796, 1976.

81. Foad, B., Litwin, A., Zimmer, H., and Hess, E.B.: Acetylator phenotype in systemic lupus erythematosus. Arthritis Rheum. 20:815, 1977.

82. Reidenberg, M.M., Levy, M., Drayer, D.E., Zylber-Katz, E., and Robbins, W.C.: Acetylator phenotype in idiopathic systemic lupus erythematosus. Arthritis Rheum. 23:569, 1980.

83. Vansant, J., Woosley, R.L., John, J.T., and Sergent, J.S.: Normal dis-

tribution of acetylation phenotypes in systemic lupus erythematosus. Arthritis Rheum. 21:192, 1978.

84. Lawson, D.H., Henry, D.A., Lowe, J., Reavey, P., Rennie, J.A.N., Solomon, A.: Acetylator phenotype in spontaneous SLE and rheumatoid arthritis. Ann. Rheum. Dis. 38:171, 1979.

85. Morris, R.J., Freed, C.R., and Kohler, P.F.L.: Drug acetylation phenotype unrelated to development of spontaneous systemic lupus erythematosus. Arthritis Rheum. 22:777, 1979.

86. Dixon, F.J.: Genetic background of murine SLE. Miescher, P.A., Bolis, L., and Torrigiani, G. (eds.): Proceedings of Menarini Foundation Symposium, July 1980. Stuttgart, Schwab Publisher, 1981, pp. 125–134.

87. Theofilopoulos, A.N., McConahey, P.J., Izui, S., Eisenberg, R.A., Pereira, A.B., and Creighton, W.D.: Comparative immunologic analysis of several murine strains with autoimmune manifestations. Clin. Immunol. Immunopathol. 15:258, 1980.

88. Raveche, E.S., Novotny, E.A., Hansen, C.T., Tijo, J.H., and Steinberg, A.D.: Genetic studies in NZB mice. V. Recombinant inbred lines demonstrate that separate genes control autoimmune phenotype. J. Exp. Med. 153:1187, 1981.

89. Murphy, E.D., and Roths, J.B.: A Y chromosome associated factor in strain BXSB producing accelerated autoimmunity and lymphoproliferation. Arthritis Rheum. 22:1188, 1979.

90. Lewis, R.M., and Schwartz, R.S.: Canine systemic lupus erythematosus: Genetic analysis of an established breeding colony. J. Exp. Med. 134:417, 1971.

91. Siegel, M., and Lee, S.L.: The epidemiology of systemic lupus erythematosus. Sem. Arthritis Rheum. 3:1, 1973.

92. Siegel, M., Lee, S.L., and Peress, N.S.: The epidemiology of drug-induced systemic lupus erythematosus. Arthritis Rheum. 10:407, 1967.

93. Durant, P.H., and Harris, R.A.: Hydrazine and lupus. N. Engl. J. Med. 303:584, 1980.

94. Beucher, W.N., Garman, R.H., and Condemi, J.J.: Familial lupus erythematosus—antibodies to DNA in household dogs. N. Engl. J. Med. 296:982, 1977.

95. Steinberg, A.D., and Reinertsen, J.L.: Lupus in New Zealand mice and in dogs. Bull. Rheum. Dis. 28:940, 1978.

96. Oxholm, P., Bendixen, G., Flagstad, A., Jansen, H., Kristensen, S., Manthorpe, R., Wiik, A.: Systemic lupus erythematosus—a zoonosis? Scand. J. Rheum. 8:222, 1979.

97. Clair, D., DeHoratius, R.J., Wolfe, J., and Halliwell, R.: Autoantibodies in human contacts of SLE dogs. Arthritis Rheum. 23:251, 1980.

98. Reinertsen, J.L., Kaslow, R.A., Klippel, J.H., Hurvitz, A.I., Lewis, R.M., Rothfield, N.F., Zvaifler, N.J., Steinberg, A.D., and Decker, J.L.: An epidemiologic study of households exposed to canine systemic lupus erythematosus. Arthritis Rheum. 23:564, 1980.

99. Messner, R.P., and DeHoratius, R.J.: Epidemiology of antilymphocyte antibodies in systemic lupus erythematosus. Arthritis Rheum. 21:S167, 1978.

100. Bluestein, H.G.: Autoantibodies to lymphocyte membrane antigens: Pathogenetic implications. Clin. Rheum. Dis. 4:643, 1978.

101. DeHoratius, R.J., and Messner, R.P.: Lymphocytotoxic antibodies in family members of patients with systemic lupus erythematosus. J. Clin. Invest. 55:1254, 1975.

102. Malave, I., Papa, R., and Layrisse, Z.: Lymphocytotoxic antibodies in SLE patients and their relatives. Arthritis Rheum. 19:700, 1976.

103. Folomeeva, O., Nassonova, V.A., Alekberova, A.S., Talal, N., and Williams, R.C., Jr.: Comparative studies of antilymphocyte, antipolynucleotide, and antiviral antibodies among families of patients with systemic lupus erythematosus. Arthritis Rheum. 21:23, 1978.

104. Raum, D., Glass, D., Soter, N.A., Stillman, J.S., Carpenter, C.B., and Schur, P.H.: Lymphocytotoxic antibodies: HLA antigen associations, disease associations, and family studies. Arthritis Rheum. 20:933, 1977.

105. Cleland, L.G., Bell, D.A., Willans, M., and Saurino, B.C.: Familial lupus: Family studies of HLA and serologic findings. Arthritis Rheum. 21:183, 1978.

106. Carr, R.I., Hoffman, A.A., and Harbeck, R.J.: Comparison of DNA binding in normal populations, general hospital laboratory personnel, and personnel from laboratories studying systemic lupus erythematosus. J. Rheum. 2:178, 1975.

107. Maddock, R.K.: Incidence of systemic lupus erythematosus by age and sex. JAMA 191:137, 1965.

108. Masi, A.T., and Kaslow, R.A.: Sex effects in systemic lupus erythematosus: A clue to pathogenesis. Arthritis Rheum. 21:480, 1978.

109. Stern, R., Fishman, J., Brusman, H., and Kunkel, H.G.: Systemic lupus erythematosus associated with Klinefelter's syndrome. Arthritis Rheum. 20:18, 1977.

110. Lahita, R.G., Bradlow, L., Fishman, J., and Kunkel, H.G.: Estrogen metabolism in systemic lupus erythematosus. Patients and family members. Arthritis Rheum. 25:843, 1982.

111. Jungers, P., Dougados, M., Pelissier, C., Kuttenn, F., Tron, F., Lesavre, P., and Bach, J.F.: Influence of oral contraceptive therapy on the activity of systemic lupus erythematosus. Arthritis Rheum. 25:618, 1982.

112. Roubinian, J.R., Papoian, R., and Talal, N.: Androgen hormones modulate auto-antibody responses and improve survival in murine lupus. J. Clin. Invest. 59:1066, 1977.

113. Roubinian, J.R., Talal, N., Greenspan, J.S., and Siiteri, P.K.: Effect of castration and hormone treatment on survival, anti-nucleic acid antibodies and glomerulonephritis in NZB/NZW F1 mice. J. Exp. Med. 147:1568, 1978.

114. Melez, K.A., Boegel, W.A., and Steinberg, A.D.: Therapeutic studies in New Zealand mice. VII. Successful androgen treatment of NZB/NZW F1 females of different ages. Arthritis Rheum. 23:41, 1980.

115. Roubinian, J.R., Talal, N., Greenspan, J.S., Goodman, J.R., and Siiteri, P.K.: Delayed androgen treatment prolongs survival of murine lupus. J. Clin. Invest. 63:902, 1979.

116. Moyes, E., and Fuchs, S.: Linkage between immune response potential to DNA and X chromosome. Nature 249:167, 1974.

117. Eisenberg, R.A., Lee, S., and Dixon, F.J.: Effect of castration on male-determined acceleration of autoimmune disease in BXSB mice. J. Immunol. 125:1959, 1980.

118. Mitchison, N.A.: Induction of immunologic paralysis with two zones of dosage. Proc. R. Soc. Lond. (Biol.) 161:275, 1966.

119. Claman, H.N., Chaperon, E.A., and Triplett, R.F.: Thymus marrow cell combinations: synergism in antibody production. Proc. Soc. Exp. Med. 122:1167, 1966.

120. Mitchell, G.F., and Miller, J.F.A.P.: Cell to cell interaction in the immune response. II. The source of hemolysin forming cells in irradiated mice given marrow and thymus or thoracic duct lymphocytes. J. Exp. Med. 128:821, 1968.

121. Allison, A.C., and Denman, A.M.: Self-tolerance and autoimmunity. Br. Med. Bull. 32:124, 1976.

122. Burnet, F.M.: The Clonal Selection Theory of Acquired Immunity. Nashville, Tenn., Vanderbilt University Press, 1959.

123. Nossal, G.J.V., and Pike, B.L.: Evidence of the clonal abortion theory of B-lymphocyte tolerance. J. Exp. Med. 141:904, 1975.

124. Bankhurst, A.D., Torrigiani, G., and Allison, A.C.: Lymphocytes binding human thyroglobulin in healthy people and its relevance to tolerance for autoantigens. Lancet 1:226, 1973.

125. Bankhurst, A.D., and Williams, R.C., Jr.: Identification of DNA-binding lymphocytes in patients with systemic lupus erythematosus. J. Clin. Invest. 56:1378, 1975.

126. Paul, W.E., and Benacerraf, B.: Functional specificity of thymus-dependent lymphocytes. Science 195:1293, 1977.

127. Rajewsky, K., Rottlander, E., Peltre, G., and Muller, B.: The immune response to a hybrid protein molecule. Specificity of secondary stimulation and of tolerance induction. J. Exp. Med. 126:581, 1967.

128. Mitchison, N.A.: Antigen recognition responsible for the induction in vitro of the secondary response. Cold Spr. Harb. Symp. Quant. Biol. 32:431, 1967.

129. Kapp, J.A., Pierce, C.W., Theze, J., and Benacerraf, B.: Modulation of immune responses by suppressor T cells. Fed. Proc. 37:2361, 1978.

130. Cosenza, H., and Kohler, H.: Specific suppression of the antibody response by antibody to receptors. Proc. Natl. Acad. Sci. USA 69:2701, 1972.

131. Habicht, G.S., Chiller, J.M., and Weigle, W.O.: Termination of acquired and natural immunological tolerance with specific complexes. J. Exp. Med. 142:312, 1975.

132. Beer, A.E., and Billingham, R.E.: Maternally acquired runt disease. Science 179:240, 1973.

133. Zinkernagel, R.M.: H2 restriction of cell mediated virus specific immunity and immunopathology: Self recognition, altered self and autoaggression. In Talal, N. (ed.): Autoimmunity. New York, Academic Press, 1977, p. 363.

134. Mitchison, N.A.: New ideas about self tolerance and autoimmunity. Clin. Rheum. Dis. 4:539, 1978.

135. Tan, E.M.: Drug-induced autoimmune disease. Fed. Proc. 33:1894, 1974.

136. Sjoberg, O., Anderson, J., and Moller, G.: Lipopolysaccharide can substitute for helper cells in the antibody response in vitro. Eur. J. Immunol. 2:326, 1972.

137. Primi, D., Smith, C.I.E., Hammarstrom, L., and Moller, G.: Polyclonal T cell activators induce immunologic responses to autologous serum protein. Cell. Immunol. 34:367, 1977.

138. Dutton, R.W., Falkoff, R., Hirst, J.A., Hoffmann, M., Kappler, J.W., Kettman, J.R., Lesley, J.F., and Vann, D.: Is there evidence for a nonantigen-specific diffusible chemical mediator from thymus-derived cells in the initiation of the immune response? Prog. Immunol. 1:355, 1971.

139. Katz, D.H.: The allogeneic effect on the immune response: Models for regulatory influences of T lymphocytes on the immune system. Transplant. Rev. 12:141, 1972.

140. Stastny, P., Stembridge, V.A., and Ziff, M.: Homologous disease in the

adult rat, a model for autoimmune disease. I. General features and cutaneous lesions J. Exp. Med. 118:635, 1963.

141. Gleichmann, E., Isaa, P., VanEleven, E.H., and Lamero, M.C.: The chronic graft versus host reaction: A lupus erythematosus-like syndrome caused by abnormal T-B cell interactions. Clin. Rheum. Dis. 4:586, 1978.

142. Failkow, P.J., Gilchrist, C., and Allison, A.C.: Autoimmunity in chronic graft versus host disease. Clin. Exp. Immunol. 13:479, 1973.

143. Katz, D.H., Graves, M., Dorf, M.E., Dimuzio, H., and Benacerraf, B.: Cell interactions between histocompatible T and B lymphocytes. VII. Cooperative responses between lymphocytes are controlled by genes in the I region of the H2 complex. J. Exp. Med. 141:263, 1975.

144. Zinkernagel, R.M., and Doherty, P.C.: Major transplantation antigens, viruses and specificity of surveillance T cells. Contemp. Top. Immunobiol. 7:179, 1977.

145. Kuntz, M.M., Innes, J.B., and Weksler, M.E.: Lymphocyte transformation induced by autologous cells. IV. Human T lymphocyte proliferation induced by autologous or allogeneic non-T lymphocytes. J. Exp. Med. 143:1042, 1976.

146. Goto, M., and Zvaifler, N.J.: Characterization of the killer cell generated in the autologous mixed leukocyte reaction. J. Exp. Med. 157:1309, 1983.

147. Weksler, M.C., Moody, C.E., and Kozak, R.W.: The autologous mixed leukocyte reaction. Adv. Immunol. 31:271, 1981.

148. Asherson, G.L., and Zembala, M.: Inhibitory T cells. Curr. Top. Microbiol. Immunol. 72:56, 1976.

149. Dutton, R.W.: Inhibitory and stimulatory effects of concanavalin A on the response of mouse spleen cell suspensions to antigen. II. Evidence for separate stimulatory and inhibitory cells. J. Exp. Med. 138:1496, 1973.

150. Goldings, E.A., Cohen, P.L., McFadden, S.F., Ziff, M., and Vitetta, E.S.: Defective B cell tolerance in adult (NZB × NZW) F1 mice. J. Exp. Med. 152:730, 1980.

151. Cohen, P.L., Zigg, M., and Vitetta, E.S.: Characterization of a B cell defect in the NZB mouse manifested by an increased ratio of surface IgM to IgD. J. Immunol. 212:973, 1978.

152. Moutsopoulos, H.M., Boehm-Truitt, M., Kassan, S.S., and Chused, T.M.: Demonstration of activation of B lymphocytes in New Zealand mice at birth by an immunoradiometric assay. J. Immunol. 119:1639, 1977.

153. Manny, N., Datta, S.K., and Schwartz, R.S.: Synthesis of IgM by cells of NZB and SWR mice and their crosses. J. Immunol. 122:1220, 1979.

154. Gershwin, M.E., Castles, J.J., Erickson, K., and Ahmed, A.: Studies of congenitally immunologic mutant New Zealand mice. II. Absence of T cell progenitor populations and B cell defects of congenitally athymic (nude) New Zealand black (NZB) mice. J. Immunol. 122:2020, 1979.

155. Ohsugi, Y., and Gershwin, M.E.: Immunologic function in nude New Zealand (NZB/W) F1 mice. Abstracts. Fourth International Congress of Immunology (Paris), 14.3.41, 1980.

156. Chused, T.M., Moutsopoulos, H.M., Sharrow, S.O., Hansen, C.T., and Morse, H.C., III: Mechanism of autoimmune disease in New Zealand black mice. In Rose, N.R., Bigazzi, P.E., and Warner, N.L. (eds.): Genetic Control of Autoimmune Disease. New York, Elsevier/North Holland, 1978, pp. 177–190.

157. Nakajima, P.B., Datta, S.K., Schwartz, R.S., and Huber, B.T.: Localization of spontaneously hyperactive B cells in NZB mice to a specific B cell subset. Proc. Natl. Acad. Sci. USA, 76:4613, 1979.

158. Romain, P.L., Cohen, P.L., Fish, F., Ziff, M., and Vitetta, E.: The specific B cell subset lacking in the CBA/N mouse is not required for autoantibody production in (CBA/N × NZB) F1 mice. J. Immunol. 125:246, 1980.

159. Taurog, J.D., Moutsopoulos, H.M., Rosenberg, Y.J., Chused, T.M., and Steinberg, A.D.: CBA/N X-linked B-cell defect prevents NZB B-cell hyperactivity in F1 mice. J. Exp. Med. 150:31, 1979.

160. Palmer, D., Dauphinee, M., Murry, E., and Talal, N.: Hyperactive T-cell function in young NZB mice: Increased proliferative responses to allogeneic cells. Clin. Exp. Immunol. 23:578, 1976.

161. Taurog, J.D., Raveche, E.S., Smothers, P.A., Glimcher, L.H., Huston, D.P., Hansen, C.T., and Steinberg, A.D.: T cell abnormalities in NZB mice occur independently of autoantibody production. J. Exp. Med. 153:221, 1981.

162. Botzenhardt, U., Klein, J., and Ziff, M.: Primary in vitro cell-mediated lympholysis reaction of NZB mice against unmodified targets syngeneic at the major histocompatibility complex. J. Exp. Med. 147:1435, 1978.

163. Klassen, L.W., Krakauer, R.S., and Steinberg, A.D.: Selective loss of suppressor cell function in New Zealand mice induced by NTA. J. Immunol. 119:830, 1977.

164. Knight, J.G., and Adams, D.D.: Failure of transferred thymus cells to suppress or prevent autoantibody production in NZB and NZB × NZW mice. J. Clin. Lab. Immunol. 1:151, 1978.

165. Roder, J., Bell, D.A., and Singhal, S.: Regulation of the immune response in autoimmune NZB/NZW F1 mice. I. The spontaneous generation of splenic suppressor cells. Cell Immunol. 29:272, 1977.

166. Huber, B., Cantor, H., Shen, F.W., and Boyse, E.A.: Independent differentiative pathways of Ly1 and Ly23 subclasses of T cells: Experimental production of mice deprived of selected T-cell subclasses. J. Exp. Med. 144:1128, 1976.

167. Gershon, R.K., Eardley, D.D., Naidorf, K., and Cantor, H.: Association of defective feedback suppressor cell activity with autoimmunity in NZB mice. Arthritis Rheum. 21:S180, 1978.

168. Cantor, H., McVay-Boudreau, L., Hugenberger, J., Naidorf, K., Shen, F.W., and Gershon, R.K.: Immunoregulatory circuits among T cell sets. II. Physiologic role of feedback in vivo: Absence in NZB mice. J. Exp. Med. 147:1116, 1978.

169. Cowdery, J.S., Taurog, J.D., and Steinberg, A.D.: Effect of CBA/N xid on spontaneous production of antibodies to DNA in MRL/1 and NZB backcross mice. Scand. J. Immunol. 12:499, 1980.

170. Theofilopoulos, A.N., Eisenberg, R.A., Bourdon, M., Crowell, J.S., and Dixon, F.J.: Distribution of lymphocytes identified by surface markers in murine strains with SLE-like syndromes. J. Exp. Med. 149:516, 1979.

171. Lewis, D.E., Giorgi, J.V., and Warner, N.L.: Flow cytometry analysis of T cells and continuous T-cell lines from autoimmune MRL/1 mice. Nature 289:298, 1981.

172. Theofilopoulos, A.N., Shawler, D.L., Eisenberg, R.A., and Dixon, F.J.: Splenic immunoglobulin-secreting cells and their regulation in autoimmune mice. J. Exp. Med. 151:446, 1980.

173. Steinberg, A.D., Roths, J.B., Murphy, E.D., Steinberg, R.T., and Raveche, E.S.: Effects of thymectomy or androgen administration upon the autoimmune disease of MRL/Mp-lpr/lpr mice. J. Immunol. 125:871, 1980.

174. Theofilopoulos, A.N., Balderas, R.S., Shawler, D.L., Lee, S., and Dixon, F.J.: Influence of thymic genotype on the systemic lupus erythematosus-like disease and T cell proliferation of MRL/Mp-lpr/lpr mice. J. Exp. Med. 153:1405, 1981.

175. Prud'Homme, G.J., Park, C.L., Fieser, T.M., Kofler, R., Dixon, F.J., and Theofilopoulos, A.N.: Identification of a B cell differentiation factor(s) spontaneously produced by proliferating T cells in murine lupus strains of the lpr/lpr genotype. J. Exp. Med. 157:730, 1983.

176. Hang, L., Izui, S., Slack, J.H., and Dixon, F.J.: The cellular basis for resistance to induction of tolerance in BXSB SLE male mice. J. Immunol. 129:787, 1982.

177. Hang, L., Izui, S., Theofilopoulos, A.N., and Dixon, F.J.: Suppression of transferred BXSB male SLE disease by female spleen cells. J. Immunol. 128:1805, 1982.

178. Smolen, J.S., Chused, T.M., Leiserson, W.M., Reeves, J.P., Alling, D., and Steinberg, A.D.: Heterogeneity of immunoregulatory T-cell subsets in systemic lupus erythematosus. Correlation with clinical features. Am. J. Med. 72:783, 1982.

179. Louie, J.S., Nies, K.M., Shoji, K.T., et al.: Clinical and antibody responses after influenza immunization in systemic lupus erythematosus. Ann. Intern. Med. 88:790, 1978.

180. Ristow, S.C., Douglas, R.C., and Condemi, J.J.: Influenza vaccination of patients with systemic lupus erythematosus. Ann. Intern. Med. 88:786, 1978.

181. Hahn, B.H., Bagby, M.K., and Osterland, C.K.: Abnormalities of delayed hypersensitivity in systemic lupus erythematosus. Am. J. Med. 55:25, 1973.

182. Rosenthal, C.J., and Franklin, D.C.: Depression of cellular-mediated immunity in systemic lupus erythematosus. Arthritis Rheum. 18:208, 1975.

183. Abe, T., and Homma, M.: Immunoreactivity in patients with systemic lupus erythematosus. Acta Rheum. Scand. 17:35, 1971.

184. Horowitz, D.A.: Impaired delayed hypersensitivity in systemic lupus erythematosus. Arthritis Rheum. 15:353, 1972.

185. Sakane, T., Steinberg, A.D., and Green, I.: Failure of autologous mixed lymphocyte reactions between T and non-T cells in patients with systemic lupus erythematosus. Proc. Natl. Acad. Sci. USA 75:3464, 1978.

186. Sakane, T., Steinberg, A.D., Arnett, F.C., et al.: Studies of immune functions of patients with systemic lupus erythematosus. III. Characterization of lymphocyte subpopulations responsible for defective autologous mixed lymphocyte reactions. Arthritis Rheum. 22:770, 1979.

187. Riccardi, P.J., Hausman, P.B., Raff, H.V., and Stobo, J.D.: The autologous mixed lymphocyte reaction in systemic lupus erythematosus. Arthritis Rheum. 25:820, 1982.

188. Morimoto, C., Reinherz, E.L., Schlossman, S.F., Schur, P.H., Mills, J.A., and Steinberg, A.D.: Alterations of immunoregulatory T cell subsets in active systemic lupus erythematosus. J. Clin. Invest. 66:1171, 1980.

189. Steinberg, A.D., Kalssen, L.W., Budman, D.R., and Williams, G.W.: Immunofluorescence studies of anti-T cell antibodies and T cells in systemic lupus erythematosus: Selective loss of brightly staining T cells in active disease. Arthritis Rheum. 22:114, 1979.

190. Delbarre, F., Go, L.A., and Kahan, A.: Hyperbasophilic immunoblasts

in the circulating blood in chronic inflammatory rheumatic and collagen diseases. Ann. Rheum. Dis. 34:422, 1975.

191. Ginsburg, W.W., Finkelman, F.D., and Lipsky, P.E.: Circulating and pokeweed mitogen-induced immunoglobulin-secreting cells in systemic lupus erythematosus. Clin. Exp. Immunol. 35:76, 1979.

192. Budman, D.R., Merchant, E.B., Steinberg, A.D., Doft, B., Gershwin, M.E., Lizzio, E., and Reeves, J.P.: Increased spontaneous activity of antibody forming cells in the peripheral blood of patients with active SLE. Arthritis Rheum. 20:829, 1977.

193. Jasin, H.E., and Ziff, M.: Immunoglobulin synthesis by peripheral blood cells in systemic lupus erythematosus. Arthritis Rheum. 18:219, 1975.

194. Nies, K.M., and Louis, J.S.: Impaired immunoglobulin synthesis by peripheral blood lymphocytes in systemic lupus erythematosus. Arthritis Rheum. 21:51, 1978.

195. Morimoto, C., Abe, T., Hara, M., and Homma, M.: In vitro TNP-specific antibody formation by peripheral lymphocytes from patients with systemic lupus erythematosus. Scand. J. Immunol. 6:575, 1977.

196. Yu, D.T.Y., Winchester, R.J., Fu, S.M., Gibofsky, A., Ko, H.S., and Kunkel, H.G.: Peripheral blood Ia-positive T cells. J. Exp. Med. 151:91, 1980.

197. Cohen, P.L., Litvin, D.A., and Winfield, J.B.: Association between endogenously activated T cells and immunoglobulin-secreting B cells in patients with active systemic lupus erythematosus. Arthritis Rheum. 25:168, 1982.

198. Bresnihan, B., and Jasin, H.E.: Suppressor function of peripheral blood mononuclear cells in normal individuals and in patients with systemic lupus erythematosus. J. Clin. Invest. 59:106, 1977.

199. Sakane, T., Steinberg, A.D., and Green, I.: Studies of immune functions of patients with systemic lupus erythematosus. I. Dysfunction of suppressor T-cell activity related to impaired generation of, rather than response to, suppressor cells. Arthritis Rheum. 21:657, 1978.

200. Fauci, A.S., Steinberg, A.D., Haynes, B.F., and Whalen, G.: Immunoregulatory aberrations in systemic lupus erythematosus. J. Immunol. 121:1473, 1978.

201. Abdou, N.I., Sagawa, A., Pascual, E., Herbert, J., and Sadeghee. S.: Suppressor T-cell abnormality in idiopathic systemic lupus erythematosus. Clin. Immunol. Immunopathol. 6:192, 1976.

202. Horwitz, D.A., and Consar, J.B.: A relationship between impaired cellular immunity, humoral suppression of lymphocyte functions and severity of SLE. Am. J. Med. 58:829, 1975.

203. Sagawa, A., and Abdou, N.I.: Suppressor-cell dysfunction in systemic lupus erythematosus. Cells involved and in vitro correction. J. Clin. Invest. 62:789, 1978.

204. Tsokos, G.C., Rook, A.H., Djeu, J.Y., and Balow, J.E.: Natural killer cells and interferon responses in patients with systemic lupus erythematosus. Clin. Exp. Immunol. 50:239, 1982.

205. Strannegard, O., Hermodsson, S., and Westberg, G.: Interferon and natural killer cells in systemic lupus erythematosus. Clin. Exp. Immunol. 50:246, 1982.

206. Katz, P., Zaytoun, A.M., Lee, J.H., Jr., Panush, R.S., and Longley, S.: Abnormal natural killer cell activity in systemic lupus erythematosus: An intrinsic defect in the lytic event. J. Immunol. 129:1966, 1982.

207. Goto, M., Tanimoto, K., and Horiuchi, Y.: Natural cell mediated cytotoxicity in systemic lupus erythematosus. Arthritis Rheum. 23:1274, 1980.

208. Mittal, K.K., Rossen, R.D., Sharp, J.T., Lidsky, M.D., and Butler, W.T.: Lymphocyte cytotoxic antibodies in systemic lupus erythematosus. Nature 225:1255, 1970.

209. Terasaki, P.I., Mottironi, V.D., and Barnett, E.V.: Cytotoxins in disease. Autocytotoxins in lupus. N. Engl. J. Med. 283:724, 1970.

210. Williams, R.C., Jr., Lies, R.B., and Messner, R.P.: Inhibition of mixed leukocyte culture responses by serum and γ-globulin fractions from certain patients with connective tissue disorders. Arthritis Rheum. 16:597, 1973.

211. Wernet, P., and Kunkel, H.G.: Antibodies to a specific surface antigen of T cells in human sera inhibiting mixed leukocyte culture reactions. J. Exp. Med. 38:1021, 1973.

212. Horwitz, D.A., and Cousar, J.B.: A relationship between impaired cellular immunity, humoral suppression of lymphocyte function and severity of systemic lupus erythematosus. Am. J. Med. 58:829, 1975.

213. Mahowald, M.L., and Dalmasso, A.P.: Lymphocyte destruction by antibody-dependent cellular cytotoxicity mediated in vitro by antibodies in serum from patients with systemic lupus erythematosus. Ann. Rheum. Dis. 41:593, 1982.

214. Pope, R.M., Keightley, R., and McDuffey, S.: Circulating autoantibodies to IgD in rheumatic diseases. J. Immunol. 128:1860, 1982.

215. Sakane, T., Steinberg, A.D., Reeves, J.P., and Green, I.: Studies of immune functions of patients with systemic lupus erythematosus. Complement-dependent immunoglobulin anti-thymus-derived cell antibodies preferentially inactive suppressor cells. J. Clin. Invest. 63:954, 1979.

216. Okudaira, K., Nakai, H., Hayakawa, T., Kashiwado, T., Tanimoto, K.,

217. Morimoto, C., Reinherz, E.L., Abe, T., Homma, M., and Schlossman, S.F.: Characteristics of anti-T-cell antibodies in systemic lupus erythematosus: evidence for selective reactivity with normal suppressor cells defined by monoclonal antibodies. Clin. Immunol. Immunopathol. 16:474, 1980.

218. Honda, M., Sakane, T., Steinberg, A.D., Kotani, H., Tsunematsu, T., Moriyama, K., and Fukase, M.: Studies of immune functions of patients with systemic lupus erythematosus: antibodies to desialized, rather than intact, T cells preferentially bind to and eliminate suppressor effector T cells. J. Clin. Invest. 69:940, 1982.

219. Sakane, T., Steinberg, A.D., Reeves, J.P., et al.: Studies of immune function in patients with systemic lupus erythematosus. T cell subsets and antibodies to T cell subsets. J. Clin. Invest. 64:1260, 1979.

220. Hahn, B.H., Pletscher, L.S., Munialn, M., and MacDermott, R.P.: Suppression of the normal autologous mixed leukocyte reaction by sera from patients with systemic lupus erythematosus. Arthritis Rheum. 25:381, 1982.

221. Okudaira, K., Searles, R.P., Goodwin, J.S., and Williams, R.C., Jr.: Antibodies in the sera of patients with systemic lupus erythematosus that block the binding of monoclonal anti-Ia to Ia-positive targets also inhibit the autologous mixed lymphocyte response. J. Immunol. 129:582, 1982.

222. Winfield, J.B., Cohen, P.L., and Litvin, D.A.: Antibodies to activated T cells and their soluble products in systemic lupus erythematosus. Arthritis Rheum. 25:814, 1982.

223. Messner, R.P., DeHoratius, R., and Ferrone, S.: Lymphocytotoxic antibodies in systemic lupus erythematosus patients and their relatives. Reactivity with the HLA antigenic molecular complex. Arthritis Rheum. 23:265, 1980.

224. Revillard, J.P., Vincent, C., and Rivera, S.: Anti-β_2 microglobulin lymphocytotoxic autoantibodies in systemic lupus erythematosus. J. Immunol. 122:614, 1979.

225. Okudaira, K., Searles, R.P., Ceuppens, J.L., Goodwin, J.S., and Williams, R.C., Jr.: Anti-Ia reactivity in sera from patients with systemic lupus erythematosus. J. Clin. Invest. 69:17, 1982.

226. Rekvig, O.P., and Hannestad, K.: Human autoantibodies that react with both cell nuclei and plasma membranes display specificity for the octamer of histones H2A, H2B, H3 and H4 in high salt. J. Exp. Med. 152:1720, 1980.

227. Searles, R.P., Messner, R.P., and Bankhurst, A.D.: Cross-reactivity of antilymphocyte and antinuclear antibodies in systemic lupus erythematosus. Clin. Immunol. Immunopathol. 14:292, 1979.

228. Von Pirquet, C.E.: Allergy. Arch. Intern. Med. 7:259, 1911.

229. Germuth, F.G., Jr.: A comparative histologic and immunologic study in rabbits of induced hypersensitivity of the serum sickness type. J. Exp. Med. 97:257, 1953.

230. Dixon, F.J., Vazquez, J.J., Weigle, W.O., and Cochrane, C.G.: Pathogenesis of serum sickness. Arch. Pathol. 65:18, 1958.

231. Cochrane, C.G., and Koffler, D.: Immune complex disease in experimental animals and man. Adv. Immunol. 16:185, 1973.

232. Wilson, C.B., and Dixon, F.J.: Antigen quantitation in experimental immune complex glomerulonephritis. I. Acute serum sickness. J. Immunol. 105:279, 1970.

233. Dixon, F.J., Feldman, J.D., and Vazquez, J.J.: Experimental glomerulonephritis. The pathogenesis of a laboratory model resembling the spectrum of glomerulonephritis. J. Exp. Med. 113:899, 1961.

234. Wilson, C.B., and Dixon, F.J.: Quantitation of acute and chronic serum sickness in the rabbit. J. Exp. Med. 134:7s, 1971.

235. Benacerraf, B., McCluskey, R.T., and Patras, D.: Localization of colloidal substances in vascular endothelium. A mechanism of tissue damage. Am. J. Pathol. 35:75, 1959.

236. Kniker, W.T., and Cochrane, C.G.: The localization of circulating immune complexes in experimental serum sickness. The role of vasoactive amines and hydrodynamic forces. J. Exp. Med. 127:119, 1968.

237. Cochrane, C.G.: Mechanisms involved in deposition of immune complexes in tissues. J. Exp. Med. 134:75s, 1971.

238. Benveniste, J., Henson, P.M., and Cochrane, C.G.: Leukocyte dependent histamine release from rabbit platelets—the role of IgE, basophils and a platelet activating factor. J. Exp. Med. 136:1356, 1972.

239. Kniker, W.T.: Amelioration of progressive complex-induced chronic glomerulonephritis by antagonists of vasoactive amines. Fed. Proc. 29:287, 1970.

240. Chused, T.M., and Tarpley, T.M., Jr.: Antagonism of vasoactive amines in NZB/W glomerulonephritis. I. Beneficial effects of methysergide. Proc. Soc. Exp. Biol. Med. 144:281, 1973.

241. Kniker, W.T.: Modulation of the inflammatory response in vivo: prevention or amelioration of immune complex disease. *In* Lepow, I.H.,

and Ward, P.H. (eds.): Inflammation, Mechanisms and Control. New York, Academic Press, 1972, p. 335.

242. Fisher, E.R., and Bark, J.: Effect of hypertension on vascular and other lesions of serum sickness. Am. J. Pathol. 39:665, 1961.

243. Cochrane, C.G., and Hawkins, D.J.: Studies on circulating immune complexes. III. Factors governing the circulating complexes to localize in blood vessels. J. Exp. Med. 127:137, 1968.

244. Weigle, W.O.: Fate and biological action of antigen-antibody complexes. Adv. Immunol. 1:283, 1961.

245. Benacerraf, B., Sebestyen, M., and Cooper, N.S.: The clearance of antigen-antibody complexes from the blood by the reticuloendothelial system. J. Immunol. 82:131, 1959.

246. Kimberly, R.P., and Ralph, P.: Endocytosis by the mononuclear phagocyte system and autoimmune disease. Am. J. Med. 74:481, 1983.

247. Takahashi, N., Takahashi, J., and Hirosi, S.: Solubilization of antigen-antibody complexes: A new function of complement as a regulator of immune reactions. Prog. Allergy 27:134, 1980.

248. Soothill, J.F., and Steward, M.W.: The immunopathologic significance of the heterogeneity of antibody affinity. Clin. Exp. Immunol. 9:193, 1971.

249. Pincus, T., Haberkern, R., and Christian, C.L.: Experimental chronic glomerulitis. J. Exp. Med. 127:819, 1968.

250. Howie, J.B., and Helyer, B.J.: The immunology and pathology of NZB mice. Adv. Immunol. 9:215, 1968.

251. Lambert, P.H., and Dixon, F.J.: Pathogenesis of the glomerulonephritis of NZB/W mice. J. Exp. Med. 127:507, 1968.

252. Ebling, F., and Hahn, B.H.: Restricted subpopulations of DNA antibodies in kidneys of mice with systemic lupus: Comparison of antibodies in serum and renal eluates. Arthritis Rheum. 23:392, 1980.

253. Mellors, R.C., Shirai, T., Toshikazu, S., Aoki, T., Huebner, R.J., and Krawczynski, K.: Wild type gross leukemia virus and the pathogenesis of the glomerulonephritis of New Zealand mice. J. Exp. Med. 133:113, 1971.

254. Dixon, F.J., Oldstone, M.B., and Tonietti, G.: Pathogenesis of immune complex glomerulonephritis of New Zealand mice. J. Exp. Med. 134:65s, 1971.

255. Nakai, Y., Maruyama, N., Ohta, K., Yoshida, H., Hirose, S., and Shirai, T.: Genetic studies of autoimmunity in New Zealand mice. Association of circulating retroviral gp70 immune complex with proteinuria. Immunol. Lett. 2:53, 1980.

256. Izui, S., McConahey, P.J., Theofilopoulos, A.N., and Dixon, F.J.: Association of circulating retroviral gp70-anti-gp70 immune complexes with murine system lupus erythematosus. J. Exp. Med. 149:1099, 1979.

257. Schur, P.H.: Complement in lupus. Clin. Rheum. Dis. 1:519, 1975.

258. Townes, A.S., Stewart, C.R., Jr., and Osler, A.G.: Immunologic studies of systemic lupus erythematosus. II. Variations of nucleoprotein-reactive gamma globulin and hemolytic serum complement levels with disease activity. Bull. Johns Hopkins Hosp. 112:202, 1963.

259. Gewurtz, H.R., Pickering, R.J., Mergenhagen, S.G., and Good, R.A.: The complement profile in acute glomerulonephritis, systemic lupus erythematosus and hypocomplementemic glomerulonephritis. Int. Arch. Allergy Immunol. 34:556, 1968.

260. Kohler, P.F., Ten Bensel, R.: Serial complement component alterations in acute glomerulonephritis and systemic lupus erythematosus. Clin. Exp. Immunol. 4:191, 1969.

261. Hunsicker, L.G., Ruddy, S., Carpenter, C.B., Schur, P.H., Merrill, J.P., Muller-Eberhard, H.J., and Austen, K.F.: Metabolism of third complement component (C3) in nephritis. N. Engl. J. Med. 281:835, 1972.

262. Sliwinski, A.F., and Zvaifler, N.J.: Decreased synthesis of the third component of complement (C3) in hypocomplementemic systemic lupus erythematosus. Clin. Exp. Immunol. 11:21, 1972.

263. Charlesworth, J.A., Gwyn Williams, D., Sherington, E., Lachmann, P.J., and Peters, D.K.: Metabolic studies of the third component of complement and the glycine-rich beta glycoprotein in patients with hypocomplementemia. J. Clin. Invest. 53:1578, 1974.

264. Ruddy, S., Carpenter, C.B., Chin, K.W., Knostman, J.N., Soter, N.A., Gotze, O., Muller-Eberhard, H.J., and Austen, K.F.: Human complement metabolism: An analysis of 144 studies. Medicine 54:165, 1975.

265. Sissons, J.G.P., Liebowitch, J., Amos, N., and Peters, D.K.: Metabolism of the fifth component of complement, and its relation to the metabolism of the third component, in patients with complement activation. J. Clin. Invest. 59:704, 1977.

266. Perrin, L.H., Lambert, P.H., and Miescher, P.A.: Complement breakdown products in plasma from patients with systemic lupus erythematosus and patients with membranoproliferative or other glomerulonephritis. J. Clin. Invest. 56:165, 1975.

267. Perrin, L.H., Lambert, P.H., Nydegger, U.E., and Miescher, P.A.: Quantitation of C3PA (Properdin factor B) and other complement components in diseases associated with a low C3 level. Clin. Immunol. Immunopathol. 2:16, 1973.

268. Wilson, M.R., Arroya, C.M., Nakamura, R.M., Vaughan, J.H., and Tan,

E.M.: Activation of the alternative complement pathway in systemic lupus erythematosus. Clin. Exp. Immunol. 26:11, 1976.

269. Lachmann, P.J., and Nichol, P.: Reaction mechanism of the alternative pathway of complement fixation. Lancet 1:465, 1973.

270. Whaley, K., Schur, P.H., and Ruddy, S.: Relative importance of C3b inactivator and beta 1H globulin in the modulation of the properdin amplification loop in systemic lupus erythematosus. Clin. Exp. Immunol. 36:408, 1979.

271. Zubler, R.H., and Lambert, P.H.: Detection of immune complexes in human diseases. Prog. Allergy 24:85, 1978.

272. Holman, H.R., and Deicher, H.R.: The reaction of lupus erythematosus (LE) cell factor with deoxyribonucleoprotein of the cell nucleus. J. Clin. Invest. 38:2059, 1959.

273. Stollar, B.D., and Levine L.: Antibodies to denatured desoxyribonucleic acid in a lupus erythematosus serum. J. Immunol. 87:477, 1961.

274. Tan, E.M., Schur, P.H., Carr, R.I., and Kunkel, H.G.: Desoxyribose-nucleic acid (DNA) and antibodies to DNA in the serum of patients with systemic lupus erythematosus. J. Clin. Invest. 45:1732, 1966.

275. Koffler, D., Carr, R., Agnello, V., Thoburn, R., and Kunkel, H.G.: Antibodies to polynucleotides in human sera: Antigen specificity and relation to disease. J. Exp. Med. 134:294, 1971.

276. Lafer, E.M., Valle, R.P.C., Möller, A., Nordheim, A., Schur, P.H., Rich, A., and Stollar, D.B.: Z-DNA-specific antibodies in human systemic lupus erythematosus. J. Clin. Invest. 71:314, 1983.

277. Shoenfeld, Y., Rauch, J., Massicotti, H., Datta, S.K., Schwartz, J.A., Stollar, B.D., and Schwartz, R.: Polyspecificity of monoclonal lupus autoantibodies produced by human-human hybridomas. N. Engl. J. Med. 308:414, 1983.

278. Tan, E.M.: An immunologic precipitin system between soluble nucleoprotein and serum antibody in systemic lupus erythematosus. J. Clin. Invest. 46:735, 1967.

279. Tan, E.M., and Kunkel, H.G.: Characteristics of a soluble nuclear antigen precipitating with sera of patients with systemic lupus erythematosus. J. Immunol. 96:464, 1966.

280. Lerner, E.A., Lerner, M., Hardin, J., Janeway, C.A., Jr., and Seitz, J.A.: Deciphering the mysteries of RNA-containing lupus antigens. Arthritis Rheum. 25:761, 1982.

281. Lerner, M.R., Boyle, J.A., Hardin, J., and Seitz, J.A.: Two novel classes of small ribonucleo proteins detected by antibodies associated with systemic lupus. Science 211:400, 1981.

282. Schur, P.H., Stollar, D., Steinberg, A.D., and Talal, N.: Incidence of antibodies to double stranded RNA in systemic erythematosus and related diseases. Arthritis Rheum. 14:342, 1971.

283. Koffler, D., Agnello, V., Thoburn, R., and Kunkel, H.G.: Systemic lupus erythematosus: Prototype of immune complex nephritis in man. J. Exp. Med. 134:169s, 1971.

284. Koffler, D., Agnello, V., Winchester, R., and Kunkel, H.G.: The occurrence of single-stranded DNA in the serum of patients with systemic lupus erythematosus and other diseases. J. Clin. Invest. 52:198, 1973.

285. Talal, N., Pillarisetty, R.J., DeHoratius, R.J., and Messner, R.P.: Immunologic regulation of spontaneous antibodies to DNA and RNA. I. Significance of IgM and IgG antibodies in SLE patients and asymptomatic relatives. Clin. Exp. Immunol. 25:377, 1976.

286. Edmonds, J.P., Johnson, G.D., Ansell, B.M., and Holborow, E.J.: The value of tests for antibody to DNA in monitoring the clinical course of SLE. A long-term study using the Farr test and the DNA counter immunoelectrophoretic method. Clin. Exp. Immunol. 22:9, 1975.

287. Holgate, S., Glass, D., Haslam, P., Maini, T., and Turner-Warwick, M.: Respiratory involvement in systemic lupus erythematosus: A clinical and immunologic study. Clin. Exp. Immunol. 24:385, 1976.

288. Leon, S.A., Green, A., Ehrlich, G.E., Poland, M., and Shapiro, B.: Avidity of antibodies in SLE. Relations to severity of renal involvement. Arthritis Rheum. 20:23, 1977.

289. Winfield, J.B., Faiferman, I., and Koffler, D.: Avidity of anti-DNA antibodies in serum and in IgG glomerular eluates in patients with systemic lupus erythematosus. Association of high avidity and high DNA antibody with glomerulonephritis. J. Clin. Invest. 59:90, 1977.

290. Halsey, J.F., Woolery, W.A., Oleinick, S., Kahaleh, M.B., and LeRoy, E.C.: DNA binding activity of serum from patients with systemic lupus erythematosus. Clin. Exp. Immunol. 35:365, 1979.

291. Schur, P.H., Monroe, M., and Rothfield, N.: The γG subclass of antinuclear and antinucleic acid antibodies. Arthritis Rheum. 15:174, 1972.

292. Beaulieu, A., Quismorio, F.P., Jr., Kitridou, R.C., and Friou, G.J.: Complement fixing antibodies to ds-DNA in systemic lupus erythematosus: A study using the immunofluorescent Crithidia luciliae method. J. Rheumatol. 6:389, 1979.

293. Frank, M.M., Lawley, T.J., Hamburger, M.I., and Brown, E.J.: Immunoglobulin G Fc receptor mediated clearance in autoimmune disease. Ann. Intern. Med. 98:206, 1983.

294. Finbloom, D.S., and Plotz, P.H.: Studies of reticuloendothelial function in the mouse with model immune complexes. II. Serum clearance, tissue

uptake and reticuloendothelial saturation in NZB/W mice. J. Immunol. 123:1600, 1979.

295. Miyakawa, Y., Yamada, A., Kosaka, K., Tsuda, F., Kosugi, E., and Mayumi, M.: Defective immune adherence (C3b) receptors on erythrocytes from patients with systemic lupus erythematosus. Lancet II:493, 1981.

296. Iida, K., Mornaghi, R., and Nussenzweig, V.: Complement receptor (CR) deficiency in erythrocytes from patients with systemic lupus erythematosus. J. Exp. Med. 155:1427, 1982.

297. Agnello, V., Koffler, D., Eisenberg, J.W., Winchester, R.J., and Kunkel, H.G.: C1q precipitins in the sera of patients with systemic lupus erythematosus and other hypocomplementemic states: Characterization of high and low molecular weight types. J. Exp. Med. 134:228S, 1971.

298. Maini, R.N., and Holborow, E.J. (eds.): Detection and measurement of circulating soluble antigen-antibody complexes and anti-DNA antibodies. Ann. Rheum. Dis. 36:(Suppl. 1), 1977.

299. Eisenberg, R.A., Theofilopoulos, A., and Dixon, F.J.: Use of conglutinin for the assay of immune complexes. J. Immunol. 118:1428, 1977.

300. Davis, J.S., Godfrey, S.M., and Winfield, J.D.: Direct evidence for circulating DNA–anti-DNA complexes in systemic lupus erythematosus. Arthritis Rheum. 21:17, 1978.

301. Bruneau, C., and Benveniste, J.: Circulating DNA: anti-DNA complexes in systemic lupus erythematosus. J. Clin. Invest. 64:191, 1979.

302. Sano, H., and Morimoto, C.: Isolation of DNA from DNA/anti-DNA immune complexes in systemic lupus erythematosus. J. Immunol. 126:538, 1981.

303. Izui, S., Lambert, P.H., and Miescher, P.A.: Failure to detect circulating DNA-anti-DNA complexes by four radioimmunological methods in patients with systemic lupus erythematosus. Clin. Exp. Immunol. 30:384, 1977.

304. Theofilopoulos, A.N., and Dixon, F.J.: Immune complexes in human sera detected by the Raji cell radioimmunoassay. In Bloom, B.R., and David, J.R. (eds.): In Vitro Methods in Cell-Mediated and Tumor Immunology. New York, Academic Press, 1976, p. 555.

305. Christian, C.L.: Immune-complex disease. N. Engl. J. Med. 280:878, 1969.

306. Christian, C.L., Hatfield, W.B., and Chase, P.H.: Systemic lupus erythematosus: Cryoprecipitation of sera. J. Clin. Invest. 42:823, 1963.

307. Hanauer, L.B., and Christian, C.L.: Studies of cryoproteins in systemic lupus erythematosus. J. Clin. Invest. 46:400, 1967.

308. Stastny, P., and Ziff, M.: Cold-insoluble complexes and complement levels in systemic lupus erythematosus. N. Engl. J. Med. 280:1376, 1969.

309. Winfield, J.B., Koffler, D., and Kunkel, H.G.: Specific concentration of polynucleotide immune complexes in the cryoprecipitates of patients with systemic lupus erythematosus. J. Clin. Invest. 56:563, 1975.

310. Winfield, J.B., Winchester, R.J., Wernet, P., and Kunkel, H.G.: Specific concentration of antilymphocyte antibodies activity in the serum cryoprecipitates of patients with SLE. Clin. Exp. Immunol. 19:399, 1977.

311. Zvaifler, N.J., and Bluestein, H.G.: Lymphocytotoxic antibody activity in cryoprecipitates from serum of patients with SLE. Arthritis Rheum. 19:844, 1976.

312. Agnello, V., Koffler, D., and Kunkel, H.G.: Immune complex systems in the nephritis of systemic lupus erythematosus. Kidney Int. 3:90, 1973.

313. Klippel, J.H., Bluestein, H.G., and Zvaifler, N.J.: Lymphocyte reactivity of antisera to cryoproteins in systemic lupus erythematosus. Clin. Immunol. Immunopathol. 12:52, 1979.

314. Bluestein, H.G., Klippel, J.H., and Zvaifler, N.J.: Antibodies to neuronal cells in antisera to SLE cryoproteins. Arthritis Rheum. 21:546, 1978.

315. Mellors, R.C., Ortega, L.G., and Holman, H.R.: Role of γ globulins in pathogenesis of renal lesions in systemic lupus erythematosus and chronic membranous glomerulonephritis, with an observation on lupus erythematosus cell reaction. J. Exp. Med. 106:191, 1957.

316. Paronetto, F., and Koffler, D.: Immunofluorescent localization of immunoglobulins, complement, and fibrinogen in human diseases. I. Systemic lupus erythematosus. J. Clin. Invest. 44:1657, 1965.

317. McCluskey, R.T., Vassalli, P., Gallo, G., and Baldwin, D.S.: An immunofluorescent study of pathogenic mechanisms in glomerular diseases. N. Engl. J. Med. 274:695, 1966.

318. Koffler, D., Agnello, V., Carr, R.I., and Kunkel, H.G.: Variable patterns of immunoglobulin and complement deposition in the kidneys of patients with systemic lupus erythematosus. Am. J. Pathol. 56:305, 1969.

319. Lewis, E.J., Busch, G.J., and Schur, P.H.: Gamma G globulin subgroup composition of the glomerular deposits in renal diseases. J. Clin. Invest. 49:1103, 1970.

320. Krishnan, C., and Kaplan, M.H.: Immunopathologic studies of systemic lupus erythematosus. II. Antinuclear reaction of γ-globulin eluted from homogenates and isolated glomeruli of kidneys from patients with lupus nephritis. J. Clin. Invest. 46:569, 1967.

321. Koffler, D., Schur, P.H., and Kunkel, H.G.: Immunological studies concerning the nephritis of systemic lupus erythematosus. J. Exp. Med. 126:607, 1967.

322. Koffler, D., Agnello, V., and Kunkel, H.G.: Polynucleotide immune complexes in serum and glomeruli of patients with systemic lupus erythematosus. Am. J. Pathol. 74:109, 1974.

323. Andres, R.A., Accinni, L., Beiser, S.M., Christian, C.L., Cinotti, G.A., Erlanger, B.F., Hsu, K.C., and Seegal, B.C.: Localization of fluorescein labelled antinucleotide antibodies in glomeruli of patients with active systemic lupus erythematosus and nephritis. J. Clin. Invest. 49:2106, 1970.

324. Brentjens, J.R., Sepulveda, M., and Balish, T.: Interstitial immune complex nephritis in patients with systemic lupus erythematosus. Kidney Int. 7:342, 1975.

325. Méry, J.P., Morel-Maroger, L., Boelaert, J., and Richet, G.: Evolution anatomo-clinique des glomérulites diffuses et focales au cours du lupus érythémateux disséminé. Nephrol. J. Urol. 79:321, 1973.

326. Rothfield, N., Ross, A., Minta, J.O., and Lepow, I.H.: Glomerular and dermal deposition of properidin in systemic lupus erythematosus. N. Engl. J. Med. 287:681, 1972.

327. Verroust, P.J., Wilson, C.B., Cooper, N.R., Edgington, T.S., and Dixon, F.J.: Glomerular complement components in human glomerulonephritis. J. Clin. Invest. 53:77, 1974.

328. Carlo, J.R., Ruddy, S., Sauter, S., and Yount, W.J.: Deposition of B 1H in renal biopsies from patients with immune renal disease. Arthritis Rheum. 22:403, 1979.

329. Biesecker, G., Katz, S., and Koffler, D.: Renal localization of the membrane attack complex in systemic lupus erythematosus nephritis. J. Exp. Med. 154:1779, 1981.

330. Hill, G.S., Hingoais, N., Tron, F., and Bach, J.F.: Systemic lupus erythematosus: Morphologic correlations with immunologic and clinical data at the time of biopsy. Am. J. Med. 64:61, 1978.

331. Donadio, J.V., Conn, D.L., Holley, K.E., and Ilsterp, D.M.: Class of immunoglobulin deposition and prognosis in lupus nephritis. Mayo Clin. Proc. 53:366, 1978.

332. Clough, J.D., and Valenzuela, R.: Relationship of renal histopathology in SLE nephritis to immunoglobulin class of anti-DNA. Am. J. Med. 68:80, 1980.

333. Couser, W.G., Jermanovich, N.B., Delok, S., Stilmant, M., and Hower, J.R.: Effect of aminonucleoside nephrosis on immune complex localization in autologous immune complex nephropathy in rats. J. Clin. Invest. 61:651, 1978.

334. Brenner, B.M., Hostetter, T.H., and Humes, D.H.: Molecular basis of proteinuria of glomerular origin. N. Engl. J. Med. 298:826, 1978.

335. Kijlstra, A., Knutson, D.W., Daha, M.R., and van Es, L.A.: Clearance and glomerular localization of preformed DNP anti-DNA immune complexes. Scand. J. Immunol. 10:421, 1979.

336. Izui, S., Lambert, P.H., and Miescher, P.A.: In vitro demonstration of a particular affinity of glomerular basement membrane and collagen for DNA. A possible basis for a local formation of DNA-anti-DNA complexes in systemic lupus erythematosus. J. Exp. Med. 144:428, 1976.

337. Izui, S, Lambert, P.H., Fournie, G.J., Turler, H., and Miescher, P.A.: Features of systemic lupus erythematosus in mice injected with bacterial lipopolysaccharides. Identification of circulating DNA and renal localization of DNA-anti-DNA complexes. J. Exp. Med. 145:1115, 1977.

338. Friend, P.S., Kim, Y., and Donadio, J.G.: Pathogenesis of membranous nephropathy in systemic lupus erythematosus: The possible role of non-precipitating DNA antibody. Br. Med. J. 1:25, 1977.

339. Ooi, Y.M., Ooi, B.S., and Pollak, V.E.: The relationship of levels of circulating immune complexes to histologic patterns of nephritis: A comparative study of membranous glomerulonephropathy and diffuse proliferative glomerulonephritis. J. Lab. Clin. Med. 90:891, 1977.

340. Hebra, F., and Kaposi, M.: On Diseases of the Skin, Including the Exanthemata. Translated and Edited by W. Tay. London, The New Sydenham Society, 1875.

341. Burnham, T.K., Neblett, T.R., and Fine, G.: The application of the fluorescent antibody technique to the investigation of lupus erythematosus and various dermatoses. J. Invest. Dermatol. 41:451, 1963.

342. Cormane, R.H.: "Bound" globulin in the skin of patients with chronic discoid lupus erythematosus and systemic lupus erythematosus. Lancet 1:534, 1964.

343. Biesecker, G., Lavin, L., Ziskind, M., and Koffer, D.: Cutaneous localization of the membrane attack complex in discoid and systemic lupus erythematosus. N. Engl. J. Med. 306:264, 1982.

344. Schrager, M.A., and Rothfield, N.F.: The lupus band test. Clin. Rheum. Dis. 1:597, 1975.

345. Burnham, T.K., and Fine, G.: The immunofluorescent "band" test for lupus erythematosus. III. Employing clinically normal skin. Arch. Dermatol. 103:24, 1971.

346. Caperton, E.M., Jr., Bean, S.F., and Dick, F.R.: Immunofluorescent skin test in systemic lupus erythematosus. Lack of relationship with renal disease. JAMA 222:935, 1972.

347. Gilliam, J.N., Cheatum, D.E., Hurd, E.R., Stastny, P., and Ziff, M.:

Immunoglobulin in clinically uninvolved skin in systemic lupus erythematosus: Association with renal disease. J. Clin. Invest. 53:1434, 1974.

348. Grossman, J., Callerame, M.L., and Condemi, J.J.: Skin immunofluorescence studies on lupus erythematosus and other antinuclear-antibody-positive-diseases. Ann. Intern. Med. 80:496, 1974.

349. Jordan, R.E., Schroeter, A.L., and Winkelmann, R.K.: Dermal-epidermal deposition of complement components and properdin in systemic lupus erythematosus. Br. J. Dermatol. 92:263, 1975.

350. Schrager, M.A., and Rothfield, N.F.: Clinical significance of serum properdin levels and properdin deposition in the dermal-epidermal junction in systemic lupus erythematosus. J. Clin. Invest. 57:212, 1976.

351. Pohle, E.L., and Tuffanelli, D.L.: Study of cutaneous lupus erythematosus by immunohistochemical methods. Arch. Dermatol. 97:520, 1968.

352. Noel, L.H., Droz, D., and Rothfield, N.: Clinical and serologic significance of cutaneous deposits of immunoglobulins, C3 and C1q, in SLE patients with nephritis. Clin. Immunol. Immunopathol. 10:381, 1978.

353. Provost, T.T., Andres, G., Maddison, P.J., and Reichlin, M.: Lupus band test in untreated SLE patients: Correlation of immunoglobulin deposition in the skin of the extensor forearm with clinical renal disease and serological abnormalities. J. Invest. Dermatol. 74:407, 1980.

354. Morris, R.J., Guggenheim, S.J., McIntosh, R.M., Rubin, R.L., and Kohler, P.F.: Simultaneous immunologic studies of skin and kidney in systemic lupus erythematosus. Clinicopathologic correlations. Arthritis Rheum. 22:864, 1979.

355. Alcocer, J., Moreno, J., Garcia-Torres, R., Gudina, J., Lavalle, C., and Fraga, A.: Immunofluorescent skin band test in the differential diagnosis of systemic lupus erythematosus. J. Rheumatol. 6:196, 1979.

356. Grishman, E., and Churg, J.: Ultrastructure of dermal lesions in systemic lupus erythematosus. Lab. Invest. 22:189, 1970.

357. Tan, E.M., and Kunkel, H.G.: An immunofluorescent study of the skin lesions in systemic lupus erythematosus. Arthritis Rheum. 9:37, 1966.

358. Gilliam, J.N.: The significance of cutaneous immunoglobulin deposits in lupus erythematosus and NZB/NZW F1 hybrid mice. J. Invest. Dermatol. 65:154, 1975.

359. Quismorio, F.P., Rea, T.H., Levan, N.E., and Friou, G.J.: Immunoglobulin deposits in lepromatous leprosy skin. Presence of deposits in apparently uninvolved skin and occurrence of serum antiepithelial antibodies. Arch. Dermatol. 111:331, 1975.

360. Davis, J.A., Weisman, M.H., and Dail, D.H.: Vascular disease in infective endocarditis. Arch. Intern. Med. 138:480, 1978.

361. Landry, M., and Sams, W.M.: Systemic lupus erythematosus: Studies of the antibodies bound to skin. J. Clin. Invest. 52:1871, 1973.

362. Thivolet, J., Beyvin, A.J., and LeMot, J.: Elution of anticorps fixés in vivo au hiveau de la peau au cours du pemphigus, de la phemphigoïde bulleuse et du lupus érythémateux. Lyon Medicate 227:241, 1972.

363. Tuffanelli, D.A.: Cutaneous immunopathology, recent observations. J. Invest. Dermatol. 65:143, 1975.

364. Wierzchowiecki, M.O., Quismorio, F.P., and Friou, G.J.: Immunoglobulin deposits in skin in systemic lupus erythematosus. Arthritis Rheum. 18:77, 1975.

365. Boart de la Faille-Kuyper, E.H.: In vivo nuclear localization of immunoglobulins in clinically normal skin in systemic and procainamide induced lupus erythematosus. Neth. J. Med. 17:58, 1974.

366. Bresnihan, B., Hale, G.M., Bunn, C.C., and Hughes, G.R.V.: Immunoglobulin classes in skin basement membrane in systemic lupus erythematosus: Clinical significance and comparison with classes of serum anti-DNA antibodies. Ann. Rheum. Dis. 38:351, 1979.

367. Wells, J.V., Webb, J., VanDeventer, M., Fry, B., Pollard, K.M., Raftos, J., Monk, W., and Nelson, D.S.: In vivo anti-nuclear antibodies in epithelial biopsies in SLE and other connective tissue diseases. Clin. Exp. Immunol. 38:424, 1979.

368. Natali, P.G., and Tan, E.M.: Experimental skin lesions in mice resembling systemic lupus erythematosus. Arthritis Rheum. 16:579, 1973.

369. Kay, D.M., and Tuffanelli, F.L.: Immunofluorescent techniques in clinical diagnosis of cutaneous disease. Ann. Intern. Med. 71:753, 1969.

370. Cripps, D.J., and Rankin, J.: Action spectra of lupus erythematosus and clinical immunofluorescence. Arch. Dermatol. 107:653, 1973.

371. Miescher, P.A., Paronetto, F., and Lambert, P.H.: Systemic lupus erythematosus. In Miescher, P.A., and Muller-Eberhard, J.H. (eds.): Textbook of Immunopathology. New York, Grune and Stratton, 1976, p. 963.

372. Mongan, E.S., Leddy, J.P., Atwater, E.C., and Barnett, E.V.: Direct antiglobulin (Coombs') reactions in patients with connective tissue diseases. Arthritis Rheum. 10:502, 1967.

373. Gilliland, B.C., Leddy, J.P., and Vaughan, J.H.: The detection of cell-bound antibody on complement-coated human red cells. J. Clin. Invest. 49:898, 1970.

374. DuBois, E.I.: Acquired hemolytic anemia as the presenting syndrome of lupus erythematosus disseminatus. Am. J. Med. 12:197, 1952.

375. Dawsset, J., and Colombani, J.: Study of leukopenias and thrombocy-

topenias by the direct antiglobulin consumption test on leukocytes and/or platelets. Blood 17:672, 1961.

376. Karpatkin, S., Strick, N., Karpatkin, M.B., and Siskind, G.: Cumulative experience in the detection of antiplatelet antibody in 234 patients with idiopathic thrombocytopenic purpura, systemic lupus erythematosus, and other clinical disorders. Am. J. Med. 52:776, 1972.

377. Lee, S.L., and Miotti, A.B.: Disorder of hemostatic function in patients with systemic lupus erythematosus. Sem. Arthritis Rheum. 4:241, 1975.

378. Karpatkin, S., Schur, P.H., Shick, N., and Siskind, F.W.: Heavy chain subclass of human anti-platelet antibodies. Clin. Immunol. Immunopathol. 2:1, 1973.

379. Henson, P.M.: Interaction of cells with immune complexes: Adherence, release of constituents, and tissue injury. J. Exp. Med. 134:114s, 1971.

380. Butler, W.T., Sharp, J.T., Rossen, R.D., Lindsley, M.D., Mittal, K.K., and Gard, D.A.: Relationship of the clinical course of systemic lupus erythematosus to the presence of circulating lymphocytotoxic antibodies. Arthritis Rheum. 15:231, 1972.

381. Utsinger, P.D.: Relationship of lymphocytotoxic antibodies to lymphopenia and parameters of disease activity in systemic lupus erythematosus. J. Rheumatol. 3:175, 1976.

382. Winfield, J.B., Winchester, R.J., and Kunkel, H.G.: Association of cold-reactive antilymphocyte antibodies with lymphopenia in systemic lupus erythematosus. Arthritis Rheum. 18:587, 1975.

383. Bluestein, H.G., and Zvaifler, N.J.: Brain-reactive lymphocytotoxic antibodies in the serum of patients with systemic lupus erythematosus. J. Clin. Invest. 57:509, 1976.

384. Bresnihan, B., Oliver, M., Grigor, G., and Hughes, G.R.V.: Brain-reactivity of lymphocytotoxic antibodies in systemic lupus erythematosus with and without cerebral involvement. Clin. Exp. Immunol. 30:333, 1977.

385. Bluestein, H.G.: Antineuronal factors in the serum of patients with systemic lupus erythematosus. Proc. Natl. Acad. Sci. (U.S.A) 75:3965, 1978.

386. Klippel, J.H., and Zvaifler, N.J.: Neuropsychiatric abnormalities in systemic lupus erythematosus. Clin. Rheum. Dis. 1:621, 1975.

387. Johnson, R.T., and Richardson, E.P.: The neurological manifestations of systemic lupus erythematosus. Medicine 47:337, 1968.

388. Estes, D., and Christian, C.L.: The natural history of systemic lupus erythematosus by prospective analysis. Medicine 50:85, 1971.

389. Ellis, S.G., and Verity, M.A.: Central nervous system involvement in systemic lupus erythematosus: A review of neuropathologic findings in 57 cases, 1955–1957. Sem. Arthritis Rheum. 8:212, 1979.

390. Bluestein, H.G.: Heterogeneous neurocytotoxic antibodies in systemic lupus erythematosus. Clin. Exp. Immunol. 35:210, 1979.

391. Simon, J., and Simon, O.: Effect of passive transfer of antibrain antibodies to a normal recipient. Exp. Neurol. 47:523, 1975.

392. Kobiler, D., Fuchs, S., and Samuel, D.: The effect of antisynaptosomal plasma membrane antibodies on memory. Brain Res. 115:129, 1976.

393. Rappaport, M.M., Karpaik, S.E., and Mahadik, S.P.: Biological activities of antibodies injected into the brain. Fed. Proc. 38:2391, 1978.

394. Bluestein, H.G., Williams, G.W., and Steinberg, A.D.: Cerebrospinal fluid antibodies to neuronal cells: Association with neuropsychiatric manifestations of systemic lupus erythematosus. Am. J. Med. 70:240, 1981.

395. Bresnihan, B., Oliver, M., Williams, B., and Hughes, G.R.V.: An antineuronal antibody cross-reactivity with erythrocytes and lymphocytes in systemic lupus erythematosus. Arthritis Rheum. 22:313, 1979.

396. Wilson, H.A., Winfield, J.B., Lahita, R.G., and Koffler, D.: Association of IgG anti-brain antibodies with central nervous system dysfunction in systemic lupus erythematosus. Arthritis Rheum. 22:458, 1979.

397. Tourtellotte, W.W.: On cerebrospinal fluid IgG quotients in multiple sclerosis and other diseases. J. Neurol. Sci. 10:279, 1970.

397a. Winfield, J.B., Shaw, M., Silverman, L.M., Eisenberg, R.A., Wilson, H.A., and Kofler, D.: Intrathecal IgG synthesis and blood-brain barrier impairment in patients with systemic lupus erythematosus and central nervous system dysfunction. Am. J. Med. 74:837, 1983.

397b. Zvaifler, N.J., and Bluestein, H.G.: The pathogenesis of central nervous system manifestations of systemic lupus erythematosus. Arthritis Rheum. 25:862, 1982.

398. Atkins, C.J., Kondon, J.J., Quismorio, F.P., and Friou, G.J.: The choroid plexus in systemic lupus erythematosus. Ann. Intern. Med. 76:65, 1972.

399. Feinglass, E.J., Arnett, F.C., Dorsch, C.A., Zizic, T.M., and Stevens, M.B.: Neuropsychiatric manifestations of systemic lupus erythematosus: Diagnosis, clinical spectrum, and relationship to other features of the disease. Medicine 55:323, 1976.

400. Sergent, J.S., Lockshin, M.D., Klimpner, M.S., and Lipsky, B.A.: Central nervous system disease in systemic lupus erythematosus, therapy and prognosis. Am. J. Med. 58:644, 1975.

401. Winfield, J., Brunner, C., and Koffler, D.: Serologic studies in patients with systemic lupus erythematosus and central nervous system dysfunction. Arthritis Rheum. 21:289, 1978.

402. Boyer, R.S., Sun, N.C.J., Verity, A., Nies, K.M., and Louie, J.S.: Im-

munoperoxidase staining of the choroid plexus in systemic lupus erythematosus. J. Rheum. 7:645, 1980.

403. Gershwin, M.E., Hyman, L.R., and Steinberg, A.D.: The choroid plexus in CNS involvement of systemic lupus erythematosus. J. Pediatr. 85:385, 1974.

404. Lampert, P.W., and Oldstone, M.B.: Immunoglobulin G and complement deposits in the choroid plexus during spontaneous immune complex disease. Science 180:408, 1973.

405. Lambert, P.W., and Oldstone, M.B.A.: Pathology of the choroid plexus in spontaneous complex disease and chronic viral infections. Vir. Arch. Path. Anat. (Berlin) 363:21, 1974.

406. Harbeck, R.J., Hoffman, A.A., Hoffman, S.A., and Shucard, D.W.: Cerebrospinal fluid and the choroid plexus during acute immune complex disease. Clin. Immunol. Immunopathol. 13:413, 1979.

407. Lampert, P.W., Garrett, R., and Lampert, A.: Ferritin immune complex deposits in the choroid plexus. Acta Neuropathol. (Berlin) 38:83, 1977.

408. Husby, G., Williams, R.C., Jr., and Wedege, E.: Huntington's disease, anti-neuronal antibodies, brain antigens, and receptors for IgG in human choroid plexus. Adv. Neurol. 23:435, 1979.

409. Hirano, T., Hashimoto, H., and Shiokawa, Y.: Antiglycolipid autoantibody detected in the sera from systemic lupus erythematosus patients. J. Clin. Invest. 66:1437, 1980.

410. Nakahara, K., Ohashi, T., Oda, T., Hirano, T., Kasai, M., Okumura, K., Tada, T.: Asialo GM$_1$ as a cell surface marker detected in acute lymphoblastic leukemia. N. Engl. J. Med. 302:674, 1980.

411. Young, W.W., Hakomor, S., Durcik, J.M., and Henny, C.S.: Identification of ganglio-N-tetraosylceramide as a new cell surface marker for murine natural killer (NK) cells. J. Immunol. 124:199, 1980.

412. Klippel, J.H., Bluestein, H.G., and Zvaifler, N.J.: Lymphocyte reactivity of antisera to cryoproteins in systemic lupus erythematosus. Clin. Immunopathol. 12:52, 1979.

413. Bluestein, H.G., and Woods, V.L., Jr.: Antineuronal antibodies in systemic lupus erythematosus. Arthritis Rheum. 25:773, 1982.

Chapter 69

Clinical Features of Systemic Lupus Erythematosus

Naomi Rothfield

INTRODUCTION

Systemic lupus erythematosus (SLE) is a connective tissue disease that is characterized by involvement of many organs. Although the disease was considered to be extremely rare in the past, SLE patients are frequently found on most medical services. The disease is characterized by marked and varied immunologic abnormalities, including a variety of autoantibodies that participate in immunologically mediated tissue injury. The cause of the disease has not been established, although recent attention has turned to genetic factors and the possibility of a viral etiology (see Chapter 68).

INCIDENCE AND PREVALENCE

The annual incidence of newly diagnosed SLE patients in a discrete population has been reported.[1] Fessel studied the incidence of SLE in a Kaiser Foundation Health Plan among members of the plan who were also resident in San Francisco City and County between July 1965 and June 1973.[1] This health plan provides complete medical care to its members, and the investigator had access to complete medical records as well as age and skin colors of the members. There were 74 new cases of SLE based on the Preliminary Criteria for the Classification of SLE[2] and for the 8-year period, during which the mean Health Plan membership was 121,444. Thus, the annual incidence of SLE was 7.6 cases per 100,000. This figure is similar to the 6.4 per 100,000 found by Nobrega and co-workers for the rural area encompassing Rochester, Minnesota.[3]

The prevalence rates for the two cities are also similar—1 case in 1969 for San Francisco and 1 case in 2400 for Rochester, Minnesota. The prevalence of SLE was also studied in Dunedin, New Zealand, which has a stable white population, and was found to be 1 case per 6780 individuals.[4]

These prevalence and incidence figures are based on the total population studied. When the incidence and prevalence in females is calculated, and when young black and white females are compared, the figures are quite different. Thus, the prevalence rate was found to be 1 case per 245 black women, aged 15 to 64 and resident in San Francisco City and County, and for all women between ages 15 and 64 the prevalence was 1 per 700. The prevalence for Dunedin, New Zealand, in all females was 1 in 4312.[4]

Race and Sex. The disease affects individuals of all races. The incidence in black females is higher than that in white females in the United States. As noted above, the prevalence of SLE in the black female between ages 15 and 64 has been estimated as 1 case per 245, whereas that for all women of the same ages is 1 per 700.[1] There have been very few reports of SLE in Africans, and a recent study of all pediatric admissions to a South African hospital during the past 20 years revealed 4 patients with SLE, all of whom were from the Indian community.[5]

A study of patients of a teaching hospital in Jamaica, West Indies, revealed that SLE was nearly as common as rheumatoid arthritis.[6] A study of cases of SLE from civilian hospitals in Hawaii revealed that there was a very high prevalence of the disease in the Oriental and Polynesian people.[7] Although no epidemiologic or case finding studies have been reported from Japan, there appears to be a very high prevalence of the disease based on the number of clinical and immunologic studies from that country now in the literature. In France, the disease appears to be more common among those who are immigrants from Portugal, Spain, North Africa, or Italy than among French-born persons. It thus appears that there is a definite difference among racial groups in the prevalence of SLE. In addition, there may be an environmental factor that affects the prevalence of the disease within racial groups. Further studies are needed to compare the HLA type and prevalence of the disease in blacks in the United States and in Africa.

SLE occurs in children and in the elderly, but the peak age of onset of the first symptom is between 15 and 25 years, and the mean age at the time of diagnosis is 30 years. Ninety percent of our own series of 433 SLE patients are females. In this group, a higher percentage of males occurred among children and the elderly SLE patients. However, in an analysis of 320 patients from his own series and from series reported by others, Maddock found that there was little correlation between the age of the male patients and the age of diagnosis.[8]

GENERAL SYSTEMIC SYMPTOMS

Fatigue. Moderate to severe fatigue was noted at the time of diagnosis in 76 percent of 209 SLE patients studied by us. An additional 5 percent of these patients did not note fatigue at the time of diagnosis but did develop fatigue later in the course of their disease. Thus, fatigue was present in 81 percent of these patients. The fatigue noted in the patients at the time of diagnosis was clearly related to the disease, since it was present prior to the onset of therapy. In most SLE patients, the fatigue disappears after the other manifestations of the disease disappear during corticosteroid therapy. In many patients, a feeling of well-being continues after the disease is treated and continues until an exacerbation of the disease occurs. In some patients, the onset of fatigue is noted prior to the onset of objective evidence of disease activity such as arthritis or rash. We have found that some patients complain of the onset of fatigue at a time when a fall in serum C3 is noted and when no other serologic or clinical evidence of activity can be detected.

It is possible to titer the amount of fatigue in these patients. The need for a morning nap or afternoon rest period in a housewife may gradually disappear as the serologic and clinical disease activity disappear. Most SLE patients are able to recognize the fatigue of the disease and to distinguish this from the fatigue felt by normal individuals. It is important to note that some SLE patients who are taking an initially high dose of corticosteroids may have extreme difficulty in sleeping because of the medication. The fatigue in these patients is clearly due to the side effect of the corticosteroids rather than to the disease.

Loss of Weight. Sixty-three percent of our 209 SLE patients state that they had lost at least 5 pounds of weight during the 3 months prior to diagnosis. Of course, patients presenting with the nephrotic syndrome would have weight gain rather than weight loss.

Fever. Eighty-three percent of SLE patients have a fever at the time of diagnosis. The fever is greater than 102° F in 41 percent. In about one third of the patients, the fever is between 101° F and 102° F, and in 12 percent the fever is less than 101° F. In an occasional patient with severe central nervous system involvement manifested by seizures and organic brain disease, a sustained high fever of more than 102° F may be noted.

Fever in a patient with the diagnosis of SLE should always suggest the presence of infection. This is true not only for the SLE patient already diagnosed and under treatment who develops a fever but also for the untreated recently diagnosed patient. The major cause of death in untreated SLE patients studied during the presteroid era was infection.[9] In a recent study of 83 febrile episodes in 63 patients, 23 percent were due to infection, and bacteremia was present in one half of these infectious episodes.[10]

It is therefore important to rule out infection as a cause of fever in SLE patients. Infection should also be considered in febrile patients at the onset of disease who have never received corticosteroid therapy.

Manifestations in the Joints and Muscles. Joint involvement is the most common manifestation of SLE. In some patients joint pain or swelling may precede the onset of multisystem disease by from 6 months to 5 years. Many SLE patients are seen by a physician during this period, and a diagnosis of rheumatoid arthritis is made. Eighty-eight percent of our 209 SLE patients seen in New York had seen a physician prior to the diagnosis of SLE and had been told they had a "rheumatic disease." Arthritis, with objective evidence of pain on motion, tenderness, or effusion, was present in 78 percent of our 365 patients at the time of diagnosis. Additional patients developed objective evidence of arthritis during the course of the disease. A total of 86 percent of our patients have had arthritis (Table 69–1). Additional patients have joint pain without objective evidence of arthritis. In our series of 365 patients, 95 percent have had either arthritis or arthralgia. This figure is similar to those reported by others.[9,11-14]

The joints most commonly involved are the proximal interphalangeal, knee, wrist, and metacarpophalangeal joints. Ankles, elbows, and shoulders are less often involved. Metatarsal joints and hips were involved in 20 percent of patients, and the distal interphalangeal joints of the hand were involved in 14 percent. The joint disease is strikingly symmetrical. Ropes found that 74 percent of 142 patients had objective involvement of more than two joints. Morning stiffness was present in 50 percent of the 209 patients in whom details of joint involvement were analyzed.

Deforming arthritis does occur in SLE patients. Typical swan neck deformities and ulnar deviation of the fingers occur in about 15 percent of SLE patients after 3 to 4 years of disease. X-rays reveal no abnormalities of the bone or cartilage, and surgical repair reveals no pannus formation or any abnormalities of the bone or cartilage.[15,16] These deformities are thought to be related to chronic involvement of the tendons of the hands and fingers and spasm of the intrinsic muscles.

Erosive arthritis occurs very infrequently in SLE patients.[15]

Table 69–1. Incidence of 14 Manifestations of the American Rheumatism Association Preliminary Criteria for the Classification of SLE[2] in 365 SLE Patients*

Manifestation	Percentage Incidence			
	ARA Series[2]	Rothfield[11]	Davis et al.[13]	Trimble et al.[12]
1. Facial erythema (butterfly rash). Diffuse erythema, flat or raised, over the malar eminence(s) and/or bridge of the nose; may be unilateral.	64	55	64	40
2. Discoid lupus. Erythematous raised patches with adherent keratotic scaling and follicular plugging; atrophic scarring may occur in older lesions; may be present anywhere on the body.	17	19	31	32
3. Raynaud's phenomenon. Requires a two-phase color reaction, by patient's history or physician's observation.	20	20	19	44
4. Alopecia. Rapid loss of large amount of the scalp hair, by patient's history or physician's observation.	43	71	64	40
5. Photosensitivity. Unusual skin reaction from exposure to sunlight, by patient's history or physician's observation.	37	41	17	28
6. Oral or nasopharyngeal ulceration.	15	36	22	16
7. Arthritis without deformity. One or more peripheral joints involved with any of the following in the absence of deformity: (a) Pain on motion. (b) Tenderness. (c) Effusion or periarticular soft tissue swelling (peripheral joints are defined for this purpose as feet, ankles, knees, hips, shoulders, elbows, wrists, metacarpophalangeal, proximal interphalangeal, terminal interphalangeal, and temporomandibular joints).	90	86	89	100
8. LE cells. Two or more classic LE cells seen on one occasion or one cell seen on two or more occasions, using an accepted published method.	92	86	75	48
9. Chronic false-positive STS. Known to be present for at least 6 months and confirmed by TPI or Reiter's tests.	12	26	8	12
10. Profuse proteinuria. Greater than 3.5 grams per day.	20	25	25	16
11. Cellular casts. May be red cell, hemoglobin, granular, tubular, or mixed.	48	34	17	16
12. One or both of the following: (a) Pleuritis, good history of pleuritic pain; or rub heard by a physician; or x-ray evidence of both pleural thickening and fluid. (b) Pericarditis, documented by EKG or rub.	60 19	54	30 19	60
13. One or both of the following: (a) Psychosis. (b) Convulsions, by patient's history or physician's observation in the absence of uremia and offending drugs.	19	16	19	20
14. One or more of the following: (a) Hemolytic anemia. (b) Leukopenia, WBC less than 4000 per cubic millimeter on two or more occasions. (c) Thrombocytopenia, platelet count less than 100,000 per cubic millimeter.	16 40 11	54	14 47 14	52

"A person shall be said to have systemic LE if any 4 or more of the above 14 manifestations are present, serially or simultaneously, during any period of observation."

*From Rothfield, N.F.: *In* McCarty, D. (ed.): Arthritis and Allied Conditions. 9th ed. Philadelphia, Lea & Febiger, 1979.

Rheumatoid nodules occur in 5 to 7 percent of patients with SLE. Hahn and co-workers described periarticular nodules in six patients with SLE.[17] Biopsies of three nodules revealed histologically typical rheumatoid nodules. Of interest was the observation that, when present in these patients, the disease was clinically active and the lesions were transient and slowly regressed along with clinical response to therapy. In two of the patients systemic disease exacerbation was associated with the reappearance of nodules, which again resolved with disease suppression.

Tenosynovitis occurs in about 8 percent of patients. Rupture of the Achilles and patellar tendons has been reported in SLE patients but is a rare occurrence.[9,18-20]

Septic arthritis may occur in SLE patients. Septic arthritis caused by *Salmonella* previously cultured from the urine has been described.[21] Gonococcal arthritis and septic arthritis resulting from other organisms have been reported.[22,23] A chronic indolent monoarticular synovitis due to meningococcus has recently been described.[24]

Synovial fluid is nearly always clear or may be slightly cloudy.[25] Viscosity is good, and a good mucin clot is noted. The white blood cell count is less than 3000 per cubic millimeter, with a predominance of mononuclear cells. On wet smear, many of the polymorphonuclear leukocytes contain cytoplasmic inclusions similar to those seen in rheumatoid arthritis.[15] Antinuclear antibodies and LE cells may be demonstrated.

Pathologic Findings. Synovium studied by light microscopy revealed superficial fibrin-like material, which did not stain for fibrin using specific stains.[15] Focal or diffuse synovial lining cell proliferation may be noted, along with a perivascular inflammation reaction consisting predominantly of mononuclear cells. Infiltration of small vessel walls consistent with a vasculitis was noted in one of six biopsies reported by Labowitz and Schumacher.[15] These investigators also described fibrinoid necrosis of small-vessel walls in another of the six patients. Although no hematoxylin bodies were noted in the synovium of the six patients, karyorrhexis and amorphous hematoxophilic material were seen in one patient. Perivascular fibrosis and obliteration of vessel lumens caused by enlarged endothelial cells, inflammatory cells, and organized thrombi were noted. It is of interest that in the study by Labowitz and Schumacher definite synovial inflammation and vascular lesions were seen in two patients who clinically had no objective signs of joint inflammation.

Electron microscopy studies reported by Labowitz and Schumacher revealed that the lining cell proliferation was composed of both phagocytic and synthetic cells and intermediate cells.[15] Red blood cells and polymorphonuclear cells were noted apparently emigrating through open gaps between venular endothelial cells. Several types of vascular endothelial inclusions were noted. Two patients of the six studied had aggregates of microtubules reminiscent of paramyxoviruses lying adjacent to endoplasmic reticulum of intact endothelium. In another patient a larger mass of similar tubular and filamentous structures was located extracellularly adjacent to a platelet-fibrin thrombus. Other venular endothelial cells had unusual, unexplained electron-dense inclusions resembling the density of nuclear chromatin. In one patient a small amount of electron-dense material, similar to the deposits described in lupus nephritis, was seen lying beneath the vascular endothelium.

Myalgia and Myositis. At the time of diagnosis one third of our patients had myalgia but pain and tenderness of muscles were less common. Myalgia, proximal muscle weakness, or muscle tenderness was present in one half of patients with active disease reported by Isbender and Snaith.[26] In contrast to the common occurrence of myalgia, significant muscle disease is uncommon. Prominent muscle involvement was noted in 18 (8 percent) of 228 patients reported by Tsokos and colleagues.[27] In 16 of these patients, the authors felt that the myositis was associated with evidence of disease activity in other systems. Extreme muscle weakness was noted in 15 percent of patients described by Ropes.[9] Some of these patients had marked atrophy and complete paralysis of the affected extremities, with flaccid muscles, absent reflexes, and marked elevation of enzyme levels. Elevation of creatine phosphokinase up to 900 units has been described in these patients. With subsidence of the disease, complete recovery is usual. In general, the aldolase level is high in patients with muscle pain and tenderness, but the creatinine phosphokinase is usually not elevated.[27]

Muscle biopsies may be entirely normal or may show lymphocytic and plasma cell perivascular infiltrates. Occasionally, chronic myositis and fibrositis have been seen. Post-mortem examination of the muscles in non–steroid-treated patients revealed abnormalities in about one quarter.[28] These lesions, noted in routine samples of muscles, consisted of perivascular and perifascicular infiltrates of lymphocytes, plasma cells, and monocytes, with occasional neutrophils and macrophages. Hyalinization and atrophy of muscle fibers were noted in about half of the involved tissue and necrosis of muscle was rare. Thus, most features characteristic of polymyositis are not found in the involved muscle of SLE patients.

Another cause for muscle weakness in SLE patients is a vacuolar myopathy.[29] This is a diffuse disease, which usually, but not always, is associated with muscle weakness or serum enzyme changes. The histologic picture is that of plump, swollen sarcolemmal nuclei, with prominent nuclei more centrally located in the muscle fiber and often found within a vacuole. This lesion has been described in untreated SLE patients. The general problem of myopathy in treated SLE patients is complicated by the fact that both steroid therapy[30] and chloroquine therapy may cause vacuolar myopathy.[31] Chloroquine myopathy has been induced in rats, and examples of chloroquine myopathy have been reported in rheumatoid arthritis, spondylosis, and sarcoid.[31-33] The chloroquine myopathy is reversible but may take many months for full recovery. Some investigators have described a unique granular deposition within the muscle fibers, which could differentiate this disorder from vacuolar myopathy caused by corticosteroids or SLE.[33,34] Muscle weakness from steroid myopathy is usually vacuolar. Although elevations of aldolase and creatine phosphokinase were not noted in steroid myopathy, elevation of serum lactic dehydrogenase has been reported. This enzyme elevation returned to normal with decreasing corticosteroid doses.[35]

Electromyography may reveal neuropathic changes or polyphasic peaks or may show no abnormalities.[27] Abnormalities suggestive of myopathy may be demonstrated even in patients with no clinical evidence of muscle disease.[36]

CUTANEOUS LESIONS

Some type of dermatologic abnormality is present in 85 percent of SLE patients (Table 69–1).

The typical erythematous blush in the butterfly area (butterfly rash) is present in about half the patients at the time of diagnosis. The rash is a very slightly edematous lesion that is located on both cheeks and across the bridge of the nose. It may be the first manifestation of the disease, preceding the onset of other manifestations by weeks or months. The rash is frequently noted after sun exposure, although many patients develop a butterfly rash without any history of sun exposure. The rash may be very intermittent and evanescent, and in fair-skinned individuals it may be brought out by alcohol ingestion or by nervousness. The rash heals well, leaving no scarring or pigmentation.

The second most common rash is an erythematous maculopapular eruption. This lesion resembles a drug eruption and may occur after exposure to sunlight (Fig. 69–1). The lesions are frequently pruritic and may be located any place on the body. Lesions occurring after sun exposure are located in the sun-exposed areas. In

Figure 69–1. Sun-sensitive eruption in a male SLE patient.

general, these lesions are above the waistline. Scattered macular lesions are also occasionally located on the fingers, palms, and, less frequently, soles of the feet. Maculopapular lesions may also be found on the scalp. The maculopapular eruption usually heals without scarring or hyperpigmentation, but in some patients the lesions persist, become crusted, and eventually develop some superficial atrophy.

Lesions of discoid lupus were present in 19 percent of our 365 SLE patients. Thirty-nine percent of the patients with these discoid lesions had had the discoid lesions more than 2 years prior to the onset of multisystem disease. In a few patients, the discoid lesions had been present for 20, 25, and 35 years before SLE was diagnosed. Half the SLE patients with discoid lesions developed the discoid lesions within 6 months of the time of diagnosis of SLE, and 8 percent developed discoid lesions after the diagnosis of SLE. We have compared the group of SLE patients with discoid lesions to the group of SLE patients without discoid lesions. The two groups did not differ, except that a significantly higher incidence of Raynaud's phenomenon and photosensitive rashes was present in the SLE patients with discoid lesions. No difference in incidence of severe renal disease (nephrotic syndrome, urinary casts) was noted. The discoid lesion usually starts with one or more raised, sharply defined papules on the butterfly area of the face. Other common locations are the scalp, ears, or forehead. The upper arms, chest, and back may also be involved. The lesion enlarges slowly and eventually becomes a typical mature lesion. Occasionally the eruption is more widespread at onset and consists of several erythematous, rapidly enlarging, slightly elevated lesions, which resemble a form of tinea. The mature discoid lesion usually consists of sharply outlined papules and plaques with bright erythema, edema, and elevation at the central

area. Eventually the central area becomes atrophic and depressed. As the plaques enlarge, the central area fades and becomes atrophic while the edges remain edematous and erythematous. The outline of the lesion is sharp and irregular. These active lesions also show telangiectasia. As the acute phase subsides, follicular scales and follicular plugging may be noted and, eventually, the central atrophy spreads outward to the edge of the lesion. Thus, there are three stages to the discoid lesion: erythema, hyperkeratosis, and atrophy. As the process burns itself out, only a white atrophic plaque remains, generally with loss of pigmentation. Hyperpigmentation is usual at the edge of the lesion (see Fig. 69–2, Plate IX, p. xliii). Leukoderma may be extensive in the affected skin of black patients. Several forms of discoid lesions have been described. The hypertrophic form consists of raised, indurated, hyperkeratotic lesions (see Fig. 69–3, Plate IX, p. xliii, and Fig. 69–4) and may be confused with hypertrophic psoriasis or with hypertrophic lichen planus. In a few instances, patients have been treated with ultraviolet light because of the mistaken diagnosis of psoriasis, leading to a severe exacerbation of the discoid lesions and of the systemic disease.

Subacute lesions are found in from 10 to 15 percent of SLE patients. These lesions are different from chronic discoid lesions in that the lesions do not lead to permanent scarring and may heal completely. Although the lesions are typically erythematous at the edges, the center of the subacute lesion is not atrophic, although there may be central depigmentation. The subacute lesions represent a midway between the chronic discoid lesion and the maculopapular eruptions seen in SLE patients. Another special feature of subacute lesions is the tendency to be annular and widespread. The widespread distribution of the lesions is similar to the widespread distribution of the rashes in SLE and is in contrast to

Figure 69–4. Hyperkeratotic and healed scarred discoid lesions in the external ear, a typical location for discoid lesions.

the lesions of chronic discoid lupus present in patients without systemic disease, which occur most often above the neck. The subacute lesions occur on the extremities, chest, and back. Patients with subacute lesions have been shown to have antibodies to Ro and La and have a very high frequency of HLA antigens B8 and Dr3.[37] The same haplotype has also been associated with a lupus subset of occult Sjögren's syndrome and is also found more frequently among patients with Graves' disease, juvenile diabetes mellitus, and chronic active hepatitis (see Chapter 46). The association between the subacute lupus lesions, HLA antigens, and the anti-Ro antigen is of interest and awaits further study to determine the relationships between clinical disease expression and the genetic markers of the immune response.

Lupus profundus or relapsing nodular nonsuppurative panniculitis occurs rarely in SLE patients. The lesions are subcutaneous nodules that appear as indurated tender or nontender lumps. We have observed these lesions in 2 of 365 SLE patients. The lesions usually occur on the extremities or on the buttocks. The overlying skin may ulcerate, and the inflammatory changes may involve the epidermis, with resulting atrophy and induration. The superficial areas overlying the nodules may become fibrotic and resemble morphea. Panniculitis may be the first manifestation of SLE.[38]

Vasculitic skin lesions may be noted in about 20 percent of patients. These lesions are commonly located on the extensor surface of the forearm and on the fingertips (see Fig. 69–5, Plate IX, p. xliii). The lesions are frequently tender, may be slightly indurated, and may ulcerate. Less commonly the vasculitic lesions may be noted on the palms, on or near the small joints of the fingers (Fig. 69–5), or on the soles of the feet. In some patients, tender vasculitic lesions occur around the lower leg near the malleoli. These lesions frequently ulcerate and lead to the formation of an exquisitely tender punched-out leg ulcer (Fig. 69–6). We have noted such

leg ulcers in 6 of our 365 patients. In two individuals, multiple lesions on the lower leg ulcerated, coalesced, and eventually led to deep ulcerations of the leg muscles. The ulcers appear during periods of disease activity and heal very gradually as the disease is suppressed with corticosteroid therapy. Grafting has been unsuccessful during the period of active disease. In all our patients, healing did occur after 6 to 8 months, leaving deep scars over the sites of the ulceration. The relationship between serologic evidence of disease activity and the appearance of leg ulcers was described in an SLE patient by Kirsner and associates.[39] In this patient there was a close correlation between ANA titer, complement, cutaneous ulcer size, and steroid dose through three exacerbations and two remissions. A similar correlation between serologic evidence of disease activity and cutaneous vasculitis was reported in 12 patients by Tuffanelli and Kay.[40]

The lesions of vasculitis may resemble palpable purpura, and the histologic appearance may be that of leukocytoclastic angiitis.

Livedo reticularis is not uncommon in SLE patients. In some, the livedo reticularis is marked at the time of diagnosis and gradually disappears over the years as the disease is suppressed with corticosteroids and the patient finally maintained in remission on little or no corticosteroid therapy. It is not uncommon for the livedo to become more marked during periods of disease exacerbation.

Splinter hemorrhages have been noted in an occasional patient with severe active disease (Fig. 69–7). A search for splinter hemorrhages should always be made in an acutely ill febrile SLE patient, since it provides evidence for cutaneous vasculitis. It is important to note that the presence of splinter hemorrhages does not necessarily indicate the presence of infection.[41] Osler's nodes have also been noted in SLE patients who did not have infection.[42]

Lesions of the fingertips or the palmar surface of the hands or toes are common in patients with active SLE.

Figure 69–6. Leg ulcer in a patient with active SLE.

Figure 69–7. Splinter hemorrhage in a nail of patient acutely ill with SLE. Note also the vasculitic lesion at the base of the nail fold.

Ropes reported such lesions in 35 percent of her 142 patients.[9]

Dilated capillaries along the base of the nail were first described by Baehr and associates.[43] We have noted periungual erythema in 10 percent of our patients. Ropes has described a similar capillary dilatation along the edges of the upper eyelids in 12 percent of her patients.[9]

Atrophic blanche lesions occasionally occur in SLE patients.[44] The lesions start as erythematous papular or infiltrated lesions and gradually develop porcelain-white centers with telangiectasias at the margins. These lesions may be found in areas of livedo reticularis and closely resemble the lesions in malignant atrophic papulosis (Degos' disease).

Bullous lesions occur occasionally in active SLE.[45] Such lesions were present in 5 percent of our patients. The lesions were subepidermal bullae. Three patients with bullous pemphigoid associated with SLE have been described.[46]

Hives or angioneurotic edema was present in 14 percent of our patients and in 13 percent of the patients described by Estes and Christian.[47] Urticaria was present at the time of diagnosis in 9 percent of our patients and was frequently associated with the presence of cryoglobulins.

Periorbital edema was noted in 14 percent of our patients prior to steroid therapy at the time of diagnosis and was noted in 22 percent of the patients studied by Ropes.[9] In some of the patients, the edema was associated with the nephrotic syndrome, while in others the edema was associated with an extensive and edematous butterfly rash. In a few of our patients and in a few of those of Ropes, the edema was present in patients without either a facial rash or the nephrotic syndrome.

Purpuric lesions were present in 14 percent of our patients and in 17 percent of those described by Estes and Christian.[47] Ropes noted purpura at some time in the course of the disease in 50 percent of her patients.[9] Purpura may be due to thrombocytopenia, but in the majority of patients the purpuric lesions are due to vasculitis.

Nail deformities occurred in 6 percent of our patients (Fig. 69–8). These changes consisted of transverse riding and pitting; in a few patients the nail became separated from its base and eventually was shed.

Musocal lesions occurred in 36 percent of our 365 patients and in 41 percent of the series described by Ropes.[9] The ulcers are most common on the hard or soft palate and range from small red areas to large, tender deep ulcerations (see Fig. 69–9, Plate IX, p. xliii).[48] In most patients, the oral ulcerations are the first manifestation of an impending exacerbation of the disease.[9] The ulcerations are usually not symptomatic and will be noted only if they are looked for. The lesions heal completely and may heal extremely rapidly within days of the onset of corticosteroid therapy at the time of diagnosis.

Nasal mucosal ulcers are not uncommon. We have noted these ulcerations in about 20 percent of patients. They occur on the lower nasal septum just within the nares or may occur slightly farther within the nose. They are usually noted on each side of the septum but may be unilateral. These ulcers heal as the disease is suppressed and other serologic and clinical evidence of disease activity subsides. The ulcerations tend to recur in future periods of disease activity in those patients in whom the ulcers were present at the time of the initial illness. We have observed nine patients with nasal septal perforation.[49] In four of these patients, the perforation was first noted within 6 months of the onset of the disease because the patients complained of a slightly bloody nasal discharge. We had not been routinely observing the nasal mucosa prior to the onset of these symptoms. The perforations in these four patients were surrounded by angry, edematous, engorged mucosal tissue. An increase in corticosteroid therapy resulted in a return of the nasal mucosal tissue to a normal appearance. With further decrease in corticosteroid therapy a few months later, the mucosal tissue was again noted to be inflamed. We have observed large perforations in other patients who have been studied only late in the course of the disease and at the time when they were in clinical remission. In these patients, the nasal mucosa appeared to be normal. Vaginal mucosal ulcers have been noted in two of our 365 patients.

Involvement of the mucosa of the upper respiratory

Figure 69–8. Nail deformities consisting of large depressions and lifting of the nail base.

tract in SLE patients may occur. We have described a patient who developed acute epiglottitis during an acute exacerbation of the disease.[50] Only two of Dubois' 520 patients developed laryngeal symptoms.[12] Necrotizing, ulcerating tracheitis was present at post-mortem examination of one of Ropes' patients.[9] We have noted a small group of patients who become hoarse during periods of disease activity, and Ropes described persistent hoarseness in 13 percent of her patients.[9] In our patient with acute epiglottitis, the symptoms were those of a sore throat, mild dysphasia, and progressive difficulty in breathing. Two hours after admission, severe stridor and upper airway obstruction occurred. Tracheostomy was carried out with relief of the respiratory difficulty. A direct laryngoscopy was then performed and revealed an epiglottis that was three times normal thickness with granular, friable inflamed mucosa. The biopsy revealed necrotic desquamating surface epithelium with necrotic connective tissue densely infiltrated with mononuclear cells. Numerous hematoxylin-like bodies were present. Immunofluorescence revealed nuclear staining in a speckled pattern.

Sun Sensitivity. A rash occurring after sun exposure was present at the time of diagnosis in 37 percent of our patients and in 34 percent of the patients reported by Ropes[9] (Fig. 69–1). Some individuals continue to have sun-sensitive eruptions throughout the course of their disease. We have observed individuals who have developed rashes on their left arms during a short (20-minute) drive to the Health Center and others who have arrived at the clinic with rashes on their lower thighs caused by the sun exposure of this area while they were wearing Bermuda shorts. Sun-sensitive rashes have been observed in patients who were skiing and have also been observed in individuals who have been behind glass windows. A small percentage of our patients have developed a sun-sensitive rash for the first time after the first year of disease. Those who have a sun-sensitive rash at the time of onset of their disease usually develop similar rashes after sun exposure during the course of the disease. It should be noted that severe urticaria and bullous lesions may occur following sun exposure. In addition, the sun-sensitive eruptions in SLE patients are not always a localized phenomenon, and many patients have objective evidence of systemic disease activation in addition to the skin lesions.

Alopecia. Alopecia was present in 58 percent of our patients at the time of diagnosis and occurred in a total of 71 percent of patients either at the time of diagnosis or later in the course of the disease. The most common form is diffuse alopecia. In some patients severe diffuse alopecia is one of the first manifestations to be noted by the patient at the onset of the disease. In many of these individuals the recurrence of alopecia may be the first manifestation of an impending flare-up of the disease and should be viewed as evidence of disease activity. Patients who lose most of their hair at the time of the first severe illness should be reassured that their hair will eventually grow back. Patchy alopecia is less common and also occurs during periods of active disease. In some patients erythematous macules may be noted

in the center of the patchy alopecia, while in others no rash is observed in the area. The new hair grows in gradually as the patient's systemic disease improves on therapy. The new hair gives the patient a ragged appearance. The duration of disease suppression in some individuals can easily be estimated by the length of the new hair. If the patient has discoid lesions in the scalp, permanent alopecia will occur owing to the healing of these lesions, with resultant atrophy and loss of the skin appendages (Fig. 69–2).

RENAL DISEASE

Clinical evidence of renal disease is present in about 50 percent of SLE patients. We have analyzed the urinalysis on 192 patients who were studied extensively at the time of diagnosis (Table 69–2). These were unselected patients studied at Bellevue Hospital at the time of admission for their previously undiagnosed systemic disease. No proteinuria on repeated examination was present in 46 percent of these patients during the first year of disease. A persistent trace was found in 6 percent, and 13 percent had no more than 1+ proteinuria during the first 6 months of disease. Twenty-nine percent of the patients had 3+ or 4+ proteinuria. Among the same group of 192 patients, hematuria (defined as greater than 2 red blood cells per high power field of the spun sediment) was present in 35 percent of patients. Thirty percent of these patients had more than five white blood cells per high power field in the spun sediment, and urinary casts were present in 23 percent. Twenty percent of the 192 patients had both hematuria and microscopic pyuria.

Although clinical evidence of renal disease is present in only 50 percent of patients, pathologic abnormalities that may be recognized using light microscopy are probably present in additional patients. Immunofluorescent studies of biopsies or of post-mortem kidneys may reveal deposits of immunoglobulins or complement proteins in nearly all patients with SLE. Therefore the definition of lupus nephritis is unclear at present, since many patients have been carefully followed for many years without any urinary abnormalities. Thirty-one percent of our patients followed for from 2 to 12 years have never had abnormal urinalysis. Additional studies of SLE patients not affected by renal abnormalities are needed to define precisely the incidence of the pathologic and immunohistologic abnormalities and their prognostic significance.

The types of lupus nephritis have been defined pathologically.[46] These are (1) focal (mild) proliferative lupus nephritis, (2) diffuse (severe) proliferative lupus nephritis, (3) membranous lupus nephritis, and (4) mesangial (minimal) lupus nephritis.[51] These are described in detail below with their clinical manifestations and course. The incidence of the various forms of lupus nephritis is difficult to estimate, since most centers do not perform renal biopsies on all SLE patients.

Mild (focal) lupus nephritis is characterized by segmental proliferation of some glomerular tufts, while oth-

Table 69-2. Renal Abnormalities at Diagnosis and During the Course of SLE*

	Within 6 Months of Diagnosis		At Diagnosis or During Course of Disease	
	Number of Patients/ Number Tested	%	Number of Patients/ Number Tested	%
Proteinuria (any)	104/192	54	141/207	78
Persistent trace	12/192	6	9/207	4
1+	26/192	13	24/207	11
2+	10/192	5	24/207	11
3+	19/192	9	27/207	13
4+	37/192	19	57/207	27
Hematuria	66/191	35	87/205	42
WBC	57/190	30	88/206	42
Casts	42/176	23	59/195	30
Fixed SG	9/165	6	15/181	8
Serum albumin < 3 grams	38/146	26	55/177	31
Serum creatinine > 1.5 mg	10/50	20	26/83	31
BUN < 21	129/176	67	119/199	59
21–35	24/176	13	38/199	19
36–50	11/176	6	13/199	6
51–70	6/176	3	9/199	4
> 70	6/176	3	20/199	10
Cholesterol 280	20/71	28	48/115	41

*From Rothfield, N.F.: Contrib. Nephrol. 7:128, 1977.

ers appear normal. By light microscopy fewer than 50 percent of glomeruli are affected by the segmental proliferation, and mesangial proliferation may be present in some glomeruli. Immunofluorescence reveals immunoglobulins and C3 in the mesangium of all glomeruli. Fine scattered granules may be noted along the capillary loops, especially in the areas of proliferations. The deposits are intermittent and scattered and are not evenly distributed along all the capillary loops. Electron microscopy reveals electron-dense deposits in the mesangium and occasional deposits in the subendothelial, subepithelial, and intrabasement membrane areas. Urinalysis in these individuals usually reveals hematuria and proteinuria, but the nephrotic syndrome is uncommon.[52,53] Renal insufficiency is either mild or not present. Many of these individuals with mild lupus nephritis have very severe extrarenal systemic disease, including involvement of the central nervous system. Thus, these patients may be acutely ill with high fevers, and serologic parameters such as antinative DNA antibodies and low serum complement levels may be noted. Treatment with adequate corticosteroids to control the systemic manifestations of the disease usually leads to a prompt clearing of the hematuria, followed by more gradual clearing of the proteinuria. Such patients do not usually develop severe renal disease in the future if the serologic abnormalities return initially to the normal range and if the patients remain in a urologic and clinical remission. Most of our patients who developed an exacerbation of the disease had a recurrence of the same focal mild nephritis that was present initially, and an increase in corticosteroid dose led to a prompt remission of the

exacerbation, including the disappearance of the urinary abnormalities. None of our patients reported earlier developed severe renal disease or died with or from renal insufficiency.[52,53]

Severe (diffuse) proliferative lupus nephritis is characterized by abnormalities of more than 50 percent of the total area of the glomerular tufts. Although proliferation is irregular, all glomeruli are involved and most of each glomerulus is abnormal. Sclerosis may or may not be present in the biopsy.

Interstitial infiltrates and deposits of immunoglobulins and complement proteins may also be noted along the tubular basement membrane, within the walls of the peritubular capillaries, or in the interstitium. Electron microscopy reveals dense deposits in the mesangium, in the subendothelial and subepithelial areas, and within the basement membrane. The deposits are not evenly distributed, and some areas show heavy clumps while granules are noted in other areas, but the deposits are located throughout the glomeruli. The immunofluorescence findings in diffuse proliferative lupus nephritis are usually quite striking, with granules and clumps of immunoglobulins and complement proteins along the peripheral capillary wall and in the mesangium.

The clinical picture in this group of patients is one of moderate to heavy proteinuria with the nephrotic syndrome, hematuria, and mild to moderately severe renal insufficiency. Red cell casts are not infrequently noted. Antibodies to native DNA and low serum C3 and C4 levels are usually present unless the pathologic lesion is inactive with significant sclerotic glomeruli. Many patients whose involved glomeruli show only sclerosis are in clinical remission and can be maintained on little, if any, corticosteroid therapy. Some of these individuals seem to have a prolonged serologic and clinical remission and do not require treatment. One of our patients with progressive sclerosis of the glomeruli has been maintained on hemodialysis for 4 years without corticosteroid therapy and a group of similar patients has recently been described.[54] The use of dialysis and transplantation in end-stage lupus renal disease is discussed elsewhere (see Chapter 70).

In general, the survival of patients with diffuse proliferative nephritis appears to be improving. In our initial report, the 5-year survival of biopsy-documented diffuse nephritis was 41 percent in the 24 patients followed prior to 1968.[52] Our current 5-year survival in the 22 patients with biopsy-proven diffuse nephritis followed since 1968 is 86 percent. It is clear that renal biopsy provides additional information besides the type of lupus nephritis. The prognosis in patients with this form of nephritis depends greatly on the degree of activity and on the degree of sclerosis and interstitial disease noted in the biopsy.

Membranous lupus nephritis appears histologically similar to idiopathic membranous glomerulonephritis. Although no proliferation is noted, a slight, irregular increase in mesangial cells and matrix may be present. Immunofluorescence reveals a striking deposit of immunoglobulins along all the basement membranes. In contrast to all the other forms of lupus nephritis, the membrane is diffusely involved, with little variation in amount or intensity of deposits from one capillary loop to another. Immunofluorescence reveals spikes of IgG, which protrude on the epithelial side of the capillary loop and correspond to the spikes seen with silver methenamine staining under light microscopy. Electron microscopy confirms the presence of subendothelial deposits.

Patients with this form of lupus nephritis have significant proteinuria and may or may not have hematuria. Hematuria is, in general, less common in patients with membranous lupus nephritis than in patients with focal or diffuse proliferative lupus nephritis. The nephrotic syndrome is usually present either at the onset of the disease or during the course of the disease. If significant extrarenal disease activity is not present, serologic evidence of disease activity may be absent, and the patient may have normal C3 and C4 levels and an absence of antibodies to native DNA.

The prognosis is quite variable but usually is good. We have followed some patients whose nephrotic syndrome has persisted along with slowly progressive renal insufficiency for as long as 10 years. We have observed progression to severe renal insufficiency 14 years after the first biopsy. Other patients have survived more than 10 years after remission of the nephrotic syndrome present at the time of diagnosis. Repeated renal biopsies have revealed a membranous lesion that was very similar to that seen at the time of diagnosis.

An additional form of lupus nephritis has been recognized because of the use of immunofluorescence and electron microscopy on specimens of renal tissue obtained from patients with no urinary abnormalities. This lesion is called mesangial (minimal) lupus nephritis. The glomeruli appear normal or may merely show a slight, irregular increase in mesangial cells and matrix on light microscopy. The diagnosis depends on the demonstration of IgG and C3 in the mesangium and occasionally along the capillary walls. Electron microscopy reveals electron-dense deposits in the mesangium. These patients have either no urinary abnormalities or transient minimal proteinuria or minimal hematuria. In a few instances, progression from the mesangial to the diffuse proliferative form has been described. In general, it is very unlikely that patients with little or no clinical evidence of renal disease at the time of diagnosis will develop progression of the renal disease if the initial episode of active systemic disease is adequately treated and initial normalization of serologic abnormalities is sustained over the course of the disease. The presence of IgG in the mesangium of these patients without renal disease is similar to the findings of IgG in the nonlesional skin of patients with clinically active systemic disease. In both situations, deposits are present without pathologic evidence of inflammation.

Pathologic Index of Activity and Sclerosis. There are two forms of proliferative nephritis as described above—focal (mild) and diffuse (severe) proliferative lupus nephritis. The activity of the proliferative lesion may be graded on a semiquantitative basis as originally suggested by Pirani and associates.[55] The following glomerular changes are considered to be signs of active glomerular lesions: fibrinoid necrosis, endocapillary proliferation, epithelial crescents, nuclear debris, hematoxylin bodies, wire-loops, and thrombi. Active interstitial lesions include cell infiltration, acute tubular epithelial lesions, and active necrotizing angiitis. Thus, there is a series of pathologic abnormalities, each of which can be graded as to presence and degree. The degree of pathologic activity may be expressed by grading each of the specific abnormalities and giving the biopsy a total score, which represents the index of activity. Similarly, the degree of sclerosis can be estimated for both glomerular sclerosis and interstitial sclerosis.

The use of the pathologic index of activity is particularly important if successive biopsies on the same patient are to be evaluated or when groups of lupus nephritis patients are to be compared. Studies of repeated sequential biopsies in 40 patients with diffuse lupus nephritis were reported by Morol-Maroger and associates.[56] These investigators found that the presence of extensive sclerosis on the first biopsy indicated a poor prognosis. High doses of prednisone did not prevent the progression of sclerosis in eight patients with severe sclerotic lesions at the time of the first biopsy. On the other hand, 15 patients with a high index of activity at the time of the first biopsy had improvement of their lesion on the second biopsy with little or no sclerosis noted.[56] In 19 of 25 patients in whom the active lesions were initially accompanied by only moderate sclerosis, the activity of the lesions was considerably decreased at the time of the second biopsy. A similar finding was reported by Striker and associates,[57] who noted a difference between active lesions, which responded to therapy, and sclerotic lesions, which did not. We and others have found that glomerular sclerosis is the finding of greatest prognostic value.[56,58-60] Thus, it is very important that the presence and degree of sclerosis be estimated in the renal biopsy report, and this information may be even more relevant to the prognosis of the patient than the mere classification of the nephritis.

The etiology of the sclerosis has recently been explored. Studies by Kant and associates have shown that sclerotic lesions may result from the presence of glomerular thrombi and that the lupus anticoagulant is more common in patients with glomerular thrombi.[61] Fifteen of 20 patients with glomerular thrombi on the initial renal biopsy had increased sclerosis on repeat biopsy, whereas increased sclerosis was found in only 2 of 17 patients who did not have glomerular thrombi on their initial biopsy. The tendency to glomerular sclerosis thus may be related to the presence of the lupus anticoagulant as suggested by these important observations. A prospective study of thrombosis in a large group of SLE patients with and without the lupus anticoagulant should be carried out in order to determine the prognostic significance of this abnormality.

The most important laboratory indicators of disease severity are an increase in serum creatinine and a decrease in serum albumin. Other factors such as the age of the patient, amount of proteinuria, degree of hematuria, and serum C3 levels may also play a role in estimation of disease severity, but there is no general agreement on their importance.

Progression of Renal Disease. It is important to note that progression from focal (mild) to diffuse lupus nephritis has been reported.[53,56,62,63] We have seen this occur in only three patients. In two of these, corticosteroid therapy had been abruptly discontinued by another physician after the patients had moved to another location. Although the patients had been in a clinical and serologic remission on low doses of corticosteroids, the abrupt discontinuation of therapy resulted in a full-blown exacerbation of the clinical and serologic disease abnormalities, and severe diffuse lupus nephritis was demonstrated. A review of 22 patients with focal nephritis by Morol-Maroger and associates described a 5-year cumulative survival rate of 82 percent from the first sign of renal involvement.[56] Deaths occurred only in patients who had normal renal function. These data are similar to those previously reported to us.[52] Morol-Maroger and associates described 81 patients with either minimal or focal lupus nephritis, of whom only six were noted to progress to diffuse lupus nephritis.[56] In two of these patients, the second biopsy showed that the initially focal lesions had become diffuse, whereas clinical symptoms remained minor at the time of the second biopsy. In the other two patients the progression to diffuse nephritis was announced by a major clinical deterioration. Progression from focal to diffuse lupus nephritis was more frequent in the series described by Ginzler and associates and by Zimmerman and associates,[62,63] in which it occurred in 9 of 31 patients and in

6 of 17 patients, respectively. Sclerosis may occur in patients with focal lupus nephritis, but the degree of sclerosis is minimal. Minimal to mild sclerosis was noted in eight of 16 patients with focal nephritis who had a stable course, and mild sclerosis was noted in the initial biopsy in half of the patients who later progressed to diffuse proliferative nephritis.[56] These studies again emphasize that classification of the glomerular lesion is not adequate and that the degree of sclerosis is a crucial element in the ultimate survival of the patients.

In general, the survival of patients with lupus nephritis has improved over the past 5 to 10 years regardless of the classification of the glomerular lesion.

Interstitial immune complex and tubular renal disease also occur in patients with SLE. The histologic findings are focal or diffuse infiltrates of inflammatory cells, tubular damage, and interstitial fibrosis. Immunoglobulins, complement proteins, or both may be noted in the peritubular capillaries, interstitium, or tubular basement membrane in a granular pattern.[64] These deposits correspond to electron-dense deposits seen by electron microscopy. We have noted an occasional patient with urinary abnormalities whose glomeruli have been normal but who has had severe interstitial and tubular renal disease. Renal tubular acidosis may occur in these patients. Microscopic calcification of the interstitial tissue has also been noted in one of our patients with severe tubular and interstitial disease who has renal tubular acidosis. It has been suggested that deposits of DNA-anti-DNA and complement are responsible for the inflammatory interstitial disease. In general, the interstitial lesions are more common in patients with diffuse proliferative lupus nephritis, but, as mentioned above, significant nonglomerular lesions may also be noted in the absence of glomerular disease.

Renal tubular acidosis has been noted in an occasional SLE patient, especially in those with severe interstitial disease. Renal tubular calcinosis is present in two of our patients with diffuse lupus nephritis and interstitial immune disease.

Hemodialysis and Transplantation. This subject is covered in Chapter 70.

VASCULAR MANIFESTATIONS

Raynaud's phenomenon was present in 20 percent of our 365 patients and in 21 percent of the patients reported by Estes and Christian[47] (Fig. 69–10). Raynaud's phenomenon was present in 16 percent of our patients at the time of diagnosis and occurred for the first time during the course of the disease in the other 4 percent of patients. In some individuals this manifestation precedes the onset of multisystem disease. In the series reported by Ropes, Raynaud's phenomenon was the first sign of the disease in 10 of 152 patients and persisted for 1 to 4 years before other manifestations of the disease occurred.[9] Cryoglobulins may be noted in patients who have Raynaud's phenomenon at the time of diagnosis. These patients usually also have nephritis. Unlike the

Figure 69–10. Raynaud's phenomenon in an SLE patient.

Raynaud's phenomenon in patients with systemic sclerosis, that present in SLE patients may gradually disappear as the disease goes into remission. In some of our patients, Raynaud's phenomenon has gradually disappeared over the course of 4 to 5 years of sustained remission. In some individuals, the Raynaud's phenomenon is severe and may result in digital gangrene with self-amputation of the distal digit (Fig. 69–11). Patients respond very poorly to sympathectomy but do respond gradually to corticosteroids. In some individuals, treatment with cyclophosphamide may be necessary to control the necrosis caused by the vasculitis.

Thrombophlebitis occurred in 7 of the 142 patients reported by Ropes[9] and in 10 percent of our patients. Recent reports have suggested that there is a relationship between deep vein thrombosis and the presence of the lupus anticoagulant;[65] however, the relationship between

Figure 69–11. Digital gangrene.

the lupus anticoagulant and thrombosis in SLE patients has not yet been evaluated. In one of our patients and in three patients reported by Ropes, pulmonary emboli were found at post-mortem examination.

Arterial occlusion is uncommon, but occlusion of medium-sized cerebral and peripheral arteries has been observed by us on arteriography in three patients. Recurrent arterial thrombosis has been reported in association with a lupus anticoagulant.[66] The exact relationship between the lupus anticoagulant and either venous or arterial thrombosis has not yet been evaluated by comparing SLE patients with and without the blood abnormality for evidence of thrombosis. Peripheral gangrene occurs rarely. One of our 365 patients developed gangrene of the leg as a result of thrombosis of the femoral artery. Recently we treated a patient with occlusion of the medium-sized arteries at mid-calf who had sudden onset of gangrene of the toes and eventually had a mid-thigh amputation.

GASTROINTESTINAL MANIFESTATIONS

Gastrointestinal manifestations are not uncommon in patients with active SLE. At the time of diagnosis during a period of clinically active disease in other systems, anorexia, nausea, or vomiting was present in 21 percent of our patients. Vomiting was present in 10 percent. Abdominal pain at the time of diagnosis was a manifestation in 10 percent of patients. Abdominal pain that persists and is associated with localizing findings on physical examination or with rebound tenderness should be viewed as an emergency. It is well documented in the literature that infarction of the small or large bowel with or without perforation may occur as a manifestation of active SLE. Mesenteric arteritis may cause ileal or colonic infarcts and perforations. In our own series, we have had three deaths from intestinal perforations among our 365 patients. Zizic and colleagues described four deaths from colonic perforations among 15 deaths in 197 SLE patients.[67] The abdominal pain in patients with perforation is colicky and well localized to the lower abdomen or infraumbilical area, whereas the pain in patients without perforations is less well localized or localized to the epigastrium or upper quadrants and may be either sharp or colicky. We noted rebound and direct tenderness in our patients with perforations, and both were present in four of the five patients reported by Zizic.[67] Rebound or localized direct tenderness was not present in our patients or in those studied by Zizic who did not have perforations.

The abdominal pain associated with bowel infarction or perforation occurs during periods of severe active SLE in other systems. It is of great importance to note that the only patients surviving colonic perforation are those who receive the earliest surgical intervention even in the face of advancing renal insufficiency.

The pathologic abnormalities found in cases with perforation are described as a necrotizing vasculitis.

Other abnormalities noted on surgical intervention in

SLE patients with abdominal pain have included regional enteritis[68-70] and erosions and ulceration.[68,71] Ropes described one patient with a severe ulcerative process extending from the terminal ileum through the entire colon and rectum; she believed the lesion was due to active SLE.[9]

It is worthwhile noting that abdominal pain in SLE patients may not be due to SLE-related abnormalities. In our series, acute onset of abdominal pain with evidence of peritoneal irritation or peritonitis occurred in 15 patients who had no evidence of active SLE at the time. Surgical intervention was prompt (within 48 hours), and ruptured ovarian cyst, perforated gastric ulcer, appendicitis, diverticulitis, and abscesses of the fallopian tubes were found. All these individuals were in remission on low doses of corticosteroids at the time of surgery, and all healed well.

Ascites was present in 4 percent of our patients at the time of diagnosis during a period of clinical disease activity prior to institution of steroid therapy. Ascites was noted in 6 of Ropes' 142 patients who were not receiving steroids and in 5 patients who were on steroid therapy.[9] In her series of 58 patients who had postmortem examinations, peritoneal involvement was present in 63 percent. The volume of fluid in these cases varied from less than 10 ml to 4000 ml. Adhesions were noted over the spleen and liver and over most of the abdominal organs. These varied from thin fibrinous and fibrous strands to firm, old adhesions and large areas of complete adhesion between the liver and the diaphragm.

Ascites associated with protein-losing enteropathy, hypoalbuminemia, and jejunal acute venulitis has been described.[72]

Dysphagia was noted in 10 percent of our patients. Barium swallow in SLE patients with dysphagia may reveal no abnormalities or slightly reduced peristalsis and slight dilatation of the lower esophagus.[73,74] Dysphagia may be due to ulcerations of the esophagus associated with arteritis. Acute esophagitis with fibrinoid necrosis and a diffuse inflammatory infiltrate has been noted at post-mortem examination.[9] As described above, ulcerations may extend into the larynx.

Pancreatitis may be noted in an occasional patient with SLE during periods of active disease. Although pancreatitis has been ascribed to the use of steroid therapy in non-SLE patients, the relationship between pancreatitis and steroid therapy in SLE patients is less clear. There have been reports of non–steroid-treated SLE patients with severe acute pancreatitis.[75,76] In some patients, the severe acute manifestations of pancreatitis have responded to steroid therapy, while in other patients death ensued, with autopsy changes of active systemic disease and acute pancreatitis with arteritis. It is of interest to note that elevations of serum amylase levels may occur in SLE patients who have active disease without abdominal pain and are not on corticosteroid therapy.[12] In these individuals, corticosteroid therapy led to a reduction in the amylase levels. In a recent retrospective analysis, elevated serum amylase was found in 26 SLE patients.[77] The diagnosis of pancreatitis was made in 20 of these patients, and in 6 patients an extrapancreatic cause for the elevation of the enzyme was present. In this study the amylase levels did not correlate with renal function or dose of corticosteroid. Four of the 20 patients with pancreatitis had no other contributory factors and were thought to have pancreatitis due to SLE. These patients recovered with steroid therapy.

LIVER DISEASE

The liver was palpable in 30 percent of our patients. Clinical jaundice is rare, occurring in only 2 percent of our 365 patients and in 1 percent of the 238 patients studied by Runyon and colleagues.[78] Hepatic insufficiency was the cause of death in one 8-year-old child followed by us. This was an acute episode, which occurred during the third year of disease and was due to massive fatty infiltration of the liver. Post-mortem examination of the liver usually reveals enlargement with moderate to marked fatty infiltration, although severe cardiac cirrhosis and healed arteritis have been reported.[9] Liver biopsies from patients with clinical liver disease or with liver enzyme abnormalities may reveal chronic active hepatitis, granulomatous hepatitis, cirrhosis, acute hepatitis, fatty change, or cholestasis.[78] A peculiar form of cholestasis in which bile firmly plugs the canaliculi has been described in 3 of 4 SLE patients with cirrhosis.[78] There is a great discrepancy between clinical and laboratory evidence of dysfunction and pathologic changes in the liver. Elevations of serum glutamic-oxaloacetic transaminase, serum alkaline phosphatase, and serum glutamic-pyruvic transaminase are common. This is found in patients who have not ingested aspirin and usually is present only at the onset of disease. These enzyme elevations return to normal with response of the disease to therapy but may remain high as long as the disease remains very active.

In most patients with biopsy-proven chronic active hepatitis associated with SLE, the liver abnormalities wax and wane along with evidence of active SLE. Thyroid disease (antithyroid antibodies, previously treated hypothyroidism or hyperthyroidism) appears to be more common in SLE patients with liver disease than in those without liver disease.[78]

SPLEEN

Slight to moderate splenomegaly is present in 20 percent of SLE patients. Splenomegaly is usually present without hemolytic anemia. The onion skin appearance of the splenic arterioles is present in 15 percent of patients and is due to concentric periarterial fibrosis. This fibrosis is thought to represent an end-stage of an earlier focal arteritis.

Lack of splenic activity has been demonstrated using technetium 99m sulphur colloid scans in three SLE patients whose peripheral blood smears suggested hyposplenism. CAT scan revealed splenic atrophy in one patient. The other patient died of pneumococcal septicemia and had no spleen when studied at autopsy.[79] The authors of this study also performed scans on 65 other SLE patients and found functional asplenism in 2 additional patients. The importance of this finding relates to the susceptibility of these individuals to infection and to the present availability of a pneumococcal vaccine.

LYMPH NODES

Lymph nodes are enlarged in about one half of SLE patients at the time of clinical disease activity. Enlargement is usually generalized but may be localized to one or two groups of nodes. One of our patients has had two episodes of active disease, each associated with massive enlargement of the occipital nodes. The enlarged nodes are usually moderately enlarged, although massive adenopathy has been noted, particularly among young children. In adolescents and young adults, the generalized lymphadenopathy may lead to an initial diagnosis of mononucleosis. Tender lymph nodes are unusual in SLE patients and should lead to a suspicion of infection. Microscopic changes in lymph nodes are nonspecific and consist of follicular hyperplasia with or without associated areas of necrosis. Three of our patients and one of Ropes'[9] had lymph node biopsies which were diagnosed as giant follicular lymphoma. Later, these patients were correctly diagnosed as having SLE and treated with corticosteroids; they are still alive 14 to 22 years after the initial biopsy.

It is common for lymph node enlargement to recur during episodes of disease activity, and lymph node enlargement may be one of the early signs of impending generalized flare of the disease in some individuals.

THYMUS

No abnormalities of the thymus have been noted in our patients or in those of Ropes.[9] Thymoma has been described in 15 SLE patients,[80] and patients with co-existent myasthenia gravis and SLE have been reported.[81-83] In nearly all of these patients SLE occurred after the diagnosis of myasthenia gravis.[82] The incidence of SLE in large series of patients with myasthenia is about 1 percent.[83] Thymectomy has been performed in a small number of SLE patients without effect on the course of the disease.[84,86] On the other hand, patients with myasthenia gravis have developed SLE after thymectomy.[87]

OCULAR MANIFESTATIONS

Conjunctivitis and episcleritis occurred in 15 percent of our patients and appeared to be associated with extensive cutaneous lesions. Subconjunctival hemorrhages have been described, and cutaneous lesions of SLE may appear on the eyelids as papules. Severe conjunctival chemosis occurred along with episcleritis and glaucoma in one of our patients.[88]

Occlusion of the central retinal artery during periods of disease activity has rarely occurred.[89] Blindness resulting from active retinal arteritis and arteriolar occlusion has been reported.[90] Cytoid bodies were noted in 8 percent of our patients and in 8 percent of the 245 SLE patients analyzed to formulate criteria for the classification of patients with SLE.[2] These are retinal exudates, which appear as hard white lesions adjacent to retinal vessels during periods of disease activity, and more widespread retinal edema, hemorrhage, and infarctions have been reported as a result of retinal artery vasculitis. The exudates gradually disappear as the disease becomes inactive. Fluorescein angiography studies in a patient with retinopathy revealed subretinal edema, and study of the eye at autopsy revealed immunoglobulins in the vascular layer of the chorid capillaries and basement membranes of the ciliary processes and bulbar conjunctiva.[91]

Loss of vision has been reported as the initial symptom of the disease[92] and was the cause for admission to the hospital of one of our patients.[88] In both of these patients, vision returned to normal after treatment with corticosteroids for the systemic disease.

We have noted an association between the presence of cytoid bodies and central nervous system disease activity (seizures and organic brain disease).

Keratoconjunctivitis sicca may occur in SLE patients but is uncommon in our series. A similar low incidence was noted by Ropes[7] and by Dubois.[93]

PAROTID GLANDS

Acute enlargement of the parotid glands occurred in 8 percent of our patients and in 6 of Dubois' 520 patients.[93] The enlargement was unilateral in half the patients and occurred during periods of disease activity. Ropes noted salivary gland enlargement in 12 percent of her patients,[9] and, as in our patients, noted that the swelling was occasionally associated with marked evidence of inflammation. In our patients, biopsies of the lip did reveal changes typical of Sjögren's syndrome. The diffuse tender parotid swelling recurred in some patients during later exacerbations of the disease after initially responding to corticosteroid therapy. The frequency of Sjögren's syndrome was very high in the study reported by Moutsopoulus and associates. In this prospective study of 24 SLE patients, clinical symptoms were present in 54 percent. It is of interest that whereas Schirmer's test was positive in only 21 percent of the patients, parotid scan was positive in 58 percent and lip biopsy in 50 percent of patients.[94]

NERVOUS SYSTEM MANIFESTATIONS

Peripheral Neuropathy. Peripheral neuropathy occurred in 14 percent of our patients, an incidence similar to that reported by others[95] (Table 69–3). The most common abnormality is sensory, but a mixed sensori-motor disturbance is present in about 5 percent of patients who have asymmetric involvement similar to that of mononeuritis multiplex. Episodes of sudden onset of peripheral neuropathy rarely occur in the absence of disease activity in other systems. Treatment of the peripheral neuropathy with corticosteroids usually leads to gradual recovery of the affected extremity. On the other hand, if the vasculitis has led to irreversible damage to the peripheral nerve, no return to normal function will result from the use of corticosteroid therapy.

An acute mixed ascending motor paralysis with variable sensory involvement typical of a Guillain-Barré syndrome rarely occurs. The peripheral neuropathy in SLE patients may be reflected in abnormalities of the cerebrospinal fluid, especially in elevation of the cerebrospinal fluid protein.

Cranial nerve involvement is less common than peripheral neuropathy. These episodes of cranial nerve involvement usually occur during episodes of active systemic disease when evidence of vasculitis is present in other systems. Extraocular movements may be due to involvement of the ophthalmic, trochlear, or abducens nerves[96,97] and may be either unilateral or bilateral. Trigeminal nerve abnormalities usually affect the sensory component of the nerve and are usually bilateral.[98,99] Facial nerve paralysis is uncommon, although we noted this in one of our SLE patients during a period when active disease was associated with organic brain disease. Optic neuritis is rare, occurring in less than 1 percent of patients. It may be the first manifestation of SLE, but more often there are other manifestations of SLE at the time and it has been reported to occur at the time that a myelopathy was also noted.[100] Treatment of the optic neuritis with corticosteroids has led to variable

outcomes, with some patients regaining normal vision and others progressing to blindness.

Paralysis. Paralysis of the extremities is very rare. We have observed only one of our patients with transverse myelitis, and the incidence in the literature is less than 4 percent.[97] Hemiparesis is usually associated with hemisensory losses, homonymous ocular field deficits, and aphasia. The lesion found on post-mortem examination is generally agreed to result from vascular lesions. The lesion of the involved vessels may be occlusive, hemorrhagic, or embolic. Two of our patients have died of intracerebral hemorrhages. Occlusion of major cerebral vessels and displacement of vessels by edematous areas of the brain have been demonstrated using angiography.[101] We have recently demonstrated occlusion of an internal carotid artery in a young man who had a cerebral vascular accident eight months after SLE had been diagnosed. He had been on tapering doses of prednisone at the time of the stroke. Another patient had a major stroke within 3 days of starting corticosteroid therapy after having had symptoms of CNS lupus for the previous month. It is of interest that thrombophlebitis was reported in two of the three patients with angiographic demonstration of major cerebral vessel occlusion reported by Trevor and associates.[101] The relationship between the presence of the lupus anticoagulant, thrombosis, and the false positive VDRL has not been established. Both the lupus anticoagulant and a false positive VDRL were present in two of our four patients with occlusion of medium-sized arteries. However, many more of our patients have the lupus anticoagulant, and few of them have had any thrombotic episodes. The etiology of the major vessel occlusions is thus obscure. Pathologic studies have revealed only a few cases of cranial arteritis and vasculitis; the majority of the abnormalities have been microinfarcts.

Paralysis resulting from lesions within the spinal cord has been described.[102] These changes may include extension to the upper thoracic or even cervical regions with resulting quadriplegia. Cerebrospinal fluid abnormalities in patients with spinal cord disease include elevated protein with paretic changes of the colloidal gold reaction and a low spinal fluid glucose.[103]

It should be noted that monoplegia and paraplegia in SLE patients are not always due to SLE. Reticulum cell sarcoma in an SLE patient treated with azathioprine was reported by Lipsmeyer,[104] and paraplegia caused by an epidural abscess from *Aspergillus fumigatus* was reported in the same patient.[104] One of our patients had evidence of meningitis and at post-mortem examination was found to have abscesses caused by the same organism.

Movement Disorders. Chorea was present in one of our 365 patients. This 12-year-old girl had persistent unilateral chorea during the 7 years of observation, and the abnormality was present during prolonged periods of sustained remission of the disease and also during periods of clinically active disease. Choreoathetoid movements may be present at any point in the course of the disease,[97] may be the first manifestation of the

Table 69–3. Neuropsychiatric Manifestations in 140 Patients with SLE*

	Manifestation	Patients
A.	SLE related	52
	Psychiatric illness	24
	Seizures	17
	Long tract signs	16
	Cranial nerve abnormalities	16
	Peripheral neuropathy	15
	Cerebellar signs	5
	Scotomas	4
	Papilledema (pseudotumor)	2
	Chorea	2
	Meningitis, myelitis	1
B.	Other cause	19†
	Psychiatric illness	13
	Meningitis	2
	Peripheral neuropathy	3
	Seizures	1

*From Feinglass, E., et al.: Medicine 55:323, 1976.

†In addition to these 19 patients, 7 patients from Group A developed other neuropsychiatric abnormalities that were due to factors not directly related to SLE.

disease, and may recur during exacerbations during the course of the disease.

Seizures. In a review of her 82 SLE patients seen before 1949 (prior to the availability of corticosteroids), Ropes noted that 17 percent of the patients had seizures and that 70 percent of those with seizures had the seizures as a terminal event.[7] In several of these patients, the seizure was the immediate cause of death. A few of her patients never regained consciousness, while others had severe respiratory distress and anoxia and died within a few hours. The information regarding the observations on this non–steroid-treated group of patients is invaluable and stresses the view that seizures are the most significant emergency in SLE patients. In our own series, seizures have been treated aggressively and immediately with high doses of corticosteroids, usually administered intravenously. We have observed repeated grand mal seizures unresponsive to the usual therapy in two patients who appeared to respond to high-dose intravenous corticosteroids.

The most commonly observed seizure is the grand mal seizure. Seizures were present at the time of diagnosis in 29 patients studied in New York. Of these, 25 patients had grand mal seizures, one had petit mal, two had psychomotor epilepsy, and two had jacksonian seizures. Additional patients developed seizures later in the course of the disease; nine additional patients had grand mal seizures, one additional patient developed petit mal, and one additional patient developed jacksonian fits. In most patients, episodes of seizures occurred along with clinical and laboratory evidence of severe systemic disease. Temporal lobe epilepsy has been observed rarely. Epilepsy is the initial manifestation of SLE in from 1 to 4 percent of patients. Whereas many of our patients survived for many years after the initial episodes of seizures at the time of diagnosis, status epilepticus is a not infrequent terminal event (see above).

Organic Brain Syndromes. One of the most serious manifestations of SLE is the presence of organic brain syndromes (OBS). The patients have impairment of orientation, perception, memory, and intellectual function.[97] In many individuals the impairment fluctuates, and during periods of relative lucidity the patients are able to communicate the fact that their thinking process is impaired. Patients may be able to recognize their physician as long as there is physical contact (hand-holding), but if the physician returns to the bedside after a few minutes absence the patient may be unable to recognize him. There is a major difficulty in orientation as to place and time. Patients who are highly educated may be unable to name the President of the United States or the Governor of the State. The patients are usually also very frightened by their inability to think. The onset of the syndrome is acute and fulminant. Complete recovery from OBS is usual, but some patients have residual impairment of mental processes such as inability to do rapid calculations. In our series of patients studied at the Bellevue Medical Psychiatric wards, most of the organic psychoses were seen early in the course of the disease. Forty-four patients had OBS at the time of

diagnosis, whereas only 16 patients had OBS during the following year and only four patients had this manifestation during the third year of disease. Eight patients were hospitalized for OBS during the fourth year, two during the fifth year, and one each during the sixth, seventh, and eighth years of disease. None of the 30 patients followed through their sixth year of the disease had OBS. It should be noted here that the presence of OBS at the time of diagnosis did not affect the 5-year survival of our patients. The 5-year survival was 71 percent for those with OBS at diagnosis as compared with 77 percent for those without OBS.[105]

SLE patients with central nervous system disease (OBS or seizures) are more likely to have evidence of vasculitis of other systems than those without central nervous system findings.[95]

Headaches. Severe headaches occurred at the time of diagnosis in 21 of our 209 patients followed in New York. In five of these patients the severe headache was associated with OBS; and in eight others, with seizures. Migraine headaches have been noted in SLE patients who had wavy or zigzag line scotomas typical of the fortification specters of migraine.[106] In some individuals, the scotomas have been noted without headaches. These phenomena occur for the first time either after the diagnosis of SLE or as an initial feature along with other manifestations of active systemic disease. Migraine headaches have occurred as isolated symptoms but at a time when serologic abnormalities of SLE were present. These headaches are important to recognize as a manifestation of SLE because they disappear when prednisone is given or when the dose is increased, and they may occur along with other manifestations of the disease during an exacerbation. A recent study revealed that there is an increased prevalence of classic migraine among SLE patients when they are compared with an age- and sex-matched control group. Twelve of the 30 SLE patients, compared with only 4 of the 30 controls, had classic migraine. In SLE patients whose classic migraine predated the diagnosis of SLE, an increase in headaches with the onset of SLE was noted in about half. We have also noted that a major flare of the disease may be associated with the reappearance of classic migraine headaches that had been present prior to the onset of SLE and disappeared during the previous period of disease inactivity owing to treatment with corticosteroids. There appears to be no association between classic migraine and Raynaud's phenomenon in SLE patients.[107]

Psychological Problems. Nonorganic syndromes (affective of functional disorders) have normal cognitive functions in contrast to the organic syndromes.[97] The most commonly observed manifestations in the SLE patients are depression and, less often, anxiety. Although severe depression may occur in a few individuals, much more often a mild depressed state occurs. The depression is nearly always a reaction to the disease and to the disfigurement caused by both the disease and the corticosteroid therapy. The young woman or teenager who has a facial rash and alopecia and then is placed on corticosteroids with the resulting cushingoid appearance and facial hair growth is very likely to become extremely depressed. The physician must provide psychologic support for the patient, and the family must be involved in helping the patient cope with the illness and the side effects of the initial therapy. In some patients, psychotherapy may be indicated during the initial stages of the illness.

It is extremely important that the reactive depression in an SLE patient not be confused with the organic brain syndrome caused by the disease. The former should be treated with reassurance and psychotherapy, whereas the latter should be treated vigorously with corticosteroid therapy.

Cerebrospinal Fluid Abnormalities. Abnormalities of the cerebrospinal fluid occurred in 32 percent of the neuropsychiatric episodes in 37 patients studied by Feinglass and associates.[95] Protein elevation was noted in about half the fluids, and in some patients an increase in protein and in numbers of white blood cells was noted. Elevations of protein may be associated with papilledema and may be modest or significant. In the series described by Feinglass and associates deaths occurred in patients with cerebrospinal fluid abnormalities, whereas none of the patients with normal cerebrospinal fluids died.[95] Spinal fluid C4 levels are lower than levels of complement proteins and will return to normal as the patient improves.[68] Unfortunately, the assay must be performed immediately, since the hemolytic activity of C4 rapidly decays.

The electroencephalogram is frequently abnormal during episodes of OBS or seizure disorders. Abnormal electroencephalograms have also been noted in patients without central nervous system (CNS) abnormalities but are more frequent in those with CNS disease.[109]

It is probably wise to obtain a brain scan in a patient with CNS disease. If it is abnormal, repeated brain scans can be performed to determine whether the abnormalities disappear as the patient recovers.[109] There have been conflicting reports in the literature regarding the correlation between clinical CNS manifestations and changes on the brain scan using both technetium-99m and oxygen-15 methods.[110,111] The latter method appears to be capable of demonstrating temporary regional ischemia but requires the use of a cyclotron, so that this technique cannot be used on a widespread basis at the present time.

Computerized axial tomography (CAT scan) is of more value in the work-up of a patient with CNS lupus. Major areas of infarction are clearly demonstrable and therefore the CAT scan should be ordered on patients with localized CNS abnormalities. The value of the CAT scan in patients without localizing findings is still unclear. The detection of diffuse cerebral abnormalities has been reported as "cerebral atrophy," which is a radiologic term describing enlargement of ventricles and cortical sulci. The cause for such enlargement may be due to a number of reasons, such as loss of water or of nerve cells. Studies on other diseases have shown that "cerebral atrophy" may be found in a variety of conditions, including alcoholism. In addition, patients on corticoste-

roid therapy for other reasons may show "cerebral atrophy." There are conflicting reports on "cortical atrophy" in SLE patients with or without any evidence of lupus cerebritis (organic brain syndrome or seizures). The frequency and degree of cerebral atrophy and the relationship of this finding to steroid therapy and the clinical manifestations of CNS lupus remain unclear at the present time.

Pathology. The neuropathologic findings in 23 patients who had seizures have been described in the literature by Ropes[9] and by Ellis and Verity.[112] Analysis of the data presented in these two reports reveals that the most common finding was microinfarcts, which was noted in 61 percent of the 23 patients. Vasculitis was found in 35 percent and intracerebral hemorrhages in 22 percent. The brains were reported as normal in 2 of the 12 patients reported by Ropes.[9] The patients reported by Ropes are essentially the same patients described by Johnson and Richardson.[96] Focal motor seizures were associated with evidence of chronic subarachnoid hemorrhage.[112] A high incidence of cortical microinfarction was noted in the much more commonly occurring grand mal seizures.

Pathologic changes found in 12 patients with hemiparesis were similar to those found in the patients with seizures with one major exception: intracerebral hemorrhage was noted in 6 of the 12 patients and was not found in patients with seizures or with cranial nerve palsies.[112]

The etiology of the cerebral hemorrhages appears to be related to the presence of vasculitis in one third of the patients.[112] Vasculitis was noted in 5 of 17 patients with subarachnoid hemorrhages, in 3 of 6 patients with intracerebral hemorrhages, and in 3 of 11 patients with microhemorrhages.

Ropes also described the abnormalities found in the brain of one patient with chorea.[9] The changes consisted of numerous microinfarcts, and several small arteries were filled with necrotic material.

It is important to note that bacterial and mycotic infections are not uncommon in SLE patients with meningitis and that the aseptic meningitis due to SLE should be diagnosed only after an extensive search for an infectious etiology. In our own series, meningitis due to tuberculosis, aspergillus, and crytococcus occurred in 3 of 209 patients followed prior to 1968 and has not been noted in over 300 patients followed since that time. On the other hand, Ellis and Verity found a significant increase in infectious meningitis in the years 1966 to 1976 compared with the period from 1955 to 1965.[112]

Changes in Ropes' eleven patients with psychoses revealed seven with microinfarcts, one with a large cerebral hemorrhage, four with vasculitis, and two with minimal changes.[9]

In the series reported by Ropes,[9] post-mortem examination of the brain was negative in 13 of the 37 patients examined. Thirty-six percent of the patients had brain infarction or definite nerve cell loss, and other abnormalities were found in 38 percent of the cases. Nineteen of the patients reported by Ropes are the same as those included in the detailed study of 24 cases reported by Johnson and Richardson.[75] These authors concluded that there was no single pathognomic lesion present in the brains of SLE patients. The prominent lesions were the result of intrinsic disease of the small vessels, especially arterioles and capillaries. Fibrinoid necrosis was found in some vessels, while others showed proliferative changes in the intima. Fibrin thrombi were occasionally observed, and a cellular inflammatory reaction within the vessel walls typical of periarteritis nodosa was seen only rarely. The authors felt that the changes observed resembled those seen in hypertensive encephalopathy, rheumatic ·fever, and thrombotic thrombocytopenic purpura (TTP). It is of interest that one of our SLE patients expired of manifestations clinically identical to those seen in TTP; on post-mortem examination of the brain, the changes were those seen in TTP. Another of our SLE patients also developed TTP but was successfully treated with high doses of corticosteroids and successive plasmaphereses.

In general, there is a correlation between the location of vascular changes in the cortex and brainstem and the patient's signs and symptoms, but there are definitely exceptions to this. Presumably the various clinical expressions represent differences in the severity and location of the lesion, and the transient nature of some of the symptoms and signs may relate to the small size of the infarcts. However, it is our experience and that of Ropes[9] that no pathologic abnormalities of the brain may be noted in the patients with severe psychosis or seizures. In addition, changes in the blood vessels alone probably do not account for the development of paraparesis or sensory neuropathy, or satisfactorily explain the diffuse disorders of the organic brain syndrome seen in some of the patients.[97]

Immunofluorescence studies of the choroid plexus have revealed deposits of IgG in patients with CNS lupus, whereas no immunoglobulins were found in the choroid plexuses from nine non–SLE-affected individuals.[113] Lampert and Oldstone described patchy granular deposits of C3 in the choroids of three SLE patients who died with CNS disease.[114] These investigators also found deposits of IgG in the choroids of 5 of 20 control patients, but no C3 was found in any of the controls. Immunoglobulins were present in the choroids of two of four SLE patients with CNS lupus and in one of three SLE patients without CNS lupus by Boyer and associates.[115] These investigators were unable to detect complement components because these proteins were destroyed by fixation. The data suggest that immunoglobulins are present in SLE patients with and without CNS disease and perhaps are also present in non–SLE-affected individuals. In a study of 36 randomly selected autopsies, IgG and C3 were not found.[116] Of interest is that the same investigators were able to demonstrate binding sites for IgG in the choroid plexus from the same subjects.[116] Future studies may lead to more information on the role of the choroid plexus as a blood-brain barrier in patients with SLE CNS disease. The number, distribution, and avidity of the choroid plexus receptors may be under genetic control or subject to environmental influences, and therefore future studies may help to explain why CNS lupus occurs only in a limited number of SLE patients with circulating immune complexes.

CARDIAC MANIFESTATIONS

Pericardium. The most frequent cardiac manifestation is pericarditis, which occurs in about 25 percent of patients. A pericardial rub is more common than the presence of a detectable amount of pericardial fluid using x-ray evaluation, although 29 percent of SLE patients have pericardial thickening on echocardiography.[117] Pericardial tamponade is very unusual. Abnormalities of the electrocardiogram are very common in SLE patients. The most common abnormality is the presence of abnormal T waves. This was present in 75 percent of the patients reported by Ropes,[9] a figure similar to those reported by other studies of the heart in SLE.[118,119] The abnormalities of the T wave disappear as the disease is treated. Pericardial involvement is present in about 80 percent at post-mortem examination. Fluid is present in less than half the patients. Microscopic abnormalities of the pericardium vary from rare foci of fibrinoid degeneration or minimal infiltration of inflammatory cells to extensive areas of fibrinous degeneration and heavy infiltration of lymphocytes, plasma cells, and monocytes. A superficial layer of fibrin is usually noted. Pericardial vessels may show proliferation of the intima, areas of fibrinous degeneration, and perivascular infiltration of inflammatory cells. In one case reported by Ropes[9] hematoxylin bodies were noted. Adhesions have been noted between the pericardium and the heart, and complete chronic adhesive pericarditis has been reported.[119,120]

Myocardium. Myocardial involvement is much less common than pericarditis. Prolonged P-R intervals were present in 10 percent of the patients described by Ropes.[9] Clinical manifestations include tachycardia, an enlarging heart, congestive heart failure, arrhythmias, and conduction defects.

Myocardial involvement was present in 42 percent of autopsies in the series described by Ropes.[9] Fibrinoid degeneration was present in nine patients, and typical Aschoff nodules in two. Myocardial abscesses have been reported.[9]

Myocardial Infarction and Coronary Artery Disease. Deaths caused by myocardial infarction from arteritis have been reported early in the course of the disease in young patients, including those in whom steroid therapy was never instituted.[9,121] Atherosclerosis of the coronary arteries was present in two patients who were not treated with corticosteroids.[122] The myocardial findings at post-mortem examination may reveal old myocardial infarctions. Ropes described a patient who died one year after a myocardial infarction and who had severe atherosclerosis of the involved vessel, but one section of the vessel adjacent to the old thrombus showed acute inflammation and necrosis in both intima and muscularis and one focus of hemorrhage and acute inflammation in the adventitia. She concluded that the vasculitis might have played a role in the infarction. Coronary arteritis with stenosis and infarction has been rarely reported.[12,119,121,123] In some of these patients, arteritis of vessels in other organs was found in addition to the coronary arteritis. A patient in whom alterations in coronary arterial anatomy occurred with angiographic improvement temporally related to the initiation of corticosteroid therapy has been reported.[123]

It should be noted that recent studies of hearts of patients dying with SLE have revealed a high incidence of coronary atherosclerosis in those treated for at least 1 year with corticosteroids,[124] and significant narrowing of the coronary arteries in patients without angina has been noted in a study of young female necropsy patients.[125] Death from myocardial infarction has been reported to occur late in the course of the disease in corticosteroid-treated patients.[126] Angina occurring late in the course of the disease in a patient without evidence of disease activity should be thoroughly investigated. Successful coronary by-pass surgery has been performed on such a patient.[123]

Coronary artery occlusion due to an embolus from an aortic valve vegetation has been reported.[127]

Valves. Systolic murmurs were heard in 30 percent of our patients, in 44 percent of the series of Harvey and associates,[71] and in 39 percent of Larson's patients.[128] In most instances, the systolic murmurs are heard equally at the apex and the base.[12] Very loud murmurs are usually associated with severe or moderately severe anemia.

Diastolic murmurs are heard very rarely. A diastolic mitral murmur was present in one of our 365 patients and was present in only 0.9 percent of the series of 540 patients described by Dubois.[93] The murmurs resemble the classic murmur of rheumatic mitral stenosis. Aortic insufficiency murmurs have been rarely described. Bernhard and associates[129] described three patients in a series of 52 whose main manifestation of SLE was aortic insufficiency, and Shulman and Christian[130] reported three cases of aortic insufficiency in SLE patients. Ropes has noted that at least two of the three patients described by Shulman and Christian were patients whose SLE was atypical and very suggestive of rheumatoid arthritis.[9] She describes one patient with definite aortic insufficiency who also had an atypical picture for SLE because of the presence of spondylitis. However, despite the aforementioned comments, it is clear that aortic insufficiency does occur in patients with typical SLE.[11,13,118,119]

The pathologic picture of the valves appears to have changed from that originally reported from studies of non–steroid-treated patients.[24] One third of the series reported in 1953 by Dubois[131] and one third of the series reported in 1954 by Harvey and associates,[71] had lesions of Libman-Sacks endocarditis. These lesions are ovoid vegetations, ranging in diameter from 1 to 4 mm; they are made up of areas of proliferating and degenerating valve tissue with fibrin and platelet thrombi. The verrucae are usually seen near the edge of the valve and less commonly on the chordae tendineae, papillary muscles, and mural endocardium. The original descriptions of the lesions by Libman and Sacks[132] and by Gross[133] emphasized that the lesions are most commonly observed on the tricuspid valve. However, recent series have shown a higher incidence on the mitral valve.[124]

The clinical significance of the presence of Libman-Sacks endocarditis has been debated. Ropes has noted that "only occasionally was the valvulitis of sufficient degree to have produced clinical signs."[9] Dubois has noted that even when the verrucae were prominent, they did not tend to involve the line of closure because they were predominantly located on the undersurface of the valve.[12] He concludes the following from a review of the literature:

It would appear that interpretation of a diastolic murmur as reflecting the development of atypical verrucous endocarditis was proven to be wrong as often as right. The circumstances that would make such an interpretation most plausible would be the development of a diastolic apical murmur de novo in a patient with SLE without heart failure, anemia, or bacterial endocarditis. This would be an exceedingly rare occurrence.[12]

Chronic disease of the valves may occur late in the course of the disease following initial treatment of endocarditis with corticosteroids. Aortic valvular insufficiency with perforations of the valves has been noted, and mitral regurgitation may rarely occur. Valve replacement has been required for severe scarring of the leaflets and ruptured chordae tendineae.[134,135]

Subacute Bacterial Endocarditis. Superimposed subacute bacterial endocarditis occasionally occurs in SLE patients. This was diagnosed clinically in two of Ropes' patients, both of whom responded to therapy.[9] Diastolic murmurs occur for the first time in SLE patients during the course of subacute bacterial endocarditis when the organisms become implanted on the leaflets previously deformed by Libman-Sacks endocarditis. A case of aortic insufficiency caused by subacute bacterial endocarditis was noted by Harvey and associates,[71] and Dubois[12] described mitral valve lesions in two of his patients resulting from subacute bacterial endocarditis.

Acute bacterial endocarditis was present on post-mortem examination in five of Ropes' patients; lesions were present on the valves and, in one, on the ventricular wall.[9] It should be noted that these patients died during the preantibiotic era.

PLEUROPULMONARY MANIFESTATIONS

Pleural Involvement. Pleuritic pain was present in 11 percent of our patients at the time of diagnosis and in 46 percent of the patients at some time during the course of the disease. The pleuritic pain was much more common than radiographic evidence of pleural effusion, which was present at the time of diagnosis in 20 percent of patients and during the course of disease in only 32 percent of patients. A pleuritic rub was heard in 22 percent of the series reported by Ropes.[9] Pleural effusions are small to moderate, although massive pleural effusions may occur occasionally. In the series reported by Ropes,[9] fluid was present in 33 patients and ranged in volume from less than 5 ml to 1500 ml. Only three of the effusions were hemorrhagic, and one fluid was grossly purulent. Most often the effusions are clearly exudates, having more than 3.0 g of protein per 100 ml.[138] The glucose concentration is more than 55 mg per 100 ml in contrast to that present in the pleural effusions of patients with rheumatoid arthritis, in whom levels of less than 20 mg per 100 ml are usually present. Typical LE cells have been identified in the pleural fluids of patients with SLE.

Pathologic abnormalities in the pleura were found in 24 percent of the 58 patients studied at post-mortem examination by Ropes[9] and in 18 percent of the 120 autopsied patients studied by Haupt and associates.[139] Changes varied from small accumulations of lymphocytes of fibrinoid necrosis with infiltrates of neutrophils and mononuclear cells. In a few patients, extensive infiltrations of inflammatory cells and fibrinous exudate were noted. In Rope's series, adhesions were present in 63 percent of the patients, and complete bilateral adhesions were noted in six cases.[9]

Lungs. *Acute Lupus Pneumonitis.* Acute pneumonitis was present in 11.7 percent of 102 patients hospitalized for SLE reported by Matthay and associates.[140] Lupus pneumonitis was present at the time of diagnosis in 6 percent of these 102 patients and in 12 percent of our 209 patients. In patients with acute pneumonitis caused by SLE, dyspnea is usually present and pleuritic chest pain may or may not occur. Cough may or may not be present. Gross hemoptysis has been noted in patients with severe acute lupus pneumonitis. Two of the patients described by Dubois died from refractory intrapulmonary bleeding.[12] On physical examination basilar rales are heard, but pleural friction rubs are uncommon. The chest roentgenograms demonstrate diffuse acinar infiltrates with a predilection for the lung bases. In the 12 patients described by Matthay and associates,[140] the infiltrates are bilateral in ten and involved only the right side in two. Pleural effusions were present in half the patients. It is of interest to note that the infiltrates may completely clear in patients who survive the acute episode, or patients may go on to develop chronic infiltrates with persistently abnormal pulmonary function tests. Pulmonary function studies on the patients with acute infiltrates reveal hypoxemia. Residual pulmonary function abnormalities in patients surviving the acute episodes have been noted even when the patients are asymptomatic. Autopsy material from patients with acute pneumonitis has revealed acute alveolar damage with interstitial edema, hyaline membranes, and, in some patients, acute alveolitis. Recently these findings have been attributed to causes other than SLE, such as congestive heart failure, oxygen toxicity, and infection.[139]

It is important to emphasize that the aforementioned description of acute pneumonitis caused by SLE relates to patients whose work-up has failed to reveal an infectious agent and in whom antibiotics fail to favorably alter the course. The recent study by Haupt revealed that the most common cause of pulmonary infiltrates is infection.[139]

Diffuse Interstitial Pneumonitis. Diffuse interstitial lung disease may occur in SLE patients. The disease is chronic, and the main symptom is dyspnea on exertion.[141] Physical findings are poor diaphragmatic movement and diminished resonance to percussion over the bases. Basilar rales are usually present, and cyanosis and clubbing may occur.[141] Pulmonary hypertension in such patients has been reported.[142] The diagnosis is based on the radiographic findings of persistent, diffuse interstitial infiltrates. These are usually of long duration, and other causes must be ruled out. Other findings in patients with diffuse interstitial lung disease include pleuritis, unilateral elevation of the diaphragm, platelike atelectasis, small pleural effusion, and localized infiltrates.[141]

Lung function in patients with diffuse interstitial pneumonia reveals a restrictive pattern with a lower than predicted vital capacity. The total lung capacity is diminished and the flow rates, maximum inspiratory flow rate, maximum expiratory flow rate, and forced expiratory volume are diminished in a degree proportional to the amount of the decrease in vital capacity. No evidence for airway obstruction is noted. Arterial oxygen tensions are diminished. Eisenberg noted that the mean alveolar-arterial difference of O_2 was 36 mm Hg, with a range from 18 to 57 mm Hg in his 18 patients with diffuse interstitial pneumonia.[141] The diffusing capacity of the lung was decreased below predicted normal values in 17 of his 18 patients. The radiographic changes in these patients consist of diffuse pulmonic interstitial infiltrates that are linear and reticulonodular. They are present throughout both lung fields but are more prominent in the lower lobe.

Pathologic examination of the chronic interstitial pneumonitis has been performed on biopsies of the lung. In the study by Haupt and associates of pulmonary lesions in 120 patients, interstitial fibrosis similar to that found in progressive systemic sclerosis was demonstrated in 5 patients.[139] Slight to moderate thickening of the alveolar walls by loose fibrous tissue, a moderate plasma cell infiltration of the interstices, slight to moderate histiocytic desquamation, and acute ulcerative and focal necrosis involving alveoli and bronchioles may be noted.[141] There is no evidence of vasculitis in the lesions obtained from the lung, although inflammatory changes are noted early in the course and fibrosis at the late stage.

Pulmonary function abnormalities have been described in SLE patients who are not dyspneic and have no radiographic abnormalities. The only abnormality found in these patients is a decreased carbon monoxide diffusing capacity.[143]

MENSTRUAL ABNORMALITIES AND PREGNANCY

A small number of SLE patients report that their disease flares at or immediately prior to the menstrual period. In some patients, the rash becomes pronounced or is noted only at the time of menses, while in other patients arthralgia or objective evidence of arthritis is noted. In about 15 percent of patients, there may be a 6- to 8-month delay in the menstrual period at the time the disease is active. Return of normal menstrual cycles is usually noted at a time when the disease has been in a sustained remission and the corticosteroid dose has been reduced to a moderate level.

Exacerbation of the disease occurs in SLE patients during pregnancy and during the post-partum period.[144] Our experience during 1950 and 1959 revealed that 24 percent of the patients had a post-partum flare of symptoms.[145] Recently, we have reviewed the experience from 1960 to 1969 at the same hospital and found that the incidence of post-partum flares was only 11 percent.[146] During the years 1970 to 1982 we have had only one significant post-partum flare (hemolytic anemia). This decrease in incidence is probably due to the fact that we had been impressed with the previous data and treated our pregnant patients aggressively during delivery and the immediate post-partum period. In another study of maternal morbidity in SLE, two deaths among seven patients who had exacerbations during the immediate (3 weeks) post-partum period was reported.[147] Neither of the two patients was treated with corticosteroids. In a recent review of 24 pregnancies, 54 percent of patients had either a clinical or serologic exacerbation during pregnancy or during the post-partum period as compared with 4 percent of the same patients during the 6 months prior to pregnancy.[148] Patients who had exacerbations during pregnancy or during the post-partum period had significant renal disease and active SLE during the 6 months prior to pregnancy. A similar correlation between exacerbation during pregnancy and the presence of active disease during the 5 months prior to pregnancy was noted in a study confined to patients with lupus nephritis.[149] Thus, patients who become pregnant while the disease is active are at a high risk of further exacerbation of their disease. In our experience, patients who are in clinical and serologic remission and taking less than 15 mg of prednisone for at least 6 months prior to pregnancy have a very slight chance of exacerbation of their disease during pregnancy or during the post-partum period.

There is little value to therapeutic abortion in SLE patients, since this may lead to an exacerbation of the disease.

We have not noted fetal abnormalities in our patients except for two children of one of our patients who were born with complete heart block.[150] Other reports have appeared in the literature describing heart block in babies born to SLE patients. Congenital lupus is described in Chapter 68.

HEMATOLOGIC ABNORMALITIES

One or more hematologic abnormalities are present in nearly all SLE patients with active disease.[151] The most common of these abnormalities is a mild to moderate normocytic normochromic anemia due to retarded erythropoiesis. Severe anemia with hematocrit values of less than 30 percent was present in half of our patients. Hemolytic anemia with reticulocytosis and low hematocrit was present in only 10 percent of our patients. It is important to note that evidence of hemolysis occurs in patients with and without positive Coombs' tests. In the series reported by Ropes[9] hemolysis occurred in 13 of 16 patients with positive Coombs' tests and in 25 of 42 patients with negative Coombs' tests. Iron deficiency may also be a cause of anemia in SLE patients.

Leukopenia is very common in SLE patients with clinical evidence of active disease. A white cell count of less than 4000 per cubic millimeter was present in only 17 percent of our 365 patients. Leukocytosis does occur in SLE patients who have no evidence of infection. However, this is a rare occurrence in the absence of steroid therapy. Ropes described a leukocyte count of greater than 20,000 in 16 percent of her patients.[9] She also states that counts above 30,000 are usually related to infection. High white blood cell counts of up to 25,000 have also been observed in SLE patients treated with high doses of corticosteroids who have no evidence of infection. Thus, the leukocytosis seen in SLE patients may be due to infection, to SLE, or to corticosteroid therapy. The presence of immature cells is suggestive of a bacterial infection. In most patients with evidence of active disease, there is an absolute lymphopenia.

Mild thrombocytopenia is present in about one third of patients. Thrombocytopenia of less than 100,000 platelets per cubic millimeter occurs much less frequently. It is of interest to note that severe thrombocytopenia may occur for the first time either early or late in the course of the disease. Thrombocytopenia occurred as an isolated event in the last trimester of pregnancy in two of our patients who had had clinically inactive disease for many years and were maintained on low doses of prednisone. An antiplatelet factor is present on the surface of platelets in the majority of SLE patients who do not have thrombocytopenia. The factor is present irrespective of the clinical status of the patients. Qualitative thrombocyte defects are also common but are not clinically significant.[151,152]

The lupus anticoagulant can be identified by the presence of a slight prolongation of the thromboplastin time, along with a more marked prolongation of the partial thromboplastin time[152] (Table 69–4). The prolongation of the partial thromboplastin time is not corrected by the addition of equal volumes of normal plasma to the patient's plasma at dilutions of 1:50, 1:100, and 1:500. The lupus anticoagulant is not clinically significant with respect to bleeding; bleeding and clotting times are normal. We have performed renal biopsies on individuals with the lupus anticoagulant without any bleeding. The

Table 69–4. Effects of Lupus Anticoagulants on Coagulation Tests*

A. Screening tests:
  1. Activated partial thromboplastin time (PTT): prolonged
  2. Prothrombin time (PT): usually slightly to moderately prolonged, occasionally normal or greatly prolonged
  3. Thrombin time: normal
B. Tests which demonstrate an inhibitor:
  1. Mixture of patient's plasma with normal plasma
    a. Prolonged activated PTT when tested immediately
    b. No further lengthening when incubated 1 hour prior to measuring activated PTT
  2. Prothrombin time with dilute thromboplastin; greater prolongation of PT for patient's plasma than for normal plasma as thromboplastin is diluted
C. Specific coagulation factor assays:
  1. Factors XII, XI, IX, and VIII by one-stage method
    a. Low values with standard dilutions of test plasma
    b. Higher values with further dilution of test plasma
  2. Factors V, VII, and X: usually within normal range
  3. Factor II (one-stage and two-stage assays)
    a. Usually normal values
    b. Abnormal values in those patients with specific prothrombin (factor II) deficiency

*From Rick, M.E., and Hoyer, L.W.: Clin. Rheum. Dis. 1:585, 1975.

lupus anticoagulant usually disappears with corticosteroid therapy treatment in newly diagnosed patients. The possible relationship between the lupus anticoagulant and thrombosis is described above.

Anticoagulant activities that specifically inactivate clotting factors are significant clinically. Factors VIII, IX, and XII are most frequently affected. It is very important to identify this anticoagulant activity, because major bleeding episodes may result from any biopsy or operative procedures. Corticosteroids reverse the action of these specific anticoagulants.[152] Bleeding problems in SLE patients with specific anticoagulants occur in patients with very active disease, especially in those with vasculitis.

False positive serologic tests for syphilis were present in 25 percent of our patients. This test is frequently positive in patients who also have the lupus anticoagulant, and it is probable that the lupus anticoagulant arises as antibody directed against the phospholipids necessary for blood coagulation. The tests for syphilis are probably positive because the antigens used in the tests are phospholipids.

The erythrocyte sedimentation rate was elevated in nearly all patients with clinical evidence of disease activity in our series of patients. Ropes has noted that the erythrocyte sedimentation rate was elevated in patients with active disease.[9] The sedimentation rate correlates well with disease activity and decreases markedly or returns to normal in remission. We have noted a small number of patients whose erythrocyte sedimentation rate has remained markedly elevated even though their initially very active, acute disease has been in remission for 5 years. We have also followed a very small number of patients whose sedimentation rate has never been

more than 20 mm (Westergren) even during episodes of severe illness.

PRECIPITATING FACTORS

The onset of the disease and the exacerbation of the disease are frequently related to specific precipitating factors. Most common among these factors are infections, sun sensitivity, operations, pregnancy, and emotional stress.

It has been our impression that disease activity frequently occurs after an infection has been documented in a patient whose disease was previously in remission. We have noted flares of clinical and serologic activity in SLE patients who have had bacterial pneumonia, viral infections, and streptococcal throat infections. The data on the relation between infection and disease exacerbation provided by Ropes clearly relate the two events. Since a large number of her patients were followed during the presteroid era and during the period prior to the availability of a wide range of antibacterial agents, these data are unique. Infections occurred in 79 percent of her 137 patients in whom data were available.[9] In 86 of the 108 patients with infections, the presence or absence of an exacerbation following the infection could be determined. Seventy-three (85 percent) of these individuals had exacerbations following the infection.

Emotional stress clearly appears to cause exacerbations of the disease. Skin rashes, including the lesion of discoid lupus, have been noted in some of our patients during a period of severe emotional stress. The illness or death of a close relative was frequently noted to precede the flare of the skin lesions. Less often a generalized exacerbation of the disease occurred.

Operations may cause an exacerbation of the disease in patients who are not adequately treated with corticosteroids prior to, during, and after the operation. In the series reported by Ropes, analysis of 126 operations revealed that exacerbations occurred in 29 patients, usually within a few days but occasionally after a few weeks.[9] It should be noted that such exacerbations have not been noted in our series of patients followed during the past 10 years. During this period we have given additional intravenous corticosteroids during the operative procedure and have continued somewhat higher doses during the 2-week postoperative period. Even with this regimen, two of our patients have had significant exacerbations. One individual developed membranous lupus nephritis within 6 months of splenectomy for thrombocytopenia, and another developed severe thrombocytopenia after a series of operations to correct the lupus deformities of the hands.

Sun sensitivity is discussed earlier in this chapter.

Pregnancy is generally accepted as one of the factors that may either precipitate the onset of the disease or cause an exacerbation of the disease. The onset of arthralgia or rashes in a previously healthy woman during the last trimester or during the post-partum period should alert the physician to the possibility of the presence of SLE. The occurrence of exacerbation of the disease in the immediate pre-partum and post-partum periods is common. Of four deliveries in our patients during 1977, mild thrombocytopenia occurred in two patients 2 weeks before delivery, and hemolytic anemia occurred in one patient a few days after delivery. In each instance, prompt remission occurred with a slight increase in corticosteroid dose.

It is important to note that exacerbations of the disease do occur after therapeutic abortion in patients who have disease activity at the time the abortion is carried out. Pregnancy should be avoided in patients with disease activity.

Precipitation of SLE by drug ingestion has been noted, as well as exacerbations of the disease following the ingestion of drugs, especially sulfonamides (Tables 69–5 and 69–6). It has been our policy to avoid using any drugs aside from those absolutely necessary in our patients. The use of the recently developed nonsteroidal anti-inflammatory agents for the treatment of arthritis in SLE patients has led to a series of reports on serious side effects in SLE patients.

Chills, fever, headache, and meningitis have been described in SLE patients taking ibuprofen.[153] Drug rechallenge under controlled conditions established the relationship between ibuprofen ingestion and meningitis.

A syndrome similar to systemic lupus erythematosus is a well-documented consequence of chronic ingestion of several drugs.[154] This syndrome has been extensively reviewed recently. In general, drug-induced lupus is milder than spontaneous SLE and occurs equally often in males and females. Arthritis and arthralgia and pulmonary and pericardial involvement are very common, whereas rashes and alopecia are much less common than in the spontaneous disease. Discoid lesions, Raynaud's phenomenon, central nervous disease, and renal disease are rare. Other manifestations seen occasionally in drug-induced lupus include hepatosplenomegaly, lymphadenopathy, and acute pancreatitis. The disease usually has its onset with arthralgia and arthritis. Drug-induced lupus resembles spontaneous systemic lupus erythematosus in elderly individuals,[155] in whom pulmonary manifestations are more common than in the younger age

Table 69–5. Drugs Capable of Activating Lupus Through Probable Pharmacological Properties (Group 1)*

Hydralazine
Procainamide
Anticonvulsants
Mephenytoin
Diphenylhydantoin
Primidone
Trimethadione
Ethosuximide
Carbamazepine
Phenylethylacetylurea
Isoniazid
Chlorpromazine

*From Alarcón-Segovia, D.: Clin. Rheum. Dis. 1:573, 1975.

Table 69–6. Other Drugs Implicated in the Causation of Systemic Lupus Erythematosus and/or Antinuclear Antibodies (Group 2)*

Aminosalicylic acid	Oxyphenisatin
Chlorthalidone†	Penicillin
D-Penicillamine	Phenylbutazone
Griseofulvin	Practolol
Guanoxan	Propylthiouracil
Isoquinazepon	Quinidine
L-Dopa	Reserpine
Methyldopa†	Streptomycin
Methysergide	Sulfonamides
Methylthiouracil	Tetracycline
Oral contraceptives	Tolazamide

*From Alarcón-Segovia, D.: Clin. Rheum. Dis. 1:574, 1975.
†May belong to Group 1.

group. In both the procainamide-induced syndrome and elderly SLE patients, renal disease is uncommon and anti-native DNA antibodies are usually absent. The immunologic abnormalities present in patients with drug-induced lupus are discussed elsewhere (Chapter 46), and the treatment is also discussed elsewhere (Chapter 70).

The three drugs that have been established as being able to induce antinuclear antibodies and the lupus syndrome are procainamide, hydralazine, and isoniazid. These three drugs have chemical and metabolic similarities in that they each contain either a primary amine or a hydrazine portion that is acetylated by the N-acetyltransferase system of the liver.[156] This enzyme is under genetic control, and there are two phenotypic expressions of the inheritance. Either individuals are homozygous for a recessive allele and termed "slow acetylators," or they are heterozygous or homozygous for the dominant allele and termed "fast acetylators."[157] The acetylator phenotype is a factor that has been shown to influence the development of drug-induced lupus after ingestion of hydralazine. The individuals who are slow acetylators are those who develop drug-induced lupus after ingestion of hydralazine.[158] Procainamide-induced antinuclear antibodies have been shown to develop sooner in individuals who are slow acetylators than in those who are fast acetylators.[159] Fifty percent of individuals who were slow acetylators developed antinuclear antibodies in 2.9 months, whereas 50 percent of the fast acetylators developed antinuclear antibodies in 7.3 months. In a retrospective study, the same investigators found that the procainamide-induced lupus syndrome occurred in 12 months in the slow acetylators, whereas the duration of therapy for the fast acetylators was significantly longer.[159]

Two other groups of drugs have been reported to induce SLE, i.e., anticonvulsants and phenothazines, but no prospective studies have been carried out. Other drugs considered to be possible inducers of SLE are quinidine, propylthiouracil, practolol, methyldopa, L-dopa, nitrofurantoin, and lithium carbonate. Even less evidence suggests that griseofulvin, phenylbutazone and oral contraceptives may induce the disease.

DIAGNOSIS AND DIFFERENTIAL DIAGNOSIS

From 1971 until 1982, the generally accepted criteria for the diagnosis of SLE was to a large extent based on the American Rheumatism Association Preliminary Criteria for the Classification of SLE[2] (see Table 69–1).

The Preliminary Criteria were used by investigators studying groups of patients with SLE. We have tested the ARA Preliminary Criteria and found that 96 percent of our recently diagnosed patients fulfilled the criteria.[160] We have used the criteria as rigidly as possible. For example, a lesion of chronic discoid lupus in the scalp is considered to provide only one manifestation, that of chronic discoid lupus, rather than providing two manifestations, i.e., discoid lupus and alopecia.

The omission of serologic manifestations such as antinuclear antibody patterns and titers, antinuclear antibodies directed at specific nuclear antigens such as anti-native DNA or anti-Sm, and levels of serum complement components were serious defects of the Preliminary Criteria, which were developed before the widespread use of these tests. In addition, the value of the study of the nonlesional skin of patients for the deposition of immunoglobulins and complement components in the diagnosis of SLE was not appreciated at the time data was collected for the Preliminary Criteria.

In 1979, a subcommittee of the American Rheumatism Association was charged with the updating and revision of the 1971 criteria. The results of this subcommittee's work were published in 1982 as "The 1982 Revised Criteria for the Classification of Systemic Lupus Erythematosus."[161] The Revised Criteria are shown in Table 69–7. This Criteria was based on a clarification of terms and was based on collection of data from 18 investigators on 10 consecutive patients thought to have SLE and on data from the next age-, race-, and sex-matched patient with a nontraumatic, nondegenerative connective tissue disease. The data on the patients and

Table 69–7. The 1982 Revised Criteria for Classification of Systemic Lupus Erythematosus

Criterion	Definition
1. Malar rash	Fixed erythema, flat or raised, over the malar eminences, tending to spare the nasolabial folds
2. Discoid rash	Erythematous raised patches with adherent keratotic scaling and follicular plugging; atrophic scarring may occur in older lesions
3. Photosensitivity	Skin rash as a result of unusual reaction to sunlight, by patient history or physician observation
4. Oral ulcers	Oral or nasopharyngeal ulceration, usually painless, observed by a physician
5. Arthritis	Nonerosive arthritis involving 2 or more peripheral joints, characterized by tenderness, swelling, or effusion
6. Serositis	(a) Pleuritis—convincing history of pleuritic pain or rub heard by a physician or evidence of pleural effusion OR (b) Pericarditis—documented by ECG or rub or evidence of pericardial effusion
7. Renal disorder	(a) Persistent proteinuria greater than 0.5 grams per day or greater than 3+ if quantitation not performed OR (b) Cellular casts—may be red cell, hemoglobulin, granular, tubular, or mixed
8. Neurologic disorder	(a) Seizures—in the absence of offending drugs or known metabolic derangements: e.g., uremia, ketoacidosis, or electrolyte imbalance OR (b) Psychosis—in the absence of offending drugs or known metabolic derangements, e.g., uremia, ketoacidosis, or electrolyte imbalance
9. Hematologic disorder	(a) Hemolytic anemia—with reticulocytosis OR (b) Leukopenia—less than 4000/mm total on 2 or more occasions OR (c) Lymphopenia—less than 1500/mm on 2 or more occasions OR (d) Thrombocytopenia—less than 100,000/mm in the absence of offending drugs
10. Immunologic disorder	(a) Positive LE cell preparation OR (b) Anti-DNA antibody to native DNA in abnormal titer OR (c) Anti-SM—presence of antibody to Sm nuclear antigen OR (d) False positive serologic test for syphilis known to be positive for at least 6 months and confirmed by *Treponema pallidum* immobilization or fluorescent treponemal antibody absorption test
11. Antinuclear antibody	An abnormal titer of antinuclear antibody by immunofluorescence or an equivalent assay at any point in time and in the absence of drugs known to be associated with "drug-induced lupus syndrome"

*The proposed classification is based on 11 criteria. For the purpose of identifying patients in clinical studies, a person shall be said to have systemic lupus erythematosus if any 4 or more of the 11 criteria are present, serially or simultaneously, during any interval of observation.

controls were stored in a computer and data analysis carried out in order to analyze relationships among variables and the sensitivity and specificity of individual criteria. In addition, combinations of variables were created and also tested for sensitivity and specificity. Potential criteria were tested on a random subset of the patients and control group. Finally, tests of contending combinations of criteria were performed on the rest of the patients and against patients with SLE, scleroderma, and dermatomyositis from the Scleroderma Criteria Cooperative Study.

The major differences between the Preliminary Criteria and the Revised Criteria are as follows: (1) The Preliminary Criteria required 4 or more of 14 manifestations, whereas the Revised Criteria requires 4 of 11 manifestations; (2) two of the 14 manifestations of the Preliminary Criteria are *not* included in the Revised Criteria, i.e., alopecia and Raynaud's phenomenon because of lack of sensitivity and/or specificity; (3) a few of the definitions have been changed; (4) manifestations that were separate in the Preliminary Criteria have been *grouped* in the Revised Criteria, i.e., 2 renal manifestations in the Preliminary Criteria are 1 manifestation in the Preliminary Criteria; (5) immunologic manifestations that were listed separately in the Preliminary Criteria (LE Prep and false positive test for syphilis) are now listed together as 1 manifestation and anti-DNA and anti-Sm are included in the immunologic manifestations; (6) a positive ANA is listed separately as a manifestation of the Revised Criteria.

Biopsies of the skin and kidney were not included in the 1982 Criteria because these were seldom performed on the patients whose data were submitted for the purpose of developing the new criteria.

The 1982 Criteria have not yet been tested on a large group of patients aside from those used for the formulation of the Criteria. We have tested the sensitivity of the Revised and the Preliminary Criteria on 156 SLE patients seen between 1980 and 1982.[162] Ninety-one percent of the patients met the Revised 1982 Criteria, whereas 88 percent met the Preliminary Criteria. Eleven percent met neither set of criteria. Eight patients who did not meet the Preliminary Criteria did meet the Revised Criteria, and this was found to be due solely to the inclusion of the antinuclear antibody as a single manifestation in the Revised Criteria. Three patients who met the Preliminary Criteria did not meet the Revised Criteria even though 1 patient had anti-DNA plus anti-Sm and another had anti-Sm. Each of the 3 patients had both Raynaud's phenomenon and alopecia, which were deleted from the Revised Criteria. The addition of anti-DNA and anti-Sm to the immunologic manifestation had little effect because only 17 of the 142 patients meeting the Revised Criteria had either anti-DNA or anti-Sm as the sole element in the immunologic manifestation, and in 16 of these 17 patients 4 or more additional manifestations of the Revised Criteria were present. Thus, our data suggest that the Revised Criteria are only slightly more sensitive than the Preliminary Criteria and that the addition of ANA rather than anti-

DNA or anti-Sm accounts for this marginally increased sensitivity.

Thus, the 1982 Criteria should be considered by the physician during the work up of a patient who might have SLE. Laboratory tests should be ordered in relation to those of the Criteria. The presence of Raynaud's phenomenon and alopecia should be considered strongly as suggestive of the diagnosis of SLE. Additional laboratory studies should be carried out even though they are not included in either Criteria because their presence is often helpful in the early diagnosis of an individual patient. The presence of other auto-antibodies, such as that determined by a Coombs' test or rheumatoid factor in a patient with arthritis or arthralgia and a butterfly rash is certainly suggestive of SLE. In addition, the presence of a lupus anticoagulant is also suggestive of SLE, although this abnormality can occur in other diseases.

There is some data to suggest that the presence of a low serum complement level (in a patient without a genetic complement deficiency) plus the presence of anti-DNA antibodies is highly specific for SLE.[163] Weinstein and associates have studied the value of anti-DNA antibodies and serum C3 levels in the diagnosis of SLE and found that high anti-DNA antibodies plus low serum C3 levels had a very high predictive value for SLE when applied in a patient population in which that diagnosis was considered.[163] The predictive value is obtained by dividing the true positives by true positives plus false positives. The sensitivity of the anti-DNA antibody was 72 percent and the specificity was 96 percent. For low serum C3 levels the sensitivity was 38 percent and the specificity was 98 percent. Analysis revealed that patients with only two or three manifestations of the Preliminary Criteria would be eligible for the diagnosis of SLE if they had either anti-DNA or low serum C3 levels.

Thus, it is clear that in the individual patient, the diagnosis of SLE should be made not only on the basis of the manifestations of the Revised Criteria but also on the basis of the presence of a low serum complement level.

More studies on the sensitivity and specificity of the Revised Criteria are needed.

The most common diagnosis made in patients before definitive diagnosis of SLE is rheumatoid arthritis or "nonspecific" arthritis. Nearly one quarter of our patients had this diagnosis made by a physician at least 1 year before the diagnosis of SLE. Other diagnoses made in our patients from 2 to 10 years before the definitive diagnosis of SLE included rheumatic fever, chronic discoid lupus, idiopathic thrombocytopenic purpura, seizure disorder, Raynaud's phenomenon, hemolytic anemia, and psychosis.

Other diseases to consider in patients with multisystem disease include subacute bacterial endocarditis, gonococcal or meningococcal septicemia with arthritis and skin lesions, serum sickness, lymphoma and leukemia, thrombotic thrombocytopenia purpura, sarcoidosis, secondary syphilis, bacterial septicemia, and leprosy.

References

1. Fessel, W.J.: Systemic lupus erythematosus in the community. Arch. Intern. Med. 134:1027, 1974.
2. Cohen, A.S., Reynolds, W.E., Franklin, E.C., Kulka, J.P., Ropes, M.L., Shulman, L.E., and Wallace, S.N.: Preliminary criteria for the classification of systemic lupus erythematosus. Bull. Rheum. Dis. 21:643, 1971.
3. Nobrega, F.T., Ferguson, R.H., Kurland, L.T., et al.: Lupus erythematosus, Rochester, Minnesota, 1950–1965. A preliminary study. *In* Bennett, P.H., and Wood, P.H.N. (eds.): Population Studies of the Rheumatic Diseases. Proceedings of the Third International Congress, Series 148. New York, Excerpta Medica Foundation, 1968, p. 259.
4. Meddings, J., and Grennan, D.M.: The prevalence of systemic lupus erythematosus in Dunedin. N.Z. Med. J. 91:205, 1980.
5. Rovers, M.J., and Coodvadia, H.M.: Systemic lupus erythematosus in children. A report of 3 cases. South African Med. J. 60:711, 1981.
6. Wilson, W.A., and Hughes, G.R.: Rheumatic diseases in Jamaica. Ann. Rheum. Dis. 38:320, 1979.
7. Serdula, M.K., and Rhoads, G.G.: Frequency of systemic lupus erythematosus in different ethnic groups in Hawaii. Arthritis Rheum. 22:328, 1979.
8. Maddock, R.K.: Incidence of systemic lupus erythematosus in age and sex. JAMA 191:149, 1965.
9. Ropes, M.W.: Systemic Lupus Erythematosus. Cambridge, Harvard University Press, 1976.
10. Stahl, N.I., Klippel, J.H., and Decker, J.L.: Fever in systemic lupus erythematosus. Am. J. Med. 67:935, 1979.
11. Armas-Cruz, R., Harnecker, J., Ducach, G., Jalil, J., and Gonzales, F.: Clinical diagnosis of systemic lupus erythematosus. Am. J. Med. 25:409, 1958.
12. Dubois, E.L.: Lupus erythematosus: A Review of the Current Status of Discoid and Systemic Lupus Erythematosus. 2nd ed. Los Angeles, University of Southern California Press, 1976.
13. Jessar, R.A., Lamont-Havers, R.W., and Ragan, C.: Natural history of lupus erythematosus disseminatus. Ann. Intern. Med. 38:717, 1953.
14. Davis, P., Atkins, B., Jesse, R.G., and Highes, G.R.V.: Criteria for classification of SLE. Br. Med. J. 3:88, 1973.
15. Labowitz, R., and Schumacher, H.R.: Articular manifestations of systemic lupus erythematosus. Ann. Intern. Med. 74:911, 1971.
16. Russel, A.S., Percy, J.S., Rigal, W.M., and Wilson, G.L.: Deforming arthropathy in systemic lupus erythematosus. Ann. Rheum. Dis. 33:204, 1974.
17. Hahn, B.H., Yardley, J.H., and Stevens, M.B.: Rheumatoid nodules in systemic lupus erythematosus. Ann. Intern. Med. 72:49, 1970.
18. Martin, J.R., Wilson, C.L., and Mathews, W.H.: Bilateral rupture of ligamenta patellae in a case of disseminated lupus erythematosus. Arthritis Rheum. 6:548, 1958.
19. Twining, R.H., Marcus, W.Y., and Garvey, J.L.: Tendon rupture in systemic lupus erythematosus. JAMA 189:377, 1964.
20. Kahn, M., and Ballou, S.P.: Tendon rupture in systemic lupus erythematosus. J. Rheumatol. 8:308, 1981.
21. Guckian, J.C., Byers, E.H., and Perry, J.E.: Arizona infection in man. Report of a case and review of the literature. Arch. Intern. Med. 119:170, 1967.
22. Edelen, J.S., Lockshin, M.D., and LeRoy, E.C.: Gonococcal arthritis in two patients with active lupus erythematosus. A diagnosis problem. Arthritis Rheum. 14:557, 1971.
23. Quismario, F.P., and Dubois, E.L.: Septic arthritis in systemic lupus erythematosus. J. Rheumatol. 2:73, 1975.
24. Schenfeld, L., Gray, R.G., Poppo, M.J., Gaylis, N.B., and Gottlieb, N.L.: Bacterial monoarthritis due to Weisseria meningitidis in Systemic Lupus Erythematosus. J. Rheumatol. 8:145, 1981.
25. Pekin, T.J., Jr., and Zvaifler, N.J.: Synovial fluid findings in systemic lupus erythematosus (SLE). Arthritis Rheum. 13:777, 1970.
26. Isbender, D.A., and Snaith, M.L.: Muscle disease in systemic lupus erythematosus: A study of its nature frequency and cause. J. Rheumatol. 8:917, 1981.
27. Tsokos, G.C., Moutsopoulos, H.M., and Steinberg, A.B.: Muscle involvement in SLE. JAMA 246:766, 1981.
28. Klemperer, P., Pollack, A.D., and Baehr, G.: Diffuse collagen disease. Acute disseminated lupus erythematosus and diffuse scleroderma. JAMA 119:331, 1942.
29. Sibrans, D.F., and Holley, H.L.: Vacuolar myopathy in a patient with positive LE cell preparations. Arthritis Rheum. 10:141, 1967.
30. Perkoff, G.T., Silber, R., Tyler, F.H., Cartwright, G.E., and Wintrobe, M.M.: Studies in disorders of the muscle. XII. Myopathy due to the administration of therapeutic amounts of 17-hydroxycorticosteroids. Am. J. Med. 26:891, 1959.
31. Eadie, M.J., and Ferrier, T.M.: Chloroquine myopathy. J. Neurol. Neurosurg. Psychiatry 29:331, 1966.

32. Hughes, J.T., Esiri, M., Oxbury, J., and Whitty, C.W.M.: Chloroquine myopathy. Q. J. Med. 40:85, 1971.
33. Itobashi, H.H., and Kokman, E.: Chloroquine neuromyopathy: A reversible granulovacuolar myopathy. Arch. Pathol. 93:209, 1972.
34. Gerard, J.M., Stovpel, N., Collier, A., and Flament-Durand, J.: Morphologic study of neuromyopathy caused by prolonged chloroquine treatment. Eur. Neurol. 9:363, 1973.
35. Kanayama, Y., Shiota, K., Horiguchi, I., Kato, N., Ohe, A., and Inove, T.: Correlation between steroid myopathy and serum lactic dehydrogenase in systemic lupus erythematosus. Arch. Intern. Med. 141:1176, 1981.
36. Vilppula, A.: Muscular disorders in some collagen diseases. A clinical electromyographic and biopsy study. Acta Med. Scand. Suppl. 540, pp. 1–47, 1972.
37. Gilliam, J.N., and Sontheimer, O.O.: Skin manifestations of SLE. Clin. Rheum. Dis. 8:207, 1982.
38. Winkelmann, R.K.: Panniculitis and systemic lupus erythematosus. JAMA 211:472, 1970.
39. Kirsner, A.B., Diller, J.G., and Sheon, R.P.: Systemic lupus erythematosus with cutaneous ulceration: Correlation of immunologic factors with therapy and clinical activity. JAMA 217:821, 1971.
40. Tuffanelli, D.L., and Kay, D.M.: Morphological and immunological studies of necrotizing vasculitis in systemic lupus erythematosus (SLE) (abstract). Clin. Res. 17:278, 1969.
41. Fraga, A., and Mintz, G.: Splinter hemorrhage in SLE. Arthritis Rheum. 9:648, 1966.
42. Rudusky, B.M.: Recurrent Osler's nodes in systemic lupus erythematosus. Angiology 20:33, 1969.
43. Baehr, G., Klemperer, P., and Schifrin, A.: A diffuse disease of the peripheral circulation usually associated with lupus erythematosus and endocarditis. Trans. Assoc. Am. Phys. 50:139, 1935.
44. Black, M.M., and Hudson, P.M.: Atrophie and blanche lesions closely resembling malignant atrophic papulosis (Degos' disease) in systemic lupus erythematosus. Br. J. Dermatol. 95:649, 1976.
45. Rothfield, N., and Weissman, G.: Bullae in systemic lupus erythematosus. Arch. Intern. Med. 107:174, 1961.
46. Jordon, R.E., Muller, S.A., Hale, W.L., and Beutner, E.H.: Bullous pemphigoid associated with systemic lupus erythematosus. Arch. Dermatol. 99:17, 1969.
47. Estes, D., and Christian, C.L.: The natural history of systemic lupus erythematosus by prospective analysis. Medicine 50:85, 1971.
48. Urman, J.D., Lowenstein, M.B., Abeles, M., and Weinstein, A.: Oral mucosal ulceration in systemic lupus erythematosus. Arthritis Rheum. 21:58, 1978.
49. Snyder, G.G., III, McCarthy, R.E., Toomey, J.M., and Rothfield, N.F.: Nasal septal perforation in systemic lupus erythematosus. Arch. Otol. 99:456, 1974.
50. Toomey, J.M., Snyder, G.G., III, Maenza, R.M., and Rothfield, N.F.: Acute epiglottitis due to systemic lupus erythematosus. Laryngoscope 84:522, 1974.
51. Pirani, C.L., and Pollak, V.E.: Systemic lupus erythematosus glomerulonephritis. *In* Andres, G.A., and McCluskey, R.T. (eds.): Immunologically Mediated Renal Disease: Criteria for Diagnosis, New York, Dekkar, 1978.
52. Baldwin, D.S., Lowenstein, J., Rothfield, N.F., Gallo, G., and McCluskey, R.T.: The clinical course of the proliferative membranous forms of lupus nephritis. Ann. Intern. Med. 73:929, 1970.
53. Rothfield, N.F.: The kidney in lupus erythematosus. Contrib. Nephrol. 7:128, 1977.
54. Coplon, N.S., Diskin, C.J., Petersen, J., and Swenson, R.S.: The long-term clinical course of systemic lupus erythematosus in end-stage renal disease. N. Engl. J. Med. 308:186, 1983.
55. Pirani, C.L., Pollak, V.E., and Schwartz, F.D.: The reproducibility of semiquantitative analyses of renal histology. Nephron 1:230, 1964.
56. Morel-Maroger, L., Mery, J.P.H., Droz, D., Godin, M., Verroust, P., Kourilsky, O., and Richet, G.: The course of lupus nephritis: Contribution of serial renal biopsies. Adv. Nephrol. 6:79, 1976.
57. Striker, G.E., Kelley, M.R., Quadracci, L.J., and Scribner, B.H.: The course of lupus nephritis: Relationship to the renal histologic findings. *In* Kincaid-Smith, P., Mathew, T.H., and Becker, L.E. (eds.): Glomerulonephritis: Morphology, Natural History and Treatment. Vol. 2. New York, John Wiley & Sons, 1973, p. 1141.
58. Baldwin, D.S., and Gallo, G.R.: Lupus nephritis. Clin. Rheum. Dis. 1:639, 1975.
59. Balow, J.E.: Clinicopathologic correlations in lupus nephritis. *In* Decker, J.L. (moderator): Systemic lupus erythematosus: Evolving concepts. Ann. Intern. Med. 91:596, 1979.
60. Zweiman, B., Kornblum, J., Cornog, J., and Hildreth, E.A.: The prognosis of lupus nephritis: Role of clinical-pathologic correlations. Ann. Intern. Med. 69:441, 1968.
61. Kant, K.S., Pollak, V.E., Weiss, M.A., Glueck, H.I., Miller, M.A., and

Hess, E.V.: Glomerular thrombosis in systemic lupus erythematosus: Prevalence and significance. Medicine (Baltimore) 60:71, 1981.

62. Ginzler, E.M., Nicastri, A.D., Chun-Juo, C., Friedman, E.A., Diamond, H.S., and Kaplan, D.: Progression of mesangial and focal to diffuse lupus nephritis. N. Engl. J. Med. 291:693, 1974.

63. Zimmerman, S.W., Jenkins, P.G., Shelp, W.D., et al.: Progression from minimal or focal to diffuse proliferative lupus nephritis. Lab. Invest. 32:665, 1975.

64. Bretjens, J.R., Sepulueda, M., Baliah, T., Bentzel, C., Erlanger, B.F., Elwood, G., Mantes, M., Hsu, K.D., and Andres, G.A.: Interstitial-immune complex nephritis in patients with systemic lupus erythematosus. Kidney Int. 7:342, 1975.

65. St. Clair, W., Jones, B., Rogers, J.S., Crouch, M., and Hrabovsky, E.: Deep venous thrombosis and a circulating anticoagulant in systemic lupus erythematosus. Am. J. Dis. Child. 135:230, 1981.

66. Carreras, L.O., Defreyn, G., Machin, S.J., Vermylen, J., Deman, R., Spitz, B., and Van Assche, A.: Arterial thrombosis intrauterine death and "lupus anticoagulant": Detection of immunoglobulin interfering with prostacyclin formation. Lancet 1:244, 1981.

67. Zizic, T.M., Shulman, L.E., and Stevens, M.B.: Colonic perforations in systemic lupus erythematosus. Medicine 54:411, 1975.

68. Tsuchiya, M., Okazaki, I., Asakura, H., et al.: Radiographic and endoscopic features of colonic ulcers in systemic lupus erythematosus. Am. J. Gastroenterol. 64:277, 1977.

69. Kurlander, D.J., and Kirsner, J.B.: The association of chronic "non-specific" inflammatory bowel disease with lupus erythematosus. Ann. Intern. Med. 60:799, 1964.

70. Shafer, R.B., and Gregory, D.H.: Systemic lupus erythematosus presenting as regional ileitis. Minn. Med. 53:789, 1970.

71. Harvey, A.M., Shulman, L.E., Tumulty, P.A., et al.: Systemic lupus erythematosus: Review of the literature and clinical analysis of 138 cases. Medicine 33:291, 1954.

72. Weiser, M.M., Andres, G.A., Birentjens, J.R., Evans, J.T., and Reichlin, M.: Systemic lupus erythematosus and intestinal venulitis. Gastroenterology 81:570, 1981.

73. Stevens, M.B., Hookman, P., Siegel, C.I., Esterly, J.R., Shulman, L.E., and Hendrix, T.R.: Aperistalsis of the esophagus in patients with connective tissue disorders and Raynaud's phenomenon. N. Engl. J. Med. 270:1218, 1964.

74. Tatelman, M., and Keech, M.K.: Esophageal motility in systemic lupus erythematosus, rheumatoid arthritis, and scleroderma. Radiology 86:1041, 1966.

75. Reifenstein, E.C., Reifenstein, E.C., Jr., and Reifenstein, G.H.: A variable symptom complex of undetermined etiology with fatal termination, including conditions described as visceral erythema group (Osler), disseminated lupus erythematosus, atypical verrucous endocarditis (Libman-Sacks), fever of unknown origin (Christian) and diffuse peripheral vascular disease (Baehr and others). Arch. Intern. Med. 63:553, 1939.

76. Seifert, G.G., Heinz, N., and Ruffman, A.: Pancreatitis in visceral lupus erythematosus. Gastroenterologia 107:317, 1967.

77. Trynolds, J.C., Inman, R.D., Kimberly, C., Chuong, J.H., Kovacs, J.E., and Walsh, M.B.: Acute pancreatitis in systemic lupus erythematosus: A report of twenty cases and a review of the literature. Medicine (Baltimore) 61:25, 1982.

78. Runyon, B.A., LaBrecque, D.R., and Anuras, S.: The spectrum of liver disease in systemic lupus erythematosus: Report of 33 histologically proved cases and review of the literature. Am. J. Med. 69:187, 1980.

79. Dillon, A.M., Stein, H.B., and English, R.A.: Splenic atrophy in SLE. Ann. Intern. Med. 96:40, 1982.

80. Cayla, J., Rondier, J., Kahan, A., Bonvarlet, J.P., Fabre, P., and Le-Brigand, H.: Thymoma and lupus (two observations and review of the literature). Rev. Rheum. 42:253, 1975.

81. Wolf, S.M., and Borrows, H.S.: Myasthenia gravis and systemic lupus erythematosus. Arch. Neurol. 14:254, 1966.

82. Chan, M.K., and Britton, M.: Comparative clinical features in patients with myasthenia gravis with systemic lupus erythematosus. J. Rheumatol. 7:838, 1980.

83. Oosterhuis, H.J.G.H., and de Haas, W.H.D.: Rheumatic diseases in patients with myasthenia gravis. Acta Neurol. Scand. 44:22, 1968.

84. Mackay, I.R., Goldstein, G., and McConchie, I.H.: Thymectomy in systemic lupus erythematosus. Br. Med. J. 2:792, 1963.

85. Makela, T.E., Ruosteenoja, R., Wager, O., Wallgren, G.R., and Jokinen, E.J.: Myasthenia gravis and systemic lupus erythematosus. Acta Med. Scand. 175:777, 1964.

86. Milne, J.A., Anderson, J.R., MacSween, R.N., Fraser, K., Short, I., Stevens, J., Shaw, G.B., and Tankel, H.I.: Thymectomy in acute systemic lupus erythematosus and rheumatoid arthritis. Br. Med. J. 1:461, 1967.

87. Alarcón-Segovia, D., Galbraith, R.F., Maldonado, J.E., and Howard, F.M., Jr.: Systemic lupus erythematosus following thymectomy for myasthenia gravis. Lancet 2:662, 1963.

88. Ayazi, S., Armstrong, W.L., and Weinstein, A.: Transient high myopia in systemic lupus associated with anasarca. Ann. Ophthalmol. 14:785, 1981.

89. Coppeto, J., and Lessell, S.: Retinopathy in systemic lupus erythematosus. 95:794, 1977.

90. Bishko, F.: Retinopathy in systemic lupus erythematosus: A case report and review of the literature. Arthritis Rheum. 15:57, 1972.

91. Aronson, A.J., Ordonez, N.G., Diddie, K.R., and Ernest, J.T.: Immune complex deposition in the eye in systemic lupus erythematosus. Arch. Intern. Med. 139:1312, 1979.

92. Wong, K., Everett, A., Jones, J.V., and Young, D.: Visual loss as the initial symptom of systemic lupus erythematosus. Am. J. Ophthalmol. 92:238, 1981.

93. Dubois, E.L.: Lupus erythematosus: A Review of the current status of discoid and systemic lupus erythematosus and their variants. New York, McGraw-Hill Book Company, 1966.

94. Moutsopoulus, H.M., Klippel, J.H., Pavilidis, N., Wolf, R.O., Sweet, J.B., Steinberg, A.D., Chu, F.C., and Tarpley, T.M.: Correlative histologic and serologic findings of sicca syndrome in patients with systemic lupus erythematosus. Arthritis Rheum. 23:36, 1980.

95. Feinglass, E.J., Arnett, F.C., Dorsch, C.A., Zizic, R.M., and Stevens, M.C.: Neuropsychiatric manifestations of systemic lupus erythematosus: Diagnosis, clinical spectrum and relationship to other features of the disease. Medicine 55:323, 1976.

96. Johnson, R.T., and Richardson, E.P.: The neurological manifestations of systemic lupus erythematosus. Medicine 47:337, 1968.

97. Klippel, J.H., and Zwaifler, N.J.: Neuropsychiatric abnormalities in systemic lupus erythematosus. Clin. Rheum. Dis. 1:621, 1975.

98. Ashworth, B., and Tait, G.B.W.: Trigeminal neuropathy in connective tissue disease. Neurology 21:609, 1971.

99. Lundberg, P.O., and Werner, I.: Trigeminal sensory neuropathy in systemic lupus erythematosus. Acta Neurol. Scand. 48:330, 1972.

100. Smith, C.A., and Pinals, R.S.: Optic Neuritis in SLE. J. Rheumatol. 9:963, 1982.

101. Trevor, R.P., Sondheimer, K.K., Fessel, W.J., and Walpert, S.M.: Angiographic demonstration of major cerebral vessel occlusion in systemic lupus erythematosus. Neuroradiology 4:202, 1972.

102. Penn, A.S., and Rowan, A.J.: Myelopathy in systemic lupus erythematosus. Arch. Neurol. 18:337, 1968.

103. Duffy, J., Andrianakos, A., Lidsky, M.D., and Sharp, J.T.: Low spinal fluid glucose in systemic lupus erythematosus with spinal cord disease (abstract). Clin. Res. 22:610A, 1974.

104. Lipsmeyer, E.A.: Development of malignant cerebral lymphoma in a patient with systemic lupus erythematosus treated with immunosuppression. Arthritis Rheum. 15:183, 1972.

105. Urman, J.D., and Rothfield, N.F.: Corticosteroid treatment in systemic lupus erythematosus: Survival studies. JAMA 238:2272, 1977.

106. Brandt, K.D., and Lessel, S.: Migrainous phenomena in systemic lupus erythematosus. Arthritis Rheum. 21:7, 1978.

107. Isenberg, D.A., Myrick, T., Snaith, M.L., McKeran, R.O., and Royston, J.P.: A study of migraine in SLE. Ann. Rheum. Dis. 41:30, 1982.

108. Hadler, N.M., Gerwin, R.D., Frank, M.M., Whitaker, J.N., Baker, M., and Decker, J.L.: The fourth component of complement in the cerebrospinal fluid in systemic lupus erythematosus. Arthritis Rheum. 16:507, 1973.

109. Bennahum, D.A., Messner, R.P., and Shoop, J.D.: Brain scan findings in central nervous system involvement by lupus erythematosus. Ann. Intern. Med. 81:763, 1974.

110. Bresnihan, B.: CNS lupus. Clin. Rheum. Dis. 8:183, 1982.

111. Bernstein, R.M., III.: Cerebral lupus: A peep into Pandora's box. J. Rheumatol. 9:817, 1982.

112. Ellis, S.G., and Verity, M.A.: Central nervous system involvement in systemic lupus erythematosus: A review of neuropathologic findings in 57 cases, 1955–1977. Sem. Arthritis Rheum. 8:212, 221, 1979.

113. Atkins, C.J., Kondan, J.J., Quismario, F.P., and Friou, G.J.: The choroid plexus in systemic lupus erythematosus. Ann. Intern. Med. 76:65, 1972.

114. Lampert, P.W., and Oldstone, M.B.A.: Pathology of the choroid plexus in spontaneous complex disease and chronic viral infections. Virchows. Arch. Pathol. Anat. 363:21, 1974.

115. Boyer, R.S., Sun, N.C., Verity, M.A., Nies, K.M., and Lovie, J.S.: Immunoperoxidase staining of the choroid plexus in systemic lupus erythematosus (abstract). Arthritis Rheum. 21:547, 1978.

116. Peress, N.S., Roxburgh, V.A., and Gelfand, M.C.: Binding components in human choroid plexus. Arthritis Rheum. 24:520, 1981.

117. Chia, G.L., Mah, E.P.K., and Feng, P.H.: Cardiovascular abnormalities in systemic lupus erythematosus. J. Clin. Ultrasound 9:237, 1981.

118. Brigden, W., Bywaters, E.G.L., Lessof, M.H., and Ross, I.P.: The heart in systemic lupus erythematosus. Br. Heart J. 22:1, 1960.

119. Hejmancik, M.R., Wright, J.C., Quint, R., and Jennings, F.F.: The cardiovascular manifestations of systemic lupus erythematosus. Am. Heart J. 68:119, 1964.

120. Yurchak, P.M., Levine, S.A., and Gorlin, R.: Constrictive pericarditis complicating disseminated lupus erythematosus. Circulation 31:113, 1965.

121. Bonfiglio, T.A., Botti, R.E., and Hagstrom, J.W.C.: Coronary arteritis, occlusion and myocardial infarction due to lupus erythematosus. Am. Heart J. 83:153, 1972.

122. Ropes, M.: Personal Communication.

123. Homcy, C.J., Liberthson, R.R., Fallon, J.T., Gross, S., and Miller, L.M.: Ischemic heart disease in systemic lupus erythematosus: Report of six cases. Am. J. Cardiol. 49:478, 1982.

124. Bulkley, B.H., and Roberts, W.C.: The heart in systemic lupus erythematosus and the changes induced in it by corticosteroid therapy: A study of 36 necropsy patients. Am. J. Med. 58:243, 1975.

125. Haider, Y.S., and Robert, W.C.: Coronary arterial disease in systemic lupus erythematosus: Quantification of degrees of narrowing in 22 necropsy patients (21 women) aged 16 to 37 years. Am. J. Med. 70:775, 1981.

126. Urowitz, M.B., Bookman, A.A.M., Loehler, B.E., Gordon, D.A., Smythe, H.A., and Ogryzio, M.A.: The bimodal mortality pattern of systemic lupus erythematosus. Am. J. Med. 60:221, 1976.

127. Lerman, B.B., Thomas, L.C., Abrams, G.D., and Pott, B.: Aortic stenosis associated with systemic lupus erythematosus. Am. J. Med. 72:707, 1982.

128. Larson, D.L.: Systemic Lupus Erythematosus. Boston, Little, Brown & Company. 1961.

129. Bernhard, G.C., Lange, R.L., and Hensley, G.T.: Aortic disease with valvular insufficiency as the principal manifestation of systemic lupus erythematosus. Ann. Intern. Med. 71:81, 1969.

130. Shulman, H.J., and Christian, C.L.: Aortic insufficiency in systemic lupus erythematosus. Arthritis Rheum. 12:138, 1969.

131. Dubois, E.L.: The effect of the L.E. cell test on the clinical picture of systemic lupus erythematosus. Ann. Intern. Med. 38:1265, 1953.

132. Libman, E., and Sacks, B.: A hitherto undescribed form of valvular and mural endocarditis. Arch. Intern. Med. 33:701, 1924.

133. Gross, L.: The cardiac lesions in Libman-Sacks disease, with a consideration of its relationship to acute diffuse lupus erythematosus. Am. J. Pathol. 16:375, 1940.

134. Murray, F.R., Fuleihan, D.S., Cornwall, C.S., and Pinals, R.S.: Acute mitral regurgitation from ruptured chordea tendineae in systemic lupus erythematosus. J. Rheumatol. 2:454, 1975.

135. Paget, S.A., Bulkley, B.H., Graver, L.E., and Seningan, R.: Mitral valve disease of systemic lupus erythematosus. A cause of severe congestive heart failure reversed by valve replacement. Am. J. Med. 59:134, 1975.

136. Rawsthorne, L., Ptacin, M.J., Hongyung, C., Olinger, G.N., and Bamrah, V.S.: Lupus vasculitis necessitating double value replacement. Arthritis Rheum. 24:561, 1981.

137. Laufer, J., Frand, M., and Milo, S.: Valve replacement for severe tricuspid regurgitation caused by Libman-Sachs endocarditis. Br. Heart J. 48:294, 1982.

138. Carr, D.T., Lillington, G.A., and Mayne, J.G.: Pleural-fluid glucose in systemic lupus erythematosus. Mayo Clin. Proc. 45:409, 1970.

139. Haupt, H.M., Moore, G.W., and Hutchins, G.M.: The lung in systemic lupus erythematosus: Analysis of the pathologic changes in 120 patients. Am. J. Med. 71:791, 1981.

140. Matthay, R.A., Schwartz, M.I., Petty, T.L., Stanford, R.E., Gupta, R.C., Sahn, S.A., and Steigerwald, J.C.: Pulmonary manifestations of systemic lupus erythematosus: Review of twelve cases of acute lupus pneumonitis. Medicine 54:397, 1974.

141. Eisenberg, H., Dubois, E.L., Sherwin, R.P., and Balchum, O.J.: Diffuse interstitial lung disease in systemic lupus erythematosus. Ann. Intern. Med. 79:37, 1973.

142. Perez, H.D., and Kramer, N.: Pulmonary hypertension in systemic lupus erythematosus. Sem. Arthritis Rheum. 11:177, 1981.

143. Huang, C.T., and Lyons, H.A.: Comparison of pulmonary function in patients with systemic lupus erythematosus, scleroderma and rheumatoid arthritis. Am. Rev. Resp. Dis. 93:865, 1966.

144. Zurier, R.B.: Systemic lupus and pregnancy. Clin. Rheum. Dis. 1:613, 1975.

145. Mund, A., Simson, L., and Rothfield, N.F.: Effect of pregnancy on the course of systemic lupus erythematosus. JAMA 183:917, 1963.

146. Zurier, R.B., Argyros, T.G., Urman, J.D., Warren, J., and Rothfield, N.F.: Systemic lupus erythematosus: Management during pregnancy. Obstet. Gynecol. 51:178, 1978.

147. Fraga, A., Mintz, G., Orozco, J., et al.: Sterility and fertility rates, fetal wastage and maternal morbidity in systemic lupus erythematosus. J. Rheumatol. 1:293, 1974.

148. Zulman, J.U., Talal, N., Hoffman, G.S., and Epstein, W.V.: Problems associated with the management of pregnancies in patients with systemic lupus erythematosus. J. Rheumatol. 7:37, 1980.

149. Jungers, P., Dougados, M., Pelissier, C., Kuttenn, F., Tron, F., Lesavre, P., and Bach, J.F.: Lupus nephropathy and pregnancy: Report of 104 cases in 36 patients. Arch. Intern. Med. 142:771, 1982.

150. Chameides, L., Truex, R.C., Vetter, V., Rashkind, W.J., Galiota, F.M., and Noonan, J.A.: Association of maternal systemic lupus erythematosus with congenital complete heart block. N. Engl. J. Med. 297:1204, 1977.

151. Budman, D.R., and Steinberg, A.D.: Hematologic aspects of systemic lupus erythematosus. Ann. Intern. Med. 86:220, 1977.

152. Rick, M.E., and Hoyer, L.W.: Hemostatic disorders in systemic lupus erythematosus. Clin. Rheum. Dis. 1:583, 1975.

153. Widener, H.L., and Littman, B.H.: Ibuprofen-induced meningitis in systemic lupus erythematosus. JAMA 239:1062, 1978.

154. Weinstein, A.: Drug-induced lupus erythematosus. *In* Schwartz, R. (ed.): Progress in Clinical Immunology. New York, Grune and Stratton. Volume 4. 1980, pp. 1–21.

155. Blomgren, S.E., Condemi, J.J., and Vaughan, J.H.: Procainamide-induced lupus erythematosus: Clinical and laboratory observations. Am. J. Med. 52:338, 1972.

156. Weber, W.W.: Acetylating, deacetylating, and amino acid conjugating enzymes. *In* Brodie, B.B., and Gillette, J.R. (eds.): Handbook of Experimental Pharmacology. Berlin, Springer-Verlag, 1971; p. 564.

157. Evans, D.A.P., Manley, K.A., and McKusick, V.A.: Genetic control of isoniazid metabolism in man. Br Med. J. 2:485, 1960.

158. Perry, H.M., Jr., Tan, E.M., Carmody, S., et al.: Relationship of acetyl transferase activity to antinuclear antibodies and toxic symptoms in hypertensive patients treated with hydralazine. J. Lab. Clin. Med. 76:114, 1970.

159. Woodsley, R.L., Drayer, E.D., Reidenberg, M.M., Nies, A.S., Carr, K., and Gates, J.A.: Effect of acetylator phenotype on the rate at which procainamide induced antinuclear antibodies and the lupus syndrome. N. Engl. J. Med. 298:1157, 1978.

160. Lie, T., and Rothfield, N.F.: An evaluation of the preliminary criteria for the diagnosis of systemic lupus erythematosus. Arthritis Rheum. 15:532, 1972.

161. Tan, E.M., Cohen, A.S., Fries, J., Masi, A.T., McShane, D., Rothfield, N.F., Schaller, J., Talal, N., and Winchester, R.: Criteria for the classification of systemic lupus erythematosus. Arthritis Rheum. 25:1271, 1982.

162. Levin, R.F., Weinstein, A., Peterson, M., Testa, M., and Rothfield, N.F.: A comparison of the sensitivity of the 1971 and the 1982 ARA Criteria for the classification of systemic lupus erythematosus. Arthritis Rheum. 27:530, 1984.

163. Weinstein, A., Bordwell, B., Stone, B., Tibbetts, C., and Rothfield, N.F.: Antibodies to native DNa and serum complement (C3) levels: Applications to the diagnosis of systemic lupus erythematosus. Am. J. Med. 74:206, 1983.

Chapter 70

Management of Systemic Lupus Erythematosus

Alfred D. Steinberg

INTRODUCTION

Systemic lupus erythematosus (SLE) is a disease without a known cure. Treatment is therefore based upon relief of symptoms, suppression of certain presymptomatic abnormalities, and prevention of future pathology. A number of medicines are capable of suppressing signs and symptoms of SLE. Unfortunately, all these drugs carry some side effects. In general, the stronger the medicine at suppressing disease, the greater the seriousness of the expected or potential side effects. Therefore, the aim of treatment is a compromise between suppressing signs and symptoms of disease and avoiding toxicities of the drugs employed. Since the severity of the disease varies greatly from person to person, therapy must be tailored to the needs of the individual.

One of the first acts in treating a patient with SLE is to educate the patient and his or her family. Too often there is an unspoken or even explicitly stated desire on the part of the family to shield the patient from knowledge of the "terrible diagnosis." Although this phenomenon is less widespread than 15 years ago, it still occurs and tends to impair rather than help the psychological health of the patient, as well as to interfere with the doctor-patient relationship and treatment. Fortunately, we can usually tell patients and their families that, despite the diagnosis of SLE, most patients can live relatively normal lives. Most of the "terrible" possibilities will not be awaiting a particular person with SLE. The outlook for long-term survival has improved in recent years to the point that many SLE patients will surely outlive their physicians.

Patients should be told that they have a chronic illness which they will have for the rest of their lives. Although considerable research is devoted to SLE, the cause of the disease remains unknown; furthermore, no cure is available. Despite this, most patients can be helped to be comfortable and to live relatively normal lives—aside from having to take medicines, periodically visit the doctor, and avoid certain stresses. It is perfectly proper to tell the patient that SLE can affect almost any organ in the body and at times can be quite serious. That is the reason the patient continues to visit the doctor and have blood and urine tests performed even when feeling well. It is also proper to tell the patient that the laboratory tests may be a guide to therapy. Through education, the patient can become a partner (though only a junior partner) in management. If the patient fully understands why certain medications are being given, as well as their potential side effects, the patient is in a better position to recognize early warning signs of toxicity or infections or disease activity, as well as reliably report to the physician and the laboratory. Furthermore, the patient is less likely to take extra pills or stop medications against the doctor's instructions.

The lay literature is capable of advancing a "new breakthrough" in SLE every few weeks. Although most of these are at best exaggerated and often groundless, the absence of effective nontoxic drug therapy makes any "new breakthrough" appealing to patients with the disease as well as to their relatives and friends. Patients should be told that what is good for one patient may not be good for another; it may even be detrimental. Each patient is different and must be treated accordingly. Nevertheless, some of the vitamin fads and other nutritional approaches to SLE may not be harmful and have not been proved to be groundless. Although they may have no scientific basis, it is best to acknowledge that their effects are unknown and could be helpful, but also could be harmful or without effect. Most important, patients should be warned that those fads are at best directed at prevention or treatment of very mild problems. They cannot replace good medical care. Through full discussion of the approaches to SLE management, the patient can avoid the disaster of clinging to a fad and avoiding the physician until it is too late to treat the problems that have developed.

The medicines used to treat SLE include nonsteroidal anti-inflammatory drugs such as aspirin and indomethacin, corticosteroids, antimalarial drugs, and in some instances cytotoxic or cytostatic (immunosuppressive) drugs. Newer forms of therapy are being developed and may replace, or be adjuncts to, current treatment programs. In addition, antihypertensive drugs, anticonvulsants, antibiotics, and others may be needed. These may be as important as the drugs given for the underlying disease process.

There is uncertainty regarding the universality of ill effects from sun exposure. In some patients, symptoms usually flare upon sun exposure; others flare at one time and at a later time do not. Some people with SLE are not worsened by sun exposure. The ill effects appear to result from two activities of ultraviolet light: induction of interleukin 1 production by keratinocytes (which augments immunity) and impairment of antigen handling by macrophages. A good principle is to restrict sun exposure most vigorously in patients with previous flares in association with sun exposure. Such people are told never to go out in direct sunlight without first applying a sun screen to exposed parts of the body. They are further instructed never to sunbathe, and to swim only in the very early morning or early evening when the sun's rays are most indirect. Finally, they are advised to cover as much of their body as possible with clothing (such as a longsleeved dress in summer) and to use a broad-brimmed hat. These precautions may be relaxed in inactive patients and in those without sun sensitivity; however, it appears prudent to advise SLE patients never to sunbathe and to wear sun screen and a hat whenever sun exposure might be excessive.It also would be sensible to advise patients not to eat foods containing psoralens, such as celery, parsnips, figs, and parsley.

The question of proper exercise and proper rest for SLE patients unnecessarily plagues many SLE families and their physicians. Patients with SLE should be advised not to exercise to the point of exhaustion. Experience suggests that this will help to avoid flares. However, if the patient is otherwise able, he or she should exercise vigorously and can partake in such sports as baseball and tennis. When the disease is active, it is usually necessary to curtail athletic activities. In addition, it appears that patients with SLE stay in better health when they get enough rest. This means a good night's sleep (which might be an hour or two longer than average) and possibly a nap or rest period in the afternoon.

Although drug administration may be very important in SLE, adjunctive treatment may be crucial for an adequate therapeutic program. Attention to the psychological needs of patients is a very important part of management. This attention is usually best supplied by the physician caring for the patient. Occasionally, a psychiatrist is needed for a short or long period; however, the physician providing primary care for the patient should be able to handle most of the psychological problems with gentle understanding, listening, and common sense advice. Additional adjunctive services include rehabilitation medicine and orthopedics for musculoskeletal problems such as hand deformities and aseptic necrosis of the hips. Finally, since SLE may affect any organ system, it may be necessary to seek help from cardiologists, neurologists, hematologists, ophthalmologists, and surgeons for specific complications.

MAJOR ORGAN INVOLVEMENT VERSUS NONMAJOR ORGAN INVOLVEMENT

Many patients with SLE never develop clinically important involvement of a major organ. These patients may have fever, rashes, alopecia, arthralgias and arthritis, pleurisy, pericarditis, and impressive serological abnormalities. They may even have moderately severe anemia and a positive Coombs test. Nevertheless, in the absence of kidney disease, central nervous system disease, lung disease, myocarditis, marked thrombocytopenia, or severe hemolytic anemia, it is usually not necessary to treat vigorously. Most patients without major organ involvement can be treated symptomatically. The usual approach is to treat systemic symptoms first with nonsteroidal anti-inflammatory drugs such as aspirin, ibuprofen, or indomethacin. Phenylbutazone is unsafe for long-term use in the treatment of SLE. Rashes, either of the discoid or systemic types, are treated with antimalarials, usually hydroxychloroquine, 200 to 600 mg per day (initially, higher doses may be used for several weeks), or chloroquine, 125 to 250 mg three to seven times per week (initially 500 mg per day may be given for a few weeks). Retinal toxicity is the major problem in antimalarial use (see below). Many patients with SLE with fever, rash, arthritis, and pleurisy can be treated successfully with aspirin and hydroxychloroquine—without corticosteroids. Some patients with active SLE develop hepatitis as a toxic reaction to aspirin treatment. In such patients it may be desirable to switch to another nonsteroidal drug, although this response may signal the need for corticosteroids. The hepatic reaction does not mean that the patient is allergic to aspirin in the usual sense; aspirin may be quite well tolerated when the disease is less active.

A patient who continues to have pleural or pericardial pain after initiation of aspirin and hydroxychloroquine may respond to the addition of indomethacin. We have found this drug particularly effective in a number of patients with pleuropericarditis as well as in patients with fever. Nevertheless, many patients without major organ involvement do not respond to nonsteroidal drugs and require corticosteroids. Although the decision to start corticosteroids should be carefully made, the dose of drug should receive equal attention. How much drug is needed depends upon the clinical situation; however, the more experienced the physician, the lower will be the initial dose. Most patients with ordinary symptoms of active SLE who have not been receiving corticosteroids will respond to 0.5 mg per kilogram per day of prednisone. Many respond to less than half that amount. It does not appear to be necessary to start with large doses (60 to 120 mg of prednisone per day) and then taper. All too often, patients "flare" during the latter part of tapering only to be raised again, thereby resulting in larger than necessary cumulative doses.

The biggest question facing the physician starting a patient with active SLE on corticosteroids is often whether to start daily or alternate-day therapy. The great advantages of alternate-day therapy include reduced chance of infection, lack of interruption of the hypothalamic-pituitary-adrenal axis, and reduced side effects of Cushing's syndrome (hypertension, appearance, osteoporosis). In practice, it is usually very difficult to control a symptomatic patient with SLE on low doses of alternate-day corticosteroids. Patients with fever, arthritis, or serositis tend to have symptoms on the day they do not receive corticosteroids, especially in the hours after midafternoon. Occasionally such symptoms may be controlled by extra nonsteroidal anti-inflammatory drugs on the alternate day. More commonly, it is necessary to administer daily steroids until the disease is under control and then try to switch (either gradually or acutely, as discussed below) to every-other day steroids. Some patients with nonmajor organ SLE will not respond to moderately low doses of corticosteroids and anti-inflammatory drugs of the nonsteroidal type. Patients with acute severe toxic lupus with serositis may require doses of prednisone as high as 1 to 2 mg per kilogram per day for a short period of time. The dose should be rapidly tapered to 0.5 mg per kilogram per day and then more slowly tapered as tolerated (see below).

The approach to patients with major organ involvement is philosophically and practically different. Here the aim of treatment is rapid restoration of an affected vital organ to good health and prevention of functional deterioration. As a result, patients with major organ involvement are usually initially treated with high doses of corticosteroids (at least 1 mg per kilogram per day of prednisone). In many cases, such treatment is based upon clinical observations suggesting that it is generally more beneficial than harmful; in other instances, it is based upon the desire not to undertreat a patient with a potentially life-threatening disease. However, in most circumstances hard data supporting this practice are not readily available. Since short-term treatment with 60 to 120 mg per day of prednisone is not very dangerous, there is often little pressure to question initiation of moderately high dose steroid treatment. When treatment must be extended over a considerable period of time, however, the side effects of the corticosteroids may soon begin to outweigh potential benefits.

TREATMENT OF NONMAJOR ORGAN SYMPTOMS

Arthritis, Arthralgias. Arthralgias are among the most common symptoms of patients with SLE, exceeded, perhaps, only by fatigue. Sometimes the arthralgias are fleeting and require no specific treatment. More often, nonsteroidal anti-inflammatory drugs are necessary to provide adequate relief. Patients with frank arthritis may respond promptly to nonsteroidal anti-inflammatory drugs. Supplementation with an antimalarial drug may result in an adequate therapeutic response without the need to administer corticosteroids. Many patients require corticosteroids for symptomatic relief. In such cases, the lowest possible dose of drug should be given. It is often possible to start low doses of daily steroids plus hydroxychloroquine, bring disease activity under control, and then taper to an every-other-day corticosteroid program under cover of the hydroxychloroquine and with the addition of a nonsteroidal anti-inflammatory drug or an increase in its dosage.

Joint pain may represent aseptic necrosis or infection rather than arthritis; these should not be treated with corticosteroids. Since some patients with SLE develop joint deformities (though without erosions), attention should be given to early mild deformities. Rehabilitation medicine, including night splints, physical therapy, and patient education, reduces the risk of severe deformities. Occasional patients may benefit from surgical correction of such deformities as dislocation of the interphalangeal joint of the thumb, by stabilization or replacement. Additional orthopedic help is often required to deal with the aseptic necrosis that frequently occurs in patients with active SLE treated with corticosteroids. Total hip replacement should not be considered lightly, especially in a young person; however, this operation has allowed previously crippled people to live almost normal lives. Newer resurfacing procedures may be the first surgical approach.

Rash. The malar erythema of patients with SLE usually does not require specific therapy. Although it often accompanies other signs of disease activity, it may occur alone in an otherwise asymptomatic patient. When it accompanies other symptoms, treatment of those should be the aim of therapy. Many patients with SLE develop more severe rashes which may require specific attention. The maculopapular eruptions and minor vasculitic lesions usually occur in patients with active disease elsewhere and indicate that control is borderline or inadequate. If they occur during steroid tapering, it may be necessary to hold the dose steady or go back to the previous dose for several weeks or longer. These eruptions are used along with other signs and symptoms and laboratory data as one indication favoring an increase in corticosteroid dosage. The vasculitic lesions usually do not signal impending disaster, and in some patients they disappear without a change in therapy or a flare. In all of the aforementioned rashes, antimalarial drugs may be very helpful; their beneficial effects often are observed in relatively short periods of time.

Discoid lesions may occur in patients with SLE and should be treated as in discoid lupus. Antimalarials and topical steroids are most effective. It usually takes such large doses of systemic corticosteroids to interfere with these lesions that it is not practical to treat them with systemic steroids. Although such treatment for other symptoms or signs may lead to some improvement in the skin disease, more often treatment with systemic corticosteroids for other symptoms is inadequate therapy for discoid lesions and specific therapy for the discoid disease must be added. Experience to date with immunosuppressive drugs is inadequate for any recommendation; however, some patients have responded to relatively nontoxic immunosuppressives such as azathioprine.

Serositis. Serositis in SLE includes pleurisy, pericarditis, and nonbacterial peritonitis. In all cases, a diagnosis of nonbacterial involvement is one of exclusion. This is most troublesome with regard to the peritoneum, where, on a statistical basis, an infectious process is as likely as SLE activity.

The treatment of serositis without major organ involvement is directed toward symptoms. Many patients with pleurisy, pericarditis, or both will respond to treatment with nonsteroidal anti-inflammatory drugs. Aspirin, alone or with indomethacin, may be sufficient to relieve symptoms. In a patient already receiving corticosteroids, but not taking high doses of nonsteroidal anti-inflammatory drugs, the addition of the latter may be adequate. In a number of patients it may be necessary to raise the corticosteroid dose or initiate such therapy. In such instances, massive doses are rarely required. As little as 15 mg per day of prednisone may be more than adequate to relieve the symptoms.

Myositis. Many patients with SLE develop myositis, not usually as an isolated problem and often resolving with treatment of the other signs and symptoms. Occasionally, myositis is an important clinical problem in a patient with an overlap syndrome. Treatment with corticosteroids in sufficient doses to suppress enzyme abnormalities is the current recommended therapy. It is desirable to switch to every-other-day therapy as soon as possible. Since the aldolase is a much more reliable measure than CPK, the former should be used in addition.[1]

Raynaud's Phenomenon. Raynaud's phenomenon, with or without esophageal motility abnormalities, occurs in a large minority of SLE patients. Patients should be encouraged to wear extra-thick, extra-warm, and an extra number of gloves. Avoiding cold and vasoconstrictors (including smoking and emotional stress) may prevent fingertip ulcers and retard atrophy. Vasodilators are helpful in some patients.[2-4]

Constitutional Symptoms and Signs: Fever, Fatigue, Alopecia. One of the most poorly defined areas of SLE therapy is the treatment of constitutional symptoms. In general, these tend to be excessively treated early in the course of illness, and inadequately treated later.

Fever must be viewed initially as due to a superimposed infection and secondary to SLE activity only after other causes have been carefully excluded. The treatment of fever in SLE is usually that of the associated symptoms and may not require specific therapy. However, many patients manifest fever despite adequate control of arthritis and other symptoms. This is particularly common during alternate-day treatment, the fever occuring only on the nonsteriod day. Many patients with fever caused by SLE activity will respond to the addition of a nonsteroidal anti-inflammatory drug to their regimen, whether the regimen be no steroids, alternate-day steroids, or daily steroids in substantial doses. If nonsteroidal drugs fail, steroids should be increased in amount or given in divided dosages. However, a second search for infection should be undertaken, and the addition of an antimalarial now considered for future coverage during reductions in steroid doses.

Fatigue occurs normally in most people, including those with SLE, at some time or other. In addition, however, fatigue appears to be an early sign of mild SLE activity. As a result, it is sometimes difficult to evaluate the symptom of fatigue, especially if it is the major complaint. If it occurs with serological changes such as rising antibody titers to DNA and falling complement levels, symptoms of fatigue, vague as they may be, should lead to consideration of therapy with higher doses of corticosteroids, especially if they have recently been tapered. On the other hand, we hardly want to recommend the treatment of ordinary, or even slightly extraordinary, fatigue with corticosteroids.

When a patient presents for the first time with a malar rash and fatigue and laboratory tests are positive for SLE, the patient is often overtreated with high doses of prednisone, apparently out of a vague fear of the "terrible" disease, SLE, even if the only symptom is fatigue. In contrast, a patient who presents with pleuropericarditis, fever, and arthritis may be treated with corticosteroids which are tapered over many months. The subsequent development of fatigue may be viewed with skepticism. In particular, there is often relief that there has been no recurrence of the previous symptoms, let alone the new development of nephritis. As a result, the fatigue may receive no attention whatsoever. The proper approach is presumably between these two extremes. Fatigue should be treated with respect as a symptom in SLE, but should not be excessively treated.

Alopecia commonly occurs during active SLE, especially after a lag period of several weeks or months of activity. It may reach its peak while the patient is responding to treatment of accompanying features of the disease, and is often incorrectly ascribed to the therapy. Usually alopecia will clear after the systemic illness is under control and does not require specific therapy. A wig may be worn while awaiting hair growth. When discoid lesions affect the scalp, treatment should be directed at them as outlined above. These latter lesions may heal with scarring, thereby resulting in varying degrees of permanent hair loss.

Overlap Syndromes. Some patients with SLE have signs and symptoms that emphasize an organ system not usually the focus of attention in SLE. Thus, a patient may have myositis out of proportion to other problems. Such a patient may appear to have polymyositis rather than SLE. Another patient may have severe deforming joint disease (usually without erosions). Others may have features of additional rheumatic diseases such as scleroderma or Sjögren's syndrome; or, several diseases may appear to coexist in a single patient. At the moment, there is no single laboratory test that well categorizes patients with SLE or SLE-like diseases or overlap syndromes into well defined, easily separable entities with relatively uniform clinical courses. However, the presence of antibodies to ribonucleoprotein antigens correlates with less kidney disease. Furthermore, the management of patients with overlap syndromes tends not to be unusually difficult. In general, these patients are less likely to develop severe renal disease; they tend to respond to corticosteroid therapy, often in low doses.[5] The treatment of such patients is as outlined above under nonmajor organ involvement.

MEASURES OF DISEASE ACTIVITY AND PROGNOSTIC FACTORS—A GUIDE TO THERAPY?

One of the major controversies in the management of the patient with SLE involves the use of prognostic factors, especially laboratory measures, as a guide to therapy. At one extreme are those who recommend that all laboratory measures and prognostic factors be ignored in favor of treatment of symptoms. At the other extreme are physicians who strongly believe that prognostic indicators and laboratory measures should be the sole guides to therapy. Unfortunately, a carefully performed clinical trial to choose between these extremes is not available; however, several are being planned. Prognostic factors for renal failure have been most widely studied; those for involvement of other organs have received much less attention. In general, evidence and theories in favor of treating a patient in the absence of symptoms, or with medicines above and beyond what is necessary to control symptoms, apply primarily to renal disease (real or potential).

Clinical and laboratory factors which suggest a good prognosis should be used to prevent the complications of excessive therapy; contrariwise, prognostic factors suggesting a bad outlook may be used to justify more vigorous therapy in an attempt to prevent major organ deterioration. Clinical factors which have suggested a relatively poor outcome include central nervous system involvement, other than a seizure during the course of early febrile lupus; renal involvement, especially with nephrotic syndrome; nonmajor organ symptoms unresponsive to high doses of corticosteroids (serositis, fevers); major organ involvement of any kind, but especially if not initially responsive to corticosteroids; and a flare occurring during steroid tapering at a relatively high steroid dose. In addition to the above, advanced age has been associated with a better outlook with regard to major organ involvement as opposed to an age of between 15 and 30 years.

Laboratory measures that are associated with a poor prognosis include biopsy showing major involvement of a major organ such as kidney or lung, azotemia, telescoped urine sediment, precipitating antibodies to DNA, prolonged severe anemia, and extremely low levels of C'3 or total hemolytic complement.

There has been an attempt to provide better immunological correlates of the prognostically poor renal biopsy picture so as to permit more frequent measurements and therefore continuous updating of prognosis. The old standby of disease activity has been the serum C3 or CH50; the lower the value, the more active the disease. Antinuclear antibodies vary greatly in their prognostic importance as well as their ability to serve as measures of disease activity. Certain antinuclear antibodies are associated with a poor outlook. This is particularly true of high titers of antibodies to native DNA, especially those with strong precipitating properties.[6,7] In contrast, antibodies to certain soluble nuclear antigens may be associated with a better outlook.[5] As a result, an antinuclear antibody titer per se is not a particularly useful prognostic sign without a more precise knowledge of the determinants with which the antibodies are reacting. The ANA pattern may help; a diffuse or rim pattern is associated with a worse prognosis and a speckled pattern with a better prognosis. Measurement of the avidity with which antibodies bind to native DNA may provide information beyond that of antibody quantity.[7,8]

How should one use prognostic factors? In general, they should probably be used more as a guide to general planning for a particular patient rather than as a formula for management. In addition, patients with SLE may be very active at one time and a year later be quite inactive with regard to the disease process. What is usually desired, in practice, is a measure of disease activity to supplement the managing physician's clinical judgment with regard to changes in medications or doses. High levels of antibodies to DNA and low levels of C3 or hemolytic complement have been used as measures of disease activity.[6] They tend toward normal as the disease becomes less active. Antibodies reactive with lymphocytes and lymphopenia follow the same pattern. Anemia is also a good correlate of disease activity. The problem with laboratory measures of disease activity is that one is often not sure of the time course of their changes or their reliability in a particular patient. Many patients have abnormal laboratory tests for years without any obvious symptoms or major organ functional deterioration. Others are symptomatic with laboratory abnormalities much less marked than those of other patients who appear quite well. Perhaps measures will be found to correlate with disease activity better than any of the current measures. Nevertheless, none will be perfectly applicable to the management of every patient. In general, the more severe the prognostic factors, the faster one should react to laboratory abnormalities with regard to stopping steroid tapering or adding to the current treatment program. Thus, a patient with diffuse glomerulonephritis on kidney biopsy and previous red cell casts who is now found to have a falling C3 and rising anti-DNA should be treated faster and more vigorously than a patient with 10 years of arthritis and intermittent serositis (without major organ involvement) with the same laboratory findings. In addition, a previous correlation of a laboratory abnormality or symptom complex preceding major flares in a particular patient would prompt more rapid therapeutic intervention than the absence of such a correlation. Nevertheless, it is not known whether or not the low C3 or high anti-DNA should be treated in the absence of symptoms. Perhaps they should in patients with previous major flares or major organ involvement. For patients who have been under observation for long periods of time and without major organ involvement, not treating such laboratory values may, in the long run, lead to less drug toxicity without seriously compromising chances for long life. In addition, the tendency of older patients with SLE to have relatively less severe disease should lead to somewhat less vigorous treatment. Finally, patients who have flared at a particular steroid dose during tapering on previous occasions should be carefully monitored during the next tapering as that dose is approached. Worsening of laboratory values at such time should indicate a halting of tapering, and perhaps a slight temporary increase in dosage.

INFECTIONS

Patients with SLE are predisposed to the development of infections of many types. Patients treated with high doses of corticosteroids and those with advanced or active renal disease are particularly predisposed to the development of bacterial infections.[9,10] Azathioprine and cyclophosphamide given in low doses have not been found to predispose to infections in patients with SLE.[10] Since it is often difficult to distinguish initially between an infection and a disease flare, it is usually necessary to search diligently for infection in patients with fever or altered symptoms. Even more frustrating in this regard is the frequent occurrence of a flare in association with (perhaps brought on by) an infection. Thus rising anti-DNA or falling complement levels do not exclude an infection.

Treatment of infections in patients with SLE is similar to that in any other patient. Since patients with SLE, especially when active, have a chance greater than one in three of developing an allergic reaction to Gantrisin, I prefer not to use sulfa drugs in the treatment of urinary tract infections when alternatives are available. Antibiotic doses may have to be reduced in renal failure or because of very low serum albumin. Steroids should be reduced to the lowest possible dose as dictated by the clinical situation; however, infections may be successfully treated despite high doses of corticosteroids.

Since patients with SLE have defective delayed hypersensitivity responses, especially to antigens of the tubercle bacillus, and since they are treated with corticosteroids, consideration of prophylaxis against tuberculosis is appropriate. Although prophylaxis is not routinely recommended, it should be considered for anyone with either previous evidence of tuberculosis or substantial exposure. Moreover, any symptoms or signs suggestive of tuberculosis should be vigorously pursued. *Pneumocystis carinii* infection is ominous in patients with SLE. Early diagnosis and intensive treatment are essential. Candida esophagitis and bacterial peritonitis also must be considered in patients with SLE and suggestive signs or symptoms.

TREATMENT OF MAJOR ORGAN INVOLVEMENT IN SLE

Kidney. One of the most heavily discussed subjects in internal medicine is the treatment of kidney disease in SLE, an excellent indication that no program is uniformly accepted. It has been the basis for a large number of trials with different corticosteroid and immunosuppressive regimens. Despite widespread interest and a large literature, the optimal treatment for kidney disease remains controversial, if not unknown. Several studies have emphasized the prognostic significance of particular biopsy patterns;[11] however, the finding that a patient may move from one biopsy category to another (with a better or worse prognosis) calls into question strict adherence to biopsy patterns as the sole prognostic and therefore therapeutic guide.[12,13] Nevertheless, histologically normal kidneys, despite urine sediment abnormalities, offer the best outlook. Disease that remains mesangial in extent also carries a good prognosis. Patients with such biopsy pictures may be better off with modest treatment, since the chance of drug toxicity may outweigh the risks from the disease. On the other hand, patients with membranoproliferative glomerulonephritis may have a sufficiently dim outlook[11] that the disease poses greater risks than the potential toxicities of vigorous therapy.

Patients with normal biopsies or membranous disease may at a later stage in their illness have the more severe diffuse biopsy picture.[12–14] In contrast, membranoproliferative disease may, with treatment, become membranous. As a result, even among subgroups of kidney biopsy pictures there is room for individualization. Finally, patients with mesangial disease may have a good outlook until the disease progresses to mesangial-proliferative and then membranoproliferative.

Since the clinical course of patients with SLE and renal disease may be quite variable, there has been a continuing search for predictive measures. Although the measures do not correlate perfectly with outcome, they are helpful in managing today's patients. Thus, renal failure,[15] heavy proteinuria,[15] light microscopic observation of diffuse proliferative glomerulonephritis,[11] and subendothelial electron dense deposits on electron microscopy[12, 16–18] have all been associated with an unfavorable long-term outcome. Glomerular hyalinization and interstitial scarring signify not only an unfavorable outlook but non-reversible damage as well. It has been suggested that the persistence of subendothelial deposits on electron microscopy of biopsy specimens taken 1 or 2 years apart implies a poor prognosis.[12] Initial presence of these deposits with subsequent dissolution or conversion to subepithelial deposits (characteristic of membranous disease) is associated with a much better prognosis.[12] Whether or not a patient should be subjected to one, let alone two, renal biopsies must be decided by the physicians for the patient on an individual basis rather than as a matter of the standard work-up for SLE kidney disease. In many instances, the information to be gained may be deemed worth the small risks involved. If the treatment will not be modified on the basis of the biopsy results, however, it can be argued that the biopsy is of academic interest only. Moreover, immunologic abnormalities have been shown to correlate with the biopsy picture of persistent subendothelial deposits.[12] Thus, persistent elevations of antibodies reactive with DNA and persistently low C3 may be considered a substitute for a repeat biopsy and suggestive of a poor outlook; in the experience of some, they would also dictate aggressive therapy.[19] The proper use of prognostic indicators with regard to management of SLE kidney disease awaits completion of adequate randomized trials.

Initial studies supporting the use of immunosuppressive drugs and high doses of corticosteroids were not randomized, and the groups of treated and nontreated patients were not comparable. Thus, the basis for "standard treatment of SLE kidney disease" with high doses of corticosteroids is shaky.[20,21] Support for treatment with low dose oral immunosuppressive drugs such as azathioprine, cyclophosphamide, chlorambucil, and methotrexate is equally tenuous; some studies suggest benefit, others do not. Some of these drugs may be of use to some patients. However, the difficulty in establishing their efficacy strongly points to their inability uniformly to treat the disease process successfully. They have impressive potential toxicities which point to the possibility that they may be more harmful than helpful.[22,23] At the moment, it is fair to say that there is no proved therapy for SLE nephritis. Corticosteroids in doses above what is needed to control symptoms are blessed more by tradition than by scientific evidence of efficacy.[20]

How then does one treat a patient with SLE and kidney disease? One way to select therapy is to enter the patient into an ongoing clinical trial to help determine which of several possible therapies is beneficial. Such trials may be available at several large medical centers[18] or at the National Institutes of Health.[24] The treatment would then become of value to the medical community and future patients as well as the particular patient under consideration. Any approach should be undertaken with the knowledge that no treatment has been proved to be effective and that mortality from SLE (and SLE kidney disease) has been declining in recent years.[25,26] In addition, dialysis and even transplantation may be available to the patient if therapy is unsuccessful. This is noteworthy since vigorous therapy for patients with advanced renal disease may produce more toxicity than benefit.[24,27] The same is true of New Zealand mice with lupus nephritis.[28]

A widely used treatment of patients with glomerulonephritis is prednisone, 40 to 50 mg per square meter per day orally for a period of about 2 months, with subsequent tapering of the drug. One would follow the general status such as hematocrit, white blood cell count, and nonrenal symptoms. The serum complement and anti-DNA determinations may be used to add to the information gained from serial analyses of urine sediment, degree of proteinuria, and a measure of renal function such as serum creatinine. Tapering of steroids should not be performed too rapidly under most circumstances (see below). Careful attention to blood pressure control and to minor infections (before they become major) is probably at least as important as the type and dosages of drugs selected for treatment of the kidney disease. The presence of hypertension in SLE is now recognized to occur before the onset of azotemia in many patients.[29] It is my opinion that the single greatest contribution to be made in the medical management of patients with SLE and kidney disease is maintenance of the blood pressure in the middle of the normal range. This opinion is based upon experience with large numbers of patients with SLE and kidney disease as well as

experiments pointing to increased renal damage when hypertension complicates immune complex disease.[30] In this regard, many physicians lose sight of the fact that the control of blood pressure is usually for a child or young adult, not an elderly person. The blood pressure of the patient may only have been 80/50 mm Hg prior to disease. Thus, a blood pressure of 145/95 might represent an enormous increase and should not be disregarded. In addition, a rise in blood urea nitrogen in association with high dose steroid therapy or a fall in renal function in patients recently started on aspirin or other nonsteroidal anti-inflammatory drugs may be related to the drug treatment rather than the underlying disease process.[31] Finally, all the other aspects of care outlined in this chapter are applicable to patients with SLE and kidney disease—with or without important nonrenal signs of disease.

Recent advances derived from randomized trials have suggested that immunosuppressive drugs may benefit patients with SLE and glomerulonephritis. Only certain subgroups of patients have been demonstrated to derive substantial benefits.[32] Young patients (< 25 years old) are at greatest risk of developing renal failure if they present with substantial renal scarring. Such patients may be benefited only by the most rigorous therapy (currently thought to be the addition of high-dose boluses of intravenous cyclophosphamide to corticosteroid therapy). Oral immunosuppressive drugs appear to benefit only those patients with minimal scarring (as opposed to none or marked) on biopsy and reasonably good renal function.[32] Further studies are necessary to determine the optimal therapy for subsets of patients with SLE and kidney disease (see Immunosuppressive Drugs, below).

Central Nervous System. The proper management of central nervous system (CNS) disease rests on even less sound scientific support than the treatment of kidney disease. Nevertheless, principles of treatment may be elaborated. Most important is the recent awareness that not all CNS problems in patients with SLE should be treated similarly. A corollary of this principle is to individualize therapy. The first aim of management of CNS problems in patients with SLE is to attempt to diagnose non-SLE causes of the symptoms. CNS infections surely should not be treated with high doses of corticosteroids in place of appropriate antimicrobial drugs. Similarly, hypertensive seizures should be treated with drugs directed at the blood pressure. Finally, steroid-induced psychosis should not be managed with prolonged use of higher doses of corticosteroids.

Since "CNS lupus" may be anything from an isolated seizure to a fatal hemorrhagic or thrombotic catastrophe,[33] it is necessary to first make some attempt to categorize the probable involvement. The most common CNS problems of SLE patients are psychological.[33] Many of these are reactions to becoming aware that one has a chronic illness which is serious and may be fatal. Family tensions may exacerbate such problems, as may the disabilities induced by the physical aspects of the disease such as arthritis, fatigue, rash, alopecia, or the therapy (cushingoid features). These psychological problems are best handled by spending considerable amounts of time with the patient—discussing the concerns and trying to impart a degree of optimism that they are likely to be temporary. A knowledgeable nurse or social worker may be a good adjunct to, but not a replacement for, such discussions. Occasionally a psychiatrist's help may be desirable or even necessary; however, these problems can often be handled by the primary physician. Many patients with SLE have psychiatric problems that go far beyond those mentioned above. Severe depression may be very temporary, but requires attention to avoid a potential suicide. Similarly, an acute schizophrenic or other psychotic episode in the life of an SLE patient should be treated in the hospital by a team of physicians, including at least the primary physician and a psychiatrist. In general, early treatment should consist of major tranquilizers (such as Thorazine) plus corticosteroids. Continued reassurance, given even to a psychotic patient, may pay dividends in a shorter period of illness and more rapid return to normal after the drugs have begun to control the symptoms. The dosages of drugs required to control such psychotic episodes vary greatly. Corticosteroid dosages as low as 30 mg per day of prednisone may be quite effective in some patients, whereas 100 mg per day may be insufficient in others. Recently, more massive doses of steroids have been giving way to greater dependence on the antipsychotic drugs in larger doses in conjunction with moderate dosages of corticosteroids. Such an approach has the dual advantage of reducing steroid side effects of infection, hypertension, and other aspects of Cushing's syndrome and also limiting the effects of the steroids themselves on the mood and personality. One of the best allies in an episode of psychosis in a patient with SLE is time, and therefore one of the greatest assets of the physician is patience. It is not necessary for the patient to return to normal within 48 hours. Many SLE patients have had weeks or months of mental disturbance with subsequent resolution and return to normal. It should be remembered that many patients with psychiatric problems cannot be relied upon to take medications. Observed pill taking and parenteral administration should be considered for such people.

Headaches may occur in patients with SLE as in large numbers of other people with the usual range of causes, e.g., tension headaches, eyestrain, sinus problems. Migraine headaches, which occur in a minority of patients with SLE, may respond to therapy with corticosteroids.[34] Hypertensive headaches should be treated with very prompt and careful attention to blood pressure control. I have the clinical impression that patients with active SLE are subject to an unusually great risk of intracranial hemorrhages at minimally elevated blood pressures. Thus, a young woman with rash, arthritis, glomerulonephritis, slightly reduced platelet count, and somewhat prolonged thrombin time with hypertensive headaches and a blood pressure of 160/100 should be viewed as being in danger of a catastrophe from the hypertension, whereas the same view would not be held of a 55-year-old individual with hypertension and no other medical problems. Finally, chronic headaches in an immunosuppressed SLE patient should prompt an investigation for cryptococcal meningitis.

Acute severe headaches should be investigated as in any other patient, and be attributed to SLE by exclusion. Although meningismus and pleocytosis on cerebrospinal fluid examination may well point to "lupus meningitis," bacterial infections, including tuberculosis, must be carefully sought. Furthermore, drugs such as azathioprine and ibuprofen may induce such a process. Sterile meningitis caused by SLE should be treated promptly with corticosteroids, with rapid tapering after clearing of signs and symptoms. In fact, the controversial areas of treatment of CNS problems in SLE involve the complications of prolonged use of very high doses of corticosteroids which predispose such patients to the risk of serious infection.[35] It is the impression of many centers that the infectious complications can be avoided without sacrificing the potential benefit of the corticosteroid therapy by use of high doses initially, followed by more rapid tapering of the drug to less worrisome dosages. Moreover, CNS involvement in SLE may occur in patients already taking large doses of corticosteroids. Some such patients respond to raising the steroid dose further, especially in daily divided doses. In a rare patient, intravenous cyclophosphamide may be effective and appropriate therapy; however, there are no controlled trials to support the anecdotal experience with this drug in SLE with CNS involvement.

A single uncomplicated seizure in a patient with active SLE may require no specific treatment. The therapy of the active disease may be sufficient. Several seizures in such a setting may respond to the addition of antiseizure medications to the corticosteroids already being given for the disease. Patients with the new onset of frequent seizures or of status epilepticus should be treated with both corticosteroids in increased dosage and antiseizure medications. In some (but by no means all) instances very large doses of corticosteroids ($\geq$240 mg per day of methylprednisolone parenterally in divided doses) may be necessary for control. Within a few days, rapid tapering should be undertaken (see Corticosteroids, below).

Movement disorders such as chorea and hemiballismus have been found to respond to increases in corticosteroid therapy; however, these problems are sufficiently uncommon as isolated symptoms in SLE that therapeutic experience is limited. It should be noted that extrapyramidal symptoms may be the result of treatment of psychosis with phenothiazines and should not, in such a context, necessarily be regarded as an indication of worsening of the patient.

Hemiparesis and other focal neurological signs such as transverse myelopathy, may occur in patients with SLE. Some patients have responded to corticosteroid therapy, some have improved without such therapy, and some have not improved despite therapy with corticosteroids with or without immunosuppressive drugs. A recommendation for corticosteroid therapy in such situations stands on shaky ground. Nevertheless, the likelihood of underlying vasculitis in some patients suggests that short-term vigorous treatment may offer some hope of benefit without the risk of intolerable complications.

Progressive dementia may occur as an isolated problem or may complicate other forms of CNS disease in SLE. The most common cause is the gradual loss of brain substance and formation of lacunae caused by small vessel disease. Corticosteroid therapy may be recommended only on the basis of a few anecdotes. Such therapy should be undertaken with periodic psychological and intellectual testing, so that potential effects of treatment may be measured. Coma secondary to SLE should be treated with very large doses of parenteral corticosteroids in divided doses. Failure to respond within 24 hours or subsequent relapse is a grave sign. An occasional patient has responded to intravenous alkylating agents; however, the experience is too small to recommend such treatment on the basis of hard data.

The efficacy of immunosuppressive drugs in the treatment of CNS disease in patients with SLE is unproved. Many patients have developed major CNS symptoms while taking azathioprine or have had their disease apparently induced by azathioprine.[33,35] In contrast, cyclophosphamide-treated patients have had a lower incidence of development of CNS disease while taking the drug. Furthermore, cyclophosphamide has been used therapeutically in uncontrolled situations with suggested success. Although immunosuppressive drugs have no current place in the standard therapy of CNS involvement in SLE, cyclophosphamide rather than azathioprine should be the drug chosen for experimental intervention.

Since the diagnosis of CNS involvement in SLE in any of its forms is largely one of exclusion, it is necessary to rule out other, especially treatable, causes of such symptoms or signs. Therefore, it would be very desirable to have a simple and reliable diagnostic test to positively make or confirm the diagnosis of CNS involvement in SLE. Unfortunately, such a test does not exist. Tests which were once thought to be helpful in the diagnosis of CNS involvement but have subsequently been shown not to be useful include the brain scan and low cerebrospinal fluid C4. Although the electroencephalogram may be abnormal, the usual pattern of diffuse slowing is not diagnostic. Serum antibodies to DNA and low serum C do not correlate with CNS disease.[36] Antibodies in the cerebrospinal fluid (CSF) have more recently been felt to correlate with active CNS disease in SLE patients. The IgG level may be moderately elevated in some patients and not in others. Recently, antibodies in the CSF reactive with lymphocytes and neurons have been found in most patients with active CNS involvement in SLE, and less frequently in patients with SLE without CNS disease.[37,38] In addition, elevated CSF cyclic GMP levels have been found in patients with CNS involvement in SLE (but also in other neurologic diseases).[39] It is hoped that such observations will lead to a test for one or more of the CNS disorders observed in patients with SLE.

For the present, we are left with clinical judgment and no specific test in the diagnosis and follow-up of patients with SLE and CNS involvement. Collective wisdom suggests that patients should be treated with as high doses of corticosteroids as it takes to control the problem (this may reach 250 to 1000 mg of methylprednisolone per day given parenterally in divided doses) but that tapering to low doses (30 mg per day) should be carried out rapidly to minimize the toxic effects of corticosteroids.

Lung. In addition to pleural disease, considered earlier, patients with SLE may develop parenchymal lung disease. In the majority of instances, the problem is secondary. Congestive heart failure, bacterial infections, uremia, pulmonary emboli, viral infections, and exotic infections all may produce signs or symptoms in the lungs. Such problems should be evaluated and treated appropriately. Thus, careful evaluation, including consideration of lung biopsy, provides a basis for a choice between antibiotics and corticosteroids. A minority of patients with SLE have pulmonary signs and symptoms which are thought to be part of the SLE diathesis.[40] This varies from a mild, self-limited infiltrate to hemoptysis and diffuse pneumonitis progressing rapidly to alveolar filling and death. The biopsy picture in SLE lung disease is not pathognomonic, and treatment is uncertain, although corticosteroids are generally used. Patients with fleeting infiltrates in association with other signs of SLE usually respond to corticosteroid therapy for the other manifestations of the disease. Those with fulminant disease often do not respond to very large doses of corticosteroid with or without the addition of immunosuppressive drugs. Some patients with acute diffuse or intermittent or chronic localized infiltrates appear to respond to corticosteroid therapy, suggesting that corticosteroids should be administered pending the results of better clinical trials. The case for immunosuppressive drugs is even more tenuous. Good supportive and nursing care with prompt treatment of superimposed infections, congestive heart failure, and fluid and electrolyte problems may allow the patient to withstand long periods of pulmonary inflammation with partial or complete symptomatic recovery.

Heart. In addition to inflammation of the pleural and pericardial membranes, the myocardium may be involved in an inflammatory process in SLE. This usually occurs in association with other signs and symptoms of active SLE, is often not specifically diagnosed, and is usually adequately treated when the other manifestations of disease are brought under control. An occasional patient may have myocardial disease as a major feature of the illness requiring therapy directed specifically at the heart. Fortunately, this is usually one of the easier manifestations of SLE to treat. In fact, it is much harder to diagnose. Such patients may have subtle signs such as mild to moderate exercise intolerance and excessive tachycardia. Since such patients may have concomitant pleuropericardial symptoms or fever, clinical and laboratory signs and symptoms may be difficult to interpret. The therapy is corticosteroids in dosages adequate to bring the signs and symptoms under control. Doses of prednisone in the range of 30 to 40 mg per square meter per day for a few weeks are usually adequate. If signs and symptoms are controlled, the dosage should be tapered.

Blood and Blood-Forming Organs. The anemia of SLE is usually one of chronic disease rather than of hemolysis. It is a very good sign of disease activity in patients with active systemic lupus. As the patient improves, the anemia generally concomitantly improves and disappears. This occasionally happens during the course of treatment with nonsteroidal anti-inflammatory drugs. More often, corticosteroid treatment is necessary to correct marked anemia in SLE patients. Large doses of corticosteroids are usually *not* necessary. Even every-other-day steroids in low doses may be adequate.

Some patients with active SLE and anemia of chronic disease have positive Coombs tests. These patients may have shortened erythrocyte survival; however, they do not have major hemolytic anemia. They can usually be treated as the patients with anemia of chronic disease. An occasional patient with SLE may have anemia primarily on the basis of hemolysis. During the course of active hemolysis, treatment should be directed at, and guided by, the laboratory abnormalities.[41] Corticosteroids in high doses are the recommended therapy. If the patient responds to corticosteroids, the dose should be reduced while following the hematologic parameters. Failure to respond to high doses of corticosteroids for a period of more than 3 weeks should lead to considerations for therapy similar to those for patients with hemolytic anemia without SLE: splenectomy and/or immunosuppressive drugs.

Thrombocytopenia in patients with SLE may be mild and transient and not require specific therapy. When more marked, the low platelet count usually dictates treatment. Corticosteroids are given in doses sufficient to raise the platelet count to near normal levels. This usually means 30 to 50 mg per square meter per day of prednisone, or more, with subsequent tapering, the platelet count serving as a guide to dosage. The drug acts both to reduce the production of antibodies reactive with platelets and to reduce splenic sequestration of antibody-bound platelets. If corticosteroids cannot adequately elevate the platelet count, splenectomy provides a means of reducing sequestration. Many patients respond initially to high doses of corticosteroids, but experience a fall in platelet count during tapering. If these patients cannot be controlled at acceptable dosages of corticosteroids, splenectomy should be considered. After splenectomy, an occasional patient may still not be adequately controlled by tolerable doses of corticosteroids. The further treatment of such patients is still experimental; oral cyclophosphamide may be helpful.[42] Intravenous cyclophosphamide has been dramatically successful in a few individuals. Plasmapheresis to remove platelet-bound antibodies, gamma globulin therapy, low doses of vincristine, and Danazol (an impeded andiogen) have all been reported to be beneficial in recent years. In addition, TTP should be treated with plasma exchange.[43]

Leukopenia, which occurs in about half of patients with SLE, should not be specifically treated. In several studies, leukopenia, especially lymphopenia, has been found to correlate with disease activity, suggesting that treatment might be appropriate. Nevertheless, many untreated patients have leukopenia or lymphopenia for years without symptoms. It therefore seems prudent to wait for studies indicating benefit before treating the laboratory finding of leukopenia. A very rare occurrence is autoimmune neutropenia of a severe degree. Treatment of such patients with corticosteroids, immunosuppressive drugs, or both, may actually increase the neutrophil count and reduce infections. More experience is necessary before precise recommendations can be given for this problem.

Fewer than 1 percent of SLE patients develop a bleeding diathesis resulting from a circulating anticoagulant. In general, the laboratory coagulation abnormalities result from antibodies (e.g., to cardiolipin) that do not alter coagulation in vivo and should not be treated. In the rare patient in whom therapy for an anticoagulant is indicated, the initial treatment of choice is high doses of corticosteroids. Failure to respond, or reactivation during steroid tapering, should lead to consideration of plasmapheresis and/or immunosuppressive drug therapy.

MARRIAGE AND PREGNANCY

The full range of ethical problems involved in communications with potential spouses of patients with a chronic and genetically conditioned disease such as SLE is far beyond the scope of this chapter. Nonetheless, experience suggests that the marriage rests on a firmer foundation and tends to last longer when the prospective spouse is more or less fully aware of the problems (real and potential) than when the spouse is kept fully in the dark until a crisis occurs. This information is usually best transmitted initially by the patient; a subsequent meeting of patient and prospective spouse jointly with the physician usually helps to alleviate anxiety more than to create problems.

Should a patient with SLE ever father a child or become pregnant? Society has not fully come to grips with parenthood for people with disease more directly genetically transmitted and with a higher degree of penetrance. Therefore, the philosophical aspects of the question are, at the moment, left up to the individual. Medically, fathering a child should not cause undue physical problems; potential physical and psychological stresses of a new child may be important in individual cases. In addition, there is a chance of passing unwanted genes to the next generation.

Pregnancy is another matter altogether.[44] The available data suggest that women with SLE cannot become pregnant at will without an increased risk of difficulty. Nevertheless, many women with SLE have successfully delivered more than one healthy child. Whether or not pregnancy should be undertaken depends upon the philosophical views of the prospective parents as well as the physical state of the prospective mother. The risks may be unacceptable in patients with active disease, with severe renal disease, with advanced cardiac disease, and with certain types of neurologic problems.

It is generally felt that pregnancy should be avoided in women with SLE during periods of active disease and in those with severe or advanced renal disease.[44] Pregnancy during active disease puts the mother at greatest risk. If the active disease includes renal involvement, worsening proteinuria and kidney function plus hypertension may be observed. Advanced cardiac disease is a contraindication to pregnancy in SLE. Pregnancy in women without renal disease and during periods of quiescence may be undertaken with the knowledge that there may be a flare, especially after an abortion (spontaneous or induced) or after delivery.[44] Such flares should be anticipated and vigorously treated with adequate steroid dosages. Spontaneous abortions are frequent in SLE mothers.[44] Nevertheless, the term births tend to be normal, aside from transient stigmata of SLE such as LE factors and tubuloreticular inclusions in cells. Unfortunately, such stigmata may be associated with subsequent SLE as the baby grows up.[45,46] The risk of the child developing an autoimmune disease or passing on the propensity to develop one has not yet been accurately calculated. The association of certain B lymphocyte antigens with SLE[47] suggests that the increased risk may ultimately be substantial, perhaps in the 1 to 10 percent range. These estimates may be falsely low for families in which autoimmunity is common and may be falsely high for others. Offspring of mother with anti-Ro (SSA) antibodies appear to be at an increased risk of congenital cardiac abnormalities (whether or not the mothers have SLE). Steroids given throughout pregnancy usually have no adverse effect on the child. However, nursing mothers will pass corticosteroids to their offspring through the milk, which would be detrimental to the child at all but the lowest doses. Thus, a pregnant woman with SLE has a very good chance of producing a normal child. If she had acute or subacute SLE at the time of pregnancy, the mother has an increased risk of dying of SLE in the postpartum period.[44] I believe that the risk can be minimized by administration of corticosteroids (or increased amounts of corticosteroids) during labor and after delivery.

Unwanted pregnancies are best avoided by birth control. There is no general agreement upon the best methods in patients with SLE. Since sex hormones can modify the expression of autoimmunity in mice,[48,49] it is possible that birth control pills may put the woman with SLE at some additional risk. Fortunately, the newer oral contraceptives contain minimal or no estrogens; these may be much safer than the older high-estrogen-containing pills. The alternative of an intrauterine device subjects the patient to a potential source of infection. Nevertheless, both forms of birth control have been used successfully by large numbers of young females with SLE. Barrier contraception is less well accepted by the young patient; but it appears to be safer, and should be highly recommended to married women with SLE and to any others who will use it. Abortion is a distinctly inappropriate method of birth control in SLE, especially since flares follow abortions as frequently as full-term deliveries. If an abortion must be performed, it should be done as early in pregnancy as possible. Generous corticosteroid coverage should be provided for the immediate postabortion period, and increased steroid therapy given for a subsequent 3- to 6-week period. During the postabortion period, the patient should be followed closely for signs or symptoms of active disease. Evidence of worsening of the clinical or laboratory picture at this time should be countered with more vigorous treatment.

Should an abortion be recommended for patients with very active disease or advanced renal disease who inadvertently become pregnant? The risks versus the benefits in these cases are best decided on an individual basis. Ironically, if the pregnancy is to be allowed to continue, the initially active disease may appear to improve. This should not lull the patient or the physician into a false sense of security; both should be mindful of the dangers of preeclampsia, and marked post-partum flare, which must be anticipated and vigorously treated. Severe active renal disease and pregnancy are a very bad combination, often resulting in a life-threatening situation for the mother and loss of the fetus late in the pregnancy. The use of immunosuppressive drugs during pregnancy is discouraged. Nevertheless, patients becoming pregnant while receiving azathioprine or subsequently treated during pregnancy have delivered normal babies. If abortion is elected, maximal disease suppressive therapy should be provided.

USE OF SPECIFIC DRUGS IN SLE

Corticosteroids (see Chapter 54 for further details). The therapeutic effects of corticosteroids are maximized by the use of high doses given daily in divided doses (e.g., every 4 hours). This therapy also is associated with the most devastating side effects.[9,10,50,51] At the other extreme, the side effects of corticosteroids are minimized by the use of short-acting preparations given once every 48 hours.[52] Treatment decisions are based upon a balance between the need for greater therapeutic drug effects and the desire to minimize toxicity. Patients with very active disease often need to be treated with high doses given daily in divided doses. As symptoms come under control, the dose should be changed to daily, reduced, and ultimately switched to alternate-day whenever possible. Milder degrees of disease activity can usually be treated with daily therapy given in a single dose. Occasional patients may respond to initiation of alternate-day treatment; however, low doses of daily drug are usually needed to bring symptoms under control, after which a gradual or abrupt switch to alternate-day treatment may be carried out. It appears that alternate-day therapy has value as prophylaxis against the acceleration of the inflammatory process; it often keeps it under control when it is smoldering. However, such treatment is usually not capable of bringing about suppression of the disease after accelerated inflammation has already taken place.

Pulses of very high doses of corticosteroids[53] given in an attempt to remove steroid toxicity must be viewed as experimental and should not be given except in the context of a randomized trial. In this manner, efficacy versus toxicity may be established. Increased long-term toxicity of such treatment in terms of arteriosclerosis, cataracts, or osteonecrosis is as likely as the possibility that such therapy will reduce steroid toxicity. Furthermore, flares of disease have been observed within several weeks of such treatment. Therefore, pulse therapy should be adequately evaluated so that it may become accepted or be discarded.

Prolonged high-dose steroid therapy for SLE patients cannot be justified on the basis of any randomized clinical trials for any sign, symptom, or organ in SLE. Nevertheless, corticosteroid drugs remain the mainstay of therapy of patients with SLE who are inadequately responsive to nonsteroidal antiinflammatory drugs such as aspirin. Most rheumatologists use prednisone, although some prefer prednisolone. Drugs with short half-lives are generally preferred so that a switch to every-other-day therapy can be made without changing the drug. Thus, dexamethasone, which is very long acting, should generally be avoided. Drug dosage should be selected such that the desired therapeutic benefits are achieved with the least risk of toxicity. In general, that means the lowest possible dose of drug. A patient with arthritis, fever, rash, and serositis despite aspirin and hydroxychloroquine therapy should be treated with corticosteroids. However, it is not necessary to start with 60 mg per day of prednisone. Most such patients will respond to lower doses of daily prednisone such as 20 to 30 mg per day or even less. An occasional patient will initially require more. Success at the lower dose may markedly reduce the total duration of daily therapy because the magnitude of the subsequent tapering will be less. The aim of treatment is always to lower the prednisone dose without allowing signs or symptoms to emerge. In general, this is best accomplished by as little manipulation of the steroid dose as possible. When tapering prednisone from daily doses of less than 30 to 40 mg per day, one should taper slowly, and below 20 mg per day very slowly. In contrast, a reduction from 200 mg per day to 80 mg per day can be accomplished in less than a week. Each physician develops his own style of steroid tapering with experience. A typical schedule for tapering from 60 mg per day might be a reduction to 50 mg per day for 5 days, 40 mg per day for 5 days, 35 mg per day for a week, 30 mg per day for a week, 27.5 mg per day for a week, 25 mg per day for a week, 22.5 mg per day for 2 weeks, 20 mg per day for 2 weeks, 17.5 mg per day for 3 weeks, 15 mg per day for a month, 15 mg alternating with 12.5 mg for 2 to 4 weeks, 15 mg alternating with 10.0 mg for 2 to 4 weeks, 15 mg alternating with 7.5 mg for a month, 15 mg alternating with 5.0 mg for a month, 15 mg alternating with 2.5 mg for

a month, 20 mg alternating with 0 for a month, 17.5 mg every other day for a month, and 15 mg every other day for 2 months. This covers a period of 1 year. If the drug was given for nonmajor organ symptoms in a patient without major organ involvement or a history of same, a somewhat faster taper might be tried. If the patient has previously flared during tapering, especially with major organ involvement, a slower taper may be in order. If a patient flares with fatigue and arthralgias during the course of tapering, it may be possible to go back to the previous dose or hold at the present dose and have the symptoms come under control. Subsequent tapering should be slower, perhaps with decrements of only 1.0 mg of prednisone. On the other hand, if the flare is severe hemolytic anemia or other major organ signs or symptoms, going to the previous dose may not be sufficient. It may be necessary to reinstitute very high doses, bring the disease under control, and then start to taper again. As a result of these problems, one should not start with more drug than is necessary. That reduces the time to get to a reasonably nontoxic dose (e.g., 10 to 15 mg of prednisone per square meter every other day). In addition, one should not taper too quickly, so as to avoid the need to interrupt the taper or actually increase the drug dose for symptoms unmasked during rapid tapering.

Although the goal is low doses of every-other-day steroids, patients with active disease, especially with fever and arthritis and serositis, usually cannot be controlled on every-other-day drug. Such patients tend to require daily drug until symptoms are brought under control. Sometimes large doses of nonsteroidal anti-inflammatory drugs such as aspirin, ibuprofen, and indomethacin will allow the taper to every other day despite arthralgias and fever on the "off day" without those drugs. In addition, the concomitant use of hydroxychloroquine may facilitate the corticosteroid taper.

Despite the fact that some patients may be successfully tapered to no prednisone, that should not necessarily be the goal of treatment. Steroids were presumably started for a logical indication. They may be necessary for disease control for many years. A taper to zero may be associated with a subsequent flare which requires reinstitution of drug in moderately high doses. It is safer to be on 20 mg of prednisone every other day for a year than on nothing for 6 months and then 20 to 30 mg daily for 6 months. Nevertheless, the patient who has weathered the taper described above and remains asymptomatic and with normal laboratory findings on 15 mg of prednisone every other day could be tapered further during the next year, and, if still in "remission" at the end of the second year, could be considered for complete withdrawal. Of course, many patients are treated unnecessarily with steroids—either with prednisone when aspirin might have been enough or with too high a dose of corticosteroid. These patients may be successfully tapered faster and to zero faster. I believe that patients with previous major organ involvement should be tapered to zero with extreme caution. If the disease was glomerulonephritis, years of inactivity would be necessary to persuade me to taper below 10 mg prednisone every other day.

A more rapid change to alternate-day therapy than that described in the aforementioned schedule is often possible and desirable. In particular, growing children are often successfully switched abruptly from 30 mg per day to 60 mg every other day. Additional patients may develop steroid psychosis at moderately high or very high drug doses. This should be treated with a combination of steroid reduction and antipsychotic drugs as required. An occasional such patient may have disease activity requiring the high steroid dose. It may be necessary to temporarily continue the high dose and add a major tranquilizer, such as Thorazine, until alternative forms of therapy can adequately be considered.

Some patients with very active disease may respond poorly to a moderately high dose of corticosteroid given once a day. A question of raising the dose arises. Many such patients will respond better to giving the drug in divided doses (e.g., every 6 hours) than to a higher daily dose. However, it must be remembered that after the disease is brought under control a change from treatment four times per day to twice a day, and then from twice a day to daily, may represent considerable taper in medication even if the total dose given in one day is unchanged. Thus, a patient receiving 20 mg every 6 hours should be changed to 15 mg every 6 hours or to 80 mg daily, but not to 60 mg daily as the first "dose reduction." Since patients with SLE are living longer and dying of or with complications of therapy with increasing frequency, restraint with regard to therapy is most desirable. It is no longer appropriate to treat every patient with active SLE with 60 to 80 mg per day of prednisone for a few months and then decide what to do.

Antimalarials (see Chapter 51 for further details). Hydroxychloroquine and chloroquine appear to provide benefit for patients with SLE in addition to their efficacy in the therapy of skin involvement in both discoid and systemic lupus. Their use often allows a lower dose of steroids to be used, every-other-day as opposed to daily steroids, or avoidance of steroids altogether. A loading dose of several tablets per day for 1 to 2 weeks (400 to 600 mg per day of hydroxychloroquine or 250 mg per day of chloroquine) should be followed by a standard daily dose (200 to 400 mg per day of hydroxychloroquine or 125 to 250 mg per day of chloroquine). When the disease is quiescent, the drug dosage can be further reduced to 200 mg of hydroxychloroquine or 125 mg of chloroquine two or three times per week and eventually stopped altogether. The major limitation in the use of these drugs is the threat of eye toxicity. Retinal accumulation is dose related, but individuals vary with regard to the dosage at which problems arise. Our own experience with hydroxychloroquine has been the observation of benefit without toxicity.

There currently is controversy regarding the usefulness of periodic tests of visual acuity, color vision, visual fields, and cone thresholds as predictors of impending toxicity. Since ocular toxicity may develop or increase after drug is withdrawn, prolonged use of these antimalarials should be carried out with care. The ophthalmologist should test color vision periodically so that early deposits may be detected. Such a practice may allow the drug to be withdrawn early enough to avoid retinal toxicity. It has been suggested that hydroxychloroquine is less likely to cause retinal toxicity; however, it is not clear if that is due to increased safety or reduced effectiveness of the usual doses given. Any suggestion on ophthalmologic examinations of impending retinal toxicity should lead to immediate and permanent withdrawal of the drug. When the cumulative dose of drug reaches 200 grams of chloroquine or 450 grams of hydroxychloroquine, termination of therapy should be considered in an attempt to avoid eye toxicity.

Immunosuppressive Drugs (see Chapter 55 for additional details). A number of cytostatic and cytotoxic drugs have been used in patients with systemic lupus. These include nitrogen mustard, azathioprine, cyclophosphamide, chlorambucil, methotrexate and vinca alkaloids. None of these should be regarded as standard therapy. They have taken a back seat to corticosteroids for several reasons: historical accident; the rapidity with which steroids work to relieve symptoms, and the longer period of time taken for the immunosuppressive drugs to have an effect on symptomatology; and the real and potential toxicities of the immunosuppressive drugs.[54] None of these reasons may be logical in a given patient, especially when steroids are neither uniformly effective nor nontoxic.

In 1949, nitrogen mustard was reported to benefit renal abnormalities in patients with glomerulonephritis.[55] Subsequently, such therapy was tried in patients with SLE renal disease with suggestive success.[56,57] Although largely replaced by corticosteroids, nitrogen mustard and other cytotoxic and cytostatic immunosuppressive drugs were given to patients with SLE throughout the 1950s and 1960s in an uncontrolled manner. In the late 1960s dissatisfaction with the cushingoid side effects of prolonged high dose corticosteroid therapy of patients with SLE led to more intensive evaluation of immunosuppressive drugs in SLE, including a series of controlled trials. In general, the uncontrolled reports tended to be very optimistic with regard to the benefits of immunosuppressive drugs in patients with SLE. One optimistic report of nitrogen mustard treatment demonstrated no impressive long-term benefit, and used outdated historical survival curves for comparison.[58] No controlled trial of this agent is available.

A number of controlled trials have been reported evaluating cyclophosphamide treatment in patients with SLE. In a randomized, but not "blinded," study, cyclophosphamide was found to be ineffective as a primary agent in SLE patients not receiving corticosteroids.[59] Although subsequent studies have demonstrated an occasional symptomatic response to cyclophosphamide alone, it has generally been found that the immunosuppressive drugs are not very effective as short-term therapy for symptomatic SLE. Thus, oral cyclophosphamide and oral azathioprine should not be considered as sole therapy for patients with symptomatic disease; corticosteroids are much more effective drugs under such circumstances. Even the nonsteroidal antiinflammatory drugs such as aspirin and ibuprofen are frequently much more effective than are the immunosuppressive drugs under such circumstances. It is possible that intravenous use of immunosuppressive drugs, such as cyclophosphamide, may provide more rapid symptomatic relief; however, the appropriate studies have not yet been performed.

Most of the controlled studies of cyclophosphamide have involved addition of the agent to corticosteroid treatment. The first such study was of 10 weeks' duration and involved a small number of patients.[60] There was no difference between placebo-treated and cyclophosphamide-treated patients with regard to creatinine clearance. However, cyclophosphamide-treated patients had improvement in proteinuria, urine sediment, anti-DNA, C3, and extrarenal symptoms as compared with placebo-treated patients. The patients with the mildest degree of renal functional impairment and those capable of taking the most drug responded best to therapy.[60] A similar subsequent study of cyclophosphamide versus azathioprine versus placebo demonstrated that cyclophosphamide was superior to azathioprine and azathioprine was superior to placebo.[61] A group of patients with SLE and glomerulonephritis treated with prednisone plus cyclophosphamide did not differ from a group treated with prednisone alone when evaluated after 6 months, but were significantly better at 24 months.[63]

The addition of oral azathioprine to a therapeutic regimen of corticosteroids has been the most popular; however, the support for such treatment is tenuous.[61,62,64,72]

A large number of uncontrolled reports support the use of chlorambucil in the treatment of SLE; however, a recent controlled international trial has not demonstrated chlorambucil to be any better than either cyclophosphamide or azathioprine.[70]

Additional studies are being performed to evaluate other immunosuppressive drugs or to evaluate the same ones in different regimens. It has been suggested that combination therapy with several drugs (such as cyclophosphamide plus azathioprine plus corticosteroids) or the use of intravenous cyclophosphamide may be more effective than treatment with oral cyclophosphamide plus corticosteroids or oral azathioprine plus corticosteroids.[71] The intravenous cyclophosphamide approach has been thought to be lifesaving in some patients. Typical doses range from 0.5 to 1.0 gram per square meter of body surface area given at intervals of between 3 weeks and 3 months.

Recent analysis of therapy in patients with SLE and glomerulonephritis has revealed information that provides a more rational approach to therapy with immunosuppressive drugs.[32,72] The degree of scarring of the kidney is a very important prognostic factor. Thus, patients with very little scarring may respond very well to therapy with corticosteroids or to therapy with corticosteroids plus oral azathioprine or cyclophosphamide. In contrast, patients with severe scarring on renal biopsy appear to respond much less well to any of those therapies; furthermore, there does not appear to be overwhelming benefit of particular therapy. Patients with a moderate degree of renal scarring had the greatest benefit from the addition of either oral azathioprine or oral cyclophosphamide to the corticosteroid regimen. Does that mean that there is no hope for patients with considerable scarring? Vigorous therapy with monthly boluses of intravenous cyclophosphamide for several months may be of benefit in retarding the progression of renal deterioration in patients with both scarring and continued disease activity. The preliminary studies are using 0.75g of cyclophosphamide per square meter of body surface area. Adequate fluid intake with half normal saline decreases the toxic effects of the metabolites on the bladder and reduces the hyponatremia associated with inappropriate ADH secretion which accompanies cyclophosphamide therapy. Some patients experience nausea and vomiting of a severe nature, which may be treated with antiemetics. The investigators who have been studying this form of therapy still regard it as experimental and have been comparing this form of bolus cyclophosphamide therapy with bolus corticosteroid therapy. The results of this comparison with regard to both effectiveness and toxicities will not be available for several years.

Occasionally a patient with SLE will present in extremis. Although the proper therapy for a patient with overwhelming SLE (without infection) is unknown, current information would suggest the following as a possible approach: a bolus of corticosteroids, immediate 4-liter plasmapheresis with protein replacement, and intravenous cyclophosphamide (0.75 to 1.0 g per square meter) followed by high doses of corticosteroids. If the patient survives, a second dose of cyclophosphamide and corticosteroid tapering at four weeks would be followed by subsequent re-evaluation of continued cyclophosphamide therapy at monthly intervals for an additinal half year. A more rapid improvement would allow faster corticosteroid tapering. Evidence of thrombotic thrombocytopenic purpura or, perhaps, very large amounts of removable circulating factors would suggest a greater emphasis on plasma exchange initially.

SYSTEMIC LUPUS ERYTHEMATOSUS IN CHILDREN

The division between child and adult is often vague. This is especially true of patients with SLE. Pediatricians often follow patients with SLE through college age, whereas "adult rheumatologists" frequently care for children with SLE from age 9 or 10. At a time when the median age of my patients with SLE in an "adult" rheumatology clinic was 15 years, I read an article from a pediatric service about children with SLE who were even older. Thus, the experience with younger patients with SLE has occurred in a variety of settings. In general, treatment of teenagers with SLE is very similar to that of young adults, with the obvious additional required attention to the special needs and problems of teenagers. The teenager is often trying to assert his or her independence from authority figures. Illness itself as well as the resultant childlike position relative to the medical community may lead to resentment and noncompliance. Special attention to these psychological needs as well as the problems of appearance, body image, and sexuality in the teenager often can turn a dangerous situation into a meaningful relationship and long-term good health. Children aged 10 to 12 years of age can often be similarly treated, except that special efforts should be made to treat with alternate-day steroids so as to avoid growth retardation as well as other steroid side effects. Although parental involvement is necessary in the care of such patients, every attempt should be made to involve the child as much as possible in discussions. The physician's relationship must be primarily with the child and only secondarily with the parent.

Children under 9 years of age are probably best handled by a physician with experience in treating children. Since long-term survival from the disease is quite good on a statistical basis, even when nephritis is present,[26] every attempt should be made to avoid prolonged use of high-dose daily steroid therapy. Although daily therapy may be initially necessary, an abrupt switch to every-other-day steroids should be attempted as soon as signs and symptoms of disease activity are minimized. Alternatively, a rapid taper to every-other-day therapy may be preferred. Flares during tapering should be treated with judicious use of additional corticosteroids and adequate doses of nonsteroidal anti-inflammatory drugs. Avoidance of excessively prolonged high dose daily steroid therapy in children cannot be overemphasized in view of the infectious and other complications observed in such patients.[26] See Chapter 82 for a more extensive discussion of the treatment of SLE in childhood.

IMMUNIZATIONS

It was once thought that immunizations would exacerbate SLE, or perhaps even induce clinical illness in an asymptomatic person with the proper genetic and immunologic abnormalities. Evidence against this notion is available for vaccination against influenza and pneumococci.[73,74] Whether or not additional immunizations will be found to be harmless remains to be determined. Common sense suggests that immunizations should be performed, whenever possible, when the patient is not taking large doses of corticosteroids or immunosuppressive drugs and when the disease activity is least marked. Since patients with SLE often have impaired primary immune responses, booster injections may be necessary to bring about an adequate immune response. A study of the use of inhibitors of vasoactive amines in association with immunization is not available to justify a practice that might have a rational basis. Perhaps such a study will soon be available.

USE OF DRUGS ASSOCIATED WITH INDUCTION OF SLE-LIKE ILLNESS IN NORMALS

A number of drugs are known to induce antinuclear antibodies and a lupus-like illness in otherwise normal people. In almost all cases, the illness eventually subsides upon withdrawal of the drug. Should such drugs be withheld from patients with known SLE? A randomized trial of addition of one of these drugs to a group of patients and an alternative drug to another has not been performed. Experience does not suggest a major problem in the use of drugs such as alphamethyldopa, Dilantin, and other agents implicated in drug-induced SLE. Low doses of hydralazine or high doses for relatively short periods of time also do not appear to be a problem. It may be prudent to use other medicines when an equally good alternative is available; however, when the alternative is inferior, the best drug should not be withheld on the basis of some theoretical objection which has no support in fact. An exception to this cavalier approach is the prolonged use of high doses of hydralazine, alternatives for which are usually available in any case.

EXPERIMENTAL FORMS OF THERAPY

Since evidence is accumulating to implicate an immune deficiency in SLE (T-lymphocyte hypofunction during active disease is well established), attempts to treat the disease with immunological stimulants or adjuvants have some rational basis. Levamisole, a drug that may augment subnormal immune responses, and could be of some benefit in preventing or helping to treat infectious complications in an SLE patient, does not appear to be as promising a major treatment modality as was hoped.

The use of antiviral drugs to treat a primary viral infection underlying SLE, or, more likely (in my view), to prevent the effects on the immune system of intercurrent viral infections (which appear to be associated with some lupus flares in our experience) has an experimental basis in the New Zealand mouse.[73] Whether or not such drugs will be effective in humans will probably not be known for several years.

Lymphoid ablative procedures such as thoracic duct drainage, leukapheresis, selected node irradiation, and early splenectomy could provide effective immunosuppression with reduced side effects. Nodal irradiation and splenectomy deserve the greatest attention; however, their efficacy must be demonstrated in good randomized trials in comparison with other effective treatments.

Since SLE is primarily an antibody-mediated disease, attempts to remove pathogenic antibodies or immune complexes have a logical basis.[76,77] Systematic plasmapheresis with protein repletion could provide for the physical removal of these serum factors without the hazards of generalized immunosuppression.[78] Since IgG antibodies are distributed outside the circulation to a greater extent than IgM molecules, it is harder to remove pathogenic IgG anti-DNA antibodies by plasmapheresis than it is to remove IgM antibodies. However, much of the lymphocytotoxic antibody activity is in the IgM class, providing an easy mechanism for removing those antibodies most implicated in the T-lymphocyte immune abnormalities. A more selective removal approach has been studied.[79,80] This involves extracorporeal circulation through solid phase attached materials that bind either anti-DNA (DNA is attached to the solid phase) or immune complexes (Clq or rheumatoid factor is bound to the solid phase) or potentially other pathogenic substances. The practicality and efficacy of this form of treatment as compared with other therapies remain to be determined.

Specific tolerance to nucleic acids has been achieved in mice and may some day have applicability to humans.[81] Treatment with suppressor substances such as prostaglandins[82] and supernatants of activated spleen cells[82] also has been effective in the New Zealand mouse model of SLE. A similar attempt to replace inadequate suppressor substances may, in the future, warrant consideration for trials in patients with SLE. Sex hormone modification of autoimmunity in intact[49] and castrated[48,49] NZB/W mice suggests possible sex hormone treatment in humans. This form of treatment is not effective in all mice with murine lupus nor is it of maximal benefit after early childhood in the mice. Therefore, it may provide no advantages (and have some disadvantages) in comparison with prednisone.

Recent studies have demonstrated that fish oil rich in eicosapentaenoic acid may reduce the progression of renal disease in NZB/W mice.[84,85] It is possible that dietary approaches to patients with SLE will one day serve as an adjunct to other therapy. Studies to test the efficacy of such treatment in humans are being planned. In addition, avoidance of certain foods or food additives that might exacerbate SLE could be important;[86] however, studies of this subject are in their infancy.

Advances in immunology suggest that self-self recognition is necessary for immune responsiveness. Much of this recognition involves Ia or DR recognition. The finding that administration of anti-Ia antibodies to mice with SLE can retard disease is therefore not surprising. Comparable anti-DR antibodies are available and could be used directly to treat patients with SLE.[87-89] Studies of autoimmune mice indicate that a single gene can prevent or retard markedly the production of autoantibodies by autoimmune-prone strains.[90,91] Moreover, such mice have prolonged survival and little kidney disease.[91] The relevant gene causes a deletion of a B-lymphocyte subset from the spleens of such mice. The B-lymphocyte subset deleted has unique surface markers. We do not know if a comparable subset of B-lymphocytes is responsible for autoantibody production in humans with SLE. If so, the development of monoclonal antibodies to such B-lymphocytes could provide a very specific treatment. Administration of such an antibody, either directly or conjugated to a toxin, might eliminate specifically the autoantibody-producing cells without altering normal immune functions.

Unless a new therapy is dramatically effective, it will be necessary to establish its usefulness in carefully performed clinical trials. The recent experiences with immunosuppressive drugs and the lack of adequate trials of corticosteroid therapy suggest that it may be many years before a new treatment could be established as being effective. Nevertheless, the prospects for minimally toxic but effective therapy for SLE have never been brighter. Basic research may yield pay-offs in this area before another decade passes.

CONCLUDING REMARKS

Systemic lupus is a disease of unknown cause. Several factors appear to contribute to illness in a given individual. The final common pathway is the production of injury-inducing autoantibodies by subpopulations of B-lymphocytes and their progeny. However, the genetic bases and environmental variables may vary substantially from one individual to another.[92] Thus, SLE might properly be viewed as a syndrome with different causes rather than a single illness. As a result, different individuals might respond differently to a given therapy and the ideal therapy for each might vary. On the other hand, an attack on the common final pathway might be similar in all individuals with SLE. It has long been hoped that understanding the pathogenesis of the disease would lead to more specific therapy. The understanding has been slow in coming, but it has been coming. Some of the pathogenic mechanisms are becoming better understood. Furthermore, the multifactorial nature of the disease, especially the contribution of genetic factors, is better appreciated. It is possible that understanding of cause will lead immediately to a logical cure. Alternatively, we may be therapeutically little better off initially. Fortunately, removal of one factor in a multifactorial disease should lead to amelioration, prevention or at least retardation of disease. It is possible that prevention of disease in a susceptible individual will be the most effective approach in the future. This may require an ability to detect susceptible but asymptomatic people and to treat them in such a manner that at least one of the disease-producing factors is reduced or eliminated. The practical and ethical problems involved are not insurmountable in view of screening currently performed for phenylketonuria and other diseases identifiable early in life, and the mandatory immunization programs which are firmly based in our society. Thus, our therapeutic armamentarium awaits refinement of knowledge of the cause(s) of SLE.

References

1. Tsokos, G.C., Moutsopoulos, H.M., and Steinberg, A.D.: Muscle involvement in systemic lupus erythematosus. JAMA 246:766, 1981.
2. Spencer-Green, G: Raynaud phenomenon. Bull. Rheum. Dis. 33:1, 1983.

3. Nilsen, K.H.: Effects of naftidrofuryl on microcirculatory cold sensitivity in Raynaud's phenomenon. Br. Med. J. 1:20, 1979.

4. Waldo, R.: Prazosin relieves Raynaud's vasospasm. JAMA 241:1037, 1979.

5. Sharp, G.C., Irvin, W.S., LaRoque, R.L., Velez, C., Daly, V., Kaiser, A.D., and Holman, H.R.: Association of autoantibodies to different nuclear antigens with clinical patterns of rheumatic disease and responsiveness to therapy. J. Clin. Invest. 50:350, 1971.

6. Schur, P.H., and Sandson, J.: Immunologic factors and clinical activity in systemic lupus erythematosus. N. Engl. J. Med. 278:533, 1968.

7. Gershwin, M.E., and Steinberg, A.D.: Qualitative characteristics of anti-DNA antibodies in lupus nephritis. Arthritis Rheum. 17:947, 1974.

8. Leon, S.A., Green, A., Ehrlich, G.E., Poland, M., and Shapiro, B.: Avidity of antibodies in SLE: Relation to severity of renal involvement. Arthritis Rheum. 20:23, 1977.

9. Staples, P.J., Gerding, D.N., Decker, J.L., and Gordon, R.S., Jr.: Incidence of infection in systemic lupus erythematosus. Arthritis Rheum. 17:1, 1974.

10. Ginzler, E., Diamond, H., Kaplan, D., Weiner, M., Schlesinger, M., and Seleznick, M.: Computer analysis of factors influencing frequency of infection in systemic lupus erythematosus. Arthritis Rheum. 21:37, 1978.

11. Baldwin, D.S., Lowenstein, J., and Rothfield, N.F.: The clinical course of the proliferative and membranous forms of lupus nephritis. Ann. Intern. Med. 73:929, 1970.

12. Hecht, B., Siegel, N., Adler, M., Kashgarian, M., and Hayslett, J.P.: Prognostic indices in lupus nephritis. Medicine 55:163, 1976.

13. Ginzler, E.M., Nicastri, A.D., Chen, C.K., Friedman, E.A., Diamond, H.S., and Kaplan, D.: Progression of mesangial and focal to diffuse nephritis. N. Engl. J. Med. 291:693, 1974.

14. Zimmerman, S.W., Jenkins, P.J., Shelp, W.D., Bloodworth, J.M.B., Jr., and Burkholder, P.M.: Progression from minimal or focal to diffuse proliferative lupus nephritis. Lab. Invest. 32:665, 1975.

15. Pollak, V.E., and Pirani, C.L.: Renal histologic findings in systemic lupus erythematosus. Mayo Clin. Proc. 44:630, 1969.

16. Grishman, E., Churg, J., Mautner, W., and Yasvnasuke, S.: Pathology of lupus nephritis. J. Mt. Sinai Hosp. 30:117, 1963.

17. Dujovne, I., Pollak, V.E., Pirani, C.L., and Dillard, M.G.: The distribution and character of glomerular deposits in systemic lupus erythematosus. Kidney Int. 2:33, 1972.

18. Hayslett, J.P., and Siegel, N.J.: Treatment of lupus nephropathy. Nephron 19:193, 1977.

19. Lange, K., Ores, R., Strauss, W., and Wachstein, M.: Steroid therapy of systemic lupus erythematosus based on immunologic considerations. Arthritis Rheum. 8:244, 1965.

20. Kagan, L.J., and Christian, C.L.: Clinicopathologic studies of SLE nephritis (abstract). Arthritis Rheum. 9:516, 1966.

21. Steinberg, A.D., and Decker, J.L.: The management of lupus nephritis. Ann. Intern. Med. 73:1035, 1970.

22. Steinberg, A.D.: An approach to the use of immunosuppressive drugs in non-malignant diseases. J. Allergy Clin. Immunol. 57:242, 1973.

23. Wagner, L.: Immunosuppressive agents in lupus nephritis: A critical analysis. Medicine 55:239, 1976.

24. Steinberg, A.D., Kaltreider, H.B., Staples, P.J., Goetzl, E.J., Talal, N., and Decker, J.L.: Cyclophosphamide in lupus nephritis: A controlled trial. Ann. Intern. Med. 75:165, 1971.

25. Estes, D., and Christian, C.L.: The natural history of systemic lupus erythematosus by prospective analysis. Medicine 50:85, 1971.

26. Fish, A.J., Blau, E.B., Westberg, N.G., Burke, B.A., Vernier, R.L., and Michael, A.F.: Systemic lupus erythematosus within the first two decades of life. Am. J. Med. 62:99, 1977.

27. Pollak, V.E., Pirani, C.L., and Kark, R.M.: Effect of large doses of prednisone on the renal lesions and life span of patients with lupus glomerulonephritis. J. Lab. Clin. Med. 57:495, 1961.

28. Steinberg, A.D., Gelfand, M.C., Hardin, J.A., and Lowenthal, D.T.: Therapeutic studies in NZB/W mice. III. Relationship between renal status and efficacy of immunosuppressive drug therapy. Arthritis Rheum. 18:9, 1975.

29. Budman, D., and Steinberg, A.D.: Relationship between hypertension and renal disease in systemic lupus erythematosus. Arch. Intern. Med. 136:1003, 1976.

30. Huttner, I., More, R.H., and Rona, G.: Fine structural evidence of specific mechanism for increased endothelial permeability in experimental hypertension. Am. J. Pathol. 61:395, 1970.

31. Kimberly, R.P., and Plotz, P.H.: Aspirin-induced depression of renal function. N. Engl. J. Med 296:418, 1977.

32. Carette, S., Klippel, J.H., Decker, J.L., Austin, H.A., Plotz, P.H., Steinberg, A.D., and Balow, J.E.: Controlled studies of oral immunosuppressive drugs in lupus nephritis. A long-term follow up. Ann. Intern. Med., 99:1, 1983.

33. Bennahum, D.A., and Messner, R.P.: Recent observations on central nervous system lupus erythematosus. Semin. Arthritis Rheum. 4:253, 1975.

34. Brandt, K.D., and Lessell, S.: Migrainous phenomena in systemic lupus erythematosus. Arthritis Rheum. 21:7, 1978.

35. Sergent, J.S., Lockshin, M.D., Klempner, M.S., and Lipsky, B.A.: Central nervous system disease in systemic lupus erythematosus. Am. J. Med. 58:644, 1975.

36. Winfield, J.B., Brunner, C.M., and Koffler, D.: Serologic studies in patients with systemic lupus erythematosus and central nervous system dysfunction. Arthritis Rheum. 21:289, 1978.

37. Williams, G.W., Bluestein, H.G., and Steinberg, A.D.: Brain reactive lymphocytotoxic antibody in the cerebrospinal fluid of patients with systemic lupus erythematosus: Correlation with central nervous system involvement. Clin. Immunol. Immunopathol. 18:126, 1981.

38. Bluestein, H.G., Williams, G.W., and Steinberg, A.D.: Cerebrospinal fluid antibodies to neuronal cells: Association with neuropsychiatric manifestations of systemic lupus erythematosus. Am. J. Med. 70:240, 1981.

39. Kassen, S.S., and Kagen, L.J.: Elevated levels of cerebrospinal fluid guanosine 3',5'-cyclic monophosphate (C-GMP) in systemic lupus erythematosus. Am. J. Med. 64:732, 1978.

40. Matthay, R.A., Schwarz, M.I., Petty, T.L., Stanford, R.E., Gupta, R.C., Sahn, S.A., and Steigerwald, J.C.: Pulmonary manifestations of systemic lupus erythematosus. Medicine 54:397, 1974.

41. Budman, D.R., and Steinberg, A.D.: Current concepts of the hematologic aspects of systemic lupus erythematosus. Ann. Intern. Med. 86:220, 1977.

42. Srichaikul, T., Boonpucknavig, S., Archararit, N., and Chaisiripumkeeree, W.: Chronic immunologic thrombocytopenic purpura-results of cyclophosphamide therapy before splenectomy. Arch. Intern. Med. 140:636, 1980.

43. Oen, K., Petty, R.E., Schroeder, M.-L., Briggs, E.J.N., and Bishop, A.J.: Thrombotic thrombocytopenic purpura in a girl with systemic lupus erythematosus. J. Rheumatol. 7:727, 1980.

44. Smolen, J.S., and Steinberg, A.D.: Systemic lupus erythematosus and pregnancy. Clinical, immunological and theoretical aspects. In Gleicher, N. (ed.): Reproductive Immunology. New York, Alan R. Liss Publishers, 1981.

45. Jackson, R., and Gulliver, M.: Neonatal lupus erythematosus progressing into systemic lupus erythematosus. A 15 year followup. Br. J. Dermatol. 101:81, 1979.

46. Fox, R.J., McCuistion, C.H., Schoch, E.P., Jr. Systemic lupus erythematosus: association with previous neonatal lupus erythematosus. Arch. Dermatol. 115:340, 1979.

47. Reinertsen, J.L., Klippel, J.H., John, A.H., Steinberg, A.D., Decker, J.L., and Mann, D.L.: B-lymphocyte alloantigens associated with systemic lupus erythematosus. N. Engl. J. Med. 299:515, 1978.

48. Roubinian, J.R., Papoian, R., and Talal, N.: Androgenic hormones modulate autoantibody responses and improve survival in murine lupus. J. Clin. Invest. 59:1066, 1977.

49. Steinberg, A.D.: Approach to the study of the role of sex hormones in autoimmunity. Arthritis Rheum. 22:1170, 1979.

50. Thorn, G.W.: The adrenal cortex. Reflections, progress and speculations. Trans. Assoc. Am. Physicians 86:65, 1973.

51. Axelrod, L.: Glucocorticoid therapy. Medicine 55:39, 1976.

52. Harter, J.G., Reddy, W.J., and Thorn, G.W.: Studies on intermittent corticosteroid dosage regimen. N. Engl. J. Med. 269:591, 1963.

53. Cathcart, E.S., Edelson, B.A., Scheinberg, M.A., and Couser, W.G.: Beneficial effects of methylprednisolone "pulse" therapy in diffuse proliferative lupus nephritis. Lancet 1:163, 1976.

54. Sharon, E., Kaplan, D., and Diamond, H.S.: Exacerbation of systemic lupus after withdrawal of azathioprine therapy. N. Engl. J. Med. 288:122, 1973.

55. Chasis, H., Goldring, W., and Baldwin, D.S.: Effect of febrile plasma, typhoid vaccine, and nitrogen mustard on renal manifestations of human glomerulonephritis. Proc. Soc. Exp. Biol. Med. 71:565, 1949.

56. Rohn, R.J., and Bond, W.H.: Some effects of nitrogen mustard and triethylene melamine in acute disseminated lupus erythematosus. Am. J. Med. Sci. 226:179, 1953.

57. Dubois, E.L.: Nitrogen mustard in treatment of systemic lupus erythematosus. Arch. Intern. Med. 93:667, 1954.

58. Dillard, M.G., Dujovne, I., Pollack, V.E., and Pirani, C.L.: The effect of treatment with prednisone and nitrogen mustard on the renal lesions and life span of patients with lupus glomerulonephritis. Nephron 10:273, 1973.

59. Fries, J.F., Sharp, G.C., McDevitt, H.O., and Holman, H.R.: Cyclophosphamide therapy in systemic lupus erythematosus and polymyositis. Arthritis Rheum. 16:154, 1973.

60. Steinberg, A.D., Kaltreider, H.B., Staples, R.J., Goetzel, E.J., Talal, N., and Decker, J.L.: Cyclophosphamide in lupus nephritis: A controlled trial. Ann. Intern. Med. 75:165, 1971.

61. Steinberg, A.D., and Decker, J.L.: A double-blind controlled trial comparing cyclophosphamide, azathioprine, and placebo in the treatment of lupus glomerulonephritis. Arthritis Rheum. 17:923, 1974.

62. Decker, J.L., Klippel, J.H., Plotz, P.H., and Steinberg, A.D.: Cyclophosphamide of azathioprine in lupus glomerulonephritis. A controlled trial—results at 28 months. Ann. Intern. Med. 83:606, 1975.

63. Donadio, J.V., Holley, K.E., Ferguson, R.H., and Ilstrup, D.M.: Progressive lupus glomerulonephritis. Treatment with prednisone and combined prednisone and cyclophosphamide. Mayo Clin. Proc. 51:484, 1976.

64. Hayslett, J.P., Kashgarian, M., and Cook, C.D.: The effect of azathioprine on lupus glomerulonephritis. Medicine 51:393, 1972.

65. Sztejnbok, M., Stewart, A., Diamond, H., and Kaplan, D.: Azathioprine in the treatment of systemic lupus erythematosus: A controlled study. Arthritis Rheum. 14:639, 1971.

66. Hahn, B.H., Kantor, O.S., and Osterland, C.K.: Azathioprine plus prednisone compared with prednisone alone in the treatment of systemic lupus erythematosus. Report of a prospective controlled trial in 24 patients. Ann. Intern. Med. 83:597, 1975.

67. Donadio, J.V., Holley, K.E., Wagoner, R.D., Ferguson, R.H., and McDuffie, F.C.: Treatment of lupus nephritis with prednisone and combined prednisone and azathioprine. Ann. Intern. Med. 77:829, 1972.

68. Donadio, J.V., Holley, K.E., Wagoner, R.D., Ferguson, R.H., and McDuffie, F.C.: Further observations on the treatment of lupus nephritis with prednisone and combined prednisone and azathioprine. Arthritis Rheum. 17:573, 1974.

69. Cade, R., Spooner, G., Schlein, E., Pickering, M., de Quesada, A., Holcomb, A., Juncos, L., Richard, G., Shires, D., Levin, D., Hackett, R., Free, J., Hunt, R., and Fregly, M.: Comparison of azathioprine, prednisone, and heparin alone or combined in treating lupus nephritis. Nephron 10:37, 1973.

70. Ivanova, M.M., Nassonova, V.A., Soloviev, S.K., Speransky, A.I., Akhnazarova, V.D., Decker, J.L., and Steinberg, A.D.: Cyclophosphamide, azathioprine or chlorambucil for systemic lupus erythematosus nephritis. Arthritis Rheum. 22:624, 1979.

71. Klippel, J.H., Steinberg, A.D., Balow, J.L., Plotz, P.H., and Decker, J.L.: Randomized study of intravenous cyclophosphamide and cyclophosphamide plus azathioprine in lupus nephritis (abstract). Arthritis Rheum. 21:570, 1978.

72. Dinant, H.J., Decker, J.L., Klippel, J.H., Balow, J.E., Plotz, P.H., and Steinberg, A.D.: Alternative modes of cyclophosphamide and azathioprine therapy in lupus nephritis. Ann. Intern. Med. 96:728, 1982.

73. Williams, G.W., Steinberg, A.D., Reinertsen, J.L., Klassen, L.W., Decker, J.L., and Dolin, R.: Influenza immunization in systemic lupus erythematosus. Ann. Intern. Med. 88:729, 1978.

74. Klippel, J.H., Karsh, J., Stahl, N.I., Decker, J.L., Steinberg, A.D., and Schiffman, G.: A controlled study of pneumococcal polysaccharide vaccine in systemic lupus erythematosus. Arthritis Rheum. 22:1321, 1979.

75. Klassen, L.W., Budman, D.R., Williams, G.W., Steinberg, A.D., and Gerber, N.L.: Antiviral agents in treatment of murine autoimmune disease. Science 195:787, 1977.

76. Branda, R.F., Tate, D.Y., McCullough, J.J., and Jacob, H.S.: Plasma exchange in the treatment of fulminant idiopathic (autoimmune) thrombocytopenic purpura. Lancet 1:688, 1978.

77. Moran, C.J., Parry, H.F., Mowbray, J., Richards, J.D.M., and Goldstone, A.H.: Plasmapheresis in systemic lupus erythematosus. Br. Med. J. 1:1573, 1977.

78. Wei, N., Klippel, J.H., Huston, D.P., Hall, R.P., Lawley, T.J., Balow, J.E., Steinberg, A.D., and Decker, J.L.: A randomized trial of plasmapheresis in systemic lupus erythematosus. Lancet 1:17, 1983.

79. Terman, D.S., Petty, D., Ogden, D., Pefley, C., and Buffaloe, G.: Specific extraction of antigens in vivo by extracorporeal circulation over antibody immobilized in collodion-charcoal. J. Immunol. 117:1971, 1977.

80. Terman, D.S., Petty, D., Harbeck, R., Carr, R.I., and Buffaloe, G.: Specific removal of DNA antibodies in vivo by extracorporeal circulation over DNA immobilized in collodion charcoal. Clin. Immunol. Immunopathol. 8:90, 1977.

81. Morimoto, C., Masuho, Y., Boren, Y., Steinberg, A.D., and Schlossman, S.F.: Selective inhibition of anti-nucleoside specific antibody production by nucleoside-recin A conjugate. J. Immunol. 131: 1762. 1983.

82. Zurier, R.B., Damjanov, I., Sayadoff, D.M., and Rothfield, N.F.: Prostaglandin E, treatment of NZB/NZW F$_1$ hybrid mice. II. Prevention of glomerulonephritis. Arthritis Rheum. 20:1449, 1977.

83. Steinberg, A.D., Krakauer, R., Reinertsen, J.L., Klassen, L.W., Ilfeld, D., Reeves, J.P., Williams, G.W., and Antonovych, T.: Therapeutic studies in NZB/W mice. VI. Age-dependent effects of concanavalin A stimulated spleen cell supernate. Arthritis Rheum. 21:204, 1978.

84. Prickett, J.D., Robinson, D.R., and Steinberg, A.D.: Dietary enrichment with the polyunsaturated fatty acid eicosapentaenoic acid prevents proteinuria and prolongs survival in NZB × NZW F$_1$ mice. J. Clin. Invest. 68:556, 1981.

85. Prickett, J.D., Robinson, D.R., and Steinberg, A.D.: Effects of dietary enrichment with eicosapentaenoic acid upon autoimmune nephritis in female (NZB × NZW) F$_1$ mice. Arthritis Rheum. 26:133, 1983.

86. Cowdery, J.S., Curtin, M.F., Jr., and Steinberg, A.D.: The effect of prior intragastric antigen administration on primary and secondary antiovalbumin responses of C57BL/6 and NZB mice. J. Exp. Med. 156:1256, 1261, 1982.

87. Adelman, N.E., Watling, D.L., and McDevitt, H.O.: J. Exp. Med. 158: 1350, 1983.

88. Steinburg, A.D., and Santoro, T.J.: Anti-Ia antibodies: A revolutionary therapy for immune mediated disease? Immunology Today 5:12, 1984.

89. Rosenberg, Y.J., Steinberg, A.D., and Santoro, T.J: The basis of autoimmunity in MRL-*lpr/lpr* mice: A role for self Ia-reactive T cells. Immunology Today 5:64, 1984.

90. Taurog, J.D., Raveche, E.S., Smathers, P.A., Glimcher, L.H., Huston, D.P., Hansen, C.T., and Steinberg, A.D.: T cell abnormalities in NZB mice occur independently of autoantibody production. J. Exp. Med. 153:221, 1981.

91. Steinberg, B.J., Smathers, P.A., Frederiksen, K., and Steinberg, A.D.: Ability of the *xid* gene to prevent autoimmunity in (NZB × NZW) F$_1$ mice during the course of their natural history after polyclonal stimulation or following immunization with DNA. J. Clin. Invest. 70:587, 1982.

92. Smolen, J.S., Chused, T.M., Leiserson, W.M., Reeves, J.P., Alling, D.W., Steinberg, A.D.: Heterogeneity of immunoregulatory T cell subsets in systemic lupus erythematosus. Correlation with clinical features. Am. J. Med. 72:783, 1982.

Chapter 71

Mixed Connective Tissue Disease and Other Overlap Syndromes

Robert M. Bennett

INTRODUCTION

Anyone who has seen half a dozen examples of common lupus and of lupus erythematosus is able with ease to distinguish one from the other . . . but let him wait awhile and see more, and he will find before long that there are examples of mixed forms of the disease which it is impossible to denote correctly without employing hybrid names.
Jonathan Hutchinson, F.R.C.S.,

British Journal, May 1880.

Some one hundred years later these words still ring true. The diagnosis of well-established rheumatoid arthritis, systemic lupus erythematosus, or scleroderma is usually clear-cut, because the characteristic presentations are well-known and are the subject of "preliminary classiciation" guidelines. However, the initial manifestations of these diseases, such as general malaise, arthralgias, and vascular instability, are often identical; a definitive diagnosis is dependent upon sequential observations for the detection of a characteristic evolution of physical findings, laboratory tests, and radiologic changes.

In most instances, the course of rheumatic disease "runs true" to established concepts. However, as Jonathan Hutchinson noted for those who see many examples of rheumatic disorders, it is not uncommon to see "mixed forms of the disease which it is impossible to denote correctly without employing hybrid names." In most instances such hybrids are characterized by the coexistence of several features usually seen in two or more well-defined rheumatic disorders, or during the course of the disease there may be the evolution of one rheumatic disease syndrome into another. Without a unifying etiology, the nosology of such overlapping syndromes must at the best remain a rather arbitrary exercise and somewhat a matter of opinion and even prejudice. Although mixed connective tissue disease (MCTD) has currently evoked most interest and provided most controversy, the occurence of other overlap syndromes will be briefly mentioned.

THE OVERLAP SYNDROMES

The classic presentations of the individual connective tissue diseases are easily recognized from the typical combinations of the clinical findings and from the serologic abnormalities. However, seldom is one clinical manifestation or one laboratory test specific to one diagnosis; rather, there is a variable degree of shared features between the individual diseases. In most instances, a period of careful follow-up will reveal an evolution that is compatible with one of the classic connective tissue disorders. In some instances such a differentiation is not seen and in such cases, a diagnosis of undifferentiated connective tissue disease seems warranted; while in other cases there will be an overlap of the arbitrary criteria used to diagnose "specific diseases," leading to such terms as "sclerodermatomyositis," "lupus," "lupoderma," and "mixed connective tissue disease."

The association of a deforming erosive arthritis, in a patient seropositive for rheumatoid factor, with unequivocal evidence of systemic lupus erythematosus (SLE) is most unusual.[1-3] In many instances of an apparent overlap between these two disorders, the finding of the LE cell phenomenon in a patient with rheumatoid arthritis prompted the report. Most of these descriptions came at a time when the lack of specificity of the LE cell test was generally appreciated.[4-6] However there are a few well-documented cases of patients with rheumatoid arthritis and a positive LE cell test who initially seemed to have untainted rheumatoid arthritis but later developed some of the characteristic features of SLE.[7-9] Although there are no large controlled series, there is a general impression that patients with rheumatoid arthritis and an associated LE cell phenomenon have a worse prognosis in comparison to LE-cell–negative patients.[3,10-13]

In a similar vein the association of SLE and scleroderma has often been observed in the older literature.[14-16,17-22] In most instances this overlap has been justified on account of the presence of LE cells in patients with scleroderma or on the basis of the occurrence of gastrointestinal changes, typical of scleroderma, in patients with SLE. An overlap of scleroderma with an inflammatory myositis has long been recognized as a not uncommon event.[23-29] Whether this represents an accentuation of the low-grade myositis that is commonly seen in scleroderma[30] or is a true overlap has not been determined. The same reservations hold for the association of SLE and polymyositis.[22,31,32] A recent report from Japan[33] describes an overlap syndrome of scleroderma, polymyositis, and SLE, which is associated with a newly described antinuclear antibody, which was designated anti-Ku (first two letters of the patient's name). Another recently described overlap is that of polymyositis and an inflammatory arthritis resembling rheumatoid disease.[34] Although the primary disease state was unequivocally polymyositis, it was suggested that the constellation of articular manifestations, namely thumb subluxations, periosteal and synovial calcification, and erosive arthritis of the small joints of the hand, should alert clinicians to the likelihood of polymyositis. A similar report of inflammatory arthritis in association with polymyositis also stressed the additional complication of interstitial lung disease.[35] A common thread running through most of these overlap syndromes in the presence of Sjögren's syndrome (sicca syndrome). This has been associated with rheumatoid arthritis, SLE, polymyositis, MCTD, primary biliary cirrhosis, necrotizing vasculitis, autoimmune thyroiditis, chronic active hepatitis, mixed cryoglobulinemia, and hypergammaglobulinemic purpura.[36] Indeed the primary form of Sjögren's syndrome has clinical, serologic, and genetic overlapping features with classical SLE,[36-40] whereas some 50 percent of patients with SLE have been reported as having a sicca syndrome.[41] This latter association may be associated with a serologic profile characterized by antibodies to SSA and a positive rheumatoid factor.[40,42]

MIXED CONNECTIVE TISSUE DISEASE

It is apparent on reading the case reports of the previously cited overlap syndromes that in some instances a diagnosis of MCTD would have been entertained if the cases had been reported subsequent to 1972. In that year, Gordon Sharp and his colleagues suggested that patients with antibodies to a ribonuclease-sensitive extractable nuclear antigen constituted an apparently distinct rheumatic disease syndrome.[43] There has been a continuing controversy over the validity of this claim to uniqueness, which is best understood in terms of an historical perspective.

The Evolving Concept of MCTD. A major milestone in the development of modern rheumatology and its intimate association with disordered immunity was the discovery of the LE cell phenomenon in 1948 by Hargraves, Richmond, and Morton.[44] Subsequent studies showed that this phenomenon was due to a plasma factor,[45] which was later identified as an immunoglobulin[46] with a reactivity towards deoxynucleoprotein.[47,48] The subsequent development of immunofluorescence techniques to readily identify antinuclear antibodies[49,50] was quickly followed by an exponential increase in both clinical and basic research efforts in the realm of SLE. Although it was initially thought that there was a single nuclear antigen responsible for positive antinuclear fluorescence, it soon became evident that just as chromatin has many components (i.e., DNA, RNA, histones, and multiple acidic nuclear proteins), the antibodies reactive with nuclei exhibit a diverse array of reactivity with these chromatin building blocks.[51,53]

Of particular relevance to the present issue was the partial purification of an extractable nuclear antigen (ENA) by Holman in 1965,[54] and the subsequent description of anti-Sm antibodies, reactive with one component of ENA, by Tan and Kunkel.[55] These initial observations paved the way for the recognition that there were clinical differences between the patients with antibodies to native DNA and those with antibodies to ENA.[56] At about the same time, Mattioli and Reichlin found a second distinctive nuclear antigen in ENA (in addition to Sm), which they designated Mo.[57] They went on to demonstrate that Sm and Mo exist in ENA as a molecular complex and that sera containing antibodies to Sm also had a very high concurrence of anti-Mo.[58] Furthermore the reactivity of certain sera with Mo could be abolished by prior RNase digestion of the ENA; subsequent studies have indicated that Mo is identical to the RNase-sensitive ENA of Sharp and colleagues,[43] and it is now usually designated as nuclear ribonucleoprotein (nRNP). There are now numerous clinical studies reporting on the clinical characteristics of patients with anti-RNP antibodies (Table 71–1). In many instances it has been shown that the *solitary* presence of high titer anti-RNP antibodies seems to modify the expression of the disease process.

The Serologic Features of MCTD. The presence of antibodies to RNP is generally considered a sine qua non for the diagnosis of MCTD. As anti-RNP antibodies produce a speckled pattern of nuclear fluorescence, which remain positive to very high serum dilutions (often > 1:10,000), the conventional ANA test is the initial screening test of choice. In most laboratories, anti-RNP antibodies are further screened by counterimmunoelectrophoresis (CIE) (Fig. 71–1), and positive sera are further identified by Ouchterlony double immunodiffusion analysis using previously characterized reference sera (Fig. 71–2).

As it has been claimed that very high titers of anti-RNP antibodies are characteristic of MCTD,[59] some laboratories further characterize the antibodies by doubling dilutions of the sera, using passive hemagglutination of ENA-coated sheep erythrocytes, as originally described by Sharp and colleagues,[43] or by diluting out to extinction in an Ouchterlony test. In each instance the presence of antibodies to RNP is verified by a control showing a reduced or absent response after digestion of the ENA with RNAse. Although many other antigen-antibody systems have now been established between ENA and sera from SLE and the connective tissue disorders, the RNase sensitivity of ENA, in the anti-RNP system, so far seems to be unique. It has become apparent, in the decade since MCTD was first described, that anti-RNP antibodies are far from exclusive to just one clinical setting, but rather are seen in a wide variety of different disorders[60-74] (see Table 71–1). Proponents of the view that MCTD is a distinct entity claim that the presence of high titer anti-RNP antibodies in the absence of other antibodies, such as anti-native DNA or anti-Sm, is the typical serologic profile.[65,67,68,71,74] Other reports have failed to find a distinctive clinical picture in association with such a serologic profile.[63,64,69,72] In making the diagnosis of a disease dependent upon a serologic abnormality it is inevitable that patients will be seen with the clinical characteristics without serologic findings. In some such cases a later development of anti-RNP antibodies has been reported,[65,76] and in other instances the emergence of anti-RNP antibodies coincided with the commencement of corticosteroid therapy.[43,77]

Furthermore, the finding of antibodies exclusive to RNP at one point in time does not imply the perpetual absence of anti-Sm, anti-dsDNA, or other antinuclear antibodies at other times.[65,78] More recent technologic refinements, using radiolabeled cell extracts with polyacrylamide gel electrophoresis of immunoprecipitated antigens, has shed important new light on the precise molecular composition of the extractable nuclear antigens[79,82] (see also under Immunopathology). These newer techniques of assaying antinuclear antibodies offer a precision not found in the conventionally utilized tests and have already yielded new information on the multiplicity of different antibodies in some patients as well as on new antibody-antigen systems.[74] Although analysis of immunoprecipitated antigens is extremely sensitive and precise, it does not yield any quantitative information. As the titer of autoantibodies, as well as the nature of their reactive antigen, is important in disease correlations, the clinical usefulness of these newer techniques remains to be established.

The appearance of free serum RNP has been described by Alarcon-Segovia's group.[83] In general they found a reciprocal relationship between free RNP and RNP antibodies, but in some cases both free RNP and anti-RNP antibodies were found simultaneously. In two patients with an overlap syndrome, free RNP but not anti-RNP was found. Such serologic findings would predict the finding of immune comlexes in MCTD; this has indeed been the case,[84-86] but in one report the complexes were not sensitive to RNase digestion.[85]

Table 71–1. Published Studies Describing Clinical Associations with Anti-RNP Antibodies

(#) Reference	Number of Patients Studied	Number with Anti-RNP Alone	Comments
(43) Sharp, G.C. et al. Am. J. Med. 52:148, 1972	25		Original report suggesting MCTD was a "distinct clinical entity".
(60) Parker, M. J. Lab. Clin. Med. 82:769, 1973	541	10	A retrospective survey of sera: 9 patients with anti-RNP had MCTD and 1 had SLE.
(71) Farber, S.J. et al. Arch. Intern. Med. 136:425, 1976	44	13	8 patients had overlaps with SLE, PSS, and PM. 11 patients had Raynaud's phenomenon. 7 had skin changes of PSS. Low incidence of nephritis.
(61) Leibfarth, J.H. et al. Arthritis Rheum. 19:851, 1976	650	16	A retrospective survey of sera. Anti-RNP antibodies associated with an overlap syndrome and less severe renal CNS disease.
(59) Sharp, G.C. et al. N. Engl. J. Med. 295:1149, 1976	272	100	In patients with RNP alone, 74% had MCTD, 12% SLE, 8% PSS, and 6% UCTD.
(67) Singsen, G.H. et al. J. Pediatr. 90:893, 1977	14	11	A description of MCTD in childhood. Supported the concept of an overlap syndrome. Associated with anti-RNP antibodies.
(70) Grennan, D.M. et al. Ann. Rheum. Dis. 36:442, 1977	63	20	A study of patients with a primary diagnosis of SLE. Anti-RNP was associated with Raynaud's phenomenon and PSS-like changes.
(73) McCain, G.A. et al. J. Rheum. 5:399, 1978	284	5	A study of patients with rheumatic diseases. The 5 patients with anti-RNP alone had MCTD (2), SLE (1), PM (1) and UCTD (1).
(63) Maddison, P.F. et al. J. Rheum. 5:407, 1978	43	43	30 patients fulfilled ARA criteria for SLE. 60% had Raynaud's phenomenon (N.B.—not a feature of later 1982 SLE criteria). Renal disease occurred in 4 patients.
(64) Gaudreau, A. et al. Ann. Rheum. Dis. 37:321, 1978	134	85	40% had SLE, PSS, PM or RA. 26% had an overlap syndrome, 28% had limited disease Raynaud's and polyarthralgias.
(75) Peskett, S.A. et al. Rheum. Rehab. 17:245, 1978	5	4	5 juveniles with MCTD. All had mild disease with Raynaud's and a nonerosive arthritis.
(66) Prystowsky, S.D. West. J. Med. 132:288, 1980	46	43	Noted a high incidence of Raynaud's phenomenon and nonerosive arthritis with little severe renal or CNS disease.
(68) Bennett, R.M. et al. Sem. Arthritis Rheum. 10:25, 1980	20	20	Supportive of a modifying clinical influence of anti-RNP antibodies, but all patients fulfilled the 1972 ARA criteria for SLE.
(65) Grant, K.D. et al. J. Rheum. 8:587, 1981	23	23	Stresses changing clinical and serological findings in patients with TD.
(69) Hockberg, M.C. Arthritis Rheum. 24:54, 1981	81	6	A survivorship study in patients with a primary diagnosis of SLE. No patient with anti-RNP alone died, but one had chronic renal failure and 2 had CNS disease.
(72) Lemmer, J.P. et al. J. Rheum. 9:536, 1982	44	44	50% had features of an overlapping syndrome. No distinct syndrome found.
(74) Matter, L. et al. Arthritis Rheum. 25:1278, 1982	54	4	A serologic study using immuno-precipitation of radiolabeled HeLa cell extracts. Patients with anti-RNP alone had features compatible with MCTD.

Figure 71–1. Counterimmunoelectrophoresis (CIE) is a rapid method of screening multiple serum samples for the presence of anti-ENA antibodies after the initial screening test (positive ANA, usually speckled pattern) has proved positive. Each pair of wells represents one test, and a band of precipitation between wells signifies the presence of anti-ENA antibodies. As can be seen in this example, several sera contain multiple antibodies. The exact specificity of the antibody system cannot be determined by this method, and positive sera are further evaluated by double immunodiffusion in agarose (see Fig. 71–2).

reports of dsDNA antibodies, as it has been shown that just a few single-stranded regions in a predominately double-stranded DNA molecule will lead to a positive result for dsDNA antibodies in a conventional Farr test.[91] These serologic changes indicate a polyclonal stimulation of B lymphocytes akin to that seen in classic SLE. Whether similar mechanisms for this immune dysregulation are the same remains to be fully elucidated (see Immunopathology). In some instances a clue to the presences of anti-RNP antibodies is obtained after submitting a skin biopsy for immunofluorescence. In MCTD the epidermal nuclei often exhibits a striking speckled pattern of immunofluorescence.[92] Whether this is due to penetration of anti-RNP antibodies during life or a fixation artifact remains to be established. The deposition of immunoglobulins and complement components at the dermal-epidermal junction of nonlesional skin (the "lupus band" test) has been reported as positive in some patients with MCTD,[93] although another study was not so conclusive.[68]

The Clinical Picture of MCTD. Whether MCTD should be considered as a "distinct rheumatic disease syndrome" as originally proposed by Sharp and his colleagues[43] remains a controversial issue. Indeed no unique pathognomonic feature has yet been reported in MCTD which would once and for all resolve this issue. The report given here, of the clinical picture of MCTD, represents a clustering of symptoms usually seen separately in scleroderma, rheumatoid arthritis, polymyositis, and SLE, having as their common bond the presence

Under certain circumstances it appears that anti-RNP antibodies may be induced by mechanical or pharmacologic manipulations. Nolph and associates have described the appearance of anti-RNP antibodies in patients undergoing long-term hemodialysis,[87] hypothesizing a sensitization by nuclear antigens released from damaged leukocytes. However, these patients did not develop any symptoms consistent with MCTD, and in most cases the levels of anti-RNP were very low and only detectable by the hemagglutination technique, which is some 1000 times as sensitive as a conventional ANA. Winfield and associates described the transient occurrence of anti-RNP antibodies in patients taking procainamide;[88] again there was no correlation with clinical findings suggestive of MCTD.

Other serologic findings that have been noted in MCTD are hyperglobulinemia,[43,54,66,68,71] lymphocytotoxic antibodies,[89,90] circulating immune complexes,[84-86] positive direct Coombs' test,[64,65,68] false positive VDRL,[65,66,68] reduced complement values,[43,64,65,68,71] and positive tests for rheumatoid factor.[43,59,65,67,68,71] Reports on the occurrence of significant levels of antibodies to dsDNA in MCTD have varied from zero[68] to 41 percent.[59] In part this is probably a reflection of "entry criteria" for MCTD, as some authors have excluded patients with dsDNA antibodies from their series while others have not done so. It seems, however, that antibodies to ssDNA are a frequent occurrence in MCTD.[66,68] This finding in itself may have led to false

Figure 71–2. An Ouchterlony plate (double immunodiffusion in agarose) of several sera that had shown positivity by screening CIE. The center well contains a soluble extract of rabbit thymus (RTE). It is seen that four sera contained anti-RNP antibodies (have merging precipitin lines—"reaction of identity"), in two sera this was the only antibody present, in the other two sera RNP antibodies were associated with anti-Sm and anti-SSB antibodies, respectively.

of anti-RNP antibodies. In this sense the concept of MCTD represents a statistically defined entity,[94] with certain overlaps occurring together more frequently than would be expected by chance.

General Features. The prevalence of MCTD is not accurately known, owing in part to the diagnostic biases of different groups. Using the definition given above, it would appear to be slightly less common than SLE but several times more prevalent than scleroderma and polymyositis. The sex ratio is similar to classic SLE, with an 8:1 female to male ratio. However, unlike classic SLE, there does not appear to be any special ethnic or racial bias. In most cases the disease starts in the second or third decade of life, but well documented cases have now been described in young children as well as elderly adults. No obvious precipitating event has been noted; although some patients have manifest photosensitivity, sun exposure is not a documented precipitating event. There is one report of a salmonella gastroenteritis causing an apparent exacerbation of MCTD.[95] Drug exposure has not been related to MCTD, although a transient appearance of anti-RNP antibodies, without symptoms, has been noted at the initiation of procainamide therapy.[88] It is unusual to see more than one patient with MCTD in any one family, although there have been several reports of a familial occurrence[96-98]; in one such family there was an association of MCTD with SLE and other connective tissue disorders.[96] In one well-studied family a brother and sister both had MCTD, and 8 out of 18 relatives had rheumatic complaints but only 2 had a positive ANA and none had anti RNP antibodies.[97] Whether there is a characteristic genotype for MCTD has not been firmly established.

Presenting Features and Evolution. As the initial description of MCTD emphasized the overlapping of features usually seen in SLE, progressive systemic sclerosis (PSS) and polymyositis (PM), it is often assumed that such an overlap is a characteristic feature of MCTD. This is not so. In fact, it is most unusual to see such an overlap during the early course of MCTD. Rather than a concurrent overlap, the additional features tend to occur sequentially, frequently at widely spaced intervals of time. The presenting features of the disease are often rather vague, with arthralgias, myalgias, fatigability, and vasospastic changes. Over a period of years or months more specific findings, such as alopecia, a discoid rash, pleurisy, classic Raynaud's phenomenon, or a deforming arthritis, may supervene. In rare cases, the presentation may take the form of a more acute problem, such as high fever, an inflammatory myopathy, aseptic meningitis, polyarthritis, digital gangrene, an acute abdomen, or trigeminal neuropathy. Thus, the presentation of MCTD can mimic several of the classic connective tissue diseases, but when followed over many years about half the patients have a picture most closely resembling PSS while the rest have a rather undifferentiated picture (UCTD) with features of both RA and SLE (Fig. 71–3). It would appear that the findings of high titer anti-RNP antibodies in a patient with a poorly defined connective tissue disease is often indicative of a later pluripotentiality of disease expression, although no one clinical syndrome can be said to be "classic" MCTD.

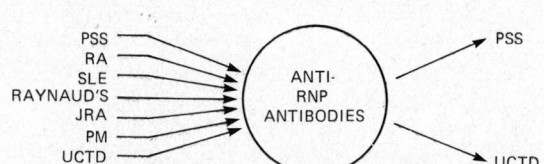

Figure 71–3. Mixed connective tissue disease will often present with symptoms suggestive of one of the classic connective tissue diseases. In many cases the presence of high titer anti-RNP antibodies *alone* seems to modify the expression of the disease in that such patients have a low incidence of severe renal disease and on follow-up over many years come to resemble patients with progressive systemic sclerosis (PSS) or remain with a relatively undifferentiated connective tissue disease (UCTD).

Specific Organ Involvement. *Systemic.* Fatigability and a general sense of malaise are common features of MCTD. Such patients often have a reduced exercise tolerance, but the extent to which this may be due to early myopathy or lung or heart involvement is not known. Fever can be a prominent feature in the absence of obvious cause; indeed MCTD has presented as a fever of unknown origin[68] (Fig. 71–4). In most cases fever can be traced to a coexistent polymyositis, aseptic meningitis, lymphadenopathy, serositis, or intercurrent infection. Significant weight loss is usually due to extensive gastrointestinal involvement with malabsorption, although lesser degrees are often unexplained. Other general symptoms that have been observed include hoarseness,[65] vascular headaches,[98] and hepatosplenomegaly.[58,65,67,68]

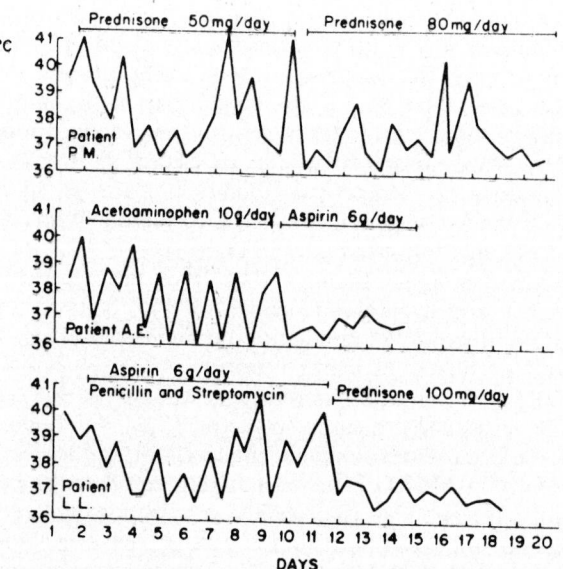

Figure 71–4. Fever patterns in three patients with MCTD. The top two patterns were associated with myositis; the bottom pattern was associated with aseptic meningitis. (From Bennett, R. and O'Connell, D.: Semin. Arthritis Rheum. 10:25, 1980.)

Figure 71–5. Puffy hands and tightness of the skin over the digits are characteristic in some patients with MCTD, but they are not exclusive to MCTD.

Figure 71–6. This 28-year-old woman had the classic clinical and serologic features of MCTD as well as the typical rash of discoid lupus erythematosus.

Skin and Mucous Membranes. Involvement of the skin is almost universal in MCTD. There is no one finding or group of findings that is characteristic. Indeed, the spectrum of changes seen includes those seen in the classic presentations of SLE, PSS, CREST (calcinosis, Raynaud's esophageal dysmotility, sclerodactyly and telangiectasia), and dermatomyositis (DM). The earliest changes are usually those of Raynaud's phenomenon and puffy hands (Fig. 71–5). About 40 percent of patients have dermal changes consistent with SLE, most commonly in the form of discoid plaques and malar eruptions (Figs. 71–6 and 71–7). There are two case reports of patients presenting with discoid LE and later developing MCTD.[68,99] Less frequent are alopecia, sclerodactyly, vitiligo, photosensitivity, urticaria, and telangiectasia. Skin changes typical of dermatomyositis are only rarely seen. Mucous membrane findings have included buccal ulceration, a sicca complex,[65,68,100] and nasal septal perforation.[101] Genital lesions have not so far been described. Other associations may be the result of chance alone. The full spectrum of reported changes is given in Table 71–2.

Skin biopsies have shown immunoglobulin deposits at the dermal-epidermal junction in some patients,[93] but the true frequency and significance of this finding is not

Figure 71–7. This patient with long-standing Raynaud's phenomenon, esophageal dysmotility, and high-titer anti-RNP antibodies has had intermittent flares of serositis, sometimes accompanied by a malar rash, as seen here.

Table 71–2. Mucocutaneous Problems that Have Been Associated with MCTD

Puffy hands	Calcinosis cutis
Raynaud's phenomenon	Skin ulceration
Alopecia	Subcutaneous nodules
Sclerodactyly	Heliotrope eyelids
Malar rash	Grotton's papules
Discoid LE	Erythema nodosum
Dyspigmentation	Lyell's disease
Telangiectasia	Buccal ulceration
Photosensitivity	Nasal septal perforation

known.[68] Scleroderma-like changes seldom extend proximal to the digits, although a scleroderma facies is occasionally seen in long-standing cases.

Joints. Virtually all patients with MCTD complain of joint pains and morning stiffness. Up to about 60 percent of patients develop an obvious arthritis. In statistical terms the arthritis of MCTD is somewhat more severe than that seen in classic SLE but generally not as destructive as rheumatoid arthritis.[102-104] Typical swan-neck deformities and ulnar deviation are not uncommon (Fig. 71–8), and boutonnière changes are occasionally seen. In a few cases a grossly destructive arthritis is seen resembling the arthritis mutilans (Fig. 71–9) of psoriatic arthritis.[68,105] Lewis and associates[106] have commented on extrinsic flexor tenosynovitis (Fig. 71–10) with tightening as a cause for hand deformities in MCTD. Flexor tightness is not a common feature of the hand in SLE,[107] and Lewis has suggested that this finding should alert one to a possible diagnosis of MCTD. As about 50 percent of patients with MCTD have a positive rheumatoid factor,[59] it is not unusual for such patients to be given an initial diagnosis of rheumatoid arthritis. In a few patients rheumatoid-like nodules have also been noted.[66,102] Significant erosions are not as common as in rheumatoid arthritis, but in contrast to classic SLE, they

do occur[108,109] and often have a well-demarcated edge, which produces a "punched out" appearance.[110] Aseptic necrosis of bone both within the joint capsule and intramedullary infarcts is another potential cause of articular symptoms.[68]

Muscle. Myalgias are a common symptom in MCTD patients.[43,58,65,68,71,92] In most cases there is no demonstrable weakness, electromyographic abnormalities, or muscle enzyme changes. Whether this symptom represents a low-grade myositis has not been determined. Muscle biopsies have sometimes demonstrated varying degrees of fiber degeneration and an interstitial and perivascular infiltrate.[43,59,111,112] Immunofluorescence staining has revealed IgG and IgM deposition in some interfascicular blood vessels (without obvious vasculitis) and around the sarcoplasmic membrane.[112] The inflammatory myopathy that occurs in some patients with MCTD is identical clinically and histologically to classic polymyositis; the skin changes that are seen in dermatomyositis are rare in this setting. In some patients there is a striking fever in association with the polymyositis,[68] and in other patients there is a history of febrile myalgias (often diagnosed as "flu"); these are generally self-limiting and last from a few days to a few weeks. In most patients the polymyositis is manifest as acute flares against the background of general disease activity. In other patients a more chronic polymyositis supervenes, with persisting muscle weakness and elevated muscle enzymes. Polymyositis in MCTD is responsive to corticosteroids, and this is the mainstay of treatment. Needless to say, iatrogenic myopathy due to the overzealous use of corticosteroids may also be seen in MCTD.

Heart. Cardiac involvement in SLE is most commonly manifest as a self-limiting pericarditis.[43,57,65,66,68] Involvement of the myocardium may be more common than initially thought. Several severe cases of myocarditis[67,111,113] have been well-documented in addition to two cases of complete heart block.[114] An association

Figure 71–8. Patients with MCTD often have a more severe form of arthritis than patients with classic SLE. The patient seen here had several of the classic findings usually seen in rheumatoid arthritis: ulnar deviation, subluxed MCP joints, and swan-neck deformities. The radiograph (*B*) shows a relative paucity of erosive disease. (From Bennett, R. and O'Connell, D.: Radiology 37:397, 1978.)

Figure 71–9. A few patients with MCTD develop a severe destructive form of arthritis (arthritis mutilans). The radiograph shown here (*B*) shows almost complete osteolysis of the carpal bones with focal osteolytic changes in several digits and bony fusion of the third DIP joint. (From Bennett, R., and O'Connell, D.: Semin. Arthritis Rheum. 10:25, 1980.)

of anti-RNP antibodies with clinically significant myocarditis has also been reported in a group of patients diagnosed as having SLE.[116] Overt cardiac failure may be secondary to renovascular hypertension or pulmonary hypertension, both being caused by scleroderma-like in-

Figure 71–10. It is thought that the nonerosive hand deformities in MCTD are a result of an extrinsic flexor tenosynovitis leading to inflammatory contractures. The pathologic specimen shown here demonstrates perivascular infiltrates, myositis, and fasciitis of a musculotendinous unit. (From Lewis, R., et al.: Hand Surg. 3:217, 1978.)

timal proliferative lesions in the kidney and lung respectively. Valvular lesions akin to Libman Sacks endocarditis have not been described, but aortic insufficiency has been documented in a child with congestive heart failure.[67] The myocardial histology has been similar to other forms of "autoimmune" myocarditis, with a prominent interstitial mononuclear infiltrate, variable fibrosis, and a perivascular cuffing.[111,117] In view of these findings it would seem reasonable to request anti-RNP antibodies in any patient with unexplained myocarditis.

Lung. Pleurisy is one of the most common clinical manifestations of MCTD.[43,59,66,67,68] It is often short lived and may well resolve spontaneously without specific treatment. Any accompanying pleural effusion is usually small; for this reason there are no good reports of pleural fluid analysis in MCTD. Interstitial parenchymal disease is often subclinical but is seen in up to about 75 percent of patients on pulmonary function tests. Most commonly there is a reduced carbon monoxide diffusing capacity and less often a reduced vital capacity. Chest radiographs may show reticulonodular shadowing at the lung bases, fleeting areas of consolidation, small effusions, and cardiac enlargement secondary to systemic or pulmonary hypertension. It has become apparent since the initial descriptions of MCTD that pulmonary hypertension (Fig. 71–11) is a potentially fatal complication.[68,117-120] It takes one of two forms: an event secondary to interstitial fibrosis[118] or a primary vascular event caused by a bland intimal proliferation of the lung arterioles[118,120,121] or by a plexogenic angiopathy.[118] When it occurs as a primary event, it may occur without warning in a patient who was previously under good control and end fatally within just a few weeks.[68] Rosenberry and colleagues reported a case of pulmonary hypertension in a child who responded to a combination of prednisone and cyclophosphamide.[120] This form of lung involvement has not generally been responsive to high-dose corticosteroids. In the immunosuppressed patient opportunistic infections are a constant hazard and have been the cause of death in MCTD.[68]

Figure 71–11. A 22-year-old female with an 8-year history of MCTD, under apparent good control, suddenly went into respiratory and cardiac failure and died within 2 weeks of fulminant pulmonary hypertension. The chest radiograph (A) shows cardiac dilatation with enlargement of the pulmonary trunk and proximal pulmonary arteries. The lung scan (B) shows multiple areas of ventilation-perfusion imbalance. (From Bennett, R., and O'Connell, D.: Semin. Arthritis Rheum. 10:25, 1980.)

Gastrointestinal. The observation that about 80 percent of patients with high-titer anti-RNP antibodies had evidence of esophogeal dysmotility was an important overlap feature with PSS in the initial descriptions of MCTD.[43,59,60,71] Cine-esophograms have revealed a pattern similar to that seen in classic PSS, with diminished amplitude of peristalsis in the lower two thirds of the esophagus and a decreased lower sphincter pressure.[68,108,122] Although significant difficulties with swallowing are rare in MCTD (about 70 percent of patients abnormal on manometric testing are asymptomatic), a history of esophageal reflux is not uncommon.[123] In the rare patient, small bowel dilatation with malabsorption due to bacterial overgrowth can be a problem.[68] Mesenteric vasculitis can cause an acute abdomen, and infarcted bowel has been a cause of death.[124] More commonly, abdominal pains are a manifestation of serositis or bowel hypomotility. Radiographically pseudodiverticula, identical to those seen in PSS may be seen on the antimesenteric border of the colon.[110,122] A rare finding is pneumatosis cystoides intestinalis.[110,122] Examples of some of these changes are shown in Figure 71–12.

Kidney. As a generalization, severe renal disease is not a feature of MCTD. Indeed, the presence of anti-RNP antibodies seems to protect against proliferative glomerular lesions whether they occur in the setting of typical SLE[60,61,63,71,72,125] or in MCTD.[43,59,65-67,126-128] The earlier concept that renal disease was rare in MCTD now needs to be modified. Up to 25 percent of MCTD patients have renal involvement, most commonly a membranous glomerulonephritis.[58] Such patients may have an overt nephrotic syndrome,[64,126,127] but this is relatively uncommon. However, inevitable exceptions do occur, and patients have died of progressive renal failure.[58] Immunofluorescence shows granular deposits of IgG, C_2, and C_4 in the glomeruli, and electron microscopy shows intramembranous and subepithelial electron-dense deposits[68,111,119,126,130] (Fig. 71–13). In a few cases a relatively acellular intimal proliferation has been described in the renal vessels.[111,131] Such patients may go on and develop a renovascular hypertensive crisis similar to scleroderma kidney.[121,127,131]

Nervous System. Neurologic involvement was not mentioned in the initial description of MCTD but has been well documented in subsequent reports. It is of interest that the most commonly described association has been a trigeminal neuropathy,[59,68,127,132] as this is also the most common neurologic problem encountered in scleroderma[133] and is a relatively rare finding in classic SLE. Trigeminal neuropathy has occasionally been the presenting symptom of MCTD.[68,134,135] In contradiction to CNS involvement in classic SLE frank psychosis and convulsion have infrequently been reported in MCTD.[65,68,132] Episodic headaches in patients with known MCTD provide an important diagnostic challenge. In the majority of patients they are probably vascular in origin with many of the components of classic migraine.[66,98] In another group of patients the headaches are accompanied by fever and sometimes myalgias, rather resembling a viral syndrome. In a small number of patients, signs of meningitis develop, and such patients have been found to have the cerebrospinal fluid changes of meningeal inflammation without infection.[67,68] Such cases of aseptic meningitis respond well to corticosteroid therapy. An interesting hypersensitivity to ibuprofen presenting as a meningitis has been documented in association with MCTD[136] and must enter into the differential diagnosis of headache. Spinal cord involvement both in the form of a transverse myelitis[137] and as a cauda equina syndrome[138] has been reported in isolated cases. The neurologic associations with MCTD are given in Table 71–3.

Autoimmune Associations. Sjögren's syndrome has been noted to occur in association with MCTD in 7 to 50 percent of patients.[59,66,68,71,100] Whether the clinical spectrum is that of primary Sjögren's syndrome, as seems to be the case regarding the association with SLE or secondary Sjögren's syndrome remains to be analyzed. An association with a Felty-like syndrome has rarely been reported.[68] Hashimoto's thyroiditis has been observed in about 5 percent of MCTD patients.[59,66,68,140] A positive direct Coombs' test is reported in 19 to 60 percent of MCTD patients;[65,66,68] a clinically significant hemolytic anemia is unusual but is occasionally seen.[65,141]

Figure 71–12. Four examples of gastrointestinal changes in patients with MCTD that resemble those seen in scleroderma. *A,* Reduced peristalsis in the lower two thirds of esophagus. *B,* Dilation of duodenal loop and proximal small bowel. *C,* Pneumatosis cystoides of the small bowel (arrows). *D,* Wide-mouthed pseudodiverticula in antimesenteric border of the colon. (From Bennett, R., and O'Connell, D.: Semin. Arthritis Rheum.: 10:25, 1980, and Br. J.. Radiology 50:620, 1977.)

Significant thrombocytopenia is rare in comparison with classic SLE but can rarely be severe,[67,141] whereas leukopenia is fairly common;[59,66-68,127] whether either of these associations is a sequela of autoimmune phenomena is not known. An interesting association of type B insulin resistance (acanthosis nigricans, circulating insulin receptor antibodies, and a connective tissue disease) in a patient with MCTD was recently reported,[142] and attention was drawn to several other possible case reports of patients with this distinctive autoimmune syndrome.[144,145]

Blood. Anemia of chronic inflammation occurs in up to 75 percent of patients with MCTD.[58,65,68,71,127] Although a positive Coombs' test is seen in up to 60 percent of patients, an overt hemolytic anemia is uncommon.[66,68] Leukopenia mainly affecting the lymphocyte series is seen in about 75 percent of patients and may correlate with disease activity.[59,65,68,71,127] Thrombocytopenia is relatively rare but may pose a major problem.[65,67,141] A false positive VDRL has been noted in about 10 percent of patients.[65,66,68,127] Whether this will be found to be associated with circulating anticoagulants, as is often the case in classic SLE, remains to be elucidated. Positive tests for rheumatoid factor have been noted in up to 50 percent of patients,[59,65-68,127] and it has been reported that this finding is associated with more severe degrees of arthritis.[102] Most patients have a hypergammaglobulinemia,[59,65,66,68,127] and it has been estimated that up to 33 percent of the IgG molecules have an anti-RNP specificity.[145] The erythrocyte sedimentation rate is intermittently elevated, and as might be expected this is usually related to disease activity.[68] By the definition of this review all MCTD patients have anti-RNP antibodies; it should be noted that their titers do not vary much with

Figure 71–13. Renal biopsy specimens from a patient with MCTD and mild proteinuria. *A,* Light microscopy shows some enlargment of the glomerulus but no increase in cellularity. The capillary walls show irregular thickening. *B,* Electron microscopy shows thickening of the capillary basement membrane with prominent intramembranous electron-dense granular deposits.

disease activity and as such the presence of anti-RNP can be viewed as a permanent "fingerprint." Antibodies to *single*-stranded DNA occurs in up to 80 percent of patients,[62,65,68] often with a standard Farr binding of greater than 75 percent. There are also reports of antibodies to *double*-stranded DNA.[59,65,78,127] Whether these do in fact occur to a significant degree in MCTD or are a technical artefact (anti-ssDNA antibodies reacting with a dsDNA contaminated with ss regions) has not been fully resolved.[91] Employing current ideas regarding the definition of MCTD, a high titer of antibodies to dsDNA is usually regarded as evidence against this diagnosis (as are anti-Sm antibodies). Reduced levels of complement components have been noted;[65-68,130] in general hypocomplementemia is not so prevalent as in classic SLE and has not been correlated with any particular clinical situation. Antilymphocytic antibodies were found in only 17 percent of MCTD patients in one study;[89,90] this compares with a prevalence of 93 percent in classic SLE.

Pregnancy. One study has addressed the issue of pregnancy in MCTD in depth; it was concluded that patients with MCTD had a reduced fertility rate and increased fetal wastage.[146] In this same study, there was an undue increase of disease onset during pregnancy, and 47 percent of MCTD patients exhibited an exacerbation of disease activity. Congenital malformations and neonatal expression of an MCTD-like disease have not been

noted. In another analysis of pregnancy in MCTD, there were 38 live births out of a total of 47. Obvious disease exacerbations during pregnancy or in the post-partum period were not noted.[68]

MCTD in Children. The occurrence of MCTD in children is now well documented.[67,75,147,148] As such it forms an important consideration in the differential diagnosis of juvenile rheumatoid arthritis, especially in children with a positive antinuclear factor. Such patients have most commonly been considered to be at risk of developing chronic iridocyclitis and arthritis or SLE. If the antinuclear staining is of a speckled pattern, there should be a heightened suspicion for a diagnosis of MCTD and further tests should be done for anti-RNP antibodies. It should be noted that in children with the iridocyclitis/arthritis picture, the ANA is usually of a homogeneous pattern.

An analysis of the reports of MCTD in childhood to date would seem to indicate that it is associated with more morbidity than in adults. Significant myocarditis, glomerulonephritis, thrombocytopenia, seizures, and aseptic meningitis have been described in the childhood variety of MCTD.[67] There is also the impression that the arthritis is often more severe in children as compared with adults. It may be that this seemingly more florid illness in children is a reflection of reports of such cases from specialized referral centers; a recent report by Peskett and associates stressed a more benign course.[75]

Course and Prognosis. There were two points made in the original description of MCTD[43] that seemed to justify its status as a distinct entity, namely ". . . its being characterized by an excellent response to corticosteroid therapy and a favorable prognosis." Over the course of the subsequent decade it has become apparent that both of these claims need to be qualified.

There seems to be a general agreement that patients with high-titer anti-RNP antibodies have a low prevalence of serious renal disease and life-threatening neurologic problems; in this sense MCTD can be favorably compared with classic SLE. In a follow-up study of the

Table 71–3. Neurological Findings That Have Been Associated with MCTD

Trigeminal neuropathy	Transverse myelitis
Aseptic meningitis	Cauda equina syndrome
Febrile headaches	Peripheral neuropathy
Vascular headaches	Neurosensory hearing loss
Seizures	Absence attacks*
Psychosis	Involuntary abdominal muscle spasm*

*Unpublished personal observations.

original 25 patients described by Sharp and colleagues, eight had died by 1980.[127] The causes of death in this report and others is given in Table 71–4. It would appear that there are at least three causes of death in MCTD that represent a different experience from classic SLE, namely, a rapidly progressive pulmonary hypertension, myocarditis, and renovascular hypertension. As more fatal cases of MCTD are being reported, pulmonary hypertension is emerging as an important cause of death.[68,117-121] Although chronic pulmonary hypertension can occur as a secondary event to chronic pulmonary interstitial disease,[118] in some fatal cases a relatively short course of a few weeks has been described.[68] Such patients present with dyspnea, a dry cough, right-sided heart failure, and a low cardiac output. So far the use of high-dose corticosteroids and immunosuppressive agents has not been successful in reversing the progression of this complication. At autopsy the major finding has been a bland intimal proliferation involving the small pulmonary blood vessels; the histologic picture is rather reminiscent of the changes seen in the kidney during a scleroderma hypertensive crisis. As in scleroderma and SLE, the prognosis ultimately depends upon the nature and severity of major organ involvement. Whether MCTD does have a better prognosis than classic SLE will only be determined by long-term follow-up studies.

At the present time it would appear misleading to tell patients with MCTD that they have an excellent prognosis. Many patients with MCTD may indeed follow a relatively benign course, but it is the development of major organ involvement that ultimately dictates the morbidity and mortality of the disease. Over the course of many years, many patients come to resemble a picture of scleroderma or rheumatoid arthritis more closely than SLE. Maybe this is due to the fact that many of the SLE-like aspects of the disease are responsive to corticosteroids whereas the sclerodermatous changes and joint deformities are unresponsive. These aspects of the course and prognosis of MCTD are in a state of flux; this is not surprising for a condition that was only recently described and attests to the need for careful prospective studies.

IMMUNOPATHOLOGY

There are many features of MCTD that suggest that a disorder of immunoregulation is of importance in its pathogenesis. Some of the features already mentioned include (i) hypergammaglobulinemia;[58,64,65,68,127] (ii) the finding of very high-titer anti-RNP antibodies during remissions as well as exacerbations of disease activity;[43,59,68,127] (iii) the demonstration of immune complex deposits in kidney biopsy specimens;[68,88,111,119,126,130] (iv) the finding of circulating immune complexes during disease activation;[84-86] (v) hypocomplementemia;[43,65,66,68,127] (vi) the demonstration of lymphocytotoxic antibodies;[89,90] and (vii) the histologic demonstration of a lymphocytic and plasma cell infiltration in synovium, intestine, heart, liver, muscle, salivary glands, and lung.[68,111,112,117,122]

Recent studies have defined the antigenic reactive site for anti-RNP antibodies, and other studies have suggested possible mechanisms for disorders of immune regulation in terms of antibody penetration into cells, abnormalities in immunoregulatory networks, and defects in Fc-mediated clearance of immune complexes. These newer findings are now discussed in greater detail.

THE ANTIGEN FOR ANTI–RNP ANTIBODIES

The early work on the nature of the antigenic site for anti-RNP antibodies had established that a complex of RNA and protein was necessary for immunologic reactivity.[58] Partial characterization of this antigenic moiety was achieved by Tan and Sharp and their colleagues.[149,150] A major breakthrough in the precise identification of the immunogenically active component of the RNP antigen has now been provided, as a result of the interest of molecular biologists in the mechanisms of transcription of active chromatin. Much of the early work on the structure of DNA and its relationship to individual amino acids was done in *E. coli* and other prokaryotes. When similar studies were attempted in mammalian cells, it became apparent that eukaryotic DNA differs from prokaryotic DNA in respect to certain base sequences between genes, which would translate into currently meaningless information. Such regions of extra nonsensical information have been called introns.

In order for messenger RNA (mRNA) to be effectively transcribed into the amino acid sequence of a particular protein it is essential that the "message" not be blocked by sequences of RNA bases which do not have a coding role. Further studies showed that the transcripton of mammalian DNA gave rise to RNA containing all the complementary sequences of the corresponding introns; this has been called heteronuclear RNA (hnRNA). However mRNA was found to be free of introns, and it became apparent that mammalian cells possessed an intricate apparatus for "splicing" out these unwanted sequences. It was subsequently found that at the end of the intragene junction of hnRNA there existed common RNA sequences, which have been called "splice junction sequences."[151,152] Futhermore it was shown that a hitherto enigmatic group of ribonucleoprotein complexes found in the nucleus, the so-called "small nuclear

Table 71–4. Reported Causes of Death in MCTD

Suicide	Pulmonary hypertension
Opportunistic infections	Renovascular hypertension
Myocarditis	Mesenteric vasculitis
Myocardial infarction*	Pulmonary embolus
Gastrointestinal hemorrhage*	Ruptured abdominal aortic aneurysm*
Acute myocardial infarction*	"Shock" lung
Cerebral hemorrhage	Unexplained ventricular Fibrillation*

*These causes of death were probably not related to MCTD.

ribonucleoproteins" (snRNPs), contained a specific sequence of RNA (called U_1) complexed to 7 proteins (MW 12,000 to 35,000), and that U_1 was complementary to the common intron-gene junction of hnRNA.[151,152]

It is now established that U_1-snRNP regulates the post-transcriptional assembly of mRNA by mediating the precise excision of nonsensical intron segments from hnRNA. The work of Lerner and colleagues[79-82] has shown that anti-RNP antibodies are reactive with U_1-snRNP (Fig. 71-14). Furthermore, in an in vitro system anti-RNP antibodies have been shown to block the post-transcriptional processing of mRNA.[153] Similar studies have now established that other ENA-reactive antibodies (anti-Sm, Ro, and La) are directed towards snRNPs other than U_1.[82,154] For instance, anti-Sm reacts with all known members of the SnRNPs (U_1, U_2, U_4, U_5, U_6), but the antigenic site on U_1 for anti-Sm is different from the site for anti-RNP.[82] It may be of relevance to the immunopathogenesis of MCTD and other similar diseases that SnRNPs are highly conserved (mice, men, sea urchins, and insects) and are present in 10^5 to 10^6 copies per nucleus.[155] Why an immune response should be mounted against such nucleic acid/protein complexes remains an enigma; nucleic acids themselves are poor immunogens, but it is now apparent that the protein component of the snRNPs is essential for the immunogenicity.[156] An attractive hypothesis is the concept of an immunologic cross-reactivity between snRNPs and exogenous RNA-protein complexes, such as those associated with certain viruses. In this respect it has been shown that anti-La antibodies are cross-reactive with RNPs of adenovirus or Epstein-Barr virus encoded RNAs.[80]

Antibody Penetration into Living Cells. There has been a generally accepted but unproven dogma[157] that antibodies do not penetrate living cells, and evidence to the contrary[158-163] was either ignored or glossed over. More recently accumulated evidence suggests that macromolecules can gain access to the inside of cells via a receptor-mediated process[164] and more specifically that the transfer of passive humoral immunity from mother to fetus seems to occur by means of antibody interiorization through Fc receptors on intestinal epithelium and the yolk sac.[165-168] In 1978 Alarcón Segovia reported that the IgG fraction obtained from the serum of a patient with a very high titer of anti-RNP antibodies could, even after adsorption of all lymphocytotoxic activity, penetrate living mononuclear cells.[169] This internalization phenomenon was dependent on the cells having intact, unoccupied Fc receptor and was arrested when cell metabolism was slowed down by cooling.

Other studies by the same group[170,171] have reported that penetration of antibodies into living cells can occur with other antibodies, and that in the case of anti-RNP antibodies, this leads to in vitro evidence of a suppressor cell loss and an arrest of the cell cycle between the S and G_2 phases.[172] The significance of these findings in vivo has yet to be established. Competition for Fc receptor by all the other IgG molecules found in vivo would certainly be expected to modulate any functionally significant effect of anti-RNP antibodies in patients with MCTD; in one study it was reported that 5.5 percent of mononuclear cells from MCTD patients contained intranuclear immunoglobulins as assessed by immunofluorescence.[173] A possible direct demonstration of a cellular penetration of anti-RNP antibodies in vivo is the finding of intranuclear immunofluorescence of epidermal cells on routine skin biopsy;[72,174] on the other hand, this observation may be artefactual, a result of sectioned cells being inadvertently exposed to MCTD plasma.

Figure 71–14. Polyacrylamide gel electrophoresis of ^{32}P-labeled nucleic acids extracted from a tissue culture of HeLa cells. Lane *T* shows the total cell content of nucleic acids and identifies in particular those RNAs (U_1, U_2, U_4, U_5, U_6) that are complexed with protein to comprise snRNPs (small nuclear RNAs can be immunoprecipitated with some of the different antibodies found in connective tissue disorders—anti-La (SSB), anti-Sm, anti-Ro (SSA) and anti-RNP. It is seen that anti-RNP antibodies react only with the snRNA that contains U1 RNA. (From Lerner, et al.: Arthritis Rheum. 25:701, 1982.)

IMMUNOREGULATORY DYSFUNCTION

The plethora of autoantibodies that are seen in classic SLE are generally thought to be a result of either an intrinsically activated population of B lymphocytes or a secondary event due to defective suppression. In the latter case a reduction in the number of suppressor T lymphocytes with a corresponding loss of suppressor activity or an abnormality of an antiidiotypic network is incriminated in the loss of B lymphocyte regulation.

Patients with MCTD likewise have a decrease in circulatory T suppressor lymphocytes and loss of suppressor cell function.[175] It is thought that both suppressor T lymphocytes and helper T lymphocytes arise from a differentiation of post-thymic precursor cells. It has furthermore been claimed that in humans the post-thymic precursor cell is similar to a cell that forms rosettes with human erythrocytes.[176,177] This has been called the autologous rosette-forming cell (Tar cells). Tar cells constitute more than 70 percent of thymocytes, are devoid of Fc receptors but have receptors for peanut agglutinin, and are very sensitive to corticosteroids.[177] In SLE the circulating Tar cells are reduced in number and have a reduced capability of generating a suppressor influence; this dysfunction is partially corrected by serum thymic factor.[178] One study in MCTD has shown an interesting difference from classic SLE, in that the number of circulating Tar cells was normal or increased, although suppression and feedback inhibition were inhibited.[179] In the case of MCTD this dysfunction was *not* corrected by serum thymic factor. It was proposed that the suppressor dysfunction in MCTD may be a result of an abnormal interaction of helper T lymphocytes with Tar cells in feedback inhibition or a defective response of helper T lymphocytes to suppressor T lymphocytes.[180]

RETICULOENDOTHELIAL DYSFUNCTION

It has been suggested that the elevated levels of circulating immune complexes observed in patients with classic SLE are partly a result of impaired clearance by the reticuloendothelial system.[181] The clearance of IgG-sensitized (anti-Rh antibody) erythrocytes has been found to be impaired in most patients with SLE, the degree of impairment being related to disease activity.[102] However, it should be stressed that IgG-sensitized erythrocytes are cleared almost exclusively by splenic macrophages possessing receptors for the Fc component of IgG. As most immune complexes are cleared predominantly by the Kupffer cells in the liver, the pathogenetic significance of impaired splenic clearance seen in SLE is not presently clear. Indeed, patients who have undergone a splenectomy have a markedly prolonged clearance of IgG-sensitized erythrocytes, but this can be nearly normalized by heavily coating the cells with IgG (fourfold the usual amount) when it is observed that clearance occurs predominantly via hepatic sequestration.[183] As patients with MCTD generally have less severe renal disease than patients with classic SLE, the question arises as to whether this may be due to a quantitative difference in the handling of immune complexes. Frank and colleagues[183] have shown in 18 patients with MCTD that the Fc-specific immune clearance of IgG-sensitized erythrocytes was only impaired in 4 patients. Furthermore, these 4 patients had a more severe form of the disease, which resembled classic SLE. It was hypothesized that the generally milder course of MCTD

compared with classic MCTD may be related to differences in immune complex clearance, due to alteration in immune complex–Fc receptor interaction or accelerated receptor generation in MCTD. It is of interest that the same group has presented preliminary evidence suggesting an association of the HLA-B8/DRw3 genotype with Fc IgG-mediated splenic clearance.

HISTOLOGIC MICROVASCULAR ABNORMALITIES

The histologic findings in MCTD have not been very thoroughly documented. Although immune complexes have been seen in the glomeruli of affected kidneys (Fig. 71–13), a florid necrotizing vasculitis, as is often seen in immune complex mediated disease, is unusual in MCTD. Rather, emerging evidence indicates that a widespread intimal proliferation affecting medium-sized arteries is the most characteristic vascular lesion in MCTD[111,118,121] (Fig. 71–15). A similar lesion has also been described in large arteries, including coronary, pulmonary, renal, and aortic in a few patients.[111] This is in contrast to classic scleroderma, in which a similar characteristic intimal proliferation is confined to the smaller vessels. Indeed, current evidence points to a generalized involvement of the microvasculature as the primary site of injury in scleroderma.[184] The finding of similar changes in patients with MCTD is therefore an important difference when comparing MCTD with classic SLE. This intimal proliferation may give rise to renovascular kidney disease and severe pulmonary hypertension in a minority of patients. In respect to the histologic findings in cases of fatal pulmonary hypertension various vascular lesions have been reported: intimal thickening with focal arteritis;[118,121] plexogenic angiopathy;[118] pulmonary interstitial fibrosis;[118] and recurrent thromboembolic hypertension[119] (Fig. 71–16). Maricq and colleagues have demonstrated an association between microvascular changes in scleroderma and characteristic changes in the capillaries of the nailfold.[185] It is of interest that about 50 percent of patients with MCTD have identical nailfold capillary changes to those observed in scleroderma[186] (see Fig. 71–17). As such, nailfold capillary changes are seldom seen in classic SLE.[186] Their presence in some patients with MCTD provides an important differential feature between one portion of the MCTD population and patients with classic SLE (Fig. 71–18). Singsen and colleagues have described an inflammatory infiltrate, mainly lymphocytes and plasma cells, in many organs, including liver, intestine, muscle, and salivary glands.[11] It was conjectured that this is the histologic counterpart of the hypergammaglobulinemia of MCTD. The same group has emphasized an asymptomatic myocardial inflammatory infiltration in children wiht MCTD (Fig. 71–19). The finding of an association between symptomatic myocarditis and anti-RNP antibodies[116] is a possible clinical counterpart of this myocardial histopathology.

Figure 71–15. Two examples of the bland, noninflammatory, intimal thickening that is seen in MCTD. *A,* A small serosal artery from the ileocecal region (× 226). *B,* A coronary artery (× 226). (From Singsen, et al.: Am. J.. Med. 68:710, 1980.)

Figure 71–16. These histologic specimens are from patients with MCTD who had pulmonary involvement. *A,* Severe intimal proliferation of a patient who died of pulmonary hypertension. (From Manthorpe, et al.: Scand. J. Rheumatol. 9:7, 1980.) *B,* Small pulmonary artery showing old recanalized thrombosis in a patient with MCTD who had fatal pulmonary hypertension. (From Jones, et al.: Am. J. Med. 65:855, 1978.) *C,* Small pulmonary artery showing a plexiform lesion with multiple vascular channels (closed arrow) in an area of intimal thickening (open arrow); patient died with pulmonary hypertension. *D,* Open lung biopsy in a 66-year-old-man with MCTD and increasing dyspnea and cough. There is distortion of the alveolar archtechture by patchy interstitial fibrosis. The muscular artery shows mild intimal thickening. (*C* and *D* from Wiener-Kronish, et al.: Am. Rev. Resp. 124:499, 1981.)

Figure 71–17. The prevalence of a scleroderma pattern of nailfold capillary changes is about 50 percent in patients diagnosed as having MCTD. *SD* = scleroderma; *RD* = Raynaud's disease (idiopathic). (From Maricq, et al.: Arthritis Rheum. 23:183, 1980.)

Figure 71–18. Different nailfold capillary patterns in health and disease. (All figures kindly provided by Dr. Maricq.) *A*, Normal pattern. (Courtesy of Microvascular Research.) *B*, Pattern in a patient with scleroderma. *C*, Pattern in a patient with MCTD (Courtesy of Clinics in Rheumatic Diseases). *D*, Pattern in a patient with acute SLE. (*B* and *D* from Maricq, H.R., et al.: Arthritis Rheum. 23:183, 1980.)

Figure 71–19. Myocardial tissue from a child with a diagnosis of MCTD who had no obvious cardiac dysfunction. There are areas of focal muscle necrosis, an inflammatory infiltrate, and increased interstitial connective tissue. (From Singsen, G.H., et al.: A. J. Med. 68:710, 1980.)

TREATMENT

The effective management of patients with MCTD in inevitably complicated by several features: the variability of specific organ involvement, the intercurrent nature of some of the problems, the ineffectiveness of current therapy for some of the specific problems, and our incomplete knowledge of the full spectrum of MCTD, its course, and its prognosis. In general the fatigability and malaise, if sufficiently bothersome, are often substantially helped by low-dose prednisone (< 10 mg per day). As the institution of corticosteroids in MCTD tends to be a long-term commitment, the concomitant use of calcium and vitamin D supplements should be considered in an effort to retard bone demineralization. Although Raynaud's phenomenon in MCTD is partly due to organic disease of the small vessels, there is a reversible component, which can often be alleviated by nifedipine (10 mg to 30 mg per day); in patients with mild Raynaud's phenomenon nifedipine can be used on a symptomatic basis during periods of cold weather. Patients with a lower esophageal motility disorder may be helped by the use of metoclopramide (10 mg three times per day); this is said to improve both lower esophogeal sphincter tone as well as peristaltic motility in the esophagus itself. In those patients suffering from persistent reflux esophagitis, the institution of cimetidine (300 mg three times per day) needs to be considered.

Symptomatically the joint pains of MCTD can often be well controlled by the judicious use of NSAIDs. The use of high to moderate doses of corticosteroids (prednisone 80 to 20 mg per day) is usually indicated in the treatment of pleuritis, pericarditis, myositis, and aseptic meningitis. Episodes of muscle inflammation may occur with explosive onset and require intensive high-dose steroids for a short course, or the inflammation may follow a low-grade indolent course over many years. In the latter case the total corticosteroid burden may well be detrimental, and the use of an immunosuppressive agent

such as azathioprine needs to be considered. Unfortunately there are no controlled studies on the use of immunosuppressives in MCTD, and their prescription is currently based on anecdotal experience. The management of aseptic meningitis is, of course, based on the exclusion of CSF infection followed by high-dose corticosteroids (prednisone about 80 mg per day) on a tapering regimen over a period of about 3 weeks. The common vascular headaches of MCTD may sometimes be reduced by the use of propranolol (40 mg twice daily). Seizures are rare in MCTD, and initial attempts at management should emphasize the use of antiepileptic medications; only if these are ineffective, should corticosteroids be instituted. Renal involvement in MCTD usually takes the form of a mild membranous glomerulonephritis and as such is not responsive to steroids.

In patients with severe renovascular disease the control of blood pressure is of paramount importance, as it is in scleroderma; in such cases the use of captopril may need to be considered. Currently there is no proven therapy for those patients with progressive pulmonary hypertension secondary to an angiopathy; apart from supportive therapy in an intensive care unit it would seem reasonable to consider intensive immunosuppression and apheresis. Patients with early interstitial pulmonary disease, as evidenced by an abnormal gallium scan or bronchioalveoler lavage, may be candidates for corticosteroids and for immunosuppression. However, there have not been any studies to definitively demonstrate that such therapy will prevent the progression to irreversible pulmonary fibrosis. Patients with myocarditis and congestive cardiac failure represent another difficult management problem for which no well defined therapy is currently available. In general, digoxin should be used with extreme caution in such patients, owing to the possibility of provoking serious rhythm disturbances. As in idiopathic myocarditis corticosteroids are seldom effective, and serious consideration needs to be given to the use of intensive immunosuppression.

Table 71–5. Responsiveness to Corticosteroids in MCTD

General Responsive Features	Generally Unresponsive Features
Myositis	Raynaud's phenomenon
Aseptic meningitis	Gastrointestinal changes
Pericarditis	Pulmonary hypertension
Arthritis	Renovascular hypertension
Fatigability	Myocarditis
Hemolytic anemia	Trigeminal neuropathy
Pleurisy	Membranous nephritis

It should be emphasized that a diagnosis of MCTD should not elicit an automatic reflex to prescribe steroids. Many patients do not need long-term corticosteroid therapy, although certain intercritical problems (e.g., pleurisy) may require a short burst of prednisone. Furthermore it is equally important to realize that only some of the clinical problems encountered in MCTD are responsive to corticosteroids (Table 71–5). In this respect, the original claim[43] of ". . . its being characterized by an excellent response to corticosteroid therapy" needs to be modified.

Lastly, the management of patients with MCTD requires continuing reassessment of an ever changing pattern of clinical problems and a constant alertness for iatrogenic problems such as infection in the immunocompromised host, interstitial renal disease, aseptic necrosis of bone, and steroid myopathy.

As with any disease of unknown etiology, the effective management of patients with MCTD represents both a therapeutic challenge and an opportunity for learning.

References

1. Mallory, T.B., and Warthin, T.A.: Case records of the Masaachusetts General Hospital. N. Engl. J. Med. 225:953, 1961.
2. Beneze, G., Lakatos, L., and Forro, L.: Correlation of rheumatoid arthritis and systemic lupus erythematosus shown by observation of a rheumatoid arthritis patient. Acta Rheum. Scand. 7:233, 1961.
3. Kantor, G.L., Bichel, Y.B., and Barrett, E.V.: Coexistence of SLE and rheumatoid arthritis: Report of a case and review of the literature with clinical, pathologic and serological observations. Am. J. Med. 47:433, 1969.
4. Haserick, J.R.: Modern concepts of SLE: A review of 126 cases. J. Chronic Dis. 1:317, 1955.
5. Toone, E.C., Jr., Irby, R., and Pierce, E.L.: The LE cell in rheumatoid arthritis. Am. J. Med. Sci. 240:599, 1960.
6. Kieviti, J.H., Goslings, J., Schmit, H.R.E., and Hijmons, W.: Rheumatoid arthritis and the positive LE cell phenomenon. Ann. Rheum. Dis. 15:211, 1956.
7. Dubois, E.L.: Lupus erythematosus, lupoid syndromes, and their relation to collagen diseases. Postgrad. Med. 32:568, 1962.
8. Debeyre, N., Kahn, M.R., Ryckewaert, E.V.: Rheumatoid arthritis with Hargraves (LE) cells. Presse Med. 74:911, 1966.
9. Blehm, G.B., Sigler, J.W., Ensign, D.C., and Rebuck, J.W.: The incidence and significance of the lupus erythematosus (LE) phenomenon in 45 rheumatoid arthritis patients observed for 10 years. Arthritis Rheum. 10:269, 1967.
10. Ross, S.W., and Clardy, E.K.: The LE test in patients presenting the clinical picture of rheumatoid arthritis. South. Med. J. 49:553, 1956.
11. Hannestad, K.: The LE factor in rheumatoid arthritis: Clinical and serological studies. Acta Rheum. Scand. 13:42, 1967.
12. Lenock, F., and Vojtisek, O.: The prevalence of LE cells in 1,000 consecutive patients with active rheumatoid arthritis. Acta Rheum. Scand. 13:313, 1967.
13. Sigler, J.W., Manter, R.W., Ensign, D.C., Wilson, G.M., Jr., Rebuck J.R. and Covett J.D.: The incidence of the LE cell phenomenon in patients with rheumatoid arthritis (a two year study) Arthritis Rheum. 1:115, 1958.
14. Beigelman, P.M., Goldner, F., and Bayles, T.B.: Progressive systemic sclerosis (scleroderma). N. Engl. J. Med. 249:45, 1953.
15. Muehrcke, R.C., Kark, R.M., Pirani, C.L., et al.: Lupus nephritis: A clinical and pathological study based on renal biopsies. Medicine (Baltimore) 36:1, 1957.
16. Rowell, N.R.: Lupus erythematosus cells in systemic sclerosis. Ann. Rheum. Dis. 21:70, 1962.
17. D'Angelo, W.A., Fries, J.F., Masi, A.T., et al.: Pathologic observations in systemic sclerosis. Am. J. Med. 46:428, 1969.
18. Dubois, E.L., Chandor, S., Friou, G.J., et al.: Progressive systemic sclerosis and localized scleroderma with positive LE cell test and unusual systemic manifestations compatible with systemic lupus erythematosus. Medicine (Baltimore) 59:199, 1971.
19. Tuffanelli, D.L., and Winkelmann, R.K.: Systemic scleroderma: A clinical study of 727 cases. Arch. Dermatol. 84:369, 1961.
20. Poirer, T.J., and Rankin, G.B.: Gastrointestinal manifestations of progressive systemic scleroderma based on a review of 364 cases. Am. J. Gastroenterol. 58:30, 1972.
21. Kampmeier, R.H.: Vascular disease due to hypersensitivity: So-called diffuse collagen disease. Am. Pract. Digest. Treat. 1:113, 1950.
22. Dubois, E.L.: In Lupus Erythematosus: A Review of the Current Status of Discoid and Systemic Lupus Erythematosus and Their Variants. 2nd ed. Los Angeles, University of Southern California Press, 1974.
23. Allan, W.: Dermatomyositis or scleroderma? Report of a case. Arch. Dermatol. Syphil. 19:265, 1929.
24. Brock, W.G.: Dermatomyositis and diffuse scleroderma: Differential diagnosis and reports of cases. Arch. Dermatol. Syphil. 30:227, 240, 1934.
25. Talbott, J.H., Gall, E.A., Consolazio, W.V., et al.: Dermatomyositis with scleroderma, calcinosis and renal endarteritis associated with focal cortical necrosis. Arch. Intern. Med. 63:476, 1939.
26. Dowling, G.B.: Generalized scleroderma. Br. J. Dermatol. Syphil. 52:242, 1940.
27. Lewis, T.: Notes on scleroderma (dermatomyositis). Br. J. Dermatol. Syphil. 52:233, 1940.
28. Seville, R.H.: Scleroderma dermatomyositis (with electronmicrographs). Br. J. Dermatol. 64:467, 1952.
29. Clark, J.A., Winkelmann, R.K., and Ward, L.E.: Serological alterations in scleroderma and sclerodermatomyositis. Mayo Clin. Proc. 46:104, 107, 1971.
30. Medsger, T.A., Rodnan, G.P., Moossy, J., and Vester, J.W.: Skeletal muscle involvement in progressive systemic sclerosis (scleroderma). Arthritis Rheum. 11:554, 1968.
31. Keil, H.: Dermatomyositis and systemic lupus erythematosus: A clinical report of transitional cases with consideration of lead as a possible etiologic factor. Arch. Intern. Med. 60:109, 1940.
32. Banks, B.M.: Is there a common denominator in scleroderma, dermatomyositis, disseminated lupus erythematosus, the Libman-Sacks syndrome and polyarteritis nodosa? N. Engl. J. Med. 225:433, 1941.
33. Mimori, T., Akizuki, M., Yamagatu, H., Inada, S., Yoshida, S., and Homna, M.: Characterization of a high molecular weight acidic nuclear protein recognized by autoantibodies in sera from patients with polymyositis-scleroderma overlap. J. Clin. Invest. 68:611, 1981.
34. Bunch, T.W., O'Duffy, J.F., and McLeod, R.A.: Deforming arthritis of the hands in polymyositis. Arthritis Rheum. 29:243, 1976.
35. Schumacher, R.H., Schimmer, B., Gordon, G.V., Bookspan, M.A., Brogadir, S., and Dorwart, B.B.: Articular manifestations of polymyositis and dermatomyositis. Am. J. Med. 67:287, 1979.
36. Moutsopolous, H.M. Sjögren's syndrome (sicca syndrome): Current issues. Ann. Intern. Med. 92:212, 1980.
37. Moutsopolous, H.M., Webber, B.C., Vlagapolous, T.P., Chussed, T.M., and Decker, J.L.: Differences in the clinical manifestations of sicca syndrome in the presence and absence of rheumatoid arthritis. Am. J. Med. 66:733, 1979.
38. Bunim, J.J.: Heberden Oration: A broader spectrum of Sjögren's syndrome and its pathogenic implications. Ann. Rheum. Dis. 20:1, 1961.
39. Shearn, M.A.: Sjögren's Syndrome. Philadelphia, W.B. Saunders Company, 1971.
40. Moutsopoulos, H.M., Klippel, J.H., Pavlidis, N., Wolf, R.O., Sweet, J.B., Steinberg, A.D., Chu, F.C., and Tarpley, T.M.: Correlative histologic and serologic findings of sicca syndrome in patients with systemic lupus erythematosus. Arthritis Rheum. 23:36, 1980.
41. Alarcón-Segovia, D., Ibánez, G., Velazquez-Forero, F., Hernández-Ortíz, J., and Gonzales-Jimenez, Y.: Sjögren's syndrome in systemic lupus erythematosus. Ann. Intern. Med. 81:577, 1974.
42. Martinez-Lavin, M., Vaughan, J.H., and Tan, E.M.: Autoantibodies and the spectrum of Sjögren's syndrome. Ann. Intern. Med. 91:185, 1979.
43. Sharp, G.C., Irvin, W.S., Tan, E.M., Gould, R.G., and Holman, H.R.: Mixed connective tissue disease: an apparently distinct rheumatic disease syndrome associated with a specific antibody to extractable nuclear antigen (ENA). Am. J. Med. 52:148, 1972.
44. Hargraves, M.M., Richmond, M., and Morton, R.: Presentation of 2

bone marrow elements: The "Tart" cell and the "LE" cell. Proc. Staff Meet. Mayo Clin. 23:25, 1948.

45. Hargraves, M.M.: Production in vitro of the LE cell phenomenon: Use of normal bone marrow elements and blood plasma from patients with acute disseminated lupus erythematosus. Proc. Staff Meet. Mayo Clin. 24:234, 1949.

46. Haserick, H.R., Lewis, L.A., and Bartz, D.W.: Blood factor in acute disseminated lupus erythematosus. 1. Determination of gamma globulin as specific plasma fraction. Am. J. Med. Sci. 219:660, 1950.

47. Holman, H.R., and Deicher, H.R.: The reaction of the lupus erythematosus (LE) cell factor with deoxyribonucleoprotein of the cell nucleus. J. Clin. Invest. 38:2059, 1959.

48. Holman, H.R., and Kunkel, H.G.: Affinity between lupus erythematosus serum factor and cell nuclei and nucleoprotein. Science (NY) 126:102, 1957.

49. Holborow, E.J., Weir, D.M., and Johnson, G.D.: A serum factor in lupus erythematosus with affinity for tissue nuclei. Br. Med. J. 2:732, 1957.

50. Friou, G.H.: Identification of the nuclear component of the interaction of lupus erythematosus globulin and nuclei. J. Immunol. 80:476, 1958.

51. Kunkel, H.G., and Tan, E.M.: Autoantibodies and disease. Adv. Immunol. 4:351, 1964.

52. Levin, L., Statler, B.D.: Nucleic acid immune systems. Prog. Allergy 12:161, 1968.

53. Tan, E.M.: An immunologic precipitation system between soluble nucleoprotein and serum antibody in SLE. J. Clin. Invest. 46:735, 1967.

54. Holman, H.R.: Partial purification and characterization of an extractable nuclear antigen which reacts with SLE sera. Ann. N.Y. Acad. Sci. 124:800, 1965.

55. Tan, E.M., and Kunkel, H.G.: Characteristics of a soluble nuclear antigen precipitation with the sera of patients with SLE. J. Immunol. 96:464, 1966.

56. Sharp, G.C., Irvin, W.S., LaRogue, R.L., Velez, C., Daly, V., Kaiser, A.D., and Holman, H.R.: Association of autoantibodies to different nuclear antigens with clinical patterns of rheumatic disease and responsiveness to therapy. J. Clin. Invest. 50:350, 1971.

57. Mattioli, M., and Reichlin, M.: Characterization of a soluble nuclear ribonucleoprotein antigen reactive with SLE sera. J. Immunol. 107:1281, 1971.

58. Mattioli, M., and Reichlin, M.: Physical association of two nuclear antigens and mutual occurence of their antibodies: The relationship of the Sm and the RNA-protein (Mu) systems in SLE sera. J. Immunol. 110:1318, 1973.

59. Sharp, G.C., Irvin, W.S., May, C.M., Holman, H.R., McDuffie, F.C., Hess, E.V., and Schmid, F.R.: Association of antibodies to ribonucleoprotein and Sm antigens with mixed connective-tissue disease, systemic lupus erythematosus and other rheumatic diseases. N. Engl. J. Med. 295:1149, 1976.

60. Parker, M.D.: Ribonucleoprotein antibodies: Frequency and clinical significance in systemic lupus erythematosus, scleroderma and mixed connective tissue disease. J. Lab. Clin. Med. 82:769, 1973.

61. Leibfarth, J.H., and Persellin, R.H.: Characteristics of patients with serum antibodies to extractable nuclear antigens. Arthritis Rheum. 19:851, 1976.

62. Hamburger, M., Hodes, S., and Barland, P.: The incidence and clinical significance of antibodies to extractable nuclear antigens. Am. J. Med. Sci. 273:21, 1977.

63. Maddison, P.J., Mogovero, H., and Reichlin, M.: Patterns of clinical disease associated with antibodies to nuclear ribonucleoprotein. J. Rheumatol. 5:407, 1978.

64. Gaudreau, A., Amar, B., Kahn, M.F., et al.: Clinical significance of antibodies to soluble extractable nuclear antigens (anti-ENA). Ann. Rheum. Dis. 37:321, 1978.

65. Grant, K.D., Adams, L.E., and Hess, E.V.: MCTD—a subset with sequential clinical and laboratory features. J. Rheum. 8:587, 1981.

66. Prystowsky, S.D.: Mixed connective tissue disease. West. J. Med. 132:288, 1980.

67. Singsen, B.H., Bernstein, B.H., Kornreich, H.K., King, K.K., Hanson, V., and Tan, E.M.: MCTD in childhood. J. Pediatr. 90:893, 1977.

68. Bennett, R.M., and O'Connell, D.J.: Mixed connective tissue disease: A clinicopathological study of 20 cases. Sem. Arthritis Rheum. 10:25, 1980.

69. Hochberg, M.C., Dorsch, C.A., Feinglass, E.J., and Stevens, M.B.: Survivorship in SLE: Effect of antibody to extractable nuclear antigen. Arthritis Rheum. 24:54, 1981.

70. Grennan, D.M., Burn, C., Hughes, G.R.V., Buchanan, W.W., and Dick, W.C.: Frequency and clinical significance of antibodies to ribonucleoprotein in SLE and other connective tissue disease subgroups. Ann. Rheum. Dis. 30:442, 1977.

71. Farber, S.J., and Bole, G.G.: Antibodies to components of extractable nuclear antigen. Clinical characteristics of patients. Arch. Intern. Med. 136:425, 1976.

72. Lemmer, J.P., Curry, N.H., Mallory, J.H., and Waller, M.V.: Clinical characteristics and course in patients with high titer anti-RNP antibodies. J. Rheum. 9:536, 1982.

73. McCain, G.A., Bell, D.A., Chodirker, W.B., and Komar, R.R.: Antibody to extractable nuclear antigen in the rheumatic diseases. J. Rheum. 5:399, 1978.

74. Matter, L., Schapper, K., Wilhelm, J.A., and Nyffenegger, T., Parisot, R.F., and DeRoberts, E.M.: Molecular characterisation of ribonucleoprotein antigens bound by antinuclear antibodies: A diagnostic evaluation. Arthritis Rheum. 25:1297, 1982.

75. Peskett, S.A., Ansell, B.M., Fizzman, P., and Howard, A.: Mixed connective tissue disease in children. Rheum. Rehab. 17:245, 1978.

76. Ellman, M.H., Pachman, L., and Medof, M.E.: Raynaud's phenomenon and initially seronegative mixed connective tissue disease. J. Rheum. 8:632, 1981.

77. Alarcón-Segovia, D.: Mixed connective tissue disease: Appearance of antibodies to ribonucleoprotein following corticosteroid treatment. J. Rheum. 6:694, 1979.

78. Alarcón-Segovia, D.: Mixed connective tissue disease: A decade of growing pains. J. Rheum. 8:535, 1981.

79. Lerner, M.R., and Steitz, J.A.: Antibodies to small nuclear RNAs complexed with proteins and produced by patients with systemic lupus erythematosus. Proc. Natl. Acad. Sci. USA 76:5495, 1979.

80. Lerner, M.R., Boyle, J.A., Hardin, J.A., and Steitz, J.A.: Two novel classes of small ribonucleoproteins detected by antibodies associated with lupus erythematosus. Science 211:400, 1981.

81. Lerner, E.A., Lerner, M.M., Janeway, C.A., Jr., and Steitz, J.A.: Monoclonal antibodies to nucleic acid containing cellular constituents: Probes for molecular biology and autoimmune disease. Proc. Natl. Acad. Sci. USA 78:2737, 1981.

82. Lerner, E.A., Lerner, M.R., Hardin, J.A., Janeway, C.A., and Steitz, J.A.: Deciphering the mysteries of RNA-containing lupus antigens. Arthritis Rheum. 25:761, 1982.

83. Fishbein, E., Ramos-Niembro, F., and Alarcón-Segovia, D.: Free serum ribonucleoproteins in mixed connective tissue disease and other connective tissue diseases. J. Rheum. 5:384, 1978.

84. Cunningham, P.H., Andrews, B.S., and Davis, J.S.: Immune complexes in progressive systemic sclerosis and MCTD. J. Rheum. 7:301, 1980.

85. Halla, J.T., Volanakis, J.E., and Schrohenloker, R.E.: Circulating immune complexes in MCTD. Arthritis Rheum. 22:484, 1979.

86. Diez-Jovanen, E., Salazar, J.F., Abud-Mendoza, C., and Alarcón-Segovia, D.: Immune complexes in autoimmune diseases: Differences in immune complexes detected by cellular receptor for complement and for Fc domains of IgG. Rev. Invest. Clin. (Mexico) 32:153, 1980.

87. Nolph, K.D., Husted, F.C., Sharp, G.C., and Siemcen, A.W.: Antibodies to nuclear antigens in patients undergoing long term hemodialysis. Am. J. Med. 60:673, 1976.

88. Winfield, J.B., Koffler, D., and Kunkel, H.G.: Development of antibodies to ribonucleoprotein following short-term therapy with procainamide. Arthritis Rheum. 18:531, 1975.

89. Schocket, A.C., and Kohler, P.F.: Lymphocytotoxic antibodies in SLE and clinically related diseases. Arthritis Rheum. 22:1060, 1979.

90. Diaz-Jovanen, E., Llorente, L., Ramos-Niembro, F., and Alarcón-Segovia, D.: Cold reactive lymphocytotoxic antibodies in mixed connective tissue disease. J. Rheum. 4:4, 1977.

91. Locker, J.D., Medof, M.E., Bennett, R.M., and Sukhupunyarksa, S.: Characterization of DNA used to assay sera for anti-DNA antibodies; determination of the specificities of anti-DNA antibodies in SLE and non-SLE rheumatic disease states. J. Immunol. 118:694, 1977.

92. Gilliam, J.N., and Prystowsky, S.D.: Mixed connective tissue disease syndrome: Ailineous manifestations of patients with epidermal nuclear staining and high titer serum antibody to ribonuclease-sensitive extractable nuclear antigen. Arch. Dermatol. 113:583, 1977.

93. Levitin, P.M., Weary, P.E., and Guilano, V.J.: The immunofluorescent band test in mixed connective tissue disease. Ann. Intern. Med. 83:53, 1975.

94. Christian, C.L.: Connective tissue disease: Overlap syndromes, the science and practice of clinical medicine. In Cohen, A.S. (ed.): Rheumatology and Immunology. Vol. 4. New York, Grove & Stratten, 1979, p. 154.

95. Davis, J.D., Parker, M.D., and Turner, R.A.: Exacerbation of mixed connective tissue disease during salmonella gastroenteritis: Serial immunological findings. J. Rheum. 5:96, 1978.

96. Ramos-Niembro, F., and Alarcón-Segovia, D.: Familial aspects of MCTD: 1. Occurrence of SLE in another member of two families and aggregation of MCTD in another family. J. Rheum. 5:433, 1978.

97. Horn, J.R., Kaper, J.J., and Walker, S.E.: Mixed connective tissue disease in siblings. Arthritis Rheum. 21:709, 1978.

98. Bronshvaz, M.M., Prystowsky, S.D., and Traviesa, D.C.: Vascular headaches in mixed connective tissue disease. Headache 18:154, 1978.

99. Gilliam, J.N., and Prystowsky, S.D.: Conversion of discoid lupus erythematosus to MCTD. J. Rheum. 4:165, 1977.

100. Alarcón-Segovia, D.: Symptomatic Sjögren's syndrome in mixed connective tissue disease. J. Rheum. 3:191, 1976.
101. Willkens, R.F., Roth, G.J., Novak, A., and Walike, J.W.: Perforation of the nasal septum in rheumatic disease. Arthritis Rheum. 19:119, 1976.
102. Ramus-Niembro, F., Alarcón-Segovia, D., and Hernández-Ortíz, J.: Articular manifestations of MCTD. Arthritis Rheum. 22:43, 1979.
103. Halla, J.M., and Hardin, J.G.: Clinical features of the arthritis of MCTD. Arthritis Rheum. 21:497, 1978.
104. Bennett, R.M., and O'Connell, D.J.: The arthritis of MCTD. Ann. Rheum. Dis. 37:397, 1978.
105. Alarcón-Segovia, D., and Uribe-Uribe, O.: Mutilans-like anthropathy in MCTD. Arthritis Rheum. 22:1013, 1979.
106. Lewis, R.A., Adams, J.P., Gerber, N.L., Decker, J.L., and Parsons, D.B.: The hand in mixed connective tissue disease. J. Hand Surg. 3:217, 1978.
107. Aptekar, R.G., Lawless, O.G., and Decker, J.L.: Deforming non-erosive arthritis of the hand in systemic lupus erythematosus. Clin. Orthop. 100:120, 1974.
108. Silver, R.M., Forler, S.S., Bole, G.G., and Martel, W.: Radiological features of MCTD and scleroderma-systemic lupus erythematosus overlap. Radiology 120:269, 1976.
109. Udoff, E.J., Genant, H.K., Kozin, F., and Ginsberg, M.: MCTD: The spectrum of radiographic manifestations. Radiology 125:613, 1977.
110. O'Connell, D.J., and Bennett, R.M.: Mixed connective tissue disease—clinical and radiological aspects of 20 cases. Br. J. Radiol. 50:620, 1977.
111. Singsen, B.H., Swanson, V.L., Bernstein, B.H., Heuser, E.T., Hanson, V., and Landing, B.H.: A histologic evaluation of mixed connective tissue disease in childhood. Am. J. Med. 68:710, 1980.
112. Oxenhandler, R., Hart, M., Corman, L., Sharp, G., and Adelstein, E.: Pathology of skeletal muscle in MCTD. Arthritis Rheum. 20:985, 1977.
113. Whitlow, P.L., Gilliam, J.N., Chubick, A., and Ziff, M.: Myocarditis in MCTD. Arthritis Rheum. 23:808, 1980.
114. Emlen, W.: Complete heart clock in MCTD. Arthritis Rheum. 22:678, 1979.
115. Rakovec, P., Kenda, M.F., Rozman, B., Semva, A., and Cibic, B.: Panconductional defect in mixed connective tissue disease. Chest 81:257, 1982.
116. Borenstein, D.G., Fye, W.B., Annett, F.C., and Stevens, M.B.: The myocarditis of systemic lupus erythematosus. Ann. Intern. Med. 89:619, 1978.
117. Parker, C., Levitt, R., Uilto, J., and Bruce, R.: Mixed connective tissue disease. Am. J. Med. 65:833, 1978.
118. Wiener-Kronish, J.P., Solinger, A.M., Warnock, M.S., Churg, A., Ordernez, N., and Golden, J.A.: Severe pulmonary involvement in mixed connective tissue disease. Am. Rev. Resp. Dis. 124:499, 1981.
119. Jones, M.B., Osterholm, R.K., Wilson, R.B., Martin, F.H., Commers, J.R., and Bachmayer, J.D.: Fatal pulmonary hypertension and resolving immune complex-glomerulonephritis in MCTD: Case report and review of the literature. Am. J. Med. 65:855, 1978.
120. Rosenberg, A.M., Petty, R.E., Cumming, G.R., and Koehler, B.E.W.: Pulmonary hypertension in a child with MCTD. J. Rheum. 5:700, 1979.
121. Manthorpe, R., Elling, H., van der Meulen, J.T., and Sorensen, S.: Two fatal cases of mixed connective tissue disease. Scand. J. Rheum. 9:7, 1980.
122. Norman, D.A., and Fleischmann, R.M.: Gastrointestinal systemic sclerosis in serologic MCTD. Arthritis Rheum. 21:811, 1978.
123. Winn, D., Gerhardt, D., Winship, D., and Sharp, G.C.: Esophageal findings in steroid treated patients with mixed connective tissue disease. Clin. Res. 24:545A, 1976.
124. Cooke, C.C., and Lurie, H.I.: Fatal gastrointestinal hemorrhage in MCTD. Arthritis Rheum. 20:1421, 1977.
125. Reichlin, M., and Mattioli, M.: Correlation of a precipitin reaction to an RNA protein antigen and a low prevalence of nephritis in patients with systemic lupus erythematosus. N. Engl. J. Med. 286:908, 1972.
126. Bennett, R.M., and Spargo, B.H.: Immune complex nephropathy in MCTD. Am. J. Med. 63:534, 1977.
127. Nimelstein, S.H., Brady, S., McShane, D., and Holman, H.R.: Mixed connective tissue disease: a subsequent evaluation of the original 25 patients. Medicine 59:239, 1980.
128. Fuller, J.J., Richmann, A.V., Auerback, D., Alexander, R.W., Lottenberg, R., and Langley, S.: Immune complex nephritis in a patient with MCTD. Am. J. Med. 62:762, 1977.
129. Mundy, T.M., Landing, B.H., Hanson, V., Bernstein, B., Kornreich, H.K., and King, K.: Renal involvement in MCTD in childhood. Arthritis Rheum. 23:724, 1980.
130. Palferman, T.G., McIntosh, C.S., and Kershaw, M.: Mixed connective tissue disease associated with glomerulonephritis and hypocomplementemia. Postgrad. Med. J. 56:177, 1980.
131. Bennett, R.M. (unpublished observation).
132. Bennett, R.M., Bong, D.A., and Spargo, B.H.: Neuropsychiatric problems in MCTD. Am. J. Med. 65:955, 1979.
133. Rodnan, G.P.: Progressive systemic sclerosis (scleroderma). In Hollander

134. Searles, R.P., Mladinick, E.K., and Messner, R.P.: Isolated trigeminal sensory neuropathy: Early manifestation of mixed connective tissue disease. Neurology 28:1286, 1978.
135. Vincent, R.M., and Van Houzen, R.N.: Trigeminal sensory neuropathy and bilateral carpal tunnel syndrome: The initial manifestation of mixed connective tissue disease. J. Neurol. Neurosurg. Psychiatry 43:458, 1980.
136. Bernstein, R.F.: Ibuprofen-related meningitis in mixed connective tissue disease. Ann. Intern. Med. 92:206, 1980.
137. Weiss, T.D., Nelson, J.S., Woolsey, R.M., Zuckner, J., and Baldassare, A.R.: Transverse myelitis in MCTD. Arthritis Rheum. 21:982, 1978.
138. Kappes, J., and Bennett, R.M.: Cauda equina syndrome in a patient with high titer anti-RNP antibodies. Arthritis Rheum. 25:349, 1982.
139. Cipoletti, J.F., Backingham, R.B., Barnes, E.L., Peel, R.L., Mahmood, K., Cisnetti, F.E., Pierce, J.M., Rabin, D.S., and Rodnan, G.P.: Sjögren's syndrome in progressive systemic sclerosis. Ann. Intern. Med. 87:535, 1977.
140. Withrington, R.H., and Seifert, M.H.: Hypothyroidism associated with mixed connective tissue disease and its response to steroid therapy. Ann. Rheum. Dis. 40:315, 1981.
141. Segond, P., Yeni, P., Jacquot, J.M., and Massias, P.: Severe autoimmune anemia and thrombopenia in mixed connective tissue disease. Arthritis Rheum. 21:995, 1978.
142. Hardin, J.G., Jr., and Siegal, A.M.: A connective tissue disease complicated by insulin resistance due to receptor antibodies: Report of a case with high titer nuclear ribonucleoprotein antibodies. Arthritis Rheum. 25:458, 1982.
143. Weinstein, P.S., High, K.A., E'Ercole, A.J., and Jennette, J.C.: Insulin resistance due to receptor antibodies: a complication of progressive systemic sclerosis Arthritis Rheum. 23:101, 1980.
144. Palini, M., Roff, S.B., Chase, R., and Gordon, E.E.: Insulin resistance and acanthosis nigricans. Ann. Intern. Med. 85:749, 1976.
145. Maddison, P.J., Reichlin, M.: Quantitation of precipitating antibodies to certain soluble nuclear antigens in SLE: Their contribution to hypergammglobulinemia. Arthritis Rheum. 20:819, 1977.
146. Kaufman, R.L., and Kitrodou, R.C.: Pregnancy in mixed connective tissue disease: comparison with systemic lupus erythematosus. J. Rheum. 9:549, 1982.
147. Baldassare, A., Weiss, T., Auclair, R., and Zuckner, J.: Mixed connective tissue disease (MCTD) in children. Arthritis Rheum. 19:788, 1976.
148. Eberhardt, K., Svantesson, H., and Svensson, B.: Follow-up study of 6 children presenting with a MCTD-like syndrome. Scand. J. Rheum. 10:62, 1981.
149. Douvas, A.S., Stumph, W.E., Reyes, P., and Tan, E.M.: Isolation and characterization of nuclear ribonucleoprotein complexes using human anti-nuclear ribonucleoprotein antibodies. J. Biol. Chem. 19:3608, 1979.
150. Takano, M., Agrus, P.F., and Sharp, G.G.: Purification and biochemical characterization of nuclear ribonucleoprotein antigen using purified antibody from the serum of a patient with mixed connective tissue disease. J. Clin. Invest. 65:1449, 1980.
151. Lerner, M.R., Boyle, J.A., Mount, S.M., Wolin, S.L., and Steitz, J.A.: Are snRNPs involved in splicing. Nature (Lond.) 183:220, 1980.
152. Rogers, J., and Wall, R.: A mechanism for RNA splicing. Proc. Natl. Acad. Sci. USA 77:1877, 1979.
153. Yang, V.W., Lerner, M.R., Steitz, J.A., and Flint, S.J.: A small ribonucleoprotein is required for splicing of adnovisel early RNA sequences. Proc. Natl. Acad. Sci. USA 78:1371, 1981.
154. Hardin, J.A., Rahn, D.R., Shen, C., Lerner, M.R., Wolin, S.L., Rosa, M.R., and Steitz, J.A.: Antibodies from patient with connective tissue diseases find specific subsets of cellular RNA-protein particles. J. Clin. Invest. 70:141, 1982.
155. Hendrick, J.P., Wolin, S.L., Rinke, J., Lerner, M.R., and Steitz, J.A.: Ro scRNP are a subclass of La RNP: Further characterization of the Ro and La small ribonucleoproteins from uninfected mammalian cells. Molec. Cell Biol. 1:1138, 1981.
156. White, P.J., Gardner, W.D., and Hock, S.O.: Identification of the immunogenically active components of the Sm and RNP antigens. Proc. Natl. Acad. Sci. USA 78:626, 1981.
157. Benacerraf, B., and Unanue, E.R.: Immunopathology. In Benacerraf, B., Unanue, E.R. (eds.): Textbook of Immunology. Baltimore, Williams and Wilkins, 1979, p. 250.
158. Coons, A.H., Leduc, E.H., and Kaplan, M.H.: Localization of antigen in tissue cells. VI. The fate of injected foreign proteins in the mouse. J. Exp. Med. 93:173, 1951.
159. Rosenkranz, H.S., Erlanger, B.F., Tanenbaum, S.W., and Beiser, S.M.: Purine and pyrimidine-specific antibodies: Effect on the fertilized sea urchin egg. Science 145:282, 1964.
160. Liebeskind, D.S.P., Hsu, K.C., Erlanger, B.F., and Beiser, S.M.: Selective inhibition of transformed cells in culture by anti-thymidine antibodies. Nature (New Biol.) 234:127, 1971.

J.L., and McCarty, D.J. (eds.): Arthritis and Allied Conditions. 8th ed. Philadelphia, Lea & Febiger, 1972.

161. Ng, C.W., and Gregory, K.F.: Antibody to lactate dehydrogenase. II. Inhibition of glycolysis and growth of tumor cells. Biochem. Biophys. Acta 130:477, 1966.

162. Ng, C.W., and Gregory, K.F.: Antibody to lactate dehydrogenase. III. Uptake, accumulation and specific intracellular action in malignant cells. Biochem. Biophys. Acta 170:45, 1968.

163. Varesio, L., Cappuccinelli, P., and Forni, G.: Inhibition of replication of virus-transformed fibroblasts by antibodies to RNA. Cancer Res. 35:3558, 1975.

164. Goldstein, J.L., Anderson, R.G.W., and Brown, M.S.: Coated pits, coated vesicles, and receptor-mediated endocytosis. Nature 279:679, 1979.

165. Kaplan, K.S., Catsoulis, E.A., and Franklin, E.C.: Maternal-fetal transfer of human immune globulins and fragments in rabbits. Immunology 8:354, 1965.

166. Tsay, D.D., and Schlamowitz, M.: Binding of IgG and papain-derived fragments to Fc receptors of the fetal rabbit yolk sac membrane. J. Immunol. 121:520, 1978.

167. Rodewald, R.: Intestinal transport of antibodies in the newborn rat. J. Cell Biol. 58:189, 1973.

168. Guyer, R.L., Koshland, M.E., and Knopf, P.M.: Immunoglobulin binding by mouse intestinal epithelial cell receptors. J. Immunol. 117:587, 1976.

169. Alarcón-Segovia, D., Ruíz-Arguelles, A., and Fishbein, E.: Antibody to ribonucleoprotein penetrates live human mononuclear cells through Fc receptors. Nature 271:67, 1978.

170. Alarcón-Segovia, D., and Ruíz-Arguelles, A.: Antibody penetration into living cells. A new mechanism of immunologically mediated damage. Rev. Invest. Clin. 31:111, 1979.

171. Alarcón-Segovia, D.: Penetration of antinuclear antibodies into immunoregulatory T cells: Pathogenetic role in connective tissue diseases. Clin. Immunol. Allergy 1:117, 1981.

172. Alarcón-Segovia, D., Llorente, L., and Ruíz-Arguelles, A.: Antibody penetration into living cells. III. Effect of antiribonucleoprotein IGG on the cell cycle of human peripheral blood mononuclear cells. Clin. Immunol. Immunopath. 23:22, 1982.

173. Alarcón-Segovia, D., Ruíz-Arguelles, A., and Fishbein, E.: Antibody penetration into living cells. I. Intranuclear immunoglobulin in peripheral blood mononuclear cells in mixed connective tissue disease and systemic lupus erythematosus. Clin. Exp. Immunol. 35:364, 1979.

174. Shu, S., Provost, T., Croxdale, M.B., Reichlin, M., and Beutner, E.H.: Nuclear deposits of immunoglobulins in skin of patients with systemic lupus erythematosus. Clin. Exp. Immunol. 27:238, 1977.

175. Alarcón-Segovia, D., and Ruíz-Arguelles, A.: Suppressor cell loss and dysfunction in mixed connective tissue disease. Arthritis Rheum. 23:314, 1980.

176. Charriere, J., and Back, J.F.: Binding of autologous erythrocytes to immature TR cells. Proc. Natl. Acad. Sci. USA 72:3201, 1975.

177. Palacios, R., Alarcón-Segovia, D., Llorente, L., Ruíz-Arguelles, A., and Diaz-Jovanen, E.: Human post-thymic precursor cells in health and disease. Immunology 42:127, 1981.

178. Palacios, R., Alarcón-Segovia, D., Llorente, L., Ruíz-Arguelles, A., and Diaz-Jovanen, E.: Human post-thymic precursor cells in health and disease. II. Their loss and dysfunction in systemic lupus erythematosus and their partial connection with serum thymic factor. J. Clin. Lab. Immunol. 5:71, 1981.

179. Alarcón-Segovia, D., and Palacios, R.: Human post-thymic precursor cells in health and disease. IV. Abnormalities in immunoregulatory T cell circuits in mixed connective tissue disease. Arthritis Rheum. 24:1486, 1981.

180. Palacios, R., and Alarcón-Segovia, D.: Human post-thymic precursor cells in health and disease. VI. Effect of serum thymic factor on the response of cells from patients with systemic lupus erythematosus or mixed connective tissue disease in autologous mixed lymphocyte reaction. Clin. Immunol. Immunopathol. 18:362, 1981.

181. Frank, M.M., Hamburger, M.I., Lawley, T.J., Kimberly, R.P., and Plotz, P.N.: Defective reticuloendothelial system Fc-receptor function in systemic lupus erythematosus. N. Engl. J. Med. 300:518, 1979.

182. Hamburger, M.I., Lawley, T.J., Kimberly, R.P., Plotz, P.H., and Frank, M.M.: A serial study of splenic reticuloendothelial system Fc receptor functional activity in systemic lupus erythematosus. Arthritis Rheum. 25:48, 1982.

183. Frank, M.M., Lawley, T.J., Hamburger, M.I., and Brown, E.J.: Immunoglobulin G Fc receptor-mediated clearance in autoimmune diseases. Ann. Intern. Med. 98:206, 1983.

184. Campbell, P.M., and LeRoy, E.C.: Pathogenesis of systemic sclerosis. Sem. Arthritis Rheum. 4:351, 1977.

185. Maricq, H.R., Spencer-Green, G., and LeRoy, E.C.: Skin capillary abnormalities as indicators of organ involvement in scleroderma, Raynaud's syndrome and dermatomyositis. Am. J. Med. 61:862, 1976.

186. Maricq, H.R., LeRoy, E.C., D'Angelo, W.A., Medsger, T.A., Rodnan, G.P., Sharp, G.C., and Wolfe, J.F.: Diagnostic potential of in vivo capillary microscopy in scleroderma and related disorders. Arthritis Rheum. 23:183, 1980.

Section VIII
Vasculitic Syndromes

Chapter 72
Necrotizing Vasculitis

Doyt L. Conn and Gene G. Hunder

INTRODUCTION

Vasculitis is a clinical and pathological process characterized by inflammation and necrosis of blood vessels. Many diseases may be associated with vascular inflammation. Inflammation may involve arteries of any size and the veins also. Vascular inflammation may be a part of various infectious diseases as a result of septicemia or embolization. Vasculitis may accompany and complicate connective tissue diseases such as rheumatoid arthritis, systemic lupus erythematosus, Sjögren's syndrome, dermatomyositis, and scleroderma.

There is a group of diseases in which the vasculitis is the primary feature of disease, and this is the group that will be discussed in detail. Vasculitis as a disease entity was first recognized in 1866 by Kussmaul and Maier when they reported a case of necrotizing arteritis and termed it "periarteritis nodosa."[1] Their patient had widespread inflammation of the small and medium-sized arteries, and in some areas there were focal inflammatory exudations, which gave rise to palpable nodular excrescences along the course of the arteries. A number of different clinical and pathological types of vasculitis have been described since then, and efforts have been made to classify these diseases. Necrotizing vasculitis in the past has been regarded as idiopathic with no known cause. However, in recent years, it has been shown that some cases of the vasculitis are associated with hepatitis B surface antigen, and there are undoubtedly other viruses and antigens yet to be found that can lead to vasculitis. The dominant mechanism of disease in many forms of vasculitis appears to involve immune complexes.

CLASSIFICATION

Although many classifications have been devised for the necrotizing vasculitides, none has been entirely satisfactory for the clinician. Zeek's classification, introduced in 1952[2], was an early standard. It has five categories, which are based on clinical and pathologic findings and the size and type of vessel involvement.

These are periarteritis nodosa, hypersensitivity angiitis, allergic granulomatous angiitis, rheumatic arteritis, and temporal arteritis.

Periarteritis nodosa in this classification conforms to the syndrome described by Kussmaul and Maier. Small and medium-sized arteries in many parts of the body can be affected. Histologically, all layers of the vessel wall are involved in varying stages of inflammation. Aneurysm formation may occur and result in nodules along the arteries.

Hypersensitivity angiitis includes by definition a history of allergy, usually allergy to a drug. Pathologically, this disease involves small arteries, arterioles, and venules, especially of the skin, heart, lungs, and kidneys. The inflammation is at the same stage in all organs.

Allergic angiitis and granulomatosis (Churg-Strauss vasculitis) always include a history of asthma that has preceded the onset of inflammation in blood vessels. Small arteries and veins are involved and are associated with extravascular granulomas and usually peripheral eosinophilia.

Rheumatic arteritis classically occurs in rheumatic fever, involves small blood vessels, especially in the heart, and includes the formation of Aschoff bodies.

Temporal arteritis is defined as a disease of older persons, with involvement of large cranial arteries. Biopsy specimens of the involved temporal artery frequently will show disruption of the arterial wall, changes of chronic inflammation, and the presence of multinucleated giant cells.

Not all cases of vasculitis fit nicely into Zeek's classification; consequently, many other classifications have been devised.[3-5] From a clinical point of view, a classification based on the size of the vessel alone is not satisfactory for several reasons. Frequently, the determination of the size of the vessel involved is dependent on the tissue sample or the technique used. For example, punch biopsy of the skin and biopsies of muscle, testicle, sural nerve, and kidney only sample small vessels. Visceral arteriography reveals pathologic changes in large and medium-sized vessels. Autopsy studies usually show an overlap in sizes of involved vessels in those cases thought to represent polyarteritis (periarteritis) nodosa or hypersensitivity angiitis. An example of varying sized vessel involvement is demonstrated in a recent case report of a patient with Churg-Strauss vasculitis and primary biliary cirrhosis. This patient initially had a small vessel vasculitis and later had a larger artery involvement, including the temporal arteries.[6]

The type of pathologic change in the vessel wall can be helpful for classification in some situations but cannot be relied on exclusively. Granulomas and giant cell formation may be seen in arteritis of large arteries, including Takayasu's arteritis and giant cell arteritis (temporal arteritis). Extravascular granulomas may be found in Wegener's granulomatosis and allergic granulomatous vasculitis. Fibrinoid necrosis of the vessel wall is seen in polyarteritis nodosa and hypersensitivity angiitis. However, frequently these typical pathologic features may not be seen because of variability of sampling and the effects of time and treatment on the pathologic picture. The type of cellular infiltration may vary depending on the stage of injury. Early in the course of vascular inflammation, polymorphonuclear leukocytes are found, whereas later a chronic mononuclear cell infiltration is predominant. Early in the case of Churg-Strauss vasculitis, the primary infiltrating cell is the eosinophil, but in the older lesions, these cells may not predominate.

It was thought that if the pathogenesis of the various vasculitides could be elucidated, this would provide a basis for establishing a rational classification. However, this has not been true thus far. For example, in vasculitis associated with hepatitis B surface antigen, immune complexes containing the virus appear to be related to the development of the vasculitis. Unfortunately, HB$_s$Ag with vasculitis is not correlated with a particular set of clinical features or involvement of vessels of a certain size. No classification has been devised that is completely satisfactory.

The classification proposed by Fauci, Haynes, and Katz is comprehensive and useful to the clinician.[7] A modification of that classification will be discussed and is shown in Table 72–1. Polyarteritis nodosa can be distinguished clinically. The term polyarteritis has been used in recent years instead of periarteritis because periarteritis implies inflammation around the arteries when in reality the entire wall of the artery is involved with the inflammation. Nodosa is still used as part of the term, but nodules in the classic Kussmaul-Maier sense are rarely found on physical examination. The term polyarteritis nodosa should be reserved for that clinical situation in which peripheral neuropathy or visceral involvement or both are the dominant features of the disease. Usually other manifestations, such as articular and cutaneous involvement, are present. Some patients have findings limited to one organ. Pathologic changes include vascular inflammation with fibrinoid necrosis and destruction of the wall of small and medium-sized arteries. The pathologic features of vascular involvement may be in various stages of inflammation and healing from acute fibrinoid necrosis to more chronic changes of intimal proliferation and fibrosis of the artery wall. This type of vasculitic disease may complicate rheu-

Table 72–1. Classification of Vasculitis

Polyarteritis (nodosa)
  Idiopathic
  Associated with hepatitis B surface antigen and other viruses
    (CMV)
  Associated with rheumatic diseases (rheumatoid arthritis,
    Sjögren's syndrome)
  Associated with malignancies (hairy cell leukemia)
Hypersensitivity vasculitis (small vessel vasculitis)
  Serum sickness (associated with drug reaction)
  Henoch-Schönlein purpura
  Mixed cryoglobulinemia
  Hypocomplementemic vasculitis
  Vasculitis associated with connective tissue disease
  Vasculitis associated with inflammatory conditions such as
    primary biliary cirrhosis
  Vasculitis associated with malignancy
Allergic angiitis and granulomatosis (Churg-Strauss vasculitis)
Wegener's granulomatosis
Lymphomatoid granulomatosis (polymorphic reticulosis)
Arteritis of large arteries
  Giant cell arteritis (temporal arteritis)
  Takayasu's arteritis
  Large artery arteritis complicating diseases such as ankylosing
    spondylitis, Reiter's syndrome, relapsing polychondritis, and
    Cogan's syndrome
Granulomatous angiitis of the central nervous system
Mucocutaneous lymph node syndrome (Kawasaki's disease)
Infectious vasculitis
Buerger's disease (thromboangitis obliterans)

matoid arthritis, Sjögren's syndrome, mixed cryoglobulinemia, vasculitis associated with HB$_s$Ag, and certain malignancies, especially hairy cell leukemia.

Hypersensitivity vasculitis is the clinical term used to indicate small vessel disease. The pathologic picture is a leukocytoclastic vasculitis in such cases. These terms can be used to describe that group of diseases in which a small vessel vasculitis of the skin is the dominant feature of the disease. In this category we include a serum sickness–like illness associated with a drug reaction, Henoch-Schönlein purpura; mixed cryoglobulinemia; hypocomplementemic vasculitis; vasculitis associated with connective tissue diseases such as rheumatoid arthritis, systemic lupus erythematosus, and Sjögren's syndrome; vasculitis associated with inflammatory conditions like inflammatory bowel disease, chronic active hepatitis, and primary biliary cirrhosis; and vasculitis associated with an underlying malignancy. This type of cutaneous involvement may be associated with other types of vasculitis such as polyarteritis nodosa and Wegener's granulomatosis.

Allergic angiitis and granulomatosis (Churg-Strauss vasculitis) forms a clinically distinct entity. The characteristic clinical features are a history of asthma, eosinophilia, and various vasculitic manifestations similar to those seen in polyarteritis nodosa. Examination of involved tissues, usually lung, reveals a necrotizing small vessel vasculitis with extravascular granulomas with eosinophilic infiltration. This disease closely resembles Wegener's granulomatosis pathologically. It is an extremely rare condition.

Wegener's granulomatosis is a recognizable clinical and pathological entity. In this disease small vessels are involved with a vasculitic and granulomatous process, appearing usually in the upper and lower respiratory tract. Other organs may be involved, and a focal necrotizing glomerulonephritis commonly occurs. Lymphomatoid granulomatosis is a disease resembling Wegener's granulomatosis. It is characterized by an angiocentric and angiodestructive vasculitis that may result in nodular lesions in the lung, kidneys, central nervous system, and skin. The cellular infiltrate is pleomorphic and may evolve into a lymphoproliferative disease. This appears to be histologically similar or identical to polymorphic reticulosis in many cases.

The next categorization is arteritis of the medium-sized and large arteries. This group of diseases can be subdivided into giant cell arteritis (temporal arteritis or cranial arteritis) and Takayasu's arteritis. Giant cell arteritis is characterized by the onset of disease in patients older than 50 years, clinical evidence of involvement of cranial arteries, frequently polymyalgia rheumatica, and a markedly elevated erythrocyte sedimentation rate. The diagnosis is made by a temporal artery biopsy, which reveals the pathologic picture of fragmentation of the internal elastica, a chronic mononuclear cell infiltration, and frequently giant cells.

Takayasu's arteritis is similar to giant cell arteritis pathologically but occurs in young adults, usually women, and there appears to be a predilection for this disease to occur in persons of an oriental background. Constitutional features appear early in the course of the disease and may include a polymyalgia-like picture, arthritis, and an elevated erythrocyte sedimentation rate. Later in the course of the disease, the symptoms are related to arterial occlusion and resulting ischemia. The diagnosis is made by demonstrating aneurysms and arterial occlusion by arteriography. There are other diseases that are associated with a large artery arteritis and specifically an aortitis, including ankylosing spondylitis, Reiter's syndrome, relapsing polychondritis, and Cogan's syndrome.

Vascular inflammation, particularly cutaneous vascular lesions, may occur in association with a variety of infectious diseases as a result of septicemia or embolization. The more common infections associated with cutaneous vascular lesions are gonococcemia, meningococcemia, viral exanthems, rickettsial diseases, staphyloccal septicemia, and pseudomonas septicemia (ecthyma gangrenosum). Septic foci may cause constitutional symptoms, and if the septic focus is a mycotic aneurysm, emboli may be released and result in distal skin lesions similar to other forms of vasculitis. Large-vessel vasculitis (aortitis) may be caused by syphilis and tuberculosis.

Infective endocarditis may closely resemble necrotizing vasculitis, and some of the features of disease in infective endocarditis are due to a vasculitis that is immune complex–induced in which the infecting organism is the inciting antigen. These patients may have Janeway lesions, Osler's nodes, purpuric lesions, glomerulonephritis, and stroke-like features of disease. The patient will usually have a significant heart murmur. Laboratory examination may reveal abnormalities that result from the immune complex disease, and these may include cryoglobulinemia, hypocomplementemia, and the presence of rheumatoid factor. The diagnosis is made by suspecting this diagnosis and obtaining the appropriate blood cultures.

There are other vasculitic diseases that have been described, including Kawasaki's disease or mucocutaneous lymph node syndrome, Berger's disease, which seems to be recognized less commonly than in the past, granulomatous angiitis of CNS, erythema nodosa, and Behçet's disease. This includes only a partial listing of the unusual types of vasculitis.

PATHOGENESIS OF VASCULITIS

Experimental Models of Vasculitis. For many years hypersensitivity mechanisms have been thought to be important in the pathogenesis of vasculitis. In the 1930s, German investigators described subendothelial hyaline necrosis in vessel walls of animals sensitized to various antigens.[8] In 1943, Rich and Gregory[9] produced lesions of polyarteritis by intravenous injection of human serum into rabbits. Subsequent studies showed that these induced vascular lesions are a result of the deposition of immune complexes in the vessel walls.[10,11] Experimental immune complex disease may be induced in several ways. The antigen and antibody may be formed in situ in the vessel wall, as in the Arthus reaction, or deposited from the circulation as in the serum sickness model. The development of experimentally induced immune complex arteritis is dependent on the continued formation of immune complexes, the size of the immune complexes, and the genetic predisposition of the experimental animal to produce only a moderate antibody response. Only large molecular weight complexes are associated with experimental serum sickness.

The site of deposition of the immune complexes from circulation depends in part upon increased vascular permeability. In the animal model this is influenced by the effects of vasoactive amines, histamine and serotonin.[12] Vasoactive amines may be released from platelets by lysis or by aggregation of platelets. This latter mechanism may occur as a result of platelet surface interaction with soluble immune complexes activating the complement cascade or platelet interaction with particulate antigens coated with antibody and early complement components.[13] An immediate hypersensitivity reaction may accompany the immune complex mechanism and influence localization. IgE plus antigen will attach to and degranulate mast cells or basophils releasing vasoactive amines and platelet-activating factor.[14]

Mechanical blood flow factors may influence localization of immune complexes. Turbulent flow at vessel bifurcation results in lesions at the bifurcation of arteries. Dependency or hydrostatic pressure may explain the location of lesions in the skin of lower legs. Induced hypertension in animals will increase the number and severity of vasculitic lesions in serum sickness in animals.[15]

The persistence of immune complexes in circulation is a factor in the development of lesions in experimental animals. Immune complexes are cleared by the reticuloendothelial system (RES), and this mechanism can be blocked by saturating the RES with immune complexes and allowing the excess immune complexes to persist in circulation.[16,17] This gives the immune complexes the opportunity to localize in tissue.

Immune complexes incite inflammation through their ability to activate complement. Activated C3 can bind to a receptor on the polymorphonuclear leukocyte (PMN) and hold the PMN to the localized immune complex.[18] Activation of the complement system releases chemotactic factors attracting PMN to the inflammatory site.[19,20] The PMN phagocytize the deposited immune complexes, leading to a series of inflammatory events involving release of lysosomal enzymes and liberation of arachidonate metabolites and free oxygen radicals, as detailed in Chapter 5.[20]

Some animal diseases resemble human polyarteritis. For example, arteritis involving muscular arteries is seen in mink with Aleutian disease.[21] In this disease there is a predilection for involvement at the bifurcation of arteries, as in the human counterpart. Immunohistochemical studies show IgG, C3, fibrin, and the Aleutian disease virus antigen in areas of fibrinoid necrosis beneath the internal elastic membrane of involved arteries. Circulating complexes of the molecular size of 22 to 25S are present in chronic Aleutian disease. Thus, the arteritis appears to be closely related to immune complexes. A similar immune complex vasculitis may be produced in mice by the lymphocytic choriomeningitis virus.[22]

Other pathologic mechanisms also may result in polyarteritis in animals. Several viruses cause arteritis by localization and growth in the vessel intima. An example is equine viral arteritis.[23] In this disease the equine virus produces vascular endothelial cell damage, which results in an arteritis of small muscular arteries, with widespread medial necrosis. Cytomegalovirus[24] and rubella virus[25] appear to damage vessels in the same fashion.

Pathogenesis of Human Disease. In the late 1930s and early 1940s, it was noted that polyarteritis appeared after injections of hyperimmune serum which were given in the treatment of pneumococcal pneumonia and after the administration of the newly discovered sulfonamides.[26] These clinical observations suggested that hypersensitivity to these substances could play a role in the development of vasculitis similar to that in animals in which the disease was induced by the administrations of various antigens. A viral antigen, hepatitis B surface antigen, has been shown to cause vasculitis in humans by an immune complex mechanism. Approximately twenty years after the association of hepatitis and polyarteritis was first noted,[27] Gocke and co-workers in 1969 demonstrated hepatitis B surface antigen and IgM in an artery wall of a patient with polyarteritis.[28] In subsequent studies, hepatitis B surface antigen has been detected in involved muscular arteries,[29] coronary arteries,[30] dermal vessels,[31] and glomeruli.[32,33] It has been found in involved small and medium-sized arteries. The findings of diminished serum complement, serum immune complexes,[34,35] and viral particles[36] in some patients has suggested that the arteritis is immune complex–induced, with hepatitis B surface antigen as the inciting antigen. However, not all studies of polyarteritis and hepatitis B antigenemia have shown the presence of immune complexes.[37] Cytomegalovirus has been associated with vasculitis in case reports and the mechanism of disease is presumed to be similar to the vasculitis induced by hepatitis B surface antigen.[38]

Vasculitis has been reported in a wide variety of underlying malignancies. Vasculitis has been associated with various types of carcinoma,[39] lymphomas, agnogenic myeloid metaplasia,[40] and immunoblastic lymphadenopathy.[41] In one case report of a patient with polyarteritis associated with carcinoma in whom the vasculitis was presumed to be immune complex induced, immune complexes were composed of antibodies and tumor antigens.[39] The mechanism of disease in these situations appears to be immune complex induced, with the tumor antigen or an opportunistic viral antigen inciting the inflammation.

The recent reports of the relationship of polyarteritis to hairy cell leukemia raises some interesting questions regarding the association and the potential mechanism causing the arteritis.[42-44] Most, but not all, of the reported cases developed their arteritis coincidental to or after the onset of hairy cell leukemia. Most patients had a malfunctioning spleen or had a splenectomy. Consequently, an impaired reticuloendothelial system might be incriminated as allowing the persistence of immune complexes, resulting in vasculitis. However, most patients have not been found to have hypocomplementemia, circulating immune complexes, or HB$_s$Ag. It is possible that other antigens such as cytomegalovirus play a role, or there may be some type of basic predisposition that allows the development of hairy cell leukemia and polyarteritis.

Immune complex mechanisms are important in certain patients with vasculitis in which the inciting antigen cannot be detected. In these patients, rheumatoid factor, diminished serum complement, and low levels of cryoglobulins have been found.[45] Immune complexes have been detected in these patients by a variety of techniques, including the monoclonal rheumatoid factor assay and the polyethylene glycol precipitation method.[46,47] Immunoglobulins, complement, and fibrin have been demonstrated in involved small and medium-sized arteries and in involved glomeruli, substantiating the immune complex mechanism of disease.[48,49] These immune deposits may not always be found even if the lesion was initially immune complex induced. This is because immune complexes may be rapidly cleared after the induction of the lesion.[50] Consequently, the duration of the disease and the treatment will influence the immunopathologic findings. It is known that certain conditions are important in the formation and persistence of circulating immune complexes. Immune complexes formed in a state of antigen excess are more likely to deposit in vessel walls. This concept was illustrated in a patient who developed vasculitis following a streptococcal infection. The patient had produced a suboptimal antibody response to the antigen.[51] Thus, this patient had circulating immune complexes in antigen excess. Other patients studied who produced greater amounts of antibody did not develop vasculitis.

Another factor influencing the pathogenicity of immune complexes is the ability of the reticuloendothelial system to clear immune complexes from circulation. It is not known whether impairment of the reticuloendothelial system frequently occurs in human systemic vasculitis. There has been one report of patients with vasculitis with altered splenic reticuloendothelial function that was reversed by plasma exchange.[52]

There are associations of vasculitis with other factors that may provide additional clues to the underlying mechanism involved. Vasculitis occurring with C2 deficiency or α_1-antitrypsin deficiency[54] suggests that absence of certain complement components or enzyme inhibitors or both may predispose the patients to development of vasculitis. Sergent and Christian reported on several adult patients in whom necrotizing vasculitis developed after an acute otitis media, which implicated a possible infectious cause.[55] However, no pathogens or evidence of an associated viral agent was found. Polyarteritis has been observed in drug abusers, particularly users of methamphetamines,[56] but other factors such as the presence of hepatitis B surface antigen may be more important in the pathogenesis of the vasculitis in these cases.[57] Allergen hyposensitization has been associated with the development of polyarteritis.[58]

Studies to detect anti–arterial wall antibodies have been negative.[59] HLA typing for A and B locus antigens has not suggested an unusual frequency of HLA antigens in patients with polyarteritis associated with hepatitis B antigenemia.[37] HLA-B8 antigens have been associated with Wegener's granulomatosis.[60] HLA-Bw52 has been associated with Takayasu's arteritis in Asians and with HLA-MB3 and HLA-DR4 in North Americans with this disease.[61] Consequently, there appears to be some genetic predisposition to certain types of vascular inflammation.

Cellular immune function has not been systematically investigated in the vasculitic diseases. A granulomatous reaction is a prominent part of the pathology in Wegener's granulomatosis and Churg-Strauss vasculitis. This type of pathologic change is usually associated with cell-mediated immunity. The granulomatous reaction may come about as a result of sensitized lymphocytes reacting with antigen and releasing mediators and recruiting macrophages to the site of injury.[62] A granulomatous reaction can be triggered by chronic immune complex disease. It is probable that many pathogenic mechanisms result in vascular inflammation with similar clinical manifestations.[63] It remains to be determined why certain vessels are involved in certain situations.

Approach to the Patient. When confronted with a patient suspected of having a vasculitis, the clinician should consider the conditions that simulate vasculitis, define the extent of the involvement of the vasculitis by a detailed history, physical examination, and appropriate laboratory examination, and then establish the vascular pathology by a biopsy and/or angiography. When possible, the patient should be studied to clarify the pathogenic mechanism involved.

The clinician must be aware of certain diseases that closely simulate necrotizing vasculitis (Table 72–2). One such disorder is left atrial myxoma.[64,65] Patients with atrial myxoma may demonstrate constitutional features of fever and weight loss; they may exhibit a purpuric rash, intermittent claudication, and Raynaud's phenomenon. Strokelike features involving the eye and central nervous system may occur. Usually auscultation of the heart will reveal a diastolic heart murmur influenced by position, but occasionally there may be no cardiac findings. These patients frequently have an elevated erythrocyte sedimentation rate and hypergammaglobulinemia. The diagnosis is made by obtaining a sector echocardiogram, which will reveal the atrial myxoma.

A variety of infections may result in septicemia or embolization that may produce a vasculitis of infectious etiology that must be differentiated from the inflammatory vasculitides.[66] Infections associated with vascular skin lesions are gonococcemia, meningococcemia, viral exanthems, rickettsial diseases, staphyloccal septicemia, and pseudomonas septicemia. Rarely, an infection of a localized area of the arterial wall, a mycotic aneurysm, can give rise to emboli, resulting in skin lesions distal to the aneurysm, producing a localized infectious vasculitis.

Infective endocarditis simulates necrotizing vasculitis, and some of the features of infective endocarditis are due to an immune complex process, with the infecting organism as the inciting antigen.[67] The manifestations may include a variety of skin lesions and a glomerulonephritis. In these situations the diagnosis can be established by obtaining the appropriate blood cultures.

Underlying malignancies may be associated with constitutional symptoms, a polymyalgia rheumatica symptom complex, and rarely actual vasculitic lesions, especially involving the skin. Consequently, this possibility must be considered when the physician is confronted with a patient with features suggestive of systemic vasculitis.

In the older individual, skin lesions of livedo reticularis and digital infarcts may result from cholesterol embolization arising from artheromatous aneurysms,

Table 72–2. Diseases Simulating Systemic Vasculitis

Atrial myxoma
Septicemia (gonococcemia, meningococcemia, Rocky Mountain spotted fever)
Infective endocarditis
Mycotic aneurysm and embolization
Malignancies—lymphoma
Cholesterol embolization from a large artery aneurysm

usually abdominal aortic aneurysms, again simulating a systemic vasculitis.[68] This diagnosis can be made by having a high index of suspicion in patients in the older age group with an aneurysm and/or peripheral vascular disease when there are no symptoms or laboratory abnormalities suggesting a systemic inflammatory process. The diagnosis can be substantiated by appropriate angiographic studies.

POLYARTERITIS

Polyarteritis, also termed "periarteritis nodosa" and "polyarteritis nodosa" (PAN), is a disease of small and medium-sized arteries. Polyarteritis may involve any organ, but the skin, joints, peripheral nerves, gut, and kidney are most commonly involved. There is a spectrum of severity from progressive fulminant disease to limited disease. Polyarteritis may also be a manifestation or complication of other diseases, such as rheumatoid arthritis, Sjögren's syndrome, mixed cryoglobulinemia,[69] and hairy cell leukemia.

Epidemiology. Polyarteritis is an uncommon disease. In one study conducted in Baltimore, a mortality rate of about 0.2 per 100,000 persons per year was found.[70] In another investigation, in which pathologic criteria were used for the diagnosis, an annual incidence rate of 0.7 per 100,000 and a prevalence of 6.3 per 100,000 population were found.[71] A recent study of the Rochester, Minnesota, population revealed an incidence of definite and probable cases of 1.8 per 100,000.[72] Polyarteritis is more common in males, and the sex ratio is about 2 to 1. All age groups may be affected, but it is more common between the ages of 40 and 60 years.

Pathology. The pathology of polyarteritis consists of focal but panmural necrotizing inflammatory lesions in small and medium-sized muscular arteries, with a predilection for involvement at the vessel bifurcation. The lesions may occur in all parts of the body, but there is usually less involvement of the pulmonary and splenic arteries.[73,74] The inflammation is characterized by fibrinoid necrosis and pleomorphic cellular infiltration, with predominantly polymorphonuclear leukocytes and variable numbers of lymphocytes and eosinophils (Fig. 72–1). The normal architecture of the vessel wall, including the elastic laminae, is disrupted. There may be thrombosis or aneurysmal dilatation at the site of the lesion (Fig. 72–2). Healed areas of arteritis show proliferation of fibrous tissue and endothelial cells, which may lead to vessel occlusion. Lesions at all stages of progression and healing may be seen pathologically if sufficient tissue is available for study.

It is difficult to determine the frequency of involvement of various organs in polyarteritis because of the heterogeneity of patients included in most studies. In autopsy series, the kidneys and heart are involved in about 70 percent of cases, liver and gastrointestinal tract in 50 percent, peripheral nerves in 50 percent, mesentery and skeletal muscle in 30 percent and central nervous system in 10 percent.[75-77] Cutaneous involvement varies from a few percent to 50 percent.[78]

Of primary importance to the clinician, however, is the ante-mortem frequency of organ involvement, particularly for those tissues available for biopsy. The tissues commonly biopsied for diagnosis are skin, skeletal muscles, peripheral nerves, kidneys, and testes. Skin involvement due to inflammation of cutaneous vessels may represent an early manifestation of disease. Small vessels in the dermis can be sampled by punch skin biopsy. Small arteries can be sampled by excisional biopsy of subcutaneous tissue or skeletal muscle.[77,79] From 30 to 50 percent of "blind" muscle biopsies performed in cases of polyarteritis may reveal evidence of arteritis.[45,77,78]

Testicular biopsies are frequently recommended for the diagnosis of polyarteritis. In autopsy studies, vascular inflammation can be found in the testes of 86 percent of patients when the entire testis is sectioned and examined thoroughly.[80] However, had a needle bi-

Figure 72–1. Polyarteritis. Right lower portion of arterial wall shows fibrinoid necrosis and formation of "microaneurysm." Intense infiltration of leukocytes is present in and about artery wall. Hematoxylin and eosin × 40. (Courtesy of Dr. J. T. Lie.)

gallbladder and appendix are involved in approximately 10 percent of cases in which other involvement of the gut is demonstrated by biopsy. Rarely, polyarteritis may manifest itself solely as cholecystitis or appendicitis.[84,85]

The vascular lesions in peripheral nerves may be widespread and may involve the entire length of an affected nerve. Small arteries, 75 to 200 μm in diameter, located in the epineurium are affected. The arterial alterations are similar to those in other organs, and a single patient may show a spectrum of pathologic changes from fibrinoid necrosis in acute lesions to intimal proliferation and perivascular fibrosis in more chronic lesions. The nerve fiber degeneration that results depends on the extent of vascular involvement. The arterial changes that occur in the peripheral nerves in patients who have rheumatoid arthritis, Wegener's granulomatosis, or allergic angiitis and granulomatosis as well as polyarteritis are indistinguishable.[86] When the sural nerve is involved clinically, biopsy may be helpful in obtaining a histologic diagnosis of polyarteritis. An entire cross-sectional segment of the nerve must be obtained to provide sufficient material for adequate sampling of epineural vessels.[87]

Arteries of the central nervous sytem may be affected but less commonly than the peripheral nerves. Inflammation may be found in the vertebral, carotid, meningeal, cerebral, and deep arteries within the brain.[88] The heart is commonly involved in polyarteritis. Autopsy findings include coronary arteritis (Fig. 72–2), myocar-

Figure 72–2. Polyarteritis involving heart. Aneurysm of proximal portion of left anterior descending coronary artery (*arrow*) formed as a result of necrotizing arteritis.

opsy been done, a diagnosis of polyarteritis would have been confirmed in about 20 percent of the patients with the disease. The biopsy must include the tunica vasculosa and the underlying parenchyma.

The kidney may be involved in 70 to 80 percent of patients with polyarteritis.[81] In autopsy studies, inflammation in the arcuate and interlobar arteries and arterioles is frequently found, all in the same kidney, along with evidence of infarction[82] (Fig. 72–3). Occasionally, perirenal and retroperitoneal hemorrhage occurs due to a hemorrhagic infarct on the surface of the kidney. This pathologic picture is diagnostic of polyarteritis. Glomerulonephritis may be present in one third of cases of polyarteritis. It may be diffuse, segmental, proliferative, or occasionally membranous. "Microscopic polyarteritis" refers to involvement of small vessels and associated segmental glomerulitis. Immunofluorescence studies of involved kidneys usually reveal IgG, IgM, C3, and fibrin in a granular pattern along capillary walls of injured lobules.[45]

On pathologic examination, arteries of the gastrointestinal tract may be involved in up to 50 percent of cases. Vessels of the liver and jejunum are most commonly affected.[83] In the liver, findings include vasculitis, along with aneurysms, infarction, and hepatitis.[76] The

Figure 72–3. Polyarteritis involving kidney. *A*, External surface of kidney shows multiple infarcts (arrowheads). *B*, Mounted microscopic slide shows aneurysmal dilatation of interlobar (*large arrowheads*) and arcuate (*small arrowheads*) arteries. *C*, Arcuate artery shows necrotizing features—fibrinoid necrosis (*large arrowhead*)—and inflammation of vessel wall (*small arrowheads*). Hematoxylin and eosin × 250. *D*, Segmental proliferation (*arrows*) and necrosis and inflammation near vascular pole (*arrowheads*). (Hematoxylin and eosin × 250.) (From Wagoner, R.D., and Holly, K.E.: Parenchymal renal disease: Clinical and pathologic features. *In* Knox, F.G. [ed.]: Textbook of Renal Pathophysiology. Hagerstown, Maryland, Harper & Row, Publishers, 1978, pp. 226–253).

dial infarction, pericarditis, and cardiac hypertrophy.[89] Rarely, cases of isolated coronary arteritis have been described.[90]

Clinical Features. The disease may present in a variety of ways. There is a spectrum of severity from mild, limited disease to fulminating and rapidly fatal forms. Virtually any organ may be affected. Typically, the patient experiences constitutional features of fever, malaise, and weight loss along with manifestations of multisystem involvement such as a skin rash, peripheral neuropathy, and asymmetric polyarthritis. Visceral involvement such as the kidney or gut may present coincidental with these features, or they may appear later. In other cases, single organ involvement may be present alone and may remain limited.[79]

Cutaneous lesions include palpable purpura, ulcerations, livedo reticularis, and ischemic changes of the distal digits (Figs. 72–4 and 72–5). Arthralgia or arthritis is present in polyarteritis in as many as 50 percent of patients.[91] An asymmetric, episodic, nondeforming polyarthritis involving the larger joints of the lower extremity may occur in 20 percent of cases and is common early in the course of the disease. Such symptoms may mimic those of rheumatoid arthritis, but as other manifestations appear, the polyarthritis usually subsides without residual joint damage. Synovial analysis is not diagnostic and

Figure 72–4. Polyarteritis involving skin of legs. Livedo reticularis is most prominent over left anterior region of thigh but is also visible over right thigh, legs below knees, and dorsum of feet. Petechiae and ulcers (*arrow*) are present on anterior and medial portions of lower legs.

shows evidence of mild inflammation, as indicated by a moderate increase in the leukocyte count.[45] Values for complement and rheumatoid factor have not been studied systematically but have been normal in the analyses done.

Peripheral neuropathy may occur in 50 to 70 percent of cases and may be the initial manifestation.[92,93] The upper and lower extremities are affected in about the same frequency. The onset may be sudden, with pain and paresthesias radiating in the distribution of a peripheral nerve, followed in hours or days by a motor deficit of the same peripheral nerve. This may progress asymmetrically to involve other peripheral nerves and produce a mononeuritis multiplex or a multiple mononeuropathy. With additional nerve damage, the final result may be a symmetrical polyneuropathy involving all sensory modalities and motor function. The presence of mononeuritis multiplex in the setting of polyarteritis does not appear to be associated with the same poor prognosis as occurs with the mononeuritis multiplex complicating rheumatoid arthritis.[91,94] Less commonly, a slowly evolving distal sensory neuropathy may occur. Brachial plexopathy has been reported.[95] Clinical manifestations suggestive of central nervous system involvement are much less common than those of peripheral nerve involvement, but the two may appear together. Features suggestive of central nervous system involvement are seizures and hemiparesis.[96]

Clinical renal involvement occurs in about 70 percent of cases. Proteinuria is common and, rarely, a nephrotic syndrome may develop. Equally common is a change in urinary sediment, with red cells and red cell casts suggestive of glomerular involvement.[82] In one series, progressive renal insufficiency was the cause of death in 65 percent of the cases.[97] Acute renal failure has been reported but is distinctly unusual.[98] Hypertension may develop as a result of renal artery or glomerular involvement and is present in about 25 percent of cases.[91,99] Patients with diffuse renal vasculitis may develop renal ischemia, secondary hyperreninemia, and hyperaldosteronism, which may result in accelerated hypertension.[100]

Abdominal pain is the most common gastrointestinal symptom and roughly correlates in location with the organ involved.[83] A patient may rarely present with abdominal pain due to localized gallbladder or appendiceal involvement. In cases of diffuse abdominal pain, mesenteric thrombosis must be considered. Abdominal distention may indicate mesenteric thrombosis with or without peritonitis. Hematemesis and melena are caused by vasculitis of the upper or lower gastrointestinal tract, respectively. Liver involvement, although common in autopsy studies, is rarely detected clinically except in those cases associated with HB$_s$ antigen. The only abnormality reflecting liver involvement may be an elevated level of alkaline phosphatase without elevated bilirubin or transaminase levels. A needle biopsy may be normal despite hepatic vascular lesions. However, an open liver biopsy may help establish the diagnosis.[101]

Cardiac involvement is common pathologically but is

Figure 72–5. Polyarteritis involving skin. Sharply circumscribed skin infarcts are 1 to 1.5 cm in diameter and are in various stages of healing.

recognized less often clinically. Myocardial infarction, when it occurs, is usually silent.[89] Congestive heart failure may develop as a result of coronary insufficiency or hypertension (or both). Tachycardia out of proportion to fever has been noted and may be unassociated with other cardiac findings.

Occasionally patients with polyarteritis have pulmonary involvement. Lung infiltrations may be diffuse and may precede the development of vascular involvement in other organs. However, pulmonary lesions are more common in patients whose findings fit better with granulomatous vasculitis (see Wegener's granulomatosis and Churg-Strauss vasculitis).

Diffuse involvement of skeletal muscle arteries may cause pain and intermittent claudication.[102] Such patients may have a favorable course. Testicular involvement is manifested by pain, but clinical involvement indicated by swelling or induration has been reported to be present in only a small percentage of patients in most series.[103] In the eye, polyarteritis may result in an exudative retinal detachment.[104] Toxic retinopathy with retinal hemorrhage or exudates is common.[105] Scleritis rarely occurs in polyarteritis unassociated with granulomatous disease of the lung.

Temporal artery involvement may occur in polyarteritis nodosa. It has not been recognized frequently and may be associated with jaw claudication. The pathologic picture in such cases reveals fibrinoid necrosis without giant cells.[106,107]

Cogan's syndrome—that is, nonsyphilitic keratitis with vestibulo-auditory dysfunction—may be associated with polyarteritis.[108] Most patients with this syndrome have symptoms that suggest a systemic process. These include myalgias, arthralgias, arthritis, and cardiovascular changes with occasional aortic insufficiency.[109] Large arteries may be affected.

Polyarteritis occurring in childhood is rare and may take two forms.[110] The infantile form occurs in children less than two years of age and may be similar to the mucocutaneous lymph node syndrome. Polyarteritis of older children is identical to adult polyarteritis. Children with the infantile form frequently have a limited number of organs involved and usually have some type of heart involvement. In childhood polyarteritis the following clinical features are common and should suggest this possibility: high fever, abdominal pain, vomiting or diarrhea, leukocytosis, proteinemia, and signs of cardiac involvement. In such a situation infection must be ruled out and then the diagnosis established either by biopsy of involved tissue or by angiography. If the child has the clinical criteria of the mucocutaneous lymph node syndrome (see that section), then a conservative management approach can be followed unless there is deterioration of major organs.

The clinical and laboratory features in patients who have HB$_s$ antigens are not different from those in patients who are antigen negative, except for variable hepatic dysfunction in some of the former patients.[37] There is no constant temporal relationship between the onset of the polyarteritis and liver disease. In addition, the activity of the arteritis does not parallel the activity of the hepatitis.[111] Clinical features of polyarteritis may be the initial manifestation or may be superimposed on the picture of chronic active hepatitis, or the polyarteritis and the acute hepatitis may occur simultaneously. Polyarteritis develops in patients who are chronic HB$_s$ antigen carriers.[112] There is a spectrum of vascular involvement in patients with associated HB$_s$ antigen, including digital vasospasm,[113] proliferative glomerulonephritis, hypertension,[114] and cryoglobulinemia.[115]

Laboratory Tests. Most tests are nonspecific and reflect the systemic inflammatory nature of the disease. An elevated erythrocyte sedimentation rate, normochromic anemia, and diminished levels of serum albumin are usually present. Neutrophilic leukocytosis, thrombocytosis and elevation of serum globulins may be found. Eosinophilia is generally associated with pulmonary involvement, particularly in allergic angiitis and granulomatosis.

Diminished concentrations of serum whole complement and C3 and C4 components may be associated with active disease[45] and may be present in about 25 percent of the cases.[91] Such cases usually have diffuse cutaneous or renal disease. Rheumatoid factor may be present in patients with hypocomplementemia and in either hepatitis B positive or negative patients.

HB$_s$ antigen has been found in 10 to 54 percent of patients, depending on the series.[45,116] In some cases the antigen is detected in the serum transiently, and serial determinations must be performed to detect it. Diminished fibrinolysis in the blood and tissue has been noted in patients with polyarteritis.[117,118] This is probably due to intravascular coagulation and fibrinolysis and is related to extensive vascular inflammation.

Immune complexes may be detected in patients with active polyarteritis by the monoclonal rheumatoid factor assay[46] and by polyethylene glycol precipitation.[47] It is not known whether these measurements are any more effective in following patients than the erythrocyte sedimentation rate. At present they should be regarded as investigational tools.

Diagnosis. Because the symptoms in polyarteritis are so diverse, the diagnosis is often difficult and delayed.[119] However, polyarteritis should be suspected in a patient with findings such as fever, chills, weight loss, fatigue, and multisystem involvement. A careful examination may reveal early cutaneous manifestations, a peripheral neuropathy, or renal involvement that might provide a clue to the diagnosis. The development of mononeuritis multiplex in a patient who has a systemic disease is highly suggestive of an underlying vasculitis. It must be remembered that the findings in patients with septicemia, infective endocarditis, malignancy, left atrial myxoma, and atherosclerosis with large artery aneurysms and cholesterol embolization may resemble patients with polyarteritis. In addition, it should be kept in mind that patients with rheumatoid arthritis, Sjögren's syndrome, and certain malignancies may have a complicating necrotizing vasculitis that may resemble polyarteritis.

Anemia, thrombocytosis, a high erythrocyte sedimentation rate, and a low level of serum albumin substantiate the systemic nature of the disease but are not helpful diagnostically. The presence of HB$_s$ antigen, diminished serum complement, or cryoglobulinemia, when coupled with suspicious clinical features, suggests the diagnosis of polyarteritis.

Evidence of vascular involvement can be established by biopsy or angiography. The likelihood of finding arteritis is greatest when clinically abnormal tissues are examined. The most accessible involved tissues are the skin, sural nerve, and kidney. Involvement of the sural nerve can be verified by electromyography.[120] Muscle biopsy may be obtained when involved tissue is not easily identified or accessible. The frequency of a positive biopsy specimen is highest when painful or tender muscles

are biopsied. In cases with abnormalities of urinary sediment or proteinuria, renal biopsy will usually reveal focal necrotizing glomerulonephritis and in about one half of the cases a small vessel vasculitis will be demonstrated.

Arteriography may be helpful diagnostically and may provide information on prognosis by defining the extent of disease. Positive findings include arterial saccular or fusiform aneurysms and narrowing or tapering of the arteries (Fig. 72–6).[121-124] This procedure is most appropriate when involved organs are not available for biopsy and in cases with evidence of intra-abdominal involvement. However, angiograms may be positive in cases without obvious visceral symptoms. Aneurysms have been found most commonly in the kidney but also occur in the liver and in mesenteric, cerebral, splenic, pulmonary, lumbar, intercostal, inferior phrenic, hypogastric, and gastroduodenal arteries. The lesions may disappear with improvement of the vasculitis.[124] There is a remote possibility of arterial rupture and hemorrhage secondary to the arteriography. Infarction of the kidney may cause a mottled appearance on nephrotomograms.

It must be remembered that other conditions may be associated with an identical or similar roentgenographic picture.[125] These conditions include Wegener's granulomatosis, acute angiitis and granulomatosis, systemic lupus erythematosis, thrombotic thrombocytopenia purpura, infective endocarditis, atrial myxoma, and metastatic malignancy involving the peritoneum.[126]

Prognosis. Polyarteritis commonly follows an acute course, and most of the deaths occur within the first year of the disease (Fig. 72–7).[78,91] Deaths occurring within the first year are usually a result of uncontrolled vasculitis. Late deaths, occurring after one year of disease, are usually either a result of complications of treatment or vascular deaths such as myocardial infarction

Figure 72–6. Superior mesenteric arteriogram in patient with polyarteritis. Several small aneurysms (*arrows*) are present in branches of superior mesenteric artery. (Courtesy of Dr. A. W. Stanson.)

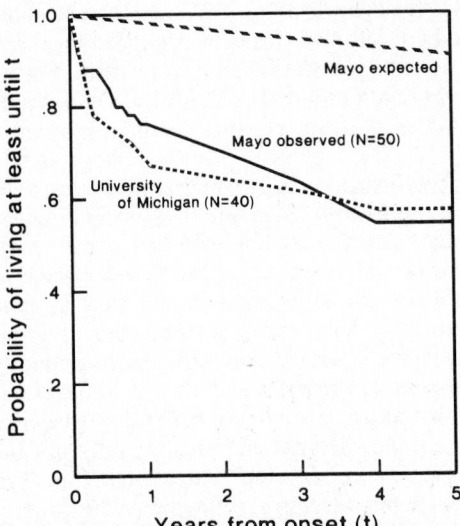

Figure 72–7. Graph showing five year survival of patients with polyarteritis. (From Cohen, R.D., Conn, D.L., and Ilstrup, D.M.: Clinical features, prognosis, and response to treatment in polyarteritis. May Clin. Proc. 55:146, 1980, and Sack, M., Cassidy, J.T., and Bole, G.G.: Prognostic factors in polyarteritis. J. Rheumatol. 2:411, 1975.)

or stroke. The prognosis of untreated polyarteritis is poor, and the 5-year survival is less than 15 percent. Improved survivorship has occurred in recent years with the use of corticosteroids, and most studies reveal a 5-year survival of between 50 and 60 percent. Recent studies indicate an even higher survival rate with the use of a combination of corticosteroids and cytotoxic agents in selected cases. It does appear that the involvement of certain organ systems has a bearing on the outcome. The involvement of the kidneys and gut and the appearance of aneurysms on visceral angiography may portend a poorer outcome. Acute oligemic renal failure associated with polyarteritis is rare—but is almost always fatal.[127]

Treatment. Corticosteroids are effective in some patients with polyarteritis, but the overall survival has not improved beyond 50 to 60 percent 5-year survival over the last 30 years. Recent retrospective studies have shown an improved survival with the addition of cyclophosphamide or azathioprine.[128,129] Other modalities of treatment have been advocated in case reports, including intravenous methylprednisolone,[130] intravenous methotrexate,[131] and plasma exchange.[132] Most deaths occur within the first year of disease, and patients with more extensive and progressive disease, particularly with gut and renal involvement, have the poorest outcome.[91] With the information available, a reasonable rational management approach can be designed.

Decisions regarding treatment of polyarteritis depend upon the extent of disease, the organs involved, and the rate of progression of disease. Consequently, patients with evidence of progressive renal, gastrointestinal, central nervous system, or heart involvement should be treated vigorously. These patients should be treated with high doses of prednisone or its equivalent, given in three or four divided doses a day and in total daily doses from 60 to 100 mg a day. If this treatment does not result in control of the disease, then one of several additional treatment modalities should be considered. Intravenous administration of methylprednisolone in doses of 1 g administered over 30 minutes can be given on three or four successive days to see if this controls the disease. Another approach would be the addition of a cytotoxic drug.

Plasma exchange could be considered in cases with rapidly progressive arteritic disease with evidence of an ongoing immune complex process as indicated by the presence of serum cryoglobulins and diminished serum complement. Plasma exchange can be performed two or three times per week depending upon the status of the patient, the patient's tolerance, and the response to this treatment. These patients should also be treated concomitantly with corticosteroids and a cytotoxic agent, preferably cyclophosphamide, in a dose of 2 mg per kg. Plasmapheresis may induce a rebound of antibody formation, which may exacerbate the disease, and this rebound can be modified by the addition of a cytotoxic drug.

In patients with involvement of the skin, peripheral nerves, musculoskeletal system, or peripheral vascular system with digital gangrene without visceral involvement, treatment should include high, divided doses of prednisone until there is control of the disease.

In some patients with polyarteritis that has involved the visceral organs and has been controlled with corticosteroids, a cytotoxic agent, either cyclophosphamide or azathioprine, in a dose of 2 mg per kg, may be added for long-term control and for a steroid-sparing effect.

The side effects of these drugs must be monitored and prevented when possible. Patients on high doses of corticosteroids are susceptible to opportunistic infections, peptic ulceration, hypertension, hypokalemia, diabetes mellitus, masking of intra-abdominal events such as perforated diverticulum, mental changes, and atrophy of the skin resulting in ecchymoses. Long-term side effects include osteoporosis with vertebral collapse, avascular necrosis, and posterior subcapsular cataract formation. Prophylactic use of calcium and vitamin D retards the development of osteoporosis.

Cyclophosphamide may be associated with alopecia, hemorrhage, cystitis, leukopenia, and gonadal dysfunction. These patients may potentially develop bladder scarring and malignancies, are susceptible to opportunistic infections, and may be susceptible to late oncogenesis.[133] Patients taking azathioprine and methotrexate may develop hepatic toxicity as well as bone marrow suppression. Consequently, the white blood cells must be monitored closely in these patients. Patients on cyclophosphamide must have their urine monitored for hematuria. Specific recommendations on the use of these agents is provided in Chapter 55.

It must be remembered that as the dose of prednisone is tapered, the hematologic toxic effects of the cytotoxic agents increase. Therefore, when tapering the prednisone, the dose of cyclophosphamide (or other cytotoxic drug) should be reduced and the white blood cell count monitored carefully. In patients successfully managed, with the disease controlled, maintenance cytotoxic treatment should continue for a year after disease control.

When the disease is controlled, the corticosteroid dose should be tapered. This can be done by keeping the dose divided and gradually reducing each of the doses. An alternative approach would be to double the dose given daily and administer it every other day in a single dose and gradually taper that dose. With the latter program, the potential exists for disease exacerbation. The reduction will be dependent upon the clinical status and the erythrocyte sedimentation rate. At times, the dose may need to be increased or stabilized for a period of time before reduction is again attempted. It should be the goal to reduce the dose to the lowest possible level.

Late complications and deaths associated with polyarteritis include renal vascular hypertension, cerebrovascular disease, and coronary artery disease.[91,128] These vascular occlusive complications may be the result of previous arterial inflammation plus the atherosclerosis-producing effects of the corticosteroids. With inflammation of the arteries there may be platelet adherence to the inflamed arterial wall, and this has the potential for causing intimal proliferation and eventual luminal occlusion.[134] Treatment with antiplatelet drugs during the course of polyarteritis should be considered, although data supporting the efficacy of this approach are not available.

Despite good management, some patients with polyarteritis develop kidney failure. Kidney transplantation has been successful in some cases after the arteritis has become inactive.[135] Patients with congestive heart failure should be managed with digoxin, and the hypertension should be vigorously controlled. Detailed attention should be given to fluid and electrolyte balance. Nonsteroidal anti-inflammatory drugs may be used as necessary for articular symptoms.

VASCULITIS ASSOCIATED WITH RHEUMATIC DISEASES

A small vessel vasculitis is intimately associated with many of the clinical manifestations seen in rheumatoid arthritis and systemic lupus erythematosus. The early development of the rheumatoid nodule is associated with a small vessel vasculitis.[136] In systemic lupus erythematosus, a small vessel vasculitis is responsible for many of the skin lesions.[137] Palpable purpura that may be seen in Sjögren's syndrome is due to a small vessel vasculitis. In each of these situations, the small vessel vasculitis is triggered by an immune complex mechanism.[138] Also, small and medium-sized arteries in the extremities, peripheral nerves, and occasionally other organs may be involved in rheumatoid arthritis.[139] It is of note that patients with rheumatoid vasculitis have a higher frequency of HLA-DR4 than those with uncomplicated rheumatoid arthritis, suggesting an inherited suscepti-

bility to this complication. Several different clinical pictures may develop.[140] Occasionally the clinical and pathologic features are similar to polyarteritis. Yet there are some significant differences clinically. The vasculitic syndromes complicating rheumatoid arthritis will be discussed.

Clinical Features. The superimposed systemic vasculitis complicating rheumatoid arthritis is uncommon. It usually occurs in rheumatoid patients who have had their disease for a number of years, usually ten or more years. Males are afflicted as commonly as females.[141] These patients have more severe rheumatoid arthritis with destructive joint disease, rheumatoid nodules, and a higher titer of rheumatoid factor.[140] Patients with Felty's syndrome are more likely to develop vasculitic complications. The rheumatoid synovitis may not be active at the time of the development of the clinical features of the systemic vasculitis. The clinical features include a variety of skin lesions: nailfold infarcts, leg ulcers, and digital gangrene (Fig. 72-8). The nailfold infarcts and leg ulcers are presumed to be due to involvement of small vessels.[142] It should be noted that not all patients with nailfold infarcts and leg ulcers go on to systemic vasculitis. Distal sensory neuropathy is another manifestation seen in vasculitis that also may occur alone without widespread vascular involvement.

The more ominous manifestations of vasculitis are the appearance of infarctions of the fingertips and a sensorimotor neuropathy.[141] If rate of appearance of new areas of involvement is rapid, this indicates widespread arterial disease. Patients also may display constitutional features, including fever. In some patients the vasculitis may extend to involve mesenteric, coronary, and cerebral arteries.

It has been thought by some that the widespread vasculitis complicating rheumatoid arthritis is caused by corticosteroids. However, patients who have never been on corticosteroids also may develop vasculitis. Wide fluctuations in corticosteroid dose, such as those caused by abruptly stopping the drug, may allow an underlying vasculitis to progress rapidly.[144] Patients with widespread vasculitic disease with three or four extremities involved with a sensorimotor neuropathy have a poor outcome.[145]

The clinical picture of systemic rheumatoid vasculitis differs from that of polyarteritis in that rheumatoid vasculitis is not associated with significant renal involvement. Patients with rheumatoid vasculitis have high titers of rheumatoid factor, low serum complement, cryoglobulins, and immune complex material in the serum.[146-148] In addition, patients with rheumatoid vasculitis will usually have an elevated erythrocyte sedimentation rate, anemia, thrombocytosis, and a diminished serum albumin.

Pathology. Study of involved vessels from patients with rheumatoid vasculitis reveals a pathologic picture identical to that seen in polyarteritis.[149] Small and medium-sized arteries are involved. In some cases the distribution of vascular lesions is like that in polyarteritis. Arterial lesions may be found in various stages of in-

Figure 72–8. Gangrene of toes and ulcerations of feet due to rheumatoid vasculitis.

flammation and healing. Early lesions will include fibrinoid necrosis of the wall with an inflammatory cell infiltrate. Chronic changes with artery wall fibrosis, occlusion, and recanalization may be seen. One pathologic difference from polyarteritis is the finding of small and medium-sized arteries involved with an occlusive intimal proliferation without much inflammation.[139] This pathologic picture is similar to that seen in scleroderma. The acute arterial lesions are immune complex induced.[143] These immune deposits are not found in the more chronic lesions as shown by the finding of immunoglobulins and complement in the involved arteries. Rather fibrin-fibrinogen is found. The fibrin may stimulate the intimal proliferative response.

Treatment. The treatment of rheumatoid vasculitis depends upon the type and the extent of the lesions. Nailfold infarcts, leg ulcers, and distal sensory neuropathy require local care and the usual program for rheumatoid arthritis, including nonsteroidal anti-inflammatory drugs. If the patient has not been on gold or penicillamine, then one of those agents should be started. Patients with fingertip infarctions and a sensorimotor neuropathy whose disease is progressive should be treated with corticosteroids in doses described in the section on polyarteritis. Cyclophosphamide should be started, to aid in control of the disease and allow smooth steroid tapering.[150] Plasma exchange can be considered for the patient resistant to the above drugs.[151]

HYPERSENSITIVITY VASCULITIS (LEUKOCYTOCLASTIC VASCULITIS)

This group includes a variety of conditions in which involvement of small blood vessels (postcapillary venules) of the skin and occasionally other organs are the prominent features of disease. Leukocytoclastic vasculitis is the term describing the pathology in which small blood vessels are infiltrated with polymorphonuclear leukocytes and there is destruction of the vessel wall and fragmentation of the PMNs. This disease was described by Zeek and colleagues and called hypersensitivity angiitis. In their description it occurred after some antigenic stimulus, such as the administration of horse serum, and all the lesions were in the same pathologic stage of development.[152] This type of disease, with primary skin involvement and a leukocytoclastic pathological picture, can be seen in a number of conditions: Henoch-Schönlein purpura, mixed cryoglobulinemia, a serum sickness–like reaction associated with drug hypersensitivity, hypocomplementemic vasculitis, vasculitis associated with certain connective tissue diseases, such as Sjögren's syndrome, vasculitis associated with other inflammatory conditions, such as hypergammaglobulinemic purpura, chronic active hepatitis, ulcerative colitis, and primary biliary cirrhosis, vasculitis associated with malignancies, and even polyarteritis and Wegener's syndrome.[153]

Pathogenesis. Allergy to drugs, a number of bacterial, parasitic and viral agents, and probably other yet undefined antigens may trigger this vasculitis. Both immune complexes and cell-mediated reactions have been implicated in the development of necrotic vascular skin lesions.[154] Hypocomplementemia may be associated with a predominantly polymorphonuclear perivenular infiltrate and normocomplementemia associated with a lymphocytic infiltrate.[155]

The inflammatory process in some of these cases is initiated by deposition of immune complexes derived from circulation which have activated complement and generated polymorphonuclear chemotaxis. The tissue necrosis occurs as a result of polymorphonuclear release of lysosomal enzymes and other noxious agents such as free radicals.[156] Complement and immunoglobulins have been demonstrated in the walls of subepidermal small vessels obtained in biopsy specimens.[157,158] The earlier the lesion, the greater the likelihood of demonstrating positive immune deposits. Similarly sized vessels in other organs may be involved to varying extents, as described below. Immune reactants have been identified in the walls of vessels in the dermis of biopsy specimens taken from clinically normal skin that is within 2 to 3 cm of an active lesion. In some studies, immunoglobulins and complement have been found in vessels in normal skin, in these cases after local injections of histamine but not in vessels in normal uninjected skin.

In hypersensitivity vasculitis, the small blood vessels, primarily the postcapillary venules, in the upper dermis and some viscera are affected. The histopathologic appearance depends on the severity of the reaction and the age of the lesion.[159] Typically, in the acute phase, endothelial swelling occurs, often with occlusion of the vessel lumen. There is infiltration of the wall and perivascular areas by polymorphonuclear leukocytes, with leukocytoclasis and fragmentation of nuclei ("nuclear dust") (Fig. 72–9). Other features include necrosis of vessel walls, fibrinoid deposits, and extravasation of red blood cells. In some cases a diffuse infiltration of polymorphonuclear leukocytes is seen with leukocytoclasis but no prominent vessel destruction. In later stages of a severe reaction, necrosis of much of the connective tissue of the dermis may be found, so that recognition of specific vessels is not possible.

Clinical Features. The manifestations usually appear abruptly with the appearance of skin lesions. In cases that are drug induced, the symptoms usually appear within a few days of initiation of drug treatment. Many drugs have been implicated. The most common are penicillin and its derivatives and sulfa drugs. The list of other drugs that may initiate hypersensitivity vasculitis would include most drugs. The fact that a patient has been on a drug for an extended time does not exclude that drug from consideration. Drug hypersensitivity is not time or dose dependent.[160]

The skin lesions appear as flat, erythematous, purpuric macules, which progress to papules or "palpable purpura."[161] The papular quality is an important feature, since it distinguishes these lesions from noninflammatory purpura. The eruption may occur on any part of the skin but is seen especially over the dependent areas, such as the lower extremities or back and gluteal regions of recumbent patients. Lesions are also commonly seen on the forearms and hands, but it is unusual to find lesions on the upper portion of the trunk or face.

Crops of cutaneous lesions may develop in episodes at irregular intervals. Individual lesions last from 1 to 4 weeks and leave hyperpigmentation and sometimes atrophic scars when they resolve. The size of the lesions varies from a millimeter to several centimeters when individual lesions coalesce. In some cases, annular lesions resembling erythema multiforme may be present. Vesicles and bullae may develop in more severe cases. They may contain bloody fluid. If the skin necrosis is severe enough, ulceration and eventual scarring may result. Smaller skin lesions rarely cause symptoms. However, larger papules, nodules, or ulcerative lesions are frequently painful. Edema of the lower part of the legs, ankles, and feet may be associated.

Constitutional symptoms, including fever, may accompany the appearance of the skin lesions. Arthralgias are present in the majority of patients. Palpable synovitis is less common. Other organs may be involved. Vasculitis can involve the kidney, and renal insufficiency may develop. Renal involvement is manifest by proteinuria and hematuria. Abdominal pain and gastrointestinal bleeding can occur. The bleeding may be severe enough to require blood transfusions. Pulmonary infiltrations, either nodular or diffuse, may be seen on chest radiographs. Pleural effusions have been described. Neurologic involvement may occur and present with headaches, diplopia, and, rarely, an organic brain syndrome. Other organ involvement is distinctly less common. A normochromic anemia and an increased erythrocyte sedimentation rate may be present during attacks and reflect the extent of the inflammatory process. Eosinophilia may be present.

Figure 72–9. Cutaneous vasculitis. Dermal vessels, probably venules, are sectioned longitudinally. Intense infiltration of inflammatory cells (primarily polymorphonuclear leukocytes) has resulted in narrowing and occlusion of vessel lumen and in necrosis of wall. Fragments of degenerated leukocyte nuclei ("nuclear dust") are visible in perivascular areas. Hematoxylin and eosin × 100.

Treatment. In every case any potential inciting drug or antigen should be discontinued or removed. In very mild cases with a brief single episode of a few scattered purpuric areas without internal organ involvement, no specific treatment is needed. If systemic symptoms are present and skin lesions are diffuse, or if internal organ involvement is present, use of corticosteroids will usually be necessary. The initial dosage can be varied, depending on the severity of the findings, and may range from 20 mg per day of prednisone, or the equivalent dose of another corticosteroid, to 40 to 60 mg per day for multisystem involvement. When the clinical abnormalities have been suppressed, the dosage should be gradually reduced to the lowest amount necessary to control the symptoms and findings. Corticosteroids are effective in most instances, but cytotoxic drugs may be considered when corticosteroids have not been successful or if hypercortisonism has developed. However, cytotoxic drugs have not yet been clearly shown to be beneficial in most patients.

The outlook is favorable in most instances. The course of an individual patient is unpredictable, however. A single episode lasting 2 to 4 weeks may be present, or the disease may be recurrent.

Special Forms of Hypersensitivity Vasculitis. *Schönlein-Henoch Purpura.* The syndrome of Schönlein-Henoch purpura has become established as a distinct clinical condition. Persons of any age may be affected, but it occurs primarily in children, with a peak incidence between 4 and 11 years of age.[162,163] The syndrome is also referred to as anaphylactoid purpura and allergic purpura because of circumstantial evidence implicating hypersensitivity to bacteria or viruses as a possible cause.

The cutaneous histopathology is as described previously. Immunofluorescence studies have shown immunoglobulins and complement deposits in cutaneous vessels and kidney, but serum complement levels are usually normal.[164,165] Immunoglobulin A is a most abundant and sometimes the only immunoglobulin found in the skin and kidney lesions. Cases of Schönlein-Henoch purpura with the congenital absence of the second component of complement have been described.[166] This finding plus the observation of IgA deposits in involved tissues suggests that the alternative complement pathway rather than the classic pathway could be involved in the pathogenesis of this disease.

The disease occurs most often in the spring and often follows an upper respiratory tract infection. The classic triad that occurs in up to 80 percent of cases is that of palpable purpura, arthritis, and abdominal pain. Skin lesions are similar to those described above, with some tendency for larger purpuric lesions to develop over the buttocks and lower extremities (Fig. 72–10). Edema of the feet and lower legs is common, and edema may also develop on the hands, scalp, and periorbital areas. The ankle and knee joints are affected most commonly and are swollen, warm, and tender. The arthritis is usually transient. Gastrointestinal lesions may cause severe cramping, abdominal pain, intussusception, hemorrhage, protein-losing enteropathy, or, rarely, perfora-

Figure 72–10. Cutaneous vasculitis—Schönlein-Henoch syndrome. Palpable purpura is most prominent over extensor surfaces of distal regions of upper and lower extremities and over buttocks. Some small skin infarcts are visible (*arrow*).

tion. Renal involvement occurs in approximately one-half the patients, and although such involvement is usually mild, persistent renal insufficiency can occur.[167,168]

For milder cases, supportive treatment alone may be adequate. In more severe instances, particularly in adults, glucocorticoids are indicated.[169]

This disease is generally self-limited; its duration varies from 6 to 16 weeks. Between 5 and 10 percent of patients recover, only to relapse weeks or months later. Such patients with persistent or recurrent renal disease may suffer significant renal impairment. The prognosis is determined mainly by the extent of renal involvement. Allen and colleagues found detectable renal impairment for at least 4 years in 28 percent of their patients.[162] Renal involvement may be more severe in adults.[167]

Hypocomplementemic Vasculitis. McDuffie and co-workers described hypocomplementemic vasculitis in 1973.[170] The incidence is unknown, but the condition is uncommon. The patients described have been young adults, predominantly women. The cause is unknown, but lesional deposits of immunoglobulins and complement and the presence of serum substances that react with Clq and monoclonal rheumatoid factor suggest that the disease is an immune complex–induced process.[171]

Skin biopsies show a polymorphonuclear leukocyte infiltration of small vessels with leukocytoclastic vasculitis.[155,170] In patients with renal involvement, renal biopsies show mild to moderate membranoproliferative glomerulonephritis, with IgG and complement deposited on the glomerular basement membrane in a lumpy, bumpy pattern.

The hallmark of this disease is an urticarial skin eruption.[172] The eruption may occur on any part of the skin, but the face, upper extremities, and trunk are involved most commonly. Urticaria typically lasts 24 to 48 hours; it has a tendency to central clearing, and it fades without leaving a residue (Fig. 72–11). The lesions may be several centimeters in diameter and are usually not pruritic. Some patients have continuous scattered areas of skin involvement, but others have episodes several times a year or more. Purpura, papules, and vesicles may be seen.

Recurrent episodes of urticaria may be associated with fever, joint pain, and abdominal pain. Peripheral joint swelling may occur, and the pattern of joint involvement is similar to that in systemic lupus erythematosus, with symmetric involvement of the small joints but without any residual deformity. The abdominal pain may be accompanied by nausea, vomiting, and tenderness, but bowel sounds are usually normal and rectal bleeding has not been reported. Renal involvement is

Figure 72–11. Cutaneous vasculitis with hypocomplementemia. Large resolving urticarial lesion on flexor surface of forearm shows central clearing.

manifest by hematuria, proteinuria, and red cell casts. Chronic obstructive pulmonary disease has been found in almost half of these cases and is associated with heavy cigarette smoking.[173]

Hypocomplementemia with low levels of both early- and late-reacting components of complement has been found and has paralleled the activity of the disease. Cryoglobulins have been absent or present in only trace amounts. Sera in these patients do not contain significant titers of antinuclear antibodies or rheumatoid factor.

The combination of urticaria and hypocomplementemia, usually accompanied by arthritis, abdominal pain, or mild renal involvement, suggests this syndrome. Skin biopsy of the involved lesion will usually reveal a necrotizing vasculitis. This syndrome resembles systemic lupus erythematosus, but it is differentiated by the absence of serum antinuclear antibodies.

Patients may be treated satisfactorily with corticosteroids. Cytotoxic agents may be used in selected instances in which the corticosteroids are not effective or cannot be lowered to reasonable dosages. The disease appears to follow a chronic course. Some patients may have renal involvement, but this has not progressed to serious renal insufficiency. The associated chronic obstructive pulmonary disease may be the major cause of serious morbidity and mortality.

Mixed Cryoglobulinemia. The syndrome of purpura, arthralgia, weakness, and mixed cryoglobulinemia described by LoSpalluto and associates[174] and Meltzer and co-workers[175] also appears to be a distinct clinical condition in which cutaneous vasculitis is a dominant feature. It is an uncommon disease and one in which there is widespread vasculitis and often progressive glomerulonephritis. It most commonly affects middle-aged females. The disease appears to be immune complex mediated. Immune deposits containing complement have been demonstrated in skin vessel walls and along the glomerular basement membrane.[176,177] The cryoglobulins are present in relatively small amounts, usually less than 100 mg per dl. They contain IgG and IgM, both of which are required for cryoprecipitation. Occasionally IgA is detected. Forty-eight hours or more at 0° C may be required for the demonstration of cryoprecipitation. The IgM component has anti-IgG (rheumatoid factor) activity.[175] Two-thirds of patients were found to be positive for HB_s antigen or its antibody when both serum and cryoprecipitates were examined.[178]

Patients with this syndrome have recurrent episodes of palpable purpura, usually involving the lower extremities, along with arthralgias and slight to moderate hepatosplenomegaly and lymphadenopathy. Some may have disease limited to the skin. A mononeuritis multiplex may occur. Diffuse glomerulonephritis may lead to terminal renal failure.[69] Rheumatoid factor activity may be directed against human but not rabbit IgG. Moderate anemia, hyperglobulinemia, and hypocomplementemia are present.

The cutaneous and histologic pictures may be identical to those of Schönlein-Henoch purpura. However, the cryoglobulins, positive rheumatoid factor, and low levels of serum complement make distinguishing between these two conditions relatively simple. Distinguishing this syndrome from systemic lupus erythematosus may be more difficult, but the absence of antibodies to double-stranded DNA and the absence of immunoglobulins at the dermal-epidermal junction aid in the diagnosis. Mixed cryoglobulinemia has also been seen in a number of other chronic autoimmune or infectious diseases (see Chapter 84).

Treatment of mixed cryoglobulinemia is dependent upon the extent of involvement. Patients with disease limited to the skin may be tried on penicillamine.[179] Patients with more extensive involvement are treated with high doses of prednisone, as described for polyarteritis. The addition of cytotoxic drugs, usually cyclophosphamide, may be required to control the disease and taper the prednisone to a reasonably low level. In some cases plasma exchange may be used in combination with prednisone and cyclophosphamide.

ALLERGIC ANGIITIS AND GRANULOMATOSIS (CHURG-STRAUSS VASCULITIS)

The association in patients of asthma, eosinophilia, vasculitis, and extravascular granulomas was termed "allergic angiitis and granulomatosis" by Churg and Strauss in 1951.[180] These authors considered allergic factors to be important in the development of the disease.

Epidemiology. This form of vasculitis is rare, although no detailed epidemiologic analyses are available. Thirty patients with this condition were found over a 25-year period.[181] In some studies, patients who have had Churg-Strauss vasculitis have been grouped with patients with polyarteritis. Thus, in Rose and Spencer's analysis of 111 patients with polyarteritis, some of the 32 patients with lung involvement had asthma and eosinophilia and probably had Churg-Strauss vasculitis.[3]

The male-to-female ratio appears to be about 2 to 1. The age at onset varies from 15 to 70 years, with a mean of about 47.

Pathogenesis. The cause of allergic angiitis and granulomatosis is not known. There is no direct evidence to suggest an infectious cause. Although Churg and Strauss reported positive *Trichinella* antibody titers in four patients, they found no evidence of parasites in the tissues. Immunoglobulins and complement have been demonstrated in vessel walls in one case.[5] Fibrinogen alone has been found in extravascular granulomas.[5] No data have been reported regarding the role of immune complexes or cell-mediated mechanisms in this disease. Elevated serum IgE concentration has been noted in several cases and may indicate a response to an inciting antigen.[45] Alternatively, the increased concentration of IgE response may reflect a defect in cellular immunity.

Pathology. The characteristic pathologic changes in this disease include small necrotizing granulomas as well as necrotizing vasculitis involving small arteries and venules[180] (Fig. 72–12). Granulomas are typically about

Figure 72–12. Churg-Strauss vasculitis. Autopsy section of lung shows intense inflammatory reaction around two small arteries, with destruction of portion of wall of lower vessel. Central area of fibrinoid necrosis (*arrow*) and surrounding infiltration of leukocytes, which were predominantly eosinophilic, resulted in obliteration of normal alveolar structures. Hematoxylin and eosin × 100. (From Kelalis, P.P., Harrison, E.G., Jr., and Greene, L.F.: 188:963, 1964. By permission of the American Medical Association.)

1 mm or more in diameter and are commonly located near small arteries or veins. They are composed of a central eosinophilic core surrounded radially by macrophages and giant cells. Inflammatory cells are also present in the granulomas, with eosinophils predominating in the early stage of development and lesser numbers being present in the healing stages. Polymorphonuclear leukocytes and lymphocytes are found in varying but smaller numbers. Macrophages and giant cells predominate in the more chronic lesions.

The vascular lesions may be seen in all stages of development. Acutely there is segmental fibrinoid necrosis with infiltration of leukocytes, predominantly eosinophils, in the vessel walls and perivascular spaces. Aneurysms or thrombosis may occur. With healing, chronic changes of endothelial proliferation, narrowing of the lumen, and reparative fibrosis of the vessel may develop. An important feature in many arterial lesions is the presence of macrophages and giant cells around necrotic areas.

Evidence of bronchial asthma is usually present. Histologically, the bronchial wall shows hyalinization of the basement membrane, increased mucus secretion, and mural eosinophilic infiltration. Parenchymal infiltration of the lungs with an eosinophilic exudate and giant cells may be present. The last-named findings are similar to those in Loeffler's pneumonia. The heart is involved more commonly than in polyarteritis. The epicardium frequently contains granulomas. Areas of interstitial eosinophilic infiltration and scattered foci of fibrosis may be found in the myocardium.

Renal biopsies may show a nonspecific focal glomerulonephritis.[181] Study of kidneys at autopsy may reveal more characteristic lesions with eosinophilic infiltration and eosinophilic granulomas. Cutaneous nodules usually show granulomas containing giant cells and eosinophils, often in a perivascular location.[182] Vasculitis and granulomas may be found in the liver, spleen, lymph nodes, and urinary tract. Peripheral nerves show inflammation of epineural vessels and pathologic changes ranging from fibrinoid necrosis with an inflammatory cell infiltration to intimal proliferation and perivascular fibrosis.[86]

Clinical Features. Respiratory manifestations are usually the first features of the disease. There is often a history of asthma or atopy (or both). Other findings include bronchitis and pneumonitis. The mean duration of asthma, the most frequent respiratory manifestation, before the onset of systemic features is 8 years.[181] The development of fever and weight loss may herald the onset of systemic disease. At this time chest roentgenograms are abnormal in approximately half the cases and show changes ranging from patchy, shifting pneumonic infiltrates (Loeffler's syndrome), through massive bilateral nodular infiltrates without cavitation, to diffuse interstitial lung disease. The symptoms of asthma often subside when the vasculitis emerges. The pneumonitis may be an eosinophilic pneumonia.[183] However, the relationship to eosinophilic pneumonitis has not been definitely established.

Cutaneous lesions occur in approximately two-thirds of the cases. Subcutaneous nodules are the most common skin manifestations. Petechiae, purpura, or skin infarctions may be seen. Peripheral neuropathy, usually mononeuritis multiplex, is found in the majority of patients. Cardiac involvement commonly results in congestive heart failure. Abdominal symptoms occur in a small percentage of cases; these may be due to granulomatous vasculitis of vessels of the stomach or small bowel, which causes infarction, ulceration, or perforation. Bloody diarrhea, simulating chronic ulcerative colitis, may be caused by ischemia of the mucosa of the large bowel. Granulomatous involvement of the bowel, liver, or omentum may produce a palpable mass.

Renal disease has been found to be frequent in some series and less common in others. Renal failure occurs infrequently. Eosinophilic granulomatous involvement of the prostate and lower urinary tract is a unique feature of this disease. It occurs in only a small percentage of cases and may cause urinary retention. Polyarthralgias are uncommon, and arthritis is unusual. Rarely, ulceration of the cornea or central nervous system manifestations such as seizures may occur.

Laboratory Tests. The characteristic laboratory abnormality is eosinophilia. In the original 13 patients of Churg and Strauss, the absolute counts ranged from 5000 to 20,000 eosinophils per mm³.[180] An initial leukocytosis with counts as high as 60,000 per mm³ has been seen. The eosinophilia often decreases as the patient improves or is treated. With active disease, anemia and an elevated erythrocyte sedimentation rate are found. Serum rheumatoid factor may be present in low titer.[181] In the few patients studied, an elevated serum IgE has been found and the serum complement has been normal.[45]

Diagnosis. The diagnosis of Churg-Strauss vasculitis is made on the basis of both clinical and pathologic features. As noted, the patient is usually middle-aged and has a history of asthma that has been present for several years. The appearance of a systemic illness in this setting should lead the clinician to consider this diagnosis. Diagnostically helpful features are noncavitary lung infiltrates, nodular skin lesions, heart failure, significant eosinophilia (usually accounting for 50 percent of the white blood count), and an elevated level of serum IgE. The diagnosis is substantiated by biopsy of involved tissues, such as the lung, the skin, or the prostate, which reveals the characteristic eosinophilic necrotizing extravascular granulomas and necrotizing small vessel vasculitis.

Churg-Strauss vasculitis must be differentiated from Wegener's granulomatosis, lymphomatoid granulomatosis (polymorphic reticulosis), sarcoidosis, bronchopulmonary aspergillosis, and eosinophilic pneumonia.[184] Eosinophilic pneumonia may represent one end of a spectrum of Churg-Strauss vasculitis, but vasculitis is rare in eosinophilic pneumonia. In broncho-pulmonary aspergillosis, peripheral eosinophilia and pulmonary infiltrates may be found, but vasculitis is absent. The diagnosis in aspergillosis can be made by culture of the organism from the bronchial secretions coupled with serologic tests for the antibody.

Treatment and Course. The treatment of choice is corticosteroids in a dosage sufficient to control the inflammatory manifestations of the disease. An initial dosage of 40 to 60 mg of prednisone a day, in divided doses, or the equivalent dosage of another corticosteroid, is usual. In some instances, the disease appears to be adequately controlled with corticosteroids. Data concerning the use of cytotoxic agents in this condition are meager. However, Churg-Strauss vasculitis closely resembles Wegener's pathologically and may respond in a similar fashion to cytotoxic agents.

The outlook may be better than that observed in patients with typical polyarteritis. Rose and Spencer noted that patients who had polyarteritis nodosa with lung involvement had a less fulminating course and that approximately one-third were living at the end of one year.[3] There were some deaths due to lung disease in this group but fewer due to renal failure than in patients without lung involvement. In a recent study of 30 patients with allergic angiitis and granulomatosis, Chumbley and co-workers noted a 90 percent 1-year survival rate and a 62 percent 5-year survival rate.[181] In this series, the most common cause of death was myocardial infarction, followed by congestive heart failure. Other causes of death were status asthmaticus, salmonella septicemia, ruptured aneurysm, renal failure, pneumonia, and small bowel infarction. Some of these deaths were direct complications of the corticosteroid treatment.

WEGENER'S GRANULOMATOSIS

Wegener's granulomatosis was initially described in the 1930s.[185-197] It is characterized by necrotizing granulomatous lesions of the respiratory tract, glomerulonephritis, and frequently vasculitis involving other organs.[188] Less extensive or limited forms of this condition have been described in which some features of the disease may be absent.[189] However, it is likely that these cases have generalized but less severe disease. Subclinical renal disease has been demonstrated by kidney biopsy.[190]

Epidemiology. The disease is uncommon, but specific incidence and prevalence data are not available. Eighty-five patients were seen at the National Institute of Health over a 21-year period.[191] Fifty patients with Wegener's granulomatosis were identified at the Mayo Clinic over the 10-year period from 1964 to 1974.[192] Consequently, it is uncommon even in referral centers. It occurs slightly more frequently in men than in women. The age at onset may range from 8 to 80 years, with a mean of approximately 45 years.

Pathogenesis. The cause of Wegener's granulomatosis is unknown, but hypersensitivity mechanisms have long been suspected of being important in its development. The clinical course of Wegener's granulomatosis, with initial respiratory tract involvement and then later glomerulonephritis, suggests a possible chain of events in which a pathogenic agent gains entry to the respiratory tract and elicits an inflammatory response that later extends to other tissues. Possible immune complex–induced inflammation has been suggested by the findings of glomerular subepithelial deposits adjacent to the basement membrane in some renal biopsies.[193] Circulating immune complexes have been reported infrequently, and

cryoglobulins are seldom detected in Wegener's granulomatosis.[194] Elevated serum immunoglobulin IgE levels have been found, which may reflect the general elevation of immunoglobulins in this disease.[195]

An alteration of cell-mediated immunity has been suggested by a discrepancy between skin reaction and polymorphonuclear migration inhibition to a number of antigens.[196] The chemotactic response of polymorphonuclear leukocytes from patients with Wegener's granulomatosis has been shown to be decreased.[197] However, peripheral blood lymphocytes, monocytes, T lymphocytes, and B lymphocytes appear to be normal in the disease.[198]

The beneficial effect of cyclophosphamide in the treatment of Wegener's granulomatosis offers indirect evidence that immunologic factors may be important in its pathogenesis.[199] Genetic susceptibility may be a factor, as indicated by the increased incidence of HLA-B8 in patients with Wegener's granulomatosis.[60]

Pathology. Pathologically, Wegener's granulomatosis is characterized by the concurrence of three features: necrotizing granulomatous lesions of the upper airway or the lower respiratory tract (or both), generalized focal necrotizing vasculitis involving both small arteries and veins in the lung and other organs, and glomerulonephritis, which is usually focal and segmental.[188,199] The involved vessels are small vessels and are often located adjacent to a granuloma. The vascular lesions show fibrinoid necrosis with mononuclear cell inflammatory cell infiltration. The walls become thickened with focal destruction of the elastic lamina, and the lumina are narrowed and obliterated (Fig. 72–13). Other areas may show healed vascular lesions. The granulomas contain a central area of necrosis surrounded by granulation tissue with palisades of fibroblasts and scattered multinucleated giant cells of the foreign-body and Langhan types.

The most common renal lesion in Wegener's granulomatosis is focal necrotizing glomerulonephritis.[190]

Figure 72–13. Wegener's granulomatosis involving lung. There is necrotizing inflammation of small blood vessel (*long arrow*), with infiltration of vascular wall by mononuclear cells. Granulomatous inflammatory reaction with multinucleated giant cells (*short arrow*) has replaced normal lung tissue.

However, the spectrum of renal involvement ranges from diffuse proliferative glomerulonephritis and interstitial nephritis to hyalinization of glomeruli. Glomerular crescent formation may be found. Granulomatous inflammation around glomeruli and a necrotizing vasculitis of small renal arteries have been reported, but they are not common.

Granulomatous involvement of the sinuses is common, and it may spread to contiguous structures such as the orbit.[200] Focal vasculitis of the eye may affect the conjunctiva, sclera, uveal tract, optic nerve, or the retinal arteries.

Granulomatous or vasculitic involvement may be present in other organs, principally the skin, central nervous system, cranial nerves, peripheral nerves, and heart. The pathologic changes found in skin lesions range from nonspecific acute and chronic inflammation to necrotizing granulomatous vasculitis.[201] The central nervous system may be involved by contiguous spread of granulomatous involvement of the sinuses, but separate granulomas may be found intracerebrally or in the meninges.[202] Vasa nervorum lesions result in mononeuritis multiplex.[203] Granulomas or vasculitis has been found in the heart in 30 percent of the autopsy cases. The pericardium, myocardium, and coronary arteries may be involved.[190] Granulomatous vasculitis may be rarely found in other sites, including the trachea, larynx, parotid gland, mastoid bone and temporal bone.

Clinical Features. The earliest complaints are usually referable to the upper respiratory tract, such as chronic sinusitis, chronic rhinitis, nasal ulceration, and serous otitis media. These may be accompanied by systemic symptoms of fever, weight loss, and anorexia. In addition, suppurative otitis, cholesteatoma, a saddle-nose defect, and hearing loss may occur. On examination, ulceration of the nasal mucosa or destructive sinusitis (or both) may be found and should suggest the possibility of Wegener's granulomatosis. Sinus roentgenograms may show mucosal thickening of the maxillary sinus and destruction of bony walls. Secondary bacterial infections often develop in the sinuses and are caused by *Staphylococcus aureus.*[191,204]

The lower respiratory tract is usually affected at some time during the course of the disease, and the initial symptoms may be related to the lungs. Symptoms are cough, hemoptysis, dyspnea, and, less commonly, pleuritic pain and tracheal obstruction. Pulmonary infiltrates are the most common roentgenologic finding. These may be transient or asymptomatic, and they may be discovered incidentally on chest roentgenograms. Cavitation may occur, but secondary infection is not common. Pleural effusion may be found in 20 percent.[205] Pulmonary function tests have revealed obstruction to airway flow in 55 percent of patients.[206] Endobronchial involvement may occur with distal atelectasis. Subglottic stenosis may occur.[207]

Renal involvement is not usually the initial finding but will eventually become clinically manifest in up to 85 percent of cases. Manifestations include proteinuria, hematuria, red blood cell casts, and renal insufficiency.

Hypertension is not common. The presence of renal lesions was used to distinguish the limited form from the generalized type. However, focal glomerulitis may be detected by renal biopsy in patients who do not have clinical evidence of renal involvement.[190]

The skin is affected in approximately half of the cases. Purpura, the most common dermatologic finding, develops over the lower extremities, but the trunk, upper extremities, and face may be included. Less commonly, the lesions become nodular or ulcerating[201] (Fig. 72–14).

Joint pains occur in up to 70 percent of the cases. They are usually present early in the course of the disease and resolve without residual effects. Synovitis is less common. A nondeforming arthritis involving the large lower extremity joints may occur. Characteristic findings on synovial fluid analysis have not been defined.

The eye is involved in approximately 60 percent of cases also. Orbital involvement may result from extension of a purulent sinusitis. This can cause dacryocystitis, proptosis, cavernous sinus thrombosis, or impaired vision. Other ocular manifestations of the vasculitis are conjunctivitis, scleritis, episcleritis, corneoscleral ulcers, uveitis, retinal artery occlusion, and optic neuritis.

About 20 percent of the cases will have nervous system involvement.[204] One half will have central nervous system involvement, including cranial nerves II, V, VII, VIII, IX, and XIII. Granulomas extending from the sinuses may affect the pituitary, resulting in diabetes insipidus. Cerebral vasculitis may occur. The other half of the cases will have vasculitis of the peripheral nerves, resulting in the multiple mononeuropathies and a symmetrical polyneuropathy.[208]

Clinical manifestations related to granulomatous or vasculitic lesions of the heart are not common. However, arrhythmias and coronary arteritis leading to death have been observed. Also pericarditis and congestive cardiomyopathy may occur. Granulomas and vasculitis may also be found in other organs, such as the gut, with clinical manifestations that reflect the site and extent of involvement.

Laboratory Tests. Normochromic, normocytic anemia, moderate leukocytosis without eosinophilia, elevated erythrocyte sedimentation rate, thrombocytosis, and hypergammaglobulinemia are common laboratory abnormalities found in Wegener's granulomatosis.[191,204] A microangiopathic hemolytic anemia may develop, with the peripheral blood smears showing schistocytes, burr cells, and a regenerative or a hemolytic picture.[209] Levels of all immunoglobulins may be elevated, but the IgA elevation has been stressed. Serum IgE levels have been elevated in a small number of patients studied.[195] Rheumatoid factor has been detected in more than 50 percent of patients and was noted most often in those with extensive disease. Antinuclear antibodies and cryoglobulins are usually absent. Serum levels of whole complement and of C3 are normal or elevated. Immune complexes are present in about half the active cases as detected by Clq binding and Raji assay.[191] Anergy to common infectious antigens and reduced lymphocyte transformation response to phytohemagglutinin have

Figure 72–14. Wegener's granulomatosis. *A*, Severe involvement of skin of head and neck, with hemorrhagic bullae and necrotic ulcers. *B*, Same patient after treatment with cyclophosphamide and corticosteroids for 2 months. Resolution of skin lesions was nearly complete.

been found in patients who have been treated with cytotoxic agents and corticosteroids.[96]

Diagnosis. The diagnosis of Wegener's granulomatosis is based on the clinical features and the histopathologic demonstration of necrotizing granulomas with vasculitis. The diagnosis should be suspected in a patient who has features of a systemic illness and the upper respiratory tract symptoms noted above. The presence of nasal mucosal ulcerations, proptosis, lung infiltrates or cavitation, proteinuria, and abnormalities in urinary sediment should further suggest this diagnosis. Anemia, an elevated erythrocyte sedimentation rate, leukocytosis, the presence of rheumatoid factor, and elevated immunoglobulin levels confirm the systemic nature of the patient's illness.

Renal biopsy will rarely be distinctive enough to be definitive. Since most of the patients with Wegener's granulomatosis have upper respiratory tract involvement early in the course of their illness, biopsy of nasal mucosal or involved sinus tissues offers the best opportunity for securing a histologic diagnosis. A generous portion of tissue must be obtained to allow adequate pathologic examination. Involved lung tissue may be obtained, preferably by open biopsy.

Lymphomatoid granulomatosis (polymorphic reticulosis), Churg-Strauss vasculitis, sarcoidosis, and lymphoma may be confused with Wegener's granulomatosis and must be considered in the differential diagnosis. Lymphomatoid granulomatosis can be distinguished on the basis of its pathologic features and the absence of glomerulonephritis. When it is localized to the upper respiratory tract, it responds favorably to radiation therapy.[210,211]

This localized form (midline granuloma) is a more destructive disease and may erode through the hard palate and the skin of the face and nose.[204,224] In Wegener's granulomatosis there may be erosion through the bones of the sinuses, but the destructive potential is less than in the midline granuloma variant or the malignant midline diseases. Churg-Strauss vasculitis is distinguished on the basis of the asthma, the eosinophilia, and the prominent presence of eosinophils in involved tissue.

Infectious granulomatous disease such as tuberculosis, actinomycosis, histoplasmosis, blastomycosis, coccidiomycosis, and syphilis must be considered.[212] Goodpasture's syndrome with pulmonary hemorrhage and glomerulonephritis may resemble Wegener's granulomatosis. The finding of the antiglomerular basement membrane antibody in Goodpasture's syndrome may be a helpful distinguishing feature. Malignancies such as lymphomas, nasopharyngeal carcinoma, and primary and secondary lung malignancies can be excluded by appropriate tissue examination.

Treatment and Course. Before the 1960s, Wegener's granulomatosis was almost uniformly fatal, and renal failure was the main cause of death.[213] Corticosteoid therapy resulted in improvement in some cases, but the overall mortality was not altered appreciably.[214] With the use of cytotoxic drugs in the treatment, the course of the disease has been altered favorably. Cyclophosphamide, azathioprine, methotrexate, chlorambucil, and nitrogen mustard have been used.[215-217] All have been relatively effective, but experience with cyclophosphamide has been the most extensive.[191] It is clear that cyclophosphamide is more effective than azathioprine in inducing a remission. It is used in doses of 2 to 4 mg per kg orally, depending upon the severity of disease.

Azathioprine may be used in maintenance therapy in those patients who have had an adverse reaction to cyclophosphamide.[191]

In patients with significant systemic features, prednisone should be given concomitantly with cyclophosphamide in a dose of 1 mg per kg in divided doses. When the systemic features of disease are controlled, then the prednisone can be tapered. The prednisone may be converted to an alternate-day regimen at this point and reduced to the lowest dose possible and eventually discontinued altogether.

Response to treatment can be judged by evaluation of the clinical features and the erythrocyte sedimentation rate. Relapses may occur and are usually successfully managed by increasing the cyclophosphamide and sometimes the prednisone, depending upon the severity of the relapse.[191] Infectious complications, such as a staphylococcal infection of the sinuses, can simulate a flare of Wegener's granulomatosis. Bacterial or viral infections can also exacerbate the inflammatory disease of Wegener's granulomatosis.[218] Maintenance cyclophosphamide should be continued for 1 year after control of symptoms, then gradually tapered.

A small percentage of patients may progress to end-stage renal failure. These patients may require hemodialysis. A number of these patients whose disease was otherwise controlled have done well after renal transplantation.[219] Intravascular coagulation and fibrinolysis can intervene in Wegener's granulomatosis, with widespread vascular involvement. This complication would be suggested by a diminished platelet count and fibrinogen level, elevated fibrin split products, and a peripheral blood smear showing schistocytes and other fragmented cells. Heparin should be considered as adjunctive therapy in such instances.

The white blood count must be monitored carefully while the patient is on cyclophosphamide. Initially the white blood count should be performed every other day until it has stabilized. There is a 7- to 10-day lag period after the initiation of treatment before the maximum leukopenic effect of cyclophosphamide is seen. The white blood count should not be allowed to drop to under 3000 to 3500 WBC per mm³. After stabilization the white blood count may be monitored every 1 to 2 weeks. The urinalysis should be followed every week to detect hematuria. Persistent hematuria should be evaluated by cystoscopy to detect any evidence of malignancy, and the cyclophosphamide should be stopped.

Cyclophosphamide is associated with significant complications. Marrow toxicity, primarily leukopenia, predisposes the patient to opportunistic infections. Herpes zoster may occur as a complication of cyclophosphamide in these patients, but fortunately visceral and central nervous system dissemination has not been reported.[220] The patients may also develop hair loss, hemorrhagic cystitis, and gonadal dysfunction. The late development of neoplasms, including bladder neoplasms, leukemia, and lymphoma, has been reported.[191,221] Hair loss has not proved to be a serious problem. Gonadal dysfunction occurs in virtually all the patients, and whether or not it is reversible is not known. Premenopausal women exhibit oligomenorrhea, and men experience decreased libido, diminished testosterone levels, and oligospermia. Thirty-four percent of the patients may show evidence of cystitis.[191]

Prednisone likewise may be associated with complications. The septic complications may be reduced by using the alternate-day regimen.[222] However, the long-term side effects of osteoporosis, cataract formation, hypertension, and diabetes mellitus may occur if a moderate dose is needed for an extended period of time.

LYMPHOMATOID GRANULOMATOSIS

This is a rare disease described by Liebow in 1972. It is characterized by an involvement of certain organs with an angiocentric and angiodestructive infiltration with atypical lymphocytoid and plasmacytoid cells.[223] It is probably identical to polymorphic reticulosis, which is the term used by Drs. Harrison, DeRemee, Weiland, and McDonald, which includes midline granuloma.[224] In the past, forms of polymorphic reticulosis localized to the upper airways were often grouped under the term midline granuloma. Lymphomatoid granulomatosis includes a spectrum of severity, and a benign form has been described—benign lymphocytic angiitis and granulomatosis.[225] The cause is not known, but this disease is closely related to the lymphoproliferative disease because a number of the patients have a disease that evolves into a lymphoma.

Pathology. The characteristic histologic feature is an angiodestructive infiltration of tissue with lymphoid or plasmacytoid cells with some atypia.[204] Veins and arteries are infiltrated to such an extent that their morphology may be unrecognizable. The following organs are affected: lung, kidney, liver, brain, spleen, adrenal gland, heart, and skin. The lung is involved in most cases. In the kidney the glomeruli are spared, and the nodular lesion appears in the interstitial space. Skin lesions have the same pathologic picture plus fat necrosis. A high percentage of the patients may progress to a malignant lymphoma.

Clinical Features. The mean age at onset of this disease is 48 years, with a range of 7 to 85 years.[226] Males are affected slightly more commonly. Patients frequently present with constitutional features of fever, malaise, and weight loss and have accompanying myalgias and arthralgias. Since the lung is involved, respiratory symptoms are a common localizing feature and include cough, chest pain, and shortness of breath. Destructive upper airway lesions may occur as well. Skin involvement may be seen in 40 percent of the patients. Erythematous macules and indurated plaques are the usual lesions. Depending upon its location, a mass lesion in the central nervous system may result in a variety of central nervous system manifestations. Cranial and peripheral neuropathies may occur but are not common. Liver, spleen, and lymph node enlargement are uncommon. Fifty percent or more of the patients develop a malignant lymphoma, which frequently causes death in these patients.

There are no characteristic laboratory abnormalities in this disease. About one half of patients have an elevated erythrocyte sedimentation rate, and a small percentage have leukopenia. The chest x-ray is helpful in demonstrating the nodular densities, which are usually present bilaterally. Pleural effusion and cavitation may be seen. Hilar adenopathy is not seen. The diagnosis is made by biopsying involved tissue and demonstrating the characteristic pathological picture.

Treatment and Course. Patients with the benign variant as well as established lymphomatoid granulomatosis should be treated with cyclophosphamide and prednisone as described for Wegener's granulomatosis. Remissions have been induced in 50 percent of the patients treated in this fashion. This approach has not proved successful in those patients who have undergone malignant transformation. This suggests the importance of early diagnosis and treatment. In the past most patients have died of the malignant progression of this disease with a mortality approaching 90 percent. The causes of death in these patients include respiratory insufficiency, pulmonary hemorrhage, progressive central nervous system disease, and opportunistic infection. Radiotherapy may be effective in treating disease localized to the upper airway.

TAKAYASU'S ARTERITIS

A few of the many other names used for this disease include aortic arch arteritis, aortitis syndrome, pulseless disease, brachiocephalic arteritis, and occlusive thromboarthropathy. Takayasu's arteritis affects large arteries and occurs primarily in children and young women. The aorta and its primary branches are involved most extensively. Varying degrees of narrowing or occlusion or dilation develop in the involved segments, leading to a wide range of symptoms.

Epidemiology. The prevalence and incidence are unknown. Cases have been described in countries all over the world. The largest number of reports, however, has come from Japan. Nasu found 100 cases in slightly fewer than 300,000 autopsies registered in Japan over a 16-year period (0.03 percent).[227] Eighty to 90 percent of cases occur in females. In the majority of instances, the onset of the disease is between the ages of 10 and 30 years.[228,229]

Pathogenesis. The cause remains obscure. Infections with spirochetes, tubercle bacilli, or streptococcal organisms have been suggested as causes, but there is little solid evidence for this. The presence of another connective tissue disease in occasional patients, elevated levels of globulins, and the finding of antiaorta antibodies in the serum of some patients with this condition have suggested an immunologic cause and possibly an autoimmune process. Ueda and co-workers found antiaorta antibodies at a titer of 1:10 or higher in 21 of 34 patients with aortitis but in only 17 of 154 patients with

other diseases.[230] Collagenase treatment of aortic tissue that was used as substrate (antigen) resulted in reduced antiaorta antibody titers. HLA studies have detected an increased frequency of HLA-Bw52 in Asians.[231] HLA-Bw52 is in linkage disequilibrium with DR4. In North Americans there is an increased frequency of MB3 and DR4 in patients with Takayasu's disease.[61] The striking association is with MB3, which was present in all ten patients studied. These findings indicate that there may be an inherited susceptibility to Takayasu's arteritis.

Pathology. The disease may be localized to the aortic arch or its branches, the ascending thoracic aorta, or the abdominal aorta, or it may involve the entire aorta.[227,228,233,234] Postmortem examinations on patients who have Takayasu's arteritis have usually shown patchy or continuous involvement of all portions of the aorta and the innominate, common carotid, and subclavian arteries.[235] Changes in the subclavian and carotid arteries may be more extensive on the left side than on the right. Other arteries commonly affected include the celiac, mesenteric, renal, pulmonary, iliac, and coronary arteries.[236] The inflammatory processes cause thickening of the arterial wall, which is most pronounced in the aortic arch and its branches. Abnormalities of the aortic valve are found in one third of autopsy cases. Aortic valve leaflets may become distorted, with the edges being rolled and contracted. The aortic ring may become dilated and cause aortic insufficiency. Atheromatous changes in the intima are common but are usually mild.[235]

Histologically, panarteritis is present in established cases. Early changes are found in the adventitia and outer part of the media. These include granulomatous inflammation with infiltration of lymphocytes and plasma cells, histiocyte cells, and occasionally polymorphonuclear leukocytes and multinucleated giant cells. Lymphocytes collect around the vasa vasorum. There may be endothelial proliferation, causing obliteration of the lumen. As the arteritis continues, the elastic fibers and smooth muscles in the media undergo fragmentation and necrosis. Pronounced intimal thickening occurs in areas with inflamed outer layers. The thickened intima and the contraction of the fibrotic media and adventitia cause narrowing or obliteration of the arterial lumen. Thrombosis commonly occurs in stenotic areas. Old areas of obstruction may recanalize. Dissections or aneurysms may form in areas where the arterial wall has been weakened by the inflammatory processes.[227,237]

Clinical Features. In the early disease (prepulseless phase), systemic symptoms such as fatigue, weight loss, and low-grade fever are common.[238] Arthralgia or mild arthritis has been noted in half of the patients.[228] Later (pulseless phase), evidence of vascular insufficiency due to large artery narrowing or obstruction becomes apparent. Important findings on examination, which are present in most patients at some time, are tenderness, diminished pulses, and bruits over one or more brachial, subclavian, or carotid arteries. The upper extremities become cool. Decreased lower extremity pulses and femoral or abdominal bruits may also be present. Claudication of the extremities develops in many patients. Occlusions of the vessels may lead to ischemic ulcers on the extremities. Frequently, there is evidence of collateral circulation about the shoulders and elsewhere.

Hypertension is found in half or more of patients and can be caused by narrowing of the thoracic or abdominal aorta, decreased elasticity of the aortic wall, or renal artery involvement.[239] Blood pressure may be difficult to assess because the arteries are narrowed or occluded. It may be measured by using a wide cuff on the legs, by ophthalmodynamometry, or by direct measurements in the ascending aorta. Pulmonary arteritis leads to dyspnea, hemoptysis, and pulmonary hypertension.[240]

As the disease progresses, the skin over the face may become atrophic, with loss of teeth and hair and with ulcers on the lips and the tip of the nose. Vertigo, syncope, convulsions, dementia, headaches, and reduced visual acuity may occur from decreased cerebral blood flow as a result of obstructed arteries in the neck or because of hypertension. Advance retinopathy with preretinal hemorrhages and arteriovenous anastomoses around the disk occurs in patients with severe narrowing or occlusion of both common carotid and vertebral arteries. Symptoms are accentuated by physical activity. Abdominal pain, diarrhea, and gastrointestinal ischemia and hemorrhage result from mesenteric artery stenosis. Angina pectoris develops from coronary artery narrowing.

Laboratory Tests. In cases of active disease, blood tests reflect the inflammatory processes.[241] In most, moderate anemia is present, which is usually normochromic but may be hypochromic. The leukocyte count tends to be normal or slightly elevated. Hypoalbuminemia and increased levels of α_2 globulin, fibrinogen, and gamma globulin are commonly found. The erythrocyte sedimentation rate is typically high early in the disease, but may be normal after the inflammatory phase.

Diagnosis. Early diagnosis may be difficult, and it is often delayed for several years because the symptoms usually are nonspecific in the prepulseless phase of the disease.[242] The diagnosis depends on the recognition of symptoms of vascular ischemia and the finding of bruits or decreased pulses, and it is confirmed by arteriography. The arteriographic changes are generally most pronounced in the region of the aortic arch and its primary branches, but instances in which changes were confined to the abdominal aorta and its branches have been reported (Fig. 72–15). Typical arteriograms show vascular segments with smooth-walled, tapered, focal, or prolonged narrowing, with other areas of dilation.[232]

Treatment and Course. Adrenocorticosteroids effectively suppress the systemic symptoms and are helpful in reversing arterial stenoses in the early stage of the disease.[241] Pulses may improve rapidly, and ischemic symptoms such as claudication may be ameliorated. A case in which hypertension was reversed has been reported.[243] After fibrous tissue has been laid down and after thrombosis has occurred, the response is diminished. An initial daily dose of 45 to 60 mg of prednisone, or the equivalent, may be given. After two to four weeks, the dosage may be gradually reduced until the minimum amount that suppresses the disease is found, as measured by the symptoms and findings and the sedimentation rate. Use of a long-term, low-maintenance-dose corticosteroid may prevent progression of the disease. Alternate-day corticosteroid therapy has not been evaluated. Anticoagulants, vasodilators, and cytotoxic drugs have been used, but the effects of these are uncertain. Salicylates may help control systemic symptoms. Digitalis preparations and antihypertensive drugs may be

Figure 72–15. Arteries of aortic arch. *A,* Angiogram shows smooth-walled, tapered narrowing of right subclavian artery (*white arrow*). Vertebral and thyrocervical trunk arteries. *B,* Abdominal aorta shows smooth-walled tubular narrowing of mid and lower portions and constriction of left common iliac artery at its origin (*arrow*).

indicated in certain instances. Arterial patch grafts or bypass grafts may be considered in late cases in which there are ischemic symptoms that are not influenced by therapy with corticosteroids.[228]

The course of Takayasu's arteritis tends to be prolonged, and there are intermittent exacerbations and an increasingly impaired circulation. After a number of years, the inflammatory component may become less active and the systemic symptoms are replaced by those of vascular ischemia—the pulseless phase of the disease. A few patients have been observed to have spontaneous remissions, but others have been followed in which there has apparently been continued activity for more than 20 years.[238] Death occurs most commonly as a result of congestive heart failure or cerebrovascular accidents. Rupture of an aneurysm is not common. In one follow-up study of 54 patients, an 83 percent 5-year survival rate was observed.[228]

KAWASAKI'S DISEASE (MUCOCUTANEOUS LYMPH NODE SYNDROME)

This disease is an acute febrile illness affecting infants and young children. It was first described in Japan in 1967.[244] Most cases have been reported among Japanese children, and the disease occurs in clusters and epidemic outbreaks.[245,246] These observations suggest a genetic predisposition and an infectious etiology. Japanese studies have shown an increase of HLA-Bw22 in patients with disease in Japan.[247] This was not found in patients involved in the epidemic in the Boston area. Rather HLA-Bw51 was found to be increased.[248] Preliminary studies have shown that a house dust mite may be a factor in the pathogenesis of Kawasaki's disease, either as an allergen or as a vector carrying a rickettsia.[249,250]

Clinical Features. The disease is slightly more common in males.[251] The peak age of the disease is 12 months, with a range of 6 weeks of age to 8 years. A rare case has been reported in an adult.[252] The illness is characterized by an abrupt onset, with fever, conjunctival injection, oropharyngeal erythema, and a strawberry tongue. The hands and feet become diffusely swollen, and palms and soles become erythematous. This may last two weeks and is followed by desquamation. A widespread erythematous rash appears several days after the onset of fever. The rash may be morbilliform and involve the face and trunk most prominently. The patients develop acute nonsuppurative enlargement of the cervical lymph nodes. A nondeforming pauciarticular arthritis may accompany this illness. Iridocyclitis may commonly occur. Cardiac involvement, specifically carditis, may be detected in 50 percent of patients early in the disease by clinical, electrocardiographic, echocardiographic, and radiographic evaluations.[253] Coronary aneurysms may be detected in 20 percent using noninvasive techniques; and up to 60 percent, by angiography.[254] There is no correlation between the presence of carditis and the eventual development of aneurysms.

Two dimensional echocardiography is a reasonable and noninvasive method for detecting coronary involvement. Hydrops of the gallbladder may occur in this disease.[255] Other unusual manifestations include diarrhea, aseptic meningitis, encephalopathy, and cranial nerve palsies.

The disease usually subsides spontaneously in 4 to 6 weeks. Despite the fact that coronary involvement can often be demonstrated in these patients, the mortality is less than 2 percent. It is possible that this coronary involvement may predispose the patient to the development of premature atherosclerosis.

Laboratory examination reveals a leukocytosis and an elevated erythrocyte sedimentation rate. There may be a mild anemia and thrombocytosis. Thrombocytopenia has been reported. The serum IgE is elevated early in the disease.[256] Urinalysis may show mild proteinuria. Because of the potential coronary involvement, an electrocardiogram and two dimensional echocardiogram should be performed.

Pathology. The coronary artery is the most common site of pathology and is always involved in necropsy studies of these patients.[257,258] Other arteries may be involved, including the aorta, celiac, carotid, subclavian, and pulmonary. It is a panarteritis with infiltration of the artery walls with granulocytes and mononuclear cells, necrosis of the wall, and in some cases aneurysm formation. Changes of endothelial proliferation may be seen. The heart may be involved with endocarditis and myocarditis. Fatalities occur when a coronary aneurysm becomes thrombosed. In cases with thrombosis of the coronary artery, the histologic features of a myocardial infarction may be present. The pathologic findings in Kawasaki's disease are probably identical to findings in infantile polyarteritis nodosa.[259]

Treatment. In most cases, this is a self-limited disease. The use of aspirin early in the course of the disease has been shown to result in regression of the aneurysms and may prevent coronary thrombosis, which may complicate the coronary artery involvement. The dose of aspirin recommended is 30 mg per kg in divided doses.[260] The use of corticosteroids is controversial. Corticosteroids are thought to predispose to aneurysm formation. However, pulse doses of corticosteroids used early in the disease have been shown to prevent coronary aneurysms.[261] Some cases require coronary bypass surgery.[262]

References

1. Kussmaul, A., and Maier, R.: Ueber eine bisher nicht beschriebene eigenthümliche Arterienerkrankung (Periarteritis nodosa), die mit Morbus Brightii und rapid fortschreitender allgemeiner Muskellähmung einhergeht. Dtsch. Arch. Klin. Med. 1:484, 1866.
2. Zeek, P.M.: Periarteritis nodosa: A critical review. Am. J. Clin. Pathol. 22:777, 1952.
3. Rose, G.A., and Spencer, H.: Polyarteritis nodosa. Q. J. Med. n.s. 26:43, 1957.
4. Alarcón-Segovia, D.: The necrotizing vasculitides; A new pathogenetic classification. Med. Clin. North Am. 61:241, 1977.
5. Hunder, G.G., and Lie, J.T.: The vasculitides. Clin. Cardiovasc. Dis. 13:261, 1983.
6. Conn, D.L., Dickson, E.R., and Carpenter, H.A.; The association of Churg-Stauss vasculitis with temporal artery involvement, primary biliary cirrhosis and polychondritis in a single patient. J. Rheumatology 9:744, 1982.

7. Fauci, A.S., Haynes, B.F., and Katz, P.: The spectrum of vasculitis: Clinical, pathologic, immunologic, and therapeutic considerations. Ann. Intern. Med. 89:660, 1978.

8. Klinge, F.: Die Eiweissüberempfindlichkeit (Gewebsanaphylaxie) der Gleneke: Experimentelle pathologisch-anatomische Studie zur Pathogenese des Gelenkrheumatismus. Beitr. Pathol. Anat. Allg. Pathol. 83:185, 1929–1930.

9. Rich, A.R., and Gregory, J.E.: The experimental demonstration that periarteritis nodosa is a manifestation of hypersensitivity. Bull. Johns Hopkins Hosp. 72:65, 1943.

10. Kniker, W.T., and Cochrane, C.G.: Pathogenic factors in vascular lesions of experimental serum sickness. J. Exp. Med. 122:83, 1965.

11. Kniker, W.T., and Cochrane, C.G.: The localization of circulating immune complexes in experimental serum sickness: The role of vasoactive amines and hydrodynamic forces. J. Exp. Med. 127:119, 1968.

12. Cochrane, C.G., and Koffler, D.: Immune complex disease in experimental animals and man. Adv. Immunol. 16:185, 1973.

13. Henson, P.M., and Cochrane, C.G.: Immunological induction of increased vascular permeability. II. Two mechanisms of histamine release from rabbit platelets involving complement. J. Exp. Med. 129:167, 1969.

14. Benveniste, J., Henson, P.M., and Cochrane, C.G.: Leukocyte-dependent histamine release from rabbit platelets. The role of IgE, basophils, and a platelet-activating factor. J. Exp. Med. 136:1356, 1972.

15. Fisher, E.R., and Bark, J.: Effect of hypertension on vascular and other lesions of serum sickness. Am. J. Pathol. 39:665, 1961.

16. Benacerraf, B., Sebestyen, M., and Cooper, N.S.: The clearance of antigen antibody complexes from blood by the reticuloendothelial system. J. Immunol. 82:131, 1959.

17. Haakenstad, A.O., and Mannik, M.: Saturation of the reticuloendothelial system with soluble immune complexes. J. Immunol. 112:1939, 1974.

18. Lay, W.H., and Nussenzweig, V.: Receptors for complement on leukocytes. J. Exp. Med. 128:991, 1968.

19. Cochrane, C.G.: Immunologic tissue injury mediated by neutrophilic leukocytes. Adv. Immunol. 9:97, 1968.

20. Cochrane, C.G., and Aiken, B.S.: Polymorphonuclear leukocytes in immunologic reactions. The destruction of vascular basement membrane in vivo and in vitro. J. Exp. Med. 124:733, 1966.

21. Porter, D.D., Larsen, A.E., and Porter, H.G.: The pathogenesis of Aleutian disease of mink. III. Immune complex arteritis. Am. J. Pathol. 71:331, 1973.

22. Oldstone, M.B.A., and Dixon, F.J.: Pathogenesis of chronic disease associated with persistent lymphocytic choriomeningitis viral infection. II. Relationship of the anti-lymphocytic choriomeningitis immune response to tissue injury in chronic lymphocytic choriomeningitis disease. J. Exp. Med. 131:1, 1970.

23. Estes, P.C., and Cheville, N.F.: The ultrastructure of vascular lesions in equine viral arteritis. Am. J. Pathol. 58:235, 1970.

24. Vogel, F.S.: Enhanced susceptibility of proliferating endothelium to salivary gland virus under naturally occurring and experimental conditions. Am. J. Pathol. 34:1069, 1958.

25. Fortuin, N.J., Morrow, A.G., and Roberts W.C.: Late vascular manifestations of the rubella syndrome: A roentgenographic-pathologic study. Am. J. Med. 51:134, 1971.

26. Rich, A.R.: The role of hypersensitivity in periarteritis nodosa: As indicated by seven cases developing during serum sickness and sulfonamide therapy. Bull. Johns Hopkins Hosp. 71:123, 1942.

27. Paull, R.: Periarteritis nodosa (panarteritis nodosa) with report of four proven cases. Calif. Med. 67:309, 1947.

28. Gocke, D.J., Hsu, K., Morgan, C., Bombardieri, S., Lockshin, M., and Christian, C.L.: Association between polyarteritis and Australian antigen. Lancet 2:1149, 1970.

29. Baker, A.L., Kaplan, M.M., Benz, W.C., Sidel, J.S., and Wolfe, H.J.: Polyarteritis associated with Australia antigen-positive hepatitis. Gastroenterology 62:105, 1972.

30. Gerber, M.A., Brodin, A., Steinberg, D., Vernace, S., Yang, C.P., and Paronetto, F.: Periarteritis nodosa, Australia antigen and lymphatic leukemia. N. Engl. J. Med. 286:14, 1972.

31. Wells, G.C.: Section of dermatology. Proc. R. Soc. Med. 69:15, 1976.

32. Kohler, P.F., Cronin, R.E., Hammond, W.S., Olin, D., and Carr, R.I.: Chronic membranous glomerulonephritis caused by hepatitis B antigen-antibody immune complexes. Ann. Intern. Med. 81:448, 1974.

33. Combes, B., Stastny, P., Shorey, J., Eigenbrodt, E.H., Barrera, A., Hull, A.R., and Carter, N.W.: Glomerulonephritis with deposition of Australia antigen-antibody complexes in glomerular basement membrane. Lancet 2:234, 1971.

34. Gocke, D.J., Hsu, K., Morgan, C., Bombardieri, S., Lockshin, M., and Christian, C.L.: Vasculitis in association with Australian antigen. J. Exp. Med. 134(Special Issue):330s, 1971.

35. Fye, K.H., Becker, M.J., Theofilopoulos, A.N., Moutsopoulos, H., Feldman, J.L., and Talal, N.: Immune complexes in hepatitis B antigen-associated periarteritis nodosa: Detection by antibody-dependent cell-mediated cytotoxicity and the Raji cell assay. Am. J. Med. 62:783, 1977.

36. Almeida, J.D., and Waterson, A.P.: Immune complexes in hepatitis. Lancet 2:983, 1969.

37. Sergent, J.S., Lockshin, M.D., Christian, C.L., and Gocke, D.J.: Vasculitis with hepatitis B antigenemia: Long-term observations in nine patients. Medicine (Baltimore) 55:1, 1976.

38. Doherty, M., and Bradfield, J.W.B.: Polyarteritis nodosa associated with acute cytomegalovirus infection. Ann. Rheum. Dis. 40:419, 1981.

39. Andrasch, R.H., Bardana, E.J., Jr., Porter, J.M., and Pirofsky, B.: Digital ischemia and gangrene preceding renal neoplasm: An association with sarcomatoid adenocarcinoma of the kidney. Arch. Intern. Med. 136:486, 1976.

40. Connelly, T.J., Abruzzo, J.L., and Schwab, R.H.: Agnogenic myeloid metaplasia with polyarteritis. J. Rheumatology 9:954, 1982.

41. Weisenburger, D., Armitage, J., and Dick, F.: Immunoblastic lymphadenopathy with pulmonary infiltrates, hypocomplementemia and vasculitis: A hyperimmune syndrome. Am. J. Med. 63:849, 1977.

42. Elkon, K.B., Hughes, G.R.V., Catovsky, D., Clauvel, J.P., Dumont, J., Seligmann, M., Tannenbaum, H., and Esdaile, J.: Hairy cell leukemia with polyarteritis nodosa. Lancet 2:280, 1979.

43. Goedert, J.J., Neefe, J.R., Smith, F.S., Stahl, N.I., Jaffe, E.S., and Fauci, A.S.: Polyarteritis nodosa, hairy cell leukemia and splenosis. Am. J. Med. 71:323, 1981.

44. Weinstein, A.: Systemic vasculitis and hairy cell leukemia. J. Rheumatol. 9:349, 1982.

45. Conn, D.L., McDuffie, F.C., Holley, K.E., and Schroeter, A.L.: Immunologic mechanisms in systemic vasculitis. Mayo Clin. Proc. 51:511, 1976.

46. Luthra, H.S., McDuffie, F.C., Hunder, G.G., and Samayoa, E.A.: Immune complexes in sera and synovial fluids of patients with rheumatoid arthritis. J. Clin. Invest. 56:458, 1975.

47. Leib, E.S., Hibrawi, H., Chia, D., Blaker, R.G., and Barnett, E.V.: Correlation of disease activity in systemic necrotizing vasculitis with immune complexes. J. Rheumatol. 8:258, 1981.

48. Mellors, R.C., and Ortega, L.G.: Analytical pathology. III. New observations on the pathogenesis of glomerulonephritis, lipid nephrosis, periarteritis nodosa, and secondary amyloidosis in man. Am. J. Pathol. 32:455, 1956.

49. Paronetto, F., and Strauss, L.: Immunocytochemical observations in periarteritis nodosa. Ann. Intern. Med. 56:289, 1962.

50. Cochrane, C.G., Weigle, W.O., Dixon, F.J.: The role of polymorphonuclear leukocytes in the initiation and cessation of the arthus vasculitis. J. Exp. Med. 110:481, 1959.

51. Parish, W.E.: Studies on vasculitis. III. Decreased formation of antibody to M protein, group A polysaccharide and to some exotoxins, in persons with cutaneous vasculitis after streptococcal infection. Clin. Allergy 1:295, 1971.

52. Lockwood, C.M., Worlledge, S., Nicholas, A., Cotton, C., and Peters, D.K.: Reversal of impaired splenic function in patients with nephritis or vasculitis (or both) by plasma exchange. N. Engl. J. Med. 300:524, 1979.

53. Friend, P., Repine, J.E., Kim, Y., Clawson, C.C., and Michael, A.F.: Deficiency of the second component of complement (C2) with chronic vasculitis. Ann. Intern. Med. 83:813, 1975.

54. Miller, F., and Kuschner, M.: Alpha$_1$-antitrypsin deficiency, emphysema, necrotizing angiitis and glomerulonephritis. Am. J. Med. 46:615, 1969.

55. Sergent, J.S., and Christian, C.L.: Necrotizing vasculitis after acute serous otitis media. Ann. Intern. Med. 81:195, 1974.

56. Citron, B.P., Halpern, M., McCarron, M., Lundberg, G.D., McCormick, R., Pincus, I.J., Tatter, D., and Haverback, B.J.: Necrotizing angiitis associated with drug abuse. N. Engl. J. Med. 283:1003, 1970.

57. Koff, R.S., Widrich, W.C., and Robbins, A.H.: Necrotizing angiitis in a methamphetamine user with hepatitis B—angiographic diagnosis, five-month follow-up results and localization of bleeding site. N. Engl. J. Med. 288:946, 1973.

58. Phanuphak, P., and Kohler, P.F.: Onset of polyarteritis nodosa during allergic hyposensitization treatment. Am. J. Med. 68:479, 1980.

59. Piomelli, S., Stefanini, M., and Mele, R.H.: Antigenicity of human vascular endothelium: Lack of relationship to the pathogenesis of vasculitis. J. Lab. Clin. Med. 54:241, 1959.

60. Katz, P., Alling, D.W., Haynes, B.F., and Fauci, A.S.: Association of Wegener's granulomatosis with HLA-B8. Clin. Immunol. Immunopathol. 14:268, 1979.

61. Volkman, D.J., Mann, D.L., and Fauci, A.S.: Association between Takayasu's arteritis and a B-cell alloantigen in North Americans. N. Engl. J. Med. 306:464, 1982.

62. Epstein, W.L.: Granulomatosis hypersensitivity. Prog. Allergy 11:36, 1967.

63. Christian, C.L., and Sergent, J.S.: Vasculitis syndromes: Clinical and experimental models. Am. J. Med. 61:385, 1976.

64. Leonhardt, E.T.G., and Kullenberg, K.P.G.: Bilateral atrial myxomas with multiple arterial aneurysms—a syndrome mimicking polyarteritis nodosa. Am. J. Med. 62:792, 1977.

65. Huston, K.A., Combs, J.J., Lie, J.T., and Giuliani, E.R.: Left atrial myxoma simulating peripheral vasculitis. Mayo Clin. Proc. 53:752, 1978.

66. Manion, W.C.: Infectious angiitis. In Orbison, J.D., and Smith, D.E. (eds.): The Peripheral Blood Vessels. Baltimore, Williams & Wilkins Company, 1963.

67. Churchill, M.A., Jr., Geraci, J.E., and Hunder, G.G.: Musculoskeletal manifestations of bacterial endocarditis. Ann. Intern. Med. 87:754, 1977.

68. Kazmier, F.J., Sheps, S.G., Bernatz, P.E., and Sayre, G.P.: Livido reticularis and digital infarcts: A syndrome due to cholesterol emboli arising from atheromatous abdominal aortic aneurysms. Vasc. Dis. 3:12, 1966.

69. Gorevic, P.D., Kassab, H.J., Levo, Y., Kohn, R., Meltzer, M., Prose, P., and Franklin, E.C.: Mixed cryoglobulinemia: Clinical aspects and long-term follow-up of 40 patients. Am. J. Med. 69:287, 1980.

70. Masi, A.T.: Population studies in rheumatic disease. Ann. Rev. Med. 18:185, 1967.

71. Kurland, L.T., Hauser, W.A., Ferguson, R.H., and Holley, K.E.: Epidemiologic features of diffuse connective tissue disorders in Rochester, Minn., 1951 through 1967, with special reference to systemic lupus erythematosus. Mayo Clin. Proc. 44:649, 1969.

72. Kurland, L.T., Chuang, T-Y., and Hunder, G.G.: The epidemiology of systemic arteritis. In: Laurence, R.E., and Shulman, L.E. (eds.): Current topics in Rheumatology: Epidemiology of the Rhuematic Diseases. New York, Gower Medical Publisher, Ltd., 1984, pp. 196–205.

73. Moskowitz, R.W., Baggenstoss, A.H., and Slocumb, C.H.: Histopathologic classification of periarteritis nodosa: A study of 56 cases confirmed at necropsy. Proc. Staff Meet. Mayo Clin. 38:345, 1963.

74. Zeek, P.M.: Periarteritis nodosa and other forms of necrotizing angiitis. N. Engl. J. Med. 248:764, 1953.

75. Arkin, A.: A clinical and pathological study of periarteritis nodosa: A report of five cases, one histologically healed. Am. J. Pathol. 6:401, 1930.

76. Mowrey, F.H., and Lundberg, E.A.: The clinical manifestations of essential polyangiitis (periarteritis nodosa), with emphasis on the hepatic manifestations. Ann. Intern. Med. 40:1145, 1954.

77. Maxeiner, S.R., Jr., McDonald, J.R., and Kirklin, J.W.: Muscle biopsy in the diagnosis of periarteritis nodosa: An evaluation. Surg. Clin. North Am., August 1952, p. 1225.

78. Sack, M., Cassidy, J.T., and Bole, G.G.: Prognostic factors in polyarteritis. J. Rheumatol. 2:411, 1975.

79. Diaz-Perez, J.L., and Winkelmann, R.K.: Cutaneous periarteritis nodosa. Arch. Dermatol. 110:407, 1974.

80. Dahl, E.V., Baggenstoss, A.H., and DeWeerd, J.H.: Testicular lesions of periarteritis nodosa, with special reference to diagnosis. Am. J. Med. 28:222, 1960.

81. Wainwright, J., and Davson, J.: The renal appearances in the microscopic form of periarteritis nodosa. J. Pathol. Bacteriol. 62:189, 1950.

82. Ralston, D.E., and Kvale, W.F.: The renal lesions of periarteritis nodosa. Proc. Staff Meet. Mayo Clin. 24:18, 1949.

83. Wold, L.E., and Baggenstoss, A.H.: Gastrointestinal lesions of periarteritis nodosa. Proc. Staff Meet. Mayo Clin. 24:28, 1949.

84. LiVolsi, V.A., Perzin, K.H., and Porter, M.: Polyarteritis nodosa of the gallbladder, presenting as acute cholecystitis. Gastroenterology 65:115, 1973.

85. Hall, J.W., Sun, S.C., and Mackler, W.: Arteritis of the appendix. Arch. Pathol. 50:240, 1950.

86. Dyck, P.J., Conn, D.L., and Okazaki, H.: Necrotizing angiopathic neuropathy: Three-dimensional morphology of fiber degeneration related to sites of occluded vessels. Mayo Clin. Proc. 47:461, 1972.

87. Stevens, J.C., Lofgren, E.P., and Dyck, P.J.: Biopsy of peripheral nerves. In Dyck, P.J., Thomas, P.K., and Lambert, E.H. (eds.): Peripheral Neuropathy. Vol. 1. Philadelphia, W. B. Saunders Company, 1975.

88. Parker, H.L., and Kernohan, J.W.: The central nervous system in periarteritis nodosa. Proc. Staff Meet. Mayo Clin. 24:43, 1949.

89. Holsinger, D.R., Osmundson, P.J., and Edwards, J.E.: The heart in periarteritis nodosa. Circulation 25:610, 1962.

90. Ahrohein, J.H.: Isolated coronary periarteritis: Report of a case of unexpected death in a young pregnant woman. Am. J. Cardiol. 40:287, 1977.

91. Cohen, R.D., Conn, D.L., and Ilstrup, D.M.: Clinical features, prognosis, and response to treatment in polyarteritis. Mayo Clin. Proc. 55:146, 1980.

92. Lovshin, L.L., and Kernohan, J.W.: Peripheral neuritis in periarteritis nodosa: A clinicopathologic study. Proc. Staff Meet. Mayo Clin. 24:48, 1949.

93. Frohnert, P.P., and Sheps, S.G.: Long-term follow-up study of periarteritis nodosa. Am. J. Med. 43:8, 1967.

94. Ferguson, R.H., and Slocumb, C.H.: Peripheral neuropathy in rheumatoid arthritis. Bull. Rheum. Dis. 11:251, 1961.

95. Allan, S.G., Smith, C.C., Towla, H.M.A., Downie, A.W., Clark, J.C.: Painful brachial plexopathy: An unusual presentation of polyarteritis nodosa. Post. Med. J. 58:311, 1982.

96. Ford, R.G., and Siekert, R.G.: Central nervous system manifestations of periarteritis nodosa. Neurology (Minneap.) 15:114, 1965.

97. Rose, G.A.: The natural history of polyarteritis. Br. Med. J. 2:1148, 1957.

98. Ladefoged, J., Nielsen, B., Raaschou, F., and Sorensen, A.W.S.: Acute anuria due to polyarteritis nodosa. Am. J. Med. 46:827, 1969.

99. Davson, J., Ball, J., and Platt, R.: The kidney in periarteritis nodosa. Q. J. Med. n.s. 17:175, 1948.

100. White, R.H., and Schambelan, M.: Hypertension, hyperreninemia, and secondary hyperaldosteronism in systemic necrotizing vasculitis. Ann. Intern. Med. 92:199, 1980.

101. Cowan, R.E., Mallinson, C.N., Thomas, G.E., and Thomson, A.D.: Polyarteritis nodosa of the liver: A report of two cases. Postgrad. Med. J. 53:89, 1977.

102. Golding, D.N.: Polyarteritis presenting with leg pains. Br. Med. J. 1:277, 1970.

103. Roy, J.B., Hamblin, D.W., and Brown, C.H.: Periarteritis nodosa of epididymis. Urology 10:62, 1977.

104. Kielar, R.A.: Exudative retinal detachment and scleritis in polyarteritis. Am. J. Ophthalmol. 82:694, 1976.

105. Wise, G.N.: Ocular periarteritis nodosa: Report of two cases. Arch. Ophthalmol. 48:1, 1952.

106. Frayha, R.A., and Abu-Haidar, F.: Polyarteritis nodosa masquerading as temporal arteritis. J. Rheumatol. 6:76, 1979.

107. Morgan, C.J., and Harris, E.D., Jr.: Non-giant cell temporal arteritis: Three cases and a review of the literature. Arthritis Rheum. 21:362, 1978.

108. Cogan, D.G.: Syndrome of nonsyphilitic interstitial keratitis and vestibuloauditory symptoms. Arch. Ophthalmol. 33:144, 1945.

109. Haynes, B.F., Kaiser-Kupper, M.I., Mason, P., and Fauci, A.S.: Cogan syndrome: Studies in thirteen patients, long-term follow-up and a review of the literature. Medicine 59:426, 1980.

110. Ettlinger, R.E., Nelson, A.M., Burke, E.D., and Lie, J.T.: Polyarteritis nodosa in childhood. Arthritis Rheum. 22:820, 1979.

111. Duffy, J., Lidsky, M.D., Sharp, J.T., Davis, J.S., Person, D.A., Hollinger, F.B., and Min, K.W.: Polyarthritis, polyarteritis and hepatitis B. Medicine (Baltimore) 55:19, 1976.

112. Drueke, T., Barbanel, C., Jungers, P., Digeon, M., Poisson, M., Brivet, F., Trecan, G., Feldmann, G., Crosnier, J., and Bach, J.F.: Hepatitis B antigen-associated periarteritis nodosa in patients undergoing long-term hemodialysis. Am. J. Med. 68:86, 1980.

113. Cosgriff, T.M., and Arnold, W.J.: Digital vasospasm and infarction associated with hepatitis B antigenemia. JAMA 235:1362, 1976.

114. Razzak, I.A., Bauer, F.W., and Itzel, W.: Hepatitis-B-antigenemia with panarteritis, diffuse proliferative glomerulitis and malignant hypertension. Am. J. Gastroenterol. 63:476, 1975.

115. Levo, Y., Gorevic, P.D., Kassab, H.J., Zucker-Franklin, D., and Franklin, E.C.: Association between hepatitis B virus and essential mixed cryoglobulinemia. N. Engl. J. Med. 296:1501, 1977.

116. Trepo, C.G., Zuckerman, A.J., Bird, R.C., and Prince, A.M.: The role of circulating hepatitis B antigen/antibody immune complexes in the pathogenesis of vascular and hepatic manifestations in polyarteritis nodosa. J. Clin. Pathol. 27:863, 1974.

117. Cunliffe, W.J.: An association between cutaneous vasculitis and decreased blood-fibrinolytic activity. Lancet 1:1226, 1968.

118. Sun, N.C.J., Conn, D.L., Schroeter, A.L., and Kazmier, F.J.: Skin fibrinolytic activity in cutaneous and systemic vasculitis. Mayo Clin. Proc. 51:216, 1976.

119. Fan, P.T., Davis, J.A., Somer, T., Kaplan, L., and Bluestone, R.: A clinical approach to systemic vasculitis. Sem. Arthritis Rheum. 9:248, 1980.

120. Wees, S.J., Sunwoo, I.N., and Oh, S.J.: Sural nerve biopsy in systemic necrotizing vasculitis. Am. J. Med. 71:525, 1981.

121. Bron, K.M., and Gajaraj, A.: Demonstration of hepatic aneurysms in polyarteritis nodosa by arteriography. N. Engl. J. Med. 282:1024, 1970.

122. Fisher, R.G., Graham, D.Y., Granmayeh, M., and Trabanino, J.G.: Polyarteritis nodosa and hepatitis-B surface antigen: Role of angiography in diagnosis. Am. J. Roentgenol. 129:77, 1977.

123. Herschman, A., Blum, R., and Lee, Y.C.: Angiographic findings in polyarteritis nodosa: Report of a case. Radiology 94:147, 1970.

124. McLain, L.G., Bookstein, J.J., and Kelsch, R.C.: Polyarteritis nodosa diagnosed by renal arteriography. J. Pediatr. 80:1032, 1972.

125. Travers, R.K., Allison, D.J., Brettle, R.P., and Hughes, G.R.V.: Polyarteritis nodosa: A clinical and angiographic analysis of 17 cases. Sem. Arthritis Rheum. 8:184, 1979.

126. Easterbrook, J.S.: Renal and hepatic microaneurysms: Report of a new entity simulating polyarteritis nodosa. Radiology 137:629, 1980.

127. Harrison, C.V., Loughridge, L.W., and Milne, M.D.: Acute oliguric renal failure in acute glomerulonephritis and polyarteritis nodosa. Q. J. Med. n.s. 33:39, 1964.

128. Fauci, A.S., Katz, P., Haynes, B.F., and Wolff, S.M.: Cyclophosphamide therapy of severe systemic necrotizing vasculitis. N. Engl. J. Med. 301:235, 1979.

129. Leib, E.S., Restivo, C., and Paulus, H.E.: Immunosuppressive and corticosteroid therapy of polyarteritis nodosa. Am. J. Med. 67:941, 1979.

130. Neild, G.H., and Lee, H.A.: Methylprednisolone pulse therapy in the treatment of polyarteritis nodosa. Postgrad. Med. J. 53:382, 1977.

131. Tannenbaum, H.: Combined therapy with methotrexate and prednisone in polyarteritis nodosa. Can. Med. Assoc. J. 123:893, 1980.

132. Chalopin, J.M., Rifle, G., Turc, J.M., Cortet, P., and Severac, M.: Immunological findings during successful treatment of HBsAg-associated polyarteritis nodosa by plasmapheresis alone. Br. Med. J. 280:368, 1980.

133. Decker, J.L.: Toxicity of immunosuppressive drugs in man. Arthritis Rheum. 16:89, 1973.

134. Fuster, V., and Chesebro, J.H.: Antithrombotic therapy: Role of platelet-inhibitor drugs. II. Pharmacologic effects of platelet-inhibitor drugs. Mayo Clin. Proc. 56:185, 1981.

135. Montalbert, C., Carvallo, A., Broumand, B., Noble, D., Anstine, L.A., and Currier, C.B., Jr.: Successful renal transplantation in polyarteritis nodosa. Clin. Nephrol. 14:206, 1980.

136. Sokoloff, L., McCluskey, R.T., and Bunin, J.J.: Vascularity of the early subcutaneous nodule of rheumatoid arthritis. Arch. Pathol. 55:475, 1953.

137. Cruickshank, B.: The basic pattern of tissue damage and pathology of systemic lupus erythematosus. *In* Dubois, E.L. (eds.): Lupus Erythematosus. Second Edition. Los Angeles, University of Southern California Press, 1974.

138. Schur, P.H.: Complement in lupus. Clin. Rheum. Dis. 1:519, 1975.

139. Bywaters, E.G.L.: Peripheral vascular obstruction in rheumatoid arthritis and its relationship to other vascular lesions. Ann. Rheum. Dis. 16:84, 1957.

140. Scott, D.G.I., Bacon, P.A., and Tribe, C.R.: Systemic rheumatoid vasculitis: A clinical and laboratory study of 50 cases. Medicine 60:288, 1981.

141. Conn, D.L., and McDuffie, F.C.: Neuropathy: The pathogenesis of rheumatoid neuropathy (Session III). *In* Organic Manifestations and Complications in Rheumatoid Arthritis (Symposium Hernstein). Stuttgart-New York, F. K. Schattauer Verlag November 2–5, 1975.

142. Douglas, W.: The digital artery lesion of rheumatoid arthritis. Ann. Rheum. Dis. 24:40, 1965.

143. Conn, D.L., McDuffie, F.C., and Dyck, P.J.: Immunopathologic study of sural nerves in rheumatoid arthritis. Arthritis Rheum. 15:135, 1972.

144. Kemper, J.W., Baggenstoss, A.H., and Slocumb, C.H.: The relationship of therapy with cortisone to the incidence of vascular lesions in rheumatoid arthritis. Ann. Intern. Med. 46:831, 1957.

145. Ferguson, R.H., and Slocumb, C.H.: Peripheral neuropathy in rheumatoid arthritis. Bull. Rheum. Dis. 11:251, 1961.

146. Weisman, M., and Zvaifler, N.: Cryoimmunoglobulinemia in rheumatoid arthritis. J. Clin. Invest. 56:725, 1975.

147. Scott, D.G.I., Bacon, P.A., Allen, C., Elson, C.J., and Wallington, T.: IgG rheumatoid factor, complement, and immune complexes in rheumatoid synovitis and vasculitis: Comparative and serial studies during cytotoxic therapy. Clin. Exp. Immunol. 43:54, 1981.

148. Hunder, G.G., and McDuffie, F.C.: Hypocomplementemia in rheumatoid arthritis. Am. J. Med. 54:461, 1973.

149. Sokoloff, L., and Bunim, J.J.: Vascular lesions in rheumatoid arthritis. J. Chron. Dis. 5:668, 1957.

150. Abel, T., Andrews, B.S., Cunningham, P.H., Brunner, C.M., Davis, J.S., and Horwitz, D.A.: Rheumatoid vasculitis: Effect of cyclophosphamide on the clinical course and levels of circulating immune complexes. Ann. Intern. Med. 93:407, 1980.

151. Scott, D.G.I., Bacon, P.A., Bothamley, J.E., Allen, C., Elson, C.J., and Wallington, T.B.: Plasma exchange in rheumatoid vasculitis. J. Rheumatol. 8:433, 981.

152. Zeek, P.M., Smith, C.C., and Weeter, J.C.: Studies on periarteritis nodosa. III. The differentiation between the vascular lesions of periarteritis nodosa and of hypersensitivity. Am. J. Pathol. 24:889, 1948.

153. Gilliam, J.N., and Smiley, J.D.: Cutaneous necrotizing vasculitis and related disorders. Ann. Allergy 37:328, 1976.

154. Soter, N.A.: Clinical presentations and mechanisms of necrotizing angiitis of the skin. J. Invest. Dermatol. 67:354, 1976.

155. Soter, N.A., Mihm, M.C., Gigli, I., Dvorak, H.F., and Austen, K.F.: Two distinct cellular patterns in cutaneous necrotizing angiitis. J. Invest. Dermatol. 66:344, 1976.

156. Sams, W.M., Jr., Thoren, E.G., Small, P., Mass, M.F., McIntosh, R.M., and Stanford, R.E.: Leukocytoclastic vasculitis. Arch. Dermatol. 112:219, 1976.

157. Sams, W.M., Jr., Claman, H.N., Kohler, P.F., McIntosh, R.M., Small,

P., and Mass, M.F.: Human necrotizing vasculitis: Immunoglobulins and complement in vessel walls of cutaneous lesions and normal skin. J. Invest. Dermatol. 64:441, 1975.

158. Schroeter, A.L., Copeman, P.W.M., Jordon, R.E., Sams, W.M., Jr., and Winkelmann, R.K.: Immunofluorescence of cutaneous vasculitis associated with systemic disease. Arch. Dermatol. 104:254, 1971.

159. Winkelmann, R.K., and Ditto, W.B.: Cutaneous and visceral syndromes of necrotizing or "allergic" angiitis: A study of 38 cases. Medicine (Baltimore) 43:59, 1964.

160. Mullick, F.G., McAllister, H.A., Jr., and Wagner, B.M.: Drug related vasculitis: Clinicopathologic correlations in 30 patients. Hum. Pathol. 10:313, 1979.

161. Cream, J.J.: Clinical and immunological aspects of cutaneous vasculitis. Q. J. Med. 45:255, 1976.

162. Allen, D.M., Diamond, L.K., and Howell, D.A.: Anaphylactoid purpura in children (Schönlein-Henoch syndrome): Review with a follow-up of the renal complications. Am. J. Dis. Child. 99:833, 1960.

163. Ansell, B.M.: Henoch-Schönlein purpura with particular reference to the prognosis of the renal lesion. Br. J. Dermatol. 82:211, 1970.

164. Levy, M., Broyer, M., Arsan, A., Levy-Bentolila, D., and Habib, R.: Anaphylactoid purpura nephritis in childhood: Natural history and immunopathology. Adv. Nephrol. 6:183, 1976.

165. Wohlfarth, B., and Asamer, H.: Symptoms and immunology of the Henoch-Schönlein syndrome. Arch. Dermatol. Res. 255:251, 1976.

166. Agnello, V.: Complement deficiency states. Medicine 57:1, 1978.

167. Cream, J.J., Gumpel, J.M., and Peachey, R.D.G.: Schönlein-Henoch purpura in the adult: A study of 77 adults with anaphylactoid or Schönlein-Henoch purpura. Q. J. Med. n.s. 39:461, 1970.

168. Koskimies, O., Rapola, J., Savilahti, E., and Vilska, J.: Renal involvement in Schönlein-Henoch purpura. Acta Paediatr. Scand. 63:357, 1974.

169. Medical Research Council Working Party: Controlled trial of azathioprine and prednisone in chronic renal disease. Br. Med. J. 2:239, 1971.

170. McDuffie, F.C., Sams, W.M., Jr., Maldonado, J.E., Andreini, P.H., Conn, D.L., and Samayoa, E.A.: Hypocomplementemia with cutaneous vasculitis and arthritis: Possible immune complex syndrome. Mayo Clin. Proc. 48:340, 1973.

171. Zeiss, C.R., Burch, F.X., Marder, R.J., Furen, N.L., Schmid, F.R., Gewurz, H.: A hypocomplementemic vasculitic urticarial syndrome. Report of four new cases and definition of the disease. Am. J. Med. 68:867, 1980.

172. Soter, N.A., Austen, K.F., and Gigli, I.: Urticaria and arthralgias as manifestations of necrotizing angiitis (vasculitis). J. Invest. Dermatol. 63:485, 1974.

173. Schewartz, H.R., McDuffie, F.C., Black, L.F., Schroeter, A.L., and Conn, D.L.: Hypocomplementemic urticarial vasculitis: Association with chronic obstructive pulmonary disease. Mayo Clin. Proc. 57:231, 1982.

174. LoSpalluto, J., Dorward, B., Miller, W., Jr., and Ziff, M.: Cryoglobulinemia based on interaction between a gamma macroglobulin and 7S gamma globulin. Am. J. Med. 32:142, 1962.

175. Meltzer, M., Franklin, E.C., Elias, K., McCluskey, R.T., and Cooper, N.: Cryoglobulinemia—a clinical and laboratory study. II. Cryoglobulins with rheumatoid factor activity. Am. J. Med. 40:837, 1966.

176. Cream, J.J.: Immunofluorescent studies of the skin in cryoglobulinemic vasculitis. Br. J. Dermatol. 84:48, 1971.

177. Golde, D., and Epstein, W.: Mixed cryoglobulins and glomerulonephritis. Ann. Intern. Med. 69:1221, 1968.

178. Levo, Y., Gorevic, P.D., Kassab, H.J., Tobias, H., and Franklin, E.C.: Liver involvement in the syndrome of mixed cryoglobulinemia. Ann. Intern. Med. 87:287, 1977.

179. Langlands, D.R., Dawkins, R.L., Matz, L.R., Cobain, T.J., Goatcher, P., Papadimitriou, J.M.: Arthritis associated with a crystallizing cryoprecipitable IgG paraprotein. Am. J. Med. 68:461, 1980.

180. Churg, J., and Strauss, L.: Allergic granulomatosis, allergic angiitis, and periarteritis nodosa. Am. J. Pathol. 27:277, 1951.

181. Chumbley, L.C., Harrison, E.G., Jr., and DeRemee, R.A.: Allergic granulomatosis and angiitis (Churg-Strauss syndrome): Report and analysis of 30 cases. Mayo Clin. Proc. 52:477, 1977.

182. Dicken, C.H., and Winkelmann, R.K.: The Churg-Strauss granuloma: Cutaneous, necrotizing, palisading granuloma in vasculitis syndromes. Arch. Pathol. Lab. Med. 102:576, 1978.

183. Cogen, F.C., Mayock, R.L., and Zweiman, B.: Chronic eosinophilic pneumonia followed by polyarteritis nodosa complicating the course of bronchial asthma: Report of a case. J. Allergy Clin. Immunol. 60:377, 1977.

184. Carrington, C.B., Addington, W.W., Goff, A.M., Madoff, I.M., Marks, A., Schwaber, J.R., and Gaensler, E.A.: Chronic eosinophilic pneumonia. N. Engl. J. Med. 280:787, 1969.

185. Klinger, H.: Grenzformen der Periarteritis nodosa. Frankfurt. Ztschr. Pathol. 42:455, 1931.

186. Wegener, F.: Über generalisierte, septische Gefäserkrankungen. Verh. Dtsch. Ges. Pathol. 29:202, 1936.

187. Wegener, F.: Über eine eigenartige rhinogene Granulomatose mit beson-

derer Beteiligung des Arteriensystems und der Nieren. Beitr. Pathol. Anat. Allg. Pathol. 102:36, 1939.

188. Godman, G.C., and Churg, J.: Wegener's granulomatosis: Pathology and review of the literature. Arch. Pathol. 58:533, 1954.

189. Carrington, C.B., and Liebow, A.A.: Limited forms of angiitis and granulomatosis of Wegener's type. Am. J. Med. 41:497, 1966.

190. Fauci, A.S., and Wolff, S.M.: Wegener's granulomatosis: Studies in eighteen patients and a review of the literature. Medicine (Baltimore) 52:535, 1973.

191. Fauci, A.S., Haynes, B.F., Katz, P., and Wolff, S.M.: Wegener's granulomatosis: Prospective clinical and therapeutic experience with 85 patients for 21 years. Ann. Intern. Med. 98:76, 1983.

192. DeRemee, R.A., McDonald, T.J., Harrison, E.G., Jr., and Coles, D.T: Wegener's granulomatosis: Anatomic correlates, a proposed classification. Mayo Clin. Proc. 51:777, 1976.

193. Horn, R.G., Fauci, A.S., Rosenthal, A.S., and Wolff, S.M.: Renal biopsy pathology in Wegener's granulomatosis. Am. J. Pathol. 74:423, 1974.

194. Howell, S.B., and Epstein, W.V.: Circulating immunoglobulin complexes in Wegener's granulomatosis. Am. J. Med. 60:259, 1976.

195. Conn, D.L., Gleich, G.J., DeRemee, R.A., and McDonald, T.J.: Raised serum immunoglobulin E in Wegener's granulomatosis. Ann. Rheum. Dis. 35:377, 1976.

196. Shillitoe, E.J., Lehner, T., Lessof, M.H., and Harrison, D.F.N.: Immunological features of Wegener's granulomatosis. Lancet 1:281, 1974.

197. Niinaka, T., Okochi, T., Watanabe, Y., Yamamura, T., and Yamamura, Y.: Chemotactic defect in Wegener's granulomatosis. J. Med. 8:161, 1977.

198. Dale, D.C., Fauci, A.S., and Wolff, S.M.: The effect of cyclophosphamide on leukocyte kinetics and susceptibility to infection in patients with Wegener's granulomatosis. Arthritis Rheum. 16:657, 1973.

199. Wolff, S.M., Fauci, A.S., Horn, R.G., and Dale, D.C.: Wegener's granulomatosis. Ann. Intern. Med. 81:513, 1974.

200. Haynes, B.F., Fishman, M.L., Fauci, A.S., and Wolff, S.M.: The ocular manifestations of Wegener's granulomatosis: Fifteen years experience and review of the literature. Am. J. Med. 63:131, 1977.

201. Hu, C.H., O'Loughlin, S., and Winkelmann, R.K.: Cutaneous manifestations of Wegener's granulomatosis. Arch. Dermatol. 113:175, 1977.

202. Sahn, E.E., and Sahn, S.A.: Wegener granulomatosis with aphasia. Arch. Intern. Med. 136:87, 1976.

203. MacFadyen, D.J.: Wegener's granulomatosis with discrete lung lesions and peripheral neuritis. Can. Med. Assoc. J. 83:760, 1960.

204. Cupps, T.R., and Fauci, A.S.: Wegener's granulomatosis. In Cupps, T.R., and Fauci, A.S. (eds.): The Vasculitides. Vol. 21. Philadelphia, W. B. Saunders Company, 1981.

205. Maguire, R., Fauci, A.S., Doppman, J.L., and Wolff, S.M.: Unusual radiographic findings in Wegener's granulomatosis. Am. J. Roentgenol. 130:233, 1978.

206. Rosenberg, D.M., Weinberger, S.E., Fulmer, J.D., Flye, M.W., Fauci, A.S., and Crystal, R.G.: Functional correlates of lung involvement in Wegener's granulomatosis. Am. J. Med. 69:387, 1980.

207. Lampman, J.H., Querubin, R., and Kondapalli, P.: Subglottic stenosis in Wegener's granulomatosis. Chest 79:230, 1981.

208. Drachman, D.A.: Neurological complications of Wegener's granulomatosis. Arch. Neurol. 8:45, 1963.

209. Crummy, C.S., Perlin, E., and Moquin, R.B.: Microangiopathic hemolytic anemia in Wegener's granulomatosis. Am. J. Med. 51:544, 1971.

210. Schechter, S.L., Bole, G.G., and Walker, S.E.: Midline granuloma and Wegener's granulomatosis: Clinical and therapeutic considerations. J. Rheumatol. 3:241, 1976.

211. Fauci, A.S., Johnson, R.E., and Wolff, S.M.: Radiation therapy of midline granuloma. Ann. Intern. Med. 84:140, 1976.

212. Smith, L.R., and Heaton, C.L.: Actinomycosis presenting as Wegener's granulomatosis. JAMA 240:247, 1978.

213. Walton, E.W.: Giant-cell granuloma of the respiratory tract (Wegener's granulomatosis). Br. Med. J. 2:265, 1958.

214. Hollander, D., and Manning, R.T.: The use of alkylating agents in the treatment of Wegener's granulomatosis. Ann. Intern. Med. 67:393, 1967.

215. Fahey, J.L., Leonard, E., Churg, J., and Godman, G.: Wegener's granulomatosis. Am. J. Med. 17:168, 1954.

216. Raitt, J.W.: Wegener's granulomatosis: Treatment with cytotoxic agents and adrenocorticoids. Ann. Intern. Med. 74:344, 1971.

217. Novack, S.N., and Pearson, C.M.: Cyclophosphamide therapy in Wegener's granulomatosis. N. Engl. J. Med. 284:938, 1971.

218. Pinching, A.J., Rees, A.J., Pussell, B.A., Lockwood, C.M., Mitchison, R.S., and Peters, D.K.: Relapses in Wegener's granulomatosis: The role of infection. Br. Med. J. 281:836, 1980.

219. Kuross, S., Davin, T., and Kjellstrand, C.M.: Wegener's granulomatosis with severe renal failure: Clinical course and results of dialysis and transplantation. Clin. Nephrol. 16:172, 1981.

220. Cupps, T.R., Silverman, G.J., and Fauci, A.S.: Herpes zoster in patients with treated Wegener's granulomatosis. Am. J. Med. 69:881, 1980.

221. Wheeler, G.E.: Cyclophosphamide-associated leukemia in Wegener's granulomatosis. Ann. Intern. Med. 94:361, 1981.

222. Fauci, A.S.: Alternate-day corticosteroid therapy. Am. J. Med. 64:729, 1978.

223. Liebow, A.A., Carrington, C.R.B., and Friedman, P.J.: Lymphomatoid granulomatosis. Hum. Pathol. 3:457, 1972.

224. DeRemee, R.A., Weiland, L.H., and McDonald, T.J.: Polymorphic reticulosis, lymphomatoid granulomatosis. Mayo Clin. Proc. 53:634, 1978.

225. Israel, H.L., Patchefsky, A.S., and Saldana, M.J.: Wegener's granulomatosis, lymphomatoid granulomatosis, and benign lymphocytic angiitis and granulomatosis of lung: Recognition and treatment. Ann. Intern. Med. 87:691, 1977.

226. Fauci, A.S., Haynes, B.F., Costa, J., Katz, P., and Wolff, S.M.: Lymphomatoid granulomatosis: Prospective clinical and therapeutic experience over 10 years. N. Engl. J. Med. 306:68, 1982.

227. Nasu, T.: Takayasu's truncoarteritis in Japan: A statistical observation of 76 autopsy cases. Pathol. Microbiol. (Basel) 43:140, 1975.

228. Ishikawa, K.: Natural history and classification of occlusive thromboaortopathy (Takayasu's disease). Circulation 57:27, 1978.

229. Lupi-Herrera, E., Sanchez-Torres, G., Marcushamer, J., Mispiretar, J., Horwitz, S., and Vela, J.E.: Takayasu's arteritis: Clinical study of 107 cases. Am. Heart J. 93:94, 1977.

230. Ueda, H., Saito, Y., Ito, I., Yamaguchi, H., Takeda, T., and Morooka, S.: Further immunological studies of aortitis syndrome. Jpn. Heart J. 12:1, 1971.

231. Isohisa, I., Numano, F., Maezawa, H., Sasazuki, T.: HLA-Bw52 in Takayasu's disease. Tissue Antigens 12:246, 1978.

232. Lande, A., and Berkmen, Y.M.: Aortitis: Pathologic, clinical, and arteriographic review. Radiol. Clin. North Am. 14:219, 1976.

233. Judge, R.D., Currier, R.D., Gracie, W.A., and Figley, M.M.: Takayasu's arteritis and the aortic arch syndrome. Am. J. Med. 32:379, 1962.

234. Nakao, K., Ikeda, M., Kimata, S., Niitani, H., Miyahara, M., Ishimi, Z., Hashiba, K., Takeda, Y., Ozawa, T., Matsushita, S., and Kuramochi, M.: Takayasu's arteritis: Clinical report of eighty-four cases and immunological studies of seven cases. Circulation 35:1141, 1967.

235. Committee on Study of Arteritis: Clinical and pathological studies of aortitis syndrome. Jpn. Heart J. 9:76, 1968.

236. Cipriano, P.R., Silverman, J.F., Perlroth, M.G., Griepp, R.B., and Wexler, L.: Coronary arterial narrowing in Takayasu's aortitis. Am. J. Cardiol. 39:744, 1977.

237. Ueda, H., Ohno, K., Ito, I., Takeda, T., Saito, Y., and Ueno, A.: Two cases of aortitis syndrome with aneurysm formation. Jpn. Heart J. 9:88, 1968.

238. Strachan, R.W.: The natural history of Takayasu's arteriopathy. Q. J. Med. n.s. 33:57, 1964.

239. Ask-Upmark, E.: On the pathogenesis of the hypertension in Takayasu's syndrome. Acta Med. Scand. 169:461, 1961.

240. Lupi, H.E., Sánchez, T.G., Horwitz, S., and Gutierrex, F.E.: Pulmonary artery involvement in Takayasu's arteritis. Chest 67:69, 1975.

241. Fraga, A., Mintz, G., Valle, L., and Flores-Izquierdo, G.: Takayasu's arteritis: Frequency of systemic manifestations (study of 22 patients) and favorable response to maintenance steroid therapy with adrenocorticosteroids (12 patients). Arthritis Rheum. 15:617, 1972.

242. Lande, A., Bard, R., Rossi, P., Passariello, R., and Castrucci, A.: Takayasu's arteritis: A worldwide entity. N.Y. State J. Med. 76:1477, 1976.

243. Kulkarni, T.P., D'Cruz, I.A., Gandhi, M.J., and Dadhich, D.S.: Reversal of renovascular hypertension caused by nonspecific aortitis after corticosteroid therapy. Br. Heart J. 36:114, 1974.

244. Kawasaki, T.: MCLS: Clinical observation of 50 cases. Jpn. J. Allergy 16:178, 1967.

245. Melish, M.E.: Kawasaki syndrome: A new infectious disease? J. Infect. Dis. 143:317, 1981.

246. Meade, R.H., and Brandt, L.: Manifestations of Kawasaki disease in New England outbreak of 1980. J. Pediatr. 100:558, 1982.

247. Kato, S., Kimura, M., and Tsuji, K.: HLA antigens in Kawasaki disease. Pediatr. 61:252, 1978.

248. Krensky, A.M., Berenberg, W., Shanley, K., and Yunis, E.: HLA antigens in mucocutaneous lymph node syndrome in New England. Pediatr. 67:741, 1981.

249. Hamashima, Y., Tasaka, K., Hoshino, T., Nagata, N., Furukawa, F., Kao, T., and Tanaka, H.: Mite-associated particles in Kawasaki disease. Lancet 2:266, 1982.

250. Fujimoto, T., Kato, H., Ichiose, E., and Sasaguri, Y.: Immune complex and mite antigen in Kawasaki disease. Lancet 2:980, 1982.

251. Melish, M.E., Hicks, R.M., Larson, E.J.: Mucocutaneous lymph node syndrome in the United States. Am. J. Dis. Child. 130:599, 1976.

252. Milgrom, H., Palmer, E.L., Slovin, S.F., Morens, D.A., Freedman, S.D., and Vaughan, J.H.: Kawasaki disease in a healthy young adult. Ann. Intern. Med. 92:467, 1980.

253. Hiraishi, S., Yashiro, K., Oguchi, K., Kusano, S., Ishii, K., and Nakazawa, K.: Clinical course of cardiovascular involvement in the muco-

cutaneous lymph node syndrome. Relation between clinical signs of carditis and development of coronary arterial aneurysm. Am. J. Cardiol. 47:323, 1981.

254. Kato, H., Ichinose, E., Yoshioka, F., Takechi, T., Matsunaga, S., Suzuki, K., and Rikitake, N.: Fate of coronary aneurysms in Kawasaki disease: Serial coronary angiography and long-term follow-up study. Am. J. Cardiol. 49:1758, 1982.

255. Liebmann, L.I., Mikelic, V., Joh, M.M., and Wilson, F.M.: Hydrops of the gallbladder in an adult with Kawasaki disease. JAMA 247:827, 1982.

256. Kusakawa, S., and Heiner, D.C.: Elevated levels of immunoglobulin E in the acute febrile mucocutaneous lymph node syndrome. Pediatri. Res. 10:108, 1976.

257. Amano, S., Hazama, F., and Hamashirma, Y.: Pathology of Kawasaki disease. I. Pathology and morphogenesis of the vascular changes. Jpn. Circ. J. 43:633, 1979.

258. Amano, S., Hazama, F., and Hamashirma, Y.: Pathology of Kawasaki disease. II. Distribution and incidence of the vascular lesions. Jpn. Circ. J. 43:741, 1979.

259. Landing, B.H., and Larson, E.J.: Are infantile periarteritis nodosa with coronary artery involvement and fatal mucocutaneous lymph node syndrome the same? Comparison of 20 patients from North America with patients from Hawaii and Japan. Pediatrics 59:651, 1977.

260. Sasaguri, Y., and Kato, H.: Regression of aneurysms in Kawasaki disease. A pathological study. J. Pediatr. 100:225, 1982.

261. Kijima, Y., Kamiya, T., Suzuki, A., Hirose, O., and Manabe, H.: A trial procedure to prevent aneurysm formation of the coronary arteries by steroid pulse therapy in Kawasaki disease. Jpn. Circ. J. 46:1239, 1982.

262. Sandiford, F.M., Vargo, T.A., and Shih, J.Y.: Successful triple coronary artery bypass in a child with multiple coronary aneurysms due to Kawasaki's disease. J. Thorac. Cardiovasc. Surg. 79:283, 1980.

Chapter 73

Giant Cell Arteritis and Polymyalgia Rheumatica

Gene G. Hunder and Brian L. Hazleman

INTRODUCTION

In recent years there has been an increasing appreciation of the close relationship between giant cell arteritis and polymyalgia rheumatica. The precise nature of the association is not known, but the two conditions affect the same patient population and frequently occur together in the same individual. Some investigators have suggested that polymyalgia rheumatica is a manifestation of arteritis, whereas others have taken the view that the two are separate entities occurring together. Because the association between giant cell arteritis and polymyalgia rheumatica has been documented by many authors, they are discussed together in this chapter.

DEFINITIONS

Giant Cell Arteritis. Giant cell arteritis[1] is also referred to as temporal arteritis,[2] cranial arteritis,[3] and granulomatous arteritis.[4] Nearly all patients are more than 50 years old when the disease develops. The inflammatory lesions in giant cell arteritis involve the cranial branches of the arteries originating from the arch of the aorta most prominently, but they may be more widespread.

Polymyalgia Rheumatica. Polymyalgia rheumatica, a term suggested by Barber,[5] is a clinical syndrome characterized by aching and morning stiffness in the proximal portions of the extremities and torso. Definitions have commonly included the presence of symptoms in two of the three commonly affected areas (shoulder girdle, hip girdle, and neck) for 1 month or more, plus evidence of a systemic reaction such as an erythrocyte sedimentation rate elevation to above 40 or 50 mm in 1 hour by the Westergren method.[6,7] Some definitions have also included a rapid response to small doses of corticosteroids such as 10 mg of prednisone daily.[8,9] The presence of another specific disease, such as rheumatoid arthritis, chronic infection, polymyositis, or malignancy, excludes the diagnosis of polymyalgia rheumatica.

EPIDEMIOLOGY

Giant cell arteritis appears to be relatively common in Europe and in the United States. Reported annual incidence rates have varied from 4.2 to 17.4 per 100,000 persons aged 50 years and older.[10-13] Among the population of Olmsted County, Minnesota, 42 cases were identified over a 25-year period,[11] these representing an average annual incidence rate of 11.7 cases per 100,000 population aged 50 years and older, and a prevalence of persons with a history of giant cell arteritis of 133 per 100,000 population aged 50 and older. The incidence increased during the 25 years of the study, from 5.1 per year in 1950 to 1959, to 17.4 in 1970 to 1974, probably reflecting an increased awareness of this disease in the later years. The age-specific rate increased from 1.4 per 100,000 in the age group 50 to 59 years to 29.6 per 100,000 in the age group 70 to 79. In Göteborg, Sweden, over the 3-year period 1973 to 1975 the average incidence of biopsy-positive giant cell arteritis was 16.8 per 100,000 persons over 50 years of age. An increased incidence with age was noted in the Swedish study similar to that in Minnesota.

Autopsy studies suggest that giant cell arteritis may be more common than is clinically apparent. Östberg found arteritis in 1.6 percent of 889 postmortem cases in which sections of the temporal artery and two transverse sections of the aorta were made.[14]

Polymyalgia rheumatica, when considered as the primary process, has been less well studied, but appears to be more common than giant cell arteritis.[15] In Olmsted County, Minnesota, over a 10-year period from 1970 through 1979, 97 cases were found, providing an average annual incidence rate of 53.7 cases per 100,000 persons aged 50 and older.[16] The prevalence of polymyalgia rheumatica (active plus remitted cases) was approximately 500 per 100,000 aged 50 and older.[16] In the Göteborg study the average annual incidence of polymyalgia rheumatica was found to be 28.6 per 100,000.

ETIOLOGY AND PATHOGENESIS

A variety of causes have been suggested for polymyalgia rheumatica and giant cell arteritis, but none have been substantiated. Although the increasing incidence of giant cell arteritis and polymyalgia rheumatica after the age of 50 implies a relationship to aging, the meaning of this observation is not understood. Several reports of familial aggregation, including a pair of identical twins and an apparent predilection of these conditions for Caucasians, suggest a genetic or hereditary predisposition.[9,17,18] In several studies of HLA antigens in polymyalgia rheumatica and giant cell arteritis no HLA-A, B, or C locus antigens have been increased consistently in frequency above controls.[19-22] However, HLA-DR4 may be associated with these conditions more commonly than expected by chance alone.[23]

Both the humoral and cellular immune systems have been implicated in the pathogenesis. The granulomatous histopathology of giant cell arteritis has suggested the presence of a cell-mediated immune reaction directed at antigens in or near elastic tissue in arterial walls.[24-26] Tests of cellular immunity in patients with giant cell arteritis and polymyalgia rheumatica have shown no consistent abnormality.[27,28]

Immunoglobulins and complement deposits have been demonstrated intracellularly and adjacent to the internal elastic lamina in some involved temporal arteries.[26,29] These deposits may represent antibodies to arterial wall antigens or immune complexes deposited from blood. However, the specificity of the deposits and correlation with the inflammatory lesions need to be defined further. Waaler, Tönder, and Milde found anti-IgG activity in biopsy specimens which showed giant cell arteritis.[30] Eghtedari and coworkers demonstrated increased numbers of circulating lymphoblasts in patients with active polymyalgia rheumatica,[31] and Malmvall and coworkers found serum immunoglobulins to be elevated slightly in similar patients.[32] These observations have been interpreted as evidence of an ongoing immune response in these patients.

Sera from patients with giant cell arteritis and/or polymyalgia rheumatica have been found to contain increased levels of circulating immune complexes during active disease.[33] Immune complex concentrations showed a positive correlation with the erythrocyte sedimentation rate and gamma globulin levels, and dropped to normal levels after treatment or resolution of the inflammatory response.

PATHOLOGY

In giant cell arteritis, inflammation is found most often in vessels that originate from the arch of the aorta, but almost any artery of the body may be affected occasionally as well as some veins.[14,34] The inflammation tends to affect the arteries in a segmental or patchy fashion, but long portions of arteries may be involved.[35] In patients who died during the active phase of giant cell arteritis, the highest incidence of severe involvement was noted in the superficial temporal arteries, vertebral arteries, and ophthalmic and posterior ciliary arteries.[25] The internal carotid, external carotid, and central retinal arteries have been affected less frequently.[25] In other post-mortem studies lesions were found commonly in the proximal and distal aorta and internal and external carotid, subclavian, brachial, and abdominal arteries.[36,37] Intracranial arteries are involved infrequently.[25] In some instances follow-up biopsy or autopsy surveys have shown persistence of mild chronic inflammation even though symptoms have resolved.[38]

In early cases or in regions of arteries with minimal involvement, collections of lymphocytes may be confined to the region of the internal or external elastic lamina or adventitia. Intimal thickening without prominent cellular infiltration is usually present. In areas with more marked involvement, all layers are affected (Fig. 73–1). Necrosis of portions of the arterial wall (including the elastic laminae) and granulomas containing multinucleated histiocytic and foreign body giant cells, his-

Figure 73–1. Giant cell arteritis. In transverse section of temporal artery, adventitia is at top of figure and intima is at central portion of bottom of figure. Multinucleated giant cell (arrow) is present at junction of media and intima. There is extensive disruption of all layers of vessel wall. Hematoxylin and eosin; × 100. (Courtesy of Dr. J. T. Lie.)

Figure 73–2. Giant cell arteritis involving the proximal aorta in a patient dying of a ruptured ascending aorta. This section of the ascending aorta is distal to the ruptured portion and shows destruction of elastic fibers (arrow). Elastic van Gieson stain; × 64. Neighboring sections stained with hematoxylin and eosin showed infiltrations of mononuclear leukocytes in the areas of disrupted fibers.

tiocytes, lymphocytes (which are predominantly T-helper cells), and some plasma cells and fibroblasts are found.[39-41] Eosinophils may be seen, but polymorphonuclear leukocytes are rare.[41] Thrombosis may develop at sites of active inflammation; later, these areas may recanalize. The inflammatory process is usually most marked in the inner portion of the media adjacent to the internal elastic lamina. Fragmentation and disintegration of elastic fibers occur, closely associated with an accumulation of giant cells (Fig. 73–2). However, giant cells are not seen in all sections and therefore are not required for the diagnosis if other features are compatible. Fibrinoid necrosis seen in necrotizing arteritis is less common.[41] The more sections that are examined in the area of arteritis, the more likely giant cells will be found.[11]

Aside from vasculitis, when present, there has been little found pathologically in polymyalgia rheumatica. Granulomatous mycarditis and hepatitis have been noted.[42-44] Muscle biopsies have been normal or showed nonspecific type II muscle atrophy.[45] However, a number of reports have shown the presence of lymphocytic synovitis in the knees, sternoclavicular joints, and shoulders and evidence of a similar reaction in sacroiliac joints.[46,47] Synovitis (mostly subclinical) has been shown in bone scans demonstrating an increased uptake of technetium pertechnetate in the joints of 24 of 25 patients with polymyalgia rheumatica.[48]

CLINICAL FEATURES

The mean age at onset of giant cell arteritis and polymyalgia rheumatica is approximately 70 years, with a range of about 50 to more than 90 years of age. Younger patients have been reported, but these are atypical. Women are affected about twice as often as men.[49]

The onset may be abrupt or insidious, but in most instances the symptoms have been present for weeks or months before the diagnosis is established. Constitutional symptoms, including fatigue, anorexia, and weight loss, are present in the majority of patients and may be an early or even an initial finding.

Giant Cell Arteritis. The majority of patients with giant cell arteritis have symptoms related to the arteries at some time during the course of the illness. However, the presenting symptoms vary widely. The initial manifestations and clinical findings in 100 patients with giant cell arteritis seen consecutively are shown in Tables 73–1 and 73–2. Headache is probably the most common symptom and is present in two thirds or more of patients.[40,50] It usually begins early in the course of the disease and is commonly an initial symptom. The pain is frequently marked, boring, or lancinating in quality and is often localized to the regions along the arteries of the scalp, but it may be less well defined. Headaches may be severe when the cranial arteries are normal to palpation and may subside even though the disease activity continues.

Scalp tenderness is a common symptom in patients and especially in those with headache. Usually tenderness is localized to the temporal or occipital arteries but may be diffuse (Fig. 73–3). Tender spots or nodules may be present for several days over any part of the scalp.

Visual symptoms are common and include diplopia, ptosis, and transient or permanent, partial or complete blindness. Visual loss is generally caused by ischemia of the optic nerve or tracts secondary to arteritis of the branches of the ophthalmic or posterior ciliary arteries,

Table 73–1. Initial Manifestation in 100 Patients with Giant Cell Arteritis*

Headache	32
Polymyalgia rheumatica	25
Fever	15
Visual symptoms without loss	7
Weakness/malaise/fatigue	5
Tenderness over arteries	3
Myalgias	4
Weight loss/anorexia	2
Jaw claudication	2
Permanent loss of vision	1
Tongue claudication	1
Sore throat	1
Vasculitis on angiogram	1
Stiffness of hands and wrists	1
Total	100

*Based on Calamia, K.T., and Hunder, G.G.: Clinical manifestations of giant cell arteritis. Clin. Rheum. Dis. 6:389, 1980.

Table 73–2. Giant Cell Arteritis: Clinical Findings in 100 Patients*

Finding	Number
Sex (female/male)	69/31
Duration of manifestations before diagnosis (months)[†]	7 (1–48)
Onset (gradual/sudden)	64/36
Weight loss or anorexia	50
Malaise, fatigue or weakness	40
Fever	42
Polymyalgia rheumatica	39
Other musculoskeletal pains	30
Synovitis	15
Symptoms related to arteries	83
Headache	68
Visual symptoms	
Transient	16
Fixed	14
Jaw claudication	45
Swallowing claudication or dysphagia	8
Tongue claudication	6
Limb claudication	4
Signs related to arteries	66
Artery tenderness	27
Decreased temporal artery pulsations	46
Erythematous, nodular, or swollen scalp arteries	23
Large artery bruits	21
Decreased large artery pulses	7
Ophthalmologic	20
Visual loss	14
Ophthalmoscopic	18
Extraocular muscle weakness	2
Raynaud's phenomenon	3
Central nervous system abnormalities	15
Sore throat	9

*Based on Calamia, K.T., and Hunder, G.G.: Clinical manifestations of giant cell arteritis. Clin. Rheum. Dis. 6:389, 1980.
[†]Shown as mean with range in parentheses

Figure 73–3 Giant cell arteritis involving temporal artery. Short segments of curved artery were erythematous and tender (long arrows). Bandage on scalp is over similar artery that was biopsied and showed giant cell arteritis. Previous biopsy of a proximal segment of right temporal artery, which was normal on physical examination, was normal histologically. Faint scar of this biopsy can be seen above and anterior to right ear (short arrows).

and less commonly is caused by occlusion of the retinal arterioles.[25,51] Rarely, arterial lesions cause infarction of the occipital cortex with visual loss. The early funduscopic appearance seen in blindness is ischemic optic neuritis with slight pallor and edema of the optic disc and scattered cotton-wool patches and small hemorrhages (Fig. 73–4). Later, optic atrophy occurs. Blindness may be the initial symptom but tends to follow other symptoms by several weeks or months and is frequently preceded by transient visual symptoms. Once established, the visual deficit is usually permanent. Visual loss may be unilateral or bilateral. If present on one side initially, involvement in the contralateral eye often occurs within one or two weeks if treatment is not started. Ophthalmoscopic examination in patients without eye involvement is generally normal. In recent reports, the incidence of blindness has been 20 percent or less.[9,15,38,50,52] Older studies often listed an incidence of 40 to 60 percent of visual loss. The lower incidence of blindness today may reflect earlier recognition (in those patients without eye symptoms) and treatment.

Intermittent claudication may occur in muscles of mastication (jaw claudication), the extremities, and occasionally the muscles of the tongue or those involved in swallowing. In the jaw muscles, the discomfort is

Figure 73–4. Ophthalmoscopic view of the acute phase of ischemic optic neuropathy as seen in patients with giant cell arteritis and loss of vision. The optic disc is pale and swollen, the retinal veins are dilated, and a flame-shaped hemorrhage is visible. (Courtesy of Dr. J. Trautmann.)

noted especially when chewing meat and may involve the muscles on one side of the mandible more than the other. In some instances, however, facial artery involvement results in spasm of the jaw muscles. More marked vascular narrowing may, rarely, lead to gangrene of an extremity, scalp, or tongue.

Clinical evidence of large artery involvement is present in 10 to 15 percent of cases.[34] The findings are upper extremity claudication, bruits over the carotid, subclavian, axillary, and branchial arteries, and/or absent or decreased pulses in the neck or arms (Fig. 73–5). In some instances aortic dissection and rupture occur. Angiographic features which suggest giant cell arteritis are smooth-walled arterial stenoses or occlusions alternating with areas of normal or increased caliber in the absence of irregular plaques and ulcerations, located especially in the carotid, subclavian, axillary, and brachial arteries.[53]

Confusion, depression, psychosis, hemiparesis, peripheral neuropathy, acute hearing loss, and brain stem strokes have been observed. Angina pectoris, congestive heart failure, and myocardial infarction secondary to coronary arteritis have been reported. A low grade fever is present in up to half the patients.[15] Approximately 15 percent of patients present with "fever of unknown origin," with a temperature frequently over 39° C.[9,44,54] Patients may experience shaking chills coincident with fever spikes.

Polymyalgia Rheumatica. As is the case in giant cell arteritis, patients are characteristically in good health before developing polymyalgia rheumatica. Systemic manifestations such as low grade fever and weight loss are present in more than half the patients and may be the initial symptoms. High spiking fevers are uncommon in polymyalgia rheumatica in the absence of giant cell arteritis, however.[16] Arthralgias and myalgias may develop abruptly or evolve insidiously over several weeks or months.[6] Malaise, fatigue, and depression along with aching and stiffness may be present for months before diagnosis is made. In the majority, the shoulder girdle is the first to become symptomatic. In the remainder, hips and neck are involved at the onset. The discomfort may begin in one shoulder or hip but usually becomes

Figure 73–5. Giant cell arteritis of large arteries. Arch aortogram. Both subclavian and axillary arteries are affected. Smooth-walled segmental constrictions alternate with areas of normal caliber or aneurysmal dilation. (From Klein, R. G., et al.: Ann. Intern. Med. *83*:806, 1975. Reprinted by permission of Annals of Internal Medicine.)

bilateral within weeks and may involve most·of the proximal limb, axial musculature, and tendinous attachments. Morning stiffness and "gelling" after inactivity are usually prominent. Morning stiffness, characteristic of that in rheumatoid arthritis, is accentuated by minimal movements of joints of affected regions. If the symptoms are severe, aching is more persistent. Although movement of the joints accentuates the pain, it is often felt in the proximal extremities rather than in the joints.[55] Pain at night is common, and movement during sleep may awaken the patient. Muscular strength is generally unimpaired, although the pain with movement makes interpretation of muscle testing difficult. Pain with movement also makes it difficult for patients to get out of bed or the bathtub. In later stages of the syndrome muscle atrophy may develop, and contracture of the shoulder capsule may result in limitation of passive motion as well as active motion.

As noted above, the presence of synovitis in polymyalgia rheumatica is being appreciated increasingly and undoubtedly is the cause for some of the findings in this condition. A careful examination may reveal transient synovitis of the knees and sternoclavicular joints. The shoulders and hips are covered by heavy muscles, and minimal effusions of slight synovitis are not palpable on physical examination. Synovitis has been documented by biopsies, synovial analysis, and joint scintiscans.[6,16,47,48,56]

RELATIONSHIP BETWEEN POLYMYALGIA RHEUMATICA AND GIANT CELL ARTERITIS

It was suggested by Paulley and Hughes that symptoms of polymyalgia rheumatica might be an expression of an underlying arteritis which was not always clinically evident.[54] Alestig and Barr supported this observation when they found temporal arteritis in patients with polymyalgia rheumatica who had no symptoms or signs of vasculitis.[57] In several reports of giant cell arteritis, polymyalgia rheumatica has been noted in about 40 to 60 percent of patients and was the initial symptom complex in 20 to 40 percent.[49] Conversely, in series of patients with polymyalgia rheumatica, giant cell arteritis has been found in 0 to 80 percent of cases.[49] The cause of this latter variability is uncertain but may be explained in part by selection of cases. In some series temporal artery biopsies were done infrequently, or only small artery segments were taken which may not have included an inflamed area. In other studies biopsies were done when giant cell arteritis was suspected on the basis of symptoms. This inevitably increased the frequency of diagnosis of arteritis. In an epidemiologic study in Olmsted County, Minnesota, in which all diagnosed cases of polymyalgia rheumatica over a 10-year period were studied, 15 percent were considered to have giant cell arteritis.[16] Although the incidence of giant cell arteritis in patients with polymyalgia rheumatica who have no symptoms or signs of arteritis may differ from one population to another, positive temporal artery biopsies will be found in perhaps 10 to 15 percent. Thus, most patients with biopsy-proved giant cell arteritis have symptoms related to artery involvement in addition to musculoskeletal aching.

Polymyalgia rheumatica may begin before, appear simultaneously with, or develop after the symptoms related to the arteries. Mild aching and stiffness may persist for months or years after other findings of giant cell arteritis have remitted. Aside from symptoms related to arteries themselves, few differences have been noted between patients with polymyalgia rheumatica who have been shown to have giant cell arteritis and those whose temporal artery biopsies are normal.[38]

Although it is tempting to conclude that the musculoskeletal symptoms are related to vasculitis, good evidence for this is lacking. Many patients with giant cell arteritis do not have polymyalgia rheumatica, even when large vessels such as the subclavian, axillary, and brachial arteries are clinically involved. In addition, the finding of joint swelling in some patients argues that polymyalgia rheumatica may be a particular form of proximal synovitis. It has been speculated that a single etiologic factor may educe two pathologic processes, both arteritis and synovitis. The varied clinical and pathological manifestations that develop (giant cell arteritis and/or polymyalgia rheumatica) would be the result perhaps of genetic susceptibility.

LABORATORY STUDIES

Except for the findings on arterial biopsy, laboratory results in polymyalgia rheumatica and giant cell arteritis are similar.[38] A mild to moderate normochromic anemia is usually present in both diseases during their active phases. Leukocyte and differential counts are generally normal. A markedly elevated erythrocyte sedimentation rate is characteristic of both. Levels of over 100 mm in 1 hour (Westergren) are common, but occasionally untreated biopsy-proved cases of giant cell arteritis may have normal or nearly normal erythrocyte sedimentation rates. Platelet counts are often increased.

Nonspecific changes in plasma proteins are often present and include a decrease in concentration of albumin and an increase in alpha-2-globulins and fibrinogen. Slight increases in gamma globulins and complement may be present.[32] Tests for antinuclear antibodies and rheumatoid factor are generally negative.

Tests measuring liver function have been found to be mildly abnormal in approximately one third of patients with giant cell arteritis and slightly less in polymyalgia rheumatica.[16,50] An abnormal Bromsulphalein retention and increased alkaline phosphatase are the most common abnormalities, but increases in glutamic-oxaloacetic transaminase and prolonged prothrombin time may also be found.[58] Liver biopsies are generally normal; granulomatous hepatitis has been observed.[43,44]

Renal function and urinalysis are usually normal. Red cell casts are found in some instances, but their presence does not correlate with clinical large artery involvement.[34]

Serum creatine kinase and other enzymes reflecting muscle damage are normal. Electromyograms have usu-

ally been reported to be normal, and muscle biopsy shows normal histology or only mild atrophy characteristic of disuse.[45]

In the relatively few synovial fluid analyses reported in giant cell arteritis or polymyalgia rheumatica, there has been evidence of mild inflammation, including a poor mucin clot and synovial fluid leukocyte counts varying from 1000 to 8000 per cubic millimeter, with 40 to 50 percent polymorphonuclear leukocytes.[6] Synovial fluid complement levels usually have been normal.[59] In some instances synovial biopsy has shown lymphocytic synovitis.[46,48]

DIAGNOSIS

The diagnosis of giant cell arteritis should be considered in any patient over the age of 50 years who has a new form of headache, transient or sudden loss of vision, polymyalgia rheumatica, unexplained prolonged fever or anemia, and high erythrocyte sedimentation rate. Because the manifestations may vary in severity or may be transient, patients suspected of having this disease must be questioned carefully about recent as well as current symptoms. The arteries of the head, neck, upper torso, and arms should be examined for tenderness, enlargement, thrombosis, and bruits. Diagnostic artery biopsy is recommended in all patients suspected of having giant cell arteritis. The temporal artery is biopsied frequently, but the occipital or facial artery can also be taken for histologic study. Because the involvement may be focal, a symptomatic or clinically abnormal segment of the artery should be chosen for biopsy (see Fig. 73-3). When the extracranial arteries are normal and giant cell arteritis is suspected, it is important to biopsy a several-centimeter segment of a temporal artery and to examine histologic sections transversely or longitudinally and consider a contralateral biopsy if the first side is normal.[35] An angiographic examination of the aortic arch and its branches should be performed in patients with symptoms or findings of large artery involvement (see Fig. 73-4).[53]

Temporal artery biopsies should be performed in most patients with polymyalgia rheumatica to determine whether giant cell arteritis is present. If clinical evidence for giant cell arteritis is absent, the decision regarding artery biopsy is often more difficult and should be based on the findings in each patient. If symptoms are mild and of recent onset, or are stable and of long duration, such as a year or longer in duration without current or previous evidence of arteritis, it may be possible to follow the patient closely without biopsy. Blindness is uncommon in such patients. Opinions are divided about the prognostic significance of a negative temporal artery biopsy.[60] In a recent study, 88 patients with negative temporal artery biopsies were followed up after a mean period of 56 months. The negative biopsy predicted the absence of clinical giant cell arteritis and the need for corticosteroid treatment in 78, or about 90 percent.[61]

Generally there is little difficulty separating giant cell arteritis from polyarteritis, hypersensitivity vasculitis, or

Wegener's granulomatosis because of the different distribution of lesions, histopathology, and organ involvement. However, in occasional cases these forms of necrotizing vasculitis appear to involve the temporal artery, and in rare instances there is some overlapping histopathology.[62,63]

Giant cell arteritis can be distinguished from isolated angiitis of the central nervous system, Takayasu's disease, and other similar arteritides by the age of the patient and distribution of lesions, even though the histopathologic findings and roentgenologic findings may be indistinguishable at times (see Chapter 72).

The diagnosis of polymyalgia rheumatica is clinical and depends on eliciting the symptoms and findings noted above. Polymyalgia rheumatica can usually be differentiated from late onset rheumatoid arthritis by the absence of prominent peripheral joint pain and swelling. In patients with polymyositis the muscular weakness is the predominant factor limiting movement, whereas in polymyalgia rheumatica pain causes limited function. In addition, in polymyositis muscle enzymes are elevated and electromyograms are abnormal. Although patients with neoplasms may have generalized musculoskeletal aching, there is no association between polymyalgia rheumatica and malignancy, and a search for an underlying tumor is not necessary unless some clinical evidence for a tumor is present. Some patients with chronic infections such as bacterial endocarditis may have findings simulating polymyalgia rheumatica, and blood cultures should be obtained in patients with fever. Patients with functional myalgias usually do not have typical morning stiffness and have laboratory tests which are normal or nearly so.

TREATMENT AND COURSE

Once the diagnosis of giant cell arteritis is established, corticosteroid treatment should be instituted. In patients strongly suspected of having giant cell arteritis, especially those with impending vascular complications such as visual loss, therapy may be started immediately or after a hemoglobin and erythrocyte sedimentation rate are obtained. Steroid treatment alters the histopathologic picture, but in most instances inflammatory changes are still recognizable for several days after corticosteroids have been started. If the temporal (or other) artery biopsies show no arteritis but the clinical suspicion of arteritis is strong as a result of vascular symptoms or findings, a trial of corticosteroid treatment still may be instituted. An initial amount of 45 to 60 mg of prednisone or equivalent, in divided daily doses, is adequate in nearly all cases. If desired, the initial dose or two can be given parenterally. If the patient does not respond promptly, the dose should be increased. The effective starting dose should be continued until all reversible symptoms and findings have gone and laboratory tests have reverted to normal. This usually occurs within 2 to 4 weeks. After that the dose can be gradually reduced by a maximum of 10 percent of the total daily dose each 1 or 2 weeks. The reduction program is gauged by the symptoms and blood tests. The erythrocyte sedimen-

tation rate is the most helpful laboratory test available to follow patients. The hemoglobin, albumin, and alpha-2-globulin concentrations may also be used but are somewhat less sensitive indicators of disease activity. At some point in the reduction program, the erythrocyte sedimentation rate may rise above normal once again and further reductions of prednisone may be temporarily interdicted. Subsequent reductions may have to be smaller and to be made at longer intervals. It is not uncommon to find that it is necessary to continue doses of 15 to 25 mg or more of prednisone daily for several months before making further reductions. Gradual reductions allow the identification of the minimum suppressive dose, and also help avoid "exacerbations" resulting from too rapid withdrawal of prednisone. Spontaneous recrudescences occur, however, in an unpredictable fashion. Generally, these occur during the first 2 years of the disease.

Giant cell arteritis runs a self-limited course over several months to several years, commonly 1 or 2 years, and eventually the corticosteroids can be reduced and discontinued in most patients.[11] A small proportion of patients appear to need low doses of prednisone for several years or more in order to control musculoskeletal symptoms. Alternate-day corticosteroid therapy is less effective than daily administration and cannot be depended upon to control acute symptoms.[50] It may be tried, however, in patients who have developed disturbing side effects from daily treatment. The effects of cytotoxic drugs, antimalarials, and penicillamine or other drugs have not been studied in a systematic fashion in this disease but may be considered in cases not responding to corticosteroids.

In patients with polymyalgia rheumatica without vascular symptoms or signs and especially in those who have temporal artery biopsies which are normal, nonsteroidal drugs may be tried. Salicylates and the new nonsteroidal anti-inflammatory drugs adequately control symptoms in some patients.[16] If the patients do not respond satisfactorily in 2 to 4 weeks, 5 to 15 mg daily doses of prednisone, or equivalent, may be started. These amounts usually result in rapid improvement of the musculoskeletal aching and stiffness, but may not suppress an underlying arteritis if it is present. Thus, the patient must be followed carefully even though he feels better. In patients with polymyalgia rheumatica, the dose should be reduced gradually as soon as symptoms permit. The erythrocyte sedimentation rate generally returns to normal more slowly with small doses of corticosteroids than is observed with 40 to 60 mg per day. If the laboratory tests become normal on the smaller doses, the likelihood of an underlying active vasculitis would seem to be much less and the risk of vascular complications smaller. However, this does not hold in all instances, because active arteritis has been observed even though the sedimentation rate has improved.[64]

References

1. Gilmour, J.R.: Giant-cell chronic arteritis. J. Pathol. Bacteriol. 53:263, 1941.
2. Horton, B.T., Magath, T.B., and Brown, G.E.: An undescribed form of

arteritis of the temporal vessels. Proc. Staff Meet. Mayo Clin. 7:700, 1932.

3. Kilbourne, E.D., and Wolff, H.H.: Cranial arteritis: A critical evaluation of the syndrome of "temporal arteritis" with report of a case. Ann. Intern. Med. 24:1, 1946.

4. McMillan, G.C.: Diffuse granulomatous aortitis with giant cells: Associated with partial rupture and dissection of the aorta. Arch. Pathol. 49:63, 1950.

5. Barber, H.S.: Myalgic syndrome with constitutional effects: Polymyalgia rheumatica. Ann. Rheum. Dis. 16:230, 1957.

6. Hunder, G.G., Disney, T.F., and Ward, L.E.: Polymyalgia rheumatica. Mayo Clin. Proc. 44:849, 1969.

7. Healey, L.A., Parker, F., and Wilske, K.R.: Polymyalgia rheumatica and giant cell arteritis. Arthritis Rheum. 14:138, 1971.

8. Dixon, A.St.J., Beardwell, C., Kay, A., Wanka, J., and Wong, Y.T.: Polymyalgia rheumatica and temporal arteritis. Ann. Rheum. Dis. 25:203, 1966.

9. Healey, L.A., and Wilske, K.R.: The Systemic Manifestations of Temporal Arteritis. New York, Grune & Stratton, 1978.

10. Hamrin, B.: Polymyalgia arteritica. Acta Med. Scan. (Suppl.) 533:1, 1972.

11. Huston, K.A., Hunder, G.G., Lie, J.T., Kennedy, R.H., and Elveback, L.R.: Temporal arteritis: A 25-year epidemiologic, clinical and pathologic study. Ann. Intern. Med. 88:162, 1978.

12. Bengtsson, B.-Å., and Malmvall, B.-E.: The epidemiology of giant cell arteritis, including temporal arteritis and polymyalgia rheumatica: Incidences of different clinical presentations and eye complications. Arthritis Rheum. 24:899, 1981.

13. Jonasson, F., Cullen, J.F., and Elton, R.A.: Temporal arteritis: A 14-year epidemiologic, clinical and prognostic study. Scot. Med. J. 24:111, 1979.

14. Östberg, G.: On arteritis with special reference to polymyalgia arteritica. Acta Pathol. Microbiol. Scand. [A] Suppl. 237:1, 1973.

15. Calamia, K.T., and Hunder, G.G.: Clinical manifestations of giant cell arteritis. Clin. Rheum. Dis. 6:389, 1980.

16. Chuang, T.-Y., Hunder, G.G., Ilstrup, D.M., and Jurland, L.T.: Polymyalgia rheumatica. A 10-year epidemiologic and clinical study. Ann. Intern. Med. 97:672, 1982.

17. Liang, G.C., Simkin, P.A., Hunder, G.G., Wilske, K.R., and Healey, L.A.: Familial aggregation of polymyalgia rheumatica and giant cell arteritis. Arthritis Rheum. 17:19, 1974.

18. Kemp, A.: Monozygotic twins with temporal arteritis and ophthalmic arteritis. Acta Ophthalmol. (Copenh.) 55:183, 1977.

19. Terasaki, P.I., Healey, L.A., and Wilske, K.R.: Distribution of HLA haplotypes in polymyalgia rheumatica (letter to the editor). N. Engl. J. Med. 295:905, 1976.

20. Hunder, G.G., Taswell, H.F., Pineda, A.A., and Elveback, L.R.: HLA antigens in patients with giant cell arteritis and polymyalgia rheumatica. J. Rheumatol. 4:321, 1977.

21. Hazleman, B., Goldstone, A., and Voak, D.: Association of polymyalgia rheumatica and giant-cell arteritis with HLA-B7. Br. Med. J. 2:989, 1977.

22. Bridgeford, P.H., Lowenstein, M., Bocanegra, T.S., Vassey, F.B., Germain, B.F., Espinoza, L.R.: Polymyalgia rheumatica and giant cell arteritis: Histocompatibility typing and hepatitis-B infection studies. Arthritis Rheum. 23:516, 1980.

23. Calamia, K.T., Moore, S.B., Elveback, L.R., and Hunder, G.G.: HLA-DR locus antigens in polymyalgia rheumatica and giant cell arteritis. J. Rheumatol. 8:6, 1981.

24. Kimmelstiel, P., Gilmour, M.T., and Hodges, H.H.: Degeneration of elastic fibers in granulomatous giant cell arteritis (temporal arteritis). Arch. Pathol. 54:157, 1952.

25. Wilkinson, I.M.S., and Russell, R.W.R.: Arteries of the head and neck in giant cell arteritis: A pathological study to show the pattern of arterial involvement. Arch. Neurol. 27:378, 1972.

26. Liang, G.C., Simkin, P.A., and Mannik, M.: Immunoglobulins in temporal arteries: An immunofluorescent study. Ann. Intern. Med. 81:19, 1974.

27. Hazleman, B.O., MacLennan, I.C.M., and Esiri, M.M.: Lymphocyte proliferation to artery antigen as a positive diagnostic test in polymyalgia rheumatica. Ann. Rheum. Dis. 34:122, 1975.

28. Papaioannou, C.C., Hunder, G.G., and McDuffie, F.C.: Cellular immunity in polymyalgia rheumatica and giant cell arteritis: Lack of response to muscle or artery homogenates. Arthritis Rheum. 22:740, 1979.

29. Park, J.R., and Hazleman, B.L.: Immunological and histological study of temporal arteries. Ann. Rheum. Dis. 37:238, 1978.

30. Waaler, E., Tonder, O., and Milde, E.-J.: Immunological histological studies of temporal arteries from patients with temporal arteritis and/or polymyalgia rheumatica. Acta Pathol. Microbiol. Scand. [A] 84:55, 1976.

31. Eghtedari, A.A., Esselinckx, W., and Bacon, P.A.: Circulating immunoblasts in polymyalgia rheumatica. Ann. Rheum. Dis. 35:158, 1976.

32. Malmvall, B.-E., Bengtsson, B.-Å., Kaijser, B., Nilsson, L.-Å, and Alestig, K.: Serum levels of immunoglobulin and complement in giant-cell arteritis. JAMA 236:1876, 1976.

33. Papaioannou, C.C., Gupta, R.C., Hunder, G.G., and McDuffie, F.C.: Circulating immune complexes in giant cell arteritis polymyalgia rheumatica. Arthritis Rheum. 23:1021, 1980.

34. Klein, R.G., Hunder, G.G., Stanson, A.W., and Sheps, S.G.: Large artery involvement in giant cell (temporal) arteritis. Ann. Intern. Med. 83:806, 1975.

35. Klein, R.G., Campbell, R.J., Hunder, G.G., and Carney, J.A.: Skip lesions in temporal arteritis. Mayo Clin. Proc. 51:504, 1976.

36. Cardell, B.S., and Hanley T.: A fatal case of giant-cell or temporal arteritis. J. Pathol. Bacteriol. 63:587, 1951.

37. Östberg, G.: Temporal arteritis in a large necropsy series. Ann. Rheum. Dis. 30:224, 1971.

38. Fauchald, P., Rygvold, O., and Øystese, B.: Temporal arteritis and polymyalgia rheumatica: Clinical and biopsy findings. Ann. Intern. Med. 77:845, 1972.

39. Parker, F., Healey, L.A., Wilske, K.R., and Odland, G.F.: Light and electron microscopic studies on human temporal arteries with special reference to alterations related to senescence, atherosclerosis and giant cell arteritis. Am. J. Pathol. 79:57, 1975.

40. Hamilton, C.R., Jr., Shelley, W.M., and Tumulty, P.A.: Giant cell arteritis: Including temporal arteritis and polymyalgia rheumatica. Medicine (Baltimore) 50:1, 1971.

41. Banks, P.M., Cohen, M.D., Ginsburg, W.W., Hunder, G.G.: Immunohistologic and cytochemical studies of temporal arteritis. Arthritis Rheum. 26:120, 1983.

42. Hamrin, B., Johsson, N., and Hellsten, S.: "Polymyalgia arteritica": Further clinical and histopathological studies with a report of six autopsy cases. Ann. Rheum. Dis. 27:397, 1968.

43. Long, R., and James, O.: Polymyalgia rheumatica and liver disease. Lancet 1:77, 1974.

44. Calamia, K.T., and Hunder, G.G.: Giant cell arteritis (temporal arteritis) presenting as fever of undetermined origin. Arthritis Rheum. 24:1414, 1981.

45. Brooke, M.H., and Kaplan, H.: Muscle pathology in rheumatoid arthritis, polymyalgia rheumatica, and polymyositis: A histochemical study. Arch. Pathol. 94:101, 1972.

46. Bruk, M.K.: Articular and vascular manifestations of polymyalgia rheumatica. Ann. Rheum. Dis. 26:103, 1967.

47. Henderson, D.R.F., Tribe, C.R., and Dixon, A.St.J.: Synovitis in polymyalgia rheumatica. Rheumatol. Rehabil. 14:244, 1975.

48. O'Duffy, J.D., Wahner, H.W., and Hunder, G.G.: Joint imaging in polymyalgia rheumatica. Mayo Clin. Proc. 51:519, 1976.

49. Hunder, G.G., and Allen, G.L.: Giant cell arteritis: A review. Bull. Rheum. Dis. 29:980, 1978–79.

50. Hunder, G.G., Sheps, S.G., Allen, G.L., and Joyce, J.W.: Daily and alternate-day corticosteroid regimens in treatment of giant cell arteritis: Comparison in a prospective study. Ann. Intern. Med. 82:613, 1975.

51. Hollenhorst, R.W., Brown, J.R., Wagener, H.P., and Shick, R.M.: Neurologic aspects of temporal arteritis. Neurology (Minneap.) 10:490, 1960.

52. Soelberg Sörensen, P., and Lorenzen, I.: Giant-cell arteritis, temporal arteritis and polymyalgia rheumatica: A retrospective study of 63 patients. Acta Med. Scand. 201:207, 1977.

53. Stanson, A.W., Klein, R.G., and Hunder, G.G.: Extracranial angiographic findings in giant cell (temporal) arteritis. Am. J. Roentgenol. 127:957, 1976.

54. Paulley, J.W., and Hughes, J.P.: Giant-cell arteritis, or arteritis of the aged. Br. Med. J. 2:1562, 1960.

55. Fernandez-Herlihy, L.: Polymyalgia rheumatica. Semin. Arthritis Rheum. 1:236, 1971.

56. Wilske, K.R., and Healey, L.A.: Polymyalgia rheumatica: A manifestation of systemic giant-cell arteritis. Ann. Intern. Med. 66:77, 1967.

57. Alestig, K., and Barr, J.: Giant-cell arteritis: A biopsy study of polymyalgia rheumatica, including one case of Takayasu's disease. Lancet 1:1228, 1963.

58. Dickson, E.R., Maldonado, J.E., Sheps, S.G., and Cain, J.A., Jr.: Systemic giant-cell arteritis with polymyalgia rheumatica: Reversible abnormalities of liver function. JAMA 224:1496, 1973.

59. Bunch, T.W., Hunder, G.G., McDuffie, F.C., O'Brien, P.C., and Markowitz, H.: Synovial fluid complement determination as a diagnostic aid in inflammatory joint disease. Mayo Clin. Proc. 49:715, 1974.

60. Allsop, C.J., and Gallagher, P.J.: Temporal artery biopsy in giant cell arteritis. A reappraisal. Am. J. Surg. Pathol. 5:317, 1981.

61. Hall, S., Persellin, S., Kurland, L., O'Brien, P.O., and Hunder, G.G.: The therapeutic impact of temporal artery biopsy. Lancet 2:1217, 1983.

62. Morgan, G.J., Jr., and Harris, E.D., Jr.: Non-giant cell temporal arteritis: Three cases and a review of the literature. Arthritis Rheum. 21:362, 1978.

63. Papaioannou, C.C., Hunder, G.G., and Lie, J.T.: Vasculitis of the gallbladder in a 70-year-old man with giant cell (temporal) arteritis. J. Rheumatol. 6:71, 1979.

64. Rynes, R.I., Mika, P., and Bartholomew, L.E.: Development of giant cell (temporal) arteritis in a patient 'adequately' treated for polymyalgia rheumatica. Ann. Rheum. Dis. 36:88, 1977.

Chapter 74
Behçet's Disease

J. Desmond O'Duffy

INTRODUCTION

In 1937 Behçet described a chronic relapsing syndrome of oral ulceration, genital ulceration, and uveitis.[1] It has been suggested that this syndrome was described by Hippocrates.[2] Besides Behçet's triad, additional features of this syndrome now recognized are synovitis, cutaneous vasculitis resembling erythema nodosum, meningoencephalitis, large artery aneurysms, and phlebitis. Diagnosis remains clinical, as there are no pathognomonic serologic or pathologic tests. The appearance of new clinical features months or years after the onset is common. The most important complications are uveitis, meningoencephalitis, and large vessel disease.

The prevalence of this disease has a peculiar distribution, as most cases have been reported from the eastern Mediterranean[2,3] countries and Japan.[4] In Japan, the prevalence is 1 per 1000,[5] and there it is considered one of the most common causes of blindness.[6] Several large series of cases have been reported from Europe and the United States.[7-10] In Olmsted County, Minnesota, the prevalence is 1 per 25,000. Males exceed females in virtually all series. However, in North America[8] and Australia,[11] females are in a majority.

DIAGNOSTIC CRITERIA

One arbitrary set of diagnostic criteria is based on the six most common clinical manifestations. It requires that three of the following six criteria be present: (1) recurrent aphthous stomatitis, (2) genital aphthous ulcers, (3) uveitis, (4) synovitis, (5) cutaneous vasculitis, and (6) meningoencephalitis.[12] Aphthous ulceration is mandatory. Incomplete forms of the syndrome may be diagnosed if recurrent aphthous ulceration coexists with one other criterion. Others have suggested alternative diagnostic formulas based on combinations of "major" and "minor" criteria.[13] The entity of aphthous stomatitis and vulvitis in adolescent females is usually self-limited and should not be labeled Behçet's disease.

CLINICAL FEATURES

The approximate frequency of the six major clinical findings is shown in Table 74–1. Phlebitis and large vessel arteritis, although less common, are equally important.

Aphthous Stomatitis. Recurrent aphthous stomatitis is virtually a sine qua non of Behçet's disease. The aphthous oral ulcers are usually the first manifestation. They resemble the lesions of uncomplicated canker sores. Like the latter, they occur on the buccal mucosa, lips,

tongue, and pharynx, but may also be found throughout the gastrointestinal tract.[14] The oral ulcers are usually multiple, occur in "crops," and are exceedingly painful. A well-developed ulcer is 2 to 10 mm in diameter, has a central yellow base, and is surrounded by a vivid red halo (Fig. 74–1; Plate X, p. xliv). Lesions heal in 3 to 30 days, usually without scarring. Aphthous ulcers may be present 50 to 100 percent of the time. Comprehensive reviews of recurrent aphthous stomatitis have been written.[15-17] It is not surprising that because of similar clinical appearances and histology some authors view recurrent aphthous stomatitis and Behçet's disease as different expressions of the same process.

Genital Ulcers. Recurrent multiple ulcers of the vulva and vagina in females (Fig. 74–2; see Plate X, p. xliv) and of the scrotum or penis in males resemble the oral aphthae. Vaginal lesions are often asymptomatic unless they are causing a discharge, but the commoner vulvar lesions are painful.[8] In most patients, recurrences of the genital ulcerations are less frequent than the oral ones; in a few they are multiple and persistent and heal with vulvar scarring.

Uveitis. Blindness from anterior uveitis with hypopyon (pus in the anterior chamber of the eye) (Fig. 74–3; see Plate X, p. xliv) was highlighted in Behçet's original report.[1] Perhaps because of topical or systemic corticosteroids, hypopyon is now seldom seen.[18] It is now clear that the posterior uveitis, embracing the vitreous body and retina, is the chief cause of visual loss (Fig. 74–4; see Plate X, p. xliv). Uveitis in Behçet's syndrome is bilateral and is seldom the initial manifestation. It occurs in about two thirds of cases and is more likely to occur in males. Typically, 6 years elapse between the first manifestation—usually aphthous ulceration—and the onset of uveitis. Ophthalmologic evaluation should include examination of the anterior chamber by biomicroscopy and of the posterior segment by biomicroscopy and indirect ophthalmoscopy.[18] Fundus photographs after intravenous fluorescein often show diffuse staining of the disc and retina, indicating vascular permeability. Keratic precipitates in the anterior chamber and vitreous cellular infiltrates indicate activity of the uveitis. In keeping with the pathologic observations of retinal

Table 74–1. Frequency of the Six Major Clinical Features of Behçet's Disease in 50 Patients

	Percent
Recurrent aphthous stomatitis	100
Genital aphthous ulcers	74
Cutaneous vasculitis	56
Uveitis	52
Synovitis	40
Meningoencephalitis	30

vasculitis,[6] venous and arterial occlusions occur.[18] In this setting, bilateral visual loss progresses, and in one series[19] blindness occurred at an average of 3.6 years after onset—in spite of corticosteroid use. In a series[18] of 21 cases of Behçet's uveitis, the three who became blind all had uveitis for longer than 8 years. The visual prognosis is distinctly improved by treatment with chlorambucil.[20-22]

Synovitis. In 50 to 60 percent of patients, there is a subacute or chronic synovitis affecting large and small joints.[8,13] Most commonly it affects the knees and ankles. It occurs during exacerbations of the disease and is steroid responsive. This synovitis rarely causes joint destruction. Synovial fluid cell counts average 5000 to 10,000 per cubic millimeter and polymorphs predominate. Arthralgia is more common but lacks diagnostic value. Rarely sacroiliitis has been noted and then only in HLA-B27 patients.

Cutaneous Lesions. The various skin lesions in Behçet's disease include pustules, nodules, and papules, all considered to be manifestations of cutaneous vasculitis. However, since cutaneous vasculitis is common in various systemic diseases, it is nonspecific. Nodular cutaneous lesions confined to the lower extremities resemble erythema nodosum. It is debated whether or not these lesions can be distinguished from erythema nodosum.[8,23] In contrast to erythema nodosum, lesions may be grouped or may become ulcerated. At times such nodules are found to represent phlebitis in superficial veins.[8] In a patient appearing to have Behçet's disease, the presence of numerous nodose leg lesions should alert the clinician to the possibility of inflammatory bowel disease.

A nonspecific skin sensitivity to simple trauma, such as needlestick, has been reported in Behçet's disease,[23] especially in its active stages. Sterile pustules have been evoked by needlestick or normal saline injections.[11,24,25] Some have not found this phenomenon to be common.[8,26]

Meningoencephalitis. In concert with crops of aphthous stomatitis, the presence of headache, fever, and stiff neck with cerebrospinal pleocytosis and focal neurologic deficit implies meningoencephalitis. In our first 25 patients this complication occurred in seven.[12] The mean interval from onset of Behçet's disease to central nervous system involvement was 1.3 years. Typically, the diagnosis is delayed while exhaustive negative microbiologic studies for this "aseptic meningitis" are performed. Clinical findings include corticospinal tract disease, cerebellar ataxia, pseudobulbar palsy, and transient ocular palsies. Successive bouts of meningoencephalitis cause extensive neurologic deficits, but at times attacks of meningitis alone occur. The cerebrospinal fluid (CSF) typically shows a lymphocytosis and a mild elevation or protein with a normal gamma globulin (in contrast to multiple sclerosis, in which it is usually raised). The meningoencephalitis is only partially responsive to high-dose steroids. Because neurologic flares tend to recur, especially as steroids are lowered, treatment with chlorambucil is now proposed for this complication.[22]

Earlier reports of central nervous system Behçet's disease indicated a grave prognosis, with a 41 percent mortality.[27] Despite one report that only two of twelve patients had lasting neurologic sequelae,[3] the weight of evidence points to a guarded prognosis. When our own series was at 37 cases, 4 of the 6 deaths had occurred in patients having central nervous system disease.[28]

Phlebitis and Arteritis. Thrombosis of large veins[3] and arteries,[29] and arterial aneurysms[30] are well described. Phlebitis of major veins can result in such divergent syndromes as Budd-Chiari syndrome, vena caval occlusion, and in the case of the dural veins, the syndrome of benign intracranial hypertension.[31,32] Diagnosis of limb or caval phlebitis may require venography and in the case of dural sinus thrombosis, digital subtraction angiography may be diagnostic. An unusual hypercoagulable state suggested in one report[33] has been confirmed.[34] Decreased fibrinolysis was suggested by prolonged euglobulin clot lysis and undetectable fibrinogen degradation products, perhaps related to low factor XII level.[34] Occlusions and aneurysms of large systemic arteries can cause life-threatening or fatal illness from limb ischemia, stroke, renovascular hypertension, or aortic aneurysm.[32] Behçet's disease is virtually alone among the vasculitides as a frequent cause of fatal aneurysms of the pulmonary arterial tree.[35,36] Such patients present with massive hemoptysis and may be diagnosed by pulmonary angiography.[36]

Other Manifestations. The relationship of Behçet's disease to inflammatory bowel disease is controversial. Virtually all the features of Behçet's disease can be seen in Crohn's disease of the colon. Most large series of Behçet's disease contain a few patients who have or will develop Crohn's disease of the colon. We have observed five patients with the Behçet-Crohn admixture.[28] Markers suggesting Crohn's colitis in such a situation are diarrhea, erythrocyte sedimentation rate > 100, erythema nodosum, and febrile systemic illness. Interestingly, colonic resection in these instances leads to amelioration of the Behçet's disease features. Discrete ulcerations of the lower ileum and right side of colon in Behçet's disease may perforate and require hemicolectomy and distal ileal resection.[37]

Pericarditis and mild nephritis have also been reported.[38]

PATHOLOGY

Microscopy of the early oral ulcers exactly resembles that of recurrent aphthae, and shows a chronic inflammatory reaction with aggregations of lymphocytes and monocytes infiltrating the basal and prickle cell layers of the epidermis.[39,40] These collections also occur around dermal vessels, but fibrinoid necrosis is not seen. Evidence of immune complex deposition is tenuous.[15,39] Similar perivascular inflammation at times, with frank necrosis of vessel walls, occurs in the skin and vulva,[8] retinal vessels,[6] and brain.[41] A non-necrotizing arteritis of the pulmonary arteries is found at autopsy of those patients dying of sudden hemoptysis.[42] However, repeated previous hemoptyses are usually on record, providing an opportunity for diagnosis by pulmonary angiography.[36] Since venous thrombosis and pulmonary artery aneurysms are common to both Behçet's disease and Hughes-Stovin syndrome,[43] it has been suggested that the latter is in fact a manifestation of Behçet's disease.[44] Secondary amyloidosis has also been described in Behçet's disease[45] with demonstration of amyloid proteins AA and AP in renal tissue.

IMMUNOPATHOGENESIS

Behçet described inclusion bodies in hypopyon fluid and oral exudates of his patients. Inoculations of CSF into rabbits,[46] and of the posterior uveal tissue into chorioallantoic membranes with subsequent passage intracerebrally into mice, causing encephalitis,[47] implicated a transmissible virus. Recent efforts to isolate a virus from lesions, CSF, and lymphocytes[48] have been fruitless.[12] Elevated sedimentation rate, mild anemia, hypergammaglobulinemia, and elevated acute phase reactants are common.

Numerous immunologic abnormalities in patients with Behçet's disease have been detected. These include circulating antibodies to human mucosal cells,[4,8,49] lymphocytoxicity to heterologous oral epithelial cells,[50] and blast transformation of patient's lymphocytes by human oral epithelial cells.[51] Lymphocytes from patients are cytotoxic to autologous oral mucous membrane cells in vitro but not to epithelial cells of patients with recurrent aphthous ulcers or of controls.[52] Although studies of T lymphocytes are normal in most patients, the similarity of the histologic lesions to those of delayed hypersensitivity suggests a disordered cellular immunity. Further scrutiny of T-lymphocyte responsiveness of patients by Sakane and colleagues[53] showed that in preactive phases of the disease both concanavalin-A–induced suppressor T-lymphocyte activity and the ability of T lymphocytes to respond in autologous mixed lymphocyte reaction to their own B lymphocytes were reduced. Furthermore, T-lymphocyte subsets OK-T4 (helper) and OK-T8 (suppressor), which are normally in a 2:1 ratio, change to a 1:1 ratio in pre-active disease.

Circulating immune complexes are found in sera of 50 to 60 percent of patients,[54] but bound complement in lesions is not.[55] Abnormalities in humoral immunity in Behçet's disease are evidenced by elevations of serum immunoglobulins A, G, and M in some patients,[8] and of C9.[56,57] Total hemolytic complement is normal or increased, but Shimada and colleagues[55] have shown that just before attacks of uveitis it drops because of activation of both the classic and C3 pathways. Occasionally, cryoprecipitates in sera of such patients are encountered,[11] especially with vasculitic flares. Interferon γ, which has functions separate from antiviral interferon α, is significantly higher in the sera of Behçet's disease patients than controls, especially in convalescent phase.[58] Increased chemotactic activity of polymorphs in Behçet's disease has been confirmed.[59,60] The polymorphs, while showing an increased directed motility response to complement-derived chemotactic factors, have no alteration in random motility, adhesion, or phagocytosis. Despite all these immunologic findings, a coherent basis for "autoimmunity" is lacking so long as the putative antigen remains unidentified.

A recent report[34] demonstrated markedly decreased levels of both free and bound secretory component (SC) of IgA in the saliva of four patients with Behçet's disease. In two patients SC deficiency was also found in jejunal fluid. Salivary IgA levels were only slightly depressed in three of four patients. There is some evidence that ingestion of certain foods, such as English walnuts, exacerbates oral ulcerations in Behçet's disease.[61] These authors observed a reduced T-lymphocyte reactivity in both Behçet's patients and controls after ingestion of 100 grams of walnuts. Besides invoking possible immunologic explanations for the flares following walnut ingestion, it is also reasonable to speculate that oral mucosal trauma by nut spicules was the inciting event.

We have found no association between HLA antigens and Behçet's disease.[62] In contrast, Japanese[63] and Turkish workers[64] have found a 3- to 4-fold increased association of HLA-B5 in Behçet's disease as compared with controls (75 vs. 20 to 30 percent). This observation also holds true in Mexican Mestizo Indians,[65] but not in British patients.[64] The B-5 antigen is about twice as common among uninvolved controls in those regions where the disease is associated with this antigen (Japan and Turkey) than in those countries where it is not associated with B-5 (United States, Britain). However, the large variation in disease prevalence is not due to B-5 antigen. A putative immune-associated antigen (Ia) with linkage dysequilibrium to HLA-B5 in some but not other races would explain this discrepancy.

TREATMENT

Inconsistent and temporary responses have been reported for such disparate agents as corticosteroids,[8,26,66] fresh blood or plasma transfusions,[67] transfer factor,[68,69] phenformin and estradiol, and colchicine.[60,70] Topical application of corticosteroids in pastes or gels palliates the pain of oral aphthae. High-dose corticosteroid therapy (up to 60 mg of prednisone daily) suppresses skin, mucosal, and joint inflammation but has only a palliative effect on posterior uveitis. Central nervous system disease, although ameliorated, seldom enters remission on corticosteroid therapy.[12] Transfer factor has been advocated. In 10 patients there were four responders, three nonresponders, and two "moderate" responders.[68] Levamisole, an immunostimulant, has been reported to benefit some patients[71] but has not been put to the test in adequate numbers of patients with active uveitis and meningoencephalitis. To really show efficacy, a given treatment should prevent blindness from active posterior uveitis and prevent recurrences of meningoencephalitis. Chlorambucil comes closest to meeting these goals.

There are encouraging reports of treating uveitis with chlorambucil orally in initial doses of 0.1 to 0.2 mg per kilogram per day.[20-22,72,73] Duration of therapy has ranged up to 4 years, and in most, visual loss and uveitis activity were arrested. Such patients require joint management by an ophthalmologist and internist. The dosage of chlorambucil is cautiously lowered as uveitis is brought under control. Relapses may require temporary dose increases. Chlorambucil in a dose of 0.1 mg per kg per day has also proved to be useful in the prevention of episodes of meningoencephalitis.[22] Among nine patients thus treated, for an average duration to date of 1.3 years, eight ceased having recurrences. Four of the nine were on corticosteroids and two of these have been able to discontinue them. Azathioprine and cyclophosphamide are probably less effective than chlorambucil. The oncogenic and cytotoxic potential of chlorambucil and other immunosuppressives must be weighed against the hazards of blindness and death from these two complications. Cytotoxic drugs are rarely indicated for the other features but would seem to be reasonable in those with major vasculitis. During chlorambucil treatment, aphthosis and other manifestations usually recede or disappear. When chlorambucil is stopped, relapses may occur. Therefore, alternative types of treatment for this disease must be sought.

References

1. Behçet H.: Über rezidivierende Aphthose, durch ein Virus verursachte Geschwüre am Mund, am Auge und an den Genitalien. Derm. Wschr. 105:1152, 1937.
2. Feigenbaum, A.: Description of Behçet's syndrome in the Hippocratic third book of endemic diseases. Br. J. Ophthalmol. 40:355, 1956.
3. Chajek, T., and Fainaru, M.: Behçet's disease. Report of 41 cases and a review of the literature. Medicine 54:179, 1975.
4. Oshima, Y., Shimizu, T., Yokohari, R., Matsumoto, T., Kano K., Kagami, T., and Nagaya, H.: Clinical studies on Behçet's syndrome. Ann. Rheum. Dis. 22:36, 1963.
5. Hirohata, T., Kuratsune, M., Nomura, A., and Jimi, S.: Prevalence of Behçet's syndrome in Hawaii with particular reference to the comparison of the Japanese in Hawaii and Japan. Hawaii Med. J. 34:244, 1975.
6. Shikano, S.: Ocular pathology of Behçet's syndrome. In Monacelli, M., and Nazzaro, P. (eds.): International Symposium on Behçet's Disease, Rome 1964. Basel, Karger, 1966, pp. 111–136.
7. Mason, R.M., and Barnes, C.G.: Behçet syndrome with arthritis. Schweiz. Med. Wschr. 98:663, 1968.
8. O'Duffy, J.D., Carney, J.A., and Deodhar, S.: Behçet's disease: Report of 10 cases, 3 with manifestations. Ann. Intern. Med. 75:561, 1971.
9. Denman, A.M., Fialkow, P.J., Pelton, B.K., Salo, A.C., Appleford, D.J., Gilchrist, C.: Lymphocyte abnormalities in Behçet's Syndrome. Clin. Exp. Immunol. 42:175, 1980.
10. Wright, V.A., and Chamerlain, V.A.: Behçet's syndrome. Bull. Rheum. Dis. 29(1–2), 1978–1979 series.
11. Cooper, D.A., and Penny, R.: Behçet's syndrome: Clinical, immunological, and therapeutic evaluation of 17 patients. Med. J. Aust. 4:585, 1974.
12. O'Duffy, J.D., and Goldstein, N.P.: Neurologic involvement in seven patients with Behçet's disease. Am. J. Med. 61:170, 1976.
13. Mason, R.M., and Barnes, C.G.: Behçet's syndrome with arthritis. Ann. Rheum. Dis. 28:95, 1969.
14. Griffin, J.W., Harrison, H.B., Tedescor, F.J., Mills, L.R.: Behçet's disease with multiple sites of gastrointestinal involvement. South. Med. J. 75:1405, 1982.
15. Rogers, R.: Recurrent aphthous stomatitis: Clinical characteristics and evidence for an immunopathogenesis. J. Invest. Dermatol. 69:499, 1977.
16. Francis, T.C.: Recurrent aphthous stomatitis and Behçet's disease. Oral Surg. 30:476, 1970.
17. Lehner, T.: Progress report: Oral ulceration in Behçet's syndrome. Gut 18:491, 1977.
18. Colvard, D.M., Robertson, D.M., and O'Duffy, J.D.: The ocular manifestation of Behçet's disease. Arch Ophthalmol. 95:1813, 1977.
19. Mamo, J.G.: The rate of visual loss in Behçet's disease. Arch. Ophthalmol. 84:451, 1970.
20. Mamo, J.G., and Azzam, S.A.: Treatment of Behçet's disease with chlorambucil. Arch. Ophthalmol. 84:446, 1970.
21. Bonnet, M.: Behçet's disease: Clinical evaluation of immunosuppressive therapy in 12 patients. Abstract No. 48, International Symposium on Behçet's Disease, Istanbul, September, 1977.
22. O'Duffy, J.D., Robertson, D.M., and Goldstein, N.P.: Chlorambucil in the treatment of uveitis and meningoencephalitis of Behçet's disease. Am. J. Med. 76:75, 1984.
23. Nazzaro, P.: Cutaneous manifestations of Behçet's disease. In Monacelli,

24. Haim, S.: Contribution of ocular symptoms in the diagnosis of Behçet's syndrome—study of 23 cases. Arch. Dermatol. 98:478, 1968.
25. Shimizu, T., Katsuta, Y., and Oshima, Y.: Immunological studies on Behçet's syndrome. Ann. Rheum. Dis. 24:494, 1965.
26. Kalbian, V.V., and Challis, M.T.: Behçet's disease: Report of 12 cases with 3 manifesting as papilledema. Am. J. Med. 49:823, 1970.
27. Wolf, S.M., Schotland, D.L., and Phillips, L.L.: Involvement of nervous system in Behçet's syndrome. Arch. Neurol. 12:315, 1965.
28. O'Duffy, J.D.: Prognosis in Behçet's syndrome. Bull. Rheum. Dis. 29:972, 1978–79.
29. Bank, H.: Thrombotic pulmonary manifestations in Behçet's syndrome. Isr. J. Med. Sci. 9:955, 1973.
30. Enoch, B.A., Castillo-Olivares, J.D., Khoo, T.C.L., Granger, R.G., and Henry, L.: Major vessel complication in Behçet's syndrome. Postgrad. Med. J. 44:453, 1968.
31. Pamir, N.M., Kansu, T., Erbengi, A., and Zileli, T: Papilledema in Behçet's syndrome. Arch. Neurol. 38:643, 1981.
32. Shimizu, T., Ehrlich, G.E., Inaba, G., and Hiyashi, K.: Behçet's disease (Behçet's syndrome). Sem. Arthritis Rheum. 4:223, 1979.
33. Cunliffe, W.K., and Menon, I.S.: Treatment of Behçet's syndrome with phenformin and ethyloestrenol. Lancet 1:1239, 1969.
34. Abdou, N.I., Schumacher, H.R., Colman, R.W., Sagawa, A., Herbert, J., Pascual, E., Carroll, E.T., Miller, M., South, M., and Abdou, N.W.: Behçet's disease: Possible role of secretory component deficiency, synovial inclusions, and fibrinolytic abnormality in the various manifestations of the disease. J. Lab. Clin. Med. 91:409, 1978.
35. Davies, J.D.: Behçet's syndrome with haemoptysis and pulmonary lesions. J. Pathol. 109:351, 1973.
36. Grenier, P. Bletry, O., Cornud, F., Godeau, P., and Nahum, H.: Pulmonary involvement in Behçet's disease. Am. J. Radiol. 137:565, 1981.
37. Baba, S., and Morioka, S.: Treatment of intestinal Behçet's disease. In Inaba, G. (ed.): Behçet's Disease: Pathogenetic Mechanism and Clinical Future. Japan Medical Research Foundation, Publication No. 18, University of Tokyo Press, 1982, pp. 559–570.
38. Herreman, G., Beaufil, S.H., Godeau, P., Cassou, B., Wechsler, B., Boujeau J., Chomette, G.: Behçet's syndrome and renal involvement: A histologic and immunofluorescent study of 11 renal biopsies. Am. J. Med. Sci. 284:10, 1982.
39. Lehner, T.: Pathology of recurrent oral ulceration and oral ulceration in Behçet's syndrome: Light, electron, and fluorescence microscopy. J. Pathol. 97:481, 1969.
40. Muller, W., and Lehner, T.: Quantitative electron microscopical analysis of leukocyte infiltration in oral ulcers of Behçet's syndrome. Br. J. Dermatol. 106:535, 1982.
41. McMenemey, W.H., and Lawrence, B.J.: Encephalomyelopathy in Behçet's disease: Report of necropsy findings in two cases. Lancet 2:353, 1957.
42. Slavin, R.E., and DeGroot, W.J.: Pathology of the lung in Behçet's disease. Am. J. Surg. Path. 5:799, 1981.
43. Hughes, J.P., and Stovin, P.G.I.: Segmental pulmonary artery aneurysms with peripheral venous thrombosis. Br. J. Dis. Chest 53:19, 1959.
44. Durieux, P., Bletry, O., Huchon, G., Wechsler, B., Chretien, J., and Godeau, P.: Multiple pulmonary artery aneurysms in Behçet's disease and Hughes-Stovin syndrome. Am. J. Med. 71:736, 1981.
45. Skinner, M.: Case records of the Massachusetts General Hospital, Case 19-1982. N. Engl. J. Med. 306:1162, 1982.
46. Alm, L., and Oberg, L.: Djuriorsok via S. K. Behçet's syndrome preliminart meddelande. Nord. Med. 25:603, 1945.
47. Sezer, F.N.: The isolation of a virus as the cause of Behçet's disease. Am. J. Ophthalmol. 36:301, 1953.
48. Yananouchi, K., Shishido, A., Kobune, F., Saka, T.A., Inaba, G.: Virologic approaches to Behçet's disease in Japan. In Behçet's Disease: Pathogenetic Mechanism and Clinical Future. Japan Medical Research Foundation Publication No. 18. University of Tokyo Press, 1982, pp. 57–63.
49. Lehner, T.: Behçet's syndrome and autoimmunity. Br. Med. J. 1:465, 1967.
50. Rogers, R.S., Sams, W., Jr., and Shorter, R.G.: Lymphocytotoxicity in recurrent aphthous stomatitis: Lymphocytotoxicity for oral epithelial cells in recurrent aphthous stomatitis and Behçet's syndrome. Arch. Dermatol. 109:361, 1974.
51. Lehner, T.: Immunologic aspects of recurrent oral ulcers. Oral Surg. 33:80, 1972.
52. Reimer, G., Steinkohl, S., Djawari, D., and Hornstein, O.P., Lytic effect of cytotoxic lymphocytes on oral epithelial cells in Behçet's disease. Br. J. Dermatol. 107:529, 1982.
53. Sakane, T., Kotani, H., Takada, S., and Tsunematso, T.: Functional aberration of T-cell subsets in patients with Behçet's disease. Arthritis Rheum. 25:1343, 1982.
54. Gupta, R.C., McDuffie, F.C., O'Duffy, M.D., Maurer, M., and Jordan, R.E.: Circulating immune complexes in active Behçet's disease. Clin. Exp. Immunol. 34:213, 1978.
55. Shimada, K., Kogure, M., Kawashima, T., and Hishioka, K.L.: Reduction

of complement in Behçet's disease and drug allergy. Med. Biol. 52:234, 1974.

56. Adinolfi, M., and Lehner, T.: Acute phase proteins and C9 in patients with Behçet's syndrome and aphthous ulcers. Clin. Exp. Immunol. 25:36, 1976.

57. Kawachi-Takahashi, S., Takahashi, M., Kogure, M., and Kawashima, T.: Elevation of serum C9 level association with Behçet's disease. Jap. J. Exp. Med. 44:485, 1974.

58. Ohno S., Kato, F., Matsuda, H., Fujii, N., and Minagawa, T.: Detection of gamma interferon in the sera of patients with Behçet's disease. Infect. Immun. 36:202, 1982.

59. Sobel, J.D., Haim, S., Obedeanu, N., Meshulam, T., and Merzbach, D.: Polymorphonuclear leucocyte function in Behçet's disease. J. Clin. Pathol. 30:250, 1977.

60. Mizushima, Y., Matsumara, N., and Mori, M.: Chemotaxis of leukocyte and colchicine treatment in Behçet's disease. J. Rheum. 6:108, 1979.

61. Marquardt, J.L., Snyderman, R., and Oppenheim, J.J.: Depression of lymphocyte transformation and exacerbation of Behçet's syndrome by ingestion of English walnuts. Cell. Immunol. 9:263, 1973.

62. O'Duffy, J.D., Taswell, H.F., and Elveback, L.R.: HL-A antigens in Behçet's disease. J. Rheumatol. 3:1, 1976.

63. Ohno, S., Narayama, E., Sugiura, S., Takura, K., Aoki, K., and Aizawa, M.: Specific histocompatibility antigens associated with Behçet's disease. Am. J. Ophthalmol. 80:636, 1975.

64. Yazici, H., Chamberlain, M.A., Schreuder, I., D'Amaro, J., Muftuoglu,

M.: HLA antigens in Behçet's disease: A reappraisal by a comparative study of Turkish and British patients. Ann. Rheum. Dis. 39:344, 1980.

65. Lavelle, C., Alorcón-Segovia, D., del Giudice-Knipping, J.A., and Fraga, A.: Association of Behçet's syndrome with HLA-B5 in the Mexican Mestizo population. J. Rheum. 8:325, 1981.

66. Breslin, H.J.: Bechet's disease: Report of a case history of seventeen years' duration. Am. J. Ophthalmol. 53:132, 1962.

67. Haim, S., and Sherb, K.: Behçet's disease: Presentation of 11 cases and evaluation of treatment. Isr. J. Med. Sci. 2:69, 1966.

68. Wolf, R.E., Rundenberg, H.H., Welch, T.M., Spitler, L.E., and Ziff, M.: Treatment of Behçet's syndrome with transfer factor. JAMA 238:869, 1977.

69. Bernhard, G.C., and Heim, L.F.: Transfer factor treatment of Bechet's syndrome (abstract). J. Rheumatol. 1:34, 1974.

70. Mizushima, Y., Matsuda, T., Ohama, N., Hoshi, K., and Takeuchi, A.: Colchicine and anti-thrombocytic drugs in the treatment of Behçet's disease. In Inaba, G. (ed.): Behçet's Disease: Pathogenetic Mechanism and Clinical future. Japan Medical Research Foundation Publication No. 18, University of Tokyo Press, 1982, pp. 513–517.

71. de Merieux P., Spitler, L.E., Paulus, H.E.: Treatment of Behçet's syndrome with levamisole. Arthritis Rheum. 24:64, 1981.

72. Tricoulis, D.: Treatment of Behçet's disease with chlorambucil. Br. J. Ophthalmol. 60:55, 1976.

73. Bonnet, M.: Immunosuppressive therapy of Behçet's syndrome. Long-term follow-up evaluation. J. Fr. Ophthalmol. 4:455, 1981.

Chapter 75

Panniculitis and Erythema Nodosum

G. James Morgan, Jr.

INTRODUCTION

The idiopathic inflammatory disorders of the subcutaneous fat, or panniculitides, are differentiated one from another by clinical and histopathologic criteria. Classification schemes rely on the development of adult subcutaneous tissue from the mesenchyme in a lobular pattern. A central nutrient artery sends multiple arterioles through an inconspicuous fibrous matrix to be drained in a peripheral system of venules located in clearly defined septa.[1] Inflammation around the central arterial system produces changes in the entire lobule (lobular panniculitis), while inflammation around the venous system gives primarily a septal inflammation (septal panniculitis), with accompanying reactions in the contiguous reticular dermis.

Erythema nodosum and its variant, subacute migratory panniculitis, provide the only clear examples of septal panniculitides, whereas pancreatic panniculitis, Weber-Christian disease, erythema induratum, and systemic vasculitis are primarily lobular panniculitides. Rare forms of panniculitis, including cold sensitivity and steroid withdrawal panniculitis, are not so readily classified, while certain infectious agents and malignancy may involve the subcutaneous tissue directly. It must be stressed that the intensity of inflammatory responses in all diseases is initiated and modified by fatty acids released by degraded lipocytes.[2] The lipodystrophies, which have been associated with rheumatic disease[3,4] and

are degenerative processes of the subcutaneous tissue, will not be discussed in this chapter.

SEPTAL PANNICULITIS

Erythema Nodosum. Erythema nodosum refers to a syndrome of crops of painful nodules occurring in a bilateral pattern on the anterior surfaces of the lower legs, and is thought to represent a hypersensitivity reaction to a variety of systemic antigens. A wider distribution of nodules is possible, but internal organs are not involved. The nodules are tender to touch, red to purple, and rarely greater than 5 cm in diameter. Inflammation of the overlying skin may cause a local warmth, and subcutaneous edema may lead to pitting on pressure. Ulceration does not occur, and healing proceeds by resorption of extravasated red blood cells (Fig. 75–1). Residual scaling and hyperpigmentation may be seen, but there is no atrophy or scarring. Recurring crops leave nodules in varying stages of development, while the entire process may last from 1 to 3 months. Chronic eruptions are most common in sarcoidosis or idiopathic erythema nodosum.[5]

The clinical picture is that of a nonspecific systemic illness with low-grade fever, malaise, arthralgias, and loss of appetite, or the patient may be entirely well save for the eruption. When there is an associated illness, this may dominate the presentation. Evidence of a specific arthritis associated with erythema nodosum per se is

Figure 75–1. Erythema nodosum. Healing subcutaneous nodules on the anterior tibial surfaces resembling multiple contusions.

rare. Nodules appearing around joints produce a picture of periarthritis. Arthritis associated with the underlying precipitating disease is often difficult to distinguish from that which has been described as occurring with erythema nodosum.[6,7] This disease may affect all ages, but there are two peaks of incidence: in childhood and in the third decade. There is a female predominance of approximately 4:1, and the disease is seldom seen in the summer. Laboratory tests show no specific abnormalities except for those related to an underlying illness. The chest x-ray may be helpful in diagnosis of an underlying tuberculosis, fungal infection, or sarcoidosis.

Erythema nodosum is considered a hypersensitivity reaction to a variety of antigenic stimuli, and thus may be seen in the course of several diseases of both known and idiopathic cause, as well as during drug therapy (Table 75–1). Patients developing erythema nodosum

Table 75–1. Diseases Associated with Erythema Nodosum

Infectious
 Coccidioidomycosis
 Histoplasmosis
 Lymphogranuloma venereum
 North American blastomycosis
 Psittacosis
 Streptococcus
 Trichophyton
 Tuberculosis
 Yersiniosis
 Leptospirosis
Unknown Etiology
 Sarcoidosis
 Regional enteritis
 Ulcerative colitis
Drugs
 Halides
 Oral contraceptives
 Sulfonamides

after a primary infection with tuberculosis, histoplasmosis, or coccidioidomycosis do so at their conversion to a positive skin test for these agents,[8,9] while children with tinea capitis develop erythema nodosum after treatment begins, apparently at the release of antigen into the circulation.[10] Also, reinjection of these agents may exacerbate the panniculitis.[11] This information supports the concept of erythema nodosum as a delayed-type hypersensitivity reaction. However, many cases occur without an identifiable systemic illness, and the actual pathophysiology of antigen-mediated tissue injury is unknown.

Acute inflammation around the veins of the septal system is characteristic. The infiltrate is primarily lymphocytic, but polymorphonuclear leukocytes may be present. Hemorrhage from the vessels occurs, and the infiltrate may extend into the fat lobule. Giant cells and histiocytes may accumulate, and a frank granulomatous reaction has been reported[2] (Fig. 75–2). Plasma cells are absent, and fat necrosis does not occur. Rarely, biopsy of lesions seemingly characteristic of erythema nodosum associated with systemic sarcoid has revealed sarcoidosis of the subcutaneous tissue.[12] In addition, two patients with disseminated histoplasmosis presented with erythema nodosum–like lesions. Both were receiving immunosuppressive therapy, and biopsy material grew *Histoplasma capsulatum*.[13] Thus, routine culture and fungal staining of all subcutaneous biopsy material are mandatory.

Treatment is aimed at identifying any underlying process. Recovery is generally the rule; bed rest with elevation and aspirin or other nonsteroidal anti-inflammatory agents are recommended. Steroids are not used, and some authors feel that they may exacerbate the erythema nodosum.

Subacute Nodular Migratory Panniculitis. Subacute nodular migratory panniculitis[14,15] is thought to be a variant of erythema nodosum[1] but deserves mention for some distinct clinical and histologic features. This process consists of a few discrete, minimally painful nodules occurring in a unilateral fashion on the anterior aspects of the leg, primarily around the ankle or knee. Single nodules expand by coalescence or peripheral extension to a size often greater than 20 cm and may show central clearing without scarring or atrophy. Their very size may lead to obstructive lymphedema, and new lesions may evolve for years and cover any portion of the integument, but internal organ involvement does not occur.

This is a syndrome primarily of Caucasian females in their fifth decade. The patients are generally well with little fever or malaise, and there is no clear relationship to specific concurrent disease as in erythema nodosum. Laboratory tests show only a mild increase in the sedimentation rate, and the etiology is unknown. Pathologically, there is a septal inflammation with marked small vessel proliferation, granulomatous tissue, and a minimal number of inflammatory cells. The prognosis is excellent, and in small uncontrolled trials potassium iodide has been helpful in treatment.[15]

Figure 75–2. Erythema nodosum. Primary septal inflammation with sparing of the fat lobule except by contiguous spread. Giant cells are evident. × 200.

LOBULAR PANNICULITIS

Pancreatic Disease. The association of pancreatic disease and fat necrosis has been noted since 1883, but its occurrence is rare.[16] To date, approximately 35 patients with an associated pancreatitis and 20 with pancreatic carcinoma have been reported. Patients with pancreatitis are predominantly males (3:1) in their third to fourth decade, with a heavy alcoholic history. However, this syndrome may occur with traumatic pancreatitis and pancreatitis secondary to stones. Acute episodes occur with single crops of painful erythematous nodules primarily on the legs, whereas chronic pancreatitis may show the evolution of new lesions over many months. Nodules are not confined to the legs and may occur over the scalp, trunk, and buttocks. Characteristically, these nodules may ulcerate, discharging a creamy, viscous material, and heal with atrophy and scarring.

Although extracutaneous sites of fat necrosis may occur in the mesentery and mediastinum, two phenomena deserve mention. (1) Periarticular fat necrosis may present as an acutely painful, asymmetrical arthritis, involving both large and small joints. Initially, the synovial fluid may be clear, with type II characteristics, but as the process progresses, creamy synovial fluid, which is positive on Sudan staining, can be obtained. The synovial membrane shows a lymphocytic infiltrate with modest synovial cell hypertrophy. Particles of unknown composition, which are small and negatively birefringent, have occasionally been noted in the synovial fluid.[17] Direct rupture of necrotic fat debris into the joint cavity has been reported.[18] (2) Intramedullary fat necrosis may present as bone pain or may be symptomless with areas of osteolysis on radiologic examination. Calcification of these bony infarcts occurs, and sites of predilection include the distal femur, proximal tibia, and the heads of the humeri and femora, leading to secondary osteoarthritis.[19]

Patients are systemically ill, and acute pancreatitis

dominates the picture. Alcoholic liver disease may also be present, but the most consistent abnormality is an elevation of serum or urinary lipase or amylase. In patients with chronic pancreatitis, urinary enzyme elevations may be the only abnormalities in laboratory evaluation.[17-19] A patient with *alpha₁-proteinase inhibitor deficiency,* pancreatitis, and panniculitis has been reported, but a second patient with alpha₁-proteinase deficiency had no obvious pancreatic disease with his disseminated panniculitis.[20]

Patients with associated carcinoma of the pancreas are usually male (7:1) and over 60 years of age.[21] The carcinoma is of the acinar type in 80 percent of cases, although this particular tumor accounts for little more than 10 percent of all pancreatic neoplasms. The clinical picture is identical to that for pancreatitis, but there may be no signs of pancreatic disease on presentation or for the life of the patient, the diagnosis being made only at autopsy.[17] Other recognized syndromes associated with adenocarcinoma of the pancreas may be present (e.g., migratory thrombophlebitis) and a striking eosinophilia has been shown in 70 percent of patients. Most authors feel that fat necrosis is secondary to the digestive action of disseminated pancreatic enzymes.[17-19,22,23] A careful immunologic study of one patient[17] revealed no abnormalities. Questions yet to be answered involve the balance between various pancreatic enzymes and inhibitors of proteinases in blood and tissues. No hypotheses about pathogenesis have explained the limited, focal nature of necrosis throughout the subcutaneous tissue.

Characteristically, foci of fat necrosis, consisting of ghost cells with thin walls and no nuclei, are seen. An infiltrate of polymorphonuclear leukocytes, lymphocytes, foam cells, and foreign body giant cells is scattered throughout the lesion. Later, calcification of damaged tissues may be seen. Treatment is aimed at the underlying disorder of the pancreas; anti-inflammatory medications and steroids are generally of little help.

Weber-Christian Disease. Since the intial description

of this lesion by Weber[24] and Christian,[25] it has been used as a generic term to encompass all types of panniculitis. Of 100 cases reported and 15 autopsies performed, a significant number have been examples of pancreatic panniculitis, and the histology of the remainder has been variable. Thus, several authors have argued that this is not a true nosological entity,[23,26] while others feel that the pathology is distinctive enough to allow classification.[27]

Patients without pancreatic disease and with relapsing nodular nonsuppurative panniculitis are usually females (3:1) in the fourth to sixth decade of life. Crops of tender nodules may occur on the thighs, trunk, and buttocks, and recur for years. There are rare cases of pericardial, mesenteric, and visceral fat necrosis.[28] Ulceration of lesions may occur, and healing leaves atrophy. Laboratory tests show no specific abnormalities, and the etiology is unknown. The pathologic process, consists initially of an acute infiltrate of polymorphonuclear leukocytes between fat cells.[27] Fat cells degenerate with histiocytic, lymphocytic, and plasma cell infiltration, and multi nucleated macrophages with foamy cytoplasm appear. Small blood vessels may show endothelial proliferation and edema of the media. Finally, there is replacement of inflammation by scar tissue. It is possible that the pathology is caused by activation of latent tissue proteinases (principally serine proteinases like those found in pancreatic secretions) which then saturate local inhibitors, begin to destroy tissue, and thereby produce inflammation.

There is no known treatment; multiple drugs have been used, but there are no clear indications that steroids or other anti-inflammatory medications are helpful. The prognosis is variable, except in those cases with visceral involvement, which have been uniformly fatal.

Erythema Induratum. Erythema induratum, or nodular vasculitis,[29] is a form of idiopathic panniculitis occurring primarily in middle-aged females. It produces brown-to-purple nodules in a bilateral distribution on the calves. Women involved with this process have legs with thickened skin, erythrocyanosis, and follicular hyperkeratosis. Individual nodules may regress with atrophy or ulcerate with chronic scarring, but there is no evidence of a systematic vasculitis and the process may evolve over years. The pathology is an inflammation of deep, small vessels with granuloma formation and marked reaction within the fat lobule. Since caseation necrosis may be seen, tuberculosis must be excluded by culture and skin testing. Also, the gummatous type of tertiary syphilis may present in a nodular fashion on the lower legs, and histologically cannot be distinguished from erythema induratum. Appropriate serologic tests should be performed and pertinent clinical history ascertained.

Systemic Vasculitis. Severe systemic vasculitis may involve the panniculus and present with subcutaneous nodules during their course (see Chapter 72). The rheumatoid nodule and its differential diagnosis will not be discussed in this chapter, but can be reviewed in an excellent clinical summary.[30] *Lupus profundus* is a rare complication of both discoid and systemic lupus erythematosus. Subcutaneous nodules often following minor trauma appear on the face, trunk, or buttocks. Although generally painless, they may last for years without change or heal with subcutaneous atrophy and scarring. Occasional lesions may ulcerate, requiring full-thickness skin grafting.[31] Histologically, a perivascular lymphocytic infiltrate predominates, with occasional plasma cells and fat-filled macrophages scattered throughout the lobule. Fibrinoid degeneration of collagen is a uniform feature. The overlying epidermis may be normal or may show a classic discoid lesion. Immunologic studies show immunofluorescence in vessel walls, suggesting a role for immune complexes.[32] Antimalarial agents and corticosteroids have been effective therapeutically.

Polyarteritis nodosa may demonstrate tender, pulsatile nodules in clusters along the course of a subcutaneous artery. These may heal spontaneously or ulcerate and scar. Biopsy shows characteristic changes of polyarteritis nodosa, and the clinical course may be dominated by internal organ involvement.[33] Among the myriad of manifestations of *Behçet's disease,* tender red nodules resembling erythema nodosum may occur. However, these lesions heal without color change or atrophy and are resistant to most therapy. Pathologically, a small vessel vasculitis predominates.[34,35] In the original descriptions of *allergic granulomatosis,* a high percentage of patients manifested cutaneous and subcutaneous nodules essentially identical to those of internal organs.[36] These consisted primarily of a granulomatous reaction with giant cells and eosinophils. Nodules were diffuse in distribution, tender, and, at times, ulcerating.

Two lesions of suspected immunologic origin that may involve the subcutaneous tissue include *Osler's nodes* and the *lepra reaction.* Osler's nodes of subacute bacterial endocarditis are red-purple, tender, subcutaneous nodules of the hands and feet, lasting hours to days. These painful nodules probably represent small vessel vasculitis induced by immune complexes and are important for their diagnostic significance.[37,38] The lepra reaction consists of a shower of indurated red nodules on the extremities, often accompanied by fever, arthritis, orchitis, lymphadenopathy, and iritis.[39] It is felt to be secondary to the release of mycobacterial antigen and occurs primarily during the first year of treatment in patients with lepromatous leprosy.[40] The unfortunate term erythema nodosum leprosum, often applied to this phenomenon, is misleading because the primary pathologic entity is a vasculitis.

MALIGNANCY AND INFECTION

Lymphoma and leukemia[41] may directly invade panniculus as a single painful nodule or may mimic erythema nodosum. The clinical course and biopsy will establish the diagnosis. A nodular, granulomatous panniculitis has been described with malignant histiocytosis.[42,43] The severity of this systemic disease, its high mortality, and a bleeding diathesis should make this diagnosis recognizable. Bone marrow and liver biopsy demonstrate malignant histiocytes and erythrophagocytosis.

Besides histoplasmosis (vida supra), atypical mycobacteria[44] may invade the subcutaneous tissue and produce a disseminated panniculitis. Other infectious granulomata, i.e., syphilis, leprosy, deep mycoses, and tuberculosis, may produce lesions in the subcutaneous tissue and mimic idiopathic panniculitides. In all cases of atypical panniculitis, appropriate fungal and mycobacterial cultures, dark-field examination, special stains, and serology should be obtained.

Miscellaneous. Acute *corticosteroid withdrawal* after long-term high-dose therapy may induce a subcutaneous inflammation consisting of tender pruritic nodules of the face, trunk, and extremities.[45] Pathology of this panniculitis consists of histiocytes and giant cells in the interstices between fat cells. The septa are uninvolved, and angiitis is not seen. Occasional clefts thought to be negative images of fatty acid crystals are present. Reinstitution of corticosteroids may be necessary, but the lesions may resolve spontaneously.[46] Some patients have localized panniculitis on *cold exposure*. A diffuse, lobular inflammation is seen and no specific etiology is known.[47-50] A nodular, nonsuppurative panniculitis has been described as a complication of *jejunoileal bypass surgery* and has resolved with reanastomosis.[51] Finally, the *iatrogenic* injection of foreign materials into the subcutaneous tissue may initiate a chronic panniculitis, both at the injection site and systemically.[52,53]

In patients with no clear clinical course and an unusual distribution of lesions, *factitial panniculitis* must be considered.[54] Dystrophic calcification on radiologic examination of soft tissues and birefringent material, as well as sinus tracts, in pathologic specimens, may be seen.[55] In one case (personal observation) the occurrence of new lesions was prevented by casting an extremity.

References

1. Reed, R.J., Clark, W.H., and Mihm, M.C.: Disorders of the panniculus adiposus. Hum. Pathol. 4:219, 1973.
2. Forstrom, L., and Winkelmann, R.K.: Granulomatous panniculitis in erythema nodosum. Arch. Dermatol. 111:335, 1975.
3. Ipp, M.M., Howard, N.H., Tervo, R.C., et al.: Sicca syndrome and total lipodystrophy. Ann. Intern. Med. 85:433, 1976.
4. Alarcón-Segovia, D., and Ramos-Niembro, F.: Association of total lipodystrophy in Sjögren's syndrome. Ann. Intern. Med. 85:474, 1976.
5. Hannerksela, M.: Erythema nodosum with special reference to sarcoidosis: A clinical study of 343 Finnish adult patients. Ann. Clin. Res. 3(Suppl. 7):5, 1971.
6. Truelove, L.H.: Articular manifestations of erythema nodosum. Ann. Rheum. Dis. 19:174, 1960.
7. James, D.G.: Erythema nodosum. Br. Med. J. 1:853, 1961.
8. Beerman, H.: Erythema nodosum. Am. J. Med. Sci. 223:433, 1952.
9. Saslaw, S., and Beman, F.: Erythema nodosum as a manifestation of histoplasmosis. JAMA 70:1178, 1959.
10. Martinez-Roig, A., Llorens-Terol, J., and Torres, J.M.: Erythema nodosum and kerion of the scalp. Am. J. Dis. Child. 136:440, 1982.
11. Favour, C.B., and Sosman, M.C.: Erythema nodosum. Arch. Intern. Med. 80:435, 1947.
12. Fitzpatrick, T.B., Arndt, K.A., Clark, W.H., et al.: Dermatology in General Medicine. New York, McGraw-Hill Book Company, 1971, p. 1475.
13. King, R.W., Jr., and Kraikpanitch, S.: Subcutaneous nodules caused by Histoplasma capsulatum. Ann. Intern. Med. 86:586, 1977.
14. Vilanova, X., and Pinol, A.J.: Subcutaneous nodular migratory panniculitis. Br. J. Dermatol. 71:45, 1959.
15. Perry, H.O., and Winkelmann, R.K.: Subcutaneous nodular migratory panniculitis. Arch. Dermatol. 89:170, 1964.
16. Mullin, G.T., Caperton, E.M., Jr., Crepsin, S.R., et al.: Arthritis and skin lesions resembling erythema nodosum in pancreatic disease. Ann. Intern. Med. 68:75, 1972.
17. Tannenbaum, H., Anderson, L.G., and Schur, P.H.: Association of polyarteritis, subcutaneous nodules and pancreatic disease. J. Rheumatol. 2:14, 1975.
18. Virshup, A.M., and Sliwinski, A.J.: Polyarthritis and subcutaneous nodules

19. Immelman, M.B., Bank, S., Krige, H., et al.: Roentgenologic and clinical features of intramedullary fat necrosis in bones in acute and chronic pancreatitis. Am. J. Med. 36:96, 1964.
20. Rubenstein, H.M., Jaffer, A.M., Kudrna, J.C., et al.: Alpha-1 antitrypsin deficiency with severe panniculitis. Ann. Intern. Med. 86:742, 1977.
21. Ona, F.V., Zamcheck, N., Dhar, P., et al.: Carcinomembryonic antigen (CEA) in the diagnosis of pancreatic disease. Cancer 31:324, 1973.
22. Moore, S.: Editorial. Syndromes resulting from dissemination of pancreatic enzymes. J. Rheumatol. 2:5, 1975.
23. Forstrom, L., Winklemann, R.K.: Acute generalized panniculitis with amylase and lipase in skin. Arch. Dermatol. 111:497, 1975.
24. Weber, F.P.: A case of relapsing nonsuppurative nodular panniculitis, showing phagocytosis of subcutaneous fat cells by macrophages. Br. J. Dermatol. 37:301, 1925.
25. Christian, H.A.: Relapsing febrile nodular nonsuppurative panniculitis. Ann. Intern. Med. 42:338, 1928.
26. Moore, S.: Relation of pancreatic disease to Weber-Christian disease. Can. Med. Assoc. J. 88:1238, 1963.
27. Lever, W.F., and Schaumburg-Lever, G.: Histopathology of the Skin. 5th ed. Philadelphia, J. B. Lippincott Company, 1975, p. 231.
28. Oram, S., and Cochrane, G.M.: Weber-Christian disease with visceral involvement. Br. Med. J. 2:281, 1958.
29. Montgomery, H., O'Leary, P.A., and Barker, N.W.: Nodular vascular disease of the legs: Erythema induratum and allied conditions. JAMA 128:335, 1945.
30. Moore, C.P., and Willkens, R.F.: The subcutaneous nodule: Its significance in the diagnosis of rheumatic disease. Semin. Arthritis Rheum. 7:63, 1977.
31. Winkelmann, R.K.: Panniculitis and systemic lupus erythematosus. JAMA 211:472, 1970.
32. Tuffanelli, D.L.: Lupus erythematosus panniculitis (profundus). Arch. Dermatol. 103:231, 1971.
33. Lyell, A., and Church, R.: The cutaneous manifestations of polyarteritis nodosa. Br. J. Dermatol. 66:335, 1954.
34. O'Duffy, J.D., Carney, J.A., and Deodhar, S.: Behçet's disease: Report of ten cases, three with new manifestations. Ann. Intern. Med. 75:561, 1971.
35. Forman, L.: Behçet's disease. Br. J. Dermatol. 63:417, 1951.
36. Strauss, L., Churg, J., and Zak, F.G.: Cutaneous lesion of allergic granulomatosis: A histopathologic study. J. Invest. Dermatol. 17:349, 1951.
37. Howard, E.J.: Osler's nodes. Am. Heart J. 59:633, 1960.
38. Lerner, P.I., and Weinstein, L.: Infective endocarditis in the antibiotic era. N. Engl. J. Med. 274:256, 1966.
39. Karat, A.B.A., Karat, S., Job, C.K., et al.: Acute exudative arthritis in leprosy-rheumatoid arthritis-like syndrome in association with erythema nodosum leprosum. Br. Med. J. 3:770, 1967.
40. Wemambu, S.N.L., Turk, J.L., Waters, M.F.R., et al.: Erythema nodosum leprosum: A clinical manifestation of the Arthus phenomenon. Lancet 2:933, 1969.
41. Sumaya, C.V., Babu, S., Reed, R.J.: Erythema nodosum-like lesions of leukemia. Arch. Dermatol. 110:415, 1974.
42. Winkelmann, R.K., and Bowie, W.: Hemorrhagic diathesis associated with benign histiocytic, cytophagic panniculitis and systemic histiocytosis. Arch. Intern. Med. 140:1460, 1980.
43. Sacher, R.A., Jacobson, R.J., Lenes, B.A., et al.: Malignant histiocytosis simulating granulomatous disease. Am. J. Clin. Pathol. 74:180, 1980.
44. Sanderson, T.L., Moskowitz, L., Hensley, G.T., et al.: Disseminated mycobacterium avium-intracellulare infection appearing as a panniculitis. Arch. Pathol. Lab. Med. 106:112, 1982.
45. Taranta, A., Mark, H., Haas, R.C., et al.: Nodular panniculitis after massive prednisone therapy. Am. J. Med. 25:52, 1958.
46. Roenigk, H.H., Haserick, S.R., and Arundell, F.D.: Post-steroid panniculitis. Arch. Dermatol. 90:387, 1964.
47. Solomon, L.M., and Berman, H.: Cold panniculitis. Arch. Dermatol. 88:265, 1963.
48. Epstein, E.H., Jr., and Oren, M.E.: Popsicle panniculitis. N. Engl. J. Med. 282:966, 1970.
49. Beacham, B.E., Cooper, P.H., Buchanan, C.S., et al.: Equestrian cold panniculitis in women. Arch. Dermatol. 116:1025, 1980.
50. Vickers, R.: Equestrian cold panniculitis in women. Arch. Dermatol. 117:315, 1981.
51. Williams, H.J., Samuelson, C.O., and Zone, J.J.: Nodular nonsuppurative panniculitis associated with jejuno-ileal bypass surgery. Arch. Dermatol. 115:1091, 1979.
52. Kossard, S., Ecker, R.I., and Dicken, C.H.: Povidone panniculitis. Arch. Dermatol. 116:704, 1980.
53. Wilkie, T.F.: Late development of granuloma after liquid silicone injections. Plast. Reconstr. Surg. 60:179, 1977.
54. Ackerman, A.B., Mosher, D.T., and Schwann, H.A.: Factitial Weber-Christian disease. JAMA 198:731, 1966.
55. Forstrom, L., and Winkelmann, R.K.: Factitial panniculitis. Arch. Dermatol. 110:747, 1974.

Section IX
Connective Tissue Diseases Characterized by Fibrosis

Chapter 76
Scleroderma (Systemic Sclerosis)

E. Carwile LeRoy

INTRODUCTION

Scleroderma (systemic sclerosis) is a multisystem and multistage disorder characterized by proliferative vascular lesions, obliterative microvascular lesions, and residual atrophy with fibrosis of multiple organs.[1-5] The characteristic hidebound fibrosis of skin is of most concern to the patient and provides the only definitive diagnostic criterion (Figs. 76–1 to 76–3). Eventual outcome, however, is due entirely to the vascular involvement of crucial viscera. Scleroderma, especially the CREST subgroup (see below), combines the chronic, indolent aspects of rheumatic disease with the sudden, life-threatening collapse of vital organs (renal scleroderma), challenging both generalist and specialist to combine compassionate, permissive long-term management with the acumen necessary for early detection of acute visceral involvement.[6-10] Optimism, always helpful in management, is justified by the fact that not all scleroderma is progressive and that intervention can prolong life in spite of incipient organ failure.[11,12] The irreversibility of late-stage scleroderma (atrophy and fibrosis) has led investigators to define the earliest possible stage of the disorder, and to intervene preferably when inflammatory and proliferative features exist without atrophy or fibrosis. Newer therapeutic approaches are closely linked to efforts to redefine scleroderma during its prefibrotic stages.

DEFINITION AND CLASSIFICATION

The term "scleroderma" has several meanings (Table 76–1). Localized (morphea) or linear areas of hidebound, scarred, and atrophic skin are designated localized scleroderma; these lesions are not associated with systemic disease and are discussed in Chapter 77. The diffuse condition scleroderma, also termed systemic sclerosis to emphasize its generalized nature, can be associated with other rheumatic disorders or can occur as an isolated condition. When combined, scleroderma is a part of overlapping or mixed syndromes, which probably represent early and as yet undifferentiated diffuse connective tissue disease; these overlapping syndromes have not yet been shown to warrant separate or independent status as rheumatic diagnoses. When isolated, scleroderma can usually be separated into rapidly developing, diffuse scleroderma, and into indolent and initially more limited forms, which historically were called acrosclerosis but which now are generally labeled the CREST syndrome (for *c*alcinosis, *R*aynaud's phenomenon, *e*sophageal hypomotility, *s*clerodactyly, and *t*elangiectasia). It must be kept in mind that after 10 to 20 years the CREST syndrome can be as generalized and as life threatening as diffuse scleroderma is in the first decade.[7,9] Many clinicians prefer to consider scleroderma as a single disorder having distinctive first decade, second decade, and third decade manifestations rather than to subdivide at all. Furthermore, the term progressive (progressive systemic sclerosis, PSS) is not used here because not all scleroderma is progressive; one may see regression of one system (e.g., subsidence of Raynaud's syndrome or softening of skin) while other organs are uninvolved, stable, or progressive. The term progressive may be misleading and is an unnecessary onus for the patient to bear.

Many investigator and patient hours have been invested in studies to establish definitive criteria for the definition of scleroderma.[13-16] These efforts are nurtured by the frustrations that stem from the broad spectrum of findings and variable rates of progression in scleroderma patients. With the variable expression of multisystem involvement and the variable rate of multistage processes such as edema, vascular compromise, and fibrosis, it is unlikely that definitive criteria encompassing all patients will ever be determined. It is reassuring that taut skin of the back of the hand represents the single major criterion, with sensitivity and specificity greater than 90 percent.

Figure 76–1. The face of a man with longstanding fibrotic scleroderma. Note the taut skin of the forehead and face and the drawn skin around the mouth which limits its ability to open.

THE CLINICAL SETTING

The representative patient destined to develop scleroderma is a female, age 30 to 40 years, who has noted pallor and/or cyanosis of the tips of the fingers or toes on cold exposure or emotional upset for months to years (Raynaud's phenomenon). She may or may not have seen a physician previously but comes now because her hands and face are puffy and full in the morning, with numbness and tingling in these areas as long as the puffiness persists.

On examination the skin may be puffy or taut, perhaps with slight pigment changes (hypo- or hyperpigmentation); there may be subungual webs and scars of the finger tufts; telangiectasia may be found on the face or the anterior chest; esophageal hypomotility and restrictive pulmonary functional abnormalities may be present; she can be expected to develop definite hidebound scleroderma of the puffy areas in weeks to months.

Less frequently but not rarely, the scleroderma patient may present with symmetrical polyarthritis resembling rheumatoid arthritis, or active myositis, or accelerated hypertension with papilledema. In this setting a careful multisystem evaluation usually confirms the suspicion of scleroderma.

THE EARLY DIAGNOSIS

Once the fibrotic features of scleroderma are present in the skin, lungs, or esophagus, the diagnosis is straight-

forward. The incidence and characteristics of fibrosis in the organ systems that are targets for involvement in scleroderma are well described in many texts and reviews.[1-5] The commanding clinical challenge of the disorder is to predict the site and extent of organ involvement prior to fibrosis.

The patient with undifferentiated, mixed, or overlapping connective tissue features (Raynaud's phenomenon, puffy hands, a variety of other features) is at risk to develop scleroderma. The term "early puffy scleroderma" has been useful to describe these patients.[139,140] With what degree of confidence can one identify the future scleroderma patient and predict the extent of involvement? Four promising areas will be discussed: (1) the extent of early system involvement; (2) antinuclear serology; (3) microvascular pattern and flow; and (4) estimates of direct vascular (intimal or endothelial) injury.

Early System Involvement. Each of the major target organs of scleroderma should be studied for the characteristic features of early involvement. Edematous thickening of the skin should be biopsied to identify the cellular phase of scleroderma recently emphasized by Fleischmajer and colleagues;[19-22] although these findings are not completely pathognomonic, they are distinctive, usually early, and prefibrotic. The characteristic findings include lymphoid and mononuclear cell infiltration of the interstitial subcutaneous tissue with perivascular

Figure 76–2. The hand of a man with scleroderma, demonstrating shiny, taut skin with limitation of finger extension. The skin has a "hidebound" feel on palpation.

Figure 76–3. The hands of a woman with scleroderma. The finger skin is taut and shiny; finger extension is limited. The skin of the hands and wrists is also taut, shiny, and partially depigmented and feels thickened and bound to underlying structures.

taneous determination of the distribution of multiple inert gases. Measurement of pulmonary hemodynamics, such as pulmonary arterial gradients in diastole and pulmonary arterial pO_2 responses to exercise, has at present investigative potential for detecting early pulmonary vascular involvement. As a routine, noninvasive, and available procedure, diffusion capacity remains the single most sensitive indicator of early pulmonary involvement in scleroderma. Initial reports of small airways disease in scleroderma patients are being evaluated to determine their sensitivity and specificity when compared with the smog-breathing and smoking population at large.[33-36] It is possible that sensitive pulmonary scans, especially the gallium scan, may become helpful in detecting the prefibrotic phase of pulmonary involvement. In preliminary studies, bronchoalveolar lavage, which has the definable risk of bronchoscopy, shows promise as a means of providing direct evidence of acute and chronic inflammatory changes both early and late in the different phases of pulmonary scleroderma.[108] Also, ventilation perfusion lung scans are being studied as po-

round cell infiltration. Immunohistological studies have generally been negative, a help in distinguishing this dermatitis and vasculitis from that of systemic lupus erythematosus. These findings provide potentially fertile soil for increased understanding of the relationship between inflammation and fibrosis. Of course the presence of fibrosis and atrophy strengthens the diagnosis of scleroderma and emphasizes the close association between edema ("puffy") and subsequent fibrosis.

Second to skin, study of the distal esophagus often provides documentation of multisystem disease in the patient suspected of having scleroderma. Even in the early puffy patient cineradiography can detect hypomotility in more than 50 percent of cases (if the technical nuances of thin barium and recumbent position are employed); sensitive manometric measurements give substantially higher yields than does radiography and can be helpful in the early diagnosis of scleroderma, even in the patient with no symptoms of dysphagia.[23-25] A sensitive use of scintigraphy to determine esophageal transit time has recently been introduced and is currently being tested.[26-32]

The lungs are a well-known target organ in scleroderma as well as in most other rheumatic syndromes. In selecting patients for further study, symptoms of breathlessness have been insensitive and late, probably because of the reduced activity of the patient. Neither has the routine chest roentgenogram been a sensitive indicator of early involvement. Functional abnormalities have been demonstrated in a majority of patients with scleroderma (and systemic lupus erythematosus) who denied having pulmonary symptoms and whose chest roentgenograms were normal. The most sensitive tests have been those detecting slight degrees of ventilation-perfusion abnormalities as measured by the alveolar-arterial oxygen difference, the diffusing capacity of carbon monoxide or helium, and potentially the simul-

Table 76–1. Classification of Scleroderma*

1. Generalized scleroderma (systemic sclerosis)
   a. Diffuse scleroderma (acute and chronic)†
   b. Limited cutaneous scleroderma (CREST syndrome: calcinosis, Raynaud's phenomenon, esophageal hypomotility, sclerodactyly, telangiectasia)
2. Localized scleroderma
   a. Morphea
   b. Linear
3. Scleroderma-like syndromes
   a. Occupational and environmental
      1. Vinyl chloride associated
      2. Vibration associated ("jackhammer disease")
      3. Silicosis associated
      4. Toxic oil syndrome (Spain)
   b. Fasciitis with eosinophilia
   c. Scleredema of Buschke (often postinfectious)
   d. Metabolic
      1. Porphyria
      2. Amyloid
   e. Immunologic
      1. Graft-versus-host reaction
   f. Drug-induced
      1. Bleomycin[206]
      2. Tryptophan and carbidopa[238]
4. Scleroderma-associated syndromes
   a. Undifferentiated overlap or mixed connective tissue syndromes
      1. Sclerolupus
      2. Sclerodermatomyositis
      3. Scleromyxedema
      4. Primary biliary cirrhosis
      5. Sjögren's syndrome
   b. Inherited
      1. Werner's syndrome
      2. Phenylketonuria
      3. Brandywine triracial isolate
   c. Tumor-associated
      1. Carcinoid syndrome
      2. Bronchoalveolar carcinoma

*Adapted from Siegel, R.C.: Med. Clin. North Am. 61:283, 1977; and Winkelmann, R.K.: Acta Derm. Venereol. 56:83, 1976.

tential noninvasive measurements of reduced pulmonary vascular capacity. These scans measure much the same capacity presently monitored by diffusion capacity, which is reduced in the great majority of scleroderma patients.[37-41]

The heart is classically a target organ in scleroderma. In practical terms one must separate coronary heart disease, hypertensive heart disease, pulmonary heart disease, pericardial effusions with subtle hemodynamic effects, and direct myocardial involvement with scleroderma (contraction band necrosis with fibrosis). One of the subtle forms of cardiac involvement in the patient with scleroderma is pericardial effusion. Since often the only clinical clue to pericardial disease in scleroderma is edema of the lower extremities, which may be non-pitting (owing to the skin changes of scleroderma) and may be attributed to cutaneous rather than cardiac causes,[42] careful echocardiography is a useful procedure for the early detection of pericardial and potentially even ventricular involvement. Arrhythmias may also be prominent in cardiac involvement in the scleroderma patient, appearing early or late in the course of the disease. In the patient with extensive pulmonary involvement who develops a cardiac arrhythmia, for example, it may be difficult to separate a cardiac cause from arrhythmia secondary to hypoxia from interstitial lung disease. Holter monitoring of patients can be useful in the precise definition of the arrhythmias, while pacemakers may be useful in their management in addition to the usual pharmacologic approaches. Dissecting the various forms of heart disease which occur in scleroderma patients can be a distinct challenge.[42-51]

Most other features of scleroderma, such as duodenal and jejunal dilatation, colonic sacculation, or trigeminal neuralgia, are not early in appearance, do not usually assist in establishing the diagnosis in the early undifferentiated patient, and can be readily documented with traditional procedures.[52-57] The present discussion includes those features which are helpful in detecting the patient with early involvement; Raynaud's phenomenon, which usually antedates all other features of connective tissue disease, will be discussed below.

Antinuclear Serology. The identification of antinuclear antibodies (ANA), using sections of liver or other organs, has permitted estimation of both pattern and titer of the immunofluorescence (IF) observed. These determinations have been widely used in patients suspected of connective tissue disease and have provided a highly sensitive technique which has some degree of diagnostic specificity.[58,59] Of the standard IF patterns, three (speckled, homogeneous, and nucleolar) are seen in some patients with early disease who are at risk to develop scleroderma. A centromere-specific pattern and Scl-70 agglutination have been described recently in scleroderma by Tan and colleagues.[60]

The homogeneous pattern, the most sensitive and least specific pattern in all rheumatic patients, occurs in a small proportion of scleroderma patients early in the disease and offers little further diagnostic information except to suggest that a rheumatic or connective tissue disorder may be present.

The speckled IF pattern is both the most common and most distinctive pattern seen in the early connective tissue patient who may develop scleroderma. It correlates well with positive agglutination tests, using the soluble or extractable nuclear antigen fraction (ENA) which has been shown to contain several antigens, primarily Sm and RNP (ribonucleoprotein). The physician's first task in patients with Raynaud's phenomenon, puffy hands, arthralgia, and a speckled IF pattern is to identify the patient who in fact has systemic lupus erythematosus (SLE). Clinically, the presence of alopecia, malar rash, pleurisy, or signs of glomerulonephritis is helpful; serologically the presence of serum autoantibodies to the Sm antigen and to DNA is also selective for SLE (see Chapters 46 and 69), as are hemolytic anemia and leukopenia. The remaining patients with a speckled IF pattern usually show high-titer agglutination of ENA; ribonuclease digestion results in a marked fall in speckled IF titer, indicating that the autoantibody is directly against the RNP antigen fraction. In some diagnostic centers these patients are often labeled as having overlap syndrome or mixed connective tissue disease because of the variety of clinical features expressed (see Chapter 71). Since a substantial proportion eventually develop scleroderma, it may be preferable to consider their condition as acute undifferentiated connective tissue syndrome (UCTS) until features of a classic syndrome develop. Thus the speckled IF pattern, coupled with Sm and RNP agglutination, can be useful in the early detection of the patient at risk for scleroderma.

The nucleolar IF pattern is considered most specific for scleroderma. It has been reported in as many as 80 percent of scleroderma patients and in as few as 20 percent of patients with other rheumatic diagnoses. In actual experience the proportion of positive sera seems less than this and the nucleolar pattern often is not present early in the syndrome when specificity is most needed. It is the relatively low yield in patients with early features which limits the usefulness of the nucleolar pattern.[61,62]

ANA determinations have been developed around observations with sera from patients with SLE. These SLE sera show strong IF patterns which are generally independent of the tissue substrate used. Scleroderma sera show much more variation in substrate specificity; this realization may explain the extremely wide discordance in the published incidence and pattern of ANA in scleroderma.

The introduction of a human esophageal carcinoma cell line with many visible mitoses as a substrate for ANA determinations (HEp 2) has led to the identification of a new ANA pattern, which at this writing seems selective for the limited cutaneous involvement group (CREST syndrome, second and third decade scleroderma). This is the anticentromere pattern. The antibody specificity is directed toward the waist of the chromosome, which is exposed only during mitosis and is called the centromere or the kinetochore, a specialized region of the centromere.

The anticentromere antibody (ACA) pattern is likely

to provide an important new tool in the selection of patients with Raynaud's phenomenon who are destined to develop any one of the scleroderma spectrum of disorders. About 15 percent of Raynaud's phenomenon patients are ACA positive; most of this 15 percent are also capillary positive (vide infra); the combination of ACA and the dilated-only capillary loop pattern strongly (90 percent) select the subject who will indolently develop the limited cutaneous form of scleroderma (CREST). Thus, the triad of Raynaud's phenomenon, ACA serology, and dilated nailfold capillary loops can be used for early selection of a very homogenous subset of scleroderma subjects, who can then be studied with controlled therapeutic trials testing the importance of several pathogenetic hypotheses.

Conversely, diffuse generalized scleroderma patients (about 20 percent of generalized scleroderma patients) are ACA negative (10 percent), have a short duration of Raynaud's phenomenon prior to "early puffy scleroderma" changes, and have a different nailfold capillary pattern (dilated capillary loops plus avascular areas with no capillary loops). It is of crucial importance to detect these patients early because of their high risk of life-threatening visceral involvement.

On this basis the ACA pattern joins the Scl-70 pattern (seen in 20 percent of scleroderma patients with as yet no further subset definition) as a highly specific ANA in the scleroderma spectrum of disorders.[60,63-67]

MICROVASCULAR ABNORMALITIES

Capillary abnormalities visible with low magnification microscopy have been observed in scleroderma patients for over 50 years. Recent refinements and extensions in the study of these abnormal capillaries have indicated their usefulness in diagnosis and prognosis of the individual patient with scleroderma.[68-75]

The most distal regions of the skin and its appendages receive nutrient blood from capillary loops which emanate from and return to a vascular plexus deeper in the skin. These capillary loops can be seen in the skinfold of the fingernail where the loop is visible over its long axis. The nailfolds thus provide direct access to skin capillaries which can be identified only by their tips in other skin areas.

Camera lucida drawings of skin capillary abnormalities in scleroderma were recorded before 1920. Descriptions of single capillary (elemental lesions) abnormalities were repeatedly documented during the period 1930 to 1970.[73,74] Maricq and colleagues expanded the field of observation (widefield capillary microscopy) and described patterns of nailfold capillary abnormalities in the rheumatic diseases. The most distinctive pattern of abnormality occurred in 90 percent of patients with scleroderma and dermatomyositis and 30 percent of patients with Raynaud's phenomenon without a connective tissue disorder or another basis for vasospastic symptoms (Fig. 76–4). This pattern was not seen in healthy or hospitalized populations and could readily be distinguished from the abnormalities observed in patients with rheumatoid arthritis or SLE.[76]

Initially, the relationship between the capillary abnormalities and the small artery lesion previously characterized in scleroderma was unclear. It was known that visceral involvement in scleroderma was closely associated and probably caused by the small artery lesion. Thus, a prospective study was undertaken to compare visceral or organ involvement (an indirect measure of small artery involvement) with capillary abnormalities in the same patient population. A strong positive correlation was shown between system involvement (skin, peripheral vascular, gut, lungs, heart, kidneys, muscles) and the severity of the scleroderma capillary pattern. The most abnormal capillary patterns (dilated, distorted capillaries adjacent to regions of absent skin capillaries) were seen in patients with the highest number of organ systems involved.[70]

Further prospective studies are in progress which suggest that patients who have only Raynaud's phenomenon, and who have definite widefield capillary pattern abnormalities, are at higher risk to develop overt connective tissue disease in the future than are patients with Raynaud's phenomenon whose capillary patterns are normal. In a multicenter study, Maricq and colleagues noted a strong positive correlation between widefield capillary abnormalities and features of scleroderma in patients classified as having mixed connective tissue disease (MCTD). Thus nailfold capillary observations may prove helpful in the early, overlapping, or mixed patient by separating the minority who ultimately develop SLE from the majority who ultimately develop scleroderma. Completion of the prospective study may help establish widefield nailfold capillary microscopy as an early diagnostic and prognostic indicator in the diffuse connective tissue diseases.[77] The capillary pattern studies are largely morphological; other approaches to the study of the microvascular bed which are promising, but still preliminary, include the estimation of rate and degree of capillary standstill of blood flow in nailfold capillaries on cooling,[75] immunopathologic studies of the microvascular bed, direct pressure measurements in microvessels,[78-80] and the monitoring of sympatholytic therapy by microvascular measurements.

Direct Vascular Damage. Since the vascular and the microvascular lesions of scleroderma occur together, it is reasonable to hypothesize a common pathogenesis (Fig. 76-5). A direct approach would be injury to the endothelial cell, which lines both vessel types.[81]

Endothelial cells provide a lining function for all blood vessels and can be isolated from vessels and propagated in culture. In vivo, endothelial cells provide a blood-compatible surface which protects erythrocytes from disruption, prevents leukocyte and platelet adherence and margination, and provides an inert surface which prevents activation of blood coagulation or the generation of vasoactive peptides (kinins). Disruption of the endothelial lining function leads to activation of blood coagulation, platelet adherence and aggregation, decreased fibrinolysis, and subsequent destruction of erythrocytes and leukocytes on the rough vascular surfaces (see Chapters 9 and 12). Clinically, evidence of intravascular coagulation, decreased fibrinolysis, and mi-

Figure 76–4. *A*, Typical nailfold capillary pattern of a normal adult. *B*, Nailfold capillary pattern of a patient with rheumatoid arthritis. Note the subpapillary plexus (SP) and the "shadow" of deeper and larger venules (V). *C*, Nailfold capillary pattern of a patient with dermatomyositis. Note the presence of large dilated capillary loops near the edge of the nailfold in both *C* and *D*. Nailfold capillary pattern of a patient with scleroderma. (From Maricq, H.R., and LeRoy, E.C.: Arthritis Rheum. 16:619, 1973.)

croangiopathic hemolysis can be taken as indirect evidence of endothelial injury.[82,83]

Endothelial cells produce several marker molecules whose plasma levels can be measured as further indirect evidence of injury. Factor VIII antigen is produced almost exclusively by endothelial cells. Plasminogen activator is produced and secreted by endothelial cells. Immunofluorescence studies have localized the site of synthesis of angiotensin converting enzyme to the endothelial cell. Measurement of these functional molecules in plasma may provide indirect estimates of the injury and repair of endothelial surfaces.[84]

Experience with direct measurements of endothelial injury and resultant platelet activation to determine the activity of the vascular and microvascular lesions is increasing. Factor VIII and von Willebrand levels are proving more reliable and technically more reproducible indicators of endothelial damage than are levels of the endothelial cytotoxic activity. Determination of plasma levels of the platelet granule proteins, beta-thromboglobulin and platelet factor 4, are also helpful in assessing the effects of failure of the endothelium to prevent platelet activation and release. The precise relationships

and sequence of these various vascular parameters remain to be discovered by future work.[85-89]

Endothelial cells in vivo are intimately associated with basement membrane structures. In vitro, these cells synthesize basement membrane components; in vivo, situations associated with endothelial damage and repair lead to reduplication and thickening of the basement membranes. It seems likely that the history of endothelial damage in a particular vessel can be estimated by the degree of duplication of its basement membrane, comparable to the duplication of the rings of a tree trunk.[90]

Endothelial cells interact not only with the blood but also with other cells of the vessel wall. On disruption of endothelial lining function, platelets adhere to the subendothelial stroma (Type III and basement membrane collagens) (see Chapter 16) and release factors that prompt smooth muscle cells in the intima and media of the vessel wall to migrate toward the damaged lumen surface, to proliferate, and to deposit connective tissue. This proliferating cell has been called a *myointimal cell*; it is considered to be the germinal cell in the development of the atherosclerotic plaque.[91] It may well be the major

PATHOGENESIS OF SCLERODERMA
(SYSTEMIC SCLEROSIS)

CYTOTOXIC STIMULUS

ENDOTHELIAL CELL INJURY

VASCULAR
PERMEABILITY

TARGET ORGAN
EDEMA AND
INFLAMMATION

SMOOTH MUSCLE
CELL MIGRATION

EDEMATOUS
PHASE

PLASMA
LEAKAGE

VASOMOTOR
INSTABILITY

FIBRIN
DEPOSITION

MICROVASCULAR
ABNORMALITIES

RENIN-ANGIOTENSIN
ACTIVATION

MICROANGIOPATHIC
HEMOLYTIC ANEMIA

CELL ACTIVATION

TARGET ORGAN
FIBROSIS

PROLIFERATIVE
ARTERIAL LESION

PROLIFERATIVE
AND FIBROTIC
PHASES

COLLAGEN SYNTHESIS

VASCULAR
CUTANEOUS
GASTRO-
INTESTINAL
PULMONARY
CARDIAC
RENAL

VASCULAR
AND MICROVASCULAR
INSUFFICIENCY

FIBROSIS

Figure 76–5. Pathogenesis of scleroderma (systemic sclerosis). A working hypothesis concerning the pathogenetic features known or thought to play a role in scleroderma. (The author thanks M.B. Kahaleh and H.R. Maricq for assistance and advice.)

cell responsible for the intimal proliferative lesions of scleroderma (Fig. 76–6). Detailed understanding of the interactions of blood, platelets, and the vascular wall is needed to design methods of intervention in the management of proliferative vascular lesions.

The aforementioned considerations provide a wealth of possibilities for the measurement of endothelial damage in scleroderma. It is reported that endothelial cells can be identified in the circulation after injury. All the factors noted above (factor VIII, plasminogen activator,

angiotensin converting enzyme, soluble basement membrane components) are potential clues of the state of the endothelial injury and repair. Systematic clinical evaluation of these factors is needed.[92]

The effects of cold exposure on the already abnormal blood vessels of patients with scleroderma have been observed in both the periphery and the viscera. Renal cortical blood flow drops dramatically after placing the hand in ice water.[12] Both the heart and the kidneys demonstrate the "no-reflow" phenomenon after cooling

Figure 76–6. A renal artery from the kidney of a woman who died of oliguric renal failure with hypertension which demonstrates the characteristic vascular lesion of scleroderma. This lesion shows intimal proliferation associated here with fibrinoid necrosis and nuclear debris. Hematoxylin and eosin × 300.

in which endothelial cell swelling impedes reperfusion after vasoconstriction.[12] Pulmonary function is decreased in cold weather, presumably because of pulmonary vasoconstriction.[36] Therefore, cold-induced vasoconstriction and vascular damage may be important in all the target organs of scleroderma.

CLINICAL CHARACTERISTICS

Peripheral Vascular–Raynaud's Phenomenon. The syndrome described by Maurice Raynaud in 1862 is characterized as episodic pallor or cyanosis on cold- or stress-induced vasoconstriction with suffusion and erythema on subsequent vasodilatation; it occurs in 90 percent of patients with the classic skin changes of scleroderma.[1] There is controversy concerning what proportion of patients with objective Raynaud's phenomenon ultimately develop scleroderma. Peripheral vascular textbooks estimate the proportion to be less than 10 percent; most rheumatologists believe that approximately 50 percent of their patients with Raynaud's phenomenon develop a connective tissue disease, that scleroderma is overwhelmingly the most likely to occur, and that a small proportion go on to SLE or rheumatoid arthritis.[8] Recently, a surgical group with a long interest in Raynaud's phenomenon reported that autoimmune and other serological abnormalities suggestive of connective tissue disease occur in 80 percent of Raynaud's patients.[93] This author believes that most Raynaud's patients ultimately develop the same visceral changes as do scleroderma patients but many develop those changes much more slowly. It is more realistic to consider the duration of Raynaud's phenomenon in the prediction of scleroderma; Birnstengl estimates that 5 percent of Raynaud's patients develop connective tissue disease *per year* of observation. This type of "per year" estimate is probably the most useful way to consider the continuum which exists between the vascular features of Raynaud's phenomenon and fibrotic features of scleroderma.[94]

A useful operational distinction among the potentially confusing terms *Raynaud's phenomenon, Raynaud's syndrome,* and *Raynaud's disease* is as follows: *Phenomenon* describes the events of pallor, cyanosis, suffusion, and tingling, which occur in an abrupt and phasic manner. When the phenomenon is associated with a known cause (scleroderma, vibration tool exposure), it is a *syndrome.* When no associated disorder has been detected, the term *disease* is appropriate. The term *disease* should probably be withheld until the phenomenon has been present for several years without apparent associated conditions. During an uncertain early phase, the term *idiopathic Raynaud's syndrome* may be useful.

The presence of Raynaud's phenomenon in scleroderma has little prognostic significance; its primary diagnostic implication is that, in the absence of Raynaud's phenomenon, another diagnosis, such as scleredema, porphyria, or amyloidosis, should be suspected. In the initial evaluation of Raynaud's phenomenon, many possible associations should be looked for but are not commonly found. These include industrial exposure to vibratory machines, vinyl chloride, or silicotic dusts;[95,96] obstruction to flow at the thoracic outlet (e.g., cervical rib, scalenus anticus); cold agglutinins or cryoglobulins, which impede microvascular flow; obliterative arterial disease; and other connective tissue syndromes (SLE, rheumatoid arthritis, mixed or overlap syndromes).[94]

Since the days of Sir Thomas Lewis, studies of the mechanism of Raynaud's phenomenon have concluded that structural abnormalities of the vessel wall predispose the digits to exaggerated vasospasm and subsequent vasodilatation. In the limited number of pathological studies of digital arteries in Raynaud's patients, vascular lesions indistinguishable from those of scleroderma have been observed.[97] Despite the structural nature of the basic lesion, most therapeutic approaches to Raynaud's phenomenon involve reducing the influence of the sympathetic nervous system by pharmacological sympatholysis. These therapeutic measures provide symptomatic relief but probably do not affect the course or frequency of developing connective tissue disease.[98-105]

Skin. Skin involvement is both the namesake and the hallmark of scleroderma, occurring in 90 to 95 percent of patients. The remaining 5 percent usually have severe gastrointestinal scleroderma without either skin involvement or Raynaud's phenomenon, an interesting subset that reminds us that although skin is by far the most common target organ in scleroderma (systemic sclerosis), skin changes are not absolutely essential for the diagnosis.

Skin involvement usually proceeds through three phases: early, classic, and late. In the *early* phase, the hands and feet are usually puffy and full-feeling in the morning and may be unremarkable for the remainder of the day. On examination a nonpitting tautness is observed which fills the fingers, toes, and dorsal hand and foot skin; epidermis and epidermal appendages remain intact. Raynaud's phenomenon and skin ulcerations are common. The face may feel taut at this stage.

In the *classic* stage of skin involvement, the puffiness subsides and is replaced, often rather suddenly, by tight, hidebound skin which is tenaciously adherent to deeper structures (tendons, joints) and impedes their easy motion. The skin may have the dry, coarse texture of wood. The epidermis becomes thin and atrophic; hair vanishes, creases disappear (a transient relief to the cosmetically concerned), and sweating is noticeably impaired. This is the full-blown, unequivocal stage of scleroderma and, frustratingly, seems to be the single specific diagnostic criterion. These changes are usually present in fingers, hands, forearms, face, and sometimes trunk. When present only in the fingers, they are called sclerodactyly and do not carry the same implications. The classic stage of skin involvement may remain unchanged for years. Measurements of skin thickness, the weight of a standardized area of skin biopsy material, and the tabulation of skin involvement by anatomic sites (total skin score) have been proposed to monitor the natural history of scleroderma subsets and to assess therapeutic interventions.[54,106,107]

At some time between 3 and 15 years after the appearance of classic skin changes, this pattern merges imperceptibly into a *late* phase. The hidebound dermis softens and becomes pliable; it may return to an almost normal state or so nearly normal that it is difficult to be certain that the patient ever had scleroderma. Although the dermis may soften, the epidermal atrophy and loss of epidermal appendages remain the best indicators of former hidebound skin changes. In the second decade of scleroderma, softening of the dermis is common. This feature of the natural history of scleroderma may explain the initial enthusiasm for a variety of therapeutic modalities which are credited with changing the course of scleroderma: the uncontrolled observation of softening skin is initially attributed to the drug; when early-stage patients are subsequently treated by other investigators, the spontaneous softening of skin may not be observed. The only safeguard for the natural softening of skin in scleroderma is the insistence on controlled therapeutic observations.

Skin biopsy results depend on the stage of cutaneous involvement. Before fibrosis, the features of subcutaneous edema, perivascular round cell infiltrates, and interstitial cellular collections are sufficiently prominent to be designated as cellular by Fleischmajer;[19-22] unfortunately, these features are not diagnostic and may be difficult to separate from lupus or other forms of dermatitis. In the classic phase, subcutaneous cellular infiltration has been replaced by subcutaneous fibrosis, which is the definitive diagnostic finding, and may extend deep in the subcutis to surround tendons, muscle bundles, and joint capsules. In the late stage the subcutaneous fibrosis may be less striking, with the thinning and loss of epidermis with abscence of epidermal appendages the major finding.

As noted above, skin involvement remains the hallmark of scleroderma and a constant reminder to the patient that he or she has a disfiguring ailment; however, the course, degree, or extent of the skin involvement appears to have little or no bearing on the outcome of the disease, which depends almost entirely on the degree of visceral involvement.[108,109]

Gut. The frequency of involvement of the gastrointestinal tract approaches that of the skin in scleroderma only because of the high incidence of esophageal hypomotility.[23-25] In contrast, involvement of the small and large intestines is distinctly uncommon.

Esophagus. Reduction in the propulsive force of the smooth muscle lining of the involuntary or lower two thirds of the esophagus can be shown to occur in 90 percent of patients with the classic skin lesions of scleroderma (if the most sensitive techniques for detection are used).[23] Probably fewer than half such patients would complain of or admit to the clinical symptoms of dysphagia (food catching, a vertical substernal pain after eating or on lying down, regurgitation, or peptic symptoms). As discussed earlier, abnormal esophageal motility can be helpful diagnostically in the early undifferentiated patient because it is commonly present and has substantial diagnostic specificity for scleroderma. Thus it is recommended that motility studies be done in the asymptomatic patient in whom a diagnosis is sought.

The standard barium swallow with fluoroscopic observation using heavy barium mixtures should probably be abandoned because it is insensitive in the detection of esophageal hypomotility. Two techniques, cineradiography and manometry, are sensitive and give slightly different types of information.

A cine-esophagram, utilizing light barium and the recumbent position, is moderately sensitive in detecting early esophageal hypomotility and has the added advantage of detecting hiatus hernia and other disorders of the esophagus which are associated with dysphagia but are not specific for scleroderma.[23] Cineradiography may also provide helpful clues to the complications of scleroderma of the esophagus, peptic esophagitis, and esophageal stricture, which follow from incompetency of the lower esophageal sphincter (LES) and from reflux of gastric acid and enzymes into the esophagus. This technique is generally available to most radiologists. Despite these advantages, cineradiography of the esophagus, even in the most experienced hands, is not as sensitive for detection of the earliest lesion, disordered esophageal motility, as is esophageal manometry.

Esophageal manometry is substantially more sensitive than any other technique known in detecting esophageal hypomotility. Loss of secondary and tertiary waves is an early finding often associated with reduced resting tone of the LES. Pharmacologic manipulations during manometry have not greatly enhanced the information gained from simple monitoring of swallowing.[25] The high sensitivity and increasing availability of manometry are its advantages; its major disadvantage is the lack of information regarding other abnormalities of the esophagus.

The pathogenesis of esophageal scleroderma is not fully understood. By inference, it should have the same basis as other visceral involvement, that of smooth muscle atrophy and fibrosis, stemming at first from intermittent and functional interruption of nutrient blood flow, and later associated with fixed vascular changes and structural devascularization. Studies of flow, morphology, or responses of the esophageal vascular or microvascular tree are needed.[26-32]

Duodenum. The most significant lesions of the gastrointestinal tract in scleroderma are duodenal-jejunal hypomotility and concomitant malabsorption, which virtually always occur in the presence of esophageal hypomotility; small bowel scleroderma occurs occasionally in the absence of cutaneous disease, posing a diagnostic dilemma (systemic sclerosis sine scleroderma); fortunately, malabsorption is present in no more than 10 percent of scleroderma patients.[30] Malabsorption should be suspected as the basis for weight loss and inanition in every scleroderma patient; it is not usually a presenting feature, and it can be detected by the standard upper gastrointestinal series showing dilatation of the third and fourth segments of the duodenum, slow transit time, and pattern changes in adjacent regions of the small bowel. The physiologic consequences of duodenal hypomotility must be assessed by measurements of absorption, of which quantitative stool fat determinations are the best indicators. Determinations of carbohydrate (xylose test) and protein absorption may be helpful as confirmatory procedures. The mechanism of these changes is probably similar to that previously described for the esophagus. Therapy is based on reduction of gut floras which compete proximally for bile salts required for fat and fat-soluble vitamin absorption.

Colon. Wide-mouth sacculations of the large bowel are distinctive lesions in scleroderma, occurring in few other disorders. They are rare, are late, seldom contribute diagnostically, and are usually of little consequence to the patient. When constipation is a problem in the scleroderma patient, sacculations are often present. They do not occur without esophageal involvement. The mechanism of their occurrence is probably the same as that of bowel involvement with scleroderma elsewhere; management is directed toward reduction of symptoms.

Lungs. Pulmonary involvement is the most underestimated organ system abnormality in the rheumatic diseases, especially in scleroderma. Such neglect is unjustified since the lungs are fourth behind skin, peripheral vasculature, and esophagus in frequency of involvement and are now recognized, concomitant with the reduction in deaths from renal scleroderma by the early use of more effective antihypertensive therapy, as the leading cause of death in scleroderma. Lack of detection of pulmonary involvement can be traced to the following points:

1. Patients with rheumatic disease, especially scleroderma, are distinctly limited in physical activity; hence they do not note dyspnea or breathlessness early.

2. The standard posteroanterior and lateral roentgenograms of the chest are insensitive indicators of early lung involvement in the rheumatic diseases, including scleroderma.

3. Both early and late involvements of the lung in scleroderma are considered to be fibrotic, progressive, irreversible, and untreatable, largely because of our dependence on autopsy studies.

4. Controlled therapeutic trials in early pulmonary scleroderma have not been conducted.

Pulmonary involvement in scleroderma consists of several types which may exist separately or in combination: pleurisy and pleural effusion (rare), pulmonary hypertension[110] with or without cor pulmonale, and diffuse interstitial lung disease with or without bronchitis. Of these, the most acute and easily detectable are pleurisy, pleural effusions, and pulmonary hypertension, the last being the most common cause of acute breathlessness in the scleroderma patient. Pulmonary hypertension can occur with or without interstitial disease and is detectable by ausculation (systolic murmur of pulmonary artery dilatation, accentuation of P2, fixed A2-P2 split), ultrasound, roentgenography, or right heart catheterization. The echocardiographic diagnosis of pulmonary hypertension is subtle but promising, since it is noninvasive.[45] The presence of pulmonary hypertension is considered prima facie evidence of active pulmonary

vascular involvement with the proliferative lesions of scleroderma. Uncontrolled observations have suggested that pulmonary hypertension, when isolated (without severe interstitial disease), is responsive to therapy with glucocorticoids, presumably reducing the inflammatory and vasculitic process.[33]

Diffuse interstitial lung disease is the most common lung involvement in scleroderma. Its onset is insidious, and early involvement may go for months to years without recognition by patient or physician. Occasionally, a dry hacking cough leads to pulmonary evaluation. Fortunately, many scleroderma patients are now being evaluated regularly with sensitive indicators of ventilation-perfusion imbalance such as tests of "diffusion," which are very helpful in detecting early lung involvement.[37-41]

The mechanism of lung involvement is incompletely understood, but probably shares features of scleroderma involvement elsewhere, including an inflammation of the vascular and microvascular elements of the lung leading to vascular thickening and ultimately to fibrosis.[33-36]

Musculoskeletal. *Muscle.* Skeletal muscle is frequently involved in scleroderma. Some patients present with acute myositis characterized by muscle weakness and tenderness (usually proximal), elevated muscle enzymes (CPK and aldolase), abnormal electromyographic findings suggestive of myositis, and mononuclear infiltrates on muscle biopsy. Since myositis is a frequent feature of rheumatoid arthritis, systemic lupus erythematosus, scleroderma, dermatomyositis, and polymyositis, it is not necessary to introduce another diagnostic label, such as overlap or mixed connective tissue disease, in these patients. In general the acute myositis which may occur at any time in the course of scleroderma is indistinguishable in its presentation, distribution, and response to therapy from myositis in any other connective tissue disease.

A more subtle form of muscle involvement is present in a larger proportion of scleroderma patients and seems to be distinctive for this disease since it is not seen in other patients with connective tissue disease.[111] This indolent or chronic myopathy, present in most patients, is characterized by mild weakness (detected primarily on muscle testing and not usually a complaint of the patient), mild atrophy in proximal muscles, slight elevations of muscle enzymes, and few or no changes on electromyography. Muscle biopsies require special histochemical stains to detect subtle differences in fiber size and composition (see Chapter 47). This mild myopathy usually persists for months to years; the slightly elevated muscle enzyme levels wax and wane and are not responsive to nonsteroidal or glucocorticoid anti-inflammatory medications. Thus, high risk therapy for the indolent myopathy of scleroderma is not indicated.

Bone. The skeleton per se may be involved in late scleroderma but is not generally a target organ in the early phases of the disease.[112] Distal tuft resorption is a relatively uncommon feature of first-decade scleroderma patients, becoming much more common in the second and third decades. Patients with longstanding Raynaud's phenomenon without connective tissue disease also resorb the distal end of their distal phalangeal tufts, independent of the presence of sclerodactyly. This resorption is not seen in other rheumatic and connective tissue diseases (in psoriasis the proximal end of the distal phalangeal tuft is resorbed first; in vinyl chloride disease the central portion of the distal phalangeal tuft is resorbed). These observations support the hypothesis that the basis for all bone resorption in scleroderma is the lack of adequate vascular supply to preserve viable bone. In a similar manner, other sites of bone resorption have been recorded in late scleroderma. Reports of mandibular resorption and of resorption of ribs and other sites have appeared periodically. The vascular basis for bone resorption is presumably similar to that for all other target organ effects of the disease.

Joints. A small proportion of patients destined ultimately to develop scleroderma present with symmetrical polyarthritis suggestive of rheumatoid arthritis. This is usually seronegative, nonerosive, and not associated with subcutaneous nodule formation. Within 6 months to 2 years, the synovitis subsides and classic cutaneous features of scleroderma develop, often appearing abruptly over 1 to 2 months. Scleroderma (systemic sclerosis) progresses in these patients, and they do not usually develop features of rheumatoid disease at a later date.

Except for this subset of scleroderma patients, representing fewer than 10 percent, the joints are not a major site of involvement.[113] After hidebound skin changes are well established, any or all joints may be limited in motion and may emit "squeaks and creaks" on movement; these phenomena may also be noticed around tendons and ligaments. True inflammatory synovitis is rare. The fibrosis so characteristic of classic scleroderma is seen in the joints on synovial biopsy; moreover, a remarkable amount of fibrin deposition is detected on the surface of the synovium. This degree of fibrin deposition may exceed in amount the fibrosis also present; such fibrin deposition is not a striking feature of other forms of synovitis and is presently poorly understood in scleroderma.[1] Joint destruction is unusual in scleroderma, and management of joint complaints is usually linked closely to therapy for maintenance of skeletal mobility in the presence of ever-tightening skin.

Kidneys. In the general clinical sense, renal involvement is not common in scleroderma patients; the kidney is, however, the most important target organ because it is the cause of death in many patients who die from this disease.[114] Estimates of renal involvement vary greatly, depending on criteria. The acute and uniformly fatal nature of renal insufficiency, once it occurs, means that few patients (usually fewer than 10 percent) in the usual clinical practice are noted to have renal scleroderma. If markers of renal involvement, such as proteinuria, hypertension, and azotemia, or signs of reduced glomerular filtration, are carefully monitored in a population with scleroderma, they are found in one third to one half, depending on the hospital-based nature of the population. Renal vascular lesions are present in most scleroderma patients examined carefully at autopsy (up to

80 percent). These three examples, clinic, hospital, and autopsy, demonstrate how the published prevalence of renal scleroderma can vary from 10 to 80 percent.[12]

There is need for specific indicators of renal involvement in scleroderma. The onset of proteinuria or hypertension during scleroderma identifies a population at substantially higher risk to develop renal scleroderma. The appearance of microangiopathic hemolytic anemia, with or without detectable evidence of intravascular coagulation or fibrinolysis, is an ominous portent of imminent renal failure.[114] Preliminary evidence suggests that the exaggerated renin response to stimulation may correlate with the silent presence of renal vascular lesions.[115] An extensive study of renal vasoactive hormone levels in 23 scleroderma patients on a fixed sodium and potassium intake revealed plasma renin to be normal in 18 and elevated in 5, while kallikrein, kinin, prostaglandin E, and aldosterone were within normal limits. This study concluded that hyper-responsiveness to normal stimuli for renin secretion may be characteristic of some, but not all, scleroderma patients.[116] The time-honored determination of renal blood flow (para-aminohippurate clearance) has been shown to be as sensitive as any known procedure for detection of renal scleroderma; unfortunately, it is not regularly used for this purpose.[12]

The therapeutic armamentarium is large, and the stakes are high. Patients with renal scleroderma can be saved from a uniformly and abruptly fatal outcome by an aggressive blockade of renin-angiotensin in both hypertensive and normotensive patients, and by vigorous peritoneal dialysis or hemodialysis.[114] Life has been sustained in this manner in several dozen patients with fully developed oliguric renal failure. Increasingly potent inhibitors of renin-angiotensin may replace the earlier use of nephrectomy for this purpose.[117,118]

Two phases in renal scleroderma are recognized: the slowly progressive arterial lesions characterized by intimal proliferation, medial thinning, and adventitial fibrosis of interlobular arteries which go undetected clinically until marked reductions of renal blood flow begin to impinge on glomerular function (Fig. 76–7); and the sudden collapse of glomerular filtration often prompted by a major event which leads to severe volume depletion, such as hemorrhage, surgery, dehydration, or diuresis (Fig. 76–8). All sudden changes in plasma volume are to be rigorously avoided in scleroderma patients with markers of renal involvement.[115,119-130]

Heart. Cardiopulmonary signs and symptoms can stem from a variety of causes in scleroderma. Atherosclerotic and hypertensive heart disease are at least as common in scleroderma patients as they are in the general population of the same age. Interstitial lung disease and pulmonary hypertension are relatively common and are discussed elsewhere.

Inflammatory and fibrotic disease of the pericardium has recently been clinically characterized in scleroderma.[42] Pericardial disease can present either as acute pericarditis with fever and a friction rub or, more commonly, as relatively silent pericardial effusion which pre-

Figure 76–7. A renal artery near a glomerulus which is totally occluded by the distinctive proliferative arterial lesion of scleroderma. Here the characteristic triad of (1) intimal proliferation with mucoid accumulation, (2) medial thinning, and (3) adventitial connective tissue deposition can be seen. Hematoxylin and eosin × 300.

sents as mild dependent edema. These effusions have been associated with subsequent renal failure in a substantial proportion of patients, suggesting that overaggressive diuretic management may be harmful in some cases.

The scleroderma heart has a venerable place in rheumatology, having been reported by Weiss and Stead in 1943.[130a] Isolated and clinically significant myocardial fibrosis is relatively uncommon in scleroderma and would seem to be a late stage of scleroderma heart disease. Recent studies of sudden death in scleroderma patients have emphasized the proliferative intimal lesion found in intramyocardial coronary vessels and associated with an unusual type of necrosis and fibrosis called "contraction band necrosis," which is considered secondary to intermittent ischemia with reperfusion.[47] This sequence of events leads ultimately to perivascular and band-like fibrosis which can be distinguished from the usual coagulation necrosis and nonreperfusion of myocardial fibrosis secondary to coronary heart disease. Studies by Bulkley and colleagues suggest an early functional stage of scleroderma heart disease which might be amenable to therapy if identified with certainty. These studies also provide support for the hypothesis that the vascular lesions are primary in scleroderma.[47]

Clinically, heart disease in scleroderma is difficult to distinguish from lung disease. Arrhythmias and ischemic pain are suggestive of myocardial disease; pericardial effusion is relatively common and can be detected by echocardiography. Cardiac enlargement may not be impressive, particularly in the presence of restrictive lung disease. It is especially important to evaluate carefully the scleroderma patient with angina and an abnormal electrocardiogram. Many such patients have normal coronary arteriograms; in these patients, it is critical to remember that scleroderma is a disease which causes severe loss of the microcirculatory bed. Thus, it is not

surprising that coronary artery bypass procedures may not help in scleroderma heart disease because the lesion is distal to the bypass and the myocardium remains underperfused because of the extensive small vessel disease.[42-47]

Nervous System. The central nervous system is not involved in scleroderma. Peripheral neuropathy can occur and is usually manifest as an entrapment neuropathy, apparently caused by fibrosis impinging on the nerve. This is usually a feature of second or third decade scleroderma; trigeminal neuralgia is the most common example of this neuropathy.[1]

Patients at risk for trigeminal neuralgia usually have had facial skin changes of scleroderma for many years. They begin to note a burning sensation localized to the face, jaw, and chin, associated with a numbness in the same area, the sensation progressing slowly over a period of years; in a small number of patients it is severe and incapacitating. It probably affects no more than 10 percent of scleroderma patients and a slightly higher proportion of the CREST subset of patients. Symptomatic relief is the mainstay of management.

In the muscle disease of scleroderma one often finds the subtle and microscopic suggestion of a mixed neuromyopathy. This impression is caused by the grouping of myopathic findings in the muscle and may be another confirmation of the primary vascular nature of the disease.[111]

Other. Male impotence is a recently described feature of scleroderma; whether this is psychogenic, the mixed impotence of chronic disease, or end organ failure on a vascular or neurovascular basis remains to be determined.[131-133] An increased frequency of chromosomal or cytogenetic aberrations has been observed in patients with scleroderma. Compound chromosomal fragmentation and rearrangement were the most common abnormalities noted. These could not be explained by drug

Figure 76–8. A renal preglomerular arteriole is shown in which fibrinoid necrosis in the vessel wall and a marginated column of erythrocytes are prominent. This patient was hypertensive; the fibrinoid is found in the hyperetensive scleroderma population but is otherwise not a consistent feature of the scleroderma artery lesion. Hematoxylin and eosin × 600.

therapy or radiation exposure and were not associated with an increased frequency of neoplasia. Both scleroderma patients and their first degree relatives were noted to have a "chromosomal breakage factor" in their serum. Thus, scleroderma is unusual because it is one of the few acquired disorders in which chromosomal aberrations are commonly found; most of the other disorders in which this is seen are clearly inherited.[134,135] The role of these observations in pathogenesis is unclear.[136,137] Whether the chromosomal aberrations have any bearing on the occasional familial clustering of scleroderma patients is also unknown.[138-143]

SCLERODERMA VARIANTS

Subsets of Scleroderma. Diffuse generalized scleroderma (systemic sclerosis) is the major and most serious systemic scleroderma syndrome (see Table 76–1). It may develop rapidly and be associated with early visceral involvement (acute diffuse) in a small proportion of patients (10 percent or less); it usually develops insidiously, and visceral involvement may be delayed (chronic diffuse) in the majority of scleroderma patients (60 to 70 percent).[144-148] A majority of patients, who live longer than patients with diffuse scleroderma and who are more likely to accumulate in practice groups, have this more slowly developing syndrome in which skin disease is often limited to fingers (sclerodactyly) and occasionally the ears and nose (acrosclerosis); in these patients, the chronic course allows time for the development of prominent calcinosis and telangiectasia. These patients also have Raynaud's phenomenon and esophageal hypomotility. This variant is called the CREST syndrome (calcinosis, *R*aynaud's phenomenon, *e*sophageal hypomotility, *s*clerodactyly and *t*elangiectasia); patients with the CREST syndrome have less obvious visceral disease in the early years.[7,149] They are not exempt from late visceral disease, however, and in the second decade may develop trigeminal neuralgia, pulmonary fibrosis with pulmonary hypertension, and, less commonly, renal and cardiac involvement. Thus the CREST syndrome may be viewed as second and third decade scleroderma, since that is when visceral lesions appear.[149,150] Because there is no selectivity of or specificity for the findings in the CREST syndrome, some have suggested that the designation be dropped. This observer finds it less useful than the concept of first, second, and third decade scleroderma; the first decade of the typical CREST patient usually consists of Raynaud's phenomenon alone.[106]

Three interesting associations with scleroderma-like disorders, which may shed light on pathogenesis, have recently been re-emphasized. The well-documented association between scleroderma and primary biliary cirrhosis as two co-existent human fibrotic disorders is provocative.[151] Careful documentation of the similarities[152] and differences[153] between scleroderma and chronic graft-vs.-host disease after marrow transplantation has been provided. And third, the scleroderma-like disorder occurring after breast augmentation with prostheses has been compared with adjuvant disease.[154]

Scleredema. Scleredema is a rare, self-limited condition in which induration of the skin without Raynaud's phenomenon often follows bacterial infection, usually of the throat.[1] The hands and fingers are spared, and skin biopsy shows accumulation of proteoglycan and glycoprotein components (PAS and alcian blue positive). Viscera, including the esophagus, are not involved. This syndrome is not difficult to distinguish from scleroderma.

A number of other syndromes which can mimic or be associated with scleroderma are listed in Table 76–1; full discussion of these disorders is beyond the scope of this chapter. One such category, the mixed connective tissue disease (MCTD) syndrome, has elements of many diffuse inflammatory diseases of connective tissue, and is distinguished by its unusual pattern of antinuclear antibody with high titer against a ribonuclear protein. Although many authorities would classify MCTD as an overlap syndrome, it is discussed in this text as a separate entity in Chapter 71.

Diffuse Fasciitis with Eosinophilia. In 1975, Shulman reported several patients with a disorder now considered a variant of scleroderma.[155] These patients were predominantly young males who noted induration of the skin of the extremities and trunk (usually sparing hands and fingers), often within days following heavy exertion. Raynaud's phenomenon was not present; the epidermis was usually preserved, and epidermal appendages were present and functioning. Induration involved the subcutaneous space and deep fascia.[156]

Laboratory evaluation included a negative test for rheumatoid factor and antinuclear antibody, prominent circulating eosinophilia (up to 50 percent of granulocytes), and hypergammaglobulinemia with elevated levels of IgG, IgA, and IgM. Biopsy of the indurated skin revealed replacement of the subcutaneous space by a cellular infiltrate of mononuclear cells (findings characteristic of scleroderma), both with and without eosinnophils and associated with the distinctive feature of thickening of the deep fascial layers with a dense fibrosis.[157]

Extensive evaluation for visceral involvement similar to that in scleroderma has been negative. Presently, the esophagus, lungs, heart, and kidneys are believed to be uninvolved in the diffuse fasciitis process.

Most patients with diffuse fasciitis have been treated with glucocorticoids, with the indurated skin exhibiting an excellent response in weeks to months. In a very few patients this syndrome subsides spontaneously with no therapeutic intervention. A longer period of observation of this disorder is necessary in order to understand the full extent of diffuse fasciitis with eosinophilia, an interesting variant of scleroderma.[158] The subsequent occurrence of aplastic anemia in several patients is fascinating but unexplained.

Longer periods of observation of patients with fasciitis and eosinophilia have revealed evidence of visceral vascular involvement identical to that of systemic sclerosis patients in a substantial proportion of fasciitis patients, suggesting that chronic fasciitis exists and is indistinguishable from scleroderma. To blur the margins even more, 20 to 25 percent of scleroderma patients have been reported to have eosinophilia,[159] which is a prominent feature of a recently described scleroderma-like disorder, the toxic oil syndrome of Spain (vide infra).

The Toxic Oil Syndrome of Spain. In May of 1981 a remarkable new disease with features of scleroderma appeared in central and northern Spain.[160] An adulterated rapeseed oil, the precise chemical composition of which remains unknown, was distributed to approximately one hundred thousand Spanish families. Within seven to ten days, young adults began to experience the abrupt onset of fever, dyspnea, malaise, myalgia, headaches, cough, and pruritus, associated with pulmonary edema without apparent heart disease; eosinophilia; exanthems; hypoxemia and, less frequently, facial edema; nausea and vomiting; abdominal pain; irritability and clouding of consciousness; purpura; and lymphadenopathy and hepatomegaly. Approximately 36,000 patients were identified over several months, two thirds of whom were hospitalized.[161-164]

Among acute patients there were slightly more men than women; the illness was distinctly unusual in children and in the elderly, providing epidemiologic confirmation of the consistently negative attempts to isolate a microbial basis for the acute interstitial pneumonitis. It was the rare occurrence of the syndrome in an infant that lead Tabuenca to make the association with toxic cooking oil.[160]

In the acute phase approximately 200 persons died of pulmonary edema with respiratory insufficiency. Treatment with cardiotonic agents and antimicrobials (e.g., erythromycin for Mycoplasma) was not helpful; glucocorticoids parenterally were associated with prompt improvement. Remarkably few if any patients developed pulmonary interstitial fibrosis, distinguishing toxic oil syndrome from paraquat or bleomycin toxicity. Fortunately the majority of acute patients recovered without major clinical sequelae.[162]

The acute histopathologic lesion was vascular and endothelial. Swelling, vacuoles, and degeneration of endothelial cells were observed throughout the pulmonary and systemic vasculature and were associated with interstitial edema and occasional mononuclear cell infiltration. Arteritis was not seen; the vascular lesion was confined to the intima.[161]

This generalized endothelial injury pattern is sufficient to account for the acute illness and for its chronic sequelae: pulmonary edema, cutaneous edema and rash, and thromboembolism in the acute phase; scleroderma-like dermal fibrosis, peripheral neuropathy, and pulmonary hypertension in the chronic phase.

Within weeks of the acute syndrome, signs of a chronic phase of the toxic oil syndrome began to emerge, predominantly in females and largely but not exclusively in known victims of the acute illness. Numbness and muscle pain were noted simultaneously with facial and limb edema, continued eosinophilia, and thrombocytopenia, and with thromboembolic episodes, which were responsible for a number of deaths in the evolving chronic phase of the disease. Weight loss and muscle atrophy became more severe, and subtle features of autoimmune disease appeared, most notably antinuclear antibodies of speckled pattern and a relative increase in HLA-DR3-4 haplotype. Ultimately the severe peripheral neuromyopathy with severe distal wasting and widespread scleroderma dominated the chronic pattern in these patients and left them completely disabled.[163]

In 10 percent or so of acute patients whose disease evolved into chronic illness, the skin became hard, taut, and shiny; the mouth and eyes were dry and irritated; motor weakness and muscle atrophy progressed; and alopecia, dysphagia, and pulmonary hypertension were noted. Respiratory disturbances reappeared, not as a result of pulmonary interstitial disease but secondary to neuromuscular disease of the respiratory muscles, which was sufficiently severe to be fatal in some patients. These features of severe neuropathy, scleroderma, and the sicca syndrome have persisted in hundreds of patients. Two years after onset, about 10 percent of chronic patients remain hospitalized with wasting, scleroderma, and malnutrition.[161,164]

For students of chronic, debilitating multisystem diseases such as the diffuse connective tissue diseases, the intriguing problem represented by the toxic oil syndrome is simply: How does an insult of limited duration (possible oleoanilides of toxic oil) result in a progressive multistage, multisystem disorder? The common denominator is endothelial injury throughout the body; the pathologic marker of the chronic phase is the continued intimal reaction, with proliferation indistinguishable from that seen in scleroderma or in chronic graft-vs.-host reaction.[161] What mechanisms selected these Spaniards for chronic illness? Is it an immune response gene linked to DR3 or DR4? Does autoimmunity to endothelial cells or basement membranes (type III or type IV collagens, fibronectin, laminin) play a role? Is the acute destruction of large molecular weight basement membrane structures, which are poorly biodegradable, an explanation for the eosinophilia and/or the elevated IgE levels (the latter found in one third of acute toxic oil patients)? Do known mechanisms, such as the enhanced platelet stickiness mediated by estrogens and seen in females, determine the preponderance of females who developed the chronic syndrome? Do these patterns of acute and chronic illness have a message for the understanding of scleroderma?

There may never be complete answers to these questions. An enhanced incidence of HLA-DR3 and DR4 subjects among chronic toxic oil syndrome patients has been reported and confirmed, and there is evidence for basement membrane autoantibodies in up to 70 percent of chronic patients. These are intriguing leads to apply to a suitable animal model which might elucidate both toxic oil syndrome and scleroderma.

The intense intimal proliferation and subsequent fibrosis of toxic oil syndrome is very similar to that seen in scleroderma; the acute pulmonary edema and the severe neuropathy of toxic oil syndrome are not components of scleroderma. Dissection of these similarities and differences remains a challenge of major international proportions.

PATHOGENESIS

Vascular and Microvascular. It is challenging to attempt to bring together the multiple factors known to be present in scleroderma.[93,165-169] One of the most appealing current concepts is that scleroderma is a reaction to repeated episodes of endothelial cell injury. When this injury occurs in small arteries, it leads to platelet aggregation, myointimal cell proliferation and migration into the damaged region, deposition of connective tissue (PAS-positive, mucoid glycoproteins, collagen and elastin fibrils which resist remodeling and resorption), and reduction in lumen diameter and changes in vessel distensibility, all of which lead to the distinctive vascular lesion of scleroderma. Endothelial damage leads to permeability changes; perhaps platelet factors activate surrounding interstitial fibroblasts, causing them to secrete collagen which forms a cuff around the adventitia

of the vessel. These intimal and adventitial reactions with reduction in medial cells (the putative source of myointimal cells) leave the media thin and atrophic. Thus the three distinctive features of the scleroderma small artery lesion (intimal proliferation with mucoid connective tissue deposition, medial thinning, and adventitial scarring) can be considered a consequence of endothelial injury to the artery.[82]

When endothelial injury occurs in the capillary bed, the changes may be substantially different. Without a population of myointimal cells, there is little proliferative response. Permeability changes may activate interstitial fibroblasts to produce more type I and type III collagens, which either inhibit new capillary budding and growth or physically exclude capillaries from areas of scar. Devascularization and atrophy occur; existing vascular channels condense and expand into the dilated capillaries observed, which ultimately become visible telangiectasia. In these altered microvessels resting flow is normally brisk; cold exposure leads to exaggerated vasoconstriction of the partially occluded lumen and taut vessel wall, resulting in standstill of capillary flow.[84]

Continued injury to the vascular endothelium leads to altered flow, to intravascular coagulation, to microangiopathic hemolysis, and to intravascular thrombosis with infarction, all of which are consistently seen, especially in renal scleroderma, in which, in addition, reduced renal blood flow leads to stimulation of renin-angiotensin, increased vasoconstriction, and further vascular damage. Whether increased permeability (with volume contraction) or reduced renal blood flow is the primary stimulus to renin-angiotensin activation is not known; hyperreninemia is a consistent finding in renal scleroderma.[12]

Because so many of the features of scleroderma are consistent with a state of vascular endothelial damage, it is tempting to carry the argument one step further and ask what prompts the endothelial injury. Several possibilities are under active investigation.

A serum component, selectivity cytotoxic for endothelial cells, has been detected in patients with scleroderma.[82] The nature of this factor is uncertain, but it does not appear to be immunoglobulin; nor is its cytotoxic activity complement dependent.[88,170]

Immune. Several indirect lines of evidence are consistent with an immune trigger mechanism leading to recurrent episodes of endothelial injury and repair.[169] A significant incidence of autoimmune phenomena (antiglobulin,[58] antinuclear,[59] and antismooth muscle antibodies[61]) is present in the sera of scleroderma patients. Clinically, scleroderma may coexist in patients with recognized autoimmune disorders such as Sjögren's syndrome and systemic lupus erythematosus.[171] Recent evidence supports a cell-mediated immune mechanism in the pathogenesis of scleroderma; tissue antigens extracted from skin and other organs induce release of lymphokines from leukocyte preparations of scleroderma patients but not of controls.[172] Direct evidence for immune reactions to basement membrane collagen (type IV) in scleroderma patients brings closer the relationship between endothelial (and its basement membrane) injury and immune perpetuation of the vascular lesion.[173] Studies have shown lymphocytes from affected subjects to be cytotoxic to cultured target cells such as fibroblasts and myoblasts. In severely ill patients, a reduction of thymus-dependent lymphocytes and reduced response to phytohemagglutinin have been observed.[174]

Perhaps the most compelling evidence for endothelial damage by immune mechanisms is the similarity between the scleroderma vascular lesion and the proliferative vascular lesion of chronic homograft rejection.[175,176] Experimentally, little has been done to study scleroderma as a form of chronic homograft rejection. An equally intriguing link between scleroderma and immune mechanisms is the scleroderma-like syndrome which develops in patients who survive for 12 to 18 months or longer after bone marrow transplants. Virtually all these patients develop features of the graft-versus-host reaction, and a substantial proportion of them develop Sjögren's syndrome and a scleroderma-like skin disease. This is a potentially fertile field for future study of the association between scleroderma and immune mechanisms.[177]

Thus both immune and nonimmune and both humoral and cellular mechanisms may be responsible for the initiation and perpetuation of endothelial injury in scleroderma. Much more precise experimental information is needed concerning the sequence of mechanisms involved.[171,172,174,178-184]

A number of tantalizing but inconclusive reports on immune abnormalities in scleroderma patients have been published.[185] Whether these abnormalities are specific or nonspecific, or primary or secondary, and how they relate to the induction of fibrosis remain unclear. They include lymphocyte hyporesponsiveness to mitogens,[186] lymphocytoxicity,[187] immunodeficiency,[188] immune complexes,[189] reduced lymphoid colony growth,[190] and other aberrations of more complex immunoregulatory networks.[191] In small groups of patients, enhanced frequencies of HLA associations have been reported but not confirmed in studies of larger patient groups.[192-197]

Connective Tissue. Pathogenetic hypotheses of scleroderma remain incomplete without consideration of the direct role of the connective tissue. The extent and widespread distribution of fibrosis in scleroderma remain virtually unique. Excessive collagen deposition has been documented in the major target organs, and cells from those organs have been shown repeatedly to synthesize increased amounts of collagen when compared with cell strains developed from control tissue.[198-200] As more evidence accumulates, this enhanced connective tissue synthesizing capacity may not be unique to scleroderma but may be a more general manifestation of inflammatory reactions.[201-209] Two methods of selection of an activated population of connective tissue synthesizing cells (fibroblasts, pericytes, endothelial, smooth muscle, and myointimal cells) can be envisioned: either a direct activation of cells in the area of stimulus or, conversely, a chronic suppression of less active cells resulting in a "selective" accumulation of less suppressible, more actively synthesizing cells. It will be important to identify

one of these two mechanisms as operative in the connective tissue defect in scleroderma.[198-209]

The Microvascular-Interstitial Continuum. Endothelial injury patterns and serum cytotoxic factors are now well documented in scleroderma. But how does vascular injury initiate and perpetuate interstitial fibrosis? Recent evidence suggests that the same sera that are cytotoxic to endothelial cells are stimulatory to the proliferation, but not to collagen synthesis, of healthy skin fibroblasts.[210,211] Furthermore, this proliferative stimulation of fibroblasts has been shown in other studies to be capable of producing or selecting a population of high-collagen-producing fibroblasts which could perpetuate fibrosis. Thus the sequence could be endothelial injury → fibioblast proliferation (myointimal cell production) → high collagen synthesis → fibrosis.[212]

The candidates for the stimulus of fibroblast activation and increased collagen synthesis are several, including lymphokines,[213] direct mononuclear leukocyte-filroblast interaction,[214] and external agents,[215] as well as glycosaminoglycans[216] or products of collagen synthesis exerting direct negative feedback[217] on collagen synthesis. Whatever the stimulus, the scleroderma fibroblast continues to be the object of fruitful study in vitro.[218-220] The possibility that distinctive patterns of collagen synthesis and deposition, such as an increased relative or absolute proportion of type III collagen, could be a marker of fibroblast activation is intriguing.[221]

THERAPY

Since no cause is known for scleroderma, no cure is available. Furthermore, management must be closely tailored to the individual patient, the system involved (skin, vascular, gut, lungs, kidney, heart), and the stage of that involvement. These factors make therapeutic generalizations meaningless. But all is not totally pessimistic, since there are many important therapeutic and management maneuvers which can sustain the activity and quality of life of the scleroderma patient.[222-226]

Raynaud's Phenomenon and Peripheral Vascular Disease. Two time-honored therapies have been largely set aside: surgical sympathectomy and direct vascular dilators (Priscoline and related drugs). These have been replaced by a group of drugs, including guanethidine, prazocin, methyldopa, reserpine (oral and intra-arterial), phenoxybenzamine,[227] and perhaps griseofulvin, which block sympathetic vasoconstriction. Although none of these agents completely relieves the signs and symptoms of Raynaud's phenomenon, they help protect digits, face, and ears from cold (winter and the air conditioner) and stress, which, in the untreated patient, can lead to tissue necrosis in the form of ulcers, reduction of digital pulp, and digital gangrene.

Experience gained from the management of patients with hypertension and oliguric renal failure suggests that aggressive blockade of the renin-angiotensin system, using large doses of effective blockers (such as captopril, enalopril, or minoxidil), not only may be lifesaving in renal scleroderma but may also have a salutary effect on sclerodermatous involvement in other organs, such as the skin and peripheral vasculature.[118] The introduction of highly selective inhibitors of angiotensin production has significantly improved the life expectancy and the quality of life in patients with renal scleroderma.[228,229] The prostaglandins E_1 and I_2, when given intravenously, provide prolonged vasodilatation, and are being used increasingly as the substantial side effects become recognized and controlled.[230,231] The vasodilator nefedipine has been used for its peripheral and pulmonary effects.[232,233] Short-term vasodilatation with topical nitroglycerine has been studied.[234]

General measures are also helpful in the management of Raynaud's phenomenon. Sensible weight, balanced meals, clothing which provides central warmth to induce peripheral vasodilation, reduction of sources of external stress, adequate sleep, and prevention of overexertion all can reduce the danger and inconvenience of Raynaud's phenomenon to the individual patient.

Skin. The taut skin of scleroderma is the most distinctive and most troublesome feature of the disease to the patient early in the illness. No therapy has yet been found which, in controlled clinical trials, softens the hidebound skin of scleroderma. Many treatments have been used; none has passed the tests of time or use by multiple investigators. One reason for enthusiastic support of various agents is the natural tendency of the skin to soften after several years of scleroderma. When this occurs while the patient is receiving a drug, enthusiasm for that agent is understandable. Specifically, salicylates and nonsteroidal anti-inflammatory agents provide only analgesic relief; glucocorticoids and corticotropin (ACTH) do not seem to affect the skin; miscellaneous agents such as EDTA, relaxin, tocopherols (vitamin E), epsilonaminocaproic acid (EACA), triiodothyronine (T_3), potassium para-aminobenzoic acid (Potaba), dimethyl sulfoxide (DMSO), penicillamine, and colchicine have been and continue to be used, but objective evidence in controlled prospective studies for changes in cutaneous or visceral involvement remains incomplete.[235-237] Immunosuppression combined with plasmapheresis has been reputed to be beneficial in further uncontrolled therapeutic trials.[238]

General skin care and avoidance of excessive skin irritation are important principles to encourage. Soaps and creams which prevent dryness and clothing which reduces exposure are helpful to the scleroderma patient. Regular movement and exercise play a significant role in the maintenance of pliability and adequate nutritional circulation to the skin. Scleroderma patients have a general tendency to immobilize affected areas. When this is superimposed on the general involutional tendency of the patient with chronic disease, immobility can be substantial. This must be changed, and the patient must be encouraged to remain active, to move all joints, and to massage all skin areas several times daily.

Skin ulcers are usually secondary to vascular insufficiency rather than to inherent skin friability. They require urgent and careful management to remove non-

viable tissue, eradicate infection, promote circulation, and ensure healing. Several preparations, other than enzymes for debridement and antibiotics, have been applied locally to aid in healing. These include nitroglycerin paste and procaine jelly for vasodilation and dimethyl sulfoxide (DMSO) on an investigational basis. Cutaneous ulcers become more of a problem in second and third decade scleroderma; unfortunately the measures mentioned above have significantly less effect as the vascular disease becomes more severe and as the structural vascular lesions become fixed. In addition to local measures, sympatholytic drugs may enhance the healing of skin ulcers.[99] Intra-arterial reserpine and local nitroglycerin paste are useful in the acute setting.

Gastrointestinal. Esophageal hypomotility is characterized clinically by dysphagia, peptic esophagitis, and occasionally esophageal stricture. Prevention of these late complications is the best therapy. All patients should be studied by cineradiography and/or manometry, whether they are symptomatic or not. Patients with esophageal hypomotility should be managed prospectively to prevent esophageal ulceration and stricture. Patients should not lie down for 4 hours after a main meal. Antacids should be taken between meals. Blocks to elevate the head of the bed and the couch are helpful. Careful chewing and the use of carbonated water and other beverages which soften food and assist its passage into the stomach are recommended. Bethanechol is occasionally helpful in assisting swallowing if given before meals. Fortunately, stricture is rare and can be dilated mechanically when it occurs; occasionally stricture dilatation is difficult in the scleroderma patient.

Duodenal hypomotility is strongly associated with malabsorption. This can be debilitating to the scleroderma patient and should be suspected in any patient in whom weight loss is otherwise unexplained. After the degree of malabsorption is determined, bacterial overgrowth should be treated by courses of antibiotics to which gut flora are usually sensitive. Antibiotics should be given intermittently and should be alternated to prevent resistant gut flora. Diet can be altered to enhance digestibility and absorption, particularly of fats with use of such preparations as medium chain triglycerides. Episodes of adynamic ileus should be prevented by careful prospective management with intermittent antibiotics and managed by intubation and decompression, without surgical intervention, when they occur.

Constipation is rarely associated with colonic sacculations in scleroderma patients. Stool softeners, adequate liquid intake, and gentle laxatives are usually adequate for relief.

Lungs. Irreversible pulmonary fibrosis is unresponsive to therapy and represents the second most frequent cause of death (after renal failure) in scleroderma.[1] Prefibrotic pulmonary lesions are difficult to identify; even more elusive is whether or not these inflammatory and vascular lesions are responsive to therapy.

One approach has been to measure pulmonary function and ventilation-perfusion ("diffusion" capacity) in all patients and to proceed with scans and occasionally open lung biopsy in the young patient with early and substantial functional abnormalities. If these studies reveal evidence of inflammatory interstitial or vascular lung disease, the patient is treated with an 8- to 12-week regimen of 40 to 60 mg of prednisone in divided doses. Modest improvements of pulmonary function have been observed in about half the patients so treated; whether fibrosis is deterred or the natural course of the disease is changed in any way is not clear.[33]

Pulmonary hypertension should be investigated in all scleroderma patients by careful auscultation, electrocardiography, echocardiography, and roentgenography. When present as an isolated entity, pulmonary hypertension should be treated immediately with prednisone. When pulmonary hypertension is associated with longstanding interstitial lung disease, glucocorticoids are usually not effective.[33]

Established interstitial lung disease in scleroderma is usually fibrotic and does not respond to any known therapy. Management must be supportive. Bronchitis and cough should be treated promptly to reduce further airway destruction. Low concentrations of oxygen can improve function dramatically. Bronchodilators and positive pressure breathing are usually not as helpful as might be expected. Optimal cardiotonic status should be maintained at all times for its secondary beneficial effect on ventilation.

Musculoskeletal and Nervous Systems. Acute myositis in the scleroderma patient is treated as it is in any rheumatic syndrome—i.e., with glucocorticoids.[1] It is usually responsive. The chronic indolent myopathy of scleroderma does not respond to any known therapy and is probably best left untreated. Symptomatic treatment seems most appropriate for the management of the entrapment neuropathies (trigeminal neuralgia) which occur in second and third decade scleroderma patients. No therapy is known to be effective for the isolated osteolysis seen in scleroderma. Nonsteroidal anti-inflammatory agents are helpful in the symptomatic control of articular symptoms. Acute synovitis is rare, except in the patient who presents with a rheumatoid pattern of symmetrical polyarthritis.

Kidneys. Early detection of impending oliguric renal failure in scleroderma is a most important aspect of therapy. Patients with renal scleroderma are usually hypertensive and are uniformly hyperreninemic, even though some are occasionally normotensive.[12] Early, aggressive blockade of renin and angiotensin is critical to the protection of the renal function remaining; once renal failure (anuria) occurs, blocking renin may be the most effective means of encouraging slow reversal of the renal vascular lesion (in conjunction with adequate dialysis, of course).[239]

Because of the rapid appearance of renal scleroderma, an important phase of its management is the identification of those scleroderma patients who are at high risk of developing renal failure. The presence of proteinuria, hypertension, azotemia, microangiopathic hemolytic anemia, a pericardial effusion, or, more specif-

ically, the abrupt appearance of any of these features places the individual patient at six times the risk of death from renal failure as compared with the patient who has none of these renal markers.[12] Once a marker is present, the patient should be carefully evaluated regarding resting and stimulated renin levels; any elevations should be blocked immediately (it is likely in the future that all patients with scleroderma will be evaluated for renin status). Patients with renal markers should be protected from sudden changes in blood volume, such as hemorrhage, surgery, intensive diuretic therapy, or dehydration. They should be warned of the signs of renal failure (headache, visual difficulties from papilledema, oliguria, dependent edema, fatigue) and instructed to seek immediate medical attention where facilities and experience are adequate to support renal failure.

Once renal failure has ensued, dialysis can be lifesaving. The problems of vascular access and efficiency of clearance can be major in scleroderma patients unless full therapeutic measures are taken to block the renin-angiotensin axis as completely as possible. More experience is needed with the renin inhibitors propanolol, clonidine, minoxidil, and others; nephrectomy provides instant elimination of renin, but it is, of course, irreversible and should be used only as a last resort. Maintenance of appropriate blood volume can be difficult, but it is essential to the management of the patient in renal failure. Renal transplantation has had limited success as an alternative to chronic hemodialysis in this setting,[114] but has largely been replaced by early, aggressive therapy with specific inhibitors of angiotensin generation.[228,229] Captopril and enalopril are the newest additions to this powerful armamentarium.

Heart. The management of coronary heart disease and congestive heart failure will not be discussed here, since their optimal management in the scleroderma patient is the same as in any other patient. However, the poor response of scleroderma patients to coronary bypass procedures, because of these patients' extensive small vessel disease, should be re-emphasized.

Pericardial effusion is frequent enough in scleroderma to warrant special mention. If the effusion is of moderate size on echocardiography, digitalis and cautious diuretics should be used under close scrutiny to reduce or eliminate the effusion. Diuretics should not be administered aggressively because of the high proportion of scleroderma patients with pericardial effusion who later develop renal failure. A persistent pericardial effusion should be managed by open pericardial window if other system involvement does not preclude this procedure and if the effusion is hemodynamically significant. Any approach which changes plasma volume is a risk to the scleroderma patient with pericardial effusion and should be made slowly and carefully.

Most myocardial lesions in scleroderma are characterized by necrosis and/or fibrosis.[46,47] It remains to be shown that these lesions are responsive to any therapy. Very rarely at autopsy, diffuse myocarditis is found in the scleroderma patient with severe myocardial disease.

If such patients can be identified early, an empirical course of glucocorticoids is a reasonable approach to management.

SUMMARY

Scleroderma is both a fascinating and a frustrating disorder. Skin involvement is its hallmark; the extent of visceral involvement determines its outcome. In each target organ, lesions can be characterized as early (cellular) or classic (fibrotic). Thus, scleroderma is both multisystem and multistage; both prognosis and response to management must be viewed in light of the system and stage of involvement of the individual patient.

The best present hypothesis of the cause of scleroderma is that injury to the endothelium of small arteries and capillaries initiates reactions which involve increased permeability of the vessels, platelet adherence, myointimal cell proliferation, intravascular coagulation, microangiopathic hemolytic anemia, luminal narrowing, and heightened sensitivity of the vessel wall. Within this altered vessel, altered structure and reactive fibrosis begin to occur. The factors which govern fibrosis in scleroderma are poorly understood. Perhaps growth factors involved in cell proliferation, altered vessel permeability, and heightened vasomotor response all play a role in the atrophy and fibrosis which ultimately develop and against which there is presently no therapeutic recourse. Detection of the many features of scleroderma at the earliest possible stage seems to offer the best hope for meaningful therapeutic intervention. Further study of the biology and pathology of the endothelial and myointimal cell, and of their interactions with blood and blood vessel, seems to offer the most direct approach to better understanding of the mechanisms of scleroderma. The potential for immune events initiating and perpetuating damage to the endothelium is strong; selective toxicity to the body's vascular lining cells seems to play a role in this poorly understood disorder.

An emphasis on immune and early vascular events in scleroderma offers many new avenues of potential therapeutic intervention. From the prevention of Raynaud's phenomenon to the blockade of the vasculotoxic effects of renin in late scleroderma, many new ideas have emerged which, for lack of an experimental model, can be tested only in the individual patient destined to develop scleroderma.

Acknowledgments

The author thanks Dr. J. K. Upshur for the histopathological illustrations and Ms. Celeste Cox for expert editorial assistance. Support for this work was provided by the National Institutes of Health, the RGK Foundation, the Charlotte and Sidney Lifschultz Foundation, and the State of South Carolina.

References

1. Rodnan, G.P.: Progressive systemic sclerosis (scleroderma). *In* Hollander, J.L., and McCarty, D.J., Jr. (eds.): Arthritis and Allied Conditions. 8th ed. Philadelphia, Lea & Febiger, 1972.
2. LeRoy, E.C.: Scleroderma (systemic sclerosis). *In* Katz, W.A. (ed.): Rheumatic Diseases, Diagnosis and Management. Philadelphia, J.B. Lippincott Company, 1977, p. 777.
3. Tuffanelli, D.L., and Winkelmann, R.K.: Systemic scleroderma: A clinical study of 727 cases. Arch. Dermatol. 84:359, 1961.
4. Siegel, R.C.: Scleroderma. Med. Clin. North Am. 61:283, 1977.
5. Campbell, P.M., and LeRoy, E.C.: Pathogenesis of systemic sclerosis: A vascular hypothesis. Sem. Arthritis Rheum. 4:351, 1975.
6. Winkelmann, R.K.: Pathogenesis and staging of scleroderma. Acta Derm. Venerol. (Stockholm) 56:83, 1976.
7. Mintz, G.: Calcinosis, Raynaud's disease, sclerodactylia and telangiectasias in progressive systemic sclerosis. Statistic analysis of contingencies. Gac. Med. Mex. 107:525, 1976.
8. Giordano, M., Ara, M., Capelli, L., Tirci, G., and Vatti, M.: Über die Vielseitigkeit und die Einstufung der klinischen Bilder der progredienten generalisierten Sklerodermie. Z. Rheumatol. 35:286, 1976.
9. Rowell, N.R.: The prognosis of systemic sclerosis. Br. J. Dermatol. 95:57, 1976.
10. D'Angelo, W.A., Fries, J.F., Masi, A.T., and Shulman, L.E.: Pathologic observations in systemic sclerosis (scleroderma). Am. J. Med. 46:428, 1969.
11. Goetz, R.H.: The pathology of progressive systemic sclerosis (generalized scleroderma) with special reference to changes in the viscera. Clin. Proc. 4:337, 1945.
12. Cannon, P.J., Hassar, M., Case, D.B., Casarella, W.J., Sommers, S.C., and LeRoy, E.C.: The relationship of hypertension and renal failure in scleroderma (progressive systemic sclerosis) to structural and functional abnormalities of the renal cortical circulation. Medicine 53:1, 1974.
13. Masi, A.T., Rodnan, G.P., Medsger, T.A., Jr., Altman, R.D., D'Angelo, W.A., Fries, J.F., LeRoy, E.C., Kirsner, A.B., MacKensie, A.H., McShane, D.J., Myers, A.R., and Sharp, G.C.: Preliminary criteria for the classification of systemic sclerosis (scleroderma). Arthritis Rheum. 23:581, 1980.
14. Merlen, J.F.: Phénomène de Raynaud et sclerodermie. Ann. de Cardiol. Angeiol. 29:333, 1980.
15. Benedek T.G., and Rodnan, G.P.: The early history and nomenclature of scleroderma and of its differentiation from sclerema neonatorum and scleroedema. Semin. Arthritis Rheum. 12:52, 1982.
16. Tan, P.L.J., Wigley, R.D., and Borman, G.B.: Clinical criteria for systemic sclerosis (letter). Arthritis Rheum. 24:1589, 1981.
17. LeRoy, E.C., Maricq, H.R., and Kahaleh, M.B.: Undifferentiated connective tissue syndromes (UCTS). Arthritis Rheum. 23:341, 1980.
18. LeRoy, E.C.: Pathogenesis of scleroderma (systemic sclerosis). J. Invest. Dermatol. 79(Suppl):87s, 1982.
19. Fleischmajer, R., Perlish, J.S., and West, W.P.: Ultrastructure of cutaneous cellular infiltrates in scleroderma. Arch. Dermatol. 113:1661, 1977.
20. Fleischmajer, R., Perlish, J.S., and Reeves, J.R.T.: Cellular infiltrates in scleroderma skin. Arthritis Rheum. 20:975, 1977.
21. Fleischmajer, R., Perlish, J.S., Shaw, K.V., and Pirozzi, D.J.: Skin capillary changes in early systemic scleroderma. Electron microscopy and "in vitro" autoradiography with tritiated thymidine. Arch. Dermatol. 112:1553, 1976.
22. Fleischmajer, R.: The pathophysiology of scleroderma. Int. J. Dermatol. 16:310, 1977.
23. Orringer, M.B., Dabich, L., Zarafonetis, C.J.D., and Sloan, H.: Gastroesophageal reflux in esophageal scleroderma: Diagnosis and implications. Ann. Thorac. Surg. 22:120, 1976.
24. Hurwitz, A.L., Duranceau, A., and Postlethwait, R.W.: Esophageal dysfunction and Raynaud's phenomenon in patients with scleroderma. Am. J. Dig. Dis. 21:601, 1976.
25. Morson, B.C., and Dawson, I.M.P.: Gastrointestinal Pathology. Oxford, Blackwell Scientific Publications, 1972, p. 584.
26. Leisner, B., Luderschmidt, C., Krieg, T., Wirsching, R., Hundecker, K., and Fink, U.: Esophagus function scintigraphy (EFS) in scleroderma. Arch. Dermatol. Res. 270:225, 1981.
27. Rajapakse, C.N.A., Bancewicz, J., Jones, C.J.P., and Jayson, M.I.V.: Pharyngo-oesphageal dysphagia in systemic sclerosis. Ann. Rheum. Dis. 40:612, 1981.
28. Clements, P.J., Kadell, B., Ippoliti, A., and Ross, M.: Esophageal motility in progressive systemic sclerosis (PSS). Comparison of cine-radiographic and manometric evaluation. Dig. Dis. Sci. 24:639, 1979.
29. Tolin, R.D., Malmud, L.S., Reilley, J., and Fisher, R.S.: Esophageal scintigraphy to quantitate esophageal transit (quantitation of esophageal transit). Gastroenterology 76:1402, 1979.

30. Cohen, S., Laufer, I., Snape, W.J. Jr., Shiau, Y.F., Levine, G.M., and Jimenez, S.: The gastrointestinal manifestations of scleroderma: Pathogenesis and management (clinical conference). Gastroenterology 79:155, 1980.

31. Russell, C.O.H., Hill, L.D., Holmes, E.R., III, Hull, D.A., Gannon, R., and Pope, C.E., II: Radionuclide transit: A sensitive screening test for esophageal dysfunction. Gastroenterology 80:887, 1981.

32. Weihrauch, T.R., and Korting, G.W.: Manometric assessment of oesophageal involvement in progressive systemic sclerosis, morphoea and Raynaud's disease. Br. J. Dermatol. 107:325, 1982.

33. Enson, Y., Thomas, H.M., III, Bosken, C.H., Wood, J.A., LeRoy, E.C., Blanc, W.A., Wigger, H.J., and Harvey, R.M.: Pulmonary hypertension in interstitial lung disease: Relation of vascular resistance to abnormal lung structure. Trans. Assoc. Am. Physicians 88:248, 1975.

34. Young, R.H., and Mark, G.J.: Pulmonary vascular changes in scleroderma. Am. J. Med. 64:998, 1978.

35. Guttadauria, M., Ellman, H., Emmanuel, G., Kaplan, D., and Diamond, H.: Pulmonary function in scleroderma. Arthritis Rheum. 20:1071, 1977.

36. Emmanuel, G., Saroja, D., Gopinathan, K., Gharpure, A., and Stuckey, J.: Environmental factors and the diffusing capacity of the lung in progressive systemic sclerosis. Chest 69:304, 1976.

37. Bjerke, R.D., Tashkin, D.P., Clements, P.J., Chopra, S.K., Gong, H., and Bein, M.: Small airways in progressive systemic sclerosis (PSS). Am. J. Med. 66:201, 1979.

38. Bagg, L.R., and Hughes, D.T.D.: Serial pulmonary function tests in progressive systemic sclerosis. Thorax 34:224, 1979.

39. König, G., Luderschmidt, C., Clocuh, Y.P., Scherer, U., and Fruhmann, G.: Klinische bedeutung der bronchoalveolären Lavage bei progressiver systemischer Sklerodermie. Deutsch. Med. Wochen. 107:723, 1982.

40. Schneider, P.D., Wise, R.A., Hochberg, M.C., and Wigley, F.M.: Serial pulmonary function in systemic sclerosis. Am. J. Med. 73:385, 1982.

41. Pisko, E., Gallup, K., Turner, R., Parker, M., Nomeir, A.-M., Box, J., Davis, J., Box, P., and Rothberger, H.: Cardiopulmonary manifestations of progressive systemic sclerosis: Associations with circulating immune complexes and fluorescent antinuclear antibodies. Arthritis Rheum. 22:518, 1979.

42. McWhorter, J.E., IV, and LeRoy, E.C.: Pericardial disease in scleroderma (systemic sclerosis). Am. J. Med. 57:566, 1974.

43. Gupta, M.P., Zoneraich, S., Zeitlin, W., Zoneraich, O., and D'Angelo, W.: Scleroderma heart disease with slow flow velocity in coronary arteries. Chest 67:116, 1975.

44. Smith, J.W., Clements, P.J., Levisman, J., Furst, D., and Ross, M.: Echocardiographic features of progressive systemic sclerosis: Correlation with hemodynamic and post mortem studies. Am. J. Med. 66:28, 1979.

45. Eggebrecht, R.F., and Kleiger, R.E.: Echocardiographic patterns in scleroderma. Chest 71:47, 1977.

46. Ridolfi, R.L., Bulkley, B.H., and Hutchins, G.M.: The cardiac conduction system in progressive systemic sclerosis. Am. J. Med. 61:361, 1976.

47. Bulkley, B.H., Ridolfi, R.L., Salyer, W.R., and Hutchins, G.M.: Myocardial lesions of progressive systemic sclerosis. A cause of cardiac dysfunction. Circulation 53:483, 1976.

48. Smith, J.W., Clements, P.J., Levisman, J., Furst, D., and Ross, M.: Echocardiographic features of progressive systemic sclerosis (PSS): Correlation with hemodynamic and postmortem studies. Am. J. Med. 66:28, 1979.

49. Roberts, N.K., Cabeen, W.R., Jr., Moss, J., Clements, P.J., and Furst, D.E.: The prevalence of conduction defects and cardiac arrhythmias in progressive systemic sclerosis. Ann. Intern. Med. 94:38, 1981.

50. Juillet, Y., Bogaert, O., Crickx, B., Fiessinger, J.N., and Housset, E.: La cardiopathie sclerodermique. Arch. Mal. Coeur 73:1019, 1980.

51. Botstein, G.R., and LeRoy, E.C.: Primary heart disease in systemic sclerosis (scleroderma): Advances in clinical and pathologic features, pathogenesis, and new therapeutic approaches. Am. Heart J. 102:913, 1981.

52. Schwarz, W., Schell, H., and Hornstein, O.P.: Serum levels of thyrotropin in progressive scleroderma. Arch. Dermatol. Res. 271:451, 1981.

53. Gordon, M.B., Klein, I., Dekker, A., Rodnan, G.P., and Medsger, T.A., Jr.: Thyroid disease in progressive systemic sclerosis: Increased frequency of glandular fibrosis and hypothyroidism. Ann. Intern. Med. 95:431, 1981.

54. Doyle, J.A., Connolly, S.M., and Winkelmann, R.K.: Cutaneous and subcutaneous inflammatory sclerosis syndromes. Arch. Dermatol. 118:886, 1982.

55. Cobden, I., Rothwell, J., Axon, A.T.R., Dixon, M.F., Lintott, D.J., and Rowell, N.R.: Small intestinal structure and passive permeability in systemic sclerosis. Gut 21:293, 1980.

56. Black, C.M.: Scleroderma. Br. J. Hosp. Med. 22:28, 1979.

57. Farrell, D.A., and Medsger, T.A., Jr.: Trigeminal neuropathy in progressive systemic sclerosis. Am. J. Med. 73:57, 1982.

58. Rothfield, N.F., and Rodnan, G.P.: Serum antinuclear antibodies in progressive systemic sclerosis (scleroderma). Arthritis Rheum. 11:607, 1968.

59. Greenwald, C.A., Peebles, C.L., and Nakamura, R.M.: Laboratory tests for antinuclear antibody (ANA) in rheumatic diseases. Lab. Med. 9(4):19, 1978.

60. Tan, E.M., Rodnan, G.P., Garcia, I., Moroi, Y., Fritzler, M.J., and Peebles, C.: Diversity of antinuclear antibodies in progressive systemic sclerosis: Anti-centromere antibody and its relationship to CREST syndrome. Arthritis Rheum. 23:617, 1980.

61. Kitridou, R.C., Fleischmajer, R., and Lagosky, P.A.: Antismooth muscle antibody in scleroderma (abstract). Arthritis Rheum. 18:526, 1975.

62. Blaszczyk, M., Beutner, E.H., Rogozinski, T., Rzesa, G., Jarzabek-Chorzelska, M., Jablonska, S., and Chorzelski, T.P.: Substrate specificity of antinuclear antibodies in scleroderma. J. Invest. Dermatol. 68:191, 1977.

63. Moroi, Y., Peebles, C., Fritzler, M.J., Steigerwald, J., and Tan, E.M.: Autoantibody to centromere (kinetochore) in scleroderma sera. Proc. Natl. Acad. Sci. USA 77:1627, 1980.

64. Mimori, T., Akizuki, M., Yamagata, H., Inada, S., Yoshida, S., and Homma, M.: Characterization of a high molecular weight acidic nuclear protein recognized by autoantibodies in sera from patients with polymyositis-scleroderma overlap. J. Clin. Invest. 68:611, 1981.

65. Bernstein, R.M., Steigerwald, J.C., and Tan, E.M.: Association of antinuclear and antinucleolar antibodies in progressive systemic sclerosis. Clin. Exp. Immunol. 48:43, 1982.

66. Brentnall, T.J., Kenneally, D., Barnett, A.J., de Aizpurua, H.J., Lolait, S.J., Ashcroft, R., and Toh, B.H.: Autoantibodies to fibroblasts in scleroderma. J. Clin. Lab. Immunol. 8:9, 1982.

67. Kleinsmith, D.M., Heinzerling, R.H., and Burnham, T.K.: Antinuclear antibodies as immunologic markers for a benign subset and different clinical characteristics of scleroderma. Arch. Dermatol. 118:882, 1982.

68. Maricq, H.R., Spencer-Green, G., and LeRoy, E.C.: Abnormal capillary patterns and systemic disease in scleroderma (progressive systemic sclerosis). Bibl. Anat. 13:248, 1975.

69. Maricq, H.R., Gordon, G., and LeRoy, E.C.: Studies in patients with connective tissue disorders. Bibl. Anat. 16:135, 1977.

70. Maricq, H.R., Spencer-Green, G., and LeRoy, E.C.: Skin capillary abnormalities as indicators of organ involvement in scleroderma (systemic sclerosis), Raynaud's syndrome and dermatomyositis. Am. J. Med. 61:862, 1976.

71. Maricq, H.R., Blume, R.S., and LeRoy, E.C.: Wide-field study of nailfold capillary bed in disorders of connective tissue. In Ditzel, J., and Lewis, D.H. (eds): Sixth European Conference on Microcirculation, Aalborg. Basel, Karger, 1971, p. 116.

72. Maricq, H.R., and LeRoy, E.C.: Patterns of finger capillary abnormalities in connective tissue disease by "wide-field" microscopy. Arthritis Rheum. 16:619, 1973.

73. Brown, G.E., and O'Leary, P.A.: Skin capillaries in scleroderma. Arch. Intern. Med. 36:73, 1926.

74. Buchanan, I.S., and Humpston, D.J.: Nail-fold capillaries in connective-tissue disorders. Lancet 1:845, 1968.

75. Maricq, H.R., Downey, J.A., and LeRoy, E.C.: Standstill of nailfold capillary blood flow during cooling in scleroderma and Raynaud's syndrome. Blood Vessels 13:338, 1976.

76. Maricq, H.R., LeRoy, E.C., D'Angelo, W.A., Medsger, T.A., Jr., Rodnan, G.P., Sharp, G.C., and Wolfe, J.F.: Diagnostic potential of in vivo capillary microscopy in scleroderma and related disorders. Arthritis Rheum. 23:183, 1980.

77. Harper, F.E., Maricq, H.R., Turner, R.E., Lidman, R.W., and LeRoy, E.C.: A prospective study of Raynaud phenomenon and early connective tissue disease: A five-year report. Am. J. Med. 72:883, 1982.

78. Kristensen, J.K.: Blood flow and blood pressure in fingers in generalized scleroderma. Int. J. Dermatol. 21:404, 1982.

79. Kristensen, J.K.: Reactive hyperemia in cutaneous tissue in generalized scleroderma. J. Invest. Dermatol. 71:269, 1978.

80. Henriksen, O., and Kristensen, J.K.: Reduced systolic blood pressure in fingers of patients with generalized scleroderma (acrosclerosis). Acta Derm. Venerol. 61:531, 1981.

81. Norton, W.L., and Nardo, J.M.: Vascular disease in progressive systemic sclerosis (scleroderma). Ann. Intern. Med. 73:317, 1970.

82. Kahaleh, M.B., Sherer, G.K., and LeRoy, E.C.: Endothelial injury in scleroderma. J. Exp. Med. 149:1326, 1979.

83. Fleischmajer, R., and Perlish, J.S.: (H-3) Thymidine labeling of dermal endothelial cells in scleroderma. J. Invest. Dermatol. 69:379, 1977.

84. Mason, R.G., Sharp, D., Chuang, H.Y.K., and Mohammad, S.F.: The endothelium. Roles in thrombosis and hemostasis. Arch. Pathol. Lab. Med. 101:61, 1977.

85. Kahaleh, M.B. Osborn, I., and LeRoy, E.C.: Increased factor VIII/vonWillebrand factor antigen and von Willebrand factor activity in scleroderma and in Raynaud's phenomenon. Ann. Intern. Med. 94:482, 1981.

86. Kazandjian, S., Fiessinger, J-N., Camilleri, J.-P., Dadoune, J.-P., and Housset, E.: Endothelial cell renewal in skin of patients with progressive systemic sclerosis (PSS): An in vitro autoradiographic study. Acta Derm. Venerol. 62:425, 1982.

87. Siebold, J.R., Iammarino, R.M., and Rodnan, G.P.: Alpha-l-antitrypsin in progressive systemic sclerosis. Arthritis Rheum. 23:367, 1980.

88. Kahaleh, M.B., and LeRoy, E.C.: Endothelial injury in scleroderma: A protease mechanism. J. Lab. Clin. Med. 1983. 101:553, 1983.

89. Kahaleh, M.B., Osborn, I., and LeRoy, E.C.: Elevated levels of circulating platelet aggregates and beta-thromboglobulin in scleroderma. Ann. Intern. Med. 96:610, 1982.

90. Vracko, R., and Benditt, E.P.: Manifestations of diabetes mellitus—their possible relationships to an underlying cell defect. Am. J. Pathol. 75:204, 1974.

91. Harker, L.A., Ross, R., and Glomset, J.A.: The role of endothelial cell injury and platelet response in atherogenesis. Thromb. Haemostas. 39:312, 1978.

92. Jaffe, E.A.: Endothelial cells and the biology of factor VIII. N. Engl. J. Med. 296:377, 1977.

93. Porter, J.M., Snider, R.L., Bardana, E.J., Rösch, J., and Eidemiller, L.R.: The diagnosis and treatment of Raynaud's phenomenon. Surgery 77:11, 1975.

94. Birnstingl, M.: The Raynaud syndrome. Postgrad. Med. J. 47:297, 1971.

95. Maricq, H.R., Johnson, M.N., Whetstone, C.L., and LeRoy, E.C.: Capillary abnormalities in polyvinyl chloride production workers. Examination by in vivo microscopy. JAMA 236:1368, 1976.

96. Ward, A.M., Udnoon, S., Watkins, J., Walker, A.E., and Darke, C.S.: Immunological mechanisms in the pathogenesis of vinyl chloride disease. Br. Med. J. 1:936, 1976.

97. Lewis, T.: Experiments relating to the peripheral mechanism involved in spasmodic arrest of the circulation in the fingers, a variety of Raynaud's disease. Heart 15:7, 1929–1931.

98. Tietjen, G.W., Chien, S., LeRoy, E.C., Gavras, I., Gavras, H., and Gump, F.E.: Blood viscosity, plasma proteins, and Raynaud syndrome. Arch. Surg. 110:1343, 1975.

99. Arnot, R.S., Boroda, C., and Peacock, J.H.: Pathophysiology of capillary circulation: Raynaud's disease. Angiology 29:48, 1978.

100. Bollinger, A., Mahler, F., and Meier, B.: Velocity patterns in nailfold capillaries of normal subjects and patients with Raynaud's disease and acrocyanosis. Bibl. Anat. 16:142, 1977.

101. Henriksen, O., Kristensen, J.K., and Wadskov, S.: Local regulation of blood flow in subcutaneous tissue in generalized scleroderma. J. Invest. Dermatol. 68:318, 1977.

102. LeRoy, E.C., Downey, J.A., and Cannon, P.J.: Skin capillary blood flow in scleroderma. J. Clin. Invest. 50:930, 1971.

103. Downey, J.A., LeRoy, E.C., Miller, J.M., III, and Darling, R.C.: Thermoregulation and Raynaud's phenomenon. Clin. Sci. 40:211, 1971.

104. Coffman, J.D., and Cohen, A.S.: Total and capillary fingertip blood flow in Raynaud's phenomenon. N. Engl. J. Med. 285:259, 1971.

105. Jahnsen, T., Nielsen, S.L., and Skovborg, F.: Blood viscosity and local response to cold in primary Raynaud's phenomenon. Lancet 2:1001, 1977.

106. Velayos, E.E., Masi, A.T., Stevens, M.B., and Shulman, L.E.: The 'CREST' syndrome. Comparison with systemic sclerosis (scleroderma). Arch. Intern. Med. 139:1240, 1979.

107. Rodnan, G.P., Lipinski, E., and Luksick, J.: Skin thickness and collagen content in progressive systemic sclerosis and localized scleroderma. Arthritis Rheum. 22:130, 1979.

108. Silver, R.M., Metcalf, J.F., Stanley, J.H., and LeRoy, E.C.: Interstitial lung disease in scleroderma. Analysis by bronchoalveolar lavage. Arthritis Rheum. In press.

109. Fisher, E.R., and Rodnan, G.P.: Pathologic observations concerning the cutaneous lesion of progressive systemic sclerosis: An electron microscopic histochemical and immunohistochemical study. Arthritis Rheum. 3:536, 1960.

110. Steckel, R.J., Bein, M.E., and Kelly, P.M.: Pulmonary arterial hypertension in progressive systemic sclerosis. Am. J. Roentgenol. Radium Ther. Nucl. Med. 124:461, 1975.

111. Clements, P.J., Furst, D.E., Campion, D.S., Bohan, A., Harris, R., Levy, J., and Paulus, H.E.: Muscle disease in progressive systemic sclerosis. Diagnostic and therapeutic considerations. Arthritis Rheum. 21:62, 1978.

112. Seifert, M.H., Steigerwald, J.C., and Cliff, M.M.: Bone resorption of the mandible in progressive systemic sclerosis. Arthritis Rheum. 18:507, 1975.

113. Resnick, D., Scavulli, J.F., Goergen, T.G., Genant, H.K., and Niwayama, G.: Intra-articular calcification in scleroderma. Radiology 124:685, 1977.

114. LeRoy, E.C., and Fleischmann, R.M.: The management of renal scleroderma. Experience with dialysis, nephrectomy and transplantation. Am. J. Med. 64:974, 1978.

115. Kovalchik, M.T., Guggenheim, S.J., Silverman, M.H., Robertson, J.S.,

and Steigerwald, J.C.: The kidney in progressive systemic sclerosis. A prospective study. Ann. Intern. Med. 89:881, 1978.

116. Oliver, J.A., Vinci, J.M., Bowden, R.E., Weinberger, A.B., Baer, L., Keiser, H.R., and Cannon, P.J.: Renal vasoactive hormones in scleroderma (progressive systemic sclerosis). Nephron 29:110, 1981.

117. Mitnick, P.D., and Feig, P.U.: Control of hypertension and reversal of renal failure in scleroderma. N. Engl. J. Med. 299:871, 1978.

118. Wasner, C., Cooke, C.R., and Fries, J.F.: Successful medical treatment of scleroderma renal crisis. N. Engl. J. Med. 299:873, 1978.

119. Lam, M., Ricanati, E.S., Khan, M.A., and Kushner, I.: Reversal of severe renal failure in systemic sclerosis. Ann. Intern. Med. 89:642, 1978.

120. Gavras, H., Gavras, I., Cannon, P.J., Brunner, H.R., and Laragh, J.H.: Is elevated plasma renin activity of prognostic importance in progressive systemic sclerosis? Arch. Intern. Med. 137:1554, 1977.

121. Merino, G.E., Sutherland, D.E.R., Kjellstrand, C.M., Simmons, R.L., and Najarian, J.S.: Renal transplantation for progressive systemic sclerosis with renal failure: Case report and review of previous experience. Am. J. Surg. 133:745, 1977.

122. Warren, B.H., and Rösch, J.: Angiography in the diagnosis of renal scleroderma. Radiol. Clin. (Basel) 46:194, 1977.

123. Woodhall, P.B., McCoy, R.C., Gunnells, J.C., and Seigler, H.F.: Apparent recurrence of progressive systemic sclerosis in a renal allograft. JAMA 236:1032, 1976.

124. Keane, W.F., Danielson, B., and Raij, L.: Successful renal transplantation in progressive sclerosis. Ann. Intern. Med. 85:199, 1976.

125. Winograd, J., Schimmel, D.H., and Palubinskas, A.J.: The spotted nephrogram of renal scleroderma. Am. J. Roentgenol. 126:734, 1976.

126. Barker, D.J., and Farr, M.J.: Resolution of cutaneous manifestations of systemic sclerosis after haemodialysis. Br. Med. J. 1:501, 1976.

127. Oliver, J.A., and Cannon, P.J.: The kidney in scleroderma. Nephron 18:141, 1977.

128. Gerber, M.A.: Immunohistochemical findings in the renal vascular lesions of progressive systemic sclerosis. Hum. Pathol. 6:343, 1975.

129. Richardson, J.A.: Hemodialysis and kidney transplantation for renal failure from scleroderma. Arthritis Rheum. 16:265, 1973.

130. McCoy, R.C., Tisher, C.C., Pepe, P.F., and Cleveland, L.A.: The kidney in progressive systemic sclerosis. Immunohistochemical and antibody elution studies. Lab. Invest. 35:124, 1976.

130a. James, T.N.: De subitaneis mortibus. VIII. Coronary arteries and conduction system in scleroderma heart disease. Circulation 50:844, 1974.

131. Lally, E.V., and Jiminez, S.A.: Impotence in progressive systemic sclerosis. Ann. Intern Med. 95:150, 1981.

132. Klein, L.E., and Posner, M.S.: Progressive systemic sclerosis and impotence (letter). Ann. Intern. Med. 95:658, 1981.

133. Davidson, R.A.: Impotence in progressive systemic sclerosis (letter). Ann. Intern. Med. 96:125, 1982.

134. Pan, S.F., Rodnan, G.P., Deutsch, M., and Wald, N.: Chromosomal abnormalities in progressive systemic sclerosis (scleroderma) with consideration of radiation effects. J. Lab. Clin. Med. 86:300, 1975.

135. Emerit, I., Housset, E., and Feingold, J.: Chromosomal breakage and scleroderma: Studies in family members. J. Lab. Clin. Med. 88:81, 1976.

136. Sherer, G.K., Jackson, B.B., and LeRoy, E.C.: Chromosome breakage and sister chromatid exchange frequencies in scleroderma. Arthritis Rheum. 24:1409, 1981.

137. Huet-Warembourg, E., Legoff, D., Jalbert, H., Sele, B., Amblard, P., Reymond, J.L., Jalbert, P., and Pison, H.: De la sclérodermie généralisée aspects cytogénétiques: Anomalies structurales et échanges de chromatides-soeurs. Ann. Genet. 25:32, 1982.

138. Greger, R.E.: Familial progressive systemic scleroderma. Arch. Dermatol. 111:81, 1975.

139. Rendall, J.R., and McKenzie, A.W.: Familial scleroderma. Br. J. Dermatol. 91:517, 1974.

140. Gray, R.G., and Altman, R.D.: Progressive systemic sclerosis in a family. Case report of a mother and son and review of the literature. Arthritis Rheum. 20:35, 1977.

141. Sasaki, S., and Yoshino, H.: Systemic scleroderma in mother and daughter (letter). Arch. Dermatol. 113:378, 1977.

142. Goel, K.M., and Shanks, R.A.: Scleroderma in childhood. Report of 5 cases. Arch. Dis. Child. 49:861, 1974.

143. Sheldon, W.B., Lurie, D.P., Maricq, H.R., Kahaleh, M.B., DeLustro, F.A., Gibofsky, A., and LeRoy, E.C.: Three siblings with scleroderma and two with Raynaud's phenomenon from a single kindred. Arthritis Rheum. 24:668, 1981.

144. Kurland, L.T., Hauser, W.A., Ferguson, R.H., and Holley, K.E.: Epidemiologic features of diffuse connective tissue disorders in Rochester, Minnesota, 1951 through 1967, with special reference to systemic lupus erythematosus. Mayo Clin. Proc. 44:649, 1969.

145. Medsger, T.A., Jr., and Masi, A.T.: Survival with scleroderma. II. A life-table analysis of clinical and demographic factors in 358 male U.S. veteran patients. J. Chron. Dis. 26:647, 1973.

146. Medsger, T.A., Jr., Masi, A.T., Rodnan, G.P., Benedek, T.G., and Ro-

binson, H.: Survival with systemic sclerosis (scleroderma). A life-table analysis of clinical and demographic factors in 309 patients. Ann. Intern. Med. 75:369, 1971.

147. Medsger, T.A., Jr., and Masi, A.T.: The epidemiology of systemic sclerosis (scleroderma) among male U.S. veterans. J. Chron. Dis. 31:73, 1978.

148. O'Leary, P.A., and Nomland, R.: A clinical study of one hundred and three cases of scleroderma. Am. J. Med. Sci. 180:95, 1930.

149. Winterbauer, R.H.: Multiple telangiectasia, Raynaud's phenomenon, sclerodactyly and subcutaneous calcinosis: A syndrome mimicking hereditary hemorrhagic telangiectasia. Bull. Johns Hopkins Hosp. 114:361, 1964.

150. Salerni, R., Rodnan, G.P., Leon, D.F., and Shaver, J.A.: Pulmonary hypertension in the CREST syndrome variant of progressive systemic sclerosis (scleroderma). Ann. Intern. Med. 86:394, 1977.

151. Miller, F., Lane, B., Soterakis, J., and D'Angelo, W.A.: Primary biliary cirrhosis and scleroderma: The possibility of a common pathogenetic mechanism. Arch. Pathol. Lab. Med. 103:505, 1979.

152. Furst, D.E., Clements, P.J., Graze, P., Gale, R., and Roberts, N.: A syndrome resembling progressive systemic sclerosis after bone marrow transplantation. A model for scleroderma? Arthritis Rheum. 22:904, 1979.

153. Janin Mercier, A., Saurat, J.H., Bourges, M., Sohier, J., Didier Jean, L., and Gluckman E.: The lichen planus–like and sclerotic phases of the graft versus host disease in man: An untrastructural study of six cases. Acta Derm. Venerol. 61:187, 1981.

154. Kumagai, Y., Abe, C., and Shiokawa, Y.: Scleroderma after cosmetic surgery: Four cases of human adjuvant disease. Arthritis Rheum. 22:532, 1979.

155. Shulman, L.E.:Diffuse fasciitis with eosinophilia: A new syndrome? Trans. Assoc. Am. Physicians 88:70, 1975.

156. Rodnan, G.P., DiBartolomeo, A., and Medsger, T.A., Jr.: Eosinophilic fasciitis. Report of six cases of newly recognized scleroderma-like syndrome (abstract). Arthritis Rheum. 18:525, 1975.

157. Kanard, R.R.: Eosinophilic fasciitis. Rocky Mt. Med. J. 74:186, 1977.

158. Bennett, R.M., Herron, A., and Keogh, L.: Eosinophilic fasciitis. Case report and review of the literature. Ann. Rheum. Dis. 36:354, 1977.

159. Giordano, M., Ara, M., Valentini, G., Chianese, U., and Bencivenga, T.: Presence of esosinophilia in progressive systemic sclerosis and localized scleroderma. Arch. Dermatol. Res. 271:411, 1981.

160. Tabuenca, J.M.: Toxic-allergic syndrome caused by ingestion of rapeseed oil denatured with aniline. Lancet 2:567, 1981.

161. Martinez-Tello, F.J., Navas-Palacios, J.J., Ricoy, J.R., Gil-Martin, R., Conde-Zurita, J.M., Colina-Ruiz Delgado, F., Tellez, I., Cabello, A., and Madero-Garcia, S.: Pathology of a new toxic syndrome caused by ingestion of adulterated oil in Spain. Virchows Arch. (Pathol. Anat.) 397:261, 1982.

162. Noriega, A.R., Gomez-Reino, J., Lopez-Encaentra, A., Martin-Escribano, P., Solis-Herruzo, J.A., and Valle-Gutierrez, J.: Toxic epidemic syndrome, Spain, 1981. Lancet 2:697, 1982.

163. Portera-Sanchez, A., Franch, O., and del Ser, T.: Neuromuscular manifestations of the toxic oil syndrome: A recent outbreak in Spain. In Battistin, L., Hashim, G., and Lajtha, A. (eds.): Clinical and Biological Aspects of the Peripheral Nervous System Diseases. New York, Alan R. Liss, Inc. 1983, p. 171.

164. Mateo, I.M., Fernandez-Dapica, M.P., Izquierdo, M., and Gomez-Reino, J.J.: Toxic epidemic syndrome: Musculoskeletal manifestations. J. Rheumatol. 11:333, 1984.

165. Gratwick, G.M., Klein, R., Sergent, J.S., and Christian, C.L.: Fibrinogen turnover in progressive systemic sclerosis. Arthritis Rheum. 21:343, 1978.

166. Tuffanelli, D.L.: Letter: Lymphangiectasis due to scleroderma. Arch. Dermatol. 111:1216, 1975.

167. Lapenas, D., Rodnan, G.P., and Cavallo, T.: Immunopathology of the renal vascular lesion of progressive systemic sclerosis (scleroderma). Am. J. Pathol. 91:243, 1978.

168. McGrath, M.A., Peek, R., and Penny, R.: Blood hyperviscosity with reduced skin blood flow in scleroderma. Ann. Rheum. Dis. 36:569, 1977.

169. Stuart, J.M., Postlethwaite, A.E., and Kang, A.H.: Evidence of cell-mediated immunity to collagen in patients with progressive systemic sclerosis (abstract). Arthritis Rheum. 18:525, 1975.

170. Cohen, S., Johnson, A.R., and Hurd, E.: Cytotoxicity of sera from patients with scleroderma. Arthritis Rheum. 26:170, 1983.

171. Cipoletti, J.F., Buckingham, R.B., Barnes, E.L., Peel, R.L., Mahmood, K., Cignetti, F.E., Pierce, J.M., Rabin, B.S., and Rodnan, G.P.: Sjögren's syndrome in progressive systemic sclerosis. Ann. Intern. Med. 87:535, 1977.

172. Kondo, H., Rabin, B.S., and Rodnan, G.P.: Cutaneous antigen-stimulating lymphokine production by lymphocytes of patients with progressive systemic sclerosis (scleroderma). J. Clin. Invest. 58:1388, 1976.

173. Mackel, A.M., DeLustro, F., DeLustro, B., Fudenberg, H.H., and LeRoy,

E.C.: Immune response to connective tissue components of the basement membrane. Conn. Tissue Res. 10:333, 1982.

174. Salem, N.B., and Morse, J.H.: Lymphocyte response to mitogens in progressive systemic sclerosis. Arthritis Rheum. 19:875, 1976.

175. Spielvogel, R.L., Goltz, R.W., and Kersey, J.H.: Scleroderma-like changes in chronic graft vs. host disease. Arch. Dermatol. 113:1424, 1977.

176. Fenyk, J.R., Jr., Warkentin, P.I., Goltz, R.W., Nesbit, M.E., Coccia, P.F., Smith, C.M., Krivit, W., Neely, J.E., Ramsay, N.K.C., and Kersey, J.H.: Sclerodermatous graft-versus-host disease limited to an area of measles exanthem. Lancet 1:472, 1978.

177. Gratwhol, A.A., Moutsopoulos, H.M., Chused, T.M., Akizuki, M., Wolf, R.O., Sweet, J.B., and Deisseroth, A.B.: Sjögren-type syndrome after allogeneic bone-marrow transplantation. Ann. Intern. Med. 87:703, 1977.

178. Rabin, B.S., Rodnan, G.P., Bassion, S., and Gill, T.J., III: Letter: HLA antigens in progressive systemic sclerosis (scleroderma). Arthritis Rheum. 18:381, 1975.

179. Birnbaum, N.S., Rodnan, G.P., Rabin, B.S., and Bassion, S.: Histocompatibility antigens in progressive systemic sclerosis (scleroderma). J. Rheumatol. 4:425, 1977.

180. Stuart, J.M., Postlethwaite, A.E., and Kang, A.H.: Evidence for cell-mediated immunity to collagen in progressive systemic sclerosis. J. Lab. Clin. Med. 88:601, 1976.

181. Hughes, P., Holt, S., Rowell, N.R., Allonby, I.D., and Dodd, J.K.: The relationship of defective cell-mediated immunity to visceral disease in systemic sclerosis. Clin. Exp. Immunol. 28:233, 1977.

182. Salyer, W.R., Salyer, D.C., and Heptinstall, R.H.: Scleroderma and microangiopathic hemolytic anemia. Ann. Intern. Med. 78:895, 1973.

183. Hughes, P., Gelsthorpe, K., Doughty, R.W., Rowell, N.R., Rosenthal, F.D., and Sneddon, I.B.: The association of HLA-B8 with visceral disease in systemic sclerosis. Clin. Exp. Immunol. 31:351, 1978.

184. Fritz, J., and Sandhofer, M.: Zelluläre Immunphänomene bei der Sklerodermie. Dermatologica 154:129, 1977.

185. Cathcart, M.K. and Krakauer, R.S.: Immunologic enhancement of collagen accumulation in progressive systemic sclerosis (PSS). Clin. Immunol. Immunopath. 21:128, 1981.

186. Baron, M., Keystone, E.C., Gladman, D.D., Lee, P., and Poplonski, L.: Lymphocyte subpopulations and reactivity to mitogens in patients with scleroderma. Clin. Exp. Immunol. 46:70, 1981.

187. Pruzanski, W., Lee, P., Willshire, A., Gladman, D., and Keystone, E.C.: Lymphocytotoxic and phagocytotoxic activity in progressive systemic sclerosis. J. Rheum. 10:55, 1983.

188. Jay, S., Helm, S., and Wray, B.B.: Progressive systemic scleroderma with IgA deficiency in a child. Am. J. Dis. Child. 135:965, 1981.

189. Siebold, J.R., Medsger, T.A., Jr., Winkelstein, A., Kelly, R.H., and Rodnan, G.P.: Immune complexes in progressive systemic sclerosis (scleroderma). Arthritis Rheum. 25:1167, 1982.

190. Winkelstein, A., Bernstein, M.L., Stevens, M.A., Rodnan, G.P., Medsger, T.A., Jr., and Dobson, S.A.: Reduced T lymphoid colony growth in patients with progressive systemic sclerosis and rheumatoid arthritis. J. Lab. Clin. Med. 100:240, 1982.

191. Morse, J.H., and Bodi, B.S.: Autologous and allogeneic mixed lymphocyte reactions in progressive systemic sclerosis. Arthritis Rheum. 25:390, 1982.

192. Lynch, C.J., Singh, G., Whiteside, T.L., Rodnan, G.P., Medsger, T.A., Jr., and Rabin, B.S.: Histocompatibility antigens in progressive systemic sclerosis (PSS; scleroderma). J. Clin. Immunol. 2:314, 1982.

193. Ercilla, M.G., Arriaga, F., Gratacos, M.R., Coll, J., Lecha, V., Vives, J., and Castillo, R.: HLA antigens and scleroderma. Arch. Dermatol. Res. 271:381, 1981.

194. Majsky, A., Kobikova, M., and Stava, Z.: HLA and scleroderma. Tissue Antigens 14:359, 1979.

195. Kallenberg, C.G., Van Der Voort-Beelen, J.M., D'Amaro, J.D., and The, T.H.: Increased frequency of B8DR3 in scleroderma and association of the haplotype with impaired cellular immune response. Clin. Exp. Immunol. 43:478, 1981.

196. Gladman, D.D., Keystone, E.C., Baron, M., Lee, P., Cane, D., and Mervest, H.: Increased frequency of HLA-DR5 in scleroderma. Arthritis Rheum. 24:854, 1981.

197. Whiteside, T., Medsger, T.A., and Rodnan, G.P.: HLA-DR antigens in progressive systemic sclerosis (scleroderma). J. Rheumatol. 10:128, 1983.

198. Buckingham, R.B., Prince, R.K., Rodnan, G.P., and Taylor, F.: Increased collagen accumulation in dermal fibroblast cultures from patients with progressive systemic sclerosis (scleroderma). J. Lab. Clin. Med. 92:5, 1978.

199. Perlish, J.S., Bashey, R.I., Stephens, R.E., and Fleischmajer, R.: Connective tissue synthesis by cultured scleroderma fibroblasts. I. In vitro collagen synthesis by normal and scleroderma dermal fibroblasts. Arthritis Rheum. 19:891, 1976.

200. LeRoy, E.C.: Increased collagen synthesis by scleroderma skin fibroblasts

in vitro: A possible defect in the regulation or activation of the scleroderma fibroblast. J. Clin. Invest. 54:880, 1974.

201. Brady, A.H.: Collagenase in scleroderma. J. Clin. Invest. 56:1175, 1975.

202. Perlish, J.S., and Fleischmajer, R.: Collagen synthesis by scleroderma fibroblasts in culture: A reply (letter). Arthritis Rheum. 20:1440, 1977.

203. Bashey, R.I., Perlish, S., Nochumson, S., Stephens, R.E., and Fleischmajer, R.: Connective tissue synthesis by cultured scleroderma fibroblasts. II. Incorporation of ³H-glucosamine and synthesis of glycosaminoglycans. Arthritis Rheum. 20:879, 1977.

204. Bashey, R.I., and Jiminez, S.A.: Increased sensitivity of scleroderma fibroblasts in culture to stimulation of protein and collagen synthesis by serum. Biochem. Biophys. Res. Commun. 76:1214, 1977.

205. Krieg, T., Müller, P.K., and Goerz, G.: Fibroblasts from a patient with scleroderma reveal abnormal metabolism. Arch. Dermatol. Res. 259:105, 1977.

206. Ko, S.D., Page, R.C., and Narayanan, A.S.: Fibroblast heterogeneity and prostaglandin regulation of subpopulation. Proc. Natl. Acad. Sci. USA 74:3429, 1977.

207. Blumenkrantz, N., and Asboe-Hansen, G.: Abnormal skin collagen in scleroderma. Acta Dermatovenerol. 58:75, 1978.

208. Ishikawa, H., Saito, Y., Yamakage, A., and Kitabatake, M.: Scleroderma-inducing glycosaminoglycan in the urine of patients with systemic scleroderma. Dermatológica 156:193, 1978.

209. Fleischmajer, R., Gay, S., Meigel, W.N., and Perlish, J.S.: Collagen in the cellular and fibrotic stages of scleroderma. Arthritis Rheum. 21:418, 1978.

210. Tan, E.M.L., Uitto, J., Bauer, E.A., and Eisen, A.Z.: Human skin fibroblasts in culture: Procollagen synthesis in the presence of sera from normal human subjects and from patients with dermal fibroses. J. Invest. Dermatol. 76:462, 1981.

211. LeRoy, E.C., Kahaleh, M.B., and Mercurio, S.: A fibroblast mitogen present in scleroderma but not control sera: Inhibition by proteinase inhibitors. Rheumatol. Int. 3:35, 1983.

212. LeRoy, E.C., Mercurio, S.M., and Sherer, G.K.: Replication and phenotypic expression of control and scleroderma human fibroblasts: Responses to growth factors. Proc. Nat. Acad. Sci. USA 79:1286, 1982.

213. Parrott, D.P., Goldberg, R.L., Kaplan, S.R., and Fuller, G.C.: The effect of lymphokines on proliferation and collagen synthesis of cultured human synovial cells. Eur. J. Clin. Invest. 12:407, 1982.

214. Hibbs, M.S., Postlethwaite, A.E., Mainardi, C.L., Seyer, J.M., and Kang, A.H.: Alterations in collagen production in mixed mononuclear leukocyte-fibroblast cultures. J. Exp. Med. 157:47, 1983.

215. Finch, W.R., Rodnan, G.P., Buckingham, R.B., Prince, R.K., and Winkelstein, A.: Bleomycin-induced scleroderma. J. Rheumatol. 7:651, 1980.

216. Fox, P.K., White, D.D., Cavanaugh, M., Davies, M.G., and Wusterman, F.: Failure to demonstrate fibrotic changes in the skin of mice injected with glycosaminoglycan fractions from the urine of scleroderma patients. Dermatologia 164:90, 1982.

217. Kreig, T., Lunderschmidt, C., Weber, L., Müller, P.K., and Braun-Falco, O.: Scleroderma fibroblasts: Some aspects of in vitro assessment of collagen synthesis. Arch. Dermatol. Res. 270:263, 1981.

218. Fleischmajer, R., Perlish, J.S., Kreig, T., and Timpl, R.: Variability in collagen and fibronectin synthesis by scleroderma fibroblasts in primary culture. J. Invest. Dermatol. 76:400, 1981.

219. Lebedev, D.A., Efimova, I.V., and Rassokhina, I.I.: Cell density, DNA, and RNA synthesis in cell cultures of fibroblasts from skin of patients with scleroderma and rheumatoid arthritis. Vopr. Med. Khim. SSSR. 28:84, 1982.

220. Gay, R.E., Buckingham, R.B., Prince, R.K., Gay, S., Rodnan, G.P., and Miller, E.J.: Collagen types synthesized in dermal fibroblast cultures from patients with early progressive systemic sclerosis. Arthritis Rheum. 23:190, 1980.

221. Fleischmajer, R., Gay, S., Perlish, J.S., Cesarini, J.-P.: Immunoelectron microscopy of type III collagen in normal and scleroderma skin. J. Invest. Dermatol. 75:189, 1980.

222. Binnick, S.A., Shore, S.S., Corman, A., and Fleischmajer, R.: Failure of dimethyl sulfoxide in the treatment of scleroderma. Arch. Dermatol. 113:1398, 1977.

223. Muers, M., and Stokes, W.: Treatment of scleroderma heart by D-penicillamine. Br. Heart. J. 38:864, 1976.

224. Taplos, G., White, J.M., Horrocks, M., and Cotton, L.T.: Plasmapheresis in Raynaud's disease. Lancet 1:416, 978.

225. Herbert, C.M., Jayson, M.I.V., Lindberg, K.A., and Bailey, A.J.: Biosynthesis and maturation of skin collagen in scleroderma, and effect of D-penicillamine. Lancet 1:187, 1974.

226. Mellstedt, H., Fagrell, B., Holm, G., and Björkholm, M.: (D)-Penicillamine treatment in systemic sclerosis (scleroderma). Scand. J. Rheumatol. 6:92, 1977.

227. Carter, S.A.: Finger systolic pressures and skin temperatures in severe Raynaud's syndrome: The relationship to healing of skin lesions and the use of oral phenoxybenzamine. Angiology 32:298, 1981.

228. Lopez-Ovejero, J.A., Saal, S.D., D'Angelo, W.A., Cheigh, J.S., Stenzel, K.H., and Laragh, J.H.: Reversal of vascular and renal crises of scleroderma by oral angiotensin-converting-enzyme blockade. N. Engl. J. Med. 300:1417, 1979.

229. Zawada, E.T., Jr., Clements, P.J., Furst, D.A., Bloomer, H.A., Paulus, H.E., and Maxwell, M.H.: Clinical course of patients with scleroderma renal crisis treated with captopril. Nephron 27:74, 1981.

230. Martin, M.F.R., Dowd, P.M., Ring, E.F.J., Cooke, E.D., Dieppe, P.A., and Kirby, J.D.T.: Prostaglandin E₁ infusions for vascular insufficiency in progressive systemic sclerosis. Ann. Rheum. Dis. 40:350, 1981.

231. Dowd, P.M., Kovacs, I.B., Bland, C.J.H., and Kirby, J.D.T.: Effect of prostaglandins I₂ and E₁ on red cell deformability in patients with Raynaud's phenomenon and systemic sclerosis. Br. Med. J. 283:350, 1981.

232. Camerini, F., Alberti, E., Klugmann, S., and Salvi, A.: Primary pulmonary hypertension: Effects of nifedipine. Br. Heart J. 44:352, 1980.

233. Dalal, J.J., Griffiths, B.E., and Henderson, A.H.: Primary pulmonary hypertension: Effects of nifedipine. Br. Heart J. 46:230, 1981.

234. Franks, A.G., Jr.: Topical glyceryl trinitrate as adjunctive treatment in Raynaud's disease. Lancet 1:76, 1982.

235. Steen, V.D., Medsger, T.A., Jr., and Rodnan, G.P.: D-Penicillamine therapy in progressive systemic sclerosis (scleroderma): A retrospective analysis. Ann. Intern. Med. 97:652, 982.

236. Gershwin, M.E.: Slow progress with scleroderma. Ann. Intern. Med. 97:776, 1982.

237. Kang, B., Veres-Thorner, C., Heredia, R., Cha, E., Bose, S., and Schwartz, M.: Successful treatment of far-advanced progressive systemic sclerosis by D-penicillamine. J. Allergy Clin. Immunol. 69:297, 1982.

238. Dau, P.C., Kahaleh, M.B., and Sagebiel, R.W.: Plasmapheresis and immunosuppressive drug therapy in scleroderma. Arthritis Rheum. 24:1128, 1981.

239. Whitman, H.H., III, Case, D.B., Laragh, J.H., Christian, C.L., Botstein, G., Maricq, H.R., and LeRoy, E.C.: Variable response to oral angiotensin-converting enzyme blockade in hypertensive Scleroderma patients. Arthritis Rheum. 25:241, 1982.

Chapter 77
Localized Scleroderma— Morphea

Steven K. Spencer

DEFINITION

Morphea (localized scleroderma, circumscribed scleroderma) is a cutaneous disease which occurs in several clinical patterns consisting of discrete sclerotic plaques, often single or few in number but occasionally generalized. In linear bandlike forms of localized scleroderma, skin and underlying muscle and bone can be involved.

EPIDEMIOLOGY

Morphea is most common in children, young adults, and females.[1,2] A few instances of familial involvement have been reported.[3] No specific racial or occupational factors have been recognized.

CLINICAL MANIFESTATIONS

Morphea. Characteristically, morphea appears as flesh-colored mildly erythematous and slightly edematous oval plaques. These well-demarcated circumscribed indurations become sclerotic with ivory-colored centers and violaceous (lilac ring) borders which represent localized inflammation (Fig. 77–1; see Plate X, p. xliv). The violaceous border is seen frequently in morphea; it is not seen in systemic scleroderma. Usually few in number, plaques range from 1 to several centimeters in diameter, and occasionally become generalized. Involved skin loses its hair and capability for perspiration. Multiple small white plaques, often spread over the upper torso, are described as guttate (droplike) and, although clinically confused with lichen sclerosus et atrophicus, can be recognized by their association with classic plaques of morphea and by characteristic histopathologic findings.

Linear Scleroderma. Bandlike lesions of linear sclerosis appear most commonly in the first and second decades of life, involve limbs usually unilaterally but occasionally bilaterally, and tend to involve underlying skin, muscle, and bone.[1,3] The extremities and scalp are involved more often than the trunk. Frontal or frontoparietal linear scleroderma (coup de sabre) forms a paramedian sclerotic band which involves the scalp and forehead and is associated with alopecia. Occasionally similar lesions involve the homolateral cheek and chin in a vertical linear band, which does not follow any dermatome (Fig. 77–2). Linear lesions occasionally remain purely cutaneous without involvement of under-lying structures (Fig. 77–3). Combinations of plaques and linear lesions can occur together. Linear lesions only rarely follow the distribution of a specific peripheral nerve, but most seem to be distributed longitudinally in the long axis of one or several spinal root zones.[4] When the hand is involved with linear scleroderma, Raynaud's phenomenon and carpal tunnel syndrome may involve the affected extremity.

Associations. In one large series of patients with morphea, migraine headaches, arthralgias, and abdominal pain occurred more often than would be expected by chance;[2] skeletal anomalies involving ribs and vertebral column have been well documented.[4] Dull pain and twitching sensations can occur following fatigue of an extremity involved with linear scleroderma.

Clinical Course. All forms of localized scleroderma have been noted to involute completely. Morphea lesions tend to soften within months to years, leaving various degrees of hyper- and hypopigmentation and atrophy. The late sequelae of linear scleroderma, which may affect fat, muscle, fascia, and bone (pansclerosis), include joint contracture, occasionally ankylosis, and calcinosis cutis. Shortening of the Achilles tendon when the heel is involved may require surgical correction. Secondary hemiatrophy is associated with linear scleroderma of the scalp and face and both skin and underlying tissues are involved (Fig. 77–4). In some children, morphea, apparently beginning in a linear pattern, has become generalized, with pansclerosis of much of the body surface, and known as disabling pansclerotic morphea of children.[5]

HISTOPATHOLOGY

Biopsy specimens of plaques of morphea resemble skin biopsies from patients with systemic scleroderma. The epidermis can be either acanthotic or atrophic with increased melanin pigmentation along the basal layer. Characteristically, the lower dermal collagen appears hyalinized with broadened collagen bundles which replace some of the subcutaneous fat and lie parallel to the skin surface. Specimens taken from the violaceous border of an early plaque have an inflammatory infiltrate of lymphocytes, histiocytes, and occasionally plasma cells around vessels in the lower dermis and in the panniculus. In late stages the adnexal structures appear to be atrophic and bound vessels show thickened walls and narrowed lumens. In linear lesions the underlying muscle may show focal edema of fibers with interstitial inflammation.

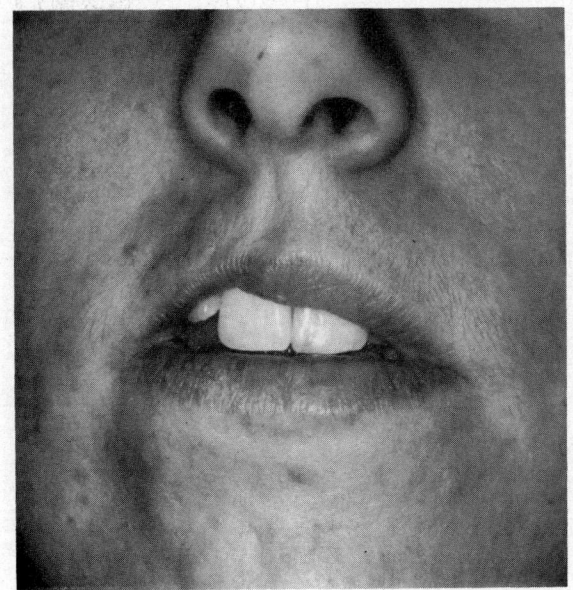

Figure 77–2. Linear morphea of right paranasal, lip, and chin areas.

ETIOLOGY AND PATHOGENESIS

The cause of the various forms of scleroderma is unknown. It has been reported that trauma can precipitate morphea; however, documentation of this is rare.[1,2,4] Various theories concerning the etiology of scleroderma are well discussed in Chapter 76. Experiments utilizing reciprocal skin autografts in scleroderma support the clinical observation that skin involvement is reversible in morphea but not in systemic scleroderma.[9,10] Grafts taken from lesional skin and placed on clinically uninvolved skin tend to resolve in morphea but not in systemic scleroderma. The occasional coexistence of nevi and vitiligo in association with linear scleroderma in a segmental (autonomic) distribution, accompanied by loss of sweating in the involved area, suggests a possible neurological or neurovascular role in pathogenesis.[11]

RELATIONSHIP OF MORPHEA TO SYSTEMIC SCLEROSIS

Whether morphea and systemic sclerosis are related processes is controversial. Several reports have indicated transition from morphea to systemic scleroderma in a small percentage of cases.[1,2,6-8] However, careful reviews of individual case histories suggest that many so-called transitions were probably instances of systemic scleroderma from the beginning, having been mistakenly called morphea initially. In one large series of patients with morphea, arthralgias, migraine, abdominal pain of unknown etiology, and Raynaud's phenomenon were reported in a few patients.[1]

Several of the patients described with disabling pansclerotic morphea of children had evidence of systemic involvement.[4] Abnormalities in decreasing frequency included hypergammaglobulinemia, peripheral eosinophilia, elevated erythrocyte sedimentation rate, decreased

Figure 77–3. Hyperpigmented "burned out" stage of linear morphea on right shoulder (*A*) and leg (*B*). Involved skin has softened, and in this instance subcutaneous tissues were not involved.

Figure 77–4. *A* and *B*, Young boy with early lesion of linear morphea on left side of chin and jawline. *C* and *D*, Same patient as in *A* and *B* 2½ years later, showing secondary hemiatrophy of face.

carbon monoxide diffusing capacity, and positive ANA tests. Perhaps morphea is a misnomer for this particular disorder; 2 of 14 patients reported have died after 4 and 9 years of progressive sclerosis.

Patients with morphea are rarely reported in the literature. Transformation of morphea to systemic scleroderma, if indeed such happens, must be extremely rare.

DIFFERENTIAL DIAGNOSIS

The differential diagnosis of morphea includes several skin diseases which either develop firm plaques or pigmentary changes and atrophy, which can closely resemble late stages of morphea. Lichen sclerosus et atrophicus

can be distinguished by surface wrinkling, delling, follicular plugging, and a distinctive histologic picture. Lesions of lichen planus, leprosy, vitiligo, and tineas have a characteristic historical onset and evolution, as well as histopathological changes which allow their differentiation from each other and from morphea. Linear melorheostotic scleroderma probably represents cutaneous changes secondary to the bony lesions of melorheostosis rather than a form of morphea.[9]

MANAGEMENT

Management of localized scleroderma should reflect the knowledge that the process is self-limited and variable in its natural history, and that no specific topical or systemic treatment has been clearly shown to alter the course or prognosis of morphea. Surgical correction of contractures and disfiguring facial deformities has been helpful. When linear scleroderma leads to significant withering and stunted growth of one leg in a growing child, epiphyseal interruption on the opposite normal limb may help to equalize limb length. At present, vigorous physical therapy and supportive care are the most important aspects of management.[13] Successful relief of a contracted knee joint in linear scleroderma has been obtained using continuous stretch applied by an extension splint. To control pain not relieved by analgesics, transepidermal nerve stimulation has been used during therapy.[14]

References

1. Curtis, A.C., and Jansen, T.G.: The prognosis of localized scleroderma. Arch. Dermatol. 78:749, 1958.
2. Christianson, H.B., Dorsey, C.S., O'Leary, P.A., and Kierland, R.R.: Localized scleroderma: A clinical study of two hundred thirty-five cases. Arch. Dermatol. 74:629, 1956.
3. Wuthrich, R.C., Roenigk, H.H., Jr., and Steck, W.D.: Localized scleroderma. Arch. Dermatol. 111:98, 1975.
4. Rubin, L.: Linear scleroderma: Association with abnormalities of the spine and nervous system. Arch. Dermatol. Syph. 58:1, 1948.
5. Diaz-Perez, J.L., Connolly, S.M., and Winkelman, R.K.: Disabling pansclerotic morphea of children. Arch. Dermatol. 116:169, 1980.
6. Jablonska, S., Bubnow, B., and Szczepanski, A.: Morphea: is it a separate entity or a variety of scleroderma? Dermatologica 125:140, 1962.
7. Tuffanelli, D.L., Marmelzat, W.L., and Dorsey, C.D.: Linear scleroderma with hemiatrophy: Report of three cases associated with collagen-vascular disease. Dermatologica 132:51, 1966.
8. Rodnan, G.P., and Fennell, R.H.: Progressive systemic sclerosis sine scleroderma. JAMA 180:665, 1962.
9. Haxthausen, H.: Studies on the pathogenesis of morphea, vitiligo and acrodermatitis atrophicans by means of transplantation experiments. Acta Derm. Venerol. 27:352, 1947.
10. Fries, J.F., Hoopes, J.E., and Shulman, L.E.: Reciprocal skin grafts in systemic sclerosis (scleroderma). Arthritis Rheum. 14:571, 1971.
11. Jablonska, S. (ed.): Scleroderma and Pseudoscleroderma. 2nd ed. New York, Academic Press, 1976.
12. Wagers, L.T., Young, A.W., Jr., and Ryan, S.F.: Linear melorheostotic scleroderma. Br. J. Dermatol. 86:297, 1972.
13. Rudolph, R.I., and Leyden, J.J.: Physiatrics for deforming linear scleroderma. Arch. Dermatol. 112:995, 1976.
14. Rizk, T.E., and Park, S.J.: Transcutaneous electrical nerve stimulation and extensor splint in linear scleroderma knee contracture. Arch. Phys. Med. Rehabil. 62:86, 1981.

Chapter 78

Localized Fibrotic Disorders

Carlo L. Mainardi and Andrew H. Kang

INTRODUCTION

Fibrotic disorders affecting vital organs are among the most common conditions with which clinicians are faced. Rheumatologists are familiar with organ fibrosis, a major component of progressive systemic sclerosis (PSS) and an accompaniment of other systemic rheumatic diseases (e.g., rheumatoid lung). Despite the frequent occurrence of diseases such as hepatic cirrhosis and the various fibrotic lung diseases, medical management of these disorders is inadequate, and our understanding of their pathogenesis is fragmentary. Rheumatologists are familiar with the sense of frustration associated with treating patients with progressive systemic sclerosis, but the localized fibrotic disorders are equally difficult to treat successfully.

In addition to PSS, there are several other sclerosing disorders that are of interest to the practice of rheumatology because of the involvement of the musculoskeletal system (Dupuytren's contracture) or because of the expression of abnormal antibodies, suggesting a relationship to immune complex disease (e.g., idiopathic pulmonary fibrosis).

It is the purpose of this chapter to elaborate on the present concepts regarding the mechanisms of tissue fibrosis, with particular focus on its relationship to tissue injury and chronic inflammation. In addition, selected clinical conditions characterized by localized sclerosis will be briefly reviewed. These disorders are related only by their end result (disruption of normal tissue architecture) and probably arrive at this stage by a variety of loosely related pathogenetic mechanisms. These represent a spectrum of conditions ranging from indolent, mild disorders such as keloids or Dupuytren's contracture to life-threatening, subacute diseases such as idiopathic pulmonary fibrosis and retroperitoneal fibrosis. In fact, the severity of any of these disorders is related to the specific organ involvement and the time required for progression to an end-stage lesion.

MECHANISMS OF PATHOGENESIS OF FIBROSIS

In studying the pathogenetic mechanisms of tissue fibrosis, one is constrained by the difficulty of conducting biochemical experiments on human subjects. Therefore, much of our insight into this topic is derived from morphologic observations of human diseases, biochemical studies of autopsy material, and careful experimentations on a spectrum of animal models with varying relevance to human diseases. Most of the specific diseases covered in this chapter share certain clinical and morphologic features with each other as well as with many pertinent animal models.

Morphologically, the end-stage of these disorders is characterized by a disruption of normal architecture with proliferation of connective tissue. In parenchymal organs such as liver and lung, this fibroproliferative process results in an abnormal cellular arrangement and is generally associated with clinically recognizable organ dysfunction. In other conditions, such as retroperitoneal fibrosis, where the process takes place in a nonvital locale (i.e., retroperitoneal fat) the normal tissue is again replaced by dense connective tissue but the clinical consequences are not as apparent in the earlier stages.

Although there may be one or two exceptions, the fibrotic reaction is generally associated with an inflammatory response and evidence indicates that the deposition of connective elements occurs in the wake of this inflammation. This implies that some injurious event occurs in the target tissue that results in an inflammatory response, which, in turn leads to a fibrotic response.

Thus, one can generalize about fibrosis and identify the following three distinct but inter-related phases of the process: (1) the phase of tissue injury; (2) the inflammatory phase; and (3) the reparative phase.

It is quite likely that these three phases are represented to some degree in all these disorders and that the apparent clinical differences can be correlated with the predominance of one or another component at a given stage of the process. Morphologic observations would support the concept of three phases, although there is significant overlap and evidence of all three phases can be found in a given tissue section.

Wound Healing: A Model of Tissue Fibrosis. Before reviewing the factors that are influential in each of these phases, a brief discussion of normal wound healing is in order. The healing process in mammals is in contrast to the regenerative response of lower vertebrates (amphibians) in which the amputation of a limb results in the growth of a new limb. Without the process of wound healing, our species would not have survived. It is tempting to speculate that fibrosis of vital organs may be an undesirable evolutionary result of the healing process, since the events in wound healing parallel those in tissue fibrosis.

Schilling has divided the wound healing process into the following four phases: (1) the wounding phase; (2) the inflammatory phase; (3) the proliferative phase; and (4) the remodeling phase.[1] This classification is similar to the one proposed above for the phases of tissue fibrosis, and the parallels between wound repair and tissue fibrosis have been previously emphasized.[2] Wounding is a specific form of tissue injury, and the reparative phase includes migration and proliferation of blood vessels and fibroblasts, with the deposition of extracellular matrix elements followed by remodeling of the matrix.

The immediate response to a wound is the activation of the coagulation system. The inflammatory phase rapidly follows and is characterized by the migration of neutrophils, eosinophils, and mononuclear cells to the wound. Neutrophils are the first to appear and are the predominant cell in the first 24 to 48 hours followed by macrophages (days 2 to 4).[3] These inflammatory cells are presumably attracted to the site by specific chemoattractants. The role of these cells appears to be complex and important to the process. Neutrophils are

felt to function primarily in the prevention of infection. It has been shown that in the absence of infection wound healing proceeded normally in guinea pigs rendered neutropenic by antineutrophil serum.[4] In subsequent studies by the same investigators, it was demonstrated that the presence of macrophage/monocytes in the wound was essential for effective healing.[5] A variety of macrophage factors influencing various components of the reparative process have been identified.[6] This is discussed in detail below.

The next stage of wound healing is the reparative phase. This includes the processes of neovascularization and fibroblast activation and occurs in the wake of the inflammatory reaction. Both these processes are probably initiated in response to signals generated during the inflammatory phase. There is evidence that implicates both the clotting system[7] and the macrophage in the generation of such signals.[8,9] Fibroblasts are attracted into the wound and are probably stimulated to proliferate and synthesize collagen and other connective tissue elements. The timing of this phenomenon is somewhat controversial. Studies from different investigators have reported conflicting results, indicating that the rate of collagen synthesis reaches maximum levels several days to 2 weeks post wounding.[10-12] A recent report has indicated that an increase in collagen synthesis begins as early as 24 hours after the injury.[13]

Once the new scar is formed, remodeling occurs. Collagenase, gelatinase, and other hydrolytic enzymes are secreted by these cells, and new matrix proteins are deposited, resulting in a healed wound. This process is essential in wound repair in the realignment of fibrous elements along tension lines. Remodeling is carefully controlled by factors that cause the release, activation, and inhibition of proteolytic enzymes balanced by the synthesis and deposition of matrix proteins. In this phase, crosslinking of collagen occurs, and this process is essential to the formation of an effective wound. If this process is inhibited by a lathyrogen, the resulting wound is weak and the collagen is more easily extractable.[14] In addition to being less easy to solubilize, crosslinked collagen is relatively resistant to degradation by collagenase.[15]

This process of wound healing is summarized in Table 78–1. It has been the subject of investigation for several decades, and this model, as briefly described above, is supported by an abundance of clinical and basic research. The pathogenesis of the localized fibrotic disorders is not as well defined, but evidence would support the concept that tissue injury, inflammation, and tissue repair are involved to some degree in most, if not all, of these conditions. In these disorders, the phases overlap considerably, and, specifically, the inflammatory component persists into the reparative phase. It is appropriate to expand on these three phases with specific focus on how they relate to the diseases discussed in this chapter.

Tissue Injury. Regardless of the nature of the fibrotic condition, it is almost certain that a specific insult initiates the process by inciting an inflammatory response.

Table 78–1. Events in Wound Healing

Event	Approximate Time Postinjury
1. Injury	
2. Coagulation	0 to 2 days
3. Inflammation	
a. PMNs	1 to 4 days
b. Monocytes	2 to 6 days
4. Repair	
a. Fibroblast migration	3 to 7 days
b. Neovascularization	6 to 10 days
c. Collagen synthesis (biochemical)	2 to 21 days
d. Collagen deposition (morphologic)	7 to 21 days
5. Remodeling and crosslinking	7 days and later

The nature of this insult is quite variable and includes infectious agents, immunologic reactions, environmental factors, drugs and toxins, tissue ischemia, and trauma. In some diseases the identity of the initiating agent is obvious, such as alcoholic cirrhosis, postnecrotic cirrhosis, silicosis, and radiation fibrosis. Unfortunately, many of these conditions are idiopathic, and the inciting agent(s) are not known.

Several of the diseases discussed in this chapter are related to drugs. It is quite likely that these agents induce fibrosis by injuring the target tissue. This is especially probable in the case of retroperitoneal fibrosis associated with ergot alkaloids. Methysergide is a vasoactive substance and may induce an inflammatory response by this mechanism.

In its early stages, retroperitoneal fibrosis is associated with an inflammatory infiltrate. The fibrotic conditions associated with the carcinoid syndrome are likely to share pathogenetic features with ergot-induced diseases, considering the structural similarities between these ergot alkaloids and serotonin. Recently, an association has been made between tissue fibrosis and certain beta-adrenergic blockers.[16-19] These drugs may, in addition, affect fibroblast function directly (see below).

The Inflammatory Response. In the wound healing model, the inflammatory response is immediate. In contrast, the diseases discussed in this chapter are not as acute, and the fibrotic process progresses over a period of weeks to years. In addition, immunologic mechanisms are not operative in wound healing but are probably central in the pathogenesis of certain fibrotic disorders.

Linking of the inflammatory response and the immune response to fibrosis has been the subject of recent investigations. There is abundant evidence indicating that soluble mediators generated during the inflammatory phase as well as cell-cell interactions influence the reparative phase and probably represent a bridge between these two phases. However, clinical observations have shown that tissue injury and inflammation do not always progress to scarring. For example, only a minority of alcoholics progress to cirrhosis, and certain bacterial infections resolve without residual fibrosis despite intense inflammation. The scientific basis for these observations is not known and may be the most compelling

question to be answered in the study of these processes. It is very likely that host factors play a role. A familial occurrence has been observed in certain of these syndromes (Dupuytren's diathesis, retroperitoneal fibrosis),[20,21] and keloids are more frequently seen in blacks. It is also probable that the intensity of the tissue destruction mediated by proteinases, oxidative products, prostaglandins, and other factors released during this phase is a determining factor in the degree to which normal architecture is disrupted by the healing phase. Furthermore, the development of delayed-type hypersensitivity and the local generation of specific modulators of fibroblast function are felt to be important in certain conditions.

The Reparative Phase. As mentioned above, scar formation occurs in the wake of inflammation in wound healing. Similarly, tissue fibrosis occurs in the wake of the inflammatory reaction. The transition to the reparative phase is generally not sharply demarcated in these diseases, and the two processes overlap considerably. Morphologic observations support this in that inflammatory infiltration and fibrosis are often seen in the same biopsy specimen.

While it is likely that events in all three phases are critical in the fibrotic process, the relative role of each step is unknown. Recent studies have suggested that the reparative process is extremely important in determining the ultimate lesion in response to a given stimulus. In one provocative study, it was shown that hamsters developed interstitial pulmonary fibrosis in response to cadmium chloride but developed bullous emphysema in response to the identical agent if the animals were rendered lathyritic by the administration of β-aminopropionitrile.[22]

The cell that is central in the reparative phase is the fibroblast. In the last decade, the complexities of this cell have been the subject of investigation of researchers of many disciplines.

FIBROBLAST FUNCTION

The fibroblast is a multifaceted cell and its various functions can be influenced by a variety of stimuli. Specifically, the fibroblast functions that are most relevant to tissue repair include (1) chemotactic migration; (2) proliferation; (3) adherence to substrata; (4) biosynthesis, processing, and deposition of the major connective tissue elements (collagen, glycosaminoglycans, elastin, and fibronectin); (5) tissue remodeling (which involves all the above in addition to the synthesis, release, and activation of proteinases that degrade these matrix proteins).

Migration and Chemoattraction of Fibroblasts. Early in the reparative phase of wound healing, local fibroblasts migrate into the site of tissue injury[23] in response to specific signals related to the inflammatory phase. Similarly, it is likely that fibroblast attraction to sites of inflammation is crucial in the pathogenesis of the fibrotic diseases. It should be pointed out that unlike other cells, which respond to certain substances by migration toward them (neutrophils and monocytes), the fibroblast is not a cell that circulates in the bloodstream. Therefore, the chemotaxis of fibroblasts results in the recruitment of local cells, and then other factors stimulating the proliferation of these cells lead to the large increase in the number of fibroblasts at the site. This is in contrast to the chemotaxis of circulating cells in which large numbers of these cells are attracted to the site of inflammation but do not proliferate locally.

Fibroblast chemoattractants are summarized in Table 78-2, and it is apparent that this process can be linked to the inflammatory phase through the coagulation system, the complement system, T lymphocytes, the macrophage, and by the degradation products of certain connective tissue proteins.[6,24-29] The relative role in the fibrotic process of each of these chemotactic factors is undetermined. The attraction of these cells to peptides derived from collagen, elastin, and fibronectin is also an important chemotactic mechanism. The inflammatory cells release their proteolytic enzymes, which debride the wound.

In view of the work of Liebovich and Ross,[5] the macrophage probably plays the major role in this process. This cell is capable of producing fibronectin, which is a fibroblast chemoattractant.[30] Furthermore, it is capable of releasing specific connective tissue–degrading proteinases into the extracellular space.[31,32] The products released by these proteinases attract the fibroblasts to deposit new matrix. In contrast, the chemotactic factors derived from T lymphocytes and C5 probably play major roles in the fibrosis associated with immunologically mediated subacute and chronic inflammation. The recent observation that platelet-derived growth factor (PDGF) is a fibroblast chemoattractant[33] is of interest for the pathogenesis of fibrosis: it confirms another link between the coagulation system and the reparative process.

Fibroblast Proliferation. In both wound healing and tissue fibrosis, the local proliferation of the migrated fibroblasts is felt to be important in the resulting scar formation. Indeed, it has been shown that fibroblasts in vitro can be stimulated to proliferate in response to

certain substances, and it can be logically assumed that these factors may play a major role in the pathogenesis of these disorders. Many investigators have been focusing on the rate of synthesis of collagen and other connective tissue elements as a function of the fibroblast in fibrotic diseases (see below), but it is possible that the proliferation of fibroblasts is more critical to the development of fibrosis than the amount of collagen synthesized per cell.

It should be stressed at this point that the systems used to study fibroblast proliferation in vitro are a source of controversy among investigators and are plagued with several variables that exert their own influence on the system. For example, it is well known that fibroblasts proliferate in vitro as a function of cell density. Furthermore, fetal calf serum is necessary to support growth of these cells, and this substance probably contains several "growth factors." Thus, experiments must be carefully designed and controlled, as one may obtain different results depending on cell density and serum concentration.

Recent observations by Stiles and his co-workers[34] have clarified some of the confusion regarding the effect of serum on fibroblast proliferation. These investigators have classified serum growth factors in two categories. Competence factors, such as platelet-derived growth factor, act early in G1 and render the cells "competent" to replicate their DNA but do not cause "progression" to S phase. Progression factors, such as the somatomedins, act later in G1 and induce "progression" to the S phase. It has been suggested that competence factors play a major role in repair growth and progression factors control developmental growth.[34]

With these considerations in mind, several factors capable of inducing the proliferation of fibroblasts have been isolated and at least partially characterized. Perhaps the best known of these is fibroblast growth factor, or FGF, which is derived from brain tissue and may be derived from myelin basic protein.[35,36] The possible role of this substance in inflammatory and fibrotic states is unclear. Another substance that is particularly germane to this topic is platelet-derived growth factor (PDGF), which is released from platelets in response to thrombin and has been extensively characterized.[37-39] PDGF may be a key factor in stimulating fibroblast proliferation in wound healing, atherosclerosis, and other conditions in which fibrosis follows aggregation of platelets and activation of the coagulation system.

Several reports have implicated mononuclear cells (both monocyte/macrophage and T lymphocytes) in the induction of fibroblast proliferation. Leibovich and Ross have found that culture supernatants from guinea pig peritoneal macrophages stimulate fibroblast growth,[40] while other investigators have found similar activity in supernatants of cultured human peripheral blood monocytes.[41] In studying the complex system of mitogen/antigen-stimulated human peripheral blood mononuclear (PBM) cells, varying results have been reported by different investigators. Korn and colleagues[42] have found that these supernatants suppressed fibroblast growth

Table 78-2. Fibroblast Chemoattractants

Source	Factor	Comments
Serum	Serum-derived chemotactic factor (SDCF)	80,000 MW, complement component, probably C5-derived[24]
Platelets	Platelet-derived growth factor (PDGF)	See Fibroblast Proliferation.[33]
T lymphocyte	Lymphocyte-derived chemotactic factor (LDCF)	22,000 MW protein[25]
Macrophage	Fibronectin[30]	
Extracellular matrix	Peptides derived from fibronectin, collagen, and elastin[26-30]	

and that this suppression was related to the production of prostaglandins by the mononuclear cells. Treatment of the PBM cells with indomethacin abrogated the suppression, while addition of exogenous PGE_2 restored the effect. Postlethwaite and his co-workers[43] fractionated these stimulated PBM supernatants and were able to identify two peaks of fibroblast growth stimulation, one with an apparent molecular weight of 60,000 and a second substance with a molecular weight of 16,000. Later studies indicated that the former substance is derived from T lymphocytes and the later substance is identical to the well-characterized monokine Interleukin I.[44-46]

The stimulation of fibroblast proliferation by T lymphocytes has been reported by other investigators using guinea pig and human T lymphocytes as well as human T lymphocyte lines.[44,45] The induction of fibroblast proliferation by Interleukin I has also been reported by Schmidt and associates.[47] Bitterman and associates have identified a substance released in vitro by stimulated human alveolar macrophages which stimulated the proliferation of noncycling human lung fibroblasts.[48] This factor was partially characterized and found to be a "progression factor" and was distinct from previously described growth factors, including Interleukin I. These investigators found no stimulation of fibroblast growth by Interleukin I. Thus, the growth factor potential of Interleukin I is controversial at this time.

Although the exact effect of monocytes and lymphocytes on fibroblast proliferation remains to be elucidated, it is almost certain that these cells exert their influence on fibroblast growth in vivo and probably play a major role in the pathogenesis of fibrotic diseases. Table 78–3 summarizes the inflammtory cell-derived mediators of fibroblast growth.

Fibroblast Adherence. It has been known for years that the fibroblast adheres to surfaces. The anchoring of the fibroblasts that migrate into sites of inflammation is probably essential in the development of fibrosis. Fibronectin is essential in this process[49] (see Chapter 14). Early studies established that fibronectin promoted the adherence and spreading of cells in vitro.[50] In addition, it was established that it was capable of binding to certain substances, including gelatin, collagen, and heparin.[49,51-53] Limited cleavage of this molecule has permitted the identification of specific domains which have different functions. The cell attachment region is located near the carboxyl terminus, whereas the gelatin(collagen)-binding region has been localized near the amino terminus.[52,53] Solubilized fragments of fibronectin could attract fibroblasts to areas of inflammation, while newly synthesized fibronectin probably serves to anchor these migrating cells.

The role of glycosaminoglycans (GAGs) in the fibrotic process is presently not well-defined. In developmental and regenerative systems, the milieu through which cells migrate is rich in hyaluronate, a GAG that is not a major component of mature tissues. The subsequent cell differentiation correlates with the enzymatic removal of hyaluronate.[54,55] In wound healing, a similar phenomenon occurs. The hyaluronate content of granulation tissue begins to decrease about 7 days after wounding, and this correlates with the presence of hyaluronidase activity.[56] The content of sulfated GAGs increases progressively from day 5 to 17 post wounding.[57]

Biosynthesis, Processing, and Deposition of Connective Tissue Elements. Having migrated to the sites of inflammation and anchored to the surrounding tissue, the fibroblast then engages in the essence of the healing process and deposits matrix substances in the extracellular space. This process is very complex and involves much more than the transcription and translation of polypeptide chains. The biosynthesis of collagen, for example, requires several post-translational processing steps in order to deposit native triple helical molecules which can be incorporated into mature fibrils. These are covered in depth in Chapter 14 and require the presence of several enzymes, which are also synthesized by the fibroblast, and the presence of certain cofactors.

As discussed in detail below, the production of collagen by fibroblasts in vitro is readily manipulated by a variety of substances. However, it is logical to ask whether the rate of production of collagen (or other matrix elements) is important in the development of fibrosis. If fibroblasts migrate into a tissue that is relatively devoid of these cells and subsequently proliferate, connective tissue matrix should accumulate even if the rate of collagen synthesis per cell is normal. Certain observations would indicate that the fibroblast synthesizes collagen at an enhanced rate in the process of fibrosis. First, in certain models of pulmonary fibrosis (bleomycin, ozone), cultured lung explants exhibit an increased rate of collagen synthesis.[58,59] Furthermore, it has been well established that scleroderma skin fibroblasts also have an enhanced rate of collagen synthesis.[60-63]

The Biochemistry of Collagen in Fibrosis. It may seem logical that the connective tissue deposited in the fibrotic states simply represents a difference in the quantity of qualitatively normal interstitium. This is not the case. In certain diseases the deviation from the norm is primarily qualitative (Table 78–4). In idiopathic pulmonary fibrosis, for example, the total collagen content of the lung is normal (as is the rate of collagen production by lung explants), but the type I/III collagen ratio is elevated and immunohistochemical studies have indicated that type V collagen is also increased.[64-66] In cirrhosis, the type I/III ratio is similarly abnormal, but the collagen content is also increased.[67] This qualitative abnormality of collagen is probably representative of fi-

Table 78–3. Inflammatory Cell Induction of Fibroblast Growth

Source	Factor
Platelet	PDGF[37-39]
T lymphocytes	60,000 MW factor[43-45]
Macrophage	(1) Interleukin I[46,47]
	(2) 18,000 MW factor from human alveolar macrophages (different from IL-I)[48]

Table 78–4. Ratio of Type I to Type III Collagen in Fibrotic States

Conditions in which ratio is elevated:
Idiopathic pulmonary fibrosis
Cirrhosis
Conditions in which ratio is normal:
PSS
Keloids (collagen synthesized by fibroblasts in vitro)
Conditions in which ratio is depressed:
Dupuytren's contracture

Table 78–5. Modulation of Fibroblast Collagen Production

Factor	Stimulate (S) or Inhibit (I)
1. Amino-terminal propeptide	I
2. Pharmacologic agents	
a. Ascorbate	S
b. Glucocorticoids	I
c. Bleomycin	S
d. Proline analogues	I
e. Factors that increase intracellular cAMP (beta-adrenergic agonists, dibutyrl cAMP)	I
f. beta-adrenergic blocking agents	?S
3. T-lymphocyte factor(s)	S and I
4. Interleukin I	I

brosis in general. There are exceptions to this. In progressive systemic sclerosis fibrotic lung contains types I and III collagen in normal ratios but increased collagen overall.[68] In Dupuytren's contracture, the thickened fascia contains a substantial amount of type III collagen, which is not present in normal palmar fascia.[69,70] These differences cannot now be explained, but they suggest different pathogenetic pathways in these diseases.

The Study of Collagen Production In Vitro. Before discussing the factors that regulate the rate of collagen synthesis, it is appropriate to briefly review the methodology employed. These studies generally utilize the incorporation of radiolabeled proline into bacterial collagenase-sensitive protein or the conversion of the labeled proline to hydroxyproline.[71,72] In the most frequently used system of fibroblast monolayers, one can measure the collagen in the cell layer, which reflects processed native collagen, and the collagen in the supernatant, which is primarily unprocessed procollagen. Generally, the overwhelming majority of collagen is found in the latter form, suggesting that in the monolayer system, the cleavage of procollagen is a rate-limiting step in the processing of the molecule. Considering the recently described feedback inhibition by the amino terminal propeptide of α chains one can question the validity of the system. This method is also clouded by two other substances that are conventionally included—fetal calf serum and ascorbic acid. Fetal calf serum increases collagen production and has been the source of some confusion. Ascorbic acid is even more of a problem. This vitamin is an essential cofactor in the hydroxylation reactions and therefore has been incorporated into culture medium as a widely accepted convention. Recent studies, however, have indicated that this substance can stimulate collagen production in vitro independent of the hydroxylation of proline and lysine.[73]

The Modulation of Collagen Synthesis. The substances that have been reported to affect this fibroblast function are many and varied (Table 78–5), and a simple classification is not possible. However, we will begin with the physiologic control of collagen synthesis and proceed to discuss the pharmacologic agents that affect this phenomenon and finally will discuss the factors that are derived from inflammatory cells.

Perhaps the most interesting observation on factors physiologically controlling collagen biosynthesis is that the amino terminal propeptide of the $\alpha1(I)$ and $\alpha1(III)$

chains (derived from the native procollagen molecules) inhibit the synthesis of collagen in a cell-free system as well as by cultured fibroblasts, suggesting that the effect is exerted at the level of mRNA translation. These extension peptides are cleaved from the procollagen molecule in the extracellular space during normal processing of collagen and thus generate feedback inhibition of collagen biosynthesis.[74,75]

As mentioned above, the effect of ascorbate on collagen production recently has been redefined. Initially considered merely an essential cofactor for the post-translational hydroxylation of proline and lysine, ascorbate has been found specifically to increase collagen synthesis in a manner independent of its well-known role in the post-translational modification of the nascent chains.[73,76] The decrease in collagen biosynthesis in animals made deficient in ascorbate has not been dissociated from the preferential decrease in collagen biosynthesis associated with weight loss.[77]

There is ample experimental evidence which would indicate that 10 to 40 percent of newly synthesized collagen can be wasted by intracellular degradation. It appears as if this event is related to lysosomal function, and this may be the site of the intracellular degradation. It has been speculated that this process may provide a mechanism for the cell to dispose of structurally imperfect collagen chains. Recent observations on the relationship between collagen production and intracellular levels of cAMP have provided some fundamental insight. Agents that increase intracellular cAMP (including dibutyryl-cAMP and beta-adrenergic agonists such as isoproterenol) cause a significant suppression of collagen production by fibroblasts.[80] This effect is linked to the rate of intracellular wastage of collagen, and this may be the major mechanism of this effect. This suppression of collagen production is type selective in that it occurs at the expense of type I collagen.[78,79] Alterations of collagen deposition mediated by intracellular cAMP may be one way in which the qualitative abnormalities of fibrosis-related collagen could be effected. One agent that stimulates intracellular cAMP is PGE_2. This is of interest because fibroblasts produce this substance, and one could hypothesize a feedback inhibition loop involving PGE_2. In fact, it has been shown that bradykinin these investigators was a rapidly progressive illness,[124] and the term IPF includes these patients as well as those with less fulminant disease.[125] The term cryptogenic fibrosing alveolitis is still commonly used in Great Britain,[126] and it reminds us of the prominent inflammatory component of the disorder. Desquamative interstitial pneumonitis (DIP) refers to an interstitial lung disease with a prominent intra-alveolar inflammatory infiltrate and contrasts with the usual interstitial pneumonitis (UIP) in which there is little inflammation but a prevalence of fibrosis.[127] Most investigators now believe that UIP and DIP are different stages in the same disease.

The disease presents subjectively with breathlessness and a nonproductive cough. These symptoms are often accompanied by systemic complaints such as weight loss, fever, malaise, and arthralgias. With the exception of digital clubbing, the physical findings are limited to the chest. Diffuse rales and rhonchi are heard in the early stages and as the disease progresses, dry, crackling rales are classically heard. In these later stages, signs of pulmonary hypertension (augmented P2) and right-sided heart failure are observed.

Laboratory evaluation reveals an elevated ESR in almost all patients. In addition, serum immunoglobulins are often elevated, and cryoglobulins are sometimes positive. Of particular interest to the rheumatologist is the significant incidence of positive antinuclear antibodies in IPF.[128] Circulating immune complexes have been found.[129] These clinical observations have led many to believe that IPF is an immune-mediated disease. Therefore, these patients are often referred to the rheumatologist to "rule out" a connective tissue disease.

Physiologically, these patients have normal indicators of airways resistance but have a depressed total lung volume and diffusion capacity. Resting hypoxia with mild hypocapnia and an exercise-induced impairment of gas exchange are the rule in IPF. Recent findings have indicated that these physiologic studies do not necessarily correlate well with the histologic features of increased cellularity and fibrosis.[130,131] Early in the disease the chest roentgenogram may have a diffuse, hazy ground-glass appearance or may have a reticulonodular pattern. In the later stages, the classic "honeycomb lung" fibrotic appearance is observed.

Open lung biopsy has been the mainstay of diagnosis in IPF. Histologic examination of lung invariably reveals thickening of the alveolar septa with fibrosis. In addition, alveolitis, manifest by infiltration of the interstitium with inflammatory cells with or without desquamation, occurs in a somewhat patchy manner.[125,131] In later stages, the inflammatory component becomes less prominent and fibrosis prevails.

Recently, investigators have emphasized the need for diagnostic procedures for the categorization and assessment of the severity of IPF. One of these is the use of bronchoscopy with lavage of the alveoli and analysis of the cellular content of the bronchoalveolar lavage fluid. The cellularity of this fluid is increased during the inflammatory phase of this disease and patients with IPF (as well as pulmonary fibrosis associated with connective tissue disease) demonstrate a relative increase in neutrophils, whereas patients with sarcoidosis and hypersensitivity pneumonitis have a relative increase in lymphocytes.[132,133] Gallium scanning has become popular in the evaluation and follow-up of these diseases. The radioisotope localizes in areas of inflammation, and methods are available for quantification of the uptake of gallium by the lung. These techniques probably do not add much to the initial evaluation of IPF but may provide a means of assessing progression of the disease and response to therapy.[125,131]

Therapy of IPF includes the early institution of glucocorticoids. Only about half the patients will experience a satisfactory response. Attempts have been made to correlate certain clinical parameters with a favorable response to steroids.[134] It seems logical that the fibrotic component is irreversible and that the effect of therapy is directed at the inflammatory component.[127] This concept is supported somewhat by the fact that patients tend to respond more frequently if therapy is initiated early in the disease and that patients with a significant amount of fibrosis are much less likely to respond. However, many patients fail to respond despite early therapy, and the reasons for this are not exactly clear. In one study, an increase in lymphocytes in the bronchoalveolar lavage fluid was associated with a favorable response, whereas an increase in neutrophils or eosinophils was associated with an unfavorable response.[135] The use of cytotoxic agents is controversial, but it is relatively common practice to add azathioprine to the regimen, and this agent has been reported to be of benefit.[136]

Pulmonary Fibrosis as a Manifestation of Systemic Connective Tissue Diseases. This is the most common setting in which the rheumatologist will encounter interstitial lung disease. It can be a manifestation of rheumatoid arthritis,[137,138] systemic lupus erythematosus,[139,140] progressive systemic sclerosis,[141,142] and dermatopolymyositis.[143,144] Most investigators agree that the interstitial pulmonary disease associated with these systemic disorders is virtually indistinguishable from IPF, as the clinical and pathologic pictures are very similar. Like IPF, the alveolitis tends to be primarily a neutrophil response.[125] The therapeutic approach is the same as for IPF, although the patients with an underlying connective tissue disease are less likely to respond to corticosteroids. Agents such as D-penicillamine and methotrexate[145,146] have been used in these conditions, although these drugs themselves have been reported to cause interstitial lung disease.[147,148] Proline analogues have been shown to have a beneficial effect on pulmonary fibrosis in animal models,[90,91] but their safety and efficacy are untested in humans. This class of compounds might eventually provide a new therapeutic approach to pulmonary fibrosis and fibrotic disorders in general.

Drug-Induced Pulmonary Fibrosis and the Rheumatologist. The spectrum of drugs reported to induce interstitial pulmonary fibrosis is vast and beyond the scope of this chapter. Certain of these drugs, however, are commonly used by rheumatologists and include gold,

D-penicillamine, methotrexate, chlorambucil, and cyclophosphamide.[147-151] Generally speaking, the clinical pattern is similar to that described above. This usually presents a perplexing problem to the clinician in that it is sometimes uncertain whether the pulmonary condition is due to the underlying disease or to the therapeutic agent. However, the withdrawal of a potentially offending agent is always warranted, considering the lack of specific therapy for the lung disease.

FIBROTIC LIVER DISEASE

The liver is the parenchymal organ most commonly diseased in a fibrotic disorder. The obvious reason for this is the prevalence of alcoholic liver disease in our society. This entity will not be discussed in this chapter. There are, however, certain chronic fibrotic disorders of the liver of special interest to rheumatologists. These include chronic active hepatitis, primary biliary cirrhosis, and sclerosing cholangitis, each of which has features in common with connective tissue diseases.[152]

Chronic Active Liver Disease. This term includes a spectrum of disorders characterized by chronic inflammation of the liver followed by a fibrotic response. Most of the cases that fall into this category are related to viral hepatitis (both hepatitis B and non-A–non-B hepatitis). A small group of patients with chronic active liver disease (CALD) have a disease characterized by chronic hepatitis, immunologic abnormalities, and extrahepatic manifestations.[153] This subgroup was once called "lupoid hepatitis," but this term has fallen into disfavor[154] and has been replaced by the terms "autoimmune chronic hepatitis" or "chronic active hepatitis of unknown etiology." These patients are mostly young and middle-aged females who present with signs and symptoms of acute hepatitis. Extrahepatic manifestations are not infrequent and arthritis/arthralgias occur in as many as 25 percent of these patients. Other manifestations include skin rash, pleuropericarditis, fever, chronic diarrhea, and interstitial pulmonary disease. Laboratory evaluation suggests an immune-mediated disease. LE cells are positive in 10 to 20 percent (hence the term "lupoid hepatitis"), and a diffuse elevation of immunoglobulins is found in most of the patients. In addition, autoantibodies, including ANA and anti–smooth muscle antibodies, are present in a majority of patients. Thus, the overlap with SLE is significant and the distinction may not be clear. The major distinguishing characteristic is the prominence of liver involvement.

If left untreated, these patients progress to fibrotic liver disease, but the response to corticosteroids is more favorable in this group when compared with other subgroups of CALD.[155]

Primary Biliary Cirrhosis. Primary biliary cirrhosis (PBC) is a progressive hepatic disease in which symptoms and signs of cholestasis result from an inflammatory and fibrotic reaction of the intrahepatic bile ducts.[156,157] The overwhelming majority of the patients are female (90 percent) and most are middle-aged. The most common presenting symptom is pruritus secondary to cholestasis. The serum cholesterol is elevated and leads to the formation of xanthomata. The disease progresses to cirrhosis with jaundice, portal hypertension, and hepatic failure.

There is an abundance of circumstantial evidence pointing toward immune mechanisms in the pathogenesis of this disease. Serum immunoglobulins (especially IgM) are elevated, and the hallmark of diagnosis is the presence of antimitochondrial antibody in the serum. Circulating immune complexes have been found, and other abnormal antibodies are often present, including ANA, rheumatoid factor, and anti–smooth muscle antibody. More circumstantial evidence is provided by the association with certain immunologic and connective tissue diseases.[156,157] Sjögren's syndrome (SS) has been reported with incidences ranging from 5 to 100 percent, and it is probable that more than half these patients have SS. In addition, a significant number of patients with PBC have either rheumatoid arthritis, PSS, or CREST syndrome.[152,156-159]

Of further interest to the rheumatologist is the frequent occurrence of metabolic bone disease. This is generally manifest as bone pain, and it has been reported that 20 percent of patients will experience vertebral collapse. Osteomalacia occurs as a result of insufficient absorption of vitamin D and calcium. Cholestasis leads to insufficient bile salts in the intestine and results in excessive intestinal fat, which complexes with calcium, preventing its absorption. The relative vitamin D deficiency is presumably due to impaired absorption (secondary to insufficient intestinal bile salts) and impaired hepatic conversion to 25-hydroxy-vitamin D.[160,161] Osteoporosis also occurs, although not as frequently as osteomalacia.

Treatment is mostly supportive, with dietary supplementation of medium-chain triglycerides and vitamin D and calcium. The pruritus is controlled with cholestyramine. Corticosteroids and azothioprine are ineffective.[162] The massive increase in hepatic copper content has led investigators to use D-penicillamine in PBC, and some benefit has been reported but side effects are limiting.[163] This agent may also act by affecting the immune system.

Sclerosing Cholangitis. This is an unusual disorder in which chronic inflammation and subsequent fibrosis occur in the extrahepatic biliary tree. More than half the cases are associated with inflammatory bowel disease (usually ulcerative proctocolitis), and there is some association with retroperitoneal fibrosis. Serum immunoglobulins (IgM) are often elevated, suggesting an immunologic role. The disease is progressive and leads to biliary cirrhosis. There is no known effective therapy.[164]

DUPUYTREN'S CONTRACTURE

This condition is characterized by a nodular thickening of the palmar fascia and contraction of the fourth and fifth digits. It is associated with alcoholic liver disease and epilepsy and often is familial. Its association with other localized fibroses (e.g., plantar fasciitis and Peyronie's disease) has led to the concept of a "Dupuytren's diathesis."[165]

Pathologically, there is a thickening of the palmar fascia, resulting in a shortened fascia without an apparent inflammatory reaction. The thickening takes the form of a firm fibrous band or of a nodular, fusiform area.[166,170] This tissue has been the subject of microscopic and biochemical analysis. The total collagen content is increased, and about 25 percent of the collagen is type III, which is not normally present in fascia. In addition, the content of hydroxylysine is elevated, as are reducible crosslinks. These observations indicate a clear-cut abnormality of the collagen present in the abnormal fascia. Of further interest is the presence of myofibroblasts (contractile smooth-muscle-like cells) in these nodules. It has been hypothesized that the contraction of the fascia is related to the presence of these contractile cells, which may be responsible for excessive production of type III collagen.[69,70,166]

KELOIDS

Keloids are exaggerated hypertropic scars seen frequently in black patients. If the steps in fibrosis parallel those in wound healing as we have proposed, then keloid formation represents wound healing in which the control mechanisms are abnormal. The dermis is hypercellular, and the collagen content is increased.[168] The rate of collagen synthesis by keloid tissue is increased.[169] There have been conflicting reports on the behavior of keloid fibroblasts in culture. Diegelmann and colleagues have found that keloid fibroblasts exhibit an enhanced rate of collagen production in vitro, but growth kinetics were not different from control cells.[170] Later studies by these investigators have characterized the relative amounts of types I and III collagen secreted by these fibroblasts and found the ratio of type I to III to be the same as that found in control dermal fibroblasts.[171] Russell and co-workers have reported that keloid fibroblasts synthesize collagen at a normal rate but exhibit an abnormal response to certain exogenous stimuli, such as the inhibition of collagen production by glucocorticoids.[172] It is an attractive hypothesis that the basic abnormality in keloid formation involves control mechanism(s) that turn off collagen synthesis.

RETROPERITONEAL FIBROSIS

Retroperitoneal fibrosis (RPF) is a disorder in which the retroperitoneal fat is the site of a subacute and chronic inflammatory reaction and is subsequently replaced by dense fibrotic tissue. It can be secondary to a malignancy (primary or metastatic retroperitoneal tumor, serotonin-producing carcinoid), retroperitoneal injury (trauma, hemorrhage, etc.), or drug ingestion (methysergide, hydralazine), or it can be idiopathic. The presentation is that of flank and abdominal pain. Systemic symptoms are common and include malaise, weight loss, and fever. As the disease progresses, the results of compression of retroperitoneal structures becomes clinically apparent and include anuria and azotemia, the Leriche syndrome, constipation, and hypertension from obstruction of the renal artery. Laboratory abnormalities include a mild anemia, marked elevation of the sedimentation rate and other acute phase reactants, hypoalbuminemia, and hyperglobulinemia. The diagnosis is made by the demonstration of a retroperitoneal mass that displaces the normal anatomic structures. Classically this is accomplished by an IVP, which reveals narrowing of the ureters at the L4-L5 level, medial displacement of the ureters, and dilatation of the calyceal system. More recently, ultrasound and computerized tomography have been used to demonstrate the anatomic abnormalities.

The natural course of the disease is variable, and spontaneous remission is not uncommon. The major therapeutic modality is surgery, with release of the ureters from the fibrotic mass. Surgery is often indicated for pathologic confirmation of the diagnosis. The use of glucocorticoids is controversial, but their benefit has been reported and a course of steroids is indicated in conjunction with the surgical procedure.[173,174]

A discussion of RPF includes the topic of drug-induced fibrotic disorders due to the association of RPF with ergot alkaloids. These drugs are infrequently used now, but fibrotic disorders have been associated with beta-adrenergic blocking agents, especially practolol.[16-19] With the increased clinical use of these agents and the introduction of new drugs within this class of agents, clinicians should be aware of this association.

OTHER LOCALIZED FIBROSES

Carcinoid tumors are associated with localized fibrosis. The pathogenesis is possibly related to the release of vasoactive substances from the tumor, but the understanding of pathogenesis is far from complete. The most familiar of these is the association of endocardial fibrosis with metastatic carcinoids. Right-sided valvular involvement occurs with liver metastases, and left-sided cardiac involvement is associated with lung metastases.[175] RPF has been associated with carcinoid tumors.[176]

Peyronie's disease is a fibrotic disorder involving the shaft of the penis that results in pain and discomfort with difficulty in sexual function. It tends to occur in conjunction with other localized fibroses (Dupuytren's contracture)[177,178] and has been associated with beta-adrenergic blocking agents.[18,179,180]

Pseudotumor of the orbit is a rare fibrotic disorder in which orbital inflammation and fibrosis result in a protrusion of the eye.[181] This disorder has also been reported to occur in association with other localized fibroses as well as with polyarteritis nodosa.[21,182,183]

Reidel's struma is a condition in which fibrotic tissue

replaces normal thyroid gland and extends beyond the thyroid to involve other strucures in the neck.[184] Like some of the diseases mentioned above, Reidel's struma occurs in association with other fibroses, including RPF,[185] sclerosing cholangitis,[186] and pseudotumor of the orbit.[182]

References

1. Schilling, J.A.: Wound healing. Surg. Clin. North Am. 56:859, 1976.
2. Shoshan, S.: Wound healing. Int. Rev. Conn. Tiss. Res. 9:1, 1981.
3. Ross, R., and Benditt, E.P.: Wound healing and collagen formation. 1. Sequential changes in components of guinea pig skin wounds observed in the electron microscope. J. Biophys. Biochem. Cytol. 11:677, 1961.
4. Simpson, D.M., and Ross, R.: The neutrophilic leukocyte in wound repair: A study with antineutrophil serum. J. Clin. Invest. 51:2009, 1972.
5. Leibovich, S.J., and Ross, R.: The role of the macrophage in wound repair: A study with hydrocortisone and antimacrophage serum. Am. J. Pathol. 78:71, 1975.
6. Diegelmann, R.F., Cohen, I.K., and Kaplan, A.M.: The role of macrophages in wound repair: A review. Plast. Reconstr. Surg. 68:107, 1981.
7. Knighton, D.R., Hunt, T.K., Thakral, K.K., and Goodson, W.H.: Role of platelets and fibrin in wound healing: An in vivo study of angiogenesis and collagen synthesis. Ann. Surg. 196:379, 1982.
8. Thakral, K.K., Goodson, W.H., and Hunt, T.K.: Stimulation of wound blood vessel growth by wound macrophages. J. Surg. Res. 26:430, 1979.
9. Polverini, P.J., Cotran, R.Z., Gimbrone, M.A., and Unanue, E.R.: Activated macrophages induce vascular proliferation. Nature (London) 269:804, 1977.
10. Madden, J.W., and Peacock, E.E., Jr.: Studies on the biology of collagen during wound healing. I. Rate of collagen synthesis and deposition in cutaneous wounds of the rat. Surgery 64:288, 1968.
11. Mussini, E., Hutton, J.J., and Udenfriend, S.: Collagen proline hydroxylase in wound healing, granuloma formation, scurvy, and growth. Science 157:927, 1967.
12. Stein, H.D., and Keiser, H.R.: Collagen metabolism in granulating wounds. J. Surg. Res. 11:277, 1971.
13. Cohen, I.K., Moore, C.D., and Diegelmann, R.F.: Onset and localization of collagen synthesis during wound healing in open rat skin. Proc. Soc. Exp. Biol. Med. 160:459, 1979.
14. Arem, A.J., Misiorowski, R., and Chvapil, M.: Effect of low-dose BAPN on wound healing. J. Surg. Res. 27:228, 1979.
15. Vater, C.A., Harris, E.D., Jr., and Siegel, R.C.: Native cross links in collagen fibrils induce resistance to human synovial collagenase. Biochem. J. 181;639, 1979.
16. Pierce, J.R., Jr., Trostle, D.C., and Warner, J.J.: Propranolol and retroperitoneal fibrosis. Ann. Intern. Med. 95:244, 1981.
17. Marshall, A.J., Bradley, H., Davies, J.D., Lee, R.F.J., Low-Beer, J.S., and Read, A.E.: A study of practolol peritonitis. Quart. J. Med. 46:135, 1977.
18. Osborne, D.R.: Propranolol and Peyronie's disease. Lancet 2:1111, 1977.
19. Musk, A.W., and Pollard, J.A.: Pindolol and pulmonary fibrosis. Br. Med. J. 2(6190):581, 1979.
20. Early, P.F.: Population studies in Dupuytren's contracture. J. Bone Joint Surg. 43B:602, 1962.
21. Comings, D.E., Skubi, K.B., Van Eyes, J., and Motulsky, A.: Familial multifocal fibrosclerosis. Ann. Intern. Med. 66:884, 1967.
22. Niewoehner, D.E., and Hoidal, J.R.: Lung fibrosis and emphysema: Divergent responses to a common injury. Science 217:359, 1982.
23. Baum, J.L.: Source of the fibroblast in central corneal wound healing. Arch. Ophthalmol. 85:473, 1971.
24. Postlethwaite, A.E., Snyderman, R., and Kang, A.H.: Generation of a fibroblast chemotactic factor from serum by the activation of complement. J. Clin. Invest. 64:1379, 1979.
25. Postlethwaite, A.E., Snyderman, R., and Kang, A.H.: The chemotactic attraction of human fibroblasts to a lymphocyte-derived factor. J. Exp. Med. 144:1188, 1976.
26. Postlethwaite, A.E., Keski-Oja, G., Balian, G., and Kang, A.H.: Induction of fibroblast chemotaxis by fibronectin: Localization of the chemotactic region to a 140,000-molecular weight non-gelatin binding fragment. J. Exp. Med. 153:494, 1981.
27. Senior, R.A., Griffin, G.L., and Mecham, R.P.: Chemotactic responses of fibroblasts to tropoelastin and elastin-derived peptides. J. Clin. Invest. 70:614, 1982.
28. Postlethwaite, A.E., Seyer, J.M., and Kang, A.E.: Chemotactic attraction of human fibroblasts to type I, II, and III collagens and collagen-derived peptides. Proc. Natl. Acad. Sci. USA 75:871, 1978.

29. Gauss-Muller, V., Kleinman, H.K., Martin, G.R., and Schiffman, E.: Role of attachment and attractants in fibroblast chemotaxis. J. Lab. Clin. Med. 96:1076, 1980.
30. Rennard, S.I., Hunninghake, G.W., Bitterman, P.B., and Crystal, R.G.: Production of fibronectin by the human alveolar macrophage. Mechanism for the recruitment of fibroblasts to sites of tissue injury in interstitial lung disease. Proc. Natl. Acad. Sci. USA 78:7147, 1981.
31. Werb, Z., and Gordon, S.: Secretion of a specific collagenase by stimulated macrophages. J. Exp. Med. 142:346, 1975.
32. Mainardi, C.L., Seyer, J.M., and Kang, A.H.: Type-specific collagenase: A type V collagen degrading enzyme from macrophages. Biochem. Biophys. Res. Comm. 97:1108–1117, 1980.
33. Seppä, H., Grotendorst, G., Seppä, S., et al.: Platelet-derived growth factor is chemotactic for fibroblasts. J. Cell Biol. 921:584, 1982.
34. Stiles, G.D., Capone, G.T., Scher, C.D., Antoniades, H.N., Van Wyk, J.J., and Pledger, W.J.: Dual control of cell growth by somatomedins and platelet-derived growth factor. Proc. Natl. Acad. Sci. USA 76:1279, 1979.
35. Lemmon, S.K., Riley, M.C., Thomas, K.A., Hoover, G.A., Maciag, T., and Bradshaw, R.A.: Bovine fibroblast growth factor: Comparison of brain and pituitary preparations. J. Cell Biol. 95:162, 1982.
36. Gospodarowicz, D., Lui, G-M., and Cheng, J.: Purification in high yield of brain fibroblast growth factor by preparative isoelectric focusing at pH 9.6. J. Biol. Chem. 257:12266, 1982.
37. Rutherford, R.B., and Ross, R.: Platelet factors stimulate fibroblasts and smooth muscle cells quiescent in plasma serum to proliferate. J. Cell Biol. 69:196, 1976.
38. Antoniades, H.N., Scher, C.D., and Stiles, G.D.: Purification of human platelet-derived growth factor. Proc. Natl. Acad. Sci. USA 76:1809, 1979.
39. Antoniades, H.N.: Human platelet–derived growth factor (PDGF): purification of PDGF-I and PDGF-II and separation of their reduced subunits. Proc. Natl. Acad. Sci. USA 78:7314, 1981.
40. Leibovich, S.J., and Ross, R.: A macrophage-dependent factor that stimulates the proliferation of fibroblasts in vitro. Am. J. Pathol. 84:501, 1976.
41. DeLustro, F., and LeRoy, E.C.: Characterization of the release of human monocyte regulators of fibroblast proliferation. J. Reticuloendothel. Soc. 31:295, 1982.
42. Korn, J.H., Halushka, P.V., and LeRoy, E.C.: Mononuclear cell modulation of connective tissue function: suppression of fibroblast growth by stimulation of endogenous prostaglandin production. J. Clin. Invest. 65:543, 1980.
43. Postlethwaite, A.E., and Kang, A.H.: Induction of fibroblast proliferation by human mononuclear leukocyte-derived protein. Arthritis Rheum. 26:22, 1983.
44. Wahl, S.M., and Gately, C.L.: Modulation of fibroblast growth by a lymphokine of human T-cell and continuous T-cell line origin. J. Immunol. 130:1226, 1983.
45. Wahl, S.M., Wahl, L.M., and McCarthy, J.B.: Lymphocyte-mediated activation of fibroblast proliferation and collagen production. J. Immunol. 121:942, 1978.
46. Postlethwaite, A.E., and Kang, A.H.: Characterization of fibroblast proliferation factor elaborated by antigen- and mitogen-stimulated guinea pig lymph node cells: Differentiation from lymphocyte-derived chemotactic factor for fibroblasts, lymphocyte mitogenic factor, and Interleukin 1. Cell. Immunol. 73:169, 1982.
47. Schmidt, J.A., Mizel, S.B., Cohen, D., and Green, I.: Interleukin 1, a potential regulator of fibroblast proliferation. J. Immunol 128:2177, 1982.
48. Bitterman, P.B., Rennard, S.I., Hunninghake, G.W., and Crystal, R.G.: Human alveolar macrophage growth factor for fibroblasts: regulation and partial characterization. J. Clin. Invest. 70:806, 1982.
49. Ruoslahti, E., Pierschbacher, M., Engvall, E., Oldberg, A., and Hayman, E.G.: Molecular and biological interactions of fibronectin. J. Invest. Dermatol. 79:65s, 1982.
50. Klebe, R.J.: Isolation of a collagen-dependent cell attachment factor. Nature(London) 250:241, 1974.
51. Hahn, L.E., and Yamada, K.M.: Isolation of a collagen-binding fragment of the adhesive glycoprotein fibronectin. Proc. Natl. Acad. Sci. USA 76:1160, 1979.
52. Hahn, L.E., and Yamada, K.M.: Isolation and characterization of active fragments of the adhesive glycoprotein fibronectin. Cell 18:1043, 1979.
53. Balian, G., Click, E.M., Crouch, E., Davidson, J.M., and Bornstein, P.: Isolation of a collagen-binding fragment from fibronectin and cold-insoluble globulin. J. Biol. Chem. 254:1429, 1979.
54. Toole, B.P., and Gross, J.: The extracellular matrix of the regenerating newt limb: Synthesis and removal of hyaluronate prior to differentiation. Dev. Biol. 25:57, 1971.
55. Toole, B.P., and Trelstad, R.L.: Hyaluronate production and removal during cornea development in the chick. Dev. Biol. 26:28, 1971.
56. Bertolami, C.N., and Donoff, R.B.: Hyaluronidase activity during open

wound healing in rabbits: a preliminary report. J. Surg. Res. 25:256, 1978.

57. Bentley, J.P.: Rate of chondroitin sulfate formation in wound healing. Ann. Surg. 165:186, 1967.

58. Collins, J.F., McCullough, B., Coalson, J.J., and Johanson, W.G., Jr.: Bleomycin-induced pulmonary fibrosis in baboons. II. Further studies on connective tissue changes. Am. Rev. Resp. Dis. 125:305, 1981.

59. Last, J.A., Greenberg, D.B., and Castleman, W.L.: Ozone-induced alterations in collagen metabolism of rat lungs. Toxicol. Appl. Pharmacol. 51:241, 1979.

60. LeRoy, E.C.: Connective tissue synthesis by scleroderma skin fibroblasts in cell culture. J. Exp. Med. 135:1351, 1972.

61. LeRoy, E.C.: Increased collagen synthesis by scleroderma skin fibroblasts in vitro. J. Clin. Invest. 54:880, 1974.

62. Uitto, J., Bauer, E.A., and Eisen, A.Z.: Increased biosynthesis of triple-helical type I and type III procollagens associated with unaltered expression of collagenase by skin fibroblasts in culture. J. Clin. Invest. 64:921, 1979.

63. Buckingham, R.B., Prince, R.K., Rodnan, G.P., and Taylor, F.: Increased collagen accumulation in dermal fibroblast cultures from patients with progressive systemic sclerosis. J. Lab. Clin. Med. 92:5, 1978.

64. Seyer, J.M., Hutcheson, E.T., and Kang, A.H.: Collagen polymorphism in idiopathic chronic pulmonary fibrosis. J. Clin. Invest. 57:1498, 1976.

65. Fulmer, J.D., Bienkowski, R.S., Cowan, M.J., Breul, S.D., Bradley, K.M., Ferrans, V.J., Roberts, W.C., and Crystal, R.G.: Collagen concentration and rates of synthesis in idiopathic pulmonary fibrosis. Am. Rev. Resp. Dis. 12:289, 1980.

66. Madri, J.A., and Furthmayer, H.: Collagen polymorphism in the lung: An immunochemical study of pulmonary fibrosis. Hum. Pathol. 11:353, 1980.

67. Seyer, J.M., Hutcheson, E.T., and Kang, A.H.: Collagen polymorphism in normal and cirrhotic human liver. J. Clin. Invest. 59:241, 1977.

68. Seyer, J.M., Kang, A.H., and Rodnan, G.: Investigation of type I and type III collagens of the lung in progressive systemic sclerosis. Arthritis Rheum. 24:625, 1981.

69. Brickley-Parsons, D., Glimcher, M.J., Smith, R., Albin, R., and Adams, J.P.: Biochemical changes in the collagen of the palmar fascia in patients with Dupuytren's disease. J. Bone Joint Surg. 63-A:787, 1981.

70. Bailey, A.J., Sims, T.J., Gabbiani, G., Bazin, S., and LeLouis, M.: Collagen of Dupuytren's disease. Clin. Sci. 53:499, 1977.

71. Peterkovsky, B., and Diegelmann, R.F.: Use of a mixture of proteinase-free collagenases for the specific assay of radioactive collagen in the presence of other proteins. Biochemistry 10:988, 1971.

72. Juva, K., and Prockop, D.J.: Modified procedure for the assay of 3H or 14C labelled hydroxyproline. Ann. Biochem. 15:77, 1966.

73. Murad, S., Grove, D., Lindberg, K.A., Reynolds, G., Sivarajah, A., and Pinnell, S.R.: Regulation of collagen synthesis by ascorbic acid. Proc. Natl. Acad. Sci. USA 78:2879, 1981.

74. Wiestner, M., Krieg, T., Horlein, D., Glanville, R.W., Fietzek, P., and Muller, P.K.: Inhibiting effect of procollagen peptides on collagen biosynthesis in fibroblast culture. J. Biol. Chem. 254:7016, 1979.

75. Paglia, L.M., Wilczek, J., Diaz de Leon, L., Martin, G.R., Horlein, D., and Muller, P.K.: Inhibition of procollagen cell-free synthesis by amino-terminal extension peptides. Biochemistry 18:5030, 1979.

76. Pinnell, S.R.: Regulation of collagen synthesis. J. Invest. Dermatol. 79:73s, 1982.

77. Chojkier, M., Spanheimer, R.G., and Peterkofsky, B.: Dissociation of the effects of in vivo ascorbate deficiency on collagen biosynthesis and proline hydroxylation. Clin. Res. 31:240A, 1983.

78. Berg, R.A., Schwartz, M.L., and Crystal, R.G.: Regulation of the production of secretory proteins: Intracellular degradation of newly synthesized "defective" collagen. Proc. Natl. Acad. Sci. 77:4746, 1980.

79. Rennard, S.I., Stier, L.E., and Crystal, R.G.: Intracellular degradation of newly synthesized collagen. J. Invest. Dermatol. 79:77s, 1982.

80. Berg, R.A., Moss, J., Baum, B.J., and Crystal, R.G.: Regulation of collagen synthesis by the β-adrenergic system. J. Clin. Invest. 67:1457, 1981.

81. Goldstein, R.H., and Polgar, P.: The effect and interaction of bradykinin and prostaglandins on protein and collagen production by lung fibroblasts. J. Biol. Chem. 257:8630, 1982.

82. Ponec, M., Klempennaar, J.A., Van Der Meulen-Van Harskamp., G.A., and Bachra, B.N.: Effects of glucocorticosteroids in cultured human skin fibroblasts. IV. Specific decrease in the synthesis of collagen but no effect on its hydroxylation. Biochem. Pharmacol. 28:2777, 1979.

83. Roskowski, R.J., Sheehy, J., and Cutroneo, K.R.: Glucocorticoid-mediated selective reduction of functioning collagen messenger ribonucleic acid. Arch. Biochem. Biophys. 210:74, 1981.

84. Verbruggen, L.A., and Abe, S.: Glucocorticoids alter the ratio of type III/type I collagen synthesis by mouse dermal fibroblasts. Biochem. Pharmacol. 31:1711, 1982.

85. Sterling, K.M., DiPetrillo, T., Cutroneo, K.R., and Prestayko, A.: Inhibition of collagen accumulation in rat lungs after intratracheal bleomycin instillation. Cancer Res. 42:405, 1982.

86. Thrall, R.S., McCormick, J.R., Jack, R.M., McReynolds, R.A., and Ward, P.A.: Bleomycin-induced pulmonary fibrosis in the rat. Am. J. Pathol. 95:117, 1979.

87. Rudders, R.A., and Hensley, G.T.: Bleomycin pulmonary toxicity. Chest 63:626, 1973.

88. Sterling, K.M., DiPetrillo, T.A., Kotch, J.P., and Cutroneo, K.R.: Bleomycin-induced increase of collagen turnover in IMR-90 fibroblasts: An in vitro model of connective tissue restructuring during lung fibrosis. Cancer Res. 42:3502, 1982.

89. Uitto, J., Tan, E.M.L., and Ryhanen, L.: Inhibition of collagen accumulation in fibrotic processes: review of pharmacologic agents and new approaches with amino acids and their analogues. J. Invest. Dermatol. 79:113s, 1982.

90. Kelley, J., Newman, R.A., and Evans, J.N.: Bleomycin-induced pulmonary fibrosis in the rat. Prevention with an inhibitor of collagen synthesis. J. Lab. Clin. Med. 96:954, 1980.

91. Riley, D.J., Kerr, J.S., Berg, R.A., Ianni, B.D., Pietra, G.G., Edelman, N.H., and Prockop, D.J.: Prevention of bleomycin-induced pulmonary fibrosis in the hamster by cis-4-hydroxy-L-proline. Am. Rev. Respir. Dis. 123:388, 1981.

92. Castor, C.W.: Synovial cell activation induced by a polypeptide mediator. Ann. N.Y. Acad. Sci. 256:304, 1975.

93. Castor, C.W., Ritchie, J.C., Scott, M.E., and Whitney, S.L.: Connective tissue activation. XI. Stimulation of glycosaminoglycan and DNA formation by a platelet factor. Arthritis Rheum. 20:859, 1977.

94. Myers, S.L., and Castor, C.W.: Connective tissue activation. XV. Stimulation of glycosaminoglycan and DNA synthesis by a polymorphonuclear leukocyte factor. Arthritis Rheum. 23:556, 1980.

95. Castor, C.W., and Pek, S.: Connective tissue activation. XX. Stimulation of prostaglandin secretion by mediators from lymphocytes (CTAP-I) and platelets (CTAP-III). Arthritis Rheum. 24:504, 1981.

96. Johnson, R.L., and Ziff, M.: Lymphokine stimulation of collagen accumulation. J. Clin. Invest. 58:240, 1976.

97. Jimenez, S.A., McArthur, W., and Rosenbloom, J.: Inhibition of collagen synthesis by mononuclear cell supernatants. J. Exp. Med. 150:1421, 1979.

98. Hibbs, M.S., Postlethwaite, A.E., Mainardi, C.L., Seyer, J.M., and Kang, A.H.: Alterations in collagen production in mixed mononuclear leukocyte-fibroblast cultures. J. Exp. Med. 157:47, 1983.

99. Wahl, S.M., Wahl, L.M., and McCarthy, J.B.: Lymphocyte-mediated activation of fibroblast proliferation and collagen production. J. Immunol. 121:942, 1978.

100. Nielson, E.G., Jimenez, S.A., and Phillips, S.M.: Cell-mediated immunity in interstitial nephritis. III. T lymphocyte–mediated fibroblast proliferation and collagen synthesis. An immune mechanism for renal fibrogenesis. J. Immunol. 125:1708, 1980.

101. Postlethwaite, A.E., Smith, G.N., Mainardi, C.L., Seyer, J.M., and Kang, A.H.: Characterization of a human lymphokine that stimulates fibroblasts to produce collagen. Arthritis Rheum. 24:S61, 1981.

102. Mizel, S.B., Dayer, J.-M., Krane, S.M., and Mergenhagen, S.E.: Stimulation of rheumatoid synovial collagenase and prostaglandin production by partially purified lymphocyte-activating factor (Interleukin 1). Proc. Natl. Acad. Sci. USA 78:2474, 1980.

103. Postlethwaite, A.E., Lachman, L.B., Mainardi, C.L., and Kang, A.H.: Interleukin 1 stimulation of collagenase production by cultured fibroblasts. J. Exp. Med. 157:801, 1983.

104. Postlethwaite, A.E., Lachman, L.B., and Kang, A.H.: Stimulation of fibroblast hyaluronate production by human Interleukin 1. Arthritis Rheum. (abstr.) 26:559, 1983.

105. Lazarus, G.S., Brown, R.S., Daniels, J.R., and Fullmer, H.M.: Human granulocyte collagenase. Science 159:1483, 1968.

106. Hibbs, M.S., Mainardi, C.L., and Kang, A.H.: Type-specific collagen degradation by eosinophils. Biochem. J. 207:621, 1982.

107. Gross, J.L., Moscatelli, D., Jaffe, E.A., and Rifkin, D.B.: Plasminogen activator and collagenase production by cultured capillary endothelial cells. J. Cell. Biol. 95:974, 1982.

108. Bauer, E.A., Stricklin, G.P., Jeffrey, J.J., and Eisen, A.Z.: Collagenase production by human skin fibroblasts. Biochem. Biophys. Res. Comm. 64:232, 1975.

109. Gadek, J.E., Kelman, J.A., Fells, G., Weinberger, S.E., Horwitz, A.L., Reynolds, H.Y., Fulmer, J.D., and Crystal, R.G.: Collagenase in the lower respiratory tract of patients with idiopathic pulmonary fibrosis. N. Engl. J. Med. 301:738, 1979.

110. Welgus, H.G., Jeffrey, J.J., and Eisen, A.Z.: The collagen substrate specificity of human skin collagenase. J. Biol. Chem. 256:9511, 1981.

111. Horwitz, A.L., Hance, A.J., and Crystal, R.G.: Granulocyte collagenase: Selective digestion of type I relative to type III collagen. Proc. Natl. Acad. Sci. USA 74:897, 1977.

112. Mainardi, C.L., Hasty, D.L., Seyer, J.M., and Kang, A.H.: Specific cleav-

age of type III collagen by human polymorphonuclear leukocyte elastase. J. Biol. Chem. 255:12006, 1980.

113. Mainardi, C.L., Dixit, S.N., Seyer, J.M., and Kang, A.H.: Type-specific collagen degradation. In Tsuchiya, M., Perez Tamayo, R., Okazaki, I., and Maruyama, K.: Collagen Degradation and Mammalian Collagenase. Amsterdam, Exerpta Medica, 1982, p. 41.

114. Okazaki, I., Maruyama, K., Kashiwazaki, K., Kamegaya, K., and Tsuchiya, M.: Hepatic collagenase activity in experimental hepatic fibrosis. Biochem. Exp. Biol. 12:129, 1976.

115. Maruyama, K., Feinman, L., Fainsilber, Z., Nakano, M., Okazaki, I., and Lieber, C.S.: Mammalian collagenase increases in early alcoholic liver disease and decreases with cirrhosis. Life Sci. 30:1379, 1982.

116. Werb, Z., Mainardi, C.L., Vater, C.A., and Harris, E.D., Jr.: Endogenous activation of latent collagenase by rheumatoid synovial cells: Evidence for a role of plasminogen activator. N. Engl. J. Med. 296:1027, 1977.

117. Werb, Z.: Biochemical actions of glucocorticoids on macrophages in culture. J. Exp. Med. 147:1695, 1978.

118. Crawford, S.W., Kang, A.H., and Mainardi, C.L.: Interstitial collagenase secretion and giant cell formation from rabbit alveolar macrophages: Effects of dexamethasone. Am. Rev. Respir. Dis. 127:46, 1983.

119. Brinckerhoff, C.E., McMillan, R.M., Dayer, J.-M., and Harris, E.D., Jr.: Inhibition by retinoic acid of collagenase production in rheumatoid synovial cells. N. Engl. J. Med. 303:432, 1980.

120. Brinckerhoff, C.E., McMillan, R.M., Fahey, J.V., and Harris, E.D., Jr.: Collagenase production by synovial fibroblasts treated with phorbol myristate acetate. Arthritis Rheum. 22:1109, 1979.

121. Delclos, K.B., and Blumberg, P.M.: Decrease in collagen production in normal and Rous sarcoma virus-transformed chick embryo fibroblasts induced by phorbol myristate acetate. Cancer Res. 39:1667, 1979.

122. Dayer, J.-M., Russell, R.G.G., and Krane, S.M.: Collagenase production by rheumatoid synovial cells: Stimulation by a human lymphocyte factor. Science 195:181, 1977.

123. Krane, S.M.: Collagenases and collagen degradation. J. Invest. Dermatol. 79:83s, 1982.

124. Hamman, L., and Rich, A.R.: Acute diffuse interstitial fibrosis of the lungs. Bull. Johns Hopkins Hosp. 74:177, 1944.

125. Crystal, R.G., Fulmer, J.D., Roberts, W.C., Moss, M.L., Line, B.R., and Reynolds, H.Y.: Idiopathic pulmonary fibrosis. Clinical, histologic, radiographic, physiologic, scintigraphic, cytologic, and biochemical aspects. Ann. Intern. Med. 85:769, 1976.

126. Turner-Warwick, M., Burrows, B., and Johnson, A.: Cryptogenic fibrosing alveolitis: clinical features and their influence on survival. Thorax 35:171, 1980.

127. Carrington, C.B., Gaensler, E.A., Coutu, R.E., FitzGerald, M.X., and Gupta, R.G.: Natural history and treated course of usual and desquamative interstitial pneumonia. N. Engl. J. Med. 298:802, 1978.

128. Nagaya, H., and Seiker, H.O.: Pathogenic mechanisms of interstitial pulmonary fibrosis in patients with serum antinuclear factor. A histologic and clinical correlation. Am. J. Med. 52:51, 1972.

129. Dreisin, R.B., Schwartz, M.I., Theophilopoulos, A.N., and Stanford, R.E.: Circulating immune complexes in idiopathic interstitial pneumonias. N. Engl. J. Med. 298:353, 1978.

130. Fulmer, J.D., Roberts, W.C., von Gal, E.R., and Crystal, R.G.: Morphologic-physiologic correlates of the severity of fibrosis and degree of cellularity in idiopathic pulmonary fibrosis. J. Clin. Invest. 63:665, 1979.

131. Crystal, R.G., Gadek, J.E., Ferrans, V.J., Fulmer, J.D., Line, B.R., and Hunninghake, G.W.: Interstitial lung disease: Current concepts of pathogenesis, staging, and therapy. Am. J. Med. 70:542, 1981.

132. Reynolds, H.Y., Fulmer, J.D., Kazmierowski, J.A., Roberts, W.C., Frank, M.M., and Crystal, R.G.: Analysis of cellular and protein content of broncho-alveolar lavage fluid from patients with idiopathic pulmonary fibrosis and chronic hypersensitivity pneumonitis. J. Clin. Invest. 59:165, 1977.

133. Weinberger, S.E., Kelman, J.A., Elson, N.A., Young, R.C., Reynolds, H.Y., Fulmer, J.D., and Crystal, R.G.: Bronchoalveolar lavage in interstitial lung disease. Ann. Intern. Med. 89:459, 1978.

134. Turner-Warwick, M., Burrows, B., and Johnson, A.: Cryptogenic fibrosing alveolitis: Response of corticosteroid therapy and its effect on survival. Thorax 35:593, 1980.

135. Rudd, R.M., Halsam, P.L., and Turner-Warwick, M.: Cryptogenic fibrosing alveolitis. Relationships of pulmonary physiology and bronchoalveolar lavage to response to treatment and prognosis. Am. Rev. Respir. Dis. 124:1, 1981.

136. Winterbauer, R.H., Hammar, S.P., Hallman, K.O., Hays, J.E., Pardee, N.E., Morgan, E.H., Allen, J., Moores, K.D., Bush, W., and Walker, J.: Diffuse interstitial pneumonitis: Clinicopathologic correlations in 20 patients treated with prednisone and azathioprine. Am. J. Med. 65:661, 1978.

137. Popper, M.S., Bogdonoff, M.L., and Hughes, R.L.: Interstitial rheumatoid lung disease: A reassessment and review of the literature. Chest 62:243, 1972.

138. Gordon, D.A., Stein, J.L., and Broder, I.: The extra-articular manifestations of rheumatoid arthritis: A systemic analysis of 127 cases. Am. J. Med. 54:445, 1973.

139. Gross, M., Esterly, J.R., and Earle, R.H.: Pulmonary alterations in systemic lupus erythematosus. Am. Rev. Respir. Dis. 105:572, 1972.

140. Eisenberg, H., Dubois, E.L., Sherwin, R.P., and Balchum, O.J.: Diffuse interstitial lung disease in systemic lupus erythematosus. Ann. Intern. Med. 79:37, 1973.

141. Spain, D.M., and Thomas, A.G.: The pulmonary manifestations of scleroderma: An anatomic-physiologic correlation. Ann. Intern. Med. 32:152, 1950.

142. Wilson, R.J., Rodnan, G.P., and Robin, E.D.: An early pulmonary physiologic abnormality in progressive systemic sclerosis (diffuse scleroderma). Am. J. Med. 36:361, 1964.

143. Songcharoen, S., Raju, S.F., and Pennebaker, J.B.: Interstitial lung disease in polymyositis and dermatomyositis. J. Rheumatol. 7:353, 1980.

144. Salmeron, G., Greenberg, S.D., and Lidsky, M.D.: Polymyositis and diffuse interstitial lung disease. A review of the pulmonary histopathologic findings. Arch. Intern. Med. 141:1005, 1981.

145. Goodman, M. and Turner-Warwick, M.: Pilot study of penicillamine therapy in corticosteroid failure patients with widespread pulmonary fibrosis. Chest 74:338, 1978.

146. Scott, G.I., and Bacon, P.A.: Response to methotrexate in fibrosing alveolitis associated with connective tissue disease. Thorax 35:725, 1980.

147. Turner-Warwick, M.: Adverse reactions affecting the lung: possible association with D-penicillamine. J. Rheumotol. 8(Suppl.7):166, 1981.

148. Weiss, R.B., and Muggia, F.M.: Cytotoxic drug-induced pulmonary disease: Update 1980. Am. J. Med. 68:259, 1980.

149. Podell, J.E., Klinenberg, J.R., Kramer, L.S., and Brown, H.V.: Pulmonary toxicity with gold therapy. Arthritis Rheum. 23:347, 1980.

150. Smith, W., and Ball, G.V.: Lung injury due to gold treatment. Arthritis Rheum. 23:351, 1980.

151. Godard, Ph., Marty, J.P., and Michel, P.B.: Interstitial pneumonia and chlorambucil. Chest 76:471, 1979.

152. Golding, P.L., Smith, M., and Williams, R.: Multisystem involvement in chronic liver disease. Studies on the incidence and pathogenesis. Am. J. Med. 55:772, 1973.

153. Boyer, J.L., and Miller, D.J.: Chronic hepatitis. In Schiff, L., and Schiff, E.R. (eds.): Diseases of the Liver. 5th ed. Philadelphia. J. B. Lippincott Co., 1982, p. 771.

154. Soloway, R.D., Summerskill, W.H.J., Baggenstoss, A.H., and Schoenfield, L.J.: "Lupoid hepatitis," a non-entity in the spectrum of chronic active liver disease. Gastroenterology 63:458, 1972.

155. Reynolds, T.B.: Chronic hepatitis: Current dilemmas. Am. J. Med. 69:485, 1980.

156. Sherlock, S.: Primary biliary cirrhosis. In Schiff, L., and Schiff, E.R. (eds.): Diseases of the Liver. 5th ed. Philadelphia. J. B. Lippincott Co., 1982, p. 979.

157. Christensen, E., Crowe, J., Doniach, D., Popper, H., Ranek, L., Rodes, J., Tygstrup, N., and Williams, R.: Clinical pattern and course of disease in primary biliary cirrhosis based on an analysis of 236 patients. Gastroenterology 78:236, 1980.

158. MacGregor, G.A.: Primary biliary cirrhosis is a dry gland syndrome. Lancet 2:535, 1980.

159. Crowe, J.P., Christensen, E., Butler, J., Wheeler, P., Doniach, D., Keenan, J., and Williams, R.: Primary biliary cirrhosis: The prevalence of hypothyroidism and its relationship to thyroid autoantibodies and sicca syndrome. Gastroenterology 78:1437, 1980.

160. Long, R.C., Wills, M.R., Skinner, R.K., and Sherlock, S.: Serum 1-25-hydroxy-vitamin D in untreated parenchymal and cholestatic liver disease. Lancet 2:650, 1976.

161. Long, R.G.: Hepatic osteodystrophy: Outlook good but some problems unsolved. Gastroenterology 78:644, 1980.

162. Crowe, J., Christensen, E., Smith, M., Cochrane, M., Ranek, L., Watkinson, G., Doniach, D., Popper, H., Tygstrup, N., and Williams, R.: Azathioprine in primary biliary cirrhosis: Preliminary report of an international trial. Gastroenterology 78:1005, 1980.

163. Dickson, E.R.: The syndrome of primary biliary cirrhosis. J. Rheumatol. 8(Suppl. 7):121, 1981.

164. Chapman, R.W.G., Arborgh, B.A.M., Rhodes, J.M., Summerfield, J.A., Dick, R., Scheuer, R.J., and Sherlock, S.: Primary sclerosing cholangitis: A review of its clinical features, cholangiography, and hepatic histology. Gut 21:870, 1980.

165. Wheeler, E.S., and Meals, R.A.: Dupuytren's diathesis: A broad-spectrum disease. Plast. Reconstr. Surg. 68:781, 1981.

166. Gelberman, R.H., Amiel, D., Rudolph, R.M., and Vance, R.M.: Dupuytren's contracture: An electron microscopic, biochemical, and clinical correlative study. J. Bone Joint Surg. 62-A:425, 1980.

167. Vande Berg, J.S., Rudolph, R., Gelberman, R., and Woodward, M.R.: Ultrastructural relationship of skin to nodule and cord in Dupuytren's contracture. Plast. Reconstr. Surg. 69:835, 1982.

168. Peacock, E.E., Jr., Madden, J.W., and Trier, W.C.: Biologic basis for treatment of keloids and hypertrophic scars. South. Med. J. 63:755, 1970.

169. Cohen, I.K., Keiser, H.R., and Sjoerdsma, A.: Collagen synthesis in human keloid and hypertrophic scar. Surg. Forum 22:488, 1971.

170. Diegelmann, R.F., Cohen, I.K., and McCoy, B.J.: Growth kinetics and collagen synthesis of normal skin, normal scar, and keloid fibroblasts in vitro. J. Cell. Physiol. 98:341, 1979.

171. Quantitative assay of types of I and III collagen synthesized by keloid biopsies and fibroblasts. Biochim. Biophys. Acta. 586:384, 1979.

172. Russell, J.D., Russell, S.B., and Trupin, K.M.: Differential effects of hydrocortisone on both cell growth and collagen metabolism of human fibroblasts from normal and keloid tissue. J. Cell. Physiol. 97:221, 1978.

173. Lepor, H., and Walsh, P.C.: Idiopathic retroperitoneal fibrosis. J. Urol. 122:1, 1979.

174. Larrieu, A.J., and Weiner, I., Abston, S., and Warren, M.M.: Retroperitoneal fibrosis. Surg. Gynecol. Obstet. 150:699, 1980.

175. Sjoerdsma, A., and Roberts, W.C.: The cardiac disease associated with the carcinoid syndrome (carcinoid heart disease). Am. J. Med. 36:5, 1964.

176. Morin, L.J., and Zuerner, R.T.: Retroperitoneal fibrosis and carcinoid tumor. JAMA 216:1647, 1971.

177. Smith, B.H.: Peyronie's disease. Am. J. Clin. Pathol. 45:670, 1966.

178. Lynd, M.: Dupuytren's contracture, fibroma plantae, periarthrosis humeri, induration penis plastica, and epilepsy, with attempt at pathogenetic valuation. Acta Psychiat. Neurol. Scand. 16:465, 1941.

179. Yudkin, J.S.: Peyronie's disease in association with metoprolol. Lancet 2:1355, 1977.

180. Wallis, A.A., Bell, R., and Sutherland, P.W.: Propranolol and Peyronie's disease. Lancet 2:980, 1977.

181. Jackson, H.: Pseudotumor of the orbit. Br. J. Ophthalmol. 42:212, 1958.

182. Arnott, E.J., and Greaves, D.P.: Orbital involvement in Reidel's thyroiditis. Br. J. Ophthalmol. 49:1, 1965.

183. Walton, E.W.: Pseudotumor of the orbit and polyarteritis nodosa. J. Clin. Pathol. 12:419, 1959.

184. Woolner, L.B., McConahey, W.M., and Beahrs, O.H.: Invasive fibrous thyroiditis (Reidel's struma). J. Clin. Endocrinol. 17:201, 1957.

185. Turner-Warwick, M., Nabarro, J.D.N., and Domiach, D.: Reidel's thyroiditis and retroperitoneal fibrosis. Proc. R. Soc. Med. 59:596, 1966.

186. Bartholomew, L.G., Cain, J.C., Woolner, L.B., Utz, D.C., and Ferris, D.O.: Sclerosing cholangitis. Its possible association with Reidel's struma and fibrous retroperitonitis: Report of two cases. N. Engl. J. Med. 269:8, 1963.

Section X
Inflammatory Diseases of Muscle

Chapter 79
Inflammatory Diseases of Muscle

Walter G. Bradley

INTRODUCTION

The inflammatory diseases of skeletal muscle are a group of conditions in which the muscles are diffusely damaged by a nonsuppurative inflammatory process in which lymphocytes predominate. This group of conditions is sometimes termed the *dermatomyositis-polymyositis complex*. It includes *dermatomyositis* (DM), in which the skeletal muscle and skin are involved, and *polymyositis* (PM), in which only the skeletal muscle is involved. Dermatomyositis or polymyositis may occur without any other disease, or may be associated with the whole range of collagen-vascular diseases, including rheumatic fever, rheumatoid arthritis, scleroderma, systemic lupus erythematosus, polyarteritis nodosa, and nonspecific mixed collagen-vascular disease. The DM-PM complex may also be associated with malignancies. Similarly, acute skeletal muscle inflammation can occur following a variety of acute viral infections, and in association with infections by a number of bacteria and parasites.

From the above it is clear that this chapter deals with a syndrome and not a single disease.[1-7] It is important to remember that the terms "dermatomyositis" and "polymyositis" are no more specific with regard to etiology than is the term "arthritis." This heterogeneity makes it difficult to determine the etiology of the condition. Inflammatory disease of muscle may present to the rheumatologist, neurologist, general internist, dermatologist, and orthopedic surgeon among others, and it is important that all physicians bear in mind the DM-PM complex. There is good, though not absolutely conclusive, evidence that these diseases respond to immunosuppressive therapy. That being so, it is a disaster if a patient is misdiagnosed as having, for instance, a muscular dystrophy.

CLASSIFICATION

Several different classifications of the DM-PM complex have been suggested. Walton and Adams[2] suggested the classification shown in Table 79–1, which has been widely used in a number of surveys.[8] This classification has been criticized by a number of authors. Rowland and associates[7] in particular emphasized that the diagnosis of PM is far less certain than that of DM as a result of the combined association of skeletal muscle and skin involvement in the latter. In their series of patients they found that DM had a worse prognosis and was associated with a high incidence of malignancy. They found that PM could be associated with all the collagen-vascular diseases, while the only collagen-vascular disease to be associated with DM was scleroderma. They also found that cardiac involvement occurred in some cases of PM, but almost never occurred in their patients with DM. These criticisms have some foundation. The difficulty of diagnosing pure PM has been emphasized by a number of authors.[5,8,9] Several studies have shown that the incidence of carcinoma is higher in adult patients with DM than with PM.[8,10] However, some series have shown no difference in the prognosis of DM and PM,[8] and there are many reports of cardiac damage in DM.[6,11,12]

The classification proposed by the Research Group on Neuromuscular Disease of the World Federation of Neurology[13] is shown in Table 79–2. This classification is, however, too lengthy and too subdivided to be easily used in surveys and therapeutic trials.

It is not clear where DM should be placed in the classifications shown in Tables 79–1 and 79–2. Walton and Adams[2,14] and DeVere and Bradley[8] restricted Group I (Table 79–1) to cases of pure PM, and found cases with combined skin and muscle involvement in

1225

Table 79–1. Classification of Dermatomyositis-Polymyositis Complex by Walton and Adams*

Group I:	Pure polymyositis, acute with myoglobinuria, subacute, or chronic; in childhood, early, middle or late life
Group II:	Polymyositis with muscle weakness the dominant feature but with evidence of an associated collagen-vascular disease; or dermatomyositis with severe muscle disability and with skin changes which are often minimal or transient
Group III:	Severe collagen-vascular disease with muscular weakness due to polymyositis of comparatively minor degree; or dermatomyositis with florid skin changes and muscle weakness of only secondary importance
Group IV:	Polymyositis or dermatomyositis in association with malignant disease

*From Walton, J.N., and Adams, R.D.: Polymyositis. Baltimore, Williams & Wilkins Company, 1958.

Table 79–2. Classification of Inflammatory Diseases of Muscle Proposed by the Research Group on Neuromuscular Diseases* and Amplified by Gardner-Medwin and Walton[†]

I. Infections of muscle
  (α) Viral (presumed)
    1. Bornholm disease
    2. Epidemic torticollis
    3. Following influenza
  (β) Bacterial
    1. Gas gangrene (*Cl. welchii*)
    2. Tetanus (*Cl. tetani*)
    3. Staphylococci and other pyogenic agents (septic myositis)
    4. Leprous myositis
    5. Tropical myositis (usually pyogenic)
  (γ) Nematode
    1. *Trichinella spiralis*
  (δ) Cestode
    1. Cysticercosis with muscle hypertrophy
    2. Cysticercosis (asymptomatic)
  (ϵ) *Trypanosomiasis cruzi*
  (ζ) Toxoplasmosis
II. Other inflammatory disorders of muscle
  (α) Polymyositis (possibly an organ-specific autoimmune disease)
    1. Acute polymyositis and myoglobinuria
    2. Subacute polymyositis
    3. Chronic polymyositis (including chronic myositis fibrosa)
  (β) Polymyositis or dermatomyositis (when occuring as one feature of what may prove to be a non-organ-specific autoimmune disease)
    1. Dermatomyositis
    2. Polymyositis in disseminated lupus erythematosus
    3. Polymyositis in rheumatic fever
    4. Polymyositis in rheumatoid arthritis
    5. Polymyositis in scleroderma and/or systemic sclerosis
    6. Scleroderma (morphea) with myopathy
    7. Ocular myositis (pseudotumor of the orbit)
    8. Muscle infarction and/or polymyositis in polyarteritis nodosa
    9. Polymyositis in Sjögren's disease
    10. Polymyopathy in Werner's disease
    11. Localized nodular myositis
  (γ) Polymyositis or dermatomyositis occurring in malignant disease
  (δ) Polymyositis with associated virus particles
III. Inflammatory disorders of muscle of unknown etiology
    1. Sarcoidosis with myopathy
    2. Granulomatous myopathy
    3. Polymyalgia rheumatica
    4. Localized myositis ossificans
    5. Fibrositis and nodular fasciitis
    6. Myopathy with relapsing panniculitis (Weber-Christian syndrome)
    7. Myositis with necrotizing fasciitis
    8. Myopathy in psoriasis
    9. Myositis with hypereosinophilic syndrome
    10. Myopathy in Reye's syndrome

*J. Neurol. Sci. 6:165, 1968.
[†]Walton, J.N.: *In* Walton, J.N. (ed.): Disorders of Voluntary Muscle. Edinburgh, Churchill Livingstone, 1981.

the three other groups. Currie and associates[15] included cases with erythematous skin rash and a history of Raynaud's phenomenon and/or arthralgia in Group II(α) (Table 79–2), provided that the skin involvement was not prominent and that there was no evidence on investigation of a widespread systemic collagen-vascular disease. They found that the peripheral blood lymphocytes in Group II(α) were cytotoxic only to muscle cultures, while those from Groups II(β) and II(γ) were also cytotoxic to fibroblast cultures.

Bohan and Peter[5] (Table 79–3) have made an attempt to overcome some of the objections to the classification of Walton and Adams,[2] while providing a relatively simple grouping. They emphasized that their classification into five groups was based not so much on convincing clinical evidence that distinctive features existed between these various groups, but on the conviction that if characteristic differences were to emerge, this would be possible only with careful subgroup analysis of the data.[6]

There are still some problems about the classification proposed by Bohan and Peter.[5] DM, defined as inflammatory myositis with the characteristic skin rash, may occur with or without association with neoplasia or one of the collagen-vascular diseases. Adult cases of DM and PM occasionally have evidence of a diffuse vasculitis similar to that in childhood DM-PM. Some authors believe that childhood DM is different from childhood PM. The Overlap Group[5] requires the presence of both clear-cut PM and a clearly defined collagen-vascular disease. This leaves it uncertain where DM-PM associated with nonspecific collagen-vascular disease should be classified. Nevertheless this classification is probably the most appropriate in our present state of knowledge.

INCIDENCE OF INFLAMMATORY DISEASES OF MUSCLE

There are a few population surveys of inflammatory diseases of muscle. Rose and Walton[16] found 89 new cases during a 12-year span between 1954 and 1965 from the northeast of England from a population of about 3.2 million. This is an annual incidence of about 2.25 new cases per million per year. Medsger and associates[17] from the United States estimated an incidence of 5 new

Table 79–3. Classification of the Dermatomyositis-Polymyositis Complex Proposed by Bohan and Peter*

Group 1: Primary idiopathic polymyositis
Group 2: Primary idiopathic dermatomyositis
Group 3: Dermatomyositis (or polymyositis) associated with neoplasia
Group 4: Childhood dermatomyositis (or polymyositis) associated with vasculitis
Group 5: Polymyositis or dermatomyositis associated with collagen-vascular disease (overlap group)

*From Bohan, A., and Peter, J.B.: N. Engl. J. Med. 292:344, 1975.

cases per million per year. This is of a similar order of magnitude to the annual incidence of new cases with muscular dystrophy. These figures are dependent upon the accuracy of diagnosis and degree of ascertainment of cases. Currie estimated that in his experience new cases of PM occurred with about one tenth the frequency of rheumatoid arthritis, about one third the frequency of systemic lupus erythematosus, one half the incidence of scleroderma, and twice the incidence of polyarteritis nodosa.[4]

PRIMARY IDIOPATHIC ADULT POLYMYOSITIS

This category includes all Group I and many of the Group II cases of Walton and Adams,[2] Rose and Walton,[16] and DeVere and Bradley,[8] with the exclusion of children. It also includes all the idiopathic PM cases of Rowland and associates[7] and all the Group I cases of Bohan and associates.[6] Patients with pure PM comprise about one third of all the reported large series of patients with the DM-PM complex.

Clinical Features. Females exceed males by about 2:1. The condition can be seen at any adult age, and some clinicians feel that there is no difference between the childhood pure PM and the adult form. In the adults

the mean age of presentation is about 50 years. The cases are usually sporadic, but rare familial cases have been reported, usually one member of a family having PM and the other DM.[18-20] I have observed a conjugal pair of cases, the wife presenting with severe DM, which proved to be due to systemic lupus erythematosus and which led to her death about 5 years later, at which time her husband presented with mild myalgia and muscle stiffness and a raised serum creatine kinase (CK).

Precipitating Factors. Insidious muscle weakness with or without myalgia usually occurs without preceding problems. However, occasional cases are preceded by a variety of febrile illnesses. Often the patient has had evidence of a "rheumatic diathesis" with Raynaud's phenomenon or occasional stiffness of joints for a number of years prior to the onset of muscle weakness. According to the classification of Walton and Adams,[2] such symptoms place the patient in Group II (see Table 79–4), but Bohan and associates[6] accept such symptoms in cases classified as primary idiopathic PM.

Symptomatology. In the typical case muscle weakness begins insidiously, either in the lower or in the upper limbs. The patient becomes aware of some difficulty in running, in climbing stairs, and in getting out of a chair. The gait becomes clumsy and waddling, and there is a tendency to fall with difficulty in arising without assistance.

Upper limb weakness is usually proximal, with difficulty in lifting heavy objects onto high shelves, which progresses to difficulty in keeping the arms up while combing the hair. In about a half of patients there is pain and tenderness in the muscles, though this symptom is often only elicited by direct questioning. Difficulty in raising the head from the pillow in bed and difficulty in chewing and swallowing are present in 10 to 20 percent of patients, though again patients often do not complain about these symptoms. Commonly the patient feels generally unwell, and has lost 1 to 12 lbs. in weight.

The typical frequencies of the various symptoms at

Table 79–4. Symptoms at Presentation with Dermatomyositis-Polymyositis*

| Symptoms | Group | | | | Total Cases (%) |
	I (%)	II (%)	III (%)	IV (%)	
Extensor neck muscle weakness	7	12	14	0	9
Upper limb weakness:					
Proximal only	48	76	77	89	67
Proximal and distal	14	22	24	0	18
Lower limb weakness:					
Proximal only	69	95	87	100	84
Proximal and distal	10	11	21	0	12
Pain:					
Bilateral symmetrical	57	70	63	67	64
Asymmetrical	17	4	11	0	9
Dysphagia	17	43	25	22	28
Dysphonia	2	3	4	0	3
Raynaud's phenomenon	0	57	66	13	35
Skin rash	0	46	30	67	36
Skin tightness	0	11	27	0	10
Joint pain	0	22	60	11	23

*Data from the survey of DeVere, R., and Bradley, W.G.: Brain 98:637, 1975.

presentation can be seen in Table 79–4, where the division of cases is according to the classification of Walton and Adams.[2]

Rate of Development of Symptoms. The symptoms have usually been present for 3 to 6 months by the time the patient comes to a physician. Rarely severe muscle weakness may develop acutely, and in this instance may be associated with myoglobinuria. At times the muscle weakness may develop insidiously over 5 to 10 years, and in this case differentiation from a progressive muscular dystrophy may be difficult. In some patients a relapsing and remitting course is seen.

Range of Severity at Presentation. The degree of muscle weakness at presentation varies considerably from patient to patient. About 4 percent of patients have significant respiratory weakness at presentation, and a similar number have bulbar muscle weakness with dysphagia and dysphonia. Occasional patients may present simply with myalgia without muscle weakness, and a diagnosis cannot be made in such circumstances without full investigations, including a muscle biopsy.

A simple scheme for classifying the degree of muscle weakness in patients with PM is given in Table 79–5 adapted from Rose and Walton.[16] It should be noted that Grades 1 to 3 are associated with minimal or no symptomatic weakness, while Grades 5 and 6 are associated with severe disability. About 4 percent of patients are unable to walk at presentation.[7] DeVere and Bradley[8] found that the mean disability grade at presentation in patients with PM was 4.5.

Clinical Signs at Presentation. The clinical signs at presentation found in the review of 118 cases of DM-PM[8] are tabulated in Table 79–6. Proximal upper limb and lower limb weakness is found to some extent in almost every patient. The distribution of weakness is usually symmetrical and diffuse, and is different from the characteristically specific pattern of muscle weakness in the muscular dystrophies. In the latter, for instance, weakness particularly affects the serratus, rhomboid, lower fibers of trapezius, supraspinatus, pectoralis major, biceps, and brachioradialis in the upper limbs with relative sparing of most of the other proximal and all the distal muscles. In PM on the other hand all the proximal muscles tend to be similarly involved, the severity of the involvement decreasing progressively in more distal muscles. However, rarely the pattern can be reversed and a distal predominance can occur.[21]

Weakness of neck flexors is present in about half the patients, and weakness of neck extensors in a smaller proportion. The muscles are frequently atrophied and tender to palpation. Contractures may be found on presentation in about a tenth of the patients, but may develop more severely as the disease progresses. Severe facial muscle weakness is uncommon, as is profound weakness of the bulbar muscles. The ocular muscles are almost never involved[22,23] unless there is associated myasthenia gravis.

By the definition of this group of pure idiopathic PM, an associated dermatomyositic skin rash is absent. The calcinosis which particularly occurs in the childhood form of DM is also not seen. However, skin tethering and acrosclerosis may be seen, though to a much lesser degree than is present in PM in association with scleroderma. Joint involvement is similarly much less than is seen in cases of PM associated with rheumatoid arthritis.

Laboratory Abnormalities. Hematologic investigations are usually normal, though the erythrocyte sedimentation rate (ESR) is raised in about half the patients, and is greater than 50 mm per hour in 20 percent of patients. There may be changes in the plasma proteins, including a rise in the gamma globulin, which are responsible for this raised sedimentation rate. Rarely clinical investigations will reveal evidence of an underlying malignancy such as leukemia, paraproteinemia, or a carcinoma, which necessitates reclassification of the patient into the category of DM-PM with neoplasia.

The urinary excretion of creatine is raised (see Chapter 47). Myoglobinuria may be present in the rare syndrome of acute PM. If this is suspected, special care should be taken to study fresh urine spectroscopically or by radioimmunoassay.

A number of skeletal muscle enzymes are released into the serum as a result of skeletal muscle damage (see Chapter 47). The raised level of these enzymes can be a helpful indicator of the extent and acuteness of the muscle fiber damage. CK is a particularly sensitive indicator of muscle fiber damage. The level of serum enzyme found in a survey of 118 patients[8] is shown in Table 79–7. The serum CK was raised in over 60 percent of the patients, occasionally being as high as 80 times normal. The mean level was about 10 times normal.

It has been emphasized[6] that serum enzyme elevation is seen in virtually all patients *at some time* during the course of their disease, if all the appropriate serum enzymes are repeatedly determined. In a series of 153 cases, in only 2 patients (1.3 percent) were all the enzymes within the normal range throughout the entire clinical course.

Serological Tests. Raised serum antibodies may be present in a number of patients with primary idiopathic PM, though the proportion is somewhat less than in the group of patients with PM-DM associated with collagen-vascular diseases. Anti-DNA antibody is rarely present, but titers of antinuclear antibody (usually homogeneous

Table 79–5. Grading of Muscle Weakness in Dermatomyositis and Polymyositis*

1. No abnormality on examination
2. No abnormality on examination, but easy fatigability and decreased exercise tolerance
3. Minimal degree of atrophy of one or more muscle groups without functional impairment
4. Waddling gait; unable to run but able to climb stairs without needing arm support
5. Marked waddling gait, accentuated lordosis; unable to climb stairs or rise from a standard chair without arm support
6. Unable to walk without assistance

*After Rose, A.L., and Walton, J.N.: Brain 89:747, 1966.

Table 79–6. Physical Signs at Presentation with Dermatomyositis-Polymyositis*

Signs	Group I (%)	II (%)	III (%)	IV (%)	Total Cases (%)
Upper limb weakness:					
Proximal only	77	97	83	89	86
Proximal and distal	24	61	25	63	39
Lower limb weakness:					
Proximal only	88	97	93	89	92
Proximal and distal	26	39	26	57	32
Neck muscle weakness:					
Flexors	37	50	54	71	47
Extensors	8	23	19	0	14
Joint involvement	0	14	40	0	22
Muscle atrophy:					
Upper limb					
Proximal only	33	46	46	22	40
Proximal and distal	10	27	17	11	17
Lower limb					
Proximal only	24	33	28	33	29
Proximal and distal	12	19	10	11	14
Muscle tenderness	34	47	46	57	43
Contractures:					
Upper limb	12	11	14	0	11
Lower limb	5	8	3	22	7
Facial weakness	2	3	7	0	4
Respiratory muscle weakness	2	11	0	0	4
Cardiac involvement	0	0	0	0	0
Bulbar weakness:					
Palate and pharynx	0	17	10	0	6
Masseters	5	3	0	13	4
Skin rash	0	46	23	67	25
Skin tethering	0	8	33	0	11
Acrosclerosis	0	41	17	22	19
Distal ulceration or clinical calcinosis	0	0	13	0	3

*Data from the survey of DeVere, R., and Bradley, W.G.: Brain 98:637, 1975.

patterns) may be high. LE cells may be found occasionally. Detailed immunological studies dealing with antibodies and lymphocytes are described under Etiology (see below).

Electrophysiology. The electromyographic findings in PM have been well described.[21,24] The characteristic changes seen in PM (see Chapter 47) consist of an increase in the insertional activity of the muscle, with numerous fibrillation potentials and positive sharp waves at rest. Motor unit action potentials show myopathic changes with decreased amplitude and duration and an increase in the proportion of polyphasic potentials. The interference pattern becomes full at mild degrees of contraction, and the overall amplitude at maximum voluntary contraction is reduced. Bizarre high frequency repetitive discharges are also a common feature. The frequency of the various electrophysiological changes found[6] in the various disease groups are recorded in Table 79–8. Almost every patient has myopathic motor units, and the majority show increased insertional activity and spontaneous activity. In the survey of DeVere and Bradley[8] about 40 percent of patients had the complete electromyographic picture of PM, and 50 percent had myopathic changes only. About 10 percent had no abnormality on EMG. It is important to sample paraspinal muscles in those without EMG abnormalities in the limb muscles.

Electromyography performed several years after presentation in patients with PM frequently shows the changes of denervation-reinnervation, with motor units of larger than normal amplitude and duration and a reduced interference pattern on maximum voluntary effort.[25] Henriksson and Stålberg[26] showed the presence of increased terminal motor nerve branching by single fiber EMG studies. The basis of these later reinnervation

Table 79–7. Serum Creatine Kinase at Presentation with Dermatomyositis-Polymyositis*

Serum CK (IU Per Liter)	Group I (%)	II (%)	III (%)	IV (%)	Total Cases (Percent)
0–50†	41	32	36	33	36
51–100	4	9	0	0	4
101–200	15	9	14	17	13
201–300	19	0	0	17	9
301–500	0	14	21	0	9
501–1000	15	9	7	0	10
1001–3000	7	14	21	17	13
>3000	0	14	0	17	6

*Data from the survey of DeVere, R., and Bradley, W.G.: Brain 98:637, 1975. †Normal level <50 IU per liter.

Table 79–8. Electromyographic Data on a Series of 153 Patients with Dermatomyositis and Polymyositis*

Electromyographic Abnormality	PM (%)	DM (%)	DM-PM Malignancy (%)	DM-PM Childhood (%)	DM-PM Overlap Group (%)	Total Patients (%)
Polyphasic units	98	100	82	100	90	90
Short small units	98	97	91	100	90	90
Fibrillations	71	76	91	67	71	74
Positive sharp waves	75	76	91	44	67	73
Irritability	75	70	91	67	67	73
High frequency discharges	33	33	36	44	43	38
Abnormalities restricted to paraspinal muscles	4	0	0	0	0	2

*From Bohan, A., et al.: Medicine 56:255, 1977.

changes is probably the damage to intramuscular nerves which can occur in PM (see below).

Muscle Biopsy. The muscle to be biopsied should be carefully selected by the clinician responsible for the care of the patient. It should be moderately weak, and neither profoundly weak and wasted nor of normal strength. PM is a very patchy process, and one area may show extensive inflammation and degeneration next to perfectly normal areas. Areas of marked inflammation may have an increased uptake of ^{99m}Tc polyphosphate,[27] but this has not proved to be of help in choosing the site for muscle biopsy. A greater diagnostic yield can be obtained by serial section of the muscle biopsy, by taking a sufficient amount of muscle for extensive study, and by taking biopsies from two muscles. It should be remembered that electromyography can produce inflammatory changes and muscle fiber damage, and muscles that have been subjected to electromyography must not be used for biopsy.

The term polymyositis implies inflammation of many muscles, and extensive inflammatory infiltrates are the diagnostic hallmark of the disease complex. The inflammatory infiltrate predominantly consists of lymphocytes, with a moderate admixture of histiocytes, plasma cells, occasional eosinophils, and polymorphs. These infiltrates are present between the muscle fibers (Fig. 79–1), and are also frequently seen around small blood vessels, particularly venules within the muscle (Fig. 79–2). Characteristically there is also damage to the skeletal muscle fibers themselves with necrosis, phagocytosis, and regeneration. Muscle fibers show focal degeneration, coagulative necrosis, and phagocytes invading the fibers. Vacuolar changes involving a small number of fibers are present in many biopsies. Regenerating fibers are small and rounded, with internal nuclei which are enlarged and vesicular with large nucleoli (Fig. 79–3). The cytoplasm of the regenerating fibers is basophilic due to the accumulation of RNA.[28] If the disease process is chronic, there is increased random variation in fiber size, rounding of the individual muscle fibers, an increased portion of internal nuclei within the fibers, and an increase in endomysial and perimysial fibrosis.

Figure 79–1. Transverse section of muscle in polymyositis showing interstitial infiltration with inflammatory cells. Hematoxylin and eosin × 160.

Figure 79–2. Longitudinal section of muscle in polymyositis showing inflammatory cell infiltration adjacent to a venule. Hematoxylin and easin × 320.

Atrophy and damage to muscle fibers is frequently concentrated at the periphery of fascicles, producing the characteristic feature of perifascicular atrophy (Fig. 79–4).[6,29-31] The reason for this is not clear, though it appears related to a decreased capillary density in these areas.

Muscle fiber atrophy is frequent, but muscle hypertrophy rarely occurs.[32] The atrophy may predominate in type 2 fibers (Fig. 79–5), and this is particularly likely to be so if myalgia, arthralgia, or long-term corticosteroid therapy has been prescribed. Small angulated atrophic fibers, rich in oxidative enzyme activity and thus highly suggestive of denervated fibers, are not infrequently seen in PM.[30] These probably result from damage to the intramuscular nerve branches.[33] In chronic PM with severe damage to the muscle, fiber type

dedifferentiation occurs, with loss of the clear separation of fiber types.

Electron microscopy shows the typical changes of skeletal muscle damage, with disruption of the sarcolemma, clumping, and overcontraction of the myofibrils, as well as lesser degrees of damage, including Z-line streaming and Z-line lysis.[34-37] Total necrosis with infiltration by phagocytes and proliferation of phospholipid membranes into spheromembranous bodies are common.[38,39] All stages of regeneration, with numerous polyribosomes and new sparse myofibrils, may be seen.

Rarely there may be a clear-cut vasculitis, with necrosis of vessels. This is much more commonly seen in childhood dermatomyositis, or in PM associated with polyarteritis nodosa or one of the other collagen-vascular

Figure 79–3. Transverse section of muscle in polymyositis showing a wedge-shaped area of regenerating muscle fibers. Hematoxylin and easin × 320.

Figure 79–4. Transverse section of muscle in polymyositis showing the marked atrophy of the peripheral fibers of the fasciculi. Myosin ATPase pH 9.4; × 30.

diseases. Occasionally in a vasculitis there are small infarcts within the muscle (Fig. 79–6).

Extensive reviews of the pathologic changes in the muscle in PM have been published at the light microscopic level,[2,28] with histochemistry,[32] and under the electron microscope.[34-40] Occasional nemaline rods and abnormal mitochondria with paracrystalline inclusions may be seen in PM, but it may well be that reports of major nemaline rod accumulation[41] and of predominant mitochondrial change[42] are in fact examples of secondary PM in cases which were primarily nemaline myopathy and mitochondrial myopathy, respectively (see Secondary PM in the Primary Myopathies, below).

The histologic changes seen at the light microscopic level in a series of patients with PM are shown in Table 79–9.[6] Muscle fiber degeneration was seen in 90 percent

of cases, and inflammation in nearly 80 percent. DeVere and Bradley[8] found the complete pathological picture of PM in half of the biopsies in pure PM, inflammatory infiltrates alone in another 15 percent, and muscle fiber destruction and regeneration without inflammatory change in about 8 percent of cases. The muscle biopsy was normal in nearly 20 percent of cases of primary idiopathic PM, an indication of the patchy nature of the pathological process.

Differential Diagnosis of Adult Polymyositis. The differential diagnosis of adult PM involves virtually every disease which can affect the skeletal muscle (see Ref. 14). A summary list of these conditions is given in Table 79–10.

The separation of polymyositis from the many conditions in this list depends both on the history and

Figure 79–5. As Figure 79–6, showing type 2 (dark) fiber atrophy. Myosin ATPase pH 9.4; × 50.

Figure 79–6. Transverse section of muscle in polymyositis in a 56-year-old man with a bronchial carcinoma. The section is stained for mitochondrial oxidative enzyme activity (NADH) and shows loss of enzyme activity in one large area which is an infarct related to a vasculitis. × 50.

clinical examination and on the results of the laboratory investigations, including the EMG and muscle biopsy. These investigations will usually be able to exclude the denervating conditions, disorders of the neuromuscular junction, and certain of the specific muscular dystrophies and myopathies. However, in view of the fact that the EMG and muscle biopsy may not be diagnostic in a moderate number of patients with polymyositis, it is important to consider every condition in Table 79–10, to study the patient's history, and to arrange appropriate investigations where indicated.

Denervating Conditions. The spinal muscular atrophies are generally autosomal recessive disorders causing progressive degeneration of the spinal anterior horn cells, with marked wasting and weakness of the effected muscles. Onset may be at all ages, but in juveniles and adults the progression is relatively slow. They may sometimes be separated clinically from PM by the specific (rather than diffuse) pattern of muscle involvement. Amyotrophic lateral sclerosis causes not only lower motor neuron denervation of muscle but also upper motor neuron signs and frequently bulbar or pseudobulbar palsy.

Neuromuscular Junction Disorders. Myasthenia gravis generally affects the extraocular and bulbar muscles, distinguishing it from PM. However, occasionally upper limb proximal muscle weakness is prominent, and then marked fatiguability may help separate this disease from PM. The Eaton-Lambert syndrome causes similar proximal muscle weakness, which becomes stronger with repeated contractions, the opposite of what is found in myasthenia gravis. Both conditions may be diagnosed by electrophysiological studies.

Muscular Dystrophies. These often have a family history of similarly effected relatives. The main types are the following:

1. *Duchenne muscular dystrophy,* which affects only males, with an X-linked inheritance. The onset of walking difficulty begins about the age of 5 years, and most children have lost the ability to walk by age 11 and die from respiratory failure by age 20. The pattern of muscle weakness is specific and stereotyped, with predominant weakness and wasting of the quadriceps, anterior tibial, biceps, and brachioradialis muscles, together with winging of the scapuli, a hyperlordic gait, and pseudohypertrophy of the calves.

Table 79–9. Muscle Biopsy Data in Biopsies of 135 Cases with Dermatomyositis and Polymyositis*

	PM (%)	DM (%)	DM-PM Malignancy (%)	DM-PM Childhood (%)	DM-PM Overlap Group (%)	Total Patients (%)
Degeneration	90	68	100	100	83	83
Inflammation	79	68	70	100	72	75
Cross-sectional diameter variation	81	68	80	88	59	73
Necrosis	69	45	80	100	41	59
Regeneration	58	33	50	50	31	44
Fibrosis	25	18	30	0	21	21
Phagocytosis	27	13	40	13	10	19
Vasculitis	0	5	0	0	7	3

*From Bohan, A., et al.: Medicine 56:255, 1977.

Table 79–10. Differential Diagnosis of Adult Polymyositis

Denervating conditions: spinal muscular atrophies,* amyotrophic
    lateral sclerosis*
Neuromuscular junction disorders: Eaton-Lambert syndrome,*
    myasthenia gravis*
The genetic muscular dystrophies: Duchenne, facioscapulohumeral,
    limb-girdle,* Becker,* Emery-Dreifuss type,* distal, ocular
Myotonic diseases: dystrophia myotonica,* myotonia congenita
Congenital myopathies: nemaline, mitochondrial, centronuclear,
    central core
Glycogen storage diseases: adult onset acid maltase deficiency.*
    McArdle's disease
Lipid storage myopathies: carnitine deficiency,* carnitine
    palmityltransferase deficiency*
The periodic paralyses
Myositis ossificans:* generalized and local
Endocrine myopathies:* hypothyroidism, hyperthyroidism,
    acromegaly, Cushing's disease, Addison's disease,
    hyperparathyroidism, hypoparathyroidism, vitamin D deficiency
    myopathy, hypokalemia, hypocalcemia
Metabolic myopathies:* uremia, hepatic failure
Toxic myopathies:* acute and chronic alcoholism; drugs including
    penicillamine,* clofibrate,* choroquine, emetine
Nutritional myopathies: vitamin E deficiency,* malabsorption*
Carcinomatous neuromyopathy:* carcinomatous cachexia
Acute rhabdomyolysis*
Proximal neuropathies: Guillain-Barré syndrome,* acute
    intermittent porphyria,* diabetic lower limb chronic
    plexopathies,* chronic autoimmune polyneuropathy
Microembolization by atheroma or carcinoma
Polymyalgia rheumatica*
Other collagen-vascular diseases: rheumatoid arthritis, scleroderma,
    systemic lupus erythematosus, polyarteritis nodosa
Infections: acute viral, including influenza, mononucleosis,
    Rickettsia, coxsackievirus rubella and rubella vaccination, acute
    bacterial including typhoid
Parasites: including *Toxoplasma, Trichinella, Schistosoma,* cysticerci,
    Sarcosporidia
Septic myositis: including *Staphylococcus, Streptococcus, Cl. welchii*
    and leprosy

* Indicates the conditions that are most commonly confused with
polymyositis.

2. *Becker muscular dystrophy* is very similar to Duchenne muscular dystrophy, including an X-linked inheritance pattern, but is more benign. Most patients continue walking beyond the age of 16 years.

3. *Limb girdle muscular dystrophy,*[88] is a relatively poorly characterized condition with autosomal recessive inheritance. Onset of proximal muscle weakness in the upper or lower limbs occurs in the second to fourth decade. The pattern of muscle involvement is similar to that seen in Duchenne muscular dystrophy.

4. *Facioscapulohumeral muscular dystrophy* is an autosomal dominant disorder with early and predominant weakness of the orbicularis oculi and obicularis oris muscles, causing a characteristic facial appearance. There is periscapular, biceps, brachioradialis, triceps, anterior tibial, and hip flexor muscle weakness. This generally has the best prognosis of all the muscular dystrophies.

Dystrophia Myotonica (Myotonic Dystrophy, Steinert's Disease). These diseases are inherited in a dominant fashion and characterized by diffuse muscle weakness and wasting involving the facial muscles and ptosis, difficulty of relaxing the grip (myotonia), frontal baldness, cataracts, and gonadal atrophy. They are very variable in their severity.

The Glycogen Storage Diseases. A number of different conditions arise as the result of deficiency of a different enzyme of the glycolytic pathway. *McArdle's disease,* or *myophosphorylase deficiency,* causes inability of the muscle to initiate the breakdown of glycogen in forced exertion, with consequent muscle pain and weakness, and occasionally rhabdomyolysis. Rarely there is a late fixed weakness and wasting, closely simulating polymyositis. The diagnosis is made by the absence of production of lactate in ischemic exercise, glycogen accumulation in the muscle fibers, and absence of myophosphorylase. *Adult acid maltase deficiency* causes accumulation of glycogen in membrane-bound lysosomes due to deficiency of this lysosomal enzyme. Patients have progressive proximal muscle weakness and wasting, with myopathic changes and often myotonia on EMG, together with glycogen accumulation in muscle fibers on biopsy.

Disorders of Muscle Lipid Metabolism. Two currently recognized disorders of muscle lipid metabolism may simulate PM. *Carnitine deficiency* causes lipid accumulation in muscle fibers because carnitine is required to transport long-chain fatty acids into mitochondria for oxidation. Patients have a proximal muscle weakness, which is often relapsing, remitting, and responsive to corticosteroid therapy. *Carnitine palmityltransferase deficiency* causes a somewhat different syndrome, with pain and weakness on exertion, often with rhabdomyolysis due to deficient ATP production from lipids during sustained exercise. A similar syndrome can result from *AMP deaminase (myoadenylate deaminase) deficiency,* an enzyme that converts AMP to IMP in exercised muscle, thus preventing the accumulation of IMP, which inhibits oxidative phosphorylation of ADP to ATP. Acute and recurrent rhabdomyolysis can result from these disorders of energy metabolism, but the metabolic basis of most cases of this syndrome is obscure.

Vitamin D deficiency of any cause (dietary, malabsorption, renal, chronic phenytoin therapy, etc.) can cause a painful proximal myopathy with a characteristic waddling gait. Chronic hypophosphatemia may cause a similar syndrome with an increased serum creatine kinase.

Proximal or diffuse muscle weakness and often wasting can have many other causes, such as endocrine disturbances, toxins, and carcinomatous neuromyopathy (see Table 79–10). Particularly difficult to separate from PM is reflex muscle weakness occurring in response to local arthritis or polymyalgia rheumatica. A mild myalgic weakness may accompany any of the collagen-vascular disorders. If weakness is severe, serum CK estimation, EMG, and muscle biopsy may be required. Myalgia without weakness rarely warrants the intense immunosuppresive therapy required for PM.

PRIMARY IDIOPATHIC ADULT DERMATOMYOSITIS

This category includes some of the group II cases of Walton and Adams,[2] Rose and Walton,[16] and DeVere and Bradley,[8] all the adult cases of dermatomyositis of

Rowland and associates,[7] and all the group 2 cases of Bohan and associates.[6] Characteristic features are the typical skin lesions and inflammatory myositis in patients older than 16 years of age. Primary idiopathic adult dermatomyositis comprises about one third of all cases of large reported series of the DM-PM complex.

Clinical Features. Females slightly outnumber males in this category. The condition may occur at any age, though the average age of presentation is about 50 years. The symptoms of the muscle and skin lesions in primary idiopathic adult dermatomyositis are identical with those seen in dermatomyositis associated with one of the other collagen-vascular diseases or with neoplasia.

The degree of skin and muscle involvement varies greatly from case to case. The skin lesions may be minimal, and may be found only after a very careful search of the characteristic areas. Conversely, patients may present with the characteristic skin lesions without any evidence of muscle involvement. A diagnosis of "autoimmune inflammatory dermatitis" should be made at this stage, though it should be recognized that such patients are very likely to develop myositis at some stage in their illness.[43]

The skin and mucous membrane lesions are variable,[44] but the typical lesions are characteristic. The areas of predisposition are the eyelids, the cheeks, the bridge of the nose (Fig. 79–7), the front and back of the chest, the extensor surfaces of the elbows and knees, the malleoli at the ankle, and the knuckles of the fingers, which develop flat plaques known as Gottron's papules. Acute untreated lesions are often bright red and become more violaceous when the patient is treated. The skin is often shiny and atrophic, but when the rash is florid there may be swelling of the skin with edema and pain. There may be scaly desquamation, and the skin may sometimes be seborrheic. Sometimes the rash is pruritic, but frequently it is asymptomatic. The nail fold may be hyperemic, and may be found under magnification to have ectatic capillaries with sludged red cells.[11] The skin may occasionally ulcerate (Fig. 79–8); see Plate XI, p. xlv) and develop calcinosis, but the latter complication is much less frequent than in childhood DM and in pro-

gressive systemic sclerosis. Not infrequently the DM skin manifestations blend into certain of the elements of progressive systemic sclerosis, with acrosclerosis, tethering, and thickening of the skin.

The clinical features of the myositis are identical with PM (above). Muscle weakness in DM may be greater than that in PM. In one series 26 percent were unable to walk, compared with only 5 percent of the PM cases. This, however, was contrary to the experience of others.[3,6,8]

Investigations. The results of laboratory investigations of DM are similar to those of PM (above), including serum enzymes, EMG, and muscle biopsy.

Skin biopsies of affected areas can be diagnostic of DM, though the changes are very similar to those of systemic lupus erythematosus. Poikilodermatous changes with epidermal atrophy, degeneration and liquefaction of the basal cell layer, and vascular dilatation were seen in 19 of 24 cases by Janis and Winkelmann.[45] The accumulation of mucin in the skin biopsy is strongly suggestive of DM. Though Janis and Winkelmann[45] found no vascular lesions in their skin biopsies, perivascular and interstitial inflammatory cell infiltration had been reported,[2,11] together with tortuosity and thrombosis of skin capillaries.[44] The skin in areas not clinically involved is much less likely to show pathognomonic histology.[45]

Differential Diagnosis. Though the skin lesions alone and the muscle lesions alone have a wide differential diagnosis, the association of the two conditions excludes virtually every disease other than dermatomyositis. The only problem that remains is to decide whether the dermatomyositis is of a primary idiopathic adult variety or of the childhood variety, or whether it is associated with another collagen-vascular disease or with neoplasia.

DERMATOMYOSITIS-POLYMYOSITIS WITH NEOPLASIA

The category of inflammatory myopathies associated with neoplasms was separated by Walton and Adams[2] (Group IV) and by Bohan and associates[6] (Group 3). An underlying neoplasm was present in about 5 to 8 percent of a large series of cases of DM-PM,[6-8] though considerably higher frequencies have been reported in smaller series in the literature. The incidence is 5 to 11 times that expected in the general population.[8,46] In childhood, however, the frequency of neoplasia is no greater than expected of the general population,[46] and thus a malignancy associated with childhood DM-PM is extremely rare. Any neoplasm can be responsible for this association, but those of the lung, ovary, breasts, and stomach are particularly common.

We are discussing here patients with major degrees of muscle weakness as a result of DM-PM, and not the cachexia seen in patients with advanced carcinoma. It is, however, possible that an inflammatory myositis may play a part in the severe muscle wasting seen in patients with advanced cancer. Usually the muscle weakness of DM-PM antedates the neoplasm by 1 to 2 years, but

Figure 79–7. The subtle hyperemic rash of the eyelids in a 21-year-old man with dermatomyositis.

in about a third of cases the neoplasm is found at the time of investigation of the muscle weakness or antedates the myositis. DM accounts for about two thirds of the cases of myositis associated with neoplasms, and PM for about a third. However, the incidence of underlying neoplasm in PM is only about 2 to 3 percent, while in DM it is about 15 to 20 percent. In patients with DM over the age of 40 and especially in males, an underlying carcinoma may be present in up to two thirds.[8,10] The clinical significance of these figures is that in a younger patient there is little worry of an underlying carcinoma, but that in an older patient, particularly with DM, it is important to search for an associated neoplasm.

Effective treatment of the underlying neoplasm may improve the degree of muscle weakness, but this response is not necessarily permanent.[6] Nevertheless presentation with DM-PM may lead to the diagnosis and treatment of a carcinoma before it becomes inoperable.

The clinical presentation and laboratory investigations in myositis associated with neoplasia are similar to those in uncomplicated myositis aside from the changes relating to the carcinoma.

DERMATOMYOSITIS-POLYMYOSITIS OF CHILDHOOD

Childhood myositis accounts for 8 to 22 percent of various large series of patients which include all age groups. Males somewhat exceed females in DM-PM in the first two decades of life. In childhood, DM exceeds PM by nearly 2:1.

Bohan and Peter[5] based their separation of childhood DM-PM from their other cases upon the widespread vasculitis which has been reported in childhood DM-PM. However, the literature on childhood DM-PM is somewhat confused, and it is necessary to discuss the prognosis here, though a fuller discussion of the prognosis in myositis is given subsequently. Rose and Walton reported that the prognosis of childhood myositis was considerably better than that of the adult;[16] no deaths occurred in 19 patients younger than 20 years of age compared with a 39 percent mortality in the adult patients. This favorable prognosis of childhood DM-PM has been found in several studies.[47-49] On the other hand in a number of the earlier surveys, approximately one third of the patients died, one third remained crippled, and one third showed remission.[11,19,23] Whether the better prognosis in the later series relates to more recent advances in therapy is not clear (see below).

Bitnum et al.[11] emphasized the frequency of vascular lesions in this childhood group, finding that one fourth of the children died with gastrointestinal hemorrhage and perforation. Banker and Victor[50] reviewed the clinical and autopsy findings in eight children who died of DM, and found widespread vasculitis causing intestinal hemorrhage and perforation in seven. Banker[51] later reported the detailed ultrastructural changes in muscle biopsies of eight patients with childhood DM, showing very widespread endothelial damage and degeneration

in arterioles, capillaries, and veins, together with platelet thrombi. These ultrastructural observations were confirmed.[52] Though similar vascular changes can occur in adult DM and PM,[53,54] they seem particularly to be a feature of the childhood form of myositis, and for this reason the condition has been separately classified.

The clinical (Fig. 79–9; Plate XI, p. xlv) and laboratory features, other than the microangiopathy, are similar to those in adult DM-PM, but the misery of the child with DM-PM is rather more striking than the verbalized malaise of the adult. The associated features of a collagen-vascular disease, including arthropathy and Raynaud's phenomenon, are seen in a small percentage of children. Calcinosis (i.e., extensive subcutaneous calcification) is seen more frequently in the childhood form than in adult DM (Fig. 79–10). The calcium deposits may be present from the onset of the illness, increase with time, and may ulcerate through the skin.

THE DERMATOMYOSITIS-POLYMYOSITIS OVERLAP GROUP

This group comprises most of Group III of Walton and Adams,[2] most of the "named PM group" of Rowland and associates,[7] and all the Group 5 cases of Bohan and associates.[6] According to the definition of Bohan and Peter,[5] cases can be included in this group when they meet the criteria for the diagnosis of an established collagen-vascular disease such as rheumatoid arthritis or scleroderma, and also meet the criteria for the diagnosis of DM or PM. This group makes up about 15 to 30 percent of large series of cases of inflammatory myositis. In the overlap group PM is more common than DM, and females outnumber males by up to 9:1.[6]

Scleroderma is the most common collagen-vascular disease associated with inflammatory myositis, with rheumatoid arthritis and systemic lupus erythematosus next in frequency. Sjögren's syndrome, polyarteritis nodosa, and myasthenia gravis may sometimes be associated with DM-PM. There is a problem in classification of patients with DM-PM and a collagen-vascular disease which does not fit exactly into one of the clear-cut categories.

The degree of skeletal muscle involvement is variable in this overlap group. Frequently the symptoms and degree of disability from the collagen-vascular disease outweigh the skeletal muscle involvement from the PM, and this is particularly true in rheumatoid arthritis and scleroderma. Less commonly there is severe inflammatory myositis and only minor manifestations of the established collagen-vascular disease. Assessment of the degree of weakness and wasting of skeletal muscle in the presence of a painful arthropathy is difficult, and this must be borne in mind in considering the diagnosis of myositis in such a patient. Also entering into the differential diagnosis in such patients is corticosteroid myopathy. It is sometimes necessary to investigate the patients with serum enzyme levels, EMG, and muscle biopsy to decide whether they have a myositis. In scle-

Figure 79–9. Views of a 15-year-old boy with severe dermatomyositis showing a very extensive skin rash of the face (*A,*) trunk(*B,*) and knuckles (*C*) in the characteristic distribution despite 3 months of treatment with prednisone (see also Fig. 79–9 *C,* Plate XI, p. xlv).

roderma the muscle may be very atrophic and fibrotic, but inflammatory infiltrates and skeletal muscle fiber degeneration may be absent as indicated by the normal levels of serum enzymes and the muscle biopsy. In this case it is probable that the diffuse fibrosis is responsible for the skeletal muscle signs rather than a true myositis. Occasionally in scleroderma there may be extensive inflammatory infiltration of the connective tissue septa without muscle fiber degeneration.

The results of the laboratory investigations of this overlap group may be indistinguishable from those of the other DM-PM.[29,55-57] However, type 2 fiber atrophy is more common in the muscle biopsy in the overlap group, and there may be the specific pathological changes of a vasculitis such as polyarteritis nodosa. Also the collagen-vascular disease may cause peripheral nerve damage, and consequently the findings of skeletal muscle denervation are more frequent in the overlap group.

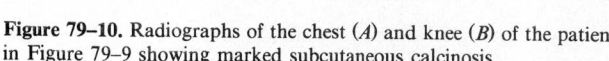

Figure 79–10. Radiographs of the chest (*A*) and knee (*B*) of the patient in Figure 79–9 showing marked subcutaneous calcinosis.

OTHER TYPES OF POLYMYOSITIS

Polymyositis with Known Infections. *Viruses.* Myalgia is commonly experienced in influenza-like illnesses and is probably due to inflammation of the skeletal muscles. An overt acute polymyositis has been recorded during and immediately following infection with influenza A and B viruses, or with virologically undetermined influenza-like illnesses.[61-64] This syndrome particularly occurs in children. The electromyogram is usually normal,[61] the serum CK is raised up to 15 times normal in two thirds of the cases,[62,65] and the muscle biopsy may show either nonspecific myopathy[61] or inflammatory cell infiltration with muscle fiber necrosis.[63]

A subacute polymyositis has also been described following rubella infection,[66] and following immunization with live attenuated rubella virus.[64] Epidemic pleurodynia (Bornholm disease) is generally due to coxsackievirus infection, and positive virological cultures from the inflamed intercostal muscles have been obtained.[67] An acute vacuolar myopathy has been reported with echovirus infection.[68]

Virus-like particles and rare instances of virological isolations have been reported in a number of cases with chronic polymyositis, as reviewed under Etiology (see below).

Bacterial Pyogenic Myositis (Pyomyositis). Particularly in tropics, but also in other regions, rare patients may develop an acute focal suppurative myositis.[69-71] This is an abscess of one or more of the proximal muscles, usually of a lower limb, and is often due to a streptococcal or staphylococcal infection. Treatment of choice is surgical drainage and administration of the appropriate antibiotic. *Clostridium welchii* infection may cause gas gangrene of the muscles, and leprosy bacilli may infect the skeletal muscle, causing an inflammatory myositis.

Parasites. Infections with a number of parasites can give symptoms similar to polymyositis and sometimes inflammatory change in muscle biopsy. These conditions include trichinosis,[72] schistosomiasis,[73] cysticercosis,[74] and sarcosporidiasis.[75]

Toxoplasmosis may also cause an acute or subacute polymyositis-like picture, and be diagnosed only by the finding of raised serum toxoplasma titers, and rarely by the findings of the organisms in muscle biopsy.[76-78] Kagen and associates[79] found an increased toxoplasma dye titer in eight of ten patients with DM-PM and raised complement fixing antibodies to toxoplasma in five of ten such patients.

Focal Nodular Myositis. Polymyositis may occasionally present with focal nodules which may wax and wane with a time course of a few days to a few weeks. In the more chronic types, the condition has to be differentiated from a skeletal muscle tumor. The histological appearance is of polymyositis, sometimes with skeletal muscle infarction. This is an uncommon condition, and appears to be a variant of PM.

Giant Cell Myositis. Muscle fibers are multinucleate syncytia. Regeneration of skeletal muscle occurs most commonly by means of mononuclear myoblasts, probably derived from satellite cells, but it can also occur by budding in continuo. The skeletal muscle buds regenerating in such instances have a superficial resemblance to multinucleate giant cells. However, they are of a different nature and significance from the multinucleate giant cells seen in such granulomatous conditions as tuberculosis, sarcoidosis, and foreign body reactions. It is important to maintain a degree of skepticism in viewing giant cells in muscle biopsies. They are only of significance if they have the characteristic structure and occur as part of a typical granuloma.

Muscle can be involved in generalized sarcoidosis. Silverstein and Siltzbach[80] reviewed their experience of a sarcoidosis clinic of 800 patients at Mt. Sinai Hospital, New York, and found one patient with severe myalgia who had myositis on muscle biopsy, two patients with a chronic progressive myopathy who had myositis on biopsy, and 8 of 25 randomly taken muscle biopsies from asymptomatic patients which showed granulomatous involvement. It is possible that cases of pure skeletal muscle sarcoidosis can occur,[81] but these require full autopsy to exclude the presence of systemic sarcoidosis.

A second condition with giant cells in the skeletal muscle is the rare but clearly defined syndrome of giant cell (granulomatous) myositis, giant cell myocarditis, and myasthenia gravis associated with a thymoma (Fig. 79–11).[82,83] The intestinal smooth muscle may also be involved.[84] This association suggests the presence of circulating myotoxic muscle antibodies as well as acetylcholine receptor antibodies in these patients, though this remains to be proved.

Secondary Polymyositis in the Primary Myopathies. The finding of inflammatory cell infiltrates in skeletal muscle biopsies is not necessarily diagnostic of DM or PM. Any focal injury, such as intramuscular injections or electromyography, may cause pathological changes suggestive of DM-PM. Also inflammatory cell infiltrates consisting mainly of lymphocytes may occasionally be found in biopsies from any of the primary degenerative muscular dystrophies, including Duchenne, Becker, limb-girdle, and particularly facioscapulohumeral muscular dystrophy.[85-88] The inflammatory infiltrate is usually interstitial, but may occasionally be perivascular. Though a rare case may improve with long-term corticosteroid therapy,[86,88] the majority show no clinical benefit despite decreased levels of serum CK.[87] It is likely that in such cases there is a secondary autoimmune inflammatory response to the chronic release of skeletal muscle fiber antigens, but only rarely is this of functional significance.

Polymyalgia Rheumatica. This condition, which is fully described in Chapter 73, may be difficult to separate from DM-PM. It usually presents in patients older than 45 years with diffuse pains in the proximal upper limbs to a greater extent than in the lower limbs. It is difficult to know if the pains come from the muscles or the joints, and there is often general malaise. Patients have no true muscle weakness, though pain may make it difficult for the patient to exert full strength. There may be some muscle wasting from disuse, but this is not severe.

Investigations show a serum CK which is almost invariably normal. The EMG may be normal or may show slight myopathic changes, and the muscle biopsy may be normal or may have type 2 fiber atrophy due to disuse. It is necessary to separate DM-PM from poly-

Figure 79–11. Muscle from a 53-year-old man with giant cell polymyositis, myasthenia gravis, and thymoma. The giant cells in this case appeared to derive from the muscle fibers. Hematoxylin and easin × 320.

myalgia rheumatica, since the latter has a better prognosis.

THE HEART AND LUNGS IN DERMATOMYOSITIS-POLYMYOSITIS.

Symptomatic cardiac involvement in DM-PM is relatively uncommon, but can occur producing dysrhythmias, congestive cardiac failure, and sometimes death.[12] More commonly there is electrocardiographic evidence of pericarditis, myocardial dysfunction, conduction defects, or arrhythmias. Clinical or electrocardiographic abnormalities are seen in 30 to 50 percent of patients with DM-PM at some time in their course.[6,8] Cardiac involvement may be seen in all the subgroups of myositis.[6,11,58] In childhood DM, Bitnum and colleagues[11] found that electrocardiographic abnormalities indicated a worse prognosis. Pathological studies show inflammatory myositis of the myocardium with muscle fiber necrosis and fibrosis.

Pulmonary fibrosis (fibrosing alveolitis) can rarely occur in DM-PM,[59,60] though it is worth remembering that certain drugs used in the treatment of myositis such as methotrexate can cause pulmonary fibrosis. In addition, muscle weakness can compromise ventilatory function, and in very ill patients in hospital the vital capacity should be measured daily. Impaired proximal pharyngeal muscle function can produce aspiration pneumonitis, which can go unnoticed on clinical examination and appear only on chest radiographs.

ETIOLOGY OF DERMATOMYOSITIS-POLYMYOSITIS

In none of the collagen-vascular diseases is the etiology completely understood, and this applies equally to DM-PM complex. Three major possibilities exist: a viral infection, an abnormal recognition of "self" by the immune system of the body, and a vasculopathy. These three possibilities are not necessarily mutually exclusive. For instance, it is conceivable that a chronic viral infection of the skeletal muscle fibers would cause an alteration in the muscle fiber antigens which would be recognized by the immunological system as "non-self," thus producing a vasculitis, and the DM-PM.

Immunological Studies. *Humoral Immunity.* The ESR is raised in about 50 percent of DM-PM, and the serum immunoglobulins are frequently raised.[89] Muscle biopsies of DM-PM show vascular deposits of immunoglobulins and complement, particularly in childhood DM,[90,91] though this has not been confirmed by all observers.[92] Similar deposits have been seen in the intramuscular blood vessels of a variety of other collagen-vascular diseases.[93] It is likely that these vascular deposits of immune complexes produce vascular damage.

However, there is conflicting evidence in the literature as to whether immunoglobulins play a significant direct role in skeletal muscle damage in DM-PM. The incidence of antibodies against skeletal muscle is similar in DM-PM and in other muscle wasting conditions.[94] Dawkins and Mastaglia[95] found that the serum of patients with DM-PM was not cytotoxic for muscle cultures in vitro. However, the serum from animals immunized with skeletal muscle is myotoxic in vivo.[96-98] Thus the evidence for the etiological role of antibodies in DM-PM is far from strong.

Cellular Immunity. When peripheral blood lymphocytes are exposed to antigens to which they are sensitized, they undergo transformation as indicated by an increased DNA synthesis leading to cell division. Several groups have found that peripheral blood lymphocytes from patients with DM-PM show much higher degrees of transformation than controls when exposed to skeletal muscle antigens,[15,99] though other studies did not confirm this.[100] Another test of lymphocyte response to antigens, the macrophage migration inhibition test, showed a higher reaction in DM-PM than in other conditions of muscle wasting.[101] The degree of lymphocyte transformation response to skeletal muscle antigens was found to be directly proportional to the degree of activity of the DM-PM, and was decreased by corticosteroid therapy.[15,99]

The peripheral blood lymphocytes from patients with DM-PM have been shown to be myotoxic in vitro, and those from Group III patients (according to the classification of Walton and Adams[2]) are toxic both to myoblasts and fibroblasts in tissue culture.[15,102,103] There is dispute whether the degree of cytotoxicity of the lymphocytes is related to disease activity and therapy.[95,104]

There appear to be two ways in which the lymphocytes damage the skeletal muscle; first, they release lymphotoxins,[95,105] and second, they directly become attached to and invade skeletal muscle fibers.[106-108]

The experimental model, experimental allergic myositis (EAM), adds support to the role of the lymphocyte in the pathogenesis of DM-PM. Animals immunized with skeletal muscle antigens and adjuvant develop an inflammatory myopathy.[109,110] It has been shown that the lymphocytes from immunized animals are cytotoxic for skeletal muscle in vitro and in vivo.[111,112] The skeletal muscle sarcolemma and myofibrillary proteins can both cause EAM.[96,113]

Thus the evidence for the role of lymphocytes in DM-PM is much stronger than that for antibodies, and it has been suggested that the DM-PM complex is a disease of cellular immunity to skeletal muscle.[114]

Virological Studies. The development of an acute or subacute polymyositis in a number of virological illnesses, including influenza and Bornholm disease, has been mentioned. This, together with the inflammatory nature of DM-PM, leads to the suggestion that the latter disease might be due to a chronic viral infection of the skeletal muscle and a secondary immunological response. There are a large number of reports of the findings of virus-like particles in DM-PM muscle studied under the electron microscope. These are of various types, including myxovirus-like particles and picornavirus-like particles.[36,38,39,115-121] However, virus-like particles have also been seen in normal autopsy muscle[122] and in the paraspinal muscles from patients with idiopathic scoliosis,[123] and thus their presence in DM-PM muscle may not be etiologically significant.

More convincing of an etiological role would be the isolation of a virus which could be shown experimentally to be myotoxic. However, no viral isolation from the skeletal muscle of a patient with typical DM-PM has ever been reported. Zweymüller[124] isolated coxsackievirus A2 from the stool of a 14-year-old patient with chronic DM, and showed that antibodies to this virus were present in the serum; no isolation of virus was obtained from the muscle, and it remains uncertain whether the fecal virus was relevant. A similar problem of interpretation exists with the report by Marcus and Bill of the isolation of an echovirus from the stool of two brothers with acute polymyositis.[68] Freudenberg and associates[125] isolated coxsackievirus from the skeletal muscle of a 6-month-old baby with myositis causing flexion contractures; the baby had been born with an antenatal fracture of the femur, and thus had a very unusual disease. Coxsackievirus B has been isolated from a child dying at the age of 1 week with myocarditis and skeletal muscle degeneration;[126] electron microscopic examination has shown picorna-like virus particles in the muscle. Coxsackievirus A9 has been isolated from the muscle of an 11-year-old girl who had had muscle weakness and physical retardation since early infancy and who died of pneumonia and respiratory muscle weakness.[127]

Thus no viral isolations have been described from the muscle of *typical* cases of subacute or chronic DM or PM, and the role of viruses in the etiology of these diseases is still uncertain.

Vasculopathy. The vasculopathy that is particularly seen in the childhood form of DM has already been described. Any diffuse vasculopathy may produce skeletal muscle ischemia, and hence necrosis of individual muscle fibers or infarctions of areas of the muscle. This may be seen in such vasculitides as polyarteritis nodosa, the microangiopathy of diabetes mellitus, and atheromatous and carcinomatous microembolization.[128,129] There is considerable evidence for a vasculopathy with endothelial cell damage and thrombosis of capillaries in DM-PM, particularly in childhood.[51] In DM and PM there may be deposition of immune complexes within the intramuscular blood vessels[90,91] and thickening and reduplication of the basement membranes of the capillaries (though similar basement membrane thickening can occur in other chronic myopathies).[51,54] There is loss of capillaries as measured by the ratio of capillaries to muscle fibers, and of number of capillaries to unit transverse area of muscle fiber in childhood DM. This is particularly marked in the perifascicular areas, which may explain the perifascicular atrophy.[52] However, Jerusalem and associates[54] found the mean capillary area to be increased in DM, SLE, and scleroderma, but not in PM.

Capillary endothelial cells of the muscle and skin of DM have been shown to contain prominent branched tubular structures (undulating tubules) of 20 to 30 nm diameter.[51,52,54,130] These were originally interpreted as virions, but have been seen in the capillary endothelial cells in many collagen-vascular diseases,[51] and probably represent specializations of the endoplasmic reticulum rather than viruses.

Summary of Etiological Studies. It is possible that a virus triggers an immunological reaction, or that a primary aberration of the immunological recognition of skeletal muscle as "self" is responsible for the disease. The immunological reaction is a cellular one and antibodies probably play a relatively minor part in pathogenesis. The lymphocytes enter the interstitial space around the muscle fibers, and there may release as yet uncharacterized lymphotoxins which directly damage the muscle fibers. The mechanism of the vasculopathy is uncertain, but this may cause widespread organ damage as in the childhood form of DM-PM, and may be related to elements of the skeletal muscle pathology in this disease complex.

TREATMENT AND PROGNOSIS OF DERMATOMYOSITIS AND POLYMYOSITIS

The treatment and prognosis of any disease are inextricably intertwined. If there is no treatment, then the prognosis is related to the intrinsic features of the disease; if there is an effective treatment, the prognosis must be improved. Unfortunately in DM-PM we have no very clear idea of the prognosis of the untreated disease, and no absolute certainty of the efficacy of the treatment.

Treatment. In view of the lymphocytic inflammatory nature of the process of DM-PM, corticosteroid therapy was tried in DM-PM.[2] Immunosuppressive therapy was similarly tried.[131,132] However, almost no control trials have been performed in DM-PM, and moreover there are very few studies of the prognosis of the disease in large series of untreated patients. This dilemma has been vigorously emphasized by Bohan and Peter,[5] who relegated to the fields of friction and fantasy the statements that corticosteroid and immunosuppressive therapy were of benefit in DM-PM. This point was taken up by Rowland and associates,[7] who reviewed the literature dealing with corticosteroids and immunosuppressive therapy in DM-PM.

Fortunately this lack of *certainty* of the benefit of corticosteroid and immunosuppressive therapy does not mean that these diseases are relegated to the category of "untreatable." Many clinicians are convinced of the efficacy of treatment in DM-PM,[2,8] and even those who express skepticism use these medications extensively.[6,7]

There is no evidence that nonsteroidal anti-inflammatory drugs are effective in treatment of DM-PM. Prednisone is the treatment of choice in the patient with acute DM-PM. The dose of prednisone needs to be as high as 60 to 100 mg per day, which may be given in four divided doses at the initiation of therapy, and may have to be continued for months to years, particularly in more chronic cases and when there has been a delay in diagnosis and treatment.[8,133] After a week of divided daily dose therapy, patients can often be changed to a single daily dose, with plans ultimately to shift to alternate day therapy when feasible. The observation that many patients may show no improvement before 3 to 6 months of prolonged high dose corticosteroid therapy is of help in supporting the resolve of both the physician and the patient when side effects of corticosteroid therapy begin to appear. The clinical state, the muscle strength, and the serum enzymes should be serially monitored throughout treatment. Though raised serum levels of CK can be reduced in a nonspecific manner by corticosteroid therapy,[87] nevertheless the serum CK is a useful monitor of disease activity in polymyositis under treatment.[8] In any patient starting corticosteroid therapy, supplemental calcium (0.5 gram Ca^{++} per day) and vitamin D (50,000 units weekly or twice weekly) may retard development of osteopenia. Potassium supplements and antacids may also be required. The risks and side effects of long-term high-dose corticosteroid therapy must always be weighed against the therapeutic benefit to be gained.

As soon as clinical improvement allows, i.e., as soon as the patient appears to have reached a plateau in improvement, the dose of prednisone can be gradually reduced, while the muscle strength and serum CK are continually monitored. It may be possible, and is certainly preferred, to change patients to a single-dose, every-other-day regimen as soon as possible. The dosage is reduced until either it has been withdrawn or clinical or chemical signs of a relapse appear. If relapse occurs, the dose of prednisone is raised until control is again achieved. Eventually approximately 75 percent of patients can stop therapy, though evidence of disease activity continues in the remainder for more than 5 years.

Dubowitz[134] treats childhood DM in a somewhat different fashion, trying to obtain remission with the relatively low dose of 1 to 1.5 mg per kilogram per day of prednisone. He then attempts to get the patient off corticosteroid therapy as soon as possible by commencing reduction of dosage as soon as signs of clinical improvement appear, without waiting for full clinical remission. However, in view of the potentially fatal vasculitis in childhood DM, it might seem better to treat this category at least as vigorously as adult DM-PM.

Immunosuppressants have been widely used in conjunction with corticosteroid therapy in DM-PM.[131,132] There seems little difference in the therapeutic effect of the two most commonly used drugs, methotrexate and azathioprine. The latter has the advantage of oral administration and a relatively slower cytotoxicity. The dosage of azathioprine should be 2 to 3 mg per kilogram per day in divided doses; monitoring with full blood count including determination of total number of lymphocytes and platelets is required. Development of malignancy (usually lymphoma) in patients receiving immunosuppressive therapy is a potential, though rare, hazard. Liver fibrosis with methotrexate therapy is a concern, but can be minimized by using weekly single dose intravenous therapy, or a dosage schedule popularized by the dermatologists for psoriasis based on intermittent oral therapy. Hepatic damage may also occur with azathioprine. It is therefore prudent to monitor liver function regularly during therapy with methotrexate or azathioprine, and perhaps to obtain 6-monthly liver biopsies in the case of methotrexate therapy.

Immunosuppressive therapy is usually added to prednisone when the latter has been found to produce an inadequate response in DM-PM after 2 to 4 months. A recent controlled trial of azathioprine in patients with DM-PM, who had been stabilized on prednisone, demonstrated that there was improvement at 1 and 3 years after starting treatment in the prednisone plus azathioprine group compared with the group receiving prednisone alone.[135] There was, however, no difference at 3 months. Personal experience suggests that patients with disease that is more severe or of longer duration will have a greater benefit if therapy with prednisone and with azathioprine is commenced simultaneously (see also Reference 136).

Side effects of therapy are not inconsequential. The frequency of significant complications ranges from 16 to 22 percent, and of fatal complications from 1 to 4 percent in recent large series.[2,6-8] All the known complications of corticosteroid therapy can occur, including diabetes mellitus, hypertension, cushingoid somatic changes, infection, delayed wound healing, hypokalemia, vertebral collapse, psychosis, gastrointestinal ulceration, hemorrhage and perforation, cataracts, and ischemic necrosis of the femoral head. Similarly the complications of immunosuppressive therapy include aplastic anemia, leukopenia, thrombocytopenia, infection, hemorrhage, pulmonary fibrosis, and liver toxicity. Corticosteroid myopathy can occur in patients receiving high dose prednisone therapy for DM-PM, and this is always a difficult diagnostic problem. It should be considered whenever a patient on long-term high dose corticosteroid therapy begins to deteriorate without an increase in the serum CK level. The diagnosis can be arrived at clinically by reducing the dose of prednisone; the muscle weakness and serum CK will increase if the problem is continuing active DM-PM, and will decrease if corticosteroid myopathy is the problem. The diagnosis of corticosteroid myopathy may be supported by investigations, including a normal CK, a muscle biopsy showing no inflammatory infiltration but simply Type 2 fiber atrophy, and an EMG which shows no increased insertional activity. However, it is important to remember that corticosteroid myopathy and DM-PM may coexist, presenting a difficult therapeutic dilemma which is best resolved by decreasing the dose of prednisone and adding or increasing the dosage of immunosuppressive therapy.

Several other elements of therapy should be mentioned. The use of penicillamine[137] needs careful monitoring in view of the increasing number of cases of PM caused by penicillamine.[138] Calcinosis is rarely more than a radiological problem, but chronic aluminum hydroxide therapy may be of help.[139] The role of physical therapy is to maintain muscle strength and range of movement without damaging regenerating muscle fibers. For that reason the following guidelines are suggested: (1) During the acute stage of severe inflammation passive range of motion to prevent soft tissue contractures should be carried out twice daily but active motion should be discouraged. (2) During recovery, or when the acute inflammation is not so severe, activity should be encouraged at a slower rate than that for inflammatory joint disease. (3) Occupational therapy should be used to aid in functions permanently lost.

Prognosis. Before the introduction of corticosteroid therapy the mortality rate in 38 patients with DM seen at the Mayo Clinic prior to 1940 was 50 percent.[22] The mortality rate was 60 percent in 291 patients collected from the literature by Schuermann.[140] Since those figures were published, antibiotics and other general medical approaches have inevitably improved the prognosis of DM-PM, and unfortunately no recent series of untreated DM-PM is available in the literature.

A number of reports since the introduction of corticosteroid therapy have indicated a prognosis only slightly better than that in the precorticosteroid era. These include a 30 percent mortality rate in childhood DM-PM,[11,19] and a 40 percent mortality rate after 5 years in adult PM.[141] Nevertheless a number of large series of childhood and adult PM-DM have shown a much better prognosis.[2,6,8,47,49] In the Newcastle series with a mean follow-up of 6 years, the mortality rate in the childhood group was 5 percent and in the overall group 28 percent.[8] In the Los Angeles series with a mean follow-up of 4.3 years, the mortality ranged from 9 to 13 percent, with the exception of the group associated with carcinoma in whom it was 54 percent.[6] Life-span tables were constructed by Medsger and associates[3] in a survey of 124 patients seen over a 22-year period from 1947 to 1968, many of whom were treated with corticosteroids. The *survival compared to an age-matched control population* was 72 percent at 2 years, 68 percent at 5 years, and 53 percent at 7 years. This should be compared with the much better prognosis in the Newcastle series of a *total survival* of 90 percent at 2 years, 80 percent at 5 years, and 77 percent at 7 years.[8]

There is also discordance in the literature concerning morbidity of DM-PM. Severe impairment of a third of cases of childhood DM,[11,19] and of 40 percent of adults[141] should be compared with the much more favorable outcome of the Newcastle series.[8] Even in the most florid cases in which all the diagnostic criteria were positive, in that series the mean disability (see Table 79-5; a level of 3 or better indicates no functional disability) fell from 5 at presentation to 4 at 1 year, 3.5 at 5 years, and 2.5 at 10 years. In the overall group of 118 patients, the mean disability fell from 4.7 at presentation to 3.4 at 1 year and 2.4 at 5 years.

It is difficult to understand the reason for the differences in the observations at different centers concerning the prognosis of DM-PM. It is possible that case material differs either intrinsically or in relation to the duration between onset and treatment, or that the treatment regimens themselves differ between different centers.

A number of prognostic features have been identified in different studies. Adults fare worse than children with regard to both morbidity and mortality.[3,8,16] Those with carcinoma have the highest mortality.[6,8,16] Those who are most severely affected at presentation have the highest morbidity and mortality.[3,6,8] The black race fares worse than the white.[3] The finding by DeVere and Bradley[8] that the overlap group fared worse with regard to morbidity and mortality was not confirmed by Bohan and associates.[6] DM as a whole has a high incidence of underlying carcinoma[8] and may thus have an increased mortality rate, though the increased morbidity of DM found by Rowland and associates[7] has not been found by others.[8] Patients with sufficient weakness of the pharyngeal muscles to cause aspiration pneumonia have a poor prognosis.[3]

Conclusions. Though it is not possible to provide hard facts to prove the therapeutic usefulness of corticosteroids in DM-PM, it is the general experience that DM-PM is a treatable group of diseases with a large amount of morbidity and mortality both from the disease and to some extent from the therapy. However, it is justified to describe DM-PM as "curable" in many cases. It is consequently important not to miss the diagnosis, and to treat patients as early and as vigorously as possible.

References

1. Eaton, L.M.: The perspective of neurology in regard to polymyositis. A study of 41 cases. Neurology 4:245, 1954.
2. Walton, J.N., and Adams, R.D.: Polymyositis. Baltimore, Williams & Wilkins Company, 1958.
3. Medsger, T.A., Robinson, H., and Masi, A.T.: Factors affecting survivorship in polymyositis. A life-table study of 124 patients. Arthritis Rheum. 14:249, 1971.
4. Currie, S.: Polymyositis and related disorders. *In* Walton, J.N. (ed.): Disorders of Voluntary Muscle. 4th ed. Edinburgh, Churchill Livingstone, 1981.
5. Bohan, A., and Peter, J.B.: Polymyositis and dermatomyositis (first of two parts). N. Engl. J. Med. 292:344, 1975.
6. Bohan, A., Peter, J.B., Bowman, R.L., and Pearson, C.M.: A computer-assisted analysis of 153 patients with polymyositis and dermatomyositis. Medicine 56:255, 1977.
7. Rowland, L.P., Clark, C., and Olarte, M.: Therapy for dermatomyositis and polymyositis. Adv. Neurol. 17:63, 1977.
8. DeVere, R., and Bradley, W.G.: Polymyositis: Its presentation, morbidity and mortality. Brain 98:637, 1975.
9. Nattrass, F.J.: Recovery from "muscular dystrophy." Brain 77:549, 954.
10. Arundell, F.D., Wilkinson, R.D., and Iläserick, J.R.: Dermatomyositis and malignant neoplasms in adults. Arch. Derm. Syph. 82:772, 1960.
11. Bitnum, S., Daeschner, C.W., Travis, L.B., Dodge, W.F., and Hopps, H.C.: Dermatomyositis. J. Pediatr. 64:101, 1964.
12. Hill, D.L., and Barrows, H.S.: Identical skeletal and cardiac muscle involvement in a case of fatal polymyositis. Arch. Neurol. 19:545, 1968.
13. Research Group on Neuromuscular Diseases of the World Federation of Neurology: Classification of the neuromuscular disorders. J. Neurol. Sci. 6:165, 1968.
14. Walton, J.N.: Clinical examination of the neuromuscular system. *In* Walton, Sir John (ed.): Disorders of Voluntary Muscle. 4th ed. Edinburgh, Churchill, Livingstone, 1981.
15. Currie, S., Saunders, M., Knowles, M., and Brown, A.E.: Immunological aspects of polymyositis: The in vitro activity of lymphocytes on incubation with muscle antigen and with muscle cultures. Quart. J. Med. 40:63, 1971.
16. Rose, A.L., and Walton, J.N.: Polymyositis: A survey of 89 cases with particular reference to treatment and prognosis. Brain 89:747, 1966.
17. Medsger, T.A., Dawson, W.N., and Masi, A.T.: The epidemiology of polymyositis. Am. J. Med. 48:715, 1970.
18. Leonhardt, T.: Familial occurrence of collagen diseases. II. Progressive systemic sclerosis and dermatomyositis. Acta Med. Scand. 169:735, 1961.

19. Cook, C.D., Rosen, F.S., and Banker, B.Q.: Dermatomyositis and focal scleroderma. Pediat. Clin. North Am. 10:979, 1963.
20. Lewkonia, R.M., and Buxton, P.H.: Myositis in father and daughter. J. Neurol. Neurosurg. Psychiat. 36:820, 1973.
21. Hollinrake, K.: Polymyositis presenting as distal muscle weakness. A case report. J. Neurol. Sci. 8:479, 1969.
22. O'Leary, P.A., and Waisman, M.: Dermatomyositis. Arch. Dermatol. 41:1001, 1940.
23. Wedgewood, R.J.P., Cook, C.D., and Cohen, J.: Dermatomyositis. Pediatrics 12:447, 1953.
24. Buchthal, F., and Pinelli, P.: Muscle action potentials in polymyositis. Neurology 3:424, 1953.
25. Mechler, F.: Changing electromyographic findings during the chronic course of polymyositis. J. Neurol. Sci. 23:237, 1974.
26. Henriksson, K.-G., and Stålberg, I.: The terminal innervation pattern in polymyositis. Muscle Nerve 1:3, 1978.
27. Spies, S.M., Swift, T.R., and Brown, M.: Increased ⁹⁹ᵐTc-polyphosphate muscle uptake in a patient with polymyositis: Case report. J. Nucl. Med. 16:1125, 1975.
28. Mastaglia, F.L., and Kakulas, B.A.: A histological and histochemical study of skeletal muscle regeneration in polymyositis. J. Neurol. Sci. 10:471, 1970.
29. Brooke, M.H., and Kaplan, H.: Muscle pathology in rheumatoid arthritis, polymyalgia rheumatica and polymyositis. Arch. Pathol. 94:101, 1972.
30. Munsat, T., and Cancilla, P.: Polymyositis without inflammation. Bull. Los Angeles Neurol. Soc. 39:113, 1974.
31. Baumli, H.-P., and Mumenthaler, M.: The perifascicular atrophy factor, an aid in the histological diagnosis of polymyositis. J. Neurol. 214:129, 1977.
32. Dubowitz, V., and Brooke, M.H.: Muscle Biopsy: A Modern Approach. London, W. B. Saunders Company, Ltd., 1973.
33. Cöers, C., Telerman-Toffet, N., and Gerard, J.F.M.: Terminal innervation ratio in neuromuscular disease. Arch. Neurol. 29:215, 1973.
34. Rose, A.L., Walton, J.N., and Pearce, G.W.: Polymyositis: An ultramicroscopic study of muscle biopsy material. J. Neurol. Sci. 5:457, 1967.
35. Shafiq, S.A., Milhorat, A.T., and Gorycki, M.A.: An electronmicroscope study of muscle degeneration and vascular changes in polymyositis. J. Pathol. 94:139, 1967.
36. Mastaglia, F.L., and Walton, J.N.: An ultrastructural study of skeletal muscle in polymyositis. J. Neurol. Sci. 12:473, 1971.
37. Hughes, J.T., and Esiri, M.M.: Ultrastructural studies in human polymyositis. J. Neurol. Sci. 25:347, 1975.
38. Chou, S.-M.: Myxovirus-like structures and accompanying nuclear changes in chronic polymyositis. Arch. Pathol. 122:649, 1968.
39. Martinez, A.J., Hooshmand, H., Mendoza, G.I., and Winston, Y.E.: Fatal polymyositis: Morphogenesis and ultrastructural features. Acta Neuropathol. 29:251, 1974.
40. Mintz, G., Gonzalez-Angulo, A., Frago, A., and Zavala, B.J.: Ultrastructure of muscle in polymyositis. Am. J. Med. 44:216, 1968.
41. Cape, C.A., Johnson, W.W., and Pitner, S.E.: Nemaline structures in polymyositis: A nonspecific pathological reaction of skeletal muscle. Neurology 20:494, 1970.
42. Chou, S.-M.: "Megacon" mitochondria observed in a case of chronic polymyositis. Neurology 17:309, 1967.
43. Krain, L.S.: Dermatomyositis in six patients without initial muscle involvement. Arch. Dermatol. 111:241, 1975.
44. Keil, H.: The manifestations in the skin and mucous membranes in dermatomyositis, with special reference to the differential diagnosis from systemic lupus erythematosus. Ann. Intern. Med. 16:828, 1975.
45. Janis, J.F., and Winkelmann, R.K.: Histopathology of the skin in dermatomyositis. Arch. Dermatol. 97:640, 1968.
46. Barnes, B.E.: Dermatomyositis and malignancy. Ann. Intern. Med. 84:68, 1976.
47. Sullivan, D.B., Cassidy, J.T., Petty, R.E., and Burt, A.: Prognosis in childhood dermatomyositis. J. Pediatr. 80:555, 1972.
48. Miller, J.J.: Late progression in dermatomyositis in childhood. J. Pediatr. 83:543, 1973.
49. Rose, A.L.: Childhood polymyositis: A follow-up study with special reference to treatment with corticosteroids. Am. J. Dis. Child. 127:518, 1974.
50. Banker, B.Q., and Victor, M.: Dermatomyositis (systemic angiopathy) of childhood. Medicine 45:261, 1966.
51. Banker, B.Q.: Dermatomyositis of childhood: Ultrastructural alterations of muscle and intramuscular blood vessels. J. Neuropathol. Exp. Neurol. 34:46, 1975.
52. Carpenter, S., Karpati, G., Rothman, S., and Watters, G.: The childhood type of dermatomyositis. Neurology 26:952, 1976.
53. Gonzalez-Angulo, A., Frago, A., Mintz, G., and Zavala, B.J.: Submicroscopic alterations in capillaries of skeletal muscles in polymyositis. Am. J. Med. 65:873, 1968.
54. Jerusalem, F., Rakusa, M., Engel, A.G., and McDonald, R.D.: Morphometric analysis of skeletal muscle capillary structure in inflammatory myopathies. J. Neurol. Sci. 23:391, 1974.
55. Bunim, J.J.: A broader spectrum of Sjögren's syndrome and its pathogenetic implications. Ann. Rheum. Dis. 20:1, 1961.
56. Wroblewski, R., and Nordemar, R.: Ultrastructural and histochemical studies of muscle in rheumatoid arthritis. Scand. J. Rheumatol. 4:197, 1975.
57. Wroblewski, R., and Nordemar, R.: Ultrastructural and histochemical studies of muscle in rheumatoid arthritis. Acta Neuropathol. 33:317, 1975.
58. Singsen, B.H., Walters, K.D., Siegel, S.E., and Hanson, V.: Lymphocytic leukemia, atypical dermatomyositis and hyperlipidemia in a 4-year-old boy. J. Pediatr. 88:602, 1976.
59. Duncan, P.E., Griffin, J.P., Garcia, A., and Kaplan, S.B.: Fibrosing alveolitis in polymyositis. Am. J. Med. 57:621, 1974.
60. Schwarz, M.I., Matthay, R.A., Sahn, S.A., Stanford, R.E., Marmorstein, B.L., and Scheinhorn, D.J.: Interstitial lung disease in polymyositis and dermatomyositis. Analysis of six cases and review of the literature. Medicine 55:89, 1976.
61. Lundberg, A.: Myalgia cruris epidemica. Acta Paediat. Scand. 46:18, 1957.
62. Middleton, P.J., Alexander, R.M., and Szymanski, M.T.: Severe myositis during recovery from influenza. Lancet 2:533, 1970.
63. Mejlszenkier, J.D., Safran, A.P., Healy, J.J., Embree, L., and Ouelletter, E.M.: The myositis of influenza. Arch. Neurol. 29:441, 1973.
64. Hanissian, A.S., Martinez, A.J., Jabbour, J.T., and Duenas, D.A.: Vasculitis and myositis secondary to rubella vaccination. Arch. Neurol. 28:202, 1973.
65. McKinlay, I.A., and Mitchell, I.: Transient acute myositis in childhood. Arch. Dis. Child. 51:135, 1976.
66. Landry, M., and Winkelmann, R.K.: Tubular cytoplasmic inclusion in dermatomyositis. Mayo Clin. Proc. 47:479, 1972.
67. Lepine, P., Desse, G., and Sautter, V.: Biopsies musculaires avec examen histologique et isolement du virus coxsackie chez l'homme attient de myalgie épidémique (maladie de Bornholm). Bull. Acad. Nat. Med. 136:66, 1952.
68. Marcus, J.C., and Bill, P.L.A.: Acute myopathy in three brothers. Neuropadiätrie 7:101, 1976.
69. Barrett, A.M., and Gresheim, G.A.: Acute streptococcal myositis. Br. Med. J. 1:347, 1958.
70. Altrocchi, P.H.: Spontaneous bacterial myositis. JAMA 217:819, 1971.
71. Rogers, D.W.: Case of pyomyositis occurring in London. Br. Med. J. 3:679, 1973.
72. Davis, M.J., Cilo, M., Plaitakis, A., and Yahr, M.D.: Trichinosis: Severe myopathic involvement with recovery. Neurology 26:37, 1976.
73. Mansour, S.E.D., and Reese, H.H.: A previously unreported myopathy in patients with schistosomiasis. Neurology 14:355, 1964.
74. Sawney, B.B., Chopra, J.S., Banerji, A.K., and Wahi, P.L.: Pseudohypertrophic myopathy in cysticercosis. Neurology 26:270, 1976.
75. McGill, R.J., and Goodbody, R.A.: Sarcosporidiosis in man with periarteritis nodosa. Br. Med. J. 2:333, 1957.
76. Rowland, L.P., and Greer, M.: Toxoplasmic polymyositis. Neurology 11:367, 1961.
77. Chandar, K., Mair, H.J., and Mair, N.S.: Case of *toxoplasma* polymyositis. Br. Med. J. 1:158, 1968.
78. Samuels, B.S., and Rietschal, R.L.: Polymyositis and toxoplasmosis. JAMA 235:60, 1976.
79. Kagen, L.T., Kimball, A.C., and Christian, C.L.: Serologic evidence of toxoplasmosis among patients with polymyositis. Am. J. Med. 56:186, 1974.
80. Silverstein, A., and Siltzbach, L.E.: Muscle involvement with sarcoidosis. Arch. Neurol. 21:235, 1969.
81. Lynch, P.G., and Bansal, D.V.: Granulomatous polymyositis. J. Neurol. Sci. 18:1, 1973.
82. Burke, J.S., Medline, N.M., and Katz, A.: Giant cell myocarditis and myositis associated with thymoma and myasthenia gravis. Arch. Pathol. 88:359, 1969.
83. Namba, T., Brunner, N.G., and Grob, D.: Idiopathic giant cell polymyositis: Report of a case and review of the syndrome. Arch. Neurol. 31:27, 1974.
84. Caquet, R., Festal, G., Deslingnères, S., Pierres, M., Lapresle, J., and Laroche, C.: Polymyosite à forme myasthénique, thymome, dégénérescence musculaire lisse. Nouv. Presse Méd. 3:743, 1974.
85. Munsat, T.L., Piper, D., Cancilla, P., and Mednick, J.: Inflammatory myopathy with facioscapulohumeral distribution. Neurology 22:335, 1972.
86. Papepetropoulos, T.A., and Bradley, W.G.: The role of secondary polymyositis in the muscular dystrophy syndrome. Excerpta Medica Int. Congr. Series No. 334. Abstract No. 211, 1974.
87. Munsat, T.L., and Bradley, W.G.: Serum creatine phosphokinase levels and prednisone-treated muscle weakness. Neurology 27:96, 1977.
88. Bradley, W.G.: The limb-girdle syndromes. *In* Vinken, P.J., and Bruyn, G.W. (eds.): Handbook of Clinical Neurology. Vol. 40. Amsterdam, Elsevier/North Holland, 1979, pp. 433–469.
89. Lisak, R.P., and Zweiman, B.: Serum immunoglobulin levels in myas-

thenia gravis, polymyositis and dermatomyositis. J. Neurol. Neurosurg. Psychiat. 39:34, 1976.

90. Whitaker, J.N., and Engel, W.K.: Vascular deposits of immunoglobulin and complement in inflammatory myopathy. Trans. Am. Neurol. Assoc. 96:24, 1972.

91. Whitaker, J.N., and Engel, W.K.: Vascular deposits of immunoglobulin and complement in idiopathic inflammatory myopathy. N. Engl. J. Med. 286:333, 1972.

92. Huntington, H.W.: Immunologic myopathy. Arch. Path. Lab. Med. 102:212, 1978.

93. Oxenhandler, R., Adelstein, E., and Hart, M.: Direct immunofluorescent study of muscle biopsies. Value in diagnosis of connective tissue disease. Lab. Invest. 34:329, 1976.

94. Caspary, E.A., Gubbray, S.S., and Stern, G.M.: Circulating antibodies in polymyositis and other muscle-wasting disorders. Lancet 2:1941, 1964.

95. Dawkins, R.L., and Mastaglia, F.L.: Cell-mediated cytoxicity to muscle in polymyositis. Effect of immunosuppression. N. Engl. J. Med. 288:434, 1973.

96. Namba, T., and Maguruma, M.: The role of skeletal muscle membrane in experimental myopathy. Neurology 22:611, 1972.

97. Korenyi-Both, A., and Kelemen, G.: Damage of skeletal muscle in rats by immunoglobulins. I. Pathophysiological data and lightmicroscopic observations. Acta Neuropathol. 34:199, 1976.

98. Korenyi-Both, A.: Damage of skeletal muscle in rats in immunoglobulins. II. Ultrastructural studies. Acta Neuropathol. 34:207, 1976.

99. Esiri, M.M., Maclennan, I.C.M., and Hazleman, B.L.: Lymphocyte sensitivity to skeletal muscle in patients with polymyositis and other disorders. Clin. Exp. Immunol. 14:25, 1973.

100. Lisak, R.P., and Zweiman, B.: Mitogen and muscle extract induced in vitro proliferative responses in myasthenia gravis, dermatomyositis and polymyositis. J. Neurol. Neurosurg. Psychiat. 38:521, 1975.

101. Caspary, E.A., Currie, S., and Field, E.J.: Sensitized lymphocytes in muscular dystrophy. J. Neurol. Neurosurg. Psychiat. 34:353, 1971.

102. Currie, S., Saunders, M., and Knowles, M.: Immunological aspects of systemic sclerosis. In vitro activity of lymphocytes from patients with the disorder. Br. J. Dermatol. 84:400, 1970.

103. Currie, S.: Destruction of muscle cultures by lymphocytes from cases of polymyositis. Acta Neuropathol. 15:11, 1970.

104. Haas, D.C.: Treatment of polymyositis with immunosuppressive drugs. Neurology 23:55, 1973.

105. Johnson, R.L., Fink, C.W., and Ziff, M.: Lymphotoxin formation by lymphocytes and muscle in polymyositis. J. Clin. Invest. 51:2435, 1972.

106. Mastaglia, F.L., and Currie, S.: Immunological and ultrastructural observations on the role of lymphoid cells in the pathogenesis of polymyositis. Acta Neuropathol. 18:1, 1971.

107. Mastaglia, F.L., Dawkins, R.L., and Papadimitriou, J.M.: Lymphocyte-muscle cell interaction in vivo and in vitro. J. Neurol. Sci. 22:261, 1974.

108. Mastaglia, F.L., Papadimitriou, J.M., and Dawkins, R.L.: Mechanisms of cell-mediated myotoxicity: Morphological observations in muscle grafts and in muscle exposed to sensitized spleen cells in vivo. J. Neurol. Sci. 25:269, 1975.

109. Pearson, C.M.: Development of arthritis, periarthritis and periostitis in rats given adjuvants. Proc. Soc. Exp. Biol. Med. 91:95, 1956.

110. Dawkins, R.L.: Experimental myositis associated with hypersensitivity to muscle. J. Pathol. 90:619, 1965.

111. Kakulas, B.A.: Destruction of differentiated muscle cultures by sensitized lymphoid cells. J. Pathol. 91:495, 1966.

112. Currie, S.: Experimental myositis: The in vivo and in vitro activity of lymph-node cells. J. Pathol. 105:169, 1971.

113. Maghani, D., Partridge, T.A., and Sloper, J.C.: The role of the myofibrillar fraction of skeletal muscle in the production of experimental polymyositis. J. Neurol. Sci. 23:489, 1974.

114. Dawkins, R.L., and Zilko, P.J.: Polymyositis and myasthenia gravis: Immunodeficiency disorders involving skeletal muscle. Lancet 1:200, 1975.

115. Chou, S.-M.: Myxovirus-like structures in a case of human chronic polymyositis. Science 158:1453, 1967.

116. Chou, S.-M., and Gutmann, L.: Picorna-like crystals in subacute polymyositis. Neurology 20:205, 1970.

117. Carpenter, S., Karpati, G., Rothman, S., and Watters, G.: The childhood type of dermatomyositis. Neurology 26:952, 1976.

118. Yunis, E.J., and Samaha, F.J.: Inclusion body myositis. Lab. Invest. 25:240, 1971.

119. Sato, T., Walker, D.L., Peters, H.A., Reese, H.A., and Chou, S.-M.: Chronic polymyositis and myxovirus-like inclusions. Arch. Neurol. 24:409, 1971.

120. Ben-Bassat, M., and Machtey, I.: Picorna-like structures in acute dermatomyositis. Am. J. Clin. Pathol. 58:245, 1972.

121. Schochet, S.S., and McCormick, W.F.: Polymyositis with intranuclear inclusions. Arch. Neurol. 28:280, 1973.

122. Caulfield, J.B., Rebeiz, J., and Adams, R.D.: Viral involvement of human muscle. J. Pathol. 96:232, 1968.

123. Webb, J.N., and Gillespie, W.J.: Virus-like particles in paraspinal muscles in scoliosis. Br. J. Med. 2:912, 1976.

124. Zweymüller, E.: Schwere Haut-Muskelerkrankung unter dem klinischen Erscheinungsbild einer Dermatomyositis mit Coxsackie-Virusbefund. Deutsche Klin. Wschr. 78:190, 1953.

125. Freudenberg, E., Roulet, F., and Nicole, R.: Kongenitale Infektion mit Coxsackie-Virus. Ann. Paediatr. 178:150, 1952.

126. Sussman, M.L., Strauss, L., and Hodes, H.L.: Fatal Coxsackie Group B virus infection in the newborn. Am. J. Dis. Child. 97:483, 1959.

127. Tang, T.T., Sedmak, G.V., Siegesmund, K.A., and McCreadie, S.R.: Chronic myopathy associated with coxsackievirus Type A9: A combined electron microscopical and viral isolation study. N. Engl. J. Med. 292:608, 1975.

128. Haygood, T.A., Fessel, W.J., and Strange, D.A.: Atheromatous microembolism simulating polymyositis. JAMA 203:423, 1968.

129. Heffner, R.R.: Myopathy of embolic origin in patients with carcinoma. Neurology 21:840, 1971.

130. Hashimoto, K., Robinson, L., Velayos, E., and Niizuma, K.: Dermatomyositis: Electronmicroscopic, immunologic and tissue culture studies of paramyxovirus-like inclusion. Arch. Dermatol. 103:120, 1971.

131. Malaviya, A.N., Many, A., and Schwartz, R.S.: Treatment of dermatomyositis with methotrexate. Lancet 2:485, 1968.

132. McFarlin, D.E., and Griggs, R.G.: The treatment of inflammatory myopathies with azathioprine. Trans. Am. Neurol. Assoc. 93:244, 1968.

133. Bradley, W.G.: Polymyositis. Br. J. Hosp. Med. 17:351, 1977.

134. Dubowitz, V.: Treatment of dermatomyositis in childhood. Arch. Dis. Child. 51:494, 1976.

135. Bunch, T.W.: Prednisone and azathioprine for polymyositis: Long-term follow-up. Arthritis Rheum. 24:45, 1981.

136. Mertens, H.G., and Lurati, M.: Immunosuppressive Behandlung der Polymyositis. Deutsche Klin. Wschr. 100:45, 1975.

137. Thomson, J., and Milne, J.A.: Two years of penicillamine for progressive systemic sclerosis: A case report. Postgrad. Med. J. (Aug. suppl.):36, 1974.

138. Schroeder, P.L., Peters, H.A., and Dahl, D.S.: Polymyositis and penicillamine. Arch. Neurol. 27:456, 1972.

139. Nassim, J.R., and Connolly, C.K.: Treatment of calcinosis universalis. Arch. Dis. Child. 45:18, 1970.

140. Schuermann, H.: Dermatomyositis. Ergeb. Inn. Med. Kunderheilkd. 10:428, 1958.

141. Riddoch, D., and Morgan-Hughes J.A.: Prognosis in adult polymyositis. J. Neurol. Sci. 26:71, 1975.

Section XI
Rheumatic Diseases of Childhood

Chapter 80
Juvenile Rheumatoid Arthritis

James T. Cassidy

INTRODUCTION

Juvenile rheumatoid arthritis (JRA) is the most frequent pediatric connective tissue disease. It is one of the more common chronic illnesses of childhood and a leading cause of disability and blindness.

JRA differs in many respects from rheumatoid arthritis in adults. Its types of onset, polyarthritis, oligoarthritis, and systemic disease, are more distinct. Acute systemic onset rarely occurs in adults, and monarthritis is unusual. The course of the disease also differs in children. At onset large joints such as the knees, wrists, and ankles are more prominently involved than small joints. There are less frequent complaints of joint pain. Pericarditis, hepatitis, and uveitis are more common. Subcutaneous nodules and rheumatoid factor seropositivity are unusual. Inflammation and ankylosis of the posterior apophyseal joints of the upper cervical spine are particularly characteristic; atlantoaxial subluxation is common, but neurologic sequelae are rare.

Management of the disease in the child is affected to a large degree by recognition of the importance of fostering normal growth patterns, both physical and psychologic. Prognosis is generally excellent. Complete recovery for properly managed children ranges from 70 to 90 percent.

HISTORICAL REVIEW

The occurrence of polyarthritis in children was first suggested in 1864 by Cornil,[1] who described a 29-year-old woman with progressive arthritis since the age of 12. Diamentberger[2] in 1890 reviewed 38 cases of rheumatoid arthritis in children. He observed that the onset was often acute, large joints were predominantly involved, the course was remittent, growth disturbances were frequent, and prognosis was good. It was not until 1897, however, when Still[3] presented a masterly description of both the acute and chronic forms of rheumatoid arthritis in children, that the disease JRA became firmly established. It is noteworthy that Still published his observations while a medical registrar at the Hospital for Sick Children, Great Ormond Street, London. He considered that JRA was so markedly different from rheumatoid arthritis in adults that it had a distinct etiology and included more than one disease. Still distinguished between acute systemic onset of disease and chronic polyarthritis. As illustrations of these distinctions, he described the character of the enlargement of the joints in children on a background of absence of cartilaginous changes, and stressed particularly 12 cases with enlargement of the lymph nodes, splenomegaly, and fever. Involvement of the serosal surfaces in this acute form of the disease was emphasized by observations of pleuritis and pericarditis. The characteristic rash of JRA was not described in his review. Today, acute systemic onset of the disease is often referred to as Still's disease.

EPIDEMIOLOGY

Few published data have centered specifically on the prevalence of JRA.[4,5] It is not a rare disease. No race or climate is excluded from its attack. It is estimated that there are one quarter of a million children with JRA in the United States.[6] A frequently quoted figure is that 5 percent of all cases of rheumatoid arthritis begin in childhood. In Michigan our data provided a minimal estimate of the incidence of the disease: 0.01 percent of children at risk per year.[7] Laaksonen in Finland reported a similar experience of approximately 0.008 percent of children under age 15 affected per year.[8]

ETIOLOGY AND PATHOGENESIS

The etiology and pathogenesis of JRA are unknown. JRA may represent not a single disease but a syndrome of diverse etiologies; or it may result from a unified etiologic event with multiple patterns of clinical involvement emerging from interaction with the host. No primary biochemical abnormality has been found. Among potential etiologic factors mentioned prominently in investigations are infection, autoimmunity, trauma, psychological stress, and heredity.

Mycoplasma and viruses have been thought to play roles in the etiology of JRA for several reasons. A similar arthritis related to these microorganisms occurs in animals. Many viral diseases of childhood, especially rubella, have an arthritis associated with their course. Chronic inflammation may be perpetuated by autoantibodies, such as antinuclear antibodies or rheumatoid factors, and the immune complexes that they form in vivo with extrinsic antigens. Finally, a serum sickness–like illness with polyarthritis may be seen as a prelude to infectious hepatitis B.

A role for overt or subtle immunodeficiency in the causation of arthritis in children is underlined by the frequent occurrence of chronic arthritis in children with selective IgA deficiency, agammaglobulinemia, or heterozygous C2 complement component deficiency. Delayed hypersensitivity may be impaired,[9,10] especially during periods of active disease. Children with JRA may also exhibit hyperreactivity of the humoral immune system.[11] Antibodies and cellular immune reactivity to type II collagen have been demonstrated.[12]

The onset of JRA can follow physical trauma to a joint, which may serve only as a localizing factor, or psychological stress within the family.

Although JRA rarely occurs in siblings, unfolding data on HLA segregation underscore the fact that there is a hereditary basis to the pathogenesis of this disease. Earlier studies of Ansell and associates[13] reported that female relatives of children with JRA had an increased frequency of seronegative erosive polyarthritis. They also found that two of five pairs of identical twins were concordant for JRA; no concordance was noted in six nonidentical pairs.[14] Baum and Fink[15] reported concordance for JRA in a pair of monozygous twins. Similar patterns of onset of JRA have been found in families.[16]

CLINICAL MANIFESTATIONS

By definition, JRA begins before the age of 16 years. Even though onset before 6 months is unusual, the age of onset is characteristically young, 1 to 3 years, with a substantial number of cases beginning throughout childhood (Fig. 80–1).[7,17] Systemic onset may be an exception with no increased frequency of occurrence at any particular age. Girls account for the majority of cases in the early peak of the distribution curve and are affected overall at least twice as often as boys, except again for systemic onset in which the sex ratio is equal.

Constitutional Signs and Symptoms. Morning stiffness, gelling following inactivity, and night pain are probably encountered as often in JRA as in adults; however, children may not directly communicate these symptoms, and their presence will be suspected only by careful observation of the child or questioning of the parent. The child's more obvious presentation may be one of increased irritability, assumption of a posture of

Figure 80–1. Age of onset (0 to 14 years) for a group of 300 children with JRA (△——△), and for girls (● – – – ●) and boys (○········○) separately. For the total group a single large peak at 1 to 2 years is observed. Age of onset for boys, however, shows a bimodal distribution, with the first peak at 2 years and the second at 9 years. Age of onset for girls does not clearly show a second peak. No accentuation in frequency of onset was seen in either sex at 10 to 14 years.

guarding the joints, or refusal to walk. Fatigue and low grade fever are common at onset of disease. Anorexia, weight loss, and failure to grow are seen in many children. Extreme degrees of inanition and muscle atrophy are sometimes encountered. Psychological regression to a more infantile pattern of adaptation is almost to be expected in children who experience moderate to severe disease.

Types of Onset. The diagnosis of JRA has been materially aided by recognition of three distinct types of onset of disease (Table 80–1). These are defined by a constellation of clinical signs and symptoms during the first 4 to 6 months of illness.[18-27] With *polyarthritis*, arthritis begins in five or more joints, usually the knees, ankles, wrists, elbows, or the small joints of the hands and feet. *Oligoarthritis* (pauciarticular disease) is defined as onset of disease in four or fewer joints; quite often only a single joint is involved, usually the knee (monarthritis). *Systemic disease* is characterized by daily spiking fevers to greater than 39° C and the appearance of a characteristic erythematous nonpruritic rash; there is usually leukocytosis and prominent involvement of viscera, including lymphadenopathy, hepatosplenomegaly, and pericarditis.

Polyarthritis. JRA begins in five or more joints in slightly less than half of the children. This articular pattern is established early within the first 6 weeks to 4 months of disease. The onset may be acute but is often insidious, with gradual development of progressive joint involvement. The arthritis is often of an indolent or remittent nature and generally involves the large rapidly growing joints of the knees, wrists, elbows, and ankles, and may include the small joints of the hands or feet either early or late in the course. The pattern of joint

Table 80–1. Types of Onset of Juvenile Rheumatoid Arthritis

	Polyarthritis	Oligoarthritis	Systemic Disease
Relative frequency	40%	50%	10%
Number of joints involved	≥ 5	≤ 4	Variable
Sex ratio (F:M)	2:1	2:1	1:1
Extra-articular involvement	Moderate	Not prominent	Prominent
Chronic uveitis	5%	20%	Rare
Seropositivity			
Rheumatoid factors	10%	Rare	Rare
Antinuclear antibodies	40%	75%*	10%
Clinical course	Systemic disease generally mild; articular involvement often unremitting	Systemic disease absent; major cause of morbidity is uveitis	Systemic disease often self-limited; arthritis chronic and destructive in 50%
Prognosis	Moderately good	Excellent	Moderate

*In girls with uveitis.

involvement is most often symmetric but may be asymmetric or may affect only one side of the body. The joints are swollen from periarticular soft tissue inflammation and edema and synovial effusions (Fig. 80–2). They are warm but are not usually erythematous. *Quite often the child does not complain of pain;* [28-30] however, the joints may be tender or painful on motion.

Synovial cysts are an unusual complication of JRA. These cysts when they present in the popliteal space may dissect into the calf of the leg (Baker's cyst). Much more rarely they develop in the antecubital area or anterior to the shoulder. In children not suspected of having JRA, these cysts may be misinterpreted as a tumor when they present unilaterally, such as in the mid-portion of the anterior upper arm (Fig. 80–3). Echography may be an aid to their correct diagnosis.

The pattern of small joint involvement of the hands is not remarkably different from that observed in adults. The terminal interphalangeal joints are affected in ap-

proximately 10 percent of children. Radial deviation at the metacarpophalangeal joints is more frequent than ulnar drift (Fig. 80–4).

Arthritis of the apophyseal joints of the spine is common in JRA. Involvement of the cervical spine is only rarely the initial site of disease but occurs eventually in half of the children with polyarthritis. The neck is usually painful and stiff; there is often an alarmingly rapid loss of extension and rotation. Occasionally a picture resembling torticollis is encountered. It is important to remember that children with cervical spine disease present special problems with intubation prior to general anesthesia. Involvement of the thoracolumbar apophyseal joints is seldom recognized clinically; however, scoliosis is increased as much as 30 times in children with JRA. [31,32] Inflammation of the sacroiliac joints may be seen in a small number of children.

Temporomandibular joint involvement is relatively common in children with polyarthritis and leads to lim-

Figure 80–2. Hands of a 2 1/2-year-old boy with systemic onset of JRA. All the small joints were swollen, warm, and painful. The terminal interphalangeal and proximal interphalangeal joints were erythematous. Generalized swelling also involved the digits between the joints. Moderate flexion contractures were already present.

Figure 80–3. Six-year-old girl who developed a brachial synovial cyst at the first manifestation of her JRA. This mass was misdiagnosed as a tumor, and an aspiration and biopsy were performed. The synovial analysis was typical of an inflammatory fluid, and there were many inclusions in the polymorphonuclear cells. The tissue showed a marked rheumatoid synovitis. Later this child developed bilateral effusions of the knees.

itation of bite and micrognathia, although ankylosis is uncommon.[33-35] Fewer than half of the children have any associated clinical findings. The remaining joints of the chest wall (acromioclavicular, sternoclavicular, and manubriosternal) are less often affected. Although we have seen involvement of the vocal cords by rheumatoid nodules causing hoarseness, cricoarytenoid arthritis is quite rare in JRA.[36]

Systemic manifestations in polyarthritis are usually not as acute or persistent as in children with systemic onset of JRA. Low grade fever and slight to moderate hepatosplenomegaly and lymphadenopathy may be present. Clinically evident pericarditis is infrequent, and chronic uveitis occurs in only 5 percent of the patients.

Oligoarthritis. The onset of JRA in half of the children involves four or fewer joints, particularly the knees, ankles, or wrists, in a low grade inflammatory process. In about half of these children this type of disease begins in only a single joint.[37] Monarthritis may occur in any joint, but the knee is especially vulnerable and is affected in 75 percent (Figs. 80–5 to 80–7). Only occasionally is another joint the initial site of involvement of monarthritis, such as a proximal interphalangeal or metacarpophalangeal joint, or the cervical spine. There is probably little value in separating a monarthric onset from oligoarthritis as types of onset, as both pursue the same general course. The hips are usually spared at least initially in this pattern of disease. Extra-articular manifestations, save for chronic uveitis, are quite unusual.[37,38]

Systemic Onset. Some children have onset of disease with severe constitutional and systemic involvement that may precede development of overt arthritis. These children make up 10 percent of the cases. Arthritis must be present for a definite diagnosis of JRA but may appear concurrent with the onset of systemic signs or many weeks to months later. The longest interval between the

Figure 80–4. Hand of a 7-year-old girl with marked inflammatory involvement of the interphalangeal joint of the thumb and the terminal interphalangeal joints of the fingers. Arthritis began as systemic disease at 5 1/2 years of age with fever, maculopapular rash, hepatosplenomegaly, and arthritis of the hands, feet, and left knee.

Figure 80–5. Massively swollen left knee of a 6-year-old boy with recent onset of monarthritis. The child was not sytemically ill and the only laboratory abnormality was a positive antinuclear antibody test. Ophthalmologic examination was negative. PPD skin test was nonreactive. Radiographs of the knees showed no alteration of the bony architecture on the left. The synovial fluid was yellow and opalescent; the white blood cell count was 10,400 per cubic millimeter, half of which were mononuclear cells. The mucin clot was good. Cultures were negative.

Figure 80–6. Radiographs of the knees of the boy in Figure 80–5, 3 years later. Now there is marked osteoporosis on the left with coarsening of the trabeculae and enlargement of the epiphyses. The joint space is narrowed laterally, and there is lengthening of the left leg with a moderate valgus deformity. Erosions are not present.

onset of systemic disease and objective signs of arthritis that we have observed was 3 years. The systemic pattern of disease generally establishes its identity at onset and does not later intervene during the course of the other types of JRA.

Figure 80–7. Pelvis of child in previous two figures. There is a quite noticeable coxa valga on the left and moderate stunting of growth of the ischium secondary to arthritis of the left knee. The hip was not involved in the inflammatory process; however, its deformity accounts in part for the ipsilateral leg length discrepancy.

A hallmark of systemic onset is the high spiking fever which in combination with the rheumatoid rash is virtually diagnostic of the disease.[39,40] The daily or twice daily temperature elevations rise to 39° C or higher with a rapid return to the baseline level (Fig. 80–8). This quotidian pattern is highly suggestive of the diagnosis of JRA. The fever may occur at any time of the day but is characteristically seen in the late afternoon to evening. The temperature may be subnormal in the morning. Chills are frequent but rigor is unusual. The children are quite often strikingly ill while experiencing the fever and surprisingly well during the rest of the time.

This intermittent fever is usually accompanied by a rheumatoid rash which is diagnostic of JRA (Fig. 80–9).[41,42] This rash consists of discrete, 2 to 5 mm erythematous morbilliform macules and is most commonly seen on the trunk, proximal extremities, and over pressure areas. It may occur on the face, palms, and soles. A signal characteristic is its evanescent nature; lesions are of short duration in any specific location and tend to be migratory. Each macule may be surrounded by a zone of pallor, and the larger lesions may show central clearing. The rash may resemble urticaria but is almost never pruritic.[43] Although seen regularly in children with systemic disease, the rheumatoid rash also occurs in patients with polyarthritis, but is rarely observed in oligoarthritis. Because of the transient nature of the rash and its usual occurrence late in the day during the febrile episodes, it is frequently missed by physicians caring for a child with "fever of unknown origin." The individual lesions may be precipitated by rubbing or scratching the

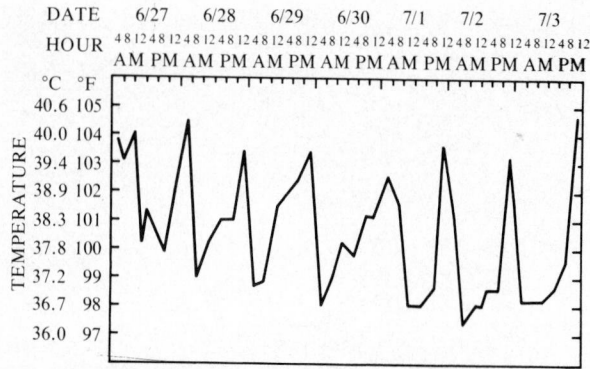

Figure 80–8. High, intermittent fever of a 3-year-old girl with systemic onset of JRA. The majority of the febrile spikes occurred in the late evening to early morning hours and were accompanied by a rheumatoid rash.

skin, the Koebner phenomenon or isomorphic response. A hot bath or psychological stress may also induce it.

Systemic onset of JRA is also accompanied by visceral lesions such as hepatosplenomegaly, lymphadenopathy, and pericarditis or other evidence of serositis. Hepatosplenomegaly and lymphadenopathy of varying degree

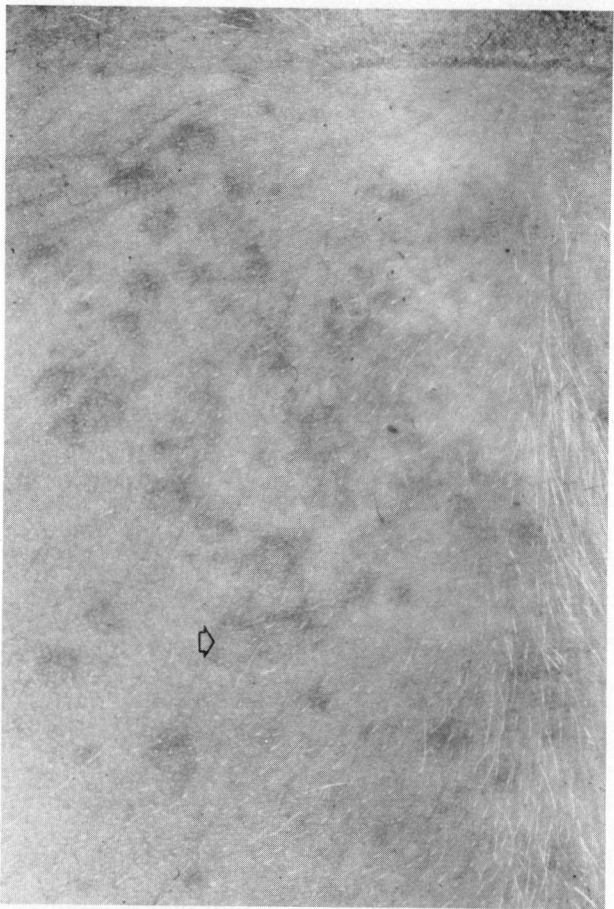

Figure 80–9. Rheumatoid rash of the patient in Figure 80–8. This was a faintly erythematous (salmon-colored), macular rash which was most prominent over the back but involved the extremities and face as well. The individual lesions were transient, appeared in crops, and conformed to a somewhat linear distribution. Some of the lesions had central clearing (arrow).

occur in most children with active systemic disease and can be striking in their development. A true hepatitis, not related to salicylate therapy, may occur; however, even massive hepatomegaly is usually associated with only mild derangement of liver function studies.[44] Hepatic disease is most common at or near the onset of JRA and regresses with time. Progressive liver disease is not seen. Occasionally a fatty liver is associated with steroid administration. Enlargement of the spleen, which occurs in a quarter of the patients, is generally most prominent within the first year of disease. The degree of splenomegaly may be extreme but is not associated with Felty's syndrome in children. Lymphadenopathy, particularly in the cervical, axillary, and epitrochlear areas, may be quite marked and is usually symmetric. The sicca complex is rarely a recognized problem in the connective tissue diseases of childhood.[45,46]

A similar pattern of systemic onset with spiking fevers, rash, and arthritis is seen occasionally in the older age groups, the so-called adult-onset Still's disease.[47,48] Some of these patients represent a recurrence of arthritis on the background of a history of JRA, and identification of hallmarks of that disease will materially aid in making a prompt, correct diagnosis. It is interesting to note that adult onset of oligoarthritis associated with chronic uveitis has not been described.[49]

Extra-articular Manifestations of the Disease. Pericarditis, which is often subclinical, is especially common in children with systemic onset of disease.[50,51] It is unusual for pericarditis to precede the development of arthritis, but it may occur at any time during the course of JRA, usually accompanied by a systemic exacerbation. It is unrelated to sex or age. Each episode generally persists for a week to 4 months; however, pericarditis may be recurrent in the face of poorly controlled disease (Fig. 80–10). Many cases develop insidiously and escape recognition. Clinically diagnosed pericarditis is estimated to occur in 7 percent of children with JRA; however, postmortem examinations in 11 fatal cases showed a 45 percent frequency of pericarditis, only one of which had been detected during life.[52] A minority of the children with pericarditis will have precordial pain, dyspnea, a friction rub, tachycardia, enlargement of the cardiac silhouette, and a diagnostic electrocardiogram. Echocardiography has been the most useful aid to diagnosis.[53] Pericardial effusion does not usually progress to tamponade and rarely results in chronic constrictive pericarditis;[54] only one case has been described. In general, children with pericarditis do not fare worse than the others.

Myocarditis is less common but may also produce cardiac enlargement and failure.[55] Valvular lesions have seldom been reported except for the early studies of Sury.[18,56] Systolic murmurs are generally functional; however, rheumatoid nodules have been described on the valve leaflets and visceral pericardium.[57]

Other extra-articular manifestations of JRA[58,59] include diffuse interstitial pulmonary fibrosis and central nervous system disease.[60-63] Rarely, a child will have a picture of idiopathic pulmonary hemosiderosis as the

Figure 80–10. Chest film showing enlargement of the cardiac silhouette in a 5-year-old girl with a pericardial effusion. Systemic onset of disease 2 years previously. This effusion persisted for about 4 months and was accompanied by fever, slight precordial discomfort, and dyspnea.

first manifestation of the disease. Pulmonary rheumatoid nodules have not been noted. Although the occurrence of CNS involvement has been described in children with JRA,[57,64-66] this complication is often related to the presence of other contributory factors such as salicylate toxicity, viral infection, fever, embolism, or other systemic disease.

A renal glomerulitis as evidenced by intermittent hematuria is apparently part of the clinical course of JRA in some children and can present real problems of differential diagnosis relative to analgesic administration or other anti-inflammatory regimens such as gold therapy. On a long-term basis as many as 45 percent of children with JRA may at one time or another show abnormalities on urinalysis.[67,68]

Tenosynovitis and myositis are manifestations of active disease. Inflammation of the tendon sheaths develops principally over the dorsa of the wrists and around the ankles. Loss of extension of the fingers can result from a stenosing synovitis of the flexor tendon sheaths, giving rise to a claw hand deformity.[69]

Subcutaneous rheumatoid nodules are not as common as in adults (5 to 10 percent vs. 35 percent).[70,71] They are associated with rheumatoid factor seropositivity in greater than three fourths of the patients and are typically seen in children with polyarthritis. They usually occur on the periosteum below the olecranon but may be found at other pressure points and in digital flexor tendon sheaths. Rheumatoid polyarteritis has been described in a few instances, usually in the older child with

rheumatoid factor seropositivity. A benign digital vasculitis probably occurs in JRA and may occasionally be associated with radiologic calcification.[72,73] We have observed a rare child with JRA who has had an associated vasculitis resembling Mucha-Habermann disease.[74]

Benign rheumatoid nodules occur in children without JRA; at least a few of these patients develop arthritis later in their course.[75,76] Granuloma annulare, a common disease in children, should not be confused with either rheumatoid or pseudorheumatoid nodules.

Chronic Uveitis. One of the most devastating complications of JRA is a chronic nongranulomatous uveitis which in many cases can lead to blindness.[77-81] Inflammation of the uveal tract usually involves only the anterior segments of the eye, the iris and ciliary body, and may be referred to as iridocyclitis. The posterior uveal tract, the choroid, is rarely affected clinically in JRA.[82] Uveitis is especially prone to occur in *young girls* of *early age of onset*[77] with *limited joint disease*[37] who have *antinuclear antibody positivity.*[83,84] It is found in over one fifth of the children with oligoarthritis.[37,85] The only hope of saving the eyesight in affected children is early and persistent use of mydriatic and corticosteroid drugs. Therefore, because the onset of chronic uveitis is usually insidious and asymptomatic, routine ophthalmologic examination must be performed at the time of diagnosis in every child with JRA and should be repeated at frequent intervals during the first years of the disease. Currently, we recommend that examinations be obtained every 3 months for the first 2 years of disease in children with oligoarthritis, and every 6 months thereafter for a period of 7 years at a minimum. In other children with JRA, slit-lamp examinations should be done at 6-month intervals for at least the first 5 years of disease. Rarely a child will have a symptomatic onset of uveitis with redness, pain, or decreased visual acuity.

Approximately two thirds of the children with uveitis have bilateral disease. If the initial involvement is unilateral, the second eye will usually be affected within a year. However, we have seen the second eye involved in a number of children after 5 to 7 years of unilateral uveitis. The earliest manifestations of inflammation are an increased number of cells in the anterior chamber of the eye or a punctate keratitic precipitate on the posterior surface of the cornea. Inflammation which is inadequately controlled results in posterior synechiae which represent adherence of the iris to the anterior surface of the lens. These changes produce an irregular or poorly reactive pupil (Fig. 80–11). Band keratopathy occurs as a degenerative lesion and is considered virtually pathognomonic of this disease. It is not as common now as formerly, perhaps because of earlier diagnosis and better treatment of the initial lesion. Complicated cataracts, secondary glaucoma, and phthisis bulbi are still encountered, however, in certain children with chronic uveitis in spite of vigorous long-term treatment of the disease. Immunosuppressive therapy is under study for the more resistant cases.

Loss of vision occurs because of any of the aforementioned changes or may be the result of amblyopia related to the formation of a secondary cataract. Extraction of a cataract is often a delicate matter of ophthalmologic judgment and experience, weighing the

risks of operating on an inflamed eye against delay and the risk of amblyopia. The use of microcryosurgical techniques has improved the chances of a successful result. Cataracts and glaucoma may also result from the steroid therapy of chronic uveitis.

Although slit-lamp examinations may return to normal soon after treatment is initiated, it is inadvisable to stop corticosteroids completely at that time because of the frequent reappearance of signs of inflammation. Indeed in our experience uveitis generally remains active for many years after onset—witness the term *chronic*—and requires long-term surveillance by an experienced ophthalmologist.

Improved prognosis for sight may be the result of the earlier detection of chronic uveitis and its prompt treatment, or may relate to relatively benign forms of the disease which are destined to remain subclinical and perhaps do not need vigorous therapy.[86] These are important questions which have not been answered by studies to date.

Growth Retardation. Disturbances of growth are characteristic features of arthritis in children. During periods of active disease linear growth is usually retarded.[87-90] Full stature will seldom be attained if chronic rheumatic activity persists for many years. There is often delayed development of secondary sexual characteristics. Although accelerated growth may occur with suppression of active disease by therapy or with a remission, we believe that it is unusual for a child who has suffered significant growth arrest to resume development within his previous auxodrome.

Growth retardation may also occur in selective areas, such as in the jaw (Fig. 80–12). Micrognathia is caused by failure of normal development of the temporomandibular growth centers or is secondary to involvement of the cervical spine.[91,92] The most extreme degrees of micrognathia result from disease of long duration which had its onset before the fourth birthday. Lesser degrees can be seen, however, with onset of JRA up to the age of 12 years.

Secondary growth deformities are frequent in children with limited joint disease involving the knee and result in unequal leg lengths. The involved leg usually grows longer. Early during active disease development of the ossification centers or epiphyses may be accelerated, and later stunting, dwarfing, and premature fusion of the involved bones may result.[93-97] Brachydactyly develops from premature closure of the epiphyseal growth plate (Fig. 80–13). Although this may be observed in isolated digits, involvement of the metatarsals or metacarpals is more characteristic. Small hands or feet may result from JRA with onset in early childhood.

Figure 80–11. Left eye of a 7-year-old boy showing an irregular pupil that resulted from adhesions of the iris to the anterior surface of the lens. Onset of polyarthritis was at 9 months of age. Chronic uveitis was first detected 2 1/2 years later in the right eye, and 5 years later in the left. The patient subsequently had cataract extractions and developed glaucoma. Eyesight remains precariously at approximately 20/200. His arthritis has progressed to severe disease with marked muscular atrophy. Antinuclear antibody tests have been persistently negative.

PATHOLOGY

JRA is characterized by many of the same histologic findings that have been identified in rheumatoid arthritis of adult onset.[98] There is villous hypertrophy of the

Figure 80–12. Micrognathia in an 11-year-old girl whose polyarthritis began at 18 months of age. There was no restriction of motion of the temporomandibular joints. Extension, rotation, and lateral binding of the cervical spine were absent, and flexion was limited to 10 degrees.

synovium and hyperplasia of the synovial lining layer. The subsynovial tissues are edematous and hyperemic, and there is often prominent vascular endothelial hyperplasia and infiltration of lymphocytes and plasma cells. Electron microscopy has confirmed the similarity of the juvenile and adult synovial response to inflam-

mation.[99,100] Pannus formation may result, and the articular cartilage, and later contiguous bone, become progressively eroded and destroyed. These events usually take place much later in the course of JRA than in adults. Many children, even after years of chronic inflammation, do not show permanent joint damage, a fact perhaps related to the greater thickness of juvenile cartilage or immunologic differences in synovial immune complexes. End-stage disease is characterized by deformity, subluxation, and fibrous or bony ankylosis.

The synovial histopathology in oligoarthritis is not distinguishable from that seen in JRA involving many joints.[101] In our experience rheumatoid nodules and necrotizing vasculitis have not been observed in synovial biopsies from children.

Rheumatoid nodules, which occur in less than 10 percent of children with JRA, probably do not differ in major pathologic characteristics from the nodules of adults, especially in seropositive patients. When seen in the seronegative child they may resemble more closely the nodules of rheumatic fever.[70] The serosal lining surfaces of the major cavities (pleura, pericardium, and peritoneum) may develop a nonspecific fibrous serositis which is characterized by pain, exudation, and effusions. Enlargement of lymph nodes is related to a nonspecific follicular hyperplasia which can simulate the picture of lymphoma, as is also true of the lymphadenopathy of adult rheumatoid arthritis. Hepatic histology usually shows a nonspecific periportal collection of inflammatory cells and hyperplasia of the Kupffer cells.[102]

The rash of JRA is one of the most characteristic clinical features of the disease. Histologically it appears as a slight infiltration of round cells surrounding capillaries and venules in the subdermal tissues.[42] A neutrophilic perivasculitis may accompany the more flagrant lesions.

Figure 80–13. Brachydactyly of the left second and fourth digits is present. There is involvement of the proximal interphalangeal joints of those fingers, the interphalangeal joints of the thumbs, and the wrists.

LABORATORY EXAMINATIONS

Many children develop a normocytic, hypochromic anemia during periods of activity of disease. This may be moderately severe in the range of 7 to 10 grams per deciliter. Hypoplastic crisis may rarely occur. Leukocytosis is common with active disease, especially in children with systemic onset. White cell counts of 30,000 to 50,000 per cubic millimeter are not uncommon; polymorphonuclear neutrophils predominate. Thrombocytosis is seen in severe disease and may also occur as a prelude to an exacerbation. Limited joint disease, such as oligoarthritis, is seldom associated with an anemia or leukocytosis.

The erythrocyte sedimentation rate is a useful acute phase reactant for following a child with active disease and is occasionally helpful in monitoring therapeutic efficacy. It has the disadvantage of being a sensitive indicator of any form of infection or inflammation and as such may not reflect the degree of activity of the arthritis. Determination of the C-reactive protein is probably a more reliable monitor of the inflammatory response. The serum protein electrophoresis as an estimate of the degree of hypergammaglobulinemia and concentration of the alpha-2 globulins is another measure of acute reactivity. Increases in the serum levels of the immunoglobulins are also correlated with activity of the disease.[103-107] Extreme degrees of hypergammaglobulinemia are seen in the sickest children and return toward normal with improvement. Serum complement components are usually elevated in children with JRA, a finding that corresponds to their role as acute phase reactants.[108-110] Accelerated complement consumption was found in children with active JRA by Pachman and associates.[111] C3b and C3c fragments were found by counter-immunoelectrophoresis as evidence of complement activation in vivo in a study by Miller and associates.[112] Serum AA protein (amyloid-like) is increased in concentration in children with JRA as a nonspecific indicator of inflammation.

Soluble immune complexes can be detected in the sera of certain children with JRA, particularly those with systemic onset of disease. In a study of circulating immune complexes in children with JRA, Rossen and associates[113] found that their presence correlated with severe disease of systemic onset. Miller and colleagues[114] demonstrated immune complexes in children with seropositive JRA who had either systemic disease or polyarthritis. Moore and associates[115] correlated the presence of immune complexes with 19S IgM rheumatoid factors, hidden rheumatoid factors, antinuclear antibodies, and the activity of the synovitis. Complexed 19S IgM rheumatoid factors and IgG were also detected in sera of nine seronegative children.

At this time the variability in assays for immune complexes and the varying results in the initial studies that have been performed do not allow one to conclude that immune complexes occupy a central part in either the systemic or synovial manifestations of JRA, and generally they are not useful in monitoring disease activity.

Viral antibody titers may be increased in some children with JRA.[116] In our experience, antibodies to rubella and rubeola viruses are usually similar to those in appropriate control groups or are associated with a general increase in serum immunoglobulin concentrations. However, there may be subtle relationships between JRA and viral antibody responses even though recent studies do not support a direct response.[117,118] In any case, we do not vaccinate children with JRA with attenuated rubella virus; at the least, a postvaccination flare of arthritis would complicate evaluation of the disease and the current therapeutic goals.

The latex fixation test or sensitized sheep cell agglutination for rheumatoid factors is positive in children less frequently than in adults.[119-121] Overall, 20 percent of children with JRA are seropositive. Rheumatoid factors tend to be present in the child of late age of onset or in the older child, and in one who has subcutaneous rheumatoid nodules or articular erosions, or who is in a poorer functional class.[122-125] We have not observed a positive latex test in a child under the age of 7. The diagnostic value of a positive rheumatoid factor test in the child with possible JRA is lessened by the frequent occurrence of seropositivity in the other connective tissue diseases of childhood such as systemic lupus erythematosus.

Children with strongly positive tests for rheumatoid factors may represent a distinct subset of disease different from the larger group of seronegative children. Although the frequency of classic rheumatoid factor seropositivity may not increase with continuing active disease of long duration, the percentage of positive patients rises progressively as the age of onset or duration of disease of the cohort group under study increases. These findings, although not unequivocal, tend to suggest that seropositivity may be a result rather than a determinative event in children with JRA who go on to unremitting, disabling disease in the early adult years.

In studies designed to demonstrate other types of antiglobulins in the sera of children with JRA, the rheumatoid rosette test was found to be frequently positive,[126] and the majority of children with seronegative JRA on the basis of the latex fixation test had IgG–anti-IgG antibodies demonstrated by immunoadsorbent techniques.[127-129] IgG and IgA antiglobulins were reported by Bianco and associates[130] and were correlated with activity of disease and the presence of IgM rheumatoid factors. On the other hand, Miller and associates[131] found few children with these antiglobulins and did not indicate that they proved helpful in the diagnosis of the disease or its course. Pepsin agglutinators, or antibodies reacting with pepsin-digested IgG, e.g., F(ab')$_2$ fragments, are found more often in JRA than are classic rheumatoid factors. They are also mainly of the IgG class.[132] Demonstration of these anti–gamma globulins has not led to a clarification of the purported distinctions between seropositive and seronegative children. Further investigations of these clinical subsets are indicated. "Hidden 19S-IgM rheumatoid factors" have been described by Moore and associates,[133-136] using acid elution–gel filtration, in the IgM-containing fractions of sera of children with JRA. With the hemolytic assay, hidden rheumatoid factors have been detected in 59 to 68 percent of children with seronegative JRA as determined by a latex fixation test. These hidden rheumatoid factors were found with all types of onset of disease and correlated best with activity of the articular disease. Other data indicate that hidden rheumatoid factors may combine with IgG as immune complexes in serum and synovial fluid.[137,138]

Tests for antinuclear antibodies are more useful diagnostically than latex agglutination and are positive in approximately 40 percent of children with JRA.[83] The pattern of fluorescent staining on mouse liver substrate is usually homogeneous or speckled, and the standardized serum dilution titer is gnerally low to moderate ($\leq 1:256$). The frequency of antinuclear antibodies increases in girls of younger age of onset and decreases in older boys and in children with systemic disease.[83,84,139-141] They reach their highest prevalence in children who have oligoarthritis and uveitis, 65 to 85 percent.[83,84] Thus antinuclear antibodies are of critical importance in the initial diagnostic program of a child suspected of having JRA, and in selecting for closer observation those children at risk for developing chronic uveitis. They are not frequently positive in other childhood illnesses except for systemic lupus erythematosus and scleroderma. Other types of antinuclear antibodies have been described (e.g., granulocyte specific), but there have been no obvious clinical correlations with these autoantibodies.[142,143] Although our studies showed that antinuclear antibodies predominantly occurred in a subclass of patients who were not seropositive for rheumatoid factors, a more recent examination of children with JRA at the University of Cincinnati for the Criteria Study suggested that antinuclear antibodies and classic rheumatoid factors were found together in two thirds of the children who were seropositive.[144]

Identifying the antigenic specificity of antinuclear antibodies has not been useful in children with JRA. Alspaugh and Miller[141] examined the sera of 77 children with JRA and found that 57 percent were positive, most commonly in a speckled pattern. Only six sera were found with the rheumatoid arthritis precipitin (RAP). These children were predominantly girls with seropositive polyarthritic disease of late onset. Antibodies to ribonucleoprotein were present in only two patients, and none was positive for SS-A, SS-B, or Sm antigens.

LE cells were apparently seen in older studies in a very small number of children with otherwise classic JRA.[22,23] This phenomenon is generally evident at onset and transient. The appearance of LE cells during the course of the disease might herald a transition to systemic lupus erythematosus. In the study by Alspaugh and Miller,[141] 3 of 35 children had antibodies to double-stranded DNA, and 2, to single-stranded DNA. Bell and associates[145] detected antibodies to double-stranded DNA in 5 of 125 children with JRA. It is our experience that anti-double-stranded DNA antibody measurements are normal in children with classic JRA.[146] The finding

of an elevated DNA-binding activity would usually indicate the supervention of active immune-complex disease of the lupus type.

Serologic typing of peripheral blood lymphocyte membrane antigens has added an important dimension to the laboratory confirmation of JRA in selected children, as the presence of HLA-B27 is characteristic of the spondyloarthropathies.[24,147-150] Current studies indicate that other HLA types display linkage dysequilibrium in certain types of onset of JRA.[151,152] Specific allotypes have already been identified that segregate with immunodeficiencies associated with JRA, as in the complement deficiencies. A specific HLA-D type, TMo, identified in mixed lymphocyte culture by homozygous typing cells from a child with JRA, has been shown to be associated with JRA.[153] Forty-six percent of children with persistent oligoarthritis typed for this antigen, which is related to the cross-reactive specificities of HLA-Dw7 and Dw11, compared to 1 percent of controls (relative risk = 68). The frequency of HLA-Dw4, the antigen characteristic of adult rheumatoid arthritis, was significantly lower in JRA, and HLA-Dw7 and Dw8 were increased. Thus typing at the D locus has provided impressive evidence of a fundamental distinction between JRA and rheumatoid arthritis in adults. While the TMo specificity has not been confirmed by the work of others, these results are encouraging to the search for more specific antisera for JRA susceptibility or clinical subtypes or a "JRA" gene. One group has mapped a putative susceptibility locus, RLA-1, centromeric to the HLA-D/DR locus in familial JRA.[154]

Our studies have shown an association of HLA-DR5, 6, and 8, both individually and in combination in certain subgroups of children with JRA, principally young girls with persistent oligoarthritis who have antinuclear antibody seropositivity.[155] Chronic uveitis was especially common in this subgroup. The strongest association appeared to be with HLA-DR8, which was present in 44 percent of the children, compared with 5 percent of controls.

Glass and associates[156] found that DR5 and DR8 were associated with the onset of oligoarthritis in young girls who eventually developed antinuclear antibody positivity and chronic uveitis and that the association with DR5 (71 percent) was stronger than that with DR8 (25 percent). (The fact that there is cross-reactivity between the DR5 and DR8 antigens has made interpretation of these associations especially difficult.) While there was a significantly increased frequency of DR5 in this study, finding this specificity in a child did not predict the future development of chronic uveitis better than the already well-recognized risk factor of a positive antinuclear antibody reaction. Suici-Foca and associates[157] reported that DR5, but not DR8, was associated with a clinical pattern of oligoarthritis and chronic uveitis. Morling and associates[158] found a normal frequency of DR5 in children with JRA. The studies of Fink[159] found an insignificant increase in DR5 and DR8 in oligoarthritis, as opposed to a greater increase in the frequency of these antigenic types in children with polyarthritis.

Although the HLA-DR5, DR6,[160] and DR8 antigens appear to be strongly associated with certain subtypes of onset and course in JRA, they are not found in increased frequency in adults with RA.

During the last decade several studies have examined in vitro cell-mediated immunity in children with JRA.[161] A few studies have been reported on cutaneous delayed hypersensitivity reactions in children with JRA and have indicated that these may be abnormal and that depression correlates with activity of the disease. In examining lymphocyte transformation to PHA, Miller and associates[162] showed that children with systemic disease and polyarthritis were more likely to have a response at three days, whereas those with oligoarthritis showed a more pronounced response at seven days.

In our own studies, both lymphocyte transformation and leukocyte migration inhibition assays were used to examine cell-mediated immunity.[163] Patients with systemic disease had markedly abnormal responses. In a few instances sera from selected children also depressed in vitro assays of lymphocytes from normal individuals. Children with oligoarthritis and polyarthritis tended to have normal lymphocyte transformation in comparison with controls. On the other hand, with leukocyte migration inhibition, children with oligoarthritis had as significant a depression of results as those with systemic disease. In both groups abnormalities were found in approximately half of the children and did not correlate with systemic manifestations of activity, as children with oligoarthritis were generally well except for their arthritis. It was concluded that abnormalities of cell-mediated immune function might be intrinsic to the pathogenesis of JRA, were in some instances related to onset type, and did not always correlate with disease activity.

It has been noted in several studies that antibodies from patients with JRA reacted with T cells of the suppressor type.[164,165] The subpopulation of cells for which these antibodies were specific would transform to concanavalin A but not to phytohemagglutinin and did not provide help in vitro for the synthesis of immunoglobulins by B lymphocytes. Further studies by this same group indicated that children with JRA who had these antibodies lacked a subset of suppressor cells and had a significantly higher proportion of B lymphocytes that were capable of secreting immunoglobulin in vitro. Morimoto and associates[166] from this same group of investigators reported that these antibodies to T lymphocytes specifically reacted with the OKT-4 cell subset identified by monoclonal antibodies and to a lesser extent with the OKT-8 suppressor T-lymphocyte population.

Williams and associates,[167] however, published investigations that suggested that these findings of the Boston group were based on the presence of high molecular weight circulating material, presumably of immune-complex type, that interfered with the E-rosette and lymphocytotoxicity assays. Ultracentrifugation of the sera diminished significantly the previously reported observations. Froelich and colleagues,[168] using flow cytometry and cytoadherence rosetting, found no increase in anti-T-lymphocyte antibodies in patients with JRA. Dobloug

and associates[169] also failed to detect in mixed lymphocyte culture any relative lack of a lymphocyte subset in children with JRA.

Wada and colleagues[170] published studies that suggested that there was an increase in a T-helper subpopulation of lymphocytes in children with JRA detected by α-naphthylacetate esterase. One study by Muraguchi[171] suggested the presence of abnormal B lymphocytes using methods that employed anti-μ antibodies.

These studies on cell populations in children with JRA are obviously in conflict. Whether children with JRA have antibodies to specific T-lymphocyte subsets, such as the inducer-suppressor population, or have immune complexes or antilymphocyte antibodies that invalidate the standard laboratory assays for T lymphocytes is presently unresolved.

Synovial fluid examination in JRA is usually typical of Group II or inflammatory fluid.[37] The white cell count does not always correlate, however, with the degree of clinical activity. Very low counts have been observed in fluids from joints clinically involved by intensively active inflammatory disease. Conversely counts in the range of infectious arthritis, e.g., 100,000 cells per cubic millimeter, have been recorded in patients with otherwise classic JRA.[172] As in adult disease, levels of glucose may be low in the synovial fluid. The complement levels are not as characteristically or uniformly depressed as in adult rheumatoid arthritis.[173] Rynes and associates,[174] in one study of synovial fluid, showed evidence of complement activation with depression of one or more components. In another study, normal levels of C3 and C4 were found in synovial fluid specimens in 20 children.[175] In concept, one would expect to find little or no rheumatoid factor seropositivity in joint fluids from patients with JRA and a less impressive number of ragocytes indicative of immune-complex phagocytosis. In actuality none of these characteristics has been sufficiently investigated in children to enable one to be unequivocal. Complexes of IgG, IgG rheumatoid factors, and complement have been described along with "hidden rheumatoid factors" in both tissues and eluates.[137,176] Martin and colleagues[175] looked at synovial fluid levels of immunoglobulins and found elevated IgM and IgG in children with oligoarthritic onset.

Urinalysis is usually normal in children with JRA, except for the proteinuria associated with fever. Persistent proteinuria is often the first indication of amyloidosis in children studied in Europe. Intermittent hematuria may occur and be evidence of a glomerulitis associated with JRA, of drug toxicity, or of the development of another disease such as lupus.

RADIOLOGIC EXAMINATION

Early radiographic changes consist of soft tissue swelling about the joints, juxta-articular osteoporosis, and, frequently, periosteal new bone formation.[93,177,178] Premature epiphyseal closure may lead to stunting of bone growth. Conversely, there may be accelerated epiphyseal development stimulated by the local inflammatory changes which leads to an increase in the length of the long bones (Fig. 80–14). A radiographic picture of marked bony overgrowth owing to enlargement of the epiphyses may occur at the interphalangeal joints (Fig. 80–15). Widening of the phalanges from periosteal new bone apposition is another characteristic roentgenographic feature in children with JRA.

Marginal erosions and narrowing of the cartilaginous space may occur in disease of long duration. We have not observed these changes to develop early in children with JRA, e.g., generally not before 2 years of active disease even in the child with polyarthritis. Indeed in some children with limited joint disease or oligoarthritis we have not seen erosions even after one or two decades of constant effusion.

Atlantoaxial subluxation is the most characteristic change in the cervical spine (Fig. 80–16). The upper limit of the atlanto-odontoid space in children is 4 mm measured on a lateral film in flexion.[179] Apophyseal joint disease of the upper cervical segments occurs and bony fusion is frequent, often observed first at the C2-C3 level. As this joint is oriented at a different angle than the other apophyseal joints, a single lateral film of the cervical spine may not be sufficient to determine the presence of ankylosis. Measuring the distance between flexion and extension at the corresponding neural spines may be helpful. The vertebral bodies at areas of fusion fail to grow normally and are smaller than contiguous vertebrae, or have an altered ratio of height to width. The intervertebral spaces at these levels are also reduced, and calcification of the discs is occasionally seen. Sacroiliac arthritis in children with JRA is not characterized by the degree of change, particularly reactive sclerosis, that is seen in juvenile ankylosing spondylitis. Late fusion occurs, particularly in children with severe disease who have been bedridden.

Fractures related to generalized osteoporosis are frequent in young children, particularly if they have had severe disease, immobilization, or corticosteroid therapy (Fig. 80–17). The metaphyseal or supracondylar area of the femur is a characteristic site of fracture, often following manipulation for contracture of the knee.[180] Vertebral compression fractures are often seen in children who have been treated with corticosteroids (Fig. 80–18).[93]

There is considerable interest in the use of objective techniques ancillary to the physical examination to document the presence of inflammation in joints. Bone scanning using radionuclides such as [133]xenon and [99m]technetium has been occasionally useful.[181] Thermography has the advantage in children of not employing an isotope and can be repeated at intervals in the difficult case.[182]

DIAGNOSIS

Classification Criteria. JRA is often a diagnosis of exclusion. Criteria for its diagnosis and classification have recently been revised (Table 80–2).[183,184] Arthritis in one or more joints for 6 weeks may be sufficient for diagnosis. Arthritis present for 3 months provides even more assurance that JRA is the correct diagnosis. The joint involvement must be persistent to meet the present concept of JRA. Objective arthritis must be distinguished from arthralgia or pain in the joints. The presence of one or more of the ancillary manifestations of the disease may help to support a preliminary impression of JRA (Table 80–3).

Except in the United States, there is no uniform agreement on the use of diagnostic terms for children with JRA.[185-188] The English clinicians in particular refer to rheumatoid-factor seropositive disease in children as juvenile rheumatoid arthritis. Seronegative disease in the larger group of patients, including children who may have rheumatoid variants such as psoriatic arthritis or juvenile ankylosing spondylitis and those with other connective tissue diseases such as systemic lupus ery-

Figure 80–14. Accelerated maturation of the left carpus in a 9-year-old girl with arthritis for 7 years. Marked osteoporosis and atrophy of soft tissues are present. Although the individual carpal bones on the left appear more mature than on the right, they are smaller and eventual growth is already stunted.

Figure 80–15. Radiograph of the left hand of a 21-year-old woman with severe polyarthritis. There is marked bony overgrowth and enlargement of the epiphyses of the interphalangeal joints. Erosive destruction of these joints is prominent, especially at the proximal ends of the proximal and middle phalanges, with invagination of the abutting bone. Additional destructive arthritis is present at the terminal interphalangeal and carpal joints with partial ankylosis evident in the latter area.

Figure 80–16. Radiograph of the cervical spine of a young girl with polyarthritis. There is an atlantoaxial subluxation (arrow) and fusion of the C2-C3 apophyseal joint. Three years later subluxation developed at the C3-C4 vertebral interspace.

thematosus, is referred to as juvenile chronic (poly)arthritis. The World Health Organization is presently studying this problem of nomenclature for the various forms of juvenile arthritis.

Exclusions for a Diagnosis of JRA. Because many of the more common types of arthritis in children may be confused with JRA, serious consideration must be given in differential diagnosis to the other rheumatic and connective tissue diseases, especially rheumatic fever, systemic lupus erythematosus, and juvenile ankylosing spondylitis (Tables 80–4 and 80–5). Particular attention must also be accorded infectious arthritis, serum sickness, Henoch-Schönlein purpura, the inflammatory enteropathies such as ulcerative colitis and regional enteritis, and hematologic diseases, especially leukemia, sickle cell anemia, and hemophilia.

A number of clinical observations are helpful in the differential diagnosis of JRA. The child with oligoarthritis will have involvement of one to four joints, generally including the knees. In this type of onset, the joint is swollen, has an effusion, but is generally not very painful, tender, or red. It is usually slightly warm. Such a child is not systemically ill. If a child with limited joint disease presents with an acutely painful and erythematous joint or systemic signs of illness, one should suspect a septic process or another disease such as acute rheumatic fever. Synovial fluid aspiration is almost always indicated in such a case to exclude a pyogenic synovitis or osteomyelitis. Synovial histopathology seldom definitively makes a diagnosis of JRA. Needle biopsy of the synovial membrane is primarily useful in monarthritis to clarify other diagnoses such as granuloma or tumor.[37,189] A negative tuberculin skin test in a child virtually excludes tuberculosis. Other types of infection may cause a monarthritis, particularly gonorrhea, and trauma may do so transiently.[190] Internal derangements of the knee are not common in children. The finding of uveitis in a child with limited joint disease will almost always indicate that the diagnosis is JRA.

Figure 80–17. Radiograph of the left knee of a 21-year-old woman who sustained a condylar fracture of the femur (arrow) following minor trauma. There is marked loss of the cartilaginous space and sclerosis of the weight-bearing surfaces of the joint.

Figure 80–18. Multiple vertebral compression fractures in a 10-year-old boy with systemic onset of JRA at age 5 years. He was treated for much of this time with steroids for recurrent fever, rash, and arthritis. T9 (arrow) is virtually destroyed.

Other causes of uveitis must be considered, however, such as sarcoidosis.

Certain tumors enter into the differential diagnosis of JRA. Among the more prominent examples are neuroblastoma, pigmented villonodular synovitis, and histiocytosis. Acute leukemia in childhood may present as an arthritis because of involvement by red marrow of the metaphyseal portions of the bones in children, or infiltration of malignant cells in the periosteum and joint capsule. The presence of bone pain on weight bearing may be a clue to its presence. In the late adolescent to early adult years red marrow ceases to occupy these areas, and therefore arthritis as a manifestation of a hematologic malignancy would not usually be seen. Sickle cell anemia because of involvement of the periosteum and microinfarcts of bones can give rise to a periarthritis or dactylitis which in many cases mimics a true arthritis. The hand-foot syndrome of this hemoglobinopathy occurs in eary infancy.

Arthritis involving either the peripheral joints or spine is seen with considerable regularity in children with regional enteritis or ulcerative colitis.[191] Although Whipple's disease has been described in children, it is very

Table 80–2. Diagnostic Criteria for the Classification of Juvenile Rheumatoid Arthritis*

1. Age of onset less than 16 years
2. Arthritis in one or more joints defined as swelling or effusion, or as the presence of two or more of the following signs: limitation of range of motion, tenderness or pain on motion, and increased heat
3. Duration of disease of 6 weeks to 3 months
4. Type of onset of disease during the first 4 to 6 months classified as:
   a. Polyarthritis—5 joints or more
   b. Oligoarthritis—4 joints or fewer
   c. Systemic disease—arthritis
             intermittent fever
             rheumatoid rash
                 visceral disease (hepatosplenomegaly, lymphadenopathy, etc.)
5. Exclusion of other rheumatoid diseases

*Modified from Brewer, E.J., Jr., et al.: Bull. Rheum. Dis. 23:712, 1972.

Table 80–3. Ancillary Manifestations of Juvenile Rheumatoid Arthritis

Morning stiffness	Cervical Spondylitis
Rheumatoid rash	Rheumatoid nodules
Intermittent fever	Tenosynovites
Pericarditis	Antinuclear antibodies
Chronic uveitis	Rheumatoid factors

Table 80–4. Diagnostic Exclusions for the Classification of Juvenile Rheumatoid Arthritis

A. Other connective tissue diseases
  1. Systemic lupus erythematosus
  2. Dermatomyositis and polymyositis
  3. Vasculitis
    a. Anaphylactoid purpura (Henoch-Schönlein)
    b. Serum sickness
    c. Polyarteritis
    d. Mucocutaneous lymph node syndrome; infantile polyarteritis
  4. Scleroderma
  5. Mixed connective tissue disease
B. The spondyloarthropathies
  1. Juvenile ankylosing spondylitis
  2. Psoriatic arthritis and spondylitis
  3. Reiter's disease
  4. Inflammatory bowel disease
    a. Regional enteritis
    b. Ulcerative colitis
C. Postinfectious arthritis
  1. Post-yersinia arthritis
  2. Acute rheumatic fever, Jaccoud's arthritis
D. Infectious arthritis
  1. Bacterial arthritis (including tuberculosis, syphilis and gonorrhea)
  2. Viral and fungal arthritides
  3. Lyme arthritis
E. Congenital anomalies and genetically determined abnormalities of the musculoskeletal system (including inborn errors of metabolism)
  1. Mucopolysaccharidoses (Morquio's disease)
  2. Spondyloepiphyseal dysplasia
  3. Ochronosis and hemochromatosis
  4. Familial Mediterranean fever
  5. Gout
  6. Gaucher's disease, Fabry's disease
  7. Hypermobility syndromes (Ehlers-Danlos)
  8. Familial flexion contractions of the fingers
  9. Diabetic cheiroarthropathy
  10. Familial carpal osteolysis
F. Nonrheumatic conditions of bones and joints
  1. Trauma
  2. Reflex sympathetic dystrophy
  3. Slipped capital femoral epiphysis
  4. Toxic synovitis of the hip
  5. Osteochondritis
  6. Chondromalacia of the patella
  7. Amyloidosis
  8. Sarcoidosis
  9. Plant thorn synovitis
  10. Rickets, scurvy
  11. Pityriasis lichenoides
G. Hematologic diseases
  1. Sickle cell anemia
  2. Hemophilia
  3. Thalassemia
  4. Leukemia and lymphoma
H. Neoplastic diseases
  1. Neuroblastoma
  2. Malignant tumors of cartilage, bone, and synovium
  3. Secondary hypertrophic osteoarthropathy
  4. Pigmented villonodular synovitis
  5. Histiocytosis
I. Rheumatic diseases associated with immunodeficiency
  1. Selective IgA deficiency
  2. Agammaglobulinemia and hypogammaglobulinemia
  3. Complement component deficiencies
J. Psychogenic rheumatism

rare. Reiter's syndrome and psoriatic arthritis have been decidedly uncommon in our clinic.[192-194]

Onset of hip disease in the very young child should be first thought of as representing a septic process or congenital dislocation of the hip. In the somewhat older child aseptic necrosis of the femoral head (Legg-Calvé-Perthes disease) is another diagnostic consideration. In the adolescent child, particularly the obese boy, a slipped capital femoral epiphysis may initially mimic JRA. Other types of aseptic necrosis, as in Osgood-Schlatter disease of the tibial tubercle, can usually be easily distinguished from involvement of the knee in JRA. Transient synovitis of the hip is a self-limited condition of uncertain origin.[195] Pain is minimal. Laboratory and radiologic studies are normal. In our opinion it is a diagnosis that is difficult to define. However, JRA rarely begins in or affects solely a hip. In our series of approximately 100 children with oligoarthritis only one had initial involvement of the hip.

Although the child with systemic onset of disease has all the manifestations of an acute infectious process, finding the rheumatoid rash or typical arthritis will point to a diagnosis of JRA. The fever in these children is of the septic type; a sustained fever readily responsive to salicylate therapy would be more characteristic of acute rheumatic fever.[39] Likewise, although many children with systemic onset of disease have pericarditis and effusion, these are isolated cardiac findings. Finding a pericardial effusion in conjunction with evidence of endocarditis such as a diastolic murmur would point away from JRA and toward a disease such as rheumatic fever or bacterial endocarditis. The onset of rheumatic fever in developed countries of the world is usually between the ages of 5 and 15 years. The arthritis is characteristically acute, painful, asymmetric, and migratory, and involves the peripheral joints without sequelae. The total duration of a single attack is usually less than 6 weeks and seldom as long as 3 months. The antistreptolysin-O titer is chronically elevated in one third of the children with JRA as a manifestation of their inflammatory disease and should not be taken as an indication of recent or current streptococcal infection.[196] During the course of rheumatic fever, one will observe a significant (two tube) rise or fall in the titer. The streptozyme test is currently regarded as more reliable in the diagnosis of acute rheumatic fever.

There are three diseases which occur with regular frequency in our clinic and which present some long-term problems in the diagnosis of JRA. These conditions are *systemic lupus erythematosus, juvenile ankylosing spondylitis*, and the arthritis of *immunodeficiency*.

Table 80–5. Frequency of the Connective Tissue Diseases in Pediatric Rheumatology

Juvenile rheumatoid arthritis	75%
Systemic lupus erythematosus	10%
Dermatomyositis	6%
Juvenile ankylosing spondylitis	5%
Scleroderma	<3%
Polyarteritis	<1%
Rheumatic fever	<1%

The child with systemic lupus erythematosus can present with an arthritis that mimics that seen in JRA, and the correct diagnosis may not be evident until one of the more characteristic clinical findings of lupus occurs later in the course of the disease. These findings include malar erythema, alopecia, Raynaud's phenomenon, central nervous system disease, and nephritis. The urinalysis in most children with JRA will not show evidence of persistent hematuria and proteinuria. The finding of an active urinary sediment in a child with JRA would strongly suggest an alternative diagnosis such as lupus, as would the occurrence of leukopenia or thrombocytopenia.

Serologic tests may confirm the presence of lupus and should always be performed when a diagnostic question arises. Hypocomplementemia, a strongly positive antinuclear antibody test with a peripheral pattern, positive LE cell tests, and high titers of anti-double-stranded DNA antibodies would be diagnostic of the active immune-complex disease of systemic lupus erythematosus.[146] In this consideration, it should be noted that the type of onset which most resembles acute lupus, systemic disease, is the one least likely to be associated with a positive antinuclear antibody test (≤ 10 percent).

Ragsdale and associates[197] have presented the course of 10 children who developed SLE after an initial diagnosis of JRA. In all cases, the anti-DNA antibody test became positive before the development of clinical symptoms characteristic of SLE.

The child with juvenile ankylosing spondylitis will usually present with arthritis of the lower extremities rather than lumbar pain or stiffness.[198,199] Pain in the groin or buttock may be an early sign. Two thirds of these individuals are boys. Remittent oligoarthritis is most frequent, and involvement of the wrists or joints of the hands is rare. Other helpful diagnostic points are onset of disease after the age of 7 to 10 years, infrequent cervical spine involvement, seronegativity for rheumatoid factors or antinuclear antibodies, and a positive family history of similar disease. Approximately 92 percent of these children will be positive for the lymphocyte surface antigen HLA-B27.[200,201] In general a negative result will be found in approximately 8 percent of children with juvenile ankylosing spondylitis, and a positive test in the same percentage of white children with JRA. The presence of HLA-B27 is, therefore, neither sufficient nor necessary for a diagnosis of juvenile ankylosing spondylitis.

A firm diagnosis of juvenile ankylosing spondylitis depends upon demonstration of the characteristic radiologic features in the sacroiliac joints. These changes are often present at onset of the disease if technically adequate, angulated views of the sacroiliac joints are obtained; however, a definite diagnosis may be delayed by months to years in unusual cases.

Children with immunologic deficiencies, particularly selective IgA deficiency,[202,203] common variable immunodeficiency and X-linked agammaglobulinemia,[204] and heterozygous C2 complement component deficiency,[205] may present with an arthritis that mimics JRA. Indeed, we hesitate at this time to separate all of these children from the larger group with JRA, as we do not know on an etiologic basis what JRA is (or are)! It is mandatory in any child with chronic arthritis to obtain studies for humoral immunologic deficiency, particularly quantitation of the serum immunoglobulins, and to determine the hemolytic complement titer.

Approximately 4 percent of the children whom we see with an arthritis that is clinically indistinguishable from JRA have selective IgA deficiency (SIgAD). This immune deficiency was first reported in 1964 in normal persons,[206] and then by us in 1966 in children with chronic arthritis.[207] Previous studies had indicated only a sporadic association of SIgAD with arthritis.[208] One investigation reported 2 of 23 children with JRA with SIgAD[209] and other publications followed.[210-211] In a paper from England,[212] 12 of 582 children with juvenile chronic polyarthritis had absent serum IgA. There was an increased oligoarthritic onset of disease in this group, but the frequency of systemic symptoms was the same as in the control group. On follow-up, nine of the 12 had developed polyarthritis. In contrast to our studies, arthritis was severe in at least one half of these affected children. The association of SIgAD with arthritis may have pathogenic significance and may represent a unique model for the study of JRA.

Table 80–6 shows some of the rheumatic diseases associated with SIgAD based upon data collected from our clinic.[202,203,213,214] The two most common are a JRA-like arthritis and "SLE." Of 477 patients with a diagnosis of JRA, 18 had absent serum IgA and undetectable secretory IgA (frequency of 3.8 percent). SIgAD has been demonstrated in SLE, rheumatoid arthritis, dermatomyositis, scleroderma, and ankylosing spondylitis. With JRA and SLE, approximate prevalence rates are 4 to 5 percent, respectively. With the other connective tissue diseases, prevalence rates have not been deter-

Table 80–6. Selective IgA Deficiency and Connective Tissue Disease

Diagnosis	Number with SIgAD	Prevalence (%)
Juvenile rheumatoid arthritis (JRA)	18	4
"Systemic lupus erythematosus"	10	5
"Dermatomyositis"	3	–
Adult chronic arthritis	4	–
"Ankylosing spondylitis"	2	–
"Scleroderma"	1	–

mined. Based upon the prevalence of SIgAD in the normal population (0.1 percent) the frequency of SIgAD in patients with rheumatic diseases is approximately 50 times higher than in a community population. An increased frequency of abnormally low levels of serum IgA in children with arthritis is also documented.[202] The diseases associated with a concurrent immune deficiency may not be the same pathogenically as those in individuals without identifiable immune deficiency; therefore, their designations have been placed in quotations.

Table 80–7 shows the characteristics of children in our study with juvenile chronic arthritis and SIgAD. As with hypogammaglobulinemia, the arthritis that developed in these children was clinically indistinguishable from JRA.[204] The sex ratio was about the same, and the age of onset was not substantially different from the young age of onset in the comparison group. The types of onset were different, however, in that most SIgAD children had an oligoarthric onset; polyarthritis occurred in only seven, systemic onset did not occur, and the majority did not have severe disease. The 22 percent in functional class III were attending school or working. We concluded from our experience that chronic arthritis in the presence of an immune deficiency was somewhat milder than that which occurred in children without immune deficiency. It also appeared, during this long period of observation, that the arthritis did not go into remission but remained active throughout most of the time. Although no discernible joint destruction occurred in most patients, articular erosions did develop in 28 percent of the children. Rheumatoid nodules occurred in two patients. Uveitis was also a frequent occurrence in this group of IgA-deficient children, perhaps related

to the oligoarthritis and high frequency of antinuclear antibody seropositivity. These antinuclear antibodies were not directed against native DNA, as is characteristic of the patient with SIgAD and SLE. The higher frequency of antinuclear antibody seropositivity in this group of children with SIgAD compared with other children with JRA may represent an increased occurrence of this autoantibody with this specific type of immune deficiency, but it is also compatible with the occurrence of chronic uveitis that was observed in this study. On the other hand, rheumatoid factors were unusual, as in JRA in general, and occurred in only one patient.

One characteristic of IgA deficiency that merits particular mention is the occurrence of anti-IgA antibodies. Three fourths of these patients had circulating antibodies to IgA (Table 80–8). These are commonly of the IgG class and have been implicated in the literature in serious transfusion reactions.[215,216] In our study of 56 individuals with SIgAD,[217,218] antibodies to IgA were not detected in patients with rheumatic diseases and normal levels of IgA, or in normal persons. Anti-IgA antibodies were found in less than one third of IgA-deficient patients with nonrheumatic diseases, in three fourths of IgA-deficient children with chronic arthritis, and in all of the IgA-deficient patients with lupus. It could be concluded that the patient with SIgAD and rheumatic disease appeared to be especially capable of developing anti-IgA antibodies and to be at risk for anaphylactoid reactions following administration of any blood products. If transfusions are indicated for a surgical procedure, it is imperative to give matched blood from an IgA-deficient donor, or, in an emergency, to give thoroughly washed red cells.

Little is known of the pathophysiology of SIgAD and connective tissue diseases. In the majority of individuals, it appears that SIgAD represents a failure of synthesis or secretion of IgA related to a functional defect in the B lymphocytes.[219] In a few patients, there may be increased T-suppressor activity that contributes to the clinical expression of this immune deficiency.[220]

SIgAD may only be the most obvious clinical expression of other associated immunologic abnormalities. In our studies, approximately 40 percent of patients with SIgAD have had defects in cell-mediated immunity by lymphocyte transformation to mitogens.[221] Patients with SIgAD may have deficiencies of specific IgG subclasses.[222] Other individuals with this abnormality may

Table 80–7. Clinical Profile of 18 Children with Chronic Arthritis and Selective IgA Deficienty

	%
Sex	
Female	75
Male	25
Age at onset	
0–4 years	50
5–9 years	45
10–12 years	5
Type of onset	
Polyarthritis	40
Oligoarthritis	60
Systemic disease	0
Functional class	
I	30
II	50
III	20
IV	0
Extra-articular manifestations	
Articular erosions	25
Rheumatoid nodules	10
Chronic uveitis	20
Laboratory findings	
Antinuclear antibodies	70
Rheumatoid factors	5
Anti-IgA antibody	80
Anti-DNA antibody	5

Table 80–8. Frequency of Anti-IgA Antibodies in Selective IgA Deficiency

Diagnosis	Number	Anti-IgA Antibodies	
		Number	%
Asymptomatic blood donors	27	5	19
Miscellaneous diseases	8	2	25
Recurrent infections	10	3	30
RA-like arthritis	4	2	50
JRA-like arthritis	13	10	77
SLE-like disease	10	10	100

have a deficiency of serum IgE[223] or of ecto-5'-nucleotidase.[224] The literature has been at odds as to whether there are specific HLA types associated with IgA deficiency.[225-227] With rare exceptions, SIgAD is congenital and permanent. Circulating immune complexes have been found in some patients with SIgAD that have included bovine antigens.[228] The levels of these complexes have also been correlated with the presence of precipitating antibodies to bovine proteins ("milk" precipitins).[229]

No specific treatment is available at this time for a child with SIgAD and arthritis. The articular disease in these patients has often responded to conventional antirheumatic therapy. Although plasma had been used experimentally in treatment, this therapy is limited by the occurrence of anti-IgA antibodies. In one instance, administration of plasma to an IgA-deficient girl with chronic erosive arthritis was followed by decreased activity of the joint disease for a long period of time.[230] Following the plasma therapy, the patient developed detectable IgA in secretions and low normal IgA levels in serum. Three and one-half years later, however, she developed antibody to native DNA and hypocomplementemia, and a diagnosis of SLE was made.

Additionally, patients with SIgAD do not generally respond to human serum immune globulin. This form of therapy might be of limited usefulness in children with SIgAD who have recurrent bacterial infections. In these instances, the clinician might be replacing a critical but missing subclass of IgG. Small amounts of IgA may be present in immune globulin and would represent a danger to any patient with anti-IgA antibodies.[231]

TREATMENT

Conservative management of JRA attempts to control the clinical manifestations of the disease and to prevent deformity.[232-235] It almost always involves a multidisciplinary team approach: rheumatologist, pediatrician, social worker, physiatrist and physical therapist, occupational therapist, nurse, and orthopedic surgeon. As JRA is characterized by recurrent inflammation of the joints and varying systemic manifestations, treatment in most children is prolonged. This long duration of therapy must be accepted ultimately by the child and his family and judged safe by the physician. Although prognosis is excellent in the majority of children with JRA, the rheumatologist is not able at onset to predict with certainty who will recover and who will have unremitting disease. Therefore, treatment must be vigorous in all cases and aimed at suppression of articular inflammation, prevention of secondary deformities, and control of systemic disease.

Acute inflammation leads to transient disability, swelling, and pain. Chronic articular inflammation may result in permanent deformity and destruction of cartilage and bone. The philosophy of management of children with JRA is to begin with the simplest, safest, and most conservative measures. If this treatment proves inadequate, the physician must choose other therapeutic modalities in an orderly fashion (Table 80–9). The potentially toxic regimens such as the immunosuppressive drugs should be employed only in life-threatening disease with full explanation of their risk-benefit ratio, and only in approved experimental protocols.

Aspirin. Aspirin is the most important pharmacologic agent and is of indispensable value in the treatment of children with JRA (Table 80–10).[236,237] It is effective in suppressing inflammation and fever in the majority of cases. Aspirin also has a proved record of long-term safety. It should be given four or five times a day with meals or at bedtime with milk. Awakening the child at night to administer aspirin is not necessary because of the prolonged half-life of salicylate after therapeutic levels are achieved.

Treatment with aspirin is started at 75 to 100 mg per kilogram per day. The higher doses are tolerated best in younger children of less than 25 kg of body weight. Salicylate levels are occasionally useful as a guide to correct dosage because of the lack of communicated signs of toxicity such as tinnitus in the preverbal child.[238-240] The appropriate serum level varies but is usually 20 to 25 mg per deciliter measured 2 hours after the morning dose. It may be difficult to reach therapeutic levels in children with systemic disease, but increasing the daily amount of aspirin beyond 130 mg per kilogram usually results in toxicity. If higher doses are required initially for control, they should be gradually reduced to maintenance levels on subsidence of the systemic manifestations. The febrile pattern will usually respond to adequate salicylate dosage in 1 to 4 weeks.

Aspirin in the young child must be used cautiously, as salicylism can occur rapidly and early signs, such as drowsiness and hyperpnea, are easily overlooked. Metabolically, the very young child develops ketosis and acidosis, whereas the older one develops respiratory alkalosis. Some children will experience abdominal pain or vomiting when given aspirin. Gastrointestinal irri-

Table 80–9. Management of Juvenile Rheumatoid Arthritis

Stage I:
   Basic program:
      Aspirin
      Local and general rest
      Physical and occupational therapy
      Education of patient, family, and school
Stage II:
   Nonsteroidal anti-inflammatory drugs
   Hydroxychloroquine
   Intra-articular steroids
Stage III:
   Hospitalization
   Gold salts
   Penicillamine
Stage IV:
   Systemic corticosteroid drugs
   Preventive surgery
Stage V:
   Reconstructive surgery
   Experimental therapy

Table 80–10. Medications Used in the Treatment of Juvenile Rheumatoid Arthritis

Drug	Dose	Indication	Toxicity
Aspirin	75–100 mg/kg/day	Control of pain, stiffness, and inflammation	Salicylism (lethargy, hyperpnea, tinnitus), gastrointestinal irritation, bleeding, hepatitis
Nonsteroidal anti-inflammatory agents	Tolmetin, 25 mg/kg/day	Control of pain, stiffness, and inflammation	Gastrointestinal irritation
Gold salts	0.75 mg/kg/month maintenance dose	Polyarthritis unresponsive to aspirin	Nephritis, dermatitis, stomatitis, bone marrow suppression
Hydroxychloroquine	5–7 mg/kg/day	Highly selective use for arthritis	Dermatitis, retinopathy, keratopathy
Corticosteroid drugs			
Systemic	Prednisone, 0.1–1 mg/kg/day (as low a dose as possible)	Life-threatening systemic disease, chronic uveitis	Growth retardation, osteoporosis, infection, Cushing's syndrome, cataracts
Ophthalmic	1–4 drops/day	Chronic uveitis	Cataracts, glaucoma
Intra-articular	10–30 mg prednisolone tertiary-butylacetate	Limited, selective use for arthritis	Infection
Pencillamine	10 mg/kg/day	Polyarthritis unresponsive to other regimens	Lupus-like syndrome, dermatitis, nephritis
Immunosuppressive agents	Varies with drug	Life-threatening systemic disease (experimental protocol)	Infection, bone marrow suppression, sterility, oncogenesis

tation can usually be controlled by prescribing salicylate with food or by use of antacids, or may be overcome by switching temporarily to a liquid preparation such as choline salicylate. In our experience peptic ulceration or obvious gastrointestinal bleeding is rare in children. A hypersensitivity rash is exceedingly uncommon.

Studies have suggested that children who chronically chew their aspirin preparations not only develop gingival inflammation but also erosions and destruction of the biting surfaces of the teeth.[241] Hence, the chewable preparations of aspirin are definitely contraindicated in the treatment of JRA. Children must be encouraged to swallow aspirin, or if they cannot, a liquid preparation may be temporarily indicated. If chewable aspirin must be used, teeth may be covered to protect against the effects of aspirin.

Some children develop a hepatitis related to salicylate therapy, although clinical manifestations of liver disease appear to be uncommon. Biopsies have shown a mild periportal round cell infiltration and scattered single cell necrosis.[242-246] This type of hepatitis occurs most frequently when the serum salicylate concentration is in the toxic range (>25 mg per deciliter), although the transaminase enzymes (SGOT and SGPT) may be intermittently increased in as many as 50 percent of the children on therapeutic levels of aspirin. Transient elevation of these enzymes in a child who is otherwise not showing signs of toxicity is not an indication for stopping the drug. If the enzymes remain elevated or the levels are high, e.g., SGOT >5 times normal, aspirin should be temporarily stopped or the dosage reduced by at least 20 percent until they return to normal. Treatment may then be reinstituted cautiously at a lower dose, which can be gradually increased if necessary.

Satisfactory treatment of the arthritis will be achieved in about 70 percent of children with aspirin alone. We generally continue salicylate therapy for 2 years after all manifestations of activity have been suppressed. When children do not respond to this program after a 6-month trial or respond inadequately, a limited number of other drugs can be considered.

Other Nonsteroidal Anti-inflammatory Agents. Most of the nonsteroidal anti-inflammatory agents have not been authorized for use in children.[247-249] They would be indicated for control of pain, stiffness, and inflammation in selected children who have been unresponsive to aspirin. Tolmetin, 25 mg per kilogram per day, has been demonstrated to be effective in children and does not interfere with salicylate administration.[250] Naproxen, 10 mg per kilogram per day divided into two or three doses, is also approved for use in children.[251,252] For patients older than 14 years, other drugs may be tried, such as fenoprofen, ≤ 2400 mg per day; sodium meclofenamate, ≤ 300 mg per day; or ibuprofen, ≤ 2400 mg per day. Indomethacin in a dose of 25 mg two to four times per day may be particularly effective for control of fever in the older patient with JRA. Phenylbutazone is seldom used in pediatric rheumatology.

The failure of one anti-inflammatory drug does not preclude successful treatment of the child with another agent. Therefore, each drug is selected in the resistant case for a trial period of 4 to 8 weeks. It is usually not considered advisable to administer the majority of these agents in combination with aspirin.

Acetaminophen in doses of 325 to 650 mg two to three times a day may be helpful for control of the temperature spikes in the systemically ill child. This drug has no anti-inflammatory action, however, and should not be used for long-term basic management of the disease. Its safety from the viewpoint of potential renal damage has been questioned. Likewise propoxyphene may be used for relief of intermittent pain but is not anti-inflammatory.

Antimalarial Drugs. Hydroxychloroquine is a useful

adjunctive agent for treatment of the older child with JRA. Its use has been restricted in the last 10 years because of concern over development of retinopathy. Stillman treated 125 of 204 children with JRA with antimalarial drugs, first chloroquine and later hydroxychloroquine.[253] The length of follow-up was up to five years. Remissions were induced in 26 children; 30 additional patients had a relapse after an initial remission when the dose of the antimalarial drug was reduced or the medication was stopped. In some children a remission could be reinstituted. Toxic effects were found in 13 patients and included macular degeneration in three. Minor side effects were noted in an additional six children. All children recovered from the toxic effects of these drugs, however, including those who had developed retinopathy. Rash, pruritus, bleaching of the hair, keratopathy, and abdominal pain were additional side effects.

The initial dose of hydroxychloroquine is 5 to 7 mg per kilogram per day (≤ 600 mg).[254] After 6 to 8 weeks dosage should be reduced, and the total period of initial treatment should probably not be prolonged beyond 1 to 2 years. An ophthalmologic examination must be performed before institution of therapy and every 3 to 6 months thereafter. Although it would be unusual for retinal toxicity to occur at these dosage levels, the drug should be discontinued permanently at any suspicion of retinopathy because its effects are cumulative.[255] Corneal deposition may occur and is an indication for lowering the dose. It should be noted that JRA is not an approved use of hydroxychloroquine. In acute overdose, especially in the very young, antimalarial drugs have no antidote and may be fatal.

Gold Salts. Gold salts are as effective in the treatment of children with JRA as in adults with rheumatoid arthritis.[256,257] Preparations which are available are gold sodium thiomalate and aurothioglucose. Gold is indicated in children whose polyarthritis has been unresponsive after 4 to 6 months to a conservative program of management. Before one of these drugs is administered, the child's basic hematologic, renal, and hepatic function must be normal. A test dose of 5 mg should be given intramuscularly on the initial visit. Weekly doses are gradually increased thereafter until approximately 0.75 mg per kilogram per week is given (≤ 50 mg). Weekly injections are continued for 20 weeks to a total dose of approximately 15 mg per kilogram (≤ 1000 mg). If satisfactory improvement or remission has been achieved, maintenance therapy is instituted every 2 weeks for 3 months and then every 3 weeks for 3 months. At that juncture, if objective signs of improvement continue, the child is placed on monthly gold injections adjusted periodically on the basis of body weight. A complete blood count and urinalysis must be obtained before each administration of gold salts, and assessment of the child for any toxicity, especially stomatitis, dermatitis, bone marrow suppression, hematuria, or proteinuria, should be done. A decrease of the white blood cell count below 5000 per cubic millimeter; a fall in the absolute neutrophil count by 50 percent; the develop-

ment of eosinophilia, proteinuria, or hematuria; or clinical signs of gold toxicity are indications for at least a temporary interruption of therapy. In selected cases therapy may be cautiously resumed at a lower dose after the child's condition returns to normal. Absolute contraindications to reinstitution of gold are severe leukopenia, neutropenia, proteinuria, or an exfoliative dermatitis. It is estimated that approximately 25 percent of children started on gold salts will not be able to complete a course of treatment because of toxicity, usually hematuria or dermatitis; 25 percent will not improve while on gold, and the remaining 50 percent will experience substantial relief or a complete remission.

Levinson reported a remission or marked improvement with gold salts in 48 percent of treated children and moderate to mild improvement in 25 percent.[258] Brewer found that children with polyarthritis responded better than those with other onset types and also concluded that gold salt therapy was useful in treating systemic disease and ameliorating concomitant fever.[259]

An initial trial of oral gold therapy with auranofin has been reported in children.[260] Safety and dosage were established in this limited study, but efficacy has not been demonstrated over a prolonged period of time.

D-Penicillamine. D-Penicillamine has not been approved for use in children. Current data suggest that it may be as effective as gold salts and no more toxic. The indications for use are the same as for gold. The maximal dose is 10 mg per kilogram per day (≤ 750 mg per day). This dose is achieved after three increments of 12 weeks each. A complete blood count and urinalysis are done once a week. Important side effects of D-penicillamine are drug-induced lupus, dermatitis, thrombocytopenia, and proteinuria.

A study of D-penicillamine therapy in children with JRA has not been completed in this country. In studies in England by Ansell,[261] there was an overall improvement in 62 percent of the children after three years of treatment with D-penicillamine. This was comparable to a 64 percent improvement demonstrated with gold-salt therapy. Four patients were withdrawn from the study because of toxic reactions. Onset of the anti-inflammatory action of D-penicillamine was found to be slow, and it was necessary to continue the drug for at least a year, and possibly up to three years, before deciding that it was ineffectual in a child. In another study, 4 of 39 severely affected children improved on D-penicillamine after failure to respond to other regimens. Proteinuria in this study was the most frequent reason for withdrawal, but was, however, often associated with the development of amyloidosis. Finally, Schairer studied 157 children on a regimen that included D-penicillamine for 3 months to 3 years.[262] Improvement was noted in this group in 63 percent and toxic reactions in 27 percent. D-Penicillamine was stopped in 11 percent of these children. Again, these findings were similar to those for comparable children that had been treated with gold salts.

Corticosteroid Agents. The corticosteroid drugs are useful in the treatment of JRA via three routes of administration. They may be given orally in life-threatening disease or in combination with ophthalmic steroid for the treatment of chronic uveitis. Intra-articular steroid is limited to use in one or two joints that continue to be actively involved in a child who has otherwise responded satisfactorily to conservative therapy, or as an aid to a physical therapy program in order to achieve a carefully selected objective. Intra-articular injections should not be given more than three times in a single joint during a restricted period of time, for example, 3 months.

Prednisone is the steroid usually chosen for use systemically. For uncontrolled systemic disease with marked disability, prednisone may be used in a single morning dose of 0.5 to 1 mg per kilogram per day (≤ 40 mg) or in divided doses. Once satisfactory control of the disease is reached or it is obvious that satisfactory control is not going to be achieved, the drug should be gradually decreased and eventually discontinued. Steroid therapy, even in high dosage, does not limit the duration of the disease, prevent extra-articular complications, or alter the eventual prognosis.[263-265] It is important that both the child, if possible, and his parents understand that total control of the signs and symptoms of JRA may not be possible and that it will be necessary to accept some degree of activity of the disease in exchange for less corticosteroid toxicity. Steroid pseudorheumatism (Slocumb's syndrome) may make even slow withdrawal of the drug difficult. Although use of steroids to suppress joint inflammation alone is to be avoided as much as possible, low-dose, every-other-day prednisone may be useful in some children with severe unresponsive polyarthritis.[266]

Growth retardation is the most significant untoward effect of steroid toxicity in children.[267-269] A dose of 5 mg per day is usually inhibitory; as little as 3 mg in the child under 25 kg of body weight may be suppressive. JRA in itself retards normal development and growth. A child may regain his loss in height with time, be it the result of either his disease or therapy, but it is our experience that this does not happen very often if a significant deficit has occurred, or is not complete in terms of resumption of the previous isodevelopmental level. Growth retardation cannot be overcome by administration of anabolic steroids or growth hormone.[270] The other frequent and important side effects of the corticosteroid medications are many: osteoporosis, an increased susceptibility to infections, pseudotumor cerebri, addisonian crisis, Cushing's syndrome, hypertension, hypokalemia, fluid retention, obesity, cataracts, and glaucoma. Prolonged administration of corticosteroids in children is associated with an appreciable mortality.[271,272] Stress doses of steroids must be given during medical emergencies. In one study of adrenocortical function in children with JRA,[273] it was found that daily corticosteroids resulted in suppression of the hypothalamic-pituitary-adrenal axis, and alternate-day or intermittent use impaired the response to a lesser degree. Even intra-articular steroids could result in a transient suppression of function. Every child on prednisone should carry a record of his therapeutic program and the amount of steroid that he is taking. As an additional precaution, children on corticosteroid drugs should not receive live virus vaccines.

It must be emphasized that systemically administered corticosteroids have no place in the treatment of a child with oligoarthritis in the absence of uveitis. These children are almost never that unwell. At the very most, persistent inflammation and effusion in one or more joints are treated by a limited course of intra-articular injections.

Primary treatment of chronic uveitis must be supervised by an ophthalmologist and usually consists of corticosteroid eye drops and a short-acting mydriatic drug to dilate the pupil and prevent posterior synechiae. It is usually advisable to use supplemental oral prednisone in low dosage (2 to 4 mg once a day). A significant proportion of children may actually require larger amounts than this to control their disease. Even ophthalmic steroid administration may result in the development of Cushing's syndrome.

Immunosuppressive Agents. Immunosuppressive and cytotoxic agents should be used in JRA only in approved experimental protocols and only for life-threatening illness. The drugs most commonly employed are azathioprine, cyclophosphamide, and chlorambucil. Leukopenia or bone marrow suppression may result from any of these agents. The potential for development of malignancy and mutagenic effects are the most critical long-term considerations in the use of these drugs. Sterility has been associated with all the immunosuppressive agents, particularly those of the alkylating variety.

There are no controlled studies that have established the usefulness of immunosuppressive drugs in children with JRA. Stoeber employed azathioprine in 321 children with severe systemic disease or uveitis and reported clinical improvement in approximately 30 percent.[274] Ansell reported that chlorambucil was useful in the treatment of children who developed amyloidosis and that it appeared to prolong survival.[275]

Other Medications. Transfer factor, after initially encouraging reports, has not been proved effective in the treatment of JRA. Newer immunoregulatory drugs such as levamisole must be approached with great caution in the treatment of children with JRA. Several children treated with this drug were reported to have developed fatal agranulocytosis or seizures.[277] Other experimental forms of treatment, such as plasmapheresis[278] and steroid IV pulse therapy,[279] are currently being evaluated for seriously ill children.

Physical and Occupation Therapy. Maintenance of function and prevention of deformity by physical therapy and splinting cannot be overemphasized and are vitally important in the total management of the child with JRA. This is particularly true for children who are initially confined to bed or wheelchair because of the activity of their disease or pain. During periods of acute inflammation of the joints, the physical therapist might best use supervised rest and range of motion in a whirlpool bath. Heat aids in the relief of joint pain and stiffness and prepares a child for the exercise program. Atrophy of the extensor muscles and later of the flexors begins early in disease, and a program should be instituted as soon as possible to strengthen these muscle groups. As weight bearing is sometimes difficult because of pain or contractures, passive and then active motion of selected joints must be begun early.

A balanced program of increased rest at night or during the day after school is advisable in many children. A child will usually best determine his own level of activity. Only rarely does encouragement beyond his present capabilities or undue restriction of daily activity profit the child. We avoid only those particular activities that have been observed to cause overtiring or joint pain. Normal play should be encouraged, and the only areas that we discuss as undersirable are those that place unacceptable levels of stress upon weight-bearing joints which are inflamed, such as basketball and certain forms of gymnastics. Tricycle riding and swimming are almost always helpful and avoid putting weight on involved joints.

Cock-up splints for the wrist and posterior night splints for the knees are used to prevent malpositioning of these joints or as aids in the long-term correction of deformity. Adequate shoes should be prescribed. Leg length discrepancy should be minimized by a lift for the shorter extremity. If the hips are involved, a prone lining board will help prevent hip flexion contractures. For severe contractures serial casting with active exercises every 4 days each time the cast is removed may be tried; forced extension should be avoided. Maintenance of reduced contractures often requires gentle stretching and the use of resting splints. Malpositioning of the cervical spine may be minimized by use of a soft collar and a desk with a tilted top on which the child can do his homework.

Orthopedic Surgery. Synovectomy does not affect the long-term course of JRA but may be useful in carefully selected children for relief of mechanical impairment of joint motion related to synovial hypertrophy, joint pain, and decreased range of motion.[280-289] Remobilization of a postsurgical joint in children is more difficult than in adults. Tenosynovectomy may be indicated to decrease the risk of tendon rupture over the dorsum of the wrist or for adhesive tenosynovitis and trigger finger. A well-thought-out plan of reconstructive surgery can be of critical importance in children who enter the late teenage years or adulthood with marked disability. Total joint replacement, particularly of the hip, might be indicated at that time when bone growth has ceased. Children with micrognathia may eventually profit cosmetically from orthodontic management.[290,291]

Education and Counseling of Family and Patient. As the prognosis for JRA is excellent, it is signally important that parents and child, if possible, understand the disease and share in its management. A considerable amount of time and effort must be expended in explaining to them the nature of JRA, reasonable expectations during the period of initial therapy, and the course of the disease. This counseling should be initiated by the physician and reinforced by the nurse and social worker. These educational efforts must be an ongoing process; it is often useful to ask a parent to write down problems and bring the list to the clinic appointments. More than half the families of children with JRA manifest psychiatrically important disruption (divorce, separation, death, or adoption) and often severe emotional disturbances.[292-300] A priority in the management of the child with JRA is to foster the formation of normal psychological and social development.[301,302] Attendance at school is strongly encouraged; only rarely is home instruction indicated.

The child's nutrition is an important aspect of the long-term management of JRA. Growth retardation almost invariably occurs during active periods of disease. This may be exacerbated by corticosteroid administration or relative inanition. Vitamin supplementation is often indicated.

COURSE OF DISEASE AND PROGNOSIS

Functional Disability. In general, 70 to 90 percent of children with JRA make a satisfactory recovery from their disease without serious disability.[303-308] A small percentage of children will have a recurrence of arthritis as adults.[309-311] Early after onset, the course of JRA is especially unpredictable. The type of onset to some extent is associated with the future unfolding of the clinical disease (Table 80-11).[312-314] After the pattern of the disease is well established, it tends to be repetitive and somewhat more predictable. The functional result in children with unremitting polyarthritis is least favorable. The child who has oligoarthritis does best from the standpoint of joint disease but worst from the risk of uveitis. Children with systemic onset are the most prone to develop life-threatening and sometimes fatal complications. Irrespective of the type of onset or pattern of disease, 83 percent of children in the 15-year series of the English clinicians were able to work.[26,315,316]

The studies of Calabro and Marchesano indicate that an excellent functional result is achieved in the majority of children; however, even after 15 years, 33 of their 100 patients continued to have active disease, and three had died.[317] Laaksonen[8] reported that complete resolution of disease was present in 30 percent of patients at reas-

Table 80-11. Types of Onset of Disease Related to Patterns of Course of Disease

Types of Onset	Course of Disease (Chronic or Intermittent)
Systemic disease	Systemic
Polyarthritis	Polyarthritis
Oligoarthritis	Oligoarthritis

sessment (which averaged 16 years from onset of disease); there was slight disability in 40 percent and incapacitation in 30 percent. Complete recovery was most common when duration of disease was ≤7 years (51 percent) and least when it was ≥16 years (10 percent).

We estimate that approximately 10 percent of children with JRA enter adulthood with severe functional disability. The child most at risk is the one with polyarthritis of late age of onset, early involvement of the small joints of the hands or feet, rapid appearance of erosions, unremitting inflammatory activity, prominent systemic manifestations, rheumatoid factor seropositivity, and subcutaneous nodules. Although the small joints may be involved in any of the various types of onset of disease, widespread symmetric involvement of the metacarpophalangeal and proximal interphalangeal joints of the hands, the so-called adult pattern of rheumatoid arthritis, is characteristically associated with a somewhat poorer prognostic outlook than disease which confines itself to large joints. Limitation of range of motion often develops early in polyarthritis related to synovial proliferation, periarticular swelling, effusion, and muscle

spasm. Later it is a direct result of contracture of soft tissue, joint destruction, and ankylosis. Hip disease, which occurs in at least half the patients, almost always begins late in the course of persistent disease and leads inexorably to destruction or abnormal development of the femoral heads and acetabula (Fig. 80–19). Subluxation, protrusio acetabuli, or fusion results.[318-321] This type of severe hip disease is a major cause of disability in JRA and is justifiably interpreted as a relatively poor prognostic sign.

The course of children with oligoarthritis may remain or become monarthritis, or may be confined to the joints of initial involvement in over one third of the children.[31] Another one third with onset of disease in a single joint will have involvement of one or two additional joints. The remaining children will progress after 4 to 6 months into an articular pattern indistinguishable from that described for polyarthritis. We have never observed a child with oligoarthritis, however, who developed acute manifestations typical of the systemic onset of the disease. We have not seen a rheumatoid rash in these children (although it is said to occur in a rare child with this

Figure 80–19. A, Pelvis at age 5 years in a boy with severe systemic disease and polyarthritis. There is bilateral hip disease, narrowing of the joint space, and remodeling of the femoral head. B, Two years later. Destructive hip disease has progressed, and there is more marked involvement of the acetabular bone with sclerosis and multiple cystic lucencies, also seen now along the margins of the femoral heads. C, One year after B. Generalized osteopenia is marked, coxa valga on the right is more extreme, and there is beginning subluxation of the right femoral head. Clinically this child had severe pain in the hips with weight bearing and virtually no rotation at those joints. Flexion contractures of approximately 35 degrees were present bilaterally.

type of disease). Because of the nature of the limited joint involvement, serious functional disability is uncommon, and these children have a generally excellent prognostic outlook if they do not develop uveitis. Osteoarthritis may occur later in the course of the disease or after clinical remission of active inflammation, particularly in the weight-bearing joints (Fig. 80–20).

The acute manifestations of the systemic form of JRA are variable in duration, lasting from weeks to months to even years, and tend to recur during the initial years of the disease, usually in association with exacerbations of the child's arthritis. About half the children with systemic onset will eventually recover completely, often after manifesting a pattern of polyarthritis for a variable period. The other half will continue to show progressive polyarthritis and moderate to severe disability. Systemic symptoms alone are not a cause of permanent disability.

Although the development of amyloidosis is rare in the United States, in certain areas of the world it occurs in approximately 5 percent of cases of JRA, usually heralded by proteinuria and the nephrotic syndrome, diarrhea, or unexplained anemia.[322] After 15 years the incidence of amyloidosis had risen to 8 percent in the English series.[323,324] It usually develops in the more severely affected children with disease activity of long duration. It is rarely seen as early as 1 year after onset and has been observed as late as 23 years. Amyloidosis has followed all types of onset of disease and is nearly always fatal. The mean duration of life after diagnosis is 8 years. A diagnosis of amyloidosis may be confirmed by rectal biopsy.

Death. Death occurs in 2 to 4 percent of children with JRA.[325-327] The major causes of death in 46 children followed at Taplow were renal failure, in half the cases associated with amyloidosis, and infections (Table 80-12). The latter are currently less prominent in this series. Excess mortality was identified at the 15-year evaluation in girls who had developed their disease early in life. The majority of the deaths associated with JRA in the United States occur in children with systemic onset of disease.

Blindness. The prognosis for sight in children with chronic uveitis is probably improving related to earlier detection and better management; however, blindness occurred previously in approximately 50 to 70 percent of children with this complication.[328,329] In the recent report by Chylack,[330] 20 percent of affected eyes had a loss in visual acuity. Kanski's review of the Taplow experience indicated that 57 percent of affected eyes had a visual acuity of 6/9 or better when last examined and 62 percent still had active inflammation.[331] Only half of the eyes that had a cataract extraction had a visual acuity of 6/9 or better.

Perspective. A child's potential for growth is an important factor working in favor of the physician and his program. To a large extent it is this endowment for future physical and psychological development that enables so much to be accomplished in the majority of children with JRA.

Figure 80–20. Radiograph of left knee of an 18-year-old woman with oligoarthritis which began in the left knee at age 3 years and involved the left ankle briefly at age 6 years. The inflammatory arthritis in the knee probably entered a remission around 14 years of age. Crepitation, momentary locking, and pain on weight bearing as symptoms of degenerative arthritis superimposed on her previous JRA were present at the time this film was obtained. Hypertrophic proliferative changes were present at the joint margins, along with extreme narrowing of the lateral joint space with sclerosis of the opposing surfaces. Another inflammatory episode occurred while she was in nursing school at age 22. Crystal synovitis and infectious arthritis such as tuberculosis were diagnostic considerations; subsequent involvement of the right knee (for the first time) confirmed the eventual impression of a flare of her JRA.

Table 80–12. Causes of Death in Juvenile Rheumatoid Arthritis*

Cause	Percent of Total Without Amyloidosis	Children with Amyloidosis
Renal failure	2	48
Infections	20	
Cardiopulmonary failure	6	4
Adrenal crisis	4	1
Cerebral hemorrhage	1	2
Hematologic disorders	3	
Neoplasms	1	
Complications of therapy	2	1
Accidents and trauma	5	

*Modified from Baum, J., and Gutowska, G.: Arthritis Rheum. 20:253, 1977; and Bywaters, E.G.L.: Arthritis Rheum. 20:256, 1977.

References

1. Cornil, M.V.: Mémoire sur des coincidences pathologiques du rhumatisme articulaire chronique. C. R. Mém. Soc. Biol. (Paris) Series 4:3, 1864.
2. Diamantberger, S.: Du rhumatisme noueux (polyarthrite déformante) chez les enfants. Paris, Lecrosnier et Babe, 1890.
3. Still, G.F.: On a form of chronic joint disease in children. Med. Chir. Trans. 80:47, 1897. (Reprinted in Arch. Dis. Child. 16:156, 1941.)
4. Baum, J.: Epidemiology of juvenile rheumatoid arthritis (JRA). Arthritis Rheum. 20:158, 1977.
5. Baum, J., Alekseev, L.S., Brewer, E.J., Jr., Dolgopolova, A.V., Mudholkar, G.S., and Patel, K.: Juvenile rheumatoid arthritis: A comparison of patients from the U.S.S.R. and U.S.A. Arthritis Rheum. 23:977, 1980.
6. Calabro, J.J., and Marchesano, J.M.: Juvenile rheumatoid arthritis—current concepts. N. Engl. J. Med. 277:696, 746, 1967.
7. Sullivan, D.B., Cassidy, J.T., and Petty, R.E.: Pathogenic implications of age of onset in juvenile rheumatoid arthritis. Arthritis Rheum. 18:251, 1975.
8. Laaksonen, A.-L.: A prognostic study of juvenile rheumatoid arthritis. Analysis of 544 cases. Acta Paediatr. Scand. (Suppl. 166) 1966.
9. Panush, R.S., Bianco, N.E., Schur, P.H., Rocklin, R.E., David, J.R., and Stillman, J.S.: Juvenile rheumatoid arthritis. Cellular hypersensitivity and selective IgA deficiency. Clin. Exp. Immunol. 10:103, 1972.
10. Höyeraal, H.M.: Impaired delayed hypersensitivity in juvenile rheumatoid arthritis. Ann. Rheum. Dis. 32:331, 1973.
11. Höyeraal, H.M., and Mellbye, O.J.: Humoral immunity in juvenile rheumatoid arthritis. Ann. Rheum. Dis. 33:248, 1974.
12. Steffen, C., Sanger, L., and Menzel, J.: Demonstration of antibodies to denatured type I and type II collagen in juvenile rheumatoid arthritis, Still's syndrome and controls by (14C) collagen radioimmunoassay. Scand. J. Rheumatol. 9:69, 1980.
13. Ansell, B.M., Bywaters, E.G.L., and Lawrence, J.S.: A family study in Still's disease. Ann. Rheum. Dis. 21:243, 1962.
14. Ansell, B.M., Bywaters, E.G.L., and Lawrence J.S.: Familial aggregation and twin studies in Still's disease (juvenile chronic polyarthritis). Rheumatology 2:37, 1969.
15. Baum, J., and Fink, C.: Juvenile rheumatoid arthritis in monozygotic twins: A case report and review of the literature. Arthritis Rheum. 11:33, 1968.
16. Rosenberg, A.M., and Petty, R.E.: Similar patterns of juvenile rheumatoid arthritis within families. Arthritis Rheum. 23:951, 1980.
17. Hanson, V., Kornreich, H.K., Bernstein, B., King, K.K., and Singsen, B.H.: Three subtypes of juvenile rheumatoid arthritis (correlations of age at onset, sex, and serologic factors) Arthritis Rheum. 20:184, 1977.
18. Sury, B.: Rheumatoid Arthritis in Children. A Clinical Study. Copenhagen, Munksgaard, 1952.
19. Edström, G.: Rheumatoid arthritis and Still's disease in children. A survey of 161 cases. Arthritis Rheum. 1:497, 1958.
20. Schlesinger, B.E., Forsyth, C.C., White, R.H., Smellie, J.M., and Stroud, C.E.: Observations on the clinical course and treatment of one hundred cases of Still's disease. Arch. Dis. Child. 36:65, 1961.
21. Grokoest, A.W., Snyder, A.L., and Schlaeger, R.: Juvenile Rheumatoid Arthritis. Boston, Little, Brown & Company, 1962.
22. Brewer, E.J., Giannini, E.H., and Person, D.A.: Juvenile Rheumatoid Arthritis. 2nd ed. Philadelphia, W. B. Saunders Company, 1982.
23. Schaller, J., and Wedgwood, R.J.: Juvenile rheumatoid arthritis: A review. Pediatrics 50:940, 1972.
24. Schaller, J.G.: Juvenile rheumatoid arthritis: Series 1. Arthritis Rheum. 20:165, 1977.
25. Stillman, J.S., and Barry, P.E.: Juvenile rheumatoid arthritis: Series 2. Arthritis Rheum. 20:171, 1977.
26. Ansell, B.M.: Juvenile chronic polyarthritis: Series 3. Arthritis Rheum. 20:176, 1977.
27. Fink, C.W.: Patients with JRA: A clinical study. Arthritis Rheum. 20:183, 1977.
28. Laaksonen, A.-L., and Laine, V.: A comparative study of joint pain in adult and juvenile rheumatoid arthritis. Ann. Rheum. Dis. 20:386, 1961.
29. Scott, P.J., Ansell, B.M., and Huskisson, E.C.: Measurement of pain in juvenile chronic polyarthritis. Ann. Rheum. Dis. 36:186, 1977.
30. Beales, J.G., Keen, J.H., and Holt, P.J.L.: The child's perception of the disease and the experience of pain in juvenile chronic arthritis. J. Rheumatol. 10:61, 1983.
31. Rombouts, J.J., and Rombouts-Lindemans, C.: Scoliosis in juvenile rheumatoid arthritis. J. Bone Joint Surg. (Br.) 56B:478, 1974.
32. Svantesson, H., Marhaug, G., and Haeffner, F.: Scoliosis in children with juvenile rheumatoid arthritis. Scand. J. Rheumatol. 10:65, 1981.
33. Martis, C.S., and Karakasis, D.T.: Ankylosis of the temporo-mandibular joint caused by Still's disease. Oral Surg. 35:462, 1973.
34. Larheim, T.A., Dale, K., and Tveito, L.: Radiographic abnormalities of the temporomandibular joint in children with juvenile rheumatoid arthritis. Acta Radiol. 22:277, 1981.
35. Larheim, T.A., Haanaes, H.R., and Dale, K.: Radiographic temporomandibular joint abnormality in adults with micrognathia and juvenile rheumatoid arthritis. Acta Radiol. 22:495, 1981.
36. Jacobs, J.C., and Hui, R.M.: Cricoarytenoid arthritis and airway obstruction in juvenile rheumatoid arthritis. Pediatrics 59:292, 1977.
37. Cassidy, J.T., Brody, G.L., and Martel, W.: Monarticular juvenile rheumatoid arthritis. J. Pediatr. 70:867, 1967.
38. Bywaters, E.G.L., and Ansell, B.M.: Monoarticular arthritis in children. Ann. Rheum. Dis. 24:116, 1965.
39. McMinn, F.J., and Bywaters, E.G.L.: Differences between the fever of Still's disease and that of rheumatic fever. Ann. Rheum. Dis. 18:293, 1959.
40. Calabro, J.J., and Marchesano, J.M.: Fever associated with juvenile rheumatoid arthritis. N. Engl. J. Med. 276:11, 1967.
41. Isdale, I.C., and Bywaters, E.G.L.: The rash of rheumatoid arthritis and Still's disease. Quart. J. Med. 25:377, 1956.
42. Calabro, J.J., and Marchesano, J.M.: Rash associated with juvenile rheumatoid arthritis. J. Pediatr. 72:611, 1968.
43. Schaller, J., and Wedgwood, R.J.: Pruritus associated with the rash of juvenile rheumatoid arthritis. Pediatrics 45:296, 1970.
44. Schaller J., Beckwith, B., and Wedgwood, R.J.: Hepatic involvement in juvenile rheumatoid arthritis. J. Pediatr. 77:203, 1970.
45. Anderson, L.G., Jackson, J., Schur, P.H., and Stillman, J.S.: Sjögren's syndrome and juvenile rheumatoid arthritis. In Jason, M.I.V. (ed.): Juvenile Chronic Polyarthritis. New York, Academic Press, 1976.
46. Athreya, B., Norman, M.E., Myers, A.R., et al.: Sjögren's syndrome in children. Pediatrics 59:931, 1977.
47. Bywaters, E.G.L.: Still's disease in the adult. Ann. Rheum. Dis. 30:121, 1971.
48. Aptekar, R.G., Decker, J.L., Bujak, J.S., and Wolff, S.M.: Adult onset juvenile rheumatoid arthritis. Arthritis Rheum. 16:715, 1973.
49. Calin, A., and Calin, H.J.: Oligoarthropathy with chronic iridocyclitis: A disease only of childhood? J. Rheumatol. 9:105, 1982.
50. Brewer, E., Jr.: Juvenile rheumatoid arthritis—cardiac involvement. Arthritis Rheum. 20:231, 1977.
51. Bernstein, B.: Pericarditis in juvenile rheumatoid arthritis. Arthritis Rheum. 20:241, 1977.
52. Lietman, P.S., and Bywaters, E.G.L.: Pericarditis in juvenile rheumatoid arthritis. Pediatrics 32:855, 1963.
53. Bernstein, B., Takahashi, M., and Hanson, V.: Cardiac involvement in juvenile rheumatoid arthritis. J. Pediatr. 85:313, 1974.
54. Scharf, J., Levy, J., Benderly, A., and Nahir, M.: Pericardial tamponade in juvenile rheumatoid arthritis. Arthritis Rheum. 19:760, 1976.
55. Miller, J.J., 3rd, and French, J.W.: Myocarditis in juvenile rheumatoid arthritis. Am. J. Dis. Child. 131:205, 1977.
56. Leak, A.M., Millar-Craig, M.W., and Ansell, B.M.: Aortic regurgitation in seropositive juvenile arthritis. Ann. Rheum. Dis. 40:229, 1981.
57. Martel, W., Cassidy, J.T., Brody, G.L., and Itabashi, H.H.: Spinal cord lesions in juvenile rheumatoid arthritis. J. Can. Assoc. Radiol. 20:32, 1969.
58. Sury, B., and Vesterdal, E.: Extra-articular lesions in juvenile rheumatoid arthritis. A survey based upon a study of 151 cases. Acta Rheumatol. Scand. 14:309, 1968.
59. Calabro, J.J.: Other extraarticular manifestations of juvenile rheumatoid arthritis. Arthritis Rheum. 20:237, 1977.
60. Brinkman, G.L., and Chaikof, L.: Rheumatoid lung disease. Report of a case which developed in childhood. Am. Rev. Respir. Dis. 80:732, 1959.
61. Jordan, J.D., and Snyder, C.H.: Rheumatoid disease of the lung and cor pulmonale. Observations in a child. Am. J. Dis. Child. 108:174, 1964.
62. Athreya, B.H., Doughty, R.A., Bookspan, M., Schumacher, H.R., Sewell, E.M., and Chatten, J.: Pulmonary manifestations of juvenile rheumatoid arthritis: A report of eight cases and review. Clin. Chest Med. 1:361, 1980.
63. Wagener, J.S., Taussig, L.M., Debenedetti, C., Lemen, R.J., and Loughlin, G.M.: Pulmonary function in juvenile rheumatoid arthritis. J. Pediatr. 99:108, 1981.
64. Sievers, K., Nissilä, M., and Sievers, U.M.: Cerebral vasculitis visualized by angiography in juvenile rheumatoid arthritis simulating brain tumor. Acta Rheumatol. Scand. 14:222, 1968.
65. Russell, A.S.: Cerebral complications in juvenile rheumatoid arthritis. Can. Med. Assoc. J. 108:19, 1973.
66. Lang, H., Anttila, R., Svékus, A., and Laaksonen, A.-L.: EEG findings in juvenile rheumatoid arthritis and other connective tissue diseases in children. Acta Paediat. Scand. 63:373, 1974.
67. Anttila, R.: Renal involvement in juvenile rheumatoid arthritis. A clinical and histopathological study. Acta Paediatr. Scand. (Suppl.) 227:3, 1972.
68. Wortmann, D.W., Kelsch, R.C., Kuhns, L., Sullivan, D.B., and Cassidy, J.T.: Renal papillary necrosis in juvenile rheumatoid arthritis. J. Pediatr. 97:37, 1980.
69. Ansell, B.M., and Bywaters, E.G.L.: Finger contractures due to tendon

lesions as a mode of presentation of rheumatoid arthritis. Ann. Rheum. Dis. 12:283, 1953.

70. Bywaters, E.G.L., Glynn, L.E., and Zeldis, A.: Subcutaneous nodules of Still's disease. Ann. Rheum. Dis. 17:278, 1958.

71. Bywaters, E.G.L., and Cardoe, N.: Multiple nodules in juvenile chronic polyarthritis. Ann. Rheum. Dis. 31:421, 1972.

72. Forsyth, C.C.: Calcification of the digital arteries in a child with rheumatoid arthritis. Arch. Dis. Child. 35:296, 1960.

73. Reid, M.M., and Fannin, T.F.: Extensive vascular calcification in association with juvenile rheumatoid arthritis and amyloidosis. Arch. Dis. Child. 43:607, 1968.

74. Ellsworth, J.E., Cassidy, J.T., Ragsdale, C.G., and Sullivan, D.B.: Mucha-Habermann disease in children—the association with rheumatic diseases. J. Rheumatol. 9:319, 1982.

75. Mesara, B.W., Brody, G.L., and Oberman, H.A.: "Pseudorheumatoid" subcutaneous nodules. Am. J. Clin. Pathol. 45:684, 1966.

76. Taranta, A.: Occurrence of rheumatic-like subcutaneous nodules without evidence of joint or heart disease. Report of a case. N. Engl. J. Med. 266:13, 1962.

77. Smiley, W.K.: Iridocyclitis in Still's disease. Prognosis and steroid treatment. Trans. Ophthalmol. Soc. UK 85:351, 1965.

78. Schaller, J., Kupfer, C., and Wedgwood, R.J.: Iridocyclitis in juvenile rheumatoid arthritis. Pediatrics 44:92, 1969.

79. Calabro, J.J., Parrino, G.R., Atchoo, P.D., Marchesano, J.M., and Goldberg, L.S.: Chronic iridocyclitis in juvenile rheumatoid arthritis. Arthritis Rheum. 13:406, 1970.

80. José, D.G., and Good, R.A.: Iridocyclitis and pauciarticular juvenile rheumatoid arthritis. J. Pediatr. 78:910, 1971.

81. Key, S.N., 3rd, and Kimura, S.J.: Iridocyclitis associated with juvenile rheumatoid arthritis. Am. J. Ophthalmol. 80:425, 1975.

82. Chylack, L.T., Jr., Bienfang, D.C., Bellows, A.R., and Stillman, J.S.: Ocular manifestations of juvenile rheumatoid arthritis. Am. J. Ophthalmol. 79:1026, 1975.

83. Petty, R.E., Cassidy, J.T., and Sullivan, D.B.: Clinical correlates of antinuclear antibodies in juvenile rheumatoid arthritis. J. Pediatr. 83:386, 1973.

84. Schaller, J.G., Johnson, G.D., Holborow, E.J., Ansell, B.M., and Smiley, W.K.: The association of antinuclear antibodies with the chronic iridocyclitis of juvenile rheumatoid arthritis (Still's disease). Arthritis Rheum. 17:409, 1974.

85. Cassidy, J.T., Sullivan, D.B., and Petty, R.E.: Clinical patterns of chronic iridocyclitis in children with juvenile rheumatoid arthritis, Arthritis Rheum. 20:224, 1977.

86. Smiley, W.K.: The eye in juvenile rheumatoid arthritis. Trans. Ophthalmol. Soc. UK 94:817, 1974.

87. Ansell, B.M., and Bywaters, E.G.L.: Growth in Still's disease. Ann. Rheum. Dis. 15:295, 1956.

88. Bernstein, B.H., Stobie, D., Singsen, B.H., King, K.K., Kornreich, H.K., and Hanson, V.: Growth retardation in juvenile rheumatoid arthritis (JRA). Arthritis Rheum. 20:212, 1977.

89. Butenandt, D.: Rheumatoid arthritis and growth retardation in children: Treatment with human growth hormone. Eur. J. Pediatr. 130:15, 1979.

90. Hollister, J.R.: Delay in motor development as a presentation of juvenile rheumatoid arthritis. J. Pediatr. 98:581, 1981.

91. Sairanen, E.: On the etiology of growth disturbance of the mandible in juvenile rheumatoid arthritis. Acta Rheum. Scand. 16:136, 1970.

92. Larheim, T.A., Haanaes, H.R., and Ruud, A.F.: Mandibular growth, temporomandibular joint changes and dental occlusion in juvenile rheumatoid arthritis: A 17-year follow-up study. Scand. J. Rheumatol. 10:225, 1981.

93. Martel, W., Holt, J.F., and Cassidy, J.T.: Roentgenologic manifestations of juvenile rheumatoid arthritis. Am. J. Roentgenol. Radium Ther. Nucl. Med. 88:400, 1962.

94. Brattström, M., and Sundberg, J.: Juvenile rheumatoid gonarthritis. I. Clinical and roentgenological study. Acta Rheum. Scand. 11:266, 1965.

95. Sundberg, J., and Brattström, M.: Juvenile rheumatoid gonarthritis. II. Disturbance of ossification and growth. Acta Rheum. Scand. 11:279, 1965.

96. Simon, S., Whiffen, J., and Shapiro, F.: Leg-length discrepancies in monoarticular and pauciarticular juvenile rheumatoid arthritis. J. Bone Joint Surg. 63A:209, 1981.

97. Maldonado-Cocco, J.A., Garcia-Morteo, O., Spindler, A.J., Hubscher, O., and Gagliardi, S.: Carpal ankylosis in juvenile rheumatoid arthritis. Arthritis Rheum. 23:1251, 1980.

98. Bywaters, E.G.L.: Pathologic aspects of juvenile chronic polyarthritis. Arthritis Rheum. 20:271, 1977.

99. Wynne-Roberts, C.R., Anderson, C.H., Turano, A.M., and Baron, M.: Light- and electron-microscopic findings of juvenile rheumatoid arthritis synovium: Comparison with normal juvenile synovium. Semin. Arthritis Rheum. 7:287, 1978.

100. Wynne-Roberts, C.R., and Anderson, C.H.: Light- and electron-micro-scopic studies of normal juvenile human synovium. Semin. Arthritis Rheum. 7:279, 1978.

101. Fletcher, M.R., and Scott, J.T.: Chronic monarticular synovitis. Diagnostic and prognostic features. Ann. Rheum. Dis. 34:171, 1975.

102. Kornreich, H., Malouf, N.N., and Hanson, V.: Acute hepatic dysfunction in juvenile rheumatoid arthritis. J. Pediatr. 79:27, 1971.

103. Houba, V., and Bardfeld, R.: Serum immunoglobulins in juvenile rheumatoid arthritis. Ann. Rheum. Dis. 27:55, 1968.

104. Salmi, T.T., Schmidt, E., Laaksonen, A.-L., Anttila, R., and Kouvalainen, K.: Levels of serum immunoglobulins in juvenile rheumatoid arthritis. Ann. Clin. Res. 5:395, 1973.

105. Goel, K.M., Logan, R.W., Barnard, W.P., and Shanks, R.A.: Serum immunoglobulin and beta 1C/beta 1A globulin concentrations in juvenile rheumatoid arthritis. Ann. Rheum. Dis. 33:35, 1974.

106. Petty, R.E., Cassidy, J.T., and Sullivan, D.B.: Serologic studies in juvenile rheumatoid arthritis: A review. Arthritis Rheum. 20:260, 1977.

107. Cassidy, J.T.: Juvenile rheumatoid arthritis: Textbook of Pediatric Rheumatology, John Wiley & Sons, Inc., New York, 1982, pp. 212–216.

108. Höyeraal, H.M., and Mellbye, O.J.: High levels of serum complement factors in juvenile rheumatoid arthritis. Ann. Rheum. Dis. 33:243, 1974.

109. Gutowska-Grzegorczyk, G., and Baum, J.: Serum immunoglobulin and complement interrelationships in juvenile rheumatoid arthritis. J. Rheumatol. 4:179, 1977.

110. Balogh, Z., Merétey, K., and Falus, A.: Serologic abnormalities in juvenile chronic arthritis: a review of 46 cases. Ann. Rheum. Dis. 39:129, 1980.

111. Pachman, L.M., Baldwin, S.M.: Assays of complement in polyarticular juvenile rheumatoid arthritis. Arthritis Rheum. 20:467, 1977.

112. Miller, J.J., Hsu, Y.P., Moss, R., Kelomaa-Sulonen, K., Osborne, C.L., and Olds-Arroyo, L.: The immunologic and clinical associations of the split products of C3 in plasma in juvenile rheumatoid arthritis. Arthritis Rheum. 22:502, 1979.

113. Rossen, R.D. Brewer, E.J., Person, D.A., Templeton, J.W., and Lidsky, M.D.: Circulating immune complexes and antinuclear antibodies in juvenile rheumatoid arthritis. Arthritis Rheum. 20:1485, 1977.

114. Miller, J.J., III, Osborne, C.L., and Hsu, Y.P.: C1q binding in serum in juvenile rheumatoid arthritis. J. Rheumatol. 7:665, 1980.

115. Moore, T.L., Sheridan, P.W., Traycoff, R.B., Zuckner, J., and Dorner, R.W.: Immune complexes in juvenile rheumatoid arthritis: A comparison of four methods. J. Rheumatol. 9:395, 1982.

116. Ogra, P.L., Chiba, Y., Ogra, S.S., Dzierba, J.L., and Herd, J.K.: Rubella-virus infection in juvenile rheumatoid arthritis. Lancet 1:1157, 1975.

117. Cassidy, J.T., Shillis, J.L., Brandon, F.B., Sullivan, D.B., and Brackett, R.G.: Viral antibody titers to rubella and rubeola in juvenile rheumatoid arthritis. Pediatrics 54:239, 1974.

118. Linnemann, C.C., Jr., Levinson, J.E., Buncher, C.R., and Schiff, G.M.: Rubella antibody levels in juvenile rheumatoid arthritis. Ann. Rheum. Dis. 34:354, 1975.

119. Toumbis, A., Franklin, E.C., McEwen, C., and Kuttner, A.G.: Clinical and serological observations in patients with juvenile rheumatoid arthritis and their relatives. J. Pediatr. 64:463, 1963.

120. Bywaters, E.G.L., Carter, M.E., and Scott, F.E.T.: Differential agglutination titre (D.A.T.) in juvenile rheumatoid arthritis. Ann. Rheum. Dis. 18:225, 1959.

121. Bywaters, E.G.L., Carter, M.E., and Scott, F.E.T.: Comparison of differential agglutination titre (D.A.T.) in juvenile and adult rheumatoid arthritis. Ann. Rheum. Dis. 18:233, 1959.

122. Cassidy, J.T., and Valkenburg, H.A.: A five year prospective study of rheumatoid factor tests in juvenile rheumatoid arthritis. Arthritis Rheum. 10:83, 1967.

123. Hanson, V., Drexler, E., and Kornreich, H.: The relationship of rheumatoid factor to age of onset in juvenile rheumatoid arthritis. Arthritis Rheum. 12:82, 1969.

124. Bluestone, R., Goldberg, L.S., Katz, R.M., Marchesano, J.M., and Calabro, J.J.: Juvenile rheumatoid arthritis: A serologic survey of 200 consecutive patients. J. Pediatr. 77:98, 1970.

125. Rudnicki, R.D., Ruderman, M., Scull, E., Goldenberg, A., and Rothfield, N.: Clinical features and serologic abnormalities in juvenile rheumatoid arthritis. Arthritis Rheum. 17:1007, 1974.

126. Prieur, A.M., Bach, J.F., Griscelli, C., Judet, C., Ballet, J.J., Bach, C., and Mozziconacci, P.: Rheumatoid rosette in juvenile rheumatoid arthritis. Arch. Dis. Child. 49:438, 1974.

127. Torrigiani, G., Ansell, B.M., Chown, E.E.A., and Roitt, I.M.: Raised IgG antiglobulin factors in Still's disease. Ann. Rheum. Dis. 28:424, 1969.

128. Panush, R.S., Biancho, N.E., and Schur, P.H.: Serum and synovial fluid IgG, IgA, and IgM anti-gamma globulins in rheumatoid arthritis. Arthritis Rheum. 14:737, 1971.

129. Florin-Christensen, A., Arana, R.M., Morteo, O.G., Roux, M.E., and Hubscher, O.: IgG, IgA, IgM, and IgD antiglobulins in juvenile rheumatoid arthritis. Ann. Rheum. Dis. 33:32, 1974.

130. Bianco, N.E., Panush, R.S., Stillman, J.S., and Schur, P.H.: Immunologic studies of juvenile rheumatoid arthritis. Arthritis Rheum. 14:685, 1971.

131. Miller, J.J., 3rd, Olds-Arroyo, L., and Akasaka, T.: Antiglobulins in juvenile rheumatoid arthritis. Arthritis Rheum. 20:729, 1977.

132. Munthe, E.: Anti-IgG and antinuclear antibodies in juvenile rheumatoid arthritis. Scand. J. Rheumatol. 1:161, 1972.

133. Moore, T., Dorner, R.W., and Zuckner, J.: Hidden rheumatoid factor in seronegative juvenile rheumatoid arthritis. Ann. Rheum. Dis. 33:255, 1974.

134. Moore, T.L., Dorner, R.W., Weiss, T.D., Baldassare, A.R., and Zuckner, J.: Hidden 19S IgM rheumatoid factor in juvenile rheumatoid arthritis. Pediatr. Res. 14:1135, 1980.

135. Moore, T.L., Dorner, R.W., Weiss, T.D., Baldassare, A.R., and Zuckner, J.: Specificity of hidden 19S IgM rheumatoid factor in patients with juvenile rheumatoid arthritis. Arthritis Rheum. 24:1283, 1981.

136. Moore, T.L., Dorner, R.W., Sheridan, P.W., Weiss, T.D. Baldassare, A.R., Osborn, T.G., and Zuckner, J.: Longitudinal study of the presence of hidden 19S IgM rheumatoid factor in juvenile rheumatoid arthritis. J. Rheumatol. 9:599, 1982.

137. Neucks, S.H., Robbins, D.L., Moore, T.L., Zuchner, J., and Dorner, R.W.: Hidden 19S IgM rheumatoid factor in synovial fluid. J. Rheumatol. 8:811, 1981.

138. Fehr, K., Velvart, M., and Rauber, M.: Production of agglutinators and rheumatoid factors in plasma cells of rheumatoid and nonrheumatoid synovial tissues. Arthritis Rheum. 24:510, 1981.

139. Miller, J.J., Henrich, V.L, and Brandstrup, N.E.: Sex difference in incidence of antinuclear factors in juvenile rheumatoid arthritis. Pediatrics 38:916, 1966.

140. Kornreich, H.K, Drexler, E., and Hanson, V.: Antinuclear factors in childhood rheumatic disease. J. Pediatr. 69:1039, 1966.

141. Alspaugh, M.A., and Miller, J.J.: A study of specificities of antinuclear antibodies in juvenile rheumatoid arthritis. J. Pediatr. 90:391, 1977.

142. Rosenberg, J.N., Johnson, G.D., Holborow, E.J., and Bywaters, E.G.L.: Eosinophil-specific and other granulocyte-specific antinuclear antibodies in juvenile chronic polyarthritis and adult rheumatoid arthritis. Ann. Rheum. Dis. 34:350, 1975.

143. Höyeraal, H.M.: Granulocyte reactive antinuclear factors in juvenile rheumatoid arthritis. Scand. J. Rheumatol. 5:84, 1976.

144. A.R.A. Subcommittee on Classification Criteria for a Diagnosis of Juvenile Rheumatoid Arthritis, unpublished observations.

145. Bell, C., Talal, N., and Schur, P.H.: Antibodies to DNA in patients with rheumatoid arthritis and juvenile rheumatoid arthritis. Arthritis Rheum. 18:535, 1975.

146. Cassidy, J.T., Walker, S.E., Soderstrom, S.J., Petty, R.E., and Sullivan, D.B.: Diagnostic significance of antibody to native deoxyribonucleic acid in children with juvenile rheumatoid arthritis and other connective tissue diseases. J. Pediatr. 93:416, 1978.

147. Edmonds, J., Morris, R.I., Metzger, A.L., Bluestone, R., Terasaki, P.I., Ansell, B., and Bywaters, E.G.L.: Follow-up study of juvenile chronic polyarthritis with particular reference to histocompatibility antigen W27. Ann. Rheum. Dis. 33:289, 1974.

148. Hall, A., Ansell, B.M., James, D.C.O., and Zylinski, P.: HL-A antigens in juvenile chronic polyarthritis (Still's disease). Ann. Rheum. Dis. 34(Suppl.):36, 1975.

149. Gibson, D.J., Carpenter, C.M., Stillman, J.S., and Schur, P.H.: Re-examination of histocompatibility antigens found in patients with juvenile rheumatoid arthritis. N. Engl. J. Med. 293:636, 1975.

150. Ohno, S., Char, D.H., Kimura, S.J., and O'Connor, G.R.: HLA antigens and antinuclear antibody titres in juvenile chronic iridocyclitis. Br. J. Ophthalmol. 61:59, 1977.

151. Oen, K., Petty, R.E., and Schroeder, M.-L.: An association between HLA-A2 and juvenile rheumatoid arthritis in girls. J. Rheumatol. 9:916, 1982.

152. Glass, D.N., and Litvin, D.A.: Heterogeneity of HLA associations in systemic onset juvenile rheumatoid arthritis. Arthritis Rheum. 23:796, 1980.

153. Stasny, P., and Fink, C.W.: Different HLA-D associations in adult and juvenile rheumatoid arthritis. J. Clin. Invest. 63:124, 1979.

154. Rossen, R.D., Brewer, E.J., Sharp, R.M., Yunis, E.J., Schanfield, M.S., Birdsall, H.H., Ferrell, R.E., and Templeton, J.W.: Familial rheumatoid arthritis: A kindred identified through a proband with seronegative juvenile arthritis includes members with seropositive, adult-onset disease. Hum. Immunol. 4:183, 1982.

155. Sher, M.R., Schultz, J.S., Ragsdale, C.G., Kapur, J.J., Sullivan, D.B., and Cassidy, J.T.: HLA-DR/MT typing identifying possible immunogenetic mechanisms for juvenile rheumatoid arthritis. Arthritis Rheum. 26:S58, 1983.

156. Glass, D., Litvin, D., Wallace, K., Chylack, L., Garovoy, M., Carpenter, C.B., and Schur, P.H.: Early onset pauciarticular juvenile rheumatoid arthritis associated with human leukocyte antigen-DRw5, iritis, and antinuclear antibody. J. Clin. Invest. 66:426, 1980.

157. Suciu-Foca, N., Godfrey, M., Jacobs, J., et al.: Increased frequency of DRw5 in pauciarticular JRA. In Terasaki, P.I. (ed.): Histocompatibility Testing 1980. UCLA Tissue Typing Laboratory, Los Angeles, 1980, pp. 953–954.

158. Morling, N., Hellesen, C., Jakobsen, B.K., Platz, P., Ryder, L.P., Svejgaard, A., and Thomsen, M.: HLA-A, B, C, D, Dr antigens and primed lymphocyte typing (PLT) defined DP-antigens in juvenile chronic arthritis. Tissue Antigens 17:433, 1981.

159. Fink, C.W.: D locus typing differences between adults and children. In Moore, T.D. (ed): Arthritis in Childhood, Report of the Eightieth Ross Conference in Pediatric Research. Columbus, Ohio, Ross Laboratories, 1981, p. 78.

160. Schaller, J.G., and Hansen, J.: Early childhood pauciarticular juvenile rheumatoid arthritis: clinical and immunogenetic studies. Arthritis Rheum. 25:S63, 1982.

161. Gershwin, M.E., Haselwood, D., Dorshkind, K., and Castles, J.J.: Altered responsiveness to mitogens in subgroups of patients with juvenile rheumatoid arthritis. J. Clin. Lab. Immunol. 1:293, 1979.

162. Miller, J.J., III, and Olds-Arroyo, L.: In vitro responses of lymphocytes in juvenile arthritis: Effects of time and concentration of PHA-P. J. Rheumatol. 8:716, 1981.

163. Ellsworth, J.E., Stein, L.D., Thebert, P.J., Ragsdale, C.G., Sullivan, D.B., and Cassidy, J.T.: Abnormalities of lymphokine generation in children with juvenile rheumatoid arthritis. Pediatr. Res. 16:221A, 1982.

164. Strelkauskas, A.J., Schauf, V., Wilson, B.S., et al.: Isolation and characterization of naturally occurring subclasses of human peripheral blood T cells with regulatory functions. J. Immunol. 120:1278, 1978.

165. Strelkauskas, A.J., Callery, R.T., McDowell, J., Borl, Y., and Schlossman, S.F.: Direct evidence for loss of human suppressor cells during active autoimmune disease. Proc. Natl. Acad. Sci. USA 75:5150, 1978.

166. Morimoto, C., Reinherz, E.L., Borel, Y., Mantzouranis, E., Steinberg, A.D., and Schlossman, S.F.: Autoantibody to an immunoregulatory inducer population in patients with juvenile rheumatoid arthritis. J. Clin. Invest. 67:753, 1981.

167. Williams, R.C., Jr., Froelich, C.J., Kilpatrick, K., Crowe, W.E., and Levinson, J.E.: T gamma subset specificity of lymphocyte reactive factors in juvenile rheumatoid arthritis and systemic lupus erythematosus sera. Arthritis Rheum. 24:585, 1981.

168. Froelich, C.J., Bankhurst, A.D., Crowe, W.E., Williams, R.C., Jr., Warner, N.L., and Levinson, J.E.: Flow cytometry and cytoadherence studies of sera from children with juvenile rheumatoid arthritis and normal controls. Arthritis Rheum. 24:457, 1981.

169. Dobloug, J.H., Chattopadhyay, C., Førre, O., et al.: Con A-induced suppressor cell activity and T-lymphocyte subpopulations in peripheral blood lymphocytes of patients with rheumatoid arthritis and juvenile rheumatoid arthritis. Scand. J. Immunol. 13:367, 1981.

170. Wada, N., Prieur, A.-M., and Griscelli, C.: Nonspecific alphanaphthyl acetate esterase activity of T lymphocytes: Study in healthy newborns and children, in immune deficiencies and juvenile rheumatoid arthritis. Pediatr. Res. 15:1266, 1981.

171. Muraguchi, A., Kishimoto, T., Kuritani, T., et al.: In vitro immune response of human peripheral lymphocytes. VII. Effect of anti-μ and anti-δ antibodies on B colony formation and detection of abnormal B cells in patients with juvenile rheumatoid arthritis. J. Immunol. 125:2638, 1980.

172. Zuckner, J., Baldassare, A., Chang, F., and Auclair, R.: High synovial fluid leukocyte counts of noninfectious etiology. Arthritis Rheum. 20:270, 1977.

173. Hedberg, H.: The total complement activity of synovial fluid in juvenile forms of arthritis. Acta Rheumatol. Scand. 17:279, 1971.

174. Rynes, R.I., Ruddy, S., Spragg, J., Stillman, J.S., and Austen, K.F.: Intraarticular activation of the complement system in patients with juvenile rheumatoid arthritis. Arthritis Rheum. 19:161, 1976.

175. Martin, C.L., and Pachman, L.M.: Synovial fluid in seronegative juvenile rheumatoid arthritis: Studies of immunoglobulins, complement, and α2-macroglobulin. Arthritis Rheum. 23:1256, 1980.

176. Munthe, E.: Complexes of IgG and IgG rheumatoid factor in synovial tissues of juvenile rheumatoid arthritis. Scand. J. Rheumatol. 1:153, 1972.

177. Sairanen, E.: On rheumatoid arthritis in children. A clinico-roentgenological study. Acta Rheum. Scand. (Suppl.)2:1, 1958.

178. Ansell, B.M., and Kent, P.A.: Radiological changes in juvenile chronic polyarthritis. Skeletal Radiol. 1:129, 1977.

179. Locke, G.R., Gardner, J.I., and Van Epps, E.F.: Atlas-dens interval (ADI) in children. A survey based on 200 normal cervical spines. Am. J. Roentgenol. Radium Ther. Nucl. Med. 97:135, 1966.

180. Badley, B.W.D., and Ansell, B.M.: Fractures in Still's disease. Ann. Rheum. Dis. 19:135, 1960.

181. Shuler, S.E., and Helvie, W.W.: Peripheral joint imaging in juvenile rheumatoid arthritis. South Med. J. 67:789, 1974.

182. Viitanen, S.M., and Laaksonen, A.-L.: Thermography in juvenile rheumatoid arthritis. Acta Rheum. Scand. 16:91, 1970.

183. Brewer, E.J., Jr., Bass, J.C., Cassidy, J.T., Duran, B.S., Fink, C.W., Jacobs, J.C., Markowitz, M., Reynolds, W.E., Schaller, J., Stillman, J.S., and Wallace, S.L.: Criteria for the classification of juvenile rheumatoid arthritis. Bull. Rheum. Dis. 23:712, 1972.

184. Brewer, E.J., Jr., Bass, J., Baum, J., Cassidy, J.T., Fink, C., Jacobs, J.,

Hanson, V., Levinson, J.E., Schaller, J., and Stillman, J.S.: Current proposed revision of JRA criteria. Arthritis Rheum. 20:195, 1977.

185. Ansell, B.M., and Bywaters, E.G.L.: Diagnosis of "probable" Still's disease and its outcome. Ann. Rheum. Dis. 21:253, 1962.

186. Bywaters, E.G.L.: Categorization in medicine: A survey of Still's disease. Ann. Rheum. Dis. 26:185, 1967.

187. Bywaters, E.G.L.: Diagnostic criteria for Still's disease (juvenile R.A.). In Bennett, P.H., and Wood, P.H.N. (eds.): Population Studies of the Rheumatic Diseases. Amsterdam, Excerpta Medica, 1968, p. 235.

188. Kvien, T.K., Höyeraal, H.M., and Kass, E.: Diagnostic criteria of rheumatoid arthritis in children: Proposed criteria for controlled clinical studies. Scand. J. Rheumatol. 11:187, 1982.

189. Jacobs, J.C., Phillips, P.E., and Johnston, A.D.: Needle biopsy of the synovium of children. Pediatrics 57:696, 1976.

190. Fink, C.W., Dick, V.Q., Howard, J., Jr., and Nelson, J.D.: Infections of bones and joints in children. Arthritis Rheum. 20:578, 1977.

191. Lindsley, C.B., and Schaller, J.G.: Arthritis associated with inflammatory bowel disease in children. J. Pediatr. 84:16, 1974.

192. Angevine, C.D., Pless, I.B., Baum, J., and Jacox, R.J.: Psoriatic arthritis in a child. Arthritis Rheum. 16:278, 1973.

193. Sills, E.M.: Psoriatic arthritis in childhood. Johns Hopkins Med. J. 146:49, 1980.

194. Shore, A., and Ansell, B.M.: Juvenile psoriatic arthritis: An analysis of 60 cases. J. Pediatr. 100:529, 1982.

195. Hellström, B.: The diagnosis and course of rheumatoid arthritis and benign aseptic arthritis in children. Acta Paediatr. (Stockholm) 50:529, 1961.

196. Sievers, K., Ahvonen, P., Aho, K., and Wager, O.: Serological patterns in juvenile rheumatoid arthritis. Rheumatism 19:88, 1963.

197. Ragsdale, C.G., Petty, R.E., Cassidy, J.T., and Sullivan, D.B.: The clinical progression of apparent juvenile rheumatoid arthritis to systemic lupus erythematosus. J. Rheumatol. 7:50, 1980.

198. Schaller, J., Bitnum, S., and Wedgwood, R.J.: Ankylosing spondylitis with childhood onset. J. Pediat. 74:505, 1969.

199. Ladd, J.R., Cassidy, J.T., and Martel, W.: Juvenile ankylosing spondylitis. Arthritis Rheum. 14:579, 1971.

200. Schaller, J.G., Ochs, H.D., Thomas, E.D., Nisperos, B., Feigl, P., and Wedgwood, R.J.: Histocompatibility antigens in childhood-onset arthritis. J. Pediat. 88:926, 1976.

201. Jacobs, J.C., Berdon, W.E., and Johnston, A.D.: HLA-B27-associated spondyloarthritis and enthesopathy in childhood: Clinical, pathologic, and radiologic observations in 58 patients. J. Pediatr. 100:521, 1982.

202. Cassidy, J.T., Petty, R.E., and Sullivan, D.B.: Abnormalities in the distribution of serum immunoglobulin concentrations in juvenile rheumatoid arthritis. J. Clin. Invest. 52:1931, 1973.

203. Cassidy, J.T., Petty, R.E., and Sullivan, D.B.: Occurrence of selective IgA deficiency in children with juvenile rheumatoid arthritis. Arthritis Rheum. 20:181, 1977.

204. Petty, R.E., Cassidy, J.T., and Tubergen, D.G.: Association of arthritis with hypogammaglobulinemia. Arthritis Rheum. 20:441, 1977.

205. Glass, D., Raum, D., Gibson, D., Stillman, J.S., and Schur, P.H.: Inherited deficiency of the second component of complement. J. Clin. Invest. 58:853, 1976.

206. Rockey, J.H., Hanson, L.A., Heremans, J.F., and Kunkel, H.G.: Beta-2A aglobulinemia in two healthy men. J. Lab. Clin. Med. 63:205, 1964.

207. Cassidy, J.T., Burt, A., Sullivan, D.B., and Dickinson, D.G.: Changes in the serum immunoglobulins in juvenile rheumatoid arthritis. Arthritis Rheum. 9:850, 1966.

208. West, C.D., Hong, R., and Holland, N.H.: Immunoglobulin levels from the newborn period to adulthood and in immunoglobulin deficiency states. J. Clin. Invest. 41:2054, 1962.

209. Huntley, C.C., Thorpe, D.P., Lyerly, A.D., and Kelsey, W.M.: Rheumatoid arthritis with IgA deficiency. Am. J. Dis. Child 113:411, 1967.

210. Panush, R.S., Bianco, N.E., Schur, P.H., Rocklin, R.E., David, J.R., and Stillman, J.S.: Juvenile rheumatoid arthritis. Cellular hypersensitivity and selective IgA deficiency. Clin. Exp. Immunol. 10:103, 1972.

211. Pelkonen, P., Savilahiti, E., Westerén, L., and Mäkelä, A-L.: IgA deficiency in juvenile rheumatoid arthritis. Scand. J. Rheumatol. Suppl. 8:4, 1975.

212. Barkley, D.O., Hohermuth, H.J., Howard, A., Webster, A.D.B., and Ansell, B.M.: IgA deficiency in juvenile chronic polyarthritis. J. Rheumatol. 6:219, 1979.

213. Cassidy, J.T., Burt, A., Petty, R.E., and Sullivan, D.B.: Prevalence of selective IgA deficiency in patients with connective tissue disease. N. Engl. J. Med. 280:275, 1969.

214. Cassidy, J.T.: Selective IgA deficiency and chronic arthritis in children. In Moore, T.D. (ed.): Arthritis in Childhood. Eightieth Ross Conference in Pediatric Research. Columbus, Ohio, Ross Laboratories, 1981, p. 82.

215. Vyas, G.N., Perkins, H.A., and Fudenberg, H.H.: Anaphylactoid transfusion reactions associated with anti-IgA. Lancet 2:312, 1968.

216. Leikola, J., Koistinen, J., Lehtinen, M., and Virolainen, M: IgA-induced analyphylactic transfusion reactions: A report of four cases. Blood 42:111, 1973.

217. Cassidy, J.T., Petty, R., Burt, A., and Sullivan, D.B.: Anti-IgA antibodies in patients with selective IgA deficiency and connective tissue diseases. Clin. Research 17:351, 1969.

218. Petty, R.E., Palmer, N.R., Cassidy, J.T., et al.: The association of autoimmune diseases and anti-IgA antibodies in patients with selective IgA deficiency. Clin. Exp. Immunol. 37:83, 1979.

219. Cassidy, J.T., Oldham, G., and Platts-Mills, T.A.E.: Functional assessment of a B-cell defect in patients with selective IgA deficiency. Clin. Exp. Immunol. 35:296, 1979.

220. Waldman, T.A., Broder, S., Krakauer, R., et al.: Defect in IgA secretion and in IgA specific suppressor cells in patients with selective IgA deficiency. Trans. Assoc. Am. Phys. 89:215, 1976.

221. Ignaczak, T.F., and Cassidy, J.T.: Cell mediated immunity in selective IgA deficiency. Clin. Res. 26:25A, 1978.

222. Van der Giessen, M., Reerink-Brongers, E.E., and Algra-van Veen, T.: Quantitation of Ig classes and IgG subclasses in sera of patients with a variety of immunoglobulin deficiencies and their relatives. Clin. Immunol. Immunopath. 5:388, 1976.

223. Kanok, J.M., Steinberg, P., Cassidy, J.T., Petty, R.E., and Bayne, N.K.: Serum IgE levels in patients with selective IgA deficiency. Ann. Allergy 41:220, 1978.

224. Edwards, N.L., Cassidy, J.T., and Fox, I.H.: Lymphocyte 5'-nucleotidase deficiency in hypogammaglobulinemia: Clinical characteristics. Clin. Immunol. Immunopath. 17:76, 1980.

225. Buckley, R.H., MacQueen, J.M., and Ward, F.E.: HLA antigens in primary immunodeficiency diseases. Clin. Immunol. Immunopath. 7:305, 1977.

226. Ambrus, M., Hernádi, E., and Bajtai, G.: Prevalence of HLA-A1 and HLA-B8 antigens in selective IgA deficiency. Immunol. Immunopath. 7:311, 1977.

227. Oen, K., Petty, R.E., and Schroeder, M.-L.: Immunoglobulin A deficiency: genetic studies. Tissue Antigens 19:174, 1982.

228. Cunningham-Rundles, C., Brandeis, W.E., Good, R.A., et al.: Bovine antigens and the formation of circulating immune complexes in selective immunoglobulin A deficiency. J. Clin. Invest. 64:272, 1979.

229. Cunningham-Rundles, C., Brandeis, W.E., Good, R.A., et al.: Milk precipitins, circulating immune complexes, and IgA deficiency. Proc. Natl. Acad. Sci. USA 75:3387, 1978.

230. Petty, R.E., Cassidy, J.T., and Sullivan, D.B.: Reversal of selective IgA deficiency following plasma transfusions in juvenile rheumatoid arthritis. Pediatrics 51:44, 1973.

231. Koistinen, J., Heikkilä, M., and Leikola, J.: Gammaglobulin treatment and anti-IgA antibodies in IgA-deficient patients. Br. Med. J. 2:923, 1978.

232. Brewer, E.J., Blattner, R.J., and Wing, H.: Treatment of rheumatoid arthritis in children. Pediatr. Clin. North Am. 10:207, 1963.

233. Calabro, J.J., and Marchesano, J.M.: Medical management of juvenile rheumatoid arthritis. Bull. Rheum. Dis. 15:378, 1965.

234. Ansell, B.M.: The management of juvenile chronic polyarthritis. (Still's disease). Practitioner 208:91, 1972.

235. Bywaters, E.G.L.: The management of juvenile chronic polyarthritis. Bull. Rheum. Dis. 27:882, 1976.

236. Orozco-Alcala, J.J., and Baum, J.: Treatment of juvenile rheumatoid arthritis — a world survey. J. Rheumatol. 1:187, 1974.

237. Lindsley, C.B.: Pharmacotherapy of juvenile rheumatoid arthritis. Pediatr. Clin. North Am. 28:161, 1981.

238. Pachman, L.M., Olufs, R., Procknal, J.A., and Levy, G.: Pharmacokinetic monitoring of salicylate therapy in children with juvenile rheumatoid arthritis. Arthritis Rheum. 22:826, 1979.

239. Mäkelä, A.-L., Yrjana, T., and Mattila, M.: Dosage of salicylates for children with juvenile rheumatoid arthritis. A prospective clinical trial with three different preparations of acetylsalicylic acid. Acta Paediatr. Scand. 68:423, 1979.

240. Doughty, R.A., Giesecke, L., and Athreya, B.: Salicylate therapy in juvenile rheumatoid arthritis. Dose, serum level, and toxicity. Am. J. Dis. Child 134:461, 1980.

241. Weaver, A.L., Sullivan R.E., and Kramer, W.S.: Iatrogenic tooth erosion in juvenile rheumatoid arthritis patients. Clin. Res. 30:810A, 1982.

242. Rich, R.R., and Johnson, J.S.: Salicylate hepatotoxicity in patients with juvenile rheumatoid arthritis. Arthritis Rheum. 16:1, 1973.

243. Zucker, P., Daum, F., and Cohen, M.I.: Aspirin hepatitis. Am. J. Dis. Child. 129:1433, 1975.

244. Athreya, B.H., Moser, G., Cecil, H.S., and Myers, A.R.: Aspirin-induced hepatotoxicity in juvenile rheumatoid arthritis. A prospective study. Arthritis Rheum. 18:347, 1975.

245. Miller, J.J., III, and Weissman, D.B.: Correlations between transaminase concentrations and serum salicylate concentration in juvenile rheumatoid arthritis. Arthritis Rheum. 19:115, 1976.

246. Bernstein, B.H., Singsen, B.H., King, K.K., and Hanson, V.: Aspirin-induced hepatotoxicity and its effect on juvenile rheumatoid arthritis. Am. J. Dis. Child. 131:659, 1977.

247. Brewer, E.J.: Nonsteroidal antiinflammatory agents. Arthritis Rheum. 20:513, 1977.

248. Barron, K.S., Person, D.A., and Brewer, E.J.: The toxicity of nonsteroidal antiinflammatory drugs in juvenile rheumatoid arthritis. J. Rheumatol. 9:149, 1982.

249. Pediatric Rheumatology Collaborative Study Group: Methodology and studies of children with juvenile rheumatoid arthritis. J. Rheumatol. 9:107, 1982.

250. Levinson, J.E., Baum, J., Brewer, E., Jr., Fink, C., Hanson, V., and Schaller, J.: Comparison of tolmetin sodium and aspirin in the treatment of juvenile rheumatoid arthritis. J. Pediatr. 91:799, 1977.

251. Mäkelä, A.-I.: Naproxen in the treatment of JRA. Scand. J. Rheumatol. 6:193, 1977.

252. Nicholls, A., Hazleman, B., Todd, R.M., Murray-Leslie, C., Kuhnen, H., and Cain, A.R.: Long-term evaluation of naproxen suspension in juvenile chronic arthritis. Curr. Med. Res. Opin. 8:204, 1982.

253. Stillman, J.S.: Antimalarials in the treatment of JRA. In Moore, T.D. (ed.): Arthritis in Childhood. Eightieth Ross Conference in Pediatric Research. Columbus, Ohio, Ross Laboratories. 1981, pp. 125–127.

254. Laaksonen, A.-L., Koskiahde, V., and Juva, K.: Dosage of antimalarial drugs for children with juvenile rheumatoid arthritis and systemic lupus erythematosus. A clinical study with determination of serum concentrations of chloroquine and hydroxychloroquine. Scand. J. Rheumatol. 3:103, 1974.

255. Sassaman, F.W., Cassidy, J.T., Alpern, M., and Masseidvaag, F.: Electroretinography in patients with connective tissue diseases treated with hydroxychloroquine. Am. J. Ophthalmol. 70:515, 1970.

256. Sairanen, E., and Laaksonen, A.-L.: The toxicity of gold therapy in children suffering from rheumatoid arthritis. Ann. Paediat. Fenn. 8:105, 1962.

257. Mäkelä, A.-L., Pehola, O., and Mäkelä, P.: Gold serum levels in children with JRA. Scand. J. Rheumatol. 7:161, 1978.

258. Levinson, J.E.: Gold salts in the rheumatic diseases. In Moore, T.D. (ed.): Arthritis in Childhood. Eightieth Ross Conference in Pediatric Research. Columbus, Ohio, Ross Laboratories, 1981, pp. 120–124.

259. Brewer, E.J., Jr., Giannini, E.H., and Barkley, E.: Gold therapy in the management of juvenile rheumatoid arthritis. Arthritis Rheum. 23:404, 1980.

260. Brewer, E.J., Giannini, E.H., and Person, D.A.: Juvenile Rheumatoid Arthritis. 2nd ed. Philadelphia, W. B. Saunders Co., 1982, p. 193.

261. Ansell, B.M.: Penicillamine, levamisole and cytotoxic drugs. In Moore, T.D. (ed.): Arthritis in Childhood. Eightieth Ross Conference in Pediatric Research. Columbus, Ohio, Ross Laboratories, 1981, pp. 127–130.

262. Schairer, H.: Long-term follow-up of 285 cases of juvenile chronic polyarthritis treated with D-penicillamine or gold. In The Care of Rheumatic Children. Eular Bulletin. Monograph Series No. 3:165. Basle, Eular Publishers, 1978.

263. Ansell, B.M., Bywaters, E.G.L., and Isdale, C.: Comparison of cortisone and aspirin in the treatment of juvenile rheumatoid arthritis. Br. Med. J. 1:1075, 1956.

264. Lindbjerg, I.F.: Juvenile rheumatoid arthritis. A follow-up of 75 cases. Arch. Dis. Child. 39:576, 1964.

265. Stoeber, E.: Juvenile chronic polyarthritis and Still's syndrome. Documenta Geigy, 1977.

266. Ansell, B.M., and Bywaters, E.G.L.: Alternate-day corticosteroid therapy in juvenile chronic polyarthritis. J. Rheumatol. 1:176, 1974.

267. Blodgett, F.M., Burgin, L., Iezzoni, D., Gribetz, D., and Talbot, N.B.: Effects of prolonged cortisone therapy on statural growth, skeletal maturation and metabolic status of children. N. Engl. J. Med. 254:636, 1956.

268. Sturge, R.A., Beardwell, C., Hartog, M., Wright, D., and Ansell, B.M.: Cortisol and growth hormone secretion in relation to linear growth: Patients with Still's disease on different therapeutic regimens. Br. Med. J. 3:547, 1970.

269. Schaller, J.G.: Corticosteroids in juvenile rheumatoid arthritis (Still's disease). J. Rheumatol. 1:137, 1974.

270. Ward, D.J., Hartog, M., and Ansell, B.M.: Corticosteroid-induced dwarfism in Still's disease treated with human growth hormone. Clinical and metabolic effects including hydroxyproline excretion in two cases. Ann. Rheum. Dis. 25:416, 1966.

271. Good, R.A., Vernier, R.L., and Smith, R.T.: Serious untoward reactions to therapy with cortisone and A.C.T.H. in pediatric practice. Pediatrics 19:95, 1957.

272. Ansell, B.M.: Problems of corticosteroid therapy in the young. Proc. R. Soc. Med. 61:281, 1968.

273. Laaksonen, A.-L., Sunell, J.-E., Westerén, H., and Mulder, J.: Adrenocortical function in children with juvenile rheumatoid arthritis and other connective tissue disorders. Scand. J. Rheumatol. 3:137, 1974.

274. Stoeber, E.: Long-term basic treatment with azathioprine in systemic juvenile chronic polyarthritis (Still's syndrome) and iridocyclitis. In The Care of Rheumatic Children. Eular Bulletin, Monograph Series No. 3:168. Basle, Eular Publishers, 1978.

275. Ansell, B.M., Eghtedari, A., and Bywaters, E.G.L.: Chlorambucil in the management of juvenile chronic polyarthritis complicated by amyloidosis. Ann. Rheum. Dis. 30:331, 1971.

276. Höyeraal, H.M., Frøland, S.S., Salvesen, C.F., Munthe, E., Natvig, J.B., Kåss, E., Blichfeldt, P., Hegna, T.-M., Revlem, E., Sandstad, B., and Hjort, N.L.: No effect of transfer factor in juvenile rheumatoid arthritis by double-blind-trial. Ann. Rheum. Dis. 37:175, 1978.

277. Prieur, A.-M., Buriot, D., Lefur, J.M., et al.: Possible toxicity of levamisole in children with rheumatoid arthritis. J. Pediatr. 93:304, 1978.

278. Brewer, E.J., Jr., Nickeson, R.W., Jr., Rossen, R.D., Person, D.A., Giannini, E.H., and Milam, J.D.: Plasma exchange in selected patients with juvenile rheumatoid arthritis. J. Pediatr. 98:194, 1981.

279. Miller, J.J., III: Prolonged use of large intravenous steroid pulses in the rheumatic diseases of children. Pediatrics 65:989, 1980.

280. Arden, G.P., and Ansell, B.M. (eds.): Surgical Management of Juvenile Chronic Arthritis. London, Academic Press, 1978.

281. Fink, C.W., Baum, J., Paradies, L.H., and Carrell, B.C.: Synovectomy in juvenile rheumatoid arthritis. Ann. Rheum. Dis. 28:612, 1969.

282. Eyring, E.J., Longert, A., and Bass, J.C.: Synovectomy in juvenile rheumatoid arthritis. Indications and short-term results. J. Bone Joint Surg. 53A:638, 1971.

283. Arden, G.P., Ansell, B.M., and Hunter, M.J.: Total hip replacement in juvenile chronic polyarthritis and ankylosing spondylitis. Clin. Orthop. 84:130, 1972.

284. Arden, G.P.: Surgical treatment of Still's disease. Ann. R. Coll. Surg. Engl. 53:288, 1973.

285. Granberry, W.M., and Brewer, E.J., Jr.: Results of synovectomy in children with rheumatoid arthritis. Clin. Orthop. 101:120, 1974.

286. Sledge, C.B.: Joint replacement surgery in juvenile rheumatoid arthritis. Arthritis Rheum. 20:567, 1977.

287. Singsen, B.H., Isaacson, A.S., Bernstein, B., Patzakis, M.J., Kornreich, H.K., King, K.K., and Hanson, V.: Total hip replacement in children with arthritis. Arthritis Rheum. 21:401, 1978.

288. Crowe, W., Hauselman, C., Shear, E., Miller, E.H., Balz, G.P., and Levinson, J.E.: Total hip arthroplasty in children with juvenile rheumatoid arthritis. Arthritis Rheum. 22:602, 1979.

289. Colville, J., and Raunio, P.: Total hip replacement in juvenile rheumatoid arthritis. Analysis of 59 hips. Acta Orthop. Scand. 50:197, 1979.

290. Larheim, T.A., and Haanaes, H.R.: Micrognathia, temporomandibular joint changes and dental occlusion in juvenile rheumatoid arthritis of adolescents and adults. Scand. J. Dent. Res. 89:329, 1981.

291. Larheim, T.A., Höyeraal, H.M., Stabrun, A.E., and Haanaes, H.R.: The temporomandibular joint in juvenile rheumatoid arthritis. Radiographic changes related to clinical and laboratory parameters in 100 children. Scand. J. Rheumatol. 11:5, 1982.

292. Cleveland, S.E., Reitman, E.E., and Brewer, E.J., Jr.: Psychological factors in juvenile rheumatoid arthritis. Arthritis Rheum. 8:1152, 1965.

293. McAnarney, E.R., Pless, I.B., Satterwhite, B., and Friedman, S.B.: Psychological problems of children with chronic juvenile arthritis. Pediatrics 53:523, 1974.

294. Calabro, J.J., Holgerson, W.B., Sonpal, G.M., and Khoury, M.I.: Juvenile rheumatoid arthritis: A general review and report of 100 patients observed for 15 years. Semin. Arthritis Rheum. 5:257, 1976.

295. Mozziconacci, P.: Pour une "prise en charge psychologique" des polyarthrites juvéniles. Ann. Pédiatr. 23:415, 1976.

296. Weil-Halpern, F., Rapoport, D., Hatt, A., Hayem, F., and Mozziconacci, P.: La polyarthrite chronique de l'enfant dans la structure hospitalière. Étude psychosociologique. I La consultation. Ann. Pédiatr. 22:499, 1975.

297. Weil-Halpern, F., Rapoport, D., Hatt, A., Griscelli, C., Hayem, F., and Mozziconacci, P.: La polyarthrite chronique juvénile dans la structure hospitalière. Étude psychosociologique. II L'hospitalisation. Ann. Pédiat. 23:420, 1976.

298. Hatt, A., Weil-Halpern, F., Rapoport, D., Hayem, F., and Mozziconacci, P.: La polyarthrite chronique juvénile dans la structure hospitalière. Étude psychosociologique. III Entretiens avec les parents. Ann. Pédiat. 23:429, 1976.

299. Rapoport, D., Hatt, A., Weil-Halpern, F., Hayem, F., and Mozziconacci, P.: La polyarthrite chronique juvénile dans la structure hospitalière. IV Étude psychologique des enfants atteints. Ann. Pédiat. 23:437, 1976.

300. Tursz, A.: La polyarthrite chronique juvénile dans la structure hospitalière. V Scolarité, vie sociale et familiale. Ann. Pédiat. 23:422, 1976.

301. Henoch, M.J., Batson, J.W., and Baum, J.: Psychosocial factors in juvenile rheumatoid arthritis. Arthritis Rheum. 21:229, 1978.

302. Miller, J.J., III, Spitz, P.W., Simpson, U., and Williams, G.F.: The social function of young adults who had arthritis in childhood. J. Pediatr. 100:378, 1982.

303. Barkin, R.E.: Clinical course of juvenile rheumatoid arthritis. Bull. Rheum. Dis. 3:19, 1952.

304. Edström, G., and Gedda, P.O.: Clinic and prognosis of rheumatoid arthritis in children. Acta Rheum. Scand. 3:129, 1957.

305. Ansell, B.M., and Bywaters, E.G.L.: Prognosis in Still's disease. Bull. Rheum. Dis. 9:189, 1959.

306. Goel, K.M., and Shanks, R.A.: Follow-up study of 100 cases of juvenile rheumatoid arthritis. Ann. Rheum. Dis. 33:25, 1974.

307. Hanson, V., Kornreich, H., Bernstein, B., King, K.K., and Singsen, B.: Prognosis of juvenile rheumatoid arthritis. Arthritis Rheum. 20:279, 1977.

308. Stoeber, E.: Prognosis in juvenile chronic arthritis. Follow-up of 433 chronic rheumatic children. Eur. J. Pediatr. 135:225, 1981.

309. Jeremy, R., Schaller, J., Arkless, R., Wedgwood, R.J., and Healey, L.A.: Juvenile rheumatoid arthritis persisting into adulthood. Am. J. Med. 45:419, 1968.

310. Ansell, B.M.: Still's disease followed into adult life. Proc. R. Soc. Med. 62:912, 1969.

311. Wilkinson, V.A.: Juvenile chronic arthritis in adolescence: Facing the reality. Int. Rehabil. Med. 3:11, 1981.

312. Ansell, B.M.: Joint manifestations in children with juvenile chronic polyarthritis. Arthritis Rheum. 20:204, 1977.

313. Cassidy, J.T., and Martel, W.: Juvenile rheumatoid arthritis: Clinicoradiologic correlations. Arthritis Rheum. 20:207, 1977.

314. Granberry, W.M., and Mangum, G.L.: The hand in the child with juvenile rheumatoid arthritis. J. Hand Surg. 5:105, 1980.

315. Ansell, B.M., and Wood, P.H.N.: Prognosis in juvenile chronic polyarthritis. Clin. Rheum. Dis. 2:397, 1976.

316. Ansell, B.M.: Rehabilitation in juvenile chronic arthritis. Rheumatol. Rehabil. Suppl. 1979, pp. 74–76.

317. Calabro, J.J., Burnstein, S.L., Staley, H.L., and Marchesano, J.M.: Prognosis in juvenile rheumatoid arthritis: A 15 year follow-up of 100 patients. Arthritis Rheum. 20:285, 1977.

318. Isdale, I.C.: Hip disease in juvenile rheumatoid arthritis. Ann. Rheum. Dis. 29:603, 1970.

319. Ansell, B.M., and Unlu, M.: Hip involvement in juvenile chronic polyarthritis. Ann. Rheum. Dis. 29:687, 1970.

320. Rombouts, J.J., and Rombouts-Lindemans, C.: Involvement of the hip in juvenile rheumatoid arthritis. A radiological study with special reference to growth disturbances. Acta Rheumatol. Scand. 17:248, 1971.

321. Bernstein, B., Forrester, D., Singsen, B., King, K.K., Kornreich, H., and Hanson, V.: Hip joint restoration in juvenile rheumatoid arthritis. Arthritis Rheum. 20:1099, 1977.

322. Calabro, J.J.: Amyloidosis and juvenile rheumatoid arthritis. J. Pediatr. 75:521, 1969.

323. Smith, M.E., Ansell, B.M., and Bywaters, E.G.L.: Mortality and prognosis related to the amyloidosis of Still's disease. Ann. Rheum. Dis. 27:137, 1969.

324. Schnitzer, T.J., and Ansell, B.M.: Amyloidosis in juvenile chronic polyarthritis. Arthritis Rheum. 20:245, 1977.

325. Baum, J., and Gutowska, G.: Death in juvenile rheumatoid arthritis. Arthritis Rheum. 20:253, 1977.

326. Bywaters, E.G.L.: Deaths in juvenile chronic polyarthritis. Arthritis Rheum. 20:256, 1977.

327. Bernstein, B.: Death in juvenile rheumatoid arthritis. Arthritis Rheum. 20:256, 1977.

328. Smiley, W.K., May, E., and Bywaters, E.G.L.: Ocular presentations of Still's disease and their treatment: Iridocyclitis in Still's disease: Its complication and treatment. Ann. Rheum. Dis. 16:371, 1957.

329. Smiley, W.K.: The visual prognosis in Still's disease with eye involvement. Proc. R. Soc. Med. 53:196, 1960.

330. Chylack, L.T., Jr.: The ocular manifestations of juvenile rheumatoid arthritis. Arthritis Rheum. 20:217, 1977.

331. Kanski, J.J.: Anterior uveitis in juvenile rheumatoid arthritis. Arch. Ophthalmol. 95:1794, 1977.

Chapter 81

Rheumatic Fever

Gene H. Stollerman

DEFINITION

Rheumatic fever is an inflammatory disease that occurs as a delayed sequel to pharyngeal infection with group A streptococci. It involves principally the heart, joints, central nervous system, skin, and subcutaneous tissues. In the acute form its common clinical manifestations are migratory polyarthritis, fever, carditis, and, less frequently, Sydenham's chorea, subcutaneous nodules, and erythema marginatum. No single symptom, sign, or laboratory test is pathognomonic of rheumatic fever, although several combinations of them are diagnostic. Although involvement of the joints justifies grouping this syndrome with the rheumatic diseases, its importance is due to involvement of the heart, which can be fatal during the acute stage of the disease or can lead to rheumatic heart disease, a chronic condition due to scarring and deformity of the heart valves.

ETIOLOGY AND PATHOGENESIS

The evidence that has established the group A streptococcus as the etiologic agent of rheumatic fever is all indirect because group A streptococci are not recoverable from the lesions and no satisfactory experimental model of the disease has been demonstrated. Nonetheless, the evidence is overwhelming and can be summarized briefly according to four main lines of observation.

Clinical Evidence. It has been recognized for more than 100 years that acute rheumatic fever (ARF) is often preceded by septic sore throat. The inconsistency of this relationship, however, has been noted repeatedly.[1] Approximately one third of patients with acute rheumatic fever deny antecedent sore throat. At the onset of the rheumatic attack cultures of the throat are usually negative and cultures of the blood are virtually always sterile. Rheumatic recurrences are even more difficult to relate to an antecedent sore throat because subclinical streptococcal infection so often reactivates the disease. On clinical grounds alone, therefore, the group A streptococcus is difficult to establish as the *only* etiologic agent.

Epidemiologic Evidence. Factors such as latitude, altitude, crowding, dampness, economic factors, and age all affect the incidence of rheumatic fever because they are related to the incidence and severity of streptococcal pharyngitis in general. Careful military epidemiologic studies over a period of 20 years show a clear sequential relationship of outbreaks of streptococcal pharyngitis or rheumatic fever. Despite epidemics caused by a variety of other respiratory pathogens, ARF is absent in the same population when streptococcal infection is controlled by chemotherapy.[2] Military recruits are healthy young adults, physically highly trained, optimally nourished, and socially and ethnically heterogeneous—yet rheumatic fever occurs among them in indiscriminate fashion except that it occurs more frequently in those with previous histories of ARF.[3]

Immunologic Evidence. Initial (primary) or recurrent (secondary) rheumatic fever does not occur without a streptococcal antibody response.[4] Furthermore, the magnitude of the antibody response is a major variable determining the attack rate of rheumatic fever following streptococcal pharyngitis.[5] This is true for both primary and secondary attacks.[6]

Prophylactic Evidence. The most convincing evidence of all is the complete prevention of rheumatic recurrences by continuous chemoprophylaxis against streptococcal infection in rheumatic subjects and the prevention of initial attacks by prompt and effective penicillin therapy of streptococcal sore throat.[7,8]

PATHOGENESIS

Despite the clear implication of the group A streptococcus as the etiologic agent of rheumatic fever, the pathogenesis of the disease remains an enigma. Four requirements for the pathogenesis seem firmly established: (1) the presence of the group A streptococcus, (2) a streptococcal antibody response indicative of actual recent infection, (3) persistence of the organism in the pharynx for a sufficient period of time, and (4) location of the infection in the throat.

The Site of Infection. Lymphatic connections between the pharynx and the heart have been pointed out and viewed with suspicion.[9] Streptococcal infections at other sites, such as in skin, wounds, puerperal sepsis, or pneumonia, have not been associated with rheumatic fever.

The Strain of Group A Streptococcus. The severity of streptococcal sore throat bears a general relationship to the attack rate of rheumatic fever, and this observation is reflected in the correlation of attack rate with the magnitude of the streptococcal antibody response.[5] Although a remarkably constant attack rate of rheumatic fever was observed in military epidemics due to a variety of M protein serotypes,[3] the actual number of such M serotypes which are now well recognized as the most common and dangerous rheumatogenic pharyngeal strains are relatively few and are not as commonly isolated now as they were previously.[7,10] As noted below in the discussion of the epidemiology of rheumatic fever, a decline in the virulence of streptococcal strains causing most current pharyngeal infections and the prevalence of strains of a wide variety of M protein serotypes not previously identified make it appear that qualitative as well as quantitative differences may exist in strains of streptococci that may relate to their rheumatogenic potential.

The Role of Toxins. Although evidence of direct *infection* is lacking,[11] a direct *toxic* effect of some streptococcal product, particularly on the heart, has not been ruled out as a pathogenic mechanism. In support of this possibility is the observation that the latent period between streptococcal pharyngitis and the onset of rheumatic fever does not shorten with rheumatic recurrences as one would expect in secondary immune responses.

Immunologic Theories. Bacterial allergy or autoimmunity is the most popular pathogenetic theory of rheumatic fever, although none of the streptococcal antibodies described to date, including those reactive with the heart, have been shown to be cytotoxic. The role of hyperimmunity is, however, supported by strong evidence because rheumatic fever patients are, in general, the population that is most intensively hyperimmune to all antigenic streptococcal products that have been tested.

Autoimmunity. The serum of patients with ARF has been known to contain autoantibodies to many tissues for more than 40 years. Of greatest interest has been the demonstration of heart antibodies, gamma globulins with specificity for cardiac components, primarily sarcolemma membranes.[12] The binding of these antibodies is also associated with the deposition of large amounts of complement component C3. Many heart antibodies in patients with rheumatic carditis can be absorbed with the patient's own atrial tissues and, therefore, are probably autoantibodies. Their role in the pathogenesis of rheumatic fever has been clouded by the growing understanding of autoantibody formation and complement activation as a general response to tissue injury. Cardiac damage by rheumatic, traumatic, or ischemic heart lesions leads to biochemical changes which are manifested by autoantibody production. It is therefore possible that heart antibodies in rheumatic carditis are the *result* rather than the *cause* of tissue injury.

Cross-Reactions Between Streptococci and Human Heart and Other Organs. In the early 1960s, Kaplan and his associates demonstrated that rabbit antisera against certain group A streptococci react with human heart preparations in the immunofluorescent test.[13,14] In the years since, additional immunologic cross-reactions have been described between streptococci and human tissues.[7,15,16] The purification of the streptococcal M proteins may now permit more incisive immunologic research concerning the pathogenetic significance, if any, of this type of autoimmune phenomenon. The concept of autoimmunity in ARF has been extended recently to Sydenham's chorea by studies demonstrating antibody to caudate and subthalamic nuclei in sera from patients with this rheumatic manifestation.[17] This antibody could be absorbed with group A streptococcal membranes which also cross-react with the sarcolemmal membranes of the heart.

There is no clear evidence for a causal relationship between cross-reactive heart antibodies and rheumatic carditis. Group A carbohydrate antibodies which cross-react with the glycoprotein of the human heart persist longer after rheumatic fever in patients with rheumatic heart disease than in those rheumatic fever patients who escape heart damage. This difference, however, could not be confirmed in a large series of patients studied with a different method. Moreover, in subsequent studies, it was found that the level of group A antibodies decreased after valvectomy but not after valvotomy, suggesting that the group A antibody persists in patients with rheumatic heart disease because of self-reimmunization with valvular components.[18]

Host Factors. The lack of evidence of clear genetic factors predisposing to rheumatic fever has been puzzling in view of the frequent observation of strong family histories. In the few adequate studies that have been made of identical twins,[19] a relatively low concordance of rheumatic fever (less than 20 percent) has been found. In addition, the incidence of ARF is remarkably similar in every race and ethnic group exposed to rheumatogenic streptococcal disease. The effect of other host variables such as sex on the frequency of certain complications of rheumatic fever suggests that host factors undoubtedly play some part. The incidence of chorea is equal among prepubescent boys and girls, but this manifestation is completely absent in the sexually mature male and exaggerated during pregnancy. Other examples of sex predilection are the increased frequency of tight mitral stenosis in the female and aortic stenosis in the male. The possible association of HLA haplotypes is under intense investigation.[20]

The Immune Response of Rheumatic Fever Patients. Virtually every immune response, humoral and cellular, to all streptococcal antigens that have been studied shows a statistically significant increase in rheumatic subjects compared with nonrheumatics recovering from streptococcal pharyngitis.[21] Rheumatic fever patients respond normally to other antigens, such as diphtheria toxoids.[22] The increased immune response may represent a greater magnitude, antigenically, of streptococcal infection in the rheumatic patient or, alternatively, more frequent or severe previous infections. The genetic control of immune responses, however, and their association with certain HLA haplotypes in other rheumatic diseases make the issue of genetic predisposition still quite viable especially with regard to certain complications such as mitral stenosis and chorea.

EPIDEMIOLOGY

Some confusion in interpreting the current epidemiology of rheumatic fever has been caused by continued high frequency of streptococcal pharyngitis in populations in which rheumatic fever has become rare. As streptococcal disease has become less epidemic and virulent, the issue of how to establish sporadic pharyngitis as truly due to a group A streptococcal infection has become more difficult to resolve. Streptococcal disease in different socioeconomic groups in different parts of the world presents confusing variables that demand precise definition of the nature of the antecedent streptococcal infections required to trigger rheumatic fever.

The Changing Pattern of Rheumatic Fever. The diminishing frequency and severity of ARF, particularly in North America, Europe and Japan has been dramatic. Although the use of antibiotics has certainly been a factor, the incidence and mortality of the disease were decreasing before antibiotics were introduced. Changes in social conditions, particularly improved housing and slum clearance, have undoubtedly contributed to the decline. Improvement in the delivery of health care in defined populations has been shown to be significant.[23] Crowding through inadequate housing is probably the chief reason for the magnified risk of streptococcal pharyngitis and rheumatic fever in certain disadvantaged populations.

The prevalence of congenital heart disease now exceeds that of rheumatic heart disease in some populations of American school children.[24,26] Notwithstanding its decline, however, rheumatic heart disease is still the leading cause of death from heart disease in the 5- to 24-year-old group in large populations of the world, and continues to be a serious public health problem, particularly in countries of the "Third World."

The Attack Rate of Rheumatic Fever. Studies on military populations in the late 1940s and early 1950s in the United States have provided the most reliable data concerning the attack rate of rheumatic fever following untreated streptococcal pharyngitis. Patients who were ill with exudative streptococcal pharyngitis caused by several common prevalent pharyngeal strains of virulent group A streptococci developed rheumatic fever at a remarkably predictable rate of approximately 3 percent regardless of their age, race, or ethnic group and regardless of the season or year in which the study was made.[27] The major variables which seemed related to this attack rate were the magnitude of the immune response and the duration of carriage of the organism.[5,28]

In contrast to these military studies, rheumatic fever occurs less frequently following the endemic, sporadic form of streptococcal disease seen in civilian practice.[29] This kind of streptococcal disease is much more difficult to diagnose and to define because of the frequency of occurrence of viral pharyngitis in patients who carry group A strains in their throats from previous episodes of infection. Without immunologic data to confirm a rising titer of streptococcal antibodies, the isolation of group A organisms from a patient's throat may be misleading. In addition, frequent mild streptococcal infections, some of them non-group A, tend to keep streptococcal antibody titers at high levels in school children and make it more difficult to detect a further increase in titer when the initial titer in acute phase serum is already high.[30]

Nonetheless, in studies of Chicago school children, the absence of rheumatic fever was noteworthy in some 300 patients who had nonexudative sore throat, a positive throat culture for group A streptococci, and a significant increase in anti-streptolysin O titer.[7] These studies raised the issue of whether the absence of rheumatic fever in these infections was a quantitative matter of "subthreshold" intensity of disease or due to a *qualitative* change in the nature of the infecting strains because the great majority of the streptococci were not M typeable with antisera available at that time.[31]

Qualitative Factors: Streptococcal Strain Variation. The decreasing frequency with which streptococcal strains can now be identified with antisera prepared against the erstwhile prevalent major serotypes has been well recognized in recent years by reference and research laboratories that type group A streptococci. The major M types that are notorious for causing epidemic rheumatic fever (e.g., types 5, 14, 19, 24) have become less prevalent, and in the past decade attention has shifted to the study of "new" M types among both pharyngeal and "skin" strains.[32] The clear demonstration that group A streptococci that cause pyoderma, with or without acute glomerulonephritis (AGN), do not cause rheumatic fever[33] has forced the recognition of the existence of "nonrheumatogenic group A streptococci"[34] because such skin strains regularly colonize the throat as well as the skin of infected individuals.

Since the pharyngeal route of infection is now accepted as a requirement for the pathogenesis of rheumatic fever (see above), the issue as to whether failure of these strains in the throat to cause the disease is a quantitative or qualitative factor is unresolved. Extensive studies of pharyngeal infections with such strains made in Memphis showed that two thirds of these sore throats were associated with streptococcal antibody increases, although the magnitude of the antibody response was not great.[35] In Trinidad, where both AGN and ARF occur concurrently in the same population with little seasonal variation, cyclic epidemics of AGN have occurred without parallel changes in the incidence of rheumatic fever. A study of the streptococcal strains in this population shows a clear distinction in the serotypes associated with AGN from those associated with rheumatic fever.[36] The studies of Widdowson, Maxted, and their colleagues[37] demonstrate the association of rheumatic fever with those streptococcal M types that cause strong immune responses to M-associated proteins. Many of the known M types which cause weaker responses are not rheumatogenic. Most recently, a group of 164 rheumatic subjects in Memphis who developed streptococcal antibody increases due to subclinical infections while under surveillance in a rheumatic fever prophylaxis clinic failed to develop rheumatic recurrences despite strong immune responses and the presence of rheumatic heart disease in many of the affected individuals.[38] The data are in striking contrast to the very high attack rates of rheumatic recurrences observed in earlier studies in New York and Chicago in rheumatic subjects with comparable antibody responses and rheumatic heart disease.[7]

Geography and Climate. Despite conflicting reports in the literature, there is the same relationship of rheumatic fever to the intensity and severity of streptococcal disease in the tropics as in the temperate climates where adequate data are available for analysis.[39] The clinical features of rheumatic fever have also been alleged to vary in different climates. In warm climates, a reported high frequency of acute rheumatic carditis in relation to other manifestations of rheumatic fever may have been due to skewed sampling. The frequency with which polyarthritis and chorea are detected depends to a large extent upon the health care system of the region and upon the interest in the disease of the physicians and health care workers.[40]

Host Factors in the Epidemiology of ARF. Once rheumatic fever is acquired, its reactivation following streptococcal infection is many times greater in rheumatic subjects than the attack rate in the general population. The recurrence rate per infection (R/I) may be as high as 50 percent during the first year and decreases sharply until 4 to 5 years after the attack when it levels off at approximately 10 percent.[41] Thereafter, it does not seem to decrease any further.[42]

PATHOLOGY

General Pathology. The earliest structural change of rheumatic inflammation is found in the collagen of the connective tissues of the heart, and is called "fibrinoid degeneration." "Mucoid edema," a basophilic-staining swelling of the ground substance, is observed most prominently in the dense collagen of the valves and endocardium. The collagen fibers themselves in these mucoid areas become swollen and eosinophilic, forming a meshwork of rigid, wax-like fibers. These changes in the myocardium are followed within a couple of weeks by the development of the most characteristic lesion of rheumatic fever, the *Aschoff nodule*. The Aschoff nodule has been described in great detail in extensive reviews of rheumatic myocarditis[43] and is the subject of considerable discussion and debate concerning its cells of origin.[7]

Fibrinoid is a complex mixture of fibrin, gamma globulin, and other constituents. By electron microscopy it seems to include both unaltered collagen fibers and granular material partially derived from degenerating collagen. Fibrinoid changes in collagen are common to many inflammatory states wherein collagen is damaged and fibrin is precipitated along with many components of the gamma globulin-complement system. Aschoff nodules, however, are virtually pathognomonic of rheumatic fever. Yet their origin, functional impact on the heart and relation to the course and severity of the rheumatic attack are still obscure. Some believe that Aschoff lesions derive from injured muscle cells,[43] but most pathologists consider them to arise from connective tissue elements.[44] Recently, it has been suggested that they may arise from terminal branches of myocardial nerve cells.[45] Whatever the origin of the Aschoff nodule, its functional role in rheumatic carditis is also controversial. Acute rheumatic myocarditis is associated with a toxic effect on the myocardium that is not always reflected in the morbid anatomy of the disease. The persistence of Aschoff nodules for many years after a rheumatic attack has been well recognized by all pathologists. Biopsies of the left atrial appendage obtained during mitral valve surgery have shown persistence of these lesions in patients who no longer have clinical or laboratory evidence of rheumatic activity. The persistence of Aschoff nodules seems to be correlated, however, with the tendency in the host to develop progressive fibrosis and stenosis of the mitral valve.[46]

Pathology of the Heart. Rheumatic carditis is characteristically a *pancarditis*; all layers of the heart are involved. On gross inspection, fresh exudative pericardial lesions, dilatation of the myocardium, and verrucous valvular lesions are almost always evident. *Pericarditis* involves both layers of the pericardium which are thickened and covered by a fibrinous exudate. Serosanguineous fluid often fills the pericardial sac. Microscopically, mucoid edema and fibrinoid changes present in other layers of the heart are also found in the pericardium. With healing, fibrosis and adhesions occur, but constrictive pericarditis is not a complication of rheumatic pericarditis.

Myocarditis is characterized by the focal cellular lesions described above, but in addition to Aschoff bodies, a diffuse cellular infiltrate is present in interstitial tissues, consisting of lymphocytes, polymorphs, histiocytes, and eosinophils. The greatest damage to myocardial fibers occurs in the vicinity of Aschoff nodules and around blood vessels, leading to myocytolysis, loss of striation, fatty degeneration, and vacuolation of muscle fibers. Despite the great frequency of delayed atrioventricular conduction in acute rheumatic fever, involvement of the bundle of His by visible anatomical changes is rare.

Endocarditis is characterized by verrucous lesions at the free borders of the valve cusps. They are amorphous masses of eosinophilic material staining as fibrin. At the base and edges of the valve, the cells line up in palisades at right angles to the base. During healing, granulation tissue develops and vascularization and progressive fibrosis take place. The annulus is involved as well as the cusps. The chordae tendineae are also frequently affected and thickened and shortened. Subendocardial scarring also occurs with the formation of very characteristic broad bands of eosinophilic granular or hyaline material which often heals as a thickened, scarred, and even calcified layer.

Rheumatic Valvulvar Deformities. Mitral incompetence or insufficiency may result from shortening of one or both cusps, from fusion and shortening of the chordae and papillary muscles, or from dilatation of the valve ring. *Mitral regurgitation* is by far the most common clinically apparent lesion of rheumatic heart disease. Such lesions often occur subclinically when extracardiac symptoms of acute rheumatic fever are absent in relatively mild attacks of the disease. Dilatation of the valve ring may occur during active carditis as a result of acute dilatation of the left ventricle, but marked regurgitation may also occur without acute ventricular dilatation when the valves are inflamed without the coexistence of severe myocarditis.

Mitral stenosis occurs with varying degrees of mitral regurgitation. When stenosis is severe, regurgitation may be hemodynamically relatively unimportant. The cusps may fuse, leaving an ovoid opening, but the cusps themselves may remain thin and pliable. In other cases the cusps become very thick, rigid, and even calcified. The remaining opening may be "funnel," "buttonhole," or "fish-mouth" in shape.

Aortic valve deformities are most commonly a combination of stenosis and incompetence. A minimal degree of aortic regurgitation occurs very frequently and often subclinically in mild rheumatic involvement. Deformity of the aortic valve results from fusion of the cusps, rigidity, shortening or "rolling" of one or more of the cusps, or combinations of these processes.

Tricuspid valve deformities almost always exist in association with mitral and aortic lesions. They occur in approximately 10 percent of patients with chronic rheumatic heart disease. *Pulmonary valve deformities* are relatively rare, and when they occur the lesions are similar to those found in the aortic valve.

Progression of Rheumatic Heart Disease. Some of the progressive changes and continued inflammation of rheumatic valvular disease do not seem to be related to the original rheumatic process or to rheumatic recurrences. Disruption of red blood cells (cardiac hemolytic anemia), rapid platelet destruction and turnover,[47] and progressive thrombosis and fibrosis can occur along with calcification. The advent of careful antistreptococcal prophylaxis and prolonged observation and follow-up of rheumatic fever-free individuals have caused pathologists and clinicians to consider that at least some of the chronic, progressive changes of rheumatic heart disease may be due to factors other than chronic or recurrent rheumatic inflammation.

Extracardiac Lesions. *Arthritis*: The characteristic feature of the pathology of the joints in rheumatic fever is the swelling and edema of the articular and periarticular structures with serous effusion into the joint space but without erosion of the joint surface and without pannus formation. The synovial membrane is reddened, thickened, and covered by a fibrinous exudate. Microscopically, the picture is one of acute exudative inflammation with focal and diffuse cellular infiltrates of polymorphs and lymphocytes. Later, focal fibrinoid lesions and histiocytic granulomas may appear, but fibrosis is absent.

Subcutaneous nodules are composed of a central zone of fibrinoid necrosis surrounded by histiocytes and fibroblasts. Lymphocytes and polymorphs collect around small blood vessels and present an appearance resembling the histology of Aschoff bodies. These lesions heal rapidly, leaving no apparent scars.

The pathology of *chorea* has caused considerable confusion for several reasons. Few patients die of "pure" chorea, whereas those who die of severe carditis may have central nervous system lesions without chorea. No single site is consistently involved; Aschoff nodules are not found in the brain. It has not been possible to correlate clinical findings with pathologic changes.[48]

CLINICAL MANIFESTATIONS

The Antecedent Streptococcal Infection. As many as one third of patients do not remember having any illness in the month preceding the onset of rheumatic fever.

Rheumatic recurrences may be preceded by asymptomatic streptococcal infections in more than 50 percent of instances. These observations on individual patients contrast with the epidemiologic and immunologic evidence that intensity and severity of streptococcal disease in a given population relate clearly to rheumatic fever attack rates. The contrast is not necessarily paradoxical. In epidemics of streptococcal pharyngitis, a significant number of patients may have red and exudative throats and cultures strongly positive for virulent strains of group A streptococci and yet may not appear very ill clinically. Streptococcal pharyngitis may be strongly immunogenic when caused by virulent strains without always producing severe symptoms. Furthermore, when streptococcal pharyngitis causes symptoms they may last for only a few days even in the absence of specific therapy.

The Latent Period. Between the onset of symptoms of pharyngitis and the onset of rheumatic fever there is always a time lag or latent period which is, on the average, approximately 18 days. It is very rarely less than 1 week or longer than 5 weeks. The latent period does not shorten with recurrent rheumatic attacks. During the latent period there is neither clinical nor laboratory evidence of active inflammation.

The Major Manifestations of the Acute Rheumatic Attack. Certain manifestations that follow streptococcal infections with a frequency far exceeding chance may occur simultaneously or in rapid succession, or singly. These *major manifestations* consist of arthritis, carditis, chorea, subcutaneous nodules, and erythema marginatum. The term "major" refers to their importance as diagnostic criteria rather than to their importance in the severity of the process, its activity, or prognosis.

Arthritis. The arthritis of rheumatic fever usually involves the large joints, particularly the knees, ankles, elbows, and wrists. The hips are less commonly involved, and the spine is only rarely affected. The smaller joints of the fingers and toes are also less commonly inflamed. Almost any joint, however, may be affected. In the classic attack, several joints are involved in quick succession and each for a brief period of time, resulting in the typical picture of migratory polyarthritis accompanied by signs and symptoms of an acute febrile illness.

Each joint remains inflamed for usually no more than a week before it begins to subside, and the inflammation usually abates spontaneously in 2 or 3 weeks. The course of the entire bout of polyarthritis is usually severe for a week in approximately two thirds of patients and for an additional week or two in the remainder, but by the end of 4 weeks it subsides with only rare exceptions. Flare-ups may occur, however, in a small percentage of patients treated with antirheumatic therapy for 4 to 6 weeks but rarely after a second 6-week course of antirheumatic treatment.

Rheumatic fever never causes permanent joint deformities with the very rare exception of the so-called Jaccoud type of deformity of the metacarpophalangeal joints.[49,50] This condition is a "postrheumatic" periarticular fibrosis and not a synovitis. Because it occurs so rarely its relationship to rheumatic fever is not clear, but it usually occurs in patients with severe rheumatic heart disease and is not associated with other evidence of active rheumatic fever.

The time of onset of rheumatic polyarthritis is very sharply defined in relation to the antecedent streptococcal infection. Acute polyarthritis virtually never occurs more than 35 days from the onset of the antecedent streptococcal infection. For that reason, it is almost always associated with a rising or peak titer of streptococcal antibodies, an association useful in identifying an isolated bout of polyarthritis as rheumatic or, more accurately, of excluding rheumatic fever as an etiology for a given bout of polyarthritis when streptococcal antibodies are not increased (see below).

Arthritis occurs in approximately three fourths of patients during the acute stage of rheumatic fever. Joint involvement becomes more common with increasing age of the patient. When arthritis is the only major manifestation of rheumatic fever, the diagnosis is most difficult, and arthritis should be carefully distinguished from arthralgia, a less specific symptom and one more difficult to assess when objective signs are lacking. Nevertheless, to the experienced physician typical migratory polyarthralgia, well-described by a reliable patient, may be quite convincing as a feature of rheumatic fever. To be acceptable as a criterion for the diagnosis of rheumatic fever, the polyarthritis should involve two or more joints, should be associated with at least two minor manifestations such as fever and increase in the erythrocyte sedimentation rate, and should be associated with high titers of antistreptolysin O or some other streptococcal antibody.

Carditis. In its most severe form, carditis causes death from acute cardiac failure. More commonly, however, it is less intense and its predominant effect is scarring of the heart valves. In contrast to the seriousness of its prognosis, rheumatic carditis most often causes no symptoms of its own. It is usually diagnosed in the course of examination of a patient with arthritis or chorea which directs the physician's attention to the heart where the murmurs of rheumatic carditis are detected. If other symptoms of rheumatic fever are absent or if the carditis is not severe enough to cause heart failure, the pain of pericarditis, or prolonged or severe fever, carditis is frequently undetected. Patients with undiagnosed carditis may later be found to have rheumatic heart disease, and they often recall no history of a previous rheumatic attack.

Cardiac involvement may occur in the mildest form of the disease. The incidence of carditis in initial rheumatic attacks varies from 40 to 51 percent in different reports. The source and selection of clinical material greatly influences the statistics.

The major *criteria* for the clinical diagnosis of carditis are (1) an organic heart murmur not previously present, (2) an enlarging heart, (3) congestive heart failure, and (4) pericardial friction rubs or signs of effusion. In a patient with active rheumatic fever, any one of the above that is unequivocal justifies the diagnosis of carditis.

The Heart Murmurs of Rheumatic Carditis. Organic murmurs are almost invariably present in clinically apparent rheumatic carditis. Involvement of the other layers of the heart is always associated with endocarditis as well. Isolated myocarditis and pericarditis do not occur in rheumatic fever.

The most common murmur is a mitral systolic one due to mitral regurgitation caused by inflammation and edema of the valve. It occurs early in the course of the disease and often with very mild cardiac involvement so that it may constitute the only evidence of the presence of carditis. For this reason, the distinction between a true mitral regurgitation murmur and the common functional murmurs heard so often in children and adolescents is of considerable importance and requires experience with auscultation of young hearts.

A murmur characteristic (but not diagnostic) of the mitral regurgitation of acute rheumatic carditis is an apical mid-diastolic low-pitched sound (Carey Coombs murmur) which begins directly after the onset of the third heart sound and ends before the first heart sound. The mid-diastolic murmur is often transient, very low-pitched, and easily missed. The presence of this murmur in association with that of mitral regurgitation makes the diagnosis of "mitral valvulitis" more definite and adds considerably to the seriousness of the prognosis for permanent valve injury.

Aortic diastolic murmurs are only one third as common as are mitral murmurs in acute carditis. The aortic diastolic blow may be audible only intermittently, depending upon cardiac output. A diastolic cooing or crying "seagull" murmur is rarely heard but can be present transiently.

Cardiac Enlargement. Cardiac enlargement resulting from dilatation of the heart, particularly the left atrium and left ventricle, is one of the most reliable expressions clinically of rheumatic myocarditis. In the presence of organic heart murmurs, the degree of enlargement generally reflects the severity of carditis.

Congestive Heart Failure. Congestive heart failure is the least common but most serious manifestation of rheumatic carditis. It has been reported in approximately 5 to 10 percent of first attacks of rheumatic carditis. Severe or fatal heart failure is encountered more commonly in recurrent than primary rheumatic attacks. Evidence of vascular congestion and patchy edema on chest x-ray may raise the question of the presence of rheumatic pneumonitis. The latter occurs in the severest forms of rheumatic fever and clinically cannot be distinguished from the aforementioned pulmonary manifestations of heart failure.

Pericarditis. Pericarditis is reported in approximately 5 to 10 percent of most large series, but its frequency of detection clinically may be increased by echocardiography. Occasionally, pericardial reaction and effusion will be more striking and prominent than the degree of myocarditis. In such cases the regression in heart size and the rate of healing of the heart can be rapid. Conversely, pericarditis may be a minor aspect of the profound heart failure due to severe myocarditis. One rarely sees tamponade without severe myocardial failure as well.

Arrhythmias. Delayed AV conduction occurs very commonly in acute rheumatic fever and does not necessarily indicate carditis. Prolongation of the PR interval occurs with similar frequency in polyarthritis which is not associated with carditis as it does in rheumatic attacks in which carditis is present.

Subcutaneous Nodules. Subcutaneous nodules are a major manifestation of rheumatic fever (Fig. 81–1). They are not pathognomonic because they also occur in rheumatoid arthritis and in systemic lupus erythematosus as well. They are associated most often with severe carditis and very rarely appear as an isolated manifestation of rheumatic fever. The nodules are round, firm, painless, freely movable subcutaneous lesions varying in size from 0.5 to 2.0 cm. They are located over bony prominences and over tendons, particularly the extensor tendons of the hands and feet. They occur in crops varying in number from one to a few dozen. One should look for them over the scalp, especially the occiput, over the vertebral spines, and over the elbows, wrists, knees, ankles, and Achilles tendons. Nodules are evanescent, disappearing often in a matter of days but usually lasting a week or

Figure 81–1. Numerous large subcutaneous nodules (sketched from life). (From Cheadle, W.B.: The Various Manifestations of the Rheumatic State. London, Smith, Elder, 1889.)

two. They tend to be much smaller, more discrete, and less persistent than rheumatoid nodules.

In line with the declining severity of rheumatic fever, rheumatic nodules are reported less commonly in patients observed with rheumatic fever during the past few decades.[7] The incidence of nodules among the major manifestations of rheumatic fever is also very low in warmer climates such as India.[40] The reason for the wide epidemiologic variations in the incidence of nodules is undetermined.

Erythema Marginatum. This rash is a less common feature of rheumatic fever than the other manifestations, but it is so characteristic as to have major diagnostic significance. It is quite useful in diagnosis when the other manifestations are equivocal. Like chorea, it is usually not associated with a clear-cut histological lesion and may persist long after other clinical signs of active inflammation have abated. Erythema marginatum is not pathognomonic of rheumatic fever, because it has been reported in sepsis, drug reactions, and glomerulonephritis, and in patients in whom no etiologic factor can be identified. Erythema marginatum appears as a bright pink ring spreading serpiginously through the skin. It is nonpruritic, nonpainful, and neither indurated nor raised; it blanches completely on pressure. It is very evanescent, changing before one's eyes. It may first appear as a pink spot, but the center then fades and the periphery forms an irregular but sharp outer line. The individual lesions appear on the trunk and the proximal parts of the extremities but not on the face. They rarely extend more peripherally than the elbows and knees.

Erythema marginatum usually occurs early in the course of rheumatic fever. It is most often associated with carditis. It may persist intermittently for months, uninfluenced by antirheumatic agents. When all other signs of rheumatic activity are gone, one can allow the patient to ambulate without fear of a relapse despite the persistence of an occasional marginating lesion.

Sydenham's Chorea (Chorea Minor, St. Vitus' Dance). Chorea is a neurological disorder characterized by involuntary, purposeless, rapid movements, muscular weakness, and emotional lability. It may be associated with other rheumatic manifestations but may also appear as the sole expression of the disease—so-called "pure" chorea. Its sex distribution is different from that of the other manifestations in that it is present after puberty exclusively in females and declines rapidly after adolescence. It is seen occasionally in adult women but never in sexually fully developed men.

Chorea has declined strikingly in frequency compared with arthritis and carditis as a sign of rheumatic fever.[7,23] The reason for the trend is not clear.

The movements of chorea are abrupt and erratic and not rhythmic or repetitive like those of athetosis. Even in the most violent attacks, all choreiform movements disappear during sleep. They are less violent with rest and sedation. The involuntary movements affect all muscles, but those in the hands, face, and feet are most apparent. The patient cannot sustain a tetanic muscular contraction for very long. His expression changes constantly as he grimaces, frowns, grins, and pouts in rapid succession. The tongue, when protruded, resembles a "bag of worms," darts in and out, and contributes to the typical choreiform speech which is staccato, halting, and explosive. Handwriting becomes clumsy or impossible to read and can be followed serially as a measure of healing. Occasionally, choreiform movement may be completely unilateral, and the muscular weakness may resemble a palsy. The inability to sustain a tetanic contraction is best demonstrated by asking the patient to squeeze the examiner's hands. This results in a repetitive, spasmodic grip, exaggerated pronation, and a sensation which has been described as "milkmaid's grip" or "the milking sign."

Personality changes and emotional lability often herald the onset of chorea. The patient becomes restless, fidgety, hyperactive, uncooperative, and cantankerous. Outbursts of anger, silliness, crying, and inappropriate behavior may be noted before chorea becomes obvious. Muscle weakness causes dropping of objects, falling, stumbling, and tripping. A typical physical sign is the pendular or "hung-up" knee jerk. Raising the arms above the head causes pronation (pronator sign) (Fig. 81–2). When the arms are extended forward, flexion of the wrists and hyperextension of the metacarpophalangeal joints cause "dishing" or "spooning" of the dorsum of the hands. The electroencephalogram frequently shows abnormal, slow waves.

Chorea may last from a week to more than 2 years but it usually runs its course in 8 to 15 weeks. It is never seen simultaneously with arthritis but often coexists with carditis. When chorea appears alone, the other minor clinical and laboratory signs of acute rheumatic fever may be absent. The erythrocyte sedimentation rate and the C-reactive protein may be normal. Even more confusing, in such cases streptococcal antibody titers may not be increased. These observations are explained by the long latent period (as long as 1 to 6 months) between the antecedent streptococcal infection and the onset of chorea.[51]

The Minor Manifestations. *Fever.* Temperature is increased in almost all rheumatic attacks and ranges from 38.4 to 40° C. Usually fever decreases in approximately a week without antipyretic treatment and becomes low grade for another week or two. It rarely lasts for more than 3 to 4 weeks.

Abdominal Pain. The abdominal pain of rheumatic fever resembles that of other conditions associated with acute microvascular mesenteric inflammation such as sepsis, endotoxin or anaphylactic shock, transfusion reactions, anaphylactoid purpura, or sickle cell crises. It usually occurs at or near the onset of the rheumatic attack so that other manifestations may not yet be present to clarify the diagnosis.

Epistaxis. Epistaxis in the past occurred most prominently and severely in patients with severe and protracted rheumatic carditis. In some studies in the 1930s its frequency was reported as high as 48 percent, but it declined to as low as 4 to 9 percent in the late 1950s and perhaps occurs even less frequently now. Although

Figure 81–2. "Spooning" or "dishing" of the hands in a patient with chorea. (From Stollerman, G.H.: Rheumatic Fever and Streptococcal Infection. New York, Grune & Stratton, 1975.)

epistaxis has been correlated in the past with the severity of rheumatic inflammation, it is difficult to assess retrospectively the possible thrombasthenic effect of large doses of salicylates administered for prolonged periods in protracted attacks.

Rheumatic Pneumonia. Rheumatic pneumonia may appear in the lung in the course of severe rheumatic carditis. As noted above, this inflammatory process is difficult or impossible to distinguish from pulmonary edema or the alveolitis associated with respiratory distress syndromes due to a variety of pathophysiologic states.[52]

LABORATORY FINDINGS

The diagnosis of rheumatic fever cannot be established by laboratory tests, but these may be helpful in two ways: demonstrating that antecedent streptococcal infection has occurred and documenting the presence or persistence of an inflammatory process. The course of carditis should be followed by serial chest x-rays, and the electrocardiogram may reflect the toxic effect of the rheumatic process on the conduction system. A variety of laboratory tests may be required to exclude the large list of conditions from which rheumatic fever must be differentiated.

Evidence of Antecedent Streptococcal Infection. Throat cultures are usually negative by the time rheumatic fever appears. When they are positive for group A streptococci, their interpretation may be difficult because the organism isolated may, indeed, represent convalescent carriage of the inciting rheumatogenic strain but could also be the result of an intercurrent infection with a different strain. Streptococcal antibodies are more useful because (1) they reach a peak titer at about the time of onset of rheumatic fever, (2) they indicate true infection rather than transient carriage, and (3) by performing several tests for different antibodies, any significant recent streptococcal infection can be detected.

The specific antibody tests which have been used to diagnose streptococcal infections most frequently are those directed against extracellular products found in the supernatant broth of streptococcal cultures. They include antistreptolysin O, anti-DNAse B, antihyaluronidase, anti-NADase (anti-DPNase), and antistreptokinase. Antistreptolysin O (ASO) has been the most widely used test and is generally available in hospitals in the United States. The methodology of these and other streptococcal antibody tests has been described in detail in recent reviews.[53]

ASO titers vary with age, season, geography, and other factors that affect the frequency and intensity of streptococcal disease. They reach peak levels in the young schoolage population. Titers of 200 to 300 Todd units per milliliter are common, therefore, in healthy children of elementary school age who live in crowded cities of the temperate zone of the USA. Following streptococcal sore throat, the antibody response peaks at about 4 to 5 weeks, which is usually during the second or third week of rheumatic fever (depending on how early it is detected). Thereafter, antibody titers fall off rapidly in the next several months, and after 6 months they decline more slowly. Evidence of increased streptococcal antibodies should be present therefore in all patients at the onset of the rheumatic attack unless the onset is ill-defined.

Anti-DNAse B tends to remain elevated longer than other streptococcal antibodies. This test, together with the ASO, has become most generally recommended for diagnosis, with antihyaluronidase a useful third. Recently, a product has been marketed which is a concentrate of extracellular streptococcal antigens (antistreptozyme [ASTZ] test). Sheep cells sensitized with this concentrate will agglutinate in the presence of streptococcal antibodies which have not yet been defined. Although the nature of the antigen(s) that adhere to and sensitize red cells is not yet clear, this slide agglutination test is a very sensitive measure of the streptococcal immune response in laboratories that have used standard lots of streptozyme.[54]

Streptococcal antibodies, when increased, support but do not prove the diagnosis of acute rheumatic fever. One should not diagnose the disease on the basis of increased titers of streptococcal antibodies alone. Streptococcal antibodies are not a measure of rheumatic activity. In the absence of intercurrent streptococcal infection, titers decline during the rheumatic attack despite the persistence or severity of rheumatic activity.

Acute Phase Reactants. Acute phase reactants is the term applied to those nonspecific laboratory tests that denote active inflammation. They include the erythrocyte sedimentation rate (ESR), C-reactive protein (CRP), serum mucoprotein or serum hexosamine levels, serum protein electrophoresis, leukocyte counts, anemia and several others. The two tests which have gained widest use are the C-reactive protein and the ESR, because both are almost invariably abnormal during the active rheumatic process if it is not suppressed by antirheumatic drugs. "Pure" chorea and persistent erythema marginatum are exceptions. CRP and ESR are not of great value when rheumatic manifestations are obvious clinically. During treatment, however, they are quite useful, especially CRP, to measure the effectiveness of the suppression of the inflammatory process. Particularly when treatment has been discontinued or is being tapered off, the CRP is very efficient in monitoring "rebounds" of rheumatic inflammation which indicate that the rheumatic process is still active. When CRP and ESR remain normal a few weeks after antirheumatic treatment has been terminated, the attack may be considered ended unless chorea appears. Even then, however, there will be no exacerbation of the systemic inflammatory component of the attack, and chorea will be present as an isolated manifestation.

Anemia. The anemia of rheumatic fever is that of the normochromic normocytic anemia of chronic infection or inflammation. It is of mild to moderate degree and is corrected partially or completely by suppression of inflammation, particularly with corticosteroids. Anemia is a useful index of the severity and chronicity of rheumatic fever.

Electrocardiography. The electrocardiogram (ECG) has no characteristic pattern in rheumatic fever, and the diagnosis of carditis should never be made on the basis of ECG changes alone. Neither the course of the acute rheumatic attack nor the subsequent development of valvular or myocardial damage can be predicted from ECG changes. Patients with abnormal ECG changes but without criteria described above for carditis recover completely without stigmata of rheumatic heart disease.

DIAGNOSIS

Manifestations of rheumatic fever that are not clearly expressed pose a dilemma because of the importance of identifying a first rheumatic attack clearly in order to establish the need for prophylaxis of recurrences (see below). Some of the isolated manifestations, particularly polyarthritis, may be difficult or impossible to distinguish from other diseases, especially at their onset. The *Jones criteria* for the diagnosis of rheumatic fever[55] have been widely utilized as a scheme to avoid the overdiagnosis of the disease whose implications for future management of the patient are so important. The currently modified criteria (Table 81-1) emphasize the importance of establishing the presence of antecedent streptococcal infection by demonstration of increased titers of streptococcal antibodies. If supported by such evidence, two major, or one major and two minor, manifestations constitute a high probability of the diagnosis of rheumatic fever. The diagnosis can be made, however, when "pure" chorea is the sole manifestation because of the rarity with which this syndrome is due to any other cause.

The *polyarthritis* of rheumatic fever when it appears as the sole major manifestation of the disease constitutes the greatest problem, especially in the adolescent and adult population in which other causes of isolated polyarthritis are so common. The exclusion of the bacteremias by appropriate blood cultures before antibiotic therapy is initiated is essential. Because gonococcal polyarthritis cannot be excluded by cultures of the joints or blood in the majority of cases, a therapeutic trial of penicillin should be used. In early cases of gonococcal polyarthritis, the prompt response to penicillin is invariable. *Subacute bacterial endocarditis* must always be considered whenever a patient with rheumatic heart disease develops polyarthritis and unexplained fever. Certain viral infections, such as *rubella,* or the persistent viremias causing immune complex disease, such as *type B hepatitis,* are often problems in a young patient who may coincidentally also have increased titers of streptococcal antibodies. The serum sickness-like syndromes, especially penicillin allergy following treatment of strep-

Table 81-1. Jones Criteria (Revised)*

Major Manifestations	Minor Manifestations
Carditis	Fever
Polyarthritis	Arthralgia
Chorea	Previous rheumatic fever or
Erythema marginatum	rheumatic heart disease
Subcutaneous nodules	Elevated ESR or positive CRP
	Prolonged PR interval

Plus supporting evidence of preceding streptococcal infection: history of recent scarlet fever; positive throat culture for group A streptococcus; increased ASO titer or other streptococcal antibodies.

*Circulation 32:664, 1965.

tococcal pharyngitis, cause diagnostic confusion. It is well to bear in mind that rheumatic fever does not cause urticaria, angioneurotic edema, or clinically overt glomerulonephritis, and that serum complement levels are increased rather than decreased in rheumatic fever. Low levels of streptococcal antibodies may be the only reliable differential diagnostic feature if other clues of immune-complex disease are absent. Antinuclear and other autoantibodies do not appear in the course of rheumatic fever, no matter how persistent the disease.

Sickle cell anemia and its variants have many of the signs and symptoms of rheumatic fever, including joint pain, fever, abdominal pain, heart murmurs, and cardiac enlargement. The coexistence of rheumatic fever and sickle cell disease is relatively rare for unknown reasons, but the two can occur in the same patient and make the etiology of the clinical manifestations of the heart disease that they cause very difficult to unravel.

Rheumatoid arthritis imitates rheumatic fever when the former begins with migratory polyarthritis of the large joints. Involvement of many small joints of the hands and feet is much more characteristic of rheumatoid arthritis, but such involvement may appear later in the course of the disease when it has become low grade and chronic with characteristic morning stiffness and fusiform swelling of the fingers. The chronic course of rheumatoid arthritis and the eventual development of joint deformities may ultimately be the only distinguishing features when streptococcal antibodies are coincidently increased at the onset of rheumatoid arthritis. The absence of rheumatoid factor (IgM–anti-IgG) in juvenile rheumatoid arthritis limits the usefulness of this test in children.

Carditis: When functional or organic murmurs are typical, there is little problem for the experienced physician in distinguishing between them. At times, however, a nondescript murmur, especially in the obese or heavy-chested individual, may defy sharp distinctions and repeated examinations and other studies may be necessary. Such murmurs are classified as "doubtful" or "questionable" when no other decision can be made. *Myocarditis* in its severe and chronic form due to other diseases may be impossible to distinguish from chronic rheumatic carditis if the heart is dilated and mitral regurgitation is prominent. This situation is encountered when rheumatic fever patients have heart failure with no associated extracardiac manifestations to provide clues. In rheumatic carditis, as the patient recovers cardiac compensation, the valvular lesions usually persist and the murmurs may become louder, whereas the reverse is true in viral and other forms of acute and subacute myocarditis.

Congenital heart disease may pose a problem when a congenital heart murmur is first discovered during a febrile illness, especially if the heart is overactive and early signs of congestive heart failure are present.

Chorea in its overt form is characteristic and easy to recognize, but multiple tics and habit spasms in a hyperactive child may be misinterpreted.

COURSE, PROGNOSIS, AND NATURAL HISTORY

The clinical course of rheumatic fever is quite variable, but in general there is a characteristic sequence of the major manifestations and a predictable duration. Most attacks begin with fever and joint symptoms. Carditis, if it is going to occur, does so early in the attack—within the first few weeks. The latent period between streptococcal infection and the onset of rheumatic fever is shortest in arthritis and erythema marginatum and longest in chorea, with carditis and subcutaneous nodules in between. The average duration of a rheumatic attack is less than 3 months. When severe carditis is present, clinical rheumatic activity may continue for 6 months or more. Less than 5 percent of attacks persist for more than 6 months, however. Such cases are classified as "chronic rheumatic fever."

The age of onset and severity of carditis influences its chronicity. Very young children, less than 3 years of age, who develop rheumatic fever have the highest incidence of carditis (more than 90 percent). The incidence of carditis declines to approximately one third in the 14- to 17-year age group. Carditis occurs occasionally after the age of 25 in what are apparently first attacks. When carditis is mild, it usually disappears rapidly. Severe carditis prolongs the attack, causes persistent cardiac enlargement and persistent valvular disease, and may produce protracted or permanent heart failure. Antirheumatic therapy "masks" rheumatic inflammation but tends to prolong rather than terminate the attack. The majority of prolonged attacks occur in patients who have had one or more previous attacks, particularly those with carditis, and the incidence of chronic rheumatic fever increases with the number of recurrences. When antirheumatic therapy is withdrawn and no "rebound" of inflammation is noted for 8 weeks or more, the attack is over and will not be reactivated without a new streptococcal infection.[56]

Prognosis. Rheumatic fever does not recur when streptococcal disease is prevented. Prognosis is excellent for the rheumatic subject who escapes carditis during the initial attack. In the United Kingdom–United States Cooperative Study on the treatment of rheumatic fever,[57,58] patients without organic murmurs during the acute attack showed virtually no evidence of the development of rheumatic heart disease on subsequent follow-up studies conducted for 5 to 10 years. In those with mild carditis, 82 percent had normal hearts who were followed for 5 years and 70 percent who were followed for 10 years showed no stigmata of rheumatic heart disease. Prognosis was poorer for those with severer carditis in the initial attack. The presence of heart failure was followed by complete healing in only 30 percent at 5 years and 40 percent at 10 years (Fig. 81–3).

Recurrences of Rheumatic Fever. First attacks of rheumatic fever following epidemics of streptococcal infection in the general population occur with a frequency of 1 to 3 percent. In contrast, the rate of reactivation

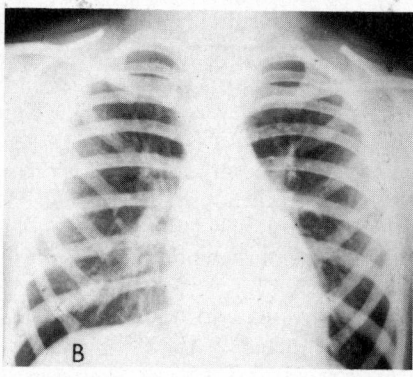

Figure 81–3. Healing of acute rheumatic carditis. *A,* Greatly enlarged heart and congestive heart failure. *B,* Same patient approximately 6 months later when the attack had subsided. (From Stollerman, G.H.: Rheumatic Fever and Streptococcal Infection. New York, Grune & Stratton, 1975.)

of rheumatic fever by streptococcal pharyngitis in patients who have had rheumatic fever previously may exceed 50 percent. In one well-known study,[6,41] the rheumatic attack rate per infection (R/I) in children decreased from 23 to 11 percent between the first and fifth year after a rheumatic attack. In adults with rheumatic heart disease, 42 infections which occurred 10 or more years after the last attack were followed by 2 recurrences (R/I = 4.8 percent).[42] Recurrence rates decline, therefore, with the time elapsed from the last attack.

The presence or absence of rheumatic heart disease is another major factor that influences the R/I of rheumatic recurrences. In the Irvington House studies in New York,[41] recurrence rates in children with rheumatic heart disease and cardiomegaly were 43 percent; in children with rheumatic heart disease and no cardiomegaly, 27 percent; and in patients without heart disease, 10 percent.

The third important factor influencing the R/I of recurrences is the severity of the streptococcal infection as reflected in the magnitude of the streptococcal immune response. Intercurrent infections causing marked antistreptolysin O increases resulted in attack rates as high as 65 percent in the heart disease group in contrast to 36 percent in those without rheumatic heart disease. Weak ASO responses caused recurrences infrequently, and no recurrences were found without evidence of immunologic response.

Rheumatic recurrences, therefore, are most likely to occur within the first several years of the rheumatic attack in those with rheumatic heart disease who are exposed to virulent streptococcal pharyngitis (Table 81–2). In the past 20 years, a remarkable decline has occurred in the frequency of rheumatic recurrences as well as in the incidence of first attacks as streptococcal pharyngitis has moderated and as streptococcal pharyngeal strains have changed in the prevalence of rheumatogenic epidemic types.[38]

The natural history of rheumatic fever is now fairly predictable once an initial rheumatic attack has abated, and a period of convalescence enables an assessment of the degree of healing of carditis. If cardiac healing is complete, prevention of recurrences should guarantee freedom from rheumatic heart disease. Persistent mild mitral regurgitation, although usually quite compatible with normal longevity if recurrences and infective en-

docarditis are prevented, must be observed continuously because of the small but significant group of patients, predominantly women, in whom mitral stenosis evolves despite careful, continuous antistreptococcal prophylaxis.[58]

TREATMENT AND MANAGEMENT

General. The manifestations and severity of the rheumatic attack will determine to a large extent the management of a given patient. In general, however, rheumatic fever is unpredictable at the onset of the attack, and patients should be put to bed for the duration of the acute, febrile phase of the illness until clinical and laboratory evidence of inflammation abates.

The administration of anti-inflammatory medicines should be withheld until the disease process is clearly expressed in order to establish the diagnosis and avoid confusion. Furthermore, in isolated polyarthritis a therapeutic trial of penicillin may be essential to eliminate the diagnosis of septic arthritis, especially of disseminated gonococcal disease in adolescents and young adults. Prompt therapeutic response to penicillin strongly suggests gonococcal polyarthritis rather than rheumatic fever. If pain must be controlled, codeine or meperidine is effective and will not mask inflammation.

Once the diagnosis is established, treatment is started with the completion of a course of penicillin adequate to eradicate pharyngeal carriage of group A streptococci. Massive penicillin therapy will not alter the course of the disease or the frequency or severity of cardiac involvement.[59] The usual penicillin regimen recommended

Table 81–2. Ratio of Rheumatic Recurrences to Streptococcal Infections in Patients Stratified for Heart Disease and for ASO Rise*

ASO Rise, in Tube Dilutions	Heart Disease	No Heart Disease
0–1	3/24 (13 %)	1/72 (1 %)
2	10/36 (28 %)	2/46 (4 %)
3	6/16 (37 %)	4/32 (13 %)
4	9/14 (65 %)	9/25 (36 %)

*From Taranta, A., et al.: Ann. Intern. Med. 60(Suppl. 5):47, 1964.

for the optimal treatment of streptococcal pharyngitis (see below) will suffice. A regimen for secondary prophylaxis, such as a monthly injection of benzathine penicillin G, should be selected and instituted along with thorough education of the patient and family concerning the importance of compliance with the program. Prophylaxis should not be delayed because the hospital environment itself may provide a high risk of streptococcal exposure. Prophylaxis during hospitalization offers the opportunity to determine tolerance of the regimen as well as education concerning its importance.

Antirheumatic Therapy. The selection of an antirheumatic agent is not critical to the outcome of most attacks of rheumatic fever. Several controlled studies have failed to show a superiority of corticosteroids over salicylates with regard to alteration of the course of the attack or prevention of cardiac stigmata.[57,58,60] These studies have been critically reviewed in detail.[7,23] Corticosteroids and salicylates can be regarded as useful symptomatic and supportive therapeutic agents, but they are not curative and may actually prolong the course of the attack. Nonetheless, they control the toxic manifestations of the disease, contribute to the comfort of the patient, and combat constitutional symptoms. In severe heart failure from rheumatic carditis, some authorities believe that such nonspecific anti-inflammatory effects may reduce the burden upon the laboring heart and occasionally may tilt the balance in favor of the survival of the critically ill patient, but such opinions are more anecdotal than established by firm data. Corticosteroids are more potent than salicylates in suppressing acute exudative inflammation, and some patients in whom salicylates fail to control the disease respond quickly to relatively large doses of corticosteroids. The effect of such doses on the course of chronic rheumatic carditis is disappointing, however, and their use in early cases of acute carditis has not been proved to decrease residual heart disease. Prolonged use of large doses of corticosteroids beyond the period of time required to control the acute manifestations is not justified.

Patients with mild arthritis or arthralgias and no carditis may be treated with analgesics only, such as codeine, as needed. This choice has two advantages: (1) the diagnosis may be established with greater certainty by a more characteristic arthritis when symptoms and signs are borderline, and (2) the course of the attack will not be prolonged by "rebounds." Most patients, however, who have frank arthritis and no evidence of carditis may be given salicylates initially as a therapeutic trial for the diagnosis of rheumatic polyarthritis because of the consistency (but not specificity) of the response to them in patients with this manifestation. Patients with mild carditis are usually given corticosteroids but without conviction that they are superior to salicylates. Patients with severe carditis are usually treated promptly with corticosteroids, particularly if heart failure is evident, and with the precaution of adequate doses of diuretics and restriction of salt intake to combat sodium retention.

Since neither corticosteroids nor salicylates or other aspirin-like compounds shorten the course of rheumatic fever, the duration of therapy must be estimated to cover the expected course of the attack. Approximately 75 to 80 percent of attacks of acute rheumatic fever subside within 6 weeks; 90 percent are over in 12 weeks; and 5 percent persist for 6 months or more. In mild attacks, therefore, one may plan a 4-week course of treatment and taper off the dose of antirheumatic drugs during the ensuing 2 weeks. It is important to taper off therapy gradually and to recognize particularly that when corticosteroids are withdrawn too abruptly, the patient will be left in a state of temporary adrenal insufficiency, making a relapse of the disease, if severe, potentially dangerous. When treatment with corticosteroids has been prolonged, their gradual withdrawal may be followed or overlapped by administration of salicylates for several weeks or months to assure suppression of inflammation until adrenocortical function is recovered.

Salicylate Therapy. An initial dose of 6 to 9 grams of acetylsalicylic acid per day is administered to patients weighing 70 kg or more, and proportionately smaller doses may be initiated in patients weighing less, but dosage should be adjusted by response more than by weight. The dose may be divided into 4- or 6-hour intervals and given until symptoms and signs of arthritis have disappeared and the temperature has returned to normal. Thereafter, the dose is decreased by one third and maintained until laboratory manifestations of inflammation have returned to normal. Subsequently, the dose may be cut back to half the starting dose for the remainder of the course of therapy. Should clinical or laboratory signs of relapse occur when doses are reduced, it is advisable to return to the previous controlling dose.

Corticosteroids. Arbitrary dosages of corticosteroids are not recommended, but a generally accepted procedure is to begin with relatively large doses of prednisone until the activity of the disease comes under control and then to reduce the dose to that level which will maintain a full suppressive effect. Thus, an initial dose of 40 to 60 mg per day in divided doses for both adults and children alike may be started and varied according to the patient's response. With other analogues of cortisol, such as triamcinolone or dexamethasone, the dose is based on their potency relative to prednisone.

Rebounds. "Rebounds" of rheumatic activity may reappear when suppressive therapy is discontinued. Such spontaneous rebounds do not occur more than 5 or 6 weeks after stopping suppressive treatment, and the great majority occur within a couple of weeks or less.

Chorea. Treatment of chorea requires special consideration because the antirheumatic agents do not directly suppress choreiform activity. However, toxic rheumatic symptoms may aggravate the process indirectly, and constitutional and other manifestations should be controlled, preferably with salicylates rather than corticosteroids. A quiet environment, understanding attendants, and an optimistic attitude should be provided the emotionally labile patient with chorea, and protection from self-injury by involuntary movements should

be ensured. Phenobarbital or tranquilizers such as chlorpromazine or diazepam, especially the latter, are useful.[61]
Haloperidol has been recommended but should be used
cautiously because toxic reactions in children have been
reported.[62] One should bear in mind that chorea
disappears completely during sleep and is easily exacerbated by excitement and that none of the psycho-
pharmacologic agents are specific for choreiform activity.

Rheumatic Carditis. Treatment of rheumatic carditis,
aside from the antirheumatic agents, is similar to that
of other forms of myocarditis. Some patients with severe
rheumatic myocarditis are inordinately sensitive to digitalis preparations, and caution is required in their use.
In most cases, however, the judicious use of digitalis is
effective treatment for heart failure of most patients
except in the most severe and protracted forms of the
disease.

Regulation of Physical Activity. All patients should
be kept in bed for the first 3 weeks of illness when
carditis will usually appear if it is going to do so at all.
Bathroom privileges and some rest in a chair may be
permitted unless arthritis or chorea is uncontrolled or
carditis is associated with cardiomegaly, tachycardia, or
incipient or frank heart failure. Following appraisal of
the course of the first 3 weeks, the degree of bed rest
should be tailored to the manifestations of the disease
and their intensity.

PREVENTION OF RHEUMATIC FEVER

The almost total absence of rheumatic fever in the
affluent sections of the cities of the western world suggests that spacious housing and noncrowding are at least
as important as good diagnosis and treatment of streptococcal sore throat in the prevention of rheumatic attacks. Nonetheless, the natural history of rheumatic
fever can be dramatically altered by the use of antimicrobials. Epidemics of streptococcal pharyngitis can be
terminated by mass penicillin prophylaxis. Proper therapy of streptococcal sore throat can abort initial attacks,
and continuous administration of appropriate antibiotics
will completely prevent recurrent attacks in rheumatic
subjects.

Secondary prophylaxis is the term used to describe
protection against rheumatic recurrences by continuous
antistreptococcal prophylaxis. Limiting prophylaxis of
recurrences to the treament of overt streptococcal infections in rheumatic subjects is hazardous, since many
such infections that reactivate rheumatic fever are subclinical. Furthermore, in contrast to the prevention of
an initial attack, it is difficult to abort a recurrence by
administering penicillin after a streptococcal sore throat
is already symptomatic.

The most effective form of continuous prophylaxis is
a single monthly injection of 1.2 million units of benzathine penicillin G.[63] Using this form of prophylaxis,
an attack rate of less than 1 recurrence per 250 patient-
years was documented in the extensive studies by the

Irvington House group[64,65] (Table 81–3). This method
circumvents the vagaries of gastrointestinal absorption
of penicillin and does not require the daily fidelity to
an oral regimen. It imposes closer surveillance upon the
patient by the managing physician. Streptococcal infections rarely occur within the first 3 weeks after the
intramuscular injection of benzathine penicillin, and
when they occur after this period the subsequent injection at 4 weeks usually serves as adequate therapy of
the infection and aborts the attack. Although the reaction rate is somewhat higher for all injectable forms
of penicillin compared with oral penicillin, reactions are
very rare after the first months of continuous prophylaxis. Furthermore, when penicillin hypersensitivity occurs it is no more severe or protracted than reactions
to other forms of parenteral penicillin. In patients who
are at highest risk to develop recurrences, especially
those with rheumatic heart disease, with recent rheumatic fever, and in a challenging environment for streptococcal exposure, monthly injections of benzathine
penicillin are undoubtly the preferred form of prophylaxis. In affluent societies and in countries in which
rheumatic fever has become very rare[66] it is unlikely that
this form of prophylaxis will be preferred by the average
managing physician except when the major risk factors
of recurrences coexist: severity of rheumatic heart disease, recency of previous attack, and exposure to streptococcal pharyngitis in locales where rheumatic fever
still occurs.

Oral prophylaxis is less reliable than repository penicillin prophylaxis. Daily doses of either sulfadiazine or
buffered penicillin G are effective, however, and should
be employed wherever the requirement for prophylaxis
is less stringent or the intramuscular form is not acceptable or feasible. The recommended dose of oral sulfadiazine is 0.5 gram once daily for patients weighing
less than 27 kg (60 lbs) and 1 gram daily for heavier
patients. Penicillin G by mouth may be given in doses
of 200,000 to 250,000 units daily. Even when oral penicillin is administered twice daily, no superiority over
sulfadiazine has been demonstrated in the prevention of
recurrences.[67]

Reaction rates are low with both oral medications
and are very rare after the first few months of prophylaxis. Group A streptococci resistant to these agents
have not appeared. For the rare patient who is sensitive
to both penicillin and sulfonamides, erythromycin may
be substituted in a dose of 250 mg twice daily.

It has been difficult to make a single arbitrary recommendation concerning the duration for which continuous prophylaxis must be maintained in all rheumatic
subjects because of the large number of variables that
influence the attack rate of recurrences following streptococcal infections (see above). Exceptions to maintaining prophylaxis should be made in adults only, and then
after assessing carefully the risk of exposure to streptococcal infection in communities in which rheumatic
fever still persists. Patients with significant rheumatic
heart disease, a history of repeated recurrences, or a
recent attack at any age require most careful consider-

Table 81–3. Prophylaxis and Attack Rates of Streptococcal Infection and Rheumatic Fever Recurrences on Three Prophylactic Regimens*

	Parenteral Benzathine Penicillin	Oral Penicillin	Oral Sulfadiazine	All Drugs
Number of patient-years	560	545	576	1681
Number and rate of all streptococcal infections	34(6.1)†	113(20.7)	138(24.0)	284(17.0)
Number and rate of all streptcoccal infections, exclusive of carrier state	24(4.3)	101(18.5)	102(17.7)	227(13.5)
Number and rate of rheumatic recurrences	2(0.4)	30(5.5)	16(2.8)	48(2.9)

*From Wood, H.F., et al.: Ann. Intern. Med. 60(Suppl. 5):6, 1964.
†Rates listed in parentheses are number per 100 patient-years.

ation before discontinuing prophylaxis, a decision that is still to be regarded as a calculated risk.

Primary prophylaxis is the term applied to the prevention of first rheumatic attacks by prompt treatment of the antecedent streptococcal infection. In classic studies in military populations, penicillin therapy of streptococcal pharyngitis causing high attack rates of rheumatic fever reduced the rate from 3 to 0.3 percent.[8] It has been more difficult to apply primary prevention to civilian populations, particularly children with sporadic or endemic streptococcal pharyngitis. Such infections are difficult to differentiate from viral pharyngitis in children who carry group A streptococci from previous streptococcal exposure (see above). Frequent, mild streptococcal exposure in this age group tends to keep streptococcal antibody titers elevated. *Throat cultures are particularly useful when they are negative in eliminating the need for intensive penicillin therapy.* When cultures are positive for group A organisms, however, the diagnosis of a current streptococcal infection may not be certain but it is still difficult to withhold therapy, particularly if pharyngeal exudate and/or tender anterior cervical nodes are present.

Effective therapy, that is, treatment adequate to prevent rheumatic fever, requires eradication of the infecting organisms rather than clinical improvement alone. To accomplish this end, penicillin must be at effective levels for 10 days. Many patients fail to extend oral therapy for 10 days because symptoms abate within a day or two. A single injection of benzathine penicillin G intramuscularly has long been known to be the most effective regimen.[63] The recommended dose is 600,000 units in children weighing less than 27 kg (60 lbs) and 1.2 million units in those who are heavier. Intramuscular benzathine penicillin G is no longer used extensively in populations in which rheumatic fever has virtually disappeared. It is still the treatment of choice, however, for those populations in which the disease is still a serious problem, (e.g., many of the "Third World" countries). If given orally, penicillin G is recommended in doses of 200,000 to 250,000 units three to four times daily. For those sensitive to penicillin, erythromycin may be substituted in doses of 250 mg four times daily or 40 mg per kil-

ogram per day in younger children. Sulfonamides, although effective in *prevention* of streptococcal infections, are not indicated for *treatment* of an established streptococcal sore throat because they do not eradicate carriage and do no prevent initial rheumatic attacks.

Bacteriologic relapse may occur in approximately 10 percent of patients adequately treated and occurs more frequently in those treated orally. Group A streptococci are more difficult to eradicate in chronic carriers than in patients with acute infection. Strains isolated from convalescent carriers tend to lose virulence as denoted by loss of M-protein typability. Individuals who harbor the same strain of streptococcus for more than a month are not likely to develop complications or to spread infection.

Mass penicillin prophylaxis is effective in populations in which streptococcal pharyngitis is epidemic. This approach is indicated in civilian or institutional epidemics only if one or more cases of rheumatic fever have occurred within a period of a week or two. Mass administration of 1.2 million units of benzathine penicillin G intramuscularly to all members of the affected population has been brilliantly effective.[2]

Recent studies have suggested that it may be possible to induce protective antibodies with small doses of purified streptococcal M protein. The M proteins of several serotypes have been purified recently to molecular homogeneity and are antigenic in laboratory animals and in humans.[68-70] Their potential for the preparation of streptococcal vaccines has been reviewed.[70] In an era in which rheumatic fever is rapidly declining or completely disappearing in some countries,[71] general recommendations for the treatment of common sore throat and for the prevention of rheumatic recurrences will have to be reassessed and may have to be tailored to particular patients and to particular populations.[72]

References

1. Zagala, J.G., and Feinstein, A.R.: The preceding illness of acute rheumatic fever. JAMA 179:863, 1962.
2. Frank, P.F., Stollerman, G.H., and Miller, L.F.: Protection of a military population from rheumatic fever. JAMA 193:775, 1965.
3. Rammelkamp, C.H., Jr.: Epidemiology of streptococcal infections. Harvey Lect. Series 51:113, 1955–56.

4. Stollerman, G.H.: The epidemiology of primary and secondary rheumatic fever. *In* Uhr, J.W. (ed.): The Streptococcus, Rheumatic Fever and Glomerulonephritis. Baltimore, Williams & Wilkins Company, 1964, pp. 311–337.

5. Stetson, C.A.: The relation of antibody response to rheumatic fever. *In* McCarty, M. (ed.): Streptococcal Infections. New York, Columbia University Press, 1954, pp. 208–218.

6. Taranta, A.: Rheumatic fever in children and adolescents. IV. Relation of the rheumatic fever recurrence rate per streptococcal infection to the titers of streptococcal antibodies. Ann. Intern. Med. 50 (Suppl. 5):47, 1964.

7. Stollerman, G.H.: Rheumatic Fever and Streptococcal Infection. New York, Grune & Stratton, 1975.

8. Wannamaker, L.W., Rammelkamp, C.H., Jr., Denny, F.W., Brink, W.R., Houser, H.B., Hahn, E.O., and Dingle, J.H.: Prophylaxis of acute rheumatic fever by treatment of the preceding streptococcal infection with various amounts of depot penicillin. Am. J. Med. 10:673, 1951.

9. Wannamaker, L.W.: The chain that links the heart to the throat. Circulation 48:9, 1973.

10. Stollerman, G.H.: The relative rheumatogenicity of strains of group A streptococci. Mod. Concepts Cardiovasc. Dis. 44:35, 1975.

11. Watson, R.F., Hirst, G.K., and Lancefield, R.C.: Bacteriological studies of cardiac tissues obtained at autopsy from eleven patients dying with rheumatic fever. Arthritis Rheum. 4:74, 1961.

12. Kaplan, M.H., Meyeserian, M., and Kushner, I.: Immunologic studies of heart tissue. IV. Serologic reactions with human heart tissue as revealed by immunofluorescent methods: Isoimmune, Wassermann, and autoimmune reactions. J. Exp. Med. 113:17, 1961.

13. Kaplan, M.H.: Immunologic relation of streptococcal and tissue antigens. I. Properties of an antigen in certain strains of group A streptococci exhibiting an immunologic cross reaction with human heart tissue. J. Immunol. 90:595, 1963.

14. Kaplan, M.H., and Suchy, M.L.: Immunologic relation of streptococcal and tissue antigens. II. Cross reactions of antisera to mammalian heart tissue with a cell wall constituent of certain strains of group A streptococci. J. Exp. Med. 119:643, 1964.

15. Zabriskie, J.B., and Freimer, E.H.: An immunological relationship between the group A streptococcus and mammalian muscle. J. Exp. Med. 124:661, 1966.

16. van de Rijn, I., Zabriskie, J.B., and McCarty, M.: Group A streptococcal antigens cross-reactive with myocardium. Purification of heart-reactive antibody and isolation and characterization of the streptococcal antigen. J. Exp. Med. 146:579, 1977.

17. Husby, G., van de Rijn, I., Zabriskie, J.B., Abdin, Z.H., and Williams, R.C.: Antibodies reacting with cytoplasm of subthalamic and caudate nuclei neurons in chorea and acute rheumatic fever. J. Exp. Med. 144:1094, 1976.

18. Ayoub, E.M., Taranta, A., and Bartley, T.D.: Effect of valvular surgery on antibody to the group A streptococcal carbohydrate. Circulation 50:144, 1974.

19. Taranta, A., Torosdag, S., Metrakos, J., Jegier, W., and Uchida, I.: Rheumatic fever in monozygotic and dizygotic twins. *In* Proceedings, Xth International Congress of Rheumatology, Torino, Minerva Medica, 1961, pp. 96–98.

20. Greenberg, L.J., Gray, E.D., and Yunis, E.J.: Association of HL-A 5 and immune responsiveness in vitro to streptococcal antigens. J. Exp. Med. 141:935, 1975.

21. Stollerman, G.H.: Hypersensitivity and antibody responses in streptococcal disease. *In* Wannamaker, L.W., and Matsen, J.M. (eds.): Streptococci and Streptococcal Diseases. Recognition, Understanding and Management. New York, Academic Press, 1972, pp. 501–513.

22. Kuhns, W.J., and McCarty, M.: Studies of diphtheria antitoxin in rheumatic fever subjects. Analysis of reactions to the Schick test and of antitoxin responses following hyperimmunization with diphtheria toxoid. J. Clin. Invest. 33:759, 1954.

23. Markowitz, M., and Gordis, L.: Rheumatic Fever. 2nd ed. Philadelphia, W. B. Saunders Company, 1972.

24. Stamler, J.: Cardiovascular diseases in the United States. Am. J. Cardiol. 10:319, 1962.

25. Smith, J.M., Stamler, J., Miller, R.A., Paul, M.H., Abrams, I., Restivo, R.M., and DeBoer, L.: The detection of heart disease in children. Results of mass field trials with use of tape-recorded heart sounds. III. The Chicago area high school study. Circulation 32:956, 1965.

26. Miller, R.A., Stamler, J., Smith, J.M., Milne, W.S., Paul, M.H., Abrams, I., Hastreiter, A.R., Restivo, R.M., and DeBoer, L.: The detection of heart disease in children. Results of mass field trials with use of tape-recorded heart sounds. II. The Michigan City Study. Circulation 32:956, 1965.

27. Rammelkamp, C.H., Denny, F.W., and Wannamaker, L.W.: Studies on the epidemiology of rheumatic fever in the armed services. *In* Thomas, L. (ed.): Rheumatic Fever. Minneapolis, University of Minnesota Press, 1952, pp. 72–89.

28. Rammelkamp, C.H., Jr.: The Lewis A. Conner Memorial Lecture. Rheumatic heart disease—a challenge. Circulation 17:842, 1958.

29. Siegel, A.C., Johnson, E.E., and Stollerman, G.H.: Controlled studies of streptococcal pharyngitis in a pediatric population. I. Factors related to the attack rate of rheumatic fever. N. Engl. J. Med. 265:559, 1961.

30. Kaplan, E.L., Top, F.H., Dudding, B.A., and Wannamaker, L.W.: Diagnosis of streptococcal pharyngitis: Differentiation of active infection from the carrier state in the symptomatic child. J. Infect. Dis. 123:490, 1971.

31. Stollerman, G.H., Siegel, A.C., and Johnson, E.E.: Variable epidemiology of streptococcal disease and the changing pattern of rheumatic fever. Mod. Concepts Cardiovasc. Dis. 34:45, 1965.

32. Top, F.H., Wannamaker, L.W., Maxted, W.R., and Anthony, G.V.: M antigens among group A streptococci isolated from skin lesions. J. Exp. Med. 126:667, 1967.

33. Wannamaker, L.W.: Medical progress. Differences between streptococcal infections of the throat and of the skin. N. Engl. J. Med. 282:23, 78, 1970.

34. Stollerman, G.H.: Nephritogenic and rheumatogenic group A streptococci. J. Infect. Dis. 120:258, 1969.

35. Bisno, A.L., Pearce, I.A., Wall, H.P., Moody, M.D., and Stollerman, G.H.: Contrasting epidemiology of acute rheumatic fever and acute glomerulonephritis. Nature of the antecedent streptococcal infection. N. Engl. J. Med. 283:561, 1970.

36. Potter, E.V., Svartman, M., Poon-King, T., and Earle, D.P.: The families of patients with acute rheumatic fever or glomerulonephritis in Trinidad. Am. J. Epidemiol. 106:130, 1977.

37. Widdowson, J.P., Maxted, W.R., Notley, C.M., and Pinney, A.M.: The antibody responses in man to infection with different serotypes of group A streptococci. J. Med. Microbiol. 7:483, 1974.

38. Bisno, A.L., Pearce, I.A., and Stollerman, G.H.: Streptococcal infections which fail to cause recurrences of rheumatic fever. J. Infect. Dis. 136:278, 1977.

39. Stollerman, G.H.: The streptococcus, rheumatic fever and rheumatic heart disease. *In* Shaper, A.G., Hutt, M.S.R., and Fejfar, Z. (eds.): Cardiovascular Disease in the Tropics. London, British Medical Associates, 1974.

40. Sanyal, S.K., Thapar, M.D., Ahmed, S.H., Hooja, V., and Tewari, P.: The initial attack of acute rheumatic fever during childhood in North India. A prospective study of the clinical profile. Circulation 49:7, 1974.

41. Taranta, A., Kleinberg, E., Feinstein, A.R., Wood, H.F., Tursky, E., and Simpson, R.: Rheumatic fever in children and adolescents. A long-term epidemiologic study of subsequent prophylaxis, streptococcal infections, and clinical sequelae. V. Relation of the rheumatic fever recurrence rate per streptococcal infection to pre-existing clinical features of the patients. Ann. Intern. Med. 60 (Suppl. 5):58, 1964.

42. Johnson, E.E., Stollerman, G.H., and Grossman, B.J.: Rheumatic recurrences in patients not receiving continuous prophylaxis. JAMA 190:407, 1964.

43. Murphy, G.E.: Nature of rheumatic heart disease with special reference to myocardial disease and heart failure. Medicine 39:289, 1960.

44. Pienaar, J.G., and Price, H.M.: Ultrastructure and origin of the Antischkow cell. Am. J. Pathol. 51:1063, 1967.

45. Hutchins, G.N., and Payne, K.T.: Possible origin of myocardial Aschoff bodies of rheumatic fever from nerves. Johns Hopkins Med. J. 132:315, 1973.

46. Virmani, R., and Roberts, W.C.: Aschoff bodies in operatively excised atrial appendages and in papillary muscles. Frequency and clinical significance. Circulation 55:559, 1977.

47. Steele, P.P., Weily, H.S., Davies, H., and Genton, E.: Platelet survival in patients with rheumatic heart disease. N. Engl. J. Med. 290:537, 1974.

48. Buchanan, D.N.: Pathologic changes in chorea. Am. J. Dis. Child. 62:443, 1941.

49. Zvaifler, N.J.: Chronic postrheumatic-fever (Jaccoud's) arthritis. N. Engl. J. Med. 267:10, 1962.

50. Meyers, O.L., and Chalmers, I.M.: Jaccoud's arthropathy. Report of seven cases. S. Afr. Med. J. 51:753, 1977.

51. Taranta, A., and Stollerman, G.H.: The relationship of Sydenham's chorea to infection with group A streptococci. Am. J. Med. 20:170, 1956.

52. Goldring, D., Behrer, M.R., Brown, G., and Elliott, G.: Rheumatic pneumonitis. Part II. Report on the clinical and laboratory findings in twenty-three patients. J. Pediatr. 53:547, 1958.

53. Bisno, A.L., and Stollerman, G.H.: Streptococcal antibodies in the diagnosis of rheumatic fever. *In* Cohen, A.S. (ed.): Laboratory Diagnostic Procedures in the Rheumatic Diseases. 2nd ed. Boston, Little, Brown & Company, 1974.

54. Bisno, A.L., and Ofek, I.: Serologic diagnosis of streptococcal infection. Comparison of a rapid hemagglutination technique with conventional antibody tests. Am. J. Dis. Child. 127:676, 1974.

55. Jones criteria (revised) for guidance in the diagnosis of rheumatic fever. Circulation 32:664, 1965.

56. Stollerman, G.H., Lewis, A.J., Schultz, I., and Taranta, A.: Relationship

of immune response to group A streptococci to the course of acute, chronic and recurrent rheumatic fever. Am. J. Med. 20:163, 1956.

57. United Kingdom and United States Joint Report on Rheumatic Heart Disease: The evolution of rheumatic heart disease in children. Five-year report of a cooperative clinical trial of ACTH, cortisone and aspirin. Circulation 22:503, 1960.

58. United Kingdom and United States Joint Report on Rheumatic Heart Disease: The natural history of rheumatic fever and rheumatic heart disease. Ten-year report of a cooperative clinical trial of ACTH, cortisone and aspirin. Circulation 32:457, 1965.

59. Vaisman, S., Guasch, J., Vignau, A., Correa, E., Schuster, A., Mortimer, E.A., Jr., and Rammelkamp, C.H., Jr.: The failure of penicillin to alter acute rheumatic vasculitis. JAMA 194:1284, 1965.

60. Combined Rheumatic Fever Study Group, 1965: A comparison of the short-term, intensive prednisone and acetylsalicylic acid therapy in the treatment of acute rheumatic fever. N. Engl. J. Med. 272:63, 1965.

61. Lockman, L.A.: Movement disorders. In Swaiman, K., and Wright, F. (eds): Practice of Pediatric Neurology. St. Louis, C. V. Mosby Company, 1975.

62. Shields, W.D., and Bray, P.F.: A danger of haloperidol therapy in children. J. Pediatr. 88:301, 1976.

63. AHA Committee on Rheumatic Fever and Bacterial Endocarditis: Prevention of rheumatic fever. Circulation 55:1, 1977.

64. Stollerman, G.H., Rusoff, J.H., and Hirschfeld, I.: Prophylaxis against group A streptococci in rheumatic fever. The use of single monthly injections of benzathine penicillin G. N. Engl. J. Med. 252:787, 1955.

65. Albam, B., Epstein, J.A., Feinstein, A.R., Gavrin, J.B., Jonas, S., Kleinberg, E., Simpson, R., Spagnuolo, M., Stollerman, G.H., Taranta, A., Tursky, E., and Wood, H.F.: Rheumatic fever in children and adolescents. A long-term epidemiologic study of subsequent prophylaxis, streptococcal infections, and clinical sequelae. Ann. Intern. Med. 60 (Suppl. 5): No. 2, Part II, 1964.

66. Land, M.A., and Bisno, A.L.: Acute rheumatic fever: A vanishing disease in suburbia. JAMA 249:895, 1983.

67. Feinstein, A.R., Wood, H.F., Spagnuolo, M., Taranta, A., Tursky, E., and Kleinberg, E.: Oral prophylaxis of recurrent rheumatic fever: Sulfadiazine vs. a double daily dose of penicillin. JAMA 188:489, 1964.

68. Beachey, E.H., Stollerman, G.H., Johnson, R.H., et al.: Human immune response to immunization with a structurally defined polypeptide fragment of streptococcal M protein. J. Exp. Med. 150:862, 1979.

69. Hasty, D.L., Beachey, E.H., Simpson, W.A., et al.: Hybridoma antibodies against protective and nonprotective antigenic determinants of a structurally defined polypeptide fragment of streptococcal M protein. J. Exp. Med. 155:1010, 1982.

70. Stollerman, G.H.: Global changes in group A streptococcal diseases and strategies for their prevention. Adv. Intern. Med. 27:373, 1982.

71. Stollerman, G.H.: Global strategies for the control of rheumatic fever. JAMA 249:931, 1983.

72. Shulman, S.T. (ed.): Pharyngitis: Management in an Era of Declining Rheumatic Fever. New York, Praeger, 1984.

Chapter 82

Systemic Lupus Erythematosus, Dermatomyositis, Scleroderma, and Vasculitides in Childhood

Virgil Hanson

INTRODUCTION

The spectrum of rheumatic disease in childhood is broad and includes the diseases that are the subject of this chapter. Both arthralgia and a true inflammatory synovitis may accompany any of the conditions described herein, but a more significant common thread is the vascular disease, usually of an inflammatory nature, found in all. Another common thread is the participation of immunologic mechanisms in their pathogenesis. In the aggregate, systemic lupus erythematosus (SLE), dermatomyositis, scleroderma, and the vasculitides are not rare in children and constitute a significant segment of childhood disease. The diseases are similar in adult and child, but there are sometimes major and sometimes subtle differences which are worthy of consideration. Systematic study of these conditions in children has really only just begun and may well yield new clues to our understanding of these often crippling and sometimes fatal disorders. Immaturity differs physiologically from maturity, and children have, for example, a highly proliferative lymphoreticular system which matures and involutes in the adolescent years and a far less complex history of antigenic exposure than that acquired

by adulthood. Maturity of gonadal function is another factor which seems to modify the expression of these diseases, as can be seen in some of the studies summarized here. In order to minimize duplication of effort, the clinical descriptions of the subject diseases in children are emphasized in this chapter with brief references to pertinent aspects of laboratory testing, pathology, treatment, and concepts of pathogenesis. These latter topics have been dealt with in detail in previous chapters, and the reader should consult these freely to gain a broader understanding of them.

SYSTEMIC LUPUS ERYTHEMATOSUS (SLE)

Clinical Considerations. Systemic lupus erythematosus (SLE) in childhood as in adult life is a multisystem disease with diverse and varied manifestations associated with antibodies to nuclear antigens in the serum. The most common presenting signs of SLE in children are fever, arthralgia, arthritis, and rash. Joint disease may be migratory or rheumatoid-like but does not result in deformity of bones or joints. The rashes of SLE in children are markedly varied in character and in distribution, and have been described as morbilliform, purpuric, bullous, ulcerative, and nodose, as well as the usual maculopapular erythematous eruptions.[1,2] Angiitic lesions on the palms and soles are not uncommon. The classic butterfly rash is evident on the face in about one third of the children at the time of diagnosis.[1] (Fig. 82–1).

Approximately 60 percent of children have laboratory evidence of renal disease at the time of diagnosis.[1] Some degree of renal involvement is probably present in all cases, but urinary changes and other laboratory signs of renal disease may be transient or may not appear for many years after onset (as long as 11 years after diagnosis in one patient reported by Meislin and Rothfield).[2] In two earlier reports 27 children had been studied at autopsy, and the histologic changes of lupus nephritis were found in six of these who had had no laboratory evidence of renal involvement during life.[3,4]

In many children the presenting symptoms and signs of SLE may be referable to organ systems other than skin, joints, or kidneys, and it may appear at first that only a single organ system is involved. Manifestations such as pleural effusion, pulmonary infiltrates, pericarditis, thrombocytopenia, abdominal pain, and convulsions or other neurologic manifestations may all be presenting signs of the disease. Lymphadenopathy and hepatosplenomegaly, particularly during the early stages, are more prominent and common in children than in adults.[1] An unusual presentation was reported by Walravens and Chase in two children who had recurrent parotid swelling as the first sign of their disease.[5] A list of the organ systems involved at the time of diagnosis in one large study is shown in Table 82–1.[1]

In a disease with such protean manifestations some guidelines or criteria are essential to define the disease for diagnostic purposes. Revised criteria for the diagnosis of SLE have been prepared by the Subcommittee on Diagnostic Criteria for Systemic Lupus Erythematosus of The American Rheumatism Association, and are shown in Chapter 69. Inclusion of any 4 of 11 listed criteria constitute the minimum requirements for the diagnosis of SLE. These criteria are as applicable to SLE in children as in adults.

SLE may occur at any age in childhood from infancy onward, but the incidence is very low under 5 or 6 years of age and rises markedly as adolescence is approached. In the second decade of life the incidence is almost as high as in any subsequent decade.[6]

The disease occurs predominantly in female children with a ratio of approximately five females to one male, but in our study of 108 children with SLE there was a significantly greater percentage of males in the children less than 12 years of age at onset.[1] Wallace and associates also reported a significantly greater percentage of males among preadolescent children.[7] Eleven studies of childhood SLE published during the last 20 years included 443 children and adolescents with onset under 18 years of age, almost all below the age of 15[1-3,5,7-14] (Table 82–2). Eighty (18.1 percent) of the 443 were male, which is a significantly higher percentage of males than the 10.9 percent reported by Dubois in a population of 520 patients of all ages at onset.[6] The data are consistent with the increasing experimental evidence that both female gender and ovarian function favor the development of SLE.[14,16]

Table 82–1. Major Systems Involved in 108 Children with SLE*

System Involvement	Percent of Patients Affected Between Onset and Diagnosis (Before Treatment)	Percent of Patients Affected After Diagnosis and Treatment (Years 1-2-5-10 and Last Visit)
Joints: Arthritis and/ or arthralgia	78.7	34.2
Cutaneous	70.4	44.4
Renal	61.1	60.2
Hematopoietic†	46.3	25.0
Lymphadenopathy	38.9	8.3
Hepatosplenomegaly	27.8	12.0
Palatal exanthem	21.3	13.0
Pulmonary	19.4	13.0
Gastrointestinal	18.5	11.1
Cardiac	16.7	16.7
Central nervous system	13.0	18.5

*From King, K.K., et al.: Arthritis Rheum. 20:287, 1977. Courtesy of the Arthritis Foundation.
†Excluding anemia and leukopenia.

Figure 82–1. Eight-year-old boy with erythematous butterfly rash of SLE. (From Kornreich, H.K.: Clin. Rheum. Dis. 2:249, 1976.)

Table 82–2. SLE in Children: Variations in Reported Sex Distribution

Study	Number of Patients	Percent Male	Percent Female
Peterson et al.[8]	22	5	95
Gribetz and Henley[9]	15	7	93
Cook et al.[3]	37	9	91
Hagge et al.[10]	41	10	90
King et al.[1]	108	17	83
Meislin and Rothfield[2]	42	19	81
Cassidy et al.[11]	58	21	79
Robinson and Williams[12]	14	21	79
Wallace et al.[7]	45	24	76
Walravens and Chase[5]	50	28	72
Zetterstrom and Berglund[14]	11	45	55
Total (80 M, 363 F)	443	18	82

Families of children with SLE have an increased incidence of this disease. King and associates found 9 of 108 children to have first degree family members with SLE and 15 of the 108 to have relatives with SLE when aunts and uncles of the probands were included.[1] Five of the 14 children reported by Robinson and Williams were siblings in two families,[12] and in a recent study an increasing number of asymptomatic relatives developed lupus related autoantibodies over a 5 year period.[13] Whether or not the increased prevalence is a result of purely genetic influences or exposure to common environmental pathogens cannot yet be stated. Children with genetic deficiencies of complement components have an increased risk of developing SLE but are probably too rare to account for the noted familial incidence.[17-20]

Infants born to mothers with known SLE have been shown to have placentally transmitted antinuclear antibody in a number of studies.[21-26] The antinuclear antibodies disappear from the serum during the first 4 to 6 months of life, as do other maternal antibodies. The most common manifestation of lupus reported in newborns has been a discoid-like rash on the face, trunk, or extremities. Other infants have had hemolytic anemia, thrombocytopenia, or leukopenia alone or in combination and with or without rash. In some cases the mother has had documented SLE at the time of birth, but in others evidence of maternal SLE was not present until weeks or months later, and in 2 patients no evidence of maternal SLE was reported. Recent reports of congenital heart disease, primarily manifested by complete heart block or endocardial fibroelastosis, in infants born to mothers with SLE are of considerable interest, but again some infants with these findings have been born to mothers with other kinds of autoimmune disease or to those with none at all.[27-30] These clinical findings in the neonate are strongly associated with antibodies to SS-A(Ro) and SS-B(La) in the sera of both mother and newborn, with or without the presence of antinuclear antibodies (ANA).[31-33]

Drugs implicated in the induction of lupus-like syndromes include hydralazine, procainamide, penicillin, isoniazid, diphenylhydantoin, mephenytoin, trimethadione, and ethosuximide. In children the most commonly implicated of these are the four last-named anticonvulsants. Twenty-four cases of SLE in children associated with the administration of these drugs have been described.[34] The most common signs and symptoms were fever, arthritis, and rash; pleural and pericardial involvement was noted in a few. Evidence of renal involvement was reported in seven, with disease progressing to death in three of these. It is possible that seizures may have been the first sign of SLE in some children with severe or persistent disease following the administration of anticonvulsants. Alternatively the anticonvulsants may have acted as a trigger in persons otherwise predisposed. Two studies of children receiving anticonvulsant medication, without evidence of disease other than their seizure disorder, showed approximately 20 percent to have positive tests for ANA in a titer of 1:10 or greater.[34,35] In one report follow-up studies 6 to 12 months after detection of ANA with continued anticonvulsant administration revealed persisting ANA in 70 percent of those positive on the first testing but no clinical evidence of SLE.[34] It would appear therefore that anticonvulsants induce formation of ANA far more commonly than clinical SLE, and that ANA positivity alone is not an indication for stopping anticonvulsant therapy.

Laboratory Findings and Pathology. The laboratory findings and histopathology of SLE in children are essentially the same as those described in Chapter 69, but a few brief comments are indicated here. Antinuclear antibodies detectable by standard immunofluorescent techniques are present in all children with active systemic lupus erythematosus.[36] The patterns of nuclear staining include the homogeneous, speckled, and rim or peripheral fluorescence, and reactions with specific nuclear antigens (nucleohistone, SM antigen, single stranded DNA, native double stranded DNA) are similar to those reported in adults.[37] Antibody to native double stranded DNA is the most specific laboratory finding in the diagnosis of SLE, but is often not detectable at low levels of disease activity.[38] LE cell preparations are positive in 90 percent of the children at some time but are cumbersome to perform and only relatively specific. Elevated immunoglobulin levels (IgG, IgM, and IgA) are found in the majority of children. Leukopenia (WBC less than 5000 per cubic millimeter) is present in only about half the children at the time of the diagnosis, but elevation of the white blood cell count above the normal range is extremely rare except during steroid therapy. IgM rheumatoid factor is present in the serum of 5 to 10 percent of children with SLE, but very high titers should raise the index of suspicion of possible mixed connective tissue disease.[2,38] Circulating anticoagulants are not uncommon and may result in difficult bleeding problems, particularly prolonged menorrhagia. In a long-term study of children with SLE depressed levels of C3 and C4 were found to be as frequently associated with exacerbations of extrarenal involvement as with advancing renal disease, and hence not always an indicator of renal change.[39]

In two patients lupus nephritis progressed slowly but inexorably to chronic renal failure with persisting normal levels of C3 and C4.

One of the most extensive discussions of the histopathology of lupus in childhood appears in the report by Cook and associates in 1960.[3] The pathologic findings in 14 children at necropsy were reviewed in this report. Among the most interesting of these was the description of the vascular lesions. The authors noted that "the single most consistent and widespread pathologic finding was the change in the arteries and arterioles which consisted of hyaline, fibrinoid necrosis of the media, proliferation and swelling of the intima, and varying degrees of periarteriolar inflammation." Changes in the coronary vessels were occasionally associated with acute myocardial damage, forecasting three later reports of myocardial infarction in childhood SLE.[7,40,41]

In the gastrointestinal tract these vascular lesions were thought to lead to areas of erosion and secondary infarction. Thrombotic occlusive arteritis was noted in the liver, spleen, and pancreas. Vascular changes in the kidneys consisted of arteriolar damage characterized by endothelial cell swelling and proliferation and proliferative and hyaline changes in the media. Obliterative periarteritic degenerative lesions of the large muscular arteries were also noted with evidence of occlusion of some of these vessels. In later experience these striking vascular changes have been less prominent, and only the occasional healing damaged artery is generally noted. These facts suggest the possibility that the more intensive treatment of later years may have altered some of the reported vascular involvement.

Cardiac enlargement was common, and Libman-Sacks valvulitis was present in seven patients. Myocardial fibrosis was prominent. In the lungs chronic pneumonia with formation of extensive hyaline membranes and hyaline necrosis in the large and small pulmonary arterial vessels was noted. Plasma cell hyperplasia was found in 10 of the 14 patients in either lymph nodes, spleen, or bone marrow.

In subsequent years increasing use of renal biopsy has helped clarify the histopathology of lupus renal disease. The histologic changes have generally been divided into three principal subtypes: focal or focal-segmental glomerulonephritis, diffuse proliferative lupus nephritis, and membranous lupus nephritis. A fourth category reported as mild glomerulitis by King and associates and as mesangial lupus nephritis by Fish and colleagues has been reported in some studies.[1,42] The last category is the mildest renal lesion but may be an early stage of diffuse proliferative nephritis in some patients. King and associates, in a study of 66 children with SLE who had renal biopsies, found diffuse proliferative nephritis to be the most common histologic subtype. Fish and colleagues found the prevalence of focal glomerulonephritis equal to that of diffuse lupus nephritis. In both studies the incidence of membranous glomerulonephritis was approximately 6 percent. In recent years the predictive value of the histologic subtypes has been increasingly challenged and the newer activity and chronicity indices have been found to be far more valuable indices of future renal function. Of these the chronicity index composed of glomerular sclerosis, fibrous crescents, interstitial fibrosis, and tubular atrophy is the most significant.[43]

Clinical Course and Prognosis. The course of SLE in children treated with corticosteroids is subject to unpredictable remissions and exacerbations, and except for improved survival and decreased morbidity, differs little from the "natural course" of SLE (without steroid therapy), described by Ropes in a study of 72 patients of all ages observed between 1932 and 1963.[44] Seventy percent of these patients had at least one remission lasting a few months to a few years. Approximately 5 to 10 percent of the patients had mild disease manifested by often widely separated remissions and exacerbations without critical episodes. SLE in a second group was characterized by a gradual onset with acute critical episodes early or late in the course of the disease. A third group of patients had acute severe onset with early fatality in many of the cases but also with long-lasting remission in many of the survivors. Signs of renal disease disappeared in 15 of 59 patients with abnormal urinalysis at the time of diagnosis, and the urine remained normal for more than 4 years in six of these.

Our experience in the study of more than 100 children with SLE, nearly all of whom were treated with steroids, includes all the phenomena noted above.[1] Five percent of the children have had mild disease, are asymptomatic most of the time, and have only occasional exacerbations without critical episodes. Even children with severe generalized lupus and marked renal involvement (4+ proteinuria, azotemia, or diffuse lupus nephritis on biopsy) at onset have gone into remissions that have been sustained for many years without corticosteroid or immunosuppressive treatment after the first year. The most common course, however, is characterized by chronic low-grade disease activity punctuated by irregular, often severe, exacerbations in which first one organ system and then another bears the brunt of attack. These episodes are often critical and may result in fatality. Only about one third of deaths in childhood SLE are attributable to lupus-renal disease.[1,2,5] Infection, heart failure, and pulmonary involvement are among the major nonrenal causes of death and serve to underline the significant involvement of other organ systems in SLE. The renal involvement may wax and wane in concert with the exacerbations and remissions but in some cases progresses slowly and asymptomatically irrespective of the occurrence of acute exacerbations, a phenomenon also noted in Ropes' study of the natural course of SLE.

In spite of the fact that contemporary therapy seems not to have altered the basic course of SLE, the reported prognosis for children has improved dramatically within the last 15 to 20 years. The estimated 75 to 80 percent mortality within the first 5 years reported in 1960 has changed to an estimated 75 to 85 percent survival after 10 years of disease in the mid-1970s.[3-5,42] How much of this improved survival can be attributed to treatment with corticosteroids and/or immunosuppressants is uncertain; but it seems likely that this treatment has at least helped the patients survive the life-threatening periods of acute severe disease characteristic of SLE. Other factors, however, must also be considered. Improved general life support in intensive care units, more effective management of hypertension, the availability of hemodialysis for patients with severely impaired renal function, and earlier detection and more effective treatment of infections are all significant elements of treatment that tend to increase survival in most serious illness and are of particular significance in the management of SLE. More frequent diagnosis of mild cases of SLE is probably another factor. Whatever the reason, it is clear that the outlook for children with SLE in 1983 is far more optimistic than 20 years ago, not only for survival but also for an acceptable quality of life, including gainful employment, advanced education, and parenthood.

Treatment. The general plan for treatment of children with SLE should take into account the natural history of the disease, the severity of disease in the individual child, the risks of treatment, and the child's need for growth and interaction with his peers. For the 5 to 10 percent of children with mild disease, aspirin or other nonsteroidal anti-inflammatory agents are indicated to suppress inflammation and reduce fever, pain, and malaise. In the experience of the author and of others, children with SLE may be prone to aspirin-induced hepatotoxicity, and modest initial doses of aspirin (60 to 80 mg per kilogram per 24 hours) with monitoring of liver enzymes are indicated. If hepatotoxicity appears, the use of other nonsteroidal anti-inflammatory agents should be considered, although there are no data to suggest that salicylates can produce chronic, significant liver dysfunction (e.g., cirrhosis or chronic active hepatitis) (see Chapter 49). It should be recognized that the associated inhibition of prostaglandin synthesis may adversely affect the function of other organ systems, including a fall in glomerular filtration rate in the kidney.[45,46]

For children who are seriously ill, or who show evidence of advancing disease on conservative therapy, prednisone, 40 to 60 mg per square meter per 24 hours in divided doses (or its equivalent in other corticosteroid), is recommended. This dosage level is generally maintained for 2 to 4 weeks when, if there has been significant improvement, the dose may be gradually consolidated into a single daily dose and then shifted in steps to an every-other-day schedule. The dose is then tapered slowly to the minimum level needed to control the signs and symptoms of disease. In general, total doses of prednisone above 60 mg per day for a child of any size should be reserved for acute life-threatening illness and maintained for the shortest possible period of time. The risks of therapy increase with both dosage and duration of treatment. The administration of methylprednisolone in a single daily pulse of 30 mg per kilogram given intravenously over 30 to 60 minutes usually for 3 successive days, with or without smaller doses of maintenance therapy, has been reported in a number of papers in recent years. The toxicity of this form of treatment appears to be low, but the effectiveness and optimum schedule of this form of treatment are not yet known.[47]

Alternate-day therapy minimizes toxicity and growth suppression, but some children cannot tolerate alternate-day therapy, and maintenance of daily therapy, sometimes in divided doses, may be necessary.[1,3,7,48,49] Daily prednisone in moderate doses suppresses growth in the majority of children, and efforts should be made to minimize this effect after the acute illness is brought under control. A very slow reduction of dosage (e.g., by 1 or 1.25 mg) every other day while maintaining or increasing the original maintenance level on the alternate days will sometimes help to achieve this effect. Adolescents frequently manifest intense concern with the disfiguring effects of corticosteroids, and noncompliance with treatment recommendations is not unusual at this age. The physician should recognize this problem as a fundamental concern of the age period, not readily dismissed by a few words or even a lecture, and work with the adolescent to minimize these adverse side effects while maintaining effective therapy.

In the postacute phase the need for continued potentially toxic levels of corticosteroid therapy may be reduced by the concomitant administration of antimalarials or other nonsteroidal anti-inflammatory drugs. Among the antimalarials, hydroxychloroquine in a dose of 200 mg per square meter per day is probably the preferred agent.[1,49] Since hydroxychloroquine is potentially toxic to the retina, the eyes should be examined by an ophthalmologist before and every 4 months during the administration of this drug. Experience with the newer nonsteroidal anti-inflammatory agents in SLE is still too limited to indicate those which, if any, might be more effective.

If the dose of corticosteroid required to control the disease remains at significantly toxic levels after the aforementioned measures, or if there are signs of advancing renal or other organ system involvement in spite of general improvement, the use of immunosuppressants may be considered. The most commonly used of these are azathioprine, cyclophosphamide, and chlorambucil, with no clear-cut evidence of superiority of one over the others at this time.[1,5,42,48,49] All are thought to have some effect while given, but none is curative. Relapse may follow cessation of apparently effective therapy with any of the three. The optimal duration of therapy is not known, but is probably greater than 1 year. All are potentially highly toxic. Severe leukopenia with the attendant danger of sepsis is the most common side effect. The theoretical though still undefined danger of induction of malignancy is associated with all three. Cyclophosphamide is associated with hemorrhagic cystitis which may be severe in some patients and may recur in severe form after the drug has been stopped. Chlorambucil- and cyclophosphamide-induced sterility in a significant number of both male and female patients and decreased ovarian function and ovarian fibrosis in females may present additional problems. Growth suppression and most other corticosteroid side effects are not associated with the administration of immunosuppressants, and hence one may be able to achieve some balance between effectiveness and toxicity with their combined use. In general, treatment with these agents is probably best left in the hands of those with special experience in their administration and well defined protocols for evaluation of effectiveness and toxicity.

General supportive measures should not be overlooked, nor their importance underestimated, in the treatment of SLE. During acute crisis fluid and electrolyte balance, maintenance of nutrition, ensuring adequate respiratory ventilation and oxygenation of tissues, management of heart failure, and detection and treatment of infections may become individually or collectively essential to the patient's survival. Control of hypertension should be vigorously pursued whenever this complication appears. Rigorous restraints on activity are probably both unnecessary and undesirable for children. Attendance at school should be encouraged whenever symptoms and strength permit. Physical education activities should be prescribed by direct contact with school authorities to match the child's strength and endurance at any given time. Participation in extracurricular activities is also desirable with reasonable precautions against excessive fatigue and overexposure to the sun. Finally, one physician or physician-led team should be responsible for the overall management of each individual child with SLE. The family, and the child when old enough, should be given all the understanding of this complex disorder and its treatment that they can manage and should be encouraged to discuss their anxieties, fears, and questions with members of the team at any time during the course of the disease. It is likely that careful attention to all the details of management has contributed as much to the current improved outlook for children with SLE as any single therapeutic regimen.

DERMATOMYOSITIS AND POLYMYOSITIS

Dermatomyositis and polymyositis in childhood are characterized by symmetrical proximal muscle weakness resulting from a chronic inflammatory myopathy of unknown cause. Dermatomyositis is distinguished from polymyositis by the presence of a characteristic rash on the face and extremities which is absent in the latter. The muscle involvement in these two forms of disease is histologically indistinguishable, and whether or not these two conditions are distinct entities remains an unsettled question. Dermatomyositis is reported 10 to 20 times more frequently than polymyositis in childhood, whereas polymyositis is the more frequent of the two in adult life.[50] Significant histopathologic and clinical differences between adult and childhood dermatomyositis have been described. Whether or not these differences are true for polymyositis is less clear[51,52] (see Chapter 79).

Dermatomyositis

Clinical Characteristics. Dermatomyositis may begin at any age in childhood with a median age of onset of 6 years. Females are more commonly affected than males in a ratio of approximately two to one.[50,53-55] The early signs of dermatomyositis are nonspecific; hence the diagnosis is often delayed until muscular weakness has become obvious, manifested by such signs as difficulty in climbing stairs or frequent falls. Malaise and easy fatigability usually precede obvious muscle weakness by days or even months. Daily temperature elevations to 38 or 38.5° C are reported in 50 to 75 percent of the children and 5 to 10 percent present with high spiking fevers to the range of 40° C.

The rash of dermatomyositis is generally evident before the onset of obvious muscle weakness, and has definite characteristics which aid in the diagnosis. Violaceous erythema is commonly observed around the eyes, over the malar eminences, and over the extensor surfaces of the elbows, metacarpophalangeal and proximal phalangeal joints, and knees (Fig. 82–2). Less commonly noted are V-shaped areas of erythema on the forehead and upper chest and extensive erythematous changes over the extensor surfaces of the arms and legs. The dermis showing such changes often has a thickened

Figure 82–2. Periorbital edema and erythema in a 4-year-old girl with dermatomyositis. There is also malar erythema, a V-shaped rash on forehead and chin. (From Hanson, V.: Clin. Rheum. Dis. 2:445, 1976.)

brawny feel owing to edema. The skin over the knuckles has a papery erythematous appearance, and paronychial erythema is often present. The facial rash in some children is often indistinguishable from that of systemic lupus erythematosus, but is characterized by greater orbital involvement. In black children the erythema may be difficult to detect, and the skin must be carefully inspected to find the more subtle changes which are nearly always present. Increased or decreased pigment in the typical areas, along with other characteristic changes such as roughening and thickening of the skin over the elbows and knees and papery thinning over the knuckles of the hands, provides helpful clues. The cutaneous changes reflect the widespread vasculitis described by Banker and Victor as characteristic of childhood dermatomyositis, and as a result small infarctions of the skin may be observed.[50,51] This vasculitis probably involves the gastrointestinal tract in a high percentage of the patients, but abdominal symptoms are not prominent except when perforation of the gut occurs. Careful inspection of the palate will frequently show mild erythema, thickening, and fine vasculitic changes more diffuse and less intense than those seen in SLE. Other organ systems are also involved but much less frequently. Evidence of renal disease, pulmonary fibrosis, and spontaneous pneumothorax have all been reported but in a very small percentage of the children.[56,57] Definite joint swelling and effusion involving small or large joints, occasionally simulating juvenile rheumatoid arthritis, is probably not rare, but the true incidence of arthritis in this syndrome is unknown.[50] Myocardial disease is rarely clinically significant, although some evidence of myocarditis has been reported in autopsy studies.[51,58]

Laboratory Studies. Measurements of the serum enzymes which reflect damage to skeletal muscle, primarily creatine kinase (CK), aldolase, and serum glutamic-oxaloacetic transaminase (SGOT), are the most important laboratory tests for the diagnosis of dermatomyositis.[51,53] These enzymes are not always abnormally elevated during active disease or all abnormal at the same time. Elevations of CK are most specifically associated with muscle disease, but it should be noted that CK can be significantly elevated in active disease of the central nervous system, pneumonia, hypothyroidism, and bronchial asthma; after intramuscular injections; and probably most commonly after greater than usual exercise stress.[59-61] Elevations of serum CK caused by disease of brain or myocardium can usually be distinguished from those caused by disease of skeletal muscle by fractionation. Other laboratory tests are of limited value. The hemoglobin and white blood cell counts are usually normal, and the sedimentation rate is normal in one third to one half the children. Antinuclear antibodies are found in about 10 percent of the children and are usually in low titer.[50,54]

Muscle biopsy is not essential to the diagnosis in patients with typical rash and proximal weakness but can provide evidence of the disease in patients with polymyositis or questionable cases. Ten percent or more of biopsies have been reported as normal, even in patients with clear-cut active disease presumably because of sampling error.[52]

Pathology. Juvenile-onset dermatomyositis is characterized by a diffuse angiopathy involving the small arteries, venules, and capillaries of skin, muscle, fat, small nerves, and gastrointestinal tissue, and in this respect it differs strikingly from the adult onset disease.[51,62] (see Chapter 79). The vascular changes result in occlusion of small vessels by intimal proliferation and microthrombi with resulting small infarctions and ulcerations. The vasculitic changes in the subcutaneous fatty tissues are often associated with necrotic tissue and calcified debris with inflammatory cells around areas of calcium deposition. The muscles show moderate to marked perivascular inflammation in some areas, and in other areas diffuse inflammatory infiltrates are present among and along the muscle fibers as shown (Figs. 82–3 and 82–4). The infiltrates are usually composed of lymphocytes, plasma cells, and macrophages but in early lesions neutrophils may be prominent. Immunofluorescent studies show deposits of IgG, IgM, and C3 in

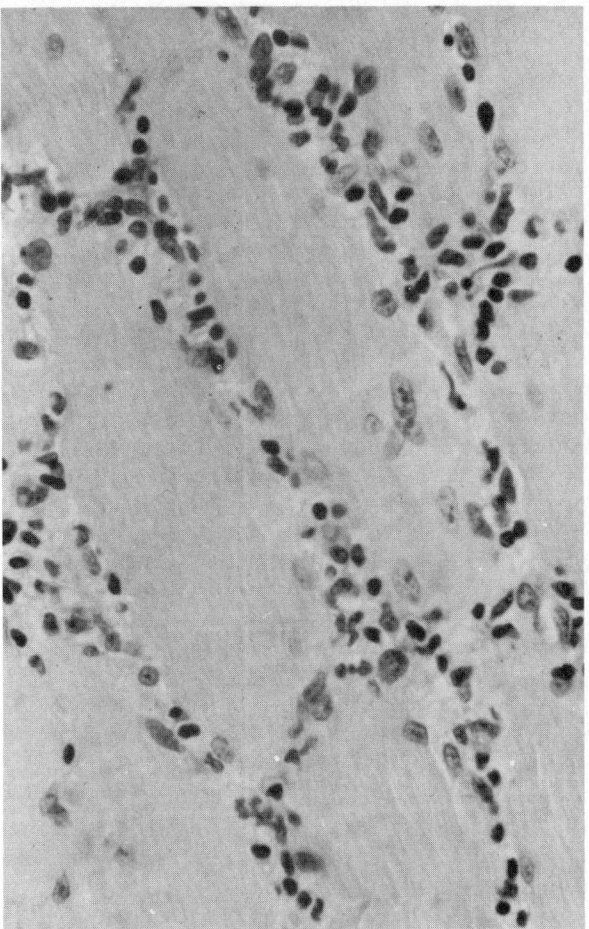

Figure 82–3. Dermatomyositis with mononuclear cell infiltrate around the muscle fibers. (From Hanson, V.: Clin. Rheum. Dis. 2:445, 1976.)

Figure 82–4. Dermatomyositis. A different field from the same section shown in Figure 82–3, showing prominent perivascular infiltrate. (From Hanson, V.: Clin. Rheum. Dis. 2:445, 1976.)

skeletal muscle blood vessel walls in a high percentage of children with dermatomyositis.[63] The muscle fibers show varied effects of injury such as loss of striations, necrosis of fibers, cystic necrosis of portions of the fibers, and evidence of regeneration.

Clinical Course and Prognosis. Dermatomyositis is a potentially fatal disease, but the mortality has decreased dramatically in recent years from 38 percent of the cases reported in the 10 years prior to 1967 to 10 percent of the cases reported in the 10 following years.[51] It is likely that this mortality can be reduced to almost 0 by early diagnosis, prompt institution of appropriate therapy, and careful supportive measures during critical periods. Recovery is associated with return to normal or near normal function in 80 to 90 percent of the children.

It is helpful to think of the course of dermatomyositis in four stages: (1) a prodromal period with nonspecific symptoms; (2) the phase of progressive muscle weakness and rash; (3) the stage of persisting weakness, rash, and active disease; and (4) the phase of recovery with or without calcinosis. The duration of each phase is quite variable.

During the prodromal period the diagnosis of dermatomyositis is often delayed for weeks or months ow-

ing to the vagueness and nonspecificity of the early symptoms. Symptoms may be initiated with an apparent respiratory infection or other viral syndrome or by a period of persisting anorexia, fatigue, and malaise lasting from a few days to a few months before definite weakness or charactistic rash makes the diagnosis readily apparent. The rash is often faint and poorly developed during this period and is frequently misdiagnosed.

The second phase begins once the weakness has been recognized. The muscle weakness then progresses in most patients within a few days or weeks to limited ability to stand or walk or raise the head and shortly thereafter may extend to weakness of respiratory and/ or pharyngeal muscles. Pneumonia is a major threat at this time because of pulmonary stasis or aspiration.

The third stage is characterized by persisting marked muscle weakness, often confinement to bed or wheel-chair, contractures, low grade fever, and marked malaise. The rash is usually prominent during this time, reflecting continuing active vasculitis. The life-threatening complications of the dermatomyositis such as gastrointestinal tract perforation and pulmonary complications are most likely to occur during the second and third stages of the disease and rarely after the first 2 years.

The onset of the fourth, or recovery, phase is marked by improving muscular strength and frequently the appearance of subcutaneous calcifications. The overall course of the disease can be subdivided into three principal types: a monocyclic course of relatively short duration without relapse, a relapsing form of the disease in which apparent complete recovery may be followed by mild to severe recurrence on one or more occasions, and a long persisting active disease which may endure for many years[64] (Figs. 82–5 and 82–6). The long persisting active disease is often compatible with relatively good function, although steroid treatment has been required for as long as 9 years before cessation of therapy. Miller and Koehler have demonstrated persisting muscle

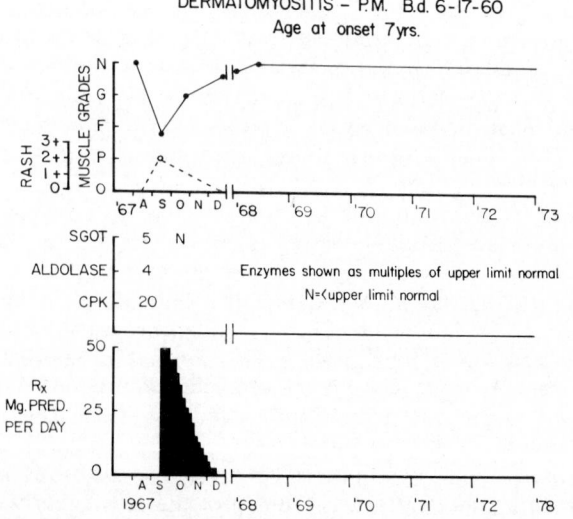

Figure 82–5. Monocyclic course with prednisone therapy and rapid recovery. (From Hanson, V.: Clin. Rheum. Dis. 2:445, 1976.)

Figure 82–6. Relapsing course with prednisone therapy and recovery after 4 years of treatment. No evidence of dermatomyositis since 1972. (From Hanson, V.: Clin. Rheum. Dis. 2:445, 1976.)

inflammation as late as 8 years after onset and progressive skeletal change up to 9 years after onset.[65]

Calcinosis detectable by physical examination develops in 40 percent or more of the children but is rarely observed before the end of the first year.[50] The most common form of calcinosis is that of discrete subcutaneous nodules prominent around major joints such as the elbows and knees (Fig. 82–7). In others, however, the calcinosis may be very extensive, appearing in armorlike plates in the skin or in diffuse sheets in fascial planes and deeper tissues, often being associated with crippling contractures (Fig. 82–8). Rarely an entire muscle group may be replaced by flocculent deposits of calcium (Fig. 82–9). Severe disability is associated with extensive calcinosis. The calcific deposits are usually slowly reabsorbed over the course of years, although a few of the subcutaneous calcific nodules may be extruded through the skin as well. Life-threatening complications are uncommon in the late stages of dermatomyositis but do

Figure 82–8. Diffuse armorlike calcinosis of the dermis in a 6-year-old boy with dermatomyositis.

occur. Rose described a patient who developed common iliac and aortic thrombosis and died in the fifth year of disease.[55] Hanson reported a patient with quiescent muscle disease but persisting active rash who developed perforation of the nasal septum and pulmonary fibrosis in the sixth year and subsequently died of the pulmonary fibrosis in the eighth year of disease.[50]

Overall it should be emphasized that the outlook for recovery of normal function in these children is good when properly treated. Some of the deaths reported in the last 10 years were associated with social factors beyond medical control, and when these cases are excluded the known mortality decreases to 6 or 7 percent at most. Present knowledge and techniques can undoubtedly reduce the percentage even further. Eighty to 90 percent of surviving children should be able ultimately to return to their usual activities and become self-supporting adults.

Treatment. No controlled studies have been carried out to establish the best form of treatment in childhood

Figure 82–7. Typical subcutaneous calcification deposit extruding through the skin in a 14-year old boy with dermatomyositis.

Figure 82–9. Calcification throughout the biceps muscle of a 14-year-old girl after 5 years of dermatomyositis.

dermatomyositis, but it seems clear from the experience of the past 10 years that corticosteroid therapy sustained over an extended period of time is the treatment of choice. A few children have very mild disease which never progresses to marked or severe weakness, and these could be managed with therapeutic aspirin levels (75 to 100 mg per kilogram per day in divided doses) if symptomatic. In asymptomatic children lower doses of aspirin on a daily basis could be considered to reduce the likelihood of microthrombi associated with their vasculitic disease. The patients with mild disease, however, should have frequent follow-up examinations to ensure that increasing muscle weakness is not overlooked.

Corticosteroid therapy is indicated in all children with dermatomyositis with significant or increasing muscle weakness. The initial dose of prednisone is 30 to 60 mg per square meter per 24 hours divided into three or four doses over the 24-hour period. A total dose of 60 mg per day should rarely be exceeded, however, and continued for only short periods when deemed necessary. Most children become more comfortable and show im-

provement in strength and muscle enzyme levels within 2 to 4 weeks, and at 6 weeks a gradual reduction of prednisone to 0.2 to 0.4 mg per kilogram per day may be begun. At this point there are different opinions, with some investigators maintaining that steroid therapy should be continued at maintenance level for all patients for 2 years and others recommending gradual cessation of treatment if there is no detectable weakness or rash, and no laboratory evidence of disease activity over a period of 2 or 3 months.[50,54,66] In this connection it should be noted that relapses occur with or without maintenance therapy. Termination of therapy should always be gradual, with careful follow-up during the tapering period and in the months immediately following.

Five to 10 percent of children are refractory to steroid therapy, and for these immunosuppressive treatment has been used by a number of investigators. Methotrexate is the most commonly used agent, but there is no clear evidence to indicate its superiority over azathioprine, cyclophosphamide, or possibly chlorambucil.[67] Treatment with these drugs should be considered to be still in the investigational phase.

Measurements of serum creatine kinase are useful in monitoring therapy and predicting relapse but should not be relied upon to the exclusion of examination of the patient. Rash may persist long after return to normal muscle function and is not of itself an indication for steroid therapy. Intensification of the erythema occurs as a result of increased heat, exertion, or emotional stress and, therefore, does not always signify exacerbation of disease.

Calcinosis resolves slowly and is the major cause of disability when extensive or severe. There is no proven treatment for this complication. Discrete calcific nodules that are painful or unsightly, interfere with function, or are subject to recurrent infection should be removed surgically. Cellulitis may develop at any time around the calcific nodules once they have appeared and usually require both antibiotics and surgical damage.

Physical therapy is even more important in children than in adults. During acute phases of the disease, thorough and gentle passive range of motion exercise must be given frequently to prevent contracture or at least minimize its severity. Active, fatiguing resistive exercise should be discouraged during the early healing phase to prevent damage to new myofibrils regenerating in areas of quiescent inflammation.

Polymyositis

Polymyositis in children is characterized by proximal muscle weakness and a clinical course similar to that of dermatomyositis except for the absence of a rash. The author's unpublished observations in four cases, however, suggest a more varied and protracted course. The histologic findings in muscle do not differ from those of dermatomyositis, and the incidence of calcinosis may be quite similar, although there are too few reported cases to firmly establish this point. The treatment for polymyositis is the same as that for dermatomyositis.

The absence of rash may reflect a less extensive and severe vasculitis and hence fewer complications, but evidence on this point is meager at present.

Whether or not polymyositis and dermatomyositis are distinct entities, it is important to recognize the occurrence of chronic myositis in children without rash. In areas of muscle where inflammation has subsided, the residual changes may be suggestive of muscular dystrophy with prominent variation in muscle fiber size. Therefore, repeat biopsies are warranted whenever there is any doubt concerning the diagnosis. Thompson reported two patients previously diagnosed as having muscular dystrophy whose condition promptly improved when the correct diagnosis was established and appropriate therapy instituted.[68]

Myositis Associated with Other Diseases

Mild myositis may occur in some patients with systemic lupus erythematosus, scleroderma, and juvenile rheumatoid arthritis but does not dominate the clinical picture, and the presence of other characteristic features aids in distinguishing these conditions from true dermatomyositis or polymyositis. Transient myositis may be associated with viral infections, particularly influenza B, and is characterized by predominantly peripheral or distal muscle involvement, particularly in the calves of the legs, rarely lasting more than a week. Elevations of creatinkinase are found in most of the patients.[69] Polymyositis due to infection of muscle with *Staphylococcus aureus* (also known as tropical myositis) has been reported with increasing frequency in temperate climes and may affect muscles singly or diffusely.[70] Proximal muscle weakness simulating polymyositis has also been described in two patients with Kawasaki disease.[71]

SCLERODERMA

Scleroderma occurs in childhood, both as systemic sclerosis and localized scleroderma. The author's experience includes 36 children with localized scleroderma and 14 with systemic sclerosis, a ratio of approximately 2.5 to 1. The combined prevalence of localized and systemic forms relative to that of juvenile rheumatoid arthritis (JRA) has been nearly constant over a 20-year period at approximately 1 to 25. Cassidy and associates reported a ratio of approximately one case of systemic sclerosis to 33 children with all forms of rheumatic disease seen in their clinic at the University of Michigan.[72] While the occurrence of these conditions in childhood is quite rare, it is important to recognize that they do occur and often with serious consequences.

Localized Scleroderma. Christianson and colleagues reported a 44 percent incidence of arthralgia in their study of 235 cases of localized scleroderma published in 1956[73] (see Chapter 77). Cook, Rosen, and Banker noted the interesting and significant finding in some children of limitation of motion of joints distant from the site of the localized sclerodermatous lesions and

without evidence of disease of the overlying skin.[53] These authors did not mention the occurrence of active synovitis. More recently this author and colleagues have confirmed the presence of active synovitis in joints both adjacent to and distant from the local skin lesions.[50,74] The synovitis occurred in 10 of 35 children in either diffuse polyarticular or oligoarticular patterns. The chronic inflammatory nature of the synovitis has been confirmed histologically in two patients and does not differ from that reported in systemic sclerosis. In addition, mononuclear cell infiltrates in muscle with muscle cell damage, and fibrosis have been found frequently when muscle has been included in diagnostic biopsy material.[50] It is apparent therefore that much more than the skin alone is involved in the localized forms of scleroderma.

While it is true that there is virtually no threat to life, complete recovery has not been observed in our patients followed as long as 20 years and new lesions have appeared as late as 14 years after onset. The late effects of patches of morphea are rarely severe (with the exception of lesions on the face), but the linear lesions are frequently associated with impaired growth of underlying bone, contractures, and progressive deformity. The concept of hemiatrophy as applied to these patients has probably been misleading. It is the deficient growth of bone under or near the localized lesions and the continuing growth of adjacent normal bone which are the major deforming factors in the childhood disease. The more benign impression obtained by Christianson and associates was probably due to the fact that 80 percent or more of the patients in that study had completed their growth at the time of onset of the disease.[73]

Morphea and Linear Scleroderma. It is customary to treat morphea and linear scleroderma as two distinct entities, but the distinctions are often difficult to make. The individual lesions are usually distinctive in appearance, but the common occurrence of characteristic lesions of each type in the same patient (40 percent or more of the children) and the not infrequent occurrence of intermediate lesions limit the usefulness of these categories for classifying individual patients.[74] In general, the linear lesions are more severe in their effects on underlying tissues and are more likely to be associated with abnormal laboratory values. Both lesions evolve slowly through the stages of edema, induration, and atrophy. In the early stage the lesion is that of sharply localized edema, occasionally slightly raised, warm to the touch, and erythematous or bluish in color. The lesion then progresses slowly to the stage of sclerosis with a firm thickened center and generally increased pigmentation at the margins and decreased pigmentation centrally (Fig. 82–10). The stage of edema is infrequently described as such, but upon questioning parents usually indicate that the first sign of the disease was a lump in the skin, sometimes described as violaceous or bluish. Lesions of the morphea type, although often multiple, do not expand beyond a few centimeters in diameter, but the linear lesions are generally described to expand from a relatively small area to involve an entire extremity

Figure 82–10. Two coalescing patches of morphea with central depigmentation and peripheral increased pigmentation.

from buttocks to toes, or shoulder to fingers (Figs. 82–10 and 82–11). In both morphea and linear scleroderma, however, mild pigmentary change without other skin involvement may extend over large areas of adjacent skin or appear in small patches distant from the major lesion. Except for occasional local pruritus or arthralgia

Figure 82–11. Linear scleroderma in an 8-year-old boy with contractures of ankle and toes and shortening of leg and foot. (From Hanson, V.: Clin. Rheum. Dis. 2: 445, 1976.)

the evolution of even the most destructive of these lesions has been essentially symptomless. The children remain active and participate in athletic activities until finally forced to desist by unmanageable contractures or marked shortening of the affected extremity.

The child is usually brought to the physician for diagnosis when the lesion or lesions have reached the stage of induration. At this stage the classic histopathology of scleroderma is found: dense collagen beneath the epidermis, atrophy of the skin appendages, and scattered foci of moderate numbers of mononuclear cells about small vessels and the skin appendages. The usual punch biopsy is superficial and shows little more than this. Immunofluorescent stains for deposition of immunoglobulins and complement are negative.

If the biopsy is extended through subcutaneous tissue to include muscle, however, it becomes clear that the disease process involves far more than the epidermis. The subcutaneous fat in relatively early stages may be heavily infiltrated with chronic inflammatory cells, seemingly an obvious forerunner of the almost universal marked subcutaneous atrophy so prominent in the third stage of the disease. Foci of mononuclear cells infiltrating muscle fibers with muscle cell injury and fibrosis were found in the muscle in the majority of children when this tissue was included in the biopsy material. Very little information is available concerning the histopathology of underlying bone, but the reader's attention is called again to the almost universal growth impairment of bone associated with the localized scleroderma lesions as a significant evidence of the depth of tissue involvement in this disease. The histopathology of the relatively common synovitis associated with the localized scleroderma has been observed too infrequently for general description except to note that the two synovial specimens which have been examined have shown a chronic nonspecific synovitis with mononuclear cell infiltrates composed of lymphocytes, macrophages, and plasma cells, not readily distinguishable from the synovitis of JRA[50,75] (Fig. 82–12). The synovial involvement is of particular interest, since it is by no means limited to tissues adjacent to the skin lesions.

Involvement of the joints may precede, or accompany, the onset of recognizable skin changes or appear after the skin disease is well established, and is as likely to be polyarticular as oligoarticular. The oligoarticular attacks are usually more transient. Residual limitation of motion may be quite marked, but in some children it seems to disappear. Evidence of cartilage damage or bony erosion has not been observed in these children.

Involvement of internal organs other than those of the musculoskeletal system has also been noted in association with the localized lesions but has not usually led to significant symptoms and is often transient. In the report by Kornreich and associates, seven children were found to have impaired esophageal peristalsis.[74] Four of these are known to have reverted to normal on subsequent studies, but the fate of the other three patients is not known. Three children with facial and scalp lesions were described who developed CNS involvement.

Figure 82–12. Synovitis in a 7-year-old male with linear scleroderma. (From Hanson, V.: Clin. Rheum. Dis. 2:445, 1976.)

Two of the patients developed unilateral seizures on the side contralateral to the side of the sclerodermatous involvement of the scalp. It could be argued that these children should be classified as having systemic sclerosis, but their localized lesions, and their limited, transient, or atypical internal organ involvement favor their continuation in the category of localized scleroderma.

Systemic Sclerosis in Childhood. Systemic sclerosis in childhood presents with essentially the same symptoms and signs as in adult life. The reported age of onset is from 3 to 14 years, with a peak incidence in the immediate preadolescent years. In three reports with a combined total of 40 children there were 34 females and 6 males, a female-to-male ratio of approximately 6 to 1.[72,74,76]

Classically, the lesions of systemic sclerosis evolve through the three stages of edema, sclerosis, and atrophy. The children are rarely seen in the edematous phase, and history of edema is rarely included in their histories. Scleroderma, however, is characterized by subtle, slow, and often symptomless progression, and it is quite possible that the evidences of edema were not recognized as such. Occasionally children are seen with diffuse swelling of the fingers ("sausage fingers," which seems a less common finding in children than in adults) or

occasionally edema of the face, as shown in Figure 82–13. The edema generally subsides as the patient enters the sclerotic or indurative phase. The most common early symptom at this time is tightening of the skin, particularly around the face and distal extremities. Constitutional symptoms such as easy fatigability, malaise, and anorexia are reported at some time in the course of the disease by most of the patients. Arthralgia and arthritis occur in some of the children, but the incidence of this organ system involvement cannot be estimated. Dysphagia is noted in one third or more of the patients, and alternating constipation and diarrhea, abdominal distention, and abdominal pain are occasionally reported.

Thickening and frequently a shiny smoothness of the skin without clear-cut demarcation of involved and normal skin are the usual findings. The changes may be most prominent on the distal extremities and face (acrosclerosis) or diffusely present over the trunk and extremities. Dermal pigmentation is altered to some extent in all cases and may be either increased or decreased, or both, and generalized or regional. In some patients a generalized bronze pigmentation suggestive of Addison's disease has been observed. Raynaud's phenomenon is present in one third to one half of the children reported and may precede the onset of other manifestations by as long as 6 years.[74,77,78] Seventy percent or more of the

Figure 82–13. Systemic sclerosis in a 12-year-old girl with edema of the face. (From Hanson, V.: Clin. Rheum. Dis. 2:445, 1976.)

children manifest Raynaud's phenomenon at some time during the course of their disease.

Cardiac and pulmonary manifestations are frequent and often of grave consequence. Cassidy and associates reported evidence of cardiac disease in four of their 15 patients, two of whom died in heart failure.[72] In this author's experience two children were first seen early in the course of their disease with severe cardiac arrhythmias, and one of these children was in heart failure at the time of presentation. Both these children survived, but death was attributed to cardiac failure in three other patients in this series.[50] Extensive myocardial fibrosis was noted in two of these at postmortem examination.[78] Pulmonary findings were also frequent, and interstitial fibrosis and pulmonary vascular sclerosis contributed to the cardiac decompensation and demise of two of the patients. Renal failure was not significant as a cause of death, and malignant hypertension as described in adult scleroderma has not been reported.

Calcinosis involving the fingers was noted in one of the patients reported by Kornreich and associates but is much less frequent than in adult onset systemic sclerosis or childhood dermatomyositis.[74] The prominent distal distribution of the calcium deposits on the hands and feet differs markedly from that seen in juvenile onset dermatomyositis.

The prognosis of juvenile onset systemic sclerosis must be considered uncertain in view of the small number of cases reported. There were 10 deaths among 40 children reported in three papers, with the earliest death at 6 months after onset and the last known death at 10 years.[72,74,76] Complete recovery from systemic sclerosis in childhood has not been reported, but significant improvement in two of the 15 children reported in one study and three of the surviving cases followed by Kornreich and associates have shown marked improvement.[72,74] One of these has now been followed 25 years and has been gainfully employed and fully self-supporting for the past 8 years.

Laboratory Findings in Localized Scleroderma and Systemic Sclerosis. The laboratory findings in both these forms of scleroderma are surprisingly similar, and any apparent differences between the two are of doubtful significance. Blood counts, sedimentation rates, and urinalyses are normal in the majority of the children.[50,72,74] Antinuclear antibodies are present in more than half, and in one study five of 16 children with localized scleroderma were found to have antibody to DNA (probably the denatured fraction), whereas none was found in six children with systemic sclerosis.[79] Rheumatoid factor in titers of 1:160 or greater is found in 30 to 40 percent of the children, but the highest titers are found in association with linear scleroderma, with titers as high as 1:20,480 reported.[80] The mean levels of IgG, IgM, and IgA are substantially higher than those of control subjects. Moderate elevations of CK and SGOT are found in about one third of the children, as could be expected from the frequent findings of muscle involvement in biopsy or necropsy studies. Although none of these findings are specific for scleroderma, they do strongly sug-

gest involvement of the immune system in the pathogenesis of scleroderma.

Treatment. No treatment at present is of proven value for either localized scleroderma or systemic sclerosis. Evaluation of therapy, however, is difficult because of the slow progression of the disease and the unpredictable equally slow improvement which occurs in some patients without therapy. Corticosteroid treatment has not been shown to alter the progress of the disease. D-Penicillamine and immunosuppressive agents have been reported to be of benefit to some patients, but both these forms of therapy should still be considered experimental.[81,82] It is important to provide physical and occupational therapeutic measures to attempt to maintain good position and function of the joints and to maintain muscle strength. Surgery can be successfully performed to correct some of the deformities or contractures in the children with localized scleroderma when the disease is relatively quiescent. Supportive therapy for the patients with systemic sclerosis is important and should not be ignored, as a patient sustained through critical periods has an excellent chance of marked improvement and subsequent long life and economic independence.

VASCULITIS

Vasculitis occurs both as primary disease and secondary to other systemic disorders in childhood. Classification of the vasculitides has been difficult, but the work of Zeek and later McCombs provided a foundation for more orderly study of these syndromes.[83,84] Recently Gilliam and Smiley proposed a useful new system of classification which with some modifications is the basis for the classification shown in Table 82–3.[85] The size and location of the affected vessels are among the major factors in the differentiation of these syndromes. Many of the primary vasculitides have distinctive patterns of involvement enabling their diagnosis without sole reliance on the exclusion process. They are often accompanied, however, by such rheumatic signs and symptoms as arthritis, arthralgia, fever, and rash. Conversely the

Table 82–3. Necrotizing Vasculitis

1. Small vessel vasculitis
   a. Henoch-Schönlein purpura
   b. Allergic vasculitis
   c. Hypocomplementemic vasculitis
   d. Vasculitis with mixed cryoglobulinemia
2. Allergic granulomatous angiitis
   a. Churg and Strauss
   b. Wegener's granulomatosis
3. Polyarteritis nodosa
   a. Classic polyarteritis nodosa
   b. Cutaneous polyarteritis
   c. Infantile polyarteritis nodosa
   d. Mucocutaneous lymph node syndrome
4. Giant cell arteritis
   a. Temporal arteritis
   b. Takayasu's arteritis
5. Vasculitis associated with the rheumatic diseases

systemic rheumatic disorders are often accompanied by prominent vasculitic manifestations. Herein lies the source of much diagnostic difficulty for the clinician. The problems of diagnosis are further complicated by common immunopathogenetic mechanisms and as a consequence shared or overlapping laboratory abnormalities. Awareness of these syndromes in children and careful attention to the details of clinical, laboratory, and pathologic findings can help in establishing the correct diagnosis in most cases.

Small Vessel Vasculitis

In this category the venules, capillaries, and small arterioles are involved with prominent perivascular infiltrates which also invade the vessel walls in many areas in association with necrotic changes. Neutrophils are the predominant infiltrating cells in the early stages but are usually accompanied by macrophages, lymphocytes, and plasma cells, particularly in the later stages. The associated skin rashes are many and vary from macules and papules to urticaria, petechiae, purpura, or ecchymoses, with usually a mixture of several forms. The high visibility of the accompanying skin rash has led some investigators to consider these vasculitides as more or less limited to the dermis. The occurrence of synovitis, nephritis, and frequently associated constitutional signs such as fever and abdominal pain suggests a more generalized and deeper involvement, however.

Anaphylactoid Purpura (Henoch-Schönlein Purpura). Anaphylactoid purpura is the best known and most common of the small vessel vasculitides in children and is characterized by nonthrombocytopenic purpura in a characteristic distribution, arthritis with often severe arthralgia, and cramping abdominal pain. While occasionally seen in adult life, it is by far more common in children, occurring from infancy to adolescence with a median age at onset of about 6 years. Seven of 131 patients reported by Allen and associates were under 1 year of age when their disease began.[86] Males are more commonly affected than females in a ratio of 2 to 1.

The skin lesions of anaphylactoid purpura have a characteristic distribution, being most prominent and numerous over the buttocks and down the backs of the legs (Fig. 82–14). Scattered purpuric spots may develop around the umbilicus, on the backs of the arms, and occasionally on the face and elsewhere on the trunk. The purpuric lesions generally begin as pink to reddish macules or maculopapules, which darken rapidly to purpuric hues as the red cells escape into the local tissue underlying the lesion. These fade within a few days to a week, leaving yellowish-brown spots caused by the residual hemosiderin. The purpuric macules vary from 2 or 3 mm to 1 cm in diameter and generally remain discrete. Angioedema occurs in half the children and is found on the extremities somewhat more commonly than on the face and scalp. It is most common in children under 3 years of age.[86]

Joint pain and swelling are significant symptoms in two-thirds of the children and are not migratory. The

Figure 82–14. Anaphylactoid purpura with prominent rash on the buttocks.

knees and ankles are most commonly affected, but fingers and elbows are also frequently involved. The joint symptoms are often severe and disabling during the acute stage of the illness. The arthritis always subsides and leaves no residual damage or deformity of the joints as sequelae.[87]

Cramping or colicky abdominal pain occurs in half to two-thirds of the children and is even more distressing to the child than the arthralgia. Blood is found in the stool in 40 to 60 percent of the children and is frequently grossly visible. Intussusception is a potentially dangerous complication, and the physician must be constantly on the alert for this problem in children with moderate or severe gastrointestinal symptoms.

In his original description Henoch emphasized the periodic nature of the disease even during the initial illness, with episodes of marked arthralgia followed by new crops of purpura and intensified abdominal symptoms lasting a few days only to gradually subside and recur.[88] During the first 2 or 3 weeks for many patients, however, these attacks merge into one almost continuous illness. With improvement the periodic pattern of new rash and pain often becomes more apparent. Most children recover within 6 weeks, but recurrent milder attacks at lengthening intervals occur in a significant percentage. These may be manifested by one or more crops of scattered purpura with or without mild to moderate abdominal pain, or as isolated bouts of hematuria.

Fever is associated with the acute illness in half to three fourths of the children and is generally sustained in elevation in contrast to the striking intermittent pattern of juvenile rheumatoid arthritis. Abnormal urinalyses are reported in 20 to 50 percent of patients in different series with hematuria the most common finding.[89-91] Evidence of renal involvement subsides with the acute illness in the majority of patients, but mild evidence of renal abnormality is found in long-term follow-up in about one fourth of the children. The incidence of severe renal disease is probably less than 2 percent.[86,90] It is of interest that some 10 to 15 percent of patients may have hypertension early in the course of their disease, but this is usually not sustained.

Laboratory Findings. There are no specific laboratory findings associated with this disease. The platelets and clotting factors are normal. The hemoglobin is normal in 90 percent or more of the patients. The white blood cell count varies, with the majority showing some elevation, which may be as high as 40,000 WBC per cubic millimeter. The sedimentation rate was normal in half the children studied by Wedgwood and Klaus and in one fourth of those reported by Allen and associates.[86,92]

Trygstad and Stiehm reported elevated serum IgA levels in 10 of 20 children with anaphylactoid purpura, all of whom had normal levels of IgG, IgM, and IgD.[93] This report is of particular interest in view of the subsequent reports of IgA deposits in the glomeruli of patients with this disease.

Pathology. The pathology of anaphylactoid purpura is typical of the small vessel angiitides with perivascular infiltration of small blood vessels and scattered areas of necrosis of the blood vessel walls. Vernier and associates noted the necrotic changes to be associated with the most marked perivascular infiltration. In his study erythrocyte extravasation and leukocyte platelet thrombi were found in many capillaries and venules but only in association with the perivascular infiltrates.[94] These infiltrates were composed of both neutrophils and mononuclear cells. The most common finding in renal biopsies consisted of focal areas of endothelial hypercellularity associated with mesangial deposits with an amorphous PAS-positive material. Normal glomeruli were noted in areas immediately adjacent to glomeruli showing typical focal lesions. Two patients without overt clinical nephritis were found to have a few glomeruli with typical focal lesions and a rare hypercellular glomerulus in renal tissue obtained at biopsy. Immunofluorescent studies by Giangiacomo and Tsai showed granular deposits of IgA along with C3 and fibrin in the mesangial regions of the glomeruli, and in the dermal capillary walls and dermal connective tissue.[95] Staining for IgG and IgM in the glomeruli was present but was much less intense in the glomeruli and rarely seen in the dermis. These observations suggest an immune complex mechanism in the pathogenesis of anaphylactoid purpura.

Treatment. There is no established therapeutic regimen for the treatment of anaphylactoid purpura, and in general aggressive measures are not indicated in view of the usually excellent prognosis. For patients who have joint symptoms as the dominant problem, the author has used aspirin in doses of 60 to 80 mg per kilogram per day in divided doses with symptomatic improvement. This therapy may have the added benefit of reducing the occurrence of the platelet thrombi noted by Vernier and associates.[94] No increase in bleeding was associated with its use. Corticosteroid therapy is indicated for children with severe colicky abdominal pain, as it may prevent the occurrence of intussusception as well as reduce the

child's marked distress. The dose is 1 to 2 mg per kilogram per day until the acute manifestations are well controlled, when it may be gradually tapered and discontinued completely within the next 7 to 10 days. Subsequent mild exacerbations are not an indication for reinstitution of the steroid therapy. There is no evidence that the outcome of the renal disease is altered by treatment with corticosteroids. The prognosis is for ultimate recovery without sequelae in 95 percent or more of the patients even though recurrent attacks may occur over a period of 2 years or more after onset.

Allergic Vasculitis. Allergic vasculitis is similar in many respects to anaphylactoid purpura with rash, fever, and frequently arthralgia, arthritis, abdominal pain, and urinary changes during the acute illness. Recurrent attacks likewise are common. The skin lesions are much more varied in type and distribution. They are as prominent on the trunk as the extremities and take the form of urticaria, macules, and papules, with occasional limited numbers of purpuric lesions[96] (Fig. 82–15). Gastrointestinal involvement is much less prominent and gastrointestinal hemorrhage unlikely. This syndrome in its clinical features in children mostly resembles that described by McDuffie and associates in adults who had varied skin lesions, including erythematous macules, urticaria, and occasional purpura, associated with necrotizing vasculitis and hypocomplementemia.[97] Soter and others described a total of 16 adult patients with a syndrome consisting of recurrent episodes of urticaria associated with arthralgias and occasionally arthritis, abdominal pain, and diffuse glomerulonephritis.[98,99] The skin lesions appeared as raised erythematous, circumscribed wheals in which the erythema blanched with the application of external pressure and occasionally areas of macular erythema, angioedema, and rarely punctate

Figure 82–15. Allergic vasculitis in a 7-year-old boy with large erythematous maculopapules.

foci of purpura. Biopsy of the skin showed endothelial swelling, fibrinoid necrosis, and infiltrates containing primarily neutrophils in and about the blood vessel walls. Eosinophils were generally absent. Hypocomplementemia was present in 7 of the 16 patients. It is worthwhile to emphasize therefore that urticaria or urticaria-like skin lesions may well be the outward sign of necrotizing vasculitis involving the small vessels. Studies have not yet been reported which related the allergic vasculitis of children to depressed complement levels or other evidence of immune complex disease, but it seems likely that such evidence will be found when these studies are carried out. The syndrome of purpura, arthralgia, and mixed cryoglobulinemia described in adults is clinically similar to anaphylactoid purpura in children but differs primarily in the reported presence of cryoglobulins and rheumatoid factor in the adult studies.[100,101]

Allergic Granulomatous Angiitis

The allergic granulomatous angiitis of Churg and Strauss is clinically a syndrome consisting of asthma, fever, hypereosinophilia, cardiac failure, renal damage, and peripheral neuropathy.[102,103] As many as 20 percent of the cases occur in the preadolescent age range. Histologically the vasculitis is manifested by fibrinoid necrosis of the media of the small arteries and veins, but arterioles and capillaries are also affected. The accompanying leukocytic infiltration is marked, with eosinophils especially prominent. The coronary arteries and pericardium are frequently involved. Granulomatous nodules consisting of central areas of fibrinoid necrosis surrounded by eosinophils, epithelioid cells, and giant cells are found in the connective tissue. Corticosteroid treatment is indicated to suppress the acute manifestations of the disease, but its long-term effect is uncertain.

Wegener's granulomatosis is characterized by necrotizing granulomatous lesions of the upper respiratory tract, bronchi, and lung and by glomerulonephritis. Eosinophilia is not characteristic of this condition. Papular erythematous lesions may be prominent on the face and less frequently present on the extremities. Eighteen cases have been reported in children.[104,105,106,107] Elevation of the sedimentation rate and anemia are usually found, but there are no diagnostic laboratory tests and diagnosis is established by biopsy. The condition progresses rapidly to death without treatment. Corticosteroid treatment seems to suppress the disease but only temporarily. Cyclophosphamide, with corticosteroids added in the early phase of treatment, is remarkably effective in the treatment of Wegener's granulomatosis and is indicated for its treatment at any age. It is not yet approved for this use by the Food and Drug Administration, however, and consultation should be sought concerning its use.

Polyarteritis Nodosa

Classic Polyarteritis Nodosa. Classic polyarteritis nodosa (PAN) in children occurs primarily in the older preadolescent and adolescent age range and is in most respects similar to PAN in adults. The male-to-female ratio is close to 1.5 to 1 in children, compared with that of 3 to 1 reported in adult life.[108-110] Varied skin rashes are reported more frequently and may be maculopapular, urticarial, petechial, purpuric, or mixed, suggesting that small vessels as well as the medium-sized arteries are frequently involved. Persistent fever, malaise, rash, abdominal pain, arthralgia, arthritis, and hypertension occur in various combination. Visible or palpable vascular nodules are uncommon except in the cutaneous form of the disease described below.

Leukocytosis (12,000 to 40,000 WBC per cubic millimeter), elevated sedimentation rate, abnormal urinalyses, anemia, and negative tests for antinuclear antibody and rheumatoid factor are the usual laboratory findings. In the patients reported by Blau and associates, and by Reimold and colleagues, high titers of antibodies to streptococcal antigens were frequently found.[108,109]

Diagnosis is facilitated by the presence of detectable nodules which may be biopsied, but blind biopsy of muscle is unlikely to be productive. Selective angiography may demonstrate typical aneurysmal changes which provide objective grounds for the diagnosis but would not exclude the diagnosis if negative. When there are signs of nephritis, renal biopsy often provides the evidence of necrotizing arteritis needed to confirm the clinical impression. There is general agreement that treatment with corticosteroids is of value in reducing morbidity and mortality. The addition of immunosuppressive agents such as cyclophosphamide has been reported to enhance the treatment of these children and to reduce the mortality in the disease.[108]

Cutaneous Polyarteritis. Cutaneous polyarteritis is a subtype of PAN that occurs in children as well as adults.[105] The arteries of the skin and subcutaneous tissue are primarily involved, although deeper lesions also occur in some patients. The skin often shows livedo reticularis and small painful nodules occurring in crops. With the lesser internal organ involvement, the prognosis for this condition is better than for those with classic PAN, and lower doses of corticosteroids are usually adequate for treatment. Verbov reported sustained remission in one patient after treatment with aspirin alone.[111]

Infantile Polyarteritis and Kawasaki's Disease (Mucocutaneous Lymph Node Syndrome). Infantile polyarteritis and Kawasaki's disease are clinically and histologically virtually indistinguishable.[112] As originally reported in the United States, IPN usually began with an apparent viral syndrome with malaise and fever, followed soon by a rash.[113] Leukocytosis was prominent and antibiotic therapy without effect. The fever was persistent, and in the case reports findings typical of Kawasaki's disease, such as conjunctivitis, swelling of the hands and feet, and desquamation of the skin were sporadically noted. Death occurred unexpectedly in these infants at an average of about 4 weeks after onset. At autopsy, death was found to be almost entirely due to coronary arteritis with prominent aneurysm formation.

Kawasaki's disease was first described in the Japanese medical literature in 1967 by Kawasaki and in the American literature by Melish, Hicks, and Larson in 1976.[114,115] The typical clinical findings are listed in Table 82–4, and these are also the diagnostic criteria recommended by the Japan MCLS Research Committee in 1974. A combination of any five of the six criteria is required for diagnosis. Any one of the three subheadings listed under the major criteria of (3) and (4) fulfill that particular criterion. Other significant findings which may be observed are myocarditis, pericarditis, diarrhea, arthralgia, or arthritis. Aseptic meningitis and evidence of mild hepatitis occur less frequently. An apparently rare but interesting complication is that of hydrops of the gallbladder. Eight cases with anterior uveitis and one case of choroidoretinitis has been reported.[116-118] The mortality rate of approximately 1.7 percent is almost entirely due to coronary arteritis with striking aneurysm formation, and myocardial infarction.

Marked leukocytosis (15,000 to 40,000), predominantly granulocytic with varying percentages of immature forms, is found in 90 percent of the children. The platelet counts usually rise to levels of 500,000 to 1,000,000 during the second to third week of the disease and are another characteristic feature.[119] Tests for antinuclear antibody and rheumatoid factor are negative. Elevated IgE levels in the majority of patients were reported in one study.[120]

Although the children appear quite ill, often severely so, during the first 2 to 3 weeks of disease, complete recovery without apparent sequelae is the rule. There are no specific clues to those who will develop coronary artery disease. The patients at greatest risk appear to be male infants under 1 year of age. A variety of nonspecific EKG changes have been found in up to 60 percent of children with Kawasaki's disease but are of uncertain predictive value for the development of coronary artery disease.

In an angiographic study of 20 surviving children by Kato and associates, 12 were shown to have aneurysms of the coronary arteries.[121] On subsequent angiography the aneurysms had completely disappeared in the two who were restudied and the coronary circulation appeared entirely normal. The incidence of coronary arteritis in Kawasaki's disease is estimated to be between 15 and 17 percent; but healing occurs in most of those so afflicted.[122,123] The arteries of other organs also may become involved and not infrequently show aneurysm formation. There are no data at present which relate Kawasaki's disease to vascular disease occurring in later life, but deaths from coronary artery disease have been documented 2 months to 10 years after the acute illness had subsided.[124,125]

The general syndrome is not rare, with approximately 10,000 cases registered in Japan in the 6 years between 1970 and 1976.[125] It is probably more common in children in Japan than in the United States, but since the first English language description appeared in 1974, numerous reports of the syndrome have been published in the American and European literature. The male-to-female ratio is 1.5 to 1 and is almost identical to that of classic IPN in childhood. Eighty percent of the patients are under 5 years of age and 20 percent less than 1 year of age at the onset of their disease.

No therapeutic regimen has yet been shown to alter the outcome of Kawasaki's disease. Early corticosteroid trials were not found to decrease the mortality in this disease and may have been detrimental in some cases.[125] Hicks recommended aspirin in therapeutic doses for antiinflammatory and antiplatelet effects.[126] In view of the reported high platelet counts, thrombosis of the coronary vessels, and the uncertainties of corticosteroid therapy in Kawasaki's disease, this conservative approach to treatment may be the wisest course to follow.

Giant Cell Arteritis

Classic giant cell arteritis or polymyalgia rheumatica is virtually unknown in childhood.[127] Atypical temporal arteritis without giant cells, however, was recently reported in two boys 7 and 8 years of age.[128] These boys had been asymptomatic except for nodules approximately 5 × 10 mm in size with no other evidence of disease. Arteritis of the temporal arteries may, therefore, occur in childhood, but its relationship to the classic giant cell arteritis of late adult life is uncertain.

Takayasu's arteritis (pulseless disease) involves the aorta and its branches and, in contrast to temporal arteritis, is well known to occur in childhood and adolescence. Twenty-five to 30 percent of the patients have the onset of their disease before age 16.[105] One case has been documented in a 7-month-old infant.[129] In children the abdominal aorta and its branches are more commonly affected than the aortic arch, in contrast to young adults in whom the aortic arch is the major site of involvement.[130] Arteries during the active phase of the disease show an inflammatory infiltration of lymphocytes and plasma cells, primarily in the media and adventitia. Giant cells are few in number. Necrosis is most pronounced in the media of the vessel, and thrombosis may occur. In the later stages, fibrosis with narrowing

---

Table 82–4. Kawasaki Disease: Clinical Criteria for Diagnosis*

1. Fever lasting 5 days or more
2. Bilateral conjunctivitis
3. Changes of lips and oral cavity
   a. Dry, red, and fissured lips
   b. Strawberry tongue
   c. Diffuse reddening of oropharyngeal mucosa
4. Changes of peripheral extremities
   a. Reddening of palms and soles
   b. Indurative edema of hands and feet
   c. Membranous desquamation from fingertips
5. Polymorphous rash, primarily on trunk
6. Acute nonpurulent swelling of cervical lymph nodes to 1.5 cm or more in diameter

*Five of the six criteria listed are required for diagnosis. One or more of the three findings listed under (3) and (5) are sufficient to establish the criterion. (Recommendations of the Japan MCLS Research Committee, 1974.)

of the vessel predominates and vascular obstruction leads to absence of pulses and associated symptoms. The early or prepulseless phase is often manifested by fever, arthralgia, arthritis, myalgia, cough, or skin rash. These symptoms usually subside after weeks or months, to be followed months to years later by occlusive vascular disease. History of the early phase of the disease is often lacking in children and, if present, may have been too vague and nonspecific to have been related to the later vascular obstruction. Hypertension is found in 70 percent or more of the patients owing to involvement of the renal arteries, and its otherwise unexplained presence in a patient with a history of rheumatic symptoms is one clue to the diagnosis. Treatment with corticosteroids is of uncertain value, particularly in the late occlusive phase of the disease.[131] Medical treatment for the hypertension is generally effective, and surgical correction of the stenotic renal arteries can be considered in those cases resistant to medical control. It is thought that vascular surgery to correct arterial insufficiency at any site should not be carried out during the acute inflammatory stage.

References

1. King, K.K., Kornreich, H.K., Bernstein, B.H., Singsen, B.H., and Hanson, V.: The clinical spectrum of systemic lupus erythematosus in childhood. Arthritis Rheum. 20:287, 1977.
2. Meislin, A.G., and Rothfield, N.: Systemic lupus erythematosus in childhood. Analysis of 42 cases with comparative data on 200 adult cases followed concurrently. Pediatrics 42:37, 1968.
3. Cook, C.D., Wedgwood, R.J.T., Craig, J.M., Hartman, J.R., and Janeway, C.A.: Systemic lupus erythematosus. Description of 37 cases in children and a discussion of endocrine therapy in 32 of the cases. Pediatrics 26:570, 1960.
4. Jacobs, J.: Systemic lupus erythematosus in childhood. Pediatrics 32:257, 1963.
5. Walravens, P.A., and Chase, H.P.: The prognosis of childhood systemic lupus erythematosus. Am. J. Dis. Child. 130:929, 1976.
6. Dubois, E.L.: Lupus Erythematosus. 2nd ed. Los Angeles, University of Southern California Press, 1974.
7. Wallace, C., Schaller, J.G., Emery, H., and Wedgwood, R.: Prospective study of childhood systemic lupus erythematosus (abstract). Arthritis Rheum. 21:599, 1978.
8. Peterson, R.D.A., Vernier, R., and Good, R.A.: Lupus erythematosus. Pediat. Clin. North Am. 10:941, 1963.
9. Gribetz, D., and Henley, W.: Systemic lupus erythematosus in childhood. J. Mt. Sinai Hosp. 26:289, 1959.
10. Hagge, W., Burke, E.C., and Strickler, G.B.: Treatment of systemic lupus erythematosus complicated by nephritis in children. Pediatrics 40:822, 1967.
11. Cassidy, J.T., Sullivan, D.B., Petty, R.E., and Ragsdale, C.: Lupus nephritis and encephalopathy. Prognosis in 58 children. Arthritis Rheum. (Suppl.) 20:315, 1977.
12. Robinson, M.J., and Williams, A.L.: Systemic lupus erythematosus in childhood. Aust. Pediatr. J. 3:36, 1967.
13. Lehman, T.J.A., Curd, J.G., Zvaifler, N.J., and Hanson, V.: The association of antinuclear antibodies, antilymphocyte antibodies, and C4 activation among the relatives of children with systemic lupus erythematosus. Arthritis Rheum. 25:556, 1982.
14. Zetterstrom, R., and Berglund, G.: Systemic lupus erythematosus in childhood: A clinical study. Acta Pediatr. Scand. 45:189, 1956.
15. Duvic, M., Steinberg, A.D., and Klassen, L.W.: Effect of the antiestrogen nafoxidine on NZB/W-autoimmune disease. Arthritis Rheum. 21:414, 1978.
16. Talal, N.: Sex steroid hormones and systemic lupus erythematosus. Arthritis Rheum. 24:1054, 1981.
17. Lahita, R., Bradlow, L., Fishman, J., and Kunkel, H.: Estrogen metabolism in systemic lupus erythematosus. Arthritis Rheum. 25:843, 1982.
18. Schaller, J.G., Gilliland, B.G., Ochs, H.D., Leddy, J.P., Lawrence, C.Y.A., and Rosenfeld, S.I.: Severe systemic lupus erythematosus with nephritis in a boy with deficiency of the fourth component of complement. Arthritis Rheum. 20:1519, 1977.
19. Day, N.K., Geiger, H., McLain, R., Michael, A., and Good, R.A.: C2 deficiency, development of lupus erythematosus. J. Clin. Invest. 52:1601, 1973.
20. Lehman, T., Curd, J., Zvaifler, J., and Hanson, V.: - The association of antinuclear antibodies, and C4 activation among the relatives of children with SLE. Arthritis Rheum. 25:556, 1982.
21. Schaller, J.G.: Lupus phenomena in the newborn. Arthritis Rheum. 20:312, 1977.
22. Bridge, R.G., and Foley, F.E.: Placental transfer of the LE factor. Am. J. Med. Sci. 227:1, 1954.
23. Mijer, F., and Olsen, R.N.: Transplacental passage of the LE factor. J. Pediatr. 52:690, 1958.
24. Seip, M.: Systemic lupus erythematosus in pregnancy with hemolytic anemia, leukopenia, and thrombocytopenia in the mother and her newborn infant. Arch. Dis. Child. 35:364, 1960.
25. Beck, J.S., and Rowell, N.R.: Transplacental passage of antinuclear antibody. Lancet 1:134, 1963.
26. Reed, W.B., May, S.B., and Tuffanelli, D.L.: Discoid lupus erythematosus in a newborn. Arch. Dermatol. 96:64, 1967.
27. Hogg, G.R.: Congenital acute lupus erythematosus associated with subendocardial fibroelastosis. Report of a case. Am. J. Clin. Pathol. 28:648, 1957.
28. Hull, D., Dinns, B.A.O., and Joyce, D.: Congenital heart block and widespread fibrosis due to maternal lupus erythematosus. Arch. Dis. Child. 41:688, 1966.
29. McCue, C.M., Mantakas, M.E., Tingelstad, J.B., et al.: Congenital heart block in newborns of mother with connective tissue disease. Circulation 56:82, 1977.
30. Chameides, L., Treux, R.C., Vetter, V., Rashkind, W.J., Galioto, F.M., and Noonan, J.A.: Association of maternal systemic lupus erythematosus with congenital complete heart block. N. Engl. J. Med. 297:1204, 1977.
31. Franco, H.L., Weston, W.H., Peebles, C., Forstot, S.L., and Phanuphak, P.: Autoantibodies directed against sicca syndrome antigens in the neonatal lupus syndrome. J. Am. Acad. Dermatol. 4:67, 1981.
32. Kephart, D.C., Hood, A.F., and Provost, T.T.: Neonatal lupus erythematosus. J. Invest. Dermatol. 77:331, 981.
33. Patrone, N.D., Kredich, D.W., and Armstrong, B.E. (Abstr.) Arthritis Rheum. 4:S71, 1983.
34. Singsen, B.H., Fishman, L., and Hanson, V.: Antinuclear antibodies and lupus-like syndromes in children receiving anticonvulsants. Pediatrics 57:529, 1976.
35. Beernink, D.H., and Miller, J.J., III: Anticonvulsant induced antinuclear antibodies and lupus-like disease in children. J. Pediatr. 82:113, 1973.
36. Lieberman, E., Heuser, E., Hanson, V., Kornreich, H.K., Donnell, G.N., and Landing, B.H.: Identical 3-year-old twins with disseminated lupus erythematosus: One with nephrosis and one with nephritis. Arthritis Rheum. 11:22, 1968.
37. Cassidy, J.T., Walker, S.E., Soderstrom, S.J., Petty, R.E., and Sullivan, D.B.: Diagnostic significance of antibody to native deoxyribonucleic acid in children with juvenile rheumatoid arthritis and other connective tissue diseases. J. Pediatr. 93:416, 1978.
38. Hanson, V., Kornreich, H.K., and Drexler, E.: Rheumatoid factor in children with lupus erythematosus. Am. J. Dis. Child. 112:28, 1966.
39. Singsen, B.H., Bernstein, B.H., King, K.K., and Hanson, V.: Systemic lupus erythematosus in childhood: Correlations between changes in disease activity and the serum complement levels. J. Pediatr. 89:358, 1976.
40. Ishikawa, S., Segar, W.E., Gilbert, E.F., Burkholder, P.M., Levy, J.M., and Viseskui, C.: Myocardial infarct in a child with systemic lupus erythematosus. Am. J. Dis. Child. 132:696, 978.
41. King, K.K.: Personal communication.
42. Fish, A.J., Blau, E.B., Westberg, N.G., et al.: Systemic lupus erythematosus within the first two decades of life. Am. J. Med. 62:99, 1977.
43. Austin, H.A. III, Muenz, L.R., Joyce, K.M., Antonovych, T.A., Kullick, M.E., Klippel, J.H., Decker, J.L., and Balow, J.E.: Prognostic factors in lupus nephritis: Contribution of renal histology. Am. J. Med. 75:382, 1983.
44. Ropes, M.W.: Observations on the natural course of disseminated lupus erythematosus. Medicine 43:387, 1964.
45. Kimberly, R.P., Bowden, R.E., Keiser, H.R., and Plotz, P.H.: Reduction of renal function by newer nonsteroidal anti-inflammatory drugs. Am. J. Med. 64:804, 1978.
46. Blum, M., Bauminger, S., Algheti, M., Kisch, E., Ayalon, D., and Aviram, A.: Urinary prostaglandin E2 in chronic renal disease. Clin. Nephrol. 15:77, 1981.
47. Ayoub, W.T., Hale, R.C., Harrington, T.M., and Torretti, D.: Adverse effects of intravenous methylprednisolone pulse therapy (PT) in systemic lupus erythematosus. (Abstract) Arthritis Rheum. 26:S34, 1983.
48. Jacobs, J.C.: Treatment of systemic lupus erythematosus in childhood. Arthritis Rheum. 20:304, 1977.

49. Kornreich, H.K.: Systemic lupus erythematosus in childhood. Clin. Rheum. Dis. 2:429, 1976.

50. Hanson, V.: Dermatomyositis, scleroderma, and polyarteritis nodosa. Clin. Rheum. Dis. 2:445, 1976.

51. Banker, B.Q., and Victor, M.: Dermatomyositis (systemic angiopathy) of childhood. Medicine 45:261, 1966.

52. Bohan, A., and Peter, J.B.: Dermatomyositis and polymyositis. A review. Part I. N. Engl. J. Med. 292:344, 1975.

53. Cook, C.D., Rosen, F.S., and Banker, B.Q.: Dermatomyositis and focal scleroderma. Pediatr. Clin. North Am. 10:979, 1963.

54. Sullivan, D.B., Cassidy, J.P., Petty, R.E., and Burt, A.: Prognosis in childhood dermatomyositis. J. Pediatr. 80:555, 1972.

55. Rose, A.L.: Childhood polymyositis: A follow-up study with special reference to treatment with corticosteroids. Am. J. Dis. Child. 127:518, 1974.

56. Bitnum, S., Daeschner, C.W., Jr., et al.: Dermatomyositis. J. Pediatr. 64:101, 1964.

57. Singsen, B.H., Tedford, J.C., Platzker, A.C.G., and Hanson, V.: Spontaneous pneumothorax: A complication of juvenile dermatomyositis. J. Pediatr. 92:771, 1978.

58. Singsen, B.H., Goldreyer, B., Stanton, R., and Hanson, V.: Childhood polymyositis with cardiac conduction defects. Am. J. Dis. Child. 130:72, 1976.

59. King, J.O., and Zapf, P.: A review of the value of creatine phosphokinase estimations in clinical medicine. Med. J. Aust. 1:699, 1972.

60. Vignos, P.J., and Goldwyn, J.: Evaluation of laboratory tests in the diagnosis and management of polymyositis. Am. J. Med. Sci. 263:291, 1972.

61. LaPorta, M.A., Linde, H.W., Bruce, D.L., and Fitzsimons, E.J.: Evaluation of creatine phosphokinase in young men after recreational exercise. JAMA 239:2685, 1978.

62. Banker, B.Q.: Dermatomyositis of childhood. Ultrastructural alteration of muscles and intramuscular blood vessels. J. Neuropathol. Exp. Neurol. 34:46, 1975.

63. Whitaker, J.N., and Engel, W.K.: Vascular deposits of immunoglobulin and complement in idiopathic inflammatory myopathy. N. Engl. J. Med. 286:333, 1972.

64. Spencer, C., Kornreich, H.K., Bernstein, B.H., King, K.K., Singsen, B.H., and Hanson, V.: Three courses of childhood dermatomyositis (CDM). Clin. Res. 27:111A, 1979.

65. Miller, J.J., III, and Koehler, P.P.: Persistence of activity in dermatomyositis of childhood. Arthritis Rheum. (Suppl.) 20:332, 1977.

66. Dubowitz, V.: Treatment of dermatomyositis in childhood. Arch. Dis. Child. 51:494, 1976.

67. Jacobs, J.C.: Treatment of dermatomyositis. Arthritis Rheum. 20:338, 1977.

68. Thompson, C.E.: Polymyositis in children. Clin. Pediatr. 7:24, 1968.

69. Middleton, P.J., Alexander, R.M., and Szymanski, R.M.: Severe myositis during recovery from influenza. Lancet 2:533, 1970.

70. Grose, C.: Staphylococcal polymyositis in South Texas. J. Pediatr. 93:457, 1978.

71. Kentras, H.: Myositis with Kawasaki's disease. Am. J. Dis. Child. 136:78, 1982.

72. Cassidy, J.T., Sullivan, D.B., Dabich, L., and Petty, R.E.: Scleroderma in children. Arthritis Rheum. 20:351, 1977.

73. Christianson, H.B., Dorsey, C.S., O'Leary, P.A., and Kierland, R.R.: Localized scleroderma: A clinical study of two hundred thirty-five cases. AMA Arch. Dermatol. 74:629, 1956.

74. Kornreich, H.K., King, K.K., Bernstein, B.H., Singsen, B.H., and Hanson, V.: Scleroderma in childhood. Arthritis Rheum. (Suppl.) 20:343, 1977.

75. Sandborg, C., Hanson, V., Kornreich, H.K., Bernstein, B.H., and King, K.K.: Arthritis, myositis, and growth defects of bone in children with localized scleroderma. (Abstract) Arthritis Rheum. 23:741, 1980.

76. Jakuboska, K.: Changes in the locomotor system in progressive systemic sclerosis in children. Mater. Med. Pol. 13:1, 1972.

77. Dabich, L., Sullivan, D.B., and Cassidy, J.T.: Scleroderma in the child. J. Pediatr. 85:770, 1974.

78. Kass, H., Hanson, V., and Patrick, J.: Scleroderma in childhood. J. Pediatr. 68:243, 1966.

79. Hanson, V., Kornreich, H.K., and Drexler, E.: Some immunologic considerations in focal scleroderma and progressive systemic sclerosis in children. Pediatr. Res. 8:806, 1974.

80. Hanson, V., Drexler, E., and Kornreich, H.K.: Rheumatoid factor (anti-gamma-globulins) in children with focal scleroderma. Pediatrics 53:945, 1974.

81. Jansen, G.T., Barraza, D.F., Ballard, J.L. Honeycutt, W.M., and Dillaka, C.J.: Generalized scleroderma. Treatment with an immunosuppressive agent. Arch. Dermatol. 97:690, 1968.

82. Bluestone, R., Grahame, R., Holloway, V., and Holt, P.J.L.: Treatment of systemic sclerosis with D-penicillamine. Ann. Rheum. Dis. 29:153, 1970.

83. Zeek, P.M.: Periarteritis nodosa and other forms of necrotizing angiitis. N. Engl. J. Med. 248:764, 1953.

84. McCombs, R.P.: Systemic "allergic" vasculitis: Clinical and pathological relationships. JAMA 194:1059, 1965.

85. Gilliam, J.N., and Smiley, J.D.: Cutaneous necrotizing vasculitis and related disorders. Ann. Allergy 37:328, 1976.

86. Allen, D.M., Diamond, L.K., and Howell, D.A.: Anaphylactoid purpura in children (Henoch-Schönlein syndrome). Am. J. Dis. Child. 99:833, 1960.

87. West, R.J.: Acute polyarthritis: Diagnosis and management. Clin. Rheum. Dis. 2:305, 1976.

88. Henoch, E.H.H.: Berl. Klin. Wochenschr. 11:641, 1874. English translation: Am. J. Dis. Child. 128:78, 1974.

89. Emery, H., Larter, W., and Schaller, J.G.: Henoch-Schoenlein vasculitis. Arthritis Rheum. 20:385, 1977.

90. Koskimies, O., Mir, S., Rapola, J., and Vilska, J.: Henoch-Schönlein nephritis: Long-term prognosis of unselected patients. Arch. Dis. Child. 56:482, 1981.

91. Meadow, S.R.: The prognosis of Henoch-Schoenlein nephritis. Clin. Nephrology 9:87, 1978.

92. Wedgwood, R.J.P., and Klaus, M.H.: Anaphylactoid purpura (Schönlein-Henoch syndrome). Pediatrics 16:196, 1955.

93. Trygstad, C.W., and Stiehm, E.R.: Elevated serum IgA globulin in anaphylactoid purpura. Pediatrics 47:1023, 1971.

94. Vernier, R.L., Worthen, H.G., Peterson, R.D., Colle, E., and Good, R.A.: Anaphylactoid purpura: I. Pathology of the skin and kidney and frequency of streptococcal infection. Pediatrics 27:181, 1961.

95. Giangiacomo, J., and Tsai, C.C.: Dermal and glomerular deposition of IgA in anaphylactoid purpura. Am. J. Dis. Child. 131:981, 1977.

96. Hanson, V., and Kornreich, H.K.: Systemic rheumatic disorders ("collagen disease") in childhood: Lupus erythematosus, anaphylactoid purpura, dermatomyositis, and scleroderma. Part I. Bull. Rheum. Dis. 17:435, 1967.

97. McDuffie, F.C., Sams, W.M., Maldonado, J.E., et al.: Hypocomplementemia with cutaneous vasculitis and arthritis: Possible immune complex syndrome. Mayo Clin. Proc. 48:340, 1973.

98. Soter, N.A., Austen, K.F., and Gigli, I.: Urticaria and arthralgias as manifestations of necrotizing angiitis (vasculitis). J. Invest. Dermatol. 63:485, 1974.

99. Soter, N.A.: Chronic urticaria as a manifestation of necrotizing venulitis. N. Engl. J. Med. 296:1440, 1977.

100. LoSpaulluto, J., Dorward, B., Miller, W., Jr., and Ziff, M.: Cryoglobulinemia based on interaction between a gamma macroglobulin and 7S gamma globulin. Am. J. Med. 32:142, 1962.

101. Meltzer, M., Franklin, E.C., Ellias, K., McCluskey, R.T., and Cooper, N.: Cryoglobulinemia—a clinical and laboratory study. II. Cryoglobulins with rheumatoid factor activity. Am. J. Med. 40:837, 1966.

102. Churg, J., and Strauss, L.: Allergic granulomatosis, allergic angiitis, and periarteritis nodosa. Am. J. Pathol. 27:277, 1951.

103. Farooki, Z.Q., Brough, A.J., and Green, E.W.: Necrotizing arteritis. Am. J. Dis. Child. 128:837, 1974.

104. Feldman, F., Fink, H., and Gruezo, Z.: Wegener's granulomatosis: Report of a case in a 13-year-old girl. Am. J. Dis. Child. 112:587, 1966.

105. Fink, C.W.: Polyarteritis and other diseases with necrotizing vasculitis in childhood. Arthritis Rheum. (Suppl.) 20:378, 1977.

106. Orlowski, J.P., Clough, J.D., and Dyment, P.G.: Wegener's granulomatosis in the pediatric age group. Pediatrics 61:83, 1978.

107. Cohen, S.R., Landing, B.H., King, K.K., and Isaacs, H.: Wegener's granulomatosis causing laryngeal and tracheobronchial obstruction in an adolescent girl. Ann. Otol. Rhinol. Laryngol. (Suppl. 52) 87:15, 1978.

108. Reimold, E.W., Weinberg, A.G., Fink, C.W., and Battles, N.D.: Polyarteritis in children. Am. J. Dis. Child. 130:534, 1976.

109. Blau, E.B., Morris, R.F., and Yunis, E.J.: Polyarteritis nodosa in older children. Pediatrics 60:227, 1977.

110. Magilavy, D.B., Petty, R.E., Cassidy, J.T., and Sullivan, D.B.: A syndrome of childhood polyarteritis. J. Pediatr. 91:25, 1977.

111. Verbov, J.: Cutaneous polyarteritis nodosa in a young child. Arch. Dis. Child. 55:569, 1980.

112. Landing, B.H., and Jarson, E.J.: Are infantile periarteritis nodosa with coronary artery involvement and fatal mucocutaneous lymph node syndrome the same? Comparison of 20 patients from North America with patients from Hawaii and Japan. Pediatrics 59:651, 1977.

113. Roberts, F.B., and Fetterman, G.H.: Polyarteritis nodosa in infancy. J. Pediatr. 63:519, 963.

114. Kawasaki, T.: MCLS: Clinical observation of 50 cases. Jap. J. Allergy 16:178, 1967.

115. Melish, M.E., Hicks, R.M., and Larson, E.J.: Mucocutaneous lymph node syndrome in the United States. Am. J. Dis. Child. 130:599, 1976.

116. Germain, B.F., Moroney, J.D., Guggino, G.S., Cimino, L., Rodriguez, C., and Bocanegra, T.S.: Anterior uveitis in Kawasaki disease. J. Pediatr. 97:780, 1980.

117. Lapointe, N., Chad, Z., Lacroix, J., Jacob, J.-L., Urbanski, P., Polomeno, R., and Kupfert, B.: Kawasaki disease: Associated with uveitis in seven patients. Pediatrics 69:376, 1982.

118. Ver hote, M., Rousseau, E., Jacob, J.L., and Lapointe, N.: An uncommon clinical sign in mucocutaneous lymph node syndrome. Acta Paediatr. Scand. 70:591, 1981.

119. Kawasaki, T., Kosaki, F., Okawa, S., et al.: A new infantile acute febrile mucocutaneous lymph node syndrome (MLNS) prevailing in Japan. Pediatrics 54:271, 1974.

120. Kusakawa, S. and Heiner, D.C.: Elevated levels of immunoglobulin E in the acute febrile mucocutaneous lymph node syndrome. Pediatr. Res. 10:108, 1976.

121. Kato, H., Koike, S., Yamamoto, M., et al.: Coronary aneurysms in infants and young children with acute febrile mucocutaneous lymph node syndrome. J. Pediatr. 86:892, 1975.

122. Chung, K.J., Brandt, L., Fulton, D.R., and Kreidberg, M.B.: Cardiac and coronary arterial involvement in infants and children from New England with mucocutaneous lymph node syndrome (Kawasaki disease). Am. J. Cardiol. 50:136, 1982.

123. Kato, H., Ichinose, E., Yoshioka, F., Takechi, T., Matsunaga, S., Suzuki, K., and Rikitake, N.: Fate of coronary aneurysms in Kawasaki disease: Serial coronary angiography and long-term follow-up study. Am. J. Cardiol. 49:1758, 1982.

124. Fujiwara, H., and Hamashima, Y.: Pathology of the heart in Kawasaki disease. Pediatrics 61:100, 1978.

125. Morens, D.M., and Nahmias, A.J.: Kawasaki disease: A "new" pediatrics enigma. Hosp. Pract. 13:109, 1978.

126. Hicks, R.M.: Mucocutaneous lymph node syndrome in Hawaii. Arthritis Rheum. 20:389, 1977.

127. Huston, K.A., Hunder, G.G., Lie, J.T., Kennedy, R.H., and Elveback, L.R.: Temporal arteritis: A 25-year epidemiologic, clinical and pathologic study. Ann. Intern. Med. 88:162, 1978.

128. Lie, J.T., Gordon, L.P., and Titus, J.L.: Juvenile temporal arteritis: Biopsy study of four cases. JAMA 234:496, 1975.

129. Gronemeyer, P.S., and deMello, D.E.: Takayasu's disease with aneurysm of right common iliac artery and iliocaval fistula in a young infant: Case report and review of literature. Pediatrics 69:626, 1982.

130. Danaraj, T.J., and Ong, W.H.: Primary arteritis of abdominal aorta in children causing bilateral stenosis of renal arteries and hypertension. Circulation 20:856, 1978.

131. Lupi-Herrera, E., Sanchez-Torres, G., Marcushamer, J., et al.: Takayasu's arteritis. Clinical study of 107 cases. Am. Heart. J. 93:94, 1977.

Section XII
Primary Disorders of Immune Function

Chapter 83
Immunodeficiency Diseases

R. Michael Blaese

INTRODUCTION

It is just three decades since Bruton described the first case of agammaglobulinemia, introducing the concept of immunodeficiency disease to clinical medicine.[1] In the ensuing 30 years, dozens of distinct disorders of immune function have been described, with pathogenic mechanisms ranging from inherited inborn errors of metabolism to congenital defects of organ development to acquired immunodeficiency states associated with infectious agents or malignancy.[2-6] Although most of these individual disorders are rare, as a group immunodeficiency diseases are common enough that every physician will encounter patients with this class of disease.

The hallmark of diseases with defects in the immune system is an increased susceptibility of the patient to infection. Immunodeficiency diseases may be associated with a myriad of other problems, including autoimmune phenomena, allergy, anemia, thrombocytopenia, malabsorption, arthritis, diarrhea, and cancer. Nevertheless the single feature common to all of these disorders is recurrent infection.

The responsibility for bodily defense against infection is shared between both specific and nonspecific mechanisms. The nonspecific elements include cells such as the polymorphonuclear leukocytes, eosinophils, mast cells, and macrophages and humoral factors, most notably serum complement. Specific defense is mediated by elements that make up the immune system. The term specific refers to the capacity of the immune system to respond uniquely to each individual foreign invader and to exhibit a memory response should that particular individual organism attempt to reinvade at a later time. The roles of the specific and nonspecific systems are closely linked. As an example, specific antibodies made by the immune system to a bacterium may utilize a nonspecific phagocyte to actually kill the organism. In turn, the phagocytic cell relies on the antibody coating the microorganism for attaching to and phagocytizing that organism.

Because literally dozens of separate immunodeficiency diseases have been reported, a systematic approach to patient evaluation is essential to help identify and appropriately treat patients with one of these frequently rare syndromes. By careful attention to the patient's history and the performance of a few simple, inexpensive laboratory tests it is quite easy to determine whether a patient has a significant disorder of immune function and to establish a limited list of diagnostic possibilities, which then may be evaluated in detail.

The immune system is usefully thought of as a dual system.[7] The B-lymphocyte or antibody system consists of bone marrow or bursa-derived lymphocytes, plasma cells, and their products, the immunoglobulins. The T-lymphocyte or cellular immune system consists of the thymus-derived lymphocytes and subpopulations of these T lymphocytes with specialized functions. From careful studies of patients with defects in one or the other of these systems, it is now known that the B-lymphocyte system and the T-lymphocyte system are each responsible for defense against different types of organisms. Humoral immune deficiency is usually associated with recurrent infections with high-grade encapsulated bacterial pathogens such as the pneumococcus and *Hemophilus influenzae*. Infections with these organisms most frequently involve the sinopulmonary tree. Deficiency of the cellular immune system is usually associated with infections by opportunistic pathogens such as *Pneumocystis carinii*, herpes viruses, and fungi. By contrast, a patient presenting with recurrent abscesses and granulomas of the skin, lungs, or internal viscera containing organisms such as *Staphylococcus aureus* or *Klebsiella* suggests that the patient has a defect in phagocytic cell function rather than a defect in the immune system.

PATIENT EVALUATION, HISTORY, AND PHYSICAL EXAMINATION

As outlined above, the types of infection the patient is experiencing provides a major clue to the type of immune defect that may exist. Bacterial meningitis, sepsis, otitis media, sinusitis, and bronchitis are the usual kinds of infections found in patients with B-lymphocyte defects. Unusual mycobacterial infections, candidiasis, systemic herpes zoster or severe varicella, disseminated cytomegalovirus infections, pneumocystis pneumonia, or generalized vaccinia following smallpox vaccination are the types of infections seen in patients with severe T cell defects (Fig. 83–1). Patients with defects in both the T- and B-lymphocyte systems will experience infections with all classes of microorganism.

"How many infections should a patient have before I work up the immune system?" Although the answer to this question is necessarily arbitrary, certainly any patient who has required hospitalization because of an infection should have a screening work-up of the immune system. In addition, any patient in whom recurrent infection has caused structural damage resulting in functional impairment such as chronic otitis media or chronic bronchitis and bronchiectasis should be evaluated for the possibility of an immunodeficiency state. The majority of patients with chronic sinopulmonary infections do not have immunodeficiency as an underlying factor, but for those patients who do, establishment of the correct diagnosis and institution of appropriate therapy may halt the progressive loss of pulmonary function, which is the leading cause of morbidity and mortality in patients with humoral immune deficiency diseases. By contrast it must be remembered that children normally have an average of six to seven upper respiratory infections each year until the early teens and if these

Figure 83–1. Cutaneous dissemination of herpes simplex in a boy with severe T lymphocyte deficiency. Disseminated infections with HSV, vaccinia, CMV, and varicella-zoster are a constant threat in patients with defective T lymphocyte immunity.

episodes are uncomplicated, no work-up of the immune system is indicated.

If the history of infections suggests immunodeficiency, certain historical details may help identify the specific disease involved. The individual features of the principal immune deficiency diseases are discussed later in this chapter, but some specific illustrations are useful. A careful family history should be obtained, particularly when the patient is an infant or child, since many of the primary immunodeficiency diseases are inherited as X-linked or autosomal recessive traits. A history of siblings, uncles, or cousins dying of infection in early childhood may be a very important clue to the specific diagnosis. In adults as well, certain disorders have a familial pattern. The age of the patient should be a major factor in directing the line of inquiry. Although some diseases, such as selective IgA deficiency or agammaglobulinemia, can initially present in either adults or children, many of the more severe immunodeficiency diseases are found only in children. Table 83–1 presents a list of some of the great variety of historical findings associated with the major immunodeficiency diseases. For example, a review of the history of immunizations may indicate the development of an anterior motor neuron paralysis after the administration of oral polio vaccine in some infants with severe forms of immunodeficiency disease. Generalized vaccinia occurring after a smallpox vaccination and generalized BCGosis after BCG immunization have also been described in infants with severe combined immune deficiency (SCID). Patients with selective IgA deficiency may present because of an unexplained blood transfusion reaction. This is a form of anaphylaxis caused by the interaction between IgA contained in the transfused normal blood and anti-IgA antibodies that some of these patients spontaneously produce. Adult patients with the acquired immune deficiency syndrome (AIDS) very frequently have severe and unexplained diarrhea in addition to suffering from recurrent infections with opportunistic pathogens such as *Pneumocystis carinii*. A polyendocrinopathy syndrome with disorders of thyroid, parathyroid, and adrenal function occurs in some patients with chronic mucocutaneous candidiasis. Patients with hemophilia and patients with a history of intravenous drug abuse have recently been found to have an increased susceptibility to the development of AIDS. Congenital rubella and congenital cytomegalovirus infections are frequently associated with a profound immune deficiency state in the affected infants, and the appearance of agammaglobulinemia in both adults and children has been described following the occurrence of a primary infection with the Epstein-Barr virus.

Physical examination provides evidence supporting a specific diagnosis in only a limited number of disorders and usually serves to confirm the consequences of recurrent infection. Table 83–1 also includes some of the key physical findings of various immunodeficiency disorders. For example, ocular telangiectasia and cerebellar ataxia are characteristics of the disorder ataxia-telangiectasia. Petechiae secondary to thrombocytopenia and

Table 83–1. Historical Features and Physical Findings in Children and Adults with Immunodeficiency Disease

System	Children	Adults
Head, Eyes, Ears, Face		
Small mouth, low set ears	DiG	
Absent tonsils	X-LA, SCID	
Premature gray hair	AT	AT
Alopecia areata	SCID with CHH	
Neurological		
Seizures	DiG	
Ataxia, choreoathetosis	AT	AT
ECHOvirus encephalitis	X-LA	X-LA
Intracranial hemorrhage	WAS	
Brain lymphoma	WAS, AT	
Skin		
Petechiae	WAS	
Eczema	WAS, X-LA	
Telangiectasia	AT	AT
Thrush	WAS, CMC, SCID, DiG	CMC
Edema	IL	IL
Vitiligo	AT	
Kaposi's sarcoma		AIDS
Endocrine/Metabolism		
Growth hormone deficiency	X-LA	
Tetany	DiG	
Polyendocrinopathy	CMC	CMC
Failure to thrive	SCID, WAS, PNP, Trans II, IL	
Insulin resistance	AT	AT
Hypogonadism	AT, CMC	AT, CMC
Gastrointestinal		
Diarrhea	SCID, WAS, Trans II, IL, CMC	CVH, AIDS, A, IL, CVH
Dysphagia	CMC, WAS, DiG	CMC
Nodular lymphoid hyperplasia	CVH	CVH
Hepatitis	CMC, AT	CMC, AT, AIDS
Cardiovascular		
Congenital heart disease	DiG	
Cor pulmonale	X-LA	CVH
Vasculitis	WAS	
Bone/Joint/Muscle		
Arthritis	WAS, X-LA	CVH, A
SLE		A
Dermatomyositis	X-LA	
Dwarfism	X-LA, SCID with CHH	
Hematologic		
Hepatosplenomegaly	WAS, CVH	CVH, Thymoma
Thrombocytopenia	WAS	CVH, Thymoma
Anemia	WAS, PNP, SCID, Trans II	CVH, Thymoma
Coombs' test +	WAS	CVH
Transfusion reaction	A	A
Transfusion-induced GVH	SCID, PNP	
Hemophilia	AIDS	AIDS
Pernicious anemia	Trans II(?), CMC	CVH, CMC
Malignancy	WAS, AT	CVH
Infectious mononucleosis	CVH, XLP	CVH
Immunization Complications		
Polio, vaccinia, BCG	SCID, PNP, WAS	
Social History		
IV drug abuse		AIDS
Promiscuous homosexual		AIDS
AIDS household contact	AIDS	
Consanquinity	AT, SCID, Trans II, ADA, PNP	
Family History		
X-linked	X-LA, WAS, SCID	
AR	AT, SCID, ADA, PNP, Trans II, A	A

Abbreviations: WAS, Wiskott-Aldrich syndrome; SCID, severe combined immunodeficiency; PNP, purine nucleoside phosphorylase deficiency; A, IgA deficiency; Trans II, transcobalamin II deficiency; AIDS, acquired immune deficiency syndrome; AT, ataxia-telangiectasia; X-LA, X-linked agammaglobulinemia; CHH, cartilage-hair hyperplasia; CVH, common variable hypogammaglobulinemia; Thymoma, thymoma and hypogammaglobulinemia; DiG, DiGeorge syndrome; IL, intestinal lymphangiectasia; CMC, chronic mucocutaneous candidiasis; XLP, X-linked lymphoproliferative syndrome.

eczema of the skin are always seen in children with the Wiskott-Aldrich syndrome. Children with X-linked agammaglobulinemia lack tonsils, and infants with the DiGeorge syndrome frequently have congenital heart disease and a characteristic facial appearance. Acute and/or chronic sinusitis and otitis media as well as chronic bronchitis and bronchiectasis are common in all patients with the various forms of B-lymphocyte defect. Hepatosplenomegaly as well as lymphadenopathy is seen in many of the different forms of immunodeficiency.

LABORATORY EVALUATION: SCREENING WORK-UP

Sophisticated techniques are available that allow a very detailed examination of the function of every facet of the immune system. Fortunately, simple and inexpensive screening tests can be used that will usually pinpoint the problem or at least allow a rational selection of additional studies. These screening tests fall into three categories: tests for humoral immunity, tests for cellular immunity, and tests for the system of nonspecific resistance (Table 83–2).

Clinically significant defects in humoral immunity can almost always be detected by two widely available laboratory tests. The first is the determination of the concentrations of serum IgG, IgA, and IgM. The range of normal values for each of these classes of immunoglobulin changes independently with age (Fig. 83–2). At birth, IgG is present at adult levels because of transplacental transport of IgG from the mother. IgA and IgM are ordinarily absent from the sera of newborns unless the infant has an infection acquired in utero. Absence of each of the immunoglobulin classes is the hallmark of the agammaglobulinemic syndromes, while dysgammaglobulinemias such as selective IgM deficiency or selective IgA deficiency are also readily diagnosed by the determination of serum immunoglobulin levels. In general the measurement of serum IgE concentrations is not useful in the diagnosis of immunodeficiency disease.

Some patients with recurrent infections with the types of organisms associated with defects in humoral immunity have immunoglobulin levels in or close to the normal range. In these cases the measurement of a functional antibody response is essential for establishing the diagnosis of an antibody deficiency syndrome. Isohemagglutinins are natural antibodies to blood group A and/or B antigens found in all normals except those with type AB red cells. By the age of three, 98 percent of normals with type A, B, or O blood will have titers of isohemagglutinins of at least 1:16. Hospital and regional blood banks routinely measure these antibodies. As an example of the usefulness of the measurement of antibodies in identifying humoral immune deficiency, patients with the Wiskott-Aldrich syndrome may have normal immunoglobulin levels and yet lack isohemagglutinins as an indication of their antibody deficiency state.

These two screening tests will be abnormal in practically all immunodeficiency diseases affecting the B-lymphocyte system. The rare exceptions that may be missed include a syndrome of recurrent infections associated with hyper-IgE[8,9] and certain patients with deficiency in one of the subclasses of IgG.[10,11] Unfortunately only a handful of laboratories in the world measure IgG subclass levels. With the recent development of monoclonal antibodies to the IgG subclasses, these measurements should become widely available within the near future.

The cellular immune system is also evaluated with two screening procedures. A white blood cell count and differential should be obtained and the absolute lymphocyte count calculated by multiplying the total white count by the percentage of lymphocytes. Children have higher absolute lymphocyte counts than adults so that age must also be considered in evaluating lymphocyte numbers. It is a useful practice to routinely perform this calculation on every WBC and differential so that low values are quickly recognized. Adults with AIDS or

Figure 83–2. Serum levels of IgG, IgA, and IgM change independently during childhood, and stable (adult) levels for each class are reached at different ages (mean and 95% normal range).

Table 83–2. Screening Tests for Defects in the Immune System

Humoral Immunity
    Serum immunoglobulins—IgG, IgA, and IgM
    Isohemagglutinin titers—at least 1:16 by age 3
Cellular Immunity
    Absolute lymphocyte count—WBC × percentage of lymphs
    Delayed hypersensitivity skin tests: tetanus toxoid, Candida, trichophyton, SKSD, diphtheria toxoid
Nonspecific Resistance
    Absolute granulocyte count—WBC × percentage of PMNs
    NBT (nitroblue tetrazolium) test
    Serum complement titer (CH$_{50}$)

intestinal lymphangiectasia or infants with severe combined immune deficiency may have fewer than 200 lymphocytes per cubic millimeter in their peripheral blood.

Functional tests of the cellular immune system are also important in screening. Delayed-type hypersensitivity skin tests are the simplest and least expensive way to screen for this function. The tests used in screening should normally be positive in a large majority of normal individuals so that negative responses have significance. Thus antigens that are often negative in normals, such as PPD and histoplasmin, are not useful as skin tests for this screening. A battery of several antigens, each of which is positive in over 90 percent of normals, should be used. Tetanus toxoid, *Candida albicans,* streptokinase, diphtheria toxoid, and Trichophyton are excellent antigens for this purpose. If a patient has severe lymphocytopenia or is anergic, additional studies will be necessary to define the defect, However, a physician can feel confident that his patient does not have a severe cellular immune deficiency disorder if these two screening procedures are normal.

This T-lymphocyte screening work-up is useful in patients old enough to have been exposed to environmental or vaccine antigens, but newborns and young infants frequently have limited exposure. In infants, the measurement of the total number of T lymphocytes using sheep erythrocyte rosetting or specific monoclonal antibodies should detect those infants with significant T-lymphocyte deficiency. Functional tests such as the proliferative response of lymphocytes in the mixed lymphocyte reaction or in response to the mitogens concanavalin A and phytohemagglutinin may also be required to detect cellular immune deficiency in the newborn.

The third set of screening procedures covers disorders of the nonspecific resistance system. Although these disorders are not immunodeficiency diseases, it is useful to keep screening tests for the major defects in mind when evaluating a patient for a defect in host defense. The polymorphonuclear leukocyte (PMN) is responsible for killing many bacterial pathogens, so that patients with neutropenia or disorders of PMN function frequently have major infections. Here again the WBC count and differential are important to rule out neutropenia as a contributor to the infection. Chronic granulomatous disease is a disorder of PMN function in which bacteria are ingested normally by the PMN but the intracellular killing mechanism of these cells is abnormal. Therefore, the ingested bacteria are not killed and they multiply intracellularly, causing abscesses and granulomas at multiple sites in the body. Chronic granulomatous disease is associated with infections by catalase-positive bacteria such as *Staphylcoccus aureus,* and most of these patients can be detected by the performance of an NBT test on the PMNs.[12]

Complement is the major serum factor contributing to the system of nonspecific resistance. Patients with certain complement deficiencies also have severe bacterial infections.[13] Curiously, *Neisseria* infection is particularly common in patients deficient in a terminal complement component. Determination of the titer of total hemolytic complement (CH50) is the best general screening test for deficiencies in this system. The measurement of serum C3 or C4 levels are not useful as a general screen of the complement system, since a clinically significant deficiency of a terminal complement component would be missed by these measurements.

ONTOGENY AND ORGANIZATION OF THE IMMUNE SYSTEM

To better understand the immunodeficiency states it is important to have an understanding of the development and organization of the immune system (see Section I for a detailed review of this topic). Figure 83–3 shows a simplified schematic representation of the differentiation pathways followed during the development of the immune system. During early embryonic life pleuripotent stem cells rise in the yolk sac and migrate to

Figure 83–3. A schematic diagram illustrating the pathways of differentiation, maturation, and cellular interactions in the immune system. Stem cells arising in the fetal yolk sac and later the bone marrow differentiate through a series of maturation steps to form competent T and B lymphocytes capable of a broad range of specific immune responses.

sites in the body where they differentiate along the hematopoietic and lymphoid lineage. When stem cells migrate to an epithelial structure derived from the third and fourth pharyngeal pouches of the embryo, the thymus, they differentiate to become T lymphocytes.

T lymphocytes are responsible for several essential immune functions. They become cytotoxic killer cells that can destroy virus-infected cells and grafts of foreign tissues. They mediate delayed hypersensitivity skin reactions and are responsible for graft-versus-host reactions. They produce biologically active humoral factors, the lymphokines, which affect the function of other cells, including B lymphocytes, macrophages, and other T lymphocytes. T lymphocytes also play an important immunoregulatory role for B-lymphocyte function. For example, T lymphocytes from agammaglobulinemic birds were shown to transfer the agammaglobulinemia when transplanted to normal recipient birds as the first demonstration of suppressor T lymphocytes involved in immunodeficiency.[14]

In avian species, pleuripotent stem cells that differentiate in the microenvironment of the bursa of Fabricius develop into lymphocytes specialized for the production of immunoglobulin, the B lymphocytes. In mammals the fetal liver appears to serve as the structural analog of the avain bursa, and it is here that the first cells of the B-lymphocyte lineage are identified in the developing embryo.[15] These cells are called pre-B lymphocytes. Pre-B lymphocytes contain cytoplasmic immunoglobulin μ heavy chains but have not yet begun to synthesize immunoglobulin light chains.[16] At the nuclear level pre-B cell DNA has rearranged the IgM heavy chain genes with the kappa and lambda light chain genes still in their germline configuration.[17] Pre-B lymphocytes do not express μ chain determinants on their surface membranes. As pre-B lymphocytes mature they acquire complete IgM molecules, which are then expressed on their surface membranes, and at this stage rearrangement of both the heavy and light chain genes is found. B lymphocytes then mature to a form that also expresses surface membrane IgD and perhaps other isotypes such as IgG and IgA in addition to IgM. More mature B lymphocytes express only a single immunoglobulin isotype. The last stage of cellular maturation in the B-lymphocyte pathway is the formation of the plasma cell.[18,19]

Many primary immunodeficiency diseases have defects that suggest that the normal pathway of lymphoid differentiation has been arrested at a premature stage. For example, patients with X-linked agammaglobulinemia are found to lack B lymphocytes, but pre-B lymphocytes may be present in normal numbers. Patients with agammaglobulinemia and thymoma lack both B lymphocytes and pre-B lymphocytes. Thus, an understanding of the normal pathway of B-lymphocyte differentiation provides a framework for a better understanding of these diseases.

In considering the potential mechanisms of disordered immunity, it is important to remember that a single phenotypic deficiency may be the result of several distinct defects. For example, agammaglobulinemia can be the result of an intrinsic defect in B-lymphocyte maturation. However, the same immunoglobulin deficiency can be the result of an active inhibition of immunoglobulin production by an extrinsic factor such as a suppressor T lymphocyte or because of the lack of an essential cofactor such as a helper T lymphocyte. Serum immunoglobulin levels may be low because of defective synthesis, but they can also be low because immunoglobulin is being lost more rapidly than normal, as in nephrosis or protein-losing gastroenteropathy. Cellular functions may be intrinsically abnormal in a certain disease, and the same function may be abnormal in another patient because of an extrinsic toxic factor such as the toxic metabolite deoxy-ATP produced in SCID patients with adenosine deaminase deficiency. There are many potential causes for immunodeficiency, and our understanding of them is certainly incomplete.

The description of the specific immunodeficiency diseases that follows is not an exhaustive listing of every type of defect that has been described. Rather it presents those diseases that are important because of their frequency or their severity or because of what they teach us about the fundamental elements of immune function and host defense.

SPECIFIC IMMUNODEFICIENCY DISEASES

Severe Combined Immune Deficiency (SCID, Reticular Dysgenesis, Swiss-type Agammaglobulinemia, Thymic Alymphoplasia). *Definition.* Severe combined immune deficiency is the most extreme form of immunodeficiency disease. It is characterized by profound defects in both humoral and cell-mediated immunity. There are a number of distinct disorders that fall into this general classification, which may have different patterns of deficiency of the immune cells and which may show either autosomal recessive or X-linked patterns of inheritance.[20,21] A positive family history is obtained in about 50 percent of cases with severe combined immunodeficiency. By definition, severe combined immune deficiency is a disorder of infants and young children. Since the immune defect in these patients is so profound, they die of infection in the first few weeks or months of life.

Clinical Features. Infants with severe combined immune deficiency present with infections during the first months of life. Recurrent pneumonia, chronic diarrhea, failure to thrive, persistent Candida infection of the oral pharnyx, skin, and esophagus and recurrent middle ear infections are common. These patients are susceptible to infections with all classes of microorganisms, but infections with opportunistic pathogens tend to dominate the clinical picture. Children with severe combined immunodeficiency regularly develop fatal generalized vaccinia following smallpox vaccination, and poliomyelitis after administration of live attenuated oral polio vaccine has also been reported. In addition to the threat of infection, many children with severe combined immune deficiency have developed graft-versus-host disease following transfusions of whole blood containing immunocompetent lymphocytes from adult donors. Graft-versus-host disease has also occurred in infants with SCID following transfer of maternal lymphocytes to the fetus during gestation or at the time of delivery.[22]

Physical examination of patients with SCID demonstrates evidence of acute and chronic infection and failure to thrive. Lymph nodes and tonsils are usually absent. On chest x-ray, the characteristic thymic shadow usually seen in infants is absent. In SCID associated with adenosine deaminase deficiency skeletal abnormalities including cupping and flaring of the ribs at the costochondral junction as well as pelvic abnormalities may be seen on x-ray.[23]

Severe combined immune deficiency has been described in association with a number of additional disorders. Reticular dysgenesis is a form of SCID occurring with neonatal agranulocytosis.[24,25] These children usually die within the first few days of life with overwhelming infection. SCID has also occurred in association with an unusual form of dysostosis, resulting in short-limbed dwarfism.[26] Partial albinism and alopecia areata may also be seen in these patients (cartilage-hair hypoplasia). A form of SCID may also be observed in infants with acrodermatitis enteropathica, and the immune deficiency in these patients may respond dramatically to zinc replacement therapy.

Immunologic Defects. Severe combined immunodeficiency is a dual system immune deficiency disease with profound defects in both humoral and cellular immune function. Laboratory evaluation, however, may reveal considerable heterogeneity with some portions of the immune system preserved essentially intact. The levels of IgG, IgA, and IgM are usually extremely low, but a few patients have been described with normal amounts of one or more of these immunoglobulin classes.[27] Antibody responses have been almost universally absent. In some patients B lymphocytes may be absent from the blood and lymphoid tissues, while other patients may have essentially normal numbers of B lymphocytes. In fact B lymphocytes may account for all of the circulating lymphocytes in some SCID patients, since extreme T-lymphocyte deficiency is usual in this disease.

All tests of cell-mediated immunity are abnormal. In 90 percent of SCID cases, less than 10 percent of the normal number of T lymphocytes are found in the peripheral blood.[28] The patients are anergic when tested with recall skin antigens and cannot be sensitized to new agents such as dinitrochlorobenzene. These patients are also unresponsive to intradermally administered phytohemagglutinin.[29] Skin allograft rejection is always abnormal in these patients. In vitro tests of T-lymphocyte function also demonstrate markedly defective responses. Absent proliferative responses to mitogens such as phytohemagglutinin are the rule.

Pathogenesis. SCID is comprised of a heterogeneous group of diseases characterized by profound dual-system immunodeficiency. Many of the immunodeficiency diseases of man appear to represent disorders of lymphocyte differentiation, and considerable evidence has been presented showing that SCID also fits this pattern. In SCID associated with agranulocytosis (reticular dysgenesis) the absence of both lymphocytes and granulocytes suggests that this disease results from a defect in the primitive hematopoietic stem cell, which is the precursor for all leukocytes. The rare form of SCID known as Swiss type agammaglobulinemia is characterized by absence of both T and B lymphocytes and normal numbers of granulocytes.[30] Here the defect in differentiation is believed to lie at the pluripotent lymphoid stem cell (position one, Fig. 83–5). Several phenotypes of SCID have been identified in which the dual-system immunodeficiency appears to result from a primary failure of T-lymphocyte differentiation with the lack of B-lymphocyte maturation occurring as a secondary event (position two, Fig. 83–5). Defects at the level of the prethymic T-lymphocyte precursor, the postthymic precursor, and the intrathymic T-lymphocyte have been demonstrated.[31,32] B lymphocytes from some of these patients will produce immunoglobulin normally when mixed with helper T lymphocytes obtained from normal donors.[33,34] In addition to defects in lymphoid cell differentiation, SCID has also been associated with the deficiency of a specific enzyme of purine metabolism, adenosine deaminase.

Adenosine Deaminase (ADA) Deficiency. SCID with ADA deficiency was the first of the primary immunodeficiency diseases in which a specific enzyme defect could be identified.[35] The disease is transmitted as an autosomal recessive trait and is usually indistinguishable clinically from SCID with normal ADA levels.[36,37] The diagnosis is confirmed by the determination of the concentration of adenosine deaminase in red blood cells. Individuals who are heterozygous for ADA deficiency can be detected with about 90 percent accuracy.

Adenosine deaminase catalyzes the conversion of adenosine to inosine and of deoxyadenosine to deoxyinosine in the normal pathway of purine catabolism (see Figure 83–4). Purine metabolites are essential, as substrates, cofactors, and regulatory molecules, for many facets of intermediary metabolism. They are required for the biosynthesis of nucleic acids, proteins, lipids, and carbohydrates and may have special regulatory role in hormone action, neurotransmission, and immunoregulation. The mechanism by which ADA deficiency results in immune deficiency is incompletely understood but is most likely to result from the accumulation of ADA substrates rather than from a deficiency of a product of ADA enzymatic action.

The ADA substrates adenosine and 2-deoxyadenosine accumulate in large amounts in the serum and urine of these patients, and both adenosine and deoxyadenosine are toxic to cultured lymphocytes.[38] Four principal mechanisms have been proposed to account for the immune deficiency seen with ADA deficiency.[39–46] In one, pyrimidine starvation, adenosine toxicity is associated with depletion of phosphoribosyl pyrophosphate, resulting in the inhibition of de novo pyrimidine biosynthesis. Lymphoid cells incubated with adenosine in vitro

Figure 83–4. The purine catabolic pathway and the positions of adenosine deaminase and purine nucleoside phosphorylase in this metabolic scheme.

excrete orotic acid, an intermediary metabolite in pyrimidine biosynthesis. Patients with ADA deficiency, however, do not appear to have excessive orotic acid in their urine. The disease orotic aciduria itself has been associated with immunodeficiency, as discussed later in this chapter.

A second proposed mechanism is the accumulation of cyclic AMP in cells from ADA-deficient patients. Increased levels of cyclic AMP can result from adenosine binding to membrane receptors and stimulating adenyl cyclase activity. The elevated cAMP levels induced by adenosine have been shown to be inhibitory to several in vitro T-lymphocyte functions. A third mechanism involves inhibition of ribonucleotide reductase and a consequent depletion of deoxy-CTP pools, leading to inhibition of DNA synthesis. 2-Deoxyadenosine is normally catabolized by adenosine deaminase. In the absence of this enzyme it becomes phosphorylated to become deoxy-ATP, a direct inhibitor of the enzyme ribonucleotide reductase. T lymphocytes appear to be considerably more sensitive to deoxyadenosine toxicity than are B lymphocytes, and thymocytes have the highest level of any cell type of a kinase that phosphorylates deoxyadenosine.

A fourth proposed mechanism for the effect of ADA deficiency on the immune system relates to inhibition of methyl transferase reactions. Adenosine is involved in methylation reactions in which S-adenosyl homocysteine is hydrolyzed to homocysteine and adenosine. This is a reversible reaction catalyzed by the enzyme S-adenosyl homocysteine hydrolase. The presence of high concentrations of adenosine can drive the reaction in the direction of S-adenosyl homocysteine synthesis. This compound is a strong inhibitor of methylation reactions. In addition, deoxyadenosine is a potent irreversible inhibitor of S-adenosyl homocysteine hydrolase, and the inhibition of this enzyme also leads to the accumulation of S-adenosyl homocysteine, with subsequent inhibition of methylation reactions and cell death.

Treatment. The search for an effective form of treatment for SCID patients has provided one of the greatest challenges for clinical immunology. In 1968, the first successful bone marrow transplantation was carried out in an infant with SCID and resulted in a cure of the patient's immunodeficiency and introduced an entirely new therapeutic approach to clinical medicine.[47] In the decade following its introduction, bone marrow transplantation was performed in over 100 patients with SCID.[48,49] When a genotypically identical HLA-matched sibling was used as the donor, over 60 percent of the SCID recipients benefited with long-lasting immunologic reconstitution. The success rate for transplants matched at HLA-D only has been considerably less (30 percent), while transplants from HLA-incompatible donors has been almost universally unsuccessful, usually resulting in the development of fatal graft-versus-host disease.

Since only a minority of patients have had an HLA-matched sibling donor available, many attempts have been made to develop transplantation techniques that would avoid graft-versus-host disease and allow the use of unrelated donors. These approaches have included the use of embryonic lymphoid tissues such as fetal liver or fetal thymus. Effective reconstitution has been achieved in a few SCID patients treated with fetal tissues (less than 20 percent), but most of these have been limited to partial T-lymphocyte reconstitution without correction of the B-lymphocyte deficiency. In another approach cultured fragments of normal thymic epithelium in which all lymphoid elements have degenerated has been used by Hong to treat 38 SCID patients.[50,51] Evidence for partial reconstitution of both T- and B-lymphocyte function has been seen in some of these patients, but this reconstitution usually did not appear until about 4 months after the transplant procedure. Perhaps because of the long interval before reconstitution was observed less than one quarter of the patients showed significant clinical benefit from this approach.[51]

Recently, reconstitution using HLA-nonidentical bone marrow treated to remove mature T-lymphocytes has shown very promising results.[52] When this approach is perfected, bone marrow transplantation will become a much more widely practicable procedure for treatment of many lymphoid and hematologic disorders.

Bone marrow transplantation has been successfully employed in the reconstitution of patients with both ADA(+) and ADA(−) forms of SCID. In a novel approach to treatment of ADA deficiency, Polmar has treated patients with this disease with repeated exchange transfusions utilizing irradiated normal red blood cells.[53]

Since erythrocytes are a rich source of adenosine deaminase, this treatment serves as a partial enzyme replacement. In about 50 percent of the cases, patient's lymphocyte function has improved, and the level of deoxy-ATP in their lymphoid cells has fallen to a normal undetectable level following transfusion therapy. Although not a curative treatment, RBC transfusions do serve as a holding action until a bone marrow transplant can be performed.

Purine Nucleoside Phosphorylase Deficiency (PNP Deficiency). Deficiency in the enzyme purine nucleoside phosphorylase is accompanied by an immunodeficiency state consisting of severely impaired T-lymphocyte function with B-lymphocyte function remaining essentially intact.[54] PNP deficiency is inherited as an autosomal recessive trait. Purine nucleoside phosphorylase is the enzyme that catalyzes the conversion of inosine to xanthine and of guanosine to guanine in the purine catabolic pathway, and this enzyme is absent or defective in patients with this disease (see Figure 83–4).

Clinical Features. About a dozen patients with PNP deficiency have been described.[54-59] In general, they presented in early childhood with recurrent infections often manifested as otitis media, pneumonia, or diarrhea. Some of the patients have received live virus vaccines and multiple blood transfusions without complication. However, other patients have died of generalized vaccinia following smallpox vaccination, and one child has died of graft-versus-host disease following a blood transfusion.[55] Some patients have had chronic cytomegalovirus infection, and others, very severe varicella. The immune deficiency in this disorder appears to be progressive in nature, with infants being relatively free of infection for the first few months of life and then infectious episodes beginning and increasing in severity and tempo.[39]

Since purine nucleoside phosphorylase catalyzes the degradation of inosine and guanosine, the principal substrates for uric acid, PNP deficiency usually results in very low levels of xanthine and uric acid. Thus a useful diagnostic screening test for this disease is the absence of uric acid in the serum or urine of these patients.

Immune Defects. Patients with PNP deficiency have characteristically had profound T-lymphocyte deficiency manifested by skin test anergy, T lymphocytopenia, and defective in vitro T-lymphocyte responses. By contrast, the patients ability to make isohemagglutinins and antibody responses is normal, as is the serum concentration of IgG, IgA, and IgM.[54] The portion of B lymphocytes in the blood is normal. All stages of precursor T-lymphocyte differentiation appear intact, as is thymic morphology.[39]

Pathogenesis. As shown in Figure 83–4, purine nucleoside phosphorylase is active in purine catabolism at the step immediately following that catabolized by adenosine deaminase. Therefore, deficiency in either of these two sequential enzymes of purine metabolism gives rise to an immune deficiency state. In purine nucleoside phosphorylase deficiency, as in adenosine deaminase deficiency, the mechanism of immune deficiency is believed to result from the accumulation of toxic deoxyribonucleotides in cells of the lymphoid system, leading to inhibition of ribonucleotide reductase and a consequent inhibition of DNA synthesis.[43-45,60,61] Deoxyguanosine is the only PNP substrate that can be phosphorylated by mammalian cells.[39] Deoxyguanosine is toxic to mammalian cells in culture after conversion to deoxy-GTP, and deoxycytidine can protect against this toxicity in vitro.

Treatment. In some patients, exchange transfusions with normal erythrocytes rich in PNP have been used to treat this disease with apparent benefit following a long period of treatment.[62] Again, however, this approach has not been effective in all cases. Preliminary attempts to treat these patients with deoxycytidine have resulted in a modest improvement in a few laboratory parameters, but deoxycytidine has not given detectable clinical improvement.

Cellular Immune Deficiency with Orotic Aciduria. Orotic aciduria is a rare inborn error of pyrimidine metabolism that is inherited as an autosomal recessive trait. The disease has been described in nine patients and is characterized by retarded growth and development and megaloblastic anemia. The enzymatic defect in this disease involves one or two sequential enzymes involved in de novo pyrimidine biosynthesis, and replacement therapy with uridine has resulted in clinical and hematologic remission in some cases. Several patients have experienced severe infections, including fatal meningitis in two patients and fatal varicella in one case.[63]

Lymphocytopenia has been a consistently reported finding in these patients. Recently Girot and associates reported the results of immunologic studies in two patients.[64] In both patients (a brother and sister) humoral immunity was normal, with normal or increased concentrations of serum IgG, IgA, and IgM and normal antibody responses to diphtheria, tetanus, polio, and pertussis and normal isohemagglutinins. By contrast, cellular immune function was defective. Both patients lacked delayed-type hypersensitivity skin test reactions and had depressed numbers of circulating T lymphocytes. In vitro lymphocyte proliferative responses to mitogens varied from low normal to strikingly depressed on different occasions. Response to allogeneic cells in mixed lymphocyte culture was generally normal, but, interestingly, cytotoxic T lymphocytes were not generated in this reaction. In addition the induction of plasma cells by pokeweed mitogen stimulation in vitro was also defective.

Although uridine therapy resulted in a hematologic improvement, no benefit to immune function was seen. No studies are as yet available to clarify the specific mechanism by which this defect in pyrimidine synthesis affects the immune system.

Thymic Hypoplasia (DiGeorge Syndrome). *Definition.* The DiGeorge syndrome[65,66] is a congenital immune deficiency disease associated with abnormalities in the development of tissues that are derived from the first through the sixth branchial pouches during embryonic development. Structures derived from the branchial pouches include portions of the ear and certain facial structures as well as portions of the aortic arch and heart, the parathyroids, the thyroid, and the thymus. It is the abnormal development of the thymus that leads to the immune deficiency that has been considered the classic example of a T-lymphocyte deficiency disease.

Clinical Features. Patients with the DiGeorge syndrome present in early infancy with symptoms usually unrelated to the immune deficiency. Congenital heart defects, including truncus arteriosis ventricular septal defect, interrupted aortic arch, and tetralogy of Fallot are common presenting problems within the first two weeks of life. Abnormal calcium homeostasis is seen in all patients, and in patients presenting after the first month of life hypocalcemic seizures are the most common initial clinical manifestation.[67] Facial abnormalities include microstomia; hypertelorism; upturned nose; small, low-set, posteriorly rotated ears with notched ear pinnae; and an anti-Mongoloid slant of the eyes. Esophageal atresia, tracheo-esophageal fistula, bifid uvula, and hypothyroidism have also been described in these patients. If the patients survive the newborn period, they will then frequently present with an increased susceptibility to infections, including recurrent pneumonia, candidiasis, and diarrhea.

Immune Defects. The DiGeorge syndrome demonstrates a marked variability in both clinical manifestations and the degree of immunodeficiency.[67-70] The immunologic defects found in this syndrome are a direct consequence of the abnormal development of the thymus. The total lymphocyte count may range from severely depressed to normal, but the percentage of T lymphocytes is more consistently depressed. Architecture of the lymph nodes and spleen is usually depleted in those areas normally populated by thymic-dependent lymphocytes. Patients with severe thymic defects have negative skin tests to recall antigens and prolonged skin allograft survival, and their lymphocytes respond very poorly when stimulated with mitogens and alloantigens in vitro. However, some patients may have normal lymphocyte numbers and normal in vitro function tests. B-lymphocyte function is preserved in most patients with this syndrome. Immunoglobulin levels are usually normal, and many patients have normal antibody responses following primary immunization. In serial studies of immune function, some patients have clearly shown spontaneous improvement in T-lymphocyte functions, while others have had definite deterioration in immune status.[67] Autopsy studies have shown that in many patients, a small residual fragment of thymus can be identified, frequently in an ectopic location. This variability in the extent of the defect in the thymus certainly contributes to the variability in clinical T-lymphocyte deficiency and may explain the occurrence of patients who manifest only the nonimmunologic features of the DiGeorge syndrome.

Pathogenesis. Between the sixth and tenth weeks of intrauterine life the thymus, parathyroids, thyroid, and certain facial and vascular structures develop from cellular elements in the first through the sixth branchial

pouch area of the developing embryo. By the twelfth week of gestation, the thymus begins to migrate towards the thorax. In the DiGeorge syndrome an intrauterine insult before the twelfth week of gestation leads to developmental abnormalities in the structures derived from these embryonic tissues (position three, Fig. 83–5). Since this disease is sporadic in nature, it is presumed to represent an environmental congenital abnormality rather than a genetic defect. It is interesting that infants with the fetal alcohol syndrome frequently have facial abnormalities similar to those seen in patients with the complete DiGeorge syndrome.[67]

Treatment. Since many of these patients present in the newborn period with the nonimmunologic complications of this syndrome, initial treatment is directed towards controlling the cardiac and metabolic abnormalities of these infants. Hypoparathyroidism with hypocalcemia has usually required prolonged treatment with vitamin D or calcium or both. Congenital heart disease may require immediate surgical intervention. Several patients with the DiGeorge syndrome have been given transplants of fetal thymic tissue with prompt improvement in their immunologic status.[71-72] However, cellular chimerism has not been demonstrated in these patients, and their rapid response may have been due to humoral thymic factors. The role of thymus transplantation in patients with this disease remains unresolved.

X-Linked Agammaglobulinemia (XLA, Bruton-Type Agammaglobulinemia). Definition. X-linked agammaglobulinemia is an immunodeficiency state limited to defects in the B-lymphocyte system characterized by the onset of recurrent infection with high-grade bacterial pathogens early in life. Principal features of this disease include low concentrations of all major classes of im-

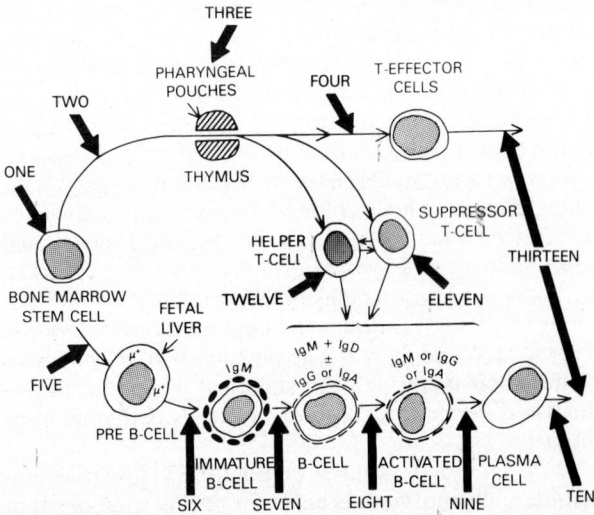

Figure 83–5. Proposed position of the defects in various immunodeficiency diseases. *One*, Reticular dysgenesis, SCID; *Two*, SCID; *Three*, DiGeorge syndrome; *Four*, AIDS, PNP deficiency; *Five*, Thymoma and hypogammaglobulinemia; *Six*, X-linked agammaglobulinemia; *Seven* through *Eleven*, Common variable immunodeficiency; *Eight*, Selective IgA deficiency; *Twelve*, Transient hypogammaglobulinemia of infancy, CVH; *Thirteen*, Intestinal lymphangiectasia.

munoglobulin, the inability to produce specific antibodies, and X-linked recessive inheritance.[73]

Clinical Features. Boys with this form of congenital agammaglobulinemia usually remain well for the first several months of life, presumably because of transplacental passage of maternal antibodies. The infants then begin to experience recurrent bacterial infections with high-grade encapsulated pathogens such as the pneumococcus, *Hemophilus influenzae*, streptococci, and meningococci. A variety of infectious processes, including septicemia and meningitis as well as infection localized to the respiratory tract, with otitis media, bronchitis, and pneumonia are particularly common. Because recurrent infections to the respiratory tract result in the development of chronic bronchitis and bronchiectasis, the principal cause of mortality in this disease is respiratory failure occurring in the third and fourth decades.

Although many patients with humoral immune deficiency have significant gastrointestinal complaints as a feature of their disorder, malabsorption and chronic diarrhea are uncommon in X-linked agammaglobulinemia. One problem that is relatively unique to these patients, however, has been the development of an indolent form of encephalomyelitis caused by various strains of ECHO virus.[74,75] This syndrome was initially described as a "dermatomyositis-like" disease and is now recognized to represent widespread tissue dissemination of ECHO virus, with destruction of central nervous system and muscle tissue. This complication has proved to be fatal in 90 percent of the patients who have acquired it, but recently success has been obtained by treating such patients with high concentrations of intravenous gammaglobulin.[76]

Immunologic Defects. X-linked agammaglobulinemia has often been considered the prototype form of humoral immune deficiency. It is characterized by a striking deficiency in serum and tissues of all classes of immunoglobulins. Lymphoid tissues lack B lymphocytes or plasma cells, and there is a failure of germinal center development in lymph nodes, spleen, tonsils, and gut associated lymphoid tissues. By contrast the lymph nodes show normal morphology in the T-lymphocyte dependent areas, and the development and morphology of the thymus are normal. As expected in patients with such a marked deficiency of immunoglobulin, there is a lack of antibodies to environmental antigens, and these patients respond poorly or not at all to immunization with vaccines or after natural infection. The number of T lymphocytes is normal, and cellular immune function is usually entirely intact in this disease.

Pathogenesis. Three phenotypic forms of X-linked hypogammaglobulinemia have been described. The principal group of these patients has been found to have no B lymphocytes in peripheral blood or lymphocyte tissues. These patients do, however, have pre-B lymphocytes in their bone marrow[77] (position six, Fig. 83–5). A second, smaller group of patients has been described in whom X-linked agammaglobulinemia is associated with the presence of circulating B lymphocytes. It is unclear whether both of these two forms of X-linked agammaglobulinemia can occur within a single family, but it has been presumed that they represent distinct genetic defects. In addition to these two forms, one family has been described in which four males had both agammaglobulinemia (without B lymphocytes) and isolated growth hormone deficiency, which was transmitted as an X-linked disorder.[78]

X-linked agammaglobulinemia is not the result of a structural gene defect, since the kappa and lambda immunoglobulin light chain genes and the immunoglobulin heavy chain genes are not located on the X chromosome but rather on chromosomes 2, 22, and 14, respectively. Furthermore, low but detectable amounts of IgG, IgA, and IgM can be demonstrated in the serum of these patients if very sensitive detection techniques are employed.

As discussed previously, many of the primary immunodeficiency diseases appear to represent disorders of lymphocyte differentiation. It has been proposed that X-linked agammaglobulinemia usually represents a block in differentiation at the stage of the transition from the pre-B lymphocyte to the B lymphocyte that expresses complete IgM molecules. Recently it has been reported that the pre-B lymphocytes from three patients with X-linked agammaglobulinemia contain an incomplete μ heavy chain.[79] The missing determinants on these μ chains are presumed to be immunoglobulin variable region gene products (V_H). This has led to the suggestion that agammaglobulinemia in these cases is caused by a failure of expression of V_H genes on chromosome 14 because of a defective regulatory gene on the X chromosome.

Treatment. Treatment of all the antibody deficiency hypogammaglobulinemia syndromes is based on replacement therapy designed to provide antibodies that the patients are incapable of producing. Several approaches have been followed. The standard method of treatment is periodic intramuscular injections of human serum immune globulin. Gamma globulin dosages are calculated for each patient at a dose of 0.7 ml per kg of body weight per month. This form of treatment does not restore immunoglobulin levels to normal but rather maintains concentrations of IgG at or above approximately 2 mg per ml. Normal serum levels of IgG average about 12 mg per ml, but control studies have shown that this dosage schedule for immunoglobulin replacement results in significant therapeutic benefits.[80]

Although effective, the intramuscular injection of gamma globulin is associated with several potential problems. The volume of gamma globulin required for each injection is large and, therefore, often painful. Furthermore, with repeated injections over many years, as required by patients with congenital antibody deficiency, significant local scarring may result at the sites of these repeated injections. Finally, administration of gamma globulin is occasionally associated with a severe shock-like syndrome, which rarely has been fatal. These reactions may be characterized by dyspnea, hypotension, cyanosis, flank pain, fever, and rash. Because these reactions have been associated with death, they must be considered a medical emergency and treated aggressively, as one would treat other forms of anaphylactic shock. The precise cause of gamma globulin reactions is still a matter of controversy, but they are probably the result of aggregates of IgG contained in the intramuscular gamma globulin preparations gaining direct access to the circulation through small capillary and venous leaks, since direct injection of this form of gamma globulin intravenously results in an identical shocklike syndrome.

Some procedures appear to lessen the probability of these reactions and make repeated injections more readily accepted by the patients. First, gammaglobulin should be warmed to room or body temperature prior to administration. The injections must be given in a deep intramuscular site, preferably in the gluteal muscles. No more than 10 ml should be given at each injection and the injections must be given very slowly. In our clinic we administer each intramuscular injection at a rate no faster than 2.5 ml per minute. Finally, in patients who have experienced reactions we have found that premedication with H-1 and H-2 antihistamines may be useful in preventing subsequent reactions. In adults we use 50 mg of diphenhydramine hydrochloride (Benadryl) and 300 mg of cimetidine given orally 1/2 hour before the gammaglobulin injection. As an additional measure we have each of our patients remain in the clinic for 30 minutes following their gamma globulin injection so that the patient will be available for immediate attention should a reaction develop. The treatment of a gamma globulin reaction, as in any form of anaphylaxis, is based on the immediate administration of epinephrine followed by supportive therapy as required.

In an attempt to obtain higher serum immunoglobulin levels than possible by intramuscular injection, various approaches to providing gamma globulin via the intravenous route have been proposed. Plasma infusions provide one mechanism, with the added benefit of also providing IgA and IgM. Plasma infusions at the rate of 10 ml per kg of body weight given intravenously on sequential days may result in a substantial increase of serum immunoglobulin levels, and such treatment has been beneficial in some patients in whom intramuscular gamma globulin was ineffective or contraindicated. Plasma infusions, however, have a number of problems that are unique to this form of therapy. First, it is often difficult to obtain hepatitis-free plasma in the large volumes required for the regular treatment of the patient. In addition, plasma will contain the antibodies from only the individual donor, whereas intramuscular gamma globulin is prepared from pools of plasma obtained from as many as 1000 donors. Therefore, these pooled sources of gamma globulin may have a much broader spectrum of protective antibodies than are found in the plasma from a single donor.

Another approach to providing a broader spectrum of protective antibodies has been the recent introduction in the United States of intravenous gamma globulin preparations. Such gamma globulin preparations have been treated chemically to largely eliminate the problems seen if an intramuscular preparation of gamma globulin were to be given intravenously. With such intravenous gamma globulin preparations much higher levels of IgG can be obtained, and the problems associated with repeated intramuscular injections are avoided. Control trials are currently in progress comparing the efficacy of intravenous gamma globulin with the intramuscular preparations. One potential drawback to the use of intravenous gamma globulin is its cost. Intravenous gammaglobulin at this time is at least 10 times as expensive per treatment than the intramuscular gamma globulin preparations, and it also requires the additional costs associated with intravenous administration. In our own clinic we have preferred to maintain patients who are clinically stable on intramuscular gamma globulin. However, if our patients begin to experience repeated infections or if they are hospitalized at any time for an infection, we supplement their intramuscular gamma globulin with the intravenous preparation to acutely raise their serum IgG levels. The recommended dose of intravenous gamma globulin is 2 cc per kilogram of body weight administered once a month by intravenous infusion. The average intravenous infusion lasts two to three hours.

A number of patients with the hypogammaglobulinemia/antibody deficiency syndromes who have developed chronic sinopulmonary disease have received significant benefit from the use of continuous or intermittent prophylactic antibiotics. The combination of trimethoprim and sulfamethoxazole has been particularly useful in many patients with agammaglobulinemia and patients with selective IgA deficiency. Bone marrow transplantation, which offers the only opportunity for cure in patients with severe cellular immune deficiency disease or combined immunodeficiency, is not indicated in patients with antibody deficiency syndromes. At this time the complications of bone marrow transplantation, including failure of engraftment and fatal or chronic graft-versus-host disease are, on balance far too risky to be considered for a disease that can be reasonably well controlled by replacement therapy with gamma globulin.

Immunodeficiency with Thymoma. Hypogammaglobulinemia associated with the occurrence of a benign thymoma has been noted in over 50 patients and is clearly a distinct syndrome. The thymoma may precede the development of the immune deficiency by several years or may follow the appearance of the immune defect by a similar margin.[81,82] Benign spindle cell tumors are the most common type of thymoma seen with this syndrome.

Patients with thymoma and hypogammaglobulinemia have clinical symptoms associated with their antibody deficiency and usually also have significant cellular immune deficiency as well. In addition, many of these patients have a significant associated hematologic abnormality. Over 50 percent of the cases have anemia and 10 percent pure red cell aplasia. About half the patients have significant leukopenia, one quarter have thrombocytopenia, and the majority of the patients have a total absence of circulating or bone marrow eosinophils.[81] Circulating basophils may also be absent from these patients.

The immunologic defects in patients with immunodeficiency and thymoma include both humoral and cellular defects. In addition to hypogammaglobulinemia many patients are anergic and have significant functional abnormalities of their T lymphocytes in vitro. Intense suppressor T-lymphocyte activity has been identified in most of these patients, with their T lymphocytes suppressing immunoglobulin production by normal B lymphocytes in tissue culture.[83,84] Despite the hypogammaglobulinemia, over 30 percent of patients have had autoantibodies to a variety of tissues, including thymus, muscle, erythrocytes, and antinuclear antibodies. The association of thymoma and hypogammaglobulinemia occurs most commonly in patients in the fifth and sixth decades and is often characterized by an exceptionally stormy course. Removal of the thymoma has had no effect on the immunodeficiency state, whereas it may have benefit in the treatment of the associated pure red cell aplasia. Thymoma and hypogammaglobulinemia represent a distinctive form of hypogammaglobulinemia in that these patients lack not only B lymphocytes but also have an absence of pre-B lymphocytes in their bone marrow and lymphoid tissues[84,85] (see position five, Fig. 83–5).

Transcobalamin II Deficiency and Hypogammaglobulinemia. A rare form of hypogammaglobulinemia that is inherited as an autosomal recessive trait has been described in a kindred of North African descent.[86] In these patients hematologic and gastrointestinal abnormalities are seen in addition to the hypogammaglobulinemia. A common feature in the patients has been an inability to produce transcobalamin II, a protein important in the transport of vitamin B_{12}. Megaloblastic anemia, granulocytopenia, and thrombocytopenia as well as failure to thrive, vomiting, and diarrhea have been observed. The patients have normal numbers of B lymphocytes but fail to develop plasma cells in their lymphoid tissues and lack circulating antibodies or immunoglobulins. Their T-lymphocyte system is intact quantitatively and qualitatively.

This genetic disorder results in the appearance of repeated infections early in childhood. It is unique in that rapid clinical improvement occurs following parenteral administration of large doses of vitamin B_{12}. Following treatment the patient's immunoglobulin levels increased to normal, and they produced antibodies to a variety of vaccine antigens. Thus, this is a form of humoral immune deficiency in which gamma globulin replacement is not required because the fundamental defect is overcome by the administration of this vitamin.

Although the mechanism by which transcobalamin II deficiency leads to immunodeficiency is not known, it is interesting that methylcobalamin is a cofactor in the remethylation of homocysteine to methionine. It is an intriguing speculation that immunoglobulin production may require S-adenosyl methionine–mediated methylation and that in ADA deficiency these reactions are inhibited by the accumulation of S-adenosyl homocysteine while in patients with deficiency of transcobalamin II there is a defect in methionine production.[39]

Common Variable Immunodeficiency (CVH, Adult-Acquired Agammaglobulinemia). *Definition.* Common variable immunodeficiency is a general diagnostic category including a heterogeneous group of disorders having in common an imparied antibody response, hypogammaglobulinemia, an increased incidence of infections, and a variable degree of cellular immunodeficiency. This diagnostic category was established by the World Health Organization to include a number of previously described syndromes for which no clear pattern of inheritance or a specific enzyme defect could be determined. These include either syndromes with no evidence for inheritable traits or ones with widely variable expression in that one individual of a family might have hypogammaglobulinemia while a related individual might present with autoimmune disease and yet another present with dysgammaglobulinemia.[87-90]

Clinical Features. Common variable immunodeficiency is characteristically associated with an increased incidence of infections with highly virulent encapsulated extracellular bacterial pathogens such as the pneumococcus or *Hemophilus influenzae*. Some patients may also have fungal or mycobacterial infections, and rare patients have had *Pneumocystis carinii* pneumonia. Patients usually have sinusitis and chronic otitis media and develop chronic lower respiratory tract disease with bronchitis and bronchiectasis. Respiratory failure is the principle cause of death.[73,87]

Patients with common variable immunodeficiency frequently have gastrointestinal symptoms, including chronic diarrhea, lactose intolerance, malabsorption, and protein-losing gastroenteropathy. Villous atrophy of the jejunum may be occasionally found, as well as a unique form of submucosal lymphoid hyperplasia known as intestinal nodular lymphoid hyperplasia.[91] *Giardia lamblia* infection of the intestinal tract is a very frequent cause of diarrhea in these patients. Overgrowth of bacteria in the upper intestinal tract has also been associated with diarrhea, as has intestinal infection with *Campylobacter* and cytomegalovirus.[6,92] Splenomegaly occurs in over one third of these patients, and anemia, leukopenia, and thrombocytopenia secondary to hypersplenism may be present.

Autoimmune hemolytic anemia, neutropenia, and thrombocytopenia as well as Graves' disease and hypothyroidism occur with increased frequency in patients with common variable immunodeficiency. Rheumatoid arthritis has been described in these patients,[93] but more commonly they develop a unique form of polyarthritis, which responds rapidly to gamma globulin therapy.[94] This disease lacks subcutaneous nodules, bony erosions, or involvement of the PIP joints of the fingers, and the joint fluid rarely contains neutrophils or immune complexes.[6] The patients most frequently complain of arthralgias that improve quickly following gamma globulin administration and often reappear about the time of the next scheduled gamma globulin injection. About 50 percent of patients have achlorhydria, but only half of these are deficient in intrinsic factor.[6] An autoimmune basis for this defect has been demonstrated in some cases.

Immunologic Defects. The most common pattern of immune defects observed is an extreme reduction of all classes of immunoglobulin and antibody deficiency. Levels of natural antibodies and isohemagglutinins are low. However, even in patients with extremely low levels of immunoglobulin there may be autoantibody production. In addition to these B-lymphocyte defects, over 50 percent of the patients exhibit cutaneous anergy. In vitro responses of T lymphocytes are also variable, with some patients demonstrating a normal proliferative response to mitogens and others showing a markedly defective response.

Pathogenesis. Within the group of disorders included in common variable immunodeficiency, several patterns of B-lymphocyte abnormality have been defined[95-97] (positions six, seven, eight, nine, and ten, Fig. 83–5). A total absence of B lymphocytes occurs in a minority of patients, while most have B lymphocytes in normal or near normal numbers.[98,99] In some cases these B lymphocytes fail to respond to all forms of stimulation in vitro, while in other patients the B lymphocytes could be induced to produce immunoglobulin normally when provided with helper T-lymphocytes from normal individuals. In these latter cases, the hypogammaglobulinemia appears to be the result of defective helper T-lymphocyte activity and occurs frequently in the syndrome of transient hypogammaglobulinemia of infancy in which delayed maturation of helper T-lymphocyte function has been described[100] (position twelve, Fig. 83–5). Still other patients with common variable immunodeficiency have B lymphocytes that can be stimulated to synthesize cytoplasmic immunoglobulin but are defective in the secretion of immunoglobulin molecules from the differentiated plasma cell (position ten, Fig. 83–5). The failure of secretion is thought to represent a defect in the glycosylation of the immunoglobulin molecules within the differentiated plasma cell in some patients.[101,102] Finally there is a group of patients whose B lymphocytes appear to be able to normally respond with immunoglobulin production but who have excessive activity of their suppressor T lymphocytes.[14,103] In these patients suppressor T lymphocytes prevent the B lymphocytes from differentiating for immunoglobulin synthesis (position eleven, Fig. 83–5). Some of these patients have developed agammaglobulinemia after infectious mononucleosis.[104] In infectious mononucleosis, intense suppressor T-lymphocyte activity appears as part of the normal defense against the B-lymphocyte activation induced by the Epstein-Barr virus.[105] The control mechanisms that regulate this suppressor T-lymphocyte response are apparently abnormal in these patients, resulting in continuous polyclonal suppression and the secondary development of agammaglobulinemia.

Treatment. The treatment for common variable immunodeficiency is based on gamma globulin replacement therapy and prophylactic antibiotics and is similar to the treatment of X-linked agammaglobulinemia. Gastrointestinal disease may require antimicrobial therapy or dietary manipulation, since gluten sensitivity is occasionally associated with this form of immune deficiency disease.

Selective IgA Deficiency. *Definition.* Selective IgA deficiency is defined as a level of serum IgA of less than 0.05 mg per ml associated with normal or elevated levels of IgG and IgM. It is the most prevalent of the immune deficiency diseases and approximately 1 in 700 normal blood donors in the United States has been found incidentally to have IgA deficiency. Most cases occur sporadically, but families have been described in which several generations are involved. Within these affected families there may also be patients with panhypogammaglobulinemia and other individuals with autoimmune disease. IgA deficiency occurs at about 10 times the normal frequency in patients with systemic lupus erythematosus.[106]

Clinical Features. Selective IgA deficiency is associated primarily with respiratory and gastrointestinal tract disease.[107] Since IgA is the predominant immunoglobulin in the external secretions, it is not surprising that these organ systems are affected by recurrent infection. Most patients with IgA deficiency, however, do not develop chronic bronchopulmonary destructive disease of the severity seen in patients with panhypogammaglobulinemia. One third of the patients with symptomatic IgA deficiency have gastrointestinal disorders. These can range from chronic diarrhea unassociated with systemic symptoms to severe malabsorption syndromes associated with progressive weight loss and intestinal villous atrophy.[108] *Giardia* is an uncommon pathogen. Allergy is also increased in patients with selective IgA deficiency, and it has been postulated that the absence of IgA in the secretions allows the systemic absorption of antigens from the gastrointestinal and respiratory tracts, promoting the development of allergic sensitization.

Immunologic Defects. Selective IgA deficiency is characterized by exceedingly low levels of IgA in the serum and external secretions. About 25 percent of patients with IgA deficiency are also deficient in IgE, and a similar number are deficient in IgG$_2$.[109] In addition, the occurrence of low molecular weight IgM (7S rather than 19S) has been seen. In spite of the deficiency in serum IgA these patients may have normal numbers of circulating B lymphocytes bearing membrane-bound IgA.[110] Importantly, IgA-deficient patients occasionally make antibodies to IgA, and these anti-IgA antibodies have been the cause of transfusion actions when these patients have required blood transfusions.[111] In addition, patients with IgA deficiency may produce antibodies directed against thyroid antigens, mitochondria, smooth muscle, collagen, and food antigens. Their production of antibodies to milk and bovine serum proteins is often associated with the appearance of circulating immune complexes following milk ingestion.[112,113] This tendency to make antibodies to bovine serum proteins also occasionally introduces an artifact in the detection of IgA deficiency when bovine antisera to IgA are used in the assay; therefore, quantitation of IgA levels is most reliably performed using rabbit or other nonbovine antibodies to human IgA.

Pathogenesis. The cause of the failure of these patients to produce IgA is unknown. Since most of these patients have B lymphocytes that bear IgA on their membranes, a defect in the structural gene encoding alpha heavy chains is not an obvious cause for this immunoglobulin deficiency. Some patients have been found to have suppressor T lymphocytes that selectively inhibit production of IgA when mixed with normal B lymphocytes, but this has been found in only a minority of these patients and is also unlikely as the primary cause of IgA deficiency.[114] Coculture studies have also shown that these patients usually have adequate helper T-lymphocyte activity that permit normal B lymphocytes to produce IgA. One study has demonstrated that the majority of IgA-bearing B lymphocytes in these patients also express surface IgM and IgD. This is the phenotype of immature B lymphocytes and has led to the hypothesis that in these patients, IgA B-lymphocyte maturation is arrested at an early stage of differentiation[115] (position eight, Fig. 83–5).

Treatment. Patients with selective IgA deficiency are usually treated symptomatically for their respiratory, gastrointestinal, allergic, and autoimmune problems. Parenteral gamma globulin preparations contain only very small amounts of IgA and so are not suitable as a source of replacement of the missing IgA molecules. Furthermore, IgA found at the mucosal surfaces is usually produced locally, and since there is no mechanism for active transport of IgA from the serum, systemically administered IgA is unlikely to reach the sites where its action would be most desirable. In a few patients with severe recurrent infection, gamma globulin or plasma therapy has been attempted, and in some of these, moderate success has been reported. Twenty percent of patients with IgA deficiency are also deficient in the IgG_2 subclass of IgG.[109] Treatment of these patients with parenteral gamma globulin has been effective in reducing the incidence of severe infections. However, the risk of an anti-IgA–mediated anaphylactic reaction must be constantly remembered in these patients. In fact, any patient with IgA deficiency who might need a blood transfusion should be very carefully monitored for the possibility of a reaction and, if possible, should be transfused with blood from another IgA-deficient individual. The American Red Cross maintains a donor file of IgA-deficient individuals for this purpose.

Ataxia-Telangiectasia. *Definition.* Ataxia-telangiectasia is an autosomal recessive disorder with an onset in childhood characterized by cerebellar ataxia, oculocutaneous telangiectasia, recurrent sinopulmonary infections, a high incidence of neoplastic disease, and a variable immunodeficiency state involving both the cellular and humoral systems.[116,117]

Clinical Features. Neurologic symptoms are the usual presenting problem in these patients. The first symptom is often ataxia, which becomes apparent when the child begins to walk. Somewhat later patients may develop chorioathetosis, myoclonic jerking, and oculomotor abnormalities. The telangiectasis characteristic of this disease initially appear after the age of 4. First appearing on the bulbar conjunctiva (Fig. 83–6), these telangiectasias later develop on the skin in exposed areas and on areas of trauma such as the nasal bridge, the ear, and flexor folds on the neck and extremities. Premature graying of the hair, vitiligo, and café au lait spots and an early loss of subcutaneous fat also develop. Endocrine abnormalities are very frequent in patients with ataxia-telangiectasia and may involve multiple organs. Glucose intolerance occurs in over half of the patients.[118] Delayed or absent development of secondary sexual characteristics associated with absent or hypoplastic ovaries is frequent in females, and male patients also demonstrate hypogonadism as a less consistent finding. Fifty percent of patients demonstrate mild hepatic dysfunction, which is usually associated with evidence of fatty infiltration and round cell accumulation in the portal areas.

An increase in the incidence of cancer is seen in several of the primary immunodeficiency diseases and is a major feature of ataxia-telangiectasia, with 10 to 15 percent of the patients ultimately dying of malignancy.[119,120] This represents an incidence 15 times that of the general population. Lymphoma accounts for the majority of cases, but brain tumors, adenocarcinoma of the stomach, and ovarian carcinoma have also been reported.

In some patients recurrent infections may be a major feature of their disease, while other patients may have no infection at all. In general there is a good correlation between the severity of the infectious illnesses and the immunologic status of an individual patient. Infections tend to be with high-grade bacterial pathogens commonly seen in patients with humoral immune deficiency, while mycobacterial and fungal infections are a less frequent cause of clinical problems. The combined effects of the neurologic disability and chronic pulmonary infections often result in pulmonary failure as a terminal event.

Immunologic Defects. Ataxia-telangiectasia has been

Figure 83–6. Striking telangiectasia of vessels on bulbar conjunctiva of a 19-year-old patient with ataxia telangiectasia. The telangiectasia usually first appears on the conjunctiva, but not until after 4 years of age.

associated with several defects in both T- and B-lymphocyte function.[116,121] However, few of the abnormalities occur in all or even in a majority of the patients. The most consistent B-lymphocyte defect is an absence of serum IgA and IgE. IgA deficiency occurs in about 75 percent of the patients and IgE deficiency in about 85 percent. The IgA and IgE deficiency may occur independently of one another, and within a family two siblings may have a different pattern of immunoglobulin deficiency. Approximately 80 percent of the patients have low molecular weight IgM (i.e., 7S). Recently a high frequency of IgG$_2$ deficiency has been reported in these patients.[122] Total B-lymphocyte numbers are normal, as are the numbers of IgA-bearing B lymphocytes. Antibody responses to antigenic challenge have been variable, but no consistent pattern of deficiency has emerged. Also, patients with ataxia-telangiectasia often have circulating autoantibodies to a variety of antigens, including immunoglobulins, mitochondria, basement membranes, muscle, and thyroid antigens.[123] Only patients with defective T-lymphocyte function appear to produce autoantibodies, suggesting a defect in immunoregulatory T-lymphocyte function as the cause.

The cellular immune system may also show variable degrees of involvement. Many patients have decreased responses to delayed hypersensitivity skin testing, and a few patients may even have delayed rejection of skin allografts. Fifty percent of patients have depressed T-lymphocyte proliferative responses to mitogens and antigens.[121] In addition, studies of antibody production in vitro have shown that some of these patients have deficient helper T-lymphocyte activity as well as poorly responsive B lymphocytes in some cases.[124]

Pathogenesis. Although the defect underlying ataxia-telangiectasia is unknown, there are several findings that have led to the development of two major hypotheses. Patients with ataxia-telangiectasia have an increased sensitivity to ionizing radiation, as do their fibroblasts in tissue culture.[125-127] Although a defect in DNA repair mechanisms has been suspected in these patients, convincing evidence for such a biochemical defect is lacking.[128] It is important to note that there is also a very high incidence of chromosomal translocation in these patients,[7,37-41] particularly involving chromosome 14.[129,130] Chromosome 14 contains the immunoglobulin heavy chain genes, and the deficiency of a factor needed for gene recombination and DNA repair could theoretically account for both the radiosensitivity and chromosomal instability in these patients as well as for the failure of activation of α and ε heavy chain genes via a switch from μ chain gene expression.

Another hypothesis first proposed nearly 20 years ago is that there is a defect in tissue differentiation in this disease.[121] At that time it was recognized that, when present, the thymus in these patients was very poorly developed and had the appearance of a fetal thymus. In addition, these patients have other defects suggesting faulty maturation of tissues dependent upon the interaction of ectodermal and mesodermal cells.[132] α-Fetoprotein is a protein produced in high concentration by the fetus and is essentially absent from serum of individuals over 6 months of age. Waldmann has found that 59 of 60 patients with ataxia-telangiectasia had substantially elevated levels of α-fetoprotein while it was not detectable in the serum of their siblings or parents or in patients with other primary immunodeficiency diseases.[133] In addition, these patients may have elevated levels of β-fetoprotein and carcinoembryonic antigen. The occurrence of ovarian agenesis is another example of tissue immaturity.

The Wiskott-Aldrich Syndrome (WAS, Immunodeficiency with Thrombocytopenia and Eczema). *Definition.* The Wiskott-Aldrich syndrome is an X-linked disease with onset in infancy or early childhood characterized by a triad of symptoms consisting of recurrent infections with all classes of microorganisms, bleeding secondary to pronounced thrombocytopenia, and eczema of the skin.[134] The Wiskott-Aldrich syndrome is also associated with a marked increased in the incidence of lymphoma, recently estimated at 128 times the rate seen in the general population.[119,135]

Clinical Features. Boys with the Wiskott-Aldrich syndrome may have a great variety of clinical problems. Their immune deficiency is second only to SCID in its severity. These boys have recurrent infections with all classes of microorganisms. Infection commonly occurs with *Hemophilus influenzae*, pneumococci, *Candida albicans*, and *Pneumocystis carinii*. These children have died of generalized vaccinia following smallpox vaccination, have developed disseminated herpes simplex infections, and chicken pox has been fatal in several cases (Fig. 83–7), particularly during periods of steroid therapy. In addition to their severe recurrent infections, these children have marked thrombocytopenia, with platelet counts ranging from 10,000 to 30,000. Approximately 20 percent ultimately die of bleeding, with intracranial hemorrhage the greatest threat.

Eczema is the third component of the triad of this disorder and is indistinguishable from the eczema found in atopic children. Another feature of the syndrome is the common occurrence of severe autoimmune disease. This autoimmune reaction may take the form of juvenile rheumatoid arthritis with hectic fevers and joint involvement. It may also include cutaneous vasculitis or vasculitis involving major blood vessels, including cerebral and coronary arteries.[136] Profound hemolytic anemia may be seen. The superimposition of an autoimmune form of thrombocytopenia on the pre-existing low platelet count also occurs, resulting in platelet counts of less than 1000.[137] The development of such an autoaggressive syndrome is an omnious clinical event and is often associated with a fatal outcome.

Immunologic Defects. The immunologic defects in this syndrome are also broad, involving humoral and cellular immune systems and the system of nonspecific resistance.[138] The children may have normal immunoglobulin levels, although a more common pattern shows low values for IgM, higher than normal values for IgA, and exceptionally high levels of IgE. In addition, each of the immunoglobulin classes in these children is being hy-

Figure 83–7. Hemorrhagic chicken pox in a boy with the Wiskott-Aldrich syndrome. The cellular immune deficiency in this disease in combination with thrombocytopenia makes this common childhood exanthem a potentially lethal complication.

percatabolized. The survival rate (T½) for IgG, IgA, and IgM is shortened to one third to one half of normal in these patients. Thus to maintain normal serum immunoglobulin levels these children are producing immunoglobulin at far greater than the normal synthetic rate.[139]

In spite of this high rate of immunoglobulin synthesis, the production of specific antibodies is often markedly impaired. Isohemagglutinins are characteristically absent, or the titer is very low.[140] Following immunization, patients respond to some antigens but are unique in being unable to make antibodies following immunization with polysaccharide antigens such as pneumococcal polysaccharide.[141,142] This observation helps to explain why these children are so susceptible to infection with high-grade encapsulated organisms such as the pneumococcus and hemophilus.

Cellular immunity is similarly involved. The children are usually anergic to all skin tests. The T lymphocytes respond quite well in vitro to stimulation with mitogens such as phytohemagglutinin or concanavalin A but respond very poorly when challenged with specific antigens such as tetanus toxoid or with foreign cells in a mixed lymphocyte reaction.[143] The patients also have a defect in cytotoxic T killer cell function and have a variety of defects in their monocytes, including a defect in the monocyte killing mechanism and an abnormality in monocyte and PMN chemotaxis.[144,145]

Pathogenesis. The fundamental defect in the Wiskott-Aldrich syndrome that causes these diverse disease manifestations is unknown. However, it is becoming increasingly apparent that many of the defects seen in these patients are secondary consequences of more fundamental problems. For example, splenectomy totally corrects the thrombocytopenia.[146] The platelets in the Wiskott-Aldrich syndrome are normally small, with a mean platelet volume of 3 μ^3 compared with the normal mean of 6.6 μ^3. This is the only disease associated with microthrombocytopenia. Following splenectomy the platelet size becomes normal, and tests of the function of these platelets are also entirely normal.[137,146] Thus one of the major components of this syndrome is a phenomenon that is a secondary consequence of a destructive process mediated by the spleen. The possibility exists that other major defects in these patients may also occur as secondary events to some as yet not understood primary disorder. Recently Parkman has described a deficiency of a specific cell membrane glycoprotein, GLP115, on the lymphocytes of patients with the Wiskott-Aldrich syndrome and another group of immune deficient patients.[147] A generalized defect in the production or expression of a critical cell membrane component could certainly account for the variety of defects found in these patients.

Treatment. Treatment of the Wiskott-Aldrich syndrome is complex because of the many problems presented by this disease. Bone marrow transplantation is the treatment of choice if a histoidentical sibling donor is available.[148,149] In the absence of a suitable donor for bone marrow transplantation a number of procedures may be useful in managing these patients. Splenectomy corrects the thrombocytopenia in essentially all patients.[146] However, splenectomy also increases patients' susceptibility to infection with high-grade pathogens, and thus it is essential that splenectomized patients be treated with prophylactic antibiotics to prevent overwhelming infection. Following splenectomy we also treat these patients with intramuscular gamma globulin. Transfer factor therapy has received a great deal of attention in recent years. Controlled studies have not been presented to demonstrate any therapeutic benefit from such treatment, and both cancer and autoimmune disease have developed while patients were receiving transfer factor. This material has no role in the therapy of the Wiskott-Aldrich syndrome.

Chronic Mucocutaneous Candidiasis. *Definition.* Chronic mucocutaneous candidiasis is a cellular immunodeficiency disorder characterized by persistent candida infection involving the mucous membranes, skin, hair, and nails.[150,151] This disease differs from most cellular immunodeficiency disorders in that the defect is usually limited to responses to *Candida albicans* and a few antigenically related fungi. Immunity to viruses, bacteria, and other microorganisms is usually intact. Antibody responses are usually entirely normal, and even most tests of cellular immunity are normal.

Clinical Features. Subgroups of chronic mucocutaneous candidiasis have been described based on variations in the clinical pattern.[151] An early form accompanied by candidal granuloma, a disfiguring eruption characterized by plaquelike hyperkeratotic scales and cutaneous horn formation of the nails and face, is the most severe type. Endocrinopathy occurs in about half of the patients with this form of the disease. Candidiasis of later onset occurs in elderly individuals and is usually quite mild, with involvement limited to the oral cavity and a few nails. Juvenile familial polyendocrinopathy syndrome with candidiasis is yet another form of this disease. This type is characterized by mild to moderate candidiasis. The endocrine abnormalities seen in these disorders include hypoparathyroidism, Addison's disease, hypothyroidism, and diabetes, and these usually appear several years after the onset of candidiasis. Autoantibodies to the affected endocrine glands are common, and associated disorders such as ovarian insufficiency, pernicious anemia, alopecia, chronic active hepatitis, and iron deficiency anemia may be found.[151]

Immune Defects. There is a heterogenous pattern of immune deficiency in patients with chronic mucocutaneous candidiasis. Some individuals have apparently normal immune function, while others might be relatively severely defective. The most characteristic abnormalities are skin anergy, impaired in vitro lymphocyte proliferative responses restricted to candida antigens, and impaired synthesis of the lymphokine migratory inhibiting factor in vitro in response to *Candidia* antigens. Antibody responses to *Candidia* and other antigens are normal, and immunoglobulin levels are normal or elevated. T- and B-lymphocyte numbers are also usually normal. Monocyte function may be severely defective.[152] The serum of some patients has been found to contain inhibitors that block lymphocyte responses to *Candidia* in vitro.[153] Interestingly, mannan from the *Candida* cell wall can be found in significant concentrations in the plasma of these patients and when mannan is added to normal plasma it also becomes inhibitory to in vitro lymphocyte responses.

Treatment. Treatment with antimycotic agents has been the principal therapy employed.[154] This is usually effective in eliminating the infection temporarily, but recurrences are common within a few weeks after therapy is discontinued. Eventually the cumulative toxicity of the antimycotic drugs limits their usefulness because repeated courses of treatment are necessary. This has led to attempts to augment the immune response of these patients to Candidia. The most widely used of these forms of immunostimulation has been transfer factor, and there is evidence that it may provide some benefit in this disease. Although not usually effective when used alone as treatment, when used in combination with amphotericin B, transfer factor may help to significantly prolong the duration of clinical remissions and thus reduce the patient's exposure to drug toxicity.[155]

Immunodeficiency Secondary to Loss of the Immunoglobulins and Lymphocytes. In addition to defects in the production of immunoglobulins and T lymphocytes found in most of the disorders already described, another major mechanism of immune deficiency is the loss of immunoglobulins and lymphocytes after they have been normally produced. In the nephrotic syndrome, for example, significant amounts of serum immunoglobulin are lost into the urine. It is uncommon, however, for enough immunoglobulin to be lost via this route to result in clinically significant hypogammaglobulinemia. A second major site of loss is the gastrointestinal tract, as seen with the protein-losing gastroenteropathies, and loss via this route can result in immune deficiency. In particular, the disorder intestinal lymphangiectasia is noteworthy for its striking association with deficiency in the immune system.

Intestinal lymphangiectasia is a disease characterized by a disorder of the lymphatics, extreme gastrointestinal protein loss, hypoalbuminemia, hypogammaglobulinemia, and generalized edema and initially affects people before the age of 30.[156] The major symptoms are edema and diarrhea. Severe diarrhea is seen in a few patients, but more will have no gastrointestinal symptoms whatever. Peripheral edema, which is also asymmetric, is almost universal, and many patients develop chylous effusions. The hallmark morphologic lesion of this disorder is dilated lymphatics in the wall of the small intestine. Striking hypoalbuminemia and hypogammaglobulinemia are found secondary to the loss of lymphatic fluid directly into the gastrointestinal lumen. In addition to the loss of lymph protein, the cells in the lymph (the lymphocytes) are also lost (position thirteen, Fig. 83–5). Thus, patients with intestinal lymphangiectasia may have profound lymphocytopenia leading to skin test anergy and even impaired rejection of allogeneic skin grafts.[157,158]

Although serum immunoglobulin levels may be very low, these patients frequently can make substantial antibody responses following immunizations, and infections with encapsulated high-grade bacterial pathogens are not a prominent clinical feature of this disease. However, mycobacterial infections and lymphoid malignancies are increased in these patients. Although intestinal lymphangiectasia is rare, more common diseases are also associated with gastrointestinal loss of lymph proteins and cells. Patients with constrictive pericarditis may present with a generalized edema and marked lymphocytopenia. In these cases, the pericardial constriction and secondary elevated venous pressure cause an increase in the pressure in the intestinal lymphatics, resulting in lymphatic leakage into the bowel. Importantly, following surgical correction of the cardiac disease in these patients the immunologic system rapidly returns to normal.[159]

AIDS (Acquired Immunodeficiency Syndrome, Gay-Related Immunodeficiency, GRID Syndrome). In the two years after its initial description in the summer of 1981, over 2000 cases of a previously unrecognized immune deficiency syndrome were reported.[160] The working definition established by the Centers for Disease Control for AIDS, for acquired immunodeficiency syndrome, includes patients under the age of 60 who develop Kaposi's sarcoma and/or opportunistic infections with no known underlying cause for immune deficiency. Over

90 percent of the reported cases have occurred in the United States, but cases have been reported from 20 other countries as well. Initially, all of the reported cases occurred in sexually promiscuous homosexual and bisexual males. Recently, however, several other high-risk groups have been identified, including male and female intravenous drug abusers and their nonaddicted sexual partners, Haitian immigrants to the United States, and patients with hemophilia A receiving maintenance clotting factor therapy, and most recently identified have been infants and children residing in households with an AIDS patient.[161-166] The disease is exceptionally severe, with only 15 percent of the patients surviving for 24 months.

Infections in these patients are caused by microorganisms for which the T-lymphocyte system has a primary defensive role: *Pneumocystis carinii*, cytomegalovirus, Epstein-Barr virus, *Candidia albicans*, *Toxoplasma*, *Cryptococcus*, *Mycobacterium avium intracellulare*, and herpes simplex virus. These infections present as pneumonia, brain abscess, esophagitis, disseminated mycobacterial or cryptococcal infections, and severe diarrhea. Kaposi's sarcoma, and to a lesser extent Burkitt's lymphoma and non-Hodgkin's lymphoma, have developed in a very high proportion of patients with AIDS. The Kaposi's sarcoma occurring in this syndrome differs markedly from that formerly described as an indolent eruption of elderly males of European Jewish and Italian extraction. The Kaposi's sarcoma in AIDS is an aggressive, metastasizing, frequently lethal tumor affecting men with a mean age of 35. It tends to involve the head, mucous membranes, trunk, and upper extremities, while "classic" Kaposi's sarcoma is usually restricted to the lower extremities[167] (Fig. 83–8).

Figure 83–8. The forearm of a 32-year-old male homosexual who initially presented with pneumocystis pneumonia. The Kaposi's sarcoma of AIDS as illustrated in the photograph is an aggressive malignant tumor, in contrast to the classic indolent eruption characteristic of Kaposi's sarcoma in elderly males. (Photograph courtesy of Dr. H. Clifford Lane, NIAID, NIH.)

Immunologically, AIDS patients often have profound lymphocytopenia and cutaneous anergy (position four, Fig. 83–5). In vitro tests of lymphocyte function reveal depressed T-lymphocyte proliferative responses. The absolute T-lymphocyte number is low in most cases, reflecting primarily a striking depression in the number of T4 antigen–bearing cells. This absolute decrease in T4 cells leads to reversal of the usual ratio of T4 to T8 cells in the peripheral blood. Most AIDS patients have polyclonal hypergammaglobulinemia with elevated titers of antibody to cytomegalovirus, herpes simplex virus, Epstein-Barr virus, and hepatitis B virus. AIDS patients also have been shown to have high levels of thymosin alpha 1 and an acid labile alpha interferon in their blood.[168,169] Hypogammaglobulinemia has also been observed infrequently. Promiscuous homosexual males and IV drug abusers commonly have chronic generalized lymphadenopathy often associated with constitutional symptoms, including weight loss and recurrent fevers. It has been suggested that this may represent a prodrome to AIDS, but the evidence for the regularity of this association is incomplete.

The etiology of AIDS has recently been claimed to be a virus. Epidemiologic studies have suggested that it is caused by an infectious agent that is transmitted in a fashion similar to hepatitis B virus: through blood products, in intravenous drug abusers who share needles, and through intimate sexual contact. There is a surprisingly high incidence of serologic responses to HTLV III (human T-lymphocyte leukemia virus) in AIDS patients, and the association between this virus and AIDS seems secure.[170-172]

CONCLUSIONS

Nature is nowhere accustomed more openly to display her secret mysteries than in cases where she shows tracings of her workings apart from the beaten paths; nor is there any better way to advance the proper practice of medicine than to give our minds to the discovery of the unusual law of nature by careful investigation of cases of rare forms of disease.

William Harvey, letter, April 24, 1657

Studies in patients with immune deficiency have indeed provided essential insights into the normal functioning of the immune system in bodily defense. Investigation of these patients has not only helped us to understand the organization and function of the host defense system, but it has also promoted the development of entirely new approaches for therapy that have benefited not only patients with immune deficiency disease but a much broader spectrum of medical disorders as well. In addition, studies of patients with these rare inborn errors of immunity have led to the development of new diagnostic tools, which have permitted a much greater understanding of the functions of the immune system in host defense and also the participation of the immune system in the pathogenesis of a variety of diseases other than immunodeficiency.

References

1. Bruton, O.C.: Agammaglobulinemia. Pediatrics 9:722, 1952.
2. Horowitz, S.D., and Hong, R.: The pathogenesis and treatment of immunodeficiency. Monographs in Allergy, Volume 10. Basel, S. Karger, 1977.
3. Seligmann, M., and Hitzig, W.H.: Primary Immunodeficiencies. Amsterdam, North Holland Biomedical Press, 1980.
4. Stiehm, E.R., and Fulginiti, V.A.: Immunologic Disorders in Infants and Children. 2nd ed. Philadelphia, W. B. Saunders Company, 1978.
5. Bergsma, D.: Immunodeficiency in Man and Animals. Sunderland, Mass., Sinauer, 1975.
6. Asherson, G.L., and Webster, A.D.B.: Diagnosis and Treatment of Immunodeficiency Diseases. Oxford, Blackwell Scientific Publication, 1980.
7. Cooper, M.D., Peterson, R.D.A., South, M.A., and Good, R.A.: The functions of the thymus system and the bursa system in chickens. J. Exp. Med. 123:75, 1966.
8. Buckley, R.H., Wray, B.B., and Belmaker, E.Z.: Extreme hyperimmunoglobulinemia E and undue susceptibility to infection. Pediatrics 49:59, 1972.
9. Hill, H.R., Ochs, H.D., Quie, P.G., Clark, R.A., Pabst, H.F., Klebanoff, S.J., and Wedgwood, R.J.: Defect in neutrophil granulocyte chemotaxis in Job's syndrome of recurrent "cold" staphylococcal abscesses. Lancet 2:617, 1974.
10. Schur, P.H., Borel, H., Gelfand, E.W., Alper, C., and Rosen, F.S.: Selective gamma-G globulin deficiencies in patients with recurrent pyogenic infections. N. Engl. J. Med. 283:631, 1970.
11. Oxelius, V.A.: Chronic infections in a family with hereditary deficiency of IgG$_2$ and IgG$_4$. Clin. Exp. Immunol. 17:19, 1974.
12. Johnston, R.B., and Baehner, R.L.: Chronic granulomatous disease: Correlation between pathogenesis and clinical findings. Pediatrics 48:730, 1971.
13. Lachmann, P.J., and Rosen, F.S.: Genetic defects in complement in man. Springer Semin. Immunopathol. 1:339, 1978.
14. Blaese, R.M., Weiden, P.L., Koski, I., and Dooley, N.: Infectious agammaglobulinemia: Transmission of immunodeficiency with grafts of agammaglobulinemia cells. J. Exp. Med. 140:1097, 1974.
15. Raff, M.C., Megson, M., Owen, J.J.T., and Cooper, M.D.: Early production of intracellular IgM by B-lymphocyte precursors in mouse. Nature 259:224, 1976.
16. Gathings, W.E., Lawton, A.R., and Cooper, M.D.: Immunofluorescent studies of the development of pre-B cells, B lymphocytes and immunoglobulin isotype diversity in humans. Eur. J. Immunol. 7:804, 1977.
17. Korsmeyer, S.J., Hieter, P.A., Ravetch, J.V., Poplack, D.G., Waldmann, T.A., and Leder, P.: Developmental hierarchy of immunoglobulin gene rearrangements in human leukemia pre-B-cells. Proc. Natl. Acad. Sci. 78:7096, 1981.
18. Melchers, F., Anderson, J., and Phillips, R.A.: Ontogeny of murine B lymphocytes: Development of Ig synthesis and of reactivities to mitogens and to anti-Ig-antibodies. Cold Spring Harbor Symp. Quant. Biol. 41:147, 1976.
19. Abey, E.R., Cooper, M.D., Kearney, J.F., Lawton, A.R., and Parkhouse, R.M.E.: Sequential expression of immunoglobulins on developing mouse B lymphocytes: A systematic survey that suggests a model for the generation of immunoglobulin isotype diversity. J. Immunol. 120:2041, 1978.
20. Hitzig, W.H.: Congenital thymic and lymphocytic deficiency disorders. In Stiehm, E.R., and Fulginiti, V. (eds.): Immunologic Disorders in Infants and Children. Philadelphia, W. B. Saunders Company, 1973.
21. Hoyer, J.R., Cooper, M.D., Gabrielson, A.E., and Good, R.A.: Lymphopenic forms of congenital immunologic deficiency diseases. Medicine 47:201, 1968.
22. Pollack, M.S., Kirkpatrick, D., Kapoor, N., Dupont, B., and O'Reilly, R.: Identification by HLA typing of intrauterine derived maternal T cells in four patients with severe combined immunodeficiency. N. Engl. J. Med. 307:662, 1982.
23. Wolfson, J.J., and Cross, V.F.: The radiologic findings in 19 patients with combined immunodeficiency. In Meuwissen, H.J., Pickering, R.J., Pollara, B., and Porter, I.H. (eds.): Combined Immunodeficiency Disease and Adenosine Deaminase Deficiency, a Molecular Defect. New York, Academic Press, Inc., 1975.
24. DeVaal, O.M., and Seynhaeve, V.: Reticular dysgenesia. Lancet 2:1123, 1959.
25. Ownby, D.R., Pizzo, S., Blackmon, L., Gall, S.A., and Buckley, R.H.: Severe combined immunodeficiency with leukopenia (reticular dysgenesis) in siblings: Immunologic and histopathologic findings. J. Pediatr. 89:382, 1976.
26. Ammann, A.J., and Fudenberg, H.H.: Immunodeficiency diseases. In Fudenberg, H.H., Stites, D.P., Caldwell, J.L., and Wells, J.V.: Basic and Clinical Immunology. 2nd ed. Los Altos, Calif., Lange Medical Publisher, 1978.

27. Pahwa, S.G., Pahwa, R.N., and Good, R.A.: Heterogeneity of B lymphocyte differentiation in severe combined immunodeficiency disease. J. Clin. Invest. 66:543, 1980.
28. Hitzig, W.H.: Protean appearances of immunodeficiencies: Syndromes and inborn errors involving other systems which express associated primary immunodeficiency. In Wedgwood, R., Rosen, F.S., and Paul, N.W. (eds.): Primary Immunodeficiency Diseases. New York, Alan R. Liss, 1983, p. 307.
29. Blaese, R.M., Weiden, P.L., Oppenheim, J.J., and Waldmann, T.A.: Phytohemagglutinin as a skin test for the evaluation of cellular immune competence in man. J. Lab. Clin. Med. 81:538, 1973.
30. Hitzig, W.H., Landolt, R., Miller, G., and Bodmer, P.: Heterogeneity of phenotypic expression in a family with Swiss-type agammaglobulinemia: Observations on the acquisition of agammaglobulinemia. J. Pediatr. 78:968, 1971.
31. Pyke, K.W., Dosch, H.M., Ipp, M.M., and Gelfand, E.W.: Demonstration of an intrathymic defect in a case of severe combined immunodeficiency disease. N. Engl. J. Med. 193:424, 1975.
32. Incefy, G.S., O'Reilly, R.J., Kapoor, N., Iwota, T., and Good, R.A.: In vitro differentiation of human marrow T cell precursors by thymic factors in severe combined immunodeficiency. Transplantation 32:299, 1981.
33. Seeger, R.C., Robins, R.A., Stevens, R.H., Klein, R.B., Waldmann, D.J., Zeltzer, P.M., and Kessler, S.W.: Severe combined immunodeficiency with B lymphocytes: In vitro correlation of defective immunoglobulin production by addition of normal T lymphocytes. Clin. Exp. Immunol. 26:1, 1976.
34. Buckley, R.H., Gilbertsen, R.B., Schiff, R.I., Ferreira, E., Sanal, S.O., and Waldmann, T.A.: Heterogeneity of lymphocyte subpopulations in severe combined immunodeficiency: Evidence against a stem cell defect. J. Clin. Invest. 58:130, 1976.
35. Giblett, E.R., Anderson, J.E., Cohen, F., Pollara, B., and Meuwissen, H.J.: Adenosine-deaminase deficiency in two patients with severely impaired cellular immunity. Lancet 2:1067, 1972.
36. Meuwissen, H.J., Pollara, B., and Pickering, R.J.: Combined immunodeficiency disease associated with adenosine deaminase deficiency. J. Pediatr. 86:169, 1975.
37. Wara, D.W., and Ammann, A.J.: Laboratory data. In Meuwissen, H.J., Pickering, R.J., Pollara, B., and Porter, I.H. (eds.): Combined Immunodeficiency Disease and Adenosine Deaminase Deficiency, a Molecular Defect. New York, Academic Press, Inc., 1975.
38. Cohen, A., Hirshhorn, R., Horowitz, S.D., Rubenstein, A., Polmar, S.H., Hong, R., and Martin, D.W.: Deoxyadenosine triphosphate as a potentially toxic metabolite in adenosine deaminase deficiency. Proc. Natl. Acad. Sci. 75:472, 1978.
39. Gelfand, E.W., and Cohen, A.: Disorders of purine metabolism and immunodeficiency. In Gallin, J.I., and Fauci, A.S. (eds.): Advances in Host Defense Mechanisms. Vol. 2. New York, Raven Press, 1983.
40. Kredick, N.M.: The Methylation Hypothesis of Adenosine Toxicity. In Ciba Foundation Symposium Series 68. Amsterdam, Elsevier, 1979.
41. Carson, D.A., Kaye, J., and Seegmiller, J.E.: Lymphospecific toxicity in adenosine deaminase deficiency and purine nucleoside phosphorylase deficiency: Possible role of nucleoside kinase(s). Proc. Natl. Acad. Sci. 24:5677, 1977.
42. Carson, D.A., Kaye, J., and Seegmiller, J.E.: Differential sensitivity of human leukemic T cell lines and B cell lines to growth inhibition by deoxyadenosine. J. Immunol. 121:1726, 1978.
43. Mitchell, B.S., Mejias, E., Daddona, P.E., and Kelley, W.N.: Purinogenic immunodeficiency diseases: Selective toxicity of deoxyribonucleosides for T cells. Proc. Natl. Acad. Sci. 75:5011, 1978.
44. Wilson, J.M., Mitchell, B.S., Daddona, P.E., and Kelley, W.N.: Purinogenic immunodeficiency diseases: Differential effects of deoxyadenosine and deoxyguanosine on DNA synthesis in human T-lymphoblasts. J. Clin. Invest. 64:1475, 1979.
45. Mejias, E., Mitchell, B., Cassidy, J., and Kelley, W.N.: Deoxyribonucleotide pools in immunodeficiency states. III. International Symposium on Purine Metabolism in Man. Clin. Res. 27:331A, 1979.
46. Hershfield, M.S., Kredich, N.M., Ownby, D.R., Ownby, H., and Buckley, R.: In vivo inactivation of erythrocyte S-adenosylhomocysteine hydrolase by 2'-deoxyadenosine in adenosine deaminase-deficient patients. J. Clin. Invest. 63:807, 1979.
47. Gatti, R.A., Allen, H.D., Meuwissen, H.J., Hong, R., and Good, R.A.: Immunological reconstitution of sex-linked lymphopenic immunological deficiency. Lancet 2:1366, 1968.
48. Bortin, M.M., and Rimm, A.A.: Severe combined immunodeficiency disease. Characterization of the disease and results of transplantation. JAMA 238:591, 1977.
49. O'Reilly, R.J., Kapoor, N., Kirkpatrick, D., Flomenberg, N., Pollack, M.S., Dupont, B., Good, R.A., and Reisner, Y.: Transplantation of hematopoietic cells for lethal congenital immunodeficiencies. In Wedgwood, R., Rosen, F.S., and Paul, N.W. (eds.): Primary Immunodeficiency Diseases. New York, Alan R. Liss, 1983, p. 307.

50. Hong, R., Santosham, M., Schutle-Wissermann, H., Horowitz, S., Hsu, S.H., and Winkelstein, J.A.: Reconstruction of B and T lymphocyte function in severe combined immunodeficiency diseases after transplantation with thymic epithelium. Lancet 2:1270, 1976.

51. Hong, R.: Thymus transplantation. In Wedgwood, R., Rosen, F.S., and Paul, N.W. (eds.): Primary Immunodeficiency Diseases. New York, Alan R. Liss, 1983, p. 259.

52. Reisner, Y., Kapour, N., Kirkpatrick, D., Pollack, M.S., Dupont, B., Rood, R.A., and O'Reilly, R.J.: Transplantation for acute leukemia with HLA-A and B identical parental marrow cells fractionated with soybean agglutinin and sheep red blood cells. Lancet 2:327, 1981.

53. Polmar, S.H., Stern, R.C., Schwartz, A.L., Wetzler, E.M., Chase, P.A., and Hirschhorn, R.: Enzyme replacement therapy for adenosine deaminase deficiency and severe combined immunodeficiency. N. Engl. J. Med. 295:1337, 1976.

54. Giblett, E.R., Ammann, A.J., Wara, D.W., Dandman, R., and Diamond, L.K.: Nucleoside phosphorylase deficiency in a child with severely defective T cell immunity and normal B cell immunity. Lancet 1:1010, 1975.

55. Stoop, J.W., Zegers, B.J.M., Hendricks, G.F.M., Siegenbeek van Heukelom, L.H., Stool, G.E.J., de Brie, P.K., Wadman, S.K., and Ballieux, R.E.: Purine nucleoside phosphorylase deficiency associated with selective cellular immunodeficiency. N. Engl. J. Med. 296:651, 1977.

56. Virelizier, J.L., Hamet, M., Ballet, J.J., Reinert, P., and Griscelli, C.: Impaired defense against vaccinia in a child with T lymphocyte deficiency associated with inosine phosphorylase defect. J. Pediatr. 92:358, 1978.

57. Hamet, M., Griscelli, C., Cartier, P., Ballay, J., de Bruyn, C., and Hasli, P.: A second case of inosine phosphorylase deficiency with severe T cell abnormalities. Adv. Exp. Med. Biol. 76A:477, 1977.

58. Gelfand, E.W., Dosch, H.M., Biggar, W.D., and Fox, I.H.: Partial purine nucleoside phosphorylase deficiency. Studies of lymphocyte function. J. Clin. Invest. 61:1071, 1978.

59. Cohen, A., Doyle, D., Martin, D.W., Jr., and Ammann, A.J.: Abnormal purine metabolism and purine overproduction in a patient deficient in purine nucleoside phosphorylase. N. Engl. J. Med. 295:1449, 1976.

60. Cohen, A., Gudas, L.J., Ammann, A.J., Sataal, G.E.J., and Martin, D.W.: Deoxyguanosine triphosphate as a possible toxic metabolite in the immunodeficiency associated with purine nucleoside phosphorylase deficiency. J. Clin. Invest. 61:1405, 1978.

61. Wortmann, R.L., Mitchell, B.S., Edwards, N.L., and Fox, I.H.: Biochemical basis for differential deoxyadenosine toxicity to T and B lymphoblasts: Role for 5'-nucleotidase. Proc. Natl. Acad. Sci. 76:2434, 1979.

62. Rich, K.C., Mejias, E., and Fox, I.H.: Purine nucleoside phosphorylase deficiency: Improved metabolic and immunologic function with erythrocyte transfusions. N. Engl. J. Med. 303:973, 1980.

63. Kelley, W.N., and Smith, L.H., Jr.: Hereditary orotic aciduria. In Stanbury, J.B., Wyngaarden, J.B., and Fredrickson, D.S. (eds.): The Metabolic Basis of Inherited Disease, 4th ed. New York, McGraw-Hill, 1978.

64. Girot, R., Hamet, M., Perignon, J.L., Guesnu, M., Fox, R.M., Cartier, P., Darandy, A., and Griscelli, C.: Cellular immune deficiency in two siblings with hereditary orotic aciduria. N. Engl. J. Med. 308:700, 1983.

65. DiGeorge, A.M.: Congenital absence of the thymus and its immunologic consequences: Concurrence with congenital hypoarathyroidism. In Bergsma, D., and Good, R.A. (eds.): Immunologic Deficiency Disease in Man. New York, The National Foundation, 1968.

66. Hitzig, W.H.: Congenital thymic and lymphocytic deficiency disorders. In Stiehm, E.R., and Fulginiti, V.A. (eds.): Immunologic Disorders in Infants and Children. Philadelphia, W.B. Saunders Company, 1973.

67. Barrett, D.J., Ammann, A.J., Wora, D.W., Cowan, M.J., Fesher, T.J., and Stiehm, E.R.: Clinical and immunologic spectrum of the DiGeorge syndrome. J. Clin. Lab. Immunol. 6:1, 1981.

68. Pabst, H.F., Wright, W.C., LeRiche, J., and Stiehm, E.R.: Partial DiGeorge syndrome with substantial cell-mediated immunity. Am. J. Dis. Child. 130:316, 1976.

69. Lischner, H.W., and DiGeorge, A.M.: Role of the thymus in humoral immunity. Observations in complete or partial congenital absence of the thymus. Lancet 2:104, 1969.

70. Kretschmer, R., Say, B., Brown, D., and Rosen, F.S.: Congenital aplasia of the thymus gland (DeGeorge's syndrome). N. Engl. J. Med. 279:1295, 1968.

71. Cleveland, W.W., Fogel, B.J., Brown, W.T., and Kay, H.E.M.: Foetal thymic transplant in a case of DiGeorge's syndrome. Lancet 2:1211, 1968.

72. Steele, R.W., Limas, C., Thurman, G.B., Schulein, M., Bauer, H., and Bellanti, J.A.: Familial thymic aplasia. Attempted reconstitution with fetal thymus in a Millipore diffusion chamber. N. Engl. J. Med. 287:787, 1972.

73. Rosen, F.S., and Janeway, C.A.: The gamma globulins. III. The antibody deficiency syndromes. N. Engl. J. Med. 275:709, 1966.

74. Wilfert, C.M., Buckley, R.H., Mohanakumar, T., Griffith, J.F., Katz, S.L., Whisnant, J.K., Eggleston, P.A., Moore, M., Treadwell, E., Oxman, M.N., and Rosen, F.S.: Persistent and fatal central nervous system echovirus infections in patients with agammaglobulinemia. N. Engl. J. Med. 296:1485, 1977.

75. Asherson, G.L., and Webster, A.D.B.: Diagnosis and Treatment of Immunodeficiency Diseases. Oxford, Blackwell Scientific Publication, 1980, p. 13.

76. Mease, P.J., Ochs, H.D., and Wedgwood, R.J.: Successful treatment of ECHO virus meningoencephalitis and myositis-fascitis with intravenous immune globulin therapy in a patient with X-linked agammaglobulinemia. N. Engl. J. Med. 304:1278, 1981.

77. Vogler, L.B., Pearl, E.R., Gathings, W.E., Lawton, A.R., and Cooper, M.D.: B lymphocyte precursors in bone marrow in immunoglobulin deficiency diseases. Lancet 2:376, 1976.

78. Fleisher, T.A., White, R.M., Broder, S., Nissley, S.P., Blaese, R.M., Mulvihill, J.V., Olive, G., and Waldmann, T.A.: X-linked hypogammaglobulinemia and isolated growth hormone deficiency. N. Engl. J. Med. 302:1429, 1980.

79. Schwaber, J.F., Molgaard, H., Orkin, S.H., Gould, H.J., and Rosen, F.: Early pre-B cells from normal and x-linked agammaglobulinemia produce Cu without an attached V_H region. Nature 304:355, 1983.

80. Working Party on Hypogammaglobulinemia: Hypogammaglobulinemia in the United Kingdom. Medical Research Council Special Report Series 310. London, Her Majesty's Stationery Office, 1971.

81. Waldmann, T.A., Strober, W., Blaese, R.M., and Strauss, A.J.L.: Thymoma, hypogammaglobulinemia and absence of eosinophils. J. Clin. Invest. 46:1127, 1967.

82. Jeunet, F.S., and Good, R.A.: Thymoma, immunologic deficits and hematologic abnormalities. In Immunologic Deficiency Diseases in Man. Birth Defects IV. National Foundation, March of Dimes, 1968.

83. Waldmann, T.A., Broder, S., Durm, M., Blackman, M., Krakauer, R., and Meade, B.: Suppressor T cells in the pathogenesis of hypogammaglobulinemia associated with thymoma. Trans. Assoc. Am. Phys. 88:120, 1976.

84. Hayward, A.R., Paolucci, P., Webster, A.D.B., and Kohler, P.: Pre-B cell suppression by thymoma patient lymphocytes. Clin. Exp. Immunol. 48:437, 1982.

85. Pearl, E.R., Vogler, L.B., Okos, A.J., Crist, W., Lawton, A.R., and Cooper, M.D.: B lymphocyte precursors in human bone marrow: An analysis of normal individuals and patients with antibody deficiency states. J. Immunol. 120:1169, 1978.

86. Hitzig, W.H., Dohmann, U., Pluss, H.J., and Vischer, D.: Hereditary transcobalamin II deficiency: Clinical findings in a new family. J. Pediatr. 85:622, 1974.

87. Hermans, P.E., Diaz-Buxo, J.A., and Stobo, J.D.: Idiopathic late-onset immunoglobulin deficiency: Clinical observations in 50 patients. Am. J. Med. 61:221, 1976.

88. Friedman, J.M., Fialkow, P.J., Davis, S.D., Ochs, H.D., and Wedgwood, R.J.: Autoimmunity in the relatives of patients with immunodeficiency diseases. Clin. Exp. Immunol. 28:375, 1977.

89. Lawrence, J.S., and Bremner, J.M.: Arthritis and hypogammaglobulinaemia: A family survey. Scand. J. Rheumatol. 5:17, 1976.

90. Soothill, J.F.: Immunoglobulins in first degree relatives of patients with hypogammaglobulinemia. Lancet 1:1001, 1968.

91. Ament, M.E., Ochs, H.D., and Davis, S.D.: Structure and function of the gastrointestinal tract in primary immunodeficiency syndromes: A study of 39 patients. Medicine 52:227, 1973.

92. Freeman, H.J., Shnitka, T.K., Piercey, J.R.A., and Weinstein, W.M.: Cytomegalovirus infection of the gastrointestinal tract in a patient with late onset immunodeficiency syndrome. Gastroenterology 73:1397, 1977.

93. Good, R.A., Rötstein, J., and Mazzitello, W.F.: The simultaneous occurrence of rheumatoid arthritis and agammaglobulinemia. J. Lab. Clin. Med. 49:343, 1957.

94. Webster, A.D., Loewi, G., Dourmashkin, R.D., Golding, D.N., Ward, D.J., and Asherson, G.L.: Polyarthritis in adults with hypogammaglobulinaemia and its rapid response to immunoglobulin treatment. Br. Med. J. 1:1314, 1976.

95. Geha, R.S., Schneeberger, E.E., Rosen, F.S., and Merler, E.: Heterogeneity of "acquired" or common variable agammaglobulinemia. N. Engl. J. Med. 291:1, 1974.

96. Platts-Mills, T.A.E., DeGast, G.C., Webster, A.D.B., Asherson, G.L., and Williams, S.R.: Two immunologically distinct forms of late-onset hypogammaglobulinemia. Clin. Exp. Immunol. 44:383, 1981.

97. Siegal, F.P., Siegal, M., and Good, R.A.: Role of helper suppressor and B cell defects in the pathogenesis of the hypogammaglobulinemias. N. Engl. J. Med. 299:172, 1978.

98. Cooper, M.D., Lawton, A.R., and Bockman, D.E.: Agammaglobulinemia

with B lymphocytes. Specific defect of plasma-cell differentiation. Lancet 2:791, 1971.

99. Preud'homme, J.L., and Seligmann, M.: Primary immunodeficiency with increased numbers of circulating B lymphocytes contrasting with hypogammaglobulinemia. Lancet 1:442, 1972.

100. Siegel, R.L., Issekutz, T., Schwaber, N., Rosen, F.S., and Geha, R.S.: Deficiency of T helper cells in transient hypogammaglobulinemia of infancy. N. Engl. J. Med. 305:1307, 1981.

101. Ciccimara, F., Rosen, F.S., Schneeberger, E.E., and Merler, E.: Failure of heavy chain glycosylation of IgG in some patients with common variable agammaglobulinemia. J. Clin. Invest. 57:1386, 1976.

102. Schwaber, J.F., and Rosen, F.S.: Somatic cell hybrids of mouse myeloma cells and B lymphocytes from a patient with agammaglobulinemia failure to secrete human immunoglobulin. J. Immunol. 122:1849, 1979.

103. Waldmann, T.A., Broder, S., Blaese, R.M., Durm, M., Blackman, M., and Strober, W.: Role of suppressor T cells in pathogenesis of common variable hypogammaglobulinemia. Lancet 2:609, 1974.

104. Provisor, A.J., Iacuone, J.J., Chilcote, R.R., Neiburger, R.G., Crussi, F.G., and Baehner, R.L.: Acquired agammaglobulinemia after a life-threatening illness with clinical and laboratory features of infectious mononucleosis in three related male children. N. Engl. J. Med. 293:62, 1975.

105. Tosato, G., Magrath, I., Koski, I., Dooley, N.J., and Blaese, R.M.: Suppressor T cell activation during Epstein-Barr virus-induced infectious mononucleosis. N. Engl. J. Med. 301:1133, 1979.

106. Cassidy, J.T., Burt, A., Petty, R., and Sullivan, D.: Selective IgA deficiency in connective tissue disease. N. Engl. J. Med. 280:275, 1968.

107. Ammann, A.J., and Hong, R.: Selective IgA deficiency: Presentation of 30 cases and a review of the literature. Medicine 50:223, 1971.

108. Anderson, K.E., Finlayson, N.D.C., and Descher, E.E.: Intractable malabsorption with a flat mucosa and selective IG deficiency. Gastroenterology 67:709, 1974.

109. Oxelius, V.A., Laurell, A.B., Lindquiest, B., Golebriowska, H., Axelsson, U., Björkander, J., and Hanson, L.A.: IgG subclasses in selective IgA deficiency: Importance of IgG$_2$-IgA deficiency. N. Engl. J. Med. 304:1476, 1981.

110. Lawton, A.R., Royal, S.A., Self, K.S., and Cooper, M.D.: IgA determinants on B-lymphocytes in patients with deficiency of circulating IgA. J. Lab. Clin. Med. 80:26, 1972.

111. Vyas, G.N., Perkins, J.A., Yang, Y.M., and Basantani, G.K.: Healthy blood donors with selective absence of immunoglobulin A: Prevention of anaphylactic transfusion reactions caused by antibodies to IgA. J. Lab. Clin. Med. 85:838, 1975.

112. Huntley, C.C., Robbins, J.B., Lyerly, A.D., and Buckley, R.H.: Characterization of precipitating antibodies to ruminant serum and milk proteins in humans with selective IgA deficiency. N. Engl. J. Med. 284:7, 1971.

113. Cunningham-Rundles, C., Brandeis, W.E., Good, R.A., and Day, N.K.: Bovine antigens and the formation of circulating immune complexes in selective immunoglobulin A deficiency. J. Clin. Invest. 64:272, 1979.

114. Waldmann, T.A., Broder, S., Krakauer, R., Durm, M., Meade, B., and Goldman, C.: Defect in IgA secretion and in IgA specific suppressor cells in patients with selective IgA deficiency. Trans. Assoc. Am. Phys. 89:215, 1976.

115. Conley, M.E., and Cooper, M.D.: Immature IgA B cells in IgA-deficient patients. N. Engl. J. Med. 305:495, 1981.

116. McFarlin, D.E., Strober, W., and Waldmann, T.A.: Ataxia-telangiectasia. Medicine 51:281, 1972.

117. Boder, E.: Ataxia-telangiectasia: Some historic, clinical and pathologic observations. In Bergsma, D., Good, R.A., Finstad, J., and Paul, N.W. (eds.): Immunodeficiency in Man and Animals. Sunderland, Mass., Sinauer Press, 1975.

118. Bar, R.S., Levis, W.R., Rechler, M.M., Harrison, L.C., Siebert, C., Podskalny, J., Roth, J., and Muggeo, M.: Extreme insulin resistance in ataxia telangiectasia: Defect in affinity of insulin receptors. N. Engl. J. Med. 298:1164, 1978.

119. Waldmann, T.A., Strober, W., and Blaese, R.M.: Immunodeficiency disease and malignancy. Ann. Intern. Med. 77:605, 1972.

120. Spector, B.D., Perry, G.S., and Kersey, J.H.: Genetically determined immunodeficiency diseases (GDID) and malignancy: Report from the Immunodeficiency-Cancer Registry. Clin. Immunol. Immunopathol. 11:12, 1978.

121. McFarlin, D.E., and Oppenheim, J.J.: Impaired lymphocyte transformation in ataxia-telangiectasia in part due to a plasma inhibitory factor. J. Immunol. 103:1212, 1969.

122. Oxelius, V.A., Berkel, A.I., and Hansen, L.A.: IgG2 deficiency in ataxia-telangiectasia. N. Engl. J. Med. 306:515, 1982.

123. Ammann, A.J., and Hong, R.: Autoimmune phenomena in ataxia telangiectasia. J. Pediatr. 78:821, 1971.

124. Waldmann, T.A., Broder, S., Goldman, C.K., Frost, K., Korsmeyer, S.J., and Medici, M.A.: Disorders of B cells and helper T cells in the pathogenesis of the immunoglobulin deficiency of patients with ataxia-telangiectasia. J. Clin. Invest. 71:282, 1983.

125. Cunliffe, P.N., Mann, J.R., Cameron, A.H., Roberts, K.D., and Ward, H.W.C.: Radiosensitivity in ataxia telangiectasia. Br. J. Radiol. 48:374, 1975.

126. Paterson, M.D., Lohman, P.H.M., Fishman, L., Smith, B.P., and Anderson, A.K.: Defective excision repair of gamma-ray-damaged DNA in human (ataxia telangiectasia) fibroblasts. Nature 20:444, 1976.

127. Kraemer, K.H.: Progressive degenerative diseases associated with defective DNA repair: Xeroderma pigmentosum and ataxia-telangiectasia. In Nochols, W.W., and Murphy, D.G. (eds.): DNA Repair Processes. Miami, Symposia Specialists, 1977.

128. Bridges, B.A.: Some DNA repair-deficient human syndromes and their implications for human health. Proc. R. Soc. Lond. B212:263, 1981.

129. Cohen, M.M., Shaham, M., Dagan, J., Shmueli, E., and Kohn, G.: Cytogenetic investigations in families with ataxia-telangiectasia. Cytogenet. Cell Genet. 15:338, 1975.

130. Oxford, J.M., Harnden, D.G., Parrington, J.M., and Delhanty, J.D.A.: Specific chromosome aberrations in ataxia-telangiectasia. J. Med. Genet. 12:251, 1975.

131. Peterson, R.D.A., Cooper, M.D., and Good, R.A.: Lymphoid tissue abnormalities associated with ataxia-telangiectasia. Am. J. Med. 41:342, 1966.

132. McReynolds, E.W., Dabbous, M.K., Hannissian, A.S., Duenas, D., and Kimbrell, R.: Abnormal collagen in ataxia-telangiectasia. Am. J. Dis. Child. 130:305, 1976.

133. Waldmann, T.A., and McIntire, K.B.: Serum alpha-fetoprotein levels in patients with ataxia telangiectasia. Lancet 2:1112, 1972.

134. Aldrich, R.A., Steinberg, A.G., and Campbell, D.C.: Pedigree demonstrating a sex-linked recessive condition characterized by draining ears, czematoid dermatitis and bloody diarrhea. Pediatrics 13:133, 1954.

135. Filipovich, A.H., Zerbe, D., Spector, B., and Kersey, J.: Lymphomas in persons with naturally occurring immune defeciency disorders. In MaGroth, I.T., O'Conner, G.T., and Ramot, B.: Pathogenesis of Leukemias and Lymphomas: Environmental Influences. New York, Raven Press, 1984, p. 225.

136. Filipovich, A.H., Krivit, W., Kersey, J.H., and Burke, B.A.: Fatal arteritis as a complication of Wiskott-Aldrich syndrome. J. Pediatr. 95:742, 1979.

137. Corash, L., Schafer, B., and Blaese, R.M.: The effects of splenectomy on platelet size, platelet function, and platelet associated immunoglobulin in the Wiskott-Aldrich syndrome. Blood, in press.

138. Blaese, R.M., Strober, W., and Waldmann, T.A.: Immunodeficiency in the Wiskott-Aldrich syndrome. In Bergsma, D. (ed.): Immunodeficiency in Man and Animals. Birth Defects. Sunderland, Massachusetts, Sinauer Associates, 1975.

139. Blaese, R.M., Strober, W., Levy, A.L., and Waldmann, T.A.: Hypercatabolism of IgG, IgA, IgM and albumin in the Wiskott-Aldrich syndrome. J. Clin. Invest. 50:2331, 1971.

140. Krivit, W., and Good, R.A.: Aldrich's syndrome (thrombocytopenia, eczema and infection) in infants. Am. J. Dis. Child. 97:137, 1959.

141. Blaese, R.M., Strober, W., Brown, R.S., and Waldmann, T.A.: The Wiskott-Aldrich syndrome. A disorder with a possible defect in antigen processing or recognition. Lancet 1:1056, 1968.

142. Cooper, M.D., Chase, H.P., Lowman, J.T., Krivit, W., and Good, R.A.: Wiskott-Aldrich syndrome: An immunologic deficiency disease involving the afferent limb of immunity. Am. J. Med. 44:499, 1968.

143. Oppenheim, J.J., Blaese, R.M., and Waldmann, T.A.: Defective lymphocyte transformation and delayed hypersensitivity in Wiskott-Aldrich syndrome. J. Immunol. 104:835, 1970.

144. Altman, L.C., Snyderman, R., and Blaese, R.M.: Abnormalities of chemotactic lymphokine synthesis and mononuclear leukocyte chemotaxis in Wiskott-Aldrich syndrome. J. Clin. Invest. 54:486, 1974.

145. Poplack, D.G., Bonnard, G.D., Holiman, B.J., and Blaese, R.M.: Monocyte-mediated antibody-dependent cellular cytotoxicity: A clinical test of monocyte function. Blood 48:809, 1976.

146. Lum, L.G., Tubergen, D.G., Corash, L., and Blaese, R.M.: Splenectomy in the management of the thrombocytopenia of the Wiskott-Aldrich syndrome. N. Engl. J. Med. 302:892, 1980.

147. Parkman, R., Kenney, D.M., Remold-O'Donnell, P. S., and Rosen, F.S.: Surface protein abnormalities in lymphocytes and platelets from patients with Wiskott-Aldrich syndrome. Lancet 2:1387, 1981.

148. Parkman, R., Rappeport, J., Geha, R., Belli, J., Cassidy, R., Levey, R., Nathan, D.G., and Rosen, F.S.: Complete correction of the Wiskott-Aldrich syndrome by allogeneic bone marrow transplantation. N. Engl. J. Med. 298:921, 1978.

149. Kapoor, N., Kirkpatrick, D., Blaese, R.M., Oleske, J., Hilgartner, M.H., Chaganti, R.S.K., Good, R.A., and O'Reilly, R.J.: Reconstitution of normal megakaryocytopoiesis and immunologic functions in Wiskott-Aldrich syndrome by marrow transplantation following myeloablation and immunosuppression with busulfan and cyclophosphamide. Blood 57:692, 1981.

150. Kirkpatrick, C.H., Rich, R.R., and Bennett, J.E.: Chronic mucocutaneous candidiasis: Model building in cellular immunity. Ann. Intern. Med. 74:955, 1971.

151. Edwards, J.E., Lehrer, R.I., Stiehm, E.R., Fischer, I.J., and Young, L.S.: Severe candidal infections: Clinical perspective, immune defense mechanisms and current concepts of therapy. Ann. Intern. Med. 89:91, 1978.

152. Snyderman, R., Altman, L.C., Frankel, A., and Blaese, R.M.: Defective mononuclear leukocyte chemotaxis: A previously unrecognized immune dysfunction. Studies in a patient with chronic mucocutaneous candidiasis. Ann. Intern. Med. 78:509, 1973.

153. Fischer, A., Ballet, J.J., and Griscelli, C.: Specific inhibition of in vitro Candida-induced lymphocyte proliferation by polysaccharide antigens present in the serum of patients with chronic mucocutaneous candidiasis. J. Clin. Invest. 62:1005, 1978.

154. Kirkpatrick, C.H., and Smith, T.K.: Chronic mucocutaneous candidiasis: Immunologic and antibiotic therapy. Ann. Intern. Med. 80:310, 1974.

155. Schulkind, M.L., Adler, W.H., III, Altemeier, W.A., III, and Ayoub, E.M.: Transfer factor in the treatment of a case of chronic mucocutaneous candidiasis. Cell. Immunol. 3:606, 1972.

156. Waldmann, T.A., Steinfeld, J.L., Dutcher, T.F., Davidson, J.D., and Gordon, R.S., Jr.: The role of the gastrointestinal system in "idiopathic hyperproteinemia." Gastroenterology 41:197, 1961.

157. Strober, W., Wochner, R.D., Carbone, P.P., and Waldmann, T.A.: Intestinal lymphangiectasia: A protein-losing enteropathy with hypogammaglobulinemia, lymphocytopenia and impaired homograft rejection. J. Clin. Invest. 46:1643, 1967.

158. Weiden, P.L., Blaese, R.M., Strober, W., Block, J.B., and Waldmann, T.A.: Impaired lymphocyte transformation in intestinal lymphangiectasia: Evidence for at least two functionally distinct lymphocyte populations in man. J. Clin. Invest. 51:1319, 1972.

159. Nelson, D.L., Blaese, R.M., Strober, W., Bruce, R.M., and Waldmann, T.A.: Constrictive pericarditis, intestinal lymphangiectasia, and reversible immunologic deficiency. J. Pediatr. 86:548, 1975.

160. Curran, J.W.: AIDS—two years later. N. Engl. J. Med. 309:609, 1983.

161. Gottlieb, M.S., Schroff, R., Schanker, H.M., et al.: Pneumocystis carinii pneumonia and mucosal candidiasis in previously healthy homosexual men: Evidence of a new acquired cellular immunodeficiency. N. Engl. J. Med. 305:1425, 1981.

162. Siegal, F.P., Lopez, C., Hammer, G.S., et al.: Severe acquired immunodeficiency in male homosexuals, manifested by chronic perianal ulcerative herpes simplex lesions. N. Engl. J. Med. 305:1439, 1981.

163. Masur, H., Michelis, M.A., and Greene, J.B., et al.: An outbreak of community-acquired Pneumocystis carinii pneumonia: Initial manifestation of cellular immune dysfunction. N. Engl. J. Med. 305:1431,1981.

164. Vieira, J., Frank, E., Spira, T.J., and Landerman, S.H.: Acquired immune deficiency in Haitians. N. Engl. J. Med. 308:125, 1983.

165. Pneumocystis carinii pneumonia among persons with hemophilia A. Morbid. Mortal. Weekly Rep. 31:365, 1982.

166. Harris, C., Butkus Small, C., and Klein, R.S.: Immunodeficiency in female sexual partners of men with the acquired immunodeficiency syndrome. N. Engl. J. Med. 308:1181, 1983.

167. Jaffe, H.W., Choi, K., and Thomas, P.A.: National case control study of Kaposi's sarcoma and Pneumocystis carinii in homosexual men: Epidemiologic results. Ann. Intern. Med. 99:145, 1983.

168. De Stefano, E., Friedman, R.M., and Friedman-Kien, A.E.: Acid-labile human leukocyte interferon in homosexual men with Kaposi's sarcoma and lymphadenopathy. J. Infect. Dis. 146:451, 1982.

169. Hersh, E.M., Reuben, J.M., and Rios, A.: Elevated serum thymosin alpha levels associated with evidence of immune deregulation in male homosexuals with a history of infectious diseases or Kaposi's sarcoma. N. Engl. J. Med. 308:45, 1983.

170. Gallo, R.C., Sarin, P.S., and Gelmann, E.P.: Isolation of human T cell leukemia virus (HTLV) in acquired immune deficiency syndrome (AIDS). Science 220:865, 1983.

171. Barre-Sinoussi, F., Chermann, J.C., and Rey, T.: Isolation of a T-lymphotrophic retrovirus from a patient at risk for acquired immune deficiency syndrome (AIDS). Science 220:868, 1983.

172. Essex, M., McLane, M.F., and Lee, T.H.: Antibodies to cell membrane associated with human T-cell leukemia virus in patients with AIDS. Science 220:859, 1983.

Chapter 84

Cryoglobulinemia and Other Dysproteinemias

Robert W. Lightfoot, Jr.

INTRODUCTION

It is appropriate to include in a text such as this a chapter on certain dysproteinemias, including those associated with cryoproteinemia, since these often either cause syndromes resembling systemic connective tissue disorders or are encountered secondarily in the course of some classic connective tissue diseases. Thus, the abnormal monoclonal proteins that occur in multiple myeloma or Waldenström's macroglobulinemia may cause a syndrome of hyperviscosity from retinal hemorrhages, cerebral vascular occlusions, and congestive failure. If they form cryoprecipitates, these proteins can result in glomerulitis, hypocomplementemia, and digital arteritis with infarcts or gangrene, as discussed below. Rheumatoid arthritis or systemic lupus erythematosus (SLE) also can be mimicked if the monoclonal dysproteinemia is associated with amyloid infiltration of the joints secondary to light-chain overproduction. On the other hand, polyclonal mixed cryoglobulinemias may occur secondarily to a host of chronic infectious and inflammatory conditions, with resultant glomerulitis, cutaneous vasculitis, vasculitic neuropathy, and occasionally arthritis, to produce a syndrome reminiscent of SLE in which the classic lupus serologies are lacking.

This chapter will deal with the clinical, pathologic, and pathophysiologic aspects of those diseases characterized by the overproduction of monoclonal or polyclonal immunoglobulin proteins, specifically multiple myeloma and macroglobulinemia, the heavy-chain diseases, and the cryoglobulinemic states, which can present clinically a syndrome suggestive of systemic connective tissue disease. The several immunodeficiency diseases characterized by an acquired or congenital lack of one or more immunoglobulin classes and associated with an increased risk of rheumatoid arthritis or SLE are discussed elsewhere in this text. As indicated below, the disease entities discussed here are not mutually exclusive, and the occasional monoclonal immunoprotein that happens to have rheumatoid factor activity may form a mixed cryoglobulin, while conversely occasional patients producing IgG rheumatoid factor secondary to patients producing IgG rheumatoid factor secondary to rheumatoid arthritis may present with a hyperviscosity syndrome as a result of self-polymerization of that abnormal protein.

THE MONOCLONAL DYSPROTEINEMIAS—MULTIPLE MYELOMA

Multiple myeloma is thought to result from the neoplastic proliferation of a single clone of plasma cells. Clinical features necessitating medical attention in this disorder result from direct invasion of bone or other structures by the proliferating tumor mass, from deposition of immunoglobulin material in tissue (e.g., amyloid arthropathy, amyloid kidney or heart), from the direct interaction of the paraprotein produced with hemostatic and immunostatic proteins present in serum, or from infection in patients with suppressed production of normal immunoglobulins secondary to the myelomatous process.

The diagnosis of myeloma requires fulfillment of specific criteria,[1] including demonstration of excessive plasmacytosis in bone marrow or tissue, the presence of a monoclonal globulin spike, or excessive light-chain excretion. While evidence of increased plasma cells is important, it must be accompanied by at least one of the other manifestations. The monoclonal component (M component) may be of any immunoglobulin type (IgG, IgA, IgD, IgE, kappa light-chain, lambda light-chain). Patients producing an IgM M component are considered to have the macroglobulinemia of Waldenström, discussed below. In only 1 percent of patients with multiple myeloma can no monoclonal component be detected in serum or urine.[3] Urinary monoclonal material is found in 70 to 80 percent of such patients, and in that 21 percent with primarily light-chain production, the urinary protein may be the only M component found.[2]

Bone pain, usually of the central skeleton, is the major manifestation in 68 percent of patients and occurs as a result of direct expansion of the marrow tumor cell mass. Although usually associated with multiple, classic "punched out" lytic lesions on radiographs, 6 percent may have only diffuse osteoporosis. Since myeloma is seen primarily beyond middle age,[3] the clinician must be careful to distinguish this from postmenopausal or senile osteoporosis. Standard technetium phosphate bone scans are usually normal in the absence of a pathologic fracture, possibly because the lesions appear to be solely osteolytic.[3] Increased bone resorption, which may be due to tumor-secreted osteoclast-activating factors, may result in impressive hypercalcemia. This can result in polyuria with dehydration, renal impairment, altered sensorium, and hypoactivity of the gastrointestinal and neurologic systems.

Infection is the most frequent cause of death in multiple myeloma. Factors increasing susceptibility to infection include deficient antibody responses, diminished synthesis of normal polyclonal immunoglobulins, and granulocytopenia secondary to the tumor or its treatment. In addition, an array of abnormalities in inflammatory response, complement activation, phagocytosis, and other granulocyte functions may contribute (reviewed in reference 3).

Beyond bone destruction, hypercalcemia, and infection, most of the clinical problems encountered in myeloma patients can be directly attributed to the overproduction of the monoclonal protein. Renal disease remains the second leading cause of death. The mechanisms contributing to renal impairment include hypercalcemia, infiltration of plasma cell tumor into the kidney, renal tubular acidosis or Fanconi syndrome, and amyloidosis, the latter occurring in 7 percent of such patients. However, the most important factor contributing to renal insufficiency appears to be Bence Jones proteinuria. Light-chain inclusion bodies have been demonstrated in proximal tubular cells in such patients in association with altered cell integrity. Atrophy of such cells correlates better with renal insufficiency than intratubular protein casts, and alterations in tubule cell function correlate closely with Bence Jones proteinuria, suggesting that these proteins have a direct nephrotoxic effect. Light chains can be reabsorbed from the tubules and catabolized by renal tubular cells.[4-6] This may also explain the significantly shorter survival in those myelomas characterized by production of lambda light-chains only.[7-11]

Paraprotein production also plays a major role in the hyperviscosity syndrome that may be seen in 4 to 9 percent of such patients.[12,13] Because IgA proteins in general tend to polymerize, IgA myeloma is particularly prone to cause the hyperviscosity syndrome. Among the IgG myelomas, hyperviscosity tends to occur when the M component is greater than 5 g per 100 ml, and especially in those of the subclass IgG_3, which tends to form concentration- and temperature-dependent aggregates.[14] Symptoms of hyperviscosity include disorders of neurologic function varying from headache and dizziness to stupor and seizures, visual loss, distention and "sausaging" of the retinal veins, retinal hemorrhages, papilledema, congestive heart failure, expanded plasma volume, and bleeding from mucosal surfaces.

Bleeding disorders may be seen even in the absence of hyperviscosity or thrombocytopenia. This has been attributed to interaction of the paraprotein with the platelet surface or with coagulation factors (reviewed in reference 1).

Amyloid infiltration of the kidneys, joints, peripheral nerves, or mesenchymal structures (heart, tongue) has been reported in 7 percent of myeloma patients.[15] In one study of patients with amyloidosis of the "primary" type, Bence Jones proteins were found in 92 percent and overt myeloma in 50 percent.[16] Such patients with amyloidosis and underlying multiple myeloma have a greatly shortened life expectancy relative to other myeloma patients, with death often resulting from cardiac amyloidosis.[17] Amyloidosis is discussed in detail in Chapter 92.

Symptoms seen in those instances in which the M component can form a cryoprecipitate are discussed under Cryoglobulins, below.

Diagnosis of Myeloma. While the typical myeloma patient presents with bone pain, osteolytic lesions or fractures, and anemia, this illness should be suspected in any older individual with unexplained musculoskeletal pain, severe osteoporosis, severe anemia, unusually high erythrocyte sedimentation rate, rouleaux on peripheral smear, or a syndrome compatible with a systemic vasculitis. Since 99 percent of patients with multiple myeloma produce a monoclonal protein, a serum protein electrophoresis, or preferably an immunoelectrophoresis, is an appropriate and sensitive screening test (Fig. 84–1). Since 20 percent of patients may have only urinary light-chain secretion, a urinary immunoelectrophoresis should also be performed when there is a high index of suspicion for myeloma or amyloidosis. When less than 1 g of protein is excreted in 24 hours, the test should be run on concentrated urine specimens.[3] Routine dipstick determinations for protein will detect most Bence Jones proteins.[18] Since the diagnostic criteria mentioned earlier require tissue or bone marrow plasmacytosis in conjunction with either lytic lesions or evidence for monoclonal protein production, immunoelectrophoresis of serum and urine should be 99 percent sensitive in detecting multiple myeloma.

Therapy of Multiple Myeloma. Therapeutic intervention in multiple myeloma has three goals. (1) The first is to ameliorate as promptly as possible potentially life-threatening rheologic and metabolic abnormalities. Since hypercalcemia can be associated both with dehydration resulting from polyuria and with renal impairment due to nephrocalcinosis and light-chain-induced tubular damage, aggressive attempts should be made to replenish intravascular and urinary volume with normal saline. Intravascular fluid volume status should be monitored in patients with pre-existing renal insufficiency. Loop diuretics may be used to promote additional calciuresis. Prednisone may suppress hypercalcemia by impairing directly the rate of bone resorption.[19] Calcitonin and mithramycin have been used in extreme instances. The hyperviscosity syndrome can usually be diagnosed at the bedside by the clinician alert enough to suspect it. Since blood viscosity increases exponentially with increasing paraprotein concentration in this disorder, a fractional reduction in paraprotein levels by manual one- or two-unit plasmapheresis may lower plasma viscosity multifold and result in prompt and dramatic amelioration of potentially life-threatening hemodynamic impairment, allowing the clinician additional time to substantiate the clinical impression. Plasmapheresis may also mitigate the interaction of the M component with platelets and coagulation factors and thus alleviate the hemorrhagic diathesis seen in some patients. (2) The next goal is to impair or reduce the proliferation of the plasma cell mass, in order to minimize bone pain and fracture, retard the contribution of bone resorption contribution to hypercalcemia, and reverse myelophthisic effects. (3) The last goal is to lower the rate of synthesis of the paraprotein and thus effect both a reduction in tissue light-chain deposition and any propensity toward hyperviscosity, complement activation, or interaction with clotting factors.

Because the tumor cell line in each myeloma patient produces its own characteristic marker in the form of an M protein, nowhere in oncology has there developed a more certain ability to quantify tumor cell mass and the kinetics of tumor cell growth. By measuring the rate of immunoglobulin synthesis in cultured myeloma cells and the turnover rate of injected radiolabeled immunoglobulins in the same patient, total myeloma cell mass can be calculated.[1] A significant correlation has been shown between tumor cell mass and extent of bone destruction, serum calcium level, degree of anemia and quantity of serum or urinary paraprotein component. Current clinical staging of multiple myeloma utilizes hemoglobin, serum calcium and urine or serum M component levels, and extent of skeletal involvement on radiographs to assign patients to one of three stages, each of which correlates with the calculated myeloma cell mass ascertained as described above.

Prior to the use of alkylating agents, median survival from diagnosis was 3.5 to 11.5 months.[20] Since the advent of melphalan and cyclophosphamide therapy, either alone or in combination with other antitumor drugs, median survival has lengthened to 24 to 30 months. Survival is in part dependent on the subtype of M protein produced, with IgG kappa myeloma associated with a better survival than those with lambda Bence Jones myeloma, for example.[21]

Durie has pointed out that response to treatment in myeloma is dependent on the clinical stage, the kinetics of myeloma cell proliferation, and the inherent susceptibility of the cell line to chemotherapeutic agents. In general, patients destined to do poorly are those with high tumor cell mass (large quantity of M component, hypercalcemia, severe anemia, extensive bone lesions),

Figure 84–1. Diagrammatic representation of immunoelectrophoretic patterns in myeloma and heavy chain disease. The troughs contain antisera specific for gamma chains in each instance. *A,* The normal immunoglobulin G precipitin arc. *B,* In IgG myeloma, the arc reveals an area of increased IgG molecules (arrow) with relatively restricted electrophoretic mobility, suggesting a monoclonal IgG increase. *C,* In gamma heavy chain disease, an incomplete gamma chain exists, often having a different electrophoretic mobility than whole IgG molecules. The spur (arrow) shows that the intact normal IgG gamma chain possesses determinants not present on the incomplete abnormal heavy chain.

those with abnormal renal function, and those with other than IgG or IgA M components. Patients with lambda Bence Jones myeloma only appear particularly prone to short remissions after therapy, perhaps because such patients have a high proportion of rapidly dividing cells and tend to have light-chain-induced renal disease, which correlates with poor prognosis.

Treatment with alkylating agents can reduce the tumor load 10- to 100-fold within several months, with the proportion of patients who achieve clinical remission approximately the same in both high and low tumor mass stages. Within several months following treatment, tumor mass, M component level, and other studies indicate a metabolically stable (plateau) stage, which may last for months or years in some patients. With relapse, cell division becomes more rapid and more refractory to therapy.[20] There have been several attempts to develop multiple drug regimens and cyclic therapy, with variable success.[21] Whether maintenance therapy is of value for patients in remission has not been established. Most patients in whom greater than 50 percent reduction in tumor load is achieved will remain in remission for an average of three years prior to relapse, and there have been reports of successful subsequent therapeutic response using drug combinations, although the rapidity and drug resistance of relapse increase with each such occurrence. Local radiation can be used to treat specific tumor masses that may be compromising neurologic or other functions.

THE MONOCLONAL DYSPROTEINEMIAS— WALDENSTRÖM'S MACROGLOBULINEMIA

Originally described by Waldenström in 1944, the monoclonal macroglobulinemic state bearing his name resembles multiple myeloma only in that it is a monoclonal dysproteinemia. It occurs generally in the sixth or seventh decade, slightly more often in males than females; is more insidious in onset; and has a much better prognosis for survival. Waldenström's macroglobulinemia would appear to present clinically less than one-twentieth as frequently as myeloma.[22] The incidence of commonly presenting symptoms is as follows: fatigue, 38 percent; epistaxis, 25 percent; weight loss, 20 percent; neurologic disturbance, 12 percent. A variety of other presenting symptoms are seen much less frequently.[22] Common physical findings are hepatomegaly in 39 to 55 percent, splenomegaly in 35 percent, ocular changes of hyperviscosity in 34 percent, lymphadenopathy in 25 to 45 percent, neurologic abnormalities in 20 percent, and purpura in 10 to 18 percent.[22,23] The circulating paraprotein is directly responsible for the majority of signs and symptoms in this illness.

Thirty-six percent of patients in one series[23] had hyperviscous serum. The serum viscosity in Waldenström's averages five times that of normal serum. Purpura and bleeding abnormalities appear to result from binding of the M component to circulating platelet membranes. Bence Jones proteinuria is seen in only 20 percent, and renal amyloidosis would appear to be much less common. While tubular disease like that seen in multiple myeloma is uncommon, several studies[24,25] have demonstrated subendothelial, nonamyloid IgM-containing glomerular thrombi in approximately half of biopsies studied, although significant proteinuria or renal impairment was uncommon. Approximately 10 percent of reported IgM monoclonal proteins have apparent antibody reactivity, most often rheumatoid factor–like. Thus, IgM rheumatoid factor-IgG (i.e., mixed) cryoglobulins may occur and cause immune complex–mediated abnormalities. Anemia is seen in 75 percent[23] and is usually attributable to chronic disease, but occasionally it results from cold hemagglutinin activity of the paraprotein. While the neurologic symptoms are occasionally attributable to the hyperviscosity syndrome or the bleeding diathesis accompanying this disease, there have been several reports of deposition of the M component between lamellae of the myelin sheaths in peripheral nerve biopsies.[26,27] This is especially interesting in view of the clear demonstration of hypocholesterolemia in half of the reported cases studied,[22] the report of depressed levels of low-density serum lipoproteins in one patient,[28] and an additional report of a very high chronic false-positive VDRL titer in the 19S proteins of a patient with this disorder.[29] These data suggest an affinity of some IgM paraproteins for lipoprotein.

Skeletal roentgenograms generally show only mild osteoporosis consistent with a patient's age, although rarely lytic lesions like those in multiple myeloma have been reported. Only 5 percent of patients reviewed by McCallister and colleagues had normal bone marrow examinations.[22] The usual marrow histopathology includes a mixture of cell types, including a modest elevation of mature plasma cells, moderate to marked (10 to 80 percent) presence of small lymphocytes, and a similar preponderance of plasmacytoid lymphocytes. On electron microscopy, the number of cells containing an endoplasmic reticulum is greater than could be accounted for by the plasma cells present, suggesting that some of the lymphocytoid forms present may be differentiating. An additional feature distinguishing this disease from multiple myeloma is the presence in marrow of increased numbers of tissue mast cells. Over one-third of patients have cryoglobulinemia, sometimes massive.[22]

Lymph node and hepatic biopsy reveal a spectrum of pathology from nearly normal or nonspecific inflammatory changes through the mixed populations described in the marrow above to a histologic picture highly suggestive of malignant lymphoma. In general, the bone marrow histopathology is abnormal more often than that of other organs. In spite of hepatomegaly, liver function tests are often normal. In one series[23] over half of the patients with an IgM paraprotein had an associated malignancy, usually a lymphoma, although a number of patients have had carcinoma of the lung, internal genitalia, bowel, kidney, or skin, in association with an IgM spike. Unlike myeloma, there tends to be little depression of the other immunoglobulin components of serum in Waldenström's macroglobulinemia.

In the review by McCallister and colleagues at least 4 percent of patients either remained asymptomatic or lived with symptoms for as long as 18 years without specific treatment. Of those with progressive disease, the average survival was 5.3 years from the onset of symptoms.

Cases with lytic bone lesions and predominantly plasmacytoid infiltrates in bone marrow might be classified by some as multiple myeloma. Factors associated with a poorer prognosis are a high concentration of IgM paraprotein, a low serum albumin, and the development of anemia. Waldenström's macroglobulinemia can be diagnosed simply with immunoelectrophoresis, as is the case in myeloma. However, if the M component is a cryoglobulin that precipitates in quantity from serum, the monoclonal component may be missed if immunoelectrophoresis is performed when the blood or serum has been stored at 4°C or lower.

Therapy of Waldenström's Macroglobulinemia. Therapy is twofold in this disorder. Plasmapheresis is the preferred initial therapy in patients with acute hyperviscosity syndrome to prevent cerebral vascular occlusion or intracranial bleeding and to relieve congestive heart failure. In view of the potentially prolonged survival in asymptomatic patients, more definitive therapy is probably indicated only in patients requiring repetitive plasmapheresis for hyperviscosity or in those who develop compromise of specific organ function as a result of infiltration by presumably malignant cells, by the deposition of the abnormal paraprotein, or in the rare instance of amyloidosis. Of the 40 patients reported by Mackenzie and Fudenberg,[23] 19, including 10 who had hyperviscosity, received treatment with alkylating agents. Forty percent of those treated experienced a decrease in serum paraprotein concentration and serum viscosity and had an average duration of survival from diagnosis of 49 months, whereas the patients who did not respond to alkylating agents lived an average of only 24.1 months. They also noted a spontaneous decrease in serum IgM levels in 4 patients unattributable to therapy and not associated with other evidence for clinical remission.

THE MONOCLONAL DYSPROTEINEMIAS—HEAVY–CHAIN DISEASES

Franklin and his associates[30] described for the first time a monoclonal dysproteinemia in a 44-year-old male with massive lymphadenopathy and a lymph node biopsy revealing a predominant reticulum cell infiltrate. Massive splenomegaly developed, and bone marrow aspirations, which had initially been normal, ultimately revealed many atypical plasmacytes. This disease was thought to represent yet another malignant condition associated with monoclonal protein production. Since then, it has become clear that the heavy-chain diseases

often occur secondary to a variety of chronic inflammatory disease states, and in some settings may represent a response to chronic infectious conditions.

Since 1964, over 50 patients have been described with gamma heavy-chain disease. The heavy-chain disease most frequently reported and studied is alpha chain disease, with more than 150 cases presently known. In contrast to these, only about 15 cases of mu chain disease have appeared since its first description in 1970.[31] The heavy-chain diseases are characterized by a much younger age of onset than is found in the previously discussed monoclonal conditions.

Because abnormal proteins may occur in a variety of conditions, the diagnosis of heavy-chain diseases requires their demonstration in serum or other body fluid using immunochemical techniques (Fig. 84–1). Standard serum electrophoresis is not sufficient to make the diagnosis, since in more than half the cases of alpha chain disease, a number of instances of gamma chain disease, and the majority of mu chain diseases, patients studied have shown no abnormalities on standard serum electrophoresis. In addition, when demonstrable, the abnormal protein often shows a broad band of distribution rather than the narrow peak suggesting monoclonality. This is especially so with those molecules prone to polymeric heterogeneity such as in alpha chain or mu chain disease. The sine qua non is the demonstration in serum of an abnormal component containing determinants reactive with antibody to gamma, alpha, or mu heavy chains but nonreactive with antisera to kappa or lambda light chains. Because most polyvalent antisera to human immunoglobulins react primarily with the light-chain-defined determinants, the use of antisera monospecific for a given heavy-chain class is essential in the demonstration. It may be difficult to confirm that the abnormal protein lacks reactivity with the light-chain antisera when the total concentration of abnormal protein is quite low. In addition, some whole myeloma proteins do not precipitate with antisera to light chains and might be misdiagnosed as heavy-chain disease. Of those patients with gamma or alpha chain disease who have been studied, the abnormal protein has belonged to a single subclass, suggesting a monoclonal origin. Proteins in each of the four IgG subclasses have been described, especially in the class IgG$_3$. Rarely, a serum monoclonal immunoglobulin belonging to a different class from that of the heavy-chain disease protein is observed concomitantly.

The abnormal protein chain does not simply represent an incompletely transcribed immunoglobulin molecule. Studies of such proteins indicate that they consist primarily of the Fc region of the appropriate heavy chain containing a normal carboxy-terminal end with internal deletions of portions of the chain toward the amino-terminal end. Of peculiar interest is the demonstration that the deletion often begins at the same point at the hinge region in the alpha, gamma, and mu heavy-chain proteins sequenced. Normal sequences occur at the beginning of constant domains toward the amino-terminal end. It is likely that this unique structure reflects abnormal assembly of heavy-chain domains as well as the occurrence of limited proteolysis after synthesis. While the lack of light-chain synthesis was originally puzzling, it is now known that well over half of patients with mu chain disease produce monoclonal light chains that are excreted as Bence Jones proteins, and that light-chain synthesis is found in a small number of cases of gamma or alpha heavy-chain disease. These data suggest that light-chain synthesis can occur in heavy-chain diseases and that a regulatory disorder in immunoglobulin synthesis is a more likely cause of the abnormal proteins than a structural genetic deletion.

Gamma Heavy-Chain Disease. The main clinical and laboratory abnormalities in gamma heavy-chain disease are similar to those in Waldenström's, including lymphadenopathy, splenomegaly, and hepatomegaly in the majority. Swelling of the uvula and tonsillar area has been an interesting unique feature in approximately one-quarter of such patients. Forty percent of cases have an underlying hematologic malignancy, which is histologically similar to Waldenström's, with a pleomorphic lymphoplasmacytoid proliferation. In 15 percent of patients, the cell type is predominantly plasmacytic. Osteolytic lesions such as are seen in multiple myeloma are rare. At least 30 percent of patients either show no histologic evidence of a malignant condition in the enlarged lymphoid organs and marrow or show no evidence of a malignant disorder whatsoever. Eighteen of 50 cases reported by Seligmann[31] had other nonmalignant diseases caused by autoimmunity, including rheumatoid arthritis, systemic lupus erythematosus, Hashimoto's disease, Sjögren's syndrome, autoimmune hemolytic anemia, vascular purpura, and myasthenia gravis.

Mu Heavy-Chain Disease. The small number of patients with mu chain disease have all presented a picture of lymphoproliferative neoplasia. Nine of 15 patients discussed by Seligmann[31] had chronic lymphocytic leukemia, although these patients tended to have more hepatosplenomegaly and less peripheral lymphadenopathy than typical chronic lymphocytic leukemia patients. In two thirds of the cases, a characteristic vacuolization of marrow plasma cells has been described. The presence of such cells or Bence Jones proteinuria in a leukemia patient should prompt a search for mu chain disease.

Alpha Chain Disease. Alpha chain disease is by far the most common heavy-chain disorder encountered. The evidence clearly suggests involvement of the IgA secretory system. The majority of cases present with a markedly uniform syndrome consisting of severe malabsorption, abdominal pain, often protein-losing enteropathy, severe weight loss, steatorrhea, and tetany. While hepatosplenomegaly and peripheral lymphadenopathy are rare, roentgenographic and gallium scintiscan studies usually demonstrate a distended abdomen with enlarged mesenteric lymph nodes, which are sometimes palpable. Bone marrow examination is usually normal, and the intestinal lesions in alpha chain disease usually predominate in the duodenum and jejunum, unlike the involvement in most digestive tract lymphomas. Seligmann, who has had the most extensive experience

with alpha chain disease, has divided it into two stages: (1) an early premalignant stage, as just described, and (2) a subsequent neoplastic stage. Since most patients have been between 10 and 30 years of age and have lived in areas with a high degree of parasitic infestation and in areas of poor hygiene and low socioeconomic achievement, it has been postulated that alpha chain disease in its first stages represents a response to some infestation. This is additionally supported by the improvement in symptoms and diminution in circulating alpha chain levels achieved in some patients with antibiotic therapy. Late in the course, the immunoblastic cell involved can be shown to possess surface alpha chains devoid of light chains, suggesting that the ultimate malignancy arises from the same B-lymphocyte lines stimulated during the early stage. The paucity of cases has not permitted a systematic approach to therapy. Unlike the previous conditions, the abnormal protein rarely is a source of pathophysiology in heavy-chain diseases. Individual cases reported in the literature have responded to a variety of agents, including nitrogen mustards, antimetabolites, and local radiation therapy. Since the mere presence of the abnormal heavy chain does not necessarily represent a malignant state, and may be an accompaniment of rheumatoid arthritis or another benign condition, and since death in these diseases is often due to infection, the decision to institute cytolytic therapy should be made with great discrimination.

THE MONOCLONAL DYSPROTEINEMIAS—IDIOPATHIC MONOCLONAL GAMMOPATHY

In a number of the conditions discussed above, the existence of a monoclonal protein is discovered inadvertently in the course of other studies. Kyle has termed these conditions monoclonal gammopathy of undetermined significance (MGUS).[32] Monoclonal gammopathies in the absence of demonstrable other disease have been described in approximately 3 percent of patients over the age of 70.[32] In a large Swedish study[33] 1 percent of patients over the age of 25 had such proteins. In a study of patients presenting with monoclonal gammopathy to the Mayo Clinic before 1971 and followed for 5 years, 9 percent had had a 50 percent or more increase in the monoclonal protein concentration or had had it appear in the urine, and 11 percent had developed either myeloma, macroglobulinemia, or amyloidosis. Nearly one-quarter of this generally elderly population had died in the 5-year interval. The progression to increasing monoclonal protein concentration or overt malignancy could not be predicted from the initial level of monoclonal material, nor was there early evidence on physical examination or routine blood count that discerned those patients destined to progress. At the end of 10 years, only 38 percent had had no progression, while 27 percent had either developed increasing dysproteinemia, dysproteinuria, or overt malignancy. Using actuarial analysis, the risk of developing an overt lympho- or mye-loproliferative malignancy at 15 years was 34 percent in this population. Factors identifying those patients who are progressing to overt malignancy are essentially those listed earlier for staging myeloma, including level of serum or urinary monoclonal protein, number of plasma cells in bone marrow, osteolytic lesions, anemia, and renal involvement.

CRYOGLOBULINEMIAS

The property of certain plasma proteins to precipitate reversibly upon exposure to cold was originally reported in 1933 by Wintrobe and Buell.[34] When the house officer performed a routine hematocrit on their patient, a woman with Raynaud's phenomenon and epistaxis, he noticed a cloudy white precipitate layered just above the packed red cells and occupying 10 percent of the blood volume. When a repeat hematocrit was performed on blood stored overnight in the refrigerator, the precipitate was found to be suspended throughout the entire supernatant plasma. Of even more interest was the fact that the precipitate disappeared 10 to 15 minutes after rewarming the mixture and could be repeatedly reprecipitated and redissolved upon alternate chilling and warming. In 1947, Lerner and Watson[35] introduced the term "cryoglobulin" to describe such cryoprecipitable proteins. This section includes an attempt to define the term "cryoglobulin," a description of the methods for its detection and quantitation, a classification of the different types of cryoglobulins into a logical system, delineation of the syndromes that they can cause, and a discussion of the treatment of these syndromes.

Definition and Detection. The initial observations of Wintrobe and Buell were made on anticoagulated blood and thus involved precipitation of proteins from plasma. Fibrinogen, a major constituent of plasma not present in serum, may form a cryoprecipitate in a variety of disease states.[36] In addition, the commonly used anticoagulant heparin may form a cold-insoluble complex with factors present in normal plasma.[37] To avoid these potential artifacts, cryoglobulin determination should always be carried out on serum. Ideally, blood should be collected free of anticoagulant in a warmed syringe and maintained at 37° C during clotting, with the serum separated by centrifugation at 37° C before cooling the specimen to permit cryoprecipitate formation. In practice it is usually sufficient to collect the specimen at room temperature and transfer it to a tube, which is then hand-carried to a 37° C waterbath to allow completion of clotting and clot retraction. Centrifugation can be carried out at room temperature, preferably in centrifuge cups prewarmed to 37° C and filled with water from the 37° C bath. The separated serum is then transferred to a conical centrifuge tube, which is then stoppered and placed in a refrigerator ($\pm$ 4° C) and inspected daily over 7 days for the presence of a precipitate. Since many normal sera will form irreversible precipitates on storage for this length of time, it is essential that the specimen be rewarmed to 37° C to establish the resolubility of the precipitate. If sufficient serum is collected initially to allow refrigeration of two tubes of serum, one can be rewarmed while the second is centrifuged at 4° C to allow quantitative and qualitative analysis of the cryoprecipitate. Since in virtually all instances the precipitate will contain only globulin components of serum, the precipitate may appropriately be referred to as a cryoglobulin. Any serum collected in the aforementioned fashion which, when chilled, forms a precipitate that is easily dissolved on rewarming can be said to contain a cryoglobulin.

Analysis of Cryoglobulins. Of the several methods for quantitating the content of a cryoglobulin, the two most commonly used determine either the packed volume of precipitate (cryocrit) expressed as a percentage or the micrograms of total protein using a colorimetric or spectrophotometric method.

In the latter method, the precipitate that is formed at the end of 7 days is centrifuged at 3000 RPM at 4° C, the supernatant serum gently removed, and the residual precipitate suspended in cold physiologic saline. This suspension is washed four times at 0 to 4° C in saline to remove nonspecifically trapped proteins and dissolved by rewarming in a measured volume of saline. Some investigators actually dissolve and reprecipitate the cryoglobulin in the first few washes by warming and rechilling.[38] Because semipurified cryoprecipitates solubilized in this way occasionally reprecipitate poorly or not at all, the author prefers to keep the precipitate cold until washing has been completed. The protein concentration of the ultimately dissolved cryoprecipitate solution can then be estimated spectrophotometrically by measuring its optical density at 280 mμ or colorimetrically using a standard assay such as the Lowry method. This method has the appeal of apparent immunochemical precision, giving results in micrograms of cryoprecipitate per milliliter of serum. However, repeated washing undoubtedly results in some loss of precipitate with each resuspension, and in the case of small cryoprecipitates this loss can be a substantial fraction of the whole. In addition, the optical density units obtained with colorimetry or spectrophotometry are expressed in terms of micrograms of a standard protein, usually IgG, analyzed by the same technique. As discussed below, the different protein constituents of the precipitate can vary considerably from case to case. Relating the optical absorbency of any given mixture of cryoprecipitated proteins to a single standard protein can introduce error, depending on the degree to which the protein used as a standard is represented in the cryoglobulin under examination.

The cryocrit method is used in the author's laboratory. In this method, a measured volume, usually 5.0 ml of serum, is pipetted into one of two identical 7-ml conical glass tubes. The second tube remains empty and is taped to the first. After 7 days at 4° C, the serum-containing tube is centrifuged at 4° C. Using a calibrated micropipette, 10 μl volumes of saline are carefully pipetted repetitively into the tip of the empty companion tube until the volume in that tube appears visually to be equivalent to that of the cryoprecipitate in the tip of the serum-containing tube. Division of the estimated volume of cryoprecipitate by the total volume of serum added yields the cryocrit, usually expressed as a percentage. For example, if 5 ml (5000 μl) of serum is added initially and the ultimate precipitate is estimated to be matched by 50 μl of saline (five 10 μl pipettings), the cryocrit is calculated as follows:

$$\frac{50}{5000} \times 100 = 1\% \text{ cryocrit}$$

Use of this method requires the undoubtedly erroneous assumption that all centrifuged proteins compact into a volume proportional to their mass. However, its one advantage over other methods is that loss of precipitate with washing is avoided. In addition, once measurement of the cryocrit has been determined, the tube can immediately be rewarmed to ascertain reversibility of precipitation, thus obviating the need for distributing the serum initially into two tubes. Gough and colleagues[39] have demonstrated that this method is extremely reproducible. While it does not yield results in customary immunochemical units, it gives similar results in patients having the same type of cryoglobulin (see below) and is extremely useful in comparing cryoglobulin levels in specimens obtained from a single patient over time. Results of cryocrit determinations in various illnesses determined by Gough are shown in Figure 84–2.

The constituent proteins in a cryoglobulin can be determined *qualitatively* by subjecting the washed, redissolved cryoglobulin to double immunodiffusion against specific antisera, including antisera to specific immunoglobulin classes, antisera to complement components, and type-specific antisera to kappa and lambda light chains. Radial immunodiffusion techniques cannot always be used reliably to *quantitate* these individual constituents, since the rationale behind these techniques assumes that the constituent being measured has a given molecular size and hence a given diffusion rate. When a protein molecule exists in complex with other proteins, as is so in some cryoglobulins, its diffusion rate may be much less than that of the uncomplexed molecule and lead to an underestimation of its concentration. However, the qualitative analysis of the individual components with a cryoprecipitate has permitted a coherent classification of cryoglobulins, as described below.

Classification of Cryoglobulins. All cryoglobulins described to date have had an immunoglobulin as their major component. The classification of cryoglobulins is outlined in Table 84–1. These cryoproteins may be classified broadly as "mixed" or "unmixed," on the basis of the immunoglobulin components they contain.

Unmixed Cryoglobulins. An unmixed cryoglobulin is one that contains only one class of immunoglobulin (e.g., IgM only, IgG only). Save for an important exception discussed below, in virtually all unmixed cryoglobulins the precipitating immunoglobulin has characteristics of a monoclonal protein, such as restricted electrophoretic mobility, single light-chain type, and, in the case of IgG, single IgG subclass.

As might be expected, these unmixed cryoglobulins are generally found in those diseases associated with monoclonal immunoglobulin production, such as myeloma, malignant lymphoma, and Waldenström's macroglobulinemia. In a recent review by Brouet and associates,[38] of 86 patients with cryoglobulins, 25 percent had unmixed monoclonal cryoglobulins, of which the majority were IgM or IgG. Approximately 6 percent of myeloma proteins studied by Brouet and associates[38] formed cryoprecipitates. Ten percent of monoclonal IgM proteins cryoprecipitated, although only slightly less than half formed unmixed cryoglobulins, the rest forming mixed cryoglobulins, as discussed below.

It is in this group with unmixed monoclonal cryoglobulins that the highest concentrations of cryoprecipitable protein are found. In Brouet's series[38] 60 percent of patients in this category had greater than 5 mg of cryoprotein per milliliter of serum. In our own experience, cryocrits greater than 3 percent are rarely found in diseases other than those associated with monoclonal protein production (Fig. 84–2 and Table 84–1). Generally the cryoprecipitates in this group form rapidly upon cooling of the serum, in some instances before the freshly drawn blood can be transferred to a waterbath. This may in part be a function of the sometimes extreme concentrations of these abnormal proteins in such sera, as discussed below.

Less than half of patients with monoclonal cryoglobulins will have symptoms resulting from the cryoprotein.[38,40] When symptoms do occur, they are a result of impairment of blood flow secondary to blood hyperviscosity or to the vasculitis that can occur with deposition of circulating immunoglobulin aggregates. The pathogenesis of specific symptomatology is discussed below.

Mixed Cryoglobulins. Mixed cryoglobulins constitute the second large category of serum cryoproteins. In this group, the cryoprecipitates contain more than one class of immunoglobulin. In virtually all instances, at least one of the immunoglobulin constituents has rheumatoid factor (RF) activity (see Chapter 44), while the other is IgG, the antigen with which rheumatoid factors react.

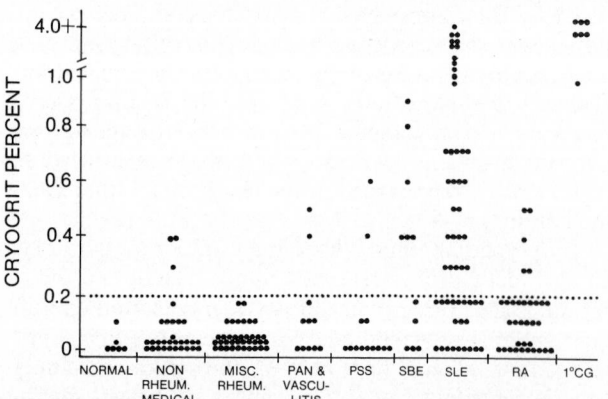

Figure 84–2. Cryocrit values in various disorders, as determined by Gough.[39] Upper limits of normal = 0.2 percent.

Table 84–1. Classification of Cryoglobulins

UNMIXED (Monoclonal)	MIXED (RF-IgG complex)	
1. Associated with myeloma 2. Associated with lymphoma 3. Associated with Waldenström's macroglobulinemia 4. Essential	**With polyclonal rheumatoid factors (IgM, IgG, and/or IgA)** 1. Associated with chronic inflammatory, infectious, or autoimmune disease 2. Essential	**With monoclonal rheumatoid factors (IgM, IgG, or IgA)** 1. Associated with lympho-/myeloproliferative state 2. Essential

This category may be subdivided further into two large subsets, those in which rheumatoid factor component is a monoclonal protein and those in which the rheumatoid factors are polyclonal.

Mixed Cryoglobulins with Monoclonal Rheumatoid Factor Component. Mixed cryoglobulins in which the rheumatoid factor was monoclonal constituted 26 percent of those in Brouet's series.[38] The rheumatoid factor component was IgM in the vast majority of these. IgG rheumatoid factors are found in less than 10 percent, and IgA rheumatoid factors are involved rarely.[38] In approximately two-thirds of cases, the cryoprotein is found in association with myeloma, Waldenström's macroglobulinemia, or malignant lymphoma,[38,40] and the monoclonal rheumatoid factor undoubtedly is the product of a single neoplastic cell line. The high incidence of anti-IgG reactivity in Waldenström's macroglobulinemia has suggested that autoantibody-producing cell clones are more prone to undergo malignant transformation.[38] An important minority of patients in this category will have a monoclonal rheumatoid factor, usually IgM, with no evidence for an underlying neoplastic disease. These patients are analogous to the patients with essential monoclonal hypergammaglobulinemia, many of whom ultimately develop clinical myeloma if followed over a several-year period. Brouet and colleagues have indicated that symptoms referable to cryoglobulins may antedate diagnosis of the underlying neoplastic process by as long as a decade.[38]

These cryoglobulins are usually present in high concentration (1 to 30 mg per milliliter),[38] and the cryoprecipitate forms rapidly in the cold. Generally, the cryocrit is somewhat less than in the case of unmixed cryoglobulins. The monoclonal component may not be detectable as a spike on routine protein electrophoresis. In addition, rheumatoid factor reactivity may not be detectable when tested in whole serum. It is likely that in some instances this results from precipitation of the cryoglobulin within the clot during routine processing of the blood specimen.

These cryoglobulins are somewhat more likely to cause symptoms suggestive of vasculitis than are the unmixed, and less likely to be associated with manifestations of hyperviscosity such as epistaxis, distal gangrene, and arterial thrombosis.[38]

Mixed Cryoglobulins with Polyclonal Rheumatoid Factor Component. The subset of mixed cryoglobulins in which the rheumatoid factor moiety is polyclonal constitutes the most common class of cryoglobulins seen by the clinician, comprising 50 percent of those reported in Brouet's series.[38] The cryoglobulin from a single patient may contain rheumatoid factors of several immunoglobulin classes, although IgM rheumatoid factors predominate.[38] Tests of whole serum for rheumatoid factor are generally positive. These cryoproteins precipitate from serum only slowly over several days of refrigeration and are usually present in such low concentrations ($<$ 1 mg per milliliter; cryocrit $<$ 1.5 percent) that they are often difficult to characterize qualitatively (Fig. 84–2). However, after isolation they precipitate rapidly even at room temperature. Their propensity to cryoinsolubility is diminished by addition of small amounts of albumin,[40] suggesting that normal serum constituents may stabilize these proteins against their cryoprecipitation in vivo.

Patients with this form of mixed cryoglobulinemia are almost always symptomatic,[38,40] usually with a syndrome resembling systemic vasculitis, as discussed below. Over three-fourths of patients with essential cryoglobulinemia will have this type of cryoprotein. However, the majority of patients with this type will have it secondary to another illness. A list of the disorders associated with cryoglobulinemia is found in Table 84–2. The list of diseases associated with mixed cryoglobulinemia is extensive and includes most of the connective tissue diseases, a number of chronic infectious diseases, and other chronic inflammatory states such as sarcoidosis and chronic liver disease. These diseases are those usually associated with rheumatoid factor formation (see Chapter 44) and all are characterized by prolonged stimulation of the immune system. It thus appears that in those diseases generally characterized by rheumatoid factor positivity, a subset of rheumatoid factors present tends to form cold-insoluble complexes with the IgG antigen. Of the illnesses in Table 84–2 associated with mixed cryoglobulin, those most extensively studied are systemic lupus erythematosus, subacute bacterial endocarditis, and essential mixed cryoglobulinemia.

Systemic Lupus Erythematosus. In SLE, both DNA and anti-DNA occur in the circulation, and deposits of immunoglobulin, complement, and DNA have been found in the renal glomerular basement membrane.[41,42] In some cases, when the glomerular antibody has been eluted, a major portion has had antinuclear antibody reactivity.[42] Mixed cryoglobulins have also been found

Table 84–2. Conditions That May Be Associated with Secondary Mixed Cryoglobulinemia

A. Connective tissue diseases
  1. Systemic lupus erythematosus
  2. Rheumatoid arthritis
  3. Polyarteritis nodosa
  4. Ankylosing spondylitis
  5. Sjögren's syndrome
B. Diseases related to an infectious agent
  1. Subacute bacterial endocarditis
  2. Post-streptococcal nephritis
  3. Cytomegalovirus mononucleosis
  4. Syphilis
  5. Toxoplasmosis
  6. Infectious mononucleosis
  7. Echinococcosis
  8. Tropical splenomegaly
  9. Leprosy
  10. Kala-azar
  11. Lymphogranuloma venereum
  12. Visceral abscesses
  13. Lyme disease
  14. Chronic hepatitis B infection
C. Other chronic diseases
  1. Sarcoidosis
  2. Intestinal bypass arthritis
  3. Ulcerative colitis
  4. Celiac disease
  5. Chronic liver disease
  6. Cutaneous plasmacytosis

in the sera from 30 to 45 percent of patients with SLE.[43,44] The IgM rheumatoid factor in such cryoproteins reacts with human IgG from a variety of sources to form a cryoprecipitate that consumes complement. In SLE, the Clq component of complement must be present for cryoprecipitation to occur.[44] Other components of complement such as C3 or C4 may be found in the cryoprecipitate as well.[43] There is a direct correlation between the presence of these cryoglobulins and hypocomplementemia in SLE, although some patients may have hypocomplementemia without cryoglobulins and vice versa. Stastny and Ziff[43] found diminished serum complement in 91 percent of patients with cryoglobulins and in 21 percent lacking cryoglobulins. They noted an increased incidence of nephritis in patients with cryoglobulins. However, in McPhaul's series,[45] the incidence of cryoglobulinemia was no different in SLE patients with and without renal disease.

An attractive hypothesis has been that chronic or repetitive exposure of the immune system to altered IgG in antigen-antibody complexes leads to the formation of the anti-immunoglobulin rheumatoid factors, which presumably react with those immune complexes. If this were so, one would expect to find the antigenic moiety of the responsible immune complex in the cryoprecipitate along with its IgG antibody and rheumatoid factor. Winfield and his associates[46] demonstrated that cryoprecipitates from sera from some patients with SLE contain anti-DNA at levels enriched up to 100-fold over those in serum. They also found DNA in these cryoprecipitates using a nonspecific colorimetric assay, although DNA was not demonstrable immunologically.

However, the significance of these findings has been clouded by the demonstration that DNA can be released into normal serum during clotting[47] and that cryoglobulins from essential mixed cryoglobulinemia, a disease in which DNA–anti-DNA complexes have not been thought to play a role, also contain DNA.[48] In SLE blood, where a variety of autoantibodies reacting with cellular constituents are found (see Chapter 68), there may be an even greater tendency toward the release of cellular constituents like DNA during clotting. Many of these sera also contain anti-DNA, and any DNA–anti-DNA complexes formed artifactually during clotting could be expected to react with rheumatoid factors present and cocryoprecipitate with them.

Subacute Bacterial Endocarditis. SBE is another illness characterized by hyperimmunization, in this case with a known infectious agent. Rheumatoid factor formation occurs in up to 70 percent,[49] and occasionally mixed cryoglobulins may be found. In a study by Gough and colleagues,[39] SBE patients with hypocomplementemia had average cryocrit levels of 0.57 percent (nl < 0.2 percent), while those with normal complements averaged 0.09 percent cryocrit (p < 0.001). The quantity of cryoglobulin correlated significantly with the severity of complement depression (r = 0.90, p < 0.001). The patients with cryoglobulinemia had a greater incidence of renal disease as well. All the aforementioned abnormalities disappear with treatment of the SBE. Efforts to demonstrate bacterial antigen within these cryoproteins have been unsuccessful.

Essential Mixed Cryoglobulinemia. Essential mixed cryoglobulinemia was first delineated in detail by Meltzer and his associates,[50] who described a group of patients with vascular purpura, arthritis, weakness, and occasionally nephritis, with mixed IgM-IgG cryoglobulins apparently unassociated with any known disease process. These patients comprised a quarter of the entire group of patients with cryoglobulinemia in Brouet's series, and 75 percent of those with mixed cryoglobulins.[38] The group that originally delineated this syndrome has subsequently reported that 87 percent of such patients have clinical or laboratory evidence of liver involvement.[51] They subsequently found that 74 percent of sera examined from such patients showed evidence of either HB_s antigen or its antibody.[52] Three of 25 sera contained HB_s antigen, and 12 had antibody. When 11 cryoprecipitates were examined, 6 had HB_s antigen and 11 had antibody. Thus, in a majority of patients with essential mixed cryoglobulinemia, the cryoprecipitate may be the result of persistent hepatitis B virus infection.

Other Diseases Associated with Mixed Cryoglobulinemia. The bulk of the remaining syndromes associated with mixed cryoglobulinemia are analogous to SBE and chronic HB antigen infection in being characterized by prolonged exposure to an infectious antigen. McIntosh and co-workers have investigated the relationship of cryoglobulinemia to the clinical course of acute poststreptococcal glomerulonephritis.[53] They found no cryoglobulin in control patients with no renal disease or with lipoid nephrosis, whereas 78 percent of patients with acute glomerulonephritis had mixed cryoglobulins. Within 3 months of initial evaluation, two-thirds of these patients had no cryoglobulin and were clinically well. The remaining one-third has persistent cryoglobulinemia, decreased renal function, and persisting urinary abnormalities. Streptococcal antigen could not be found in the cryoprecipitate.

In a group of patients with echinococcosis studied by Bombardieri and his associates,[54] 83 percent of patients with cysts containing live protoscolices had cryoglobulins, while none of the patients with calcified cysts did. Steere and his associates[55] have reported cryoglobulins in 18 of 30 patients with Lyme disease, an epidemic disease resulting from a spirochete. In this disease, a unique skin rash, erythema chronicum migrans, often precedes the development of synovitis, following which both skin and joint symptoms defervesce. Eighty percent of patients with active skin or joint disease had cryoglobulins, whereas none were found in patients whose disease had become inactive.

"Unmixed" Mixed Cryoglobulins. A unique form of mixed cryoglobulinemia occurs when an IgG rheumatoid factor reacts with its antigen, the IgG molecule. While these may contain one class of immunoglobulin, they are in fact mixed cryoglobulins in the sense that the IgG rheumatoid factor can react with IgG from a variety of sources.[56,57] Data from several investigators[56,57] have indicated a tendency of IgG rheumatoid factors to react with themselves in a "head-to-tail" fashion. When cryo-IgG rheumatoid factor was digested to $F(ab')_2$ fragments to preclude this self-association, the rheumatoid factor could still form complexes with intact nonrheumatoid factor IgG, but no cryoprecipitation occurred.[56] This self-associating propensity of IgG rheumatoid factors has been reported to cause the hyperviscosity syndrome.[58]

PATHOGENETIC MECHANISMS AND SYMPTOMATOLOGY IN CRYOGLOBULIN–INDUCED DISEASE

As mentioned earlier, many patients with cryoglobulinemia may be asymptomatic. In those with symptoms, the resulting manifestations can be roughly divided into those secondary to the rheologic effects of the cryoproteins and those resulting from activation of inflammatory mediators by the cryoglobulin. An understanding of the factors predisposing to cryoprecipitation of proteins will assist in understanding the pathophysiology of the resulting clinical syndromes. These factors have been reviewed thoroughly by Grey and Kohler.[59]

Factors Affecting Cryoprecipitability. Cryoprecipitation appears to be dependent upon noncovalent interactions between protein molecules, as extremes of pH, high ionic strength, and the presence of dissociating molecules such as urea all inhibit cryoprecipitation.[40] The single most important factor in precipitation of cryoglobulins in general is protein concentration.[40] When purified cryoglobulin is present in high concentration, cryoprecipitation occurs more readily and at higher temperatures than when the same cryoglobulin is present in dilute concentrations. Cryoprecipitability does not seem to result from a unique amino acid composition.[59] Several lines of evidence suggest, however, that certain molecular species are subject to cryoprecipitation more readily than others. Grey and Kohler[59] pointed out that 52 of 54 monoclonal IgM cryoglobulins reported in the literature contained kappa light chain types, an incidence out of proportion to the expected. This predisposition does not apparently hold for IgG cryoglobulins.[59] However, molecules of the heavy-chain subclass IgG_3 seem to be over-represented in the IgG cryos. Thirty-eight percent of IgG cryoglobulins reviewed by Grey and Kohler were IgG_3, whereas this subclass occurred in only 7 percent of noncryoprecipitating IgG monoclonal proteins. The fact that cryoprecipitation is not confined exclusively to one light- or heavy-chain subclass, however, suggests that properties of the variable (i.e., non-subclass-specific) region play an important role. The work of Saha and his associates[60] showed that the $F(ab')_2$ (i.e., variable) fragment of a nonrheumatoid factor IgG cryoglobulin could self-associate to precipitate in the cold. Reduction and alkylation have usually abolished cryoprecipitability of monoclonal IgM cryoproteins, with variable results on IgG and IgA cryoproteins.

Other factors seem to play a role in the mixed cryoglobulins, where the Fc portion of IgG always represents the antigen toward which the involved rheumatoid factors are directed. There are no clear indications that these rheumatoid factors react preferentially with a certain IgG subclass. However, several investigators have reported the presence in a mixed cryoglobulin of IgG molecules deficient in the negatively charged sialic acid moiety present in normal IgG.[38,61] In one instance, reaction of the IgM component with normal IgG was greatly enhanced following digestion of the normal IgG with neuraminidase.

Dissociation of the IgM component into 7S monomers by sulfhydryl reagents has destroyed its ability to cryoprecipitate with IgG.[40,59] This ability was fully restored if the disulfide bonds were allowed to reform.[40] However, if reassociation occurred in the presence of 7S IgM monomers from a noncryoprotein IgM molecule, cryoprecipitability of the reformed 19S hybrid pentamer was impaired.

In general the rheumatoid factors in mixed cryoglobulins show a more restricted reactivity than do noncryoglobulin rheumatoid factors. Usually both cryoprecipitating and noncryoprecipitating IgM rheumatoid factors react preferentially with human IgG. However, some noncryoprecipitating rheumatoid factors react preferentially with rabbit gamma globulin, a property not found in IgM rheumatoid factors from mixed cryoglobulins. IgG rheumatoid factors in mixed cryoglobulins appear to react *only* with primate IgGs. As mentioned earlier, the presence of certain complement components may be necessary to effect cryoprecipitation in some instances.

In summary, the reason for the cold-insolubility of most cryoglobulins cannot be specifically discerned and is probably the result of a combination of the factors outlined above.

Pathogenesis of Symptomatology in Cryoglobulin-Induced Disease. As mentioned above, the proteins forming monoclonal cryoglobulins appear to self-associate via largely nonimmunologic interactions. Perhaps as a result, they appear to be relatively poor activators of the complement system. This may explain why they do not cause symptoms generally until present in quite high concentrations. The symptoms, therefore, are frequently a result of alterations in blood viscosity induced by the cryoglobulin protein. In 1972 Pruzanski and Watt[62] reviewed 32 patients with IgG myeloma and hyperviscosity. These proteins tended to form high molecular weight polymers. In 6 of the 32, a cryoprecipitate or cryogel was found. Patients with monoclonal IgM cryoglobulins are even more likely to have symptoms related to hyperviscosity, since the higher intrinsic viscosity of IgM compared with IgG is greatly amplified by cryoprecipitation. Symptoms suggestive of hyperviscosity seen in the monoclonal cryoglobulinemias include severe Raynaud's phenomenon, fingertip necrosis, distal gangrene or ulceration, congestive heart failure, arterial thromboses, and hemorrhagic phenomena. Renal biopsies in such patients may show massive intracapillary deposits of the paraprotein.[38]

While these proteins are not generally very efficient activators of inflammatory mediators, they may occasionally promote the activation of the complement sequence, depending upon their absolute quantity and thermal properties. When hypocomplementemia is found in such a serum, it is important to ascertain the degree of decomplementation that has occurred in vitro. This requires keeping the serum at 37° C from the moment it is collected until the complement assay has been completed. The author has seen sera in which massive cryoprecipitation associated with depletion of complement occurred at temperatures as high as 30° C. Possibly because of the anticomplementary activity exhibited by these cryoproteins when present in adequate concentration, symptoms in some patients will resemble those of immune complex vasculitis, immunofluorescent studies showing immunoglobulin and complement deposition in the glomerular basement membrane and cutaneous vessels.

The mixed cryoglobulins, especially those with polyclonal rheumatoid factor components, are generally found in somewhat lower concentrations than the monoclonal cryoproteins. They therefore rarely cause hyperviscosity syndromes. Conversely, because they represent a true immune complex of rheumatoid factor, its antigen, and frequently complement, the symptoms exhibited are usually those of immune complex vasculitis. Rother and associates have demonstrated that the activation of complement by cryoprotein tends to be a bithermic event.[63] Cryoprecipitation of mixed cryoglob-

ulins is marginal at temperatures greater than 22° C. On the other hand, activation of the complement sequence is negligible below that temperature. Thus, the inflammatory potential of such cryoglobulins is probably negligible at both very cold and very warm temperatures, and most probably maximal at intermediate temperatures such as those found in the distal extremities.

Cutaneous manifestations are the most common in the mixed cryoglobulinemias, 70 percent in Brouet's series exhibiting vascular purpura[38] (Fig. 84–3). Skin biopsy has shown an acute necrotizing vasculitis, and immunofluorescent studies have shown deposition of IgM, IgG, and C3 in arterial walls.[50] Less common cutaneous manifestations include livedo and urticaria, which may be transferred to normal recipients by injection of isolated cryoglobulin.[64] The second most common symptom of mixed cryoglobulinemia is joint pain. This is usually a mild arthralgia unaccompanied by swelling, redness, or joint destruction. Neurologic symptoms occur in 25 percent of the patients with mixed cryoglobulinemia. This virtually always presents as a peripheral neuropathy characterized initially by paresthesia and numbness and leading ultimately to deficiencies in motor function. Central nervous system symptoms are rare,

Figure 84–3. Vascular purpura of the lower extremity in a patient with mixed cryoglobulinemia.

and when present, are generally secondary to arterial occlusion occurring in the hyperviscosity syndrome rather than cerebral vasculitis. Glomerulonephritis is seen in 20 to 35 percent of patients with mixed cryoglobulinemia. Immunofluorescent studies show the deposition of IgM, IgG, and complement.[38] Renal histology may show focal or diffuse proliferative glomerulitis or predominantly membranous disease. In Brouet's series, patients with both monoclonal unmixed and both varieties of mixed cryoglobulins had diffuse glomerulonephritis. Eight of 17 biopsied patients showed diffuse proliferative disease, and 5 had large membranous deposits without cell proliferation.[38]

Intestinal vasculitis has been reported in mixed cryoglobulinemia.[65] Anemia was a common feature noted in the original series by Meltzer and his associates.[50] An interesting artifact occurring in cryoglobulinemic states is pseudoleukocytosis. This occurs if the leukocyte count is performed in an electronic particle-counting instrument, when particles of suspended cryoprecipitate are mistaken for leukocytes.[65,66]

TREATMENT OF THE CRYOGLOBULINEMIA SYNDROMES

Principles of therapy in the cryoglobulinemic states are similar to those in myeloma and Waldenström's macroglobulinemia and include attempts to remove the cryoprotein, use of pharmacologic agents to inhibit mediators of inflammation, and administration of cytotoxic drugs to diminish the synthetic rate of offending proteins.

In those patients with severe hyperviscosity syndrome, plasmapheresis of only 1 to 2 units of plasma may have dramatic and immediate effects, for the reasons outlined earlier. A reduction in the concentration of the abnormal protein by just a few percent may reduce the blood viscosity severalfold. The use of long-term high-volume plasma exchange in the definitive treatment of immune complex diseases is currently in vogue. The exact role of this form of therapy in managing cryoglobulinemia is far from established. It would seem to have the greatest potential for good (1) in cryoglobulinemia in which large amounts of IgM are present, since IgM is distributed predominantly within the vascular space, and (2) in mixed cryoglobulinemia in which, for example, several molecules of IgG and complement can combine with IgM in complex. Since the association at equilibrium is in part dependent on the product of the concentrations of the individual components, halving the concentration of each of three components could theoretically reduce the concentration of the complex eightfold.

In those cryoglobulinemic patients in whom hypocomplementemia, vasculitis, and intravascular immune complex deposition seem to be playing a role, especially if glomerulonephritis is present, a trial of aggressive corticosteroid therapy is indicated. Although the immune complex vasculitis of SLE typically responds dramatically to this therapy, treatment of essential mixed cryoglobulinemia with prednisone has met with limited success. In the nonessential (i.e., secondary) cryoglobulinemias, treatment should be directed primarily at the underlying disease process. In the monoclonal cryoglobulinemias, steroids are less likely to be effective than agents cytotoxic for the cell line producing the abnormal protein. Beneficial effects of steroids appear to be primarily a result of their anti-inflammatory properties and not due to cytolytic effects. Steroids are marginally effective in controlling fever, skin lesions, and musculoskeletal symptoms but have no effect on circulating cryoprotein levels.[67-68]

The effectiveness of cytotoxic drugs in treating the monoclonal cryoglobulinemias is generally identical to that achieved in typical myeloma or Waldenström's macroglobulinemia. Cytotoxic drug regimens have been used with variable success in treating the essential mixed cryoglobulinemias. Regimens employed successfully include chlorambucil,[70] cyclophosphamide,[71] and melphalan/prednisone.[72] The rarity with which the cryoglobulinemic syndromes are seen by the average physician, the protean manifestations of these syndromes, and their extremely variable clinical course have prevented the development of a consensus regarding optimal therapy in these diseases.

References

1. Paredes, J.M., and Mitchell, B.S.: Multiple myeloma: Current concepts in diagnosis and management. Med. Clin. North Am. 64:729, 1980.
2. Williams, R.C., Brunning, R.D., and Wallheim, F.C.: Light chain disease: An abortive variant of multiple myeloma. Ann. Intern. Med. 65:471, 1966.
3. Early, A.P., Ozer, H., and Henderson, E.S.: Multiple myeloma. N.Y. State J. Med. 81:883, 1981.
4. Defronzo, R., Cooke, R.C., Wright, J.R., and Humphrey, R.L.: Renal function in patients with multiple myeloma. Medicine (Balt.) 57:151, 1978.
5. Levi, D.F., Williams, R.C., and Lindstrom, F.D.: Immunofluorescent studies of the myeloma kidney with special reference to light chain disease. Am. J. Med. 44:922, 1968.
6. Waldman, T., Strober, W., and Mogielnicky, P.: The renal handling of low molecular weight proteins. J. Clin. Invest. 51:2162, 1972.
7. Alexanian, R., Balcerzak, S., Bonnet, J.D., Gehan, E.A., Haut, A., Hewlett, S.J., and Monto, R.W.: Prognostic factors in multiple myeloma. Cancer 36:1192, 1975.
8. Medical Research Council's Working Party for Therapeutic Trials in Leukemia: Report on the first myelomatosis trial. Part I. Analysis of presenting features of prognostic importance. Br. J. Haematol. 24:123, 1973.
9. Bergsagel, D.E., Migliore, P.J., and Griffith, K.M.: Myeloma proteins and the clinical response to melphalan therapy. Science 148:376, 1965.
10. Shustik, C., Bergsagel, D.E., and Pruzanski, W.: Kappa and lambda light chain disease: Survival rates and clinical manifestations. Blood 48:41, 1976.
11. Bergsagel, D.E., Bailey, A.J., Langley, G.R., MacDonald, R.N., White, D.F., and Miller, A.B.: The chemotherapy of plasma cell myeloma and the incidence of acute leukemia. N. Engl. J. Med. 301:743, 1979.
12. Preston, F.E., Cooke, K.B., Foster, M.E., Winfield, D.A., and Lee, D.: Myelomatosis and the hyperviscosity syndrome. Br. J. Haematol. 38:517, 1978.
13. Pruzanski, W., and Watt, J.B.: Serum viscosity and hyperviscosity syndrome in IgG multiple myeloma. Ann. Intern. Med. 77:853, 1972.
14. Capra, J.D., and Kunkel, H.G.: Aggregation of IgG3 proteins: Relevance to the hyperviscosity syndrome. J. Clin. Invest. 49:610, 1970.
15. Kyle, R.A.: Multiple myeloma: Review of 869 cases. Mayo Clin. Proc. 50:29, 1975.
16. Kyle, R.A., Maldonado, J.E., and Bayrd, E.D.: Idiopathic Bence-Jones proteinuria: A distinct entity? Am. J. Med. 55:222, 1973.
17. Kyle, R.A., and Bayrd, E.D., Amyloidosis: Review of 236 cases. Medicine (Balt.) 54:271, 1975.
18. Smith, J.K.: The significance of the "protein error" of indicators in the diagnosis of Bence-Jones proteinuria. Acta Haematol. 30:144, 1963.

19. Lazor, M., and Rosenberg, L.: Mechanism of adrenal-steroid reversal of hypercalcemia in multiple myeloma. N. Engl. J. Med. 270:749, 1964.

20. Durie, B.G.M.: Staging and kinetics of multiple myeloma. Clin. Haematol. 11:3, 1982.

21. Durie, B.G.M., and Salmon, S.E.: The current status and future prospects of treatment for multiple myeloma. Clin. Haematol. 11:181, 1982.

22. McCallister, B.D., Bayrd, E.D., Harrison, E.G., Jr., and McGuckin, W.F.: Primary macroglobulinemia: Review with a report on thirty-one cases and notes on the value of continuous chlorambucil therapy. Am. J. Med. 43:394, 1967.

23. Mackenzie, M.R., and Fudenberg, H.H.: Macroglobulinemia: Analysis of forty patients. Blood 39:874, 1972.

24. Morel-Maroger, L., Basch, A., Danon, F., Verroust, P., and Richet, G.: Pathology of the kidney in Waldenström's macroglobulinemia. Study of sixteen cases. N. Engl. J. Med. 283:123, 1970.

25. Zlotnick, A., and Rosenmann, E.: Renal pathologic findings associated with monoclonal gammopathies. Arch. Intern. Med. 135:40, 1975.

26. Julien, J., Vital, C., Vallat, J.M., Lagueny, A., Deminiere, C., and Darriet, D.: Polyneuropathy in Waldenström's macroglobulinemia. Deposition of M component on myelin sheaths. Arch. Neurol. 35:423, 1978.

27. Kahn, S.N., Smith, I.S., Eames, R.A., Thomas, P.K., and Lacey, B.W.: IgM paraproteinemia and autoimmune peripheral neuropathy. N. Engl. J. Med. 304:1430, 1981.

28. Strisower, E.H., and Galleto, A.T.: Waldenström's macroglobulinemia. Differential diagnosis, lipoprotein study, and case report. Am. J. Med. 32:304, 1962.

29. Drusin, L.M., Litwin, S.D., Armstrong, D., and Webster, B.P.: Waldenström's macroglobulinemia in a patient with a chronic biologic false-positive serologic test for syphilis. Am. J. Med. 56:429, 1974.

30. Franklin, E.C., Lowenstein, J., Bigelow, B., and Meltzer, M.: Heavy chain disease: A new disorder of serum γ-globulins. Am. J. Med. 37:332, 1964.

31. Seligmann, M., Mihaesco, E., Preud'homme, J.L., Danon, F., and Brouet, J.C.: Heavy chain diseases: Current findings and concepts. Immunological Rev. 48:145, 1979.

32. Kyle, R.A.: Monoclonal gammopathy of undetermined significance (MGUS): A review. Clin. Haematol. 11:123, 1982.

33. Axelsson, U., Bachmann, R., and Hallen, J.: Frequency of pathological proteins (M-components) in 6995 sera from an adult population. Acta. Med. Scand. 179:235, 1966.

34. Wintrobe, M.M., and Buell, M.V.: Hyperproteinemia associated with multiple myeloma; with report of a case in which an extraordinary hyperproteinemia was associated with thrombosis of the retinal veins and symptoms suggesting Raynaud's disease. Bull. Johns Hopkins Hosp. 52:156, 1933.

35. Lerner, A.B., and Watson, C.J.: Studies of cryoglobulins. I. Unusual purpura associated with the presence of high concentration of cryoglobulin (cold precipitable serum globulin). Am. J. Med. Sci. 214:410, 1947.

36. Smith, S.B., and Arkin, C.: Cryofibrinogenemia: Incidence, clinical correlations, and a review of the literature. Am. J. Clin. Pathol. 58:524, 1972.

37. Stathakis, N.E., and Mosesson, M.W.: Interactions among heparin, cold-insoluble globulin, and fibrinogen in formation of the heparin-precipitable fraction of plasma. J. Clin. Invest. 60:855, 1977.

38. Brouet, J.C., Clauvel, J.P., Danon, F., Klein, M., and Seligmann, M.: Biological and clinical significance of cryoglobulins. A report of 86 cases. Am. J. Med. 57:775, 1974.

39. Gough, W.W., Lightfoot, R.W., Jr., and Christian, C.L.: Cryoglobulins and complement in immune complex disease. VI Pan-American Congress on Rheumatic Diseases, Toronto, Canada, 1974.

40. Meltzer, M., and Franklin, E.C.: Cryoglobulinemia—a study of twenty-nine patients. I. IgG and IgM cryoglobulins and factors affecting cryoprecipitability. Am. J. Med. 40:828, 1966.

41. Mellors, R.C., Ortega, L.G., and Holman, H.R.: Role of gamma globulins in pathogenesis of renal lesions in systemic lupus erythematosus and chronic membranous glomerulonephritis, with an observation on the lupus erythematosus cell reaction. J. Exp. Med. 106:191, 1957.

42. Koffler, D., Schur, P.H., and Kunkel, H.G.: Immunological studies concerning the nephritis of systemic lupus erythematosus. J. Exp. Med. 126:607, 1967.

43. Stastny, P., and Ziff, M.: Cold-insoluble complexes and complement levels in systemic lupus erythematosus. N. Engl. J. Med. 280:1376, 1969.

44. Christian, C.L., Hatfield, W.B., and Chase, P.H.: Systemic lupus erythematosus: Cryoprecipitation of serum. J. Clin. Invest. 42:823, 1963.

45. McPhaul, J.J., Jr.: Cryoimmunoglobulinaemia in patients with primary renal disease and systemic lupus erythematosus. Clin. Exp. Immunol. 31:181, 1978.

46. Winfield, J.B., Koffler, D., and Kunkel, H.G.: Specific concentration of polynucleotide immune complexes in the cryoprecipitates of patients with systemic lupus erythematosus. J. Clin. Invest. 56:563, 1975.

47. Steinman, C.R.: Free DNA in serum and plasma from normal adults. J. Clin. Invest. 26:512, 1975.

48. Bluestone, R., Goldberg, L.S., Cracchiolo, A., III, and Barnett, E.V.: Detection and characterization of DNA in mixed (IgG-IgM) cryoglobulins. Int. Arch. Allergy 39:16, 1970.

49. Williams, R.C., and Kunkel, H.G.: Rheumatoid factor, complement and conglutinin aberrations in patients with subacute bacterial endocarditis. J. Clin. Invest. 41:666, 1962.

50. Meltzer, M., Franklin, E.C., Elias, K., McCluskey, R.T., and Cooper, N.: Cryoglobulinemia—a clinical and laboratory study. II. Cryoglobulins with rheumatoid factor activity. Am. J. Med. 40:837, 1966.

51. Levo, Y., Gorevic, P.D., Kassab, H.J., Tobias, H., and Franklin, E.C.: Liver involvement in the syndrome of mixed cryoglobulinemia. Ann. Intern. Med. 87:287, 1977.

52. Levo, Y., Gorevic, P.D., Kassab, H.J., Zucker-Franklin, D., and Franklin, E.C.: Association between hepatitis B virus and essential mixed cryoglobulinemia. N. Engl. J. Med. 196:1501, 1977.

53. Barnett, E.V., Bluestone, R., Cracchiolo, A., Goldberg, L.S., Kantor, G.L., and McIntosh, R.M.: Cryoglobulinemia and disease. Ann. Intern. Med. 73:95, 1970.

54. Bombardieri, S., Teichner, A., and Vicaro, G.: Cryoglobulinemia with echinococcosis. Proc. Soc. Exp. Biol. Med. 142:941, 1973.

55. Steere, A.C., Hardin, J.A., and Malawista, S.E.: Erythema chronicum migrans and Lyme arthritis: Cryoimmunoglobulins and clinical activity of skin and joints. Science 196:1121, 1977.

56. Grey, H.M., Kohler, P.F., Terry, W.D., and Franklin, E.C.: Human monoclonal γG-cryoglobulins with anti-γ-globulins and clinical activity. J. Clin. Invest. 47:1875, 1968.

57. Pope, R.M., Teller, D.C., and Mannik, M.: The molecular basis of self-association of antibodies to IgG (rheumatoid factors) in rheumatoid arthritis. Proc. Natl. Acad. Sci. USA. 71:517, 1974.

58. Pope, R. M., Mannik, M., Gilliland, B.C., and Teller, D.C.: The hyperviscosity syndrome in rheumatoid arthritis due to intermediate complexes formed by self-association of IgG-rheumatoid factors. Arthritis Rheum. 18:97, 1975.

59. Grey, H.M., and Kohler, P.F.: Cryoimmunoglobulins. Sem. Hematol. 10:87, 1973.

60. Saha, A., Chowdhury, P., Sambury, S., Smart, K., and Rose, B.: Studies on cryoprecipitation. IV. Enzymatic fragments of a human cryoglobulin. J. Biol. Chem. 245:2730, 1970.

61. Zinneman, H.H., and Caperton, E.: Cryoglobulinemia in a patient with Sjögren's syndrome, and factors of cryoprecipitation. J. Lab. Clin. Med. 89:483, 1977.

62. Pruzanski, W., and Watt, J.G.: Serum viscosity and hyperviscosity syndrome in IgG multiple myeloma. Ann. Intern. Med. 77:853, 1972.

63. Rother, U., Rother, K., Flad, H.D., and Miescher, P.A.: Bithermic complement activation in cryoglobulinaemic serum. Eur. J. Clin. Invest. 2:59, 1972.

64. Constanzi, J.J., and Coltman, C.A.: Kappa chain cold precipitable immunoglobulin IgG associated with cold urticaria. Clin. Exp. Immunol. 2:167, 1967.

65. Reza, M.J., Roth, B.E., Pops, M.A., and Goldberg, L.S.: Intestinal vasculitis in essential mixed cryoglobulinemia. Ann. Intern. Med. 81:632, 1974.

66. Emori, H.W., Bluestone, R., and Goldberg, L.S: Pseudoleukocytosis associated with cryoglobulinemia. Am. J. Clin. Pathol. 60:202, 1973.

67. Grossman, J., Abraham, G.N., Leddy, J.P., and Condemi, J.L.: Cryoglobulinemia. Ann. Intern. Med. 77:395, 1972.

68. Volpe, R., Bruce-Robertson, A., Fletcher, A.A., and Charles, W.B.: Essential cryoglobulinemia: Review of the literature and a report of a case treated with ACTH and cortisone. Am. J. Med. 20:533, 1956.

69. Lapes, M.J., and Davis, J.S. IV: Arthralgia-purpura-weakness-cryoglobulinemia. Arch Intern. Med. 126:287, 1970.

70. Golde, D., and Epstein, W.: Mixed cryoglobulins and glomerulonephritis. Ann. Intern. Med. 69:1221, 1968.

71. Mathison, D.A., Condemi, J.J., Leddy, J.P., Callerame, M.L., Panner, B.J., and Vaughan, J.H.: Purpura, arthralgia, and IgM-IgG cryoglobulinemia with rheumatoid factor activity: Response to cyclophosphamide and splenectomy. Ann. Intern. Med. 74:383, 1971.

72. Brody, J.I., and Samitz, M.H.: Cutaneous signs of cryoparaproteinemia: Control with burst Alkeran and prednisone. Am. J. Med. 55:211, 1973.

Chapter 85

Complement Deficiencies and the Rheumatic Diseases

Shaun Ruddy

INTRODUCTION

Deficiencies of individual proteins of the complement or properdin system are of clinical importance for two reasons: (1) Homozygous deficiency of the early-reacting components, for example, C1, C4, or C2, is clearly associated with an increased frequency of diseases such as systemic lupus erythematosus, polymyositis, vasculitis, and glomerulonephritis.[1,2] (2) Homozygous deficiency of any of the constituents of the membrane attack complex, for example, C5, C6, C7, C8 or C9, predisposes to recurrent *Neisserial* infections, including recurrent gonococcal arthritis.[3,4]

This chapter reviews the inherited deficiencies of complement proteins that have been found together with rheumatic diseases, the clinical features of such diseases, and the possible reasons for their association. Details of the biochemistry and immunobiology of the complement and properdin systems are given in Chapter 7, and more general information about control of complement protein synthesis is contained in reviews elsewhere.[5-7]

METHODS OF MEASURING COMPLEMENT

Total Hemolytic Complement (CH50). The traditional technique for the determination of the complement in serum measures the ability of the test specimen to lyse 50 percent of a standard suspension of sheep erythrocytes coated with rabbit antibody (EA) in a reaction that includes the entire classic reaction sequence.

$$EA + \frac{test}{material} \xrightarrow[37°C]{Mg^{++}, Ca^{++}} lysis$$

The outcome of this reaction is the result of the interaction of the EA with all nine of the complement components and the normal (or any abnormal) inhibitors contained in the test sample. Because of this inclusiveness, the CH50 is the procedure of choice for detecting deficiency states.

EA are incubated with varying dilutions of the test specimen for a time sufficient to complete the reaction, the mixtures centrifuged, and the percent hemolysis determined from spectrophotometric measurements of hemoglobin released into the supernatant fluid by the lysed cells. The actual number of CH50 units (U) per milliliter obtained is a function of the number of EA in the test system and the relative concentrations of the reactants. Either of two systems is commonly employed in clinical laboratories: the method of Kent and Fife,[8] which measures the lysis of 0.6 ml of a 1 percent suspension of EA in a total volume of 1.5 ml; or the method of Mayer, which uses 1.0 ml of EA at a concentration of 5×10^8 per milliliter in a total volume of 7.5 ml.[9] Although the precise limits of a normal population must be determined by assaying in the laboratory where the test is being performed, normal CH50 values for the Kent and Fife method are usually in the range of 125 to 300 U per milliliter and for the Mayer method, 25 to 50 U per milliliter.

Effective Molecule Component Titrations. The availability of purified components and stable intermediate complexes of the immune hemolytic sequence has permitted the development of assays specific for the activities of individual components of complement.[10] Stoichiometric titrations are available only in research laboratories because they require such highly specialized techniques and uneconomical reagents.

Immunochemical Assays. Monospecific antibodies have been prepared against all of the complement and properdin proteins as well as the control proteins and are commercially available for most of them. Using such antibodies, the concentrations of complement proteins in plasma or other body fluids may be measured by their antigenic reactivity in immunoassays. The most widely used technique is radial immunodiffusion;[11] kits providing all of the necessary reagents in easy-to-use form are marketed by a number of suppliers. When "complement levels" are requested in most hospitals, the clinical pathology laboratory usually measures C3 and C4 by radial immunodiffusion. In this technique, monospecific antibody directed against a complement protein is incorporated into an agarose gel, holes are punched in the gel, and test samples or known standards are placed in the holes. As the antigenic complement protein diffuses into the gel and encounters its specific antibody, a precipitin ring forms around the hole. At equilibrium, the area enclosed by the precipitin ring is proportional to the concentration of complement antigen placed in the hole. From the size of rings produced by samples of known concentration, a standard curve is constructed, and the concentration of the complement antigen in the test sample determined. The coefficient of variation of this method is usually between 5 and 10 per cent.

Electroimmunodiffusion, in which the sample is unidirectionally electrophoresed into antibody-containing gel, yielding a set of "rockets," whose height is proportional to concentration, is more rapid and slightly more sensitive than radial immunodiffusion.[12] Immunonephelometry measures light scattering due to the formation of complexes between detecting antibody and complement antigen. Sensitivity is enhanced by using a highly collimated laser light source, which allows detection of light scattered at a narrow angle to the transmitted beam.[13,14] Both endpoint (equilibrium) and kinetic (rate of increase in scattering) analyses are in use.

Comparison of Methods. Since the CH50 is widely available and its use preceded specific component assays by about 50 years, it has the advantage that many observations relating complement levels in human disease are based on it. The CH50 continues to be a useful screening procedure for the detection of deficiency states. A normal CH50 does not, however, exclude all complement abnormalities; heterozygous deficient individuals often have normal levels. When the CH50 is subnormal, specific component measurements are required to determine the precise nature of the abnormality.

Functional assays are extremely sensitive, a distinct advantage at concentrations corresponding to fewer than 5 micrograms per milliliter, at which measurements by immunoassay are not sensitive. Most importantly, effective molecule titrations measure the active component, whereas immunodiffusion, which measures the component as antigen, does not distinguish between active complement protein and that which is inactive due to an error of synthesis. Certain kindreds with hereditary angioedema due to C1 inhibitor deficiency synthesize antigenically intact nonfunctional inhibitor protein.[15] Individuals deficient in C8 activity due to absence of the β chain of C8 have immunoreactive α-γ chains in their plasma.[16] In either case immunoassay might yield near normal concentrations and a "false-negative" result, and functional assays would be required to make the correct diagnosis.

Because radial immunodiffusion does not require the elaborate preparation of reagents and is easily performed using commercially available kits, this technique is most commonly used. Nephelometry requires a heavy capital investment in equipment and the use of antisera that have been specially prepared and are, therefore, quite expensive. Nephelometry is clearly more sensitive, and its precision may be greater than that of radial immunodiffusion, since it does not depend on the skill of the operator. Automation, with continuous-flow design and computerized data reduction, analysis, and reporting of results, affords greatly increased efficiency for centers where large numbers of measurements must be made.

Detection of Deficiency States. For the classic activation pathway (C1, C4, C2) or the terminal sequence (C5-C9), the CH50 performed with sheep erythrocytes coated with rabbit antibody is a reliable screen for homozygous deficiencies. For the alternative activation pathway, lysis of rabbit erythrocytes in the absence of exogenous antibody[17] is the screening test of choice. Homozygous deficiencies of all nine of the classic components, three of the four control proteins, and one of

the three alternative pathway factors have been described; to date, absence of C4 binding protein, factor D, and factor B have not been reported.

Because of the wide range of normal for most complement proteins, detection of the heterozygous deficient state is difficult. Even in populations that are carefully checked for the absence of recent infections, ingestion of medications, or other factors that might influence the level of complement proteins, values for normals often do not have a Gaussian distribution and the 95 percent confidence limits of the population approximate $\pm$ 50 of the mean or median value.[18] Heterozygous deficient individuals usually have levels that range between 30 and 70 per cent of the normal mean, so that for any single individual, confidence about heterozygosity cannot be great. Careful family studies demonstrating reduced levels in relatives consistent with autosomal codominant inheritance increase the confidence of ascertaining heterozygosity;[19] the presence in the pedigrees of a homozygous deficient individual greatly increases it. As a matter of routine, studies of the genetics of complement deficiencies should be supported by analyses of erythrocyte or leukocyte (HLA) antigens, which verify the pedigree obtained by history.

SPECIFIC DEFICIENCY STATES FOUND WITH RHEUMATIC DISEASES

C1q Deficiency. Following an initial report of selective deficiency of the C1q subcomponent of C1 in a young Turkish male with skin disease and nephritis,[20] complete absence of this protein was demonstrated in the sera of three siblings who also had renal and cutaneous lesions.[21] Renal biopsies showed mesangioproliferative glomerulonephritis with deposits of IgM and C3. The skin disease had both clinical and pathological features of congenital poikiloderma (Rothmund-Thompson syndrome). In a third kindred, one child had a severe lupus-like syndrome while the other was normal; a dysfunctional C1q molecule, which was antigenically deficient and devoid of activity, was found.[22]

C1r Deficiency. The first patient to be described with C1r deficiency was a female with chronic glomerulonephritis which progressed to end-stage renal disease and required transplantation.[23] The second kindred had for its propositus a 16-year-old Puerto Rican boy with a lupus-like syndrome, including fever, malar rash, arthralgias, and subacute focal membranous glomerulonephritis. Although immunoglobulins and C3 were demonstrated by immunofluorescence as deposited along the glomerular basement membrane, studies of biopsies of the skin lesions, which were typical of discoid lupus erythematosus, failed to reveal similar deposits of immunoglobulin and C3 usually observed in such lesions. Serology for antinuclear antibodies and LE cells was negative.[24] The 24-year-old sister of the proband had arthralgias and skin ulcers and was said to have had a malar rash. Her skin biopsy was also negative for deposits of immunoglobulins and C3. Two other siblings had died in infancy of gastroenteritis of unknown cause; a third had died at age 12 of "lupus erythematosus."[25]

Affected individuals have no detectable total hemolytic complement activity or immunochemical C1r. Levels of C1s are approximately 40 percent of normal, but all other components, including C1q, are normal or elevated. Family studies have identified heterozygotes with 60 to 90 percent of normal mean C1r levels, indicating an autosomal recessive mode of inheritance. Appropriate studies have excluded linkages between C1r deficiency gene and the HLA loci.[26]

C1s Deficiency. A 6-year-old girl with cutaneous manifestations of SLE was the first reported case of C1s deficiency.[27] Tests for antinuclear antibody and for deposits of immunoglobulin in the skin were both positive. Subsequently, a second kindred containing two individuals with C1s deficiency and a lupus-like disease manifested by polyarthritis, alopecia, discoid lupus, Raynaud's phenomenon, and a positive antinuclear antibody test has been reported.[28] Another sibling with the same syndrome had normal complement levels; two others with C1s deficiency were well.

C1̄ Inhibitor Deficiency. Inherited absence or reduced levels of this important control protein are regularly associated with the clinical syndrome of hereditary angioedema, manifested by recurrent swellings of the subepithelial areas of the skin and upper respiratory and gastrointestinal tracts.[29] The diagnosis, pathogenesis, and treatment of this disease are reviewed elsewhere[30] and are beyond the scope of this chapter. Of importance for the interpretation of the association between complement deficiencies and rheumatic diseases, however, are the occurrences of systemic or discoid lupus in individuals with C1̄ inhibitor deficiency. In one kindred,[31] a mother with systemic lupus erythematosus and C1̄ inhibitor deficiency gave birth to identical twin boys who had discoid lupus. Although C4 measurements of antinuclear antibody were not available for the mother's serum, she did have a false-positive VDRL and a negative LE cell test. The twins both had weakly positive antinuclear antibody tests with antibodies to single- but not double-stranded DNA. Measurements of metabolism indicated the profoundly depressed serum levels and increased fractional catabolic rates for this component usually found in C1̄ inhibitor deficiency.

Another set of twins has one member with symptoms of hereditary angioedema since the age of 6 who developed classic SLE with positive antinuclear antibodies and antibodies to double-stranded DNA at the age of 14.[32] Her C4 levels before the onset of SLE were less than 4 percent of normal. The twin without symptoms of hereditary angioedema did not develop SLE; her C4 levels ranged between 10 and 15 percent of normal.

Three other unrelated patients with C1̄ inhibitor deficiency and lupus-like disease, manifested predominantly as rash, have been reported.[33] Among 220 patients with C1̄ inhibitor deficiency, the occurrence of lupus erythematosus-like disease was approximately 2 percent, a figure considerably in excess of the usual estimates of the frequency of this disease (0.1 to 0.01 percent).[33]

C4 Deficiency. Like the other proteins in the major histocompatibility complex to which it is linked, including the leukocyte antigens HLA-A, B, and D and the complement proteins C2 and factor B, C4 is highly polymorphic. This polymorphism is complicated by the existence of two adjacent loci, C4A and C4B, which correspond to two separate structural genes. At both of these loci, null (Q0) alleles are common, and serum levels roughly correspond to the number of expressed C4 genes.[34] Individuals homozygous for null alleles at both loci (C4AQ0, BQ0/C4AQ0, BQ0) and who are totally deficient are rare, but those with one, two, or three null alleles and serum levels equal to ¾, ½, or ¼ of the normal mean occur more frequently. While nearly all those with complete deficiency have manifested one or another rheumatic disease syndrome, the disease consequences of partial deficiency are less clear.[35] Certain polymorphic variants of C4 are in linkage disequilibrium with certain HLA antigens, and associations of specific C4 allotypes with diseases such as multiple sclerosis, insulin-dependent diabetes mellitus, and systemic lupus erythematosus have been reported.[36,37] Thus far none of these diseases has been more closely associated with a particular C4 allotype than with the corresponding HLA-D antigen with which the C4 allotype was in linkage disequilibrium.

Homozygous C4 deficiency was first described in an 18-year-old girl with cutaneous and renal involvement typical of SLE.[38] Serologic tests for antinuclear antibodies and DNA binding were negative, and immunofluorescent studies of skin did not demonstrate binding of immunoglobulins or complement components. The patient's mother had approximately half normal levels of C4. A second kindred had for its propositus a 5-year-old boy with rash, fever, arthralgias, and hepatosplenomegaly who subsequently developed diffuse proliferative glomerulonephritis.[39] Antinuclear antibodies were present and DNA binding was increased with the onset of the glomerlonephritis. Both in this kindred and in the earlier one, linkage of the C4 deficiency to the major histocompatibility complex was demonstrated. Subsequent reports have included patients with SLE and renal involvement,[40] lupus-like disease,[41] Henoch-Schönlein purpura,[42] Sjögren's syndrome,[43] and SLE with pulmonary infection.[44]

C2 Deficiency. This is by far the most frequent of the complement component deficiencies in man.[45,46] It is inherited as an autosomal codominant, heterozygotes having levels between 30 to 70 percent of the normal mean. Based on the finding of six possible heterozygotes in a population of 509 normal blood donors[47] and a single homozygote among 10,000 others, the gene frequency appears to be approximately 1 percent.[5] Levels of other components are usually normal with the exception of properdin factor B, which has been found to be moderately depressed in several homozygous deficient individuals; this may be a secondary phenomenon, reflecting overutilization of the alternative pathway in individuals who lack the classic one.

Although the probands of the first two kindreds with

C2 deficiency appeared to be normal,[48,49] those of the subsequently reported kindreds have had diseases such as systemic lupus erythematosus, discoid lupus erythematosus, polymyositis, glomerulonephritis, Henoch-Schönlein purpura, Hodgkin's disease, or vasculitis. In a recent tabulation, 14 of 38 homozygous C2 deficient individuals had either systemic or discoid lupus erythematosus.[45] The female:male ratio for such individuals was consistent with the predominance of females generally seen in these diseases. Although a few patients with florid lupus, including fulminant renal disease, have been described,[50] attention has been called to the somewhat atypical features of the disease present in most such patients.[45] Five of eight patients with SLE had weak or absent antibodies to native double stranded DNA. Five of seven tested had no immunoglobulins or complement deposited in the skin, and the remaining two had only IgG present. The frequency of discoid lupus is also quite high. The lesions may be the typical erythematosus raised scaly rash, beginning first on the malar area and later spreading, and be aggravated by the sun. Immunofluorescent studies of such lesions often fail to demonstrate presence of immunoglobulin or complement along the epidermal-dermal junction which are typical of the usual form of this disease.

Retrospective analysis of patients referred for rheumatic diseases (and *not* for complement deficiency) has revealed an increased frequency of heterozygous C2 deficiency among such patients when compared with normal blood bank donors.[47] Among 509 normal blood bank donors, six heterozygous C2 deficients were found. Significant increases above this proportion were found in patients with juvenile rheumatoid arthritis (10 of 274, 3.7 percent) and systemic lupus erythematosus (8 of 137, 5.9 percent). As in the earlier studies, patients with C2 deficiency and SLE tended to have lower titers of antinuclear antibody.

C2 deficiency was the first of the complement component deficiencies to be linked to the HLA loci[51] and has subsequently been found to be in linkage dysequilibrium with the haplotype HLA-A10, B18, D2,[52] and with C4A4 and C4B2 allotypes.[53]

C3 Deficiency. Homozygous deficiency of C3 is usually associated with profound defects in host defenses, consistent with the pivotal role of this component in both the classic and alternative activation pathways.[54-57] Recurrent infections with both pyogenic gram-positive and gram-negative bacteria result in severe furunculosis, pneumonia, meningitis, and septic arthritis. Syndromes resembling systemic lupus have also been observed, however.[58] Vasculitis with circulating immune complexes has been found in a Dutch family with complete C3 deficiency,[59] as well as in familial partial deficiency.[60] A 34-month-old male with fever, skin rash, and arthralgias had homozygous C3 deficiency and improved dramatically following transfusion therapy.[61]

Other Deficiencies. Although more frequently associated with recurrent *Neisserial* infections,[62-64] complete deficiency of C5 has been found in a patient with systemic lupus erythematosus manifested by Raynaud's phenomenon, arthritis, hemolytic anemia, and membranous glomerulonephritis.[65,66] Antinuclear antibodies and anti-DNA were present as well as typical immunofluorescent deposits on skin biopsy. A 10-year-old half-sister also had 1 to 2 percent of normal C5 levels and recurrent pyogenic infections, including two episodes of pneumonia. One of two propositi of C7 deficient kindreds has been found to have severe Raynaud's phenomenon and sclerodactyly.[67] Both systemic lupus erythematosus[68] and rheumatoid arthritis have also been described in homozygous C7 deficient individuals; in the patient with rheumatoid arthritis, platelet aggregation induced by thrombin was found to be impaired.[69] Absence of C8 has been found in a patient with systemic lupus erythematosus manifested by membranous glomerulonephritis, photosensitivity, and a positive LE cell test.[70]

Significance of Association between Complement Deficiencies and Rheumatic Diseases. Although the list of deficiency states with diseases compiled in Table 85-1 is long, some of the associations may be artifacts of sampling—"ascertainment bias"—reflecting the fact that patients with rheumatic disease or nephritis tend to have their complement levels determined more fre-

Table 85-1. Rheumatic Diseases Associated with Complement Deficiencies

Protein	Disease
C1q	Glomerulonephritis and poikiloderma congenita
C1r	Glomerulonephritis; lupus-like syndrome
C1s	Lupus-like syndrome
C1INH	Discoid lupus; systemic lupus; lupus-like syndrome
C4	Systemic lupus; Sjögren's syndrome
C2	Systemic lupus; discoid lupus; polymyositis; Henoch-Schönlein purpura; Hodgkin's disease; vasculitis; glomerulonephritis; common variable hypogammaglobulinemia
C3	Vasculitis: lupus-like syndrome; glomerulonephritis
C5	Systemic lupus; *Neisseria* infection
C6	*Neisseria* infection
C7	Systemic lupus; rheumatoid arthritis; Raynaud's phenomenon and sclerodactyly; vasculitis; *Neisseria* infection
C8	Systemic lupus; *Neisseria* infection
C9	*Neisseria* infection

quently than do normal individuals. Even if there were no true association with rheumatic diseases, deficiency states would be found more frequently among such patients simply because their levels are more frequently measured. One example of such an artifact is the finding that the probands of the first two kindreds with C2 deficiency were both immunologists,[48,49] another group which has its complement levels measured more frequently than normal because of proximity and availability to the measuring laboratory. Only prospective determinations of the occurrence of complement deficiency and rheumatic disease in a randomly sampled population would serve to establish such an association beyond all doubt; because of the low frequency of both of these events, the large sample size required prohibits such a study. In the next best thing, a case-control study, the prevalence of C2 deficiency in a group of patients with rheumatic diseases has been compared with that of a group of control blood donors.[47] The increase in C2 deficiency in patients with systemic lupus erythematosus or juvenile rheumatoid arthritis was highly significant. From large population surveys,[71,72] the gene frequency for C2*Q0 is about 1 percent, in good agreement with the results of the case control study, and supporting the conclusion that the association between C2 deficiency and rheumatic diseases has not occurred by chance alone. Given the small numbers of cases and the absence of reliable estimates of gene frequencies for deficiencies of the other complement proteins, the significance of their association with rheumatic diseases is less certain. One tabulation indicated that 7 percent of patients with deficiencies of the late-acting (C5-C9) components had SLE or a related illness.[68]

Mechanism for Increased Frequency of Rheumatic Diseases. Since the genes for C4, C2, and factor B are located in the major histocompatibility complex, the same region that contains immune response genes, the association of complement deficiency and rheumatic diseases may reflect inheritance of an impaired immune response. This seems unlikely because (1) deficiency states with increased susceptibility include several components that are not linked to the MHC and (2) the range of diseases is such that a single etiologic agent is probably not responsible for all of them. Since virtually all of the diseases described have in common the finding of circulating immune complexes, impairment of the clearance or processing of such complexes may be involved. In some instances this may reflect faulty opsonization of the complexes for clearance by the phagocytic systems. In patients with hereditary angioedema who have low levels of C4 and no detectable C2 the survival of IgM-coated erythrocytes is grossly prolonged, essentially equivalent to that of erythrocytes never exposed to antibody. The clearance is normalized by prior exposure of the IgM-coated erythrocytes to a source of normal serum,[73] and is correlated with the deposition of C3b on the cell membranes. Patients with systemic lupus erythematosus also have defective clearance of antibody-coated erythrocytes, although this phenomenon seems more likely to be a result than a cause of their disease.[74]

Alternatively, the predisposition of complement-deficient individuals to immune complex diseases may reflect the function of complement in solubilizing such complexes.[75] This in vitro phenomenon is related to partial dissociation of the complexes by intercalation of C3b into the antigen-antibody lattice and is dependent on the function of the alternative pathway.[76] Sera from individuals deficient in the early-reacting components, in whom the overall prevalence of SLE was 41 percent, were ineffective in solubilizing immune complexes, whereas those with C5, C6, C7, or C8 deficiency, in whom the prevalence of SLE is much lower, were normally active in this regard.[68] The in vivo correlate of these in vitro findings with the pathogenesis of the disease remains to be demonstrated.

RECURRENT NEISSERIAL INFECTIONS IN DEFICIENCY OF MEMBRANE ATTACK COMPONENTS

Although not usually considered a "rheumatic" disease, recurrent or disseminated gonococcal infection is frequently encountered by the practicing rheumatologist. Although the capacity of serum to kill gram-negative bacteria in vitro had been known since the beginning of the century, only during the mid-1970s was the clinical correlate of this identified, namely increased *Neisseria* infections in individuals deficient in constituents of the membrane attack complex (C5-C9). The first such instance occurred in an 18-year-old female with chills, polyarthralgia, painful fingertip lesions, and a history of gonococcal arthritis some 13 months earlier; C6 deficiency was found.[77] The first patient with C8 deficiency also had recurrent gonococcal infection.[78] Both the C6- and the C8-deficient serum had no bactericidal activity against *N. gonorrhoeae,* but addition of the appropriate purified components restored this activity to normal. Patients with C5 deficiency or C7 deficiency have also been described with disseminated *Neisseria* infections.[64,79] Perhaps because C9 is not absolutely required for bacteriolysis, but merely accelerates the process,[80] only some cases of C9 deficiency have had problems with infection.[4] Among 24 cases of homozygous deficiency of C6, C7, or C8, 13 had at least one episode and usually two or more episodes of *Neisseria* meningitidis or *Neisseria* gonorrhoeae bacteremia, or both.[3] Even among sporadic cases of meningococcal disease, 3 of 20 patients had deficiencies of either C6 or C8, and 3 others had depletion of multiple complement proteins associated with underlying systemic lupus erythematosus.[81]

The striking association of late component deficiencies with recurrent infections, specifically *Neisseria* infections, has two implications. First, formation of the membrane attack complex and subsequent bacterial lysis has a central and probably critical role in host defense against serum-sensitive *Neisseria* organisms, particularly in preventing dissemination. Second, and most importantly for the rheumatologist, any patient with recurrent gonococcal infections should be screened for a deficiency of the late complement components by measurement of total hemolytic complement (CH50). Measurements most commonly available in clinical pathology laboratories, namely immunodiffusion tests for C3 and C4, will *not* detect deficiencies of the late-reacting components important in defense against *Neisseria*. While most complement-deficient individuals with *Neisseria* infections have responded promptly to appropriate antibiotic therapy, transfusions with fresh plasma might prove lifesaving when response to the more common therapeutic modalities remains unsatisfactory.

SUMMARY AND CONCLUSIONS

Deficiencies of individual complement proteins may be accompanied by systemic lupus erythematosus or related syndromes. Most commonly, deficiencies of the classic activation pathway are involved, including those induced secondarily by the disease hereditary angioedema. In the case of C2, the evidence is strong that this association occurs more frequently than would be expected by chance. Often the clinical picture differs from classic SLE. There is an increased frequency of skin involvement, a decreased frequency of renal disease, low or absent levels of antibody to native DNA, and infrequent deposits of immunoglobulins and complement in the skin. The mechanism for the association may involve impaired solublization of the immune complexes, a phenomenon dependent on the alternative pathway but also shown to be enhanced by the classic pathway. Disseminated and/or recurrent *Neisseria* infections are common in patients lacking the constituents of the terminal membrane attack complex.

REFERENCES

1. Agnello, V., de Bracco, M.M.E., and Kunkel, H.G.: Hereditary C2 deficiency with some manifestations of systemic lupus erythematosus. J. Immunol. 108:837, 1972.
2. Ruddy, S.: Complement, rheumatic diseases and the major histocompatibility complex. Clin. Rheum. Dis. 3:215, 1977.
3. Petersen, B.H., Lee, T.J., Snyderman, R., and Brooks, G.F.: *Neisseria* meningitidis and *Neisseria* gonorrhoeae bacteremia associated with C6, C7, or C8 deficiency. Ann. Intern. Med. 90:917, 1979.
4. Fine, D.P., Gewurz, H., Griffiss, M., and Lint, T.F.: Meningococcal meningitis in a woman with inherited deficiency of the ninth component of complement. Clin. Immunol. Immunopathol. 28:413, 1983.
5. Lachmann, P.J., and Rosen, F.S.: Genetic defects of complement in man. Springer Semin. Immunopathol. 1:339, 1978.
6. Colten, H.R., Alper, C.A., and Rosen, F.S.: Genetics and biosynthesis of complement proteins. N. Engl. J. Med. 304:653, 1981.
7. Colten, H.R.: Molecular genetics of the major histocompatibility linked complement genes. Springer Semin. Immunopathol. 6:149, 1983.
8. Kent, J.F., and Fife, E.H.: Precise standardization of reagents for complement fixation. Am. J. Trop. Med. 12:103, 1963.
9. Mayer, M.M.: Complement and complement fixation. *In* Kabat, E.A., and Mayer, M.M. (eds.): Experimental Immunochemistry. Springfield, Ill., Charles C. Thomas, 1961.
10. Ruddy, S., and Austen, K.F.: Complement and its components. *In* Cohen, A. (ed.): Laboratory Diagnostic Procedures in the Rheumatic Diseases. 2nd ed. Boston, Little, Brown & Company, 1975.
11. Mancini, G., Vaerman, J.P., Carbonara, A.O., and Heremans, J.F.: Single radial-diffusion method for immunological quantitation of protein. *In* Peeters, H. (ed.): Colloquium on the Protides of Biological Fluids. Proc. 10/11th Colloquium, Bruges 1962/1963. Amsterdam, Elsevier 2:370.

12. Laurell, C.B.: Quantitative estimation of proteins by electrophoresis in agarose gel containing antibodies. Anal. Biochem. 15:45, 1966.
13. Alexander, R.L., Jr.: Comparison of radial immunodiffusion and laser nephelometry for quantitating some serum proteins. Clin. Chem. 26:314, 1980.
14. Guiguet, M., Padieu, P., Mack, G., and Dalebroux, M.: Laser nephelometric measurement of seven serum proteins compared with radial immunodiffusion. J. Clin. Chem. Clin. Biochem. 21:217, 1983.
15. Rosen, F.S., Charache, P., Pensky, J., and Donaldson, V.: Hereditary angioneurotic edema: Two genetic variants. Science 148:957, 1965.
16. Tschopp, J., Esser, A.F., Spira, T.J., and Muller-Eberhard, H.J.: Occurrence of an incomplete C8 molecule in homozygous C8 deficiency in man. J. Exp. Med. 154:1599, 1981.
17. Platts-Mills, T.A., and Ishizaka, K.: Activation of the alternate pathway of complement by rabbit cells. J. Immunol. 113:348, 1974.
18. Hapke, M., and Patil, K.: The establishment of normal limits for serum proteins measured by the rate nephelometer. Concepts of normality revisited. Hum. Pathol. 12:1011, 1981.
19. Schur, P.H.: Genetics of complement deficiencies associated with lupuslike syndromes. Arthritis Rheum. 21:5153, 1978.
20. Izzet-Berkel, A., Sanal, O., Thesen, R., and Loos, M.: A case of selective C1q deficiency. Turk. J. Pediatr. 19:101, 1977.
21. Mampaso, F., Ecija, J., Fogue, L., Moneo, I., Gallego, N., and Leyva-Cobian, F.: Familial C1q deficiency in 3 siblings with glomerulonephritis and Rothmund-Thomson syndrome. Nephron 28:179, 1981.
22. Chapuis, R.M., Hauptmann, G., Grosshans, E., and Isliker, H.: Structural and functional studies in C1q deficiency. J. Immunol. 129:1509, 1982.
23. Pickering, R.J., Naff, G.B., Stroud, R.M., Good, R.A., and Gewurz, H.: Deficiency of C1r in human serum: Effects on the structure and function of macromolecular C1. J. Exp. Med. 131:803, 1970.
24. Moncada, B., Day, N.K.B., Good, R.A., and Windhorst, D.B.: Lupus-erythematosus-like syndrome with a familial defect of complement. N. Engl. J. Med. 286:689, 1972.
25. Day, N.K., Geiger, H., Stroud, R., de Bracco, M., Mancado, B., Windhorst, D., and Good, R.A.: C1r deficiency: An inborn error associated with cutaneous and renal disease. J. Clin. Invest. 51:1102, 1972.
26. Mittal, K.K., Wolski, K.P., Lim, D., Gewurz, A., Gewurz, H., and Schmid, F.R.: Genetic independence between the HLA-A system and deficits in the first and sixth component of complement. Tissue Antigens 7:97, 1976.
27. Pondman, K.W., Stoop, J.W., Cormane, R.H., and Hannema, A.J.: Abnormal C1 in a patient with systemic lupus erythematosus (abstract). J. Immunol. 101:811A, 1968.
28. Chase, P.H., Barone, R., Blum, L., and Wallace, S.L.: "Lupus-like" syndrome associated with deficiency of C1s: Family studies. Ann. R. Coll. Phys. Surg. 9:93, 1976.
29. Donaldson, V.H., and Evans, R.R.: A biochemical abnormality in hereditary angioneurotic edema. Absence of serum inhibitor of C'1-esterase. Am. J. Med. 35:37, 1963.
30. Ruddy, S., and Austen, K.F.: Inherited abnormalities of the complement system in the human. *In* Stanbury, J.B., Wyngaarden, J.B., and Fredrickson, D.S. (eds.): The Metabolic Basis of Inherited Disease. 4th ed. New York, McGraw-Hill Book Company, 1978.
31. Kohler, P.F., Percy, J., Campion, W.M., and Smyth, C.: Hereditary angioedema and "familial" lupus erythematosus in identical twin boys. Am. J. Med. 56:406, 1974.
32. Rosenfeld, G.B., Partridge, R.E.H., Bartholomew, W., Murphey, W.H., and Singleton, C.M.: Hereditary angioneurotic edema (HANE) and systemic lupus erythematosus (SLE) in one of identical twin girls. J. Allergy Clin. Immunol. 53:68, 1974.
33. Donaldson, V.H., Hess, E.V., and McAdams, A.J.: Lupus erythematosus-like disease in three unrelated women with hereditary angioneurotic edema. Ann. Intern. Med. 86:312, 1977.
34. Awdeh, Z.L., Ochs, H.D., and Alper, C.A.: Genetic analysis of C4 deficiency. J. Clin. Invest. 67:260, 1981.
35. Fielder, A.H., Walport, M.J., Batchelor, J.R., Rynes, R.I., Black, C.M., Dodi, I.A., and Hughes, G.R.: Family study of the major histocompatibility complex in patients with systemic lupus erythematosus: Importance of null alleles of C4A and C4B in determining disease susceptibility. Br. Med. J. 286:425, 1983.
36. Schroder, R., Zander, H., Andreas, A., and Mauff, G.: Multiple sclerosis: Immunogenetic analyses of sib pair double case families. II. Studies on the association of multiple sclerosis with C2, C4, BF, C3, C6, and GL0 polymorphisms. Immunobiology 164:160, 1983.
37. McCluskey, J., McCann, V.J., Kay, P.H., Zilko, P.J., Christiansen, F.T., O'Neill, G.J., and Dawkins, R.L.: HLA and complement allotypes in Type 1 (insulin dependent) diabetes. Diabetologia 24:162, 1983.
38. Hauptmann, G., Grosshans, E., and Heid, E.: Lupus érythémateux aigus et déficits héréditaires en complement. À propos d'un cas par déficit complet en C4. Ann. Dermatol. Syphil. 101:479, 1974.
39. Ochs, H.D., Rosenfeld, S.I., Thomas, E.D., Giblett, E.R., Alper, C.A., du Pont, B., Schaller, J.G., Gilliladd, B.C., Hansen, J.A., and Wedgwood, R.J.: Linkage between the gene (or genes) controlling synthesis

of the fourth component of complement and the major histocompatibility complex. N. Engl. J. Med. 296:470, 1977.

40. Tappeiner, G., Hintner, H., Scholz, S., Albert, E., Linert, J., and Wolff, K.: Systemic lupus erythematosus in hereditary deficiency of the fourth component of complement. J. Am. Acad. Dermatol. 7:66, 1982.
41. Ballow, M., McLean, R.H., Yunis, E.J., Awdeh, Z.L., O'Neill, G.J., Einarson, M., and Alper, C.A.: C4 polymorphism and HLA linkage: Studies in a family with hereditary C4 deficiency. Clin. Immunol. Immunopathol. 20:354, 1981.
42. Tappeiner, G.: Personal communication.
43. Hersey, P., Lawrence, S., Prendergast, D., Bindon, C., Benson, W., and Valk, P.: Association of Sjögren's syndrome with C4 deficiency, defective reticuloendothelial function and circulating immune complexes. Clin. Exp. Immunol. 52:551, 1983.
44. Mascart-Lemone, F., Hauptmann, G., Goetz, J., Duchateau, J., Delespesse, G., Vray, B., and Dab, I.: Genetic deficiency of C4 presenting with recurrent infections and an SLE-like disease. Genetic and immunologic studies. Am. J. Med. 75:295, 1983.
45. Agnello, V.: Complement deficiency states. Medicine 57:1, 1978.
46. Rynes, R.I.: Inherited complement deficiency states and SLE. Clin. Rheum. Dis. 8:29, 1982.
47. Glass, D., Raum, D., Gibson, D., Stillman, J.S., and Schur, P.H.: Inherited deficiency of the second component of complement. Rheumatic disease associations. J. Clin. Invest. 58:853, 1976.
48. Klemperer, M.R., Woodworth, H.C., Rosen, F.S., and Austen, K.F.: Deficiency of the second component of complement (C2) in man. J. Clin. Invest. 45:880, 1966.
49. Klemperer, M.R., Austen, K.F., and Rosen, F.S.: Hereditary deficiency of the second component of complement (C2) in man: Further observations of a second kindred. J. Immunol. 98:72, 1967.
50. Day, N.K., Geiger, H., McLean, R., Michael, A., and Good, R.A.: C2 deficiency. Development of lupus erythematosus. J. Clin. Invest. 52:1601, 1973.
51. Fu, S.M., Kunkel, H.G., Brusman, H.P., Allen, F.H., Jr., and Fotino, M.: Evidence for linkage between HL-A. Histocompatibility genes and those involved in the synthesis of the second component of complement. J. Exp. Med. 140:1108, 1974.
52. Raum, D., Glass, D., Carpenter, C.B., Alper, C.A., and Schur, P.H.: The chromosomal order of genes controlling the major histocompatibility complex, properdin factor B, and deficiency of the second component of complement. J. Clin. Invest. 58:1240, 1976.
53. Hauptmann, G., Tongio, M.M., Goetz, J., Mayer, S., Fauchet, R., Sobel, A., Griscel, C., Berthoux, F., Rivat, C., and Rother, U.: Association of the C2 deficiency gene (C2Q*0) with the C4A*4, C4B*2 genes. J. Immunogenet. 9:127, 1982.
54. Alper, C.A., Colten, H.R., and Rosen, F.S.: Homozygous deficiency of C3 in a patient with repeated infections. Lancet 2:1179, 1972.
55. Ballow, M., Shira, J.E., Harden, L., Yang, S.Y., and Day, N.K.: Complete absence of the third component of complement in man. J. Clin. Invest. 56:703, 1975.
56. Davis, A.E., III, Davis, J.S., Rabson, A.R., Osofsky, S.G., Colten, H.R., Rosen, F.S., and Alper, C.A.: Homozygous C3 deficiency: Detection of C3 by radioimmunoassay. Clin. Immunol. Immunopathol. 8:543, 1978.
57. Hsieh, K.H., Lin, C.Y., and Lee, T.C.: Complete absence of the third component of complement in a patient with repeated infections. Clin. Immunol. Immunopathol. 20:305, 1981.
58. Sano, Y., Nishimukai, H., Kitamura, J., Nagaki, K., Inai, S., Hamasaki, Y., Maruyama, I., and Igata, A.: Hereditary deficiency of the third component of complement in two sisters with systemic lupus erythematosus-like symptoms. Arthritis Rheum. 24:1255, 1981.
59. Toord, J.J., Daha, M., Kuis, W., Verbrugh, H.A., Verhoef, J., Zegers, B.H., and Stoop, J.W.: Inherited deficiency of the third component of complement associated with recurrent pyogenic infections, circulating immune complexes, and vasculitis in a Dutch family. Pediatrics 71:81, 1983.
60. McLean, R.H., Weinstein, A., Chaptitis, J., Lowenstein, M., and Rothfield, N.F.: Familial partial deficiency of the third component of complement

(C3) and the hypocomplementemic cutaneous vasculitis syndrome. Am. J. Med. 68:549, 1980.
61. Osofsky, S.G., Thompson, B.H., Lint, T.F., and Gewurz, H.: Hereditary deficiency of the third component of complement in a child with fever, skin rash and arthralgias, and response to whole blood transfusion. J. Pediatr. 90:180, 1977.
62. Snyderman, R., Durack, D.T., McCarty, G.A., Ward, F.E., and Meadows, L.: Deficiency of the fifth component of complement in human subjects. Clinical, genetic and immunologic studies in a large kindred. Am. J. Med. 67:638, 1979.
63. Haeney, M.R., Thompson, R.A., Faulkner, J., Mackintosh, P., and Ball, A.P.: Recurrent bacterial meningitis in patients with genetic defects of terminal complement components. Clin. Exp. Immunol. 40:16, 1980.
64. Peter, G., Weiger, M.B., Bissel, A.R., Gold, R., Kreutzer, D., and McLean, R.H.: Meningococcal meningitis in familial deficiency of the fifth component of complement. Pediatrics 67:882, 1981.
65. Rosenfeld, S.I., Kelly, M.E., and Leddy, J.P.: Hereditary deficiency of the fifth component of complement in man. I. Clinical immunochemical and family studies. J. Clin. Invest. 57:1626, 1976.
66. Rosenfeld, S.E., Baum, J., Steigbigel, R.T., and Leddy, J.P.: Hereditary deficiency of the fifth component of complement in man. II. Biological properties of C5 deficient human serum. J. Clin. Invest. 57:1635, 1976.
67. Boyer, J.T., Gall, E.P., Norman, M.E., Nilsson, U.R., and Zimmerman, T.S.: Hereditary deficiency of the seventh component of complement. J. Clin. Invest. 56:905, 1975.
68. Zeitz, H.J., Miller, G.W., Lint, T.F., Ali, M.A., and Gewurz, H.: Deficiency of C7 with systemic lupus erythematosus: Solubilization of immune complexes in complement deficient sera. Arthritis Rheum. 24:87, 1981.
69. Alcalay, M., Bontoux, D., Wautier, J.I., Vilde, J.M., Vial, M.C., and Peltier, A.P.: Déficit héréditaire en 7e composant du complément avec trouble de l'agrégation plaquettaire, associé à une polyarthrite rhumatoïde. Une observation. Nouv. Presse Med. 9:2147, 1980.
70. Jasin, H.E.: Absence of the eighth component of complement in association with systemic lupus erythematosus-like disease. J. Clin. Invest. 60:709, 1977.
71. Hässig, Von A., Borel, J.F., Ammann, P., Thoni, M., and Butler, R.: Essentielle hypokomplementämie. Pathol. Microbiol. 27:542, 1964.
72. Torisu, M., Arata, M., and Majima, H.: Low reactivity of human complement in healthy adults. Japan J. Exp. Med. 36:251, 1966.
73. Atkinson, J.P., and Frank, M.M.: Studies on the in vivo effects of antibody: Interaction of IgM antibody and complement in the immune clearance and destruction of erythrocytes in man. J. Clin. Invest. 54:339, 1974.
74. Frank, M.M., Hamburger, M.I., Lawley, T.J., Kimberley, R.P., and Plotz, P.H.: Defective reticuloendothelial system Fc receptor function in systemic lupus erythematosus. N. Engl. J. Med. 300:518, 1979.
75. Miller, G.W., and Nussenzweig, V.: A new complement function: Solubilization of antigen antibody aggregates. Proc. Natl. Acad. Sci. USA 72:418, 1975.
76. Takahashi, M., Takahashi, S., and Hirose, S.: Solubilization of antigen antibody complexes: a new function of complement as a regulator of immune reactions. Prog. Allergy 27:418, 1975.
77. Leddy, J.P., Frank, M.M., Gaither, T., Baum, J., and Klemperer, M.R.: Hereditary deficiency of the sixth component of complement in man: I. Immunochemical, biologic and family studies. J. Clin. Invest. 53:544, 1974.
78. Petersen, B.H., Graham, J.A., and Brooks, G.F.: Human deficiency of the 8th component of complement. The requirement of C8 for serum Neisseria gonorrhoeae bactericidal activity. J. Clin. Invest. 57:283, 1976.
79. Lee, T.J., Utsinger, P.D., Snyderman, R., Yount, W.J., and Sparling, P.F.: Familial deficiency of the seventh component of complement associated with recurrent bacteremic infections due to Neisseria. J. Infect. Dis. 138:359, 1978.
80. Lint, T.F., Zeitz, H.J., and Gewurz, H.: Genetic aspects of deficiency of the ninth component of complement in man. Immunobiology 15:107, 1980.
81. Ellison, R.T., Kohler, P.F., Curd, J.G., Judson, F.N., and Reller, L.B.: Prevalence of congenital or acquired complement deficiency in patients with sporadic meningococcal disease. N. Engl. J. Med. 308:913, 1983.

Section XIII
Crystal-Induced Synovitis

Chapter 86

Gout and Related Disorders of Purine Metabolism

William N. Kelley and Irving H. Fox

INTRODUCTION

"Gout is a term representing a heterogeneous group of diseases found exclusively in man, which in their full development are manifest by (a) an increase in the serum urate concentration; (b) recurrent attacks of a characteristic type of acute arthritis, in which crystals of monosodium urate monohydrate are demonstrable in leukocytes of synovial fluid; (c) aggregated deposits of nosodium urate monohydrate (tophi) occurring chiefly in and around the joints of the extremities and sometimes leading to severe crippling and deformity; (d) renal disease involving glomerular, tubular, and interstitial tissues and blood vessels; and (e) uric acid urolithiasis. These manifestations can occur in different combinations."[1]

HISTORY

Gout has been called the "king of diseases" and the "disease of kings." Several excellent narrative and pictorial histories of gout have appeared.[2-10] The major events in the history of gout are summarized in Table 86–1.

EPIDEMIOLOGY

A true serum urate value above 7.0 mg per 100 ml is abnormal: in physiochemical terms it represents supersaturation; in epidemiologic terms it carries an increased risk of gout or renal stones. This value corresponds to a concentration of 7.5 to 8.0 mg per 100 ml as determined by chemical methods and automatic analyzers.

A variety of factors appear to be associated with higher mean serum urate concentration. Studies of several indigenous Pacific peoples have disclosed populations with mean serum urate levels significantly higher than those in Caucasian populations.[1] Serum urate values show positive correlations with weight and with surface area in peoples of widely differing races and cultures throughout the world,[12] although specific exceptions do exist. For example, in epidemiologic studies body bulk (as estimated by body weight, surface area, or ponderal index) has proved to be one of the most important predictors of hyperuricemia.[13] Numerous studies have also described an association of higher serum urate values with greater intelligence, drive, achievement, leadership, range of activities, and/or education.[1] In commenting upon these associations, Acheson and Chan[13] have expressed the situation well by stating, "The associates of a high uric acid are the associates of plenty."

The serum urate concentration varies with the age and sex of the patient.[14] Children of both sexes normally have a serum urate concentration in the range of 3 to 4 mg per 100 ml. At puberty, males exhibit a further elevation in the serum urate concentration of 1 to 2 mg per 100 ml, which is generally sustained throughout life, while females exhibit little if any change in the serum urate concentration at this time; at menopause, however, the serum urate concentration rises and begins to approach the value for adult males.

Physiologic determinants of serum urate levels in adolescence include sexual and skeletal maturation in early stages and body composition (skin-fold thickness and body mass index), blood pressure, and hematocrit in later stages.[15] In adults serum urate levels correlate strongly with serum creatinine, body weight, height, age, urea nitrogen, blood pressure, and alcohol intake.[16-18]

The incidence of gout in populations varies from 0.20 to 0.35 per 1000, with an overall prevalence of 2 to 2.6 per 1000.[18-20] The prevalence seems to increase substantially with age and increasing serum urate concentration.[17,18] For example, the prevalence was 15 per 1000 in males in the 35 to 44 age range.[17]

CLINICAL FEATURES

In the full development of its natural history, gout passes through four stages, termed asymptomatic hyperuricemia, acute gouty arthritis, intercritical gout, and chronic tophaceous gout.

Table 86–1. Major Events in the History of Gout

Date	Event	Author(s)	Reference
5th century B.C.	Aphorisms on gout	Hippocrates	11
1st century A.D.	Familial nature	Seneca	475
3rd century	Tophi described	Galen	476
13th century	The term gout originated	de Vielehardouin	2
1679	Crystals in gouty tophi	van Leeuwenhoek	477
1776	Uric acid in stones	Scheele	478
1797	Urate in tophi	Wollaston	479
1814	Specificity of colchicine in acute gout	Want	480
1848	Hyperuricemia in gout	Garrod	481
1899	Urate crystals cause gouty arthritis	Freudweiler	300
1950	Introduction of effective uricosuric agents	Talbott	482
		Gutman and Yu	483
1963	Introduction of allopurinol	Rundles et al.	484
1967	First specific enzyme defect described in patients with gout	Kelley et al.	248

Asymptomatic Hyperuricemia

Asymptomatic hyperuricemia is that stage in which the serum urate level is raised but arthritic symptoms, tophi, or uric acid stones have not yet appeared. In male subjects at risk from the classic form of primary gout this stage begins at puberty, whereas in females at risk hyperuricemia is usually delayed until menopause. By contrast, in patients with hyperuricemia secondary to a specific enzyme deficiency, this trait is present from birth.

Asymptomatic hyperuricemia usually lasts throughout the lifetime of the individual with no recognizable consequences. The tendency toward acute gout increases with the height of the serum urate concentration value. The risk of nephrolithiasis increases with the height of the serum urate value and with the magnitude of the daily uric acid excretion.[1] The approach to the patient with asymptomatic hyperuricemia is discussed in Chapter 33.

The phase of asymptomatic hyperuricemia ends with the first attack of gouty arthritis or of urolithiasis. In most instances gout comes first and usually after at least 20 to 30 years of sustained hyperuricemia. However, between 10 and 40 percent of gouty subjects will have had one or more attacks of renal colic prior to the first articular event, sometimes more than a decade earlier. A diagnosis of gout should be reserved for the disease marked by urate crystal deposition and an associated inflammatory tissue response and not used to describe the patient with hyperuricemia and/or renal stones.

Acute Gouty Arthritis

The basic pattern of clinical gout is one of acute attacks of exquisitely painful arthritis, at first usually monarticular and associated with few constitutional symptoms, later often polyarticular and febrile, lasting a variable but limited period of time and separated by intervals of complete freedom from all symptoms. Attacks recur at shorter intervals and eventually resolve incompletely, leaving chronic arthritis which progresses slowly to a crippling disease upon which acute exacerbations are superimposed with decreasing frequency and severity. The peak age of onset of acute gouty arthritis is between the fourth and sixth decades[21-24] in various studies. There is a marked predominance for males with a peak age of onset at 50 years.[25] Onset before the age of 30 should raise the question of an unusual form of gout, perhaps related to a specific enzymatic defect that leads to marked overproduction of purines, or rarely to an unusual form of parenchymal renal disease.

In about 85 to 90 percent of first attacks a single joint will be involved. In at least one half of initial acute attacks the first metatarsophalangeal joint will be the site of the paroxysm (podagra). In Scudamore's[26] series of 516 cases collected in 1817, 60 percent of initial attacks involved the great toe of one foot only. Both great toes were involved simultaneously in 5 percent of subjects in the first attack. The percentage of patients in whom the initial attack is polyarticular varies from 3 to 14 percent.

Ninety percent of gouty patients experience acute attacks in the great toe at some time during the course of their disease. Next in order of frequency as sites of initial involvement are the insteps, ankles, heels, knees, wrists, fingers, and elbows. Acute gout is predominantly a disease of the lower extremity, but any joint of any extremity may be involved. Acute attacks may affect the shoulders, hips, spine, sacroiliac, and sternoclavicular and mandibular joints, but attacks at such sites are very rare. The more distal the site of involvement, the more typical is the character of the attack. Acute gouty bursitis occurs and mainly involves the prepatellar or olecranon bursa.[27]

Some patients report numerous short trivial episodes of "ankle sprains," or sore heels, or twinges of pain in the great toe, prior to the first dramatic gouty attack, sometimes going back over several years. The patient may "walk these off" in a few hours. However, in most patients the initial visitation of the gout occurs with explosive suddenness during apparent excellent health.

Commonly the first attack begins at night. In some patients symptoms are first detected when the foot is placed on the floor after awakening. In others, the pain awakens the victim. Within a few hours the affected joint becomes hot, dusky red, and extremely tender. Initially, the joint is only slightly swollen, but signs of inflammation may progress to resemble a bacterial cellulitis, and on occasion the joint is incised by an unwary physician intent on draining pus. Occasionally, lymphangitis may be evident. Systemic signs of inflammation may include leukocytosis, fever, and elevation of the erythrocyte sedimentation rate.

It is difficult to improve upon Sydenham's[28] classic description of the acute attack:

The victim goes to bed and sleeps in good health. About two o'clock in the morning he is awakened by a severe pain in the great toe; more rarely in the heel, ankle or instep. This pain is like that of a dislocation, and yet the parts feel as if cold water were poured over them. Then follow chills and shivers and a little fever. The pain, which was at first moderate, becomes more intense. With its intensity the chills and shivers increase. After a time this comes to its full height, accommodating itself to the bones and ligaments of the tarsus and metatarsus. Now it is a violent stretching and tearing of the ligaments—now it is a gnawing pain and now a pressure and tightening. So exquisite and lively meanwhile is the feeling of the part affected, that it cannot bear the weight of bedclothes nor the jar of a person walking in the room. The night is passed in torture, sleeplessness, turning of the part affected, and perpetual change of posture; the tossing about of the body being as incessant as the pain of the tortured joint, and being worse as the fit comes on. Hence the vain effort by change of posture, both in the body and the limb affected, to obtain an abatement of the pain.

The course of untreated acute gout is highly variable. Mild attacks may subside in several hours or persist for only a day or two, and never reach the intensity described by Sydenham. Severe attacks may last days to weeks. The skin over the joint may desquamate as the attack subsides. Upon recovery the patient will re-enter an asymptomatic phase termed the intercritical period. Resolution is usually complete, and the patient is once again perfectly well.

Provocative factors may include trauma, alcohol ingestion, certain drugs, surgery, dietary excess, hemorrhage, venisection, foreign protein therapy, infections, and x-ray therapy.

Intercritical Gout

The intervals between gouty attacks are called intercritical periods. Some patients never have a second attack. In others, the next attack occurs after an intercritical period of 5 to 10 years. In most patients a second attack occurs within 6 months to 2 years. In Gutman's[29] series, 62 percent had recurrences within the first year, 16 percent in 1 to 2 years, 11 percent in 2 to 5 years, 4 percent in 5 to 10 years, and 7 percent no recurrence in 10 or more years. The frequency of the gouty attacks usually increases with time in the untreated patients. Later attacks are often polyarticular, more severe, longer, and perhaps febrile. Roentgenographic changes may develop, and the attacks may abate more gradually than before, but the joints may nevertheless recover complete symptomless function.

One third of patients with late polyarticular attacks report that their initial attack was also polyarticular.[30] In polyarticular gout, 83 percent of all joints involved are of the lower extremity. Curiously, in one third of patients with this form of gout the foot is spared. Various joints may be involved in sequence in a migratory attack, which may include subdeltoid or olecranon bursitis, Achilles tendon involvement, or affliction at other para-articular sites. Eventually the patient may enter a phase of chronic polyarticular gout with no pain-free intercritical periods. At this stage gout may be easily confused with rheumatoid or degenerative arthritis.

The course described above is the usual one. If the patient is seen late in the disease, a clear and detailed description of the initial attacks and of the completely asymptomatic intervals between attacks of sudden onset and rapid offset can usually be obtained, and is exceedingly valuable in pointing toward the correct diagnosis. However, not all patients will have followed this course. Rarely the disease may run a fulminant febrile course. In addition, a percentage of patients will progress directly from the initial acute attack into a subchronic and then chronic illness, with no remissions and early development of tophi and incapacity.

The diagnosis of gout in a hyperuricemic patient with a past history of acute attacks of monarthritis may be difficult or inconclusive during the intercritical phase. However, aspiration of an asymptomatic metatarsophalangeal joint may be a useful adjunct in the diagnosis of gout if extracellular urate crystals are demonstrated.[31,32] In renal failure this test is limited by false-positive results. Crystals have also been observed in the asymptomatic knee joints of patients with tophaceous gout.[33]

Chronic Tophaceous Gout

The duration of time from the initial attack to the beginning of chronic symptoms of visible tophaceous involvement was highly variable in the untreated patient, ranging in the experience of Hench[34] from 3 to 42 years, with an average of 11.6 years. Ten years after the first acute attack about half were still nontophaceous and most of the remainder still had only minimal deposits. Thereafter the proportion of nontophaceous patients slowly declined to 28 percent after 20 years. The percentage of patients with severe crippling disease reached appreciable proportions (24 percent) only some 20 years after the initial attack.

The principal determinant of the rate of urate deposition in and about the joints is the serum urate level. In Gutman's[35] series, the mean serum urate concentration was 9.1 mg per 100 ml (uricase method) in 722 nontophaceous patients, 10 to 11 mg per 100 ml in 456 patients with minimal to moderate tophaceous deposits, and greater than 11.0 mg per 100 ml in 111 patients with extensive tophaceous involvement. The rate of formation of tophaceous deposits in primary gout is thus a direct function of the degree and duration of hyperuricemia. The rate of formation of tophi is also correlated with the severity of renal disease, which in turn is related to the duration of hyperuricemia as well as being a factor in determining its degree.[36] The ability to control hyperuricemia in recent years has been associated with a striking reduction in the frequency with which tophi develop in the gouty population. The decreasing incidence of tophi in patients with gout is shown in Table 86–2. Tophaceous gout has been observed in as few as 9.2 percent of a large gouty population.[25]

Tophaceous gout is a consequence of the progressive inability to dispose of urate as rapidly as it is produced. The urate pool expands and crystalline deposits of urate appear in cartilage, synovial membranes, tendons, soft tissues, and elsewhere. Occasionally, palpable tophi may be present at the time of the initial acute attack. This is very unusual in primary gout, but was recorded by Yu[37] in nearly 0.5 percent of subjects with gout secondary to myeloproliferative disease, and may also occur in juvenile gout, for example complicating glycogen storage disease[38] or the Lesch-Nyhan syndrome.[39]

A classic location of tophi is the helix or, less commonly, the antihelix of the ear (Fig. 86–1 and 86–2). Tophaceous deposits may produce irregular asymmetrical, moderately discrete tumescences of fingers (Fig. 86–3), hands (Figs. 86–4, and 86–5) knees, or feet (Fig. 86–6), requiring larger gloves or shoes. The classic gouty shoe is one with a window cut to accommodate an irregularly prominent joint, usually the first metatarsophalangeal. Tophi commonly form lumps along the ulnar surface of the forearm, or saccular distentions of olecranon bursae (Figs. 86–7 and 86–8), or fusiform or lumpy enlargements of the Achilles tendon (Fig. 86–9). Occasionally they develop subcutaneously along the tibial surface.

As tophi and renal disease advance, acute attacks recur less frequently and are milder; late in the illness they may disappear altogether. Those that occur may be superimposed on the indolent soreness of an involved joint, or may seek out new locations of previously uninvolved sites.

The process of tophaceous deposition advances insid-

Figure 86–1. Tophus of the helix of the ear adjacent to the auricular tubercle.

iously, and although the tophi themselves are relatively painless, there is often progressive stiffness and persistant aching of affected joints. Eventually extensive destruction of joints and large subcutaneous tophi may lead to grotesque deformities, particularly of hands and feet, and to progressive crippling. The tense, shiny thin skin overlying the tophus may ulcerate and extrude white chalky or pasty material composed of myriads of fine needlelike crystals. Bony ankylosis may rarely occur.[40]

Rarely, tophi suppurate; they may produce a marked limitation of joint movement by the direct involvement of the joint structure or of tendons serving the joint.

Table 86–2. Changing Trend in the Incidence of Tophi in Primary Gout*

Years	Patients (No.)	Tophi	
		No.	%
1948–1953	165	88	53
1954–1958	369	154	42
1959–1963	522	172	33
1964–1968	355	112	32
1969–1973	289	49	17
Total	1700	575	—

*From Yu, T.-F.: Am J. Med. 56:676, 1974. Reproduced by permission of the American Journal of Medicine.

Figure 86–2. Multiple tophi of the helix of the ear.

Figure 86–3. Tophus of fifth digit, with smaller tophus over fourth proximal interphalangeal joint.

Any joint may be involved, although those of the lower extremity are chiefly affected. Spinal joints do not escape urate deposition, but acute gouty spondylitis is very unusual. Symptoms related to spinal cord compression by tophi have been rarely observed.[41,42] Tophi may also occur in myocardium, mitral valve, cardiac conduction system, and various parts of the eye, as well as the larynx. Prior to the advent of antihyperuricemic agents, 50 to

Figure 86–4. Tophi of dorsal aspects of index and second fingers, over distal interphalangeal joints. Subcutaneous urate deposits are easily visible. (From Zollner, N.: *In* Heilmeyer, L., et al. (eds.): Ergebnisse der innern Medizin und Kinderheilkunde. 14th ed. Berlin, Springer-Verlag, 1960, p. 376.)

Figure 86–5. Chronic tophaceous gout of severe degree, with bulbous enlargements of several fingers. Note sparing of fourth finger of right hand. (Courtesy of Dr. R. Wayne Rundles, Duke University Medical Center.)

70 percent of gouty patients developed visible tophi, permanent joint changes, or chronicity of symptoms.[43,44]

Radiologic Findings

Soft tissue swelling, osteopenia, and aseptic necrosis may occur as nonspecific x-ray manifestations early in the disease. More typical radiologic changes, particularly erosions (sharply marginated lucent pockets), occur with the development of tophi. Other radiologic findings observed include lace pattern, intracortical lesions, subchondral compressions, chondrocalcinosis, and intraosseus calcifications.[45-47] See Chapter 39 for further discussion.

Figure 86–6. Chronic gouty arthritis of feet, with enlargement of right metatarsophalangeal joint, enlargement of two toes, and a draining sinus of a third.

Figure 86–7. Lumpy tophi of olecranon bursa, ulnar surface, and wrist.

Associated Conditions

Obesity. The association of gout with obesity and overeating has been recognized for hundreds of years.[6,48-51] In 6000 subjects in Tecumseh, Michigan, hyperuricemia was found in only 3.4 percent of those with a relative weight at or below the twentieth percentile, in 5.7 percent of those between the twenty-first and seventy-ninth percentile, and in 11.4 percent of those at or above the eightieth percentile.[52] Other recent population studies have also demonstrated a positive correlation between serum urate and weight or body surface area.[53-57]

As expected from the data cited above, obesity is also common in subjects selected because of hyperuricemia or gout. Gouty patients show body weights above ideal values for age and height in a large percentage of subjects. Emmerson and Knowles[58] noted that subjects with primary gout were an average of 17.8 percent overweight (compared with patients with lead gout who were an average of 1.3 percent overweight). Brochner-Mortensen[59] found that 78 percent of his gouty subjects were more than 10 percent overweight and 57 percent more than 30 percent overweight. Grahame and Scott[60] noted that 48 percent of 355 patients with gout were more than 15 percent overweight. Obesity seems to be the common factor relating diabetes,[61-63] hyperlipidemia,[64] hypertension,[65] and atherosclerosis.[52]

Diabetes Mellitus. Hyperuricemia has been reported in 2 to 50 percent of patients with diabetes, whereas gouty arthritis has been reported in from less than 0.1 percent to 9.0 percent of diabetic subjects.[66] Abnormal

Figure 86–8. Saccular tophaceous enlargements of olecranon bursae, with small cutaneous deposits of overlying skin.

Figure 86–9. Tophi of Achilles tendons and their insertions in a black patient with gout.

glucose tolerance tests have been noted in 7 to 74 percent of patients with gout,[66-70] depending, in part, on the criteria used. When overt clinical diabetes is present in such patients, it tends to be mild. Engelhardt and Wagner[61] called attention to obesity as an integral part of a triad with gout and diabetes; others have since noted this association.[61,63] Thus obesity may predispose to both hyperuricemia and hyperglycemia.

Despite the apparent high incidence of hyperuricemia in patients selected for diabetes, and of glucose intolerance in patients selected for gout, epidemiologic studies have not demonstrated any relation between gout and diabetes or between serum urate and blood glucose concentrations.[52,66,71] In such studies the mean serum urate concentration is actually lower in patients with overt diabetes. This has been attributed to the apparent uricosuric effect of high blood glucose levels.[72-74]

Hyperlipidemia. Hypertriglyceridemia has been reported in 75 to 84 percent of patients with gout[49,69,75-77] and hyperuricemia in up to 82 percent of patients with hypertriglyceridemia.[77] A rank order correlation of serum urate and serum triglyceride values has been described[77] but also disclaimed.[64] The gouty patients who drank alcohol excessively had a mean serum triglyceride level that was higher than that of their obesity-matched controls and that of nondrinking gouty patients. It appears that diet and possibly defective clearance of triglyceride may be the etiologic factors associated with elevated triglycerides and lipoprotein concentrations in gouty individuals.[78] Since these lipid abnormalities are not present in first-degree relatives of gouty subjects, the abnormalities appear to be more a reflection of the lifestyle of the patient than genetic factors.[79]

Although individual gouty subjects are frequently hypercholesterolemic,[80,81] many studies have failed to show a correlation between serum urate and cholesterol values.[49,58,76,77,82,83] Gibson and Grahame[64] reported that serum cholesterol values of their gouty patients did not differ significantly from either weight-matched or unmatched controls.

Hypertension. Hyperuricemia has been reported in 22 to 38 percent of untreated hypertensives.[84-86] This is significantly greater than the prevalence of hyperuricemia expected in an unselected population. When therapy and renal disease are not excluded, the prevalence increases to 47 to 67 percent.[84-88] The overall prevalence of gout in hypertension has been variously reported as 2 to 12 percent.[85,87]

The prevalence of hyperuricemia in the general population rises with increases of diastolic or systolic blood pressure in both males and females. However, there is no consistent pattern relating hyperuricemia to the interaction of diastolic and systolic blood pressures. Furthermore, when serum urate values are standardized for population variables of weight, age, and anthropometric measurements, there is only random variation of hyperuricemia and diastolic and systolic pressures in relation to one another.[60] In the population study of 6000 residents of Tecumseh, Michigan, Myers and associates[52] found no correlation between serum urate concentrations adjusted for age, sex, and relative body weight, and levels of blood pressure.

Hypertension is present in one fourth to one half of patients with classic gout.[89-92] The incidence of both moderate and severe hypertension was unrelated to duration of gout, but that of moderate hypertension rose with increasing age of onset. The incidence of severe hypertension was greatest in the group with onset of gout in the second decade. Moderate hypertension was more common in obese than in nonobese subjects.

The serum urate concentration correlates inversely with renal blood flow and urate clearance, and directly with renal vascular and total resistance.[93-96] Therefore, the association between hypertension and hyperuricemia may be related to reduction of renal blood flow in the former condition. Furthermore, it has been proposed that an elevation of the serum urate concentration may be an indicator of renal vascular involvement in essential hypertension.

Atherosclerosis. In 1951 Gertler and coworkers[50] noted a statistically significant excess of hyperuricemia in a group of young patients with coronary heart disease. Several other reports have noted the association of hyperuricemia with the manifestations of atherosclerosis[97-101] and hyperuricemia has been proposed as a risk factor for coronary heart disease.[102] In the Tecumseh study,[52,103] there was no clear association between levels of blood pressure, blood sugar, or serum cholesterol and serum urate concentrations when adjustments were made for effects of age, sex, and relative weight. When these variables were taken into account, the figures showed that the serum urate levels of persons with coronary heart disease were not significantly different from the mean of the population. Myers and associates[52] concluded that an elevated serum urate concentration value could not be taken as an attribute associated with coronary heart disease.

In a retrospective study on the cause of death in patients with gout treated with antihyperuricemic drugs,[104] however, cerebrovascular disease and cardiovascular disease accounted for more than 50 percent of the mortality. The majority of these patients had either hypertension or hyperlipidemia. It seems likely that in patients with hyperuricemia, clinical correlates such as hypertension, diabetes mellitus, hyperlipidemia, and obesity[104-109] may all contribute to the observed association between elevated serum urate concentration and arteriosclerosis.

Negative Disease Associations. A negative association appears to exist between gout and specific rheumatologic disorders such as systemic lupus erythematosus,[110-112] rheumatoid arthritis,[113-116] and amyloidosis.[117,118] The basis for the decreased concurrence of these disorders, however, is unclear. In the former two diseases there is a disparity of the population that each disease affects. There may be difficulty in distinguishing acute gout from a flare of the other diseases; the low synovial fluid complement occurring in these diseases may inhibit the expression of clinical gout; and treatment with full doses of aspirin is often used, which would delay or prevent the onset of gout due to the uricosuric effect of high doses of aspirin.

Parenchymal Renal Disease

Two types of parenchymal renal damage have been associated with hyperuricemia. Urate nephropathy is due to the deposition of sodium urate crystals in the renal interstitial tissue and the resulting inflammatory reaction. This condition appears to be associated with chronic hyperuricemia. Uric acid nephropathy is due to the formation of uric acid crystals in the collecting tubules, pelvis, or ureter, and the resulting blockade of urine flow. This condition is related to hyperuricaciduria and may be subdivided into two types, acute uric acid nephropathy and uric acid stones. Thus, these two pathologic processes have very different pathogeneses. Each type of lesion appears in a sufficiently distinctive setting to allow a presumptive diagnosis on clinical grounds. Rarely the two lesions may occur simultaneously in the same kidney.

Urate Nephropathy. Chronic renal disease is the second most common manifestation of gout.[90,119,120] Progressive renal failure accounted for 17 to 25 percent of deaths in the gouty population prior to the use of chronic hemodialysis.[120-124] In a more recent study 15 percent of 1700 patients with gout had nephropathy and approximately 9 percent of deaths in this group were related directly to renal failure.[125]

A common manifestation of urate nephropathy is albuminuria, which occurs in 20 to 40 percent of patients with gout.[120] Usually the proteinuria is mild and often it is intermittent. Inability to generate a maximally concentrated urine may be one of the earliest manifestations of urate nephropathy.[120] Hypertension occurs in about one third of the gouty population and often contributes to the renal disease. Urate nephropathy may, in turn, aggravate the hypertensive state. As the renal disease progresses, azotemia appears and renal failure with acidosis may ensue. When a patient is seen for the first time at this stage of illness, it may be difficult to decide whether renal failure is a consequence of hyperuricemia and urate nephropathy, or whether hyperuricemia is a result of the renal disease. A history of gouty arthritis suggests that urate nephropathy may be the underlying disease, since gout is rare in chronic renal failure of other etiologies[126-128] and the extent of urate nephropathy is usually correlated with the severity of gouty arthritis.[120]

There has been considerable controversy over the years concerning the pathogenesis of the lesions of urate nephropathy. Part of this confusion has no doubt been due to the multiple factors that may produce renal disease in the gouty subject. Nonetheless, there is a distinctive histologic finding characteristic of the gouty kidney, namely the deposit of urate crystals in the interstitium of the medulla and pyramids with surrounding giant-cell reaction (Fig. 86–10).[129] The traditional view has been that the renal lesion arises from the deposition of urate salts in the collecting ducts with secondary obstruction of the more proximal nephron leading to dilatation, atrophy, necrosis of tubular cells, erosion of crystals into the interstitium, and finally fibrosis.[122,130-132] More recently investigators have concluded that the initial lesion is damage of the tubular epithelium of the loop of Henle and juxtaposed interstitial tissue.[133,134] The available evidence favors the latter hypothesis.

In addition to changes produced in the tubules and interstitium, vascular changes in the glomerular capillary bed and larger blood vessels may be prominent.[133,134] These consist of hyalinization of the glomeruli and hy-

Figure 86–10. *A*, Urate deposit in the medulla of the kidney as seen in alcohol-fixed section stained with hematoxylin and eosin (×250). *B*, Adjacent section of deposit shown in *A*, stained with methenamine silver (×250). *C*, Adjacent section of deposit shown in *A* as seen with polarized light (×250).

pertrophy of the intima and some portions of the media of the arterioles.

Crystals present in the interstitium of kidney obtained from patients with gout have proved on x-ray diffraction analysis to be a urate salt, and not uric acid.[135] Crystals of calcium oxalate or phosphate may also occur in renal tissue, and these crystals can be confused with crystals of sodium urate or uric acid when viewed by light microscopy alone. However, oxalate crystals tend to be predominantly cortical in location as contrasted with the medullary site of urate crystals.

Although it is clear that renal disease is associated with gout, it has not been evident to what extent this is related to hyperuricemia only and to the deposition of monosodium urate in the renal tissue. Indeed, it appears at this time that hyperuricemia per se causes little if any harmful effect on renal function.[105,136-139] Other factors, such as coexistant hypertension, chronic lead exposure, ischemic heart disease, or primary pre-existent renal insufficiency may be more important than urate in the pathogenesis of the lesion previously considered to be "urate" nephropathy.[8,13,138-141] Although increasing age does lead to deterioration of renal function in both gouty and control populations,[136-139] the aging phenomenon appears to be accentuated in the gouty patients,[136] especially in the presence of hypertension, ischemic heart disease, or pre-existent renal disease.[139] On the other hand, extreme hyperuricemia in excess of 13 mg per dl in males or 10.0 mg per dl in females may be implicated in the etiology of renal damage.[105] These extremes of hyperuricemia may exist in the presence of inherited enzyme deficiencies, leading to urate overproduction, fulminating gout, and blood dyscrasias with oliguria and urolithiasis.[139] Indeed, the gouty kidney, as described by Garrod,[142] may be rare at the present time.

More recently, the uniqueness of renal monosodium urate deposition to gout has been questioned. Two studies have documented a substantial incidence of urate deposition not associated with clinical gout.[143,144] In one study, 17 of 62 patients dying of renal insufficiency had renal medullary tophi, which were attributed to the hyperuricemia of chronic renal insufficiency;[143] however, only 4 of these patients had attacks of articular gout. In another study, medullary microtophi were found in 8 percent of unselected autopsies.[144] While these deposits were most frequently associated with a history of gout or the presence of pre-existing, nongouty renal disease, in 26 percent of patients there was no etiology evident. Each of these studies suggests that, in some instances, urate deposition in the renal medulla may be a consequence rather than a direct cause of renal failure. In addition, factors other than hyperuricemia, which are unclear at present, contribute to urate deposition in the kidney.

Uric Acid Nephropathy. *Acute Uric Acid Nephropathy.* A severe form of acute renal failure resulting from the precipitation of uric acid crystals in collecting ducts and ureters may occur in hyperuricemic subjects, most commonly in patients with leukemia or lymphoma subjected to aggressive chemotherapy[145,146] but also (1) in patients with gout and markedly accelerated purine synthesis, (2) following severe exercise in poorly conditioned individuals,[147] or (3) after epileptic seizures.[148] Each of these disorders produces marked hyperuricemia and increased uricaciduria; the latter two are also associated with acidosis and strongly acid urines, thus reducing uric acid solubility.

It is important to recognize the clinical settings in which this type of acute renal failure develops because the complication is preventable, and may be reversible with prompt appropriate management. Since treatment has become more aggressive, mortality has dropped from 47 percent[146] to close to zero.[149] The usual patient has acute leukemia or chronic leukemia that has entered a "blastic" or uncontrolled stage. In the patient with lymphoma the disease is usually widespread and rapidly progressive.[145,146] In both leukemia and lymphoma there is a marked increase in cell turnover and in uric acid production.[146,149,150] In addition, patients with these disorders are likely to be receiving aggressive radiation therapy or chemotherapy in hopes of controlling the underlying process. Such cytotoxic therapy increases the load of uric acid presented to the kidneys. Furthermore, the patients are often severely ill and may be dehydrated from the anorexia that accompanies the underlying disease and its therapy. This leads to low urine volumes of high concentration. Finally, acidosis is not uncommon in this setting and the urine becomes more acidic under these circumstances. The combination of a three- to five-fold increase in uric acid excretion,[146] a highly concentrated urine, and a low urine pH provides an ideal setting for the precipitation of un-ionized uric acid in the collecting tubules.

Pathogenesis. Acute renal failure in uric acid nephropathy is due to the precipitation of un-ionized uric acid in the collecting ducts with secondary blockage of the tubules. Rieselbach and colleagues[146] have demonstrated that renal failure in this syndrome is correlated with the amount of uric acid excreted and not with the serum urate. The initial pathologic event is the precipitation of uric acid in the collecting ducts. Dilatation of the more proximal nephron occurs as a consequence of tubular obstruction by the precipitates. Alterations in tubular epithelium occur as late events. Studies in experimental models support the concept that acute uric acid nephropathy is caused by the mechanical obstruction of the tubule with precipitates of un-ionized uric acid.[151] Marked hyperphosphatemia and hyperkalemia during cancer chemotherapy may also contribute to the toxicity of this syndrome.[152] This may be particularly true for the precipitation of phosphate.

Clinical Features and Diagnosis. There are several features of this syndrome that are quite distinctive. Hyperuricemia may be marked. In 16 cases, Kjellstrand and associates[149] recorded a mean serum urate of 20 mg per 100 ml with a range from 12 to 36 mg per 100 ml. Serum urate concentrations in excess of 80 mg per 100 ml have been reported.[153] Oliguria and azotemia are common features. Anuria occurs if complete bilateral obstruction develops at the ureteral level. Urinary gravel or sand may be noted by the patients. Extremely heavy uric acid crystalluria may be observed in the urine sediment. In other patients uric acid crystalluria may be completely absent.[149] The most distinctive feature of this syndrome is the amount of uric acid excreted in the urine in subjects who are not completely anuric. In most cases of renal failure from other causes, total urinary uric acid excretion is normal or reduced.[154] The uric acid to creatinine ratio is usually less than 1.0. For example, in patients with acute renal failure examined by Kelton and associates[155] this ratio averaged 0.43 ± 0.28. In individuals with acute uric acid nephropathy the uric acid to creatinine ratio is typically > 1.0.[155] Thus, the diagnosis can be confirmed by demonstrating a high level of uric acid excretion in the face of acute renal failure. Once this diagnosis is made, therapy must be initiated at once.

Uric Acid Stones. Uric acid stones account for 5 to 10 percent of all stones in the United States.[156] The percentage is lower in the "stone belts" of the southeastern United States where calcium oxalate and phosphate stones predominate.[157-159] In other parts of the world they range from 5 (Great Britain) to 40 percent (Israel) of all stones.[156] The overall prevalence of uric acid stones in the population of the United States is about 0.01 percent.[160] An etiologic classification of uric acid nephrolithiasis is presented in Table 86–3.[161]

Prevalence in Primary Gout. In patients with gout the prevalence of stones ranges from 10 to 25 percent, except in Israel where 75 percent of gouty subjects are afflicted with stones.[156] This prevalence of renal stones is at least 1000 times greater than in the general population. One of the best studied groups of patients is that of Yu and Gutman.[161,162] The prevalence of stones in 1228 patients with primary gout was 22 percent (Table 86–4). The yearly risk for the development of urolithiasis in estab-

Table 86–3. Etiologic Classification of Uric Acid Nephrolithiasis*

Idiopathic uric acid nephrolithiasis
  1. Sporadic
  2. Genetically transmitted
Uric acid nephrolithiasis associated with hyperuricemia due to
  1. Inborn errors of metabolism
    a. Primary gout (at least one attack of arthritis)
    b. Lesch-Nyhan syndrome
    c. Glycogen storage diseases
  2. Myeloproliferative and other neoplastic diseases
  3. Undetermined causes
Uric acid nephrolithiasis associated with dehydration due to excessive extrarenal loss of water
  1. By way of the skin
  2. By way of the gastrointestinal tract
Uric acid nephrolithiasis associated with hyperuricosuria without significant hyperuricemia due to
  1. Uricosuric drugs
  2. Overindulgence in purines and proteins
  3. Inherent or acquired defect in tubular reabsorption of uric acid

*From Gutman, A.B., and Yu, T.-F.: Am. J. Med. 45:756, 1968. Reproduced by permission of the American Journal of Medicine.

Table 86–4. Relationship of Serum Urate Concentration to Prevalence of Urolithiasis in Gout*

Serum Urate (mg/100 ml)	Primary Gout				Secondary Gout			
	Total Patients		Patients with Urolithiasis		Total Patients		Patients with Urolithiasis	
	No.	%	No.	%	No.	%	No.	%
5.1–6.0[†]	9	1[‡]	0		0		0	
6.1–7.0	74	6	9	12[§]	2	3	0	
7.1–8.0	181	15	31	17	2	3	1	50[§]
8.1–9.0	291	24	56	19	7	12	2	29
9.1–10.0	295	24	64	22	5	9	4	80
10.1–11.0	196	16	59	30	12	21	5	42
11.1–12.0	99	8	21	21	5	9	1	20
12.1–13.0	45	4	20	44	4	7	3	75
13.1–14.0	28	2	15	54	6	11	3	50
14.1	10	1	5	50	14	25	5	36
Total	1228		280		57		24	

*From Yu, T.-F., and Gutman, A.B.: Ann. Intern. Med. 67:1133, 1967. Reproduced by permission of the Annals of Internal Medicine.
†The patients with serum urate of 5.1 to 6.0 mg per 100 ml were women.
‡Percentage in relation to the total number of patients.
§Percentage in relation to the number of patients with the same urate level.

lished gouty arthritis is about 1 percent in all studies recently examined.[105,162,163] The risk in asymptomatic hyperuricemia is substantially smaller, at 0.2 percent per year.[105]

Factors that modify the risk of uric acid calculi include the serum urate level and the urinary uric acid excretion.[161,162] The prevalence increased with the height of the serum urate concentration, reaching 50 percent at serum urate values of 13 mg per 100 ml or above. However, in another study the initial serum urate level was not significantly different in those in whom stones ultimately developed than in the rest of the patients.[105] In 40 percent of the patients stones preceded the development of gouty arthritis, by more than a decade in 14 percent. In 84 percent the stones were pure uric acid, in 4 percent uric acid and calcium oxalate, in 8 percent calcium oxalate alone, and in 4 percent calcium phosphate. The mean age of onset in the series of Yu and Gutman[162] was 44 years, 2 years later than the mean age of the first attack of acute gouty arthritis.

Uric acid stones also occur in patients with no history of gouty arthritis. Approximately 20 percent of the patients in this group are hyperuricemic.[164,165] If not treated with antihyperuricemic agents, some of these patients would very likely go on to develop acute gouty arthritis. Other disorders associated with the development of uric acid stones, particularly in normouricemic subjects, are discussed later in this chapter.

Prevalence in Secondary Gout. Yu and Gutman[162] reported a prevalence of renal calculi of 42 percent in 57 patients with gout secondary to myeloproliferative diseases associated in most instances with hyperuricaciduria. In this group the prevalence was not correlated with the height of the serum urate value. Urolithiasis tended to occur after vigorous cytolytic therapy.

By contrast, renal stones are not common in gout secondary to lead nephropathy. Emmerson[166] recorded no renal calculi in 34 patients with lead gout compared with a prevalence of 28 percent in patients with primary gout. The mean urinary uric acid excretions in the two groups were 232 and 585 mg per day, respectively. In 96 patients with crystal-proved gout at Duke University only 7 percent had renal calculi, and none of these occurred in the 55 patients with a history of heavy ingestion of unbonded alcohol.[167]

Pathogenesis. Factors that predispose toward uric acid nephrolithiasis in gout include increased urinary excretion of uric acid, undue acidity of the urine, increased urine concentration, and perhaps qualitative or quantitative abnormalities of urinary constituents which affect solubility of uric acid. According to Dulce[168] and Boshamer,[169] uric acid stones are formed only when supersaturation prevails and when there is a crystallization nucleus of organic matrix. Sperling and associates[170,171] concluded that urine is invariably supersaturated with uric acid when the pH is below 5.5 to 5.7.

The most important factor leading to the high prevalence of uric acid stones in patients with gout appears to be an increased concentration of this compound in urine. In most gouty patients the increased concentration of uric acid is due to its increased production. Yu and Gutman[162] noted a prevalence of stones of 11 percent in patients with a urinary uric acid excretion of less than 300 mg per day, of 21 percent with uric acid excretion values between 300 and 700 mg per day, of 35 percent in patients with uric acid excretion values between 700 and 1100 mg per day, and of 50 percent with uric acid excretion rates in excess of 1100 mg per day Table 86–5). The higher prevalence of stones in patients with higher serum urate values probably depends on the influence of serum urate values on urinary uric acid excretion.

An increase in the clearance of uric acid may lead to an increased concentration of uric acid in the urine. Uricosuric agents produce a transient increase in the concentration of uric acid which may accelerate the formation of uric acid stones. Yu and Gutman[162] noted that 16 percent of stones in their patients occurred after the

Table 86–5. Relationship of Urinary Uric Acid Excretion to Prevalence of Urolithiasis in Gout*

Urinary Uric Acid Excretion (mg/24 hr)	Primary Gout				Secondary Gout			
	Total Patients		Patients with Urolithiasis		Total Patients		Patients with Urolithiasis	
	No.	%	No.	%	No.	%	No.	%
<300	36	4†	4	11‡	0		0	
300–499	324	37	68	21	4	11†	0	
500–699	317	36	66	21	13	37	2	15†
700–899	154	17	53	34	7	20	3	43
900–1099	39	4	15	38	7	20	4	57
>1100	18	2	9	50	4	11	2	50
Total	888		215		35		11	

*From Yu, T.-F., and Gutman, A.B.: Ann. Intern. Med. 67:1133, 1967. Reproduced by permission of the Annals of Internal Medicine.
†Percentage in relation to the total number of patients.
‡Percentage in relation to the number of patients with the same urinary uric acid excretion.

administration of uricosuric agents, although in many instances these occurred in the early days of availability of these drugs, before adequate precautionary measures against stones had been introduced. A sudden increase in uric acid clearance may also be an important factor in patients who are given a drug for other reasons, e.g., x-ray contrast agents, which have a substantial uricosuric effect. Correction of a condition or removal of a drug producing uric acid retention could have a similar consequence.

Reduced urine volume is another important factor leading to increased urinary concentration of uric acid. Loss of water through the skin in subjects living in a hot dry climate may account for the frequent occurrence of uric acid stones in Israel. The sweat does not contain uric acid. Similarly, patients with fever or volume depletion are at increased risk for developing uric acid stones. This is perhaps best documented in patients with ileostomies.[172,173]

As described in Chapter 21, uric acid is a weak acid which ionizes at the N-9 position with a pK_a of 5.75.[174] Thus, uric acid is half-ionized (urate) and half-unionized (uric acid) at a pH equal to the pK_a, or 5.75. At a pH of 4.75, 91 percent of uric acid is un-ionized. Similarly, at a pH of 6.75, 91 percent is ionized. This principle is relevant to the problem of uric acid precipitation since uric acid is considerably less soluble than urate. At a temperature of 37° C, urine is saturated with uric acid (in the presence of an equivalent amount of sodium) at concentrations of 15 mg per 100 ml at pH 5.0, 22.0 mg per 100 ml at pH 6.0, 158 to 200 mg per 100 ml at pH 7.0, and 1520 mg per 100 ml at pH 8.0.[175,176]

Gouty patients have a tendency toward unusually acid urine both in fasting morning specimens and throughout the day.[177-182] There is also a substandard rise of urinary pH in response to oral alkali. Gutman and Yu[182] noted that a preprandial morning urine sample had a pH less than 5.0 in 48 percent of gouty patients with stones, in 36 percent of gouty patients without stones, and in 15 percent of control subjects. In the three fourths of gouty subjects whose urinary uric acid excretion values fall within the normal range, the high prevalence of renal stones is probably in part related to low urinary pH.

The persistently acid urine in gouty subjects is due to a low ratio of NH_4^+ to titratable acidity, attributed by some to a subnormal ammonium excretion at a given acid load or pH[178,179,183] and by others to high values of titratable acidity.[181,184-186] The deficit of ammonium excretion, when present, has been assigned to the effects of occult or measurable renal damage,[185,187] aging,[188] or high purine intake[189] by some authors, but is regarded as an intrinsic defect in the production of ammonia, presumably from glutamine, by Gutman and Yu.[161,182,190]

In idiopathic uric acid nephrolithiasis, by definition occurring in patients with normal plasma and urinary uric acid values, a tendency toward a low urine pH is also a consistent finding. Henneman,[178] Woeber,[179] and Rapoport[191] and their associates have reported reduced ammonium excretion and normal or increased titratable acidity in such patients, whereas Metcalfe-Gibson and associates[185] found normal ammonium excretion in relation to pH, except in patients with overt renal damage. In the latter patients ammonium excretion per unit of glomerular filtration rate was normal.

A familial form of uric acid lithiasis is found in Israel, in which patients are normouricemic but may have unusually acid urines in the absence of other abnormalities of renal function. Frank and associates[184] and Barzel and associates[186] found normal rates of ammonium excretion and elevated values for titratable acidity in these subjects. The excretion of ammonium, with or without administration of an acid load, was not lower than that in control subjects of equivalent age.[188] There was no apparent deficiency of urinary "solubilizers" of uric acid.[192] This disorder appears to be an inherited disease distinct from gout with an autosomal dominant mode of inheritance and high penetrance in both sexes.[180]

Patients with chronic acidosis resulting from renal disease or chronic diarrhea may also maintain a persistently acid urine and may be oliguric, and thus be susceptible to development of uric acid stones. The prevalence of stones in patients with colon resection and ileostomy for inflammatory bowel disease ranges from 7.4 to 12.5 percent. Most of the stones produced by these patients are composed of uric acid.[173,193-196] Patients with ileostomies exhibit increased renal conservation of sodium, a decreased urinary Na/K ratio, increased urinary acid excretion, low urinary pH values, and low urine volumes.[173,195]

Since uric acid stones are unusual even when urine is saturated with uric acid,[170,192] the role of solubilizing factors has been considered. The Tamm-Horsfall mucoprotein of urine helps maintain uric acid in a supersaturated state.[197] Uric acid stone formers have a normal urinary uric acid solubility and a normal capacity to form supersaturated urine.[171,192,197]

The solubility of urate is inversely related to the concentration of sodium while the solubility of uric acid is unaffected by the sodium concentration. Thus, sodium content is a critical factor in the precipitation of urate within the kidney, but its importance for the precipitation of uric acid is negligible.

Calcium Stones. Gouty subjects also have an increased prevalence of calcium-containing stones.[164,198] The overall prevalence of calcium stones in the population is about 0.1 percent. In subjects with primary gout, the prevalence of calcium stones that do not contain a detectable nidus of uric acid is about 1 to 3 percent.[162] The responsible mechanism(s) remains unknown.

Urinary uric acid excretion values may be normal[199] or increased[199,200] in patients with idiopathic calcium stone disease. A careful analysis of ten patients with recurrent calcium stones revealed that (1) as a group they had a significantly greater consumption of dietary purines than normal subjects, (2) three of the ten excreted a greater than normal quantity of uric acid ex-pressed as milligrams per kilogram per day after 7 days of purine restriction, and (3) nine of the ten excreted a given quantity of uric acid at a lower serum urate concentration and therefore were mildly hyperuricosuric.[200]

Hyperuricosuria and idiopathic hypercalciuria coexisted in 12 percent of 230 patients with calcium stones studied by Coe and Kavalach.[200]

Others. Stones composed of xanthine, oxipurinol, or orotic acid may occur rarely in patients with gout treated with allopurinol.[1]

CLASSIFICATION AND PATHOGENESIS OF HYPERURICEMIA AND GOUT

The biochemical hallmark and prerequisite of gout is hyperuricemia. The concentration of uric acid in body fluids is determined by the balance between rates of production and elimination of urate. The development of hyperuricemia may be due to an excessive rate of uric acid production, a decrease in the renal excretion of uric acid, or a combination of both events.

Hyperuricemia and gout may be classified as primary, secondary, or idiopathic (Table 86–6). Primary hyperuricemia or gout refers to those cases which appear to be innate, that are neither secondary to another acquired disorder nor a subordinate manifestation of an inborn error that leads initially to a major disease unlike gout. While some cases of primary gout will have a genetic basis, others do not. Secondary hyperuricemia or gout refers to those cases that develop in the course of another

Table 86–6. Classification of Hyperuricemia and Gout

Type	Metabolic Disturbance	Inheritance
Primary		
Molecular defects undefined		
Underexcretion (90% of primary gout)	Not established	Polygenic
Overproduction (10% of primary gout)	Not established	Polygenic
Associated with specific enzyme defects		
PP-ribose-P synthetase variants; increased activity	Overproduction of PP-ribose-P and of uric acid	X-linked
Hypoxanthine-guanine phosphoribosyltransferase deficiency, partial	Overproduction of uric acid; increased purine biosynthesis de novo driven by surplus PP-ribose-P	X-linked
Secondary		
Associated with increased purine biosynthesis de novo		
Glucose 6-phosphatase deficiency or absence	Overproduction plus underexcretion of uric acid; glycogen storage disease, type I (von Gierke)	Autosomal recessive
Hypoxanthine-guanine phosphoribosyltransferase deficiency, "virtually complete"	Overproduction of uric acid; increased purine biosynthesis do novo driven by surplus PP-ribose-P; Lesch-Nyhan syndrome	X-linked
Associated with increased nucleic acid turnover	Overproduction of uric acid	Most not familial
Associated with decreased renal excretion of uric acid	Decreased filtration of uric acid; inhibited tubular secretion of uric acid; or enhanced tubular reabsorption of uric acid	Some autosomal dominant; some not familial; most unknown
Idiopathic		Unknown

disease or as a consequence of drugs. Finally, idiopathic hyperuricemia or gout represents those cases in which a more precise classification cannot be assigned. Further subdivisions within each major category are based on the identification of overproduction or underexcretion or both as responsible for the hyperuricemia.

Primary Gout

Renal Handling of Uric Acid in Primary Gout. Over a century ago, Garrod proposed that diminished excretion of uric acid by the kidneys was one of the possible causes of hyperuricemia. A careful comparison of uric acid clearances and excretion rates over wide but comparable ranges of filtered loads of urate indicates that most gouty subjects have a lower C_{urate}/C_{inulin} ratio than nongouty subjects.[201-207] This ratio increases in gouty subjects as in normal controls when the plasma urate level is raised by feeding of RNA or by infusion of lithium urate, but higher plasma urate values are required in gouty subjects to achieve a given clearance ratio.[208,209] When the data from these studies are plotted as rates of uric acid excretion at various serum urate levels, the curve of excretion rates has the same form in gouty subjects as in nongouty controls, and the capacity of the excretory mechanism for uric acid is not reduced in gout (Fig. 86-11). However, the excretion curve is

Figure 86–11. Rate of uric acid excretion at various plasma urate levels in nongouty (solid symbols) and gouty (open symbols) subjects. Large symbols represent mean values; small symbols represent individual data of a few mean values selected to illustrate the degree of scatter within groups. Studies were conducted under basal conditions, after RNA feeding, and after infusions of lithium urate. ▲, △, Nugent and Tyler;[202] ▼, ▽, Seegmiller et al.;[203] ●, ○, Yu et al.;[204] ■, □, Latham and Rodnan.[152] (From Wyngaarden, J.B.: Adv. Metabol. Dis. 2:2, 1965. Reproduced by permission of Academic Press.)

shifted such that gouty subjects require serum urate values 2 or 3 mg per 100 ml higher than those of controls in order to achieve equivalent uric acid excretion rates. Perhaps 75 to 90 percent of patients with primary gout will exhibit the renal defect as defined by this abnormal substrate-velocity curve. Patients with gout due to one of the specific enzymatic defects usually exhibit a normal uric acid/inulin (or creatinine) clearance ratio.[203]

Theoretically, the shift in the substrate-velocity curve in gouty subjects could be due to (1) reduced filtration of uric acid, (2) enhanced reabsorption, or (3) decreased secretion. Attempts to localize the site of the defect of uric acid transport in the nephron have been thwarted by the limitations of available techniques. At present there are no unequivocal data to establish any one of these three mechanisms.

Glomerular Filtration. Enchanced binding of urate to proteins in gouty subjects could result in precisely the abnormal substrate-velocity curve described above. While such an abnormality has been proposed in the hyperuricemic Maori,[210] it has yet to be confirmed. Reduced urate binding to proteins has also been described in some gouty subjects by two different groups of investigators.[211,212]

Tubular Reabsorption. Increased reabsorption of uric acid as a cause of the altered substrate-velocity curve has not received serious consideration in the past. Since reabsorption of secreted urate occurs, the extent of reabsorption in the nephron may be well in excess of 100 percent of the filtered urate. Thus, increased reabsorption could be an important factor in the pathogenesis of hyperuricemia.

There is increasing evidence to suggest that uric acid, sodium, and other solute excretion may be related and that uric acid should be added to the growing list of solutes that respond to changes in "physical factors." It is possible that the abnormality in uric acid excretion in some patients with gout may involve an alteration in these "physical factors" which affects reabsorption of solutes in general, including that of uric acid.

Tubular Secretion. Rieselbach and associates[213] have postulated diminished renal urate secretion *per nephron* as a basis for hyperuricemia in some patients with primary gout without demonstrable overproduction of uric acid. The evidence for this was based on the pyrazinamide suppression test, the reliability of which has now been questioned. According to the current interpretation of the test by Steele,[214] the data presented in support of decreased secretion in these patients would now be reinterpreted as enhanced reabsorption distal to the urate secretory site. Nevertheless, decreased secretion could lead to the abnormal substrate-velocity curve and should be considered further. If one assumes that benzbromarone selectively inhibits tubular reabsorption of secreted urate,[215,216] then maximum uricosuria induced by this drug could be equated with the minimal secretory rate. Using this measure, gouty patients with normal production hyperuricemia had a significantly lower secretory rate in comparison with patients with an overproduction of uric acid.[215,216]

There are several mechanisms whereby an alteration in the transport of an organic acid could be related to a defect of urate secretion in gouty subjects. Certain organic acids may share a secretory site in the nephron with uric acid. An increased secretion of an organic acid sharing such a transport system could competitively inhibit the tubular secretion of uric acid. Alternatively, the reduced secretion of an organic acid could reflect a defective secretory system, which might also reduce uric acid secretion.

A number of naturally occurring organic acids reduce the renal excretion of uric acid presumably by inhibiting its tubular secretion. Elevated concentrations of lactate and β-hydroxybutyrate are important causes of secondary hyperuricemia, as will be discussed later. These observations led to the proposal that the renal defect in uric acid transport could be related to a subtle abnormality in organic acid metabolism in some patients with gout. Kramer and associates[217] found a normal excretion of total organic acids in the urine in 32 gouty subjects. However, analysis of Krebs cycle organic acids in 12 of these patients revealed a decreased excretion of citrate in all 12, an increased excretion of lactate in five, and an increased excretion of succinate-fumarate in three. Unfortunately, plasma concentrations could not be measured so the renal handling of these compounds could not be estimated. Citrate does have a uricosuric effect, and thus its reduced presence could lead to uric acid retention.

Other renal functional abnormalities in gouty patients include reduced renal clearances of serine, threonine, and glutamine,[218,219] reduced excretion of dehydroepiandrosterone,[220-223] androsterone, and etiocholanolone,[223] and reduced ammonia excretion.[134,182,185,186,224-226]

Hyperuricemia and gout are well recognized complications of chronic lead intoxication. While a renal defect appears to be present, it has not been well defined. Recently, Campbell and associates[141] have reported that patients with primary gout have elevated blood lead levels when compared to age- and sex-matched controls despite the absence of a history of overt lead exposure. This suggests that occult chronic lead intoxication could play an etiologic role in some patients with primary gout. In addition, increased quantity of mobilizable lead in patients with gout who had renal impairment as compared to gouty patients with normal renal function suggests an important potential role for lead in the pathogenesis of gouty nephropathy.[140] On the other hand, no correlation was found between extent of depression in urate or creatinine clearance and amount of lead excretion following EDTA infusion.[226a] Factors other than lead nephropathy, such as obesity, ethanol consumption, hypertension, and hereditary traits, may be responsible for the decreased urate clearance observed in over 70 percent of the gouty patients studied, many of whom had ingested moonshine.

Several families have been reported in which there is (1) a high incidence of hyperuricemia with gout beginning at an unusually young age, (2) involvement of females or involvement of both sexes with hypertension, and (3) progressive renal disease leading to death before the age of 40.[227-235] Although hyperuricemia and gout may be familial and may be associated with progressive renal disease, it is unusual for renal disease to be the cause of early death in primary gout. In addition, although hyperuricemia may eventually occur in renal disease of any type, it is rare for the hyperuricemia of chronic renal failure to be associated with gout. Usually the patients described with familial urate nephropathy do not exhibit features suggestive of hereditary renal disease,[236,237] such as deafness, retinitis pigmentosa, skin lesions, renal calculi, aminoaciduria, or markedly enlarged kidneys. Specific diagnosis may be relevant since stabilization of renal function has occurred in some patients following allopurinol therapy.[234] In one family the renal insufficiency was due to medullary cystic disease[231] and the possibility cannot be overlooked that the renal disease is the primary event in other families as well. Whatever the disease in each family, it often appears to be inherited in an autosomal dominant manner.

Overproduction of Uric Acid in Primary Gout. Determination of the 24-hour urinary uric acid excretion is essential in defining the role of uric acid overproduction as a cause of hyperuricemia. Before and during the collection period, the patient should not be taking medications that alter the metabolism or excretion of uric acid. For adults on a purine-free diet, up to 600 mg per day is considered within the normal range, with a mean value of about 425 mg per day or 5.6 mg per kg per 24 hours.[238,239] Under usual circumstances, however, it is not practical to place patients on a purine-free diet for 3 to 5 days before the collection of a 24-hour urine sample. With patients on a regular purine diet, a value in excess of 1000 mg per day is clearly abnormal, while 800 to 1000 mg per day is considered a borderline value.

It has been suggested recently that an overproduction of uric acid can be assessed simply by determining the ratio of uric acid to creatinine in the urine or the ratio of the uric acid clearance to the creatinine clearance.[240] Comparison of these two ratios with the 24-hour urine acid excretion, however, reveals a poor correlation between the urinary uric acid excretion in 24 hours in most patients and these ratios.[241] This is largely because of a striking diurnal variation in the excretion of uric acid. Only specific enzymatic deficiencies lead to such a substantial increase in uric acid production that the ratio of uric acid to creatinine in the urine is consistently greater than 0.75. It is necessary, therefore, in most gouty patients to measure the 24-hour uric acid excretion before proper classification of the patient is possible. Attempts to correlate de novo purine synthesis in circulating lymphocytes with clinical assessment of uric acid production status also has been unsuccessful.[242] Therefore, the measurement of purine synthesis in vitro will not predict urate overproduction.

Patients classified as exhibiting an overproduction of uric acid probably represent 10 percent or less of the gouty population. In these patients with primary gout caused by an overproduction of uric acid there is an acceleration in the rate of purine biosynthesis de novo.

Three specific defects which appear to be important as a cause of uric acid overproduction include hypoxanthine-guanine phosphoribosyltransferase deficiency, PRPP synthetase overactivity, and glucose-6-phosphatase deficiency; these are discussed below. Recently Hers and Van Den Berghe have proposed that abnormalities of AMP deaminase could lead to accelerated nucleotide degradation, increased production of uric acid, and gout.[243] In addition, a deficiency in adenylosuccinate synthetase in cultured cells leads to overexcretion of purine metabolites and increased de novo purine synthesis.[244] These observations predict that a similar deficiency in humans could lead to increased synthesis of uric acid.

Hypoxanthine-Guanine Phosphoribosyltransferase Deficiency.

In 1967, Seegmiller, Rosenbloom, and Kelley described a virtually complete deficiency of an enzyme of purine metabolism, hypoxanthine-guanine phosphoribosyltransferase (HPRT) (Fig. 86–12), in erythrocyte lysates from three children and in cultured skin fibroblasts from a fourth patient with the Lesch-Nyhan syndrome,[245] a disorder characterized by choreoathetosis, striking growth and mental retardation, spasticity, self-mutilation, and marked hyperuricemia, with excessive uric acid production and uric acid crystalluria (Fig. 86–13).[246] The enzyme defect was subsequently confirmed in other tissues, as well as in cultured skin fibroblasts and erythrocytes from many similarly affected subjects.[247] Adolescent and adult patients were then described with a "partial" rather than a "complete" deficiency of HPRT (Fig. 86–14).[248] These patients presented with uric acid calculi or gouty arthritis and did not have the devastating neurological and behavioral features characteristic of children with the complete enzyme defect.[249]

Partial HPRT deficiency is considered to be a form of primary hyperuricemia since the major clinical manifestations are a direct result of the hyperuricemia and hyperuricaciduria. Patients with the Lesch-Nyhan syndrome and a virtually complete deficiency of HPRT are considered to have secondary hyperuricemia since their major clinical manifestations are unrelated to hyperuricemia per se.

Figure 86–12. Reactions catalyzed by hypoxanthine-guanine phosphoribosyltransferase.

Clinical Features. Patients with a partial deficiency of HPRT typically exhibit a markedly increased production of uric acid and, accordingly, the daily urinary excretion of uric acid is high when expressed on the basis of body weight. Values range from 10 to 36 mg per kilogram per day in patients with a "partial" deficiency of HPRT.[249] The upper limits of normal in children and adults are 18 and 10 mg per kilogram per day, respectively.[250]

Because of the increased quantity of uric acid in the urine, most patients experience uric acid crystalluria at some time. Some patients develop symptomatic uric acid nephrolithiasis which may lead eventually to obstructive uropathy with severe and unrelenting azotemia. The older the patient prior to institution of proper therapy, the more likely that uric acid concretions will develop. Nineteen of the initial 28 patients described with partial HPRT deficiency had a history of uric acid calculi. In at least nine, this was the initial symptom prompting the patient to seek medical care.[249] The hyperuricaciduria may also lead to pitressin-resistant polyuria.[251]

The serum urate concentration may range from 7 to as high as 18 mg per 100 ml in the absence of renal insufficiency. In an occasional patient, particularly before puberty, a random value will fall within the normal range.[252-254] The serum urate concentration may provide an initial clue to the diagnosis; however, it is not an infallible screening test because of its variability, especially in the younger patients. A history of gouty arthritis was present in 20 of the initial 23 patients with the partial defect who were older than 13 before effective antihyperuricemic therapy was instituted.[249] Over half of this latter group had developed tophi. The likelihood that gouty arthritis or tophi will develop reflects the duration and severity of hyperuricemia prior to antihyperuricemic therapy.

Six of the initial 28 patients with a partial deficiency of HPRT had evidence of neurologic dysfunction.[249,255-257] In four of these, the neurological features suggested a forme fruste relationship to the devastating neurological disease found in patients with the Lesch-Nyhan syndrome. Two siblings had a spinocerebellar syndrome characterized by nystagmus, hyperreflexia, and an inability to perform heel-to-toe walking. Another patient had a delayed onset of speech as a child and a lifelong history of spasticity. A fourth patient had a long history of a seizure disorder. Three of these four patients were mildly retarded, with IQ values ranging from 67 to 75 by formal testing. However, most patients with partial HPRT deficiency are normal neurologically.

A number of investigators have confirmed the presence of macrocytic erythrocytes in the peripheral blood and megaloblastic changes in the bone marrow in patients with partial HPRT deficiency.[258-260] Such changes may be present even in the absence of overt anemia. The cause of the megaloblastic changes remains unclear.

Biochemical Features—Nature of the Enzyme Defect. The level of HPRT activity in erythrocytes from patients with the partial enzyme defect is the same within a family but often differs between families with values ranging

Figure 86–13. *A*, Patient H. D. *B*, Note agitated appearance and the attempt by the patient to bite his fingers after the wrapping is removed from his hands.

from 0.01 to nearly 30 percent of normal (Table 86–7).[249,255-257] This and a series of other observations suggest that separate mutations on the structural gene for HPRT are responsible for the enzyme defect. Detailed studies of highly purified erythrocyte enzyme from five unrelated patients have provided direct evidence for the existence of at least four different mutations of hypoxanthine-guanine phosphoribosyltransferase.[261-265] In fact, a major advance in understanding the basis for this enzyme deficiency has been the definition of specific amino acid substitutions in the deficient enzymes (Table 86–8). The importance of increased activity in erythrocytes of several enzymes, including adenine phosphoribosyltransferase, inosinic acid dehydrogenase, orotate phosphoribosyltransferase, orotidine 5′-phosphate decarboxylase, and possibly PRPP synthetase, in these patients remains unclear.[1]

The excessive production of uric acid characteristic of partial HPRT deficiency results from an accelerated rate of purine biosynthesis de novo. There are at least three

Figure 86–14. Three brothers in one family with "partial" hypoxanthine-guanine phosphoribosyltransferase deficiency.

Table 86–7. Specific Activity of Hypoxanthine-Guanine Phosphoribosyl-transferase (HPRT) in Erythrocyte Hemolysates in Families in Which Two or More Members Partially Deficient in HPRT Were Discovered*

	PRT Activity (m μmoles/mg. prot./hour)		
	Hypoxanthine	*Guanine*	*Adenine*
Normal	103±18	103±21	31.3±6.0
J. family			
F.J.	1.3	0.6	46
R.J.	1.5	0.8	43
T.J.	1.8	0.8	56
L. family			
M.L.	8.7	0.5	64
F.L.	11.8	0.5	74
G. family			
J.G.	9.4	8.8	32
R.G.	9.2	7.5	38
T. family			
R.T.	0.06	0.07	36
M.W.	0.06	0.05	29
R.L.	0.09	0.10	44
N. family			
C.N.	0.3	0.3	35
E.S.	0.4	0.3	39

*From Kelley, W.N., et al.: Ann. Intern. Med. 70:155, 1969.

possible mechanisms by which a deficiency of HPRT could result in excessive purine synthesis. First, the deficiency could lead to enhanced purine synthesis by virtue of decreased concentrations of either IMP or GMP, since these nucleotides are normally important inhibitors of de novo purine biosynthesis.[266,267] Attempts to measure intracellular levels of IMP and GMP in these cells have been of only limited value, partly because of the very low intracellular concentration of these compounds under normal conditions.[268,269] Second, the increased concentration of PP-ribose-P characteristic of HPRT deficiency could increase de novo purine biosynthesis by providing more substrate for the enzyme which catalyzes the presumed limiting step of this pathway, amidophosphoribosyltransferase (see Chapter 21). The altered concentration of PP-ribose-P appears to be the more important factor responsible for the accelerated rate of purine biosynthesis de novo occurring with HPRT deficiency. Third, a decreased reutilization of hypoxanthine occurs in hypoxanthine-guanine phosphoribosyltransferase deficiency,[270,271] where the loss of enzyme activity leaves hypoxanthine only one pathway of metabolism, i.e., oxidation to uric acid. The loss of hypoxanthine reutilization leads to decreased consumption of phos-

phoribosylpyrophosphate and increased intracellular concentrations of this compound.

Genetic Features. The familial nature of partial HPRT deficiency was recognized in the original report of this disease.[248] Major clinical manifestations occur in affected males, with evidence of transmission through carrier females. The X-linked nature of the inheritance has been confirmed by studies in cell culture.[272] Recent experiments have resulted in the cloning of the DNA sequences from the hypoxanthine-guanine phosphoribosyltransferase gene.[273,274]

Several observations indicate that heterozygotes for a deficiency of HPRT exhibit subtle biochemical abnormalities in vivo, even though they are generally asymptomatic clinically. An elevated serum urate concentration has been noted in a number of such patients, and at least four have had recurrent monarticular arthritis thought clinically to represent gout. In addition, several obligate heterozygotes have excreted greater than normal quantities of uric acid in their urine.[275,276] Finally, studies on the incorporation of ^{14}C-glycine into urinary uric acid in heterozygous individuals have demonstrated a moderate increase in the rate of purine synthesis de novo.[249,277,278] Based on the data cited above, some cases of gout in the female occurring after menopause may be related to heterozygosity for HPRT deficiency.

Increased PRPP Synthetase Activity. Sperling and colleagues[279] demonstrated a markedly accelerated rate of PP-ribose-P synthesis in two gouty brothers with flamboyant overproduction of urate, and showed[280] that this was a consequence of altered kinetic properties of PP-ribose-P synthetase (Fig. 86–15). Subsequently, at least two additional families have been discovered in which excessive rates of PP-ribose-P synthesis can be

Table 86–8. Structural and Functional Abnormalities in Mutant Forms of Human HPRT*

| Mutant Enzyme | Clinical Presentation | Mutation | | Functional Abnormalities | | | |
| | | Amino Acid Substitution | Position | Intracellular Concentration | Maximal Velocity | Michaelis Constants | |
						Hypoxanthine	PP-Ribose-P
HPRT$_{Toronto}$	Gout	Arg→Gly†	50	Decreased	Normal	Normal	Normal
HPRT$_{London}$	Gout	Ser→Leu	109	Decreased	Normal	↑5-fold	Normal
HPRT$_{Ann Arbor}$	Nephrolithiasis	ND	ND	Decreased	Normal	Normal	Normal
HPRT$_{Munich}$	Gout	Ser→Arg	103	Normal	↑20-fold	↑100-fold	Normal
HPRT$_{Kinston}$	Lesch-Nyhan Syndrome	Asp→Asn	193	Normal	Normal	↑200-fold	↑200-fold

*From Wilson, J.M., Young, A.B., and Kelley, W.N.: N. Engl. J. Med. 309:900, 1983.
†Arg denotes arginine; Gly, glycine; Ser, serine; Leu, leucine; Asp, asparagine; Asn, aspartic acid; ND, not determined; and the arrow, "is replaced by."

attributed to abnormalities of this enzyme. The exact molecular alteration of the enzyme is different in each of the three families.[281-286] Affected male subjects had clinical gout. Age of onset of gout has ranged from 21 to 39 years. Three of the patients had a history of renal calculi, with onset as early as age 18 in one. None of the patients had tophi. Hyperuricemia ranged from 9.6 to 13.6 mg per 100 ml and urinary uric acid excretion values ranged from 950 to 2400 mg per day.

The enzyme is now known to be coded by DNA in the X chromosome,[287] and thus males are affected through asymptomatic carrier females. Recent studies suggest mosaicism in female family members and X-linked dominant transmission of this trait.[288]

While the biochemical cause of the increased PRPP synthetase activity is different in each family, the net result of all three types of defects is an excessive rate of generation of PP-ribose-P. There is little question now that increased PP-ribose-P synthetase activity represents a specific genetic subtype of gout. This class of defects is probably rare. Several hundred additional gouty overproducers have been screened for abnormal PP-ribose-P synthetase activity in several laboratories in this country, in Europe, in Japan, and in Israel with discovery of only a few other possible examples.

Secondary Gout

Renal Handling of Uric Acid in Secondary Gout. Numerous secondary causes of hyperuricemia and gout can be attributed to a decrease in the renal excretion of uric acid. A reduction in the glomerular filtration rate leads to a decrease in the filtered load of uric acid and thus to hyperuricemia; patients with renal disease will be hyperuricemic on this basis. Other factors, such as decreased secretion of uric acid, have been postulated

in patients with some types of renal disease, e.g., polycystic kidney disease and lead nephropathy. Gout is a rare complication of the secondary hyperuricemia resulting from renal insufficiency.

Diuretic therapy currently represents one of the most important causes of secondary hyperuricemia in man. Diuretic-induced volume depletion leads to enhanced tubular reabsorption of uric acid as well as a decreased filtered load of uric acid. Decreased secretion of uric acid has also been postulated as a possible mechanism in diuretic-induced hyperuricemia. A number of other drugs lead to hyperuricemia by a renal mechanism, although the nature of the abnormality remains less clear; these agents include low dose aspirin, pyrazinamide, nicotinic acid, ethambutol, and ethanol.

Decreased renal excretion of uric acid is thought to be an important mechanism for the hyperuricemia associated with several disease states. Volume depletion may be an important factor in patients with hyperuricemia associated with adrenal insufficiency and nephrogenic diabetes insipidus. An accumulation of organic acids on any basis is thought to competitively inhibit uric acid secretion and, thus, lead to hyperuricemia on that basis. This is the case in patients with starvation, alcoholic ketosis, diabetic ketoacidosis, maple syrup urine disease, and lactic acidosis of any cause: e.g., hypoxemia, respiratory insufficiency, chronic beryllium disease, and acute alcohol intoxication. The renal basis of the hyperuricemia in conditions such as chronic lead intoxication, hyperparathyroidism, hypoparathyroidism, pseudohypoparathyroidism, and hypothyroidism remains unclear.

Overproduction of Uric Acid in Secondary Gout. There are many causes of secondary hyperuricemia associated with an increased production of uric acid. In some, the increased excretion of uric acid is related, as it is in primary gout, to an accelerated rate of purine biosynthesis de novo. Patients with glucose-6-phosphatase deficiency (von Gierke's glycogen storage disease) uniformly exhibit an increased production of uric acid as well as an accelerated rate of purine biosynthesis de novo. A major cause of increased uric acid synthesis results from an accelerated breakdown of ATP. This occurs during hypoglycemia-induced glycogen degra-

D–Ribose 5'–Phosphate

α 5–Phospho–D–Ribosyl–1–Pyrophosphate (PP–Ribose–P)

Figure 86–15. Reaction catalyzed by PP-ribose-P synthetase.

dation with the subsequent elevated concentrations of phosphorylated sugars in the liver in glucose-6-phosphatase deficiency.[271] Indeed, the acceleration of purine synthesis de novo observed in this disorder is secondary to a primary depletion of the adenine nucleotide pool. Patients with the Lesch-Nyhan syndrome, which is due to a virtually complete deficiency of hypoxanthine-guanine phosphoribosyltransferase, also uniformly exhibit a profound overproduction of uric acid and an accelerated rate of purine biosynthesis de novo. In these patients, as in those with gout caused by a partial deficiency of hypoxanthine-guanine phosphoribosyltransferase, the basic mechanism is thought to be related to a decreased consumption of PRPP and perhaps to decreased reutilization of hypoxanthine.

In the majority of patients with secondary hyperuricemia caused by an overproduction of uric acid, the predominant abnormality appears to be an increased turnover of nucleic acids. A number of diseases, including the myeloproliferative and lymphoproliferative disorders, multiple myeloma, secondary polycythemia, pernicious anemia, certain hemoglobinopathies, thalassemia, other hemolytic anemias, infectious mononucleosis, and some carcinomas, may be associated with increased marrow activity or increased cell turnover at other sites and an associated increased turnover of nucleic acids. The increased turnover in nucleic acids leads in turn to hyperuricemia, hyperuricaciduria, and a compensatory increase in the rate of purine biosynthesis de novo.

An important cause for overproduction of uric acid in secondary hyperuricemia appears to be related to the acceleration of ATP degradation to uric acid. Hyperuricemia observed in acutely ill patients may be related to the accelerated degradation of ATP.[271,289] Patients with myocardial infarction, acute smoke inhalation, respiratory failure, and status epilepticus appear to fall into this category. Strenuous exercise leads to the excessive degradation of muscle ATP to uric acid.[290] This can lead to increased serum urate levels, which can be substantial with extreme exercise, as seen in status epilepticus.[147,148] Excessive alcohol consumption, although associated with hyperlacticacidemia, also appears to be associated with increased synthesis of uric acid due to accelerated degradation of ATP.[291] Finally, the hyperuricemia of glycogen storage disease type I, described above, is related to this mechanism.

GENETICS OF GOUT

Gout has been recognized as a familial disorder since antiquity. Garrod[292] found the ancestral trait to be almost 80 percent among his patients, and commented that "breed is stronger than pasture." A familial incidence of gout of 50 to 80 percent has been reported by English observers,[293] but these contrast with figures as low as 11 percent in Denmark.[22] In the United States the familial incidence has generally ranged from 6 to 18 percent,[294,295] but figures up to 75 percent[296] have been

obtained after persistent questioning. In two large series from clinics with a special interest in gout, one English[60] and one American,[297] about 40 percent of the gouty subjects gave a positive family history of gout. These wide discrepancies may be attributed in part to variations of diligence in pursuing genealogic data. Population studies of families suggested the highest correlations between the mothers' serum urate and their children's, mainly their sons'.[18] These data suggest that the mothers' serum urate level has a strong influence on their children's levels.

When all available data are considered, they suggest that serum uric acid concentrations are controlled by multiple genes.[298] The probability of isolating an apparently dominant genetic factor increases when the basis of selection is racial, when the group is an isolate, or when the study concerns several generations of families in which gout occurs. Evidence for polygenic control will be more prominent when the population is heterogeneous or when only sibs of gouty subjects are studied.

The modes of inheritance of known rare subtypes of primary gout were described above. These include X-linked inheritance of both HPRT deficiency and PRPP synthetase overactivity and autosomal inheritance of glucose-6-phosphatase deficiency and some types of gout associated with a renal defect and a high incidence of renal disease.

ACUTE GOUTY ARTHRITIS

The Role of the Urate Crystal in the Acute Attack

Garrod[299] proposed in 1859 that the acute gouty paroxysm was triggered by precipitation of sodium urate crystals in the joint or neighboring tissues: "The deposited urate of soda may be looked upon as the cause, and not the effect, of the gouty inflammation." In 1899, Freudweiler[300] reproduced acute gouty attacks by injection of microcrystals of sodium urate and also of other crystals such as those of hypoxanthine or xanthine.[301] Subcutaneous injection of urate crystals was followed by evolution of a histologically characteristic tophus.[302] Freudweiler also proposed a central role for the urate crystal in the genesis of the acute gouty attack. In 1961 a study of joint fluid by McCarty and Hollander[303] led to a renewed interest in crystals of sodium urate in gouty effusions,[304] and particularly in the diagnostic value of large numbers of negatively birefringent crystals within synovial fluid leukocytes during the acute attack as demonstrated with the use of polarized light.[305,306] Urate crystals are virtually constant in acute gouty arthritis.[307,308] At the height of the response, the majority of the crystals are intracellular, though the extracellular proportion increases as inflammation subsides. Urate crystals may also occur in synovial fluid in a spherulite form.[309] The large "beach ball"-like structures are negatively birefringent and are digestible with the addition of uricase to the slide. Since the simultaneous occurrence of gout and infection in the same joint has been observed,[310,311] the identification of urate crystals does not rule out a concommitant septic arthritis. The importance and use of urate crystals in the diagnosis of gouty arthritis is reviewed in Chapter 38.

In 1962 Faires and McCarty[312] and Seegmiller and associates[313-315] rediscovered the capacity of microcrystals of sodium urate to evoke an inflammatory response in skin, subcutaneous tissues, and joints of animals and man. In both normouricemic and gouty man, the inflammatory response strikingly resembles the acute gouty attack. It may be successfully treated with[316] or prevented by[317] colchicine. The response is not limited to crystals of sodium urate but may also be evoked by calcium oxalate,[312] calcium pyrophosphate dihydrate,[318] sodium orotate,[313] and certain steroids,[313] but not by diamond dust.[319]

Synovial Membrane Tophi in Acute Gout. Agudelo and Schumacher[320] have observed urate crystals and microtophi in the synovial membrane 2 days after the onset of the first attack of acute gout. This finding as well as others suggests that acute gout may be superimposed on a joint in which urate deposition and low-grade chronic inflammation may have developed silently at an earlier time. The crystals of the synovium are often in a superficial location near the joint space. Thus, it seems possible that crystals could flake off the synovial membrane and enter the joint space, there to trigger an inflammatory attack when engulfed by polymorphonuclear or synovial cells of the synovial fluid.

Mechanism of Crystal Formation. The factors leading to precipitation of monosodium urate crystals in tissue and the mechanisms by which these crystals induce inflammation are complex and poorly understood. The mystery of crystal deposition in some tissues and not others is not yet satisfactorily explained, but some interesting clues are emerging from studies of the chemistry of cartilage. A relationship between the process by which the acute attack is triggered and that by which visible urate deposits form is not yet established, but both processes involve crystal formation and it is reasonable to surmise that a pathogenetic connection exists. This link too may reside in the behavior of certain cartilage constituents.

Supersaturation of serum or synovial fluid with monosodium urate is a necessary but not sufficient precondition for the development of acute gouty arthritis. To be sure, there is a correlation between the degree of hyperuricemia and the prevalence of gouty arthritis,[321] but it is also true that most hyperuricemic subjects never develop gout, and that those who do are often hyperuricemic for years before an attack supervenes. In addition, subjects with a history of gout may develop acute gouty arthritis at a time when their serum urate concentration is well below saturation. Perhaps the best example of this phenomenon is the occurrence of acute gouty arthritis in the patient recently started on antihyperuricemic therapy.

In subjects with gouty synovitis the concentration of urate in the synovial fluid is usually equal to its concentration in serum.[322,323] Urate has less of a tendency to precipitate in plasma than synovial fluid, since plasma is a significantly better solvent for monosodium urate than synovial fluid.[324] Thus, an important question is what makes monosodium urate crystals form in some subjects but not in others despite a similarity in serum urate concentrations. Specific factors in gouty synovial fluid may enhance urate crystallization. Addition of synovial fluids from gout patients to a supersaturated solution of sodium urate under physiological conditions greatly enhanced urate nucleation, whereas fluids from degenerative joint disease patients moderately enhanced nucleation, and fluids from rheumatoid patients had only a slight effect.[325]

Role of Proteoglycans. In 1892, Roberts[304] incubated pig tarsal bones in a saturated solution of sodium urate, and after 3 days noted the encrustation of tophaceous-like material on the cartilaginous articulating surface. At that time little was known of the macromolecules of cartilage, but its electrolyte composition had been determined. He proposed that precipitation occurred because of relatively high sodium concentration in connective tissues as compared to serum and parenchymal organs.

The connective tissue sites of urate deposition are rich in polysaccharides.[129] These polysaccharides are covalently bound to protein and hence are called protein-polysaccharides, or more recently "proteoglycans." Cartilage and synovial fluid contain a series of proteoglycans, composed of protein and chondroitin sulfate or keratan sulfate. The linear polysaccharides are attached to the protein core like bristles on a brush. Certain of these markedly enhance the solubility of urate in buffers having molarities and hydrogen ion concentrations similar to those of most body fluids.[326] The integrity of the proteoglycan molecule is essential: unbound chondroitin sulfate or proteoglycans digested by trypsin effects no significant augmentation of urate solubility. These proteoglycan macromolecules also inhibit the crystallization of urate from a supersaturated solution. Although the mechanism of this solubilizing phenomenon has not been investigated, some type of physical or chemical binding of urate is proposed.

There is a continuous turnover of proteoglycan molecules and this may be relevant to the genesis of the acute attack. Katz and Schubert[326] suggest that when proteinpolysaccharide is enzymatically destroyed as a result of normal or accelerated connective tissue turnover, its binding capacity for urate is reduced. Because the tissue is relatively avascular, degradation will result in a sudden local increase in the concentration of free sodium urate. Crystals may precipitate from the supersaturated tissue fluids, with silent deposition in cartilage, bone, or tendon, or with activation of an acute synovitis. Perhaps destruction of connective tissue also releases bound sodium, resulting in an even greater increase in sodium activity and an enhanced tendency toward crystal formation through common ion effects, as first proposed by Roberts.[304] This formulation postulates that connective tissue storage of bound urate precedes crystallization and the acute attack. This point has not been critically examined in the laboratory, although it is known that cartilage has an affinity for absorbing urate in vitro.[327] This hypothesis does not readily account for the poor correlation of urate crystal formation with the serum or synovial fluid urate concentration. In addition, it assumes that the postulated increase in urate concentration is localized to the layer of synovial fluid in intimate contact with cartilage, since the concentration of urate measured in synovial fluid samples is not greater than the serum concentration in gout. This notion is consistent with a growing body of knowledge of the behavior of "unstirred layers" in physiological fluids.[328] Thus, a possible contributory role of connective tissue proteoglycans to urate storage and crystal formation is an attractive hypothesis. The proteoglycans of serum migrate as α_1-α_2-globulins.[329] In contrast to the aforementioned studies, Perricone and Brandt[330] have recently provided data to suggest that proteoglycans may not be an important factor for urate solubility in vivo, since these solubilizing effects are not sustained. The urate-solubilizing properties of proteoglycan molecules are related to a cation exchange function of the glycosaminoglycans within the proteoglycan molecule.[331] These molecules can exchange potassium for sodium of the urate molecule, leading to the formation of highly soluble potassium urate.

Reduced binding of urate in gouty subjects could lead to the precipitation of crystals at lower than usual plasma concentrations of urate. While exceptions may exist,[212] most subjects with gout exhibit normal binding of urate to plasma proteins. In addition, patients with chronic renal insufficiency have hyperuricemia and reduced binding of urate to plasma protein,[332] yet the incidence of acute gouty arthritis in renal insufficiency is very low. Whatever the case, in patients with gout, urate binding to plasma protein now appears so weak that it is of little significance.[333,334]

Temperature Differentials and Urate Solubility. Several other factors may contribute to the initial precipitation of urate. Loeb[335] has emphasized the possible role of temperature in the precipitation of urate crystals. The maximal equilibrium concentration of urate in the presence of a physiologic concentration of sodium drops from 6.8 mg per 100 ml at 37° C to 4.5 mg per 100 ml at 30° C.[335] A gradient exists between central body temperature and intra-articular temperatures of extremity joints. Hollander and colleagues[336-338] have measured joint temperatures with a filamentous copper-constantin thermocouple inserted through the bore of an aspiration needle. The intra-articular temperature of the normal knee joint is approximately 32° C. The temperature of peripheral joints increases during exercise.[338]

Acute gout often begins at night, and may follow greater than usual exercise. Perhaps cooling of extremity joints during rest is a contributing factor in acute gout. Loeb[335] suggests that the cooler peripheral extracellular fluids may be supersaturated with sodium urate even at plasma urate concentration values usually considered normal. The phenomenon would be even more striking

in the patient with basal hyperuricemia. A temperature effect could explain the tendency of urate to crystallize in more distal or peripheral parts of the body, such as joints of the foot or the ears. In addition, Loeb proposes that the heat associated with inflammation may help limit the process by enhancing the solubility of the urate crystals. In the chronically gouty joint with moderately active inflammation, temperatures of 35.5 and 35.6° C have been recorded, while in the acutely inflamed gouty knee temperatures may rise to as high as 37.0° C.[337]

Dysequilibrium. Simkin[339] has proposed that urate may crystallize owing to a transient increase in concentration when extracellular fluid is reabsorbed from the joint space at a faster rate than urate. This factor may contribute to urate precipitation in gouty subjects, but direct confirmatory demonstration is lacking.

Trauma and Aging. Trauma is often thought to play a role in acute gout, and has been implicated as a factor in the predisposition of joints of the lower extremity to gout. Acute gout often begins at night or after exposure out of doors (e.g., "pheasant hunter's toe"[170]). The most frequently affected site is the first metatarsophalangeal joint of the great toe, a site that is subjected during walking to the greatest stress, in kilograms of weight per square centimeter of area, of any joint in the body. Mechanical damage to connective tissue might be a factor in the mechanism proposed by Katz and Schubert.[326] Trauma might also help flake off urate crystals from an articular crust and serve to trigger an attack. Other factors favoring crystal formation may include age-related changes in connective tissue and in the microvascular circulation. Any reduction in blood flow would be expected to affect the rate of dissipation of a local increase in tissue urate concentration, and also to contribute to the temperature differentials postulated above.

The Role of pH. Although a decrease in pH, resulting from production of lactic acid during anaerobic glycolysis of leukocytes, has been postulated to play a role in the propagation of the acute attack of gout,[314,315] there is little evidence to support this hypothesis. In fact, monosodium urate is more soluble at pH 6.0 or 6.5 than at pH 7.4.[170] A decrease in pH would increase the likelihood of uric acid (rather than monosodium urate) precipitation. Since the crystals present in synovial leukocytes during an acute attack are monosodium urate, this pH change would seem to be unimportant. In addition, the pH changes actually observed during the acute attack of gout are small. The maximal pH drop is only 0.5 unit,[340,341] probably inconsequential in terms of its effect on urate solubility,[170] though perhaps significant in activating proteins of the inflammatory process.[342]

Mediation of the Inflammatory Response. The urate crystal itself can activate Hageman factor of synovial fluid.[343,344] Urate crystals cause a proteolytic cleavage of Hageman factor into fragments, which indicate activation. The Hageman factor cleaved on urate crystals may either remain crystal associated or be released into joint fluid.[345] This may initiate a series of reactions leading to the development of permeability enhancing activity, kallikrein, and kinins.[342,346] The concentration of kinin-like peptides in synovial fluid may rise as much as 50-fold during crystal-induced attacks in man, as it does during spontaneous attacks of gout, but this response is not specific for gout and also occurs in other inflammatory states such as rheumatoid arthritis.[347] These factors can induce vasodilation, increased vascular permeability, and leukocyte margination and emigration through the vessel wall. However, an inflammatory response to urate can also occur in the absence of this system. Phelps and associates[348] found in dogs that arthritis induced with urate crystals was not prevented by carboxypeptidase injected directly into the joint space or into the arterial supply to the joint. Carboxypeptidase inactivates bradykinin, but not kallikrein. In addition, Spilberg[349] has shown that monosodium urate crystals can induce an acute inflammatory synovitis in the chicken stifle joint even though these animals lack Hageman factor and do not have detectable kinin activity in their synovial fluid. Finally, at least one patient has been described with classic gout and Hageman factor trait.[350] These studies suggest that the kallikrein-kinin system is not an obligatory mediator of the inflammatory response of acute gout.

The complement systems may be involved in the acute inflammatory response to urate crystals as a concomitant or alternative activator. Naff and Byers[351] found that incubation of urate crystals with serum led to marked reduction of activity of C4, C2, C3, and C5, but to only a slight decrease in C1. Heat-stable chemotactic activities consistent with C5a and C567 are also generated during incubation. The reaction does not appear to require properdin or Hageman factor. Recent studies have shown that the activation of C3 occurs through the classic pathway.[352,353]

Complement levels in synovial fluid obtained from patients during an acute attack of gouty arthritis are normal[354,355] or low[356] and activated complement components may be seen in gouty synovial fluid.[356] Depletion of C3 and C5 in rabbits and dogs by injection of purified cobra venom factor does not diminish the leukocyte response to urate crystals in synovial fluid.[352,354] It appears that the inflammatory response to urate crystals does not show an obligatory dependence on complement.[357]

Leukotrienes, especially leukotriene B$_4$, have been implicated as mediators in acute crystal-induced synovitis.[358,359] Monosodium urate stimulates the formation of leukotrienes from endogenous sources of arachidonate. In addition, the biologic deactivation of leukotriene B$_4$ was inhibited by crystals of monosodium urate. Therefore, urate crystals may stimulate the production of an important chemical mediator and help lead to its persistence.

The platelet may be an important source of mediators of the acute inflammatory response. Monosodium urate crystals activate platelet secretion of biogenic amines and nucleotides as well as prostaglandins and their intermediates.[360-362] This platelet stimulation is mediated by membrane proteins[362] and is a true example of platelet secretion.[361] The relative importance of this component in the pathogenesis of the inflammatory reaction remains to be established.

Binding of protein to the surface of monosodium urate crystals may be important for initiating and perpetuating inflammation. IgG and Clq bind to crystal surfaces.[363,364] The Fc portion of IgG is fully exposed, suggesting that the site of attachment may reside on the Fab moiety of IgG.[364] The presence of cell surface IgG enhances the stimulation of platelets and leukocytes.[360,365,366] The additional adsorption of lysosomal enzymes to monosodium urate crystals[367] could damage the cell that phagocytizes these crystals.

The multiplicity of factors identified in the acute inflammation associated with monosodium urate crystals make it difficult to identify those that are critical from those that may be playing a facilitating role. Other factors may be involved in mediating the chronic inflammation and joint destruction that occur in gout. The release of latent collagenase and PGE$_2$ from cultured synovial fibroblasts may have a role in the latter process.[368] Synovial lining cells may also produce a chemotactic factor.[369]

Role of the Leukocyte

The inflammatory response to urate crystals depends on the presence of polymorphonuclear leukocytes. In dogs rendered leukopenic with vancomycin[370] or with antipolymorphonuclear leukocyte serum,[371] urate crystals fail to induce an inflammatory response; responsiveness is restored by cross circulation with replacement of leukocytes[370] or when time for recovery is allowed.[371]

Chemotactic Factor. Phelps[372,373] has shown that leukocytes release a factor chemotactic for other leukocytes within 11 minutes after phagocytosis of urate crystals. The generation of this urate-induced chemotactic factor is markedly diminished when the polymorphonuclear leukocytes are exposed to monosodium urate crystals in the presence of inhibitors of RNA synthesis such as actinomycin D[374] or in the presence of colchicine.[375] Physical characterization of this chemotactic factor is incomplete; however, it has a molecular weight of approximately 8400 and is located predominantly in the lysosomal fraction of the polymorphonuclear leukocytes.[370,376] The protein is rich in glycine, serine, aspartic acid, glutamic acid, and alanine.[369] A specific binding site for the chemotactic factor has been identified on the surface of human neutrophils.[377] The equilibrium dissociation constant is 0.5 μM and there are 6.4 $\times$ 10^5 binding sites per cell. There appears, therefore, to be a relationship between a specific binding site on neutrophils and the ability to be chemotactically activated. The generation of this chemotactic factor may be a general response of the neutrophil to the phagocytosis of foreign particles, since it is released in response to monosodium urate, calcium pyrophosphate dihydrate, diamond dust or heat-aggregated human gamma globulin.[378,379] This chemotactic substance supplies a mechanism whereby more leukocytes can be attracted into the joint space in response to the phagocytosis of monosodium urate crystals.

Crystal Ingestion. Protein-coated crystals of sodium urate are taken up within the phagosomes of the polymorphs. Phagosomes merge with primary lysosomes, and crystals come to lie within secondary lysosomes. A direct interaction of urate crystals with lysosomes takes place, perhaps by hydrogen bonding to cholesterol-rich, testosterone-containing membranes. The organelle perforates, injury results to the cell in general, and escape of leukocyte contents induces tissue injury and inflammation. Urate crystals absorb a variety of proteins, including lysosomal enzymes,[367,380] and this protein adsorption modulates the ability of the crystal to disrupt the lysosome.[381,382] Monosodium urate mediates the production of superoxide anions by human neutrophils either during phagocytosis[365] or upon exposure without phagocytosis.[383] The latter is stimulated by IgG coating of the crystals. Superoxide radical generation may also occur in response to chemotactic factor alone.[384] The superoxide anion therefore may contribute substantially to local inflammation in acute gouty arthritis.

Disruption of the membrane around the crystals leads to a release into the cytoplasm of the crystal along with the lysosomal enzymes.[385,386] The crystals may then be available to be engulfed by other leukocytes, thus perhaps contributing to the perpetuation of the inflammatory response. Urate in solution may potentiate this process by inhibiting the formation of a protective protein coat about the crystal.[387] This protein coat must ordinarily be dissolved before the crystal can interact with the cell membrane. Finally, activation of prostaglandin E_2 synthesis may contribute to the severity of the inflammation as well as its chronicity.[366]

Considerable destruction of ingested urate crystals is also routinely observed by light microscopy within the lysosome. This has been attributed to enzymatic digestion by leukoperoxidases of the leukocyte.[388-391] So far as is known, this is the only uricolysis occurring within the tissues of man, and it accounts for less than 1 percent of the urate turnover of the human body.

The Role of Lysosomal Enzymes. By whatever intermediary mechanisms are involved, it appears that lysosomal enzymes released in this process play a key role in both the acute inflammatory reaction and the destructive changes of gout, as they do in other forms of joint disease.[385,386] Lysosomes are viewed as components of a "common final pathway" of tissue damage.[392] In joints, lysosomes are found in synovial lining cells, cartilage cells, wandering and fixed macrophages, the pericytes of blood vessels, and the polymorphonuclear leukocytes which enter joint spaces from the blood.[393] Leukocyte lysosomes contain a cationic protein that induces inflammation by disrupting mast cell granules, a proteinase which induces capillary permeability, and acid proteinases capable of breaking down cartilage proteinpolysaccharide[394] and of cleaving C5 to C5a.[395] Perhaps a further breakdown of proteoglycans in cartilage could lead to further urate crystallization. Synovial cells also contain a collagenase capable of attacking whole articular cartilage. The cleavage of collagen by synovial collagenase may be the rate-limiting step in cartilage degradation. The collagenase of rheumatoid synovium is four times as active at 36° C as at 33° C[396] and may thus be activated in this setting. Other factors such as the prostaglandins and cAMP may also play a role in the pathogenesis of the acute attack, but evidence at present is fragmentary.

Unexplained Features

Self-Limited Nature of the Attack. While it is not known why acute gouty arthritis is self-limited, several contributing factors may be postulated: (1) The increased heat of inflammation may increase urate solubility, diminishing the tendency toward new crystal formation, and favoring dissolution of existing crystals. (2) The increased blood flow may help transport urate away from the joint and lessen the tendency toward formation of local regions of supersaturation. (3) Some of the ingested urate crystals may be destroyed by the myeloperoxidase of the leukocytes, thus diminishing the load of crystals released by ruptured cells and capable of perpetuating the inflammatory response. (4) Adrenal cortical hormones secreted as a part of the alarm reaction of acute attack may suppress the inflammatory process.

Crystals Present with Minimal Inflammation. The work of McCarty[305] and others[307,308] has shown that urate crystals are a virtually constant finding in the synovial fluid during an acute attack, and a great deal of work has been directed toward the mechanism or mechanisms by which urate crystals may trigger the attack. However, urate crystals are also often found in the joints of patients with chronic gout at times when there is only indolent soreness of low intensity. Also, as mentioned above, urate crystals may be present in the synovium of joints during the quiescent phase between acute attacks. Clearly, more than the presence of crystals is involved in the pathogenesis of the gouty paroxysm.

TREATMENT OF GOUT

The therapeutic aims in gout are (1) to terminate the acute attack as promptly and gently as possible; (2) to prevent recurrences of acute gouty arthritis; (3) to prevent or reverse complications of the disease resulting from deposition of sodium urate crystals in joints, kidneys, or other sites; (4) to prevent or reverse associated features of the illness which are also deleterious, such as obesity, hypertriglyceridemia, or hypertension; and (5) to prevent formation of uric acid kidney stones.

In considering these aims, an important distinction must be made between the means employed in the management of the acute inflammatory manifestations on the one hand, and the control of hyperuricemia (and hyperuricaciduria) on the other. With one possible exception, those agents which are so highly effective in the treatment of acute gout are of no value in the control of hyperuricemia. Conversely, those drugs useful in the control of hyperuricemia are of no immediate or direct value in the treatment of the acute gouty attack.

Asymptomatic Hyperuricemia

There are relatively few indications for institution of drug therapy in patients with asymptomatic hyperuricemia, for the incidence of gout is low. Since advice on the indications for drug therapy of asymptomatic hyperuricemia is so often solicited, this is reviewed in Chapter 33.

Acute Gouty Arthritis

The affected joint should be placed at rest and suitable therapy instituted as soon as possible. The pharmacology of agents of value in the treatment of acute gout has been considered in Chapters 50 and 57. The acute gouty attack may be effectively terminated by any of several drugs. For practical purposes the choice is among colchicine, indomethacin, and phenylbutazone or its analogue oxyphenbutazone. The newer nonsteroidal antiinflammatory agents are also effective in acute gout, but experience is still limited.

Drugs that affect the serum urate concentration should not be changed, i.e., started or stopped, during an acute attack. Just as sudden fluctuations in serum urate levels may tend to precipitate an acute attack, an inflammatory reaction already in progress may be made substantially worse by a major change in the urate concentration. Antihyperuricemic drug therapy should not be instituted until an attack has resolved. Antihyperuricemic drugs already in place should not be stopped unless the drug has just been started and has itself contributed to the attack.

If an appropriately treated attack has not begun to resolve within 48 hours, one should consider the possibility that another disease, such as infection,[397] may be contributing to the inflammatory process. If no other disease can be incriminated, one should then consider changing the medication. For example, in protracted attacks phenylbutazone will sometimes succeed where colchicine has failed. If after several days the attack is still disabling and inflammation does not abate, intraarticular corticosteroids may be indicated.

Colchicine. *Oral Administration.* Colchicine is usually administered orally in a dose of 0.5 or 0.6 mg (one tablet) at hourly intervals until the joint symptoms ease, the patient develops nausea, vomiting, or diarrhea, or he has taken a maximum of 12 doses (6 mg). In most patients the side effects precede or coincide with improvement in joint symptoms. If the attack is treated within the first few hours, a favorable response can be predicted over 90 percent of the time.[398] If treatment is delayed beyond 12 hours, only 75 percent of patients with acute gouty arthritis treated in this manner will respond within 12 to 48 hours.[398] Diseases other than gout reported to improve on this regimen are serum sickness,[399] pseudogout,[400] hydroxyapatite calcific tendinitis,[401] sarcoid arthritis,[402] erythema nodosum,[403] rheu-

matoid arthritis,[404] and familial Mediterranean fever.[405] Only rarely will the response in any of these diseases meet the criteria set forth by Wallace and associates[398] for an acceptable response in gout. The near specificity of colchicine in acute gout has been confirmed by many observers. The major disadvantage of the oral colchicine regimen is that 50[406] to 80 percent[407] of patients treated in the usual manner develop increased peristalsis, cramping abdominal pain, diarrhea, nausea, or vomiting before relief from gout occurs, thus making some compromise with the ideal dose necessary. Generally, we use oral colchicine when the diagnosis of gout is uncertain and the patient's response will be of diagnostic help. In the gouty patient with an established diagnosis, we use indomethacin, colchicine intravenously, or phenylbutazone.

Intravenous Administration. Colchicine has been used intravenously since at least 1951.[407,408] When used properly the drug abolishes the acute attack without the high incidence of gastrointestinal side effects observed with oral administration. In addition, response to the drug given intravenously may be more specific for gouty arthritis than when used orally.

An initial dose of 2 mg is followed, if prompt relief is not obtained, by an additional 1 mg every 6 hours to a maximum dose of 4 to 5 mg during the treatment period. The colchicine should be diluted with 20 ml of normal saline prior to administration to minimize sclerosis of the vein. In addition, oral colchicine should be discontinued in order to reduce the likelihood of gastrointestinal intolerance.

The use of intravenous colchicine is associated with some risk. The most common complication is local extravasation during or immediately after injection. This can lead to inflammation and necrosis which may be painful. In addition, we have observed cases of median nerve neuritis of the injected arm on this basis. The presence of small veins which are difficult to inject represents a relative contraindication to intravenous use of this drug. Since one loses gastrointestinal symptoms as an indicator of toxicity, bone marrow suppression may be the first complication. The drug should be used sparingly, if at all, in patients who are neutropenic. In addition the total dose should be reduced if the patient has been receiving oral colchicine chronically or if he has significant liver or renal disease. Although serious toxicity has been rare, it has occurred when these factors have not been considered.[229] However, not every fatality attributed to colchicine can clearly be related to this agent.[409]

Indomethacin. Indomethacin was first shown to be effective in the treatment of acute gouty arthritis in 1963.[410-412] This response has subsequently been confirmed by many investigators. The drug may be effective in doses as low as 25 mg given four times a day. We recommend an initial dose of 50 to 75 mg followed by 50 mg every 6 hours with a maximum dose of 200 mg in the first 24 hours. In most instances substantial relief will have occurred within this time. In order to prevent relapse it is reasonable to continue this dose for an additional 24 hours, then taper to 50 mg every 8 hours for 24 hours, and then 25 mg every 8 hours for 24 hours.

Contraindications to the use of indomethacin include active peptic ulcer disease, regional enteritis, ulcerative colitis, severe infection, and mental disease. Inflammatory bowel disease is considered a relative contraindication because of reports[413,414] of bowel perforation occurring after indomethacin in this setting. Indomethacin also should be used with caution in patients with impaired renal function or coronary artery disease. Although it may cause a transient rise of blood urea nitrogen and creatinine, severe azotemia may result in patients with diminished glomerular filtration rate from congestive heart failure.[415] Acute renal failure has occasionally been observed in patients with normal renal function.[416] Indomethacin decreases coronary blood flow and increases coronary vascular resistance in patients with coronary artery disease.[417] These properties are probably related to inhibition of prostaglandin synthesis; these side effects, therefore, are not unique to indomethacin, but may occur with other nonsteroidal drugs and salicylates.[415,418]

Phenylbutazone. Phenylbutazone has been used in the treatment of acute gouty arthritis since the early 1950's. The drug is effective in this setting, with 75 to 90 percent of patients with acute gouty arthritis showing dramatic improvement.[419-422] The initial dose is 200 to 600 mg followed by 100 to 200 mg three to four times the first day with a maximum dose of 600 mg per day. After 24 hours the dose can usually be tapered to 100 mg four times a day for the next 2 days, and then discontinued. Oxyphenbutazone can also be used. The dose is the same as that of phenylbutazone, and side effects are similar.

This type of program is associated with side effects in less than 10 percent[406,423] of the patients so treated. Although phenylbutazone may lead to serious or even lethal bone marrow suppression, toxicity is rare with short-term use of the drug for less than 1 week. The major complications noted with this program are sodium retention, peptic ulcer disease, and serum sickness. Accordingly, the presence of active peptic ulcer disease and states of severe sodium retention represent contraindications to the use of phenylbutazone.

Phenylbutazone is tightly bound to serum proteins and may displace other compounds from albumin. By this mechanism the agent potentiates the effect of many drugs in common use such as the oral anticoagulants and the oral hypoglycemic agents. The drug should therefore be used with caution in patients receiving these drugs.

Naproxen. Cuq[424] treated 20 patients with acute gouty arthritis with naproxen, and recorded a response in 75 percent. Minor reactions occurred in four patients but in no case did these necessitate discontinuation of the drug. He recommends a dose of 500 mg initially followed by 250 mg every 8 hours for the acute attack. Wilkens and Case[425] treated 12 patients with acute gouty arthritis using an initial dose of naproxen of 600 mg followed by 300 mg every 8 hours for a total duration of 48 hours. A "majority" of those treated within 48 hours of the onset of symptoms responded well. Sturge and associates[426] found that naproxen, 750 mg as the initial dose, followed by 250 mg three times per day, was as effective in the treatment of acute gouty arthritis as phenylbutazone, 200 mg four times per day.

Fenoprofen. Several recent studies document the effectiveness of fenoprofen in the treatment of acute gouty arthritis. Ridolfo[427] noted good or excellent response in seven of ten patients, whereas Wallace[428] noted at least a good response in seven of ten patients. Wanasukapunt[429] treated 27 patients with gouty arthritis with fenoprofen, 800 mg every 6 hours, until improvement occurred followed by taper of the drug. Nineteen patients had a good response within 48 hours. Three patients noted possible side effects.

Ibuprofen. Ten patients with acute gouty arthritis were treated with ibuprofen, 800 mg every 8 hours orally.[430] With resolution the dose was reduced to 400 mg every 6 hours for an additional 24 to 72 hours. All ten patients showed complete resolution within 72 hours.

Indoprofen. Caruso and associates[431] treated 17 patients with acute gouty arthritis with indoprofen, 200 mg intravenously, followed by continuous infusion at a rate of 100 mg per hour for 2 to 4 hours and then 200 to 600 mg per day orally. Most patients were essentially free of symptoms within 24 hours.

Sulindac. In comparative studies the efficacy of sulindac, 400 mg daily, was found to be similar to that of phenylbutazone, 600 mg daily.[432]

Piroxicam. The administration of piroxicam, 40 mg per day for 5 days, is an effective therapy in acute gout.[433,434] The dose of 40 mg per day is more effective than 20 mg per day in that a higher percentage of patients received faster and complete relief within 5 days (53 versus 28 percent).[434] Substantial improvement is seen by 24 hours and most patients are improved or free of symptoms by 5 days.

Corticosteroids. Triamcinolone hexacetamide injected intra-articularly into the involved joint is useful in treating acute gout limited to a single joint or bursa; relief from pain is usually prompt and complete within 12 hours.[435] When this local measure was accompanied by administration of colchicine or phenylbutazone, no recurrence was noted. Steroid hormones are not recommended for parenteral or systemic use in acute gout, as the effects are inconsistent and rebound attacks are frequent.[436]

Choice of Agents

While many of the newer nonsteroidal anti-inflammatory agents appear to show promise, the choice of a drug for the treatment of acute gouty arthritis can still be narrowed at this time essentially to colchicine, indomethacin, or phenylbutazone. With time and more experience in using the drugs, some of the newer nonsteroidal anti-inflammatory drugs may prove equally effective while causing fewer acute side effects than any of these three. The time of initiation of therapy may be as important as the choice of drug. With any of these agents, the sooner the drug is started the more likely the patient is to have a rapid and complete response. We use and recommend intravenous colchicine for the hospitalized patient and oral colchicine for the ambulatory patient in whom the diagnosis of gouty arthritis is not clearly established. For most patients in whom the diagnosis is secure, the acute attack should be treated with indomethacin or phenylbutazone. We tend not to use oral colchicine to manage acute gout because of its gastrointestinal side effects and the potency of other drugs available.

Results of studies comparing the effectiveness of indomethacin and phenylbutazone in the management of gouty arthritis are divided. Some have favored phenylbutazone,[437,438] others indomethacin,[406,439,440] and still another has found no difference in the effectiveness of the two drugs.[423] Although the immediate side effects seem to be more frequent with indomethacin, the response may be a little faster with this drug. We tend to favor indomethacin because it does not have uricosuric properties. The latter, a characteristic of phenylbutazone, may modify the serum urate and urinary uric acid excretion and make a subsequent workup of altered uric acid levels more difficult to interpret.

Patients with established gout should have their preferred anti-inflammatory agent immediately available to them, and they should be instructed to start taking the drug at the first "twinge" of an acute attack. The attack may often be aborted with less than a full therapeutic dose of the drug. Some patients can terminate an incipient acute attack with a single dose of 50 to 100 mg of indomethacin, or of 400 mg of phenylbutazone.

The anti-inflammatory agents are reviewed extensively in Chapters 50 and 57.

Prophylaxis

The practice of giving small daily doses of colchicine as prophylaxis against acute attacks of gout was introduced by Cohen in 1936,[441] and advocated by Talbott and Coombs in 1938.[442] In 1952 Gutman and Yu[53] reported that 18 of 31 patients who ingested colchicine daily for 18 months or more experienced a conspicuous reduction in the frequency of acute attacks. This program enabled restoration of full employment for 13 patients who had been virtually incapacitated because of frequent episodes of gout.

Gutman[443] reported observations in 260 patients who were given 0.5 to 2 mg of colchicine a day (in 66 percent the dose was 1.0 mg) over a mean period of 6.4 years. Colchicine was given alone in 117 patients; the remainder received uricosuric agents in addition. In 74 percent there was complete or virtually complete cessation of attacks; in 20 percent the response was satisfactory, and in 6 percent the regimen was a failure. In patients who received both uricosuric drugs and colchicine, discontinuance of colchicine alone was sometimes followed by recurrence of attacks, whereas this did not happen in patients in whom uricosuric drug alone was stopped.

The effectiveness of prophylactic colchicine has been confirmed by Paulus and associates.[444]

In the rare patient unable to tolerate even one colchicine tablet per day, indomethacin has been used prophylactically at a dose of 25 mg two times per day with some subjective success.

A program of maintenance colchicine or indomethacin may make the difference between frequent incapacitation and uninterruped daily activites. If for a period of a year the serum urate value has been maintained within the normal range and there have been no acute attacks, maintenance colchicine may be discontinued. Here, again, it is advisable to warn the patient that this alteration in the therapeutic program may be followed by an exacerbation of acute gouty arthritis.

Control of Hyperuricemia and Monosodium Urate Deposition

Based on our current concepts, the first episode of acute gouty arthritis represents the initial clinical evidence of urate deposition in most patients. Control of hyperuricemia with antihyperuricemic agents can prevent and, in fact, reverse urate deposition. A spectrum of opinion exists as to when in the course of gout antihyperuricemic therapy should be started, and how important maintenance of normal serum urate levels may prove to be in the absence of renewed symptoms. Some physicians regard the first gouty attack as already a late event in a disorder marked by years of antecedent silent deposition of microcrystalline deposits of urate in cartilage and other connective tissue. There is some morphologic evidence for this,[320] and we subscribe to this point of view.

Others take the position that since tophi and symptomatic chronic gouty arthritis develop only in a minority of cases of gout—ordinarily very slowly after many years of recurrent acute attacks—unnecessary or premature medication can be avoided, without demonstrable penalty, by withholding antihyperuricemic drugs until there is an indication that recurrent attacks cannot be prevented by a prophylactic program alone or that tophaceous deposits are indeed forming.[445] For example, some patients will never have a second attack even in the absence of therapy. The probability of such a course is greatest in patients with only minimally elevated serum urate values and with normal 24-hour urinary uric acid values. In the Framingham population study,[321] intervals between attacks were longer early in the course of the disease and in subjects with serum urate values under 8 mg per 100 ml as compared to those with higher values. In the experience of Yu and Gutman[446] only 62 percent of patients experienced a second attack of acute gout within 1 year, and 78 percent within 2 years. Seven percent had no further attacks for 10 years or more even without antihyperuricemic drugs or maintenance colchicine therapy.

Antihyperuricemic drugs provide a definitive method for controlling hyperuricemia. While it is important to treat and prevent acute attacks of gouty arthritis with anti-inflammatory agents, it is the long-term control of hyperuricemia that ultimately modifies the manifestations of the gouty diathesis. In general, the aim of antihyperuricemic therapy is to reduce the serum urate concentration to below the concentration at which monosodium urate saturates extracellular fluid (6.4 mg per dl). When this is achieved, urate deposits will resolve (Figs. 86–16 and 86–17). Reduction to these levels may be achieved pharmacologically at present by the use of uricosuric agents or allopurinol. Antihyperuricemic drugs generally do not have anti-inflammatory properties. Uricosuric agents reduce the serum urate concentration by enhancing the renal excretion of uric acid. While a large number of drugs exhibit this property, the most effective agents available in the United States today are probenecid and sulfinpyrazone. These two drugs are effective in lowering the serum urate in 75 to 80 percent of patients with hyperuricemia and gout. The prototypic drug available to decrease uric acid synthesis is allopurinol. Allopurinol inhibits xanthine oxidase, the enzyme which catalyzes the oxidation of hypoxanthine to xanthine and xanthine to uric acid. These agents are discussed extensively in Chapter 56.

The choice of an antihyperuricemic drug should have a rational basis because the treatment of hyperuricemia in gout is ordinarily carried on indefinitely. In those patients with gout who excrete less than 700 mg of uric acid per day, a reduction in serum urate concentration can be achieved equally well with allopurinol or a uricosuric drug such as probenecid or sulfinpyrazone. Each

Figure 86–16. Roentgenograms of hands of W. L., taken on June 23, 1965 *(A)*, and July 11, 1968 *(B)*. Note the extensive resolution of soft-tissue tophi and modest reduction in size of bony erosions, with some recalcification. (Courtesy of Dr. R. Wayne Rundles, Duke University Medical Center.)

Figure 86–17. Roentgenograms of right foot of W. L., taken on June 23, 1965 (*A*), and July 11, 1968 (*B*). Note virtually complete resolution of soft-tissue tophi and extensive repair and recalcification of bone, especially of the first metatarsophalangeal joint. (Courtesy of Dr. R. Wayne Rundles, Duke University Medical Center.)

of these agents may prevent the deterioration of renal function in patients with primary gout.[447-454] There is no clear-cut evidence that uricosuric drugs are superior to the inhibitors of xanthine oxidase or vice versa in preventing renal damage from hyperuricemia in subjects with a normal excretion of uric acid and no history of renal calculi. All other things being equal, a uricosuric drug might be tried first, since these agents are not known to influence purine or pyrimidine metabolism as allopurinol does,[455,456] and they are known to be relatively safe after more than a quarter century of clinical use. As more experience is gained with allopurinol, factors such as cost or convenience may become the more important concerns. In general, the candidate for uricosuric agents at present is the gouty patient under 60 years old with normal renal function (creatinine clearance greater than 80 ml per minute), uric acid excretion of less than 700 mg per 24 hours on a general diet, and no history of renal calculi. There is very little to lead one to choose either probenecid or sulfinpyrazone over the other. Our personal choice is usually the latter because of its added antiplatelet effect.

There are certain situations in which an inhibitor of xanthine oxidase is clearly the drug of choice in the gouty patient (Table 86–9). Gouty individuals with a history of renal calculi of any type should be treated

with an inhibitor of xanthine oxidase. Likewise, patients with tophi should receive allopurinol to decrease the load of uric acid that must be handled by the kidney. Patients with gout and renal insufficiency can be tried on either type of agent, but uricosuric drugs would not be expected to work when the GFR is less than 30 ml per minute.[457] A final indication for allopurinol is the failure of uricosuric drugs to produce a serum urate of less than 7.0 mg per 100 ml or patient intolerance of the uricosuric agent. Occasionally, allopurinol and a uricosuric drug may be used in combination when the patient has tophaceous gout and it is not possible to reduce the serum urate below 7.0 mg per 100 ml with allopurinol alone.

Table 86–9. Indications for Allopurinol

Hyperuricemia Associated with Increased Uric Acid Production
    Urinary uric acid excretion of 1000 mg or more in 24 hours
    Hyperuricemia associated with HPRT deficiency or PP-ribose-P
        synthetase overactivity
    Uric acid nephropathy
    Nephrolithiasis
    Prophylaxis prior to cytolytic therapy
Intolerance or Reduced Efficacy of Uricosuric Agents
    Gout with renal insufficiency (GFR < 60 ml per minute)
    Allergy to uricosurics

A somewhat less clear indication for allopurinol therapy in the hyperuricemic patient relates to the level of uric acid excretion. The incidence of renal calculi is greater than 34 percent in patients with primary gout who excrete more than 700 mg per day of uric acid.[162] Likewise, it is the magnitude of uric acid excreted per day that correlates best with the development of acute uric acid nephropathy.[458] Therefore, these individuals run a risk of developing renal disease. They are also at greater risk for developing uric acid stones or acute uric acid nephropathy upon initiation of uricosuric therapy. The logical choice of therapy in these patients is, therefore, an agent, such as allopurinol, which decreases uric acid synthesis. For the same reason, patients with certain neoplastic diseases that are associated with hyperuricemia caused by increased nucleotide catabolism with increased uric acid synthesis may be treated with allopurinol. (See Chapter 33.) The effectiveness of allopurinol as an antihyperuricemic agent is illustrated in Figure 86–18.

The antihyperuricemic drugs are reviewed in detail in Chapter 56.

Management of Nephrolithiasis

In potential formers of stones of any type the first rule is to maintain a large urinary volume by the liberal ingestion of fluids, about 2 or 3 liters per day. This is particularly important in those hyperuricemic subjects whose daily urinary uric excretion is excessive; these patients constitute about 20 to 25 percent of the total. In gouty subjects with persistently acid urine, regular use of suitable alkalinizing agents may be required to adjust urine pH up to 6.0 to 6.5, which will shift uric acid to its more soluble urate form.

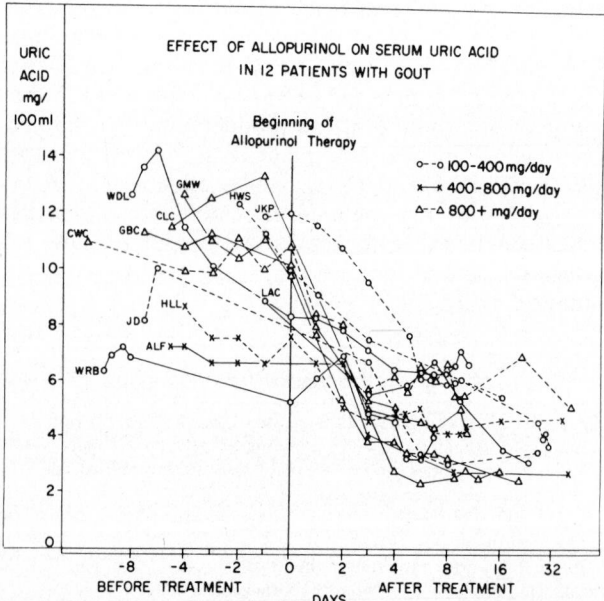

Figure 86–18. Reductions in serum urate concentrations in patients receiving allopurinol. (From Wyngaarden, J.B., and Kelley, W.N.: Gout and Hyperuricemia. New York, Grune & Stratton, 1976.)

The treatment of choice in nephrolithiasis of gout is allopurinol, which lowers both serum and urinary uric acid values. Allopurinol has greatly ameliorated the uric acid stone problem in gout. There is also evidence that its use reduces the rate of recurrence of calcium stones in hyperuricemic subjects.[200]

Ancillary Factors

In addition to anti-inflammatory agents, colchicine prophylaxis, and antihyperuricemic therapy, other factors may be decisive in determining whether recurrent attacks, chronic arthritis, stone, or nephropathy will develop.

Role of the Diet. *Weight Reduction.* Many gouty patients are overweight, and restoration of ideal weight through regulated caloric restriction is to be advocated strongly. Crash weight-reduction programs are to be avoided, as these may precipitate attacks of gout. Some gouty subjects respond to gradual weight loss with a reduction in serum urate concentration and urinary uric acid excretion;[459,460] others do not.[461]

Alcohol Ingestion. Many gouty patients consume liberal amounts of alcohol. Acute excesses may lead to exacerbations of hyperuricemia, in large part secondary to the temporary hyperlacticacidemia found during inebriation. Chronic ingestion of alcohol may stimulate increased purine production, resulting in increased hyperuricemia and hyperuricaciduria.[291,462] The added purine load resulting from regular ingestion of beer may also be detrimental. The gouty patient should be instructed in the deleterious effects of too liberal use of alcoholic beverages.

Avoidance of Acute Attack. Some gouty subjects are susceptible to acute attacks following use of alcoholic beverages, especially heavy wines and champagnes, or of rich foods, notably those high in purines, proteins, or fats. Others describe idiosyncratic responses, such as acute gout following eating of asparagus, but such relationships are rare and questionable. In gouty subjects the dietary indiscretions of holidays, feast days, and weddings are especially prone to end in gouty arthritis. A diet designed to avoid indiscretions known to be associated with the precipitation of an acute gouty attack in a particular individual may suffice, of itself, to avoid such attacks, but in general additional therapy is required.

Reduction in Body Load of Purines. In the pursuit of this objective by dietary means one may limit the ingestion of preformed purines that add to the burden of the uric acid pool and urinary disposal, as well as the ingestion of dietary constituents that promote endogenous production of purines. The introduction of potent uricosuric agents in the management of gout led to a general loss of attention to the purine content of the diet on the part of both physician and patient. While the use of rigid purine restriction is indeed superseded by the use of uricosuric agents, and now also allopurinol, the neglect of dietary factors in gout has been a disservice to some patients. It is still prudent to avoid excessive intake of purines in the average gouty patient. A diet restricted in purine content will reduce the urinary excretion of uric acid by 200 by 400 mg per day, and lower the mean serum urate value about 1 mg per 100 ml.[53] In some patients the reduction is even greater.[213] Severe dietary purine restriction is not often necessary, unless renal function is very poor and the control of hyperuricemia with drugs is unsatisfactory. The purine content of certain foods is summarized in Table 86–10, and several low purine diets are proposed in Table 86–11.

In both normal and gouty man, the rate of endogenous purine production is somewhat greater on a high protein than on a more moderate protein diet.[463] It may be desirable to limit the intake of nitrogenous precursors of uric acid by restriction of dietary proteins to levels of 70 or 80 grams per day. However, the benefits of dietary protein restriction are small compared with those of purine restriction. Excessive loads of dietary fructose may result in sudden acceleration of adenyl nucleotide catabolism and accelerated rates of uric acid synthesis,[464,465] and should also be avoided.

Control of Hypertriglyceridemia. Seventy-five percent or more of patients with primary gout have hypertriglyceridemia, which may be related to ethanolism in some, but in others appears to be independent of alcohol ingestion. The initial step in management of hypertriglyceridemia is reduction to ideal weight. If triglycerides are still over 300 mg per 100 ml after 6 weeks of appropriate dietary regulation and weight reduction, clofibrate (2 grams per day) may be tried. Unfortunately, it is not effective in about half of patients with hypertriglyceridemia. In addition, in view of the recent demonstration of serious effects on mortality,[466,467] clofibrate should be used with caution. In unresponsive patients, nicotinic acid (1.5 to 3.0 grams per day), less pleasant to take, will usually lower triglycerides, although if caloric restriction and weight maintenance do not return the triglycerides to completely normal values, drugs rarely will, and control, not "cure," becomes the highest expectation.[468] The hyperuricemic effect of nicotinic acid should not prevent its use in the patient with gout so long as anti-hyperuricemic therapy is modified accordingly.

Management of Hypertension. About one third of gouty subjects are hypertensive. The complications of hypertension are potentially more serious than those of hyperuricemia, and one should not hesitate to use whatever drugs are necessary to control the hypertension.

Many hypertensive gouty patients will require a thiazide diuretic. If needed in order to control hypertension, one should not hesitate to use one and to adjust the antigout program. The combined control of hypertension and hyperuricemia (and hyperlipidemia if present) should give the patient the best possible outlook with respect to avoidance of gouty attacks, preservation of renal function, and maintenance of cardiovascular and cerebrovascular status.

Table 86–10. Purine Content of Certain Foods[*][†]

List 1.	Foods that contain very large amounts (150–1000 mg) of purine bodies in 100 grams:					
	Heart, sheep	174	Meat extracts	236–356	Smelts	168
	Herring	172	Mussels	154	Sweetbreads	426
	Herring roe	484	Sardines	234	Yeast	570–990

List 2. Foods that contain a large amount (75–150 mg) of purine bodies in 100 grams: anchovies, bacon, codfish, goose, grouse, haddock, liver, kidneys, mackerel, mutton leg, partridge, pheasant, pigeon, salmon, scallops, trout, turkey, veal, venison

List 3. Foods that contain a moderate amount (up to 75 mg) of purine bodies in 100 grams: asparagus, bass, beef, bouillon, brains, chicken, crab, duck, eel, halibut, ham, kidney beans, lentils, lima beans, liverwurst, lobster, mushrooms, mutton chop, navy beans, oysters, peas, plaice, pork, rabbit, roe, shrimp, spinach, tongue, tripe

List 4. Foods that contain an insignificant amount of purine or no purine:

1. Beverages
   Carbonated
   Chocolate
   Cocoa
   Coffee
   Fruit juices
   Postum
   Tea
2. Butter[‡]
3. Breads and breadstuffs (refined and whole grain)
4. Caviar
5. Cereals (refined and whole grain)
6. Miscellaneous cereal products
   Arrowroot
   Hominy
   Macaroni
   Noodles
   Sago
   Spaghetti

7. Cheese of all kinds[‡]
8. Eggs
9. Fats of all kinds (but eat in moderation)[‡]
10. Fruits of all kinds
11. Gelatin
12. Milk
    Buttermilk
    Condensed milk
    Malted milk
13. Nuts of all kinds
    Peanut butter
14. Pies (except mincemeat)[‡]
15. Sugar and sweets
16. Vegetables (except those in List 3)
17. Vegetables and cream soups (to be made with allowed vegetables and without meat stock)
18. Vitamin concentrates
    Cod liver oil
    Halibut oil

*Source: Hench, P.S.: *In* Cecil, R.L., and Loeb, R.F. (eds.): Textbook of Medicine. 9th ed. From Bridges, M.A.: Food and Beverage Analyses. 3rd ed. Philadelphia, Lea & Febiger, 1950, pp. 188–192; and Dirr, K., and Decker, P.: Biochem. Z. 316:239, 1944.

†To calculate the purine or "purine bodies" in a given food, the purine nitrogen is multiplied by 3: for example, 200 mg of purine nitrogen equals 600 mg of purine bodies.

‡These foods are high in fat.

Table 86–11. Purine Free Diet: Sample Menu (2500 Calories, 70 grams Protein)*

	Household Measure	Gram Weight
Breakfast		
Orange juice	1 cup	240
Cream of wheat	1 cup	240
2% Milk	1 cup	240
Egg	1	55
Toast	2 slices	45
Margarine	2 teaspoons	10
Jelly	1 tablespoon	20
Sugar	2 teaspoons	10
Coffee (decaffeinated)		
Lunch		
Grilled Cheese Sandwich		
bread	2 slices	45
cheese	2 ounces	60
margarine	2 teaspoons	10
Tomato soup		
Apple	1 medium	150
Celery sticks	1 large stalk	50
Sugar cookie	2	43
Sugar	1 teaspoon	5
Coffee (decaffeinated)		
Supper		
Spaghetti		
tomato sauce	½ cup	135
spaghetti noodles	1 cup	150
Broccoli	⅔ cup	100
Tossed salad		
lettuce	1 serving	100
tomato	½ small	50
Italian dressing	2 tablespoons	30
French bread	1 slice	20
Margarine	2 teaspoons	10
Peaches, canned	½ cup	100
2% Milk	1 cup	240
Sugar	1 teaspoon	5
Coffee decaffeinated)		
Snack		
Banana	1 medium	150

*Typical diet used for research purposes at the Clinical Research Center, University Hospital, University of Michigan, Ann Arbor, Michigan. (Courtesy of Constance Hydrich, Head Dietitian).

Figure 86–19. Reaction catalyzed by adenine phosphoribosyltransferase.

OTHER RELATED DISORDERS OF PURINE METABOLISM

Adenine phosphoribosyltransferase catalyzes the conversion of adenine to AMP (Fig. 86–19). In 1968, Kelley and associates[469] described a deficiency of adenine phosphoribosyltransferase in one family. These subjects were heterozygous for a deficiency of the enzyme and had no associated disease. In subsequent years, it became apparent that heterozygosity for this enzyme deficiency may occur commonly in the population, perhaps as often as one in a hundred.[470] A homozygous deficiency of adenine phosphoribosyltransferase has now been described in three patients with a history of renal stones composed of 2,8-dihydroxyadenine (Fig. 86–20).[471,472] Because of their chemical similarity, 2,8-dihydroxyadenine may be confused with uric acid, and in each of these patients a diagnosis of uric acid nephrolithiasis was incorrectly made initially.

Xanthine oxidase catalyzes the oxidation of hypoxanthine to xanthine, xanthine to uric acid, and adenine to 2,8-dihydroxyadenine (Fig. 86–21). The disease, xanthinuria, the first inborn error of purine metabolism to be defined at the enzyme level, is due to a deficiency of xanthine oxidase.[473,474] As a direct result of this enzy-

Figure 86–20. Kidney stones composed of 2,8-dihydroxyadenine obtained from a patient with complete adenine phosphoribosyltransferase deficiency. (Courtesy of Dr. Anne Simmonds, Guys Hospital, London.)

XANTHINE OXIDASE

Figure 86–21. Conversion of hypoxanthine and xanthine to uric acid in the reaction catalyzed by xanthine oxidase.

matic defect, patients with xanthinuria have hypouricemia and hypouricaciduria as well as an increased urinary excretion of the oxypurines, hypoxanthine and xanthine. About 50 percent of the patients with xanthinuria are asymptomatic, and about one third have urinary xanthine stones. Several patients have been noted to have polyarthritis. Precipitation of xanthine has been proposed as an important factor in the development of each of these clinical manifestations.

Disorders of purine metabolism associated with altered immune function are discussed in Chapter 83.

References

1. Wyngaarden, J.B., and Kelley W.N.: Gout and Hyperuricemia. New York, Grune & Stratton, 1976.
2. Copeman, W.S.C.: A Short History of the Gout. Berkeley, University of California Press, 1964.
3. Neuwirth, E.: Milestones in the diagnosis and treatment of gout. Arch. Intern. Med. 72:377, 1943.
4. Schnitker, M.A.: A history of the treatment of gout. Bull. Inst. Hist. Med. 4:89, 1936.
5. Talbott, J.H.: Gout. 3rd ed. New York, Grune & Stratton, 1967, p. 5.
6. Rodnan, G.P.: A gallery of gout. Being a miscellany of prints and caricatures from the 16th century to the present day. Arthritis Rheum. 4:27, 1961.
7. Rodnan, G.P., and Benedek, T.G.: Cotton Mather and the gout. Arthritis Rheum. 6:789, 1963.
8. Rodnan, G.P., and Benedek, T.G.: Ancient therapeutic arts in the gout. Arthritis Rheum. 6:317, 1963.
9. Bywaters, E.G.L.: Gout in the time and person of George IV: A case history. Ann. Rheum. Dis. 21:325, 1962.
10. Strauss, M.B.: Familiar Medical Quotations. Boston, Little, Brown & Company, 1968, p. 186.
11. Hippocrates: The Genuine Works of Hippocrates, Vols. I and II. Translated from the Greek with a preliminary discourse and annotations by Francis Adams. New York, Wood, 1886.
12. Evans, J.G., Prior I.A.M., and Harvey, J.P.B.: Relation of serum uric acid to body bulk, haemoglobin and alcohol intake in two South Pacific Polynesian populations. Ann. Rheum. Dis. 27:319, 1968.
13. Acheson, R.M., and Chan, Y.K.: The prediction of serum uric acid on haemoglobin and other factors in the general population. Lancet 2:777, 1966.
14. Mikkelsen, W.M., Dodge, H.J., and Valkenburg, H.: The distribution of serum uric acid values in a population unselected as to gout or hyperuricemia: Tecumseh, Michigan, 1959–1960. Am. J. Med. 39:242, 1965.
15. Harlan, W.R., Cornoni-Huntley, J., and Leaverton, P.E.: Physiologic determinants of serum urate levels in adolescence. Pediatrics 63:569, 1979.
16. Kuntz, D., Chretien, J.M., Ryckewaert, A., et al.: Distribution and correlations of serum uric acid in two French adult populations. Semin. Hop. Paris 55:241, 1979.
17. Zalokar, J., Lellouch, J., and Claude, J.R.: Serum urate and gout in 4663 young male workers. Semin. Hop. Paris 57:664, 1981.
18. Nishioka, K., and Mikanagi, K.: Hereditary and environmental factors influencing on the serum uric acid throughout ten years population study in Japan. Adv. Exp. Med. Biol. 122A:155, 1980.

19. Currie, W.J.C.: Prevalence and incidence of the diagnosis of gout in Great Britain. Ann. Rheum. Dis. 38:101, 1979.
20. Akizuki, S.: A population study of hyperuricaemia and gout in Japan: Analysis of sex, age and occupational differences in thirty-four thousand people living in Nagano Prefecture. The Ryumachi 22:201, 1982.
21. Delbarre, F., Braun, S., and St. George-Chaumet, F.: Lagoutte feminine (analyse de quarante observations). Semin. Hop. Paris 43:623, 1967.
22. Arnold, W.J., and Gröbner, W.: Clinical manifestations of hyperuricemia. Clin. Rheum. Dis. 3:51, 1977.
23. Grahame, R., and Scott, J.T.: Clinical survey of 354 patients with gout. Ann. Rheum. Dis. 29:461, 1970.
24. Harth, M., and Robinson, C.E.G.: Gouty arthritis in a D.V.A. hospital. A retrospective study. Med. Serv. J. Can. 18:671, 1962.
25. Nishioka, N., Mikanagi, K.: Clinical features of 4,000 gouty subjects in Japan. Adv. Exp. Med. Biol. 122A:47, 1980.
26. Scudamore, C.: A Treatise on the Nature and Cure of Gout and Rheumatism, Including General Considerations on Morbid States of the Digestive Organs: Some Remarks on Regimen, and Practical Observations on Gravel. 2nd ed. London, Longman, 1817.
27. Canoso, J.J., and Yood, R.A.: Acute gouty bursitis: report of 15 cases. Ann. Rheum. Dis. 38:326, 1979.
28. Sydenham, T.: The Works of Thomas Sydenham, translated from the Latin by R.G. Lathan, Vol. II. London, New Sydenham Society, 1850, p. 124.
29. Gutman, A.B.: Gout. In Beeson, P.B., and McDermott, W. (eds.): Textbook of Medicine. 12th ed. Philadelphia, W.B. Saunders Company, 1958, p. 595.
30. Hadler, N.M., Franck, W.A., Bress, N.M., et al.: Acute polyarticular gout. Am. J. Med. 56:715, 1974.
31. Weinberger, A., and Schumacher, H.R.: Urate crystals in asymptomatic metatarsophalangeal joints. Ann. Intern. Med. 91:56, 1979.
32. Rouault, T., Caldwell, D.S., and Holmes, E.W.: Aspiration of the asymptomatic metatarsophalangeal joint in gout patients and hyperuricemic controls. Arthritis Rheum. 25:209, 1982.
33. Gordon, T.P., Bertouch, J.V., Walsh, B.R., and Brooks, P.M.: Monosodium urate crystals in asymptomatic knee joints. J. Rheumatol. 9:967, 1982.
34. Hench, P.S.: The diagnosis of gout and gouty arthritis. J. Lab. Clin. Med. 220:48, 1936.
35. Gutman, A.B.: The past four decades of progress in the knowlege of gout, with an assessment of the present status. Arthritis Rheum. 16:431, 1973.
36. Gutman, A.B., and Yu, T-F: Renal function in gout with a commentary on the renal regulation of urate excretion and the role of the kidney in the pathogenesis of gout. Am. J. Med. 23:600, 1957.
37. Yu, T-F.: Secondary gout associated with myeloproliferative diseases. Arthritis Rheum. 8:765, 1965.
38. Smythe, C.M., and Cutchin, J.H.: Primary juvenile gout. Am. J. Med. 32:799, 1962.
39. Wood, M.H., Fox, R.M., Vincent, L., et al.: The Lesch-Nyhan syndrome: Report of three cases. Aust. N.Z. J. Med. 1:57, 1972.
40. Good, A.E., and Rapp, R.: Bony ankylosis: A rare manifestation of gout. J. Rheumatol. 5:335, 1978.
41. Sequeira, W., Bouffard, A., Salgia, K., et al.: Quadriparesis in tophaceous gout. Arthritis Rheum. 24:1428, 1981.
42. Magid, S.K., Gray, G.E., and Anand, A.: Spinal cord compression by tophi in a patient with chronic polyarthritis: Case report and literature review. Arthritis Rheum. 24:1431, 1981.
43. Bauer, W., and Klemperer, F.: Gout. In Duncan, G.G. (ed.): Diseases of Metabolism. 2nd ed. Philadelphia, W.B. Saunders Company, 1947, p. 611.
44. Bartels, E.C., and Matossian, G.S.: Gout: Six year follow-up on probenecid (Benemid) therapy. Arthritis Rheum. 2:193, 1959.
45. Bloch, C., Hermann, G., and Yu, T.-F.: A radiologic reevaluation of gout: A study of 2,000 patients. Am. J. Radiol. 134:781, 1980.
46. Resnick, D., and Broderick, T.W.: Intraosseous calcifications in tophaceous gout. Am. J. Radiol. 137:1157, 1981.
47. Stockman, A., Darlington, L.G., and Scott, J.T.: Frequency of chondrocalcinosis of the knees and avascular necrosis of the femoral heads in gout: A controlled study. Ann. Rheum. Dis. 39:7, 1980.
48. Krizek, V.: Serum uric acid in relation to body weight. Ann. Rheum. Dis. 25:456, 1966.
49. Benedek, T.G.: Correlations of serum uric acid and lipid concentrations in normal, gouty, and atherosclerotic men. Ann. Intern. Med. 66:851, 1967.
50. Gertler, M.M., Garn, S.M., and Levine, S.A.: Serum uric acid in relation to age and physique in health and in coronary artery disease. Ann. Intern. Med. 34:1421, 1951.
51. Acheson, R.M., and Florey, C. du V.: Body-weight, ABO blood groups, and altitude of domicile as determinants of serum-uric-acid in military recruits in four countries. Lancet 2:391, 1969.
52. Myers, A., Epstein, F.H., Dodge, H.J., et al.: The relationship of serum

uric acid to risk factors in coronary heart disease. Am. J. Med. 45:520, 1968.

53. Gutman, A.B., and Yu, T-F.: Gout, a derangement of purine metabolism. Adv. Intern. Med. 5:227, 1952.

54. O'Brien, W.M., Burch, T.A., and Bunim, J.J.: Genetics of hyperuricemia in Blackfeet and Pima Indians. Ann. Rheum. Dis. 25:117, 1966.

55. Acheson, R.M., and O'Brien, W.M.: Dependence of serum uric acid on haemoglobin and other factors in the general population. Lancet 2:777, 1966.

56. National Center for Health Statistics, Harlan, W.R., Hull, A.L., Schmouder, R.P., et al.: Dietary intake and cardiovascular risk factors Part II. Serum urate, serum cholesterol and correlates. United States, 1971-75, Vital and Health Statistics Series 11, No. 227, DHHS Pub No. (PHS) 83-1677. Public Health Service. Washington, U.S. Government Printing Office, March, 1983.

57. Brauer, G.W., and Prior, I.A.M. A prospective study of gout in New Zealand Maoris. Ann. Rheum. Dis. 37:466-472, 1978.

58. Emmerson, B.T., and Knowles, B.R.: Triglyceride concentrations in primary gout of chronic lead nephropathy. Metabolism 20:721, 1971.

59. Brochner-Mortensen, K.: 100 gouty patients. Acta Med. Scand. 106:81, 1941.

60. Grahame, R., and Scott, J.T.: Clinical survey of 354 patients with gout. Ann. Rheum. Dis. 29:461, 1970.

61. Englehardt, H.T., and Wagner, E.L.: Gout, diabetes mellitus and obesity, a poorly recognized syndrome. South. Med. J. 43:51, 1950.

62. Prior, I.A.M., Rose, B.S., Harvey, H.P.B., et al.: Hyperuricaemia, gout, and diabetic abnormality in Polynesian people. Lancet 1:333, 1966.

63. Healey, L.A., and Hall, A.P.: The epidemiology of hyperuricemia. Bull. Rheum. Dis. 20:600, 1970.

64. Gibson, T., and Grahame, R.: Gout and hyperlipidaemia. Ann. Rheum. Dis. 33:298, 1974.

65. Kahn, H.A., Medalie, J.H., Newfeld, H.N., et al.: The incidence of hypertension and associated factors: The Israel ischemic heart disease study. Am. Heart J. 84:171, 1972.

66. Mikkelsen, W.M.: The possible association of hyperuricemia and/or gout with diabetes mellitus. Arthritis Rheum. 8:853, 1965.

67. Denis, G., and Launay, M.P.: Carbohydrate intolerance in gout. Metabolism 18:770, 1969.

68. Bernheim, C., Ott, H., Zahnd, G., et al.: Goutte et diabète. 1. La goutte et ses relations avec le diabète. Schweiz Med. Wochenschr. 98:33, 1968.

69. Berkowitz, D.: Gout, hyperlipidemia and diabetes interrelationships. JAMA 197:77, 1966.

70. McKechnie, J.K.: Gout, hyperuricemia and carbohydrate metabolism. S. Afr. Med. J. 38:182, 1964.

71. Herman, J.B., Mount, F.W., Medalie, J.H., et al.: Diabetes prevalence and serum uric acid: Observations among 10,000 men in a survey of ischemic heart disease in Israel. Diabetes 16:858, 1967.

72. Padova, J., Patchefsky, A., Onesti, G., et al.: The effect of glucose loads on renal uric acid excretion in diabetic patients. Metabolism 13:507, 1964.

73. Herman, J.B., and Keynan, A.: Hyperglycemia and uric acid. Isr. J. Med. Sci. 5:1048, 1969.

74. Skeith, M.D., Healey, L.A., and Cutler, R.E.: Urate excretion during mannitol and glucose diuresis. J. Lab. Clin. Med. 70:213, 1967.

75. Barlow, K.A.: Hyperlipidemia in primary gout. Metabolism 17:289, 1968.

76. Feldman, E.B., and Wallace, S.L.: Hypertriglyceridemia in gout. Circulation 29:508, 1964.

77. Berkowitz, D.: Blood lipid and uric acid interrelationships. JAMA 190:856, 1964.

78. Naito, H.K., and Mackenzie, A.H.: Secondary hypertriglyceridemia and hyperlipoproteinemia in patients with primary asymptomatic gout. Clin. Chem. 25:371, 1979.

79. Darlington, L.G., Slack, J., and Scott, J.T.: Family study of lipid and purine levels in gout patients. Ann. Rheum. Dis. 41:253, 1982.

80. Harris-Jones, J.N.: Hyperuricemia and essential hypercholesterolemia. Lancet 1:857, 1957.

81. Salvini, L., and Verdi, G.: Statistical study on correlation between blood level of cholesterol beta/alpha lipoprotein ratio and uric acid of normal and arteriosclerotic subjects. Gerontologia 3:327, 1959.

82. Jensen, J., Blankenhorn, D.H., and Dornerup, V.: Blood-uric acid levels in familial hypercholesterolemia. Lancet 1:298, 1966.

83. Strejcek, J., and Kucerova, L.: Idiopathic hyperlipidemia and gout. Acta Rheumatol. Scand. 14:95, 1968.

84. Cannon, P.J., Stason, W.B., Demartini, F.E., et al.: Hyperuricemia in primary and renal hypertension. N. Engl. J. Med. 275:457, 1966.

85. Breckenridge, A.: Hypertension and hyperuricemia. Lancet 1:15, 1966.

86. Garrick, R., Bauer, G.E., Ewan, C.E., et al.: Serum uric acid in normal and hypertensive Australian subjects: From a continuing epidemiological survey on hypertension commenced in 1955. Aust. N.Z. J. Med. 2:351, 1972.

87. Dollery, C.T., Duncan, H., and Schumer, B.: Hyperuricemia related to treatment of hypertension. Br. Med. J. 2:832, 1960.

88. Simon, N.M., Smucker, J.E., O'Conor, J., Jr., et al.: Differential uric acid excretion in essential and renal hypertension. Circulation 39:121, 1969.

89. Kuzell, W.C., Schaffarzick, R.W., Naugler, W.E., et al.: Some observations on 520 gouty patients. J. Chronic Dis. 2:645, 1955.

90. Barlow, K.A., and Beilin, L.J.: Renal disease in primary gout. Quart. J. Med. 37:79, 1968.

91. Rapado, A.: Relationship between gout and arterial hypertension. In Sperling, O., DeVries, A., and Wyngaarden, J.B. (eds.): Purine Metabolism in Man. Vol. 41B. New York, Plenum Press, 1974, p. 451.

92. Weiss, T.E., and Segaloff, A.: Gouty Arthritis and Gout. Springfield, Ill., Charles C Thomas, 1959, p. 74.

93. Messerli, F.H., Frohlich, E.D., Dreslinski, G.R., et al.: Serum uric acid in essential hypertension: An indicator of renal vascular involvement. Ann. Intern. Med. 93:817, 1980.

94. Prebis, J.W., Gruskin, A.B., Polinsky, M.S., et al.: Uric acid in childhood essential hypertension. J. Pediatr. 98:702, 1981.

95. Simon, N.M., Smucker, J.E., O'Connor, V.J., Jr., et al.: Differential uric acid excretion in essential and renal hypertension. Circulation 39:121, 1969.

96. Saito, I., Saruta, T., Kondo, K., et al.: Serum uric acid and the renin-angiotensin system in hypertension. J. Am. Geriatr. Soc. 26:241, 1978.

97. Upmark-Ask, E., and Adner, L.: Coronary infarction and gout. Acta Med. Scand. 139:1, 1950.

98. Kramer, D.W., Perilstein, P.K., and DeMedeiros, A.: Metabolic influences in vascular disorders with particular reference to cholesterol determinations in comparison with uric acid levels. Angiology 9:162, 1958.

99. Dreyfuss, F.: The role of hyperuricemia in coronary heart disease. Dis. Chest 38:332, 1960.

100. Eidlitz, M.: Uric acid and arteriosclerosis. Lancet 2:1046, 1961.

101. Hansen, O.E.: Hyperuricemia, gout and atherosclerosis. Am. Heart J. 72:570, 1966.

102. Kohn, P.M., and Prozan, G.B.: Hyperuricemia—relationship to hypercholesterolemia and acute myocardial infarction. JAMA 17:1909, 1959.

103. Editorial: Serum uric acid and coronary heart disease. Lancet 1:358, 1969.

104. Nishioka, K., and Mikanagi, K.: A retrospective study on the cause of death, in Japan, of patients with gout. The Rymuchi 21(Suppl.):29, 1981.

105. Fessel, W.J.: Renal outcomes of gout and hyperuricemia. Am. J. Med. 67:74, 1979.

106. Johnson, M.W., and Mitch, W.E.: The risks of asymptomatic hyperuricemia and the use of uricosuric diuretics. Drugs 21:220, 1981.

107. Tweddale, M.G., and Fodor, J.G.: Elevated serum uric acid: A cardiovascular risk factor. Nephron 23:3, 1979.

108. Fessel, W.J.: High uric acid as an indicator of cardiovascular disease, independence from obesity. Am. J. Med. 68:401, 1980.

109. Wyngaarden, J.B., and Kelley, W.N.: Gout and Hyperuricemia. New York, Grune & Stratton, 1976.

110. Lally, E.V., Parker, V.S., and Kaplan, S.R.: Acute gouty arthritis and systemic lupus erythematosus. J. Rheumatol. 9:308, 1982.

111. Moidel, R.A., and Good, A.E.: Coexistent gout and systemic lupus erythematosus. Arthritis Rheum. 24:969, 1981.

112. Wall, B.A., Agudelo, C.A., Weinblatt, M.E., et al.: Acute gout and systemic lupus erythematosus: Report of 2 cases and literature review. J. Rheumatol. 9:305, 1982.

113. Jessee, E.F., Toone, E., Owen, D.S., et al.: Coexistent rheumatoid arthritis and chronic tophaceous gout. Arthritis Rheum. 23:244, 1980.

114. Atdjian, M., and Fernandez-Madris, F.: Coexistence of chronic tophaceous gout and rheumatoid arthritis. J. Rheumatol. 8:989, 1981.

115. Rizzoli, A.J., Trujeque, L., and Bankhurst, A.D.: The coexistence of gout and rheumatoid arthritis: Case reports and a review of the literature. J. Rheumatol. 7:316, 1980.

116. Wallace, D.J., Klineberg, J.R., Morhaim, D., et al.: Coexistent gout and rheumatoid arthritis. Arthritis Rheum. 22:81, 1979.

117. Rubinow, A., and Sonnenblick, M.: Amyloidosis secondary to polyarticular gout. Arthritis Rheum. 24:1425, 1981.

118. Levo, Y., Shalev, O., Rosenmann, E., et al.: Gout and amyloidosis. Ann. Rheum. Dis. 39:589, 1980.

119. Wyngaarden, J.B.: The role of the kidney in the pathogenesis and treatment of gout. Arthritis Rheum. 1:191, 1958.

120. Talbott, J.H., and Terplan, K.L.: The kidney in gout. Medicine 39:405, 1960.

121. Mayne, J.G.: Pathological study of the renal lesions found in 27 patients with gout (abstract). Ann. Rheum. Dis. 15:61, 1965.

122. Brown, J., and Mallory, G.K.: Renal changes in gout. N. Engl. J. Med. 243:325, 1950.

123. Epstein, W.: Die Natur und Behandlung der Gight. Berlin and New York, Springer-Verlag (Bergmann), 1906.

124. Umber, F.: Ernahrung und Stoffwechselkrankheiten. Vienna, Corban und Schwarzenberg, 1914.

125. Yu, T.-F., and Berger, L.: Renal disease in primary gout. Semin. Arthritis Rheum. 3:293, 1975.

126. Sorensen, L.B.: The pathogenesis of gout. Arch. Intern. Med. 109:379, 1962.
127. Richet, G., Ardaillou, R., DeMontera, H., et al.: Étude de 31 cas de nephropathie associée à la goutte. J. Urol. Nephrol. 67:1, 1961.
128. Sarre, H., and Mertz, D.D.: Sekundare Gicht bei Niereninsuffizienz. Klin. Wochenschr. 43:1134, 1965.
129. Sokoloff, L.: The pathology of gout. Metabolism 6:230, 1957.
130. Fahr, T.: Handbuch der Speziellen Pathologischen Anatomie and Histologie, Vol. I by Heake, F., and Lubarsch, O. Berlin and New York, Springer-Verlag, 1926.
131. Bell, E.T.: Renal Diseases. 2nd ed. Philadelphia, Lea & Febiger, 1950, p. 413.
132. Modern, F.W.S., and Meister, L.: The kidney of gout, a clinical entity. Med. Clin. North Am. 36:941, 1952.
133. Greenbaum, D., Ross, J.G., and Steinberg, V.L.: Renal biopsy in gout. Br. Med. J. 1:1502, 1961.
134. Gonick, H.C., Rubini, M.E., Gleason, I.O., et al.: The renal lesion in gout. Ann. Intern. Med. 62:667, 1965.
135. Seegmiller, J.E., and Frazier, P.D.: Biochemical considerations of the renal damage of gout. Ann Rheum. Dis. 25:668, 672, 1966.
136. Gibson, T., Highton, J., Potter, C., et al.: Renal impairment and gout. Ann Rheum. Dis. 39:417, 1980.
137. Berger, L., and Yu, T.-F.: Renal function in gout. IV. An analysis of 524 gouty subjects including long-term follow-up studies. Am. J. Med. 59:605, 1975.
138. Yu, T.-F., Berger, L., Dorph, D.J., et al.: Renal function in gout. V. Factors influencing renal hemodynamics. Am. J. Med. 67:766, 1979.
139. Yu, T.-F., and Berger, L.: Renal function in gout: Its association with hypertensive vascular disease and intrinsic renal disease. Am. J. Med. 72:95, 1982.
140. Batuman, V., Maesaka, J.K., Haddad, B., et al.: The role of lead in gout nephropathy. New Engl. J. Med. 304:520, 1981.
141. Campbell, B.C., Moore, M.R., Goldberg, A., et al.: Subclinical lead exposure: A possible cause of gout. Br. Med. J. 2:1403, 1978.
142. Garrod, A.B.: A Treatise on Gout and Rheumatic Gout. 3rd edition, London, Longman, Green and Co., 1876.
143. Verger, D., Leroux-Robert, G.P., and Richet, G.: Depots d'urate intrarenaux chez les insuffisants renaux chroniques hyperuricemiques. Urol. Nephrol. 73:314, 1967.
144. Linnane, J.W., Burry, A.F., and Emmerson, B.T.: Urate deposits in the renal medulla: Prevalence and associations. Nephron 29:216, 1981.
145. Frei, E., Bentzel, C.J., Rieselbach, R.E., and Block, R.B.: Renal complications of neoplastic disease. J. Chronic Dis. 16:757, 1963.
146. Rieselbach, R.E., Bentzel, C.J., Cotlove, E., et al.: Uric acid excretion and renal function in the acute hyperuricemia of leukemia. Am. J. Med. 37:872, 1964.
147. Knochel, J.P., Dotin, L.N., and Hamburger, R.J.: Heat stress, exercise and muscle injury: Effects on urate metabolism and renal function. Ann. Intern. Med. 81:321, 1974.
148. Warren, D.J., Leitch, A.G., and Leggett, R.J.E.: Hyperuricaemic acute renal failure after epileptic seizures. Lancet 2:385, 1975.
149. Kjellstrand, C.M., Campbell, D.C., von Hartitzsch, B., et al.: Hyperuricemic acute renal failure. Arch. Intern. Med. 133:349, 1974.
150. Lilje, E.: Hyperurikaemi og akut nyriensufficiens. Ugeskr. Laeg. 132:12, 1970.
151. Stavric, B., Johnson, W.J., and Grice, H.C.: Uric acid nephropathy: An experimental model. Proc. Soc. Exp. Biol. Med. 130:512, 1969.
152. Cohen, L.F., Balow, J.E., Poplack, D.G., et al.: Acute tumor lysis syndrome: A review of 37 patients with Burkitt's lymphoma. Am. J. Med. 68:486, 1980.
153. Deger, G.E., and Wagoner, R.D.: Peritoneal dialysis in acute uric acid nephropathy. Mayo Clin. Proc. 47:189, 1972.
154. Steele, T.H., and Rieselbach, R.E.: The contributions of residual nephrons within the chronically diseased kidney to urate homeostasis in man. Am. J. Med. 43:876, 1967.
155. Kelton, J., Kelley, W.N., and Holmes, E.W.: A rapid method for the diagnosis of acute uric acid nephropathy. Arch. Intern. Med. 138:612, 1978.
156. Atsmon, A., DeVries, A., and Frank, M.: Uric Acid Lithiasis. Amsterdam, Elsevier, 1963.
157. Hughes, J., Coppridge, W.M., Roberts, L.C., et al.: Oxalate urinary tract stones. JAMA 172:774, 1960.
158. Nicholas, H.O.: Urinary calculi. II. Further observations on calculi from patients in the southeast Texas area. Clin. Chem. 7:175, 1961.
159. Leonard, R.H.: Quantitative composition of kidney stones. Clin. Chem. 7:546, 1961.
160. Boyce, W.H., Garvey, F.K., and Strawcutter, H.E.: Incidence of urinary calculi among patients in general hospitals, 1948 to 1952. JAMA 161:1437, 1956.
161. Gutman, A.B., and Yu, T-F.: Uric acid nephrolithiasis. Am. J. Med. 45:756, 1968.
162. Yu, T.-F., and Gutman, A.B.: Uric acid nephrolithiasis in gout. Predisposing factors. Ann. Intern. Med. 67:1133, 1967.
163. Currie, W.J., and Turner, P.: The frequency of renal stones within Great Britain in a gouty and non-gouty population. J. Urol. 51:337, 1979.
164. Talbott, J.H.: Gout. New York, Grune & Stratton, 1957, p. 205.
165. Armstrong, W.A., and Greene, L.F.: Uric acid calculi with particular reference to determinations of uric acid content of blood. J. Urol. 70:545, 1953.
166. Emmerson, B.T.: The clinical differentiation of lead gout from primary gout. Arthritis Rheum. 11:623, 1968.
167. Holmes, E.W., and Kelley, W.N.: Unpublished data.
168. Dulce, H.J.: Biochemie der Harnsteinbildung. Urol. Int. 7:137, 1958.
169. Boshamer, K.: Morphologie und Genese der Harnsteine. Handbuch der Urologie, Vol. X, Die Steinerkrankungen. Berlin and New York, Springer-Verlag, 1961, p. 549.
170. Sperling, O., Kedem, O., and DeVries, A.: Etiologie de la lithiase urique. I. Solubilité de l'acide urique et de l'urate de sodium en solution tampon. Rev. Fr. Étud. Clin. Biol. 11:40, 1966.
171. Sperling, O., and DeVries, A.: Studies on the etiology of uric acid lithiasis. Part 2. Solubility of uric acid in urine specimens from normal subjects and patients with idiopathic uric acid lithiasis. J. Urol. 92:331, 1964.
172. Wilmore, D.W.: The etiology of uric acid urolithiasis following ileostomy. Arch. Surg. 99:421, 1969.
173. Clarke, A.M., and McKenzie, R.G.: Ileostomy and the risk of urinary uric acid stones. Lancet 2:395, 1969.
174. Bergmann, F., and Dikstein, S.: Relationship between spectral shifts and structural changes in uric acids and related compounds. J. Am. Chem. Soc. 77:691, 1955.
175. Peters, J.P., and Van Slyke, D.D.: Quantitative Clinical Chemistry, Vol. 1. 2nd ed. Baltimore, Williams & Wilkins Company, 1946, p. 953.
176. Klinenberg, J.R., Goldfinger, S., Miller, J., et al.: The effectiveness of a xanthine oxidase inhibitor on the treatment of gout. Ann. Intern. Med. 62:639, 1965.
177. Serane, J., and Lederer, J.: Contribution a l'étude du rein des goutteux. Presse Méd. 63:335, 1955.
178. Henneman, P.H., Wallach, S., and Dempsey, E.F.: The metabolic defect responsible for uric acid stone formation. J. Clin. Invest. 41:537, 1962.
179. Woeber, K.A., Ricca, L., and Hills, A.G.: Pathogenesis of uric acid urolithiasis (abstract). Clin. Res. 10:45, 1962.
180. DeVries, A., Frank, M., and Atsmon, A.: Inherited uric acid lithiasis. Am. J. Med. 33:880, 1962.
181. Delbarre, F., Auscher, C., and DuLac, Y.: Documents pour l'étude du rein goutteux. IV. Documents sur le pH-urinaire et ses variations. Rein Foie 6:53, 1964.
182. Gutman, A.B., and Yu, T.-F.: Urinary ammonium excretion in primary gout. J. Clin. Invest. 44:1474, 1965.
183. Gutman, A.B., and Yu, T.-F.: On the nature of the inborn metabolic error(s) of primary gout. Trans. Assoc. Am. Physicians 76:141, 1963.
184. Frank, M., deVries, A., Atsmon, A., et al.: Urinary pH, ammonia and calcium excretion in renal uric acid stone patients, Isr. Med. J. 12:299, 1960.
185. Metcalfe-Gibson, A., McCallum, F.M., Morrison, R.B.I., et al.: Urinary excretion of hydrogen ion in patients with uric acid calculi. Clin. Sci. 28:325, 1965.
186. Barzel, U.S., Sperling, O., Frank, M., et al.: Renal ammonium excretion and urinary pH in idiopathic uric acid lithiasis. J. Urol. 92:1, 1964.
187. Pak Poy, R.K.: Urinary pH in gout. Aust. Ann. Med. 14:35, 1965.
188. Sperling, O., Frank, M., and deVries, A.: L'excretion d'ammoniac au cours de la goutte. Rev. Fr. Etud. Clin. Biol. 11:401, 1966.
189. Plante, G.E., Durivage, J., and Lemieux, G.: Renal excretion of hydrogen in primary gout. Metabolism 17:377, 1968.
190. Gutman, A.B., and Yu, T.-F.: An abnormality of glutamine metabolism in primary gout. Am. J. Med. 35:820, 1963.
191. Rapoport, A., Crassweller, P.O., Husdan, H., et al.: The renal excretion of hydrogen ion in uric acid stone formers. Metabolism 16:176, 1967.
192. Sperling, O., deVries, A., and Kedem, O.: Studies on the etiology of uric acid lithiasis. IV. Urinary non-dialyzable substances in idiopathic uric acid lithiasis. J. Urol. 94:286, 1965.
193. Deren, J.J., Porush, J.G., Levitt, M.F., et al.: Nephrolithiasis as a complication of ulcerative colitis and regional enteritis. Ann. Intern. Med. 56:843, 1962.
194. Bennett, R.C., and Jepson, R.P.: Uric acid stone formation following ileostomy. Aust. N.Z. J. Surg. 36:153, 1966.
195. Gigax, J.H., and Leach, J.R.: Uric acid calculi associated with ileostomy for ulcerative colitis. J. Urol. 105:797, 1971.
196. Reisner, G.S., Wilansky, D.L., and Schneiderman, C.: Uric acid lithiasis in the ileostomy patient. Br. J. Urol. 45:340, 1973.
197. Alvasker, J.O.: Uric acid in human plasma. IV. Investigations on the interactions between urate and the macromolecular fraction in plasma from healthy individuals and patients with diseases associated with hyperuricemia. Scand. J. Clin. Lab. Invest. 17:476, 1965.

198. Prien, E.L., and Prien, E.L., Jr.: Composition and structure of urinary stone. Am. J. Med. 45:654, 1968.
199. Smith, M.J.V., Hunt, L.D., King, J.S., et al.: Uricemia and urolithiasis. J. Urol. 101:637, 1969.
200. Coe, F.L., and Kavalach, A.G.: Hypercalcemia and hyperuricosuria in patients with calcium nephrolithiasis. N. Engl. J. Med. 291:1344, 1974.
201. Gutman, A.B., and Yu, T.-F.: Renal function in gout with a commentary on the renal regulation of urate excretion, and the role of the kidney in the pathogenesis of gout. Am. J. Med. 23:600, 1957.
202. Nugent, C.A., and Tyler, F.H.: The renal excretion of uric acid in patients with gout and in nongouty subjects. J. Clin. Invest. 38:1890, 1959.
203. Seegmiller, J.E., Grayzel, A.I., Howell, R.R., et al.: The renal excretion of uric acid in gout. J. Clin. Invest. 41:1094, 1962.
204. Yu, T.-F., Berger, L., and Gutman, A.B.: Renal function in gout. II. Effect of uric acid loading on renal excretion of uric acid. Am. J. Med. 33:829, 1962.
205. Lathem, W., and Rodnan, G.P.: Impairment of uric acid excretion in gout. J. Clin. Invest. 41:1955, 1962.
206. Houpt, J.B., and Ogryzlo, M.A.: Persistence of impaired uric acid excretion in gout during reduced synthesis with allopurinol (abstract). Arthritis Rheum. 7:316, 1964.
207. Snaith, M.L., and Scott, J.T.: Uric acid clearance in patients with gout and normal subjects. Ann. Rheum. Dis. 30:285, 1971.
208. Wyngaarden, J.B.: Gout. Adv. Metabol. Dis. 2:2, 1965.
209. Nugent, C.A., MacDiarmid, W.D., and Tyler, F.H.: Renal excretion of urate in patients with gout. Arch. Intern. Med. 113:115, 1964.
210. Campion, D.S., Olsen, R.W., Caughey, D., et al.: Does increased free serum urate concentration cause gout? (abstract). Clin. Res. 23:109A, 1974.
211. Alvasker, J.O.: Uric acid in human plasma. V. Isolation and identification of plasma proteins interacting with urate. Scand. J. Clin. Invest. 18:227, 1966.
212. Klinenberg, J.R., and Kippen, I.: The binding of urate to plasma proteins determined by means of equilibrium dialysis. J. Lab. Clin. Med. 75:503, 1970.
213. Rieselbach, R.E., Sorensen, L.B., Shelp, W.D., et al.: Diminished renal urate secretion per nephron on a basis for primary gout. Ann. Intern. Med. 73:359, 1970.
214. Steele, T.H.: Urate secretion in man: The pyrazinamide suppression test. Ann. Intern. Med. 79:734, 1973.
215. Levinson, D.J., and Sorensen, L.B.: Renal handling of uric acid in normal and gouty subject: Evidence for a 4-component system. Ann. Rheum. Dis. 39:173, 1980.
216. Levinson, D.J., Decker, D.E., and Sorensen, L.B.: Renal handling of uric acid in man. Ann. Clin. Lab. Sci. 12:73, 1982.
217. Kramer, H.J., Lu, E., and Gonick, H.C.: Organic acid excretion patterns in gout. Ann. Rheum. Dis. 31:137, 1972.
218. Yu, T.-F., Alder, M., Bobrow, E., et al.: Plasma and urinary amino acids in primary gout, with special reference to glutamine. J. Clin. Invest. 48:885, 1969.
219. Kaplan, D., Diamond, H., Wallace, D.L., et al.: Amino acid excretion in primary hyperuricaemia. Ann. Rheum. Dis. 28:180, 1969.
220. Sonka, J., Gregorova, I., and Krizek, V.: Dehydroepiandrosterone. Steroids 4:843, 1964.
221. Pittman, J.A., Starnes, W.R., Beetham, W.P., et al.: Dehydroepiandrosterone excretion and gout (abstract). Clin. Res. 14:66, 1966.
222. Casey, J.H., Hoffman, M.M., and Solomon, S.: The excretion of urinary dehydroepiandrosterone in gout. Arthritis Rheum. 11:444, 1968.
223. Sparagana, M., and Phillips, G.: Dehydroepiandrosterone (3,β-hydroxy-5-androsten-17-one) metabolism in gout. Steroids 19:477, 1972.
224. Henderson, L.J., and Palmer, W.W.: On the several factors of acid excretion in nephritis. J. Biol. Chem. 21:37, 1915.
225. Hilton, J.G., Goodbody, M.F., Jr., and Kruesi, O.R.: The effect of prolonged administration of ammonium chloride on the blood acid-base equilibrium of geriatric subjects. J. Am. Geriat. Soc. 3:697, 1955.
226. Falls, W.F., Jr.: Comparison of urinary acidification and ammonium excretion in normal and gouty subjects. Metabolism 21:433, 1972.
226a. Reynolds, P.P., Knapp, M.J., Baraf, H.S.B., and Holmes, E.W.: Moonshine and lead: Relationship to the pathogenesis of hyperuricemia in gout. Arthritis Rheum. 26:1057, 1983.
227. Duncan, H., and Dixon, A.S.: Gout, familial hyperuricemia and renal diseases. Quart. J. Med. 113:127, 1960.
228. Bennett, R.M., Chait, A., and Lewis, B.: Familial hyperuricemia and hypertriglyceridemia. Ann. Rheum. Dis. 32:497, 1973.
229. Carr, A.A.: Colchicine toxicity. Arch. Intern. Med. 115:29, 1965.
230. Rosenbloom, F.M., Kelley, W.N., Carr, A.A., et al.: Familial nephropathy and gout in a kindred. Clin. Res. 15:270, 1967.
231. Thompson, G.R., Weiss, J.J., Goldman, R.T., et al.: Familial occurrence of hyperuricemia, gout and medullary cystic disease. Arch. Intern. Med. 138:1614, 1978.
232. Massari, P.U., Hsu, C.H., Barnes, R.V., et al.: Familial hyperuricemia and renal disease. Arch. Intern. Med. 140:680, 1980.

233. Simmonds, H.A., Cameron, J.S., Potter, C.F., et al.: Renal failure in young subjects with familial gout. Adv. Exp. Med. Biol. 122A:15, 1980.
234. Simmonds, H.A., Warren, D.J., Cameron, J.S., et al.: Familial gout and renal failure in young women. Clin. Nephrol. 14:176, 1980.
235. Stapleton, F.B., Nyhan, W.L., Borden, M., et al.: Renal pathogenesis of familial hyperuricemia: Studies in two kindreds. Pediatr. Res. 15:1447, 1981.
236. Whalen, R.E., and McIntosh, H.D.: The spectrum of hereditary renal diseases. Am. J. Med. 33:282, 1962.
237. Perkoff, G.R.: The hereditary renal diseases. N. Engl. J. Med. 277:79, 1967.
238. Kavalich, A.G., Moran, E., and Coe, F.L.: Dietary purine consumption by hyperuricosuric calcium oxalate stone formers and normal subjects. J. Chronic Dis. 29:745, 1976.
239. Seegmiller, J.E., Grayzel, A.I., and Howell, R.R.: The renal excretion of uric acid in gout. J. Clin. Invest. 41:1094, 1962.
240. Simkin, P.A., Hoover, P.L., Paxson, C.S., et al.: Uric acid excretion: Quantitative assessment from spot, midmorning serum and urine samples. Ann. Intern. Med. 91:44, 1979.
241. Wortmann, R.L., and Fox, I.H.: Limited value of uric acid to creatinine ratios in estimating uric acid excretion. Ann. Intern. Med. 93:822, 1980.
242. Gordon, R.B., Counsilman, A.C., Cross, S.M.C., and Emmerson, B.T.: Purine synthesis de novo in lymphocytes from patients with gout. Clin. Sci. 63:429, 1982.
243. Hers, H.-G., and Van Den Berghe, G.: Enzyme defect in primary gout. Lancet 1:585, 1979.
244. Ullman, B., Wormsted, M.A., Cohen, M.B., et al.: Purine oversecretion in cultured murine lymphoma cells deficient in adenylosuccinate synthetase: Genetic model for inherited hyperuricemia and gout. Proc. Natl. Acad. Sci. USA 79:5127, 1982.
245. Seegmiller, J.E., Rosenbloom, R.M., and Kelley, W.N.: An enzyme defect associated with a sex-linked human neurological disorder and excessive purine synthesis. Science 155:1682, 1967.
246. Lesch, M., and Nyhan, W.L.: A familial disorder of uric acid metabolism and central nervous system function. Am. J. Med. 36:561, 1964.
247. Kelley, W.N.: Hypoxanthine-guanine phosphoribosyltransferase deficiency in the Lesch-Nyhan syndrome and gout. Fed. Proc. 27:1047, 1968.
248. Kelley, W.N., Rosenbloom, E.M., Henderson, J.F., et al.: A specific enzyme defect in gout associated with overproduction of uric acid. Proc. Natl. Acad. Sci. USA 57:1735, 1967.
249. Kelley, W.N., Greene, M.L., Rosenbloom, J.F., et al.: Hypoxanthine-guanine phosphoribosyltransferase deficiency in gout. Ann. Intern. Med. 70:155, 1969.
250. Michener, W.M.: Hyperuricemia and mental retardation with athetosis and self-mutilation. Am. J. Dis. Child 133:195, 1967.
251. Marie, J., Royer, P., and Rappaport: Hyperuricemie congenitale avec troubles neurologiques, renaux et sanguins. Arch. Fr. Pediat. 23:970, 1966.
252. van Bogaert, L., Damme, J.V., and Verschueren, M.: Sur un syndrome professif d'hypertonie extrapyrimidale avec ostéoarthropathies goutteuses chez deux frères. Rev. Neurol. 114:15, 1966.
253. Riley, J.D.: Gout and cerebral palsy in a three-year-old boy. Arch. Dis. Child. 35:293, 1960.
254. Berman, P.H., Balis, M.E., and Dancis, J.: Congenital hyperuricemia: An inborn error of purine metabolism associated with psychomotor retardation athetosis, and self-mutilation, Arch. Neurol. 20:44, 1969.
255. Kogut, M.D., Donnell, G.N., Nyhan, W.L., et al.: Disorder of purine metabolism due to partial deficiency of hypoxanthine-guanine phosphoribosyltransferase: A study of a family. Am. J. Med. 48:148, 1970.
256. Sperling, O., Frank, M., Ophir, R., et al.: Partial deficiency of hypoxanthine-guanine phosphoribosyltransferase associated with gout and uric acid lithiasis. Eur. J. Clin. Res. 15:942, 1970.
257. Delbarre, F., Cartier, P., Auscher, C., et al: Gouttes enzymopathiques: Dyspurinies par défict en hypoxanthineguanine phosphoribosyltransférase. Fréquence et caractères cliniques de l'anenzymose. Presse Med. 78:729, 1970.
258. Marie, J., Royer, P., and Rappaport, R.: Hyperuricemie congenitale avec troubles neurologiques, renaux et sanguins. Arch. Fr. Pediat. 24:501, 1967.
259. Manzke, H.: Hyperuricamie mit cerebralparese Syndrome eines hereditaren Purinstoffwechselleidens. Helv. Paediat. Acta 22:258, 1967.
260. van der Zee, S.P.M., Schretlen, E.D.A.M., and Monnens, L.A.H.: Megaloblastic anemia in the Lesch-Nyhan syndrome (letter to the editor). Lancet 1:1427, 1968.
261. Wilson, J.M., Baugher, B.W., Landa, L., et al.: Human hypoxanthine-guanine phosphoribosyltransferase: Purification and characterization of mutant forms of the enzyme. J. Biol. Chem. 256:10306, 1981.
262. Wilson, J.M., Baugher, B.W., Mattes, P.M., et al.: Human hypoxanthine-guanine phosphoribosyltransferase: Demonstration of structural var-

iants in lymphoblastoid cells derived from patients with a deficiency of the enzyme. J. Clin. Invest. 69:706, 1982.

263. Wilson, J.M., Tarr, G.E., and Kelley, W.N.: Human hypoxanthine-guanine phosphoribosyltransferase: A single amino acid substitution in a mutant form of the enzyme isolated from a patient with gout. Proc. Natl. Acad. Sci. 80:870, 1983.

264. Wilson, J.M., and Kelley, W.N.: The molecular basis of hypoxanthine-guanine phosphoribosyltransferase deficiency in a patient with the Lesch-Nyhan syndrome. J. Clin. Invest 71:1331, 1983.

265. Wilson, J.M., Young, A.B., and Kelley, W.N.: Hypoxanthine-guanine phosphoribosyltransferase deficiency: The molecular basis of the clinical syndrome. N. Engl. J. Med. 309:900, 1983.

266. Holmes, E.W., McDonald, J.A., McCord, J.M., et al.: Human glutamine phosphoribosylpyrophosphate amidotransferase: Kinetic and regulatory properties. J. Biol. Chem. 248:144, 1973.

267. Holmes, E.W., Wyngaarden, J.B., and Kelley, W.N.: Human glutamine phosphoribosylpyrophosphate amidotransferase: Two molecular forms interconvertible by purine ribonucleotides and phosphoribosylpyrophosphate. J. Biol. Chem. 248:6035, 1973.

268. Rosenbloom, F.M., Henderson, J.F., Caldwell, I.C., et al.: Biochemical bases of accelerated purine biosynthesis denovo in human fibroblasts lacking hypoxanthine-guanine phosphoribosyltransferase. J. Biol. Chem. 243:1166, 1968.

269. Nuki, G., Lever, J., and Seegmiller, J.E.: Biochemical characteristics of 8-azaguanine resistant human lymphoblast mutants selected in vitro. In Sperling, O., DeVries, A., and Wyngaarden, J.B. (eds.): Purine Metabolism in Man. New York, Plenum, 1974, p. 255.

270. Edwards, N.L., Recker, D.P., and Fox, I.H.: Overproduction of uric acid in hypoxanthineguanine phosphoribosyltransferase deficiency: Contribution of impaired purine salvage. J. Clin. Invest. 63:922, 1979.

271. Fox, I.H.: Metabolic basis for disorders of purine nucleotide degradation. Metabolism 30:616, 1981.

272. Rosenbloom, F.M., Kelley, W.N., Henderson, J.F., et al.: Lyon hypothesis and X-linked disease. Lancet 2:305, 1967.

273. Brennand, J., Chinault, A.C., Konecki, D.S., et al.: Cloned cDNA sequences of the hypoxanthine-guanine phosphoribosyltransferase gene from a mouse neuroblastoma cell line found to have amplified genomic sequences. Proc. Natl. Acad. Sci. USA 79:1950, 1982.

274. Jolly, D., Esty, A.C., Bernard, H.U., and Friedmann, T.: Isolation of a genomic clone partially encoding human hypoxanthine phosphoribosyltransferase. Proc. Natl. Acad. Sci. USA 79:5038, 1982.

275. Hoefnagel, D., Andrew, E.D., Mireault, N.G., et al.: Hereditary choreoathetosis, self-mutilation, and hyperuricemia in young males. N. Engl. J. Med. 273:130, 1965.

276. Shapiro, S.L., Sheppard, G.L., Jr., Dreifuss, F.E., et al.: X-linked recessive inheritance of a syndrome of mental retardation with hyperuricemia. Proc. Soc. Exp. Biol. Med. 122:609, 1966.

277. Emmerson, B.T., and Wyngaarden, J.B.: Purine metabolism in heterozygous carriers of hypoxanthine-guanine phosphoribosyltransferase deficiency. Science 166:1533, 1969.

278. Emmerson, B.T.: Urate metabolism in heterozygotes for HGPRTase deficiency. In Sperling, O., DeVries, A., and Wyngaarden, J.B. (eds.): Purine Metabolism in Man. New York, Plenum, 1974, p. 287.

279. Sperling, O., Eilam, G., Persky-Brosh, S., et al.: Accelerated erythrocyte 5'-phosphoribosyl-1-pyrophosphate synthesis. A familial abnormality associated with excessive uric acid production and gout. Biochem. Med. 6:310, 1972.

280. Sperling, O., Perksy-Brosh, S., Boer, P., et al.: Human erythrocyte phosphoribosylpyrophosphate synthetase mutationally altered in regulatory properties. Biochem. Med. 7:389, 1973.

281. Becker, M.A., Meyer, L.J., Wood, A.W., et al.: Purine overproduction in man associated with increased phosphoribosylpyrophosphate synthetase activity. Science 179:1123, 1973.

282. Becker, M.A., Meyer, L.J., and Seegmiller, J.E.: Gout with purine overproduction due to increased phosphoribosylpyrophosphate synthetase activity. Am. J. Med. 55:232, 1973.

283. Becker, M.A., Kostel, P.J., Meyer, L.J., et al.: Human phosphoribosylpyrophosphate synthetase: Increased enzyme specific activity in a family with gout and excessive purine synthesis. Proc. Natl. Acad. Sci. USA 70:2749, 1973.

284. Becker, M.A., Meyer, L.J., Dostel, P.J., et al.: Increased 5-phosphoribosyl-1-pyrophosphate (PRPP) synthetase activity and gout: Diversity of structural alterations of the enzyme (abstract). J. Clin. Invest. 53:4a, 1974.

285. Akaoka, I., Fujimori, S., Kamatani, N., et al.: A gouty family with increased phosphoribosylpyrophosphate synthetase activity: Case reports, familial studies, and kinetic studies of the abnormal enzyme. J. Rheumatol. 8:563, 1981.

286. Becker, M.A., Losman, M.J., Itkin, P., et al.: Gout with superactive phosphoribosylpyrophosphate synthetase due to increased enzyme catalytic rate. J. Lab. Clin. Med. 99:495, 1982.

287. Yen, R.C.K., Adams, W.B., Lazar, C., and Becker, M.A.: Evidence for

x-linkage of human phosphoribosylpyrophosphate synthetase. Proc. Natl. Acad. Sci. USA 75:482, 1978.

288. Takeuchi, F., Hanaoka, F., Yano, E., et al.: The mode of genetic transmission of a gouty family with increased phosphoribosylpyrophosphate synthetase activity. Hum. Genet. 58:322, 1981.

289. Woolliscroft, J.O., Colfer, H., and Fox, I.H.: Hyperuricemia in acute illness: A poor prognostic sign. Am. J. Med. 72:58, 1982.

290. Sutton, J., Toews, C.J., Ward, G.R., and Fox, I.H.: Purine metabolism during strenous muscular exercise in man. Metabolism 29:254, 1980.

291. Faller, J., and Fox, I.H.: Ethanol-induced hyperuricemia: Evidence for increased urate production by activation of adenine nucleotide turnover. N. Engl. J. Med. 307:1598, 1982.

292. Garrod, A.B.: A Treatise on Gout and Rheumatic Gout (Rheumatic Arthritis). 3rd ed. London, Longmans, Green, 1876, p. 584.

293. Cohen, H.: Gout. In Copeman, W.S.C. (ed.): Textbook of the Rheumatic Diseases. Edinburgh, Livingstone, 1955, p. 361.

294. Neel, J.V.: The clinical detection of the genetic carriers of inherited disease. Medicine 26:115, 1947.

295. Rosenberg, E.F.: Gout and male hermaphroditism: Report of a case. Ann. Rheum. Dis. 2:273, 1941.

296. Talbott, J.G.: Gout. J. Chronic Dis. 1:338, 1955.

297. Yu, T.-F.: Milestones in the treatment of gout. Am. J. Med. 56:676, 1974.

298. Morton, N.E.: Genetics of hyperuricemia in families with gout. Am. J. Med. Genet. 4:103, 1979.

299. Garrod, A.B.: The Nature and Treatment of Gout and Rheumatic Gout. London, Walton and Maberly, 1859.

300. Freudweiler, M.: Experimentelle Untersuchungen über das Wesen der Gichknoten. Dtsch. Arch. Klin. Med. 63:266, 1899.

301. Freudweiler, M.: Experimentelle Untersuchungen über die Entstehung der Gichtknoten. Dtsch. Arch. Klin. Med. 69:155. 1901. (English translation: Experimental investigations into the origin of gouty tophi. Arthritis Rheum. 8:270, 1965.)

302. His, W.J.: Schicksal und Wirkungen des sauren harnsauren Natrons in Bauch und Gelenkohle des Kaninchens. Dtsch. Arch. Klin. Med. 67:81, 1900.

303. McCarty, D.J., Jr., and Hollander, J.L.: Indentification of urate crystals in gouty synovial fluid. Ann. Intern. Med. 54:452, 1961.

304. Roberts, W.: The Croonian Lectures. On the chemistry and therapeutics of uric acid gravel and gout. Br. Med. J. 2:61, 1892.

305. McCarty, D.J., Jr.: Phagocytosis of urate crystals in gouty synovial fluid. Am. J. Med. Sci. 243:288, 1962.

306. Phelps, P., Steele, A.D., and McCarty, J.D., Jr.: Compensated polarized light microscopy. JAMA 203:508, 1968.

307. Zvaifler, N.J., and Pekin, T.J.: Significance of urate crystals in synovial fluids. Arch. Intern. Med. 111:99, 1963.

308. Seegmiller, J.E., Laster, L., and Howell, R.R.: Biochemistry of uric acid and its relation to gout. N. Engl. J. Med. 268:712, 1963.

309. Fiechtner, J.J., and Simkin, P.A.: Urate spherulites in gouty synovia. JAMA 245:1533, 1981.

310. Hamilton, M.E., Parris, T.M., Gibson, R.S., et al.: Simultaneous gout and pyarthrosis. Arch. Intern. Med. 140:917, 1980.

311. Itzkowitch, D.F., Famaey, J.-P., and Appelboom, T.: Crystal arthropathy as a complication of septic arthritis. J. Rheumatol. 8:3, 1981.

312. Faires, J.S., and McCarty, D.J., Jr.: Acute synovitis in normal joints of man and dog produced by injections of microcrystalline sodium urate, calcium oxalate and corticosteroid esters (abstract). Arthritis Rheum. 5:295, 1962.

313. Malawista, S.E., Howell, R.R., and Seegmiller, J.E.: Factors modifying the inflammatory response to injected microcrystalline sodium urate (abstract). Arthritis Rheum. 5:307, 1962.

314. Seegmiller, J.E., and Howell, R.R.: The old and new concepts of acute gouty arthritis. Arthritis Rheum. 5:616, 1962.

315. Seegmiller, J.E., Howell, R.R., and Malawista, S.E.: Inflammatory reaction to sodium urate: Its possible relationship to genesis of acute gouty arthritis. JAMA 180:469, 1962.

316. Seegmiller, J.E., Howell, R.R., and Malawista, S.E.: A mechanism of action of colchicine in acute gouty arthritis (abstract). J. Clin. Invest. 41:1399, 1962.

317. Malawista, S.E., and Seegmiller, J.E.: The effect of pretreatment with colchicine on the inflammatory response to injected microcrystalline monosodium urate: A model for gouty inflammation. Ann. Intern. Med. 62:648, 1965.

318. McCarty, D.J., and Gatter, R.A.: Pseudogout syndrome. Bull. Rheum. Dis. 14:331, 1964.

319. Tse, R., and Phelps, P.: Polymorphonuclear leukocyte motility in vitro: V. Release of chemotactic activity following phagocytosis of calcium pyrophosphate crystals, diamond dust and urate crystals. J. Lab. Clin. Med. 76:403, 1970.

320. Agudelo, C.A., and Schumacher, H.R.: The synovitis of acute gouty arthritis: A light and electron microscopic study. Hum. Pathol. 4:265, 1973.

321. Hall, A.P., Barry, P.E., Dawber, T.R., et al.: Epidemiology of gout and hyperuricemia: A long-term population study. Am. J. Med. 42:27, 1967.

322. Ropes, M.W., and Bauer, W.: Synovial Fluid Changes in Joint Disease. Cambridge, Mass., Harvard University Press, 1953, p. 150.

323. Seegmiller, J.E.: Serum uric acid. In Cohen, A.S. (ed.): Laboratory Diagnostic Procedures in the Rheumatic Diseases. 2nd ed. Boston, Little, Brown & Company, 1974, p. 216.

324. Dorner, R.W., Weiss, T.D., Baldassare, A.R., et al.: Plasma and synovial fluid as solvents for monosodium urate. Ann. Rheum. Dis. 40:70, 1981.

325. Tak, H.-K., Cooper, S.M., and Wilcox, W.R.: Studies on the nucleation of monosodium urate at 37°C. Arthritis Rheum. 23:574, 1980.

326. Katz, W.A., and Schubert, M.: The interaction of monosodium urate with connective tissue components. J. Clin. Invest. 49:1783, 1970.

327. Brugsch, T., and Citron, J.: Ueber die Absorption der Harnsaure Durch Knorpel. Z. Exp. Pathol. Ther. 5:401, 1908.

328. Dainty, J., and House, C.R.: "Unstirred layers" in frog skin. J. Physiol. 182:66, 1966.

329. Katz, W.A., and Ehrlich, G.E.: The solubility of monosodium urate in serum and connective tissue fractions. Arthritis Rheum. 11:492, 1968.

330. Perricone, E., and Brandt, K.D.: Enhancement of urate solubility by connective tissue. I. Effect of proteoglycan aggregates and buffer cation. Arthritis Rheum. 21:453, 1978.

331. Perricone, E., and Brandt, K.D.: Enhancement of urate solubility by connective tissue. II. Inhibition of sodium urate crystallization by cation exchange. Ann. Rheum. Dis. 38:467, 1979.

332. Postlethwaite, A.E., Gutman, R.A., and Kelley, W.N.: Salicylate-mediated increase in urate removal during hemodialysis: Evidence of urate binding to protein in vivo. Metabolism 23:771, 1974.

333. Kovarsky, J., Holmes, E., and Kelley, W.N.: Absence of significant urate binding to human serum proteins. J. Lab. Clin. Med. 93:85, 1979.

334. Roch-Ramel, F., Diezi-Chomety, F., Rougemont, D., et al.: Renal excretion of uric acid in the rat: A micro-puncture and microperfusion study. Am. J. Physiol. 230:768, 1976.

335. Loeb, J.N.: The influence of temperature on the solubility of monosodium urate. Arthritis Rheum. 15:189, 1972.

336. Horvath, S.M., and Hollander, J.L.: Intra-articular temperature as a measure of joint reaction. J. Clin. Invest. 28:469, 1949.

337. Hollander, J.L., Stoner, E.K., Brown, E.M., Jr., et al.: Joint temperature measurements in the evaluation of antiarthritic agents. J. Clin. Invest. 30:701, 1951.

338. Hollander, J.L., and Horvath, S.M.: The influence of physical therapy procedures on intra-articular temperature of normal and arthritic subjects. Am. J. Med. Sci. 218:543, 1949.

339. Simkin, P.A.: Concentration of urate by differential diffusion: A hypothesis for initial urate deposition. In Sperling, O., DeVries, A., and Wyngaarden, J.B. (eds.): Purine Metabolism in Man. New York, Plenum, 1974, p. 547.

340. Howell, D.S.: Preliminary observations on local pH in gout tophi and synovial fluid. Arthritis Rheum. 8:736, 1965.

341. Spilberg, I., Tanphaichitr, D., and Kantor, O.: Synovial fluid pH in acute gouty arthritis (letter). Arthritis Rheum. 20:142, 1977.

342. Kellermeyer, R.W.: Hageman factor and acute gouty arthritis. Arthritis Rheum. 11:452, 1968.

343. Kellermeyer, R.W., and Breckenridge, R.T.: The inflammatory process in acute gouty arthritis. I. Activation of Hageman factor by sodium urate crystals. J. Lab. Clin. Med. 65:307, 1965.

344. Kellermeyer, R.W., and Breckenridge, R.T.: The inflammatory process in acute gouty arthritis. II. The presence of Hageman factor and plasma thromboplastin antecedent in synovial fluid. J. Lab. Clin. Med. 67:455, 1966.

345. Ginsberg, M.H., Jaques, B., Cochrane, C.G., et al.: Urate crystal-dependent cleavage of Hageman factor in human plasma and synovial fluid. J. Lab. Clin. Med. 95:497, 1980.

346. Kellermeyer, R.W.: The inflammatory process in acute gouty arthritis. III. Vascular permeability enhancing activity in normal human synovial fluid; induction by Hageman factor activators and inhibition by Hageman factor antiserum. J. Lab. Clin. Med. 70:372, 1967.

347. Melmon, K., Webster, M.E., Goldfinger, S.E., et al.: The presence of a kinin in inflammatory synovial effusion from arthritides of varying etiologies. Arthritis Rheum. 10:13, 1967.

348. Phelps, P., Prokop, D.J., and McCarty, D.D.: Crystal induced inflammation in canine joints. III. Evidence against bradykinin as a mediator of inflammation. J. Lab. Clin. Med. 68:433, 1966.

349. Spilberg, I.: Urate crystal arthritis in animals lacking Hageman factor. Arthritis Rheum. 17:143, 1974.

350. Green, D., Arsever, C.L., Grumet, K.A., et al.: Classic gout in Hageman factor (factor XII) deficiency. Arch. Intern. Med. 142:1556, 1982.

351. Naff, G.B., and Byers, P.H.: Complement as a mediator of inflammation in acute gouty arthritis. I. Studies on the reaction between human serum complement and sodium urate crystals. J. Lab. Clin. Med. 81:747, 1973.

352. Hasselbacher, P.: C3 activation by monosodium urate monohydrate and other crystalline material. Arthritis Rheum. 22:571, 1979.

353. Giclas, P.C., Ginsberg, M.H., and Cooper, N.R.: Immunoglobulin G independent activation of the classical complement pathway by monosodium urate crystals. J. Clin. Invest. 63:759, 1979.

354. Pekin, T.J., and Zwaifler, N.J.: Hemolytic complement in synovial fluid. J. Clin. Invest. 43:1372, 1964.

355. Fostiropoulus, K., Austen, K.F., and Block, K.J.: Total hemolytic complement and second component of complement activity in serum and synovial fluid. Arthritis Rheum. 8:219, 1965.

356. Hasselbacher, P.: Immunoelectrophoretic assay for synovial fluid C3 with correction for synovial fluid globulin. Arthritis Rheum. 22:243, 1979.

357. Spilberg, I.: Current concepts of the mechanism of acute inflammation in gouty arthritis. Arthritis Rheum. 18:129, 1975.

358. Rae, S.A., Davidson, E.M., and Smith, M.J.H.: Leukotriene B₄, an inflammatory mediator in gout. Lancet 2:1122, 1982.

359. Serhan, C.N., Lundberg, U., Abramson, S., et al.: Formation of leukotrienes and hydroxy acids by human leukocytes exposed to monosodium urate. Clin. Res. 31:521A, 1983.

360. Ginsberg, M.H., and Kozin, F.: Mechanisms of cellular interaction with monosodium urate crystals: IgG-dependent and IgG-independent platelet stimulation by urate crystals. Arthritis Rheum. 21:896, 1978.

361. Ginsberg, M., Henson, P., Henson, J., et al.: Mechanisms of platelet response to monosodium urate crystals. Am. J. Pathol. 94:549, 1979.

362. Jaques, B.C., and Ginsberg, M.H.: The role of cell surface proteins in platelet stimulation by monosodium urate crystals. Arthritis Rheum. 25:508, 1982.

363. Kozin, G., and McCarty, D.J.: Molecular orientation of immunoglobulin G adsorbed to microcrystalline monosodium urate monohydrate. J. Lab. Clin. Med. 95:49, 1980.

364. Hasselbacher, P.: Binding of IgG and complement protein by monosodium urate monohydrate and other crystals. J. Lab. Clin. Med. 94:532, 1979.

365. Simchowitz, L., Atkinson, J.P., and Spilberg, I.: Stimulation of the respiratory burst in human neutrophils by crystal phagocytosis. Arthritis Rheum. 25:181, 1982.

366. McMillan, R.M., Hasselbacher, P., Hahn, J.L., et al.: Interactions of murine macrophages with monosodium urate crystals: Stimulation of lysosomal enzyme release and prostaglandin synthesis. J. Rheumatol. 8:555, 1981.

367. Ginsberg, M.H., Kozin, F., Chow, D., et al.: Adsorption of polymorphonuclear leukocyte lysosomal enzymes to monosodium urate crystals. Arthritis Rheum. 20:1538, 1977.

368. Hasselbacher, P.: Stimulation of synovial fibroblasts by calcium oxalate and monosodium urate monohydrate: A mechanism of connective tissue degradation in oxalosis and gout. J. Lab. Clin. Med. 100:977, 1982.

369. Phelps, P., Andrews, R., and Rosenbloom, J.: Demonstration of chemotactic factor in human gout: Further characterization of occurrence and structure. J. Rheumatol. 8:889, 1981.

370. Phelps, P., and McCarty, D.J., Jr.: Crystal induced inflammation in canine joints. II. Importance of polymorphonuclear leukocytes. J. Exp. Med. 124:115, 1966.

371. Chang, Y.-H., and Gialla, E.J.: Suppression of urate crystal-induced canine joint inflammation by heterologous antipolymorphonuclear leukocyte serum. Arthritis Rheum. 11:145, 1968.

372. Phelps, P.: Polymorphonuclear leukocyte motility in vitro. III. Possible release of a chemotactic substance after phagocytosis of urate crystals by polymorphonuclear leukocytes. Arthritis Rheum. 12:197, 1969.

373. Phelps, P.: Appearance of chemotactic activity following intraarticular injection of monosodium urate crystals. Effect of colchicine. J. Lab. Clin. Med. 76:622, 1970.

374. Spilberg, I., Mandell, B., and Wochner, R.D.: Studies on crystal induced chemotactic factor. I. Role of protein synthesis and neutral protease activity. J. Lab. Clin. Med. 83:56, 1974.

375. Phelps, D.: Polymorphonuclear leukocyte motility in vitro: IV. Colchicine inhibition of chemotactic activity formation after phagocytosis of urate crystals. Arthritis Rheum. 13:1, 1970.

376. Spilberg, I., Gallacher, A., Mehta, J.M., and Mandell, B.: Urate crystal-induced chemotactic factor. Isolation and partial characterization. J. Clin. Invest. 58:815, 1976.

377. Spilberg, I., and Mehta, J.: Demonstration of a specific neutrophil receptor for a cell-derived chemotactic factor. J. Clin. Invest. 63:85, 1979.

378. Spilberg, I., Mehta, J., and Simchowitz, L.: Induction of a chemotactic factor from human neutrophils by diverse crystals. J. Lab. Clin. Med. 100:399, 1982.

379. Zigmond, S.H., and Hirsch, J.G.: Leukocyte locomotion and chemotaxis. New methods for evaluation and demonstration of a cell-derived chemotactic factor. J. Exp. Med. 137:387, 1973.

380. Kozin, F., and McCarty, D.J.: Protein adsorption to monosodium urate, calcium pyrophosphate dihydrate, and silica crystals. Relationship to the pathogenesis of crystal induced inflammation. Arthritis Rheum. 19:433, 1976.

381. Wallingford, W., and McCarty, D.J.: Differential membranolytic effects of microcrystalline sodium urate and calcium pyrophosphate dihydrate. J. Exp. Med. 133:100, 1971.

382. Skosey, J.L., Kozin, F., Ginsberg, M.H., et al.: Protein adsorption to monosodium urate crystals: Differential responses of human peripheral blood neutrophils. Second International Symposium on Purine Metabolism in Man, 1976.

383. Abramson, S., Hoffstein, S.T., and Weissmann, G.: Superoxide anion generation by human neutrophils exposed to monosodium urate: Effect of protein adsorption and complement activation. Arthritis Rheum. 25:174, 1982.

384. Simchowitz L., Mehta, J., and Spilberg, I.: Chemotactic factor-induced superoxide radical generation by human neutrophils: Requirement for proteinase (esterase) activity. J. Lab. Clin. Med. 94:403, 1979.

385. Weissmann, G.: Crystals, lysosomes, and gout. Adv. Intern. Med. 19:239, 1974.

386. Rajan, K.T.: Lysosomes and gout. Nature 210:959, 1966.

387. Malawista, S.E., Van Blaricom, G., Cretella, S.B., et al.: The phlogistic potential of urate in solution: Studies of the phagocytic process in human leukocytes. Arthritis Rheum. 22:728, 1979.

388. Ratti, G.: Sull esistenza di una attivita, uricolitica nell'uomo. Reumatiso 10(Suppl. 2):33, 1958.

389. Agner, K.: Crystalline myeloperoxidase. Acta Chem. Scand. 12:89, 1958.

390. Howell, R.R., and Seegmiller, J.E.: Uricolysis by human leukocytes. Nature 196:482, 1962.

391. Howell, R.R., and Wyngaarden, J.B.: On the mechanism of peroxidation of uric acids by hemoproteins. J. Biol. Chem. 225:3544, 1960.

392. Zwaifler, N.: A speculation on the pathogenesis of joint inflammation in rheumatoid arthritis. Arthritis Rheum. 8:289, 1965.

393. Weissmann, G.: Lysosomes. N. Engl. J. Med. 273:1084, 1143, 1965.

394. Weissmann, G., and Spilberg, I.: Breakdown of cartilage protein polysaccharide by lysosomes. Arthritis Rheum. 11:162, 1968.

395. Ward, P.A., and Hill, J.H.: C5 chemotactic fragments produced by an enzyme in lysosomal granules of neutrophils. J. Immunol. 104:535, 1970.

396. Harris, E.D., Jr., and McCroskery, P.A.: The influence of temperature and fibril stability on degradation of cartilage collagen by rheumatoid synovial collagenase. N. Engl. J. Med. 290:1, 1974.

397. Hess, R.J., and Martin, J.H.: Pyarthrosis complicating gout. JAMA 218:592, 1971.

398. Wallace, S.L., Bernstein, D., and Diamond, H.: Diagnostic value of the colchicine therapeutic trial. JAMA 199:525, 1967.

399. Mugler, A., Wackenheim, A., and Grappe, J.: Nouvelles observations de maladies allergiques traitées par la colchicine par voie intraveineuse. Bull. Mem. Soc. Med. Hôp. Paris 67:821, 1951.

400. McCarty, D.J., Jr.: Crystal-induced inflammation; syndromes of gout and pseudogout. Geriatrics 18:467, 1963.

401. Thompson, G.R., Ming Ting, Y., Riggs, G.A., et al.: Calcific tendinitis and soft-tissue calcification resembling gout. JAMA 203:464, 1968.

402. Kaplan, H.: Further experience with colchicine in the treatment of sarcoid arthritis. N. Engl. J. Med. 268:761, 1963.

403. Blomgren, S.E.: Conditions associated with erythema nodosum. N.Y. State J. Med. 72:2302, 1972.

404. Zuckner, J.: Colchicine therapeutic trial responses in rheumatoid arthritis (abstract). Arthritis Rheum. 5:329, 1962.

405. Goldfinger, S.E.: Colchicine for familial Mediterranean fever. N. Engl. J. Med. 287:1302, 1972.

406. Boardman, P.L., and Hart, F.D.: Indomethacin in the treatment of acute gout. Practitioner 194:560, 1965.

407. Davis, J.S., Jr.: Guest editorial. V. Med. Mon. 78:335, 1951.

408. Davis, J.S., Jr., and Bartfield, H.: The effect of intravenous colchicine on acute gout. Am. J. Med. 16:218, 1954.

409. Stemmermann, G.N., and Hayashi, T.: Colchicine intoxication. A reappraisal of its pathology based on a study of three fatal cases. Hum. Pathol. 2:321, 1971.

410. Smyth, C.J., Velayos, E.E., and Amoroso, C.: A method for measuring swelling of hands and feet. II. Influence of new anti-inflammatory drug, indomethacin in acute gout. Acta Rheumatol. Scand. 9:306, 1963.

411. Hart, F.D., and Boardman, P.L.: Indomethacin: A new non-steroid antiinflammatory agent. Br. Med. J. 2:965, 1963.

412. Norcross, B.M.: Treatment of connective tissue diseases with a new nonsteroidal compound (indomethacin) (abstract). Arthritis Rheum. 6:290, 1963.

413. Shack, M.E.: Drug-induced ulceration and perforation of the small bowel. Ariz. Med. 23:517, 1966.

414. O'Brian, W.M.: Indomethacin: A survey of clinical trials. Clin. Pharmacol. Ther. 9:94, 1968.

415. Simon, L.S., and Mills, J.A.: Medical Intelligence: Nonsteroidal antiinflammatory drugs. N. Engl. J. Med. 302:1179, 1980.

416. Gary, N.E., Dodelson, R., and Eisinger, R.P.: Indomethacin-associated acute renal failure. Am. J. Med. 69:135, 1980.

417. Friedman, P.L., Brown, E.J., Gunther, S., et al.: Coronary vasoconstrictor effect of indomethacin in patients with coronary-artery disease. N. Engl. J. Med. 305:1171, 1981.

418. Kimberly, R.P., Bowden, R.E., Keiser, H.R., et al.: Reduction of renal function by newer nonsteroidal anti-inflammatory drugs. Am. J. Med. 64:804, 1978.

419. Wallace, S.L.: The treatment of gout. Arthritis Rheum. 15:317, 1972.

420. Kuzell, W.C., Schaffarzick, R.W., Brown, B., et al.: Phenylbutazone (Butazolidin) in rheumatoid arthritis and gout. JAMA 149:729, 1952.

421. Kidd, E.G., Boyce, K.C., and Freyberg, R.H.: Clinical studies of phenylbutazone (Butazolidin) and butapyrine (Irgapyrine) in rheumatoid arthritis, rheumatoid spondylitis and gout. Ann. Rheum. Dis. 12:20, 1953.

422. Johnson, H.P., Engleman, E.P., Forsham, P.H., et al.: Effects of phenylbutazone in gout. N. Engl. J. Med. 250:665, 1954.

423. Smyth, C.J., and Percy, J.S.: Comparison of indomethacin and phenylbutazone in acute gout. Ann. Rheum. Dis. 32:351, 1973.

424. Cuq, P.: Experience francaise du traitement de la crise de goutte aigue par le naproxen-C 1674. Scand. J. Rheumatol. Suppl. 2:64, 1973.

425. Wilkens, R.F., and Case, J.B.: Treatment of acute gout with naproxen. Scand. J. Rheumatol. 2(Suppl. 2):69, 1973.

426. Sturge, R.A., Scott, J.T., Hamilton, E.B.D., et al.: Multicentre trial of naproxen and phenylbutazone in acute gout. Ann. Rheum. Dis. 36:80, 1977.

427. Ridolfo, A.S.: Personal communication.

428. Wallace, S.L.: Colchicine and new anti-inflammatory drugs for the treatment of acute gout. Arthritis Rheum. (Suppl.) 18:847, 1975.

429. Wanasukapunt, S., Lertratanakul, Y., and Rubinstein, H.M.: Effect of fenoprofen calcium on acute gouty arthritis. Arthritis Rheum. 19:933, 1976.

430. Schweitz, M.C., Nashel, D.J., and Alepa, F.P.: Ibuprofen in the treatment of acute gouty arthritis. JAMA 239:34, 1978.

431. Caruso, I., Fumagalli, M., Marcolongo, R., and Sacchetti, G.: Indoprofen for acute gouty arthritis. Arthritis Rheum. 20:1438, 1977.

432. Brogden, R.N., Heel, R.C., Speight, T.M., and Avery, G.S.: Sulindac: Review of its phamacologic properties and therapeutic efficacy. Drugs 16:97, 1978.

433. Widmark, P.H.: Piroxicam: Its safety and efficacy in the treatment of acute gout. Am. J. Med. 72:63, 1982.

434. Bluestone, R.H.: Safety and efficacy of piroxicam in the treatment of gout. Am. J. Med. 72:66, 1982.

435. Hollander, J.L.: Intra-articular hydrocortisone in arthritis and allied conditions. J. Bone Joint Surg. 35A:983, 1953.

436. Gutman, A.B., and Yu, T.-F.: Current principles of management in gout. Am. J. Med. 13:744, 1952.

437. Barnes, C.G.: The treatment of gout. J.R. Coll. Physicians Lond. 1:427, 1967.

438. Boland, E.W.: Gout and gouty arthritis—current concepts and management. Calif. Med. 105:249, 1966.

439. Moyano, A.G., Jr.: Tratamiento de la gota con indometacina. Galicia Clin. 37:749, 1965.

440. Reiner, J.C.: Etude clinique de l'indomethacine. Arch. Med. D'angers 66:51, 1965.

441. Cohen, A.: Gout. Am. J. Med. Sci. 192:448, 1936.

442. Talbott, J.H., and Coombs, F.S.: Metabolic studies on patients with gout. JAMA 110:1977, 1938.

443. Gutman, A.B.: Treatment of primary gout: The present status. Arthritis Rheum. 8:911, 1965.

444. Paulus, H.E., Schlosstein, L.H., Godfrey, R.G., et al.: Prophylactic colchicine therapy of intercritical gout. A placebo-controlled study of probenecid-treated patients. Arthritis Rheum. 17:609, 1974.

445. Gutman, A.B.: Medical management of gout. Postgrad. Med. 51:61, 1972.

446. Yu, T.-F., and Gutman, A.B.: Efficacy of colchicine prophylaxis. Prevention of recurrent gouty arthritis over a mean period of five years in 208 gouty subjects. Ann. Intern. Med. 55:179, 1961.

447. Rundles, R.W., Metz, E.N., and Silberman, H.R.: Allopurinol in the treatment of gout. Ann. Intern. Med. 64:220, 1966.

448. Robinson, W.D.: The present status of colchicine and uricosuric agents in management of gout. JAMA 173:1076, 1960.

449. Emmerson, B.T.: The use of the xanthine oxidase inhibitor, allopurinol, in the control of hyperuricemia, gout and uric acid calculi. Aust. Ann. Med. 16:205, 1967.

450. Levin, N.W., and Abrahams, O.L.: Allopurinol in patients with impaired renal function. Ann. Rheum. Dis. 25:681, 1966.

451. Ogryzlo, M.A., Urowitz, M., Weber, H.M., and Haupt, J.B.: Effects of allopurinol on gouty and nongouty uric acid nephropathy. Ann. Rheum. Dis. 25:673, 1966.

452. Stoberg, K.-H.: Allopurinol therapy of gout with renal complications. Ann. Rheum. Dis. 25:688, 1966.

453. Rundles, R.W.: Allopurinol in gouty nephropathy and renal dialysis. Ann. Rheum. Dis. 25:694, 1966.

454. Wilson, J.D., Simmonds, H.A., and North, J.D.K.: Allopurinol in the treatment of uremic patients with gout. Ann. Rheum. Dis. 26:136, 1967.

455. Fox, R.M., Royse-Smith, D., and O'Sullivan, W.J.: Orotidinuria induced by allopurinol. Science 168:861, 1970.

456. Kelley, W.N., and Beardmore, T.D.: Allopurinol: Alteration in pyrimidine metabolism in man. Science 169:388, 1970.

457. Gutman, A.B., and Yu, T.-F.: Protracted uricosuric therapy in tophaceous gout. Lancet 2:1258, 1957.

458. Rieselbach, R.E., Bentzel, C.J., Cotlove, F., Frei, E., and Driereich, E.J.: Uric acid excretion and renal function in the acute hyperuricemia of leukemia. Am. J. Med. 37:872, 1961.

459. Emmerson, B.T.: Alteration of urate metabolism by weight reduction. Aust. N.Z. J. Med. 3:410, 1973.

460. Heyden, S.: Risikofaktoren fur das Herz. Ergebnisse und Konsequenzen der post-Framingham-Studien. Boehringer Manheim GmbH, 1974, p. 53.

461. Nicholls, A., and Scott, J.T.: Effect of weight-loss on plasma and urinary levels of uric acid. Lancet 2:1223, 1972.

462. MacLachlan, M.J., and Rodnan, G.P.: Effect of food, fast and alcohol on serum uric acid and acute attacks of gout. Am. J. Med. 42:38, 1967.

463. Bien, E.J., Yu, T.-F., Benedict, J.D., et al.: The relation of dietary nitrogen consumption to the rate of uric acid synthesis in normal and gouty man. J. Clin. Invest. 32:778, 1953.

464. Perheentupa, J., and Raivio, K.: Fructose-induced hyperuricemia. Lancet 2:528, 1967.

465. Maenpaa, P.H., Raivio, K.O., and Kekomaki, M.P.: Liver adenine nucleotides: Fructose-induced depletion and its effect on protein synthesis. Science 161:1253, 1968.

466. Oliver, M.F., Heady, J.A., Morris, J.N., et al.: A cooperative trial in the primary prevention of ischaemic heart disease using clofibrate. Report from the committee of principal investigators. Br. Heart J. 40:1069, 1978.

467. Oliver, M.F., Heady, J.A., Morris, J.N., et al.: The world health organization cooperative trial on primary prevention of ischaemic heart disease using clofibrate to lower serum cholesterol: Mortality follow-up. Report of the committee of principal investigators. Lancet 2:379, 1980.

468. Fredrickson, D.S., and Levy, R.I.: Familial hyperlipoproteinemia. In Stanbury, J.B., Wyngaarden, J.B., and Fredrickson, D.S. (eds.): The Metabolic Basis of Inherited Disease. 3rd ed. New York, McGraw-Hill Book Company, 1972, p. 545.

469. Kelley, W.N., Levy, R.I., Rosenbloom, R.M., et al.: Adenine phosphoribosyltransferase deficiency: A previously undescribed genetic defect in man. J. Clin. Invest. 47:2281, 1968.

470. Fox, I.H., Lacroix, S., Planet, G., and Moore, M.: Partial deficiency of adenine phosphoribosyltransferase in man. Medicine 56:515, 1977.

471. Cartier, M.B., and Hamet, M.: Une nouvelle maladie metabolique: Le deficit complet en adeninephosphoribosyltransferase avec lithiase de 2,8-dihydroxyadenine. C.R. Acad. Sci. Paris 270:883, 1974.

472. Simmonds, H.A., and Van Acker, K.J.: Adenine phosphoribosyl-transferase deficiency: 2,8-dihydroxyadenine lithiasis. In Stanbury, J.B., Wyngaarden, J.B., Fredrickson, D.S., Goldstein, J.L., and Brown, M.S. (eds.): The Metabolic Basis of Inherited Disease. New York, McGraw-Hill Book Company, 1983.

473. Engleman, K., Watts, R.W.E., Klinenberg, J.R., et al.: Clinical, physiological and biochemical studies of a patient with xanthinuria and pheochromocytoma. Am. J. Med. 37:839, 1964.

474. Wyngaarden, J.B., and Kelley, W.N.: Hereditary xanthinuria. In Gout and Hyperuricemia. London, Grune & Stratton, 1976, p. 397.

475. Garrison, F.H.: An Introduction to the History of Medicine: With Medical Chronology, Suggestions for Study and Bibliographic Data. 4th ed. Philadelphia, W. B. Saunders Company, 1929.

476. Galen, C.: Opera Omina, ed. by Kuhn. Leipzig, 1821–1883.

477. McCarty, D.J.: A historical note: Leeuwenhoek's description of crystals from a gouty typhus. Arthritis Rheum. 13:414, 1970.

478. Scheele, K.W.: Examen chemicum calculi urinarii. Opuscula 2:73, 1776.

479. Wollaston, W.H.: On gouty and urinary concretions. Philos. Trans. R. Soc. Lond. 87:386, 1797.

480. Want, J.: The use of Colchicum autumnale in rheumatism. Med. Physiol. J. Lond. 32:312, 1814.

481. Garrod, A.B.: Observations on certain pathological conditions of the blood and urine in gout, rheumatism and Bright's disease. Trans. M-Chir. Soc. Edinburgh 31:83, 1848.

482. Talbott, J.H., Bishop, C., Norcross, B.M., et al.: The clinical and metabolic effects of Benemid in patients with gout. Trans. Assoc. Am. Physicians 64:372, 1951.

483. Gutman, A.B., and Yu, T.F.: Benemid (P-(di-n-propylsulfamyl)-benzoic acid) as uricosuric agent in chronic gouty arthritis. Trans. Assoc. Am. Physicians 64:279, 1951.

484. Rundles, R.W., Wyngaarden, J.B., Hitchings, G.H., et al.: Effects of a xanthine oxidase inhibitor on thiopurine metabolism, hyperuricemia and gout. Trans. Assoc. Am. Physicians 76:126, 1963.

485. Hench, P.S.: Gout and gouty arthritis. In Cecil, R.L., and Loeb, R.F. (eds.): Textbook of Medicine. 9th ed. Philadelphia, W. B. Saunders Company, 1955, p. 643.

486. Smyth, C.J.: Diagnosis and treatment of gout. In Hollander, J.L., and McCarty, D.J. (eds.): Arthritis and Allied Conditions, 8th ed. Philadelphia, Lea & Febiger, 1972, p. 1112.

487. Zollner, N.: Modern Gichtprobleme: Atiologie, Pathogenese, Klinik. In Heilmeyer, L., Schoen, R., and DeRudder, B. (eds.): Ergebnisse der inneren Medizin und Kinderheilkunde. 14th ed. Berlin, Springer-Verlag, 1960, p. 76.

Chapter 87

Diseases Due to the Deposition of Calcium Pyrophosphate and Hydroxyapatite

David S. Howell

CLINICAL FEATURES OF CALCIUM PYROPHOSPHATE DEPOSITION DISEASE (CPDD)

Intrasynovial crystal deposition of calcium pyrophosphate dihydrate ($Ca_2P_2O_7 \cdot 2H_2O$) (CaPPi) was discovered in 1961 by McCarty and Hollander[1] and Kohn and associates[2] during a study of patients believed to have gout. In the midst of identifying intrasynovial urate crystals by polarizing light microscopy and x-ray diffraction analysis,[1,2] they found crystals with different peg-holing characteristics from those of urate and labeled the disease related to the new crystals *pseudogout*.[3] The term *crystal synovitis* was then devised to describe joint inflammation generated from urate or CaPPi crystal forms and later to include iatrogenic crystals of injected corticosteroid. It was apparent that the disease *chondrocalcinosis familiaris* described by Zitnan and Sitaj in 1958[4] was linked to *pseudogout* because of similar attacks of acute synovitis. The term *calcium pyrophos-*

phate deposition disease (CPDD) was coined to designate the total disease state caused by CaPPi deposition,[2] i.e., a synonym for pseudogout including acute and chronic inflammatory as well as degradative joint lesions. The term chondrocalcinosis referred to the detection, usually by roentgenograms or autopsy studies, of calcium (Ca) mineral salts in the articular fibrous or hyaline cartilages.[3] With few exceptions (see below), in all clinically expressed disease in which chondrocalcinotic mineral has been examined, the mineral has proved to be composed of CaPPi.

The predominant detectable mineral in normal cartilage or bone is a prototype of hydroxyapatite.[5,6] Thus the finding of CaPPi ($Ca_2P_2O_7 \cdot 2H_2O$) in most cases of human chondrocalcinosis is an extraordinary event, since to make this salt in vitro from ordinary calcium phosphates requires heating to high temperatures (hence the origin of the term pyrophosphate). How this salt might be made biologically has aroused much interest, as discussed below.

Despite the importance of polarized light microscopy in clinical diagnoses (see Chapter 38), the usage of x-ray diffraction has been the principal tool used in studying and sorting out the different crystal structures present in chondrocalcinosis.[7] In this latter method a beam of x-rays is passed into either a single large crystal or multiple small ones (as usually encountered in clinical samples), providing the so-called powder diagram (Fig. 87–1). Interaction of a specific wavelength of x-ray with the specific atomic and molecular structures and diffraction of x-rays by sheets of atoms is registered on x-ray film or on a strip chart recorder as a template of the internal atomic structure (Fig. 87–1). The distinct maxima of the pattern measured by intensity and associated d spacings (linear distance on film from the primary x-ray beam to the diffraction maxima) provide a fingerprint of the unknown crystal, which is then compared with relevant standards. In chondrocalcinosis one finds predominantly $Ca_2P_2O_7 \cdot 2H_2O$ triclinic crystals[2] (unit cells with three obtuse angles) and monoclinic crystals (unit cells with one obtuse and two right angles). There have been case reports on chondrocalcinosis wherein brushite, $CaHPO_4 \cdot 2H_2O$[8] or hydroxyapatite $Ca_5(PO_4)_3OH$[9] were the predominant minerals detected

in the deposits, as discussed in detail elsewhere.[9] Evidence for the presence of these minerals in synovial fluid and intracellularly, suggesting phlogistic action, as well as the nature of crystal deposits in cartilage and surrounding membranes is discussed later in the chapter.

CPDD is important to the differential diagnosis of septic arthritis and gout because of its frequent association with certain metabolic diseases, because of a possible familial form with severe crippling, and finally because of the high incidence of associated osteoarthritis. Less is known concerning the etiology and pathogenesis of CPDD than of urate gout, yet similarities between the two diseases are obvious. In both there is a chronic variable progression with an accumulation of crystal deposits in joint tissues with sporadic appearance of crystals in synovial fluid similar to those deposited in the solid tissues. As with gout, there is an acute episodic synovitis characterized by influx of leukocytes and phagocytosis of crystals. Also in both diseases, high local concentrations of the relevant ions, urate or pyrophosphate (PPi), are present and there is tissue damage resulting from the massive deposits of crystals in the tissues: in addition, acute attacks are provoked by trauma, surgery, or ischemic heart disease in both diseases.

Prevalence and Clinical Presentation of CPDD. Data on one large series of 300 patients studied over 13 years[10] provide the first major characterization of this disease and substantiate categorization of clinical expression based on the first 80 cases[11] (Tables 87–1 and 87–2). The usefulness of this segregation of clinical patterns has been confirmed in the studies of Menkes and associates[12] and Okazaki and associates.[13] These characterizations provide reassurance that the same disease in Japan,[13] Paris,[12] and Chicago[10] was under scrutiny, i.e., a predominantly sporadic form of CPDD (Table 87–1). Although no data on clinical overall prevalence exist, there was one rough estimation that in McCarty's clinic about two gouty patients were under care for each CPDD patient.[10] In the author's Miami arthritis clinic the frequency of CPDD-to-gout ratio is somewhat less, 1:3 of symptomatic patients with occasional observation of all the presentations of joint disease as described by McCarty. It is likely, based on the Hôpital Cochin series

Figure 87–1. X-ray diffraction analysis provides proof of the nature of the mineral phases deposited in cartilage. Each plot of amplitude versus Bragg angle (degrees 2θ) can be identified by comparison with literature values and/or known standards. Graph A shows a portion of a wide-angle x-ray diffraction pattern obtained by examination of a calcified meniscus of a patient with CPDD. The pattern corresponds to that of calcium pyrophosphate dihydrate. Graph B shows the same region of a wide angle x-ray diffraction pattern obtained during examination of a rotator cuff calcification. This pattern is characteristic of hydroxyapatite. (Courtesy of A.L. Boskey and A. Posner, Hospital for Special Surgery, Cornell Medical College.)

DEGREES (2Θ)

Table 87–1. General Classification of CPDD

I. Sporadic (Table 87–2)
   A. Associated with osteoarthritis
   B. Inflammatory syndrome resembling rheumatoid
      arthritis
   C. Destructive pseudoneuropathic (no known
      proprioceptive neural deficit)
   D. Destructive in presence of diseases with known
      proprioceptive neural deficits
   E. Post-traumatic
II. Associated with metabolic disease "secondary"
   A. Hemochromatosis
   B. Hyperparathyroidism
   C. Associations suspected but difficult to establish in
      varying degrees
      1. Gout
      2. Diabetes mellitus
      3. Hypophosphatasia
      4. Wilson's disease
      5. Ochronosis
III. Hereditary
   A. HLA association, frequent spinal syndromes (Czech)
   B. Autosomal—male-to-male transmission (Dutch,
      Chilean)

and others, that prevalence of forms secondary to metabolic diseases are 10 percent or less of the total,[12] and familial forms at present are rare, possibly because of difficulty of detection.[14] At the Mayo Clinic per 1000 registrants (1970-71), the frequency of pseudogout admissions was 0.9 versus 1.5 to 2.2 (over a wider period) for gout.[15] At autopsy, several statistical series studied for the presence of cartilaginous mineral in the knee joint indicate that about 5 percent of the adult population have CPDD there at the time of death.[10] Interestingly out of line with these autopsy data is detection in an aged Jewish population by Ellman and Levin of 27 percent chondrocalcinosis among those tested radiologically for articular calcifications.[16] In the majority of Ellman and Levin's series the patients were asymptomatic.

Sporadic Form. Common Presentations. The approximate percentage distribution of the different types of presentation was roughly the same reported from Chicago,[10] Paris,[12] and Japan,[13] with the exception that destructive arthropathy comprised a surprisingly high portion of the Parisian series.[12] With regard to the sporadic and associated or "secondary" forms (Tables 87–1 and 87–2), the predominant age of onset is in the sixth and seventh decades with a significantly lower mean age of onset in the secondary than in the sporadic form. In four separate series of cases from different centers, sex incidence favored female to male by 2 to 3:1 in three of the studies[13,17,18] and a male predominance of 1.4:1 in the fourth study.[10] There were five principal categories of sporadic disease presentation (Table 87–2): (1) pseudogout, (2) pseudorheumatoid arthritis, (3) pseudoosteoarthritis with superimposed acute attacks, (4) pseudo-osteoarthritis without acute attacks, and (5) an asymptomatic, so-called "lanthenic" form. In most series, severe destructive forms of osteoarthritis were recognized in only a very small number of cases. These

could be categorized as those having a true suspected proprioceptive deficit—i.e., history of syphilis, tertiary or latent[10]—and those without such a history but in whom ischemic necrosis or other causes of mutilating osteoarthritis were suspected.[12] Clinical criteria used to make the diagnoses in most of these patients are given in Table 87–3 and include polarized light microscopic crystal identification as well as the finding on x-rays of chondrocalcinosis.[19]

In the presence of acute attacks there was swelling, pain, stiffness, and local heat over the offending joint. In general, acute episodes are not as intense as those found in gouty arthritis. Symptoms and signs reached a maximum severity in ½ to 2½ days. Attacks lasted from ½ day to a month or longer with an average of about 9 days.[10] Many patients had what McCarty described as "petite" or subclinical attacks in which transient stiffness or aching and small amounts of synovial fluid, if any, were obtainable. When found, synovial fluid showed CaPPi crystals and active phagocytosis. Attacks often occurred in clusters, with one or several joints around the initially inflamed joint becoming involved. Systemic findings included a small fever of 1 to 2° Fahrenheit, leukocytosis of moderate degree, and left shift as well as high sedimentation rates.

The knees were by far the most frequent site of acute arthritis, but hips, shoulders, elbows, ankles, wrists, and several bursae, including the space between the superficial and deep medial collateral ligaments and calcaneal cuboid joints, were involved. Occasionally the bunion joint and smaller joints of the hands and feet were symptomatic.

Type B presentation, which resembled mild rheumatoid arthritis, revealed affliction of multiple joints, including the wrists, elbows, and shoulders. There was often some morning stiffness and pain on weightbearing. Flexion contractures at the knees and wrists with atrophy of related musculature were found. High sedimentation rate and weakly positive rheumatoid factor in 10 percent of patients were noted in this category. Often both knees or both wrists were involved with chondrocalcinosis; the acute involvement was "out of phase," i.e., not symmetrically inflamed as in rheumatoid arthritis. Type C was distinguished from type B by a negative rheumatoid factor; also, only one or two joints at most at a time were involved, whereas in type B almost continuous acute episodes occurred in a number of joints. In type C there was progressive chronic arthritis of larger weight-bearing joints, particularly in the knee, hip, and lower spine with less frequent superimposed episodes. In type D, the chronic arthritis was present just as in type C, but there were no acute attacks. Particularly in type D, women predominated. However, consignment to a given category at one point over the period of years of observation was often not a permanent designation, since in subsequent studies some of these patients shifted to other categories. For example, type E asymptomatic cases might become symptomatic at later dates.[10]

Uncommon Presentations. Less common clinical pres-

Table 87–2. The More Common Types of Clinical Presentation in CPDD

Type	Appropriate Proportion of Cases in Series (%)	Nature of Clinical Manifestations	Duration of Clinical Manifestations	Predominant Joint Distribution	Deformity	Associated Conditions
A. Isolated pseudogout	25, males predominatly	Attack provoked by surgery (9.4% of cases) or severe medical illness (24%); 50% attacks in knees, 10% in first carpometacarpal joints	Acute or subacute self-limited attacks, 1–28 days; often as severe as gout; pain-free between attacks; inflammation spreads from mother joint (e.g., wrist) to daughter joints	One or a few appendicular joints	None or mild with a few exceptions	Hyperuricemia 20%, urate gout 5% (same as normal controls)
B. Pseudorheumatoid arthritis	5	Morning stiffness, fatigue common; localized pitting edema over joints; loss of joint motion, synovial thickening, flexion contractures elevated; erythrocyte sedimentation rates; positive rheumatoid factor in 10% of cases in low titer as in urate gout	Attacks lasting 4 weeks to several months	Wrists, elbows, metacarpo phalangeals, knees, and shoulders	Contractures; in this and other forms, metacarpo phalangeal joints may have hooklike osteophytes, squared bone ends and subchondral cysts	True RA in 3 cases (1%); "true RA" present at frequency level found in general population (not lower, as in urate gout)
C. Pseudoosteoarthritis with episiodic superimposed acute attacks	25	Involvement is generally bilaterally symmetrical; varus deformities, flexion contracture, and osteophytes common	Chronic over period of months or years	Knees predominantly; wrists, metacarpophalan geal joints, hips, shoulders, elbows, and ankles in decreasing order of frequency		Common stigmata of associated primary osteoarthritis, e.g., Heberden's and Bouchard's nodes
D. Pseudoosteoarthritis without acute attacks	25	Progressive degeneration of multiple joints; crystal synovitis occasional in joints showing no radiologically detectable chondrocalcinosis	Same as C	Same as C		Same as C
E. Asymptomatic (lanthenic) and less common types of clinical presentation	20			By radiological study same as B or C		

Table 87–3. Diagnostic Criteria for CPDD (Pseudogout)*

Criteria

I. Demonstration of CaPPi crystals (obtained by biopsy, necropsy, or aspirated synovial fluid) by definitive means (e.g., characteristic "fingerprint" by x-ray diffraction powder pattern or by chemical analysis)

II. (a) Identification of monoclinic and/or triclinic crystals showing none or a weakly positive birefringence by compensated polarized light microscopy
   (b) Presence of *typical* calcifications in roentgenograms†

III. (a) Acute arthritis, especially of knees, hips, wrists, carpus, elbow, shoulder, and metacarpophalangeal joints with or without concomitant hyperuricemia
   (b) Chronic arthritis, especially of knees and hips and if accompanied by acute exacerbations

Categories

A. Definite—Criteria I or II (a) plus (b) must be fulfilled
B. Probable—Criteria II (a) or II (b) must be fulfilled
C. Possible—Criteria III (a) or (b) should alert the clinician to the possibility of the diagnosis

---

*From McCarty, D.J.: *In* McCarty, D.J. (ed.): Arthritis and Allied Conditions. 9th ed. Philadelphia, Lea & Febiger, 1979, p. 1282.
†Occasionally faint and/or atypical calcifications may be the result of $CaHPO_4 \cdot 2H_2O$ deposits or vascular mineralization.

entations of CPDD involve a tabetic-like joint destruction, with or without signs of a proprioceptive defect (pseudotabes). Among the latter, trauma was a factor in some cases. There have been a few reports on an oligo- or polyarticular destructive arthropathy associated with CPDD (reviewed in reference 12) without proprioceptive deficit disease. One of the most well documented studies is that of Menkes and associates.[12] Of their 15 patients, 14 were women. Knees and shoulders were afflicted most frequently, with hips, wrists, and ankles involved less often. The arthropathy had the appearance, as in other reported cases, of severe osteoarthritis. The majority had chronic hydrarthrosis, and 21 of 38 joints had undergone destructive change in the series. Pseudogout attacks occured in eight of the patients. Large subchondral bone cysts without condensation around them radiologically coexisted with joint demineralization. Osteophytosis was exuberant, and osteochondromatosis was also a common occurrence. At the shoulder, tendon avulsions and rotary cuff tears occurred and subluxations were frequent. The disease evolution was quite slow; yet when bone destruction occurred, lesions progressed rapidly within a few months. CaPPi microcrystals in synovial fluid or membranes were found. Symptoms of polyarthralgia were particularly severe at night and severe disability resulted.

Essentially indistinguishable from this destructive arthropathy is that of a few patients in whom there was evidence of latent syphilis or tabes dorsalis as reported by Jacobelli and colleagues.[20] In four consecutive patients, these authors reported that CaPPi crystals were deposited in the damaged knee joints, and it was suggested that the crystal deposition and neuropathy might be acting synergistically to produce a neuropathic joint.[10,20]

In regard to trauma, it was noted by Mandl in 1927 that nodules of mineral salt were found in menisci of young men who had received traumatic injury to the knee.[21] Rubinstein and Shah related trauma to pseudogout of the knee in two patients,[22] and Bjelle and Sunden noted that five of their 50 patients had a history of knee joint trauma.[23] Monoarticular chondrocalcinosis was present in two of these five cases. In an arthoscopic study of knees, Altman described five cases with x-ray-diagnosed chondrocalcinosis confined to a knee previously injured, and a history of trauma in nine other cases with more than one knee involved.[24] McCarty described a possible relationship of trauma to production of chondrocalcinosis[10] antecedent to these other reports. For further discussion of trauma, see Hydroxyapatite Arthropathy below.

Hereditary Form. Hereditary forms of CPDD have been documented in small numbers from a few centers.[4,26-31] Studies performed in widely separated geographic sites revealed a familial nature of the disease with certain features in common. Most or all of the patients with familial chondrocalcinosis received medical workups by the respective authors and were believed not to have any significant associated diseases which might contribute to mineral deposition.

Czechoslovakian Series. Zitnan and Sitaj[27] have described 20 years' experience with respect to 33 patients followed at least 10 years. There were 20 females to 13 males with an age range of 38 to 95 years. Acute crystal synovitis and arthritis lasting several weeks and recurrent attacks of pseudogout predominated in the younger patients—fourth to sixth decades—and symptoms of associated osteoarthritis in the decades thereafter. A mild form of the disease characterized by oligoarthritis and chondrocalcinotic involvement of fibrocartilages of the large joints was distinguished from a second much more severe form with chondrocalcinosis and polyarthritis involving almost every joint in the body. The severe form started at a younger age and was characterized by more intense and frequent attacks of crystal synovitis. This group eventually developed severe crippling, contractures at the wrists, knees, and elbows, and muscle atrophy. Hallux valgus deformities and ulnar drift of the fingers were found.[28]

In addition to chondrocalcinosis, radiological studies of these patients revealed osteoarthritis in peripheral joints as well as those of the spine with periostotic calcifications, large spurs, cartilage destruction, and subchondral cysts. Ankylosing hyperostosis of the calcified intervertebral discs was often found.

Despite diligent study of lineage, the hereditary features of this series were not clear, but there was no evidence of male-to-male transmission. The finding of a significantly increased number of patients with HLA-2 and W18 histocompatibility antigens as compared with a control population might be considered more likely to simply represent evidence of inbreeding rather than a marker specific for CPDD per se.

Chiloe Islands Series. Reginato reported on 10 years' experience following 44 females and 36 males aged 25 to 84 years with hereditary CPDD; all patients were natives of the Chiloe Islands and of Spanish descent, traced in some families to the sixteenth century.[28,29] Except for a few with the expected incidence, e.g., small numbers with diabetes mellitus or hypertension, there were no associated diseases. As with the Czech series, there was an oligoarthritis of a milder nature starting in the fifth decade and following a milder course in subsequent years. With onset prior to the fifth decade, there was a much more severe polyarthritic form characterized by frequent attacks of pseudogout or continuing active inflammation. These patients had heavy joint calcification and subsequent cartilage destruction leading in a few patients to bony ankylosis. The nature of the hereditary pattern of transmittance was unclear, but there was male-to-male transmission present. No increased incidence of any histocompatibility antigens was found in a later study.[29]

For further details on features of the Czechoslovakian, Chiloe Island, Dutch, French, Spanish, and Swedish series, the original literature should be consulted.[4,26-32] No clear-cut pattern of hereditary transmission is common to all these families, and widely variable clinical features are encountered in respect to age of onset, severity of symptoms, and tissue damage.[4,26-32] Biochemical changes (see below) in cartilage were recently studied by Bjelle.[32]

CPDD Associated with Metabolic and Other Diseases. There is a considerable literature on possible associations of CPDD and a wide variety of diseases. For example, in the largest reported series with a mean age of 72 years,[19,33] the disease associations listed in 238 cases were diabetes mellitus 40 to 60 percent, hypertension 25 to 40 percent, atherosclerosis 35 to 50 percent, azotemia 34 percent, hyperuricemia 34 percent, gynecomastia 7 percent in 142 males, hyperparathyroidism 7.2 percent, renal stones 7.5 percent, classic gout with crystal identification 5 percent, hyperthyroidism 3 percent, inflammatory bowel disease 2.1 percent, and Paget's disease of bone 3.4 percent. There have been other reported associations, including osteoarthritis, Wilson's disease, neuropathic joints, acromegaly, rheumatoid arthritis, hemochromatosis, ochronosis, hypophosphatasia,[33] carpal tunnel syndrome,[34] chondromatosis, and amyloid deposits.[35]

The most common single associated disease is osteoarthritis, which has been discussed in various portions of this chapter, and the frequency range in different series is from 40 to 70 percent.[33] Unfortunately, it is impossible to determine whether this frequency is greater than in a control population. It seems likely that, at the least, the most severe forms of CPDD lead de novo to secondary osteoarthritis and that milder forms, for reasons discussed under Pathogenesis, contribute to worsening of already present osteoarthritis.

Diabetes Mellitus. Among ten studies cited,[33] two large series of CPDD patients showed a high frequency, but two small matched control studies showed no increased frequency.[10,36] The range of reported frequencies was 8 to 73 percent.[33]

Gouty Arthritis. Cited frequency was 0 to 8 percent in six reports,[33] but one matched control study showed no greater frequency in the CPDD group.[36] While in one study of 31 gouty patients, one third were reported to have chondrocalcinosis,[37] subsequent questions have been raised as to the clinical validity of the technique used; in many of the reported cases the diagnosis of gout was subject to doubt.

In a review of 138 patients with urate gout, 8 patients had concurrent evidence of chondrocalcinosis of the knees, whereas none of the controls revealed demonstrable chondrocalcinosis, supporting the association of gout with chondrocalcinosis.[38] It is possible, however, that accompanying cartilage degradation accounts for this association.

Rheumatoid Arthritis. One study reporting an increased frequency was performed by Moskowitz and Garcia, who found 28 percent with rheumatoid arthritis in 43 CPDD patients.[39] Also, Bywaters reported CPDD in three of 34 patients with rheumatoid arthritis consecutively collected.[40] However, in an aforementioned controlled study, the incidence was only 8 percent, insignificantly higher than in the control group.[36] It is of interest that of all these common diseases, doubt concerning an increased association (except for severe forms of CPDD with osteoarthritis) still exists.

More convincing evidence of disease association has occurred in studies of uncommon and rare diseases in which a substantial number or proportion of reported cases of such a disease manifest chondrocalcinosis.

Hyperparathyroidism. Increased association has been described in at least nine cited reports.[33] The frequency of chondrocalcinosis in a total of 22 of 116 cases of primary hyperparathyroidism was far above the conjectured normal incidence of 5 percent chondrocalcinosis.[33] Also, the mean age of patients with hyperparathyroidism and chondrocalcinosis was significantly greater than without chondrocalcinosis.[33] Furthermore, the frequency of hyperparathyroidism in CPDD in four reports on 336 cases ranged 5 to 15 percent, whereas at the Mayo Clinic the frequency of hyperparathyroidism ranged one in 1000 to one in 2000 admissions.[33] Considerable interest was also aroused by the findings of Phelps and Hawker of an elevated immunoreactive parathyroid hormone (PTH) level in ten of 26 patients with CPDD.[41] However, patients with osteoarthritis also had an elevated PTH level.[41] Slight increases of PTH level resulting from associated degenerative arthritis and bony remodeling or problems with assay methodology may have accounted for these results.

Hemochromatosis. In two well-studied series of hemochromatosis, 41 percent of 61 patients and 44 percent of 54 patients showed chondrocalcinosis, respectively.[33] Also, chondrocalcinosis was reported in secondary hemochromatosis resulting from hereditary spherocytosis.[33] These cases had a striking feature in that an arthropathy was frequently found in the metacarpophalangeal joints with special reference to the second and third,[33] presumably related to the hemochromatosis itself (see Chapter 94). Otherwise, knees, wrists, hips, symphysis pubis, and lumbar spine were affected as in other forms.

Hypothyroidism. Dorwart and Schumacher reported

in a series of patients with hypothyroidism synovial effusions with CaPPi crystals present.[42] Acute pseudogout attacks occurred only after the patients were started on treatment with thyroid replacement.[42]

Neuropathic Joints. The aforementioned studies of Jacobelli and associates[20] and classifications (Table 87–2) assumed the association of tabetic joints with CPDD. Avascular necrosis might be synergistic with CPDD to explain the mutilating lesions of the destructive arthropathy of Menkes and associates.[12] A possibility also exists that the destructive arthropathy itself leads to the calcium pyrophosphate deposition.

Wilson's Disease. Feller and Schumacher found chondrocalcinosis in two of 17 cases, aged 26 and 31, both in the upper end of the age range for his series.[43]

Hypophosphatasia. Three patients with CPDD in this disease have been noted.[44,45] Elevated plasma PPi and urinary PPi levels were found.[44] An x-ray diffraction pattern of CaPPi was obtained from tissue at a symphysis pubis biopsy.[44]

Ochronosis. CaPPi deposition was found in synovium of peripheral joints in four cases of ochronosis;[33] CaPPi was found in intervertebral discs as well as apatite by x-ray diffraction.[9] For most of these diseases, the number or proportion of patients with CPDD is insufficient to make valid comparisons, and only a tentative association can be assigned.

Precipitation of Acute Attacks. The finding that acute attacks of CPDD characterized by fever, warm or hot and swollen joints, synovial effusions, and crystal synovitis confirmed by synovianalysis are precipitated by a variety of specific factors has been well documented.[15] A common precipitating agent is surgery, involving a wide variety of operative procedures, e.g., knee or hip arthroplasty, prostatectomy, cholecystectomy. Attacks developed at a median of 3 days postoperatively in O'-Duffy's series with predilection for the attack in the knees regardless of operative site.[15] Cases were either sporadic or the form secondary to hyperparathyroidism, but precipitation of attacks by surgery of the familial form has also been noted.

In addition, nonsurgical events may trigger attacks of crystal synovitis caused by CPDD as evidenced in one study by 31 such attacks in 16 nonsurgical patients with cerebral infarction, ischemic heart disease, thrombophlebitis, popliteal artery thrombosis, trauma, and other entities.[15] Attacks may follow congestive heart failure or use of diuretics.

As for a possible cause of acute attacks, in O'Duffy's series measurement of serial serum Ca during and after operation for parathyroid adenoma indicated that acute attacks in those cases studied developed at the nadir (lowest level) of serum Ca.[15] Moreover, not the absolute level but the fall per se was important in relation to both parathyroid- and nonparathyroid-related disease. Clowes and Simeone showed that after major surgery of the abdomen or thorax there is an 11 percent mean postoperative transient decrement of serum Ca below preoperative levels,[46] a finding confirmed by O'Duffy.[15]

Integrating all these observations has led to the conclusion that "crystal shedding into intra-articular space occurs when deposits are loosened within their deposit sites by erosion of the margins of these deposits."[10] Erosion results from solubilization of PPi ions taken from the solid phase, a process enhanced vastly by lowering the PPi ion concentration in extracellular fluid bathing the deposits, a process that follows any abrupt fall in serum Ca. In regard to experimental studies that support this view, Bennett and associates found in man that removal of synovial fluid PPi by lavage with magnesium salts, instead of improving the patient, caused acute crystal synovitis attacks.[47]

These results provide another striking analogy to urate gout and the urate crystal synovitis provoked by surgical operations and similar medical illness,[10] wherein the concept of crystal shedding[10] also applies as described in Chapter 86.

Diagnostic Measures for CPDD. Blood studies are usually of no avail except to detect associated diseases. Except in CPDD secondary to hypophosphatasia wherein plasma PPi is elevated, no tests to date show any significant abnormality. Serum Ca, P, and alkaline phosphatase are within normal limits.[19]

Synovianalysis. The less specific findings include in acute crystal synovitis highly elevated leukocyte levels and in chronic crystal synovitis slightly elevated leukocyte levels averaging 21,350 and 1800 cells per cubic millimeter, respectively.[19]

In 98.9 percent of acute synovial effusions, using a polarizing light microscope, McCarty specifically identified CaPPi crystals (Fig. 87–2), but in chronic effusion this percentage dropped to 73.8 percent.[19] In contrast to sodium (Na) urate crystals, which polarize light strongly, CaPPi crystals polarize light weakly. Overall, CaPPi crystals are less numerous than in gouty arthritis, and diligent search for a "period of time" is necessary to exclude the presence of these crystals.[22] As to method, after delivery of a fresh drop of synovial fluid onto a cleaned slide and application of a coverslip, the slide is first inspected thoroughly at high dry magnification without use of the polarizer and with the light constricted. On finding a crystal (Fig. 87–2), light intensity is increased to the maximum and the polarizer brought into use.[22] Crystals are usually irregular or rhomboid and 2 to 25 μm in length[19] (Fig. 87–2). Crystals with a needle shape like urate are sometimes encountered. Although such crystals are most often intracellular (Fig. 87–2), clusters or clumps of extracellular crystals may be observed.[22]

By use of the red compensator plate in the optical system, the birefringence signs positive or negative can be ascertained; the observation of weakly positive birefringence distinguishes the CaPPi crystals from Na urate, which is strongly negatively birefringent.[22] Use of the plate is most important when needle-shaped CaPPi crystals are present or when both urate and CaPPi crystals are encountered in the same synovial sample.[22] Iatrogenic corticosteroid and other crystal types must

Figure 87–2. CaPPi crystal within leukocyte in synovial fluid from a patient with chondrocalcinosis. 450 × magnification of wet film examination. (From Rodnan, G.P. [ed.]: Primer on the rheumatic diseases. Reprinted from JAMA 224: No. 5, 1973.)

sometimes be distinguished in the search. Alizarin red staining may be useful as a screening technique for calcium minerals. See Hydroxyapatite Arthropathy.

Radiological Studies. These comprise the second sine qua non of diagnosis (Table 87–3). Findings are in three categories: chondrocalcinosis per se, associated osteoarthritis, and pseudotabes tissue destruction. The mineral appears in hyaline and fibrocartilage as coalescent or stippled calcifications in lines or bands paralleling the subchondral bone border. Mineral by x-ray viewing is detected in sporadic CPDD most frequently in knee menisci, trangular disc hyaline articular cartilages (of the wrist), and the symphysis pubis.[49] Use of type M industrial film for small joints and magnification techniques of Genant (Figs. 87–3 and 87–4) for large joints have been superior to conventional x-ray methodology in sensitivity of mineral detection.[49]

In most cases of CPDD and spinal involvement, calcification of intervertebral discs is hard to demonstrate with only a slight increase of radiodensity, in contrast to the dense calcification of multiple discs observed in ochronosis. In the vast majority of cases reported, there is radiologically demonstrable chondrocalcinosis.[49] In many sporadic cases and in a substantial fraction of familial cases studied, radiologically detectable chondrocalcinosis appears in a majority of joints of the appendicular skeleton.[49] However, small numbers of patients with CaPPi crystal synovitis have been diagnosed without evidence of chondrocalcinosis either in the symptomatic or other joints.[50]

The associated radiological changes are similar to those described for primary osteoarthritis with three distinctive features. First, in general, in sporadic, secondary, and familial forms the more severe the crystal synovitis and the more heavy and widespread the crystal deposits, the more severe are the osteoarthritic changes. Second, there are distinctive features in distribution of radiologically identified degenerative joint changes found by Resnick and associates[51] and Martel and

Figure 87–3. *A,* Fine lines of meniscal and articular calcification in magnified radiograph of articular and fibrocartilage of the knee. Osteoarthritic spurs are visible. Such thin lines of mineral would no doubt be missed by conventional radiographic methods. *B,* Chondrocalcinosis of the triangular disc as well as linear calcification of hyaline cartilage from a patient with CPDD and hemochromatosis. There is diffuse osteopenia. (From Genant, H.K.: *In* McCarty, D.J. [ed.]: Proceedings of the Conference on Pseudogout and Pyrophosphate Metabolism. Arthritis Rheum. 19: Suppl. 3, May–June, 1976.)

Figure 87–4. Punctate and linear mineral deposition in the fibrocartilage of the lateral meniscus as well as in hyaline articular cartilage, demonstrated by the magnification technique of Genant. (From Genant, H.K.: *In* McCarty, D.J. [ed.]: Proceedings of the Conference on Pseudogout and Pyrophosphate Metabolism. Arthritis Rheum. 19: Suppl. 3. May–June, 1976.)

associates[52] in CPDD compared to osteoarthritic patients. These differences include (1) involvement of carpal bones other than the first carpometacarpal joint, elbow, or metacarpophalangeal joints, all sites rarely afflicted with primary osteoarthritis; (2) a significantly higher frequency of subchondral bone cysts, patellofemoral osteoarthritis, and trabecular bony fractures consistent with an overlying cartilage stiffened by mineral;[51] and (3) peculiar metacarpophalangeal joint osteophytes (hook-shaped nodes are found in some cases).[52] Third, there may be severe joint destructive changes of pseudotabes, and changes in the familial forms as described above.

PATHOGENESIS

Cause of Tissue Injury. During the last two decades, information, albeit fragmentary, has accumulated on pathogenic pathways in production of CPDD. At the least, the pathogenic pathways involved seem complex, even if one considers only the sporadic type of CPDD. At present most researchers in this field believe that for all forms the single causative agent for the disease is the CaPPi crystal; this crystal, insofar as is known at present, instigates all its injurious effects at local tissue sites rather than in production of systemic disease manifestations—with a few minor exceptions related to an inflammatory response. These direct local effects are mediated, first, through the phlogistic action of crystals in the intrasynovial space and membranes and, second, by development of large crystal deposits containing altered connective tissue components.

Role of CPDD Production in Crystal-Induced Inflammation. Much of the information on this subject has been secured in the same studies aimed at identifying the phlogistic properties of Na urate. In general for the agents causing the three known crystal-induced diseases, Na urate gout, CPDD, and silicosis (caused by alpha quartz in the lungs), the CPDD crystal is perhaps the least phlogistic.[7,53] Much of what is known about crystal phlogism derives from studies in animals or in vitro using the monosodium urate (MSU) and CPDD crystals prepared synthetically to show morphologic and crystallographic similarity to natural counterparts.[7,53] Injection of either synthetic Na urate or CaPPi crystals into normal human or dog joints was followed by crystal phagocytosis and an acute inflammatory reaction typified by its being dose related, reversible, and apparently not specific with respect to host species or to chemicals.[54,55]

Pathogenic pathways in these experimental crystal reactions have been studied. Activation of Hageman factor by CPDD or urate was demonstrated in vitro.[56] Subsequent generation of kinins and bradykinin activation of plasminogen to plasmin and activation of complement pathways must be considered as possible mediators of acute inflammation through the well-documented effects of these factors described in Chapters 7 and 8. The question as to whether these pathways were essential to crystal-induced inflammation arose from studies of Phelps, Prockop, and McCarty.[57] In the latter study, a critical role for either complement or activation of Hageman factor was brought into question, but increasing knowledge of these pathways renders an important role still likely.[58] Inasmuch as an absolutely essential ingredient for induction of inflammation is recruitment of polymorphonuclear (PMN) leukocytes,[59] other factors that might be involved in recruitment were therefore sought. Studies by Phelps,[60,61] using the Boyden chamber in vitro with regard to leukocyte motility, indicated that PMN leukocytes per se release a non-dialyzable chemotactic factor after either MSU or CPDD crystal phagocytosis. This factor has been further characterized in Spilberg's laboratory.[62-64] The same leukotactic glycopeptide was generated by CaPPi crystals as by Na urate[62,63] crystals, and the alleviation of acute attacks of CPDD by intravenous colchicine further supported the role of this peptide in both diseases.[64]

Yet, explanations have been sought for the lesser severity of acute attacks of CPDD than of urate gout. Studies by Schumacher and associates in vitro indicated that in the presence of PMN leukocytes, synthetic CaPPi was phagocytosed more slowly and in lesser amounts than Na urate.[65] In addition, the urates were membranolytic within the lysosomes, whereas CPDD was much less so.[65] Urates and to a much lesser extent CPDD are membranolytic on erythrocyte membranes and PMN leukocyte lysosomes, as well as on artificial lipid membranes comprising liposomes.[66] It was postulated that hydrogen bonding was important in the process of the membranolytic effect, inasmuch as H^+ acceptors such as polyvinylpyridine-N-oxide (PVPNO) blocked the reaction.[67] Again, the crystals of CPDD seemed considerably less reactive than urates as hydrogen bonding agents. However, studies of Mandel[53] indicated that other hydrogen bonding crystals have no phlogistic action in vitro. Thus, the hydrogen bonding theory alone could not explain the membranolysis. These authors showed in an analysis of atomic packing at the surfaces of a series of different crystalline chemicals tested for phlogistic action that those with smooth surfaces were not phlogistic, whereas those with atomically irregular cavities and projections were phlogistic. These irregularities are postulated to provide sites for hydrogen bonding contact and electrostatic interactions with head groups in the lysosomal membranes. In any event, the lysosomal membrane lysis permitted release of hydrolytic enzymes into the cell cytoplasm followed by PMN autolysis, thereby magnifying the inflammation. Possible roles of superoxide generation, activation of complement components, and interrelations to the extrinsic clotting pathway are reviewed in Chapters 7, 8, and 9.

An important additional observation has been the recent demonstration that plasma proteins and, more specifically, IgG are adsorbed to various crystals.[68] This adsorption is more complete in the case of urate than CaPPi. It has been postulated that the IgG in synovial fluid binds to the crystals and that the IgG Fc sites may combine with Fc receptors on leukocytes and thereby

stimulate phagocytosis.[68] Once the crystal is contained in the phagosome, the coating of protein would have to be removed enzymatically prior to any interaction of the crystal with the lysosomal membrane.

As above, the acute attack of CPDD is probably due to rupture of preformed clusters of CaPPi from local vascular cartilage into the adjacent synovial cavity. Depending on the amount of crystals released and the rate at which they appear, severity and duration of inflammation are probably governed. Evidence that CaPPi crystals are not precipitated in the synovial fluid during an attack will be discussed later. As the inflammatory response proceeds, crystals are found not only in the synovial fluid PMN leukocytes engulfed in phagosomes (Figs. 87–5B and 87–6A) but also in mononuclear leukocyte phagosomes.[69] In addition, lining synovial cells revealed by electron microscopy evidence of crystals with phagosomes (Fig. 87–6B). In some of the synovial membranes, mononuclear cell infiltrates are found in internal stages of the disease. In what may be analogous to chronic inflammation, in vivo crystals may cause mononuclear cells and synoviocytes to undergo a phagocytic response, with elaboration of prostaglandins E_2 and F_2 and collagenase production with inhibition by cyclooxygenase inhibitors.[70,71] Wear particles from accompanying osteoarthritis may also contribute to this

Figure 87–5. *A*, Light microscopic histological section of articular cartilage from the knee of a patient with chondrocalcinosis and hyperparathyroidism. Stained with hematoxylin, eosin, and von Kossa techniques. × 250. Note large granular deposits not only in central zone of the articular cartilage but scattered also in the tangential zone. (Courtesy of Dr. Eric Bywaters, Professor Emeritus, Hammersmith Hospital, London, England.) *B*, Interior of the cryofractured exudative neutrophil from the synovial fluid of a patient with CPDD. When viewed by the scanning electron microscope, intact neutrophil granules and nuclear lobe and numerous crystals of CaPPi and different arrangements are displayed three dimensionally. × 14,000. (Courtesy of Jeanne M. Riddle, Ph.D., Director of Rheumatological Research, Henry Ford Hospital, Detroit, Michigan.)

Figure 87–6. *A*, Crystal holes (*C*) from which crystals were dislodged and fibrin-like material (*F*) in synovial fluid neutrophil phagosomes from a patient with CPDD. Original magnification × 27,000. *B*, Electron micrograph of CaPPi crystal site in a phagosome of a phagocytic synovial lining cell. Original magnification × 15,000. (From Schumacher, H.R.: *In* McCarty, D.J. [ed.]: Proceedings of the Conference on Pseudogout and Pyrophosphate Metabolism. Arthritis Rheum. 19: Suppl. 3, May–June, 1976.)

process.[72] Often the inflammatory cell infiltrates are more severe in the hereditary form.[28] Whether the more intense chronic phlogistic responses seen in severe hereditary forms of CPDD are due to the nature and amount of crystals released into the joint space or to the presence of other factors not yet identified remains to be determined. Also, little is known concerning initiating factors in the acute crystal synovitis of CPDD of all types (Table 87–1). The bouts of inflammation may also be associated not only with adsorption to

crystals of IgG but possibly also with its denaturation. This event has been postulated as possibly provoking the low-titer rheumatoid factor seen in about 10 percent of patients with CPDD as well as urate gout.[68]

The Nature of Mineral Deposits and Their Influence on Structure and Function. Studies at autopsy and in living patients with CPDD have indicated that, in general, only articular cartilage and closely associated synovial, tendinous, or ligamentous structures contain CaPPi.[10] Although hydroxyapatite was found in 1.3 percent and dicalcium phosphate dihydrate (DCPD) was identified in 2.3 percent of a series of 215 anatomic cadavers involving 800 menisci studied by x-ray diffraction, more menisci showed CaPPi (3.4 percent).[73] It appeared that the normal bone salt, a prototype of hydroxyapatite, was confined to blood vessels supplying the menisci.[73] Much less often, tendinous origins of adductor muscles of the thighs, Achilles tendon insertion sites, and areas adjacent to intervertebral discs are involved.[74] Even in patients with CaPPi in the joints, mineral deposits in aortic plaques and costal cartilage consisted of hydroxyapatite.[10] Among several exceptions to exclusive joint deposition was the finding of monoclinic CaPPi in the dura mater of a patient with hyperparathyroidism, pseudogout, and gout.[75] Interestingly, there is no evidence that the rather insoluble CaPPi is ever selectively reabsorbed substantially from chondrocalcinotic cartilage,[15] except for transient surface solubilization, which has already been discussed under precipitation of acute attacks (Fig. 87–5*A*).[15] Parathyroidectomy has failed to reduce over a period of years the presence of CaPPi in afflicted cartilages of the secondary type CPDD.[15] In contrast, hydroxyapatite mineral may be removed in calcified cartilage about the tidemark during recurrent capillary invasion from bone marrow at the site of calification, with influx of chondroclasts active in mineral resorption in secondary osteoarthritis.[76,77]

The ill effects of the mineral CaPPi, deposited as it is in an unnatural location for apatite mineral development, must have a deleterious effect on biomaterial properties of the articular cartilage. It has been shown that hydroxyapatite mineral deposition in animal models is inhibited by proteoglycans largely in the form of proteoglycan aggregates[78] and promoted by proteoglycan degradation. It is unknown whether such proteoglycans are inhibitory to growth of CaPPi crystals. Reduced alcian blue staining, a stain relatively specific for proteoglycans in cartilage, has been found in the area of mineral deposition at light microscopic studies of CPDD cartilages. However, some alcian blue and saffranin O staining matrix is retained around the crystals as shown by Schumacher.[79] It has been postulated that proteoglycans might also be degraded or removed mechanically in the course of fissure formation at sites of heavy weight bearing, impact loading, and shearing forces that afflict the hip and knee. This result should hypothetically heighten the number and severity of acute and chronic inflammatory attacks related to crystal release in these large weight-bearing joints compared to more protected appendicular joints. The stiffened cartilage from chondrocalcinosis also should make these heavy weight-bearing sites more vulnerable to breakdown, whereas similar reduced elasticity of appendicular articular cartilage might not be sufficient in many cases to provoke a degenerative reaction. Increased frequency of subchondral microfractures in osteoarthritic cartilage may be a sign of an additional hazard. Radin has proposed that stiffened subchondral bone occurs as a result of microfracture in osteoarthritis.[80] This stiffening of subchondral bone should have deleterious effects on cartilage wear. The high incidence of associated osteoarthritis (70 percent) in a sporadic series[10] and mutilating osteoarthritis of varying degrees in the familial forms[29] is probably related to these variables and many more not yet documented. For the various hypothetical pathways of osteoarthritis production, once cartilage injury has occurred, see Chapter 88.

Disturbance in PPi Metabolism. *Normal PPi Metabolism.* To comprehend the pathogenesis of CPDD entails a brief review of PPi metabolism in both normal and abnormal cartilage.

PPi is composed of two molecules of orthophosphate joined with the loss of one molecule of water; this reaction takes place in the chemical synthesis of PPi and in vitro requires unphysiological high temperatures, $2H_3PO_4 \rightarrow H_4P_2O_7 + H_2O$.[44] The principal source of PPi biologically is probably pyrophosphorolysis of nucleotide triphosphates or related compounds such as uridine diphosphoglucose, particularly in cartilage. Most macromolecular materials made by the cells in general and cartilage in particular involve release of PPi. Thus, PPi is produced at one or more steps in biochemical pathways that cause synthesis of proteins, lipids, phospholipids, nucleotides, nucleic acid, steroids, structural proteoglycans, and glycogen.[44]

Because PPi is a product of so many biosynthetic reactions, the amount of PPi formed within tissues is probably large and has been estimated in adult man to represent several kilograms of PPi per day.[44] It seems almost a certainty that the PPi produced by these biosynthetic reactions must be rapidly hydrolyzed to orthophosphate within the local tissue cells. Certainly PPiases capable of catalyzing such a hydrolysis have been detected in all tissues so far studied.

However, there is a small but definite leakage of PPi into the general circulation as indicated by a low concentration, i.e., 1 to 6 μM in plasma, saliva, and synovial fluid, 3 to 13 μM in serum and 10 to 100 μM in urine.[44] In studies of Russell in dogs, labeled PPi injected into the blood stream showed a turnover time in plasma of 1.4 to 2.6 minutes.[44] Only 10 percent of the label appeared in the urine from the plasma compartment. Rapid hydrolysis by cells lying on or within the peripheral vascular system was postulated.[44]

Metabolic studies of PPi in man have indicated that PPi does not appear to be absorbed from the intestinal tract, hydrolysis probably occurring in the intestine prior to absorption perhaps caused by alkaline phosphatase in the brush border of intestinal mucosal cells. The PPi

that appears in human urine has been shown to be of endogenous origin. The precise source of this endogenous PPi in urine and plasma is unknown, but it could be derived from nonspecfic leakage from several different tissues, such as the liver, active in biosynthesis.[44] Clearance values of PPi in the kidneys suggest that only 5 to 10 percent of the filtered load is excreted as intact PPi. The remainder is probably reabsorbed or hydrolyzed within the kidney.[44]

A route of catabolism of PPi considered to be physiologically important is uptake on bony surfaces of ions derived from both the circulation and local tissue sources. It has long been known that PPi ions in vitro inhibit precipitation of calcium phosphate (CaPi)* mineral salts and retard conversion of precursory CaPi to crystalline hydroxyapatite. In addition, PPi retards dissolution of apatite crystals placed in solutions containing low Ca and Pi concentrations.[44] Such CaPi minerals can adsorb PPi so completely from solution that even when present in micromolar concentrations, large amounts of PPi adsorb on the surface of these salts. In bone and dentin it has been found that PPi occurs in up to 1 percent of the total Pi in the mineral.[44] It has been suggested that Pi may regulate onset of calcification and rates of entry influx and efflux of mineral ions from these calcified tissues.[44] In the body such adsorbed PPi is removed by local PPiases, and a group of compounds, the diphosphonates, in which a PCP bond replaces the POP bond, have been developed to resist enzymatic hydrolysis[44] and to inhibit mineral growth in Paget's disease[44] and myositis ossificans progressiva as well as other conditions.[44]

PPi Alterations in Endocrine Disorders. The importance of the postulated regulatory role of PPi as an inhibitor of mineral formation growth remains controversial. Consistent with its possible regulatory role is the finding of consistently elevated serum plasma PPi levels and urine outputs of PPi in the inherited disorder, hypophosphatasia.[44] Lack of alkaline phosphatase could hypothetically permit PPi to accumulate and inhibit the calcification found in this disease.[44] Similarly, plasma PPi was increased in patients with osteomalacia resulting from vitamin D deficiency.[44] PPi levels are also increased in serum and plasma in some patients with chronic renal failure, but the amount of unmineralized osteoid in bone biopsies has failed to correlate positively with the PPi concentration in plasma.[44] In chronic renal failure and in acromegaly, increases of PPi appear to correlate more with raised plasma Pi than to show a close relationship to failure of mineralization.

Concentrations of PPi in CPDD in Synovial Fluid and Kinetics of Removal from the Joint. Early studies on PPi levels indicated that plasma alone must be analyzed, since release of a large content of PPi from platelets during clotting can vitiate the results,[44] and recently use of a tourniquet has been shown to cause platelet release of PPi, spuriously raising plasma levels. Serum pyro-

---

*CaPi-General class of calcium phosphates.

phosphate concentration seems to be maintained under homeostatic control, inasmuch as values varied slightly per 24-hour period for a 10-day study.[81] Exercise raised the venous pyrophosphate of the lower but not the upper extremities.

Russell was the first to observe in CPDD that CaPPi deposition is associated with elevated PPi levels in synovial fluid but not in plasma.[44] Silcox and McCarty[82] confirmed the findings of Altman and associates[83] in regard to elevated levels of PPi in synovial fluid from patients with osteoarthritis; for example, the former investigators reported values for PPi of 8.86 μM $\pm$ 1.4 in CPDD, 8.40 μM $\pm$ 1.27 in osteoarthritis, and 4.20 μM $\pm$ 0.57 in rheumatoid arthritis.[82] In CPDD, the concentrations of PPi in synovial fluid appeared higher in those with chronically symptomatic joints and lower in patients with acutely inflamed joints as compared to normal.[10] PPi was not elevated in synovial fluid of several other disease controls or normal synovial fluid. Whether the elevated PPi level found in synovial fluid from an occasional patient with gout or rheumatoid arthritis may be due to concurrent osteoarthritis remains to be determined.[83] *All these studies strongly suggest a local disorder in PPi metabolism leading to deposition of CaPPi crystals and are in contrast to the aforementioned metabolic bone disease wherein adsorbed PPi ions prevent growth of mineral (apatite) crystals.*

The elevated concentration of PPi in synoval fluid of CPDD may be due to (1) an accelerated rate of biosynthesis of PPi, (2) leakage from adjacent cartilage or synovial membrane, (3) reduced rate of PPi catabolism, or (4) a reduced disappearance of intact PPi from the joint into the venous blood and lymphatics. Analysis of this problem is complicated by presence of CaPPi crystals in synovial fluids of CPDD patients. In regard to reduced catabolism of PPi, the situation remains controversial. While early studies indicate reduction of inorganic PPiases in synovial fluid of a few patients with CPDD, later studies failed to confirm these findings.[10,44] In an important study by Camerlain and associates the rate of ^{32}P-PPi degradation by normal and CPDD synovial fluids was determined in vitro and in vivo.[84] It was found that crystals exchanged PPi ions, and fluid PPi breakdown was extremely slow in comparison to the rapid turnover of PPi found in vitro.[84] Although data of Bennett, Lehr, and McCarty suggested that the synovial fluid is undersaturated with respect to CaPPi crystals,[47] current evidence suggests that most of the CaPPi crystals in synovial fluid eventually deposit in the lining synovial membrane.[85] In fact, labeled CaPPi crystals were cleared from human joints more slowly and more variably than from rabbit joints.[86] The smaller crystals were cleared more rapidly. Labeled disodium etidronate (EHDP) binding used to semiquantitate mineral particles was absent in inflammatory joint fluids but present in 29 percent of noninflammatory joint fluids.[87] Such binding was greatest in the presence of CaPPi crystals and x-ray evidence of cartilage degeneration. It is still possible that phosphatase degradation of CaPPi in the synovial space is important, and that intrasynovial fluid precipitation of CaPPi crystals occurs under unclarified conditions.

Sites of Initial CaPPi Crystal Deposition. Because of the results described above, studies have been devoted to searching for evidence of increased PPi production by joint tissues.[86,87] If PPi production were high, it must be within the joint tissues per se, inasmuch as no systemic metabolic disturbance has been found. For example, red cell PPiase from CPDD patients was identical to that of normal controls.[88] The initial deposits of CaPPi, according to McCarty, appear in rims around cartilage cells; larger deposits are associated with cell necrosis in the periphery. Ultrastructural studies of synovium have indicated deposits only at sites of surface phagocytic cells and adjacent interstitium.[79] Thus, histological evidence would favor cartilage as the initiating site, although initiation in synovium has not been excluded. Appearance of crystals in the synovial fluid, therefore, would seem to be a "shedding phenomenon" of preformed crystals rather than spontaneous precipitation from supersaturated solutions, regardless of tissue origin, inasmuch as the state of supersaturation has not been found.[47] Yet supersaturation in respect to the product of Ca $\times$ Pi may occur by current knowledge of crystal formation at sites where the CaPPi aggregates develop in cartilage, unless mineral forms through a mechanism of heterogeneous nucleation.[78] Conceivably higher concentrations of PPi and/or Ca could be found in microscopic sites in cartilage than those levels found in synovial fluid of CPDD patients.

Howell and associates studied the production of PPi by cartilage taken at biopsy or surgery from patients with osteoarthritis and chondrocalcinosis and incubated immediately after removal in synthetic media. Human ulcerated osteoarthritic cartilage as well as cartilage from two patients with chondrocalcinosis extruded PPi into the medium.[86] Normal synovial membrane and articular cartilage as well as that from patients with avascular necrosis, rheumatoid arthritis, and femoral neck fractures failed to cause PPi elaboration.[86] Incubates of rabbit articular and growth plate cartilages elaborated PPi; this PPi was postulated to be a precursor of Pi liberated at sites of new mineralization.[86] Rabbit synovial membrane failed to elaborate PPi,[86] but hyaline cartilage did extrude it in a recent study.[87] The amount of PPi elaborated by the osteoarthritic cartilage when extrapolated for total cartilage in a human knee could account for the PPi turnover found by Camerlain and associates.[84] In all human and rabbit samples alkaline phosphatase activity was extruded into the media along with the PPi but not extruded by any of the control tissues. Neutral PPiase activity was elaborated substantially from growth plate incubates but absent from chondrocalcinotic incubates. Also, the PPi was hydrolyzed over 8 hours in the growth plate incubates, but not the chondrocalcinotic ones.[86] These data were interpreted to indicate that the growth of CaPPi crystals or apatite crystals depends on the local tissue environment (Fig. 87-7), predomi-

Figure 87–7. Clusters of needle-shaped mineral crystals (*M*) resembling hydroxyapatite among articular cartilage matrix vesicles (*MV*) from a patient with CPDD. Much larger crystals of CaPPi were found in the neighborhood closely adjacent to these sites (not shown). Original magnification × 80,000. (From Schumacher, H.R.: *In* McCarty D.J. [ed.]: Proceedings of the Conference on Pseudogout and Pyrophosphate Metabolism. Arthritis Rheum. 19: Suppl. 3, May–June, 1976.)

nantly the supply of unhydrolyzed PPi. Low content but no qualitative biochemical defect of pyrophosphatase in CPDD was detectable.[89,90]

Generation of PPi from ATP by membrane-bound phosphatases from articular cartilage of patients with chondrocalcinosis was greater than that observed with osteoarthritic or normal cartilage.[90,91] This finding of a new enzyme in cartilage which hydrolyses nucleotides to release pyrophosphate was definitively documented,[90,91] and its presence as an ectoenzyme (NTP pyrophosphohydrolase) has recently been shown.[92] The ratio of 5'-nucleotidase to pyrophosphatase is high in chondrocalcinotic cartilage[90] and the generation of a PPi ion gradient necessary for precipitation of CaPPi might occur if the former ectoenzyme were exposed to nucleotides, e.g., ATP, GTP, or UTP.[90,91] The recent controversy over whether ATP is physiologically transferred through cell plasma membranes has been reviewed.[93] Nevertheless, chondrocyte injury as may occur in osteoarthritis or excessive synthetic functions (growth plates) were postulated to create nucleotide leakage with generation of PPi in cartilage.[94] The ratio of the activity of this enzyme to neutral pyrophosphatase was high in CPDD and osteoarthritis compared with normal articular cartilages (Table 87–4). These findings support the

hypothesis that a final common pathway in chondrocalcinosis may require two phases: (1) midzonal cartilage cellular modulation to form a mineral phase and (2) failure of adequate hydrolysis of PPi in the environment of the newly formed mineral seeds in extracellular matrix vesicles (Fig. 87–7) such that CaPPi crystals rather than hdroxyapatite are grown.

Other workers[44] question whether the limited number of cells (about 10 percent of adult human articular knee cartilage volume) could continuously support the PPi gradient required for making crystal aggregates of the size actually found in CPDD. It is particularly hard to explain the most common sites of CPDD mineral deposition, the symphysis pubis and the triangular cartilage of the wrist, where cellularity is probably even less than in other areas. The histologically granular appearance of the matrix around CaPPi deposits has raised speculation that a special nucleational compound for CaPPi salts, as opposed to hydroxyapatite, may be produced in the course of modulation of these cells to invoke mineral formation. Certainly such an agent would seem to be necessary if the synovial fluid and adjacent hypocellular cartilage are undersaturated with respect to Ca × PPi ions. It is not clear how PPi could be delivered to the matrix if one subscribes to the cellular elaboration

Table 87–4. Distribution of Enzyme Activities Between Superficial Layers of Articular Cartilage in Patients with Osteoarthritis and CPDD, Compared with Normal Articular and Growth Plate Cartilage*

No. of Subjects and Study	Cartilage Site	Neutral Pyrophosphatase†	5′-Nucleotidase†	NTP-Pyrophospho-hydrolase†	Cell Counts per Mg Wet Weight
CPDD[8]	Superficial layers	0.4 ± 0.1	150 ± 27	31.5 ± 7.8	$3.5 \pm 9 \times 10^3$
Normal Articular (Human)[6]					
Growth Plates (Rabbit) Normal[6]	Total tissue	0.03 ± 0.01	151 ± 53	17.2 ± 5	3.8×10^{-3}
Growth Plates	Total tissue	144 ± 0.2	351 ± 20	118 ± 21	$12.8 \pm 2.6 \times 10^3$

*The high ratio of (ecto) NTP pyrophosphohydrolase to neutral pyrophosphatase in CPDD cartilage in comparison with growth plates supports the possibility of nucleotide hydrolysis and generation of pyrophosphate ions from leakage of nucleotides in CPDD cartilage. In growth plates also shown to extrude PPi, only hydroxyapatite-type minerals are formed.

†x $\pm$ S.D., units/g wet weight

theory, especially inasmuch as cultured CPDD fibroblasts have failed to export PPi despite elevated intracellular PPi content in both nonhereditary[95] and hereditary[96] forms. Most of the PPi present in cells in vivo exists as magnesium complexes, which do not diffuse through the cellular limiting membrane. Whether transport may occur in vesicles or whether there is leakage of nucleotides as mentioned earlier remains controversial. It is unlikely that cell surface adenylcyclases, which can generate PPi, are involved.[92,94]

Another view that commands some interest does not demand that a PPi gradient be established by uncalcified midzonal cartilage cells; rather it suggests that PPi is derived from the subchondral bone plate. Certainly, the growth plate-like cells of the calcified cartilage and overlying basal uncalcified cartilage cells can become activated to assume a growth plate function. It was shown by Lane, Villacin, and Bullough[77] that the frequency of capillary invasion up to the tidemark at weight-bearing sites in major joints such as the hip and knee increases with increasing age from 50 to 70 years. The capillary invasions are associated with increased calcification in the basal articular cartilage with reduplication of the tidemark. Histologically, cells bordering the tidemark have an increased level of alkaline phosphatase.[97,98] These channels are believed to precede the lesions of osteoarthritis in some cases.[77] Perhaps PPi is deposited in the calcified cartilage zone either through local cell production or from entering through the subchondral circulation. This would provide a reservoir for PPi either at rest, during the remodeling process mentioned above, or during mechanical abrasion from bone-on-bone contact in the osteoarthritic ulcers.[86] This mechanism alone, however, fails to explain the predominant midzonal cartilage location of the CaPPi mineral deposition in CPDD. The cartilage remodeling in osteoarthritic ulcers, consistent output of phosphatase and PPi in incubates of osteoarthritic ulcer tissue, and sporadic high alkaline phosphatase content in total tissue[98] also provide a rationale for the existence of hydroxyapatite arthropathy[99] described below.

Finally, deposition of the CaPPi crystals may be a response secondary to abnormal metabolism of chondrocytes from various causes as evidenced in a study of

Bjelle. In cartilage biopsies from four patients with hereditary CPDD, chemical properties of the matrix were compared with those of cartilage from 13 control "normal" subjects.[32] Low hydroxyproline, a low ratio of keratan sulfate to chondroitin sulfate, and a low ratio of chondroitin-4-sulfate to chondroitin-6-sulfate were found in diseased versus control cartilages.[32] Total glycosaminoglycan levels were normal, and no relation of biochemical changes to tissue degeneration was seen. This was considered evidence for a calcium pyrophosphate deposition pathway separate from that postulated to evolve in the presence of severe osteoarthritis.[32]

Possibly such pathways exist for the hereditary or familial forms of CPDD or even the late old age form encountered by Pritzker, in which osteoarthritis was minor and mineral deposition was extensive in patients with femoral neck fractures.[33] Otherwise nonfamilial CPDD seems, just as hydroxyapatite arthropathy, to express itself in relationship to the severity of accompanying osteoarthritis or post-traumatic arthritis, as studied by Halverson and associates,[87] Dieppe and associates,[100] and Schumacher and associates.[101]

ETIOLOGICAL CONSIDERATIONS

In sporadic disease there are few clues. Occult hyperparathyroidism, chondrocytic abiotrophy with modulation to mineral formation, and subtle genetic factors in midzonal joint cartilage not yet understood could hypothetically turn on mineral production at abnormal sites and, at least in man, produce an abnormal mineral.

In the form of CPDD with associated metabolic diseases, one could postulate that abnormal storage products cause chondrocyte injury, breakdown of proteoglycan mineral inhibitors, and subsequent exposure of collagen nucleational sites. However, the reason for switching on of cellular machinery for mineral production in hyaline or adjacent calcified cartilage remains unknown. In hemochromatosis, although some Fe salts are good nucleating agents, the Fe deposits do not seem to coincide with those of mineral.[44] The possible role of intracellular stored Fe in hemochromatosis, Cu in Wilson's disease, and Ca in hyperparathyroidism as inhibitors of intracellular PPiase has been speculated upon by McCarty and Pepe.[88] Such speculations are supported by their study on the inhibitory effect of these metal ions on erythrocyte phosphatases.

Current and future research in familial disease may provide clues to the switching on of mineral production. Also, the capacity to induce midzonal apatite chondrocalcinosis in young rabbits,[102] resembling what they develop spontaneously in old age, provides for the first time an animal model to investigate etiological mechanisms.

MANAGEMENT OF CPDD

Acute attacks have often been treated successfully by aspiration of synovial fluid and injection of long-acting corticosteroid preparation.[11] For severe acute attacks, phenylbutazone, 150 to 200 mg four times a day, seems most useful, whereas other nonsteroidal anti-inflammatory agents can be used efficaciously and more safely for milder attacks of chronic inflammation on a long-term basis. For those with peptic ulcer disease or other contraindications to the use of phenylbutazone, the use of intravenous colchicine provides an approach which is rapid, potent, and consistent, especially when contrasted to its sporadic action per os. The remainder of the treatment program is the same as for the associated diseases such as osteoarthritis, hyperparathyroidism, or diabetes mellitus. Patients with "pseudotabes" without neural deficits have a far superior result following total joint replacement than those with a neural deficit.[12]

HYDROXYAPATITE ARTHROPATHY

In patients with subacute or acute synovitis and osteoarthritis studied by Dieppe and associates the aspirated knee effusions upon centrifugation showed a major component of the solid phase in the pellet to be a CaP mineral.[103] The mineral was also present in inflammatory cells. Similar clinical findings were also recorded by Schumacher et al. in 1976[104] in patients with what also appeared clinically to be primary osteoarthritis. Stimulated by these findings, Schumacher et al. injected dogs intra-articularly with a solution containing synthetic CaP mineral of the apatite class. The injections caused swelling and heat in the dog joints similar to crystal synovitis[104] caused by CaPPi. PMN leukocytes from human synovial effusions were studied by electron probe analysis and found to contain a high concentration of Ca and P consistent with their inclusion of apatite or amorphous CaPi.[104] Inasmuch as the dimensions of hydroxyapatite crystals in man are about 200×30 to 70 Å, only aggregates of crystals could be seen in these electron microscopic studies, and apparently aggregates were necessary to produce a phlogistic effect.

Overall, these findings suggested that hydroxyapatite

aggregates per se produced serious joint disease similar to that of CPDD. Subsequently McCarty[105] described a group of patients with glenohumoral osteoarthritis and bilateral rotator cuff defects, joint stiffness and instability.[106-108] These patients also had interesting synovial fluid findings: hydroxy crystals clumps, synovial collagenolytic activity, neutral proteases, and presence of collagen type I, II, and III in an almost acellular synovial fluid. Synovial tissue from these joints showed typical chondromatosis, and transmission electron microscopic views revealed clumps of crystals leaking into the joint space through histologic regions denuded of synoviocytes. Some crystal aggregates were found in the synovia per se. Cartilage and bony destruction and synovial proliferation as well as tendon erosion were not unlike the arthropathy with chondrocalcinosis described by Menkes.[12]) Instead of bands of calcium-mineral deposits confined to articular cartilage, however, there were exuberant deposits of mineral in the capsule. These cases referred to earlier, designated "Milwaukee shoulder," manifested evidence on x-ray of upward dislocation of humoral heads against the acromium or downward dislocation on hyperextension.[106-108] Both types of arthropathy (i.e., "Milwaukee shoulder" and arthropathy of Menkes[12]) are characterized by mineral deposition in joint tissues, chronic proliferative synovitis, cartilage degeneration, and tendon erosion.

A feature shared by and common to "Milwaukee shoulder,"[106-108] hydroxyapatite arthropathy, and nonfamilial CPDD is the presence of concurrent osteoarthritis in the same and other joints. Inasmuch as histologic evidence of tissue breakdown may antedate radiologic or clinical signs, most cases of chondrocalcinosis might have this association. Could it be in all three of these disorders, and possibly multiple subsets not yet studied in detail, that osteoarthritis may precede apatite deposition or chondrocalcinosis and that the mineral formation is a consequence of disarrayed cartilage metabolism as a spinoff or secondary effect of osteoarthritis?

Consistent with this viewpoint have been the data accrued by Schumacher and colleagues in which over half of their autopsy series consisted of cases in which osteoarthritic lesions were found by light microscopy to have signs of mineral deposition in the deep radial zone of articular cartilage.[101] They found a positive correlation between severity of lesions and presence of mineral. Also, Schumacher's group examined osteoarthritic joint effusions from 100 patients fulfilling standard criteria for oestoarthritis, and excluding any patients with leukocyte counts over 2000 per mm³. Sixty percent have had evidence for either apatite or CPDD crystals in synovial fluid. Thirty percent of those with crystals revealed hydroxyapatite; 27 percent, CPDD; and 43 percent, both types of crystals.[101] Patients with these findings were older and had more prolonged osteoarthritis and more severe osteoarthritis than patients lacking crystals. Only 29 percent of patients with "mild" osteoarthritis had crystals, while 100 percent of those with severe osteoarthritis displayed crystals.[101]

Furthermore, a clear-cut association of chondrocalcinosis with premature osteoarthritis in hypermobility has been described.[109] Dieppe and Doherty[100] studied 100 consecutive patients who had undergone unilateral meniscectomy at least 19 years previously. Knee radiographs of these patients and of 100 age- and sex-matched controls were graded similarly. Chondrocalcinosis was present in 20 percent of operated and in only 4 percent of unoperated knees. Three percent of the control group had chondrocalcinosis. Radiologic evidence of calcium salt deposition was found in unstable joints and in postmeniscectomy patients who had no evidence of chondrocalcinosis elsewhere and no other obvious predisoposing causes. The nature of the mineral in these studies has been pursued lately with electron microscopic techniques.

Increasing evidence by electron microscopic examinations from Ali's[110] and Schumacher's[101] laboratories indicates frequent intracartilaginous collections of mineral registering as hydroxyapatite or as a prototype mineral with carbonate substitution. The data suggest that without electron microscopic study and simply with isolation of larger mineral desposits necessary to register in x-ray powder diagnosis one selects patients with principally $Ca_2P_2O_7 \cdot 2H_2O$ deposition[7] and that other types of crystal deposition may be overlooked. On the other hand, demonstrating the nature and site of deposition of minute amounts of mineral in a histologic section requires cautious interpretation with respect to changes in crystal phase and location related to[3] fixation and embedding techniques. Accurate crystal analysis in histologic sites is improved by recent advances in electron diffraction and Fourier transform infrared spectroscopy.[7] These approaches should eventually converge on an accurate version of the in vivo frequency and distribution of crystal deposition disease.

Diagnosis is still hampered by the difficulty of reliably preparing biologic samples free of artifactual mineral phase from translocated ions in the lymph or by spontaneous precipitation during preparations for microscopic studies. The need for instant freezing of samples and the maintenance of deep frozen temperatures throughout processing are difficult problems to be faced in studies of these patients' cellular inclusions of apatite.

Management of Hydroxyapatite Apatite Arthropathy. Orthopedic and physiatric consultation is advised for possible splinting, non-weight-bearing exercise programs, arthrotomy, as well as partial or total joint replacement.

Attempts to remove mineral already deposited by methods that are successful in tophaceous gout have largely failed. "Chemical lysis" has been attempted experimentally by intra-articular infusion of solutions high in Mg content. Mobilization of crystals (crystal shedding) associated with fresh severe acute attacks of synovitis or failure to mobilize mineral[47] was encountered. Extracartilaginous mineral can be excised when present abundantly as in "Milwaukee shoulder," but the deposits are often too small to warrant such extirpation.

REFERENCES

1. McCarty, D.J., and Hollander, J.L.: Identification of urate crystals in gouty synovial fluid. Ann. Intern. Med. 54:452, 1961.
2. Kohn, N.N., Hughes, R.E., McCarty, D.J., and Faires, J.S.: The significance of calcium phosphate crystals in the synovial fluid of arthritic patients: The pseudogout syndrome. II. Identification of crystals. Ann. Intern. Med. 56:738, 1962.
3. McCarty, D.J., Kohn, N.N., and Faires, J.S.: The significance of calcium phosphate crystals in the synovial fluid of arthritis patients: The "pseudogout syndrome." I. Clinical aspects. Ann. Intern. Med. 56:711, 1962.
4. Zitnan, D., and Sitaj, S.: Mnohopocetna familiarna kalcifikacia ortikularnyck chrupick. Bratisl. Lek. Listy 38:217, 1958.
5. Glimcher, M.J.: Handbook of Physiology. Baltimore, Williams & Wilkins, 1976, p. 25.
6. Boskey, A.L.: Current concepts of the physiology and biochemistry of calcification. Clin. Orthop. Rel. Res. 157:225, 1981.
7. Mandel, N.S., and Mandel, G.S.: Structures of crystals that provoke inflammation. In Weissmann, G. (ed.): Advances in Inflammation Research. Vol. 4. New York, Raven Press, 1982, p. 73.
8. Faure, G., Netter, P., Malaman, B., et al.: Monocrystalline calcium hydrogen phosphate dihydrate in destructive arthropathies of chondrocalcinosis. Lancet ii:142, 1977.
9. Crystalline deposits in human tissues. In Pritzker, K.P.H. (ed.): Symposium on Crystallography. J. Rheumatol. 8:997, 1981.
10. McCarty, D.J.: Calcium pyrophosphate dihydrate deposition disease—1975. Arthritis Rheum. 19:275, 1976.
11. McCarty, D.J.: Pseudogout, articular chondrocalcinosis. In Hollander, J.L. (ed.): Arthritis and Allied Conditions. 7th ed. Philadelphia, Lea & Febiger, 1966, p. 947.
12. Menkes, C.J., Simon, F., Delrieu, F., Forest, M., and Delbarre, F.: Destructive arthropathy in chondrocalcinosis articularis. Arthritis Rheum. 19:329, 1976.
13. Okazaki, T., Saito, T., Mitomo, T., and Siota, Y.: Pseudogout: Clinical observations and chemical analyses of deposits. Arthritis Rheum. 19:293, 1976.
14. Russell, R.G.G.: Discussion: Session II. Genetics of CPPD deposition. Arthritis Rheum. 19:410, 1976.
15. O'Duffy, J.D.: Clinical studies of acute pseudogout attacks. Comments on prevalence, predispositions, and treatment. Arthritis Rheum. 19:349, 1976.
16. Ellman, M.H., and Levin, B.: Chondrocalcinosis in elderly persons. Arthritis Rheum. 18:43, 1975.
17. Moskowitz, R.W., and Katz, D.: Chondrocalcinosis and chondrocalsynovitis (pseudogout syndrome). Analysis of twenty-four cases. Am. J. Med. 43:322, 1967.
18. Skinner, M., and Cohen, A.S.: Calcium pyrophosphate dihydrate deposition disease. Arch. Intern. Med. 123:636, 1969.
19. McCarty, D.J.: Pseudogout: Articular chondrocalcinosis. Calcium pyrophosphate crystal deposition disease. In Hollander, J.L. and McCarty, D.J. (eds.): Arthritis and Allied Conditions. 8th ed. Philadelphia, Lea & Febiger, 1972, p. 1140.
20. Jacobelli, S., McCarty, D.J., Silcox, D.C., et al.: Calcium pyrophosphate dihydrate crystal deposition in neuropathic joints. Four cases of polyarticular involvement. Ann. Intern. Med. 79:340, 1973.
21. Mandl, F.: Zur Pathologie und Therapie der zwischen Knorpelerkrankungen des Kniegelenks. Arch. Klin. Chir. 146:149, 1927.
22. Rubenstein, H.M., and Shah, D.M.: Pseudogout. Semin. Arthritis Rheum. 2:259, 1972–1973.
23. Bjelle, A., and Sunden, G.: Pyrophosphate arthropathy: A clinical study of fifty cases. J. Bone Joint Surg. 56B:246, 1974.
24. Altman, R.D.: Arthroscopic findings of the knee in patients with pseudogout. Arthritis Rheum. 19:286, 1976.
25. Bjelle, A.: Morphological study of articular cartilage in pyrophosphate arthropathy (chondrocalcinosis articularis or calcium pyrophosphate dihydrate crystal deposition disease). Ann. Rheum. Dis. 31:449, 1972.
26. van der Korst, J.K., Geerards, J., and Driessens, F.C.M.: A hereditary type of idiopathic articular chondrocalcinosis. Survey of a pedigree. Am. J. Med. 56:307, 1974.
27. Zitnan, D., and Sitaj, S.: Natural course of articular chondrocalcinosis. Arthritis Rheum. 19:363, 1976.
28. Reginato, A.J., Hollander, J.L., Martinez, V., et al.: Familial chondrocalcinosis in the Chiloe Islands, Chile. Ann. Rheum. Dis. 34:260, 1975.
29. Reginato, A.J., Schiapachasse, V., Zmyjiwsky, C., Schumacher, H.R., Fuentes, C., and Galdamez, M.: HLA antigens and ankylosing chondrocalcinosis. A rthritis Rheum. 22:928, 1979.
30. Rodriguez-Valverde, V., Tinture, T., Zuniga, M., Pena, J., and Gonzalez, A.: Familial chondrocalcinosis. Prevalence in northern Spain and clinical features in five pedigrees. Arthritis Rheum. 23:471, 1980.
31. Gaucher, A., Faure, G., Netter, P., Pourel, J., Raffoux, C., Streiff, F.,

Tongio, M.-M., and Mayer, S.: Hereditary diffuse articular chondrocalcinosis. Scand. J. Rheumatol. 6:217, 1977.

32. Bjelle, A.: Cartilage matrix in hereditary pyrophosphate arthropathy. J. Rheumatol. 8:959, 1981.

33. Hamilton, E.B.D.: Disease associated with CPPD deposition disease. Arthritis Rheum. 19:353, 1976.

34. Gerster, J.C., Lagier, R., Boivin, G., and Schneider, C.: Carpal tunnel syndrome in chondrocalcinosis of the wrist. Clinical and histologic study. Arthritis Rheum. 23:926, 1980.

35. Teglbjaerg, P.S., Ladefoged, C., Sorenson, K.H., and Christensen, H.E.: Local articular amyloid deposition in pyrophosphate arthritis. Histological aspects. Acta Path. Microbiol. Scand. 87:307, 1979.

36. Good, A.E., and Rapp, R.: Chondrocalcinosis of the knee with gout and rheumatoid arthritis. N. Engl. J. Med. 277:286, 1967.

37. Dodds, W.J., and Steinbach, H.L.: Gout associated with calcification of cartilage. N. Engl. J. Med. 275:745, 1966.

38. Stockman, A., Darlington, L.G., and Scott, J.T.: Frequency of chondrocalcinosis of the knees and avascular necrosis of the femoral heads in gout: a controlled study. Ann. Rheum. Dis. 39:7, 1980.

39. Moskowitz, R.W., and Garcia, F.: Chondrocalcinosis articularis. Arch. Intern. Med. 132:87, 1973.

40. Bywaters, E.G.L.: Calcium pyrophosphate deposits in synovial membrane. Ann. Rheum. Dis. 31:219, 1972.

41. Phelps, P., and Hawker, C.D.: Serum parathyroid hormone levels in patients with calcium pyrophosphate crystal deposition disease (chondrocalcinosis, pseudogout). Arthritis Rheum. 16:590, 1973.

42. Dorwart, B.B., and Schumacher, H.R.: Joint effusions. Chondrocalcinosis and other rheumatic manifestations in hypothyroidism. A clinicopathologic study. Am. J. Med. 59:780, 1975.

43. Feller, E.R., and Schumacher, H.R.: Osteoarticular changes in Wilson's disease. Arthritis Rheum. 15:259, 1972.

44. Russell, R.G.G.: Metabolism of inorganic pyrophosphate (PPi). Arthritis Rheum. 19:465, 1976.

45. O'Duffy, J.D.: Hypophosphatasia associated with calcium pyrophosphate dihydrate deposits in cartilage. Arthritis Rheum. 13:381, 1970.

46. Clowes, G.H.A., Jr., and Simeone, F.A.: Acute hypocalcemia in surgical patients. Ann. Surg. 146:530, 1957.

47. Bennett, R.M., and Lehr, J.R., and McCarty, D.J.: Factors affecting the solubility of calcium pyrophosphate dihydrate crystals. J. Clin. Invest. 56:1571, 1975.

48. Paul, H., Reginato, A.J., and Schumacher, H.R.: Alizarin red S staining as a screening test to detect calcium compounds in synovial fluid. Arthritis Rheum. 26:191, 1983.

49. Genant, H.K.: Roentgenographic aspects of calcium pyrophosphate dihydrate crystal deposition disease (pseudogout). Arthritis Rheum. 19:307, 1976.

50. Pachas, W.N.: Pseudogout without chondrocalcinosis. A clinical, radiologic and pathologic study of eighteen cases. Arthritis Rheum. 15:121, 1972.

51. Resnick, D., Niwayama, G., Georgen, T., et al.: Clinical radiographic and pathologic abnormalities in calcium pyrophosphate deposition disease: An analysis of 85 patients. Radiology 122:1, 1977.

52. Martel, W., Champion, C.K., Thompson, G.R., et al.: A roentgenologically distinctive arthropathy in some patients with pseudogout syndrome. Am. J. Roentgenol. Radium Ther. Nucl. Med. 109:587, 1970.

53. Mandel, N.S.: The structural basis of crystal-induced membranolysis. Arthritis Rheum. 19:439, 1976.

54. Faires, J.S., and McCarty, D.J.: Acute arthritis in man and dog after intrasynovial injection of sodium urate crystals. Lancet 2:682, 1962.

55. McCarty, D.J., Phelps, P., and Pyenson, J.: Crystal-induced inflammation in canine joints. I. An experimental model with quantification of the host response. J. Exp. Med. 124:99, 1966.

56. Kellermeyer, R.W.: Hageman factor and acute gouty arthritis. Arthritis Rheum. 11:452, 1968.

57. Phelps, P., Prockop, D.J., and McCarty, D.J.: Crystal-induced inflammation in canine joints. III. Evidence against bradykinin as a mediator of inflammation. J. Lab. Clin. Med. 68:433, 1966.

58. Ginsberg, M.H., Jaques, B., Cochrane, C.G., and Griffin, J.H.: Urate crystal-dependent cleavage of Hageman factor in human plasma and synovial fluid. J. Lab. Clin. Med. 95:497, 1980.

59. Phelps, P., and McCarty, D.J.: Crystal-induced inflammation in canine joints. II. Importance of polymorphonuclear leukocytes. J. Exp. Med. 124:115, 1966.

60. Phelps, P.: Polymorphonuclear leukocyte motility in vitro. III. Possible release of a chemotactic substance after phagocytosis of urate crystals by polymorphonuclear leukocytes. Arthritis Rheum. 12:197, 1969.

61. Tse, R.L., and Phelps, P.: Polymorphonuclear leukocyte motility in vitro. V. Release of chemotactic activity following phagocytosis of calcium pyrophosphate crystals, diamond dust and urate crystals. J. Lab. Clin. Med. 76:403, 1970.

62. Spilberg, I., Gallacher, A., and Mandell, B.: Calcium pyrophosphate

dihydrate (CPPD) crystal-induced chemotactic factor: Subcellular localization role of protein synthesis and phagocytosis. J. Lab. Clin. Med. 89:817, 1977.

63. Spilberg, I., Mandell, B., Mehta, J., Simchowitz, L., and Rosenberg, D.: Mechanism of action of colchicine in acute urate crystal-induced arthritis. J. Clin. Invest. 64:775, 1979.

64. Spilberg, I., McLain, D., Simchowitz, L., and Berney, S.: Colchicine and pseudogout. Arthritis Rheum. 23:1062, 1980.

65. Schumacher, H.R., Fishbein, P., Phelps, P., et al.: Comparison of sodium urate and calcium pyrophosphate crystal phagocytosis by polymorphonuclear leukocytes. Effects of crystal size and other factors. Arthritis Rheum. 18:783, 1975.

66. Wallingford, W.R., and McCarty, D.J.: Differential membranolytic effects of microcrystalline sodium urate and calcium pyrophosphate dihydrate. J. Exp. Med. 133:100, 1971.

67. Weissman, G.W., and Rita, G.A.: A molecular basis of gouty inflammation. Nature 240:167, 1972.

68. Kozin, F., and McCarty, D.J.: Protein absorption to monosodium urate, calcium pyrophosphate dihydrate, and silica crystals. Relationship to the pathogenesis of crystal-induced inflammation. Arthritis Rheum. 19:433, 1976.

69. Solnica, J., Mitrovic, D., and Kahn, M.-F.: L'interet de la mise en evidence des formations cristallines dans le liquide synovial. Semin. Hop. Paris 43-2573, 1967.

70. Hasselbacher, P.: Microcrystalline material stimulates secretion of collagenease and PGE$_2$ by synovial fibroblasts. In Pritzker, K.P.H. (ed.): Symposium on Crystalline Deposits in Human Tissues. J. Rheumatol. 8:1013, 1981.

71. Cheung, H.S., Halverson, P.B., and McCarty, D.J.: Release of collagenase, neutral protease, and prostaglandins from cultured mammalian synovial cells by hydroxyapatite and calcium pyrophosphate dihydrate crystals. Arthritis Rheum. 24:1338, 1981.

72. Evans, C.H.: Cellular mechanisms of hydrolytic enzyme release in osteoarthritis. Semin. Arthritis Rheum. 11:93, 1981.

73. McCarty, D.J., Hogan, J.M., Gatter, R.A., and Grossman, M.: Studies on pathological calcifications in human cartilage. I. Prevalence and types of crystal deposits in the menisci of two hundred and fifteen cadavers. J. Bone Joint Surg. 48A:309, 1966.

74. Pritzker, K.P.H.: Aging and degeneration in the lumbar intervertebral disc. Orthop. Clin. North Am. 8:65, 1977.

75. Grahame, R., Sutor, D.J., and Mitchener, M.B.: Crystal deposition in hyperparathyroidism. Ann. Rheum. Dis. 30:597, 1971.

76. Johnson, L.C.: Kinetics of osteoarthritis. Lab. Invest. 8:1223, 1959.

77. Lane, L.B., Villacin, A., and Bullough, P.G.: A study of endochondral ossification in the adult: A mechanism for continuous joint remodelling. J. Bone Joint Surg. 57A:576, 1975.

78. Howell, D.S., and Pita, J.C.: Calcification of growth plate cartilage with special reference to studies on micropuncture fluids. Clin. Orthop. 118:208, 1976.

79. Schumacher, H.R.: Ultrastructural findings in chondrocalcinosis and pseudogout. Arthritis Rheum. 19:413, 1976.

80. Radin, E.L., and Paul, I.L.: Response of joints to impact loading. I. In vitro wear. Arthritis Rheum. 14:356, 1971.

81. Ryan, L.M., Kozin, F., and McCarty, D.J.: Quantification of human plasma inorganic pyrophosphate. II. Biologic variables. Arthritis Rheum. 22:892, 1979.

82. Silcox, D.C., and McCarty, D.J.: Elevated inorganic pyrophosphate concentrations in synovial fluids in osteoarthritis and pseudogout. J. Lab. Clin. Med. 83:518, 1974.

83. Altman, R.D., Muniz, O., Pita, J.C., et al.: Microanalysis of inorganic pyrophosphate (PPi) in synovial fluid and plasma. Arthritis Rheum. 16:171, 1973.

84. Camerlain, M., McCarty, D.J., Silcox, D.C., et al.: Inorganic pyrophosphate pool size and turnover rate in arthritic joints. J. Clin. Invest. 55:1373, 1975.

85. McCarty, D.J., Palmer, D.W., and James, C.: Clearance of calcium pyrophosphate dihydrate crystals in vivo. Arthritis Rheum. 22:1122, 1979.

86. Howell, D.S., Muniz, O., Pita, J.C., and Enis, J.: Extrusion of pyrophosphate into extracellular media by osteoarthritic cartilage incubates. J. Clin. Invest. 56:1473, 1975.

87. Ryan, L.M., Cheung, H.S., and McCarty, D.J.: Extrusion of inorganic pyrophosphate by normal mammalian articular hyaline and fibrocartilage in organ culture. Arthritis Rheum. 24:1522, 1981.

88. McCarty, D.J., and Pepe, P.F.: Erythrocyte neutral inorganic pyrophosphatase in pseudogout. J. Lab. Clin. Med. 79:277, 1972.

89. Tenenbaum, J., Muniz, O., Good, A., Schumacher, H.R., and Howell, D.S.: Further observations on cartilage phosphatases in osteoarthritis and chondrocalcinosis. Arthritis Rheum. 21:597, 1978.

90. Tenenbaum, J., Muniz, O., Schumacher, H.R., Good, A.E., and Howell, D.S.: Comparison of phosphohydrolase activities from articular car-

tilage in calcium pyrophosphate deposition disease and in primary osteoarthritis. Arthritis Rheum. 24:492, 1981.

91. Howell, D.S., Muniz, O.E., and Morales, S.: 5'Nucleotidase and pyrophosphate (PPi)-generating activities in articular cartilage extracts in calcium pyrophosphate deposition disease (CPDD) and in primary osteoarthritis (OA). *In* Peyron, J.G. (ed.): Epidemiology of Osteoarthritis. Paris, Ciba-Geigy, 1980, p. 99.

92. Ryan, L.M., Wortmann, R.L., Karas, B., and McCarty, D.J.: Nucleoside triphosphate (NTP) pyrophosphohydrolase activity in canine articular cartilage. Arthritis Rheum. 25:S30, 1982.

93. Chandry, I.H.: Does ATP cross the cell plasma membrane? Yale J. Biol. Med. 55:1, 1982.

94. Howell, D.S., Pelletier, J., Martel-Pelletier, J., and Morales, S.: Nucleoside pyrophosphohydrolases in human osteoarthritic and chondrocalcinotic cartilage. Arthritis Rheum. 26:S41, 1983.

95. Lust, G., Nuki, G., and Seegmiller, J.E.: Inorganic pyrophosphate and proteoglycan metabolism in cultured human articular chondrocytes and fibroblasts. Arthritis Rheum. 19:479, 1976.

96. Lust, G., Faure, G., Netter, D., and Seegmiller, J.E.: Increased pyrophosphate in fibroblasts and lymphoblasts cultured from patients with hereditary diffuse articular chondrocalcinosis. Science 214:809, 1981.

97. Stockwell, R.A., and Meachim, G.: The chondrocytes. *In* Freeman, M.A.R. (ed.): Adult Articular Cartilage. Oxford, Isaac Pitman and Sons, 1973, p. 51.

98. Ali, S.Y., and Bayliss, M.T.: Enzymic changes in human osteoarthrotic cartilage. *In* Normal and Osteoarthrotic Articular Cartilage. London, Institute of Orthopaedics, 1974, p. 189.

99. Howell, D.S.: Crystal deposition disease. *In* Wright, V. (ed.): Topical Reviews in Rheumatic Disorders. Bristol, John Wright and Sons, 1982, Chapter 2.

100. Dieppe, P., and Doherty, M.: Which comes first: Crystals or osteoarthritis? *In* Cooke, T.D. (ed.): Clinical Patterns and Pathological Features in Osteoarthritis. J. Rheumatol. (Suppl. 9), 1983.

101. Schumacher, H.R.: Implication of crystal deposition in osteoarthritis. *In* Cooke, T.D. (ed.): Clinical Patterns and Pathological Features in Osteoarthritis. J. Rheumatol. (Suppl. 9), 1983.

102. Reginato, A.J., Schumacher, H.R., and Brighton, C.T.: Experimental hydroxyapatite (HA) articular calcification. Arthritis Rheum. 21:585, 1978.

103. Dieppe, P.A., Crocker, P., Huskisson, E.C., et al.: Apatite deposition disease. A new arthropathy. Lancet 1:266, 1976.

104. Schumacher, H.R., Tse, R., Reginato, A., Miller, J., and Maurer, K.: Hydroxyapatite-like crystals in synovial fluid cell vacuoles: A suspected new cause for crystal-induced arthritis. Arthritis Rheum. 19:821, 1976.

105. McCarty, D.J., and Gatter, R.A.: Recurrent acute inflammation associated with focal apatite crystal deposition. Arthritis Rheum. 9:804, 1966.

106. McCarty, D.J., Halverson, P.B., Carrera, G.F., et al.: "Milwaukee Shoulder"—Association of microspheroids containing hydroxyapatite crystals, active collagenase and neutral protease with rotator cuff defects. I. Clinical aspects. Arthritis Rheum. 24:464, 1981.

107. Halverson, P.B., Cheung, H.S., McCarty, D.J., et al.: "Milwaukee Shoulder"—Association of microspheroids containing hydroxyapatite crystals, active collagenase and neutral protease with rotator cuff defects. II. Synovial fluid studies. Arthritis Rheum. 24:474, 1981.

108. Garancis, J.C., Cheung, H.S., Halverson, P.B., et al.: "Milwaukee Shoulder"—Association of microspheroids containing hydroxyapatite crystals, active collagenase and neutral protease with rotator cuff defects. III. Morphologic and biochemical studies of an excised synovium showing chondromatosis. Arthritis Rheum. 24:484, 1981.

109. Bird, H.A., Tribe, C.R., and Bacon, P.A.: Joint hypermobility leading to osteoarthrosis and chondrocalcinosis. Ann. Rheum. Dis. 37:203, 1978.

110. Ali, S.Y., and Griffiths, S.: New types of calcium phosphate crystals in arthritic cartilage. Osteoarthritis Symposium. Semin. Arthritis Rheum. XI(Suppl. 1): 124, 1981.

Section XIV

Degenerative Joint Disease and Other Primary Diseases of Cartilage

Chapter 88

Pathogenesis of Osteoarthritis

Kenneth D. Brandt

Chapter 89 details the descriptive pathology of osteoarthritis (OA) and emphasizes the two principal morphologic changes associated with the disease: (1) progressive focal disintegration of the articular cartilage and (2) formation of new bone in the floor of the cartilage lesion and at the joint margins (osteophytes). The sequence of these pathologic changes, their inter-relationship, and their pathogenesis are not yet well understood. In this field today most workers hold the concept that the pathologic changes of OA are the consequence of a wide variety of etiologic factors that cause mechanical injury to the joint, evoking a response that results in breakdown of the articular cartilage.[1-3]

Although it has been proposed that the primary abnormality in OA may occur in the synovium[4] or subchondral bone,[5] most of the current theories on its pathogenesis focus upon primary alterations in the articular cartilage.[1-3] A brief review of the molecular organization of normal joint cartilage and of the biomechanics of the joint may help indicate major structure-function relationships and provide some background for discussion of the changes related to the disease.

NORMAL ARTICULAR CARTILAGE

Biochemical Composition. The cartilage covering the ends of the bones within diarthrodial joints has two essential mechanical functions: (1) It is a bearing surface that permits smooth gliding of the osseous structures over each other during movement of the joint, and (2) it supports load. The biochemical properties that permit articular cartilage to subserve these functions depend upon the chemical composition and macromolecular organization of its extracellular ground substance, or matrix; the cells constitute only about 5 percent of the total volume of adult articular cartilage.[6] The matrix consists chiefly of two macromolecular species—collagen and proteoglycans (PGs; formerly designated proteinpoly-saccharides)—which account for about 50 percent and 10 percent, respectively, of the dry weight of joint cartilage.

Glycosaminoglycans and Proteoglycans. The glycosaminoglycans (GAGs) (formerly designated mucopolysaccharides) of articular cartilage are keratan sulfate and chondroitin sulfate. The latter exists in two isomeric forms, with the sulfate moiety residing in the 4- or 6-position, respectively, of the galactosamine residue. In normal adult articular cartilage, chondroitin 6-sulfate predominates, whereas immature cartilage contains chiefly chondroitin 4-sulfate.[7] In addition to these sulfated GAGs, cartilage contains small quantities of hyaluronic acid (less than 1 percent of the total uronic acid of the tissue), which plays an essential role in aggregation of the PGs[8,9] (see Chapter 15).

The relative proportions of chondroitin sulfate and keratan sulfate vary throughout the depth of articular cartilage, with keratan sulfate constituting a relatively larger proportion of the total GAG content in deeper layers. The topographic distribution of the GAGs exhibits much individual variation,[10] which does not correlate with age or sex but may be genetically determined (i.e., the "fingerprint" of the cartilage)[11] or may reflect stresses. Thus, the biochemical composition of the matrix may reflect local biomechanical requirements.

Several reports have suggested a causal relationship between the GAG content of connective tissue and the mechanical stress to which it is subjected. The chondroitin sulfate content of weight-bearing areas of cartilage is greater than that of non-weight-bearing regions of the same joint.[12] Similarly, GAGs constitute a higher proportion of the dry weight of weight-bearing sites than of non-weight-bearing sites of dermis.[13] A study of the GAG content in the rabbit flexor digitorum profundus tendon is also relevant to this concept.[14] This tendon contains a thickened region that is normally subjected to compressive forces at the point at which it is in contact with the calcaneus. In this thickened region, the GAG content is 15-fold greater than in the non-pressure-bearing (tension-transmitting) portion. Dermatan sulfate is the predominant GAG in the tensional areas, whereas a twofold to threefold increase in the proportion of chondroitin sulfate occurs in the pressure-bearing region, with a concomitant decrease in dermatan sulfate. When forces were reversed by translocation of the tendon, the GAG content in the original tension-transmitting region increased, and the original pressure-bearing region showed a rapid loss of GAG.[15] Replacement of the tendon to its normal position restored the GAG content to normal levels in both areas. In a more direct test of the effect of mechanical stress on GAG metabolism, cultured smooth muscle cells from aorta showed an increase in GAG synthesis when subjected to high gravity (g) forces by centrifugation.[16]

Static compressive loading (at physiologic stresses) of calf and human articular cartilage slices in vitro reversibly reduced sulfur-35 (^{35}S) incorporation into GAGs.[17] Defined static and cyclic compressive stresses of physiologic magnitudes suppress or stimulate, respectively, GAG synthesis in organ cultures of normal canine knee cartilage.[18]

Traumatic loading in vivo has also been shown to affect cartilage metabolism. Thus, rabbit knee cartilage subjected to repetitive impulse loading of physiologic magnitude showed a transient increase in GAG synthesis in vivo.[19] Also, canine patellar cartilage showed a transient increase in water and uronic acid content following a single traumatic impact load delivered by a drop tower in vivo.[20] Thus, the evidence suggests a good correlation between compressive stress and the GAG content of joint cartilage in vivo.

Chondroitin sulfate and keratan sulfate do not exist free in cartilage, but are covalently linked to proteins to form PGs.[21] On average, some 50 to 100 chains of chondroitin sulfate are appended to each PG protein molecule,[22,23] which represents about 10 percent of the weight of the molecule and is situated internally with respect to the GAG chains, thus creating a molecule with a bottle-brush configuration (Figs. 15-3 and 15-4) in Chapter 15. The average molecular weight (MW) of a single chondroitin sulfate chain is about 15,000 to 20,000 daltons[24] and the average MW of the protein core is about 200,000 daltons, so that articular cartilage PGs have average molecular weights of 1 to 3 million daltons.[25,26]

A discussion of the molecular structure of cartilage PGs, and of their macromolecular organization in articular cartilage, is provided in Chapter 15. In brief, because of their structure the PGs are extremely hydrophilic, and they account for the fact that water represents some 70 to 80 percent of the total weight of articular cartilage.[10] This high degree of hydration provides the tissue with its elastic resistance to compression.[27] Conversely, the molecular structure of the PG renders it especially vulnerable to degradation by proteolytic enzymes; cleavage of only one or two peptide bonds on the protein core may totally destroy the molecule.[21] Most of the PGs in cartilage exist in noncovalent association

with hyaluronic acid and specific link glycoproteins, in enormous aggregates with molecular weights of 100 million daltons or greater.[8,9,28,29] The purpose of this PG aggregation is unknown, but it may help constrain individual PGs in the collagen meshwork of cartilage and provide the PGs with some protection from proteolytic degradation.[28] In addition, aggregation may help sustain the stiffening of the interacting network of PG molecules produced by shear forces.[30]

Collagen. Whereas the PGs impart elasticity to articular cartilage and resistance to compression, collagen affords tensile strength[31] and serves to constrain the PGs. In the superficial layer of the cartilage (lamina splendens) most of the collagen fibers are oriented parallel to the joint surface, protecting it like a skin against the abrasive forces generated during joint motion. In contrast, the collagen fibers in the deeper layers extend upward toward the surface and downward through the zone of calcified cartilage to embed in subchondral bone.

Collagen is not evenly distributed throughout the depth of the cartilage; its content diminishes progressively from the superficial layer to the deeper zones. Enormous individual variation occurs in the collagen content of the superficial layer, which may range from 90 percent in some cases to 45 percent in others.[31] The basis for this variation is unclear, but as discussed previously in relation to variations in GAG distribution, it appears to be characteristic of each individual cartilage.[11] Cartilage that contains more collagen in the superficial zone may be better able to withstand the stresses of impact loading and abrasive forces during joint movement than can cartilage that contains less collagen.

Collagen is an important determinant of the form of the cartilage. Thus, when cartilage was treated with trypsin or hyaluronidase so that most of the PGs were degraded with little loss of collagen, the tissue's shape was unchanged though its resistance to compression was markedly reduced. In contrast, although the tissue showed relatively little change in its ability to resist compression after treatment with collagenase, its thickness was diminished.[32]

The collagen of normal articular cartilage is phenotypically unique (type II) and consists of three identical α-chains [α I(II)]$_3$, which differ in amino acid composition and primary sequence from the α-chains of other collagens in the body, such as those in skin, tendon, or bone.[33,34] The most striking feature of type II collagen is its high content of hydroxylysine and glycosidically bound carbohydrate, which is five times as great as that of type I collagen. In addition, type II collagen is more resistant to digestion with collagenase than is type I collagen.[35] Ionic association may occur between ε-amino groups of the lysine and hydroxylysine residues of collagen and the negatively charged moieties of the GAGs, and these interactions may be further stabilized by hydrogen bonding to the glucosyl-galactosyl residues of the collagen.[36]

Collagenous proteins that are distinct from the α_1(II) chain of type II collagen have been described in normal articular cartilage.[37] Type I collagen has been identified in the superficial zone of joint cartilage,[38] and the minor collagens, type A and type B, have been found in the pericellular zone,[39] in which they are interwoven with hyaluronate and PGs to form a "capsule" that may serve to shield the chondrocyte from stress. Because of their pericellular location, these minor collagens will come in contact with newly synthesized PGs as they are secreted by the cell, and may thus be of great importance in organizing the immediate pericellular matrix. Chondronectin, a noncollagenous protein recently identified in articular cartilage, may be important in establishing an interaction between the chondrocytes and the surrounding collagen.[40,41]

In vitro, chondrocytes may synthesize type I or type III collagen.[42-44] Furthermore, when aspirin was fed to normal dogs while cartilage atrophy was being induced by immobilization of a leg, type I collagen was synthesized in vivo,[45] although the bulk of the collagen remained type II. Notably, no type I collagen could be seen in atrophic cartilage of dogs that were not fed aspirin, or after aspirin administration to normal dogs.

In general, interactions between collagen and PGs in cartilage are not well understood. The PGs appear to give the fibers mechanical stability, since the shrinkage temperature of collagen in the deeper zones of normal human articular cartilage is as high as 90° C, whereas that of skin collagen is about 56° C. Significant correlations have been found between the shrinkage temperature of cartilage collagen and the hexosamine (i.e., PG) content of the tissue, which would explain why the shrinkage temperature of collagen in OA cartilage, in which the PG content is diminished, is as low as that of dermal collagen.[46] PGs may also have a functional role in determining the size or organization, or both, of collagen fibrils in the tissue, since even in very low concentrations they retard precipitation of collagen fibrils from physiologic solutions.[47] This may account for the observation that collagen fibrils in cartilage of mutant chondrodysplastic C57 BL1/Fr mice, which suffer from a genetic defect in PG synthesis,[48] are thicker than normal.

Metabolism of Normal Cartilage Matrix (see Chapter 15). The PGs, collagen, link proteins, and hyaluronic acid of cartilage are all synthesized by the chondrocyte, which also regulates their degradation. In addition, a number of other noncollagenous proteins are present in articular cartilage and appear to be synthesized by the chondrocyte. They include proteolytic enzymes,[49-51] enzyme inhibitors,[52] lysozyme,[53] insoluble structural glycoproteins,[54,55] chondronectin, and a number of[66] matrix proteins,"[56-60] whose functions are unknown. This complex composition may influence the organization of the PGs in the matrix.

Normal adult cartilage is avascular; the chondrocyte receives its nutrients from the synovial fluid.[61] Some intermittent joint motion (or load-bearing), which provides compression, may be necessary to distribute nutrients through the cartilage and to remove catabolites. This may explain why PG synthesis was decreased by 40 percent in articular cartilage of a normal dog whose

leg had been immobilized in a cast for only 6 days.[62] In that study, following 3 weeks of restraint, atrophy of the cartilage was noted, and PG aggregation was no longer demonstrable. Although these changes were rapidly reversible when casts were removed after a few weeks,[62] longer periods of immobilization produced irreversible changes in the joint, with atrophy of the synovium, complete cartilage destruction, and ankylosis.[63] In contrast, continuous passive motion of the joint has been shown to facilitate healing of cartilage injury.[64]

Matrix Synthesis. The collagen in normal joint cartilage has been considered to be extremely stable metabolically, and most of the collagen appears to have an infinite half-life.[65] However, a fraction of the collagen of normal rabbit knee cartilage has been shown to have a half-life of only a few months.[66] The PGs turn over more rapidly than the collagen, though they exhibit considerable metabolic heterogeneity. Mankin and Lippiello estimated that a fraction of the GAGs in adult rabbit cartilage had a half-life of only 8 days,[67] whereas other data have indicated that the mean half-life of the sulfated GAGs synthesized in cartilage of immature rabbits is about 45 days and that the half-life of those synthesized in human cartilage is 250 to 600 days.[68] The disappearance rate of radionuclide tracers of PG synthesis appears to be similar throughout the depth of the cartilage,[69] providing no indication that cartilage surface is being shed selectively. This turnover of PGs reflects, instead, a normal remodeling process enzymatically mediated within the tissue. The processes required for synthesis of PGs and collagen appear to be independent, since interference in the synthesis of one does not affect the other.[70,71]

The chondrocytes are highly responsive to changes in their extracellular milieu. Thus, when the matrix of chick embryonic cartilage was depleted in vitro by enzymatic digestion, it was resynthesized by the cells in only a few days.[72] Removal of 80 percent of the chondroitin sulfate by digestion with hyaluronidase caused the cells to synthesize five times as much PG as was noted in controls.[73] The newly synthesized PGs, however, had a lower uronic acid:protein ratio than normal, whereas their chondroitin sulfate chain lengths were normal. This would indicate that the core protein contained fewer chondroitin sulfate chains than normal, suggesting that the capacity of the chondrocyte for repair of the matrix may be limited.

The factor or factors—chemical, mechanical, or other—effecting the metabolic response of the chondrocyte to changes in its extracellular milieu are largely unknown. However, hyaluronic acid, when added to the culture medium, has been shown to be a potent inhibitor of PG synthesis by chondrocytes from adult[74] and embryonic[75] cartilage. This effect of hyaluronate appears to be as specific as its interaction with PGs in aggregation (see Chapter 15), and it is similarly inhibited by oligosaccharides of hyaluronic acid.[75] Inhibition of PG synthesis by hyaluronic acid requires the attachment of the latter to the cell surface; the inhibition is not seen if the cell surface is perturbed by mild trypsinization prior to the addition of hyaluronate, or if the hyaluronic acid is not free but rather is present in PG aggregates. Handley and Lowther have suggested that hyaluronic acid may suppress synthesis of the PG core protein or of the glycosyltransferase involved in the initiation of synthesis of chondroitin sulfate chains.[76]

Matrix Catabolism. Since the collagen and PGs in normal cartilage are not metabolically inert, mechanisms for their degradation must exist. Although collagenase activity could not be demonstrated in normal human cartilage,[77] with the use of fluorescein-labeled specific anticollagenase antiserum, immunoreactive enzyme was found to be widely distributed throughout normal articular cartilage.[78] This suggests that an inhibitor may play an important regulatory role in collagen metabolism in the normal joint or that collagenase may be present in the form of proenzyme. Kuettner has isolated a low-MW (11,000 daltons) cationic protein[79] from normal articular cartilage, which inhibits collagenase and may play a role in preventing the invasion of cartilage by blood vessels.[80]

The PGs in articular cartilage may be degraded by a variety of mechanisms. When large doses of vitamin A were administered to rabbits, articular cartilage matrix was digested, owing to the release of enzymes with papain-like activity from the chondrocytes.[81] As indicated previously, the molecular structure of the PG makes the protein core particularly vulnerable to digestion by proteases. Considerable attention has been directed toward the lysosomal proteinases of cartilage, particularly cathepsins, D, B1, and F,[82] all of which degrade cartilage PGs. Since the cathepsins have acid rather than neutral pH optima, and since they are inactive at pH 7 (the pH of the matrix), they probably exert their effects intracellularly and in the immediate vicinity of the cell surface. A metalloproteinase that degrades PGs at a neutral pH is also present in normal human joint cartilage.[83] Although it is present in much smaller quantities than the acid proteinases, it could account for digestion of the matrix between cells. In addition, the synovium may have an indirect effect on the breakdown of cartilage matrix. Synovial tissue, explanted at a distance from living cartilage but grown in the same culture dish, causes depletion of both PGs and collagen in the cartilage. Since the effect is not seen with dead cartilage, the results suggest that it is not enzymatic and is mediated by activation of chondrocytes.[84] This activity has been named "catabolin"; it appears to be released by mononuclear cells and stimulates the chondrocyte to synthesize and release collagenese and other neutral proteases.[85,86] The degradative effects of the neutral proteinases and cathepsins may be balanced in vivo and may be modulated by small proteins that are native to the cartilage and exhibit antiproteinase activity.[87]

The enzymes that can degrade the chondroitin sulfate chain can be classified as exo- or endoglycosidases. The former attack only the terminal nonreducing sugar and are not capable of cleaving *within* an intact poly- or oligosaccharide. The latter, in contrast, will cleave the intact GAG. Because of the very great differences in substrate level, any given degree of digestion of a GAG chain requires much more exo- than endoenzyme.

Hyaluronidase, an endoglycosidase that degrades chondroitin sulfate chains to oligosaccharides (and for which the hyaluronic acid in the PG aggregate would also serve as substrate), has an acid pH optimum similar to that of the cathepsins, suggesting that it, too, is most active intracellularly. Although it is present in synovial membrane and synovial fluid, hyaluronidase had not been found in joint cartilage[88] until recently when hyaluronidase activity, which appeared to be lysosomal in origin (its pH optimum was about 3), was identified in normal articular cartilage.[89] Notably, the activity appeared to be specific for hyaluronate and could not be demonstrated when chondroitin was employed as a substrate. No other enzyme with endoglycosidase activity has yet been demonstrated in adult articular cartilage. Normal chondrocytes contain exoglycosidases, for example, exo-β-n-D-hexosaminidase and exo-β-D-glucuronidase,[90] that will digest oligosaccharides (such as would result from hyaluronidase-like activity) to monosaccharides. The extent to which they perform this function in adult articular cartilage is unclear, since intravenously injected chondroitin sulfate chains, which are rapidly degraded to monomers,[91] are broken down in the liver rather than in cartilage.[92] Arylsulfatases are present, but an enzyme has not yet been identified in cartilage that can cleave sulfate from undegraded chondroitin sulfate or keratan sulfate chains.

As already indicated, aggregation provides the PG with relative resistance to proteolytic digestion.[28] The size of aggregates, and hence their susceptibility to degradation, may be regulated by lysozyme,[93] which is present in cartilage in large amounts. Like the tissue inhibitors of collagenase and other proteases already described, lysozyme is a small (MW 14,000 daltons) cationic protein. It has enzymatic activity and specifically cleaves the linkage between *N*-acetylmuramic acid and *N*-acetylglucosamine, which, notably, is present only in cell walls of certain bacteria. Whether it functions as an enzyme in cartilage is unknown; no substrate for lysozyme in mammalian tissue has been identified. Cartilage lysozyme shows a marked increase in activity after electrophoresis, suggesting that it may be associated with an inhibitor in the tissue. It appears to play an important role in calcification of growth cartilage[94] by dissociating PG aggregates, an effect that seems to be restricted to the aggregates of largest size (60 S or greater). Since these superaggregates inhibit precipitation of calcium phosphate, this action of lysozyme leads to matrix mineralization. The molecular mechanism by which lysozyme regulates the size of PG aggregates is not clear. A decrease in the sedimentation velocity of hyaluronic acid has been noted in the presence of lysozyme,[95] but other studies have not supported a hyaluronidase-like action for the molecule,[96] and whether or not it is a regulator of PG aggregation in normal adult cartilage requires further study.

Biomechanical Consequences of the Macromolecular

Organization of Normal Articular Cartilage. Weight-bearing joints are obviously subjected to repeated, localized high loads. Although the soft tissues (e.g., capsule and muscles) and subchondral bone play major roles in dissipating the energy of weight-bearing, considerable mechanical force is nonetheless transmitted to the cartilage. Normal joint cartilage dissipates this force by virtue of its special properties (e.g., compressibility, elasticity, self-lubrication), all of which are attributable to its chemical composition and to the interactions that occur among collagen, PGs, and other molecular constituents. If it were not for this effect of the cartilage, bone would be quickly worn away by the frictional forces within the joint.

Because of its high GAG content, cartilage has low hydraulic permeability,[97] which limits the amount of interstitial fluid lost from the surface when it is loaded in compression. Thus, when load is applied, the pressure within the cartilage rises immediately, but the cartilage deforms gradually and reversibly as water is surrendered to the joint surface. When the load is removed, the layer of exuded fluid on the surface is reimbibed.

As noted, the high fixed negative charge density of the PGs allows them to hold enormous amounts of water, so that constraint of the PGs by the collagen meshwork creates considerable swelling pressure in the tissue.[98] This pressure—in the absence of load—has been calculated to be greater than 3 atmospheres.[99] Nonetheless, normal cartilage does not swell when placed in solution, implying that the high swelling pressure of the PGs is counteracted by strong tensile forces within the collagen network.

In weight-bearing, the collagen network is subjected to even greater tensile stresses. When compressive load is applied to cartilage, the flow of water will be impeded by the high interstitial swelling pressure and low hydraulic permeability of the tissue, but the aqueous PG gel will attempt to move away from the loaded region. However, the pressure gradient will restrict upward flow, and the subchondral bone will oppose downward flow. Flow will therefore occur mainly in a lateral direction, at which point it will be restricted by the collagen network. The network will therefore receive forces acting radially from the center of the applied load, whose main vector will be parallel to the joint surface. It has been shown that tensile strength of articular cartilage is greater in this direction than in a plane perpendicular to the surface.

It should be understood that the functional collagen network of cartilage consists not only of the collagen fibers but also of substances that cement them together[100] to help inhibit slippage of adjacent fibers over each other. These substances have not been defined but presumably consist, at least in part, of the PGs that are closely associated with the collagen. Although the collagen fibers themselves are held together by very strong covalent peptide bonds that should resist any of the mechanical forces transmitted to the matrix, the cementing substances may be vulnerable to mechanical damage, and this may be a proximate or contributing factor in de-

generation of joint cartilage in OA (see later discussion).

OSTEOARTHRITIC CARTILAGE

The principal biochemical change that occurs in OA cartilage appears to be a loss in the tissue content of PGs, which occurs while the collagen content remains normal.[101-103] The factors that lead to depletion of the matrix PGs, and the biomechanical consequences of the PG deficiency, are central to the pathogenesis of OA.

Changes in PGs. The following changes are typical of OA: (1) a decrease in the tissue content of PGs;[101-103] (2) a decrease in PG aggregation, so that the cartilage contains a larger proportion of unaggregated PGs, and aggregates that are present are smaller than normal;[105] (3) an increase in the extractability of the PGs from the cartilage;[105] (4) a decrease in the chondroitin sulfate chain length;[106] and (5) a change in GAG composition, so that the PGs tend to contain a much lower proportion of keratan sulfate than chondroitin sulfate, and a much higher proportion of chondroitin 4-sulfate than chondroitin 6-sulfate.[6]

In some cases of OA the aggregation defect appears to be due to a functional abnormality of the hyaluronate-binding region of the PG core protein. In these instances when PGs isolated from the diseased tissue are incubated in vitro with high-MW hyaluronic acid, no evidence of PG-hyaluronate interaction is observed. In other cases in which the severity of the aggregation defect may be indistinguishable from the preceding, PGs isolated from the OA cartilage undergo extensive aggregation with hyaluronic acid in vitro, implying that the aggregation defect in vivo may have been due to an abnormality in the hyaluronic acid rather than in the PGs.[107,108] Whatever its cause, the aggregation defect may account for the fact that PGs are more readily extractable from the matrix of OA cartilage than normal cartilage,[104] but the latter could also indicate an abnormality in PG-collagen interactions within OA cartilage.

The increased ratios of chondroitin sulfate:keratan sulfate and of chondroitin 4-sulfate:chondroitin 6-sulfate in OA cartilage were initially presumed to represent synthesis of a more immature type of cartilage by the chondrocyte.[6] Metabolic studies,[109] however, have shown that patterns of synthesis of keratan sulfate, chondroitin 4-sulfate, and chondroitin 6-sulfate were the same in OA cartilage as in normal cartilage. This suggested that the altered GAG composition of OA cartilage is due not to an alteration in synthesis but to a change in GAG degradation, with enzymatic cleavage of the PG core protein, splitting off a fragment poor in chondroitin 4-sulfate and rich in keratan sulfate,[109] which is rapidly broken down. This may result in diminished PG-collagen interaction in the cartilage, since the 6-sulfate moiety projects out farther from the GAG chain than the 4-sulfate group does.[110]

It has been suggested that the decrease in chondroitin sulfate chain length in OA is due to digestion of chondroitin sulfate chains by synovial fluid hyaluronidase,[106] which may diffuse into the cartilage once the disease process has been initiated. Chondroitin-sulfate degrading activity has not been demonstrated in cartilage, however, and an abnormality in GAG synthesis has not been excluded in OA.

Despite the decrease in the tissue content of PGs in the early stages of OA, PG synthesis, as well as that of protein and DNA (indicating cell replication), is increased.[111] Furthermore, PG synthesis continues to rise in proportion to the severity of the lesion until the disease, by morphologic criteria, is far advanced. When the disease becomes sufficiently severe, however, PG synthesis falls off sharply—that is, the chondrocyte "fails."[111] The fall in the tissue content of PGs that occurs in the face of an increase in PG synthesis must indicate an even greater increase in PG catabolism. Numerous studies point to the fact that the activity of endogenous acid and neutral proteinases is increased in OA cartilage in comparison with normal cartilage. Since OA cartilage appears to be deficient in its content of endogenous proteinase inhibitor,[87] an imbalance may exist between the proteoglycanases of cartilage and their inhibitors, a factor that could be important in the pathogenesis of the cartilage breakdown. Glynn has proposed[4] that a deficiency of proteinase inhibitors, synthesized not by the chondrocytes but by the B lymphocytes in the synovial lining, may underlie the development of OA. This possibility warrants further study.

Changes in Collagen. Collagen synthesis in OA cartilage[115] is also substantially greater than normal, and it increases progressively with the severity of the disease until the lesion becomes sufficiently severe that collagen synthesis falls, which is associated with chondrocyte failure. Collagenolytic activity has been demonstrated in human OA cartilage,[77] and it appeared to be caused by an enzyme that was bound to a trypsin-sensitive inhibitor.

As noted, normal articular cartilage contains type II collagen.[33,34] Although cartilage from an osteoarthritic femoral head has been reported to contain type I as well as type II[116] collagen, suggesting that collagen synthesis by the OA chondrocyte underwent a phenotypic change, other studies have shown only type II collagen in fibrillated OA cartilage.[46,117] When an immunofluorescence technique[118] was applied to the study of collagen in OA cartilage, some type I collagen was found around chondrocyte clusters in fibrillated cartilage, but antibody to type I collagen did not localize to the bulk of the diseased tissue.

The Earliest Matrix Changes. How does OA begin? The early stages of naturally occurring OA cannot be readily studied because onset of the disease cannot be determined accurately. Some experimental animal models of OA, such as the rabbit partial meniscectomy model[119] and the dog model produced by section of the anterior cruciate ligament,[120] fortunately simulate all the progressive morphologic changes of naturally occurring OA and afford an opportunity to study the earliest changes of the disease. Both represent models of "sec-

ondary" OA produced by internal derangement of the knee joint.

Particular attention has been paid to the initial biochemical changes in the dog model, in which the very first alteration appears to be an increase in the water content of the cartilage. This is detectable within days after transection of the cruciate ligament[121,122] and, at first, occurs focally in cartilage of the tibial plateau and femoral condyle. Soon, however, it spreads to the entire cartilage of the joint. A similar increase in water content has been noted in human OA cartilage.[106]

The PG content of the canine cartilage is not diminished in the initial stages, but the PGs are more readily extractable from the matrix than under normal conditions. This enhanced extractability of the PGs is also seen in spontaneously occurring OA in dogs[122] and steers[105] and in experimentally induced OA in rabbits.[123] It may be attributed to the increase in tissue water content, which permits greater permeability of the extracting solvent.[126]

The proximate cause of the increase in water content of OA cartilage is not known, but the increase implies a failure in the elastic restraint of the collagen network, enabling the PGs to swell to a higher degree of hydration than normal.[124] Studies of the cartilage ultrastructure in the early stages of OA show a loss of orientation of the collagen fibers near the surface, with individual fibers being more widely separated than normal.

Very shortly after the increase in cartilage water, the newly synthesized PGs in the canine model show a change in their GAG composition and contain a higher proportion of chondroitin sulfate and a lower proportion of keratan sulfate than normal.[121] Aggregation may be impaired in the earliest stages.[125]

It should be noted that all the aforementioned changes in the dog model occur throughout the entire articular cartilage before fibrillation or other morphologic change is evident and while the tissue PG content is normal. They provide an explanation for the generalized decrease in stiffness that occurs in visibly normal cartilage taken from sites adjacent to fibrillated areas.[126] With progression of the disease in subsequent months, focal cartilage ulcerations develop in which losses of PG are seen, accompanied by worsening of the PG aggregation defects, persistence of the abnormalities in GAG composition, and decreases in chondroitin sulfate chain length. As the loss of PG becomes sufficiently great, the water content, which initially increased, falls below normal. Thus, the sequence of events in this experimental model suggests that the first change may occur in the collagen meshwork, permitting swelling of the tissue, followed very shortly by a change in the type of PG synthesized by the chondrocyte and a change in PG aggregation.

The operational concept of pathogenesis that has been held by many workers since it was proposed by Bollet in 1967[127] is that physical (mechanical) stresses injure the chondrocyte, causing it to release enzymes that cause fibrillation and matrix breakdown. In contrast, and as proposed by Freeman,[100] mechanical effects may initially damage the collagen network rather than the cell. Thus, although fibrillated cartilage from OA samples undoubtedly shows a reduction in PG content, it is not clear at this time whether PG depletion precedes fibrillation or results from it.

Biomechanical Alterations Resulting from the Biochemical Changes in OA. The loss of PGs from the matrix in OA cartilage leads to a loss of compressive stiffness and elasticity of the cartilage and to an increase in its hydraulic permeability. The former can be expected to lead to transmission of increased mechanical force to the chondrocytes. The latter, among other effects, will result in loss of interstitial fluid and an increased diffusion of molecules through the cartilage. Pathogenetically, this may be particularly relevant to the diffusion of degradative enzymes and their inhibitors into the cartilage from the synovial fluid and through the cartilage away from the border of the chondrocyte that has synthesized them. As already noted, the loss of cartilage PGs will affect cartilage self-lubrication by impairing generation of the surface "squeeze-film." Figure 88–1 is a servodiagram that shows the relationship of these factors to other events in the pathogenesis of OA.

Osteophytes and Bony Proliferation in OA. It is obvious from the foregoing discussion that much attention has been directed to the mechanisms of cartilage breakdown in OA. Less attention has been focused on the pathogenesis of the bony proliferation that occurs at the joint margins and in the floor of the cartilage lesions, which may be responsible for restriction of motion of the OA joint and for some of the pain. Osteophytes from human osteoarthritic joints synthesize sulfated PGs that are similar to those of normal adult human cartilage with respect to monomer size and their predominance of chondroitin 6-sulfate, but that are relatively deficient in keratan sulfate and tend not to interact with hyaluronic acid.[128]

The relationship of osteophytes to cartilage degeneration in OA is not entirely clear. In experimentally induced OA, osteophytes may develop while the cartilage is still normal.[129] By increasing the amount of joint surface available for load-bearing, in some cases they may be associated with a tendency to remission.[130] It has been suggested that osteophytes occur as a result of the proliferation of blood vessels into sites of degenerating cartilage.[131] The vascular ingrowth may occur, alternatively, during healing of fractures of subchondral trabeculae (see earlier discussion) near the joint margins.[132] In experimentally induced OA caused by section of the cruciate ligament in dogs, periarticular osteophyte formation was noted to commence in the marginal zone at the point at which synovium merges with fibrocartilage as early as 3 days after induction of instability.[133] Bone hyperplasia occurred also beneath nonarticulating cartilage and was thus not confined to development of the osteophyte. An increase in vascularity was associated with the development of new bone at the earliest stages, both in the osteophyte and internally at sites of bony remodeling.

Other studies have shown that bony proliferation may result from venous congestion.[134] In humans with OA of the hip, venography has demonstrated a marked alteration in the pattern of venous drainage,[135] presumably due to changes in the medullary sinusoids, which may be compressed by subchondral cysts and thickened subchondral trabeculae, leading to formation of medullary varices. The subchondral cysts of OA may be caused by entry of synovial fluid under pressure through defects in the diseased cartilage,[136] or they may develop in necrotic areas of the subchondral bone. The increased venous pressure caused by the cysts and remodeled trabeculae probably accounts for some of the pain in OA.

Marginal osteophytes have also been produced in dog knee joints by repeated injections of autogenous cartilage homogenates.[137] The osteophytic change was preceded by thickening of the cartilage at the chondrosynovial junction, and it was suggested that the pluripotential cells at this site were stimulated to form osteophytes by the prolonged presence of cartilage debris. By analogy, the slough of cartilage from the joint surface may be a factor in the cause of the low-grade synovitis in OA, and perhaps also of osteophyte formation. Chondroitin sulfate has been shown to activate Hageman factor (factor XII),[138] leading to triggering of the kinin pathway. If this also occurs in vivo, it may account for the mononuclear cell infiltration of the synovium and the vascular hyperplasia of the OA membrane. The low-grade synovitis leads to capsular thickening and fibrotic shortening, which may cause pain and muscle spasm.[139]

Whatever the cause of osteophytes, immobilization of the joint appears to effectively prevent their formation,[140,141] and injections of triamcinolone acetonide, 3 mg per week for 6 weeks, markedly decreased the prevalence of osteophytes in a rabbit model of experimentally induced OA, though femoral cartilage ulcerations were unaffected.[142]

Etiologic Factors in OA. The previous parts of this chapter have focused on mechanisms of cartilage damage in OA (i.e., on *pathogenetic* factors). It is likely that there is no single "cause" of OA—that no *one* factor triggers the processes that result in cartilage destruction. Furthermore, since changes in any of the constituents of the joint (e.g., collagen, PG, chondrocytes, subchondral bone, synovial membrane) may affect the other constituents, the degeneration process in the articular cartilage may be initiated in a variety of ways.

Clinically, it is useful to classify OA into "primary" and "secondary" forms. This emphasizes the relationship to OA of certain diseases (e.g., chondrocalcinosis, alkaptonuria), whose presence at times may not be immediately apparent. The following portion of this chapter considers some of the etiologic factors implicated in OA. It is written from these three perspectives: (1) that the morphologic changes of OA are the consequences of altered cartilage physiology; (2) that not all of the etiologies of OA can legitimately be viewed as "diseases," but that some represent, instead, states of altered physiology; and (3) that, in this sense, all OA is "secondary."

The two concepts of OA etiology most widely held by both lay people and physicians are (1) that it is a "wear and tear" disease, and (2) that it is an inevitable concomitant of aging. What is the supporting evidence for each of these views?

Wear-and-Tear. Repeated use of a joint could theoretically break down cartilage by two mechanisms: (1) abrasion from repeated oscillation of the moving surfaces or (2) degeneration from repetitive impact loading.

Oscillatory Stress on the Joint. Articular cartilage is remarkably resistant to damage by shear forces.[143] When joints are subjected to repeated oscillation in vitro, the cartilage does not wear, even under the maximal constant loads that can be borne by subchondral bone.[144] For joints not to wear under these conditions, the joint surfaces must be kept apart. The subject of joint lubrication has received extensive attention; the evidence suggests that multiple mechanisms serve to prevent cartilage-on-cartilage wear.

Cartilage Lubrication Under High Load Conditions. Under high loading, lubrication is provided chiefly by a film of fluid squeezed out of the cartilage in areas adjacent to the zone of impending contact.[145] Since the flow of fluid in cartilage is restricted by the subchondral plate and the highly hydrophilic PGs, when cartilage is compressed its interstitial fluid is instantly pressurized and takes much of the load. This pressurization of the tissue prevents the lubricating fluid film that has seeped out of the cartilage from flowing back into it. In addition, the elasticity of the cartilage in the moving joint (also attributable to the PGs) causes stenosis at the margins of the zone of contact, trapping the "squeeze film" between the opposing cartilage surfaces. Under high loads, this trapped "squeeze film" keeps the surfaces apart, preventing damage to the cartilage from shear.

Cartilage Lubrication Under Low Load Conditions. Generation of the "squeeze film" in this self-pressurized lubricating mechanism depends on the presence of a high load on the joint. Under low loads it would be ineffective, and another mechanism—boundary lubrication—which is dependent on the synovial fluid rather than on the cartilage interstitial fluid, is more important.[146]

Boundary lubrication in the joint is due to the presence of a molecular monolayer film that binds to opposing cartilage surfaces and facilitates sliding of one surface over the other. Boundary lubrication may fail under high loads, which may shear the lubricating monolayer off the cartilage surface, but, as noted previously, the high loads will generate an effective "squeeze film."

A glycoprotein that serves as the boundary lubricant has been identified in synovial fluid.[147] This glycoprotein (LGP-1) has a molecular weight of 227,500 daltons and consists of approximately equal proportions of protein and carbohydrate, with about 20 percent of the latter being accounted for by sialic acid. It is absent from serum and articular cartilage and is presumably synthesized by the synovial membrane, though its site of origin has not yet been identified.[148] Whether LGP-1 alone provides all the cartilage-on-cartilage boundary lubrication exhibited by synovial fluid or whether other constituents of the fluid influence its interaction with the cartilage surface is not yet clear.

Hyaluronic acid, which accounts for the viscosity of synovial fluid, is not an effective lubricant in cartilage-on-cartilage systems. Digestion with hyaluronidase, which reduces the viscosity of joint fluid to nearly that of water, does not reduce its lubricating ability in this system.[148] However, hyaluronic acid does provide effective boundary lubrication in the synovium and periarticular soft tissues, in which most of the resistance to joint motion arises.

Joint Lubrication in OA. There is no evidence of a defect in boundary lubrication in OA, even in advanced lesions.[146] Pathologic synovial fluids have been found to be as effective in cartilage-on-cartilage lubrication as fluids from normal joints,[100] although in a latex-glass system[146] one specimen from a patient with a large noninflammatory knee effusion associated with massive edema showed poor lubricating ability, raising the possibility that the lubricating moiety could be diluted out in large effusions. The molecular weight of hyaluronic acid from pathologic synovial fluid is sufficiently great so as not to impair its effectiveness as a lubricant for the synovial soft tissues.[149] Although boundary lubrication may be normal in OA, it is likely that mechanisms for generation of a pressurized lubricating "squeeze film" may be impaired as the disease progresses because of the loss of PGs from OA cartilage and the consequent decrease in elasticity of the tissue.

Stress from Impact Loading. In contrast to its resistance to wear from repeated oscillation under constant load, articular cartilage is highly vulnerable to repetitive impact loading, which will reproducibly cause the joint to wear out. It is likely that this accounts for the high frequency of OA related to joint overload, for example, in shoulders and elbows of pneumatic drill operators and baseball pitchers, ankles of ballet dancers, metacarpophalangeal joints of boxers, and knees of basketball players.

Quantitatively, the major forces on articular cartilage result not from weight-bearing but from contraction of the muscles that stabilize or move the joint.[150] In normal walking (an example par excellence of repetitive impact loading) four to five times the body weight may be transmitted through the knee joint, and in squatting up to ten times the body weight may be transmitted.[61] Considerable attention has recently been directed toward understanding the mechanisms that protect the joint under conditions of physiologic impact loading, since evidence suggests that the articular cartilage itself is too thin to be an effective shock absorber.[151]

The major factors that attenuate shock delivered to the joint appear to be joint motion and the associated lengthening of muscles under tension,[152] as well as deformation of the subchondral bone under load.[5] Seemingly minor, but unanticipated, impulsive loads (e.g., misstepping off a curb, slipping on a stair) have been viewed by some as a major etiologic factor in "idiopathic" joint degeneration. It has been shown that the reaction time required to prepare the neuromuscular apparatus reflexly for an impulse load is about 75 msec.[153] Therefore, unexpected falls of only about 2 cm. allow insufficient time to bring protective reflexes into play and would be associated with transmission of the load to joint structures. In contrast, in falls from higher distances, energy is absorbed by the lengthening of muscles that surround the joint and by motion of joint structures. Obviously, factors that lead to muscle fatigue would tend to impair this shock-absorbing mechanism, as would muscle atrophy or myopathy.

The cancellous subchondral bone, by virtue of its elasticity, functions as a major shock attenuator.[152] Normally, the opposing surfaces of a joint are not congruous in the unloaded condition. Under loading, both the cartilage and bone deform so that a larger proportion of the opposing surfaces comes into contact. This increase in congruity serves to distribute the load over the largest possible area.[154] Excessive loads cause microfractures of the subchondral trabeculae, which heal with callus formation and remodeling. The remodeled trabeculae may be stiffer than normal and less effective as shock absorbers. They cannot, under those conditions, deform normally with load, so that congruity of the joint surfaces with loading is reduced, causing forces to be concentrated at certain sites on the articular cartilage.

A variety of indirect evidence supports the view that physical changes in the subchondral bone may be important in OA. Clinically, an increased incidence of healing microfractures is seen in patients with OA,[155] whereas osteoporosis of the femur, which is associated with softening and greater compliance of the subchondral bone, appears to protect the joint from OA of the hip.[156] Furthermore, in the laboratory, stiffening of the cancellous bone with methacrylate, thereby abolishing its ability to deform, leads promptly to cartilage degeneration under conditions of repetitive impact loading.[157]

It has been suggested[5] that trabecular microfractures may be the *primary* cause of the cartilage degeneration in OA (i.e., that OA is more likely to develop in individuals who have accumulated more microfractures in their lifetime than in those who have not). The evidence for this is not clear, however. When the articular surface of a bone was subjected to repeated impact loading in vitro, fibrillation of the cartilage and ultrastructural changes in the chondrocytes occurred *prior* to changes in the mechanical properties of the subchondral plate.[158]

In summary, with respect to the role of "wear-and-tear" as an etiologic factor in OA, a failure of lubrication does not appear to be at fault, but changes in the subchondral bone produced by accumulated microtraumata may affect its ability to absorb the energy of longitudinal impulse loading of the joint and may thereby lead to cartilage degeneration. The bony changes may contribute significantly—even if they are not primary—to cartilage breakdown in OA.

Neuropathic Joint Degeneration. The degeneration of a joint that results from a disturbance in its sensory innervation (Charcot arthropathy) provides an excellent example of the effects of trauma on articular cartilage. Loss of pain is not necessarily present clinically in such cases, and the abnormality may be due to impairment of nerve impulses from the joint's mechanoreceptors.[159,160] These highly specialized nerve endings, which are located in the capsule, menisci, and ligaments, are

sensitive to joint position and movement. They initiate reflexes that control the tone of the muscles around the joint and check excessive, potentially damaging movement, thus protecting the joint from the ever-present microtrauma incurred in daily activity. If abnormalities in the function of the mechanoreceptors resulted in increased muscle tone, they would increase the load across the joint, and thus could be of pathogenetic importance in the cartilage breakdown in neuropathic joint disease.

The following example indicates that this may indeed occur: When the posterior articular nerve (a purely sensory nerve that supplies capsule, meniscus, and cruciate ligaments and carries mechanoreceptor input) of the knee of normal dogs was transected external to the capsule, within 3 weeks the water content of articular cartilage from the joint increased to a level 16 percent greater than that of controls, and the extractability of the PGs from the cartilage rose so that almost all (92 percent) of the PGs were solubilized from the matrix with guanidinium chloride.[161] These changes, which occurred in the presence of normal histologic conditions, are the same as those that occur in the earliest stages of OA that is produced by section of the cruciate ligament (see earlier discussion). They imply that the microtrauma incurred following deafferentation of a joint causes loosening of the collagen network in the cartilage.

Aging. It has been considered that OA may be the consequence of "aging," that is, intrinsic senescence of articular cartilage—an inevitable "running down" of its machinery. It is possible to define "aging" in another way, however—that is, as the accumulation with time of an ever-increasing number of mechanical insults to the joint. Thus, the distinction between "wear-and-tear" and aging may be somewhat blurred.

What is the evidence that cartilage ages? A number of studies point to the fact that *nonarticular* (e.g., costal, laryngeal) cartilage undergoes a variety of progressive physical and biochemical changes with age, such as a decrease in collagen and water content and an increase in the proportion of keratan sulfate relative to chondroitin sulfate. In sharp contrast, following cessation of growth and development, *articular* cartilage exhibits a more constant biochemical composition. After skeletal maturity is achieved, no progressive change with age occurs in the water, collagen, hexosamine, chondroitin sulfate, sulfur, ash, or total nitrogen[162] content of articular cartilage. The chain length of chondroitin sulfate in joint cartilage has also been found not to vary with age. The polysaccharide attachment region of the PGs, however, does show some variation with age; PGs from younger cartilage appear to have a longer chondroitin sulfate attachment region than do those from older cartilage.[163] This would account for some increase in the relative proportion of keratan sulfate to chondroitin sulfate with aging. The solubility of collagen, as well as its amino acid composition, was found to be no different in articular cartilage of 70-year-old people than in that of younger people,[164] implying a relative constancy in the degree of crosslinking of the fibers. However, although the reducible crosslinks of cartilage collagen do not change with age, the tissue content of nonreducible hydroxypyridinium crosslinks has been shown to increase with age.[165]

Although a progressive decrease in cell density (based on analysis of histologic sections or on measurements of DNA concentration) occurs with age in articular cartilage of several species, in human cartilage no reduction in cellularity occurs after maturity, and the cells remain metabolically active.[166] Sulfate uptake (incorporation into PGs) by articular cartilage chondrocytes is also not affected by age,[167] and protein synthesis, which in rabbit cartilage decreases for the first 6 months of life, has been shown to remain constant thereafter.[168] Thus, regardless of age, the chondrocytes in normal articular cartilage are capable of maintaining constancy in the composition of the extracellular ground substance.

Whether or not changes in the macromolecular organization of the cartilage are a feature of aging is less clear. In a study of morphologically normal hip cartilage from aged humans (69 to 81 years) with recent femoral neck fractures but without prior joint disease, PG aggregation was found to be defective.[169] The PGs were not complexed with hyaluronic acid, and link glycoproteins were not found in association with the PGs. After incubation with hyaluronic acid in vitro, minimal augmentation of the hydrodynamic size of the PGs occurred, indicating that hyaluronate-PG interaction had not taken place. The data suggested that aggregation was diminished because of a defect in the core protein of the PGs, which impaired their ability to interact with hyaluronic acid. Since aggregation has been found to be normal in cartilage from other apparently normal aged individuals, it is unclear whether the aggregation defect in these specimens (which was indistinguishable from that seen in typical OA) was a feature of aging itself, represented "preosteoarthritic" change, or was due to some other factor. Notably, PG aggregation in pig laryngeal (nonarticular) cartilage has also been shown to diminish with age.[170]

Weightman[171] has shown that the ability of articular cartilage to withstand fatigue testing (i.e., to resist fracture) diminishes progressively with age. When vertical cleft formation was induced in apparently normal femoral heads by repeated cyclical application of small loads (which would not produce any change in the cartilage if applied only once) in vitro, fissuring occurred. No apparent loss of PGs from the cartilage occurred, suggesting that the damage occurred in the collagen. Furthermore, the orientation of the clefts suggested that the fatigue defect was probably due not to fracture of individual collagen fibers, which are held together by strong peptide bonds, but to loosening or separation of the collagen network in the cartilage (see preceding discussion). The molecular defect that accounts for the experimentally induced fatigue fractures in these femoral heads has yet to be identified.

Heredity. The influence of genetic factors on the development of OA is complex. In some cases, the genetic defect causes a change in joint structure and therefore affects congruity of the joint surfaces; this seems to be particularly common in the hip (e.g., acetabular dys-

plasia and congenital dislocation).[123,172] This also appears to account for the prevalence of OA of the knee in inbred male STR/ORT mice, in which a strong correlation exists between the arthritis and spontaneous medial dislocation of the patella. It was shown recently that surgical stabilization of the patellae of young male STR/ORT mice prevented the normal development of OA, whereas surgically produced dislocation of the patella in non-arthritis-prone CBA/ORT mice produced OA.[173]

It has been claimed that Heberden's nodes occur on a hereditary basis,[174] though other variables, such as joint use, may be a major factor. Since most of the load across joints is derived from the contraction of the muscles crossing the joint, the stress (force per unit area) on the cartilage of the distal interphalangeal joint, especially in "feminine" forms of grasp or pinch,[175] probably approximates that on the cartilage of weight-bearing joints. Cultural characteristics, rather than genetic factors, may also account for the lower prevalence of OA of the hip in Orientals than in Caucasians.[176] Is this attributable to the common practice in Asia of squatting, which distributes load across a broader area of the femoral head than standing upright? Or is it attributable to the fact that cement sidewalks are less common in Asia or that high-heeled shoes are less commonly worn there?

In another sense, genetic influences may enter into the development of OA through systemic metabolic effects such as in ochronosis. Compositional differences between apparently normal joints exist which could predispose to DA, but nothing is known about the basis for these differences. For example, is the collagen content of the superficial layer of articular cartilage, which varies from 50 to 90 percent among various individuals, genetically determined? Similarly, do these conditions have a genetic basis, namely, the levels of lysosomal hydrolases synthesized by chondrocytes, the cell's capacity to augment synthesis of matrix components in its attempt to "repair," or the synthesis of PGs that are unable to undergo normal interaction with hyaluronic acid to form aggregates in the ground substance?

Obesity. It is self-evident that excessive body weight will increase the load borne by weight-bearing joints. As pointed out by Sokoloff,[62] obesity may also cause changes in posture and gait and in overall locomotor activity, which must be taken into account in considering the joint biomechanics. It seems clear that obesity in humans is associated with an increase in symptomatic OA of the knee,[177] although not of the hip.[178] The majority of obese patients exhibit varus knee deformities,[179] presumably representing a compensatory attempt to bring the feet under the center of gravity when the thighs are separated by adiposity.[5] Load is therefore concentrated on the cartilage of the medial compartment—the point at which degenerative changes most commonly develop in the knees of obese people.

Whether metabolic, genetic, or other factors, as well as mechanical ones, contribute to the OA changes in obesity is unsettled. The data are contradictory as to whether obesity is associated with an increased prevalence of OA in non-weight-bearing joints. In mice fed a diet enriched with lard, a saturated fat, the frequency and severity of OA was increased,[180] but this was not confirmed in another study, and a diet supplemented with vegetable (unsaturated) fat did not influence the development of OA lesions in mice, despite the development of obesity.[181] In STR/IN mice, which develop hyperlipidemia and become obese on an ordinary diet, these changes are genetically dissociated from the development of OA,[182] suggesting the importance of hereditary factors.

Altered Congruity of Joint Surfaces. Bone remodeling is normal and probably occurs in response to normal stresses.[183] It has been proposed that abnormal remodeling, caused by uneven distribution of pressure within the joint, is a factor in the pathogenesis of OA.[184] In general, the earliest progressive degenerative changes in the joint occur at the site that bears the greatest pressure.

Subtle incongruity has been considered to account for a number of cases of "idiopathic" OA in the human hip. In this joint a thin piece of fibrocartilaginous tissue exists at the zenith of the acetabulum as a normal anatomic variant.[185] In some individuals younger than 50 years of age who have hips possessing this thin area of tissue, contact between the femoral head and the thin area does not occur, or does so at low pressures. However, in hips of older persons, presumably as a consequence of the normal remodeling changes that occur with age, contact does occur, resulting in pressures up to four times higher than those seen in hips of younger persons. Murray has suggested that developmental defects may be the major cause of hip OA in humans and that some 80 percent of all cases of "idiopathic" or "primary" hip OA may be due to excessive joint congruity stemming from such defects.[172]

The basis for the joint degeneration that results from overcongruity is not entirely clear. It could be due to mechanical "fatigue failure" of the cartilage[99] or to interference with nutrition of the chondrocyte, which in the adult is derived principally from the synovial fluid. Conversely, some incongruity may be important for the pumping of nutrients from the synovial fluid into the cartilage. This could explain the development of OA in non-weight-bearing joints, in non-weight-bearing areas of joints that bear weight at other sites,[186] and in the cartilage degeneration and ankylosis seen with prolonged immobilization.[64]

Inflammatory Joint Disease. OA itself is generally not associated with much synovitis. Scattered foci of lymphocytes are seen in the synovial membrane, and the synovial fluid leukocyte count is usually less than 2000 cells per mm³. Pannus, as seen in the rheumatoid joint, does not occur in OA. To the extent that inflammation does occur in OA, it may be the result of crystal-induced synovitis (either calcium apatite or calcium pyrophosphate dihydrate) or the removal of cartilage breakdown products, which provoke synovial inflammation,[137] perhaps via activation of Hageman factor.[138]

Wear particles, representing material derived from the articular surface as a result of mechanical or enzymatic destruction of the cartilage in OA, or both, have been found in synovial fluid[187] and have been shown to cause the release of collagenase and other hydrolytic enzymes from synovial cells and macrophages.[188]

Deposits of immunoglobulin and complement can be found in the collagenous latticework of the superficial zone of the articular cartilage, suggesting that deposition of immune complexes, perhaps containing breakdown products of the cartilage matrix as antigen, may play a role in the chronicity of OA.[189]

The recently documented "Milwaukee shoulder syndrome" (chronic tendinitis-capsulitis) represents a form of destructive OA with some evidence of inflammation in the synovial membrane but with minimal synovial fluid leukocytosis. Severe OA of the shoulder is present, with hydroxyapatite crystal deposition in the synovial membrane and rotator cell degeneration.[190]

Although consideration of the pathogenetic significance of inflammation in idiopathic, or primary, OA is receiving much current attention, it is apparent that secondary OA may develop as a sequela to any of a variety of inflammatory joint diseases, such as rheumatoid arthritis, acute bacterial joint infection, or tuberculous arthritis. Initial damage to the cartilage in these cases is probably chiefly enzymatic, with breakdown of the cartilage matrix by degradative enzymes released from the synovial membrane or from leukocytes within the joint space. In addition, studies by Herman have shown that lymphocytes may produce factors that suppress PG synthesis by the chondrocyte or accelerate PG degradation.[191,192] The extent to which impaired chondrocyte nutrition, resulting from immobility or lack of weight-bearing, might contribute to the initiation of cartilage breakdown in inflammatory arthritis is unknown, but it could be an additional factor in initiating OA.

Deposition Diseases of Cartilage. This category includes several diseases that lead to OA, including hemochromatosis, Wilson's disease, ochronotic arthropathy, gouty arthritis, and calcium pyrophosphate dihydrate (CPPD) crystal deposition disease. In these cases hemosiderin, copper, homogentisic acid polymers, or crystals of monosodium urate or CPPD, respectively, deposit within the articular cartilage matrix and cause cartilage degeneration directly via chondrocyte injury or indirectly by increasing the stiffness of the matrix and thereby leading to alterations in load forces. Whether biochemical or physicochemical changes in the matrix precede the deposition of the aforementioned substances in cartilage is uncertain. Notably, PG aggregates have been shown to inhibit precipitation of calcium salts[92] and monosodium urate,[193] whereas disaggregated PGs do not. As already noted, a defect in PG aggregation is among the earliest changes to develop in OA.

In particular, the relationship of CPPD deposition disease to OA is complex. First, the other metabolic disorders mentioned as examples of cartilage deposition diseases (e.g., hemochromatosis, Wilson's disease, gout, alkaptonuria) may all be associated with deposition of CPPD in articular cartilage—with clinical attacks of pseudogout. In addition, active calcification occurs in OA cartilage; thus, the basal zones stain strongly for alkaline phosphatase,[194] and matrix vesicles, indicating cartilage calcification, are seen by electron microscopy.[113] When human OA cartilage is cultured in vitro, large quantities of alkaline phosphatase and pyrophosphate (PPi), which are produced by the chondrocytes during active matrix synthesis, are recovered from the medium.[195] Analogously, the levels of PPi in OA synovial fluids are very high,[196] mimicking the synovial fluid levels in CPPD, and they correlate directly with the severity of the OA as judged radiologically.[197] Howell and associates have shown that normally young or proliferating chondrocytes are a major source of PPi secretion, whereas resting chondrocytes from normal adult cartilage secrete little PPi.[198] Thus, the increased PPi secretion in OA cartilage may reflect the increased activity of the cells in their attempt at matrix "repair" (see earlier discussion). Such observations raise the question of whether a disturbance in mineral metabolism exists as an integral component of OA.

It has been recently shown that PPi is generated from adenosine triphosphate (ATP) in cartilage, which can be accounted for by the presence of the exoenzyme nucleoside pyrophosphohydrolase in extracts of cartilage from patients with CPPD and OA.[199] If ATP or other nucleoside triphosphates were extensively hydrolyzed to PPi and the monophosphate by-product in vivo, increased activity of 5' nucleotidase, which has been documented in CPPD,[200] could drive the reaction and increase the rate of PPi production. If increased removal of PPi did not occur, resulting from a relative deficiency of extracellular pyrophosphatase, as shown in human OA and CPPD large incubates, the increased PPi would be available for mineralization. Since DNA contents of cartilage from patients with CPPD are no higher than those from patients with OA, the marked increase in 5' nucleotidase levels, relative to those of alkaline phosphatase and other enzymes, presumably reflects a greater mass of limiting membrane per cell in CPPD or a special functional role for the nucleotidase.[199] It is thus possible that the increased PPi in the OA joint precipitates in cartilage as CPPD when other factors, such as the concentration of ionized calcium and the physical state of the matrix (disaggregation of PGs), exist. The deposition of CPPD into the cartilage could then, by altering its physical and mechanical properties, lead to accelerated matrix breakdown.

References

1. Bollet, A.J.: An essay on the biology of osteoarthritis. Arthritis Rheum. 12:152, 1969.
2. Lee, P., Rooney, P.J., Sturrock, R.D., Kennedy, A.C., and Dick, W.C.: The etiology and pathogenesis of osteoarthrosis: A review. Semin. Arthritis Rheum. 3:189, 1974.
3. Howell, D.S., Sapolsky, A.I., Pita, J.C., and Woessner, J.F.: The pathogenesis of osteoarthritis. Semin. Arthritis Rheum. 5:365, 1976.
4. Glynn, L.E.: Primary lesions in osteoarthrosis. Lancet 1:574, 1977.
5. Radin, E.L.: The physiology and degeneration of joints. Semin. Arthritis Rheum. 2:245, 1972–1973.
6. Mankin, H.J., and Brandt, K.D.: Biochemistry and metabolism of cartilage. *In* Moskowitz, R.W., Howell, D.S., Goldberg, V.M., and Man-

7. kin, H.J. (eds.): Osteoarthritis—Diagnosis and Management. Philadelphia, W.B. Saunders Company. 1984.
7. Mankin, H.J., and Lippiello, L.: The glycosaminoglycans of normal and arthritic cartilage. J. Clin. Invest. 50:1712, 1971.
8. Hascall, V.C., and Heinegard, D.: Aggregation of cartilage proteoglycans. I. The role of hyaluronic acid. J. Biol. Chem. 249:4232, 1974.
9. Hardingham, T.E., and Muir, H.: Hyaluronic acid in cartilage and proteoglycan aggregation. Biochem. J. 139:565, 1974.
10. Muir, H., Maroudas, A., and Wingham, J.: The correlation of fixed negative charge with glycosaminoglycan content of human articular cartilage. Biochim. Biophys. Acta 177:494, 1969.
11. Muir, H.: Cartilage structure and metabolism and basic changes in degenerative disease. Aust. N.Z. J. Med. 8:1, 1978.
12. Matthews, M.B.: Collagen chondroitin sulfate ratio of human articular cartilage related to function. Br. Med. J. 2:1295, 1952.
13. Gillard, G., Reilly, H., Bell-Booth, P., and Flint, M.: A comparison of the glycosaminoglycans of weight-bearing and non-weight-bearing human dermis. J. Invest. Derm. 69:257, 1977.
14. Gillard, G., Merrilees, M., Bell-Booth, P., Reilly, H., and Flint, M.: The proteoglycan content and axial periodicity of collagen in tendon. Biochem. J. 163:145, 1977.
15. Gillard, G., Reilly, H., Bell-Booth, P., and Flint, M.: The influence of mechanical forces on the glycosaminoglycan content of the rabbit flexor digitorium profundus tendon. Connec. Tissue Res. 7:37, 1979.
16. Merrilees, M.J., Merrilees, M.A., Birnbaum, P., Scott, P., and Flint, M.: The effect of centrifugal force on glycosaminoglycan production by aortic smooth muscle cell in culture. Atherosclerosis 27:259, 1977.
17. Jones, I., Klampfeldt, A., and Sandstrom, T.: The effect of continuous mechanical pressure upon the turnover of articular cartilage proteoglycans in vitro. Clin. Orthop. 165:283, 1982.
18. Palmoski, M., and Brandt, K.: Effects of static and cyclic pressure on joint cartilage in vitro. Clin. Res. 31:453A, 1983.
19. Radin, E., Boyd, R., Martin, R., Goodwin, C., and Brandt, K.: Relationship between bone and cartilage changes after impulsive-loading. Trans. Orthop. Res. Soc. (Abstract) 7:214, 1982.
20. Donohue, J.M., Oegema, T., Thompson, R.C., and Buss, D.: Morphological and biochemical changes in adult articular cartilage following indirect blunt trauma. Trans. Orthop. Res. Soc. (Abstract) 8:243, 1983.
21. Muir, H.: The nature of the link between protein and carbohydrate of a chondroitin sulfate complex from hyaline cartilage. Biochem. J. 69, 1958.
22. Mathews, M.B., and Lozaityte, I.: Sodium chondroitin sulfate-protein complexes of cartilage. I. Molecular weight and shape. Arch. Biochem. Biophys. 74:158, 1958.
23. Partridge, S.M., Davis, H.F., and Adair, G.S.: The chemistry of connective tissues. 6. The constitution of the chondroitin-sulphate-protein complex in cartilage. Biochem. J. 79:15, 1961.
24. Brandt, K.D., and Muir, H.: Characterization of protein-polysaccharides of articular cartilage from mature and immature pigs. Biochem. J. 114:871, 1969.
25. Luscombe, M., and Phelps, C.F.: The composition and physicochemical properties of bovine nasal-septa protein-polysaccharide complex. Biochem. J. 102:110, 1967.
26. Rosenberg, L., Hellmann, W., and Kleinschmidt, A.K.: Macromolecular models of protein-polysaccharides from bovine nasal cartilage based on electron microscopic studies. J. Biol. Chem. 245:4123, 1970.
27. Kempson, G.E., Muir, H., Swanson, S.A.V., and Freeman, M.A.R.: Correlations between the compressive stiffness and chemical constituents of human articular cartilage. Biochim. Biophys. Acta 215:70, 1970.
28. Heinegard, D., and Hascall, V.C.: Aggregation of cartilage proteoglycans. III. Characteristics of the proteins isolated from trypsin digests of aggregates. J. Biol. Chem. 249:4250, 1974.
29. Muir, H., and Hardingham, T.E.: Structure of proteoglycans. *In* Whelan, W.J. (ed.): MTP International Review of Science, Biochemistry of Carbohydrates. Vol. 5. London, Butterworths, 1975, pp. 153–222.
30. Mak, A.F., Mow, V.C., and Lai, W.M.: Predictions of the number and strength of the proteoglycan-proteoglycan interactions from viscometric data. Trans. Orthop. Res. Soc. 10:3, 1983.
31. Kempson, G.E., Muir, H., Pollard, C., and Tuke, M.: The tensile properties of the cartilage of human femoral condyles related to the content of collagen and glycosaminoglycans. Biochem. Biophys. Acta 297:456, 1973.
32. Harris, E.D., Jr., Parker, H.G., Radin, E.L., and Krane, S.M.: Effects of proteolytic enzymes on structural and mechanical properties of cartilage. Arthritis Rheum. 15:497, 1972.
33. Miller, E.J., and Matukas, V.J.: Chick cartilage collagen: A new type of alpha 1 chain not present in bone or skin of the species. Proc. Natl. Acad. Sci. 64:1264, 1969.
34. Miller, E.J.: Isolation with characterization of a collagen from chick cartilage containing three identical alpha chains. Biochemistry 10:1652, 1971.

35. McCroskery, P.A., Richards, J.F., and Harris, E.D., Jr.: Purification and characterization of a collagenase from rabbit tumours. Biochem. J. 152:131, 1975.

36. Nimni, M.E.: Collagen: Its structure and function in normal and pathological connective tissues. Semin. Arthritis Rheum. 4:95, 1974.

37. Burgeson, R.E., and Hollister, D.W.: Collagen heterogeneity in human cartilage: identification of several new collagen chains. Biochem. Biophys. Res. Commun. 87:1124, 1979.

38. Stanescu, V., Stanescu, R., and Maroteaux, P.: Répartititon differénte du collagène de type I et du collagène de type II dans la zone superficielle et dans la zone intermédiare du cartilage articulaire. C.R. Hebd. Seances Acad. Sci. Ser. D 283:279, 1976.

39. Rhodes, R.K., and Miller, E.J.: Physicochemical characterization and molecular organization of the collagen A and B chains. Biochemistry 17:3447, 1978.

40. Hewitt, A.T., Kleinman, H.K., Pennypacker, J.P., and Martin, G.R.: Identification of an adhesion factor for chondrocytes. Proc. Natl. Acad. Sci. U.S.A. 77:385, 1980.

41. Kleinman, H.K., Hewitt, A.T., Murray, J.S., Liotta, L.A., Rennard, S.E., Pennypacker, J.P., McGoodwin, E.M., Martin G.R., and Fishman, P.H.: Cellular and metabolic specificity in the interaction of adhesion proteins with collagen and with cells. J. Supramol. Struct. 11:69, 1979.

42. Benya, P.D., Padilla, S.R., and Nimni, M.E.: The progeny of rabbit articular chondrocytes synthesize collagen types I and III and type I primer but not type II: verifications by cyanogen bromide peptide analysis. Biochemistry 16:805, 1977.

43. Mayne, R., Vail, M.S., Mayne, P.M., and Miller, E.J.: Changes in type of collagen synthesized as clones of chick chondrocyte grow and eventually lose division capacity. Proc. Natl. Acad. Sci. U.S.A. 73:1674, 1976.

44. Norby, D.P., Malemud, C.J., and Sokoloff, L.: Differences in collagen metabolism between normal and osteoarthritic human articular cartilage. Science 181:751, 1973.

45. Gay, S., Gay, R., Brandt, K., and Palmoski, M.: Aspirin causes chondrocytes in atrophic articular cartilage to synthesize Type I collagen in vivo. Arthritis Rheum. 25:540, 1982.

46. Herbage, D., Huc, A., Chabrand, D., and Chapuy, M.C.: Physicochemical study of articular cartilage from healthy and osteoarthritic human hips. Biochim. Biophys. Acta 271:339, 1972.

47. Oegema, T.R., Jr., Laidlaw, J., Hascall, V.C., and Dziewiatkowski, D.D.: The effect of proteoglycans on the formation of fibrils from collagen solutions. Arch. Biochem. Biophys. 170:698, 1975.

48. Seegmiller, R., Ferguson, C.C., and Sheldon, H.: Studies on cartilage. VI. A genetically determined defect in tracheal cartilage. J. Ultrastruct. Res. 38:288, 1972.

49. Poole, A.R., Hembry, R.M., and Dingle, J.T.: Cathepsin D in cartilage: The immunohistochemical demonstration of extracellular enzyme in normal and pathological conditions. J. Cell Sci. 14:139, 1974.

50. Bayliss, M.T., and Ali, S.Y.: Studies on cathepsin B in human articular cartilage. Biochem. J. 171:149, 1978.

51. Sapolsky, A.I., Keiser, H., Howell, D.S., and Woessner, J.F., Jr.: Metalloproteases of human articular cartilage that digest cartilage proteoglycan at neutral and acid pH. J. Clin. Invest. 58:1030, 1976.

52. Kuettner, K.E., Hiti, J., Eisenstein, R., and Harper, E.: Collagenase inhibition by cationic proteins derived from cartilage and aorta. Biochem. Biophys. Res. Commun. 72:40, 1976.

53. Greenwald, R.A.: Connective tissue lysozyme in health and disease. Semin. Arthritis Rheum. 6:35, 1976.

54. Shipp, D.W., and Bowness, J.M.: Insoluble non-collagenous cartilage glycoproteins with aggregating sub-units. Biochim. Biophys. Acta 379:282, 1975.

55. Bowness, J.M.: Comparison of structural glycoproteins with matrix proteins and fibronectin. Can. J. Biochem. 59:181, 1981.

56. Choi, H.U., Tang, L-H., Johnson, T.L., Pal, S., Rosenberg, L.C., Reiner, A., and Poole, A.R.: Isolation and characterization of a 35,000 molecular weight subunit fetal cartilage matrix protein. J. Biol. Chem. 258:655, 1983.

57. Kleine, T.O., and Singh, A.: Isolation and characterization of glycoproteins in proteoglycan aggregates of calf rib cartilage. Connec. Tissue Res. 9:145, 1982.

58. Chaminade, F., Stanescu, V., Stanescu, R., Maroteaux, P., and Peyron, J.G.: Noncollagenous proteins in cartilage of normal subjects and patients with degenerative joint disease. A gel electrophoretic study. Arthritis Rheum. 25:1078, 982.

59. Paulsson, M., and Heinegard, D.: Purification and structural characterization of a cartilage matrix protein. Biochem. J. 197:367, 1981.

60. Fife, R.S., D'Anniballe, L.J., and Brandt, K.D.: Cartilage matrix protein in articular cartilage. Trans. Orthop. Res. Soc. 29th Annual Meeting, p. 145, 1983.

61. Sokoloff, L.: The Biology of Degenerative Joint Disease. Chicago, University of Chicago Press, 1969.

62. Palmoski, M., Perricone, E., and Brandt, K.D.: Development and reversal

63. Enneking, W.F., and Horowitz, M.: The intra-articular effects of immobilization on the human knee. J. Bone Joint Surg. 54A:973, 1972.

64. Salter, R.B., Simmonds, D.F., Malcolm, B.W., Rumble, E.J., MacMichael, D., and Clements, N.D.: The biological effect of continuous passive motion on the healing of full-thickness defects in articular cartilage. J. Bone Joint Surg. 62A:1232, 1980.

65. Mankin, H.J.: The structure, chemistry and metabolism of articular cartilage. Bull. Rheum. Dis. 17:447, 1967.

66. Repo, R.U., and Mitchell, N.: Collagen synthesis in mature articular cartilage of the rabbit. J. Bone Joint Surg. 53B:541, 1971.

67. Mankin, H.J., and Lippiello, L.: The turnover of adult rabbit articular cartilage. J. Bone Joint Surg. 51A:1591, 1969.

68. Maroudas, A.: Transport through articular cartilage and some physiological implications. In Ali, S.Y., Elves, M.W., and Leaback, D.H. (eds.): Normal and Osteoarthrotic Articular Cartilage. London, Institute of Orthopaedics, 1974, pp. 33–47.

69. Mankin, H.J., and Lippiello, L.: The turnover of adult rabbit articular cartilage. J. Bone Joint Surg. 63A:131, 1981.

70. Bhatnagar, R.S., and Prockop, D.J.: Dissociation of the synthesis of sulphated mucopolysaccharides and the synthesis of collagen in embryonic cartilage. Biochim. Biophys. Acta 130:383, 1966.

71. Dondi, P., and Muir, H.: Collagen synthesis and deposition in cartilage during disrupted proteoglycan production. Biochem. J. 160:117, 1976.

72. Fitton Jackson, S.: Environmental control of macromolecular synthesis in cartilage and bone. Proc. R. Soc. Series B 175:405, 1970.

73. Hardingham, T.E., Fitton Jackson, S., and Muir, H.: Replacement of proteoglycans in embryonic chick cartilage in organ culture after treatment with testicular hyaluronidase. Biochem. J. 129:101, 1972.

74. Wiebkin, O.W., Hardingham, T.E., and Muir, H.: The interaction of proteoglycans and hyaluronic acid and the effect of hyaluronic acid of proteoglycan synthesis by chondrocytes of adult cartilage. In Burleigh, P.M.C., and Poole, A.R. (eds.): Dynamics of Connective Tissue Macromolecules. Amsterdam, North-Holland, 1975, pp. 81–104.

75. Toole, B.P.: Hyaluronate and hyaluronidase in morphogenesis and differentiation. Am. Zool. 13:1061, 1973.

76. Handley, C.J., and Lowther, D.A.: Inhibition of proteoglycan biosynthesis by hyaluronic acid in chondrocytes in cell culture. Biochim. Biophys. Acta 444:69, 1976.

77. Ehrlich, M.G., Mankin, H.J., Jones, H., Wright, R., Crispen, C., and Vigliani, G.: Collagenase and collagenase inhibitors in osteoarthritis and normal human cartilage. J. Clin. Invest. 59:226, 1977.

78. Sakamoto, M., Sakamoto, S., Goldhaber, P., and Glimcher, M.J.: Immunocytochemical studies of collagenase localization in normal mouse tissues with special reference to cartilage and bone. Trans. Orthop. Res. Soc. 24th Annual Meeting, February 21–23, 1978, p. 141.

79. Kuettner, K.E., Hiti, J., Eisenstein, R., and Harper, E.: Collagenase inhibition by cationic proteins derived from cartilage and aorta. Biochem. Biophys. Res. Commun. 72:40, 1976.

80. Kuettner, K.E., Soble, L., Croxen, R.L., Marczynska, B., Hiti, J., and Harper, E.: Tumor cell collagenase and its inhibition by a cartilage-derived protease inhibitor. Science 196:653, 1977.

81. Thomas, L., McCluskey, R.T., Potter, J.L., and Weissman, G.: Comparison of the effects of papain and vitamin A on cartilage. I. The effects in rabbits. J. Exp. Med. 111:705, 1960.

82. Dingle, J.T.: Studies on the mechanism of cartilage erosion. In Ali, S.Y., Elves, M.W., and Leaback, D.H. (eds.): Normal and Osteoarthrotic Articular Cartilage. London, Institute of Orthopaedics, 1974, pp. 65–71.

83. Sapolsky, A.I., Howell, D.S., and Woessner, J.F., Jr.: Neutral proteases and cathepsin D in human articular cartilage. J. Clin. Invest. 53:1044, 1974.

84. Fell, H.B., and Jubb, R.W.: The effect of synovial tissue on the breakdown of articular cartilage in organ culture. Arthritis Rheum. 20:1359, 1977.

85. Dingle, J.T.: The role of catabolin in arthritic damage. Agents and Actions 7:79, 1980.

86. Ridge, S., Oronsky, A.L., and Kerwar, S.S.: Induction of the synthesis of latent collagenase and latent neutral protease in chondrocytes by a factor synthesized by activated macrophages. Arthritis Rheum. 23:448, 1980.

87. Kuettner, K.E., Harper, E., and Eisenstein, R.: Protease inhibitors in cartilage. Arthritis Rheum. (Suppl.) 20:S124, 1977.

88. Bollet, A.J., Bonner, M.W., Jr., and Nance, J.L.: The presence of hyaluronidase in various mammalian tissues. J. Biol. Chem. 238:3522, 1963.

89. Stack, M.T., and Brandt, K.D.: Identification and characterization of articular cartilage hyaluronidase. Arthritis Rheum. 25:S100, 1982.

90. Leaback, D.H.: Studies on some glycosidases from the chondrocytes of articular cartilage and from certain other cells and tissues. In Ali, S.Y., Elves, M.W., and Leaback, D.H. (eds.): Normal and Osteoarthrotic Cartilage. London, Institute of Orthopaedics, 1974, pp. 73–83.

91. Hardingham, T.E., and Muir, H.: The excretion and degradation of

chondroitin 4-sulphate administered to guinea pigs as free chondroitin sulphate and as proteoglycan. Biochem. J. 130:597, 1972.

92. Wood, K.M., Wusteman, F.S., and Curtis, C.G.: The degradation of intravenously injected chondroitin 4-sulphate in the rat. Biochem. J. 134:1009, 1973.

93. Kuettner, K.E., Pita, J.C., Howell, D.S., Sorgente, N., and Eisenstein, R.: The possible function of lysozyme in cartilage metabolism. Ann. Rheum. Dis. (Suppl.) 34:69, 975.

94. Kuettner, K.E., Sorgente, N., Croxen, R.L., Howell, D.S., and Pita, J.C.: Lysozyme in preosseous cartilage. VII. Evidence for physiological role of lysozyme in normal endochondral calcification. Biochim. Biophys. Acta 372:335, 1974.

95. Howell, D.S., Pita, J.C., Sorgente, N., and Knettner, K.: Possible role of lysozyme in degradation of osteoarthritic cartilage. Trans. Assoc. Am. Physicians 87:169, 1974.

96. Greenwald, R.A.: Lack of effect of lysozyme on cartilage proteoglycans. Arch. Biochem. Biophys. 175:520, 1976.

97. Maroudas, A.: Physicochemical properties of cartilage in the light of ion exchange theory. Biophys. J. 8:575, 1968.

98. Maroudas, A.: Balance between swelling pressure and collagen tension in normal and degenerate cartilage. Nature 260:808, 1976.

99. Maroudas, A.: Fluid transport in cartilage. Ann. Rheum. Dis. (Suppl.) 34:77, 1975.

100. Freeman, M.A.R.: Discussion on pathogenesis of osteoarthrosis. In Ali, S.Y., Elves, M.W., and Leaback, D.H. (eds.): Normal and Osteoarthrotic Articular Cartilage. London, Institute of Orthopaedics, 1974, pp. 301–319.

101. Matthews, B.F.: Composition of articular cartilage in osteoarthritis. Br. Med. J. 2:660, 1953.

102. Bollet, A.J., Handy, J.R., and Sturgill, B.C.: Chondroitin sulfate concentration and protein-polysaccharide composition of articular cartilage in osteoarthritis. J. Clin. Invest. 42:853, 1963.

103. Mankin, H.J., and Lipiello, L.: Biochemical and metabolic abnormalities in articular cartilage from osteoarthritic human hips. J. Bone Joint Surg. 52A:424, 1970.

104. Brandt, K., and Palmoski, M.: Organization of ground substance proteoglycans in normal and osteoarthritic knee cartilage. Arthritis Rheum. 19:209, 1976.

105. Brandt, K.D.: Enhanced extractability of articular cartilage proteoglycans on osteoarthrosis. Biochem. J. 143:475, 1974.

106. Bollet, A.J., and Nance, J.L.: Biochemical findings in normal and osteoarthritic articular cartilage. II. Chondroitin sulfate concentration and chain length, water and ash contents. J. Clin. Invest. 45:1170, 1966.

107. Brandt, K.D., Palmoski, M.J., and Perricone, E.: Aggregation of cartilage proteoglycans. II. Evidence for the presence of a hyaluronate binding region on proteoglycans from osteoarthritic cartilage. Arthritis Rheum. 19:1308, 1976.

108. Brandt, K.D.: Proteoglycans: Structure and metabolism. Arthritis Rheum. (Suppl.) 20:S109, 1977.

109. Mankin, H.J.: Biochemical abnormalities in articular cartilage in osteoarthritis. In Ali, S.Y., Elves, M.W., and Leaback, D.H. (eds.): Normal and Osteoarthrotic Cartilage. London, Institute of Orthopaedics, 1974, pp. 153–172.

110. Atkins, E.D.T.: Molecular architecture of the animal and some microbial extracellular polysaccharides. In Walton, A.G. (ed.): Proceedings of the First Cleveland Symposium on Macromolecules. Amsterdam, Elsevier Scientific, 1977.

111. Mankin, H.J., Dorfman, H., Lippiello, L., and Zarins, A.: Biochemical and metabolic abnormalities in articular cartilage from osteoarthritic human hips. J. Bone Joint Surg. 53A:523, 1971.

112. Sapolsky, A.I., Altman, R.D., and Howell, D.S.: Cathepsin D activity in normal and osteoarthritic human cartilage. Fed. Proc. 32:1489, 1973.

113. Ali, S.Y., and Bayliss, M.T.: Enzymic changes in human osteoarthrotic cartilage. In Ali, S.Y., Elves, M.W., and Leaback, D.H. (eds.): Normal and Osteoarthrotic Cartilage. London, Institute of Orthopaedics, 1974, pp. 189–205.

114. Sapolsky, A.I., Matsuka, K., Woessner, J.F., and Howell, D.S.: Metal-dependent neutral proteoglycans from normal and ulcerated human articular cartilage. Trans. Orthop. Res. Soc. 3:71, 1978.

115. Lippiello, L., Hall, D., and Mankin, H.J.: Collagen synthesis in normal and osteoarthritic human cartilage. J. Clin. Invest. 59:593, 1977.

116. Nimni, M.E., and Deshmukh, K.: Differences in collagen metabolism between normal and osteoarthritic human articular cartilage. Science 181:751, 1973.

117. Eyre, D.R., McDevitt, C.A., and Muir, H.: Experimentally induced osteoarthrosis in the dog. Ann. Rheum. Dis. (Suppl. 2) 34:137, 1975.

118. Gay, S., Muller, P.K., Lemmen, C., Remberger, K., Matzen, K., and Kuhn, K.: Immunohistological study on collagen in cartilage-bone metamorphosis and degenerative osteoarthrosis. Klin. Wochenschr. 54:969, 1976.

119. Moskowitz, R.W., Davis, W., Sammarco, J., Martens, M., Baker, J.,

Mayor, M., Burstein, A.H., and Frankel, V.H.: Experimentally induced degenerative joint lesions following partial meniscectomy in the rabbit. Arthritis Rheum. 16:397, 1973.

120. Muir, H.: Molecular approach to the understanding of osteoarthrosis. Ann. Rheum. Dis. 36:199, 1977.

121. McDevitt, C.A., Muir, H., and Pond, M.J.: Biochemical events in early osteoarthrosis. In Ali, S.Y., Elves, M.W., and Leaback, D.H. (eds.): Normal and Osteoarthrotic Cartilage. London, Institute of Orthopaedics, 1974, pp. 207–217.

122. McDevitt, C.A., and Muir, H.: Biochemical changes in the cartilage of the knee in experimental and natural osteoarthritis in the dog. J. Bone Joint Surg. 58B:94, 1976.

123. Moskowitz, R.W., Howell, D.S., Goldberg, V.M., Muniz, O., and Pita, J.C.: Cartilage proteoglycan alterations in an experimentally induced model of rabbit osteoarthritis. Arthritis Rheum. 22:155, 1979.

124. Maroudas, A.: Physico-chemical properties of articular cartilage. In Freeman, M.A.R. (ed.): Adult Articular Cartilage. London, Pitman Medical, 1973, pp. 131–170.

125. Brandt, K., Palmoski, M., and Clayton, R.: Unpublished manuscript.

126. Kempson, G.E., Spivey, C.J., Swanson, S.A.V., and Freeman, M.A.R.: Patterns of cartilage stiffness on normal and degenerate human femoral heads. J. Biomech. 4:597, 1971.

127. Bollet, A.J.: Connective tissue polysaccharide metabolism and the pathogenesis of osteoarthritis. Adv. Intern. Med. 13:33, 1967.

128. Malemud, C.J., Goldberg, V.M., Moskowitz, R.W., Getzy, L.L., Papay, R.S., and Norby, D.P.: Biosynthesis of proteoglycan in vitro by cartilage from human osteochondrophytic spurs. Biochem. J. 206:329, 1982.

129. Marshall, J.L., and Olsson, S.E.: Instability of the knee: a long term study in dogs. J. Bone Joint Surg. 53A:1561, 1971.

130. Danielsson, L.G.: Incidence and prognosis of coxarthrosis. Acta Orthop. Scand. (Suppl.) 66:1, 1964.

131. Trueta, J.: Studies of the Development and Decay of the Human Frame. Philadelphia, W.B. Saunders Company, 1968.

132. Swanson, S.A.V., and Freeman, M.A.R.: The mechanics of synovial joints. In Simpson, D.C. (ed.): Modern Trends in Biomechanics. Vol. 1. London, Butterworths, 1970, p. 239.

133. Gilbertson, E.M.M.: The development of periarticular osteophytes in experimentally induced osteoarthritis in the dog. Ann. Rheum. Dis. 34:12, 1975.

134. Bernstein, M.A.: Experimental production of arthritis by artificially produced passive congestion. J. Bone Joint Surg. 15:661, 1933.

135. Phillips, R.S.: Phlebography in osteoarthritis of the hip. J. Bone Joint Surg. 48B:280, 1966.

136. Landells, J.W.: The bone cysts of osteoarthritis. J. Bone Joint Surg. 35B:643, 1953.

137. Chrisman, O.D., Fessel, J.M., and Southwick, W.O.: Experimental production of synovitis and marginal articular exostoses in the knee joints of dogs. Yale J. Biol. Med. 37:409, 1965.

138. Moskowitz, R.W., Schwartz, H.J., Michel, B., Ratnoff, O.D., and Astrup, T.: Generation of kinin-like agents by chondroitin sulfate, heparin, chondroitin sulfate, and human articular cartilage: Possible pathophysiologic implications. J. Lab. Clin. Med. 76:790, 1970.

139. Lloyd-Roberts, G.C.: The role of capsular changes in osteoarthritis of the hip joint. J. Bone Joint Surg. 35B:627, 1953.

140. Palmoski, M.J., and Brandt, K.D.: Immobilization of the knee prevents osteoarthritis after anterior cruciate ligament transection. Arthritis Rheum. 25:1201, 1982.

141. Williams, J.M., and Brandt, K.D.: Immobilization ameliorates chemically induced articular cartilage damage. Arthritis Rheum. 27:208, 1984.

142. Moskowitz, R.W., Goldberg, V.M., Rosner, I.A., Getzy, L., and Malemud, C.J.: Specific drug therapy of experimental osteoarthritis. Semin. Arthritis Rheum. 11 (Suppl. 1):127, 1981.

143. Linn, F.C., and Radin, E.L.: Lubrication of animal joints. III. The effect of certain chemical alterations of the cartilage and lubricant. Arthritis Rheum. 11:674, 1968.

144. Radin, E.L., and Paul, I.L.: The response of joints to impact loading. I. In vitro wear. Arthritis Rheum. 14:356, 1971.

145. Radin, E.L., and Paul, I.L.: A consolidated concept of joint lubrication. J. Bone Joint Surg. 54A:607, 1972.

146. Davis, W.H., Jr., Lee, S.L., and Sokoloff, L.: Boundary lubricating ability of synovial fluid in degenerative joint disease. Arthritis Rheum. 21:754, 1978.

147. Swann, D.A., and Radin, E.L.: The molecular basis of articular lubrication: Purification and properties of a lubricating fraction from bovine synovial fluid. J. Biol. Chem. 247:8069, 1972.

148. Swann, D.A.: Macromolecules of synovial fluid. In Sokoloff, L. (ed.): The Joints and Synovial Fluid. I. New York, Academic Press, 1978, pp. 407–435.

149. Swann, D.A., Radin, E.L., Nazimiec, M., Weisser, P.A., and Lewinnek, G.: The role of hyaluronic acid in joint lubrication. Ann. Rheum. Dis. 33:318, 1974.

150. Reilly, D.T., and Mertens, M.: Experimental analysis of the quadriceps

muscle force and patello-femoral joint reaction force for various activities. Acta Orthop. Scand. 43:126, 1972.

151. Radin, E.L., and Paul, I.L.: Does cartilage compliance reduce skeletal impact loads? The relative force attenuating properties of articular cartilage, synovial fluid, peri-articular soft-tissues and bone. Arthritis Rheum. 13:139, 1970.

152. Hill, A.V.: Production and absorption of work by muscle. Science 131:897, 1960.

153. Jones, C.M., and Watt, D.G.D.: Muscular control of landing from unexpected falls in man. J. Physiol. 219:729, 1971.

154. Bullough, P., Goodfellow, J., and O'Connor, J.: The relationship between degenerative changes and load-bearing in the human hip. J. Bone Joint Surg. 55B:746, 1973.

155. Todd, R.C., Freeman, M.A.R., and Pirie, C.J.: Isolated trabecular fatigue fractures in the femoral head. J. Bone Joint Surg. 54B:723, 1972.

156. Foss, M.V.L., and Byers, P.D.: Bone density, osteoarthrosis of the hip and fracture of the upper end of the femur. Ann. Rheum. Dis. 31:259, 1972.

157. Radin, E.L.: Mechanical aspects of osteoarthrosis. Bull. Rheum. Dis. 26:862, 1975–1976.

158. Mankin, H.: Discussion of paper by L. Sokoloff. *In* Ali, S.Y., Elves, M.W., and Leaback, D.H. (eds.): Normal and Osteoarthrotic Articular Cartilage. London, Institute of Orthopaedics, 1974, p. 123.

159. Freeman, M.A.R., and Wyke, B.: The innervation of the knee joint. An anatomical and histological study in the cat. J. Anat. 101:505, 1967.

160. Dee, R.: The innervation of joints. *In* Sokoloff, L. (ed.): The Joints and Synovial Fluid. I. New York, Academic Press, 1978, pp. 177–204.

161. Palmoski, M., O'Connor, B., and Brandt, K.: Sectioning of articular nerves impairs the integrity of articular cartilage. Clin. Res. 27:473A, 1979.

162. McDevitt, C.A.: Biochemistry of articular cartilage. Nature of proteoglycans and collagen of articular cartilage and their role in aging and in osteoarthrosis. Ann. Rheum. Dis. 32:364, 1973.

163. Heinegard, D., Paulsson, M., and Sonmarin, Y.: Proteoglycans and matrix proteins in cartilage. Prog. Clin. Biol. Res. 110B:35, 1983.

164. Miller, E.J., Van der Korst, J.K., and Sokoloff, L.: Collagen of human articular and costal cartilage. Arthritis Rheum. 12:21, 1969.

165. Eyre, D.R.: Collagen: molecular diversity in the body's protein scaffold. Science 207:1315, 1980.

166. Meachim, G., and Collins, D.H.: Cell counts of normal and osteoarthritic cartilage in relation to the uptake of sulphate ($^{35}SO_4$) in vitro. Ann. Rheum. Dis. 21:45, 1962.

167. Collins, D.H., and Meachim, G.: Sulphate ($^{35}SO_4$) fixation by human articular cartilage compared in the knee and shoulder joints. Ann. Rheum. Dis. 20:117, 1961.

168. Mankin, H.J., and Baron, P.A.: The effect of aging on protein synthesis in articular cartilage of rabbits. Lab. Invest. 14:658, 1965.

169. Perricone, E., Palmoski, M.J., and Brandt, K.: Failure of proteoglycans to form aggregates in morphologically normal aged human hip cartilage. Arthritis Rheum. 20:1372, 1977.

170. Tsiganos, C.P., and Muir, H.: Proteoglycan aggregation in different types of cartilage and its dependence on age. *In* Vogel, H.G. (ed.): Connective Tissue and Aging. Amsterdam, Excerpta Medica, 1973, pp. 132–137.

171. Weightman, B.: In vitro fatigue testing of articular cartilage. Ann. Rheum. Dis. 34 (Suppl. 2):108, 1975.

172. Murray, R.O.: The aetiology of primary osteoarthritis of the hip. Br. J. Radiol. 38:810, 1965.

173. Walton, M.: Patella displacement and osteoarthrosis of the knee joint in mice. J. Pathol. 127:165, 1979.

174. Stecher, R.M.: Heberden's nodes: A clinical description of osteoarthritis of the finger joints. Ann. Rheum. Dis. 14:1, 1955.

175. Radin, E.L., Parker, H.G., and Paul, I.L.: Pattern of degenerative arthritis. Preferential involvement of the distal finger-joints. Lancet 1:377, 1971.

176. Byers, P.D., Hoaglund, F.T., Purewal, G.S., and Yau, A.C.M.C.: Arti-

cular cartilage changes in Caucasian and Asian hip joints. Ann. Rheum. Dis. 33:157, 1975.

177. Kellgren, J.H., Lawrence, J.S., and Bier, F.: Genetic factors in generalized osteoarthritis. Ann. Rheum. Dis. 22:237, 1963.

178. Saville, P.D., and Dickson, J.: Age and weight in osteoarthritis of the hip. Arthritis Rheum. 11:635, 1968.

179. Leach, R.E., Baumgard, S., and Broom, J.: Obesity: Its relationship to osteoarthritis of the knee. Clin. Orthop. Rel. Res. 93:271, 1973.

180. Silberberg, M., and Silberberg, R.: Osteoarthrosis in mice fed diets enriched with animal or vegetable fat. Arch. Pathol. 70:385, 1960.

181. Sokoloff, L., and Mickelsen, O.: Dietary fat supplements, body weight and osteoarthritis in DBA/2JN mice J. Nutr. 85:117, 1965.

182. Sokoloff, l., Crittenden, L.B., Yamamoto, R.S., and Jay, G.E.: The genetics of degenerative joint disease in mice. Arthritis Rheum. 5:531, 1962.

183. Johnson, L.C.: Kinetics of osteoarthritis. Lab. Invest. 8:1223,1959.

184. Johnson, L.C.: Joint remodeling as the basis of osteoarthritis. J. Am. Vet. Med. Assoc. 131:1237, 1962.

185. Swanson, S.A.V., Freeman, M.A.R., and Day W.H.: Contact pressures in the loaded cadaver human hip. Ann. Rheum. Dis. 34 (Suppl. 2):114, 1975.

186. Goodfellow, J.W., and Bullough, P.G.: The patterns of aging of the articular cartilage of the elbow joint. J. Bone joint Surg. 49B:175, 1967.

187. Evans, C.H., Mears, D.C., and McKnight, J.L.: A preliminary ferrographic study of the wear particles in human synovial fluid. Arthritis Rheum. 24:912, 1981.

188. Evans, C.H.: Cellular mechanisms of hydrolytic enzyme release in osteoarthritis. Semin. Arthritis Rheum. 11 (Suppl.):93, 1981.

189. Cooke, T.D.: Immune deposits in osteoarthritic cartilage: their relationship to synovitis and disease site pattern. In press.

190. McCarty, D.J., Halverson, P.B., and Carresa, G.F. Brewer, B.J., and Kozin, F.: Milwaukee shoulder: association of microspheroids containing hydroxyapatite crystals, active collagenase and neutral protease with rotator cuff defects. Arthritis Rheum. 24:464, 1981.

191. Herman, J.H., Mowery, C.S. Koo, K.H., and Dennis, M.V.: Lymphokines: potential role in the immunopathogenesis of osteoarthritis. Semin. Arthritis Rheum. 11 (Suppl.1):104, 1981.

192. Herman, J.H., Musgrave, D.S., and Dennis, M.V.: Phytomitogen-induced, lymphokine-mediated cartilage proteoglycan degradation. Arthritis Rheum. 20:922, 1977.

193. Perricone, E., and Brandt, K.D.: Enhancement of urate solubility by connective tissue. I. Effect of proteoglycan aggregates and buffer cation. Arthritis Rheum. 21:453, 1978.

194. Freeman, M.A.R.: Adult Articular Cartilage. New York, Grune & Stratton, 1972.

195. Howell, D.S., Muniz, O., Pita, J.C. and Enis, J.E.: Extrusion of pyrophosphate into extracellular media by osteoarthritic cartilage incubates. J. Clin. Inves. 56:11473, 1975.

196. Altman, R.D., Muniz, O., Pita, J.C., and Howell, D.S.: Articular chondrocalcinosis. Microanalysis of pyrophosphate (PPi) in synovial fluid and plasma. Arthritis Rheum. 16:171, 1973.

197. Silcox, D.C., and McCarty, D.J., Jr.: Elevated inorganic pyrophosphate concentrations in synovial fluids in osteoarthritis and pseudogout. J. Lab. Clin. Med. 83:518, 1974.

198. Howell, D.S., Muniz, O., Pita, J.C., and Enis, J.E.: Pyrophosphate release by osteoarthritic cartilage incubates. Arthritis Rheum. 19(Suppl. 3):488, 1976.

199. Howell, D.S., Muniz, O,E., and Morales, S.: 5' Nucleotidase and pyrophosphate (PPi)-generating activities in articular cartilage extracts in calcium pyrophosphate deposition disease (CPPD) and in primary osteoarthritis (OA). *In* Peyron, J.G. [ed.]: Epidemiology of osteoarthritis. Paris, Ciba-Geigy, 1980, p. 99.

200. Tenenbaum, J., Muniz, O., Schumacher, H.R., Jr., Good, A.E., and Howell, D.S.: Comparison of pyrophosphohydrolase activities for articular cartilage in calcium pyrophosphate deposition disease and in primary osteoarthritis. Arthritis Rheum. 24:492, 1981.

Chapter 89

Osteoarthritis: Clinical Patterns and Pathology

Kenneth D. Brandt

INTRODUCTION

Terminology. The term osteoarthritis (OA) is used interchangeably with osteoarthrosis and degenerative joint disease. Less commonly, the condition may also be called hypertrophic arthritis. None of these terms is wholly adequate. Osteoarthritis implies that the primary event is inflammatory. Most students of OA do not accept this, although some degree of secondary synovitis is usually apparent and may be clinically significant. On the other hand, osteoarthrosis fails to take into account the presence of inflammation. The suffix implies increase or overproduction, reflecting the reactive changes in cartilage and bone and the osteophyte formation seen in OA. The term degenerative joint disease may be criticized on the grounds that degeneration implies deterioration, senescence, aging, or breakdown. Clinically, however, the disease may not be progressive.[1,2] Furthermore, active anabolic processes are at work in the disease[3] and presumably reflect a repair attempt by the articular cartilage (see Chapter 88). The term hypertrophic arthritis is a poor one, since it describes only one aspect of the disease, the overgrowth of bone and cartilage.

Classification: Primary versus Secondary OA. In primary (idiopathic) OA no predisposing factors (e.g., trauma or antecedent inflammatory disease) are apparent, and breakdown of the joint is presumed to be due to intrinsic factors (see Chapter 88). In secondary OA the disease is attributed to an obvious underlying cause (Table 89–1). Recent data suggest that this classification may be artificial; thus, many cases that have been considered to be primary OA of the hip may, in fact, arise on the basis of subtle joint incongruities (e.g., acetabular dysplasia or slipped femoral epiphysis). Notably, the prevalence of an underlying mechanical defect in patients with "so-called" idiopathic hip OA has been reported to be as high as 90 percent,[4] casting doubt on the very existence of primary OA in this joint.[5]

Historical Background. OA is the most common joint disease in man and other vertebrates. Osteophytes, sometimes leading to ankylosis, were common in giant dinosaurs.[6] OA has been observed in all mammalian species, including whales and dolphins, as well as in fish, birds,[7] and some amphibia. It occurs in all races of man. OA was first identified as a distinct entity, however, only in the 20th century. In 1904, Goldthwaite distinguished hypertrophic arthritis from atrophic arthritis,[8] and Garrod, in 1907, described OA as a clinical entity.[9]

Table 89–1. Classification of Osteoarthritis

Primary
1. Idiopathic
2. Generalized osteoarthritis
3. Erosive osteoarthritis

Secondary
1. Due to mechanical incongruity of joint
   a. Congenital or developmental defects
      i. Hip dysplasia
      ii. Legg-Calvé-Perthes disease
      iii. Slipped femoral capital epiphysis
      iv. Femoral neck abnormalities
      v. Protrusio acetabuli
      vi. Multiple epiphyseal dysplasia
      vii. Osteochondritis
      viii. Morquio's syndrome
   b. Post-traumatic
2. Due to prior inflammatory joint disease
   a. Rheumatoid arthritis and variants
   b. Chronic gouty arthritis or pseudogout
   c. Infectious arthritis
3. Endocrinopathies
   a. Diabetes mellitus
   b. Acromegaly
   c. Sex hormone abnormalities
   d. Iatrogenic hyperadrenocorticism
4. Metabolic disorders
   a. Hemochromatosis
   b. Ochronosis
   c. Wilson's disease
   d. Chondrocalcinosis
   e. Paget's disease
5. Miscellaneous
   a. Avascular necrosis
   b. Hemarthrosis associated with blood dyscrasias

Recognition of the distinct clinical syndromes of OA was not common until recently, and even today the differential diagnosis between certain types of OA (e.g., erosive osteoarthritis) and seronegative rheumatoid arthritis may be difficult clinically.

Epidemiology. OA is the single most frequent cause of rheumatic complaints and results in the greatest loss of time from work.[10,11] Based on radiologic evidence, more than 80 percent of people over the age of 55 have OA. The prevalence of the disease rises with increasing age, but OA is by no means exclusively a disease of the elderly. Indeed, one radiologic survey showed a 10 percent prevalence of OA in patients 15 to 24 years old.[12] Another survey found evidence of OA in the hands or feet of over 40 million Americans (33 percent of the target population), although symptoms or disability occurred only in about 5 million.[13,14] Differences between blacks and whites with respect to the prevalence of OA have been noted, and differences in patterns of joint involvement have been related to race.[15,16] Whether these differences are genetic or are attributable to differences in lifestyle and use of joints is not clear. People in China and India have a lower prevalence of OA of the hip than Caucasians.[17,18] Whether this is related to differences in use of joints (e.g., increased squatting), less use of high-heeled shoes, fewer sidewalks, or other factors is not known. Among the Chinese, a lower frequency of pre-disposing factors, such as congenital dysplasia of the hip and slipped capital femoral epiphysis, may account for some of these differences.[18] On the other hand, the prevalence of OA in distal interphalangeal joints and its association with multiple joint involvement was reported to be similar in Caucasians and Chinese. In other population studies, OA was more prevalent in American Indians than in the general population.[19]

When all age groups are considered, men and women in the United States are equally affected by OA. However, in people less than 45 years old, the prevalence of OA is greater in men, while in those over 45 years of age, it is greater in women.[13,19,20] In Great Britain, both the number of joints involved by OA and the radiologic severity were similar in men and women under the age of 55,[21] while in older individuals the disease in women was more severe than that in men and involved more joints. The pattern of joint involvement in men and women under age 55 was similar, but in older people involvement of the distal and proximal interphalangeal joints and the first carpometacarpal joint was more common in women, while hips were more frequently involved in men. Differences in joint involvement may be affected by prior vocational and avocational usage of the joints.[22]

CLINICAL FEATURES OF OSTEOARTHRITIS

Signs and Symptoms. The clinical features of OA depend upon the joint(s) involved and the duration and severity of the disease. The predominant symptom is a deep ache, usually localized to the involved joint. Typically, the pain occurs following use of the joint and is relieved by rest (Table 89–2). With progression of the disease, however, pain may be present with minimal use at rest and may even interfere with sleep. Pain is a relatively late feature of OA. It does not originate in the articular cartilage, which is aneural, but pain may arise from the joint capsule, synovium, ligaments, tendons, muscle, and bone. Often, the pain of OA is aggravated by dampness or changes in barometric pressure.

The joints involved most commonly are the distal and proximal interphalangeal joints of the hands, the first carpometacarpal joint, knees, hips, cervical and lumbar spine, and the metatarsophalangeal joint of the great toe. Most other joints are spared in primary OA, so that if they are involved, secondary OA should be suspected. Morning stiffness and stiffness following disuse during the day are common. Stiffness is usually of brief duration (lasting only 15 minutes or less) and is confined

Table 89–2. Typical Clinical Features of Osteoarthritis

Usually in elderly
Monoarthritis or oligoarthritis
Joints most frequently involved:
   Distal interphalangeal joints of fingers
   Proximal interphalangeal joints of fingers
   First carpometacarpal joint
   First metatarsophalangeal joint
   Hips
   Knees
   Cervical spine
   Lumbar spine
Joints spared:
   Metacarpophalangeal joints
   Wrists
   Elbows
   Shoulders
   Ankles
No systemic manifestations
Characteristics of joint discomfort:
   Aggravated by joint use; relieved by rest (but pain also at rest with severe disease)
   Jelling sensation
   Morning stiffness absent, or present for less than 30 minutes
Signs on joint examination:
   Local tenderness
   Bony and/or soft tissue swelling (joint enlargement)
   Crepitus
   Effusions
Characteristics of synovial fluid:
   High viscosity
   Good mucin test
   Mild leukocytosis ($<$ 2000 wbc/mm^3), predominantly mononuclear cells

to the involved joint. Limitation of motion develops due to loss of congruity of the articular surfaces, muscle spasm, flexion contractures, capsular fibrosis, intra-articular loose bodies, and/or development of large buttressing osteophytes.

Physical findings include tenderness, crepitus, and enlargement of the joint (Table 89–2). Synovial effusions and flexion contractures may occur. The tenderness often appears to be associated with active synovitis. Crepitus may be found during both active and passive motion and is due to surface incongruities. When cartilage has been completely destroyed and the subchondral bone becomes thick with an ivory-like surface (i.e., eburnation), the crepitus transmits a distinct sensation to the examiner's fingers. Enlargement of the joint may be due to the thickening of synovium and capsule, effusion, or proliferation of cartilage and bone (osteophytes). With progression, gross deformity occurs, with subluxation and gross bony hypertrophy. Periarticular muscle atrophy is common but is usually less marked than in rheumatoid arthritis. Joints may be warm, due to associated inflammation, but the overlying skin is usually not erythematous, except in the acute flares associated with Heberden's nodes.

Laboratory Studies. No specific clinical laboratory abnormalities occur in primary osteoarthritis. The erythrocyte sedimentation rate is generally normal, as are routine clinical tests, such as complete blood counts, urinalyses, and serum chemistry studies. The synovial fluid shows only a slight increase in the total leukocyte count, high viscosity, a normal mucin test, and a normal or only slightly increased total protein concentration.[23] Fragments of cartilage and/or bone (wear particles) may be present in the fluid.[24] The inorganic pyrophosphate concentration of the joint fluid is increased in OA, and the level correlates with radiologic severity[25] of the disease. In secondary OA associated with an underlying metabolic disorder or endocrinopathy (Table 89–1), specific laboratory studies may help pinpoint the underlying condition.

Radiologic Characteristics. In early OA radiographs may be normal (see Chapter 39). With progressive loss of articular cartilage, narrowing of the joint space develops (Fig. 89–1). Widening of the space, however, may be seen occasionally in the presence of a synovial effusion. Sclerosis of subchondral bone (eburnation) is characteristic, as are marginal osteophytes. Subchondral cysts develop, surrounded by a rim of dense bone, and must be differentiated from the juxta-articular erosions of rheumatoid arthritis, which are generally associated with defects in the cortical bone (Fig. 89–2).

Late in the disease, subluxation and gross deformity may develop (Fig. 89–1). True ankylosis is rare.[26] The radiologic criteria for diagnosis of OA, as defined in the Atlas of Standard Radiographs,[27] are shown in Table 89–3.

It should be emphasized that there is often great disparity between the severity of the radiologic changes of OA and the severity of symptoms. Thus, although over 90 percent of people over the age of 40 have radiologic evidence of OA in weight-bearing joints,[28] only about 30 percent will complain of symptoms.[29] Even though most people with radiologic evidence of OA are asymptomatic, it has been shown that radiologic evidence of asymptomatic OA predisposes the patient to develop symptomatic disease in the affected joint, except for the apophyseal joints of the lumbar spine.[2] Similarly, Gresham and Rathey[30] noted a positive correlation between radiographic evidence of OA in the knee and clinical symptoms. The poor correlation between radiographic changes and symptoms observed in some studies may relate to the criteria employed for the radiologic diagnosis of OA. It is clear from prospective studies, for example, that osteophytes alone—in the absence of other radiologic criteria of OA (see Table 89–2)—may be related to aging, rather than to cartilage damage, and that their presence (at least in hip and knee roentgenograms) has no prognostic significance with respect to the subsequent development of other radiologic features of OA, such as joint space narrowing, subchondral sclerosis, or cysts.[31,32]

Pathology. In the earliest stages of osteoarthritis, localized areas of softening are present in the articular cartilage, which exhibits a pebbled texture of the surface at these sites. The cartilage is disrupted along the planes of the collagen fibrils. When this occurs tangential to the surface layer, the process is referred to as flaking. When disruption procedes perpendicular to the surface, in which case it may extend down to the tidemark just above subchondral bone, it is referred to as fibrillation (Fig. 89–3). With joint motion, the fibrillated cartilage

Figure 89–1. The evolution of osteoarthritis—hip. *Left*, Age 55, mild osteoarthritis. Note joint space narrowing in weight-bearing area and some acetabular lip osteophytes. *Middle*, Age 60, moderate osteoarthritis. See joint space narrowing more advanced and extensive and the appearance of medial acetabular osteophyte. *Right*, Age 65, severe osteoarthritis. Total obliteration of joint space. numerous cysts in acetabulum and femoral head, and a large medial acetabular osteophyte with secondary lateral subluxation of femoral head. The shape of the femoral head in this male patient, the "pistol-grip deformity," suggests that a mild slipped capital femoral epiphysis occurred during childhood, making the osteoarthritis *secondary* to a childhood hip deformity.

Figure 89–2. The gross pathology of osteoarthrosis—hip. The advanced osteoarthrotic changes depicted in the radiograph are reflected in the pathologic changes of the gross specimen. There is complete loss of articular cartilage in the area of weight bearing: small cysts communicate with the eburnated surface, and a small rim of osteophytes has formed at the margin of the femoral head.

is abraded, and the underlying bony cortex is exposed. Progressive destruction of the joint surface occurs in those areas of the joint that are habitually loaded (Fig. 89–2). On the other hand, it is the habitually unloaded regions of the joint that show the earliest changes of fibrillation (e.g., the infrafoveal portion of the femoral head.)[33] These changes in the unloaded area, which are virtually ubiquitous, are, however, not progressive or associated with symptoms or with radiologic changes. They have mistakenly been called OA by some pathologists, resulting in the erroneous impression that OA is essentially universal in every diarthrodial joint in people over the age of 30 or 40 years.

In parallel with the cartilage changes, new bone formation occurs in the marrow subjacent to the cartilage and at the joint margins. The marginal osteophytes protrude into the joint space or extend into the capsular and ligamentous attachments at the joint margins. The osteophytes are often capped by a layer of new hyaline cartilage. Proliferation of subchondral bone is most apparent at sites in which the overlying articular cartilage has been eroded. In these areas, repeated motion leads to a polishing of the bone, which takes on the glistening appearance of ivory, so that the process is referred to as "eburnation" (Fig. 89–4).

Marginal osteophytes in OA may be due to stimulation of cells in the chondrosynovial junction by breakdown products of the articular cartilage.[33a] Osteophytes

may occur, however, without articular cartilage damage. Thus, in dogs that had undergone anterior cruciate ligament transection, osteophyte development was noted as early as 3 days following surgery, prior to any morphologic changes in the articular cartilage.[33b] Mechanical instability itself may be important, since osteophytes do not develop after cruciate ligament transection in the dog if the unstable knee is immobilized,[33c] or in tendons of osteolathyritic rats if the muscles or their motor nerves are transected.[33d, 33e]

Subchondral cysts are areas of rarefaction in the bone commonly seen beneath the eburnated surface in the hip (Fig. 89–5) but are much less frequent in other locations. Such cysts occur on both the femoral and acetabular components. Uncommonly, they may be present before narrowing of the joint spaces is apparent.[34] Pathologic examination shows bone necrosis,[35,36] with disappearance of the trabeculae in the affected area, and fibromyxomatous degeneration of the marrow. Dead bone, cartilage and amorphous material are often also present within the cavity. Eventually, a rim of reactive new bone and fibrous tissue surrounds the cavity. Tiny gaps in the overlying cortex, due to microfractures, are frequently noted at the apex of the pseudocysts, suggesting that transmission of pressure from the articular space into the underlying subchondral marrow occurred, compressing blood vessels in the marrow and leading to death of subchondral bone and the subsequent resorptive changes which result in cyst formation. Only rarely do the cavities contain pockets of mucoid fluid. Thus, they are usually not true cysts but rather "pseudocysts."

New bone formation occurs not only in the cyst margins and osteophytes but also focally at the base of the articular cartilage as a result of metaplasia of osteoblasts there. This leads to fragmentation and duplication of the tidemark.

Much of the joint deformity in OA seen by gross and radiologic exam results from collapse of the joint surface. The remodeling processes described above have been studied extensively in the femoral head, where they have been shown to result in obliteration of the original landmarks as they are replaced by osteophytic cartilage, which, itself, then degenerates. Thus, in most surgically

Table 89–3. Criteria for Radiologic Diagnosis of Osteoarthritis*

1. Formation of osteophytes in the joint margins or at ligamentous attachments, e.g., tibial spine
2. Periarticular ossicles, mainly distal and proximal interphalangeal joints
3. Narrowing of joint space associated with sclerosis of subchondral bone
4. Cystic areas with sclerotic walls situated in the subchondral bone
5. Altered shape of bone end, e.g., head of the femur

*The following five-step grading system is used according to the number of criteria present: 0 = no OA; 1 = doubtful OA; 2 = minimal OA; 3 = moderate OA; 4 = severe OA.

Figure 89–3. Early fibrillation of articular cartilage.

resected specimens of OA femoral heads, little of the native articular cartilage remains.

PRIMARY OSTEOARTHRITIS

Heberden's Nodes. The most common manifestation of primary OA is the Heberden's node,[37] which represents collagenous, bony, synovial, and capsular enlargement of the distal interphalangeal joint. Similar nodes occur in the proximal interphalangeal joints, where they are referred to as Bouchard's nodes (Fig. 89–6). Heberden's nodes produce firm swelling on the dorsolateral and dorsomedial aspects of the distal interphalangeal joints of the fingers and are often associated with flexion and lateral deviation of the distal phalanx. Analogous lesions do not occur in the feet, presumably because the flexor and extensor tendons do not insert into the distal phalanx. Heberden's nodes usually develop slowly and are not often painful. They may be single but are usually multiple and are approximately 10 times more common in women than in men.[38] They generally develop after age 45 but are not uncommon earlier.

Although Heberden's nodes are often associated with little discomfort and may go unnoticed by the patient for years, in some cases they present with an acute onset, associated with redness, swelling, and pain. A history of recent prior trauma to the digit may be elicited. Some loss of dexterity of the involved joints is common. Multiple distal interphalangeal joints may be involved simultaneously or sequentially.

During the acute stage, gelatinous cysts, which may be painful and tender, may occur on the dorsolateral and/or dorsomedial aspects of the distal interphalangeal joint. They represent mucoid transformation of periarticular fibroadipose tissue and are associated with proliferation of fibroblasts producing glycosoaminoglycan. Fluid aspirated from the cysts contains hyaluronic acid.[40] The gelatinous cysts may persist or may recede spontaneously. The cysts communicate with the distal interphalangeal joint space,[39] although the communication may not persist. They are associated with underlying osteophytes and, if removed, are likely to recur unless the osteophyte is also removed.[39,41]

A strong hereditary tendency underlies the development of Heberden's nodes. Based on the studies of Stecher, this is particularly obvious in females.[42] Thus, Heberden's nodes were twice as common in mothers, and three times as common in sisters, of affected women than they were in the general population. If they occur in men, it is likely that both parents will exhibit Heberden's nodes; if they occur in women, only one parent

Figure 89–4. A femoral head with osteoarthritic changes is pictured on the left. The flattened, eburnated weight-bearing surface and dense subchondral bone under this surface can be seen on the right.

Figure 89–5. Patterns of osteoarthritis—hip. An example of bilateral primary osteoarthritis, with two distinct patterns of development in the same individual. Right hip: Note concentric joint space narrowing, slight protrusio, few cysts, and large acetabular lip osteophyte, but no medial acetabular and few femoral head osteophytes. Left hip: Joint space is most narrowed over the weight-bearing dome, with multiple small cysts in superior segment of the femoral head, marked femoral head subluxation, and large medial acetabular osteophyte displacing the femoral head laterally.

typically exhibits the abnormality. Stecher concluded that the abnormality was inherited as a single, autosomal gene, which was dominant in females and recessive in males.[43] Other studies, however, suggest that various modes of transmission may occur.

Pathologic study of Heberden's nodes has indicated that in some cases their appearance is different from that of osteoarthritis in other locations.[44] Thus, the articular

cartilage has been found to be hypertrophic rather than fibrillated and eroded. The bony swelling was found to be due to ossific transformation of the insertion of the tendons into the joint capsule. Smythe[45] has suggested that thickening of the insertion of the extensor tendon precedes development of bony or cystic swelling in Heberden's nodes, and that shortening of the tendon insertions as well as thickening occurs, resulting in restricted distal interphalangeal joint flexion. Action of the powerful finger flexor muscles against this normal resistance would produce compressive forces, which would act on the cartilage and subchondral bone to produce crush deformities. Asymmetrical resistance may lead to deviation as well as flexion. Attacks of pain, redness, swelling and effusion, characteristic of the acute Heberden's node, may follow excessive use and may be associated with bony deformation and reactions to crush fractures.

Primary Generalized Osteoarthritis (GOA). This condition, which was described initially by Haygarth in 1805,[46] was further characterized by Cecil and Archer in 1926[47] and was given its present name in 1952 by Kellgren and Moore.[48] GOA is marked by involvement in three or more joints or groups of joints (the proximal and distal interphalangeal joints and the metacarpophalangeal joints are each considered as a group).

As described by Kellgren and Moore,[48] GOA occurs predominantly in middle-aged postmenopausal women. The distal and proximal interphalangeal joints of the hands and the first carpometacarpal joint are most often involved. Knees, hips, the first metatarsophalangeal joint, and joints of the spine are also commonly involved.[48] Other joints are usually spared. Joint hypermotility has been noted in a number of patients.[49]

Symptoms are episodic, and are often accompanied by signs of inflammation (warmth, effusion) in the involved joints, with elevation of the erythrocyte sedi-

Figure 89–6. *A.* An 85-year-old female with primary osteoarthritis of the right hand. The distal interphalangeal joints are involved, producing the bulbous deformities called Heberden's nodes: the proximal interphalangeal joints are involved to a lesser extent, resulting in milder deformities called Bouchard's nodes: and the carpometacarpal joint of the thumb is involved, making abduction of the thumb difficult and producing the square hand often seen in this form of OA. *B.* Osteoarthritis of the distal and proximal interphalangeal joints. Heberden's and Bouchard's nodes, as well as characteristic involvement of the first carpometacarpal joint and the scaphotrapezoid joints.

A   B

mentation rate. The inflammatory phase may be the presenting feature of GOA. The titer of serum rheumatoid factor is not elevated.

No significant increase in the prevalence of Heberden's nodes was noted in a prospective study of patients with hip or knee OA.[50] Similarly, a recent study by Solomon[51] showed that only 21 percent of patients with OA of the hip had polyarticular disease when the OA was due to excessive mechanical stress on previously normal cartilage. In contrast, 81 percent of those with OA of the hip due to some intrinsic cartilage defect (which increased the vulnerability of the cartilage to normal mechanical stress, e.g., chondrocalcinosis) had polyarticular disease. This suggests the importance of systemic factors in most cases of GOA.

Many epidemologic data support the concept of GOA. Thus, patients with OA in one joint tend to have more OA in other joints than matched controls.[52] A population survey in the United States has shown that the prevalence of OA in finger joints is correlated with its prevalence in other joints, especially in women, suggesting the presence of a systemic factor.[51] Similar results were obtained in an analysis of patients with GOA confined to 5 or more locations[53] and suggested that, depending upon the site of finger involvement, two types of GOA could be defined on the basis of clinical and epidemiologic features.

The *nodal* type, marked by distal interphalangeal joint involvement (Heberden's nodes) predominated in women and was marked by familial aggregation. The *non-nodal* type was marked by proximal, rather than distal, interphalangeal joint involvement and was only slightly more common in women. Familial clustering was much less obvious than in the nodal type. However, prior episodes of inflammatory polyarthritis and elevation of the erythrocyte sedimentation rate were common, as was obesity. The data suggested that heredity played an important role in nodal forms of GOA, whereas prior inflammation was more important in the non-nodal type.[54]

Certain radiologic differences exist between GOA and the much more common form of idiopathic OA.[48] The knees exhibit joint space narrowing and flowing "molten wax" osteophytes rather than the usual more sharply tapered osteophyte. In the spine, the articular facets, spinous processes, and neural arches may show striking enlargement. Radiologic studies of the progression of the disease[55] suggest that the initial changes do not occur in the articular cartilage (as in idiopathic primary OA), but in subchondral bone, resulting in proliferation at the base of the cartilage and exophytic growth at the joint margins.

Erosive Osteoarthritis. This disease chiefly affects the distal and/or proximal interphalangeal joints of the hands; occasionally, the metacarpophalangeal joints may also be affected.[56] Symptoms are often episodic and associated with local inflammation. Gelatinous cysts (similar to those associated with Heberden's nodes), which may be painful and tender, may develop around involved joints. Acute painful flare-ups may recur for

years. Roentgenograms of the involved joints show loss of joint space, osteophytes, and subchondral sclerosis. Bony erosions and collapse of the subchondral plate (which are not usually noted in primary OA) are seen. Joint deformity may be severe. In many cases bony ankylosis, which occurs rarely in Heberden's nodes,[26] develops and may be due to pannus, healing of eroded cartilage surfaces, or coalescence of adjacent osteophytes.[2] Ankylosis is generally attended by relief of pain as the disease "burns itself out." Erosive osteoarthritis has a predilection for postmenopausal women. Tests for rheumatoid factor are negative, and despite the clinical and pathologic (see below) evidence of inflammation, the erythrocyte sedimentation rate is normal or only slightly elevated. Microscopically, the synovium is extensively infiltrated with lymphocytes and monocytes.[57,58] Pannus may be seen.

Whether the marked inflammatory reaction in the synovium represents an exuberant response to joint detritus in an unusually destructive form of OA, or whether the cartilage and bony changes are a consequence of primary synovial inflammation, is unclear. Notably, Ehrlich found that 15 percent of 170 patients who presented with erosive osteoarthritis subsequently developed rheumatoid arthritis.[59]

Diffuse Idiopathic Skeletal Hyperostosis (DISH). This syndrome is considered by some to be a variant of OA. DISH[60] occurs chiefly in men over the age of 50 and produces back pain and stiffness with characteristic radiologic changes. It must be differentiated from both spondylosis and ankylosing spondylitis. The condition has also been designated Forestier's disease,[61] senile ankylosing hyperostosis of the spine, spondylitis ossificans ligamentosa, and spondylosis hyperostotica. The term DISH, however, which was coined by Resnick,[62] is preferable to the other labels, since it emphasizes the widespread manifestations of the disease which, in some instances, may be more marked at extraspinal sites than in the spine.[63]

The diagnosis is made radiologically.[60,62] Roentgenograms show exuberant flowing spinal osteophytes, which are larger and more numerous than those usually seen in OA of the spine. Furthermore, the height of the intervertebral discs is not reduced in DISH, and neither vacuum signs nor sclerosis of the vertebral end plates are present. The spinal changes are most marked in the lower thoracic region, although any level of the spine may be affected. Ligamentous changes occur, with calcification and ossification most prominent in the anterior spinal ligament. A lucent line is often apparent between the ossified anterior spinal ligament and the subjacent vertebral body (Fig. 89–7). The diagnosis of DISH requires flowing calcification or osseous bridging of four or more contiguous vertebrae, in the absence of changes in the apophyseal and sacroiliac joints (to exclude ankylosing spondylitis, which DISH may resemble radiologically).[64] The degree of ossification in DISH, moreover, is typically greater than in ankylosing spondylitis.

Clinically, most patients with DISH are asymptomatic; the majority of cases are detected during radio-

Figure 89–7. Diffuse idiopathic skeletal hyperostosis of the cervical spine, Note the linear "flowing bone," areas of radiolucency between the cortex of the vertebral body and the new bone, remarkable preservation of the intervertebral disc spaces, and absent vacuum phenomenon. These bony changes differ strikingly from osteophytes of osteoarthritis.

logic screening for unrelated problems. However, complaints of back pain or stiffness may be present, although spinal motion is generally relatively painless and, surprisingly, often shows little restriction. In addition to spinal pain, recurrent tendinitis may be seen, associated with prominent osseous spurs at sites where tendons or ligaments attach to bone (e.g., olecranon process, calcaneus, iliac crest, trochanters). Ligamentous ossification may occur (e.g., sacrotuberous and iliolumbar ligaments). Patients with DISH are often obese and exhibit glucose intolerance.[65,66]

The etiology of DISH is unknown. HLA typing has not revealed predominance of any haplotype,[67] including HLA-B27, although earlier studies had reported the presence of HLA-B27 in 34 percent of patients with DISH.[68]

Most patients with this condition require no treatment other than reassurance and simple analgesics. Occasionally, local corticosteroid injections may be useful for periarticular complaints or pain related to spurs.

It has been suggested that DISH represents an ossification diathesis, leading to excessive bone formation at sites of stress at tendinous and ligamentous insertions into bone. Consistent with this view is the evidence that patients with DISH develop ossification in response to surgery or in association with coexisting diseases such as rheumatoid arthritis.

The earliest pathologic changes consist of a mild inflammatory reaction with fibrosus extending from the annulus fibrosus.[69] With progression, new bone is deposited locally, involving the annulus fibrosus, anterior longitudinal ligament, and perivertebral space. Cartilage degeneration is not a feature, so that pathologically, as well as radiologically, the disease is clearly distinct from OA.

OSTEOARTHRITIS OF SPECIFIC SITES

OA of the Hip (Malum Coxae Senilis; Morbus Coxae Senilis). This condition is more common in men than in women and more often unilateral than bilateral. Some 20 percent of patients with unilateral hip degeneration, however, developed OA of the other hip during an 8-year follow-up period.[70] The disease has been regarded as secondary to congenital or developmental defects in up to 80 percent of cases.[71,72]

Congenital dysplasia (Fig. 89–8), Legg-Calvé-Perthes disease and slipped capital epiphysis, multiple epiphyseal dysplasia, iliac horn syndrome (arthro-onychodysplasia), and nail-patella syndrome may all lead to premature

Figure 89–8. Secondary osteoarthritis—hip. Bilateral congenitally dislocated hips, reduced, with residual dysplastic, shallow acetabula. Advanced OA of the right hip with characteristic radiographic changes associated with dysplasia, including joint space narrowing very localized to the weight-bearing dome, large cysts in this area, marked subluxation of the femoral head, and few osteophytes.

OA. Although x-ray studies of the contour of the hip joint have suggested to some investigators that acetabular dysplasia is the basis for most cases of OA of the hip, this view may be questionable because subluxation has been documented radiologically to occur as a late manifestation of OA.

In congenital hip dysplasia, with inadequate development of the acetabulum, a shallow cavity exists which is directed laterally and anteriorly, with insufficient coverage for the femoral head. The femoral head may subluxate in childhood, causing a limp. In other instances, symptoms may not appear until the teenage years, or the dysplasia may present first as OA in the middle years of life. Hip dysplasia is more common in women than in men.

Slipped capital femoral epiphysis tends to occur in the 10- to 15-year-old individual, causing pain in the groin, buttock, thigh, or knee. The pain is often accompanied by a limp. Some individuals may remain asymptomatic until OA develops in middle age or later.

Legg-Calvé-Perthes disease is avascular necrosis of the proximal capital femoral epiphysis. Its peak incidence occurs between 4 and 8 years of age. The condition is more common in boys than in girls. The softened femoral head is distorted, and the surface incongruities lead to development of OA.

Clinically, symptoms of hip OA include pain in the groin or inguinal region. Occasionally, pain may be situated in the trochanteric region, lateral buttock, or proximal thigh. In some 20 percent of patients, OA of the hip presents with pain in the distal thigh or knee. Referral to the knee occurs because the obturator nerve supplies both the hip joint and subsartorial plexus. On examination, hip motion evokes discomfort. In the early stages flexion may be painless, but internal rotation and, less often, extension may produce pain. Hip pain can be reproduced clinically by moving the hip through its range of motion without moving the knee joint. Loss of motion is seen first with internal rotation, followed by extension, adduction, and flexion. Most patients will show limitation of flexion, external rotation, and adduction (FABER test). Adduction and/or flexion contractures may lead to shortening of the ipsilateral limb. Shortening may also result from lateral and upward subluxation of the femoral head into the supralateral area of the acetabulum. The quadriceps muscle is often atrophic. An antalgic gait, with the trunk lurching to the affected side in the stance phase (to minimize abductor contraction that causes pain), or a Trendelenburg gait, with the pelvis dropping on the opposite side during the stance phase, or both, may result.

OA of the Knee. Primary OA of the knee[1] is common and may involve the medial or lateral femoral tibial compartments, patellofemoral compartment, or both. As with OA in other joints, pain is aggravated by motion and relieved by rest. Localized tenderness may occur on palpation. Bony enlargement due to osteophytes may be visible as well as palpable. Effusions are usually not very large. Crepitus is common with flexion of the knee. In OA involving the patellofemoral compartment, if the patella is compressed against the femur with the quadriceps muscle relaxed, and the patient then contracts the muscle, severe pain is often elicited (shrug sign). Limitation of joint motion may occur, and atrophy of the quadriceps muscles is common. OA in the medial compartment results in genu varus; degeneration in the lateral compartment produces genu valgus (Fig. 89–9).

Chondromalacia patellae is a clinical syndrome seen typically in young adults. It is more common in females than in males. The clinical syndrome is associated with a softening of the articular cartilage of the patella. The lesion is located on the midportion of the patella between the lateral and medial facet, and between the medial and "odd" facet, the sites where the patella comes into contact with the femur in midflexion of the knee. The anatomic lesions are indistinguishable from those of early OA, with swelling of the cartilage, an increase in water content, and fibrillation. The pathologic changes are, however, usually nonprogressive (i.e., ulceration of the cartilage extending as deep as the subchondral bone is uncommon),[73] although in some cases the condition appears to be a precursor of typical OA of the knee. The lesion is considered to develop in response to microtrauma in an area of articular cartilage subject to compressive as well as to shear forces, as the patella glides over the trochlea of the femur.[74]

OA of the Spine. Degeneration of the spine may occur in either of two discrete articulations: the diarthrodial (apophyseal) joints and the synchondroses (intervertebral discs).[75] The term spinal osteoarthritis should be restricted to changes in the apophyseal joints, while spondylosis deformans should be used to refer to degenerative disc disease. Commonly, both sites are involved concurrently, although on adjacent rather than the same vertebra.[76]

The progressive changes that occur in the nucleus pulposus in spondylosis deformans follow a pathologic sequence similar to that which occurs in the articular cartilage in OA: fissuring of the nucleus occurs, and the hyaline cartilage endplates (through which it is anchored to the vertebral bodies) fibrillate and eventually disintegrate, leading to eburnation of the subchondral bony plate. Nodules of cartilage and fibrous tissue beneath the vertebral subchondral plates (Schmorl's nodes) represent displacement of the nucleus pulposus into the vertebral body.[77] Marginal osteophytes arise as a result of tractional forces due to horizontal pulsion of the annulus fibrosis and its periosteal attachments, caused by spreading of the degenerating nucleus pulposus.[75] Marginal osteophytes develop on the anterolateral aspects of the vertebral bodies. Posterior osteophytes may also occur and may impinge on the spinal cord or nerve roots (Fig. 89–10). Osteophytes in the joints of Luschka (uncovertebral, neurocentral joints) may compromise the vertebral arteries.

Symptoms of OA of the spine include localized pain and stiffness and radicular pain. The former presumably originates in the joint capsules, periosteum, ligaments, and perispinous muscles. Radicular pain results from nerve root compression by osteophytes or may represent

Figure 89–9. *A,* Osteoarthritis—knee. A common pattern of osteoarthritis of the knee, often associated with a bow-legged deformity, is depicted in the radiograph. There is marked joint space narrowing of the medial compartment, with sparing of the lateral compartment and patellofemoral joint. This pattern is reflected in the gross pathologic changes, which consist of complete loss of cartilage and the presence of eburnated bone over the medial femoral condyle and mild degenerative changes in the remainder of the joint. There is a remarkable contrast between the advanced destruction of the medial compartment and the virtual sparing of the lateral compartment of this knee. *B,* A 70-year-old female with a severe *varus* (bow-legged) deformity of the left knee. This deformity is associated with advanced osteoarthritis of the medial compartment of the knee, illustrated in the standing anteroposterior radiograph. Patients with severe *valgus* (knock-knee) deformities develop osteoarthritis of the *lateral* compartment of the knee. Thus, osteoarthritis of the knee frequently reflects the uneven stress placed upon it by the developmental configuration of the joint.

referred pain. Nerve roots may be compromised by osteophytes impinging on the neural foramina, by prolapse of a degenerated disc, or by narrowing of the neural foramina as a result of apophyseal joint subluxation. Pressure on the nerve root may cause pain, parasthesias, loss of reflexes, and muscle weakness in the distribution of the affected nerve root. Nerve root compression due to OA is most common in the cervical spine but may occur in other areas.

Large anterior osteophytes in the cervical region may cause dysphagia.[78] Large posterior osteophytes or posterior protusion of the degenerated disc may compress the spinal cord, producing long tract signs. Compression of the anterior spinal artery may occur. If the vertebral arteries are compromised,[79] a syndrome of basal artery insufficiency may develop, with vertigo, diplopia, scotomata, nystagmus, and ataxia. The vascular insufficiency may be intermittent and related to the position of the neck.

OA of the First Carpometacarpal and First Metatarsophalangeal Joints. Primary OA of the first carpometacarpal joint is common. Clinically, swelling, pain, and tenderness at the base of the first metacarpal may be observed, and the joint may have a squared appearance. Motion is painful and restricted and may be accompanied by palpable and audible crepitus.(Fig. 89–6).

The metatarsophalangeal joint of the great toe is an extremely common site of primary OA. Pain, stiffness, and swelling usually begin insidiously. Inflammation of the bursa overlying the medial aspect of the joint (bunion) may occur. Bony enlargement of the joint is palpable and joint motion may produce crepitus.

SECONDARY OSTEOARTHRITIS

Metabolic Diseases. *Ochronosis.* Metabolic disorders, such as ochronosis, may be associated with severe generalized OA.[80] Hyaline articular cartilage and nucleus pulposus, as well as other connective tissue, are the sites of deposition of a brownish-black pigment, a polymer of homogentisic acid. Chondrocyte necrosis is prevalent. Material properties of the tissues are altered by the pigment, so that the articular cartilage becomes brittle and numerous shards break off the cartilage surface. Severe degenerative disease of the spine is common in ochronosis, and radiologic demonstration of calcification of intervertebral discs at multiple levels is characteristic. This may represent ossification of degenerated pigmented tissue rather than dystrophic calcification of the nucleus pulposus itself. Similarly, radiodense loose bodies occur in the peripheral joints and represent osteochondromatous reaction of the synovium to the articular debris. Except for the radiologic evidence of these osteochondral bodies, and more severe degeneration of shoulders and sacroiliac joints, the x-ray changes in ochronosis resemble those of primary OA, although os-

Figure 89–10. *A.* A lateral radiographic view of the cervical spine in which the black arrows point to posterior osteophytes and the white arrows to anterior osteophytes at the C5–6 and C6–7 level. Note increased density of the subehendral bone in the vertebral plates as well as the apophyseal joints at C5–6 and C6–7. *B.* An anteroposterior view illustating the osteophytes and narrowing of the joint spaces in the joints of Luschka and also at the C5–6 and C6–7 levels. *C.* An oblique view illustrating encroachment by osteophytes of the joints of Luschka on the C5–6 and C6–7 intervertebal foramina.

teophytes tend to be much less prominent in ochronotic arthropathy. Synovial fluid may contain numerous particles of debris, resembling ground pepper.[81] Synovial fluid from patients with ochronotic arthropathy has been shown to contain crystals of calcium pyrophosphate dihydrate (CPPD).[82-84] Although calcification of the joint capsule was present in one case, chondrocalcinosis has not been reported, and the relationship between alkaptonuria and CPPD deposition is unclear (however, see Neuropathic Joint Disease, below).

Hemochromatosis. The arthropathy of hemochromatosis, described by Schumacher in 1964,[85] affects 20 to 50 percent of patients with this disease and generally resembles OA. Occasionally, the joint disease may antedate other clinical features of hemochromatosis.[86,87] The joint disease is progressive and involves, in particular, metacarpophalangeal joints, knees, hips, and shoulders. Joint pain, swelling, and stiffness occur, without warmth. Attacks of acute arthritis, related to deposition of CPPD crystals, may be superimposed on the chronic, progressive OA-like disease. Hemosiderin granules are present in the synovial lining cells or in perivascular macrophages.[88] CPPD crystals may be seen in the synovium[5,6] and articular cartilage.[89,90] Radiologic changes in the involved joints include joint space narrowing, subchondral sclerosis, osteophytes, and subchondral cysts, which may be large. Joints that are not involved commonly in OA are affected in hemochromatosis (as they are in CPPD deposition disease); the most characteristic sites of involvement in hemochromatotic arthropathy are the second and third metacarpophalangeal joints.[91] Midcarpal and radiocarpal joints, elbows, and glenohumeral joints are also affected frequently.

The pathogenesis of the joint degeneration in hemochromatosis is unclear. Iron is present only in very low quantities in the affected cartilage.[90] Moreover, arthropathy is rarely a feature of transfusional siderosis,[92,93] suggesting that factors other than iron deposition may underlie the cartilage damage. In vitro, iron inhibits pyrophosphatase.[94] If such inhibition also occurred in vivo, it could facilitate CPPD deposition. However, arthropathy occurs in hemochromatosis in patients who fail to reveal cartilage calcifications.

Wilson's Disease. The arthropathy of Wilson's disease[95] (hepatolenticular degeneration) may occur in 50 percent of adults with the disease but is unusual in children. Although pain and swelling may occur, joint abnormalities are frequently asymptomatic. Multiple joints may be involved, including metacarpophalangeal joints, wrists, elbows, shoulders, knees, and hips.[96] Subchondral cysts and sclerosis and cortical irregularities occur and have been considered to represent premature OA. Some radiologic features of Wilson's disease help differentiate it from primary OA, however, such as radiodense lesions, which occur centrally and at the joint margins,[97] and focal areas of bone fragmentation, which do not appear to be related to the presence of tremor.[98] Synovial biopsies have shown mild cell lining hyperplasia and inflammation with vasculitis.[99] No increase in copper content of the synovial tissue was noted, and CPPD crystals were not observed. On the other hand, articular cartilage calcification has been observed in patients with Wilson's disease,[97] although this has not been shown to be due to CPPD. It is of interest that copper ion inhibits pyrophosphatase,[94] which could account for an increase in CPPD in patients with Wilson's disease. Joint space narrowing, confined to the patellofemoral compartment and resembling the patellofemoral arthropathy of CPPD deposition disease, has been noted in Wilson's disease.[96]

Crystal Deposition Diseases. Crystals are commonly found in articular cartilage and synovium of osteoarthritic joints. CPPD and/or hydroxyapatite (HA) can be identified in the synovial fluid in about 30 percent of patients with OA.[100] It has been considered, on the one hand, that crystal deposition may be a primary factor leading to joint damage in OA and, on the other hand, that crystal deposition may occur secondary to the development of OA.[101]

Evidence in support of the view that crystal deposition can lead to premature OA comes from studies indicating a progression from early chondrocalcinosis to definite OA in cases of familial CPPD deposition,[102] and from the observation that the OA associated with CPPD deposition is clinically distinct from primary OA, e.g., with involvement of the metacarpophalangeal joints and wrists.[103] Furthermore, it has been shown that collagenase and other enzymes may be released from synovial cells following phagocytosis of CPPD crystals.[104]

Electromicroscopic studies of articular cartilage biopsies from clinically and radiologically normal joints of young individuals with proven familial CPPD deposition disease in other joints have shown degenerative changes in chondrocytes, even in the absence of gross or histologic abnormalities in the cartilage or crystal deposition.[105] This would suggest that cellular changes in the cartilage may antedate the deposition of crystals.

This view is supported by a recent study of patients who had undergone meniscectomy.[106] OA changes, as expected, were more frequent and severe in the operated than in the unoperated knees. Chondrocalcinosis was present in 20 percent of the operated knees, but in only 4 percent of the unoperated knees of these patients and in 3 percent of knees of an age- and sex-matched control group. These data thus suggest that previously damaged joint tissues are predisposed to crystal deposition.

On the other hand, a lack of association between OA and CPPD deposition has also been noted.[107] CPPD crystals were observed in only 2 percent of 95 femoral heads with OA and in 19 percent of femoral heads that were removed surgically because of fracture. The mean age for the OA group as a whole was 63 years, while for the CPPD group it was 81 years. CPPD crystals were found in both the fibrillated hyaline cartilage and regenerative fibrocartilage, and in osteophytes, ligamentum teres, and joint capsule.

A recent study showed that 30 percent of patients with OA had apatite crystals in their synovial fluid, and an additional 43 percent had both apatite and CPPD crystals.[100] Autopsy studies support the correlation between the severity of OA and the presence of crystals.[109] X-ray evidence of periarticular calcifications and perichondrocytic staining of cartilage with the von Kossa's stain, both of which suggest increased apatite deposition, are more common with increasing severity of OA. In rheumatoid arthritis, the presence of apatite crystals correlates with the severity of secondary OA.[110]

Apatite and CPPD crystals are associated with the degenerative changes in cartilage in patients with hemachromatosis and OA, and in patients who have OA associated with endocrine disorders, such as hyperparathyroidism, hypothyroidism, and acromegaly. Furthermore, HA deposits have been identified in joints that are extensively destroyed,[111] and HA has been shown in vitro to be capable of releasing collagenase and other proteases from synovial cells following phagocytosis.[104]

Paget's Disease. OA may develop in patients with Paget's disease, in whom it occurs most often in the hip and knee.[112,113] Hypervascularity and rapid bone turnover in Paget's disease may lead to increased endochondral bone formation, with encroachment on the articular cartilage. In addition, enlargement of the femoral head and incongruities resulting from deformities (e.g., protrosio acetabuli, femoral bowing) may produce abnormal loading of the articular cartilage, leading to secondary OA.

Chronic Trauma. Chronic joint trauma, such as that related to occupational activities, appears clearly to cause OA in some individuals. Thus, there is an increased prevalence of OA in elbows of foundry workers[114] and in the spine and knees of miners.[20]

Neuropathic Joint Disease (Charcot Arthropathy). This is a form of severe progressive OA affecting one or more peripheral or axial joints, in which both the degenerative and hypertrophic components are grossly exaggerated by trauma, due to a loss of the normal sensory innervation of the joint[115] (Table 89–4). The

Table 89–4. Causes of Neuropathic (Charcot) Arthropathy

Tabes dorsalis
Diabetic neuropathy
Alcoholic neuropathy
Leprosy
Syringomyelia
Spina bifida with meningomyelocele
Pernicious anemia (subacute combined with degeneration of the spinal cord)
Spinal cord tumors
Spinal cord trauma
Arachnoiditis after spinal anesthesia or meningitis
Hemiplegia or paraplegia
Amyloidosis
Congenital indifference to pain
Peroneal muscle atrophy (Charcot-Marie-Tooth disease)
Repeated intra-articular corticosteroid injections
Idiopathic
Familial dysautonomia (Riley-Day syndrome) and other hereditary neuropathies (e.g., Dejerine-Sottas disease)

condition was first described in tabes dorsalis by Charcot in 1868,[116] in syringomyelia by Sokoloff in 1892,[117] and in diabetes mellitus by Jordan in 1936.[118] It is generally believed that loss of proprioception or pain, or both, underlies development of the Charcot joint. However, other data suggest that the loss of muscular reflexes, which protect articular and periarticular tissues from excessive excursion during joint motion, may be important.[119,120] A neurovascular (rather than neurotraumatic) pathogenesis for the neurotrophic joint has also been suggested,[121] with osteoclastic bone resorption occuring in hyperemic areas which are devoid of vasoconstrictive activity.[122] The sensory deficits in neurophic jont disease are usually clinically obvious; they may, however, be subclinical or difficult to detect,[123,124] raising the possibility that some cases of primary OA may arise on a neuropathic basis.

Previous efforts to produce a Charcot joint in animals have frequently been unsuccessful. Eloesser[119] found, for example, that cat's joints that had been rendered anesthetic by dorsal rhizotomy remained intact unless they were subjected to additional (thermal) damage. Similarly, no joint disease developed in dogs followed for as long as 16 months after dorsal ganglionectomy (L4-S1). Notably, knee cartilage ulcerations (i.e., secondary OA) in dogs with anterior cruciate ligament transection who had been subjected to prior dorsal ganglionectomy were more severe, and developed more rapidly, than in neurologically intact dogs who had undergone cruciate ligament transection.[120] Thus, some significant (?traumatic) initiating factor may be required for development of Charcot arthropathy in a denervated joint.

In the early stages, x-ray findings in Charcot arthropathy may be normal. In more advanced cases, however, the x-rays show varying degrees of destructive and hypertrophic change, with loss of articular cartilage, fragmentation and loss of subchondral bone, and exuberant marginal new bone formation (Fig. 89–11). Para-articular tissues are thickened and may exhibit abundant calcification or ossification, representing fragments of fractured bone and/or metaplastic change. Joint dislocations and fractures are common.

Jacobelli and associates[125] have described chondrocalcinosis due to deposition in neuropathic joints. It may be hypothesized that trauma to the denervated joint leads to proliferation of chondrocytes, resulting in release of inorganic pyrophosphate (PPi) from the dividing cells and subsequent deposition of CPPD in the matrix. Howell and associates have shown that proliferating chondrocytes are a rich source of PPi, whereas resting chondrocytes from normal adult cartilage secrete little PPi.[126] The presence of CPPD in the matrix alters the mechanical properties of the cartilage and leads to further degeneration. The shedding of CPPD crystals from the cartilage into the joint space may contribute to the synovitis in the traumatized joint.

Excessive Intra-articular Injection of Adrenal Corticosteroids. In 1959, Chandler and associates[127] described a patient with Charcot-like arthropathy which developed following frequently repeated injections of

Figure 89–11. Acute Charcot's arthropathy off the knee. Example of acute neuropathic arthropathy secondary to severe and extensive chondrocalcionosis and pseudogout, with resulting extensive destruction of the tissues within the joint, loss of bony substance, large intra-articular fragments, and early secondary OA.

hydrocortisone into an osteoarthritic hip. The condition may progress very rapidly, with severe osseous and cartilaginous destruction, and may be associated with a variety of underlying articular disorders, for example, rheumatoid arthritis or osteoarthritis.[128,129] It has been suggested that the analgesic effect of the steroid results in overuse of the previously damaged joint, with joint destruction aggravated, perhaps, by associated steroid-induced osteoporosis. A direct effect of the drug on the articular cartilage may also be important. Repeated injection of corticosteroid into the knee joints of normal rabbits results in cartilage degeneration,[130] with suppression of proteoglycan and collagen synthesis by the cartilage.[131] Although little histologic change was seen in non–weight-bearing joints, weight-bearing cartilage developed fibrillation and cystic degeneration.

Avascular (Aseptic) Necrosis of Bone. When avascular necrosis occurs subjacent to the joint, fracture of the necrotic bone may lead to collapse of the articular surface. The surface incongruities may then lead to secondary OA.[132] This is most common in the hip following femoral neck fracture. This form of secondary OA may occur also in the knee and other joints, however, when avascular necrosis occurs due to trauma, systemic corticosteroid administration, Caisson's disease, sickle cell disease, and so on.

As noted above, necrosis of the superficial eburnated bone, presumably due to friction, and of the bone surrounding enlarging subchondral cysts, is common in the advanced stages of primary OA.[35,36] However, there is little evidence that bone necrosis is important in the early stages of primary OA.

Hemophilic Arthropathy. The arthropathy that follows repeated hemorrhages into a joint in hemophilia,[133] and other congenital bleeding disorders that cause hemarthrosis, may resemble OA. In the later stages of he-

mophilic arthropathy, however, much more joint destruction occurs than in OA.[134] Erosion of the articular cartilage occurs early, followed by eburnation and marginal osteophytes. Subchondral pseudocyts occur and are filled with hemorrhagic material.

Kashin-Beck Disease. This condition is endemic in northeast Asia (Manchuria, eastern Siberia, North Korea). Enchondral bone growth is affected, leading to epiphyseal and metaphyseal dystrophic changes, resulting in severe osteoarthritic changes in multiple peripheral joints and in the spine.[135] The disease appears to be due to nutritional factors. A toxin from a parasitic fungus infecting food grains has been implicated.

Endocrine Disorders. The arthropathies associated with various endocrine disorders are discussed in detail in Chapter 102. In some instances, joint changes resulting from the endocrinopathy may lead to secondary OA. For example, an association between diabetes mellitus and OA has been suggested.[136-138] Waine claimed that in the diabetic individual OA tended to develop earlier and to be more severe than in the nondiabetic person.[139] The data, however, are not sufficiently strong to assure that the association is more than fortuitous. As noted above, joint degeneration may occur as a result of diabetic neuropathy (Charcot joint).

The association between acromegaly and OA,[140,141] on the other hand, seems more clear-cut. The OA changes develop while the articular cartilage is still thickened, owing to the action of somatomedin on the chondrocytes. Development of osteophytes in the presence of a widened joint space is suggestive of acromegaly. With progression of the joint disease, however, fibrillation and joint space narrowing ensue, accompanied by subchondral cysts and sclerosis and progressive osteophytosis, a development that is indistinguishable from primary OA.

The arthropathy of myxedema has been described by Bland and Frymoyer.[142] It appears that uncommonly a destructive arthropathy resembling OA may occur. However, since CPPD deposition, which itself may produce a destructive arthropathy (see above), may be seen in hypothyroidism,[143] the pathogenesis of this manifestation of myxedema is unclear.

Although data exist with respect to the effects of estrogens and androgens on development of OA in animals,[144-147] the results are conflicting, and whether changes in sex hormones are an important factor in OA in humans is unclear.

Estradiol has been shown to inhibit proteoglycan synthesis and degradation in a rabbit model of secondary OA,[147] while testosterone had no effect. Tamoxifen, an antiestrogen, diminished cartilage ulceration and pitting in this model when given to female rabbits after oophorectomy.[147]Estrogen, however, had no beneficial effect on the disease process[148] and reduced synthesis of glycosaminoglycans in the cartilage.

As noted above, primary generalized osteoarthritis occurs predominantly in women.[48] A trial of estrogen therapy in 20 middle-aged women with OA was found to produce no subjective or objective benefit.[48]

References

1. Forman, M.D., Malamet, R., and Kaplan, D.: A survey of osteoarthritis of the knee in the elderly. J. Rheum. 10:282, 1983.
2. Lawrence, J.S., Brenner, J.M., and Bier, F.: Osteoarthritis. Ann. Rheum. Dis. 25:1, 1966.
3. Mankin, H.J., Dorfman, H., Lippiello, L., et al.: Biochemical and metabolic abnormalities in articular cartilage from osteoarthritic human hips. J. Bone Joint Surg. 53A:523, 1971.
4. Solomon, L.: Pathogenesis of osteoarthritis. Lancet 1:1072, 1972.
5. Harris, W.H.: Primary osteoarthritis of the hip: A vanishing diagnosis. J. Rheum. 10 (Suppl. 9):64, 1983.
6. Blumberg, B.S., and Sokoloff, L.: Coalescence of caudal vertebrae in the giant dinosaur diplodocus. Arthritis Rheum. 4:592, 1961.
7. Sokoloff, L.: Degenerative joint disease in birds. Lab. Invest. 12:531, 1963.
8. Goldthwait, J.E.: The differential diagnosis and treatment of the so-called rheumatoid diseases. Boston Med. Surg. J. 151:529, 1904.
9. Garrod, A.E.: Rheumatoid arthritis, osteoarthritis, arthritis deformans. In Albutt, T.C., and Radleston, H.D. (eds.): A System of Medicine. London, Macmillan and Company, 1907, 3:3–43.
10. Lawrence, J.S.: Surveys of rheumatic complaints in the population. In Dixon, A.S.J (ed.): Progress in Clinical Rheumatology. London, J. and A. Churchill, 1966, p. 1.
11. Wood, P.H.N.: Rheumatic complaints. Br. Med. Bull. 27:82, 1971.
12. Lawrence, J.S., Bremner, J.M., and Bier, F.: Osteoarthrosis prevalence in the population and relationship between symptoms and x-ray changes. Ann. Rheum. Dis. 25:1, 1966.
13. Gordon, T.: Osteoarthrosis in U.S. adult. In Bennett, Ph., and Wood, P.H.N. (eds.): Population Studies of the Rheumatic Diseases. New York, Excerpta Medica Foundation, 1968, pp. 391–397.
14. Disease Control Program—Arthritis. U. S. Department of Health, Education and Welfare, 1966.
15. Bremner, J.M., Lawrence, J.S., and Mioll, W.E.: Degenerative joint disease in a Jamaican rural population. Ann. Rheum. Dis. 27:326, 1968.
16. Solomon, L., Beighton, P., and Lawrence, J.S.: Rheumatic disorders in the South African negro. S. Afr. Med. J. 49:1737, 1975.
17. Byers, P.D., Hoagland, F.T., Purewol, G.S., et al.: Articular cartilage changes in caucasian and Asian hip joints. Ann. Rheum. Dis. 33:157, 1974.
18. Hoagland, F.T., Yau, A.C.M.C., and Wong, W.L.: Osteoarthritis of the hip and other joints in southern China and Hong Kong. J. Bone Joint Surg. 55A:545, 1973.
19. Roberts, J., and Burch, T.A.: Prevalence of Osteoarthritis in Adults by Age, Sex, Race, and Geographic Area, United States—1960–1962. Public Health Service, Publ. No. 1,000, Series 11, No. 15, 1966.
20. Kellgren, J.H., and Lawrence, J.S.: Osteoarthrosis and disc degeneration in an urban population. Ann. Rheum. Dis. 17:388, 1958.
21. Kellgren, J.H., Lawrence, J.S., and Bier, F.: Genetic factors in generalized osteoarthritis. Ann. Rheum. Dis. 22:237, 1963.
22. Hadler, N.M.: The variable of usage in the epidemiology of osteoarthrosis. In J.G. Peyron (ed.): Epidemiology of Osteoarthrosis. Geigy, 1981, p. 164.
23. Cohen, A.S., Brandt, K.D., and Krey, P.: Synovial fluid. In Cohen, A.S. (ed.): Laboratory Diagnostic Procedures in the Rheumatic Diseases. 2nd ed, Boston, Little, Brown and Co., 1975, pp. 1–62.
24. Evans, C.H., Mears, D.C., and McKnight, J.L.: A preliminary ferrographic survey of the wear particles in human synovial fluid. Arthritis Rheum. 24:912, 1981.
25. McCarty, D.J.: Calcium pyrophosphate dihydrate deposition diseases—a current appraisal of the problem. In Holt, P.J.L. (ed.): Current Topics in Connective Tissue Disease. New York, Churchill and Livingstone, 1975, pp. 181–197.
26. Smukler, N.M., Edeiken, J., and Giviliano, V.J.: Ankylosis in osteoarthritis of the finger joints. Radiology 100:525, 1971.
27. CIOMS: The epidemiology of chronic rheumatism. In Vol.2 Atlas of Standard Radiographs of Arlhritis, Vol.2. Oxford, Blackwell Press, 1963.
28. Lowman, E.W.: Osteoarthritis. JAMA 157:487, 1955.
29. Cobb, S., Merchant, W.R., and Rubin, T.: The relation of symptoms to osteoarthritis. J. Chron. Dis. 5:197, 1957.
30. Gresham, G.E., and Rathey, U.K.: Osteoarthritis in knees of aged persons. Relationship between roentgenographic and clinical manifestations. JAMA 233:168, 1975.
31. Danielson, L.G.: Incidence and prognosis of coxarthrosis. Acta. Orthop. Scand. Suppl. 66:9, 1964.
32. Hernborg, J., and Nilsson, B.E.: The relationship between osteophytes in the knee joint, osteoarthritis and aging. Acta. Orthop. Scand. 44:69, 1973.
33. Bullough, P., Goodfellow, J., and O'Connor, J.: The relationship between degenerative changes and load-bearing in the human hip. J. Bone Joint Surg. 55B:746, 1973.
33a. Chrisman, O.D., Fessel, J.M., and Southwick, W.O.: Experimental pro-

duction of synovitis and marginal articullar exostoses in the knee joints of dogs. Yale J. Biol. Med. 37:409, 1965.
33b. Gilbertson, E.M.M.: Development of perarticullar osteophytes in experimentally induced osteoarthritis in the dog. Ann. Rheum. Dis. 34:12, 1975.
33c. Palmoski, M.J., and Brandt, K.D.: Immobilization of the knee prevents osteoarthritis after anterior cruciate ligament transection. Arthritis Rheum. 25:1201, 1982.
33d. Hamre, C.J., and Yeager, V.L.: Influence of muscle section on exostoses of lathyritic rats. Arch. Pathol. 64:426, 1957.
33e. Hamre, C.J., and Yeager, V.L.: Influence of denervated muscles on exostoses of rats fed a sweet-pea diet. Arch. Pathol. 65:215, 1958.
34. Eggers, G.W.N., Evans, E.B., Blumel, J., et al: Cystic change in the iliac acetabulum. J. Bone Joint Surg. 45A:669, 1963.
35. McCarthy, E.F.: The relationship of osteonecrosis to osteoarthritis. J. Rheum. 10(Suppl. 9):46, 1983.
36. Milgram, J.W.: Morphological alterations of the subchondral bone in advanced degenerative arthritis. Clin. Orthop. 73:293, 1983.
37. Heberden, W.: Commentaries on the History and Cure of Diseases. 2nd ed. London, T. Payne, 1803, p. 148.
38. Stecher, R.M., and Hauser, H.: Heberden's nodes. VII. The roentgenological and clinical appearance of degenerative joint disease of the fingers. Am. J. Roentgenol. 59:326, 1948.
39. Eaton, R.G., Dobranski, A.I., and Littler, J.W.: Marginal osteophyte excision in treatment of mucous cysts. J. Bone Joint Surg. 55A:570, 1973.
40. Jackson, D.S., and Kellgren, J.H.: Hyaluronic acid in Heberden's nodes. Ann. Rheum. Dis. 16:238, 1957.
41. Kleinert, H.E., Kutz, J.E., Fishman, J.H. et al.: Etiology and treatment of the so-called mucous cyst of the finger. J. Bone Joint Surg. 54A:1455, 1972.
42. Stecher, R.M.: Heberden's nodes. Heredity in hypertrophic arthritis of the finger joints. Am. J. Med. Sci. 201:801, 1941.
43. Stecher, R.M., Hersh, A.H., and Hauser, H.: Heberden's nodes. The family history and radiographic appearance of a large family. Am. J. Hum. Genet. 5:46, 1953.
44. Collins, D.H.: The Pathology of Articular and Spinal Diseases. London, E. Arnold, 1949.
45. Smythe, H.A.: Digital extensor tendon thickening: The primary lesion of Heberden's and Bouchard's nodes. Arthritis Rheum. 23:249, 1980.
46. Haygarth, J.: A clinical history of diseases. London, Cadell, 1805.
47. Cecil, R.L., and Archer, B.H.: Classification and treatment of chronic arthritis. JAMA 87:741, 1926.
48. Kellgren, J.H., and Moore, R.: Generalized osteoarthritis and Heberden's nodes. Br. Med. J. 1:181, 1952.
49. Rubens-Duval, A., Villiaumey, J., Kaplan, G., et al.: Aspects cliniques de la maladie arthrosique. Rev. Rhum. Mal. Osteoartic. 37:129, 1970.
50. Yazici, H., Saville, P.D., Salvata, E.A. et al.: Primary osteoarthrosis of the knee or hip. Prevalence of Heberden's nodes. JAMA 231:1260, 1975.
51. Solomon, L.: Osteoarthritis, local and generalized: a uniform disease? J. Rheum. 10 (Suppl. 9):13, 1983.
52. Roh, Y.S., Dequeker, J., and Mulier, J.C.: Osteoarthrosis at the hand skeleton in primary osteoarthrosis of the hip and in normal controls. Clin. Orthop. 90:90, 1973.
53. Acheson, R.M., and Collart, A.B.: New Haven survey of joint diseases. XVII. Relationships between some systemic characteristics and osteoarthrosis in a general population. Ann. Rheum. Dis. 34:379, 1975.
54. Lawrence, J.S., and Sebo, M.: The geography of osteoarthrosis. In Nuki, G. (ed.): The Etiopathogenesis of Osteoarthritis. London, Pitman, 1980, p. 155.
55. Kellgren, J.H.: Primary generalized osteoarthritis. Bull. Rheum. Dis. 4:63, 1954.
56. Ehrlich, G.E.: Inflammatory osteoarthritis. I. The clinical syndromes. J. Chron. Dis. 25:317, 1972.
57. Goldie, I.: Erosive osteoarthritis of the distal finger joints. Acta Orthop. Scand. 43:469, 1972.
58. Marmor, L., and Peter, J.B.: Osteoarthritis of the hand. Clin. Orthop. 64:164, 1969.
59. Ehrlich, G.E.: Osteoarthritis beginning with inflammation definitions and correlations. JAMA 232:157, 1975.
60. Forestier, J., and Rotes-Querol, J.: Senile ankylosing hyperostosis of the spine. Ann. Rheum. Dis. 9:321, 1950.
61. Forestier, J., and Lagier, R.: Ankylosing hyperostosis of the spine. Clin. Orthop. 74:65, 1971.
62. Resnick, J., Shaul, S.R., and Robins, J.M.: Diffuse idiopathic skeletal hyperostosis (DISH): Forestier's disease with extraspinal manifestations. Radiology 115:513, 1975.
63. Utsinger, P.D., Resnick, D., and Shapiro, R.: Diffuse skeletal abnormalities in Forestier disease. Arch. Intern. Med. 136:763, 1976.
64. Resnick, J., Shapiro, R.F., Wiesner, K.B. et al.: Diffuse idiopathic skeletal hyperostosis DISH (ankylosing hyperostosis) of Forestier and Rotes-Querol. Semin. Arthritis Rheum. 7:153, 1978.

65. Littlejohn, G.V., and Smythe, H.A.: Marked hyperinsulinemia after glucose challenge in patients with diffuse idiopathic skeletal hyperostosis. J. Rheumatol. 8:965, 1981.

66. Gray, R.J., and Gottlieb, N.L.: Rheumatic disorders associated with diabetes mellitus: a literature review. Semin. Arthritis Rheum. 6:19, 1976.

67. Perry, J.D., Wolf, H., Festernstein, J., et al.: Ankylosing hyperostosis: A study of HLA A, B and C antigens. Ann. Rheum. Dis. 38:72, 1979.

68. Shapiro, R.F., Wiesner, K.B., Bryan, B.L., et al.: HLA-B27 and modified bone formation. Lancet 1:230, 1976.

69. Vernon-Roberts, B., Pirie, C.J., and Trenwith, V.: Pathology of the dorsal spine in ankylosing hyperostosis. Ann. Rheum. Dis. 33:281, 1974.

70. Evarts, C.M.: Challenge of the aging hip. Geriatrics 24:112, 1969.

71. Solomon, L.: Patterns of osteoarthritis of the hip. J. Bone Joint Surg. 58B:176, 1976.

72. Murray, R.O.: The aetiology of primary osteoarthritis of the hip. Br. J. Radiol. 38:810, 1965.

73. Goodfellow, J., Hungerford, D.S., and Woods, C.: Patellofemoral joint mechanics and pathology. J. Bone Joint Surg. 58B:291, 1976.

74. Goodfellow, J., Hungerford, D.S., and Zindel, M.: Patellofemoral joint mechanics and pathology. Functional anatomy of the patello-femoral joint. J. Bone Joint Surg. 58B:287, 1976.

75. Collins, D.H.: The Pathology of Articular and Spinal Disease. London, E. Arnold, 1949.

76. Friedenberg, Z.B., Edeiken J., Spencer, H.N., et al.: Degenerative changes in the cervical spine. J. Bone Joint Surg. 41A:61, 1959.

77. Schmorl, G., and Junghanns, H.: The Human Spine in Health and Disease. 2nd ed. New York, Grune and Stratton, 1971.

78. Prince, D.S., Luna, R.F., Cohn, M.H. et al.: Osteophyte-induced dysphagia. JAMA 234:77, 1975.

79. Dutton, C.B., and Riley, L.H.: Cervical migraine: Not merely a pain in the neck. Am. J. Med. 47:141, 1969.

80. O'Brien, W.M., La Du, B.N., and Bunim, J.J.: Biochemical, pathologic and clinical aspects of alkaptonuria, ochronosis and ochronotic arthropathy. Am. J. Med. 34:813, 1963.

81. Hunter, T., Gordon, D.A., and Ogryzlo, M.A.: The ground pepper sign of synovial fluid: A diagnostic feature of ochronosis. J. Rheumatol. 1:45, 1974.

82. Reginato, A.J., Schumacher, H.R., and Martinez, V.A.: Ochronotic arthropathy with calcium pyrophosphate crystal deposition. A light and electron microscopic study. Arthritis Rheum. 16:1705, 1973.

83. Bywaters, E.G.L., Dorling, J., and Sutor, J.: Ochronotic densification. Ann. Rheum. Dis. 29:563, 1970.

84. Lagier, R., and Steiger, U.: Hip arthropathy in ochronosis: Anatomical and radiological study. Skel. Radiol. 5:91, 1980.

85. Schumacher, H.R., Jr.: Hemochromatosis and arthritis. Arthritis Rheum. 7:41, 1964.

86. Angevine, C.D., and Jacox, R.F.: Unusual connective tissue manifestations of hemochromatosis. Arthritis Rheum. 17:477, 1974.

87. Gordon, D.A., Clarke, P.V., and Ogryzlo, M.A.: The chondrocalcific arthropathy of iron overload. Relationship to hemochromatosis. Arch. Intern. Med. 134:21, 1974.

88. Schumacher, H.R.: Ultrastructural characteristics of the synovial membrane in idiopathic hemochromatosis. Ann. Rheum. Dis. 31:465, 1972.

89. Hamilton, E., Williams, R., Barlow, K.A., et al.: The arthropathy of idiopathic hemochromatosis. Q. J. Med. 37:171, 1968.

90. Mitrovic, D., Mazabraud, A., Jaffries, R., et al.: Etude histologique et histochemique des lesions articularies de la chondrocalcinese survenant au cours d'une hemochromatose. Arch. Anat. Pathol. 14:264, 1966.

91. Hirsch, J.H., Killien, C., and Troupin, R.H.: The arthropathy of hemochromatosis. Radiology 118:591, 1976.

92. Dymock, I.W., Hamilton, E.B.D., Laws, J.W., et al.: Arthropathy of haemochromatosis: Clinical and radiological analysis of 63 patients with iron overload. Ann. Rheum. Dis. 29:469, 1970.

93. Sella, E.J., and Goodman, A.H.: Arthropathy secondary to transfusion hemachromatosis. J. Bone Joint Surg. 55A:1077, 1973.

94. McCarty, D.J., and Pepe, P.F.: Erythrocyte neutral inorganic pyrophosphatase in pseudogout. J. Lab. Clin. Med. 79:277, 1972.

95. Boudin, G., Pepin, B., Barbizet, J., et al.: Les arthropathies de la maladie de Wilson. Rev. Rhum. 31:594, 1964.

96. Golding, D.N., and Walshe, J.M.: Arthropathy of Wilson's disease. Study of clinical and radiological features in 32 patients. Ann. Rheum. Dis. 36:99, 1977.

97. Feller, E.R., and Schumacher, H.R.: Osteoarticular changes in Wilson's disease. Arthritis Rheum. 15:259, 1972.

98. Roesenoer, V., and Michell, R.C.: Skeletal changes in Wilson's disease (hepatolenticular degeneration). Br. J. Radiol. 32:805, 1959.

99. Kaklamanis, P., and Spengos, M.: Osteoarticular changes and synovial biopsy findings in Wilson's disease. Ann. Rheum. Dis. 32:422, 1973.

100. Dieppe, P.A., Crocker, P.R., Corke, C.F., et al.: Synovial fluid crystals. Q. J. Med. 48:533, 1979.

101. Dieppe, P.A.: Crystal-induced arthropathies and osteoarthritis. *In* Buchanan, W.W., and Dick, W.C. (eds.): Recent Advances in Rheumatology. Edinburgh, Churchill Livingstone, 1981, p. 1.

102. Zitnan, D., and Sitaj, S.: Natural course of articular chondrocalcinosis. Arthritis Rheum. 19:363, 1976.

103. Menkes, C.K., Simon, F., and Delrieu, F.: Destructive arthropathy in chondrocalcinosis articularis. Arthritis Rheum. 19:329, 1976.

104. McCarty, D.J., Halverson, P.B., Carrera, G.F., et al.: Milwaukee shoulder. Arthritis Rheum. 24:464, 1981.

105. Reginato, A.J., Schumacher, H.R., and Martinez, V.: The articular cartilage in familial chondrocalcinosis: Light and electron microscopic study. Arthritis Rheum. 17:974, 1974.

106. Doherty, M., Watt, I., and Dieppe, P.A.: Localised chonrocalcinosis in post-meniscectomy knees. Lancet,1:12207, 1982

107. Pritzker, K.P.H., Renlund, R.C., and Cheng, P.-T.: Which comes first: Crystals or osteoarthritis? Study of surgically removed femoral heads. J. Rheum. 10(Suppl. 9):38, 1983.

108. Gibilisco, P.A., Schumacher, H.R., Sieck, M., et al.: Studies on the role of synovial fluid apatite and calcium pyrophosphate crystals in osteoarthritis. Arthritis Rheum. 25:543, 1982.

109. Schumacher, H.R., Gordon, G., Paul, M., et al.: Osteoarthritis, crystal deposition and inflammation. Semin. Arthritis Rheum. 11:116, 1981.

110. Reginato, A.J., Paul, H., and Schumacher, H.R.: Hydroxyapatite crystals in rheumatoid arthritis synovial fluid. Clin. Res. 30:662A, 1982.

111. Halverson, P.B., and McCarty, D.J.: Identification of hydroxyapatite crystals in synovial fluid. Arthritis Rheum. 22:389, 1979.

112. Roper, B.A.: Paget's disease of the hip with osteoarthrosis: results of intertrochanteric osteotomy. J. Bone Joint Surg. 53B:660, 1971.

113. Graham, J., and Harris, W.H.: Paget's disease involving the hip joint. J. Bone Joint Surg. 53B:650, 1971.

114. Mintz, G., and Fraga, A.: Severe osteoarthritis of the elbow in foundry workers. Arch. Environ. Health 27:78, 1973.

115. Bruckner, F.E., and Howell, A.: Neuropathic joints. Semin Arthritis Rheum. 2:47, 1972.

116. Charcot, J.M.: Sur quelques arthropathies qui paraissent d'ependre d'une l'esion du cerveau ou de la moelle 'epini'ere. Arch. Physiol. Norm. Pathol. 1:161, 1868.

117. Sokoloff, L.: Beitrag zur Casuistik der Erkrankungen der Gelenke bei Giomatose des Ruckenmarkes (Syringomyelia). Deutsche Ztschr. fur Chir. 51:506, 1892.

118. Jordan, W.R.: Neuritic manifestations in diabetes mellitus. Arch. Intern. Med. 57:307, 1936.

119. Eloesser, L.: On the nature of neuropathic affections of joints. Ann. Surg. 66:201, 1917.

120. O'Connor, B.L., Palmoski, M.J., and Brandt, K.D.: Neurogenic acceleration of degenerative arthropathy. Trans. 30th Ann. Orthop. Res. Soc. Mtg. 9:237, 1984.

121. Brower, A.C., and Allman, R.M.: Pathogenesis of the neurotrophic joint: neurotraumatic vs. neurovascular. Radiology 139:349, 1981.

122. Johnson, L.C.: Discussion of: Williams, L.E., Bland, J.H., and Lipson, R.L.: Cervical spine subluxation and massive osteolysis in the upper extremities in rheumatoid arthritis. Arthritis Rheum. 9:348, 1966.

123. Dyck, P.J., Stevens, J.C., O'Brien, P.E., et al.: Neurogenic arthropathy and recurring fractures with subclinical inherited neuropathy. Neurology 33:357, 1983.

124. Johnson, J.T.H.: Neuropathic fractures and joint injuries. Pathogenesis and rationale of prevention and treatment. J. Bone Joint Surg. 49A:1, 1967.

125. Jacobelli, S., McCarty, D.J., Silcox, D.C., et al.: Calcium pyrophosphate crystal deposition in neuropathic joints: Four cases of polyarticular involvement. Ann. Intern. Med. 79:340, 1973.

126. Howell, D.S., Muniz, O., Pita, J.C., et al.: Pyrophosphate release by osteoarthritic cartilage incubates. Arthritis Rheum. 19(Suppl. 3):488, 1976.

127. Chandler, G.N., Jones, D.T., Wright, V., et al.: Charcot's arthropathy following intra-articular hydrocortisone. Br. Med. J. 1:952, 1959.

128. Steinberg, C.L., Duthe, R.B., and Piva, A.E.: Charcot-like arthropathy following intra-articular hydrocortisone. JAMA 181:851, 1962.

129. Bentley, G., and Goodfellow, J.W.: Disorganization of the knees following intra-articular hydrocortisone injections. J. Bone Joint Surg. 51B:498, 1969.

130. Moskowitz, R.W., Davis, W., Sammarco, J., et al.: Experimentally induced corticosteroid arthropathy. Arthritis Rheum. 134:236, 1970.

131. Behrens, F., Shepard, H., and Mitchell, N.: Alteration of rabbit articular cartilage by intra-articular injections of glucocorticoids. J. Bone Joint Surg. 58A:1157, 1976.

132. Bullough, P.G.: Osteonecrosis in surgically replaced osteoarthritic hips. J. Rheum. 10(Suppl. 9):51, 1983.

133. Arnold, W.D., and Hilgartner, M.W.: Hemophilic arthropathy: Current concepts in pathogenesis and management. J. Bone Joint Surg. 59A:287, 1977.

134. Gilchrist, G.S., Hagedorn, A.B., and Stouffer, R.N.: Severe degenerative joint disease: Mild and moderately severe hemophilia. JAMA 238:2883, 1977.

135. Neslerov, A.I.: The clinical course of Kashin-Beck disease. Arthritis Rheum. 7:29, 1964.

136. Silberberg, R., and Silberberg, M.: Pathogenesis of osteoarthritis. Pathol. Microbiol. 27:447, 1964.

137. Ghanem, M.H., and Said, M.: Diabetes mellitus and osteoarthritis. Egypt Rheum. 4:1, 1967.

138. Blanchi, V., and Ricci, G.: The role of various factors in the etiology of osteoarthritis: Observations on 500 subjects. Rheumatismo (Milano) 19:146, 1967.

139. Waine, H., Nevinny, D., Rosenthal, J., et al.: Association of osteoarthritis and diabetes mellitus. Tufts Folia Med. 7:13, 1961.

140. Kellgren, J.H., Ball, J., and Tutton, G.K.: The articular and other limb changes in acromegaly. A clinical and pathological study of 25 cases. Q. J. Med. 21:405, 1952.

141. Bluestone, R., Bywaters, E.G.L., Hartog, M., et al.: Acromegalic arthropathy. Ann. Rheum. Dis. 30:243, 1971.

142. Bland, J.H., and Frymoyer, J.W.: Rheumatic syndromes of myxedema. N. Engl. J. Med. 282:1171, 1970.

143. Dorwart, B.B., and Schumacher, H.R.: Joint effusions, chondrocalcinosis and other rheumatic manifestations in hypothyrodisim. A clinicopathologic study. Am. J. Med. 59:780, 1975.

144. Silberberg, M., and Silberberg, R.: Role of sex hormones in the pathogenesis of osteoarthrosis of mice. Lab. Invest. 12:285, 1963.

145. Silberberg, M., and Silberberg, R.: Modifying action of estrogen on the evolution of osteoarthrosis in mice of different ages. Endocrinology 72:449, 1963.

146. Sokoloff, L., Varney, D.A., and Scott, J.F.: Sex hormones, bone changes and osteoarthritis in DBA/2JN mice. Arthritis Rheum. 8:1027, 1965.

147. Moskowitz, R.W., Goldberg, V.M., Rosner, I.A., et al.: Specific drug therapy of experimental osteoarthritis. Sem. Arthritis Rheum. 11(Suppl. 1):127, 1981.

148. Rosner, I.A., Goldberg, V.M., Getzy, L., et al.: Effects of estrogen on cartilage in experimentally induced osteoarthritis. Arthritis Rheum. 22:52, 1979.

Chapter 90

Management of Osteoarthritis

Kenneth D. Brandt

THE CORRECT DIAGNOSIS

Optimal management of osteoarthritis requires an accurate diagnosis. Since the diagnosis is dependent upon the presence of typical radiologic features (e.g., joint space narrowing, subchondral sclerosis, osteophytosis) that commonly occur in asymptomatic individuals,[1] the clinical significance of the x-ray findings must be interpreted in light of the patient's history and physical examination. Furthermore, before the physician considers therapeutic options for the patient with joint pain and radiologic evidence of osteoarthritis, the following question must be considered: Is osteoarthritis responsible for the patient's pain?

The question is not always easily answered. Two problems compound the issue. First, rheumatic diseases are not mutually exclusive. Thus, gout, pseudogout, bacterial joint infection, or some other condition may be the proximate cause of joint pain in such a patient, rather than osteoarthritis. On the other hand, the patient's symptoms may be due to soft tissue rheumatism. For example, the patient with radiologic evidence of osteoarthritis of the knee may suffer from knee pain that results not from the intra-articular disease but from anserine bursitis; the patient with osteoarthritis of the acromioclavicular joint may present with shoulder pain caused by coincidental bicipital tendinitis; the patient with osteoarthritis of the first carpometacarpal joint may have pain in the thumb due to an unrelated carpal tunnel syndrome or de Quervain's disease. In each case, accurate diagnosis and treatment of the soft tissue problem may produce gratifying relief of pain, even though nothing has been done to affect the patient's osteoarthritis.

COMPONENTS AND GOALS OF THE TREATMENT PROGRAM

The components of a treatment program for the patient with osteoarthritis may include drugs, physical measures, surgery, and patient education—and when appropriate, education of family members and advisors. Although no medical cure exists today for osteoarthritis, much can be done to relieve the patient's pain, maintain or improve mobility, and minimize disability.

How aggressively should the patient be treated? Salicylates and other nonsteroidal anti-inflammatory drugs are useful in producing symptomatic relief, since they are analgesic and also reduce the synovitis that is present. However, none of the these drugs will arrest the pathologic changes in cartilage or bone. Indeed, some may contribute to degenerative changes in the articular cartilage and bone (see later discussion).[2-5] Measures that protect the involved joint from mechanical damage (e.g., instructing the patient in the use of assistive devices and patterns of joint usage to avoid excessive loading of the articular cartilage, strengthening the supporting muscles to increase joint stability) are important in diminishing pain and discomfort. In many patients with osteoarthritis of the knee, a program of isometric quadriceps exercises may eliminate the patient's pain within weeks. Although no evidence is available to indicate that such physical measures are prophylactic, it is logical to consider that they may retard or prevent progression of the disease by preventing further cartilage damage. This important question requires study.

Furthermore, the view, widely held by patients and their doctors, that osteoarthritis is inevitably progressive, requires closer examination. In a survey of 682 elderly people, the prevalence and severity of signs and symptoms suggestive of osteoarthritis of the knee did not increase with age but remained constant in the seventh, eighth, and ninth decades of life.[6] Similarly, in another study of symptomatic individuals with "non-rheumatoid" arthritis older than 54 years of age with significant radiologic evidence of osteoarthritis, the percentage with the most marked abnormalities did not increase with age.[7] Radiologic evidence of osteophytosis, in particular, is not a diagnostic criterion or a prognostic indicator of osteoarthritis, but appears to be related to age. Thus, in patients who had osteophytes as the sole radiologic abnormality in the hip x-ray, less than 1 percent had developed joint space narrowing and other changes of osteoarthritis after 10 years.[8] Similar results were obtained in a study of the significance of osteophytosis in the knee. Clinically important progressive cartilage damage occurred in only a minority of patients.[9]

In view of the preceding, treatment of osteoarthritis should be tailored to fit the clinical severity of the disease. For patients with only mildly symptomatic disease, instruction in principles of joint protection, reassurance, and occasional analgesics may be all that is required. The importance of reassurance should not be minimized, however. Many patients with clinically mild osteoarthritis in one or two joints worry greatly that their disease will become widespread and ultimately incapacitating, dooming them to years of pain, uselessness, restricted mobility, and dependency. The physician can help considerably by pointing out that such a fate is very unlikely. In contrast, for the patient who has more severe disease, with impaired function and significant disability, a comprehensive, aggressive approach is warranted.

ATTENTION TO FACTORS CAUSING EXCESSIVE JOINT LOADING

Poor body mechanics may cause or aggravate osteoarthritis. Pronated feet, genu varum, and genu valgum all create excessive loading on the knee, and may be corrected with orthotics, or by osteotomy. Poor posture should be corrected, and supports for the pendulous abdomen or breasts or the excessively lordotic lumbar spine may be helpful:

Instructing the patient in the principles of joint protection is usually indicated. For patients with significant osteoarthritis of the interphalangeal or the first carpometacarpal joints, the following measures may be helpful:*

1. Use electric appliances (scissors, can openers, knives, mixers, power tools) whenever possible. Try to select multipurpose tools with controls that are easy to reach and operate.

2. Use lightweight utensils, such as those made of aluminum and plastic, rather than those made of glass or heavy materials.

3. Large handles are easier to hold than small handles. Wrap a piece of foam rubber around eating utensils, toothbrushes, pens, irons, and other items with narrow handles.

4. Pinching a small zipper tab may be difficult. To pull the zipper more easily, use a ring or loop of string on the zipper tab, and place a finger through the loop.

5. Replace buttons with Velcro fasteners. Secure cuff buttons with elastic thread to eliminate the need for buttoning.

6. Use easy-to-reach kitchen storage to avoid the strain of reaching deeply into cupboards. Lazy Susans, slide-out shelves, and pegboard wall storage are good alternatives.

7. Allow dishes to air dry or use an automatic dishwasher.

8. Use a single-lever type of faucet, rather than one that requires twisting or turning.

9. Use a wall-mounted jar-opener that allows you to grasp the jar with both hands while twisting to open.

10. Whenever possible, slide objects to move them instead of lifting them. To transport heavy objects, use a cart with wheels.

11. When you must lift a heavy item, do not attempt to pick it up in one hand. Get under the object and lift with the palms of both hands.

Patients may use the following measures to reduce stress on the hips and knees:*

1. Do not walk or jog as an exercise. Swimming is an excellent alternative.

2. Avoid stairs whenever possible.

3. Sit rather than stand. Use high stools when working at a counter.

4. Use higher chairs rather than low sofas.

5. Avoid kneeling or squatting.

6. Before rising from a chair, sit at the edge of the seat with your legs under your body. Use the arm rests to push yourself up from the seat.

If there is significant osteoarthritis of the lumbar spine, the patient may be instructed in the following measures:*

1. Avoid lifting heavy objects.

2. Keep your back straight while lifting; lift by bending the knees.

3. Do not lift objects above the level of your waist.

4. Avoid reaching to grasp an object, as when leaning into a car trunk.

5. Always stand close to your work.

6. Avoid standing for prolonged periods.

7. Push, do not pull, objects.

8. Avoid leaning over a desk or work surface for prolonged periods.

9. When driving, move the seat forward enough to

---

*From form used by Occupational Therapy Department, University Hospital, Indianapolis, Indiana.

*Adapted from form used by Physical Therapy Department, University Hospital, Indianapolis, Indiana.

keep the knees bent and to decrease the arch in your back.

The preceding should be viewed as measures not only to diminish pain but also to prevent further joint damage.

For all patients with osteoarthritis, an analysis of vocational and avocational use of the arthritic joint is important. The pattern of usage may clearly determine the development of osteoarthritis in a given joint, as shown in an interesting clinical and radiologic analysis of the hands of burlers, winders, and spinners in a worsted mill in rural Virginia.[10] Burling is a task that calls for a predominance of precision pinch in the right hand; winding is a bimanual task requiring a repetitive power grip; and spinning requires predominantly precision pinch with the right hand. Results showed that the localization of impairment and x-ray evidence of osteoarthritis correlated nicely with the demands placed on the joints by these occupational tasks.

Activities that cause excessive loading of the involved joint should be avoided when possible. For example, it will be helpful for the patient with osteoarthritis of the hip or knee if the work place can be modified to permit sitting instead of standing and if requirements for kneeling or squatting can be eliminated. Rest periods in a chair or bed for 30 to 60 minutes in the morning and the afternoon may diminish discomfort in lower extremity joints or the lumbar spine. Several shorter periods of standing or walking are more desirable than a single prolonged one. Temporary use of a cervical collar may be helpful for the patient who is acutely symptomatic with cervical spondylosis, but immobilization of the painful joint or complete bed rest is rarely required.

The osteoarthritic patient may have difficulty accepting the recommendation that use of the affected joint be reduced, because of fear that the joint will stiffen unless used continuously. The sensation of jelling that many of these individuals experience following periods of inactivity or prolonged sitting (as during an automobile or plane ride) contributes to this concern. Instructing the patient to put the involved joint through its range of motion every 15 to 20 minutes during such periods may minimize this discomfort. Also, informing the patient that prescribed exercises (see section on Physical Therapy) will be an important component of the treatment program will help reassure the individual who resists curtailment of activities that stress the diseased joint.

The patient with painful osteoarthritis of the hip or knee may benefit from a cane (to be used in the contralateral hand) or, if symptoms are bilateral, crutches or a walker. Such ambulation aids pose fewer problems for the patient with osteoarthritis than for the individual with rheumatoid arthritis, who is more likely to encounter difficulty with their use because of concomitant involvement of hands, wrists or shoulders, or all of these. Many patients with osteoarthritis, however, are psychologically unprepared to accept an ambulatory aid. In this case, education of the patient concerning the mechanical advantages to be derived from the device, a

trial of usage to permit the patient to experience the relief of discomfort afforded by the device, and emphasis on the possible slowing of disease progression to be derived from its use are all warranted. The collaboration of a physical therapist in these efforts is usually desirable.

DIET

No one will take issue with the recommendation that the obese patient with osteoarthritis should lose weight. The excess weight contributes to the abnormal loading of articular cartilage in weight-bearing joints. However, *most* of the loading of articular cartilage results not from ponderal mass but from the contraction of the muscles that span the joint and help to stabilize it.[11]

There is no good evidence that obesity itself *causes* osteoarthritis in lower extremity joints except, perhaps, in the individual who is so massively obese that it is not possible to appose the thighs; genu varum may develop from trying to maintain the feet under the center of gravity. In this case degeneration of the medial compartment of the knee may develop.[12] Notably, data from the United States Health and Nutrition Examination Survey (HANES) demonstrated an association between obesity and osteoarthritis of hands and knees, but not of hips or ankles.[13]

Even though obesity may not cause osteoarthritis, it may *aggravate* symptoms and accelerate cartilage breakdown in the lumbar spine and the lower extremity joints. For these reasons, the obese osteoarthritic patient should be instructed in a weight reduction diet and urged to strive to normalize body weight. However, this goal, although laudable, is not likely to be achieved. Because of the degree of inactivity imposed by the arthritis, and a caloric requirement that is often low, weight loss is difficult for these individuals. If the patient is sufficiently motivated, participation in a mutual support group (e.g., Weight Watchers, TOPS) may be helpful.

The preceding measures, to the extent that they diminish joint loading, not only provide symptomatic relief but also may reduce the synovial inflammation that is attributed to cartilage breakdown. Cartilaginous wear particles, shown by ferrography to be indicative of cutting wear and rubbing wear, have been demonstrated in human synovial fluid aspirates.[14] Such particles are capable of eliciting the release from macrophages and synovial cells of neutral proteases capable of releasing glycosaminoglycans and hydroxyproline from cartilage.[15]

PSYCHOLOGICAL COPING

Yet another problem may confront the physician who advises patients to diminish their levels of physical activity. Patients with osteoarthritis often develop techniques to help maintain normalcy in their daily activities and in their interactions with others. They are similar to the techniques used by patients with other chronic conditions.[16] Two approaches commonly emerge—"keeping up" (i.e., maintaining the previous level of activity) and "covering up" (i.e., hiding the illness from the public).

Many patients with osteoarthritis attempt to keep up with whatever they perceive as normal activities, despite the likelihood that this may increase their joint pain. Some engage in excessive keeping up to prove their ability or to recapture their identity. For example, a patient with osteoarthritis of the knee may refuse to seek a feasible modification of the situation at work by asking for a job that would permit sitting instead of standing because of the perceived need to maintain an image of health for co-workers or the employer. Keeping up may be possible during work hours, but at the end of the day, in the privacy of their own homes, these patients collapse on the couch with pain and fatigue.

Covering up involves masking the disability and pain. Patients with osteoarthritis often relate that they reply, "I'm fine," when someone asks how they are, even when they are experiencing considerable joint pain. They are often unwilling to reveal visible symbols of their disability, for example, a cane or walker. They may refuse to face a trip to the shopping center because it hurts too much to walk without their cane.

For the physician to advise patients to abandon these techniques is not always helpful.[17] Through experience, most patients already know that they suffer when they overdo activities. Many know that it is illogical to refuse to accept their need for a cane or walker but have not overcome their need to hide their physical problems from the public.

Patients with osteoarthritis who take great care to mask their discomfort or disability may wonder why their families or friends are not more helpful or sympathetic. Patients are sometimes proud because "no one knows" yet distressed because "no one cares."[16] Because osteoarthritis is often not a visible illness, and because many still consider arthritis to be a minor disease, lack of understanding by others can be a problem even to the patient who is not keeping up or covering up. It is often useful to suggest to patients that the price they may pay for covering up or keeping up is the loss of potential support, help, and understanding. It may be pointed out that no matter how much others may care for the patient, they cannot read minds. This may help the patient decide when and where to keep up and cover up.

SEXUALITY

Osteoarthritis may significantly affect sexual function. This may be a particular problem for patients with osteoarthritis of the hips, knees, or spine. Results of a survey of 121 patients with osteoarthritis revealed that the most frequently mentioned causes of sexual difficulties were pain (40 percent), stiffness (75 percent), and loss of libido (22 percent).[18] Of the 81 patients who expressed sexual difficulties resulting from their disease,

23 percent felt that these difficulties were the cause of marital unhappiness. Surgical treatment of osteoarthritis of the hip resulted in complete or considerable improvement in sexual function for 34 percent of the 70 patients who underwent surgery.

It is appropriate for the physician or other health care professional to initiate discussion of sexual concerns, insofar as the patient may be reluctant to do so.[19] This may often be accomplished as a natural component of the evaluation for hip disease, during which the physician may ask about sexual problems while ascertaining the effects of the disease on other aspects of function, such as ability to rise from a sofa or toilet seat.[20] One might ask, "Has your disease caused a change in your sexual function?" and, if indicated, "Does this change concern you?" The cause of the sexual concern should be ascertained, as well as what the patient thinks might improve the problem and how the partner feels about the problem. At times, arthritis is an excuse for, not the cause of, the sexual problem. If the patient is unaware of how the partner feels about the problem, poor communication is likely to be contributory. In either case, in-depth marital counseling may be appropriate.

For the patient with limited spine or hip mobility, or both, a side-by-side position for intercourse may be preferable to one requiring the patient to be supine. Physicians should encourage couples to try a variety of positions to discover which is most comfortable for sexual activity. The Arthritis Foundation's excellent pamphlet, "Living and Loving with Arthritis," which contains suggestions for resolving a variety of sexual problems, is a valuable educational resource for arthritic patients.[21]

PHYSICAL THERAPY

Physical therapy holds a prominent position in the treatment of osteoarthritis and involves principally the use of heat or cold and an appropriate exercise program. It is generally useful to precede each exercise session with applications of moderate heat for 15 to 20 minutes to relieve pain and diminish stiffness. Patients should be cautioned to remove any liniment from the skin prior to heat application and to avoid lying on the heat source, since this may cause local compression of circulation and lead to a burn. Application of diathermy or ultrasound to joints that have undergone arthroplasty, and contain metal components, is contraindicated, since this may lead to deep thermal burns.

A variety of forms of heat may be used, for example, hydrocollator packs, electric pads, ultrasound, infrared bakers, diathermy, and paraffin baths. Patients often find moist heat to be more effective than dry heat. Practicality and cost should be considered in prescribing the particular modality to be employed. A warm bath or shower often proves to be the most convenient form of heat treatment. For deep-seated joints (e.g., hips, spine), ultrasound or diathermy may be particularly effective, although they often afford no greater benefit than less expensive, simpler forms of heat application.

Occasionally, heat may increase the patient's pain, and ice packs prove to be a more effective analgesic. Although controlled studies have not been performed in osteoarthritis, the efficacy of cryotherapy has recently been shown in patients with rheumatoid arthritis, in whom it increased range of motion and decreased pain through a mechanism apparently related to endorphin release.[22]

The exercise program should be designed to preserve or improve range of motion and to strengthen the involved muscles. Periarticular muscle atrophy, which has been shown to be selective for type II fibers,[23] is common in osteoarthritis and is presumably due to decreased activity as a consequence of joint pain. Isometric exercises are preferable to isotonic ones, since they minimize joint stress. Exercises should be initiated with three or four sessions daily. A small number of repetitions should be prescribed initially and gradually increased to the desired maximum. The following describes two types of isometric quadriceps exercises (quadriceps setting and straight leg raises).*

Quadriceps Setting Exercise

1. Lie on your back with legs stretched out straight.
2. Keeping your knee straight, press your knee down into the bed, tightening the big muscle on the front of your thigh above your knee.
3. Hold the muscle tight for 5 seconds (count one thousand and one, one thousand and two, one thousand and three, and so forth).
4. Relax the muscle for 5 seconds.
5. Repeat ten times.
6. Perform three times daily (ten repetitions each time).
7. Gradually increase until you are performing this exercise ten times daily (10 to 15 repetitions each time).
8. Note: This exercise can also be performed while sitting in a chair with legs stretched out straight. Simply press the heels into the floor, tightening the thigh muscle as already described.

Straight Leg Raises

1. Lie on your back in bed.
2. To exercise the right leg, first bend the left knee, placing the left foot flat. (This will prevent any back strain during the exercise.)
3. Tighten the big muscle about the right knee and slowly lift the right leg straight up as high as it will go. If the knee bends, do not lift further.
4. Now slowly lower the leg and hold about 6 in. off the bed for 5 seconds (count one thousand and one, one

thousand and two, one thousand and three, and so forth).
5. Lower the leg to the bed.
6. Repeat five to ten times.
7. Perform two to three times daily.

Note: If you have severe pain during exercise, or pain that lasts more than 15 minutes to 20 minutes following the exercise, temporarily decrease the number of repetitions by one half.

DRUG THERAPY

Drug therapy in osteoarthritis today is symptomatic. It should be recognized that many patients with this condition have only minimal symptoms and may be managed with the physical measures described previously, without medications. However, in others, symptomatic relief requires the use of analgesic or anti-inflammatory drugs, or both.

The fact that drug therapy is "symptomatic" does not mean that it is not important or that it may not be helpful. Notably, patients with severe osteoarthritis rated their satisfaction with life lower than did patients undergoing chronic hemodialysis.[24] Although this may have been related in part to factors such as living alone and duration of unemployment, chronic pain may well be a significant factor in the decreased satisfaction in life among patients with osteoarthritis. Pain in osteoarthritic patients may be ascribed to a number of factors, for example, microfractures in subchondral trabeculae, irritation of periosteal nerve endings, ligamentous stress due to bone deformity or effusion, venous congestion caused by remodeling of subchondral bone,[25] associated soft tissue rheumatism (see previous discussion), and muscle strain. Since the articular cartilage itself is aneural, pain does not arise from the degenerating cartilage. Synovial inflammation does occur commonly in osteoarthritis and may be a significant source of pain. A recent symposium dealt extensively with the topic of inflammation in osteoarthritis.[26] Usually, the synovitis is much less intense than that seen in rheumatoid arthritis; for example, the synovial fluid leukocyte counts are normal or only slightly increased (2000 cells/mm³). The synovial membrane may contain foci of infiltrating lymphocytes, but pannus does not occur. Given the pathologic changes discussed here, it is not surprising that anti-inflammatory drugs may afford greater symptomatic relief than that provided by simple analgesics.

The anti-inflammatory drugs that are useful for treatment of osteoarthritis include salicylates and other nonsteroidal anti-inflammatory drugs. Notably, the latter were designed principally for use in rheumatoid arthritis and without consideration of the pathophysiology of osteoarthritis.

Although aspirin administration in a nonblinded study was reported to prevent chondromalacia in patients with recurrent dislocation of the patella,[27] a prospective double-blind clinical study of 29 patients with

---

*Adapted from form used by Physical Therapy Department, University Hospital, Indianapolis, Indiana.

chondromalacia patellae diagnosed by arthroscopy showed no changes in signs, symptoms, or macroscopic appearance of the cartilage either in patients treated with aspirin or in those given placebo.[28] Unfortunately, the condition of the patella prior to aspirin administration in that study was not ascertained.

Only recently have attempts been made to design pharmacologic agents that take into account the disease process in osteoarthritis. Compounds that, for example, stimulate chondrocyte metabolism or inhibit the enzymes capable of degrading articular cartilage matrix are receiving current attention.[29] Unfortunately, none has yet been shown in controlled studies to affect the natural history of osteoarthritis in humans. The development of such compounds is in its infancy, however, and the area warrants much additional effort.

Salicylates and Other Nonsteroidal Anti-inflammatory Drugs. Salicylates, in doses of about 650 mg qid and, if needed, acetaminophen or propoxyphene hydrochloride (Darvon) are all useful as simple analgesics in the treatment of osteoarthritis. Codeine or other narcotics are rarely indicated. If required, they should be used only briefly. If pain is not alleviated by analgesics, or if clinical signs of inflammation are present (e.g., warmth, synovial effusion, erythema), anti-inflammatory drugs are indicated. They include salicylates in higher doses, or one of the newer nonsteroidal anti-inflammatory agents. In the elderly, however, salicylate ototoxicity may develop at relatively low doses, precluding achievement of anti-inflammatory levels of the drug. Furthermore, the elderly may exhibit gastrointestinal intolerance to salicylates more frequently than do younger patients. Buffered preparations, enteric-coated salicylates, or formulations that provide slow, sustained release of salicylate may produce less dyspepsia than generic acetylsalicylic acid. Much of the problem of salicylate-induced dyspepsia can be circumvented by instructing the patient to take the medication with or after meals.

It should be emphasized that salicylate intoxication may be atypical in its presentation and difficult to recognize in the elderly patient with osteoarthritis.[30] The older individual with salicylate intoxication may have no gastrointestinal complaints or ototoxicity (or may have decreased auditory acuity for other reasons). In such patients confusion, agitation, hyperactivity, slurring of speech, or seizures may be the presenting features of salicylate toxicity. Since such neurologic abnormalities suggest other diagnoses, it is particularly important to consider the possibility of salicylate intoxication when these abnormalities are present in the elderly. Routine electrolyte determinations (anion gap) will be helpul, since acid-base disturbances are invariably present.

The renal effects of salicylates may also cause problems in the elderly. Any drug that significantly inhibits prostaglandin synthetase, such as aspirin, may diminish renal blood flow. Although this is not of clinical importance in patients with normal kidneys, full doses of salicylate may lead to a rise in blood urea nitrogen (BUN) and creatinine levels in patients with intrinsic renal disease, such as nephrosclerosis, a common problem in the elderly. In patients who are hypertensive or who have incipient or frank congestive heart failure, this may present a significant clinical problem.

Fortunately, for the patient who is unable to tolerate salicylates, one of the other nonsteroidal anti-inflammatory drugs currently available (e.g., ibuprofen, tolmetin sodium, naproxen, fenoprofen, sulindac, piroxicam) is likely to provide a satisfactory alternative. Each of these drugs, when taken in the full daily dosage recommended on the package insert for rheumatoid arthritis, is equivalent in its anti-inflammatory effect to 12 to 15 aspirin tablets per day.

The preceding drugs are generally well tolerated and produce less dyspepsia than salicylates. A strong case can be made, therefore, that they may be the drugs of choice for the elderly patient with osteoarthritis. Furthermore, the average daily dose required for the patient with osteoarthritis may be only one half to one third that required for optimal management of rheumatoid arthritis. Nonetheless, the fact that the average cost of one of the newer agents may be seven to eight fold greater than that of a comparable dose of aspirin is of consideration for both patient and physician.

All the nonsteroidal anti-inflammatory drugs inhibit prostaglandin synthetase to some extent, and they are all thus relatively contraindicated in the patient who has an active peptic ulcer, a past history of ulcer disease, or a bleeding disorder. In such patients, nonacetylated salicylate preparations, for example, choline salicylate (Arthropan) or choline magnesium trisalicylate (Trilisate), which have no effect on platelet aggregation, are more reasonable alternatives than any of the nonsteroidal anti-inflammatory drugs mentioned previously.

Phenylbutazone and Indomethacin. These two drugs should be considered separately from those already discussed because they are more potent and may present either an increased incidence or severity of side effects.

Phenylbutazone is a potent anti-inflammatory drug and may be particularly effective in management of acute flareups of the disease. A dosage of 100 mg tid or qid, with meals, of phenylbutazone (Butazolidin) or its derivative, oxyphenbutazone (Tandearil), may be given for a few days, and then tapered, so that therapy is terminated in 7 to 10 days. When given for brief periods of time in this fashion, the ulcerogenic potential of the drug is seldom a problem. However, the hematologic side effects (agranulocytosis and aplastic anemia), although uncommon, are idiosyncratic and are not related to the dosage or to the duration of therapy. Hence, they may develop after only a brief course of therapy, considerably limiting the usefulness of phenylbutazone in the treatment of osteoarthritis.

Indomethacin is also an effective drug in osteoarthritis. However, gastrointestinal and neurologic side effects are considerably more frequent than with the other nonsteroidal anti-inflammatory drugs mentioned, and they restrict its usefulness in the chronic treatment of osteoarthritis. For patients with nocturnal pain, however, a single dose of 25 to 50 mg, taken at bedtime, may produce gratifying relief. Newer formulations of indomethacin, which avoid abrupt peaks in serum concentrations, are currently under study. This may eliminate the undesirable gastrointestinal and neurologic side effects of indomethacin, while retaining the clinical efficacy of the drug.

Indomethacin has been considered to be particularly effective in providing pain relief in osteoarthritis of the hip. If true, it is unknown why it should be especially efficacious in this joint as opposed to other joints. In a double-blind study in which indomethacin was found to be superior to placebo for osteoarthritis of the hip, no effect on disease progression was noted over a 5-year period.[31] The effective mean daily dose at the onset of the study was 85 mg and rose to 155 mg at the conclusion of the study. In another study, the clinical efficacy of indomethacin, 150 mg daily, was comparable to that of 1.3 g of aspirin in patients with osteoarthritis of the hip or knee.[32]

In contrast to this double-blind study, which found no effect of indomethacin on the progression of osteoarthritis, a recent retrospective analysis of the radiographic progression of osteoarthritis of the hip led to the conclusion that indomethacin administration was associated with greater joint destruction than seen in controls.[33] Although it is arguable that the symptomatic relief produced by indomethacin was sufficiently effective that the patients incurred further damage to their osteoarthritic joints by overuse, the drug, via its effects on prostaglandin synthetase, may interfere with the repair of microfractures in subchondral bone.[34] This may have accounted for the increases in cyst formation and joint destruction observed radiologically.

Other studies suggest that salicylates and several other nonsteroidal anti-inflammatory drugs may suppress proteoglycan biosynthesis in articular cartilage.[2-4] Salicylates have been shown to worsen the degenerative changes in osteoarthritic[3] and atrophic[4] canine articular cartilage in vivo, whereas they apparently do not affect normal cartilage. Although these effects in animals suggest that chronic administration of salicylates and some other nonsteroidal anti-inflammatory drugs may be injurious to articular cartilage, it is not possible to deduce from animal studies the effects of these drugs on the pathophysiology of the human osteoarthritic joint.

Adrenal Corticosteroid Therapy. Systemic corticosteroid treatment or administration of adrenocorticotrophic hormone is not indicated in treatment of osteoarthritis. Beneficial effects are equivocal and the side effects associated with prolonged use of these agents, especially in the elderly, far outweigh any possible benefits. Conversely, intra-articular injection of corticosteroids may be of benefit. Hollander and colleagues[35] reported marked to complete relief of symptoms in 87 percent of 231 patients who received repeated injections over a 20-year period. Similar results were noted by the same author in a subsequent review of nearly 1000 patients with osteoarthritis of the knee who received intraarticular steroid injections as needed over a 9-year period.[36] In that series nearly 60 percent no longer had sufficient pain to require further injections, about 20

percent were still receiving injections, and about 20 percent had not benefited from the injections or had been lost to follow-up.

The preceding data must be viewed alongside results of other studies, however, which have shown similar benefits following single injections of 1 percent procaine,[37] isotonic saline,[37] or the suspending vehicle.[38]

Symptomatic improvement following intra-articular steroid injection is likely to be temporary. Although pain relief after intra-articular injection was significantly greater after 1 week with steroids than with a control injection (the suspending vehicle), by 4 weeks after the injection the response of patients who received the steroid was indistinguishable from that of the controls.[39] The mechanism of pain relief with intra-articular steroids in osteoarthritis may be associated with decreases in synovial permeability, even when they produce an increase in synovial fluid leukocytosis[40] (presumably due to postinjection synovitis, caused by the microcrystalline preparation).[41] The masking of pain by intra-articular steroid injections may lead to overuse, with subsequent breakdown and instability.[42,43]

Steroids may also damage cartilage directly. Weekly injections into rabbit joints for 4 to 9 weeks produced histologic evidence of cartilage degeneration[44] and depressed synthesis of collagen and proteoglycans, leading to a decrease in proteoglycan concentration in the cartilage.[45] Although little histologic change was seen in non-weight-bearing joints, weight-bearing cartilage developed surface fissures and cystic degeneration. It is of interest, in view of the preceding, that some evidence also exists that intra-articular corticosteroids may ameliorate the pathologic changes of osteoarthritis. Thus, repeated injections of triamcinolone acetate, 3 mg per kg, diminished osteophyte formation in rabbits with secondary osteoarthritis.[46] In another study, utilizing a somewhat different rabbit model of osteoarthritis, a single injection of 1 mg of triamcinolone hexacetonide, a long-acting glucocorticoid, provided significant protection against articular cartilage degeneration.[47] In humans, however, no evidence exists that steroids favorably influence the pathologic changes in the articular cartilage or that they influence osteophyte formation.

Because of the stated concerns, intra-articular steroids are generally not employed more frequently than once every 4 to 6 months for any given joint. It appears advisable to caution the patient to minimize joint loading for a period of time following the injection, even though no controlled data are available to prove that this is helpful in humans. Injection of steroids into painful pericapsular sites and ligaments may also produce symptomatic relief and is not associated with the potential dangers of intra-articular injection.

ORTHOPEDIC SURGERY

Surgical procedures are generally reserved for patients with more severe disease, persistent pain, and significantly impaired function. Osteotomies to correct malalignment (e.g., tibial or femoral osteotomy in the patient with knee osteoarthritis and genu varum or genu valgum) may be of greatest benefit, however, when the disease is only moderately advanced. By altering stresses of load-bearing, and bringing more normal cartilage surfaces into opposition, such surgery may provide effective relief of pain. Debridement of the joint, with removal of free cartilage fragments (joint mice), may prevent locking, eliminate pain, and prevent rapid wear of the joint surfaces. Surgical removal of large osteophytes may also increase range of motion, although by buttressing the joint the constraining osteophytes may, at times, serve to diminish breakdown of the articular surface. In advanced disease, arthroplasty (partial or total) or arthrodesis may be required and can generally be expected to relieve pain; often arthroplasty will improve range of motion as well. In weight-bearing parts, such as the hip and knee, arthrodesis is generally avoided, but in patients whose future activities will require heavy usage of the involved joint, making failure of an arthroplasty likely, arthrodesis may be the procedure of choice, even though it permanently eliminates joint motion.

TREATMENT OF OSTEOARTHRITIS AT SPECIFIC SITES

The Hand. Although Heberden's nodes often develop insidiously and may be present without symptoms, in some patients they develop rapidly with localized swelling, erythema, marked tenderness, and pain. In such instances Heberden's nodes may be particularly sensitive to pressure or to accidental trauma. Patients with Heberden's nodes require reassurance that they do not have a crippling form of arthritis or a form that is likely to progress to involve other joints. They should be reassured that the nodes will eventually become painless, and they need support in accepting the resulting cosmetic changes. For relief of pain, heat—in the form of contrast baths, hot soaks, or paraffin baths—is usually effective. If the symptoms are severe, analgesic or nonsteroidal anti-inflammatory drugs, or both, may be helpful. Local injections of corticosteroids into or around the affected joint may be helpful, especially in the unusually painful, acutely inflamed node, which is accompanied by a large, painful mucinous cyst. Trauma, which may aggravate pain and the deformity, should be avoided. Instruction of the patient in joint protection principles (see previous list) is indicated. Nylon-spandex stretch gloves, worn at night, have been reported to relieve pain and morning stiffness.[48]

Osteoarthritis at the base of the thumb, in the first carpometacarpal joint, may also be benefited by judicious use of intra-articular steroids and by splinting. A slip-on hand splint to immobilize the first carpometacarpal and metacarpophalangeal joints of the thumb can reduce pain during functional activities.[49] If severe pain persists, arthroplasty or arthrodesis may be indicated. Arthroplasty will allow retention of motion but will compromise grip strength. Arthrodesis will preserve good grip strength but will eliminate motion.

The Hip. Diminished loading on the involved joint should be accomplished by use of an ambulatory aid (e.g., cane, crutch, walker). If a cane or crutch is prescribed, it should be used on the uninvolved side. Practical measures to reduce stress on the joint should be discussed (see previous list). If obesity is present, the patient should be encouraged to reduce to ideal weight. Rest periods, the use of heat, analgesic and anti-inflammatory drugs, and non-weight-bearing exercises to strengthen supporting muscles and maintain normal range of motion are indicated. Attempts should be made to prevent flexion contractures by having the patient lie prone for periods of 30 minutes two or three times daily. Patients should be advised to use higher chairs, or seat cushions, rather than low chairs or sofas. Elevated toilet seats are helpful.

Applications of heat will help relieve muscle spasm. However, if spasm is severe, traction may be required. In many patients with osteoarthritis of the hip, limitation of motion results from capsular contractures. Exercises to improve adduction, extension, and external rotation are therefore indicated. Intra-articular injections of steroids may be helpful when pain is severe. However, they are often ineffective, perhaps because of the difficulty in assuring that the injection is actually placed within the joint space.

With advanced disease, surgery should be considered. Total hip arthroplasty is generally the procedure of choice and, in most cases, provides excellent pain relief and restores hip motion to a level approaching normal. Intertrochanteric osteotomy has been reported to produce lasting benefit in at least 85 percent of patients.[50,51] Although it may have a role in the treatment of younger patients, later conversion to a total hip replacement may be difficult. Thus, the place of this procedure may be somewhat limited.

The Knee. The general measures already described will usually provide effective relief of pain and stiffness. As is the case with osteoarthritis of the hip, weight reduction is indicated if the patient is obese. Other measures to decrease joint loading should also be recommended (see previous list). Jogging and participation in racket sports should be discouraged. The patient should be instructed not to rest with pillows placed behind the knees, which may lead to flexion contractures. Isometric quadriceps exercises are indicated (see previous list). Elastic supports or knee cages (hinged braces that lace up the front) increase stability and may protect against stress.

Flareups are not uncommon in osteoarthritis of the knee and are marked by increased pain, often with joint effusion and increased warmth and tenderness of the joint. Elimination of weight-bearing is usually effective treatment for the flareup. Aspiration of the effusion and intra-articular administration of steroid are often helpful. Steroid injections into tender periarticular ligaments may also provide relief. Often, the patient with knee osteoarthritis may be symptomatic because of an associated anserine bursitis. In this case, injection of corticosteroid into the tender area, by localizing the bursitis, will often produce marked relief of pain.

Locking of the knee suggests a torn meniscus or the

presence of joint mice, which should be removed surgically or arthroscopically. As already described, surgery may be of great benefit. Total knee arthroplasty has not enjoyed the same rate of success as total hip arthroplasty because of the greater complexity of the biomechanics of the knee, but nonetheless may afford excellent pain relief, increased mobility, and improved function.

The Spine. Symptoms caused by osteoarthritis of the cervical spine generally respond to the measures described previously; that is, rest, heat, and analgesics or anti-inflammatory drugs, or both. A cervical pillow may be helpful. To decrease stress on the cervical spine, the patient should be advised not to maintain the neck in extension or flexion for prolonged periods, as when shampooing or sitting near the screen in a movie theater. Prolonged periods of rotation may also increase discomfort, as when watching television while lying on a sofa, or watching a tennis match from a midcourt seat. Symptoms caused by nerve root irritation may be relieved by a cervical collar. Occasionally, severe muscle spasm or nerve root compression may require cervical traction. This may be accomplished in the home under a physician's guidance. In patients with neurologic complications whose symptoms are unresponsive to the preceding measures, surgery may be indicated.

Symptoms resulting from osteoarthritis of the lumbar spine also will usually respond to rest, heat, and medications as described, and simple measures for joint protection (see previous list). A lumbosacral corset with abdominal support, and weight reduction if the patient is obese, may be helpful. A firm mattress, or bedboard placed beneath the mattress, is often beneficial. Muscle spasm may be alleviated with muscle relaxants, local heat, or massage. Exercises to strengthen the anterior abdominal muscles and to correct poor posture should be instituted when acute symptoms subside in order to minimize the likelihood of recurrences. Surgery, such as laminectomy, discectomy, or fusion, may be required when symptoms are severe or neurologic deficits are present.

The Feet. Osteoarthritis of the first metatarsophalangeal joint may produce pain, limitation of motion, and marked proliferation of osteophytes in the joint margins. In early cases, relief may be obtained by metatarsal pads or metatarsal bars, or by stiffening the sole of the shoe with metal to minimize dorsiflexion at this joint during walking. If the condition is advanced and chronically painful, and the preceding measures are ineffective, surgery may be required. Inflammation and swelling of the bursa medial to the first metatarsophalangeal joint may be treated by a local steroid injection. Osteoarthritis of the subtalar joint is often resistant to the general measures outlined. Reduction of weight-bearing by use of a cane or crutches may be helpful. In severe cases, arthrodesis may be indicated.

VOCATIONAL REHABILITATION

At times, a change in occupation may be desirable. Although assistance from vocational rehabilitation counselors may be helpful, a recent survey of 86 counselors in the Indiana Department of Rehabilitation Services, which is presumably representative of similar departments in other states, showed that 80 percent of the counselors had had no on-the-job orientation about arthritis, 72 percent had had no formal education about arthritis in college, and 70 percent had not participated in a continuing education program about arthritis within the previous 2 years.[52] It is thus incumbent on the physician to inform the counselor about the patient's limitations, disease prognosis, and so forth. It should be pointed out, however, that even the most enlightened vocational rehabilitation counselor may encounter great difficulty in finding suitable employment for the arthritis patient, who is competing in a "buyer's market."

SOCIAL SECURITY DISABILITY

The disabled patient with osteoarthritis may be more concerned about the ability to provide financially for self and family than about the disease itself. Patients who are unable to continue working may be eligible for Social Security Disability Insurance (DI) or Supplemental Security Income (SSI) disability benefits. Both DI and SSI disability require that the disabling condition last, or be expected to last, continuously for at least 12 months. To be eligible for DI, the disabled worker must have contributed to the Social Security trust fund for a specified length of time, which is dependent on age at onset of disability. For example, workers older than 31 years of age must have contributed to the Social Security trust fund for 20 of the preceding 40 quarter-years. For younger workers, progressively fewer quarters are required. In contrast to DI, SSI is funded through general tax revenues and does not require contributions to the trust fund.

The Social Security Administration has published a "Listing of Impairments" that is used to determine whether the applicant's impairment significantly limits his ability to perform basic work activities. If the applicant's clinical findings meet the listed criteria the impairment will be considered severe enough to be disabling and benefits will be awarded. Since the criteria are not specific to osteoarthritis, findings that are equivalent in severity to those in the following* list will also qualify for determination of disability.

I. Arthritis of a major weight-bearing joint. With history of persistent joint pain and stiffness with signs of severe limitation of motion of the affected joint on current physical examination. With

A. Gross anatomic deformity of hip or knee (e.g., subluxation, contracture, bony or fibrous ankylosis, instability) with x-ray evidence of either severe joint space narrowing or significant bony

---

*Adapted from Disability Evaluation Under Social Security: A Handbook for Physicians. U.S. Department of Health and Human Services, Social Security Administration, Publication No. (SSA) 79-10089, August, 1979.

destruction and severely limiting ability to walk and stand or

    B. There was reconstructive surgery or surgical arthrodesis of a major weight-bearing joint, and return to full weight-bearing status did not occur, or is not expected to occur, within 12 months of onset.

II. Arthritis of one major joint in each arm. With history of persistent joint and stiffness, signs of severe limitation of motion of the affected joints on current physical examination, and x-ray evidence of either severe joint space narrowing or significant bony destruction. With

    A. Abduction and forward flexion (elevation) of both arms at the shoulders, including scapular motion, restricted to less than 90 degrees; or

    B. Gross anatomic deformity and enlargement or effusion of the affected joints.

III. Disorders of the spine.

    A. Arthritis manifested by ankylosis or fixation of the cervical or dorsolumbar spine at 30 degrees or more of flexion measured from the neutral position with x-ray evidence of

        1. Calcification of the spinal ligaments or

        2. Bilateral ankylosis of the sacroiliac joints with abnormal apophyseal articulation.

    B. Osteoporosis, generalized (established by x-ray), manifested by pain and limitation of back motion and paravertebral muscle spasm with x-ray evidence of nontraumatic vertebral compression fracture or fractures.

    C. Other vertebrogenic disorders (e.g., herniated nucleus pulposus, spinal stenosis) with the following persisting for at least 3 months, despite prescribed therapy, and expected to last 12 months. With

        1. Pain, muscle spasm, and significant limitation of motion in the spine and

        2. Appropriate radicular distribution of significant muscle weakness and sensory and reflex loss.

If the applicant's impairment does not meet or equal the criteria mentioned in the preceding list, but is severe, the individual may still be eligible for DI or SSI disability benefits. Thus, in determining eligibility, Social Security also considers the applicant's "residual functional capacity," that is, the applicant's ability to perform work-related tasks despite physical or mental limitations, or both. Work-related tasks that are considered include walking, standing, lifting, carrying, pushing, pulling, reaching, handling, and so forth. Pain and fatigue may be considered in determining the residual functional capacity if accompanied by objective medical evidence.

The Social Security Administration has prepared a booklet for physicians describing in detail the content of the previous list.[53] To reduce the likelihood that patients legitimately disabled by osteoarthritis will be denied benefits, the physician must be as specific as possible about the claimant's ability to perform work-related tasks and must provide documentation of the patient's objective clinical findings.[54]

References

1. Linholm, R.V., Koivisto, E., and Punto, L.: Radiologic signs of hip and knee joint degeneration. Postgrad. Med. 65:155, 1979.
2. Palmoski, M., and Brandt, K.: Effects of some nonsteroidal anti-inflammatory drugs on articular cartilage proteoglycan metabolism and organization. Arthritis Rheum. 23:1010, 1980.
3. Palmoski, M., and Brandt, K.: *In vivo* effect of aspirin on canine osteoarthritic cartilage. Arthritis Rheum. 26:994, 1983.
4. Palmoski, M., and Brandt, K.: Aspirin aggravates the degeneration of canine joint cartilage caused by immobilization. Arthritis Rheum. 25:1333, 1982.
5. Ronningen, H., and Langeland, N.: Indomethacin treatment in osteoarthritis of the hip joint. Acta Orthop. Scand. 50:169, 1979.
6. Forman, M.D., Malamet, R., and Kaplan, D.: A survey of osteoarthritis of the knee in the elderly. J. Rheum. 10:282, 1983.
7. Lawrence, J.S., Brenner, J.M., and Bier, F.: Osteoarthritis. Ann. Rheum. Dis. 25:1, 1966.
8. Danielsson, L.G.: Incidence and prognosis of coxarthrosis. Acta Orthop. Scand. (Suppl.) 66:9, 1964.
9. Hernborg, J., and Nilsson, B.E.: The relationship between osteophytes in the knee joint, osteoarthritis and aging. Acta Orthop. Scand. 44:69, 1973.
10. Hadler, N.M.: The variable of usage in the epidemiology of osteoarthrosis. *In* Peyron, J.G. (ed.): Epidemiology of Osteoarthrosis. Ciba-Geigy, 1981, p. 164.
11. Reilly, D.T., and Martens, M.: Experimental analysis of the quadriceps muscle force and patello-femoral joint reaction force for various activities. Acta Orthop. Scand. 43:126, 1972.
12. Leach, R.E., Baumgard, S., and Broom, J.: Obesity: its relationship to osteoarthritis of the knee. Clin. Orthop. 93:271, 1973.
13. Acheson, R.M.: Epidemiology and the arthritides. Ann. Rheum. Dis. 41:325, 1982.
14. Evans, C.H., Mears, D.C., and McKnight, J.L.: A preliminary ferrographic survey of the wear particles in human synovial fluid. Arthritis Rheum. 24:912, 1981.
15. Evans, C.H., Mears, D.C., and Cosgrove, J.L.: Release of neutral proteinases from mononuclear phagocytes and synovial cells in response to cartilaginous wear particles in vitro. Biochim. Biophys. Acta 677:287, 1981.
16. Wiener, C.L.: The burden of rheumatoid arthritis: tolerating the uncertainty. Soc. Sci. Med. 9:97, 1975.
17. Gross, M.: Psychosocial aspects of arthritis: helping patients cope. Health Soc. Work 6:40, 1981.
18. Currey, H.L.F.: Osteoarthrosis of the hip joint and sexual activity. Ann. Rheum. Dis. 29:488, 1970.
19. Ferguson, K., and Figley, B.: Sexuality and rheumatic disease: a prospective study. Sexual. Disabil. 2:130, 1979.
20. Ehrlich, G.E.: Sexual problems of the arthritic patient. *In* Erlich, G.E. (ed.): Total Management of the Arthritic Patient. Philadelphia, J.B. Lippincott Company, 1973, pp. 193–208.
21. Arthritis Foundation: Living and Loving: Information About Sex. Atlanta, Georgia, 1982.
22. Utsinger, P.D., Bonner, F., and Hogan, N.: Efficacy of cryotherapy (CR) and thermotherapy in the management of rheumatoid arthritis (RA) pain: evidence for an endorphin effect. Arthritis Rheum. 25:S113, 1982.
23. Sirca, A., and Susec-Michieli, M.: Selective Type II fibre muscular atrophy in patients with osteoarthritis of the hip. J. Neurol. Sci. 44:149, 1980.
24. Laborde, J.M., and Powers, M.J.: Satisfaction with life for patients undergoing hemodialysis and patients suffering from osteoarthritis. Res. Nurs. Health 3:19, 1980.
25. Lempberg, R.K., and Arnoldi, C.C.: The significance of intraosseous pressure in normal and diseased states with special reference to intraosseous engorgement pain syndrome. Clin. Orthop. 136:143, 1978.
26. Howell, D.S., and Talbott, J.H. (eds.): Osteoarthritis Symposium. Florida, Palm Aire, October 20–22, 1980. Semin. Arthritis Rheum. 11 (Suppl. 1), 1981.
27. Chrisman, O.D., Snook, G.A., and Wilson, T.C.: The protective effect of aspirin against degeneration of human articular cartilage. Clin. Orthop. 84:193, 1972.
28. Bentley, G., Leslie, I.J., and Fischer, D.: Effect of aspirin treatment on chondromalacia patellae. Ann. Rheum. Dis. 40:37, 1981.
29. Fife, R.S., and Brandt, K.D.: Experimental modes of therapy in osteoarthritis. *In* Moskowitz, R.W., Howell, D.S., Goldberg, V.M. and Mankin, H.J. (eds.): Osteoarthritis Diagnosis and Management. Philadelphia, W.B. Saunders, Co., 1984.
30. Anderson, R.J., Potts, D.E., Gabow, P.A., Rumack, B.H., and. Schrier, R.W. Unrecognized adult salicylate intoxication. Ann. Intern. Med. 85:745–748, 1976.

31. Hodgkinson, R., and Woolf, D.: A five-year clinical trial of indomethacin in osteoarthrosis of the hip. Practitioner 210:372, 1974.

32. Harth, M., and Bondy, D.C.: Indomethacin and acetylsalicylic acid in the treatment of osteoarthritis of the hips and knees. Can. Med. Assoc. J. 101:311, 1969.

33. Ronninger, H., and Langeland, N.: Indomethacin treatment in osteoarthritis of the hip joint. Does the treatment interfere with the natural course of the disease? Acta Orthop. Scand. 50:169, 1979.

34. Sudmann, E., Dregelid, E., Bessesen, A., and Morland, J.: Inhibition of fracture healing by indomethacin in rats. Eur. J. Clin. Invest. 9:333, 1979.

35. Hollander, J.L.: Intraarticular hydrocortisone in arthritis and allied conditions. J. Bone. Joint Surg. 35A:983, 1953.

36. Hollander, J.L.: Treatment of osteoarthritis of the knees. Arthritis Rheum. 3:564, 1960.

37. Traut, E.F.: Procaine and procaineamide hydrochloride in skeletal pain. J.A.M.A. 150:785, 1952.

38. Wright, V., Chandler, G.N., Morrison, R.A.H., and Hartfall, S.J.: Intraarticular therapy in osteoarthritis. Comparison of hydrocortisone acetate and hydrocortisone tertiary butylacetate. Ann. Rheum. Dis. 19:257, 1960.

39. Friedman, D.M., and Moore, M.A.: The efficacy of intraarticular corticosteroid for osteoarthritis of the knee. Arthritis Rheum. 21:556, 1978.

40. Eymontt, M.J., Gordon, G.V., Schumacher, H.R., and Hansell, J.R.: The effects on synovial permeability and synovial fluid leukocyte counts in symptomatic osteoarthritis after intraarticular corticosteroid administration. J. Rheum. 9:198, 1982.

41. McCarty, D.J., and Hogan, J.M.: Inflammatory reaction after intrasynovial injection of microcrystalline adrenocorticosteroid esters. Arthritis Rheum. 7:359, 1964.

42. Alarcon-Segovia, D., and Ward, L.E.: Marked destructive changes occurring in osteoarthritic finger joints after intraarticular injection of corticosteroids. Arthritis Rheum. 9:443, 1966.

43. Miller, W.T., and Restifo, R.A.: Steroid arthropathy. Radiology 86:652, 1966.

44. Moskowitz, R.W., Davis, W., Sammarco, J., Mast, W., and Chase, S.W.: Experimentally induced corticosteroid arthropathy. Arthritis Rheum. 134:236, 1970.

45. Behrens, F., Shepard, H., and Mitchell, N.: Alteration of rabbit articular cartilage by intra-articular injections of glucocorticoids. J. Bone Joint Surg. 58A:1157, 1976.

46. Moskowitz, R.W., Goldberg, V.M., Schwab, W., and Berman, L.: Effects of intraarticular corticosteroids and exercise in experimental models of inflammatory and degenerative arthritis. Arthritis Rheum. 18:417, 1975.

47. Butler, M., Columbo, C., Hickman, L., O'Byrne, E., Steele, R., Steinetz, B., Quintavalla, J., and Yokoyama, N.: A new model of osteoarthrosis in rabbits: III. Evaluation of antiarthrotic effects of selected drugs administered intraarticularly. Arthritis Rheum. 26: 1380, 1983.

48. Ehrlich, G., and DiPierro, A.M.: Stretch gloves: nocturnal use to ameliorate morning stiffness in arthritic hands. Arch. Phys. Med. Rehabil. 52:479, 1971.

49. Melvin, J.L.: Rheumatic Disease, Occupational Therapy and Rehabilitation. 2nd ed. Philadelphia, F.A. Davis Company, 1982, p. 345.

50. Mogensen, B.A., Zoega, H., and Marinko, P.: Late results of intertrochanteric osteotomy for advanced osteoarthritis of the hip. Acta Orthop. Scand. 51:85, 1980.

51. Langlais, F., Roure, J-L., and Maquet, P.: Valgus osteotomy in severe osteoarthritis of the hip. J. Bone Joint Surg. 61B:424, 1979.

52. Potts, M., and Brandt, K.: Educational needs of vocational rehabilitation counselors working with clients who have arthritis. J. Appl. Rehabil. Counsel. 15:22, 1984.

53. Disability evaluation under Social Security: a handbook for physicians. U.S. Department of Health and Human Services, Social Security Administration, Publication No. (SSA) 79-10089, August, 1979.

54. Meenan, R.F., Liang, M.H., and Hadley, N.M.: Social Security disability and the arthritis patient. Bull. Rheum. Dis. 33:1, 1983.

Chapter 91

Polychondritis

Jerome H. Herman

CHARACTERIZATION OF DISEASE

Relapsing polychondritis is an infrequently recognized, though not necessarily uncommon, episodic systemic disorder that is characterized by recurrent, widespread, and potentially destructive inflammatory lesions involving cartilaginous structures, the cardiovascular system, and organs of special sense, such as the eyes and ears. Although the etiology is unknown and its pathogenesis is incompletely understood, experimental evidence strongly suggests that immunologically mediated mechanisms are operative. The increasing awareness of its clinically distinct, and at times more subtle, modes of presentation has resulted in recognition of approximately 350 reported cases.

Clinical Manifestations. The disease occurs predominantly in Caucasians but has been reported in all races. There is an equal sex prevalence and no apparent familial predisposition. Time of onset has varied from birth to the ninth decade of life—the majority of cases appearing between the ages of 40 and 60 years (Fig. 91–1). The frequency of system involvement at the onset and in the subsequent course of illness is shown in Table 91–1.

The most prevalent symptoms are rather sudden onset of pain, tenderness, and a violaceous erythematous swelling confined, in a patchy or diffuse distribution, to the cartilaginous portions of one or both external *ears*. Inflammatory encroachment upon the external auditory meatus may lead to narrowing that is sufficient to cause impairment of hearing. A clear serous discharge can occur, and inflammation can extend to the retroauricular soft tissues. Attacks tend to vary in severity, with duration spanning several days to weeks before subsiding spontaneously. Protracted or recurrent episodes of inflammation may lead to permanent loss of cartilaginous structural integrity, resulting in a flabby or drooping appearance to the ears (Fig. 91–2).

Although infrequent at the onset, *internal ear disease* characterized by auditory or vestibular dysfunction, or both, subsequently appears in 40 percent of patients.[1] Auditory impairment may result not only from external meatal narrowing but also from middle ear inflammation, serous otitis media, eustachean tube obstruction secondary to chondritis of the nasopharyngeal segment, or neurosensory abnormalities presumably caused by vasculitis of the internal auditory artery or its cochlear branch. The latter may be acute or insidious in onset. Arteritis of the internal auditory artery or its vestibular

Figure 91–1. Age of onset of polychondritis in 290 patients.

Figure 91–2. Distortion and collapse of the external ear in a patient having polychondritis.

branch may result in episodes of vertigo, ataxia, nausea, and vomiting.

Sixty-eight percent of patients develop *nasal chondritis,* which often occurs suddenly and is associated with inflammation that resolves over several days. Repeated attacks may result in cartilage collapse and a characteristic saddle nose deformity. Low-grade inflammation may produce cartilage destruction and nose deformity in the absence of overt inflammation. The inflammation and deformity often produce nasal stuffiness or fullness,

crusting, rhinorrhea, and epistaxis. *Ocular inflammation* may be a presenting feature, appearing subsequently in 59 percent of patients.[2] Its manifestations include episcleritis, scleritis, conjunctivitis, and iritis. Less common features are proptosis, ophthalmoplegia, keratitis, keratoconjunctivitis sicca, scleromalacia, chorioretinitis, retinal artery thrombosis, panophthalmitis, retinal de-

Table 91–1. Predominant Clinical Manifestations of Relapsing Polychondritis*

	Frequency (Percent of Patients)	
	Features Observed at Onset of Illness	*Features Presenting During Course of Illness*
Auricular inflammation	32	84
Arthropathy (total)	26	76
Peripheral joints		69
Costochondral-manubriosternal		30
Nasal cartilage inflammation	18	68
Ocular inflammation (total)	15	59
Scleritis-episcleritis	13	37
Conjunctivitis	6	31
Iritis-chorioretinitis	4	19
Laryngotracheal-bronchial disease	15	54
Internal ear involvement (total)	6	40
Auditory		35
Vestibular		19
Cardiovascular disease (total)		25
Systemic vasculitis		13
Valvular insufficiency		8
Aneurysm		4
Cutaneous lesions		18

*Compiled from established reviews[11,45,54,55] and new case presentations totaling 292 patients. The figures presented should be regarded as approximations based upon the incomplete reporting of case material in subspecialty journals.

tachment, optic neuritis, and an increased prevalence of cataracts. Blindness may follow.

The *arthropathy* of relapsing polychondritis is the second most common presenting feature, eventually appearing in 76 percent of patients. It varies clinically from transient arthralgias to a mono-, pauci-, or polyarticular symmetric or asymmetric synovitis involving both large and small peripheral joints and parasternal articulations (costochondral, sternomanubrial, sternoclavicular). Its classic presentation is that of an episodic, asymmetric, nonerosive, and nondeforming arthritis of several days' to several weeks' duration, resolving spontaneously or upon response to anti-inflammatory measures.[3] Occasionally, there may be cervical, dorsal, or lumbar spine pain. Transient tenosynovitis has been described. Costochondral involvement may be manifested by chest pain and tenderness; destruction of these articulations is rare but can cause a flail chest. Joint effusions may occur. Synovial fluid analyses reported in the absence of concurrent connective tissue disease have been noninflammatory. No correlation exists between joint involvement and disease activity appearing elsewhere. Although aortitis, iritis, and, rarely, sacroiliitis and involvement of the symphysis pubis are features of polychondritis, the frequency of HLA-B27 in these patients is no more common than in the general population.[4] Joint radiographs may reveal demineralization of juxta-articular bone and, on occasion, joint space narrowing without erosion. The disease may appear in conjunction with pre-existing articular destructive disorders, such as adult and juvenile rheumatoid arthritides, Reiter's disease, psoriatic arthritis, Sjögren's syndrome, and ankylosing spondylitis.

Laryngotracheal bronchial involvement is an indicator of a poor prognosis.[5] Hoarseness and tenderness over the thyroid cartilage and anterior trachea are common presenting symptoms of involvement here. A nonproductive cough, dyspnea, aphonia, inspiratory stridor or, rarely, hemoptysis can develop. Glottic, subglottic, and laryngeal inflammation with concomitant edema may necessitate tracheostomy in severe cases. Collapse of tracheal and bronchial rings, inflammation, edema, and cicatrization have led to severe focal or diffuse airway narrowing in which tracheostomy was ineffectual in reestablishing adequate ventilation. Recurrent attacks may cause permanent loss of structural support, and death can occur from asphyxiation. Secondary infections of both upper and lower parts of the respiratory system are common. The few available detailed assessments of pulmonary function have demonstrated varying degrees of obstructive airway impairment, with bronchodilators exhibiting no significant effect. Arterial oxygen saturation is usually normal. Studies of the maximal expiratory and inspiratory flow-volume loop and airway resistance may provide useful information as to the site and nature of the obstructive process.[6]

Cardiovascular complications appear in 25 percent of patients and can cause death. Most ominous is the development (predominantly in males) of aortic insufficiency secondary to progressive dilatation of the aortic ring and ascending aorta, or at times the destruction of the valve cusps without annulus dilatation.[7] Mitral and tricuspid valvular insufficiencies occur less frequently. Such valvular involvement may arise as early as 6 months or as late as 17 years following the onset of disease and bears little temporal relationship to other manifestations. Successful valvuloplasty and valve replacements have been reported. In addition, aneurysms involving the ascending, thoracic, and abdominal aorta, and the subclavian artery have developed, leading to death from rupture (Fig. 91–3).[8] Less frequently, pericarditis, myocarditis with conduction disturbances, endocarditis, and myocardial infarction develop.

Medium and large vessel disease can develop independently of cardiac involvement.[9] In addition to aneurysm formation, thrombosis secondary to vasculitis has been reported, involving the descending and abdominal aorta, and the subclavian, intracerebral, hepatic, superior mesenteric, and peripheral arteries. Cases of associated temporal arteritis, polyarteritis, Wegener's granulomatosis, allergic granulomatosis, and Takayasu's disease have been described. The vasculitis may be focal or diffuse, indolent or fulminant, and rapidly fatal.

Although dermal involvement occurs in 18 percent of patients, no distinctive cutaneous features characteristic of polychondritis have been identified. Lesions have varied from biopsy-documented leukocytoclastic vasculitis to livedo reticularis, erythema nodosum, and keratodermia blennorrhagica. Hyperpigmentation over sites of cartilage involvement, alopecia, retarded nail growth, and subcutaneous fat necrosis have been reported.

Further clinical manifestations may include fever and myalgias. Renal disease is uncommon. When present, it usually reflects concurrent systemic vasculitis or other associated disease. Crescentic glomerulonephritis is being reported with increased frequency.[10] Minor liver function abnormalities are observed on occasion.

Coexistent Disease. As shown in Table 91–2, there is a significant coexistence of polychondritis with diverse forms of connective tissue disease. In most cases these diseases antedate the onset of polychondritis by months or years. On the basis of our present state of knowledge, it is impossible to ascertain whether such associations represent the independent coexistence of two separate entities, connective tissue disease features arising in a particular subset of polychondritis, or polychondritis appearing as a specific manifestation in genetically distinct subsets of such connective tissue diseases. There also is an association of polychondritis with thyroid disease (4 percent) presenting as Graves' disease, goiter, hypothyroidism, or Hashimoto's disease. Ulcerative colitis has been reported in six cases. Malignancy has been reported in eight cases, the latter including carcinomas of the stomach, pancreas, and prostate, a cerebral ependymoma, Hodgkin's disease, and leukemia.

Laboratory Features. There are no laboratory tests specific for polychondritis. The principal abnormalities are shown in Table 91–3. Most often there is an elevated sedimentation rate and modest leukocytosis, which to a large measure correlate with disease activity. Throm-

91–3. Aortograms. *Left,* An abdominal aortogram demonstrating a 9 by 3.5 cm fusiform aneurysm of the abdominal aorta below the renal arteries. *Right,* Thoracic aortogram in the left anterior oblique projection demonstrating a 5 cm saccular aneurysm in the proximal descending thoracic aorta. (From Cipiano, P.R., et al.: Am. J. Cardiol. 37:1097, 1976.)

bocytosis and eosinophilia may be seen. A normocytic, normochromic anemia of a mild to moderate degree frequently occurs. Although serum iron and iron binding capacity have been reported to be low, normal bone marrow iron stores have been observed. Hemolytic anemia is a rare occurrence. Serologic studies have detected rheumatoid factor and antinuclear antibody activity, the latter usually demonstrating a diffuse staining pattern. A false-positive serologic test result for syphilis may occur. Total hemolytic complement and C3 and C4 determinations are usually normal but are on occasion

Table 91–2. Connective Tissue Diseases Coexistent with Polychondritis (292 Cases)

Disease	Number of Reported Occurrences
Systemic vasculitis	28
Juvenile-adult rheumatoid arthritis	13
Sjögren's syndrome	8
Systemic lupus erythematosus	8
Reiter's disease–psoriatic arthritis	3
Progressive systemic sclerosis	2
Ankylosing spondylitis	2
Behçet's disease	1
Polymyalgia rheumatica	1
Retroperitoneal fibrosis	1

elevated, reflecting an acute-phase response. Transient elevations of IgG and IgA have been reported. Cryoglobulins have occasionally been detected. Circulating immune complexes have been increasingly identified using C1q precipitation and solid phase assays. Serum protein electrophoresis may show nonspecific abnormalities consisting of diminished serum albumin and elevated levels of α_1 and gamma globulins.

Roentgenographic Abnormalities. Roentgenographs are useful in delineating complications of polychondritis. The most common findings reflect evidence of cartilaginous destruction. Tracheal tomograms, cinebronchography, and computed tomography (CT) scans may show stenosis and bronchial tree narrowing. Chest films may reveal atelectasis, pneumonia, aortic arch widening, or prominence of the ascending or descending aorta.

Cartilaginous calcification of the pinna, the nose, the trachea, and the larynx has been observed. The calcification of ear cartilage is not specific for polychondritis and occurs following trauma and in adrenal insufficiency, ochronosis, acromegaly, hyperthyroidism, hyperparathyroidism, diabetes mellitus, hypertension, and hypervitaminosis A.

X-ray changes occurring in peripheral joints have been discussed. Spine films are usually normal, but there have

Table 91–3. Principal Laboratory Abnormalities in Polychondritis

	Number of Reported Cases	Number Positive	Percent Positivity
Sedimentation rate elevation	193	168	87
Anemia	183	104	57
Leukocytosis	176	58	33
Elevated ASO titer	32	8	25
Antinuclear antibody	128	30	23
Rheumatoid factor	139	25	18
Eosinophilia	132	15	11
Serologic testing for syphilis	84	5	6
LE cell preparation	109	8	7

been occasional reports of severe kyphosis, joint space narrowing, and erosion of vertebral endplates and the symphysis pubis as well as erosive irregularities and partial obliteration of the sacroiliac joints.

Differential Diagnosis. Conspicuous inflammatory lesions involving cartilage of the ear, nose, and laryngobronchial system distinguish polychondritis from other diseases. A variety of external auricular diseases may cause diagnostic confusion. Infectious perichondritis associated with external otitis may occur as a complication of mastoid surgery or may appear as a result of trauma. Acute streptococcal inflammation of the pinna must be differentiated from deeper cartilage inflammation, as must chronic infections such as lupus vulgaris, fungal disease, syphilis, and leprosy. Chondrodermatitis nodularis chronica helicis, which is believed to stem from a developmental vascular insufficiency accentuated by aging and repetitive trauma, is characterized by circumscribed inflammatory and degenerative changes that resemble changes found in longstanding polychondritis. Auricular inflammation induced by trauma, irritant chemicals, and frostbite must be excluded.

Inflammation and destructive changes involving nasal cartilage require differentiation from Wegener's granulomatosis, lymphomatoid granulomatosis, lethal midline granuloma, granulomatous lesions secondary to syphilis, tuberculosis, and leprosy, as well as from carcinoma and lymphosarcoma. Biopsy and culture often facilitate clarification. A saddle nose deformity may rarely be associated with rheumatoid arthritis lacking other features of polychondritis.

Necrotizing scleritis, keratitis, polyarthritis, and otitis media with potential audiovestibular dysfunction may also occur in polyarteritis and Wegener's granulomatosis. Pulmonary and renal parenchymal and central and peripheral neurologic lesions occurring in the latter help to distinguish it from polychondritis. Cogan's syndrome is characterized by a nonsyphilitic interstitial keratitis and audiovestibular disease, but it is not a generalized chondropathy. The coexistence of ocular inflammation, arthritis, and valvular or myocardial heart disease requires differentiation from rheumatoid arthritis, Behçet's disease, sarcoidosis, and the seronegative spondyloarthropathies. The mucosal lesions of Behçet's syndrome and the hilar adenopathy of sarcoidosis are not components of polychondritis. Patients with rheumatoid arthritis and ocular inflammation usually have erosive, symmetric arthritis that precedes the ocular disease.

Rheumatoid factor titers are usually high in these patients in contrast to polychondritis.

The lesions of aortitis and aortic aneurysms require differentiation from syphilis, Marfan's syndrome, Ehlers-Danlos syndrome, idiopathic medial cystic necrosis, and arteriosclerosis. More benign thoracic cage syndromes, such as idiopathic or traumatic costochondritis, Tietze's syndrome, chondrodynia costosternalis, and the xiphoid cartilage syndrome, have no systemic manifestations. Isolated bronchial stenosis has been reported in conjunction with the use of β blockers.

Proposed Diagnostic Criteria. In previous years the diagnosis of polychondritis was based upon detection of recurrent inflammation involving two or more cartilaginous sites (with at least one such site affecting an organ of special sense) in conjunction with compatible histologic findings derived from biopsy of involved cartilage.[11] More recently, McAdams and associates have proposed the diagnostic criteria listed in Table 91–4.

PATHOLOGY

The pathologic findings in involved cartilage tend to be similar.[12] The earliest manifestation is a focal or diffuse loss of basophilic staining of matrix, which is indicative of glycosaminoglycan depletion in conjunction with variable polymorphonuclear and prominent lymphocyte and plasma cell infiltration in perichondral tis-

Table 91–4. Proposed Diagnostic Criteria for Polychondritis*

Clinical Manifestations
Bilateral auricular chondritis
Nonerosive, seronegative inflammatory polyarthritis
Nasal chondritis
Ocular inflammation (conjunctivitis, keratitis, scleritis-episcleritis, uveitis)
Respiratory tract chondritis (laryngeal or tracheal cartilages, or both)
Cochlear or vestibular dysfunction, or both (neurosensory hearing loss, tinnitus, vertigo)
Plus†
Cartilage biopsy confirmation of compatible histologic picture

---

*Derived from McAdam, L. P., et al.: Medicine 55:193, 1976. To establish definitive diagnosis, three or more of the above clinical features are required.

†If the diagnosis is clinically obvious, it is unnecessary to obtain a biopsy for confirmation. Biopsy can be derived from the ear, nose, or respiratory tract.

sue (Fig. 91–4). The process may continue relentlessly from the periphery to the deeper layers of cartilage. Chondrocyte degeneration, dedifferentiation, and dissolution soon become apparent. Granulation tissue subsequently invades and replaces regions of cartilage, creating sequestered islands of degenerating cells and proteoglycan-depleted matrix. An overabundance of such granulation tissue is responsible for the development of auricular nodules and, in part, tracheal narrowing. Fibrosis eventually ensues, and cystic spaces containing gelatinous material become evident. Focal regions of calcification and bone formation may occur.

By electron microscopy,[13,14] chondrocytes in the superficial and deeper layers of pathologic specimens have been shown to contain large quantities of lysosomes, lipid, and glycogen. Such cells and adjacent collagen and elastic fibers may be destroyed or replaced by small electron-dense granules and vesicles that vary in size, shape, and density. Cytoplasmic processes containing such material have been observed extending into regions immediately surrounding cells. It has been suggested that such particles are products of chondrocytes and represent extruded lysosomes, matrix vesicles, or cell debris. Viable chondrocytes may be seen phagocytosing degraded material. Diffuse, finely granular electron-dense material has also been described on the surface of cartilage and coating elastic fibers.[15]

Sections of involved aorta show patchy vascularization of the media with inflammatory cell infiltration, decreased collagen and glycosaminoglycan content, and fragmentation of elastic fibers. Lymphocyte cuffing may appear around the vasa vasorum. Secondary fibrosis of the intima and adventitia occurs. The aortic ring appears stretched or dilated, whereas the valve leaflets can be normal or thickened. Endothelial proliferation observed in syphilitic aortitis is not evident, nor is the pooling in the media of periodic acid-Schiff (PAS) positive material characteristic of medial cystic necrosis. The loss of aortic

elastic tissue is similar to that encountered in Marfan's syndrome, but the glycosaminoglycan content of the aortic root is not depleted in the latter disease. Destruction of muscle fibers can lead to aneurysm formation.

The tracheal mucosa frequently appears edematous. Cartilaginous rings of the trachea show changes ranging from mild inflammation to total resorption by granulation tissue. Large- and medium-sized bronchi show patchy widening of the lumens resembling bronchiectasis. There may be extensive narrowing and dissolution of these airway components. The histologic changes involving cartilage are identical to those already described. The lesions may be discrete and localized or may involve the entire upper airway.

A chronic synovitis with edematous changes, vessel dilatation, and infiltration with chronic inflammatory cells may be seen histologically.[12] An increase in lining cells primarily of phagocytic type A cells has been reported.

Ocular pathologic changes have revealed a loss of basophilia and the fragmentation of elastic tissue at the scleroconjunctival angle. Scattered mast cells, plasma cells, and lymphocytes have been observed around episcleral vessels. The corneal stroma may be edematous and necrotic, with an inflammatory cell infiltrate occurring in peripheral regions. Infiltration of the iris with lymphocytes, plasma cells, and granulation tissue has been described.

ETIOLOGIC AND PATHOPHYSIOLOGIC CONSIDERATIONS

The etiology of polychondritis is unknown. Theories have incriminated excessive alcoholic intake, trauma, infection, allergy, biosynthetic defects in mesenchymally derived cells, enhanced enzymatic proteolysis, autoimmunity, and connective tissue disease manifested by vas-

Figure 91–4. Biopsy of the external ear revealing a necrotizing chondritis with inflammatory cell infiltrate, chondrocyte degeneration, and fibrosis. (Left, × 197; right, × 150.)

culitis that is confined to tissues high in glycosaminoglycan content. A perichondritis involving laryngeal and thyroid cartilage can occur in a variety of infectious processes, including syphilis, tuberculosis, diphtheria, typhus, actinomycosis, varicella, and rubella, yet generalized destructive cartilaginous changes do not ensue. The failure to culture an infectious agent and the lack of response to antibiotic treatment point away from an infectious etiology. The generalized loss of all forms of glycosaminoglycans, the distortion of normal chondrocyte architecture and distribution, the retention of normal-appearing cartilage in segregated islands, and the lack of uniform involvement of cartilaginous structures throughout the body are factors distinctly against a generalized defect in biosynthesis.

The clinical and pathologic features of polychondritis strongly suggest a primary acquired disease in which an inflammatory response is mounted against tissues rich in proteoglycans. Unlike other inflammatory joint diseases in which synovial inflammation occurs first, polychondritis is unique in possibly being the direct result of a primary inflammatory response against cartilage.

Proteinases—The Mediators of Cartilage Degradation. There is experimental evidence supporting enzymatic proteolysis in the induction of such matrix dissolution. The intravenous injection of crude papain into young rabbits has been shown to cause collapse of normally rigid ears within 4 hours.[16] Histologic studies have demonstrated a diffuse loss of metachromasia and basophilia—not only of auricular matrix but also in the ribs, larynx, trachea, epiphyses, and joints. There is a substantial increase of sulfated glycosaminoglycans in the serum and urine. Some animals show respiratory distress secondary to collapse of the trachea or bronchi, or both. However, the absence of inflammation and the limited course of disease are conspicuous differences from polychondritis. Following a single intravenous injection of crude papain, focal plaque lesions have been described in the ascending aorta and arch secondary to connective tissue alterations in the media, which may proceed to metaplastic changes leading to cartilage and bone formation.[17] Comparable changes have been noted in polychondritis. The potential importance of endogenous chondrocyte enzymes in inducing matrix destruction is suggested by the observations that administration of large doses of retinol (an agent that promotes lysosomal enzyme release from chondrocytes) to rabbits or its introduction into in vitro cultures of embryonic bone rudiments may induce histologic changes similar to papain-mediated amorphous matrix depletion.[18,19]

The description of characteristics and substrate specificities of proteinases found in chondrocytes and polymorphonuclear (PMN) leukocytes are detailed in Chapter 12. The capacity for complete cartilage destruction can be expressed by both of these cell types. It is likely that cartilage matrix degradation is in part dependent upon a local proteinase-antiproteinase imbalance. Recent studies have shown that conditioned media of activated rabbit peritoneal macrophages contain a factor capable of inducing synthesis and release de novo of latent collagenase and neutral proteinase by chon-

drocytes.[20] It is probable, but unproved, that in polychondritis such potential products of the inflammatory response or the phagocytosis of degraded matrix components, or both, stimulate chondrocytes to release proteinases that supplement enzymes released by inflammatory cells present in the milieu of destruction.

Immunobiology of Cartilage. As has been discussed, there is a disproportionately high coexistence of relapsing polychondritis and connective tissue diseases that are known to have immunologic mechanism functioning in a direct or indirect manner in their pathogenesis. The predominant lymphocytic and plasma cell infiltrate observed at pathologic sites in polychondritis provides additional circumstantial evidence supporting the potential role of immunologic mechanisms.[12]

The proteoglycans and collagen of cartilage matrix are antigenic.[21] Yet antigenicity is to a measure masked in the native state, resulting in part from conformational structure.[22] Chondrocytes also manifest histocompatibility and tissue-specific surface antigens, but they are normally sequestered from the immune system by being surrounded by a matrix impervious to antibody diffusion or the entrance of immunocompetent cells.[23] Thus avascular cartilage may be regarded as a truly immunologically privileged tissue. Should there be an insult to its structural integrity, irrespective of inciting factors, there may be release of or de novo exposure to intrinsic determinants that are capable of host sensitization, with resultant activation of humoral and cell-mediated immunologic mechanisms that are sufficient to generate inflammation. The consequences may be widespread based upon the sharing of cartilage proteoglycan antigenicity with the sclera, the anterior uveal tract, the endoneurium and the perineurium of the optic nerve, the endothelial cells of blood vessels, the interfibrillar material within the aortic media and intima, the heart valves, the myocardial sarcolemma, the tracheal submucosal basement membrane, the synoviocytes, and the renal glomerular and the tubular basement membranes.[21,24] Similarly, the antigenicity of vitreous collagen is similar to type II cartilage collagen and it has been shown to have arthritogenic potential.[25]

Several groups have shown that intra-articularly or intravenously administered homologous or autologous hyaline cartilage preparations and antiproteoglycan antisera can induce a chronic synovitis, cartilaginous degenerative changes, or perichondritis, or all of these.[21] Antiproteoglycan antisera can suppress chondrocyte proteoglycan synthesis. In vitro studies have shown that antibodies having cell-membrane antigen specificity have induced a reversible, complement-dependent cartilage matrix dissolution in chick limb bud rudiments.[26] Following mitogen or homologous and autologous cartilage proteoglycan and collagen antigen stimulation, T lymphocytes have been shown to release lymphokines having the capacity to (1) induce cartilage proteoglycan degradation via macrophage activation and (2) reversibly suppress, in the absence of a macrophage requirement, synthesis of glycosaminoglycan, collagen, protein, and nucleic acid by chondrocytes.[27-31]

Cytokines derived from lectin-stimulated human and

porcine mononuclear cells can induce chondrocyte proteoglycanase and collagenase release.[32-34] The inducing cytokines appear to represent a monokine or monokines (e.g., interleukin 1) that have a direct catabolic effect, and a lymphokine or lymphokines that are released by monokine-lectin–triggered T lymphocytes,[32] or both of these.[32] Native and component α-chains of type II collagen have been shown to produce a dose-dependent activation of the alternative pathway of complement and to induce macrophage proteinase release.[35] Humoral and cell-mediated immune responses to proteoglycan and collagen antigenic determinants have been identified in experimental models of antigen-induced arthritis.[36,37]

The intradermal injection of cartilage-specific type II collagen can induce a destructive arthropathy in rats and mice (see Chapter 14).[38] Response appears linked to Ir regions of the major histocompatability loci and is strain specific.[39,40] Antibodies specific for conformational determinants of native type II collagen and cell-mediated immune responses lacking conformational or collagen-type specificity appear. Passive transfer of disease has been achieved using both cells and serum. It is of interest that rats so immunized (9 to 14 percent) may develop an intense chondritis and immunofluorescent localization of IgG and C3 in lesions.[41,42] Electron-dense deposits observed in the proximity of chondrocytes correspond with IgG and C3 deposition. Auricular involvement occurs significantly later and is independent of the development of arthritis. Ocular, tracheobronchial, and cardiovascular lesions did not occur. Although a humoral immune response to a cartilage matrix antigen or antigens is present, its role in the pathogenesis of chondritis remains unclear. The specificity of the localized IgG is unknown. Is it representative of entrapped immune complexes, or does it reflect antibody binding in situ to matrix determinants? Could it function in induction of complement- or cell-mediated cytotoxic responses? Does strain restriction reflect epitope specificity of autoantibody?

Cartilage degradation may be mediated not only by a direct immunologic insult but also indirectly in the role of an "innocent bystander" effect. In antigen-induced experimental models of chronic synovitis, antigen retention occurs in a patchy distribution in the superficial layers of articular cartilage, presumably in the form of immune complexes bound to collagen.[43] Similarly, the deposition of immunoglobulin and complement has been observed in rheumatoid, and to a lesser degree osteoarthritic, articular collagenous tissues.[44] The insoluble deposits may attract inflammatory cells that release proteinases following attempts at phagocytosis of the fixed complexes.

Immunologic Studies. There have been relatively few studies attempting to incriminate immunologic mechanisms in the pathogenesis of polychondritis. Several investigators have identified circulating anticartilage antibodies using indirect immunofluorescence.[11,45] In limited studies, antibodies to proteoglycan aggregates and subunit and link protein fractions have been identified by hemagglutination.[46] These antibodies, however, are not unique to polychondritis. They can be shown in patients having cartilage destruction that is associated with diverse diseases. Antibodies specific for type II collagen have been reported in polychondritis, with the antibody and its titer correlating with activity and early disease.[47-49] In some instances antibodies appeared to be directed against the native collagen molecule only, suggesting that the potential of their formation may be a primary event in pathogenesis rather than an epiphenomenon of inflammation. Using direct immunofluorescence, coarsely granular deposits of IgG, IgA, and C3 have been demonstrated at the chondrofibral junction of auricular biopsies, suggesting potential immune complex deposition.[50] Similar deposits have at times been observed throughout the cartilage matrix. Circulating immune complexes are being reported with increased frequency.[49] A report of decreased total hemolytic complement in the inflammatory effusion of an affected ear suggests local activation.[51] Such observations raise the potential of either a direct immunologically mediated cartilage insult or an immune complex–associated indirect "innocent bystander" effect, or both, being operative in pathogenesis.

Cell-mediated immune responses to cartilage proteoglycans and other products of chondrocyte synthesis have been demonstrated in patients having polychondritis.[52,53] Positive responses have been shown to correlate with periods of overt disease activity but, again, lack specificity for polychondritis. Thus, autosensitization to constituents inherent to cartilage matrix occurs in this disease. More comprehensive studies are required to delineate the relative significance of the observations discussed.

Pathogenesis—A Hypothesis. The initial manifestation of disease is apparently a patchy depletion of the proteoglycans of cartilaginous structures, large arteries, and other tissues rich in such matrix content. Although the triggering mechanism and genetic susceptibility remain unknown, it appears clear that matrix degradation is mediated enzymatically, with enzymes originating through immunologically and nonimmunologically triggered mechanisms from chondrocytes and infiltrating cells. Alterations in the integrity of connective tissue matrix may, in turn, result in autoimmunization to proteoglycan, collagen, elastin, and perhaps chondrocyte antigenic determinants. The humoral (direct or immune complex, or both) and cell-mediated immune responses that follow may both induce and perpetuate inflammation, resulting in further tissue damage at local, and possibly at more distant sites sharing such matrix component antigenicity.

CLINICAL COURSE, PROGNOSIS, AND TREATMENT

The clinical course of polychondritis is highly variable. It is characterized by episodic flareups of activity, or smoldering disease of ever-changing severity, or it can be fulminant with a rapid downhill course. Prognosis is difficult because the diagnosis is essentially a clinical one. The disease frequently goes unrecognized or is misdiagnosed. Only the most florid cases are usually reported.

There have been 51 deaths recorded in the 286 cases analyzed (18 percent), with mean survivals from time of onset varying from 4.2 to 5.2 years in established reviews.[54,55] Fatality has primarily resulted from respiratory tract involvement (airway collapse, 16 cases; pneumonia, 5 cases) and cardiovascular complications (aneurysmal rupture, 3 cases; vasculitis, 4 cases; valvular heart disease, 3 cases). Three deaths have occurred from renal failure, and six deaths from concurrent malignancy have been reported. The outlook is far from being completely ominous. Symptoms may often be completely controlled by therapeutic measures, and total recovery has at times been noted.

Less severe manifestations of disease can usually be controlled with the use of aspirin and the newer nonsteroidal anti-inflammatory compounds. Based upon its capacity to inhibit lysosomal enzyme-mediated cartilage degradation induced by hypervitaminosis A along with its immunomodulatory potential, dapsone, 50 to 200 mg per day, has been used increasingly with some measure of success.

Although evidence that corticosteroids alter the natural course of disease is lacking, they are often effective in suppressing acute manifestations and are capable of reducing the frequency and severity of recurrences. Initially a program of 30 to 60 mg of prednisone or its equivalent is instituted in daily divided doses with subsequent gradual tapering to a maintenance dose of 5 to 25 mg, dependent upon clinical response. Doses as high as 80 mg to 100 mg may be required in particularly severe acute stages in which laryngotracheal, bronchial, ocular, or inner ear involvement is present. Alternate-day schedules are not recommended. Pulse therapy has not been evaluated. If disease progression occurs despite such measures, a trial of immunosuppressive agents is warranted. Cyclophosphamide, 6-mercaptopurine, and azathioprine have been used with some measure of success, and a steroid-sparing effect has been evident.[54,55]

At any indication of severe respiratory tract distress, one should be ready to perform a tracheostomy rather than procrastinate with endoscopy and intubation. Surgical resection of a perichondrial inflammatory mass causing airway narrowing followed by airway reconstruction has been reported. Valve replacement or valvuloplasty should be considered in intractable heart failure secondary to valvular insufficiency. Aortic aneurysms have been successfully resected. The key to optimal management is individualized therapy with a careful, prolonged followup period.

References

1. Cody, D.T.R., and Sones, D.A.: Relapsing polychondritis: Audiovestibular manifestations. Laryngoscope 81:1208, 1971.
2. McKay, D.A.R., Watson, P.G., and Lyne, A.J.: Relapsing polychondritis and eye disease. Br. J. Opthalmol. 58:600, 1974.
3. O'Hanlan, M., McAdam, L.P., Bluestone, R., and Pearson, C.M.: The arthropathy of relapsing polychondritis. Arthritis Rheum. 19:191, 1976.
4. Luthra, H.S., McKenna, C.H., and Terasaki, P.I.: Lack of association of HLA-A and B locus antigens with relapsing polychondritis. Tissue Antigens 17:442, 1981.
5. Gibson, G.J., and Davis, P.: Respiratory complications of relapsing polychondritis. Thorax 29:726, 1974.
6. Mohsenifar, Z., Tashkin, D.P., Carson, S.A., and Bellamy, P.E.: Pulmonary function in patients with relapsing polychondritis. Chest 81:711, 1982.
7. Owen, D.S., Jr., Irby, R., and Toone, E.: Relapsing polychondritis with aortic involvement. Arthritis Rheum. 13:877, 1970.
8. Cipriano, P.R., Alonso, D.R., Baltaxe, H.A., Gay, W.A., Jr., and Smith, J.P.: Multiple aortic aneurysms in relapsing polychondritis. Am. J. Cardiol. 37:1097, 1976.
9. Esdaile, J., Hawkins, D., Gold, P., Freedman, S.O., and Duguid, W.P.: Vascular involvement in relapsing polychondritis. Can. Med. Assoc. J. 116:1019, 1977.
10. Neild, G.H., Cameron, J.S., Lessof, M.H., Ogg, C.S., and Turner, D.R.: Relapsing polychondritis with cresentic glomerulonephritis. Br. Med. J. 1:743, 1978.
11. Dolan, D.L., Lemmon, G.B., Jr., and Teitelbaum, S.L.: Relapsing polychondritis. Analytical literature review and studies on pathogenesis. Am. J. Med. 41:285, 1966.
12. Mitchell, N., and Shepard, N.: Relapsing polychondritis. An electron microscopic study of synovium and articular cartilage. J. Bone Joint. Surg. 54A:1235, 1972.
13. Hashimoto, K., Arkin, C.R., and Kang, A.H.: Relapsing polychondritis. An ultrastructural study. Arthritis Rheum. 19:91, 1977.
14. Dryll, A., Lansaman, J., Meyer, O., Bardin, T., and Ryckewaert, A.: Relapsing polychondritis. An ultrastructural study of elastic and collagen fibres degradation revealed by tannic acid. Virchows Arch. (Pathol. Anat.) 390:109, 1981.
15. Shaul, S.R., and Schumacher, H.R.: Relapsing polychondritis. Electron microscopy of ear cartilage. Arthritis Rheum. 18:617, 1975.
16. McCluskey, R.T., and Thomas, L.: The removal of cartilage matrix in vivo by papain. J. Exp. Med. 108:371, 1958.
17. Tsaltas, T.T.: Metaplasia of aortic connective tissue to cartilage and bone induced by the intravenous injection of papain. Nature (Lond.) 196:1006, 1962.
18. Thomas, L., McCluskey, R.T., Potter, J.L., and Weissman, G.: Comparison of the effects of papain and vitamin A on cartilage. I. The effects in rabbits. J. Exp. Med. 111:705, 1960.
19. Fell, H.B., and Thomas, L.: Comparison of the effects of papain and vitamin A on cartilage. II. The effects on organ cultures of embryonic skeletal tissue. J. Exp. Med. 111:719, 1960.
20. Deshmukh-Phadke, K., Nanda, S., and Lee, K.: Macrophage factor that induces neutral protease secretion by normal rabbit chondrocytes. Eur. J. Biochem. 104:175, 1980.
21. Herman, J.H., and Carpenter, B.A.: Immunobiology of cartilage. Semin. Arthritis Rheum. 5:1, 1975.
22. Herman, J.H., and Dennis, M.V.: Polydispersity of human articular cartilage proteoglycan antigens. J. Rheumatol. 3:390, 1976.
23. Malseed, Z.M., and Heyner, S.: Antigenic profile of the rat chondrocyte. Arthritis Rheum. 19:223, 1976.
24. Poole, A.R., Pidoux, I., Reiner, A., Coster, L., and Hassell, J.R.: Mammalian eyes and associated tissues contain molecules that are immunologically related to cartilage proteoglycan and link protein. J. Cell Biol. 93:910, 1982.
25. Stuart, J.M., Cremer, M.A., Dixit, S.N., Kang, A.H. and Townes, A.S.: Collagen-induced arthritis in rats. Comparison of vitreous and cartilage derived collagens. Arthritis Rheum. 22:347, 1979.
26. Lackmann, P.J., Coombs, R.R.A., Fell, H.B., and Dingle, J.T.: The breakdown of embryonic (chick) cartilage and bone cultivated in the presence of complement sufficient antiserum. III. Immunological analyses. Int. Arch. Allergy Appl. Immunol. 35:469, 1969.
27. Herman, J.H., Musgrave, D.S., and Dennis, M.V.: Phytomitogen-induced, lymphokine-mediated cartilage proteoglycan degradation. Arthritis Rheum. 20:922, 1977.
28. Taplits, M.S., Crissman, J.D., and Herman, J.H.: Histologic assessment of lymphokine-mediated suppression of chondrocyte glycosaminoglycan synthesis. Arthritis Rheum. 22:19, 1979.
29. Herman, J.H., Herzig, E.B., Crissman, J.D., Dennis, M.V., and Hess, E.V.: Idiopathic chondrolysis—an immunopathologic study. J. Rheumatol. 7:694, 1980.
30. Herman, J.H., Nutman, T.B., Nozoe, M., Mowery, C.S., and Dennis, M.V.: Lymphokine-mediated suppression of chondrocyte glycosaminoglycan and protein synthesis. Arthritis Rheum. 24:824, 1981.
31. Herman, J.H., Khosla, R.C., Mowery, C.S., and Appel, A.M.: Modulation of chondrocyte synthesis by lymphokine-rich conditioned media. Arthritis Rheum. 25:668, 1982.
32. Herman, J.H., Greenblatt, D., Khosla, R.C., and Appel, A.M.: Cytokine modulation of chondrocyte proteinase release. Arthritis Rheum. 27:79, 1984.
33. Jasin, H.E., and Dingle, J.T.: Human mononuclear cell factors mediate cartilage matrix degradation though chondrocyte activation. J. Clin. Invest. 68:571, 1981.
34. Saklatvala, J., and Sarsfield, S.J.: Lymphocytes induce resorption of cartilage by producing catabolin. Biochem. J. 202:275, 1982.

35. Hanauske-Abel, H.M., Pontz, B.V., and Schorlemmer, H.U.: Cartilage specific collagen activates macrophages and the alternative pathway of complement: evidence for an immunopathogenic concept of rheumatoid arthritis. Ann. Rheum. Dis. 41:168, 1982.

36. Glant, T., Hadas, E., and Nagy, M.: Cell-mediated and humoral immune responses to cartilage antigenic components. Scand. J. Immunol. 9:39, 1979.

37. Champion, B.R. and Poole, R.A.: Immunity to homologous cartilage proteoglycans in rabbits with chronic inflammatory arthritis. Coll. Res. 5:453, 1981.

38. Trentham, D.E., Townes, A.S., and Kang, A.H.: Autoimmunity to Type II collagen: An experimental model of arthritis. J. Exp. Med. 146:857, 1977.

39. Stuart, J.M., Townes, A.S., and Kang, A.H.: Nature and specificity of the immune response to collagen in type II collagen-induced arthritis in mice. J. Clin. Invest. 69:673, 1982.

40. Griffiths, M.M., Eichwald, E.J., Martin, J.H., Smith, C.B., and DeWitt, C.W.: Immunogenetic control of experimental type II collagen-induced arthritis. 1. Susceptibility and resistance among inbred strains of rats. Arthritis Rheum. 24:781, 1981.

41. Cremer, M.A., Pitcock, J.A., Stuart, J.M., Kang, A.H., and Townes, A.S.: Auricular chondritis in rats. An experimental model for relapsing polychondritis induced with type II collagen. J. Exp. Med. 154:535, 1981.

42. McCune, W.S., Schiller, A.L., Dynesius-Trentham, R.A., and Trentham, D.E.: Type II collagen-induced auricular chondritis. Arthritis Rheum. 25:266, 1982.

43. Cooke, T.D., Hurd, E.R., Ziff, M., and Jasin, H.E.: The pathogenesis of chronic inflammation in experimental antigen-induced arthritis. J. Exp. Med. 135:323, 1972.

44. Ohno, O., and Cooke, T.D.: Electron microscopic morphology of immu-noglobulin aggregates and their interactions in rheumatoid articular collagenous tissues. Arthritis Rheum. 21:516, 1978.

45. Hughes, R.A.C., Berry, C.L., and Seifert, M.: Relapsing polychondritis. Three cases with a clinico-pathologic study and literature review. Q. J. Med. 61:363, 1972.

46. Herman, J.H.: Unpublished observations.

47. Foidart, J.M., Abe, S., Martin, G.R., Zizic, T.M., Barnett, E.V., Lawley, T.J., and Katz, S.I.: Antibodies to type II collagen in relapsing polychondritis. N. Engl. J. Med. 299:1203, 1978.

48. Ebringer, R., Rook, G., Swana, G.T., Bottazzo, F., and Doniach, D.: Autoantibodies to cartilage and type II collagen in relapsing polychondritis and other rheumatic diseases. Ann. Rheum. Dis. 40:473, 1981.

49. Ueno, Y., Chia, D., and Barnett, E.V.: Relapsing polychondritis associated with ulcerative colitis. Serial determinations of antibodies to cartilage and circulating immune complexes by three assays. J. Rheumatol. 8:456, 1981.

50. Valenzuela, R., Cooperrider, P.A., Gogate, P., Deodhar, S.D., and Berfeld, W.F.: Relapsing polychondritis. Immunomicroscopic findings in cartilage of ear biopsy specimens. Hum. Pathol. 11:19, 1980.

51. McKenna, C.H., Luthra, M.S., and Jordon, R.E.: Hypocomplementemic ear effusions in relapsing polychondritis. Mayo Clin. Proc. 51:495, 1976.

52. Herman, J.H., and Dennis, M.V.: Immunopathologic studies in relapsing polychondritis. J. Clin. Invest. 52:549, 1973.

53. Rajapakse, D.A., and Bywaters, E.G.L.: Cell-mediated immunity to cartilage proteoglycan in relapsing polychondritis. Clin. Exp. Immunol. 16:497, 1974.

54. Arkin, C.R., and Masi, A.T.: Relapsing polychondritis: Review of current status and case report. Semin. Arthritis Rheum. 5:41, 1975.

55. McAdam, L.P., O'Hanlan, M.A., Bluestone, R., and Pearson, C.M.: Relapsing polychondritis: Prospective study of 23 patients and a review of the literature. Medicine 55:193, 1976.

Section XV
Infiltrative Systemic Diseases

Chapter 92
Amyloidosis

Edgar S. Cathcart and Thomas F. Ignaczak

INTRODUCTION

Definition of Amyloidosis. Amyloidosis is a syndrome characterized by the deposition of an insoluble proteinaceous material in the extracellular matrix of one or several organs. These deposits encroach upon parenchymal tissues, compromise organ function, and produce diverse clinical manifestations. Amyloidosis is pertinent to the rheumatic diseases because it occurs as a potentially fatal complication of longstanding or poorly controlled inflammation, or it mimics more common rheumatic problems in its presentations.

Until recently, amyloidosis was characterized chiefly by its histologic properties. The diagnosis was seldom made by the clinician, since it was, and in fact remains, a morphologically defined entity. The key to the modern approach to amyloidosis in all its forms has been the discovery of a characteristic and unique fibrillar ultrastructure of amyloid deposits from any source, clinical or experimental.[1,2] The rigid, nonbranching filament of about 100 Å diameter became the very definition of amyloidosis and provided a unifying concept of a disease that otherwise took on so many forms that it raised the suspicion that it was really a collection of unrelated entities. The unifying concept was further refined with the discovery that the amyloid fibril is composed of a protein arranged in a β-pleated sheet,[3] a configuration first described by Pauling and Corey.[4] It is this unusual molecular arrangement that is responsible for the diagnostic staining properties of amyloid, specifically the green birefringence when stained with Congo red (Table 92–1).

History of Amyloidosis Research. The history of amyloid research can be traced to 1700, when T. B. Bonet reported on two postmortem cases of splenic infiltration with amyloid-like material.[5] Subsequent sporadic reports were consistent with amyloid infiltration of liver or spleen, but elucidation of the morbid anatomy was not accomplished until the early nineteeth century by pathologists investigating the waxy or lardaceous enlargement of abdominal viscera. Portal (1813), Lobstein (1829), Hodgkin (1832), Abercrombie (1830), and Carswell (1838) described lardaceous degeneration of liver or spleen compatible with modern-day amyloid depo-

sition.[5] In 1842, Rokitansky distinguished lardaceous infiltrations of the liver from other types of waxy or fatty degeneration and affirmed the association of a lardaceous liver with debilitating illnesses.[6] He further described splenic infiltration associated with hepatic disease, which implied the systemic nature of the disorder.[6]

In 1854, Virchow initiated over a century of controversy regarding the chemical nature of the lardaceous deposits when he called the cerebral corpora amylacea deposits "amyloid" (starchlike) based on their staining with iodine and acid.[7] He similarly believed that splenic deposits of amyloid material contained starch, despite their atypical tinctorial properties.[8] Meckel refuted the cellulose origin of amyloid, but accepted amyloid as a morphologic designation.[9] In 1859, Schmidt[10] and Friedreich and Kekulé[11] emphasized the "albuminoid" nature of amyloid material. The proteinaceous nature of amyloid deposits has since been confirmed by numerous investigators.

Early twentieth century amyloid research resulted in the development of experimental animal models for the disease,[12,13] the recognition of the unique optical properties of amyloid deposits following Congo red staining,[14,15] and the gradual incrimination of the immune system in amyloidogenesis. In 1931, Magnus-Levy noted the frequent association of amyloidosis and Bence Jones proteinuria, and implicated the abnormal proteins in the pathogenesis of the amyloid tissue infiltrates.[16] Apitz, in 1940, reported an atypical bone marrow plasmacytosis in amyloidosis and suggested a causal association.[17] Osserman[18] further strengthened the circumstantial links among bone marrow plasmacytosis, circulating paraproteinemia, and amyloidosis. These observations fell short of proving the immunologic basis of amyloidosis, however, and inconclusive immunofluorescent studies left further cause to doubt the immunoglobulin origin of amyloidosis. With the discovery of the amyloid fibril in 1959, it became possible to attempt isolation and chemical characterization of amyloid. The first proteins to be analyzed by Glenner and co-workers[19] were from patients with primary amyloidosis. Amino acid sequence data revealed these proteins to be homologous to the variable region of immunoglobulin light chains. Shortly thereafter, Benditt and Eriksen discovered the extracel-

Table 92–1. Characteristics of Amyloid

Method of Study	Findings
Light microscopy	Eosinophilia
	Green birefringence with Congo red stains*
	Metachromasia with methyl violet and crystal violet stains
	Faint autofluorescence
	Fluorescence with thioflavine stains
Electron microscopy	Rigid, nonbranching fibrils of approximately 100 Å diameter*
	Pentagonal units (P-component)
X-ray diffraction	Antiparallel β-pleated-sheet conformation*

*Definitive criteria for amyloid.

lular protein that appears to be the major constituent of secondary amyloid deposits.[20] This substance, now called amyloid A (AA) protein, has a molecular weight of 8500 daltons and is composed of 76 amino acids in a sequence that is not related to that of any previously identified proteins.[21,22] Thus, after many years of frustration, biochemical investigations had succeeded in answering the question "What is amyloidosis?" though leaving unsolved the equally important questions as to how and why it occurs in the first place.

AMYLOID DEPOSITS

Light Microscopy of Amyloid Deposits. Amyloid deposits from various human and animal sources appear similar and amorphous under light microscopy. These accumulations stain eosinophilically with hematoxylin and eosin, exhibit metachromasia with crystal violet,[23] and demonstrate an affinity for Congo red.[14] The most useful histochemical procedure for detecting amyloid deposits involves polarization microscopy of Congo red–

stained specimens, which produces a pathognomonic green birefringence.[24-26] Amyloid deposits also fluoresce after staining with thioflavin dyes, but this reaction is less specific than Congo red–induced green birefringence.[5,27,28]

Ultrastructure of Amyloid Deposits. Amyloid deposits have been shown by electron microscopy to contain two distinct formed elements: a fibrillar component[1,2,29,30] and a pentagonal unit (P-component).[31-33] Both constituents have been present in all human or animal amyloid preparations studied to date. The fibrils are characteristically thin, rigid, nonbranching, and approximately 100 Å wide. They have a tendency toward lateral aggregation in order to form fibers (Fig. 92–1).[29] Individual fibrils are composed of two to five 25- to 30-Å wide filaments, arranged essentially parallel to the long axis of the fibril in a twisted-ribbon fashion. This configuration produces a hollow core profile on cross section of the fibril.[34]

Amyloid fibrils are dispersed in the extracellular space. Fibrils distant from cellular elements are arranged almost randomly, whereas fibrils in proximity to cells may be oriented perpendicularly or parallel to the plasma membrane.[35] Fibrils adjacent to cells often appear to merge with the membrane. Amyloidlike fibrils have been demonstrated in the intracellular milieu of several types of phagocytic mononuclear cells,[36,37] but these intracellular fibrils are not morphologically identical to the extracellular fibrils.[38] Furthermore, these fibrils could be lying in the extracellular compartment in invaginations of the plasma membrane. Regardless, the close morphologic relationship of amyloid fibrils and phagocytic cells suggests that these cells are intimately involved in the synthesis or processing of amyloid fibrils.[39]

X-ray crystallography of amyloid fibril concentrates reveals that the fibrils consist of polypeptide chains arranged perpendicularly to the long axis of the fibril with a cross β-pleated sheet conformation.[40,41] Infrared spec-

Figure 92–1. Amyloid fibrils. Electron microscopic appearance of 100Å wide fibrils isolated from amyloid deposits. A tendency to aggregate laterally is evident. (Courtesy of H. A. Bladen and G. G. Glenner, Bethesda, Maryland.)

troscopy further indicates that the polypeptide chains are folded in an antiparallel fashion.[3,42] The β-pleated sheet conformation has been found in all amyloid proteins investigated and may explain certain characteristics of amyloid deposits. Congo red–induced green birefringence of amyloid deposits implies that the dye molecules are regularly arranged with their long axes parallel to the long axes of the fibrils.[43] The twisted β-pleated sheet conformation of amyloid fibrils facilitates appropriate alignment of the Congo red dye molecules, which are then bound by nonionic forces to the polypeptide chains.[44] The resistance of amyloid deposits to digestion by most mammalian enzymes may also be related to the β-pleated structure, which is rare in mammalian systems. Finally, certain polypeptides undergo a conformational change to a β-pleated sheet conformation following thermal or enzymatic denaturation in vitro; with this change, they assume the tinctorial or physical properties of amyloid fibrils.[45,46]

The P-component is a normal plasma protein that was discovered by its crossreactivity with antisera raised against saline extracts of human amyloid deposits.[47] No differences have yet been found between P-component isolated from serum (SAP) and P-component obtained from amyloid-laden tissues (AP), and their amino acid sequences are identical.[48,49] SAP has a doughnut-like structure composed of five globular subunits surrounding a central cavity.[31-33] It is 80 Å in diameter with a tendency to aggregate into rods with a 40-Å periodicity (Fig. 92–2). The observation that SAP and AP undergo calcium-dependent binding to agarose[50] has greatly facilitated the isolation and purification of these proteins in humans and in other animals. AP has an intimate association with all types of amyloid deposits,[51] with the possible exception of cerebral amyloid plaques.[52] It does not appear to be of pathogenetic significance in amyloidosis and may be nonspecifically absorbed from the plasma onto the amyloid fibrillar network. In the mouse, SAP behaves as a true acute-phase reactant, its concentration in the serum starting to rise 8 hours after an acute physical or chemical injury and reaching a peak after 24 hours to 48 hours.[53] A remarkable homology between SAP and CRP (C-reactive protein) with respect to structure and function[54] supports the theory that SAP has been stably conserved during vertebrate evolution, possibly even to a greater extent than CRP.[55] The recent finding that P-component is a normal constituent of human basement membrane and of elastic fiber microfibrils[56] has opened an exciting new area of study in the CRP-SAP family of acute phase reactants.

Amyloid Deposits of Immunoglobulin Light Chain Origin (AL Proteins). The solubilization of amyloid fibril preparations under denaturing conditions has facilitated the isolation of purified amyloid fibrillar proteins for biochemical characterization.[57] The first two amyloid proteins studied by automated amino acid sequence analysis were homogeneous and homologous to the variable regions of immunoglobulin κ light chains (Table 92–2). Four additional amyloid fibrillar proteins with "blocked amino termini had amino acid compositions consistent with immunoglobulin λ light chains.[58] Based on these and other experimental data, it is concluded that some amyloid fibrils have as their major protein component an intact immunoglobulin light chain (rare), an amino terminal fragment of a light chain, or a homogeneous light chain and its amino terminal fragments.[59] Several laboratories have since confirmed the immunoglobulin light chain origin of certain amyloid proteins.[60-62]

Immunochemical studies substantiate the derivation

Figure 92–2. Amyloid P-component. 80 Å diameter, doughnut-like structure composed of five globular subunits (pentraxins) (Courtesy of H. A. Bladen and G. G. Glenner, Bethesda, Maryland.)

Table 92–2. Partial Amino Acid Sequences of Selected Amyloid Proteins and Human CRP

Type	Amino Acid Sequence
AA	Arg-Ser-Phe-Phe-Ser-Phe-Leu-Gly-Glu-Ala-
AL (κ I)	Asp-Lle-Gln-Met-Thr-Gln-Ser-Pro-Ser-Ser-
AL (κ II)	Asp-Lle-Val-Met-Thr-Gln-Ser-Pro-Leu-Ser-
AL (λ VI)	Asp-Phe-Met-Leu-Thr-Glu-Pro-His-Ser-Val-
AF (prealbumin)	Gly-Pro-Thr-Gly-Thr-Gly-Glu-Ser-Lys-Cys-
AP	His-Thr-Asp-Leu-Ser-Gly-Lys-Val-Phe-Val-
CRP	PCA-Thr-Asp-Met-Ser-Arg-Lys-Ala-Phe-Val-

of amyloid fibrillar proteins from immunoglobulin light chains and further demonstrate that a component antigenically related to the tissue protein can be found in the serum of many amyloidosis patients.[63] Detection of these antigenically related serum light-chain components may be hampered by their low concentrations and restricted antigenicity. In one case of primary amyloidosis in which a serum component could not be found by standard immunoelectrophoretic techniques, a homogeneous polypeptide light chain was extracted from serum by immunoabsorbent chromatography.[59] These serum components are presumed to be the precursors of the tissue fibrillar proteins and could derive from several sources. Synthesis of a mutant immunoglobulin polypeptide light chain fragment, analogous to the heavy chain diseases, is one potential source of an amyloid precursor moiety.[64] Disordered assembly of heavy and light polypeptide chains and synthetic disequilibrium of these polypeptide chains are other potential sources of free serum light chains that could function as amyloid precursors.[65-67]

Clinical observations and experimental data indicate that some but not all immunoglobulin light chains are capable of being converted to amyloid fibrils. It is postulated that the primary structure of these light chains renders them susceptible to undergo conformational changes to a β-pleated sheet structure; that is, they are "amyloidogenic" light chains.[59] Conversion may be spontaneous upon entrance into the extracellular milieu, or it may be triggered by proteolytic degradation of a precursor molecule to an amyloidogenic fragment. The concept of amyloidogenic light chains is strengthened by (1) a disproportionately high ratio of λ to κ Bence Jones proteins in amyloidosis relative to normal subjects and uncomplicated multiple myeloma; (2) the differential electrophoretic mobility of Bence Jones proteins in amyloidotic and nonamyloidotic myeloma; (3) the restricted distribution of λ amyloid proteins in two variable region subclasses of λ light chains; (4) the selective in vitro transformation of some Bence Jones proteins to amyloidlike fibrils following pepsin degradation; and (5) the presence of unique amino acid substitutions in amyloid proteins and Bence Jones proteins from amyloidosis patients.

Amyloid Deposits of Protein Origin (AA Proteins). A class of amyloid fibrillar proteins distinct from immunoglobulin has been isolated from tissue deposits in cases of secondary amyloidosis and familial Mediterranean fever.[21,22] AA proteins from different tissue and patient sources range in molecular weight from 5000 to 9000 daltons, but they have remarkably similar amino acid compositions and sequences (see Table 92–2). The amino acid sequence of AA protein is unique among recognized animal proteins. Amyloid fibrils derived from the AA protein are morphologically indistinguishable from fibrils derived from the AL protein. An immunoglobulin light chain invariably constitutes a minor portion of fibrils derived from AA protein.[21,63,68] AA protein, however, is no longer felt to be a constituent of amyloid deposits of immunoglobulin origin.[69,70]

A serum component antigenically related to the AA protein (SAA) has been detected by immunodiffusion and radioimmunoassay procedures.[71-74] SAA has an α-β electrophoretic mobility and an apparent molecular weight of 160,000 to 180,000 daltons,[71,72] resulting from an association with serum high-density lipoprotein.[75] It can be broken down with guanidine, formic acid, or sodium dodecyl sulfate to a 12,000-dalton component (SAAL or apoSAA) that has an identical amino acid sequence to the smaller tissue AA protein.[72,74,76] Apo-SAA proteins isolated from human, rabbit, and mouse sera demonstrate hetereogeneity,[77-79] although the hypothesis that only certain types of SAA can form amyloid fibrils has not been proved.

There is now ample evidence that several acute-phase reactants, including SAA, are synthesized in the liver.[80,81] Although there are scattered reports of SAA synthesis in granulocytes, connective tissue fibroblasts, and spleen, it is unlikely that these sites can account for the acute-phase concentrations obtained after injury.[82] In the mouse, SAA is synthesized by hepatocytes after stimulation by a monocyte-derived factor sharing very similar or identical properties to interleukin I.[82,83] The principal function of SAA protein is not known; Benson and associates have shown it to be a nonspecific supressor of antibody responses in mouse spleen cell cultures and human peripheral blood lymphocytes.[84] In mice, rapid clearance from plasma of native apoSAA compared to with apolipoprotein A-1[85] suggest a special function, possibly related to clearance by the mononuclear phagocytic system.

SAA can be detected in low levels in normal individuals and in cord blood. Elevated levels of SAA are found in aged individuals as well as in a variety of acute and chronic infectious, inflammatory, and neoplastic disorders. Among them are secondary amyloidosis, primary amyloidosis, multiple myeloma, benign monoclonal gammopathy, leprosy, tuberculosis, acute viral illnesses, connective tissue diseases, leukemias, and familial Mediterranean fever.[73,74,84,87] In acute illnesses, SAA levels fluctuate analogous to acute-phase reactants.[88] SAA levels are not high in the familial amyloid neuropathy of Finland or in medullary carcinoma of the thyroid with amyloid deposits.[87,88] The kinetics of SAA production closely resemble another acute-phase reactant, CRP, after a standard inflammatory insult in normal volunteers.[89] At this time, the detection or quantitation of SAA has no recognized diagnostic or prognostic value.

Endocrine Amyloid Deposits (AE Proteins). The amyloid deposits found in neoplastic or degenerative disorders of endocrine glands appear to contain an amyloid fibrillar protein derived from locally synthesized polypeptides. Deposits from seven endocrine tumors studied by Pearse and associates do not contain tryptophan, a feature that distinguishes them from AL or AA proteins.[90] Immunofluorescent studies indicate that calcitonin-like material is present in amyloid deposits from medullary carcinoma of the thyroid.[91] A polypeptide chain with a molecular weight of 5700 daltons has been isolated as the major fibrillar protein from this tumor, and has an amino acid composition consistent with procalcitonin or a fragment of procalcitonin.[92] It appears that the medullary carcinoma cells synthesize an amyloidogenic calcitonin precursor that is converted to a β-pleated sheet fibril. Local histiocytic cells may be important in this transformation.[93] Insulin has been demonstrated in the amyloid deposits of human pancreatic islets, although chemical identification of the fibrillar proteins is lacking.[94] Amyloid-like fibrils can be synthesized in vitro from glucagon and insulin.[41,95] P-component has been detected in amyloid deposits of endocrine origin.[96]

Amyloid deposits are also present in bronchial carcinoids, carotid body tumors, parathyroid adenomas, pheochromocytomas, pituitary adenomas, and gastrinomas.[90,97,98] They are presumed to be locally synthesized. This class of amyloid proteins was previously called APUD amyloid, based on the common histochemical properties of the cells involved.

Senile Amyloid Deposits (AS Proteins). Trace deposits of amyloid can be demonstrated in the great vessels, pancreatic islets, cardiac tissue, and cerebral vessels of an aged population.[99] These deposits are microscopic, rarely produce clinical symptoms, and are usually diagnosed at necropsy examination. Their prevalence tends to increase with age, and some authors feel they are pathogenetically related to the aging process.[5,100]

Senile cardiac amyloid deposits are usually clinically insignificant, but extensive infiltration of myocardium and conduction tissues can occur in a minority of cases.[101] These deposits are resistant to degradation by oxidation and proteolysis, which suggests they are distinct from secondary amyloid deposits.[102] Fibril preparations in two instances contain a 6000-dalton subunit that has a similar amino acid composition in each case but is distinct from AL or AA proteins. This subunit (A_{SCA}) can be converted to congophilic fibrils in vitro.[103]

Amyloid has been found in the neuritic plaque, the neurofibrillary tangle, and the microangiopathy that occur in the brains of Alzheimer's presenile dementia and senile dementia of Alzheimer's type.[104] Electron microscopic studies have revealed that there are two different types of fibrillar structures in these brain lesions: (1) typical amyloid fibrils that are 100 Å wide and (2) paired helical filaments (PHF) that are 200 Å wide and twisted at about 800-Å intervals. The neurofibrillary tangles are composed of PHFs; the small blood vessel lesions of amyloid fibrils and the neuritic plaques usually contain both fibrillar types.[105-108] Immunocytochemical studies have shown reactivity of all three lesions with antibodies to polyclonal immunoglobulin,[109-112] vasoactive intestinal polypeptide,[113] and human prealbumin,[114] respectively. Although these findings are difficult to interpret at the present time, the association with prealbumin may be of the most significance in that this protein has been identified in other forms of amyloidosis associated with aging.

A protein obtained from amyloidosis in familial Portuguese neuropathy, a syndrome first described by Andrade,[114] is immunochemically identical to serum prealbumin but shows chemical heterogeneity.[115] This protein is called AF, and recent reports of prealbumin-related amyloid deposits in patients of Japanese, Swedish, and Jewish ancestry suggest a common pathogenesis for this entire class of hereditary amyloidosis.[116]

Pathogenesis of Amyloidosis. It has been suggested that proteolytic enzymes play a key role in the pathogenesis of primary (type AL) amyloidosis.[117] Epstein and colleagues[118] demonstrated the formation of amyloid fibrils in vitro by the action of human kidney lysosomal enzymes on Bence Jones proteins, and it has recently been shown that cultured bone marrow cells from a patient with multiple myeloma caused de novo synthesis of amyloid fibrils within a 14-day culture period.[119] There was morphologic evidence of Bence Jones protein synthesis by the myeloma cells (with prominent rough endoplasmic endothelium), subsequent processing of these proteins in macrophage lysosomes, and eventual secretion of the amyloid fibrils. Although the macrophages may have also ingested some amyloid material, the presence of well-oriented tufts of amyloid fibrils at the invagination sites beside packed lysosomes indicated a predominantly secretory process. Unlike amyloidosis of immunoglobulin origin, many steps in the genesis of secondary or type AA amyloidosis are unsettled. Human monocytes can degrade SAA protein, apparently by a surface-associated protease[120] with some properties of an elastase.[121] When normal persons and amyloid patients were compared, all amyloid patients showed an AA-sized intermediate that was noted during breakdown by mononuclear cells, but it appeared in only some of the controls. These results have suggested that variation in the handling of SAA protein may underlie the variable incidence of amyloidosis in different disease populations. Polymorphonuclear leukocytes (PMN) can also degrade SAA in vitro through a pathway that is blocked by an elastase inhibitor.[122] In these studies, PMN and monocytes were equivalent in their ability to process SAA, demonstrating that various cell lines may be responsible for amyloid formation, as suggested by extensive morphologic evidence. Furthermore, it was shown that lysosomal enzymes capable of SAA degradation were released from PMNs by zymosan. These results are intriguing in the light of previous electron microscopic studies suggesting lysosomal production of amyloid.[123,124] It is likely, therefore, that amyloid fibril deposition may occur at several intracellular or extracellular locations, depending on local factors in various organs or sites of inflammation.

Investigations on the chemistry and pathogenesis of human amyloidosis are paralleled by a vast body of work in experimental animals that was begun in the early years of this century. The induction of systemic amyloidosis in the mouse, rabbit, and guinea pig by serial injections of casein has been the most extensively used mode.[125] It has been verified that this model is an exact chemical analogy for human amyloidosis of the AA type,[126] and it has permitted investigations of immune function and the mononuclear phagocytic system that would not be possible in human subjects. Using a radioimmunoassay to follow SAA levels during the induction of amyloidosis, no differences were found between the amyloid-susceptible CBA and the amyloid resistant A mouse strains.[127] It was also noted that SAA levels were the same in casein-treated mice as in those treated with a nonamyloidogenic regimen of bovine serum albumin. Although heterogeneity of SAA proteins could explain these results,[128] it was concluded that other factors beyond SAA production are necessary for amyloidogenesis. Indeed, the results tend to support the tacit assumption held by some that treatment with an amyloid-inducing substance initiates a pathologic cellular response terminating in secondary amyloidosis.

Extensive morphologic evidence at the electron microscopic level incriminating reticuloendothelial cells in the synthesis of amyloid made the mononuclear phagocytic system (MPS) a prime candidate for functional studies. In 1927, Smetena used India ink to effect blockade of the MPS in experimental animals and concluded from the observed decrease in the rate of amyloid formation that reticuloendothelial cells were involved in amyloidogenesis.[129] He further noted that though amyloid appeared in proximity to these cells, those tissue areas with the most abundant amyloid showed no uptake of India ink. He suggested that amyloid appeared as reticuloendothelial cells were altered or destroyed. Many years later, it was shown in both mice and rabbits that amyloid induction is associated with an initial increase in the ability of the MPS to clear particulate matter from the bloodstream, followed by a decline at the time of amyloid deposition.[130,131]

The concept that emerges from these and other studies is that amyloidosis is a biphasic process, both morphologically and functionally.[132,133] Since the amyloid fibril appears to be the product of aberrant processing of normal proteins, amyloid disease can be thought of as a metabolic defect, hereditary or acquired.[134] The best evidence put forward to date points to the macrophage as the site of this defect (Fig. 92–3). In some cases, as in tumors or focal deposits, the local degradative system may simply be overloaded.[135] When the problem is systemic, particularly in secondary amyloidosis, a wide range of factors comes into play. Judging from experi-

Figure 92–3. Theoretical pathways in the genesis of amyloidosis.

mental animal data, they include macrophage activation via endotoxins[136] and other potent inflammatory stimuli,[137] immunosuppressive agents,[138] hereditary defects,[139] and aging.[140,141] Although the laying down of amyloid deposits is usually a long, drawnout process, the time course may be accelerated by "transfer factors"[142,143] or by lowering the normal concentration of serum protease inhibitors.[144] In secondary amyloidosis, the accessory role of PMNs and their lysosomal enzymes needs to be determined whereas in Alzheimer's disease and familial polyneuropathy, the affinity of serum prealbumin for certain elements of nerve tissue needs further study.[145]

CLINICAL AMYLOIDOSIS SYNDROMES

Classification of Amyloidoses. Clinical amyloidosis syndromes occur as acquired or hereditary illnesses. The acquired amyloidoses have traditionally been designated primary, secondary, or myeloma-associated, dependent upon organ distribution of amyloid deposits and the presence or absence of associated illnesses.[145] The following list provides a classification of these syndromes.

I. Nonhereditary
   A. Systemic
      1. Primary amyloidosis
      2. Secondary amyloidosis
      3. Amyloidosis in overt plasma cell dyscrasias (multiple myeloma, macroglobulinemia, heavy chain disease, or plasmacytoma)
      4. Amyloidosis in agammaglobulinemia
   B. Localized
      1. Endocrine amyloid deposits (thyroid, pancreas, and so forth)
      2. Senile amyloid deposits (cardiac, capsular, or cerebral)
      3. Isolated nodular amyloid deposits (cutaneous, pulmonary, or genitourinary)
II. Hereditary
   A. Systemic
      1. Neuropathic amyloidosis

a. Type I amyloid neuropathy (Portuguese type)
b. Type II amyloid neuropathy (Indiana-Maryland type)
c. Type III amyloid neuropathy (Iowa type)
d. Type IV amyloid neuropathy (Finland type)
2. Nephropathic amyloidosis
   a. Familial Mediterranean fever amyloidosis
   b. Amyloid nephropathy of Ostertag
   c. Amyloid nephropathy of Muckle-Wells
3. Cardiomyopathic amyloidosis
   a. Amyloid cardiomyopathy (Denmark)
   b. Amyloid cardiomyopathy with persistent atrial standstill
B. Localized
   1. Cerebral amyloid deposits (cerebral hemorrhage of Iceland)
   2. Cutaneous amyloid deposits (lichen or nodular)
   3. Ocular amyloid deposits (corneal or conjunctival)

Table 92-3. Classification of Amyloidosis

Current Clinical Classification	Terminology for Amyloid Fibril Proteins	Probable Precursor Protein
Primary and myeloma-associated	AL κ or AL λ	Ig L chains
Secondary and familial Mediterranean fever–associated	AA	SAA
Familial type I neuropathy and	AFp or AFs	Prealbumin
familial cerebral hemorrhage of Iceland	AFi	Serum γ-trace protein
Endocrine tumor	AEt	Thyrocalcitonin
Senile cardiac and senile brain	ASc or ASb	Prealbumin
Dermal	AD	Not known

Although new classifications based on biochemical knowledge are being developed, the older schemes retain their clinical usefulness, and, in fact, their outlines are still visible in the new formulations.

Primary amyloidosis best refers to those amyloidosis syndromes that occur in the absence of an associated infectious, inflammatory, or non-B-lymphocyte neoplastic disorder. This designation implies the presence of an associated plasma cell dyscrasia and amyloid deposits of immunoglobulin origin. Multiple myeloma-associated amyloidosis is closely related to primary amyloidosis, except for the severity of the underlying plasma cell dyscrasia.

Secondary amyloidosis applies to those syndromes occurring as a consequence of longstanding or poorly controlled inflammatory or neoplastic diseases. It implies amyloid deposits of unknown origin, with AA protein as the major fibrillar protein, provided a monoclonal paraprotein cannot be found in serum or urine. In the presence of coexistent paraproteinemia and chronic debilitating disease, the amyloid deposits could obviously contain either AL or AA proteins. Only biochemical characterization of the fibrillar proteins would resolve that question. SAA may be elevated in secondary amyloidosis, but the ubiquitous nature of SAA in health and disease states renders this finding nondiscriminatory. A correlation of clinical amyloidosis syndromes with fibrillar protein composition is presented in Table 92–3.

Hereditary amyloidosis syndromes are distinguished by their clinical presentations and the distribution of organ system infiltration. They are usually divided into neuropathic and non-neuropathic forms. The non-neuropathic forms can be further subdivided into cardiopathic and nephropathic types. Biochemical classification of the hereditary syndromes is in progress. As already noted, amyloid deposits in type I neuropathy

have a prealbumin origin, whereas the major protein extracted from the brains of Icelandic patients with hereditary cerebral hemorrhage has been identified as serum gamma trace.[146]

Finally, it should be noted that the β-pleated sheet fibrils are emerging as the common feature that links together these diseases of remarkable chemical and clinical heterogeneity. Any future revisions of amyloidosis classification should consider the central role of the β-pleated sheet fibrils.[3]

Primary Amyloidosis. Primary amyloidosis is a disease of middle and advanced age, with a mean age at diagnosis of 55 years and 62 years in two recent series.[147,148] It has been recognized as early as the second decade of life.[147] Men are affected significantly more often than women, and Caucasians are affected more than non-Caucasians. Virtually all patients with primary amyloidosis demonstrate a monoclonal immunoglobulin protein in their serum or urine, or both, and a bone marrow plasmacytosis. The clinical manifestations of primary amyloidosis are protean, but certain symptom complexes suggest its presence: (1) idiopathic, sensorimotor, peripheral neuropathy with autonomic neuropathy;[149,150] (2) restrictive cardiomyopathy with a low-voltage electrocardiogram and conduction disturbances in the absence of other recognized causes;[151] (3) nonthrombocytopenic purpura with cutaneous induration, "pinch purpura," or "postproctoscopic purpura";[152] (4) rheumatoidlike arthritis with little inflammation and prominent large joint involvement (shoulder-pad sign);[153] (5) macroglossia;[154] (6) hemorrhagic diathesis secondary to isolated acquired factor X deficiency;[155,156] (7) idiopathic nephrotic syndrome;[157] and (8) idiopathic carpal tunnel syndrome in a man.[158,159] Demonstration of paraproteinemia or Bence Jones proteinuria in conjunction with these clinical syndromes strongly suggests primary amyloidosis.

Secondary Amyloidosis. Although the precise incidence of secondary amyloidosis is difficult to estimate, many authors now feel that rheumatoid arthritis is the most frequent predisposing factor.[160] From postmortem series, the approximate frequency of amyloidosis complicating rheumatoid arthritis is 26 percent and 14 percent.[161,162] In a careful study comparing the necropsy prevalence of amyloidosis in rheumatoid and nonrheumatoid subjects, deposits typical of secondary amyloidosis were found in only one case of rheumatoid arthritis; senile amyloid deposits in cerebral, aortic, cardiac, and pancreatic tissues were present in 13 of 47 arthritis patients and in 19 of 47 control subjects.[99]

Rectal biopsies in 115 consecutive rheumatoid patients with longstanding disease showed an ante-mortem amyloidosis prevalence of 5.2 percent (six cases).[163] A similar study using gingival biopsy revealed amyloid deposits in 9 of 192 unselected rheumatoid patients, for a prevalence of 5 percent.[164] Renal biopsy (4 amyloidosis in 32 rheumatoid patients) and subcutaneous fat aspiration have also been employed to estimate the prevalence of amyloidosis in rheumatoid arthritis.[165-167] Secondary amyloidosis usually appears after several years of rheumatoid arthritis and is uncommon within the first 2 years of its diagnosis. Insidious proteinuria, nephrosis, and hepatosplenomegaly are the most frequent clinical presentations of amyloidosis in rheumatoid arthritis.

Secondary amyloidosis is recognized as an important cause of morbidity and mortality in juvenile rheumatoid arthritis. It occurred in 16 of 389 (4.1 percent) juvenile rheumatoid patients in one series and caused almost 33 percent of the deaths during a 10-year period.[168] Onset of secondary amyloidosis is at a mean of 8.2 years following the onset of juvenile rheumatoid arthritis. Of 1272 cases with juvenile chronic polyarthritis, a diagnostic category that encompasses juvenile rheumatoid arthritis, psoriatic arthritis, and ankylosing spondylitis, 51 (4 percent) have secondary amyloidosis.[169] Of 243 such patients who have had arthritis for at least 15 years, 18 (7.4 percent) have developed amyloidosis. One half of the patients with secondary amyloidosis die within 10 years of the diagnosis.[169]

Secondary amyloidosis has also been reported in ankylosing spondylitis, Reiter's syndrome, psoriatic arthritis, chronic rheumatic heart disease, dermatomyositis, scleroderma, Behçet's syndrome, and, rarely, systemic lupus erythematosus.[170-174]

Systemic infections remain a significant worldwide cause of secondary amyloidosis.[175] One hundred fifty of 200 patients with renal amyloidosis reported from India have underlying tuberculosis.[176] Twenty of 37 patients from a Scottish series and 7 of 22 patients from an American series had tuberculosis, although it was inactive in most instances.[147,175] Estimates for amyloidosis complicating leprosy range as high as 31 percent.[177] Amyloid deposits have been detected in rectal biopsy specimens from 16 of 190 leprosy patients in Papua, New Guinea. Secondary amyloidosis characteristically occurs either in lepromatous subjects with recurrent attacks of erythema nodosum leprosum or in nonlepromatous subjects with chronic trophic ulcers.[177] SAA levels rise in parallel with the acute nodular lesions in

patients with lepromatous leprosy, and are also elevated in nonlepromatous patients with chronic trophic ulcers.[178] Amyloidosis frequently complicates paraplegia, probably as a result of chronically infected decubitus ulcers and chronic pyelonephritis.[179] Bronchiectasis, osteomyelitis, inflammatory bowel diseases, and chronically infected burns are other commonly cited predispositions to amyloidosis. Parenteral drug abuse has emerged as a new causative factor in secondary amyloidosis.

Hypernephroma and Hodgkin's disease are the neoplasms most frequently associated with secondary amyloidosis.[180-182] Secondary amyloidosis has also been recognized in carcinomas of the gastrointestinal tract, lung, and genitourinary tract, and in non-Hodgkin's lymphomas and malignant melanomas.[182-184] Elevated serum levels of SAA are present in most of the patients with these neoplasms, but the chemical nature of amyloid deposits has been ascertained only for Hodgkin's disease (AA protein).[22] The tumor-localized amyloid deposits associated with endocrine neoplasms are probably distinct from the secondary amyloidosis seen with other carcinomas. Localized amyloid deposits have also been seen in odontogenic tumors.[185]

Multiple Myeloma–Associated Amyloidosis. Multiple myeloma–associated amyloidosis closely resembles primary generalized amyloidosis in its age distribution, sex predilection, and clinical presentations. Six to 15 percent of myeloma patients develop amyloidosis.[161,183] The majority of patients with myeloma-associated amyloidosis demonstrate an intact immunoglobulin paraprotein in serum, but also have Bence Jones proteinemia or proteinuria, or both.[186-188] Excessive free light chain synthesis may be intimately related to the dissemination and formation of amyloid deposits. The ratio of κ to λ light chains in myeloma-associated amyloidosis may differ from the ratio in primary amyloidosis, in which lambda Bence Jones proteins predominate. In two recent reports on myeloma-associated amyloidosis, the κ to λ ratio was 9:3 and 3:4.[65,148] The detection of amyloidosis in 7 of 35 patients with light chain myeloma supports the concept that light chain paraproteinemia per se is not sufficient to cause amyloidosis,[65] qualitative differences in light chains are important in amyloidosis of myeloma.

Mean survival is reduced in myeloma complicated by amyloidosis compared with nonamyloidotic cases.[189] Treatment directed at myeloma has variable effects on the progression of amyloidosis.

Familial Neuropathic Amyloidosis Syndromes. The first well-substantiated example of a hereditary neuropathic amyloidosis syndrome came from Portugal.[114] A similar neuropathic disease has since been found in Portuguese subjects in Brazil, France, and Africa, and in non-Portuguese subjects from the United States, Germany, Japan, Sweden, and Great Britain.[190-193] This disease, designated type I neuropathy or Portuguese neuropathy, is inherited in an autosomal dominant manner with equal sex predilection and a high penetrance.[194] Symptoms characteristically begin in the third or fourth decade of life with a distal sensory neuropathy in a "stocking" distribution.[114] Upper extremity and truncal sensory deficits appear later. Motor deficits occur in advanced disease. Signs and symptoms of autonomic neuropathy (i.e., impotence, postural hypotension, gastrointestinal motility disturbances, and hypohidrosis) are prominent.[114,195] Visual findings include irregular pupillary margins, sluggish light reflexes, and vitreous opacities.[195] Renal failure, carpal tunnel syndrome, macroglossia, and heart failure are not manifestations of the type I neuropathy. A recently reported American kindred of Swedish origin with peripheral neuropathy and systemic amyloidosis bears a phenotypic resemblance to type I neuropathy cases, but is associated with significant renal disease.[196]

Type II amyloid neuropathy is characterized by the carpal tunnel syndrome and a diffuse neuropathy that is especially prominent in the upper extremities. The disease is inherited in an autosomal dominant fashion. Large kindreds have been described in Indiana (Swiss origin) and Maryland (German origin).[197-199] Symptoms of carpal tunnel syndrome usually appear in the fourth or fifth decade of life, and progression of disease is slow. After several years or decades of carpal tunnel symptoms, evidence of diffuse neuropathy develops, and eventually, the legs are involved. Vitreous opacities,[200] electrocardiographic abnormalities, congestive heart failure, and hepatic, gastrointestinal, and diffuse vascular infiltration may occur, but macroglossia and uremia are rare. Plasma lipoprotein abnormalities seen in this syndrome are of uncertain significance.[197] The composition of the fibrils is unknown.

Type III neuropathy, initially described in an Iowa family of Scottish, English, and Irish descent, is characterized by upper and lower extremity neuropathy, duodenal ulcer, and nephropathy.[201,202] Inherited as an autosomal dominant disease, it becomes manifest in the third or fourth decade of life with lower extremity neuropathy. Concomitant upper extremity neuropathy is usually present. Autonomic symptoms may be prominent, and cerebrospinal fluid protein is usually elevated. Duodenal ulcer is apparently common, but the ulcer crater does not contain amyloid on biopsy.[201] Renal involvement progresses at variable rates to uremia and death from renal insufficiency. No vitreous opacities have been described. The chemical nature of the deposits is unknown.

Type IV neuropathy is manifested by corneal lattice dystrophy, cranial nerve palsies, cutis laxa, and an autosomal dominant inheritance pattern.[203-205] Lattice dystrophy usually appears in the third decade of life, but no vitreous opacities are detected.[204] Visual acuity tends to be preserved to old age, but corneal ulcerations can be troublesome in patients more than 40 years old. Upper facial paresis is a regular feature in older patients.[203,205] Dermal changes begin in the fifth decade of life, with upper facial and scalp thickening. Past the seventh decade of life, the skin over the rest of the body may become atrophic and pendulous. Amyloid deposits are prominent around lattice lines and diseased peripheral nerves and in dermal appendages.[203] Localized forms of lattice corneal dystrophy are recognized and may be distinguishable from systemic varieties by histologic and clinical criteria.

Familial Nephropathic Amyloidosis Syndromes. Familial Mediterranean fever is an autosomal recessive disease affecting primarily Sephardic Jews, Armenians, and Arabs. Familial Mediterranean fever is characterized by acute, self-limited febrile episodes that are accompanied by peritonitis, pleuritis, arthritis, or erysipelaslike erythema.[206-208] Generalized amyloidosis with prominent renal involvement occurs in many patients younger than the age of 40 years.[209] Microscopic deposits of amyloid are present in vessels throughout the body, but are most significant in the renal glomeruli.[210] Death results from renal failure, and spontaneous remissions are unknown.[209] Colchicine has proved effective prophylaxis for the acute febrile paroxysms and is reported to favorably influence the course of renal amyloidosis.[211-214] Protein AA has been demonstrated in familial Mediterranean fever amyloid deposits.[21] SAA levels fluctuate with the acute episodes of familial Mediterranean fever.[73]

Amyloid nephropathy of Muckle-Wells is a rare syndrome characterized by nerve deafness, urticaria, limb pain, and extensive amyloid deposits in the kidneys, adrenal cortices, and spleen. Fewer than 30 cases have been reported in the literature.[215-217] Amyloid nephropathy of Ostertag is characterized by chronic nephropathy, hypertension, and hepatosplenomegaly, with amyloid deposits in kidneys, adrenal glands, and liver.[218] It is also rare.

Familial Cardiopathic Amyloidosis Syndromes. An amyloidotic cardiomyopathy has been reported in five members of a Danish sibship.[219] Symptoms of congestive heart failure develop in the fourth decade of life with progression to death over 2 years to 6 years. Hemodynamic studies are consistent with a restrictive cardiomyopathy. Three cases of persistent atrial standstill have been reported in another sibship.[220] The patients present with bradycardia, absent P waves, cardiac enlargement, and modest congestive heart failure. Amyloid has been found in the right atrial appendage in one case.

AMYLOID INFILTRATION OF ORGAN SYSTEMS

Pathophysiologic Considerations. Amyloid infiltration of tissues results in pressure atrophy of parenchymal cells and organ dysfunction or failure. The effects of significant accumulation in any given organ system are similar whether the underlying amyloidosis syndrome is primary, secondary, myeloma-associated, or familial in nature. For example, significant myocardial amyloid infiltration presents as a restrictive cardiomyopathy in any type of amyloidosis syndrome. In some instances symptoms also develop as the result of amyloid deposits in nutrient arteries or nerves. For example, the malabsorption seen in amyloidosis is largely the result of an autonomic neuropathy and motility disturbances rather than direct gastrointestinal infiltration. Likewise, arterial obstruction by amyloid deposits in the superior mesenteric system can cause ischemic necrosis of bowel.

Cutaneous Amyloid Deposits. The skin is involved in up to 40 percent of cases of systemic amyloidosis, and is more likely to be affected in primary or myeloma-associated amyloidosis than in secondary amyloidosis.[221-222] Cutaneous amyloid deposition has an unexplained predilection for the face and upper trunk. Waxy, indurated papules, purpura, or tumefactions are the most frequent dermatologic signs. Excessive accumulations in the dermis occasionally produce marked skin thickening with an orange peel effect that mimics scleroderma or myxedema (Fig. 92–4). Cutaneous purpura can often be induced by gently stroking the involved skin 20 or 30 times with the examining finger or by gentle pinching.[152] Induced purpura will be resorbed within a few days. Valsalva maneuver or proctoscopic examination will occasionally produce periorbital purpura.[189] Alopecia can be prominent. Histologically, amyloid deposits are found in dermal and subcutaneous vessel walls or throughout the dermis with a predilection for the dermal appendages (Fig. 92–5).

Figure 92–5. Cutaneous amyloidosis. Nodular deposit of amyloid material in upper dermis from patient shown in Figure 92–4. Crystal violet stain. (Courtesy of C. R. Arkin and J. Holbert, Memphis, Tennessee.)

Figure 92–4. Cutaneous amyloidosis. Scleroderma-like infiltration of skin in a patient with primary generalized amyloidosis. Punch biopsy site is apparent. Patient had extensive amyloid deposition in chin area. (Courtesy of C. R. Arkin and J. Holbert, Memphis, Tennessee.)

Two main types of localized cutaneous amyloidosis exist, namely, (1) lichen, including macular amyloidosis, and (2) nodular amyloidosis. Lichen amyloidosis is a syndrome of middle-aged patients, in which coalescent papules form a lichenoid eruption that is especially prominent over the extensor surfaces of the legs and thighs. Amyloid deposits are restricted to the pericapillary areas of the papillary dermis, and are not seen in vessel walls or in other organs.[223] Papular mucinosis (scleromyxedema) is an infiltrative skin disorder of sun-exposed areas that clinically resembles cutaneous amyloidosis and is associated with a monoclonal gammopathy; however, excess mucopolysaccharides, and not amyloid, are deposited in the dermis.

Amyloid Arthropathy. One of the least common but most striking clinical manifestations of primary and myeloma-associated amyloidosis is a chronic symmetric arthropathy, mainly involving the shoulders, wrists, knees, and fingers.[134,224,225] It is often accompanied by severe constitutional symptoms of morning stiffness and fatigue, and these features—plus the physical findings of joint tenderness, limitation of motion, and soft tissue swelling—may lead to an erroneous diagnosis of rheumatoid arthritis. Soft tissue contractures of the interphalangeal joints may appear rather early in the illness. Joint swelling tends to be less inflammatory than in rheumatoid disease, and a grittiness or unusual firmness can often be appreciated on joint examination.[224,225] Subcutaneous nodules are present in more than half the cases and may be mistaken for rheumatoid nodules. Infiltration of the glenohumeral articulation and the surrounding muscles produces the characteristic "shoulder-pad sign" (Fig. 92–6).[153] Microscopic amyloid deposits may be localized in articular cartilage, and macroscopic lesions in bone simulate neoplasms and may lead to pathologic fractures.

Many of the patients with amyloid arthropathy develop a carpal tunnel syndrome. Since this syndrome may also be the initial manifestation of type II familial neuropathy, amyloidosis should be suspected in cases of idiopathic carpal tunnel syndrome occurring in middle-aged and elderly men. An association between calcium pyrophosphate dihydrate deposition disease (CCPD or chondrocalcinosis) and amyloidosis has recently been found in elderly patients. Focal amyloid deposits have

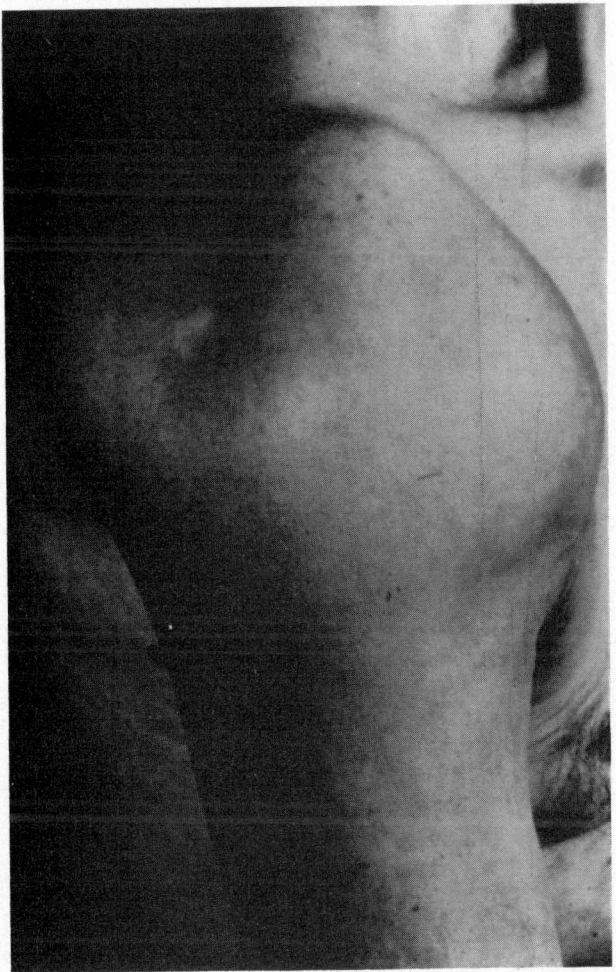

Figure 92–6. Amyloid arthropathy. Shoulder-pad sign. (Courtesy of G. C. White, Chapel Hill, North Carolina, and G. G. Glenner, Bethesda, Maryland.)

also been described in the fibrous capsules of hips and knee joints requiring surgery for advanced degenerative joint disease.[226] In primary amyloid arthropathy synovial fluid analysis usually reveals a noninflammatory fluid with predominantly mononuclear cells. The fluid may be xanthochromic, and mucin clot tests give variable results. Inspection of centrifuged, Congo red–stained sediments from synovial fluid under polarization microscopy reveal amyloid deposits in fragments of synovial villi.[227] X-rays show osteoporosis, lytic lesions, or soft tissue swelling.

Amyloid Neuropathy. Peripheral neuropathy occurs in certain hereditary and acquired forms of the illness. Patterns of neural involvement in the various familial syndromes can be distinctive.[145] The acquired neuropathic cases usually present as "idiopathic," painful, predominantly sensory polyneuropathies with associated autonomic dysfunction.[228,229] Pain and temperature sensation are affected more than other sensory modalities.[149] Motor dysfunction affecting the lower extremities develops later in the course of the illness. Carpal tunnel syndrome and significant weight loss are frequently concomitant complaints.[149]

Amyloid deposits are located in dural blood vessels, autonomic ganglia, spinal nerve roots, and peripheral nerves, sparing the brain and spinal cord parenchyma. Ultrastructurally, a severe loss of unmyelinated fibers of peripheral nerves is seen.[230] Amyloid deposits in peripheral nerves rarely seem large enough to cause pressure atrophy of tissue, which supports an ischemic or toxic-metabolic origin of the neuropathy.[149] Amyloid deposits can often be found in vessel walls and connective tissue in frozen sections of muscle biopsies from amyloid polyneuropathy patients. Sural nerve biopsy is also diagnostic in most cases.[149]

An associated overt or occult plasma cell dyscrasia has been demonstrated in virtually all well-studied cases of nonhereditary amyloid polyneuropathy, which is compatible with an immunoglobulin origin of these deposits.[149,150] Paraproteins in this syndrome have predominantly κ-type light chains.[149,224] Treatment with melphalan and prednisone has had no demonstrable benefit in neuropathy cases.[149] Carbamazepine has produced significant relief of painful paresthesias in a single case.[231]

Amyloid Nephropathy. Renal involvement occurs in almost every type of systemic amyloidosis. Proteinuria is the most common presentation and progresses at a variable rate to nephrotic syndrome and uremia.[147] Hematuria is unusual in renal disease itself, but can result from amyloid infiltration in the lower urinary tract. Although hypertension was once felt to be uncommon in renal amyloidosis, it has recently been found in 50 percent of such patients.[232] Renal vein thrombosis is a recognized complication of renal amyloidosis.

Amyloid deposits are most pronounced in the renal glomeruli (Fig. 92–6) and arteriolar walls, but can also be detected along the tubular basement membrane.[233] Peritubular deposits are apparently responsible for one case of nephrogenic diabetes insipidus in amyloidosis.[234] Glomerular deposits tend to localize to the mesangial and subendothelial regions, but can be seen in subepithelial locations as well.[233] Renal involvement is suspected in cases of idiopathic proteinuria or nephrotic syndrome, especially in the presence of a chronic inflammatory disease. It is diagnosed by renal biopsy and appropriate histochemical studies. Amyloid-like fibrils can be demonstrated in the urine sediment from some renal amyloidosis patients, but similar fibrils are also found in nonamyloidotic nephrotic patients.[235-237] Radiographic findings in renal amyloidosis are also nonspecific. Enlarged kidneys may be seen, but normal-sized or contracted kidneys are more prevalent. Renal size can decrease with progression of disease.[238] Renal angiography is frequently abnormal with irregular narrowing and tortuosity of interlobar arteries, an indistinct corticomedullary junction, and nonvisualization of cortical arteries.[238,239]

Renal disease is the most common cause of death in several large series of amyloidosis. A variety of therapeutic modalities have been applied to halt the progression of renal insufficiency, and considerable experience with chronic hemodialysis and renal transplantation is now available (see later discussion).

Amyloid Cardiomyopathy. Cardiac infiltration occurs in primary, secondary, and hereditary forms of amyloidosis. The diagnosis of amyloidosis should be suspected in very old patients with idiopathic restrictive cardiomyopathy,[240] especially if other cardiac diseases such as atherosclerosis are minimal or absent.[100] Signs and symptoms of failure of the right side of the heart may dominate the early clinical picture, with a resemblance to constrictive pericarditis.[151] Chest x-ray may show only minimal cardiomegaly; hemodynamic studies demonstrate a "dip and plateau" pattern. Electrocardiograms reveal low voltage in the limb leads, conduction disturbances, arrhythmias, poor R-wave progression in the precordial leads, and patterns that simulate acute myocardial infarctions.[151] Echocardiography shows symmetrically increased left ventricular wall thickness, hypokinesia, and decreased systolic thickening of the interventricular septum and left ventricular wall, and a small or normal-sized left ventricular cavity.[241] The findings on M-mode echocardiographic analysis, as well as a virtually diagnostic "granular sparkling" appearance on two-dimensional echocardiogram have been described. Another study found that an analysis combining echocardiographic information with data obtained on a standard electrocardiogram identified characteristic findings of amyloid heart disease.[242]

Amyloid deposits can be seen in all layers of the cardiac wall.[151] They are most pronounced in the myocardium at which point they encroach on muscle fibers. Although conduction and rhythm disturbances are frequent in cardiac amyloidosis, direct amyloid infiltration does not account for the majority of these disturbances.[243] Valvular deposits are quite common in aged individuals, but they rarely produce hemodynamically significant changes. Transvenous endocardial biopsy has been employed safely in several patients to establish an antemortem diagnosis.[244]

Treatment of cardiac amyloidosis is symptomatic. Digitalis is ineffective in most restrictive myocardiopathies, and it may be associated with a high incidence of sudden death in amyloidosis patients.[245] Diuretics should be used judiciously to avoid dehydration.

Respiratory Tract Amyloid Deposits. Amyloid deposits can occur at any level of the respiratory tract, from the nasopharynx to the alveolar-capillary bed. Respiratory amyloidosis is most prevalent as an isolated organ system involvement or as a component of systemic disease. Amyloid deposits in the upper nasal passages present as mass lesions with hemorrhage or perforation. Isolated, submucosal accumulations in the vocal cord structures appear as single or multiple nodules and can cause hoarseness. These presentations usually indicate isolated disease restricted to the upper airways, without concomitant systemic amyloidosis.[246]

Five types of lower respiratory tract involvement are recognized:[247-251] (1) Isolated nodular deposits of the tracheobronchial tree. They may be asymptomatic or may cause hemorrhage and signs of airway obstruction. (2) Diffuse tracheobronchial infiltration. Extensive submucosal deposits may cause wheezing and dyspnea as early manifestations. Chest x-ray is usually normal. This form may be seen as a localized disease or as a component of systemic amyloidosis. Repeated bronchoscopy to remove symptomatic deposits may be necessary. (3) Hilar adenopathy. (4) Isolated nodular pulmonary amyloidosis, either solitary or multiple. Nodules are present in parenchymal tissue and often contain giant cells; these nodules cannot be differentiated radiographically from neoplastic processes. This form of disease is usually asymptomatic, and prognosis is good with surgical removal of symptomatic nodules. (5) Diffuse pulmonary parenchymal amyloidosis. This form is usually seen with primary amyloidosis and may lead to life-threatening alveolar-capillary block within months of detection.

Gastrointestinal Amyloidosis. Any level of the gastrointestinal tract may be affected by amyloid deposition. In the nonhereditary syndromes, gastrointestinal involvement can be found in approximately 50 percent of cases.[144,184] Gingival and tongue infiltrations are the hallmarks of oral cavity amyloidosis. The tongue is firm to palpation and may be massively enlarged from amyloid deposits.[154] Macroglossia may interfere with speech, deglutition, and respiration.

The hypopharyngeal muscles and voluntary muscles of the upper one third of the esophagus are prone to amyloid infiltration. Deposits may impair deglutition and cause pooling of x-ray contrast material in the piriform recess during upper gastrointestinal studies.

Amyloid deposits may also present as tumefaction in the esophagus or as diffuse infiltrates that produce a rigid, aperistaltic segment.[252] Gastric accumulations can result in motility disturbances, hemorrhage, obstruction, achlorhydria, and vitamin B_{12} deficiency, and can mimic gastric carcinoma.[147,253,254] Radiographic findings are nonspecific in gastric amyloidosis, but gastroscopic examination may be highly suggestive of amyloid infiltration.[255,256] A positive biopsy result for amyloid deposits is definitive. Small bowel amyloidosis may present as motility disturbances with diarrhea or constipation, malabsorption (which may be related to motility disorders), hemorrhage, protein-losing enteropathy, perforation, or ischemic necrosis.[257-258] X-ray changes are, again, nonspecific, but biopsy can be diagnostic. Amyloid deposits are most pronounced in the submucosal layer and in the vasculature.[259] Cases of isolated intestinal amyloidosis have been reported.[68,259]

Hepatic infiltration, which is present in almost 75 percent of generalized, nonhereditary amyloidosis, can produce massive organomegaly, but rarely causes portal hypertension or hepatic insufficiency.[147,260] Liver function tests are usually normal, although sulfobromophthalein sodium retention may be increased, and alkaline phosphatase levels may be mildly elevated. In the rare case of primary amyloidosis, intrahepatic cholestasis with severe jaundice is a poor prognostic sign.[261] Preliminary scintigraphic studies suggest that hepatic uptake of technetium or gallium isotopes may be abnormal in amyloidotic livers and inversely related to the quantity of amyloid deposits.[262,263] Splenic infiltration can occasionally result in castastrophic splenic rupture.

DIAGNOSIS OF AMYLOIDOSIS

Biopsy Sites. The diagnosis of amyloidosis is established by demonstration of the characteristic apple-green birefringence of Congo red–stained tissue specimens under polarization microscopy (Fig. 92–7). Virtually any organ can be biopsied to establish this diagnosis. As a general rule, a biopsy should be taken from an organ suspected of being infiltrated with amyloid material. If this cannot be done for any reason, rectal biopsy is the preferred technique. Rectal biopsy results are positive for amyloid deposits in 75 percent to 85 percent of cases of generalized amyloidosis if adequate submucosal tissue is obtained for microscopic examination.[189,264] Percutaneous renal biopsy is also a relatively safe, high-yield diagnostic procedure in amyloidosis.[145] Liver biopsy has produced fatal complications, but is generally safe in patients without massive hepatomegaly.[265] Bone marrow biopsy, small bowel biopsy, splenic aspiration, "punch" skin biopsy, subcutaneous fat aspiration, and endomyocardial biopsy, have all been used to diagnose amyloidosis.[266-268] Arthrocentesis and examination of Congo red–stained sediment under polarizing conditions can show amyloid in synovial villous fragments.[227] Amyloidlike fibrils in urinary sediments examined electron microscopically are not specific for amyloidosis.[235,236] Echography, angiography, and scintigraphy are helpful diagnostic adjuncts.

Immunologic Studies. All patients with systemic amyloidosis should be evaluated for evidence of an associated plasma cell dyscrasia. Evaluation includes serum and urine electrophoresis and immunoelectrophoresis. Urine samples are tested unconcentrated and after 50- and 100-fold concentration. Quantitative serum immunoglobulin assays are also indicated. Bone marrow aspiration and

Figure 92–7. Glomerular amyloid deposits. Birefringent material within glomerulus showed characteristic apple-green color of amyloid deposits. On black and white photomicrograph this cannot be distinguished from birefringent collagen fibers in glomerular capsule.

biopsy are performed to exclude multiple myeloma. Bone marrow samples are also cultured for mycobacterial and fungal agents. Skeletal radiographic survey is carried out to search for osteolytic lesions.

Homogeneous immunoglobulins, especially Bence Jones proteins, can be detected in the serum or urine, or both, of most patients with primary amyloidosis.[187,188] Serum concentrations of the paraproteins in primary amyloidosis are generally lower than in multiple myeloma. Nonparaprotein immunoglobulin levels in both primary amyloidosis and multiple myeloma are depressed; they tend to be higher in secondary amyloidosis. Quantitative B (bursa equivalent) and T (thymus-dependent) peripheral blood lymphocyte counts are normal in all patients with primary and secondary amyloidosis tested to date.[269] Lymphocyte proliferative responses to phytohemagglutinin and pokeweed mitogen is normal in primary and secondary amyloidosis, but responses to concanavalin A are significantly reduced.[269] More profound aberrations of cellular immunity are seen during the induction phase of amyloidosis in the murine casein model.[270]

TREATMENT OF AMYLOIDOSIS

Prognosis. Amyloidosis is almost invariably fatal. Renal failure and cardiac disease are the most frequent causes of death. In primary amyloidosis survival from the time of diagnosis approximates 14 months.[148,189] In multiple myeloma–associated amyloidosis, survival may be even shorter, with a recent estimate of 4 months from diagnosis. This is considerably shorter than the mean survival for nonamyloidotic myeloma patients in the same study (20 months).[189] Prognosis in secondary amyloidosis is dependent upon the nature of the underlying disorder as well as the rate of progression of amyloidosis. In several instances in which the underlying disease could be controlled, clinical recovery from amyloidosis has been noted.[232,271-273]

It is difficult to document the regression of amyloid deposits. Serial biopsies are helpful, but considerations of sampling error make it impossible to state that deposits have truly "regressed" in any case. Clinical improvement in amyloidosis is certainly proved and is assumed to parallel resorption of deposits. Experimental data and newer concepts of amyloidogenesis imply that phagocytic cells are involved in the resorption of amyloid fibrils as well as in their deposition, and that an equilibrium between synthesis and dissolution of deposits might exist.

Therapeutic Approaches. The goals of therapy in amyloidosis are to prevent further deposition of amyloid material and to promote or accelerate its resorption. Recent insights into the pathogenesis of amyloidosis suggest several approaches to treatment of primary amyloidosis or myeloma-associated amyloidosis. First, the underlying B-lymphocyte disorder could be treated with cytotoxic agents to reduce the serum concentration of amyloid-precursor light chains. Second, dissemination of amyloid-precursor light chains could be interrupted by plasmapheresis or extracorporeal perfusion through immunoabsorbent materials. Third, the processing of precursors to fibrillar components could be prevented by agents that interfere with lysosomal uptake or degradation of the polypeptide chain or aggregation of the fibril precursors. Another therapeutic approach that holds promise for the future is the administration of thymic hormones. When given to mice receiving multiple casein injections thymosin reduced the incidence of amyloidosis while maintaining T lymphocyte function.[274]

Chemotherapeutic Measures. There are sporadic case reports that suggest that primary amyloidosis occasionally responds to treatment with cytotoxic agents. This improvement may be accompanied by diminution in paraprotein levels. Cytotoxic drugs will sometimes lower paraprotein levels although the amyloidosis progresses. Kyle and Bayrd observe some improvement in 17 patients with primary amyloidosis on melphalan; two developed a rapidly fatal leukemia after 4 years of treatment.[189] Missmahl reported improvement in eight patients with mild to moderate amyloidosis being treated with methotrexate and chloroquine, although not all his patients had primary amyloidosis.[275] Trotter and associates recently noted the failure of cytotoxic therapy to affect the course of amyloid neuropathy.[149] Because of the grave prognosis in primary amyloidosis, a trial of a cytotoxic agent may be warranted if an associated plasma cell dyscrasia can be documented.

Cytotoxic agents have also been used in the management of amyloidosis secondary to connective tissue diseases. In amyloidosis secondary to juvenile chronic polyarthritis, daily chlorambucil therapy for at least 1 year brings the arthritis under control rapidly and appears to improve survival from amyloidosis.[169] Severe viral infections complicate this therapeutic regimen.

Recent experience with colchicine has shown that divided doses of 1.0 to 1.5 mg per day decrease the frequency and severity of acute febrile attacks of familial Mediterranean fever.[211,212] It is hoped, but not yet proved, that chronic colchicine therapy will prevent amyloidosis in familial Mediterranean fever patients. Intraperitoneal injections of colchicine significantly reduce the development of amyloid deposits in casein-induced murine amyloidosis, a model for secondary amyloidosis.[276,277] Ravid and colleagues report that colchicine-induced clinical remissions occurred in three patients with familial Mediterranean fever amyloid nephropathy and appeared to reduce the size of amyloid deposits.[214] In one "primary amyloidosis" patient with no demonstrable paraprotein, similar improvement is noted. It is not yet clear which patients are likely to respond to colchicine, but trials are warranted in patients with familial Mediterranean fever amyloidosis and secondary amyloidosis.

Dimethyl sulfoxide (DMSO), when used in massive doses, causes a partial or total disappearance of amyloid deposits in casein-treated mice when compared with control mice. DMSO also promotes the excretion of amyloid precursor material in the urine of the amyloidotic mice.[278] Single intravenous or oral doses of DMSO given to human subjects result in the transient excretion of congophilic, amyloid-like fibrils in the urine. The urinary fibrils may represent fragments of amyloid fibrillar subunits dislodged from renal amyloid deposits.[279]

The use of glucocorticoids in amyloidosis is controversial; these drugs can accelerate amyloid deposition under certain experimental conditions, and a similar effect has been suggested in humans.[173] At present, there is not sufficient evidence to withhold glucocorticoids when they are indicated in the management of an underlying inflammatory or neoplastic disease.

Supportive Measures. Since amyloidosis may be a fatal disease, the patient and his family should be accorded the necessary professional counseling and psychological support. A variety of unique problems can be encountered in systemic amyloidosis, and they demand good supportive medical care. Congestive heart failure in amyloidosis does not usually respond to digitalis. Also, a number of reports document a high incidence of sudden death and cardiac arrhythmia in amyloidosis patients who take digitalis.[151,245] Digitalis preparations should be administered in a hospital setting when other measures to manage heart failure have proved inadequate. Diuretics must also be used judiciously to avoid dehydration and cardiovascular collapse. Postural hypotension can result from volume depletion (secondary to diuretics, decreased fluid intake, or protein-osmotic diuresis), adrenal insufficiency, autonomic neuropathy, or low-output cardiac failure. Mineralocorticoids can reverse volume depletion from adrenal insufficiency. Elastic stockings may remedy neuropathic hypotension. Malabsorption syndromes, often the result of bacterial overgrowth secondary to visceral motility disturbances, respond to broad-spectrum antibiotics in many cases. Macroglossia may interfere with deglutition, necessitating supplemental gastrotomy feeding. Compromise of the upper airways by an enlarged tongue may necessitate tracheostomy. Hemorrhagic diatheses caused by isolated factor X deficiency do not respond to fresh frozen plasma, but may respond transiently to factor IX concentrate.[280] Carbamazepine has provided symptomatic relief for one patient with polyneuropathy.[281] Bronchoscopy with curettage of bronchial amyloid deposits can provide significant palliation in some types of respiratory tract amyloidosis. Administration of immunoglobulin may ameliorate severe infections in patients with immunoglobulin deficiencies secondary to amyloidosis.[173]

In patients with end-stage renal failure resulting from amyloidosis, the choice at present lies between maintenance dialysis and renal transplantation. The results of maintenance dialysis in such patients are not as good as in patients with nonsystemic diseases. European experience of hospital dialysis patients shows a cumulative patient survival of 75.8 percent for all patients at 2 years compared with 50 percent for diabetic patients, 53 percent for patients with amyloidosis, and 65 percent for patients with systemic lupus erythematosus. The number of patients with amyloidosis on dialysis was 212.[281] The results of renal transplantation in 21 patients with renal amyloidosis has been reported.[282] Five patients survived for more than 3 years, and of these one lived for 7 years and two lived for 10 years. Amyloidosis of other organ systems seems to be a slow process and probably does not influence the outcome, though cardiac involvement may be troublesome in older patients. The limiting factor in these patients appears to have been rejection rather than recurrence of amyloid disease, though this did happen in one patient.[282] Although they seem not to do so well as other patients treated either by regular dialysis or transplantation, patients with amyloidosis should not be excluded from consideration for these treatments.

References

1. Cohen, A.S., and Calkins, E.: Electron microscopic observation on a fibrous component in amyloid of diverse origins. Nature 183:1202, 1959.
2. Spiro, D.: The structural basis of proteinuria in man. Electron microscopic studies of renal biopsy specimens from patients with lipid nephrosis, amyloidosis, and subacute and chronic glomerulonephritis. Am. J. Pathol. 35:47, 1959.
3. Glenner, G.G.: Amyloid deposits and amyloidosis. The β-Fibrilloses. N. Engl. J. Med. 302:1283, 1980.
4. Pauling, L., and Corey, P.B.: Configuration of polypeptide chains with favored orientation around single bonds: two new pleated sheets. Proc. Natl. Acad. Sci. (U.S.A.) 37:729, 1951.
5. Schwartz, P.: Amyloidosis: Cause and Manifestation of Senile Deterioration. Springfield, Ill., Charles C Thomas, 1970, pp. 5–20.
6. Rokitansky, K.F. von: Handbuch der Pathologischen Anatomie 3. Vienna, Braumuller and Seidel, 1842.
7. Virchow, R.: Ueber eine im Gehirn und Ruckenmark des menochen aufgefundene Substanz mit der chemischen Reaction der Cellulose. Virchow-Reinhardt Arch. Path. Anat. 6:135, 1854.
8. Virchow, R.: Zur Cellulose-frage. Virchow Arch. Path. Anat. 6:416, 1854.
9. Meckel, H.: Die Speck- oder Cholestrinkrankheit. Ann. Charité-Krankenhauses 4:264, 1853.
10. Schmidt, M.B.: Uber das sogennante thierische Amyloid. Ann. Chem. Pharm. 110:250, 1859.
11. Friedreich, N., and Kekulé, A.: Zur Amyloidfrage. Arch. Pathol. Anat. Physiol. Klin. Med. 16:50, 1859.
12. Kuczynski, M.H.: Neue Beiträge zur Lehre vom Amyloid. Klin. Wschr. 2:727, 1923.
13. Kuczynski, M.H.: Weitre Beiträge zur Lehre vom Amyloid. 3. Mitteilung. Über die Rückbildung des Amyloids. Klin. Wschr. 2:2193, 1923.
14. Bennhold, H.: Eine spezifische amyloid Färburg mit Kongorot. München Med. Wschr. 69:1537, 1922.
15. Divry, P., and Florkin, M.: Sur les propriétés optiques de l'amyloide. C. R. Soc. Biol. 97:1808, 1927.
16. Magnus-Levy, A.: Bence Jones Eiweiss und Amyloid. Z. Klin. Med. 116:510, 1931.
17. Apitz, K.: Die Paraproteinosin. Über die Störung des Eiweisstoffwechsels bei Plasmocytom. Virchows Arch. Pathol. Anat. Physiol. 306:631, 1940.
18. Osserman, E.F.: Plasma-cell myeloma. II. Clinical aspects. N. Engl. J. Med. 261:1006, 1959.
19. Glenner, G.G., Terry, W., Harada, M., Isersky, C., and Page, D.: Amyloid fibril proteins: Proof of homology with immunoglobulin light chains by sequence analysis. Science 172:1150, 1971.
20. Benditt, E.P., Eriksen, N., Hermodson, M.A., and Ericsson, L.H.: The major proteins of human and monkey amyloid substance: Common properties including unusual N-terminal amino acid sequences. FEBS Lett. 19:169, 1971.
21. Levin, M., Franklin, E.C., Frangione, B., and Pras, M.: The amino acid sequence of a major nonimmunoglobulin component of some amyloid fibrils. J. Clin. Invest. 51:2773, 1972.
22. Sletten, K., and Husby, G.: The complete amino acid sequence of nonimmunoglobulin amyloid fibril protein AS in rheumatoid arthritis. Eur. J. Biochem. 41:117, 1974.
23. Pras, M., and Schubert, M.: Metachromatic properties of amyloid in solution. J. Histochem. Cytochem. 17:258, 1969.
24. Stoker, G.: An improved Congo red method for amyloid. Med. Lab. Sci. 33:79, 1976.
25. Bordin, G.M.: Natural green birefringence of amyloid. Am. J. Clin. Pathol. 65:417, 1976.
26. Puchtler, H., and Sweat, F.: Congo red as a stain for fluorescence microscopy of amyloid. J. Histochem. Cytochem. 13:693, 1965.
27. Vassar, P.S., and Culling, C.F.A.: Fluorescent stains, with special reference to amyloid and connective tissues. Arch. Pathol. 68:487, 1959.
28. Waldrop, F.S., Puchtler, H., and Valentine, L.S.: Fluorescence microscopy of amyloid using mixed illumination. Arch. Pathol. 93:37, 1972.
29. Shirahama, T., and Cohen, A.S.: High resolution electron microscopic analysis of the amyloid fibril. J. Cell. Biol. 33:679, 1967.
30. Sorenson, G.D., and Finke, E.: The ultrastructure of amyloid. In Mandema, E., Ruinen, L., Scholten, J.H., and Cohen, A.S. (eds.): Amyloidosis. Amsterdam, Excerpta Medica, 1968, p. 184.
31. Bladen, H.A., Nylen, M.U., and Glenner, G.G.: The ultrastructure of human amyloid as revealed by the negative staining technique. J. Ultrastruct. Res. 14:449, 1966.
32. Glenner, G.G., and Bladen, H.A.: Purification and reconstitution of the periodic fibril and unit structure of human amyloid. Science 154:271, 1966.
33. Cathcart, E.S., Shirahama, T., and Cohen, A.S.: Isolation and identification of a plasma component of amyloid. Biochim. Biophys. Acta 147:392, 1967.
34. Glenner, G.G., Ignaczak, T.F., and Page, D.L.: The inherited systemic amyloidoses and localized amyloid deposits. In Stanbury, J.B., Wyngaarden, J.B., and Fredrickson, D.S. (eds.): The Metabolic Basis of Inherited Disease. 4th ed. New York, McGraw-Hill Book Company, 1978, p. 1308.
35. Heefner, W.A., and Sorenson, G.D.: Experimental amyloidosis. I. Light and electron microscopic observations of spleen and lymph nodes. Lab. Invest. 11:585, 1962.
36. Ben-Ishay, Z., and Zlotnick, A.: The cellular origin of amyloid. Electron microscopic study in a case of amyloidosis. Isr. J. Med. Sci. 4:987, 1968.
37. Ranlov, P., and Wanstrup, J.: Ultrastructural investigations on the cellular morphogenesis of experimental mouse amyloidosis. Acta Pathol. Microbiol. Scand. 71:575, 1967.

38. Zucker-Franklin, D., and Franklin, E.: Intracellular localization of human amyloid by fluorescence and electron microscopy. Am. J. Pathol. 59:23, 1970.

39. Glenner, G.G., and Page, D.L.: Amyloid, amyloidosis, and amyloidogenesis. Int. Rev. Exp. Pathol. 15:1, 1976.

40. Eanes, E.D., and Glenner, G.G.: X-ray diffraction studies of amyloid filaments. J. Histochem. Cytochem. 16:673, 1968.

41. Glenner, G.G., Eanes, E.D., Bladen, H.A., Linke, R.P., and Termine, J.D.: β-Pleated sheet fibrils: A comparison of native amyloid with synthetic protein fibrils. J. Histochem. Cytochem. 22:1141, 1974.

42. Termine, J.D., Eanes, E.D., Ein, D., and Glenner, G.G.: Infrared spectroscopy of human amyloid fibrils and immunoglobulin proteins. Biopolymers 11:1103, 1972.

43. Romhanyi, G.: Über die submikroskopische Struktur des Amyloids. Schweiz Z. Pathol. (Pathol. Microbiol.) 12:253, 1949.

44. Cooper, J.H.: Selective amyloid staining as a function of amyloid composition and structure. Lab. Invest. 31:232, 1974.

45. Glenner, G.G., Ein, D., Eanes, E.D., Bladen, H.A., Terry, W., and Page, D.: The creation of "amyloid" fibrils from Bence Jones proteins in vitro. Science 174:712, 1971.

46. Glenner, G.G., Eanes, E.D., and Page, D.L.: The relations of the properties of Congo red-stained amyloid fibrils to the β-conformation. J. Histochem. Cytochem. 20:821, 1972.

47. Cathcart, E.S., Comerford, F.R., and Cohen, A.S.: Immunologic studies on a protein extracted from human secondary amyloid. N. Engl. J. Med. 273:143, 1965.

48. Skinner, M., Cohen, A.S., Shirahama, T., and Cathcart, E.S.: P-component (pentagonal unit) of amyloid: Isolation, characterization, and sequence analysis. J. Lab. Clin. Med. 84:604, 1974.

49. Anderson, J.K., and Mole, J.E.: Large scale isolation and partial primary structure of human plasma P-component. Ann. N.Y. Acad. Sci. 389:216, 1982.

50. Pepys, M.B., Dash, A.C., Munn, E.A., Feinstein, A., Skinner, M., Cohen, A.S., Gewurtz, H., Osmand, A.P., and Painter, R.H.: Isolation of amyloid P component (protein AP) from normal serum as a calcium dependent binding protein. Lancet 1:1029, 1977.

51. Cathcart, E.S., Skinner, M., and Cohen, A.S.: Immunogenicity of amyloid. Immunology 20:945, 1971.

52. Westermark, P., Shirahama, T., Skinner, M., Brown, A., Cameron, R., and Cohen, A.S.: Immunohistochemical evidence for the lack of amyloid P component in some intracerebral amyloids. Lab. Invest. 46:457, 1982.

53. Pepys, M.B., Baltz, M., Gomer, K., Davies, A.J.S., and Doenhoff, M.: Serum amyloid P component is an acute phase reactant in the mouse. Nature 278:259, 1979.

54. Osmand, A.P., Friedenson, B., Gewurtz, H., Painter, R.H., Hoffman, T., and Shelton, E.: Characterization of C-reactive protein and the complement subcomponent C1t as homologous proteins displaying cyclic pentameric symmetry (pentraxins). Proc. Natl. Acad. Sci. (U.S.A.) 74:739, 1977.

55. Pepys, M.B., Baltz, M.L., de Beer, F.C., Dyck, R.F., Holford, S., Breathnach, S.M., Black, M.M., Tribe, C.R., Evans, D.J., and Feinstein, A.: Biology of serum amyloid P component. N.Y. Acad. Sci. 389:286, 1982.

56. Dyck, R.F., Lockwood, M., Kershaw, M., McHugh, N., Duance, V., Baltz, M.L., and Pepys, M.B.: Amyloid P component is a constituent of normal human glomerular basement membrane. J. Exp. Med. 152:1162, 1980.

57. Glenner, G.G., Harada, M., and Isersky, C.: The purification of amyloid fibril proteins. Prep. Biochem. 2:39, 1972.

58. Kimura, S., Guyer, R., Terry, W.D., and Glenner, G.G.: Chemical evidence for γ-type amyloid fibril proteins. J. Immunol. 109:891, 1972.

59. Glenner, G.G., Terry, W.D., and Isersky, C.: Amyloidosis: Its nature and pathogenesis. Semin. Hematol. 10:65, 1973.

60. Skinner, M., Benson, M.D., and Cohen, A.S.: Amyloid fibril protein related to immunoglobulin γ-chains. J. Immunol. 114:1433, 1975.

61. Sletten, K., Husby, G., and Natvig, J.B.: N-Terminal amino acid sequence of amyloid fibril protein AR, prototype of a new γ-variable subgroup, VγV. Scand. J. Immunol. 3:833, 1974.

62. Solomon, A., Frangione, B., and Franklin, E.C.: Bence Jones proteins and light chains of immunoglobulins. J. Clin. Invest. 70:453, 1982.

63. Isersky, C., Ein, D., Page, D.L., Harada, M., and Glenner, G.G.: Immunochemical cross-reactions of human amyloid-proteins with immunoglobulin light polypeptide chains. J. Immunol. 108:486, 1972.

64. Pruzanski, W., Katz, A., Nyburg, S.C., and Freedman, M.H.: In vitro production of an amyloid-like substance from γ₃ heavy chain disease protein. Immunol. Commun. 3:469, 1974.

65. Stone, M.J., and Frenkel, E.P.: The clinical spectrum of light chain myeloma. A study of 35 patients with special reference to the occurrence of amyloidosis. Am. J. Med. 58:601, 1975.

66. Terry, W.D., Page, D.L., Kimura, S., Isobe, T., Osserman, E.F., and Glenner, G.G.: Structural identity of Bence Jones and amyloid fibril proteins in a patient with plasma cell dyscrasia and amyloidosis. J. Clin. Invest. 52:1276, 1973.

67. Putnam, F.W., Whitley, E.J., Paul, C., and Davidson, J.N.: Amino acid sequence of a κ Bence Jones protein from a case of primary amyloidosis. Biochemistry 12:3763, 1973.

68. Westermark, P., Natvig, J.B., Anders, R.F., Sletten, K., and Husby, G.: Coexistence of protein AA and immunoglobulin light-chain fragments in amyloid fibrils. Scand. J. Immunol. 5:31, 1976.

69. Husby, G., Sletten, K., Michaelsen, T.E., and Natvig, J.B.: Amyloid fibril protein subunit, 'protein AS': Distribution in tissue and serum in different clinical types of amyloidosis including that associated with myelomatosis and Waldenström's macroglobulinaemia. Scand. J. Immunol. 2:395, 1973.

70. Husby, G., Natvig, J.B., and Sletten, K.: New, third class of amyloid fibril protein. J. Exp. Med. 139:773, 1974.

71. Levin, M., Pras, M., and Franklin, E.C.: Immunologic studies of the major nonimmunoglobulin protein of amyloid. Identification and partial characterization of related serum component. J. Exp. Med. 138:373, 1973.

72. Linke, R.P., Sipe, J.D., Pollock, P.S., Ignaczak, T.F., and Glenner, G.G.: Isolation of a low molecular weight serum component antigenically related to an amyloid fibril preparation of unknown origin. Proc. Natl. Acad. Sci. 72:1473, 1975.

73. Rosenthal, C.J., and Franklin, E.C.: Variation with age and disease of an amyloid A protein-related serum component. J. Clin. Invest. 55:746, 1975.

74. Ignaczak, T.F., Sipe, J.D., Linke, R.P., and Glenner, G.G.: Immunochemical studies on the nature of the serum component (SAA) related to secondary amyloidosis. J. Lab. Clin. Med. 89:1092, 1977.

75. Benditt, E.P., and Eriksen, N.: Amyloid protein SAA is associated with high density lipoprotein from human serum. Proc. Natl. Acad. Sci. (U.S.A.) 74:4025, 1977.

76. Anders, R.F., Natvig, J.B., Michaelsen, T.E., and Husby, G.: Isolation and characterization of amyloid-related serum protein SAA as a low molecular weight protein. Scand. J. Immunol. 4:397, 1957.

77. Bausserman, L.L., Herbert, P.N., and McAdam, K.P.W.J.: Heterogeneity of human serum amyloid proteins. J. Exp. Med. 152:641, 1980.

78. Tobias, P.S., McAdam, K.P.W.J., and Ulevitch, R.J.: Interactions of bacterial lipopolysaccharide with acute-phase rabbit serum and isolation of two forms of rabbit serum amyloid A. J. Immunol. 128:1420, 1982.

79. Benditt, E.P., Eriksen, N., and Hanson, R.H.: Amyloid protein SAA is an apoprotein of mouse plasma high density lipoprotein. Proc. Natl. Acad. Sci. (U.S.A.) 76:4092, 1979.

80. Benson, M.D., and Kleiner, E.: Synthesis and secretion of serum amyloid protein A (SAA) by hepatocytes in mice treated with casein. J. Immunol. 124:495, 1980.

81. Selinger, M.J., McAdam, K.P.W.J., Kaplan, M.M., Sipe, J.D., Vogel, N., and Rosenstreich, D.L.: Monokine-induced synthesis of serum amyloid A protein by hepatocytes. Nature 285:498, 1981.

82. McAdam, K.P.W.J., Li, J., Knowles, J., Foss, N.T., Dinarello, C.A., Rossenwasser, L.J., Selinger, M.J., Kaplan, M.M., and Goodman, R.: The biology of SAA. Identification of the inducer, in vitro synthesis and heterogeneity demonstrated with monoclonal antibodies. Proc. N.Y. Acad. Sci. 389:137, 1982.

83. Sipe, J.D., Vogel, S.N., Sztein, B., Skinner, M., and Cohen, A.S.: The role of interleukin I in acute phase serum amyloid (SAA) and serum amyloid P(SAP) bisynthesis. Proc. N.Y. Acad. Sci. 389:137, 1982.

84. Benson, M.D., and Aldo-Benson, M.A.: SAA suppression of in vitro antibody response. Proc. N.Y. Acad. Sci. 389:121, 1982.

85. Hoffman, J.S., and Benditt, E.P.: Changes in high density lipoprotein content following endotoxin administration in the mouse. J. Biol. Chem. 257:10510, 1982.

86. Benditt, E.P., Hoffman, J.S., Eriksen, N., Parmelee, D.C., and Walsh, K.A.: SAA, an apoprotein of HDL: its structure and function. Ann. N.Y. Acad. Sci. 389:183, 1982.

87. Meretoja, J., Natvig, J.B., and Husby, G.: Amyloid-related serum protein (SAA) in patients with inherited amyloidosis and certain viral conditions. Scand. J. Immunol. 5:169, 1976.

88. Gorevic, P.D., Rosenthal, C.J., and Franklin, E.C.: Amyloid-related serum component (SAA)—studies in acute infections, medullary thyroid carcinoma and postsurgery. Clin. Immunol. Immunopathol. 6:83, 1976.

89. McAdam, K.P.W.J., Elin, R.J., Sipe, J.D., and Wolff, S.M.: Changes in human serum amyloid A and C-reactive protein after etiocholanalone-induced inflammation. J. Clin. Invest. 61:390, 1978.

90. Pearse, A.G.E., Ewen, S.W.B., and Polak, J.M.: The genesis of apudamyloid in endocrine polypeptide tumours: Histochemical distinction from immune amyloid. Virchows Arch. Abt. B. Zellpathol. 10:93, 1972.

91. Tashjian, A.H., Wolfe, H.J., and Voelkel, E.F.: Human calcitonin. Immunologic assay, cytologic localization and studies on medullary thyroid carcinoma. Am. J. Med. 56:840, 1974.

92. Sletten, K., Westermark, P., and Natvig, J.B.: Characterization of amyloid fibril proteins from medullary carcinoma of the thyroid. J. Exp. Med. 143:993, 1976.

93. Schober, L., and Nelson, D.: Fine structure and origin of amyloid deposits in pituitary adenoma. Arch. Pathol. 99:403, 1975.

94. Westermark, P.: On the nature of amyloid in human islets of Langerhans. Histochemistry 38:27, 1974.

95. Burke, M.J., and Rouguie, M.A.: Cross-B protein structures. I. Insulin fibrils. Biochemistry 11:2435, 1972.

96. Westermark, P., Skinner, M., and Cohen, A.S.: The P-component of amyloid of human islets of Langerhans. Scand. J. Immunol. 4:95, 1975.

97. Anderson, T.J., and Ewen, S.W.B.: Amyloid in normal and pathological parathyroid glands. J. Clin. Pathol. 27:656, 1974.

98. Bilbao, J., Horveth, E., Hudson, A.R., and Kovacs, K.: Pituitary adenoma producing amyloid-like substance. Arch. Pathol. 99:411, 1975.

99. Ozdemir, A.I., Wright, J.R., and Calkins, E.: Influence of rheumatoid arthritis on amyloidosis of aging. Comparison of 47 rheumatoid patients with 47 controls matched for age and sex. N. Engl. J. Med. 285:534, 1971.

100. Pomerance, A.: The pathology of senile cardiac amyloidosis. J. Pathol. Bacteriol. 91:357, 1966.

101. Wright, J.R., and Calkins, E.: Amyloid in the aged heart: Frequency and clinical significance. J. Am. Geriat. Soc. 23:97, 1975.

102. Romhanyi, G.: Differences in ultrastructural organization of amyloid as revealed by sensitivity or resistance to induced proteolysis. Virchows Arch. Pathol. Anat. 357:29, 1972.

103. Westermark, P., Natvig, J.B., and Johansson, B.: Characterization of an amyloid fibril protein from senile cardiac amyloid. J. Exp. Med. 146:631, 1977.

104. Terry, R.D., Gonatas, N.K., and Weiss, M.: Ultrastructural studies in Alzheimer's presenile dementia. Am. J. Pathol. 44:269, 1964.

105. Narang, H.K.: High resolution electron microscopic analysis of amyloid fibril in Alzheimer's disease. J. Neuropathol. Exp. Neurol. 39:621, 1980.

106. Terry, R.D., and Wisniewski, H.: The ultrastructure of the neurofibrillary tangle and the senile plaque. In Wolstenholme, G.E.W., and O'Connor, M. (eds.): Alzheimer's Disease and Related Conditions. London, J&A Churchill, 1970, p. 145.

107. Torack, R.M.: Congophilic angiopathy complicated by surgery and massive hemorrhage. A light and electron microscopic study. Am. J. Pathol. 81:349, 1975.

108. Wisniewski, H.M., Narang, H.K., and Terry, R.D.: Neurofibrillary tangles of paired helical filaments. J. Neurol. Sci. 27:178, 1976.

109. Ishii, T., Seiji, H., and Shimizu, F.: Identification of components of immunoglobulins in senile plaques by means of fluorescent antibody technique. Acta Neuropathol. 32:157, 1975.

110. Powers, J.M., and Skeen, J.T.: An immunoperoxidase study of neuritic plaques. J. Neuropathol. Exp. Neurol. 40:310, 1981.

111. Torack, R.M., and Lynch, R.G.: Cytochemistry of brain amyloid in adult dementia. Acta Neuropathol. 53:189, 1981.

112. Johnson, A.B., Cohen, S.A., Said, S.I., and Terry, R.D.: Neuritic plaque amyloid, microangiopathy and Alzheimer neurofibrillary tangles: Do they share a common antigen? J. Neuropathol. Exp. Neurol. 40:310, 1981.

113. Shirahama, T., Skinner, M., Westermark, P., Rubinow, A., Cohen, A.S., Brun, A., and Kemper, T.L.: Senile cerebral amyloid. Prealbumin as a common constituent in the neuritic plaque, in the neurofibrillary tangle, and in the microangiopathic lesion. Am. J. Pathol. 107:47, 1982.

114. Andrade, C.: A peculiar form of peripheral neuropathy. Familial atypical generalized amyloidosis with special involvement of the peripheral nerves. Brain 75:408, 1952.

115. Costa, P.P., Figueira, A.S., and Bravo, F.R.: Amyloid fibril protein related to pre-albumin in familial amyloidotic polyneuropathy. Proc. Natl. Acad. Sci. U.S.A. 75:4499, 1978.

116. Benson, M.D.: Partial amino acid sequence homology between an heredofamilial amyloid protein and human plasma prealbumin. J. Clin. Invest. 67:1035, 1981.

117. Linke, R.P., Zucker-Franklin, D., and Franklin, E.C.: Morphologic, chemical and immunologic studies of amyloid-like fibrils formed from Bence Jones protein by proteolysis. J. Immunol. 111:10, 1973.

118. Epstein, W.V., Tan, M., and Wood, I.S.: Formation of amyloid fibrils in vitro by action of human kidney lysosomal enzymes on Bence Jones proteins. J. Lab. Clin. Med. 84:107, 1974.

119. Durie, B.G.M., Persky, B., Soehnlen, B.J., Grogan, T.M., and Salmon, S.E.: Amyloid production in human myeloma stem-cells with morphologic evidence of amyloid secretion by associated macrophages. N. Engl. J. Med. 307:1689, 1982.

120. Lavie, G., Zucker-Franklin, D., and Franklin, E.C.: Degradation of serum amyloid protein A by surface associated enzymes of human blood monocytes. J. Exp. Med. 148:1020, 1978.

121. Lavie, G., Zucker-Franklin, D., and Franklin, E.C.: Elastase-type proteases on the surface of human blood monocytes: possible role in amyloid formation. J. Immunol. 125:175, 1980.

122. Silverman, S.L., Cathcart, E.S., Skinner, M., and Cohen, A.S.: The degradation of serum amyloid A protein by activated polymorphonuclear leucocytes: participation of elastase. Immunology 46:737, 1982.

123. Shirahama, T., and Cohen, A.S.: Intralysosomal formation of amyloid fibrils. Am. J. Pathol. 81:101, 1975.

124. Gueft, B., and Ghidoni, J.J.: The site of formation and ultrastructure of amyloid. Am. J. Pathol. 43:837, 1963.

125. Cohen, A.S. and Cathcart, E.S.: Casein-induced experimental amyloidosis. I. Review of cellular and immunologic aspects. Methods Achiev. Exp. Pathol. 6:207, 1972.

126. Skinner, M., Cathcart, E.S., Cohen, A.S., and Shirahama, T.: Isolation and sequence analysis of experimentally induced guinea pig amyloid fibrils. J. Exp. Med. 140:871, 1974.

127. Benson, M.D., Scheinberg, M.A., Shirahama, T., Cathcart, E.S., and Skinner, M.: Kinetics of serum amyloid protein A in casein-induced murine amyloidosis. J. Clin. Invest. 59:412, 1977.

128. Gorevic, P.D., Levo, Y., Frangione, B., and Franklin, E.C.: Polymorphism of tissue and serum amyloid A (AA and SAA) proteins in the mouse. J. Immunol. 121:138, 1978.

129. Smetana, H.: The relation of the reticulo-endothelial system to the formation of amyloid. J. Exp. Med. 45:619, 1927.

130. Shearing, S., Comerford, F.R., and Cohen, A.S.: Effect of an amyloid inducing regimen on phagocytosis of carbon particles. Proc. Soc. Exp. Biol. Med. 119:673, 1966.

131. Ranlov, P.: Phagocytosis in experimental mouse amyloidosis. Acta Pathol. Microbiol. Scand. 68:19, 1966.

132. Teilum, G.: Pathogenesis of amyloidosis; the two phase cellular theory of local secretion. Acta Pathol. Microbiol. Scand. 61:21, 1964.

133. Sipe, J.D., McAdam, K.P.W.J., and Uchino, F.: Biochemical evidence for the biphasic development of experimental amyloidosis. Lab. Invest. 38:110, 1978.

134. Cathcart, E.S., and Wohlgethan, J.R.: Amyloidosis. In Panayi, G.S. (ed.): Scientific Basis of Rheumatology. Edinburgh, Churchill Livingston, 1982, p. 131.

135. Cathcart, E.S., Mullarkey, M., Cohen, A.S.: Amyloidosis: an expression of immunological tolerance? Lancet 2:639, 1970.

136. Barth, W.F., Gordon, J.K., and Willerson, J.T.: Amyloidosis induced in mice by Escherichia coli endotoxin. Science 162:694, 1968.

137. Lazzari, A.A., Wohlgethan, J.R., and Cathcart, E.S.: Azocasein and endotoxin responses in amyloid resistant strains of mice. In Bacon, P.A., and Tribe, C.R. (eds.): Proc. Eur. Amyloid Symp. Bristol, John Wright and Sons, in press.

138. Hardt, F.: Acceleration of casein-induced amyloidosis in mice by immunosupressive agents. Acta Pathol. Microbiol. Scand. 79:61, 1971.

139. Wohlgethan, J.R., and Cathcart, E.S.: Amyloid resistance in the A/J mouse is determined by a single gene. Nature 278:453, 1979.

140. Scheinberg, M.A., Cathcart, E.S., Eastcott, J.W., Skinner, M., Benson, M.D., Shirahama, T., and Bennett, M.: The SJL mouse. A new model for spontaneous age-associated amyloidosis. Lab. Invest. 35:47, 1976.

141. Higuchi, K., Matsumura, A., Hashimoto, K., Honma, A., Takeshita, S., Hosokawa, M., Yasuhira, K., and Takeda, T.: Isolation and characterization of senile amyloid-related antigenic substance (SASsam) from mouse serum. J. Exp. Med. 158:1600, 1983.

142. Werdelin, O., and Ranlov, P.: Amyloidosis in mice produced by transplantation of spleen cells from casein-treated mice. Acta Pathol. Microbiol. Scand. 68:1, 1966.

143. Wehlgethan, J.R., and Cathcart, E.S.: Amyloid resistance in A/J mice. Studies with a transfer model. Lab. Invest. 42:663, 1980.

144. Maury, C.P., and Teppo, A.M.: Mechanisms of reduced amyloid-A-degrading activity in serum of patients with secondary amyloidosis. Lancet 2:234, 1982.

145. Cohen, A.S.: Amyloidosis. N. Engl. J. Med. 277:522, 574, 968, 1967.

146. Cohen, D. H., Feiner, H., Jensson, O., and Frangione, B.: Amyloid fibril in hereditary cerebral hemorrhage with amyloidosis (HCHWA) is related to the gastroentero-pancreatic neuroendocrine protein, gamma trace. J. Exp. Med. 158:623, 1983.

147. Brandt, K., Cathcart, E.S., and Cohen, A.S.: A clinical analysis of the course and prognosis of 42 patients with amyloidosis. Am. J. Med. 44:955, 1968.

148. Pruzanski, W., and Katz, A: Clinical and laboratory findings in primary generalized and multiple-myeloma-related amyloidosis. Can. Med. Assoc. J. 114:906, 1976.

149. Trotter, J.L., Engel, W.K., and Ignaczak, T.F.: Amyloidosis with plasma cell dyscrasia. An overlooked cause of adult onset sensorimotor neuropathy. Arch. Neurol. 34:209, 1977.

150. Benson, M.D., Brandt, K.D., Cohen, A.S., and Cathcart, E.S.: Neuropathy, M components and amyloid. Lancet 1:10, 1975.

151. Buja, L., Khoi, N.B., and Roberts, W.C.: Clinically significant cardiac amyloidosis. Am. J. Cardiol. 26:394, 1970.

152. Barth, W.F., Glenner, G.G., Waldmann, T.A., and Zelis, R.F.: Primary amyloidosis. Ann. Intern. Med. 69:787, 1968.

153. Katz, G.A., Peter, J.B., Pearson, C.M., and Adams, W.S.: The shoulder-

pad sign—a diagnostic feature of amyloid arthropathy. N. Engl. J. Med. 288:355, 1973.

154. Akin, R.K., Barton, K., and Walters, P.J.: Amyloidosis, macroglossia and carpal tunnel syndrome associated with myeloma. J. Oral Surg. 33:690, 1975.

155. Furie, B., Greene, E., and Furie, B.: Syndrome of acquired factor X deficiency and systemic amyloidosis. In vivo studies of the metabolic fate of factor X. N. Engl. J. Med. 297:81, 1977.

156. Glenner, G.G.: Factor X deficiency and systemic amyloidosis. N. Engl. J. Med. 297:108, 1977.

157. Jones, N.F., Hilton, P.J., Tighe, J.R., and Hobbs, J.R.: Treatment of primary renal amyloidosis with melphalan. Lancet 2:616, 1972.

158. Bastian, F.O.: Amyloidosis and the carpal tunnel syndrome. Am. J. Clin. Pathol. 61:711, 1974.

159. Lambird, P.A., and Hartmann, W.H.: Hereditary amyloidosis, the flexor retinaculum and the carpal tunnel syndrome. Am. J. Clin. Pathol. 52:714, 1969.

160. Husby, G.: Amyloidosis in rheumatoid arthritis. Ann. Clin. Res. 7:154, 1975.

161. Calkins, E., and Cohen, A.S.: Diagnosis of amyloidosis. Bull. Rheum. Dis. 10:215, 1960.

162. Missen, G.A.K., and Tailor, J.D.: Amyloidosis in rheumatoid arthritis. J. Pathol. Bacteriol. 71:179, 1956.

163. Arapakis, G., and Tribe, C.R.: Amyloidosis in rheumatoid arthritis investigated by means of rectal biopsy. Ann. Rheum. Dis. 22:256, 1963.

164. Bland, J.H.: Clinical incidence of renal amyloidosis in rheumatoid arthritis. J. Maine Med. Assoc. 56:251, 1965.

165. Brun, C., Olsen, T.S., Raaschou, F., and Sörensen, A.W.S.: Renal biopsy in rheumatoid arthritis. Nephron 2:65, 1965.

166. Westermark, P., and Stenkvist, B.: A new method for the diagnosis of systemic amyloidosis. Arch. Intern. Med. 132:522, 1973.

167. Stenkvist, B., Westermark, P., and Wibell, L.: Simple method of diagnostic screening for amyloidosis. Ann. Rheum. Dis. 33:75, 1974.

168. Smith, M.E., and Bywaters, E.G.L.: Mortality and prognosis related to the amyloidosis of Still's disease. Ann. Rheum. Dis. 27:137, 1968.

169. Schnitzer, T.J., and Ansell, B.M.: Amyloidosis in juvenile chronic polyarthritis. Arthritis Rheum. (Suppl.) 20:245, 1977.

170. Tiku, M.L., Mathai, N., Chakrabarti, A.K., Johnson, S.C., and Bhaktaviziama, A.: Amyloidosis complicating ankylosing spondylitis. J. Assoc. Phys. Ind. 23:391, 1975.

171. Caughey, D.E., and Wakem, C.J.: A fatal case of Reiter's disease complicated by amyloidosis. Arthritis Rheum. 16:695, 1973.

172. Qureshi, M.S., Sandle, G.I., Kelly, J.K., and Fox, H.: Amyloidosis complicating psoriatic arthritis. Br. Med. J. 2:302, 1977.

173. Zilko, P.J., and Dawkins, R.L.: Amyloidosis associated with dermatomyositis and features of multiple myeloma: The progression of amyloidosis associated with corticosteroid and cytotoxic drug therapy. Am. J. Med. 59:448, 1975.

174. Schleissner, L.A., Sheehan, W.W., and Orselli, R.C.: Lupus erythematosus in a patient with amyloidosis, adrenal insufficiency, and subsequent immunoblastic sarcoma. Arthritis Rheum. 19:249, 1976.

175. Kennedy, A.C., Burton, J.A., and Allison, M.E.M.: Tuberculosis as a continuing cause of renal amyloidosis. Br. Med. J. 2:795, 1974.

176. Rizvi, S.N.A., Gulati, P.D., and Vaishnava, H.: Tuberculosis and renal amyloidosis. Br. Med. J. 4:657, 1974.

177. Williams, R.C., Jr., Cathcart,, E.S., Calkins, E., Fite, G.L., Rubio, J.B., and Cohen, A.S.: Secondary amyloidosis in lepromatous leprosy. Possible relationship of diet and environment. Ann. Intern. Med. 62:1000, 1965.

178. Kronvall, G., Husby, G., Samuel, D., Bjune, G., and Wheate, H.: Amyloid related serum component (protein ASC) in leprosy patients. Infect. Immunol. 11:969, 1975.

179. Brownstein, M.H., and Helwig, E.B.: Secondary systemic amyloidosis: analysis of underlying disorders. South. Med. J. 64:491, 1971.

180. Penman, H.G., and Thomson, K.J.: Amyloidosis and renal adenocarcinoma; a post-mortem study. J. Pathol. 107:45, 1972.

181. Rigdon, R.H.: Occurrence and association of amyloid with diseases in birds and mammals including man: A review. Texas Rep. Biol. Med. 32:665, 1974.

182. Kimball, K.G.: Amyloidosis in association with neoplastic disease; report of an unusual case and clinicopathological experience at Memorial Center for Cancer and Allied Diseases during eleven years (1948–1959). Ann. Intern. Med. 55:958, 1961.

183. Dahlin, D.C.: Classification and general aspects of amyloidosis. Med. Clin. North Am. 34:1107, 1950.

184. Foroughi, E.: Amyloid producing malignant melanoma. J. Med. Soc. N.J. 73:153, 1976.

185. Buchner, A., and David, R.: Amyloid-like material in odontogenic tumors. J. Oral Surg. 34:320, 1976.

186. Osserman, E.F., Takatsuki, K., and Talal, N.: The pathogenesis of "amyloidosis." Studies on the role of abnormal gammaglobulins and gammaglobulin fragments of the "primary" and "secondary" amyloidosis associated with plasma cell myeloma. Semin. Hematol. 1:3, 1964.

187. Isobe, T., and Osserman, E.F.: Patterns of amyloidosis and their association with plasma-cell dyscrasia, monoclonal immunoglobulins and Bence Jones proteins. N. Engl. J. Med. 290:473, 1974.

188. Cathcart, E.S., Ritchie, R.F., Cohen, A.S., and Brandt, K.: Immunoglobulins and amyloidosis. An immunologic study of sixty two patients with biopsy-proved disease. Am. J. Med. 52:93, 1972.

189. Kyle, R.A., and Bayrd, E.D.: Amyloidosis: Review of 236 cases. Medicine 54:271, 1975.

190. Julião, O.F., Queiroz, L.S., and Loped de Faria, J.: Portuguese type of familial amyloid polyneuropathy: Anatoclinical study of a Brazilian family. Eur. Neurol. 11:180, 1974.

191. Dyck, P.J., and Lambert, E.H.: Dissociated sensation in amyloidosis: Compound action potential, qualitative histologic and teased-fiber, and electron microscopic studies of sural nerve biopsies. Arch. Neurol. 20:490, 1969.

192. Kito, S.: A new focus of familial amyloid polyneuropathy. Nippon Rinsho 31:170, 1973.

193. Andersson, R., and Hofer, P.A.: Primary amyloidosis with polyneuropathy: Some aspects on the histopathological diagnosis antemortem based on studies of biopsy specimens from 30 familial and non-familial cases. Acta Med. Scand. 196:115, 1974.

194. Andrade, C.: Familial amyloidotic polyneuropathy. In Mandema, E., Ruinen, L., Scholten, J.H., and Cohen, A.S. (eds.): Amyloidosis. Amsterdam, Excepta Medica, 1968, p. 377.

195. Silva Horta, J.D., Filipe, I., and Duarte, S.: Portuguese polyneuritic familial type of amyloidosis. Pathol. Microbiol. 27:809, 1964.

196. Benson, M.D., and Cohen, A. S.: Generalized amyloid in a family of Swedish origin. A study of 426 family members in seven generations of a new kinship with neuropathy, nephropathy and central nervous system involvement. Ann. Intern. Med. 86:419, 1977.

197. Rukavina, J.G., Block, W.D., Jackson, C.E., Falls, H.F., Carey, J.H., and Curtis, A.C.: Primary systemic amyloidosis: A review and an experimental genetic and clinical study of 29 cases with particular emphasis on the familial form. Medicine 35:239, 1956.

198. Andrade, C., Araki, S., Block, W.D., Cohen, A.S., Jackson, C.E., Kuroiwa, Y., McKusick, V.A., Nissim, J., Sohar, E., and Van Allen, M.W.: Hereditary amyloidosis Arthritis Rheum. 13:902, 1970.

199. Mahloudji, M., Teasdell, R.D., Adamkiewicz, J.J., Hartmann, W.H., Lambird, P.A., and McKusick, V.A.: The genetic amyloidosis: With particular reference to hereditary neuropathic amyloidosis Type II (Indiana or Rukavina type). Medicine 48:1, 1969.

200. Falls, H.F., Jackson, J., Carey, J.H., Rukavina, J., and Block, W.D.: Ocular manifestations of hereditary primary systemic amyloidosis. AMA Arch. Ophthalmol. 54:660, 1955.

201. Van Allen, M.W., Frolich, J.A., and Davis, J.R.: Inherited predisposition to generalized amyloidosis. Neurology 19:10, 1969.

202. Gimeno, A., Garcia-Alix, D., Segovia de Arana, J.M., Mateos, F., and Sotelo, M.T.: Amyloidotic polyneuritis of Type III (Iowa-Van Allen). Eur. Neurol. 11:46, 1974.

203. Meretoja, J.: Familial systemic paramyloidosis with lattice dystrophy of the cornea, progressive cranial neuropathy, skin changes and various internal symptoms: A previously unrecognized heritable syndrome. Ann. Clin. Res. 1:314, 1969.

204. Meretoja, J.: Comparative histopathological and clinical findings in eyes with lattice corneal dystrophy of two different types. Ophthalmologica 165:15, 1972.

205. Meretoja, J.: Genetic aspects of familial amyloidosis with corneal lattice dystrophy and cranial neuropathy. Clin. Genet. 4:173, 1973.

206. Siegal, S.: Familial paroxysmal polyserositis. Analysis of fifty cases. Am. J. Med. 36:893, 1964.

207. Reimann, H.A., Moadie, J., Semerdijian, S., and Sahyoun, P.F.: Periodic peritonitis–heredity and pathology: Report of seventy-two cases. JAMA 154:1254, 1954.

208. Heller, H., Gafni, J., Michaeli, D., Shahin, N., Sohar, E., Erlich, G., Karten, I., and Sokoloff, L.: The arthritis of familial Mediterranean fever (FMF). Arthritis Rheum. 9:1, 1966.

209. Sohar, E., Gafni, J., Pras, M., and Heller, H.: Familial Mediterranean fever. Am. J. Med. 43:227, 1967.

210. Blum, A., Gafai, J., Sohar, E., and Heller, H.: Amyloidosis as the sole manifestation of familial Mediterranean fever (FMF). Ann. Intern. Med. 57:795, 1962.

211. Goldfinger, W.E.: Colchicine for familial Mediterranean fever (letter). N. Engl. J. Med. 287:1302, 1972.

212. Goldstein, R.C., and Schwabe, A.D.: Prophylactic colchicine therapy in familial Mediterranean fever: A controlled, double-blind study. Ann. Intern. Med. 81:792, 1974.

213. Zemar, D., Pras, M., Sohar, E., and Gafni, J.: Colchicine in familial Mediterranean fever. N. Engl. J. Med. 294:170, 1976.

214. Ravid, M., Robson, M., and Kedar, I.: Prolonged colchicine treatment in four patients with amyloidosis. Ann. Intern. Med. 87:568, 1977.

215. Muckle, T.J., and Wells, M.: Urticaria, deafness and amyloidosis: A new heredofamilial syndrome. Q. J. Med. 31:235, 1962.

216. Black, J.T.: Amyloidosis, deafness, urticaria and limb pains: A hereditary syndrome. Ann. Intern. Med. 70:989, 1969.

217. LaGrue, G., Vernant, J.P., Revuz, J., Touraine, R., and Weil, B.: Syndrome de Muckle et Wells. Cinquième observation familiale. Nouv. Presse Med. 1:2223, 1972.

218. Weiss, S.W., and Page, D.L.: Amyloid nephropathy of Ostertag: Report of a kindred. Birth Defects 10:67, 1974.

219. Frederiksen, T., Gφtzsche, H., Harboe, N., Kiaer, W., and Mellangaard, K.: Primary familial amyloidosis with severe amyloid heart disease. Am. J. Med. 33:328, 1962.

220. Allensworth, D.C., Rice, G.J., and Lowe, G.W.: Persistent atrial standstill in a family with myocardial disease. Am. J. Med. 47:775, 1969.

221. Franklin, E.C.: Amyloid and amyloidosis of the skin. J. Invest. Dermatol. 67:451, 1976.

222. Goltz, R.W.: Systematized amyloidosis: A review of the skin and mucous membrane lesions and a report of two cases. Medicine 31:381, 1952.

223. Moschella, S.L.: Amyloidosis. In Moschella, S.L., Pillsbury, D.M., and Hurley, H.L.: Dermatology. Philadelphia, W. B. Saunders Company, 1975, p. 1285.

224. Wiernik, P.H.: Amyloid joint disease. Medicine 51:465, 1972.

225. Gordon, D.A., Pruzanski, W., Ogryzlo, M.A., and Little, H.A.: Amyloid arthritis simulating rheumatoid disease in five patients with multiple myeloma. Am. J. Med. 55:142, 1974.

226. Christensen, H.E., and Sorensen, K.H.: Local amyloid formation of capsule fibrosa in arthritis coxa. Acta. Path. Scand. [A] 233:128, 1972.

227. Gordon, D.A., Pruzanski, W., and Ogryzlo, M.: Synovial fluid examination for the diagnosis of amyloidosis. Ann. Rheum. Dis. 32:428, 1973.

228. Munsat, T.L., and Poussaint, A.F.: Clinical manifestations and diagnosis of amyloid polyneuropathy. Report of three cases. Neurology 12:413, 1962.

229. Sullivan, J.F., Twitchell, T.E., Gherardi, G.J., and Vanderlaan, W.P.: Amyloid polyneuropathy. Neurology 5:847, 1955.

230. Thomas, P.K., and King, R.H.M.: Peripheral nerve changes in amyloid neuropathy. Brain 97:395, 1974.

231. Bada, J.L.: Carbamazepine for amyloid neuropathy. N. Engl. J. Med. 296:396, 1977.

232. Triger, D.R., and Joekes, A.M.: Renal amyloidosis—a fourteen year follow-up. Q. J. Med. 42:15, 1973.

233. Watanabe, T., and Saniter, T.: Morphological and clinical features of renal amyloidosis. Virchows Arch. A. Path. Anat. Histol. 366:125, 1975.

234. Carone, F.A., and Epstein, F.H.: Nephrogenic diabetes insipidus caused by amyloid disease. Am. J. Med. 29:539, 1960.

235. Derosena, R., Koss, M.N., and Pirani, C.L.: Demonstration of amyloid fibrils in urinary sediment. N. Engl. J. Med. 293:1131, 1975.

236. Shirahama, T., Skinner, M., Cohen, A.S., and Benson, M.D.: Uncertain value of urinary sediments in the diagnosis of amyloidosis. N. Engl. J. Med. 297:821, 1977.

237. Linke, P.P.: Urinary amyloid fibrils in the absence of amyloidosis. Br. Med. J. 2:1259, 1976.

238. Ekelund, L.: Radiologic findings in renal amyloidosis. Am. J. Roentgenol. 129:851, 1977.

239. McCormick, T.L., and Cho, K.J.: Angiographic findings in renal amyloidosis. Am. J. Roentgenol. 129:855, 1977.

240. Chew, C., Ziady, G.M., Raphael, M.J., and Oakley, C.M.: The functional defect in amyloid heart disease. The "stiff heart" syndrome. Am. J. Cardiol. 36:438, 1975.

241. Child, J.S., Levisman, J.A., Abbasi, A.S., and MacAlpin, R.N.: Echocardiographic manifestations of infiltrative cardiomyopathy. A report of 7 cases due to amyloid. Chest 70:726, 1976.

242. Carroll, J.D., Gaasch, W.H., and McAdam, K.P.W.J.: Amyloid cardiomyopathy: Characterization by a distinctive voltage/mass relation. Am. J. Cardiol. 49:9, 1982.

243. Rudolfi, R.L., Bulkley, B.H., and Hutchins, G.M.: The conduction system in cardiac amyloidosis. Am. J. Med. 62:677, 1977.

244. Schroeder, J.S., Billingham, M.E., and Rider, A.K.: Cardiac amyloidosis. Diagnosis by transvenous endomyocardial biopsy. Am. J. Med. 59:269, 1975.

245. Cassidy, J.T.: Cardiac amyloidosis: Two cases with digitalis sensitivity. Ann. Intern. Med. 55:989, 1961.

246. Celli, B.R., Rubinow, A., Cohen, A.S., and Brody, J.S.: Patterns of pulmonary involvement in systemic amyloidosis. Chest 74:543, 1978.

247. Wilson, S.R., Sanders, D.E., and Delarue, N.C.: Intrathoracic manifestations of amyloid disease. Radiology 120:283, 1976.

248. Lee, S.C., and Johnson, H.A.: Multiple nodular pulmonary amyloidosis. Thorax 30:178, 1975.

249. Bonfils-Roberts, E., Marx, A.J., and Nealon, T.F.: Primary amyloidosis of the respiratory tract. Ann. Thorac. Surg. 19:313, 1975.

250. Poh, S.C., Tjia, T.S., and Seah, H.C.: Primary diffuse alveolar septal amyloidosis. Thorax 30:186, 1975.

251. Rubinow, A., Celli, B.R., Cohen, A.S., Rigden, B.G., and Brody, J.S.: Localized amyloidosis of the lower respiratory tract. Am. Rev. Resp. Dis. 118:603, 1978.

252. Battle, W.H., Rubin, M.R., Cohen, S., and Snape, W.J.: Gastrointestinal motility dysfunction in amyloidosis. N. Engl. J. Med. 301:24, 1979.

253. Schnider, B.I., and Burka, P.: Amyloid disease of the stomach stimulating gastric carcinoma. Gastroenterology 28:424, 1955.

254. Jarnum, S.: Gastrointestinal hemorrhage and protein loss in primary amyloidosis. Gut 6:14, 1965.

255. Legge, D.A., Carlson, H.C., and Wollaeger, E.E.: Roentgenologic appearance of systemic amyloidosis involving gastrointestinal tract. Am. J. Roentgenol. Rad. Ther. Nucl. Med. 11:406, 1970.

256. Rivera, R.A.: Endoscopic findings in gastroduodenal amyloidosis. Endoscopy 17:137, 1971.

257. Brody, I.A., Wertlake, P.T., and Laster, L.: Causes of intestinal symptoms in primary amyloidosis. Arch. Intern. Med. 113:512, 1964.

258. Mallory, A., Struthers, J.E., and Kern, F.: Persistent hypotension and intestinal infarction in a patient with primary amyloidosis. Gastroenterology 68:1587, 1975.

259. Griffel, B., Man, B., and Kraus, L.: Selective massive amyloidosis of small intestine. Arch. Surg. 110:215, 1975.

260. Levine, R.A.: Amyloid disease of liver: Correlation of clinical, functional and morphologic features in forty-seven patients. Am. J. Med. 33:349, 1962.

261. Rubinow, A., Koff, R., and Cohen, A.S.: Severe intrahepatic cholestasis in primary amyloidosis. Am. J. Med. 64:937, 1978.

262. Sostre, S., Martin, N.D., Lucas, R.N., and Strauss, H.W.: Scintigraphic findings in primary amyloidosis. Radiology 115:675, 1975.

263. Georgen, T.G., Taylor, A., and Alazrake, N.: Lack of gallium uptake in primary hepatic amyloidosis. Am. J. Roentgenol. 126:1246, 1976.

264. Gafni, J., and Sohar, E.: Rectal biopsy for the diagnosis of amyloidosis. Am. J. Med. Sci. 240:332, 1960.

265. Stauffer, M.H., Gross, J.B., Foulk, W.T., and Dahlin, D.: Amyloidosis: Diagnosis with needle biopsy of liver in 18 patients. Gastroenterology 41:92, 1961.

266. Pasternack, A.: Fine needle aspiration biopsy of spleen in diagnosis of generalized amyloidosis. Br. Med. J. 2:20, 1974.

267. Stenkvist, B. Westermark, P., and Wibell, L.: Simple method of diagnostic screening for amyloidosis. Ann. Rheum. Dis. 33:75, 1974.

268. Krause, J.R.: Value of bone marrow biopsy in the diagnosis of amyloidosis. South. Med. J. 70:1072, 1977.

269. Scheinberg, M.A., and Cathcart, E.S.: Comprehensive study of humoral and cellular immune abnormalities in 26 patients with systemic amyloidosis. Arthritis Rheum. 19:173, 1976.

270. Scheinberg, M.A., and Cathcart, E.S.: New concepts in the pathogenesis of primary and secondary amyloidosis. Clin. Exp. Immunol. 33:185, 1978.

271. Lowenstein, J., and Gallo, G.: Remission of the nephrotic syndrome in renal amyloidosis. N. Engl. J. Med. 282:128, 1970.

272. Fitchen, J.H.: Amyloidosis and granulomatous ileocolitis: Regression after surgical removal of the involved bowel. N. Engl. J. Med. 292:352, 1974.

273. Dikman, S.H., Kahn, T., Gribetz, D., and Churg, J.: Resolution of renal amyloidosis. Am. J. Med. 63:430, 1977.

274. Scheinberg, M.A., Goldstein, A.L., and Cathcart, E.S.: Thymosin restores T cell function and reduces the incidence of amyloid disease in casein-treated mice. J. Immunol. 116:156, 1976.

275. Missmahl, H-P.: Follow-up studies for a 30-year period on patients with amyloidosis; diagnostic methods; treatment. In Mandema, E., Ruinen, L., Scholten, J.H., and Cohen, A.S. (eds.): Amyloidosis. Amsterdam, Excerpta Medica, 1968, p. 429.

276. Kedar, I., Ravid, M., Sohar, E., and Gafni, J.: Colchicine inhibition of casein-induced amyloidosis in mice. Isr. J. Med. Sci. 10:787, 1974.

277. Shirahama, T., and Cohen, A.S.: Blockage of amyloid induction by colchicine in an animal model. J. Exp. Med. 140:1102, 1974.

278. Kedar, I., Greenwald, M., and Ravid, M.: Treatment of experimental murine amyloidosis with dimethyl sulphoxide. Eur. J. Clin. Invest. 7:149, 1977.

279. Ravid, M., Kedar, I., and Sohar, E.: Effects of a single dose of dimethyl sulphoxide on renal amyloidosis. Lancet 1:730, 1977.

280. Spero, J.A., Lewis, J.H., Hasiba, U., and Ellis, I.D.: Treatment of amyloidosis associated factor X deficiency. Thromb. Haemostas. 35:377, 1975.

281. Gurland, H.J., Brunner, F.P., Chantler, C., Jacobs, C., Scharer, K., Selwood, N.H., Spies, G., and Wing, A.J.: Combined report on regular dialysis and transplantation in Europe. VI Proc. Eur. Dial. Transplant. Assoc. 13:3, 1977.

282. Advisory Committee to the Royal Transplant Registry: Renal transplantation in congenital and metabolic diseases. A report from the ASC/NIH renal transplant registry. J.A.M.A. 232:148, 1975.

Chapter 93

The Rheumatic Manifestations of Sarcoidosis

William J. Arnold

INTRODUCTION

Sarcoidosis is a puzzling multisystem disorder of unknown etiology and pathogenesis that is characterized by the presence of noncaseating granulomas in biopsy specimens from clinically involved or uninvolved organs.[1,2] The disease usually begins in the third or fourth decade of life and involves both sexes with equal frequency. Sarcoidosis predominantly affects young adults, presenting most frequently with bilateral hilar lymphadenopathy, pulmonary infiltration, and skin and eye lesions.[3,4] Peripheral lymphadenopathy, hepatosplenomegaly, cardiac, renal, and skeletal muscle involvement, bone and joint lesions, and central and peripheral nervous system involvement may occur in addition to the more prominent clinical manifestations. In the United States, a higher prevalence of sarcoidosis has been noted in Blacks, but individuals of any racial or ethnic origin may be affected.[5] Sporadic instances of familial sarcoidosis have been reported.[6] The Kveim test has been found to be positive in 79 percent of 3676 patients with sarcoidosis studied in a large worldwide series.[3] However, the specificity of this test for sarcoidosis has been questioned.[7] Histologic examination of tissues from patients with sarcoidosis reveals the presence of numerous granulomas composed primarily of epithelioid cells with occasional giant cells in the absence of caseation necrosis.[2] Recent studies have suggested that the epithelioid cells in the sarcoid granuloma are metabolically active in the synthesis of angiotensin-I-converting enzyme and 1,25 dihydroxyvitamin D.[8-10a] Crystalline or Schaumann conchoidal inclusion bodies can frequently be found in the cytoplasm of the giant cells within the granulomas, particularly if the disease is of long duration. The sarcoid granuloma may resolve spontaneously or may slowly undergo hyaline fibrosis. Histologically similar granulomas may be found in chronic berylliosis, tuberculosis, histoplasmosis, coccidioidomycosis, lymphoma, Hodgkin's disease, bronchogenic carcinoma, foreign body granuloma, drug reactions, schistosomiasis, syphilis, and leprosy.[1,2]

CLINICAL FEATURES

Pulmonary involvement detected by chest x-ray is found in at least 90 percent of patients with sarcoidosis.[3,4] Bilateral hilar adenopathy, with or without parenchymal involvement, is the most frequent pulmonary finding. The prognosis of sarcoidosis is best predicted by the roentgenographic stage of the pulmonary disease present at the time of diagnosis.*[3,4,11] Total resolution of stage 1 disease occurs in approximately 60 percent of patients. Stage 2 disease has a less favorable course, with a resolution rate of about 46 percent. Stage 3 disease is frequently associated with bullae, dense fibrosis, pulmonary insufficiency, and cor pulmonale and has an expected incidence of resolution of only about 12 percent. The overall mortality in a large series of patients with sarcoidosis from several centers around the world was 6 percent.[4] Approximately 90 percent of the fatalities could be directly related to sarcoidosis.

Skin lesions, other than erythema nodosum, are asymptomatic and appear as hyperpigmented papules that most commonly occur around the mouth, eyes, ears, and nape of the neck (Fig. 93–1*A*). Skin lesions, including erythema nodosum, are found in approximately 30 percent of patients.[3,4] The incidence of erythema nodosum in sarcoidosis varies markedly with ethnic background and geographic location and appears most commonly in, Irish females in London and Puerto Ricans in New York City.[3]

Eye involvement occurs in approximately 20 percent of patients. Although a wide spectrum of ocular abnormalities can be found, the uveal tract is affected in 75 percent of these patients. Thirteen percent of patients with uveitis may develop total blindness.

IMMUNOLOGY AND BIOCHEMISTRY

The pathogenesis of pulmonary sarcoidosis is related to the proliferation of activated T lymphocytes in the lung.[12] Recent studies have shown that this proliferation may be due to the release of interleukin-2 by lung T lymphocytes.[13] Conversely, most previous studies of skin and peripheral blood found depressed parameters of cellular immunity in patients with sarcoidosis. Although cutaneous anergy to purified protein derivative (PPD) occurs in 64 percent of patients, anergy to a battery of four antigens (PPD, mumps, Candida and streptokinase-streptodornase [SK-SD] occurs in no more than 20 per-

---

*Stage 0 = Clear chest x-ray
Stage 1 = Bilateral hilar adenopathy
Stage 2 = Bilateral hilar adenopathy with infiltrates
Stage 3 = Pulmonary infiltrates without hilar adenopathy

Figure 93-1. Osseous sarcoidosis. *A,* Typical papular skin lesions of lupus pernio located on the external nares, malar eminences, eyelids, and corners of the mouth in a patient with chronic (Stage III) sarcoidosis. *B,* Hands in the same patient. The scaling lesions located on the second and fourth fingers of the left hand are the site of a soft tissue biopsy, which revealed noncaseating granulomas. *C,* X-ray of the patient's left hand taken in the anteroposterior (on the left) and semioblique positions. In addition to the soft tissue swelling, numerous lytic and destructive lesions are present, primarily in the heads of the proximal and middle phalanges.

cent of patients.[14] The total peripheral blood lymphocyte count in most patients with sarcoidosis is significantly depressed when compared with a normal control population.[15-17] The absolute number and percentage of T lymphocytes have been found to be either normal or depressed.[14-17] Also, in vitro stimulation of peripheral blood lymphocytes with phytohemagglutinin, concanavalin A, and pokeweed mitogen has been either depressed or normal and was not always correlated with cutaneous anergy.[18] It is now clear that studies of uninvolved tissues, such as peripheral blood, do not reflect the ongoing immune process at the site of granuloma formation.[12]

Several biochemical abnormalities have been described in patients with sarcoidosis. Hypercalcemia and hypercalciuria have been found in 3 percent to 28 percent of patients with sarcoidosis.[4] Recent reports have documented elevated levels of 1,25-dihydroxyvitamin D in hypercalcemic sarcoid patients even after bilateral nephrectomy, suggesting that the increased levels of calcium are due to enhanced synthesis or reduced catabolism of

this active vitamin D metabolite.[9] Hyperuricemia has been noted in from 10 percent to 50 percent of patients in whom it has been measured.[19,20] One author has concluded that hyperuricemia in sarcoidosis is seen only in patients with renal failure; however, this inference is clearly not supported in other studies.[19,21] Although clinical sequelae of hyperuricemia occur rarely in sarcoidosis, it has been reported that several patients have had the triad of gout, psoriasis, and sarcoidosis.[22,23]

Lieberman first reported elevated levels of serum angiotensin-converting enzyme (ACE) in patients with sarcoidosis.[24] Elevated levels occurred in 60 percent of patients and appeared to be related to active disease, whereas patients who were in remission or who were receiving steroids had normal ACE levels.[24,26-28] Subsequent studies have demonstrated that serum ACE levels correlate best with the amount and activity of pulmonary parenchymal involvement in sarcoidosis.[25,26] Although elevated serum ACE levels are also found in Gaucher's disease and in leprosy, other diseases that can be confused with sarcoidosis but have normal serum ACE levels include Wegener's granulomatosis, lymphomatoid granulomatosis, and tuberculosis.[27]

Gallium citrate binds to the surface of mononuclear cells presented at inflammatory sites and gallium scans are reported to be abnormal in 97 percent of patients with active sarcoidosis.[28] This increased uptake in the pulmonary parenchyma on gallium scanning is significantly correlated with an elevated serum ACE level.[28] Although an abnormal gallium scan is not specific for sarcoidosis, if pulmonary uptake of gallium is accompanied by parotid uptake or by an elevated serum ACE level, the diagnosis of sarcoidosis is much more likely.[28-30] Pulmonary gallium accumulation, but not serum ACE levels, correlated with the percentage of lymphocytes in bronchoalveolar lavage (BAL) fluid,[31,32] and an increased number of lymphocytes, T lymphocytes, and activated T lymphocytes are found in BAL specimens from patients with active versus inactive sarcoidosis.[12] Finally, gallium scanning may be useful both to stage the activity and to guide the therapy of sarcoidosis.

Pulmonary talc granulomatosis is the only other illness besides sarcoidosis that is associated with the combination of an elevated serum ACE level, a positive gallium scan, and an increased percentage of lymphocytes in BAL fluid.[33] The diagnosis of pulmonary talc granulomatosis is established by the finding of birefringent talc particles with examination of the BAL fluid by polarizing microscopy.

RHEUMATIC MANIFESTATIONS

Sarcoid Arthritis. Arthritis is the most frequent rheumatic manifestation of sarcoidosis, occurring in 5 to 37 percent of patients.[20,21,34] Sarcoid arthritis is two- to three-fold more common in females. Two distinct clinical patterns of sarcoid arthritis have been recognized in adults.[20,26,35] The most common form of arthritis occurs acutely and is often the initial manifestation of sarcoidosis. Frequently, erythema nodosum and bilateral hilar adenopathy are associated with the arthritis (Löfgren's syndrome). The clinical features of acute sarcoid arthritis are identical in patients with or without erythema nodosum.[36] Periarthritis and tenosynovitis also commonly accompany the arthritis and can appear without arthritis. Acute sarcoid arthritis is best characterized as a symmetric, migratory, additive polyarthritis most frequently involving the knees, ankles, proximal interphalangeal joints, wrists, and elbows.[20,21] Monoarticular acute sarcoid arthritis is extremely unusual. The arthritis reaches maximal intensity within 3 days of onset and may last from 2 weeks to 4 months. Pain and limitation of motion are the primary signs of inflammation in acute sarcoid arthritis. Synovial effusions are usually minimal. Joint deformity or destruction does not occur in acute sarcoid arthritis.

The erythrocyte sedimentation rate and C-reactive protein (CRP) are elevated in 80 and 60 percent of patients with acute sarcoid arthritis, respectively.[20] Approximately 15 percent of the patients will have rheumatoid factor detected in the serum by either the latex fixation technique or the sheep cell agglutination technique.[20] In one series, hyperuricemia was noted in 25 percent of 24 patients with acute sarcoid arthritis.[20] Chest x-rays of patients with acute sarcoid arthritis reveal bilateral hilar adenopathy, with or without interstitial changes, in greater than 90 percent of the patients.[20,21] Roentgenograms of involved joints reveal only soft tissue swelling.

Synovial biopsy results have not been reported in patients with acute sarcoid arthritis. However, tendon sheath biopsies from patients with tenosynovitis that is associated with acute sarcoid arthritis have revealed noncaseating granulomas with multinucleated giant cells.[20] Synovial fluid analysis has revealed an inflammatory effusion in one patient with acute sarcoid arthritis.[37]

Sarcoidosis should be suspected in any young adult presenting with acute polyarthritis or periarthritis, particularly in the presence of erythema nodosum. The diagnosis of rheumatoid arthritis is frequently suggested by the symmetric pattern of joint involvement and the finding of rheumatoid factor in the serum. In the early stages of acute sarcoid arthritis, acute rheumatic fever may be considered because of the migratory nature of the arthritis. Histoplasmosis may also present with bilateral hilar adenopathy and joint pain.[38] In this instance, the diagnosis is based on the isolation of *Histoplasma capsulatum* from blood and bone marrow cultures. Finally, the rapid development of the articular inflammation in a patient with hyperuricemia would raise the possibility of gouty arthritis. The clinical findings of bilateral hilar adenopathy, erythema nodosum, and synovianalysis with polarizing microscopy would differentiate acute sarcoid arthritis from the aforementioned possibilities.

Chronic sarcoid arthritis may begin early or late in the course of the disease and may occur with acute exacerbations over a period of years. Rarely, chronic sarcoid arthritis may have an insidious onset and produce polyarticular joint destruction and disability, suggestive of the diagnosis of rheumatoid arthritis.[39] In chronic sarcoid arthritis mono- or oligoarticular involvement in the knees and ankles is frequent.[40,41] Chronic destructive sarcoid arthritis of the temporomandibular joint has also recently been reported.[42] The diagnosis of infectious arthritis, particularly tuberculous arthritis and sporotrichosis, should be considered in patients with chronic sarcoid arthritis.[43] Synovial fluid analysis in patients with chronic sarcoid arthritis has revealed characteristics of a group II inflammatory fluid.[21] Therefore, the diagnosis of infectious arthritis is best excluded by negative synovial fluid cultures and the finding of noncaseating granulomas in synovial biopsy specimens.[20,21]

In children, sarcoid arthritis begins before age 4 years and is manifested by painless, boggy synovial proliferation and effusions of tendon sheaths and joints.[44,44a] Destructive articular changes and pulmonary disease are also unusual in these children with sarcoid arthritis, though skin and ocular abnormalities occur frequently. Circulating immune complexes may participate in the pathogenesis of acute sarcoid arthritis. Immune complexes have been found in the serum of patients with sarcoidosis, erythema nodosum, and polyarthritis.[45-47] In addition, the presence in serum of C3 activation products has been reported in this group of patients.[46] Membranous glomerulonephritis associated with electron dense subepithelial immune deposits has been described in a patient with sarcoidosis,[48] and the presence of circulating immune complexes has been documented in a patient with coexistent systemic lupus erythematosus and sarcoidosis.[49]

An inherited predisposition for patients with sarcoidosis to develop arthritis has been suggested by the finding of an increased incidence of HLA-B8 in patients with sarcoid arthritis.[50]

The choice of therapy for sarcoid arthritis will depend on the severity and chronicity of the patient's symptoms. No therapy is indicated for mild, transient arthritis. In patients with moderately severe, acute sarcoid arthritis, therapy with salicylates should be attempted first. A daily total of 3.6 g of aspirin administered in divided doses has been adequate in some patients. Oral colchicine therapy has been reported to be effective in patients with acute or chronic sarcoid arthritis of moderate severity.[35,51,52] The same therapy may be effective for sarcoid periarthritis, which is characterized by warm, red, tender areas of skin overlying the joints but not involving the synovium.[53] One colchicine tablet (0.6 mg) should be administered at hourly intervals until relief is obtained or side effects such as diarrhea and nausea and vomiting occur. Although 7 mg of colchicine is the maximum recommended oral dose for an attack, it is of note that as much as 9.6 mg of oral colchicine has been required for relief.[51] In patients with severely symptomatic acute or chronic sarcoid arthritis or patients who have not responded to aspirin or colchicine, prednisone administered orally as a single daily dose of 15 to 40 mg has been effective in suppressing articular inflammation until spontaneous resolution occurs. Longterm therapy with 7.5 to 15 mg of prednisone administered on alternate days may be effective in the treatment of recurrent acute or indolent sarcoid arthritis. Finally, anecdotal reports of the effectiveness of chloroquine and methotrexate suggest that these agents should be reserved for treatment of severe sarcoid arthritis that is resistant to prednisone therapy.

Osseous Sarcoidosis. Bone lesions occur in 3 to 9 percent of patients with sarcoidosis.[3,4,19] The lesions are frequently asymptomatic and most commonly occur in the bones of the hands and feet.[19] A striking association between the occurrence of bone lesions and chronic skin lesions has been noted (see Fig. 93–1A).[19] When osseous sarcoid extensively involves the hands, a diffuse "spongy" thickening of the fingers and thumb may be noted (see Fig. 93–1B). Although radiographic characteristics of osseous sarcoid are variable, lytic lesions are the most common abnormality (see Fig. 93–1C).[19] They may appear as minute cortical defects or cysts in phalangeal or metatarsal heads. Less frequent x-ray changes include thickening of cortical bone with a fine lacy re-

ticular alteration of the trabecular pattern, sclerosis of the distal phalanges, or gross destructive changes of bone that may secondarily produce joint destruction. Scanning techniques utilizing ^{99m}Tc-pyrophosphate[54] may be a more sensitive indicator than routine x-rays of early osseous sarcoidosis.[55]

Although osseous sarcoid is most common in the hands and feet, involvement of the skull, nasal bones, vertebrae, and long bones has been reported. Sarcoid of the skull is perhaps the rarest of all osseous involvements.[56] The lesions appear as multiple lytic defects and may be associated with overlying soft tissue masses that contain granulomas. A total of 11 patients have been described with vertebral sarcoidosis. Vertebral involvement presents radiographically as extensive lytic and sclerotic changes of one or more vertebrae in any area of the spine.[57] Vertebral sarcoidosis may clinically present with either back pain or neurologic deficits resulting from spinal cord compression. Since involvement of the pedicles and disc space may occur, biopsy is needed for definitive diagnosis. An unusual patient with vertebral sarcoidosis and ligamentous ossification suggestive of ankylosing spondylitis has recently been reported.[58] Although involvement of long bones is rare, pathologic fractures have been noted secondary to osseous sarcoid.[59] Although lytic lesions are characteristic of osseous sarcoid, osteosclerotic lesions have also been reported.[60]

The diagnosis of osseous sarcoidosis is seldom difficult, since abnormal chest x-rays and chronic skin lesions are also present in greater than 70 percent of these patients.[19] In addition, 54 percent of patients with osseous sarcoid have concomitant ocular abnormalities. However, an isolated case of sarcoidosis limited to the hands and feet has been reported.[61] In this case, the diagnosis was made by the demonstration of noncaseating granulomas in a bone biopsy specimen.

If osseous sarcoidosis is asymptomatic, therapy is not indicated. However, if pain, disability, or deformity is present, the drug of choice for osseous sarcoid at any site appears to be steroids. Documented healing of cystic and destructive lesions has occurred during steroid therapy.[19,56,57,60,61]

Sarcoidosis of Muscle. Skeletal muscle sarcoidosis is usually asymptomatic.[62-64] First described by Myers and associates, involvement of skeletal muscle in patients with sarcoidosis is reliably detected only by examining serial sections of generous muscle biopsy specimens.[65] From 50 to 80 percent of muscle biopsy specimens obtained from patients who have had sarcoidosis for less than 2 years will contain typical noncaseating granulomas (Fig. 93–2).[63,65] Thus, in a patient suspected of having sarcoidosis, a random muscle biopsy specimen may be useful in confirming the diagnosis.

Symptoms of skeletal muscle involvement in patients with sarcoidosis may consist of acute muscle pain and weakness or chronic muscle wasting and weakness.[62-64,66] Acute skeletal muscle sarcoidosis may be indistinguishable from idiopathic polymyositis, since weakness of proximal muscles is prominent and the electromyogram reveals nonspecific myositis.[66,67] Although myopathy

Figure 93–2. Skeletal muscle sarcoidosis. *A*, Longitudinal section of a gastrocnemius muscle biopsy specimen obtained from a patient with stage II sarcoidosis and acute muscle weakness and pain. Multiple noncaseating granulomas with giant cells and a sparse lymphocytic infiltrate are located between apparently normal muscle fibers. (Original magnification $\times$ 250.) *B*, Higher magnification demonstrates the epithelioid cells abutting a vacuolated muscle fiber that has retained its cross-striations. (Original magnification $\times$ 400.)

could occur as an isolated manifestation of the disease, the diagnosis of sarcoidosis is usually obvious because of concomitant multisystem involvement.[68] Rarely, acute skeletal muscle sarcoidosis may be present as tender, palpable muscle nodules or pseudohypertrophy.[64] Biopsy of these nodules has revealed typical noncaseating granulomas. Typically, chronic skeletal muscle sarcoidosis occurs in patients with longstanding multisystem disease who may have palpably "hard" muscles.[69]

A puzzling aspect of sarcoidosis of skeletal muscle is the pathogenesis of symptomatic skeletal muscle disease. Since muscle biopsy specimens are similar in both the asymptomatic and symptomatic forms, factors other than the presence and distribution of the noncaseating granulomas must be operative.

Involvement of cardiac muscle is also most frequently asymptomatic and may be present in up to 20 percent of patients at autopsy.[70,71] Symptomatic cardiac muscle involvement has been found in 5 to 13 percent of patients and most frequently presents as a disturbance of cardiac rhythm. A direct relation between skeletal and cardiac muscle sarcoidosis has been suggested by the finding of a high coincidence between the presence of skeletal and cardiac muscle granulomas at autopsy.

Asymptomatic sarcoidosis of skeletal muscle requires no therapy. Administration of steroids to patients with symptomatic muscular sarcoidosis is recommended by most authors, but others have questioned the effectiveness of this therapy.[66] Steroids are most effective in acute myopathy and are of little benefit in chronic myopathy.

REFERENCES

1. Mitchell, D.N., and Scadding, J.G.: Sarcoidosis. Am. Rev. Resp. Dis. 110:774, 1974.
2. Mitchell, D.N., Scadding, J.G., Heard, B.E., and Hinson, K.F.: Sarcoidosis: Hisopathological definition and clinical diagnosis. J. Clin. Pathol. 30:395, 1977.
3. Siltzbach, L.E., James, D.G., Neville, E., et al.: Course and prognosis of sarcoidosis around the world. Am. J. Med. 57:847, 1974.
4. James, D.G., Neville, E., Siltzbach, L.E., et al.: A worldwide review of sarcoidosis. Ann. N.Y. Acad. Sci. 278:321, 1976.

5. Sartwell, P.E.: Racial difference in sarcoidosis. Ann. N.Y. Acad. Sci. 278:368, 1976.

6. Sharma, O.P., Neville, E., Walker, A.N., and James, D.G.: Familial sarcoidosis: A possible genetic influence. Ann. N.Y. Acad. Sci. 278:386, 1976.

7. Israel, H.L., and Goldstein, R.A.: Relation of Kveim-antigen reaction to lymphadenopathy. N. Engl. J. Med. 284:345, 1971.

8. Silverstein, E., Friendland, J., Lyons, H.A., and Gourin, A.: Markedly elevated angiotensin converting enzyme in lymph nodes containing nonnecrotizing granulomas in sarcoidosis. Proc. Natl. Acad. Sci. U.S.A. 73:2137, 1976.

9. Barbour, G., Coburn, J., Slatopulsky, E., et al: Hypercalcemia in an anephric patient with sarcoidosis: Evidence for extrarenal generation of 1,25-dihydroxyvitamin D. N. Engl. J. Med. 305:440, 1981.

10. Maesaka, J., Bautman, V., Pablo, N., and Shakamuri, S.: Elevated 1,25-dihydroxyvitamin D levels—occurrence with sarcoidosis with end-stage renal disease. Arch. Intern. Med. 142:1206, 1982.

10a. Mason, R.S., Frankel, T., Chan, Y., et al.: Vitamin D conversion by sarcoid lymph node homogenate. Ann. Intern. Med. 100:59, 1984.

11. Wurm, K., and Rosner, R.: Prognosis of chronic sarcoidosis. Ann. N.Y. Acad. Sci. 278:732, 1976.

12. Crystal, R.G., Roberts, W., Hunninghake, G., et al.: Pulmonary sarcoidosis: A disease characterized and perpetuated by activated lung T-lymphocytes (NIH Conference). Ann. Intern. Med. 94:73, 1981.

13. Pinkston, P., Bitterman, P.B., Crystal, R.G.: Spontaneous release of interleukin-2 by lung T-lymphocytes in active pulmonary sarcoidosis. N. Engl. J. Med. 308:793, 1983.

14. Tannenbaum, H., Rocklin, R.E., Schur, P.H., and Sheffer, A.L.: Immune function in sarcoidosis. Clin. Exp. Immunol. 26:511, 1976.

15. Kataria, Y.P., LoBuglio, A.F., Bromber, P.A., and Hurtubise, P.E.: Sarcoid lymphocytes: B- and T-cell quantitation. Ann. N.Y. Acad. Sci. 278:69, 1976.

16. Daniele, R.P., and Rowland, D.T., Jr.: Lymphocyte subpopulations in sarcoidosis: Correlation with disease activity and duration. Ann. Intern. Med. 85:593, 1976.

17. Hedfors, E., Holm, G., and Pettersson, D.: Lymphocyte subpopulations in sarcoidosis. Clin. Exp. Immunol. 17:219, 1974.

18. Goldstein, R.A., Janicki, B.W., Mirro, J., and Foellmer, J.W.: Cell-mediated immune responses in sarcoidosis. Am. Rev. Respir. Dis. 117:55, 1978.

19. Neville, E., Carstairs, L.S., and James, D.G.: Bone sarcoidosis. Ann. N.Y. Acad. Sci. 278:475, 1976.

20. Spilberg, I., Siltzbach, L.E., and McEwen, C.E.: The arthritis of sarcoidosis. Arthritis Rheum. 12:126, 1969.

21. Siltzbach, L.E., and Duberstein, J.L.: Arthritis in sarcoidosis. Clin. Orthop. Rel. Res. 57:31, 1968.

22. Simmer, J.G., and Demis, D.J.: Associations between gout, psoriasis and sarcoidosis. Ann. Intern. Med. 64:786, 1966.

23. Bunim, J.J., Kimberg, D.V., Thomas, L.B., et al.: Syndrome of sarcoidosis, psoriasis and gout. Ann. Intern. Med. 57:1018, 1962.

24. Lieberman, J.: Elevation of serum angiotensin-converting enzyme (ACE) level in sarcoidosis. Am. J. Med. 59:365, 1975.

25. Rohatgi, P.K., Ryan, J., and Lindeman, J.: Value of serial measurement of angiotensin converting enzyme in the management of sarcoidosis. Am. J. Med. 70:44, 1981.

26. Rohrback, M.S., and DeRemee, R.A.: Pulmonary sarcoidosis and serum angiotensin-converting enzyme. Mayo Clin. Proc. 57:64, 1982.

27. Katz, P., Fauci, A.S., Yeager, H., and Reen, B.: Serum angiotensin-converting enzyme and lysozymel in granulomatous disease of unknown cause. Ann. Intern. Med. 94:359, 1981.

28. Gupta, R., Bekerman, C., Sicilian, L., et al.: Gallium 67 citrate scanning and serum angiotensin converting enzyme levels in sarcoidosis. Radiology 144:895, 1982.

29. Wiener, S.N., and Patel, B.: 67 GA-Citrate uptake by the parotid glands in sarcoidosis. Nucl. Med. 130:763, 1979.

30. Nosal, A.D., Schleissner, L.A., Mishkin, F.S., and Lieberman, J.: Angiotensin-1-coverting enzyme and gallium scan in noninvasive evaluation of sarcoidosis. Ann. Intern. Med. 90:328, 1979.

31. Rossman, M.D., Dauber, J.H., Cardello, M.E., and Daniele, R.P.: Pulmonary sarcoidosis: correlation of serum angiotensin-converting enzyme with blood and bronchoalveolar lymphocytes. Am. Rev. Resp. Dis. 125:266, 1982.

32. Line, B.R., Hunninghake, G.W., Keogh, B.A., et al.: Gallium 67 scanning to stage the alveolitis of sarcoidosis: correlation with clinical studies, pulmonary function studies and bronchoalveolar lavage. Am. Rev. Resp. Dis. 124:440, 1981.

33. Farber, H.W., Fairman, R.P., and Glauser, F.L.: Talc granulomatosis: laboratory findings similar to sarcoidosis. Am. Rev. Resp. Dis. 125:258, 1982.

34. Mayock, R.L., Bertrand, P., Morrison, C.E., and Scott, J.H.: Manifestations of sarcoidosis. Am. J. Med. 35:67, 1963.

35. Kaplan, H.: Sarcoid arthritis. Arch. Intern. Med. 112:924, 1963.

36. Pennec, Y., Youinou, P., LeGoff, P., et al: Comparison of the manifes-

37. Varkey, B.: Synovial fluid in sarcoid arthritis. Ann. Intern. Med. 81:557, 1974.

38. Thornberry, D.K., Wheat, L.J., Brandt, K.D., and Rosenthal, J.: Histoplasmosis presenting with joint pain and hilar adenopathy. Arthritis Rheum. 25:1396, 1982.

39. Boyd, R.E., and Andrews, B.S.: Sarcoidosis presenting as cutaneous ulceration, subcutaneous nodules and chronic arthritis. J. Rheum. 8:311, 1981.

40. Turek, S.L.: Sarcoid disease of bone at the ankle joint. J. Bone Joint Surg. 35:465, 1953.

41. Bjarnason, D.F., Forrester, D.M., and Swezey, R.L.: Destructive arthritis of the large joints. J. Bone Joint Surg. 55:618, 1973.

42. Schwartz, H.C.: Sarcoid temporomandibular arthritis. Oral Surg. 30:588, 1981.

43. Boehm, D., Lynch, J.M., Hodges, G.R., et al.: Case report. Disseminated sporotrichosis presenting as sarcoidosis: electron microscopic and immunologic studies. Am. J. Med. Sci. 283:71, 1982.

44. North, A.F., Fink, C.W., Gibson, W.M., et al.: Sarcoid arthritis in children. Am. J. Med. 48:449, 1970.

44a. Rosenberg, A.M., Yee, E.H., and MacKenzie, J.W.: Arthritis in childhood sarcoidosis. J. Rheumaltol. 10:987, 1983.

45. Hedfors, E., and Norberg, R.: Evidence for circulating immune complexes in sarcoidosis. Clin. Exp. Immunol. 16:493, 1974.

46. Jones, J.V., Cumming, R.H., Asplin, C.M., et al.: Circulating immune complexes in erythema nodosum and early sarcoidosis. Lancet 1:153, 1976.

47. Gupta, R.C., Kueppers, F., DeRemee, R.A., et al.: Pulmonary and extrapulmonary sarcoidosis in relation to circulating immune complexes. Am. Rev. Resp. Dis. 116:261, 1977.

48. Taylor, T.K., Senekjian, H.O., Knight, T.F., et al.: Membranous nephropathy with epithelial crescents in a patient with pulmonary sarcoidosis. Arch. Intern. Med. 139:1183, 1979.

49. Needleman, S.W., Silber, R.A., Von Brecht, J.H., and Gocken, J.A.: Systemic lupus erythematosus complicated by disseminated sarcoidosis. Am. J. Clin. Pathol. 78:105, 1982.

50. Brewerton, D.A., Cockburn, C., James, D.C., James, D.G., and Neville, E.: HLA antigens in sarcoidosis. Clin. Exp. Immunol. 27:227, 1977.

51. Kaplan, H.: Sarcoid arthritis with a response to colchicine. N. Engl. J. Med. 263:778, 1960.

52. Kaplan, H.: Further experience with colchicine in the treatment of sarcoid arthritis. N. Engl. J. Med. 268:761, 1963.

53. Harris, E.D., Jr., and Millis, M.: Treatment with colchicine of the periarticular inflammation associated with sarcoidosis: A need for continued appraisal. Arthritis Rheum. 14:130, 1971.

54. McBrine, C.S., and Fisher, M.S.: Acrosclerosis in sarcoidosis. Radiology 115:279, 1975.

55. Reginato, A.J., Schiappaccase, U., Guzman, L., and Claure, H.: ^{99m}Tc-pyrophosphate scintiphotography in bone sarcoidosis. J. Rheumatol. 3:426, 1976.

56. Franco-Saenz, R., Ludwig, G.D., and Henderson, L.W.: Sarcoidosis of the skull. Ann. Intern. Med. 72:929, 1970.

57. Baldwin, D.M., Roberts, J.G., and Croft, H.E.: Vertebral sarcoidosis. J. Bone Joint Surg. 56:629, 1974.

58. Perlman, S.G., Damergis, J., Witorsch, P., et al.: Vertebral sarcoidosis with paravertebral ossification. Arthritis Rheum. 21:271, 1978.

59. Watson, R.C., and Cahen, I.: Pathological fracture in long bone sarcoidosis. J. Bone Joint Surg. 55:613, 1973.

60. Marcove, R.C., Rooney, R., and Weis, L.D.: Osteosclerotic lesions in sarcoidosis. Clin. Orthop. Rel. Res. 129:248, 1977.

61. Schriber, R.A., and Firooznia, H.: Extensive phalangeal cystic lesions—limited sarcoidosis. Arthritis Rheum. 18:123, 1975.

62. Silverstein, A., and Siltzbach, L.E.: Muscle involvement in sarcoidosis. Arch. Neurol. 21:235, 1969.

63. Wallace, S.L., Lattes, R., Malia, J.P., and Ragan, C.: Muscle involvement in Boeck's sarcoid. Ann. Intern. Med. 48:497, 1958.

64. Douglas, A.C., Macleod, J.G., and Matthews, J.D.: Symptomatic sarcoidosis of skeletal muscle. J. Neurol. Neurosurg. Psychiat. 36:1034, 1973.

65. Myers, G.B., Gottlieb, A.M., Mattman, P.E., et al.: Joint and skeletal muscle manifestations in sarcoidosis. Am. J. Med. 12:161, 1952.

66. Thorpe, C.G.: Muscle weakness due to sarcoid myopathy. Neurology 22:917, 1972.

67. Hinterbuchner, C.N., and Hinterbuchner, L.P.: Myopathic syndrome in muscular sarcoidosis. Brain 87:355, 1964.

68. Lynch, P.G., and Banasal, D.V.: Granulomatous polymyositis. J. Neurol. Sci. 18:1, 1973.

69. Delaney, P.: Neurologic manifestations in sarcoidosis. Ann. Intern. Med. 87:336, 1977.

70. Fleming, H.A., Gresham, G.A., and Stovin, P.G.I.: Myocardial sarcoidosis. Br. Heart J. 34:769, 1972.

71. Roberts, W.C., McAllister, H.A., Jr., and Ferrans, W.: Sarcoidosis of the heart. Am. J. Med. 63:86, 1977.

Chapter 94

Arthropathy with Iron Storage Disease

Irving H. Fox

INTRODUCTION

Iron storage disease refers to a group of disorders characterized by an increased accumulation of iron in tissues. Hemosiderosis is a state of increased iron stores, particularly in cells of the reticuloendothelial system, with localization in only a few organs, such as the liver and bone marrow. There are no characteristic pathologic changes of tissue structure or function. Hemochromatosis is a "disorder of the control of iron absorption in which iron is admitted by the intestine irrespective of the requirement for iron. The excess iron is deposited in tissue to their ultimate detriment so that patients develop cirrhosis, diabetes, sterility, myocardial incompetence, or other ailments.[1] Primary hemochromatosis refers to an idiopathic familial form of iron overload. Secondary hemochromatosis refers to an iron overload from increased intake or accumulation, which results from some other disorder. The following list provides a classification of excess iron stores:

Primary hemochromatosis
    Latent (precirrhotic phase)
    Cirrhotic stage
Secondary hemochromatosis
    Transfusion iron overload
    Increased absorption
        Chronic refractory anemia with hemolysis
        Increased dietary intake
        Pre-existing cirrhosis, especially with portacaval shunt
    Impaired iron transport
        Congenital transferrin deficiency
    Other
        Zellweger syndrome

Although a clear pathologic distinction has been drawn between hemochromatosis and hemosiderosis, it has been suggested from recent studies that these two disorders may represent a continuum of disease in familial hemochromatosis encompassing the "precirrhotic stage" and the fully manifested disorder.[2-4]

ETIOLOGY

Family studies have indicated that the metabolic abnormality in primary hemochromatosis is inherited.[1-5] The discovery of a significant association between primary hemochromatosis and HLA-A3 and HLA-B14 antigens has provided further data supporting a genetic basis for the disease.[6,7] HLA-A3 is found in 78 percent of patients, whereas HLA-B14 is found in 26 percent of patients. These data suggest that a hemochromatosis gene is closely linked to the HLA-A locus. In fact, studies of families indicate that a gene for idiopathic hemochromatosis is located close to the genes for HLA on the short arm of chromosome 6, since this gene is inherited together with the adjacent HLA haplotype.[6,8] Therefore, homozygosity and autosomal recessive inheritance for the disease has been established, since a gene for idiopathic hemochromatosis and a linked HLA group is contributed by each parent to the affected offspring.[9] HLA-A3-B14 is the most common haplotype. The abnormal gene has a frequency as high as 0.056.[10] The homozygous state may occur in 1 per 1000 people and may progress to overt tissue damage in approximately 1 per 5000 people.[11,12] Although there is strong evidence for a genetic basis in the primary form of the disease, data suggest that the expression of the clinical features is modified by environmental factors, including the quantities of alcohol intake and iron ingestion.[1-5]

Although the molecular basis for primary HLA-related hemochromatosis remains undefined, most studies have demonstrated an abnormal increase in the intestinal absorption of iron.[5] Increased uptake of iron by the mucosal cells of the duodenum has been demonstrated.[13] The internal distribution of excess iron in HLA-related iron overload appears to favor the parenchymal cells, with very little hemosiderin deposited in the reticuloendothelial system.[14] It has been proposed that intestinal and reticuloendothelial cells have defective iron storage, leading to an increased delivery of iron by the plasma to hepatocytes and other parenchymal cells.[15]

In other types of iron overload, large amounts of iron are present in reticuloendothelial cells, with variable involvement of the liver and other organs.[15] Secondary hemochromatosis and hemosiderosis are often associated with transfusion iron overload or excessive dietary intake (see preceding list).[5] In alcoholic cirrhosis, the associated hematologic complications, an increased dietary intake of iron, and an ethanol-mediated enhancement of ferric ion absorption[16] are factors that may predispose to secondary hemochromatosis. Alcohol intake and iron overload appear to contribute to the mild to moderate siderosis of porphyria cutanea tarda.[17] Increased absorption of iron from a normal dietary intake and a resultant excess iron storage are observed in anemia with erythroid hyperplasias and intramedullary hemolysis. Hematologic abnormalities, iron administration, and the HLA antigens associated with iron overload predispose hemodialysis patients to severe hemosiderosis.[18,19] Congenital transferrin deficiency results in the accumulation of unneeded iron.[20]

IRON DEPOSITION AND MUSCULOSKELETAL DISEASE

Clinically apparent disease usually results when 20 to 50 g of iron are present. This usually requires several decades, and most patients become symptomatic after the age of 40. The disease is ten times more frequent in males, since females are protected by the iron losses associated with menstruation, pregnancy, and lactation. In patients with primary hemochromatosis, an abnormality in the iron kinetics involves a 10- to 20-fold increase in the movement of iron from plasma into storage. This results in a massive increase in storage iron.

The mechanism by which an elevated concentration of storage iron ultimately causes tissue damage is unclear. The earliest detectable abnormalities in hereditary hemochromatosis include an increase in hepatic parenchymal cell-stainable iron, hepatic iron concentration, transferrin saturation, serum iron concentration, and serum ferritin concentration.[2-5] The transport protein for iron becomes saturated, and iron stores are increased. Ferritin is the primary and most readily available iron storage protein and functions as an alternative pathway for iron during iron absorption and heme synthesis. It is a compound formed from a variable number of hydrous ferric oxide–phosphate micelles that adhere to the inner spherical surface of apoferritin, a high molecular weight protein. Serum ferritin concentration is directly proportional to reticuloendothelial ferritin. The synthesis of ferritin is similar in normal subjects and in idiopathic hemochromatosis patients,[21] indicating that no defect can be linked to this compound.

Hemosiderin, a storage form of iron, is an insoluble compound that is formed from the denaturation of ferritin, with the associated loss of apoferritin, and micellar aggregation. It is only slowly mobilized. Transferrin is a plasma protein with an electrophoretic mobility of β_1-globulin. It is the carrier protein for iron. This single polypeptide has two iron-binding sites, so that it may exist as apoferric, monoferric, or diferric transferrin.[22] The transferrin-iron complex interacts with specific membrane receptors to deliver iron to tissues.[23]

Tissue damage is correlated with the location of iron in cells other than those of the reticuloendothelial system over long periods of time. Marked and persistent enlargement of the chelatable iron pool and saturation of the intracellular iron carrier result in deposition of iron and cellular damage. Excessive iron storage in patients is associated with an arthropathy that resembles degenerative arthritis with calcium pyrophosphate dihydrate deposition disease. The relationship between the degenerative arthritis and excessive iron stores is obscure. The

data suggest that iron deposition is responsible for producing the articular changes. Arthropathy occurs in half the patients with hemochromatosis and is associated with hemosiderin deposits in synovial membrane[24,25] and chondrocytes. The development of arthropathy in secondary hemochromatosis[24,26,27] or cartilage degeneration in immature rabbits overloaded with parenteral iron[28] further supports an etiologic role for iron. Ionic iron is toxic to cultured chondrocytes[29] and decreases the rate of clearance of calcium pyrophosphate dihydrate crystals from rabbit knee joints.[30]

The metabolic basis for these toxic properties is unclear, but there are a few clues from recent observations. Ionic iron uptake by synovial fibroblasts is accompanied by increased production of latent collagenase and prostaglandin E_2.[31] In addition, ferrous iron inhibits synovial tissue pyrophosphatase.[32] The latter may explain calcium pyrophosphate dihydrate deposition in cartilage. However, the data do not account for the continued progression of the articular disorder after iron removal by venesection therapy. Other speculations suggest that articular damage may result from an iron-mediated alteration of mucopolysaccharide complexes,[33] or an increase of lipid peroxidation, with membrane and lysosomal damage.[34-36]

Pathologic changes in hemochromatosis are characterized (Fig. 94–1) by increased amounts of hemosiderin in the synovial lining cells,[24,25,27,33,37-42] predominantly in the type B synthetic cells.[24] Hemosiderin is also present in lacunae and chondrocytes in cartilage,[33,40-42] although it has not been observed in all studies.[25,43] The amount of synovial iron deposition is directly related to the total body iron overload.[25] Synovial hemosiderosis is not specific for iron storage disorders, since it can be seen in other diseases, including rheumatoid arthritis.[24] Although synovial thickening may occur, there is little or no evidence of synovial inflammation. The cartilage from joints, which are radiologically abnormal, contains mineral deposits that have been characterized as calcium pyrophosphate;[33,43,44] these deposits are found in the superficial layer initially. Calcium phosphate deposits also may occasionally be present in synovium.[33] Other cartilage changes are similar to osteoarthritis.

Only limited data are available concerning the pathologic changes of iron overload secondary to blood transfusion.[27,40] The features appear to be similar to primary hemochromatosis. One possible exception to this may be a proximal myopathy that develops in iron-overloaded patients undergoing maintenance hemodialysis.[19] Proximal muscle biopsies showed iron deposition in either macrophages or muscle fibers. In iron overload associated with idiopathic hemochromatosis, proximal myopathy is not a common feature, although skeletal muscle iron deposition in the sarcoplasm and endomysium occurs in 45 percent of patients.[45]

Complex metabolic abnormalities from vitamin deficiencies may explain the osteoporosis that frequently occurs in hemochromatosis. These patients have reduced intestinal absorption of calcium and reduced plasma levels of 25-hydroxyvitamin D.[46] In addition, iron ov-

Figure 94-1. Iron stain of cartilage and synovium. These photographs show black granular material between nuclei. This represents the iron pigment. There is iron deposition in chondrocytes of hyaline cartilage (*A*) and in synovial lining cells and the underlying stroma (*B*). (Photographs were provided by Dr. Victor Fornasier, The Ontario Cancer Institute, Toronto, Canada.)

erload leads to ascorbic acid depletion by accelerating the oxidation of ascorbic acid to oxalic acid.[47-52] Frank scurvy has been observed during iron overload.[47-53] The association among iron overload, chronic ascorbic acid deficiency, and osteoporosis has been confirmed experimentally.[54]

CLINICAL FEATURES

Primary Hemochromatosis. Most patients with primary hemochromatosis first see a physician when they are between the ages of 40 and 60 years, with initial symptoms that are related to cirrhosis, darkening of the skin to a bronze or slate-gray color, diabetes, hypopituitarism, and arthropathy.

Early recognition of iron overload is now possible because of the recent advances in the understanding of the genetics of the disorder. By using HLA genotyping of siblings of patients with hemochromatosis, it has been possible to identify affected individuals before clinical manifestations develop and even before significant iron loading occurs.[55] It is now clear that joint pain occurs in more than 50 percent of patients and is the most frequent symptom of hemochromatosis at the time of presentation.[55] In one study the age of onset of arthralgias was 45 to 63 years, except for four persons in a single sibship in whom the onset occurred at 30 to 35 years of age.[55] Arthralgias were present an average of 4 years (1 to 15 years) before hemochromatosis was diagnosed. X-ray abnormalities were generally evident at the time of diagnosis. Therefore, a chronic arthropathy may provide the first clinical clue for occult iron storage disease.[41,42,56] Other presenting symptoms include intermittent pain of the right side of the upper abdomen, impotence, weakness, and fatigue.[55] Hepatomegaly and skin pigmentation were the most common abnormalities on physical examination and occurred in about 50 percent of patients.

The clinical features of the arthropathy associated with hemochromatosis have been extensively studied,[24,26,33,38,39,41-44,56-60] after the initial descriptions by Schumacher[37] and by Delbarre[57] in 1964. About 50 percent of patients with idiopathic hemochromatosis have an arthropathy. The earliest and usually the first joints to be affected by arthritic changes are the small joints of the hands, especially the second and third metacarpophalangeal joints.[26,33,37,41,42,44,58,59] This frequently observed arthropathy causes increasing stiffness of fingers, pain in hands with excessive use, slight bony swelling, and an inability to flex the metacarpophalangeal joints completely. With further progression, there is increased swelling and involvement of interphalangeal joints with restricted wrist movement. In many patients, there is a more generalized arthropathy involving wrists, shoulders, elbows, hips, knees, ankles, and spine. This can resemble degenerative arthritis with accompanying joint tenderness.[26,33,37,41-44,56-58] In 15 to 50 percent of patients, acute episodes of inflammatory arthritis are superimposed upon this chronic progressive arthritis. These acute episodes of arthritis are the same as acute pseudogout and result from a crystal-induced synovitis related to the presence of calcium pyrophosphate dihydrate crystals.[26,33,37,43,44,58]

Radiologic features include cystic changes and sclerosis in the subchondral bone, loss of articular cartilage, and chondrocalcinosis of articular cartilage.[26,33,37,41-44,57]

Characteristic changes are observed in the hands, with abnormalities of the second and third metacarpophalangeal joints (Fig. 94–2). The most common abnormalities include 1- to 3-mm cysts with sclerotic margins in the subarticular area of the metacarpal heads and at the base of the adjacent phalanges. The carpal joints are frequently abnormal. Cyst formation, usually in the distal end of the ulna and radius, occurs often with a loss of cartilage. In the hips, there may be subarticular cysts and a decrease of the cartilage space (Fig. 94–3). A loss of cartilage space and lipping at joint margins may be evident in the knees. Chondrocalcinosis may occur in up to half the patients with arthropathy,[26,33,37,41,43,44,56,57] including some patients with hemochromatosis with no symptomatic arthropathy.[26,43] The joints affected with chondrocalcinosis in this disease, in a decreasing order of frequency, include knee (menisci and articular cartilage), wrist (fibrocartilage of the triangular ligament), hips, and symphysis pubis. Chondrocalcinosis may also occur in the spine (intervertebral disc), Achilles tendon, and plantar fascia. Finally, osteoporosis is present in 25 to 50 percent of patients, although it is usually asymptomatic.[33,37]

It is unclear whether the arthropathy associated with primary hemochromatosis is specific for that disorder. Although this controversy is not resolved,[61] many features of this arthropathy are indistinguishable from the arthritis associated with calcium pyrophosphate dihydrate deposition disease. Evidence for increased iron stores occurred in 3 of 44 patients in two series describing the latter disorder.[59,62] The radiologic features correspond with the description of the arthropathy accompanying pseudogout syndrome by Martel and colleagues[63] or calcium pyrophosphate dihydrate crystal deposition disease by Utsinger and colleagues.[64]

Figure 94–2. Arthropathy of iron storage disease. This radiograph demonstrates advanced changes in the metacarpophalangeal joints that may accompany iron storage disease. Note the narrowing, sclerosis, spurring, and cystic changes most pronounced in the second and third metacarpophalangeal joints. More subtle degenerative changes are evident in the proximal and distal interphalangeal joints and the first carpometacarpal joints. (This radiograph was provided by Dr. Edward Keystone, Wellesley Hospital, Toronto, Canada.)

Figure 94–3. Arthropathy of iron storage disease. This radiograph demonstrates degenerative changes in both hip joints that may accompany iron storage disease. The changes are more pronounced in the left hip. Note the sclerosis on the weight-bearing surface of the acetabulum and the flattening, spurring at the lower part, and cystic changes of the left femoral head. The latter has given a mottled appearance to the left femoral head. (This radiograph was provided by Dr. Edward Keystone, Wellesley Hospital, Toronto, Canada.)

Secondary Hemochromatosis. Little information is available concerning the arthropathy associated with secondary causes of iron overload. In transfusion-induced iron overload, ankles, knees, and wrists are abnormal, but there is no report of metacarpophalangeal joint disease.[27,40] An arthropathy of small and large joints occurred in two patients with sideroblastic anemia and iron overload.[65]

Recent studies of acquired transfusion iron overload in adults indicate that the pattern of organ involvement resembles that encountered in idiopathic hemochromatosis, although the musculoskeletal system was not examined.[66] An iron-overload-associated myopathy characterized by proximal muscle weakness has been observed in patients on maintenance hemodialysis.[19]

An arthritis secondary to excess iron intake in drinking water occurs in Kashin-Beck disease.[67,68] Shortened long bones, deformity of joints, an arthropathy similar to primary hemochromatosis, and premature closure of epiphyses are seen in this disease in endemic areas.

In pediatric practice, a disorder of iron storage may occur in Zellweger syndrome.[68] This complex of multiple congenital anomalies includes developmental abnormalities of the brain, hepatomegaly, renal cortical cysts, retinopathy, congenital stippled epiphyses, enlargement of the patellae with serpentine calcification, and a characteristic facies.

LABORATORY FEATURES

The plasma iron concentration and total iron binding capacity are useful screening tests when the diagnosis of hemochromatosis is suspected. Symptomatic patients with primary hemochromatosis have an elevated plasma iron concentration of 175 to 275 μg per dl, a total iron binding capacity less than 300 μg per dl and a transferrin saturation greater than 75 percent. In patients with transfusion hemochromatosis, the plasma iron concentration is similarly elevated, but the total iron binding capacity is usually greater than 300 μg per dl. The plasma iron concentration in uncomplicated liver cirrhosis is usually within the normal range.

Serum ferritin concentration is a useful indicator of iron stores and has been found to be elevated in many untreated patients with primary hemochromatosis.[69-71] Serum ferritin is believed to be a product of the reticuloendothelial system and is proportional to reticuloendothelial iron. In one study of subjects who were homozygous for the hemochromatosis alleles, serum ferritin levels were elevated among most of them, and a few of the heterozygous family members also exhibited elevated levels.[9] An elevated ferritin level may be even more useful for secondary forms of hemochromatosis. However, it should be noted that ferritin levels also may be elevated secondary to hepatic damage or inflammation.[72] A normal value for ferritin concentration in "precirrhotic hemochromatosis" with a small amount of iron excess indicates some limitation of sensitivity for this test.[71,73,74] Importantly, however, less than 5 percent of patients with iron overload have normal ferritin values.[75]

The most accurate method for estimating tissue iron stores is by phlebotomy,[76] with retarded hematopoiesis as an end point. Iron stores also may be estimated by chelating agents using deferoxamine or diethylenetriaminopenta-acetic acid.[77-80] Normal iron stores in an adult male average 687 mg with a range of 130 to 1900 mg.[77] Urinary iron mobilized by chelation correlates directly with liver parenchymal iron rather than reticuloendothelial iron[78] and correlates linearly with iron mobilization by phlebotomy.[77,79] Postdeferoxamine urinary iron excretion exceeding 2200 μg per 24 hours dependably indicates iron excess.

Liver biopsy represents the definitive method for diagnosing excess iron storage; large stores of parenchymal iron occur in hemochromatosis. Iron stores may be demonstrated by staining or measuring hepatic iron concentrations. Grade 2 (on a scale of 0 to 4) parenchymal iron concentration or greater, or a hepatic iron concentration in excess of 40 μg per 100 mg wet weight represents an abnormally high value. Biopsy of other tissues such as bone marrow, intestinal mucosa, or synovium may be helpful if abnormal.

New noninvasive measurements of hepatic iron have a relatively high correlation with the quantity of iron in the liver.[81] These techniques include computed tomography,[82,83] nuclear resonance scattering of γ rays,[84] and magnetic susceptibility.[85] These latter methods, however, do not distinguish reticuloendothelial from parenchymal iron overload.

DIAGNOSIS

The finding of an arthropathy in a male with slate-gray skin, cirrhosis, diabetes, hypopituitarism, and congestive heart failure provides a characteristic picture for diagnosis of a disorder of excess iron storage. It may be a challenge, however, to diagnose the arthropathy correctly in the early stages of disease before these gross abnormalities of organ function are evident. This can only be done with a high index of suspicion, especially in patients presenting with a typical arthropathy.[42] A serum iron concentration, a plasma iron binding capacity, and a serum ferritin determination are useful screening tests. If these tests are abnormal, a deferoxamine loading test and a liver biopsy will establish the diagnosis (Table 94–1).

Iron overload arthropathy must be distinguished from rheumatoid arthritis, since the early features of both diseases may include metacarpophalangeal joint disease and a positive latex fixation test. The occurrence of sclerosis near affected joints, the lack of marginal erosions, and the absence of ulnar deviation—together with an elevated serum iron concentration, a decreased plasma iron binding capacity, increased ferritin levels, and excessive liver parenchymal iron—will establish the distinction. These latter features will also help distinguish the arthropathy of excess iron storage from primary calcium pyrophosphate dihydrate deposition disease and osteoarthritis. Other arthropathies associated with hepatic disease should be differentiated from the

excess iron storage states. Hepatic function abnormalities, abnormal serologic findings, and a characteristic biopsy picture may indicate chronic active hepatitis or primary biliary cirrhosis. Hepatic dysfunction, accompanying the transient acute immune complex arthritis of viral hepatitis or the arthritis associated with infectious mononucleosis, will be easily separated from the hepatic abnormalities and arthropathy of iron excess.

TREATMENT

Treatment for the arthropathy and for the iron overload must be separated in patients with hemochromatosis because removal of excess iron does not apparently improve the associated arthropathy, and continued progression of the joint disease may be anticipated. It is unclear whether treatment earlier in the disease might modify the natural history of arthropathy. Aspirin or other nonsteroidal anti-inflammatory drugs can be effective in managing the chronic arthritis. Acute episodes of pseudogout may be managed with oral indomethacin or phenylbutazone as well as with joint aspiration and use of intra-articular glucocorticoids. Other conservative measures involving physiotherapy and various appliances may be useful. With progressive joint deterioration, surgical intervention will be appropriate in selected instances.

Excess body iron is usually removed by a weekly or twice weekly phlebotomy of 500 ml of blood. This removes 10 to 20 g or iron each year. The hemoglobin should be maintained at or above 11 g per dl, and the hematocrit should remain at or above 34 percent. The end point of phlebotomies is usually indicated by an inability of the patient to maintain a constant hemoglobin level and by a normal serum ferritin level, and normalization of the serum iron and total iron binding capacity. Depletion of iron stores should be confirmed by liver biopsy. A maintenance program to prevent reaccumulation of excess iron is necessary, using the same end points. Phlebotomy of 500 ml of blood every 4 to 6 weeks is usually adequate for a maintenance program.

Phlebotomy is not helpful for secondary causes of iron overload when anemia is a problem.[7] Recent advances in chelation therapy using continuous parenteral deferoxamine appear to be helpful.[86-92] Overnight continuous subcutaneous infusion with a small infusion pump appears to be the optimal mode of therapy.[5] In-

Table 94–1. Diagnosis of Arthropathy of Excess Iron Storage

Arthropathy	Other Associated Disorders	Family History	Laboratory Values
Second and third metacarpophalangeal disease Degenerative changes Acute pseudogout Chondrocalcinosis	Hepatic dysfunction Slate-gray color Diabetes mellitus Hypogonadism Congestive heart failure	Similar disease Excess iron intake Excess alcohol ingestion	Elevated serum iron (175 μg– 275 μg/dl) TIBC (300 μg/dl; 75% saturation) Serum ferritin (300 ng/dl) Liver biopsy (+4 parenchymal iron) Synovial biopsy (positive for hemosiderin)

hibition of dietary iron absorption with tea or other inhibitors may provide additional management.[89] The use of ascorbic acid to enhance iron excretion is somewhat more controversial. Mobilization of iron from reticuloendothelial cells appears to result from ascorbic acid administration and may be associated with a deterioration of parenchymal organ function.[53,90] If ascorbic acid is to be administered, the current recommendation is to give the oral dose of ascorbic acid 1 hour or 2 hours after deferoxamine infusion is started and adequate blood levels of the latter are achieved. Finally, treatment with hemofiltration and deferoxamine chelation therapy effectively mobilized iron in a dialysis patient with hemosiderosis.[92]

Appropriate management of primary iron overload includes examination of family members for evidence of this disease, which is a treatable genetic disorder. All male sibs of the involved patient older than 10 years of age should be tested for HLA type and iron status.[5] Plasma iron levels, transferrin saturation, and plasma ferritin concentrations should be measured. The finding in a sib of HLA haplotypes identical to those of the patient probably indicates a homozygous status and a high risk for having or developing iron overload and the associated tissue damage. If no evidence of iron overload is found in sibs with identical haplotypes, the iron status should be evaluated every 2 to 3 years to detect early disease.[5]

References

1. Crosby, W.H.: Hemochromatosis: The unsolved problems. Semin. Hematol. 14:135, 1977.
2. Rowe, J.W., Wands, J.R., Mezey, E., Waterbury, L.A., Wright, J.R., Tobin, J., and Andres, R.: Familial hemochromatosis: Characteristics of the precirrhotic stage in a large kindred. Medicine 56:197, 1977.
3. Feller, E.R., Pont, A., Wands, R.R., Carter, E.A., Foster, G., Kourides, I.A., and Isselbacher, K.J.: Familial hemochromatosis; physiologic studies in the precirrhotic stage of the disease. N. Engl. J. Med. 296:1422, 1977.
4. Edwards, C.Q., Carroll, M., Bray, P., and Cartwright, G.E.: Hereditary hemochromatosis diagnosis in siblings and children. N. Engl. J. Med. 297:7, 1977.
5. Bothwell, T.H., Charlton, R.W., and Motulsky, A.G.: Idiopathic hemochromatosis. In Stanbury, J.B., Wyngaarden, J.B., Fredrickson, D.S., Goldstein, J., and Brown, M. (eds.): The Metabolic Basis of Inherited Disease. 5th ed. New York. McGraw-Hill Book Company, 1983.
6. Simon, M., Bourel, M., Genetet, B., and Faucher, R.: Idiopathic hemochromatosis: Recessive inheritance and early detection of HLA typing. N. Engl. J. Med. 297:1017, 1977.
7. Editorial: Idiopathic haemochromatosis. Br. J. Med. 2:1242, 1977.
8. Kravitz, K., Skolnick, M., Cannings, C., Carmelli, D., Baty, B., Amos, B., Johnson, A., Mendel, N., Edwards, C., and Cartwright, G.: Genetic linkage between hereditary hemochromatosis and HLA. Am. J. Hum. Genet. 31:601, 1979.
9. Beaumont, C., Simon, M., Fauchet, R., Hespel, J.P., Brissot, P., Genetet, B., and Bourel, M.: Serum ferritin as a possible marker of the hemochromatosis allele. N. Engl. J. Med. 301:169, 1979.
10. Cartwright, G.E., Edwards, C.Q., Kravitz, K., Skolnick, M., Amos, D.B., Johnson, A., and Buskjaer, L.: Hereditary hemochromatosis. Phenotypic expression of the disease. N. Engl. J. Med. 301:175, 1979.
11. Finch, C.A., and Huebers, H.: Perspectives in iron metabolism. N. Engl. J. Med. 306:1520, 1982.
12. Finch, S.C., and Finch, C.A.: Idiopathic hemochromatosis, an iron storage disease. A. Iron metabolism in hemochromatosis. Medicine (Baltimore) 34:381, 1955.
13. Cox, T.M., and Peters, T.J.: In vitro studies of duodenal iron uptake in patients with primary and secondary iron storage disease. Q. Med. J. 49:249, 1980.
14. Brink, B., Disler, P., Lynch, S., Jacobs, P., Charlton, R., and Bothwell,

15.   T.: Patterns of iron storage in dietary iron overload and idiopathic hemochromatosis. J. Lab. Clin. Med. 88:725, 1977.
15. Bothwell, T.H., Charlton, R.W., Cook, J.D., and Finch, C.A.: Iron metabolism in man. Oxford, Blackwell Scientific, 1979.
16. Charlton, R.W., Jacobs, P., Seftel, H., and Bothwell, T.H.: Effect of alcohol on iron absorption. Br. Med. J. 2:1427, 1964.
17. Hines, J.D.: Effects of alcohol on inborn errors of metabolism: Porphyria cutanea tarda and hemochromatosis. Semin. Hematol. 17:113, 1980.
18. Ali, M., Fayerri, A.O., Rigolosi, R., Frascino, J., Marsden, T., and Malcolm, D.: Hemosiderosis in hemodialysis patients: An autopsy study of 50 cases. JAMA 244:343, 1980.
19. Bregman, H., Gelfand, M.C., Winchester, J.F., Manz, H.J., Knepshield, J.H., and Schreiner, G.E.: Iron-overload-associated myopathy on maintenance hemodialysis: A histocompatibility-linked disorder. Lancet 2:882, 1980.
20. Goya, N., Miyazaki, S., Kodate, S., and Uschio, B.: A family of congenital atransferrinemia. Blood 40:239, 1972.
21. Basset, M.L., Halliday, J.W., and Powell, L.W.: Ferritin synthesis in peripheral blood monocytes in idiopathic hemochromatosis. J. Lab. Clin. Med. 100:137, 1982.
22. Huebers, H., Josephson, B., Huebers, E., Csiba, E., and Finch, C.: Uptake and release of iron from human transferrin. Proc. Natl. Acad. Sci. U.S.A. 78:2572, 1981.
23. Aisen, P.: The transferrins. In Jacobs, A., and Wowood (eds.): Iron in Biochemistry and Medicine. II. London, Academic Press, 1980.
24. Schumacher, H.R., Jr.: Ultrastructural characteristics of the synovial membrane in idiopathic haemochromatosis. Ann. Rheum. Dis. 31:465, 1972.
25. Walker, R.J., Dymach, I.W., Ansell, I.D., Hamilton, E.B.D., and Williams, R.: Synovial biopsy in haemochromatosis arthropathy. Ann. Rheum. Dis. 31:98, 1974.
26. Dymach, I.W., Hamilton, E.B.D., Laws, J.W., and Williams, R.: Arthropathy of haemochromatosis. Ann. Rheum. Dis. 29:469, 1970.
27. Abbott, D.F., and Gresham, G.A.: Arthropathy in transfusional siderosis. Br. Med. J. 1:418, 1972.
28. Brighton, C.T., Bigley, F.C., Jr., and Smolenski, B.I.: Iron induced arthritis in immature rabbits. Arthritis Rheum. 13:849, 1970.
29. Choi, Y., Hough, A.J., Morris, G.M., and Sokoloff, L.: Experimental siderosis of articular chondryocytes cultured in vitro. Arthritis Rheum. 24:809, 1981.
30. McCarty, D.J., Palmer, D.W., and Garancis, J.C.: Clearance of calcium pyrophosphate dihydrate crystals in vivo: III. Effects of synovial hemosiderosis. Arthritis Rheum. 24:706, 1981.
31. Okazaki, I., Brinkerhoff, C.E., Sinclair, J.F., Sinclair, P.R. Bonkowsky, R.,H.L., and Harris, E.D., Jr.: Iron increases collagenase production by rabbit synovial fibroblasts. J. Lab. Clin. Med. 97:396, 1981.
32. McCarty, D.J., and Pepe, P.F.: Erythrocyte neutral inorganic pyrophosphatase in pseudogout. J. Lab. Clin. Med. 79:277, 1972.
33. De Seye, S., Solnica, J., Mitrovic, D., Miraret, L., and Dorfmann, H.: Joint and bone disorders and hypoparathyroidism in hemochromatosis. Semin. Arthritis Rheum. 2:71, 1972.
34. Jacobs, A.: Iron overload—clinical and pathologic aspects. In Muller-Eberhard, U., Miescher, P.A., and Jaffe, E.R. (eds.): Iron Excess: Aberrations of Iron and Porphyrin Metabolism. New York, Grune & Stratton, 1977.
35. Peters, T.J., and Seymour, C.A.: Acid hydrolase activities and lysosomal integrity in liver biopsies from patients with iron overload. Clin. Sci. Mol. Med. 50:75, 1976.
36. Peters, T.J., Selden, C., Seymour, C.A.: Lysosomal disruption in the pathogenesis of hepatic damage in primary and secondary haemochromatosis. In Jacobs, A. (ed.): Iron Metabolism, Ciba Foundation Symposium 51 (new series). Amsterdam, Elsevier/North Holland, 1977, p. 317.
37. Schumacher, H.R., Jr.: Hemochromatosis and arthritis. Arthritis Rheum. 7:41, 1964.
38. Kra, S.J., Hollingsworth, J.W., and Finch, S.C.: Arthritis with synovial iron deposition in a patient with hemochromatosis. N. Engl. J. Med. 272:1268, 1965.
39. Wardle, E.N., and Patton, J.T.: Bone and joint changes in haemochromatosis. Ann. Rheum. Dis. 28:15, 1969.
40. Sella, E.J., and Goodman, A.H.: Arthropathy secondary to transfusion hemochromatosis. J. Bone Joint Surg. 55A:1077, 1973.
41. Gordon, D.A., Clarke, P.V., and Ogryzlo, M.A.: The chondrocalcific arthropathy of iron overload. Arch. Intern. Med. 134:21, 1974.
42. McSeffar, A., Fornasier, V.L., and Fox, I.H.: Arthropathy as the major clinical indicator of occult iron storage disease. J.A.M.A. 238:1825, 1977.
43. Bywaters, B.G.L., Hamilton, E.G.O., and Williams, R.: The spine idiopathic haemochromatosis. Ann. Rheum. Dis. 30:453, 1971.
44. Hamilton, E., Williams, R., Barlow, K.A., and Smith, P.M.: The arthropathy of idiopathic haemochromatosis. Q. J. Med. 37:171, 1968.
45. Sheldon, J.H.: Haemochromatosis. London, Oxford University Press, 1935.
46. Monnier, L.H., Colette, C., Claude, R., Mion, C., and Mirouze, J.: Evidence for 25-hydroxyvitamin D deficiency as a factor contributing to osteopenia in diabetic patients with idiopathic haemochromatosis. Eur. J. Clin. Invest. 10:183, 1980.

47. Seftel, H.C., Malkin, C., Schaman, A., Abrahams, C., Lynch S.R., Charlton, R.W., and Bothwell, T.H.: Osteoporosis, scurvy and siderosis in Johannesburg Bantu. Br. Med. J. 1:642, 1966.

48. Lynch, S.R., Seftel, H.C., Torrance, J.D., Charlton, R.W., and Bothwell, T.H.: Accelerated oxidative catabolism of ascorbic acid in siderotic Bantu. Am. J. Clin. Nutr. 20:641, 1967.

49. Hankes, L.V., Jansen, C.R., and Schmaeler, M.: Ascorbic acid catabolism in Bantu with hemosiderosis (scurvy). Biochem. Med. 9:244, 1974.

50. Modell, C.B., and Beck, J.: Long-term desferrioxamine therapy in thalassemia. Ann. N.Y. Acad. Sci. 232:210, 1974.

51. O'Brien, R.T.: Ascorbic acid enhancement of desferrioxamine-induced urinary iron excretion in thalassemia major. Ann. N.Y. Acad. Sci. 232:221, 1974.

52. Brissot, P., Deugnier, Y., LeTreut, A., Regnouard, F., Simon, M., and Bourel, M.: Ascorbic acid status in idiopathic hemochromatosis. Digestion 17:479, 1978.

53. Cohen, A., Cohen, I.J., and Schwartz, E.: Scurvey and altered iron stores in thalassemia major. N. Engl. J. Med. 304:158, 1981.

54. Wapnick, A.A., Lynch S.R., Seftel, H.C., Charlton, R.W., Bothwell, T.H., and Jowsey, J.: The effect of siderosis and ascorbic acid depletion on bone metabolism, with special reference to osteoporosis in the Bantu. Br. J. Nutr. 25:367, 1971.

55. Edwards, C.Q., Cartwright, G.E., Skolnick, M.H., and Amos, B.: Homozygosity for hemochromatosis. Ann. Intern. Med. 93:519, 1980.

56. Angevine, C.D., and Jacox, R.F.: Unusual connective tissue manifestations of hemochromatosis. Arthritis Rheum. 17:477, 1974.

57. Delbarre, P.F.: Les manifestations osteo-articulaires de l'hemochromatose. Presse Med. 72:2973, 1964.

58. Dorfmann, H., Solnica, J., DiMenza, C., and Sez, S. de: Les arthropathies des hemochromatoses—resultats d'une enquete prospective portant sur 54 malades. Semin. Hop. Paris. 45:516, 1969.

59. Atkins, C.J., MacIvor, J., Smith, P.M., Hamilton, E., and Williams, R.: Chondrocalcinosis and arthropathy: Studies in haemochromatosis and idiopathic chondrocalcinosis. Q. J. Med. 39:71, 1970.

60. Webb, J., Corrigan, A.B., and Robinson, R.G.: Haemochromatosis and "pseudogout." Med. J. Aust. 2:24, 1972.

61. Hamilton, E.B.D.: Diseases associated with CPPD deposition disease. Arthritis Rheum. (Suppl.)19:353, 1976.

62. McCarty, D.J., Silcox, D.C., Coe, F., Jacobelli, S., Reiss, E., Genant, H., and Ellman, M.: Diseases associated with calcium pyrophosphate dihydrate crystal deposition. Am. J. Med. 56:704, 1974.

63. Martel, W., Champion, C.K., Thompson, G.R., and Carter, T.L.: A roentgenologically distinctive arthropathy in some patients with the pseudogout syndrome. Am. J. Roentgenol. Rad. Ther. Nuc. Med. 109:587, 1970.

64. Utsinger, P.D., Zvaifler, N.J., and Resnick, D.: Calcium pyrophosphate dihydrate deposition disease without chondrocalcinosis. J. Rhuematol. 2:258, 1975.

65. Fitzcharles, M.A., Kirwan, J.R., Colvin, B.T., and Currey, H.L.F.: Sideroblastic anemia with iron overload presenting as an arthropathy. Ann. Rheum. Dis. 41:97, 1982.

66. Schafer, A.I., Cheron, R.G., Dluhy, R., Cooper, B., Gleason, R.E., Soeldner, J.S., and Bunn, H.F.: Clinical consequences of acquired transfusional iron overload in adults. N. Engl. J. Med. 304:319, 1981.

67. Hiyeda, K.: The cause of Kaschin-Beck's disease. Jpn. J. Med. Sci. 4:91, 1936.

68. O'Brien, R.T.: Iron overload: Clinical and pathological aspects in pediatrics. In Muller-Eberhard, U., Miescher, P.A., and Jaffe, E.R. (eds.): Iron Excess: Aberations of Iron and Porphyrin Metabolism. New York, Grune & Stratton, 1977.

69. Jacobs, A., and Worwood, M.: Serum ferritin. N. Engl. J. Med. 294:900, 1976.

70. Powell, L.W., and Halliday, J.W.: Serum ferritin in hemochromatosis. N. Engl. J. Med. 294:1185, 1976.

71. Walsh, J.R., Rowe, J.A., Mezey, S.E., Waterbury, L.A., Wright, J.R., Halliday, J.W., Isselbacher, K.J., and Powell, L.W.: Normal serum ferritin concentrations in precirrhotic hemochromatosis. N. Engl. J. Med. 294:301, 1976.

72. Lipschitz, D.F.A., Cook, J.D., and Finch, C.A.: A clinical evaluation of serum ferritin as an index of iron stores. N. Engl. J. Med. 290:1213, 1974.

73. Crosby, W.H.: Editorial: Serum ferritin fails to indicate hemochromatosis—nothing gold can stay. N. Engl. J. Med. 294:333, 1976.

74. Crosby, W.H.: Normal serum ferritin in precirrhotic hemochromatosis. N. Engl. J. Med. 296:1116, 1977.

75. Wands, J.R., Rowe, J.A., Mezey, S.E.: Normal serum ferritin concentrations in precirrhotic hemochromatosis. N. Engl. J. Med. 294:302, 1976.

76. Haskins, D., Stevens, A.R., Jr., Finch, S., and Finch, C.A.: Iron stores in man as measured by phlebotomy. J. Clin. Invest. 31:543, 1952.

77. Balcerzak, S.P., Westerman, M.P., Heinle, E.W., and Taylor, F.H.: Measurement of iron stores using deferoxamine. Ann. Intern. Med. 68:518, 1968.

78. Harler, L.A., Fund, D.D., and Finch, C.A.: Evaluation of storage iron chelates. Am. J. Med. 45:105, 1968.

79. Zimelman, A.P., Edelstein, A., and Miller, A.: Storage iron measurement in hemochromatotic patients reaccumulating iron. Clin. Res. 25:352A, 1977.

80. Baldus, W.P., Fairbanks, V.F., Dickson, E.R., and Baggenstoss, A.H.: Deferoxamine-chelatable iron in hemochromatosis and other disorders of iron overload. Mayo Clin. Proc. 53:157, 1978.

81. Finch, C.A.: The detection of iron overload. N. Engl. J. Med. 307:1702, 1982.

82. Houang, M.T.W., Arozena, X., Skalicka, A., Huehns, E.R., and Shaw, D.G.: Correlation between computed tomographic values and liver content in thalassaemia major with iron overload. Lancet 1:1322, 1979.

83. Chapman, R.W.G., Williams, G., Bydder, G., Dick, R., Sherlock, L., and Kreel, L.: Computed tomography for determining liver iron content in primary haemochromatosis. Br. Med. J. 280:440, 1980.

84. Vartsky, D., Ellis, K.J., Hull, D.M., and Cohn, S.H.: Nuclear resonant scattering of gamma rays: A new technique for in vivo measurement of body iron stores. Phys. Med. Biol. 24:689, 1979.

85. Brittenham, G.M., Farrell, D.E., Harris, J.W., Feldman, E.S., Danish, E.H., Muir, W.A., Tripp, J.H., and Bellow, E.M.: Magnetic-susceptibility measurement of human iron stores. N. Engl. J. Med. 307:1671, 1982.

86. Propper, R.D., Surin, S.B., and Nathan, D.G.: Reassessment of the use of desferrioxamine B in iron overload. N. Engl. J. Med. 294:1421. 1976.

87. Weatherall, D.J., Pippard, M.J., and Callender, S.T.: Iron loading and thalassemia—experimental success and practical realities. N. Engl. J. Med. 297:445, 1977.

88. Cooper, B., Bunn, H.F., Propper, R.D., Nathan, D.G., Rosenthal, D.S., and Maloney, W.C.: Treatment of iron overload in adults with continuous parenteral desferrioxamine. Am. J. Med. 63:958, 1977.

89. DeAlarcon, P.A., Donovan, M., Forbes, G.B., Landaw, S.A., and Stockman, J.A.: Iron absorption in the thalassemia syndromes and its inhibition by tea. N. Engl. J. Med. 300:5, 1979.

90. Nienhuis, A.W.: Vitamin C and iron. N. Engl. J. Med. 304:170, 1981.

91. Weatherall, D.J., Pippard, M.J., and Callender, S.T.: Iron loading in thalassemia: Five years with the pump. N. Engl. J. Med. 308:456, 1983.

92. McCarthy, J.T., Libertin, C.R., Mitchell, J.C., III, and Fairbanks, V.F.: Hemosiderosis in a dialysis patient: Treatment with hemofiltration and deferoxamine chelation therapy. Mayo Clin. Proc. 57:439, 1982.

Chapter 95

Multicentric Reticulohistiocytosis

William W. Ginsburg and J. Desmond O'Duffy

INTRODUCTION

Multicentric reticulohistiocytosis is a rare systemic disease of unknown etiology that is characterized by an infiltration of lipid-laden histiocytes and multinucleated giant cells into various tissues. Skin nodules and a destructive polyarthritis are the most common findings. There are fewer than 100 cases reported in the literature, the most comprehensive papers being reviews by Barrow and Holubar in 1969[1] and Chevrant-Breton in 1977.[2] Various other names have been used to describe this disorder, including lipoid dermatoarthritis, reticulohistiocytosis, giant cell reticulohistiocytoma, and normocholesterolemic xanthomatosis. In 1954, Goltz and Layman introduced the term multicentric reticulohistiocytosis to describe patients demonstrating the typical skin lesions as well as definite arthritis.[3]

CLINICAL FEATURES AND COURSE

The mean age of onset in reticulohistiocytosis is 43 years, but the disease has occurred in patients 11 to 71 years of age. Females predominate over males by a ratio of 3 to 1. In approximately 60 percent of cases, polyarthritis is the presenting symptom, followed by the nodular skin eruption. Diagnosis is initially very difficult without the accompanying skin nodules, which do not appear until an average of 3 years after the arthritis. In 20 percent of cases, the skin eruption is the initial symptom, and in the remaining cases there is a simultaneous presentation. The skin nodules can range in number from a few to hundreds, and are light copper to reddish-brown in color. They vary in size from several millimeters to 2 cm and characteristically involve the dorsum of the fingers, including nail folds, and the face, ears, and chest (Fig. 95–1; see Plate XI, p. xlv). A leonine facies can result from extensive facial and paranasal nodulation. Occasionally, nodules may occur over the olecranon process, causing confusion with the subcutaneous nodules of rheumatoid arthritis (Fig. 95–2). Mucosal surfaces are also frequently involved, and lesions can occur on the lips, nasal septum, tongue, gingiva, and pharynx. In approximately 30 percent of cases, severe pruritus is the first complaint, even before nodules are present. Confluent nodules on the face or trunk may present a cobblestone texture. Like the arthritis, the skin lesions may regress spontaneously. Some patients may experience weight loss and fever.[1,4,5]

The polyarthritis tends to be symmetric, most commonly involving the interphalangeal joints of the fingers, followed in frequency by the knees, shoulders, wrists, hips, ankles, feet, elbows, and spine. Atlantoaxial and temporomandibular joints may also be affected.[1,6] Morning stiffness occurs, and examination may reveal warm, swollen, and tender joints. Common involvement of the distal interphalangeal joints helps distinguish this condition from rheumatoid arthritis, but, unless the characteristic skin nodules are present, distinction is most difficult.

In 40 to 50 percent of cases, the arthritis progresses over a 7- to 8-year period to an arthritis mutilans. In the fingers this can produce the "main en lorgnette" or opera glass deformity of the hand. However, the natural history of the disease is not well defined, and some patients have mild disease, sometimes even with spontaneous remission.[1]

Multicentric reticulohistiocytosis is not limited to involvement of the skin and joints. Cases of myositis, pleural effusions, gastric ulcers, and pericarditis secondary to histiocytic and multinucleated giant cell infiltration have been reported. Infiltration into bronchial lymph nodes, bone marrow, and endocardium has also been reported.[5,7-11]

LABORATORY AND ROENTGENOGRAPHIC FEATURES

Joint fluid analysis has been reported in six patients.[7,9,12-14] Leukocyte counts are usually less than 30,000 per mm^3, and two patients had counts less than 4000 per mm^3. Three patients had predominantly polymorphonuclear cells, and two patients had high numbers of monocytes (40 and 53 percent), whereas one of these patients also had foam cells present. Synovial biopsy has revealed numerous lipid-laden histiocytes and multinucleated giant cells, such as those seen on skin biopsy.[7,9,14] Electron microscopy reveals that these cells contain vacuoles and inclusions that contain a flocculent material.[14]

There are no specific laboratory abnormalities in multicentric reticulohistiocytosis, although about half the patients have a slightly elevated erythrocyte sedimentation rate and a mild anemia. About 30 percent have slight to moderate hypercholesterolemia. Normal values are reported for serum uric acid, thyroxine, glucose, triglycerides, and creatinine levels, as well as for serol-

Figure 95–2. Nodular infiltrates on extensor surface of forearm can simulate clusters of rheumatoid nodules.

Figure 95–3. Radiograph of hand demonstrating distal interphalangeal joint erosion as well as cutaneous nodules.

ogic tests for syphilis. Tests for rheumatoid factor, antinuclear antibody, and LE cells are usually negative. A positive rheumatoid factor as reported in four cases could cause confusion in the diagnosis especially if the arthritis precedes skin manifestations.[15] There are no abnormalities noted on serum protein electrophoresis. Bone marrow examinations have been normal, and patients have been shown to have intact delayed hypersensitivity by skin tests to *Candida,* mumps, and tuberculin.[1,5]

Roentgenographic findings may show erosive changes that are very similar to those of rheumatoid arthritis. As in rheumatoid arthritis, they tend to be bilaterally symmetric. However, circumscribed erosions often spread from the synovial reflections over the articular surface, resulting in widening of joint space, loss of cartilage, and absorption of subchrondral bone. These changes are to be found especially in the proximal and distal interphalangeal joints. Osteoporosis is relatively mild despite the severe erosive destruction, and there is absent or minimal periosteal reaction. Hand radiographs often show well-defined extra-articular nodules (Fig. 95–3). Rarely, atlantoaxial involvement, as is seen in rheumatoid arthritis, may develop.[6,16,17]

ASSOCIATED DISORDERS

Approximately 50 percent of patients are tuberculin positive. In one patient with both tuberculosis and multicentric reticulohistiocytosis, treatment of the tuberculosis brought a complete resolution of the multicentric reticulohistiocytosis.[12] Active tuberculosis has not been found in other cases. Approximately one third of the patients have xanthelasma.[1,5]

Twenty to 30 percent of patients with multicentric reticulohistiocytosis have been reported to have malignant disease.[1,15] The meaning of this association is unknown, although it is interesting that the mononuclear phagocytic system, which includes the histocyte or tissue macrophage, is important in immune surveillance. Associated malignancies have included three cases each of carcinoma of the bronchus, the stomach, the breast, and the cervix, and malignant lymphoma. Isolated cases of ovarian and colon carcinoma and sarcoma have also been reported. There is no clear relationship between the onset of malignancy and multicentric reticulohistiocytosis. In some cases, the malignancy has appeared many years after the onset of multicentric reticulohistiocytosis. Treatment of the malignancy may or may not lead to improvement of the multicentric reticulohistiocytosis.[15]

PATHOLOGY AND ETIOLOGY

The diagnosis of multicentric reticulohistiocytosis is made on skin or synovial biopsy that demonstrates the characteristic aggregates of multinucleated giant cells and histiocytes, which have a granular ground-glass appearance (Fig. 95–4). The giant cells can be as large as 50 to 100 μ in diameter, and up to 20 nuclei have been observed. In the skin, the nodular infiltrate can occupy the entire dermis, and it is encapsulated. Histochemical staining reveals that the ground-glass cytoplasm contains a Periodic acid-Schiff (PAS)-reactive material. The PAS-reactive material, which can be completely removed by digestion with pepsin but not with diastase, has been the subject of much investigation and conflicting opinions, but it is currently thought to represent a mucoprotein or glycoprotein. Sudan black–reactive material is also found, which suggests the presence of phospholipids, and neutral fats are present as detected by positive staining with oil red O, Nile blue, Scharlach R, and Sudan III and Sudan IV. Multicentric reticulohistiocytosis was at one time thought to represent a lipid storage disease, but no consistent abnormality of the serum or intracellular lipids has been found.[1,4,5,14] Various histochemical stains are not consistently positive in all patients, and it has recently been suggested that the histiocytes and giant cells contain a nonspecific accumulation of lipids. It is still unclear whether the lipid accumulation is a primary or secondary event in the pathogenesis of the disease. In two reports, cells were found to contain intact and degraded collagen fibers by electron microscopy.[18,19] The significance of this finding is unknown. Electron microscopy of the histiocytes has also shown large membrane-bound vacuoles with lipid accumulations in some cases.[1,14]

It has also been postulated that multicentric reticulohistiocytosis represents a histiocytic granulomatous reaction. Numerous cytoplasmic electron dense granules resembling lysosomes are seen by electron microscopy. Ultracytochemical studies demonstrate that these granules stain positive for acid phosphatase, which is considered an enzymatic marker for lysosomes.[19,20] The PAS-positive material was also located in these granules.[20] Activated histiocytes contain numerous primary and secondary lysosomes. The release of neutral protease and acid hydrolase from these cells may induce tissue destruction and the inflammation seen in multicentric reticulohistiocytosis.[21,22]

DIFFERENTIAL DIAGNOSIS

Besides rheumatoid arthritis, the differential diagnosis must exclude lepromatous leprosy, sarcoidosis, xanthomatosis, generalized eruptive histiocytoma, and histiocytosis X, all of which can have skin nodules and bone changes on roentgenography.

Figure 95–4. Skin biopsy demonstrating multinucleated giant cells with ground glass cytoplasm (hematoxylin and eosin × 400).

TREATMENT

Treatment for multicentric reticulohistiocytosis has consisted of trials of low-fat diets, clofibrate, prednisone, azathioprine, and isoniazid.[1,12,14] None of these agents has consistently been shown to be of any benefit for the arthritis or skin lesions. One patient had marked improvement of skin lesions after topical nitrogen mustard therapy.[23] There are also several case reports of improvement after cyclophosphamide administration, but as in rheumatoid arthritis, protracted spontaneous remissions make treatment evaluation difficult.[15,23,24] Accordingly, symptomatic relief with salicylates or nonsteroidal agents should be sought first. If not successful, glucocorticoids may be added to these. Only in very severe disease should immunosuppressive treatment be considered, particularly because there is an increased risk of malignancy associated with these agents. The rarity of the disease seems to preclude the possibility of a well-planned double-blind control study in one center.

References

1. Barrow, M.V., and Holubar, K.: Multicentric reticulohistiocytosis, a review of 33 patients. Medicine 48:287, 1969.

2. Chevrant-Breton, J.: La Réticulo-histiocytose multicentrique: Revue de la littérature récente (depuis 1969). Ann. Derm. Vénéréol. (Paris) 104:745, 1977.
3. Goltz, R.W., and Layman, C.W.: Multicentric reticulohistiocytosis of the skin and synovia. Arch. Dermatol. Syph. 69:717, 1954.
4. Albert, J., Bruce, W., Allen, A.C., et al.: Lipoid dermatoarthritis. Am. J. Med. 28:661, 1960.
5. Orkin, M., Goltz, R.W., Good, R.A., et al.: A study of multicentric reticulohistiocytosis. Arch. Dermatol. 89:640, 1964.
6. Martel, W., Abell, M.R., and Duff, I.F.: Cervical spine involvement in lipoid dermato-arthritis. Radiology 77:613, 1961.
7. Ehrlich, G.E., Young, I., Nosheny, S.Z., and Katz, W.A.: Multicentric reticulohistiocytosis, a multisystem disorder. Am. J. Med. 52:830, 1972.
8. Fast, A.: Cardiopulmonary complications in multicentric reticulohistiocytosis. Arch. Dermatol. 112:1139, 1976.
9. Flam, M., Ryan, S.C., Mah-poy, G.L., et al.: Multicentric reticulohistiocytosis: Report of a case with atypical features and electron microscopic study of skin lesions. Am. J. Med. 52:841, 1972.
10. Waren, R.P., Evans, C.D., Hewitt, M., et al.: Reticulohistiocytosis. Br. Med. J. 1:1387, 1957.
11. Anderson, T.E., Carr, A.J., Chapman, R.S., et al.: Myositis and myotonia in a case of multicentric reticulohistiocytosis. Br. J. Med. 80:39, 1968.
12. Gold, K.D., Sharp, J.T., Estrada, R.E.: Relationship between multicentric reticulohistiocytosis and tuberculosis. J.A.M.A. 237:2213, 1977.
13. Taylor, D.R.: Multicentric reticulohistiocytosis. Arch. Dermatol. 113:330, 1977.
14. Krey, P.R., Comerford, F.R., and Cohen, A.S.: Multicentric reticulohistiocytosis, fine structural analysis of the synovium and synovial fluid cells. Arthritis Rheum. 17:615, 1974.
15. Catterall, M.D.: Multicentric reticulohistiocytosis: A review of eight cases. Clin. Exp. Dermatol. 5(3):267, 1980.
16. Gold, R.H., Metzger, A.L., and Mirra, J.M.: Multicentric reticulohistiocytosis, an erosive polyarthritis with distinctive clinical roentgenographic and pathologic features. Am. J. Roentgenol. Rad. Ther. Nucl. Med. 124:610, 1975.
17. Schwarz, E., and Fish, A.: Reticulohistiocytoma: A rare dermatologic disease with roentgen manifestations. Am. J. Roentgenol. Rad. Ther. Nucl. Med. 83:692, 1960.
18. Caputo, R., Alessi, E., and Berti, E.: Collagen phagocytosis in multicentric reticulohistiocytosis. J. Invest. Dermatol. 76(5):342, 1981.
19. Coode, P.E., Ridgway, H., and Jones, D.B.: Multicentric reticulohistiocytosis: Report of two cases with ultrastructure, tissue culture and immunology studies. Clin. Exp. Dermatol. 5(3):281, 1980.
20. Tani, M., Hori, K., Nakanishi, I., Iwasaki, I., Ugawa, Y., and Jimbo, I.: Multicentric reticulohistiocytosis. Electron microscopic and ultracytochemical studies. Arch. Dermatol. 117(8):495, 1981.
21. Davies, P.A., and Allison, A.C.: Secretion of macrophage enzymes in relation to the pathogenesis of chronic inflammation. In Nelson, D.S. (ed.): Immunobiology of the macrophage. New York, Academic Press, Inc., 1976, p. 427.
22. Nishi, K.: Possible role of lysosomes in cells of "the epitheloid cell system." Acta Histochem. 11:252, 1978.
23. Brandt, F., Lipman, M., Taylor, J.R., Halprin, K.M.: Topical nitrogen mustard therapy in multicentric reticulohistiocytosis. J. Am. Acad. Dermatol. 6(2):260, 1982.
24. Hanauer, L.B.: Reticulohistiocytosis: Remission after cyclophosphamide therapy. Arthritis Rheum. 15:636, 1972.

Section XIV

Arthritis Associated with Recognized Infectious Diseases

Chapter 96

Septic Arthritis Caused by Bacteria

Allen R. Myers

INTRODUCTION

Despite the ready availability of potent antibacterial agents, acute infectious arthritis remains a serious medical problem. Although joint sepsis accounts for only approximately 0.02 percent of hospital admissions,[1,2] there appears to be no decrease in its frequency over the past two to three decades.[3-5] The major changes that seem to have occurred with this entity over the past quarter century or more appear to be a shift in hosts and organisms. However, the basic clinical problem remains the same: delay in diagnosis leading to poorer long-term results. Therefore, acute bacterial arthritis is a true medical emergency that requires early recognition and aggressive treatment in order to prevent joint destruction and permanent disability.

Previously, septic arthritis was a disease primarily of children, but more recent studies note a significant occurrence in the elderly, the chronically ill, and patients with impaired host resistance.[5,6] Furthermore, whereas staphylococci are the overwhelmingly predominant organisms causing nongonococcal suppurative arthritis, gram-negative bacterial infections have become increasingly prevalent.[6-8] The prevalence and recognition of disseminated gonococcal infection has led to a definite predominance of that organism as a cause of infectious arthritis in most institutions. The epidemiology, clinical features, pathogenesis, and therapy of disseminated gonococcal infection are sufficiently different from other forms of acute bacterial arthritis to merit detailed, separate consideration.

PREDISPOSING FACTORS

One of the enigmas concerning acute nongonococcal bacterial arthritis is why there are not more cases of this entity when bacteremia and septicemia are relatively so common. The explanation has been that in an immunocompetent host a normal joint can be readily cleared of invading bacteria by the phagocytic capabilities of synovial cells. Although occasionally an essentially normal individual may develop joint sepsis, the majority of patients who experience this disease demonstrate altered host resistance, local joint abnormalities, or even both of those features.

Systemic Disease. A variety of systemic or debilitating illnesses appear to predispose patients to acute infectious arthritis. Diabetes mellitus,[9] alcoholism with or without cirrhosis of the liver,[2,10] malignancies (including solid tumors and myeloproliferative disorders),[11,12] uremia,[2] and rheumatoid arthritis[13] are common substrates for superimposed joint sepsis. Less common entities include systemic lupus erythematosus[14] (Fig. 96–1) and sickle cell disease.[15,16] More recently, intravenous drug abusers[17-19] and immunosuppressed patients[11] have become increasingly important repositories for suppurative arthritis. Inherent in the association of systemic diseases with complicating infectious processes is the problem of relating the susceptibility to a basic host abnormality associated with the disease or more specifically with its treatment. In the case of diabetes mellitus, it appears that specific host defense defects exist which may predispose to infection.[20,21] These, combined with the well-known propensity of diabetics to develop skin and urinary tract infections, provide a fertile soil for hematogenous bacterial dissemination and subsequent joint localization. While alcoholic patients characteristically may develop infections primarily as a result of aspiration, trauma, or exposure, they do appear to demonstrate defects in leukocyte mobilization and chemotaxis as well.[22,23] Typically, pneumococcal pneumonia and/or meningitis provides the focus for dissemination in the alcoholic patient. Myeloproliferative diseases, particularly multiple myeloma and leukemias (i.e., B-lymphocyte disorders), commonly become superinfected, and life-threatening gram-negative infections are a well

Figure 96–1. Radiographs of knee of patient with systemic lupus erythematosus who presented acutely with *Salmonella choleraesuis* septic arthritis. *A*, Anteroposterior projection of knee showing medial femoral condylar halo-shaped lesion similar to osteonecrosis. *B*, Lateral projection of same. Surgical exploration revealed golf ball–sized cavity.

known complication.[24] Additionally, corticosteroid, immunosuppressive, and cytotoxic therapies are frequently employed and further compromise the host. Myeloma patients typically may develop pneumococcal infections, while leukemia patients seem to be predisposed to a variety of gram-negative organisms. In systemic lupus erythematosus, underlying host problems and therapy both appear to contribute to the susceptibility to infection.[25-27] Sickle cell disease patients exhibit an opsonic defect,[28] which leads to a high incidence of pneumococcal infections but remarkably only occasionally results in septic arthritis[15] (Fig. 96–2). Intravenous drug abusers experience a high incidence of infectious complications which include endocarditis, osteomyelitis, phlebitis, and abscesses as well as arthritis. The common denominator in these cases is the introduction of infectious agents into the intravascular space, whereupon hematogenous spread to the joints occurs. Specific host defects do not seem to play a role here, but the organisms are somewhat unusual in that they include mostly gram-negative agents such as *Serratia* and *Pseudomonas* species. Another example of hematogenous dissemination from an intravascular source is that which occurs in patients undergo-

ing chronic hemodialysis.[29] In this group, in addition to ready vascular access for bacteria, uremia and chronic illness impair the host's defenses.

The role of systemic steroid therapy in predisposing to pyarthrosis is complicated. It is clear that patients on high dose steroids have a striking incidence of bacterial and fungal infections,[30] and dissemination to synovium would not be surprising.[31] However, low or moderate dose steroid treatment may not actually lead to septic arthritis, but predisposition may be related to the primary disease process (see below). On the other hand, immunosuppressive agents act to enhance susceptibility to infection by bone marrow element suppression.

The problem of superimposed joint sepsis in rheumatoid arthritis is well recognized[1,2,6,9,13,32-37] (Fig. 96–3). Many factors may contribute to the rheumatoid patient's susceptibility to septic arthritis. General factors include chronic illness and debility and use of systemic corticosteroids or immunosuppressive agents. Intra-articular factors include diminished polymorphonuclear leukocyte chemotaxis,[38] defective polymorphonuclear leukocyte phagocytosis,[39] decreased synovial fluid bacteriolytic activity,[40] and perhaps low synovial fluid comple-

Figure 96–2. Bilateral septic arthritis of hips caused by *Enterobacter* in a 50-year-old female with hemoglobin S-C disease. *A,* Hip film, 8/3/76, obtained at initial presentation of symptoms demonstrating loss of left hip joint space. *B,* Hip film, 2/3/78, reveals significant resorption of femoral heads bilaterally.

ment. Intrasynovial injections of corticosteroids may enhance this susceptibility as well (see below).

Local Factors. Local joint pathology certainly appears to be one of the significant predisposing factors to bacterial arthritis.[9] Rheumatoid arthritis is by far the most common predisposing local anatomic derangement, but almost any underlying joint disease may be implicated. Degenerative joint disease,[6] trauma,[41] gout,[42,43] pseudogout,[43-45] and Charcot's arthropathy[46] have all been reported. While the association may be apparent, the mechanisms are unclear except for perhaps rheumatoid arthritis, in which several contributing factors have been recognized (see above).

Joint sepsis may be introduced directly into the joint by direct penetration of the joint membrane (Fig. 94–6). While this may rarely occur through trauma, the most common mode is via intra-articular corticosteroid injection (Fig. 96–5). Although Hollander suggests sepsis is a very rare complication of this procedure,[47] the fact that any sepsis after arthrocentesis did occur should lead to extreme caution with the technique. Specific reports of infection following joint injection, however, are numerous.[48-50]

PATHOGENESIS OF ACUTE INFECTIOUS ARTHRITIS

Acute infectious arthritis results most frequently from hematogenous dissemination from a primarily infected site. However, joints may become infected by direct inoculation (see above) or local extension. Local extension may occur from adjacent infected soft tissue or result from spread from contiguous osteomyelitis.[51] Once having arrived at the joint, the bacteria migrate from the vascular compartment into the interstitial space of the synovium, a phenomenon demonstrated with experimental pneumococcal infection.[52] The inflammatory response in the joint to bacterial invasion of the synovium is apparently related to factors produced by the organism as well as factors generated by the host, the virulence and quantity of inoculum of the organism and the status of the host defense mechanisms.[53] Microbial factors include exotoxins (e.g., staphylococcal hemolysins), endotoxins, and enzymes (e.g., staphylococcal kinase, which activates plasmin). Endotoxins have been shown to stimulate synovial fibroblast function[54] and prostaglandin production.[55] In addition, bacteria may

Figure 96–3. Radiographic demonstration of knee with *Pseudomonas aeruginosa* septic arthritis in a patient with rheumatoid arthritis. Poor response to therapy required eventual fusion of knee.

produce chemotactic factors directly or as a result of interactions leading to complement activation. Furthermore, bacterial debris (e.g., bacterial envelopes and peptidoglycanpolysaccharides) clearly has phlogistic properties.[56]

Once a virulent organism establishes an infectious focus in a joint, unless it is eradicated early, joint destruction will generally ensue. The pathogenesis of the joint lesion caused by septic arthritis involves a complex series of events which results in cartilage destruction.[57] The latter may occur even after infection itself is controlled. The study of the pathophysiology of suppurative arthritis dates back more than half a century when Phemister initiated studies in which he incubated articular cartilage in vitro with staphylococcal pus, a staphylococcal suspension, and tuberculous pus, each at 55°C. Only the articular cartilage incubated with staphylococcal pus demonstrated significant digestion within 3 to 24 hours.[58] The staphylococcal suspension and the tuberculous pus showed no gross changes in the cartilage during the incubation period. Phemister concluded that the chondrolysis was caused by enzymes in the pus probably derived from the polymorphonuclear leukocytes. Further studies performed by Keefer and associates[59] demonstrated that the incubation of cartilage at 37°C and 56°C with polymorphonuclear leukocyte autolysates resulted in cartilage alterations only at a temperature of 56°C. At physiological body temperatures (37°C) no significant changes were identified. Subsequently, it was demonstrated that products of bacterial infection may activate proteolytic enzymes that are es-

pecially destructive to cartilage. Plasmin, which may be activated by kinases produced by staphylococci or streptococci, attacks the proteoglycans of the cartilage matrix, leading to chondrolysis.[60] Inflammatory cellular products also lead to enzymatic degradation of the ground substance of cartilage.[61] In depth studies performed by Curtiss and Klein both in vitro and in vivo[62,63] indicated that the removal of the collagen content was required for visible gross destruction of the cartilage. Elastase, found in granules of polymorphonuclear leukocytes, has the capability of degrading proteoglycans by attacking the protein core. The acute inflammation accompanying sepsis also leads to synovial cell proliferation, and it may well be that enzymes released by the proliferating, activated synovial cells are responsible in large part for cartilage degradation in septic arthritis.

From these and other detailed studies,[64-66] of septic arthritis in vitro and in vivo, three stages of articular cartilage destruction can be identified. The initial stage involves the release of proteolytic enzymes into the joint by the activated polymorphonuclear leukocytes. These enzymes are augmented by synovial lysosomal enzymes and lead to a relatively rapid removal of a significant amount of proteoglycan from articular cartilage. In addition, the invading bacteria may participate in the cartilage matrix depletion.[67] This early stage is reversible as long as the chondrocytes are not damaged. The proteoglycan matrix can be restored within days to weeks if the process can be arrested early in this period. During the second stage, the physical properties of the articular cartilage are seriously compromised. The compressive

Figure 96–4. Staphylococcal infection of interphalangeal joint of thumb resulting in destructive arthritis. The problem arose following a puncture wound. (Generously provided from the Philadelphia General Hospital X-Ray Teaching File at the Mütter Museum of the College of Physicians of Philadelphia.)

Figure 96–5. Progressive destructive arthritis of knee caused by staphylococcal arthritis following an intra-articular steroid injection. *A,* Radiograph of knee (anteroposterior) at time of acute presentation reveals only mild degenerative arthritis and patchy osteoporosis. *B,* Radiograph of knee (anteroposterior) 1 year later revealing severe destructive changes.

strength provided by the proteoglycan components is altered, and the chondrocytes within the articular cartilage receive increased mechanical stresses. In addition, altered diffusion of nutrients contributes to chondrocyte injury, leading to an impaired capacity for matrix reconstitution. In the last stage, the synovium proliferates at the periphery of the affected joint. Collagenase, elastase, and cathepsins released by the polymorphonuclear leukocytes and the synovium gradually destroy the collagen and residual proteoglycans. Mechanical aberrations and stresses further injure the collagen network, and, with time, the collagen is distorted and destroyed. Only with the destruction of the collagen superstructure does the articular cartilage show gross deformation. In the presence of chondrocyte death, the third stage may be entered even after the infection has been curtailed. Chondrocytes do not have ability to re-establish the cartilage collagen (type II) superstructure within the matrix, although in the presence of active inflammation, they may release both proteinases and collagenase.

Histochemical staining of the cartilage with Safranin-O, a dye bound to the repeating sulfide units of the keratan sulfate and chondroitin sulfate oligosaccharide chains, is lost rapidly within days after the onset of septic arthritis.

It can be concluded from these studies that the complete restitution of normal articular cartilage requires the cessation of the septic process during the first stage before chondrocyte death or collagen loss occurs. Only with intact chondrocytes can the proteoglycans be reconstituted. Continuous removal of the activated polymorphonuclear leukocytes is crucial during treatment of acute bacterial arthritis, for their presence even in the absence of viable bacteria will perpetuate the articular destruction. It has been estimated that with synovial fluid polymorphonuclear leukocyte counts greater than 50,000 per cubic millimeter, natural inhibitors of proteinases present in the synovial fluid are saturated, and free enzymes may work on unprotected proteoglycans or collagen substrates.[68]

CLINICAL FEATURES

Generally, the patient with acute septic arthritis presents with the cardinal findings of inflammation: swelling, pain, and heat. Erythema is present less frequently. Limitation of active and passive motion of the joint is characteristic. These signs and symptoms are most frequently confined to a single joint, but polyarticular involvement is well described.[4-9] Any joint may become infected, but the larger weight-bearing joints of the lower extremity are involved most often.[3-9] While the hip may have been more commonly involved previously, perhaps related to the prevalence of acute infectious arthritis in children, the knee is now the primary site of involvement. Other involved areas include the ankle, elbow, wrist, and shoulder, while rarely small joints of hands and feet are affected. Systemic signs and symptoms usually include fever, although it is frequently low grade

(< 100°F). Chills are uncommon. Except for gonococcal arthritis, men appear to be afflicted more often than women. As noted above, persons with previous joint damage, particularly rheumatoid arthritis, are especially susceptible to superimposed joint sepsis. Since those patients exhibit inflammatory joint findings routinely, how may a septic joint be distinguished? In that case, a joint that is out of proportion to the general level of activity of the disease or disproportionate to other joint findings with or without low grade fever should be a clue to complicating suppurative arthritis.

General laboratory studies are of little help in establishing the diagnosis of infectious arthritis. Peripheral leukocytosis occurs in one half to two thirds of patients, and elevation of erythrocyte sedimentation rate is usual. Unfortunately, these tests are not specific, and the absence of the former should not dissuade one from an appropriate diagnosis.

The differential diagnosis of monarticular acute bacterial arthritis may include crystal-induced synovitis (gout, pseudogout, or hydroxyapatite), traumatic arthritis, viral arthritis, toxic synovitis, and acute hemarthrosis. Monarticular rheumatoid arthritis, Reiter's syndrome, a peripheral manifestation of ankylosing spondylitis, or monarticular juvenile rheumatoid arthritis might be considered, but generally these do not have as abrupt an onset. If the presentation is polyarticular, the differential could include acute rheumatic fever, acute gout, serum sickness, and viral arthritis. Acute rheumatoid arthritis or sero-negative arthropathies would be less likely due to the more insidious onset.

DIAGNOSTIC STUDIES

The key to the diagnosis of acute bacterial arthritis is clinical suspicion, and it is confirmed by synovial fluid analysis and culture. The typical pyarthrosis reveals a thick, purulent effusion with a mean synovial fluid white blood cell count of greater than 50,000 cells per cubic millimeter and more than 90 percent polymorphonuclear leukocytes.[6,41] However, it should be recognized that while synovial fluid cell counts frequently may be greater than 100,000 to 200,000 per cubic millimeter, occasionally only modest increases in cell counts (i.e., 5,000 to 10,000 per cubic millimeter) may be associated with intra-articular infection.[5] Characteristically, the mucin clot is poor.[6] Synovial fluid glucose may be low,[6,41] but this is a variable finding. The usual simultaneously drawn plasma-synovial fluid glucose differential obtained in a fasting state is < 40 mg per deciliter,[69] and frequently this difference exceeds 90 mg per deciliter in acute infectious arthritis.[6,41] Unfortunately, synovial fluid glucose may be quite low in rheumatoid arthritis, thus diminishing its usefulness diagnostically in that particular situation. Furthermore, little is known about the kinetics of glucose transport into synovial fluid in the nonfasting or diabetic states; hence values obtained under those conditions may be uninterpretable. Polarizing microscopy should be performed routinely, since in elderly people the differential diagnosis may include crystal-induced arthritis. Occasionally, both septic arthritis and crystal-induced synovitis will be present concurrently.[42-45]

Gram stain and culture of the synovial fluid are mandatory when infection is suspected. The Gram stain may be positive in one half[5] to two thirds[6] of patients subsequently culturally proved to have septic arthritis and can provide a basis for rapid institution of treatment. The joint fluid culture is the definitive study and provides the basis for specific antibiotic treatment, including sensitivity assays. However, even in frank nongonococcal infectious arthritis, cultures may occasionally be negative, especially if antibiotic treatment had been instituted prior to arthrocentesis. The yield for positive cultures increases in relation to the care with which cultures are obtained. Routinely, cultures should be planted immediately at the bedside or rushed to the microbiology laboratory while maintaining a warmed syringe. Aerobic and anaerobic cultures should be obtained customarily. (Special cultural techniques for the gonococcus and other fastidious organisms will be described under specific organisms.)

Since the overwhelming majority of pyogenic arthritis cases occur from hematogenous dissemination, a portal of entry should always be sought. Routine blood, urine, sputum, stool, wound, and nasopharyngeal cultures should be obtained prior to the introduction of antibiotic therapy. Blood cultures are essential, since they may be positive in almost three quarters of patients.[9] Primary infectious foci leading to suppurative arthritis may involve any site but generally include upper and lower respiratory tracts, genitourinary tract, soft tissues, skin, and gastrointestinal tract. However, as may be expected, a number of unusual primary sites of infection leading to septic arthritis have been reported, and therefore ex-

treme diligence may be necessary in isolating the portal of entry. In particular, pyarthrosis has occurred following perforation of abdominal organs[70] (Fig. 96–6), from use of a intrauterine device,[71] or even following contact with animals.[72]

Radiographic evaluation for the diagnosis of acute infectious arthritis is generally unrewarding, especially early in the course.[73,74] However, radiographic studies should be performed routinely in order to serve as a baseline for follow-up studies. If underlying joint disease such as rheumatoid arthritis is present, superimposed radiographic changes secondary to sepsis may be obscured. The earliest radiographic finding in septic arthritis is synovial effusion, and frequently adjacent soft tissue swelling is visible. Rarely are there any other findings within the first 7 to 10 days except for juxta-articular osteopenia, a nonspecific finding. If the infection is untreated or is unresponsive to therapy, joint space narrowing will develop (Fig. 96–7). Subchondral bone destruction is a late radiographic manifestation. Subluxation of the hip may be a relatively early finding in suppurative arthritis of that joint in infants or children owing to the anatomic configuration in the presence of a large effusion. This may occasionally occur in the shoulder in adults as well.[75] An unusual radiologic feature of acute pyogenic arthritis caused by *E. coli* is gas in the joint and periarticular tissues.[76,77] Anaerobic infections may produce a similar occurrence.[76] The gas formation occurs as a result of glucose fermentation. Rarely, periarticular calcification may occur as a late complication of infectious arthritis.[78] It was suggested that this may result from rupture through the joint capsule with extravasation into the soft tissues and subsequent necrosis and calcification. Another radiographically demonstrable late complication of septic arthritis of the shoulder has been tears of the rotator cuff.[75] This

Figure 96–6. *E. coli* septic arthritis of left hip. *A,* Hip radiograph taken for mild hip pain in patient with fever of unknown source. Destruction of articular surfaces and loss of joint space are evident. *B,* Left hip radiograph 6 weeks later detailing progressive destruction of femoral head and acetabulum. The source of this infection was an intra-abdominal abscess that extended into the hip.

Figure 97–7. Progressive destructive radiographic changes in an ankle secondary to staphylococcal arthritis. *A,* Baseline radiograph of involved ankle revealing normal joint space. Incidental bone infarct is noted. *B,* Ankle radiograph 2 months later detailing marked destruction of articular surfaces and obliteration of joint space. (Generously provided from the Philadelphia General Hospital X-Ray Teaching File at the Mütter Museum of the College of Physicians of Philadelphia.)

may be revealed by contrast arthrography and is caused by extra-articular extension of the septic destruction.

Special Diagnostic Techniques. A variety of clinical laboratory studies have been proposed as reliable diagnostic tools for acute infectious arthritis. These studies are intended to speed diagnosis or confirm an infectious etiology when cultures may be negative for unknown reasons or as a result of inadequate bacteriologic techniques or partial treatment. Gas chromatography may be employed to detect microbial metabolites and can provide very rapid results (e.g., 4 hours) even when cultures are negative.[79] Lactic acid assayed by this technique reportedly can distinguish septic from nonseptic arthritis and differentiate nongonococcal arthritis from gonococcal arthritis. In a refinement of this technique, other investigators found that the presence of lactic acid correlated with septic arthritis only when present in concentrations greater than 250 mg per dl. The specificity of this finding is enhanced if succinic acid in a concentration of greater than 0.2 mg per dl is found as well.[80] These findings are present in synovial fluids infected with either gram-positive or gram-negative organisms. The detection of succinic acid may be particularly helpful in patients previously treated with antibiotics. However, specificity and sensitivity must still be confirmed. The major disadvantages of the procedure include its cost and the complexity of the technique. A much simplified and rapid method for the determination of lactic acid in synovial fluid is available, and it is suggested that inflammatory and septic fluids can be

differentiated.[81] However, some overlap was recognized, and further studies are indicated.

Counterimmunoelectrophoresis is a rapid (e.g., 1 to 2 hours), specific, and sensitive technique for the detection of bacterial antigens in synovial fluid.[82] Like gas chromatography, it may be positive even in the absence of viable organisms by culture. Counterimmunoelectrophoresis combines the features of double immunodiffusion in gel and electrophoresis and requires only specific antiserum to the bacteria in question. It has been successfully employed for pneumococcal,[83] meningococcal,[84] and *Hemophilus influenzae*[85] synovial infections. Of course, antibodies as well as antigens may be searched for by counterimmunoelectrophoresis, but the problem that is raised when a positive antibody titer is detected is that of the determination of recency of infection. Bacterial antigens also may be searched for by the use of monoclonal antibodies,[86] but little specific information is available as yet in suppurative arthritis.

Of interest have been the recent observations of localization of specific areas of septic involvement by scintigraphy[87] (see Chapter 40). While radionuclide imaging of the musculoskeletal system is not routinely necessary for the diagnosis of acute infectious arthritis, it may provide localization of unsuspected sites of involvement,[88] help to differentiate overlying cellulitis from infectious synovitis or osteomyelitis,[89] define localization and perhaps degree of activity of osteomyelitis,[89, 90] and aid in evaluating the presence of superimposed joint infection in patients with underlying joint disease such as rheumatoid arthritis. Standard radioisotopes utilized include technetium phosphate compounds or gallium citrate. In some instances, the two techniques may complement each other.[89]

Sacroiliac joint suppurative arthritis, a disease especially seen in children, appears to be a situation in which joint scintigraphy is particularly helpful.[88] These patients often present with pain in adjacent areas to the sacroiliac joint, and routine roentgenograms are usually unremarkable, especially early in the course of the illness. Computerized axial tomography of the sacroiliac joints may demonstrate abnormalities before radiographs are positive.[91]

Finally, for the sake of completeness in regard to diagnostic studies of acute bacterial arthritis, the synovial biopsy should be mentioned. While not specifically diagnostic, the technique may be helpful in obtaining tissue for culture. Histopathologic changes are uniformly marked by an extensive polymorphonuclear leukocyte infiltration in the synovial membrane and frequently by a modest synovial lining cell hyperplasia.[92]

SPECIFIC INFECTIOUS AGENTS IN SEPTIC ARTHRITIS CAUSED BY BACTERIA

While virtually any organism can produce septic arthritis, certain infectious agents appear to be more common than others. Awareness of this epidemiology can provide helpful diagnostic and therapeutic clues. In adults, *Neisseria gonorrhoeae* is responsible for the overwhelming proportion of all septic arthritis, especially in younger healthy hosts. In fact, in most large general hospitals in the United States, presently for every case of nongonococcal infectious arthritis diagnosed, two to three cases caused by *N. gonorrhoeae* will be seen.[93] The staphylococcus accounts for approximately two thirds of all acute nongonococcal septic arthritis (Table 96–1), while streptococci and pneumococci are responsible for

another 15 to 20 percent. Gram-negative organisms appear to be accounting for an increasing proportion of cases of suppurative arthritis,[6-8] and polymicrobial joint infections occur more often than as an occasional oddity (Table 96–1).[96] The spectrum of organisms differs markedly for children, especially for those less than 2 years of age, and because of this and other unique characteristics this topic will be discussed separately.

Gram-Positive Organisms. As noted in Table 96–1, gram-positive organisms account for 80 to 90 percent of acute nongonococcal suppurative arthritis, and staphylococci are responsible for one half to three quarters of those cases. This is a uniform finding throughout most reported series and an important fact to consider when confronted with a suspected acute septic arthritis that is Gram stain negative and lacks the features of disseminated gonococcal infection. Appropriate therapy should be directed at the most likely agent, which is the staphylococcus. Unfortunately, however, it appears that penicillin-resistant staphylococci causing septic arthritis have increased significantly over the past 30 years,[5] and this knowledge must be incorporated into the therapeutic approach.

Streptococci account for up to one quarter of cases of nongonococcal pyarthrosis (Table 96–1), but there are no apparent unique features of the organisms or hosts that result in the illness. Streptococcal arthritis usually results from hematogenous spread from upper respiratory or skin infections, but unusual sources have been described.[71,97] Pneumococci (now referred to as *Streptococcus pneumoniae* instead of *Diplococcus pneumoniae*) are less significant causes of acute nongonococcal suppurative arthritis but account for approximately 6 percent of cases despite their absence as an etiologic agent in some large series (Table 96–1). Septic arthritis caused by pneumococci generally results from bacteremic spread from a primary pulmonary source or, less commonly, from meningeal, upper respiratory, or endocardial sites.[98] Frequently, the hosts are predisposed to pneumococcal infections such as in al-

Table 96–1. Etiologies of Nongonococcal Septic Arthritis in Adults

Studies	Number with Positive Joint Culture	Staphyl-ococci	Strepto-cocci	Pneumo-cocci	Gram-Negative	Multiple Organisms
Watkins et al. (1956)[3]	22	10	5	3	0	4
Ward et al. (1960)[41]	18	11	4	0	3	0
Willkens et al. (1960)[2]	15	10	0	3	1	1
Baitch (1962)[94]	27	15	5	4	3	0
Argen et al. (1966)[9]	42	25	6	9	2	0
Lidgren and Lindberg (1973)[95]	22	17	1	0	4	0
Kelly (1975)[4]	141	108	5	1	22	5
Newman (1976)[5]	104	80	13	0	7	4
Goldenberg and Cohen (1976)[6]	47	15	13	5	11	3
Sharp et al. (1976)[7]	51	24	11	3	13	0
Manshady et al. (1980)[8]	50	28	8	2	12	0
Totals:	539	343 (64%)	71 (12%)	30 (6%)	78 (15%)	17 (3%)

coholics,[10] and occasionally there may be polyarticular involvement. Other gram-positive organisms are extremely rare as a cause of acute bacterial arthritis.

Gram-Negative Organisms. Gram-negative bacteria cause approximately 12 percent of cases of acute nongonococcal infectious arthritis (Table 96–1).[6,12] The apparent reasons for the increasing prevalence of this type of infectious arthritis are related primarily to host factors. In addition to drug addiction,[17,18] underlying chronic diseases such as diabetes or neoplasia, use of agents that suppress the bone marrow, and the presence of intra-articular pathology predispose to infectious articular complications with gram-negative organisms.[12] *Escherichia coli,*[2] *Pseudomonas aeruginosa,*[17,18] and *Serratia marcescens*[99] are the most frequent offending organisms. *E. coli* and *Proteus mirabilis* most commonly originate from the urinary tract, from which they spread hematogenously to joints. By contrast, *Pseudomonas* and *Serratia* joint infections generally result from intravenous drug abuse.

However, gram-negative pyarthrosis is not limited to those organisms described above. There is, in fact, a broad spectrum of gram-negative organisms that have produced suppurative arthritis, and it includes *Salmonella* species,[100] *Hemophilus influenzae,*[101] *Aeromonas hydrophila,*[102,103] anaerobic bacteria,[104] *Arizona hinshawii,*[105] *Vibrio fetus,*[106,107] and *Yersinia enterocolitica.*[108,109] *Salmonella* and *Hemophilus influenzae* infections primarily occur in children, but adult infections, particularly by *H. influenzae,* seem to be increasingly prevalent.[110] Interestingly, *S. choleraesuis* is more likely to be associated with septic arthritis than are other *Salmonella* organisms.[100] *Aeromonas hydrophila* septic arthritis appears to be almost uniquely found with acute myelogenous leukemia. Anaerobic bacterial suppurative arthritis, while rare, nevertheless occurs with enough frequency to require careful culture of any suspected septic arthritis with anaerobic cultures.[111] Suppurative arthritis caused by *Y.enterocolitica* is a more recently recognized illness, although a reactive type of polyarthritis associated with intestinal disease had been well known previously. A further gram-negative organism well-recognized outside of the United States that produces both septic and reactive arthritis is *Brucella* species. While studies of synovial fluid are limited, in some instances of those patients presenting with peripheral arthritis as a manifestation of brucellosis, cultures may be positive.[112]

DISSEMINATED INFECTION BY *N. GONORRHOEAE*

Because of the distinctive clinical picture and marked predominance of gonococcal arthritis over other forms of acute infectious arthritis, special emphasis on this syndrome is indicated. Figures for the prevalence of articular disease complicating gonorrheal infection in the present era are difficult to obtain but appear to be in the range of 1.0 to 3.0 percent.[113-115] The increasing frequency of primary gonococcal infections over the past two decades has led to a striking increase in the number of cases of gonococcal arthritis presenting to physicians and hospitals.[115]

General Clinical Features. Prior to the antibiotic era, gonococcal arthritis was generally recognized as a disease of males that frequently produced residual joint damage.[116] However, recent reports emphasize a female preponderance[114,115,117-121] and a more benign course. Typically, the patients are young (i.e., less than 40 years of age),[119,121] but children[122] and older adults[123] can be afflicted so that the diagnosis must always be kept in mind in the appropriate clinical setting. The presumed reason for the female predominance in this illness is that women constitute the largest reservoir of asymptomatic and untreated gonococcal infection.

In addition to genital sources for dissemination of the gonococcal infection, rectal[115] and pharyngeal[124] sites are playing increasingly important roles as primary foci of infection. It is particularly important to culture the pharynx and anogenital sites in suspected gonococcal infection, as these may be the only sources of a positive culture.

Interestingly, an association between pregnancy or menstruation and the subsequent development of gonococcal arthritis has been repeatedly identified.[113-115,125] In most series reported, females presenting with acute gonococcal arthritis frequently do so during pregnancy or within 1 week of the onset of menses. The essence of the association remains unclear, but physiologic factors (e.g., pH of vaginal secretions) may have an important role.

Systemic features of disseminated gonococcal infection such as fever, chills, and leukocytosis may be present. Fever may be absent, low grade,[119] or significantly elevated.[115] It is especially likely to occur in patients with bacteremia.[114,115,118] Chills occur in one quarter[119] to one half[118] of patients. Peripheral blood leukocyte counts may be normal or mildly elevated;[118,119] striking increases are unusual.

Articular Manifestations. Arthritis is a cardinal manifestation of disseminated gonococcal infection and is often the major clinical feature leading patients to seek medical care. Classically, gonococcal arthritis presents as a migratory polyarthritis which subsequently may localize in one or more joints.[113,119] Monarticular involvement as a presenting sign has generally been found to be uncommon,[115,120] although exceptions have been noted.[119] The most frequently involved joints are the knees and wrists.[117,119] Ankles and the small joints of the hands are less often infected, but any joint may be involved, including the temporomandibular joint.[124] Synovial fluid analyses reveal generally inflammatory joint fluids with mean white blood cell counts of 35,000 to 60,000 per cubic millimeter, of which 90 percent are polymorphonuclear leukocytes.[119] However, occasionally synovial fluid leukocyte counts are normal or only mildly inflammatory.[119] There is apparently no correlation between the level of the synovial fluid leukocyte count and the yield from synovial fluid culture.[118]

Tenosynovitis has long been recognized as a significant component of this syndrome,[116] and many modern series[113,114,117,119] have emphasized its presence. In fact, tenosynovitis was present in 68 percent of all patients in one large study and thus was recommended as a major diagnostic feature of the syndrome.[119] The tenosynovial involvement commonly includes the dorsum of the hands and feet, wrists, or Achilles tendons. Periarthritis or periarticular pain out of proportion to clinical evidence of joint involvement is a less well recognized feature of disseminated gonococcal infection.[119]

Skin Manifestations. The skin lesions that accompany disseminated gonococcal infection may be considered almost pathognomonic for the disease, especially if they occur along with other suggestive clinical features.[126] Several characteristic types of skin lesions may be seen: vesicopustular lesions on an erythematous base, hemorrhagic papules, or hemorrhagic bullae[115] (Fig. 96–8). The lesions are typically tender but sparse in number and tend to be distributed on the distal aspects of the extremities. Occasionally, the patient may be unaware of the presence of these lesions, and attention must be given to a careful skin examination in view of the virtually diagnostic nature of the findings. Histologically, the lesions reveal small vessel vasculitis in the dermis and subcutis, fibrinoid necrosis, dense cellular infiltrate, leukocytoclasis, and hemorrhage.[120] Gram stains and immunofluorescent techniques have often demonstrated the presence of gonococci.[120,127] Direct cultures of the lesions are rarely positive, even in the presence of a positive Gram stain.[114]

Figure 96–8. Skin lesions of disseminated gonococcal infection. The major lesion is vesicopustular, surmounting a hemorrhagic base. The other two, smaller lesions appear more necrotic and probably represent older lesions.

The only skin eruption that may present in a similar fashion is chronic meningococcemia. However, in the presence of an acute onset of arthritis, especially migratory and polyarticular and complicated by tenosynovitis, these skin lesions uniformly suggest disseminated gonococcal infection rather than meningococcal disease.

Miscellaneous Features. Patients with disseminated gonococcal infection may have multiple other organ system manifestations as a result of bacteremia. The most serious are endocarditis, meningitis, and myocarditis.[115] Fortunately, these are relatively uncommon.[119] Hepatic involvement in the form of a perihepatitis may result from gonococcal peritonitis arising from a pelvic focus (Fitz-Hugh–Curtis syndrome),[128] but more commonly is a consequence of gonococcal bacteremia producing a subclinical hepatitis.[115] Gonococcal conjunctivitis is ordinarily the result of direct inoculation rather than hematogenous spread.

Pathogenesis. The pathogenesis of disseminated gonococcal infection has been the subject of controversy, especially since the organism is so infrequently cultured from synovial fluid or skin. If that were not the case, most could readily accept the concept of a direct toxic effect by the bacteria on the various tissues.[115] However, in the absence of that type of evidence, investigators have raised questions of a hypersensitivity mechanism or immune complex interaction. The former postulate would invoke a response to the gonococcus much like the response in patients who develop carditis and arthritis (e.g., rheumatic fever) after group A streptococcal infection.[115,129] Recent experimental studies contributing to this type of hypothesis have involved the intra-articular introduction of *N. gonorrhoeae* and have demonstrated an acute purulent synovitis followed by a chronic synovitis. Significantly, no organisms could be recovered after 24 hours, whereas viable *S. aureus* could be recovered indefinitely.[130] Furthermore, a nonviable bacterial cell wall component, the gonococcal lipopolysaccharide, can produce a similar picture, suggesting a "reactive" type of arthritis. Investigations for the presence of immune complexes in the sera and synovial fluids of active patients with disseminated gonococcal infection have yielded varying results, depending upon the assay employed.[131-133] Immune mechanisms may play a role in other ways, such as in the production of skin lesions, in which complement activation has been shown to occur through the alternate complement pathway by gonococcal endotoxic lipopolysaccharide.[134]

Based upon the present body of knowledge, it appears that the peripheral manifestations of disseminated gonococcal infection are more often related to a "reactive" or "postinfectious" arthritis than to a classic septic arthritis. Why dissemination occurs is unclear, but it has been shown that gonococci causing the arthritis-dermatitis syndrome are resistant to the bactericidal action of normal human serum[135] and the clinical manifestations may be linked to this property.[136] Resistant organisms also have unique nutritional requirements[137] and there is evidence that they bind IgG, which acts as a blocking antibody and competes with the bactericidal action of normal human serum.[138] Furthermore, it has been recognized that susceptibility to *Neisseria* infections is enhanced in individuals with a homozygous deficiency of the sixth, seventh, or eighth components of complement.[139]

On the basis of clinical studies, two apparently distinct forms of gonococcal arthritis have been described.[114] The first or bacteremic form is manifested by fever, chills, vesiculopustular skin lesions, polyarthralgias, tenosynovitis, and positive blood cultures. In this form, synovial effusions are rare. The second or septic form is characterized by monoarthritis with effusion but lacks fever, chills, skin lesions, or positive blood cultures. This concept was expanded by others so that a spectrum was recognized and a transition phase was noted that was marked by both positive joint fluid cultures and hemotogenous manifestations.[140-142] However, other clinical studies challenge that concept based upon their review of patterns of diseases and clinical response to therapy.[118,119] It remains to be clarified as to whether sequential stages or significant overlapping of clinical features is the clinical rule.

Diagnosis. The diagnosis of disseminated gonococcal infection depends upon clinical suspicion and cultural documentation. However, even in the absence of positive cultures, the syndrome may be so highly suspected that a therapeutic trial may be justified.[119] The acute onset of migratory polyarthritis, tenosynovitis, and/or typical skin lesions in a young sexually active female should clearly lead one to consider disseminated gonococcal infection as the cause of the illness. Fever, pharyngitis, urethritis, proctitis, and vaginal discharge, while helpful in diagnosis, often are not present. Cultures should be obtained from cervix or urethra, blood, involved joints, rectum, and pharynx.[119] Gram stains should be performed on urethral material, joint fluid, and fresh skin lesions. If gram-negative intracellular diplococci are seen in the appropriate clinical setting, treatment should be instituted.

The gonococcus is a very fastidious organism and requires extra care for effective cultures. In noncontaminated areas such as blood, skin lesions, or synovial fluid, chocolate agar (heated blood enriched with a thermolabile yeast extract) is the most widely used medium. For contaminated areas such as cervix, rectum, and pharynx, Thayer-Martin medium is advised in order to reduce growth of normal bacterial flora.[143] This medium contains vancomycin, colistin, and nystatin plus other supplements in addition to conventional chocolate agar. With either medium, plates should be warmed immediately prior to use and cultures plated at the bedside. Conditions for culture growth should include increased humidity, increased carbon dioxide tension, and optimal pH. However, even under the most optimal circumstances, synovial fluids yield less than 50 percent growth of the organism.[119] Therefore, in the appropriate clinical setting a positive culture from any of the cultured sites may be considered as confirmatory for diagnosis. Note should be made of the recovery of *N. gonorrhoeae* from a "sterile" synovial fluid in a patient with gonococcal

arthritis by using an overlay medium containing a high sucrose concentration. It was presumed that the organisms existed in a cell-wall-deficient osmotically fragile state and thus could not be grown on conventional media.[144]

In addition to routine diagnostic studies, fluorescent antibody techniques have been successfully applied in disseminated gonococcal infection in order to identify the organism.[127] Counterimmunoelectrophoresis of serum and synovial fluid has had varying results, but it may be a promising technique.[132] Gonococcal serologic studies as presently performed cannot distinguish between recent and distant infections and therefore provide little diagnostic aid for the acute situation.

Treatment. Treatment of disseminated gonococcal infection with arthritis includes appropriate antibiotics, joint drainage, and immobilization of the involved joint(s). Acutely, analgesics may be necessary, but this will become unnecessary as response to therapy ensues. The most widely recommended antibiotic program for disseminated gonococcal infection includes 10 million units of aqueous penicillin G intravenously daily until symptoms subside, followed by oral ampicillin, 2 grams daily up to a total of 10 days.[121] Other regimens, including oral ampicillin alone, low-dose parenteral penicillin G, oral tetracycline, or parenteral cephalosporins, appear to result in adequate responses.[121] Of interest, a low-dose regimen of penicillin (procaine penicillin G, 600,000 units intramuscularly every 12 hours for 10 days) has been shown to be as effective as high-dose penicillin therapy in the treatment of disseminated gonococcal infection.[145] In fact, even short-term (3 days) parenteral therapy with aqueous penicillin G has been shown to be effective in this syndrome.[146] In the pregnant penicillin-allergic woman, oral erythromycin (500 mg every 6 hours) has been effective.[147] However, it should be clear that unreliable patients or patients with complicated problems such as purulent synovial effusions should never have their treatment continued on an ambulatory basis. They require further hospitalization for supervision of parenteral therapy and supportive care.[121] Clearly, if endocarditis or meningitis is present, prolonged intravenous therapy of 10 million to 20 million units per day is required. If penicillin allergy exists, treatment should consist of oral tetracycline or erythromycin.

Joint drainage can generally be accomplished by repeated needle aspirations (see Management of Acute Infectious Arthritis) and should be continued until the effusion is minimal. Joint rest will reduce pain and may be accomplished by temporary splinting. As soon as joint symptoms subside, passive range of motion exercises may be instituted preparatory to active exercises or weight-bearing.

The therapeutic response is generally brisk and occurs within 2 days.[119,121] Occasionally, very purulent effusions resolve more slowly. The response to therapy is uniformly so clear that is has been employed as a diagnostic feature when a therapeutic trial has been initiated.[119] One may attempt a therapeutic trial of penicillin therapy if the clinical picture is strongly suggestive of disseminated gonococcal infection but only after appropriate cultures have been obtained. Unfortunately, gonococcal arthritis due to penicillin-resistant organisms has been recognized recently[148] and vigilence in this regard is suggested for the future. Parenteral cefoxitin appears to be effective against penicillinase-producing gonococci.

Neisseria meningitidis **Arthritis.** Since meningococcal arthritis may closely resemble gonococcal arthritis, it requires a separate review in order to contrast it with the more common syndrome. Arthritis complicates meningonococcal infection in between 2 and 10 percent of cases.[149–50] It is usually oligoarticular and appears as the meningeal infection is improving,[149] but may present as an acute polyarthritis[151] or may even mimic disseminated gonococcal infection.[152] Skin lesions may be indistinguishable from those seen with gonococcemia,[126] and the diagnosis may only be made bacteriologically.[152,153] Tenosynovitis does not appear to occur or is rare with meningococcal infection and hence, if present, may provide a differentiating point. The effusions may be mildly inflammatory or purulent[149,151] but are usually sterile upon culture. Joints involved primarily include the knee, ankle, and elbow. The pathogenesis of the arthritis (and cutaneous lesions) is believed to be a hypersensitivity phenomenon. Evidence for this has included the demonstration of circulating antibody and reduced serum complement, and deposits of meningococcal antigen, immunoglobulin, and complement in synovium and synovial fluid leukocytes.[154] Circulating immune complexes have been detected in one case.[155]

Diagnostic principles are similar to that for disseminated gonococcal infection. In addition to the routine studies, counterimmunoelectrophoresis of synovial fluid has been diagnostically helpful in meningococcal infection.[84] Routine cerebrospinal fluid examination should be performed if the diagnosis is suspected or made without meningeal signs being present. Treatment consists of high dose penicillin therapy.

MANAGEMENT OF ACUTE INFECTIOUS ARTHRITIS

The management of acute nongonococcal infectious arthritis should begin immediately after reasonable suspicion of the diagnosis or certainly following confirmation of that diagnosis. Of all the clinical adages concerning septic arthritis, the one that stands out as incontestable is the fact that early treatment leads to the best long-term results, whereas conversely, delay in institution of treatment leads to the poorest long-term results[4-6,9,156,157] (Table 96–2). Basically, the treatment of septic arthritis includes appropriate antibiotic therapy and adequate drainage. In the following discussion these various aspects of medical treatment will be reviewed and the role of surgical intervention will be examined. Generally it may be stated that most cases may be controlled with medical therapy alone, but sufficient exceptions exist such that early consultation with an orthopedic surgeon may be indicated, even if surgical intervention is subsequently obviated.

Medical therapy of acute suppurative arthritis begins with the choice of antibiotic agents. Antibiotic therapy should be routinely administered parenterally in an effort to provide maximal serum and synovial fluid concentrations. The initial choice of antibiotic should be based upon results of culture, findings on Gram stain, or greatest clinical likelihood (in that order). If the organism is known, the choice of antibiotic is obvious, especially if drug sensitivities are available. Alternative choices of antibiotics may be necessary (Table 96–3) if the patient is allergic to the drug of choice. In the absence of a positive culture, the physician must rely upon the

Table 96–2. General Approach to Acute Bacterial Arthritis

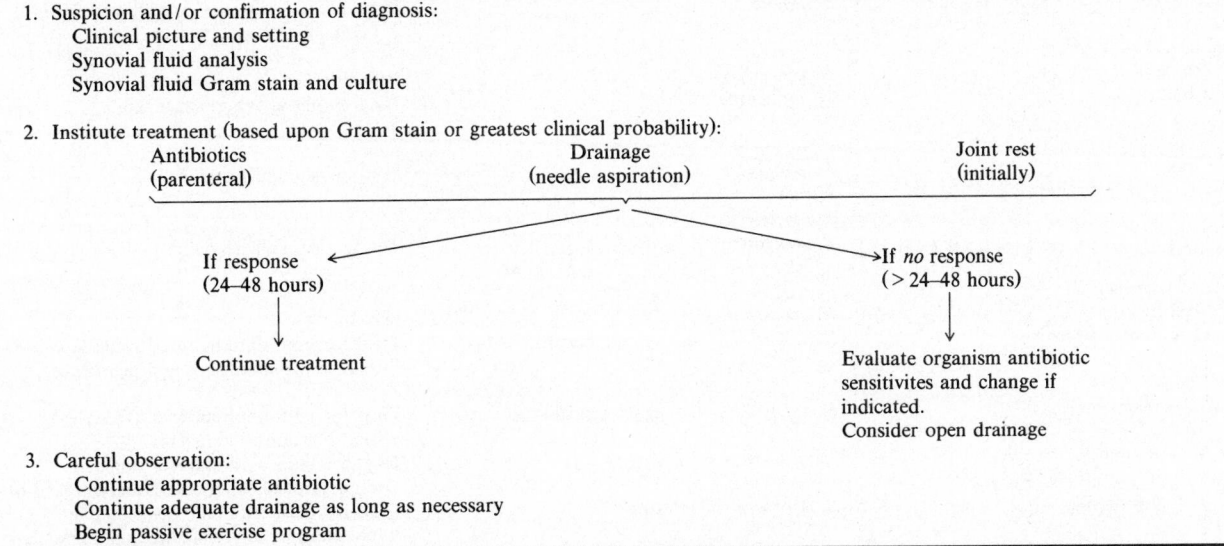

1. Suspicion and/or confirmation of diagnosis:
   Clinical picture and setting
   Synovial fluid analysis
   Synovial fluid Gram stain and culture

2. Institute treatment (based upon Gram stain or greatest clinical probability):
   Antibiotics (parenteral)   Drainage (needle aspiration)   Joint rest (initially)

   If response (24–48 hours)   If *no* response (>24–48 hours)

   Continue treatment   Evaluate organism antibiotic sensitivites and change if indicated.
   Consider open drainage

3. Careful observation:
   Continue appropriate antibiotic
   Continue adequate drainage as long as necessary
   Begin passive exercise program

Table 96–3. Antibiotic Therapy of Acute Infectious Arthritis of Known Cause in Adults

Infecting Organism	Initial Choice	Alternative Choices		Duration of Treatment
Neisseria gonorrhoeae	Penicillin G 10 million units/ day (q 6 hours)	Tetracycline Erythromycin	2 g/day (p.o) 2 g/day (p.o)	10–14 days
Staphylococcus aureus	Nafcillin 8–12 g/day (q 4–6 hours)	Cefazolin Clindamycin Vancomycin	3 g/day 1–2 g/day 2 g/day	3–4 weeks
Streptococcus pyogenes *Streptococcus pneumoniae*	Penicillin G 10 million units/ day (q 6 hours)	Vancomycin	2 g/day	2–3 weeks
Escherichia coli (and *Proteus* species) *Pseudomonas aeruginosa* *Serratia marcescens*	Tobramycin 5 mg/kg/day (q 8 hours) and Ticarcillin 20 g/day	Gentamicin Amikacin	5 mg/kg/day 15 mg/kg/day	4–6 weeks

Gram stain for guidance in antibiotic therapy. Gram-positive cocci will generally indicate *Staphylococcus aureus* infection; and since an increasing percentage of these are due to penicillin-resistant organisms,[5] a penicillinase-resistant penicillin should be employed (Table 93–3). Gram-negative cocci on smear indicate a gonococcal infection, except in infants and children in whom they are more likely to be related to *H. influenzae* infection (see below). Gram-negative bacilli in joint fluids of adults usually indicate infection caused by *E. coli, P. aeruginosa,* or *S. marcescens.* These organisms are generally sensitive to a combination of tobramycin and ticarcillin. (Table 96–3). In those patients in whom the diagnosis of acute septic arthritis is suspected but the synovial fluid Gram stain is negative, antibiotic treatment must be based upon probabilities. This should take into account the age of the patient, clinical presentation, and presence of underlying disease (Tables 96–4 and 96–5). In previously healthy adults, *N. gonorrhoeae* is the most likely causative organism, especially if typical skin lesions and/or tenosynovitis is present. Penicillin G is the definitive therapy. If the patient is an adult and has an underlying chronic disease, initial antibiotic coverage should include a penicillinase-resistant penicillin for possible *S. aureus* and tobramycin for possible gram-negative bacillary infection (Table 96–4). Neonates initially must be treated for gram-negative bacillary and *S. aureus* infections, whereas infants and children with negative smears must be treated for both *H. influenzae* and *S. aureus* (Table 96–4). Patients with rheumatoid arthritis, diabetes mellitus, or myeloproliferative disorders or those who are alcoholics or drug abusers have a predisposition to particular infections (Table 96–5), and this information may be helpful in directing treatment if septic arthritis supervenes in such patients.

There is abundant evidence that parenterally administered antibiotics penetrate the synovial membrane and achieve sufficient concentrations in joint fluid that are many times greater than the minimal inhibitory concentration necessary for most pathogenic bacteria invading joints.[158-165] This is true for most commonly used antibiotics except for perhaps erythromycin[159] and there-

Table 96–4. Choice of Initial Antibiotic Therapy Based Upon Gram Stain and Age

Gram Stain	Presumed Organism	Agent
Gram-positive cocci (adult or child)	*S. aureus*	Penicillinase-resistance penicillin (nafcillin or methicillin)
Gram-negative cocci		
Adolescent or adult	*N. gonorrhoeae*	Penicillin G
Child	*H. influenzae*	Chloramphenicol and ampicillin
Gram-negative bacilli		
Adult	*P. aeruginosa* *E. coli* *S. marcescens*	Tobramycin and ticarcillin
Child	*P. aeruginosa*	Tobramycin and ticarcillin
Negative smear		
Healthy adult	*N. gonorrhoeae*	Penicillin G
Compromised host	*S. aureus* or gram-negative bacilli	Treat for both until cultures available (nafcillin, tobramycin, and ticarcillin)
Child		
Neonate	*S. aureus* or gram-negative bacilli	Treat for both until cultures available (nafcillin and tobramycin)
1–18 months	*H. influenzae* or *S. aureus*	Treat for both until cultures available (chloramphenicol, nafcillin and ampicillin)
>18 months	*S. aureus* or *H. influenzae*	Treat for both until cultures available (chloramphenicol, nafcillin and ampicillin)

Table 96–5. Most Likely Causes of Acute Bacterial Arthritis Related to Underlying Disease

Disease	Agents	Comments
Rheumatoid arthritis	S. aureus	Usual joint sites; may be polyarticular
Alcoholism and/or cirrhosis	Gram-negative bacilli	Usual joint sites
	S. pneumoniae	
Drug abusers	P. aeruginosa	Usual plus unusual sites (sternoclavicular and sacroiliac joints)
	S. marcescens	
Myeloproliferative disorders	Gram-negative bacilli	Treatment of underlying disease may produce immunosuppression and further decrease host resistance
	Aeromonas hydrophila	
Diabetes mellitus	Gram-positive and negative	Diabetes frequently out of control

fore allows for reliable treatment of acute infectious arthritis with systemic antibiotics. The use of intra-articular antibiotics is therefore unnecessary and even contraindicated. Intra-articular injection of antibiotics appears to produce a chemical synovitis[9] and additionally offers the risk of introducing superinfection. Assuming that the antibiotic employed reaches the joint, one potential problem still exists. This concerns aminoglycoside antibiotics and is related to the significant reduction of their antibacterial activity by lowered pH that results from the acidosis associated with significant leukocytosis.[166] Whether this phenomenon is clinically important or not is unclear, but adequate drainage and antibacterial monitoring are of paramount importance in gram-negative septic arthritis treated with these agents.

The antibacterial activity of the synovial fluid during systemic antibiotic therapy may be monitored by a simple tube-dilution procedure, and simultaneous assessment of serum activity should also be obtained.[159] This type of determination is most useful in more recalcitrant joint sepsis such as gram-negative bacillary infections but may even be considered for routine management of acute nongonococcal bacterial arthritis.

Assuming adequate drainage, the duration of systemic antibiotic therapy is the next prime consideration. As noted, gonococcal articular infections may be treated systemically until symptoms and signs clear (several days usually) and be followed by oral antibiotic therapy for up to 10 to 14 days. However, other bacterial joint infections require more prolonged treatment (Table 96–3). Pneumococcal and streptococcal arthritis should be treated for 2 to 3 weeks, while staphylococcal pyarthrosis requires at least 3 to 4 weeks of therapy. Gram-negative bacillary suppurative arthritis necessitates a minimum of 4 to 6 weeks of antibiotic treatment.

It is necessary to consider acute infectious arthritis similar to any other closed-space infection.[167] As noted previously, purulent effusions may accelerate the destruction of articular cartilage because of increased pressure and enzymatic activity. Thus, adequate drainage is essential in the management of this suppurative process. The issue of closed needle aspiration versus open surgical drainage as the initial mode of drainage has been hotly debated for many years. Since most early series (preantibiotic era) were collected by orthopedic surgeons, open surgical drainage was primarily used. With the development of the specialty of Rheumatology and the ready access to sterile disposable equipment, closed needle

aspiration became a reasonable alternative. On subsequent review of some more recent series, the superiority of one form of drainage over the other was not obvious.[3-5,9] Goldenberg and associates specifically looked at that question, albeit in a retrospective study, and concluded that needle aspiration was in fact superior to surgical drainage. This was in spite of a greater prevalence of adverse host factors existing in the medically treated group.[168] Similar results have been recorded by Rosenthal and associates.[169] The only significant exception may be the hip, for which there are few data with regard to the relationship of outcome to needle drainage. Joint aspiration with a large bore needle can be easily performed in superficial joints such as the knee, shoulder, wrist, or ankle. It should be carried out once or twice daily for as long as a significant purulent exudate is present.

The septic joint that responds within 48 hours to high-dose parenteral antibiotic administration and daily complete aspiration of the proteolytic pus does not require surgical drainage. Nevertheless, surgical drainage of the infected joint has specific indications. A persistent febrile course, purulent accumulation in spite of frequent aspirations and effective serum levels of antibiotic determined by tube dilution studies, unsuccessful complete aspiration of viscous pus through a large bore needle, and inaccessibility to the joint (e.g., hip and sacroiliac joint) are all indications for surgical drainage. The method of decompression of the joint depends on the stage of infection and the accessibility of the joint. Surgical decompression is performed as soon as the conditions for surgical intervention have been established in order to prevent further joint destruction and pathological dislocation.

The principles of surgical decompression include adequate exposure of the joint, representative material removed for culture, copious irrigation of the articular cartilage surface, and synovectomy. The capsule is closed around temporary closed-suction drainage. Perfusion with isotonic solutions without dextrose have been utilized since this type of closed system irrigation and drainage permits continuous debridement of the joint. There is both clinical and experimental suggestion[170,171] that this type of technique may be helpful in the treatment of septic arthritis, but controlled human studies are not available. However, as noted previously, antibiotic instillation into the closed suction irrigation is not necessary, because adequate joint concentrations are reached through intravenous antibiotic administration. Postoperatively the septic joints should be splinted in a position of function. After 10 days following initiation of treatment, a program of guided mobilization should be started. Synovitis may persist, and long-term rehabilitation programs are necessary to gain adequate motion.

The prognosis for septic arthritis that requires surgical decompression is related to the chronicity of the disease, presence of osteochondral destruction, and extent of synovitis at the time of decompression. When bony destruction occurs as a result of septic arthritis, specific surgical approaches to the individual joints may be indicated subsequently.

In addition to systemic antibiotic therapy and drainage, initially, the acute pyogenic joint should be immobilized in an effort to decrease pain and reduce trauma to the articular cartilage. When subsidence of pain occurs, usually after approximately 48 to 72 hours, passive range of motion exercises should be initiated. This entails movement of the joint through as much of its range of motion as tolerated by the patient once or twice daily. As convalescence progresses and the inflammation further subsides, active assisted exercises should begin in order to regain mobility and increase strength. Finally, when able, the patient may begin active resistive exercises in order to further improve strength. Of note, it has been demonstrated that early active motion in the treatment of pyogenic arthritis of the knee may have significant advantages.[172]

In summary, appropriate systemic antibiotic therapy coupled with adequate joint aspiration appears to produce results that are equal or superior to surgical decompression in the treatment of acute bacterial arthritis. With the exception of the hip joint of the infant or young child and the sacroiliac joint, this nonoperative form of management should be instituted initially. The earlier the recognition of the diagnosis occurs and treatment is instituted, the better the results. However, if some clinical response does not occur in 48 to 72 hours or adequate drainage is not accomplished, surgical decompression should then be immediately considered. A cooperative approach to septic arthritis between the rheumatologist and orthopedist should result in maximal patient care and minimal morbidity.

SPECIAL PROBLEMS

Childhood Septic Arthritis. Acute suppurative arthritis occurs in all age groups in children and is often seen in those under 2 years of age.[173] Notably, it is two to three times more common in males.[174] The most common joint involvement occurs in the hip, with the knee and elbow following in order of frequency. Rarely, multiple joints are involved.

Three routes of entry of bacteria have been postulated in the pediatric population: (1) Hematogenous seeding of the synovium via the blood from a distant focus. This is the most common pathogenesis of childhood septic arthritis. These infections arise most commonly from the middle ear, the upper respiratory tract, or infected abrasions or furuncles. (2) Direct extension of a bacterial organism from an adjacent focus such as osteomyelitis. Osteomyelitis uniformly occurs in the metaphysis at the site of vascular invasion of the hypertrophied zone of the epiphyseal plate, a site of sluggish blood flow and poor reticuloendothelial defenses. Bacterial osteomyelitis may be the origin for pyarthrosis primarily in the hip and occasionally in the shoulder, elbow, and knee, since the metaphysis anatomically is within the joint capsule in these joints. Extension of the metaphyseal infection beyond the boundary of the cortex would lead to direct spread into the joint. (3) Direct inoculation of bacteria by accidental wounds such as a puncture wound[175] or as a complication of femoral venipuncture.[176]

The causative organism in suppurative arthritis in the pediatric population is significantly related to the age group (Table 96–4). Nelson,[173] in an in-depth study of 221 patients, did not find a single case of staphylococcal septic arthritis in children between the ages of 1 month and 18 months of age, although others have.[177,178] However, his small group of neonatal pyarthroses included *Staphylococcus aureus* as well as a variety of other agents, a finding similar to a more recent study.[179] In an earlier study, Nelson and Koontz[180] had called attention to the previously unrecognized frequency of *Hemophilus influenzae* as a causative agent of acute pyogenic arthritis in children. This occurred primarily in the age group from 1 to 24 months of age and uniformly was due to Type b *Hemophilus* organisms. Rarely *H. influenzae* may cause acute suppurative arthritis in the neonate.[181] Group B streptococcal infections appear to be emerging as an important etiologic agent in septic arthritis of infants less than 2 months of age, and these infants usually have an associated osteomyelitis.[182]

A history of antecedent infection or of recent injury may be obtained in many pediatric patients. The onset of symptoms is usually abrupt, although it may be insidious, and the affected limb is generally the focus of the presenting complaint. If the lower extremity is involved, the child will walk with an antalgic gait; the youngest infants will refrain from utilizing the limb and cry when it is touched or moved. Temperature may be significantly elevated, although in a newborn infant systemic manifestations may be sparse. Physical examination of the involved joint will show it to be warm and swollen and held in a position that would maximize the capsular volume (the hip in abduction, flexion, and external rotation; the knee in 45 degrees of flexion). The child is quite sensitive to the slightest motion about the joint. Laboratory abnormalities such as leukocytosis or elevation of erythrocyte sedimentation rate may be present but are nonspecific findings. Early radiographic findings include only joint capsular distention. If the hip joint is involved, subluxation or joint space widening may be seen. Late stage radiographic abnormalities may include dislocation and/or separation or even disappearance of the epiphyseal plate.[183] Signs of underlying osteomyelitis may be present, particularly in the hip joint. Arthrography of the hip, especially in infants, may help distinguish the late sequelae of bacterial infection from avascular necrosis.[184]

As previously noted, the diagnosis of infectious arthritis depends upon direct aspiration of the joint and identification of the etiologic agent. Suspected sites of seeding should be cultured, particularly the throat, sputum, and skin, in addition to blood cultures. Direct aspiration of the hip may be difficult, and fluoroscopic control is essential even in a well sedated child. A large bore needle is necessary to adequately obtain the viscous pus. In addition to diagnosis, hip aspiration immediately reduces the pressure on the tenuous retinacular vessels and removes degradative enzymes.

Because of the great variety of bacterial agents involved in childhood septic arthritis, precise diagnosis is imperative. Gram stains of joint fluid may be helpful in initiating appropriate antibiotic therapy. In the neonate, if gram-positive cocci are seen in direct stains of joint fluid, nafcillin therapy should be initiated. Should the infecting agent turn out to be a streptococcus, penicillin G is adequate therapy. If gram-negative rods are seen, tobramycin and ticarcillin should be utilized. If the smear is negative in this age group and septic arthritis is suspected, both nafcillin and tobramycin should be utilized until culture results are available. In the 1- to 18-month age group, *Hemophilus influenzae* or *S. aureus* is usually involved, and nafcillin and ampicillin plus chloramphenicol are recommended for those patients with a negative smear. When treating suspected *H. influenzae* infection, initial therapy should include both ampicillin and chloramphenicol because of the emergence of ampicillin-resistant strains.[185] In the pediatric age group beyond 2 years, the most common organisms are *S. aureus* or *H. influenzae* and appropriate treatment is rendered on that basis unless the Gram stain is particularly revealing. In all cases once the etiologic agents and sensitivities have been established, the safest agent with the narrowest spectrum should be administered parenterally. It has been demonstrated[160] that in children, as in adults, antibiotic concentrations in septic joint effusions approach or exceed serum levels, and intra-articular administration is unnecessary and even contraindicated. Joint aspiration should be performed frequently to remove pus. The limb should be immobilized initially to help control the associated synovitis and for relief of pain. Parenteral antibiotic therapy should be continued for at least 2 weeks for *Hemophilus*, pneumococci, and streptococci. A minimum of 3 weeks of therapy is indicated for staphylococcal and coliform organisms. Evidence for underlying osteomyelitis would require more prolonged periods of antibiotic therapy.

Surgical drainage of an affected joint should be considered in the presence of a persistent febrile course in spite of adequate antibiotic coverage (48 hours) and/or difficulty in providing adequate joint drainage. Septic arthritis of the hip, however, presents a special problem. Because of the vulnerability of the vascular supply by the retinaculum vessels in the hip, maximal decompres-sion of the joint is required. Inaccessibility of the hip joint to repeated percutaneous aspiration uniformly ne-cessitates surgical drainage. Postoperatively, the affected limb should be fixed in a spica cast in a position of abduction and slight flexion to prevent dislocation.

The prognosis of infantile and childhood septic arthritis is primarily related to the duration of disease prior to institution of treatment. Other prognostic factors include site of joint involvement, virulence of the organism, and presence or absence of associated osteomyelitis.[174,186,187] As noted, the infantile hip is particularly vulnerable to long-term complications which include persistent dislocation, subluxation, femoral head and neck deformity, osteonecrosis, shortening of extremity, and fusion.[186-190] Early diagnosis and institution of appropriate antibiotic treatment and surgical decompression of the hip joint should help prevent these complications.

Sacroiliac Joint Septic Arthritis. Pyogenic infection of a sacroiliac joint is a rare and frequently misdiagnosed form of septic arthritis.[88,191-194] It is characterized by buttock pain often complicated by upper sciatica and limping, and usually occurs in late childhood or adolescence. However, pyogenic sacroiliitis has been recognized more recently as a problem encountered in parenteral drug abusers.[195,196] The presence of fever is variable, and clinical findings may be obscured, leading to delay in diagnosis unless care is taken to consider the entity. Because of the buttock symptoms and limp, hip disease is usually contemplated; but careful examination discloses the presence of sacroiliac tenderness, along with a positive straight leg raise, a positive Gaenslen test, and pain on pelvic compression. X-rays may be negative initially, but radionuclide bone scintigraphy is very helpful for diagnosis,[88,196] as may be computerized axial tomography.[91] The majority of cases in non–drug abusers are due to staphylococcal infection, and the primary source is the skin. In drug abusers, the usual etiology is a gram-negative bacillus, especially *Pseudomonas aeruginosa*. Diagnosis may be confirmed by needle aspiration[195] or operative biopsy of the sacroiliac joint. Blood cultures are frequently positive. Treatment, if discovered early, consists of parenteral antibiotics and immobilization only. Surgical drainage and debridement are required only for chronic infections. The prognosis is quite good.

It appears that intravenous drug abusers have a predilection for septic arthritis of fibrocartilagenous joints, as noted above.[19,195,196] These include the sacroiliac and sternoclavicular joints as well as intervertebral discs. To this may be added the pelvic symphysis.[197] *P. aeruginosa* was found to be the etiologic agent, and patients presented with suprapubic pain. Early recognition and treatment, including parenteral antibiotics and debridement, produce a rapid response.

Septic Bursitis. Septic bursitis is an uncommon but easily treated form of musculoskeletal infection.[198] It involves the olecranon and prepatellar and infrapatellar bursae primarily and occurs as a result of direct inno-culation. Whereas chronically ill or immunocompro-mised individuals are the usual hosts for suppurative arthritis, septic bursitis generally occurs in healthy individuals who are predisposed to trauma. Although septic bursitis is not associated ordinarily with intra-articular infection, rare examples of such an association have been reported.[199] Septic bursitis can readily be distinguished from pyarthrosis by careful examination. The most frequent diagnostic problem is its misinterpretation as a nonseptic or traumatic bursitis. The diagnosis is suspected from the history of acute painful bursal swelling and skin erythema over the involved bursa. Fluid aspiration and analysis ordinarily reveal a significant leukocytosis with polymorphonuclear cell predominance. Confirmation of the diagnosis occurs with culture proof of infection, which is invariably staphylococcal. Therapy includes antibiotics (which reach the bursal fluid readily) and closed drainage, which usually results in an excellent prognosis.[200] In contrast to septic arthritis, late complications are extremely rare.

Postinfectious Synovitis. A feature of treated septic arthritis that has received relatively little attention but occasionally provides clinical confusion is the phenomenon of postinfectious synovitis.[9] The entity consists of the development of a sterile effusion and synovitis which occurs after the acute infectious arthritis has been controlled. The synovitis is unrelated to the severity of infection or previous status of the involved joint. The joint is warm and tender, and an effusion with leukocytosis is present. Unfortunately, this synovitis may be misinterpreted as a recrudescence of infection and aggressive therapy instituted. Biopsy of the synovial membrane reveals the characteristics of a more chronic inflammation with synovial lining cell hyperplasia and mononuclear cell as well as striking polymorphonuclear leukocyte infiltration.[92] Argen and associates[9] have related this phenomenon to intra-articular antibiotic injection, but clearly this does not account for all or perhaps even most cases. The role of bacterial debris in this process is unknown, but bacterial cell envelopes clearly have phlogistic properties[56] and may be involved in this sequela of acute infectious arthritis. Once confirmed as a noninfectious problem, anti-inflammatory therapy may be introduced.

References

1. Kellgren, J.H., Ball, J., Fairbrother, R.W., and Barnes, K.L.: Suppurative arthritis complicating rheumatoid arthritis. Br. Med. J. 1:1193, 1958.
2. Willkens, R.F., Healey, L.A., and Decker, J.L.: Acute infectious arthritis in the aged and chronically ill. Arch. Intern. Med. 106:354, 1960.
3. Watkins, M.B., Samilson, R.L., and Winters, D.M.: Acute suppurative arthritis. J. Bone Joint Surg. 38A:1313, 1956.
4. Kelly, P.J.: Bacterial arthritis in the adult. Orthop. Clin. N. Am. 6:973, 1975.
5. Newman, J.H.: Review of septic arthritis throughout the antibiotic era. Ann. Rheum. Dis. 35:198, 1976.
6. Goldenberg, D.L., and Cohen, A.S.: Acute infectious arthritis. A review of patients with nongonococcal joint infections (with emphasis on therapy and prognosis). Am. J. Med. 60:369, 1976.
7. Sharp, J.T., Lidsky, M.D., Duffy, J., and Duncan, M.W.: Infectious arthritis. Arch. Intern. Med. 139:1125, 1979.
8. Manshady, B.M., Thompson, G.R., and Weiss, J.J.: Septic arthritis in a general hospital, 1966–1977. J. Rheumatol. 7:523, 1980.
9. Argen, R.J., Wilson, C.H., and Wood, P.: Suppurative arthritis. Clinical features of 42 cases. Arch. Intern. Med. 117:661, 1966.
10. Kauffman, C.A., Watanakunakorn, C., and Phair, J.P.: Pneumococcal arthritis. J. Rheumatol. 3:409, 1976.
11. Douglas, G.W., Levin, R.U., and Sokoloff, L.: Infectious arthritis complicating neoplastic disease. N. Engl. J. Med. 270:299, 1964.
12. Goldenberg, D.L., Brandt, K.D., Cathcart, E.S., and Cohen, A.S.: Acute arthritis caused by gram-negative bacilli: A clinical characterization. Medicine 53:197, 1974.
13. Myers, A.R., Miller, L.M. and Pinals, R.S.: Pyarthrosis complicating rheumatoid arthritis. Lancet 2:714, 1969.
14. Quismorio, F.P., and Dubois, E.L.: Septic arthritis in systemic lupus erythematosus. J. Rheumatol. 2:73, 1975.
15. Palmer, D.W.: Septic arthritis in sickle cell-thalassemia: Pathophysiology of impaired response to infection. Arthritis Rheum. 18:339, 1976.
16. Ebong, W.W.: The treatment of severely ill patients with sickle cell anemia and associated arthritis. Clin. Orthop. 149:145, 1980.
17. Gifford, D.B., Patzaikis, M., Ivler, D., and Swezey, R.L.: Septic arthritis due to Pseudomonas in heroin addicts. J. Bone Joint Surg. 57A:631, 1975.
18. Bayer, A.S., Chow, A.W., Louie, J.S., and Guze, L.B.: Sternoclavicular pyoarthrosis due to gram-negative bacilli. Arch. Intern. Med. 137:1036, 1977.
19. Roce, R.P., and Yoshikawa, T.T.: Primary skeletal infections in heroin users: A clinical characterization, diagnosis and therapy. Clin. Orthop. 144:238, 1979.
20. Mowat, A.G., and Baum, J.: Chemotaxis of polymorphonuclear leukocytes from patients with diabetes mellitus. N. Engl. J. Med. 284:621, 1971.
21. Bagdade, E.A., Root, R.K., and Bulger, R.J.: Impaired leukocyte function in patients with poorly controlled diabetes. Diabetes 23:9, 1974.
22. Brayton, R.G., Stokes, P.E., Schwartz, M.S., and Louria, D.B.: Effect of alcohol and various diseases on leukocyte mobilization, phagocytosis and intracellular bacterial killing. N. Engl. J. Med. 282:123, 1970.
23. VanEpps, D.E., Strickland, R.G., and Williams, R.G.: Inhibitors of leukocyte chemotaxis in alcoholic liver disease. Am. J. Med. 59:200, 1975.
24. Twomey, J.J.: Infections complicating multiple myeloma and chronic lymphocytic leukemia. Arch. Intern. Med. 132:562, 1973.
25. Myers, A.R., Mills, J.A., and Ropes, M.W.: The problem of infection in systemic lupus erythematosus. Arthritis Rheum. 10:300, 1967.
26. Staples, P.J., Gerding, D.N., Decker, J.L., and Gordon, R.S.: Incidence of infection in systemic lupus erythematosus. Arthritis Rheum. 17:1, 1974.
27. Ginzler, E., Diamond, H., Kaplan, D., Weiner, M., Schlesinger, M., and Seleznick, M.: Computer analysis of lupus erythematosus. Arthritis Rheum. 21:37, 1978.
28. Winkelstein, J.A., and Drachman, R.H.: Deficiency of pneumococcal serum opsonizing activity in sickle-cell disease. N. Engl. J. Med. 279:459, 1968.
29. Mathews, M., Shen, F., Lindner, A., and Sherrard, D.J.: Septic arthritis in hemodialyzed patients. Nephron 25:87, 1980.
30. Fauci, A.S., Dale, D.C., and Balow, J.E.: Glucocorticoid therapy: Mechanisms of action and clinical considerations. Ann. Intern. Med. 84:304, 1976.
31. Mills, L.C., Boylston, B.F., Green, J.A., and Moyer, J.H.: Septic arthritis as a complication of orally given steroid therapy. JAMA 164:1310, 1957.
32. DeAndrade, J.R., and Tribe, C.R.: Staphylococcal septicemia with pyoarthrosis in rheumatoid arthritis. Br. Med. J. 1:1516, 1962.
33. Rimoin, D.L., and Wennberg, J.E.: Acute septic arthritis complicating chronic rheumatoid arthritis. JAMA 196:617, 1966.
34. Karten, I.: Septic arthritis complicating rheumatoid arthritis. Ann. Intern. Med. 70:1147, 1969.
35. Russell, A.S., and Ansell, B.M.: Septic arthritis. Ann. Rheum. Dis. 31:40, 1972.
36. Gristina, A.G., Rovere, G.D., and Shoji, H.: Spontaneous septic arthritis complicating rheumatoid arthritis. J. Bone Joint Surg. 56A:1180, 1974.
37. Mitchell, W.S., Brooks, P.M., Stevenson, R.D., and Buchanan, W.W.: Septic arthritis in patients with rheumatoid disease: A still undiagnosed complication. J. Rheumatol. 3:124, 1976.
38. Mowat, A.G., and Baum, J.: Chemotaxis of polymorphonuclear leukocytes from patients with rheumatoid arthritis. J. Clin. Invest. 50:2541, 1971.
39. Turner, R.A., Schumacher, H.R., and Myers, A.R.: Phagocytic function of polymorphonuclear leukocytes in rheumatic diseases. J. Clin. Invest. 52:1632, 1973.
40. Pruzanski, W., Leers, W.D., and Wardlow, A.C.: Bacteriolytic and bactericidal activity of sera and synovial fluid in rheumatoid arthritis and in osteoarthritis. Arthritis Rheum. 17:207, 1974.
41. Ward, J., Cohen, A.S., and Bauer, W.: The diagnosis and therapy of acute suppurative arthritis. Arthritis Rheum. 6:522, 1960.
42. Hess, R.J., and Martin, J.H.: Pyarthrosis complicating gout. JAMA 218:592, 1971.
43. McConville, J.H., Pototsky, R.S., Calia, F.M., and Pachas, W.N.: Septic and crystalline joint disease. JAMA 231:841, 1975.
44. Smith, J.R., and Philips, P.: Septic arthritis, gout, pseudogout in knee of a patient with multiple myeloma. Arthritis Rheum. 15:89, 1972.

45. Mayer, J.W., DeHoratius, R.J., and Messner, R.P.: *Serratia marcescens—*caused arthritis with negative and positive birefringent crystals. Arch. Intern. Med. 136:1323, 1976.

46. Martin, J.R., Root, H.S., Kim, S.O., and Johnson, L.G.: Staphylococcus suppurative arthritis occurring in neuropathic knee joints. A report of four cases with a discussion of the mechanisms involved. Arthritis Rheum. 8:389, 1965.

47. Hollander, J.L.: Intrasynovial corticosteroid therapy in arthritis. Maryland State Med. J. 19:62, 1970.

48. Bunn, P.: Pyoarthrosis: Its treatment and role of adrenal steroids in its pathogenesis. Trans. Am. Clin. Climatol. Soc. 69:9, 1957.

49. Tondreau, R.L., Hodes, P.J., and Schmidt, E.R., Jr.: Joint infections following steroid therapy: Roentgen manifestations. Am. J. Roentgenol. Rad. Ther. Nucl. Med. 82:258, 1970.

50. Gowans, J.D.C., and Granieri, P.A.: Septic arthritis, its relation to intraarticular injections of hydrocortisone acetate. N. Engl. J. Med. 261:502, 1959.

51. Atcheson, S.G., and Ward, J.R.: Acute hematogenous osteomyelitis progressing to septic synovitis and eventual pyarthrosis. The vascular pathway. Arthritis Rheum. 21:968, 1978.

52. Lewis, G.W., and Cluff, L.E.: Synovitis in rabbits during bacteremia and vaccination. Johns Hopkins Hosp. Med. J. 116:175, 1965.

53. Tesar, J.T., and Dietz, F.: Mechanisms of inflammation in infectious arthritis. Clin. Rheum. Dis. 4:51, 1978.

54. Buckingham, R.B., and Castor, C.W.: The effect of bacterial products on synovial fibroblast function: Hypermetabolic changes induced by endotoxin. J. Clin. Invest. 51:1186, 1972.

55. Yaron, M., Yaron, I., Smetana, O., Eylan, E., and Zor, U.: Stimulation of prostaglandin E production by bacterial endotoxins in cultured human synovial fibroblasts. Arthritis Rheum. 23:921, 1980.

56. Hadler, N.M., and Granovetter, D.A.: Phlogistic properties of bacterial debris. Semin. Arthritis Rheum. 8:1, 1978.

57. Curtiss, P.H., Jr.: The pathophysiology of joint infections. Clin. Orthop. 96:129, 1973.

58. Phemister, D.B.: The effect of pressure on articular surfaces in pyogenic and tuberculosis arthritides and its bearing on treatment. Ann. Surg. 80:481, 1924.

59. Keefer, C.S., Holmes, W.F., Jr., and Myers, W.K.: The inhibition of tryptic digestion of cartilage by synovial fluid from patients with various types of arthritis. J. Clin. Invest. 14:131, 1935.

60. Lack, C.H.: Chondrolysis in arthritis. J. Bone Joint Surg. 41B:384, 1959.

61. Ziff, M., Gribetz, H.J., and Lospalluto, J.: Effect of leukocyte and synovial membrane extracts on cartilage mucoprotein. J. Clin. Invest. 39:405, 1960.

62. Curtis, P.H., Jr., and Klein, L.: Destruction of articular cartilage in septic arthritis. I. In vitro studies. J. Bone Joint Surg. 45A:797, 1963.

63. Curtiss, P.H., Jr., and Klein, L.: Destruction of articular cartilage in septic arthritis. II. In vivo studies. J. Bone Joint Surg. 47A:1595, 1965.

64. Bardenheier, J.A., Morgan, H.C., and Stamp, W.G.: Treatment and sequelae of experimentally produced septic arthritis. Surg. Gynecol. Obstet. 90:249, 1966.

65. Johnson, A.H., Campbell, W.G., Jr., and Callahan, B.C.: Infection of rabbit knee joints after intra-articular injection of *Staphylococcus aureus.* Am. J. Pathol. 60:165, 1970.

66. Schurman, D.J., Mirra, J., Ding, A., and Nagel, D.A.: Experimental *E. coli* arthritis in the rabbit. A model of infectious and post-infectious inflammatory synovitis. J. Rheumatol. 4:118, 1977.

67. Smith, R.L., Merchant, T.C., and Schurman, D.J.: In vitro cartilage degradation by *Escherichia coli* and *Staphylococcus aureus.* Arthritis Rheum. 25:441, 1982.

68. Harris, E.D., Jr., Faulkner, C.J., II, and Brown, F.E.: Collagenolytic systems in rheumatoid arthritis. Clin. Orthop. 110:34, 1975.

69. Ropes, M.W., and Bauer, W.: Synovial Fluid Changes in Joint Disease. Cambridge, Mass., Harvard University Press, 1953.

70. Smith, W.S., and Ward, R.M.: Septic arthritis of the hip complicating perforation of abdominal organs. JAMA 195:1148, 1966.

71. Brosseau, J.D., and Mazza, J.J.: Group A streptococcal sepsis and arthritis. Origin from an intrauterine device. JAMA 238:2178, 1977.

72. Barth, W.F., Healey, L.A., and Decker, J.L.: Septic arthritis due to *Pasteurella multocida* complicating rheumatoid arthritis. Arthritis Rheum. 11:294, 1968.

73. Butt, W.P.: Radiology of the infected joint. Clin. Orthop. 96:136, 1973.

74. Dalinka, M.K., Lally, J.F., Koniver, G., and Koren, G.S.: The radiology of osseous and articular infection. CRC Crit. Rev. Clin. Radiol. Nucl. Med. 7:1, 1975.

75. Master, R., Weisman, M.H., Armbuster, T.G., Slivka, J., Resnick, D., and Georgen, T.G.: Septic arthritis of the glenohumeral joint. Arthritis Rheum. 20:1500, 1977.

76. Bliznack, J., and Ramsey, J.: Emphysematous septic arthritis due to *Escherichia coli.* J. Bone Joint Surg. 58A:138, 1976.

77. Meredith, H.C., and Rittenberg, G.M.: Pneumoarthropathy: An unusual radiographic sign of gram-negative septic arthritis. Radiology 128:642, 1978.

78. Shawaker, T.H., and Dennis, J.M.: Periarticular calcification in pyogenic arthritis. Am. J. Roentgenol. Rad. Ther. Nucl. Med. 113:650, 1971.

79. Brook, I., Reza, M.J., Bricknell, K.S., Bluestone, R., and Finegold, S.M.: Abnormalities in synovial fluid of patients with septic arthritis detected by gas liquid chromatography. Ann. Rheum. Dis. 39:168, 1980.

80. Borenstein, D.G., Gibbs, C.A., and Jacobs, R.P.: Gas-liquid chromatographic analysis of synovial fluid. Arthritis. Rheum. 25:947, 1982.

81. Behn, A.R., Mathews, J.A., and Phillips, I.: Lactate UV-system: A rapid method for diagnosis of septic arthritis. Ann. Rheum. Dis. 40:489, 1981.

82. Rytel, M.W.: Microbial antigen detection in infectious arthritis. Clin. Rheum. Dis. 4:83, 1978.

83. Dorff, G.J., Ziolkowski, J.S., and Rytel, M.W.: Detection by counterimmunoelectrophoresis of pneumococcal antigen in synovial fluid from septic arthritis. Arthritis Rheum. 18:613, 1975.

84. Feldman, S.A., and DuClos, T.: Diagnosis of meningococcal arthritis by immunoelectrophoresis of synovial fluid. J. Appl. Microbiol. 25:1006, 1973.

85. Merritt, K., Boyle, W.E., Jr., Dye, S.K., and Porter, R.E.: Counterimmunoelectrophoresis in the diagnosis of septic arthritis caused by *Hemophilus influenza.* J. Bone Joint Surg. 58A:414, 1976.

86. Polin, R.A., and Kennett, R.: Use of monoclonal antibodies in an enzymelinked inhibition assay for rapid detection of streptococcal antigen. J. Pediat. 97:540, 1980.

87. Rosenthal, L., and Hawkins, D.: Radionuclide joint imaging in the diagnosis of synovial disease. Semin. Arthritis Rheum. 7:49, 1977.

88. Miller, J.H., and Gates, G.F.: Scintigraphy of sacroiliac pyarthrosis in children. JAMA 238:2701, 1977.

89. Lisbona, R., and Rosenthal, L.: Observations on the sequential use of ^{99m}Tc-phosphate complex and ^{67}Ga imaging in osteomyelitis, cellulitis, and septic arthritis. Radiology 123:123, 1977.

90. Handmaker, H., and Leonards, R.: The bone scan in inflammatory osseous disease. Semin. Nucl. Med. 6:95, 1976.

91. Morgan, G.J., Schlegelmilch, J.G., and Spiegel, P.K.: Early diagnosis of septic arthritis of the sacroiliac joint by use of computed tomography. J. Rheumatol. 8:979, 1981.

92. Goldenberg, D.L., and Cohen, A.S.: Synovial membrane histopathology in the differential diagnosis of rheumatoid arthritis, gout, pseudogout, systemic lupus erythematosus, infectious arthritis and degenerative joint disease. Medicine 57:239, 1978.

93. Garcia-Kutzbach, A., and Masi, A.T.: Acute infectious agent arthritis (IAA): A detailed comparison of proved gonococcal and other bloodborne bacterial arthritis. J. Rheumatol. 1:13, 1974.

94. Baitch, A.: Recent observations of acute suppurative arthritis. Clin. Orthop. 22:157, 1962.

95. Lidgren, L., and Lindberg, L.: Twenty-nine cases of bacterial arthritis. A prospective study. Acta Orthop. Scand. 44:263, 1973.

96. Esposito, A.L., and Gleckman, R.A.: Acute polymicrobial septic arthritis in the adult: Case report and literature review. Am. J. Med. Sci. 267:251, 1974.

97. Good, A.E., Hague, A.M., and Kauffman, C.A.: Streptococcal endocarditis initially seen as septic arthritis. Arch. Intern. Med. 138:805, 1978.

98. Kluge, R., Schmidt, M., and Barth, W.F.: Pneumococcal arthritis. Ann. Rheum. Dis. 32:21, 1973.

99. Donovan, T.L., Chapman, M.W., Harrington, K.D., and Nagel, D.A.: Serratia arthritis: Report of seven cases. J. Bone Joint Surg. 58A:1009, 1976.

100. David, J.R., and Black, R.L.: Salmonella arthritis. Medicine 39:385, 1960.

101. Hoaglund, F.T., and Lord, G.P.: *Hemophilus influenza* septic arthritis in adults. Arch. Intern. Med. 119:648, 1967.

102. Dean, H.M., and Post, R.M.: Fatal infection with *Aeromonas hydrophila* in a patient with acute myelogenous leukemia. Ann. Intern. Med. 66:1177, 1967.

103. Chmel, H., and Armstrong, D.: Acute arthritis caused by *Aeromonas hydrophila,* Clinical and therapeutic aspects. Arthritis Rheum. 19:169, 1976.

104. Ziment, I., Davis, A., and Finegold, S.M.: Joint infection by anaerobic bacteria: A case report and review of the literature. Arthritis Rheum. 12:627, 1969.

105. Smilack, J.D., and Goldberg, M.A.: Bone and joint infection with *Arizona hinshawii:* Report of a case and a review of the literature. Am. J. Med. Sci. 270:503, 1975.

106. King, S., and Bronsky, D.: *Vibrio fetus* isolated from a patient with localized septic arthritis. JAMA 175:1045, 1961.

107. Kilo, C., Hageman, P.O., and Marzi, J.: Septic arthritis and bacteremia due to *Vibrio fetus.* Am. J. Med. 38:962, 1965.

108. Spira, T.J., and Kabins, S.A.: *Yersinia enterocolitica* septicemia with septic arthritis. Arch. Intern. Med. 136:1305, 1976.

109. Taylor, B.G., Zahir-Zafarzi, M., Humphreys, D.W., and Manfredi, F.: Nodular pulmonary infiltrates and septic arthritis associated with *Yersinia enterocolitica* bacteremia. Am. Ref. Respir. Dis. 116:525, 1977.

110. Ho, G., Jr., Gadbow, J.J., Jr., and Glickstein, S.L.: Hemophilus influenza septic arthritis in adults. Semin. Arthritis Rheum. 12:314, 1983.

111. Fitzgerald, R.M., Jr., Rosenblatt, J.E., Tenney, J.H., and Bourgault, A.: Anaerobic septic arthritis. Clin. Orthop. 164:141, 1982.

112. Gotuzzo, E., Alarcon, G.S., Bocanegra, T.S., Carillo, C., Guerra, J.C., Rolando, I., and Espinoza, L.R.: Articular involvement in human brucellosis: A retrospective analysis of 304 cases. Semin. Arthritis Rheum. 12:245, 1982.

113. Goobar, J.E., and Clark, G.M.: Rheumatologic manifestations of gonorrhea. Arch. Interam. Rheum. 7:1, 1964.

114. Keiser, H., Ruben, F.L., Wolinsky, E., and Kushner, I.: Clinical forms of gonococcal arthritis. N. Engl. J. Med. 279:234, 1968.

115. Holmes, K.K., Counts, G.W., and Beaty, H.N.: Disseminated gonococcal infection. Ann. Intern. Med. 74:979, 1971.

116. Spink, W.W., and Keefer, C.S.: Diagnosis, treatment and end results in gonococcal arthritis: Study of seventy cases. N. Engl. J. Med. 218:453, 1938.

117. Cooke, C.L., Owen, D.S., Jr., Irby, R., and Toone, E.: Gonococcal arthritis. JAMA 217:204, 1971.

118. Brandt, K.D., Cathcart, E.S., and Cohen, A.S.: Gonococcal arthritis. Arthritis Rheum. 17:503, 1974.

119. Brogadir, S.P., Schimmer, B.M., and Myers, A.R.: Spectrum of the gonococcal arthritis-dermatitis syndrome. Semin. Arthritis Rheum. 8:177, 1979.

120. Seifert, M.H., Warin, A.P., and Miller, A.: Articular and cutaneous manifestations of gonorrhoea. Ann. Rheum. Dis. 33:140, 1974.

121. Handsfield, H.H., Wiesner, P.J., and Holmes, K.K.: Treatment of the gonococcal arthritis-dermatitis syndrome. Ann. Intern. Med. 84:661, 1976.

122. Fink, C.W.: Gonococcal arthritis in children. JAMA 194:123, 1965.

123. Straus, S.E., Vest, J.V., and Glew, R.H.: Gonococcal arthritis in the elderly. South. Med. J. 71:214, 1978.

124. Metzgar, A.L.: Gonococcal arthritis complicating gonorrheal pharyngitis. Ann. Intern. Med. 73:267, 1970.

125. Taylor, H.A., Bradford, S.A., and Patterson, S.P.: Gonococcal arthritis in pregnancy. Obstet. Gynecol. 27:776, 1966.

126. Ackerman, A.B.: Hemorrhagic bullae in gonococcemia. N. Engl. J. Med. 282:793, 1970.

127. Barr, J., and Danielsson, D.: Septic gonococcal dermatitis. Br. Med. J. 1:482, 1971.

128. Reichert, J.A., and Valle, R.F.: Fitz-Hugh-Curtis syndrome. JAMA 236:266, 1976.

129. Goldenberg, D.L.: "Postinfectious" arthritis. New look at an old concept with particular attention to disseminated gonococcal infection. Am. J. Med. 74:925, 1983.

130. Goldenberg, D.L., Chisholm, P.L., and Rice, P.A.: Experimental models of bacterial arthritis: A microbiological and histopathological characterization of the arthritis after intraarticular injections of *Neisseria gonorrhoeae, Staphylococcus aureas,* group A streptococci, and *Escherichia coli.* J. Rheumatol. 10:5, 1983.

131. Walker, L.C., Ahlin, T.D., Tung, K.S.K., and Williams, R.C., Jr.: Circulating immune complexes in disseminated gonorrheal infection. Ann. Intern. Med. 89:28, 1978.

132. Ludivico, C.L., and Myers, A.R.: Survey for immune complexes in disseminated gonococcal arthritis-dermatitis syndrome. Arthritis Rheum. 22:19, 1979.

133. Manicourt, D.H., and Orloff, S.: Gonococcal arthritis-dermatitis syndrome. Study of serum and synovial fluid immune complex levels. Arthritis. Rheum. 25:574, 1982.

134. Scherer, R., and Braun-Falco, O.: Alternative pathway complement activation: A possible mechanism inducing skin lesions in benign gonococcal sepsis. Br. J. Dermatol. 95:303, 1976.

135. Schoolnik, G.K., Buchanan, T.M., and Holmes, K.K.: Gonococci causing disseminated gonococcal infection are resistant to the bactericidal action of normal human serum. J. Clin. Invest. 58:1163, 1976.

136. Rice, P.A., and Goldenberg, D.L.: Clinical manifestations of disseminated infection caused by *Neisseria gonorrhoeae* are linked to differences in bactericidal reactivity of infecting strains. Ann. Intern. Med. 95:175, 1981.

137. Knapp, J.S., and Holmes, K.K.: Disseminated gonococcal infections caused by *Neisseria gonorrhoeae* with unique nutritional requirements. J. Infect. Dis. 132:204, 1975.

138. McCutchan, J.A., Katzenstein, D., Norquist, D., Chikami, G., Wunderlich, A., and Braude, A.I.: Role of blocking antibody in disseminated gonococcal infection. J. Immunol. 121:1884, 1978.

139. Peterson, B.H., Lee, T.J., Snyderman, R., and Brooks, G.F.: *Neisseria meningitidis* and *Neisseria gonorrhoeae* bacteremia associated with C6, C7, or C8 deficiency. Ann. Intern. Med. 90:917, 1979.

140. Gelfand, S.G., Masi, A.T., and Garcia-Kutzbach, A.: Spectrum of gonococcal arthritis: Evidence for sequential stages and clinical subgroups. J. Rheumatol. 2:83, 1975.

141. Eisenstein, G.I., and Masi, A.T.: Disseminated gonococcal infection (DGI) and gonococcal arthritis (GCA): I. Bacteriology, epidemiology, host factors, pathogen factors, and pathology. Sem. Arthritis Rheum. 10:155, 1981.

142. Masi, A.T., and Eisenstein, B.I.: Disseminated gonococcal infection (DGI) and gonococcal arthritis (GCA): II. Clinical manifestations, diagnosis, complications, treatment, and prevention. Sem. Arthritis Rheum. 10:173, 1981.

143. Thayer, J.D., and Martin, J.E., Jr.: Improved medium selective for cultivation of *N. gonorrhoeae* and *N. meningitidis.* Public Health Rep. 81:559, 1966.

144. Holmes, K.K., Gutman, L.T., Belding, M.E., and Twick, M.: Recovery of *Neisseria gonorrhoeae* from "sterile" synovial fluid in gonococcal arthritis. N. Engl. J. Med. 284:318, 1971.

145. Trentham, D.E., and McCravey, J.W., and Masi, A.T.: Low dose penicillin for gonococcal arthritis: A comparative therapy trial. JAMA 236:2410, 1976.

146. Blankenship, R.M., Holmes, R.K., and Sanford, J.P.: Treatment of disseminated gonococcal infection. N. Engl. J. Med. 290:269, 1974.

147. Thompson, S.E., Jacobs, N.F., Zacarias, F., Rein, M.F., and Shulman, J.A.: Gonococcal tenosynovitis-dermatitis and septic arthritis. Intravenous penicillin vs. oral penicillin. JAMA 244:1101, 1980.

148. Rinaldi, R.Z., Harrison, W.O., and Fan, T.F.: Penicillin-resistant gonococcal arthritis. A report of four cases. Ann. Intern. Med. 97:43, 1982.

149. Pinals, R.S., and Ropes, M.W.: Meningococcal arthritis. Arthritis Rheum. 7:241, 1964.

150. Schaad, U.B.: Arthritis in disease due to Neisseria meningitidis. Rev. Infectious Dis. 2:880, 1980.

151. Pinals, R.S.: Meningococcemia presenting as acute polyarthritis. J. Rheumatol. 4:420, 1977.

152. Young, E.J., and Morton, G.L.: Meningococcal arthritis stimulating gonococcemia. South. Med. J. 68:636, 1975.

153. Byeff, P.D., and Suskiewicz, L.: Meningococcal arthritis. JAMA 235:2752, 1976.

154. Greenwood, B.M., Whittle, H.C., and Bryceson, A.D.M.: Allergic complications of meningococcal disease. II. Immunological investigations. Br. Med. J. 2:737, 1973.

155. Larson, H.E., Nicholson, K.G., Lowei, G., and Tyrrell, D.A.J.: Arthritis after meningococcal meningitis. Br. Med. J. 1:618, 1977.

156. Orchard, R.A., and Sampt, W.C.: Early treatment of induced suppurative arthritis in rabbit knee joints. Clin. Orthop. 59:287, 1968.

157. Mielants, H., Dhondt, E., Goethals, L., Verbruggen, G., and Veys, E.: Long-term functional results of the non-surgical treatment of common bacterial infections of joints. Scand. J. Rheumatol. 11:101, 1982.

158. Hirsh, H.L., Feffer, H.L., and O'Neil, C.B.: A study of the diffusion of penicillin across the serous membranes of joint cavities. J. Lab. Clin. Med. 31:535, 1946.

159. Parker, R.H., and Schmid, F.R.: Antibacterial activity of synovial fluid during therapy of septic arthritis. Arthritis Rheum. 14:96, 1971.

160. Nelson, J.D.: Antibiotic concentrations in septic joint effusions. N. Engl. J. Med. 284:349, 1971.

161. Baciocco, E.A., and Iles, R.L.: Ampicillin and kanamycin concentrations in joint fluid. Clin. Pharmacol. Ther. 12:858, 1971.

162. Chow, A., Hecht, R., and Winters, R.: Gentamicin and carbenicillin penetration into the septic joint. N. Engl. J. Med. 285:178, 1971.

163. Lorber, B.: Penetration of antimicrobial agents into synovial fluid: Is there a blood-joint barrier? *In* Lowenthal, D.T., and Major, D.A. (eds.): Clinical Therapeutics. New York, Grune & Stratton, 1978.

164. Schurman, D.J., and Wheeler, R.: Gram negative bone and joint infection: Sixty patients treated with amikacin. Clin. Orthop. 134:268, 1978.

165. Fraser, G.L.: Treatment of nongonococcal bacterial septic arthritis. Drug Intell. Clin. Pharm. 15:531, 1981.

166. Ward, T.T., and Steigbigel, R.T.: Acidosis of synovial fluid correlates with synovial fluid leukocytosis. Am. J. Med. 64:933, 1978.

167. Schmid, F.R., and Parker, R.H.: Ongoing assessment of therapy in septic arthritis. Arthritis Rheum. 12:529, 1969.

168. Goldenberg, D.L., Brandt, K.D., Cohen, A.S., and Cathcart, E.S.: Treatment of septic arthritis. Comparison of needle aspiration and surgery as initial modes of joint drainage. Arthritis Rheum. 18:83, 1975.

169. Rosenthal, J., Bole, G.G., and Robinson, W.D.: Acute nongonococcal infectious arthritis. Evaluation of risk factors, therapy and outcome. Arthritis Rheum. 23:889, 1980.

170. Compere, E.L., Metzger, W.I., and Mitra, R.N.: The treatment of pyogenic bone and joint infections by closed irrigation (circulation) with a non-toxic detergent and one or more antibiotics. J. Bone Joint Surg. 49A:614, 1967.

171. Daniel, D., Akeson, W., Amiel, D., Ryder, M., and Boyer, J.: Lavage of septic joints in rabbits: Effects of chondrolysis. J. Bone Joint Surg. 58A:393, 1976.

172. Ballard, A., Burkehalter, W.E., Wayfield, G.W., Dehne, E., and Brown, P.W.: The functional treatment of pyogenic arthritis of the adult knee. J. Bone Joint Surg. 57A:1119, 1975.

173. Nelson, J.D.: The bacterial etiology and antibiotic management of septic arthritis in infants and children. Pediatrics 50:437, 1972.

174. Morrey, B.F., Bianco, A.J., and Rhodes, K.H.: Septic arthritis in children. Orthop. Clin. North Am. 6:923, 1975.

175. Chusid, M.J., Jacobs, W.M., and Sty, J.R.: Pseudomonas arthritis following puncture wounds of the foot. J. Pediat. 94:429, 1979.
176. Asnes, R.S., and Arendar, G.M.: Septic arthritis of the hip: A complication of femoral venipuncture. Pediatrics 38:837, 1966.
177. Almquist, E.E.: The changing epidemiology of septic arthritis in children. Clin. Orthop. 68:96, 1970.
178. Gillespie, R.: Septic arthritis of childhood. Clin. Orthop. 96:152, 1973.
179. Pittard, W.B., Thullen, J.D., and Fanaroff, A.A.: Neonatal septic arthritis. J. Pediat. 88:621, 1976.
180. Nelson, J.D., and Koontz, W.C.: Septic arthritis in infants and children: A review of 117 cases. Pediatrics 38:966, 1966.
181. Granoff, D.M., and Nankervis, G.A.: Infectious arthritis in the neonate caused by *Haemophilus influenzae*. Am. J. Dis. Child 129:730, 1975.
182. Memon, I.A., Jacobs, N.M., Yeh, T.F., and Lilean, L.D.: Group B streptococcal osteomyelitis and septic arthritis. Its occurrence in infants less than 2 months old. Am. J. Dis. Child. 133:921, 1979.
183. Wood, B.P.: The vanishing epiphyseal ossification center: A sequal to septic arthritis of childhood. Radiology 134:387, 1980.
184. Glassberg, G.B., and Ozonoff, M.B.: Arthrographic findings in septic arthritis of the hip in infants. Radiology 128:151, 1978.
185. Chang, M.J., Controni, G., and Rodgriguez, W.J.: Ampicilin-resistant hemophilus influenzae type B septic arthritis in children. Clin. Pediatr. 20:139, 1981.
186. Morrey, B.F., Bianco, A.J., and Rhodes, K.H.: Suppurative arthritis of the hip in children. J. Bone Joint Surg. 58A:388, 1976.
187. Howard, J.B., Highgenboten, C.L., and Nelson, J.D.: Residual effects of septic arthritis in infancy and childhood. JAMA 236:932, 1976.
188. Petersen, S., Knudson, F.U., Andersen, E.A., and Egeblad, M.: Acute hematogenous osteomyelitis and septic arthritis in childhood. A 10-year review and follow-up. Acta. Orthop. Scand. 51:451, 1980.
189. Hallel, T., and Salvati, E.A.: Septic arthritis of the hip in infancy. End result study. Clin. Orthop. 132:115, 1978.
190. Lunseth, P.A., and Heiple, K.G.: Prognosis in septic arthritis of the hips in children. Clin. Orthop. 139:81, 1979.
191. Delbarre, F., Rondier, J., Delrieu, F., Evrard, J., Cayla, J., Menkes, C.J., and Amor, B.: Pyrogenic infection of the sacro-iliac joint. Report of thirteen cases. J. Bone Joint Surg. 57A:819, 1975.
192. Coy, J.T., Wolf, C.R., Brouner, T.D., and Winter, D.G.: Pyogenic arthritis of the sacro-iliac joint. J. Bone Joint Surg. 58A:845, 1976.
193. Dunn, E.J., Bryan, D.M., Nugent, J.T., and Robinson, R.A.: Pyogenic infections of the sacro-iliac joint. Clin. Orthop. 118:113, 1976.
194. Schaad, U.B., McCracken, G.H., Jr., and Nelson, J.D.: Pyogenic arthritis of the sacroiliac joint in pediatric patients. Pediatrics 66:375, 1980.
195. Miskew, D.B., Block, R.A., and Witt, P.F.: Aspiration of infected sacro-iliac joints. J. Bone Joint Surg. 61A:1071, 1979.
196. Gordon, G., and Kabins, S.A.: Pyogenic sacroliitis. Am. J. Med. 69:50, 1980.
197. Sequeiria, W., Jones, E., Siegel, M., Lorenz, M., and Kallick, C.: Pyogenic infections of the pubic symphysis. Ann. Intern. Med. 96:604, 1980.
198. Ho, G., Jr., Tice, A.D., and Kaplan, S.R.: Septic bursitis in the prepatellar and olecranon bursae. An analysis of 25 cases. Ann. Intern. Med. 88:21, 1978.
199. Viggiano, D.A., Garrett, J.C., and Clayton, M.L.: Septic arthritis presenting as olecranon bursitis in patients with rheumatoid arthritis. J. Bone Joint Surg. 62-A:1011, 1980.
200. Ho, G., Jr., and Su, E.Y.: Antibiotic therapy of septic bursitis. Its implication in the treatment of septic arthritis. Arthritis Rheum. 24,905, 1981.

Chapter 97

Mycobacterial and Fungal Infections of Bones and Joints

Gary S. Hoffman

INTRODUCTION

Mycobacteria and fungi are among the major pathogens responsible for chronic bone and joint infections. Involvement of skeletal structures is characterized by a slow evolution of objective physical and radiographic findings. The inflammatory processes produced by these agents may spontaneously exacerbate and remit, remaining dormant but potentially harmful for many years.[1] Consequently, aggressive or invasive diagnostic approaches tend not to be considered until roentgenographic signs of destruction and permanent injury occur. In the case of *Mycobacterium tuberculosis,* constitutional symptoms are usually absent, and an average of 19 months has been known to elapse from the onset of symptoms (usually pain) to diagnosis.[2-4] Similar experiences abound with skeletal infections caused by atypical mycobacteria and fungi.

TUBERCULOUS SKELETAL DISEASE

At least half of all patients with skeletal involvement have normal chest radiographs.[3-7] Tuberculin skin tests are usually positive with bony disease and should therefore be part of the evaluation of any undiagnosed bone or joint lesion. Anergic immunocompromised patients (e.g., renal transplant recipients) represent an exception to the usually positive skin test.[8] On occasion, even apparently otherwise healthy persons with tuberculosis (TB) may show negative results on PPD (purified protein derivative) tests.[3,9-11]

About 1.3 percent of all TB patients in the United States have skeletal involvement, much of which is recognized only at post-mortem examination. Whereas *M. tuberculosis* is responsible for a relatively small number of all cases of skeletal infections in North America, it remains a major cause of osteomyelitis and septic arthritis in parts of Asia, Africa, and South America. Tuberculosis affecting extremities occurs primarily within joints.[12] Although any bone, joint, bursa,[13] or tendon[14] may be involved, there is a definite predilection for the vertebrae and weight-bearing surfaces (hip ≥ knee ≥ ankle). Multiple lesions have been noted in up to one third of cases.

Many months may pass prior to development of focal areas of osteopenia or articular erosions. In weight-bearing joints, especially the knee and hip, subchondral erosion often precedes cartilaginous destruction. Sequestration of subchondral bone may follow, and joint space

Figure 97–1. Large primary sequestrum of capitulum humeri. Articular cartilage intact. (From Luck, J.V.: Bone and Joint Diseases. Springfield, IL, Charles C Thomas, 1950.)

narrowing tends to occur late in the course of events. Thus, infection may be advanced without significant loss of the joint space (Fig. 97–1).[13,15,16] In some patients radiographic changes may be less suggestive of TB and be indistinguishable from other causes of chronic joint infection or even chronic noninfectious synovitis (e.g., rheumatoid arthritis).[7,17] Osteomyelitis may involve long bones secondary to a contiguous tuberculous synovitis or, conversely, tuberculous osteomyelitis may lead to a septic joint. In children the short tubular bones of the hands and feet may be infected (tuberculous dactylitis), a phenomenon very rarely seen in adults. Granulomatous reaction within the diaphyses causes expansion of the medullary cavity, lytic lesions, and lamellation of periosteal bone (Fig. 97–2).[6,7,12,18,19] Solitary lytic lesions of long bones requires distinction from primary bone tumors (e.g., osteoblastoma).[7]

Vertebral tuberculosis occurs more often in the thoracolumbar spine than in the cervical and sacral spine. It is seen in 50 percent of all cases of skeletal involvement. Early changes usually occur at the anterior vertebral borders and discs, causing disc space narrowing and eventually anterior collapse. A hump or gibbous deformity of the spine may result. Any part of the vertebral body may become involved; rarely, posterior changes are the first to be appreciated.[6,7,12,19,20] Multiple contiguous sites of destruction may occur owing to direct extension from a paravertebral abscess, or skip lesions may indicate a hematogenous mechanism. Destructive changes in ribs usually arise by anterior extension from paravertebral abscesses. Rarefied bony lesions may later be followed by varying degrees of calcification and new bone formation, leading to a mixed lytic-sclerotic picture.[6,13] Attempts to identify features that are radiographically unique to tuberculosis of the axial skeleton have failed,[9] indicating the necessity for histologic and culture examination of involved tissue to distinguish these lesions from those of malignancy and atypical mycobacterial or fungal infections. The choice of open or closed biopsy will depend upon the location of the lesion and the surgeon's personal preferences.

The presence of granulomas within synovial tissue may or may not be associated with caseation necrosis. In either case, the finding of granulomatous synovitis makes tuberculosis highly suspect. However, such findings are also compatible with atypical mycobacterial and fungal infections. Synovial biopsies from patients with culture-proven mycobacterial and fungal arthritis may also reveal only nonspecific inflammatory changes, without granulomata or necrosis.[7,21,22] Thus, classifying these agents under the heading of organisms that cause granulomatous infections emphasizes the classic histopathology but is potentially misleading. *The absence of granulomas does not rule out fungal or mycobacterial infection.*

With continued growth of synovial pannus and extravascular formation of fibrin, amorphous fragments —"rice bodies"—may separate from the margins of synovial granulation tissue (Fig. 97–3). Rice bodies were first described in 1895 by Riese[23] in a case of tuberculous

Figure 97–2. Tuberculous dactylitis (spina ventosa) of the index and fifth fingers. The fifth finger developed a sinus. Note the periosteal bone and the fusiform enlargement of the involved fingers. (From Luck, J.V.: Bone and Joint Diseases. Springfield, IL, Charles C Thomas, 1950.)

arthritis. They have since been seen in rheumatoid disease and other chronic arthritides.[3,24] The histopathologic appearance and the culture of tissue from open synovial biopsies have been diagnostic in more than 90 percent of cases.[4] Synovial biopsies obtained by arthroscopy promise to be of great diagnostic value and may save the patient from more extensive procedures.

Tuberculous synovial fluid is usually cloudy and yellow. Protein content is elevated, and white blood cell (WBC) counts are quite variable, averaging between 10,000 and 20,000 per mm³. Counts may range from less than 1000 to greater than 100,000 per mm³, with the percentage of neutrophils being greater at higher WBC counts. Sixty-one percent of reported cases have had blood sugar–synovial fluid sugar differences of *less than* 50 mg per dl. Thus, one cannot include or exclude tuberculous arthritis in the differential diagnosis of monoarticular or pauciarticular arthritis on the basis of synovial fluid WBC count, sugar, or protein. Acid-fast stains of synovial fluid from tuberculous joints have

Figure 97–3. *A,* Rice bodies removed from the knee of a patient with systemic lupus erythematosus and *Mycobacterium avium* infection. *B,* Low power ($\times$ 35) microscopic view of a rice body separating from granulomatous synovial tissue. The rice body may be caused by fibrin formation in inflammatory exudate, leading to ischemic necrosis of the distal tips of synovial villi and resolution of the fibrin-cellular debris into a discrete, compact, free-floating mass.

revealed organisms in 20 percent of specimens. Synovial fluid cultures have been positive in 80 percent of specimens.[4]

During the predrug era for tuberculosis, osseous disease was treated with immobilization and bed rest, in some centers averaging up to 13 months. When progression was apparent, local incision and drainage, excision, joint fusion, or amputation was added.[1] Since then it has been shown that antituberculous drugs may be curative for most osseous disease and that surgery should be reserved for drainage of abscesses and fusion of unstable spines.[25]

Disagreement exists regarding the number of drugs that are necessary and the duration of therapy. Although some authors feel that two agents may be adequate for mild to moderate osseous disease, others feel that skeletal disease implies more widespread occult dissemination and always requires three drugs, with reduction to two following initial improvement.[26] The Medical Research Council Working Party has published 5-year followup results of therapy for thoracolumbar spinal tuberculosis in Korean children.[27] All patients received 18 months of chemotherapy with isoniazid (INH) and para-aminosalicylic acid (PAS). About half of the children initially received daily streptomycin for 3 months. *The third drug did not significantly improve results.* In addition, no extra benefit appeared to be obtained from an initial 6-month period of bed rest or plaster thoracolumbar immobilization jackets. At 5-year followup, 89 percent of 295 patients were capable of full physical activity.

Data regarding large numbers of patients with severe pulmonary disease have indicated that the combination of INH and rifampin is at least as effective as all other drug combinations, including INH, rifampin, and streptomycin. These protocols, used for 6 months, produced cure rates for severe pulmonary tuberculosis that were comparable to those achieved with standard 18-month three-drug protocols.[28,29] Whether or not rifampin and INH can be as effective for osseous disease is uncertain. For the moment it would seem prudent to continue treatment of osseous TB with at least two agents for a minimum of 18 months. If surgery is necessary, ideally it should be carried out after chemotherapy has been undertaken. Such an approach would theoretically minimize the risk of bacteremia and subsequent new foci of infection.

Table 97–1 summarizes the commonly used antituberculous drugs and their properties.

MUSCULOSKELETAL INFECTIONS DUE TO ATYPICAL MYCOBACTERIA

Atypical mycobacteria have been recognized as being distinct from *M. tuberculosis* since the late nineteenth century.[33,34] Although atypical organisms were once thought to be harmless saprophytes, increasing numbers of reports demonstrate their pathologic potential in the lungs, lymphatics, meninges, skin, bone, joints, and tendons. Occasionally, widely disseminated disease occurs.

To date, no convincing evidence of human to human transmission of atypical mycobacteria exists. The wide distribution of these organisms in nature (e.g., in soil, fresh and salt water) has led to the strong belief that transmission occurs from environment to humans.[34,35] Although the lungs are frequently foci for atypical mycobacterial infections (especially *M. kansasii* and *M. avium–M. intracellulare*), only rarely are signs of pulmonary disease present in patients with skeletal involvement.[24]

The pathologic lesions produced by the tubercle bacilli and the atypical organisms are usually indistinguishable.[28,34] Specific diagnosis requires isolation of the organism and subsequent analysis of growth characteristics and biochemical and serologic properties. Atypical organisms grow readily on Lowenstein's medium, as well as on other standard media for tubercle bacilli. *M. tuberculosis* produces colorless colonies in culture, whereas the photochromogenic (group I) and scotochromogenic (group II) atypical mycobacterial are colored[34,36] (Table 97–2). Unlike *M. tuberculosis,* the atypical organisms are relatively insensitive to antituberculous drugs when tested in vitro; they lack guinea pig pathogenicity; and they do not produce niacin. Resistance to antituberculous drugs in vivo was emphasized by Dutt and Stead[37] in a study of 90 patients with *M. avium* and *M. intracellulare* infections. All received medical therapy (usually three to five drugs), and after 3 years, only about 45 percent had apparently inactive disease.

The atypical mycobacteria undergo systemic dissemination much less often than does *M. tuberculosis.* Consequently, skeletal disease is rare. When lesions occur, they are either single or few in number. Multiple sites occur more often with osteomyelitis[38,39] than with septic arthritis or periarthritis.[24] These generalizations are less reliable in immunocompromised hosts, including renal transplant recipients and hemodialysis patients[8] as well as in homosexuals and drug abusers.[40]

Since Runyon[36] described the classification scheme for atypical mycobacteria in 1959, more than 50 cases of presumed articular infection with these organisms have been reported.[24] However, at the time of surgical exploration, most of these patients were noted to have only periarticular disease.[41-50] Some patients had both periarticular and articular infections.[51] Atypical myobacterial septic arthritis was present in about 40 percent of cases.[24,33,42,43,51-58] In 15 percent of the cases, diagnoses were made by culture of joint or bursal fluid.[52,56-62] Definitive diagnosis depended on surgically obtained tissue in 85 percent of patients. The most common sites of periarticular involvement were around the wrists, fingers, and bursae. Articular disease most often affected digital joints and knees. The septic process was usually insidious, leading to delays in diagnosis of up to 3 to 8 years.[42,43,58,63] At least 40 percent of reported patients had received intra-articular corticosteroid injections prior to definitive diagnosis.

About 90 percent of patients in whom details of treatment have been reported received either surgery alone or surgery plus antituberculous drugs. Almost all pa-

Table 97–1. Antituberculous Drugs used in Initial Therapy*

	Agent	Route	Dose (mg/kg/day) Average Daily Dose	Toxicity	Miscellaneous	References
1.	Isoniazid (INH)	Oral	(3 to 5), 300 mg once daily, up to 600 mg qd for life-threatening disseminated infections	Elevations of SGOT in 10 to 20%; overt hepatitis in 1.5%; increased risks: age, alcoholism, malnutrition; lupus-like syndromes; peripheral neuritis; psychosis; seizures.	Single most important agent in treatment of tuberculosis. Bactericidal.	30, 31
2.	Rifampin	Oral	(10), 600 mg once daily	Thrombocytopenia, flulike syndrome, hepatitis; decreases effect of warfarin.	Relatively expensive; very active agent; sweat, urine, feces, saliva, sputum, and tears may become red-orange. Bactericidal.	31, 32
3.	Streptomycin	Intramuscular	(15), 1 g once daily for 1 month; after improvement 1 g twice weekly; may stop after 2 to 6 months	Vestibular 10 to 25%; decrease in high-frequency hearing 5 to 15%; rash 5%; renal excretion. Renal impairment and age over 50 years are relative contraindications.	First major antituberculous drug; resistance emerges rapidly. Bactericidal.	26, 32
4.	Ethambutol	Oral	(15 to 25), 1.5 to 2 g once daily	Visual acuity and loss of green color vision; no other major toxicity; good patient acceptance, hyperuricemia. Minor gastrointestinal symptoms.	Poor activity used alone, but very effective with INH; ophthalmology followup is desirable. Bacteriostatic.	31

*Most efficacious combinations: 1 + 2 or 1 + 4 + 3 (optional). Patient compliance represents a major problem with all protocols. 1 + 2 increases risk of hepatitis compared with either one alone. Ethambutol has replaced PAS in current programs.

tients with either periarticular or articular disease have had apparent arrest and possible cure of infection when surgical excision and chemotherapy have been combined. The fact that chemotherapy alone may be of value, in spite of in vitro resistance, is demonstrated by the therapeutic response of occasional patients receiving only drug therapy and the response of infections that were surgical failures to the later addition of chemotherapy.[24,58,63]

The relative resistance in vitro of atypical mycobacteria to antituberculous drugs has led to serious concern about the adequacy of chemotherapy for these infections.[33,35,36,64] Both this concern and the failure to make a diagnosis without biopsy material probably explain why 90 percent of reported patients have had surgery as part of their therapy. Because of relative drug resistance, Runyon[36] recommends that the use of chemotherapy depend heavily on in vitro susceptibility studies.

Table 97–2. Classification of Atypical Mycobacteria*

Group	Growth Rate	Color	Members
Photochromogens	3 to 4 weeks	Yellow-orange when exposed to light while being grown	M. kansasii M. marinum (balnei)
Scotochromogens	3 to 4 weeks	Yellow-orange in the dark; become more reddish in light	M. scrofulaceum M. szulgai
Nonchromogens	3 to 4 weeks	None or light yellow	M. battey M. avium–M. intracellulare M. triviale M. ulcerans
Rapid growers	1 to 3 days	Usually none, occasionally variable color	M. fortuitum

*Abstracted from Runyon, E.H.: Med. Clin. North Am. 43:273, 1959 and Fogan, L.: Medicine 49:243, 1970.

In most surgical cases, only partial excision of involved synovial tissue is possible, which provides an opportunity for later relapse. The rate of relapse from pulmonary infection with *M. intracellulare* has been described as being 2 to 7 percent per year, with a cumulative rate of 19.6 percent after 5 years of treatment.[64] These data suggest that caution be applied in interpreting the therapeutic response seen with atypical organisms. "Clinically inactive" and "quiescent" disease are terms to be preferred to "cure." Such patients require continuous followup surveillance.

MYCOTIC INFECTIONS OF BONES AND JOINTS

Osteomyelitis is the most common type of mycotic skeletal disease. Septic joints may arise by direct extension from such bony foci. Less often synovial infections occur directly by hematogenous dissemination. One or more sites may be involved simultaneously. Except for the frequent association of mandibular osteomyelitis and *Actinomyces israelii*, the location of bony involvement is of little differential diagnostic value. The only reliable method of definitive diagnosis remains culture of involved tissues. Although the data for fungal arthritis area necdotal, it appears that yields with culture of synovial fluid are inferior to those with culture of synovial biopsy tissue.[65-67] Synovial analyses are quite variable and, depending on the stage of disease, can include WBC counts ranging from noninflammatory (< 1000 per mm^3)[68] to markedly inflammatory ($> 100,000$ per mm^3).[66] Most cases have had WBC counts of 10,000 to 60,000, with a predominance of granulocytes at the more inflammatory end of the spectrum.

Acute fungal arthritis is distinctly uncommon but has been reported, particularly with blastomycoses and *Candida* organisms.[68,69] It is the indolent course of most fungal joint infections that has led to delays in diagnosis, even for many years. The first several months of undiagnosed chronic illness are usually associated with normal radiographs, which later develop lucent and lytic changes, and still many months later show a mixed lytic-sclerotic picture.[70] Undiagnosed patients often undergo inappropriate treatment, particularly with intra-articular and systemic steroids for "nonspecific synovitis." This is usually followed by little to no improvement, and finally surgery is sought for diagnostic and therapeutic assistance. In many such cases, fungal arthritis may still not be considered, and synovectomy may be followed by recurrent problems.[65,71]

Familiarity with fungal epidemiology and extraskeletal manifestations of disease may provide vital diagnostic clues (Table 97–3).

The Superficial Mycoses. Mycotic infections can conveniently be grouped into those *usually* causing "superficial" (cutaneous) disease and those producing more severe "deep" (visceral) pathology. Among the superficial mycoses that can cause bone or joint infections, or both, are *Sporothrix schenckii*, *Candida* species, and the maduromycoses, which are more accurately infections with different fungi (*Allescheria boydii*, *Nocardia*, and *Aspergillus* species), and even bacteria.[70,72] *Nocardia* is actually not a fungus. It is a gram-positive, partially acid-fast aerobic filamentous bacterium whose clinical manifestations resemble those of fungi and mycobacteria. It may be particularly difficult to distinguish this organism from the rapid grower *M. fortuitum*.[73] Apart from its role in mycetomas, *Nocardia* is an extremely uncommon cause of skeletal disease.[74]

The maduromycoses are responsible for mycetomas of the distal lower extremities. They are localized infections of skin, subcutaneous tissues, and bone, associated with sinus tracts, swelling, and disfigurement. Because of its prevalence in the Madura province of India, the term "maduromycosis" has come to be used synonymously with mycetoma. However, an even greater number of cases have been reported from the Sudan in Africa.

Sporotrichosis occurs worldwide and is caused by *Sporothrix schenckii*, a dimorphic, aerobic fungus existing as a yeast in infected tissues and as a mycelium in nature. Its environmental habitat includes areas of high humidity such as soil, decaying vegetation, gardening supplies (sphagnum moss), and the sawed timbers of mines.[75,100] Although cutaneolymphatic infection of the upper extremities is an occupational hazard of gardeners, floral workers, farmers, and miners, it has also been observed in patients without such obvious risk factors.[65,75] Extracutaneous sporotrichosis is rare. Most cases have been associated with the skin as the primary site of infection. Extension of infection from the soft tissues of the hand can produce arthritis and tenosynovitis.

Rarely, inhalation and pulmonary infection have led to disseminated disease. When hematogenous dissemination occurs, about 80 percent of cases will have bone or joint involvement.[100] Crout and associates[65] report the unusual experience of diagnosing seven cases of sporotrichosis arthritis. Among them, six lacked evidence of prior skin or lung disease. An average of 25 months passed from the onset of symptoms to the time of diagnosis. This delay led to irreversible joint damage in four of seven persons. Six of seven patients had been treated with intra-articular steroids before diagnosis, and four received systemic steroids as well. Altner and Turner[75] have noted similar problems with misdiagnosis and mistreatment among 6 of their own patients and 24 patients reviewed from the literature. Fifteen (62 percent) presented with bone or joint involvement of the lower extremity only. Others have noted polyarticular presentations,[65,76,101] and rarely symmetric polyarthritis has mimicked rheumatoid disease.[102] The most commonly affected joints have been knees, ankles, wrists, and elbows, and the most common site of osteomyelitis has been the tibia.[65,75,76] Although lymphocutaneous disease has usually responded to potassium iodide therapy, intravenous amphotericin B has been necessary for extracutaneous forms of sporotrichosis. In spite of the fact that fungicidal levels of amphotericin B have been demonstrated in joint fluid during intravenous therapy,[65,66] some patients finally responded only after repeated in-

Table 97–3. Fungi Causing Infections of Bones and Joints

Fungus	Mode of Infection	Geographic Distribution	Frequency of Septic Bone and Joint Involvement
Superficial "maduromycoses"	Fungus enters via local injury to uncovered foot	Worldwide, especially in tropical climates where inhabitants do not wear shoes; rare in United States	Usual; soft tissue infection leading to osteomyelitis[70,74]
Sporothrix schenckii	Fungus enters via local injury to skin—direct implantation of plant material carrying fungus; alcoholism and myeloproliferative diseases are predisposing factors[104]	Worldwide, especially areas of high humidity; South Africa, France, and Mexico are most common areas	80% of cases of systemic sporotrichosis[75,76]
Candida albicans and rarely *C. stellatoidea*[77] *C. tropicalis*[66,84,85] *C. guilliermondi*[86] *C. parapsilosis*[86a,115]	Endogenous: in premature infants and other compromised hosts having malignancies, indwelling catheters, hyperalimentation, immunosuppressive therapies, multiple antibiotics; drug addicts (especially heroin)	Worldwide	Rare[78-83]
Actinomyces israelii (anaerobic bacterium)	Endogenous—host may or may not be compromised; focal cervicofacial disease or disseminated bacteremia; may follow oral trauma such as tooth extractions	Worldwide	Common in facial bones[70,83,87]
Deep *Aspergillus fumigatus*	Inhalation or endogenous infection in a compromised host; dissemination via respiratory tree and blood; rarely via gastrointestinal tract	Worldwide	Rare[88]
Histoplasma capsulatum	Inhalation; aerosol from soil rich in bird droppings (especially chickens, starlings) and bat feces	Worldwide; in United States most concentrated in Midwest, Ohio and Mississippi River valleys	Rare[89,90]
H. duboisii	Uncertain	Africa	About 66% with disseminated disease[91]
Cryptococcus neoformans	Inhalation, often compromised host as well as normal persons	Worldwide; no regional concentration in United States	5 to 10%[89,92-95,120]
Coccidioides immitis	Inhalation, especially during dry, dusty months	Southwestern United States, Central and South America, especially arid dusty regions	10 to 20% cases with disseminated disease[10,67,70,71,89,96]
Blastomyces dermatitidis	Usually inhalation; very rarely inoculation into traumatized skin. Most common among persons repeatedly exposed to soil. 9 males:1 female[149]	United States: Mississippi, Ohio River basins, middle Atlantic states, Canada, Africa, Europe, northern South America[149]	25 to 50% disseminated blastomycoses cases[14,70,87,89,97-99]

stillations (intra-articular or intrabursal, or both) of this agent.[76,102] Still others also required surgery for both diagnosis and treatment.[65,75,101]

Candida species are ubiquitous in humans. Environmental acquisition of disease is unlikely. It is believed that *Candida* is acquired by human to human or animal to human transmission, a unique property among the mycoses affecting humans.[105] *C. albicans* has been found in about 50 percent of secretions from the oropharynx and gastrointestinal tract of healthy individuals. In about 2 percent of people the skin may be colonized.[69,105,106] Although *Candida* species are among the "superficial" fungi, usually inhabiting mucocutaneous body surfaces, they can behave like the "deep" mycoses in the compromised host, in whom the incidence of colonization and subsequent infection is greatly enhanced.[85] Susceptible populations include premature ba-

bies, diabetic patients, intravenous drug abusers, and patients with malignancies associated with immunologic disequilibrium, immunosuppressive therapies, multiple antibiotics, and prolonged periods of intravenous feedings. Nine different species have been associated with human candidiasis, the most virulent being *C. albicans* and *C. tropicalis*.[85] Hematogenous dissemination has occurred most often with *C. albicans*, producing disease in any tissue but having a definite preference for the kidneys. Nonspecific arthralgias and myalgias have occasionally been noted during periods of fungemia.[85] Bone and joint infections have been rare, with initial foci being either in bone or synovium. Knees have been most often involved,[65,78,79,84,86,107-110] and occasionally contiguous osteomyelitis is also noted.[79,111-113] Onset may be acute, subacute, or chronic.[114,115] The rarity of *Candida* arthritis-osteomyelitis, variations in host immunoincompetence, and differences in severity of infection in reported cases have precluded unanimity among therapeutic protocols. Many patients have responded to intravenous amphotericin B and closed drainage only,[69,108,111,112] whereas others did not seem to respond until surgical debridement,[66,77,79] intra-articular amphotericin B,[84,110] or 5-fluorocytosine[78,79,113] was added. Crucial to the success of therapy is the ability to diminish factors that compromise the patient's immunologic defenses (e.g., immunosuppressive drugs, indwelling catheters, concurrent infections).

Actinomycoses. The *Actinomyces* are strictly anaerobic bacilli with Gram stain–positive appearance. Branching properties give them a funguslike morphology that has led to misclassification within the mycoses (actinomycosis: Greek = branching fungus). Although several species have been associated with human infections, *Actinomycosis israelii* is by far the most common.[116,117] Because clinical behavior resembles that of the mycoses, *A. israelii* is discussed here. One of its major distinctions from the fungi is its sensitivity to antibiotics such as penicillin and tetracycline. *A. israelii* exists as a commensal in the crypts and crevices of the tonsils and gingiva. Its anaerobic requirements are particularly well supported by infected carious teeth, oral injuries associated with small necrotic foci, and breaks in the mucous membranes (e.g., dental extractions). Isolation of the bacilli from such sites is not equivalent to infection, which is best proved by demonstrating tissue invasion. The most common form of bone disease involves direct extension from the mouth to the mandible. Further extension into the maxilla, orbit, and paranasal sinuses can occur.[70,87,116,118,119] Abscess formation and draining sinus tracts may follow. Aggregates of branching organisms, held together by protein-polysaccharide, may form yellowish macroscopic particles ("sulfur granules") that can be found in sinus drainage.[120] Cervicofacial disease is most often mistaken for cancer[116] when classic clinical findings are absent.

Pulmonary actinomycosis may be complicated by invasion of the pleura, chest wall, and dorsal vertebrae, mimicking malignancy. An unresolving pneumonia with contiguous bone involvement suggests malignancy or actinomycosis. Although the vertebral bodies may be extensively involved and associated with paravertebral abscesses, the vertebrae rarely collapse and the disc is usually spared, helping distinguish this process from tuberculous involvement.[87,118,119,121,122] Similar involvement of the lumbar spine may occur from direct extension of a gastrointestinal focus. Hematogenous dissemination resulting in bony or articular lesions of the extremities is extremely rare. When the limbs are involved, the initial lesion is usually in the soft tissues, which may then extend to bone.[70,123] Remembering to include *anaerobic cultures* in the assessment of unusual osseous lesions, especially those of the head and neck, is essential to making a diagnosis of actinomycosis. Because actinomyces thrive in relatively avascular regions, large doses of penicillin are required for effective treatment (e.g., penicillin G, 100 to 150 mg per kg of body weight in four divided doses daily). In the penicillin-allergic patient, tetracycline, clindamycin, cefoxitin, chloramphenicol, or erythromycin would be an acceptable alternative for treatment. Treatment may be required for several months,[116,118,124] although the ideal duration of treatment is unknown.

The Deep Mycoses. The organisms responsible for "deep" mycotic infections include *Cryptococcus neoformans, Coccidioides immitis, Histoplasma capsulatum, Blastomyces dermatitidis,* and *Aspergillus fumigatus.* Systemic fungal infections are most often acquired by inhalation and are frequently asymptomatic or mild. Serious clinical consequences occur in a minority of cases. The severity of fungal disease is often greatest in the compromised host, but many otherwise normal persons can be infected as well.

Aspergillus species are the most commonly encountered fungi in the environment of humans and exist in soil, water, and decaying vegetation throughout the world. Spores have been recovered from the upper atmosphere, from snow in the Antarctic, and from the sand and winds over the Sahara Desert![125] *A. fumigatus* has a low degree of virulence for normal humans. It may exist as a commensal organism in the respiratory tree, external auditory canal, oral cavity, and gastrointestinal tract. Sputum colonization is especially common in patients with chronic obstructive lung disease. The range of disease produced includes focal infection within previously damaged pulmonary parenchyma (fungus ball), hypersensitivity responses (bronchopulmonary aspergillosis), and invasion and dissemination, which often follows a fulminant course. Systemic disease is almost always seen in immunologically impaired patients. In this population, *Aspergillus* ranks second only to *Candida* species as a common opportunistic fungus. *More than 50 percent of cases are associated with concurrent or prior bacterial infections, leading to diagnostic confusion and delays in diagnosis.*[125] Dissemination involves the kidneys and central nervous system in about two thirds of cases. Other systems, including the skeleton, are involved less often.[126] Osteomyelitis has been described in the vertebral column, skull, sinuses, and ribs, but septic arthritis caused by this organism is rare.[88,125,127] In a recent review of *Aspergillus* skeletal disease Tack and colleagues[128] describe 19 patients (7 children and 12 adults), of whom only 3 were not immunocompromised. Sites of involvement included vertebrae (12), ribs (2), sternum (1), tibia (2), pelvis (2), knee (1), and wrist (1). In children, bone disease was usually from a contiguous pulmonary focus, whereas adults more often experienced hematogenous seeding of bones and joints.

H. capsulatum is acquired by humans via inhalation of airborne spores. It is most often responsible for a mild self-limiting pulmonary illness. Symptoms may be indistinguishable from the common cold or influenza. About 500,000 cases occur per year in the United States.[120] In about 5 to 10 percent of cases, acute histoplasmosis may be associated with polymyalgias, polyarthralgias, and, rarely, nonseptic arthritis.[90,129-133] Such patients often have erythema nodosum or erythema multiforme, or both. In most, joint symptoms resolve within 4 to 6 weeks, although more prolonged courses are also known.[131-133] If initial presentation is associated with hilar adenopathy, one is at risk of confusing acute, and less often, chronic histoplasmosis with sarcoidosis.[131,134] Osteomyelitis occurs more often as part of chronic disseminated disease, and even in this setting it is quite rare.

This clinical picture is almost the opposite of that seen with *H. duboisii* or African histoplasmosis, in which pulmonary infection has not been documented and bone disease occurs in about two thirds of cases.[91] The primary focus of infection is uncertain, although skin trauma is suspect. Pleomorphic skin lesions exist in almost all cases. Such lesions may be followed by direct extension to underlying tissues and lymphatic-hematogenous dissemination. Skeletal disease has been found in essentially all bones, large and small. Multiple foci of osteomyelitis are common and often have associated lytic lesions.

C. neoformans, like *H. capsulatum*, is found in nature associated with avian feces. Human acquisition most likely occurs by inhalation. Pigeon droppings appear to be particularly favorable for propagation and maintenance of the cryptococcus. However, many patients with well-established cryptococcosis lack a history of exposure to bird droppings and may not have findings of pulmonary disease.[92,135] Cryptococcosis occurs in both immune-compromised and competent hosts. As would be expected, the former group is particularly prone to severe and fatal infections. This is particularly true of patients with lymphoma, leukemia, and leukopenia whose therapy includes steroids.[120] Pulmonary infection may lead to hematogenous dissemination, with central nervous system seeding being the most dreaded complication. Other organ systems are less vulnerable, and skeletal disease occurs in only 5 to 10 percent. The organism does not produce a marked inflammatory response in any affected tissue. Thus, early lesions tend to be primarily composed of gelatinous masses of budding yeast. With long standing lesions, granulomas may appear, but only rarely is this followed by caseation and calcification. For these reasons, crytococcosis is somewhat unique among the fungal osteomyelitides in remaining a predominantly lytic process, even when chronic (Fig. 97–4). The distinction of such lesions from malignant ones may only become apparent after biopsy and culture.[22,136] The axial skeleton, long bones, skull, and ribs are the most frequent sites of infection. Sinus formation and septic arthritis are uncommon.[93,94,119] When septic arthritis has occurred, the knee has been the most frequent joint affected.[129] Cryptococcal arthritis is usually secondary to extension of adjacent osteomyelitis. Patients have been treated, with variable success, with amphotericin B alone or together with 5-fluorocytosine. The timing for surgical intervention must be determined for each patient based on the general state of health and the response to initial therapy. Because spontaneous remissions and relapses are known to occur, the evaluation of therapy for skeletal disease remains difficult.[93]

Figure 97–4. Cryptococcosis of bone. Note osteolytic lesions of the fifth metatarsal. (From Conant, N., et al.: Manual of Clinical Mycology, 3rd ed. Philadelphia, W.B. Saunders Company, 1971.)

Coccidioides immitis is a highly infectious organism that has been shown, by skin test studies, to infect 80 percent of people living in endemic areas (see Table 97–3) within 5 years. At least three fourths of those infected have lacked symptoms or clinical signs of coccidioidomycosis.[137] When symptoms occur, they may resemble those of an acute viral upper respiratory infection. About 5 percent of cases develop chronic progressive pulmonary disease, and in only 0.1 to 0.2 percent does dissemination occur.[67,96] In contrast to patients with *Candida, Aspergillus,* and *Cryptococcus* infections, those with coccidioidal and blastomycotic disease have generally been in prior good health.[138] Two forms of arthritis are seen with *C. immitis* infection. Among patients with acute symptomatic infection, one third will experience arthralgias, and an occasional patient may have overt signs of synovitis. These features, like erythema nodosum and erythema multiforme, resolve within days to weeks and probably represent a hypersensitivity response to fungal proteins similar to that noted in acute histoplasmosis. However, actual septic bone and joint disease does occur in one fifth of patients with dissemination.[10,67,71,137] Although septic arthritis is usually an extension of osteomyelitis,[87,139,140] a growing number of primary joint infections are being reported.[67,141-143] Bone and joint lesions are often multiple[144-146] and are said by some authors to have a predilection for skeletal prominences such as elbows, knees, and malleoli[96,140] (Fig. 97–5). The value of this diagnostic clue has been questioned by McGahan and co-workers,[145] who did not find such a predilection in their experience with 43 patients. In as many as 40 to 80 percent of cases the bone or joint problems, or both, may be the only signs of apparent infection.[141,147] Thus, in endemic areas and in persons having traveled to such areas, the differential diagnosis of chronic monoarticular or pauciarticular arthritis, with or without osteomyelitis, should always include coccidioidomycosis. A recent review of coccidioidal synovitis demonstrated a mean interval of 4.5 years between the time of initial symptoms and definite diagnosis.[138] Therapeutic protocols for osseous and articular disease have varied, as was noted for other fungi. Intravenous amphotericin B and surgery remain the foundations for treatment, with the role of intra-articular chemotherapy needing to be further defined.[67,148]

In the United States, *Blastomyces dermatitidis* infections are endemic in the Mississippi and Ohio River basins, Middle Atlantic states, and Southeast.[149] Although the fungus is probably acquired by inhalation from the environment, most attempts to isolate it from soil have been unsuccessful.[150] With the exception of one well-documented case,[151] it has not been associated with avian feces.[152] In endemic regions dogs are frequently infected with *B. dermatitidis*. However, in only two instances has transmission of infection from dog to human been documented. In each case a bite had produced a digital infection.[153,154] Most infections are probably asymptomatic or resemble colds or influenza. Self-limiting arthralgias and myalgias may accompany these symptoms, as was noted for acute histoplasmosis and coccidioidomycosis.[149] Bone or joint infection, or both, occur in up to half of all patients with systemic disease. Although most joint infections arise from an osteomyelitic focus, some occur only in the synovium. About 50 to 90 percent of persons with skeletal involvement have had concomitant lung or skin disease, or both.[68,87,97,155] Skin lesions are usually secondary to hematogenous spread or extension from an underlying osteomyelitis.[156] The skin is rarely involved as a primary traumatic lesion. Any part of the skeleton can be involved, although lesions in ribs, vertebrae, long bones, and skull are most common.[87,97,156,157] Joint infection is most common in a single knee or ankle. Unlike patients with synovitis from other deep mycoses, those with blastomycotic infection may have acute septic joints.[10,68] They appear more toxic,

Figure 97–5. *A* and *B*, Chronic coccidioidal arthritis. The amount of bone erosion and destruction that can occur is striking. The deep marginal erosions strongly resemble those of tuberculous or hemophilic joint disease. (From Rosen, R.S.: Semin. Roentgenol. 1:370, 1966. Reproduced by permission.)

and their course tends to be more rapid than is noted in other fungal infections. Blastomycotic arthritis is also unique in having a high incidence (88 percent) of positive synovial fluid wet mounts for fungal organisms.[158] Approaches to therapy mirror those noted for the other deep mycoses.

THERAPY

In 1956, Gold and co-workers at Squibb Pharmaceuticals isolated amphotericin from a soil streptomycote. The original material was found to be a mixture of two substances, amphotericin A and B. Amphotericin B is a potent polyene antibiotic that has substantially decreased the mortality and morbidity from systemic mycotic infections.[159] Binding of polyene antibiotics to sterols within cell membranes results in altered cell permeability, leakage of cytosol, and subsequent cell death. Amphotericin B preferentially binds ergosterol, a major sterol in fungal membranes. Cholesterol, the major sterol in animal cell membranes, is bound to a lesser extent by amphotericin B, thereby providing a net effect that usually favors the patient. The development of other polyene antibiotics has been in part limited by not being able to take better advantage of this important difference in cell membranes.[160]

The goals of antifungal chemotherapy are often limited by drug toxicity. Table 97–4 presents guidelines for treatment. The initial intravenous dose of amphotericin B should be 1 to 5 mg and, if tolerated, should be doubled on subsequent days until a maintenance dose of 0.5 to 1 mg per kg per day is obtained. Following unequivocal clinical response, some authors would then switch to alternate-day therapy in an attempt to minimize toxicity.[161] Amphotericin B may cause headaches, nausea, vomiting, and fever, which require either diminution of the daily dose or switching to alternate-day therapy. Thrombophlebitis at the site of intravenous administration is a common problem. Extended infusion times (≥ 6 hours), intravenous drug concentrations of less than 0.1 mg per ml, and adding 100 U of heparin and 25 to 50 mg of hydrocortisone to each infusion[161,162] may also minimize these side effects. Anemia is common after several weeks of treatment; leukopenia and thrombocytopenia are rare. Azotemia will eventually develop in most patients. This may be associated with renal tubular acidosis, hypokalemia, or hypomagnesemia. A serum creatinine level of 2 mg per dl or more should also lead to less vigorous drug therapy.[105,160-162]

There are no controlled studies that examine optimal duration of amphotericin B treatment in these disorders. Empirically derived programs have led to treatment with a total dose of about 2 g given over a 6- to 12-week period. This has been modified to take into account the particular organism, the extent of infection, the initial clinical response, and toxicity.[161]

5-Fluorocytosine, a very well-absorbed oral agent, was initially synthesized by Roche Laboratories, with the hope of being efficacious in cancer chemotherapy.

Table 97–4. Treatment Guidelines for Chemotherapy of Fungi

Antifungal Agent	Route of Administration	Daily Dose*
Amphotericin B	IV in 5% dextrose	0.6–1.0 mg/kg
5-Fluorocytosine†	Oral	75–150 mg/kg in four divided doses

*Adjustments to be made based on renal function. Duration of treatment will vary with severity of disease, initial response, adjunctive therapy (surgery, intra-articular chemotherapy), and toxicity. Most patients require several months of treatment.

†*H. capsulatum, B. dermatitidis, C. immitis,* and some *Candida* species are often resistant, and other fungi may become resistant. Sensitivity testing is essential.[31,86,160,161]

Although it was found to be a virtually useless drug for that purpose, it was shown in 1963 to have antifungal properties.[159] As an antimetabolite it interferes with fungal RNA and DNA synthesis. However, it is limited by natural or acquired resistance, or both, occurring in *H. capsulatum, B. dermatitidis, C. immitis,* and some *Candida* species.[31,86,159-163] Nonetheless, 5-fluorocytosine has proved to be a useful agent in selected cases of candidiasis, aspergillosis, and cryptococcosis. Most authorities recommend that because of the potential for acquired drug resistance, 5-fluorocytosine should *not* be used alone for serious infections, but instead should be used in combination with amphotericin B.[159-162] In such cases the daily dose of amphotericin should be reduced to about 0.3 mg per kg.[161]

Much has been written in the past few years about the antifungal properties of new imidazole derivatives (clotrimazole, miconazole, ketoconazole). Some of these agents have proved to be excellent for mucocutaneous, cutaneous, and vaginal mycoses. However, their role in the treatment of systemic infections is questionable. In one study of musculoskeletal coccidioidomycosis treated with miconazole, only 34 percent of 31 patients responded, more than half of whom later relapsed.[146,163] Trials with ketoconazole have been similarly disappointing. Although initial response rates were noted in 50 to 88 percent of patients,[142,143,164,165] more than half of them relapsed either during therapy or after its discontinuation, which in many cases exceeded 6 to 12 months. Both miconazole and ketoconazole appear to suppress rather than eradicate fungi.[142,143] Studies to date have not combined the use of ketoconazole and amphotericin B. Because ketoconazole inhibits ergosterol synthesis, there is concern that it would diminish the effectiveness of amphotericin.[142] Thus, in spite of its shortcomings, amphotericin B remains the mainstay of medical therapy for systemic mycotic infections.

References

1. LaFond, E.M.: An analysis of adult skeletal tuberculosis. J. Bone Joint Surg. 40:346, 1958.
2. Walker, G.F.: Failure of early recognition of skeletal tuberculosis. Br. Med. J. 1:682, 1968.
3. Davidson, P.T., and Horowitz, I.: Skeletal tuberculosis. A review with patient presentations and discussion. Am. J. Med. 48:77, 1970.
4. Wallace, R., and Cohen, A.S.: Tuberculous arthritis. A report of two

cases with a review of biopsy and synovial fluid findings. Am. J. Med. 61:277, 1976.

5. Tuberculosis—United States, 1980. Morbidity Mortality Weekly Report 30:325, 1981.

6. Nathanson, L., and Cohen, W.: A statistical and roentgen analysis of two hundred cases of bone and joint tuberculosis. Radiology 36:550, 1941.

7. Chapman, M., Murray, R.D., and Stoker, D.J.: Tuberculosis of bones and joints. Semin. Roentgenol. 14:266, 1979.

8. Lloveras, J., Peterson, P.K., Simmons, R.L., and Najarian, J.S.: Mycobacterial infections in renal transplant recipients. Seven cases and a review of the literature. Arch. Intern. Med. 142:888, 1982.

9. Paus, B.: Tumour, tuberculosis and osteomyelitis of the spine. Acta Orthop. Scand. 44:372, 1973.

10. Goldenberg, D.L., and Cohen, A.S.: Arthritis due to tuberculous and fungal microorganisms. Clin. Rheum. Dis. 4:211, 1978.

11. Konstam, P.G., and Konstam, S.T.: Spinal tuberculosis in Southern Nigeria. J. Bone Joint Surg. 40B:26, 1958.

12. Luck, J.V.: Tuberculous osteomyelitis and arthritis. In Bone and Joint Diseases. Springfield, Illinois, Charles C Thomas, 1950, pp. 75–103.

13. Pomeranz, M.M.: Roentgen diagnosis of bone and joint tuberculosis. Am. J. Roentgenol. 29:253, 1933.

14. Adams, R., Jones, G., and Marble, H.C.: Tuberculous tenosynovitis. 223:706, 1940.

15. Phemister, D.B.: Changes in the articular surfaces in tuberculous and pyogenic infections of joints. Am. J. Roentgenol. Rad. Ther. 12:1, 1924.

16. Golding, F.C.: Tuberculosis of joints. In Shanks, S.C., and Kerley, P. (eds.): A Textbook of X-ray Diagnosis. 4th ed. London, H.K. Lewis & Company, Ltd., 1971, pp. 307–316.

17. Versfeld, G.A., and Soloman, A.: A diagnostic approach to tuberculosis of bones and joints. J. Bone Joint Surg. 64B:446, 1982.

18. Namey, T.C., and Halla, J.T.: Radiographic and nucleographic techniques. Clin. Rheum. Dis. 4:95, 1978.

19. Steinbach, H.L.: Infections of bones. Semin. Roentgenol. 1:337, 1966.

20. Bell, D., and Cockshott, W.P.: Tuberculosis of the vertebral pedicles. Radiology 99:43, 1971.

21. Newton, P., Sharp, J., and Barnes, K.L.: Bone and joint tuberculosis in Greater Manchester 1969–1979. Ann. Rheum. Dis. 41:1, 1982.

22. Hammerschlag, M.R., Domingo, J., Halber, J.O., and Papayanopulos, D.: Cryptococcal osteomyelitis. Report of a case and review of the literature. Clin. Pediatr. 21:109, 1982.

23. Riese, H.: Die Reishorperchen in tuberculos Erkrankten. Synovalsachen. Deutsch. Z. Chir. 42:1, 1895.

24. Hoffman, G.S., Myers, R.L., Stark, F.R., and Thoen, C.O.: Septic arthritis associated with Mycobacterium avium: A case report and literature review. J. Rheumatol. 5:2, 1978.

25. Hodgson, A.R., and Stock, F.E.: Anterior spine fusion for treatment of tuberculosis of the spine. J. Bone Joint Surg. 42A:295, 1960.

26. Golden, H.E., and Parker, R.H.: Mycobacterial and fungal forms of arthritis. Mod. Treatment 6:1117, 1969.

27. Fifth report of the Medical Research Council Working Party on Tuberculosis of the Spine. A five year assessment of controlled trials of inpatient and outpatient treatment and of plaster-of-Paris jackets for tuberculosis of the spine in children on standard chemotherapy. J. Bone Joint Surg. 58B:399, 1976.

28. East African/British Medical Research Councils: Controlled clinical trial of four short-course (6 months) regimens of chemotherapy for treatment of pulmonary tuberculosis. Lancet 1:7816, 1973.

29. East African/British Medical Research Councils (Second): Controlled clinical trial of four short-course (6 month) regimens of chemotherapy for treatment of pulmonary tuberculosis. Lancet 2:1100, 1974.

30. Mitchell, J.R., Zimmerman, H.J., Ishak, K.G., et al.: Isoniazid liver injury: Clinical spectrum, pathology and probable pathogenesis. Ann. Intern. Med. 84:181, 1976.

31. Clarke, J.T.: The antibiotic therapy of septic arthritis. Clin. Rheum. Dis. 4:133, 1978.

32. Chapman, P.T., and Eichoff, T.C.: Tuberculosis. In Top, F.H., and Wehrle, P.F. (eds.): Communicable and Infectious Diseases. 8th ed. St. Louis, C.V. Mosby Company, 1976.

33. Chapman, J.S.: Atypical mycobacterial infections. Med. Clin. North Am. 51:503, 1967.

34. Fogan, L.: Atypical mycobacteria. Medicine 49:243, 1970.

35. Owens, D.W.: General medical aspects of atypical mycobacteria. South. Med. J. 67:39, 1974.

36. Runyon, E.H.: Anonymous mycobacteria in pulmonary disease. Med. Clin. North Am. 43:273, 1959.

37. Dutt, A.K., and Stead, W.W.: Long-term results of medical treatment in Mycobacterium intracellulare infection. Am. J. Med. 67:449, 1979.

38. Chicoine, L., LaPointe, N., Simoneau, R., et al.: "Anonymous" mycobacterial infection causing disseminated osteomyelitis and skin lesions. Can. Med. Assoc. J. 98:1059, 1968.

39. Lincoln, E.M., and Gilbert, L.A.: Disease in children due to mycobacteria other than Mycobacterium tuberculosis. Am. Rev. Respir. Dis. 105:683, 1972.

40. Greene, J.B., Sidhu, G.S., Lewin, S., Levine, J.F., Masur, H., Simberkoff, M.S. et al.: Mycobacterium avium-intracellulare: a cause of disseminated life-threatening infection in homosexuals and drug abusers. Ann. Intern. Med. 97:539, 1982.

41. Cohen, M.J., Matz, L.R., and Elphick, H.R.: Infection of the soft tissues of the ankle by a group II atypical mycobacterium (scotochromogen). Med. J. Aust. 2:679, 1976.

42. Kelly, P.J., Karlson, A.G., Weed, L.A., et al.: Infection of synovial tissue by mycobacteria other than Mycobacterium tuberculosis. J. Bone Joint Surg. 49A:1521, 1967.

43. Kelly, P.J., Weed, L.A., and Lipscomb, P.R.: Infections of tendon sheaths, bursae, joints and soft tissue by acid-fast bacilli other than tubercle bacilli. J. Bone Joint Surg. 45A:323, 1963.

44. Gofton, J.P.: Mycobacterium marinum infection in a finger. J. Rheumatol. 3:324, 1976.

45. Aaronson, C.M., and Park, C.H.: Sporotrichoid infection due to Mycobacterium marinum: Lesion exacerbation by corticosteroid infiltration. South. Med. J. 67:117, 1974.

46. Herndon, J.H., Dantzker, D.R., and Lanque, A.M.: Mycobacterium fortuitum infections involving the extremities. Report of three cases. J. Bone Joint Surg. 54A:1279, 1972.

47. Aronson, J.D.: Spontaneous tuberculosis in salt water fish. J. Infect. Dis. 39:315, 1926.

48. Philpott, J.A., Woodburne, A.R., Philpott, O.S., et al.: Swimming pool granuloma—study of 290 cases. Arch. Dermatol. 88:158, 1963.

49. Pekin, T.J., and Zvaifler, N.J.: Synovial fluid findings in systemic lupus erythematosus. Arthritis Rheum. 13:777, 1970.

50. Dixon, J.: Non-tuberculous mycobacterial infection of the tendon sheaths of the hand. Report of six cases. J. Bone Joint Surg. 1981.

51. Williams, C.S., and Riordan, D.C.: Mycobacterium marinum infections of the hand. J. Bone Joint Surg. 55A:1042, 1973.

52. Molony, J., and Connolly, K.: Knee arthropathy secondary to Mycobacterium scrofulaceum. Ann. Rheum. Dis. 32:69, 1973.

53. Godwin, M.C.: Infection of knee joint by Mycobacterium kansasii. JAMA 194:88, 1965.

54. Girard, D.E., Bagby, G.C., and Walsh, J.R.: Destructive polyarthritis secondary to Mycobacterium kansasii. Arthritis Rheum. 16:665, 1973.

55. Klinenberg, J.R., Grimley, P.M., and Seegmiller, J.R.: Destructive polyarthritis due to photochromogenic mycobacterium. N. Engl. J. Med. 272:190, 1965.

56. Owen, D.S., and Toone, E.: Soft tissue infection by group I atypical mycobacteria. South. Med. J. 63:116, 1970.

57. Dechairo, D.C., Kittredge, D., Myers, A., et al.: Septic arthritis due to Mycobacterium triviale. Am. Rev. Respir. Dis. 108:1224, 1973.

58. Cheatum, D.E., Hudman, V., and Jones, S.R.: Chronic arthritis due to Mycobacterium intracellulare. Sacroiliac, knee and carpal tunnel involvement in a young man and response to chemotherapy. Arthritis Rheum. 19:777, 1976.

59. Kelly, P.J., and Karlson, A.G.: Granulomatous bacterial arthritis. Clin. Orthop. Rel. Res. 96:165, 1973.

60. Marks, J., and Jenkins, P.A.: Mycobacterium szulgai—a new pathogen. Tubercle 53:210, 1972.

61. Koenig, M.G., Collins, R.D., and Heyssel, R.M.: Disseminated mycobacteriosis caused by Battey type mycobacteria (addendum). Ann. Intern. Med. 64:145, 1966.

62. Winter, F.E., and Runyon, E.H.: Prepatellar bursitis caused by Mycobacterium marinum (balnei). J. Bone Joint Surg. 47A:375, 1965.

63. Gunther, S.F., and Elliot, R.C.: Mycobacterium kansasii. Infection in the deep structures of the hands. Report of two cases. J. Bone Joint Surg. 58A:140, 1976.

64. Yeager, H., and Raleigh, J.W.: Pulmonary disease due to Mycobacterium intracellulare. Am. Rev. Respir. Dis. 108:547, 1973.

65. Crout, J.E., Brewer, N.S., and Tompkins, R.B.: Sporotrichosis arthritis. Am. J. Med. 60:587, 1976.

66. Murray, H.W., Fialk, M.A., and Roberts, R.B.: Candida arthritis. Am. J. Med. 60:587, 1976.

67. Greenman, R., Becker, J., Campbell, C., et al.: Coccidioidal synovitis of the knee. Arch. Intern. Med. 135:526, 1975.

68. Fountain, F.F.: Acute blastomycotic arthritis. Arch. Intern. Med. 132:684, 1973.

69. Noyes, F.R., McCabe, J.D., and Fekety, F.R.: Acute candida arthritis. J. Bone Joint Surg. 55A:169, 1973.

70. Rosen, R.S., and Jacobson, G.: Fungus disease of bone. Semin. Roentgenol. 1:4, 1966.

71. Bayer, A.S., Yushikawa, T.T., Galpin, J.E., et al.: Unusual syndromes of coccidioidomycosis: Diagnostic and therapeutic considerations. Medicine 55:131, 1976.

72. Hayden, G., Lapp, C., and Loda, F.: Arthritis caused by Monosporium

apiospermum treated with intra-articular amphotericin B. Am. J. Dis. Child. 131:927, 1977.

73. Staneck, J.L., Frame, P.T., Altemeier, W.A., and Miller, E.H.: Infection of bone by *Mycobacterium fortuitum* masquerading as *Nocardia asteroides*. Am. J. Clin. Pathol. 76:216, 1981.

74. Curry, W.A.: Human nocardiosis. Arch. Intern. Med. 140:818, 1980.

75. Altner, P.C., and Turner, R.R.: Sporotrichosis of bones and joints. Clin. Orthop. Rel. Res. 68:138, 1970.

76. Wilson, D.E., Mann, J.J., Bennett, J.E., et al.: Clinical features of extracutaneous sporotrichosis. Medicine 46:265, 1967.

77. Holzman, R.S., and Bishko, F.: Osteomyelitis in heroin addicts. Ann. Intern. Med. 75:693, 1971.

78. Lertratanakul, Y., Glassford, G.H., and Rubinstein, H.M.: Arthritis and osteomyelitis due to *Candida albicans*. A case report. J. Rheumatol. 4:317, 1977.

79. Lindstrom, F.D., and Lindholm, T.: *Candida albicans* arthritis treated with flucytosine. Ann. Intern. Med. 79:131, 1973.

80. Klein, J.D., Yamauchi, T., and Horlick, S.P.: Neonatal candidiasis, meningitis and arthritis. J. Pediatr. 81:31, 1972.

81. Hutter, R.V.P., and Collins, H.S.: The occurrence of opportunistic fungus infections in a cancer hospital. Lab. Invest. 11:1035, 1962.

82. Curry, C.R., and Quie, P.G.: Fungal septicemia in patients receiving parenteral hyperalimentation. N. Engl. J. Med. 285:1221, 1971.

83. Hart, P.D., Russell, E., Jr., and Remington, J.S.: The compromised host and infection. J. Infect. Dis. 120:169, 1969.

84. Poplack, D.G., and Jacobs, S.A.: Candida arthritis treated with amphotericin B. J. Pediatr. 87:989, 1975.

85. Wingard, J.R., Merz, W.G., and Saral, R.: *Candida tropicalis*: A major pathogen in immunocompromised patients. Ann. Intern. Med. 91:539, 1979.

86. Umber, J., Chapman, M.W., and Drutz, D.J.: Candida pyarthrosis. J. Bone Joint Surg. 56A:1520, 1974.

86a. MacGregor, R.R., Schimmer, B.M., and Steinberg, M.E.: Results of combined amphotericin B-5-fluorocytosine therapy for prosthetic knee joint infected with *Candida parapsilosis*. J. Rheumatol. 6:451, 1979.

87. Reeves, R.J., and Pederson, R.: Fungus infection in bone. Radiology 62:55, 1954.

88. Grossman, M.: Aspergillosis of bone. Br. J. Radiol. 48:57, 1975.

89. Ajello, L.: The medical mycological iceberg. Proc. Int. Symp. Mycoses 205:3, 1970.

90. Class, R.N., and Cascio, F.S.: Histoplasmosis presenting as acute polyarthritis. N. Engl. J. Med. 287:1133, 1972.

91. Cockshott, W.P., and Lucas, A.O.: Radiological findings in *Histoplasma duboisii* infections. Br. J. Radiol. 37:653, 1964.

92. Hoeprich, P.D.: Cryptococcosis. *In* Hoeprich, P. (ed.): Infectious Diseases. 2nd ed. New York, Harper & Row, 1977, Chap. 114.

93. Gosling, H.R., and Gilmer, W.S.: Skeletal cryptococcosis (torulosis). J. Bone Joint Surg. 38A:660, 1956.

94. Cowen, N.J.: Cryptococcosis of bone. Clin. Orthop. Rel. Res. 66:174, 1969.

95. Levinson, D.J., Silcox, D.C., Rippon, J.W., et al.: Septic arthritis due to nonencapsulated *Cryptococcus neoformans* with coexisting sarcoidosis. Arthritis Rheum. 17:1037, 1974.

96. Dalinka, M.K., and Greendyke, W.H.: The spinal manifestations of coccidioidomycosis. J. Can. Assoc. Radiol. 22:93, 1971.

97. Gehweiler, J.A., Capp, M.P., and Chick, E.W.: Observations on the roentgen patterns in blastomycosis of bone. Am. J. Roentgenol. 108:497, 1970.

98. O'Neill, R.P., and Penman, R.W.B.: Clinical aspects of blastomycosis. Thorax 25:708, 1970.

99. Sanders, L.L.: Blastomycosis arthritis. Arthritis Rheum. 10:91, 1967.

100. Utz, J.P.: Sporotrichosis. *In* Hoeprich, P. (ed.): Infectious Diseases. 2nd ed. New York, Harper & Row, 1977, Chap. 104.

101. Dehaven, K.E., Wilde, A.H., and O'Duffy, J.D.: Sporotrichosis arthritis and tenosynovitis. J. Bone Joint Surg. 54A:874, 1972.

102. Weitzner, R., Mak, E., and Lerthratanakul, Y.: Articular sporotrichosis. Ann. Intern. Med. 87:382, 1977.

103. Molstad, B., and Strom, R.: Multiarticular sporotrichosis. JAMA 240:556, 1978.

104. Bayer, A.S., Scott, V.J., and Guze, L.B.: Fungal arthritis. III. Sporotrichal arthritis. Semin. Arthritis Rheum. 9:66, 1979.

105. Goldstein, E., and Hoeprich, P.D.: Candidosis. *In* Hoeprich, P. (ed.): Infectious Diseases. 2nd ed. New York, Harper & Row, 1977, Chap. 37.

106. Silva-Hutner, M., and Cooper, B.H.: Yeasts of medical importance. *In* Lennette E.H. et al. (eds.): Manual of Clinical Microbiology. Washington, D.C., American Society for Microbiology, 1980.

107. Pittard, W.B., Thullen, J.D., and Fanaroff, A.A.: Neonatal septic arthritis. J. Pediatr. 88:621, 1976.

108. Fitzgerald, E., Lloyd-Still, J., and Gordon, S.L.: Candida arthritis. Clin. Orthop. Rel. Res. 106:143, 1975.

109. Ide, A., Jacobelli, S., and Zenteno, G.: Candida arthritis associated with

110. Marmor, L., and Peter, J.B.: Candida arthritis of the knee joint. Clin. Orthop. Rel. Res. 118:133, 1976.

111. Adler, S., Randall, J., and Plotkin, S.A.: Candidal osteomyelitis and arthritis in a neonate. Am. J. Dis. Child. 123:595, 972.

112. Noble, H.B., and Lyne, E.D.: Candida osteomyelitis and arthritis from hyperalimentation therapy. J. Bone Joint Surg. 56A:825, 1974.

113. Businco, L., Iannaccone, G., Del Principe, D., et al.: Disseminated arthritis and osteitis by *Candida albicans* in a two month old infant receiving parenteral nutrition. Acta Paediatr. Scand. 66:393, 1977.

114. Bayer, A.S., and Guze, L.B.: Fungal arthritis. I. Candida arthritis. Semin. Arthritis Rheum. 8:142, 1978.

115. Yarchoan, R., Davies, S.F., Fried, J., and Mahowald, M.L.: Isolated *Candida parapsilosis* in a heroin addict. J. Rheumatol. 6:447, 1979.

116. Richtsmeier, W.J., and Johns, M.E.: Actinomycosis of the head and neck. CRC Crit. Rev. Clin. Lab. Sci. 11:175, 1979.

117. Schaal, K.P., Schofield, G.M., and Pulverer, G.: Taxonomy and clinical significance of Actinomycetaceae and Proprionibacteriaceae. Infection (Suppl.) 8:122, 1980.

118. Goldsand, G.: Actinomycosis. *In* Hoeprich, P. (ed.): Infectious Diseases. 2nd ed. New York, Harper & Row, 1977, Chap. 36.

119. Wang , Y.: Critical Reviews in Clinical Radiology and Nuclear Medicine. Boca Raton, Fla., CRC Press, Inc., 1975.

120. Kinderlehrer, D.A., and Reese, R.E.: Fungal infections. *In* Reese, R.E., and Douglas, R.G., Jr., (eds.): A Practical Approach to Infectious Diseases. Boston/Toronto, Little, Brown and Co., 1983, Chap. 19.

121. Rhangos, W.C., and Chick, E.W.: Mycotic infections of bone. South. Med. J. 57:664, 1964.

122. Lane, T., Goings, S., Fraser, D.W., Ries, K., Pettrozzi, J., and Abrutyn, E.: Disseminated actinomycosis with spinal cord compression: Report of two cases. Neurology 29:890, 1979.

123. Sherer, P.B., and Dobbins, J.: Actinomycosis arthritis: A case report. Med. Ann. (D. C.) 43:66, 1974.

124. Schaal, K.P., and Pape, W.: Special methodological problems in antibiotic susceptibility testing of fermentative actinomycetes. Infection (Suppl.) 8:176, 1980.

125. Bardana E.J., Jr.: The clinical spectrum of aspergillosis. *In* Batsakis J., and Savory, J.E. (eds.): CRC Critical Reviews in Clinical Laboratory Sciences. Boca Raton, Fla., CRC Press Inc., 1981.

126. Utz, J.P.: Aspergillosis. *In* Hoeprich, P. (ed.): Infectious Diseases. 2nd ed. New York, Harper & Row, 1977, Chap. 41.

127. Corall, C.J., Merz, W.G., Rekedal, K., and Hughes, W.T.: Aspergillus osteomyelitis in an immunocompetent adolescent. A case report and review of the literature. Pediatrics 70:455, 1982.

128. Tach, K.J., Rhame, F.S., Brown, B., and Thompson R.C., Jr.: Aspergillus osteomyelitis. Report of four cases and review of the literature. Am. J. Med. 73:295, 1982.

129. Bayer, A.S., Choi, C., Tillman, D.B., and Guze, L.B.: Fungal arthritis. V. Cryptococcal and histoplasmal arthritis. Semin. Arthritis Rheum. 9:218, 1980.

130. Wheat, L.J., Slama, T.G., Eitzen, H.E., Kohler, R.B., French, L.V., and Biesecker, J.L.: A large urban outbreak of histoplasmosis: Clinical features. Ann. Intern. Med. 94:331, 1981.

131. Thornberry, D.K., Wheat, L.J., Brandt, K.D., and Rosenthal, J.: Histoplasmosis presenting with joint pain and hilar adenopathy. Arthritis Rheum. 25:1396, 1982.

132. Sellers, T.F., Price, W.N., and Newberry, W.M.: An epidemic of erythema multiforme and erythema nodosum caused by histoplasmosis. Ann. Intern. Med. 62:1244, 1963.

133. Medeiros, A.A., Marty, S.D., Tosh, F.E., and Chin, T.D.Y.: Erythema nodosum and erythema multiforme as clinical manifestations of histoplasmosis in a community outbreak. N. Engl. J. Med. 274:415, 1966.

134. Dismukes, W.E., Royal, S.A., and Tynes, B.S.: Disseminated histoplasmosis in corticosteroid-treated patients. JAMA 240:1495, 1978.

135. Paterson, P.Y.: Infection in the compromised host. *In* Youmans, G.P., Paterson, P.Y., and Sommers, H.M. (eds.): The Biological and Clinical Basis of Infectious Diseases. Philadelphia W. B. Saunders Company, 1975, Chap. 43.

136. Fialk, M.A., Marcove, R.C., and Armstrong, D.: Cryptococcal bone disease: A manifestation of disseminated cryptococcosis. Clin. Orthop. Rel. Res. 158:219, 1981.

137. Youmans, G.P.: Histoplasmosis, coccidioidomycosis, blastomycosis. *In* Youmans, G.P., Paterson, P.Y., and Sommers, H.M. (eds.): The Biological and Clinical Basis of Infectious Diseases. Philadelphia, W. B. Saunders Company, 1975, Chap. 26.

138. Bayer, A.S., and Guze, L.B.: Fungal arthritis. II. Coccidioidal synovitis. Semin. Arthritis Rheum. 8:200, 1979.

139. Carter, R.A.: Infectious granulomas of bones and joints, with special reference to coccidioidal granuloma. Radiology 23:1, 1934.

140. McMaster, P.E., and Gilfillan, C.: Coccidioidal osteomyelitis. JAMA 112:1233, 1939.

141. Winter, W.G., Larson, R.K., Honnegar, M.M., et al.: Coccidioidal arthritis and its treatment—1975. J. Bone Joint Surg. 57A:1152, 1975.

142. DeFelice, R., Galgiani, J.N., Campbell, S.C., Palpant, S.D., Friedman, B.A. et al.: Ketoconazole treatment of nonprimary coccidioidomycosis. Am. J. Med. 72:681, 1982.

143. Catanzaro, A., Einstein, H., Levine, B., Ross, J.B., Schillaci, R. et al.: Ketoconazole for treatment of disseminated coccidioidomycosis. Ann. Intern. Med. 96:436, 1982.

144. Boddicker, J.H., Fong, D., Walsh, T.E., Schillaci, R.F., Moniot, A.L., and Catanzaro, A.: Bone and gallium scanning in the evaluation of disseminated coccidioidomycosis. Am. Rev. Respir. Dis. 122:279, 1980.

145. McGahan, J.P., Graves, D.S., Palmer, P.E.S., Stadalnik, R.C., and Dublin, A.B.: Classic and contemporary imaging of coccidioidomycosis. AJR 136:393, 1981.

146. Deresinski, S.C., and Stevens, D.A.: Bone and joint coccidioidomycosis treated with miconazole. Am. Rev. Respir. Dis. 120:1101, 1979.

147. Birsner, J.W., and Smart, S.: Osseous coccidioidomycosis: A chronic form of dissemination. AJR 76:1052, 1956.

148. Aidem, H.P.: Intraarticular amphotericin B in the treatment of coccidioidal synovitis of the knee. J. Bone Joint Surg. 50A:1663, 1968.

149. Sarosi, G.A., and Davies, S.F.: Blastomycosis. Am. Rev. Respir. Dis. 120:911, 1979.

150. Tenenbaum, M.J., Greenspan, J., and Kerkering, T.M.: Blastomycosis. CRC Crit. Rev. Microbiol. 9:139, 1982.

151. Sarosi, G.A., and Serstock, D.S.: Isolation: of *Blastomyces dermatitidis* from pigeon manure. Am. Rev. Respir. Dis. 114:1179, 1976.

152. Utz, J.P.: Blastomycosis. *In* Hoeprich, P. (ed.): Infectious Diseases. 2nd ed. New York, Harper & Row, 1977, Chap. 40.

153. Gnann J.W., Jr., Bressler, G.S., Bodet, C.A., and Avent, C.K.: Human blastomycosis after a dog bite. Ann. Intern. Med. 98:48, 1983.

154. Jaspers, R.H.: Transmission of blastomycosis from animals to man. J. Am. Vet. Assoc. 164:8, 1974.

155. Cush, R., Light, R.W., and George, D.B.: Clinical and roentgenographic manifestations of acute and chronic blastomycosis. Chest 69:345, 1976.

156. Witorsch, P., and Utz, J.P.: North American blastomycosis: A study of 40 patients. Medicine 47:169, 1968.

157. Bassett, F.H., and Tindall, J.P.: Blastomycosis of bone. South. Med. J. 65:547, 1972.

158. Bayer, A.S., Scott, V.J., and Guze, L.B.: Fungal arthritis. IV. Blastomycotic arthritis. Semin. Arthritis Rheum. 9:145, 1979.

159. Holt, R.J.: Progress in antimycotic chemotherapy 1945–1980. Infection (Suppl.) 8:284, 1980.

160. Medoff, G., and Kobayashi, G.S.: Strategies in the treatment of systemic fungal infection. N. Engl. J. Med. 302:145, 1980.

161. Cohen, J.: Antifungal chemotherapy. Lancet 2:532, 1982.

162. Hermans, P.E.: Antifungal agents used for deep-seated mycotic infections. Mayo Clin. Proc. 52:687, 1977.

163. Bennett, J.E., and Remington, J.S.: Miconazole in cryptococcosis and systemic candidiasis: a word of caution. Editorial. Ann. Intern. Med. 94:708, 1981.

164. Dismukes, W.E., Stamm, A.M., Graybill, J.R., Craven, P.C., Stevens, D.A., Stiller, R.L., et al.: Treatment of systemic mycoses with ketoconazole: emphasis on toxicity and clinical response in 52 patients. Ann. Intern. Med. 98:13, 1983.

165. Graybill, J.R., Craven, P.C., Donovan, W., and Matthew, E.B.: Ketoconazole therapy for systemic fungal infections. Inadequacy of standard dosage regimens. Am. Rev. Respir. Dis. 126:171, 1982.

166. Hoeprich, P.D.: Ketoconazole in systemic mycoses. Editorial. Ann. Intern. Med. 98:105, 1983.

Chapter 98

Viral Arthritis

Thomas J. Schnitzer

INTRODUCTION

Arthritis is a frequent accompaniment to a number of common viral illnesses in humans (type B hepatitis, rubella, alphavirus infection). It also occurs, but at a lower incidence, in association with a wide range of other viral infections (mumps, enteroviruses, adenoviruses, herpesviruses). Rheumatic manifestations are believed to arise either as a result of actual viral infection of synovial tissues (e.g., rubella) or as a consequence of the immunologic response of the host to the viral infection with the formation and deposition of immune complexes in synovial tissues (e.g., type B hepatitis). Generally, rheumatic symptoms first become apparent during the prodrome or at the onset of the clinical illness and are often temporally associated with the appearance of a characteristic skin rash. Different patterns of joint and soft tissue involvement are observed with each of the infectious agents. However, in most viral-related arthritides, joint symptoms occur suddenly, are of brief duration, and do not recur, although notable exceptions have been documented (e.g., rubella, alphavirus infections). Routine laboratory studies are not helpful in establishing the etiology of the arthritis, but specific serologic tests are available to confirm the diagnosis of a viral infection. In all instances the arthritis is non-destructive and does not lead to any currently recognized form of chronic joint disease.

Several mechanisms exist[1-8] by which viruses may initiate rheumatic diseases in general and joint signs and symptoms in particular. The simplest and most obvious mechanism is by direct infection of synovial tissues, a process believed to occur during rubella and rubella vaccine virus infection in humans. If the interaction between the virus and the host cell is a lytic one, the attendant tissue destruction and inflammatory response may be responsible both for the joint symptoms and for the ultimate resolution of the infection.[1] When viruses cause persistent or latent infections, however, cell destruction may be mediated by immunologic mechanisms that are directed either toward viral or host membrane-associated antigens or toward viral products released into the joint fluid or systemic circulation.[1,7,8]

Although ultimately protective, the immunologic response to viral infection can itself give rise to rheumatic manifestations.[1-6] Clearance of virus from the circulation following the onset of viremia may be associated with the development of virus-antibody complexes. In some individuals, these immune complexes may be deposited in synovial tissues in which activation of complement pathways can lead to an inflammatory response. With viruses able to cause a persistent infection in synovial

Table 98–1. Rheumatic Manifestations of Viral Diseases

Viral Disease	Prevalence of Rheumatic Manifestations	Joint Involvement*					Comments
		Symmetric	Asymmetric	Small	Large	Duration	
Hepatitis B	10–25% Male = female	++++	+	++++	++ knees	7–21 days	Onset during prodrome Often coincident with rash
Rubella	15–30% of adult women 1–6% of adult men Uncommon in children	++++	+	++++	+++ knees	3–14 days	Tendinitis and carpal tunnel syndromes common Rash often precedes arthritis
Rubella vaccine–induced	1–5% of children Adult women > adult men	++++	+	+++	+++ knees	1–5 days	Arthralgias > arthritis Prolonged course and recurrences observed
Alphavirus infections							
Ross River	Majority of adults	+	+++	++++	+	7–28 days	Pain may persist for weeks to months
Chikungunya	Majority of adults	+++	+	++	++	3–7 days	Joint swelling uncommon Arthralgias precede rash
O'nyong-nyong	Majority of adults	+	+++	+	+++	7–14 days	
Mumps	0.4% Males > females	++	++	++	++ knees	10–15 days	Parotitis precedes arthritis by 1–2 weeks High incidence of orchitis
Enterovirus infections	≥ 0.13%	++	++	++	++ knees		Salicylates provide little relief Diagnosis difficult to confirm because of multiple immunotypes
Smallpox	0.25–0.5% 2.5% of children < 10 years old	++	+	+	++++	Weeks	Onset 10–30 days after rash Secondary to osteomyelitis
Adenovirus infections	Case reports	++	++	++	++	7–35 days	Can be seen after vaccinia infection
Herpesvirus infections	Case reports	+	+++	+	++++	Variable, 7 days to 1 month	VZV: female predominance noted
Erythema infectiosum	Variable: up to 74% of adults, 5% of children	++	++	+	++++ knees	4–10 days	Infectious etiology inferred by epidemiology

*+++++ = predominant, +++ = marked, ++ = common, + = infrequent

tissues, immune complexes can be formed locally and released into the joint fluid, in which the inflammatory response generated will give rise to the clinical signs and symptoms of arthritis.

In some persistent and latent infections, viral particles are not released from infected cells, but viral antigens are inserted into the cellular membranes, where they are recognized as foreign. Interaction at the cell surface between these viral antigens and host antigens can generate new, yet immunologically related (cross-reactive), antigenic determinants recognized by the host as "altered-self." These new determinants, as well as the original determinants found on uninfected normal host cells, will then be the target of immunologic responses leading to cell destruction.[1,3,7,8] Thus, for the initiation of autoimmune diseases, viral infection and expression of viral antigens need not persist but can occur transiently, triggering the immune response, which will be maintained by the continued presence of the original but now cross-reactive determinants of the unaltered host antigens. In the event that such antigens are tissue specific, subsequent symptoms will present as distinct syndromes or diseases.

A final mechanism that can give rise to rheumatic disease is direct viral infection of elements of the immune system.[1,3,5] Many viruses are known to be able to infect lymphocytes (e.g., Epstein-Barr virus, cytomegalovirus, measles, rubella) and can persist in such cells as well. Alteration of the immune response may arise either as a consequence of direct lysis of a particular subset of immune cells (e.g., T helper or suppressor lymphocytes, B lymphocytes) or, more likely, by a virus-induced modulation of surface components (e.g., receptors), leading to alteration in the recognition of and reaction to both host and foreign antigens.

HEPATITIS B VIRUS

Virology. The recognition by Blumberg, Prince, and others[9-12] of "Australia antigen" as a marker of hepatitis B virus (HBV) infection permitted identification of the etiologic agent in the serum of patients in the early 1970s.[12] Its physicochemical properties, antigenic determinants, genome structure, and protein composition have been extensively characterized, resulting in identification of HBV as the prototype of a new class of viruses, the "hepadnaviruses" (hepatitis-DNA-virus).[10-18]

The complete hepatitis B virion (Fig. 98–1) has been shown to consist of a 42-nm particle (Dane particle) composed of a 27-nm nucleocapsid surrounded by a 7-nm coat (HBsAg).[10-18] When the coat is synthesized in excess of nucleocapsid, HBsAg is released from infected cells and forms the 22-nm-diameter spherical and filamentous particles lacking nucleic acid that are commonly seen by electron microscopy in the sera of patients with HBV infection. The nucleocapsid is composed of a number of different elements, including two antigenically distinct constituents—the hepatitis B core antigen

1. HBsAg:
   Particles with HBsAg (a, d/y, w/r) on their surfaces.

   42 nm   15-25 nm

   20 x 20-200 nm

   "Dane particle"

   non-ionic detergent (NP 40)

2. HBcAg:
   Dane particle core with HBcAg on its surface and DNA polymerase activity.

   28 nm

   "Dane particle" core

   strong detergent (SDS)

3. DNA and DNA Polymerase:
   Circular, double stranded Dane particle DNA with a single stranded gap up to 1/3 of circle length. DNA polymerase reaction makes the single stranded region double stranded.

   mw - 2.0 x 10^6 daltons

4. HBeAg:
   ~ 3 x 10^5 dalton protein antigenically and physically distinct from HBsAg and HBcAg.

Figure 98–1. Composition of hepatitis B viral structures found in the blood of infected patients. (From Robinson, W.S.: Ann. N.Y. Acad. Sci. 354:372, 1980.)

(HBcAg) and the hepatitis B e antigen (HBeAg), one molecule of partially double-stranded DNA, and an associated DNA polymerase activity that is capable of completing the synthesis of the shorter DNA strand.[10-18]

The events that occur upon infection of a cell with HBV are not yet well understood. Viral replication is believed to proceed through an RNA intermediate and to involve reverse transcription[17] (i.e., RNA-directed DNA synthesis), both processes being unique among DNA viruses. In addition, HBV has been shown to be able to integrate into host cellular DNA, perhaps in a site-specific manner.[16,17,19-20]

Clinical Disease. The majority of people exposed to HBV experience an acute, self-limited infection. Most often this process is not clinically apparent but does result in the development of an antibody response to HBsAg (anti-HBs). However, in 5 to 10 percent of cases, the acute HBV infection proceeds to a chronic phase that is characterized by the persistence of one or more of the serologic markers of viral presence (HBeAg, HBcAg, anti-HBcAg, anti-HBs) or the infectious virus itself.[11-15] In approximately 30 percent of these cases clinical illness is present (chronic active hepatitis), whereas in the remainder either evidence exists of chronic persistent hepatitis or no biochemical nor pathologic abnormalities are found.[11,12,14]

The clinical presentation of acute icteric HBV infection has been well described.[11-15] After an incubation period of 40 to 180 days, symptoms of headache, fatigue, anorexia, nausea, vomiting, abdominal pain, and fever appear and generally precede the development of icterus by 2 to 14 days. With the onset of jaundice these symptoms abate, and resolution of clinical disease occurs in adults over the ensuing 3 to 4 weeks. The sequence of serologic events[10-15] in this type of HBV infection is shown in Figure 98–2. The earliest sign of infection is the appearance of HBsAg, which is followed by the detection of anti-HBc. Free HBcAg is not found in the serum. HBeAg appears just prior to clinical illness, is present during the period of maximum infectivity, and leads to the production of anti-HBe shortly thereafter. Anti-HBs generally appears only late in the course of the disease, not until some weeks after HBsAg has disappeared from the circulation. The reason for such a delayed appearance of anti-HBs is not known, but once present this antibody persists for years as a marker of past infection.

Hepatocyte damage is believed to occur primarily by cell-mediated immune responses directed against both HBV antigens in infected cells and tissue-specific host antigens in uninfected hepatocytes.[10,14,19-21]

Pathogenesis of Arthritic Symptoms. In those patients who develop joint involvement during HBV infection, an antibody response to HBsAg occurs not as shown in Figure 98–2 but earlier in the course of the disease prior to the onset of clinical symptoms.[11,13,22-26] Since HBsAg levels are high at this time, anti-HBs production results in the formation of soluble immune complexes. The tissue deposition of these HBsAg-anti-HBs complexes is believed to be responsible for the initiation of the inflammatory processes, which result in the joint manifestations observed.[27-33] Cryoprecipitates containing HBsAg, anti-HBs, C3, C4, and C5 have been detected in patients with arthritis associated with HBV infection,[22,32] and longitudinal studies have confirmed the sequence of serologic events outlined in Figure 98–2 and have demonstrated complement consumption (Fig. 98–3).[22-26]

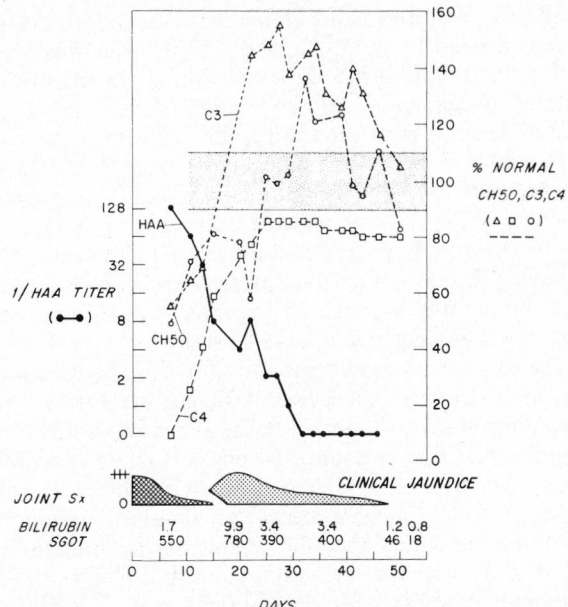

Figure 98–3. Relationship of HBsAg (HAA) titers to serum levels of C3, C4 and CH$_{50}$ during the course of HBV hepatitis and associated arthritis. (From Alpert, E., Schur, P.H., and Isselbacher, K.J.: N. Engl. J. Med. 287:103, 1972. Reprinted by permission of the New England Journal of Medicine.)

In those people with chronic HBV infection, persistent viral antigenemia can occur,[10-15] and immune complex formation may take place later after infection. Under these circumstances not only may arthritis be apparent but a variety of clinical presentations may also occur (see later discussion), including polyarteritis nodosa,[12,14,15,22,34-43] glomerulonephritis,[12,14,15,40,44-47] and mixed essential cryoglobulinemia.[12,48,49]

Rheumatologic Manifestations. Although first remarked upon by Graves in 1843,[50] only recently has it been appreciated that joint symptoms may be a prominent manifestation during the prodromal phase of both icteric and anicteric liver disease caused by HBV.[31,32,51-53] Similar musculoskeletal involvement has not been demonstrated in patients with type A or non-A, non-B hepatitis.[12,54] A frequency of joint symptoms (arthralgias and arthritis) in 10 to 25 percent of patients with HBV infections reflects the findings of the majority of studies.[11,14,15,31,51,52,55] Occasional "outbreaks" of HBV infection have been associated with significantly higher joint attack rates, suggesting the existence of "arthritogenic" strains of HBV.[51,56,57]

The age range of patients with HBV infection who demonstrate joint manifestations is quite broad (13 to 72 years old), but few cases of this association in children have been reported. Women tend to be more at risk of developing arthritis than are men, but the difference is not great and is not apparent when arthralgia is considered as well.[25,52] Joint symptoms are typically present during the prodromal phase of acute HBV infection and may precede clinical jaundice by days to weeks (up to 18 weeks in one report). Some of the other more commonly associated prodromal symptoms of hepatitis such

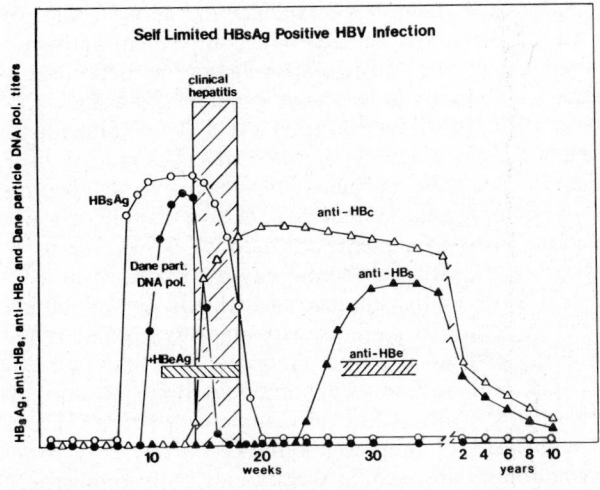

Figure 98–2. Diagrammatic representation of the temporal evolution of viral markers detectable in the blood of patients during self-limited HBsAg-positive HBV infection. (From Robinson, W.S.: Hepatitis B virus. *In* Mandell, G.L., Douglas, R.G., Jr., and Bennett, J.E. (eds.): Principles and Practice of Infectious Diseases. New York, John Wiley & Sons, 1979, p. 1398.)

as nausea, vomiting, and abdominal discomfort occur in only a minority (approximately 25 percent) of people with joint involvement. Fever is present in about 25 percent of patients with arthralgias and in 50 percent of those with arthritis and tends to be moderate, between 100° F and 102° F, in most cases.[31,32,52] Skin involvement [31,51,52,58,59] is frequently present in people having joint symptoms and often appears at the onset of the arthritis. Urticarial and maculopapular eruptions involving primarily the lower extremities are most common, but nonthrombocytopenic purpura, petechiae, and angioneurotic edema may also be seen.

The onset of articular symptoms is usually quite rapid, and joint pain may be severe. Articular involvement is generally symmetric and occurs in either an additive or migratory fashion, but simultaneous polyarticular symptoms may also be exhibited. The small joints of the hands, (metacarphophalangeal, proximal interphalangeal) and the knees are most frequently symptomatic, followed by wrists, ankles, shoulders, and elbows.[31,52,58] Although most patients present with both large and small joint involvement, large joint involvement alone is not uncommon. Early morning stiffness is often a prominent manifestation of this stage of the disease. Subcutaneous nodules, clinically and histologically similar to those seen in rheumatoid arthritis, have been reported[33,59,60] but are rare.

Once present, joint symptoms persist for several days to weeks with a mean duration of 1 to 3 weeks in most reported series.[12,13,15,22,31,52] Typically, arthralgias and arthritis resolve with the onset of jaundice, but in approximately 5 percent of cases the two occur simultaneously. In patients who develop chronic active hepatitis (CAH) or who demonstrate chronic HBV antigenemia, arthralgias and arthritis may be present or may recur over long periods of time.[23,57]

Other Syndromes Associated with HBV Infection. Two other well-defined rheumatologic disorders, polyarteritis nodosa[12,14,15,22,34-43] and mixed essential cryoglobulinemia,[12,14,48,49] have been associated with HBV infection and are believed to arise as a consequence of the persistent antigenemia that occurs with subacute or chronic HBV infection. In both conditions the deposition of immune complexes containing immunoglobulin, complement and HBV antigen in vessel walls has been demonstrated. These two disorders differ primarily in the size of the vessels involved. This may reflect differences in the sizes or types of immune complexes formed, which, in turn, are a function of factors such as the level of antigenemia as well as the quality and quantity of the host immune response. In polyarteritis nodosa that is associated with HBV infection, free HBsAg is commonly found in the serum—a condition of antigen excess that results in the formation of soluble complexes.[22,30,34-36] Conversely, in mixed essential cryoglobulinemia free HBsAg is often not detectable or is present only at low levels, the antigen being greatly concentrated in the cryoprecipitate. These findings reflect either a lower level of synthesis of viral antigen or a more efficient host immune response.[48,49,61]

Renal and nervous system involvement are well-recognized manifestations of immune complex–mediated disease and are often a prominent finding in patients with polyarteritis nodosa or mixed essential cryoglobulinemia. In most cases, evidence of vasculitis involving multiple organs exists, and the finding of single organ involvement in an immune complex–mediated disease is uncommon. However, patients presenting with isolated membranous glomerulonephritis as a consequence of HBV infection have been reported,[44-47] and HBsAg, immunoglobulin, and complement have been demonstrated in the glomerular capillaries and mesangium of the involved kidneys. One case of a severe peripheral polyneuropathy[62] has also been seen in association with CAH secondary to HBV infection. Appreciation of such presentations should lead to appropriate serologic and biochemical testing in these settings to confirm the relationship with HBV infection.

Laboratory Investigations. The diagnosis of HBV infection is made by demonstrating the presence of one or more of the antigenic determinants of HBV, or the antibodies to these components, in the serum of patients affected.[10-15,31,32,52] Confirmation of this diagnosis can require repeated testing, particularly if only HBsAg is sought, because antigenemia may be transient or may occur only at low levels, or free antigen may not be present, being completely bound in antigen-antibody complexes. Typically, however, during the period of joint involvement free HBsAg is present in the serum (often at high titer) in the absence of detectable anti-HBsAg. With the onset of jaundice and resolution of arthritic symptoms, the HBsAg titer falls and may become undetectable concomitant with the appearance of anti-HBsAg.[13,22-26] Generally, liver function tests are mildly abnormal during the period of joint involvement, which helps support the diagnosis, though some patients with normal liver function tests have been reported.[13,24,31]

As already mentioned, evidence of the activation of both the classic and the alternate complement pathways exists. CH_{50} and C3 and C4 levels may be depressed—either individually or in concert—but a substantial number of patients will have normal levels.[22-26,31-33] Since complement levels are often elevated in inflammatory liver disease, even these normal values may reflect activation of the complement system and relative complement depletion. In many patients, cryoglobulins have been reported.[13,22,40] Although commonly associated with liver disease even in the absence of arthritis, cryoglobulins that are found in patients with joint symptoms differ by being present in greater amounts, by containing C3, C4, C5, and occasionally immunoglobulin A, and by often being composed of the complement-fixing G1 and G3 subclasses of immunoglobulin G. Furthermore, these cryoglobulins are capable of activating both complement pathways in vitro, whereas those from patients without joint symptoms lack this ability.[22]

Most commonly the synovial fluid appears inflammatory in nature with a protein content of more than 2 g per dl and a high leukocyte count.[26] Either mononuclear cells or polymorphonuclear leukocytes may predominate. Glucose levels are almost always normal, even in the presence of large numbers of leukocytes, and help distinguish this synovial effusion from that seen in septic arthritis. Hepatitis antigen and antibody may be found in the joint fluid, and synovial fluid complement levels have been reported to be depressed, which is consistent with the hypothesis that immune complex deposition is responsible for the joint findings.[26,31,49,64]

Management. As for all virus-associated arthritides, no specific therapy is available. Restriction of activity and the institution of salicylate therapy have been found to be effective in the majority of patients.[31] In those patients with acute hepatitis, joint symptoms are self-limited and have never been associated with chronic joint disease or permanent joint damage.

RUBELLA

Virology. Rubella, a member of the Togaviridae family (genus *Rubiviridae*), is a spherically shaped structure with a diameter of 50 to 70 nm that is composed of an outer lipoprotein envelope surrounding a 30- to 40-nm-diameter nucleocapsid that contains the single-stranded RNA genome.[65-69] The envelope contains 5- to 6-nm surface projections that constitute the viral hemagglutinin. Other viral antigens have been defined, of which the complement-fixing antigen is perhaps the most widely utilized for clinical and epidemiologic purposes (see further on).

Clinical Presentation. Rubella virus causes a mild acute exanthematous illness that is marked clinically by a characteristic maculopapular rash and significant lymphadenopathy. The incidence of subclinical disease is high (25 to 50 percent of those infected), though the range reported is quite broad (10 to 90 percent).[65,66,68-70] The incubation period of rubella averages 18 days (range 12 to 23 days), with the virus replicating initially in pharyngeal tissues and regional lymph nodes and then spreading via a viremic phase to other organs.[65-70] In children there typically is no prodrome. In adults, however, nonspecific symptoms of an upper respiratory infection (sore throat, headache, lymphadenopathy, low-grade fever, myalgias, chills, nausea, vomiting) and eye pain, which may be severe, often precede the appearance of rash by 1 to 5 days. In both children and adults, adenopathy involving primarily the posterior auricular, posterior cervical, and suboccipital lymph nodes usually develops 4 to 10 days before the rash and may persist for several weeks.[65,66,68,69] The rash itself[65-70] is short-lived. It begins on the face as a light pink maculopapular eruption and spreads centrifugally (often disappearing quickly from previously affected areas) to involve the trunk, hands, and feet, while sparing the palms, soles, and scalp. The rash is generally not confluent; in adults it is often pruritic and may be mistaken for an allergic reaction. Low-grade fever can be present at the onset of the rash but rarely persists beyond the first 24 hours, at which time most of the other prodromal manifestations have likewise resolved.

The clinical diagnosis of rubella may be confirmed either by direct viral isolation (most successfully undertaken by cultures obtained from the nasopharynx) or by serologic methods employing hemagglutination inhibition (HI) or complement fixation (CF) assays.[65-70] During the rash detectable HI titers appear first, peak 1 to 2 weeks later, and then decline to a stable level by 4 to 12 months, remaining positive for life. The CF assay is less sensitive and shows positive results only 4 to 8 weeks following infection (Fig. 98–4). Recently both a solid-phase radioimmunoassay and an enzyme-linked immunosorbent assay have been developed that are more sensitive than the HI assay and can specifically distinguish IgM from IgG responses.[67]

Pathogenesis of Arthritic Symptoms. Because of the unusually high frequency of arthritic symptoms following infection with either the wild-type rubella virus or the various vaccine strains (see further on), rubella virus is believed to have a particular predilection, or tropism, for growth in joint tissues. The reports of virus isolation from joint aspirates tend to lend further support to the belief that active viral replication in synovial tissues may be responsible for producing the symptoms and signs of arthritic disease.[71-75]

This proposed pathogenetic mechanism must be balanced against the fact that immune complexes have also been isolated from involved joints. The finding of virus in the joint does not prove that viral replication either is occurring or is responsible for the inflammatory response. Indeed, in studies of the pathogenesis of the rash of rubella, infectious virus is found not only in involved but also in uninvolved skin.[65,66,68,70] Additionally, the onset of both the rash and the arthritis is coincident with the period when rubella-specific antibody is first detected in the serum (Fig. 98–4) and virus is being actively cleared from the circulation.[65,66,68-70] Furthermore, serum complement levels can also be depressed during this time.[76] Thus, the deposition of immune complexes in which virus particles serve as the antigenic component may initiate an acute inflammatory response in the joint.

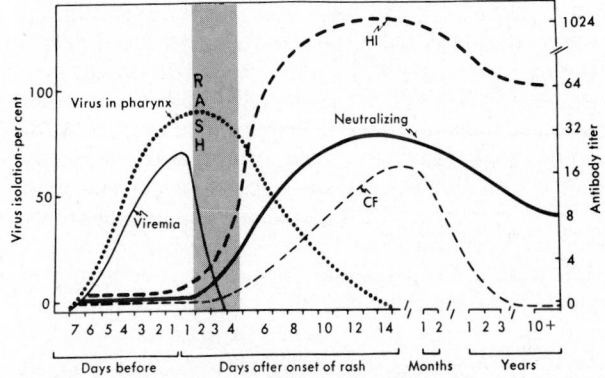

Figure 98–4. Pattern of viral excretion and antibody response during postnatal rubella infection. Arthritis is generally observed in close temporal relation to the rash but may occur from as early as 6 days prior to as late as 6 days after the onset of the rash. (From Krugman, S., and Katz, S.L.: Rubella. *In* Infectious Diseases of Children. 7th ed. St. Louis, The C.V. Mosby Company, 1981, p. 319.

Recently, rubella virus has been isolated from lymphocytes of patients who had experienced either rubella- or rubella vaccine–associated arthritis years earlier.[71,77,78] If confirmed, these findings would suggest that rubella virus could alter the immune response itself by direct infection of elements of the immune system. Furthermore, the fact that virus persists in these cells for prolonged periods of time means that there exists a source for later direct viral seeding of the joint or for antigen release and subsequent immune complex formation.

Rheumatologic Manifestations. Unlike typical rubella infection, which has a peak incidence in the 15- to 19-year-old age group and affects both sexes equally, rubella infection associated with joint symptoms is most commonly seen in women who are 20 to 40 years old, with the youngest patient reported being 1 year and the oldest 82 years of age.[73, 79-87] Approximately 30 percent of females and 6 percent of males with rubella have joint symptoms.[83,88-90]

Symptoms of joint involvement have most often been recognized during epidemics of rubella infection, probably because of the clustering of a large number of cases.[80,87,91-96] The onset of joint symptoms is usually rapid and may occur as early as 6 days prior to or as long as 6 days after the appearance of the characteristic maculopapular rash of rubella. Although several joints are often affected simultaneously, typically in a bilaterally symmetric distribution, joint involvement may progress in a migratory, additive fashion not unlike that seen in rheumatic fever.[83,85,88-90,97] Articular symptoms evolve over a 3- to 13-day period. Although generally short-lived, they may persist for as long as 52 days.[80,83,92,97]

The joints most commonly involved are the small joints of the hands (proximal interphalangeal, metacarpophalangeal), the knees, and the wrists, followed by the ankles and the elbows. The larger joints (shoulders, hips) may also occasionally be affected.[83,85,89,90,92,97] Arthralgias are more common than frank arthritis, and significant stiffness is often associated with these joint complaints; often it is a presenting complaint. Periarthritis with swelling and redness around the affected joint is common,[80] and involvement of synovial linings outside the joints themselves can lead to the development of tenosynovitis[83, 98] and the carpal tunnel syndrome,[83,97,99-103] which are both well-recognized complications of rubella infection. Symptoms may persist for extended periods of time, with arthralgias occasionally being present for more than 1 year, but chronic joint disease or evidence of rheumatoid arthritis or other rheumatic disorders does not occur.[83,90,92]

Laboratory Investigations. The laboratory values of patients with joint symptoms are not significantly different from the laboratory values of patients whose rubella infection is uncomplicated by these complaints. In general there are no distinctive laboratory abnormalities.[99-105]

In the two cases in which joint fluid has been examined,[83,97] the synovial fluid has been described as yellow and viscous, with a protein content ranging between 1.9 and 3.4 g per dl, and containing 14,000 to 27,000 leukocytes per mm³. The differential counts in the two studies available were contradictory, one reporting 90 to 98 percent polymorphonuclear leukocytes[97] and the other describing such cells as rare with mainly macrophage and synovial cells present.[83] These differences may relate to the stage of the arthritis during which the samples were collected. The mucin clot has been reported to be fair to poor. Isolation of rubella virus from the joint fluid has been reported only rarely.[71-73] Synovial tissue from an affected joint has been examined on one occasion and was reported to show active, nonspecific synovitis.[97]

RUBELLA VACCINE VIRUS

Virology. Three vaccine strains are now licensed for use in the United States: the Cendehill strain cultured in rabbit kidney, the HP77 strain propagated in duck embryo culture, and the RA 27/3 strain grown in WI38 cells derived from human embryonic lung.[106-108] The RA 27/3 vaccine, which has been shown to be more immunogenic than either the duck-grown HP77 or the Cendehill vaccine,[65-69,108-113] is the only strain available in the United States. Approximately 95 percent of individuals receiving this vaccine demonstrate serologic evidence of infection, and local antibody production is also stimulated.

Clinical Presentation. In rare instances a rubella-like rash and lymphadenopathy occur after vaccination.[67-69,75,114] Fever is even less common. Transient polyneuropathies have also been reported following both rubella and rubella vaccine virus infection (see later on).[67-69,115-117]

Rheumatologic Manifestations. A variety of musculoskeletal complaints are associated with the clinical use of rubella vaccines and include myalgias, arthralgias, arthritis, and paresthesias.[118-126] As with natural rubella, signs and symptoms of musculoskeletal involvement are most often observed in women. In children, the frequency of joint manifestations is about 1 to 5 percent.[118-120,125-127]

Joint symptoms are most common; patients complain primarily of stiffness or arthralgia of involved joints, and approximately 10 to 20 percent of the latter group will have frank arthritis on examination.[118-122,126-129] The distribution of joint involvement is generally similar to that seen in natural rubella infection, but in several studies the knee has been reported to be the most frequently involved joint followed by the small joints of the fingers (proximal interphalangeal, metacarpophalangeal), ankles, and wrists. Symptoms first become apparent approximately 2 weeks (range 8 to 45 days) after vaccination, a time that just precedes or is coincident with seroconversion and the ability to isolate rubella from the pharynx of inoculated people.[128,130] Symptoms are short-lived, lasting from 1 to 5 days in general,[118,119,124,126,128,130,131] though more prolonged involvement does occur and has been associated on several occasions with the isolation of rubella vaccine virus from the involved joint, even as late as 3 months after inoculation.[74,128] Furthermore, unlike natural rubella, recurrences of joint symptoms are not uncommon,[74,118,127,130,132-135] having been observed in approximately 1.3 percent of people with joint symptoms, a frequency that represents 0.1 percent of all children inoculated. The frequency and severity of recurrent attacks have been found to decrease with time, and despite careful long-term examination most studies have failed to demonstrate the development of any form of chronic arthritis, and rheumatoid arthritis in particular, in people demonstrating such recurrent joint symptoms.[120,133-137]

In addition to arthritis and arthralgias, paresthesias involving the fingers, hands, and arms have also been associated with the administration of rubella vaccine.[118,126,127] In most instances, the clinical presentation is most compatible with carpal tunnel syndrome, but a characteristic form of brachial radiculoneuritis may also develop in recipients of rubella vaccine.[138-140] A second form of radiculoneuropathy involving the lumbar plexus[138-140] has been described after rubella vaccination and results in what has been described as the "catcher's crouch" or "catcher's leg" syndrome. Typically, affected children awake with early morning aching centered on the popliteal fossa and assume the characteristic crouching posture. Both forms of radiculoneuropathy occur 4 to 6 weeks following inculation (range 7 to 99 days) and persist for approximately 2 weeks (range 2 to 35 days). No evidence of permanent neurologic damage has been reported.

ALPHAVIRUSES

Virology and Epidemiology. The alphaviruses, members of the Togoviridae,[141-144] include at least 20 serologically related but distinguishable viruses, of which five—chikungunya, O'nyong-nyong, Mayaro, Ross River, and Sindbis—cause disease in which rheumatic complaints are a major feature. Alphavirus particles are spherical, 60 to 65 nm in diameter, and consist of a nucleoprotein core containing the single-stranded RNA genome surrounded by a lipoprotein envelope into which are inserted at least two viral-specified glycoproteins.[141-144] The latter are the major antigens to which the host serologic response is mounted, and they permit diagnosis by standard HI, CF, and neutralization assays.

Although closely related antigenically and structurally, and in the type of clinical disease produced, the five alphaviruses associated with arthritic illnesses are found in different ecologic settings and have distinct epidemiologic features. Chikungunya virus[145-153] was first isolated in East Africa. Its name was derived from a local description of the illness meaning "that which bends up," and it has subsequently been reported in India, Southeast Asia, and the Philippines. In rural Africa the virus is maintained in a cycle involving wild primates and forest mosquitoes; in an urban setting transmission is likely by *Aedes aegypti* in a human to mosquito to human cycle. The disease tends to appear suddenly, affect a large part of the susceptible population, and then disappear.

O'nyong-nyong virus[143,151,154,155] is seen in the same area of Africa as chikungunya and produces a similar disease, as its name attests (meaning "joint breaker"). It is the only arthropod-borne virus to be transmitted by anopheline mosquitoes and was associated with a major epidemic in East Africa between 1959 and 1962 involving several million people. Since that time only sporadic cases have been reported. Because of the similarity in geographic distribution and clinical presentation between O'nyong-nyong and chikungunya, differentiation between the two is often difficult and may require appropriate serologic testing.

Ross River virus,[143,150,156-164] endemic in Australia, New Zealand, and a large number of South Pacific Islands, gives rise to a disease recognized as "epidemic polyarthritis." In Australia the virus is limited primarily to rural locations, existing in a wild vertebrate to mosquito cycle, and affects mainly travelers to these areas during the summer and autumn. However, on various South Pacific Islands epidemics of disease have been reported, with up to 40 to 50 percent of the local populace, as well as tourists, being affected. In these instances, human to mosquito to human transmission probably occurs.

Mayaro virus[143-165] has been reported from Trinidad, Surinam, Brazil, Colombia, and Bolivia, where disease is seen primarily among men working in the tropical forests. As with Ross River virus, a wild animal to mosquito cycle is believed to exist. Sindbis virus,[143,150,160,166-169] in distinction to the preceding four alphaviruses, has a wider geographic distribution, which includes Europe, Asia, Africa, Australia, and the Philippines. Human infection is uncommon, however, and the virus is maintained primarily in a wild bird to mosquito cycle.

Clinical Presentation. The illnesses arising from infection by these five viruses share a great number of clinical features, of which fever, arthritis, and rash are the most constant and characteristic. However, the spectrum of disease is wide, and patients may experience any one or two of these signs in the absence of the others, making diagnosis in nonepidemic settings difficult. The incubation period ranges from 2 to 10 days and, in the case of chikungunya and O'nyong-nyong, is followed by the abrupt appearance of joint pain as the presenting manifestation of disease.[143,147,148,151,155,159,170-172] The other viruses result in illnesses that evolve more gradually, often with a prodromal period of 1 to 3 days that is marked by fever, malaise, and nonspecific constitutional symptoms followed by the appearance of joint manifestations.[158,159,162,167,168,173,174] Males and females are generally equally affected, though in occasional epidemics females have been found to predominate. The peak incidence of disease has been reported in the 10- to 39-year-old age group.[143,151,156,157,159]

Fever in patients with O'nyong-nyong, Ross River, and Sindbis infections is mild, rarely exceeding

103° F,[143,155,157,158,162,163,167,168,174,175] whereas patients with chikungunya and Mayaro infections typically appear significantly more ill, often with temperatures as high as 104° F to 105° F.[143,147-149,151,165,171,172,176,177] Frequently there will be a biphasic or "saddleback" profile to the fever with an initial temperature elevation lasting 1 to 6 days, followed by a 1- to 3-day period of normal temperature, and then the recurrence of fever for a shorter period of time. The rash[143,148,149,151,155,157-159,162,163,165,167,168,171-174] seen in association with these illnesses generally appears 3 to 4 days after the onset of the joint symptoms. It is maculopapular or morbilliform in character, lasts 3 to 4 days (range 2 to 10 days), and involves predominantly the face, flexor surfaces of the extremities, and the trunk. The palms, soles, and scalp can be affected. In the case of Sindbis infection, vesicles may also be seen.[143,167,168] The rash may be mildly pruritic; desquamation does not occur, but a transient brown discoloration of the skin may remain after resolution of the exanthem.[143,157-159,162,168]

A range of other symptoms, including headache, retro-orbital pain, mild pharyngitis, conjunctivitis, myalgias, anorexia, nausea, and vomiting may accompany these illnesses but are not major features of the diseases. Mild lymphadenopathy is observed in all five disorders, but patients with O'nyong-nyong may demonstrate particularly striking enlargement of the posterior cervical nodes.[143,148,151,155,157,159,162,172,174] A life-threatening hemorrhagic state has been documented in patients with chikungunya from the Far East but rarely in those from Africa.[143,151,177] Other serious complications, however, have not been reported in these self-limited disorders.

Diagnosis is most often made clinically and may be confirmed either by isolation of virus from the blood of affected individuals, a procedure that is successful only during the first several days of the illness, or by demonstration in paired sera of a fourfold or greater rise in HI, CF, or neutralizing antibody titers.[143,147-151,156-158,163-169,172,176-179] A number of other mosquito-borne viruses (West Nile, dengue, Bunyamwera) can also give rise to syndromes characterized by fever, rash, and arthralgias, though not arthritis. Therefore, appropriate serologic testing is indicated, particularly in nonepidemic conditions, to confirm the diagnosis.

Pathogenesis of Arthritic Symptoms. No evidence exists to implicate either direct viral infection of the joints or immune complexes in the pathogenesis. Virus can be isolated from the blood during the first several days of illness but has never been reported in joint fluid.[143,147,148,152,167,171,172,176-178] Complement levels have been recorded in numerous patients with Ross River virus infection, and they are normal or elevated rather than depressed.[143,152,180] Recent studies have demonstrated T lymphocyte activation and depressed natural killer cell activity during clinical disease.[181]

Rheumatologic Manifestations. Arthritis can be severe, particularly in adults. The joints most frequently affected include the small joints of the hands, as well as the wrists, elbows, knees, ankles, and small joints of

the feet.[143,148-152,155,157-159,162,168,172-174,178,182] Previously injured joints are particularly prone to involvement. The arthritis is generally symmetric and polyarticular, although the distribution and pattern of appearance of joint symptoms are quite variable. Typically, affected joints are hot and swollen, and there may be significant periarticular soft tissue swelling and tendonitis as well. In patients with chikungunya, subcutaneous nodules clinically similar to those observed in patients with rheumatoid arthritis have been described. In the majority of alphavirus infections, joint symptoms generally resolve over a 3- to 7-day period but may recur. A variable number of patients continue to have joint pain and swelling for weeks to months and in some patients infected by chikungunya, joint symptoms have been documented that persist for more than 1 year.[148,151,152,157,158,174,182] In no instance, however, has there been evolution to a more chronic form of arthritis, and no evidence of permanent joint damage has been presented.

Laboratory Investigations. A mild leukopenia with a relative lymphocytosis is often seen during the first week of illness but need not be present.[151,155,159,162,165-168,171-177] Platelet counts are usually normal, though significant thrombocytopenia has been recorded in cases of chikungunya and Mayaro infections.[151,171] Complement values are normal or elevated,[143,152,180] and neither antinuclear antibodies nor rheumatoid factors are generally found.[152] In one study of Ross River disease, a greater than expected incidence of symptomatic disease in patients with HLA-DR7 as well as the heterozygous Gm phenotype a$^+$x$^+$b$^+$ was observed.[183]

Joint fluids have been examined from a small number of patients with Ross River infection.[180,181,184] Synovial fluid cell counts have ranged from 1500 per mm^3 to 14,200 per mm^3 with a marked predominance of mononuclear cells. Viral antigens have been detected by immunofluorescence in these cells shortly after the onset of the arthritis, but infectious virus has never been recovered from joint fluids.

MUMPS

Virology. Mumps virus, a member of the Paramyxoviridae family, consists of an irregular, spherically shaped particle with a mean diameter of 140 nm (range 90 to 300 nm) composed of a helical nucleocapsid containing the single-stranded RNA genome surrounded by a lipoprotein envelope covered with spikelike projections.[70,185-189] Associated with the outer coat are both the hemolytic and neuraminidase activities of the virus as well as the viral hemagglutinin. The V (viral) antigen detected by CF has been correlated with the viral coat, whereas the S (soluble) antigen is found in the nucleocapsid.[185-188]

Clinical Presentation. Subclinical infection with mumps is common (20 to 40 percent of those infected), and any of the clinical features of mumps infection may precede, follow, or occur in the absence of clinically apparent parotitis.[70,186,188,189] The incubation period averages 16 to 18 days (range 2 to 4 weeks) and is followed by a short prodrome of 24 to 48 hours characterized by nonspecific symptoms (low-grade fever, anorexia, malaise, headache, myalgia). Complaints of earache and tenderness over the adjacent parotid gland ensue, and parotid swelling and pain reach their peak during the next 1 to 3 days. In 75 percent of people the contralateral parotid is similarly affected 1 to 5 days later.

Although mumps is a generalized infection, the virus demonstrates a particular predilection for grandular and nervous tissues. Epididymo-orchitis[185,186,189] is the most common extrasalivary gland manifestation of mumps infection in adult men, reported in 20 to 30 percent of postpubertal males. Involvement is bilateral in 15 to 25 percent of cases, but sterility is a rare complication. Other glandular involvement includes oophoritis, seen in approximately 5 percent of postpubertal women, and less commonly mastitis, prostatitis, and thyroiditis. Central nervous system infection is common, encephalitis being reported in 1 of every 6000 cases of mumps.[185] Clinical meningitis is seen in 1 to 10 percent of people with parotitis, although subclinical disease determined by cerebrospinal fluid pleocytosis has been reported in as many as 62 percent of those with mumps.[185,188,189] Among patients with meningitis, a distinct male predominance has been noted. Cardiac involvement (myocarditis) may also occur and is most often subclinical, but EKG changes may be seen in up to 15 percent of people examined.[185,190]

The diagnosis of mumps is most often made clinically, but in patients with atypical presentations or subclinical disease, mumps infection can be confirmed by viral isolation or by demonstration of a specific serologic response.[185,188] Antibody directed against the S antigen appears early and may be present at the onset of clinical disease. It rises rapidly and then declines over the next several weeks. Antibody to the V antigen is detected later; it peaks at 2 to 4 weeks after the onset of clinical disease and persists for years. Neutralizing antibody generally first appears during convalescence. An HI assay for detection of antibody to mumps does exist but is not specific because cross-reactivity with many of the other paramyxoviruses occurs and false-positive results have been reported.[185]

It is currently recommended that at 15 months of age all children be given a live mumps virus vaccine grown in chick embryo culture. Ninety-five percent of recipients have been shown to develop protective levels of neutralizing antibody after vaccination, although these levels are lower than those seen after natural infection.[70,185,189]

Pathogenesis of Arthritic Symptoms. Many of the manifestations occurring in close temporal relation to the onset of parotitis have been documented to be due to mumps infection of the affected tissues.[185,187-189] Similarly, joint inflammation may arise as a consequence of active viral replication within synovial tissues, although mumps virus has never been isolated from an involved joint. An immune complex–mediated arthropathy cannot be excluded, particularly since the joint symptoms occur at an appropriate time for immune complex formation in relation to the serologic response to infection.[185,189]

Rheumatologic Manifestations. Although fewer than 50 cases of arthritis associated with mumps have been reported in the world's literature, Maisondieu observed 6 people with this complication among 1334 with clinical evidence of disease.[191] Young adult males are most commonly affected (6:1 male to female ratio), with the highest incidence of this complication being seen among those in the third decade of life (age range 5 to 47 years).[192-194] Symptoms, which include morning stiffness and arthralgias as well as the typical signs of arthritis, may precede the onset of parotitis but most commonly occur 1 to 3 weeks (mean of 10 days) after the disease becomes clinically evident.[185-189,192,194,195] Two cases of arthritis have been reported in patients serologically shown to have been acutely infected by mumps but who failed to demonstrate parotitis.[196,197] Since up to 40 percent of mumps infections may be subclinical (i.e., without parotitis), a significant number of cases of unexplained self-limited acute arthritis may occur as a consequence of infection by this virus.

Three modes of presentation of the rheumatic symptoms have been reported: (1) most commonly, patients complain of a migratory polyarthritis that involves principally the large joints (shoulders, hips, knees, ankles) although small joints (metacarpophalangeal, proximal interphalangeal) may also frequently be symptomatic; (2) arthralgias alone may occur, without signs of arthritis; and (3) a monoarticular arthritis may also be observed.[190,192,194,195,198,199] Tenosynovitis, though not common, may occur as part of this syndrome. Patients with arthritis are almost invariably febrile at the time of the onset of joint involvement, with generally modest temperature elevations (100° F to 102° F), but occasional patients have had temperatures in excess of 105° F.[194,195] The duration of symptoms is highly variable (2 days to 6 months), but in the majority of patients joint involvement has cleared within 2 weeks of its onset.[194,197] No residual joint damage has been observed in patients with mumps-associated arthritis. Interestingly, the incidence of orchitis (60 percent) in patients with arthritis is approximately three times the expected rate,[194,195] suggesting that the mechanism responsible for joint involvement (see earlier) may also lead to involvement of other organs.

Laboratory Investigations. Patients with joint involvement during mumps infection demonstrate a moderate leukocytosis (10,000 to 15,000 WBC per mm^3) but may have a normal WBC count in mild cases. The erythrocyte sedimentation rate is invariably elevated, occasionally markedly so.[192-195,198,201] Rheumatoid factor is usually absent from the serum of these patients.[194] In the only study to examine these parameters, serum complement levels were found to be normal, and immune complexes were not detectable during clinically active arthritis.[197] When positive, the CF test for antibodies to mumps virus is useful to confirm the clinical diagnosis.[185,188,193,194,198]

Joint fluid has been examined in only two patients with mumps-associated arthritis, and in both instances the fluid was described as yellow and clear.[192,196] One fluid specimen was said to contain numerous polymorphonuclear leukocytes, but no quantitation was provided. Virus has never been isolated from an affected joint.[193,197]

ENTEROVIRUSES: COXSACKIEVIRUS AND ECHOVIRUS

Virology.[202-204] Coxsackieviruses and echoviruses, along with polioviruses, are members of the *Enterovirus* genus of the Picornaviridae family. They consist of icosahedron-shaped particles that are 20 to 30 nm in diameter and have an outer protein capsid composed of 60 capsomeres which encloses a linear, single-stranded RNA genome. Currently it is possible to distinguish 67 species (immunotypes) of enteroviruses: polioviruses types 1 to 3; group A coxsackieviruses, types 1 to 24; group B coxsackieviruses, types 1 to 6; echoviruses, types 1 to 34; and the newer enteroviruses, types 68 to 71 (four earlier assignments having been mistaken or redundant).

Clinical Presentation.[202-208] Infection by enteroviruses is worldwide in distribution, has a peak incidence during the summer and fall in temperate climates, and has a prevalence that varies inversely with socioeconomic levels. The prevalence of any given immunotype varies markedly, one or two types predominating each year within restricted geographic areas. Epidemics are not unusual and have provided much of the basis for our understanding of the clinical expression of infection by individual immunotypes of enteroviruses.

The spectrum of clinical disease produced by different enteroviruses is remarkably broad and shows a tremendous overlap among the different immunotypes, and the frequency of clinical disease among infected individuals is highly variable. Even though infections with the same immunotype of virus may produce an extraordinarily wide range of symptoms, certain enterovirus immunotypes are commonly associated with characteristic clinical presentations, e.g., particular immunotypes of group A coxsackieviruses with herpangina and of group B coxsackieviruses with myopericarditis.

The incubation period of enterovirus infection ranges from 2 to 15 days, but generally it is 3 to 5 days. The most common clinical expression of infection by these viruses is a mild febrile illness that has an abrupt onset without a prodrome. Temperature elevations usually range from 101° F to 104° F and are associated with headache and malaise. Anorexia, sore throat, nausea, vomiting, and myalgias may occasionally be seen. The illness typically lasts 2 to 4 days but may be biphasic, resolving after several days only to recur shortly thereafter. Other common manifestations of infection include mild pharyngitis, various gastrointestinal symptoms (abdominal pain, nausea, vomiting, diarrhea), conjunctivitis, and aseptic meningitis. Enterovirus infections are often accompanied by a maculopapular rash, particularly in younger individuals.

Since intercurrent infection with these viruses is common and generally asymptomatic, the finding of enterovirus in a random stool specimen, or even the observation of rising antibody titers to an enterovirus, need not be evidence of a causal relation with illness in an individual. Definitive diagnosis requires viral isolation from a site of active disease (e.g., pharynx, skin vesicle) or from more than one location (e.g., blood and stool) at the same time. Serologic screening for infection is not a particularly useful means of confirming the diagnosis of enterovirus infection because of the large number of serotypes.

Pathogenesis of Arthritic Symptoms.[202-206,209] The pathogenesis of the arthritis is not known. Virus has not been recovered from joint fluids in the limited number of studies reported, and no evidence for the involvement of immune complexes has been presented.

Rheumatologic Manifestations.[202,206-209] When specifically sought, arthritis has been found to be an uncommon but definite manifestation of enterovirus infections. During one surveillance study involving 7075 individuals from whom enteroviruses were isolated, 9 cases of "rheumatic disease" were reported, including 6 with arthritis. In a further investigation in which serologic evidence (fourfold or greater rise in neutralizing antibody titer) of infection by coxsackievirus A9 and coxsackieviruses B1 through B6 was specifically sought in individuals with the presenting complaint of acute inflammatory arthropathy, six cases of self-limited arthritis were identified.[209] The arthritis was accompanied by fever in all patients, sore throat and pleuritic pain in five patients, and rash in three patients. One had accompanying myocarditis.

In addition to these patients with coxsackievirus infection, three cases of an acute, self-limited arthritis believed to be associated with echovirus infection have been reported in adults.[207,208] In these patients, both large and small joints were affected, and significant knee effusions were noted in one patient. An evanescent maculopapular rash appeared early in the course of the arthritis. Joint symptoms resolved spontaneously over a 10- to 15-day period.

Laboratory Investigations.[207,209] Leukocytosis, an elevated erythrocyte sedimentation rate, and raised antistreptolysin O titers have been reported in approximately half of the patients studied. Examination of joint fluids from five patients has demonstrated cell counts ranging from 2500 to 46,000 per mm^3 with 45 to 90 percent neutrophils and a protein content of 2.9 to 4.5 g per dl. Synovial biopsy has revealed only nonspecific inflammatory changes. Virus has never been recovered from synovial fluids.

SMALLPOX AND VACCINIA

Virology.[210-212] As members of the genus *Orthopoxvirus,* variola virus (smallpox) and vaccinia virus, a derivative of smallpox and cowpox, share a common brick-shaped morphology and measure 250 to 300 nm × 200 to 250 nm × 100 nm. Each also contains a genome consisting of double-stranded DNA. Vaccinia virus is antigenically identical to variola but may be distinguished by in vitro growth properties.

Clinical Presentation.[210,211,213,214] Smallpox has an incubation period of 7 to 17 days that is terminated by the abrupt onset of high fever (102° F to 105° F), headache, and prominent myalgias. Two to four days later the characteristic rash appears on the face and spreads centrifugally to the trunk and extremities. The rash is initially macular and evolves in stages—first to papules, then to vesicles by day 4, to pustules by day 6, and finally to dry crusts by the tenth day. The mortality varies greatly by geographic location (1 to 30 percent), probably reflecting differences in the virulence of viral strains.

Pathogenesis of Arthritic Symptoms.[210,211,213,214-216] Joint involvement in all nonseptic cases arises secondary to the development of viral osteomyelitis (osteomyelitis variolosa), which involves the metaphyseal ends of the long bones, seeded at the time of the secondary viremia. The localization of virus to this growth area explains the age distribution observed (see later on).

Rheumatologic Manifestations and Laboratory Investigations.[210-215,217,219,220] Joint symptoms are a well-recognized manifestation of smallpox, reported in 0.25 to 0.50 percent of patients in one smallpox epidemic. Involvement is limited almost exclusively to children less than 10 years of age, with an incidence within this group of 2 to 5 percent of those at risk. Typically, joint pain and swelling arise 10 to 30 days after the onset of the rash. The elbows are almost invariably the first joints involved. In about 50 percent of the patients the arthritis then evolves in an additive, symmetric fashion to affect the wrists, ankles, or knees. Radiographic examination at this stage reveals changes of osteomyelitis involving the underlying metaphyseal bone. Spontaneous resolution of the arthritis ensues over the following weeks, but significant bone deformities and interference with the normal growth patterns are common sequelae. Joint aspiration during the period of acute arthritis may reveal fluid containing the characteristic elementary bodies of variola.

Arthritis has also been reported as a rare accompaniment of vaccinia infection,[217,219,220] occurring 12 days after immunization in the single well-documented case.[219] The synovial fluid of the involved knee was inflammatory in nature, and vaccinia virus was recovered upon culture. The swelling resolved spontaneously after 11 days, but arthralgias persisted for several months. No radiographic changes of the involved joint were observed at any time during the course of the illness.

ADENOVIRUS

Although the spectrum of disease caused by adenovirus[221,222] is quite broad, arthritis is a rare manifestation of infection, reported for the first time in 1974.[223] The initial case involved a military recruit who presented with myalgias, meningeal signs, and an upper respiratory illness. Shortly thereafter, a rash, arthralgias of the hands and wrists, and frank arthritis of the knees developed. Arthrocentesis revealed a joint fluid that was straw-colored, gave a good mucin clot, and contained 4.5 g protein per dl and 24,800 WBC per mm³, with a predominance of neutrophils (89 percent). Synovial biopsy demonstrated an inflammatory synovitis. Over the next 3 weeks the joint symptoms resolved completely. The diagnosis of adenovirus type 7 infection was made serologically, but it was not possible to isolate adenovirus. Since this initial case, four additional patients[209,224] have been reported to have arthritis associated with serologically documented adenovirus infection. As in the initial case, arthritis developed in the majority of these patients 3 to 8 days after the onset of a nonspecific upper respiratory illness and involved both large and small joints of the upper and lower extremities. In two patients joint fluid examination demonstrated WBC counts of less than 4000 per mm³, with a predominance of mononuclear cells, whereas in a third patient the synovial fluid contained 8500 leukocytes per mm³, with a predominance of neutrophils. Virus was not recovered from synovial fluid. Serum complement levels were depressed in two of three patients, and cryoproteins and immune complexes were demonstrated in both the serum and the joint fluid of all three patients.

VARICELLA-ZOSTER VIRUS

Arthritis has been reported as a rare complication of infection by each of the viruses of the Herpetoviridae family: herpes simplex virus, varicella-zoster virus (VZV), Epstein-Barr virus, and cytomegalovirus.[225] Although arthritis has been commented upon as a complication of chickenpox from as early as 1931,[226-238] it was not until the 1970s that individual case reports appeared in the medical literature. Since that time, ten children (age range 5 to 11 years) and one adult (age 20 years)[209] have been observed with aseptic arthritis, and four children (age range 1.5 to 4 years) have been seen with septic arthritis complicating chickenpox. None of the patients demonstrated the more serious systemic complications of VZV infection nor did they have generalized disease. In cases of aseptic arthritis, joint symptoms began 1 to 5 days after the onset of rash and were associated with swelling, significant pain, and limitation of movement. Monoarticular swelling of the knee was the most common rheumatologic presentation, although two cases of polyarticular involvement have been reported.[209,230] A distinct female predominance has been noted. In all instances the joint symptoms resolved spontaneously within one week of onset, and no sequelae were observed.

The finding of an acute monoarthritis in a patient with chickenpox should not automatically be interpreted to represent an associated aseptic (virus-induced) arthritis because several cases of joint infection by bacteria have been reported in these patients. Patients with septic arthritis differ from those with aseptic arthritis by being younger (less than 5 years old), by displaying involvement of joints other than the knee, and by having synovial fluids with a predominance of polymorphonuclear cells rather than mononuclear cells. Distinction between these two conditions ultimately requires a culture of synovial fluid. In those instances in which the diagnosis is not apparent after examination of the joint fluid, antibiotic therapy should be initiated until the bacteriology results have been obtained.

Synovial fluid analysis has been reported in several cases of VZV-associated aseptic arthritis. In general, the fluid is clear and straw-colored and gives a fair to poor mucin clot. The synovial fluid leukocyte count is usually low but may be elevated, occasionally strikingly so (one case > 50,000 leukocytes per mm³), and most often demonstrates a majority of mononuclear cells. However, early in the course of the arthritis polymorphonuclear leukocytes may predominate. Virus has been isolated from the joint on one occasion.[232]

EPSTEIN-BARR VIRUS

Arthritis is an extremely rare complication of Epstein-Barr (EB) virus infection,[239-244] having been reported in fewer than 10 cases of either presumed or proven infectious mononucleosis.[245-248] In two recent and well-documented cases,[245,248] a monoarticular arthritis involving the knee and ankle, respectively, developed shortly after the onset of clinical disease and resolved over the course of days to weeks without sequelae. Arthrocentesis revealed inflammatory joint fluids (elevated leukocyte counts with a predominance of either neutrophils or monocytes and elevated protein levels). In the one patient in whom complement levels were determined, synovial fluid C3 and C4 levels were lower than those in the serum but higher than expected for an immune complex–mediated process. Synovial tissue has been biopsied from patients with arthritis complicating infectious mononucleosis and is said to have shown a nonspecific subacute synovitis.[215]

HERPES SIMPLEX VIRUS

Two serologically, biologically, and biochemically distinct types of herpes simplex virus (HSV) have been described: (1) HSV type 1 (HSV-1), which is associated primarily with oral infections; and (2) HSV type 2 (HSV-2), which is the predominant form in genital infections.[249-251] Generalized or disseminated disease is a well-recognized, although uncommon, manifestation of HSV infection that is seen most often in immunocompromised individuals, but is occasionally observed in otherwise normal people. Two cases of arthritis associated with HSV infection have been reported, and both have occurred in normal individuals with generalized HSV-1 disease.[252] In one patient, acute monoarticular arthritis

of the knee developed coincident with the appearance of a diffuse vesicular rash 1 week after the patient had wrestled with an individual having similar skin lesions. The involved joint was described as warm, tender, and swollen. The synovial fluid was cloudy and had a normal viscosity, a good mucin clot, and a cell count of 10,000 per mm³ with the majority being mononuclear leukocytes or synovial lining cells. Synovial biopsy demonstrated nonspecific inflammatory changes but no evidence of viral infection of the synovial tissues. Culture of the fluid, however, did result in isolation of HSV-1. Over the ensuing 10 days both the skin lesions and the arthritis resolved spontaneously without sequelae. In the second patient, acute monoarticular arthritis of the ankle occurred in conjunction with an illness characterized by fever and a diffuse, vesicular rash. Results of throat and skin lesion cultures were positive for HSV-1. No joint fluid could be obtained for examination. Serum complement levels were reported to be normal. Joint symptoms and swelling persisted for 3 months but resolved by the fourth month.

CYTOMEGALOVIRUS

Arthritis associated with cytomegalovirus (CMV) infection has been documented in a single case.[252] In this immunosuppressed individual, generalized CMV infection occurred 12 weeks after renal transplantation and was associated with the development of an erythematous, warm, painful, and swollen knee. Initial arthrocentesis revealed a clear yellow fluid containing fewer than 100 WBCs per mm³ with 40 percent neutrophils. Ten days later the joint fluid was cloudy, contained 1200 WBCs per mm³ with 93 percent neutrophils, and yielded CMV when cultured in vitro. The arthritis persisted, and at 1 month the synovial fluid leukocyte count had risen to 37,000 per mm³ with 53 percent neutrophils. A synovial biopsy at that time revealed no inflammatory response within synovial tissues, but particles morphologically consistent with CMV were observed in cells from the synovial fluid. No resolution of the arthritis occurred prior to the patient's death several months later.

ERYTHEMA INFECTIOSUM

Erythema infectiosum is a mild illness of childhood that presents with a characteristic rash. It is of presumed viral etiology, although no infectious agent has been isolated. Arthritis was noted to occur in association with erythema infectiosum as early as 1905,[253] but most subsequent reports of epidemics have failed to note this manifestation.[254-260] This may be a consequence of the fact that joint involvement in children is uncommon, occurring primarily in adults. In one well-documented, more recent epidemic of erythema infectiosum,[261] arthralgias were noted in 77 percent and arthritis in 60 percent of 57 adult patients (age 20 years and older), whereas in 176 children less than 10 years of age the frequency of joint pain was 5 percent, and the frequency of arthritis was 3 percent. The arthritis was said to involve only the large joints, particularly the wrists and knees. No sequelae were noted.

References

1. Oldstone, M.B.A., and Dixon, F.J.: Immunopathology of viral infections. *In* Miescher, P.A., and Muller-Eberhard, H.J. (eds.): Textbook of Immunopathology. 2nd ed. New York, Grune & Stratton, 1976.
2. Oldstone, M.B.A., and Dixon, F.J.: Immune complexes in chronic viral infections. J. Exp. Med. 134:32s, 1971.
3. Stevens, J.G., Todaro, G.J., and Fox, C.F.: Persistent Viruses. ICN-UCLA Symposia on Molecular and Cellular Biology. Vol. 11. New York, Academic Press, 1978.
4. Oldstone, M.B.A., Buchmeier, M.J., and Doyle, M.V.: Immunobiology of persistent virus infections. *In* Stevens, J.G., Todaro, G.J., and Fox, C.F.: Persistent Viruses, ICN-UCLA Symposia on Molecular and Cellular Biology, Vol. 11. New York, Academic Press, 1978.
5. Fulginiti, V.A.: Virus and virus vaccine–induced immunologic injury. *In* Talmage, D.W., Rose, B., Austen, K.F., and Vaughan, J.H.: Immunological Diseases. 3rd ed. Boston, Little, Brown & Company, 1978.
6. Editorial.: Arthritis and Immune Complexes. Br. Med. J. 1:4, 1972.
7. Burns, W.H., and Allison, A.C.: Surface antigens of virus-infected cells. *In* Poste, G., and Nicolson, G.L. (eds.): Virus Infection and the Cell Surface. Amsterdam, North Holland Publishing Company, 1977.
8. Blanden, R.V., Pang, T.E., and Dunlop, M.B.C.: T cell recognition of virus-infected cells. *In* Poste, G., and Nicolson, G.L. (eds.): Virus Infection and the Cell Surface. Amsterdam, North Holland Publishing Company, 1977.
9. Blumberg, B.S., Alter, H.J., and Visnich, S.: A "new" antigen in leukemia sera. JAMA 292:541, 1965.
10. Zuckerman, A.J.: Immunology of hepatitis viruses. *In* Nahmias, A.J., and O'Reilly, R.J. (eds.): Immunology of Human Infection. New York, Plenum Medical Book Company, 1982.
11. Maynard, J.E.: Hepatitis, type B. *In* Wehrle, P.F., and Top, F.H., Jr. (eds.): Communicable and Infectious Diseases. 9th ed. St. Louis, C. V. Mosby Company, 1981.
12. Krugman, S., and Katz, S.L.: Viral hepatitis. *In* Infectious Diseases of Children. 7th ed. St. Louis, C. V. Mosby Company, 1981.
13. Aach, R.D.: Viral hepatitis. *In* Feigen, R.D., and Cherry, J.D. (eds.): Textbook of Pediatric Infectious Diseases. Philadelphia, W. B. Saunders Company, 1981.
14. Robinson, W.S.: Hepatitis B virus. *In* Mandell, G.L., Douglas, R.G., Jr., and Bennett, J.E. (eds.): Principles and Practice of Infectious Diseases. New York, John Wiley & Sons, 1979.
15. Robinson, W.S., and Greenberg, H.: Hepatitis B. *In* Hoeprich, P.D. (ed.): Infectious Diseases. 2nd ed. New York, Harper & Row Publishers, Inc., 1977.
16. Tiollasi, R., Charnay, P., and Vyas, G.N.: Biology of hepatitis B virus. Science 213:406, 1981.
17. Summers, J., and Mason, W.S.: Properties of the hepatitis B–like viruses related to their taxonomic classification. Hepatology 2:61S, 1982.
18. Robinson, W.S.: Genetic variation among hepatitis B and related viruses. Ann. N.Y. Acad. Sci. 354:371, 1980.
19. Brechot, C., Pourcel, C., Hadchouel, M., Dejean, A., Louise, A., Scotto, J., and Tiollais, P.: State of hepatitis B virus DNA in liver diseases. Hepatology 2:27S, 1982.
20. Thomas, H.C., Montano, L., Goodall, A., deKoning, R., Oladapo, J., and Wiedman, K.H.: Immunological mechanisms in chronic hepatitis B virus infection. Hepatology 2:116S, 1982.
21. Eddleston, A.L.W.F., Mondelli, M., Mieli-Vergani, G., and Williams, R.: Lymphocyte cytotoxicity to autologous hepatocytes in chronic hepatitis B virus infection. Hepatology 2:122S, 1982.
22. Wands, J.R., Mann, E., Alpert, E., and Isselbacher, K.J.: The pathogenesis of arthritis associated with acute hepatitis-B surface antigen-positive hepatitis. J. Clin. Invest. 55:930, 1975.
23. Alpert, E., Isselbacher, K.J., and Schur, P.H.: The pathogenesis of arthritis associated with viral hepatitis. N. Engl. J. Med. 285:185, 1971.
24. Alpert, E., Schur, P.H., and Isselbacher, K.J.: Sequential changes of serum complement in HAA related arthritis. N. Engl. J. Med. 287:103, 1972.
25. Segool, R.A., Lejtenyi, C., and Taussig, L.M.: Articular and cutaneous prodromal manifestations of viral hepatitis. J. Pediatr. 87:709, 1975.
26. Onion, D.K., Crumpacker, C.S., and Gilliland, B.C.: Arthritis of hepatitis associated with Australia antigen. Ann. Intern. Med. 75:29, 1971.
27. Dixon, F.J., Vazquez, J.J., Weigle, W.O., and Cochrane, C.: Pathogenesis of serum sickness. Arch. Pathol. 65:18, 1958.
28. Shulman, N.R., and Barker, L.F.: Virus-like antigen, antibody, and an-
tigen-antibody complexes in hepatitis measured by complement fixation. Science 165:304, 1969.
29. Almeida, J.D., and Waterson, A.P.: Immune complexes in hepatitis. Lancet 2:983, 1969.
30. Cochrane, C.G., and Hawkins, D.: Studies on circulating immune complexes. J. Exp. Med. 127:137, 1968.
31. Duffy, J., Lidsky, M.D., Sharp, J.T., Davis, J.S., Person, D.A., Hollinger, F.B., and Min, K.W.: Polyarthritis, polyarteritis, and hepatitis B. Medicine 55:19, 1976.
32. Shumaker, J.B., Goldfinger, S.E., Alpert, E., and Isselbacher, K.J.: Arthritis and rash. Arch. Intern. Med. 133:483, 1974.
33. Wenzel, R.P., McCormick, D.P., Busch, H.J., and Beam, W.E., Jr.: Arthritis and viral hepatitis. Arch. Intern. Med. 130:770, 1972.
34. Gocke, D.J., Hsu, K., Morgan, C., Bombardieri, S., Lockshin, M., and Christian, C.L.: Association between polyarteritis and Australia antigen. Lancet 1:1148, 1970.
35. Gerber, M.A., Brodin, A., Steinberg, D., Vernace, S., Yang, C.P., and Paronetto, F.: Periarteritis nodosa, Australia antigen, and lymphatic leukemia. N. Engl. J. Med. 286:14, 1972.
36. Sergent, J.S., Lockshin, M.D., Christian, C.L., and Gocke, D.J.: Vasculitis and hepatitis B antigenemia. Medicine 55:1, 1976.
37. Trepo, C., and Thivolet, J.: Hepatitis associated antigen and periarteritis nodosa (PAN). Vox. Sang. 19:410, 1970.
38. Fye, K.H., Becker, M.J., Theofilopoulos, A.N., Moutsopoulos, H., Feldman, J., and Talal, N.: Immune complexes in hepatitis B antigen-associated periarteritis nodosa. Am. J. Med. 62:783, 1977.
39. Trepo, C.G., Zuckerman, A.J., Bird, R.C., and Prince, A.M.: The role of circulating hepatitis B antigen/antibody immune complexes in the pathogenesis of vascular and hepatic manifestations in polyarteritis nodosa. J. Clin. Pathol. 27:863, 1974.
40. McIntosh, R.M., Koss, M.N., and Gocke, D.J.: The nature and incidence of cryoproteins in hepatitis B antigen (HBsAg) positive patients. Q. J. Med. 177:23, 1976.
41. Trepo, C.G., Thivolet, J., and Prince, A.M.: Autralia antigen and polyarteritis nodosa. Am. J. Dis. Child. 123:390, 1972.
42. Gocke, D.J., Hsu, K., Morgan, C., Bombardieri, M.L., and Christian, C.L.: Vasculitis in association with Australia antigen. J. Exp. Med. 134:330S, 1971.
43. Christian, C.L., and Sergent, J.S.: Vasculitis syndromes: Clinical and experimental models. Am. J. Med. 61:385, 1976.
44. Combes, B., Stastny, P., Shorey, J., Eigenbrodt, E.H., Barrera, A., Hull, A.R., and Carter, N.W.: Glomerulonephritis with deposition of Australia antigen-antibody complexes in glomerular basement membranes. Lancet 2:234, 1971.
45. Kohler, P.F., Cronin, R.E., Hammond, W.S., Olin, D., and Carr, R.I.: Chronic membranous glomerulonephritis caused by hepatitis B antigen-antibody immune complexes. Ann. Intern. Med. 81:448, 1974.
46. Knieser, M.R., Jenis, E.H., Cowenthal, D.T., Bancroft, W.H., Burns, W., and Shalhoub, R.: Pathogenesis of renal disease associated with viral hepatitis. Arch. Pathol. 97:193, 1974.
47. Myers, B.D., Griffel, B., Naveh, D., Jankielowitz, T., and Klajuman, A.: Membrano-proliferative glomerulonephritis associated with persistent viral hepatitis. Am. J. Clin. Pathol. 59:222, 1973.
48. Levo, Y., Gorevic, P.D., Kassab, H.J., Tobias, H., and Franklin, E.C.: Liver involvement in the syndrome of mixed cryoglobulinemia. Ann. Intern. Med. 87:287, 1977.
49. Levo, Y., Gorevic, P.D., Kassab, H.J., Zucker-Franklin, D., and Franklin, E.C.: Association between hepatitis B virus and essential mixed cryoglobulinemia. N. Engl. J. Med. 296:1501, 1977.
50. Graves, R.J.: Clinical Lectures on the Practice of Medicine. Dublin, Fannin and Company, 1843.
51. Steigman, A.J.: Rashes and arthropathy in viral hepatitis. Mt. Sinai Med. J. 40:752, 1973.
52. Alarcon, G.S., and Townes, A.S.: Arthritis in viral hepatitis: Report of two cases and review of the literature. Johns Hopkins Med. J. 132:1, 1973.
53. Stevens, D.P., Walker, J., Crum, E., Roth, H.P., and Moskowitz, R.W.: Anicteric hepatitis presenting as polyarthritis. JAMA 220:687, 1972.
54. Chang, L.W., and O'Brien, T.F.: Australia antigen serology in the Holy Cross football team hepatitis outbreak. Lancet 2:59, 1970.
55. Klemola, E., and Torma, S.: Arthralgia and arthritis caused by infectious hepatitis. Ann. Med. Intern. Fenn. 38:161, 1949.
56. Mirick, G.S., and Shank, R.E.: An epidemic of serum hepatitis studied under controlled conditions. Am. Clin. Climat. Assoc. 71:176, 1959.
57. McCarty, D.J., and Ormiste, V.: Arthritis and HB Ag-positive hepatitis. Arch. Intern. Med. 132:264, 1973.
58. Fernandez, R., and McCarty, D.J.: The arthritis of viral hepatitis. Ann. Intern. Med. 74:207, 1971.
59. Koff, R.S.: Immune-complex arthritis in viral hepatitis? N. Engl. J. Med. 285:229, 1971.
60. Wenzel, R.P., and McCormick, D.P.: Arthritis and hepatitis. N. Engl. J. Med. 285:805, 1971.

61. Crowley, J.P., and Lewis, E.J.: Multiple organ involvement in hepatitis. N. Engl. J. Med. 285:579, 1971.

62. Farivar, M., Wands, J.R., Benson, G.D., Dienstag, J.L., and Isselbacher, K.J.: Cryoprotein complexes and peripheral neuropathy in a patient with chronic active hepatitis. Gastroenterology 71:490, 1976.

63. Schumacher, H.R., and Gall, E.P.: Arthritis in acute hepatitis and chronic active hepatitis. Am. J. Med. 57:655, 1974.

64. McKenna, P.J., O'Brian, J.T., Scheinman, H.Z., Delaney, W.E., Pellecchia, C., and Lepore, J.J.: Hepatitis and arthritis with hepatitis-associated antigen in serum and synovial fluid. Lancet 2:214, 1971.

65. Gershon, A.A.: Rubella virus. In Mandell, G.L., Douglas, R.G., Jr., and Bennett, J.E. (eds.): Principles and Practice of Infectious Diseases. New York, John Wiley & Sons, 1979.

66. Cherry, J.D.: Rubella. In Feigen, R.D., and Cherry, J.D. (eds.): Textbook of Pediatric Infectious Diseases. Philadelphia, W. B. Saunders Company, 1981.

67. Top, F.H., Jr.: Rubella. In Wehrle, P.F., and Top, F.H., Jr. (eds.): Communicable and Infectious Diseases. 9th ed. St. Louis, C. V. Mosby Company, 1981.

68. Marcy, S.M., and Kibrick, S.: Rubella. In Hoeprich, P.D. (ed.): Infectious Diseases. 2nd ed. New York, Harper & Row Publishers, Inc., 1977.

69. Krugman, S., and Katz, S.L.: Rubella (German measles). In Infectious Diseases of Children, 7th ed. St. Louis, C. V. Mosby Company, 1981.

70. Frenkel, L.D., and Bellanti, J.A.: Immunology of measles, mumps, and rubella viruses. In Nahmias, A.J., and O'Reilly, R.J. (eds.): Immunology of Human Infection. New York, Plenum Medical Book Company, 1982.

71. Grahame, R., Armstrong, R., Simmons, N.A., Mims, C.A., Wilton, J.M.A., and Laurent, R.: Isolation of rubella virus from synovial fluid in five cases of seronegative arthritis. Lancet 2:649, 1981.

72. Smith, M.F., Haydock, G.B., and Grahame, R.: Rubella and juvenile chronic arthritis. Arch. Dis. Child. 56:310, 1981.

73. Hildebrandt, H.M., and Maassab, H.F.: Rubella synovitis in a one-year-old patient. N. Engl. J. Med. 274:1428, 1966.

74. Swartz, T.A., Kingberg, W., and Goldwasser, R.A.: Clinical manifestations according to age, among females given HPV-77 duck embryo vaccine. Am. J. Epidemiol. 94:246, 1971.

75. Weibel, R.E., Stokes, J., Buynak, E.B., and Hilleman, M.R.: Live rubella vaccines in adults and children. Am. J. Dis. Child. 118:226, 1969.

76. Panush, R.S.: Serum hypocomplementemia with rubella arthritis. Case report. Milit. Med. 140:117, 1975.

77. Chantler, J.K., Ford, D.K., and Tingle, A.J.: Rubella-associated arthritis: rescue of rubella virus from peripheral blood lymphocytes two years postvaccination. Infect. Immunol. 32:1274, 1981.

78. Chantler, J.K., Ford, D.K., and Tingle, A.J.: Persistent rubella infection and rubella-associated arthritis. Lancet 2:1323, 1982.

79. Austin, S.M., Altman, R., Barnes, E.K., and Dougherty, W.J.: Joint reactions in children vaccinated against rubella. Am. J. Epidemiol. 95:53, 1972.

80. Loudon, I.S.L.: Polyarthritis in rubella. Br. Med. J. 1:1388, 1953.

81. Johnson, R.E., and Hall, A.P.: Rubella arthritis. Report of cases studied by latex tests. N. Engl. J. Med. 258:743, 1958.

82. Lee, P.R., Barnett, A.F., Scholer, J.F., Bryner, S., and Clark, W.H.: Rubella arthritis. A study of twenty cases. Calif. Med. 93:125, 1960.

83. Chambers, R.J., and Bywaters, E.G.L.: Rubella synovitis. Ann. Rheum. Dis. 22:263, 1963.

84. Osler, W.: The Principles and Practice of Medicine. 6th ed. New York, Appleton and Company, 1906.

85. Bennett, R.A., and Copeman, W.S.C.: Notes on rubella with special reference to certain rheumatic sequelae. Br. Med. J. 1:924, 1940.

86. Geiger, J.C.: Epidemic of German measles in a city adjacent to an army cantonment. JAMA 70:1818, 1918.

87. Lewis, G.W.: Polyarthritis in rubella. Rheumatism 10:66, 1954.

88. Hope-Simpson, R.E.: Rubella and polyarthritis. Br. Med. J. 1:830, 1940.

89. Smith, D., and Guzowska, J.: Arthritis complicating rubella. Med. J. Aust. 1:845, 1970.

90. Kantor, T.G., and Tanner, M.: Rubella arthritis and rheumatoid arthritis. Arthritis Rheum. 5:378, 1962.

91. Branch, K.G., and Taylor, J.H.: Rubella in 1962. Br. Med. J. 2:1325, 1962.

92. Miller, W.H., and Curl, O.J.: Arthritis complicating rubella in a recent epidemic. Practitioner 190:515, 1963.

93. Green, R.H., Balsamo, R.R., Giles, J.P., Krugman, S., and Mirick, G.S.: Studies of the natural history and prevention of rubella. Am. J. Dis. Child. 110:348, 1965.

94. Ritchken, J.: Rubella rheumatism. Cent. Afr. J. Med. 2:85, 1956.

95. Smith, D., and Guzowska, J.: Arthritis complicating rubella. Med. J. Aust. 1:845, 1970.

96. Lewis, G.W.: Polyarthritis in rubella. Br. Med. J. 2:149, 1953.

97. Yanez, J.E., Thompson, G.R., Mikkelsen, W.M., and Bartholomew, L.E.: Rubella arthritis. Ann. Intern. Med. 64:772, 1966.

98. Johnston, I.N.L.: Complications of rubella. Br. Med. J. 2:414, 1962.

99. Heathfield, K.W.G.: Carpal-tunnel syndrome. Br. Med. J. 2:58, 1962.

100. Hodges, E.M.: Brachial neuritis following rubella. Br. Med. J. 1:548, 1940.

101. Fry, J., Dillane, J.B., and Fry, L.: Rubella, 1962. Br. Med. J. 2:833, 1962.

102. Ellis, W.: Rubella arthritis. Br. Med. J. 4:549, 1973.

103. Robertson, P.W., and Bell, S.M.: Prolonged rubella IgM antibody response. Med. J. Aust. 2:857, 1974.

104. Dresner, E., and Trombly, P.: The latex-fixation reaction in non-rheumatic diseases. N. Engl. J. Med. 261:981, 1959.

105. Robitaille, A., Cockburn, C., James, D.C.O., and Ansell, B.M.: HLA frequencies in less common arthropathies. Ann. Rheum. Dis. 35:271, 1976.

106. Meyer, H.M., Parkman, P.D., and Panos, T.C.: Attenuated rubella virus. N. Engl. J. Med. 275:575, 1966.

107. DuPan, R.M., Huygelen, C., Peetermans, J., and Prinzie, A.: Clinical trials with a live attenuated rubella virus vaccine. Am. J. Dis. Child. 115:658, 1968.

108. Plotkin, S.A., Farquhar, J.D., Katz, M., and Buser, F.: Attenuation of RA 27/3 rubella virus in WI-38 human diploid cells. Am. J. Dis. Child. 118:178, 1969.

109. Fogel, A., Moshkowitz, A., Rannon, L., and Gerichter, Ch.B.: Comparative trials of RA 27/3 and Cendehill rubella vaccines in adult and adolescent females. Am. J. Epidemiol. 93:392, 1971.

110. Marshall, W.C.: Rubella vaccination in adult and adolescent females. Can. J. Pub. Health 62:58, 1971.

111. Tobin, J.O.H.: Rubella vaccination of postpartum women and of adolescents in the northwest of England. Can. J. Pub. Health 62:64, 1971.

112. LeBouvier, G.L., and Plotkin, S.A.: Precipitin responses to rubella vaccine RA 27/3. J. Infect. Dis. 123:220, 1971.

113. Ogra, P.L., Kerr-Grant, D., Umana, G., Dzierba, J., and Weintraub, B.: Antibody response in serum and nasopharynx after naturally acquired and vaccine-induced infection with rubella virus. N. Engl. J. Med. 285:1333, 1971.

114. Rowlands, D.F., and Freestone, D.S.: Vaccination against rubella of susceptible school girls in Reading. J. Hyg. 69:579, 1971.

115. Simpson, R.E.H.: Rubella and polyarthritis. Br. Med. J. 1:830, 1940.

116. Harrison, B.L.: Neuritis following rubella. Br. Med. J. 1:637, 1940.

117. Moylan-Jones, R.J., and Penny, P.T.: Complications of rubella. Lancet 2:355, 1962.

118. Cooper, L.Z., Ziring, P.R., Weiss, H.J., Matters, B.A., and Krugman, S.: Transient arthritis after rubella vaccination. Am. J. Dis. Child. 118:218, 1969.

119. Dudgeon, A.J., Marshall, W., and Peckham, C.: Rubella vaccine trials in adults and children. Am. J. Dis. Child. 118:237, 1969.

120. Center for Disease Control: Rubella virus vaccine. Ann. Intern. Med. 75:757, 1971.

121. Grand, M.G., Shelby, A.W., Gehlbach, S.H., Landrigan, P.J., Judelsohn, R.G., Zendel, S.A., and Witte, J.J.: Clinical reactions following rubella vaccination. JAMA 220:1569, 1972.

122. Horstmann, D.M., Liebhaber, H., and Kohorn, E.I.: Postpartum vaccination of rubella-susceptible women. Lancet 1:1003, 1970.

123. Plotkin, S.A., Farquhar, J.D., and Ogra, P.L.: Immunologic properties of RA 27/3 rubella virus vaccine. JAMA 225:585, 1973.

124. Farquhar, J.D., and Curretjer, J.E.: Clinical experience with Cendehill rubella vaccine in mature women. Am. J. Dis. Child. 118:266, 1969.

125. Rogers, K.D., Ramirez, G., Cortez, M., Michaels, R., Savin, M., Montgomery, R., Welty, T., Taylor, F., and Hingson, R.A.: Clinical response to immunization with Cendehill strain rubella vaccine. Pediatrics 47:7, 1971.

126. Spruance, S.L., and Smith, C.B.: Joint complications associated with derivatives of HPV-77 rubella vaccine. Am. J. Dis. Child. 122:105, 1971.

127. Thompson, G.R., Ferreyra, A., and Brackett, R.G.: Acute arthritis complicating rubella vaccination. Arthritis Rheum. 14:19, 1971.

128. Weibel, R.E., Stokes, J., Jr., Buynak, E.B., and Hilleman, M.R.: Rubella vaccination in adult females. N. Engl. J. Med. 280:682, 1969.

129. Gold, J.A., Prinzie, A., and McKee, J.: Adult women vaccinated with rubella vaccine. Am. J. Dis. Child. 118:264, 1969.

130. Lerman, S.J., Nankervis, G.A., Heggie, A.D., and Gold, E.: Immunologic response, virus excretion, and joint reactions with rubella vaccine. Ann. Intern. Med. 74:67, 1971.

131. Ogra, P.L., and Herd, J.K.: Arthritis associated with induced rubella infection. J. Immunol. 107:810, 1971.

132. Spruance, S.L., Klock, L.E., Jr., Bailey, A., Ward, J.R., and Smith, C.B.: Recurrent joint symptoms in children vaccinated with HPV-77 DK12 rubella vaccine. J. Pediatr. 80:413, 1972.

133. Thompson, G.R., Weiss, J.J., Eloise, M.L., Shillis, J.L., and Brackett, R.G.: Intermittent arthritis following rubella vaccination. Am. J. Dis. Child. 125:526, 1973.

134. Griffiths, M.M., Spruance, S.L., Ogra, P.L., Thompson, G.R., and DeWitt, C.W.: HLA and recurrent episodic arthropathy associated with rubella vaccination. Arthritis Rheum. 20:1192, 1977.

135. Spruance, S.L., Metcalf, R., Smith, C.B., Griffiths, M.M., and Ward, J.R.: Chronic arthropathy associated with rubella vaccination. Arthritis Rheum. 20:741, 1977.

136. Deinard, A.S., and Bilka, P.J.: Joint involvement following vaccination for rubella. Minn. Med. 54:337, 1971.

137. Chiba, Y., Sadeghi, E., and Ogra, P.L.: Abnormalities of cellular immune response in arthritis induced by rubella vaccination. J. Immunol. 117:1684, 1976.

138. Gilmartin, R.C., Jr., Jabbom, J.T., and Duenas, D.A.: Rubella vaccine myeloradiculoneuritis. J. Pediatr. 80:406, 1972.

139. Kilroy, A.W., Schaffner, W., Fleet, W.F., Jr., Lefkowitz, L.B., Jr., Karzon, D.T., and Fenichel, G.M.: Two syndromes following rubella immunization. Clinical observations and epidemiological studies. JAMA 214:2287, 1970.

140. Schaffner, W., Fleet, W.F., Kilroy, A.W., Lefkowitz, L.B., Herrmann, K.L., Thompson, R.N., and Karzon, D.T.: Polyneuropathy following rubella immunization. Am. J. Dis. Child. 127:684, 1974.

141. Schlesinger, R.W. (ed.): The Togaviruses. New York, Academic Press, 1980.

142. Russell, P.K.: Alphavirus (Eastern, Western, and Venezuelan equine encephalitis). In Mandell, G.L., Douglas, R.G., Jr., and Bennett, J.E. (eds.): Principles and Practice of Infectious Diseases. New York, John Wiley & Sons, 1979.

143. Tesh, R.B.: Arthritides caused by mosquito-borne viruses. Ann. Rev. Med. 33:31, 1982.

144. Calisher, C.H., Shope, R.E., Brandt, W., Casals, J., Karabatsos, N., Murphy, F.A., Tesh, R.B., and Wiebe, M.E.: Proposed antigenic classification of registered arboviruses (Togaviridae, Alphavirus). Intervirology 14:229, 1980.

145. Lumsden, W.H.R.: An epidemic of virus disease in southern province, Tanganyika territory, in 1952–53. II. General description and epidemiology. Trans. R. Soc. Trop. Med. Hyg. 49:33, 1955.

146. Robinson, M.C.: An epidemic of virus disease in southern province, Tanganyika territory, in 1952–53. I. Clinical features. Trans. R. Soc. Trop. Med. Hyg. 49:28, 1955.

147. Ross, R.W.: The Newala epidemic. III. The virus: Isolation, pathogenic properties and relationship to the epidemic. J. Hyg. (Camb.) 54:177, 1956.

148. de Ranitz, C.M., Myers, R.M., Varkey, M.J., Isaac, Z.H., and Carey, D.E.: Clinical impressions of chikungunya in Vellore gained from study of adult patients. Ind. J. Med. Res. 53:756, 1965.

149. Moore, D.L., Reddy, S., Akinkugbe, F.M., Lee, V.H., David-West, T.S., Causey, O.R., and Carey, D.E.: An epidemic of chikungunya fever in Ibadan, Nigeria, 1969. Ann. Trop. Med. Parasitol. 68:59, 1974.

150. Tesh, R.B., Gajdusek, D.C., Garruto, R.M., Cross, J.H., and Rosen, L.: The distribution and prevalence of group A arborvirus neutralizing antibodies among human populations in southeast Asia and the Pacific Islands. Am. J. Trop. Med. Hyg. 24:664, 1975.

151. Gear, S.H.S.: Arboviruses of Southern Africa. In Feigin, R.D., and Cherry, J.D. (eds.): Textbook of Pediatric Infectious Diseases. Philadelphia, W. B. Saunders Company, 1981.

152. Kennedy, A.C., Fleming, J., and Solomon, L.: Chikungunya viral arthropathy: a clinical description. J. Rheum. 7:231, 1980.

153. Weinberg, M.P., Haddow, A.J., and Williams, M.C.: The occurrence of chikungunya virus in Uganda. Trans. R. Soc. Trop. Med. Hyg. 52:253, 1958.

154. Haddow, A.J., Davies, C.W., and Walker, A.J.: O'nyong-nyong fever: An epidemic virus disease in East Africa. I. Introduction. Trans. R. Soc. Trop. Med. Hyg. 54:517, 1960.

155. Shore, H.: O'nyong-nyong fever: An epidemic virus disease in East Africa. III. Some clinical and epidemiological observations in the northern province of Uganda. Trans. R. Soc. Trop. Med. Hyg. 55:361, 1961.

156. Doherty, R.L., Barrett, E.J., Gorman, B.M., and Whitehead, R.H.: Epidemic polyarthritis. Occurrence in eastern Australia 1959–1970. Med. J. Aust. 1:5, 1971.

157. Clarke, A.J., Marshall, I.D., and Gard, G.: Annually recurrent epidemic polyarthritis and Ross River virus activity in a coastal area of New South Wales. Am. J. Trop. Med. Hyg. 22:543, 1973.

158. Seglenicks, Z., and Moore, B.W.: Epidemic polyarthritis in South Australia: Report of an outbreak in 1971. Med. J. Aust. 2:552, 1974.

159. Anderson, S.G., and French, E.L.: An epidemic exanthem associated with polyarthritis in the Murray Valley, 1956. Med. J. Aust. 1:113, 1957.

160. Doherty, R.L., Gorman, B.M., Whitehead, R.H., and Carley, J.G.: Studies of arthropod-borne virus infections in Queensland. V. Survey of antibodies to group A arboviruses in man and other animals. Aust. J. Exp. Biol. Med. Sci. 44:365, 1966.

161. Gard, G., Marshall, I.D., and Woodroofe, G.M.: Annually recurrent epidemic polyarthritis and Ross River virus activity in a coastal area of New South Wales. II. Mosquitoes, viruses, and wildlife. Am. J. Trop. Med. Hyg. 22:551, 1973.

162. Halliday, J.H., and Horan, J.P.: An epidemic of polyarthritis in the Northern Territory. Med. J. Aust. 2:293, 1943.

163. Clarke, J.A., Marshall, J.D., and Gard, G.: Annually recurrent epidemic polyarthritis and Ross River virus activity in a coastal area of New South Wales. Am. J. Trop. Med. Hyg. 22:543, 1973.

164. Tesh, R.B., McLean, R.G., Shroyer, D.A., Calisher, C.H., and Rosen, L.: Ross River virus (Togaviridae: Alphavirus) infection (epidemic polyarthritis) in American Samoa. Trans. R. Soc. Trop. Med. Hyg. 75:426, 1981.

165. Pinheiro, F.P., Freitas, R.B., Travassos da Rosa, J.F., Gabbay, Y.B., Mello, W.A., and LeDuc, J.W.: An outbreak of Mayaro virus disease in Belterra, Brazil. Am. J. Trop. Med. Hyg. 30:674, 1981.

166. Taylor, R.M., Hurlbut, H.S., Work, T.H., Kingston, J.R., and Frothingham, T.E.: Sindbis virus: A newly recognized arthropod-transmitted virus. Am. J. Trop. Med. Hyg. 4:844, 1955.

167. Malherbe, H., Strickland-Cholmley, M., and Jackson, A.L.: Sindbis virus infection in man. Report of a case with recovery of virus from skin lesions. S. Afr. Med. J. 37:547, 1963.

168. McIntosh, M., McGillivray, G.M., Dickinson, D.B., and Malherbe, H.: Illness caused by Sindbis and West Nile viruses in South Africa. S. Afr. Med. J. 38:291, 1964.

169. Skogh, M., and Espmark, A.: Ockelbo disease: epidemic arthritis-exanthema syndrome in Sweden caused by Sindbis-virus like agent. Lancet 1:795, 1982.

170. Fraser, J.R.E., and Cunningham, A.L.: Incubation time of epidemic polyarthritis. Med. J. Aust. 1:550, 1980.

171. Jadhav, M., Namboodripad, M., Carman, R.H., Carey, D.E., and Myers, R.M.: Chikungunya disease in infants and children in Vellore: A report of clinical and hematological features of virologically proven cases. Ind. J. Med. Res. 53:764, 1965.

172. Deller, J.J., and Russell, P.K.: Chikungunya disease. Am. J. Trop. Med. Hyg. 17:107, 1968.

173. Sibree, E.W.: Acute polyarthritis in Queensland. Med. J. Aust. 2:565, 1944.

174. Dowling, P.G.: Epidemic polyarthritis. Med. J. Aust. 1:245, 1946.

175. Fuller, C.W., and Warner, P.: Some epidemiological and laboratory observations on an epidemic rash and polyarthritis occurring in the upper Murray region of South Australia. Med. J. Aust. 2:117, 1957.

176. Anderson, C.R., Downs, W.G., Wattley, G.H., Ahin, N.W., and Reese, A.A.: Mayaro virus: A new human disease agent. Am. J. Trop. Med. Hyg. 6:1012, 1957.

177. Nimmannitya, S., Halstead, S.B., Cohen, S.N., and Margiotta, M.R.: Dengue and chikungunya virus infection in man in Thailand, 1962–1964. I. Observations on hospitalized patients with hemorrhagic fever. Am. J. Trop. Med. Hyg. 18:954, 1969.

178. Doherty, R.L., Carley, J.G., and Best, J.C.: Isolation of Ross River virus from man. Med. J. Aust. 1:1083, 1972.

179. Lim, T.W., Burhamuddin, M., and Abbas, A.: A case of Sindbis virus infection in Kuala Lumpur. Med. J. Malaysia 27:147, 1972.

180. Clarris, B.J., Doherty, R.L., Fraser, J.R.E., French, E.L., and Muirden, K.D.: Epidemic polyarthritis: A cytological, virological, and immunochemical study. Aust. N.Z. J. Med. 5:450, 1975.

181. Aaskov, J.G., Fraser, J.R.E., and Dalglish, D.A.: Specific and non-specific immunological changes in epidemic polyarthritis patients. Aust. J. Exp. Biol. Med. Sci. 59:599, 1981.

182. Mudge, R.: Epidemic polyarthritis in South Australia. Med. J. Aust. 2:823, 1974.

183. Fraser, J.R.E., Tait, B., Aaskov, J.G., and Cunningham, A.L.: Possible genetic determinants in epidemic polyarthritis caused by Ross River virus infection. Aust. N.Z. J. Med. 10:597, 1980.

184. Fraser, J.R.E., Cunningham, A.L., Clarris, B.J., Aaskov, J.G., and Leach, R.: Cytology of synovial effusions in epidemic polyarthritis. Aust. N.Z. J. Med. 11:168, 1981.

185. Baum, S.G., and Litman, N.: Mumps virus. In Mandell, G.L., Douglas, R.G., and Bennett, J.E. (eds.): Principles and Practice of Infectious Diseases. New York, John Wiley & Sons, 1979.

186. Brunell, P.A.: Mumps. In Feigin, R.D., and Cherry, J.D. (eds.): Textbook of Pediatric Infectious Diseases. Philadelphia, W. B. Saunders Company, 1981.

187. Brunell, P.A.: Mumps. In Wehrle, P.F., and Top, F.H., Jr. (eds.): Communicable and Infectious Diseases. 9th ed. St. Louis, C. V. Mosby Company, 1981.

188. Marcy, S.M., and Kilbrick, S.: Mumps. In Hoeprich, P.D. (ed.): Infectious Diseases. 2nd ed. New York, Harper & Row Publishers, Inc., 1977.

189. Krugman, S., and Katz, S.L.: Mumps (epidemic parotitis). In Infectious Diseases of Children. 7th ed. St. Louis, C. V. Mosby Company, 1981.

190. Magida, M.G.: Epidemic parotitis complicated by pericarditis and serositis. Ann. Intern. Med. 35:218, 1957.

191. Maisondeau, P.: Etude des manifestations articulaires des orcillons, thesis Jouve. Paris. 1924.

192. Appelbaum, E., Kohn, J., Steinman, R.E., and Shearn, M.A.: Mumps arthritis. Arch. Intern. Med. 90:217, 1952.

193. Lass, R., and Shephard, E.: Mumps arthritis. Br. Med. J. 2:1613, 1961.
194. Caranasos, G.J., and Felker, J.R.: Mumps arthritis. Arch. Intern. Med. 119:394, 1967.
195. Ghosh, S.K., and Reddy, T.A.: Arthralgia and myalgia in mumps. Rheumatol. Rehabil. 12:97, 1973.
196. Solem, J.H.: Mumps arthritis without parotitis. Scand. J. Infect. Dis. 3:173, 1971.
197. Gordon, S.C., and Lauter, C.B.: Mumps arthritis: unusual presentation as adult Still's disease. Ann. Intern. Med. 97:45, 1982.
198. Filpi, R.G., and Houts, R.L.: Mumps arthritis. JAMA 205:216, 1968.
199. Bryer, D., and Routhwaite, F.J.: Cricoarytenoid arthritis due to mumps. Laryngoscope 83:372, 1973.
200. Gold, H.E., Boxerbaum, B., and Leslie, H.J., Jr.: Mumps arthritis. Am. J. Dis. Child. 116:547, 1968.
201. Tracey, J.P., and Riggenbach, R.D.: Mumps arthritis associated with positive latex fixation reaction. South. Med. J. 63:1122, 1970.
202. Cherry, J.D.: Nonpolio enteroviruses: coxsackieviruses, echoviruses and enteroviruses. In Feigin, R.D., and Cherry, J.D. (eds.): Textbook of Pediatric Infectious Diseases. Philadelphia, W. B. Saunders Company, 1981.
203. Johnson, K.M.: Enteroviruses: coxsackievirus and echovirus infections. In Wehrle, P.F., and Top, F.H., Jr. (eds.): Communicable and Infectious Diseases. 9th ed. St. Louis, C. V. Mosby Company, 1981.
204. Young, N.A.: Picornaviridae. Introduction. In Mandell, G.L., Douglas, R.G., Jr., and Bennett, J.E. (eds.): Principles and Practice of Infectious Diseases. New York, John Wiley & Sons, 1979.
205. Young, N.A.: Coxsackievirus and echovirus. In Mandell, G.L., Douglas, R.G., Jr., and Bennett, J.E. (eds.): Principles and Practice of Infectious Diseases. New York, John Wiley & Sons, 1979.
206. Morens, D.M., Zweighaft, R.M., and Bryan, J.M.: Non-polio enterovirus disease in the United States. Int. J. Epidemiol. 8:49, 1979.
207. Blotzer, J.W., and Myers, A.R.: Echovirus-associated polyarthritis. Arthritis Rheum. 21:978, 1978.
208. Sandford, J.P., and Sulkin, S.E.: The clinical spectrum of ECHO-virus infection. N. Engl. J. Med. 261:1113, 1959.
209. Rahal, J.J., Millian, S.J., and Noriega, E.R.: Coxsackie and adenovirus infection. JAMA 235:2496, 1976.
210. Wehrle, P.F.: Smallpox (variola). In Feigin, R.D., and Cherry, J.D. (eds.): Textbook of Pediatric Infectious Diseases. Philadelphia, W. B. Saunders Company, 1981.
211. Benenson, A.S.: Smallpox. In Wehrle, P.F., and Top, F.H., Jr. (eds.): Communicable and Infectious Diseases. 9th ed. Philadelphia, W. B. Saunders Company, 1981.
212. Neff, J.M.: Poxviridae. Introduction. In Mandell, G.L., Douglas, R.G., Jr., and Bennett, J.E. (eds.): Principles and Practice of Infectious Diseases. New York, John Wiley & Sons, 1979.
213. Neff, J.M.: Variola virus (smallpox). In Mandell, G.L., Douglas, R.G., Jr., and Bennett, J.E. (eds.): Principles and Practice of Infectious Diseases. New York, John Wiley & Sons, 1979.
214. Cockshott, P., and MacGregor, M.: Osteomyelitis variolosa. Q. J. Med. 27:369, 1958.
215. Ansell, B.M.: Infective Arthritis. In Scott, J.T. (ed.): Textbook of the Rheumatic Diseases. 5th ed. Edinburgh, Churchill Livingstone, 1978.
216. Sewall, S.: Vaccinia osteomyelitis. Bull. Hosp. Joint Dis. 10:59, 1949.
217. Neff, J.M.: Vaccinia virus (cowpox). In Mandell, G.L., Douglas, R.G., Jr., and Bennett, J.E. (eds.): Principles and Practice of Infectious Diseases. New York, John Wiley & Sons, 1979.
218. Nitzkin, J.L., Anderson, L., Skaggs, J.W., and Hernandez, C.: Complications of smallpox vaccination in Kentucky in 1968. J. Ky. Med. Assoc. 69:184, 1971.
219. Silby, H.M., Farber, R., O'Connell, C.J., Ascher, J., and Marine, E.J.: Acute monoarticular arthritis after vaccination. Ann. Intern. Med. 62:347, 1965.
220. Holtzman, C.M.: Postvaccination arthritis. N. Engl. J. Med. 280:111, 1969.
221. Baum, S.G.: Adenovirus. In Mandell, G.L., Douglas, R.G., Jr., and Bennett, J.E. (eds.): Principles and Practice of Infectious Diseases. New York, John Wiley & Sons, 1979.
222. Spencer, M.J., and Cherry, J.D.: Adenoviral infections. In Feigin, R.D., and Cherry, J.D. (eds.): Textbook of Pediatric Infectious Diseases. Philadelphia, W. B. Saunders Company, 1981.
223. Panush, R.S.: Adenovirus arthritis. Arthritis Rheum. 17:534, 1974.
224. Utsinger, P.D.: Immunologic study of arthritis associated with adenovirus infection (abstract). Arthritis Rheum. 20:138, 1977.
225. Douglas, R.G., Jr.: Herpetoviridae. Introduction. In Mandell, G.L., Douglas, R.G., Jr., and Bennett, J.E. (eds.): Principles and Practice of Infectious Diseases. New York, John Wiley & Sons, 1979.
226. Brunell, P.A.: Varicella-zoster virus. In Mandell, G.L., Douglas, R.G., Jr., and Bennett, J.E. (eds.): Principles and Practice of Infectious Diseases. New York, John Wiley & Sons, 1979.

227. Brunell, P.A.: Chickenpox. In Wehrle, P.F., and Top, R.G., Jr. (eds.): Communicable and Infectious Diseases. 9th ed. St. Louis, C. V. Mosby Company, 1981.
228. Brunell, P.A.: Varicella-zoster infections. In Feigin, R.D., and Cherry, J.D. (eds.): Textbook of Pediatric Infectious Diseases. Philadelphia, W. B. Saunders Company, 1981.
229. Ward, J.R., and Bishop, B.: Varicella arthritis. JAMA 242:1954, 1970.
230. Friedman, A., and Naveh, Y.: Polyarthritis associated with chickenpox. Am. J. Dis. Child. 122:179, 1971.
231. Mulhern, L.M., Friday, G.A., and Perri, J.A.: Arthritis complicating varicella infection. Pediatrics 48:827, 1971.
232. Priest, J.R., Urick, J.J., Groth, K.E., and Balfour, H.H., Jr.: Varicella arthritis documented by isolation of virus from joint fluid. J. Pediatr. 93:990, 1978.
233. Atkinson, L.S., Halford, J.G., Jr., Burton, O.M., and Moorhead, S.R., Jr.: Septic and aseptic arthritis complicating varicella. J. Fam. Pract. 12:917, 1981.
234. Brook, I.: Varicella arthritis in childhood. Clin. Pediatr. 16:1156, 1977.
235. Diliberti, J.H., Bartel, S.J., Humphrey, T.R., and Pang, A.W.: Acute monoarticular arthritis in association with varicella. Clin. Pediatr. 16:663, 1977.
236. Pascual-Gomez, E.: Identification of large mononuclear cells in varicella arthritis. Arthritis Rheum. 23:519, 1980.
237. Sekanina, M., and Frana, L.: The case of acute polyarthritis complicating chickenpox. Cesk. Pediatr. 28:253, 1973.
238. Tezner, O.: Ergebnisse der inheren Medizin and Kinderheilkunde, Varicellen. Berlin, Springer-Verlag, 1931.
239. Bernstein, A.: Infectious mononucleosis. Medicine 19:98, 1940.
240. Hoagland, R.J.: Infectious mononucleosis. Am. J. Med. 13:158, 1952.
241. Schooley, R.T., and Dolin, R.: Epstein-Barr virus (infectious mononucleosis). In Mandell, G.L., Douglas, R.G., Jr., and Bennett, J.E. (eds.): Principles and Practice of Infectious Diseases. New York, John Wiley & Sons, 1979.
242. Evans, A.S.: Mononucleosis, infectious. In Wehrle, P.F., and Top, F.H., Jr. (eds.): Communicable and Infectious Diseases. 9th ed. St. Louis, C. V. Mosby Company, 1981.
243. Lange, D.J.: Infectious mononucleosis (Epstein-Barr virus). In Feigin, R.D., and Cherry, J.D. (eds.): Textbook of Pediatric Infectious Diseases. Philadelphia, W. B. Saunders Company, 1981.
244. Evans, A.S.: Infectious mononucleosis in University of Wisconsin students. Am. J. Hyg. 71:342, 1960.
245. Pollack, S., Enat, R., and Barzilai, D.: Monoarthritis with heterophil-negative infectious mononucleosis. Arch. Intern. Med. 140:1109, 1980.
246. Sauter, S. van H., and Utsinger, P.D.: Viral arthritis. Clin. Rheumatol. Dis. 4:225, 1978.
247. King, K.: Infectious mononucleosis. A summary of fourteen cases and review of the literature. N.C. Med. J. 26:110, 1965.
248. Adebonojo, F.O.: Monoarticular arthritis: An unusual manifestation of infectious mononucleosis. Clin. Pediatr. 11:549, 1972.
249. Hirsch, M.S.: Herpes simplex virus. In Mandell, G.L., Douglas, R.G., Jr., and Bennett, J.E. (eds.): Principles and Practice of Infectious Diseases. New York, John Wiley & Sons, 1979.
250. Lang, D.J.: Postnatal herpesvirus hominis (herpes simplex). In Feigin, R.D., and Cherry, J.D. (eds.): Textbook of Pediatric Infectious Diseases. Philadelphia, W. B. Saunders Company, 1981.
251. Nahmias, A.J., and Kohl, S.: Herpes simplex. In Wehrle, P.F., and Top, F.H., Jr. (eds.): Communicable and Infectious Diseases. 9th ed. St. Louis, C. V. Mosby, 1981.
252. Friedman, H.M., Pincus, T., Gibilisco, P., Baker, D., Glazer, J.P., Plotkin, S.A., and Schumacher, H.R.: Acute monoarticular arthritis caused by herpes simplex virus and cytomegalovirus. Am. J. Med. 69:241, 1980.
253. Shaw, H.L.K.: Erythema infectiosum. Am. J. Med. Sci. 129:16, 1905.
254. Smith, E.H.: An epidemic of erythema infectiosum. Arthritis Pediatr. 46:456, 1929.
255. Coe, N.C., and Kelly, F.L.: Erythema infectiosum. Calif. West. Med. 34:39, 1932.
256. Kerr, P.S., and Marsh, E.H.: Outbreak of erythema infectiosum in Elmsford, N.Y. Am. J. Public Health 23:1271, 1933.
257. Chargin, L., Sobel, N., and Goldstein, N.: Erythema infectiosum. Arch. Dermatol. Syph. 47:467, 1943.
258. Condon, F.J.: Erythema infectiosum. Report of an area-wide outbreak. Am. J. Public Health 49:528, 1959.
259. Auriemma, P.R.: Erythema infectiosum: Report on a familial outbreak. Am. J. Public Health 44:1450, 1954.
260. Balfour, N.N., Jr., May, D.B., Rotte, T.C., Phelps, W.R., and Schiff, G.M.: A study of erythema infectiosum: Recovery of rubella virus and echovirus-12. Pediatrics 50:285, 1972.
261. Ager, E.H., Chin, T.D.Y., and Poland, J.D.: Epidemic erythema infectiosum. N. Engl. J. Med. 275:1326, 1966.

Chapter 99

Lyme Disease

Allen C. Steere and Stephen E. Malawista

INTRODUCTION

Lyme disease, originally called Lyme arthritis, was recognized in 1975 because of close geographic clustering of children in Old Lyme, Connecticut affected with what was thought to be juvenile rheumatoid arthritis.[1] The illness is now known to be a complex multisystem disorder. It usually begins in summer with erythema chronicum migrans (ECM) and associated symptoms,[2,3] is sometimes followed weeks to months later by neurologic[4] or cardiac abnormalities,[5] and is often followed weeks to years later by arthritis.[2,6,7] Lyme disease is caused by a newly recognized spirochete,[8-10] which is transmitted by *Ixodes dammini* or related ixodid ticks.[11-13] The disorder is associated with characteristic immune abnormalities,[14-17] and patients with severe and prolonged illness often have the B lymphocyte alloantigen, DR2.[6,18] Early in the illness when ECM is present, tetracycline or penicillin therapy shortens the duration of the skin lesion and often prevents or attenuates subsequent arthritis.[19,20] Later stages respond to high-dose intravenous penicillin.[21,22] The known geographic distribution of the disease includes at least 14 states,[11,23] Europe,[24-27] and Australia.[28]

CLINICAL CHARACTERISTICS

Early Manifestations

Erythema chronicum migrans, the unique clinical marker for Lyme disease, begins as a red macule or papule that expands to form a large, annular lesion (as big as 50 cm), usually with a bright red outer border, partial central clearing, and an indurated center (Fig. 99–1 and Table 99–1).[2,3] Although the lesion can be located any place, the thigh, groin, and axilla are particularly common sites. The lesion is hot to touch but often not painful. The histologic appearance is compatible with that of an arthropod bite—epidermal and dermal involvement at the center, with only dermal involvement in the periphery. About 30 percent of patients remember a tick bite at the site of the lesion 3 days to 32 days before it forms.

Within several days after onset of the initial skin lesion (ECM), almost half of patients develop multiple annular secondary lesions (see Table 99–1).[2,3] Although their appearance is similar to the initial lesions, they are generally smaller, migrate less, and lack indurated centers. In addition, they are not associated with previous tick bites. During this period, some patients develop malar rash or conjunctivitis or, rarely, diffuse urticaria. ECM and secondary lesions usually fade within 3 to 4 weeks (range 1 day to 14 months). However, during or soon after their resolution patients may develop new, evanescent lesions, consisting of small (2 to 3 cm) red circles and blotches, for several more weeks. Any of the dermatologic manifestations of the illness may recur.

Skin involvement is often accompanied by malaise and fatigue, headache, fever and chills, generalized achiness, and regional lymphadenopathy (Tables 99–1 and 99–2).[2,3] In addition, patients sometimes have evidence of meningeal irritation, mild encephalopathy, migratory musculoskeletal pain, hepatitis, generalized lymphadenopathy or splenomegaly, sore throat, nonproductive cough, or testicular swelling. Except for fatigue and lethargy, which are often constant, the early signs and symptoms are typically intermittent and changing. For example, a patient might experience predominantly headache and stiff neck for several days. After a few days of improvement, musculoskeletal pain might begin. Associated symptoms may occur several days before ECM, and conversely may last for months (particularly fatigue and lethargy) after the skin lesions have disappeared.

Later Manifestations

Neurologic. Symptoms suggestive of meningeal irritation may occur at the beginning of the illness when ECM is present.[4] Such individuals often have episodic attacks of excruciating headache and neck pain, stiffness, or pressure, which typically lasts hours. During the first 1 week or 2 weeks of illness, such symptoms are not associated with spinal fluid pleocytosis or objective neurologic deficit. However, after several weeks to months, about 15 percent of patients develop frank neurologic abnormalities, including meningitis, encephalitis, chorea, cranial neuritis (including bilateral facial palsy), motor and sensory radiculoneuritis, mononeuritis multiplex, or myelitis, in various combinations. The usual pattern is fluctuating meningoencephalitis with superimposed cranial (particularly facial palsy) and peripheral radiculoneuropathy (Fig. 99–2). However, facial palsy may occur alone. At this time, a lymphocytic pleocytosis (about 100 cells per mm³) is found in cerebrospinal fluid, and often there is diffuse abnormal slowing on electroencephalograms. However, on examination, such patients usually have neck stiffness only on extreme flexion, and Kernig's and Brudzinski's signs are negative. Neurologic abnormalities typically last for months but usually resolve completely. They may recur.

Heart. Within several weeks after the onset of illness, about 8 percent of patients develop cardiac involvement.[5] The commonest abnormality is fluctuating degrees of atrioventricular block (first-degree, Wencke-

Figure 99–1. Two patients are seen, one with erythema chronicum migrans *(A)*, the other with secondary annular lesions *(B)*. The lesions began as red macules that expanded to form large rings. In *A*, the "outer border is an intense red, the middle shows partial clearing, and the center is indurated. In *B*, the outer rims are red, and centers show nearly complete clearing. The lesions were hot to touch. (From Steere AC, et al.: Ann. Intern. Med. 86:685, 1977.)

bach, or complete heart block). However, some patients have evidence of more diffuse cardiac involvement, including electrocardiographic changes compatible with acute myopericarditis, radionuclide evidence of mild left ventricular dysfunction, or, rarely, cardiomegaly (Fig. 99–3). None have had heart murmurs. The duration of cardiac involvement is usually brief (3 days to 6 weeks), but it may recur.

Arthritis. Within a few weeks to 2 years after the onset of illness, about 60 percent of patients develop arthritis.[2,6,7] If joint involvement occurs early in the illness, the typical pattern is one of migratory musculoskeletal pain in joints, tendons, bursae, muscles, or bones, often without joint swelling. The pain tends to affect only one or two sites at a time and usually lasts a few hours to several days in a given location. Frank arthritis with marked joint swelling usually does not begin until months after the onset of the illness. At that time, patients often experience intermittent attacks of joint swelling and pain, primarily in large joints (especially the knee), usually one or two joints at a time (Fig. 99–4). Affected knees are commonly much more swollen than they are painful and are often hot but rarely red. Baker's cysts may form and rupture early. However,

Table 99–1. Early Signs of Lyme Disease

	No. of Patients	
	N = 314	*%*
Erythema chronicum migrans	314	100*
Multiple annular lesions	150	48
Lymphadenopathy		
Regional	128	41
Generalized	63	20
Pain on neck flexion	52	17
Malar rash	41	13
Erythematous throat	38	12
Conjunctivitis	35	11
Right upper quadrant tenderness	24	8
Splenomegaly	18	6
Hepatomegaly	16	5
Muscle tenderness	12	4
Periorbital edema	10	3
Evanescent skin lesions	8	3
Abdominal tenderness	6	2
Testicular swelling	2	1

*ECM was required for inclusion in this study. (From Steere, A.C., et al.: Ann. Intern. Med. 99:76, 1983.

Table 99–2. Early Symptoms of Lyme Disease

	No. of Patients	
	N = 314	*%*
Malaise, fatigue, lethargy	251	80
Headache	200	64
Fever and chills	185	59
Stiff neck	151	48
Arthralgias	150	48
Myalgias	135	43
Backache	81	26
Anorexia	73	23
Sore throat	53	17
Nausea	53	17
Dysesthesia	35	11
Vomiting	32	10
Abdominal pain	24	8
Photophobia	19	6
Hand stiffness	16	5
Dizziness	15	5
Cough	15	5
Chest pain	12	4
Ear pain	12	4
Diarrhea	6	2

(From Steere, A.C., et al.: Ann. Intern. Med. 99:76, 1983.

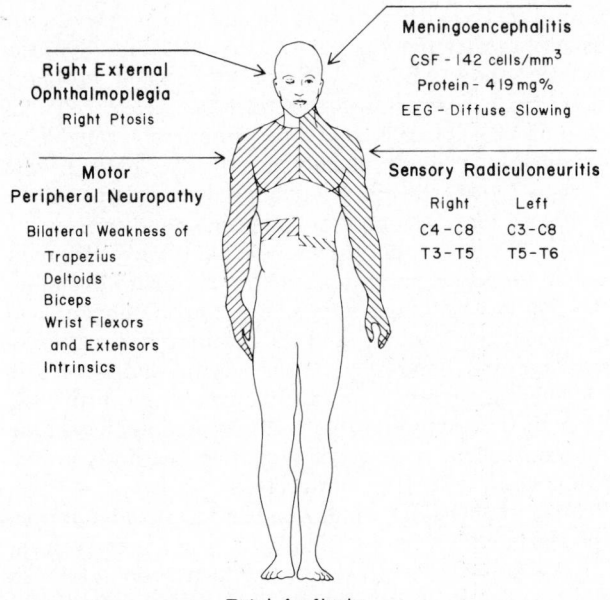

Right External
Ophthalmoplegia
Right Ptosis

Meningoencephalitis

CSF - 142 cells/mm^3
Protein - 419 mg%
EEG - Diffuse Slowing

Motor
Peripheral Neuropathy

Bilateral Weakness of
 Trapezius
 Deltoids
 Biceps
 Wrist Flexors
  and Extensors
 Intrinsics

Sensory Radiculoneuritis

Right	Left
C4-C8	C3-C8
T3-T5	T5-T6

Total Areflexia

Figure 99–2. A 49-year-old man with neurologic abnomalities of Lyme disease. Five weeks after the onset of erythema chronicum migrans, the patient developed meningoencephalitis, followed by right external ophthalmoplegia, right ptosis, and bilateral motor and sensory radiculoneuropathy. The patient was totally areflexic.

Figure 99–4. A 32-year-old man with Lyme arthritis. Fifteen months after erythema chronicum migrans, the patient began to have intermittent attacks of arthritis, primarily in his knees. At the time of this picture, the patient had had such attacks for 6 years.

both large and small joints may be affected, and a few patients have had symmetric polyarthritis. Attacks of arthritis, which generally last from a few weeks to months, typically recur for several years. In 10 percent of patients with arthritis, involvement in large joints may become chronic, with erosion of cartilage and bone.[6,7] Late in the illness, fatigue is common with active joint involvement, but fever or other symptoms are unusual.

LABORATORY FINDINGS

Etiologic Agent. Lyme disease is now known to be caused by a newly recognized spirochete that has characteristics of both treponemes and borreliae.[8,9] Since an exact classification is currently lacking, we use the more

general name, *I. dammini* spirochete. The organism has been recovered from patient specimens of blood[9,10] and skin (ECM) early in the illness and from cerebrospinal fluid when neurologic abnormalities were present.[9] Thus, we believe that the spirochete is either injected into the skin or bloodstream in tick saliva[12] or is deposited in fecal material on the skin.[8] We suspect that after an incubation period of 3 to 32 days, the organism migrates outward in the skin (ECM), is spread in lymph (regional adenopathy), or is disseminated in blood to organs (e.g., brain and presumably liver or spleen) or other skin sites (secondary annular lesions). Later in the illness, the fate of the organism is unclear, but therapeutic[22] and immunologic[17] evidence suggest that it is still alive when arthritis is present, and probably in affected joints.

Figure 99–3. Chest roentgenograms of a 22-year-old man with cardiac abnormalities of Lyme disease. Three weeks after the onset of erythema chronicum migrans, the patient developed syncopal episodes, which were found to be due to complete heart block. *Left,* On admission to the hospital, he had cardiomegaly and evidence of pulmonary venous hypertension. *Right,* Five days after treatment with intravenous penicillin and prednisone the chest roentgenogram was normal. (These films were obtained by courtesy of Drs. George A. Jacoby and Theresa McCloud, Massachusetts General Hospital, Boston, Mass.)

Antibody Titers. Specific IgM antibody titers against the *I. dammini* spirochete usually reach a peak between the third week and the sixth week after the onset of disease; specific IgG antibody titers rise slowly and are generally highest months later when arthritis is present.[9] Among 40 patients with early disease only (ECM), 90 percent had elevated IgM titers (≥ 1:128) determined by indirect immunofluorescence (Fig. 99–5), between the ECM and convalescence 2 to 3 weeks later. Among 95 patients with later manifestations (nervous system, heart, or joint involvement), 94 percent had elevated titers of IgG (≥ 1:128), and all 60 patients with arthritis had such titers. In contrast, of 40 healthy control subjects and 40 control patients with infectious mononucleosis or various rheumatic diseases, none had elevated IgG titers, and only 3 of 20 control patients with infectious mononucleosis had elevated IgM titers. Thus, the presence of antibody titers against the *I. dammini* spirochete are particularly useful in differentiating Lyme disease from other rheumatic syndromes.

Immunologic Characteristics. Several findings support the hypothesis that Lyme disease begins as a systemic, immune-mediated disorder that may become localized and propagated in joints. At the beginning of the illness, when ECM is present, many patients have circulating immune complexes.[16,17] At that time, the finding of elevated serum IgM levels and cryoglobulins containing IgM, which correlate directly, predicts subsequent nervous system, heart, or joint involvement.[14,15] Serial determinations of serum IgM are often the single most helpful laboratory indicator of disease activity. These abnormalities tend to persist during neurologic or cardiac involvement. However, later in the illness, when arthritis is present, serum IgM levels are more often normal. At that time, immune complexes and cryoglobulins are usually lacking in serum, though they are found uniformly in joint fluid, as in rheumatoid arthritis. Throughout the illness, C3 and C4 levels are generally normal or elevated. Tests for rheumatoid factor or antinuclear antibodies are usually negative.

The development of later complications is associated with a particular genetic susceptibility.[6,18] In a study of 45 patients at the two ends of the clinical spectrum of Lyme disease, those with severe and prolonged illness (ECM followed by meningoencephalitis or chronic arthritis) had an increased frequency of the B cell alloantigen, DR2 (67 percent of patients), compared with 36 percent of those with mild and brief illness (ECM alone) (relative risk equals 3.4) or 25 percent of those in a normal population (relative risk equals 6). Thus, Lyme disease seems to fit within a pathogenetic framework that is thought to be important in several rheumatic diseases, namely, that in genetically susceptible individuals, certain infectious agents may trigger a characteristic immune response that leads to arthritis.

Joint Findings. Joint fluid white cell counts range from 500 to 110,000 cells per mm³, with an average of about 25,000 cells per mm³, most of which are polymorphonuclear leukocytes.[2] Total protein ranges from 3 to 8 g per dl. C3 and C4 levels are generally greater than one third that of serum, and glucose levels are usually greater than two thirds that of serum. Synovial biopsies show villous hypertrophy, vascular proliferation, and a heavy infiltration of mononuclear cells, including plasma cells that are presumably capable of producing antibody locally.[2,6,7] In one patient with chronic Lyme arthritis, synovium grown in tissue culture produced large amounts of collagenase and prostaglandin E$_2$.[7] Thus, in Lyme disease, the joint fluid cell counts, the immune reactants (except for rheumatoid factor), the synovial histologic appearance, the amounts of synovial enzymes released, and the resulting destruction of cartilage and bone may be similar to what is seen in rheumatoid arthritis. These findings support the hypothesis that many possible agents, including the *I. dammini* spirochete, may trigger a common pathway in synovium leading to joint destruction.

Other Laboratory Findings. The most common nonspecific laboratory abnormality, particularly early in the illness, is a high erythrocyte sedimentation rate.[2,3] In addition, patients may be mildly anemic early in the illness and may occasionally have elevated white cell counts, with shifts to the left in the differential count. When ECM is present, about 20 percent of patients have an increased serum glutamic oxaloacetic transaminase (SGOT) level.[3] These patients usually also have increased levels of serum glutamic pyruvic transaminase (SGPT) and lactate dehydrogenase (LDH), but none has had abnormal creatine phosphokinase (CPK) levels. The enzyme levels generally return to normal within several weeks. A few patients have had microscopic hematuria, sometimes with mild proteinuria (dipstick), whereas values for creatinine and blood urea nitrogen (BUN) have been normal.

EPIDEMIOLOGY

Vector of Transmission. The vector of Lyme disease is the minute tick, *I. dammini,* or related ixodid ticks.[11-13] Of 314 patients examined from 1976 through 1982, 31 percent recalled having had a tick bite at the same skin site at which ECM developed 3 to 32 days later.[3] In addition, the histologic appearance of ECM is compatible with that of an arthropod bite.[2,3] In concomitant studies of patients and arthropods on both sides of the Connecticut River, the incidence of Lyme disease was almost 30 times as great,[12] and the number of *I. dammini* on preferred hosts (mice and deer) was more than 12 times as great on the east side (where Old Lyme is) as on the west side of the river.[13] With direct immunofluorescence, spirochetes were found in more than 20 percent of nymphal and adult *I. dammini* ticks in selected areas of Connecticut,[9] and in a study on Shelter Island, New York, the prevalence was 60 percent.[8] These prevalences of infected ticks are high for any vector-borne disease, but are consistent with the large number of cases and their close geographic clustering in affected areas.

Demographic Characteristics. Although the overall frequency of Lyme disease is unknown, currently 444

Figure 99–5. Antibody titers are shown against the *I. dammini* spirochete in serum samples from 135 patients with different clinical manifestations of Lyme disease and from 80 control subjects. The heavy bar shows the geometric mean titer for each group; the shaded areas indicate the range of titers generally observed in control subjects. (From Steere AC, et al.: N. Engl. J. Med. 308:733, 1983, reprinted with permission.)

of the 12,000 residents of the Old Lyme area are known to have had it—a cumulative frequency of 4 percent,[9] and 858 individuals have participated in Lyme disease studies at Yale. The earliest case that we know of occurred in Old Lyme, Connecticut, in 1965.[11] Each year, there have been more affected patients than in the preceding year. In our studies, the age of patients has ranged from 2 to 88 years (median 28 years), and the sex ratio is nearly 1:1.[3] Age-adjusted attack rates show that the risk of acquiring this illness is similar in all age groups through the fourth decade of life; thereafter, the risk drops, presumably because older residents are less likely to be exposed to tick-infested areas.[29]

Lyme disease seems to occur primarily in three distinct foci in the United States: (1) in the Northeast from Massachusetts to Maryland, (2) in the Midwest in Wisconsin and Minnesota, and (3) in the West in California and Oregon.[11,23] However, cases have also been reported in other states,[23] as well as in Germany,[24] Switzerland,[25] France,[26,27] and Australia.[28] The occurrence of cases in the United States correlates closely with the known distribution of *I. dammini* in the Northeast and Midwest and with *I. pacificus* in the West. Both species are members of the *I. ricinus* complex, which is the tick that is thought to transmit ECM in Europe. Onset of the illness is generally between May 1 and November 30; the ma-

jority of onsets are in June or July, the peak questing period of *I. dammini* nymphs.

OTHER SPIROCHETAL DISEASES

Lyme disease has similarities and differences when compared with other spirochetal infections, such as leptospirosis, syphilis, or relapsing fever. Like them, Lyme disease has different clinical stages with remissions and exacerbations. Although the stages may overlap or occur alone, the illness usually begins with ECM and associated symptoms (stage 1), followed weeks to months later by neurologic or cardiac abnormalities (stage 2), and weeks to years later by arthritis (stage 3). The early symptoms—headache, stiff neck, conjunctivitis, muscle and joint pain, profound weakness—and the neurologic and heart abnormalities are reminiscent of other spirochetal infections.[30-32] In addition, frank arthritis has been described as a rare feature of leptospirosis,[33,34] syphilis,[35-37] and relapsing fever.[32] However, the dermatologic manifestations of Lyme disease, particularly ECM, and the late manifestations, which consist primarily of intermittent or chronic arthritis, seem to be unique.

DIFFERENTIAL DIAGNOSIS

ECM is the unique clinical marker for Lyme disease (see Fig. 99–1). When this lesion is present in its classic form, there is little else that might be confused with it. However, in some patients, the lesion expands little and resembles the red papule that may follow an uninfected arthropod bite. In others, the lesion remains an even red as it expands, as in streptococcal cellulitis, or the center becomes vesicular or necrotic, as in tularemia. Patients with secondary lesions might be thought to have erythema multiforme; however, we have not observed blistering, mucosal lesions, or involvement of the palms and soles in Lyme disease. A malar rash, as seen in systemic lupus erythematosus, may occur. Instead of the typical secondary lesions, several patients have had a pruritic, urticarial rash, perhaps suggesting hepatitis B infection or serum sickness. As earlier lesions fade, some patients continue to have evanescent red blotches and circles. Evanescent lesions may resemble erythema marginatum, but those of Lyme disease do not expand.

The early manifestations of Lyme disease may be confused with viral infections, especially when ECM is absent or missed or is not the first manifestation. The severe headache and stiff neck may be reminiscent of aseptic meningitis; abdominal symptoms may be suggestive of hepatitis; and generalized, tender lymphadenopathy and splenomegaly may resemble infectious mononucleosis. As in infectious mononucleosis, profound fatigue is sometimes a major symptom in Lyme disease, and often the most persistent one.

The later manifestations of Lyme disease may mimic several immune-mediated disorders. Like rheumatic fever, Lyme disease may be associated with sore throat followed by migratory polyarthritis and carditis. However, we have not seen valvular involvement in Lyme disease. Migratory pain in tendons and joints may also suggest disseminated gonococcal infection. A few patients with neurologic involvement of Lyme disease have evidence of myelitis, which may be confused with multiple sclerosis, or symmetric peripheral neuropathy, reminiscent of the Guillain-Barré syndrome. In adults with Lyme disease, the large joint effusions, most commonly in knees, resemble those in Reiter's syndrome, and a few patients have had symmetric polyarthritis, which is suggestive of rheumatoid arthritis. In children, the attacks of arthritis in Lyme disease, though generally shorter, may be identical to those seen in the oligoarticular form of juvenile arthritis. However, we have not seen iridocyclitis in Lyme disease.

TREATMENT

During 1980 and 1981, we compared the efficacy of phenoxymethyl penicillin, erythromycin, and tetracycline in 108 patients with ECM.[20] In each instance the dosage was 250 mg four times per day for 10 days. At these dosages, the order of efficacy was tetracycline, penicillin, and erythromycin, but with each antibiotic,

treated patients did much better than untreated patients in an earlier study.[19] With tetracycline and penicillin, 18 and 15 percent of patients, respectively (generally those with more severe disease), had a Jarisch-Herxheimer–like reaction (higher fever, redder rash, or greater pain) during the first 24 hours after the start of antibiotic therapy. This happened less frequently with erythromycin (7 percent). ECM and its associated symptoms resolved significantly faster in penicillin- or tetracycline-treated patients than in those patients given erythromycin (mean duration, 5.4 and 5.7 days for penicillin and tetracycline, respectively, versus 9.2 days for erythromycin). In addition, fewer patients given penicillin (5 percent) or tetracycline (8 percent) than those treated with erythromycin (17 percent) required retreatment (10 more days of antibiotic therapy) because of persistence of symptoms or immediate relapse. More important, none of the 39 patients given tetracycline developed major late complications (myocarditis, meningoencephalitis, or recurrent attacks of arthritis) compared with 3 of 40 penicillin-treated patients (8 percent) and 4 of 29 given erythromycin (14 percent) (p = 0.07). In 1982, all 49 adult patients were given tetracycline, and again, none of them developed major complications.

Regardless of the antibiotic agent given, nearly 50 percent of patients had minor late complications—recurrent episodes of headache, or pain in joints, tendons, bursae, or muscles, often accompanied by lethargy.[20] However, except for five patients who had pain on motion of a joint or tendon or mild joint effusion, their examinations were normal. Symptoms were reminiscent of those experienced at the beginning of the illness, but were generally briefer and less severe. In a given attack, pain usually occurred in one or two sites and lasted from hours to days. With frequent attacks, the pain was often migratory. In 17 of 45 patients (38 percent), attacks occurred within the first year only after ECM; the remaining 28 patients had them for one or two years.

The pathogenesis of these symptoms is unclear. A severely depleted number of live spirochetes might continue to produce these less serious but sometimes debilitating symptoms. However, they occurred with equal frequency with each antibiotic given, and two patients with such symptoms did not respond to high-dose intravenous penicillin. It is also possible that late symptoms do not require the persistence of an intact organism.

Recommendations. When patients are early in the illness, we recommend treatment with oral tetracycline, 250 mg four times per day, for at least 10 days and up to 20 days if symptoms persist or recur. Phenoxymethyl penicillin, 500 mg four times per day, for the same duration, or 2.4 million U of benzathine penicillin intramuscularly may be theoretically as effective as the recommended tetracycline regimen, but these treatment schedules have not yet been tested in Lyme disease. In children, we recommend phenoxymethyl penicillin 50 mg per kg per day (not less than 1 g per day or more than 2 g per day) in divided doses for 10 days to 20 days, or in case of penicillin allergy, erythromycin, 30 mg per kg per day, in divided doses for 15 or 20 days. These doses of penicillin or erythromycin are high and may not be tolerated by all patients. Even with them, physicians should remain alert to the possibility of relapse or major late complications.

In patients who develop frank meningitis, spinal fluid pleocytosis, and cranial or peripheral neuropathies, intravenous penicillin G, 20 million units a day in divided doses for 10 days, is effective therapy.[21] Headache, stiff neck, and radicular pain usually begin to subside by the second day of therapy and are often gone by 7 to 10 days, but motor deficits frequently require 7 to 8 weeks for complete recovery.

Established Lyme arthritis can also be treated successfully with high-dose penicillin.[22] In a double-blind, placebo-controlled trial, 7 of 16 patients who received intramuscular benzathine penicillin remained well afterwards, but all 20 patients given saline coninued to have attacks of arthritis (p = 0.001). In a subsequent study, 13 of 20 patients given penicillin G, 20 million U a day intravenously for 10 days, have remained well, including both patients who were benzathine penicillin failures.

References

1. Steere, A.C., Malawista, S.E., Snydman, D.R., Shope, R.E., Andiman, W.A., Ross, M.R., and Steele, F.M.: Lyme arthritis: An epidemic of oligoarticular arthritis in children and adults in three Connecticut communities. Arthritis Rheum. 20:7, 1977.
2. Steere, A.C., Malawista, S.E., Hardin, J.A., Ruddy, S., Askenase, P.W., and Andiman, W.A.: Erythema chronicum migrans and Lyme arthritis: The enlarging clinical spectrum. Ann. Intern. Med. 86:685, 1977.
3. Steere, A.C., Bartenhagen, N.H., Craft, J.E., Hutchinson, G.J., Newman, J.H., Rahn, D.W., Sigal, L.H., Spieler, P.N., Stenn, K.S., and Malawista, S.E.: The early clinical manifestations of Lyme disease. Ann Intern. Med. 99:76, 1983.
4. Reik, L., Steere, A.C., Bartenhagen, N.H., Shope, R.E., and Malawista, S.E.: Neurologic abnormalities of Lyme disease. Medicine 58:281, 1979.
5. Steere, A.C., Batsford, W.P., Weinberg, M., Alexander, J., Berger, H.J., Wolfson, S., and Malawista, S.E.: Lyme carditis: Cardiac abnormalities of Lyme disease. Ann. Intern. Med. 93:8, 1980.
6. Steere, A.C., Gibofsky, A., Patarroyo, M.E., Winchester, R.J., Hardin, J.A., and Malawista, S.E.: Chronic Lyme arthritis: Clinical and immunogenetic differentiation from rheumatoid arthritis. Ann. Intern. Med. 90:286, 1979.
7. Steere, A.C., Brinckerhoff, C.E., Miller, D.J., Drinker, H., Harris, E.D., Jr., and Malawista, S.E.: Elevated levels of collagenase and prostaglandin E$_2$ from synovium associated with erosion of cartilage and bone in a patient with chronic Lyme arthritis. Arthritis Rheum. 23:591, 1980.
8. Burgdorfer, W., Barbour, A.G., Hayes, S.F., Benach, J.L., Grunwaldt, E., and Davis, J.P.: Lyme disease—A tick-borne spirochetosis? Science 216:1317, 1982.
9. Steere, A.C., Grodzicki, R.L. Kornblatt, A.N., Craft, J.E., Barbour, A.G., Burgdorfer, W., Schmid, G.P., Johnson, E., and Malawista, S.E.: The spirochetal etiology of Lyme disease. N. Engl. J. Med. 308:733, 1983.
10. Benach, J.L., Bosler, E.M., Hanrahan, J.P., Coleman, J.L., Habicht, G.S., Bast, T.F., Cameron, D.J., Ziegler, J.L., Barbour, A.G., Burgdorfer, W., Edelman, R., and Kaslow, R.A.: Spirochetes isolated from the blood of two patients with Lyme disease. N. Engl. J. Med. 308:740, 1983.
11. Steere, A.C., Malawista, S.E.: Cases of Lyme disease in the United States: Locations correlated with distribution of Ixodes dammini. Ann. Intern. Med. 91:730, 1979.
12. Steere, A.C., Broderick, T.E., and Malawista, S.E.: Erythema chronicum migrans and Lyme arthritis: Epidemiologic evidence for a tick vector. Am. J. Epidemiol. 108:312, 1978.
13. Wallis, R.C., Brown, S.E., Kloter, K.O., and Main, A.J., Jr.: Erythema chronicum migrans and Lyme arthritis: Field study of ticks. Am. J. Epidemiol. 108:322, 1978.
14. Steere, A.C., Hardin, J.A., and Malawista, S.E.: Erythema chronicum migrans and Lyme arthritis. Cryoimmunoglobulins and clinical activity of skin and joints. Science 196:1121, 1977.
15. Steere, A.C., Hardin, J.A., Ruddy, S., Mummaw, J.G., and Malawista, S.E.: Lyme arthritis: Correlation of serum and cryoglobulin IgM with activity and serum IgG with remission. Arthritis Rheum. 22:471, 1979.
16. Hardin, J.A., Walker, L.C., Steere, A.C., Trumble, T.C., Tung, K.S.K., Williams, R.C., Jr., Ruddy, S., and Malawista, S.E.: Circulating immune complexes in Lyme arthritis: Detection by the ^{125}I-C1q binding, C1q solid phase and Raji cell assays. J. Clin. Invest. 63:468, 1979.
17. Hardin, J.A., Steere, A.C., and Malawista, S.E.: Immune complexes and the evolution of Lyme arthritis: Dissemination and localization of abnormal C1q binding activity. N. Engl. J. Med. 301:1358, 1979.
18. Steere, A.C., Gibofsky, A., Hardin, J.A., Winchester, R.J., and Malawista, S.E.: Lyme arthritis: Immunologic and immunogenetic markers (abstract). Arthritis Rheum. 22:662, 1979.
19. Steere, A.C., Malawista, S.E., Newman, J.H., Spieler, P.N., and Bartenhagen, N.H.: Antibiotic therapy in Lyme disease. Ann. Intern. Med. 93:1, 1980.
20. Steere, A.C., Hutchinson, G.J., Rahn, D.W., Sigal, L.H., Craft, J.E., DeSanna, E.T., and Malawista S.E.: Treatment of the early manifestations of Lyme disease. Ann. Intern. Med. 99:22, 1983.
21. Steere, A.C., Pachner, A., and Malawista, S.E.: Neurologic abnormalities of Lyme disease: Successful treatment with high-dose intravenous penicillin. Ann Intern. Med. 99:767, 1983.
22. Steere, A.C., Green, J., Hutchinson, G.J., Rahn, D.W., Schoen, R., Sigal, L.H., and Malawista, S.E.: Curing Lyme arthritis: Successful antibiotic therapy of established joint involvement (abstract). Arthritis Rheum. 27:S26, 1984.
23. Centers for Disease Control: Lyme disease. MMWR 31:367, 1982.
24. Ackermann, R., Runne, U., Klenk, W., and Dienst, C.: Erythema chronicum migrans mit Arthritis. Dtsch. Med. Wochenschr. 105:1779, 1980.
25. Gerster, J.C., Guggi, J., Perroud, H., and Bovet, R.: Lyme arthritis appearing outside the United States: A case report from Switzerland. Br. Med. J. 283:951, 1981.
26. Illouz, G., and Hewitt, J.: A propos de l'arthrite de Lyme: Polyarthrite inflammatoire après un érythème annulaire migrant. Revue du Rheumatisme 48:813, 1981.
27. Mallecourt, J.M., Landurean, M., and Wirth, A.M.: Lyme's disease: a clinical case observed in Western France. Nouv. Presse Med. 11:39, 1982.
28. Stewart, A., Glass, J., Patel, A., Watt, G., Cripps, A., and Clancy, R.: Lyme arthritis in Hunter Valley. Med. J. Aust. 1:139, 1982.
29. Steere, A.C., and Malawista, S.E.: The epidemiology of Lyme disease. In Lawrence, R.C., and Schulman, L.E. (eds.): The Epidemiologic Study of the Rheumatic Diseases. Proceedings of the Fourth International Conference. New York, Gower Medical Publishing Limited, 1983, pp. 33–42.
30. Edwards, G.A., and Domm, B.M.: Human leptospirosis. Medicine 39:117, 1960.
31. Perine, P.L.: Immunology of syphilis. In Nahmias, A.J., and O'Reilly, R.J. (eds.): Immunology of Human Infection Part I: Bacteria, Mycoplasmae, Chlamydiae, and Fungi. New York, Plenum Medical Book Company, 1981, pp. 391–413.
32. Southern, P.M., Jr., and Sanford, J.P.: Relapsing fever: A clinical and microbiological review. Medicine 48:129, 1969.
33. Johnson, D.W.: The Australian leptospiroses. Med. J. Aust. 2:724, 1950.
34. Sutliff, D.W., Shepard, R., and Dunham, W.B.: Acute Leptospira pomona arthritis and myocarditis. Ann. Intern. Med. 39:134, 1953.
35. Wile, U.J., and Senear, F.E.: A study of the involvement of the bones and joints in early syphilis. Am. J. Med. Sci. 153:689, 1916.
36. Hench, P.S., Bauer, W., Boland, E.W., et al.: Rheumatism and arthritis: Review of American and English literature of recent years. Ann. Intern. Med. 28:66, 1948.
37. Reginato, A.J., Schumacher, H.R., Jimenez, S., and Maurer, K.: Synovitis in secondary syphilis: Clinical, light, and electron microscopic studies. Arthritis Rheum. 22:170, 1979.

Section XVII

Arthritis as a Manifestation of Other Systemic Diseases

Chapter 100

Hemophilia and Arthritis

Carlo L. Mainardi and Peter H. Levine

INTRODUCTION

Interference with the normal regulatory mechanisms of hemostasis can lead to spontaneous hemorrhage into joints, which can, in turn, lead to chronic arthritis and irreversible joint damage. Spontaneous hemarthrosis can occur in a variety of inherited disorders of coagulation[1-3] and has been a reported complication of anticoagulation therapy.[4] Hemophilia is the disorder in which recurrent hemarthrosis occurs most frequently, though chronic arthropathy has been reported in severe cases of von Willebrand's disease.[5] Bleeding into the joints is in fact the hallmark of the hemophilias and in the past has invariably led to chronic arthropathy and disability.

The term "hemophilia" refers to two disorders, hemophilia A and hemophilia B, in which a functional deficiency of a clotting factor—factor VIII and factor IX, respectively—leads to spontaneous hemorrhage.[1] They are both inherited as X-linked recessive disorders; however, there may be no family history of them in as many as 25 percent of cases.[6] In these diseases, the functional defect is in the intrinsic pathway of coagulation. The extrinsic, tissue factor–dependent pathway is functional in these patients[7] and presumably represents the major system regulating hemostasis in hemophiliacs. It is of interest that synovial tissue as well as cultures of synovial fibroblasts have been found to be deficient in tissue factor, and this may explain the marked propensity toward joint hemorrhage in these patients.[8,9]

CLINICAL FEATURES

The severity of hemophilia, as determined by the functional level of factor VIII or factor IX varies from patient to patient, but it remains constant in a single individual. The incidence and severity of joint disease are directly related to the severity of the coagulation defect. Ramgren has reported that nearly all patients with moderate or severe hemophilia (less than 5 percent activity of the deficient factor) had experienced hemarthrosis, whereas

less than half the patients with mild disease (greater than 5 percent activity) had ever bled into their joints.[10] The patients with mild disease only rarely had disability resulting from chronic arthropathy.[11] The joints most frequently involved were the knee, elbow, ankle, hip, and wrists.[12] According to a recent study, involvement of the small joints of the hands and feet occurs much more frequently than previously recognized.[13]

The first episode of acute hemarthrosis usually occurs during childhood but is very rare before the child begins to walk. The patient often senses a prodrome just before the acute episode. After several hours, mild discomfort and slight limitation of motion are noted. The joint is warm, a tense effusion is present, and the joint is generally held in flexion. Once bleeding has stopped, the blood is reabsorbed and the joint can return to normal. However, an episode of bleeding into a joint predisposes that joint to further episodes of hemarthrosis. There are two factors that may account for this phenomenon: (1) synovial proliferation with hypervascularity of the synovial membrane, and (2) atrophy of the periarticular musculature and a subsequent compromise in the protection provided by these muscles. Recurrent hemarthrosis leads to a condition in which abnormalities persist despite the absence of major bleeding episodes. In this stage, called subacute or chronic arthritis, the joint is characteristically painless with prominent synovial thickening, and an effusion is often present. A mild flexion deformity and mild limitation of motion are frequent findings at this stage. It is not clear whether this phenomenon is due to repeated minor hemorrhages or is related to irreversible synovial proliferation induced by previous hemarthrosis. However, it is this clinical picture that leads to the joint destruction seen in the advanced lesion.

The end stage of hemophilic arthropathy has features in common with both degenerative joint disease and longstanding rheumatoid arthritis. Joint function is lost, and motion is severely restricted. There is often an associated flexion deformity, and when ankylosis occurs it is generally fibrous and not bony. Subluxation, joint laxity, and alignment abnormalities are not uncommon.

Bleeding into muscles and soft tissues is also a common occurrence in hemophilia. There are a few specific syndromes with which rheumatologists should be familiar. The first of these is iliopsoas hemorrhage, which is associated with an acute onset of groin pain along with a flexion contracture of the hip. However, rotation of the hip is not limited, and this may help distinguish iliopsoas hemorrhage from acute hemorrhage in the hip joint. This lesion, if left untreated, can progress to the point of causing a compression neuropathy of the femoral nerve.[14,15] Other frequent sites of soft tissue bleeding are the forearm and the gastrocnemius. Bleeding into the forearm can cause a deformity resembling Volkmann's ischemic contracture. Bleeding into the gastrocnemius can cause a talipes equinus deformity.[14]

A rare skeletal complication of hemophilia is the development of a pseudotumor. This is a progressive cystic swelling involving soft tissues and adjacent bones and generally occurs following an inadequately treated major hematoma that becomes organized and highly vascular. Two types have been described: (1) the adult type that occurs proximally, usually in the pelvis or femur, and (2) a childhood type that generally occurs distal to the knee or elbow and carries a better prognosis than does the adult type. A period of correction of the coagulopathy is indicated but usually fails to resolve the tumorous lesion. If there is a progression of the lesion despite conservative therapeutic measures, surgery is indicated to avoid serious complications such as perforation, fistula formation, or fracture of adjacent bone. Aspiration of the pseudotumor is contraindicated.[6]

ROENTGENOGRAPHIC FEATURES

The earliest roentgenographic findings in hemophilic arthropathy are seen in the setting of acute hemarthrosis. The joint capsule is distended, and there is an increased hazy density caused by the intra-articular blood. With recurrent hemarthrosis and synovial thickening, there is often an increase in soft tissue density. During childhood, there are definite changes in the epiphyses. Initially, the epiphyses demonstrate overgrowth and irregularity, and this may be associated with lengthening of the affected extremity. Occasionally, premature closure of the epiphyses occurs.

As chronic proliferative synovitis progresses, marginal erosions develop, the joint space narrows, and irregularities appear along the surfaces of the subchondral bone. Chondrocalcinosis has been reported in association with chronic hemophilic arthropathy.[17] Subchondral bone cysts develop and can be quite large. These bony cysts are characteristic of hemophilic arthropathy. Osteophyte formation and bony overgrowth are common, whereas bony ankylosis is rare. In advanced cases, osteophyte formation, loss of joint space, and eburnation are seen and may be indistinguishable from degenerative joint disease.

The aforementioned changes are characteristic of hemophilic arthropathy but are not specific (Fig. 100–1A). Several findings are quite characteristic of the arthropathy seen in hemophilia. They include widening of the intercondylar notch of the femur, squaring of the distal margin of the patella in the lateral projection, and enlargement of the proximal radius (Fig. 100–1B). Hip involvement prior to puberty has features similar to those seen in Legg-Perthes disease, whereas a postpubertal patient has a lesion most closely resembling degenerative joint disease.[18] Flattening of the talus is somewhat characteristic of hemophilic arthritis, and bony ankylosis seems to occur more frequently in the ankle than in other joints.[19] A system of classification of the severity of hemophilic arthropathy by the degree of radiographic abnormality has been proposed.[20]

PATHOLOGIC FEATURES

Pathologic studies of hemophilic arthropathy have been limited to autopsy specimens and specimens obtained at surgery. Therefore, such studies have been scant, and observations may represent the advanced lesion only. However, well-conducted studies on dogs with hemophilia A have greatly improved our knowledge of the evolution of this lesion.[21] Clinical and pathologic observations would support the concept that canine hemophilia is an acceptable model for the human disease.

A single hemorrhage induces changes in the synovial membrane.[22] There is a varying inflammatory reaction, which includes the presence of polymorphonuclear leukocytes, lymphocytes, and mononuclear cells. Iron pigment begins to accumulate within synovial cells, and hyperplasia of synovial tissue occurs early. With concurrent hemarthrosis and chronic synovitis, villous hypertrophy of the synovium is prominent, and inflammatory cells are generally scanty (Fig. 100–2). The superficial cells are laden with hemosiderin, and the synovium is grossly pigmented. The subsynovial layer is thickened and fibrotic, and there are often macrophages present. The proliferative synovium eventually organizes into a pannus and begins to invade and erode the cartilage at its margin.[23]

The articular cartilage is also grossly abnormal. In addition to the marginal erosions caused by the hyperplastic synovium, changes similar to degenerative joint disease are apparent. Alcian blue staining has demonstrated a patchy distribution, indicating loss of glycosaminoglycan from the matrix. The chondrocytes are morphologically abnormal, displaying intracytoplasmic hemosiderin deposits, and the cells are often arranged in pairs and clusters. The iron pigment is primarily concentrated in the chrondrocytes. As fibrillation and fissuring occur, the cartilage thins and central erosions appear at weight-bearing surfaces.[24,25]

Bony changes include marginal osteophyte formation and subchondral bone cysts. The cysts are lined with synovial cells and communicate with the joint space.[21]

Figure 100–1. Roentgenographic changes of hemophilic arthropathy. *A,* Early arthritis of the knee, showing soft tissue swelling, widening of the femoral condyles and tibial plateau, irregularity of the distal femoral epiphysis, and a few subchondal bone cysts. *B,* More advanced arthritis involving the elbow, demonstrating almost complete loss of joint space and extensive subchondral cyst formation. The widening of the proximal radius is characterisic of hemophilic arthropathy.

Figure 100–2. Proliferative synovitis of hemophilia. Villous hypertrophy of synovium with pigment deposition in superficial cells. The reaction is mainly synovial cell hyperplasia. Infiltrating inflammatory cells are scarce. (Hematoxylin and eosin. × 250.)

PATHOGENESIS

It has seemed logical to attribute these striking pathologic changes to the recurrent hemarthrosis experienced by these humans and dogs. Numerous authors have tried to prove this relationship by injecting blood into the joint of a laboratory animal. Earlier studies of experimental hemarthrosis produced synovial changes identical to those seen in hemophilia, but the articular cartilage remained normal.[26-28] In 1967, however, Hoaglund produced articular cartilage changes characteristic of hemophilic arthropathy by repeatedly injecting blood into the knees of mongrel puppies for 18 weeks. In addition to synovial hypertrophy and pigmentation, cartilage fibrillation, pannus formation, and enlargement of the distal femoral epiphyses were noted.[29] Because of these studies, it can now be stated that hemophilic arthropathy in humans arises as a result of recurrent untreated joint hemorrhage.

Roy and Ghadially made some ultrastructural observations on specimens of synovium obtained from humans who had recently experienced hemarthrosis.[22] They reported evidence of villous hypertrophy as early as 4 days posthemorrhage with an increase in synovial type B cells and intermediate cells. They noted whole erythrocytes within the cytoplasm of synovial cells, suggesting that the cells were capable of phagocytosing whole red blood cells. Siderosomes were also seen in the cytoplasm of synovial cells and were evident as early as 4 days posthemorrhage. In further studies, these changes were reproduced by experimentally inducing hemarthrosis in adult rabbits.[30] In addition, these studies revealed large siderosomes in subsynovial macrophages. The hemosiderin deposits in the synovium persisted for 6 months after the last injection of blood.

It has been suggested that in rheumatoid arthritis the synovium consists of "activated" cells that, under the influence of various factors, release proteolytic enzymes capable of degrading the articular connective tissue. Hilgartner found elevated levels of acid phosphatase and cathepsin D in hemophilic synovial tissues.[31] Although these enzymes may be markers for an activated "state" of the cells, they are relatively inactive at neutral pH, and therefore are not likely to contribute to the extracellular degradation of connective tissue.[32] It has subsequently been demonstrated that both hemophilic synovium and adherent synovial cells isolated from hemophilic synovium release a neutral proteinase presumably capable of degrading the protein core of the glycosaminoglycan component of cartilage. Of perhaps greater importance was the observation that these cultures also released a collagenase in quantities equal to those reported from similar cultures of rheumatoid synovium.[33] Furthermore, it has been shown that when rabbit synovial fibroblasts were cultured in the presence of ionic iron, collagenase and prostaglandin$_2$ production were increased, and this increase correlated with the intracellular accumulation of iron.[34] This supports the hypothesis that repeated intra-articular hemorrhage can lead to the accumulation of iron in the synovial lining cells and alter the biology of these cells, resulting in the release of substances that contribute to connective tissue breakdown.

There is also evidence that would indicate that the destructive changes are due, at least in part, to the direct effect of intra-articular hemorrhage on the biology of cartilage. The pathologic similarities to degenerative joint disease would support this concept. Hough and colleagues studied human cartilage obtained from patients with hemophilia and found iron deposits in the chondrocytes and degradation of the ground substance surrounding these cells.[35] Further studies have shown that iron cultured with chondrocytes or cartilage slices accumulated in the cytoplasm of the cells and that this effect resulted in cytotoxicity.[36] It has also been shown that recurrent hemarthrosis in dogs was associated with a linear decrease in the hexosamine content of the cartilage and an associated loss of compressive stiffness.[37] These observations would suggest that joint hemorrhage may directly alter the biology of the chondrocyte and the biochemical composition of the cartilage, thereby rendering it less resistant to normal stresses placed on the joint.

The implication of these observations is that both chemical (enzymes and oxidants) and mechanical factors, perhaps working synergistically, contribute to the joint destruction seen in hemophilic arthropathy.

LABORATORY DIAGNOSIS

The diagnosis of hemophilia is generally made by the pediatrician or hematologist, and the rheumatologist is usually consulted for the management of difficult joint problems. Modern laboratory techniques have permitted accurate quantification of the factor deficiency and subsequent classification of the severity of the clotting defect. According to current practice, a factor VIII level of 100 percent is defined as the amount found in fresh frozen plasma obtained from many normal donors and pooled together. In more recent terminology, such reference plasma is defined as containing 1 U of factor VIII per ml. An individual with severe hemophilia—a factor VIII assay of 1 percent of normal—can also be said to have a factor VIII level of 0.01 U per ml of plasma. The factor VIII or factor IX level in a normal person on a given day may range between 50 percent and 200 percent (0.5 U to 2 U per ml).

Individuals with factor VIII or factor IX levels of ≤ 1 percent of normal (≤ 0.01 U per ml) will have joint and muscle hemorrhages requiring therapy three to four times per month on the average, though the range is large and the episodes are irregularly spaced. Such patients are classified as severe hemophiliacs. Individuals with factor VIII or factor IX levels of greater than 5 percent of normal (> 0.05 U per ml) are considered mild hemophiliacs, and usually hemorrhage only with trauma or at surgery. Occasionally, "spontaneous" hemarthrosis may occur in such patients, especially in joints damaged by previously undertreated hemorrhage. Patients whose factor VIII levels fall between the two ranges given are considered moderately severe, and their clinical picture falls someplace between the two extremes. If such patients have had multiple untreated or inadequately treated hemarthroses with subsequent joint damage, the anatomic instability of these joints will cause frequent and severe bleeding, and the patient's condition will appear clinically more severe than the factor VIII assay would suggest.

The treatment for each of the aforementioned disorders is unique to the disorder and is generally ineffectual for the others. "A unit of fresh frozen plasma" is no longer acceptable treatment for bleeding caused by any of these conditions, unless the disorder is unusually mild and the bleeding is trivial. For these reasons, adequate treatment requires a precise diagnosis, including (1) identification of the deficient factor (or factors), (2) precise quantitation of the factor level to allow accurate prognosis and calculation of replacement doses, and (3) determination of the presence or absence of an acquired inhibitor antibody against factor VIII or factor IX in patients with hemophilia A or hemophilia B.

THERAPY OF HEMARTHROSIS

Unlike most conditions in medical practice, hemophilia should be treated at the earliest symptoms suggestive of joint hemorrhage, long before the development of any physical findings. Only in this way can the long-term disabling sequelae be prevented.

The keystone of therapy in hemophilia is to provide the patient with access to immediate and adequate correction of the hemostatic defect at the earliest symptom suggestive of hemorrhage. For the majority of severe and moderately severe hemophiliacs, the achievement of this goal results from a combination of intensive education of the patient and the family and the institution of a carefully supervised home therapy program.

Most patients—except those with inhibitor antibodies, those that are highly unreliable or are unstable, or children less than 3 years of age—are candidates for home therapy, often with the support of family members or close friends. All suitable candidates should first undergo an initial detailed history and physical examination and a battery of appropriate laboratory and radiographic studies. The patient and the family are seen by two physicians who independently attempt to identify family members with the greatest potential competence, and these members are selected for further training. Since hemophilia treatment centers now exist in all areas of the United States and Canada, such training usually takes place at a major hemophilia center. The day to day supervision of the patient may often be provided by a physician in the patient's immediate geographic vicinity, with subsequent yearly visits to the center for longterm evaluation and comprehensive care.

At most centers, all patients and selected family members receive an individual half-day course on the pathophysiology, diagnosis, and therapy of hemophilia. Patients are taught the possible symptoms and signs of some of the major lesions of hemophilia and how much factor VIII or factor IX is needed for various types of bleeding. The patient and the family are then taught intravenous technique, and family members perform several venipunctures on each other. Special attention is also paid to the indications for making contact with their physician or the hemophilia center, which include the occurrence of any major hemorrhage or failure of a minor hemorrhage to resolve with two infusions at home.

The first several infusions are made under observation. If the patient demonstrates proficiency in self-infusion and a good grasp of basic principles, maximum independence is then allowed.

Patients are instructed to raise their factor VIII or factor IX level with home infusion at the first suggestion of joint or muscle hemorrhage. Prophylactic infusions are used for brief periods in occasional patients—as part of a therapy program for recurrent monarticular hemarthrosis or when a child is mastering a new physical activity such as bicycle riding.

All patients should attend yearly comprehensive evaluation sessions as a minimum mandatory requirement for continuation of the program. At this comprehensive clinic, a decision is made whether interim visits will be necessary during the ensuing year and whether changes in supportive health care measures are required. During the course of these evaluations, each patient is personally interviewed and examined by a hematologist, an or-

thopedic surgeon, or a rheumatologist, or all of them. The patient is also seen by a nurse practitioner, a medical social worker, a psychologist, an oral surgeon, a physical therapist, a vocational counselor, and, when indicated, a genetic counselor.

It should be emphasized that the least important aspect of self-therapy is teaching venipuncture. The program achieves its dramatic results through patient education plus the systematic application of the skills of a variety of appropriate medical personnel who can address (and usually prevent) the longterm problems of this lifelong disease.

Replacement Therapy

Factor VIII Replacement. The half-life of factor VIII in vivo is between 8 hours and 12 hours. Although the minimum plasma level necessary to achieve hemostasis will depend on the location, severity, and duration of hemorrhage, a level of 30 percent (0.30 U per ml) is generally sought for most acute hemorrhages. Early bleeding into muscles or joints will be arrested by a single infusion to attain this level in 95 percent of episodes. For advanced joint or muscle bleeding, a factor VIII level of 50 percent should be achieved.

The therapeutic material will contain a certain number of factor VIII units. One unit is equivalent to the factor VIII found in 1 ml of pooled fresh frozen plasma. For factor VIII, the replacement formula is as follows:

Each unit of factor VIII infused per kilogram
of body weight yields a 2 percent rise in
plasma VIII level (0.02 U per ml)

To achieve a 50 percent level in vivo, a 70-kg man with an advanced hemarthrosis would require 25 kg × 70 kg, or approximately 1750 U of factor VIII, assuming a starting point of essentially 0 percent of factor VIII. This calculation demonstrates why fresh frozen plasma cannot be used in hemophilia; it would require 1750 ml of this material just to achieve the initial desired level, and volume overload would likely result.

If a given minimum level is to be maintained over several days, it can be achieved by (1) giving an initial infusion to twice the desired minimum; (2) giving one half this dose every 12 hours, assuming a 12-hour half-life; or (3) performing factor VIII assays every several days for more precise dose adjustments. For example, a 50-kg boy has undergone arthroscopy of the knee, requiring that his levels of factor VIII be kept above 30 percent until healing is complete. An initial infusion is given to attain the 60 percent level—30 kg × 50 kg, or 1500 units of factor VIII. He then receives 750 U every 12 hours thereafter for 7 to 10 days.

Wet frozen cryoprecipitate was the replacement product of choice several years ago and is still used as such in some centers. It should preferentially be used when the patient has mild hemophilia and seldom requires exposure to blood products, in order to minimize the risk of hepatitis. The plasma product requirements of patients with moderately severe or severe hemophilia will be such that clinical or subclinical hepatitis appears to be as frequent with cryoprecipitate as with commercial concentrates, according to several recent studies. The average bag of cryoprecipitates from the average blood center should be assumed to contain approximately 70 U of factor VIII for purposes of calculation. Thus, the hemophiliac who requires 1500 U of factor VIII should receive 21 bags of cryoprecipitate.

At least eight different commercial factor VIII concentrates are now available. They are made from large pools of normal plasma and are sold in lyophilized form. When reconstituted, one can administer 1000 U of factor VIII in 30-ml to 100-ml volume, depending on the product used. Each vial is labeled with the number of units it contains, and such figures are quite accurate. These products not only allow accurate dose calculations but also are convenient for home use, are stable at home refrigerator temperature for months to years and at room temperature for weeks to months, and can be rapidly prepared for self-administration. The major disadvantage is cost. Current prices are in the range of $0.07 to $0.12 per factor VIII U ($17.50 to $27.50 per 250-U vial) wholesale cost. These materials have made early and intensive home therapy possible, however, and thus overall costs of health care have greatly declined for patients treated with these materials.

Occasional patients develop allergic reactions to cryoprecipitate, usually manifested as urticaria, pruritus, or low-grade fever. Rarely, bronchospasm or serious anaphylactoid reactions have been reported. Allergic reactions to commercial concentrate are quite infrequent and very mild.

The major side effect with either cryoprecipitate or factor VIII concentrate is hepatitis, which may be either type A or type B, or type non-A or type non-B. Hemophiliacs also have high titers of cytomegalovirus antibody, and this virus or other viruses may also contribute to liver dysfunction. In most series, the great majority of treated hemophiliacs will have plasma levels of hepatitis B surface antibody, and a significant minority (2 to 5 percent) will carry hepatitis B surface antigen. Presumably because of their extensive exposure to plasma products from an early age, the incidence of overt clinical hepatitis in moderately severe or severe hemophiliacs who receive pooled commercial concentrate is very low.

A newly recognized problem in hemophilia is the development of acquired immune deficiency syndrome (AIDS), reported in a small number of individuals and presumed to be transmitted or induced by exposure to blood products.[38] This frequently fatal disorder is characterized by recurrent opportunistic infections such as *Pneumocystis carinii* pneumonia, candidiasis, cytomegalovirus, toxoplasmosis or atypical mycobacterium; Kaposi's sarcoma; generalized lymphadenopathy; cutaneous anergy; reduced helper T lymphocytes and increased suppressor T lymphocytes, with inverted helper:suppressor (T4:T8) ratios; decreased natural killer cell activity, and hyperglobulinemia. It has also been noted that repeated exposure to pooled plasma derivatives can lead to abnormal T4:T8 ratios in hemophilia.[39,40] The significance of this finding is unclear at this time.

The development of inhibitor antibody occurs only after exposure to factor VIII, but is not related to the source of replacement product or to the frequency or intensity of exposure. Recent data suggest that there may be a familial predisposition to the development of this dreaded complication. Because bleeding cannot be reliably controlled in patients with inhibitor antibodies, elective surgery should not be considered in such patients. The treatment of patients with inhibitor antibodies will be discussed later in this chapter.

Factor IX Replacement. Factor IX is not found in either cryoprecipitate or factor VIII concentrate; these two materials are totally ineffective for the treatment of hemophilia B.

The half-life of factor IX *in vivo* is between 20 hours and 24 hours. Although the plasma level necessary to achieve hemostasis will depend on the location, severity, and duration of hemorrhage, the minimum hemostatic level appears to be somewhat less than that needed for factor VIII. A minimum level of 20 percent (0.20 U per ml) is generally sought for most acute hemorrhages. Early bleeding into muscles or joints will be permanently arrested by a single infusion to attain this level in 95 percent of episodes. For more advanced joint or muscle bleeding, a factor IX level of 40 percent should be achieved.

The therapeutic material will contain a number of factor IX units. One unit is equivalent to the factor IX found in 1 ml of pooled fresh frozen plasma. The replacement formula for factor IX is as follows:

Each unit of factor IX infused per kilogram of body weight yields a 1 percent rise in plasma IX level (0.01 unit per l)

To achieve a 20 percent level in vivo in a 70-kg man with an early hemarthrosis would require 20 kg × 70 kg, or approximately 1400 U of factor IX, assuming a starting point of essentially 0 percent of factor IX. Because factor IX has a significantly longer half-life than does factor VIII, and because lower in vivo minimum levels appear necessary for hemostasis, fresh frozen plasma is still sometimes used in hemophilia B. However, for patients with moderately severe or severe hemophilia, or for prolonged or major bleeding, factor IX concentrate is generally preferred.

If a given minimum level is to be maintained over several days, it can be achieved by methods similar to those described for factor VIII, except that the half-life of 24 hours (as compared with approximately 12 hours for factor VIII) indicates the need for either lower or less frequent subsequent doses by a factor of 50 percent. Factor IX assays should be monitored every few days for adequate control.

There are two commercially available factor IX concentrates at present. Both products contain factors II, VII, IX, and X, but because of the high risk of hepatitis for individuals not frequently exposed to blood products previously, these products should probably be used only for the treatment of hemophilia B. In addition to the allergic and infectious side effects already listed for factor VIII concentrate, factor IX may also predispose to deep venous as well as other types of thrombosis. Such thrombosis has generally been associated with very large doses of factor IX given in the setting of general anesthesia and surgery, or in patients with clinically overt hepatic dysfunction. Some physicians recommend the addition of small doses of heparin to the factor IX concentrate or directly to the recipient in cases of large-dose factor IX replacement for surgery. Thrombosis has not been recorded in the home therapy of routine acute hemorrhage in hemophilia.

Inhibitor Antibodies. Inhibitor antibodies in factor VIII–deficient hemophiliacs have a highly unpredictable natural history. At times, very low titer and clinically weak antibodies are easily neutralized by factor VIII and are found not to undergo anamnestic rises in titer after multiple factor VIII challenges. Such antibodies may unexpectedly become high in titer. Other patients will develop rising antibody titers after each exposure to factor VIII. Still other patients appear to have spontaneously lost their antibody despite multiple subsequent factor VIII challenges. The type of antibody response to factor VIII infusion and the patient's clinical response will dictate therapy. The therapy of patients with inhibitor ranges from total avoidance of all exposure to factor VIII in some centers to aggressive megadose factor VIII replacement in others. Possibly because of factor X concentrate's variable contamination with activated factor VII or factor X, it is thought to be efficacious by some, and is usually given in large doses, for example, 50 U to 100 U of factor IX activity per kilogram of body weight. The use of immunosuppressives or corticosteroids had been abandoned in most centers owing to lack of efficacy in this condition and to serious side effects.

In our experience, patients with low-titer antibodies that remain low in titer after repeated therapy often do well with standard but repeated doses of factor VIII concentrate. For those patients who fail to benefit or who have higher titers of antibodies, factor IX concentrate is used. Both groups of patients are often on home therapy, and bleeding is more likely to be arrested when treatment is applied at once than if it is delayed.

Purposefully, activated factor IX concentrate has recently been shown useful in certain patients with inhibitor antibodies who are treatment failures, or for surgical emergencies, but such agents are not always effective.[41]

Inhibitor antibody against factor IX is exceedingly rare. There is no generally accepted efficacious therapy. Treatment is usually reserved for severe episodes and usually includes large and frequent doses of factor IX concentrate.

Because bleeding cannot be reliably controlled in patients with inhibitor antibodies, elective surgery should not be considered in such patients.

Acute Hemarthrosis. The single most important measure in the therapy of acute hemarthrosis is prompt correction of the clotting abnormality by administration of the deficient factor. Some investigators have advocated the use of a short course of oral corticosteroids (5 days) at the time of particularly severe or advanced acute episodes, though this practice remains controversial.[42] Arthrocentesis with evacuation of the joint is generally accepted as beneficial if done within the first 24 hours and after the deficient factor has been administered. Pain relief is often accomplished by the administration of analgesics and by splinting the affected joint. Immobilization should be limited to about 2 days in order to avoid muscle atrophy. At this point, passive range of motion and isometric exercises should be initiated.

Chronic Hemophilic Arthropathy. Along with several weeks or months of regular, prophylactic infusions of factor VIII or factor IX a variety of conservative maneuvers can bring remarkable benefit. These include (1) intensive physical therapy for muscle building and increased joint stability; (2) periods of avoiding weight bearing to allow regression of synovitis; (3) correction of flexion contractures by wedging casts, night splints, or the judicious use of traction, and (4) training in sports to allow future maintenance of muscle mass. In modern treatment programs, aspiration of joints is rarely necessary, but it can be accomplished following appropriate hemostatic correction when very large acute joint hemorrhages are encountered.

Chronic joint effusions more frequently reflect an underlying synovitis, and arthrocentesis is seldom of lasting benefit. Chronic synovitis should first be treated with a period of intensive factor VIII or factor IX replacement plus conservative orthopedic and physical therapy measures. Many clinicians advocate aspirating the joint dry initially, as well as the use of intra-articular corticosteroid in a single dose and several days of oral corticosteroids at the start of the period of conservative therapy for chronic synovitis.

The value of nonsteroidal anti-inflammatory drugs (NSAID) in hemophilia is unproved, and these agents should be used with caution considering their potential effect on platelet function and their propensity to cause gastrointestinal bleeding. Recent studies have suggested that choline magnesium trisalicylate and ibuprofen can be safely administered to hemophiliacs and afford some symptomatic relief, though the abatement of symptoms may be related to the analgesic effect of these agents.[43,44] When it seems clear that chronic joint pain is due to degenerative arthropathy rather than to bleeding, a period of NSAID therapy may be tried and will sometimes cause excellent symptomatic relief. An occasional patient may be particularly sensitive to these drugs, and measurement of bleeding times and close followup for an increased rate of new hemorrhages are recommended.

Surgery in Hemophilia

Despite the highly successful home therapy programs for hemophiliacs, patients may still experience chronic proliferative synovitis that fails to regress with intensive replacement therapy. These are the patients who are often considered as surgical candidates. The availability of factor VIII concentrates and accurate laboratory monitoring has made surgery in the hemophiliac a rather commonplace occurrence. Surgical synovectomy has been performed on numerous patients with refractory proliferative synovitis, and the results have been mixed.[45-47] The potential benefits of this procedure include a decrease in the frequency of hemarthrosis (at least in the short-term) and a general improvement in joint function. However, these benefits must be weighed against the high cost of hospitalization and replacement therapy, the high rate of postoperative complications, and the long rehabilitation period. Total knee replacement has also been performed on hemophiliacs.[45,48,49] The results have been generally favorable after brief followup. The true value of these surgical procedures will require longterm followup of operated patients.

The following general requirements should be met before surgery is undertaken: (1) a hematologist and diagnostic coagulation laboratory should be available; (2) the surgeon should be familiar with the handling of a patient with a coagulation disorder; (3) there should be a blood bank capable of providing adequate supplies of appropriate replacement material; (4) there should be an appropriate rehabilitation team for postoperative management; and (5) no inhibitor antibody should be present. The last point should be rechecked a few days before surgery.

As orthopedic, general, oral, and other kinds of surgery become increasingly commonplace in the hemophiliac, certain guidelines require re-emphasis. Both physician and patient should consider the following points in an orderly and systematic manner before surgery is undertaken.

1. Will the lesion recur postoperatively? If the lesion developed because of inadequate medical control of hemophilia, it may well recur. This principle is of special importance with respect to orthopedic surgery in hemophilia. Orthopedic surgery will often fail when the patient has demonstrated unreliability in adhering to a conservative regimen. For this reason, elective orthopedic surgery should be preceded by a period of intensive nonsurgical management. This will emphasize to the patient the importance of basic medical principles (e.g., immediate infusion at the first sign of hemorrhage, appropriate physical therapy). It will also test the patient's ability to adhere to the regimen.

2. Have the patient avoid antiplatelet medication before and after surgery. Aspirin and aspirin-containing medications such as Darvon Compound, Empirin, or Percodan, can inhibit platelet function for as long as 10 days. The effect of non-aspirin-containing, nonsteroidal anti-inflammatory drugs on clotting mechanisms is of shorter duration after they are discontinued (1 day to 2 days).

3. Schedule the surgery for Monday or Tuesday. This allows the best availability of laboratory services for factor assays and the best access to consultants during the first few days after surgery.

4. Check the supply of replacement therapeutics. Calculate the expected dose of material needed for a period of at least 2 weeks, multiply by 2, and notify the blood bank or pharmacy of your need. Ask them to confirm the arrival of the material; do not proceed with surgery until such confirmation has been received.

5. Consider multiple procedures. Because of the great expense of hospitalization and replacement therapy, it makes sense to perform minor procedures such as dental extractions or excision of cutaneous lesions at the same time as major ones. These should be performed a day or two prior to the major surgery in some cases. For example, oral surgery with its transient bacteremia might increase the risk of osteomyelitis if done on the same day as elective orthopedic surgery.

6. Schedule a preoperative conference among the patient, the family, and the physicians involved. This can often be conveniently done on the day of admission to the hospital. The benefits of such communications are obvious. Many patients or family members may have an unstated fear of fatal bleeding, and will respond dramatically to reassurance on this issue.

7. In the order book write: "Hemophiliac: IM medications contraindicated. Patient may not be given aspirin in any form, including Darvon Compound, Empirin, or Percodan. Avoid prescription of any compound medicine to avoid unnoticed aspirin. Joint or muscle pain may indicate hemorrhage — notify physician at once for possible coagulation factor infusion." These same instructions should be taped to the cover of the patient's chart holder, to ensure that they are seen by all house officers, medical students, medical consultants, and nursing staff.

For major surgery, the factor VIII levels should be brought to the 80 percent to 100 percent range just prior to the surgery, and then should be kept at more than 30 percent for 10 to 14 days. For extensive orthopedic surgery, 4 to 6 weeks of replacement may be required. For example, a 50-kg boy will require major surgery. To achieve an 80 percent factor VIII level, give 40 U per kilogram, or 2000 factor VIII U (e.g., 30 bags of cryoprecipitate averaging 70 U per bag, or two vials of factor VIII concentrate averaging 1000 U per vial). Twelve hours later, his factor VIII level will have fallen to approximately 40 percent. One could then give 1000 factor VIII units every 12 hours to keep in the desired range. For the factor IX–deficient patient, initial levels of approximately 60 percent should be achieved. Given the possible development of thromboembolic complications and the current use of concomitant heparin in these patients, a hematologist should design the specific program for each factor IX–deficient patient. A recent development in therapy is the use of arginine vasopressin (DDAVP) to raise the factor VIII level in patients with mild hemophilia A or von Willebrand's disease.[50]

The best therapy for hemophilic arthropathy remains its prevention, and prevention is now clearly attainable. With a combination of early and aggressive replacement therapy, patient education, application of comprehensive care, and emphasis on the importance of physical activity to maintain muscle mass, new or progressive arthropathy can usually be reduced to nil.

References

1. Houghie, C.: Hemophilia and related conditions—congenital deficiencies of prothrombin (factor II), factor V, and factors VII and XII. *In* Williams, W.J., Beutler, E., Erslev, A.J., et al. (eds.): Hematology. 2nd ed. New York, McGraw-Hill Book Co., 1977.

2. Larrieu, J.M., Caen, J.P., Meyer, D.O., et al.: Congenital bleeding disorders with long bleeding time and normal platelet count. II. Von Willebrand's disease (report of thirty-seven patients). Am. J. Med. 45:354, 1968.

3. Egbring, Von R., Andreassy, K., Egli, H., et al.: Disgnostische and therapeutische Probleme bei congenitaler Afribrinogenämie. Blut 22:175, 1971.

4. Wild, J.H., and Zvaifler, N.J.: Hemarthrosis associated with sodium warfarin therapy. Arthritis Rheum. 19:98, 1976.

5. Ahlberg, A., and Silwer, J.: Arthropathy in von Willebrand's disease. Acta Orthop. Scand. 41:539, 1970.

6. Ramgren, O., Nilsson, I.M., and Blomback, M.: Haemophilia in Sweden. IV. Hereditary investigations. Acta Med. Scand. 171:759, 1962.

7. Astrup, T., and Brakman, P.: Tissue repair and vascular disease in hemophilia. *In* Brinkhous, K.M., and Hemker, H.C. (eds.): Handbook of Hemophilia. Part I. New York, American Elsevier Publishing Co., Inc., 1975.

8. Astrup, T., and Sjolin, K.E.: Thromboplastic and fibrinolytic activity of the synovial membrane and fibrous capsular tissue. Proc. Soc. Exp. Biol. Med. 97:852, 1958.

9. Green, D., Ryan, C., Malandruccuolo, N., et al.: Characterization of the coagulant activity of cultured human fibroblasts. Blood 37:47, 1971.

10. Ramgren, O.: Hemophilia in Sweden. III. Symptomatology, with special reference to differences between hemophilia A and B. Acta Med. Scand. 171:237, 1962.

11. Ahlberg, A.: Hemophilia in Sweden. VII. Incidence, treatment, and prophylaxis of arthropathy and other musculoskeletal manifestations of hemophilia A and B. Acta Orthop. Scand. (Suppl.) 77:38, 1965.

12. Jordan, H.H.: Hemophilic Arthropathies. Springfield, Ill. Charles C Thomas, 1958.

13. Pavlon, H., Goldman, A.B., and Arnold, W.D.: Hemophilic arthropathy in the joints of the hands and feet. Br. J. Radiol. 52:173, 1979.

14. Gilbert, M.S.: Musculoskeletal manifestations of hemophilia. Mt. Sinai J. Med. 44:339, 1977.

15. Goodfellow, J., Fearn, B.D., and Matthews, J.M.: Iliacus hematoma. J. Bone Joint Surg. 49B:748, 1967.

16. Ahlberg, A.: On the natural history of hemophilic pseudotumor. J. Bone Joint Surg. 57A:1133, 1975.

17. Jensen, P.S., and Putman, C.E.: Chondrocalcinosis and hemophilia. Clin. Radiol. 28:401, 1977.

18. Winston, M.E.: Hemophiliac arthropathy of the hip. J. Bone Joint Surg. 34B:412, 1952.

19. Schreiber, R.R.: Musculoskeletal system—radiologic findings. *In* Brinkhous, K.M., and Hemker, H.C. (eds.): Handbook of Hemophilia. Part I. New York, American Elsevier Publishing Co. Inc., 1975.

20. Patterson, H., Ahlberg, A., and Nilsson, M. A radiologic classification of hemophilic arthropathy. Clin. Orthop. 149:153, 1980.

21. Swanton, M.C., and Wysocki, G.P.: Pathology of joints in canine hemophilia A. *In* Brinkhous, K.M., and Hemker, H.C. (eds.): Handbook of Hemophilia. Part I. New York, American Elsevier Publishing Co., 1975.

22. Roy, S., and Ghadially, F.N.: Ultrastructure of synovial membrane in human hemarthrosis. J. Bone Joint Surg. 49A:1636, 1967.

23. Van Creveld, S., Hoedemaker, P.J., Kingman, M.J., et al.: Degeneration of joints in hemophiliacs under treatment by modern methods. J. Bone Joint Surg. 53B:296, 1971.

24. Hoedemaker, P.J., and Wagenvoort, C.A.: Pathological changes in patients

25. Stein, H., and Duthie, R.B.: The pathogenesis of chronic haemophilic arthropathy. J. Bone Joint Surg. 63B:601, 1981.

26. Key, J.A.: Experimental arthritis. The reaction of joints to mild irritants. J. Bone Joint Surg. 11:705, 1929.

27. Young, J.M., and Hudacek, A.C.: Experimental production of pigmented villonodular synovitis in dogs. Am. J. Pathol. 30:799, 1954.

28. Wolf, C.R., and Mankin, H.J.: The effect of experimental hemarthrosis on articular cartilage of rabbit knee joints. J. Bone Joint Surg. 47A:1203, 1965.

29. Hoaglund, F.T.: Experimental hemarthrosis. J. Bone Joint Surg. 49A:285, 1967.

30. Roy, S., and Ghadially, F.N.: Synovial membrane in experimentally produced chronic hemarthrosis. Ann. Rheum. Dis. 28:402, 1969.

31. Hilgartner, M.W.: Hemophilic arthropathy. Adv. Pediatr. 21:139, 1975.

32. Barrett, A.J.: Cathepsin D and other carboxyl proteinases. *In* Barrett, A.J. (ed.): Proteinases in Mammalian Cells and Tissues. Amsterdam, North-Holland Publishing Co., 1977.

33. Mainardi, C.L., Levine, P.H., Werb, Z., et al.: Proliferative synovitis in hemophilia. Biochemical and morphologic observations. Arthritis Rheum. 21:137, 1978.

34. Okazaki, I., Brinckerhoff, C.E., Sinclair, J.F., et al.: Iron increases collagenase production by rabbit synovial fibroblasts. J. Lab. Clin. Med. 97:396, 1981.

35. Hough, A.J., Banfield, W.G., and Sokoloff, L.: Cartilage in hemophilic arthropathy. Arch. Pathol. Lab. Med. 100:91, 1976.

36. Choi, Y-C., Hough, A.J., Morris, G.M., et al.: Experimental siderosis of articular chondrocytes cultured *in vitro*. Arthritis Rheum. 24:809, 1981.

37. Convery, F.R., Woo, S.L-Y., Akeson, W.F., et al.: Experimental hemarthrosis in the knee of the mature canine. Arthritis Rheum. 19:59, 1976.

38. Update on acquired immunodeficiency syndrome (AIDS) among patients with hemophilia A. Morbidity Mortality Weekly Report 31:644–646; 652, 1982.

39. Lederman, M.M., Ratnoff, O.D., Scillian, J.J., et al.: Impaired cell-mediated immunity in patients with classic hemophilia. N. Engl. J. Med. 308:79, 1983.

40. Menitove, J.E., Aster, R.H., Casper, J.T., et al.: T-lymphocyte subpopulations in patients with classic hemophilia treated with cryoprecipitate and lyophilized concentrates. N. Engl. J. Med. 308:83, 1983.

41. Lusher, J.M., Shapiro, S.S., Palascak, J.E., et al. Efficacy of prothrombin complex concentrates in hemophiliacs with antibodies to factor VIII. N. Engl. J. Med. 303:421, 1980.

42. Kisker, C.T., and Burke, C.: Double-blind studies on the use of corticosteroids in the treatment of acute hemarthrosis in patients with hemophilia. N. Engl. J. Med. 282:639, 1970.

43. Thomas, P., Hepburn, B., Kim, H.C., et al.: Nonsteroidal anti-inflammatory drugs in the treatment of hemophilic arthropathy. Am. J. Hematol. 12:131, 1982.

44. McIntyre, B.A., Philp, R.B., and Inwood, M.J.: Effect of ibuprofen on platelet function in normal subjects and hemophiliac patients. Clin. Pharmacol. Ther, 24:616, 1978.

45. McCollough, N.C., Enis, J.E., Lovitt, J., et al.: Synovectomy or total replacement of the knee in hemophilia. J. Bone Joint Surg. 61A:69, 1979.

46. Sneppen, O., Beck, H., and Holsteen, V.: Synovectomy as a prophylactic measure in recurrent haemophilic haemarthrosis. Acta Paediatr. Scand. 67:491, 1978.

47. Kay, L., Stainsby, D., Buzzard, B., et al.: The role of synovectomy in the management of recurrent haemarthroses in haemophilia. Br. J. Haematol. 49:53, 1981.

48. Marmor, L.: Total knee replacement in hemophilia. Clin. Orthop. Rel. Res. 125:192, 1977.

49. Goldberg, V.M., Heiple, K.G., Ratnoff, O.D., et al.: Total knee arthroplasty in classic hemophilia. J. Bone Joint Surg. 63A:695, 1981.

50. Manucci, P.M.: DDAVP in haemophilia. Lancet 2:1171, 1977.

Chapter 101

Arthritis Associated with Sickle Cell Disease and Other Hemoglobinopathies

H. Ralph Schumacher, Jr.

INTRODUCTION

A variety of musculoskeletal manifestations have been described in sickle cell disease. Most problems can be seen not only in homozygous sickle cell (hemoglobulin SS) disease but also in sickle C hemoglobin disease, sickle-thalassemia disease and sickle F hemoglobin disease. Rheumatic manifestations appear to be rare in sickle trait (hemoglobin AS) but have been reported in β-thalassemia.

Hemoglobin S, which is most common in blacks, results from the substitution of a single amino acid in the β-chain of hemoglobin.[1] Normally present glutamic acid is replaced by valine. This change produces severe systemic disease, which is manifested by sickling. When this sickling occurs in small vessels it is the presumed basis for the painful crises. Abnormal interactions between sickled erythrocytes and endothelium have recently received emphasis.[2] Other manifestations are hemolytic anemia, hyposthenuria, leg ulcers, hyporegenerative crises, increased infections—especially with salmonellae, and the bone and joint problems to be discussed further on. Diagnosis is suspected when sickled cells are identified in vitro through the use of reducing agents such as metabisulfite. Diagnosis of the homozygous disease is established by starch or cellulose acetate hemoglobin electrophoresis showing 76 percent to 100 percent hemoglobin S. The altered charge in the mutant form of hemoglobin allows distinctive changes in migration in the electric field.

Hemoglobin C disease is less common and is caused by the substitution of lysine for glutamic acid in the β-chains. The pure disease produces some hemolysis and many target cells, but this abnormal hemoglobin is most important when combined with hemoglobin S. Hemoglobin SC has generally been associated with a high frequency of aseptic necrosis of bone. A recent review however, suggests that this, and bone disease in general, is not as common as in homozygous sickle cell disease, although thromboembolic problems are more common with SC hemoglobin.[3] More than 300 human hemoglobin variants have been discovered; most are caused by mutations in single amino acids.[4] The great majority are of no known clinical significance. Other abnormal hemoglobins can be associated with hemoglobin S, but there is little information about their musculoskeletal manifestations.

β-thalassemia refers to another inherited disorder that is especially common in persons of Mediterranean background. β-chains are reduced, producing a very unstable hemoglobin with formation of Heinz bodies. There are high levels of hemoglobin F. Patients with β-thalassemia have hemolytic anemia, splenomegaly, and hyperplastic bone marrows, producing changes on skeletal x-rays. Patients with a combination of β-thalassemia with hemoglobin S often have increased hemoglobin A2. This hemoglobinopathy clinically combines features of thalassemia and homozygous sickle cell disease.

SICKLE CELL DISEASE

Bone Trabecular Changes Associated With Expansion of the Bone Marrow. Sickle cell disease and other hemoglobinopathies asociated with hemolysis cause characteristic expansion of the bone marrow. Marrow expansion produces wider intertrabecular spaces with coarser trabeculations that are most evident in the axial skeleton in which red (hematopoietic) marrow is most plentiful (Fig. 101–1). In sickle cell patients, red marrow also persists more peripherally in the long bones near joints and even in the small tarsal and carpal bones, often causing some thinning of cortical bone with widening of the medulla. Total width of the bone may be increased. Radiographic signs of marrow expansion vary widely and can be quite subtle.

In patients with SC hemoglobin, hemolysis tends to be less, and there are fewer bone trabecular changes.[5] Scattered increased densities can interrupt trabecular patterns and are probably due to areas of marrow infarction (see later discussion).

Skull x-rays can show thickening of the diploë with a granular texture. Occasionally in severe sickle cell disease the coarse trabeculae are arranged perpendicular to the curvature of the vault, giving "hair-on-end" or "porcupine quill" trabeculae. This is more common in thalassemia major than in sickle cell disease[6] and has not been seen in SC hemoglobin disease.[7]

Vertebral bodies may also have characteristic alterations. Coarsened trabeculae are most often vertical, and the bodies of the vertebrae can have a characteristic deep central cuplike indentation[6,8] (Fig. 101–2). Vertebral compression can occur with resulting accentuated dorsal kyphosis and lumbar lordosis. Osteophytes occasionally

Figure 101–1. Radiograph showing coarsened trabeculae from marrow expansion in severe sickle cell anemia. Some focal densities may be a result of bone infarctions.

Figure 101–2. Cuplike indentation of vertebral body in radiograph in sickle cell disease.

develop, and even fusion of vertebrae has been seen (see later). Bone changes in sickle cell patients caused by increased hematopoiesis appear to be asymptomatic except when secondary mechanical problems develop.

Protrusio acetabuli has been reported in 14 of 155 adults with sickle cell disease and pelvic radiographs. This did not correlate with changes in the femoral head and was felt to be a result of softening of acetabuar bone.[8a]

The Hand-Foot Syndrome. Children from 6 months to 2 years of age may develop the hand-foot syndrome. This consists of dramatic, diffuse, symmetric, very tender, warm swelling of the hands (Fig. 101–3) or feet, or both.[9,10] This can be the first manifestation of sickle cell disease. Hematologic signs and fever may be absent, or fever may be present with peripheral blood leukocytosis up to 55,000 per mm^3.[11] Swelling lasts 1 week to 3 weeks. Infarction of marrow, cortical bone, periosteum, and periarticular tissues appears most likely to be the underlying mechanism. Espinoza and associates[12] considered that there was an arthritis of the fingers but did not document this.

X-rays may be normal, especially during the first week, but later show marrow densities, lytic areas, or periosteal elevation. Most of the periosteal changes are no longer identifiable in 1 month to 4 months. Rarefaction of the medulla can occur. Hematopoiesis occurring in the small finger and toe bones of children, but not in adults even with SS hemoglobin disease, is presumably a factor in the restriction of this syndrome to childhood.

The incidence varies from 17 percent in a study of American blacks to 80 percent in a group of Congolese children.[8] Venous stasis in the extremities of African children strapped to their mothers' backs has been suggested as a factor to explain the increased frequency in Africa.[10] Exposure to cold is not a factor.[11] Five examples have been described in Saudi Arabians with SS hemoglobin, reminding us that the various manifestations of sickle cell disease are not restricted to blacks.[13]

Although hand-foot syndrome is characteristic of SS hemoglobin disease, it has also been reported in children with SC hemoglobin disease and S thalassemia.[9,14] Involvement of hands and feet alone, as well as together, has been seen with sickle thalassemia as well as with homozygous sickle disease.[14] Metatarsal lysis was seen in one case.[11] Osteomyelitis can also occur in children and must always be kept in mind.

Usually only analgesics have been used for therapy.

Hyperuricemia and Gout. Approximately 40 percent of adults with sickle cell disease are hyperuricemic (most often 6.5 mg per dl to 11 mg per dl), whereas only occasional affected children under 13 years of age have elevated serum uric acid levels. Overproduction of uric acid associated with increased red cell turnover does occur and seems initially to be associated with hyperuricosuria.[14-17] In young people, urate clearance maintains a normal serum uric acid concentration, but in older patients uric acid excretion often diminishes and results in hyperuricemia.[15,17,18] Decreases in urate clearance are reported by Diamond and colleagues[18] to occur in association with other evidence of impaired renal function.

Clinical diagnoses of acute gouty arthritis have been reported[19,20] in patients with sickle hemoglobin. Typical

Figure 101–3. Diffusely swollen hands as seen in the hand-foot syndrome of young children with sickle cell disease.

crystals of monosodium urate have been found less often.[15] Actual, proven acute gouty arthritis has therefore been rare but may be seen more with the increasing longevity of sickle cell patients.

Osteomyelitis. Patients with sickle cell disease are especially susceptible to bacterial infection. The frequency of osteomyelitis, caused by a variety of organisms (but predominantly salmonellae), is more than 100 times that seen in normal populations.[21] Reasons for the increased incidence of infections may include tissue damage from sickling and infarcts, increased hospital exposure to infection, impaired clearing of bacteria after splenic fibrosis, impaired phagocytosis at low oxygen tensions,[21] and impaired opsonic activity.[22,23] A deficiency of properdin factor B has been demonstrated; this appears to be due to complement activation.[24] More than 80 percent of hematogenous osteomyelitis in persons without hemoglobinopathies is due to staphylococci, but more than 50 percent of osteomyelitis in sickle cell patients is caused by salmonellae.[21] Other organisms causing osteomyelitis in sickle cell disease have included staphylococci, pneumococci, serratia, *Escherichia coli*, and hemophilus. Gram-negative organisms seem most common.[25]

Multiple sites of osteomyelitis may be seen in infected patients. Onset may not be dramatic, and bone infection has apparently been overlooked for years.[25] Osteomyelitis may be very difficult to distinguish radiographically from the results of bone infarction. Progression or other signs of infection are needed for diagnosis. Osteomyelitis most often begins in the medullary cavity of long bones but can involve any bone.

Osteomyelitis may become evident only weeks or months after a known bacteremia. Both crisis and infection present with bone pain, fever, and leukocytosis. Persistent fever must increase the concern about osteomyelitis. Infection rarely extends from bones into joints. Abscess and sinus formation may develop. Bone destruction with periosteal elevation, progressive massive

longitudinal intracortical diaphyseal fissuring, and involucrum formation are seen. Exploration or demonstration of the organism from a draining site is needed for diagnosis.

Treatment generally includes splinting severely involved bones to prevent pathologic fracture.[10] Salmonella bone infection seems to respond well to chloramphenicol without much development of chronic osteomyelitis.[25] Surgical drainage has not been necessary in most cases. Salmonella osteomyelitis has also been seen in sickle-thalassemia disease.[26] Engh and colleagues[25] found osteomyelitis in patients with SC hemoglobin and S thalassemia disease but not sickle trait.

Septic Arthritis. Septic arthritis may be seen[23] but fortunately is not especially common.[21,27,28] Septic arthritis is much less frequent than osteomyelitis. Multiple joints have been involved in some cases.[23] A variety of organisms have been seen, including staphylococci, *E. coli*, *Enterobacter*, and salmonellae. Impaired synovial capillary flow caused by sickling has been suggested as a factor in poor responses to therapy in two patients, and exchange transfusion was suggested as an adjunct to treatment.[27,29]

Joint Effusions. Far more common than gout or septic arthritis are other joint effusions that appear to be due to sickle cell disease. Effusions are often, but not invariably, associated with fever, leukocytosis, and other manifestations of crises.[28] There is generally warmth and tenderness that may also involve the periarticular areas.

Knees have been by far the most commonly involved joints, but effusions have also often been found in elbows and other joints. Usually only one or two joints are involved. Effusions generally subside in 2 to 14 days.

X-rays in most of these patients at the time of effusion have shown only the results of previous cortical or medullary infarcts. One should not expect to see roentgenographic evidence of aseptic necrosis or joint space narrowing, and the acute effusions are clearly not purely a mechanical result of severe degenerative changes. Radioisotope scans,[30] using technetium sulfur colloid, have shown areas of decreased marrow uptake adjacent to many effused joints, suggesting small marrow infarctions. Sequential roentgenographic and scan studies are still limited.

Synovial effusions have usually been "noninflammatory," that is, clear, with most synovial fluid leukocyte counts less than 1000 per cu/mm[29] and with a low percentage of polymorphonuclear leukocytes. Similar "noninflammatory" effusions have been seen in sickle-thalassemia.[28,31]

A few reported effusions in sickle cell disease have been cloudy and have contained higher leukocyte counts in the inflammatory range.[12,32] Effusions with leukocyte counts of 33,000[33] and 126,000[34] with 90 percent to 97 percent polymorphonuclear cells have been described. Crystals or organisms were not found, but both of the latter patients were given antibiotics. Diggs[7] has noted "purulent exudates" in knee joints, which produced negative results for bacteria on direct examination and culture. No mechanism is yet evident for these inflammatory effusions. Synovial fluid complement has not been depressed,[12] and synovial fluid glucose levels have been normal.[28,32,33]

The only inflammatory effusion studied so far by our group contained 29,000 leukocytes per mm³, with 94 percent polymorphonuclear cells. No crystals were found on a careful 30-minute search with compensated polarized light. Aspiration of the same joint the next day yielded 50,100 leukocytes with 50 percent of cells containing negatively birefringent crystals typical of monosodium urate. The explanation for this is not clear, but gout thus cannot be excluded by one synovianalysis.

Sickled erythrocytes can be seen in effusions, but this only shows that the patient has sickle hemoglobin,[28] since sickled cells can also be seen in individuals with sickle cell trait and arthritis of other causes. Some effusions are dark colored because of the patient's hyperbilirubinemia.[28]

Needle synovial biopsies at the time of acute joint effusions have shown only mild focal lining cell proliferation and a few chronic inflammatory cells in two of five biopsies. Small vessels have been congested in some areas, but in four patients there has also been definite microvascular thrombosis (Fig. 101–4). Perivascular fibrosis is also seen.[28]

Electron microscopy of synovium in the author's laboratory has confirmed the presence of occluded vessels, with some vessel lumens containing erythrocytes with the characteristic 180 Å–diameter rods or "tactoids" of typical sickled hemoglobin. No electron-dense deposits have been found in vessel walls. These morphologic studies suggest synovial microvascular obstruction as a likely factor in the noninflammatory effusions.[28] Infarction of bone adjacent to joints with effusions[30] or pain[35] may also contribute to joint manifestations.

No specific treatment has been required for the effusions. Local steroids are not useful. Treatment of crises generally involves the use of analgesics, including occasional narcotics, plus hydration. Limited exchange transfusion can eliminate many abnormal cells and help terminate prolonged crises.[36] Alkali can be given to prevent acidosis that can aggravate sickling. Other measures that have been tried, but are not recommended, include intravenous urea, steroids, anticoagulants, dextran, and cyanate.

Bloody synovial fluid is not common in sickle cell disease, although this might be expected in some severely destroyed joints resulting from aseptic necrosis. The only hemarthrosis in the patients we have studied proved to be due to a small fracture into the knee joint.[30] Casey and Cathcart[37] have suggested that sickle cell trait might have contributed to the development of hemoarthrosis in a patient who also had rheumatoid arthritis. Hemarthrosis has been briefly noted in a patient with sickle cell disease[31] and as a feature of two inflammatory effusions examined by Hanissian and Silverman.[32]

Erosions and Chronic Inflammation. Occasional chronic synovitis with cartilage destruction or erosion

Figure 101–4. Synovium in sickle cell disease. The synovial lining layer (SL) here shows slightly increased cellularity, but most importantly the vessels (V) are occluded with cellular thrombi.

has been mentioned in patients with sickle cell disease and no other evident cause for arthritis.[39,40] Erosions have been described in uncontrolled studies at wrists, metacarpal heads, and calcanei.[40] Lymphocytic and plasma cell infiltration of synovium was seen in one report.[39] Although chronic inflammation is nonspecific and can, for example, be a response to crystals of several types, immunologic mechanisms might possibly be involved. Immune complexes have been implicated as factors in the nephropathy of sickle cell disease[41,42] and in the leg ulcers.[43] Johnston and associates[44] noted an abnormality of the alternative pathway of complement activation in sickle cell disease. Defects in cell-mediated immunity have also been reported with decreased numbers of T lymphocytes[45] and abnormal circulating suppressor lymphocytes.[46] Sickle cell disease and rheumatoid or other arthritis can occur in the same patient

Bone Infarctions. Bone infarctions occur most commonly in individuals with SS hemoglobin, but they may also be seen in SC hemoglobin disease and S thalassemia.[47]

Localized deformities and failure of bone growth can result from infarction of the epiphyseal plate of growing children.[5,6] This is common in both SS hemoglobin and SC hemoglobin disease. The chronic anemia itself can cause some general retardation of growth.[48]

Infarctions in cortical bone are thought to be the cause of periosteal elevation, irregular cortical thickening, and sclerosis. Infarctions in the bone marrow produce fibrosis, lysis, sclerosis, new bone formation, and calcified dense marks on radiographs. X-rays taken at the time of acute bone pain do not show changes from that infarction; small infarcts may never produce roentgenographic changes.

Radioisotope studies[35] using technetium colloid have shown areas of decreased marrow uptake at sites of bone pain, whereas x-rays were normal. This suggests decreased marrow perfusion. Strontium scans have shown increased uptake in the adjacent cortical bone.

The basis for bone infarcts is presumed to be sickling and thrombosis in small vessels. The bone pains in sickle cell crises are felt to be largely a result of such infarctions. Those infarcts involving only the medulla often produce pains without local tenderness.

Aseptic Necrosis (Avascular Necrosis). When bone infarction occurs from occlusion of end arteries so that necrotic bone is at the articular margin, collapse of the periarticular bone and cartilage occurs. Although necrosis of bone in the shaft is also "aseptic" unless accompanied by infection, the term "aseptic necrosis" is usually used in reference to that necrosis associated with joint disease (see Chapter 107).

Pathologic specimens have not been obtained at the time of initial infarction, so the mechanism remains presumptive based on other findings in sickle cell disease. From pathologic studies after hip disintegration, Sherman[49] suggested that both small hemorrhages and local damage to small blood vessels were significant factors. Although most occlusion does seem to be in the microvasculature, some reports[50] suggest that large vessel obliteration can also occur.

Aseptic necrosis of the head of the femur is a common finding and is the most disabling musculoskeletal complication of sickle cell disease. Similar aseptic necrosis occurs at the humeral head, tibial condyles, and occasionally at other sites. Fragments of necrotic bone and cartilage can break loose into the joint cavity. The major joint incongruity leads to further secondary degenerative changes.

Radiographs are similar to those of aseptic necrosis from other causes unless the other bony changes described are noted. Initially there is local sclerosis near the joint margin. Patchy lucencies then develop and may include a lucency between the sclerotic bone and the intact bone. Flattening, separation of the necrotic fragment, and secondary osteoarthritis may later be seen.

Radioisotope studies can suggest infarction occasionally before the development of detectable aseptic necrosis.[30] Technetium pyrophosphate bone scans show increased uptake at sites of infarction. Marrow scans with colloids may show decreased uptake. Protection of a femoral head, known by such studies to be a site of infarction, may help prevent progression.

Aseptic necrosis of the femoral head is rare in children, probably because the artery in the ligamentum teres is patent, giving the femoral head a dual blood supply.

Early treatment can be attempted with prevention of weight bearing, which may allow healing without the resultant distortion of bone. Young people seem better able to replace their necrotic bone. Replacement of the femoral head with a prosthesis or total hip replacement has now been performed in many patients, and this seems the treatment of choice once articular breakdown has become well established.[51] Osteotomies have also been used to try to alter the line of weight bearing.[51] Bone marrow decompression procedures that are being tried in other types of aseptic necrosis have not been systematically evaluated in sickle cell disease.

Aseptic necrosis of the humeral head produces much less difficulty and often needs no treatment. Shoulder prostheses have been inserted in two patients with good early results.[51] Total knee joint prosthetic replacements have been rarely required after aseptic necrosis, but good results were reported on short-term followup.[52] Preoperative transfusions have been used to diminish the chances of sickling. Tourniquets can be avoided to reduce anoxia and stasis. Good hydration and special efforts during anesthesia to avoid hypoxia and acidosis are merited.[52]

As noted above, aseptic necrosis can occur in SC hemoglobin disease and has been felt by some to be even more common than in SS hemoglobin disease.[53] This is possibly because many patients with SS hemoglobin have had earlier deaths from other complications. Diggs[7] has also explained the prominence of infarcts in SC hemoglobin disease on the basis of greater viscosity of the blood. Aseptic necrosis has also been reported in S thalassemia, with SF hemoglobin[53] as well as in sickle cell trait (see later discussion).

Other Musculoskeletal Aspects. Bony ankylosis of hips[7] and spine[54] has been reported, but it is not certain if it was caused by sickle cell disease only or whether infection also played a role.

Irregular sclerosis of sacroiliac joints superficially mimicking the changes of ankylosing spondylitis has been reported[28,55] and is probably a result of bone infarctions at the joint.

Acute muscle pain and localized muscle swelling can be seen with crises.[56] Myonecrosis has been demonstrated and has even required fasciotomy for pain relief. Some sickle cell patients have been described with long, slender arms and legs and tapered fingers, but there is no strong evidence that this is really a manifestation of the hemoglobinopathy.[7] Disproportionate elongation of extremities was not seen in SC hemoglobin disease or S thalassemia.[47]

Leukemia has occasionally occurred in patients with sickle cell disease.[39,57] One such case had elbow pain due to leukemic infiltration.[57]

Sickle Cell Trait. Sickle cell trait (hemoglobin AS) can be associated with systemic sickling under conditions of low oxygen tension. Aseptic necrosis has been reported in patients with sickle cell trait,[58-60] but a recent study[61] found no greater incidence of aseptic necrosis in patients with hemoglobin AS than in age-matched controls with AA hemoglobin. There was a slightly increased history of past transient bouts of unexplained joint symptoms in the patients with sickle cell trait. Otherwise unexplained noninflammatory knee effusions were recently reported in a patient with sickle cell trait and diaphyseal bone infarctions.[61a]

THALASSEMIA

In β-thalassemia (major, intermedia, and occasionally minor) there is increased erythrocyte destruction, causing osteopenia, wide medullary spaces, coarse trabeculations, and thin cortices, much as in sickle cell disease. However, aseptic necrosis is not characteristic. In a series of 50 thalassemic patients,[62] 25 patients (ages 5 to 33 years) had ankle pain that was exacerbated by weight bearing and relieved by rest. Ankles were severely painful in seven patients; there was diffuse ankle and foot tenderness and occasional ankle effusions. X-rays of the ankles of one patient showed subchondral sclerosis suggesting microfractures. Pathologic studies on two autopsy specimens and on a specimen obtained from a femoral osteotomy showed expansion of hematopoietic marrow into the small bones, osteopenia, increased osteoid, and a striking number of microfractures. All these patients studied by Gratwick and colleagues[62] had received multiple transfusions, and iron deposition was prominent in the marrow, in osteoid, at cement lines, and in synovial lining cells. Iron was not mentioned in osteocytes or chondrocytes, but slight articular cartilage erosion was reported.

The ankle problems thus appeared to be due largely to the underlying bone disease, with marrow expansion and osteomalacia also involved. Since serum calcium and phosphorus levels were normal, Gratwick and colleagues[62] speculated that there might be abnormal vitamin D conversion in iron-laden tissues. No therapy has yet been found effective, though rest gives temporary relief.

One patient with thalassemia and repeated transfusions has developed an arthropathy with iron deposition in the synovium,[63] as occurs in idiopathic hemochromatosis.[64] This degenerative arthropathy, which typically involves the second to third metacarpophalangeal joints, hips, knees, and other joints with firm swelling and stiffness, may be complicated by chondrocalcinosis or pseudogout. Other examples of secondary hemochromatosis have been seen in hypoplastic anemia, spherocytosis, and sideroblastic anemia,[65] but so far not in other hemoglobinopathies. Hyperuricemia with gout[66] and septic arthritis[67] can occur in thalassemia. In patients such as these receiving multiple transfusions, the arthritis of viral hepatitis should be considered.

There are reports of aseptic necrosis in thalassemia minor[68,69] but there is no evidence that this is more than coincidental. Schlumpf studied seven patients with thalassemia minor (trait) and noted pain without effusions at ankles and also at wrists and elbows.[68] Recently two other reports of otherwise unexplained mono- or oligoarticular disease in thalassemia minor have appeared. Joint effusions have been noninflammatory[70] or mildly inflammatory.[71] Large and small joints have been involved. Most cases have not had radiographic evidence of adjacent bone disease, so mechanisms of this arthropathy are still unclear. The sicca syndrome has been reported in thalassemia major; iron overload of the salivary glands was demonstrated and presumably resulted from repeated transfusions.[72]

References

1. Dean, J., and Schedchter, A.N.: Sickle cell anemia: Molecular and cellular bases of therapeutic approaches. N. Engl. J. Med. 299:752;804;863, 1978.
2. Klug, P.P., Kaye, N., and Jensen, W.N.: Endothelial cell and vascular damage in the sickle cell disorders. Blood Cells 8:175, 1982.
3. Ballas, S.K., Lewis, C.N., Noone, A.M., et al.: Clinical, hematological and biochemical features of SC disease. Am. J. Hematol. 13:37, 1982.
4. Winslow, R.M., and Anderson, W.F.: The hemoglobinopathies. In Stanbury, J.B., et al. (eds.): The Metabolic Basis of Inherited Disease. 5th ed. New York, McGraw-Hill Book Co., 1983, pp. 1666–1697.
5. Barton, C.J., and Cockshott, W.P.: Bone changes in hemoglobin SC disease. Am. J. Roentgenol. 88:523, 1962.
6. Reynolds, J.: Re-evaluation of the "fish-vertebra" sign in sickle cell haemoglobinopathy. Am. J. Roentgenol. 97:693, 1966.
7. Diggs, L.W.: Bone and joint lesions in sickle cell disease. Clin. Orthop. 52:119, 1967.
8. Lagundoye, S.B.: Radiological features of sickle cell anemia and related hemoglobinopathies in Nigeria. Afr. J. Med. Sci. 1:315, 1970.
8a. Martinez, S., Apple, J.S., Baber, C., Putman, C.E., and Rosse, W.F.: Protrusio acetabuli in sickle-cell anemia. Radiology 151:43, 1984.
9. Haggard, M.E.: Sickle cell anemia in the first two years of life. J. Pediatr. 58:785, 1961.
10. Cockshott, W.P.: Dactylitis and growth disorders. Br. J. Radiol. 36:19, 1963.
11. Watson, R.J., Burko, H., Megas, H., and Robinson, M.: Hand-foot syndrome in sickle cell disease in young children. Pediatrics 31:975, 1963.
12. Espinoza, L.R., Spilberg, I., and Osterland, C.K.: Joint manifestations of sickle cell disease. Medicine 53:295, 1974.
13. Perrine, R.P., Pembry, M.E., John, P., Perrine, S., and Shoup, F.: Natural history of sickle cell anemia in Saudi Arabs. A study of 270 subjects. Ann. Intern. Med. 88:1, 1978.
14. Karpathios, T., Nicolaidou, P., Korkgs, A., and Thomaidis, T.: The hand-foot syndrome in sickle cell beta thalassemia disease. J.A.M.A. 238:1540, 1977.
15. Reynolds, M.D.: Gout and hyperuricemia associated with sickle-cell anemia. Semin. Arthritis Rheum. 12:404, 1983.
16. Walker, B.R., and Alexander, F.: Uric acid excretion in sickle cell anemia. J.A.M.A. 215:255, 1971.
17. Diamond, H.S., Meisel, A., Sharon, E., Holden, D., and Cacatian, A.: Hyperuricosuria and increased tubular secretion of urate in sickle cell anemia. Am. J. Med. 59:796, 1975.
18. Diamond, H.S., Meisel, A.D., and Holden, D.: The natural history of urate overproduction in sickle cell anemia. Ann. Intern. Med. 90:752, 1979.
19. Aquilina, J.T., Moynihan, J.W., Bissell, G.W., and Talbott, J.H.: Gout in sickle cell anemia. Arch. Interam. Rheumatol. 1:708, 1968.
20. Gold, M.S., Williams, J.C., Spivack, M., and Grann, V.: Sickle cell anemia and hyperuricemia. J.A.M.A. 206:1572, 1968.
21. Barrett-Connor, E.: Bacterial infection and sickle cell anemia. An analysis of 250 infections in 166 patients and a review of the literature. Medicine 50:97, 1971.
22. Hand, W.L., and King, N.L.: Serum opsonization of salmonella in sickle cell anemia. Am. J. Med. 64:388, 1978.
23. Ebong, W.W.: The treatment of severely ill patients with sickle-cell anemia and associated septic arthritis. Clin. Orthop. 149:145, 1980.
24. Wilson, W.A., Thomas, E.J., and Sissons, J.G.P.: Complement activation in asymptomatic patients with sickle cell anemia. Clin. Exp. Immunol. 36:130, 1979.
25. Engh, C.A., Hughes, J.L., Abrams, R.C., and Bowerman, J.W.: Osteomyelitis in the patient with sickle cell disease. Diagnosis and management. J. Bone Joint Surg. 53:1, 1971.
26. Weiss, H., and Katz, S.: Salmonella paravertebral abscess and cervical osteomyelitis in sickle thalassemia disease. South. Med. J. 63:339, 1970.
27. Palmer, D.W.: Septic arthritis in sickle-cell thalassemia. Pathophysiology of impaired response to infection. Arthritis Rheum. 18:339, 1975.
28. Schumacher, H.R., Andrews, R., and McLaughlin, G.: Arthropathy in sickle cell disease. Ann. Intern. Med. 78:203, 1973.
29. Palmer, D.W., and Ellman, M.H.: Septic arthritis and Reiter's syndrome in sickle cell disorders: Case reports and implications for management. South. Med. J. 69:902, 1976.
30. Alavi, A., Schumacher, H.R., Dorwart, B.B., and Kuhl, D.E.: Bone marrow scan evaluation of arthropathy in sickle cell disorders. Arch. Intern. Med. 136:436, 1976.
31. Crout, J.E., McKenna, C.H., and Petit, R.M.: Symptomatic joint effusion

in sickle cell-beta-thalassemia disease. Report of a case. J.A.M.A. 235:1878, 1976.

32. Hanissian, A.S., and Silverman, A.: Arthritis of sickle cell anemia. South. Med. J. 67:28, 1974.

33. Goldberg, M.A.: Sickle cell arthropathy: Analysis of synovial fluid in sickle cell anemia with joint effusion. South. Med. J. 66:956, 1973.

34. Orozco-Alcala, J., and Baum, J.: Arthritis during sickle cell crisis. N. Engl. J. Med. 288:420, 1973.

35. Hammell, C.F., DeNardo, S.J., DeNardo, G.L., and Lewis, J.P.: Bone marrow and bone mineral scintigraphic studies in sickle cell disease. Br. J. Haematol. 25:593, 1973.

36. Brody, J.I., Goldsmith, M.H., Park, S.K., and Soltys, H.D.: Symptomatic crises of sickle cell anemia treated by limited exchange transfusion. Ann. Intern. Med. 72:327, 1970.

37. Casey, D.J., and Cathcart, E.S.: Hemarthrosis and sickle cell trait. Arthritis Rheum. 13:882, 1970.

38. Saheb, F.: Arthropathy in sickle cell disease. N. Engl. J. Med. 288:971, 1973.

39. Schumacher, H.R., Dorwart, B.B., Bond, J., Alavi, A., and Miller, W.: Chronic synovitis with early cartilage destruction in sickle cell disease. Ann. Rheum. Dis. 36:413, 1977.

40. Rothschild, B.M., and Sebes, J.I.: Calcaneal abnormalities and erosive bone disease associated with sickle cell anemia. Am. J. Med. 71:427, 1981.

41. Walker, B.R., Alexander, R., Birdsall, T.R., and Warren, R.L.: Glomerular lesions in sickle cell nephropathy. J.A.M.A. 215:437, 1971.

42. Strauss, J., Koss, M., Griswold, W., Chernack, W., Pardo, V., and McIntosh, R.M.: Cryoprecipitible immune complexes, nephropathy and sickle cell disease (letter). Ann. Intern. Med. 81:114, 1974.

43. Morgan, A.G., Venner, A-M.: Immunity and leg ulcers in homozygous sickle cell disease. J. Clin. Lab. Immunol. 6:51, 1981.

44. Johnston, R.B., Newman, S.L., and Struth, A.G.: An abnormality of the laternate pathway of complement activation in sickle cell disease. N. Engl. J. Med. 288:803, 1973.

45. Glassman, A.B., Deas, D.V., Berlinsky, F.S., et al.: Lymphocyte blast transformation and peripheral lymphocyte percentages in patients with sickle cell disease. Ann. Clin. Lab. Sci. 10:9, 1980.

46. Kaur, P., Cooper, R., Alexander, J., et al.: Impaired cell mediated immunity in sickle cell disease. Clin. Res. 30:513A, 1982.

47. Smith, E.W., and Conley, C.L.: Clinical features of the genetic variants of sickle cell disease. Bull. Johns Hopkins Hosp. 94:289, 1954.

48. Serjeant, G.R.: Delayed skeletal maturation in sickle cell anemia in Jamaica. Johns Hopkins Med. J. 132:95, 1973.

49. Sherman, M.: Pathogenesis of disintegration of the hip in sickle cell anemia. South. Med. J. 52:632, 1959.

50. Stockman, J.A., Nigro, M.A., Mishkin, M.M., and Oski, F.: Occlusion of large cerebral vessels in sickle cell anemia. N. Engl. J. Med. 287:846, 1972.

51. Chung, S.M.K., Alavi, A., and Russell, M.O.: Management of osteonecrosis in sickle cell anemia and its genetic variants. Clin. Orthop. 130:158, 1978.

52. Haberman, E.T., and Grayzel, A.I.: Bilateral total knee replacement in a patient with sickle cell disease. Clin. Orthop. 100:211, 1974.

53. Chung, S.M.K., and Ralston, E.L.: Necrosis of the femoral head associated with sickle cell anemia and its genetic variants. J. Bone Joint Surg. 51A:33, 1969.

54. Kanyerezi, B.R., Ndugwa, C., Owor, R., Singabual, S.N., Masembe, J., Nzaro, E., and Bosa, J.L.: The spinal column in sickle cell disease. J. Rheumatol. (Suppl.)1(1):21, 1974.

55. Tanaka, K.R., Clifford, G.O., and Axelrod, A.R.: Sickle cell anemia (homozygous S) with aseptic necrosis of the femoral head. Blood 11:998, 1956.

56. Dorwart, B.B., and Gabuzda, T.G.: Symmetric myonecrosis: A previously undescribed vaso-occlusive complication of sickle cell anemia (abstract). Clin. Res. 27:140A, 1979.

57. Ludmerer, K.M., and Kissane, J.M.: Left elbow pain and death in a young woman with sickle-cell anemia. Am. J. Med. 73:268, 1982.

58. Ratcliff, R.B., and Wolfe, M.D.: Avascular necrosis of the femoral head associated with sickle cell trait (AS hemoglobin). Ann. Intern. Med. 57:299, 1962.

59. Keeling, M.M., Lockwood, W.B., and Harris, E.A.: Avascular necrosis and erythrocytosis in sickle cell disease. N. Engl. J. Med. 290:442, 1977.

60. Nachamie, B.A., and Dorfman, H.D.: Ischemic necrosis of bone in sickle cell trait. Mt. Sinai J. Med. 41:527, 1974.

61. Dorwart, B.B., Goldberg, M.A., Schumacher, H.R., and Alavi, A.: Absence of increased frequency of bone and joint disease with hemoglobin AS and AC. Ann. Intern. Med. 86:66, 1977.

61a. Lally E.V., Buckley W.M., and Claster S.: Diaphyseal bone infarctions in a patient with sickle cell trait. J. Rheum. 10:813, 1983.

62. Gratwick, G.M., Bullough, P.G., Bohne, W.H.O., Markenson, A.L., and Peterson, C.M.: Thalassemic arthropathy. Ann. Intern. Med. 88:494, 1978.

63. Sella, E.J., and Goodman, A.H.: Arthropathy secondary to transfusion hemochromatosis. J. Bone Joint Surg. 55A:1077, 1973

64. Schumacher, H.R.: Hemochromatosis and arthritis. Arthritis Rheum. 7:45, 1964.

65. Abbott, D.F., and Gresham, G.A.: Arthropathy in transfusional siderosis. Br. Med. J. 1:418, 1972.

66. Paik, C.H., Alavi, I., Dunca, G., and Weiner, L.: Thalassemia and gouty arthritis. JAMA 213:296, 1970.

67. Schlumpf, U., Gerber, N., Bunzli, H., Elsasser, U., Pestalozzi, A., and Boni, A.: Arthritiden bei Thalassemia minor. Schwiez. Med. Wochenschr. 107:1156, 1977.

68. Schlumpf, U.: Thalassemia minor and aseptic necrosis, a coincidence? Arthritis Rheum. 21:280, 1978.

69. Abourizk, N.N., Nasr, F.W., and Frayha, R.A.: Aseptic necrosis in thalassemia minor. Arthritis Rheum. 20:1147, 1977.

70. Dorwart, B.B., and Schumacher, H.R.: Arthritis in beta thalassemia trait: clinical and pathological features. Ann. Rheum. Dis. 40:185, 1981.

71. Gerster, J-C., Dardel, R., and Guggi, S.: Recurrent episodes of arthritis in thalassemia minor. J. Rheum. 11:352, 1984.

72. Borgna-Pignatti, C., Cammareri, V., DeStefano, P. and Magrini, V.: The sicca syndrome in thalassaemia major. Brit.Med.J. 288:668, 1984.

Chapter 102

Arthropathies Associated with Endocrine Disorders

James L. McGuire

INTRODUCTION

The systemic manifestations of endocrine disorders reflect the diverse but specialized control that hormones exert on target organs. The list of cells possessing various hormone receptors is rapidly expanding. Many are not in endocrine organs. The monocyte-macrophage line, lymphocyte subpopulations, fibroblasts, and bone cells are recent additions to this list.

Historically, the untreated adult endocrine disorders of acromegaly, primary hyperparathyroidism (PHP), and myxedema were initially classified within the rheumatic diseases. Moreover, the overlap of the multisystem complaints, both constitutional and musculoskeletal, have served to link the endocrine syndromes with connective tissue disease. The rheumatologist usually encounters endocrine disease in one of three ways. First, a patient with a defined endocrine disorder can present with a specific rheumatologic complaint. Second, the presentation of endocrine disease as an undiagnosed systemic illness involving joints, muscles, or skin may suggest a vasculitis or connective tissue disease. Finally, a nonspecific problem such as carpal tunnel syndrome or a pseudogout attack may warrant a specific endocrine test, which may result in the early recognition of an endocrine disease.

Table 102–1 is an abbreviated list of symptoms and signs that are suggestive of endocrine disease in patients seeking help from a rheumatologist.

The clinical presentations of the classic endocrine disorders such as primary hyperparathyroidism (PHP), acromegaly, and Cushing's disease have dramatically changed during the last decade because of early and accurate detection. This, in turn, results in appropriate therapeutic intervention before the complete syndrome evolves. PHP, for example, is often diagnosed by finding hypercalcemia on a routine laboratory screen in a patient without "moans, groans, stones, or bones." The rheumatologist must be aware of these changing faces of a classic disease.

Pediatricians constantly observe the action of hormonal regulation of skeletal growth during the evaluation of children with short stature, bony deformities, and joint hypermobility. Disorders of growth hormone production, vitamin D resistance, and PHP of childhood must be added to the differential diagnoses of abnormal skeletal growth, which have included achondroplasia, osteogenesis imperfecta, and Ehlers-Danlos syndrome. In some diseases, the hormonal and connective tissue abnormalities are strongly associated but inherited independently. Patients with classic pseudohypoparathyroidism have hypocalcemia due to parathyroid hormone (PTH) resistance and a skeletal deformity (short 4th metacarpal), called Albright's hereditary osteodystrophy (AHO), which may not be related to the hypoparathyroid state. Both conditions may be inherited separately (pseudohypoparathyroidism without AHO or AHO with normal serum calcium). The latter is often referred to as pseudo-pseudohypoparathyroidism.

Finally, the appearance of an endocrine disorder during the course of an existing connective tissue disease can dramatically alter the symptoms. The concomitant development of hyperthyroidism in a patient with rheumatoid arthritis often results in joint complaints that are out of proportion to the physical findings. The dramatic aggravation or amelioration of connective tissue diseases during different stages of pregnancy has been well described. The iatrogenic Cushing's syndrome during steroid therapy results in a diagnostic dilemma when muscle weakness reappears during the clinical course of polymyositis with stable muscle enzymes. The appearance of PHP in a patient with active Paget's disease of bone can result in massive, rapid resorption of bone. The effects of sex and other steroid hormones on the immune response is as fascinating to the immunologist, as is the "autoimmune" attack on an endocrine gland, resulting in stimulation (e.g., hyperthyroidism), inhibition (e.g., acanthosis nigricans and diabetes), or destruction (e.g., Hashimoto's disease), to the endocrinologist.

DIABETES MELLITUS

Diabetes mellitus is a heterogeneous disorder that is classified according to insulin dependence, degree of insulin resistance, and age of onset.[1] Clinical studies in this chronic disease must incorporate not only the type of diabetes but age- and weight-matched controls. Attention to these variables may be reflected in the recent clinical reports that have not confirmed the traditional association of diabetes with the rheumatic disorders of gout, CPPD crystal disease, osteoporosis, and osteoarthritis. On the other hand, the association of diffuse idiopathic spinal hyperostosis (DISH) and maturity onset diabetes has been supported.[2]

Although many reports in the literature have supported an association between diabetes and osteoporosis (see Chapter 105), a recent well-controlled retrospective study demonstrated no difference in clinical fractures.[3,4] Nevertheless, patients with poorly controlled diabetes excrete more urinary calcium,[5] and bone formation in the growing skeleton requires insulin.[6]

The relationship of osteoarthritis to diabetes is suggested by the accelerated destruction of articular cartilage in diabetic Chinese hamsters[7] and in rats with streptozocin-induced diabetes.[8] Osteoarthritis is more common in patients with maturity-onset diabetes than in age-matched controls, but the lack of controls for obesity makes any unique association questionable.[9,10] In a similar fashion, obesity is an important factor in patients with maturity-onset diabetes who have hyperuricemia and gout[11] (see Chapter 86). Finally, controlled studies of the frequency of pseudogout in the diabetic population have not confirmed the initially reported association.[12]

The "stiff-hand" syndrome has been observed in ap-

Table 102–1. Clinical Findings Common to Both Rheumatologic and Endocrine Disorders

Skin	*Periarticular*
Thickening	Fibrositis
Local	Tenosynovitis
Diffuse	Bursitis
Alopecia	*Neurologic*
Vitiligo	Carpal tunnel
Easy bruisability	Depression
Vascular	*Bone*
Leg ulcers	Osteopenia
Raynaud's phenomenon	Abnormal Stature
Muscle	Deformities
Weakness and pain	*Hand Radiograph Abnormalities*
(with or without	Distal tufts
muscle enzyme	CPPD
elevation)	Joint space
Arthritis	Osteopenia
Pseudogout	*Laboratory*
Seronegative rheumatoid	Positive rheumatoid factor
arthritis	
Diffusely swollen hands	Antinuclear antibody
Premature osteoarthritis	Elevated creatine kinase

proximately 30 percent of type I (juvenile) diabetics.[13] Flexion contractures in the fingers are attributed to the thickened tight skin around the MCP and PIP joints. The natural progression of this disorder is not well-characterized, but an association with other microangiopathic complications of diabetes has been suggested.[14] The stiff-hand syndrome must be distinguished from the increased prevalence of flexor tenosynovitis, causing trigger fingers,[15] and Dupuytren's contractures of the palmar fascia.[16] All three conditions are observed in approximately one third of the patients with juvenile-onset diabetes. Moreover, the role of hyperlipidemia in the pathogenesis of the multiple tendon problems described in the diabetic population is not known. Calcific peritendonitis and bursitis of the shoulder are well described in the diabetic population.[17,18] Moreover, an association of this condition, which may be bilateral, with reflex sympathetic dystrophy (RSD) can result in all clinical patterns of the shoulder-hand syndrome.[19]

A variety of rheumatic complaints are directly related to the neuropathy of diabetes mellitus. Actual infarction of the nerve may be caused by involvement of the vasonervorum.[24] The median nerve may be particularly vulnerable to the mild compression caused by RSD or obesity. The presence of nocturnal paresthesias in any of the first four fingers or of thenar muscle wasting should suggest the carpal tunnel syndrome.[20] RSD itself may need the background of the dysautonomia of diabetes for full expression in the setting of calcific bursitis or cervical spine osteoarthritis.[16] Peripheral neuropathies account for the high frequency of undetected foreign objects embedded in the "diabetic foot." Osteomyelitis is a common complication in this setting, especially with coexistent peripheral vascular disease.[21] An acute mononeuritis can present as a confusing clinical picture. Involvement of the femoral nerve can cause pain and weakness, which can simulate either a herniated disc or a greater trocanteric bursitis.[22]

In some patients with diabetes and peripheral neuropathy, a classic Charcot arthropathy involving the tarsus and ankle results in painless deformities of the foot[23] (Figs. 102–1 and 102–2). Similar involvement of the knee, with surprising preservation of function, and the spine has been described.[24] The pathogenesis of this destructive arthropathy is not completely understood but may involve chronic CPPD crystal shedding.[25] A dramatic osteolysis of the bones of the forefoot is peculiar to patients with diabetes[26] (Fig. 102–3). The terms

Figure 102–1. Neuropathic arthropathy involving the right tarsus in diabetes mellitus. The left tarsus is normal.

resorptive osteodystrophy, osteolysis of the forefoot, and diabetic osteopathy have been used interchangeably for this condition.[27] The progression from patchy osteopenia to complete resorption of the distal metatarsals and proximal phalanges can be rapid. The pathophysiology of this resorptive process is unknown. Overt peripheral vascular disease and severe neuropathy are not characteristically present.[28]

Diffuse idiopathic spinal hyperostosis (DISH) is associated with diabetes mellitus, especially in obese patients with maturity-onset diabetes.[29,30] There is some preliminary evidence that nondiabetics with DISH have an abnormal insulin response to induced hyperglycemia .[2] DISH is usually a radiographic diagnosis, to be distinguished from ankylosing spondylitis by the preservation of sacroiliac joints and predominantly right-sided syndesmophytes.

Skin disorders in diabetes mellitus have been diagnosed as scleroderma. Abnormalities of subcutaneous fat have been observed in patients with insulin-depend-

Table 102–2. Rheumatologic Disorders in Diabetes Mellitus

Direct Complications	Indirect Complications	Possible Associations
Diabetic osteolysis	Forestier's disease (DISH)	Gout
Septic arthritis		CPPD crystal disease
Neuropathic joint	Dupuytren's contracture	Osteoporosis
Stiff hand syndrome	Frozen shoulder	Osteoarthritis
	Carpal tunnel syndrome	
	Reflex sympathetic dystrophy	

Figure 102–2. *A* and *B*, Radiographs of the ankle joint in a patient with diabetes mellitus and severe chronic peripheral neuropathy. Note the extensive destruction of the joint with fluffy new bone formation. The patient presented with only a slightly painful swelling of the ankle region.

ent diabetes. Lipoatrophy at the site of repeated insulin injections is common. Changing to a monocomponent insulin is reported to reverse the process. A rare condition called total lypodystrophy is characterized by an absence of subcutaneous fat. It is commonly associated with severe insulin resistance, acanthosis nigricans, and the sicca syndrome.[31,32] A wide variety of diabetic skin changes related to vascular abnormalities can occur over the anterior tibial area. Necrobiosis lipoidica diabeticorum may suggest a small vessel vasculitis by histopathology demonstrating an obliterative endarteritis.[33]

The rheumatologic disorders commonly associated with diabetes mellitus are summarized in Table 102–2.

HYPERPARATHYROIDISM

The bone disease of primary hyperparathyroidism (PHP) is discussed in Chapter 106. Several additional rheumatic conditions are commonly encountered in this disease and should be discussed here.

First, a painless proximal muscle weakness suggestive of a myopathy has been described. The muscle enzymes CPK and aldolase are normal. The EMG is characteristically abnormal; some patients have a myopathic pattern and others demonstrate a neuropathic picture. The

latter is supported by muscle biopsies consistent with denervation. Following the removal of the parathyroid adenoma, the neuromuscular disorder and the abnormal EMG improve dramatically.[34]

Second, an inflammatory arthritis associated with erosions and chondrocalcinosis has been described in patients with PHP.[35] One form of this arthropathy is thought to be induced by crystals. The common association of hyperuricemia and PHP supported urate as the important pathogenetic crystal, but the demonstration of calcium pyrophosphate dihydrate crystals in synovial fluid popularized this crystal as the driving force behind the chronic inflammation. Although larger, age-matched studies are needed, the literature supports the chronic pseudogout model as a cause of the arthropathy of PHP.[36–38] However, the demonstration of both calcium apatite and calcium oxalate crystals[39] in patients with secondary hyperparathyroidism due to chronic renal disease suggests that further evaluation is needed before naming any one crystal as the cause of this arthritis.

The erosive arthritis described by Bywaters and associates was referred to as osteogenic synovitis to emphasize the primary role of the bone disease in the acquired articular disorder.[40] Subchondral thinning of bone resulted in collapse and eventual loss of cartilage (Fig. 102–4). The resultant osteoarthritic changes were

Figure 102–3. Radiograph of forefoot showing diabetic osteolysis of metatarsals and phalanges. *A,* Some sharply outlined juxta-articular erosions and early subluxations of first, second, and third metatarsophalangeal joints are evident. *B,* A variable degree of bony dissolution has resulted in tapering of bone ends and a telescoping deformity of the toes. (*B* from Bluestone, R.: Clin. Rheum. Dis. 1:95, 1975.)

consistent with the radiographic findings (Fig. 102–5). It is interesting to note that the destructive bone disease of osteitis fibrosa cystica, the first pathology linking PHP and bone, has all but disappeared from the current descriptions of bone histopathology in patients with PHP[41] (Chapter 106).

The secondary hyperparathyroidism of chronic renal disease frequently causes bony abnormalities similar to osteitis fibrosa cystica of classic PHP.[42] This form of renal osteodystrophy is associated with erosions of both ends of the clavicle and sacroiliac joints[43,44] (Fig. 102–6). In addition to subcutaneous calcifications,[45,46] calcium crystal–induced inflammation of tendon and joints has been described.[47] Whether these mechanisms are operative in the pathogenesis of arthritis in PHP is suggested but unproved at this time.

Although hyperuricemia, gout, and PHP have been reported together in some patients,[48] no strong association of gout and PHP has been confirmed. The earlier studies may reflect a different presentation of PHP than the current early, more mild disease being diagnosed and have generally predated the description of CPPD-induced pseudogout. The possible association of ankylosing spondylitis and PHP has not been fully confirmed in a large study.[49] Ectopic calcifications in skin and tendons can present as unexplained firm nodules and acute periarticular disease, respectively.[50]

In addition to the rheumatic complaints and kidney stones, recent studies have emphasized the importance of asymptomatic hypercalcemia, generalized osteoporosis, and fever of unknown origin (FUO) as presentations of PHP.[51,52]

HYPOPARATHYROIDISM

Patients with hypocalcemia due to hypoparathyroidism can now be separated into groups according to the levels of immunoreactive parathyroid hormone (iPTH). Undetectable levels are found in idiopathic hypoparathyroidism (IH) and in patients who have had surgical removal of the parathyroids, whereas normal to elevated levels are found in patients with pseudohypoparathyroidism with target organ resistance.

Idiopathic hypoparathyroidism is rare. The principal muscular symptom of fatigue is directly related to the degree of hypocalcemia. A spondylitis similar to DISH has been described in patients with IH.[53] The restricted spinal movement is caused by extensive nonmarginal syndesmophytes along the anterior vertebral ligaments.[54] There is neither sacroiliac joint narrowing nor vertebral body squaring, so that ankylosing spondylitis can be excluded. A subgroup of IH has a particular susceptibility to superficial *Candida* infections involving the nails and skin.[55,56] Defects in cell-mediated immunity, including cutaneous anergy, have been described in this group.[57,58] IH has been associated with other endocrinopathies, such as Addison's disease, Hashimoto's dis-

Figure 102–4. Right knee showing outer part of lateral (*A*) and medial (*B*) condyle of tibia (coronal slice) from a patient with primary hyperparathyroidism. Radiograph (above) and photomicrograph (below) × 4.5. Note collapse of bone trabeculae and of cartilage with secondary osteoarthritic change and osteophytes. (From Bywaters, E.G.L., et al.: Ann. Rheum. Dis. 22:171, 1963.)

ease, and hypothyroidism. The acronym HAM is used to refer to the syndrome of IH, Addison's disease, and moniliasis.[59,60] Interestingly, an association of IH with other connective tissue diseases usually found on the "autoimmune" list has not been emphasized.

Pseudohypoparathyroidism is generally associated with the skeletal deformities of a short fourth metacarpal and diminished overall stature. The condition of hormone resistance can occur independently of the somatic defects, which have been termed Albright's hereditary osteodystrophy (AHO).[61] Patients with pseudohypoparathyroidism and AHO have a deficiency in the cell membrane–associated guanine nucleotide regulatory protein (G unit), which may explain the association of this endocrine disorder with other hormone-resistant states possessing the same defect in the G unit.[62]

The short metacarpals are the result of premature epiphyseal closure. AHO can be suggested by a routine exam of the hands. With a clenched fist, the so-called "knuckle, knuckle, dimple, knuckle" sign emphasizes the short fourth metacarpal. Deformities involving the hips, pelvis, and knees have been also described in patients with AHO[63,64] (Fig. 102–7).

Ectopic ossifications in the subcutaneous and soft tis-

Figure 102–5. Right knee before (*A*) and 1 year after (*B*) removal of parathyroid adenoma. Collapse and erosion of lateral condyles of tibia and femur, present earlier, were partially repaired. (From Bywaters, E.G.L., et al.: Ann. Rheum. Dis. 22:171, 1963.)

Figure 102–6. Abnormalities of the sacroiliac joint in a patient with secondary hyperparathroidism. *A,* On a coronal section, loss of the ilial cartilage (arrowheads) can be noted. The sacral cartilage is relatively intact. Focal intra-articular fibrous adhesions (straight arrow) and subchondral sclerosis (curved arrow) are present. *B,* Macerated coronal section reveals extensive fraying along the ilial side of the joint (arrowheads), with associated trabecular thickening (straight arrow). Note similar but mild abnormality of the inferior aspect of the sacrum (curved arrow) and sclerosis of ilial subperiosteal bone (open arrow). *C,* The sectional radiograph outlines erosion (*e*) and sclerosis (*scl*) of subchondral bone in the ilium. Slight ossification of the interosseous ligament (lig) is apparent. *D,* In the photomicrograph (× 2), trabecular thickening and substitutive fibrosis are prominent in the ilium (straight arrow). Subperiosteal sclerosis along the inferior aspect of the ilium is also apparent (curved arrows). Note the intra-articular adhesions (arrowhead). *E,* At higher magnification (× 124), disruption and disappearance of the ilial cartilage are readily apparent (arrowhead). Resorption of bone, replacement with fibrous tissue and thickening of remaining trabeculae can be noted in the subchondral region of the ilium (arrows). (From Resnick, D., and Niwayama, G.: Radiology 118:315, 1976.)

sues are preferentially deposited around the weight-bearing joints in patients with pseudohypoparathyroidism. Whereas ectopic calcification of the basal ganglia occurs in all forms of chronic hypoparathyroidism, subcutaneous deposits of bone in the lower extremities have been described almost exclusively in patients with pseudohypoparathyroidism.[65]

HYPERTHYROIDISM (GRAVES' DISEASE)

The suggestion that Graves' disease, Hashimoto's thyroiditis, and hypothyroidism are separate disease entities has been questioned. Pretibial myxedema, lymphocytic

Figure 102–7. Albright's hereditary osteodystrophy in pseudohypoparathyroidism. The "knuckle-knuckle-dimple-knuckle" sign has its radiological equivalent in the short fourth metacarpal. (Courtesy of Neil Breslau, M.D.)

Figure 102–8. Radiograph of a fifth metacarpal from a patient with thyroid acropachy. Note the fluffy periostitis along the ulnar aspect of the bone. (From Bluestone, R.: Clin. Rheum. Dis. 1:95, 1975.)

infiltration of the thyroid gland, thyroid-specific antibodies, and association with other "autoimmune" diseases have been described in all three classic thyroid diseases. It is possible that the clinical expression of hyperthyroidism, hypothyroidism, or euthyroid goiter just reflects the predominate immunologic influence at the time. Support of this theory is based on the transition of hyperthyroid to hypothyroid stages of Hashimoto's disease and euthyroid Graves' disease with ophthalmopathy.[66-68]

In the pathogenesis of Graves' disease, the antibody thyroid-stimulating immunoglobulin (TSI) develops against the thyroid-stimulating hormone (TSH) receptor on the follicular cell. Rather than inhibiting hormone production, however, in a manner similar to that seen in other antireceptor antibody diseases, such as myasthenia gravis and acanthosis nigricans with diabetes, TSI stimulates the thyroid cell to produce excessive thyroxine.[69,70] The role of long-acting thyroid stimulator (LATS) in human thyrotoxicosis, acropachy, and opthalmopathy is not understood.

Thyroid acropachy is an uncommon manifestation of Graves' disease consisting of a clinical constellation of distal soft tissue swelling, clubbing, and periostitis, especially of the metacarpals (Fig. 102–8). The symptoms may first occur after a euthyroid state is achieved and are often associated with exophthalmus and pretibial myxedema.[71]

Two skin problems described in patients with Graves' disease can be confused with other connective tissue diseases. First, onycholysis, an elevation of the nail from the nail bed, is also found in patients with Reiter's disease and psoriatic arthritis. Second, pretibial myxedema can present with nodules over the calves and shins. The pink plaques of hyaluronic acid can be confluent and simulate morphea[72] (see Chapter 77). In the nodular form, erythema nodosum enters the differential diagnosis (see Chapter 75). Pretibial myxedema is a classic

component of Graves' disease. The cause is unknown, but site-specific fibroblasts, taken from the pretibial skin, were induced to produce excessive glycosaminoglycans when exposed to serum from patients with Graves' disease. Fibroblasts from other areas did not.[73]

Painless proximal muscle weakness without muscle enzyme elevation has been described in approximately 70 percent of patients with hyperthyroidism. The myopathy is rapidly reversible with corrective therapy.[74]

The true incidence of adhesive capsulitis of the shoulder and fibrositis in patients with hyperthyroidism is debated. Early descriptions emphasized restricted painful shoulders in approximately 25 percent of patients.[75]

The osteoporosis associated with hyperthyroidism is described in Chapter 106. Organ cultures of bone suggesting augmented bone resorption are consistent with the bone histology of increased numbers of osteoclasts.[76] Additionally, impaired intestinal calcium absorption may contribute to the osteopenia.[77]

Although the incidence of rheumatoid arthritis in patients with Graves' disease is not increased, high titers of rheumatoid factor have been described.[78] The occurrence of systemic lupus erythematosus (SLE) in a patient with Graves' disease has been described.[79] Additionally, the appearance of a drug-induced lupus syndrome in patients with Graves' disease taking propylthiouracil has been reported.[80] An association of Graves' disease with giant cell arteritis has been reported.[81]

Finally, the significance of the routine demonstration

of antibodies to thyroglobulin in synovial fluid of patients with a wide variety of arthropathies, including osteoarthritis and gout, cannot be explained at this time.[82]

HYPOTHYROIDISM

In the United States, hypothyroidism is usually caused by either Hashimoto's disease or the long-term effects of thyroid ablation by radioactive iodine for Graves' disease. The rheumatic manifestations occupy a central role in the clinical picture of myxedema.

Myxedematous arthropathy has several distinctive features. First, the synovial fluid is extremely viscous because of the markedly increased hyaluronic acid content (Fig. 102–9). Examination of an involved knee may produce a characteristic slow fluid wave (bulge sign). Second, the link between CPPD crystals and this form of metabolic arthritis seems firmly established. Although CPPD crystals can be demonstrated continuously, the joint fluid is surprisingly noninflammatory.[83,84] Joint swelling and stiffness are the usual presenting features of this arthritis. Effusions in the knee associated with ligamentous laxity and synovial thickening have been emphasized. The symmetric involvement of the small joints of the hands and feet, especially the metacarpophalangeal and metatarsophalangeal, can simulate rheumatoid arthritis. Similarly, the demonstration of CPPD crystals often results in the general diagnosis of chronic pseudogout.[85] Despite the persistent effusions, morning stiffness is not remarkable.

The myopathy of hypothyroidism may present with proximal muscle pain and stiffness. Moreover, despite elevations of muscle enzymes, weakness may not be a prominent symptom.[86-88] Muscle biopsies are usually normal, although occasional fiber destruction and mucinous infiltrates have been reported in some patients. The peculiar nature of this myopathy could suggest

Figure 102–9. Semigelatinous synovial fluid from myxedematous patients often required several seconds to begin vertical fall from a syringe, even with greater than usual pressure on the plunger. If allowed to "stringout" vertically from a Pasteur pipette, unbroken streams of greater than 45 cm occurred in these fluids. (From Dorwart, B.B., and Schumacher, H.R.: Am. J. Med. 159:780, 1975.)

either polymyalgia rheumatica (when stiff, painful muscles predominate[89,90]) or polymyositis (when the creatine kinase (CK) is elevated).

Carpal tunnel syndrome (CTS) has been noted in approximately 7 percent of patients with myxedema. Compression of the median nerve by the extraneural accumulation of mucinous material in the tunnel has been implicated as the cause. An intrinsic neuropathy similar to that found in patients with diabetes and acromegaly may play a contributing role. Although carpal tunnel syndrome should be considered in the myxedematous patient presenting with pain or paresthesias in any one of the first four fingers, other causes, such as flexor tenosynovitis, should be ruled out.[91]

Osteonecrosis of the hip has been described in patients with myxedema.[92] Whether this mechanism accounts for some patients who experience collapse of the tibial plateau is not clear. Additionally, the hypercholesterolemia associated with hypothyroidism has been proposed as a contributing factor for both the avascular necrosis of bone and the arthropathy.[93,94]

The diagnosis of hypothyroidism should be entertained in all patients with unexplained CTS, seronegative rheumatoid arthritis (RA), polymyalgia rheumatica with a normal sedimentation rate, and polymyositis with a normal muscle biopsy. The dramatic reversal of all of these rheumatic manifestations with thyroxine therapy emphasizes the importance of including myxedema in the differential diagnosis.

Hashimoto's disease is a thyroiditis characterized by lymphocytic infiltration and enlargement of the gland. Eventually, primary hypothyroidism ensues, although the disease may pass through a hyperthyroid phase. In addition to the presence of antimicrosomal antibodies and antithyroglobulin antibodies, specific abnormalities have been identified in cell-mediated immunity, including diminished T-suppressor populations and the demonstration of increased migration inhibition factor (MIF) lymphokines in Hashimoto's as well as Graves' disease.[95,96] Finally, Hashimoto's disease is associated with Sjögren's syndrome, SLE, RA, and other "autoimmune" endocrinopathies.[97,98] The increased prevalence of HLA-B8, Aw30, and DR3 in patients with Hashimoto's disease is consistent with its inclusion in this list.[99,100]

CUSHING'S SYNDROME

Cushing's syndrome due to excess glucocorticoids can be either naturally occurring or iatrogenic. The advanced syndrome is easily diagnosed by the characteristic moon facies, buffalo hump, acne, hypertension, and osteoporosis.[101]

Proximal muscle weakness without muscle enzyme elevation occurs in some patients with the natural disease. Additionally, certain steroid preparations have a greater propensity to cause the myopathy.[102-104] Osteoporosis is characteristic of both well-established disease and long-term daily steroid administration. Poor wound healing, easy bruisibility, and blue striae have all been attributed to inhibition of collagen, elastin, and matrix synthesis by fibroblasts.

Iatrogenic Cushing's syndrome is generally associated with single daily dosages of prednisone of 10 mg or greater. At lower doses, preservation of the hypothalamo-pituitary-adrenal axis and intestinal calcium absorption are maintained.[105,106] The symptoms of the iatrogenic syndrome parallel the natural disease except for the higher frequencies of avascular necrosis (see Chapter 106) and cataract formation (see Chapter 54).

The appearance of new symptoms in a patient with active connective tissue disease who is receiving high doses of steroids poses a difficult diagnostic problem. Two common situations illustrate this point. First, the reappearance of weakness in a patient with polymyositis (PM) on steroid therapy could mean either reactivation of the disease or steroid-induced myopathy. This differential diagnosis is especially trying if abnormal muscle enzymes persist unchanged or no further increments in their levels are observed. Attempts to evaluate this dilemma by urinary creatine levels has not been satisfactory.[107] Second, when psychotic behavior is apparent in a patient with SLE receiving steroids, steroid-induced psychosis or CNS lupus must be considered.

The tapering of glucocorticoids after the desired therapeutic effect has been achieved can be associated with a withdrawal syndrome. Low-grade fever, lethargy, intense myalgias, and arthralgias are common. Moreover, these symptoms can occur when absolute levels of cortisol are within the normal range. The withdrawal syndrome can be confused with reactivation of the primary disease.[108,109] Finally, a rare but somewhat specific syndrome of panniculitis occurring in patients with acute rheumatic fever who have been tapered off steroids has been described.[110,111]

Addison's disease itself is usually not associated with specific rheumatic complaints. However, it has been associated with Sjögren's syndrome and other "autoimmune" endocrinopathies.[112,113]

ACROMEGALY

Acromegaly is the result of oversecretion of growth hormone (GH) by an adenoma, usually acidophilic, of the anterior pituitary gland. The insidious progression of symptoms over several years characteristically escapes clinical detection. The skeletal effects of growth hormone, mediated by production of somatomedins in the liver, is responsible for the well-coordinated growth of the epiphyseal plate during puberty.[114] The chronic overstimulation of bone cells, fibroblasts, and chondrocytes in the adult skeleton can cause a variety of musculoskeletal manifestations.

Premature osteoarthritis has been described in the weight-bearing joints of patients with acromegaly. The overgrowth of cartilage may cause a particular susceptibility to fissuring and ulceration and the development of osteophytes (Figs. 102–10 and 102–11). The simul-

Figure 102–10. Femur in acromegaly, showing undercut ulcer on weight-bearing area of medial condyle. (From Bluestone, R., et al.: Ann. Rheum. Dis. 30:243, 1971.)

taneous response of fibroblast proliferation in periarticular tissue often results in ligamentous laxity. The osteoarthritic process in the knee can be aggravated by chronic shedding of CPPD crystals, which can generate attacks of pseudogout. Moreover, the rapid enlargement of components of this joint may predispose to internal derangements, especially tears in the meniscus. Finally, osteoarthritic involvement of the temporomandibular joint has been described.[115,116]

Joint space widening, caused by overgrowth of articular cartilage, can be observed radiographically (Figs.

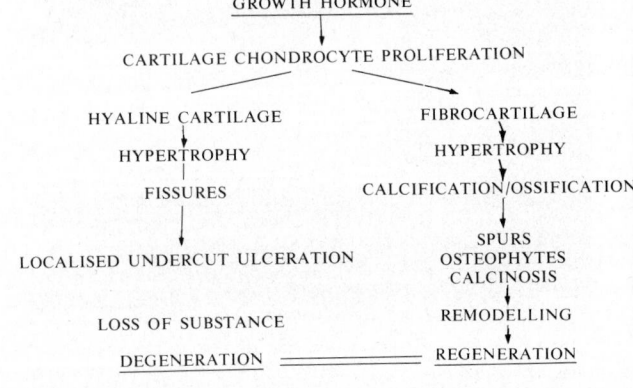

Figure 102–11. Schematic representation of the pathophysiology of acromegalic arthropathy. (From Bluestone, R.: Clin. Rheum. Dis. 1:95, 1975.)

Figure 102–12. Radiograph of the forefoot in a patient with acromegaly. Note the greatly widened metatarsophalangeal joint spaces, reflecting cartilage hyperplasia; there is remodeling of metatarsal and phalangeal bones.

102–12 and 102–13). As the osteoarthritis progresses, joint space narrowing, eburnation, osteophytes, and chondrocalcinosis make the radiographic changes of acromegaly indistinguishable from those produced by other causes of osteoarthritis, including early neuropathic arthropathy. The acquired bowing of the tibia and femur in patients with acromegaly must be differentiated from Paget's disease, rickets, and postfracture repair.

The proposed pathophysiology of acromegalic arthropathy emphasizes the role of both cartilage and bone (Table 102–3.) The altered cartilage growth results in easy fissuring, CPPD accumulation, and ultimately, loss of cartilage. The bone produced by activated osteoblasts may explain the subchondral rigidity and osteophyte formation (see Chapters 87 and 88).

Approximately one-half of patients with acromegaly have nonradiating low back pain. The physical examination characteristically reveals normal reversal of the lumbar lordosis and an intact neurologic system. In addition, hypermobility of the spine has been described in some patients. Radiographically the intervertebral disc spaces may be increased, and large anterior osteophytes with ligamentous calcification are common.[117] The roles of osteopenia (see Chapter 105) and the acquired kyphoscoliosis in the evaluation of this symptom must be considered.[118] In summary, the back pain of patients with acromegaly is probably the result of mechanical, metabolic, and degenerative processes. This complex interaction may explain the disappointing results often obtained with conservative measures such as physical therapy, rest, and nonsteroidal anti-inflammatory drugs.

Carpal tunnel syndrome has been described in approximately one-half of patients with acromegaly.[119] Neural enlargement and excessive soft tissues contribute to the compression of the median nerve at the flexor retinaculum of the wrist.

Painless proximal muscle weakness is well documented in acromegaly. Muscle enzymes and EMG are characteristically normal. A biopsy of a weak muscle does not demonstrate inflammation. The cause of the myopathy is largely unknown but may reflect the effects of GH on the enlarging muscle mass.[120,121]

Figure 102–13. Histology of distal interphalangeal joint in acromegaly, showing hypertrophied cartilage, marginal fibrocartilage calcification of capsular insertion, and on the other side ossification of this. Hematoxylin and eosin × 6. (From Bluestone, R., et al.: Ann. Rheum. Dis. 30:243, 1971.)

Table 102–3. Pathoradiographic Features of Acromegalic Arthropathy

Pathology	Radiology
Cartilage hypertrophy	Widened joint/disc space
Capsular calcification	Periarticular calcinosis
Exuberant marginal new bone formation	Large bridging osteophytes
New bone formation at tendinous/membranous insertions	Bone and joint remodeling
Eventual cartilage fragmentation and ulceration	Loss of joint space

The exaggerated skin folds, deep furrows, and hyperelasticity should suggest the diagnosis of acromegaly in patients with characteristic acral changes. In the early phases of the disease, some of the facial features can simulate pretibial myxedema. Later on, the differentiating acromegaly from pachydermatoperiostitis becomes difficult.[122] Finally, approximately one third of patients with acromegaly have Raynaud's phenomenon.[117]

The diagnosis of acromegaly can be confirmed by a lack of GH level suppression during the early phases of a glucose tolerance test (GTT). When available, comparison photographs taken a decade apart can dramatize the changes in facial features. Despite all the clinical manifestations of acromegaly, some patients are not diagnosed until the enlarging pituitary adenoma causes neurologic symptoms. Headaches and visual loss (usually bitemporal hemianopsia) are the most common.

For the rheumatologist, hand roentgenograms can suggest the diagnosis. Four signs are common. First, the soft tissues are greatly increased. Second, the distal tufts are characteristically spadelike. Third, the well-described joint space widening is noted. Finally, chondrocalcinosis of the wrist and ligamentous calcification have been described.[123]

PREGNANCY

The interaction of hormones with the immune and musculoskeletal systems during pregnancy results in several rheumatic conditions. Moreover, the course of existing connective tissue disease may be dramatically altered.

Carpal tunnel syndrome, presenting with nocturnal paresthesias of the first four digits, is common during the last trimester. Wrist splints and local steroid injections usually produce an excellent result, and prolonged oral medicines or decompressive surgery is avoided.[124]

Low back pain in the last trimester is almost universal and is attributed to the multifactorial interaction of posture abnormalities (lordosis) caused by the enlarging fetus with the excess mobility of the synarthrial joints of the pelvis. Estrogen, progesterone, and relaxin have been implicated in this articular laxity. The condition

of osteitis condensans ilii, which radiographically can be confused with sacroiliitis, is more common in women with multiple pregnancies.[125]

Swollen tender ankles and pedal edema are common complaints during the last trimester. No case of crystal-induced synovitis has been described.

During the last two trimesters both sedimentation rate and complement levels gradually increase.[126,127]

Depression of neutrophil chemotaxis[128] and cell-mediated immunity[129,130] have been observed during the third trimester and early post-partum period. The elevated levels of estrogen, progesterone, prolactin, and, of course, cortisol have each been implicated, but the rapid fluctuations of these levels during pregnancy do not permit the assignment of a causal role to any one.

Female NZB mice demonstrate a severe glomerulonephritis at an earlier age than male littermates. This model of immune complex–mediated disease emphasizes the control exerted by sex hormones on the immune response and immune complex clearance.[131]

Exacerbations and remissions in certain patients with existing connective tissue disease are common during pregnancy. Approximately three quarters of patients with established rheumatoid arthritis (RA) have improvement in their symptoms.[132] However, a return to pregravid disease activity is characteristic after delivery. Finally, RA appears for the first time during the second and third trimesters in a small percentage of pregnancies.[133]

Patients with SLE present with a different problem. Classically, exacerbation of the disease was the rule, but recent studies reflect the complexity of this generalization. First, mild flare-ups are common throughout the entire pregnancy, especially in the third trimester and the post-partum period. Second, remissions have been described in all trimesters but at a lower rate than exacerbations. Finally, patients with active problems at the onset of pregnancy can be expected to have persistent disease throughout[134,135] (see Chapter 70).

The determination of a major or minor flare-up can itself be difficult. The skin disease of SLE must be differentiated from the common dermatologic problems of pregnancy. The butterfly rash can be confused with melasma, the so-called "mask of pregnancy," in the malar region. Melasma can be caused by both estrogen and progesterone. Dramatic hair loss due to the telogen phase predominance during the post-partum period must be distinguished from the alopecia of SLE.[136] Finally, palmar erythema is common in both but involves the fingertips only in SLE.[44]

Severe conditions such as glomerulonephritis and CNS lupus can also be difficult to diagnose during pregnancy. A low serum complement level is a helpful indicator of active disease because complement is usually elevated in normal pregnancy.[137,138]

The administration of birth control pills, especially those with high estrogen content, causes effects that are similar to pregnancy. Melasma, carpal tunnel syndrome, exacerbation of SLE, and amelioration of RA have all been reported with their use.[139] Additionally, erythema nodosum and a soft tissue "inflammation" similar to fibrositis have been described.[140]

Estrogen deficiency states, especially natural menopause, is associated with osteoporosis[141] (see Chapter 105). The X chromosome monosomy (XO) of Turner's syndrome results in gonadal dysgenesis. Invariably, these females have short stature and progressive osteoporosis. Whereas the osteopenia is the result of estrogen lack and is improved with conjugated estrogen therapy, the short stature and other somatic stigmata are not dependent on estrogen for their expression.[142]

SUMMARY

In summary, the endocrine disorders occupy a central position in the differential diagnosis of many common rheumatic conditions. This may seem surprising because the specific cellular mechanisms and target organ of each hormone can differ so widely.

Carpal tunnel syndrome has been well described in hypothyroidism, acromegaly, diabetes, pregnancy, and primary hyperparathyroidism. A component of neural entrapment is common to all. Additionally, an intrinsic neuropathy may contribute to the first three.

Muscle weakness without enzyme elevation is common to the endocrinopathies. Cushing syndrome, steroid therapy, hyperthyroidism, acromegaly, and primary hyperparathyroidism share this presentation. On the other hand, the mypopathy of hypothyroidism is often associated with moderate to marked elevations of creatine kinase. The weak, myxedematous patient has many clinical features in common with the patient with dermatomyositis.

The pathogenetic association of CPPD and premature (secondary) osteoarthritis has been described in a variety of metabolic disorders. Inborn errors of metabolism (ochronosis, Wilson's disease), increased urate synthesis (gout), and iron overload states (hemochromatosis) can be added to the endocrinopathies as probable causes. The association of acromegaly, PHP, and hypothyroidism with CPPD seems more certain than in patients with diabetes (see Chapters 87 and 88).

In a similar fashion, some patients with diabetes and primary hypoparathyroidism meet the radiologic criteria for DISH, whereas the spinal hyperostosis of acromegaly does not (see Chapter 89).

The growing list of diseases associated with avascular necrosis include Cushing's syndrome, myxedema, and hyperlipidemia. The "osteogenic synovitis" of primary hyperparathyroidism may have some component of avascular necrosis (see Chapter 106).

The changes in the soft tissues and blood vessels produced by endocrine disorders can be confused with classic connective tissue syndromes. First, onycholysis is well described in thyrotoxicosis and must be added to Reiter's disease, psoriatic arthritis, and fungal dermatoses when this nail finding is encountered. Additionally,

the distal nail changes of primary hypoparathyroidism may be confused with onycholysis.

Second, a variety of subcutaneous nodules are present in the endocrinopathies. Calcific nodules are described in pseudohypoparathyroidism and PHP. The firm nodules of pretibial myxedema are found in some patients with hyperthyroidism. A lobular panniculitis is associated with acute and chronic disorders of the exocrine pancreas (see Chapters 75 and 77).

Third, Raynaud's phenomenon may be a component of the vasomotor symptoms of acromegaly.

Finally, hyperextensible joints have been described in acromegaly and primary hyperparathyroidism of childhood. In certain clinical settings, confusion with Ehlers-Danlos and Marfan's syndromes may be noted.

In addition to the edematous phase of scleroderma and reflex sympathetic dystrophy (RSD), the differential diagnosis of the unilateral or bilateral diffusely swollen hand or hands must include certain endocrine disorders and their articular sequelae. Moreover, RSD is associated with calcific peritendonitis in the diabetic population. The stiff-hand syndrome of juvenile diabetes characteristically has swollen hands with flexed finger contractures. Subacute pseudogout of the wrist can simulate reflex sympathetic dystrophy. Finally, in myxedema and acromegaly, the soft tissues of the hands can be dramatically increased.

The suggestion of an endocrine disorder by specific rheumatic manifestation should prompt ordering of one or more of the following laboratory tests: *initial screen*—thyroxine (T_4); T_3 resin uptake (T_3U); fasting blood sugar (FBS); serum calcium; serum phosphate; serum albumin; alkaline phosphatase; creatine kinase; and *specific tests*—TSH (thyroid-stimulating hormone); growth hormone during glucose tolerance test; parathyroid hormone; a.m. cortisol.

References

1. National Diabetes Data Group: Classification and diagnosis of diabetes mellitus. Diabetes 28:1039, 1979.
2. Julkunen, H., Heinonen, O.P., and Pyorala, K.: Hyperostosis of the spine in an adult population: Its relationship to hyperglycemia and obesity. Ann. Rheum. Dis. 30:605, 1971.
3. Heath, H.H., Melton, L., Joseph, L.J., and Chu, C-P.: Diabetes mellitus and the risk of skeletal fracture. N. Engl. J. Med. 303:567, 1980.
4. Levin, M.E., Boisseau, V.C., and Avioli, L.V.: Effects of diabetes mellitus on bone mass in juvenile and adult onset diabetes. N. Engl. J. Med. 294:241, 1976.
5. Raskin, P., Stevenson, M.R.M., Barilla, D.E., and Pak, C.Y.C.: The hypercalciuria of diabetes mellitus: Its amelioration with insulin. Clin. Endocrinol. 9:329, 1978.
6. Wettenhall, R.E.H., Schwartz, P.L., and Bornstein, J.: Actions of insulin and growth hormone on collagen and chondroitin sulfate synthesis in bone organ culture. Diabetes 18:280, 1969.
7. Silberberg, R., Gerritsen, G., and Hasler, M.: Articular cartilage of diabetic Chinese hamsters. Arch. Pathol. Lab. Med. 100:50, 1976.
8. Silberberg, R., Hirshberg, G.E., and Lesker, P.: Enzyme studies in the articular cartilage of diabetic rats and of rats bearing transplanted pancreatic islets. Diabetes 26:732, 1977.
9. Waine, H., Nevinny D., Rosenthal, J., et al.: Association of osteoarthritis and diabetes mellitus. Tufts Folio Med. 7:13, 1961.
10. Caterson, B., Baker, J.R., Christner, J.E., Pollok, B.A., and Rostand, K.S.: Diabetes and osteoarthritis. Alabama J. Med. Sci. 17:292, 1980.
11. Buchanan, K.D.: Diabetes mellitus and gout. Semin. Arthritis Rheum. 2:157, 1972.

12. McCarty, D.J., Silcox, D.C., and Coe, F.: Diseases associated with calcium pyrophosphate dihydrate crystal deposition. Am. J. Med. 56:704, 1974.

13. Grgic, A., Rosenbloom, A.L., Weber, F.T., Giordano, B., Malone, J., and Shuster, J.J.: Joint contracture: A common manifestion of childhood diabetes mellitus. J. Pediatr. 88:584, 1976.

14. Rosenbloom, A.L., Silverstein, J.H., Lezotte, D.C., et al.: Limited joint mobility in childhood diabetes mellitus indicates increased risk for microvascular disease. N. Engl. J. Med. 305:191, 1981.

15. Mackenzie, A.H.: Final diagnosis in 63 patients presenting with multiple palmar flexor tenosynovitis (MPFT). Arthritis Rheum. 18:415, 1975.

16. Holt, P.J.: Rheumatological manifestations of diabetes mellitus. Clin. Rheum. Dis. 7:723, 1981.

17. Brigdeman, J.F.: Periarthritis of the shoulder and diabetes mellitus. Ann. Rheum. Dis. 31:67, 1972.

18. Kaklamanis, P., Rigas, A., Giannatos, J., Matsas, S., and Economou, P.: Calcification of the shoulders and diabetes mellitus. N. Engl. J. Med. 293:1266, 1975.

19. Lequesne, M., Dang, N., Benasson, M., and Mery, C.: Increased association of diabetes mellitus with capsulitis of the shoulder and shoulder-hand syndrome. Scand. J. Rheumatol. 6:53, 1977.

20. Phelen, G.S.: Reflections on 21 years' experience with the carpal tunnel syndrome. JAMA 212:1365, 1970.

21. Meltzer, A.D., Skversky, N., and Ostrum, B.J.: Radiographic evaluation of soft tissue necrosis in diabetics. Radiology 90:300, 1968.

22. Child, D.L., and Yates, D.A.H.: Radicular pain in diabetes. Rheum. Rehab. 17:195, 1978.

23. Sinha, S., Munichoodoppa, C.S., and Kozak, G.P.: Neuropathic (Charcot) joints in diabetes mellitus (clinical study of 101 cases). Medicine (Baltimore) 51:191, 1972.

24. Feldman, P., Johnson, A.M., and Walter, J.F.: Diabetes and axial neuroarthropathy. Radiology 111:1, 1974.

25. Jacobelli, S., McCarty, D.J., Silcox, D.C., et al.: Calcium pyrophosphate dihydrate crystal deposition in neuropathic joints: Four cases of polyarticular involvement. Ann. Intern. Med. 79:340, 1973.

26. Bluestone, R.: Rheumatological complications of some endocrinopathies. Clin. Rheum. Dis. 1:95, 1975.

27. Clause, M.E., Gramm, H.F., Legg, M., and Flood, R.: Diabetic osteoarthropathy: Clinical and roentgenographic observations in 90 cases. Am. J. Roentgenol. Rad. Ther. Nucl. Med. 121:22, 1974.

28. Lither, F., and Hietala, S.O.: Skeletal lesions of the feet in diabetics and their relation to cutaneous erythema with and without necrosis in the feet. Acta. Med. Scand. 200:155, 1976.

29. Resnick, D., Shapiro, R.F., Wiesner, K.E., et al.: Diffuse idiopathic skeletal hyperostosis (DISH): Ankylosing hyperostosis of Forestier and Rotes-Querol. Semin. Arthritis Rheum. 7:153, 1978.

30. Harris, J., Carter, A.R., Glick, E.N., and Story, E.O.: Ankylosing hyperostosis. I. Clinical and radiologic features. Ann. Rheum. Dis. 33:210, 1974.

31. Ipp, M.M., Howard, N.J., Tervo, R.C., and Gelfand, E.W.: Sicca syndrome and total lipodystrophy: A case in a fifteen-year-old female patient. Ann. Intern. Med. 85:443, 1976.

32. Braverman, I.M.: Endocrine and metabolic diseases. In Braverman, I.M. (ed.): Skin Signs of Systemic Disease. Philadelphia, W.B. Saunders Company, 1981, p. 666.

33. Ullman, S., and Dahl, M.V.: Necrobiosis lipoidica: An immunofluorescence study. Arch. Dermatol. 113:161, 1977.

34. Frame, B., Heinze, E.G., Block, M., and Manson, G.A.: Myopathy in primary hyperparathyroidism: Observations in 3 patients. Ann. Intern. Med. 68:1022, 1968.

35. Resnick, D.L.: Erosive arthritis of the hand and wrist in hyperparathyroidism. Radiology 110:263, 1974.

36. Rynes, R.I., and Merzig, E.G.: Calcium pyrophosphate crystal deposition disease and hyperparathyroidism: A controlled prospective study. J. Rheumatol. 5:460, 1978.

37. Pritchard, M.H., and Jessop, J.D.: Chondrocalcinosis in primary hyperparathyroidism. Ann. Rheum. Dis. 36:146, 1977.

38. Alexander, G.M., Dieppe, P.A., Doherty, M., and Scott, D.G.I.: Pyrophosphate arthropathy: A study of metabolic associations and laboratory data. Ann. Rheum. Dis. 41:377, 1982.

39. Hofmann, G.S., Schumacher, H.R., and Paul, H.: Calcium oxalate microcrystalline-associated arthritis in end stage renal disease. Ann. Intern. Med. 97:36, 1982.

40. Bywaters, E.G.L., Dixon, A.S.J., and Scott, J.T.: Joint lesions of hyperparathyroidism. Ann. Rheum. Dis. 22:171, 1963.

41. Bland, J.H., Frymoyer, J.W., Newberg, A.H., Revers, R., and Norman, R.J.: Rheumatic syndromes in endocrine disease. Semin. Arthritis Rheum. 9:23, 1979.

42. Debnam, J.W., Bates, M.L., Kopelman, R.C., and Teitelbaum, S.L.: Radiological/pathological correlations in uremic bone disease. Radiology 125:653, 1977.

43. Resnick, D., Dwosh, J.L., and Niwayama, G.: Sacro-iliac joint in renal

osteodystrophy: Roentgenographic-pathologic correlation. J. Rheumatol. 2:287, 1975.

44. Teplick, J.G., Eftekhari, F., and Haskin, M.E.: Erosion of the sternal ends of the clavicle: A new sign of primary and secondary hyperparathyroidism. Radiology 113:323, 1974.

45. Contiguglia, S.R., Alfrey, A.C., Miller, M.L., Runnetts, D.E., and Legeras, R.Z.: Nature of soft tissue calcification in uremia. Kidney Int. 4:229, 1973.

46. Kuzela, D.C., Hoffer, W.E., Conger, J.D., Winter, S.D., and Hammond, W.S.: Soft tissue calcification in chronic dialysis patients. Am. J. Pathol. 86:403, 1977.

47. Mirahmadi, K.S., Coburn, J.W., and Bluestone, R.: Arthritis and periarticular inflammation associated with calcification in patients treated with regular hemodialysis. JAMA 223:548, 1973.

48. Scott, J.T., Dixon, St. J., and Bywaters, E.G.L.: Association of hyperuricemia and gout with hyperparathyroidism. Br. Med. J. 1:1070, 1964.

49. Goldin, R., Brickman, A.S., Massry, S.G., and Bluestone, R.: Ankylosing Spondylitis and hyperparathyroidism. JAMA 240:759, 1978.

50. Hilbish, T.F., and Bartler, F.C.: Roentgen findings in abnormal deposition of calcium in tissues. Am. J. Roentgenol. 87:1128, 1962.

51. Dauphine, R.T., Riggs, B.L., and Scholz, D.A.: Back pain and vertebral crush fractures: An unemphasized mode of presentation for primary hyperparathyroidism. Ann. Intern. Med. 83:365, 1975.

52. Blair, D.C., and Fekety, R.F.: Primary hyperparathyroidism presenting as fever of unknown origin with unremitting headaches. Ann. Intern. Med. 91:575, 1979.

53. Chaykin, L.B., Frame, B., and Sigler, J.W.: Spondylitis: A clue to hypoparathyroidism. Ann. Intern. Med. 70:995, 1969.

54. McEwan, C., Ditata, D., Lingg, C., Porini, A., Good, A., and Rankin, T.: Ankylosing spondylitis and spondylitis accompanying ulcerative colitis, regional enteritis, psorasis and Reiter disease. Arthritis Rheum. 14:291, 1971.

55. Hung, W., Migeon, C.J., and Parrott, R.H.: A possible autoimmune basis for Addison's disease in three siblings, one with idiopathic hypoparathyroidism, pernicious anemia and superficial moniliasis. N. Engl. J. Med. 269:658, 1963.

56. Sjoberg, K.H.: Moniliasis an internal disease? Three cases of idiopathic hypoparathyroidism and moniliasis, steatorrhea, primary amenorrhea, and pernicious anemia. Acta. Med. Scand. 179:157, 1966.

57. Arulanatham, K., Dwyer, J.M., and Genel, M.: Evidence for defective immunoregulation in the syndrome of familial candidiasis endocrinopathy. N. Engl. J. Med. 300:164, 1979.

58. Chilgren, R.A., Quie, P.G., Meuwissen, H.J., Good, R.A., and Hong, R.: The cellular immune defect in chronic mucocutaneous candidiasis. Lancet 1:1286, 1969.

59. DiGeorge, A.M., and Paschkis, D.: The syndrome of Addison's disease, hypoparathyroidism, and superficial moniliasis. Am. J. Dis. Child. 94:476, 1957.

60. Eisenbarth, G.S., Wilson, P.W., Ward, F., Buckley, C., and Lebovitz, H.: The polyglandular failure syndrome: Disease inheritance, HLA type, and immune function. Ann. Intern. Med. 91:528, 1979.

61. Mann, J., Allerman, S., and Hills, A.G.: Albright's hereditary osteodystrophy comprising pseudohypoparathyroidism and pseudopseudohypoparathyroidism. Ann. Intern. Med. 56:315, 1962.

62. Levine, M.A., Downs, R.W., Moses, A.M., Breslau, N.A., Marx, S.J., Lasker, R.D., Rizzoli, R.E., Aurbach, G.D., and Spiegel, A.M.: Resistance to multiple hormones in patients with pseudohypoparathyroidism: Association with deficient activity of guanine nucleotide regulatory protein. Am. J. Med. 74:545, 1983.

63. Poznanski, A.K., Werder, E.A., Giedion, A., Martin, A., and Shaw, H.: The pattern of shortening of the bones of the hand in PHP and PPHP: A comparison with brachydactyly E., Turner syndrome, and acrodyostosis. Radiology 123:707, 1977.

64. Steinbach, H.L., Rudhe, U., Jonsson, M., and Young, D.A.: Evolution of skeletal lesions in pseudohypoparathyroidism. Radiology 85:670, 1965.

65. Nagant de Deuxchaisnes, C., and Krane, S.M.: Hypoparathyroidism. In Avioli, L.V., and Krane, S.M. (eds.): Metabolic Bone Disease. Vol. II. New York, Academic Press, 1978, p. 393.

66. Brown, J., Solomon, D.H., Beall, G.N., et al.: Autoimmune thyroid diseases—Graves' and Hashimoto's. Ann. Intern. Med. 88:379, 1978.

67. Volpe, R.: The role of auto-immunity in hypoendocrine and hyperendocrine function. Ann. Intern. Med. 87:86, 1977.

68. Strakosch, G.R., Wenzel, B.E., Row, V.V., and Volpe, R.: Immunology of autoimmune thyroid diseases. N. Engl. J. Med. 307:1499, 1982.

69. Strakosch, C.R., Joyner, D., and Wall, J.R.: Thyroid-stimulating antibodies in patients with autoimmune disorders. J. Clin. Endocrinol. Metab. 47:361, 1978.

70. Zakarija, M., McKenzie, J.M., and Banovac, K.: Clinical significance of assay of thyroid-stimulating antibody in Graves' disease. Ann. Intern. Med. 93:28, 1980.

71. Gimlette, T.M.D.: Thyroid acropathy. Lancet 1:22, 1960.

72. Gorman, C.A.: Unusual manifestations of Graves' disease. Mayo Clin. Proc. 47:926, 1972.

73. Cheung, H.S., Nicoloff, J.T., Kamiel, M.B., Spotler, L., and Nimni, M.E.: Stimulation of fibroblast biosynthetic activity by serum of patients with pretibial myxedema. J. Invest. Dermatol. 71:12, 1978.

74. Ramsey, I.D.: Muscle dysfunction in hyperthyroidism. Lancet 2:931, 1966.

75. Skillern, P.G.: The association of periarthritis of the shoulder with hyperthyroidism. In Transactions of the American Goiter Association. Springfield, Ill., Charles C Thomas, 1953, p. 100.

76. Mundy, G.R., Shapiro, J.L., Bandelin, J.G., Canalis, E.M., and Raisz, L.G.: Direct stimulation of bone resorption by thyroid hormone. J. Clin. Invest. 58:529, 1976.

77. Avioli, L.V.: Osteoporosis pathogenesis and therapy. In Avioli, L.V., and Krane, S.M. (eds.): Metabolic Bone Disease. Vol. I. New York, Academic Press, 1977, p. 347.

78. Silverberg, J., and Volpe, R.: Rheumatoid factors in Graves' disease. Ann. Intern. Med. 88:216, 1978.

79. Librik, L., Sussman, L., Bejar, R., and Clayton, G.W.: Thyrotoxicosis and collagen-like disease in three sisters of American Indian extraction. J. Pediatr. 76:64, 1970.

80. Amrheim, J.A., Kenny, F.M., and Ross, D.: Granulocytopenia, lupus-like syndrome and other complications of propylthiouricil therapy. J. Pediatr. 76:54, 1970.

81. Thomas, R.D., and Croft, D.N.: Thyrotoxicosis and giant cell arteritis. Br. Med. J. 2:408, 1974.

82. Blake, D.R., McGregor, A.M., Stansfield, E., and Rees Smith, B.: Antithyroid antibody activity in the synovial fluid of patients with various arthritides. Lancet 2:224, 1979.

83. Dorwart, B.B., and Schumacher, H.R.: Joint effusions, chondrocalcinosis and rheumatic manifestations of hypothyroidism. Am. J. Med. 59:780, 1975.

84. Bland, J.H., and Fryomyer, J.W.: Rheumatic syndromes of myxedema. N. Engl. J. Med. 282:1171, 1970.

85. Alexander, G.J.M., Scott, D.G.I., and Dieppe, P.A.: Pyrophosphate arthropathy: A study of metabolic associations and laboratory data. Ann. Rheum. Dis. 4:377, 1981.

86. Goldman, J., Matz, R., Mortimer, R., and Freeman, R.: High elevations of creatine phosphokinase in hypothyroidism. JAMA 238:325, 1977.

87. Hochberg, M.C., Edwards, C.Q., Barnes, H.V., Arnette, F.C., and Koppes, G.M.: Hypothyroidism presenting as a polymyositis-like syndrome. Arthritis Rheum. 19:1363, 1976.

88. Fessel, W.J.: Myopathy of hypothyroidism. Ann. Rheum. Dis. 27:590, 1968.

89. How, J., Bowsher, P.D., and Walker, W.: Giant cell arteritis and hypothyroidism. Br. Med. J. 2:99, 1977.

90. Golding, D.N.: Hypothyroidism presenting with musculoskeletal symptoms. Ann. Rheum. Dis. 29:10, 1970.

91. Frymoyer, J.W., and Bland, J.: Carpal tunnel syndrome in patients with myxedematous arthropathy. J. Bone Jt. Surg. 55A:78, 1973.

92. Seedat, Y.K., and Randeree, M.: Avascular necrosis of the hip joint in hypothyroidism. S. African Med. J. 49:2071, 1975.

93. Rubinstein, H.M., and Brooks, M.H.: Aseptic necrosis of bone in myxedema. Ann. Intern. Med. 87:580, 1977.

94. Siegelman, S.S., Schossberg, I., Becker, N.H., and Sachs, B.A.: Hyperlipidemia with skeletal lesions. Clin. Orthop. 87:228, 1972.

95. Okita, N., Row, V.V., and Volpe, R.: Suppressor T-lymphocyte deficiency in Graves' disease and Hashimoto's thyroiditis. J. Clin. Endocrinol. Metab. 52:528, 1981.

96. Okita, N., Topliss, D., Lewis, M., Row, V.V., and Volpe, R.: T-lymphocyte sensitization in Graves' and Hashimoto's disease confirmed by an indirect migration factor test. J. Clin. Endocrinol. Metab. 52:523, 1981.

97. Whaley, K., Webb, J., McAvoy, B.A., Hughes, G.R.C., Lee, P., MacSween, R.N.U., and Buchanan, W.W.: Sjögren's syndrome: Two clinical associations and immunological phenomena. Quart. J. Med. 42:513, 1973.

98. Becker, K.L., Ferguson, R.H., and McConahey, W.M.: The connective tissue diseases and symptoms associated with Hashimoto's thyroiditis. N. Engl. J. Med. 268:277, 1963.

99. Forid, N.R., and Bear, J.C.: The major histocompatibility complex and endocrine disease. Endocrinol. Rev. 2:50, 1981.

100. Eisenbarth, G.S., Wilson, P.W., Ward, F., Buckley, C., and Lebovitz, H.: The polyglandular failure syndrome: Disease inheritance, HLA type and immune function. Ann. Intern. Med. 91:528, 1979.

101. Urbanic, R.C., and George, J.M.: Cushing's disease—18 years' experience. Medicine 60:14, 1981.

102. Muller, R., and Kugelberg, E.: Myopathy in Cushing's syndrome. J. Neurol. Neurosurg. Psych. 22:304, 1959.

103. Afifi, A.K., Bergman, R.A., and Harvey, J.C.: Steroid myopathy: Clinical histologic and cytologic observations. Johns Hopkins Med. J. 123:158, 1968.

104. Lane, R.J., and Mastaglia, F.L.: Drug-induced myopathies in man. Lancet 2:562, 1978.

105. Axelrod, L.: Glucocorticoid therapy. Medicine 55:39, 1976.

106. Danowski, T.S., Boness, J.V., Sabeh, G., Sulton, R.O., Webster, M.V., and Sarver, M.E.: Probabilities of pituitary-adrenal responsiveness after steroid therapy. Ann. Intern. Med. 61:11, 1964.

107. Askari, A., Vignos, P.J., and Moskowitz, R.W.: Steroid myopathy in connective tissue disease. Am. J. Med. 61:485, 1976.

108. Dixon, R.B., and Nicholas, P.C.: On the various forms of corticosteroid withdrawal syndrome. Am. J. Med. 68:224, 1980.

109. Byyny, R.L.: Withdrawal from glucocorticoid therapy. N. Engl. J. Med. 295:30, 1976.

110. Smith, R.T., and Good, R.A.: Sequelae of prednisone treatment of acute rheumatic fever. Clin. Res. Proc. 4:156, 1956.

111. Spagnuolo, M., and Tranta, A.: Post-steroid panniculitis. Ann. Intern. Med. 54:1181, 1963.

112. Neufeld, M., MaClaren, N.K., and Blizzard, R.U.: Two types of autoimmune Addisons' disease associated with different polyglandular (PGA) syndromes. Medicine 60:355, 1981.

113. Williamson, J., Patterson, R.W.W., and McGavin, D.D.M.: Sjögren's syndrome in relation to pernicious anemia and idiopathic Addison's disease. Br. J. Opthalmol. 54:31, 1970.

114. Daughaday, W.H.: The Adenohypophysis. In Williams, R.H. (ed.): Textbook of Endocrinology. Philadelphia, W.B. Saunders Company, 1981, p. 89.

115. Bluestone, R., Bywaters, E.G.L., Hartog, M., Holt, P.J.L., and Hyde, S.: Acromegalic arthropathy. Ann. Rheum. Dis. 30:243, 1971.

116. Sledge, C.B.: Growth hormone and articular cartilage. Fed. Proc. 30:243, 1971.

117. Holt, P.J.L.: Locomotor abnormalities in acromegaly. Clin. Rheum. Dis. 7:689, 1981.

118. Riggs, B.L., Randell, R.V., Wahner, H.W., Jowsey, J., Kelly, P.J., and Singh, M.: The nature of the metabolic bone disorder in acromegaly. J. Clin. Endocrinol. 34:911, 1972.

119. O'Duffy, J.D., Randell, R.V., and MacCarty, C.S.: Median neuropathy (carpal tunnel syndrome) in acromegaly. Ann. Intern. Med. 78:379, 1973.

120. Nagulesparen, M., Trickey, R., Davies, M.T., and Jenkins, J.S.: Muscle changes in acromegaly. Br. Med. J. 2:914, 1976.

121. Mastalgia, F.L., Bawick, D.D., and Hall, R.: Myopathy in acromegaly. Lancet 2:907, 1976.

122. Mills, J.A.: Connective tissue disease associated with malignant neoplastic disease. J. Chronic Dis. 16:797, 1963.

123. Steinbach, H., Feldman, R., and Goldberg, M.B.: Acromegaly. Radiology 72:535, 1959.

124. Phalen, G.S.: Reflections on 21 years' experience with the carpal tunnel syndrome. JAMA 212:1365, 1970.

125. Forrester, D.M., Brown, J.C., and Nesson, J.W.: The spine, the sacroiliac joint, and the symphysis pubis. In Forrester, D.M., Brown, J.C., and Nesson, J.W. (eds.): The Radiology of Joint Disease. Philadelphia, W.B. Saunders Company, 1978, p. 534.

126. Baines, M.G., Miller, K.G., and Mills, P.: Studies of complement levels in normal human pregnancy. Obstet. Gynecol. 43:806, 1974.

127. Cecere, F.A., and Persellin, R.H.: The interaction of pregnancy and the rheumatic diseases. Clin. Rheum. Dis. 7:747, 1981.

128. Persellin, R.H., and Liebforth, J.K.: Studies of the effects of pregnancy serum on polymorphonuclear leukocyte functions. Arthritis Rheum. 21:316, 1978.

129. Sridana, V., Pancini, F., Yank, S.L., Moawad, A., Reilly, M., and GeGroot, L.J.: Decreased levels of helper T cells: A possible cause of immunodeficiency in pregnancy. N. Engl. J. Med. 307:353, 1982.

130. Fugisaki, S., Mori, N., Sasaki, T., and Maeyama, M.: Cell mediated immunity in human pregnancy. Microbiol. Immunol. 23:899, 1979.

131. Roubanian, J.R., Talal, N., Greenspan, J.S., Goodman, J.R., and Siiteri, P.K.: Effect of castration and sex hormone treatment on survival, antinucleic acid antibodies, and glomerulonephritis in NZB/NZW F-1 mice. J. Exp. Med. 147:1568, 1978.

132. Cecere, F.A., and Persellin, R.H.: The interaction of pregnancy and the rheumatic diseases. Clin. Rheum. Dis. 7:747, 1981.

133. Persellin, R.H.: The effect of pregnancy on rheumatoid arthritis. Bull. Rheum. Dis. 27:922, 1977.

134. Fine, L.G., Barnett, E.V., and Danovitch, G.B.: Systemic lupus erythematosus in pregnancy. Ann. Intern. Med. 94:667, 1981.

135. Zulman, J.I., Talal, N., Hoffman, G.S., and Epstein, W.V.: Problems associated with the management of pregnancy with systemic lupus erythematosis. J. Rheumatol. 7:37, 1980.

136. Schiff, B.L., and Kern, A.B.: A study of postpartum alopecia. Arch. Dermatol. 35:323, 1960.

137. Tozman, E.C.S., Urowitz, M.B., and Gladman, D.D.: Systemic lupus erythematosus and pregnancy. J. Rheumatol. 7:624, 1980.

138. Devoe, L.D., and Taylor, R.L.: Systemic lupus erythematosus in pregnancy. Am. J. Obstet. Gynecol. 135:473, 1979.

139. Bole, G.G., Jr., Friedlander, M.H., and Smith, C.K.: Rheumatic symptoms and serological abnormalities induced by oral contraceptives. Lancet 1:323, 1969.
140. Blomgren, S.E.: Erythema nodosum. Semin. Arthritis Rheum. 4:1, 1974.
141. Praeger, L., et al.: Roentgenographic abnormalities in phenotypic females with gonadal dysgenesis: A comparison of chromatin positive patients

and chromatin negative patients. Am. J. Roentgenol. Rad. Ther. Nucl. Med. 104:899, 1968.
142. Grumbach, M.M., and Conte, F.A.: Disorders of sex differentiation. *In* Williams, R.L. (ed.): Textbook of Endocrinology. Philadelphia, W.B. Saunders Company, 1981, p. 458.

Chapter 103
Hypertrophic Osteoarthropathy

Roy D. Altman and Jerry Tenenbaum

INTRODUCTION

Hypertrophic osteoarthropathy may be defined as a syndrome of (1) chronic proliferative periostitis of the long bones, (2) clubbing of fingers or toes, or both, and (3) oligo- or polysynovitis.

Clubbing is not a new disorder, having been described in the writings of Hippocrates, circa 400 B.C.; hence the label "Hippocratic fingers."[1] The association among clubbing, arthritis, and chronic lung and chronic heart disease was later elaborated by von Bamburger (1889)[2] and Marie (1890).[3] Subsequently a familial form of hypertrophic osteoarthropathy was described predominantly in young men.[4] More recently, the triad of periostitis, clubbing, and arthritis has been associated with numerous extrathoracic diseases (Table 103–1).

CLASSIFICATION (Table 103–1)

Hypertrophic osteoarthropathy may be primary or secondary. The primary form is most often hereditary. However, occasional idiopathic cases have been reported in adults. The secondary form of hypertrophic osteoarthropathy is most often associated with neoplastic or infectious diseases. The condition is most often bilaterally symmetric.

Isolated clubbing, not associated with periostitis or polyarthritis, deserves special consideration.[7,55] It is not certain whether this familial condition is a separate entity or simply an incomplete expression of hypertrophic osteoarthropathy. There are certain conditions that may be associated with clubbing alone; these are indicated by an asterisk (*) in Table 103–1.

Thyroid acropachy, a rare condition seen in patients with longstanding hyperthyroidism, is a unique form of hypertrophic osteoarthropathy and will be discussed separately.[53,54]

CLINICAL SYNDROMES

Pachydermoperiostosis. The primary form of hypertrophic osteoarthropathy occurs most often within families. It is referred to as pachydermoperiostosis or Touraine-Solente-Golé syndrome. Symptoms usually begin in adolescent males, but may appear in both sexes, either before or after puberty.[56] Pedigree studies suggest that it is transmitted by an autosomal dominant gene with variable expression. Symptoms are usually limited to one or two decades, and the condition can be detected in other family members.

Most commonly, there is insidious development of clubbing with "spadelike" enlargement of hands and feet during adolescence. Complaints are most often directed at cosmetic unsightliness and to decreasing dexterity or awkwardness when using the fingers. Symptoms may include vague pains in the joints and along the bones.[5] Joint pain and swelling may be exacerbated by alcohol.[57]

On examination there is marked clubbing with cylindric thickening of forearms and legs involving bones and soft tissues corresponding to radiologic periosteal changes.[4,5] Recurrent joint effusions may occur[58] but rarely cause pronounced discomfort. Acrolysis may occur with excessive resorption of distal phalanges of both hands and feet.[59] The syndrome is associated with thickening and furrowing of the facial features with deep nasolabial folds and corrugated scalp (Fig. 103–1), revealing "leoninelike" features. The skin of the face and scalp are often "greasy." There is often excessive sweating, particularly of the hands and feet. The facial features, greasy skin, and sweating are uncommonly seen in secondary hypertrophic osteoarthropathy. Some patients demonstrate gynecomastia, female hair distribution, striae, and acne vulgaris. Cranial suture defects have been associated with hypertrophic osteoarthropathy.[60]

Laboratory findings of pachydermoperiostosis are discussed further on.

Clubbing. Clubbing is a descriptive term pertaining to the appearance of the fingers or toes, or both (Figs. 103–2 and 103–3). The presence of clubbing does not distinguish its origin as familial or idiopathic. Clubbing should be distinguished from the syndrome of hypertrophic osteoarthropathy. Clubbing may be a feature of hypertrophic osteoarthropathy, but periostitis and polysynovitis do not invariably accompany clubbing.

The clinical characteristics of clubbing are as follows:
1. Initially there is fluctuance and *softening of the nail*

Table 103–1. Classification of Hypertrophic Osteoarthropathy

I. Primary
  A. Pachydermoperiostosis[5]
  B. Idiopathic[5]
  C. Clubbing*
    1. Familial[6]
    2. Idiopathic[7]
II. Secondary
  A. Pulmonary
    1. Neoplasms
      a. Bronchogenic carcinoma[8]
      b. Pleural tumors[9]
      c. Lymphosarcoma of mediastinum[10]
    2. Infections
      a. Bronchiectasis[11]
      b. Chronic bronchitis*[7]
      c. Lung abscess[8]
      d. Empyema[12]
      e. Pulmonary tuberculosis[13]
      f. Hydatid disease of the lung[14]
    3. Other
      a. Cystic fibrosis[15]
      b. Bronchogenic cyst[10]
      c. Pulmonary hemangioma*[16]
      d. Pneumoconiosis*[7]
      e. Diffuse infiltrating diseases of the lung*
        (e.g, causes of diffuse interstitial pulmonary fibrosis)[7]
      f. Sarcoidosis[17]
  B. Cardiovascular
    1. Bacterial endocarditis*[18]
    2. Cyanotic congenital heart disease[19]
    3. Patent ductus arteriosus[20]
    4. Aortic aneurysm*[16]
    5. Cardiac rhabdomyosarcoma[21]
    6. Abdominal aortic prosthesis[22] (infected)[23]
  C. Gastrointestinal
    1. Neoplasms
      a. Small intestinal carcinoma[24]
      b. Carcinoma of liver[25]
      c. Carcinoma of esophagus[26]
      d. Carcinoma of colon[7]

    2. Infections
      a. Amebic colitis[7]
      b. Bacillary dysentery[7]
      c. Intestinal tuberculosis[7]
      d. Whipworm infestation*[27]
      e. Subphrenic abscess[28]
    3. Hepatobiliary
      a. Cholangiolitic biliary cirrhosis[7]
      b. Cirrhosis[29,30]
      c. Secondary hepatic amyloidosis*[7]
      d. Biliary atresia[30a]
    4. Other
      a. Inflammatory bowel disease[31]
      b. Polyposis of colon[7]
      c. Sprue[7,10]
      d. Esophageal polyps[32]
      e. Pseudomembranous colitis[33]
  D. Neoplasms (often with intrathoracic metastases)
    a. Carcinoma of the nasopharynx[34]
    b. Chronic myelogenous leukemia[10]
    c. Neurilemmoma[35]
    d. Thymoma[36]
    e. Hodgkin's disease[37]
    f. Lymphoma[38]
    g. Secondary myelofibrosis[39]
    h. Renal carcinoma[40,41]
    i. Malignant melanoma[42]
    j. Endometrial carcinoma[43]
    k. Osteosarcoma[44]
    l. Ovarian carcinoma[44a]
  E. Miscellaneous
    a. Myxedema[45]
    b. Polyarteritis nodosa[46]
    c. Pregnancy[47]
    d. Hyperparathyroidism*[48]
    e. Purgative abuse*[49]
    f. Systemic lupus erythematosus[50]
    g. Thalassemia[51]
    h. Lymphomatoid granulomatosis*[52]
  F. Thyroid acropathy[53,54]

*Associated with clubbing alone; rarely associated with periostitis and polyarthritis.

bed. There is often a "rocking" sensation to palpation of the nail bed accompanied by periungual erythema, often with noticeable telangiectasia.

2. There is *loss of the normal 15-degree angle* between the nail and the soft tissue of the nail bed (cuticle).

3. There is *accentuated convexity* of the nail itself.

4. A *clubbed* appearance of the fingertip is accompanied by local warmth and sweating.

5. Finally, "shining" or "glossy" changes of the *nail and adjacent skin* with longitudinal striations of the nail may occur. This is followed by eponychia, paronychia, "hangnails," and breaking of the nail with accelerated nail or cuticle growth. The distal interphalangeal joint may become hyperextensible.

Aside from occasional cosmetic unsightliness, congenital clubbing causes no symptoms. Frequently, similar changes occur in the toes.

Methods have been proposed for the early detection of clubbing. In one method, the diameter of the index finger at the base of the nail is divided by the diameter at the distal interphalangeal joint. This should yield a ratio of one or less. A ratio of greater than one signifies clubbing.[61] Another method proposes a shadowgram technique[62] for measurement of the hyponychial angle.The most recent proposal for measurement is a technique by Schamroth. He proposed placing the dorsal surfaces of contralateral fingers together, using particularly the ring finger (Figure 103–4).[63] A gap appears normally at the nail bed. As the nail bed expands, the gap fills.

Familial clubbing is common and may reflect an incomplete expression of pachydermoperiostosis.[6,7] A genetic pattern has not yet been established.

Similarly, idiopathic or secondary clubbing may in some instances be a *forme fruste* of hypertrophic osteoarthropathy, but more likely it is unrelated.

Clubbing frequently emerges insidiously over a period of months or years without symptoms (see Table 103–1). Most cases of isolated clubbing are idiopathic. Idiopathic clubbing may simply be hereditary with delayed expression. More rapid onset of clubbing in the adult is more often associated with chronic infections, for example, bacterial endocarditis.[18] Clubbing related to bacterial endocarditis has become less common, probably because of earlier detection and therapy of endocarditis.

Unilateral clubbing is unusual but has been reported

Figure 103–1. Facies and hands in pachydermoperiostosis.

Figure 103–3. Clubbing. On lateral view, the index finger demonstrates loss of the normal 15 degree angle between the nail and the cuticle, accentuated convexity of the nail, enlargement of the distal finger pad, and shininess of the nail and adjacent skin.

with aneurysmal dilatation of the large arteries of the chest in addition to isolated reports of its occurrence[7] with apical lung neoplasms, axillary neoplasms, recurrent subluxation of the shoulder, aortic insufficiency with venous incompetence of the arm, and hemiplegia. Unidigital clubbing is most often related to trauma.[7]

Secondary Hypertrophic Osteoarthropathy. The secondary form of the syndrome of periostitis, clubbing, and polyarthritis most often presents in the adult, with age and sex distribution corresponding to the underlying disease.[64]

The onset of symptoms in secondary hypertrophic osteoarthropathy is often insidious, but disease progression is often more rapid than in the primary form.

Most often, the underlying disease is already apparent. However, clinical manifestations of hypertrophic osteoarthropathy may precede symptoms of the underlying associated disease by as much as 18 months.[8]

Periostitis usually causes relatively acute, increasing, and often severe burning and deep-seated pain of the distal extremities. The pain is particularly severe in the legs and is characteristically accentuated by dependency. This discomfort is often relieved by elevation. It is not uncommon to observe the patient reversed in a hospital bed with feet elevated at the head of the bed[65] (Figs. 103–5 and 103–6). In addition, the patient may complain of heat and swelling over the feet and legs. Clubbing is most often symptomatic only by its unsightliness. There may be occasional dysesthesia of the fingers with heat and sweating associated with clumsiness and stiffness of the hands. Joint symptomatology ranges from mild arthralgia to severe articular pain, the latter of which is

Figure 103–2. Clubbing. On this dorsal view of the hand, the fingertips are widened, replacing the normally tapered appearance of the digits.

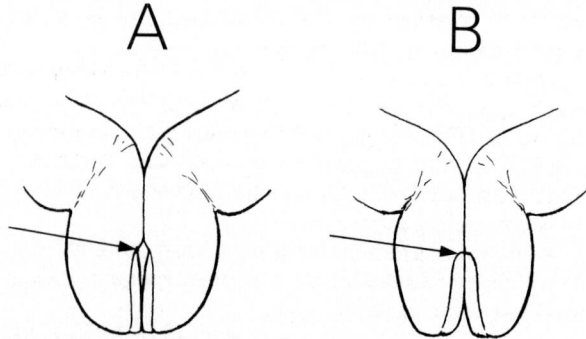

Figure 103–4. Schamroth test for clubbing[62]: Apposition of dorsal surfaces of contralateral digits demonstrates the proximity of the nail beds (arrows). The normal digits (*A*) demonstrate a gap . In early clubbing (*B*) the gap is lost and the convexity of the nail is more obvious.

Figure 103–5. Symptoms of periostitis are often aggravated by dependencey and relieved in part by elevation of the lower extremities. While reclined, patients are frequently more comfortable in a reversed position with the feet elevated at the head of the bed.

frequently symmetric and involves metacarpophalangeal joints, wrists, elbows, knees, and ankles.[64] There is occasional pain over the temporomandibular joints or clavicles. The patient may be aware of a low grade fever. Muscular weakness may accompany the acute presentation.

On examination, a broadened appearance of the distal parts of the extremities is often produced by a firm, mildly pitting edema. There is often warmth and tenderness to pressure over the feet and legs, the distal shin (tibia), the radius, and the ulna. Glistening thickened skin, perspiration, and erythema are often observed. The clinical appearance of clubbing is readily apparent (see Figs. 103–2 and 103–3). The periungual tissues become edematous, erythematous, and warm. There may be a dusky discoloration of the tips of the digits. The nails may rock, loosen, or break as clubbing progresses. Severely clubbed fingers and toes may resemble drumsticks. Mildly symptomatic joints are cool with small effusions and no palpable pannus. More symptomatic joints may be warm, tender, and swollen with definite effusions and limited range of motion. The symmetric involvement of hands, wrists, knees, and ankles with insidious onset gives the patient a rheumatoid appearance.[66] In far-advanced cases, ankylosis of joints may occur. The subcutaneous tissues around the active joints may be thickened and indurated with hypopigmented skin suggestive of scleroderma.[67] Functional assessment often reveals clumsiness of hand function and an awkward gait. Occasional patients have gynecomastia.[68]

The insidious emergence of clubbing over months or years, followed or accompanied by asymptomatic or mildly symptomatic bone and joint pain, is more often associated with the infectious diseases. Rapid progression of clubbing accompanied by fairly severe bone and joint symptoms is more commonly associated with malignant disease. However, as already noted, signs and symptoms of hypertrophic osteoarthropathy may precede any pulmonary symptom of neoplasia so that the assessment must include a chest x-ray.

Figure 103–6. Symptoms of periostitis are often relieved by elevation of the legs. This extreme example demonstrates a patient who could achieve enough pain relief to sleep only while standing on his head in the corner of the room. Note the comfortably placed pillow.

In childhood, secondary hypertrophic osteoarthropathy is often related to pulmonary infections,[69] congenital heart disease,[19] or osteosarcoma metastatic to lung. Hypertrophic osteoarthropathy caused by cyanotic congenital heart disease has been reported in up to 31 percent of cases, and is directly related to the degree of bypass of the lungs.[70]

In the adult, infections or neoplastic intrathoracic conditions are most common. Hypertrophic osteoarthropathy was observed in 9.2 percent of 1879 patients with pulmonary neoplasms, with bronchogenic carcinoma being the most common.[8,71,72] In a series of localized pleural mesotheliomas, hypertrophic osteoarthropathy and clubbing were noted only in the benign variant.[73] These tumors are usually peripheral in the lung fields. Relatively few case reports associate hepatobiliary and gastrointestinal diseases with hypertrophic osteoarthropathy.

Of interest is the occurrence of clubbing alone or hypertrophic osteoarthropathy that is present only in the lower extremities in patients with patent ductus arteriosus who have developed right to left shunting of blood flow secondary to pulmonary hypertension.[20] Hypertrophic osteoarthropathy of the lower extremeties has been reported with aortic grafts that are infected[23] or associated with intra-abdominal fistula formation.[22] Rarely, hypertrophic osteoarthropathy has begun during pregnancy and remitted post partum. These patients most often have other illnesses that have been associated with hypertrophic osteoarthropathy.[47] Although not reported in rheumatoid arthritis per se, clubbing has been noted in 9 of 12 patients with diffuse interstitial pulmonary fibrosis associated with rheumatoid arthritis.[74]

Thyroid Acropachy. Thyroid acropachy is an uncommon condition characterized by clubbing of the fingers and asymptomatic periosteal proliferation of the bones of the hands and feet.[52,54] It is associated with previous (or present) hyperthyroidism. It occurs concomitantly with exophthalmos, pretibial myxedema, and localized myxedema (nonpitting soft tissue swelling of the extremities).

The history is usually of a patient with Graves' disease who progresses to pronounced exophthalmos and pretibial myxedema. After months or, more often, years, clubbing may be noticed, and periostitis is discovered by x-ray. There are seldom other symptoms. The periosteal new bone formation is irregular and is associated with formation of small, rounded radiolucent areas, producing a bubbled or spiculated appearance. This reaction occurs in the midportion and diaphyseal regions of the metacarpals and phalanges, giving the shafts of these short bones a fusiform contour. Thyroid acropachy rarely involves long bones such as forearms and legs. This irregular periosteal thickening and appearance is in contrast to the relatively uniform, smooth periosteal new bone formation of primary or secondary hypertrophic osteoarthropathy.

The interval between hyperthyroidism and the onset of thyroid acropachy is occasionally quite long, obscuring their relationship. Hormones associated with hyperthyroidism, such as thyroid stimulating immunoglobulin, have been implicated and studied. However, there is no present evidence to support this relationship.

The abnormality of clubbing appears to be the only overt manifestation of thyroid acropachy. Treatment of hyperthyroidism has no effect upon the syndrome. No specific therapy is indicated for thyroid acropachy.

LABORATORY FINDINGS

The laboratory findings in primary and secondary hypertrophic osteoarthropathy are similar. Blood and urine tests are normal with the exception of the eryth-rocyte sedimentation rate (ESR), which may be increased in pachydermoperiostosis.[44] The ESR is also often elevated in secondary hypertrophic osteoarthropathy. Serum complement levels (total complement, C3, C4) are normal in cases of secondary hypertrophic osteoarthropathy.[75] The latex fixation test for rheumatoid factor and the fluorescent antinuclear antibody test have been found to be negative.[58,76] With sufficient active periosteal new bone formation, the serum alkaline phosphatase level may be increased.

Synovial fluid in pachydermoperiostosis and secondary hypertrophic osteoarthropathy is noninflammatory, and is clear and yellow in appearance. The viscosity is normal and the leukocyte count is low, demonstrating predominantly lymphocytes and monocytes. The total protein in the synovial fluid is low, and complement levels (C3, C4) are normal.[58,75]

RADIOGRAPHS AND RADIONUCLIDE SCANNING

The x-ray findings of hypertrophic osteoarthropathy may occur in the absence of any clinical findings in both the primary and the secondary forms. A consistent finding is periosteal thickening along the shafts of long and short bones, appearing first in the area of musculotendinous insertion, in the distal diaphyseal regions of the long bones and less often of the phalanges (Fig. 103–7). Periosteal changes appear as a continuous, thin sclerotic line of new bone at the distal end of the diaphysis of the long bones. This new finding is separated from the bony cortex by a narrow radiolucent line. The periosteal new bone formation then becomes thicker and fuses with the cortex. This symmetric involvement progresses proximally with prominence of subperiosteal new bone. Still later, the cancellous portion of the involved bone may become osteoporotic, and the cortex may become thin. These changes most often occur symmetrically in the tibia, radius, ulna, fibula, femur, and occasionally the clavicles.[7]

X-rays of the hands may reveal flaring of the terminal process and osteophytosis in more advanced stages of clubbing. The distal interphalangeal joints may or may not appear normal. On rare occasions, x-rays are normal in the presence of florid clinical disease.[77] Angiography demonstrates hypervascularization of the fingerpads associated with anteriovenous anastomoses and rapid filling of veins.[78]

Radionuclide bone scan utilizing a polyphosphate bone scanning agent is often helpful in documenting hypertrophic osteoarthropathy[79] (Figs. 103–8 and 103–9). Scans demonstrate a pericortical linear concentration of nuclide along the radial, femoral, and tibial shafts along with periarticular uptake of the radionuclide, emphasizing the presence of synovitis. The clubbed phalanges may also accumulate nuclide, giving the digital tips a "string of lights" appearance (Fig. 103–9).[65] Unusual sites of periosteal activity may be revealed, such as the mandible, scapula, patella, and clavicle.[36] The bone scan may be positive prior to the development of symptoms.

Figure 103–7. X-ray in hypertrophic osteoarthropathy. Periosteal new bone formation is demonstrated by arrowheads at the distal portions of the radius and ulna (*A*) as well as the tibia (*B*).

PATHOLOGY

Periosteum. The basic lesion is subperiosteal cancellous new bone formation at the level of the distal diaphysis of tubular bones. Initially there is subperiosteal edema with resultant periosteal elevation. Subsequently there is deposition of new osteoid beneath the periosteum. This osteoid mineralizes, causing a new layer of bone around the predominantly distal portions of the long bones. With time, the process advances proximally. There is associated increased osteoclastic activity and weakening of the subperiosteal bone. In a few extreme cases, pathologic fractures have occurred. These pathologic changes occur at the distal ends of the metacarpals, metatarsals, tibiae, fibulae, radii, ulnae, femora, humeri, and clavicles. Occasionally the scapulae, pelvis, malar bones, and ribs are involved. Similar round cell infiltration and edema occur in the adjacent subcutaneous tissues.[80]

Synovium. Synovial involvement is often continuous with the subperiosteal changes. The findings of light microscopy have ranged from apparently normal synovium to pannus formation with erosion and destruction of cartilage.[80] The synovial tissues may reveal thickening

Figure 103–8. Total body radionuclide bone scan in hypertrophic osteoarthropathy. Note localization of the nuclide to the periosteal areas of the tibiae and ulnae (closed arrows). The primary lesion, a brochogenic carcinoma, also accumulated the nuclide (open arrow).

of the subsynovial blood vessels and mild synovial cellular hyperplasia. The synovium becomes edematous and mildly infiltrated with lymphocytes, plasma cells, and occasional polymorphonuclear leukocytes.[58,75,76] Electron microscopic studies in secondary hypertrophic osteoarthropathy reveal occasional electron-dense subendothelial deposits in vessel walls[75,76] with hyaline-like material on the synovial surface, in the interstitium, and in some of the dense deposits.[76] Many endothelial cells exhibit swollen cytoplasm. There is a concentric increase in basement membrane–like lamellae with intervening pericytic cytoplasmic processes and occasional endothelial cell gaps. Thickened and concentric multilamination of capillary basement membranes[75] (Fig. 103–10)

Figure 103–9. Bone scan of foot in hypertrophic osteoarthropathy. Note accumulation of the isotope in the clubbed distal tufts (arrows).

Figure 103–10. Electron microscopy of synovium in hypertrophic osteoarthropathy. Synovial capillary lumen (*CL*) is surrounded by normal endothelial cells (*En*). The basal lamina (*BL*) is thickened and multilayered ($\times$ 5250). Occasional dense deposits are seen in the basal lamina (inset—arrowheads; $\times$46,500). Uranyl acetate and lead citrate stains.

can be seen and is similar to that described for pachydermoperiostosis.[58] In pachydermoperiostosis no electron-dense deposits are found in vessel walls.[58]

Immunologic studies of secondary hypertrophic osteoarthropathy synovium do not suggest a recent immunologically mediated injury. In three cases, immunohistologic studies failed to reveal immunoglobulin, C3, C4, or fibrinogen.[75,81]

Clubbing. The clubbed distal portion of the digits results from an increase in the connective tissue of the nail bed as well as a proliferation of all the distal digital soft tissues. The collagen bundles in the dermis are swollen with enlargement of the rete pegs and narrowing of the epidermal papillae. There are round cell infiltrates and fibroblastic proliferation with dilatation and thickening of blood vessel walls.[7,80]

DIFFERENTIAL DIAGNOSIS

Whenever hypertrophic osteoarthropathy is diagnosed, it is crucial to search for an associated disease. This process should begin with a chest x-ray. Evaluation should include assessment of the cardiopulmonary and gastrointestinal systems. When clubbing, periostitis, and arthritis are present in association with a primary pulmonary lesion, the disorder is easily recognized. However, these features may appear in different combinations separated by intervals of time.

As mentioned, isolated clubbing may present as a prodrome of hypertrophic osteoarthropathy or may represent a separate entity. One must be aware of the family history and length of time the patient has been aware of the clubbing. Even when these findings are suggestive of a familial factor, one should be alert to a possible

associated disease (see Table 103–1). Spooning of the nails associated with hypochromic anemia should be differentiated from clubbing. Clubbing should also be differentiated from acromegaly. Calcific deposits in the distal digital pads may give the finger a clubbed appearance in the patient with scleroderma.[65]

The periostitis of hypertrophic osteoarthropathy is usually characteristic, but one should consider periostitis of other causes such as bone tumor, osteomyelitis, subperiosteal hemorrhage, juvenile polyarthritis, syphilis, Reiter's syndrome, psoriasis, lymphangitis, and scurvy. Leg pain may suggest peripheral neuritis, Paget's disease of bone, or radiculopathy. The pretibial edema may suggest thrombophlebitis, venous stasis, or pretibial myxedema and must be considered in light of the general presentation. Simultaneous presentation of synovial metastases with hypertrophic osteoarthropathy has been reported.[82]

When the primary presenting complaint is polyarthritis, the picture may strongly resemble rheumatoid arthritis. The history of discomfort of the lower extremities, periosteal tenderness, clubbed digits, and benign synovial fluid findings suggest hypertrophic osteoarthropathy.

Pachydermoperiostosis can usually be differentiated from secondary hypertrophic osteoarthropathy because of the family history, age and sex at onset, and the nature of the periostitis. In pachydermoperiostosis the periostitis is less symptomatic and is radiographically more thick, smooth, and dense than in hypertrophic osteoarthropathy.

Thyroid acropachy is associated with longstanding hyperthyroid findings, such as exophthalmos. Periostitis is limited to the phalanges in spite of the associated pretibial myxedema.

ETIOLOGY AND PATHOGENESIS

The etiology of hypertrophic osteoarthropathy is unknown. Intrathoracic lesions of a malignant or infectious nature compose the majority of the associated systemic diseases. The most commonly related disease is bronchogenic carcinoma. The role that these lesions play in precipitation or production of hypertrophic osteoarthropathy is speculative.

The reversal of hypertrophic osteoarthropathy by vagotomy, both in patients[83] and in a dog model,[84] suggests that in some cases the association between pulmonary hypertrophic osteoarthropathy and intrathoracic disease is a reflex one, with afferent fibers from the lesion traveling via the vagus nerve.[84] Thus, the organs that are the site of the causative disease have a common feature— parts of their afferent innervation have a common nucleus of termination, accounting for a common afferent arc as an integral part of the pathogenic mechanism. Thoracotomy alone was ineffective.

Further proposed hypotheses include absorption of toxic material from neoplasms, peripheral concentration of toxic products by venous stasis, and peripheral hyperemia caused by compression of lung capillaries;[7,55] there is at present little evidence for these mechanisms. Extensive vascular anastomoses, both locally in the lungs and peripherally in the limbs, have been proposed as a reflex response to ischemia.[86] The finding that overgrowth of vascular connective tissue is the earliest demonstrable abnormality in hypertrophic pulmonary osteoarthropathy supports this hypothesis. Adrenergic blockade to reverse the hypervascularity was somewhat successful in one study.[86]

Increased vascularity of the clubbed digits has been demonstrated and provides evidence for a pathogenic role of a local circulatory abnormality.[7,78] A circulating vasodilator that appears to act on local vessels has been demonstrated in some patients.[87]

Theories proposing elevated growth hormone levels as being of etiologic importance arise from the finding of growth hormone elaboration from lung tumors in patients with hypertrophic pulmonary osteoarthropathy.[88] However, though elevation of growth hormone levels was found, there was no correlation between abnormalities of growth hormone metabolism and the pathologic changes of hypertrophic osteoarthropathy.[89]

The presence of gynecomastia coexistent with hypertrophic osteoarthropathy and increased urine estrogen excretion (to twice control levels) in a series of patients with hypertrophic osteoarthropathy suggests a role for estrogen.[68,90] This is supported by the occurrence of hypertrophic osteoarthropathy in pregnancy,[47] biliary cirrhosis, and Laennec's cirrhosis,[29] all of which show increased levels of circulating estriols. However, investigation fails to delineate a role for estrogen in this condition, and there is no direct evidence that excess levels of circulating estriols give rise to bony changes of hypertrophic osteoarthropathy.[91]

One theory of hypertrophic osteoarthropathy relates etiology to circulating tumor immune complexes that have been found in a variety of tumors, including pulmonary carcinoma. Although electron microscopic findings were suggestive, immunologic and complement studies failed to support such a hypothesis.[75]

Pachydermoperiostosis does not have an underlying chromosomal abnormality, though there was an earlier report of XYY trisomy.[92]

A role for prostaglandins $F_{2\alpha}$ and E in the development of clubbing has been suggested.[93]

MANAGEMENT

The most effective therapy for the pain and discomfort of secondary hypertrophic osteoarthropathy is ablation or cure of the underlying condition. Infectious diseases most often can be controlled by antibiotics or drainage. Removal or effective suppressive therapy (e.g., chemotherapy) for the primary tumor most often results in prompt remission of symptoms of hypertrophic osteoarthropathy, sometimes within hours or days.[8] Radiotherapy to the primary tumor[94] or to the metastatic lesion[95] may result in relief of joint symptoms. Even though there may be progression of the tumor with recurrent metastases, joint symptoms may not recur after initial relief. Vagotomy has been successful in some instances,[83] and percutaneous block of the vagus nerve was also successful in a series of patients.[96] Benefit may be achieved with chemical vagotomy by atropine[97] and possibly with propantheline bromide.[98,99]

Anti-inflammatory agents have been quite beneficial in reducing the discomfort of hypertrophic osteoarthropathy. Aspirin in modest doses is frequently effective.[44] The propionic acid derivatives may be helpful. Indomethacin is quite effective,[65] and adrenocortical steroids[66] may be helpful. Symptoms may resolve with successful therapy of bacterial endocarditis.[100]

Familial hypertrophic osteoarthropathy and clubbing are most often asymptomatic and rarely require therapy. Salicylates should be sufficient if therapy is needed.

COURSE AND PROGNOSIS

The course of primary hypertrophic osteoarthropathy is one of adolescent onset and self-limited disease, though recurrent joint effusions may occur.[58] The course of secondary hypertrophic osteoarthropathy varies greatly, reflecting the activity of the underlying disease and depending on the nature of the primary condition. Symptoms may wax and wane with exacerbations and remissions of the primary condition. After the resection of a lung tumor (or in some cases, after palliative treatment by resection of metastases in the lung) or a lung abscess, the symptoms and signs of arthropathy may subside rapidly over several hours or within a day. X-ray abnormalities usually remit more slowly over weeks or months.[64] Without treatment of the primary condition, symptoms of hypertrophic osteoarthropathy may result in a chronically painful demise.

References

1. Hippocrates: The book of prognostics. *In* The Genuine Works of Hippocrates, translated by F. Adams. London, Sydenham Society, 1849, Vol. 1.
2. von Bamberger, E.: Über Knochenveränderungen bei chronischen Lungenund Herzkrankenheiten. Ztschr. Klin. Med. 18:193, 1890–1891.
3. Marie, P.: De l'ostéo-arthropathie hypertrophiante pneumique. Rev. Med. (Paris) 10:1, 1890.
4. Touraine, A., Solente, G., and Golé, L.: Un syndrome ostéodermopathique: La pachydermie plicaturée avec pachypériostose des extrémités. Presse Méd. 43:1820, 1935.
5. Vogl, A., and Goldfischer, S.: Pachydermoperiostosis: Primary or idiopathic hypertrophic osteoarthropathy. Am. J. Med. 33:166, 1962.
6. Seaton, D.R.: Familial clubbing of fingers and toes. Br. Med. J. 1:614, 1938.
7. Mendlowitz, M.: Clubbing and hypertrophic osteoarthropathy. Medicine 21:269, 1942.
8. Vogl, A., Blumenfeld, S., and Gutner, L.B.: Diagnostic significance of pulmonary hypertrophic osteoarthropathy. Am. J. Med. 18:51, 1955.
9. Polley, H.F., Claggett, O.T., McDonald, J.R., and Schmidt, H.W.: Articular reactions associated with localized fibrous mesothelioma of the pleura. Ann. Rheum. Dis. 11:314, 1952.
10. Temple, H.L., and Jaspin, G.: Hypertrophic osteoarthropathy. Am. J. Roentgenol. 60:232, 1948.
11. Wierman, W.H., Clagett, O.T., and McDonald, J.R.: Articular manifestations in pulmonary diseases: Analysis of their occurrence in 1,024 cases in which pulmonary resection was performed. JAMA 155:1459, 1954.
12. Compere, E.L., Adams, W.E., and Compere, C.L.: Generalized hypertrophic pulmonary osteoarthropathy. Surg. Gynecol. Obstet. 61:312, 1935.
13. Corper, H.J., Cosman, P., Gilmore, W.M., and Black, L.T.: Hypertrophic osteoarthropathy in pulmonary tuberculosis. Am. Rev. Tuberc. 5:357, 1921–1922.
14. Thiodet, J., Fourrier, A., Chevrot, L., and Massonot, J.: Echinococcose pulmonaire et ostéo-arthropathie hypertrophiante pneumique de Pierre Marie. Bull. Soc. Méd. Hôp. Paris 66:1769, 1950.
15. Matthay, M.A., Matthay, R.A., Mills, D.M., Lakshiminarayan, S., and Cotton, E.: Hypertrophic osteoarthropathy in adults with cystic fibrosis. Thorax 31:572, 1976.
16. Shapiro, S.: Hypertrophic osteoarthropathy. AMA Arch. Intern. Med. 98:700, 1956.
17. West, S.G., Gilbreath, R.E., and Lawless, O.J.: Painful clubbing and sarcoidosis. JAMA 246:1338, 1981.
18. Cotton, T.F.: Clubbed fingers as a sign of subacute infective endocarditis. Heart 9:347, 1921–1922.
19. McLaughlin, G.E., McCarty, D.J., and Downing, D.F.: Hypertrophic osteoarthropathy associated with cyanotic congenital heart disease. Ann. Intern. Med. 67:579, 1967.
20. Williams, B., Ling, J., Leight, L., and McGaff, C.J.: Patent ductus arteriosus and osteoarthropathy. Arch. Intern. Med. 111:346, 1963.
21. Pascuzzi, C.A., Parkin, T.W., Bruwer, A.J., and Edwards, J.E.: Hypertrophic osteoarthropathy associated with primary rhabdomyosarcoma of the heart. Mayo Clin. Proc. 32:30, 1957.
22. Stein, H.B., and Little, H.A.: Localized hypertrophic osteoarthropathy in the presence of an abdominal aortic prosthesis. Can. Med. Assoc. J. 118:947, 1978.
23. Sorin, S.B., Askari, A., and Rhodes, R.S.: Hypertrophic osteoarthropathy of the lower extremities as a manifestation of arterial graft sepsis. Arthritis Rheum. 23:768, 1980.
24. Hollis, W.C.: Hypertrophic osteoarthropathy secondary to upper gastrointestinal tract neoplasm. Ann. Intern. Med. 66:125, 1967.
25. Morgan, A.G., Walker, W.C., Mason, M.D., Herlinger, H., and Losowsky, M.S.: A new syndrome associated with hepatocellular carcinoma. Gastroenterology 63:340, 1972.
26. Peirce, T.H., and Weir, D.G.: Hypertrophic osteoarthropathy associated with a non-metastasizing carcinoma of the oesophagus. J. Ir. Med. Assoc. 66:160, 1973.
27. Bowie, M.D., Morison, A., Ireland, J.D., and Duys, P.J.: Clubbing and whipworm infestation. Arch. Dis. Child. 53:411, 1978.
28. Gay, R.J., Shaw, K.M., and Watson, G.: Case report: Hypertrophic osteoarthropathy secondary to sub-phrenic abscess. Ir. J. Med. Sci. 144:330, 1975.
29. Buchan, D.J., and Mitchell, D.M.: Hypertrophic osteoarthropathy in portal cirrhosis. Ann. Intern. Med. 66:130, 1967.
30. Epstein, O., Dick, R., and Sherlock, S.: Prospective study of periostitis and finger clubbing in primary biliary cirrhosis and other forms of chronic liver disease. Gut 22:203, 1981.
30a. Rothberg, A.D., and Boal, D.K.: Hypertrophic osteoarthropathy in biliary atresia. Pediatr. Radiol. 13:44, 1983.
31. Kitis, G., Thompson, H., and Allan, R.N.: Finger clubbing in inflammatory bowel disease: Its prevalence and pathogenesis. Br. Med. J. 2:825, 1979.
32. Melvin, K.E.W.: Oesophageal polyp with hypertrophic osteoarthropathy. Proc. R. Soc. Med. 58:576, 1965.
33. Ueno, Y., Cassell, S., and Barnett, E.V.: Hypertrophic osteoarthropathy and pseudomembranous enterocolitis. J. Rheumatol. 8:825, 1981.
34. Martin, C.L.: Complications produced by malignant tumors of the nasopharynx. Am. J. Roentgenol. 41:377, 1939.
35. Trivedi, S.A.: Neurilemmoma of the diaphragm causing severe hypertrophic pulmonary osteoarthropathy. Br. J. Tuberc. Dis. Chest 52:214, 1958.
36. Ali, A., Tetalman, M.R., Fordham, E.W., Turner, D.A., Chiles, J.T., Patel, S.L., and Schmidt, K.D.: Distribution of hypertrophic pulmonary osteoarthropathy. Am. J. Radiol. 34:771, 1980.
37. Lofters, W.S., and Walker, T.M.: Hodgkin's disease and hypertrophic pulmonary osteoarthropathy. West Indian Med. J. 28:227, 1978.
38. McNeil, M.M., Sage, R.E., and Dale, B.M.: Hypertrophic osteoarthropathy complicating primary bone lymphoma—association with invasive phycomyosis and Aspergillus infections. Aust. N.Z. J. Med. 11:71, 1981.
39. Mason, B.A., Kressel, B.R., Cashdollar, M.R., Bernath, A.M., and Schechter, G.P.: Periostitis associated with myelofibrosis. Cancer 43:1568, 1979.
40. Solimbu, C., Marchetta, P., Firooznnia, H., and Rafu, M.: Hypertrophic osteoarthropathy in metastatic renal cell carcinoma. J. Urol. 22:669, 1983.
41. Allison, N.L., Stote, R.M., Rai, R., Roy, R.H., and Dubb, J.W.: Pulmonary osteoarthropathy preceding evidence of metastases from hypernephroma. Lancet 1:950, 1981.
42. Arlson, K.S., and Naidoo, A.: Hypertrophic osteoarthropathy. Mayo Clin. Proc. 59:208, 1979.
43. Margolick, J., Bonom, P., Fordham, E., Yordan, E., and Slayton, R.: Hypertrophic osteoarthropathy associated with endometrial carcinoma. Gynecol. Oncol. 13:399, 1982.
44. Lokich, J.J.: Pulmonary osteoarthropathy; association with mesenchymal tumor metastases to the lungs. JAMA 238:37, 1977.
44a. Lester, W.M., and Robertson, D.I.: Hypertrophic osteoarthropathy complicating metastatic ovarian adenocarcinoma. Can. J. Surg. 24: 520-523, 1981.
45. Chremos, A.M.: Relentless localized myxedema with exophthalmos, clubbing of the fingers and hypertrophic osteoarthropathy. Am. J. Med. 38:954, 1965.
46. Lovell, R.R.H., and Scott, G.B.D.: Hypertrophic osteoarthropathy in polyarteritis. Ann. Rheum. Dis. 15:46, 1956.
47. Borden, E.C., and Holling, H.E.: Hypertrophic osteoarthropathy and pregnancy. Ann. Intern. Med. 71:577, 1969.
48. Souders, C.R., and Manuell, J.L.: Skeletal deformities in hyperparathyroidism. N. Engl. J. Med. 250:594, 1954.
49. Armstrong, R.D., Crisp, A.J., and Grahame, R.: Hypertrophic osteoarthropathy and purgative abuse. Br. Med. J. 282:1836, 1981.
50. Mackie, R.M.: Lupus erythematosus in association with finger-clubbing. Br. J. Dermatol. 89:533, 1973.
51. Sinniah, D., White, J.C., Omar, A., Murugasu, R., and Iyngkaran, K.: Digital clubbing—a clinical sign in thalassemia. J. Pediatr. 92:597, 1978.
52. Prabhu, R., Berger, H.W., Subietas, A., and Lee, M.: Lymphomatoid granulomatosis, report of a patient with severe anemia and clubbing. Chest 77:883, 1980.
53. Kinsella, R.A., and Back, D.K.: Thyroid acropathy. Med. Clin. North Am. 52:393, 1968.
54. Rothschild, B.M., and Yoon, B.H.: Thyroid acropathy complicated by lymphatic obstruction. Arthritis Rheum. 25:588, 590, 1982.
55. Fischer, D.S., Singer, D.H., and Feldman, S.M.: Clubbing, a review, with emphasis on hereditary acropathy. Medicine 43:459, 1965.
56. Rimoin, D.L.: Pachydermoperiostosis (idiopathic clubbing and periostosis): Genetic and physiologic considerations. N. Engl. J. Med. 272:923, 1965.
57. Mueller, M., and Trevarthen, D.: Pachydermoperiostosis: Arthropathy aggravated by episodic alcohol abuse. J. Rheumatol. 8:862, 1981.
58. Lauter, S.A., Vasey, F.B., Huttner, I., and Osterland, C.K.: Pachydermoperiostosis: Studies on the synovium. J. Rheumatol. 5:85, 1978.
59. Fam, A.G., Chin-Sang, H., and Ramsay, J.: Pachydermoperiostosis: scintographic, plethysmographic, and capillaroscopic observations. Ann. Rheum. Dis. 42:98, 1983.

60. Reginato, A., Jr, Schinpachasse, Y., and Guerrero, R.: Familial idiopathic hypertrophic osteoarthropathy and cranial suture defects in children. Skeletal Radiol. 8:105, 1982.
61. Sly, R.M., Ghazanshahi, S., Buranakul, B., Paupan, P., Gupta, S., Warren, R., and Waring, W.: Objective assessment for digital clubbing in Caucasian, Negro, and Oriental subjects. Chest 64:687, 1973.
62. Sinniah, D., and Omar, A.: Quantitation of digital clubbing by shadowgram technique. Arch. Dis. Child. 54:145, 1979.
63. Schamroth, L.: Personal experience. S. Afr. Med. J. 50:297, 1976.
64. Shulman, L.E.: Hypertrophic osteoarthropathy. Bull. Rheum. Dis. 7:135, 1957.
65. Altman, R.D.: Personal observation.
66. Sega, A.M., and MacKenzie, A.H.: Hypertrophic osteoarthropathy: a ten year retrospective analysis. Semin. Arthritis Rheum. 12:220, 1982.
67. Gray, R.G., and Gottlieb, N.L.: Pseudoscleroderma in hypertrophic osteoarthropathy. JAMA 246:2062, 1981.
68. Ginsburg, J., and Brown, J.B.: Increased oestrogen excretion in hypertrophic pulmonary osteoarthropathy. Lancet 2:1274, 1961.
69. Cavanaugh, J.J.A., and Holman, G.H.: Hypertrophic osteoarthropathy in childhood. J. Pediatr. 66:27, 1965.
70. Martinez-Lavin, M., Bobadilla, M., Casanova, J., Attie, F., and Martinez, M.: Hypertrophic osteoarthropathy in cyonotic congenital heart disease. Arthritis Rheum. 25:1186, 1982.
71. Stenseth, J.H., Clagett, O.T., and Woolner, L.B.: Hypertrophic pulmonary osteoarthropathy. Dis. Chest 52:62, 1967.
72. Calabro, J.J.: Cancer and arthritis. Arthritis Rheum. 10:553, 1967.
73. Okike, N., Bernatz, P.E., and Woolner, L.B.: Localized mesothelioma of the pleura: Benign and malignant variants. J. Thorac. Cardiovasc. Surg. 75:363, 1978.
74. Walker, W.C., and Wright, V.: Pulmonary lesions and rheumatoid arthritis. Medicine 47:501, 1968.
75. Vidal, A.F., Altman, R.D., Pardo, V., and Schultz, D.: Structural and immunologic changes of synovium of hypertrophic osteoarthropathy. Arthritis Rheum. 20:139, 1977.
76. Schumacher, H.R.: Articular manifestations of hypertrophic pulmonary osteoarthropathy in bronchogenic carcinoma. Arthritis Rheum. 19:629, 1976.
77. Horn, C.R.: Hypertrophic osteoarthropathy without radiographic evidence of new bone formation. Thorax 35:479, 1980.
78. Jajic, I., Pecina, M., Kostulovic, B., Kovacevic, D., Pavicic, F., and Spaventi, S.: Primary hypertrophic osteoarthropathy (PHO) and changes in the joints. Scand. J. Rheumatol. 9:89, 1980.
79. Rosenthall, L., and Kirsh, J.: Observations on radionuclide imaging in hypertrophic pulmonary osteoarthropathy. Radiology 120:359, 1976.
80. Gall, E.A., Bennett, G.A., and Bauer, W.: Generalized hypertrophic osteoarthropathy: A pathologic study of seven cases. Am. J. Pathol. 27:349, 1951.
81. Awerbuch, M.S., and Brook, P.M.: Role of immune complexes in hypertrophic osteoarthropathy and nonmetastatic polyarthritis. Ann. Rheum. Dis. 40:470, 1981.
82. Fam, A.G., and Cross, E.G.: Hypertrophic osteoarthropathy, phalangeal

and synovial metastases associated with bronchogenic carcinoma. J. Rheumatol. 6:680, 1979.
83. Yacoub, M.H.: Cervical vagotomy for pulmonary osteoarthropathy. Br. J. Dis. Chest 59:28, 1965.
84. Holling, H.E., and Brody, R.S.: Pulmonary hypertrophic osteoarthropathy. JAMA 178:977, 1961.
85. Carroll, K.B., and Doyle, L.: A common factor in hypertrophic osteoarthropathy. Thorax 29:262, 1974.
86. Reardon, G., Collins, A.J., and Bacon, D.A.: The effect of adrenergic blockade in hypertrophic pulmonary osteoarthropathy (HPOA). Postgrad. Med. J. 52:170, 1976.
87. Shneerson, J.M.: Digital clubbing and hypertrophic osteoarthropathy: The underlying mechanisms. Br. J. Dis. Chest 75:113, 1981.
88. Dupont, B., Hoyer, I., Borgeskov, S., and Nerup, J.: Plasma growth hormone and hypertrophic osteoarthropathy in carcinoma of the bronchus. Acta Med. Scand. 188:25, 1970.
89. Ennis, G.C., Cameron, D.P., and Burger, H.G.: On the aetiology of hypertrophic pulmonary osteoarthropathy in bronchogenic carcinoma: Lack of relationship to elevated growth hormone levels. Aust. N.Z. J. Med. 3:157, 1973.
90. Jao, J.Y., Barlow, J.J., and Krant, M.J.: Pulmonary hypertrophic osteoarthropathy, spider angiomata, and estrogen hyperexcretion in neoplasia. Ann. Intern. Med. 70:581, 1969.
91. Holling, H.E.: Pulmonary hypertrophic osteoarthropathy. Ann. Intern. Med. 66:232, 1967.
92. Susmano, A., Shah, P., Krompotic, E., and Tashima, C.: Normal sex-chromosome complement in the case of familial osteoarthropathy. Lancet 2:131, 1967.
93. Lemen, R.J., Gates, A.J., Mathé, A.A., Waring, W.W., Hyman, A.L., and Kadowitz, P.D.: Relationships among digital clubbing, disease severity and serum prostaglandins $F_{2\alpha}$ and E concentrations in cystic fibrosis patients. Am. Rev. Respir. Dis. 117:639, 1978.
94. Steinfeld, A.D., and Munzenrider, J.E.: The response of hypertrophic pulmonary osteoarthropathy to radiotherapy. Radiology 113:709, 1974.
95. Rao, G.M., Gurupoakash, G.H., Poulose, K.P., and Blaskar, G.: Improvement in hypertrophic pulmonary osteoarthropathy after radiotherapy to metasasis. Am. J. Radiol. 133:944, 1979.
96. Dam, W.H., and Hagelsten, J.O.: Blocking of the vagus nerve relieving osteoarthropathy in lung disease. Dan. Med. Bull. 11:131, 1964.
97. Lopez-Enriquez, E., Morales, A.R., and Robert, F.: Effect of atropine sulfate in pulmonary hypertrophic osteoarthropathy. Arthritis Rheum. 23:822, 1980.
98. Schwartz, H.A.: Pro-Banthine for hypertrophic osteoarthropathy. Arthritis Rheum. 23:1588, 1980.
99. Deal, C.L., and Canoso, J.J.: Minimal response to propantheline bromide therapy in hypertrophic pulmonary osteoarthropathy: A double blind controlled case study. J. Rheumatol. 10:165, 1983.
100. Shapiro, C.M., and Mackinnon, J.: The resolution of hypertrophic pulmonary osteoarthropathy following treatment of subacute bacterial endocarditis. Postgrad. Med. J. 56:513, 515, 1980.

Chapter 104

Musculoskeletal Syndromes Associated with Malignancy

David S. Caldwell

INTRODUCTION

Malignancy may produce a variety of manifestations, most often owing to tumor interference with the function of the organ system involved. Less frequently the presentation may be a so-called paraneoplastic syndrome, that is, alteration in the function of an organ system unrelated to tumor mass or invasion. An estimated 15

percent of patients hospitalized with advanced malignancy will have a clinically apparent paraneoplastic syndrome. Careful search in this group will often reveal the existence of an equal number of subclinical syndromes. The chance of a paraneoplastic syndrome arising over the life span of a patient with cancer may reach 50 to 75 percent.[1]

Endocrine syndromes secondary to ectopic hormone

production are most commonly seen, accounting for one third of all paraneoplastic syndromes. Connective tissue, hematologic, and neuromuscular syndromes account for the majority of the remaining syndromes, occur with approximately equal frequency, and are presumably humorally mediated.[1,2]

The existence of a causal relationship between malignancy and connective tissue disease is firmly established for some entities such as hypertrophic osteoarthropathy, in which resection of the primary process has been followed by dramatic resolution of the presenting musculoskeletal symptoms. A variety of other musculoskeletal syndromes may be the presenting manifestation of an occult neoplastic process. Conversely, malignancy in the setting of a pre-existing connective tissue disease may occur. Whether a true relationship exists in all such cases is a point of contention, as both processes may commonly occur and the clinical expression may simply represent the chance occurrence of two disease processes. It is also possible that the common feature is not that one produces the other, but that they share the same unknown etiology. Whether the relationship is casual or causal, it would seem that the importance of their possible relationship is twofold: (1) The awareness that an underlying malignancy may produce musculoskeletal symptoms may allow for earlier recognition of an otherwise occult, potentially curable malignancy. Conversely, knowledge that a connective tissue process may predispose to cancer may provide early recognition of a predictable malignancy. (2) The association of cancer and musculoskeletal syndromes may ultimately provide insight regarding the etiology of rheumatic disorders and malignancy.[3]

DIRECT ASSOCIATIONS BETWEEN MUSCULOSKELETAL SYNDROMES AND MALIGNANCY

The mechanisms by which malignant disease may simulate a musculoskeletal syndrome by direct involvement are depicted in Table 104–1. Tumors involving joints are discussed in more detail in Chapter 105. Several clinical presentations are of particular importance in view of their similarity to the paraneoplastic processes.

Metastatic Disease. Arthritis associated with metastatic carcinoma is most commonly monarticular, with the knee being involved most often followed by the hip. Involvement of the ankle, wrist, hand, and foot occurs less frequently. Carcinoma of the breast and lung are the primary neoplasms in the majority of patients.[4–11] Polyarthritis resulting from metastatic skeletal invasion is usually asymmetric in distribution.[12] Symmetric polyarthritis is more often secondary to a paraneoplastic process such as hypertrophic osteoarthropathy or carcinoma polyarthritis.

Although bone metastases occur in 33 percent of bronchogenic carcinoma, they rarely involve the small bones. Rarer still is the situation of small bone metastases heralding underlying bronchogenic carcinoma.

Table 104–1. Direct Pathologic Mechanisms by Which Malignancy May Present as a Musculoskeletal Syndrome

1. Metastatic disease
   a. Bone
   b. Synovium
   c. Meninges
2. Primary malignant disease
   a. Synovium
      (1) Primary involvement
      (2) Systemic tumor with synovial infiltration
          (a) Leukemia
          (b) Lymphoma
   b. Bone (juxta-articular)
      (1) Primary lymphoma
      (2) Osteogenic sarcoma
      (3) Chondrosarcoma

However, approximately half the metastatic hand lesions reported have had a pulmonary primary neoplasm, the others originating from a primary source within the breast, kidney, colon, or parotid glands.[13] Metastases should be considered when x-ray films suggest a particularly destructive process.[14]

Symmetric metastatic finger deposits may resemble rheumatoid arthritis.[15] The true etiology of such a clinical picture may be further concealed by the reported incidence of rheumatoid factor in up to 20 percent of patients with malignancy,[16] as well as in older persons with no obvious illnesses.[17] Conversely, upon the development of malignancy, rheumatoid factor has disappeared from the serum of patients with rheumatoid arthritis, Sjögren's syndrome, or systemic lupus erythematosus.[18]

Phalangeal metastases may also simulate the clinical appearance of an acute synovitis, such as gout, osteomyelitis, or tenosynovitis,[14,19–21] by direct synovial implantation or involvement of the juxta-articular bone.[22,23] Spread to synovium from subchondral bone has also been described.[24,25] It is unclear why synovial tissue, with its large surface area and rich blood supply, is not involved more often. Malignant bursal involvement rarely occurs.[26] A constellation of clinical features should suggest possible underlying metastasis[27,28] (Table 104–2).

Although the majority of patients with metastatic disease simulating a primary musculoskeletal disorder have had pulmonary malignancies, a variety of nonpulmonary neoplasms have been reported, including melanoma.[5,6,10,11,29–32] The diagnosis of underlying malignancy, although not initially suspected, can generally be made by appropriate studies, including x-rays, bone scans, and local biopsy.[33] Synovial fluid exfoliative cy-

Table 104–2. Frequent Features of Arthritis Resulting From Metastatic Carcinoma

1. Presence of constitutional symptoms
2. Prior history of malignancy
3. Protracted clinical course
4. Negative culture results, negative crystal analysis
5. Medical therapeutic failure
6. Rapid reaccumulation of hemorrhagic noninflammatory effusion
7. Radiologic evidence of destructive process

tology may also be of value in the early recognition of metastatic carcinomatous arthritis.[34]

Involvement of the axial skeleton by tumor may mimic spondylosis with or without radiculopathy.[35] Radiographic evidence of tumor may be lacking.[36,37]

Leukemia. The musculoskeletal manifestations of leukemia include symmetric or occasional migratory polyarthritis, arthralgias, and bone pain and tenderness. Large peripheral joints are involved most often. Sternal tenderness is known to occur in chronic myelogenous leukemia.[12,38,39] Arthritis is the presenting feature in 13.5 percent of patients with leukemia, the majority of whom have acute leukemia.[40-44]

Polyarthritis may be the presenting complaint in children with leukemia. Joint manifestations have been attributed to leukemic synovial infiltration; hemorrhage into joint or periarticular structures; synovial reaction to adjacent bony, periosteal, or capsular lesions; and crystal-induced synovitis.[44,45] Back pain mimicking a radiculopathy may be caused by diffuse leukemic infiltrate of the meninges.

Distinguishing points in patients with polyarthritis secondary to leukemia include hematologic abnormalities and severe joint pain that are disproportionate to the apparent degree of arthritis.[45] The initial peripheral blood smear is often diagnostic. Less often, radiographic changes suggestive of leukemia (metaphyseal rarefaction, osteolytic or periosteal reactions) may be demonstrated.[45-49] The sedimentation rate may be of no help in distinguishing this group of patients.[45] Rheumatoid factor and rheumatoid-like nodules have been reported in patients with leukemia.[50,51] Response to therapy may also confuse the diagnosis, as joint complaints in leukemic patients may be partially or temporarily relieved by salicylates or nonsteroidal anti-inflammatory agents. Disappearance of bone and joint involvement often occurs promptly after induction of therapy for leukemia and may be one of the first indications of the drug's effectiveness.[42,47]

Lymphoma. Patients with lymphoma may also have musculoskeletal manifestations as the presenting feature. Bone pain is the most common symptom attributable to osseous involvement.[52] Synovial reaction is rarely caused by direct invasion; it is most often attributed to adjacent bone disease.[12,24,53] Articular symptoms are less frequent than one might expect in view of the frequency of skeletal invasion.[54] Both monarticular and polyarticular involvement attributed to lymphoma has been reported.[55-58]

Synovial Reaction to Juxta-articular Bone Tumors. Synovial reaction produced by adjacent tumor should always be considered in the evaluation of patients with monarticular arthritis.[11,24] This reaction is nonspecific and may occur with malignant or benign tumors such as osteoid osteoma.[59,60] If radiographs of joints involved in a monarticular, low-grade inflammation suggest any irregularity of adjacent bones, tomography or radionuclide scans and serum enzyme studies (e.g., alkaline phosphatase), or all of these, should determine whether an independent bone lesion exists.[24]

INDIRECT ASSOCIATIONS BETWEEN MUSCULOSKELETAL SYNDROMES AND MALIGNANCY

The indirect associations between musculoskeletal syndromes and malignancy are depicted in Table 104–3. The true paraneoplastic syndromes are divided into the myopathies, arthropathies, and a host of miscellaneous presentations described in the literature. The myopathies are extensively reviewed in Chapter 79 and will not be reviewed here. Hypertrophic osteoarthropathy (Chapter 103), amyloidosis (Chapter 92), and secondary gout (Chapter 86) are also reviewed elsewhere in this text. It is important to remember that because both acquired connective tissue disease and malignancy are common in older populations, many times it is impossible to tell whether the occurrence of both in the same individual is coincidental or causally related.

Carcinoma Polyarthritis. A polyarthritis, generally resembling rheumatoid arthritis, may be the presenting manifestation of malignancy.[3,12,61-71] This is a distinct entity not to be confused with hypertrophic osteoarthropathy or with symmetric metastatic implants alluded to earlier. Although most often confused with rheumatoid disease, it has been mistaken for adult Still's disease when associated with unexplained fever.[68] Mechanisms for this process are not known, although several authors have considered alterations in cellular immunity[72] and circulating immune complexes[73-77] as possible clues to the etiology of carcinoma polyarthritis.

The possibility that the arthritis and the malignancy share a common but unknown etiology certainly exists, but the incidence of malignancy in patients with rheumatoid arthritis has not been greater than that found in the general population, ranging from 2 to 24 percent.[78-82]

Determining the true frequency of polyarthritis resembling rheumatoid disease that occurs as a manifes-

Table 104–3. Indirect Associations Between Musculoskeletal Syndromes and Malignancy: Paraneoplastic Syndromes

1. Myopathy (dermatomyositis–polymyositis)
2. Arthropathy
   a. Hypertrophic osteoarthropathy
   b. Amyloidosis
   c. Secondary gout
   d. Carcinoma polyarthritis
3. Miscellaneous presentations
   a. Lupus syndrome
   b. Necrotizing vasculitis
   c. Cryoproteins
   d. Immune complex disease
   e. Reflex sympathetic dystrophy syndrome
   f. Scleroderma (progressive systemic sclerosis)
   g. Polyarteritis
   h. Polymyalgia rheumatica
   i. Panniculitis
   j. Polychondritis
   k. Lupus antibody syndrome
   l. Pyogenic arthritis
   m. Osteomalacia

tation of an occult or overt neoplasm is obviously difficult and is made more so by the early reports, which do not always exclude hypertrophic pulmonary osteoarthropathy. It is quite possible that periosteal reaction that would be diagnostic of the latter condition was not detected.[67]

More recent reviews suggest that a syndrome clinically inseparable from rheumatoid disease may occur in association with malignancy with a frequency similar to that of hypertrophic osteoarthritis and dermatomyositis.[63] Although they are not diagnostic, several typical features suggest the possibility of malignancy underlying the musculoskeletal syndrome (Table 104–4).[63,83]

Although no predominant type of malignancy has been reported in association with carcinoma polyarthritis, 80 percent of the women with this syndrome have had breast carcinoma.[83] Serologic studies in carcinoma polyarthritis are generally negative.[63,85,86] In one series of 53 elderly patients with polyarthritis, 26 had malignancy, and 25 of those 26 patients had a negative rheumatoid factor test. Of the 27 patients without malignancy, 26 had a positive test for rheumatoid factor.[86] In most patients in whom the antinuclear antibody titer was elevated, there appeared to be a definite inflammatory connective tissue disease unrelated to the malignancy. Positive antinuclear antibodies, however, have been described in association with malignancy.[87] A "lupus antibody syndrome" including not only positive antinuclear antibody but also elevated anti-double-stranded DNA antibody has been described in association with several tumors.[88–90] Similarly, lupus erythematosus (LE) cells have been noted in patients with lymphoma.[91] The sedimentation rate is often markedly increased (greater than 100 mm per hr) in malignancy,[92] but this is nonspecific and is not helpful diagnostically. Although comprehensive data on synovial fluid analysis in carcinoma polyarthritis are lacking, one patient with carcinoma polyarthritis had an inflammatory effusion devoid of crystals.[70] Conversely a characteristic noninflammatory synovial fluid is described in patients with hypertrophic osteoarthropathy.[93] Distinctive radiographic features for carcinoma polyarthritis have not been described.

In addition to solid tumor–related arthritis, joint symptomatology has been widely reported in several hematologic neoplasms.[40,45,94–103] A few reports of arthropathy occurring in conjunction with reticuloendothelial tumors have also appeared in the literature.[54,58,96] In a review of 1000 patients with lymphoma, 22 patients had significant rheumatic complaints. Ten of these patients had predominant musculoskeletal symptoms, and 12 had connective tissue disease.[96] However, in a post-mortem study of 1102 patients with Hodgkin's disease, there were no reports of arthritic symptoms during the course of the disease.[97]

Available data indicate that when the cancer is successfully treated, the connective tissue symptoms frequently resolve.[63,83] Conversely, relapse of the articular symptoms often heralds recurrence of primary or metastatic tumor.[63,83]

In summary, several observations would suggest that in some situations the association of malignancy and polyarthritis is more than fortuitous: (1) a close temporal relationship between the onset of a low-grade, seronegative polyarthritis and discovery of the malignancy, (2) improvement in the connective tissue syndrome with treatment of the underlying tumor, and (3) recurrence of the connective tissue syndrome when the tumor reappears.

Definite proof of a causal relationship is lacking, as in the mechanism or mechanisms to explain the association. Tumors may synthesize mediators that provoke a connective tissue reaction.[2] The possibility of cross-reactivity with shared determinants between synovium and immunologically foreign neoplastic tissue or its products is speculative.[104] Equally plausible is the possibility of autoimmune phenomena arising in lymphocytes that originate in hyperplastic nodes that drain tumor sites.[96] Other host factors in reaction to tumor may play a role in damaging natural bearers, allowing for the evolution of a connective tissue process.[63] A common host defect may exist, the expression of which results in neoplasia and rheumatic disease. A specific antigen-antibody system may be operative in the pathogenesis of the rheumatic disease, with antigen being either tumor-associated antigen, re-expressed fetal antigen, viral antigen, or autologous nontumor antigen.[76] Circulating immune complexes have been demonstrated in association with a variety of malignancies and may contain tumor-specific antibodies. However, other factors must be considered in view of the relatively high incidence of circulating immune complexes and the infrequent occurrence of immune complex–mediated disease in this particular setting.[64–66]

A variety of miscellaneous musculoskeletal syndromes have been described as the manifestation of an underlying malignancy, ranging from transient periarticular inflammation to more dramatic, classic presentations such as systemic lupus erythematosus and the reflex sympathetic dystrophy syndrome. Acute monarticular arthritis, migratory tenosynovitis, transitory arthralgias, localized acute, transient, periarticular inflammation, and fibromyalgia syndrome without other signs of rheumatoid disease or hypertrophic osteoarthropathy have all been noted to occur unrelated to metastatic disease; presumably they are paraneoplastic manifestations of underlying malignancy.

Table 104–4. Features of Carcinoma Polyarthritis

1. Close temporal relationship (10 months) between onset of arthritis and malignancy
2. Late age of onset of arthritis
3. Asymmetric joint involvement
4. Explosive onset
5. Predominant lower extremity involvement with sparing of wrists and small joints of hands
6. Absence of rheumatoid nodules
7. Absence of rheumatoid factor
8. No family history of rheumatoid disease
9. Nonspecific histopathologic appearance of synovial lining

Lupuslike Syndrome. A syndrome similar to systemic lupus erythematosus (SLE) has been described in several series in association with underlying malignancies.[63,68,105,106] Characteristically, the malignancy had been diagnosed previously and treated, with response to therapy, although in one report malignancy was not diagnosed until autopsy.[106] A syndrome compatible with SLE has then developed, characterized by nondeforming polyarthritis, pneumonitis, pleural effusion, positive antinuclear antibody titers, and LE cell preparations.[105] In some patients, appearance of the connective tissue disease has preceded the occurrence of metastatic disease.[63] In one patient the connective tissue disease responded to the treatment given for the underlying primary malignancy.[67] Thus, when patients with known tumors have presenting complaints of pleural effusions, pericarditis, and respiratory distress, the possibility of a potentially reversible lupuslike illness should be considered along with the more common possibilities of metastatic tumor and radiation-induced changes.[105] Patients with SLE who have not been treated with immunosuppressive therapy do not have a recognized increased incidence of malignancy.[107]

Necrotizing Vasculitis. This condition may occur prior to or with the onset of malignancy. It has been described in association with lymphoreticular disorders,[108–110] a lymphomalike entity, and immunoblastic lymphadenopathy, as well as other tumor types.[112–114] Christianson and Fine describe the findings of vasculitis or panniculitis, or both, in six patients with lymphoma or related disease such as leukemia, reticulum cell sarcoma, and multiple myeloma. In each case, the former developed as an initial or early sign of the latter[108] (Fig. 104–1). Earlier studies had noted the occasional association of erythema nodosum with lymphoreticular malignancy;[115,116] some of these patients were atypical for erythema nodosum and possibly had vasculitis.[108] In a review of 72 patients with systemic allergic vasculitis, 5

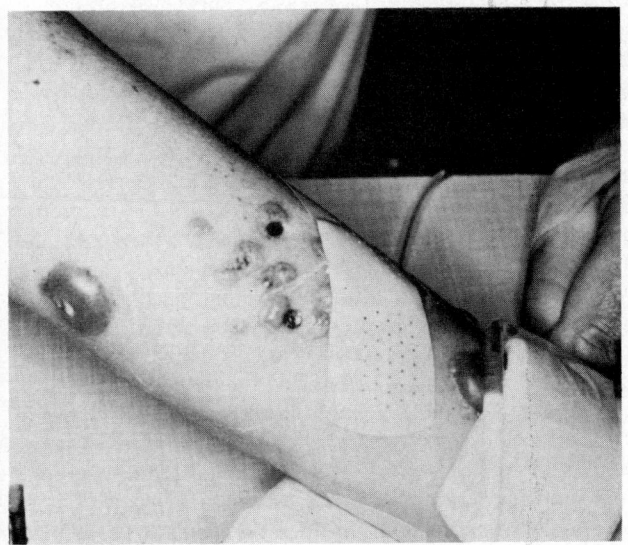

Figure 104–1. Cutaneous vasculitis involving the upper extremity in a patient with lymphoma.

patients with a lymphoproliferative disorder were noted. Four of these patients had chronic leukemia and one had a lymphoma.[117] Acute febrile neutrophilic dermatosis (Sweet's syndrome), which is a recurrent skin disorder that is characterized by inflammatory papules, fever, arthralgias, and leukocytosis, and resembles vasculitis, may be associated with leukemia.[118,119] Another remote effect of cancer related to vasculitis may be mononeuritis multiplex.[120] Although a definite causal relationship between lymphoreticular malignancy and vasculitis cannot be established, and the possibility of a drug-induced reaction presenting with vasculitis is often difficult to exclude,[121] substantial evidence suggests that vasculitis can be a feature of this group of malignancies. Endogenous antigens, such as tumor antigens, may serve as a sensitizing antigen and provoke host reactions identical to the more classic hypersensitivity vasculitides.[122] Perhaps the patient with a chronic, unexplained, necrotizing vasculitis should be observed for malignancy, particularly of the lymphoreticular type. When systemic vasculitis develops in the patient who has apparently had a successfully treated malignancy, tumor recurrence should be considered. Systemic evaluation for a recurrent tumor is essential prior to immunosuppressive therapy because such therapy could potentially enhance tumor growth by suppressing immune surveillance.[113]

Cryoproteins. Many tumors are associated with dysproteinemia, and many abnormal proteins have the capacity to cause peripheral vascular disease, especially those characterized by cryoglobulins (see Chapter 84) or those circulating as immune complexes. Peripheral gangrene secondary to the presence of circulating cryoglobulins or cryofibrinogens may occur prior to recognition of a tumor by the usual diagnostic methods.[123,124] Cryoglobulinemia, with symptoms of Raynaud's phenomenon, purpura, circulatory impairment, and at times occlusion in gangrene following cold exposure, is frequently associated with plasma cell dyscrasias—particularly plasma cell myeloma.[125–128] Purpura, often cold induced, thromboembolic phenomena, and a hemorrhagic diathesis may be seen with high levels of cryofibrinogen. Other manifestations include retinal hemorrhage and retinal vein thrombosis. Most commonly an increased level of cryofibrinogen is associated with metastatic malignancy.[128–130]

Immune Complex Disease. Evidence for the presence of circulating immune complexes in malignancy has been reported by several investigators using a variety of techniques.[76,131–136] Over a 3-year period, Teshima and colleagues observed that 10 percent of patients with various cancers were hypocomplementemic.[111,131] More than 50 percent of patients with cancer appear to have circulating immune complexes. The quantity of complexes in the patients studied was sometimes as great as that detected in patients with SLE.[131] One patient with chronic lymphocytic leukemia had marked hypocomplementemia associated with recurrent, nonhereditary angioedema and cryoglobulinemia.[137] Immune complexes consisting of IgM antilymphocyte antibody and lymphocyte membrane antigen were present in the serum of this patient, and antilymphocyte antibody was specifically enriched in the cryoglobulin.[131] Circulating immune complexes have also been reported in Hodgkin's disease.[138–144] Granular deposits of IgG and C3 are found in the glomerular capillaries on renal biopsy at staging laparotomy in 10 to 20 percent of these patients. Although the majority have no clinical evidence of glomerulonephritis,[143] one patient has been described who had Hodgkin's disease with a simultaneous onset of the nephrotic syndrome.[144] Further study of immune complexes in cancer patients may improve our understanding of the immune response to tumor antigens and of immunotherapy, and possibly lead to early detection of recurrence of tumor. It is also tempting to postulate a pathogenic mechanism for a variety of musculoskeletal manifestations on the basis of circulating immune complexes.

Reflex Sympathetic Dystrophy Syndrome. Steinbrocker and associates listed 35 possible conditions that could be associated with reflex sympathetic dystrophy, and the list has continued to expand to include brain tumors.[145–147] Bremer reported a patient with the classic shoulder-hand syndrome refractory to high-dose steroids.[147] Five months after presentation, carcinoma of the ovary, with extensive involvement of the peritoneum and adjacent structures, was diagnosed. Radiation therapy resulted in regression of the neoplasm with coincident improvement in the shoulder-hand syndrome. Medsger and others described six postmenopausal women with bilateral shoulder and hand pain and limited motion as well as prominent palmar fasciitis and polyarthritis. Rheumatic signs preceded diagnosis of ovarian adenocarcinoma by 5 to 25 months. Nonresectable tumor was found in all patients, and no consistent improvement of the musculoskeletal syndrome was seen after either corticosteroid therapy or chemotherapy. Death followed 2 to 17 months after the diagnosis of neoplasm.[148]

Upper extremity pain simulating cervical nerve root irritation or the painful phase of shoulder-hand syndrome may also be seen with tumors of the lung that are localized to the superior sulcus, the so-called Pancoast's syndrome.[35] This entity should always be considered in a setting of unilateral shoulder girdle–arm pain.

Scleroderma. Scleroderma may appear as the initial manifestation of malignancy.[62] Sclerodermatous changes occasionally supervene in patients with dermatomyositis associated with cancer. Christian, Brunsting, and Perry reviewed 125 patients with systemic sclerosis and 235 patients with localized scleroderma, finding 8 malignancies in the first group and 4 in the second.[149] Of the eight patients with systemic sclerosis and carcinoma, seven were female, and four had carcinoma of the breast and two had carcinoma of the uterus.[149] The author has observed one patient whose presenting complaints were sclerodermatous changes in the extremities and immunoblastic lymphadenopathy.

In an analysis of patients with coexisting scleroderma and malignant disease, the majority of neoplasms were of two varieties: adenocarcinoma and carcinoid tumors.

Women were affected three times as often as men, and although all patients had cutaneous manifestations of scleroderma, less than half had proven systemic sclerosis.[150] Asboe-Hansen postulated that in those patients with carcinoid tumors and scleroderma, serotonin may stimulate fibrous tissue proliferation by its ability to produce overhydration of connective tissue[151] (see Chapter 8).

Polyarteritis. In view of the fact that circulating immune complexes occur in malignancy, it would seem that polyarteritis would occur more frequently than is generally appreciated. Polyarteritis has been described with Hodgkin's disease[97] and with hairy cell leukemia.[98–101] In the latter group the vasculitis was typical of polyarteritis clinically and radiologically except for two patients with non-giant-cell temporal arteritis. Histologically the vasculitis was characterized by arterial wall necrosis and infiltration with mononuclear cells. The reason for the association of hairy cell leukemia and polyarteritis remains unclear.[102] Lansbury, reviewing the connective tissue manifestations of leukemia, noted that recurrent infiltrations into muscles may occasionally mimic the localized tender swellings found in polyarteritis.[3] Atrial myxoma may mimic symptoms of polyarteritis nodosa, as illustrated by one such patient whose symptoms largely resolved after myxoma resection[103]

Polymyalgia Rheumatica. Polymyalgia rheumatica has rarely been associated with malignancy. In a series in which 42 patients with temporal arteritis were identified in a 25-year period, the cause of death was attributed to carcinoma of the breast in two patients. However, there was no association of temporal arteritis in this series with any other disease.[152] Sheon and colleagues described six patients with polymyalgia rheumatica syndrome in association with malignancy. Malignancy occurred within 3 months of the onset of polymyalgia rheumatica in five patients, whereas in one patient the onset of polymyalgia rheumatica coincided with the appearance of metastases. There was no common type of malignancy, with primary sites involving ovary, colon, prostate, kidney, blood, and lymphatic tissue.[83] Cranial arteritis has also been described as the initial manifestation of malignant histiocytosis.[84]

Panniculitis. There are multiple types of pannicular inflammation,[153–156] as reviewed in Chapter 75. The first report of subcutaneous fat necrosis and arthritis associated with carcinoma of the pancreas appeared in 1908.[157] Since then a number of similar cases have appeared.[158–172] Subcutaneous nodules and arthritis may appear simultaneously and may precede abdominal pain or other signs and symptoms suggestive of pancreatic disease.[172] In Hughes' series of patients with pancreatic carcinoma, the most common presenting complaints were skin nodules (65 percent) and joint pain (35 percent); only 12 percent of these patients complained initially of abdominal pain.[158] The arthropathy, which is secondary to periarticular fat necrosis (biopsy proven in two cases),[167,168] may be monarticular or polyarticular (Fig. 104–2).[172] Eosinophilia (5 to 20 percent) occurred

Figure 104–2. Subcutaneous fat necrosis of the lower extremity in a patient with pancreatic carcinoma. (Courtesy of Dr. Robert Gilgor.)

in 65 percent of the 17 cases of subcutaneous fat necrosis with associated carcinoma of the pancreas, compared with a 19 percent incidence in 36 patients with subcutaneous fat necrosis and pancreatitis. The subcutaneous fat necrosis has been attributed to the local action of blood-borne trypsin and lipase.[158] The extrapancreatic inflammatory manifestations may be related to an increased concentration of free fatty acids within the joint space.[159]

Histopathologic features described by Szymanski and Bluefarb, consisting of foci of fat necrosis with "ghost-like" cells having thick, shadowy walls and no nuclei, are pathognomonic.[160] Granular material that appears basophilic is located within and around necrotic fat cells. An inflammatory zone—consisting of polymorphonuclear leukocytes, eosinophils, lymphocytes, histiocytes, foam cells, and foreign body giant cells—surrounds the foci of necrosis. Hemorrhage may also be seen.[158]

Therapy for this process with a variety of anti-inflammatory drugs, including corticosteroids, is ineffective.[161,172,173] The possibility of subcutaneous fat necrosis should be considered in otherwise unexplained cases of polyarthritis or monarticular arthritis with subcutaneous nodules, particularly when occurring in older men. Diagnostic studies should include nodule biopsy and serum lipase determinations.[158,172] Erythema nodosum has also been noted with lymphoproliferative diseases.[174]

Polychondritis. Relapsing polychondritis is a rare syndrome that is characterized by inflammation of cartilage, specifically of the ear and nose, and is often associated with ocular and cardiac involvement as well as a number of other concomitant disorders.[175] It has been rarely associated with malignancy. In each patient reported, polychondritis preceded the diagnosis of malignancy.[176,177]

Pyogenic Arthritis. Pyogenic arthritis caused by intestinal flora has been reported as a late complication in patients with advanced neoplastic disease,[178] and more recently has been reported as the presenting feature of carcinoma of the colon.[179] Whenever an unusual enteric bacteremia or its complications develop, the clinician should consider the possibility of a malignant source.[179]

Osteomalacia. Osteomalacia, characterized by bone pain, muscle weakness, and failure of newly formed bone matrix to calcify, may be associated with solid tissue tumors.[180] Osteomalacia secondary to neoplasia, or oncogenic osteomalacia, has the unique feature of resolution after complete tumor removal.[180] Two mechanisms have been proposed by which neoplastic tissue may give rise to osteomalacia.[181] Regardless of the mechanism, however, diligent, careful search for tumor should be undertaken in all patients with vitamin D–resistant osteomalacia.[181]

PRE-EXISTING CONNECTIVE TISSUE DISEASE

The association of musculoskeletal syndromes with malignancy also includes the development of malignancy in the setting of pre-existing connective tissue disease (Table 104–5). The type of connective tissue disorder and the organ system involved often dictate the type of malignancy expected in that particular setting. The initial event may be tissue alteration induced by the connective tissue disease.[61] Malignancy arising in patients with a pre-existing connective tissue disease may also be a result of the therapy administered for the connective tissue disease, or an immunologic disorder may be causing both the malignancy and the connective tissue proc-

Table 104–5. Clinical Settings of Pre-existing Connective Tissue Disease Associated with Malignancy

1. Disease related
   a. Lupus erythematosus
      (1) Systemic
      (2) Discoid
   b. Sjögren's syndrome
   c. Rheumatoid arthritis
   d. Scleroderma (progressive systemic sclerosis)
   e. Sarcoidosis
   f. Osteomyelitis
   g. Paget's disease
   h. Eosinophilic fasciitis
   i. Lymphomatoid granulomatosis
2. Complications of therapy
   a. Immunosuppressive therapy
   b. Radiation therapy

ess.[182,186,187] One particular type of malignant lymphoma, so-called B-lymphocyte immunoblastic sarcoma, has been described as characteristic of lymphoid neoplasia arising in connective tissue disease.[188,189] Banks and colleagues, however, have suggested that the appearance of lymphoid neoplasia after the development of connective tissue disease does not show any distinctive morphologic features.[190]

Systemic Lupus Erythematosus. New Zealand (NZB and NZB/NXW F1) mice spontaneously develop serologic abnormalities, including LE cells, antinuclear antibodies, antibodies to nucleic acids (DNA and RNA), autoimmune hemolytic anemia, and immune complex glomerulonephritis, as well as antibodies to murine leukemia viral antigens. In addition, they develop lymphoid infiltration of many organs, and with aging, monoclonal macroglobulinemia and lymphoid malignancies.[191-196] Thus, they provide an animal model not only for human SLE but also for the relationship between SLE and malignancy. The spectrum of disease in the New Zealand mouse, ranging from autoimmune disease to lymphoid malignancy, can be seen as a progressive escape of B-lymphocyte function from T-lymphocyte regulation, ultimately manifested by B-lymphocyte malignancy. Although the propensity to the development of lymphoreticular malignancy may be due predominantly to the B-lymphocyte proliferation, older New Zealand mice also demonstrate markedly deficient T-lymphocyte effector function, as revealed in part by their impaired capacity to reject malignant tumors.[196] Furthermore, carcinogens or immunosuppressive drugs may increase the frequency of lymphoid malignancies.[197,198] Both of these mechanisms likely function through impairment of immune tumor surveillance. This theory may also explain the high incidence of malignancies seen in immunodeficiency states.

The association of connective tissue disease, particularly SLE, with lymphoreticular disorders and less frequently with solid tumors is now well established.[12,67,91,96,97,104,199-215] Canoso and Cohen reviewed their experience in a consecutive series of 70 patients with SLE;[200] over a median interval of 6 years and 8 months, 11.4 percent of their patients developed malig-

nancy, including cases of reticulum cell sarcoma, multiple myeloma, Bowen's carcinoma of the skin, and carcinoma of the cervix. Six of these patients had received corticosteroids, which in two cases was combined with azathioprine therapy.[200] Agudelo and co-workers presented four patients with non-Hodgkin's lymphoma in SLE. None received immunosuppressive therapy except for low-dose prednisone in one patient, suggesting that lymphoma may be related to SLE or to factors causing both the lymphoma and the SLE, more than to therapy. They suggested that non-Hodgkin's lymphoma should be considered in patients with SLE who develop adenopathy or masses.[214] Lymphomas,[96,104,199,203-205] leukemia,[206] and epithelial tumors[207-210] have also been described. Despite this well-established relationship, Oleinick found no greater frequency of death from these malignancies in patients with SLE (or rheumatoid arthritis) than in the general population.[216]

Discoid Lupus Erythematosus. Epitheliomas occasionally may appear in healed scars of discoid lupus erythematosus. These are usually found in the oldest plaques, developing 20 years or more after the onset of the discoid lesion, and they occur primarily in men between the ages of 30 and 60 years.[217-219] They are almost always of the squamous cell variety. Although the pathogenesis is unclear, it possibly relates to the chronic inflammatory process or to the scarring itself.[220,221]

Sjögren's Syndrome. Sjögren's syndrome is a chronic inflammatory disease process affecting principally the exocrine glands and is frequently associated with a connective tissue disorder, most often rheumatoid disease (see Chapter 64).[222] It may closely resemble the New Zealand mouse model with development of salivary gland lymphoid infiltrates, generalized lymphoproliferation, autoantibodies, monoclonal IgM, and lymphoma.[193] In 1951, Rothman and associates reported the association of Sjögren's syndrome with lymphoblastoma and hypersplenism.[223] In 1964, Talal and Bunim reported the development of extrasalivary lymphoma in 3 of 58 patients with Sjögren's syndrome that pre-existed for 4 to 8 years.[202] Since that time a number of similar reports and reviews have appeared.[199,201,224-232] A spectrum of lymphoproliferation occurs in the setting of Sjögren's syndrome—from benign lymphoid infiltration that is confined to glandular tissue to widespread lymphoreticular malignancy. In the middle of these extremes exists a condition characterized by nonmalignant, extraglandular extension of lymphoproliferation (Figs. 104–3 and 104–4). This "pseudolymphoma" may regress in response to appropriate therapy or may progress to frank neoplasia, either macroglobulinemia or lymphoma.[226,227] Clues to the progression from "pseudolymphoma" to lymphoma may be a decline in the level of serum IgM and the disappearance of rheumatoid factor, both of which may be elevated in "pseudolymphoma."[227] (See Chapter 64.)

The normal functioning state of the immune system depends on appropriate regulation of suppression as well as of effector T and B lymphocytes. It is likely that a defect in cell function ultimately leads to the clinical

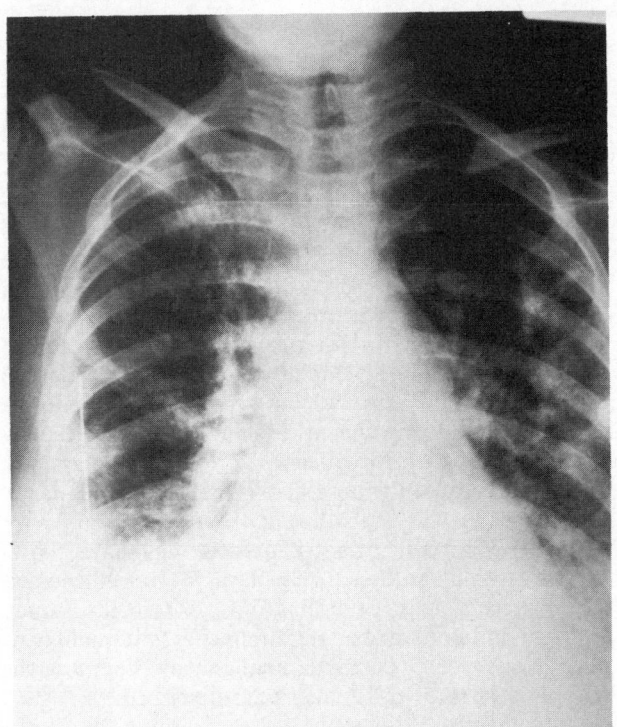

Figure 104–3. Chest x-ray revealing pulmonary involvement in a patient with Sjögren's syndrome and pseudolymphoma.

expression of both autoimmunity and malignancy in Sjögren's syndrome and possibly in other connective tissue diseases. Autoimmune diseases may be accompanied by decreased T suppressor activity with uncontrolled T helper function and augmented humoral immunity. Conversely, in some cases failure of immune surveillance may be due to inhibition of effector T lymphocytes by abnormally active suppressor cells.[229] Pa-

tients with Sjögren's syndrome have not been found to have decreased suppressor T-lymphocyte function.[228] It is likely that an immunoregulatory disturbance results in increased activity of some types of suppressor cells and decreased activity of others. With the putative escape of autoimmune and potential neoplastic B-lymphocytes, the features of an autoimmune disorder then appear. The fact that malignancy is a rare and late event in many of these situations is consistent with the concept that malignancy develops only after a long sequence of transitions and selection of mutant populations.[233,234]

Rheumatoid Arthritis. The reported incidence of malignancy in rheumatoid disease has ranged from 2 to 24 percent. Several investigators have shown, however, that the incidence of malignancy, including lymphoreticular disorders, is no greater in rheumatoid disease than that found in the general population. Too few patients with rheumatoid arthritis preceding malignancy have been reported to postulate any causal relationship with a particular cancer type.[235-237] However, Mackenzie and Scherbel described four patients with longstanding rheumatoid disease in whom arthritis suddenly became rapidly progressive and refractory to additional therapy (including corticosteroids) 4 to 6 months prior to the discovery of a neoplasm. Such a refractory flare in the appropriate setting may therefore suggest an underlying malignancy.[63]

Scleroderma (Progressive Systemic Sclerosis). The first report of the association of scleroderma and cancer appeared in 1953 when Zatuchni and associates described three individuals who had scleroderma with lung involvement and at autopsy were found to have not only pulmonary fibrosis but also terminal bronchiolar (alveolar cell) carcinoma.[238] A variety of tumors have subsequently been described either preceding or following scleroderma.[239-253] Fibrosing changes of specific internal

Figure 104–4. Lung biopsy specimen from the patient depicted in Figure 104–3, revealing characteristic findings of pseudolymphoma.

organs have generally preceded the development of a malignant lesion.[250,252] Among all malignancies reported in scleroderma, there is a predominance of lung neoplasia, with an even more striking predominance of alveolar cell carcinoma within this group (Figs. 104–5 to 104–7). More than 50 percent of the lung tumors that appear in patients with progressive systemic sclerosis were of the alveolar cell type, whereas this condition generally encompasses less than 4 percent of all primary lung neoplasms.[254] Collins and associates, in reporting a patient with scleroderma who developed alveolar cell carcinoma in a setting of pulmonary fibrosis and honeycomb lung, proposed the following pathologic sequence of events: scleroderma, pulmonary fibrosis, honeycomb lung, adenomatosis, and carcinoma.[240] Thus, alveolar cell carcinoma in progressive systemic sclerosis may be the result of metaplasia following, or superimposed upon, fibrosis rather than a direct consequence of systemic sclerosis.[250] The fact that inhaled oncogenic factors are poorly eliminated by a sclerodermatous lung may be an added stimulus to malignant transformation in regenerating cells.[251] The naturally occurring disease *jaagsiekte*, or "drive sickness," provides an interesting animal model for the proposed pathologic sequence.[255-258] In spite of these reports, a comparable incidence of cancer was noted by Masi and D'Angelo in 32 scleroderma patients who died and 60 matched controls.[259]

Werner's syndrome is a rare autosomal recessive connective tissue disorder that is characterized by juvenile cataracts, sclerodermalike skin changes, and accelerated aging. In addition there is a high incidence of neoplasm, often of connective tissue origin.[260] The syndrome should not be confused with progressive systemic sclerosis, but

should be regarded as a cutaneous marker of internal malignancy.[261]

Sarcoidosis. Sarcoidosis is a systemic disease of unknown etiology that is characterized pathologically by the appearance of noncaseating granulomas in multiple organs. The impairment of a cell-mediated hypersensitivity reaction is a well-recognized characteristic of this process. A consequence of this impairment may be decreased immunologic surveillance, resulting in an increase in neoplasia.[262] Brincker and Wilbek reported a 50 percent higher incidence of malignancy occurring in patients with sarcoid than in the sex- and age-matched general population. The higher incidence was accounted for entirely by patients with lung cancer and lymphoma, as there were no significant differences between the expected and observed frequencies for other neoplasms.[263] However, because the observed incidence of malignancy in this series was high during the first 4 years after diagnosis of sarcoid, the granulomas may have represented sarcoid reaction to neoplasm.[262] Indeed, noncaseating granulomas resembling those of sarcoidosis may be found in lymph nodes that drain sites with malignant neoplasms.[264,265] Documented malignancy preceding the diagnosis of sarcoid has also been described.[263,266,267]

Osteomyelitis. Squamous cell carcinoma is a complication of chronic osteomyelitis, with an estimated incidence of between 0.2 and 1.7 percent.[268-271] Fitzgerald and colleagues, reviewing the Mayo Clinic experience, reported 25 patients with squamous cell carcinoma and 3 patients with sarcoma at the site of chronic osteomyelitis.[272] They postulated that the squamous cell carcinoma probably arises in the proliferating edges of the cutaneous ulcer and then invades the bone.[272]

Paget's Disease of Bone. Persistent, severe pain may

Figure 104–5. Chest x-ray of a patient with scleroderma and lung involvement. Biopsy of the nodular lesion revealed alveolar cell carcinoma. (Courtesy of Dr. Herbert Baraf.)

Figure 104–6. Alveolar cell carcinoma. Characteristic low power "papillary" appearance along the periphery of an alveolar cell carcinoma (right) invading normal lung tissue. (Courtesy of Dr. Michael Ehrie.)

alert the clinician to the most dreaded complication of Paget's disease—the development of osteogenic sarcoma.[273] The frequency of this process is probably less than 1 percent.[280] In a study of 553 patients with osteogenic sarcoma, 33 cases were found to arise in bones involved in Paget's disease. However, in patients older than 40 years of age with osteogenic sarcoma, the incidence of sarcoma arising from pagetic bone rose to 19 percent. Tumors most frequently involved the femur, humerus, skull, face, and pelvis. Survival after diagnosis is usually less than 1 year.[281] Swelling and bone destruction in the setting of Paget's disease may be due to other types of malignancy as well.[273]

Neoplastic skeletal invasion may sometimes present with a clinical picture similar to Paget's disease. Although several clinical signs have been noted to aid the clinician in distinguishing between the two, the ultimate diagnosis may require biopsy.[273]

Eosinophilic Fasciitis. Diffuse fasciitis with eosinophilia is a disorder that is characterized by sclerodermalike skin changes, hypereosinophilia, hypergammaglobulinemia, an elevated sedimentation rate, and the characteristic biopsy revealing mononuclear cells and plasmacytes infiltrating the deep fascia, which becomes very thickened (see Chapter 78). Eosinophils may or may not be present.[274,275] Serious hematologic complications, including aplastic anemia and thrombocytopenia, have been reported during long-term follow-up,

Figure 104–7. Alveolar cell carcinoma. Characteristic high power view with columnar-shaped tumor cells growing along the supportng framework of the lung, lining the alveolar spaces. (Courtesy of Dr. Michael Ehrie.)

presumably on the basis of an immunologic disorder.[276,277] Michaels has reported a patient with eosinophilic fasciitis complicated by Hodgkin's disease, suggesting that eosinophilic fasciitis may be the result of an abnormal lymphoplasmacytic proliferation and that these patients should therefore be followed closely for development of serious hematologic disorders, including lymphoid malignancies.[278]

Lymphomatoid Granulomatosis. This disorder is an unusual form of vasculitis with a granulomatous reaction that is characterized by an angiotropic and angiodestructive infiltration of various tissues, particularly lung. The cellular infiltrate, which is composed of atypical lymphocytoid and plasmacytoid cells, has lymphoproliferative characteristics, and clear-cut lymphomas evolve in at least 13 percent of patients.[279]

MALIGNANCY AS A COMPLICATION OF TREATMENT

Immunosuppressive Therapy. Immunosuppressive drugs are being increasingly utilized on a long-term basis for transplant recipients and for patients suffering from nonmalignant diseases such as rheumatoid arthritis, SLE, psoriasis, and polymyositis-dermatomyositis. An alarming complication of chemotherapy is the development of neoplasm. Reimer and associates noted that patients with ovarian carcinoma who received alkylating agent chemotherapy had a 21-fold to 36-fold increased risk of developing acute leukemia. For patients living longer than 2 years after initiation of therapy, the risk increased from 66.7-fold to 171.4-fold.[282] These findings are supported by animal studies that have demonstrated a carcinogenic potential of alkylating agents.[283] Purine antimetabolites, such as azathioprine, have also been associated with the development of malignancy, particularly lymphomas and squamous cell carcinomas. In contrast, the pyrimidine antagonists—methotrexate and 5-fluorouracil—have little carcinogenic effect in animals and have likewise not been implicated in humans.[284]

There is relatively little information on the development of tumors in patients treated with antineoplastic drugs for nonmalignant conditions. Most of these disorders have been in the connective tissue category, predominantly SLE and rheumatoid arthritis.[285,286] The increased incidence of cervical atypia in women with SLE who receive chemotherapy suggests that such patients should have cervical smears taken regularly.[287] The actual incidence of a neoplastic complication is difficult to determine because the number of patients receiving such drugs is not available.[197] Because impairment of immune surveillance with subsequent proliferation of mutant malignant clones may already occur in the altered immune state, immunosuppressive therapy in this setting may be a very serious therapeutic maneuver, possibly further enhancing the potential for malignant growth.[288]

Several patients with rheumatoid arthritis that was treated with immunosuppressive drugs have developed malignancy.[182,186] In one series this occurred shortly after exposure to azathioprine, suggesting that the role of azathioprine may have been to permit acceleration of tumor growth rather than to induce malignant transformation.[186] In another series of patents with rheumatoid arthritis that was treated with immunosuppressive agents the incidence of malignancy was 1.3 percent compared with an estimated incidence in the population of 0.009 percent.[182]

Several other isolated reports may be instructive. Cutaneous dissemination of Kaposi's sarcoma occurred in a patient with temporal arteritis that was treated with corticosteroids. Reduction of steroids was followed by tumor regression.[183] A single incidence of tumor (diffuse histiocytic lymphoma) was noted in a large group of cyclophosphamide-treated Wegener's granulomatosis patients during a 21-year period. The patient had required maintenance cyclophosphamide and developed cancer in his ninth year of therapy.[184] After 37 months of high-dose penicillamine therapy, acute lymphoblastic leukemia developed in a patient with Wilson's disease, suggesting that penicillamine-induced alterations in host immunity may predispose to certain malignancies.[185]

The decision to use immunosuppressive drugs in a patient with a nonmalignant disease must be carefully made given the increased risk of malignancy.[289,290] Informed consent in such a situation obviously places a great burden on the patient faced with the alternatives of morbid and mortal complications of the underlying disease.

Radiation Therapy. Deep x-ray therapy was formerly used in the treatment of ankylosing spondylitis, which is a potentially disabling disorder with no known primary association with malignancy.[291,292] Court Brown and Doll studied a group of spondylitic patients after x-ray therapy to determine the possible late effects of such therapy.[293] These patients were found to have a statistically significant higher mortality from several types of cancer with no particular type predominating. The increase in malignancy was greater for sites that had been heavily irradiated than for cancer of other sites, and excess deaths appeared about 6 to 8 years after treatment and increased in incidence thereafter until 15 years following irradiation or longer, suggesting a cause-effect relationship between the radiotherapy and the cancer.[293]

A later study utilizing the same population base reported that patients with ankylosing spondylitis who were not treated with radiotherapy had increased mortality from malignancy, suggesting a disease-related mortality factor.[294] A Canadian study concurred that in men with ankylosing spondylitis, survival is less than expected; however, men who did not receive radiotherapy had a normal life span. Patients requiring radiotherapy may have more aggressive disease, increasing the likelihood of death from disease complications.[295] Thus radiotherapy may be an additional, rather than the sole, risk factor in the patient with ankylosing spondylitis. Basal cell carcinoma in the lumbosacral area may be a late complication of radiotherapy for ankylosing spondylitis.[296] The skin at sites of previous irradiation should be carefully examined.

References

1. Hall, T.C.: The paraneoplastic syndromes. *In* Rubin, P. (ed.): Clinical Oncology for Medical Students and Physicians. 4th ed. Rochester, N.Y., University of Rochester, 1974.
2. Odell, W.D., and Wolfsen, A.R.: Hormones from tumors: Are they ubiquitous? Am. J. Med. 68:317, 1980.
3. Lansbury, J.: Connective tissue manifestations of neoplastic disease. Geriatrics 9:319, 1954.
4. Murray, G.C., and Persellin, R.H.: Metastatic carcinoma presenting as monarticular arthritis: A case report and review of the literature. Arthritis Rheum. 23:95, 1980.
5. Weinblatt, M.E., and Karp, G.I.: Monarticular arthritis: Early manifestation of a rhabdomyosarcoma. J. Rheumatol. 8:685, 1981.
6. Speerstra, F., Boerbooms, A.M.Th., Van De Putte, L.B.A., Kruls, H.J.A., Van Haelst, U.J.G.M., and Vooijs, G.P.: Arthritis caused by metastatic melanoma. Arthritis Rheum. 24:223, 1982.
7. Goldberg, I., Nudelman, J., and Yosipovitch, Z.: Frozen shoulder as a presenting symptom of lung cancer: A report of three cases. Contemp. Orthop. 4:689, 1982.
8. Benedek, T.G.: Lysis of the patella due to metastatic carcinoma. Arthritis Rheum. 8:560, 1965.
9. Gall, E.P., Didizian, N.A., and Park, Y.: Acute monarticular arthritis following patellar metastasis: A manifestation of carcinoma of the lung. JAMA 229:188, 1974.
10. Moutsopoulos, H.M., Fye, K.H., Pugay, P.I., and Shearn, M.A.: Monarthric arthritis caused by metastatic breast carcinoma: Value of cytologic study of synovial fluid. JAMA 234:75, 1975.
11. Shenberger, K.N., and Morgan, G.J., Jr.: Recurrent malignant melanoma presenting as monarthritis. J. Rheumatol. 9:328, 1982.
12. Calabro, J.J.: Cancer and arthritis. Arthritis Rheum. 10:553, 1967.
13. Bunkis, J., Mehrhof, A.I., and Stayman, J.W., III: Metastatic lesions of the hand and foot. Orthop. Rev. 9:97, 1980.
14. Vaezy, A., and Budson, D.C.: Phalangeal metastases from bronchogenic carcinoma. JAMA 239:226, 1978.
15. Karten, I., and Bartfeld, H.: Bronchogenic carcinoma simulating early rheumatoid arthritis. Metastases to the fingers. JAMA 179:162, 1962.
16. Bartfeld, H.: Incidence and significance of seropositive tests for rheumatoid factor in non-rheumatoid diseases. Ann. Intern. Med. 52:1059, 1960.
17. Heimer, R., Levin, F.M., and Rudd, E.: Globulins resembling rheumatoid factor in serum of the aged. Am. J. Med. 35:175, 1963.
18. Cobau, C.D., Sheon, R.P., and Kirsner, A.B.: Immunosuppressive drugs and acute leukemia. Ann. Intern. Med. 79:131, 1973.
19. Mulvey, R.B.: Peripheral bone metastases. Am. J. Roentgenol. Radium Ther. Nucl. Med. 91:155, 1964.
20. Jacox, R.F., and Tristan, T.A.: Carcinoma of breast metastatic to bones of foot: Case report. Arthritis Rheum. 3:170, 1960.
21. Nause, W., and Sundstrom, W.R.: Lung carcinoma: Juxtaarticular disease resembling bursitis and tenosynovitis. J. Rheumatol. 7:106, 1980.
22. Benedek, T.G.: Lysis of the patella due to metastatic carcinoma. Arthritis Rheum. 8:560, 1965.
23. Lang, F.J., and Thurner, J.: Erkrankugen der Gelenke. Lehrbuch der speziellen pathologischen Anatomie. II Band, 4 Teil, 7 Lieferung. Berlin, W. de Gruyter and Co., 1962.
24. Lagier, R.: Synovial reaction caused by adjacent malignant tumors: anatomicopathological study of three cases. J. Rheumatol. 4:65, 1977.
25. Milch, R.A., and Changus, G.W.: Response of bone to tumor invasion. Cancer 9:340, 1956.
26. Jaleel, K.A.: Personal communication: Metastatic carcinoma synovitis associated with malignant bursitis. April 6, 1981.
27. Wu, K.W., Winkelman, N.Z., and Guise, E.R.: Metastatic bronchogenic carcinoma to the finger simulating acute osteomyelitis. Orthopaedics 3:25, 1980.
28. Naib, Z.M.: Cytology of synovial fluids. Acta Cytol. 17:299, 1973.
29. Roques, C.F., Amigues, H., Puget, J., et al.: Metastase synoviale du genou, premier symptôme d'un cancer de l'estomac. Rev. Méd. Toulouse 10:235, 1974.
30. Goldenberg, D.L., Kelley, W., and Gibbons, R.B.: Metastatic adenocarcinoma of synovium presenting as an acute arthritis. Arthritis Rheum. 18:107, 1975.
31. Bevan, D.A., Ehrlich, G.E., and Gupta, V.P.: Metastatic carcinoma simulating gout. JAMA 237:2746, 1977.
32. Wu, K.K., and Guise, E.R.: Metastatic tumors of the foot. South. Med. J. 71:807, 1978.
33. Meals, R.A., Hungerford, D.S., and Stevens, M.B.: Malignant disease mimicking arthritis of the hip. JAMA 239:1070, 1978.
34. Fam, A.G., Kolin, A., and Lewis, A.J.: Metastatic carcinomatous arthritis and carcinoma of the lung. A report of two cases diagnosed by synovial fluid cytology. J. Rheumatol. 7:98, 1980.
35. Pancoast, H.K.: Superior pulmonary sulcus tumor; tumor characterized by pain, Horner's syndrome, destruction of bone and atrophy of hand muscles. JAMA 99:1391, 1932.
36. Klier, I., and Santo, M.: Low back pain as a presenting symptom of chronic granulocytic leukemia. Orthop. Rev. 11:111, 1982.
37. Rosen, S.T., Aisner, J., Makuch, R.W., Matthews, M.J., Ihde, D.C., Whitacre, M., Glatstein, E.J., Wiernik, P.H., Lichter, A.S., and Bunn, P.A., Jr.: Carcinomatous leptomeningitis in small cell lung cancer: A clinicopathologic review of the National Cancer Institute experience. Medicine 61:45, 1982.
38. Quesada, J.R., Keating, M.J., Libshitz, H.I., and Llamas, L.: Bone involvement in hairy cell leukemia. Am. J. Med. 74:228, 1983.
39. Luzar, M.J., and Sharma, H.M.: Leukemia and arthritis: Including reports on light immunofluorescent and electron microscopy of the synovium. J. Rheumatol. 10:132, 1983.
40. Spilberg, I., and Meyer G.J.: The arthritis of leukemia. Arthritis Rheum. 15:630, 1972.
41. Fink, C.W., Windmiller, J., and Sartain, P.: Arthritis as the presenting feature of childhood leukemia. Arthritis Rheum. 15:347, 1972.
42. Douer, D., Weinberger, A., Djaldetti, M., Pinkhas, J., and deVries, A.: Successful treatment of severe bone pain and acute arthritis in chronic myelomonocytic leukaemia by cytosine-arabinoside. Ann. Rheum. Dis. 36:192, 1977.
43. Van Soesberger, R.M., Feltkamp-Vroom, T.M., Feltkamp, C.A., Somers, R., and Van Beek, W.P.: T-cell leukemia presenting as chronic polyarthritis. Arthritis Rheum. 25:87, 1982.
44. Weinberger, A., Schumacher, H.R., Schimmer, B.M., Myers, A.R., and Brogadir, S.P.: Arthritis in acute leukemia: clinical and histopathological observations. Arch. Intern. Med. 141:1183, 1981.
45. Schaller, J.: Arthritis as a presenting manifestation of malignancy in children. J. Pediatr. 81:793, 1972.
46. Silverman, F.N.: The skeletal lesions in leukemia: Clinical and roentgenographic observations in 103 infants and children, with a review of the literature. Am. J. Roentgenol. Radium Ther. Nucl. Med. 59:819, 1948.
47. Thomas, L.B., Forkner, C.E., Jr., Frei, E., III, Besse, B.E., Jr., and Stabenau, J.R.: The skeletal lesions of acute leukemia. Cancer 14:608, 1961.
48. Silverstein, M.N., and Kelly, T.J.: Leukemia with osteoarticular symptoms and signs. Ann. Intern. Med. 59:637, 1963.
49. Willson, J.K.V.: The bone lesions of childhood leukemia: A survey of 140 cases. Radiology 72:672, 1959.
50. Poynton, F.J., and Moncrieff, A.: Subcutaneous nodules in the scalp in fatal cases of glandular enlargements with mononucleosis. Lancet 2:812, 1929.
51. Sherry, M.G.: The incidence of positive RA tests in Hodgkin's disease and leukemia. Am. J. Clin. Pathol. 50:398, 1968.
52. Reimer, R.R., Chabner, B.A., Young, R.C., Reddick, R., and Johnson, R.E.: Lymphoma presenting in bone: Results of histopathology, staging, and therapy. Ann. Intern. Med. 87:50, 1977.
53. Sutro, C.J.: Lymphosarcoma of the patella; Radical excision without repair of the extensor apparatus of the leg. Bull. Hosp. Joint Dis. 24:68, 1973.
54. Hench, P.K., Mayne, J.G., Kiely, J.M., and Dockerty, M.B.: Clinical study of rheumatic manifestations of lymphoma. Arthritis Rheum. 5:301, 1962.
55. Hustu, H.O., and Pinkel, D.: Lymphosarcoma, Hodgkin's disease, and leukemia in bone. Clin. Orthop. 52:83, 1967.
56. Martin, V.M., Bennett, R.M., Hughes, G.R.V., and Holt, P.J.L.: Lymphosarcomatous arthropathy. Ann. Rheumatol. Dis. 32:162, 1973.
57. Adunsky, A., Yaretzky, A., and Klajman, A.: Malignant lymphoma presenting as sternoclavicular joint arthritis. Arthritis Rheum. 23:1330, 1980.
58. Gottlieb, M., Hoppe, R.T., Calin, A., and Strober, S.: Arthritis in a patient with mycosis fungoides: complete remission after radiotherapy. Arthritis Rheum. 22:424, 1979.
59. Lejeune, E., and Brun Ney, P.: Les formes rhumatismales de l'ostéome ostéoide. Journées Rhumatol. (Montpellier) 3-4, Octobre 1975.
60. Spjut, H.J., Dorfman, H.D., Fechner, R.E., et al.: Tumors of bone and cartilage. Atlas of Tumor Pathology, 2nd Series, Fasc. 5. Armed Forces Institute of Pathology, 1971.
61. Mills, J.A.: Spectrum of organ systems that respond to cancer: The joints and connective tissue. Ann. N.Y. Acad. Sci. 230:443, 1974.
62. Mills, J.A.: Connective tissue disease associated with malignant neoplastic disease. J. Chronic Dis. 16:797, 1963.
63. Mackenzie, A.H., and Scherbel, A.L.: Connective tissue syndromes associated with carcinoma. Geriatrics 18:745, 1963.
64. Awerbuch, M.S., and Brooks, P.M.: Role of immune complexes in hypertrophic osteoarthropathy and non-metastatic polyarthritis. Ann. Rheum. Dis. 40:470, 1981.
65. Samayoa, E.A., McDuffie, F.C. Nelson, A.M., et al.: Immunoglobulin complexes in sera of patients with malignancy. Int. J. Cancer 19:12, 1977.
66. Robins, R.A., and Baldwin, R.W.: Immune complexes in cancer. Cancer Immunol. Immunother. 4:1, 1978.
67. Lansbury, J.C.: Collagen disease complicating malignancy. Ann. Rheum. Dis. 12:301, 1953.

68. Bennett, R.M., Ginsberg, M.H., and Thomsen, S.: Carcinoma polyarthritis. The presenting symptom of an ovarian tumor and association with a platelet activating factor. Arthritis Rheum. 19:953, 1976.

69. Leonard, J.W.: Rheumatoid-like arthritis preceding brain tumor. Arch. Intern. Med. 141:139, 1981.

70. Simon, R.D., Jr., and Ford, L.E.: Rheumatoid-like arthritis associated with a colonic carcinoma. Arch. Intern. Med. 140:698, 1980.

71. Caldwell, D.S.: Carcinoma polyarthritis manifestations and differential diagnosis. Medical Grand Rounds 1:378, 1982.

72. Wybran, J., and Fudenberg, H.H.: Thymus derived rosette forming cells in human disease states: Cancer, lymphomas, viral and bacterial infections, and other diseases. J. Clin. Invest. 52:1026, 1973.

73. Lee, J.C., Yamauchi, H., and Hopper, J.: The association of cancer and the nephrotic syndrome. Ann. Intern. Med. 64:41, 1966.

74. Husby, G., Sletten, K., Michaelsen, T.E., et al.: Blocking of lymphocyte-mediated cytotoxicity for rat hepatoma cells by tumor specific antigen-antibody complexes. Nature (New Biol.) 238:185, 1972.

75. Hellstrom, I., Sjögren, H.O., Warner, G., et al.: Blocking of cell mediated tumor immunity by sera from patients with growing neoplasms. Int. J. Cancer 7:226, 1971.

76. Jermanovich, N.B., Giammarco, R., Ginsberg, S.J., Tinsley, R.W., and Jones, D.B.: Small cell anaplastic carcinoma of the lung with mesangial proliferative glomerulonephritis. Arch. Intern. Med. 142:397, 1982.

77. Barton, C.H., Vaziri, N.D., and Spear, G.S.: Nephrotic syndrome associated with adenocarcinoma of the breast. Am. J. Med. 68:308, 1980.

78. Ragan, C., and Snyder, A.I.: Rheumatoid arthritis. DM 11:2, 1955.

79. Owen, D.S., Jr., Waller, M., and Toone, E.: Rheumatoid disease and malignancy. Arthritis Rheum. 10:302, 1967.

80. Uddin, J., Kraus, A.S., and Kelly, G.H.: Survivorship and death in rheumatoid arthritis. Arthritis Rheum. 13:125, 1970.

81. Moesmann, G.: Malignancy and mortality in subacute rheumatoid arthritis in old age. Acta Rheum. Scand. 15:193, 1969.

82. Litwin, S.D., Allen, J.C., and Kunkel, H.G.: Disappearance of the clinical and serologic manifestations of rheumatoid arthritis following a thoracotomy for a lung tumor. Arthritis Rheum. 9:865, 1966.

83. Sheon, R.P., Kirsner, A.B., Tangsintanapas, P., Samad, F., Garg, M.L., and Finkel, R.I.: Malignancy in rheumatic diseases: Interrelationships. J. Am. Geriat. Soc. 25:20, 1977.

84. Hammoudeh, M., and Khan, M.A.: Cranial arteritis as the initial manifestation of malignant histiocytosis. J. Rheumatol. 9:443, 1982.

85. Spilberg, I., and Meyer, G.J.: The arthritis of leukemia. Arthritis Rheum. 15:630, 1972.

86. Strandberg, B., and Jarlov, N.V.: Cancer, arthritis and rheumatoid arthritis. Rheumatism 17:45, 1961.

87. Husian, M.N., Neff, J., Darby, E., et al.: Antinuclear antibodies: Clinical significance of titers and fluorescence patterns. Am. J. Clin. Pathol. 61:59, 1974.

88. Marcus, R.M., and Grayzel, A.I.: A lupus antibody syndrome associated with hypernephroma. Arthritis Rheum. 22:1396, 1979.

89. Byrd, W.E., Matthews, O.P., and Hunt, R.E.: Left atrial myxoma presenting as a systemic vasculitis. Arthritis Rheum. 23:240, 1980.

90. Salem, N.B.: Lupus antibody syndrome with intestinal lymphoma. Arthritis Rheum. 23:613, 1980.

91. Howqua, J., and Mackay, I.R.: LE cells in lymphoma. Blood 22:191, 1963.

92. Zacharski, L.R., and Kyle, R.A.: Significance of extreme elevation of erythrocyte sedimentation rate. JAMA 202:264, 1967.

93. Ropes, M.W., and Bauer, W.: Synovial Fluid Changes in Joint Disease. Cambridge, Harvard University Press, 1953, p. 89.

94. Aisner, M., and Hoxie, T.B.: Bone and joint pain in leukemia simulating acute rheumatic fever and subacute bacterial endocarditis. N. Engl. J. Med. 238:733, 1948.

95. Falchi, G., and Gerlini, F.: Le manifestazioni articolari in corso di leukemia o forma rheumatoide della leukemia. Arch. Ital. Pediatr. 19:272, 1959.

96. Cammarata, R.J., Rodnan, G.P., and Jensen, W.N.: Systemic rheumatic disease and malignant lymphoma. Arch. Intern. Med. 111:330, 1963.

97. Razis, D.V., Diamond, H.D., and Craver, L.F.: Hodgkin's disease associated with other malignant tumors and certain non-neoplastic diseases. Am. J. Med. Sci. 238:327, 1959.

98. Elkon, K.B., Hughes, G.R.V., and Catovsky, D.: Hairy cell leukemia with polyarteritis nodosa. Lancet 2:280, 1979.

99. Goedert, J.J., Neefe, J.R., Smith, F.S., Stahl, N.I., Jaffe, E.S., and Fauci, A.S.: Polyarteritis, hairy cell leukemia, and splenosis. Am. J. Med. 71:323, 1981.

100. Pope, A., Lazarchick, J., Hoyer, L., and Weinstein, A.: Hairy cell leukemia and vasculitis. J. Rheumatol. 7:895, 1980.

101. LePogamp, P., Ghandour, C., and LePrise, P.Y.: Hairy cell leukemia and polyarteritis nodosa. J. Rheumatol. 9:441, 1982.

102. Weinstein, A.: Systemic vasculitis and hairy cell leukemia (editorial). J. Rheumatol. 9:349, 1982.

103. Thomas, M.H.: Myxoma masquerading as polyarteritis nodosa. J. Rheumatol. 8:133, 1981.

104. Cammarata, R.J., et al.: Association of systemic rheumatic disease and malignant lymphoma. Clin. Res. 9:329, 1961.

105. Wallach, H.W.: Lupus-like syndrome associated with carcinoma of the breast. Arch. Intern. Med. 137:532, 1977.

106. Pierce, D.A., Stern, R., Jaffe, R., Zulman, J., and Talal, N.: Immunoblastic sarcoma with features of Sjögren's syndrome and systemic lupus erythematosus in a patient with immunoblastic lymphadenopathy. Arthritis Rheum. 22:911, 1979.

107. Harvey, A.M., Shulman, L.E., Tumulty, P.A., Conley, C.L., and Schoenrich, E.H.: Systemic lupus erythematosus: A review of the literature and clinical analysis of 138 cases. Medicine 33:291, 1954.

108. Christianson, H.B., and Fine, R.M.: Vasculitis with or without panniculitis in leukemia, lymphoma and multiple myeloma. South. Med. J. 60:567, 1967.

109. Sams, W.M., Jr., Harville, D.D., and Winkelmann, R.K.: Necrotizing vasculitis associated with lethal reticuloendothelial diseases. Br. J. Dermatol. 80:555, 1968.

110. Greco, F.A., Kolins, J., Rajjoub, R.K., and Brereton, H.D.: Hodgkin's disease and granulomatous angiitis of the central nervous system. Cancer 30:2037, 1976.

111. Weisenberger, D., Armitage, J., and Dick, F.: Immunoblastic lymphadenopathy with pulmonary infiltrates, hypocomplementemia and vasculitis. Am. J. Med. 63:849, 1977.

112. Cairns, S.A., Mallick, N.P., Lawler, W., and Williams, G.: Squamous cell carcinoma of bronchus presenting with Henoch-Schönlein purpura. Br. Med. J. 2:474, 1978.

113. Cupps, T.R., and Fauci, A.S.: Neoplasm and systemic vasculitis: A case report. Arthritis Rheum. 25:475, 1982.

114. Friedman, S.A., Bienenstock, H., and Richter, I.H.: Malignancy and arteriopathy: A report of 2 cases. Angiology 20:136, 1969.

115. Pinski, J.B., and Stanisfer, P.D.: Erythema nodosum as the initial manifestation of leukemia. Arch. Dermatol. 89:339, 1964.

116. Bluefarb, S.M., Wallk, S., and Gecht, M.L.: Acute monocytic leukemia with erythema nodosum. Case presentation, Chicago Dermatological Society. Arch. Dermatol. 75:596, 1957.

117. McCombs, R.P.: Systemic "allergic" vasculitis: Clinical and pathological relationships. JAMA 194:1059, 1965.

118. Spector, J.I., Zimbler, H., Levine, R., Ross, J.S., Valigorsky, J.M., and Cole, L.M.: Sweet's syndrome, association with acute leukemia. JAMA 244:1131, 1980.

119. Chmel, H., and Armstrong, D.: Acute febrile neutrophilic dermatosis: Sweet's syndrome. South. Med. J. 71:1350, 1978.

120. Johnson, P.C., Rolak, L.A., Hamilton, R.H., and Laguna, J.L.: Paraneoplastic vasculitis of nerve: A remote effect of cancer. Ann. Neurol. 5:437, 1979.

121. Sams, W.M., Jr., Harville, D.D., and Winkelmann, R.K.: Necrotizing vasculitis associated with lethal reticuloendothelial diseases. Br. J. Dermatol. 80:555, 1968.

122. Alarcón-Segovia, D.: The necrotizing vasculitides. A new pathogenic classification. Med. Clin. North Am. 61:24, 1977.

123. Bergevin, P.R.: The increasing problem of malignancy in the elderly. Med. Clin. North Am. 60:1241, 1976.

124. Ioachim, N., McKenna, P.J., Delaney, W.E., Toth, I., and Chung, F.J.: Cryoglobulinemia and amyloidosis associated with intestinal lymphoma. Arch. Intern. Med. 138:1158, 1978.

125. Lerner, A.B., and Watson, C.J.: Studies of cryoglobulins. I. Unusual purpura associated with presence of high concentration of cryoglobulin (cold precipitable serum globulin). Am. J. Med. Sci. 214:410, 1947.

126. Watson, C.J., and Lerner, A.B.: Clinical significance of cryoglobulinemia. Acta Med. Scand. Suppl. 196:489, 1947.

127. Brouet, J.C., Claunel, J.P., Danow, F., et al.: Biological and clinical significance of cryoglobulins: A report of 86 cases. Am. J. Med. 57:775, 1974.

128. Scully, R.E., Galdabini, J.J., and McNeely, B.U.: Case records of the Massachusetts General Hospital. Case 11-1979. New Engl. J. Med. 300:610, 1979.

128a. Korst, D.R., and Kratochvil, C.H.: "Cryofibrinogen" in a case of lung neoplasm associated with thrombophlebitis migrans. Blood 10:945, 1955.

129. McKee, P.A., Kalbfleisch, J.M., and Bird, R.M.: Incidence and significance of cryofibrinogenemia. J. Lab. Clin. Med. 61:203, 1963.

130. Zlotnick, A., Shanim, W., and Rachmilewitz, E.A.: Studies in cryofibrinogenemia. Acta Haematol. 42:8, 1969.

131. Teshima, H., Wancbo, H., Pinsky, C., and Day, N.K.: Circulating immune complexes detected by ^{125}I-C1q deviation test in sera of cancer patients. J. Clin. Invest. 59:1134, 1977.

132. Theofilopoulos, A.N., Wilson, C.B., and Dixon, F.J.: The Raji cell radioimmune assay for detecting immune complexes in human sera. J. Clin. Invest. 57:169, 1976.

133. Rosen, R.D., and Barnes, B.C.: Measuring serum immune complexes in cancer. Ann. Intern. Med. 88:570, 1978.

134. Rosen, R.D., Reisberg, M.A., Hersh, E.M., and Gutterman, J.U.: The C1q binding test for soluble immune complexes: Clinical correlations

obtained in patients with cancer. J. Natl. Cancer Inst. 58:1205, 1977.

135. Cano, P., Jerry, L.M., Lewis, M.G., Hartmann, D., Phillips, T., Capek, A., Shibata, H., and Mansell, P.W.: Circulating immune complexes in human malignant melanoma (abstract). Proceedings of the 12th Annual Meeting of the American Society of Clinical Oncology. Cancer Res. 17:74, 1976.

136. Samayoa, E.A., McDuffie, F.C., Nelson, A.M., et al.: Immunoglobulin complexes in sera of patients with malignancy. Int. J. Cancer 19:12, 1977.

137. Day, N.K., Winfield, J., Gee, T., Winchester, R., Teshima, H., and Kunkel, H.G.: Evidence for immune complexes involving antilymphocyte antibodies associated with hypo-complementaemia in chronic lymphocytic leukemia (CLL). Clin. Exp. Immunol. 76:189, 1976.

138. Long, J.C., Hall, C.L., Brown, A., Stamatos, C., Weitzman, S.A., and Carey, K.: Binding of soluble immune complexes in serum of patients with Hodgkin's disease to tissue cultures derived from the tumor. N. Engl. J. Med. 297:295, 1977.

139. Amlot, P.L., Slaney, J.M., and Williams, B.D.: Circulating immune complexes and symptoms in Hodgkin's disease. Lancet 1:449, 1976.

140. Kávai, M., Berényi, E., Pálkovi, S.G., et al.: Immune complexes in Hodgkin's disease. Lancet 1:1249, 1976.

141. Plager, J., and Stutzman, L.: Acute nephrotic syndrome as a manifestation of active Hodgkin's disease. Am. J. Med. 50:56, 1971.

142. Routledge, R.C., Hann, I.M., and Morris Jones, P.H.: Hodgkin's disease complicated by the nephrotic syndrome. Cancer 38:1735, 1976.

143. Sutherland, J.C., Markham, R.V., Ramsey, H.E., et al.: Subclinical immune complex nephritis in patients with Hodgkin's disease. Cancer Res. 34:1179, 1974.

144. Brown, C.A., Hall, C.L., Long, J.C., Carey, K., Weitzman, S.A., and Aisenberg, A.C.: Circulating immune complexes in Hodgkin's disease. Am. J. Med. 64:289, 1978.

145. Steinbrocker, O.: The shoulder-hand syndrome. Am. J. Med. 3:402, 1947.

146. Steinbrocker, O., Freidman, H.H., and Lapin, L.: The shoulder-hand syndrome: Reflex neurovascular dystrophy of the upper extremity. Postgrad. Med. 16:46, 1954.

147. Bremer, C.: Shoulder-hand syndrome: A case of unusual aetiology. Ann. Physical Med. 9:168, 1966.

148. Medsger, T.A., Jr., Dixon, J.A., and Garwood, V.F.: Palmar fasciitis and polyarthritis associated with ovarian carcinoma. Ann. Intern. Med. 96:424, 1982.

149. Christianson, H.B., Brunsting, L.A., and Perry, H.D.: Dermatomyositis: Unusual features, complications and treatment. Arch. Dermatol. 74:581, 1956.

150. Basten, A., and Bonnin, M.: Scleroderma in carcinoma. Med. J. Aust. 1:452, 1966.

151. Asboe-Hansen, G.: Scleroderma in carcinoid syndrome. Acta Dermatol. Venereol. 39:270, 1959.

152. Huston, K.A., Hunder, G.G., Lie, J.T., Kennedy, R.H., and Elveback, L.R.: Temporal arteritis. A 25-year epidemiologic, clinical and pathologic study. Ann. Intern. Med. 88:162, 1978.

153. Niemi, K.M., Förström, L., Hannuksela, M., Mustakallio, K.K., and Salo, O.P.: Nodules on the legs. A clinical, histological and immunohistological study of 82 patients representing different types of nodular panniculitis. Acta Dermatal. Venereol. 57:145, 1977.

154. MacDonald, A.: A review of the concept of Weber-Christian panniculitis with a report of 5 cases. Br. J. Dermatol. 80:355, 1968.

155. Blomgren, S.E.: Erythema nodosum. Semin. Arthritis Rheum. 4:1, 1974.

156. Förström, L., and Winkelman, R.K.: Acute, generalized panniculitis with amylase and lipase in skin. Arch. Dermatol. 111:497, 1975.

157. Berner, O.: Subkutane Fettgewebsnekrose. Virchows Arch. Pathol. Anat. 193:510, 1908.

158. Hughes, P.S.H., Apisarnthanarax, P., and Mullins, J.F.: Subcutaneous fat necrosis associated with pancreatic disease. Arch. Dermatol. 111:506, 1975.

159. Simkin, P.A., Brunzell, J.D., Wisner, D., Fiechtner, J.J., Carlin, J.S., and Willkens, R.F.: Free fatty acids in the pancreatitic arthritis syndrome. Arthritis Rheum. 26:127, 1983.

160. Szymanski, F.J., and Bluefarb, S.M.: Nodular fat necrosis and pancreatic disease. Arch. Dermatol. 83:224, 1961.

161. Robertson, J.C., and Eeles, G.H.: Syndrome associated with pancreatic acinar cell carcinoma. Br. Med. J. 2:708, 1970.

162. Auger, C.: Acinous cell carcinoma of the pancreas with extensive fat necrosis. Arch. Pathol. 43:400, 1947.

163. Osborne, R.R.: Functioning acinous cell carcinoma of the pancreas accompanied with widespread focal fat necrosis. Arch. Intern. Med. 85:933, 1950.

164. Jackson, S.H., Savidge, R.S., Stein, L., et al.: Carcinoma of the pancreas associated with fat necrosis. Lancet 268:962, 1952.

165. Belsky, H., and Cornel, N.W.: Disseminated focal fat necrosis following radical pancreaticoduodenectomy for acinous carcinoma of the head of the pancreas. Am. Surg. 141:556, 1955.

166. Hegler, C., and Wohlwill, F.: Fettgewebnekrosen in Subcutis und Kno-

chemark durch Metastasen eines Carcinoms der Pankreas Schwanzes. Virchows Arch. Pathol. Anat. 274:784, 1930.

167. Titone, M.: Über ungewohnlich ausgebriete Fettgewebs und Gewebschekrosen bei Pankreaskrebs. Virchows Arch. Pathol. Anat. 297:416, 1936.

168. Schmid, M.: Über das Syndrom des sekototorich Aktiren, metastasierenden exokrinen Pancreas Adenomas. Z. Klin. Med. 154:439, 1954.

169. Wuketich, S., and Pavlik, F.: Syndrome des metastasierenden lipasebildenen Pancreasadenoms Zugliesch ein Beitrag zur differential Diagnose der Pfeifer-Weber-Christianchen-Krankheit. Arch. Klin. Exp. Derm. 216:412, 1963.

170. Lievre, J.A., May, V., Bénichou, C., et al.: Stéatonécrose disséminée, ostéolyse stéatonécrotique et cancer du pancréas. Discussion du syndrome de Weber-Christian. Bull. Soc. Med. Hôp. Paris 115:755, 1964.

171. De Graciansky, P., Paraf, A., Rautureau, J., et al.: Panniculite nodulaine aiguë fébrile récidivante au cours d'un cancer acineux du pancréas. La problème de la maladie de Weber-Christian. Soc. Med. Hôp. Paris 116:261, 1965.

172. Virshup, A.M., and Sliwinski, A.J.: Polyarthritis and subcutaneous nodules associated with carcinoma of the pancreas. Arthritis Rheum. 16:388, 1973.

173. Swerdlow, A.B., Berman, M.E., Gibbel, M.I., et al.: Subcutaneous fat necrosis associated with acute pancreatitis. JAMA 173:765, 1960.

174. Pinski, J.B., and Stanisfer, P.D.: Erythema nodosum as the initial manifestation of leukemia. Arch. Dermatol. 89:339, 1966.

175. Dolan, D.L., Lemmon, G.B., Jr., and Teitelbaum, S.L.: Relapsing polychondritis. Am. J. Med. 41:285, 1966.

176. Odkuist, L.: Relapsing polychondritis. Acta Otolaryngol. 70:448, 1970.

177. Miller, S.B., Donlan, C.J., and Roth, S.B.: Hodgkin's disease presenting as relapsing polychondritis. A previously undescribed association. Arthritis Rheum. 17:598, 1974.

178. Douglas, G.W., Levin, R.H., and Sokoloff, L.: Infectious arthritis complicating neoplastic disease. N. Engl. J. Med. 270:299, 1964.

179. Lyon, L.J., and Nevins, M.A.: Carcinoma of the colon presenting as pyogenic arthritis. JAMA 241:2060, 1979.

180. Linovitz, R.J., Resnick, D., Keissling, P., et al.: Tumor-induced osteomalacia and rickets: A surgically curable syndrome. J. Bone Joint Surg. 58:419, 1976.

181. Parker, M.S., Klein, I., Haussler, M.R., and Mintz, D.H.: Tumor-induced osteomalacia, evidence of a surgically correctable alteration in vitamin D metabolism. JAMA 245:492, 1981.

182. Seidenfeld, A.M., Smythe, H.A., Ogryzlo, M.A., Urowitz, M.B., and Dotten, D.A.: Acute leukemia in rheumatoid arthritis treated with cytotoxic agents. J. Rheumatol. 3:294, 1976.

183. Leung, F., Fam, A. G., and Osoba, D.: Kaposi's sarcoma complicating corticosteroid therapy for temporal arteritis. Am. J. Med. 71:320, 1981.

184. Fauci, A.S., Haynes, B.F., Katz, P., and Wolff, S.M.: Wegener's granulomatosis: prospective clinical and therapeutic experience with 85 patients for 21 years. Ann. Intern. Med. 98:76, 1983.

185. Gilman, P.A., and Holtzman, N.A.: Acute lymphoblastic leukemia in a patient receiving penicillamine for Wilson's disease. JAMA 248:467, 1982.

186. Pinals, R.S.: Azathioprine in the treatment of chronic polyarthritis: Longterm results and adverse effects in 25 patients. J. Rheumatol. 3:140, 1976.

187. Black, K.A., Zilko, P.J., Dawkins, R.L., Armstrong, B.K., and Mastaglia, G.L.: Cancer in connective tissue disease. Arthritis Rheum. 25:1130, 1982.

188. Lukes, R.J., and Collins, R.D.: Immunologic characterization of human malignant lymphomas. Cancer 34:1488, 1974.

189. Lukes, R.J., and Collins, R.D.: The Lukes-Collins classification and its significance. Cancer Treat. Rep. 61:971, 1977.

190. Banks, P.M., Witrak, G.A., and Conn, D.L.: Lymphoid neoplasia following connective tissue disease. Mayo Clin. Proc. 54:104, 1979.

191. Howie, J.B., and Helyer, B.J.: The immunology and pathology of NZB mice. Adv. Immunol. 9:215, 1968.

192. Howie, J.B., and Simpson, L.O.: Autoimmune disease in NZB mice and their hybrids. In Dubois, E.L. (ed.): Lupus Erythematosus, 2nd ed. Los Angeles, University of Southern California Press, 1974.

193. Sugai, S., Pillarisetty, R., and Talal, N.: Monoclonal macroglobulinemia in NZB/NZW F₂ mice. J. Exp. Med. 138:989, 1973.

194. Mellors, R.C.: Autoimmune and immunoproliferative diseases of NZB mice and hybrids. Int. Rev. Exp. Pathol. 5:217, 1966.

195. East, J.: Immunopathology and neoplasms in New Zealand Black (NZB) and SJL mice. Prog. Exp. Tumor Res. 13:84, 1970.

196. Talal, N., Fye, K., and Moutsopoulos, H.: Autoimmunity. In Fudenberg, H.H., Stites, D.P., Caldwell, J.L., and Wells, J.V. (eds.): Basic and Clinical Immunology. Los Altos, Cal., Lange Medical Publications, 1976.

197. Steinberg, A.D.: Efficacy of immunosuppressive drugs in rheumatic diseases. Arthritis Rheum. 16:92, 1973.

198. Walker, S.E., and Anver, M.R.: Accelerated appearance of neoplasms in

female NZB/NZW mice treated with high-dose cyclophosphamide. Arthritis Rheum. 22:1338, 1979.

199. Miller, D.G.: The association of immune disease and malignant lymphoma. Ann. Intern. Med. 66:507, 1967.

200. Canoso, J.J., and Cohen, A.S.: Malignancy in a series of 70 patients with systemic lupus erythematosus. Arthritis Rheum. 17:383, 1974.

201. Talal, N., Sokoloff, L., and Barth, W.F.: Extrasalivary lymphoid abnormalities in Sjögren's syndrome (reticulum cell sarcoma, "pseudolymphoma," macroglobulinemia). Am. J. Med. 43:50, 1967.

202. Talal, N., and Bunim, J.J.: The development of malignant lymphoma in the course of Sjögren's syndrome. Am. J. Med. 36:529, 1964.

203. Smith, C.K., Cassidy, J.T., and Bole, G.G.: Type I dysgammaglobulinemia, systemic lupus erythematosus, and lymphoma. Am. J. Med. 48:113, 1970.

204. Fernandez-Herlihy, L., and Kott, S.: Connective tissue disease and lymphomas: Case report and review. Lahey Clin. Found. Bull. 16:165, 1967.

205. Lipsmeyer, E.A.: Development of malignant cerebral lymphoma in a patient with systemic lupus erythematosus treated with immunosuppression. Arthritis Rheum. 15:183, 1972.

206. Deaton, J.G., and Levin, W.C.: Systemic lupus erythematosus and acute myeloblastic leukemia. Report of their coexistence and a survey of possible associating features. Arch. Intern. Med. 120:345, 1967.

207. Delmas-Marsalet, Y., Leduc, M., and Lerche, B.: Tumeur du thymus et lupus érythémateux disséminé. Étude anatomoclinique et considérations physio-pathologiques. Presse Med. 77:821, 1969.

208. Joseph, R.R., and Zarafonetis, C.J.D.: Clinical onset of lupus erythematosus in the older age group. J. Am. Geriat. Soc. 12:789, 1964.

209. Kahn, M.F., Ryckewaert, A., and Cannat, A.: Systemic lupus erythematosus and ovarian dysgerminoma: Remission of the systemic lupus erythematosus after extirpation of the tumor. Clin. Exp. Immunol. 1:355, 1966.

210. Tripp, C.D.: Auto-immune disease with neoplasm. N.Y. State J. Med. 67:1907, 1967.

211. Schleissner, L.A., Sheehan, W.W., and Orselli, R.C.: Lupus erythematosus in a patient with amyloidosis, adrenal insufficiency, and subsequent immunoblastic sarcoma. Demonstration of the LE phenomenon in the lung. Arthritis Rheum. 19:249, 1976.

212. Andreev, V.V., and Zlatkov, N.B.: Systemic lupus erythematosus and neoplasia of the lymphoreticular system. Br. J. Dermatol. 89:503, 1968.

213. Lea, A.J.: An association between the rheumatic diseases and the reticuloses. Ann. Rheum. Dis. 23:480, 1964.

214. Agudelo, C.A., Schumacher, R., Glick, J.H., and Molina, J.: Non-Hodgkin's lymphoma in systemic lupus erythematosus. Report of 4 cases with ultra-structural studies in 2. J. Rheumatol. 8:69, 1981.

215. Goodwin, J.S.: Remission in systemic lupus erythematosus after combination chemotherapy for Hodgkin's disease. JAMA 244:1962, 1980.

216. Oleinick, A.: Leukemia or lymphoma occurring subsequent to autoimmune disease. Blood 29:144, 1967.

217. Andreasen, J.O., and Poulsen, H.E.: Oral discoid and systemic lupus erythematosus. I. Clinical investigation. Acta Odont. Scand. 22:295, 1964.

218. Ryan, C.: Epithelioma complicating lupus erythematosus. Br. Med. J. 2:334, 1947.

219. Wolstenholme, G.E.W.: Epithelioma arising on lupus erythematosus. Br. J. Dermatol. 61:126, 1949.

220. Beeson, B.B., and Ebert, M.H.: Lupus erythematosus plus epithelioma. Urol. Cutan. Rev. 38:785, 1934.

221. Epstein, J.H., and Tuffanelli, D.L.: Discoid lupus erythematosus. In Dubois, E.L. (ed.): Lupus Erythematosus. 2nd ed. Los Angeles, University of Southern California Press, 1974.

222. Mason, A.M.S., Gumpel, J.M., and Golding, P.L.: Sjögren's syndrome—a clinical review. Semin. Arthritis Rheum. 2:30, 973.

223. Rothman, S., Block, M., and Hauser, F.V.: Sjögren's syndrome associated with lymphoblastoma and hypersplenism. Arch. Dermatol. Syph. 63:642, 1951.

224. Talal, N.: Sjögren's syndrome. Bull. Rheum. Dis. 16:404, 1966.

225. Hornbaker, J.H., Jr., Foster, F.A., Williams, G.S., and Davis, J.S., IV: Sjögren's syndrome and nodular reticulum cell sarcoma. Arch. Intern. Med. 118:449, 1966.

226. Cummings, N.A., Schall, G.L., Asofsky, R., Anderson, L.G., and Talal, N.: Sjögren's syndrome—newer aspects of research, diagnosis, and therapy. Ann. Intern. Med. 75:937, 1971.

227. Anderson, L.G., and Talal, N.: The spectrum of benign to malignant lymphoproliferation in Sjögren's syndrome. Clin. Exp. Immunol. 9:199, 1971.

228. Moutsopoulos, H.M., and Fauci, A.S.: Immunoregulation in Sjögren's syndrome: influence of serum factors on T cell subpopulation. J. Clin. Invest. 65:519, 1980.

229. Kennealey, G.T., Kaetz, H.W., and Smith, G.J.: Sjögren's syndrome with pseudolymphoma 13 years after Hodgkin's disease. Arch. Intern. Med. 138:635, 1978.

230. Diaz-Jouanen, E., Ruiz-Argüelles, G.J., Vega-Ortiz, J.M., Villareal, G., and Alarcón-Segovia, D.: From benign polyclonal to malignant monoclonal lymphoproliferation in a patient with primary Sjögren's syndrome. Arthritis Rheum. 24:850, 1981.

231. Aizawa, Y., Zawadzki, Z.A., Micolonghi, T.S., McDowell, J.W., and Neiman, R.S.: Vasculitis and Sjögren's syndrome with IgA-IgG cryoglobulinemia terminating in immunoblastic sarcoma. Am. J. Med. 67:160, 1979.

232. Fye, K.H., Daniels, T.E., Zulman, J., Michalski, J.P., Jaffe, R., and Talal, N.: Aplastic anemia and lymphoma in Sjögren's syndrome. Arthritis Rheum. 23:1321, 1980.

233. Talal, N., and Schnitzer, B.: Lymphadenopathy and Sjögren's syndrome. Clin. Rheum. Dis. 3:421, 1977.

234. Nowell, P.C.: The clonal evolution of tumor cell populations. Science 194:23, 1976.

235. Conley, C.L., Misiti, J., and Laster, A.J.: Genetic factors predisposing to chronic lymphocytic leukemia and to autoimmune disease. Medicine 59:323, 1980.

236. Fam, A.G., Lewis, A.J., and Cowan, D.H.: Multiple myeloma and amyloid bone lesions complicating rheumatoid arthritis. J. Rheumatol. 8:845, 1981.

237. Crofts, M.A., Sharp, J.C., and Joyner, M.V.: Rheumatoid arthritis and hairy cell leukemia. Lancet 2:203, 1979.

238. Zatuchni, J., Campbell, W.N., and Zarafonetis, C.J.D.: Pulmonary fibrosis and terminal bronchiolar ("alveolar cell") carcinoma in scleroderma. Cancer 6:1147, 1953.

239. Caplan, H.: Honeycomb lungs and malignant pulmonary adenomatosis in scleroderma. Thorax 14:89, 1959.

240. Collins, D.H., Darke, C.S., and Dodge, O.G.: Scleroderma with honeycomb lungs and bronchiolar carcinoma. J. Pathol. Bacteriol. 76:531, 1958.

241. Jonsson, S.M., and Houser, J.M.: Scleroderma (progressive systemic sclerosis) associated with cancer of the lung. Brief review and report of a case. N. Engl. J. Med. 255:413, 1956.

242. Richards, R.L., and Milne, J.A.: Cancer of the lung in progressive systemic sclerosis. Thorax 13:238, 1958.

243. Schenkel, J.P.: The sclerodermal lung. Ann. Anat. Pathol. 5:32, 1960.

244. Batsakis, J.G., and Johnson, H.A.: Generalized scleroderma involving lungs and liver with pulmonary adenocarcinoma. Arch. Pathol. 69:633, 1960.

245. Montgomery, R.D., Stirling, G.A., and Hamer, N.A.J.: Bronchiolar carcinoma in progressive systemic sclerosis. Lancet 1:586, 1964.

246. Ezzo, J.A., and Davis, D.K.: Progressive systemic sclerosis (scleroderma) with adenocarcinoma of the lung: Report of a case. Dis. Chest 47:235, 1965.

247. Szymczyk, E., and Klott, M.: A case of generalized scleroderma and alveolar carcinoma. Gruźlica 35:159, 1967.

248. Tomkin, G.H.: Systemic sclerosis associated with carcinoma of the lung. Br. J. Dermatol. 81:213, 1969.

249. Neto, R.P.D., Steinberg, A., Kron, S.D., and Rachman, R.: Breast carcinoma in a patient with scleroderma. Postgrad. Med. 44:161, 1968.

250. Talbott, J.H., and Barrocas, M.: Progressive systemic sclerosis (PSS) and malignancy pulmonary and non-pulmonary. Medicine 58:182, 1979.

251. Trotta, F., Potena, A., Marchi, M., Corte, R.L., and Cavazzini, L.: Progressive systemic sclerosis and pulmonary malignancy. J. Rheumatol. 9:970, 1982.

252. Talbott, J.H., and Hoch-Ligeti, C.: Cancer associated with collagenvascular disease. South. Med. J. 72:127, 1979.

253. Katz, A.L., Nashel, D.J., Goard, C.P., and Bauer, H.: Pemphigus vulgaris and lymphoma in a patient with scleroderma. South. Med. J. 72:1463, 1979.

254. Spencer, H., and Raeburn, C.: Pulmonary (bronchiolar) adenomatosis. J. Pathol. Bacteriol. 71:145, 1956.

255. Theiler, A.: 7th and 8th Reports of Director of Veterinary Research. Department of Agriculture, Union of South Africa, p. 59.

256. Cowdry, E.V.: Studies on the etiology of jaagsiekte. J. Exp. Med. 42:323, 1925.

257. Dungal, N.: Experiments with jaagsiekte. Am. J. Pathol. 22:737, 1946.

258. Nobel, T.A., and Perk, K.: Animal model of human disease. Bronchioloalveolar cell carcinoma. Am. J. Pathol. 90:783, 1978.

259. Masi, A.J., and D'Angelo, W.A.: Epidemiology of fatal systemic sclerosis (diffuse scleroderma). A 15-year survey in Baltimore. Ann. Intern. Med. 66:870, 1967.

260. Epstein, C.J., Martin, G.M., and Schultz, A.L.: Werner's syndrome: A review of its symptomatology, natural history, pathologic features, genetics and relationship to natural aging process. Medicine 45:177, 1966.

261. Hrabko, R.P., Milgrom, H., and Schwartz, R.A.: Werner's syndrome with associated malignant neoplasms. Arch. Dermatol. 118:106, 1982.

262. Israel, H.L.: Sarcoidosis, malignancy, and immunosuppressive therapy. Arch. Intern. Med. 138:907, 1978.

263. Brincker, H., and Wilbek, E.: The incidence of malignant tumors in patients with respiratory sarcoidosis. Br. J. Cancer 29:247, 1974.

264. Nadel, E.M., and Ackerman, L.V.: Lesions resembling Boeck's sarcoid. Am. J. Clin. Pathol. 20:952, 1950.

265. Gregorie, H.B., Jr., Othersen, H.B., Jr., and Moore, McK. P., Jr.: The significance of sarcoid-like lesions in association with malignant neoplasms. Am. J. Surg. 104:577, 1962.

266. Sybert, A., and Butler, T.P.: Sarcoidosis following adjuvant high-dose methotrexate therapy for osteosarcoma. Arch. Intern. Med. 138:488, 1978.

267. Israel, H.L.: Effects of chlorambucil and methotrexate in sarcoidosis. *In* Levinsky, L., and Wacholda, F. (eds.): Proceedings of the Fifth International Conference on Sarcoidosis. Prague, Karlova University Press, 1971, pp. 632–634.

268. Benedict, E.B.: Carcinoma in osteomyelitis. Surg. Gynecol. Obstet. 53:1, 1931.

269. Hobart, M.H., and Miller, D.S.: Unusual complications of osteomyelitis. Am. J. Surg. 45:53, 1939.

270. Lovell, W.W., King, R.E., and Alldredge, R.: Carcinoma in skin, sinuses, and bone following chronic osteomyelitis. South. Med. J. 50:266, 1957.

271. McAnally, A.K., and Dockerty, M.B.: Carcinoma developing in chronic draining cutaneous sinuses and fistulas. Surg. Gynecol. Obstet. 88:87, 1949.

272. Fitzgerald, R.H., Jr., Brewer, N.S., and Dahlin, D.C.: Squamous-cell carcinoma complicating chronic osteomyelitis. J. Bone Joint Surg. 58A:1146, 1956.

273. Harris, E.D., and Krane, S.M.: Paget's disease of bone. Bull. Rheum. Dis. 18:506, 1968.

274. Shulman, L.E.: Diffuse fasciitis with hypergammaglobulinemia and eosinophilia: A new syndrome? Abstract. J. Rheumatol. (Suppl.) 1:46, 1974.

275. Moutsopoulos, H.M., Webber, B.L., Paulidis, N.A., et al.: Diffuse fasciitis with eosinophilia. A clinicopathologic study. Am. J. Med. 68:701, 1980.

276. Shulman, L.E., Hoffman, R., Dainiak, N., et al.: Antibody mediated aplastic anemia and thrombocytopenia purpura in diffuse eosinophilic fasciitis. Abstract. Clin. Res. 27-514A, 1979.

277. Littlejohn, G., and Keystone, E.: Eosinophilic fasciitis and aplastic anemia. J. Rheumatol. 7:730, 1980.

278. Michaels, R.M.: Eosinophilic fasciitis complicated by Hodgkin's disease. J. Rheumatol. 9:473, 1982.

279. Liebow, A.A., Carrington, C.R.B., and Friedman, P.J.: Lymphomatoid granulomatosis. Hum. Pathol. 3:457, 1972.

280. Porretta, C.A., Dahlin, D.C., and Janes, J.M.: Sarcoma in Paget's disease of bone. J. Bone Joint Surg. 39A:1314, 1957.

281. McKenna, R.J., Schwinn, C.P., Soong, K.Y., and Higinbotham, N.L.: Osteogenic sarcoma arising in Paget's disease. Cancer 17:42, 1964.

282. Reimer, R.R., Hoover, R., Fraumeni, J.F., et al.: Acute leukemia after alkylating-agent therapy of ovarian cancer. N. Engl. J. Med. 297:177, 1977.

283. Sieber, S.M., and Adamson, R.H.: Toxicity of antineoplastic agents in man: Chromosomal aberrations, antifertility effects, congenital malformations, and carcinogenic potential. Adv. Cancer Res. 22:57, 1975.

284. Chabner, B.A.: Second neoplasm—a complication of cancer chemotherapy. N. Engl. J. Med. 297:213, 1977.

285. Love, R.R., and Sowa, J.M.: Myelomonocytic leukemia following cyclophosphamide therapy of rheumatoid disease. Ann. Rheum. Dis. 34:534, 1975.

286. Silvergleid, A.J., and Schrier, S.L.: Acute myelogenous leukemia in two patients treated with azathioprine for non-malignant diseases. Am. J. Med. 57:885, 1974.

287. Nyberg, G., Eriksson, O., and Westberg, N.G.: Increased incidence of cervical atypia in women with systemic lupus erythematosus treated with chemotherapy. Arthritis Rheum. 24:648, 1981.

288. Potolsky, A., and Creger, W.P.: Radiation and drug therapies, and leukemia. Ann. Rev. Med. 24:75, 1973.

289. Decker, J.L.: Toxicity of immunosuppressive drugs in man. Arthritis Rheum. 16:89, 1973.

290. Fahey, J.L.: Cancer in the immunosuppressed patient. Ann. Intern. Med. 75:310, 1971.

291. Whitfield, A.G.W.: Ankylosing spondylitis. J. R. Coll. Physicians Lond. 11:107, 1976.

292. Radford, E.P., Doll, R., and Smith, P.G.: Mortality among patients with ankylosing spondylitis not given X-ray therapy. N. Engl. J. Med. 297:572, 1977.

293. Court Brown, W.M., and Doll, R.: Mortality from cancer and other causes after radiotherapy for ankylosing spondylitis. Br. Med. J. 2:1332, 1965.

294. Radford, E.P., Doll, R., and Smith, P.G.: Mortality among patients with ankylosing spondylitis not given x-ray therapy. N. Engl. J. Med. 297:572, 1977.

295. Kaprove, R.E., Little, A.H., Graham, D.C., and Rosen, P.S.: Ankylosing spondylitis. Survival in men with and without radiotherapy. Arthritis Rheum. 23:57, 1980.

296. Good, A.E., Diaz, L.A., and Bowerman, R.A.: Basal cell carcinomas following roentgen therapy of ankylosing spondylitis. Arthritis Rheum. 23:1065, 1980.

Section XVIII

Diseases Associated with Abnormalities of Structural Proteins

Chapter 105

Diseases Associated with Abnormalities of Structural Proteins

David W. Rowe and Jay R. Shapiro

INTRODUCTION

The heritable disorders of connective tissue are the result of a defect in the quantity or structure of the collagen, elastin, or other matrix proteins. With the application of newer techniques in molecular biology and more established methods of protein chemistry, we are on the threshold of understanding the basis of many of these diseases at the structural and genetic level. The major objective here will be to relate clinical and biochemical data in order to provide a foundation for interpreting future studies related to connective tissue diseases. It is assumed that the reader will be familiar with the basic elements of collagen biochemistry and collagen gene structure as presented in Chapter 14.

BIOCHEMICAL AND MOLECULAR ASPECTS OF HERITABLE DISORDER CONNECTIVE TISSUE

Experiments of nature in the form of inherited disease give insight into those elements that are essential for normal synthesis and structure of collagen and elastin. It is instructive to begin this chapter by pointing out biochemical features that appear to be critical for normal connective tissue function.

Tissue-Specific Distribution of Collagen Types. Specific types of collagen have evolved for specialized functions of the various connective tissues.[1,2] Each collagen type is a distinct gene product that will produce a different clinical disorder when it is abnormal. Type I collagen is located primarily in tissues that provide a high tensile strength such as tendon, skin, sclera, and bone.

Thus, an abnormality in type I collagen will result in lax joints, thin skin, and bowing or fracturing of bone.

Type II collagen is the primary constituent of hyaline cartilage. It also plays an important morphologic role, since the cartilage anlagen precedes endochondral bone growth. Many of the heritable disorders of chondrogenesis and the spondyloepiphyseal dysplasias may ultimately reflect an abnormality of type II collagen.[3] Since these disorders are not yet understood at the biochemical level, they will not be discussed in this chapter.

Type III collagen is found in tissues lining hollow viscera and vascular tissue. During fetal development and the first year of life it is a prominent component of skin and may provide the scaffold for type I collagen deposition.[4,5] Type III collagen may play a similar role in wound healing, since it precedes the synthesis of type I collagen following trauma.[6] Its structural role appears to impart an elastic resistance to extensible organs. A frequent catastrophic consequence of a deficiency of type III collagen (Ehlers-Danlos, type IV) is the rupture of the aorta, bowel, or uterus.

Type IV collagen is a principal component of basement membrane,[7,8] whereas type V collagen has a pericapillary and pericellular location.[9,10] Although these types of collagen play an important role in cell to cell interactions, morphogenesis, and cell migration, heritable abnormalities in their formation have not been recognized.

Collagen Synthesis and Maturation. The steps of collagen synthesis, assembly, secretion, and fiber formation are probably similar for all collagen types, though they have been best characterized for type I (Fig. 105–1). The type I collagen genes for the α_1 and α_2 collagen chains are present as one allele per haploid set of chromo-

1621

1. GENE

    Transcription
    Start Site
Promotor   Exon   Intron

TRANSCRIPTION

2. NUCLEAR
   mRNA

SPLICING

3. PROCESSED
   mRNA

POLYADENYLATION
CAPPING

4. CYTOPLASMIC
   mRNA

LEADER   ROUGH
                   ER

TRANSLATION
HYDROXYLATION
CHAIN ASSEMBLY

5. INTRACELLULAR
   PROCOLLAGEN   GOLGI

SECRETION   CELL
                  MEMBRANE

PROPEPTIDE
SCISSION

N-PROPEPTIDE   C-PROPEPTIDE

6. EXTRACELLULAR
   COLLAGEN

FIBRIL FORMATION
CROSSLINKAGE

7. INSOLUBLE
   COLLAGEN

Figure 105–1. Steps fo collagen biosynthesis relevant to the heritable diseases of collagen. The structure of the gene (step 1) is represented by darkened squares for the exons and by a line for the introns. The RNAs (steps 2 to 4) are represented by open squares. See text for the narrative description of the figure.

somes.[11-16] Both alleles of the collagen gene appear to be active because in certain dominantly inherited disorders both normal and abnormal populations of collagen chains are observed. The gene has proved to be one of the largest and most complex yet described, The $\alpha 1(I)$ gene contains 51 exons and 50 introns within an 18-kilobase region, while the $\alpha 2(I)$ gene is composed of 50 exons and 49 introns within a 38-kilobase region. In contrast, the globin genes contain three exons and two introns extending 1.8 kilobases. The promoter region of the $\alpha 1$ and $\alpha 2$ collagen gene, the region of the gene preceding the beginning of the coding sequence that controls transcription of the gene, has been sequenced.[17] It resembles other eukaryotic promoters.[18]

The initial transcribed messenger RNA (mRNA) is an exact copy of the gene containing both introns and exons (see Fig. 105–1, step 2). The intervening sequences are removed through a splicing mechanism similar to other eukaryotic mRNAs.[19,20] There appears to be a recognition sequence at each side of the intron-exon junction that is complementary to a small nuclear RNA

(U_1RNA), which may act to bring the ends of the introns into alignment for removal and subsequent joining of the adjacent exons. Any abnormality in the gene that alters the structure of the promoter or interferes with the process of splicing would have an adverse effect on the quantity of mRNA and subsequently the protein being synthesized.[21-23] Thus, these "regulatory" mutants would produce low amounts of collagen, but the collagen that was produced from the remaining normal allele would be structurally normal.

Upon reaching the rough endoplasmic reticulum, mRNA is translated into a polypeptide chain. Abnormalities in the primary sequence of the mRNA that would result in a translationally inactive mRNA include a base change that codes for a stop codon prior to the end of the coding region or that shifts the reading frame. In the former case the mRNA codes for a truncated protein, whereas in the latter case all the amino acids beyond the frame shift mutation would be inappropriate.[24,25] In both cases the amount of normal protein produced would be reduced and would reflect the activity of the remaining normal allele.

As the collagen mRNA is translated, certain prolyl residues in the third position of the (gly-X-Y) triplet become hydroxylated, and specific lysines are hydroxylated and then glycosylated (see Fig. 105–1, step 4). The function of the hydroxyproline residues appears to enhance the stability of the collagen triple helix at physiologic temperatures.[26] Although prolylhydroxylation is an essential modifying step in the formation of collagen, there is no direct evidence showing it is rate limiting.[27] The fact that mutants of prolylhydroxylase have not been described may imply that a half-normal level of the enzyme is sufficient to mediate normal hydroxylation, whereas a complete deficiency of the enzyme is lethal. Both prolyl and lysyl hydroxylase act on nascent procollagen chains and are unable to hydroxylate once the procollagen chain assumes the helical conformation. Excessive lysyl hydroxylation is observed in association with α-chain mutations, which impair the rate of the helix formation.[28,29] Lysyl hydroxylation is important for the formation of stable interchain crosslinks. The function of the glycosylated hydroxylysine or the heterosaccharide unit of the C-terminal propeptide is uncertain.[30,31]

Within the Golgi apparatus, the individual procollagen chains initiate self-assembly from the C-terminal propeptide toward the N-terminus (see Fig. 105–1, step 5).[32,33] There is a highly conserved region within the C-terminal propeptide in all the collagen α-chains.[34,35] It is assumed that this region is essential for initial chain alignment and subsequent assembly. It can be anticipated that a defect in this region of the molecule would inhibit incorporation of the abnormal chain into the triple helix. This defect in chain assembly would reduce collagen synthesis or lead to improper alignment within the helix. In the latter case, the malaligned helix would be unstable at body temperatures or would be more susceptible to cellular and tissue proteases. Besides mutations in the C-terminal propeptide, a point mutation within the collagen helix, particularly one affecting the glycine residues, would also be expected to interfere with the integrity of the helical region. Glycine residues permit the polypeptide chain to maintain the tight helical conformation. Molecules containing a loopout or loosening of the helix have increased susceptibility to tissue proteases. Mutations of this type can lead to enhanced intracellular or interstitial degradation of collagen α-chains and thus a lower net rate of collagen production. Such structural defects, in contrast to "regulatory" mutants, would manifest normal collagen mRNA levels. Thus cytoplasmic mRNA content can be used to determine whether low collagen production was secondary to a regulatory mutation or to a mutation that produced an unstable collagen chain that was degraded.

The assembled procollagen molecule is secreted by an exocytotic process.[36,37] There appear to be determinants within the procollagen molecule that are necessary for secretion, since there are diseases involving both type I and type III collagen in which the abnormal collagen molecules are retained within the cell.[29,38] Removal of the N- and C-terminal propeptides in the extracellular space is essential for normal fiber assembly.[39] Genetic defects involving the N-terminal propeptide region have been defined in both humans and animals. In this situation, failure to cleave the N-terminal propeptide interferes with the organization of the collagen fiber.[40] Genetic defects involving removal of the C-terminal propeptide have not been defined.

The final step in the formation of a stabilized collagen fiber is the assembly of the individual molecules into the collagen polymer and its subsequent stabilization by inter- and intramolecular crosslinks (see Fig. 105–1, step 7). The assembly process appears to be directed by information within exposed areas of the triple helical molecule, since fiber formation can occur in vitro.[39] However, the formation of the microfibril can be modified by the presence of proteoglycans. Detailed analysis of the formation of microfibrils has been difficult to define biochemically, but it is an area of extreme importance because the alignment of microfibrils is essential for normal crosslink formation between adjacent molecules.[41-43] Agents that block crosslink formation (e.g., penicillamine, or β-aminoproprionitrile) result in enhanced tissue friability, bowing of the bones, and aortic aneurysms (lathyrism). Besides enzymatic defects affecting lysyl oxidase, a failure in the proper alignment of adjacent molecules or the absence of appropriately placed lysine residues would limit the number of crosslinks that could form within the microfibril.

Molecular Biologic Tools Used to Define Defects in the Structure or Regulation of the Collagen Gene. As the gap narrows between advances in molecular biology and their application to clinical medicine, it will become important for the clinician to have a better understanding of the following methods, since they are the foundation for interpreting and understanding these disorders.

DNA Cloning.[44,45] The ability to amplify DNA sequences using plasmid or viral vectors has been the single

most important technique for understanding these connective tissue abnormalities at the gene level (Fig. 105–2a). Complementary DNAs (cDNAs) are exact copies of mRNA sequences, whereas genomic DNA is obtained from fragments of chromosomal DNA. The primary difference between a genomic probe and a cDNA probe is that the former contains not only sequences complementary to coding regions but also regions that are complementary to the intervening sequences. In either case the genomic or cDNA will specifically hybridize to mRNA or genomic sequences coding for a specific protein. With these radioactive probes one is able to assess both the function and structure of a gene.

Assessment of Gene Activity. The activity of a gene can be assessed by measuring the steady state levels of mRNA that accumulates in the cytoplasm and the rate at which the gene is transcribed (Fig. 105–2b). The

Figure 105–2. Common procedure used by the molecular biologist to define genetic defects. The control sample (lane C) has four restriction sites within the region of the genes that yield four distinct bands that hybridize with the probe. The sample in lane X1 has lost a restriction site between fragment 1 and produces a new fragment that migrates ahead of fragment 3. The sample in lane X2 has a deletion within fragment 4, which increases the mobility of this fragment but has no effect on the other fragments. In panel d, X1 represents a DNA sample with a loss of a restriction enzyme site, producing a DNA band with increased mobility.

steady state mRNA levels are most conveniently assessed by the dot hybridization technique.[46,47] In this method, RNA is serially diluted and dotted onto nitrocellulose paper in parallel with RNA from a standard source. The nitrocellulose paper is then hybridized with the radioactive probes, and the intensity of the radioactive spots is measured and related to the standard RNA preparation. The transcriptional activity of a gene is measured by incubating isolated nuclei from the cells in the presence of highly radioactive uridine triphosphate.[48] All of the radiolabeled RNAs are extracted and hybridized to nitrocellulose paper containing a nonradioactive DNA probe. With suitable controls one is able to detect the fraction of total radioactivity that hybridized specifically to the filter-bound DNA. The combination of measuring steady state levels of mRNA and the rate of nuclear transcription allows one to differentiate between cells with a low content of a specific mRNA resulting from low gene activity (gene deletion or inactive gene) and cells with an unstable mRNA.

Assessment of Gene Structure. The DNA probes are of great value in defining structural abnormalities in either the mRNA or its gene (see Fig. 105–2c). To determine abnormalities at the mRNA level, RNA extracted from the cytoplasm is separated by size on an agarose gel then is transferred and irreversibly bound to nitrocellulose paper. The DNA probe is then hybridized to the binding matrix, and the radioactive bands containing complementary sequences are identified by exposure to x-ray film. This procedure is referred to as a northern hybridization.[49] In comparing the pattern of hybridization with the control RNA, a deletion of coding material within the mRNA is detected by the presence of two bands rather than one. The two bands would represent mRNA that had been coded for by each α-chain allele.

The discovery and application of restriction endonucleases, enzymes derived from bacteria that cleave specifically recognized DNA sequences, have made possible the mapping of genes according to the size of enzyme-generated DNA fragments (see Fig. 105–2d). In this procedure, referred to as a Southern hybridization, DNA is digested with a specific endonuclease and the resulting fragments are separated by size with agarose gel electrophoresis.[50] The DNA is then transferred and fixed to nitrocellulose paper and subsequently hybridized with a specific DNA probe. The gene can be mapped in relation to the size and position of a series of specific restriction enzyme sites. Knowing the fine structure of the gene allows one to localize deletions and occasionally even point mutations within the gene. Thus, if a point mutation inactivates a restriction site, the resulting radioactive band will migrate more slowly than the control, since two fragments were not generated (lane X1). In contrast a deletion can result in increased electrophoretic mobility of a known DNA fragment identified by the DNA probe (lane X2).

One of the most useful applications of the Southern hybridization technique, as applied to connective tissue disease, is the concept of linkage polymorphisms.[51-53] In this procedure, genomic DNA is cut with a variety of restriction enzymes and the DNA is hybridized with DNA probes that include or are adjacent to the collagen gene. This strategy recognizes a pattern of bands, indicating changes in restriction sites that are normally present within the population. These restrictive patterns are allelic, and the haplotype can be followed through generations within a specific family. Since many of the connective tissues diseases are dominantly inherited, one can determine whether or not the disease is linked to a specific collagen gene if there is segregation of a specific polymorphic haplotype (restriction enzyme cleavage pattern) in those individuals with the disease. Such an approach has been successful with the human α₂ collagen gene.[54] Linkage polymorphism will be important in deciding whether a collagen gene or the gene for another structural protein is causative in a dominantly inherited connective tissue disease.

CLINICAL EVALUATION OF HERITABLE CONNECTIVE TISSUE DISORDERS

The heritable disorders of connective tissue are the result of mutations that impair the normal synthesis of one of the components of the extracellular matrix. Clinical and genetic heterogeneity are characteristic of each syndrome. It is best to consider these diseases in terms of pleiotropy, variable expressivity, and genetic heterogeneity.[55] Pleiotropy refers to the phenotypic expression of a single gene mutation in multiple organ systems. Although the mechanisms underlying this process are unknown, a host of tissue-specific factors will determine the final expression of a mutant gene in one or another organ. Variable expression or penetrance refers to the qualitative and quantitative aspects of gene expression. Penetrance as applied to connective tissue disorders is always questionable because we lack the techniques to accurately measure the extent that certain physical findings (lax joints, extensible skin) deviate from normal in affected populations. Variable expression is a characteristic feature of dominantly inherited disorders. Genetic heterogeneity refers to the fact that similar phenotypes are produced by different mutations. For example, several of the syndromes to be described include mitral valve prolapse and hyperextensible joints. It is because there is considerable overlap in phenotype that ultimate resolution of variants within a syndrome must await definition of the underlying biochemical lesion.

Marfan's Syndrome and Related Variants

In its most typical form, Marfan's syndrome includes dislocations of the lens (ectopia lentis), dilation of the ascending aorta with aortic regurgitation, tall stature, and arachnodactyly. Marfan's syndrome includes patients with either asthenic or nonasthenic habitus who are distinct from patients with the marfanoid hypermobility syndrome, congenital contractural arachnodactyly, and homocystinuria.[56] The assumption is that a separate gene defect underlies each clinical phenotype.

Classic (Asthenic Form of Marfan's Syndrome). This is defined by McKusick as patients who are excessively tall with long, thin extremities (dolichostenomelia) and diminished subcutaneous fat.[57] The nonasthenic form refers to subjects with a more normal habitus who nevertheless carry other stigmata associated with the complete syndrome. However, the nonasthenic form may reflect pleiotropy rather than a separate mutation, since both phenotypes have been observed in the same kindred.[58]

Marfan's syndrome has been reported in 2 to 6 per 100,000 persons.[59,60] However, the real prevalence may exceed these numbers if mild cases go unrecognized. Since Marfan's syndrome is inherited as an autosomal dominant trait, 50 percent of offspring are at risk. In 15 percent of cases both parents appear normal; in this situation the disease is assumed to represent a new mutation. The phenotype is equally prevalent in males and females.

Patients with the classic form of the syndrome tend to be excessively tall. Arm span frequently is 8 cm or more in excess of height. Disproportionately long limbs cause the lower trunkal segment (LS, pubis to heel) to be longer (more than 2 inches) than the upper segment (US, pubis to crown), producing a US:LS ratio of less than 0.85. The ratio is 0.93 in normal white males.[57] However, both arm and leg length discrepancies are present in up to 10 percent of the normal population and may be normal for blacks.[61] Therefore, neither excessive height nor lengthened arm span and longer lower segment can be relied upon to confirm the diagnosis of Marfan's syndrome.

Arachnodactyly occurs in 90 percent of patients with the asthenic form, but this is not diagnostic, since elongation of hands and feet may occur in otherwise normal individuals. Confirmation of arachnodactyly may be sought using the following clinical tests: (1) the thumb or Steinberg test, which is positive when the thumb, enclosed in the clenched fist, extends beyond the hypothenar border;[62] (2) the wrist (Walker-Murdoch) sign, in which there is overlap of the thumb and fifth digit as they encircle the opposite wrist;[63] and (3) the metacarpal index, which is the mean value of the lengths divided by the midpoint widths of the second, third, and fourth metacarpals. In normal subjects, the metacarpal index ranges from 5.4 to 7.9, whereas in Marfan's syndrome it ranges from 8.4 to 10.4.[61]

Skeletal abnormalities include dolichocephaly (long, narrow face with prognathism), a high arched palate, loss of normal cervical curve, kyphoscoliosis, pectus excavatum and carinatum, funnel-shaped deformities of the chest, and spondylolisthesis. These patients are subject to slipped epiphyses, talipes equinovarus, and long, unstable feet with pes planus.[58] Hallux valgus and contractures of the toes are common. Joint laxity tends to

be variable but may appear marked in some patients, causing genu recurvatum and recurrent dislocations. Hyperextensibility leads to joint pain and effusions. Although the prevalence of osteoporosis is unknown, there are reports of vertebral rarefaction or collapse.[61]

Spinal abnormalities include increased interpeduncular distance of nonrotated vertebrae, vertebral inversion (flattening of the normal kyphosis at the dorsal level and kyphosis or disappearance of the physiologic lordosis at the lumbar level), and vertebral dysplasia (dolichospondylea), wherein vertebral bodies may be elongated with increased concavity, particularly in the lumbar area. Scoliosis constitutes one of the major management problems in the Marfan syndrome. In one series the average age of onset of spinal curves was 10.5 years (range 3 to 15 years) with rapid progression during adolescence.[64] If mechanical bracing or physical therapy fails to halt progression, spinal fusion should be considered, particularly when the curvature exceeds 45 to 50 degrees. Experimental protocols have been devised to limit skeletal growth and thus progression of scoliosis by means of estrogen administration to adolescent females.[59]

Ectopia lentis occurs in 50 to 80 percent of patients with Marfan's syndrome. Subluxation of the lens is usually bilateral and appears by the age of 5 years. Although the lens is typically displaced upward, displacement may occur into any quadrant. Visual acuity is diminished in a large proportion of patients with Marfan's syndrome because of lens subluxation or secondary acute glaucoma. Vision is also impaired because of the increased axial length of the globe, which can lead to severe myopic degeneration of the retina. Retinal detachment may occur following surgery to remove the subluxated lens. The decision as to whether a displaced lens should be removed must be individualized; usually removal is not required.[65]

Cardiovascular abnormalities are responsible for the majority of deaths from Marfan's syndrome. The average life span is approximately 32 years. The most frequent lesions are mitral valve prolapse with mitral regurgitation and aneurysmal dilatation of the ascending aorta with regurgitation and aortic rupture. Auscultatory evidence of mitral and aortic valve disease exists in approximately 60 percent of affected patients. Widespread use of echocardiography shows valve involvement to be more frequent (80 percent). Therefore, the chest x-ray should not be relied upon to establish the presence of aortic root disease.[66] Involvement of the aortic root may be discovered at any age from the first to sixth decades of life and is gradually progressive. The diameter of the aorta slowly increases giving the ascending aorta a characteristic "sausage shape" on angiography. Careful echocardiographic monitoring of the diameter of the ascending aorta is required so that surgical intervention may be considered at the appropriate age. Baseline measurements of the aortic root should be obtained in all family members at risk.

Roberts and Honig have provided excellent clinical-pathologic correlation of the cardiovascular lesions.[67] Patients were divided into the following three groups: (1) those with chronic aortic regurgitation, (2) those with aortic dissection, and (3) those with isolated mitral regurgitation. Patients in group 1 suffered periodic chest pain and showed evidence of mitral regurgitation in 50 percent of the cases. Cause of death included aneurysmal rupture, chronic congestive heart failure, and postoperative death following valve replacement. Histologic examination revealed severe elastic fiber degeneration in the aorta, with increased amounts of acid mucopolysaccharides in aortic and mitral valve cusps. Group 2 subjects experienced sudden chest pain as a result of dissection that occurred in the absence of preceding enlargement of the aorta. Except for the tear, the histologic appearance of the aorta was not abnormal. Group 3 patients showed cardiac enlargement caused by mitral regurgitation or rupture of chordae tendinae, or both, in the absence of previous aortic dilatation.

Aortic regurgitation, dissection, and rupture occur most commonly when the aorta dilates to 6 cm or more in adults. To monitor gradual enlargement of the aorta, echocardiography is recommended once a year until the size exceeds 50 percent of normal for the body surface area, at which time studies are repeated every 6 months.[59] The use of propranolol to retard aortic dilatation is currently under study. Although vigorous activity should be discouraged, pregnancy appears to be safe if the aortic dilatation is not present.[68] Antibiotic prophylaxis should be instituted in all patients with mitral or tricuspid valve prolapse caused by an increased incidence of infective endocarditis. The outlook for surgical correction of Marfan's syndrome defects of the aortic root has improved considerably during the past decade.[69] In the series reported by McDonald and colleagues involving valve graft placement, there were no hospital deaths, and survival at 3 years was 61 percent.[70]

Pulmonary function may be compromised by kyphoscoliosis and malformations of the sternum and ribs. The spectrum of pulmonary lesions in Marfan's syndrome includes congenital malformations, cystic disease, emphysema, spontaneous pneumothorax, and increased susceptibility to respiratory infections.[71-73] Patients with Marfan's syndrome may develop inguinal or femoral herniae at an early age. Striae of the skin (striae distensae) occur in the pectoral areas and over the lower back and buttocks.

Asthenic Versus Nonasthenic Forms of the Marfan Syndrome. This distinction was proposed by McKusick to draw attention to an obvious difference in phenotype within families and among isolated patients.[58] Although the nonasthenic patient may be considered as representing a forme fruste of the syndrome, Pyeritz and McKusick emphasized that those with few or mild signs of the disease harbor the same gene as more affected relatives.[59] Emanuel and colleagues studied 18 families in which individual members had severe aortic regurgitation and dilatation of the ascending aorta but no other stigmata of Marfan's syndrome.[74] Although one or more stigmata of Marfan's syndrome were present in

37.3 percent of first-degree relatives, none had classic features of the syndrome. While this study casts doubt on the significance of the term "forme fruste," in that there was no obvious relationship with classic Marfan's syndrome, it served to illustrate the importance of the variable expression of a mutant gene.

Molecular Pathology. There is a significant body of biochemical data suggesting that an abnormality in the crosslinks of collagen or elastin, or both, underlies Marfan's syndrome.[75,76] Increased solubility of skin collagen, of radiolabeled collagens produced by cultured fibroblasts, and of elastin from aortic tissue has been found in individuals with Marfan's syndrome.[77-79] This data is consistent with a deficiency in the extent of collagen or elastin crosslinking. However, diminished activity of lysyl oxidase has not been demonstrated.[41]

There is more direct evidence for a cross-linking defect independent of lysyl oxidase in the observation of a decreased content of the multifunctional crosslink 3-hydroxypyridinium, along with a normal or elevated content of the bifunctional crosslink dihydroxylysinonorleucine, in skin samples from patients with Marfan's syndrome.[80] The data suggests that although lysine-derived aldehydes and adequate lysyl oxidase activity are present, there is a block in the age-related progression from bifunctional to mature multifunctional crosslinks.

Since Marfan's syndrome is inherited as a dominant trait, a defect in a structural protein that affects the maturation of crosslinks is a likely abnormality. Evidence for this includes:

1. One patient with Marfan's syndrome has been found to have a structural abnormality of the α_2-chain of type I collagen. The abnormal chain appears to contain a 20 amino acid insertion in the midhelical region.[81] The extra chain length may have the effect of displacing specific lysine residues so that multifunctional crosslinks cannot be formed. It is likely that point mutations affecting a specific lysine residue within either the α_1 or the α_2 chain could produce a similar abnormality.

2. The aortic content of desmosine, the multifunctional crosslink of elastin, is low in patients with Marfan's syndrome who have aortic dilatation. Elastin derived from these aortas has shown an increased hydroxyproline content, which, it is postulated, interferes with the formation of the multifunctional elastin crosslink.[79] The mechanism for the excess hydroxyproline content of elastin is not understood. It may reflect a structural mutation that interferes with the rate at which the elastin is synthesized or assembled.

3. Excessive accumulation of hyaluronic acid in aortic tissue[82,83] and in fibroblasts obtained from individuals with Marfan's syndrome[84,85] may affect the formation of multifunctional collagen and elastin crosslinks.

Thus Marfan's syndrome, and some of its variants, may be a syndrome complex reflecting an abnormality in either of the three connective tissue components having in common a block in the production of mature crosslinks. Identification of the specific defect will require finding biochemical markers of the disease, preferably in cultured fibroblasts. Until a specific biochemical marker can be identified, linkage polymorphisms to the collagen or elastin gene may permit the association of one phenotype to a single gene.

Marfanoid Hypermobility Syndrome. Patients in this category have many stigmata of classic Marfan's syndrome plus the added feature of hyperelastic skin and markedly hyperextensible joints. The patient reported by Cotton and colleagues was tall, with arachnodactyly, ectopia lentis, and a history of spontaneous pneumothorax.[86] In addition, his skin was velvety, hyperelastic, and had "cigarette paper" scars as seen in the Ehlers-Danlos syndrome. There was hyperextension at the elbow and genu recurvatum. Aortic valve replacement was eventually required. These patients have obvious features of both the Ehlers-Danlos and Marfan's syndromes and therefore are considered to represent a distinct syndrome.[87,88]

Congenital Contractual Arachnodactyly (CCA). First described by Marfan in 1896, this syndrome includes an autosomal dominant inheritance, tall stature, arachnodactyly, dolichostenomelia, and multiple contractures involving large joints.[89,90] There is a characteristic "crumpled ear" deformity due to a flattened helix, prominent crura, and partial obliteration of the concha.[91,92] Osteopenia occurs frequently. The diaphysis is narrow in tubular bones. Marked deformity of the chest cage also occurs, and scoliosis may be progressive and severe. For unknown reasons, the contractures tend to lessen in severity with age. The ocular and typical cardiac lesions of classic Marfan's syndrome are absent. The observation that dolichostenomelia and arachnodactyly may occur in relatives lacking the marfanoid habitus suggests variable expression of the CCA gene.[93] However, heterogeneity is suggested by the observation of both mitral regurgitation and cystic medial necrosis of the aorta in isolated cases of CCA.[94]

Homocystinuria. This disorder is included here, since it shares certain clinical features with Marfan's syndrome.[95,96] These patients become tall and slender (marfanoid) by adolescence and have disproportionately long, slender extremities. They have a fair complexion, brittle hair, and thin skin. The facial expression is characterized by protrusion of crowded upper teeth, a high-arched palate, and a prominent malar flush. There is iridodonesis (iris flutter) caused by dislocation of the lens, which is typically located inferonasally but may be found in any quadrant. Ectopia lentis occurs from actual disruption of zonular fibers that connect the lens to the ciliary body. Subluxation of the lens, which usually occurs by 8 years of age, is associated with myopia and astigmatism, which worsens after the lens dislocates. As with the Marfan's syndrome, dislocation may induce acute glaucoma. Retinal detachment and chronic glaucomatous changes of the retina may occur. Table 105–1 contrasts the clinical features of homocystinuria with those of the Marfan's syndrome.[97]

Chest wall deformity occurs as a result of pectus carinatum or pectus excavatum, and kyphoscoliosis is common. Although joint extensibility is usually mild, humerus valgum, genu valgum, and pes planus occur

frequently. In occasional patients one sees limited supination of the forearms and fixed flexion of fingers caused by contractures.[98] Arachnodactyly is occasionally present. The dominant skeletal finding is osteoporosis, which affects most patients and may be present by 5 years of age. Both the vertebrae and extremities are demineralized. Vertebral fractures, causing the classic "cod fish" deformity, occur during the first decade of life or by adolescence. However, unlike what is seen with postmenopausal osteoporosis, the endplate depressions tend to be located posteriorly rather than centrally.[99] This finding has been attributed to thrombosis of nutrient vessels. Other radiographic findings include metaphyseal spicules, enlargement of carpal bones, and elongation of the talus. Widening of the metaphysis and epiphysis of long bones, with actual bowing may occur.[100]

Homocystinuric patients are subject to thrombotic and embolic occlusion of major arteries or veins; for this reason, relatively few patients reach adulthood. Myocardial infarction, mesenteric or renal thrombosis and infarction, cerebrovascular accidents, and pulmonary embolism occur during infancy and adolescence. Any vessel may be involved and may lead to sudden death. Thrombi are particularly likely to occur following surgery.[101] Unlike Marfan's syndrome, aortic dissection does not occur in homocystinuria. Livedo reticularis, which causes erythematous mottling of the extremities, occurs in approximately 50 percent of patients.

Mental retardation may occur in 80 percent of homocystinuric patients and may constitute the presenting symptom. The remainder have normal or near-normal intelligence. Developmental delay and mental retardation are apparent during childhood, but their severity varies among sibships. Seizures occur in 15 percent of cases and may be the result of vascular thrombosis.

Molecular Pathology. Homocystinuria as a clinical entity may be caused by the following biochemical lesions:

1. A deficiency of cystathionine B synthetase, the enzyme that catalyzes the condensation of serine and homocysteine to form cystathionine. Pyridoxal-5′-phosphate is the cofactor for this reaction. Typically, patients with this enzymatic deficiency have elevated plasma methionine and homocystine concentrations and increased urinary excretion of homocysteine. This is the most common and severe form.[102,103]

Table 105–1. Contrasting Features of Marfan's Syndrome and Homcystinuria

	Marfan's Syndrome	Homocystinuria
Inheritance	autosomal dominant	autosomal recessive
Lens dislocation	superior	inferior
Osteoporosis	absent	present
Widened metaphysis and epiphysis	absent	present
Codfish vertebrae	absent	present
Scoliosis	severe	mild
Mental retardation	uncommon	common
Vascular thrombosis	absent	present
Aortic dissection	present	absent

2. Defective remethylation of homocysteine to methionine.[102] Homocysteine accumulates in blood, and homocystine (the oxidized disulfide) spills in the urine, since the conversion of homocysteine to methionine is blocked. Patients with these lesions have homocysteinemia and homocystinuria but low blood levels of methionine and folic acid.[95] Defective methyl transfer may limit formation of the active form of vitamin B_{12}.

The prevalence of homocystinuria as estimated from worldwide screening of millions of infants is about 1 per 200,000.[104] The disease is inherited as an autosomal recessive trait. Obligate heterozygotes have less than 50 percent of the mean value for cystathionine synthetase activity in liver, cultured fibroblasts, and phytohemagglutin-stimulated lymphocytes.[105] Biochemical definition of the defect in the individual patient is advisable in view of the favorable prognosis when appropriate therapy is started at an early age.

Vascular lesions in homocystinuria are characterized by marked intimal thickening and fibrosis, with fraying of elastic fibers in the media and splitting and fraying of muscle fibers.[96] Platelet adhesiveness is increased in homocystinuria; the addition of homocysteine to normal blood will increase platelet adhesiveness.[106,107] In addition, homocysteine may directly damage endothelial cells, which could promote platelet-mediated intimal proliferation.[108] Homocysteine also interferes with the normal crosslinking of collagen and elastin.[109] Decreased aldehyde precursors and diminished bifunctional crosslinks found by Kang and Trelstad in collagen from two patients were attributed to the binding of reactive aldehydes by excess sulfhydryl groups.[110]

Approximately 50 percent of cystathionine synthetase–deficient patients respond to therapy with oral pyridoxine if it is started early.[111] The responsive patient will be essentially cured with an average pyridoxine dose of 500 mg per day. This not only prevents mental retardation but relieves the tendency to intravascular thrombosis and promotes normal skeletal development.[112,113] Patients with homocystinuria that is unresponsive to pyridoxine can be treated with a low methionine, cystine-supplemented diet. An infant with the tetrahydrofolate reductase deficiency was successfully treated using methionine, folinic acid, pyridoxine, and vitamin B_{12}.[114] High doses of the active form of vitamin B_{12}, hydroxycyanocobalamin-1, may benefit those patients whose homocystinuria results from an inability to form the active vitamin. Recent studies suggest that the addition of reagents that promote remethylation of homocysteine, such as betaine, potentiate the benefits of enhanced therapy used for the pyridoxine-unresponsive patient.[115] The use of various antiplatelet anticoagulants may be considered to lessen the risk of vascular thrombosis.[116]

The Ehlers-Danlos Syndrome

The connective tissue disorders grouped as the Ehlers-Danlos syndromes (EDS) illustrate the genetic and clinical variability that is so characteristic of these diseases. Patients having one of the EDS may demonstrate dominant, recessive, or sex-linked inheritance. A classification based on inheritance will be used here in order to emphasize the character and site of the putative biochemical gene defects (Table 105–2).

Dominantly Inherited EDS. The autosomal dominant forms of the disease account for 90 percent of the reported cases.[117] Clinically, they are the most difficult to separate because of a sizable overlap in phenotype. It should be pointed out that up to 50 percent of individuals with clinical signs of EDS do not fit into the current classification.

EDS I and II (Gravis and Mitis Forms). These forms of EDS (Figure 105–3) are characterized by marked

Table 105–2. Ehlers-Danlos Syndrome

Mode of Inheritance	Distinguishing Clinical Features	Molecular Abnormality	General Comments
Autosomal dominant			
I	Excessive joint laxity and skin hyperextensibility	Unknown	Fraying of collagen fibers
II	Less severe than type I	Unknown	Differentiation between milder forms of EDS can be difficult
III	Lax joints with normal skin	Unknown	
IV	Thin skin, rupture of blood vessels and viscera	Defective type IV collagen production	Sporadic cases occur and represent new mutations or genetic compounds
VII	Recurrent joint dislocation in childhood	Procollagen accumulation in tissues	Recessive inheritance also occurs but probably is less common
VIII	Periodontitis	Unknown	Skin and joint findings similar to EDS I or EDS II
Autosomal recessive			
VI	Scoliosis, ocular rupture	Lysyl hydroxylase deficiency	Clinically and biochemical heterogeneity
X	Bruising	Possible fibronectin deficiency	Only one case reported
X-linked recessive			
V	Hyperextensible skin	Unknown	Reports of lysyl oxidase deficiency not confirmed
IX	Occipital horns and bladder neck obstruction	Low lysyl oxidase activity; low serum copper levels	This form may overlap with X-linked cutis laxa

Figure 105–3. EDS I. Tissue elasticity, joint hypermobility, and tissue fragility are demonstrated by the patient's ability to extend her tongue to the tip of the nose (Gorlin's sign), by hyperextensibility at the knee (genu recurvatum), and by characteristic "cigarette paper" or papyraceous scars of the knees and tibial skin. (Courtesy of V. McKusick, M.D.)

hyperextensibility of large and small joints and are the classic forms of EDS.[118] Infants may be born prematurely to affected mothers because of early rupture of membranes and are found to be hypotonic and floppy with articular hyperextensibility. Bilateral inguinal hernias have been recognized in the newborn period. Respiratory insufficiency is a serious complication, which is perhaps secondary to abnormal chest wall mechanics, and in the occasional infant may necessiate intubation and mechanical ventilation.[119] Thin, fragile skin and tissues may complicate the surgical repair of hernias or rectal prolapse, which occurs in many affected infants. As these children grow, their muscle strength tends to improve, although decreased strength can be demonstrated in many adults.

Characteristically, the patients with EDS I have parrotlike facies, broad nasal root, and epicanthal folds that are secondary to lateral displacement of the inner canthus. The patient may be floppy eared, and traction on the ears or elbow will reveal skin hyperextensibility. The contour of the skull and the dentition are normal. The skin has a velvety, smooth, and warm texture that can be best appreciated on the volar surface of the forearm or across the back. A gaping "fishmouth" wound may

appear when skin is traumatized. Thin, atropic, corrugated, and hyperpigmented scars are found on the forehead and lower extremities (papyraceous or "cigarette paper" scars). Typically, skin lesions heal slowly after surgery or trauma. The ability to touch the tip of the tongue to the nose (Gorlin's sign) is also evidence of tissue hyperelasticity. Molluscoid pseudotumors, violaceous subcutaneous tumors ranging in size from 0.5 cm to 3 cm, may be palpated in the tissue over the forearms and lower extremities. Pseudotumors are calcified fat-containing cysts and are found over pressure points and may be visualized on x-ray film. Although many patients claim to bruise easily, ecchymoses distributed over the extremities are found only in patients with the more severe forms of the disease. Severe bilateral varicose veins are a common problem even in the milder forms of EDS.[120] In addition to the occurrence of inguinal and umbilical hernias, diverticulae of the gastrointestinal tract, hiatus hernia, and eventration of the diaphragm may occur.

Examination of the chest may reveal evidence of spontaneous pneumothorax, pneumomediastinum, and subpleural blebs.[121] Mitral valve prolapse and tricuspid valve insufficiency may complicate EDS I. Echocardiography is essential for complete cardiographic diagnosis, since auscultatory evidence of either mitral valve or tricuspid valve prolapse may be absent. Leier and colleagues have described the spectrum of cardiac lesions common to EDS, types I and III.[122] In the severe forms, 47 percent of the patients had cardiovascular abnormalities that fell into two general categories: (1) lesions associated with the connective tissue defects such as dilatation of the aortic root, the sinus of Valsalva, and the main pulmonary artery and (2) congenital abnormalities, such as intracardiac shunts and conduction defects. Aortic dissection is a rare, but reported, complication. Cupo and associates have described a variant of EDS I that is associated with panacinar emphysema, aneurysms of the sinus of Valsalva, and myocardial infarction that is associated with intractable ventricular fibrillation.[123]

The criteria for measuring joint hyperextensibility are illustrated in Figure 105–4.[124] This hyperextensibility is marked in EDS I and is mild and limited to the hands and feet in EDS II. At times, it may be difficult to decide if limited hyperextensibility is present in an older sibling or parent, since joint laxity decreases with increasing age. Recurrent joint dislocations, periodic joint effusion related to trauma, and the eventual appearance of osteoarthritis pose significant management problems.[125,126] Bilateral synovial thickening has been observed in EDS along with the accumulation of small masses of crystalline material in synovial villi. Osborn has observed that EDS, types II and III were found to constitute 5 percent of a pediatric arthritis clinic population.[127]

The spectrum of skeletal findings in EDS I and II has been summarized by Coventry.[128] They include thoracolumbar kyphoscoliosis, a long giraffelike neck, downward sloping of the ribs of the upper part of the thorax, and a tendency to reversal of the normal cervical, tho-

Figure 105–4. Maneuvers that may be used to establish the presence of clinically significant joint laxity. Examples of joint laxity found in the Ehlers-Danlos syndrome. It is not unusual to find extreme laxity of the small joints and less laxity in large joints. Laxity decreases with age, so that the dominant nature of most of these syndromes may not be appreciated when examining older family members. Figure redrawn and modified from Wynne-Davies.[124]

racic, and lumbar curves. Anterior wedging of thoracic vertebral bodies may occasionally be seen; however, there has been no systematic study of bone mineral content in EDS. Although the coexistence of EDS I and osteogenesis imperfecta has been reported, presumably in the form of a genetic compound, fractures of the extremities are no more frequent than in the normal population.[129]

EDS III (Benign Hypermobility Syndromes). In 1967, Kirk and colleagues applied the term "hypermobility syndrome" to patients having generalized joint laxity associated with musculoskeletal complaints.[130] Also apparent was a strong familial tendency with dominant inheritance and variable expression. Although the majority of individuals with this syndrome are asymptomatic, there are many with rheumatologic complaints that pose problems in diagnosis and therapy. In addition, there is the added anxiety about the relationship of physical activity to joint trauma, which may adversely limit a patient's life style.

The extent of joint laxity may be measured in terms of the following criteria:[124] (1) passive approximation of the thumb toward the forearm with the wrist in flexion, (2) passive hyperextension of digits, (3) active hyperextension of the elbow more than 10 degrees, (4) active hyperextension of the knee more than 10 degrees, (5) passive and excessive dorsiflexion of ankle and eversion of foot, and (6) the ability to touch the floor with palms without bending knees (Fig. 105–4). Generalized hyperextensibility may be considered to be present if three of six joint pairs test positive. It may be diagnostically important in evaluating the heritable disorders of connective tissue to carefully differentiate small as opposed to both large and small joint extensibility.

Using a goniometer, Boone and co-workers measured the arcs of active joint motion in males between the age of 18 months and 54 years and found that joint laxity diminishes with age in the normal population.[131] Most

children have lax joints at the age of 2 or 3 years but by 6 and 12 years, only 5 percent and 10 percent of normal children, respectively, demonstrate joint laxity. Others have found mobility of the upper limb joints to be a continuously distributed variable that is subject to age, ethnic factors, and the particular joint being tested.[132,133]

By definition, patients with the hypermobility syndrome lack the excessive skin laxity and the other stigmata of EDS or the Marfan syndrome. Females tend to be more frequently affected. Although hypermobility is usually apparent in early childhood, patients generally become symptomatic and seek medical advice during their 20s and 30s.[134] Finsterbush documented musculoskeletal complaints in 100 cases of generalized joint hypermobility, of which 51 were female and 49 were male.[135] Age at presentation for treatment varied from 4 to 37 years. Hypermobile joints were found in 65 percent of first-degree relatives. Fifty-six patients had localized complaints, and 44 patients had more generalized musculoskeletal complaints, including episodic acute knee pain, patellar dislocation, and patellofemoral arthritis with effusion. Bilateral ankle instability, progressive scoliosis with back pain, and pain due to hyperextension at the elbow were also seen. Recurrent dislocation at several joints—sternoclavicular, shoulder, and hip—was particularly frequent in infants. In the severely affected kindred described by Horton and colleagues as "familial joint instability," chronic sequelae included hypoplasia of the femoral heads and acetabulae with the formation of pseudoacetabulae.[136]

Grahame and co-workers have observed an increased incidence of mitral value prolapse in hypermobile patients.[137] Conversely, hypermobile joints were found to be more common in patients with mitral valve prolapse.[138] Patient selection may influence the outcome of such studies, since Jessee and colleagues failed to find an increased incidence of mitral valve prolapse in patients with the hypermobile joint syndrome.[139] Because mitral valve prolapse is relatively common, its association with joint laxity and its relation to a generalized connective tissue lesion remain speculative.

EDS VIII. The characteristics of this syndrome, as reported by McKusick, Hollister, and others, include (1) a severe resorptive periodontitis that leads to early loss of teeth in the absence of intrinsic tooth disease and (2) marked fragility of the skin in the absence of hyperelasticity, which leads to dystrophic scarring.[140,141] Joint hypermobility is mild. Mitral valve prolapse has been observed. Even the limited number of cases reported to date suggest that clinical variability as occurs in the other variants will also be seen in EDS VIII. The dental findings, however, have been rather uniform. There is early loss of primary dentition by age 5 or 6 years. Gum resorption becomes apparent in the second decade of life and is followed by periodontitis with acute episodes of inflammation leading to resorption of alveolar bone and loosening of teeth.[142]

Molecular Pathology. Little progress has been made in understanding the underlying molecular basis for dominantly inherited EDS.[143] Larger dermal collagen fibrils have been noted, but this may not be specific.[144-146] Factors involved in the orientation and lateral growth of collagen fibers are areas of active investigation. Of primary importance may be the hydrophilic and charge differences on the surface of the triple helical collagen molecule and also the nonhelical N- and C-terminal extension peptides. These topographic features are determined by the primary sequence of the α-chains and are probably modified by other extracellular substances such as fibronectin and proteoglycan. Since primary protein studies of collagen from EDS fibroblasts have not shown an α-chain abnormality, the approach in the future will be directed toward linkage polymorphisms of collagen genes within dominant families. Once localized to a specific collagen allele, DNA sequencing of the abnormal gene or mRNA may pinpoint the primary abnormality. If a linkage polymorphism cannot be identified, a collagen-modifying protein or proteoglycan that alters collagen fiber formation will need to be investigated.

Therapy. Obviously there is no specific therapy directed at the molecular defect in the dominantly inherited forms of EDS. Supportive therapy, however, is essential to preserve normal joint function. Planned exercise programs and muscle strengthening exercises are useful and do much to maintain a positive outlook in these individuals, who may have a poor prognosis if joint stability and articular surfaces are compromised by excessive activity or chronic trauma.[147]

The following should be considered in regard to management of the hypermobile patient: (1) reassurance that they do not have an inevitably crippling disease; (2) strengthening exercises for better control of affected joints, including fingers and abdominal muscles; and (3) instructions to protect susceptible joints. For example, avoidance of sitting with crossed legs, flexing the knees slightly when standing if genu recurvatum is present,

and minimizing repetitive motion such as knitting or typing in order to avoid finger injury. Use of built-in or flexible arch supports may relieve the discomfort of pes planus and add stability to the ankle.[148]

The presence of multiple ecchymoses will raise concern of a bleeding diathesis, particularly at the time of elective surgery. Although no consistent basis for the hemorrhagic tendency in EDS I has been identified, caution is advised in the patient with a strong history of easy bruisability.[149] The fact that infective endocarditis may complicate mitral valve prolapse necessitates appropriate antibiotic prophylaxis and requires that each relative at risk for valve prolapse be identified.

EDS VII (Arthrochalasis Multiplex Congenita Form). This form of EDS (Fig. 105–5) is marked by pronounced joint hypermobility, moderate cutaneous elasticity, moderate bruising, and short stature. Clinically, these patients experience multiple joint dislocations involving large joints such as the hips. Their tissues are very friable, which complicates orthopedic procedures.[143]

Molecular Pathology. EDS VII, along with the bovine and ovine homolog dermatosporaxis,[40,150] has provided insight into the process of normal fiber formation. The initial observation was an accumulation of procollagen within the dermis of affected children.[151] With subsequent recognition that procollagen had both N- and C-terminal extension propeptides and that there were separate enzymes responsible for their removal,[152] the syndrome has become more sharply defined as an accumulation of procollagen with the N-terminal peptides still attached (pN collagen). Interference by the extension propeptide to normal fiber formation probably accounts for the clinical disorder.

Figure 105–5. EDS VII: This variant is marked by the presence of short stature and round facies. Joint hypermobility and skin laxity are severe, and recurrent dislocations may requre surgical repair. (Courtesy of V. McKusick, M.D.)

At present, two distinctly different genetic abnormalities result in procollagen accumulation. The first is an inactive N-terminal procollagen peptidase, a condition that has recessive inheritance.[151] The extent of procollagen accumulation is a reflection of the degree of the enzyme inactivity. The second and probably more common abnormality is a resistance of a procollagen chain to the action of the N-terminal procollagen peptidase. The resistance probably results from an amino acid substitution or deletion in the pro-α_1- or pro-α_2-chain leading to half of the pro α-chains containing an abnormal N-terminal extension.[153] This one dose of the abnormal gene deranges collagen structure sufficiently to be recognized as a dominant trait.

EDS IV (Ecchymotic or Arterial Form). The clinical characteristic in EDS IV is repeated arterial rupture, commonly involving iliac, splenic, or renal arteries, or the aorta, resulting in either massive hematomas or death. These patients have thin, soft, and transparent skin through which a prominent venous pattern is seen. Venous varicosities are present in the lower extremities. They are also susceptible to rupture of internal viscera and may experience repeated rupture of diverticulae on the antimesenteric border of the large bowel. Abdominal scars consequent to colon repair or colon removal performed to control episodes of rupture are a characteristic finding. Uterine rupture may complicate pregnancy, although in many instances delivery may be uneventful.[154,155]

In contrast to the other forms of EDS, these patients do not have hyperextensible joints and although their skin is thin, it is not hyperelastic. EDS IV includes, as a subgroup, patients who have been described as acrogyric.[156] These patients have a characteristic thin facies, prominent eyes, and thin extremities that lack subcutaneous fat—features that give the appearance of premature aging. Both dominant and recessive inheritance have been reported in the acrogyric form of EDS IV. The dominant form tends to be less severe than the recessive form, with a life expectancy of 30 to 50 years; longevity in the recessive form varies from 15 to 30 years. Byers has collected information on 20 affected individuals in eight families with EDS IV. Causes of death included gastrointestinal rupture in three cases, peripartum uterine rupture in two cases, and rupture of the hepatic artery in one case.[157] Spontaneous pneumothorax and mitral valve prolapse occur frequently.[158]

Surgical repair of ruptured vessels or internal viscera is extremely difficult because of friable tissues. Wesley and associates have discussed both anesthetic and surgical difficulties related to intubation, spontaneous arterial bleeding during surgery, and the ligation of vessels that tear under pressure. These authors stress the danger of performing arteriography in patients with this severe form of the disease.[159]

Molecular Pathology. Although EDS, IV, was clinically recognized as a disorder distinct from the other forms of EDS, the findings by Pope that tissues from these individuals were deficient in type III collagen clearly distinguished this as a separate form of EDS.[160]

Subsequent studies have shown both clinical and biochemical heterogeneity.[156,161] Most of the cases studied have a dominant pedigree consistent with a primary defect in one of the type III collagen alleles. However, in certain sporadic cases, recessive inheritance has been suggested. In the latter forms, the biochemical findings have not differed from those of the dominant forms, suggesting that the lack of a dominant family history was secondary to a new mutation in the type III collagen gene or to decreased reproductive fitness of the affected individual.

Two general types of biochemical defects have been observed in cultured dermal fibroblasts.[143] The first is a decreased or absent production of an electrophoretically normal type III procollagen molecule.[157] Future studies of type III collagen mRNA should differentiate among abnormalities that diminish the stability of mRNA (splicing or frame shift mutations), abnormalities that affect the transcriptional activity of the gene, and a mutation that blocks incorporation of the abnormal $\alpha1$ (III)-chain into the helix. The second category of defects is found in cells that make an electrophoretically abnormal $\alpha1$ (III) molecule that is inefficiently secreted by the fibroblast.[143] These cells are derived from individuals with dominantly inherited, severe disease. Their fibroblastic cells contain dilated rough endoplasmic reticulum, probably secondary to the retained type III procollagen. It is likely that the underlying defect is a primary structural abnormality in one of the collagen alleles that alters the processing and secretion of those type III molecules containing one or more of the abnormal chains.

Recessively Inherited EDS. Although the recessive forms of EDS represent a small portion of the spectrum of EDS, these variants are sufficiently well characterized to be recognized as distinct syndromes. The recessive forms tend to be clinically more severe than those that are dominantly inherited.

EDS VI (Ocular Form). The first example of a biochemical mutant of collagen biosynthesis was described in 1972 by Pinnell and colleagues.[162] This report described hydroxylysine-deficient collagen in two sisters with severe scoliosis, recurrent joint dislocation, and hyperextensible skin and joints. Premature rupture of fetal membranes had occurred at the birth of one of the children. Both were floppy at birth with poor respiratory movements and subsequent bouts of penumonia. Spinal deformity was apparent, as was easy bruisability. Early growth and motor development were delayed, and muscle mass was diminished. Their skin was described as pale, translucent, and velvety, and it showed the typical gaping, fishmouth wound after trauma.

The range of clinical manifestations of EDS VI (Fig. 105–6) as summarized by Krane, are broadly representative of those of EDS.[163] One exception has been involvement of the ocular tissues, with microcornea, retinal detachment, and glaucoma. The eye is particularly susceptible to trauma, often leading to enucleation. Blue sclerae may be present, as in other types of EDS. In contrast to other forms of EDS, kyphoscoliosis may be

Figure 105–6. EDS VI. The occular-scoliotic form of EDS includes severe scoliosis at an early age, thin hyperelastic skin (tibial scars), and hyperextensible joints with recurrent dislocations. (Courtesy of V. McKusick, M.D.)

severe. Mild arachnodactyly, chest wall deformity associated with narrow shoulders, molluscoid pseudotumors, thin atrophic scars, and easy bruisability also occur. Hyperextensibility of joints is marked, which may lead to severe pes planus or a varus deformity. A narrow, high-arched palate has been observed. Although not mentioned in other reports, the siblings described by Steinmann and colleagues were extremely osteoporotic, with narrow diaphysis and broad metaphyses seen in tubular bones.[164]

Molecular Pathology. In the original description of EDS VI, Pinnell found that the hydroxylysine content of collagen in skin and tendons was less than 1 residue per 1000 total amino acids, in contrast to 4 residues per 1000 in control tissue.[162] The hydroxylysine content was somewhat less than normal in bone and was normal in cartilage. Subsequently, a number of investigators demonstrated low lysyl hydroxylase activity in fibroblasts obtained from individuals with this form of EDS.[165,166] The mechanism for the low activity was shown to result from an altered affinity (K_m) for ascorbic acid, the cofactor of the enzyme.[167] These studies suggested that at higher levels of ascorbic acid, enzyme activity would increase. There is one report of improved wound healing and muscle strength in two children with EDS VI during treatment with ascorbic acid.[168]

Despite these encouraging reports, there are a number of inconsistencies that may represent heterogeneity within this syndrome. For example, not all affected individuals have been shown to have a reduced level of hydroxylysine in their tissues.[169] Furthermore, there is not a good correlation between the reduction in lysyl hydroxylase and reduced hydroxylysine content in cell culture or in tissues.[165] Detailed studies of the enzyme kinetics for lysyl hydroxylase have shown that not all the mutants have an altered K_m for ascorbate.[170] Now that the human enzyme has been purified, it will be possible to combine immunologic and biochemical studies from various patients, and in this way differentiate between different mutations within the lysyl hydroxylase enzyme complex.[170] This approach will be necessary before evaluation of vitamin therapy or other treatments can be undertaken.

The consequence of deficient hydroxylysine content of collagen is related to the role of this amino acid in crosslink formation. Hydroxylysine-containing crosslinks are able to undergo a stabilizing change (Amidori rearrangement), which is particularly common to the types of crosslinks found in bone. Although individuals with EDS VI do form reducible crosslinks, a significant proportion appear to lack the hydroxylysine residue.[171] Of particular note is the anomalous chromatographic elution of hydroxypyridinium crosslinks from bone and cartilage in EDS VI, despite the fact that total hydroxylysine content in these tissues is normal.[42] By some mechanism that is not yet appreciated, it would seem that a larger proportion of the nonhydroxylated lysine residues are participating in formation of this multifunctional crosslink.

EDS X. In the original case report of EDS X by Arneson and associates in 1980, the proband was a 28-year-old woman with hypermobile joints, easy bruising, fishmouth scars on her extremities, and mitral valve prolapse.[172] Although this patient clinically resembled EDS II or EDS III, there were significant differences. The characteristic velvety feel of the skin was absent, as were striae. Her three brothers had similar skin and joint findings, but they lacked the history of bruising or unusual bleeding. Platelets obtained from this patient revealed resistance to aggregation in response to collagen and adenosine diphosphate (ADP), whereas the responses to serotonin, thrombin, and epinephrine were diminished. Since normal plasma or cryoprecipitate were found to correct the clotting defect, it was suggested that a qualitative deficiency of fibronectin caused the abnormality. Fibronectin is a serum protein that is known to interact with collagen as a cell attachment factor in the extracellular matrix.

X-Linked EDS—EDS V and EDS IX (Occipital Horn Syndrome). These forms of EDS are the least well-characterized, but they are distinguished by their inheritance pattern. X-linked inheritance in EDS V was suggested by the report of DiFerrante in which the propositus and two male cousins (maternal) were similarly affected.[173] These patients had strikingly extensible skin and bruisability with molluscoid pseudotumors. Dermal scarring was moderate in severity. Although joint mobility was mild, they experienced recurrent dislocations.

EDS IX is characterized by skeletal dysplasia, occipital horns, diarrhea, and obstructive uropathy.[141,174] The propositus noted had an unusual facial appearance and had undergone repair of bladder neck obstruction at age 5 years. The propositus and two maternal uncles had unusually long, narrow faces with high foreheads. Mild hyperextensibility of the small joints was present, but cutaneous elasticity was normal. A remarkable finding was the presence of two symmetric bony spurs projecting inferiorly from the occiput. The existence of skeletal dysplasia was also evident by virtue of modeling defects seen in the distal ulna, fusion of the capitate-hamate, and generalized osteoporosis. Both the propositus and his uncles complained of chronic diarrhea.

Molecular Pathology. Initial reports of decreased lysyl oxidase activity in EDS V were not verified with the use of more specific enzyme assays.[41] Furthermore, a reduction in the crosslink content was not demonstrated. However, low lysyl oxidase activity and increased collagen solubility have been found in cultured fibroblasts from individuals with a phenotype suggestive of EDS IX (see discussion of lysyl oxidase and copper metabolism in section on Menkes' kinky hair syndrome).[175] To date, lysyl oxidase is the only protein related to collagen synthesis localized to the X chromosome. Thus, the underlying molecular abnormality in all the X-linked forms of EDS remains unknown.

Osteogenesis Imperfecta

Osteogenesis imperfecta (OI) refers to a generalized disorder of connective tissue that predominately affects the skeletal system.[176] It is estimated to affect approximately 10,000 persons in the United States. The gene prevalence of OI is calculated as 5 per 100,000.[177-179] These estimates may fall short of its true prevalence because of the number of very mild cases that are either undiagnosed or diagnosed late in life. For example, some cases of postmenopausal osteoporosis may actually be OI, unmasked by menopausal estrogen deficiency. Approximately 60 percent of OI is inherited as an autosomal dominant trait, 15 to 20 percent is inherited as an autosomal recessive trait, whereas approximately 25 percent appears to represent a new mutation. Because the definition of the obligate heterozygote is uncertain at this time, it is difficult to determine whether a new case represents a fresh mutation or a genetic compound.

The traditional designation of OI congenita and OI tarda should be discarded. There are patients who have fractures at birth, yet have a relatively mild course, whereas a small number will have no fracture during birth but will develop severe deformities thereafter. Obviously the rate at which the individual patient develops fractures depends on factors apart from the severity of the genetic disorder. Of particular concern is the effect of early immobilization (as with a body spica cast) when an infant has repeatedly fractured one extremity. This is not an infrequent event and puts the child at even greater risk when ambulation finally occurs because of the detrimental effect immobilization osteopenia has on bone strength.

In the discussion to follow, the authors have merged the clinical classification of Sillence[179] with more recent information concerning the locus of the molecular defect in each clinical variant (Table 105–3). This is meant to emphasize the molecular basis for each variant and to illustrate that genetic heterogeneity lessens the value of a strictly clinical classification.

Mild OI Associated with Diminished Type I Collagen Production (Sillence Type I). These individuals have OI of mild to moderate severity both in terms of their clinical course and the radiologic appearance of the peripheral skeleton (Fig. 105–7*A*). The disease is usually inherited as an autosomal dominant trait but may infrequently be sporadic. Length and weight are normal at birth. These patients have a characteristic triangular facial shape caused by mild prominence of the frontal bones in association with a class III malocclusion of the jaw and a narrow anterior mandible.[180] Sclerae are almost uniformly blue, with the tint varying from a deep hue to pale blue-gray. Patients have observed that the color of their sclerae may vary over time; in general, deeper hues are seen in children. Arcus senilis that is not related to lipid abnormalities occurs in many patients during the middle years. Although we have not observed the occurrence of dentinogenesis imperfecta (DI) in this group, a subgroup of patients having DI has been noted by Levin and colleagues.[181]

Auditory function is intact in most OI patients during their early years. However, during the second and third decades of life, a characteristic high-frequency, sensorineural or mixed, hearing loss can be detected.[182] Hypermetabolism, in association with elevated serum thyroid levels, has been reported, but the existence of "uncoupling" or oxidative metabolism has not been confirmed.[183] Careful physical examination and determination of thyroid levels before and after stimulation with thyrotropin-releasing hormone (TRH) failed to reveal a consistent abnormality in the pituitary-thyroid axis.[184] Although instances of mitral valve prolapse and aortic root enlargement have been reported, overall the incidence of mitral valve prolapse is not increased in these patients.[185,186] However, individual kindreds have been observed in whom increased diameter of the aortic root has been found on echocardiography; their pulmonary function is normal. Presenting complaints may include both umbilical and inguinal hernias. Scar formation and wound healing are usually normal, but occasional patients will develop keloids at the site of previous surgery.

Mildly affected patients usually do not have fractures at birth, although there is occasionally a fracture of a clavicle or of an extremity during delivery. Prenatal diagnosis by ultrasound is not helpful in the mild form because intrauterine fractures are uncommon. A fracture occurs, most frequently in the upper femur, either in the newborn nursery with daily handling or as the infant starts to crawl. The frequency of fracture thereafter depends, in part, on the child's activity, the need for immobilization, and the attitudes of the family toward independent activity. In general, these patients have 5 to 15 fractures prior to puberty, although they may

Table 105–3. Characteristics of Osteogenesis Imperfecta, Based on the Clinical Classification of Sillence*

Sillence Classification	Clinical Features	Variant Frequency	Inheritance	Estimated Average No. of Fractures	Scleral Color	Presence of DI	Biochemical Abnormality
I	No major skeletal deformities	50%	Dominant, occasionally sporadic	5–15	Blue	25%	Marked decrease in type I synthesis; normal $\alpha1{:}\alpha2$ ratio
II	Lethal; severely deformed	5%	Recessive or new mutation	Multiple in utero and at birth	Blue	Occurs, but prevalence is uncertain	Failure to secrete type I collagen; insertions and deletions of $\alpha1(I)$ and $\alpha2(I)$
III	Major skeletal deformities, very osteopenic, usually not ambulatory	20%	Recessive; may be genetic compound	30–60	Usually white, occasionally blue	25%	No abnormalities in type I collagen have been found. Molecular defect unknown
IV	Moderate severity of osteopenia and bony deformities, scoliosis may be prominent; usually ambulatory but with mechanical support	25%	Sporadic or dominant; may be a genetic compound or new mutation	10–25	Blue; may lighten with age	25%	Variable decrease in type I synthesis; abnormalities in $\alpha2(I)$ structure or production

*Based on Sillence, D.O., and Danks, D.M.: J. Med. Genet. 16:101, 1979.

Figure 105–7. These radiographs illustrate skeletal differences among variants of osteogenesis imperfecta. *A,* Dominant, mild, with minimal deformity; *B,* Moderate OI, mild epiphyseal dysplasia; *C,* Severe OI, marked diaphyseal narrowing and widening of the metaphysis with severe epiphyseal dysplasia. Lethal OI is not illustrated.

experience several minor traumatic fractures of the digits or the small bones of their feet. Poor alignment or repeated immobilization leads to recurrent fractures at one site, which may induce bowing and subsequent disturbance of gait. Osteopenia is observed in both the spine and the peripheral skeleton and tends to progress with age. It is remarkable that in spite of multiple fractures, the long bones heal with no residual deformity. These children almost never require the insertion of intramedullary rods and almost never develop nonunion at a fracture site. As occurs in other variants, the frequency of fractures diminishes markedly after puberty, an observation that is not explained by the level of activity or the child's ability to protect against trauma. Although osteopenia, moderate coarsening of trabeculae, and cortical thinning are observed in x-rays, many cases are so mild as to be missed on routine examination (see Fig. 105–4A). In fact, the diagnosis may first be suspected when a parent with unrecognized disease is found to have an affected child. This situation has led to the accusation of child abuse on several occasions.[187]

The skin of the patient with mild OI has normal elasticity but is occasionally thin and somewhat smooth in texture. Although many patients complain of easy bruising, only rarely has this been of clinical significance. Detailed studies of clotting function in OI patients have not revealed a consistent abnormality.[188] Many patients are found to have hyperextensible joints as children, but this tends to be less marked in adults. Only occasionally will the OI patient have genu recurvatum, but many have pes planus.

It is our experience that there is relatively little phenotypic variability within an affected kindred. Sibships in which a severely affected infant has been born to mildly affected parents have been reported but are the exception rather than the rule. It is now recognized, however, that relatives who have not had fractures may have subtle manifestations of the disease, such as hyperextensible joints, scoliosis, or audiologic disturbances.

Molecular Pathology. Cultured fibroblasts from these individuals synthesize low amounts of type I collagen, whereas type III collagen production is normal.[189] Therefore, the ratio of type III to type I collagen is elevated in both cultured cells[190] and collagens extracted from skin biopsies.[191] Consistent with the low production is a bone collagen fiber diameter that is significantly smaller than that of controls.[192] The underproduction of a normal type I collagen molecule may explain the recurrent fractures that occur during periods of rapid growth and bone remodeling when the demand for collagen production is high. The fall in fracture rates after puberty would then be explained by the ability of the osteoblast to match the decreased demand for collagen production.

The molecular basis for the low production of type I collagen appears to be related to diminished activity of one of the $\alpha 1(I)$ collagen alleles, since the rate of $\alpha 1(I)$ production is half of that expected.[189] Because collagen molecules composed of more than one $\alpha 2$ chain are unstable, the rate of $\alpha 1$ chain synthesis determines the rate of type I collagen production. Alpha 2 chains in excess of $\alpha 1$ are degraded.[193] The level of $\alpha 1(I)$ collagen mRNA is also half of that expected, suggesting a nonfunctional $\alpha 1$ collagen gene or instability of its mRNA.[194] Although a gene deletion could account for these findings, the experience from similar types of molecular mutation in β-thalassemia suggests a single base mutation that alters the activity of the promoter, the reading frame, or the site for splicing an intron. Since collagen has 50 such intervening sequences, the number of mutations that could result in diminished $\alpha 1$ mRNA accumulation is staggering.[195]

Lethal OI Associated with Failure to Secrete Type I Collagen (Silence Type II). About 10 percent of OI patients have this form of the disease, which is incompatible with survival. Studies have yielded a segregation ratio consistent with recessive inheritance,[177,196] but biochemical evidence for new dominant mutations has been presented.[197] Infants are born with severe bone fragility and experience multiple intrauterine fractures. X-ray of these children reveals a characteristic beading of the ribs representing callus over multiple fractures and an "accordian type" deformity of the extremities, which appear crumpled, foreshortened, and broad. There is little ossification of the cranium (wormian bones), and the skull appears large in comparison with the short and deformed extremities.[198] An occasional fetus will be mascerated at the time of delivery, and dismemberment has occurred. The sclerae are typically deep blue, and the skin is thin and transparent. Respiratory reserve is very limited, and death ensues usually within a week.

Prenatal diagnosis by ultrasound is possible starting at about the 16th week of pregnancy. Termination of an affected pregnancy has been reported.[199,200] The family must be counseled that the chance for recurrence is as high as 25 percent.[201]

Molecular Pathology. The biochemical abnormality common to the lethal form of OI appears to be an impaired ability to synthesize or secrete type I collagen.[202] As a result, the type I collagen of bone is low, whereas the minor collagen types, III and V, are relatively high.[203] Bone collagen fibers are distinctly smaller than the fibers from age-matched normal infants.[192] Retained collagen within dilated endoplasmic reticulum has been observed.[204]

The biochemical basis for the lack of collagen secretion appears to reside within the primary structures of either the $\alpha 1(I)$ chains or the $\alpha 2$ chains. A number of structural mutations, both deletions and insertions, within both chains have been observed.[205,206] Intracellular procollagen also shows evidence for excessive post-translational modifications that would be expected if the mutation delayed the rate of helix formation.[28] However, other cases of lethal OI do not have large alterations of the protein or mRNA, suggesting that point mutations may also affect chain assembly and secretion.

Severe, Nonlethal OI Associated with Normal Production of Type I Collagen (Silence Type III). This variant is the classic form of OI and accounts for about 20 percent of cases. The disease is inherited as an autosomal recessive trait. Several families have now been reported with more than one affected child, normal parents, and an absence of consanguinity. This variant is characterized by severe deformity of the limbs, marked kyphoscoliosis, and marked growth retardation.[175] Although termed "progressive deforming" by Sillence, the deformities are fully established by the age of 5 years and remain relatively unchanged until the middle years, when kyphoscoliosis may worsen. The extent of growth retardation is remarkable in that many patients may not surpass 3 ft (90 to 100 cm) in height. Measurements of the skull are normal, although the skull may appear proportionately large for the small trunk. Molding occurs in utero and infancy, producing frontal bossing and a characteristic occipital "overhang" termed the "helmet deformity." Wormian bones and delayed closure of fontanelles may be observed. Platybasia may cause the external ear canals to slant upward as the base of the skull, softened by defective ossification, sinks on the cervical vertebrae.[207] This may lead to hydrocephalus, cranial nerve palsy, and upper and lower motor neuron lesions. Third-degree malocclusion of the mandible is common. The majority of patients in this category have white sclerae as adults, although bluish discoloration is apparent in childhood. Arcus senilis is commonly seen. Approximately 25 percent of these patients have DI (vide infra), necessitating constant dental care through childhood. Severe hearing impairment occurs in 10 percent of patients, although milder degrees of hearing loss are more common. An unusual and characteristic feature of this group is a high-pitched voice.

The skeleton is quite soft and deforms easily, particularly prior to puberty, leading to scoliosis and severe deformity of the sternum. Displacement of the cardiac borders occurs, which may be associated with flow murmurs. However, in our study of patients at the National Institutes of Health, the incidence of mitral valve prolapse was not increased when compared with normal controls. Aortic root diameter may be increased in certain kindreds.[184] Pulmonary function is diminished because of distortion of the spine and chest cage and may worsen in adulthood.

Deformities of the limbs constitute a remarkable feature of this disease. Even at birth limbs may be twisted into near pretzel shape, depending on the effect of muscle pull in utero. A saber deformity of the distal tibia is very common. Spontaneous fractures occur with little stress so that the infant may experience 20 or more fractures during the first 2 or 3 years of life. These children tend to be hypotonic and have lax joints so that head control and motor development are delayed. It is obvious from the first year of life that the limbs will probably not support weight and, for that reason, patients with this variant are usually wheelchair-bound for most of their lives. Radiographs of the skeleton reveal marked osteopenia, narrowing of the diaphysis, and widening of the metaphysis, which merges into a dysplastic epiphyseal zone filled with whorls of partially calcified cartilage (popcorn deformity) (Fig. 105–7C).[208] Bowing of the extremities produces severe deformity, whereas

osteopenia causes collapse of vertebral endplates. Lack of weight-bearing increases the severity of osteoporosis and increases the risk of fracture. In spite of this, spontaneous fractures do not regularly occur after puberty. However, trauma, such as an auto accident or falling from a wheelchair, can have disastrous results. In spite of these multiple complications, we have seen patients survive with gainful employment into their 60s.

Molecular Pathology. Despite the dramatic clinical features of this form of OI, little insight has been gained into the molecular basis for the disease. At this time no specific abnormalities of collagen synthesis have been reported.[190] The bone collagen fibers are of normal size, although disaggregation has been observed.[192] We have found delayed α-chain migration on acrylamide gel electrophoresis,[190] and others have reported excessive mannosylation of the C-terminal heterosaccharide unit,[209] but these findings have been difficult to reproduce. Thus, it is yet to be shown that this form of OI is a collagen abnormality. Rather, it may be a defect in a collagen modifier such as a proteoglycan or a noncollagen matrix protein.

OI of Moderate Severity Associated with Abnormal α2 Chain Production (Sillence Type IV). Clinically, these patients overlap with those having mild disease; however, occasional patients may be more severely affected. Inheritence in this group is frequently sporadic, although dominant mutations or the formation of a genetic compound is suspected in some. Their sclerae tend to be blue, although others have observed families in which sclerae are blue at birth but lighten to white with age. In our limited series they appear to have more moulding of the skull, and an occipital overhang may be palpable. Kyphoscoliosis is present, and during adolescence progressive spinal deformity may occur. As a corollary, one sees hyperextensible joints and pes planus. The majority of fractures occur in childhood and recur in postmenopausal women. Following each fracture there tends to be long bone deformity and inequality of the length; thus gait disturbances occur more frequently than in the mildly affected patient. Radiographs of the long bones and vertebral bodies demonstrate marked osteopenia and vertebral collapse, which leads to back pain and restricted pulmonary function. Although there is marked cortical thinning, bowing, and coarsening of trabeculae, the overall architecture of bone remains intact (see Fig. 105–7B). The presence of moderate degrees of skeletal deformity eventually requires that these patients resort to the use of a cane or a walker; at times they may be forced to use a wheelchair.

DI has been observed in variable numbers of patients in several of the groups already described, and it is used as one of the criteria in separating individual patients within categories I and IV.[181] When present, it is inherited as a dominant trait. The authors have observed DI in only 25 percent of individuals in groups III and IV. Studies are now in progress to determine if patterns of collagen synthesis differ between patients with and without DI. The relationship between OI and DI is not yet precisely defined. Both deciduous and permanent teeth have an opalescent or translucent appearance, which tends to darken with age. The enamel of these teeth is normal; however, the dentin is dysplastic, so that chipping of enamel occurs and the teeth are thus subjected to erosion and breakage. The formation of dentin is seen to be irregular by scanning electron microscopy, and dentinal tubules are oriented in a random rather than regular manner and are decreased in number.[210] On x-ray there is an exaggerated constriction at the coronal junction and obliteration of pulpal spaces. Early consideration should be given to capping affected teeth to minimize wear and breakage.

Molecular Pathology. This form of OI represents a heterogenous grouping both clinically and biochemically. Current studies suggest that abnormalities of the α2 chain production are present in this form of OI.[190] The types of molecular abnormalities of the α2 chain are similar to those of the α1(I) found in type I and type II OI, for example, regulatory and structural, occurring as either a single or compound mutation. Of particular value in studying families with dominant pedigrees is the use of restriction length polymorphisms. Tsipoouras has demonstrated an Eco RI restriction polymorphism that occurs in sufficient frequency within the general population to be useful as a genetic marker for the alleles of the α2 gene.[54] Its value has been demonstrated in a family with type IV OI. However, the marker does not give insight into the underlying molecular abnormality.

Nichols and associates described a child who failed to incorporate α2 chain into type I collagen in cell culture or skin.[211] Subsequent work indicated that the mRNA for the α2 chain was present in the cells and was capable of generating an α2 chain in a cell-free translation system.[212] Intracellular α2 chains could also be found after a brief radiolabeling pulse, indicating that α_2 chains were being synthesized but were being rapidly degraded. The best explanation for these findings is a structural mutation in the C-terminal propeptide region of the α2 molecule essential for chain assembly. The parents of this child, who do not have OI and who are first-degree relatives, were found to have an elevated α1(I):α2 chain ratio, suggesting that one inactive α2 allele is tolerated without clinical effect.

The second type of defect in this form of OI occurs when a structural abnormality of the α2 chain is incorporated into the molecule. The initial patient who demonstrated this situation contained a 15 to 30 amino acid deletion in the N-terminal helical region of the α2 chain.[213] It should be anticipated that a point mutation within the α2 chain, particularly at any of the glycine residues, could have a similar effect.

The third situation is the sporadic case of OI in which a history of mild connective tissue symptoms may be present on both sides of the family.[214] Thus, a slightly increased frequency of fracture or joint laxity may be found without frank manifestations of OI. Preliminary evidence suggests that the affected child, a sporadic case, in fact represents a genetic compound having inherited two α-chain defects. These defects can be either regulatory or structural, which when present in one copy are well tolerated. However, when two abnormal alleles are combined, the result is OI. Clearly the challenge in the future will be to differentiate the sporadic case as either a genetic compound or a new dominant mutation.

In all forms of OI, interpretation of the histopathologic appearance of bone is subject to the age of the patient, the severity of the disease, and the site from which the bone was obtained. Specimens obtained at the time of surgery are frequently not representative of nontraumatized bone. Osteopenia, fewer bony trabeculae, and thin cortices are the rule. As the severity of the disease increases, one sees fewer trabeculae and more primitive organization of osteoid and calcified matrix (woven bone). The appearance of osteoblasts and osteoclasts in OI bone is normal.[204,215] As a rule, bone biopsy does not aid in the diagnosis of OI.

Therapy. There have been multiple attempts at treatment with a variety of hormones and drugs, none of which has been successful. The list includes administration of mineral supplements, fluoride, calcitonin, androgenic steroids, ascorbic acid, and vitamin D.[216,217] The rationale for the use of each of these has not always been clear, and as a result many of these trials have been inconclusive. In the future, agents that promote bone growth, such as growth hormone and low-dose anabolic steroids, may play a role in treating OI when underproduction of a normal type I collagen can be demonstrated. However, unless the abnormal gene product can be substantially modified, merely enhancing production of defective collagen chains may have little beneficial effect on bone strength.

The use of surgery to correct deformities and to facilitate weight-bearing has been the subject of several recent reviews.[218,219] Intramedullary rods have been placed in many children with salutory effects, both cosmetic and functional.

Every child with OI will benefit from appropriate rehabilitative therapy.[220] Bracing with new lightweight plastics can be accomplished as the child begins to walk in order to minimize microfracture and bowing of the upper femurs.[221] Muscle strengthening exercises are essential as primary care and following immobilization for fracture. Perhaps the most beneficial programs have been developed around swimming, preferably in heated pools, as part of a planned program of rehabilitative medical care.

Heritable Disorders of Elastin

The inclusion of the following disorders as elastin-specific diseases is somewhat artificial, since collagen may also be abnormal. However, the more prominent clinical and pathologic features are related to disordered elastin production. Thus the Marfan syndrome was classified as a collagen disorder, since the major phenotypic changes are due to alteration in collagen, although there are also abnormalities within elastin. The overlap between the collagen and elastin abnormalities in these diseases probably relate to common cofactors and enzymes that modify these structural proteins, particularly those that are x-linked.

Cutis Laxa. This term refers to a group of generalized connective tissue disorders in which the common clinical feature is lax, redundant, and inelastic skin. The skin in these patients is wrinkled and sags in loose folds, imparting a prematurely aged appearance. The disease is exceedingly rare. Cutis laxa may be inherited as an autosomal dominant, autosomal recessive, or sex-linked disease.[222-224] Acquired cutis laxa may follow ingestion of penicillamine,[225] inflammatory skin disease, or a nonspecific febrile illness.[226]

The autosomal dominant form is mild, largely limited to the dermis, and thus compatible with a normal life span. Dermal changes may be present in infancy but usually are not marked until the second or third decade of life when facial tissues loosen. The nose develops a hooked appearance with a hanging tip, and the ears sag. There may be marked drooping of the eyelids, with ectropion, eversion of the nostrils, and elongation of the upper lip. Skin is also redundant on other parts of the body, particularly over the elbows and knees. Unlike EDS, the skin in cutis laxa does not recoil when stretched. Several patients have been found to harbor bronchiectasis or mild pulmonary emphysema. Aside from pulmonary infections in childhood and the occurrence of inguinal hernias, these patients remain in good health. The joints are not hyperextensible in this disease.

The recessive variety is more severe, as evidenced by diagnosis at birth or shortly thereafter and the early development of severe cardiopulmonary complications.[227] Characteristic facies, a hoarse cry, and a large umbilical hernia may be present at birth. The vocal cords tend to be elongated and lax, leading to aspiration and upper airway obstruction. Eventration of the diaphragm, and paraesophageal, inguinal, or femoral hernias may require surgery during the first months of life. Multiple diverticulae involving the entire bowel impair digestion, and diverticulae of the urinary bladder lead to bouts of urinary tract obstruction, hydroureter, and hydronephrosis.[228]

Different cardiac murmurs have been observed in the severe forms of cutis laxa.[229] On angiographic examination there may be evidence of segmental pulmonary artery branch stenosis associated with pulmonary artery hypertension.[230] X-ray evidence of severe emphysema may be evident in these patients at an early age, along with cardiomegaly and cor pulmonale. Angiographic studies have demonstrated tortuous, narrow, and kinked (corkscrew) distal pulmonary arteries,[231] changes that resemble those found in Menkes' syndrome. Severely affected infants do poorly and may succumb to pulmonary infections or right ventricular failure.

The X-linked variety of cutis laxa appears to be intermediate in severity between the autosomal recessive and dominant forms.

Molecular Pathology. Microscopic examination of the dermis reveals alterations in both elastic fibers and collagen. Fine elastic fibers that normally rise into the dermal papillae may be absent. Individual elastic fibers that vary greatly in diameter are short and globular in outline and less compact; the elastica may be more abundant at deeper levels of the dermis.[232] Globular, fragmented, and clumped elastic fibers have also been observed in the lung and aorta.

Although no information regarding the abnormality in elastin structure and biosynthesis is currently available, the dominant form should yield to techniques of molecular biology, once human elastin cDNA and gene probes are developed. Byers and associates studied fibroblasts from two male cousins with the X-linked form of cutis laxa. Lysyl oxidase activity was found to be low, whereas collagen extractibility was enhanced, and the amount of lysyl-derived aldehydes and collagen crosslinks was diminished.[223] Serum levels of copper and ceruloplasmin were also low in these patients (see later discussion).

Therapy. Treatment is limited to plastic surgery, which can significantly improve the patient's appearance. Unlike EDS, surgery is not complicated by excessive bleeding or tissue fragility.

Menkes' Kinky Hair Syndrome. First described by Menkes in 1962, this is a sex-linked disorder of copper metabolism that involves connective tissue by affecting metalloenzymes essential to collagen and elastin synthesis.[233] The disease begins in utero and is apparent at birth. These infants have a chubby, expressionless, and cherubic face and a depressed nasal bridge and are hypotonic, lethargic, and hypothermic. Hyperbilirubinemia is common. Pale skin and depigmented hair are attributed to a defect in tyrosinase, a copper-dependent enzyme. The syndrome derives its name from the kinky (pilitorti), beaded, and brittle sparse hair, which is evident by the first month of life. Poor head control, reflex abnormalities, seizures, and spasticity occur in association with mental retardation.[234]

The histopathologic appearance reveals both cerebral and cerebellar atrophy as well as loss of myelin, gliosis, and degeneration of the spinocerebellar tracts. Electroencephalographic findings, which vary with age, eventually show slow-wave activity with admixed paroxysmal features.[235] Skeletal demineralization occurs. Angiographic studies show a characteristic corkscrew tortuosity of intracerebral, renal, and intestinal vessels. Because of failure to thrive, the severely affected infants are susceptible to respiratory infections.

Infants with Menkes' syndrome have low serum copper, low serum ceruloplasmin, and diminished white cell cytochrome-C oxidase activity.[236] Trace mineral analysis of post-mortem specimens reveal marked reductions in hepatic and brain copper content, but elevated renal, skeletal muscle, and placental copper content.[237,238] Attempts to increase longevity with administration of oral or intravenous copper have not been successful.[237]

Molecular Pathology. Although the X-linked connective tissue syndromes have little clinical similarity, there may be a common biochemical link. Lysyl oxidase and its cofactor, copper, are important for the initial steps of collagen crosslinking.[41] From studies of the aneurysm-prone mottled mouse and Menkes' kinky hair syndrome, either the enzyme or copper transport, or both, are linked to the X chromosome. Similarly, X-linked cutis laxa has been shown to have low immunologic and enzymatic activity for lysyl oxidase.[223] The aneurysm-prone mice have low serum copper levels and diminished enzyme activity.[239] It is not known if the enzyme is absent or deficient in activity because of the copper abnormality. In Menkes' syndrome, abnormal cellular copper transport results in low levels of serum copper. In contrast, a high intracellular copper content is present in cultured fibroblasts. High levels of zinc and cadmium plus the protein that binds these metals, metallothionein, are also found in these cells.[240] Thus, a possible lesion may be an inability to transfer copper to cellular enzymes, resulting in the neurologic and connective tissue syndromes.

Pseudoxanthoma Elasticum (PXE). A rare disorder, PXE is characterized by degeneration and calcification of elastic fibers in the skin, retina, and blood vessels.[241,242] The estimated incidence of PXE varies from 1 per 70,000 to 1 per 160,000 live births; however, the true incidence may be obscured by milder cases that go unrecognized. PXE affects females twice as frequently as it does males. In most kindreds, PXE is inherited as an autosomal recessive trait, although autosomal dominant inheritance has been reported.[243,244]

In its classic form, PXE is recognized by the presence of asymptomatic, symmetric, yellowish-white papules in flexural skin folds, which, in the dominant variant, appear during the second or third decade of life but appear earlier in recessive forms. The papules, which have an xanthomatoid appearance, initially involve the skin of the neck and axilla, and progress to the periumbilicus, antecubital fossa, and inguinal areas, and there they coalesce to give a redundant, thickened, doughy appearance.[245] Thus, PXE may present a similar facial appearance to cutis laxa, with sagging, redundant folds of skin. Mucocutaneous lesions may also occur on the oral and buccal mucosae and other mucous membranes.[246]

Angioid streaks of the retina are radially oriented, resembling vessels, and are the result of a break in Bruch's membrane.[247] Although they occur in approximately 85 percent of patients, they are not specific to this syndrome and may be found in a variety of systemic diseases, including Paget's disease, sickle cell anemia, EDS, and acromegaly. Retinal lesions may be demonstrated with fluorescence angiography, which shows transmitted choroidal hyperfluorescence indicative of the pigmentary alteration. There is also retinal hyperpigmentation with the formation of atypical druzen within the posterior pole and periphery, which eventually involve the optic nerve and macula. Visual loss in PXE may vary from mild to legal blindness and is the result of maculopathy and retinal hemorrhage, which lead to neovascularization and retinal detachment.

Progressive dyspnea may signal either pulmonary or cardiac involvement. The lesions in the lung include vascular calcification and intimal fibrosis due to damage of the elastic laminae in arteries, arterioles, and venules. Calcific deposits occur in alveolar lumen and may be visualized in radiographs.[248]

Involvement of the heart may cause angina, dyspnea, and arrhythmias suggestive of a cardiomyopathy.[249] Small ventricular size and elevated end diastolic pressure result from a diffuse endocardial fibroelastosis.[250] Endomyocardial biopsy and post-mortem specimens have revealed fragmented and mineralized elastic fibers similar to those seen in the skin. Intimal fibrosis may compromise the coronary circulation. Heart muscle appears to be spared, except for foci of fibrosis secondary to the small vessel arteriopathy. Mitral valve prolapse was found in 71 percent of one series of 14 patients, but there was no association between the severity of skin lesions and valve dysfunction.[251] Angiography of peripheral vessels may show evidence of a diffuse obliterative arteriopathy. Hypertension may effect 75 percent of patients and is perhaps secondary to renal involvement.

Both genitourinary and uterine bleeding complicate the clinical course of PXE. Arteries of the gastrointestinal tract are particularly susceptible to rupture, which occurred in 14 percent of one series.[252] Gastroscopy has shown nodular or linear yellowish lesions in the colonic mucosa of patients with lower gastrointestinal bleeding.[253] Wound healing is generally normal in PXE until late in the course of the disease when dermal calcification may be extensive. Hyperextensibility may lead to dislocations of both large and small joints.

Molecular Pathology. Dermal elastic fibers are frayed, swollen, and clumped and appear to be increased in number. The centers of elastin fibers are replaced by an electron-dense material, which appears to disrupt the fiber, leading to calcification. Nonaffected skin in PXE has also been shown to contain increased quantities of this dense material, and elastic fibers are microscopically normal in PXE.[254] No information regarding the nature of the abnormality of elastic structure or synthesis is currently available. Since heterogeneity is present in this syndrome, a wide spectrum of structural or regulatory defects, or both, can be anticipated.[255]

References

1. Bornstein, P., and Sage, A.: Structurally distinct collagen types. Ann. Rev. Biochem. 491:957, 1980.
2. von der Mark, K.: Localization of collagen types in tissues. Int. Rev. Conn. Tiss. Res. 9:269, 1981.
3. Rimoin, D.L., and Sillence, D.O.: Chrondro-osseous morphology and biochemistry in the skeletal dysplasias. Birth Defects 17:249, 1981.
4. Epstein, E.H.: Alpha 1(III) human skin collagen release by pepsin digestion and preponderance in fetal life. J. Biol. Chem. 249:3225, 1974.
5. Shuttleworth, C., and Forrest, L.: Changes in guinea-pig dermal collagen during development. Eur. J. Biochem. 55:391, 1975.
6. Bailey, A.J., Sims, T.J., Lelous, M., and Vazin, S.: Collagen polymorphism in experimental granulation tissue. Biochem. Biophys. Res. Commun. 66:1160, 1975.
7. Sage, H., Woodbury, R.G., and Bornstein, P.: Structural studies on human type IV collagen. J. Biol. Chem. 254:9899, 1979.
8. Crouch, E., Sage, H., and Bornstein, P.: Structural basis for apparent heterogeneity of collagen in human basement membranes: Type IV procollagen contains two distinct chains. Proc. Natl. Acad. Sci. 77:745, 1980.
9. Kumamoto, C.A., and Fessler, J.H.: Biosynthesis of A, B procollagen. Proc. Natl. Acad. Sci. 77:6434, 1980.
10. Alitalo, K., Myllyla, R., Sage, H., Pritzl, P., Vah Eri, A., and Bornstein, P.: Biosynthesis of type V procollagen in A204, a human rhabdomyosarcoma cell line. J. Biol. Chem. 257:9016, 1982.
11. Chu, M.L., Myers, J.C., Bernard, M.P., Ding, J.F., and Ramirez, F.:

Cloning and characterization of five overlapping cDNAs specific for the human proα₁(I) collagen chain. Nucleic Acids Res. 10:5925, 1982.

12. Lehrach, H., Frischauf, A., Hanahan, D., Wozine, Y.J., Fuller, F., and Boedtker, H.: Construction and characterization of proα₁ collagen complementary deoxyribonucleic acid clones. Biochemistry 18:3146, 1979.

13. Myers, J.C., Chu, M.L., Faro, S.H., Clark, W.J., Prockop, D.J., and Ramirez, F.: Cloning a cDNA for the proα₂ chain of human type I collagen. Proc. Natl. Acad. Sci. 78:3516, 1981.

14. Wozney, J., Hanahan, D., Douglastate, V., Boedtker, H., and Doty, P.: Structure of the proα₂(I) collagen gene. Nature 294:129, 1981.

15. Dalgeleish, R., Trapnell, B.C., Crystal, R.G., and Tolstoshev, P.: Copy number of a human alpha₂(I) collagen gene. J. Biol. Chem. 257:13816, 1982.

16. Vogeli, G., Ohkubo, H., Sobel, M.E., Yamata, Y.S., Pastan, I., and deCrombrugghe, B.: Structure of the promoter for chicken alpha 2 type I collagen gene. Proc. Natl. Acad. Sci. 78:5334, 1981.

17. Chu, M.L., deWet, W., Bernard, M., Ding, J.F., Morabito, M., Myers, J., Williams, C., and Ramirez, F.: Structure of the human proα1(I) collagen gene: Evolutionary conservation of functional domain. Submitted for publication.

18. McKnight, S.I., and Kingsbury, R.: Transcriptional control signals of a eukaryotic protein-coding gene. Science 217:316, 1982.

19. Sharp, P.A.: Speculations on RNA splicing. Cell 23:643, 1981.

20. Rogers, J., and Wall, R.: A mechanism for RNA splicing. Proc. Natl. Acad. Sci. 77:1877, 1980.

21. Treisman, R., Proudfoot, J., Shander, M., and Maniatis, T.: A single-base change at a splice site in a β°-thalassemic gene causes abnormal RNA splicing. Cell 29:903, 1982.

22. Moschonas, N., DeBoer, E., Grosveld, F.G., Dahl, H.H.M., Wright, S., Shewmaker, C.K., and Flavell, R.A.: Structure and expression of a cloned β°-thalassaemia globin gene. Nucleic Acids Res. 9:1391, 1981.

23. Westaway, D., and Williamson, R.: An intron nucleotide sequence variant in a cloned β⁺-thalassemia globin gene. Nucleic Acids Res. 9:1777, 1981.

24. Orkin, S.H., and Goff, S.C.: Nonsense and frameshift mutations in beta-globin O-thalassemia detected in cloned beta-globin genes. J. Biol. Chem. 256:9782, 1981.

25. Pergolizzi, R., Spritz, R.A., Spense, S., Goossens, M., Waikan, Y., and Bank, A.: Two cloned thalassemia genes are associated with amber mutations at codon 39. Nucleic Acid Res. 9:7065, 1981.

26. Jimenez, S.A., Harsch, M., Murphy, L., and Rosenbloom, J.: Effects of temperature on conformation, hydroxylation, and secretion of chick tendon procollagen. J. Biol. Chem. 249:4480, 1974.

27. Kruse, N.J., Rowe, D.W., Fujimoto, W.Y., and Bornstein, P.: Effect of glucocorticoids on collagen synthesis in the sponge granuloma of the mouse. Biochem. Biophys. Acta 548:101, 1978.

28. Trelstad, R.L., Rubin, D., and Gross, J.: Osteogenesis imperfecta congenita: Evidence for a generalized molecular disorder of collagen. Lab. Invest. 36:501, 1977.

29. Byers, P.H., and Barsh, G.S.: Reduced secretion of structurally abnormal type I procollagen in a form of osteogenesis imperfecta. Proc. Natl. Acad. Sci. 78:5142, 1981.

30. Kivirikko, K.I. and Myllyla, R.: Collagen glycosyl transferases. Int. Rev. Conn. Tiss. Res. 8:23, 1979.

31. Clark, C.C., and Kefalides, N.A.: Localization and partial composition of the oligosaccharide units on the propeptide extension of type I procollagen. J. Biol. Chem. 253:47, 1978.

32. Bruckner, P., Eikenberry, E.F., and Prockop, D.J.: Formation of the triple helix of type I procollagen in cellulo: A kinetic model based on cis-trans isomerization of peptide bonds. Eur. J. Biochem. 118:607, 1981.

33. Rosenbloom, J., Endo, R., and Harsch, M.: Termination of procollagen chain synthesis by puromycin: Evidence that assembly and secretion require a C007-terminal extension. J. Biol. Chem. 255:2070, 1976.

34. Bernard, M.P., Myers, J.C., Chu, M-L., Ramirez, F., Eikenberry, E.F., and Prockop, D.J.: Structure of a cDNA for the proα2 chain of human type I procollagen. Comparison with chick cDNA for proα2(I) identifies structurally conserved features of the protein and the gene. Biochemistry 22:1139, 1983.

35. Showalter, A.M., Pesciotta, D.M., Eikenberry, E.F., Yamamoto, T., Pastan, I., deCrombrugghe, B., Fietzek, P.P., and Olsen, B.: Nucleotide sequence of a collagen cDNA-fragment coding for the carboxyl end of proα1(I) chains. FEBS Lett. 111:61, 1980.

36. Diegelmann, R.F., and Peterkofsky, B.: Inhibition of collagen secretion from bone and cultured fibroblasts by microtubular descriptive drugs. Proc. Natl. Acad. Sci. 69:892, 1972.

37. Uchida, N., Smilowitz, H., and Tanzer, M.L.: Monovalent ionophoreses inhibit secretion of procollagen and fibronectin from cultured human fibroblasts. Proc. Natl. Acad. Sci. 76:1868, 1979.

38. Byers, P.H., Holbrook, K.A., Barsh, G.S., Smith, L.T., and Bornstein, P.: Altered secretion of type III procollagen in a form of type Ehler-Danlos syndrome. Biochemical studies in cultured fibroblasts. Lab. Invest. 44:336, 1981.

39. Trelstad, R.L.: Multistep assembly of type I collagen fibrils. Cell 28:197, 1982.

40. Lenaers, A., Ansay, M., Nusgens, B.V., and Lapiere, C.M.: Collagen made of extended α chains, procollagen, in genetically-defective dermatosparatic calves. Eur. J. Biochem. 23:533, 1971.

41. Siegel, R.C.: Lysyl Oxidase. Int. Rev. Conn. Tis. Res. 8:73, 1979.

42. Eyre, D.R.: Collagen cross-linking. In Akeson, W.H., Bornstein, P., and Glimcher, J.J. (eds.): Heritable Disorders of Connective Tissue. St. Louis, The C.V. Mosby Company, 1982, p. 43.

43. Eyre, D.R., and Oguchi, H.: The hydroxypyridinium crosslinks of skeletal collagens: their measurement, properties and proposed pathway of formation. Biochem. Biophy. Res. Commun. 92:440, 1980.

44. Miller, W.L.: Medical progress recombinant DNA and the pediatrician. J. Pediatr. 99:1, 1981.

45. Vosberg, H-P.: Molecular cloning of DNA: An introduction into techniques and problems. Hum. Genet. 40:1, 1977.

46. Thomas, P.A.: Hybridization of denatured RNA and small DNA fragments transferred to nitrocellulose. Proc. Natl. Acad. Sci. 77:5201, 1980.

47. Kafatos, F.C., Jones, W.C., and Estratiadis, A.: Determination of nucleic acid sequence homologies and relative concentrations by a dot hybridization procedure. Nucleic Acid Res. 7:1541, 1979.

48. McKnight, G.S., and Palmiter, R.D.: Transcriptional regulation of the ovalbumin and conalbumin genes by steroid hormones in chick oviduct. J. Biol. Chem. 254:9050, 1979.

49. Adams, S.L., Alwine, J.C., deCrombrugghe, B., and Pastan, I.: Use of recombinant plasmids to characterize collagen RNAs in normal and transformed chick embryo fibroblasts. J. Biol. Chem. 254:4935, 1972.

50. Southern, E.M.: Detection of specific sequences among DNA fragments separated by gel electrophoresis. J. Mol. Biol. 98:503, 1975.

51. Orkin, S.H., Kazazian, H.H., Antonarakis, S.E., Goff, S.C., Boehm, C.D., Sexton, J.P., Waber, P.G., and Giardina, P.J.: Linkage of β-thalassaemia mutations and β-globin gene polymorphisms with DNA polymorphisms in human β-globin gene cluster. Nature 296:627, 1982.

52. Boehm, D.C., Antonarakis, S.E., Phillips, J.A., Stelten, G., and Kazazian, H.H.: Prenatal diagnosis using DNA polymorphism. N. Engl. J. Med. 308:1034, 1983.

53. Pyeritz, R.E., and McKusick, V.A.: Basic defects in the Marfan syndrome. New Engl. J. Med. 305:1011, 1981.

54. Tsipouras, P., Myers, T.C., Ramirez, F., and Prockop, D.J.: Restriction fragment length polymorphism associated with the proα2(I) gene of human type I procollagen. J. Clin. Invest. 72:1262, 1983.

55. Pyeritz, R.: The Marfan phenotype: pleiotropy and variability as clues to genetic heterogeneity. In Akeson, W.H., Bornstein, P., and Glimcher, M.J. (eds.): Heritable Disorders of Connective Tissue. St. Louis. The C.V. Mosby Company, 1980, p. 114.

56. Beighton, P.: Inherited Disorders of the Skeleton. Edinburgh, Churchill Livingstone, 1978, p. 222.

57. McKusick, V.A.: The Heritable Disorders of Connective tissue. St. Louis. The C.V. Mosby Company, 1979, p. 70.

58. McKusick, V.A.: The classification of heritable disorders of connective tissue. Birth Defects. Original article series 1116:7, 1975.

59. Pyeritz, R., and McKusick, V.A.: The Marfan syndrome: Diagnosis and management. New Engl. J. Med. 300:772, 1958.

60. Lynas, M.A., and Merretl, J.D.: Data on linkage in man, Marfan's syndrome in Northern Ireland. Ann. Hum. Genet. 22:310, 1958.

61. Sinclair, R.J.G., Kitchen, A.H., and Turner, R.W.D.: The Marfan syndrome. Q. J. Med. 113:19, 1960.

62. Steinberg, I.: A simple screening test for the Marfan syndrome. Am. J. Roentgen. 97:118, 966.

63. Walker, B.A., and Murdock, J.L.: The wrist sign: A useful physical finding in the Marfan syndrome. Ann. Intern. Med. 126:276, 1970.

64. Savini, R., Cervellati, S., and Beroaldo, E.: Spinal deformities in Marfan's syndrome. Ital. J. Orthop. Traumatol. 1:19, 1980.

65. Maumenee, I.H.: The eye in the Marfan syndrome. Trans. Am. Ophthalmol. Soc. 79:684, 1981.

66. Spangler, R.D., Nora, J.J., Lortscher, R.H., Wolf, R.R., and Okin, J.R.: Echocardiography in Marfan's syndrome. Chest 69:72, 1976.

67. Roberts, W.C., and Honig, H.S.: The spectrum of cardiovascular disease in the Marfan syndrome: A clinico-morphologic study of 18 necropsy patients. Am. Heart J. 104:115, 1982.

68. Pyeritz, R.E.: Maternal and fetal complications of pregnancy in the Marfan syndrome. Am. J. Med. 71:784, 1981.

69. Donaldson, R.M., Emanuel, W.W., Olsen, J.G.E., and Rosse, D.N.: Management of cardiovascular complications in the Marfan syndrome. Lancet 2:1178, 1980.

70. McDonald, G.K.R., Schaff, H.V., Pyeritz, R.E., McKusick, V.A., and Gott, V.L.: Surgical management of patients with the Marfan syndrome and dilation of the ascending aorta. J. Thorac. Cardiovasc. Surg. 81:180, 1981.

71. Berliner, S., Dean, H., and Pinkhas, J.: Spontaneous pneumothorax in a patient with Marfan syndrome. Respiration 42:127, 1981.

72. Gawkrodger, D.J.: Marfan's syndrome presenting as bilateral spontaneous pneumothorax. Postgrad. Med. 57:240, 1981.

73. Reye, R.D., and Bale, P.M.: Elastic tissue in pulmonary emphysema in Marfan syndrome. Arch. Pathol. 96:427, 1973.

74. Emanuel, R., Marcomichelakis, E., Mores, C., Jefferson, K., Macfaul, P.A., and Withers, R.: Formes fruste of Marfan's syndrome presenting with severe aortic regurgitation. Clinicogenetic study of 18 families. Br. Heart J. 39:190, 1977.

75. Barron, M.W., Simpson, C.F., and Miller, E.S.: Lathyrism: A review. Q. Rev. Biol. 49:101, 1974.

76. Carner, W.H.: Copper and connective tissue metabolism. Int. Rev. Conn. Tissue Res. 4:197, 1968.

77. Priest, R.E., and Moinuddin, J.F.: Collagen of Marfan syndrome is abnormally soluble. Nature 245:264, 1973.

78. Francis, G., Donnelly, P.V., and DiFerrante, N.: Abnormally soluble collagen produced in fibroblasts in cultures. Experientia 326:691, 1976.

79. Abraham, P.A., Perejda, A.J., Carnes, W.H., and Uitto, J.: Marfan syndrome demonstration of abnormal elastin in aorta. J. Clin. Invest. 70:1245, 1982.

80. Boucek, R.J., Noble, N.L., Gunja-Smith, Z., and Butler, W.T.: The Marfan syndrome: A deficiency in chemically stable collagen crosslinks. N. Engl. J. Med. 305:989, 1982.

81. Byers, P.H., Siegel, R.C., Peterson, K.E., Rowe, D.W., Holbrook, K.A., Smith, L.T., Chang Y-H, and Fu, J.C.: Marfan's syndrome: Abnormal α_2 chain in type I collagen. Proc. Natl. Acad. Sci. 78:7745, 1981.

82. Saruk, M., and Eisenstein, R.: Aortic lesion in Marfan syndrome. Arch. Pathol. Lab. Med. 101:74, 1977.

83. Schlatmann, T.J.M., and Becker, A.E.: Pathogenesis of dissecting aneurysm of aorta comparative histopathologic study of significance of medical changes. Am. J. Cardiol. 39:21, 1977.

84. Lamsberg, S.I., and Dorfman, A.: Synthesis and degradation of hyaluronic acid in cultured fibroblasts of Marfan's disease. J. Clin. Invest. 52:2428, 1973.

85. Appel, A.B., Horowitz, A.L., and Dorfman, A.: Cell-free synthesis of hyaluronic acid in Marfan syndrome. J. Biol. Chem. 254:12199, 1979.

86. Cotton, D.J., and Brandt, K.: Cardiovascular abnormalities in the Marfanoid hypermobility syndrome. Arthritis Rheum. 19:763, 1976.

87. Walker, B.A., Beighton, P., and Murdoch, J.L.: The Marfanoid hypermobility syndrome. Ann. Intern. Med. 71:349, 1969.

88. Schuttle, J.E., Gaffney, F.A., Blend, L., and Blumquist, C.G.: Distinctive anthropometric characteristics of women with mitral valve prolapse. Am. J. Med. 71:533, 1981.

89. Goodman, R.M., Baba, N., and Wooley, C.: Observations on the heart in a case of combined Ehlers-Danlos and Marfan's syndromes. Am. J. Cardiol. 24:734, 1969.

90. Marfan, A.B.: Un cas de déformation des quatre membres, plus prononcé aux extremités, charaterisée par l'allongement des as avec un certain degré d'amincement. Bull. Mem. Soc. Med. Hôp. (Paris) 13:220, 1896.

91. Beals, R.K., and Hecht, I.: Congenital contractual arachnodactyly. J. Bone Joint Surg. 53A:987, 1971.

92. Epstein, C.J., Graham, C.B., Hodgkin, W.F., Hecht, F., and Motulsky, A.G.: Hereditary dysplaysia of bone with kyphoscoliosis, contractures, and abnormally shaped ears. J. Pediatr. 73:379, 1968.

93. Meinecke, P.: Marfan-like features and congenital contractural arachnodactyly. J. Pediatr. 100:1006, 1982.

94. Bass, H.N., Sparkes, R.S., Crandall, B.F., and Marcy, M.S.: Congenita contractural arachnodactyly, keratoconus and probably Marfan syndrome in the same pedigree. J. Pediatr. 94:591, 1981.

95. Mudd, S.H., and Levy, H.L.: Disorders of transsulfuration. *In* Stanbury, J.B., et al. (eds.): The Metabolic Basis of Inherited Disease, New York, McGraw-Hill Book Company, 1983, p. 533.

96. Carson, N., Dent, C., Field, C., and Gaull, G.: Homocystinuria—clinical and pathological review of ten cases. J. Pediatr. 66:565, 1965.

97. Brenton, D.P., Dow, C.J., James, J.I.P., Hay, R.L., and Wynne-Davies, R.: Homocystinuria and Marfan's syndrome. A comparison. J. Bone Joint Surg. 54B:277, 1972.

98. Brenton, D.: Skeletal abnormalities in homocystinuria. Postgrad. Med. J. 53:488, 1977.

99. Westerman, M., Greenfield, G., and Wong, P.: "Fish vertebrae," homocystinuria and sickle cell anemia. JAMA 230:8, 1980.

100. Schedewie, H., Willich, E., Grobe, H., Schmidt, H., and Muller, K.M.: Skeletal findings in homocystinuria: a collaborative study. Pediatr. Radiol. 1:12, 1973.

101. Regenbogen, L., Ilie, S., and Elian, I.: Homocystinuria—a surgical and anaesthetic risk. Metabol. Ophthalmol. 4:209, 1980.

102. Schulman, J., Mudd, H., Schneider, J., Spielberg, S., Boxer, L., Oliver, J., Corash, L., and Sheetz, M.: Genetic disorders of glutathione and sulfur amino-acid metabolism. Ann. Intern. Med. 93:330, 1980.

103. Fowler, K.B., Kraus, J., Packman, S., and Rosenberg, L.: Evidence for three distinct classes of cystathionine beta-synthase mutants in cultured fibroblasts. J. Clin. Invest. 61:645, 1978.

104. Pullon, D.H.H.: Homocystinuria and other methionunemias. *In* Bickel, H., Guthrie, R., Hammerson, G. (eds.): Neonatal screening for inborn errors of metabolism. Berlin, Springer Verlag, 1980, p. 29.

105. Goldstein, J.L., Campbell, B.K., and Gartler, S.M.: Cystathionine synthase activity in human lymphocytes. Induction by phytohemagglutin. J. Clin. Invest. 51:1034, 1972.

106. McDonald, L., Bray, C., Field, C., Love, F., and Davies, B.: Homocystinuria, thrombosis and the blood platelets. Lancet 1:745, 1964.

107. Barber, G.W., and Spaeth, G.L.: The successful treatment of homocystinuria with pyridoxine. J. Pediatr. 75:463, 1969.

108. Harker, L.A., Ross, R., Slichter, S.J., and Scott, C.R.: Homocysteine induced arteriosclerosis: the role of endothelial cell injury and platelet response in its genesis. J. Clin. Invest. 58:731, 1976.

109. Harris, E.D., and Sjoerdsma, A.: Collagen profiles in various clinical conditions. Lancet 2:707, 1966.

110. Kang, A., and Trelstad, R.: A collagen defect in homocystinuria. Clin. Invest. 52:2571, 1973.

111. Kelly, T., Wilson, W., and Squillaro, E.: Homocystinuria: need for early diagnosis and therapy. Vir. Med. 109:392, 1982.

112. Grobe, H.: Homocystinuria (cystathionine synthase deficiency). Results of treatment in late-diagnosed patients. Eur. J. Pediatr. 135:199, 1980.

113. Thomas, P., and Carson, N.: Homocystinuria: the evolution of skeletal changes in relation to treatment. Ann. Radiol. 21:95, 1978.

114. Harpey, J., Rosenblatt, K.D., Cooper, C.R., and Lafourcade, J.: Homocystinuria caused by 5, 10-methylenetetrahydrofolate reductase deficiency: a case in an infant responding to methionine, folinic acid, pyridoxine, and vitamin B12 therapy. J. Pediatr. 98:275, 1981.

115. Wiliken, D.E., Wiliken, B., Dudman, N.P., and Tyrrell, P.A.: Homocystinuria—the effects of betaine in the treatment of patients not responsive to pyridoxine. N. Engl. J. Med. 309:448, 1983.

116. Schulman, J.D., Agarival, B., Mudd, S.W., and Shulman, N.R.: Pulmonary embolism in a homocystinuric patient during treatment with dipyridamole and acetyl salicylic acid. N. Engl. J. Med. 229:661, 1978.

117. Hollister, D.W.: Heritable disorders of connective tissue: Ehler-Danlos syndrome. Pediatr. Clin. North Am. 25:575, 1978.

118. McKusick, V.A.: Heritable Disorders of Connective Tissue. St. Louis. The C.V. Mosby Company, 1972, p. 292.

119. McEntyre, R.L., and Raffensberger, J.G.: Surgical complications of Ehlers-Danlos syndrome in children. J. Pediatr. Surg. 12:531, 1977.

120. Beighton, P.: The Ehlers-Danlos syndrome. London, William Heinemann Medical Books, Ltd., 1970.

121. O'Neill, S., Sweeney, J., Walker, F., and O'Dwyer, W.F.: Pneumothorax in the Ehlers-Danlos syndrome. Irish J. Med. Sci. 150:43, 1981.

122. Leier, C.V., Call, T.D., Tulkerson, P.K., and Woolery, C.F.: The spectrum of cardiac defects in the Ehlers-Danlos syndrome types I and III. Ann. Intern. Med. 92:171, 1980.

123. Cupo, L.N., Pyeritz, R.E., Olson, J.L., McPhee, S.J., Hutchins, G.M., and McKusick, V.: Ehlers-Danlos syndrome with abnormal collagen fibrils, sinus of Valsalva aneurysms, myocardial infarction, panacinar emphysema and cerebral heterotopia. Am. J. Med. 71:1051, 1981.

124. Wynne-Davies, R.: Acetabular dysplasia and familial joint laxity: Two etiological factors in congenital dislocation of the hip. A review of 589 patients and their families. J. Bone Joint Surg. 52B:704, 1970.

125. Beighton, P., and Horan, F.: Orthopedic aspects of the Ehlers-Danlos syndrome. J. Bone Thorac. Surg. 51B:444, 1969.

126. Bird, H.A., Tribe, C.R., and Bacon, P.A.: Joint hypermobility leading to osteoarthrosis and chondrocalcinosis. Bull. Rheum. Dis. 37:203, 1978.

127. Osborn, T.G., Lichenstein, J.R., Moore, T.L., Weiss, T., and Zuckner, J.: Ehlers-Danlos syndrome presenting as rheumatic manifestations in the child. J. Rheumatol. 8:79, 1981.

128. Coventry, M.B.: Some skeletal changes in the Ehlers-Danlos syndrome. J. Bone Joint Surg. 43A:855, 1961.

129. Biering, A., and Iversen, T.: Osteogenesis imperfecta associated with the Ehlers-Danlos syndrome. Acta Paediatr. 44:279, 1955.

130. Kirk, J.A., Ansell, B., and Bymators, E.G.L.: The hypermobility syndrome. Ann. Rheum. Dis. 26:419, 1967.

131. Boone, D.C., and Azen, S.P.: Normal range of motion of joints in male subjects. J. Bone Joint Surg. 61A:756, 1979.

132. Wood, P.H.N.: Is hypermobility a discrete clinical entity. Proc. Roy. Soc. Med. 64:30, 1971.

133. Green, F.A., Wood, P.H.N., and Sackett, D.L.: The effect of age, body weight, and use on joint movement in a random population study. Arthritis Rheum. 8:444A, 1965.

134. Beighton, P., Grahame, R., and Bird, H.: Hypermobility of Joints. Berlin, Springer-Verlag, 1983, pp. 61, 66 and 150.

135. Finsterbush, A., and Pogrund, H.: The hypermobility syndrome. Clin. Orthop. 168:124, 1982.

136. Horton, W.A., Collins, D.L., De Smet, A.A., Kennedy, J.A., and Schimke, R.N.: Familial joint instability syndrome. Am. J. Med. Genet. 6:221, 1980.

137. Grahame, R., Pitcher, E.D., Gabell, A., and Harvey, W.: A clinical and echocardiographic study of patients with hypermobility syndrome. Am. Rheum. Dis. 40:541, 1981.

138. Pitcher, D., and Grahame, R.: Mitral valve prolapse and joint hyper-

mobility: evidence for a systemic connective tissue abnormality. Ann. Rheum. Dis. 41:352, 1982.

139. Jessee, E.F., Owen, D.S., and Sagar, K.B.: The benign hypermobile joint syndrome. Arthritis Rheum. 23:1053, 1980.

140. Stewart, R.E., Hollister, P.W., and Rimoin, D.C.: A new variant of Ehlers-Danlos syndrome: An autosomal dominant disorder of fragile skin, abnormal scarring and generalized peridontitis. Birth Defects XIII (38):85, 1977.

141. Hollister, D.W.: Clinical features of Ehlers-Danlos syndromes types VIII and IX. *In* Akeson, W.H., Bornstein, P., Glimcher, V.M.J. (eds.): AAOS Symposium on Heritable Disorders of Connective Tissue. St. Louis. The C.V. Mosby Company, 1982, p. 102.

142. Hernandez, A., Acquirre-Negrete, S., Liparoli, J.C., and Cantu, J.M.: Third case of a distinct variant of the Ehlers-Danlos syndrome. Clin. Genet. 20:222, 1981.

143. Byers, P.H., Barsh, G.S., and Holbrook, K.A.: Molecular mechanisms of connective tissue abnormalities in the Ehlers-Danlos syndrome. Coll. Res. 5:475, 1981.

144. Holbrook, K.A., and Byers, P.H.: Structural abnormalities in the dermal collagen and elastin matrix from the skin of patients with inhibited connective tissue disorders. J. Invest. Dermatol. 79:7s, 1982.

145. Vogel, A., Holbrook, K.A., Steinman, B., Gitzelman, R., and Byers, P.H.: Abnormal collagen fibril structure in the gravis form (type I) of Ehlers-Danlos syndrome. Lab. Invest. 40:201, 1979.

146. Sevenich, M., Schultz-Ehrenburg, U., and Orfanos, C.E.: Ehlers-Danlos syndrome: Eine fibroblasten-und kollagen krankheit. Arch. Dermatol. Res. 267:237, 1980.

147. Bilkey, W.J., Baxter, T.L., Kottke, F.J., and Mundale, M.D.: Muscle function in Ehlers-Danlos syndrome. Arch. Phys. Med. Rehabil. 62:444, 1981.

148. Sheon, R.P., Kursner, A.B., Farber, S.V., and Finkel, R.I.: The hypermobility syndrome. Postgrad. Med. 71:199, 1982.

149. Uden, A.: Collagen and bleeding diathesis in Ehlers-Danlos syndrome. Scand. J. Haematol. 28:425, 1982.

150. Becker, U., Timpl, R., Helle, O., and Prockop, D.: NH₂-terminal extensions on skin collagen from sheep with a genetic defect in conversion of procollagen into collagen. Biochemistry 15:2853, 1976.

151. Lichtenstein, J.R., Martin, G.R., Kuhn, L.D., Byers, P.H., and McKusick, V.A.: Defect in conversion of procollagen to collagen in a form of Ehlers-Danlos syndrome. Science 183:298, 1973.

152. Leung, M.K., Fessler, L.I., Greenberg, D.B., and Kessler, J.H.: Separate amino and carboxyl procollagen peptidase in chick embryo tendons. J. Biol. Chem. 254:224, 1979.

153. Steinmann, B., Tuderman, L., Peltonen, L., Martin, G.R., McKusick, V.A., and Prockop, D.J.: Evidence for a structural mutation of procollagen type I in a patient with the Ehlers-Danlos Syndrome type VII. J. Biol. Chem. 255:8887, 1980.

154. Barabas, A.P.: Heterogenity of the Ehlers-Danlos syndrome: Description of three clinical types and a hypothesis to explain the basic defects. Br. Med. J. 2:612, 1967.

155. Beighton, P.: Lethal complications of the Ehlers-Danlos syndrome. Br. Med. J. 3:656, 1968.

156. Pope, F.M., Nicholls, A.C., Jones, P.M., Wells, R.S., and Lawrence, D.: EDS IV (acrogyria): New autosomal and dominant types. J. Roy. Soc. Med. 73:180, 1980.

157. Byers, P.H., Holbrook, K.A., and Barsh, G.S.: Ehlers-Danlos syndrome type IV: Disorders of type III collagen metabolism. *In* Akeson, W.H., Bornstein, P., and Glimcher, V.M.J. (eds.): AAOS Symposium on Heritable Disorders of Connective Tissue. St. Louis. The C.V. Mosby Company, 1982, p. 76.

158. Jaffe, A.S., Getman, E.M., Rodney, G.E., and Uitto, J.: Mitral valve prolapse: A consistent manifestation of type IV Ehlers-Danlos syndrome. Circulation 64:121, 1981.

159. Wesley, J.R., Mattour, G.H., and Woolley, M.M.: Multiple surgical problems in two patients with Ehlers-Danlos syndrome. Surgery 87:319, 1980.

160. Pope, F.M., Martin, G.R., Lichtenstein, J.R., Penttinen, R., Gerson, B., Rowe, D.W., and McKusick, V.A.: Patients with Ehler's Danlos syndrome type IV lack type III collagen. Proc. Natl. Acad. Sci. 72:1314, 1975.

161. Byers, P.H., Holbrook, K.A., McGillivray, B., MacLeod, P.M., and Lowry, R.B.: Clinical and ultrastructural heterogeneity of type IV Ehlers-Danlos syndrome. Hum. Genet. 47:141, 1979.

162. Pinnell, S.R., Krane, S.M., Kenzora, J.E., and Glimcher, M.J.: A heritable disorder of connective tissue: Hydroxylysine-deficient collagen disease. N. Engl. J. Med. 286:1013, 1972.

163. Krane, S.M.: Hydroxylysine-deficient collagen disease: A form of Ehlers-Danlos syndrome. *In* Akeson, W.H., Bornstein, P., and Glimcher, V.M.J. (eds.): AAOS Symposium on Heritable Disorders of Connective Tissue. The C.V. Mosby Company, 1982, p. 61.

164. Steinmann, B., Gitzelman, R., Vogel, A., Grant, M.E., Harwood, R., and Sear, C.H.J.: Ehlers-Danlos syndrome in two siblings with deficient lysyl hydroxylase activity in cultured skin fibroblasts but only mild hydroxylysine deficit in skin. Helv. Pediatr. Acta 30:255, 1975.

165. Krane, S.M., Pinnell, S.R., and Erbe, R.W.: Lysyl-protocollagen hydroxylase deficiency in fibroblasts from siblings with hydroxylysine-deficient collagen. Proc. Natl. Acad. Sci. 69:2899, 1972.

166. Sussman, M., Lichtenstein, J.R., Nigra, T.P., Martin, G.R., and McKusick, V.A.: Hydroxylysine-deficient skin collagen in a patient with a form of the Ehlers-Danlos syndrome. J. Bone Joint Surg. 56A:1228, 1974.

167. Quinn, R.S., and Krane, S.M.: Abnormal properties of collagen lysyl hydroxylase from skin fibroblasts of siblings with hydroxylysine-deficient collagen. J. Clin. Invest. 57:83, 1976.

168. Elsas, L.J., Miller, R.L., and Pinnell, S.P.: Inherited human collagen lysyl hydrolylase deficiency: Ascorbic acid response. J. Pediatr. 92:378, 1978.

169. Judisch, G.F., Waziri, M., and Krachmer, J.H.: Ocular Ehlers-Danlos syndrome with normal lysyl hydroxylase activity. Arch. Ophthalmol. 94:1489, 1976.

170. Turpeenniemi-Hujanen, T.M., Puistola, U., and Kivirikko, K.A.I.: Human lysyl hydroxylase: Purification to homogenity, partial characterization and comparison of catalytic properties with those of a mutant enzyme from Ehlers-Danlos Syndrome I-VI fibroblasts. Coll. Rel. Res. 1:355, 1981.

171. Eyre, D.R., and Glimcher, M.J.: Reducible crosslink in hydroxylysine-deficient collagens of a heritable disorder of connective tissue. Proc. Natl. Acad. Sci. 69:2594, 1972.

172. Arneson, M.A., Hammerschmidt, D.E., Furcht, L.T., and King, R.A.: A new form of Ehlers-Danlos syndrome. JAMA 244:144, 1980.

173. DiFerrante, N., Leachman, R.D., Angelini, P., Donnelly, P.V., Francis, G., Almazan, A., Guiseppe, S., and Franzblau, C.: Ehlers-Danlos Type V (X-linked form): A lysyl oxidase deficiency. Conn. Tissue Res. 3:49, 1975.

174. Lazoff, S.G., Rybak, J.J., Parker, B.R., and Lyzzatti, L.: Skeletal dysplasia, occipital horns, diarrhea and obstructive uropathy—a new hereditary syndrome. Birth Defects 9:71, 1975.

175. Kuivaniemi, H., Peltonen, L., Palotie, A., Kaitila, I., and Kivirikko, K.I.: Abnormal copper metabolism and deficient lysyl oxidase activity in a heritable connective tissue disorder. J. Clin. Invest. 69:730, 1982.

176. Shapiro, J.R., Kaiser-Kupfer, M.I., Pikus, A., and Rowe, D.W.: Osteogensis imperfecta: Current clinical research. *In* Akeson, W.J., Bornstein, P., and Glimicher, M.J. (eds): AAOS Symposium on Heritable Disorders of Connective Tissue. St. Louis, The C.V. Mosby Company, 1982, p. 238.

177. Wynne-Davies, R., and Gormley, J.: Clinical and genetic patterns in osteogenesis imperfecta. Clin. Orthop. 159:26, 1981.

178. Gunnear, S.: Osteogenesis Imperfecta. Sweden, Stockholm University Books, 1961.

179. Sillence, D.O., and Danks, D.M.: Genetic heterogeneity in osteogenesis imperfecta. J. Med. Genet. 16:101, 1979.

180. Bergstrom, L.: Osteogenesis imperfecta, otologic and maxillofacial aspects. Laryngoscope 87(Suppl. 6):1, 1977.

181. Levin, L.S.: The dentition in the osteogenesis imperfecta syndromes. Clin. Orthop. 159:64, 1981.

182. Shapiro, J.R., Pikus, A., Weiss, G., and Rowe, D.W.: Hearing and middle ear function in osteogenesis imperfecta. JAMA 247:2120, 1982.

183. Brown, D.M.: Biochemical abnormalities in osteogenesis imperfecta. Clin. Orthop. 159:75, 1981.

184. Shapiro, J.R., Levine, J., and Bercu, B.: The thyroid-pituitary axis is normal in osteogenesis imperfecta. In preparation.

185. Cohen, I.M., Vieweg, W.V.R., Alpert, J.S., Kaufman, J.A., and Hagan, A.D.: Osteogenesis imperfecta tarda; cardiovascular pathology. West. J. Med. 126:228, 1977.

186. Shapiro, J.R., Tsipouras, P., Maron, B., and Hartrop, J.: Echocardiographic findings in osteogenesis imperfecta. Submitted for publication.

187. Patterson, C.R.: Osteogenesis imperfecta in the differential diagnosis of child abuse. Arch. Dis. Child. 52:808, 1977.

188. Siegel, B.M., Friedman, I.A., and Schwarts, S.P.: Hemorrhage disease in osteogenesis imperfecta. Am. J. Med. 22:315, 1957.

189. Rowe, D.W., Shapiro, J.R., Poirier, M., and Schlesinger, S.: Segregation of a defect in type I collagen biosynthesis in a family with dominantly inherited Osteogenesis imperfecta. Submitted for publication.

190. Rowe, D.W., Poirier, M., and Shapiro, J.R.: Osteogenesis imperfecta: a genetic probe to study type I collagen synthesis. *In* Veis, A., and Butler, W.T. (eds.): Chemistry and Biology of Mineralized Matrix. New York, Elsevier-North Holland Press, 1981, p. 213.

191. Sykes, B., Francis, N.J., and Smith, R.: Altered relation of two collagen types in osteogenesis imperfecta. N. Engl. J. Med. 296:1200, 1977.

192. Shapiro, J.R., Ahlgren, A., Triche, T., McDonald, D., and Rowe, D.W.: Light and electronmicroscopic abnormalities of bone and collagen in osteogenesis imperfecta. In preparation.

193. Barsh, G.S., David, K.E., and Byers, P.H.: Type I osteogenesis imperfecta: A non-functional allele for proα₁(I) chains of type I procollagen. Proc. Natl. Acad. Sci. 79:3838, 1982.

194. Rowe, D.W., Stover, M.L., Poirier, M., Genovese, C., and Shapiro, J.R. : Low type I collagen mRNA in type I osteogenesis imperfecta. In preparation.

195. Shapiro, J.R., and Rowe, D.W.: Collagen genes and brittle bones. Ann. Intern. Med., 99:700, 1983.

196. Lubs, H.A., and Traver, H.: Genetic counseling in osteogenesis imperfecta. Clin. Orthop. 159:36, 1981.

197. Williams, C.J., and Prockop, D.J.: Synthesis and processing of a type I procollagen containing shortened proα_1(I) chains by fibroblasts from a patient with osteogenesis imperfecta. J. Biol. Chem. 258:5915, 1983.

198. Cremin, B., Goodman, H., Prax, M., Spranger, J., and Beighton, P.: Wormian bones in osteogenesis imperfecta and other disorders. Skeletal Radiol. 8:35, 1982.

199. Milsom, I., Mattsson, L.A., and Dahlen-Nilsson, I.: Antenatal diagnosis of osteogenesis imperfecta by real time ultrasound: two case reports. Br. J. Radiol. 55:310, 1982.

200. Shapiro, J.E., Byers, P.H., Levin, S.L., Barsh, G.S., and Goldstein, P.: Prenatal diagnosis of lethal perinatal osteogenesis imperfecta (OI type II). J. Pediatr. 100:127, 1982.

201. Tsipouras, P., Shields, E.P., Silbergerg, D., and Fraser, F.C.: Genetics of osteogenesis imperfecta type II. Pediatr. Res. 15:570, 1981.

202. Barsh, G.S., and Byers, P.H.: Abnormal secretion of type I procollagen in a variety of osteogenesis imperfecta. Proc. Natl. Acad. Sci. 78:5142, 1981.

203. Pope, F.M., Nicholls, A.C., Eggleton, C., Narcissi, P., Heg, E.N., and Parkin, J.M.: Osteogenesis imperfecta (lethal) bones contain type III and V collagen. J. Clin. Pathol. 33:534, 1980.

204. Sillence, D.O., and Rimoin, D.L.: Morphological studies in osteogenesis imperfecta. In Ackeson, W.J., Bornstein, P., and Glimcher, M.J. (eds.): AAOS Symposium on Heritable Disorders of Connective Tissue. The C.V. Mosby Company, 1982, p. 259.

205. Chu, M.L., Williams, C.J., Pepe, G., Hirsch, J., Prockop, D.J., and Ramierz, F.: Internal deletion in a collagen gene in a perinatal lethal form of osteogenesis imperfecta. Nature 304:48, 1983.

206. Prockop, D.J., William, C., deWet, W., Lippola, M., Uitto, J., and Pihlajaniemi, T.: Shortening and lengthening of proα chains of type I procollagen in osteogenesis imperfecta. Clin. Res. 31:533A, 1983.

207. Frank, E., Berger, T., and Tew, J.M.: Basilar impression and platybasia in osteogenesis imperfecta tarda. Surg. Neurol. 17:116, 1982.

208. Bullough, P.G., Davidson, D.D., and Lorenzo, J.C.: The morbid anatomy of the skeleton in osteogenesis imperfecta. Clin. Orthop. 159:42, 1981.

209. Peltonen, L., Palotie, A., and Prockop, D.J.: A defect in the structure of type I procollagen in a patient who had osteogenesis imperfecta: Excess mannose in the COOH-terminal propeptide. Proc. Natl. Acad. Sci. 77:6179, 1980.

210. Levin, L.S., Brady, J.M., and Melnick, M.: Scanning electron microscopy of teeth in dominant osteogenesis imperfecta. Support for genetic heterogeneity. Am. J. Med. Genet. 5:189, 1980.

211. Nicholls, A.C., and Pope, F.M.: Biochemical heterogeneity of osteogenesis imperfecta: A new variant. Lancet 1:1193, 1979.

212. Chu, M.L., Nicholls, A.R., Pope, F.M., Rowe, D.W., and Prockop, D.J.: Presence of mRNA for proα2(I) chains in fibroblasts from a patient with osteogenesis imperfecta whose type I collagen does not contain α1(I) chains. Submitted for publication.

213. Byers, P.H., Shapiro, J.R., Rowe, D.W., Holbrook, K., and David, K.E.: An abnormal α2 chain in type I collagen from a patient with a form of osteogenesis imperfecta. J. Clin. Invest. 71:689, 1983.

214. Rowe, D.W., Shapiro, J.R., Poirier, M., and Schlessinger, S.: Type I collagen synthesis in a family with sporadically inherited osteogenesis imperfecta. Pediatr. Res. 17:218A, 1983.

215. Albright, J.P., Albright, J.A., and Crelin, E.S.: Osteogenesis imperfecta tarda: The morphology of rib biopsies. Clin. Orthop. 108:204, 1975.

216. Albright, J.P.: Systemic treatment of osteogenesis imperfecta. Clin. Orthop. 159:88, 1981.

217. Smith, R., Francis, M.J.O., and Houghton, G.R.: The brittle bone syndrome, osteogenesis imperfecta. Kent, Butterworths, 1982, p. 141.

218. Moorefield, W.G., and Miller, G.R.: Aftermath of osteogenesis imperfecta, the disease of adulthood. J. Bone Joint Surg. 62A:113, 1980.

219. Rodriquez, R.P., and Bailey, R.W.: Internal fixation of the femur in patients with osteogenesis imperfecta. Clin. Orthop. 159:126, 1981.

220. Bleck, E.E.: Nonoperative treatment of osteogenesis imperfecta. Clin. Orthop. 159:111, 1981.

221. Shapiro, J.R., Gerber, N.L., and Binder, H.: The use of lightweight splints to facilitate early ambulation in osteogenesis imperfecta. In preparation.

222. Beighton, P.: The dominant and recessive forms of cutis laxa. J. Med. Genet. 9:216, 1972.

223. Byers, P.H., Siegel, R.C., Holbrook, K., Narayanan, S.A., Bornstein, P., and Hall, J.G.: X-linked cutis laxa; defective crosslink formation due to decreased lysyl oxidase activity. New Engl. J. Med. 202:61, 1980.

224. Uitto, J., Ryhanen, L., Abraham, P.A., and Perejda, A.J.: Elastin in diseases. J. Invest. Dermatol. 79:160s, 1982.

225. Linares, A., Zarranz, J.J., Rodriquez-Alarcon, J., and Diaz-Perez, S.L.: Reversible cutis laxa due to maternal D-penicillamine treatment. Lancet 2:43, 1974.

226. Marshall, J., Heyl, T., and Weber, H.: Postinflammatory elastolysis and cutis laxa. S. Afr. Med. J. 40:1016, 1966.

227. Hajjer, B.A., and Jayner, E.N.: Congenital cutis laxa with advanced cardiopulmonary disease. J. Pediatr. 73:116, 1968.

228. Goltz, R.W., Hult, A.M., Goldfarb, M., and Gorlin, R.W.: Cutis laxa a manifestation of generalized elastolysis. Arch. Dermatol. 92:373, 1965.

229. Weir, K.E., Jaffe, H.S., Blaufuss, A.H., and Beighton, P.: Cardiovascular abnormalities in cutis laxa. Eur. J. Cardiol. 5:253, 1977.

230. Merten, D.F., and Roonery, R.: Progressive pulmonary emphysema associated with generalized elastolysis (cutis laxa). Radiology 13:691, 1974.

231. Meine, R., Grasman, H., Forman, W., and Jackson, D.: The radiographic findings in congenital cutis laxa. Radiology 113:687, 1974.

232. Marchase, P., Holbrook, R., and Pinnell, S.R.: A familial cutis laxa syndrome with ultra-structural abnormalities of collagen and elastin. J. Invest. Dermatol. 75:399, 1980.

233. Menkes, J.H., Alter, M., Steigledur, G.K., Weakley, D.R., and Sung, J.H.: A sex-linked recessive disorder with retardation, peculiar hair, and facial cerebral and cerebellar degeneration. Pediatrics 29:764, 1962.

234. Wheeler, M.E., and Roberts, P.F.: Menkes' steely hair syndrome. Arch. Dis. Child. 51:269, 1976.

235. Troost, D., Van Rossum, A., Straks, W., and Willemse, J.: Menkes' kinky hair disease. II: a clinicopathologic report of three cases. Brain Rev. 4:115, 1982.

236. Willemse, J., Van deu Hamer, C., Prins, H.W., and Jonker, P.L.: Menkes' kinky hair disease. I. Comparison of classical and unusual clinical and biochemical features in two patients. Brain Rev. 4:105, 1982.

237. Williams, D.M., and Arthur, C.L.: Tissue copper concentrations of patients with Menkes' kinky hair disease. Am. J. Dis. Child. 135:375, 1981.

238. Camakaris, J., Danks, D., Ackland, L., Cartwright, E., Borger, P., and Colton, R.G.H.: Altered copper metabolism in cultured cells from human Menkes' syndrome and mottled mouse mutants. Biochem. Genet. 18:117, 1980.

239. Rowe, D.W., McGoodwin, E.B., Martin, G.H., and Grahn, D.: Lysyl oxidase activity in the aneurysm-prone mottled mouse. J. Biol. Chem. 252:939, 1977.

240. Labadie, G.V., Hirschhorn, K., Katz, S., and Beratis, N.: Increased copper metallothionein in Menkes cultured skin fibroblasts. Pediatr. Res. 15:257, 1981.

241. McKusick, V.: Pseudoxanthoma elasticum. In McKusick, V.: Heritable Disorders of Connective Tissue. St. Louis, The C.V. Mosby Company, 1972, p. 475.

242. Goodman, R.M., Smith, E.W., and Paton, D.: Pseudoxanthoma elasticum; a clinical and histopathological study. Medicine 42:297, 1963.

243. Berlyne, G.M., Bulmer, M.G., and Platt, R.: The genetics of pseudoxanthoma elasticum. Q. J. Med. 30:201, 1961.

244. Pope, F.M.: Historical evidence for the genetic heterogeneity of pseudoxanthoma elasticum. Br. J. Dermatol. 92:493, 1975.

245. Altman, L.K., Fialkow, P.J., Parker, F., and Sagebiel, R.W.: Pseudoxanthoma elasticum. Arch. Intern. Med. 134:1048, 1974.

246. Goette, D.K., and Carpenter, W.M.: The mucocutaneous marker of pseudoxanthoma elasticum. Oral Surg. 51:68, 1981.

247. Carr, R.E., and Noble, K.: Angioid streaks. Ophthalmology 87:263, 1980.

248. Jackson, A., and Loh, C.: Pulmonary calcification and elastic tissue damage in pseudoxanthomas elasticum. Histopathology 4:607, 1980.

249. Przybojewski, J.Z., Maritz, F., Tiedt, F.A.C., and Van der Walt, J.J.: Pseudoxanthoma elasticum with cardiac involvement. S. Afr. Med. J. 59:268, 1981.

250. Navrro-Lopez, F., Llorian, A., Ferrer-Roca, O., Betriv, A., and Sanz, G.: Restrictive cardiomyopathy in pseudoxanthoma elasticum. Chest 78:113, 1980.

251. Lebwohl, M., Distefano, K., Prioleau, P.G., Uram, M., Yannuzzi, L.A., and Fleischmajer, R.: Pseudoxanthoma elasticum and mitral prolapse. N. Engl. J. Med. 307:228, 1982.

252. Meislik, J., Neldner, K., Reeve, E., and Ellis, P.: Laser treatment in the maculopathy of pseudoxanthoma elasticum. Can. J. Ophthalmol. 13:210, 1978.

253. Cunningham, J.R., Lippman, S.M., Reine, W.A., Francomano, C.A., Maumenee, I.H., and Pyeritz, R.E.: Pseudoxanthoma elasticum: Treatment of gastrointestinal hemorrhage by arterial embolization and observations on autosomal dominant inheritance. Johns Hopkins Med. J. 147:168, 1980.

254. Huang, S., et al.: Ultrastructural changes of elastic fibers in pseudoxanthomas elasticum: A study of histogenesis. Arch. Pathol. 83:108, 1967.

255. Uitto, J.: Biochemistry of the elastic fibers in normal connective tissues and its alterations in diseases. J. Invest. Dermatol. 72:1, 1979.

Section XIX
Metabolic Bone Disease

Chapter 106
Metabolic Bone Disease

Frederick R. Singer

INTRODUCTION

A metabolic bone disease can be defined as a skeletal disorder in which the pathologic process is generalized.[1] The generalized nature of the disorder may be readily apparent, as in patients with the recessive form of osteopetrosis, or it may be more subtle, as in patients with primary hyperparathyroidism who have a secondary lesion such as a brown tumor, which may obscure the milder generalized abnormality.

Occasionally disorders of a localized nature, such as Paget's disease of bone, may be confused with a metabolic bone disease because of a widespread distribution of the lesions. Careful appraisal of the skeleton in these cases always reveals the presence of normal bone in some regions.

CLINICAL EVALUATION

The History and Physical Examination

Although the definitive diagnosis of a metabolic bone disease is dependent upon demonstrating the appropriate biochemical, radiologic, and histologic abnormalities, these parameters may not be examined until the information obtained from a careful history and physical examination is appreciated.

Some of the general clinical features that suggest an underlying metabolic bone disease are listed in Table 106–1. Bone pain and symmetrical deformity are prominent features in patients with rickets and osteomalacia. The presence of short stature is a clue to the time of onset of the disease. Muscle weakness and tenderness are frequently associated with rickets and osteomalacia. Tetany reflects the presence of hypocalcemia of any cause. The presence of pathologic fractures is usually an indication of underlying osteoporosis but may also occur in rickets and osteomalacia. Corneal and scleral calcification are found in primary hyperparathyroidism or secondary hyperparathyroidism resulting from renal failure. A large variety of constitutional symptoms often mistaken for "psychoneurotic" complaints may be present in patients with primary hyperparathyroidism or in hypocalcemic states.

Clinical Biochemistry

If possible, blood for analysis should be taken in the fasting state to avoid dietary influences. This is best done in the morning, both in normal subjects whose samples define the normal range of a test and in patients undergoing evaluation, since random sampling may cause greater variation in test results because of the known circadian rhythm of ions such as phosphate. Urinary samples can be obtained in short timed collections after an overnight fast or during a 24-hour period. It is useful to place the patient on a known calcium and phosphorus intake for 3 to 5 days prior to urine collection if urinary studies are to be done.

Serum Calcium. The estimation of the total serum calcium concentration can now be accomplished by several precise techniques that are in close agreement. The most commonly used are atomic absorption spectrophotometry and the automated Technicon Auto-Analyser method. The mean normal serum concentration is approximately 9.5 mg per dl. Ionized calcium represents approximately 50 percent of the total; measurement of this fraction is performed now by a number of commercial laboratories and measures directly the biologically active calcium in blood. Approximately 10 percent of the total serum calcium is present in the form of complexes to phosphate, citrate, and bicarbonate. The biologic role of these complexes is unknown. Since approximately 40 percent of the calcium in serum is bound to proteins (mainly albumin), care should be taken in the sampling of blood.[2] Prolonged use of a tourniquet to obtain the sample can elevate serum albumin concentration and produce a spurious elevation of calcium concentration. Plasma proteins may also increase after changing from the supine to the erect state. It is advisable to obtain a serum albumin determination simultaneously with the initial serum calcium determination even if a proper blood sampling technique is used, since a variety of medical disorders can alter serum albumin concentration. A crude correction factor can then be applied to compensate for the aberrant protein concentration. For every 1 g per dl above or below the normal mean serum albumin concentration in the particular laboratory, 0.8 g per dl should be subtracted or added to the calcium concentration. In general, this maneuver will

1645

Table 106–1. Signs and Symptoms Associated with Metabolic Bone Disease

1. Bone pain
2. Bone deformity
3. Short stature
4. Muscle weakness (proximal)
5. Tetany
6. Fractures
7. Corneal and scleral calcification
8. Vague constitutional symptoms
   a. Malaise
   b. Arthralgias
   c. Irritability
9. Radiographic evidence of osteopenia

give a reasonable estimate of the actual extracellular calcium concentration. In such situations, measurement of the ionized calcium gives a direct measure of the biologically active component.

The finding of an elevated or a diminished serum calcium concentration may indicate the presence of an underlying bone disease such as hyperparathyroidism or osteomalacia, although it must be kept in mind that a normal calcium concentration does not rule out bone disease. Severe generalized osteoporosis and polyostotic Paget's disease of bone usually are associated with the normocalcemic state.

Serum Inorganic Phosphate. The serum inorganic phosphate concentration ranges from 2.5 mg per dl to 4.5 mg per dl in normal adults and may attain levels up to 8.5 mg per dl in normal children.[3] With aging, the concentration tends to rise in females and fall in males. It is particularly important to obtain blood for phosphate determination in the fasting state, since phosphate intake will raise the serum concentration and carbohydrate intake in the absence of phosphate will lower the serum concentration. A circadian variation has been noted with the highest concentrations in the afternoon and evening. False elevations of serum phosphate concentration may result from hemolysis or from prolonged standing of blood prior to separation of cells from serum. Only about 10 percent of the serum inorganic phosphate is bound to plasma proteins.[2]

Serum Alkaline Phosphatase. It is generally accepted that skeletal alkaline phosphatase is important in the mineralization of bone. Although the physiologic role of alkaline phosphatase has yet to be defined completely, this enzyme can serve as a marker of the state of metabolic activity of bone. Histochemical techniques reveal that it is found in abundance in osteoblasts and in some osteocytes but not in osteoclasts.[4] In disorders in which increased numbers of osteoblasts are present in bone, there is usually an elevation of serum alkaline phosphatase activity. It is not certain whether the enzyme is liberated from living or degenerating cells.

Numerous methods have been developed for the estimation of alkaline phosphatase activity.[4] Since the units are not interchangeable, care should be taken to note the normal range for each assay. It should also be appreciated that serum alkaline phosphatase activity is two- to threefold greater in normal children and adolescents than in adults.

A variety of tissues could contribute to the pool of alkaline phosphatase in the circulation. The hepatobiliary system, the intestine, and the placenta are known to release the enzyme into the circulation. Kidney cells and white blood cells also contain alkaline phosphatase, but it is not known if the enzyme escapes these cells. Certain malignant tumors may also be a source of increased serum alkaline phosphatase activity.

Alkaline phosphatase from the skeleton can be distinguished from that of other tissues by a variety of laboratory techniques, but none of them is routine. A simple method of distinguishing the skeletal isoenzyme from that found in the serum of patients with hepatobiliary disease is to determine the enzyme activity that remains after heating the serum at 56° C for 15 minutes. The skeletal isoenzyme activity will fall by 85 to 95 percent, as compared with a 30 to 40 percent decrease in serum enzyme activity in hepatobiliary disease.

Urinary Calcium Excretion. The mean 24-hour urinary calcium on a free diet is approximately 200 mg; males excrete about 20 percent more calcium than do females.[5] The most important determinant of urinary calcium excretion is the filtered load of calcium. Hypercalcemia is usually associated with hypercalciuria and hypocalcemia is associated with hypocalciuria. Parathyroid hormone is an important modulator of renal calcium handling through its action of stimulating renal tubular reabsorption of calcium in the distal tubules.

In disorders in which the rate of bone resorption is in significant excess of the rate of bone formation, hypercalciuria may be considerable. This may be assessed by measuring the 24-hour urinary excretion of calcium or the calcium:creatinine ratio after a 12-hour fast. The latter test can be obtained from a spot urine collection after the bladder has been emptied of the overnight urine. The upper limit of normal is 0.16 when both calcium and creatinine are expressed in the same units. This test primarily reflects the degree of bone resorption and avoids for the most part the influence of dietary calcium. Measurement of 24-hour urinary calcium excretion should be carried out while the patient is on a known dietary calcium intake. This is particularly important in patients who hyperabsorb dietary calcium. In such patients a low calcium intake (400 mg or less per day) may result in a relatively normal urinary excretion of calcium, whereas a normal calcium intake (800 to 1000 mg) will produce hypercalciuria. Sodium intake is also an important determinant of urinary calcium excretion as are diuretic agents. Thiazide diuretics lower urinary calcium excretion, and other diuretics, such as furosemide, raise calcium excretion.

Urinary Phosphate Excretion. A large variety of factors can influence urinary phosphate excretion, but in normal subjects the dominant factor is the dietary phosphate intake.[6] This observation accounts for the relative lack of diagnostic value in the measurement of 24-hour urinary phosphate levels.

Measurement of renal handling of phosphate is a useful test in assessing patients with certain bone disorders. Impairment of tubular reabsorption of phosphate may reflect excessive levels of parathyroid hormone or an inherited or acquired primary renal tubular defect in phosphate reabsorption. This is best assessed by determining the maximal transport capacity for phosphate ($tmPO_4$) above which any increase in filtered load is excreted. Because $tmPO_4$ is proportional to the glomerular filtration rate (GFR), the most appropriate means of expressing tubular reabsorption of phosphate is $tmPO_4$:GFR. This can be determined without infusing phosphate by the following method: (1) after an overnight fast the patient should void and discard the urine; (2) a urine sample should be collected over a 1- to 2-hour period, and blood should be drawn; (3) phosphate and creatinine determinations should be done on the urine and serum specimens; and (4) after calculation of C_{PO_4}/C_{creat}

$$\frac{(U_{PO_4} \times S_{creat})}{S_{PO_4} \times U_{creat}}$$

or tubular reabsorption of phosphate

$$\frac{(1 - C_{PO_4})}{C_{creat}}$$

the nomogram in Figure 106–1 can be used to estimate $tmPO_4$:GFR. The justification for this derivation of $tmPO_4$:GFR. is found in a paper by Walton and Bijvoet.[7]

Urinary Hydroxyproline Excretion. Hydroxyproline is an amino acid that is an important constituent of collagen. It is also found in elastin and circulates as a constituent of C1q in blood. In normal subjects hydroxyproline is excreted into the urine primarily in the form of hydroxyproline-containing peptides of up to 10,000 molecular weight.[8] It is uncertain in normal subjects what the relative contribution of each collagen-containing organ is to the total urinary hydroxyproline excreted daily. However, it has been shown that in patients with bone disease there is a good correlation between urinary hydroxyproline excretion and estimates of the rate of bone resorption. In normal adults on a low-gelatin diet the 24-hour urinary hydroxyproline excretion is less than 40 mg. The highest levels are found in patients with polyostotic Paget's disease, in whom the excretion of more than 2000 mg in 24 hours has been reported.

Serum Parathyroid Hormone. The development of radioimmunoassays for parathyroid hormone during the past 20 years has led to a major advance in the evaluation of patients with metabolic bone disease. The differential diagnosis of hypercalcemic and hypocalcemic states has been aided by the emergence of assays for parathyroid hormone in a number of commercial laboratories. It is no longer necessary to rely on indirect tests of parathyroid function to evaluate the activity of the parathyroid glands. This will be discussed further in the section on Primary Hyperparathyroidism.

Nomogram for derivation of renal threshold phosphate concentration.

Figure 106–1. To derive Tm_{PO_4}/GFR, calculate C_{PO_4}/C_{creat} or T.R.P. (as indicated in text) on a 1 to 2 hour urine collection after an overnight fast. A straight line through the appropriate values of [PO_4] and T.R.P. or C_{PO_4}/C_{er} passes through the corresponding value of Tm_{PO_4}/GFR. Tm_{PO_4}/GFR and [PO_4] are expressed in the same units. Two scales have been chosen: the 0.0 to 2.0 scale estimates Tm_{PO_4}/GFR close to the normal range expressed in S.I. units (0.80 to 1.35 mmol per liter), and the 0.0 to 5.0 scale estimates values expressed in mass units (2.5 to 4.2 mg per deciliter). The scale for [PO_4] and Tm_{PO_4}/GFR can be multiplied or divided by any number, provided that the same number is used for both scales. (From Walton, R.J., and Bijvoet, O.L.M.: Lancet 2:309, 1975.)

Vitamin D Metabolite Assays. Assays for circulating 25-hydroxyvitamin D and 1α,25-dihydroxyvitamin D levels have recently become available in commercial laboratories. Measurement of serum 25-hydroxyvitamin D concentration is the best index of overall vitamin D status. Serum 1α,25-dihydroxyvitamin D levels are of greatest value in evaluating patients with suspected abnormalities of vitamin D metabolism. Use of these assays will be discussed in the sections concerning Primary Hyperparathyroidism and Osteomalacia.

Radiology

Roentgenographic evaluation of the skeleton is a valuable noninvasive means of determining the nature and severity of bone disease in many patients. An appreciation of the most common sites of abnormality is important, as it will reduce the amount of radiation a patient is exposed to and limit the expense of the evaluation.

The "metabolic bone survey" generally consists of a lateral skull radiograph, hand radiographs, lateral thoracic and lumbar spine radiographs, and a pelvic radiograph. In the majority of patients with a generalized bone disease, an abnormality in one or more of these sites would be apparent. If hyperparathyroidism is suspected, films of the lamina dura or clavicles might also be revealing. Areas in which bone pain or deformity is present are also liable to demonstrate roentgenographic abnormality.

Some roentgenographic features that should be looked for in patients with suspected metabolic bone disease include a reduction in bone density, an abnormality of bone texture, widening of the epiphyseal cartilage growth plate, thinning or thickening of the cortex, endosteal scalloping, periosteal new bone formation, fractures or pseudofractures, and abnormalities in the size and shape of bone.

Assessment of the density of bone in patients with osteoporosis has proved to be a difficult task and will be further discussed under Osteoporosis.

The development of high-resolution scanning equipment and technetium-labeled disphosphonates has brought about major improvements in the quality and safety of bone scans in recent years. The main use of the bone scan is to determine if skeletal tracer uptake is symmetric or not. The test is particularly useful in assessing the activity of specific lesions of Paget's disease and in determining the presence of occult metastases in hypercalcemic patients. There has been little use made of bone scans in most metabolic bone diseases, but it has been demonstrated that quantitation of isotope uptake by the skeleton is a good index of skeletal metabolic activity.[9,10]

Bone Biopsy and Microanatomy of Bone

The use of bone biopsies in the evaluation of patients with suspected metabolic bone disease has not been a widely accepted practice in the United States. This has come about because of an insufficient number of physicians who are trained in obtaining iliac crest bone biopsies and because routine pathology departments seldom have the appropriate equipment to process the biopsy specimens properly.

Until recent years most bone biopsies were obtained from a rib by conventional surgical techniques. The design of a trocar by Bordier and colleagues made it possible to obtain iliac crest biopsies with minimal pain.[11] Bone biopsies could then be carried out under local anesthesia on outpatients. Jowsey has extensively reviewed the several bone biopsy methods subsequently developed.[12]

To appreciate the pathology of the metabolic bone diseases it is necessary to have some knowledge of the normal microanatomy of bone. This is reviewed in Chapter 17.

Routine histological assessment of bone in most pathology departments is initiated by decalcifying the bone after fixation and embedding it in paraffin. After sectioning the paraffin block hematoxylin and eosin staining is carried out. This type of preparation allows identification of the various bone cells that are present and evaluation of the overall structure of the bone. A serious drawback of this technique is the inability to distinguish mineralized from nonmineralized bone because of the obligatory decalcification step. A much more satisfactory technique, which is available in a few laboratories, is the preparation of undecalcified bone specimens for histologic evaluation. In this technique after fixation of the specimen it is embedded in plastic and sectioned with a special microtome. A variety of specialized stains can then be used to demonstrate the amount of unmineralized bone in the specimen.[13] This type of technique is critical in demonstrating the presence of osteomalacia, particularly in mild cases (Fig. 106-2). An alternative method for the evaluation of the amount of unmineralized bone in appropriately demineralized specimens is the azan stain.[14]

Another important technique that gives dynamic information concerning the state of bone is the use of tetracycline to label the sites of mineralization in os-

Figure 106–2. The accumulation of wide osteoid seams (light gray) in an iliac crest bone biopsy of a patient with Paget's disease treated with disodium etidronate, 20 mg per kilogram, for 6 months. Undecalcified, solochrome cyanin R × 750. (Provided by Professor Pierre Meunier.)

Figure 106–3. The uptake of demethylchlortetracycline demonstrated by fluorescent microscopy. The two fluorescent lines reflect 2 days of drug ingestion, 12 days without the drug, and 4 days of drug ingestion prior to a bone biopsy. The space between the two lines reflects the amount of bone formed during the 12-day period. Undecalcified, unstained, × 750. (Provided by Professor Pierre Meunier.)

teoid.[15] This was made possible by the discovery that ultraviolet light causes fluorescence of the tetracycline antibiotics, and that these compounds localize in areas of newly formed bone. The procedure is carried out by giving the patient two separate courses of tetracycline (0.5 g, 2 to 3 days) interrupted by a 10- to 14-day period without the drug. A bone biopsy is then obtained and examined by fluorescent microscopy. In a normal person, two bands of fluorescence will be found (Fig. 106–3). The band found deepest within the bone matrix represents the first labeling dose and the outer band the second. The rate of bone formation can be calculated by measuring the average width between the tetracycline bands and by dividing by the number of days between tetracycline labeling. In normal adults this is 1 micron per day. In patients with osteomalacia a characteristic feature is an impaired uptake of tetracycline by the bone.

The primary indication for iliac crest bone biopsy in clinical practice is to determine the presence of osteomalacia in patients in whom the diagnosis is not certain. Another indication is in the follow-up evaluation of therapy for bone disorders such as renal osteodystrophy.

PRIMARY HYPERPARATHYROIDISM

Parathyroid Hormone

Knowledge of the physiology and biochemistry of parathyroid hormone has increased tremendously during the past 20 years. In many instances this information has been beneficially applied to clinical practice. A brief review of selected aspects of the advances in parathyroid basic science follows.

Parathyroid hormone is a polypeptide consisting of 84 amino acids. The amino acid sequences of bovine, porcine, and human parathyroid hormone are similar but not identical[16] (Fig. 106–4). Studies of the biosynthesis of the hormone have identified two precursor peptides, proparathyroid hormone and preproparathyroid hormone.[17] The latter has an additional 31 peptides on the amino-terminal region of the molecule and is the

Figure 106–4. Amino acid sequences of human, bovine, and porcine parathyroid hormone. The backbone sequence represents the human structure. Added residues indicate sequence changes found in the bovine and porcine hormones. (From Keutmann, H.T., *In* De Groot, L. (eds.): Endocrinology, Vol. 2, New York, Grune & Strattonn, 1979.)

Figure 106–5. A proposed intracellular pathway of the biosynthesis of parathyroid hormone (PTH). Preproparathyroid hormone (Pre ProPTH), the initial product of synthesis on the ribosomes, is converted into proparathyroid (ProPTH) by removal of (1) the NH₂-terminal methionyl residues and (2) the NH₂-terminal sequence (-29 to -7) of 23 amino acids during and/or within seconds after synthesis, respectively. The conversion of Pre-ProPTH probably occurs during transport of the polypeptide into the cisterna of the rough endoplasmic reticulum. By 20 minutes after synthesis, ProPTH reaches the Golgi region and is converted into PTH by (3) removal of the NH₂-terminal hexapeptide. PTH is stored in the secretory granule until released into the circulation in response to a fall in the blood calcium concentration. The time needed for these events is given below the schema. (From Habener, J.F., Kemper, B.W., Rich, A., and Potts, J.T., Jr.: Recent Prog. Horm. Res. 33:249, 1977.)

initial biosynthetic product. Cleavage of the 25 amino-terminal amino acids of preproparathyroid hormone produces the 90 amino acid proparathyroid hormone. The amino-terminal hexapeptide of this precursor is highly susceptible to cleavage by trypsin. The function of the precursors is not known, but the hydrophobic properties of preproparathyroid hormone suggest that its function is to facilitate transport of the peptide across the rough endoplasmic reticulum membrane (Fig. 106–5).

The dominant factor in the control of secretion of parathyroid hormone is the concentration of ionized calcium which perfuses the parathyroid glands.[18] The hormone is secreted in response to a decrease in ionized calcium. Hypercalcemia, hypermagnesemia,[18,19] and severe magnesium deficiency[19] decrease parathyroid secretion. A variety of other agents, including beta-adrenergic agonists,[20] prostaglandin E₂,[21] and secretin,[22] have been shown to stimulate parathyroid hormone secretion, but their physiologic role is unkown. Direct suppression of parathyroid hormone secretion by vitamin D metabolites has been reported in animals,[23] but in man their role in parathyroid secretory control is uncertain.

Parathyroid hormone is the dominant factor in the prevention of hypocalcemia. It acts directly or indirectly on three organs to maintain the extracellular calcium concentration within a narrow range.[24] The hormone stimulates osteoclastic bone resorption and osteocytic osteolysis of bone, both of which release calcium from skeletal stores. The effect of the hormone on the kidney is to stimulate tubular reabsorption of calcium. An increased intestinal absorption of calcium also may be found in hyperparathyroid states. This probably occurs because of a stimulation of renal metabolism of vitamin D by parathyroid hormone. Elevated $1\alpha,25$-dihydroxyvitamin D levels in the circulation of some patients with primary hyperparathyroidism have been reported.[25]

The action of parathyroid hormone is mediated, in part, by stimulation of membrane-bound adenylate cyclase in the target organs.[26] In support of this is the observation that dibutyryl cyclic AMP can mimic the actions of the hormone in bone and in the kidney. An additional mediator of parathyroid hormone action may be an influx of calcium intracellularly.[27]

Parathyroid hormone in the circulation is present in a heterogeneous state.[28] Intact hormone is found but in a much smaller concentration than carboxyl-terminal fragments of the hormone. Amino-terminal fragments of parathyroid hormone have not been consistently found. Parathyroid fragments appear to arise during the metabolism of the hormone. In animal studies both the liver and the kidney have been demonstrated to cleave the hormone and release fragments into the circulation.[28] Evidence for the direct secretion of carboxyl-terminal fragments has also been reported.[29] The biologic significance of the fragments is not known, but the biologic activity of parathyroid hormone resides within the amino-terminal 27 amino acids.[16] Therefore much of the parathyroid-related peptides in the circulation appear to have no function. In man metabolic clearance of intact parathyroid hormone occurs in the liver, kidney, and extremities (presumably by bone).[30] Animal studies have demonstrated that only the kidney is capable of clearing carboxyl-terminal fragments of parathyroid hormone.[28] This accounts for the particularly high concentration of these fragments in the circulation of patients with renal failure.[31]

Clinical Features

Epidemiology. The true incidence of primary hyperparathyroidism in the general population has not been established, primarily because many affected individuals are asymptomatic. The most extensive survey was carried out in Rochester, Minnesota.[32] After the introduction of routine chemical screening into clinical practice, the average annual incidence rose from 7.8 ± 1.2 (mean $\pm$ S.D.) cases per 100,000 population to 51.1 ± 9.6.

Women develop primary hyperparathyroidism more commonly than men; a ratio of 2 or 3 to 1 is found in most series. The disorder is particularly prominent in postmenopausal women; 188 cases per 100,000 were found in women of 60 years or greater in Rochester.[32] The reduction in estrogen secretion appears to allow an accelerated rate of bone resorption and unmasks subclinical hyperparathyroidism.

There is no evidence to suggest an unusual geographic distribution of primary hyperparathyroidism. The disease does occur with an increased incidence in certain families. The affected members of a kindred may have hyperparathyroidism alone[33] or may have a variety of endocrine neoplasia. Two syndromes have been recognized, multiple endocrine neoplasia type I with pituitary and pancreatic neoplasia,[34] and multiple endocrine neoplasia type II with medullary thyroid carcinoma and pheochromocytoma.[35] The inheritance of familial hyperparathyroidism is of an autosomal dominant type.

Recent epidemiologic studies have uncovered an important finding that might explain the origin of the disease in some patients.[36] In several studies a high percentage of patients had radiation therapy during childhood or adolescence. The radiation was used in the treatment of facial acne, thymic enlargement, tonsillar hypertrophy, and tuberculous adenitis.

Signs and Symptoms. In Table 106–2 are listed the signs and symptoms that may be associated with hyperparathyroidism. They can be categorized into three groups: those arising from the direct effect of parathyroid hormone, those from hypercalcemia, and those from complicating disorders. The most definite symptom resulting from a direct hormonal effect is bone pain. Hypercalcemia is responsible for numerous abnormalities, including anorexia, nausea, vomiting, constipation, renal colic, polyuria, mental changes, and calcification of the eye. Abdominal pain may arise from peptic ulcer disease or pancreatitis, and joint pain and effusion may reflect gout or pseudogout.

Biochemistry. The most common abnormality that suggests the presence of primary hyperparathyroidism is hypercalcemia. The level and persistence of hypercalcemia is quite variable. Almost all patients at some time can be demonstrated to have a calcium concentra-

Table 106–2. Signs and Symptoms Associated with Primary Hyperparathyroidism

1. Systemic: fatigue, weakness, malaise
2. Musculoskeletal: bone pain, arthralgia, joint effusion, myalgia, muscle weakness
3. Genitourinary: polyuria, nocturia, renal colic
4. Neuropsychiatric: impaired concentration, lethargy, confusion, depression, obtundation, coma, hyporeflexia
5. Gastrointestinal: anorexia, nausea, vomiting, polydipsia
6. Cardiovascular: hypertension
7. Ophthalmologic: conjunctival and corneal calcification

tion above the upper limit of normal. Rarely a patient with primary hyperparathyroidism will have calcium concentrations consistently below 10.5 mg per deciliter. In such patients measurement of the ionized calcium concentration may reveal an abnormality.[37]

Serum phosphate concentration is below normal in about 50 percent of hyperparathyroid patients. This occurs because of the phosphaturic effect of parathyroid hormone.[17] Since hypophosphatemia may also be present in patients with nonparathyroid hypercalcemia,[38] it is not of great value in the differential diagnosis of hypercalcemia.

A mild metabolic acidosis is common in patients with hyperparathyroidism.[39] This develops as a result of renal bicarbonate wasting. A serum chloride concentration of 107 mEq per liter or above coupled with a serum bicarbonate concentration of 23 mEq per liter or less is suggestive of hyperparathyroidism in a hypercalcemic patient. Non–parathyroid-mediated hypercalcemia is generally associated with a mild metabolic alkalosis resulting from suppression of parathyroid hormone secretion.[39]

The development of radioimmunoassays for parathyroid hormone has significantly simplified the evaluation of the hypercalcemic patient.[24] Most assays in clinical use depend on the cross-reactivity of antibovine parathyroid hormone antisera with human parathyroid hormone. The heterogeneity of parathyroid hormone in the circulation complicates the interpretation of these assays, since each antiserum recognizes different antigenic sites in the hormonal molecule. Antisera whose dominant recognition sites are in the amino-terminal region mainly estimate the amount of intact hormone in the circulation. Carboxyl-terminal and mid-region antisera measure both intact hormone, and mid-region and carboxyl-terminal fragments; these antisera are most often utilized clinically. Because of this situation estimates of the concentration of immunoreactive parathyroid hormone in the circulation, unlike most peptide hormones, are highly variable from laboratory to laboratory. The clinician must become familiar with the results of a given laboratory in order to properly interpret the results of parathyroid hormone assays. In the majority of laboratories most patients with primary hyperparathyroidism have a concentration of the hormone in the circulation above the normal range. However, it should be stressed that 10 to 20 percent of patients may have a normal concentration. In these patients it is the combination of hypercalcemia and a clearly detectable (albeit normal) level of hormone which points to the diagnosis. Patients with nonparathyroid hypercalcemia should have either undetectable or low normal hormone levels.

Serum uric acid concentrations may be elevated in patients with primary hyperparathyroidism resulting from increased tubular reabsorption of uric acid.[40] Serum potassium and magnesium may be decreased in some patients owing to renal losses of these ions.

Urinary calcium excretion may be normal in patients with mild hypercalcemia or markedly elevated if the serum calcium is quite high. However, at any level of hypercalcemia patients with nonparathyroid hypercalcemia are likely to excrete significantly more calcium.[41] This is explained by an increase in tubular reabsorption of calcium induced by parathyroid hormone and a reduction in tubular reabsorption in patients with suppressed parathyroid secretion.

Urinary phosphate excretion is primarily dependent on dietary intake in patients with normal renal function. If renal tubular handling of phosphate is evaluated, a good discrimination from normal subjects is found. Patients with primary hyperparathyroidism will generally have a tmPO$_4$ of less than 2.5.[6] However, this reduced threshold for phosphate excretion is not specific for hyperparathyroidism. Hypercalcemia of any cause can inhibit renal tubular reabsorption of phosphate.

A test of more recent vintage which reflects the biologic activity of parathyroid hormone is estimation of urinary cyclic AMP excretion.[43] This is best expressed at present by calculating the urinary cyclic AMP per 100 ml glomerular filtrate. The test can be meaningfully carried out on urine obtained during a short collection period or on a 24-hour sampling. Urinary cyclic AMP excretion is elevated in primary hyperparathyroidism and decreased in hypoparathyroidism, although there is an overlap with the excretion of normal subjects (Fig. 106–6). This test unfortunately is not specific for parathyroid hormone activity, since patients with localized or metastatic carcinomas may also excrete increased amounts of cyclic AMP.[44] One study indicated that intravenous or oral calcium load rapidly reduced urinary cyclic AMP in normal subjects but not in patients with hyperparathyroidism.[45] It has been suggested that such a dynamic test of parathyroid suppressibility would prove valuable in the evaluation of patients with mild hyperparathyroidism and/or intermittent hypercalcemia, since serum parathyroid hormone concentrations may not be elevated in all patients.

However, in a subsequent study, the reliability of an oral calcium tolerance test in distinguishing normal subjects from patients with mild primary hyperparathyroidism was poor.[45]

Radiology. The radiologic features of primary hyperparathyroidism are well known but are found with less frequency at present because of earlier diagnosis of the disease.

The skeletal changes induced by primary hyperparathyroidism produce a variety of radiologic lesions. The earliest and most common change is that of subperiosteal bone resorption (Fig. 106–7). A lacelike appearance of the outer margin of the cortex is best appreciated at the radial aspects of the middle phalanges. Other sites in which this finding can be sought are the medial aspect

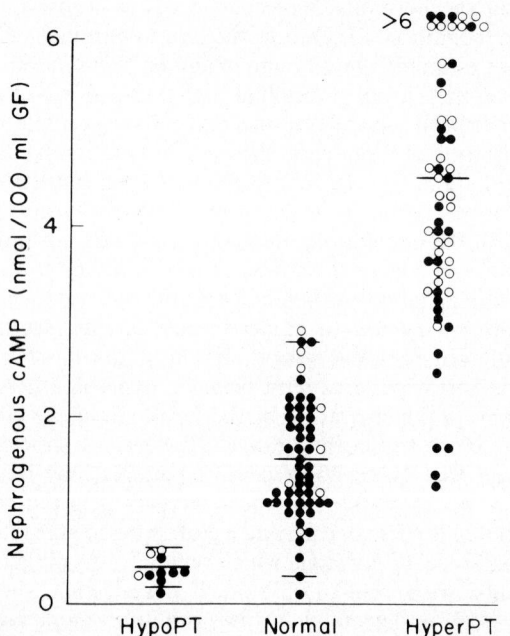

Figure 106–6. Urinary cyclic MP, expressed in nmol per 100 ml GF in normocalcemic control subjects and in patients with hypoparathyroidism and primary hyperparathyroidism. The open circles depict the subjects and patients with renal impairment (mean GFR ≤ 80 ml per minute). The horizontal bars represent the mean values for the patients with hypoparathyroidism and primary hyperparathyroidism, and the control group is shown as mean ±2S.D. (From Broadus, A.E. Mahaffey, J.E., Bartter, F.C., and Neer, R.M.: J. Clin. Invest. 60:771, 1977.)

Figure 106-7. Subperiosteal resorption of phalanges in a patient with primary hyperparathyroidism. Note the marked resorption of the distal phalanges.

Figure 106–8. "Salt and pepper" skull of a patient with primary hyperparathyroidism.

of the proximal tibia, the proximal humerus, the distal radius and ulna, the superior margins of the ribs, the pubis, and the ischium. A later abnormality is the presence of endosteal scalloping. A total loss of cortical bone may occur after prolonged exposure to high concentrations of parathyroid hormone in the circulation. Resorption of the terminal tufts of the phalanges may occur and give the appearance of clubbing of the fingers.

Other evidence of an increased rate of bone resorption is provided by the absence of the lamina dura; by resorption of the distal clavicles, symphysis pubis, and sacroiliac joints; and by a loss of density of the skull, which gives a "salt and pepper" appearance (Fig. 106–8). Occasionally, generalized osteopenia without the classic radiologic features of primary hyperparathyroidism may be present.

Solitary lesions of variable size may develop which are expansile and lightly trabeculated (Fig. 106–9*A*). They may be found in any bone but are more likely to involve the pelvis, ribs, mandible, and long bones. These lesions are either brown tumors or cysts and cannot be distinguished by their radiologic features before treatment of the disease. After cure of the disease there is

Figure 106–9. *A*, Brown tumor in the left ulna of a patient with primary hyperparathyroidism. Note the expansile and lightly trabeculated quality of the lesion. *B*, Almost complete healing of the lesion seen in *A* 4 years after parathyroidectomy.

demonstrable healing of brown tumors but not of cysts (Fig. 106–9*B*).

Paradoxically, an increase in the density or size of a bone may be observed. Such osteosclerosis may rarely be apparent at the end plates of vertebral bodies (Fig. 106–10). The appearance of horizontal stripes of increased density alternating with bands of lesser density has been termed the "rugger jersey" spine. The calvarium of the skull may thicken in some patients.

Calcification of various tissues is a feature of primary hyperparathyroidism and occasionally may lead to the diagnosis. Calcification of articular cartilages, menisci, joint capsules, and periarticular structures by deposition of calcium pyrophosphate dihydrate is discussed in Chapter 39 and 87. Calcification of medium and large arteries may be found, but it is not certain that the incidence in primary hyperparathyroidism is higher than in an age-matched population. Diffuse nephrocalcinosis and nephrolithiasis are generally associated with high levels of urinary calcium excretion. Calcifications in the pancreas, salivary glands, and prostate may occur. Soft tissue calcification is uncommon and much less frequent than in secondary hyperparathyroidism.

Bone Pathology. Von Recklinghausen first recognized the differences between the skeletal abnormalities of osteomalacia and hyperparathyroidism in 1891.[47] The pathologic changes found in advanced disease came to be known as generalized osteitis fibrosa cystica. Although many patients with primary hyperparathyroidism have little or no evidence of clinical bone disease, a bone biopsy almost always will have some abnormal features.

The most characteristic findings are increased numbers of osteoclasts within Howship's lacunae, plump osteoblasts in the process of repairing the resorbed bone, and a dense fibrovascular marrow with numerous fibroblasts (Fig. 106–11). In severe disease cysts may occur with a well-defined fibrous lining. The cysts may be empty or may show evidence of old or recent hemorrhage. Brown tumors are composed of a connective tissue stroma containing spindle cells and multinucleated giant cells which may have 100 or more nuclei on cross section (Fig. 106–12). The brown color is imparted by hemosiderin, which is apparently deposited after hemorrhage occurs.

Evidence of osteocytic osteolysis, or perilacunar enlargement around osteocytes, has been found by several investigators. This can be discerned only by quantitative histologic techniques.[48]

In most patients the structure of bone is entirely lamellar in character, but in patients with severe disease woven or primitive bone may be found. Rarely a pagetoid appearance may develop, with numerous cement lines intersecting to produce a mosaic pattern.

Although there may be an increased surface area of bone covered with osteoid, bone mineralization is normal in uncomplicated primary hyperparathyroidism.

Differential Diagnosis

Since the classic skeletal lesions of primary hyperparathyroidism are seldom observed any more, the differential diagnosis of primary hyperparathyroidism is usually identical to that of hypercalcemia. Table 106–3

Figure 106–10. Osteosclerosis of lumbar vertebral bodies in a patient with primary hyperparathyroidism. Note the dense endplates of the vertebrae.

Figure 106–11. Histologic features of severe primary hyperparathyroidism: numerous osteoclasts in Howship's lacunae, fibrovascular bone marrow, and osteoblasts repairing partially resorbed bone. Decalcified, hematoxylin and eosin × 200.

lists the numerous disorders that can cause hypercalcemia. Those that are likely to give the most difficulty in diagnosis are malignancies without bone invasion, familial hypocalciuric hypercalcemia, sarcoidosis, and chronic renal failure with intermittent hypercalcemia.

Approximately 15 percent of patients with a malignancy and hypercalcemia have no evidence of skeletal metastases.[49] These patients often have bone lesions indistinguishable from those of primary hyperparathyroidism save for excessive osteoblasts, cysts, and brown tumors. Parathyroid hormone, prostaglandin E_2, and other, as yet unidentified humoral hypercalcemic agents have been implicated as the factors produced by the neoplasms. If the serum parathyroid hormone concentration is elevated in such a patient, selective venous catheterization of the tumor and parathyroid venous drainage should be done to assess the origin of the parathyroid hormone, since a variety of malignancies may be found in association with functional parathyroid adenomas.[50]

Familial hypocalciuric hypercalcemia is an autosomal dominant disorder in which hypercalcemia of moderate

Figure 106-12. Brown tumor from a patient with primary hyperparathyroidism demonstrating dense connective tissue stroma, spindle cells, and numerous multinucleated giant cells. Decalcified, hematoxylin and eosin, × 500.

Table 106–3. Differential Diagnosis of Hypercalcemia

1. Malignancies
   a. With skeletal invasion
   b. Without skeletal invasion (humoral hypercalcemia of
      malignancy)
2. Primary hyperparathyroidism
   a. Sporadic
   b. Familial
      (1) Hyperparathyroidism alone
      (2) Multiple endocrine neoplasia Type I with pituitary and
          pancreatic neoplasia
      (3) Multiple endocrine neoplasia Type IIa with medullary
          thyroid carcinoma and pheochromocytoma
3. Familial hypocalciuric hypercalcemia
4. Other endocrine disorders
   a. Acromegaly
   b. Hyperthyroidism
   c. Hypothyroidism (children)
   d. Pheochromocytoma
   e. Acute adrenal insufficiency
5. Renal failure
   a. Diuretic phase of acute renal failure
   b. Chronic
   c. Postrenal transplantation
6. Iatrogenic
   a. Vitamin D excess
   b. Vitamin A excess
   c. Milk-alkali syndrome
   d. Calcium salts
   e. Total parenteral nutrition
   f. Chlorothiazide diuretics
   g. Lithium?
7. Granulomatous disorders
   a. Sarcoidosis
   b. Tuberculosis
   c. Coccidioidomycosis
   d. Histoplasmosis
   e. Berylliosis
8. Idiopathic hypercalcemia of infancy
9. Immobilization
10. Hypophosphatasia
11. Increased serum proteins
    a. Hemoconcentration
    b. Hyperglobulinemia due to multiple myeloma

degree probably is present from birth.[51] The pathogenesis of the hypercalcemia appears related to an increased renal tubular reabsorption of calcium. The 24-hour excretion of calcium may be 100 mg or lower. What factor accounts for this and the simultaneous increased renal tubular reabsorption of magnesium is uncertain. Because serum parathyroid hormone concentrations in the patients are almost invariably normal or low, it has been suggested that the underlying abnormality may be a sensitivity to the hormone. Urinary cyclic AMP excretion is intermediate between normal levels and those generally found in hyperparathyroidism. Another unexplained feature of this disorder is the fact that it is highly uncommon for these patients to be symptomatic or to exhibit functional abnormalities of any organ system.

In sarcoidosis, hypercalcemia occurs in about 20 percent of patients.[52] Although radiographic evidence of bone involvement by sarcoid granulomas is not rare, an increase in intestinal absorption of calcium is the dominant factor responsible for hypercalcemia. Recent studies have indicated that hypercalcemic sarcoidosis pa-

tients have elevated levels of $1\alpha,25$-dihydroxyvitamin D in the circulation, which is restored to normal by glucocorticoid therapy.[53] The source of the excess $1\alpha,25$-dihydroxyvitamin D may be the macrophages associated with the sarcoid granuloma.[54] The hypercalcemia of sarcoidosis can be readily distinguished from that of primary hyperparathyroidism because hypercalcemic sarcoidosis patients have suppressed parathyroid hormone levels[52] and have reversible hypercalcemia if glucocorticoids are administered.[53]

Patients with end-stage renal failure may occasionally develop hypercalcemia of a generally intermittent type. This may occur because of massive hyperplasia of the parathyroid glands. As these patients often have severe renal osteodystrophy, subtotal parathyroidectomy may be the only effective therapy.

Treatment

Primary hyperparathyroidism is unequivocally a disease treated best by surgery. Unless it is decided to withhold treatment in an asymptomatic elderly patient or if there are contraindications to surgery, it is preferable to undertake appropriate surgery rather than attempt medical control of the disease. This is the case because there is no medical treatment effective in completely neutralizing the effects of parathyroid hormone.

The surgical management of hyperparathyroidism requires close collaboration between the surgeon and pathologist during the course of the surgery. This is mandatory because of the heterogeneity of parathyroid pathology.[55] Approximately 80 percent of patients have a single parathyroid adenoma, which is usually composed primarily of chief cells and almost devoid of fat. A rim of normal tissue is also a characteristic feature. Perhaps 1 percent of patients have two adenomas. Chief cell or, much less frequently, clear cell hyperplasia of all four glands occurs in 15 percent of patients. Parathyroid carcinoma affects 3 percent or less of patients. Little or no fat is also found in hyperplastic and carcinomatous glands. Only histologic examination of a gland can give a definitive answer as to what type of lesion is present. In some cases the differentiation of an adenoma from a hyperplastic gland is difficult, because not all adenomas have a discernible rim of normal tissue. Adding to the difficulty is the possibility of asymmetric hyperplasia of four glands. One or more may not be frankly enlarged but simply be devoid of fat. Because of this it is imperative to biopsy or even remove a second gland for frozen section once one abnormal gland is resected. If the second gland is normal, it is highly likely that removal of the abnormal gland will result in permanent cure. If two glands are abnormal, then three and a portion of the fourth should be resected. In most cases this will effectively treat the parathyroid hyperplasia. A silver clip can be attached to the remaining gland to allow easy localization if continuing hyperplasia leads to recurrent hyperparathyroidism.

In patients with clinical bone disease surgical correction of hyperparathyroidism may be followed postoperatively by a long period of hypocalcemia and/or hypophosphatemia.[1] This "hungry bone" syndrome develops as a result of the great requirement for calcium and phosphorus in the healing phase of the disease. Supplemental calcium, phosphate, and vitamin D are often needed for months after surgery. Another cause of hypocalcemia following surgery is unsuspected magnesium deficiency. Postoperative hypoparathyroidism is quite uncommon and can be diagnosed by serum immunoreactive parathyroid hormone measurement.

Chronic medical treatment of primary hyperparathyroidism can be reasonably effective when the disease is relatively mild. Oral phosphate therapy is particularly effective in patients who have increased intestinal calcium absorption associated with elevation of serum 1α,25-dihydroxyvitamin D levels.[56] The dose required is between 1 and 3 grams of elemental phosphorus given in four divided doses daily. In patients with renal failure the dose should be reduced. If the serum phosphate concentration is high normal or elevated, phosphate therapy should not be given. Phosphate therapy may control the calcium concentration in serum for years, but there is little evidence to prove that the deleterious effects of parathyroid hormone on the skeleton are prevented.

In severely hypercalcemic patients intravenous fluids may be necessary to restore extracellular volume. Occasionally intravenous saline and furosemide therapy must be given to reduce the calcium concentration in patients whose mental function is impaired.[57] After restoration of a normal mental status oral phosphate therapy could be instituted.

An alternative approach to phosphate therapy can be undertaken in postmenopausal women with primary hyperparathyroidism. Physiologic estrogen replacement therapy can lower serum calcium concentration up to 2 mg per dl; the usual decrease is 0.5 to 1 mg per dl.[58] Concomitant with the fall in serum calcium concentration, the urinary calcium falls. As little as 0.3 mg conjugated estrogens daily for 3 weeks each month can be effective hypocalcemic therapy. The action of estrogenic hormones is to reduce parathyroid hormone–induced bone resorption as evidenced by the reduction in urinary hydroxyproline excretion observed in the treated patients. A disadvantage of this therapy is the possibility of an increased incidence of uterine carcinoma in estrogen-treated postmenopausal women. The addition of a progestational agent, such as medroxyprogesterone acetate, during the last 10 days of each 3-week estrogen administration may make this complication much less likely.

OSTEOPOROSIS

Definition

Osteoporosis is a disorder of bone that can arise from a variety of underlying pathologic processes (Table 106–4). It is characterized in all instances by a decreased

Table 106–4. Classification of Osteoporosis

1. Aging
2. Endocrine abnormality
   a. Estrogen deficiency
   b. Testosterone deficiency
   c. Glucocorticoid excess
   d. Thyrotoxicosis
   e. Diabetes mellitus
   f. Primary hyperparathyroidism
3. Immobilization or weightlessness
4. Genetic
   a. Osteogenesis imperfecta
   b. Homocystinuria
   c. Ehlers-Danlos syndrome
   d. Menkes' syndrome
   e. Marfan's syndrome
5. Juvenile osteoporosis
6. Rheumatoid arthritis
7. Scurvy
8. Heparin therapy
9. Systemic mastocytosis
10. Hematologic malignancy
    a. Multiple myeloma
    b. Leukemia
    c. Lymphoma
11. Liver disease
12. Alcoholism

mass of normally mineralized bone. The existence of such a condition may not be appreciated clinically until such time as the bone mass is insufficient to provide adequate mechanical support.

Osteoporosis is the most common bone problem of a nontraumatic nature and as such constitutes a major health problem in the elderly female and in patients treated for a long time with glucocorticosteroids.

Clinical Features

Signs and Symptoms. A prolonged subclinical phase undoubtedly occurs in many patients prior to the recognition of the disorder. The most common complaint is that of back pain. This may begin suddenly and with great intensity. It is sharp in character, is aggravated by movement and weight bearing, and reflects an underlying compression fracture of a vertebral body. The twelfth thoracic and first lumbar vertebrae are most often affected. After healing occurs, the pain may completely resolve. Residual pain may reflect spasm of the paravertebral muscles.

Deformity of the spine may slowly evolve in the absence of back pain. A progressive loss in height occurs as a result of compression of the vertebral bodies. Dorsal kyphosis may be a severe manifestation of longstanding spinal osteoporosis. The deformity may cause the lower ribs to touch the iliac crests.

Fractures of the femoral neck, distal radius, and ribs are prone to develop after apparently trivial trauma.

Clinical Biochemistry. Frank abnormalities of the calcium, phosphate, or alkaline phosphatase concentrations in the circulation are unusual. Only in the least common disorders associated with osteoporosis are abnormalities noted with any frequency. In thyrotoxicosis serum calcium, phosphate, and alkaline phosphatase may all be elevated.[59] Hypercalcemia and hyperphosphatemia may complicate the immobilization of patients under 25 years of age.[60] Alkaline phosphatase may rise slightly if a fracture of an extremity bone occurs.

Consistent abnormalities of immunoreactive parathyroid hormone concentration in the circulation have not been found. In postmenopausal women both low and high levels have been reported.[61,62]

A 30 percent decrease in plasma $1\alpha,25$-dihydroxyvitamin D has been reported in postmenopausal osteoporotic females as compared with normal age-matched women.[63] The reduced vitamin D metabolite levels correlate with a reduction in intestinal calcium absorption.

Evidence for impaired calcitonin secretion has also been reported in postmenopausal women with osteoporosis.[64] Calcium infusion failed to elicit a rise in plasma calcitonin levels in osteoporotic subjects. Normal age-matched women did have a small response. An entire reassessment of the potential role of calcitonin in osteoporosis will be necessary, utilizing assays for the biologically active monomer of calcitonin.[65]

In patients whose rate of bone resorption exceeds that of bone formation, hypercalciuria may be observed. This is particularly likely to be present in immobilized or hyperthyroid patients. The measurement of the fasting calcium:creatinine ratio in the urine avoids the contribution of dietary calcium in most patients and is therefore preferable to the measurement of 24-hour urinary calcium excretion.[66]

Urinary hydroxyproline excretion may also be elevated in states of increased bone resorption. The fasting hydroxyproline:creatinine ratio avoids the influence of dietary gelatin.[66]

Radiology. The cardinal radiologic feature of osteoporosis is a decreased density of bone. This is most readily visualized in studies of the spine. Marked thinning of the cortex and loss of transverse trabeculation are characteristic features. A paradoxical accentuation of the density of the cortex and vertical trabeculae may result. Ballooning of the nuclei pulposi into the vertebral bodies produces the classic biconcave or "codfish" deformity (Fig. 106–13). A localized herniation of a nucleus pulposus into a vertebral body, termed Schmorl's node, may occasionally be present. Anterior wedging of the vertebrae generally occurs with extreme loss of bone mineral, although trauma may produce a compression fracture at an earlier stage of osteoporosis.

Manifestations of osteoporosis at other sites include a patchy loss of density of the calvarium, decreased cortical density of long bones, and vertical striation of long bones. Bowing of long bones occurs in patients with osteogenesis imperfecta but not in other forms of the disorder.

Although routine radiologic examination of the skeleton is of use in evaluating patients with osteoporosis, until recently most physicians were unable to obtain precise quantitation of the severity of the disorder in their patients. This was not for a lack of noninvasive methods of estimating bone mass.[67] Trabecular bone

Figure 106–13. "Codfish" deformities of the lumbar spine in a 54-year-old male with osteoporosis resulting from multiple myeloma.

density is most commonly assessed by visually examining lateral radiographs of the spine, but this cannot be considered a precise method even in the hands of highly experienced radiologists. Morphometric measurements of vertebral biconcavity or the degree of anterior wedging of the vertebral bodies are also of limited value because of difficulty in reproducing the appropriate views of the spine. Radiographic densitometric measurements of the spine have been described but are not widely used. A common means of quantitating trabecular bone density in research units is by photon beam absorptiometry of the distal radius. Both dual-photon absorptiometry and computerized tomography are widely available methods of quantitating trabecular bone density and have dramatically improved the ability to discern osteoporosis in an earlier stage and to evaluate therapeutic intervention.

Assessment of cortical bone density has been made by a variety of techniques (see also Chapter 19). Photon beam absorptiometry of the midshaft of the radius and cortical thickness of the second metacarpal and proximal radius have most often been utilized. However, abnormalities at these sites do not accurately reflect the degree of osteoporosis at other more clinically relevant sites.[68]

Bone Pathology. The histologic features of osteoporosis are quite variable and depend upon the underlying etiology. Two findings are always present: a decrease in bone volume and normal mineralization of the bone matrix.

Quantitative histology of iliac crest biopsies from patients with postmenopausal osteoporosis has been reported by several laboratories. Jowsey and colleagues utilized quantitative microradiography, a technique which evaluates the density of the mineral phase of the bone.[66] They found that resorptive surfaces were increased as compared to normal subjects and that bone-forming surfaces were usually normal. However, assessment of active bone resorptive surfaces as judged by the presence of osteoclasts has led to the opposite conclusion by other investigators.[68,69] In these studies trabecular bone did not appear to be affected by increased osteoclastic resorption, but there was evidence of decreased bone formation.[69] Bone formation was also found to be reduced in a study of rib cortical bone utilizing tetracycline labeling.[70] The reason for the discrepancies between these studies is not entirely clear, but Teitelbaum and colleagues have stressed the heterogeneity of an osteoporotic population.[62] They observed a subpopulation of patients who had increased cortical osteoclasts but no increased trabecular osteoclasts. These patients also had a greater percentage of trabecular surface area covered by osteoid than normal. Serum immunoreactive parathyroid hormone was elevated in this group and was thought to account for the histologic findings. However, a follow-up study of this group reported no correlation between morphologic parameters and any biochemical parameters, including parathyroid hormone.[73] The pathogenesis of postmenopausal osteoporosis based on quantitative bone histomorphometry is yet to be resolved.

In patients with Cushing's syndrome resulting from adrenal disease or costicosteroid therapy, both quantitative microradiography[74] and quantitative histology of bone biopsies[75,76] have shown increased rates of bone resorption and decreased bone formation.

In patients with hyperthyroidism the histologic findings document a marked increase in bone remodeling.[59] Numerous osteoclasts and osteoblasts and a fibrous bone marrow may be present. The percentage of trabecular bone covered with osteoid is increased, but the osteoid seams are not widened and the mineralization rate is normal. A decrease in cortical and trabecular bone becomes apparent after the rate of bone resorption exceeds that of bone formation for an appropriate period of time. Hyperthyroid bone disease can be distinguished from that of hyperparathyroidism by the size of the periosteocytic lacunae. There is no increase in this parameter in patients with hyperthyroidism.

Osteoporosis resulting from immobilization is associated with an increase in osteoclastic bone resorption as well as marked suppression of osteoblastic activity.[77]

In the rare disorder of idiopathic juvenile osteoporosis an increase in bone resorption surfaces as determined by quantitative microradiography has been reported.[78] Bone formation surface was normal.[78] In a second study quantitative histomorphometry confirmed an increase in bone resorption surface area, but as there were few osteoclasts and few osteoblasts observed, it was proposed that the primary abnormality was impaired bone formation.[79]

The pathologic findings in patients with osteogenesis imperfecta are unlike those in any other form of osteoporosis.[80] There is a persistence of primitive woven bone and a failure to develop well-organized haversian systems. Osteoclasts are not prominent and osteoblasts are spindle-shaped and flattened, a feature of inactive cells.

Pathogenesis and Treatment

The treatment of osteoporosis is most likely to be successful if the pathogenesis of the disorder in a particular patient is fully understood. The various types of osteoporosis and their specific therapies will now be discussed.

Aging. In both women and men over the age of 75, cortical and trabecular bone loss is so pronounced as to account for the high incidence of vertebral and femoral fractures.[81] It has been suggested that this might be accounted for by a decrease in bone formation by senescent osteoblasts coupled with the presence of secondary hyperparathyroidism due to the age-related decrease in intestinal calcium absorption.[81] It is conceivable that the osteoporosis of aging could be prevented, to some extent, by maintaining a continuous program of weight-bearing exercise and by ingesting enough calcium to avoid negative calcium balance (1500 mg/day) in the postmenopausal female).

Gonadal Hypofunction. The largest group of patients who develop osteoporosis are postmenopausal women whose menses ceased at least 10 years previously. The pathogenesis of this form of osteoporosis is not agreed upon. One viewpoint is that the development of symptomatic bone disease in the elderly woman arises from a failure to develop a normal skeletal mass during the growth period.[82] This might arise from poor nutrition, severe illness, inadequate exercise or prolonged immobilization, or genetic influences controlling collagen synthesis. The universal loss of bone mass that inevitably occurs during the menopause in estrogen-deficient women may then cause symptomatic osteoporosis in those women who had a reduced bone mass prior to the menopause.

An alternative concept of the pathogenesis of postmenopausal osteoporosis is that one or more factors can lead to accelerated loss of bone mass in a proportion of women who, after a decade or more, experience the clinical syndrome of pathologic fractures and bone pain. The factor usually implicated in these patients is estrogen deficiency.[83] Estrogen deficiency has been postulated to impair calcium homeostasis in several ways. Lack of estrogens may sensitize the skeleton to the actions of parathyroid hormone on bone. Supporting evidence for this is provided by the observation that estrogen replacement in postmenopausal women with primary hyperparathyroidism reduces serum and urinary calcium levels and urinary hydroxyproline excretion.[58] A mild reduction in 1α,25-dihydroxyvitamin D levels in the circulation of postmenopausal females has also been reported.[63] This could arise indirectly from a slight decrease in circulating parathyroid hormone concentration and could account for the documented calcium malabsorption and negative calcium balance in these patients.[63] A direct effect of estrogen on conversion of 1α,25-hydroxycholecalciferol to 1α,25-dihydroxycholecalciferol has also been postulated.[84] Other factors such as reduced levels of exercise and poor nutrition might also contribute to bone loss.

Albright postulated that bone loss in the postmenopausal woman occurred because of diminished osteoblastic activity.[1] However, subsequent studies of a wide variety have stressed the concept of increased bone resorption as the underlying mechanism of bone loss in these patients.[61,63,85] Nevertheless, quantitative bone histology utilizing tetracycline labeling has demonstrated a reduction of bone formation in postmenopausal women.[72]

Those who stress the concept that osteoporosis in postmenopausal women develops primarily in those women who did not attain normal skeletal mass during the growth phase believe that the emphasis of treatment should be on prevention of the disorder during childhood and adolescence. Proper nutrition and exercise would seem to be the appropriate means to attempt to prevent the future development of bone disease.

In the woman who is entering the menopause there are two modes of therapy that may also prevent future symptomatic bone disease. It has now been demonstrated by several techniques that estrogen replacement therapy given during the 5 to 10 years following the menopause can retard loss of bone[85-87] (Fig. 106–14) and reduce the risk of fracture by 50% or more.[88] Relatively modest doses of estrogens, 0.2 mg ethinyl estradiol, 0.625 mg conjugated equine estrogens, or 5 mg diethylstilbesterol, given 3 weeks each month are effective in preventing loss of bone mass. The mechanism by which this is achieved is not fully understood, but it is likely that inhibition of bone resorption is a factor. This could occur as a consequence of an increase in calcitonin secretion, since estrogen replacement has been demonstrated to raise serum calcitonin levels.[89] However, assay of monomeric calcitonin in pre- and postmenopausal women reveals no difference in calcitonin concentrations[65] and leaves open the question of whether estrogen influences calcitonin secretion. Estrogen therapy has also been reported to produce enhancement of intestinal calcium absorption. This appears to result from an increase in levels of 1α,25-dihydroxyvitamin D in the circulation.[90]

A second means of inhibiting bone loss during the postmenopausal years is to increase calcium intake to 1500 mg daily.[91] This has been demonstrated to be ef-

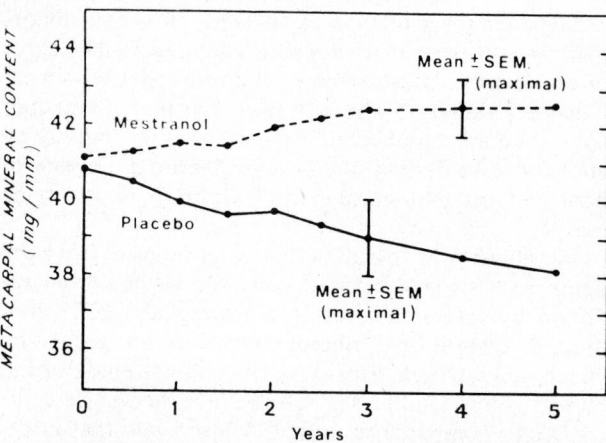

Figure 106–14. Mean metacarpal mineral content during 5-year follow-up of patients observed from 3 years after bilateral oophorectomy (zero time). Patients given a placebo lost bone mass at an average rate of 0.7 mg per $mm^{-1}\ yr^{-1}$, the mean fall becoming significant after 1.5 years. Patients given mestranol (average daily dose, 24.8ug) gained bone mass for first 3 years (p < 0.001) and had little increase thereafter. Treatment groups are significantly different (p < 0.01) after only 1 year's treatment. (From Lindsay, R., Hart, D.M., Aitken, J. M., MacDonald, E.B., Anderson, J.B., and Clarke, A.C.: Lancet 1:1038, 1976.)

fective in at least partially offsetting the expected bone loss in postmenopausal women. The need for this large calcium intake to prevent a negative calcium balance arises from a reduced efficiency of intestinal calcium absorption in these patients. The impaired intestinal calcium absorption can be related to decreased circulating 1α,25-dihydroxyvitamin D levels.[63,90]

In patients with symptomatic osteoporosis the use of estrogen replacement and/or supplemental calcium may retard bone loss, but a sustained positive calcium balance has not been observed. In one study, during the initial 6 months of estrogen treatment a small positive balance ensued because of a reduction in bone resorption, but following this bone formation fell and no further gain in skeletal mass was observed.[92] However, an increase of metacarpal cortical bone was observed in postmenopausal women treated with high doses of estradiol.[93]

A number of disturbing problems may occur in patients on estrogen therapy. Vaginal bleeding may occur at times other than after hormone withdrawal and require dilatation and curettage. The question of induction of uterine carcinoma remains controversial, but administration of medroxyprogesterone acetate on the last 10 days of estrogen therapy may reduce the likelihood of this complication. Fluid retention, hypertension, and vascular thrombosis are other problems that may be encountered.

Other modes of therapy have been proposed as possible inducers of bone formation. Anabolic steroids, calcitonin, vitamin D metabolites, and sodium fluoride should still be considered experimental drugs, although they are readily obtainable by practitioners. The most promising of these drugs is sodium fluoride, which at a dose of 50 mg daily can stimulate significant bone formation.[94] The quality of the bone formed has been questioned, since it is known that endemic fluorosis can lead to osteomalacia with secondary hyperparathyroidism.[95] For this reason it is necessary to give supplemental calcium, 1000 to 1500 mg per day. This combination therapy apparently prevents formation of inadequately mineralized bone. Side effects that may occur in patients treated with fluoride include epigastric distress, arthralgias and/or osteophytosis, and skin rash.

Few reports of osteoporosis in hypogonadal males have appeared. A moderate increase in bone resorption and a more severe impairment of bone formation have been described. Testosterone treatment for 6 months in one patient produced a striking increase in the rate of bone formation.[96]

Glucocorticoid Excess. Rheumatologists not infrequently will encounter patients with severe osteoporosis that arises as a consequence of chronic corticosteroid therapy of disorders such as rheumatoid arthritis and systemic lupus erythematosus. Spontaneous Cushing's syndrome may also produce severe osteoporosis, but this is seldom encountered because of the rarity of the disorder.

The deleterious effects of corticosteroids on the skeleton are particularly evident in children in whom not only osteoporosis but also decreased bone growth may develop.[97] This may occur because of inhibition of cartilage growth,[98] as well as from an impairment of bone collagen synthesis and bone formation.[99] The inhibition of bone formation may be mediated through the antianabolic effect of the steroid glucocorticoids on existing bone cells and by interference with mesenchymal cell differentation into osteoblasts and osteoclasts.[100]

Another contribution to the pathogenesis of osteoporosis involves the anti–vitamin D effects of glucocorticoids. Intestinal absorption of calcium is reduced by glucocorticoids, although the mechanism by which this occurs is not certain.[101] Measurement of vitamin D metabolites in the circulation of patients with either endogenous or exogenous excess of glucocorticoids has produced conflicting results. Both normal[102-105] and low[76,106] levels of 25-hydroxyvitamin D have been reported. Similar confusion exists in the studies of 1α,25-dihydroxyvitamin D in the circulation. Normal levels were found in two studies,[104,105] although high normal levels fell to lower levels after removal of ACTH-producing tumors in one study.[104] In a third study of prednisone-treated adolescents with systemic lupus erythematosus, serum 1α,25-dihydroxyvitamin D levels were low.[107] Even if impaired metabolism of vitamin D is a factor in the pathogenesis of steroid-induced osteoporosis, it is also likely that glucocorticoids directly inhibit intestinal calcium transport. In the rat, administration of 1α,25-dihydroxyvitamin D is unable to fully correct impaired calcium absorption produced by cortisone.[108] A role for parathyroid hormone in the development of osteoporosis has also been proposed. Elevated or high normal levels of parathyroid hormone have been found in four studies;[76,104,109,110] and normal levels, only in one study.[103] The finding of increased trabecular osteoclastic resorption surfaces in glucocorticoid-treated patients[76]

is probably a manifestation of secondary hyperparathyroidism.

Finally it must be kept in mind that patients who are sufficiently ill to require glucocorticoid therapy may frequently be unable to exercise or maintain a well-balanced diet. Some investigators feel that these factors may be the prime deteminants of whether a patient will develop osteroporosis.

The treatment of glucocorticoid-induced osteoporosis is difficult unless it is possible to discontinue or reduce the dose of steroid. Successful treatment of patients with endogenous Cushing's syndrome has been followed by an unequivocal healing process in the abnormal bone.[76] Unfortunately, changing from daily to alternate day doses of glucocorticoids does not seem to reduce the degree of bone loss in rheumatic patients who need to remain on therapy.[111]

Recent studies have demonstrated that near-physiologic doses of 1α,25-dihydroxycholecalciferol (0.4 μg daily) can increase calcium absorption in patients receiving high-dose glucocorticoid therapy.[106] Treatment with 25-hydroxycholecalciferol has produced a similar effect on calcium absorption and significantly increased bone density.[112] At this time these drugs have yet to be approved by the Food and Drug Administration for use in patients with osteoporosis. An alternative available drug for which there are few guidelines in use is vitamin D_2. Doses ranging from 50,000 units per week to 50,000 units daily have been recommended for patients with glucocorticoid-induced osteoporosis. Should the highest doses be used, careful monitoring of the serum and urinary calcium levels is imperative to avoid hypercalcemia and/or hypercalciuria. Dietary and/or supplemental calcium intake should be 1000 to 1500 mg daily. If the urinary calcium exceeds 300 mg per day, the dietary calcium intake should be reduced to a level that maintains calcium excretion below this amount. In some patients reduction of vitamin D_2 dosage may be necessary.

The beneficial effects of exercise on stimulating bone formation should be kept in mind. A judicious exercise and physical therapy program may be more beneficial to the patients than any other therapy.

Thyrotoxicosis. Osteoporosis is an uncommon complication of thyrotoxicosis. It will develop in the severely affected patient only after a long period of untreated disease. Although thyroid hormone induces increased bone formation as well as bone resorption, in patients with osteoporosis the rate of bone resorption has clearly been greater. It is not known why this occurs.

The treatment of osteoporosis resulting from thyrotoxicosis is the restoration of a euthyroid state by radioiodine ablation, antithyroid drug therapy, or thyroidectomy. An increase in bone mass can be demonstrated after successful treatment, but it is less evident in postmenopausal women.[113] Propranolol has been shown to rapidly correct the hypercalcemia sometimes seen in thyrotoxic patients.[114] It probably directly inhibits the effect of thyroid hormone on bone cells. However, chronic use of propranolol in the management of thyrotoxic bone disease is not recommended, since a 3-month trial in 17 patients failed to produce any benefit.[115]

Diabetes Mellitus. Osteoporosis may develop in patients with diabetes mellitus, probably as a result of impaired bone formation.[116] Insulin therapy in juvenile diabetics appears to exert a protective effect on the skeleton.

Primary Hyperparathyroidism. As discussed in the section on Primary Hyperparathyroidism, some patients may present with generalized osteopenia. This feature would be a strong indication for parathyroidectomy.

Immobilization. Severe osteoporosis is a complication in patients confined to bed for prolonged periods as a result of trauma or neuromuscular disorders. Bone biopsies reveal an increase in osteoclastic bone resorption and reduced osteoblastic activity.[77] The factors responsible for the often dramatic bone loss are thought to be local as well as systemic. In most studies of hypercalcemic immobilized patients circulating parathyroid hormone is suppressed.[60] The lack of muscular activity produces the localized bone loss in an unknown manner. A similar phenomenon occurs during space flight and is not prevented by exercise.

Successful treatment of osteoporosis caused by immobilization can be achieved by mobilizing the patient as soon as possible. In patients who develop hypercalcemia, usually under age 25, calcitonin therapy is effective in controlling hypercalcemia.[60] However, there is no evidence that osteoporosis can be prevented or corrected by calcitonin therapy.

Genetic Disorders. A variety of rare genetic disorders may be associated with osteoporosis.[116] These include osteogenesis imperfecta, homocystinuria, Menkes' syndrome, Ehlers-Danlos syndrome, and Marfan's syndrome. Defects in collagen synthesis probably account for the bone disease in these conditions.

Little has proved useful in the treatment of these disorders, although preliminary studies have suggested a beneficial effect of calcitonin in patients with osteogenesis imperfecta.[117]

Juvenile Osteoporosis. In prepubertal children a virulent form of generalized osteoporosis may rarely occur and result in pathologic fractures of many bones. No evidence of hormonal abnormality has been found in these patients. In most a spontaneous remission occurs coincident with the onset of puberty.

Rheumatoid Arthritis. Osteoporosis is a common complication in patients with rheumatoid arthritis. It is most apparent in periarticular areas (See Chapter 39), but it may be present in a generalized distribution.[118] In patients who have received glucocorticoids chronically and/or have impaired mobility, osteoporosis would be a likely consequence. However, it has been suggested that disordered calcium homeostasis with a state of hyperparathyroidism may be a feature of the disease unrelated to these factors. Hyperparathyroidism could not be confirmed in a study utilizing an extremely sensitive bioassay for parathyroid hormone.[119] It will require bone biopsy analysis as well as further biochemical studies to define the pathogenesis of osteoporosis in rheumatoid arthritis.

MISCELLANEOUS

Osteoporosis has been reported to occur in patients on chronic heparin therapy, in patients with systemic mastocytosis or scurvy, in patients with liver disease (and/or alcoholism), and in patients with hematologic malignancies.[116] The successful treatment of bone disease in these patients has seldom been documented.

OSTEOMALACIA

Definition

Osteomalacia is a disorder of diverse etiology characterized by an excess of unmineralized bone resulting from an impairment of bone mineralization. In children the disorder is associated with rickets, which has the additional feature of epiphyseal dysfunction leading to retardation of longitudinal growth and typical skeletal deformities.

Vitamin D Metabolism

To have a full appreciation of the pathogenesis and treatment of osteomalacia and rickets, an understanding of the complex metabolism of vitamin D is necessary (Fig. 106–15). A brief review of this subject will follow.

Figure 106–15. Metabolism of vitamin D_3 and some of its metabolites. The heavy arrows indicate the pathway of greatest biologic significance. The synthetic analogue $1\alpha,25$-hydroxyvitamin D_3 can also be converted to 1α-dihydroxycholecalciferol by the liver. The trihydroxylated derivative of vitamin D_3, $1\alpha,24R,25$-trihydroxy-vitamin D_3 can be produced under experimental conditions, but its biologic role is unknown. (From Haussler, M.R., and McCain. T.A.: N. Engl. J. Med. 297:974, 1977.)

Vitamin D_3 is a sterol that is synthesized in the skin from 7-dehydrocholesterol under the influence of ultraviolet light. Recent evidence indicates that an intermediary molecule, previtamin D_3, is formed subsequent to vitamin D_3.[120] A major advance in the knowledge of vitamin D action was the discovery that the parent molecule required metabolic activation before it could have any biological effect.[121-123] Enzymes in the liver, vitamin D_3-25-hydroxylase, and in the kidney, 25-hydroxyvitamin $D_3$1α-hydroxylase, are responsible for adding hydroxyl groups to the 25 and 1 positions, respectively, of the vitamin D_3 molecule. A third enzyme, 25-hydroxyvitamin D_3-24-hydroxylase, is present in the kidney, intestine, bone, and cartilage and is responsible for synthesis of 24R,25-dihydroxyvitamin D_3.[124] The liver enzyme is found in the microsomes, whereas the renal and cartilage enzymes are confined to mitochondria. Numerous other vitamin D metabolites have been identified in recent years, but their physiologic role has not been established.[124]

Vitamin D_2, irradiated ergosterol, is a synthetic form of vitamin D that is used to supplement a number of foods in the United States in order to provide a dietary source of vitamin D. This form of vitamin D appears to be metabolized in the same manner as the natural vitamin D_3 and has the same biological effects.

The regulation of vitamin D metabolism appears to depend primarily on the regulation of the renal hydroxylases of vitamin D.[124] The liver hydroxylase does not appear to be tightly regulated, since the concentration of 25-hydroxyvitamin D in the circulation correlates well with the intake of vitamin D over a wide range of doses.[125]

In the presence of a calcium deficient diet synthesis of 1α,25-dihydroxyvitamin D increases. This appears to be mediated by the action of increased parathyroid hormone secretion on the renal 25-hydroxyvitamin D_3-1α-hydroxylase rather than by hypocalcemia, since parathyroidectomy abolishes this phenomenon.[124] Another strong influence on the synthesis of 1α,25-dihydroxyvitamin D_3 is the level of phosphate in the extracellular fluid. Hypophosphatemia stimulates and hyperphosphatemia suppresses the synthesis of this potent vitamin D metabolite.[124] MacIntyre et al. have proposed that there are two main categories of regulators of renal vitamin D metabolism.[126] The first group is thought to control production of 1α,25-dihydroxyvitamin D during times of increased need for calcium: growth, pregnancy, and lactation. The proposed regulators include growth hormone, prolactin, placental lactogen, the circulating calcium concentration, and parathyroid hormone. The second type of regulation is thought to modulate 1α,25-dihydroxyvitamin D production in the face of varying amounts of the substrate 25-hydroxyvitamin D. It has been shown that both 25-hydroxyvitamin D_3 and 24,25-dihydroxyvitamin D_3 can suppress 25-hydroxyvitamin D_3-1α-hydroxylase activity in vitro.[126] Since 25-hydroxyvitamin D_3 is present in highest concentration in the circulation, it is possible that the concentration of this vitamin D metabolite acts to maintain a constant level of 1α,25-dihydroxyvitamin D in order to offset varying sun exposure, dietary vitamin D intake, and variable hepatic metabolism of vitamin D. There is also evidence that 1α,25-dihydroxyvitamin D_3 inhibits its own synthesis by suppressing renal 25-hydroxyvitamin D_3-α-hydroxylase.[127]

In animals who have been experimentally depleted of vitamin D, treatment with vitamin D_3 or D_2 produces an increase in intestinal calcium and phosphate absorption, restoration of normal bone mineralization, resolution of hyperplastic parathyroid glands, and an increase in the rate of growth. While it is accepted that 1α,25-dihydroxyvitamin D_3 is the critical metabolite in the control of intestinal calcium and phosphate absorption, the role of this and other metabolites in the expression of the other actions of vitamin D_3 is not certain.[124] For example, there is evidence that 24R,25-dihydroxyvitamin D_3 is involved in the mineralization of bone[128] and in the modulation of parathyroid function,[23] but this concept has been challenged by experiments that demonstrate that an analogue of vitamin D that cannot be hydroxylated at the 24 position has full biological activity.[124]

Another uncertain aspect of vitamin D action is whether 1α,25-dihydroxyvitamin D_3 is a physiologic regulator of bone resorption. It is a highly potent agent in inducing bone resorption in vitro and is quite effective in the treatment of hypoparathyroidism in man.[129] However, the latter response is primarily dependent upon increased intestinal absorption of calcium. Another possible site of direct vitamin D action is the kidney. There is evidence that 1α,25-dihydroxyvitamin D_3 increases renal tubular reabsorption of calcium.[124]

Clinical Features

Signs and Symptoms. Bone pain is the most common symptom of osteomalacia. It may be experienced in the pelvis, the lower extremities, the spine, and the ribs. In weight-bearing bones the pain is worsened by activity. Tenderness may be present upon palpation of the affected bones. Muscle weakness and tenderness, particularly of the proximal muscles of the lower extremity, may sometimes be dramatic features of the disorder. Tentany may occasionally reflect the presence of hypocalcemia.

Skeletal deformities are seldom encountered in adults who acquire the disorder after growth has ceased. In patients with severe osteomalacia of long duration, abnormal spinal curvature, a bell-shaped thorax, or pelvic deformity may develop. The child with rickets typically manifests the disorder with enlargement of the costochondral junctions (rachitic rosary) and bowing of the lower extremities.

Clinical Biochemistry. The biochemical abnormalities found in patients with osteomalacia can be classified into two types.[130] In those patients who develop osteomalacia as a consequence of an abnormality in vitamin

D homeostasis, the serum calcium and phosphate concentrations are generally low. In patients with hypophosphatemia as the etiologic factor serum calcium levels are almost always normal. Serum alkaline phosphatase concentrations are usually elevated in both types of patients. Serum parathyroid hormone levels are elevated in the hypocalcemic patients but seldom in the hypophosphatemic group.

The renal phosphate threshold is reduced in both groups. Aminoaciduria of a generalized nature is found in vitamin D deficient patients, whereas normal amino acid excretion or renal wasting of a single amino acid may be found in hypophosphatemic individuals. The generalized aminoaciduria is a consequence of secondary hyperparathyroidism. Urinary calcium excretion is markedly reduced in hypocalcemic patients and may be less so in the hypophosphatemic group. Urinary hydroxyproline excretion may be moderately increased in vitamin D deficient patients,[8] another reflection of secondary hyperparathyroidism.

Assays of vitamin D metabolites have recently been applied to the assessment of normal subjects and patients with osteomalacia.[131] The concentration of 25-hydroxyvitamin D (25-hydroxyvitamin D_3 + D_2) in normal subjects ranges from 10 to 80 ng per milliliter in most studies and varies with sun exposure and dietary vitamin D intake. 24,25-Dihydroxyvitamin D circulates at concentrations about 5 to 10 percent of the liver metabolite and 1α,25-dihydroxyvitamin D at approximately 0.1 percent of 25-hydroxyvitamin D. As would be expected, 25-hydroxyvitamin D and 24,25-dihydroxyvitamin D are found in low concentrations in the circulation of patients with classic vitamin D deficient osteomalacia. An unexpected finding has been the presence of normal levels of 1α,25-dihydoxyvitamin D in some patients with nutritional osteomalacia.[132] Depending on the pathogenesis of osteomalacia, other types of abnormalities of the circulating metabolites of vitamin D have been described. These will be discussed individually under Pathogenesis.

Radiology. The radiologic features of osteomalacia to a great extent mimic those of osteoporosis.[133] A generalized loss of bone density with thinning of the cortex is indistinguishable from that found in osteoporosis. Occasionally the trabecular pattern of the bone is thickened, and mottled radiolucent areas may be apparent. Paradoxically, osteosclerosis may be an unusual finding in isolated bones, particularly the vertebral bodies. This is much more likely to be found during the healing phase of the disease.

In patients with vitamin D deficiency radiologic evidence of secondary hyperparathyroidism may be manifested by subperiosteal resorption of the phalanges, cysts, or brown tumors and widening of the spaces at the symphysis pubis and at the sacroiliac joints.

The most characteristic radiologic feature of osteomalacia is the presence of pseudofractures,[134] also termed Looser zones or Milkman fractures (Fig. 106–16). These narrow zones of rarefaction are most often found in the shafts of long bones but may also affect flat bones. They

Figure 106–16. A pseudofracture at the lateral border of the proximal right femur in a 65-year-old woman with osteomalacia resulting from renal tubular acidosis.

are often bilaterally symmetric. Common sites at which they are found include the femoral neck and shaft, the ulna and radius, the pubic and ischial rami, the scapula, the clavicle, the ribs, and the metacarpals, metatarsals, and phalanges. Sclerosis of the borders of a pseudofracture is sometimes seen in severe longstanding cases.

Deformity of the skeleton is a feature which is helpful in distinguishing osteomalacia or rickets from osteoporosis. In adults and children kyphoscoliosis of the spine, a "bell-shaped" thorax, a triangular shape of the pelvic lumen, and bowing of the lower extremities are characteristic findings, although more common in children. Knock knees (genu valgum) may occur in children.

The radiologic signs of rickets are easier to discern at the metaphyses which are most rapidly growing. During the first year of life the upper extremities and limbs grow rapidly and exhibit the most significant abnormality. Subsequently the lower extremities are most likely to exhibit changes caused by rickets. The radiologic features of rickets include a widening of the growth plates, a variable deficiency of the zones of provisional calci-

Figure 106–17. *A* Roentgenograms of the knees in a 13-month-old child with rickets resulting from vitamin D deficiency. Note the wide growth plates, the irregular ends of the metaphyses, and the wide metaphyses. *B*, Almost complete healing of rickets after 5 months of treatment with vitamin D.

fication, an irregular appearance of the ends of the metaphyses, and metaphyseal cupping and widening (Fig. 106–17). The healing process begins with mineralization of the epiphyseal cartilage, which appears as a dense line adjacent to the metaphysis. In patients in whom there is a fluctuating degree of the activity of rickets, transverse lines termed Harris lines may be apparent across the shafts of long bones.

Bone Pathology. A bone biopsy may occasionally be required to confirm a suspected diagnosis of mild osteomalacia. The criteria used to judge the presence of osteomalacia are both an excess of unmineralized osteoid and a decrease in the rate of bone mineralization as determined by labeling with tetracycline. The increase in osteoid is reflected by the greater extent of osteoid seams covering cortical and trabecular bone surfaces and by an increased width of the seams. Numerous osteoblasts are usually present. An excess surface area of osteoid may also occur in such disorders as thyrotoxicosis, primary hyperparathyroidism, and Paget's disease, in which an increased rate of bone formation and a normal rate of mineralization are present. In these disorders the width of the osteoid seams is usually not increased. An unusual subset of patients with bone disease associated with total parenteral nutrition exhibit atypical histologic findings.[135] Increased osteoid and im-

paired uptake of tetracycline are found, and osteoblasts are absent.

In patients with vitamin D deficiency, histologic evidence of secondary hyperparathyroidism may be manifested by an increase in the number of osteoclasts and by a fibrovascular marrow. These features are usually not present in patients with osteomalacia caused by hypophosphatemia. In hypophosphatemic osteomalacia the increase in osteoid and impaired mineralization is indistinguishable from that found in vitamin D deficiency. It has been reported that a decrease in mineral surrounding osteocyte lacunae is a feature of hypophosphatemic osteomalacia, but this has subsequently been observed in other types of osteomalacia.[13]

Pathogenesis and Treatment

Osteomalacia or rickets may develop as an isolated pathologic entity or as a feature of a disease state of a more general nature. A classification of these disorders is listed in Table 106–5. It can be seen from this classification that the majority of patients will have an abnormality of vitamin D metabolism or action, or will have hypophosphatemia. The latter abnormality leads to bone disease, because phosphate is an essential constituent of hydroxyapatite.

Table 106–5. Classification of Osteomalacia and Rickets

1. Reduction of circulating vitamin D metabolites
   a. Vitamin D deficiency due to inadequate ultraviolet light and dietary lack
   b. Vitamin D malabsorption
      (1) Postgastrectomy
      (2) Small intestinal disease
      (3) Pancreatic insufficiency
      (4) Insufficient bile salts
   c. Abnormal vitamin D metabolism
      (1) Liver disease
      (2) Chronic renal failure
      (3) Vitamin D dependent rickets (25-hydroxyvitamin D-1α-hydroxylase deficiency)
      (4) Mesenchymal tumors
      (5) Anticonvulsant drugs
      (6) Glutethimide
   d. Renal loss
      Nephrotic syndrome
2. Peripheral resistance to vitamin D
      (1) Chronic renal failure
      (2) Anticonvulsant drugs
      (3) Vitamin D dependent rickets Type II
3. Hypophosphatemia
   a. Malnutrition
   b. Malabsorption due to gastrointestinal disease or phosphate binding antacids
   c. Chronic dialysis
   d. Renal phosphate wasting
      (1) Hypophosphatemic rickets
         (a) Familial X-linked
         (b) Autosomal recessive
         (c) Sporadic
      (2) Hypophosphatemic osteomalacia
         (a) Familial X-linked
         (b) Sporadic
      (3) Familial renal phosphate leak with hypercalciuria, nephrolithiasis, and osteomalacia
      (4) Fanconi syndrome
      (5) Mesenchymal tumors, prostatic carcinoma, fibrous dysplasia, and epidermal nevus syndrome
      (6) Primary hyperparathyroidism
4. Miscellaneous
   a. Inhibitors of calcification
      (1) Sodium fluoride
      (2) Disodium etidronate
   b. Calcium deficiency
   c. Hypophosphatasia
   d. Fibrogenesis imperfecta ossium
   e. Total parenteral nutrition
   f. Systemic acidosis

Vitamin D Deficiency. Classic vitamin D deficiency is seldom found in the United States at present. To develop this deficiency state requires not only avoidance of sunshine but also an inadequate intake of vitamin D–supplemented food. Prevention of vitamin D deficiency can be accomplished through dietary means by providing a recommended intake of 400 IU (10 μg) daily for children and 100 IU (2.5 μg) daily for adults. In patients with established bone disease these doses would be adequate to produce full healing. However, to hasten the clinical course toward more rapid recovery, as much as two- to tenfold higher doses have been given.[134] Adequate dietary calcium and phosphorus intake must also be maintained to optimize the healing process. Dihydrotachysterol, a potent analogue of vitamin D, is highly effective in treating hypocalcemia but is not recom-

mended for treating osteomalacia, since it has little antirachitic activity.

With the initiation of vitamin D therapy the earliest biochemical change that can be documented is a rise in plasma phosphate concentration within 3 to 4 days.[133] Plasma calcium may decline and alkaline phosphatase rise initially, but after weeks both move toward normal levels. Care must be taken to avoid vitamin D intoxication in those patients receiving pharmacologic doses. This can be avoided by measuring the plasma calcium every 2 to 4 weeks, as well as by obtaining appropriate radiographs to assess the rate of healing in children with rickets (Fig. 106–17). The dose should be reduced gradually toward maintenance levels once radiographic improvement is noted.

Vitamin D Malabsorption. The malabsorption of dietary vitamin D may occur as a result of impaired gastrointestinal function, pancreatic insufficiency, or inadequate bile salts. Despite this, the key factor in the development of osteomalacia in these patients appears to be failure of adequate exposure to ultraviolet light.[136]

The treatment of severe vitamin D malabsorption is dependent upon the ability of the physician to correct the underlying disease. For example, appropriate therapy of gluten-sensitive enteropathy will in itself lead to correction of bone disease. In irreversible disorders pharmacologic doses of vitamin D or a metabolite may be required. In rare patients parenteral vitamin D administration may be necessary to achieve sufficient levels of vitamin D metabolites in the circulation.

Abnormal Vitamin D Metabolism. Impairment of 25-hydroxylation of vitamin D has been suggested to occur in patients with parenchymal liver disease as evidenced by the finding of decreased concentrations of 25-hydroxyvitamin D in the circulation.[137] The low levels of this vitamin D metabolite may also arise from poor nutrition and lack of sunshine. Treatment with vitamin D_2 in pharmacologic doses has been demonstrated to raise 25-hydroxyvitamin D levels in cirrhotic patients.[137] This suggests that a defect in 25-hydroxylation may not be present in all patients with parenchymal liver disease.

Patients on long-term anticonvulsant therapy may develop rickets and/or osteomalacia.[138] This is associated with low levels of 25-hydroxyvitamin D thought to result from increased metabolism of this metabolite to more polar metabolites. Both normal[139] and low[140] levels of plasma 1α,25-dihydroxyvitamin D and low levels of 24,25-dihydroxyvitamin D have been reported.[140] Prophylactic administration of vitamin D_2 has been reported to prevent or reduce the severity of anticonvulsant-induced bone disease. Doses of 3000 units or greater per week have been used. Higher doses of vitamin D (up to 15,000 units daily) may be required for full healing of established bone disease. Lower doses of 25-hydroxycholecalciferol may be effective.[138]

Chronic renal failure is associated with a reduction in both 1α,25-dihydroxyvitamin D and 24,25-dihydroxyvitamin D in the circulation. Treatment of patients with 1α,25-dihydroxycholecalciferol does not always heal the bone disease which is commonly found in patients with end-stage renal failure. This will be discussed further under Renal Osteodystrophy.

Reduction of circulating 1α,25-dihydroxyvitamin D has also been reported in patients with vitamin D dependent rickets, an autosomal recessive state.[131] Physiologic doses of 1α,25-dihydroxycholecalciferol are capable of healing the bone disease of these patients who appear to be deficient in renal 25-hydroxyl-1α-hydroxylase.[141]

Systemic acidosis has been proposed as another factor in producing 1α,25-dihydroxyvitamin D deficiency. Both in vivo and in vitro studies have demonstrated impairment of production of this renal metabolite of vitamin D in the presence of a low ambient pH.[142,143] However, a study in 10 patients with renal tubular acidosis revealed no abnormalities of 1α,25-dihydroxy vitamin D in the circulation.[144] In chronic renal failure and Fanconi syndrome correction of the acidosis may be helpful in controlling associated osteoma lacia or rickets.

Decreased levels of 1α,25-dihydroxyvitamin D have also been reported in rare patients with mesenchymal tumors who have hypophosphatemia and osteomalacia,[145] in patients with prostatic carcinoma,[146] and in patients with pseudohypoparathyroidism who may have subclinical osteomalacia.[147] The pathogenesis of this apparent deficiency of 1α,25-dihydroxyvitamin D is unclear, and the need for therapy with this potent metabolite is not well established in each of these disorders.

Renal Loss. Evidence of renal loss of vitamin D_3, 25-hydroxyvitamin D_3, 24,25-dihydroxyvitamin D_3, and 1α,25-dihydroxyvitamin D_3 associated with low blood levels has been reported in patients with nephrotic syndrome.[148,149] In one study bone biopsies revealed subtle osteomalacia and secondary hyperparathyroidism.[150] In a second study normal serum ionized calcium and parathyroid hormone levels were found in a group of patients who had less severe nephrotic syndrome based on biochemical parameters.[149]

Peripheral Resistance to Vitamin D. In chronic renal failure evidence has been presented which suggests that higher than physiologic doses of 1α,25-dihydroxycholecalciferol are required to increase intestinal calcium absorption.[151]

Normal levels of 1α-25-dihydroxyvitamin D are present in some patients with rickets or osteomalacia who have been treated on a long-term basis with anticonvulsant drugs.[139] This is consistent with the hypothesis that these drugs inhibit the peripheral action of 1α,25-dihydroxyvitamin D. There is in vitro evidence of impairment of the action of this vitamin D metabolite on bone and intestine in the presence of diphenylhydantoin or phenobarbital.[138]

Patients with hypocalcemia, secondary hyperparathyroidism, osteomalacia, osteitis fibrosa, and elevated serum 1α,25-dihydroxyvitamin D levels have been reported.[131] A subset of these rare patients have alopecia totalis and skin fibroblasts that exhibit defective nuclear uptake of 1α,25-dihydroxycholecalciferol.[131] The syndrome has been termed vitamin D dependent rickets type II. Successful therapy requires pharmacologic doses of vitamin D_2, 25-hydroxycholecalciferol, or 1α,25-dihydroxycholecalciferol.

Hypophosphatemia. Chronic hypophosphatemia, a manifestation of phosphate deficiency, may lead to osteomalacia and rickets through several routes. Less commonly it may develop as a result of poor nutrition or because of impairment of dietary phosphate absorption in patients with gastrointestinal diseases or in those who ingest large amounts of phosphate-binding antacids.[152] Treatment of such patients should provide dietary or supplemental phosphate sufficient to correct the hypophosphatemia. This is easier to achieve if underlying gastrointestinal disease can be improved and if the offending antacids are discontinued. Hypophosphatemia has also been associated with reversible bone disease in a few patients undergoing chronic dialysis.[153] The most frequent pathogenesis of hypophosphatemic bone disease is through the mechanism of renal phosphate wasting.

Renal Phosphate Wasting. The most common cause of rickets in the United States is X-linked vitamin D resistant or hypophosphatemic rickets, a disorder first described by Albright in 1937.[154] Since then it has been appreciated that hypophosphatemic bone disease associated with a renal phosphate "leak" in children and adults is heterogeneous in character.

X-Linked Hypophosphatemic Rickets. This disorder is a dominantly inherited disease in which the phenotypic trait of hypophosphatemia is transmitted by the X chromosome.[155] In males bone disease and short stature are invariable, whereas in heterozygous females there is great variability of penetrance of these somatic traits.

The pathogenesis of hypophosphatemia is related to a severe impairment of phosphate transport by the renal tubules. The exact nature of the abnormality in transepithelial phosphate transport is as yet undetermined. It is clearly not due to excessive parathyroid hormone secretion, since parathyroid hormone levels in the circulation are usually normal[156] or only slightly elevated.[157] In a small number of patients abnormalities in intestinal absorption of phosphate have also been described. However, this is not an invariable finding.[155]

Evidence for an abnormality in vitamin D metabolism in patients with hypophosphatemic rickets has accumulated in recent years.[131] Serum 1α,25-hydroxyvitamin D levels are normal or low; the lower values are generally found in vitamin D–treated patients. Since hypophosphatemia is a potent stimulator of renal synthesis of 1α,25-dihydroxyvitamin D, it has been suggested that a normal level of this metabolite represents a relative deficiency. Further evidence of impaired synthesis of 1α,25-dihydroxyvitamin D in this syndrome was found when exogenous parathyroid hormone produced a blunted response in circulating levels of this vitamin D metabolite.[158] The fact that 1α,25-dihydroxycholecalciferol treatment of patients with x-linked hypophosphatemic rickets does not fully correct the hypophosphatemia suggests that an abnormality in renal metabolism of vitamin D is not the primary defect in these patients.

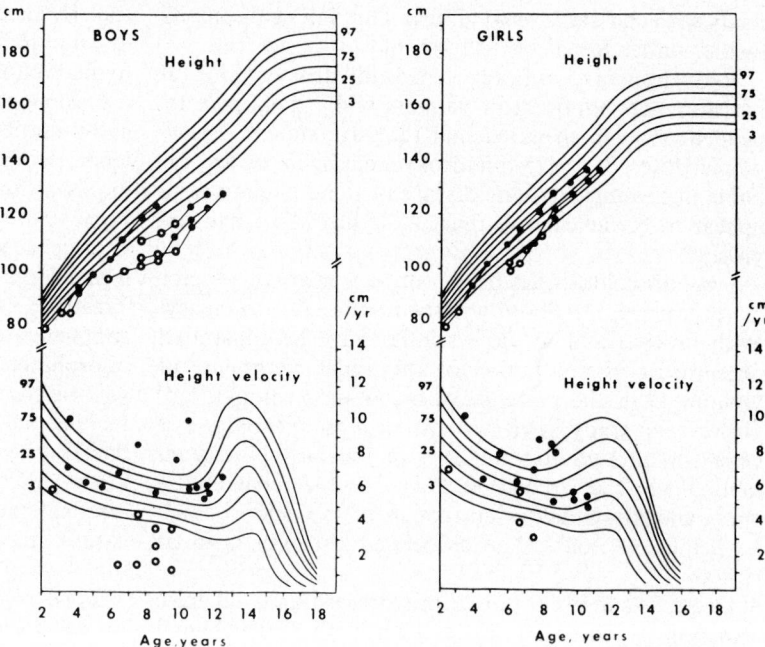

Figure 106–18. Growth charts for boys and girls with X-linked hypophosphatemic rickets before (open circles) and during (closed circles) phosphate supplementation. Vitamin D alone was the major form of treatment given before the combined regimen was begun. The upper graphs show growth as a linear measurement related to age. The lower graphs indicate the rate of growth (gain in height per year). Graphs show percentiles for a normal reference population. (From Glorieux, FH., Scriver, C.R., Reade, T.M., Goldman, H., and Roseborough, A.: N. Engl. J. Med. 287: 481, 1972.)

The earliest treatment of X-linked hypophosphatemic rickets was with pharmacologic doses of vitamin D or dihydrotachysterol. These drugs were often used at near toxic levels, which led to hypercalciuria and hypercalcemia in some patients. Healing of rickets occurred in some patients, but significant improvement of short stature was seldom observed. A major advance in the therapy of this disorder occurred when it was appreciated that supplemental phosphate could produce dramatic clinical benefits.[159] If the serum phosphate concentration can be maintained near 4 mg per dl during most of the 24 hours, a remarkable increase in the linear growth velocity of patients can be achieved (Fig. 106–18). If appropriate treatment is begun at an early age, it is conceivable that prevention of dwarfism and severe rachitic deformities can be achieved. The amount of phosphate supplementation required for such an effect is empiric. Initial treatment should be with smaller amounts of a buffered phosphate solution. Fraser and Scriver[155] recommend the following schedule in 1-year-old children: 0.125 g phosphate three times a day on day 1, 0.25 g three times a day on day 2, 0.25 g four times a day on day 3, and 0.25 g every 4 hours five times a day on day 4 and succeeding days. Adjustment of the dose will depend on the clinical response. It may require as much as 5 g of elemental phosphorus to control the disease. The most common side effect of the treatment is diarrhea, but this is seldom a persistent problem after several weeks. The main difficulty with this therapy is compliance. The cooperation of the parents is critical in assuring that the night dose as well as the other doses are taken. The need for frequent ingestion of phosphate is dictated by observations that the peak serum phosphate concentration is reached about 1½ hours after a dose and that 4 hours later the level is back to baseline.

Optimal therapy of X-linked hypophosphatemic rickets requires the addition of pharmacologic doses of vitamin D. This is necessary because phosphate therapy alone will reduce the ionized calcium concentration by increasing bone calcium deposition and induce a state of secondary hyperparathyroidism.[159] This can be treated or prevented with doses of vitamin D up to 50,000 units daily. Occasionally higher doses may be required.

Although growth may be stimulated by phosphate and vitamin D therapy of X-linked hypophosphatemic rickets, bone mineralization may not be improved.[131] A combination of phosphate salts and 1α,25-dihydrocholecalciferol appears to produce the best result in regard to healing the osteomalacia of trabecular bone.[160] Persistence of a low calcification rate in the cortical bone of most patients despite this therapy suggests that there may be a primary osteoblast defect in some patients.[161]

After full growth is achieved in a treated patient, the need for vitamin D can be re-evaluated, since a fully mineralized skeleton should protect against hypocalcemia induced by phosphate therapy alone.

In patients with skeletal deformities of the lower extremities surgical intervention may be needed to improve mobility and prevent the long-term complication of degenerative joint disease. After adequate metabolic control of the disease, procedures such as osteotomy or epiphyseal stapling may greatly improve the immediate and future status of a patient.

Autosomal Recessive Hypophosphatemic Rickets. Autosomal recessive inheritance of hypophosphatemic rickets is quite rare. Two families have been described in which the features of X-linked hypophosphatemic rickets were present but the genetics of the disorder could be explained only on the basis of autosomal recessive inheritance.[162,163] A particularly prominent feature of the patients was gross osteosclerosis.

Sporadic Hypophosphatemic Rickets. Hypophosphatemia accompanied by classic rickets uncommonly may occur in the absence of abnormal phosphate levels and/or bone disease in any family member. This disorder may arise from the same mutation that is responsible for X-linked hypophosphatemic rickets and is clinically indistinguishable from the latter problem. Treatment with vitamin D and phosphate has been demonstrated to increase the growth rate and heal the rickets and osteomalacia.

Hypophosphatemic Osteomalacia. There are two forms of hypophosphatemic osteomalacia in adults. Most commonly it is a sporadic condition in which renal phosphate wasting occurs to the same degree as in patients with familial X-linked rickets.[164] The osteomalacia can be healed by phosphate supplementation alone, but vitamin D in large doses is usually required to prevent the complication of secondary hyperparathyroidism.

A familial form of hypophosphatemic osteomalacia has been described in a single large kindred.[165] The inheritance of the disorder was X-linked. The patients were identical to those with familial X-linked hypophosphatemic rickets, with the major difference of no rachitic deformities in the kindred with adult onset of bone disease.

Familial Renal Phosphate Leak with Hypercalciuria, Nephrolithiasis and Osteomlacia. An apparently autosomal dominant syndrome of renal phosphate wasting, hypercalciuria, nephrolithiasis, and osteomalacia has been described in a Jewish Yemenite family.[166] The exact pathogenesis of bone disease in this family is unclear, since evidence of hyperabsorption of both calcium and phosphorous was found.

Fanconi Syndrome. In the variety of disorders classified under the general term Fanconi syndrome, renal phosphate wasting may be significant enough to produce bone disease.[164] Since these patients have a generalized impairment of function of the proximal renal tubules, urinary losses of bicarbonate leading to systemic acidosis may also contribute to the development of bone disease.[167] Optimal therapy of these patients may require a combination of phosphate, vitamin D, and alkali.

Mesenchymal Tumor, Prostatic Carcinoma, Fibrous Dysplasia, and Epidermal Nevus Syndrome. Rickets and/or osteomalacia may develop in patients with a variety of benign or malignant mesenchymal tumors[167] (Table 106–6), as well as in patients with prostatic carcinoma,[146] fibrous dysplasia,[168] and epidermal nevus syndrome.[169] These patients have in common the findings of hypo-

Table 106–6. Types of Tumors Associated with Osteomalacia

1. Giant cell tumor, malignant or benign
2. Reparative giant cell granuloma
3. Hemangioma
4. Hemangiopericytoma
5. Angiosarcoma
6. Nonossifying fibroma
7. Mesenchymal tumors, unclassified, malignant or benign
8. Malignant neurilemmoma
9. Prostatic carcinoma

phosphatemia, increased renal phosphate clearance, normal or slightly decreased serum calcium concentrations, usually normal serum parathyroid hormone concentrations, and reversal of all abnormalities after successful removal of pathologic tissue. In a patient with a giant cell tumor of bone and in patients with prostatic carcinoma, serum $1\alpha,25$-dihydroxyvitamin D levels were low.[145,146] The significance of this observation in regard to the pathogenesis of this syndrome is unclear. It is more likely that an unknown phosphaturic factor secreted by the abnormal tissue is responsible for the renal and skeletal findings. In one study a phosphaturic response in dogs was produced by an extract of a fibroangioma.[169]

Phosphate and vitamin D therapy in patients with tumors has been generally disappointing. Surgery is clearly the treatment of choice. In patients with fibrous dysplasia and hypophosphatemic osteomalacia or rickets vitamin D therapy has been effective.[168]

Primary Hyperparathyroidism. The phosphaturic effect of parathyroid hormone is responsible for the finding of hypophosphatemia in about 50 percent of patients with primary hyperparathyroidism. It is conceivable that a secondary form of osteomalacia could develop in patients with severe hypophosphatemia. Quantitative morphometry of bone biopsies from some patients with primary hyperparathyroidism has revealed a reduction in calcification rate but no increase in the width of the osteoid seams.[170] No correlations with serum phosphate concentrations were made. It is conceivable that phosphate therapy in patients with primary hyperparathyroidism may produce a beneficial effect on bone mineralization, but this has not been studied adequately enough to allow any conclusions to be reached.

Miscellaneous. *Inhibitors of Calcification. Sodium Fluoride.* In areas of endemic fluorosis[95] or in osteoporotic patients treated with sodium fluoride, inhibition of bone mineralization may occur. An excess of osteoid can be seen in histologic sections, and pseudofractures may be found on radiologic examination. If supplemental calcium is administered with sodium fluoride to patients with osteoporosis, the mineralization defect is prevented.

Disodium Etidronate. Diphosphonates are synthetic analogues of pyrophosphate, a natural inhibitor of bone formation and resorption. The diphosphonate disodium etidronate is an effective suppressor of the activity of Paget's disease of bone and of postoperative heterotopic ossification. However, at administered doses of 10 to 20 mg per kg of body weight it may inhibit mineralization and lead to pathologic fractures in patients with Paget's disease.[167] At doses of 5 mg per kg suppression of disease activity is maintained without diffuse evidence of increased osteoid. Recently, focal osteomalacia has been demonstrated in patients treated with 5 mg/per kg.[171]

Calcium Deficiency. Radiologic evidence of rickets[172] and histologic evidence of osteomalacia[173] have been documented in children with low dietary intakes of calcium. The features of the disease were identical to classic vitamin D deficient rickets; hypocalcemia, hypophosphatemia, elevated serum alkaline phosphatase, secondary hyperparathyroidism, and typical radiologic features of rickets were present. The patients had been on an inadequate calcium intake but were not vitamin deficient. Levels of plasma or serum 25-hydroxyvitamin D were normal. The rickets healed when adequate dietary calcium intake was provided. No change in vitamin D intake was made. It is not known whether calcium deficiency can cause osteomalacia in adults.

Hypophosphatasia. Hypophosphatasia is a disorder that is inherited primarily as an autosomal recessive trait, although in some families an autosomal dominant inheritance seems likely.[174] The disorder is characterized by a failure of calcification of osteoid and epiphyseal cartilage probably because of a deficiency of alkaline phosphatase. It is postulated that the deficiency of alkaline phosphatase leads to elevated plasma and urine levels of inorganic pyrophosphate and phosphorylethanolamine. Inorganic pyrophosphate is a substrate for alkaline phosphatase and is felt to be an important intermediary in the initiation of bone mineralization by extracellular matrix vesicles. The role of phosphorylethanolamine in bone mineralization is unknown, but this ester is hydrolyzed by alkaline phosphatase.

In children other features of hypophosphatasia may include premature synostosis of the cranial vault, premature loss of deciduous teeth, and unexplained hypercalcemia and nephrocalcinosis. Adults appear to have a milder form of the disorder in many instances. Hypercalcemia is seldom found, and the skeletal abnormalities are often less severe.

Treatment of this disorder with vitamin D has been ineffective. Oral phosphate therapy has been reported to improve the calcification of bone as determined by radiographic survey.

Fibrogenesis Imperfecta Ossium. Fibrogenesis imperfecta ossium is a rare disorder which occurs in males over age 50 who were previously healthy.[175] The patients develop progressive skeletal pain and tenderness and may become completely incapacitated. The radiologic findings are striking in that there is a generalized increase in bone density with a lack of trabeculation and a mottled appearance. Pseudofractures may be present. Bone histology reveals an increase in the amount of osteoid and impaired mineralization as evidenced by abnormal uptake of tetracycline. The absence of a normal lamellar arrangement of the collagen fibers has led to the speculation that there is an underlying collagen defect. This is consistent with the observations of normal serum calcium and phosphorus concentrations. The serum alkaline phosphatase activity is increased.

Because of the rarity of this disorder there is little experience concerning therapy. Some improvement with vitamin D or dihydrotachysterol therapy has been reported.

Total Parenteral Nutrition. Patients on long-term total parenteral nutrition may develop bone disease characterized by pain, patchy osteomalacia, reduced serum levels of 1α,25-dihydroxyvitamin D and parathyroid hormone, hypercalciuria, and intermittent hypercalcemia.[135,176] A possible relationship of this syndrome to aluminum excess from casein hydrolysate has been hypothesized,[176] but the syndrome also occurs in patients who receive free amino acids instead of casein hydrolysate.[177] Withdrawal of vitamin D from the parenteral solutions inexplicably improved the disorder in the latter group of patients.

RENAL OSTEODYSTROPHY

Definition

Renal osteodystrophy is the general term used to describe the variable constellation of skeletal abnormalities which may be encountered in patients with chronic renal failure. One or more of the following metabolic bone disorders may be encountered in a single patient: osteomalacia, secondary hyperparathyroidism, osteoporosis, and osteosclerosis.

Clinical Features

Signs and Symptoms. The clinical presentation of patients with renal osteodystrophy is quite similar to that of patients with rickets and/or osteomalacia. Bone pain and muscle weakness are prominent features in adults, whereas short stature and skeletal deformities are additional problems encountered in children.

Soft tissue calcification may affect a variety of sites in patients with severe renal failure.[178] Corneal and conjunctival calcifications are most common. Acute conjunctival inflammation may give rise to a "red eye." Arterial calcification may rarely cause gangrene, usually involving the fingers or toes. Tumoral calcinosis around large joints may occasionally occur. Calcinosis cutis is usually associated with intense pruritus. Muscle calcification may reach massive proportions. Cardiac and pulmonary calcifications may impair function of these organs to such an extent as to be fatal.

Clinical Biochemistry. The patient with renal osteodystrophy may present with a wide variety of abnormal biochemical parameters. Serum calcium concentration may be low, normal, or even slightly elevated.[179] Serum phosphorus is almost always elevated. Alkaline phosphatase activity occasionally is normal but often is elevated. Serum parathyroid hormone concentration is usually slightly to markedly elevated, although there is a small group of patients with osteomalacia unresponsive to vitamin D therapy who have low levels.[180] These latter patients comprise a group of hemodialysis patients who have high bone aluminum concentrations.[181] Serum 1α,25-dihydroxyvitamin D[131] and 24,25-dihydroxyvitamin D[182] levels are low, whereas 25-hydroxyvitamin D is normal if dietary intake is adequate.[183] Urinary cyclic AMP excretion is usually elevated, reflecting a state of secondary hyperparathyroidism. For the same reason the renal tubular maximum for phosphorus is reduced. Urinary calcium excretion per 24 hours is reduced because of a decreased filtered load of calcium. Increased bone resorption is reflected by elevated plasma hydroxyproline levels, although this may not be a precise index, since renal failure per se raises the concentration also.[179]

Radiology. The radiologic findings which may be present in patients with renal osteodystrophy reflect the presence of osteomalacia, secondary hyperparathyroidism, osteosclerosis, or osteoporosis. Pseudofractures may develop in children or adults, whereas skeletal deformites mainly are found in children. Subperiosteal bone resorption, "salt and pepper" skull, and other lesions of hyperparathyroidism are commonly seen. Osteosclerosis is also a common finding, most often seen in the spine. The "rugger jersey" spine is characterized by sclerosis of the inferior and superior portions of the vertebral bodies. Sclerosis may also be found in the skull and long bones. Generalized osteopenia is an uncommon feature of renal osteodystrophy.

Soft tissue calcifications are a dramatic feature in some patients. Arterial calcification as well as calcification in a variety of organs may occasionally be the first indication of the presence of chronic renal failure (Fig. 106–19).

Bone Pathology. The histologic abnormalities found in the bone of patients with renal osteodystrophy are usually divided into two types: those of osteomalacia and those of hyperparathyroidism.[184] Patients who exhibit osteomalacia as the dominant abnormality will have widened osteoid seams, which cover an increased percentage of the trabecular surface of the bone, and impairment of uptake of tetracycline. Numerous osteoblasts are usually present, and there may be evidence of hyperparathyroidism as manifested by increased numbers of osteoclasts and marrow fibrosis.

In patients with hyperparathyroidism as the dominant feature, increased areas of osteoclastic bone resorption and marrow fibrosis are present. In these patients there is increased new bone formation as indicated by the presence of many osteoblasts, by an increased trabecular surface area of osteoid, and by studies utilizing tetracycline labeling.

A small percentage of hemodialysis patients have an unusual form of osteomalacia.[180] These patients exhibit the typical histologic findings of osteomalacia but have no evidence of secondary hyperparathyroidism in bone biopsies or by measurement of serum parathyroid hormone concentrations. In these patients high bone aluminum concentrations are found and correlate directly with the amount of unmineralized osteoid.[181]

Osteosclerosis, which is commonly found in the axial skeleton,[178] is characterized by an increased volume of bone. Although widened osteoid seams are present, the total amount of mineralized bone is increased. Woven bone may also be a feature of the lesions.

Decreased bone volume may complicate renal osteodystrophy. This least common complication of renal failure is always accompanied by the histologic features of osteomalacia and/or secondary hyperparathyroidism.

Pathogenesis and Treatment

The pathogenesis of osteomalacia in patients with renal osteodystrophy to a great extent is related to impairment of vitamin D metabolism. Low levels of $1\alpha,25$-

Figure 106–19. Severe arterial calcification in a patient with end-stage renal failure.

dihydroxychlolecalciferol are a consequence of a reduced functional renal mass and perhaps, in part, of hyperphosphatemia. Impaired intestinal calcium absorption and hypocalcemia are corrected by treatment with 1α,25-dihydroxycholecalciferol in physiologic or near-physiologic doses.[151] 25-Hydroxycholecalciferol also is highly effective in near-physiologic amounts. It has been suggested that osteomalacia in patients with renal failure primarily occurs in patients with poor dietary vitamin D intake, a state which is reflected by low levels of the hepatic metabolite in the circulation.[183] If this is so, it is not clear why vitamin D_2 must be used in pharmacologic amounts to treat patients effectively. Dihydrotachysterol is more potent than vitamin D_2 because it does not require renal metabolism to be active, but has not been widely studied. It has been suggested that 25-hydroxycholecalciferol is the preferred drug to treat the osteomalacia of renal failure because it is more likely to cause a significant improvement in bone mineralization.[185] For reasons which are poorly understood, bone mineralization is not always corrected by 1α-25-dihydroxycholecalciferol therapy.[186] It is conceivable that 25-hydroxycholecalciferol itself or conversion of the metabolite to 24,25-dihydroxycholecalciferol may be necessary for effective bone mineralization to occur. However an alternative possibility is that suboptimal regimens of 1α,25-dihydroxycholecalciferol have been used in some patients.

The failure of 1α,25-dihydroxycholecalciferol therapy in a group of patients with renal osteodystrophy has led to the characterization of a syndrome resembling osteomalacia but apparently unrelated to vitamin D.[180] This syndrome occurs in uremic patients undergoing regular dialysis and is histologically characterized by widened osteoid seams and a lack of features of secondary hyperparathyroidism. Serum parathyroid hormone levels are normal or low in the presence of normal or slightly elevated serum calcium concentrations. Treatment with vitamin D_2, dihydrotachysterol, or 1α,25-dihydroxycholecalciferol fails to improve mineralization. Treatment with 1α,25-dihydroxycholecalciferol often causes frank hypercalcemia. In one patient renal transplantation improved the skeletal abnormality. It is not known whether the excretory or endocrine function of the kidney was the responsible factor in the improvement of this patient. Other factors which could conceivably be involved in the pathogenesis of this subgroup of renal osteodystrophy are acidosis, aluminum toxicity, hypophosphatemia caused by antacid therapy, and hypermagnesemia. Recent evidence points to an excess of aluminum in bone as the important factor.[181]

The development of secondary hyperparathyroidism in patients with renal failure has been attributed to a variety of mechanisms. Phosphate retention, impaired vitamin D metabolism, and skeletal resistance to parathyroid hormone have all been proposed as the underlying cause of secondary hyperparathyroidism.[179] It is likely that all these factors contribute to the pathogenesis of hyperparathyroidism in an interrelated fashion. Impaired vitamin D metabolism leading to a vitamin D deficient state is at least partially responsible for skeletal resistance to parathyroid hormone. The latter can be significantly but not completely corrected by 1α,25-dihydroxycholecalciferol therapy in uremic dogs and rats.[179] It is possible that an unknown uremic "toxin" is also partially responsible for parathyroid hormone resistance.

In hyperparathyroid patients with a low or normal serum calcium concentration excellent therapeutic results with 1α,25-dihydroxycholecalciferol have been achieved.[179] Suppression of parathyroid hormone secretion, healing of the lesions of osteitis fibrosa on bone biopsy and x-ray (Fig. 106–20), and marked improvement of bone pain and muscle weakness have been observed in a high percentage of patients. Resolution of soft tissue calcification may also occur. Such success has not been the case in patients with secondary hyperparathyroidism who have a high normal or slightly elevated serum calcium concentration before treatment. These patients are quite sensitive to the effects of small doses of 1α,25-dihydroxycholecalciferol and may develop severe hypercalcemia shortly after onset of therapy. For this reason a trial of any form of vitamin D is contraindicated. Because most of these patients have massive parathyroid hyperplasia, subtotal parathyroidectomy is the treatment of choice.[179] In some centers transplantation of the residual parathyroid tissue into forearm muscles has been done in order to simplify future therapy. If significant parathyroid hyperplasia recurs, the excessive tissue can be removed under local anesthesia.

The pathogenesis of osteosclerosis in patients with chronic renal failure is unclear. It has been suggested that it occurs primarily in patients with severe secondary hyperparathyroidism and may reflect an anabolic effect of parathyroid hormone.[178] It is presumed that successful suppression of parathyroid hormone secretion will lead to reversal of osteosclerosis, but this has not been documented in the literature.

Osteoporosis cannot be considered a direct consequence of chronic renal failure, but rather a reflection of associated problems such as a poor dietary intake, relative immobilization, and estrogen deficiency during the menopause. Attention to these peripheral aspects of patient care may improve the state of the skeleton over and above that achieved by specific therapy of renal osteodystrophy.

The prevention of renal osteodystrophy is now coming under more investigative scrutiny. At present the objectives should be (1) to maintain the serum calcium and phosphorus concentrations as close to normal as possible and (2) to correct acidosis. This can be achieved by maintaining an adequate calcium intake (1000 mg or more if necessary), controlling phosphorus intake[187] (or utilizing antacids) to prevent hyperphosphatemia, and administering alkali as needed. In patients on dialysis the dialysate calcium concentration should be 6 to 7 mg per deciliter. It is likely that prophylactic administration of physiologic doses of 1α,25-dihydroxycholecalciferol will help prevent some of the manifestations of renal osteodystrophy, but this is now under investigation.

PRE - TREATMENT
13 Aug., 1973
A

TREATMENT (6 mos)
1 July, 1974
B

Figure 106–20. *A*, "Salt and pepper" skull of a patient with renal osteodystrophy. *B*, Healing of the lesions after 6 months of treatment with 1α,25-dihydroxycholecalciferol. (Provided by Jack W. Coburn, M.D.)

OSTEOPETROSIS

Osteopetrosis is a rare inherited disorder characterized by increased skeletal density.[188] Other terms applied to the disorder are Albers-Schönberg's disease, marble bone disease, and osteosclerosis fragilis generalisata. Patients with osteopetrosis can be categorized into two types. The severe form is inherited as an autosomal recessive trait. Common features of this dramatic disorder include optic atrophy, hepatosplenomegaly, impaired growth, enlarged head, fractures, hearing loss, lymphadenopathy, anemia, and osteomyelitis. The mild form is usually inherited as an autosomal dominant trait, although patients with mild disease have been described whose pedigree analysis reveals an autosomal recessive inheritance.[189] About half of the patients with this form of the disorder have no symptoms. Fractures, cranial nerve palsies, bone pain, and osteomyelitis occur in some patients with mild osteopetrosis. Serum calcium, phosphorus, and alkaline phosphatase concentrations are usually normal, but hypocalcemia, hypophosphatemia, and elevated alkaline phosphatase occasionally are present. Serum acid phosphatase is more likely to be elevated.

A recently recognized syndrome of autosomal recessive osteoporosis, type I renal tubular acidosis and basal ganglia calcification has been found to be associated with carbonic anhydrase II deficiency.[190]

The striking radiological features of osteopetrosis include markedly increased skeletal density (Fig. 106–21), absent marrow cavities, "clublike" deformities of the long bones, and a "bone within a bone" appearance of the vertebral bodies.

Histologic examination of the bone reveals remnants of fetal calcified cartilage and woven bone. The volume of bone is increased. During childhood osteomalacia may be present. Numerous osteoclasts may be present but do not appear to be engaged in the resorption of bone. In one patient evidence for increased bone formation rate was obtained by tetracycline labeling.[191] Parameters of bone resorption were normal.

In recent years new information concerning the pathogenesis and treatment of osteopetrosis has evolved in several centers. Clinical studies were stimulated by the dramatic studies of Walker, which demonstrated that impaired bone resorption in osteopetrotic mice could be restored by transplants of normal bone marrow and spleen cells.[192] It now appears that in man transplantation of bone marrow from a closely related donor to an affected individual can also produce remarkable improvement in the clinical course of the disease.[193,194] Within months of bone marrow infusion a dramatic remodeling of bones toward a more normal structure has been observed. Resolution of anemia has also been found in concert with the appearance of marrow cavities. Bone histology reveals that an active level of osteoclastic bone resorption has been induced. These early studies suggest that a normal hematopoietic cell has been lacking in the osteopetrotic subjects and that there has been fusion of these putative osteoclast precursors with the patients' defective osteoclasts. Long-term evaluation of these and other patients treated similarly will be necessary to establish whether a reasonably normal life can be expected in some patients with severe osteopetrosis. A possible alternative to this form of therapy is treatment with high-dose $1\alpha,25$-dihydroxycholecalciferol.[195] In one patient up to 32 ug daily of this agent produced an increase in bone resorption. The treatment period was too short to determine if clinical benefit would occur.

FIBROUS DYSPLASIA

Fibrous dysplasia of bone is a disorder of unknown etiology and does not appear to have a genetic basis.[196] It does occur more commonly in girls. Clinical recognition of the disorder usually occurs between the ages of 3 and 10. A triad of abnormalities is often present: bone lesions, precocious puberty (primarily in girls), and "café au lait" skin lesions with serrated edges. The bone lesions most commonly are found to involve the femur, the tibia, the pelvis, the feet, the hands, the ribs, the humerus, and the skull. Deformity, pain, and pathological fractures are the main manifestations of the underlying bone disease. A variety of malignant bone tumors may arise in the lesions of fibrous dysplasia.[197]

Serum calcium and phosphorus concentrations are usually normal in patients with this disorder, but serum alkaline phosphatase activity and urinary hydroxyproline excretion may be considerably elevated, a reflection of accelerated bone turnover.[198] As discussed under Osteomalacia, hypophosphatemia and osteomalacia or rickets have been found to affect patients with fibrous dysplasia.[168]

The radiologic features of fibrous dysplasia are dominated by the ground glass appearance of the lesions (Fig. 106–22). Focal cortical thinning, expansion of the diaphysis, and a multilocular appearance of the lesions are other features. Gross deformities such as shepherd's-crook deformity of the femur, coxa vara, tibial bowing, and protrusio acetabuli are common. Increased radiodensity of the base of the skull as well as thickening of the occiput are common abnormalities. Involvement of facial bones is also frequently observed.

The histology of the lesions of fibrous dysplasia, as

Figure 106–21. Roentgenogram of the lumbar spine of a patient with osteopetrosis. Marked sclerosis of the vertebral end plates gives the appearance of a rugger jersey.

Figure 106–22. Roentgenogram of a lower extremity of a patient with fibrous dysplasia. Note the expansion of the fibula, the ground glass appearance, and the cortical thinning.

the term implies, features the presence of fibrous tissue within which are found the bony trabeculae.[196] The bone is of the woven type with random distribution of the collagen fibers. The collagen fibers of the bone appear to extend into the surrounding fibrous tissue. Numerous osteoblasts may be seen in areas of active new bone formation. Some areas have widened osteoid seams with few osteoblasts. Osteoblasts can be found in areas adjacent to new bone formation. Occasionally islands of cartilage may be found. Fluid-filled cysts appear to develop in areas of previous surgery or trauma. After recent fracture the callus may be poorly formed.

The pathogenesis of fibrous dysplasia remains a complete mystery. It is unclear as to whether the disorder has an underlying metabolic basis, since patients with monostotic disease have been observed. Although the

histologic finding of increased osteoclasts in the lesions suggests that calcitonin might be an effective therapy, the few patients treated have not had significant improvement.[198]

HEREDITARY HYPERPHOSPHATASIA

Hereditary hyperphosphatasia[199] is a rare autosomal recessive disorder which has been described by a variety of terms, including hyperostosis corticalis deformans juvenilis, chronic idiopathic hyperphosphatasia, osteochalasia desmalis familiaris, familial osteoectasia, juvenile Paget's disease, chronic progressive osteopathy with hyperphosphatasia, and hereditary bone dysplasia with hyperphosphatasemia.[200] The disease is usually manifested during infancy. Bowing of the extremities with pathological fractures and enlargement of the skull and facial bones are commonly present. Skin temperature over affected bones may be increased. Bone pain and pathologic fractures are common. Serum alkaline phosphatase activity and urinary hydroxyproline excretion are characteristically elevated to extreme levels.

The radiologic abnormalities in patients with hereditary hyperphosphatasia are generalized and to a great extent resemble those of Paget's disease, a localized disorder. There is loss of the normal cortical architecture with a loss of distinct separation of the cortex and medullary cavity. There may be expansion of the diaphysis resulting in its having a greater diameter than the metaphysis. The calvarium may be strikingly increased in thickness with patchy "cotton-wool" lesions typical of Paget's disease.

The histologic findings in patients with this disorder have been somewhat heterogeneous, possibly indicating that classification of patients is imperfect. All studies of bone histology do report the presence of numerous osteoblasts and a fibrovascular bone marrow. Both woven and lamellar bone have been reported to predominate. The bone is laid down in a chaotic fashion indistinguishable from the "mosaic" pattern of bone found in patients with Paget's disease. A point of some controversy is whether increased osteoclastic activity is mainly responsible for the increased rate of bone resorption in patients with hereditary hyperphosphatasia. In several reports numerous osteoclasts were found in bone specimens,[199] whereas in one report of two siblings osteoclasts were rarely found.[200] Instead it appeared that a marked degree of osteocytic osteolysis was responsible for the increased bone resorption. Study of the ultrastructure of bone cells in several patients with this disorder has revealed the presence of intramitochondrial microcrystalline bodies within osteocytes and osteoblasts.[201] These are presumed to be calcium deposits of unknown significance.

The pathogenesis of hereditary hyperphosphatasia is unknown. Despite this, recent studies indicate that remarkable clinical improvement can be achieved with human calcitonin therapy.[200-202] During treatment suppression of serum alkaline phosphatase activity and urinary hydroxyproline excretion, as well as improvement of the radiologic abnormalities, has been observed. A decrease in bone pain and a reduction in the number of fractures sustained have also been documented. Bone biopsies taken during treatment have revealed a more normal type of lamellar bone being laid down, as well as a reduction in the degree of osteocytic osteolysis.

PAGET'S DISEASE OF BONE

Paget's disease of bone is a localized disorder of bone which Sir James Paget described in exquisite detail more than 100 years ago.[203] He termed the disease osteitis deformans because of the severe deformity of the affected bones and because he felt the disease process was inflammatory in nature. Although Paget's disease is not considered a metabolic disease of bone, it is often included in a consideration of metabolic bone diseases because in its polyostotic form the level of metabolic activity of the skeleton is as high as that of any bone disease.

Clinical Features

Signs and Symptoms. A significant proportion of patients with Paget's disease have no outward signs of symptoms of the disease.[204] The diagnosis in these patients results from the chance findings of abnormalities on radiologic examination or blood chemistry screening.

The most common complaints of patients with Paget's disease are pain and skeletal deformity. In most patients both occur simultaneously, although either complaint can be present in the absence of the other.

The pain associated with Paget's disease may be of bone, joint, or nerve origin.[205] Bone pain is usually of mild to moderate degree and is characterized by a deep boring quality. It may be slightly worsened by weight bearing if present in a weight-bearing bone. Joint pain is often moderate to severe, particularly if the hip joint is affected. Weight bearing worsens the severity of the pain considerably. Impingement of nerve tissue by deformed vertebrae produces the most excruciating pain, which may be felt in the back or may radiate to the lower extremity. It is possible that a combination of two or more types of pain may exist in a single patient.

The skeletal deformities of Paget's disease are characterized by both abnormal shape and increase in size of the affected bones. The skull, clavicles, and long bones are most readily appreciated as abnormal on physical examination.

There is a characteristic increase in skin temperature over affected extremity bones in many patients. This is most frequently encountered over the tibia. It is explained by an increase in blood flow to the soft tissues surrounding the bone.[206]

In approximately 50 percent of patients with Paget's disease involving the skull, loss of auditory acuity is present. This is usually of a combined conductive and sensorineural type.

Angioid streaks of the retina, which represent disruptions of Bruch's membrane, are found in a small percentage of patients. Loss of visual acuity because of retinal abnormalities is quite uncommon.

Clinical Biochemistry. The markedly elevated rate of bone turnover in patients with polyostotic Paget's disease is reflected by the high concentration of serum alkaline phosphatase and by the excretion of large amounts of urinary hydroxyproline. The former reflects the number of osteoblasts, and the latter is an index of osteoclastic activity. In patients with monostotic disease involving a small bone such as a clavicle, both parameters are likely to be normal. Since the rate of bone formation is usually similar to the rate of bone resorption in patients with Paget's disease, the serum calcium concentration and urinary calcium excretion are almost always normal.[207] In patients who become immobilized for any reason the rate of bone resorption will be considerably greater than that of bone formation. Hypercalcemia and/or hypercalciuria is then likely to reflect this uncoupling of resorption and formation. Serum phosphorus and immunoreactive parathyroid hormone concentrations are normal[208] in the absence of complications such as immobilization, vitamin D deficiency, or primary hyperparathyroidism. Serum uric acid concentration may be elevated in males with extensive disease, perhaps reflecting increased purine turnover in the numerous bone cells.[205]

Radiographic Evaluation. The earliest manifestation of Paget's disease that can be recognized on radiologic examination is a localized osteolytic lesion (Fig. 106–23). Since such patients are often asymptomatic for years, this type of abnormality is not often encountered. It is most commonly discovered in the skull and long bones. The descriptive term, osteoporosis circumscripta, has been aptly applied to early skull lesions. The osteolytic lesion typically is found at either end of a long bone and advances as a V-shaped osteolytic front (Fig. 106–24).

It has been observed that the evolution of osteolytic

Figure 106–23. The early radiologic appearance of Paget's disease involving the skull, osteoporosis circumscripta.

Figure 106–24. The advancing osteolytic front of Paget's disease in a distal femur.

lesions into the late osteoblastic phase may take many years. In the skull there is a thickening of the calvarium with a loss of definition of the outer and inner tables. A patchy increase in bone density is common and has been termed a "cotton wool" appearance (Fig. 106–25). Occasionally a "honeycomb" appearance of the skull may occur when patchy deposition of new bone occurs in a focus of osteoporosis circumscripta. In far advanced disease platybasia or basilar invagination may occur. Osteoblastic lesions involving vertebrae may produce a homogeneous increase in density or, more commonly, may result in a "picture frame" appearance (Fig. 106–26). Compression fractures and adjacent large osteophytes are also common. In the long bones the osteolytic lesion is replaced by a coarsened trabecular pattern of bone with loss of corticomedullary differentiation. Bowing of the femur and tibia is common, and incomplete fissure fractures are sometimes seen on the convex surface of the femur. Involvement of the bones adjacent to the hip joint may result in protrusio acetabuli.

The skeletal uptake of bone-seeking radioisotopes such as technetium disphosphonate may be an important test in the assessment of certain patients with Paget's disease (see Chapter 40). In patients with localized disease the bone scan may be the only objective measurement of the activity of the disease, since biochemical parameters may be normal with a limited abnormality.[209] In some patients bone pain may be present in the absence of radiologic abnormalities. In the presence of typical radiologic lesions at other sites, a positive bone scan in a "normal" area of the skeleton can lead to a presumptive diagnosis of Paget's disease in that area.[210] Finally, a radiologic abnormality in association with a normal scan suggests that the disorder is no longer active at that site.

Figure 106–25. "Cottonwool" appearance of the skull in the osteoblastic phase of Paget's disease.

Figure 106–26. Involvement of multiple vertebral bodies by Paget's disease. Note the marked osteophyte formation.

Bone Pathology. The earliest pathologic abnormality discernible in biopsies of Paget's disease is an increased number of osteoclasts.[211] These large multinucleated bone-resorbing cells may contain up to 100 nuclei in a single cross-section of a cell, a number rarely seen in the osteoclasts of any metabolic bone disease (Fig. 106–27). The osteoclasts are usually found in Howship's lacunae but sometimes are found to be at some distance from a bone spicule. Since most pathologic specimens of Paget's disease are obtained at a later stage of the disease, it is quite likely that large numbers of active osteoblasts will be found forming bone at sites of previous osteoclastic resorption. Associated with the intense osteoclastic and osteoblastic activity in active Paget's disease is a dense fibrovascular bone marrow containing numerous fibroblasts and cells, which are thought to be osteoprogenitor cells. It has been proposed that osteocytic osteolysis plays a major role in the accelerated bone resorption of Paget's disease, but this has not been generally accepted. In the final or "burned-out" phase of Paget's disease the number of bone cells is markedly reduced and the marrow contains primarily fat cells.

The bone matrix in Paget's disease is characterized by the chaotic "mosaic" pattern of lamellar bone (Fig. 106–28). Woven bone may also be interspersed between the incomplete osteons, and occasionally woven bone may be the dominant feature in a focus of Paget's disease. The mineralization of osteoid is usually normal in Paget's disease, and tetracycline uptake often reveals an increased rate of bone formation.

Ultrastructural studies of the bone cells of Paget's disease have revealed that the osteoclasts of all patients contain nuclear and cytoplasmic inclusions consisting of numerous microfilamentous structures (Fig. 106–29).[212] The inclusions most closely resemble viral nucleocapsids of the Paramyxoviridae family. These structures are not found in the osteoblasts or osteocytes of Paget's disease

Figure 106–27. Several large multinucleated osteoclasts in Howship's lacunae. More than 50 nuclei are present in the osteoclast at the far left, a common finding in Paget's disease. Note the numerous osteoblasts at the lower surface of the bone matrix. Decalcified, hematoxylin and eosin × 500.

Figure 106–28. The mosaic pattern of Paget's disease. There is predominantly lamellar bone, which is in a disorganized pattern. Decalcified, hematoxylin and eosin × 80.

or in any bone cells from patients with a wide variety of metabolic bone diseases. Immunohistologic studies of bone specimens from Paget's disease have revealed that the osteoclasts harbor measles virus antigens[212] and respiratory syncytial virus antigens.[213,214]

Complications

In Table 106–7 are listed some complications that may occur in patients with Paget's disease.

Pathological fractures of the vertebral bodies, femur, and tibia are not uncommon. Healing of the long bones may be somewhat delayed, but nonunion is not a major problem.

A variety of neoplasms may develop in patients with Paget's disease.[204] The most deadly are the sarcomas, particularly osteogenic sarcoma. Their presence should be suspected when there is an increase in pain or deformity of relatively sudden onset in a previous lesion of Paget's disease. Radiologic features include cortical destruction and a discernible soft tissue mass which may show patchy calcification. It is fortunate that these tumors occur in fewer than 1 percent of patients, since they are almost uniformly fatal within 1 year of diagnosis.

Giant cell tumors of bone, usually benign, may also arise in the lesions of Paget's disease. Most commonly these tumors are found in the skull and facial bones. In

Figure 106–29. Ultrastructure of an osteoclast showing characteristic nuclear inclusions of Paget's disease. The arrows indicate nuclear inclusions composed of 125 to 150 nm tubules in groups which are not membrane bound or attached to the nucleolus. The chromatin is condensed and marginated in these nuclei. The cytoplasm contains vacuoles and mitochondria, but the cell membrane is disrupted and the cell appears to be degenerating. × 648 (Provided by Barbara G. Mills, M.D.)

Table 106–7. Complications of Paget's Disease

1. Pathological fractures
2. Neoplasms
   a. Sarcoma
   b. Giant cell tumor
   c. Multiple myeloma
   d. Metastatic carcinoma
   e. Parathyroid adenoma
3. Rheumatologic
   a. Degenerative arthritis
   b. Calcific periarthritis
   c. Gout and hyperuricemia
   d. Rheumatoid arthritis and variants?
   e. Chondrocalcinosis and pseudogout?
4. Neurologic
   a. Decreased auditory acuity
   b. Vertigo
   c. Brainstem compression
   d. Nerve root or spinal cord compression
   e. Vascular "steal" syndrome
5. Hypercalcemia and/or hypercalciuria associated with immobilization
6. Increased cardiac output
7. Arterial calcification?

patients without Paget's disease the giant cell tumors are found chiefly in the extremities. It has been suggested that giant cell reparative granulomas may also arise in Paget's disease,[215] and that these lesions can be mistaken for giant cell tumors.

Multiple myeloma and metastatic carcinoma appear to be chance complications of Paget's disease.

It has been reported that the incidence of parathyroid adenomas is higher in patients with Paget's disease than in the general population.[215] The possible relationship between these disorders is unexplained.

Rheumatologic abnormalities are a common finding in patients with Paget's disease, and in some patients the dominant clinical feature is joint pain.[205] This is most likely to arise from degenerative arthritis affecting the hip, the spine, or the knee. Calcific periarthritis is also a commonly found cause of painful swollen joints.

A variety of significant neurologic abnormalities may occur.[208] The most common is loss of auditory acuity.

Gout and hyperuricemia were reported to be frequent occurrences in male patients with polyostotic Paget's disease.[205] It has been suggested that this might arise from an increase in nucleic acid turnover due to the large number of metabolically active bone cells in patients with generalized disease. Rheumatoid arthritis and its variants and chondrocalcinosis and pseudogout have been reported in patients with Paget's disease but not with great frequency.

Hypercalcemia seldom occurs in patients with Paget's disease in the absence of marked immobilization.[207] Urinary calcium excretion also is usually within the normal range, although renal stones have been reported in as many as 15 percent of patients. Other explanations such as prostatic hypertrophy in elderly males probably account for the development of stones in Paget's disease.

The marked vascularity of the bone lesions and surrounding soft tissues gives rise to an increased cardiac output in patients whose disease affects 35 percent or more of the skeleton.[216] This could contribute to the development of congestive heart failure and myocardial infarction, but such patients appear to respond well to the standard therapeutic measures.

Arterial calcification of the Mönckeberg type has been reported to be present in almost 50 percent of patients.[217] The significance of this observation is unclear, since no control studies have been reported.

Pathogenesis and Treatment

A variety of hypotheses have been proposed to explain the pathogenesis of Paget's disease.[208] It has been suggested that the disorder results from an abnormality of hormone secretion, from an autoimmune process, from an abnormality of the vascular supply of bone, from an inborn error of connective tissue metabolism, or from a neoplastic process. There is little evidence to support any of these hypotheses.

Since the earliest lesion of the disease is a proliferation of osteoclasts, it is likely that the key to understanding the disease will be found in these bone-resorbing cells. The recent finding of nuclear inclusions resembling viral nucleocapsids in the osteoclasts of all patients with Paget's disease has led to speculation that the disorder may be a slow virus infection analogous to subacute sclerosing panencephalitis. The characteristics of a slow virus infection as originally described by Sigurdsson include a long clinically latent period, involvement of a single organ, and the lack of an inflammatory response. Additional features include the presence of intranuclear inclusions and giant cells. Each of these characteristic features of a slow virus infection is found in patients with Paget's disease. The disorder is often present for years or even decades prior to diagnosis, only the skeleton is definitely affected, inflammatory cells are not a major feature of the pathology, intranuclear inclusions are always present in osteoclasts, and giant osteoclasts are common in pathologic specimens. The findings of Paramyxoviridae antigens in the osteoclasts lends further support to the concept of a viral etiology of Paget's disease.[212,214] The exact nature of the virus that would account for the immunohistologic data is unknown, since there is no known antigenic cross-reactivity between measles and respiratory syncytial virus. As yet, attempts to isolate an infectious virus from cultured bone cells of Paget's disease have been unsuccessful.[218]

The treatment of Paget's disease has been dramatically improved during the past decade as a result of the development of drugs that inhibit both proliferation and activity of bone cells.[208] The first drug to become available for general use was calcitonin. This peptide hormone acutely inhibits bone resorption in Paget's disease by altering the function of osteoclasts. Within 30 minutes of injection osteoclasts are less likely to be attached to a trabecula, there is disruption of the ruffled border, and there is a reduction in the number of osteoclasts.[219] Coincident with these histologic findings there is a reduction in serum calcium, phosphorus, and serum and urinary hydroxyproline—biochemical changes that reflect decreased mineral and matrix resorption. Long-term administration of the hormone reduces both bone resorption and formation on histologic examination; the biochemical parameters reflecting these processes, urinary hydroxyproline excretion and serum alkaline phosphatase activity, respectively, are also modified.

Salmon calcitonin is the species of hormone currently approved for use in the United States. Porcine and human calcitonin are also used in several other countries. Salmon calcitonin is generally administered by subcutaneous injection at a dose of 50 to 100 MRC units daily. Occasionally higher doses may be required to induce maximal radiologic improvement.[220] Relief of bone pain is usually found after 2 to 6 weeks of treatment in a high percentage of patients. A reduction in skin temperature over affected extremities may also be noted during this period. Other clinical observations which have been reported during calcitonin therapy are a decrease in cardiac output, stabilization of auditory acuity, improvement of neurological disability, absence of complications during and after orthopedic surgery, and healing of osteolytic bone lesions on radiological survey. The last-named observation is particularly striking, as it can be demonstrated within several months after the onset of therapy (Fig. 106-30).

Chronic treatment with calcitonin results in an av-erage reduction of 50 percent of both serum alkaline phosphatase activity and urinary hydroxyproline excretion (Fig. 106-31). The maximal reduction is usually observed within 3 to 6 months; the fall in hydroxyproline begins during the first day of treatment, whereas alkaline phosphatase activity does not usually decrease during the first week or two. Side effects occur in approximately 10 percent of patients treated with salmon calcitonin and include nausea, a metallic taste sensation, facial flushing, and rarely vomiting or diarrhea. Allergic reactions have rarely been observed.

In more than 50 percent of patients treated with salmon calcitonin, antibodies appear in the circulation.[221] High titers of antibodies can inactivate the effect of the calcitonin and produce a state of hormone resistance. This should be suspected if a patient has a decrease in biochemical parameters during the initial period of therapy followed by a return to pretreatment levels despite continuous treatment with the same dose of hormone. In the largest series so far reported, resistance to salmon calcitonin developed in 26 percent of 85 patients with Paget's disease.[221] Human calcitonin therapy has been uniformly effective in patients resistant to the salmon hormone as manifested by high antibody titers.[221,223]

The leading indications for treatment with calcitonin include bone pain, preparation for orthopedic surgery,

Figure 106–30. *A*, Osteolytic lesions in cortices of right femur of a patient with Paget's disease. *B*, Healing of osteolytic lesions after 1 year of daily treatment with 0.5 mg human calcitonin.

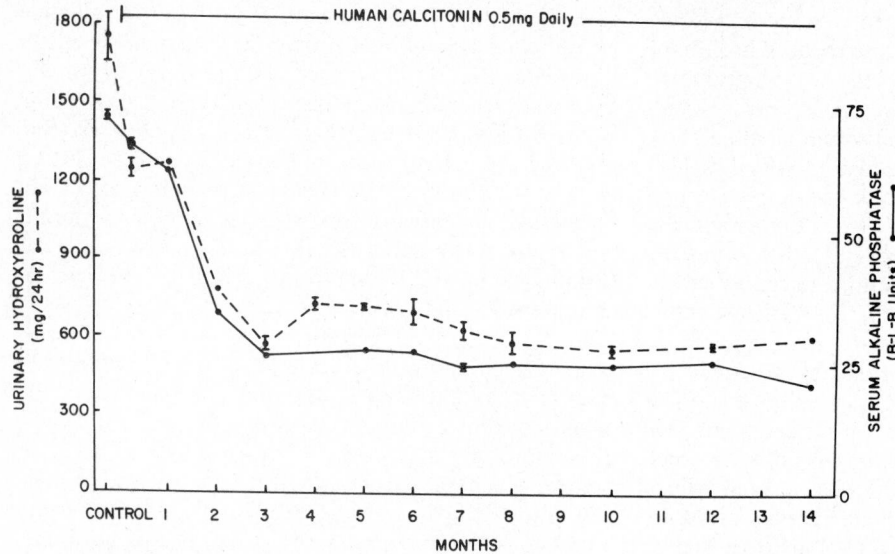

Figure 106–31. The effect of long-term treatment with subcutaneous human calcitonin on the biochemical parameters of a patient with polyostotic Paget's disease. Both serum alkaline phosphatase (normal 1 to 3) and urinary hydroxyproline excretion (normal < 40) fell more than 50 per cent of baseline values.

treatment or prevention of hypercalcemia resulting from immobilization, neurological deficits, and perhaps the prevention of future complications.

It has not been determined what the optimal duration of treatment should be. In one series of patients treated for an average of 22 months, there was still evidence of suppressed metabolic activity 1 year after stopping therapy.[224] In patients with an advancing osteolytic front, calcitonin therapy clearly produces radiologic healing, but cessation of therapy is followed by reactivation of the osteolytic front.[220] It seems appropriate to continue such patients on therapy indefinitely. In patients in the osteoblastic phase of the disease the treatment may be discontinued after 1 or 2 years, or the dose can be reduced to 50 MRC units three times a week with persistence of the clinical benefits in most patients.

The diphosphonates are analogues of pyrophosphate (P-O-P), a component of bone felt to be important in bone metabolism. These agents have been shown to suppress both bone resorption and formation.[225] Disodium etidronate (disodium ethane-1-hydroxyl-1,1-diphosphonate) has been approved for the treatment of Paget's disease and the prevention of heterotopic ossification following orthopedic surgery.

Disodium etidronate is administered orally. Gastrointestinal absorption is variable. Following absorption it is mainly localized to bone or excreted in the urine. In general the clinical effects of the drug are similar to calcitonin with some important differences. Suppression of the activity of the disease, in many patients, is greater with the diphosphonate than with calcitonin, and alkaline phosphatase activity may fall by more than 50 percent.[226] This is particularly true with higher doses, i.e., 10 to 20 mg per kilogram of body weight. Unfortunately high doses of disodium etidronate induce a mineralization defect which may lead to pathological fractures.[226,227] For this reason it is best to begin therapy with a daily dose of 5 mg per kg, as this dose produces effective biochemical suppression without inducing a generalized excess of unmineralized osteoid. Focal os-

teomalacia from this dose has been reported.[171] It has also been observed that disodium etidronate may produce a paradoxical increase in bone pain in about 10 percent of patients. This decreases with cessation of therapy and may not return if treatment is resumed. In most patients bone pain is relieved. One other difference from the effect of calcitonin therapy is that radiologic healing of osteolytic lesions has seldom been reported to result from therapy with disodium etidronate. Actual progression of osteolytic lesions has been observed despite biochemical improvement.[220]

The incidence of side effects is low. Loose bowel movements may occasionally develop. Hyperphosphatemia has also been observed, particularly in patients given high doses. It has been recommended that a 6-month course of treatment be given initially. A prolonged suppression of biochemical parameters is common after stopping treatment.[226] Once symptoms recur, the drug can then be readministered for another 6-month period. It will require further experience to determine if this is an optimal type of management.

Disodium etidronate has been administered in combination with calcitonin with evidence of excellent biochemical suppression of the disease, but healing of osteolytic lesions was less apparent than with calcitonin therapy alone.[220] Newer diphosphonate compounds may prove to be more effective than disodium etidronate but have not been released for general use.[225]

Mithramycin, a cytotoxic antibiotic used in cancer therapy, has also been used to treat Paget's disease.[228] The drug is a potent inhibitor of RNA synthesis and acutely inhibits the action of osteoclasts. This property has led to its use in the treatment of severe hypercalcemia.

Mithramycin has been administered intravenously at a dose of 15 to 50 μg per kg of body weight, utilizing a variety of treatment schedules. Initially it was infused daily for up to 10 days intermittently. More recently it has been given weekly.[229] Marked suppression of the activity of the disease as well as relief of bone pain has been reported. However, side effects and toxicity are significant features in the use of this drug. Nausea and malaise are frequently encountered and may last for days. Platelet abnormality leading to hemorrhage is the most serious toxic effect. Transient elevation of liver enzymes is common, and occasionally renal function may be impaired. The latter is usually reversible. The availability of calcitonin and disodium etidronate for treatment of Paget's disease make it unlikely that mithramycin will be a commonly used drug in the future. It has not been approved for treatment of Paget's disease in the United States.

A combination of oral calcium supplementation and chlorthalidone has been used by one group of investigators in an attempt to stimulate endogenous calcitonin secretion and suppress parathyroid hormone secretion.[230] This relatively inexpensive regimen was reported to relieve bone pain in most patients and to reduce serum alkaline phosphatase activity and urinary hydroxyproline excretion by about 30 percent. Radiologic improvement of osteolytic lesions was not observed.

The benefits of elective surgery in the management of Paget's disease should not be overlooked.[208] Neurosurgery may be required in patients with severe basilar impression and neurologic deficit or in patients who have nerve compression from vertebral involvement. Orthopedic surgery is often needed in patients who develop severe degenerative arthritis of the hip. A total hip replacement can result in pain-free normal ambulation. Severe bowing of the tibia may cause difficulty in ambulation not only because of the deformity but also as a result of stress on the knee joint. Arthralgia and effusions may be recurrent problems. Tibial osteotomy can correct the deformity and allow much improved ambulation.[231]

All surgery on bones affected by Paget's disease ideally should be done only after treatment with a drug which suppresses the activity of the disease. In a series of patients undergoing tibial osteotomy, treatment with calcitonin prior to surgery appeared to prevent excessive hemorrhage and postoperative hypercalcemia.[231] If possible, drug treatment should be given for a minimum of 1 to 2 months before surgery.

References

1. Albright, F.A., and Reifenstein, E.C., Jr.: The Parathyroid Glands and Metabolic Bone Disease. Baltimore, Williams & Wilkins Company, 1948, p. 81.
2. Marshall, R.W.: Plasma fractions. In Nordin, B.E.C. (ed.): Calcium, Phosphate and Magnesium Metabolism. Edinburgh, Churchill Livingstone, 1976, p. 162.
3. Robertson, W.G.: Plasma phosphate homeostasis. In Nordin, B.E.C. (ed.): Calcium, Phosphate and Magnesium Metabolism. Edinburgh, Churchill Livingstone, 1976, p. 217.
4. McComb, R.B., Bowers, G.N., and Posen, S.: Alkaline Phosphatase. New York, Plenum Press, 1979.
5. Robertson, W.G.: Urinary excretion. In Nordin, B.E.C. (ed.): Calcium, Phosphate and Magnesium Metabolism. Edinburgh, Churchill Livingstone, 1976, p. 113.
6. Bijvoet, O.L.M.: Kidney function in calcium and phosphate metabolism. In Avioli, L.V., and Krane, S.M. (eds.): Metabolic Bone Disease, Vol. I. New York, Academic Press, 1977, p. 50.
7. Walton, R.J., and Bijvoet, O.L.M.: Nomogram for derivation of renal threshold phosphate concentration. Lancet 2:309, 1975.
8. Kivirikko, K.I.: Urinary excretion of hydroxyproline in health and disease. In Hall, D.A., and Jackson, D.S. (eds.): International Review of Connective Tissue Research, Vol. 5. New York, Academic Press, 1970, p.93.
9. Fogelman, I., Bessent, R.G., Turner, J.G., Citrin, D.L., Boyle, I.T., and Greig, W.R.: The use of whole-body retention of Tc-99m diphosphonate in the diagnosis of metabolic bone disease. J. Nucl. Med. 19:270, 1978.
10. Caniggia, A., and Vattimo, A.: Kinetics of ^{99m}technetium-tin-methylenediphosphonates in normal subjects and pathological conditions: A simple index of bone metabolism. Calcif. Tissue. Int. 30:5, 1980.
11. Bordier, P., Matrajt, H., Miravet, L., and Hioco, D.: Mesure histologique de la masse et de la résorption des travées osseuses. Path. Biol. 12:1238, 1964.
12. Jowsey, J.: The Bone Biopsy. New York, Plenum Medical Books, 1977.
13. Byers, P.D.: The diagnostic value of bone biopsies. In Avioli, L.V., and Krane, S.M. (eds.): Metabolic Bone Disease, Vol I. New York, Academic Press, 1977, p. 183.
14. Bartelheimer, H., and Schmitt-Rohde, J.M.: Die Biopsie des Knochens als differentialdiagnostische klinische Methode. Klin. Wschr. 35:429, 1957.
15. Frost, H.M.: Tetracycline-based histological analysis of bone remodeling. Calc. Tiss. Res. 3:211, 1969.
16. Keutmann, H.J.: Chemistry of parathyroid hormone. In De Groot, L.J. (ed.): Endocrinology, Vol. 2. New York, Grune & Stratton, 1979, p. 593.
17. Habener, J.F., Kemper, B.W., Rich, A., and Potts, J.T., Jr.: Biosynthesis of parathyroid hormone. Recent Prog. Horm. Res. 33:249, 1977.
18. Mayer, G.P.: Parathyroid hormone secretion. In De Groot, L.J. (ed.): Endocrinology, Vol. 2. New York, Grune & Stratton, 1979, p. 607.
19. Rude, R.K., Oldham, S.B., Sharp, C.F., Jr., and Singer, F.R.: Parathyroid hormone secretion in magnesium deficiency. J. Clin. Endocrinol. Metab. 47:800, 1978.
20. Fischer, J.A., Blum, J.W., and Binswanger, U.: Acute parathyroid hormone response to epinephrine in vivo. J. Clin. Invest. 52:2434, 1973.
21. Gardner, D.G., Brown, E.M., Windeck, R., and Aurbach, G.D.: Prostaglandin E_2 stimulation of adenosine 3',5'-monophosphate accumulation and parathyroid hormone release in dispersed bovine parathyroid cells. Endocrinology 103:577, 1978.
22. Windeck, R., Brown, E.M., Gardner, D.G., and Aurbach, G.D.: Effect of gastrointestinal hormones on isolated bovine parathyroid cells. Endocrinology 103:2020, 1978.
23. Canterbury, J.M., Lerman, S., Claflin, A.J., Henry, H., Norman, A., and Reiss, E.: Inhibition of parathyroid hormone secretion by 25-hydroxycholecalciferol and 24,25-dihydroxycholecalciferol in the dog. J. Clin. Invest. 61:1375, 1978.
24. Habener, J.F., and Potts, J.T., Jr.: Parathyroid physiology and primary hyperparathyroidism. In Avioli, L.V., and Krane, S.M. (eds.): Metabolic Bone Disease, Vol. II. New York, Academic Press, 1978, p. 1.
25. Kaplan, R.A., Haussler, M.R., Deftos, L.J., Bone, H., and Pak, C.Y.C.: The role of 1α,25-dihydroxyvitamin D in the mediation of intestinal hyperabsorption of calcium in primary hyperparathyroidism and absorptive hypercalciuria. J. Clin. Invest. 59:756, 1977.
26. Aurbach, G.D., and Chase, L.R.: Cyclic nucleotides and biochemical actions of parathyroid hormone and calcitonin. In Aurbach, G.D. (ed.): Handbook of Physiology, Section 7, Endocrinology, Vol. VII, Parathyroid Gland. Washington, D.C., American Physiological Society, 1976. p. 353.
27. Parsons, J.A., Neer, R.M., and Potts, J.T., Jr.: Initial fall of plasma calcium after intravenous injection of parathyroid hormone. Endocrinology 89:735, 1971.
28. Segre, G.V.: Heterogeneity and metabolism of parathyroid hormone. In De Groot, L.J. (ed.): Endocrinology, Vol 2. New York, Grune & Stratton, 1979, p. 613.
29. Flueck, J.A., Di Bella, F.P., Edis, A.J., Kehrwald, J.M., and Arnaud, C.D.: Immunoheterogeneity of parathyroid hormone in venous effluent serum from hyperfunctioning parathyroid glands. J. Clin. Invest. 60:1367, 1977.
30. Oldham, S.B., Finck, E., and Singer, F.R.: Parathyroid hormone clearance in man. Metabolism 27:993, 1978.
31. Freitag, J., Martin, K.J., Hruska, K.A., Anderson, C., Conrades, M., Ladenson, J., Klahr, S., and Slatopolsky, E.: Impaired parathyroid hormone metabolism in patients with chronic renal failure. N. Engl. J. Med. 298:29, 1978.
32. Heath, H., III, Hodgson, S.F., and Kennedy, M.A.: Primary hyperparathyroidism: Incidence, morbidity, and potential enconomic impact in a community. N. Engl. J. Med. 302:189, 1980.
33. Marx, S.J., Powell, D., Shimkin, P.M., Wells, S.A., Ketcham, A.S., McGuigan, J.E., Bilezikian, J.P., and Aurbach, G.D.: Familial hyperparathyroidism. Ann. Intern. Med. 78:371, 1973.
34. Wermer, P.: Endocrine adenomatosis and peptic ulcer in a large kindred. Inherited multiple tumors and mosaic pleiotropism in man. Am. J. Med. 35:205, 1963.

35. Heath, H., III, Sizemore, G.W., and Carney, J.A.: Preoperative diagnosis of occult parathyroid hyperplasia by calcium infusion in patients with multiple endocrine neoplasia, type 2a. J. Clin. Endocrinol. Metab. 43:428, 1976.

36. Prinz, R.A., Paloyan, E., Lawrence, A.M., Pickleman, J.R., Braithwaite, S., and Brooks, M.H.: Radiation-associated hyperparathyroidism: A new syndrome? Surgery 82:296, 1977.

37. Transbøl, I.: On the diagnosis of so-called normocalcemic hyperparathyroidism. Acta Med. Scand. 202:481, 1977.

38. Schussler, G.C., Verso, M.A., and Nemoto, T.: Phosphaturia in hypercalcemic cancer patients. J. Clin. Endocrinol. Metab. 35:497, 1972.

39. Wills, M.R.: Value of plasma chloride concentration and acid-base status in the differential diagnosis of hyperparathyroidism from other causes of hypercalcemia. J. Clin. Pathol. 24:219, 1971.

40. Scott, J.T., Dixon, A.S.J., and Bywaters, E.G.L.: Association of hyperuricemia and gout with hyperparathyroidism. Br. Med. J. 1:1070, 1964.

41. Broadus, A.E., Horst, R.L., Lang, R., Littledike, E.T., and Rasmussen, H.: The importance of circulating 1,25-dihydroxyvitamin D in the pathogenesis of hypercalciuria and renal stone formation in primary hyperparathyroidism. N. Engl. J. Med. 302:421, 1980.

42. Transbøl, I., Hornum, I., Hahnemann, S., Hasner, E., Øhlenschlaeger, H., Diemer, H., and Lockwood, K.: Tubular reabsorption of calcium in the differential diagnosis of hypercalcemia. Acta Med. Scand. 188:505, 1970.

43. Broadus, A.E., Mahaffey, J.E., Neer, R.M., and Bartter, F.C.: Nephrogenous cyclic AMP as a parathyroid function test. J. Clin. Invest. 60:771, 1977.

44. Rude, R.K., Sharp, C.F., Jr., Fredericks, R.S., Oldham, S.B., Elbaum, N., Link, J., Irwin, L., and Singer, F.R.: Urinary and nephrogenous adenosine 3',5'-monophosphate in the hypercalcemia of malignancy. J. Clin. Endocrinol. Metab. 52:765, 1981.

45. Broadus, A.E., Horst, R.L., Littledike, E.T., Mahaffey, J.E., and Rasmussen, H.: Primary hyperparathyroidism: Serial observations and simple diagnosis by means of an oral calcium tolerance test. Clin. Endocrinol. 12:225, 1980.

46. Madvig, P., Young, G., and Marcus, R.: Assessment of adenosine 3', 5'-monophosphate excretion and an oral calcium tolerance test in the diagnosis of mild primary hyperparathyroidism. J. Clin. Endocrinol. Metab. 58: 480, 1984.

47. von Recklinghausen, F.: Die Fibröse oder deformierende Ostitis, die Osteomalacie und die osteoplastische Carcinose in ihren gegenseitigen Beziehungen. In Festschrift für Rudolf Virchow. Berlin, G. Reimer, 1891.

48. Meunier, P., Vignon, G., Bernard, J., Edouard, C., and Courpron, P.: Quantitative bone histology as applied to the diagnosis of hyperparathyroid states. In Frame, B., Parfitt, A.M., and Duncan, H. (eds.): Clinical Aspects of Metabolic Bone Disease. Amsterdam, Excerpta Medica, 1972, p. 215.

49. Singer, F.R., Sharp, C.F., Jr., and Rude, R.K.: Pathogenesis of hypercalcemia in malignancy. Mineral Electrolyte Metab. 2:161, 1979.

50. Samaan, N.A., Hickey, R.C., Hill, C.S., Jr., Medellin H., and Gates, R.B.: Parathyroid tumors. Preoperative localization and association with other tumors. Cancer 33:933, 1974.

51. Marx, S.J., Spiegel, A.M., Brown, E.M., Koehler, J.O., Gardner, D.G., Brennan, M.F., and Aurbach, G.D.: Divalent cation metabolism. Familial hypocalciuric hypercalcemia versus typical primary hyperparathyroidism. Am. J. Med. 65:235, 1978.

52. Sharma, O.P.: Sarcoidosis. A Clinical Approach. Springfield, Illinois, Charles C Thomas, 1975.

53. Bell, N.H., Stern, P.H., Pantzer, E., Sinha, T.K., and DeLuca, H.F.: Evidence that increased circulating 1α,25-dihydroxyvitamin D is the probable cause for abnormal calcium metabolism in sarcoidosis. J. Clin. Invest. 64:218, 1979.

54. Adams, J.S., Sharma, O.P., Gacad, M.A., and Singer, F.R.: Metabolism of 25-hydroxyvitamin D₃ by cultured pulmonary macrophages in sarcoidosis. J. Clin. Invest. 72:1856, 1983.

55. Castleman, B., and Roth, S.I.: Tumors of the Parathyroid Glands. Washington, D.C., Armed Forces Institute of Pathology, 1978.

56. Broadus, A.E., Magee, J.S., Mallette, L.E., Horst, R.L., Lang, R., Jensen, P.S., Gertner, J.M., and Baron, R.: A detailed evaluation of oral phosphate therapy in selected patients with primary hyperparathyroidism. J. Clin. Endocrinol. Metab. 56:953, 1983.

57. Suki, W.N., Yium, J.J., Von Minden, M., Saller-Hebert, C., Eknoyan, G., and Martinez-Maldonado, M.: Acute treatment of hypercalcemia with furosemide. N. Engl. J. Med. 283:836, 1970.

58. Gallagher, J.C., and Wilkinson, R.: The effect of ethinylestradiol on calcium and phosphorus metabolism of postmenopausal women with primary hyperparathyroidism. Clin. Sci. Mol. Med. 45:785, 1973.

59. Meunier, P.J., Bianchi, G.G.S., Edouard, C.M., Bernard, J.C., Courpron, P., and Vignon, G.E.: Bony manifestations of thyrotoxicosis. Orthop. Clin. North Am. 3:745, 1975.

60. Rosen, J.F., Wolin, D.A., and Finberg, L.: Immobilization hypercalcemia

after single limb fractures in children and adolescents. Am. J. Dis. Child. 132:560, 1978.

61. Riggs, B.L., Jowsey, J., Kelly, P.J., Hoffman, D.L., and Arnaud, C.D.: Studies on pathogenesis and treatment in postmenopausal and senile osteoporosis. Clin. Endocrinol. Metab. 22:317, 1973.

62. Teitelbaum, S.L., Rosenberg, E.M., Richardson, C.A., and Avioli, L.V.: Histological studies of bone from normocalcemic postmenopausal osteoporotic patients with increased circulatory parathyroid hormone. J. Clin. Endocrinol. Metab. 42:537, 1976.

63. Gallagher, J.C., Riggs, B.L., Eisman, J., Hamstra, A., Arnaud, S.B., and DeLuca, H.F.: Intestinal calcium absorption and serum vitamin D metabolites in normal subjects and osteoporotic patients. Effects of age and dietary calcium. J. Clin. Invest. 64:729, 1979.

64. Taggart, H.M., Chestnut, C.H., III, Ivey, J.L., Baylink, D.J., Sisom, K., Huber, M.B., and Roos, B.A.: Deficient calcitonin response to calcium stimulation in postmenopausal osteoporosis? Lancet 1:475, 1982.

65. Body, J.-J., and Heath, H., III: Estimates of circulating monomeric calcitonin: Physiological studies in normal and thyroidectomized man. J. Clin. Endocrinol. Metab. 57:897, 1983.

66. Aaron, J.: Diagnostic procedures. In Nordin, B.E.C. (ed.): Calcium, Phosphate and Magnesium Metabolism. Edinburgh, Churchill Livingstone, 1976, p. 469.

67. Mazess, R.B.: The noninvasive measurement of skeletal mass. In Peck, W.A. (ed.): Bone and Mineral Research. Annual 1. Amsterdam, Excerpta Medica, 1983, p. 223.

68. Riggs, B.L., Wahner, H.W., Dunn, W.L., Mazess, R.B., Offord, K.P., and Metton, L.J., III: Differential changes in bone mineral density of the appendicular and axial skeleton with aging. J. Clin. Invest. 67:328, 1981.

69. Jowsey, J., Kelly, P.J., Riggs, B.L., Bianco, A.J., Jr., Scholz, D.A., and Gershon-Cohen, J.: Quantitative microradiographic studies of normal and osteoporotic bone. J. Bone Joint Surg. 47:785, 1965.

70. Meunier, P., Courpron, P., Edouard, C., Bernard, J., Bringuier, J., and Vignon, G.: Physiological senile involution and pathological rarefaction of bone. Clin. Endocrinol. Metab. 2:239, 1973.

71. Rasmussen, H., and Bordier, P.: The Physiological and Cellular Basis of Metabolic Bone Disease. Baltimore, Williams & Wilkins Company, 1974, p. 272.

72. Wu, K., and Frost, H.M.: Bone formation in osteoporosis. Arch. Pathol. 88:508, 1969.

73. Whyte, M.P., Bergfeld, M.A., Murphy, W.A., Avioli, L.V., and Teitelbaum, S.L.: Postmenopausal osteoporosis. A heterogeneous disorder as assessed by histomorphometric analysis of iliac crest bone from untreated patients. Am. J. Med. 72:193, 1982.

74. Riggs, B.L., Jowsey, J., and Kelly, P.J.: Quantitative microradiographic study of bone remodeling in Cushing's syndrome. Metabolism 15:773, 1966.

75. Jowsey, J., and Riggs, B.L.: Bone formation in hypercortisonism. Acta Endocrinol. 63:21, 1970.

76. Bressot, C., Meunier, P.J., Chapuy, M.C., Lejeune, E., Edouard, C., and Darby, A.J.: Histomorphometric profile, pathophysiology and reversibility of corticosteroid-induced osteoporosis. Metab. Bone Rel. Res. 1:3303, 1979.

77. Minaire, P., Meunier, P., Edouard, C., Bernard, J., Courpron, P., and Bouret, J.: Quantitative histological data on disuse osteoporosis: Comparison with biological data. Calcif. Tiss. Res. 17:57, 1974.

78. Jowsey, J., and Johnson, K.A.: Juvenile osteoporosis: Bone findings in seven patients. J. Pediatr. 81:511, 1972.

79. Smith, R.: Idiopathic osteoporosis in the young. J. Bone Joint. Surg. 62-B:417, 1980.

80. Jaffe, H.L.: Metabolic, Degenerative, and Inflammatory Diseases of Bones and Joints. Philadelphia, Lea & Febiger, 1972, p. 162.

81. Riggs, B.L., and Melton, L.J., III: Evidence for two distinct syndromes of involutional osteoporosis. Am. J. Med. 75:899, 1983.

82. Morgan, D.B.: Osteomalacia, Renal Osteodystrophy, and Osteoporosis. Springfield, Ill., Charles C Thomas, 1973, p. 248.

83. Avioli, L.V.: Osteoporosis. In Peck W.A. (ed.): Bone and Mineral Research. Annual 1. Amsterdam, Excerpta Medica, 1983, p. 280.

84. Tanaka, Y., Castillo, L., and DeLuca, H.F.: Control of renal vitamin D hydroxylases in birds by sex hormones. Proc. Natl. Acad. Sci. USA 23:2701, 1976.

85. Heaney, R.P., Recker, R.R., and Saville, P.D.: Menopausal changes in bone remodeling. J. Lab. Clin. Med. 92:964, 1978.

86. Meema, S., Bunker, M.L., and Meema, H.E.: Preventive effect of estrogen on postmenopausal bone loss. Arch. Intern. Med. 135:1436, 1975.

87. Lindsay, R., Hart, D.M., Aitken, J.M., MacDonald, E.B., Anderson, J.B., and Clarke, A.C.: Long-term prevention of postmenopausal osteoporosis by oestrogen. Lancet 1:1038, 1976.

88. Weiss, N.S., Ure, C.L., Ballard, J.H., Williams, A.R., and Daling, J.R.: Decreased risk of fractures of the hip and lower forearm with postmenopausal use of estrogen. N. Engl. J. Med. 303:1195, 1980.

89. Morimoto, S., Tsuji, M., Okada, U., Onishi, T., and Kumahara, U.: The

effects of oestrogens on human calcitonin secretion after calcium infusion in elderly female subjects. Clin. Endocrinol. 13:135, 1980.

90. Lund, B., Sorensen, O.H., Lund, B., and Agner, E.: Serum 1,25-dihydroxyvitamin D in normal subjects and in patients with postmenopausal osteopenia. Influence of age, renal function and oestrogen therapy. Horm. Metab. Res., 14:271, 1982.

91. Recker, R.R., Saville, P.D., and Heaney, R.P.: Effects of estrogens and calcium carbonate on bone loss in postmenopausal women. Ann. Intern. Med. 87:649, 1977.

92. Riggs, B.L., Jowsey, J., Goldsmith, R.S., Kelly, P.J., Hoffman, D.L., and Arnaud, C.D.: Short and long-term effects of estrogen and synthetic anabolic hormone in postmenopausal osteoporosis. J. Clin. Invest. 51:1659, 1972.

93. Horsman, A., Jones, M., Francis, R., and Nordin, C.: The effect of estrogen dose on postmenopausal bone loss. N. Engl. J. Med. 309:1405, 1983.

94. Riggs, B.L.: Treatment of osteoporosis with sodium fluoride: An appraisal. In Peck, W.A. (ed.): Bone and Mineral Research. Annual Bone and Mineral Research. Annual 2. Amsterdam, Elsevier, 1984, p. 366.

95. Teotia, S.P.S., and Teotia, M.: Secondary hyperparathyroidism in patients with endemic skeletal fluorosis. Br. Med. J. 1:637, 1973.

96. Baran, D.T., Bergfeld, M.A., Teitelbaum, S.L., and Avioli, L.V.: Effect of testosterone therapy on bone formation in an osteoporotic hypogonadal male. Calcif. Tiss. Res. 26:103, 1978.

97. Blodgett, F.M., Burgin, L., Jezzoni, D., Gribetz, D., and Talbot, N.B.: Effects of prolonged cortisone therapy on the statural growth, skeletal maturation and metabolic status of children. N. Engl. J. Med. 254:636, 1956.

98. Barrett, A.J., Sledge, C.B., and Dingle, J.T.: Effect of cortisol on the synthesis of chondroitin sulfate by embryonic cartilage. Nature 211:83, 1966.

99. Peck, W.A., Brandt, J., and Miller, I.: Hydrocortisone-induced inhibition of protein synthesis and uridine incorporation in isolated bone cells in vitro. Proc. Natl. Acad. Sci. USA 57:1599, 1967.

100. Jett, S., Wu, K., Duncan, H., and Frost, H.M.: Adrenal corticosteroid and salicylate actions on human and canine haversian bone formation and resorption. Clin. Orthop. Rel. Res. 68:301, 1970.

101. Harrison, H.E., and Harrison, H.C.: Transfer of Ca^{45} across intestinal wall in vitro in relation to action of vitamin D and cortisol. Am. J. Physiol. 199:265, 1960.

102. Hahn, T.J., Halstead, L.R., and Haddad, J.G., Jr.: Serum 25-hydroxyvitamin D concentrations in patients receiving chronic corticosteroid therapy. J. Lab. Clin. Med. 90:399, 1977.

103. Slovik, D.M., Neer, R.M., Ohman, J.L., Lowell, F.C., Clark, M.B., Segre, G.V., and Potts, J.T., Jr.: Parathyroid hormone and 25-hydroxyvitamin D levels in glucocorticoid-treated patients. Clin. Endocrinol. 12:243, 1980.

104. Findling, J.W., Adams, N.D., Lemann, J., Jr., Gray, R.W., Thomas, C.J., and Tyrrell, J.B.: Vitamin D metabolites and parathyroid hormone in Cushing's syndrome: Relationship to calcium and phosphorus homeostasis. J. Clin. Endocrinol. Metab. 54:1039, 1982.

105. Rickers, H., Deding, A., Christiansen, C., Rodbro, P., and Naestoft, J.: Corticosteroid-induced osteopenia and vitamin D metabolism. Effect of vitamin D_2, calcium phosphate and sodium fluoride and administration. Clin. Endocrinal. 16:409, 1982.

106. Klein, R.G., Arnaud, S.B., Gallagher, J.D., DeLuca, H.F., and Riggs, B.L.: Intestinal calcium absorption in exogenous hypercortisonism. J. Clin. Invest. 60:253, 1977.

107. O'Regan, S., Chesney, R.W., Hamstra, A., Eisman, J.A., O'Gorman, A.M., and DeLuca, H.F.: Reduced serum 1,25(OH)₂ vitamin D_3 levels in prednisone-treated adolescents with systemic lupus erythematosus. Acta Paediatr. Scand. 68:109, 1979.

108. Favus, M.J., Walling, M.W., and Kimberg, D.V.: Effects of 1,25-dihydroxycholecalciferol on intestinal calcium transport in cortisone treated rats. J. Clin. Invest. 52:1680, 1973.

109. Fucik, R.F., Kukreja, S.C., Hargis, G.K., Bowser, E.N., Henderson, W.J., and Williams, G.A.: Effect of glucocorticoids on function of the parathyroid glands in man. J. Clin. Endocrinol. Metabol. 40:152, 1975.

110. Lukert, B.P., and Adams, J.S.: Calcium and phosphorus homeostasis in man. Arch. Intern. Med. 136:1249, 1976.

111. Gluck, O.S., Murphy, W.A., Hahn, T.J., and Hahn, B.: Bone loss in adults receiving alternate day glucocorticoid therapy: A comparison with daily therapy. Arthritis Rheum. 24:892, 1981.

112. Hahn, T.J., Halstead, L.R., Teitelbaum, S.L., and Hahn, B.H.: Altered mineral metabolism in glucocorticoid-induced osteopenia. Effect of 25-hydroxyvitamin D administration. J. Clin. Invest. 64:655, 1979.

113. Mosekilde, L., and Melsen, F.: Effect of antithyroid treatment on calcium-phosphorus metabolism in hyperthyroidism, II: Bone histomorphometry. Acta Endocrinol. 87:751, 1978.

114. Rude, R.K., Oldham, S.B., Singer, F.R., and Nicoloff, J.T.: Treatment of thyrotoxic hypercalcemia with propranolol. N. Engl. J. Med. 294:431, 1976.

115. Mosekilde, L., Jastrup, B., Melson, F., Lund, B., Lund, B., Sorensen, O.H., Nielsen, H.E., and Yde, H.: Effect of propranolol treatment on bone mass, bone mineral content, bone remodelling, parathyroid function and vitamin D metabolism in hyperthyroidism. Eur. J. Clin. Invest. 14:96, 1984.

116. Avioli, L.V.: Osteoporosis: Pathogenesis and therapy. In Avioli, L.V., and Krane, S.M. (eds.): Metabolic Bone Disease, Vol. I. New York, Academic Press, 1977, p. 307.

117. Castells, S., Inamdar, S., Baker, R.K., and Wallach, S.: Effects of porcine calcitonin in osteogenesis imperfecta tarda. J. Pediatr. 80:757, 1972.

118. Kennedy, A.C., and Lindsay, R.: Bone involvement in rheumatoid arthritis. Clin. Rheum. Dis. 3:403, 1977.

119. Dunham, J., Bourke, B.E., Bitensky, L., Chayen, J., Loveridge, M., and Scott, J.T.: Circulating levels of biologically active parathyroid hormone in rheumatic diseases. Ann. Rheum. Dis. 41:569, 1982.

120. Holick, M.F., Frommer, J.E., McNeill, S.C., Richtand, N.M., Henley, J.W. and Potts, J.T., Jr.: Photometabolism of 7-dehydrocholesterol to previtamin D_3 in skin. Biochem. Biophys. Res. Commun. 76:107, 1977.

121. Blunt, J.W., Tanaka, Y., and DeLuca, H.F.: The biological activity of 25-hydroxycholecalciferol, a metabolite of vitamin D_3. Proc. Natl. Acad. Sci. USA 61:717, 1968.

122. Fraser, D.R., and Kodicek, E.: Unique biosynthesis of a biologically active vitamin D metabolite. Nature 228:764, 1970.

123. Norman, A.W., Myrtle, J.F., Midgett, R.J., Nowicki, H.G., Williams, V., and Popjak, G.: 1,25-Dihydroxycholecalciferol: Identification of the proposed active form of vitamin D_3 in the intestine. Science 173:51, 1971.

124. DeLuca, H.F.: Metabolism and mechanism of action of vitamin D-1982. In Peck, W.A. (ed.): Bone and Mineral Research. Annual 1. Amsterdam, Excerpta Medica, 1983, p. 7.

125. Gertner, J.M., and Domenech, M.: 25-Hydroxyvitamin D in patients treated with high-dosage ergo- and cholecalciferol. Clin. Pathol. 30:144, 1977.

126. MacIntyre, I., Arnett, T.R., Brown, D.J., Galan, F., Girgis, S.I., Rogers, R.M., Spanos, E., Stevenson, J.C., and Bone, Q.: The interrelation of the calcium regulating hormones: Some recent findings. In MacIntyre, I., and Szelke, M. (eds.): Molecular Endocrinology. Amsterdam, Elsevier, 1979, p. 193.

127. Larkins, R.G., MacAuley, S.J., and MacIntyre, I.: Feedback control of vitamin D metabolism by a nuclear action of 1,25-dihydroxycholecalciferol. Nature 252:412, 1974.

128. Ornoy, A., Goodwin, D., Noff, D., and Edelstein, S.: 24,25-Dihydroxyvitamin D is a metabolite of vitamin D essential for bone formation. Nature 276:517, 1978.

129. Rosen, J.R., Fleischman, A.R., Finberg, L., Eisman, J., and DeLuca, H.F.: 1,25-Dihydroxycholecalciferol: Its use in the long-term management of idiopathic hypoparathyroidism in children. J. Clin. Endocrinol. Metab. 45:457, 1977.

130. Dent, C.E., and Stamp, T.C.B.: Vitamin D, rickets and osteomalacia. In Avioli, L.V., and Krane, S.M. (eds.): Metabolic Bone Disease, Vol. I. New York, Academic Press, 1977, p. 237.

131. Chesney, R.W.: Current clinical applications of vitamin D metabolite research. Clin. Orthop. 161:285, 1981.

132. Eastwood, J.B., DeWardener, H.E., Gray, R.W., and Lemann, J.L., Jr.: Normal plasma 1,25-(OH)₂-vitamin-D concentrations in nutritional osteomalacia. Lancet 1:1377, 1979.

133. Mankin, H.J.: Rickets, osteomalacia and renal osteodystrophy. J. Bone Joint Surg. 56A:101, 1974.

134. Frame, B., and Parfitt, A.M.: Osteomalacia: Current concepts. Ann. Intern. Med. 89:966, 1978.

135. Klein, G.L., Targoff, C.M., Ament, M.E., Sherrard, D.J., Bluestone, R., Young, J.H., Norman, A.W., and Coburn, J.W.: Bone disease associated with total parenteral nutrition. Lancet 2:1041, 1980.

136. Dibble, J.B., Sheridan, P.; and Losowsky, M.S.: A survey of vitamin D deficiency in gastrointestinal and liver disorders. Quart. J. Med. 53:119, 1984.

137. Imawari, M., Akanuma, Y., Itakura, H., Muto, Y., Kosaka, K., and Goodman, D.S.: The effects of diseases of the liver on serum 25-hydroxyvitamin D and on the serum binding protein for vitamin D and its metabolites. J. Lab. Clin. Med. 93:171, 1979.

138. Hahn, T.J., and Avioli, L.V.: Acquired (noninherited) disorders of vitamin D function. In De Groot, L.J. (ed.): Endocrinology, Vol. 2. New York, Grune & Stratton, 1979, p. 809.

139. Jubiz, W., Haussler, M.R., McCain, T.A., and Tolman, K.G.: Plasma 1,25-dihydroxyvitamin D levels in patients receiving anticonvulsant drugs. J. Clin. Endocrinol. Metab. 44:617, 1977.

140. Christensen, C.K., Lund, B., Lund, B.J., Sorensen, O.H., Neilsen, H.E., and Mosekilde, L.: Reduced 1,25-dihydroxyvitamin D and 24,25-dihydroxyvitamin D in epileptic patients receiving chronic combined anticonvulsant therapy. Metab. Bone. Dis. Rel. Res. 3:17, 1981.

141. Delvin, E.E., Glorieux, F.H., Marie, P.J., and Pettifor, J.M.: Vitamin D

dependency: Replacement therapy with calcitriol. J. Pediatr. 99:26, 1981.

142. Sauveur, B., Garabedian, M., Fellot, C., Mongin, P., and Balsan, S.: The effect of induced metabolic acidosis on vitamin D_3 metabolism. Calcif. Tiss. Res. 23:121, 1977.

143. Lee, S.W., Russell, J., and Avioli, L.V.: 25-Hydroxycholecalciferol to 1,25-dihydroxycholecalciferol: Conversion impaired by systemic metabolic acidosis. Science 195:994, 1977.

144. Chesney, R.W., Kaplan, B.S., Phelps, M. and DeLuca, H.F.: Renal tubular acidosis does not alter circulating values of calcitriol J. Pediatr. 104:51, 1984.

145. Drezner, M.K., and Feinglos, M.N.: Osteomalacia due to 1α,25-dihydroxycholecalciferol deficiency: Association with a giant cell tumor of bone. J. Clin. Invest. 60:1046, 1977.

146. Lyles, K.W., Berry, W.R., Haussler, M., Harrelson, J.M., and Drezner, M.K.L.: Hypophosphatemic osteomalacia: Association with prostatic carcinoma. Ann. Intern. Med. 93:275, 1980.

147. Drezner, M.K., Neelon, F.A., Haussler, M., McPherson, H.T., and Lebovitz, H.E.: 1,25-Dihydroxycholecalciferol deficiency: The probable cause of hypocalcemia and metabolic bone disease in pseudohypoparathyroidism. J. Clin. Endocrinol. Metab. 42:621, 1976.

148. Schmidt-Gayk, H., Schmitt, W., Grawunder, C., Ritz, E., Tschoepe, W., Pietsch, V., Andrassy, K., and Bouillon, R.: 25-hydroxy-vitamin-D in nephrotic syndrome. Lancet 2:105, 1977.

149. Lambert, P.W., De Oreo, P.B., Fu, I.Y., Kaetzel, D.M., vonAhn, K., Hollis, B.W., and Roos, B.A.: Urinary and plasma vitamin D_3 metabolites in the nephrotic syndrome. Metab. Bone Dis. Rel. Res. 4:7, 1982.

150. Malluche, H.H., Goldstein, D.A., and Massry, S.G.: Osteomalacia and hyperparathyroid bone disease in patients with nephrotic syndrome. J. Clin. Invest. 63:494, 1979.

151. Brickman, A.S., Coburn, J.W., and Massry, S.G.: 1,25-dihydroxyvitamin D_3 in normal man and patients with renal failure. Ann. Intern. Med. 80:161, 1974.

152. Dent, C.E., and Winter, C.E.: Osteomalacia due to phosphate depletion from excessive aluminium hydroxide ingestion. Br. Med. J. 1:551, 1974.

153. Ahmed, K.Y., Varghese, Z., Wills, M.R., Meinhard, E., Skinner, R.K., Baillod, R.A., and Moorhead, J.F.: Persitent hypophosphatemia and osteomalacia in dialysis patients not on oral phosphate binders: Response to dihydrotachysterol therapy. Lancet 2:439, 1976.

154. Albright, F., Butler, A.M., and Bloomberg, E.: Rickets resistant to vitamin D therapy. Am. J. Dis. Child. 54:529, 1937.

155. Fraser, D., and Scriver, C.R.: Disorders associated with hereditary or acquired abnormalities in vitamin D function: Hereditary disorders associated with vitamin D resistance or defective phosphate metabolism. In De Groot, L.V. (ed.): Endocrinology, Vol. 2. New York, Grune & Stratton, 1979, p. 797.

156. Arnaud, C., Glorieux, F., and Scriver, C.R.: Serum parathyroid hormone in X-linked hypophosphatemia. Science 173:845, 1971.

157. Reitz, R.E., and Weinstein, R.L.: Parathyroid hormone secretion in familial vitamin-D-resistant rickets. N. Engl. J. Med. 289:941, 1973.

158. Lyles, K.W., Clark, A.G., and Drezner, M.K.: Serum 1,25-dihydroxyvitamin D levels in subjects with X-linked hypophosphatemic rickets and osteomalacia. Calcif. Tissue Int. 34:125, 1982.

159. Glorieux, F.H., Scriver, C.R., Reade, T.M., Goldman, H., and Roseborough, A.: Use of phosphate and vitamin D to prevent dwarfism and rickets in X-linked hypophosphatemia. N. Engl. J. Med. 287:481, 1972.

160. Glorieux, F.H., Marie, P.J., Pettifor, J.M., and Devlin, E.E.: Bone response to phosphate salts, ergocalciferol, and calcitriol in hypophosphatemic vitamin D-resistant rickets. N. Engl. J. Med. 303:1023, 1980.

161. Marie, P.J., and Glorieux, F.H.: Stimulation of cortical bone mineralization and remodeling by phosphate and 1,25-dihydroxyvitamin D in vitamin D-resistant rickets. Metab. Bone Dis. Rel. Res. 3:159, 1981.

162. Stamp, T.C.B., and Baker, L.R.I.: Recessive hypophosphatemic rickets, and possible etiology of the 'vitamin D-resistant' syndrome. Arch. Dis. Child. 51:360, 1976.

163. Perry, W., and Stamp, T.C.B.: Hereditary hypophosphatemic rickets with autosomal recessive inheritance and severe osteosclerosis. J. Bone Joint Surg. 60B:430, 1978.

164. Nagant De Deuxchaisnes, C., and Krane, S.M.: The treatment of adult phosphate diabetes and Fanconi syndrome with neutral sodium phosphate. Am. J. Med. 43:508, 1967.

165. Frymoyer, J.W., and Hodgkin, W.: Adult-onset vitamin D-resistant hypophosphatemic osteomalacia. A possible variant of vitamin D-resistant rickets. J. Bone Joint Surg. 59A:101, 1977.

166. Arie, R., Samuel, R., Halabe, A., and Liberman, U.A.: Hereditary familial symdrome of renal phosphate leak with hypercalciuria, nephrolithiasis and bone lesions. In Silbermann, M., and Slavkin, H.C. (eds.): Current Advances in Skeletogenesis. Amsterdam, Excerpta Medica, 1982, p. 537.

167. Goldring, S.R., and Krane, S.M.: Disorders of calcification: Osteomalacia and rickets. In De Groot, L. (ed.): Endocrinology, Vol. 2. New York, Grune & Stratton, 1979, p. 853.

168. Dent, C.E., and Gertner, J.M.: Hypophosphatemic osteomalacia in fibrous dysplasia. Quart. J. Med. N.S. 45:411, 1976.

169. Aschinberg, L.C., Solomon, L.M., Zeis, P.M., Justice, P., and Rosenthal, I.M.: Vitamin D-resistant rickets associated with epidermal nevus syndrome: Demonstration of a phosphaturic substance in the dermal lesions. J. Pediatr. 91:56, 1977.

170. Bressot, C., Courpron, P., Edouard, C., and Meunier, P.: Histomorphometrie des Osteopathies Endocriniennes. Lyon, Association Corporative des Etudiants en Medecines de Lyon, 1976, p. 117.

171. Boyce, B.F., Smith, L. Fogelman, I., Johnston, E., Ralston, S., and Boyle, I.T.: Focal osteomalacia due to low-dose diphosphonate therapy in Paget's disease. Lancet 1:821, 1984.

172. Kooh, S.W., Fraser, D., Reilly, B.J., Hamilton, J.R., Gall, D.G., and Bell, L.: Rickets due to calcium deficiency. N. Engl. J. Med. 297:1264, 1977.

173. Marie, P.J., Pettifor, J.M., Ross, F.P., and Glorieux, F.H.: Histological osteomalacia due to dietary calcium deficiency in children. N. Engl. J. Med. 307:584, 1982.

174. Rasmussen, H.: Hypophosphatasia. In Stanbury, J.B., Wyngaarden, J.B., Fredrickson, D.S., Goldstein, J.L., and Brown, M.S., (eds.): The Metabolic Basis of Inherited Disease. 5th ed. New York, McGraw-Hill Book Company, 1983, p. 1497.

175. Frame, B., Frost, H.M., Pak, C.Y.C., Reynolds, W., and Argen, R.J.: Fibrogenesis imperfecta ossium. A collagen defect causing osteomalacia. N. Engl. J. Med. 285:769, 1971.

176. Klein, G.L., Alfrey, A.C., Miller, N.L., Sherrard, D.J., Hazlet, T.K., Ament, M.E., and Coburn, J.W.: Aluminum loading during total parenteral nutrition. Am. J. Clin. Nutr. 35:1425, 1982.

177. Shike, M., Sturtridge, W.C., Tam, C.S., Harrison, J.E., Jones, G., Murray, T.M, and Jeejeebhoy, K.H.: A possible role of vitamin D in the genesis of parenteral-nutrition-induced metabolic bone disease. Ann. Intern. Med. 95:560, 1981.

178. Avioli, L.V.: Renal osteodystrophy. In Avioli, L.V., and Krane, S.M. (eds.): Metabolic Bone Disease, Vol. II. New York, Academic Press, 1978, p. 149.

179. Coburn, J.W., Kurokawa, K., and Llach, F.: Altered divalent ion metabolism in renal disease and renal osteodystrophy. In Maxwell, M.H., and Kleeman, C.R. (eds.): Clinical Disorders of Fluid and Electrolyte Metabolism. New York, McGraw-Hill Book Company, 1980, p. 1153.

180. Hodsman, A.B., Sherrard, D.J., Wong, E.G.C., Brickman, A.S., Lee, D.B.N., Alfrey, A.C., Singer, F.R., Norman, A.W., and Coburn, J.W.: Vitamin D-resistant osteomalacia in hemodialysis patients lacking secondary hyperparathyroidism. Ann. Intern. Med. 94:629, 1981.

181. Hodsman, A.B., Sherrard, D.J., Alfrey, A.C., Ott, S., Brickman, A.S., Miller, N.L., Maloney, N.A., and Coburn, J.W.: Bone aluminum and histomorphometric features of renal osteodystrophy. J. Clin. Endocrinol. Metab. 54:539, 1982.

182. Horst, R.L., Shepard, R.M., Jorgensen, N.A., and DeLuca, H.F.: The determination of 24,25-dihydroxyvitamin D and 25,26-dihydroxyvitamin D in plasma from normal and nephrectomized man. J. Lab. Clin. Med. 93:277, 1979.

183. Eastwood, J.B., Harris, E., Stamp, T.C.B., and De Wardener, H.E.: Vitamin D deficiency in the osteomalacia of chronic renal failure. Lancet 2:1209, 1976.

184. Sherrard, D.J., Baylink, D.J., Wergedahl, J.E., and Maloney, N.: Quantitative histological studies on the pathogenesis of uremic bone disease. J. Clin. Endocrinol. Metab. 39:119, 1974.

185. Eastwood, J.B., Stamp, T.C.B., De Wardener, H.E., Bordier, P.J., and Arnaud, C.D.: The effect of 25-hydroxy vitamin D_3 in the osteomalacia of chronic renal failure. Clin. Sci. Mol. Med. 52:499, 1977.

186. Bordier, P., Zingraff, J., Gueris, J., Jungers, P., Marie, P., Pechet, M., and Rasmussen, H.: The effect of 1α(OH)D_3 and 1α,25(OH)$_2D_3$ on the bone in patients with renal osteodystrophy. Am. J. Med. 64:101, 1978.

187. Maschio, G., Tessitore, M., D'Angelo, A., Bonucci, E., Lupo, A., Valvo, E., Loschiavo, C., Fabris, A., Morachiello, P., Previato, G., and Fiaschi, E.: Early dietary phosphorus restriction and calcium supplementation in the prevention of renal osteodystrophy. Am. J. Clin. Nutr. 33:1546, 1980.

188. Jaffe, H.L.: Metabolic, Degenerative, and Inflammatory Diseases of Bones and Joints. Philadelphia, Lea & Febiger, 1972, p. 178.

189. Kahler, S.G., Burns, J.A., and Aylsworth, A.S.: A mild autosomal recessive form of osteopetrosis. Am. J. Med. Gen. 17:451, 1984.

190. Sly, W.S., Hewett-Emmett, D., Whyte, M.P., Yu, Y.S.L., and Tashian, R.E.: Carbonic anhydrase II deficiency identified as the primary defect in the autosomal recessive syndrome of osteopetrosis with renal tubular acidosis and cerebral calcification. Proc. Natl. Acad. Sci. USA 80: 2752, 1983.

191. Manzke, E., Gruber, H.E., Hiness, R.W., and Baylink, D.J.: Skeletal remodelling and bone related hormones in two adults with increased bone mass. Metabolism 31:25, 1982.

192. Walker, D.G.: Bone resorption restored in osteopetrotic mice by transplants of normal bone marrow and spleen cells. Science 190:784, 1975.

193. Ballet, J.J., and Griscelli, C.: Lymphoid cell transplantation in human osteopetrosis. In Horton, J.E., Tarpley, T.M., and Davis, W.F. (eds.): Mechanisms of Localized Bone Loss. Special Supplement to Calcified Tissue Abstracts, 1978, p. 399.

194. Coccia, P.F., Krivit, W., Cervenka, J., Clawson, C., Kersey, J.H., Kim, T.H., Nesbit, M.E., Ramsay, N.K.C., Warkentin, P.I., Teitelbaum, S.L., Kahn, A.J., and Brown, D.M.: Successful bone-marrow transplantation for infantile malignant osteopetrosis. N. Engl. J. Med. 302:701, 1980.

195. Key, L., Carnes, D. Cole, S., Holtrop, M., Bar-Shavit, Z., Shapiro, F., Arceci, R., Steinberg, J., Gundberg, C., Kahn, A., Teitelbaum, S., and Anast, C.: Treatment of congenital osteopetrosis with high-dose calcitriol. N. Engl. J. Med. 310:409, 1984.

196. Harris, W.H., Dudley, H.R., Jr., and Barry, R.J.: The natural history of fibrous dysplasia. An orthopaedic, pathological and roentgenographic study. J. Bone Joint Surg. 44A:207, 1962.

197. Schwartz, D.T., and Alpert, M.: The malignant transformation of fibrous dysplasia. Am. J. Med. Sci. 247:35, 1964.

198. Bell, N.H., Avery, S., and Johnston, C.C.: Effects of calcitonin in Paget's disease and polyostotic fibrous dysplasia. J. Clin. Endocrinol. Metab. 31:283, 1970.

199. Thompson, R.C., Jr., Gaull, G.E., Horwitz, S.J., and Schenck, R.K.: Hereditary hyperphosphatasia. Studies of three siblings. Am. J. Med. 47:209, 1969.

200. Whalen, J.P., Horwith, M., Krook, L., MacIntyre, I., Mena, A., Viteri, F., Torun, B., and Nunez, E.A.: Calcitonin treatment in hereditary bone dysplasia with hyperphosphatasemia: A radiographic and histologic study of bone. Am. J. Roentgenol. 129:29, 1977.

201. Nunez, E.A., Horwith, M., Krook, L., and Whalen, J.P.: An electron microscopic investigation of human familial bone dysplasia. Inhibition of osteocytic osteolysis and induction of osteocytic formation of elastic fibers following calcitonin treatment. Am. J. Pathol. 94:1, 1979.

202. Doyle, F.H., Woodhouse, N.J.Y., Glen, C.A., Joplin, G.F., and MacIntyre, I.: Healing of the bones in juvenile Paget's disease treated by human calcitonin. Br. J. Radiol. 47:9, 1974.

203. Paget, J.: On a form of chronic inflammation of bones (osteitis deformans). Med. Chir. Trans. 60:27, 1877.

204. Barry, H.C.: Paget's Disease of Bone. Baltimore, Williams & Wilkins Company, 1969.

205. Franck, W.A., Bress, N.M., Singer, F.R., and Krane, S.M.: Rheumatic manifestations of Paget's disease of bone. Am. J. Med. 56:592, 1974.

206. Heistad, D.D., Abboud, F.M., Schmid, P.G., Mark, A.L., and Wilson, W.R.: Regulation of blood flow in Paget's disease of bone. J. Clin. Invest. 55:69, 1975.

207. Nagant de Deuxchaisnes, C., and Krane, S.M.: Paget's disease of bone: Clinical and metabolic observations. Medicine 43:233, 1964.

208. Singer, F.R.: Paget's Disease of Bone. New York, Plenum Medical Book Company, 1977.

209. Waxman, A.D., Ducker, S., McKee, D., Siemsen, J.K., and Singer, F.R.: Evaluation of 99mTc diphosphonate kinetics and bone scans in patients with Paget's disease before and after calcitonin treatment. Radiology 125:761, 1977.

210. Khairi, M.R.A., Wellman, H.N., Robb, J.A., and Johnston, C.C., Jr.: Paget's disease of bone (osteitis deformans): Symptomatic lesions and bone scan. Ann. Intern. Med. 79:348, 1973.

211. Singer, F.R., Mills, B.G., and Terry, R.: Bone resorbing cells in Paget's disease. In Horton, J.E., Tarpley, T.M., and Davis, W.F. (eds.): Mechanisms of Localized Bone Loss. Special Supplement to Calcified Tissue Abstracts, 1978, p. 365.

212. Rebel, A., Basle, M., Pouplard, A., Malkani, K., Filmon, R., and Lepatezour, A.: Bone tissue in Paget's disease of bone. Ultrastructure and immunocytology. Arthritis Rheum. 23:1104, 1980.

213. Mills, B.G., Singer, F.R., Weiner, L.P., and Holst, P.A.: Immunohistological demonstration of respiratory syncytial viral antigens in Paget's disease of bone, Proc. Natl. Acad. Sci. USA 78:1209, 1981.

214. Mills, B.G., Singer, F.R., Weiner, L.P., Suffin, S.C., Stabile, E., and Holst, P.: Evidence for both respiratory syncytial and measles virus antigens in the osteoclasts of patients with Paget's disease of bone. Clin. Orthop. 183: 303, 1984.

215. Posen, S., Clifton-Bligh, P., and Wilkinson, M.: Paget's disease of bone and hyperparathyroidism: Coincidence or causal relationship? Calcif. Tiss. Res. 26:107, 1978.

216. Howarth, S.: Cardiac output in osteitis deformans. Clin. Sci. 12:271, 1953.

217. O'Reilly, T.J., and Race, J.: Osteitis deformans. Quart. J. Med. 25:471, 1932.

218. Mills, B.G., Singer, F.R., Weiner, L.P., and Holst, P.A.: Long term culture of cells from bone affected by Paget's disease. Calcif. Tiss. Int. 29:79, 1979.

219. Singer, F.R., Melvin, K.E.W., and Mills, B.G.: Acute effects of calcitonin on osteoclasts in man. Clin. Endocrinol. 5:333s, 1976.

220. Nagant de Deuxchaisnes, C., Maldague, B., Malghem, J., Devogelaer, J.P., Huaux, J.P., and Rombouts-Lindemans, C.: The action of the main therapeutic regimes on Paget's disease of bone, with a note on the effect of vitamin D deficiency. Arthritis Rheum. 23:1215, 1980.

221. Singer, F.R., Fredericks, R.S., and Minkin, C.: Salmon calcitonin therapy for Paget's disease of bone. The problem of acquired clinical resistance. Arthritis Rheum. 23:1148, 1980.

222. Rojanasathit, S., Rosenberg, E., and Haddad, J.G., Jr.: Paget's bone disease: Response to human calcitonin in patients resistant to salmon calcitonin. Lancet 2:1412, 1974.

223. Singer, F.R.: Human calcitonin treatment of Paget's disease of bone. Clin. Orthop. Rel. Res. 127:86, 1977.

224. Avramides, A., Flores, A., De Rose, J., and Wallach, S.: Paget's disease of bone: Observations after cessation of long-term synthetic salmon calcitonin treatment. J. Clin. Endocrinol. Metab. 42:459, 1976.

225. Fleisch, H.: Bisphosphonates: Mechanisms of action and clinical applications. In Peck, W.A. (ed.): Bone and Mineral Research. Annual 1. Amsterdam, Excerpta Medica, 1983, p. 319.

226. Khairi, M.R.A., Altman, R.D., De Rosa, G.P., Zimmerman, J., Schenk, R.K., and Johnston, C.C.: Sodium etidronate in the treatment of Paget's disease of bone. A study of long-term results. Ann. Intern. Med. 87:656, 1977.

227. Canfield, R., Rosner, W., Skinner, J., McWhorter, J., Resnick, L., Feldman, F., Kammerman, S., Ryan, K., Kunigonis, M., and Bohne, W.: Diphosphonate therapy of Paget's disease of bone. J. Clin. Metab. 44:96, 1977.

228. Ryan, W.G., Schwartz, T.B., and Northrop, G.: Experiences in the treatment of Paget's disease of bone with mithramycin. JAMA 213:1153, 1970.

229. Lebbin, D., Ryan, W.G., and Schwartz, T.B.: Outpatient treatment of Paget's disease of bone with mithramycin. Ann. Intern. Med. 81:635, 1974.

230. Evans, R.A., Dunstan, C.R., Wong, S.Y.P., and Hills, E.: Long-term experience with a calcium-thiazide treatment for Paget's disease of bone. Mineral Elec. Metabol. 8:325, 1982.

231. Meyers, M., and Singer, F.R.: Osteotomy for tibia vara in Paget's disease under cover of calcitonin. J. Bone Joint Surg. 60A:810, 1978.

Section XX

Disorders of Bone of Uncertain Etiology

Chapter 107

Avascular Necrosis of Bone

Thomas M. Zizic and David S. Hungerford

INTRODUCTION

Avascular necrosis (AVN) and osteonecrosis are the more commonly used terms for an entity that is also referred to as aseptic necrosis, osteochondritis dissecans, and ischemic necrosis of bone. Pathologically, it is characterized by death of cells in bone resulting from an interruption of blood supply to bone. Evidence demonstrates that the extent and location of the circulatory disturbance determines the magnitude of the resulting osseous necrosis.[1]

Although the knees and shoulders are frequently involved, the hips are the favorite target. More rarely the tarsal navicular, the body of the talus, and the carpal scaphoid and navicular are affected.

There are a number of primary diseases that are associated with the development of ischemic bony changes. The Johns Hopkins experience collected over the past 10 years is listed in Table 107–1. In general, predisposing diseases can be grouped into the following three major categories: (1) conditions that are generally accepted to be contributory to the development of AVN, such as trauma, hemoglobinopathies, decompression sickness, Gaucher's disease, hypercortisonism, and irradiation; (2) conditions that are believed to be commonly associated with AVN, such as alcoholism, pancreatitis, hyperuricemia, and gout; and (3) the so-called idiopathic group, in which there is no discernible underlying disease.

EPIDEMIOLOGY

A population survey in a small Swiss village revealed a prevalence of AVN of 0.1 percent of the general population. Two to three percent of all patients with chronic hip disease at the clinic in that village had idiopathic ischemic necrosis of the femoral head.[2] In the United States, of over 2000 patients undergoing total hip replacement at the Mayo Clinic in the 1970s, 5 percent were diagnosed as having aseptic necrosis as the underlying pathologic process leading to arthritis of the hip.[3] In most series of idiopathic AVN of the femoral head, the sex ratio is 4 to 5 males to 1 female, with a peak incidence between the ages 30 and 60; in 33 to 72 percent of the patients the disease is bilateral.[4-12] Male preponderance is not present in SLE. Spontaneous idiopathic osteonecrosis of the knee, unassociated with AVN elsewhere, usually affects elderly females.[13-15]

A number of conditions that are radiologically similar to AVN affect the apophyses and epiphyses of children and adolescents. The most important of these is Legg-Calvé-Perthes disease, believed by many to be a result of primary aseptic necrosis.[16] This and other epiphyseal osteochondroses of childhood are beyond the scope of this text and will not be discussed.

DISEASE ENTITIES ASSOCIATED WITH DEVELOPMENT OF AVN AND PATHOGENESIS OF AVN

Trauma. Necrosis of a large volume of bone following trauma is nearly always confined to anatomic sites with few arterial anastomoses.[17] Although AVN has been described in the carpal lunate and navicular and in the tarsal navicular, the most common sites of post-traumatic AVN are the femoral and humeral heads, the body of the talus, and the carpal scaphoid. All four latter sites are similar in that the portion of bone that becomes avascular is intra-articular and has a limited attachment of soft tissue. Because of the similarities in the pathogenesis of AVN following trauma to different bones, the hip will be used as an illustrative example.

In childhood and early adulthood, fractures of the proximal femur are usually the result of a violent injury, but in the elderly a simple fall is a frequent cause. Because of the contribution of postmenopausal osteoporosis with structural weakening of the skeleton, these fractures are two to five times more common in women than in men.[18-20] The incidence of these fractures in women doubles for each decade over the age of 45 years.[18] The principal source of blood to the adult femoral head is the profunda femoris artery by way of its circumflex femoral branches.[21] A more variable source

1689

Table 107-1. Diseases in Patients with
Avascular Necrosis

Associated Disease	Number Patients
Systemic lupus erythematosus	82
Rheumatoid arthritis	26
Renal transplant	14
Hemoglobinopathy	12
Trauma	11
Alcoholism	10
Solid tumors	5
Hodgkin's disease	3
Leukemia	2
Gout	9
Asthma	8
Polyarthritis—unknown etiology	7
Poly(dermato)myositis	4
Undifferentiated connective tissue disease	3
Inflammatory bowel disease	4
Giant cell arteritis/polymyalgia rheumatism	3
Arteritis—unspecified	2
Sarcoidosis	2
Cushing's syndrome	2
Progressive systemic sclerosis	1
Raynaud's disease	1
Idiopathic thrombocytopenia	1
Caisson's disease	1
Gaucher's disease	1
Juvenile rheumatoid arthritis	1
Ankylosing spondylitis	1
Sjögren's syndrome	1
Other steroid	4
Nonassociated diseases	61
Ischemic necrosis of bone only	91
	373

comes to the femoral head along the vessels of the ligamentum teres, which enter the bone of the fovea capitis. The late complication of avascular necrosis following trauma is probably determined by the relative contribution of the arteries to the total femoral head blood supply and the extent of anastomoses between them, which varies from individual to individual. Although the amount of blood flow through the ligamentum teres vessels may be minimal, blood flow into the foveal area is important, as it may provide a source of revascularization when the remainder of the femoral head is avascular.[22] Intertrochanteric or extracapsular fractures rarely develop avascular necrosis and late segmental collapse. Transcervical or subcapital fractures, on the other hand, result in a high incidence of avascular necrosis, presumably as a result of injury to the superior retinacular vessels near their point of entry into the bone.

Despite a multitude of devices for internal fixation of femoral neck fractures, the incidence of avascular necrosis and late segmental collapse ranges from 11 to 45 percent and does not appear to be related to the type of fixation device.[19,20,23-25]

The cause of avascular necrosis after hip dislocations is interruption of the circulation, due to tears of the ligamentum teres and joint capsule, which compromise the vessels lying in the capsular reflections. Posterior dislocations are not only more frequent than anterior ones but are associated with an incidence of avascular

necrosis of 10 to 26 percent as opposed to an incidence of 3 to 9 percent in anterior dislocations.[26-28] In one series 52 percent of hips that remained dislocated longer than 12 hours developed AVN, while only 22 percent of those reduced within 12 hours had a similar bad outcome.[28]

Decompression Sickness. Osteonecrosis is the major late complication of exposure to high pressure environments. Men working in caissons or in tunnels built through water-bearing ground requiring compressed air to prevent water seepage are at risk. The first published radiographs of aseptic necrosis in adults were in compressed air workers described in 1911.[29] Prevalence has ranged from 12 to 35 percent.[30-32] Bony lesions do not occur unless the workers are exposed to pressures of greater than 17 pounds per square inch.[31,33,34] In Europe and America avascular necrosis is much more common in compressed air workers than in divers, but in Japan, the prevalence of osteonecrosis is predominant in divers, ranging from 38 to 77 percent.[35] Pathogenesis is related to appearance during decompression of bubbles of intravascular nitrogen, which obstruct capillaries, and extravascular bubbles within fatty marrow encased in bone, which can compress intraosseus vessels.[34] In several patients dying within hours after acute decompression sickness, air bubbles were present in bone marrow cavities of the femoral heads.[36] In addition, it is postulated that arteriolar spasm may contribute to bone marrow ischemia.[36]

Sickle Cell Anemia and Allied Hemoglobinopathies. There are multiple bone changes that occur with sickle cell anemia and its allied hemoglobinopathies like thalassemia, Hb C, Hb D, and Hb E anemias (see Chapter 101). At the University of Kinshas, 20 percent of the consultations in sickle cell disease were for bone crises compared with 13 percent for anemia and 17 percent for gastroenteritis.[37] Aseptic necrosis occurs only when there is an S gene to cause the sickling phenomenon. In thalassemia and Hb E/thalassemia, bone infarction does not occur.[38] The incidence in SS disease ranges from 4 to 12 percent.[37,39,40] In SC disease, the incidence of bone necrosis varies from 20 to 68 percent.[37] It is possible that avascular necrosis is more common in SC and S thalassemia than in SS patients because the latter do not live long enough to show such changes. Vascular blockage due to sickled cells in the capillaries and sinusoids of the red marrow may occur in any bone of the body, producing painful and febrile crises.[41,42] Infarction may occur in the subarticular zone or in the shaft of a bone (Fig. 107-1). The signs and symptoms, the progress of lesions, the roentgenologic appearance, and the anatomic findings are characterized by variability.[37,38,41,42] In the early phase there is frequently a paucity of radiograpic findings despite dramatic symptoms of recurrent aching, episodes of acute pain, and exaggeration of pain after strenous activity. The rate of progression of anatomic changes after the initial onset of pain is also variable and unpredictable. Eventually, classic changes develop on routine radiographs (Fig. 107-2).

As in other causes of AVN, abnormal bone marrow

Figure 107–1. A 30-year-old black male with sickle cell anemia with femoral shaft infarcts producing "bone on bone sign." (Courtesy of Dr. Peter Holt.)

pressures and venography are helpful in detecting pre-radiologic disease, which can be confirmed by core biopsy.[37] Early diagnosis may be particularly important in these patients for two reasons. First, the sites of bone ischemia and infarction seem particularly susceptible to *Salmonella* osteomyelitis, which can be documented by the core biopsy and treated appropriately with antibiotics. Secondly, the minor procedure of core biopsy is better tolerated than major procedures and may obviate the necessity for subsequent joint arthroplasty.

Gaucher's Disease and Metastatic Carcinoma. In Gaucher's disease the metabolic disorder consists of a deficiency in the enzyme glucocerebrosidase resulting in an abnormal accumulation of glucorerebroside (an analoque of kerasin) in macrophages. The glucocerebroside-laden macrophages accumulate in the liver, spleen, and bone marrow, where accumulated masses may produce cortical thinning and expansion, particularly at the lower end of the femur (Fig. 107–3), or the Gaucher's cells may pack the marrow spaces of the femoral head, resulting in necrosis (Fig. 107–4). Masses of Gaucher's cells may compress the intraosseous sinusoids, or perhaps the lumina may be blocked by the macrophages.[43] A similar mechanism may apply to ischemic necrosis of bone associated with metastatic cancer involving bone; AVN was noted in 46 of 80 cases of lung cancer metastatic to bone.[44]

Glucocorticoids. Glucocorticoids were first implicated in the development of AVN over 25 years ago.[45] The more frequent diagnosis of avascular necrosis coincides with the introduction and widespread availability of cortisone and its derivatives.[46-53] Individuals with systemic lupus erythematosus and renal allograft recipients treated with steroids are the two groups with the highest reported prevalence of AVN, and they will be discussed separately.

Systemic Lupus Erythematosus (SLE). Avascular necrosis is the dominant orthopedic problem in patients with SLE and occurs in 5 to 40 percent of patients with this disease.[46-48,54-58] Diagnosis of "preradiographic" disease, the increased survival of patients with SLE,[59] and the reliance upon glucocorticoids for effective therapy

Figure 107–2. Same patient as in Figure 107–1. Clinical picture characterized by progressive hip pain at rest with night pain and markedly increased discomfort with walking which is limited to one block. Core biopsy decompression revealed extensive avascular necrosis.

Figure 107–3. Characteristic in Gaucher's disease is expansion from the diaphysis to the metaphysis of the distal femur with thinning of the bony cortex, producing the "Erlenmeyer flask sign."

Figure 107–4. Subchondral fracture and collapse of the right femoral head in a patient with Gaucher's disease.

allow emergence of late-stage complications such as AVN with greater frequency.

At Johns Hopkins, 54 patients with SLE were studied prospectively. Twenty-eight developed AVN at 93 bony sites, 26 did not develop AVN.[60] Demographically and clinically, including duration of disease and glucocorticoid therapy, patients with AVN were similar to the others except that 24 (86 percent) of 28 were clinically cushingnoid as compared with 4 (15 percent) of the 26 without bony lesions ($p < 0.0001$). The mean prednisone dose for the highest single month as well as for the highest consecutive 3, 6, and 12 months of therapy is a useful predictive parameter. A significant correlation was also found between higher mean prednisone dose at all of the above time intervals and an increased number of bone sites involved.[60]

It is unlikely that corticosteriod dosages are the only factor determining the development of AVN in SLE.[61] In a series of patients with poly(dermato)myositis treated with steriods 2 (50 percent) of the 4 patients with AVN had vasculitis as compared with 5 (7 percent) of 72 poly(dermato)myositis patients without ischemic bones ($p < 0.05$). Vasculitis and Raynaud's syndrome are more frequent in SLE patients who develop AVN[55,56,58]; in our prospective study, a lower mean dose of prednisone was required to produce AVN in SLE patients with Raynaud's syndrome.[60] These findings support the hypothesis that vascular abnormalities and high glucocorticoid dosage for a month or more as well as individual variation of biologic response of lipocytes to glucocorticoids are all of pathogenetic significance in the development of AVN in SLE and perhaps in other diseases as well.

Renal Transplantation. Avascular necrosis following renal transplantation was first reported 20 years ago.[62,63] Since then necrosis of bone following transplantation has been reported to occur in up to 40 percent of patients.[63-69] As in AVN in SLE, the hips, knees, and shoulders are most frequently affected, although occa-

sionally other sites such as the talus are involved; and the majority of renal allograft recipients have multiple bony sites involved.[49,66,68-70] The interval between transplantation and onset of symptoms of AVN ranges from 1 to 126 months, with a mean of 16 months.[66,69,70] In a prospective study of children with renal transplantation, 9 (25 percent) of 36 developed avascular necrosis.[64] There were no patients under the skeletal age of 10 or without episodes of rejection reaction who developed this complication.

In most of the reports in which adequate information on dosage is available there is a statistically significant positive correlation between the mean daily prednisone dosage during the first month following transplantation and the subsequent development of avascular necrosis.[49,65,71-73] The prevalence of AVN is high in patients given doses in excess of 100 mg per day during the first month following transplantation[49,65,71,74,79] and uncommon in recipients given less than this dosage.[49,73,74] Additional evidence in favor of the importance of glucocorticoids are the reports of a significant reduction in the incidence of AVN when the mean steroid dosages were lower following transplantation.[49,73,74] As in the experience with SLE,[60] it appears that high glucocorticoids for relatively short periods are more important than the cumulative dose or total duration of therapy.

Several studies have indicated that there are lower serum phosphate levels in renal graft recipients who develop avascular necrosis.[70,75,76] Patients with hypophosphatemia after renal transplantation tend to develop osteomalacia.[77] A lower bone density has also been demonstrated in graft recipients who subsequently develop AVN.[78,79] Recently it has been shown that a reduction in renal bone disease with better dialysis techniques (increasing ionized calcium in dialysate) and medical management significantly reduced the incidence of AVN in two groups of renal transplant patients who were nearly identical in regard to transplant technique and immunosuppression protocols.[80]

Miscellaneous Glucocorticoid-Treated Patients. In 169 patients with AVN seen at Johns Hopkins, 88 (52 percent) had received glucocorticoids. Excluding patients with SLE and renal allografts, steroids were given for a variety of diseases, including asthma, polymyalgia rheumatica, rheumatoid arthritis, sarcoidosis, giant cell arteritis, Bell's palsy, polymyositis, scleroderma, hepatitis, inflammatory bowel disease, psoriatic arthritis, nephrotic syndrome, hemolytic anemia, and malignancies (Table 107–1). Slightly more than half of our miscellaneous steroid-treated patients were female, in contrast to the male preponderance in idiopathic AVN. Almost 60 percent were less than 50 years of age at the time of diagnosis of AVN. One of our patients developed bilateral AVN of the hips, knees, and shoulders after only 3 weeks of prednisone, which was given for viral pneumonitis.

Alcoholism. In reported series of patients with idiopathic avascular necrosis, 17 to 39 percent of the patients had a significant alcoholic history.[10,12,81] In 26 patients with alcohol-associated AVN, nineteen (73 percent) either presented with bilateral disease or eventually developed it.[82] These features as well as a striking male predominance have been found by others.[1,12] The femoral head is most frequently involved, followed by the humeral head, proximal tibia, and distal femur. In one series, 7 of 9 livers examined histologically had fatty metamorphosis, and evidence of systemic fat embolism was found in 9 of 19 patients; in two of these probable intravascular fat globules in resected femoral heads were observed.[1]

Pancreatic Disease. Pancreatitis and pancreatic carcinoma have been reported to be associated with necrosis of the fatty marrow and bone trabeculae as well as soft tissue fat necrosis. Juxta-articular necrosis of the femoral and humeral heads as well as medullary necrosis are seen.[12,83,84] Lipase and other enzymes liberated during these processes presumably break down the fat from marrow cells into fatty acids which take up calcium. If marrow necrosis is extensive, death of bone may result.[5] In 269 patients with AVN, 11 (4 percent) had clinically documented pancreatitis; however, 9 were alcohol abusers and 2 also had sickle cell trait, which may have played an additional pathogenetic role.[12]

Irradiation. The occurrence of avascular necrosis presumably caused by fibrosis or endothelial proliferation with endarteritis and vascular compromise following irradiation has been reported.[85-88] With the improved survival of patients with lymphomas, osteonecrosis is a treatment complication associated with considerable morbidity and incapacity.[87,88] The prevalence of avascular necrosis in patients with malignant lymphoma has varied between 1.3 and 10 percent of treated patients.[87,88] AVN is more common in Hodgkin's disease than in non-Hodgkin's lymphoma. A common denominator in these patients with AVN and lymphomas is combination chemotherapy, including intermittent moderate to high doses of glucocorticoids, and often local radiotherapy. Local irradiation of the site of subsequent AVN was given in 30 (81 percent) of 37 patients.[87,88] It is unusual for the humeral head to be involved in the absence of other sites, and 3 of 4 patients with isolated humeral involvement had mantle radiotherapy which encompassed the humeral heads.[87]

Gout and Hyperuricemia. In two series of idiopathic AVN the prevalence of hyperuricemia has been 22 to 50 percent and that of gout has been 15 to 25 percent.[7,12] Uric acid crystals were demonstrated in the synovium from the hips of 8 patients with clinical gout, 3 patients with hyperuricemia, and 1 patient with neither.[7] Some of the patients in both studies were alcoholics and/or received glucocorticoids.[7,12] Other large series do not show the same prevalence, and in the Johns Hopkins experience gout was diagnosed in 2 percent of our patients with AVN (Table 107-1). In our opinion, there is as yet no definite relationship between AVN and gouty arthritis or hyperuricemia.

Idiopathic. In 269 patients, there were 22 patients without either demonstrable hyperlipidemia or coexistent disorders known to be associated with AVN.[12] Approximately one out of four patients seen at Johns Hopkins had no other disease and would appear to fall into the truly idiopathic category (Table 107-1).

PATHOGENESIS

Lipocyte Hypertrophy in Man and Experimental Models. Younger and very old persons are less frequently affected by idiopathic ischemic necrosis, which peaks in the 5th and 6th decades.[89] Infarction occurs only in fat marrow, which increases with maturity. In youth even the marrow which is rich in fatty tissue contains many scattered hematopoietic foci that can be compressed without significant embarrassment of the microcirculation. In the elderly, the turgor of the yellow marrow decreases, and the fat cells become smaller and the space between them is increasingly filled with a loose reticulum and a mucoid fluid. Within this so-called gelatinous marrow the hemodynamic conditions for infarction are no longer fulfilled, even in the presence of considerable pressure in the marrow. The interstitial fluid can always escape into the vessels, leaving the spaces free to absorb the pressure.[90]

Despite the fact that cortisone-treated rabbits lose as much as 30 percent of their body weight as compared with controls, intramedullary lipocytes increase in size by approximately 25 percent.[91] Not only is bone blood flow decreased in animals exposed to compressed air, but lipocytes exposed to similar conditions increase in size.[92] In adult ponies treated with intramuscular dexamethasone (equivalent to 15 mg of prednisone per 100 pounds) daily for 4 months, the intramedullary lipocytes increased in size and this was accompanied by elevated bone marrow pressure with marrow edema and fatty marrow necrosis.[93] These same changes are characteristic of early AVN in patients with alcoholism and in those receiving high-dose glucocorticoids; the mean intramedullary fat cell size was increased by 69 percent in patients with AVN as compared with those with osteoarthritis.[94] Moreover, microscopically there was a notable absence of vascular sinusoids in the fatty marrow in patients with AVN, and intraosseous pressures were elevated.

Venous Stasis and Intraosseous Hypertension. It is probably of pathogenetic significance that venographic abnormalities, particularly venous stasis, and increased bone marrow pressure are present in the majority of bones with AVN regardless of which type of associated disease is present or not.[56,81,94-99] Also significant is the fact that it is present in early disease before radiologic abnormalities appear and even in asymptomatic bones in which the increased bone marrow pressure may be of predictive value.[100] Since veins are more susceptible to compression as a result of the increased pressure, venous stasis is produced.

The fact that abnormal pressures and venography can be demonstrated in the trochanteric region demonstrates that the circulatory abnormality is widespread and at a distance from the femoral head itself. Histologic studies demonstrate that the necrotic lesions are not localized in the upper part of the femoral head but are usually diffuse lesions of the entire upper end of the femur.[96]

Summary and Postulated Pathogenesis. Avascular necrosis of bone, like infarction in other organ systems, results from a significant reduction in or obliteration of the affected area's blood supply. In AVN following fractures or dislocations, it is generally agreed that the initiating event is due to interruption of arterial inflow to bone by disruption of the macrovasculature. In the nontraumatic or idiopathic situation, one of the fundamental questions is whether the death of bone cells results from an interruption of blood supply to the tissue and subsequent loss of nutrition and oxygen for the cells. The superior portion of the femoral head, which becomes necrotic and collapses, is not superimposed on an area irrigated by one or more large vascular trunks. The irregularities of its limits and the persistence of zones of living tissue within the area are opposed to the hypothesis of the obliteration of large vascular trunks.[101] There is a merging of numerous juxtaposed necrotic foci, which correspond to the irrigation zones of the arterioles and small arteries. The arterioles are difficult to find and appear to be contracted. This suggests microcirculatory difficulties. Frequently histologic studies demonstrate islands of viable bone between necrotic foci, which is another fact that mitigates against the view that osteonecrosis is due to the interruption of the main arteries to the femoral head.[4] It now appears probable that in nontraumatic avascular necrosis the microvascular anatomy of the subchondral region of bone is responsible for the lesion as we recognize it.[102] The blood vessels extend into sinusoids in the subchondral area and are at all times enclosed within a rigid shell of bone, which makes it difficult for collaterals to develop and makes them vulnerable to increased pressure in the bony compartment. Marrow is more sensitive to ischemia than bony tissue. The disappearance of hematopoiesis followed by the atrophy of fat cells and the disappearance of intercellular circulation, and finally the development of a reticulofibrillosis are indicative of ischemia by stasis of increasing severity.[101] The ischemia of the necrosed area does not occur suddenly; it is gradual.

It is obvious that the same morphologic appearances have had widely different interpretations with regard to the preceding pathogenetic events.[5] It is most likely that avascular necrosis of bone is caused by multiple pathogenetic factors acting concomitantly and in some cases sequentially. Important facts to be considered are the following: (1) there is general agreement that the lesions are a result of ischemia; (2) the lesions primarily occur in long bones in the subcortical areas, which are supplied by terminal end-artery circulation, which has little possibility for the development of significant collateral circulation and is prone to embolic injury; (3) these bony sites have extensive fatty marrow, which has narrower capillary circulation than more hematopoietically active marrow; and (4) because of its rigidity, increased pressure within bone as an organ may have more devastating effects on the microcirculation than it would have in the more elastic compressible soft tissue organs.

We believe that the initial ischemic episode can be produced by either extraosseous and/or intraosseous circulatory disturbances (Fig. 107–5). Trauma with severance of major vessels, vasculitis, or vasospasm, such as seen in Raynaud's syndrome or decompression sickness can result in ischemia by interference with the extraosseous macrovasculature. Intraosseously, the sinusoidal microcirculation can be obstructed by sickled red cells, thrombi, nitrogen bubbles, or emboli. Compression of the microcirculation can occur by intramedullary lipocyte hypertrophy or expanding nitrogen bubbles or by abnormal cells such as metastic tumor or Gaucher's cells filling up the marrow space. In the weight-bearing area of the bone, increased compression of the capillary circulation by the transmitted pressure tends to accentuate the problem. The subchondral bone just beneath the cartilage is denser than the deeper layers, and the pressure is transmitted to them. In fatty marrow there are narrow capillaries which are compressed even further

Figure 107–5. Postulated pathogenesis of osteonecrosis. The etiology of osteonecrosis is multifactorial with numerous methods by which bone marrow pressure may be elevated directly or via ischemia with resultant cellular damage and edema. The final common pathway appears to be elevated bone marrow pressure, which produces increased resistance to flow and ischemia, with subsequent cellular damage and edema, leading to further increase in the intraosseous pressure. If uninterrupted, this vicious amplification cycle results in bone necrosis and collapse, particularly with continued weight-bearing.

Figure 107–6. Twelve months after impacted valgus fracture of the femoral neck, the *new* weight-bearing area is collapsing. Arrow marks the position of the acetabular margin before the fracture. (From Hungerford, D.S., and Zizic, T.M.: Pathogenesis of ischemic necrosis of the femoral head. *In* Hungerford, D.S. (ed.): The Hip. St. Louis, C.V. Mosby Company, 1983.)

by the only slightly compressible adipose tissue.[90] This produces ischemia in areas of high pressure that can result in infarction. Weight bearing alone is not a sufficient cause, because non–weight bearing will not prevent the collapse, as has been previously documented. Consequently, we believe that it is the continued increased bone marrow pressure compressing the microvasculature in the rigid osseous compartment in concert with weight bearing that produces the eventual collapse. Even with trauma in which interruption of the macrovasculature initiates the circulatory disturbance, it appears that increased bone marrow pressure and progressive ischemia produce the eventual collapse. We have now evaluated four patients with fractures resulting in subsequent valgus deformities (Fig. 107–6). If the "infarct" is a direct result of only the trauma, and occurred at one point in time, the anatomical superolateral portion of the femoral head should collapse. It does not, but the *new* functional weight-bearing area does (Fig. 107–6). This suggests that progressive ischemia in combination with weight bearing produces the eventual collapse.

PATHOLOGY

Gross Appearance. Grossly, the cancellous bone in the femoral head shows irregular areas of yellow necrosis extending up to within several millimeters of the articular cartilage; the individual trabeculae remain intact. With progression, a patchy zone of softening develops

in the necrotic cancellous bone at the interface with living bone.

There is a line of trabecular fractures running across the dead bone which partially separates an articular sequestrum.[5] Subsequent to the trabecular fracture, there is generally some collapse of the load-bearing segment of the head. Breaks in the smooth contour become visible, most often at the superior margin of the fovea and beneath the acetabular lip.[5] The covering cartilage is generally alive. It retains normal thickness, and chondrocytes have a normal appearance.[11,103] Once collapse of the articular surface of the femoral head has occurred, the gross pathologic changes visible are a yellowish, opaque mass of dead tissue beneath the articular cartilage and a greyish, glistening line of fibrous tissue beneath the mass of dead tissue.[5] Following the collapse and resultant incongruity, marginal osteophytes begin to form as progressive degenerative changes occur.

Microscopic Appearance. The first cells to be affected are the less well-differentiated blood and mesenchymal cells and the young osteoblasts. Eventually the fat and bone cells die and undergo lysis.[5,22,103] The earliest microscopic signs of ischemia appear at 48 hours in the hematopoietic areas of the bone marrow. Ovoid spaces, presumably filled with fat, are surrounded by cells that lose normal nuclear staining and eventually become eosinophilic ghost cells (Fig. 107–7). Similar changes occur in the sparsely cellular fatty marrow, with loss of nuclei and evidence of blood vessel necrosis by about the fifth day.[22] Only after several weeks is histologic recognition of bone death evident by loss of basophilia followed by the disappearance of osteocytes from bone lacunae.[22]

The evolution of osteonecrotic lesions has been divided into several phases, including the phase of cell necrosis, described above, followed by the repair of the coarse cancellous bone.[104] At the junction of the necrotic zone and live marrow there is a proliferation of capillaries accompanied by macrophages and fibroblasts, which advance into the dead tissue.[5] As the blood supply is more completely restored by the revascularization, osteoclasis of dead bone occurs and viable woven bone is laid down on the surface of dead bone and, less frequently, as new trabeculae in the marrow spaces (Fig. 107–8). This phase of repair affects the compact bone and articular cartilage differently in that new bone resorption rather than bone formation occurs first.[104] New bone formation fails to keep pace with bone resorption, resulting in a significant loss of the subchondral plate. In the process of revascularization, capillaries and pericapillary cells fail to stop at the osteochondral junction and invade and resorb the calcified cartilage and the deeper parts of the uncalcified articular cartilage, particularly in the peripheral portion, especially in the lateral aspect of the femoral head.[103] This cartilaginous capillary penetration and resorption are most extensive following collapse of the head; and in late stages in patients with marked osteoarthritis, most of the cartilage mass may be lost.

If revascularization and appositional new bone formation are incomplete, late collapse may occur. The cause of incomplete revascularization remains specula-

Figure 107–7. *A*, Fat necrosis in an early phase of osteonecrosis. (H & E × 600) *B*, Fat necrosis with lipophages phagocytizing the dead marrow fat. (H & E × 390) *C*, Extensive marrow necrosis with dead bony trabeculae with empty lacunae. (H & E × 180) *D*, High-powered view of *C* with vacant lacunae. (H & E × 600) (Courtesy of Dr. Donald W. Edlow.)

tive, but perhaps there is a critical size beyond which a bone infarct fails to revascularize completely.[5] This explanation may be more tenable in fractures than in non-traumatic situations in which continued and progressive ischemia due to increased intraosseous pressure and compression of the microcirculation may be of critical importance.

Pathologic Variations. In patients with AVN following trauma, there is convincing evidence that the whole head had been necrotic.[105] Thus it appears that while femoral head collapse is late and segmental, the necrosis is early and complete. The appositional new bone in necrotic femoral heads following subcapital fracture is most often woven while that in nontraumatic avascular necrosis is more lamellar in character.[103]

Some investigators report no specific pathologic differences in steroid-treated patients as compared with other cases with idiopathic AVN.[9,10] Others have suggested that the femoral heads in their steroid-treated patients were histologically more porotic and that disintegration was more rapidly progressive.[85] In AVN associated with glucocorticoids there is a decreased dif-

ferentiation of the mesenchymal cells to osteoblasts and less appositional new bone formation, with osteopenia and reduction in the thickness and number of trabeculae in all but 2 of 25 bones.[66]

CLINICAL SYMPTOMS AND SIGNS

There may be a delay from several months up to 5 years between the onset of symptoms and the development of radiographic abnormalities.[1,96] Consequently, if early diagnosis and effective therapy are to be achieved, a high index of suspicion must be maintained in populations at high risk, even if radiographs are negative. Certainly, patients with the associated conditions described above who present with pain—particularly in the hips, knees or shoulders—should be aggressively evaluated for the possibility of AVN. Those at highest risk are patients who already have AVN in one bone (in our first 169 patients, 97 (57 percent) had multiple sites of involvement). Bilateral involvement is present in 42 to 72 percent of patients and increases with the du-

Figure 107–8. *A*, Early repair phase with capillary proliferation and small amount of appositional new bone formation. (H & E × 480) *B*, Later repair phase with more extensive appositional new bone formation on a dead trabeculum. (H & E × 400) *C*, As part of the repair process fibroblastic activity with resultant marrow fibrosis can occur. (H & E × 625)

ration of follow-up.[2,6,8,10,12] Involvement of the second bone usually follows the first bone within several years but may occur as long as 3 to 5 years later.[2,6]

Certain clinical signs should alert the physician to the possibility of avascular necrosis following traumatic fractures. The most important is increased pain and limp instead of the usual continued improvement seen in the first year following fractures.

In femoral head necrosis the insidious initial symptom is usually pain in the groin with intermittent radiation down the anteromedial thigh.[1] At times the pain is of a

pseudoradicular character, is increased by coughing, and occurs at night.[106] A remarkable feature in many cases is that the symptoms start suddenly; many patients remember the day and hour when they first felt a sudden, severe, and incapacitating pain.[9] The vast majority of patients have "mechanical" pain induced by standing, walking, moving, or other mechanical stress but eased by rest. Approximately two-thirds have pain at rest and about 40 percent have pain at night, which may be accompanied by prolonged morning pain and stiffness.[89] Some patients, after mild intermittent pain for several months, will note a sudden increase in pain and a distinct clicking with changes in position, particularly when arising from the sitting position. This may be accompanied by an antalgic gluteus medius limp or limited motion (particularly flexion, abduction, and internal rotation), and a click may be elicited by external rotation of the flexed abducted hip (Fig. 4 sign).[107] Instability of the hip as defined by a positive Trendelenburg sign was present in the majority of hips affected and was significantly more frequent than in control patients with radiologic changes of osteoarthritis of the hip.[89] It should be kept in mind, however, that early in the disease there is frequently a clear dissociation of pain, which can be considerable, and limitation of movement, which can be minimal.

Idiopathic osteonecrosis of the knee in elderly people is associated with pain of sudden onset with no preceding trauma.[15] It is usually localized to the medial side of the knee. On examination there is tenderness over the medial femoral condyle, and in one third of patients there is a mild to moderate effusion. At times fluid accumulation in the knees is sufficient to require aspiration to increase mobility. The differential diagnosis of osteonecrosis and osteoarthritis of the knee is helped by the sudden onset and rapid development of the former, with primary involvement of bone rather than cartilage. Obviously, in a young patient with one of the clinical conditions associated with avascular necrosis, this differentiation is even easier.[14]

It is probable that many instances of avascular necrosis of the humeral head go undetected because usually the shoulder is not a weight-bearing joint and symptoms may be transient or minimal. Even with extensive cyst formation and sclerosis, the humeral head may be relatively asymptomatic. It is unusual for the humeral head to be involved without other sites of involvement.[108] Generally pain in the shoulder is insidious in onset, is aggravated by activity, and radiates to the deltoid tuberosity of the humerus. The major complaint is pain on motion, which may progress to the point of pain on very slight movement. There is generally a very early and serious limitation of active motion, with preservation of passive motion until late in the course when capsular adhesions may occur.[108]

In the first 169 AVN patients at Hopkins with 310 involved bones, 263 (85 percent) of the sites were symptomatic; 47 (15 percent) were asymptomatic. The manifestations in symptomatic sites with respect to the most frequently involved joints are listed in Table 107-2. Interestingly, except for less frequent limitation of motion of the knees, these clinical findings are fairly consistent when hips, knees, and shoulders are compared.

DIAGNOSIS

Since certain patient populations are at increased risk to develop AVN and most physicians agree that early diagnosis, certainly before segmental collapse occurs, is essential to effective treatment, these patients might ben-

Table 107–2. Manifestations in Symptomatic Sites

Manifestation	Site of Involvement		
	Hips	Knees	Shoulders
Pain on motion (active)	$\frac{205}{208}$ (99%)	$\frac{40}{40}$ (100%)	$\frac{13}{13}$ (100%)
Pain at rest	$\frac{119}{179}$ (66%)	$\frac{26}{36}$ (72%)	$\frac{5}{18}$ (63%)
Night pain	$\frac{53}{144}$ (37%)	$\frac{9}{24}$ (38%)	$\frac{3}{7}$ (43%)
Pain on motion (exam)	$\frac{178}{197}$ (90%)	$\frac{27}{40}$ (68%)	$\frac{10}{13}$ (77%)
Limitation of motion (exam)	$\frac{132}{205}$ (64%)	$\frac{10}{40}$ (25%)	$\frac{9}{14}$ (64%)

efit by diagnostic screening. Methods presently available for diagnosis of AVN include routine radiography, tomography, radionuclide scans, bone marrow pressure measurements, intraosseous venography, and core biopsy.

Radiography. There may be a considerable delay between the onset of symptoms and radiographic abnormalities. In 20 patients with histologically confirmed avascular necrosis, symptoms were present from 1 to 5 years prior to roentgenographic findings.[96] In the experience at Johns Hopkins 58 (20 percent) of 310 ischemic bones were radiologically normal.[109] Occasionally, the converse occurs. In 11 asymptomatic hips diagnosed roentgenographically, the interval between diagnosis and the onset of symptoms was 5 months to 6 years, with two thirds of the silent hips becoming symptomatic within 2 years.[107]

There are four important parameters in the radiologic evaluation of AVN: (1) the shape and contour of the juxta-articular bone; (2) the presence of generalized or local areas of radiographic densities and lucencies; (3) the fine structure and organization of the bony trabeculae; and (4) the evaluation of the joint space and degenerative changes in the opposing bones in the joint involved. In terms of technique, probably the greatest fault lies in underpenetration of radiographs. Because of this, trabecular detail is not clearly seen and consequently small dense areas close to the joint surface will not be identified.[34]

We find it helpful to classify avascular bones by radiographic stages, particularly for the comparison of various diagnostic and treatment techniques.

Stage I. At this stage the radiographs are normal, or at most there may be minimal osteoporosis present in certain situations. When a bone is immobilized, there is an increase in osteoclastic activity, leading to excessive bone resorption, so that the total mass of bone is reduced. When sufficient bone has been lost (usually about one third), the reduction of bone density can be demonstrated radiologically. Obviously, the diagnosis at this stage must be made by biopsy with histologic confirmation.

Stage II. In idiopathic AVN of the femoral head the first radiographic sign is usually a patchy mottled sclerosis in the superolateral part of the head related to viable new appositional bone formation occurring on the surface of dead trabeculae.[5,11,103,105,107] Layers of new bone are deposited around necrotic trabeculae, and new fibrous bone is formed, which is manifested on radiographs by a coarsening of the structural pattern of the cancellous bone. The trabeculae in such areas can be considerably thickened in caliber, and the interspaces are generally enlarged. The main cause of the increased radiodensity is the formation of abnormally thickened trabeculae in the revascularized area and not calcification of the marrow fat.[105] Beneath the area of fibrous revascularization, the living marrow is hyperemic with the revascularization, and attempted healing of the necrotic bone may be associated with areas of reduced density radiographically.[9] Thus, the characteristic radiographic features in stage II AVN are patchy osteoporosis and osteosclerosis (which may be wedge shaped with the base situated in the superolateral portion of the head), while the shape, size and contour of the juxta-articular bone is normal, as is the joint line (Fig. 107–9).

Stage III. A translucent subcortical band appears as a fine line immediately under the articular cortex and parallel to it. This has been described as the "radiolucent crescent sign" and repesents a fracture line. The fracture line occurs just below the subchondral plate for most of its length, but at its lateral and superior peripheral margin it may extend into the subchondral plate and into the articular cartilage as well.[103] Sometimes the subchondral cortex remains connected to the cartilage and is separated from the underlying spongy tissue by a horizontal fissure corresponding to the "egg-shell" x-ray picture.[11] Early collapse may be apparent, in which case there may be a widening of the joint space (Fig. 107–10.

Stage IV. Progression of AVN is characterized radiographically by a loss of contour of the femoral head

Figure 107–10. Although the radiographic changes are more subtle, the subchondral plate is definitely irregular and therefore structurally no longer intact. This therefore represents stage III disease.

manifested by either a flattening of a segment of the head or a discrete discontinuity ("joint step"), both of which are caused by the subchondral collapse. In its terminal phases there may be a complete separation of the superior fragment from the underlying femoral head, or the detached fragment may be depressed into the femoral head.[103] At times small pieces of cartilage may be completely free in the joint and grow into fairly large, oval joint "mice." At times subchondral cysts are seen on radiographs and represent local regions of bone resorption replaced by fibrous tissue and fibrocartilage.[110] With extensive destruction and collapse, the resultant incongruity leads to progressive degenerative changes, with marginal osteophyte formation, narrowing of the joint space, and in the hip secondary acetabular changes (Fig. 107–11). Radiographic changes in the humeral heads parallel those seen in the femoral heads.[108] In the humeral head, flattening, fragmentation, and collapse most often occur in the central dome of the head. In osteonecrosis of the knee the x-rays are usually normal during the initial month or two, but at times there may be a slight flattening of the weight-bearing portion of the medial femoral condyle.[15] Although the typical lesion of a radiolucency surrounded by a typical sclerotic halo may appear as early as 2 months after the onset of pain, it is often present much later. The majority of patients eventually develop secondary osteoarthritis.

Radiographic Variability. Signs of bone repair are frequent in the area below the necrotic zone of the femoral head. They might, however, be minimal or absent in patients on continuous glucocorticoid therapy.[2] In avascular necrosis associated with glucocorticoids, the first radiologic manifestation may be the slightly irregular, radiolucent subchondral line ("crescent sign")

Figure 107–9. In spite of considerable patchy osteosclerosis throughout the femoral head, it remains spherical with an intact subchondral plate and a normal joint space; the criteria for designation of stage II.

Figure 107–11. The anteroposterior x-ray (left) shows nearly complete obliteration of the joint line indicating the acetabular involvement characterizing stage IV disease. The frogleg view of the hip (right) shows the magnitude of the femoral head destruction.

caused by fracture through dead subchondral bone.[103] This occurs because bone formation is markedly decreased, and local absorption of compact subchondral bone continues. Structural failure with subchondral fracture and mechanical (opposed to biologic) compaction of the weight-bearing portion of the femoral head is the major cause of the increased radiodensity and the loss of fine structure observed radiographically.[103] In this situation, some degree of flattening of the femoral head is invariably detectable as well. In patients with avascular necrosis following renal transplantation, some patchy areas of demineralization are seen, but they do not begin in the subchondral area. Although they may progress in size and extent, there is less frequent collapse despite extensive changes.[108]

Tomography. Tomography, with hypocycloidal technique if possible, can be of help in determining the extent and the detailed structure of the bony changes. Although the subtle mottled densities scattered in the anterosuperior region of the femoral head may be seen on the anteroposterior roentgenogram, they might be missed and tomograms may be of considerable help. In the femoral head, detail is obscured in standard projections by the overlying acetabulum, and consequently lesions at this site are identified much more readily with tomography or a "frog lateral" projection.[34] Tomography or a "frog lateral" projection helps with further definition.[42] Similarly, in the shoulder, difficulties in inter-

pretation arise from malrotation of the joint, resulting in the superior border of the greater tuberosity appearing as a dense layer, which could be misinterpreted as osteonecrosis. In these situations, in which detail is obscured by overlying bone, tomography may be immensely helpful in improving definition.

Radionuclide Scanning Techniques. Radionuclide scans have definite advantages over roentgenograms in allowing earlier diagnosis prior to the appearance of significant morphologic changes when the bone is most amenable to therapeutic intervention[56,103,111-116] (see Chapter 40). Abnormalities in bone scans may precede radiographic changes by 2 to 18 months.[116,117]

Scintigraphy is graphic representation of the counting rate in the form of various degrees of blackening of the film, which sacrifices precision and resolution. Since the primary data consist of digital analogs, the digital readout or scintimetry permits statistical analysis, which yields increased precision.[116] One of the advantages of the currently used radiopharmaceuticals that label organic phosphates and diphosphonates with ^{99m}technetium is a relatively low dose of radiation. The skeletal radiation dose is 500 mrad and the whole body radiation dose is 120 mrad for a 15 mCi injection, compared with 2000 mRad for a single lateral lumbar spine radiograph, for example.[118]

The bone scan findings depend on the length of time the study is performed after onset of the disease, the activity of the reparative process, and the resultant morphologic derangement of the joint. The bone scan can become positive 3 weeks after a vascular insult. In the very early phase (days to weeks) following a vascular insult with subsequent development of AVN, the involved area may rarely appear "cold" on the scintiscan, owing to absent blood supply in the avascular segment.[114,118] This picture usually precedes the radiographic changes of sclerosis and collapse.[118] If the zone of infarction is very narrow, hyperemia and revascularization of the surrounding living bone may mask any cold spot. Subsequently (weeks to months), revascularization and appositional new bone formation will produce "hot" areas due to increased uptake of the radioisotope until repair is completed.[114] Late in the course of the disease, bone scans may revert to normal or demonstrate abnormalities that cannot be differentiated from those of degenerative osteoarthritis. False-negative qualitative scans occur in some patients with bilateral involvement because the uptake, although symmetrical, is in reality increased bilaterally, or if it is asymmetrical, the more severely affected side makes the less involved side look normal by comparison. Quantitative scintimetry, on the other hand, detected 73 to 89 percent of early (preradiologic) AVN.[109,115]

With use of techniques employing three-phase bone scans, 37 (92 percent) of 40 knees with spontaneous osteonecrosis were detected.[119] With more experience in nontraumatic AVN, the precise value of three-phase radionuclide scanning in the early detection of avascular necrosis will be established.

Bone Marrow Pressure Measurements. Increased bone marrow pressure (BMP) has been found to be a sensitive and reliable indicator of AVN even in the preradiologic stage.[37,56,81,82,94,95,109] The technique of measuring BMP involved tapping a wide-bore, slightly conical cannulae into the bone to insure a watertight seal. Following removal of the obturator, the intraosseous trocar is filled with heparinized saline and connected via a three-way stopcock and saline-filled semirigid cannula to a pressure transducer and pen recorder. The BMP fluctuates normally up to 6 mm Hg with arterial pulsations. The absence of visible pulsations indicates mechanical obstruction, and the needle should be carefully flushed with saline or pushed forward a few millimeters.[120]

Despite highly significant differences in diseased versus normal bones, it is clear that individual pressure values overlap considerably.[120] The following are BMPs (in millimeters of mercury) in presumably normal bones adjacent to nonosteoarthritic joints: greater trochanter, mean 17.2 (range 12 to 26);[97] femoral neck, mean 18.7 (range 12.9 to 23.5);[121] femoral head, mean 24 (range 20 to 30);[98] proximal tibia, mean 29.1 (range 17 to 34);[122] and distal femur, 19.9 ± 1.8.[123] After baseline BMPs are determined, 5 ml of saline can be injected intraosseously as a stress test. In normal bones, the BMP increases by less than 10 mm Hg in response to the stress test, while in those with AVN there is an elevation of more than 10 mm Hg that persists for longer than 5 minutes.[56,82,95] Normal and abnormal baseline bone marrow pressures and stress tests are illustrated in Figures 107–12 and 107–13.

The value of combined baseline BMPs and stress tests is illustrated in Table 107–3, in which 48 (19 percent) of bones with radiographic or histologic documentation of AVN would be missed if only baseline pressures were measured. There is a highly significant statistical difference in the baseline BMPs and stress tests in all four radiographic stages of AVN as compared with control bones (Table 107–4). These differences remain significant regardless of AVN site except for the ankles, as only two pressure determinations have been done in the talus (Table 107–5). The true incidence of false-positive bones is not yet known. Of the first 270 bones in which we documented increased pressures, 224 (83 percent) had radiographic or histologic evidence of AVN and 46 (17 percent) did not. Over a 3-year period, 15 of these 46 patients who were radiographically negative have subsequently developed AVN. Thus, in our hands, the maximum false-positive incidence is now 11 percent, and this may be decreased even further with continued follow-up of these patients. This relates to one of the most exciting aspects of hemodynamic measurements in radiographically normal bones: predictive value potential. We have followed 57 patients with AVN who had bone marrow pressure measurements performed on the asymptomatic and radiologically normal contralateral side.[100] As can be seen in Table 107–6, 15 (43 percent) of 35 bony sites with increased baseline BMPs and/or abnormal stress tests developed AVN subsequently as compared with only 2 (9 percent) of 22 with normal hemodynamics ($p < 0.025$).

Intraosseous Venography. Intraosseous venography is a procedure in which iodized contrast medium is injected into spongy bone and the projection and evacuation are followed with serial x-rays. In our hands, following bone marrow pressure measurements, the same needle and access are utilized to inject the contrast medium. Phlebography has revealed the presence of impaired venous

Figure 107–12. Normal bone marrow pressure averages 20 mm Hg with narrow pulse pressure. Injection of 5 ml of saline (arrow) through the recording trocar does not significantly elevate the intramedullary pressure.

Figure 107–13. Elevated baseline bone marrow pressure with hypertensive response to saline injection (arrow) in a patient with Stage I disease. (From Hungerford, D.S., and Zizic, T.M.: Pathogenesis of Ischemic Necrosis of the Femoral Head. *In* Hungerford, D.S., The Hip. St. Louis, C.V. Mosby, 1983.)

drainage in the upper end of the femur, even at the stage when no pathologic changes can be demonstrated on the standard x-ray.[56,82,95,96,98,100,109] Intraosseous phlebography, therefore, seems to be an excellent means of early diagnosis. In unaffected hip joints, dislocated hips, and femoral neck fractures with a partially functioning venous system, there is no increased resistance to injection of contrast medium; and the extraosseous veins are filled if the dye is injected into the femoral head.[99] In idiopathic ischemic necrosis there is increased resistance to injection of the contrast medium, and a "trabeculary" contrast picture, with filling of the marrow meshes of the spongious bone, is invariably seen. Most of the contrast medium drains through the medullary sinus towards the periphery, there is delayed drainage of the medium, and the regional draining venous system collapses almost completely. The reflux of the contrast medium into the diaphysis may fill part of the large central sinus of the diaphysis. It is not necessarily of pathologic significance if the injection is made at the junction of the metaphysis and the diaphysis, in which case there may be partial filling of the large central diaphyseal sinus in normals.[96] If the injection is made in the trochanteric part of the femur, diaphyseal reflux is a frequent and reliable indication of avascular necrosis.

In summary, in AVN intraosseous venography demonstrates certain characteristic abnormalities, such as (1) a delay in evacuation by the efferent veins, which is present on the 5-minute postinjection film but may persist for hours; (2) abnormal persistence of contrast medium in the metaphyseal cancellous bone and diaphyseal reflux; and (3) poor filling and visualization of some of the efferent veins. The characteristic pictures of intraosseous venography in normals as compared with bones with AVN are illustrated in Figures 107–14 and 107–15.

In our hands, maximum diagnostic sensitivity is achieved by the combined use of baseline BMPs, saline stress tests, and intraosseous venography. Of 219 proven AVN bones studied, 145 (66 percent) had elevated baseline pressures, 129 (59 percent) were abnormal on stress testing, and 193 (88 percent) had abnormal intraosseous venograms.[109] Table 107–7 delineates the combination of venographic abnormalities seen in our experience, and Table 107–8 looks at the venographic abnormalities with respect to the status of baseline BMPs and stress tests.

When all three of these diagnostic procedures were used, 209 (96 percent) of 219 AVN sites were detected. Most importantly, of the 10 sites missed only four of the bones had preradiologic disease; thus, 215 (99 percent) of the AVN bones were detected, including those with radiographically evident disease.

Long-term follow-up after femoral neck fractures has revealed that avascular necrosis occurs within 2 years in approximately 90 percent of cases lacking drainage of the contrast medium through the extraosseous veins, while in about 85 percent, sufficient blood supply in the femoral head fragment is guaranteed when the venous drainage system is intact.[99] Combining abnormal pressure studies with abnormal venograms has enhanced the predictive value for the subsequent development of nontraumatic AVN. Forty-four patients with unilateral AVN had BMPs and intraosseous venograms performed

Table 107–4. Baseline BMPs and Stress Tests in AVN Versus Controls

AVN Stage	No. Sites	Baseline BMP Mean (Range)	No. Sites	Stress Test Mean (Range)
I	43	45 (15–110)	43	54 (13–110)
II	98	38 (14–92)	96	53 (12–112)
III	76	39 (8–115)	75	55 (10–130)
IV	8	28 (15–50)	8	49 (20–95)
Totals	225	39 (8–115)	222	54 (10–130)
Controls	14	17 (8–28)*	14	18 (8–26)*

*All four stages significantly different from controls with $p < 0.001$ using one-way analysis of variance.

Table 107–3. Results of Baseline BMPs and Stress Tests

Measurement Results		Number AVN Bones
↑ Baseline and ↑ stress test	=	109 (42%)
↑ Baseline and normal stress	=	63 (24%)
Normal baseline and ↑ stress	=	48 (19%)
Normal baseline and normal stress	=	39 (15%)
Total	=	259 (100%)

Table 107–5. Baseline BMPs and Stress Tests by AVN Site

AVN Site	No. Bones	Baseline BMP Mean (Range)	No. Bones	Stress Test Mean (Range)
Hips	180	41 (10–115)*	178	54 (12–118)*
Knees	34	32 (8–78)*	34	51 (10–110)*
Shoulders	14	39 (12–80)*	13	57 (20–130)*
Ankles	2	26 (25–26)	2	75 (70–80)
Controls	14	17 (8–28)	14	18 (8–26)

*Significantly different from controls with $p < 0.001$ using one-way analysis of variance.

Table 107–6. Predictive Value of Bone Marrow
Pressures

BMP Measurement	No. Bones	Subsequent AVN	Follow-up (Months) Mean (Range)
Increased BMP*	35	15 (43%)	34 (3–87)
Normal BMP	22	2 (9%)	32 (1–83)

*$p < 0.025$.

on the asymptomatic and radiologically normal side.[100] Of 22 bones with abnormal pressure studies and venography, 11 (50 percent) subsequently developed AVN, as compared with none of 11 in which both studies were normal. ($p < 0.01$).

Core Biopsy. In stage I and even in stage II, there is some hope of saving the ischemic bone, but diagnosis is essential if collapse and irreversible damage are to be avoided.[56,94,95,106,124] The diagnosis can be made by core biopsy, which also has significant therapeutic value, particularly in these early stages of disease (vide infra). Core biopsy has allowed us to make the diagnosis of 49 (23 percent) of 211 AVN bones treated by core decompression.[125] Malignant fibrous histiocytomas and osteogenic sarcomas have occasionally been shown to be associated with bone infarcts.[12,43] Despite the fact that the small numbers of cases preclude the establishment of a causal relationship, disproportionate pain or fracture (or both) through the site of infarction suggests this complication and warrants biopsy and histologic evaluation. In addition, malignancy in the form of primary bone tumors or metastases may present with symptoms suggestive of AVN. The patient with hip pain, a negative radiograph, and a positive bone scan deserves a complete evaluation, including core biopsy.

Core biopsy has some limitations in the early diagnosis of preradiologic lesions in that there is a sampling error, since the specimen removed is generally several centimeters in length and slightly less than a centimeter in diameter. There is in addition some variation in the

Figure 107–15. *A,* Metaphyseal veins fill poorly, and marked diaphyseal reflux and stasis on the 5-minute film *(B)* characterize this abnormal venogram from a patient with Stage I bone necrosis and SLE (from Zizic, T.M., Hungerford, D.S., and Stevens, M.B.: Ischemic necrosis in systemic lupus erythematosus. Medicine 59:134, 1980.)

histologic appearance of tissue from different types of osteonecrosis (e.g., traumatic versus steroid associated), in different specimens in the same type, and also from region to region within the same femoral head.[104] Although generally there is a zone of osseous necrosis extending over several millimeters, at times these may be more scattered, particularly in early lesions where they may be at a distance from the supporting pole of the head of the femur.[106] Thus, one must be cautious in rejecting the diagnosis of AVN in histologically negative specimens, particularly in early disease with significant symptoms and signs and especially if scintigraphy and hemodynamic studies are abnormal.

Figure 107–14. *A,* Normal venogram at termination of injection showing excellent filling of metaphyseal veins. *B,* Five minutes after injection, most of the dye has cleared the bone. (From Zizic, T.M., Hungerford, D.S., and Stevens, M.B.,: Ischemic necrosis in systemic lupus erythematosus. Medicine 59:134, 1980.)

Table 107-7. Venographic Abnormalities in AVN

Venographic Results	No. AVN Bones
Stasis + reflux	47 (22%)
Stasis + reflux + poor venous filling	39 (18%)
Reflux + poor venous filling	33 (15%)
Reflux only	26 (12%)
Stasis only	20 (9%)
Stasis + poor venous filling	19 (9%)
Poor venous filling	9 (4%)
Completely normal venogram	26 (12%)
Total	219 (100%)

TREATMENT

On the basis of pathobiologic and clinical data, it is believed that the processes in idiopathic osteonecrosis are progressive and will inevitably result in destruction of the joint. Consequently, surgical intervention during an early phase should be strongly considered.[110] Once the disease is evident radiologically, it is generally progressive, leading to serious joint dysfunction in the hips and knees and to a lesser degree in the shoulders.

One of the major problems is that AVN frequently affects young, otherwise physically active individuals. The long-term success of total joint replacement based on initial reports in patients over age 65 has not been realized in younger, more active individuals.[126] Because of the number of surgical revisions that have been required in young patients, there is a growing conviction that total joint replacement is not compatible with unrestricted vigorous activity. Consequently, ways of salvaging ischemic bones short of replacement arthroplasty continue to be sought.

In evaluating the success of various treatment modalities, there are two important parameters to consider. First, radiographic staging must be included in reporting the results of any treatment. In a recent study there were significant differences between the postoperative scores of the groups classified by the stage of the lesion.[13] The earlier the stage at the time of operation, the higher the statistically significant improvement. Second, since the majority of untreated patients will have radiologic pro-

gression within 2 years, it is suggested that this minimal follow-up interval be used to evaluate whether a given procedure will prevent the natural progression of the disease.[26,107]

Non-Weight Bearing. Conservative treatment consisting primarily of non-load bearing in an attempt to prevent collapse while repair is completed. In a Swiss multicenter study group, 46 patients were treated by nonsurgical means with non-weight bearing for 8 to 36 months in 5, physiotherapy in 20, analgesic and anti-inflammatory drugs in 18, and a combination of physiotherapy and drugs in 5 patients The results were very poor in all but one of the hips, and the authors concluded that much valuable time was wasted by expecting spontaneous healing to occur in response to non-weight bearing alone.[127] In another study, although about one-quarter of the patients improved spontaneously and have a tolerable disability, some degree of collapse of the head occurred eventually in 90 percent and was accompanied by the development of a progressive arthrosis.[6] Nonoperative treatment by avoidance of weight bearing, with analgesics and decrease of steroid therapy in renal allograft recipients with AVN carries a prolonged morbidity as well as an increase in the risk of rejection.[69] Thus, attempts to protect the necrotic femoral head without surgical intervention have been for the most part unsuccessful.[10,69,127,128] Prolonged non-weight bearing yielded only a 2 to 17 percent success rate.[10,127]

Once radiographic changes occur in AVN the patient requires surgical therapy in order to have a chance of maintaining reasonable hip joint function. Conservative treatment of the shoulder, however, is more successful. In 19 patients with glucocorticoid-related avascular necrosis of the humeral heads, conservative treatment, consisting of maintenance of motion through a vigorous program of pendulum exercises and a decrease in forces acting across the shoulder by avoidance of abduction, resulted in excellent results in 9 (47 percent) with respect to range of motion and the patients' success in returning to most normal activities.[102] In 6 patients (32 percent), results were somewhat satisfactory, but all of these had some limitation of motion, particularly in abduction and external rotation, and all had some limitation of activities that they could perform comfortably. Five (26 per-

Table 107-8. Venographic Abnormalities in AVN with Respect to Bone Marrow Pressure (BMP) Determinations

BMP	Normal	Stasis	Reflux	↓ Venous Filling	Stasis + Reflux	Stasis + ↓ Venous Filling	Reflux + ↓ Venous Filling	Stasis + Reflux + ↓ Venous Filling	Totals
NL base + NL stress	9	2	6	0	6	3	3	3	32
NL base + ABN stress	2	5	3	1	10	1	4	10	36
ABN base + NL stress	6	4	3	4	13	4	8	6	48
ABN base + ABN stress	8	8	12	3	17	10	16	20	94
NL base + stress N.D.	1	0	0	1	0	0	0	0	2
ABN base + stress N.D.	0	0	0	0	0	0	2	0	2
Neither base nor stress done	0	1	2	0	1	0	0	0	4

Abbreviations: NL-normal; ABN-abnormal; N.D.-not done.

cent) had severe pain and almost absent external rotation. These all had hemiarthroplasties with excellent results.

Bone Grafting. Cortical bone grafts were conceived to provide mechanical support to the subchondral bone and articular cartilage in an attempt to prevent collapse as the femoral head revascularizes.[4,26,129] Subsequently, in 116 patients treated by drilling and tibial bone grafting for avascular necrosis with or without union of the fractured femoral neck, 91 (78 percent) had a successful outcome.[130] One of the advantages of this conservative method is that when it fails, a salvage operation, such as mold arthroplasty or prosthetic replacement, may still be done, as it was in 12 of the 25 hips with unsatisfactory results in this series. In addition to more complications other disadvantages of bone grafting as compared with core decompression are that the intraoperative time is about 2 hours, and three-point crutch-walking is extended from 6 to 24 months, with an average of 12 months.[130] Others have had more discouraging results with this technique.[107,128,131] Reasonable results in most hands are obtained only if bone grafting is done early in the disease before collapse and secondary acetabular changes occur (stage I and II disease).

Osteotomy. The principle underlying the various osteotomy procedures is to alter the mechanics of the joint to redistribute the maximal load-bearing forces in an attempt to prevent collapse and deformation of the femoral head. In several reports this was accomplished with varus or valgus rotational osteotomies.[6,19,127] In 59 osteotomies applied prior to collapse (stage II) or with minimal collapse (early stage III), there was good to excellent results with respect to pain relief.[9] However, from that same institution, a 6-year follow-up of 47 oblique or transverse osteotomies revealed that 47 percent had painless hips, that good functional results were present in only 32 percent, and that further collapse of the head occurred in 42 percent. Secondary arthrosis was present in 90 percent, and altogether 40 percent of the cases could be considered as failures, either immediate (18 percent), early (7 percent), or late (18 percent).[6] The authors concluded that a successful osteotomy depended upon a suitable size and location of the necrotic area and the ability to change the position of the femoral head enough to relieve the pressure on the necrotic parts of the head. Best results were achieved if there was healthy bone superolaterally as well as posteriorly.

Transtrochanteric anterior rotation osteotomy of the femoral head has been utilized to reduce the weight-bearing forces on the necrotic area and to transfer shear forces to the intact posterior cartilage.[132] There was complete relief of pain and no collapse of the femoral heads of 17 of 18 patients with early x-ray changes. Recurrence of symptoms and progressive collapse occurred in 5 (22 percent) of 23 hips with stage III and IV radiologic changes. The advantage of transtrochanteric anterior rotational osteotomy is that it appears to be more effective for cases with extensive lesions in the femoral head than simple adduction or abduction osteotomy, and there is no additional difficulty for prosthetic re-

placement in the future because the anatomic shape of the subtrochanteric area is unchanged.[132] A disadvantage is the long period of non–weight bearing followed by crutch gait.

Thirty-seven knees with osteonecrosis were treated by high tibial osteotomy either alone (in 14) or in combination with drilling (in 17) or bone grafting (in 6).[13] At the final follow-up, which averaged 61 months and ranged from 24 to 102 months, 21 patients had complete relief of pain; 13, moderate relief; and 2, minimum relief. The prognosis of the osteonecrotic lesions was significantly better in the 23 knees treated by osteotomy and bone grafting or drilling than in the 14 knees treated by osteotomy alone.

Core Decompression. Although drilling of the neck and the head of the femur has been used for over 50 years in the treatment of chronic hip disease, it has been used in the treatment of AVN for the past two decades.[133] In addition, by replacing the solid drill with a hollow trephine this therapeutic measure can also be used as a means of diagnosis in preradiologic disease.[134] Together with the trephine the cylinder of bone is extracted so it can be examined histologically (Fig. 107–16).

The rationale for this procedure is that by removing an 8- to 11-mm core of cancellous bone out of the ischemic segment, there is a decrease in the intraosseous pressure (decompression), which reduces the forces compressing the capillary and sinusoidal microcirculation. This interrupts the cycle of the increased pressure that leads to decreased blood flow that produces ischemia and edema, resulting in further increased pressure, decreased blood flow, and progressive ischemia (vide supra). It is likely that the stimulation of the living adjacent bone by core biopsy and drilling may induce the formation of new capillaries and progenitor cells as well as create avenues for revascularization and repopulation of the dead portions of the bone.

An additional rationale for use of methods, such as core decompression, that allow for earlier mobilization is the preservation of articular cartilage. Diffusion of solutes to the deepest cartilage cells has been shown to be promoted by agitation of synovial fluid in vitro.[37] Intermittent weight bearing in vivo may be vital in providing nutrition to the articular cartilage (see Chapter 16).

Figure 107–16. Core specimen obtained with special hollow trocar. The left portion comes from the femoral head and "looks" ischemic.

The primary indication for core decompression is in the diagnosis and treatment of symptomatic and radiologically normal bones in patients with AVN at another site or in patients in whom an underlying associated disease makes the clinician suspect the possibility of AVN. Not only can the diagnosis be confirmed by histologic examination of the removed specimen, but in our hands and others', it is highly effective in relieving pain, preventing further x-ray progression, and avoiding the requirement for major surgery.[37,94,124,125] Recently, we have reported results that would suggest that core decompression alters the natural history of preradiologic AVN.[135] Of 64 patients with normal radiographs but increased bone marrow pressure, 49 (77 percent) were symptomatic and treated with core decompression and 15 were asymptomatic and untreated. Each of these latter 15 were studied hemodynamically because they had definite AVN in the corresponding contralateral bone. The comparative course to date in these two subgroups is shown in Table 107–9. Despite more advanced (i.e., symptomatic) disease, the core decompression group has significantly less frequent new or recurrent symptoms, less frequent radiographic progression, and less need for major surgery.

During the past 8 years, core decompressions have been carried out in our institution on 211 avascular bones (Table 107–10). AVN bones in both stage I and stage II had significantly less recurrence of symptoms and less need for major surgery than stage III bones. Consequently, our experience is that stage II disease is also a primary indication for core decompression. Since it is a simple procedure with a short incision, operating time, and hospitalization and significantly less requirement for postoperative non–weight bearing than procedures such as bone grafting or osteotomy, we also feel it is an excellent palliative procedure for stage III and IV disease. Even in advanced disease approximately half the patients were without recurrent symptoms, and only 40 to 43 percent have required further major surgery, with a mean follow-up of about 3 years (Table 107–10). Particularly since core decompression does not interfere with any surgical procedures that may be necessary subsequently, we believe it should be included in the armamentarium for the management of AVN in young patients and in those who are poor surgical risks for more major procedures.

Complications have been minimal. We have had two fractures occur through the core site because the patients did not use their crutches for the required minimum of 6 weeks post surgery. No infections or deaths occurred in our patients nor in a reported series of 800 interventions.[37] One of our patients developed a postoperative ipsilateral thrombophlebitis, but no pulmonary embolus occurred. In one series, thrombophlebitis occurred in 6 cases out of the first 100 patients, with one of these having a pulmonary embolism.[134]

Miscellaneous Procedures. Recently there has been a report of a small series of patients with muscle pedicle grafting to the necrotic segment through a window in the posterior neck using the quadratus femoris and its attachment to the intertrochanteric crest.[4] The necrotic segment of the femoral head is debrided and packed with cancellous bone chips from the ilium with the musculopedicle graft impacted through the window and fixed in place with a single screw. In 23 cases followed for up to 4 years, 13 were rated good, 1 fair, and 9 poor. Still highly experimental is the replacement of collapsed segments by fresh osteochondral allografts.[4] In 5 hips in young vigorous patients treated by this method the results are encouraging, but the follow-up has only been from 6 months to just over 2 years.

Arthrodesis is a good method to use to obtain a painless and stable hip through occasionally a pseudoarthrosis may necessitate a reoperation.[127] It should also be kept in mind that in up to 80 percent of patients the disease is bilateral and subsequent involvement of the other side may severely interfere with the patient's activity. Other procedures such as tenotomy, spongioplasty, and Girdlestone and Milk-Bachelor procedures have been used in small numbers of patients, but the results are not very encouraging.[127]

Endoprosthetic Arthroplasty. Once there is flattening of the femoral head and a subchondral lucent line (stage III), some recommend prosthetic replacement of the femoral head without acetabuloplasty (usually an endoprosthesis in view of the patient's age).[6,107] As long as the acetabulum is normal (even early stage IV), they feel this is the procedure of choice. In 46 replaced necrotic femoral heads with a metallic prosthesis, which have been followed for 3 to 10 years, the functional results were classified as excellent in only 3, good in 16, fair in 12, and poor in 15.[6] Two prostheses were removed for sepsis, and 5 had to have total hip replacements because of pain. Many of the failures appeared to be caused by deterioration of the acetabulum, even in half of the patients who had a normal or increased joint space prior to surgery.

Eighty hips were treated with "adjusted cup" arthroplasty and followed for 1 to 6 years.[6] There was complete or nearly complete success in two-thirds of the cases,

Table 107–9. Core Decompression and the Course of Preradiologic Avascular Necrosis of Bone

| Clinical Status | No. Bones | Subsequent Course | | Major Surgery | Mean Follow-up (Months) |
		Symptoms	Positive X-ray		
Asymptomatic, untreated	15	14 (93%)	13 (87%)	5 (33%)	44
Symptomatic, cored	49	15 (31%)	15 (31%)	2 (4%)	32
P value		<0.00001	<0.0001	<0.01	

Table 107–10. The Treatment of Avascular Necrosis of Bone (AVN)
by Core Decompression

X-ray Stage	No. Bones	Course Subsequent to Core			Mean Follow-Up (Months)
		Recurrent Symptoms	X-ray Progression	Major Surgery	
I	49	15 (31%)	15 (31%)	2 (4%)*	32
II	90	29 (32%)	36 (40%)	21 (23%)†	32
III	65	37 (57%)*	20 (31%)	26 (40%)	37
IV	7	3 (43%)	—	3 (43%)	36
Total	211	84 (40%)	71 (35%)	52 (25%)	34

*p < 0.005.
† p < 0.05.

and another 16 percent were improved but with residual pain. In this situation, as well as with osteotomy, it is recommended that if at arthrotomy the necrosis involves the posterior slope of the femoral head, total joint replacement should be undertaken. If the necrosis is limited to the anterior part of the head with sparing of an arc of at least 20 percent of the lateral part, either an osteotomy, bringing the shaft into adduction and flexion, or an adjusted cup arthroplasty is indicated. The latter requires only one month of non–weight bearing in contrast to 3 to 4 months for the osteotomy.

Joint Replacement. Total hip replacement, although effective, is not without greater risk than the more conservative procedures. In a large series, there was about an 8 percent incidence of pulmonary embolism, which was fatal in 1.5 percent.[136] Other complications include dislocation, infection, and loosening of the prosthesis. Although it is often recommended in patients over 60 years of age, many believe young patients should be treated by procedures that offer a chance to preserve their femoral head. Surgery performed on 15 patients with AVN in renal allograft recipients included 25 total joint replacements, 21 hips, 3 knees, and 1 ankle.[60] Although this resulted in relief of symptoms in the majority of patients, a few experienced pain following exercise. Total joint replacement itself may be a hazard in kidney transplant patients, as the loss of a functioning renal allograft at the time of, and presumably secondary to, total hip arthroplasty has been reported.[137]

Total shoulder replacement has been reported to give satisfactory or excellent results in avascular necrosis of the humeral head.[139] This is a more difficult procedure than total hip replacement, in which bone supplies stability, and total knee replacement, in which the ligaments are important for stability. Since the muscles are so critical for both stability and movement, optimum functional results require as much skill in the reconstruction of the rotator cuff and deltoid muscles as in the orientation of the implants.[138]

Other Measures. Obviously the best treatment is prevention of the disease in the first place. Although this is not entirely possible at this point, progress is being made. Stricter adherence to decompression schedules and pre-employment screening for additional risk factors such as hemoglobinopathies have decreased the incidence of bone necrosis in decompression sickness.

The prevalence of AVN in renal allografts has been markedly decreased by improved preoperative dialysis and management of renal hyperparathyroidism and osteomalacia and by significantly decreasing the amount of glucocorticoids used postoperatively.[110] Because of the association of hypophosphatemia and avascular necrosis in renal transplant recipients, antacids that deplete phosphates should be used in moderation and replaced by agents, such as aluminum phosphate, that have a smaller phosphate-binding capacity. In some cases it may be prudent to normalize the serum phosphate level by supplementation.

The recent reports on the glucocorticoid regimens and added risk that Raynaud's imposes on the AVN in SLE patients may begin to decrease the frequency of bone problems in SLE and other steroid-associated conditions.[56,60] Since the risk of the subsequent development of AVN in patients with lymphoma appears to be related to the amount of radiation exposure to the involved bones as well as to high levels of glucocorticoid therapy, the design of the overall treatment program should take these factors into consideration.

In situations in which the disorder cannot be prevented, it is clear that early diagnosis and treatment can have a significant effect on the final outcome. Fortunately, quantitative scintimetry, bone marrow pressure measurement, and intraosseous venography are able to diagnose all but a few patients even prior to radiographic change. Our latest data convince us that without question symptomatic preradiologic disease should be treated and suggest that perhaps asymptomatic patients should be treated as well.[135] Since the incidence of bilateral AVN is as high as 80 percent, others have also suggested treating the asymptomatic or silent side as well.[107,128]

In some situations, one of the most important aspects of treatment is selecting the procedure based on the age of the patient and the associated disease. For example, treatment by core decompression is especially helpful in patients in whom general anesthesia may be hazardous, for example, in hemoglobinopathies. In these patients it is essential to maintain adequate oxygenation and prevent dehydration and acidosis. Failure to accomplish this may lead to sudden death due to systemic sickling of erythrocytes.,

In renal allograft recipients, the tendency toward generalized osteoporosis makes prolonged immobilization inadvisable and the frequency of bilateral involved weight-bearing joints makes prolonged walking with minimal weight bearing impractical.[49] Consequently, we feel that core decompression is an ideal procedure in this situation.

The less than certain results with endoprosthesis, cup arthroplasty, and osteotomy and the long-term durability of total hip arthroplasty in younger patients warrant consideration of more conservative procedures such as bone grafting and particularly core decompression. One of the major disadvantages of bone grafting is that patients generally have to be non–weight bearing for 6 months (average 4 to 8 months) and partially bear weight for an average of another 6 months (range 2 to 14 months).[107]

In summary, core decompression in early disease is not only simple and effective but requires significantly less postoperative protective weight bearing than other surgical interventions, allowing for better compliance and quicker return to more normal activities.

References

1. Jones, J.P., Jr.: Alcoholism, hypercortisonism, fat embolism and osseous avascular necrosis. In Zinn, W.N. (ed.): Idiopathic ischemic necrosis of the femoral head in adults. Stuttgart, Georg Thieme, 1971.
2. Zinn, W.N.: Introduction. In Zinn, W.N. (ed.): Idiopathic ischemic necrosis of the femoral head in adults. Stuttgart, Georg Thieme, 1971.
3. Coventry, M.B.: 2,012 total hip arthroplasties, a study of post operative course and early complications. J. Bone Joint Surg. 56A:273, 1974.
4. Meyers, M.H.: The treatment of osteonecrosis of the hip with fresh osteochondral allografts and with the muscle pedicle graft technique. Clin. Orthop. 130:202, 1978.
5. Catto, M.: Pathology of aseptic bone necrosis. In Davidson, J.K. (ed.) Aseptic necrosis of bone. Amsterdam, Excerpta Medica, 1976.
6. Kerboul, M., Thomine, J., Postel, M., and Merle D'Aubigne, R.: The conservative surgical treatment of idiopathic aseptic necrosis of the femoral head. J. Bone Joint Surg. 56B:291, 1974.
7. McCollum, D.E., Mathews, R.S., O'Neil, M.T., and Pickett, P.T.: Gout hyperuricemia and aseptic necrosis of the femoral head. In Zinn, W.N. (ed.): Idiopathic ischemic necrosis of the femoral head in adults. Stuttgart, Georg Thieme, 1971.
8. Boettcher, W.G., Bonfiglio, M., and Smith, K.: Non-traumatic necrosis of the femoral head. Part II. Experiences in treatment. J. Bone Joint Surg. 52A:322, 1970.
9. Merle D'Aubigne, R.M., Postel, M., Mazabraud, A., Massias, P., and Geugen, J.: Idiopathic necrosis of the femoral head in adults. J. Bone Joint Surg. 47B:612, 1965.
10. Patterson, R.J., Bickel, W.H., and Dahlin, D.C.: Idiopathic avascular necrosis of the head of the femur. A study of fifty-two cases. J. Bone Joint Surg. 46A:267, 1964.
11. Welfing, J.: Primary necrosis of the femoral head. Current state of the subject in French medical opinion. In Zinn, W.N. (ed.): Idiopathic ischemic necrosis of the femoral head in adults. Stuttgart, Georg Thieme, 1971.
12. Jacobs, B.: Epidemiology of traumatic and nontraumatic osteonecrosis. Clin. Orthop. 130:51, 1978.
13. Koshino, T.: The treatment of spontaneous osteonecrosis of the knee by high tibial osteotomy with and without bone-grafting or drilling of the lesion. J. Bone Joint Surg. 64A:47, 1982.
14. Ahback, S., Bauer, G.C.H., and Bohne, W.H.: Spontaneous osteonecrosis of the knee. Arthritis Rheum. 11:705, 1968.
15. Bauer, G.C.: Osteonecrosis of the knee. Clin. Orthop. 130:210, 1978.
16. Caffey, J.: The early roentgenographic changes in essential coxa plana. Am. J. Roentgenol. 103:620, 1968.
17. Graham, J., and Wood, S.K.: Aseptic necrosis of bone following trauma. In Davidson, J.K. (ed.): Aseptic necrosis of bone. Amsterdam, Excerpta Medica, 1976.
18. Knowlden, J., Buho, A.J., and Dunbar, O.: Incidence of fractures in persons over 35 years of age. Bn J. Prev. Soc. Med. 18:130, 1964.
19. Frangatiis, E.K.: Intracapsular fractures of the neck of the femur. Fractures influencing non-union and ischemic necrosis. J. Bone Joint Surg. 48B:17, 1966.
20. Barnes, R., Brown, J.T., Garden, R.S., and Nicoll, E.A.: Subcapital fractures of the femur: A prospective review. J. Bone Joint Surg. 58B:2, 1976.

21. Graham, J., and Wood, S.K.: Aseptic necrosis of bone following trauma. In Davidson, J.K. (ed.): Aseptic necrosis of bone. Amsterdam, Excerpta Medica, 1976.
22. Catto, M.: A histological study of avascular necrosis of the femoral head after transcervical fracture. J. Bone Joint Surg. 47B:749, 1965.
23. Fielding, J.W.: The telescoping Pugh Nail in the surgical management of the displaced intracapsular fracture of the femoral neck. Clin. Orthop. 152:123, 1980.
24. Simon, W.H., and Wyman, E.T.: Femoral neck fractures. Clin. Orthop. 70:152, 1970.
25. Meyers, M.H., Harvey, J.P., and Moore, T.M.: Treatment of displaced subcapital and transcervical fractures of the femoral neck by muscle pedicle bone graft and internal fixation. J. Bone Joint Surg. 55A:257, 1973.
26. Bonfiglio, M., and Bardenstein, M.B.: Treatment by bone-grafting of aseptic necrosis of the femoral head and non-union of the femoral head (Phemister technique). J. Bone Joint Surg. 40A:1329, 1958.
27. Epstein, H.C.: Traumatic dislocations of the hip. Clin. Orthop. 92:116, 1973.
28. Brav, E.A.: Traumatic dislocation of the hip. J. Bone Joint Surg. 44A:1115, 1962.
29. Burstein A., and Plate E.: Uber Chronische Gelenkveranderungen, enstanden durch Pressluftkrankung. Fortschr. Geb. Roengenstr. 18:197, 1911/12.
30. Golding, F.C., Griffiths, P., Hempleman, H.V., Paton, W.D.M., and Walder, D.N.: Decompression sickness during construction of the Dartford Tunnel. Br. J. Indust. Med. 17:167, 1960.
31. Nellen, J.R., and Kindwall, E.P.: Aseptic necrosis of bone secondary to occupational exposure to compressed air: roentgenologic findings in 59 cases. Am. J. Roentgenol. 115:512, 1972.
32. McCallum, R.I., Walder, D.N., Barnes, R., Catto, M.E., Davidson, J.K., Fryer, D.I., Golding, F.C., and Paton, W.D.M.: Bone lesions in compressed air workers with special reference to men who worked on the Clyde Tunnels 1958 to 1963. J. Bone Joint Surg. 48B:207, 1966.
33. Jones, J.P., and Behnke, A.R.: Prevention of dysbaric osteonecrosis in compressed air workers. Clin. Orthop. 130:118, 1978.
34. Davidson, J.K.: Dysbaric osteonecrosis. In Davidson, J.K. (ed.): Aseptic necrosis of bone. Amsterdam, Excerpta Medica, 1976.
35. Ohta, Y., Maatsunaga, H.: Bone lesions in divers. J. Bone Joint Surg. 56B:3, 1974.
36. Kawashima, M., Torisu, T., Hayashim, K., and Kitano, M.: Pathological review of osteonecrosis in divers. Clin. Orthop. 130:107, 1978.
37. Ficat, R.P., Arlet, J., and Hungerford, D.S.: Ischemia and necrosis of bone. Baltimore, Williams and Wilkins, 1980.
38. Middlemiss, H.: Aseptic necrosis and other changes occurring in bone in the hemoglobinapathies. In Davidson, J.K. (ed.): Aseptic necrosis of bone. Amsterdam, Excerpta Medica, 1976.
39. Chung, S.M.K., and Ralston, E.L.: Necrosis of the femoral head associated with sickle-cell anemia and its genetic variants. A review of the literature and study on thirteen cases. J. Bone Joint Surg. 51A:33, 1969.
40. Tanaka, K.R., Clifford, G.O., and Axelrod, A.R.: Sickle cell anemia with asceptic necrosis of the femoral head. Blood 11:998, 1956.
41. Diggs, L.W.: Sickle cell crisis. Am. J. Clin. Pathol. 44:1, 1965.
42. Diggs, L.W., and Anderson, L.D.: Aseptic necrosis of the head of the femur in sickle-cell disease. In Zinn, W.M. (ed.): Idiopathic ischemic necrosis of the femoral head in adults. Stuttgart, Georg, Thieme, 1971.
43. Jaffe, H.L.: Metabolic, Degenerative and Inflammatory Diseases of Bones and Joints. Philadelphia, Lea and Febiger, 1972.
44. Cramer, S.F., Fried, L., and Carter, K.J.: The cellular basis of metastatic bone disease in patients with lung cancer. Cancer 48:2649, 1981.
45. Pietrogrande, V., and Vastomarino, R.: Osteopatia da prolungato frattamento cortisonico. Ortop e Travmatol 25:791, 1957.
46. Dubois, E.L.: Lupus Erythematosus. 2nd ed. Los Angeles, University of Southern California Press, 1974, pp. 332 and 424.
47. Bergstein, J.M., Wiens, P., Fish, A.J., et al.: Avascular necrosis of bone in systemic lupus erythematosus. J. Pediatr. 85:31, 1974.
48. Hurley, R.M., Steinberg, R.H., Patriquin, H., et al.: Avascular necrosis of the femoral head in childhood systemic lupus erythematosus. Can. Med. Assoc. J. 111:781, 1974.
49. Harrington, K.D., Murray, W.R., Kountz, S.L., and Belzer, F.O.: Avascular necrosis of bone after renal transplantation. J. Bone Joint Surg. 53A:203, 1971.
50. Diamant, J., Gingler, E.M., Diamond, H.S., et al.: Computer analysis of factors influencing the appearance of aseptic necrosis in patients with SLE. J. Rheumatol. 5:136, 1978.
51. Abeles, M., Urman, J.D., and Rothfield, N.: Aseptic necrosis of bone in systemic lupus erythematosus: Relationship to corticosteroid therapy. Arch. Intern. Med. 138:750, 1978.
52. Hungerford, D.S., Zizic, T.M., and Moore, R.: Steroid associated ischemic necrosis of the knee (abstr.). Arthritis Rheum. 22:624, 1979.
53. Zizic, T.M., Hungerford, D.S., Dansereau, Y.-V., and Stevens, M.B.:

Corticosteroid associated ischemic necrosis of bone in SLE (abstr.). Arthritis Rheum. 1:952, 1979.

54. Dubois, E.L., and Cozen, L.: Avascular (aseptic) bone necrosis associated with systemic lupus erythematosus. JAMA 174:966, 1960.

55. Klipper, A.R., Stevens, M.B., Zizic, T.M., and Hungerford, D.S.: Ischemic necrosis of bone in systemic lupus erythematosus. Medicine 55:251, 1976.

56. Zizic, T.M., Hungerford, D.S., and Stevens, M.B.: Ischemic bone necrosis in systemic lupus erythematosus. The early diagnosis of ischemic necrosis of bone. Medicine 59:134, 1980.

57. Klippel, J.H., Gerber, L.H., Pollak, L., and Decker, J.L.: Avascular necrosis in SLE. Am. J. Med. 67:83, 1979.

58. Smith, E.F., Sweet, D.E., Brunner, C.M., et al.: Avascular necrosis in systemic lupus erythematosus: An apparent predilection for young patients. Ann. Rheum. Dis. 35:227, 1976.

59. Feinglass, E.J., Arnett, F.C., Dorsch, C.A., Zizic, T.M., and Stevens, M.B.: Neuropsychiatric manifestations of systemic lupus erythematosus. Medicine 55:323, 1976.

60. Zizic, T.M., Marcoux, C., Hungerford, D.S., Dansereau, J.Y., Hochberg, M.C., and Stevens, M.B.: Steroids, Raynauds and ischemic necrosis of bone (INB) in SLE (abstr.). Arthritis Rheum. 26:S34, 1983.

61. Marcoux, C., Zizic, T.M., Feldman, D., Hochberg, M.C., Hungerford, D.S., and Stevens, M.B.: Vasculitis in ischemic necrosis of bone (INB) in adult poly(dermato)myositis (PDM) (abstr.). Arthritis Rheum. 26:547, 1983.

62. Jones, J.P., Engleman, E.P., Steinbach, H.L., Murray, W.R., and Rambo, O.N.: Fat embolism as a possible mechanism producing avascular necrosis. Arthritis Rheum. 8:449, 1965.

63. Starzl, T.E., Marchioro, T.L., Porter, K.A., Moore, C.A., Rifkind, D., and Waddell, W.R.: Renal homotransplantation, late function and complications. Ann. Intern. Med. 61:470, 1964.

64. Stern, P.J., and Watts, H.G.: Osteonecrosis after renal transplantation in children. J. Bone Joint Surg. 61A:851, 1979.

65. Hawking, K.M., Van Den Bosch, B.F., and Wilmink, J.M.: Avascular necrosis of bone after renal transplantation. N. Engl. J. Med. 294:397, 1976.

66. Ibels, L.L., Alfrey, A.C., Huffer, W.E., and Weil, R.: Aseptic necrosis of bone following renal transplantation. Medicine 47:25, 1978.

67. Braud, J.F, Herman, J.H., and Smyth, C.H.: Musculoskeletal disorders after renal homotransplantation. Ann. Intern. Med. 66:89, 1967.

68. Bravo, J.J.: Musculoskeletal disorders after renal homotransplant. Ann. Intern. Med. 66:87, 1967.

69. Susan, L.P., Braun, W.E., Banowsky, L.H., Straffon, R.A., Bergfeld, J.A.: Avascular necrosis following renal transplantation: Experience with 449 allografts with and without high-dose steroid therapy. Urology 11:225, 1978.

70. Elmstedt, E.: Avascular bone necrosis in the renal transplant patients: A discriminant analysis of 144 cases. Clin. Orthop. 158:149, 1981.

71. Harris, R.R., Wieman, K.M.W., and Diethelm, A.G.: Skeletal complications after renal transplantation. South Med. J. 67:1016, 1974.

72. Pierides, A.M., Simpson, W., Stainsby, D., Alvarez Vde, F., Uldall, P.R.: Avascular necrosis of bone following renal transplantation. Q. J. Med. 44:459, 1975.

73. Nelson, C.L., Evarts, C.M., and Popowniak, K.: Musculoskeletal complication of renal transplantation. Surg. Clin. North Am. 51:1205, 1971.

74. Murray, W.R.: Hip problems associated with organ transplants. Clin. Orthop. 90:57, 1973.

75. Briggs, W.A., Hampers, C.L., Merritt, J.P., Hager, E.B., Wilson, R.E., Birtch, A.G., and Murray, J.E.: Aseptic necrosis in the femur after renal transplantation. Ann. Surg. 175:182, 1972.

76. Potter, D.E., Genant, H.K., and Salvatierra, O.: Avascular necrosis of bone after renal transplantation. Am. J. Dis. Child. 132:1125, 1978.

77. Moorhead, J.F., Wills, M.R., Ahmed, K.Y., Bailrod, R.A., Varghese, Z., and Tatler, G.I.V.: Hypophosphatemic osteomalacia after cadaveric renal transplantation. Lancet 1:694, 1974.

78. Lindsay, R., McPherson, S.G., Anderson, J.B., and Smith, D.A.: The value of bone density measurements in predicting the risk of developing avascular necrosis following renal transplantation. Calcif. Tiss. Res. 21:242, 1976.

79. Melsen, R., and Nielson, H.F.: Osteonecrosis following renal allotransplantation. Acta Pathol. Microbiol. Scan. Sect. A85:99, 1977.

80. Kenzora, J.E., and Glimcher, M.J.: The role of renal bone disease in the production of transplant osteonecrosis. Orthopedics 4:305, 1981.

81. Hungerford, D.S.: Pathogenic considerations in ischemic necrosis of bone. Can. J. Surg. 24:583, 1981.

82. Hungerford, D.S., and Zizic, T.M.: Alcohol associated ischemic necrosis of the femoral head. Clin. Orthop. 130:144, 1978.

83. Gerle, R.D., Walker, L.A., Achard, J.L., and Weens, H.S.: Osseous changes in chronic pancreatitis. Radiology 85:330, 1965.

84. Immelman, E.J., Bank, S., Krige, M., and Marks, I.N.: Roentgenologic

85. Hastings, D.E., and Macnab, I.: Spontaneous avascular necrosis of the femoral head: A clinical and pathological review. Can. J. Surg. 8:68, 1965.

86. Looney, W.B.: Late effects (twenty-five to forty years) of the early medical and industrial use of radioactive materials: Their relation to the more accurate establishment of maximum permissible amounts of radioactive elements in the body. Part II. J. Bone Joint Surg. 38A:175, 1956.

87. Engel, I.A., Sraus, D.J., Lacher, M., Lane, J., and Smith, J.: Osteonecrosis in patients with malignant lymphoma: A review of twenty-five cases. Cancer 48:1245, 1981.

88. Thorne, J.C., Evans, W.K., Alison, R.E., and Fournasier, V.: Avascular necrosis of bone complicating treatment of malignant lymphoma. Am. J. Med. 71:751, 1981.

89. Zinn, W.N.: II. Clinical picture and laboratory findings. Results of a Swiss Multi-Center study. In Zinn, W.N. (ed.): Idiopathic Ischemic Necrosis of the Femoral Head in Adults. Stuttgart, Georg Thieme, 1971.

90. Riniker, P., and Huggler, A.: Idiopathic necrosis of the femoral head. A further patho-anatomical study. In Zinn, W.N. (ed.): Idiopathic ischemic necrosis of the femoral head in adults. Stuttgart, Georg Thieme, 1971.

91. Wang, G.J., Sweet, D.E., Reger, S.I., and Thompson, R.C.: Fat cell changes as mechanism of avascular necrosis of the femoral head in cortisone treated rabbits. J. Bone Joint Surg. 59A:729, 1977.

92. Pooley, J., and Walder, D.N.: Reduction in bone marrow blood flow during simulated divers: Investigation of the mechanism. J. Bone Joint Surg. 62B:535, 1980.

93. Nasseri, D., Hungerford, D.S., White, K.K., and Jones, L.L.: Equine model of ischemic necrosis of bone (abstr.). Arthritis Rheum. 25:533, 1982.

94. Solomon, L.: Idiopathic necrosis of the femoral head: Pathogenesis and treatment. Can. J. Surg. 24:573, 1981.

95. Hungerford, D.S.: Early diagnosis of ischemic necrosis of the femoral head. Johns Hopkins Med. J. 137:270, 1975.

96. Arlet, J.: Pertrochanteric phlebography in primary necrosis of the femoral head in the initial stage (stage I). In Zinn, W.N. (ed.): Idiopathic Ischemic Necrosis of the Femoral Head in Adults. Stuttgart, Georg Thieme, 1971.

97. Arlet, J., Ficat, P., and Sebbag, D.: Intéret de la mesure de la pression intra-médullaire dans la massif trochantérien chez l'homme, en particulier pour le diagnostic de l'ostéonécrose fémoro-capitale. Rev. Rhum. Mal. Osteoartic. 35:250, 1968.

98. Arlet, J., Ficat, P., Lartiguie, G., and Tran, M.A.: Recherches cliniques sur la pression intra-osseuse dans la métaphyse et l'épiphyse fémorales supérieures chez l'homme. Application du diagnostic des ischémies et nécroses. Rev. Rhum. Mal. Osteoartic. 39:717, 1972.

99. Eberle, H.: Venographic differences in traumatic hip affections and in idiopathic femoral head necrosis. In Zinn, W.N.: Idiopathic Ischemic Necrosis of the Femoral Head in Adults. Stuttgart, Georg Thieme, 1971.

100. Zizic, T.M., Marcoux, C., Hungerford, D.S., and Stevens, M.B.: Predictive value of hemodynamic studies in ischemic necrosis of bone (INB) (abstr.). Arthritis Rheum. 26:537, 1983.

101. Jacqueline, F., and Rutishauser, E.: Pathology. Part A. Idiopathic necrosis of the femoral head. Anatomo-pathologic study. In Zinn, W.M. (ed.): Idiopathic Ischemic Necrosis of the Femoral Head in Adults. Stuttgart, Georg Thieme, 1971.

102. Cruess, R.L.: Experience with steroid-induced avascular necrosis and etiologic considerations regarding osteonecrosis of the hip. Clin. Orthop. 130:86, 1978.

103. Glimcher, M.J., and Kenzora, J.E.: The biology of osteonecrosis of the human femoral head and its clinical implications: II. The pathological changes in the femoral head as an organ and in the hip joint. Clin. Orthop. 139:283, 1979.

104. Glimcher, M.J., and Kenzora, J.E.: The biology of osteonecrosis of the human femoral head and its clinical implications: I. Tissue biology. Clin. Orthop. 138:284, 1979.

105. Catto, M.: The histologic appearances of late segmental collapse of the femoral head after transcervical fracture. J. Bone Joint Surg. 47B:777, 1965.

106. Arlet, J., and Ficat, P.: Biophy drilling as a means of early diagnosis. In Zinn, W.M. (ed.): Idiopathic ischemic necrosis of the femoral head in adults. Stuttgart, Georg Thieme, 1971.

107. Marcus, N.D., Enneking, W.F., and Massam, R.A.: The silent hip in idiopathic aseptic necrosis. Treatment by bone grafting. J. Bone Joint Surg. 55A:1351, 1973.

108. Cruess, R.L., Blennerhasset, J., MacDonald, F.R., MacLeon, L.D., and Dossiter, J.: Aseptic necrosis following renal homotransplantation. J. Bone Joint Surg. 50A:1577, 1968.

109. Zizic, T.M., Marcoux, C., Hungerford, D.S., and Stevens, M.B.: Radiography, scintigraphy, and hemodynamics: Diagnosis of ischemic necrosis of bone (INB) (abstr.). Arthritis Rheum. 26:S37, 1983.

110. Glimcher, M.S., and Kenzora, J.E.: The biology of osteonecrosis of the human femoral head and its clinical implications. III. Discussion of the etiology and genesis of the pathological sequelae: Comments on treatment. Clin. Orthop. 140:273, 1979.

111. Conklin, J.J., Dansereau, J.-Y., Alderson, P.O. Zizic.T.M., Hungerford, D.S., and Wagner, H.N., Jr.: Bone scans in steroid-treated patients with systemic lupus erythematosus (abst.). J. Nucl.Med. 21:6, 1980.

112. Zizic, T.M. Conklin, J.J., Hungerford D.S., Dansereau, J.-Y, Alderson, P.D., Golber, A., Wagner, H.N., and Stevens, M.B.: Sensitivity of quantitative scintigraphy in the early detection of ischemic necrosis of bone (abstr.). Arthritis Rheum. 24:4, p. 1981.

113. Deutsch, S.D., Gundsman E.J., and Sproragen, S.C.: Quantitative regional blood-flow analysis and its clinical application during routine bone-scanning . J. Bone Joint Surg. 63A:295, 1981.

114. D'Ambrosia, R.D., Shoji, H., Riggins, R.S., Staddlnik, R.C., and DeAardo, G.L.: Scintigraphy in the diagnosis of osteonecrosis. Clin. Orthop. 130:139, 1978.

115. Conklin, J.J., Alderson, P.O., Zizic, T.M., Hungerford, D.S., Dansereau, J.Y., Gober, A., and Wagner, H.W.: Comparison of bone scan and radiograph sensitivity in detection of steroid-induced ischemic necrosis of bone. Radiology 147:991, 1983.

116. Bauer, G.C.: The use of radionucleides in orthopedics. Part IV. Radionuclide scintimetry of the skeleton. J. Bone Joint Surg. 50A:1681, 1709, 1968.

117. Cameron, R.B.: Strontium-85 scintimetry in nontraumatic necrosis of the femoral head. Clin. Orthop. 65:243, 1969.

118. Greyson, W.D.: Radionuclide bone and joint imaging in rheumatology. Bull. Rheum. Dis. 30:1034, 1980.

119. Greyson, N.D., Lotem, M.M., Gross, A.E., and Houpt, J.B.: Radionuclide evaluation of spontaneous femoral osteonecrosis. Radiology 142:729, 1982.

120. Lemlperg, R.K., and Arnoldi, C.C.: The significance of intraosseous pressure in normal and diseased states with special reference to the intraosseous engorgement-pain syndrome. Clin. Orthop. 136:143, 1978.

121. Arnoldi, C.C., Lemperg, R., and Linderholm, H.: Immediate effect of osteotomy on the intramedullary pressure of the femoral head and neck in patients with degenerative osteoarthritis. Acta Orthop. Scand. 42:357, 1971.

122. Lynch, J.A.: Venous abnormalities and intraosseous hypertension associated with osteoarthritis of the knee. *In* Ingwesen, O.S. (ed.): The Knee Joint. Proceedings of the International Congress. Rotterdam, Sept. 13–15, 1973. Amsterdam, Excerpta Medica, 1974.

123. Arnoldi, C.C., Lemperg, K., and Linderholm, H.: Intraosseous hypertension and pain in the knee. J. Bone Joint Surg. 57b:360, 1975.

124. Hungerford, D.S., and Zizic, T.M.: Ischemic bone necrosis in systemic lupus eythematosus. The treatment of ischemic necrosis of bone. Medicine 59:143, 1980.

125. Zizic, T.M., Marcoux, C., Hungerford, D.S., and Stevens, M.B.: The treatment of ischemic necrosis of bone (INB) by core decompression (abstr.). Arthritis Rheum. 26:S38, 1983.

126. Chandler, H.P., Reineck, F.T., and Watson, R.L.: A five year review of total hip replacements in patients under the age of 30—with emphasis on loosening. Orthop. Trans. 3:303, 1979.

127. Romer, V., and Wettstein, P.: Results of treatment of eighty-one Swiss patients with 11NFH. *In* Zinn, W.N. (ed.): Idiopathic Ischemic Necrosis of the Femoral Head in Adults. Stuttgart, Georg Thieme, 1971.

128. Springfield, D.S., and Enneking, W.J.: Surgery for aseptic necrosis of the femoral head. Clin. Orthop. 130:175, 1978.

129. Phemister, D.B.: Treatment of the necrotic head of the femur in adults. J. Bone Joint Surg. 31A:55, 1949.

130. Bonfiglio, M., Voke, E.M.: Aseptic necrosis of the femoral head and non-union of the femoral neck: Effect of treatment by drilling and bone-grafting (Phemister technique). J. Bone Joint Surg. 50A:48, 1968.

131. Dunn, A.W., and Grow, T.: Aseptic necrosis of the femoral head. Treatment with bone grafts of doubtful value. Clin. Orthop. 122:249, 1977.

132. Sugioka, Y.: Transtrochanteric anterior rotational osteotomy of the femoral head in the treatment of osteonecrosis affecting the hip. A new osteotomy operation. Clin. Orthop. 130:191, 1978.

133. Arlet, J., and Ficat, P.: Diagnostic et traitement de l'osteonecrose primitive femoro-capitale de l'adulte av début. Apport du forage-biopsie. Rev. Med. (Paris) 1:19, 1965.

134. Arlet, J., and Ficat, P.: Biopsy drilling as a means of early diagnosis. *In* Zinn, W.N. (ed.) Idiopathic Ischemic Necrosis of the Femoral Head in Adults. Stuttgart, Georg Thieme, 1971.

135. Zizic, T.M., Marcoux, C., Hungerford, D.S., and Stevens, M.B.: Core decompression and the course of pre-radiologic ischemic necrosis of bone (abstr.). Arthritis Rheum. 26:S37, 1983.

136. Charnley, J.: Total hip replacement by low-friction arthroplasty. Clin. Orthop. 72:7, 1970.

137. Zimmerman, C.E., and Yett, H.S.: Renal transplant infarction during total hip arthroplasty. Clin. Orthop. 165:195, 1982.

138. Neer, C.S., Watson, K.C., and Stanton, F.J.: Recent experience in total shoulder replacement. J. Bone Joint Surg. 64A:319, 1982.

Section XXI
Tumors Involving Joints

Chapter 108
Tumors and Tumor-Like Lesions Involving Joints

Alan L. Schiller

INTRODUCTION

As true neoplasms of the joint are rare and the majority of tumor-like conditions associated with synovial tissue may not be neoplastic in nature but are nonetheless of great importance in differential diagnosis, this chapter will cover those lesions of the synovium of joints, tendon sheaths, and bursae that arise as masses and may behave locally as neoplasms. Obviously non-neoplastic lesions such as synovial and meniscal cysts will not be considered. The more common of the lesions to be discussed, such as synovial chondromatosis, pigmented villonodular synovitis, and localized nodular tenosynovitis, and diseases of unknown etiology and their possible neoplastic-like nature are still a matter of debate.

Except for a single case of angiosarcoma of the knee,[1] for all practical purposes, there are no other proved cases of a malignant neoplasm arising within synovial tissue. The whole concept of tenosynovial sarcomas, which are often closely associated with synovial tissue, is still controversial because of the uncertainties regarding the tissue of origin for these relatively rare but malicious malignant tumors.

FATTY LESIONS OF THE SYNOVIUM

A true benign lipoma of a joint is extremely rare. There are a few scattered cases of knee or ankle joint involvement, a bilateral case involving the knees, and a few cases involving tendon sheaths of the hands, feet, and ankles, usually of the extensor more often than the flexor tendons.[2-4] True lipomas are lobulated fatty masses, either sessile or stalked, and histologically resemble lipomas elsewhere in the body. Some may present with knee pain if they twist on their stalk. There is, however, another, more common lesion, which, although not a true lipoma, has been termed lipoma arborescens. This is a benign, fatty intra-articular mass that is found in the knee or, less commonly, the elbow and is almost always associated with some degenerative arthritis. When in the knee, it is usually located in the suprapa-tellar or lateral pouches (Fig. 108–1). Grossly, the lesion consists of a localized or diffuse fatty polypoid mass covered by a thin membranous layer of normal synovium.[5,6] (Fig. 108–2). Histologic examination shows normal fatty tissue with some accentuated vascularity. It is unclear whether lipoma arborescens is primary or secondary to the associated degenerative arthritis or to some type of joint irritation. Pain, locking, or limitation of motion and a clear, watery effusion usually bring the patient to a physician for evaluation. Radiographs are often unrewarding, and either arthroscopy or surgical intervention is needed for the diagnosis. Another entity to be considered here is Hoffa's disease, a condition in which the subsynovial fat tissue of the knee joint, which is normally adjacent to the patellar ligament, becomes hyperemic, inflamed, and hypertrophied and may also simulate a fatty tumor.[6]

VASCULAR LESIONS OF SYNOVIUM

True hemangiomas of the synovium or joint capsule are rare, and most are associated with soft tissue vascular abnormalities, particularly arteriovenous malformations or skin vascular lesions (40 percent), including patients with Klippel-Trenaunay syndrome (bone and soft tissue hypertrophy, cutaneous hemangiomas, and varicose veins). One reported case[7] had bilateral knee involvement associated with Kasabach-Merritt syndrome (capillary hemangiomas, purpura, and decreased clotting factors). Symptoms invariably begin before the age of 30, and most patients (75 percent) are females who are under 16 years of age at the time of diagnosis and have had symptoms dating into childhood. The most common symptoms include unilateral, intermittent joint pain and enlargement with subsequent limitation of motion, locking, or buckling, especially following minor trauma. Classically, the affected joint reduces in size if elevated sufficiently to allow the blood to drain. The areas most commonly involved are the knee or, more rarely, the elbow, ankle, tarsometatarsal joints, and synovial tendon sheaths of the wrist or ankle.[2,3,5-10] The joint is

Figure 108–1. Lipoma arborescens presenting as a suprapatellar mass; it is easily seen on flexion of the knee. (Courtesy of Drs. C. Rowe and B. Zarins.)

swollen and doughy and yields bloody fluid on aspiration. Radiographic examination may show nothing more than a vague soft tissue shadow indicative of a swollen synovium and distended joint capsule. Radiopaque phleboliths may be apparent, however, and are more often associated with a soft tissue arteriovenous malformation with secondary joint involvement than with an isolated intra-articular hemangioma[7] (Fig. 108–3). Arthrography may demonstrate intra-articular filling defects, and arteriography may show localized dye collection in the tumor.

There appear to be two forms of benign vascular abnormalities that occur within joints: a circumscribed or true hemangioma, and a diffuse angiomatous type resembling an arteriovenous malformation. The circum-

Figure 108–2. Lipoma arborescens represented as a diffuse, fatty polypoid mass covered by a thin, glistening synovium.

scribed hemangioma is typically a small sessile or stalked lesion arising near the infrapatellar fat pad and must be distinguished from pigmented villonodular synovitis. Larger lesions up to 8.0 cm have occasionally been seen.[6] Infrequently, bone invasion may be present secondary to pressure atrophy by the hemangioma and may mimic the radiographic changes of hemophilia unless phleboliths are present to confirm the diagnosis of a vascular mass (Fig. 108–4). Microscopically, the hemangioma is usually of the cavernous type, with large, dilated, blood-filled channels lined by prominent but benign-appearing endothelial cells. In the diffuse form, which is invariably associated with soft tissue arteriovenous malformations, the entire synovium may be edematous and beefy red with enlarged, tortuous, blood-filled channels that are contiguous with the joint capsule and soft tissue (Fig. 108–5). Often the surgeon will describe these vessels as extending beyond the surgical field both proximally and distally, making surgical resection an impossibility. Microscopic examination of the diffuse lesion shows large, intermixed venous and arterial-like vascular channels with prominent smooth muscle walls and intermediate-type vessels which communicate between the venous and arterial channels, a finding that is typical for arteriovenous malformations. The adjacent normal synovium may be blood stained and may contain hemosiderin secondary to repeated intra-articular bleeding episodes.

Therapy for a localized hemangioma of the joint is excision of the tumor, which yields a good result. However, those lesions associated with soft tissue vascular malformations may have poor therapeutic results with recurrences, since the vascular abnormality may extend along tendon sheaths as well as fascial planes, and surgical extirpation is often not possible. Radiation therapy has been advocated in such cases with mixed results.[2]

Figure 108–3. Arteriogram of an arteriovenous malformation in the soft tissues of the thigh and leg with involvement of the knee joint. The extensive vascular blush in the knee indicates aberrant synovial and capsular vasculature.

Recently we reported on an angiosarcoma arising in the knee of a 76-year-old man.[1] This single case is the only one we know of in which a malignant tumor has been proved to arise from the synovium. The tumor filled the entire joint cavity as friable, red-brown, papillary and nodular masses and extended along all the synovial recesses of the joint (Fig. 108–6). The tumor extended into the subchondral regions of the femur and tibia, particularly subjacent to the cruciate ligament attachments, and extended along the subperiosteal regions without involving any soft tissues. The lower limb was amputated, but the patient died 8 months later with microscopic lung metastases. Microscopic examination showed characteristic vascular spaces with malignant endothelial cell proliferation and reactive fibrosis, a typical picture for angiosarcoma.

There are no reports of vascular lesions in bursae.

Figure 108–4. A localized synovial hemangioma with phleboliths prominently seen in the joint. The patient was 16 years old with many years' history of painful swelling when standing and relief of this pain when the knee was flexed.

INTRA-ARTICULAR OSSICLES

Small bony nodules frequently occur in the knees of some rodents[11] and other mammals and may rarely occur in man, with a total of only about 15 cases having been reported.[12] In rodents, they are constantly found in the anterior portions of the joint and frequently in the posterior portions as well. The clinician should be aware of such structures, since a patient may present with symptoms of a loose body and yet none may be found at

Figure 108–5. A diffuse form of hemangioma of the synovium with an edematous beefy synovium and large dilated vascular channels. In life these channels were filled with blood and the synovium was markedly thickened.

Figure 108–6. Angiosarcoma arising in the knee of a 76-year-old man as friable red-tan tissue replacing the synovium, crawling over the patella, and filling up all synovial recesses. The patient died 8 months later with microscopic lung metastases.

exploration or arthroscopy. Because the ossicles are embedded within the menisci, they are discovered only when the menisci are palpated or carefully examined.

Microscopy reveals that the ossicles form within the fibrocartilaginous matrix of the meniscus and have either a fibrocartilage or hyaline cartilage envelope surrounding trabeculae of lamellar and/or woven bone embedded in a loose fibrous or fatty marrow (Fig. 108–7). Often osteoblastic and osteoclastic cellular activity is evident.

Figure 108–7. An intra-articular ossicle embedded in the fibrocartilage of the meniscus. The bone is lamellar and the marrow is fatty. The interface between the fibrocartilage and bone resembles a tendinous insertion including Sharpey's fibers. (Hematoxylin and eosin × 25)

The exact etiology of such structures is unknown, although most probably they either are true sesamoid bones, as seen in rodents, or represent ossification secondary to local injury. A history of past knee trauma was present in a number of the reported cases. The symptoms are usually pain after some sort of exertion such as walking or prolonged standing, with relief when the knee is at rest. Radiographs of the involved knee may reveal what appears to be a loose body after multiple views are examined. The differential diagnosis to be considered should include a loose body and a torn meniscus. At surgery, however, the joint surface will be intact and neither loose body nor torn meniscus will be found, but either the lateral or medial meniscus will have a small (about 1.0 cm in diameter) palpable bony nodule which should be excised along with the meniscus itself. Symptoms disappear when the ossicle is removed.

SYNOVIAL CHONDROMATOSIS

Synovial chondromatosis is an uncommon, benign, often self-limiting condition of unknown etiology involving joints, bursae, or even tendon sheaths of young and middle-aged adults.[2,3,6,13-15] This disease is characterized by the formation of numerous nodules of metaplastic cartilage within the synovial tissue and their subsequent release into the joint space as free-floating cartilage bodies. If there is endochondral ossification within some of the cartilage masses, the term synovial osteochondromatosis is more appropriate. Although the masses may have focal cellular atypicality, this lesion is not considered sarcomatous, for it never metastasizes and generally remains within the confines of the involved joint space. The prognosis is good after removal of the involved synovium and free bodies, although there may be local recurrences.

Location. This is a disease primarily of large diarthrodial joints. The most common joint involved is the knee, which is affected in at least half of all cases, usually as a monarticular condition. The next most common sites include the hip, elbow,[16,17] shoulder[18] and ankle.[19] Sometimes involvement of the small joints of the hands and feet, e.g., metacarpophalangeal joints,[20] as well as of the tendon sheaths of the fingers and toes is seen, with the latter form perhaps being better termed "extra-articular synovial chondromatosis." At times multiple fingers or toes may be affected simultaneously. Isolated cases involving the distal radioulnar joint[21] and temporomandibular joint are also reported.[22-27] In about 10 percent of all cases bilateral involvement occurs.

Age and Sex. The condition is twice as common in young and middle-aged males as in females,[13] although, interestingly, middle-aged females are more likely to develop temporomandibular involvement. The age range is 7 to 67 years, with an average in the fifth decade. In the case of hand or foot involvement, however, there seems to be an equal distribution of the sexes, and this form of the disease is usually seen in elderly people, most often in the sixth decade.

Symptoms and Signs. Symptoms are related to the presence of the many intra-articular loose bodies and may persist for many years (average duration, 3 to 8 years) before the patient seeks medical help. Complaints commonly include pain, joint swelling, stiffness, joint crepitance, and limitation of joint motion with a locking or grating feeling upon movement of the joint. If the temporomandibular joint is involved, pain and tenderness over the joint more often occur. The question of a relationship between diabetes mellitus and synovial chondromatosis has been raised by French investigators, since in a series of 40 patients with synovial chondromatosis 17 had non-insulin-dependent diabetes mellitus.[28] Another interesting association has been seen in the temporomandibular joint, where two cases of synovial chondromatosis with simultaneous pigmented villonodular synovitis have been reported.[29]

Radiographic Findings. The radiographic findings depend mainly upon whether there is calcified cartilage or bone present in either the synovium or the loose bodies. In most cases of synovial chondromatosis, calcified intra-articular free-floating bodies are seen and appear as discrete dot-like radiopacities associated with synovial thickening or intra-articular soft tissue masses (Fig. 108–8). There is a substantial minority of cases, however, in which no calcification is apparent and the joint may appear normal.[30] Occasionally, the entire joint contour is outlined with calcification because calcified cartilage and/or bone is visible on the radiograph (Fig. 108–9). In some cases, bone erosion by direct pressure from the swollen cartilage-filled joint is present, particularly in the femoral neck when the hip is involved, and may in fact lead to secondary degenerative changes of the joint.[30] In cases of temporomandibular joint involvement, joint space widening is usually present on radi-

ographs with or without the additional findings of calcific loose bodies, irregularity of the joint surfaces, and sclerosis of the glenoid fossa and mandibular condyle.[24] In those cases in which the tendon sheath of a finger is involved, there may be a linear arrangement of small calcific densities aligned along the sheath spanning a number of joints for the whole length of the involved ray and sparing joints. The differential radiologic diagnosis of synovial chondromatosis includes osteochondritis dissecans, osteoarthritis with loose bodies, tuberculosis, hemopathic arthropathies, and pseudogout with extensive synovial calcification.[31] In most cases, the clinical story and radiographic picture should lead the clinician to the proper diagnosis of synovial chondromatosis, particularly if a thickened synovial lining is seen on radiographs. There are many instances, however, in which the radiographic picture is not particularly helpful and the clinical story is rather vague, so that only arthroscopy and biopsy will remove all doubts about the patient's condition.

Gross Pathology. Synovial chondromatosis has the very characteristic gross appearance of a thickened synovial lining with innumerable shiny, blue-white glistening cartilage nodules (generally) 0.1 to 0.5 cm in diameter) either embedded within the substance of the lining or attached along the surface in a cobblestone pattern (Fig. 108–10). The synovium is usually moist, often papillated and thrown into folds, and sometimes hyperemic. If there are bony foci, they are apparent as tiny areas of gritty trabeculae, which may be associated with yellow marrow (Fig. 108–11). There are almost always many loose bodies, sometimes hundreds. These are similar to the embedded cartilage nodules, although they are often larger (1 to 2 cm in diameter) and are found coating the synovial surface, from which they are

Figure 108–8. Radiographs of the wrist with prominent multiple calcified bodies of varying sizes present in the soft tissues of the wrist and extending along the forearm. These bodies have a smooth surface and a lucent center, some of which have a trabeculated pattern rather than an amorphous densely calcified center. The diagnosis is synovial osteochondromatosis.

Figure 108–9. Synovial osteochondromatosis of the knee with narrowing of the joint space and multiple large calcified bodies filling the joint space and suprapatellar pouch.

easily detached when touched. Traditionally, most pathologists would expect to see at least four loose bodies before resting on the diagnosis of synovial chondromatosis.

Microscopic Features. The diagnostic feature of this disease is the metaplastic cartilage, often arranged in layers, being formed within the synovial lining (Fig. 108–12). In contrast to osteochondritis dissecans or a loose body of osteoarthritis, in which a fragment of articular hyaline cartilage implants in the synovium, synovial chondromatosis presents a histologic spectrum in which mesenchymal tissue of the synovium gives rise to chondroblasts and chondrocytes, which ultimately blend into nodules of hyaline cartilage (Fig. 108–13). If these structures are still attached to the synovium, there may be vascular ingrowth, resulting in endochondral ossification with woven and lamellar bone formation. A medullary

cavity filled with fatty marrow may eventually result (Fig. 108–14). If these nodules break away from their synovial attachments, they will continue to increase in size, since the cartilage can still derive its nourishment from synovial fluid, although the osseous portion will die. The adjacent synovium without cartilage nodules usually appears totally normal. In those lesions involving the hands or feet, small foci resembling localized nodular tenosynovitis may be seen adjacent to some cartilage nodules.[32]

An important point to emphasize concerns the focal atypicality that may be seen in the metaplastic cartilage nodules. Despite the presence of binucleate cells and cells with slight nuclear enlargement, both of which are commonly observed, the majority of chondrocytes are small and uniform, with dark round nuclei, militating against the diagnosis of something more ominous such

Figure 108–10. Synovial chondromatosis with innumerable cartilage nodules forming a cobblestone-like appearance of the synovial lining. (Courtesy of Dr. C. Campbell.)

Figure 108–11. Synovial osteochondromatosis. The smooth-surfaced nodules are seen merging with the synovium rather than appearing as implanted pieces of cartilage which may easily separate from the synovium and have irregular roughened surfaces. Prominent bone trabeculae and a fatty marrow are easily seen within each nodule.

Figure 108–12. Synovial chondromatosis with metaplastic hyaline cartilage nodules in the synovium. The adjacent noncartilaginous synovium is normal. (Hematoxylin and eosin × 36)

Figure 108–14. Synovial osteochondromatosis with a metaplastic hyaline cartilage nodule near the synovial surface and bony nodules deeper in the synovium. Note the fatty marrow inside the osseous nodules. (Hematoxylin and eosin × 23)

as chondrosarcoma (Fig. 108–15). The few ultrastructural studies performed on this disease further support the benign nature of the cartilage, since there are many similarities between the cartilage nodules and articular cartilage.[33]

Clinical Course and Prognosis. The treatment of choice for synovial chondromatosis is excision of the involved synovium and removal of all loose bodies from the joint. The prognosis is very good, although there may be recurrences if removal is incomplete. More rarely, in the case of loose bodies embedded in fat or muscle, spontaneous regression of the disease has been seen even after incomplete removal. The loose bodies in these cases are thought to have herniated through a capsular defect or perhaps to have formed secondary to a previous surgical procedure rather than by extra-articular or capsular cartilage metaplasia.[34]

Instances of malignant degeneration of synovial chondromatosis to chondrosarcoma or a de novo intra-

articular chondrosarcoma have been reported in a few isolated rare cases.[13,35,36] It is difficult to decide whether these cases represent a primary process arising from adjacent bone with joint invasion or whether they are indeed primary lesions of the joint, since all cases have had bone, soft tissue, and joint involvement by tumor.

The etiology of synovial chondromatosis is not known. Although trauma has been implicated in some instances, it is difficult to prove cause and effect. In an attempt to better understand the evolution of this entity, three stages or phases have been described.[37] The first stage is an active or florid stage in which the formation and presence of the cartilage nodules are strictly confined to the synovial lining. The hyperemic, papillary, edematous synovium seen grossly corresponds to this stage. The second or intermediate stage is a transition phase in which loose bodies and synovial cartilage nodules are both present. The third, late, or final stage occurs when only loose bodies are present with virtually no new

Figure 108–13. A higher view of chondromatosis illustrating the continuity between synovial tissue and metaplastic hyaline cartilage nodules. (Hematoxylin and eosin × 160)

Figure 108–15. Synovial chondromatosis with mild cellular atypicality and binucleate cells, common features of such lesions; but the majority of chondrocytes are small, round, and uniform. (Hematoxylin and eosin × 400)

metaplastic cartilage masses in the synovium. The disease becomes self-limiting and may "burn out" or regress, and the synovium in this stage has been restored to a normal state. The chance of recurrence, therefore, may rest largely on what stage the disease is in at the time of surgery. It is possible, for example, that surgery carried out during the final or late stage will not be followed by recurrence, since no new cartilage nodules are being formed. On the other hand, intra-articular loose bodies may persist and grow larger after synovectomy, necessitating more surgery for their removal even though there may be no new intrasynovial lesions.

INTRACAPSULAR OR PERIARTICULAR CHONDROMA

Intracapsular or periarticular chondroma is an extremely rare lesion. It is thought to occur as a true benign neoplasm of hyaline cartilage and is solitary, extrasynovial, and often well circumscribed. There may be partial ossification of the cartilage mass. It has been seen in the knee as a well-delineated mass, 5 cm or more in diameter, without any history of prior trauma, and may produce mild symptoms of pain, local discomfort, or locking of the joint.[6] If it is excised, there is no recurrence. Chondromas are usually infrapatellar and can be attached to the meniscus (Fig. 108–16). A very large (8 × 5 × 3 cm) partially ossified mass has been reported in the knee of an 86-year-old man and was classified as an intra-articular osteochondroma,[38] although it may represent an intra-articular chondroma. Interestingly, this patient had a history of trauma 39 years before surgery with subsequent joint effusions. At surgery the mass seemed to be nourished by a thin synovial pedicle, and there were no cartilage nodules elsewhere in the joint.

Solitary chondromas have also been described in or near tendon sheaths of the fingers and toes.[39,40] The fingers are more commonly involved (64 percent), particularly the thumb, but lesions in the toes (20 percent) are also seen.[40] The chondromas usually range between 1 and 2 cm in diameter and occur most often in the third and fourth decades. They are usually single, but multiple nodules along a tendon sheath have been described. This latter picture is difficult or impossible to distinguish from tenosynovial chondromatosis and raises the question of whether the chondroma is really a variant of synovial chondromatosis of the fingers or toes. The treatment of choice is local excision; although a recurrence may result, conservative re-excision is still advocated, since these tumors do not metastasize.[33,40]

A variation of solitary chondroma may be the cases of intracapsular chondromas that have been reported in the knees of three members of a family with familial dysplasia epiphysealis hemimelica.[41] There are two other cases in which cartilaginous hamartomas of the volar plates of the proximal and distal interphalangeal joints of the hands and feet were described and were associated

Figure 108–16. An intra-articular solitary chondroma of the knee in the infrapatellar region and represented as a well delineated mass with amorphous dense calcification suggesting mineralized cartilage. (Courtesy of Dr. C. Campbell.)

with peculiar hypertrophic skin lesions of the hand and hemihypertrophy of the limb.[42,43] It is possible that these peculiar cartilaginous lesions represent enzymatic abnormalities in which primitive cartilage tissue persists in joint sites very much akin to the involvement of bones in multiple enchondromatosis (Ollier's disease). Apparently, however, these joint lesions are benign and are completely cured by excision.

VILLONODULAR SYNOVITIS

Villonodular synovitis comprises a group of idiopathic lesions that affect the synovial surface lining joints, tendon sheaths, and bursae through the production of tumor-like growths. Although these lesions may not be true neoplasms, their locally aggressive behavior and capacity to invade bone, joint capsules, tendons, and adjacent soft tissues simulate a neoplastic condition. Despite their destructive tendencies, however, they never metastasize. Included in this group are pigmented villonodular synovitis (localized or diffuse types), localized nodular tenosynovitis, and the rare localized nodular bursitis.

The common histologic denominator of these lesions is the exuberant proliferation of synovial lining cells, both as a surface phenomenon and as a downward invasion into the subsynovial tissue. Such cell growth results in a markedly papillary synovial lining with innumerable finger-like projections, villi, and folds. These projections often fuse into nodules and form confluent lobulated masses admixed with a tangle of hair-like villi. The lesion may be a local phenomenon involving only part of the synovial lining, or it may be extensive with the whole synovial surface affected. Grossly, the lesion most commonly is stained red-brown secondary to extensive hemorrhage with mottled yellow-orange areas caused by lipid-containing macrophages. Since microscopy reveals fibroblasts, polyhedral phagocytic or histiocytic cells, giant cells, and often a mild inflammatory component, some pathologists have called these lesions benign fibrous histiocytomas arising from a synovial lining.[44] However, the prevailing trend is to refrain from using this term because it clearly implies a neoplastic state. As the current terminology is already well accepted by clinicians, the use of this new term would cause undue fear among those not familiar with recent tumor taxonomy.

The etiology of villonodular synovitis is totally unexplained. Experimental models are not convincing, since, although histologically the lesions produced may somewhat resemble the human condition, biologically they are self-limited and resolve when the inducing factor, usually a blood serum component or iron, is stopped. Therefore, the role of simple trauma and subsequent bleeding, leading to the formation of villonodular synovitis, is probably not important. Also, neither hemophiliac patients nor those people with other bleeding disorders have an associated villonodular synovitis despite frequent bouts of joint bleeding and the subsequent development of osteoarthritis with joint destruction. The question of a benign but locally aggressive neoplasm may indeed be a true representation of such lesions, but there is no substantial experimental data confirming this. Furthermore, Jaffe[6] (among others) felt that these lesions were a reactive synovitis to some unknown factor, and he described three sequential stages in their development, confirming, for him at least, their non-neoplastic, reactive nature. According to Jaffe, the earliest lesion is that of synovial cell proliferation causing synovial hypertrophy with villous overgrowth as a beard-like mass which replaces the normal synovial lining. These delicate villi become fused by clotted blood lying in the joint from previous bleeding episodes and subsequent clot organization and fibrosis. The net result is the formation of nodules and matted, confluent synovial projections. Ultimately, the synovial cellular proliferation wanes, and fibrosis with hyalinization occurs, resulting in fibrous nodules firmly adherent to synovial structures. More often than not, all stages of cellular activity are seen in various parts of the involved synovium, although a pre-dominant pattern may be seen in various lesions and may have clinical and radiographic importance. What is implied here is that the fibrous-like stage may represent an end stage of the disease and, therefore, during this period radiographic studies may be unrewarding, clinical signs and symptoms will be minimal, and synovectomy will more than likely be curative. Conversely, according to this viewpoint, if the disease were in an active stage at the time of surgery, recurrences might be more likely. However, basic observations of this type have not been extensive enough to confirm or refute such a clinicopathologic correlation.

Pigmented Villonodular Synovitis. (*Synonyms*: Synovial xanthoma, synovial fibroendothelioma, synovial endothelioma, benign fibrous histiocytoma, xanthomatous giant cell tumor.)

The prototype of the villonodular synovitis group is pigmented villonodular synovitis, which diffusely involves a joint or tendon sheath. However, the term localized nodular synovitis (see below) is used if the disease is confined to one clearly delineated focus of a joint or tendon sheath.

Age and Sex. This form of the disease occurs mostly in young adults.[2,3,5,6,13,44,45] There is an equal distribution between males and females, but some series report either male or female predominance.

Sites. Unilateral involvement of the knee joint is most commonly seen and occurs in about 80 percent of cases.[46] The next most common sites are the hip, ankle, calcaneocuboid joint, elbow, and tendon sheaths of fingers and sometimes toes. Occasionally involvement is seen in the hand, sole of the foot, rather unusual sites such as the temporomandibular joint,[47] and even, rarely, along the posterior elements of the cervical spine. Bursae are rarely involved and no anatomic site in particular is predilected,[6] although the popliteal and iliopectineal bursae and the bursa anserina have been implicated. A diffuse form of the disease seems to be the more common lesion in bursae. The diffuse form may also be seen in the common flexor sheaths of the hand or in the so-called radial and ulnar bursae. There are two reported cases involving the temporomandibular joint in which synovial chondromatosis coexisted with pigmented villonodular synovitis.[29] Occasionally, the disease affects larger tendon sheaths proximal to the ankle or wrist and presents as a soft tissue mass adjacent to a large joint. Of eleven such cases, seven involved the lower extremity and four the upper limb, primarily in middle-aged males.[48] It was thought that the lesions dissected through either a joint capsule or tendon sheath and extended along fascial planes as a soft tissue mass. Apparently surgical excision was curative in these cases, since there were no recurrences over a 2- to 9-year follow-up. If there is extensive hemorrhage in similar soft tissue extensions of pigmented villonodular synovitis, they are often misdiagnosed as vascular hamartomas.[49] Invasion of bone on either side of a joint can also be seen with intra-articular, bursal, or tendon sheath involvement.[50] Rarely, only one bone may be invaded by an intra-articular lesion and may mimic a primary bone tumor on radiographs.[51] Bone erosion can be seen in virtually any site adjacent to pigmented villonodular synovitis.

Clinical Data. The main complaints include pain and mild, intermittent, or repeated bouts of swelling over a long period of time, ranging from many months to as long as a few years, before the patient seeks medical assistance. Sometimes acute, severe pain may occur with locking of the joint and a concurrent effusion. Joint aspiration will yield dark bloody fluid. There is usually no history of trauma or of a bleeding disorder. Repeated episodes of joint effusion with bloody fluid in a young individual are highly suggestive of pigmented villonodular synovitis. Arthroscopic examination is often diagnostic.

Radiologic Features. In at least two thirds of cases, a soft tissue density, which is due to either the lesion or the effusion or both, can be seen on a plain film.[52] Calcification is not found in this entity. Arteriograms are usually striking owing to the prominent vascularity of the lesion. However, cases in which there is essentially no hypervascularity may be seen. Interestingly such a case when examined histologically consists mostly of densely collagenized tissue with few active cellular areas and little vasculature. Bone erosion is uncommon but, if the lesion is intra-articular, usually involves both sides of the joint[51] and typically consists of lytic clusters of well marginated, cyst-like lucencies (Fig. 108–17). In the knee, the intercondylar areas are most frequently involved. Adjacent osteopenia, significant joint destruc-

tion, and periosteal reaction are rare. The joint space is usually preserved until late in the course. However, bone erosion of one side of a joint, particularly the hip and, more rarely, the knee, may be seen and should not be misdiagnosed as a primary bone tumor[51] (Fig. 108–18). The differential diagnosis of a given case might include tuberculosis, which generally has more osteopenia and joint destruction; hemophilia with its more extensive joint destruction; synovial chondromatosis, which may have calcified radiopaque bodies; and rheumatoid arthritis, which has more osteopenia and joint narrowing.

Pathology. Grossly, the synovium in pigmented villonodular synovitis is red-brown to mottled orange-yellow and looks like a plush angora rug. Matted masses of villous projections and synovial folds are prominent and are admixed with sessile or pedunculated, rubbery to soft nodules (0.5 to 2 cm in diameter) enmeshed within the synovial tissue. The synovial membrane is thick and succulent, and is often coated with thin wisps of fibrinous exudate. Fragments of bone and/or cartilage are not present in the synovial lining. Although other conditions such as hemochromatosis and hemosiderosis may similarly stain the synovium, the nodular component is usually absent, and, in addition, microscopic features are definitive for separating these entities (see below). Red-brown or golden-brown tissue may extend deep into

Figure 108–17. Pigmented villonodular synovitis involving the small joints of the foot with multiple bone erosions. There is no calcification present in the lesion.

Figure 108–18. Pigmented villonodular synovitis involving the tibiofibular joint with an adjacent extensive soft tissue mass and eccentric erosion of both bones. The knee joint is normal.

subsynovial structures or invade the joint capsule. If a tendon sheath is involved, a sausage-shaped mass may be evident as the sheath is distended by proliferating synovium. If the joint capsule or tendon sheath is invaded, adjacent soft tissue structures, including nerves and vessels, may be coated by wispy, red-brown tissue. If there is bone erosion, similar tissue may be present near the chondro-osseous junction or wrapped around vascular and ligamentous attachments to bone surfaces, representing entrance points into the bone interior.[51] If there is extensive soft tissue invasion, the lesion may present as a soft to rubbery, red-brown mass with foci of hemorrhagic cysts (Fig. 108–19).

Microscopic examination reveals a marked synovial cell hyperplasia with surface proliferation and, more important, subsynovial invasion by masses of polygonal or round cells with pink cytoplasm and round nuclei (Fig. 108–20). Included within these invasive synovial cells are giant cells (of the osteoclast Touton, or foreign body type), hemosiderin-laden macrophages, and fibroblasts. Hemosiderin can also be seen between cells, in synovial lining cells, and in polygonal cells. Foci of hemorrhage are common and are surrounded peripherally by the giant cells and macrophages. Scattered collections of foamy macrophages (xanthoma cells) filled with lipid are also common (Fig. 108–21). The above-described cells fill the distended synovial villi and cause them to fuse with adjacent villi. The nodules also consist of similar tissue, presumably representing affected villi that have been fused by fibrin plugs and subsequent fibrosis. Slits or clefts between villi are present owing to the persistence of some areas that have not been fused and are still lined by the remaining synovial cells. In some nodules, there may be massive collagen deposition with interlacing bands of fibroblasts and hyalinized foci with little cellular activity except for a few scattered giant cells and macrophages. Often a scant, diffuse

Figure 108–20. A low power view of a synovium that is thickened and thrown into papillary folds by invading synovial lining cells, a characteristic feature of pigmented villonodular synovitis. (Hematoxylin and eosin × 16)

chronic inflammatory component is seen, particularly near hemorrhagic foci. Although pigmented villonodular synovitis is a proliferative lesion, there are very few mitoses present in the synovial cells, and cytologic criteria for malignancy are absent. The differential microscopic features include the fact that in synovial hemochromatosis pigment is found in the synovial lining cells only, and in synovial hemosiderosis secondary to trauma pigment is found only in the synovial lining cells and in macrophages. Furthermore, collections of foam cells, giant cells, and, most importantly, the invasive synovial cells are absent in hemosiderosis and hemochromatosis.

If there is bone erosion, the lesion enters the bone along perivascular foramina or ligamentous attachments to the bone. It is also possible that the chondro-osseous junction at the peripheral portions of the joint is another area of easy access to the bony interior via perivascular paths and soft tissue attachment sites. Pigmented villonodular synovitis may also cause pressure erosion.[51] A biopsy taken from an intraosseous focus may cause

Figure 108–19. The gross specimen of this case shows a large bulky soft tissue mass which is mottled from red to yellow, soft, and focally hemorrhagic. The lesion totally obscures the fibular head and pushes into the soft tissue as a lobulated mass.

Figure 108–21. Pigmented villonodular synovitis with polygonal and round synovial-type cells, hemosiderin-laden macrophages, prominent vascularity, and scattered foam cells (macrophages). (Hematoxylin and eosin × 160)

much confusion, since giant cell tumor of bone may be offered as a diagnostic possibility. This diagnosis should be ruled out by clinical suspicion coupled with the absence of the histologic features typical of giant cell tumor such as random distribution of osteoclastic-type giant cells, the characteristic stromal cells, and the similarity of the nuclei of the giant cells and stromal cells.

Therapy. Total synovectomy should be done whenever possible. Incomplete excision (16 to 48 percent of cases) often leads to recurrences.[46] Recurrent lesions seem to grow faster than the original lesion.[3] Occasionally, radiotherapy (1500 to 3000 r) has been done for extensive lesions with some success because of vascular scarring and fibrosis of the lesion.[3] However, recurrent lesions may necessitate more radical surgery such as ray resection or even amputation, especially if vital structures such as nerves and vessels are surrounded by tumor.

Localized Nodular Synovitis. (*Synonyms*: benign giant cell synovioma, benign synovioma.)

This entity is the localized or focal expression of pigmented villonodular synovitis in which only one area of the synovium is involved. Histologically, it is identical to the nodules of pigmented villonodular synovitis, with the same cellular population, although fibrosis is usually more pronounced. The main difference is that the prominent synovial villi seen in pigmented villonodular synovitis are absent and the localized form is usually represented as a single, large, sessile, or pedunculated, sometimes lobulated nodule or mass (1 to 8 cm in diameter) (Fig. 108–22). It is most common as a unilateral lesion of the knee in mature adults of both sexes.[53]

Symptoms are similar to those of pigmented villonodular synovitis but may be more prolonged and extend over many years. Since it is a focal disease, knee locking may be a prominent feature. Effusions are usually present, and the fluid tends to be less bloody than that in pigmented villonodular synovitis and may even be clear. Radiographs may show a soft tissue density in the joint (Fig. 108–23). In the knee joint, the junction between the capsule and meniscus is a frequent site as well as the intercondylar fossa adjacent to the patella.[6] Occasionally, the mass may twist on its stalk, become infarcted, and present with sudden, acute knee pain (Fig. 108–24). There is usually no bone invasion. A simple excision of the lesion is curative, and, with the increasing use of the arthroscope, the surgical excision may be done through the arthroscope if the lesion is small. The so-called "synovial fibroma" may represent a collagenized and fibrosed localized nodular synovitis.

Localized Nodular Tenosynovitis. (*Synonyms*: giant cell tumor of the tendon sheath, fibroxanthoma of tendon sheath.)

This lesion is almost wholly confined to the tendon sheaths of the hands and feet, with hand involvement being the more common. In fact, the most common mass of the hand is probably localized nodular tenosynovitis (Fig. 108–25). Grossly, it is identical to localized nodular synovitis, while histologically it is virtually identical to pigmented villonodular synovitis.

Localized nodular tenosynovitis occurs mostly in young and middle-aged women (20 to 40 years), often on the flexor surface of the middle or index finger.[3,6,45,54] It also may present on the lateral aspect of a finger or even as a nodular mass on the flexor surface of the wrist, metacarpophalangeal joint, ankle, or toe. If the lesion grows to a large size, any aspect of the finger or toe may be involved. Although multiple lesions may occur, they are distinctly uncommon. Occasionally there is underlying bone erosion (10 percent of cases), since these lesions arise from the synovial tissue lining the tendon sheath.[13] Radiographs generally reveal a soft tissue mass in the region of the tendon. If there is bone involvement, the bone underlying the lesion shows a scooped-out

Figure 108–22. Localized nodular synovitis on cross section with mottled hemorrhagic and yellow soft tissue, similar to a nodule of pigmented villonodular synovitis, with a long stalk. This is typical for this lesion. (Courtesy of Dr. C. Campbell.)

Figure 108–25. Localized nodular tenosynovitis of the distal flexor surface of the fourth finger. Note the distended flattened overlying skin. The mass straddles the distal interphalangeal joint. (Courtesy of Dr. C. Campbell.)

Figure 108–23. Localized nodular synovitis involving the suprapatellar portion of the knee. The lesion is seen as a large elliptical intra-articular soft tissue density.

Figure 108–24. An infarcted localized nodular synovitis which twisted on its stalk. Histologically it was of dense collagen and necrotic hemorrhagic tissue. Grossly the lesion was bright red.

extrinsic excavation rimmed by a sclerotic margin[46] (Fig. 108–26). Symptoms are usually related to the appearance of a slowly enlarging mass which is generally nontender. If large enough, the overlying skin will be stretched and shiny, and there may be some loss of function in the involved digit. If the lesion occurs in a pregnant woman, it may grow more rapidly and be of great concern to the patient.

The gross pathology is that of a multinodular round, rubbery mass, generally not larger than 5 cm in diameter, which is firmly attached but easily peeled off the involved tendon. At surgery the lesion may "pop out" of the incision as an "encapsulated mass," although careful attention should be paid to the external surface of the mass because the lesion may infiltrate the adjacent structures and not be truly encapsulated. Lesions in the ankle or foot tend to be larger than those occurring in the hand. The cut surface ranges from hues of yellow to orange-brown, depending upon the amount of lipid and blood pigments. Often there are cross bands and septa of white fibrous tissue traversing softer, yellow foci, and there may be foci of hemorrhage as well. Cyst-like spaces are unusual. The histology is virtually identical to that of pigmented villonodular synovitis, although there may be more fibrosis and a rare mitosis may also be seen (Fig. 108–27). Electron microscopic findings and cell

Figure 108–26. A localized nodular tenosynovitis of the middle second phalanx with pressure erosion of the flexor aspect of the middle phalanx. There is a scalloped, well marginated bone lesion, including a more distal subcortical cyst.

Figure 108–27. A low power view of localized nodular tenosynovitis to emphasize the relatively good delineation of the mass from adjacent soft tissue and the broad bands of collagen transversing the lesion. Note the scattered osteoclast-type giant cells. (Hematoxylin and eosin × 160)

cultures suggest that these lesions develop from synovial and extrasynovial histiocytes.[54,55] The differential diagnosis includes the possibility of pigmented villonodular synovitis, since the latter may extend along tendon sheaths from a nearby joint and should be ruled out by clinical, radiographic, and surgical observations. If there are multiple lesions, especially if the Achilles and extensor tendons have multiple masses, xanthoma tuberosum multiplex with associated hypercholesterolemia must be ruled out.

The treatment of choice is conservative surgical excision, which is usually curative. These lesions can recur, however, if incompletely excised (16 to 48 percent of cases), although they never metastasize.[46]

Recently, an entity termed "fibroma of tendon sheath" has been described from the files spanning 30 years at the Armed Forces Institute of Pathology[45,56] These lesions (77 cases) are well circumscribed masses composed of dense fibrous stroma with hyaline foci and prominent dilated vessels. They occur at any age but mostly in the third and fourth decades (age 4 to 63, with a median age of 30) and mostly in males by more than 3 to 1 (59 males, 18 females). The sites of involvement include the fingers (48 percent), wrist (25 percent), forearm (10 percent), and feet and ankles (8 percent). They present as slow-growing, usually asymptomatic masses which have been present from 3 weeks to 6 years (average 8 months) and are easily removed by local excision with about a 5 percent recurrence rate. At present, it is unclear whether this is truly a new lesion or is a variant of neurofibroma, nodular fasciitis, fibromatosis, or localized nodular tenosynovitis with extensive fibrosis.

TENOSYNOVIAL SARCOMA

In virtually all discussions dealing with tumors of joints there is mention of various types of rather rare malignant soft tissue neoplasms, particularly synovial sarcoma. This confusion occurs because (as the name implies) these tumors are thought to arise from the synovium lining joints, bursae, or tendon sheaths. However, joint involvement, when it occurs, is rare and is always from a primary tumor of the adjacent soft tissue which has extended into the joint or tendon sheath. In other words, such malignant tumors have never definitively been demonstrated to arise within a joint or tendon sheath, and, in fact, rarely involve these structures. Furthermore, the histogenesis of these neoplasms has never been proved to be from synovial lining tissue, and, therefore, their classification is based on some morphologic similarities to synovial cells. Thus, such names as synovial sarcoma and various tendon sheath sarcomas may be misnomers. Included in the tenosynovial sarcoma group of tumors are three main subtypes of sarcomas, called synovial sarcoma (which can be further classified into biphasic tumors and monophasic spindle and epithelial-like tumors), clear cell sarcoma, and epithelioid sarcoma. This group is best discussed under the inclusive term of tenosynovial sarcomas, since they have similar histologic, electron microscopic, tissue culture, histochemical, and biologic features and often arise near tendons, joints, bursae, fascia, and aponeuroses.[57] The term tenosynovial sarcoma has an additional advantage, since many soft tissue tumors are not easily classified but share some features with the various subtypes subsumed under this term. The prevailing thought is that a primitive mesenchymal cell with the ability to modulate into any one of a number of soft tissue components with similar functions and cellular composition, such as tendon sheath lining cells, is the histogenic cell of these neoplasms. Therefore, the histologic pattern of these tumors varies over a wide spectrum from an undifferentiated monophasic cellular pattern at one end to a biphasic differentiated pattern at the other.

There are some biologic features of tenosynovial sarcomas that are worth emphasizing before discussing each tumor subtype.[58] The overall 5-year survival rate is about 40 percent. The prognosis is better if the tumor is small so that almost 75 percent of the patients with small tumors (less than 5 cm) survive 5 years and only 25 percent of patients with large sarcomas survive 5 years. Children and elderly patients have a more favorable prognosis. However, there is also a 60 percent recurrence rate after wide excision. A peculiar feature of these tumors is their propensity to metastasize to regional lymph nodes (15 percent) and bone (10 percent). Patients who die of their disease, usually within 2 years of diagnosis, develop massive pulmonary metastases. Those patients who have a biphasic tumor or epithelioid sarcoma tend to have a slightly better prognosis than those who have monophasic undifferentiated tumors with 5-year survivals for the former group approaching 60 percent, although their 10-year survival is only about 25 percent. The most common sites include the extremities, particularly the lower extremity (90 percent), but the neck, back, pelvis, and groin can also be involved. Biphasic tumors tend to occur near big joints such as the knee, and monophasic tumors are more likely to be deep soft tissue tumors. Most epithelioid and clear cell sarcomas are superficially located on a limb. Prognosis is also influenced by the duration of symptoms; the longer the symptoms, the worse the prognosis, so that those patients with symptoms greater than 1 year have a grave prognosis. The majority of patients, about 50 percent, are between 16 and 36 years of age, and although there is slight predominance of males, female patients predominate in the first and seventh decades. Furthermore, female patients tend to do slightly better than males, since they have mostly superficially located tumors.

The treatment of choice seems to be a team approach, using preoperative radiation therapy followed by surgery consisting of either a wide en bloc local excision or amputation. Although these tumors may have regional node metastases, regional node dissections do not seem to significantly affect prognosis. A re-excision or amputation of recurrent tumor tends to better the prognosis for both small and large tumors. There is recent evidence that resection of pulmonary metastases may prolong

survival as well.[59] The most important factor influencing prognosis is the initial treatment of the tumor. The symptoms are invariably those of a slow-growing painless mass which may be present for months before the patient seeks medical help. Unfortunately, there is a common trap which leads to an all-too-familiar pattern of inadequate initial therapy. The lesion is incompletely excised because it looks very innocuous at surgery, often being well delineated and easily "shelled out" from its site. It is only after this procedure that the diagnosis is made by the pathologist, and the realization that tumor tissue is left behind then prompts further treatment. However, some clinicians may delay any further treatment and the patient might be followed until the appearance of recurrences, which will invariably develop, and only then will more extensive surgery be performed. Therefore, most tenosynovial sarcomas have had initially incomplete surgical therapy, which condemns the patient to a poor prognosis and recurrent tumor. Ideally, a soft tissue tumor should be biopsied soon after its appearance in such a manner that the biopsy tract can be excised with the tumor. After the pathologist makes the diagnosis, radiation therapy and early definitive surgery should be carried out. The surgeon's *suspicion* and *awareness* of the existence of such tumors before any therapy is administered are likely to be the best insurance for a better prognosis.

Recently a new system for the surgical staging of soft tissue sarcomas has been introduced.[60] Such a system will standardize the type of surgery performed and evaluate such pretreatment features as the grade of tumor (degree of cytologic atypicality), site of lesion, and biologic behavior (presence or absence of metastases) before surgery is to be performed. As illustrated in Table 108–1, all tumors are graded according to their histologic grade (low grade, G_1, or high grade, G_2), anatomic site (intracompartmental, T1, or extracompartmental, T2), and presence of metastases (M_0, no metastases, or M_1, metastatic disease). Therefore, a low-grade, intracompartmental tumor without metastases is a stage IA tumor. However, if it extends into another anatomic compartment it becomes a stage IB lesion. All high-grade tumors are a stage II lesion, and if any lesion has metastatic foci, it becomes a stage III tumor regardless of grade or site.

The surgical procedures for soft tissue tumors are divided into four categories based on the surgical margin to the neoplasm. These are summarized in Table 108–2. It is hoped that with this systematic approach, joining

Table 108–1. Surgical Stages*

Stage	Grade	Site
IA	Low (G_1)	Intracompartmental (T_1)
IB	Low (G_1)	Extracompartmental (T_2)
IIA	High (G_2)	Intracompartmental (T_1)
IIB	High (G_2)	Extracompartmental (T_2)
III	Any (G) regional or distant metastasis	Any (T)

*Reprinted Clin. Ortho. Rel. Res. 153:106, 1980.

Table 108–2. Surgical Margins*†

Type	Plane of Dissection	Result
Intralesional	Piecemeal debulking or curettage	Leaves macroscopic disease
Marginal	Shell out en bloc through pseudocapsule or reactive zone	May leave either "satellite" or "skip" lesions
Wide	Intracompartmental en bloc with cuff of normal tissue	May leave "skip" lesions
Radical	Extracompartmental en bloc with entire compartment	No residual lesions

*Reprinted from Clin. Ortho. Rel. Res. 153:106, 1980.
†The plane of dissection used to achieve a particular margin is shown as well as the result of that margin in terms of residual lesion remaining in the wound.

otherwise standard surgical procedures as well as linking radiotherapy and chemotherapy with this staging system, will support the development of a universal language for staging and treatment so that accurate evaluations of tenosynovial tumors will be forthcoming.

SYNOVIAL SARCOMA

(*Synonyms*: Malignant synovioma, monophasic synovial sarcoma, biphasic synovial sarcoma.)

The synovial sarcoma is the best known and described neoplasm included in the tenosynovial sarcoma group, but is still a rare lesion, accounting for 3 to 10 percent of soft tissue sarcoma.[61-64] This lesion is the prototype for neoplasms of synovial cell origin, and classically has a biphasic pattern, which to some pathologists is reminiscent of early joint development with large polygonal cells secreting hyaluronic acid and lining a microscopic joint space, together with spindle-shaped stromal cells representing more primitive undifferentiated cells. Since either one of these two cell populations may predominate, synovial sarcoma is now further subdivided into a monophasic spindle cell type and a monophasic epithelioid type. Earlier descriptions of this tumor attest to its wide range of morphology because such names as adenosarcoma and synovial fibrosarcoma were used until the term synovial sarcoma was first introduced in 1936.[65]

Age and Sex. These tumors occur equally in each sex and are a disease of young adults. The majority of people afflicted (75 percent) are less than 50 years old, with a mean age of 32 years, but the tumors occur at virtually any age, including in children. A single congenital case has also been reported.[44]

Sites. Synovial sarcoma is almost exclusively (95 percent) found on the extremities, especially the lower limb (70 percent) and frequently near large joints, particularly the popliteal area of the knee and the foot.[2,3,5,44,45] Regions of the thigh, hand, leg, and even digits may be affected, however, and in these regions the tumors often are adjacent to joint capsules and/or tendon sheaths. On the upper limb, distal involvement is more common than arm or elbow sites. Tumors are less commonly seen in the neck,[66,67] torso, nasopharynx, chest, abdominal wall, retroperitoneal region,[62] orbit,[67] tongue[67] and soft palate,[68] and at the bifurcation of the carotid artery.[69] These rarer sites suggest an undifferentiated mesenchymal cell origin for these tumors, since they are not near joints or synovium. Interestingly, most of the synovial sarcomas in the neck tend to occur in the late teenage years and in the early third decade.[66,68]

Clinical Data. The most common complaint is the awareness of a painless, slow-growing mass that has been present from a period of months to 2 to 3 years, but in some cases the tumor has been present for as long as 26 years.[70] Pain or tenderness may occur in 25 to 60 percent of cases. If the tumor is located within the deeper portions of the soft tissues, the delay in diagnosis and treatment is longer than with the more superficial and clinically noticeable lesions. In some cases involving the knee region, vague mild pain over several months may occur before a mass is appreciated. Head and neck lesions produce symptoms related to their specific sites such as hoarseness and breathing or swallowing difficulties. If the tumor is large, limitation of motion may finally occur. Rarely, a patient may present with symptoms secondary to pulmonary metastases, such as hemoptysis.[63] The mean survival time from the appearance of symptoms to death is about 7 years.

Radiographic Findings. Synovial sarcoma is one of the few primary soft tissue tumors that may have speckled calcifications on radiographs, and these are present in about a third of the cases (Fig. 108–28). The radiologic differential diagnosis should include soft tissue chondrosarcoma, mesenchymal chondrosarcoma, hemangioma, lipoma, and even synovial chondromatosis. It is typically a well-delineated, homogeneous soft tissue mass, 2 to 20 cm in diameter, which may erode into an adjacent bone (10 percent of cases) or stimulate a mild periosteal bone reaction (Fig. 108–29). To assess the size of the tumor, however, arteriography and xerography may be more helpful, although arteriography may not be particularly rewarding in some cases since these tumors have a variable amount of vascularity. The adjacent joint is almost always normal.

Pathology. The gross pathology of synovial sarcoma is invariably a well-demarcated, pink to yellow, rather fleshy mass that easily detaches or "shells out" from its tumor bed. This "pseudoencapsulation" often leads the surgeon down the path of false security, and an incomplete excision is performed as the initial therapy. The cut surface is usually uniform, gray-yellow, and rubbery. If calcification is present, the tumor may be gritty. In larger tumors, areas of hemorrhage and/or necrosis with cystification and gelatinous breakdown of tissue may also be seen. Occasionally infiltrating tumors are seen with interdigitating tongues of tumor between tendons, muscle, and fascial planes or wrapped around neurovascular bundles (Fig. 108–30). Extension into a joint is rare.

Figure 108–28. Synovial sarcoma in the soft tissues of the calf represented in these multiple views as a large soft tissue density with amorphous speckled and nodular calcifications. There is slight pressure erosion of the medial aspect of the fibula.

Synovial sarcoma is subtyped into three patterns based on the predominant microscopic findings. These types are monophasic spindle cell synovial sarcoma, monophasic epithelial-like or pseudoglandular synovial sarcoma, and biphasic synovial sarcoma. Obviously, there is some subjectivity in the use of such a classification system, since many of these tumors have a variable histologic picture, and this has prompted some pathologists to abandon any subtyping of these tumors. Furthermore, some pathologists will not make the diagnosis of monophasic synovial sarcoma, particularly since the spindle cell type is often indistinguishable from a fibrosarcoma. However, a useful differential observation is that marked cellular pleomorphism and atypia

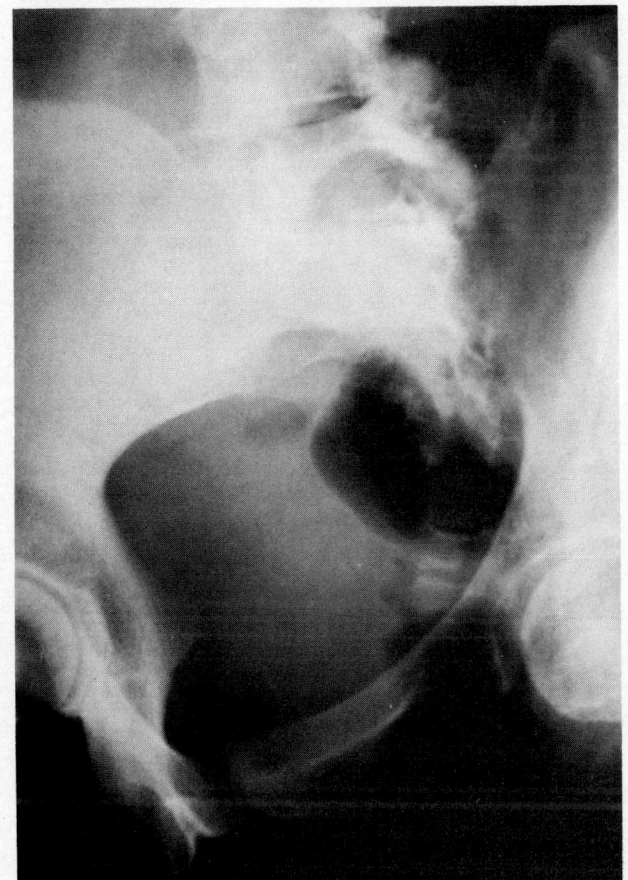

Figure 108–29. Another synovial sarcoma involving the sacrum and ilium on both sides of the sacroiliac joint. The large soft tissue component is not well seen. In contrast to the previous case, there are no soft tissue calcifications.

Figure 108–30. Low power view of a synovial sarcoma to point out the highly cellular tongues of tumor that push out into the soft tissue. If this lesion were "shelled-out," a recurrence surely would follow. (Hematoxylin and eosin × 36)

are usually not present in synovial sarcoma and, when present, tend to point to some other type of neoplasm such as a high grade fibrosarcoma. Electron microscopy and tissue culture observations indicate some unifying and common features to both cell types composing synovial sarcoma.[66,71] These include a distinct basal lamina between epithelial and stromal cells and specialized cell junctions, such as desmosomes and maculae adherentes, which are present mostly between epithelial cells but also between some stromal cells. The epithelial cells may also have microvilli, intercellular spaces, free ribosomes, arrays of endoplasmic reticulum, prominent Golgi apparatuses, and small vesicles (Figs. 108–31 and 108–32). The spindle cells secrete amorphous extracellular fibrils without periodicity and possess microfibrils. There are usually few recognizable collagen fibrils. Since most of these features are nonspecific and may be found in many cells of the body, as such they do not necessarily support the view that synovial sarcoma represents a neoplasm of a primitive ancestor cell committed to modulate into synovial tissue. In tissue culture, both cell types make mucopolysaccharides, a feature that synovium shares with other mesenchymal tissues.[13]

Monophasic spindle cell synovial sarcoma is a tumor composed of whirling interdigitating bundles of elongated cells with little cytoplasm and large elliptical nuclei. There is usually little atypia, mitoses may be plentiful, and a small amount of collagen production is evident (Fig. 108–33). Rarely, small, narrow slit-like spaces or clefts may be present which are not lined by cells. Such spaces are thought to represent primitive joint spaces and may stain positively for hyaluronic acid with periodic acid–Schiff (PAS), alcian blue (acidic pH), or mucicarmine stains. This staining disappears with hyaluronidase digestion.

Figure 108–32. Higher power electron microscopic print of synovial sarcoma. The abutting cell borders have frequent junctions. The cytoplasm contains a background of free ribosomes and scattered microfilaments. Moderate numbers of mitochondria and cisternae of rough endoplasmic reticulum are usually localized in one end of the cell, and cisternae are slightly dilated and contain a material of medium electron density. ($\times$ 4300)

Figure 108–31. Lower power electron microscopic print of a synovial sarcoma. The neoplastic cells are polygonal and slightly elongate and have abutting cell borders. There is a high nuclear-cytoplasmic ratio, and prominent nucleoli are sometimes visible. ($\times$ 3260)

Figure 108–33. Synovial sarcoma, monophasic spindle cell type, with interdigitating fascicles of spindle cells. The cells have plump nuclei, little cytoplasm, and very little collagen production. (Hematoxylin and eosin $\times$ 400)

Monophasic epithelial-like or pseudoglandular synovial sarcoma is made up of large polygonal or oval cells with a poorly defined cytoplasm. The single nucleus is large, oval, and pale staining. Cellular pleomorphism is frequently prominent (Fig. 108–34). The cells are arranged in nests or small sheets and line slits, tubules, and gland-like spaces that lack basement membranes, and are often filled with mucicarmine and PAS-positive fluid, which no longer stains by these methods after hyaluronidase digestion. Similar intracellular granules are also seen.

The biphasic synovial sarcoma is a mixture of the aforementioned two cellular patterns (Fig. 108–35). All subtypes of synovial sarcomas may show small foci of calcification as well as blood vessel invasion, scattered giant cells, focal necrosis, and a scattered mast cell infiltration among the tumor cells.

Prognosis and Therapy. The overall 5-year survival rate for all types of synovial sarcoma is about 36 percent[72] and is slightly higher (47 percent) for tumors in the neck.[66] The 10-year survival rate is more distressing, however, since only 10 to 27 percent of patients remain alive for that length of time.[65] The clinical course is one of recurrent tumor and, ultimately, metastases to regional lymph nodes (12 to 37 percent), lungs, pleuropericardium, chest wall, bones (lytic lesions, usually of the axial skeleton), skin, and brain.[73] Interestingly, liver metastases are distinctly unusual. About 10 percent of patients die within 1 year after diagnosis with metastatic disease, 90 percent of whom will have massive pulmonary metastases.

There are a number of factors that may influence prognosis. The histologic type of synovial sarcoma seems to be of considerable importance. The monophasic spindle cell type has the best 5-year survival (56 to 59 percent), followed by the biphasic type (29 to 50 percent). The worst prognosis is found with the monophasic epithelial type (12 to 36 percent).[65] There does not seem

Figure 108–35. Synovial sarcoma with a biphasic pattern of spindle cells and epithelial-like cells arranged around gland-like spaces. Mitoses are evident and the lumens of the pseudoglands contain hyaluronic acid. (Hematoxylin and eosin × 400)

to be any correlation with the relative amounts of the two cell types in the biphasic tumors. Histologic grading of these tumors, not usually done by pathologists, also seems to play a prognostic role. Grading based on cell maturation, cellular atypism, mitotic index, and cellularity indicates that most patients with high-grade tumors die within 5 years, whereas those with low-grade lesions have better survivals. As noted above for tenosynovial sarcomas as a group, small tumor size, a peripheral site, and prompt recognition of the tumor with subsequent wide excision or amputation in conjunction with radiotherapy are factors that favorably alter the prognosis. As stated earlier, however, the greatest factor influencing prognosis is the long delay between symptoms and treatment and the inadequate initial surgery which leads to recurrent tumor and vascular invasion.

CLEAR CELL SARCOMA

The clear cell sarcoma was first described in 1965 as a tumor thought to arise from tendons and aponeuroses.[74] It is a rare tumor that occurs at any age, although mostly in the third decade, and is equally divided among the sexes. It primarily affects the extremities, particularly the lower limb, with parts of the foot being the most commonly involved (heel, toes, ankle). The tumor grows as a painless, slowly enlarging lump over months to years. The hallmark of this lesion is a cell population of clear, fusiform to polygonal cells with pale nuclei and prominent acidophilic nucleoli. The cells are arranged in nests or clusters and are surrounded by fine reticulum (Fig. 108–36). Scattered giant cells may be found. About two thirds of the tumors are positive for intracytoplasmic glycogen, and a substantial number have been demonstrated to contain melanin granules.[8] Incomplete excision is common owing to the tumor's propensity to invade tendons and extend along fascial planes, and the

Figure 108–34. Synovial sarcoma, monophasic epithelial-like cells with sheets of polygonal or oval cells with indistinct cytoplasmic borders. There is slight nuclear pleomorphism. (Hematoxylin and eosin × 400)

Figure 108–36. Clear cell sarcoma with a rather uniform population of polygonal cells, each with clear cytoplasm, a pale oval nucleus, and a prominent nucleolus. (Hematoxylin and eosin × 400)

clinical course is most often characterized by recurrences and/or metastases over several years and, ultimately, death.

Since the description of this unusual tumor many investigators have reported similar cases with particular attention paid to the presence of melanin granules.[75-80] Electron microscopic findings confirm the presence of melanosomes and point to a neural crest origin for these tumors. Implicit in this idea is the possibility that these lesions may represent soft tissue malignant melanomas since they have melanosomes. If one looks at all the data related to these tumors, however, including their histologic features, one is struck by the great similarities between these tumors and synovial sarcoma, particularly the monophasic epithelial-like subgroup. Those tumors that produce melanin probably represent malignant melanoma, either metastases from skin lesions which are not apparent or primary soft tissue melanomas of neural crest origin.

EPITHELIOID SARCOMA

Another recently described (1961) soft tissue malignant tumor is epithelioid sarcoma.[81] The name is derived from the microscopic findings, which at first glance resemble epithelioid cells seen in granulomatous reactions.[82] This tumor is also thought to arise from synovial tissue lining tendons, since it is intimately associated with tendons and aponeuroses. It rarely invades into joints. Electron microscopic findings suggest that the tumor is also a variant of synovial sarcoma.[83,84] Such findings include the presence of two cell types similar to the epithelial and spindle cells of synovial sarcoma with such structures as desmosomes and maculae adherentes, the production of mucopolysaccharide, and the existence of light and dark cells like those seen in normal synovial tissue. This tumor occurs mostly on the hand, wrist, or forearm. Rare cases elsewhere have been re-

ported (penis, scalp, neck, vulva, abdomen).[84] The vast majority of cases (63 percent) occur between the ages of 20 and 40, with an average age of 29 at the time the patient presents to a physician with symptoms.[85] The tumor seems to be slightly more common in males. The clinical course is one of insidious but relentless, painless growth of a mass or a series of lumps culminating in loss of function of the affected anatomy, e.g., finger movements. Some tumors will cause overlying skin ulceration, and this feature coupled with the histology of large epithelioid cells often leads to the erroneous diagnosis of squamous cell carcinoma. A linear pattern of subcutaneous lumps may also be seen in longstanding lesions, indicating either invasion along tendons or vascular and/or lymphatic extension. Deep and large lesions may extend into adjacent bone.

The microscopic pattern characteristic of this tumor is one of multiple nodules with central necrosis (Figs. 108–37 and 108–38). The nodules are composed of oval to polyhedral cells with well-defined borders and dense eosinophilic cytoplasm which may be vacuolated. The nuclei are vesicular with prominent nucleoli; mitoses are uncommon. Binucleate and multinucleate giant cells are present in half of the cases. The so-called malignant giant cell or large cell tumors of tendon sheath represent epithelioid sarcomas with a prominent giant cell population[86,87] and ultrastructural features similar to synovial sarcoma.[87] Spindle cells and some clear cells resembling elements of the biphasic synovial sarcoma are also admixed in clusters or arranged in single file cords of cells like those seen with carcinoma cells. Calcification may be present (25 percent of cases). Recurrent tumors tend to have more pleomorphism and higher mitotic counts. Factors that adversely affect prognosis include blood vessel invasion, the appearance of recurrent tumors, and the presence of regional lymph node metastases. In general, the overall 5-year survival rate is about 60 percent, but the 10-year survival is about 27 percent, approximately equal to that of synovial sar-

Figure 108–37. Epithelioid sarcoma with the characteristic nodular and scarring pattern and central necrosis resembling superficially a granulomatous reaction. (Hematoxylin and eosin × 46)

Figure 108–38. Epithelioid sarcoma with cellular pleomorphism, mitoses, spindle and epithelial-like cells with vesicular nuclei, and focal scarring. (Hematoxylin and eosin × 375)

coma. The average time between symptoms and death is 7 years.

Between 67 and 92 percent of cases will have recurrent tumors secondary to incomplete initial surgical excision, and at least half of these cases will have multiple recurrences.[85] A third of cases will develop metastases to regional lymph nodes and/or lungs. The worst single finding among those which adversely affect prognosis is vascular invasion. Therefore, the recommended therapy is early radical surgery consisting of either a wide en bloc excision or amputation.

SECONDARY TUMORS OF SYNOVIUM AND "PSEUDOTUMORS"

The synovium, like other highly vascular tissues, may be the site of metastatic carcinoma. The relative rarity of such a finding may reflect the fact that only clinical cases in which joint symptoms prevail are reported, since at autopsy joints are usually not examined routinely. Metastatic adenocarcinoma from the colon that simulated an acute arthritis has been described, as well as metastatic carcinoma from the breast and lung.[88-90] Lymphoproliferative diseases, including leukemia, may also invade the synovium and mimic other conditions such as rheumatoid arthritis.[91] Primary bone tumors such as osteogenic sarcoma, chondrosarcoma, and giant cell tumor can directly invade the joint capsule and synovium as a late event in their clinical course. Virtually any of the tenosynovial sarcomas may invade a joint by direct extension from the soft tissues, but this is an uncommon event.

There are occasions when the clinical signs and symptoms point to an intra-articular mass and at surgery a hemorrhagic boggy synovial mass is found. Such cases invariably occur after some traumatic event with subsequent joint swelling. The knee is particularly suscep-

tible to this process, and often the "tumor" is a hemorrhagic mass of fat tissue which was dislocated and wedged between the articular surfaces.[92] However, even the small joints of the hands may have post-traumatic synovial hemorrhage simulating a synovial mass.[93] Also, it is worth recalling that torsion of a nodule of pigmented villonodular synovitis or localized nodular synovitis with subsequent infarction can lead to hemorrhage and worsening of symptoms, prompting a hasty and frantic visit to the physician. The pathologist may see only necrotic hemorrhagic tissue with only the vaguest outline of the underlying architecture needed to make the correct diagnosis. Other conditions that may cause concern and confusion with joint masses are pseudogout, various synovial cysts, para-articular ganglia, and tumoral calcinosis, all of which have characteristic microscopic features that should be recognized by the competent pathologist.

References

1. Case Records of the Massachusetts General Hospital: Case 43-1983. N. Engl. J. Med. 309:1042, 1983.
2. Lichtenstein, L.: Bone Tumors. 2nd ed. St. Louis, C. V. Mosby Company, 1959.
3. Rodnan, G.P.: Tumors of synovial joints, bursae and tendon sheaths. In Hollander, J.E. (ed.): Arthritis and Allied Conditions. A Textbook of Rheumatology. 7th ed. Philadelphia, Lea & Febiger, 1966.
4. Pudlowski, R.M., Gilula, L.A., and Kyriakos, M.: Intra-articular lipoma with osseous metaplasia: Radiographic-pathologic correlation. Am. J. Roentgenol. 132:471, 1979.
5. Collins, D.H.: Pathology of Bone. London, Butterworths, 1966.
6. Jaffe, H.L.: Tumors and Tumorous Conditions of the Bones and Joints. Philadelphia, Lea & Febiger, 1958.
7. Resnick, D., and Oliphant, M.: Hemophilia-like arthropathy of the knee associated with cutaneous and synovial hemangioma. Diag. Radiol. 114:323, 1975.
8. Zvantseva, V.A.: Hemangioma of the synovial membrane of the knee joint. Vestn. Khir. 1178:52, 1976.
9. Mulder, J.W.: Hemangioma in the knee joint. Arch. Chir. Neerl. 24:135, 1972.
10. Larsen, E.: Synovial hemangioma in the elbow joint. Ugeskr. Laeger 137:1199, 1975.
11. Cooper, G., and Schiller, A.L.: Anatomy of the Guinea Pig. Cambridge, Mass., Harvard University Press, 1975.
12. Symeonides, P.P., and Ioannides, G.: Ossicles in the knee menisci. Report of three cases. J. Bone Joint Surg. 54A:1288, 1972.
13. Spjut, H.J., Dorfman, H.D., Fechner, R.E., and Ackerman, L.V.: Tumors of Bone and Cartilage, Atlas of Tumor Pathology, Fascicle 5. Washington, D.C., Armed Forces Institute of Pathology, 1971.
14. Murphy, F.P., Dahlin, D.C., and Sullivan, C.R.: Articular synovial chondromatosis. J. Bone Joint Surg. 44:77, 1962.
15. Dahlin, D.C.: Bone Tumors. General Aspects and Data on 6,221 Cases. 3rd ed. Springfield, Ill. Charles C Thomas, 1978.
16. Jacob, R.A., Campbell, W.P., and Niemann, K.M.W.: Synovial chondrometaplasia. A case report. Clin. Orthop. 109:152, 1975.
17. Giustra, P.E., Furman, R.S., Roberts, L., and Killoran, P.J.: Synovial osteochondromatosis involving the elbow. Am. J. Roentgenol. 127:347, 1976.
18. Varma, B.P., and Ramakrishna, Y.J.: Synovial chondromatosis of the shoulder. Aust. N. Z. J. Surg. 46:14, 1976.
19. Holm, C.L.: Primary synovial chondromatosis of the ankle. A case report. J. Bone Joint Surg. 58A:878, 1976.
20. Szepesi, J.: Synovial chondromatosis of the metacarpophalangeal joint. Acta Orthop. Scand. 46:926, 1975.
21. Lyritis, G.: Synovial chondromatosis of the inferior radio-ulnar joint. Acta Orthop. Scand. 47:373, 1976.
22. Lomba, J.A., Cabanas, R., and Marrero, I.: Synovial chondrometaplasia of the temporomandibular joint: Report of case. J. Oral Surg. 35:674, 1977.
23. Rosen, P.S., Pritzkey, P.H., Greenbaum, J., Holgate, R.C., and Noyek, A.M.: Synovial chondromatosis affecting the temporomandibular joint. Case report and literature review. Arthritis Rheum. 20:736, 1977.
24. Noyek, A.M., Holgate, R.C., Fireman, S.M., Rosen, P., and Pritzker,

K.P.: The radiologic findings in synovial chondromatosis (chondrometaplasia) of the temporomandibular joint. J. Otolaryngol. 6:45, 1977.

25. Tasanen, A., Lamberg, M.A., and Kotilainen, R.: Osteochondromatosis of the temporomandibular joint. Report of a case. Oral Surg. 38:845, 1974.

26. Jokinen, K., Stenback, F., Palva, A., and Sutinen, S.: Benign cartilaginous tumor of the temporomandibular joint. J. Laryngol. Otol. 90:299, 1976.

27. Ballard, R., and Weiland, L.H.: Synovial chondromatosis of the temporomandibular joint. Cancer 30:791, 1972.

28. Schiano, A., Acquaviva, P., and Serratrice, G.: Diabetes and synovial chondromatosis (author's translation). Diabete Metab. 2:183, 1976.

29. Raibley, S.O.: Villonodular synovitis with synovial chondromatosis. Oral Surg. 44:279, 1977.

30. Christensen, J.H., and Poulsen, J.O.: Synovial chondromatosis. Acta Orthop. Scand. 46:919, 1975.

31. Ellman, M.H., Krieger, M.I., and Brown, N.: Pseudogout mimicking synovial chondromatosis. J. Bone Joint Surg. 57A:863, 1975.

32. Dahlin, D.C., and Salvador, A.H.: Cartilage tumors of the soft tissues of the hands and feet. Mayo Clin. Proc. 49:721, 1974.

33. Alled, C.D. and Gondos, B.: Ultrastructure of synovial chondromatosis. Arch. Pathol. Lab. Med. 106:688, 1982.

34. Dunn, A.W., and Whisler, J.H.: Synovial chondromatosis of the knee with associated extracapsular chondromas. J. Bone Joint Surg. 55A:1747, 1973.

35. Richter, K.J., Freeman, N.S., and Quick, C.A.: Chondrosarcoma of the temporomandibular joint: Report of a case. J. Oral Surg. 32:777, 1974.

36. Milgram, J.W., and Addison, R.G.: Synovial osteochondromatosis of the knee. Chondromatous recurrence with possible chondrosarcomatous degeneration. J. Bone Joint Surg. 58A:264, 1976.

37. Milgram, J.W.: Synovial osteochondromatosis: A histologic study of 30 cases. J. Bone Joint Surg. 59A:792, 1977.

38. Sarmiento, A., and Elkins, R.W.: Giant intra-articular osteochondroma of the knee. J. Bone Joint Surg. 57A:560, 1975.

39. Someren, A., and Merritt, W.H.: Tenosynovial chondroma of the hand. A case report with a brief review of the literature. Hum. Pathol. 9:476, 1978.

40. Chung, E.B., and Enzinger, F.M.: Chondroma of soft parts. Cancer 41:1414, 1978.

41. Hensinger, R.N., Cowell, H.R., Ramsey, P.L., and Leopold, R.G.: Familial dysplasia epiphysealis hemimelica associated with chondromas and osteochondromas. Report of a kindred with variable presentations. J. Bone Joint Surg. 56A:1513, 1974.

42. Heiple, K.G., and Elmer, R.M.: Chondromatous hamartomas arising from the volar digital plates. A case report. J. Bone Joint Surg. 54A:393, 1972.

43. Hensinger, R.N., and Rhyne, D.H.: Multiple chondromatous hamartomas. Report of a case. J. Bone Joint Surg. 56A:1068, 1974.

44. Stout, A.P., and Lattes, R.: Tumors of the Soft Tissues, Atlas of Tumor Pathology, Fascicle, 1. Washington, D.C., Armed Forces Institute of Pathology, 1967.

45. Enzinger, F.M., and Weiss, S.W.: Soft Tissue Tumors. St. Louis, C.V. Mosby, 1983.

46. Byers, P.D., Cotten, R.E., Deacon, O.W., Lowy, M., Newman, P.H., Sissons, H.A., and Thomas, A.D.: The diagnosis and treatment of pigmented villonodular synovitis, J. Bone Joint Surg. 50B:290, 1968.

47. Miyamoto, Y., Tani, T., and Hamaya, K.: Pigmented villonodular synovitis of the temporomandibular joint. Case report. Plast. Reconstr. Surg. 59:283, 1977.

48. Arthand, J.B.: Pigmented nodular synovitis. Report of 11 lesions in nonarticular locations. Am. J. Clin. Pathol. 58:511, 1972.

49. Burnett, R.A.: A cause of erroneous diagnosis of pigmented villonodular synovitis. J. Clin. Pathol. 29:17, 1976.

50. Kindbloom, K.G., and Gunterverg, B.: Pigmented villonodular synovitis involving bone. Case report. J. Bone Joint Surg. 60A:830, 1978.

51. Jergensen, H.E., Mankin, H.J., and Schiller, A.L.: Diffuse pigmented villonodular synovitis mimicking primary bone neoplasm. A report of 2 cases. J. Bone Joint Surg. 60A:830, 1978.

52. Smith, J.H., and Pugh, D.G.: Roentgenographic aspects of articular pigmented villonodular synovitis. Am. J. Roentgenol. 87:1146, 1962.

53. Fraire, A.E., and Fechner, R.E.: Intra-articular localized nodular synovitis of the knee. Arch. Pathol. 93:473, 1972.

54. Eisenstein, R.: Giant cell tumor of tendon sheath; Its histogenesis as studied in the electron microscope. J. Bone Joint Surg. 50A:476, 1968.

55. Ozello, L., Stout, A.P., and Murray, M.R.: Cultural characteristics of malignant histocytomas and fibrous xanthomas. Cancer 16:331, 1963.

56. Chung, E.B., and Enzinger, F.M.: Fibromas of tendon sheath (abstract). Lab. Invest. 36:333, 1977.

57. King, E.S.J.: Tissue differentiation in malignant synovial tumors. J. Bone Joint Surg. 34B:97, 1952.

58. Hajdu, S.I., Shiu, M.H., Fortner, J.G.: Tendosynovial sarcoma. A clinicopathologic study of 136 cases. Cancer 39:1201, 1977.

59. Shiu, M.H., McCormack, P.M., Hajdu, S.I., and Fortner, J.G.: Surgical treatment of tendosynovial sarcoma. Cancer 43:889, 1979.

60. Euneking, W.F., Spanier, S.E., and Goodman, M.A.: A system for the surgical staging of musculoskeletal sarcoma. Clin. Ortho. Rel. Res. 153:106, 1980.

61. Stout, A.P.: Sarcomas of the soft tissues. Cancer 11:231, 1961.

62. Ariel, I.M., and Pack, G.T.: Synovial sarcoma. Review of 25 cases. N. Engl. J. Med. 268:1272, 1963.

63. Cadman, N.L., Soule, E.H., and Kelly, P.J.: Synovial sarcoma: An analysis of 134 tumors. Cancer 18:613, 1965.

64. Suit, H.D.: Sarcoma of soft tissue. CA 28:284, 1978.

65. Moberger, G., Nilsonne, U., and Friberg, S.: Synovial sarcoma. Acta Orthop. Scand. Suppl. No. 11, 1968.

66. Roth, J.A., Enzinger, F.M., and Tannenbaum, M.: Synovial sarcoma of the neck. A follow-up study of 24 cases. Cancer 35:1243, 1975.

67. Jacobs, L.A., and Weaver, A.W.: Synovial sarcoma of the head and neck. Am. J. Surg. 128:527, 1974.

68. Massarelli, G., Tanda, F., and Salis, B.: Synovial sarcoma of the soft palate. Report of a case. Hum. Pathol. 9:341, 1978.

69. Golomb, H.M., Gorny, J., Powell, W., Graff, P., and Utmann, J.E.: Cervical synovial sarcoma of the bifurcation of the carotid artery. Cancer 35:483, 1975.

70. Thunold, J., and Bang, G.: Synovial sarcoma. A case report. Acta Orthop. Scand. 47:231, 1976.

71. Gabbiani, G., Kaye, G.I., Lattes, R., and Majno, G.: Synovial sarcoma. Electron microscopy of a typical case. Cancer 28:1031, 1971.

72. Gerner, R.E., and Moore, G.E.: Synovial sarcoma. Ann. Surg. 8:22, 1975.

73. Kaufman, J., and Tsukada, Y.: Synovial sarcoma with brain metastases. Report of a case responding to super voltage irradiation and review of the literature. Cancer 38:96, 1976.

74. Enzinger, E.M.: Clear cell sarcoma of tendons and aponeuroses. An analysis of 21 cases. Cancer 18:1163, 1965.

75. Chung, E.B., and Enzinger, F.M.: Clear cell sarcoma of tendons and aponeuroses: Further observations. (abstract). Lab. Invest. 38:8, 1978.

76. Tsuneyoshi, M., Enjoji, M., and Kubo, T.: Clear cell sarcoma of tendons and aponeuroses. A comparative study of 13 cases with subgrouping into melanotic and synovial types. Cancer 42:243, 1978.

77. Bearman, R.M., Noe, J., and Kempson, R.L.: Clear cell sarcoma with melanin pigment. Cancer 36:977, 1975.

78. Hoffman, G.J., and Carter, D.: Clear cell sarcoma of tendons and aponeuroses with melanin. Arch. Pathol. 95:22, 1973.

79. Boudreaux, D., and Waisman, J.: Clear cell sarcoma with melanogenesis. Cancer 41:1387, 1978.

80. Alitalo, K., Paavolainen, P., Franssila, K., and Ritsila, V.: Clear cell sarcoma of tendons and aponeuroses. Report of 2 cases. Acta Orthop. Scand. 48:241, 1977.

81. Laskowski, J.: Sarcoma aponeuroticum. Nowotwory 11:61, 1961.

82. Enzinger, F.M.: Epithelioid sarcoma. A sarcoma simulating a granuloma or a carcinoma. Cancer 26:1029, 1970.

83. Gabbiani, G., Fu, Y.-S., Kaye, O.I., Lattes, R., and Majno, G: Epithelioid sarcoma. A light and electron microscopic study suggesting a synovial origin. Cancer 30:486, 1972.

84. Bloustein, P.A., Silverberg, S.G., and Waddell, W.R.: Epithelioid sarcoma. Case report with ultrastructural review, histigenic discussion and chemotherapy data. Cancer 39:2390, 1976.

85. Prat, J., Woodruff, J.M., and Marcove, R.C.: Epithelioid sarcoma. An analysis of 22 cases indicating the prognostic significance of vascular invasion and regional lymph node metastases. Cancer 41:1472, 1978.

86. Bliss, B.O., and Reed, R.J.: Large cell sarcomas of tendon sheath, malignant giant cell tumor of tendon sheath. Am. J. Clin. Pathol. 49:776, 1968.

87. Kahn, L.B.: Malignant giant cell tumor of the tendon sheath. Ultrastructural study and review of the literature. Arch. Pathol. 95:203, 1973.

88. Goldenberg, D.L., Kelley, W., and Gibbons, R.B.: Metastatic adenocarcinoma of synovium presenting as an acute arthritis. Diagnosed by closed synovial biopsy. Arthritis Rheum. 18:107, 1975.

89. Khan, F.A., Garterhouse, W., and Khan, A.: Metastatic bronchogenic carcinoma: An unusual case of localized arthritis. Chest 67:738, 1975.

90. Moutsopoulos, H.M., Fye, K.H., Pugay, P.I., and Shearn, M.A.: Monarthritic arthritis caused by metastatic breast carcinoma. Value of cytologic study of synovial fluid. JAMA 234:75, 1975.

91. Emkey, R.D., Ragsdale, B.D., Ropes, M.W., and Miller, W.: A case of lymphoproliferative disease presenting as juvenile rheumatoid arthritis. Am. J. Med. 54:825, 1973.

92. Cameron, H.U., Gillespie, R., and Mancer, K.: Torsion of a tumor within 0103suprapatellar pouch. Report of a case. J. Bone Joint Surg. 58A:266, 1976.

93. Hoeffel, J.C., Rolain, G., Preaut, J., Rauber, G., and Hoeffel, G.: Pseudotumoral aspect of post-traumatic digital synovitis. Am. J. Surg. 134:416, 1977.

Section XXII
Medical Orthopedics

Chapter 109
Recreational Musculoskeletal Injuries

Arthur L. Boland

INTRODUCTION

Injuries resulting from recreational activities are among the most common problems confronting physicians in their offices and hospital emergency rooms. Acute traumatic injuries to ligaments and musculotendinous units may occur in any age group and lead to functional disability if not promptly diagnosed and appropriately treated. Likewise, repetitious athletic and occupational activities may insidiously cause damage to periarticular tendons and bursae, producing pain, gradual restriction of motion, and troublesome limitation of motion. In order to accurately recognize and manage these traumatic and overuse syndromes, one must be familiar with the specific anatomical features of the involved joints, the common mechanisms of injury, the physical demands of athletic activities, the relevance of the clinical signs and symptoms, and the acceptable treatment options. It is important to realize that pain experienced near one joint may be referred from the spine or an adjacent joint. Musculotendinous or capsular contractures about the hip, for example, may elicit pain in the thigh or knee; whereas, tightness of the gastrocnemius/soleus muscle complex may produce symptoms in the foot and ankle. These facts illustrate that care must be taken to regain flexibility and strength throughout the body, not just at the level of injury. Following immobilization, troublesome weaknesses and contractures develop not just in the involved extremity but also in the contralateral limb. These changes, when either overlooked or unsuspected, can lead to recurrent or related problems as the patient attempts to return to his preinjury activity. Thus, it is frequently inadequate rehabilitation that results in persistent disability.

GENERAL ANATOMICAL CONSIDERATIONS

Joint function and stability are dependent upon a number of complex interrelated factors. These include (1) the specific bony joint geometry and associated interarticular structures (meniscus, labrum), (2) the static ligamentous support, (3) the dynamic musculotendinous units, (4) the neurovascular structures, and (5) developmental abnormalities. Each joint has a degree of static stability determined both by its bony joint geometry plus its capsular and ligamentous support. Thus, the hip and elbow joints with their relatively stable articulations are less prone to ligamentous strain and subsequent instability than are the loosely constrained shoulder and knee joints. The major joint ligaments are oriented to guide joints through a functional range of motion, resisting the extremes of rotational stress as well as flexion/extension and varus/valgus forces.[1,2] Unfortunately, the collagen structure of these ligaments allows only a few millimeters of elongation before the ligaments become taut.[3,7] Forces applied to these ligaments beyond their tensile strength result in ligamentous *sprains* and, at times, complete disruption. An appreciation of which specific ligaments resist which forces applied to a joint is essential in order to diagnose joint laxities and estimate potential functional loss. The examining physician must know not only where to locate these ligaments but also in which position to place the joint when applying clinical stress tests to assess the degree of ligamentous damage. The evaluation of ligamentous injuries is one of the most difficult clinical tasks for physicians examining patients with acute athletic injuries.

Damage to interarticular structures, such as the mensci and glenoid labrum, results in significant functional disabilities. These structures assist not only in stabilizing joints but also in reducing joint compressive loads by distributing the impact uniformly over a larger surface area.[8,10] In doing so, they protect the articular cartilage from unphysiologic loads. During joint motion they also assist in lubrication by dispersing the joint fluid uniformly over the articular surface. Consequently, joint stability, nutrition, and biomechanics are adversely affected by injuries to these important interarticular structures.

The musculotendinous units dynamically control joint motion. Sudden overloads to these structures produce disruption of their fibers, most frequently at the musculotendinous junction. Classified as strains, they result in hemorrhage and necrosis, followed by an inflammatory repair process. Severe muscle strains can cause residual muscle weakness and fibrous contractures, which significantly affect joint function during strenuous activities.[11] Loss of flexibility, for example, in the hamstrings or the quadriceps muscle may result in abnormal loads through the patellofemoral joint, producing degenerative changes in the articular cartilage, increased subchondral pressure, and patellofemoral pain. Repetitious activities such as rowing, running, and throwing can produce acute tenosynovitis and bursitis. The subsequent inflammatory response results in swelling, tenderness, and crepitus. Among the major etiologic factors leading to bursitis and tendonitis are the lack of flexibility and inadequate muscle strength to withstand repeated athletic demands.[12]

Neurovascular injuries resulting from direct trauma or entrapment are troublesome diagnostic problems.[13,14] A thorough evaluation of these conditions may require EMGs, nerve conduction times, compartment pressure evaluations, and arteriograms.

Finally, joint function can be significantly affected by unrecognized developmental congenital malformations.[15,16] Scoliosis, leg length inequality, rotational deformities of the extremities, subtalar coalitions, and pronated feet may go undetected until symptoms develop following strenuous athletic or occupational activities. These conditions, which significantly alter joint biomechanics, must be considered in evaluating individuals with acute and chronic pain syndromes. To avoid diagnostic errors, one must therefore be aware of the interarticular, ligamentous, musculotendinous, neurovascular, and developmental factors that affect joint function.

THE SHOULDER

Specific Injuries

Glenohumeral Subluxation. *History.* Glenohumeral subluxations occur commonly in young adults and often lead to significant disability.[17-19] The mechanism of injury is similar to that of an anterior shoulder dislocation or a fall or contact injury with the arm in abduction and external rotation. The patient describes a "slipping" in his shoulder accompanied by sudden pain. Often a clicking sensation is noted in the shoulder with abduction. Frequently the patient does not seek medical advice after his initial injury. The pain subsides shortly, and he has little trouble until he is again required to use his arm with force in the abducted externally rotated position. Activities such as throwing, serving a tennis ball, and swimming lead to recurrent subluxation, pain, and more capsular laxity. The anterior-inferior and anterior-middle glenohumeral capsular ligaments are the major restraints that prevent subluxation (Fig. 109–1).

Physical Exam. If the patient is seen shortly after an episode of subluxation, there will be tenderness anteriorly over the joint capsule. As the arm is passively brought into abduction and external rotation, the patient experiences apprehension and resists further motion in that plane. Crepitus in the anterior capsule is often noted when the shoulder is abducted. One must be careful to evaluate the axillary nerve to rule out neuropraxia. Injuries to the axillary nerve result in weakness of the deltoid and loss of sensation over the lateral shoulder.

Diagnostic Tests. Routine x-rays are frequently normal. However, occasionally a small avulsion fracture is noted along the anterior/inferior rim of the glenoid (Fig. 109–2). An arthrogram[20-22] may show enlargement of the capsular recesses anteriorly and inferior to the coracoid process.

Treatment. Treatment of the acute primary subluxation is immobilization of the arm in a sling for 3 weeks to allow the capsular tissues to heal. Following immobilization, a rehabilitation program should be initiated to strengthen the rotator cuff muscles, especially the subscapularis muscle. Since the rate of recurrence is extremely high even when proper treatment has been given, the patient should be advised to avoid strenuous activities in the abducted and externally rotated position. Those individuals who have functional disability from recurrent subluxation may require surgical correction. At the time of the surgery, damage to the glenoid labrum, loose bodies, and attenuation of the anterior capsule are commonly encountered. Results of surgical correction are predictably good, although the patient may have some restriction of external rotation postoperatively, depending upon the specific procedure carried out.[18]

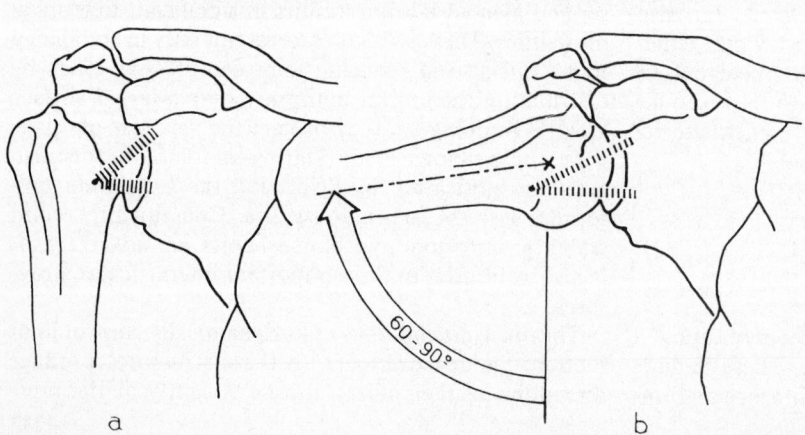

Figure 109–1. The anterior inferior and anterior middle glenohumeral ligaments are relaxed when the shoulder is in neutral (*a*) and become taut in abduction (*b*). (Reproduced with permission from Kapandji, *The Physiology of the Joints*, E&S Livingstone, London, 1970.)

Figure 109–2. Axillary lateral view of the shoulder, demonstrating bony changes along the anterior rim of the glenoid in a patient with recurrent anterior subluxations.

On rare occasions one may encounter an individual who subluxes posteriorly.[23] This is common in teenage athletes and must be carefully evaluated, since it may be voluntary or habitual. A physical therapy program that includes strengthening of the rotator cuff muscles, particularly the external rotators, is advised.[11]

Acromioclavicular Separations. *History.* Acromioclavicular (AC) separations result from a fall or blow on the top the shoulder.[24-26] As the shoulder girdle descends, the clavicle is restrained by the first rib, resulting in damage to the acromioclavicular and coracoclavicular ligaments. The first degree, or mild AC, separation is characterized by injury only to the AC capsule and no detectable separation of the AC joint clinically or radiographically. However, there is marked tenderness and some soft tissue swelling over the AC joint. When the involved arm is adducted, pain is reproduced at the injury site. In the more severe injuries, the coracoclavicular ligaments as well as the acromioclavicular capsule are disrupted. In the second and third degree separations, the distal end of the clavicle is elevated above

the level of the acromion. These deformities are quite obvious when compared with the uninjured side. Careful assessment of the neurovascular structures around the shoulder should be conducted to exclude these potential complications.

Diagnostic Tests. X-rays should always be obtained to rule out a fractured clavicle.[32] Comparison films of the uninjured shoulder are necessary to detect minor subluxations.

Treatment. Treatment of the first-degree AC separation is symptomatic and includes ice, compression pad, and a sling. When the pain and swelling have begun to subside in 5 or 6 days, the patient can begin a rehabilitation program. This initially consists of range of motion exercises, begun in a supine position to avoid the force of gravity. When motion is regained, a strengthening program can be initiated to restore power to the entire shoulder region.

The more severe second-degree and third-degree AC separations require a more prolonged period of immobilization or surgery.[26,27] If the separation can be reduced with a shoulder harness, immobilization should continue for 6 weeks. However, if the reduction cannot be maintained or if the patient remains symptomatic, surgical correction is indicated.[30,31] Symptomatic degenerative changes can develop in the AC joint following even minor AC separations.[28,29] Follow-up x-rays may show joint narrowing or erosive changes in the distal clavicle (Fig. 109–3).[33] Pain is experienced when the arm is used in the adducted and forward flexed position. Excision of the distal portion of the clavicle is indicated in these cases.

Overuse Syndromes

Anatomic Considerations. The strenuous and repetitious shoulder motions required to throw, serve a tennis ball, and swim frequently result in damage to the capsule, the rotator cuff tendons, and bursa in the subdeltoid region of the shoulder.[16,35-43] Impingement syn-

Figure 109–3. X-ray demonstrating A-C joint narrowing and subchondral cystic changes in the distal clavicle.

dromes, rotator cuff injuries, bicipital tendonitis, and chronic subdeltoid bursitis have been discussed in Chapter 29. The pathologic changes described in that chapter occur also in athletes who are involved in those sports in which the arm is repeatedly brought first into abduction, extension, and external rotation followed by a forceful acceleration into forward flexion, adduction, and internal rotation. The throwing mechanism is divided into the cocking, acceleration, and follow-through phases[19,46,64] (Fig. 109–4). In the initial cocking motion, the external rotators, postdeltoid fibers and rhomboids abduct, extend, and externally rotate the shoulder. Injuries to the infraspinatous and teres minor musculotendinous units can occur as the arm is brought suddenly back into this position. The anterior capsule and subscapularis muscle are relaxed during the cocking phase and are placed under considerable passive stretch. As this motion is repeated, the anterior capsule may become attenuated, allowing the shoulder to sublux anteriorly.[44] Injuries to the glenoid labrum and to the interarticular portion of the biceps tendon, which assists in stabilizing the humeral head in the glenoid, can occur with these transient subluxations. As the arm comes rapidly forward during the later acceleration phase of throwing, the subscapularis muscle actively contracts to bring the arm into forward flexion, adduction, and internal rotation. Simultaneously, the external rotators are reflexly inhibited, and they, along with the posterior capsule, are passively stretched. Tearing of the posterior capsule, with transient posterior subluxation, may occur during this phase of throwing.[45] Consequently, injuries to the capsular attachment, the musculotendinous units, and the interarticular components of the joint can result from this vigorous throwing activity.

Another mechanism of injury to the arm as it is brought from the abducted, externally rotated position into the forward flexion and internal rotation is the impingement of the subdeltoid bursa and rotator cuff tendons, particularly the supraspinatous, under the overlying coracoacromial arch.[36-39] The anterolateral aspect of the acromion and the firm coracoacromial ligament form the superior restraints above the humeral head. Repeated impingement upon these structures may produce recurrent microtrauma causing hemorrhage and edema, followed by an inflammatory reaction, fibrosis and eventually rupture of the rotator cuff tendons. Throwing and swimming the freestyle and butterfly strokes produce a very forceful adduction motion. During this phase the blood supply to the distal attachment of the rotator cuff tendons is impaired.[37] Vascular injection studies of the surpaspinatous muscle reveal that it receives its blood supply from vessels coming from the muscle proximally and extending distally into its tendinous component.[47,48] These studies clearly illustrate that when the arm is in the adducted position, pressure from the humeral head below produces an obstruction to normal blood flow into the distal tendinous segment. Consequently, in swimming and throwing there is not only repeated impingement of the supraspinatous and subdeltoid bursa under the coracoacromial arch, but also a brief repetitious ischemia to these vulnerable tendons. These mechanical and vascular factors contribute significantly to the pathologic changes that result in these painful shoulder syndromes in athletes.

History. The overuse shoulder injuries are usually characterized by the insidious onset of pain. The symptoms are experienced initially after practice or participation in the activity. As the changes become more severe, the pain is present during the activity and eventually becomes disabling, preventing participation. Characteristically, the patient has difficulty localizing the exact site of the pain. Not infrequently the discomfort is experienced over the anterior/superior aspect of the shoulder and later appears in the posterior capsule. At other times it may radiate down toward the humeral attachment of the deltoid. Occasionally the athlete will perceive a clicking or crepitation within the shoulder. Attempts should be made by questioning the individual to determine in which phase of motion the pain is most severe. This may give the physician a clue as to the exact location of the inflammatory response. The variable location and intensity of the pain are frustrating for the patient and physician, but in fact this variability is typical and therefore helpful in making the diagnosis.

Physical Examination. On physical examination the shoulder should be inspected for asymmetry, especially as a result of atrophy of the deltoid or infraspinatous muscle groups. Occasionally, axillary[13] and/or suprascapular[14] nerve entrapments can result in obvious weakness and wasting of the deltoid and external rotator group. A careful palpation of the anterior and posterior capsules of the shoulder and of the attachment of the

THE PITCHING ACT

(a) Cocking Phase

(b) Acceleration Phase: 1st stage

(c) Acceleration Phase: 2nd stage

(d) Follow-through Phase

Figure 109–4. Diagram depicting the cocking (*a*), acceleration (*b* and *c*) and follow-through (*d*) phases of the throwing act. (Reproduced with permission from Woods, G.W., Tullos, H.S., and King, J.W.: The throwing arm. J. Sports Med. 4:00, 1973.)

specific rotator cuff muscles as well as the bicipital groove while gently rotating the humerus is tedious but rewarding in localizing tenderness. There is typically a painful arc between 70 and 120 degrees of abduction and forward flexion.[36,37] Resistance to abduction and forward flexion exacerbates the pain. Moving the arm passively into forward flexion and internal rotation frequently elicits pain and occasionally crepitus as the subdeltoid structures impinge upon one another under the coracoacromial arch. A very careful neurological exam should be carried out to exclude referred pain or weakness from cervical spine injuries and to determine whether there is any specific weakness in rotator cuff units.

Diagnostic Tests. Routine x-rays are frequently normal, especially in younger age groups. However, in middle-aged and older athletes, degenerative changes in the acromioclavicular joint, osteophytes under the acromion, sclerosis at the humeral tuberosities, and traction spurs or avulsion fracture around the glenoid may be observed[49] (Fig. 109–5). Double-contrast arthrography[20-22] can help define partial or complete rotator cuff tears (Fig. 109–6), and tomographic[50] studies performed simultaneously can assist in detecting loose bodies or degenerative changes within the glenohumeral joint (Fig. 109–7). CAT scans can outline interarticular pathology.[51]

Treatment. The treatment of overuse syndromes about the shoulder is symptomatic and dictated by the extent of the injury. In first-degree and mild second-degree injuries in which symptoms occur only after practice and do not affect performance during participation, the treatment should consist primarily of rest, with a reduction of the offending motion. These individuals may be able to tolerate shorter practice sessions with a less

Figure 109–6. Arthrogram of a patient with chronic impingement and rotator cuff tear demonstrating extension of contrast into the subacromial space.

vigorous workout. Ice should be applied for 15 to 20 minutes following each practice and oral nonsteroidal anti-inflammatory agents are recommended. In the more severe second- and third-degree injuries in which the pain is disabling, total rest from the offending activities is necessary. In addition to the nonsteroidal oral anti-inflammatory agents and ice, ultrasound treatments and injections of local anesthetics and steroids are helpful. It is important to realize that steroid injections into tendons produce local tissue necrosis.[52-56] Therefore, following injections, athletes should be required to rest for at least 2 weeks to allow adequate regeneration of the tissue. It is much safer and therapeutically more beneficial to inject the subdeltoid bursa and not the tendons. Most often these conditions will respond to conservative management, especially if the treatment can be started early. An important part of the rehabilitation is strengthening of the shoulder musculature, particularly the rotator cuff group.[57,58] Many swimmers and throwers exhibit relative weakness in the external rotator muscle group, a finding that may be a significant etiologic factor. Gentle pendulum exercises are initiated first, followed by progressive resistance exercises to the rotator cuff groups and the deltoid. Since a biomechanically poor swimming, throwing, and serving technique may contribute to the onset of the problem, a coach or instructor should be consulted before allowing the participant to return to practice. Correction of potentially harmful techniques is necessary to avoid recurrences.

In patients who do not respond to conservative treatment, arthroscopy can be helpful in locating rotator cuff tears, injuries to the glenoid labrum, bicipital tendonitis, and loose bodies within the glenohumeral joint. Those individuals with rotator cuff tears and advanced impingement syndromes may require corrective surgery.[39,59,60] Excision of the coracoacromial ligament, par-

Figure 109–5. X-ray demonstrating degenerative changes in the A-C joint, osteophytes inferiorly on the acromion and sclerosis of the humeral tuberosities in a patient with symptoms of chronic impingement syndrome.

Figure 109–7. Arthrogram demonstrating narrowing of the anterior glenohumeral joint and a large loose fragment with inferior capsule.

tial anterior acromionectomy, repair of the rotator cuff lesions, and occasionally arthrotomy of the glenohumeral joint for removal of the loose bodies and correction of subluxation may be necessary.

THE ELBOW

Humeral Epicondylitis/Tennis Elbow

Anatomic Considerations. Athletic[61-64] and occupational activities may produce painful injuries to the soft tissue about the elbow. Lateral epicondylitis, or tennis elbow, is perhaps the most common syndrome encountered by physicians treating recreational athletes. However, trauma or repetitive activities, such as using a screwdriver, may also initiate these complaints. Similar pathologic changes and symptoms may also develop on the medial epicondyle from repetitious throwing activities that produce a valgus force through the elbow.

The various etiologic factors responsible for tennis elbow are still unclear and controversial.[65-72] The most widely accepted theory is that there is a mechanical overload placed on the common extensor muscle tendon at its attachment on the lateral epicondyle. Repeated contraction of these muscles, producing wrist extension and supination, causes small tears of the extensor aponeurosis followed by inflammatory response. Although some authors feel that the diagnosis is periostitis, routine x-rays rarely reveal periosteal reaction around the lateral epicondyle. Entrapment of the recurrent branch of the radial nerve to the joint has also been considered as a possible cause of lateral epicondylitis.[71,72]

Mechanism of Injury. Many recreational tennis players note that the backhand stroke reproduces their pain.[65] Improper technique, particularly leading with a flexed elbow, has therefore been incriminated as a major cause of lateral epicondylitis. Poor tennis hitting techniques, improper size of the racquet grip, excessive tension on the racquet strings, and improper weight of the racquet are all factors that have been discussed and are very difficult to analyze and evaluate objectively. Most recreational tennis players, however, have relative weakness of their extensor muscle groups compared with the flexor mass, making overload of the extensors more likely in these inadequately conditioned players. Evaluation of experienced professional tennis players on the other hand reveals a much higher incidence of medial epicondylitis.[77] Medial injuries are associated with the serve, which resembles the throwing motion. In both of these activities there is a significant valgus force through the elbow, placing the medial collateral ligament and the flexor musculotendinous units under considerable tension.

History. Epicondylitis may develop insidiously or from an acute overload. The pain is clearly localized to either the medial or lateral epicondyles with occasional radiation into the forearm. Shaking hands, opening doors, and direct contact all reproduce the pain.

Physical Examination. On examination there is localized tenderness over the involved medial or lateral epicondyle. When the lateral side is involved, resistance to wrist extension and supination reproduces the pain. When the medial epicondyle is involved, resistance to wrist flexion and pronation often produces pain. Since there is an inflammatory response within the extensor aponeurosis resulting in contracture of the muscle unit, passive extension of the elbow when the wrist is held in flexion and pronation will maximally stretch the extensor group and produce pain. Similarly, extension of the elbow with the wrist supinated and extended will often reproduce symptoms of medial epicondylitis.

A careful neurologic examination should be performed to rule out entrapment of either the median or ulnar nerves. Pronator teres syndrome can be encountered, in which the median nerve is entrapped as it passes through that muscle. This condition often produces sensory and motor changes distally in the hand similar to those noted with carpal tunnel syndrome. EMGs and nerve conduction times may be required to confirm this diagnosis. Patients with medial epicondylitis from throwing or serving a tennis ball may also have entrapment of the ulnar nerve.[77,78] The valgus overload may produce subluxation of the ulnar nerve from its groove or simply mechanical impingement and inflammation without subluxation. There may be local tenderness over the ulnar groove with dysesthesias extending into the forearm and hand. An examination should be made for weakness of the intrinsic hand muscles and sensory changes in the fourth and fifth fingers. Whereas collateral ligament injuries of the lateral side of the elbow are uncommon, repeated valgus forces through the elbow in throwing and serving a tennis ball may produce an acute or chronic strain of the medial collateral ligament. It is difficult to diagnose this injury, since the flexor muscle mass overlies the medial collateral ligament. If the tenderness appears to be deep to the flexor mass and if there is pain on valgus stress of the elbow, one can more confidently entertain a diagnosis of medial collateral ligament injury. The injuries may coexist and should be suspected.

Diagnostic Tests. X-ray examination for lateral epicondylitis is most frequently negative. However, in cases of medial epicondylitis in growing children, one must look carefully for widening or separation of the medial epicondylar apophysis. "Little league elbow" is characterized by separation of this medial epicondylar apophysis from valgus forces (Fig. 109–8) and chondral and osteochondral defects in the radial capitellar joint from compressive loads.[73-76] In the mature individual with chronic medial epicondylitis, particularly the baseball pitcher, degenerative changes may be noted in the elbow joint with loose bodies near the olecranon and traction spurs along the medial size of the trochlea. Arthrotomograms and CAT scans may be helpful in localizing loose bodies and chondral injuries within the joint.

Treatment. The treatment of tennis elbow is conservative, with rest being the most important component initially. When the pain is severe, splinting the elbow in 90 degrees of flexion for 3 to 5 days will help reduce the acute inflammation and pain. Prolonged immobilization, however, should be discouraged. Oral nonsteroidal anti-inflammatory drugs, ultrasound, and ice will also assist in relieving the inflammatory response. Local injections of bupivacaine hydrochloride and steroids can be useful when the pain is acute and well localized. One should again keep in mind the complications of steroid injections. Subcutaneous fat necrosis can result in unsightly and painful scars around the elbow.

When local pain and tenderness have subsided, a muscle strengthening and flexibility program is essential to avoid recurrence.[65] Isometric wrist extension and flexion exercises should be initiated as soon as they can be performed painlessly. Passive stretching of the extensor groups by extending the elbow with the wrist flexed and pronated is also essential. Gradual progressive resistance exercises should be continued with weights until the extremity has returned to a normal functional level of strength. The patient should return to activity gradually, first hitting against the backboard for 5 to 10 minutes and then progressively increasing this time over the next several days until he is confident that he can hit all strokes comfortably to avoid recurrence. Application of ice after participation is encouraged along with a conscientious stretching program.

Since factors of technique and equipment may be related to tennis and throwing injuries, patients with these injuries who want to resume these sports should consult with an instructor to determine if their tennis racquet and techniques are appropriate. The use of a forearm band may be helpful in reducing the tension through the extensor muscle mass.[65] With early and proper conservative treatment of tennis and throwing injuries of the elbow, there is rarely need for surgery. However, in the occasional incapacitating chronic epicondylitis that is unresponsive to conservative treatment, release of the extensor aponeurosis, exploration of the joint with removal of loose bodies, or partial synovectomy may be indicated.

Olecranon Bursitis

Acute traumatic olecranon bursitis may result from a direct blow to the elbow, resulting in marked swelling from hemorrhage within the bursal sac. Aspiration will

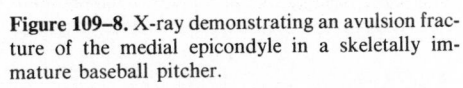
Figure 109–8. X-ray demonstrating an avulsion fracture of the medial epicondyle in a skeletally immature baseball pitcher.

relieve the swelling and discomfort. When the aspirant is not bloody, cell counts and cultures should be obtained. One must consider gout, rheumatoid arthritis, and sepsis in the differential diagnosis of acute or chronic bursitis. Following aspiration, a compressive Ace bandage is usually sufficient to keep the bursa decompressed. Special pads may be constructed to protect the elbow and prevent recurrences. Cases of recurrent chronic olecranon bursitis with fibrosis of the bursa may require surgical excision.

THE HIP

Trochanteric Bursitis

Anatomic Considerations. Acute trochanteric bursitis produces pain over the lateral side of the hip and proximal thigh. This bursa lies over the lateral aspect of the greater trochanter and under the tensor fascia lata muscle. The gluteus maximus muscle posteriorly and the tensor fascia lata muscle anteriorly combine to form a bipennate muscle mass, which then extends distally as the iliotibial band.[2] This band eventually attaches to the lateral aspect of the tibia.

History. With prolonged sitting or repeated hip flexion and extension, the tensor fascia is compressed over the greater trochanter, producing a mechanical inflammation of the underlying bursa. At times it is associated with a snapping sensation as the band slips over the bony prominences of the trochanter. Sitting in a deep chair or car seat often exacerbates the pain. The discomfort often radiates along the lateral aspect of the thigh producing symptoms suggestive of sciatica. In acute severe cases, motion of the hip is so painful that the condition can mimic an acute septic arthritis or synovitis of the hip.

Examination. Examination reveals maximum tenderness laterally over the greater trochanter with extension of the tenderness distally for a few inches below the trochanter. With the hip in extension, gentle internal and external rotation of the hip is less painful than that experienced with a septic hip or acute synovitis of the hip. Hip flexion and rotation will be painful in trochanteric bursitis, and the patient may not be able to bear weight.

Diagnostic Tests. A normal white blood count, sedimentation rate, and temperature help exclude an infectious process. Routine anteroposterior and lateral x-rays of the hip may show some soft tissue swelling lateral to the trochanter, but the hip capsule should not be distended, as is seen in intra-articular conditions of sepsis or synovitis. In young children, one must always consider early osteomyelitis developing in the metaphyseal bone near the trochanter. Appropriate laboratory tests and the clinical course are helpful in diagnosing this condition.

Stress fractures[79-81] (Fig. 109–9) and avulsion fractures (Fig. 109–10) should be considered in athletes presenting with hip pain. Discomfort in the anterior hip and groin in runners can be secondary to stress fractures of the femoral neck, pubic rami, or subtrochanteric region of the femur. X-rays are typically negative during the first 2 to 3 weeks following the onset of symptoms. Bone scans,[82] however, are positive early in the clinical course and should be ordered if this diagnosis is suspected. Children sustain avulsion fractures of the lesser trochanter, anterior iliac spine, and ischial apophysis more frequently during running and jumping activities. Although often the result of an acute injury with sudden onset of pain, these injuries may develop slowly, particularly the very serious slipped femoral capital epiphysis. These patients have painful limitation of hip motion, especially internal rotation, and often complain of pain extending down toward the knee. Comparison x-rays of the asymptomatic hip may be necessary to detect these conditions.

Treatment. The treatment of acute trochanteric bursitis is rest, application of ice, nonsteroidal oral anti-inflammatory agents, and often an interbursal injection of a local anesthetic agent and steroid. Ultrasound treatments may also be helpful in relieving inflammation. A

Figure 109–9. Radiograph of a jogger demonstrating a stress fracture of the inferior pubic ramus.

Figure 109–10. X-ray of a young soccer player demonstrating an avulsion fracture of the lesser trochanter.

partial weight-bearing crutch gait is suggested until the patient can walk comfortably without assistance.

One must be diligent in looking for an underlying biomechanical cause of the trochanteric bursitis. Leg length inequalities, producing a pelvic obliquity and prominence of the trochanter on the long side, result in increased mechanical pressure from the overlying fascia lata. Jogging can cause contractures of the tensor fascia lata muscle, resulting in snapping of the iliotibial band over the trochanter. These contractures must be stretched out with a proper physical therapy program to avoid recurrence of the bursitis.[83] Those individuals with leg length discrepancies should be balanced by a lift placed in the appropriate shoe. With prompt and proper symptomatic treatment combined with the correction of any contractures with physical therapy, patients with trochanteric bursitis recover satisfactorily. However, on rare occasions surgical release of the tight fascia over the trochanter may be indicated.

THE KNEE

The common knee joint injuries sustained in athletic activities involve the interarticular structures (menisci and articular cartilage), the major capsular ligaments, and the periarticular musculotendinous units and bursae. Frequently there is a combination of both inter- and extra-articular damage compounding the diagnostic and therapeutic problems.

Meniscal Tears

Anatomic Considerations. The semilunar cartilages attach to the tibia peripherally by the coronary ligament and the deep meniscal tibial component of the capsular ligaments.[2] Although the anterior and posterior horns of the menisci in the intercondylar notch are firmly attached, the peripheral fixation allows enough laxity to permit the menisci to move forward and backward with flexion and extension. Since the axis of knee rotation is through the medial femoral condyle, the lateral femoral

condyle rotates through a larger arc than the medial condyle.[1] To accommodate for this motion, the lateral meniscus is also more mobile than the medial meniscus. Because the concave contour of the menisci articulates with the convexity of the femoral condyles, the menisci also add stability to the knee. The menisci distribute the compressive loads through the joint over a wider area of the opposing femoral and tibial surfaces.[8-10] The menisci assist in dispersing the synovial joint fluid over the femoral articular cartilage, thus assisting in joint lubrication and nutrition. These multiple functions of the menisci attest to their importance for normal joint activity.

Mechanism of Injury. The menisci are torn by compressive, rotational, and sheering forces through the knee joint.[16,84] Twisting into a deep knee position often results in a vertical tear through the mid substance of the meniscus. Valgus external rotation forces that occur when the knee is struck on the lateral side may produce a tear in the body of the meniscus, but more frequently cause a peripheral separation of the meniscus from its capsular attachments posteromedially. Horizontal cleavage tears are more common in the older age groups and may result from relatively trivial compressive and rotational injuries.[85] Both traumatic and degenerative horizontal tears near the periphery of the menisci, especially in the lateral meniscus, may develop cystic degeneration, resulting in a visible and palpable soft tissue mass.

History. At the time of an acute injury, the patient often describes a tearing or popping sensation within his knee. A similar sensation can be experienced with ligamentous tears and subluxation of the patella. The time of onset of swelling and the extent of swelling are important facts. Since swelling that occurs within the first 6 to 10 hours usually represents a hemarthrosis, one should suspect in these cases a tear of the vascular peripheral portion of the meniscus rather than the avascular mid substance. Other common causes of acute hemarthrosis include tears of the anterior cruciate ligament, partial injuries to the medial collateral ligament, subluxation of the patella, and osteochondral fractures. Any of these injuries may occur from contact or noncontact activities. A sudden pivoting motion or a twisting injury when landing from a jump are common mechanisms of meniscal tears, ligamentous injuries, and osteochondral fractures. If the patient can clearly recall that he could not fully extend his knee prior to the onset of his effusion or hemarthrosis, the diagnosis of a displaced tear of the meniscus should be strongly considered. Loose bodies, as seen in osteochondritis dessicans, or an avulsion of the tibial eminence in association with an anterior cruciate tear will also produce a mechanical block to extension. Meniscal tears usually produce pain localized over the joint line. Complaints of buckling and locking, which are the result of interference with normal joint motion by the displaced fragment, are common. Meniscal tears may produce swelling from synovitis, resulting in a sensation of fullness in the popliteal and suprapatellar areas as well as stiffness and loss of flexibility.

Physical Examination. Joint swelling or a displaced meniscus will result in the inability to fully extend the knee in stance and gait. Local swelling anterior to the fibular collateral ligament should alert the physician to a diagnosis of cystic degeneration of the lateral meniscus. Tenderness is most frequently along the joint line, with increased discomfort on the extremes of flexion and extension. A clicking sensation may be felt when the knee is compressed and rotated during a valgus or varus stress test (positive McMurray test). Careful examination of the collateral and cruciate ligaments, as well as the patellofemoral joint, should be carried out to exclude injuries to these structures. Acute meniscal tears in athletes under 30 are rarely isolated lesions; in older patients, isolated degenerative tears may occur with minimal trauma.

Diagnostic Tests. Routine anteroposterior, lateral, and tunnel views of the knee joint plus a 30-degree sunrise view of the patellofemoral joint should be taken to exclude osteochondral fractures of the patella, tibial plateau fractures, avulsions of the tibial spine, and os-

Figure 109–12. Arthrogram demonstrating a horizontal tear extending into the avascular portion of the medial meniscus.

teochondritis dissecans. Arthrography[21,22] is extremely helpful in localizing meniscal tears, particularly in the medial compartment (Figs. 109–11 to 109–14). Diagnostic arthroscopy[86,87] may be indicated when the routine x-rays and arthrograms are inconclusive and the knee remains symptomatic.

Treatment. Acute meniscal tears that result in a locked knee require prompt diagnosis and management. Although not a true emergency, the knee should not be allowed to remain locked for more than 7 to 14 days or unnecessary quadriceps weakness and joint contractures will develop. If the knee is not locked and the examiner is confident that there is no ligamentous or osteochondral damage, the knee can be immobilized in a splint and compressive bandage to keep swelling to a minimum. The application of ice and the use of crutches are also recommended. When the swelling and tenderness have begun to recede in the first 3 to 5 days, an early rehabilitation program consisting of active range of motion exercises, isometric quadriceps strengthening,

Figure 109–11. Arthrogram demonstrating a vertical tear in the vascular peripheral portion of the medial meniscus.

Figure 109–13. Arthrogram demonstrating a vertical tear in the avascular portion of the medial meniscus (Bucket-handle tear).

Figure 109–14. Arthrogram demonstrating a long oblique tear in the medial meniscus.

tomy, medial meniscectomy in a varus knee, lateral meniscectomy in a valgus knee, residual quadriceps weakness, a retained posterior horn, and a total meniscectomy as opposed to partial removal.

With the introduction of arthroscopy, which has assisted the surgeon in making a more accurate diagnosis, there has been a more selective and conservative approach to meniscectomy by orthopedists.[93-95] Some tears are now being left alone, particularly the small degenerative tears in the degenerative knee and the stable meniscal tears in the ligamentously unstable knee. Partial meniscectomy is recommended for bucket handle (Fig. 109–13) and flap tears. Peripheral separations (Fig. 109–14) are being repaired rather than removed.[97-99] Unfortunately, there are still complex meniscal tears that will require total meniscectomy. It is hoped with this more conservative approach to meniscal problems that the disability from these injuries can be reduced significantly in the future.

Ligamentous Injuries

Anatomic Considerations. It is not the function of this chapter to describe the complex classification of ligamentous injuries about the knee.[100,101] This is available in the literature for those who want to pursue it in more detail. However, certain basic concepts are essential in order to accurately diagnose acute and chronic instabilities of the knee.

The deep capsule forms a sleeve, which encircles the knee, extending from the femur above to the peripheral margin of the menisci and then down to the tibia. The tibial collateral ligament, which runs from the medial femoral condyle down to the tibia, primarily resists valgus forces; however, because it extends distally and anteriorly to attach on the tibia, it also prevents excessive external rotation of the tibia on the femur. This ligament is thus frequently injured by a valgus external rotation force, as seen in the football clipping maneuver. The lateral collateral ligament runs from the lateral femoral condyle to the fibular head. It is lax in flexion and tight in extension and is often damaged by a blow to the medial side of the knee, producing a varus force. The anterior and posterior cruciate ligaments originate on the anterior and posterior aspects of the tibia respectively and extend parallel to each other through the intercondylar notch to attach on the femur posteriorly and anteriorly, respectively. Because of their central location within the knee joint, they form the axis around which the knee joint rotates. These ligaments tighten as the femur rotates on the tibia.[1,2,102]

Mechanism of Injury. In contact injuries in which there is a valgus force through the knee, the medial collateral is the first line of defense. After this ligament fails, the deep medial capsular ligament is the next to rupture.[103-105] These injuries are frequently associated with a peripheral separation of the medial meniscus. After the tibial collateral and medial capsular ligaments have been disrupted, the anterior cruciate will tear with further valgus force. However, the mechanism of injury that most commonly damages the anterior cruciate lig-

and progressive partial weight bearing is recommended. When there is a very tense, painful effusion or hemarthrosis, the joint may be aspirated. This will reduce the pain and allow a more complete and accurate evaluation of the knee. If a hemarthrosis is aspirated, one should observe the aspirate for fat droplets, which indicate an osteochondral fracture. Tears through the avascular portion of the meniscus do not heal spontaneously. Consequently, the patient should be alerted to the possibility of recurrent symptoms of internal derangement when he returns to activity.

The details of the surgical management of meniscal tears are not the purpose of this chapter. However, rheumatologists may be consulted by patients seeking information about the consequences of the meniscal pathology and the potential benefits of surgery. In discussing these topics, the physician must be aware that the meniscus is a very important structure and that there are several factors that may contribute to an unsatisfactory prognosis. Experimental work clearly suggests that meniscal tears in laboratory animals will produce degenerative joint disease.[88-90] This corresponds with the clinical evidence of degenerative changes seen in patients who have had recurrent pain, swelling, buckling, and locking from meniscal tears. The degree of degenerative joint disease at the time of meniscectomy appears to be related to the duration of symptoms and to the extent of the meniscal damage.[91,92] On the other hand, laboratory experiments show that meniscectomy also leads to degenerative joint disease.[89] The long-term clinical follow-up studies of patients having had meniscectomies indicate that 60 percent of these patients have symptomatic knees 10 to 15 years following their surgery.[91,92] Fairbank[96] originally described the radiologic changes of joint space narrowing, flattening of the femoral condyle, and hypertrophic spurring in the joint in patients following meniscectomy. Some of the factors that seem to contribute to the poor results include associated ligamentous laxity, degenerative changes at the time of meniscectomy, prolonged symptoms prior to meniscecament is a noncontact privoting motion. Since the anterior cruciate tightens around the posterior cruciate with internal rotation around the lateral condyle in external rotation, and is compressed under the roof of the intercondylar notch with hyperextension, both hyperextension and rotational injuries sustained in jumping and pivoting may result in complete disruption of this important ligament. These noncontact injuries to the anterior cruciate may show little evidence of damage to the collateral or capsular ligaments.[106,107] The posterior cruciate ligament is commonly torn in two different ways: by a hyperextension injury or a blow over the tibia to the flexed knee which drives the tibia posteriorly. Lateral collateral ligament tears result from a blow to the medial side of the knee causing a varus deformity.

History. An accurate diagnosis can often be made by history alone. The mechanism of injury, the degree and location of pain, the time of onset and the amount of swelling, and the presence of a popping or snapping sensation are all very helpful clues. Contact injuries to the medial or lateral side of the knee frequently result in collateral ligament injuries and associated cruciate ligament tears. Noncontact pivoting and jumping injuries commonly produce "isolated" tears in the anterior cruciate ligament. The most severe grade III tears of the medial collateral ligament have less pain and less swelling than the incomplete grade I and II sprains. This is due to the complete disruption of the capsular sleeve, which extends peripherally around the joint. When this occurs the hemarthrosis is decompressed into the soft tissues below the joint.

It is the tense hemarthrosis of the incomplete injury that produces the most marked pain and the most visible joint distention. If the swelling occurs within the first 8 to 10 hours following a twisting injury, one should consider this a hemarthrosis and suspect the diagnosis of anterior cruciate ligament tear, subluxation of the patella, incomplete tear of the medial collateral ligament, peripheral separation of the meniscus, or an osteochondral fracture. Swelling that develops 24 hours following the injury is most often an effusion associated with a meniscal tear in the avascular portion, a chondral injury to the patella or femur, or a mild sprain of the medial collateral ligament.

Physical Examination. The uninjured knee should be examined first to document normal range of motion, especially the presence of hyperextension and generalized ligamentous laxity. With this as a baseline, one can better appreciate subtle differences on the injured side. The degree and location of the swelling should be carefully documented. Tenderness and swelling below the knee joint over the proximal tibia medially indicate an injury to the tibial collateral ligament at its attachment three to four finger breadths below the joint line. Tenderness along the joint line suggests damage to the meniscus or to the deep capsular ligaments. A marked hemarthrosis or effusion will produce lateral tilting of the patella, suggesting patellofemoral subluxation. This condition can occur simultaneously with medial collateral ligament disruption. The most common site of tenderness in medial collateral ligament sprains is on the femoral attachment above the joint line.

Pain and hamstring spasm make examination of the ligaments difficult in acute cases. However, if the thigh is allowed to remain resting on the examining table, the lower leg can be supported and flexed gently over the side of the table. In this position, the knee can be stressed into valgus and varus. The medial collateral ligament should be stressed in full extension and in 30 degrees of flexion. In the former position, the posterior capsule and posterior cruciate ligaments as well as the medial collateral ligament are tight. Significant laxity in this position suggests that all of these tissues may be damaged, since the medial collateral ligament can be completely disrupted and the knee will appear stable in full extension if the posterior capsule and posterior cruciate are still intact.[101] However, when the knee is flexed 30 degrees, the posterior capsule and posterior cruciate are relaxed and one can isolate and assess the integrity of the medial collateral ligament. The lateral collateral ligament is also tested in both flexion and extension. The anterior cruciate is perhaps the most difficult to evaluate in acute injuries. The standard anterior Drawer test done with the knee flexed 90 degrees and the tibia pulled forward is generally impossible to perform because of the pain associated with this maneuver. However, an anterior Drawer test in 15 degrees of flexion (Lachman test) is very helpful and consistently reliable in evaluating acute anterior cruciate disruptions.[107,108] A positive posterior Drawer sign or posterior sag noted when the knee is flexed 90 degrees and observed from the side indicates a posterior cruciate ligament tear (Fig. 109–15). Careful neurovascular examination is essential, particularly in posterior cruciate ligament injuries, to exclude damage to the popliteal vessels. In addition, neuropraxia of the peroneal nerve is frequently associated with lateral collateral ligament injury.

Diagnostic Tests. Routine anterior, posterior, lateral, tunnel, and 30-degree sunrise views should be obtained. The anterior cruciate ligament, particularly in young individuals, may avulse from the tibia, elevating an osteochondral fragment.[109] Valgus and varus stress films can be very helpful in assessing the degree of collateral

POSTERIOR
DRAWER
TEST

Figure 109–15. Inspection of the knee from the side reveals a posterior drawer or posterior sag, indicating damage to the posterior cruciate ligament.

ligament laxity; however, this procedure may be difficult and misleading if the patient is experiencing pain and hamstring spasm. Aspiration of the knee joint to remove a tense hemarthrosis or examination under anesthesia may be necessary to accurately document the degree of ligamentous damage. Arthrography[21,22] is generally not necessary in chronic ligamentous instabilities but can be helpful in diagnosing acute anterior cruciate tears. When the diagnosis remains in doubt, examination under anesthesia and arthroscopy will allow extremely accurate diagnosis.[106,107] It is important to note that during arthroscopy of knees with complete capsular disruption, one can have complications from the extravasation of the fluid posteriorly into the soft tissues, resulting in compression of the popliteal vessels and nerves.[110]

Treatment. Incomplete injuries to the medial collateral ligament can be successfully treated conservatively.[111] Following 3 to 5 days of immobilization at 30 degrees of flexion in a splint or knee support, the soft tissue swelling and tenderness will begin to recede. Early range of motion exercises and protective weight bearing may be allowed. Crutches should be continued until the patient can fully extend the knee and flex at least 95 degrees. Ice is applied during the first 48 to 72 hours. During the rehabilitation period, warm whirlpools may be beneficial. It is essential to regain adequate strength in the hamstrings and quadriceps muscles in addition to a full range of joint motion. Weakness and contractures of the ipsilateral hip can occur following periods of immobilization for a knee injury and the hip must be rehabilitated along with the injured joint.

When there is disruption of two or more ligaments, for example the medial collateral and anterior cruciate ligaments, the problem is best treated surgically and ideally operated upon within the first two weeks to obtain the best results.[101] Delaying the procedure results in retraction and fibrosis of the ligamentous structures, making identification and proper reapproximation of the tissues exceedingly difficult, if not impossible.

The treatment of acute anterior cruciate ligament tears is still controversial. Since they frequently have associated but unsuspected meniscal tears or chondral fractures, these injuries may result in significant functional disability.[107] Consequently, in the competitive athlete who wants to return to his high-risk activity, prompt diagnosis and surgical treatment of the anterior cruciate and the related injuries is justified. However, in the recreational athlete, a more conservative approach may be justified utilizing a brace for activities after a thorough rehabilitation with appropriate strengthening program is completed. It is essential to maintain maximum strength of the hamstrings and quadriceps muscle to safely resume recreational or competitive athletic pursuits.[11]

Tendonitis/Bursitis

History. Patella tendonitis (jumper's knee)[112,113] is a disabling inflammation of the attachment of the patella tendon into the inferior pole of the patella. Commonly seen in young, recreational or competitive athletes, it is precipitated by jumping, hurdling, and running. Climbing or descending stairs and deep knee bends may exacerbate the pain. The pain is localized to the area below the patella.

Examination. On examination there is local tenderness along the inferior pole of the patella. This is best identified by depressing the superior pole of the patella. This tilts the inferior pole up and allows the tenderness to be more easily located. These patients often have tight hamstrings, as evidenced by limitation of straight leg raising. The quadriceps mechanism can also be contracted. This is best noted by placing the patient prone on the examining table, flexing the knee, and demonstrating limited knee flexion. Although routine x-rays are usually normal, irregular calcifications at the inferior pole of the patella may be present. This is similar to the changes noted at the tibial tubercle in Osgood-Schlatter's disease.

Treatment. Treatment consists of ice, restriction of activity, and avoidance of jumping and climbing stairs. Immobilization in a splint is helpful if the lesion is symptomatic with walking. Oral anti-inflammatory drugs are suggested; however, corticosteroid injections are generally not necessary. If corticosteroid injections are employed, one must realize that these substances produce focal tissue necrosis of the tendon and render the tendon subject to spontaneous rupture if the quadriceps mechanism is stressed.[52]

The most important component of the treatment of patella tendonitis is adequate rest until the tenderness has begun to subside. The rehabilitation program should consist of strengthening and stretching of both the quadriceps and the hamstring muscle group. Persistent contractures in these areas will lead to a recurrence of pain when the athlete resumes his participation. A gradual warm-up period with adequate stretching followed by the application of ice compresses for 15 to 20 minutes following competition can be very helpful procedures.

Prepatellar Bursitis (Housemaid's Knee)

Prepatellar bursitis is commonly seen in contact sports such as wrestling.[114] Traumatic in origin, the swelling of the prepatellar bursa produces the sensation of stiffness and limitation of motion. The swelling is localized to the bursa and does not involve the knee joint itself. When marked swelling occurs, aspiration, followed by compression with a foam rubber pad and Ace bandage is indicated. Compression should be maintained for 3 to 5 days, since reaccumulation of fluid in the bursa is common. Protective padding for this area could be worn when the individual resumes participation.

Pes Anserinus Tendonitis/Bursitis

The medial hamstring group consists of the sartorius, gracilis, and semitendinosis tendons. These attach below the flare of the tibial metaphysis approximately four finger breadths below the joint line. The pes anserinus bursa surrounds these tendons and allows them to glide smoothly over the bony prominence of the tibial metaphysis. Running and jogging activities may result in acute inflammation of these tendons.[79] The pain is felt along the medial side of the knee but can radiate up along the posteromedial aspect of the thigh. This is often seen in individuals after just beginning a jogging program. In addition to the local tenderness over the tendons and bursa, the patient may experience pain when hamstring contractions are resisted and the tendons palpated. One should look for predisposing factors, such as hamstring contractures with limited straight leg raising, genu valgum, out-toeing gait (external tibial torsion), and a history of beginning a jogging program without adequate time to gradually build up endurance, strength, and flexibility. Occasionally the semimembranosis, which attaches to the posteromedial aspect of the tibia, is involved and produces pain that can mimic a meniscal injury.

The treatment is symptomatic, utilizing oral anti-inflammatory agents, local applications of ice, reduction of activity, and occasionally ultrasound treatments. Local corticosteroid injections may be helpful in the acute stages. When the pain and tenderness have subsided, a rehabilitation program to regain flexibility and strength in the hamstrings is essential.

Lateral Band Syndrome

Recreational athletes, particularly runners, frequently develop disabling pain on the lateral aspect of the knee as the result of friction from a tight iliotibial band.[79,83,115]

The iliotibial band is a thick fibrous structure and is an extension of the fascia lata proximally in the thigh. It courses over the femoral condyle and attaches to the tibia at Gerdy's tubercle. With repeated knee flexion and extension, this tight band produces mechanical impingement and inflammation of the synovial tissues at the lateral femoral condyle (Fig. 109–16). Predisposing factors include tightness of the hip abductor muscles, bowlegs, running regularly on sloping surfaces, and excessive pronation of the feet. The tenderness is localized to the area of the lateral femoral condyle.

Treatment. Treatment consists of oral anti-inflammatory agents, ice, ultrasound treatments, stretching of the hip abductors and fascia lata, and longitudinal arch supports to reduce pronation. Local injections of corticosteroids may be helpful, but correction of any biomechanical factors or training errors is essential for the prevention of recurrences.

These various overuse syndromes about the knee are particularly difficult to diagnose and treat. They develop insidiously and may be the result of several factors. Careful neurologic evaluation should be carried out to exclude the possibility of sciatica from chronic disc disease, SI joint arthritis, or spondylolisthesis. Leg length inequalities, contractures about the hip, tightness of the hamstrings and quadriceps muscle groups, valgus and varus malalignments of the knee, excessive tibial torsion, and foot deformities may all participate in producing the abnormal forces that cause "runner's knees."[116] One can certainly localize the site of tenderness by examining the knee only; however, a complete examination of the entire lower extremity and spine is necessary to evaluate all possible etiologic factors.

Iliotibial "Band" Friction Syndrome

Tensor fasciae latae

Iliotibial tract

Vastus lateralis

Lateral epicondyle of femur

Insertion of iliotibial tract to tibia

Diagram showing friction of iliotibial tract on lateral femoral epicondyle as fascial tract glides backward and forward with flexion and extension of knee

Area of diffuse pain and tenderness

Figure 109–16. Diagram of how the iliotibial band produces mechanical inflammation of the lateral femoral epicondyle. (Reproduced with permission from Brody, D.M.: Running injuries. CIBA Clinical Symposia 32, No. 4, 1980.)

Patellofemoral Pain Syndrome/ Chondromalacia Patella

Pain originating about the patellofemoral joint is generally diagnosed as chondromalacia of the patella. Although chondromalacia is indeed a cause of disabling patellofemoral pain, it should be diagnosed only when the physician is confident that there is retropatellar articular cartilage degenerative changes. The etiology and classification of chondromalacia of the patella have been described in the literature[117,118] and should be reviewed by those interested in pursuing the subject in detail. It is important to recognize that there is a spectrum of patients with patellofemoral pain, some of whom have not developed the true pathologic changes to justify the diagnosis of chondromalacia. Although chondral injuries and subluxations of the patellofemoral joint may result from direct trauma, most of the patellofemoral pain syndromes, including chondromalacia, are the result of chronic abnormal biomechanical forces producing malalignment of the patellofemoral joint. Therefore, to accurately diagnose the condition, one must understand the anatomic features and biomechanical forces about this complex joint.

Anatomic Considerations. The patella is a large sesamoid bone and articulates with the femoral trochlea groove and femoral condyles. The contact areas and the amount of compressive force through this joint increase with flexion and with contraction of the quadriceps muscle.[117] Activities performed in flexion, such as running, ascending and descending stairs, squatting, and jumping all dramatically increase the load through this joint. The stability of the joint is determined both by the shape of the patella and femoral trochlea and also by the muscular control through the quadriceps. Thus, developmental abnormalities, such as shallow trochlea groove, and abnormally flat or small patella, excessive genu valgum, patella alta, and excessive hyperextension of the knee may all result in instability of the patella. The dynamic control of the patella is through the quadriceps muscles. However, the vastus medialis, particularly its distal oblique fibers, is the most important stabilizing component of this muscle group, since only they pull the patella medially. Weakness or dysplasia of the vastus medialis coupled with an overdeveloped vastus lateralis may produce a lateral subluxation of the patella. Excessive genu valgum or external tibial torsion also place the patella tendon attachment lateral to the normal axis of alignment and can contribute to lateral subluxation and abnormal compressive forces.

Symptoms. Early in the clinical course, patellofemoral pain syndrome is characterized by a vague, poorly localized discomfort or ache. It is made worse by activities such as sitting (positive theater sign) and descending and ascending stairs and is relieved by placing the knees in extension. Clicking and crepitus is often described when the patient arises from a chair or extends his knees through the last 30 degrees of extension. Buckling or pseudolocking, resulting from the incongruity, transient subluxation, or pain in the patellofemoral joint is also a common symptom. Pivoting motions may precipitate buckling and pain and make one entertain the diagnosis of meniscal tear. Swelling can occur with acute lateral subluxations as the capsular attachments to the medial side of the patella are attenuated. However, chronic swelling with the sensation of stiffness and limitation of motion strongly suggest that there are degenerative changes on the articular suface of the patella or femur, with disruption of the collagen structure and release of lysosomal enzymes into the joint causing a chemical synovitis.

Physical Examination. The contour of the lower extremity should be inspected in stance, gait, supine, and sitting positions. The presence of atrophy of the vastus medialis, the height of the patella, the presence of genu valgum or external tibial torsion, and the appearance of a lateral tilting patella should be noted. With the patient sitting with the legs flexed 90 degrees over the edge of the table, one should observe the path of the patella as the knee is brought into full extension. The patient may complain of pain during the last 30 degrees of extension. Manual resistance to knee extension and compression of the patella may reproduce the pain. Tenderness is often noted along the medial facette of the patella and crepitus detected with flexion and extension. The alignment of the quadriceps mechanism in extension (Q angle) should be observed and recorded with and without isometric quadriceps contraction. Passive compression of the patella laterally often produces apprehension as the patient experiences a sensation of pending subluxation. The buckling that these patients experience can result in injuries to the menisci and the ligamentous structures. Thus, careful palpation of the joint line and careful assessment of the integrity of the collateral and cruciate ligaments are important. Static contractures of the hamstrings and quadriceps, evidenced by limitation of straight leg raising and limited knee flexion with the hip extended, respectively, may be contributing factors.

X-rays. Standing anteroposterior and lateral x-rays of the knee joint will help in assessing the valgus/varus alignment of the leg. The lateral x-ray will demonstrate the presence of patella alta or patella baja. Insall's technique of comparing the length of the patella to that of the patella tendon is a reliable method of determining the height of the patella.[121] A sunrise view taken at 20 to 30 degrees of flexion will reveal the contour of the patellofemoral joint.[119,120] In chronic lateral compression of the patella, there may be excessive lateral tilt with sclerosis noted in the subchondral bone of the lateral facette and osteoporosis evident in the medial portion of the patella (Fig. 109–17). Chronic subluxation of the patella may result in avulsion fractures or traction spurs along the medial facette of the patella. Tomograms can be helpful in defining osteochondral fractures or irregularities of the patella and femoral surfaces. Although diagnostic arthroscopy is perhaps the most accurate way of visualizing defects in the patellofemoral joint, arthrography can also be of assistance.[21,22]

Treatment. Accurate diagnosis is essential in planning the proper treatment program for patellofemoral pain

Figure 109–17. Tangential view of the patella, demonstrating lateral patellar subluxation, narrowing of the lateral patello-femoral joint, subchondral sclerosis of the lateral facet, and relative osteoporosis of the medial facet in a patient with patello-femoral pain syndrome.

syndrome. Patients with associated displaced osteochondral fractures of the patella or femoral condyle will require prompt surgical intervention to reduce or excise these fragments and to prevent incongruity, which may cause chronic instability or degenerative arthrosis. However, most of the patients with patellofemoral pain syndromes are young females with minimal changes on x-ray, who require a conservative therapeutic program. Oral anti-inflammatory agents, isometric quadriceps strengthening exercises, hamstring stretching, and a reduction in activities such as bending, stair climbing, running, and sitting in a deep knee position should be encouraged. Follow-up studies indicate that 80 percent of the patients with this condition can be managed by these conservative measures.[121,122] Patella restraining braces with a felt padding along the lateral side of the patella can minimize lateral subluxation.[123] The most important component of the program is strengthening of the quadriceps muscles, especially the vastus medialis obliquus and correction of all musculotendinous contractures in the hamstring, quadriceps, and hip abductor musculature by diligent stretching. Patients with persistent disability from recurrent subluxation or from degenerative changes on the articular surface of the patella may require surgical debridement of the patella and realignment of the extensor mechanism. The details of the surgical treatment are not the purpose of this chapter. However, since good surgical results are highly dependent upon the patient's faithful adherence to a prolonged supervised physical therapy program in the postoperative period, operative intervention should be considered only when the physician is convinced the patient has conscientiously tried the similar preoperative conservative rehabilitation program.

LOWER LEG PAIN

With the recent interest in fitness and running, physicians are called upon to diagnose troublesome leg pains in these dedicated and determined athletes. The most common problems include shin splints, stress fractures, Achilles tendonitis, and compartment syndromes.

Shin Splints. This condition is more accurately termed posterior tibial stress syndrome.[124,125] Although the exact etiology is still debated, the pain and tenderness appear to be localized over the posterior medial border of the middle third of the tibia, along the course of the posterior tibial tendon. Whether this represents a tendonitis or periostitis is still debated. It is often associated with excessive pronation of the feet, which results in mechanical stress on the posterior tibial tendon as it courses behind the medial malleolus into the arch of the foot. Many of these patients have associated tight Achilles tendons. Gradual in onset, this condition is often disabling and resistant to treatment. X-rays and bone scans are negative. The treatment consists of oral anti-inflammatory agents, rest, and proper orthotics to correct any excessive pronation of the feet. Ultrasound treatments and heel cord stretching exercises are helpful. Proper running shoes and training techniques are important. The patient should be referred to one of the many books that describe acceptable training and conditioning programs.

Stress Fractures. Stress fractures are the result of the excessive demands placed upon the lower extremities before the athlete has taken sufficient time for proper conditioning.[79,80] Bone density and strength increase in response to progressive increases in physical training (Wolff's law).[126] Thus, stress fractures are seen often in the beginning runner or in the individual who has suddenly increased his mileage in preparation for a competition. Stress fractures commonly occur in the proximal tibia and distal fibula. Tenderness and induration may be noted over the fracture site. Other etiologic factors may include a tight heel cord and limitation of flexibility in the subtalar joint (cavovarus deformities). Adequate subtalar motion is essential for absorption of compressive weight-bearing forces in gait.

X-rays. Routine x-rays will not demonstrate the stress fracture for at least 2 to 3 weeks following the onset of symptoms. Bone scans[82] are positive early in the clinical course and extremely helpful.

Treatment. Although no immobilization is necessary to treat these fractures, rest is essential. Usually within 6 to 8 weeks the individuals are comfortable and able to resume training. The underlying biomechanical problems must be corrected with stretching exercises or orthotics and the training modified with a more gradual increase in distance to prevent recurrence of injury.

Achilles Tendonitis. Achilles tendonitis is characterized by pain and swelling along the tendon sheath proximal to its insertion at the os calcis. This condition comprises a spectrum of pathologic changes, from simple tenosynovitis involving the peritenon to interstitial disruption of the Achilles tendon fibers.[127,128] Usually gradual in onset, at times it can appear suddenly. The patient notices limitation of motion in the ankle and pain with attempts to drive off the ball of the foot. On physical examination there is tenderness and crepitus along the distal third of the Achilles tendon in those with acute tenosynovitis. In chronic injuries an indurated or nodular tendon may be palpable. Routine x-rays are negative; however, CT scans may show soft tissue thickening of the tendon.

If the patient is symptomatic when walking, treatment should include crutches, with either a minimal weight-bearing gait or a period of immobilization in a short leg cast. Oral anti-inflammatory agents, ultrasound treatments, and contrast ice and warm whirlpools may be helpful. Corticosteroid injections should be given with caution and only around the tendon. Subcutaneous atrophy and scarring secondary to these injections can be particularly severe complications in this area. Although a heel lift may be helpful in relieving the tension on the Achilles tendon, stretching is an essential part of the rehabilitation program to regain flexibility in the gastroc-soleus complex. Strengthening exercises, particularly raising up on toes and lowering over the edge of a stair, are helpful in regaining both power and flexibility.

Compartment Syndromes. The muscles of the anterior, lateral, and posterior compartments of the lower leg are surrounded peripherally by a tight fascial sheath and internally by the tibia, fibula, and intermuscular septum. Consequently, with the repeated muscular activity of athletic events, the muscles may hypertrophy beyond the normal volume of their respective compartments. This results initially in venous obstruction with edema and subsequently ischemia of the muscles and nerves.[129,131] The ischemic pains subside when the individual stops running but recurs when the activity is repeated. When these individuals are examined shortly after running, there is often tenderness and induration over the involved compartment. If the patient attempts to run through the pain, there may be severe pain with associated dysesthesias and paresthesias suggesting neurologic involvement. The anterior compartment is most frequently involved. Routine x-rays are negative. A definitive diagnosis can be made by measuring the compartment pressure, using the technique described by Whiteside.[132,133]

Unfortunately, this condition is difficult to treat conservatively. Those individuals who insist on continuing with their athletic activities may require surgical decompression by fasciotomy. A less common form of claudication can occur in runners as the result of entrapment of branches of the popliteal artery as they course through the muscles or over the fascial layers in the back of the calf. These conditions are rare and require arteriography to diagnose accurately.

Tennis Leg. Middle-aged individuals involved in running, jumping, and racquet sports often sustain an acute disruption of the Achilles tendon. Most commonly this occurs at the distal portion of the Achilles tendon above its attachment to the os calcis. The patient often claims he had been kicked by someone or struck by an object. This is followed by an inability to stand on the ball of the foot or to toe off in normal gait. On physical examination there may be a palpable defect in the Achilles tendon and marked weakness on plantar flexion. Because the tendinous connection with the gastrocnemius muscle is disrupted, squeezing the gastrocnemius muscle fails to produce the normal plantar flexion response (Thompson test).[135] Acceptable treatment for acute ruptures of the Achilles tendon includes surgical reattachment or immobilization in a long leg cast, depending on the personal preference of the physician. Both will give satisfactory results.

Another form of tennis leg is characterized by sudden pain in the calf in an area more proximal to the sight of the classical Achilles tendon ruptures. Frequently referred to as a torn plantaris, this actually results from disruption of the musculotendinous junction of the medial head of the gastrocnemius muscle.[134] This may be as dramatic and painful as a ruptured Achilles tendon but is considerably less serious. There is tenderness and swelling along the medial portion of the gastrocnemius muscle. A defect may be palpable if the patient is seen before the swelling occurs or after it has subsided. These patients are also unable to walk on their toes because of pain and weakness. The treatment, however, does not require surgery or prolonged immobilization. A posterior splint for 3 to 5 days followed by a partial weight-bearing gait thereafter is recommended. When pain and swelling have subsided sufficiently to allow a rehabilitation program to begin, the patient should start by strengthening and stretching the gastrocnemius complex to regain normal function. Although it takes several weeks to regain full strength and flexibility after these injuries, the patient can anticipate a good functional result.

ANKLE SPRAINS

Ankle sprains may be the most neglected musculoskeletal injury. Unfortunately, patients who have sustained significant injuries to the lateral ligaments of the ankle may have residual disability from inadequate treatment and rehabilitation.

Anatomic Considerations. The lateral ankle ligaments are much more commonly injured than the medial deltoid ligament. The anterior inferior tibiofibular ligament stablizes the fibula to the tibia and is disrupted as the talus forces the fibula laterally with inversion or eversion stress. The anterior talofibular ligament courses anteriorly from the fibula to attach on the talus laterally. This ligament is tight in plantar flexion and is most frequently torn with plantar flexion and inversion. The anterior talofibular ligament prevents the anterior translation of the talus from under the tibia. The calcaneal fibular ligament runs distally from the fibula to attach on the calcaneus. It is tight in dorsiflexion and may be disrupted in this position in combination with marked inversion. The posterior talofibular ligament is rarely torn except in total dislocations of the ankle. The large medial deltoid ligament is disrupted with eversion and dorsiflexion injuries and is frequently associated with fractures of the fibula.[1,2]

History. A history of a sudden inversion injury is the most common mechanism of lateral ligament injuries. Dorsiflexion, eversion injuries involving the deltoid ligament, are quite severe and frequently result from step-

Figure 109–19. Anteroposterior x-ray, demonstrating an osteochondral injury to the superior lateral aspect of the talus following an ankle injury.

Figure 109–18. Lateral x-ray, demonstrating a fracture of the posterior aspect of the talus following a plantar flexion injury to the ankle.

ping on another individual's foot, which then forces the injured foot into dorsiflexion and eversion. The pain is severe in all of the injuries and often associated with a popping or tearing sensation. Swelling usually occurs promptly over the site of the injury, and the patient has difficulty bearing weight.

On physical examination it is important to examine the normal ankle first to obtain an appreciation of the degree of flexibility in the patient. One should begin the examination by palpating along the course of the fibula from its proximal portion down to the ankle. Ankle sprains may be associated with proximal fibular fractures. Local tenderness or swelling over the fibula or tibia should alert one to the diagnosis of a fracture.

Figure 109–20. Stress x-ray of the ankle, revealing excessive anterior subluxation of the talus in the lower left film and instability on inversion in the lower right film. The normal contralateral ankle is depicted under stress in the upper two films.

Although there may be a diffuse hemarthrosis, there is generally more swelling over the site of the ligamentous damage. The anterior talofibular ligament and anterior tibular-fibular ligaments are the most common sites of pain and tenderness. Limitation of dorsiflexion and plantar flexion will be present secondary to joint swelling and pain. The inversion[138,139] and anterior Drawer[136,137] laxity tests are painful and difficult to assess in acute cases. A predisposing factor is an acquired or developmental limitation of subtalar motion.[15] This is important when assessing the normal side and also when reviewing the x-rays for a subtalar coalition.

Routine x-rays include anteroposterior, lateral, and mortise views. In addition to fractures of the distal and proximal fibula and the medial malleolus, on the lateral film one should look carefully at the posterior articular surface of the talus (Fig. 109–18) and distal tibia, where vertical compression fractures or avulsion fractures are possible. In addition, the mortise film may show an osteochondral fracture on the articular surface of the talus (Fig. 109–19). Stress films may be obtained in those cases in which significant instability is suspected (Fig. 109–20). A positive anterior Drawer stress film indicates damage to the anterior talofibular ligament[136,137] and a positive talar tilt film is indicative of disruption of the calcaneal fibular ligament.[138,139] It is important to obtain comparative stress films of the normal ankle, since it is the degree of change compared with the uninjured ankle that is significant. Ankle arthrograpy[21,22] is very helpful in defining ligament tears, chondral fractures of the talus, and loose bodies (Fig. 109–21).

Treatment. Mild ankle sprains exhibiting little or no laxity can be successfully managed by ice, elevation, compression bandage, crutches, and early mobilization encouraging partial weight bearing and progressive strengthening exercises. With prompt and proper treatment most patients with ankle sprains can be participating in normal activities in 6 to 7 days. The prevention of swelling with compression and ice and early rehabilitation prevent weakness and stiffness, which are the major disabilities from ankle injuries.

The treatment of severe combined sprains of the anterior talofibular ligament and calcaneal fibular ligament remains controversial, with the choices including early functional mobilization and rehabilitation, cast immobilization for 6 weeks, and surgical repair.[140-142] Satisfactory results can indeed be obtained by any of these methods. However, the unsatisfactory results, regardless of the method of original treatment, have as their common denominator inadequate rehabilitation.[11] Prolonged immobilization in plaster with or without operative procedures can result in troublesome joint contractures and residual weakness of the peroneal muscle groups. These problems need to be corrected by vigorous strengthening programs and flexibility exercises, particularly for the Achilles tendon.[143] Loss of proprioception[141] is also an important cause of disability and can be corrected by using a properly designed proprioceptive exercise program on a tilt board.[145] Protective taping and bracing and the use of high-top athletic shoes have also been found effective in preventing reinjury.[144]

In this section I have discussed a variety of acute, traumatic, and chronic overuse athletic injuries. Unfortunately, reinjury remains one of the most frequent problems. The most common cause of reinjury is not failure to properly diagnose and treat the condition initially but failure to rehabilitate the patient completely. Restoration of adequate strength, endurance, and flexibility is essential for a safe return to recreational or competitive athletics. The practicing physician must give this goal as much dedication and interest as he expends in formulating an accurate diagnosis and treatment plan for the acute injury.

Figure 109–21. Arthrotomogram of the ankle, demonstrating a defect in the articular cartilage on the superior lateral aspect of the talus following an ankle sprain.

References

1. Kapanji, I.A.: The Physiology of Joints. Vols. I and II. Edinburgh and London, E. & S. Livingston, 1970.
2. Goss, C.M.: Gray's Anatomy of the Human Body. 28th ed. Philadelphia, Lea & Febiger, 1966.
3. Noyes, F.R., Torvik, P.J., Hyde, W.B., and DeLucas, J.L.: Biomechanics of ligament failure. J. Bone Joint Surg. 56A:1406, 1974.
4. Noyes, F.R., DeLucas, J.L., and Torvik, P.J.: Biomechanics of anterior cruciate failure, J. Bone Joint Surg. 56A:236, 1974.
5. Tipton, C.M., James, S.L., Mergner, W., et al.: Influence of exercise on strength of medial collateral ligament of dogs. Am. J. Physiol. 218:894, 1970.
6. Tipton, C.M., Matthes, R.D., Maynard, J.A., et al.: The influence of physical activity on ligaments and tendons. Med. Sci. Sports 7:165, 1975.
7. Weisman, G., Pope, M.H., and Johnson, R.J.: Cyclic loading in knee ligament injuries. Am. J. Sports Med. 8:24, 1980.
8. Walker, P.S., and Erkman, M.J.: The role of the menisci in force transmission across the knee. Clin. Orthop. (109):184, 1975.
9. Maquet, P.G., and VanDeBerg, A.J.: Femorotibial weight bearing areas. J. Bone Joint Surg. 57A:766, 1978.
10. Kurosawa, H., et al.: Load-bearing mode of the knee joint: Physical behavior of the knee joint with and without menisci. Clin. Orthop. (149):283, 1980.
11. Allman, F.L., Jr.: Rehabilitation of the injured athlete. In Ryan, A.J., and Allman, F.L., Jr. (eds.): Sports Medicine. New York, Academic Press, 1974.

12. Clancy, W.G.: Tendinitis and plantar fasciitis in runners. *In* D'Ambrozia, R., and Drez, D., Jr. (eds.): Prevention and Treatment of Running Injuries. Thorofare, N.J., Charles B. Slack, Inc., 1982.
13. Cahill, B.R.: Quadrilateral space syndrome. *In* Omer, G.E., Jr., and Spinner, M.D., (eds.): Management of Peripheral Nerve Injuries. Philadelphia, W.B. Saunders Company, 1980.
14. Drez, D., Jr.: Suprascapular neuropathy in the differential diagnosis of rotator cuff injuries. Am. J Sports Med. 4:43, 1976.
15. Snyder, R.B., Lipscomb, A.B., and Johnston, R.K.: The relationship of tarsal coalitions to ankle sprains in athletes. Am J. Sports Med. 9:313, 1981.
16. O'Donoghue, D.H.: Treatment of Athletic Injuries. 3rd ed. Philadelphia, W.B. Saunders Company, 1976.
17. Blazina, M.E., and Saltzman, J.S.: Recurrent Subluxations of the Shoulder in Athletes. Proceedings of The American Academy of Orthopedic Surgeons. J. Bone Joint Surg. 51A, 1969.
18. Rowe, C.R., and Zarins, B.: Recurrent subluxation of the shoulder. J. Bone Joint Surg. 63A:863, 1981.
19. Bateman, J.E.: The Shoulder and Neck. 2nd ed. Philadelphia, W.B. Saunders Company, 1978.
20. Neviaser, J.S.: Arthrography of the Shoulder. Springfield, Ill., Charles C Thomas, 1975.
21. Freiberger, R.H., and Kaye, J.: Arthrography. New York, Appleton-Century-Crofts, 1979.
22. Arndt, R.D., Horns, J.W., and Gold, R.H.: Clinical Arthrography. Baltimore, Williams and Wilkins Co., 1981.
23. Fowler, P.J.: Posterior Subluxation of the Shoulder in Swimmers. Presented at the annual meeting of the American Orthopedic Society for Sports Medicine, Lake of the Ozarks, Missouri, July 1982.
24. Hoyt, W.A., Jr.: Etiology of shoulder injuries in athletes. J. Bone Joint Surg. 49A:755, 1967.
25. Moseley, H.F.: Shoulder Lesions. 3rd ed. Baltimore, Williams and Wilkins Company, 1969.
26. Allman, F.L., Jr.: Fractures and ligamentous injuries of the clavicle and its articulation. J. Bone Joint Surg. 49A:744, 1967.
27. Vrist, M.R.: Complete dislocations of the acromioclavicular joint. J. Bone Joint Surg. 45A:1750, 1963.
28. Bergfeld, J.A., Andrish, J.T., and Clancy, W.G.: Evaluation of the acromioclavicular joint following first and second degree sprains. Am. J. Sports Med. 6:153, 1978.
29. Cox, J.S.: The fate of the acromioclavicular joint in athletic injuries. Am. J. Sports Med. 9:50, 1981.
30. Browne, J.E., Stanley, R.F., and Tullos, H.S.: Acromioclavicular joint dislocations: Comparative results following operative treatment with and without primary clavisectomy. Am. J. Sports Med. 5:258, 1977.
31. Glick, J.M., Milburn, L.J., Haggerty, J.F., et al.: Dislocated acromioclavicular joint: Followup study of 35 unreduced acromioclavicular dislocations. Am. J. Sports Med. 5:264, 1977.
32. Alexander, O.M.: Radiology of the acromioclavicular articulation. Med. Radiogr. Photogr. 30:34, 1954.
33. Jacobs, P.: Post-traumatic osteolysis of the outer end of the clavicle. J. Bone Joint Surg. 46B:705, 1964.
34. Mumford, E.B.: Acromioclavicular dislocation: A new operative treatment. J. Bone Joint Surg. 23:799, 1941.
35. Bennett, G.E.: Shoulder and elbow lesions distinctive of baseball players. Ann. Surg. 126:107, 1947.
36. Hawkins, R.J., and Kennedy, J.C.: Impingement syndromes in athletes. Am. J. Sports Med. 3:151, 1980.
37. Kennedy, J.C., and Hawkins, R.T.: Swimmer's shoulder. Physician Sports Med. 2:35, 1974.
38. Priest, J.D., and Nagel, D.A.: Tennis shoulder. Am. J. Sports Med. 4:28, 1976.
39. Jackson, D.W.: Chronic rotator cuff impingement in the throwing athlete. Am. J. Sports Med. 4:231, 1976.
40. Bateman, J.E.: Cuff tears in athletes. Orthop. Clin. North Am. 4:721, 1973.
41. Neer, C.S., and Welsh, R.P.: The shoulder in sports. Orthop. Clin. North Am. 8:583, 1977.
42. Richardson, A.B., Jobe, F.W., and Collins, H.R.: The shoulder in competitive swimming. Am. J. Sports Med. 8:159, 1980.
43. Barnes, D.A., and Tullos, H.S.: An analysis of 100 symptomatic baseball players. Am. J. Sports Med. 6:62, 1978.
44. Norwood, L.A., DelPizzo, W., Jobe, F.W., and Kerlan, R.K.: Anterior shoulder pain in baseball pitchers. Am. J. Sports Med. 6:103, 1978.
45. Lombardo, S.J., Jobe, F.W., Kerlan, R.K., et al.: Posterior shoulder lesions in throwing athletes. Am. J. Sports Med. 5:106, 1977.
46. Tullos, H.S., and King, J.W.: Throwing mechanism in sports. Orthop. Clin. North Am. 4:709, 1973.
47. Rathbun, J.B., and MacNab, I.: The microvascular pattern of the rotator cuff. J. Bone Joint Surg. 52B:540, 1970.
48. Moseley, H.F., and Goldie, I.: The arterial pattern of the rotator cuff. J. Bone Joint Surg. 45B:780, 1963.
49. Weiner, D.S., and MacNab, I.: Superior migration of the humeral head: A radiological aid in the diagnosis of tears of the rotator cuff. J. Bone Joint Surg. 52B:524, 1970.
50. Braunstein, E.M., and O'Connor, G.: Double contrast arthrotomography of the shoulder. J. Bone Joint Surg. 64A:192, 1982.
51. Danzig, L., Resnik, D., and Greenway, G.: Evaluation of shoulders by computed tomograph. Am. J. Sports Med. 10:138, 1982.
52. Kennedy, J.C., and Willis, R.B.: The effects of local steroid injections on tendons: A biomechanical and microscopic correlative study. Am. J. Sports Med. 4:11, 1976.
53. Ismail, A.M., Balakishnan, R., and Rajakumar, M.K.: Rupture of patellar tendon after steroid infiltration. J. Bone Joint Surg. 51B:503, 1969.
54. Malmed, E.P.: Spontaneous bilateral rupture of the calcaneal tendon during steroid injection. J. Bone Joint Surg. 47B:104, 1965.
55. Unverferth, L.J., and Olix, M.L.: The effects of local steroid injections on tendon. J. Sports Med. 1:31, 1973.
56. Wrem, R.N., Goldner, J.L., and Markee, J.L.: An experimental study of the effects of cortisone on the healing process and tensile strength of tendons. J. Bone Joint Surg. 36A:588, 1954.
57. Jobe, F.W., and Moynes, D.R.: Delineation of diagnostic criteria and a rehabilitation program for rotator cuff injuries. Am. J. Sports Med. 10:336, 1982.
58. Boland, A.L.: Rehabilitation of the injured athlete. *In* Strauss, R.H. (ed.): Sports Medicine and Physiology. Philadelphia, W. B. Saunders Company, 1979.
59. Neer, C.S.: Anterior acromioplasty for the chronic impingement syndrome in the shoulder: A preliminary report. J. Bone Joint Surg. 54A:41, 1972.
60. Codman, E.A.: The Shoulder—Rupture of the Supraspinatous Tendon and Other Lesions in and About the Subacromial Bursa. Boston, Thomas Todd Company, 1934.
61. Bennett, G.E.: Elbow lesions of baseball players. Am. J. Surg. 98:484, 1959.
62. Slocum, D.B.: Classification of elbow injuries from baseball pitching. Tex. Med. 64:48, 1968.
63. King, J.W., Brelsford, H.J., and Tullos, H.S.: Analysis of the pitching arm of the professional baseball pitcher. Clin. Orthop. 67:116, 1969.
64. Woods, G.W., Tullos, H.S., and King, J.W.: The throwing arm: Elbow joint injuries. Am. J. Sports Med. 4:43, 1977.
65. Nirschl, R.P.: The etiology and treatment of tennis elbow. J. Sports Med. 2:308, 1975.
66. Goldie, I.G.: Epicondylitis lateralis humeri. Acta Chir. Scand. Suppl. 339:1–114, 1961.
67. Conrad, R.W., and Hooper, W.R.: Tennis elbow: Its course, natural history, conservative and surgical management. J. Bone Joint Surg. 55A:1177, 1973.
68. Garden, R.S.: Tennis elbow. J. Bone Joint Surg. 43B:100, 1961.
69. Stack, J.K.: Acute and chronic bursitis in the region of the elbow joint. Surg. Clin. North Am. 29:155, 1949.
70. Trethowan, W.H.: Tennis elbow. Br. Med. J. 2:1218, 1929.
71. Kaplan, E.B.: Treatment of tennis elbow (epicondylitis) by denervation. J. Bone Joint Surg. 41A:147, 1959.
72. Roles, N.C., and Maudsley, R.H.: Radial tunnel syndrome: Resistant tennis elbow as a nerve entrapment. J. Bone Joint Surg. 54B:499, 1972.
73. Gugenheim, J.J., Stanley, R.T., Woods, G.W., and Tullos, H.S.: The Little League survey: The Houston study. Am. J. Sports Med. 4:189, 1976.
74. Larson, R.L., Singer, K.N., and Nagel, D.A.: The Little League survey: The Eugene study. Am. J. Sports Med. 4:201, 1976.
75. Adams, J.E.: Bone injuries in the very young athlete. Clin. Orthop. 58:129, 1968.
76. Tullos, H.S., and King, J.W.: Lesions of the pitching arm in adolescents. JAMA 220:264, 1972.
77. Priest, J.D., Jones, H.H., and Nagel, D.A.: Elbow injuries in the highly skilled tennis players. Am. J. Sports Med. 2:137, 1974.
78. DelPizzo, W., Jobe, F.W., and Norwood, L.: Ulnar nerve entrapment syndrome in baseball players. Am. J. Sports Med. 5:182, 1977.
79. D'Ambrosia, R., and Drez, D.J.: Prevention and Treatment of Running Injuries. Thorofare, N.J., Charles B. Slack, Inc., 1982.
80. McBryde, A.M., Jr.: Stress fractures in athletes. J. Sports Med. 3:212, 1975.
81. Kaltsas, D.S.: Stress fractures of femoral neck in young adults: Report of 7 cases. J. Bone Joint Surg. 63B:33, 1981.
82. Siddiqui, A.R.: Bone scans for early detection of stress fractures. N. Engl. J. Med. 298:1033, 1978.
83. Brody, D.M.: Running injuries. Clinical Symposia-CIBA 32(4), 1980.
84. Smillie, I.S.: Injuries of the Knee Joint. 4th ed. Baltimore, Williams and Wilkins Company, 1970.
85. Müller, W.: The Knee. Form, Function and Ligament Reconstruction. New York, Springer-Verlag, 1983.
86. Dandy, D.J.: Arthroscopic Surgery of The Knee. London, Churchill Livingstone, 1981.

87. Johnson, L.L.: The Comprehensive Examination of the Knee. St. Louis, C. V. Mosby Co., 1977.

88. King, D.: The function of semilunar cartilages. J. Bone Joint Surg. 18:1069, 1936.

89. Cox, J.S., Nye, C.E., et al.: The degenerative effects of partial and total resection of the medial meniscus in dog's knees. Clin. Orthop. (109):178, 1975.

90. Shapiro, F., and Glimcher, M.J.: Induction of osteoarthritis in the rabbit knee joint. Clin. Orthop. (147):287, 1980.

91. Tapper, E.M., and Hoover, N.W.: Late results after meniscectomy. J. Bone Joint Surg. 51A:517, 1969.

92. Johnson, R.J., Kettlekamp, D.B., Clark, W., and Leaverton, P.: Factors affecting late results after meniscectomy. J. Bone Joint Surg. 56A:719, 1974.

93. McGinty, J.B., Geuss, L.F., and Marvin, R.A.: Partial or Total Meniscectomy. J. Bone Joint Surg. 59A:763, 1977.

94. Jackson, R.W.: The results of partial arthroscopic meniscectomy in patients over 40 years of age. J. Bone Joint Surg. 64B:481, 1982.

95. Dandy, D.J., and Jackson, R.W.: The diagnosis of problems after meniscectomy. J. Bone Joint Surg. 57B:349, 1975.

96. Fairbank, T.J.: Knee joint changes after meniscectomy. J. Bone Joint Surg. 30B:664, 1948.

97. Cabaud, H.E., Rodkey, W.G., and Fitzwater, J.E.: Medial meniscus repairs: An experimental and morphologic study. Am. J. Sports Med. 9:3, 129, 1981.

98. Cassidy, R.E., and Shaffer, A.J.: Repair of peripheral meniscus tears: A preliminary report. Am. J. Sports Med. 9:209, 1981.

99. DeHaven, K.E.: Selective approach to meniscectomy. Presented at the American Academy of Orthopedic Surgeon's Knee Injury Course. Boston, May 1983.

100. Slocum, D.B., and Larson, R.L.: Rotary instability of the knee. J. Bone Joint Surg. 50A:211, 1968.

101. Hughston, J.C., Andrews, J.R., et al.: Classification of knee ligament instabilities. J. Bone Joint Surg. 58A:159, Part I, 58A:173, Part II, 1976.

102. Brantigan, O.C., and Voshell, A.F.: Ligaments of the knee joint, J. Bone Joint Surg. 28:66, 1946.

103. Warren, L.F., Marshall, J.L., and Girgis, F.: The prime static stabilizer of the medial side of the knee. J. Bone Joint Surg. 56A:665, 1974.

104. Kennedy, J.C., and Fowler, P.J.: Medial and anterior instability of the knee: An anatomical and clinical study using stress machines. J. Bone Joint Surg. 53A:1257, 1971.

105. Kennedy, J.C., et al.: Tension studies of human knee ligaments, yield point, ultimate failure and disruption of the cruciate and tibial collateral ligaments. J. Bone Joint Surg. 58A:350, 1976.

106. DeHaven, K.E.: Diagnosis of acute knee ligament injuries with hemarthrosis. Am. J. Sports Med. 8:9, 1980.

107. Noyes, F.R., Bassett, R.W., Grood, E.S., and Butler, D.L.: Arthroscopy in acute traumatic hemarthrosis of the knee: Incidence of anterior cruciate tears and other injuries. J. Bone Joint Surg. 62A:687, 1980.

108. Torg, J.S., Conrad, W., and Kalen, V.: Clinical diagnosis of anterior cruciate ligament instability in the athlete. Am. J. Sports Med. 4:84, 1976.

109. Kennedy, J.C.: The Injured Adolescent Knee. Baltimore, Williams and Wilkins Company, 1979.

110. Noyes, F.R., and Spievack, E.S.: Extraarticular fluid dissection in tissues during arthroscopy. Am. J. Sports Med. 10:346, 1982.

111. Clancy, W.G., Bergfeld, J., O'Connor, G.A., and Cox, J.A.: Symposium: Functional rehabilitation of medial collateral ligament sprains. Am. J. Sports Med. 7:206, 1979.

112. Blazina, M.: Jumper's knee. Orthop. Clin. North Am. 4:665, 1973.

113. Roels, J., Martens, M., et al.: Patellar tendinitis (jumper's knee) Am. J. Sports Med. 6:362, 1978.

114. Estwanik, J.J., Bergfeld, J., and Canty, T.: Report of injuries sustained during the Olympic wrestling trials. Am. J. Sports Med. 6:335, 1978.

115. Renne, J.W.: The iliotibial band friction syndrome. J. Bone Joint Surg. 57A:1110, 1975.

116. James, S.L., Bates, B.T., and Osternig, L.R.: Injuries to runners. Am J. Sports Med. 6:40, 1978.

117. Ficat, R.P., and Hungerford, D.S.: Disorders of the Patellofemoral Joint. Baltimore, Williams and Wilkins Company, 1977.

118. Outerbridge, R.E.: The etiology of chondromalacia patella. J. Bone Joint Surg. 43B:752, 1961.

119. Laurin, C.A., et al.: The abnormal lateral patellofemoral angle. J. Bone Joint Surg. 60A:55, 1978.

120. Merchant, A.C., Mercer, R.L., et al.: Roentgenographic analysis of patellofemoral congruence. J. Bone Joint Surg. 56A:139, 1964.

121. Insall, J., and Salvati, E.: Patella position in the normal knee joint. Radiology 101:101, 1971.

122. Henry, J.H., and Crosland, J.W.: Conservative treatment of patellofemoral subluxations. Am. J. Sports Med. 7:12, 1979.

123. Palumbo, P.M.: Dynamic patellar brace: A new orthosis in the management of patellofemoral disorders. Am. J. Sports Med. 9:45, 1981.

124. Slocum, D.B.: The shin splint syndrome: Medical aspects and differential diagnosis. Am. J. Surg. 114:875, 1967.

125. Mubarak, S.J., Gould, R.N., et al.: The medial tibial stress syndrome: A cause of shin splints. Am. J. Sports Med. 10:201, 1982.

126. Baker, J., Frankel, V.H., et al.: Fatigue fractures: Biomechanical considerations. J. Bone Joint Surg. 54A:1345, 1972.

127. Clancy, W.G., Neidhart, D., and Brand, R.L.: Achilles tendinitis in runners: A report of five cases. Am. J. Sports Med. 4:46, 1976.

128. Puddu, G., Ippolito, E., and Postacchini, F.: A classification of Achilles tendon disease. Am. J. Sports Med. 4:145, 1976.

129. Reneman, R.S.: The anterior and the lateral compartmental syndrome of the leg due to intensive use of muscles. Clin. Orthop. 113:69, 1975.

130. Mubarak, S.J., Owen, C.A., Garfin, S.R., et al.: Acute exertional superficial posterior compartment syndrome. Am. J. Sports Med. 6:287, 1978.

131. Snook, G.A.: Intermittent claudication in athletes. Am. J. Sports Med. 3:71, 1975.

132. Whitesides, T.E., Haney, T.C., et al.: Tissue pressure measurements as a determinant for the need of fasciotomy. Clin. Orthop. 113:43, 1975.

133. Mubarak, S.J., Hargens, A.R., Owen, C.A., et al.: The wick catheter technique for measurement of intramuscular pressure: A new research and clinical tool. J. Bone Joint Surg. 58A:1016, 1976.

134. Miller, W.A.: Rupture of the musculotendinous junction of the medial head of the gastrocnemius muscle. Am. J. Sports Med. 5:191, 1977.

135. Thompson, T.C.: A test for rupture of the tendo Achilles. Acta Orthop. Scand. 32:461, 1962.

136. Seligson, D., Gassman, J., and Pope, M.: Ankle instability: Evaluation of the lateral ligaments. Am. J. Sports Med. 8:39, 1980.

137. Frost, H.M., and Hanson, C.A.: Technique for testing the drawer sign in the ankle. Clin. Orthop. 123:49, 1977.

138. Laurin, C., and Mathiew, J.: Sagittal mobility of the normal ankle. Clin. Orthop. 108:99, 1975.

139. Cox, J.S., and Hewes, T.F.: "Normal" talar tilt angle. Clin. Orthop. 140:37, 1979.

140. Freeman, M.A.: Treatment of ruptures of the lateral ligaments of the ankle. J. Bone Joint Surg. 47B:661, 1965.

141. Freeman, M.A.: The etiology and prevention of functional instability of the foot, JBJS 47B: 678, 1965.

142. Staples, O.S.: Ruptures of the fibular collateral ligaments of the ankle: Result study of immediate surgical treatment. J. Bone Joint Surg. 57A:101, 1975.

143. McClusky, G.M., et al.: Prevention of ankle sprain. Am. J. Sports Med. 4:151, 1976.

144. Garrick, J.C., and Requa, R.K.: Role of external supports in the prevention of ankle sprains. Med. Sci. Sports 5:200, 1973.

145. Glick, J.M., Gordon, R.B., and Nishimoto, D.: The prevention and treatment of ankle injuries. Am. J. Sports Med. 4:136, 1976.

Chapter 110
Entrapment Neuropathies

Kenneth K. Nakano

INTRODUCTION

Entrapment neuropathies occur commonly, and the clinician must possess a method of assessment and treatment of patients with these syndromes. The term entrapment describes the mechanical irritation by which a specific peripheral nerve becomes locally injured in a vulnerable anatomic site. Nerve compression can occur at any point where a peripheral nerve passes through an opening in fibrous tissue or through an osseofibrous canal. Table 110–1 lists the nerves encountered in entrapment syndromes.

A thorough familiarity with the anatomy of the peripheral nerves is essential, and the reader should familiarize himself with standard texts.[1-6] Table 110–2 provides certain characteristic clinical features associated with nerves commonly involved in entrapment syndromes. Differential findings in lower motor neuron (anterior horn cells of the spinal cord, nerve roots, peripheral nerves, neuromuscular junction, and muscle) weakness are summarized in Table 110–3.

In addition to a neurologic examination, the evaluation of every patient with an entrapment neuropathy should include electromyography (EMG), motor and sensory nerve conduction velocity studies, and appropriate radiographs. EMG and nerve conduction velocity measurements provide localizing information often necessary in the early diagnosis of a compressive neuropathy and reliably document the severity and extent of nerve entrapments.[7,8]

INTERPRETATION OF ELECTRODIAGNOSTIC STUDIES

Various EMG and nerve conduction patterns help differentiate the normal from a diffuse polyneuropathy, focal entrapment neuropathy, radiculopathy or nerve root compression syndrome, myopathy, disorder of the neuromuscular junction, and anterior horn cell disease (Table 110–4). No one feature of the EMG (except true myotonia) alone gives a diagnosis; rather it becomes the summated information of insertional activity, spontaneous activity, and recruitment (both minimal and maximal), as well as nerve conduction values which the clinician utilizes in the evaluation of his patient. For example, in both an L5 nerve root compression and a peroneal neuropathy, increased insertion, fibrillations, positive waves, long duration polyphasic motor units, and a decreased interference pattern may be seen in the anterior tibial, extensor hallucis longus, and peroneal muscles. However, in L5 nerve root compression the

nerve conduction velocities remain normal and EMG changes follow a dermatome (e.g., paraspinal L5 muscles).

Clinicians are faced with the problem of diagnosis of muscular weakness. Weakness may be secondary to disease within the muscle, nerve, neuromuscular junction, or upper motor neuron (spinal cord, cerebrum). The need for more definitive treatment, including surgery, can be established when the physician is aware of the cause, extent, and prognosis of the weakness. Evaluation of the electrical activity of muscle tissue and muscle response to nerve stimulation solves many of these problems.

UPPER LIMBS

Median Nerve. The median nerve derives from nerve root fibers C6, C7, C8, and T1 (Fig. 110–1). It arises in two heads, an outer and inner, which are derived from the upper and lower secondary trunks of the brachial plexus. The median nerve controls the following movements: pronation of the forearm by the pronator quadratus and pronator teres; flexion of the hand by the flexor carpi radialis and palmaris longus; flexion of the thumb and index and middle fingers by the superficial and deep flexors; and opposition and abduction of the thumb (Table 110–5). The sensory supply of the median nerve covers the radial side of the palm of the hand and the palmar surface of the thumb, index, middle, and neighboring half of the ring finger (Fig. 110–1). Except for articular branches to the elbow joint, the median nerve has no branches above the elbow. Because associated lesions involve blood vessels, vasomotor disturbances occur with median nerve lesions. Causalgic syndromes frequently result after median nerve lesions.

Carpal Tunnel Syndrome. The carpal tunnel syndrome is the most commonly encountered entrapment neuropathy in the patient with rheumatoid arthritis. This entrapment occurs in the carpal tunnel of the hand where the median nerve passes in company with the flexor tendons of the fingers (Fig. 110–1). Since the transverse carpal ligament is a strong structure which forms the roof of the tunnel, flexor tenosynovitis in this area often produces pressure on the median nerve. Various disease states may be found in association with the carpal tunnel syndrome,[9] and in the evaluation of patients with this syndrome the physician must consider the following disorders: rheumatoid arthritis,[10] hypothyroidism,[11] amyloid,[12] gout,[13] acromegaly,[14] and other inflammatory reactions involving the tendons and connective tissue in the wrist.[4,15,16]

Table 110–1. Peripheral Entrapment Neuropathies*

Nerve	Entrapment Syndrome
Upper Limbs	
Median	Carpal tunnel
	"Pseudo-carpal tunnel (sublimis)"
	Digital nerve
	Anterior interosseous nerve
	Pronator teres
	Ligament of Struthers
	"Double crush"
Ulnar	Guyon's canal
	Digital nerve
	Cubital canal
	"Tardy ulnar palsy"
	"Double crush"
Radial	Saturday night palsy
	Posterior interosseous nerve
	"Tennis elbow"
Musculocutaneous	Coracobrachialis
Suprascapular	Suprascapular foramen
	Infraspinatus branch
Dorsal scapular	Scalenus medius
Brachial plexus	Thoracic outlet
	Scalenus-anticus
	Costoclavicular
	Hyperabduction
Lower Limbs	
Sciatic	Piriformis
	Popliteal (Baker's) cyst
Common peroneal	Hereditary compression neuropathy
	Ganglion
	Leprosy
	Popliteal (Baker's) cyst
Posterior tibial	Popliteal (Baker's) cyst
	Tarsal tunnel
	Medial and lateral plantar nerve
	Interdigital nerve
Femoral	Pressure by space limiting process
Saphenous	Subsartorial (Hunter's) canal
Lateral femoral cutaneous	Meralgia paresthetica
Obturator	Obturator canal
	Osteitis pubis
Ilioinguinal	Anterior superior iliac spine
Genitofemoral	Adhesions after surgery

*From Nakano, K.K.: Neurology of Musculoskeletal and Rheumatic Disorders. Boston, Houghton Mifflin, 1979.

Table 110–2. Characteristic Features Associated with Various Nerves*

Nerve	Clinical Involvement
Median	Thumb and thenar eminence
Anterior interosseous	Flexor pollicis longus, pronator quadratus, flexor digitorum profundus to index and middle fingers; normal sensation
Ulnar	Small finger and hypothenar eminence
Musculocutaneous	Biceps
Radial	Wrist drop; sensory loss in dorsum of thumb
Posterior interosseous	Wrist drop; normal sensation
Femoral	Absent knee jerk; weak knee extension and hip flexion
Peroneal	Foot drop; sensory loss in dorsum of foot
Posterior tibial	Sensory loss in medial heel; weakness in intrinsic muscles of foot
Sciatic	Pain down lateral thigh; often absent ankle jerk; foot drop
Sural	Sensory loss over lateral foot

*From Nakano, K.K.: Neurology of Musculoskeletal and Rheumatic Disorders. Boston, Houghton Mifflin, 1979.

majority of cases.[9] Hyperextension of the hand (*reverse Phalen* maneuver) may also produce symptoms in certain cases. In addition, patients complain of either hypesthesia (with greater touch than pain loss) or hyperpathia (especially to pinprick testing) in the median supply but sparing part of the thenar eminence (the palmar cutaneous branch arises proximal to the carpal tunnel) and varying degrees of thenar weakness and atrophy, depending on the duration of the entrapment.

In the majority of cases a prolonged distal median nerve motor latency is demonstrated by nerve conduction testing. However, the single most sensitive test for the carpal tunnel syndrome is the sensory conduction study.[17] In over 90 percent of the patients there is a delayed sensory latency across the wrist. It is customary to measure both motor and sensory nerve conduction velocities, and also to carry out EMG of the thenar and upper limb muscles. If the patient demonstrates only sensory symptoms and mild changes on electrodiagnostic studies, treatment with wrist splints, anti-inflammatory-analgesic medications, and local injection would be indicated. On the other hand, if weakness or significant changes on electrodiagnostic tests occur, then hand surgery would be recommended. Occasionally patients with cervical radiculitis of the C6 and C7 (and possibly C5) roots or a thoracic outlet syndrome may present with clinical symptoms similar to those of the carpal tunnel syndrome.

Usually a careful neurologic examination as well as cervical spine and thoracic outlet radiographs and nerve conduction velocity along with EMG will help differentiate other entities from the "pure" carpal tunnel syndrome. If a patient treated for documented carpal tunnel syndrome does not improve over a period of 6 to 9 weeks, the possibility of inadequate treatment versus a

Since the median nerve is a mixed sensorimotor nerve, one finds both sensory and motor symptoms in patients with the carpal tunnel syndrome. Numbness or paresthesias of the thumb, index, middle, and one half of the ring finger usually precede weakness and atrophy of the thenar muscles. Characteristically, the patient states that the discomfort worsens at night and often awakens him from sleep. Frequently the entrapment is bilateral, although the symptoms usually begin in and are of greater intensity in the dominant hand. If severe, the carpal tunnel syndrome may produce retrograde pain to the forearm and, less commonly, to the shoulder and neck regions. Examination of the patient reveals a positive *Tinel* sign (percussion of the nerve at the volar wrist causes paresthesias) and reproduction of pain and paresthesia with the *Phalen* maneuver (the examiner flexes the patient's hand at the wrist for over 1 minute) in the

Table 110–3. Differential Diagnosis of Neuropathy, Myopathy, Neuromuscular Junction Syndromes, Upper Motor Neuron Disease, and Functional States*

Localization of Clinical Condition	Weakness	Sensory Loss	Deep Tendon Reflex	CPK	NCV	EMG	Tensilon Test	CSF	Muscle Biopsy	Nerve Biopsy
Nerve root	Nerve root pattern	Dermatome	Decreased, normal	Normal	Normal	Abnormal	Normal	Normal	Normal or focal change	Normal
Neuropathy	Distal	1. Distal 2. Peripheral nerve distribution	Decreased, absent	Normal, slight increase	Slow	Abnormal	Normal	Increased protein or normal	Grouped atrophy	Abnormal
Guillain-Barré	Proximal and distal	None	Decreased, absent	Normal	Slow	Abnormal	Normal	Increased protein	Abnormal	Abnormal
Myopathy	Proximal	None	Normal	Increased	Normal	Abnormal	Normal	Normal	Normal	Normal
Neuromuscular junction	Fatigue; may have ocular weakness	None	Normal	Normal	Normal	Abnormal	Positive, corrects weakness	Normal	Normal	Normal
Anterior horn cell (ALS)	Variable	None	Decreased, normal	Normal, slight	Normal or slight delay	Abnormal	Normal	Normal	Grouped atrophy	Normal
Upper motor neuron: Brain	Hemiparesis, monoparesis	Hemisensory, monosensory (rare)	Increased	Normal	Normal	Normal	Normal	Normal or increased protein	Normal	Normal
Spinal cord	Bilateral below level	Bilateral below level	Increased below level	Normal	Normal	Normal	Normal	Often increased protein	Normal	Normal
Multiple sclerosis (MS)	Multiple	Multiple, variable	Increased	Normal	Normal	Normal	Normal	Normal protein, increased globulin	Normal	Normal
Psychiatric	Nonanatomic collapsing	Nonanatomic	Normal	Normal	Normal	Normal	Normal	Normal	Normal	Normal

*From Nakano, K.K.: Neurology of Musculoskeletal and Rheumatic Disorders. Boston, Houghton Mifflin, 1979.

Table 110–4. Summary of the EMG-NCV Findings by Location of Disease in the Motor Unit*

		Location					
		Nerve Root					
Study	Spinal Cord: Anterior Horn Cell	*Anterior Motor Root*	*Dorsal Ganglion* Pre-	*Dorsal Ganglion* Post-	Peripheral Nerve	Neuromuscular Junction	Muscle
MNCV	N	N	N	N	+	N	N
SNAP	N	N	N	±	+	N	N
EMG	+	+	N	N	+	±	+
Repetitive stimulation	±	N	N	N	±	+	N
F wave	+	+	N	N	+	N	N
H reflex	+	+	+	+	+	N	N
SER	N	N	+	+	+	N	N

*From Nakano, K.K.: Neurology of Musculoskeletal and Rheumatic Disorders. Boston, Houghton Mifflin, 1979.

N	=	Normal.	MNCV	=	Motor nerve conduction velocity.
+	=	Abnormal.	SNAP	=	Sensory nerve action potential.
±	=	Occasional abnormality.	EMG	=	Electromyography.
			SER	=	Somatosensory evoked response.

"pseudo-carpal tunnel (sublimis) syndrome" produced by the lateral border of the sublimis muscle belly[18] versus a "double crush" syndrome should be considered (see below).

Anterior Interosseous Nerve Syndrome. The anterior interosseous nerve (AIN) is a pure motor branch of the median nerve and supplies the flexor pollicis longus (FPL), pronator quadratus (PQ), and flexor digitorum profundus of the index and middle fingers (FDP 1,2) (Fig. 110–2). In the AIN syndrome patients often complain of a nonspecific pain in the forearm or elbow, and on examination they demonstrate weakness of the FPL, PQ, and FDP 1,2 muscles (Fig. 110–3). Sometimes only

Figure 110–1. Diagram of the course and distribution of the median nerve. The field of sensory innervation in the hand is marked by stipple. The branch of the median nerve indicated by 1 goes to the abductor pollicis brevis muscle; that by 2, to the opponens pollicis; that by 3, to the superficial head of the flexor pollicis brevis; and those by 4, to the first and second lumbrical muscles. (From Nakano, K.K.: Orthop. Clin. North Am. 6:837, 1975.)

Figure 110–2. Diagram of the anterior interosseous nerve, which is a pure motor branch of the median nerve in the forearm. The anterior interosseous nerve supplies the flexor digitorum profundus to the index and middle fingers (FDP 1,2), flexor pollicis longus (FPL), and pronator quadratus muscles. (From Nakano, K.K., Lundergan, C., and Okihiro, M.M.: Arch. Neurol. 34:477, 1977.)

Figure 110–3. A patient with an anterior interosseous nerve syndrome. Note the characteristic pinch attitude, with hyperextension of the thumb at the metacarpophalangeal joint and weakness of the flexor pollicis longus and flexor digitorum profundus to the index fingers. (From Nakano, K.K., Lundergan, C., and Okihiro, M.M.: Arch. Neurol. 34:477, 1977.)

the flexor pollicis longus or flexor digitorum profundus of the index finger may be involved.[5] In the latter situation one must rule out tendon ruptures of the flexor pollicis longus or flexor digitorum profundus to the index finger, which occasionally develops in rheumatoid arthritis.[10] In the AIN syndromes, routine motor and sensory nerve conductions of the radial, median, and ulnar nerves will be normal.[19] However, the latency and duration of the evoked action potential from elbow to pronator quadratus will be prolonged.[20] EMG may show evidence of denervation in the pronator quadratus, flexor pollicis longus, and flexor digitorum profundi to the index and middle fingers (Fig. 110–4). Surgery may not

be necessary unless there is evidence of a penetrating injury, significant entrapment, or certain fractures (specifically forearm or supracondylar). AIN syndromes occasionally happen bilaterally.[20] Spontaneous recovery may take from 6 weeks to 18 months in AIN syndromes.

Double Crush Syndrome of the Median Nerve. Degenerative cervical spine disease with variable degrees of spondylosis is a common condition. When such a patient becomes symptomatic as a result of the cervical spine process and develops a carpal tunnel syndrome concomitantly, one can conveniently refer to the entire clinical picture as the "double crush" syndrome.[21] By use of newer techniques and more frequent EMG and nerve conduction studies, this syndrome can be readily ascertained. Generally, the patient responds only if one treats both processes (i.e., cervical collar, exercises, and analgesics for the cervical spine symptoms and therapy for the carpal tunnel syndrome).

In the differential diagnostic possibilities, thoracic outlet syndromes should also be considered, for this entity may simulate cervical spine disease or the carpal tunnel syndrome, or both. For this reason, nerve conduction velocity studies should be performed from Erb's point (supraclavicular fossa region) to the elbow, and from elbow to wrist. EMG examination of the hand as well as proximal and paraspinal muscles should be performed in most cases of carpal tunnel and more proximal syndromes. Although the median nerve is most frequently involved in the "double crush" syndrome, occasionally the ulnar nerve becomes entrapped instead.

Ulnar Nerve. The ulnar nerve is the major branch of the lower secondary trunk of the brachial plexus, and its fibers arise from the C8 and T1 segments (Fig. 110–5). It has both motor and sensory functions. Motor functions provided by the ulnar nerve include flexion and abduction of the wrist and flexion of the ring and fifth fingers, abduction and opposition of the fifth finger,

Figure 110–4. Evoked response (bottom) upon stimulation of the median nerve at the elbow and recording with a concentric needle in the pronator quadratus muscle. In the anterior interosseous nerve syndrome the evoked action potential has a delayed latency and prolonged duration.

Flexor carpi ulnaris

Flexor digitorum profundus

Dorsal cutaneous branch

6
7

1
2
3
4
5

Dorsal
cutaneous branch

CUTANEOUS
INNERVATION

Dorsal
cutaneous branch

Palmar branch

Dorsal digital
nerves

Palmar digital
nerves

Posterior

Anterior

Figure 110–5. Diagram of the course and distribution of the ulnar nerve. The numbered branches supply the following muscles: 1, palmaris brevis; 2, abductor digiti minimi; 3, opponens digiti minimi and flexor digiti minimi; 4, third and fourth lumbricals; 5, palmar and dorsal interosseous muscles; 6, adductor pollicis; and 7, flexor pollicis brevis (deep head). (From Nakano, K.K.: Orthop. Clin. North Am. 6:837, 1975.)

adduction of the thumb, and adduction and abduction of the fingers (Table 110–5). The sensory portion of the ulnar nerve supplies the skin on the palmar and dorsal surfaces of the fifth finger, inner half of the ring finger, and ulnar side of the hand.

Dissociated paresis of the muscles supplied by the ulnar nerve results with partial lesions of the nerve in the arm or forearm. Irritative lesions may be accompanied by pain, but injuries to the ulnar nerve infrequently produce causalgia.

The diagnosis of ulnar nerve lesions requires clinical findings limited to the distribution of the ulnar nerve, while EMG and nerve conduction studies localize the precise area of entrapment and the degree of abnormality (e.g., presence of denervation potentials). Results of therapy can best be monitored by serial electrodiagnostic studies.

Ulnar Nerve Entrapment at the Wrist in Guyon's Canal. Ulnar nerve entrapment in Guyon's canal occurs less frequently than at the elbow.[22] Anatomically there are no tendons passing through Guyon's canal, and therefore there should be no potential tenosynovium to entrap the nerve. Rarely the tenosynovium within the

carpal tunnel can bulge and compress the ulnar nerve proximal to the canal, resulting in symptoms. Clinically this may simulate an ulnar nerve neuropathy at the elbow. However, on examination one finds normal motor function of the flexor carpi ulnaris and the flexor digitorum profundus to the fourth and fifth fingers. Additionally, the sensory loss is confined to the palmar branch while the dorsum of the hand has normal sensation (the dorsal cutaneous branch is proximal to the wrist). The diagnosis is confirmed by delayed motor and sensory terminal latencies of the ulnar nerve in the hand. Most commonly a ganglion would produce this picture; other entities include trauma, rheumatoid arthritis, and long distance bicycling.[23] Surgery produces good results in cases caused by a ganglion and some selected cases of trauma and rheumatoid arthritis.

Ulnar Nerve Entrapment at the Elbow in the Cubital Fossa. Ulnar neuropathy secondary to compression at the cubital fossa produces a clinical picture in which there is weakness of the flexor carpi ulnaris, flexor digitorum profundus of the fourth and fifth fingers, and intrinsic hand muscles (Table 110–5 and Fig. 110–5). In addition, the sensory loss extends to the dorsum of the ulnar aspect of the hand. Electrodiagnostic testing localizes the area of entrapment. If the patient has significant compression from severe rheumatoid arthritis, decompression and elbow synovectomy may be necessary.[10]

Double Crush Syndrome of the Ulnar Nerve. As in the case of the median nerve, the ulnar nerve may become entrapped concomitantly with lower cervical spine disease (C8-T1) or in the thoracic outlet syndrome. Thus cervical spine and thoracic outlet x-ray films, EMG, and complete nerve conduction velocity studies along the entire course of the ulnar nerve from Erb's point to the wrist should be obtained in all patients suspected of an ulnar nerve entrapment syndrome with symptoms referable to the neck. In most instances of the double crush syndrome involving the ulnar nerve, the patient improves only when the cervical spine disorder and the more distal ulnar entrapments are adequately treated.

Radial Nerve. The radial nerve arises from the posterior secondary trunk of the brachial plexus (C5-C8) (Fig. 110–6); it is predominantly a motor nerve and innervates the extensors of the forearm, wrist, and fingers as well as supinator of the forearm (Table 110–5). The sensory supply of the radial nerve includes a small area on the posterior radial surface of the hand and the first and second metacarpals of the thumb and index and middle fingers. Entrapments of the radial nerve or its branches in the forearm or wrist result in clinical findings according to the site of the lesion.

Radial Nerve Entrapment in Axilla (Saturday Night Palsy). This syndrome occurs usually after pressure from crutches in the axilla or in alcoholics and drug addicts.[24] Frequently the alcoholic or drug addict falls asleep in a stuporous state with his arm over the back of a chair or against some hard surface. This produces pressure on the radial nerve in the axilla and causes weakness of the triceps, brachioradialis, and extensors of the hand,

Table 110–5. Median, Ulnar, and Radial Nerve Muscle Innervation of the Upper Limbs*

Division	Nerve		
	Median	*Ulnar*	*Radial*
Muscular branches			
In arm	None	None	Triceps
			Anconeus
			Brachioradialis
			Extensor carpi radialis longus
In forearm	Pronator teres	Flexor carpi ulnaris	From posterior interosseous nerve:
	Flexor carpi radialis	Flexor digitorum profundus	Extensor carpi radialis brevis
	Flexor digitorum sublimis	(medial half)	Supinator
	Palmaris longus		Extensor digitorum
	Flexor pollicis longus†		Extensor digiti quinti
	Flexor digitorum profundus†		Extensor carpi ulnaris
	From anterior interosseous nerve:		Abductor pollicis longus
	Flexor pollicis longus		Extensor pollicis longus
	Flexor digitorum profundus		Extensor pollicis brevis
	(lateral half)		Extensor indicis
	Pronator quadratus		
In hand	Abductor pollicis brevis	Palmaris brevis	None
	Opponens pollicis	Abductor digiti quinti	
	Flexor pollicis brevis (superficial or	Opponens digiti quinti	
	outer head)	Flexor digiti quinti	
	First, second lumbricals	Third, fourth lumbricals	
		Interossei	
		Flexor pollicis brevis (deep inner	
		head)	
		Adductor pollicis	
Cutaneous branches			
In arm	None	None	Posterior cutaneous nerve of arm
			Lower lateral cutaneous nerve of
			arm
			Posterior cutaneous nerve of
			forearm
In hand	Palmar branch (occasionally	Dorsal branch	Dorsal digital nerve
	absent)		
	Palmar digital nerves	Palmar branch	
		Superficial terminal branch	

*From Nakano, K.K.: Orthop. Clin. North Am. 6:837, 1975.
†Frequently.

wrist, and fingers, as well as supinator muscles. With a complete lesion in the axilla, paralysis of the triceps and abolition of the triceps reflex will be noted. If the lesion occurs in the posteromedial surface of the arm, one or more branches to the triceps may be spared so that weakness of extension of the forearm is minimal. Atrophy of the paralyzed muscles follows a complete lesion of the radial nerve. Unless a vascular lesion develops, vasomotor or trophic disturbances rarely are seen. Infrequently causalgia follows a partial radial nerve lesion. One observes a sensory loss in the characteristic dorsal portion of the hand, including the web interspace. Usually this pressure neuropathy resolves over 6 to 8 weeks. If pressure has been exerted in the axilla, appropriate splinting and therapy with the hand in the position of function will be indicated. EMG and nerve conduction velocities will show a proximal location of the deficit. Stimulation from Erb's point to the above-elbow segment will demonstrate a delayed or absent response. Stimulation distal to the block will produce normal nerve conduction of the radial nerve. Saturday night palsy should be differentiated from a fracture of the humerus that can injure the radial nerve; therefore, radiographs of the upper limb and shoulder, as well as the neck, may

be indicated in patients without a clear-cut history of pressure alone. One can ascertain the level of injury by EMG and nerve conduction studies. Early recognition is essential, as unattended fracture may sever the radial nerve in the upper arm.

Posterior Interosseous Nerve Syndrome. The posterior interosseous nerve (PIN) is a pure motor branch of the radial nerve in the forearm (Fig. 110–6). PIN paralysis is uncommon but is a well documented neuropathy associated with rheumatoid arthritis.[25] In other instances trauma, fractures, or vascular malformations may produce this picture. In rheumatoid arthritis the PIN syndrome is due to a bulging elbow synovitis, which compresses the PIN as it dives into the supinator muscle (Fig. 110–7). PIN paralysis usually results in partial or, less frequently, complete inability to extend the digits at the metacarpophalangeal joints. In certain cases extensor paralysis in the long, ring, and fifth digits with extension preserved in thumb and index fingers has been noted. The findings are similar to those with extensor tendon rupture, and in fact patients have been operated upon for extensor tendon rupture only to find the tendons intact.

The proper diagnosis of the PIN syndrome can be

extensor tendons are intact. In patients with ruptured extensor tendons, the ends of the tendons are distal to the wrist, and therefore one will have a negative tenodesis. The most important physical finding is radial deviation of the wrist on dorsiflexion resulting from noninvolvement of the extensor carpi radialis longus and extensor carpi radialis brevis, with paralysis of the extensor carpi ulnaris. Also one finds that even with partial paralysis, the digits that extend show marked weakness. EMG confirms the diagnosis. There will be denervation changes in the muscles supplied by the PIN which include the extensor digitorum communis, extensor carpi ulnaris, extensor digiti minimi, extensor indicis proprius, abductor pollicis longus, extensor pollicis brevis, and extensor pollicis longus.

Regarding therapy, if there has been pressure or trauma in that area without severance of the nerve, recovery will occur over weeks. In rheumatoid arthritis, steroid injections into the elbow joint may be helpful. In refractory cases, elbow synovectomy and decompression of the PIN may be necessary. In cases with permanent denervation, tendon transfer may be necessary.

Thoracic Outlet Syndromes. Bony, fascial, and muscular structures potentially interfere with functions of the neurovascular bundle located in the thoracic outlet (Fig. 110–8). In addition to the vascular and neurologic examinations, diagnostic procedures such as venography, arteriography, and electrodiagnostic studies will help arrive at a diagnosis and assess the need for surgery.[26-29]

Contributing factors predisposing to the thoracic outlet syndrome include anatomical, congenital, traumatic, and vascular disorders. Usually there is a wide range of motion in the components of the shoulder joint. A moderate range of motion takes place at the sternoclavicular articulation. The acromioclavicular articulation permits the inferior angle of the scapula to move laterally (approximately 45 degrees) during elevation of the arm. These movements involve changes in relative position of regional structures and may result in compression under

Figure 110–6. Diagram of the course and distribution of the radial nerve. Wrist drop (bottom) is a sign of a proximal radial nerve lesion. (From Nakano, K.K.: Orthop. Clin. North Am. 6:837, 1975.)

established by clinical examination and electrodiagnosis. The patient shows evidence of elbow synovitis in rheumatoid arthritis with pain, limitation of movement, and elbow spasm. A positive tenodesis effect is noted with PIN paralysis. When the wrist is passively flexed, the metacarpophalangeal joints extend, showing that the

Figure 110–7. The posterior interosseous nerve (1) is a motor branch of the radial nerve in the forearm. The posterior interosseous nerve may be compressed by synovium as it enters the arcade of Frohse (2) and the supinator muscle in cases of rheumatoid arthritis. (From Millender, L.H., Nalebuff, E.A., and Holdsworth, D.E.: J. Bone Joint Surg. 55A:753, 1973.)

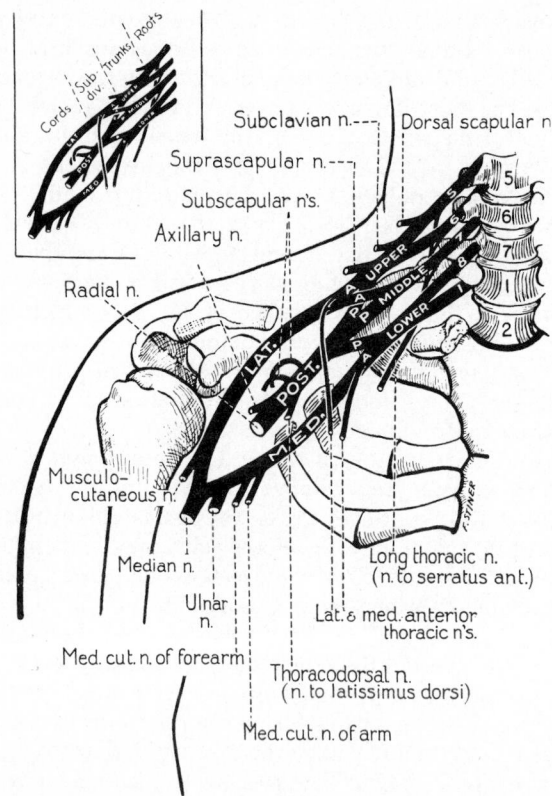

Figure 110–8. Diagram of nerves to the upper limb, including a view through the thoracic outlet. (From Haymaker, W., and Woodhall, B.: Peripheral Nerve Injuries, Philadelphia, W. B. Saunders Company, 1953.)

arm, and shoulder, as well as paresthesias which frequently are perceived in the distribution of C8 and T1. Numbness in a similar distribution may be noted. Ischemic symptoms secondary to intermittent compression of the subclavian artery include numbness, coldness, weakness, and discoloration.

Other Conditions Causing Pain and Paresthesia in the Upper Limbs. Herniated cervical discs, cervical osteoarthritis, cervical radiculitis, and spinal cord tumors may produce symptoms which, on superficial consideration, may suggest one of the syndromes of the thoracic outlet or a peripheral neuropathy. Usually the neurologic manifestations of the compression syndromes of the thoracic outlet confine themselves to involvement of the C8 and T1 roots.

Other conditions which may cause confusion with the thoracic outlet and entrapment neuropathy syndromes include Hodgkin's disease, thromboangiitis obliterans, frostbite, migratory thrombophlebitis, vasculitis, reflex sympathetic dystrophy, post-traumatic osteoporosis, herpes zoster, post–hemiplegic dystrophy, sclerodactyly associated with myocardial ischemia, causalgia, syringomyelia, Dupuytren's contracture, dermatomyositis, and nodular panniculitis. Appropriate laboratory studies (e.g., CPK, sedimentation rate, ANA, complement), radiography, EMG and nerve conduction studies, and eventual arteriography and venography will differentiate between the aforementioned conditions.

Conservative measures should be employed initially in most patients with the thoracic outlet syndrome.

LOWER LIMBS

Sciatic Nerve. The sciatic nerve originates from undivided primary rami L4, L5, S1, S2, and S3, and can be divisible into component parts: tibial, common peroneal, and nerve to hamstring muscles (Fig. 110–9). As a single trunk the sciatic nerve leaves the pelvis by traversing the greater sciatic foramen. After emerging in the gluteal region, it courses laterally and then downward to lie in the hollow midway between the ischial tuberosity and the greater trochanter, where it is under cover of the gluteus maximus muscle. In the thigh region the sciatic nerve is at the inferior aspect of the buttock, where it occupies a superficial position and descends in the plane between the adductor magnus and the hamstring muscles. Above the popliteal fossa, the sciatic nerve terminates into the tibial and common peroneal nerves. In the medial side of the sciatic trunk is the nerve to the hamstrings, which innervates the adductor magnus, semimembranosus, semitendinosus, and long head of the biceps femoris muscles. The short head of the biceps is supplied by the common peroneal nerve (Table 110–6).

The sural nerve originates from an anastomotic branch of the tibial nerve, which joins the peroneal anastomotic nerve and extends down the back of the leg to the outer side of the foot. At the upper level of the soleus muscle the tibial nerve becomes the posterior

either blood vessels or nerves or both. When the arm is in full hyperabduction above the head, the axillary artery is bent 180 degrees from its position when the arm is at the side. This motion pulls the vessels across the coracoid process and head of the humerus as across a pulley. Increase in muscular bulk in the thoracic outlet may occur because of vigorous exercise or work. This may reduce the space in which the artery, vein, and nerves pass. The presence of a cervical rib, a bifid clavicle, or a bony protuberance on the first rib may cause pressure on the vessels or nerves when the arm is in certain positions. There may be a fascial band behind the scalenus anticus muscle or an abnormal insertion of the scalenus medius muscle in the first rib. Fracture of the clavicle and subacromial dislocation of the humeral head can cause thoracic outlet syndromes. A crushing injury of the upper thorax may stretch part of the brachial plexus and/or thrombose the artery or vein. Inflexible arteriosclerotic arteries may not tolerate excess activity and potentially contribute to thoracic outlet syndromes.

The way in which a patient with these syndromes will present depends upon the frequency, duration, and degree of compression of the subclavian or axillary vessels and the lower cords of the brachial plexus. The character of the symptoms in themselves does not differentiate these syndromes from other conditions. Most often the symptoms include pain in the fingers, hand, forearm,

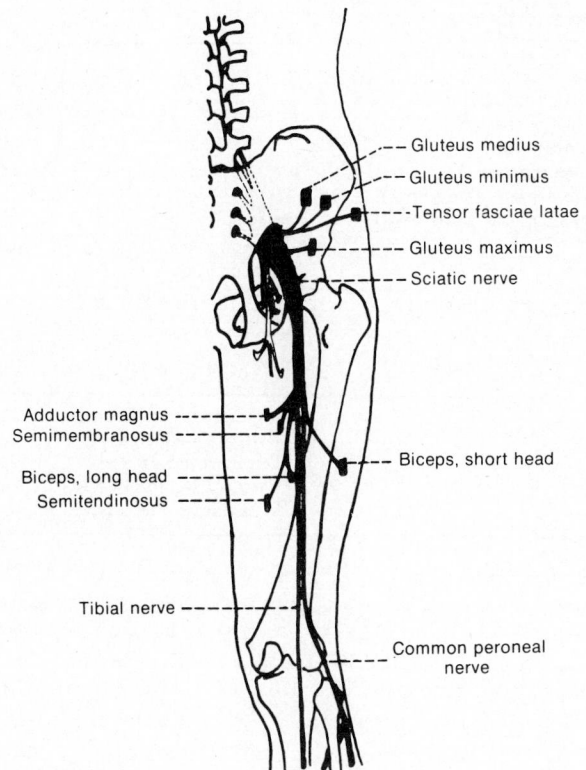

Gluteus medius
Gluteus minimus
Tensor fasciae latae
Gluteus maximus
Sciatic nerve

Adductor magnus
Semimembranosus

Biceps, long head
Semitendinosus

Biceps, short head

Tibial nerve

Common peroneal
nerve

Figure 110–9. Diagram of the course and distribution of the component parts of the sciatic nerve (common peroneal, tibial, and nerve to the hamstring muscles). (From Nakano, K.K.: Orthop. Clin. North Am. 6:837, 1975.)

tibial nerve, which, on reaching the sole of the foot, divides into medial and lateral plantar nerves. The common peroneal nerve divides into the superficial peroneal and deep peroneal nerves; both nerves ultimately reach the dorsum of the foot.

Entrapments of the proximal sciatic nerve occur infrequently. More often pressure on the nerve caused by immobility or intramuscular injections into or near the nerve can produce a sciatic neuropathy. Hip surgery and insertion of prostheses may also cause sciatic nerve injury. A potential entrapment point for the sciatic nerve exists where the sciatic trunk leaves the pelvis through the greater sciatic notch and crosses its sharp lower edge. If the piriformis muscle entraps the sciatic nerve at the aforementioned location, this becomes the "piriformis syndrome."[2] This syndrome presents with distal motor and sensory signs and may simulate a lumbar disc syndrome. When a high sciatic neuropathy is suspected by clinical examination, appropriate documentation by EMG and nerve conduction studies is indicated. In the piriformis syndrome EMG will demonstrate normal activity of the gluteus medius and minimus and tensor fasciae latae muscles, while the innervation below this will document abnormalities, including those in the gluteus maximus muscles. Additionally, in the piriformis syndrome EMG of the paravertebral lumbosacral muscles will be normal, while in lumbar disc disease EMG usually demonstrates abnormalities of muscle innervated by both anterior and posterior rami of the affected nerve

root. In difficult clinical cases, myelography and spinal fluid analysis may become necessary. Conservative measures should first be tried in a piriformis syndrome. Rarely will surgical exposure of the sciatic notch for neurolysis be necessary.[2]

Infrequently, unilateral sciatic nerve entrapment secondary to prolonged squatting may result where the sciatic nerve runs between the ischial tuberosity and the trochanter major or where it reaches the thigh between the adductor magnus and the hamstring muscles.[30] Rarely, the sciatic nerve may be stretched from standing for hours in an awkward position (e.g., with a strongly bent trunk and legs fully stretched).[31]

When the gastocnemius-semimembranous bursa communicates with the knee joint, an effusion may produce a popliteal (Baker's) cyst. Popliteal cysts can produce symptoms by pressure, rupture, and dissection and can clinically simulate thrombophlebitis (including a positive Homan sign). Baker's cysts can rarely entrap the lower sciatic nerve (Fig. 110–10). This has been reported in patients with rheumatoid arthritis.[10,32] The peroneal nerve, the tibial nerve, or the sural nerve, or all three, may be involved. Patients with Baker's cysts have a palpable enlargement in the popliteal area, which is best appreciated when the knee is extended.[32] A knee arthrogram with contrast material will document the extent of the cyst (Fig. 110–11). Other modalities of documentation include technetium radionuclear material injected into the cyst with subsequent radioisotope scanning. Echo scanning of the popliteal area can also document the extent of Baker's cysts. EMG and nerve conduction studies may be utilized to determine whether an impairment of the tibial or peroneal nerves exists.[32] If the common peroneal nerve is involved, neurologic and electrodiagnostic examination demonstrates involvement of the peroneal muscles, tibialis anterior, extensor hallucis longus, extensor digitorum longus, and extensor digitorum brevis (Table 110–6). The sensory loss will be over the lateral leg and dorsum of the foot, including the web interspace of the first and second toes. With tibial nerve involvement the patient will have weakness of the gastrocnemius, soleus, tibialis posterior, flexor digitorum longus, flexor hallucis longus, and intrinsic muscles of the foot, associated with a sensory defect of the plantar aspect of the foot, including the heel and the posterolateral aspect of the calf (Table 110–6). Drainage of the popliteal cyst or steroid injections have been successful in most cases; however, a synovectomy may be necessary in refractory or recurrent cases.[10,32]

Common Peroneal Nerve. Pressure palsy of the common, deep or superficial peroneal nerves secondary to trauma or undue pressure can be seen in both medical or surgical patients. An entrapment infrequently causes a peroneal palsy. The most vulnerable spot for compression occurs where the nerve winds around the neck of the fibula just about where it divides into the deep and superficial peroneal nerves (Fig. 110–10). The peroneal nerve may be involved in hereditary compression neuropathy[33] and entrapment by a ganglion[34] or leprosy.[35]

Table 110–6. Sciatic Nerve and Its Branches*

Division	Sciatic Nerve		
Muscular branches		Hamstring muscles	
		Adductor magnus	
		Semimembranosus	
		Semitendinosus	
		Biceps femoris (long head)	
		Biceps femoris (short head)	
In leg	Tibial nerve		Common peroneal nerve
	Gastrocnemius		Superficial peroneal nerve
	Plantaris		Peroneus longus
	Soleus		Peroneus brevis
	Popliteus		
	Posterior tibial nerve		Deep peroneal nerve
	Tibialis posterior		Tibialis anterior
	Flexor digitorum longus		Extensor digitorum longus
	Flexor hallucis longus		Extensor hallucis longus
			Peroneus tertius
In foot	Lateral plantar nerve		Extensor digitorum brevis
	Abductor digiti quinti		First dorsal interosseous
	Flexor digitorum accessorius		
	Flexor digiti quinti brevis		
	Adductor hallucis		
	Interossei		
	Second, third, and fourth lumbricals		
	Medial plantar nerve		
	Flexor digitorum brevis		
	Abductor hallucis		
	Flexor hallucis brevis		
	First umbrical		
Cutaneous branches			
In leg	Sural nerve		Common peroneal nerve
	(Anastomosis from tibial and peroneal nerves)		Lateral cutaneous nerve of calf
			Superficial peroneal nerve
			Medial cutaneous branch
			Lateral cutaneous branch
In foot	Medial and lateral calcaneal nerves		Deep peroneal nerve
			Dorsal digital cutaneous nerve

*From Nakano, K.K.: Orthop. Clin. North Am. 6:837, 1975.

Neurologic examination in cases of peroneal neuropathy reveals weakness or paralysis of extension of the foot and toes and eversion of the foot (Table 110–6). The ankle reflex and inversion of the foot remain intact. A sensory deficit can be found in the area of the superficial and deep peroneal nerves.

One must consider and differentiate peroneal pressure palsy from mononeuritis multiplex, Baker's cyst, sciatic neuropathy, or the anterior tibial compartment syndrome. Neurologic examination, as well as EMG, nerve conduction studies, and appropriate radiographs, will help differentiate between these entities. In the anterior tibial compartment syndrome (an ischemic muscle lesion most often seen after heavy exertion in poorly trained persons),[36] one finds a foot drop, severe pain, and swelling in the anterior tibial, extensor hallucis, and extensor digitorum muscles. Palpation of the dorsalis pedis artery reveals an absent pulse, and the syndrome requires surgery (fasciotomy) to decompress the involved muscles. Sciatic nerve or lumbosacral nerve root lesions manifest with foot drop; however, the ankle jerk diminishes or vanishes, and there is weakness of the posterior tibial muscle (inversion of the foot).

Posterior Tibial Nerve. *Tarsal Tunnel Syndrome.* The tarsal tunnel syndrome is a rare cause of entrapment neuropathy.[37,38] The posterior tibial nerve becomes entrapped in a flexor retinaculum along the medial malleolus of the ankle (Fig. 111–10). Painful dysesthesias and intrinsic foot weakness are prominent features. Usually the patient complains of "burning feet," especially at night, and has difficulty with intrinsic muscles of the foot (Table 110–6). This syndrome can occur with trauma or active peripheral joint disease and rheumatoid arthritis, as well in other conditions (e.g., leprous neuritis[39]) that may compromise the retinaculum. A ganglion arising from the subtalar joint has been noted in a few cases.[40,41] One makes a diagnosis by the neurologic examination and EMG and nerve conduction velocity studies that show denervation in the distribution of the posterior nerve supply (Table 110–6) and a delay or block of the posterior tibial nerve terminal latency into the foot. Local steroid injections have been helpful in many cases. If the symptoms and findings persist beyond 6 weeks, surgery would be indicated.

Medial and Lateral Plantar Nerve Syndrome. A partial tarsal tunnel syndrome (i.e., either a medial or lateral

Figure 110–10. Diagram of the course and distribution of the sciatic, peroneal, tibial, femoral, and obturator nerves. (From Kendall, H.O., Kendall, F.P., and Wadsworth, G.E.: Spinal Nerve and Motor Point Chart. Trunk and Lower Extremity, Huntington, N.Y., Kreiger Publishing Co., Inc., 1970.)

Figure 110–11. Knee arthrogram (anteroposterior view) of a patient with a large popliteal cyst who clinically presented with a foot drop. (From Nakano, K.K.: Orthop. Clin. North Am. 6:837, 1975.)

plantar nerve deficit in the foot) alerts the clinician to the possibility of a process distal to the flexor retinaculum (Fig. 110–10). Patients with a medial or lateral plantar nerve syndrome complain of weakness and burning of the feet. Neurologic examination shows the process to be distal to the ankle. Sensation of the heel is preserved, whereas the plantar aspect of the foot shows decreased touch and pinprick sensation. Nerve conduction velocity studies and EMG are useful in confirming the level of the block. Therapy consists of steroid injection into the appropriate area. Surgery should be considered if the symptoms or signs progress, or if the exact level of compression is not certain.

Femoral Nerve. The femoral nerve arises from the L2, L3, and L4 nerve roots, traverses the psoas muscle in a lateral direction, and then, in the pelvis, pursues its way in the fossa between the psoas and iliacus muscles (Fig. 110–10). The motor branches of the femoral nerve innervate the quadriceps (rectus femoris, vastus medialis, vastus lateralis, vastus intermedius), sartorius, and pectineus muscles. Sensory branches divide as the anterior femoral cutaneous nerve (supplies the anterior aspect of the thigh), the medial femoral cutaneous nerve (innervates part of the medial aspect of the thigh), and the long saphenous nerve (along with the infrapatellar

branch, supplies the medial tibial surface of the leg, reaching to the medial malleolus and medial edge of the foot).

Femoral nerve syndromes develop infrequently, and actual entrapments of this nerve occur rarely. The more common causes of femoral neuropathy include trauma (penetrating, blunt, and stretch injuries), diabetes, and vascular disease.[43] Pressure on the femoral nerve can be produced by a psoas abscess, tumors of the pelvis, lymphoma, aneurysms (external iliac and femoral arteries), and hematomas (in hemophiliacs or those receiving anticoagulation medication).

Clinically, a femoral nerve lesion is characterized by one or more of three findings: (1) motor weakness, (2) sensory loss, and (3) reduced or absent knee jerk. Frequently, pressure on the groin or stretching the nerve will elicit pain in the patient with a femoral neuropathy. In the differential evaluation, high lumbar nerve root disorders, a lumbar plexus deficit, and herpes zoster should be considered. EMG will show neurogenic changes in the quadriceps (rectus femoris, vastus medialis, vastus lateralis, vastus intermedius), sartorius, and pectineus muscles. Motor nerve conduction velocities serve to document slowing of the femoral nerve (the contralateral femoral nerve and additional lower limb nerves should also be tested for comparison). Treatment depends on the accurate diagnosis of the causative process (e.g., stopping anticoagulants in a hematoma-induced neuropathy).

Lateral Femoral Cutaneous Nerve (Meralgia Paresthetica). The lateral femoral cutaneous nerve is derived from the L2, L3 lumbar nerve roots and emerges from the lateral border of the psoas major muscle to run down laterally to cross the iliacus muscle. It goes forward to the lateral end of the inguinal ligament and at first lies under the iliacus fascia. It then enters in and runs between the fascial layers just before going through a tunnel in the lateral attachment of the inguinal ligament to the anterior superior iliac spine. Beyond its opening in the inguinal ligament, the nerve is beneath the deep fascia of the upper thigh for a short portion of its course, piercing it to reach its final sub- and intracutaneous position. About 12.5 cm below the anterior superior iliac spine, the nerve divides into anterior and posterior branches. The anterior branch innervates the skin of the anterior and lateral aspects of the thigh as far as the knee. The posterior branch innervates the skin over the lateral and posterior portions of the thigh from the trochanteric region to the middle of the thigh.

The lateral femoral cutaneous nerve becomes entrapped at the anterior superior iliac spine where the nerve passes to the lateral end of the inguinal ligament. The bending point of the nerve occurs at this position. Beyond this point the nerve is held down, where it pierces the fascia lata. Usually, in lateral femoral cutaneous nerve syndromes, burning pain and paresthesias develop in the lateral thigh area.[43] Clinical examination will show decreased or absent sensation in the lateral thigh region (Fig. 110–12).

Meralgia paresthetica can be produced by direct

Figure 110–12. Distribution of sensory alteration in a patient with a lateral femoral cutaneous nerve entrapment (meralgia paresthetica.)

trauma and can result after a fracture of the anterior portion of the ilium. Pelvic tilt, either by a shift of the trunk or by a shortened lower extremity, can result in meralgia paresthetica. Adduction at the opposite hip is caused by a shortened lower extremity, and this stretches the deep fascia and the nerve against the entrapment point. Diabetes causes meralgia paresthetica, and systemic disease states should be suspected in individuals without other obvious etiologies.

In the diagnosis of meralgia paresthetica the characteristic distribution of sensory findings without motor weakness will present little difficulty for the clinician. In addition, sensory nerve conduction velocities of the lateral femoral cutaneous nerve provide useful information.

Treatment of the lateral femoral cutaneous neuropathies includes symptomatic measures (rest, analgesics). In cases of pelvic tilt, a heel lift on the contralateral shoe would be recommended. If no relief of symptoms follows conservative measures, operation would be indicated. A neurolysis has been advocated in refractory cases. It is important to realize that patients complaining of pain originating near the lateral aspect of the buttock and radiating down the lateral aspect of the thigh to the knee may have lumbar spine abnormalities. In lumbar spine disease tenderness is elicited along the medial lateral aspect of the buttock and down the course of the fascia lata, and in this situation there are no sensory findings as seen with a lateral femoral cutaneous neuropathy. In lumbar nerve root syndrome EMG of the paraspinal muscle often shows neurogenic abnormalities,

while EMG remains normal in L2, L3 innervated muscles in the lateral femoral cutaneous nerve syndrome.

COMPARTMENT SYNDROMES

Compartment syndromes (CS) occur in specific clinical situations in which locally increased tissue pressure within a closed muscle compartment compromises local circulation (capillary blood perfusion) and neuromuscular function.[44,45] The increased prevalence of CS correlates with the frequency of limb trauma, drug and alcohol abuse, limb surgery, limb ischemia, and overuse (physical exertion) of limb muscles. The frequency of the aforementioned entities may, in turn, depend on community and geographic factors.

The underlying pathophysiology of the CS includes increased tissue pressure, which, in turn, compromises tissue blood flow, oxygenation, and function. The time required to produce functional abnormalities relates to the severity of the pressure-induced circulatory compromise. Factors that reduce the tolerance of limbs for increased tissue pressure include hypotension, hemorrhage, arterial occlusion, and limb elevation.

Clinical features of CS include (1) tense compartment envelope, (2) severe pain in excess of that clinically expected for the specific condition, (3) pain on passive stretch of the muscles in the compartment, (4) muscle weakness within the compartment, and (5) altered sensation in the distribution of the nerves coursing through the compartment. Anatomic locations within the body in which the CS may occur include (1) *Leg*—anterior, lateral, posterior (superficial and deep); (2) *Thigh*—quadriceps; (3) *Buttock*—gluteal; (4) *Hand*—interosseous; (5) *Forearm*—dorsal, volar; and (6) *Arm*—deltoid, biceps.

Treatment of the CS aims at minimizing neurologic deficits by promptly restoring local blood flow. Nonoperative measures include eliminating external envelopes and maintaining local arterial pressures. The objective of surgery is decompression of limiting envelopes and débridement of nonviable tissue.

Other medical conditions that may be confused with CS include infection or inflammation, arterial occlusion, and primary nerve injury or entrapment. Careful clinical examination, tissue pressure measurements, direct nerve stimulation, EMG–nerve conduction velocities, doppler, arteriography, and venography will assist in differentiating between these conditions and the various compartment syndromes.

CONCLUSION

As a clinical rule the patient with rheumatoid arthritis experiences an insidious onset of symptoms relating to nerve entrapment. In most patients with compression, neuropathies diagnosis can be effected early if a careful neurologic examination as well as roentgenographic and electrodiagnostic studies (EMG–nerve conduction) are performed at the time the patient initially complains of symptoms from his neuropathy (Table 110–2). When the diagnosis of the patient's entrapment neuropathy or "double crush" syndrome is established at the outset, therapy can be gratifying.

References

1. Haymaker, W., and Woodhall, B.: Peripheral Nerve Injuries. 2nd ed. Philadelphia, W. B. Saunders Company, 1953.
2. Kopell, H.P., and Thompson, W.A.L.: Peripheral Entrapment Neuropathies. Baltimore, Williams & Wilkins Company, 1963.
3. Medical Research Council: Aids to the Investigation of Peripheral Nerve Injuries. War Memorandum No. 7. 2nd ed. London, His Majesty's Stationery Office, 1943.
4. Sunderland, S.: Nerves and Nerve Injuries. Edinburgh, Churchill Livingstone, 1968.
5. Spinner, M.L.: Injuries to the Major Branches of Peripheral Nerves of the Forearm. Philadelphia, W. B. Saunders Company, 1972.
6. Nakano, K.K.: Neurology of Musculoskeletal and Rheumatic Disorders. Boston, Houghton Mifflin, 1979.
7. Goodgold, J., and Eberstein, A.: Electrodiagnosis of Neuromuscular Diseases. Baltimore, Williams & Wilkins Company, 1972.
8. Smorto, M.P., and Basmajian, J.V.: Clinical Electroneurography. Baltimore, Williams & Wilkins Company, 1972.
9. Phalen, G.S.: The carpal tunnel syndrome: Seventeen years' experience in diagnosis and treatment of 654 hands. J. Bone Joint Surg. 48A:211, 1966.
10. Nakano, K.K.: The entrapment neuropathies of rheumatoid arthritis. Orthop. Clin. North Am. 6:837, 1975.
11. Scarpalezos, S., Lygidakis, C., Papageorgiou, C., et al.: Neural and muscular manifestations of hypothyroidism. Arch. Neurol. 29:140, 1973.
12. Cohen, A.S.: Amyloidosis. N. Engl. J. Med. 277:522, 574, 628, 1967.
13. Committee of the American Rheumatism Association, Section of the Arthritis Foundation: Section 32, Carpal tunnel syndrome. In Rodman, G.P. (ed.): Primer on the Rheumatic Diseases. JAMA 224:No. 5 (Suppl.) 1973, p. 89.
14. O'Duffy, J.D., Randall, R.V., and MacCarty, C.S.: Median neuropathy (carpal-tunnel syndrome) in acromegaly. A sign of endocrine overactivity. Ann. Intern. Med. 78:379, 1973.
15. Sidiq, M., Kirsner, A.B., and Sheon, R.P.: Carpal tunnel syndrome. First manifestation of systemic lupus erythematosus. JAMA 222:1416, 1972.
16. Valenta, L.F.: Hyperparathyroidism due to parathyroid adenoma and carpal tunnel syndrome. Ann. Intern. Med. 82:541, 1975.
17. Buchthal, F., Rosenfalk, A., and Trojaborg, W.: Electrophysiological findings in entrapment of the median nerve at wrist and elbow. J. Neurol. Neurosurg. Psychiatry 37:340, 1974.
18. Gardner, R.C.: Confirmed case and diagnosis of pseudocarpal tunnel (sublimis) syndrome. N. Engl. J. Med. 282:858, 1970.
19. O'Brien, M.D., and Upton, A.R.M.: Anterior interosseous nerve syndrome. A case report with neurophysiological investigation. J. Neurol. Neurosurg. Psychiatry 35:531, 1972.
20. Nakano, K.K., Lundergan, C., and Okihiro, M.M.: Anterior interosseous nerve (AIN) syndrome. Diagnostic methods and alternative therapies. Arch. Neurol. 34:477, 1977.
21. Upton, A.R.M., and McComas, A.J.: The double crush in nerve entrapment syndromes. Lancet 2:359, 1973.
22. Shea, J.D., and McClain, E.J.: Ulnar nerve compression syndromes at and below the wrist. J. Bone Joint Surg. 51A:1095, 1969.
23. Eckman, P.B., Perlstein, G., and Altrocchi, P.H.: Ulnar neuropathy in bicycle riders. Arch. Neurol. 32:130, 1975.
24. Trojaborg, W.: Rate of recovery in motor and sensory fibers of the radial nerve: Clinical and electrophysiological aspects. J. Neurol. Neurosurg. Psychiatry 33:625, 1970.
25. Millender, L.H., Nalebuff, E.A., and Holdsworth, D.E.: Posterior interosseous nerve syndrome secondary to rheumatoid synovitis. J. Bone Joint Surg. 55A:753, 1973.
26. Nelson, R.M., and Davis, R.W.: Thoracic outlet compression syndrome. Ann. Thorac. Surg. 8:437, 1969.
27. Adams, J.T., DeWeese, J.A., Mahoney, E.B., et al.: Intermittent subclavian vein obstruction without thrombosis. Surgery 63:147, 1968.
28. Roos, D.B., and Owens, J.C.: Thoracic outlet syndrome. Arch. Surg. 93:71, 1966.
29. Urschell, H.C., and Razzuk, M.A.: Management of the thoracic outlet syndrome. N. Engl. J. Med. 286:1140, 1972.
30. Singh, A., and Jolly, S.S.: Wasted leg syndrome (a compression neuropathy of the lower limbs). J. Assoc. Phys. India 11:1031, 1963.
31. Bertrand, L., Labauge, R., and Vergues, J.: Paralysie de posture bilatérale et régressive du nerf sciatique chez une jeune vendangeuse. Montpellier Med. 67:87, 1965.
32. Nakano, K.K.: Entrapment neuropathy from Baker's cyst. JAMA 239:135, 1978.
33. Staal, A., Weerdt, C.J., and Went, L.N.: Hereditary compression syndrome of peripheral nerves. Neurology 15:1008, 1965.
34. Stack, R.E., Bianco, A.J., and MacCarty, C.S.: Compression of the common peroneal nerve by ganglion cysts. Report of nine cases. J. Bone Joint Surg. 47A:773, 1965.
35. Browne, S.G.: Some less common neurologic findings in leprosy. J. Neurol. Sci. 2:253, 1965.
36. Leach, R.E., Zohn, D.A., and Strijker, W.S.: Anterior tibial compartment syndrome. Clinical and electromyographic aspects. Arch. Surg. 88:187, 1964.
37. Keck, C.: The tarsal tunnel syndrome. J. Bone Joint Surg. 44A:180, 1962.
38. Goodgold, J., Kopell, H.P., and Spielholz, N.I.: The tarsal tunnel syndrome. N. Engl. J. Med. 273:742, 1965.
39. Enna, C.D., and Callaway, J.C.: The tarsal tunnel syndrome. Case report: Posterior tibial leprous neuritis associated with tendon sheath ganglion. Int. J. Leprosy 32:279, 1964.
40. Brooks, D.M.: Nerve compression by simple ganglia. A review of thirteen collected cases. J. Bone Joint Surg. 34B:391, 1952.
41. MacFarlane, I.J.A., and DuToit, S.N.: A ganglion causing tarsal tunnel syndrome. S. Afr. Med. J. 48:2568, 1974.
42. Biemond, A.: Femoral neuropathy. In Vinken, P.J., and Bruyn, G.W. (eds.): Handbook of Clinical Neurology, Vol. 8, Diseases of Nerves, Part II. New York, American Elsevier Publishing Company, 1970, pp. 303–310.
43. Kopell, H.P., and Thompson, W.A.L.: Peripheral entrapment neuropathies of the lower extremity. N. Engl. J. Med. 262:56, 1960.
44. Matsen, F.A., III: Compartmental Syndromes. New York, Grune & Stratton, 1980.
45. Mubarak, S.J., and Hargens, A.R.: Compartment Syndromes and Volkmann's Contracture. Philadelphia, W. B. Saunders, 1981.

Section XXIII
Rehabilitation

Chapter 111
Rehabilitation of Patients with Rheumatic Diseases

Lynn H. Gerber

INTRODUCTION

Rehabilitation is that process that renders a broad range of treatments designed to help patients achieve their maximal potential for normal living.[1] During the past decade, there has been an increased interest in what rehabilitation can offer patients with rheumatic disease and an increased awareness of significant improvements that have resulted from rehabilitation interventions, both of which help to place the specialty on a more rational basis.[2-4] Whereas rheumatology is dedicated to the understanding of and control of disease activity, rehabilitation medicine aims to maintain or restore function or prevent dysfunction by means of physical therapy, occupational therapy, physical medicine, and vocational counseling. The tools used in providing comprehensive rehabilitation evaluation and treatment include exercises, heat, cold, ultrasound, electricity, counseling, splints, sophisticated engineering, adaptive aids, and motion analysis systems. This chapter will discuss what constitutes a rehabilitation evaluation, the scope of treatment options used in rehabilitation, and how these are applied to the problems seen in patients with rheumatic diseases. This approach will reflect current practice and incorporate principles of the physiology of muscle and joint action as well as principles of human behavior upon which treatments in this discipline are based. A review of measurement outcomes useful in the evaluation of treatment will be included, as will a section discussing those rehabilitation techniques and materials likely to be of use to the practicing rheumatologist.

EVALUATION

The ability to formulate an appropriate treatment plan is based upon a thorough evaluation, which includes data from the physical, psychosocial, and vocational aspects of patients' lives.

The physical evaluation usually concentrates on the musculoskeletal system, including a neurologic exam, and identifies problems of range; strength; deformity; number of hot, swollen joints; trigger points; and whether the problems are partly or totally remediable. Level of pain is often determined. In addition to static measures, the physicians and therapists must evaluate how well the patient ambulates and attends to daily living and work needs. They assess whether deficits are due to weakness, deformity, limitation in range of motion, or lack of stamina or motivation. A joint count is only one small part of the assessment. Joint range of motion (ROM) is a standard, highly reproducible and valid measurement tool.[5] Much of what is learned from ROM is useful in predicting functional impairment; for example, if one is unable to obtain 110 degrees of elbow flexion, it is likely that there will be grooming and feeding abnormalities because of an inability to get the hand to the mouth or head.

The psychosocial evaluation identifies depression and adaptive or maladaptive behavior to illness, and tries to assess whether a patient needs assistance other than physical to continue to perform important life functions, ranging the full gamut from sleep to sex to exercise. Occasionally, family members need to participate in the evaluation. Finally, a vocational assessment or educational evaluation is performed to estimate what the economic sequelae of the disease may be and to identify needs for adaptive devices or removal of environmental barriers.

Physical Assessment. Intra-articular pressure is influenced by joint position,[6] and those positions associated with lower intra-articular pressure are frequently assumed by arthritics: flexion and external rotation of the hip and 40 degrees of flexion of the knee,[7,8] and 90 degrees of flexion of the elbow. While patients assume these positions to relieve pain, they are not those of optimal function. Early intervention can often reverse a contracture, but by 8 weeks of fixed positioning, dense capsular adhesions are formed and a contracture less amenable to straightening is likely to have developed. Clearly one form of intervention is to give instruction in exercises to preserve ROM in order to maintain the extremities in positions of maximal function and to maximize joint alignment. Another is to educate the patient about proper joint positioning and to reinforce its importance. Normal joint alignment is necessary for preserving the ability of the joint to transmit stress uniformly and to minimize articular cartilage fibrillation and fraying. Intermittent compression of articular cartilage is essential for normal delivery of nutrients to this tissue. However, when ROM exercises and positioning exercises fail to preserve joint congruity and mechanical alignment, measures directed at reducing the load across a joint should be taken. This may take the form of a gait aid for lower extremity problems or use of more proximal joints for lifting in upper extremity work.

Patients with rheumatic disease are at risk for losing range of joint motion. Soft tissue contractures are quite common in early rheumatoid arthritis (RA), mixed connective tissue disease (MCTD), and scleroderma or progressive systemic sclerosis (PSS). True bony ankylosis occurs in advanced RA, juvenile arthritides, spondyloarthropathies, and advanced osteoarthritis (OA). Although deformity is common in systemic lupus erythematosus (SLE), this is not usually associated with contracture, and the deformity is usually reducible. Knowledge of these differences may result in selection of the appropriate treatment regimen (e.g., exercise or surgery).

In addition to ROM, the physical examination must include an assessment of pain and edema. A painful, edematous joint inhibits smooth gliding movement. Effusion is often associated with ligamentous laxity and joint instability and inefficiency of muscle contraction. Pain inhibits motion and potentiates deformity.[9] The ability to distinguish between a joint that has potential for change and one that does not is important. Intervention to reduce rubor, calor, and tumor, including the modalities of heat, cold, and electricity in the form of galvanic stimulation and transcutaneous nerve stimulation (TENS), and ultrasound (a form of deep heat) is frequently used. Useful help can be obtained in estimating the reversibility of joint deformity from radiographs. For example, contracture in the presence of apparently normal cartilage thickness and minimal loss of periarticular bone is a better prognosis than a similarly contracted joint with associated loss of cartilage, subchondial bone erosions, and osteopenia.

Strength, as measured by a manual muscle examination, is another determination essential to the physical examination. The muscle is graded on a scale from 0 to 5. Zero indicates no muscle action, 1 indicates trace contraction, 2 denotes a poor contraction (visible but unable to overcome gravity), 3 indicates a fair contraction (able to overcome gravity and can take minimal resistance), 4 indicates good strength (able to take resistance), and 5 means that the evaluator is unable to overcome the contracted muscle. Muscle testing does not measure a sustained contraction, nor can it be used as an indicator of stamina or endurance. These are influenced by a number of factors including cardiovascular status and voluntary effort expended, which influences strength by increasing the number of motor units recruited to perform the task.[10] Muscle fiber types have different physiologic properties, and each responds differently to exercise. For example, there is an increase in the ratio of type I to type II fibers with bicycling and a disproportional decrease in type II with disuse.[11] Strength does not seem to be directly proportional to muscle bulk; the amount of contractile protein increases with training.[12] Conversely, atrophy does not imply functional loss, and exercise programs in patients with rheumatic disease should be designed not to increase muscle bulk but to restore or preserve function.

Almost all rheumatic diseases are associated with abnormalities of strength. Most commonly heard are complaints of fatigue and decrease in stamina, an almost universal complaint that is difficult to quantify. Polymyositis is associated with decreased proximal muscle strength. Milder degrees of weakness are seen in SLE, RA, and PSS, and the distribution varies, but often includes distal musculature. Polymyalgia rheumatica is associated with pain and stiffness in the proximal musculature, often interfering with the ability to accurately evaluate strength but rarely causing true weakness. Vasculitides and amyloidosis may be associated with weakness because of stroke in the former or polyneuropathy in either.

Pain and stiffness induced by inflammation are frequent complaints of patients with rheumatic diseases. Painful states are responsible for significant morbidity and usually require intervention. The rehabilitation interventions are usually not pharmacologic, hence minimizing the likelihood of substance abuse. When pain is a result of an underlying biomechanical or inflammatory process, treatment is directed at correcting the problem.

New techniques that provide analgesic control include transcutaneous electrical nerve stimulation (TENS), a superficial means of applying electric current, and acupressure techniques, manual pressure over some of the acupuncture points. Stimulation of large somatosensory afferents may block the noxious stimuli of small fibers and prevents their ascent to the CNS. Pressure on the acupuncture points may release endorphins and other endogenous opiates at the CNS level.[12a]

Quantification of pain is difficult, although the descriptive terms mild, moderate, and severe are commonly used, as are visual analog scales. These are simply lines upon which a dot is placed indicating where the patient believes his pain falls with respect to a maximum and minimum intensity as described by the length of the bar. A number can be assigned to the value by determining into which segment of 10 equal segments the dot falls.[13]

Static measures are necessary but not sufficient in the comprehensive evaluation. Kinematics, the study of human motion, presents a dynamic picture of how a patient is moving and helps round out the picture. Major strides in this area have been made within the last decade, mainly in the evaluation of gait. A variety of analyses are available. A highly organized system for the observation of gait has been developed and is now quite widely applied;[14] and video tape analysis, using both visual and computer evaluation, has been used to guide surgical treatment and resolve biomechanical problems.[15,16] Pressure mats and foot pads with pressure transducers have been used to study weight-bearing patterns in children and adults with RA.[17] The information obtained from these systems includes joint angle motion and ground reaction forces. Stride length, cadence, weight acceptance pattern, and percent of gait cycle on single or double limb support are measurable from the foot switch system. In addition, dynamic electromyography, which provides a recording of a muscle's electrical activity during movement, can be used to identify which muscles are firing during which phases of gait. No defined relationship, however, has been made between electrical activity of a muscle and the force it generates during movement.

Normal gait is a complex series of events designed to move the body from one point to another.[18] At normal walking speeds, little energy is consumed, and the limb segment motions are smooth. At increased or decreased walking speeds energy requirements are increased.[19] Arthritics walk at a significantly decreased speed, which may partially explain their extreme fatigue and decreased stamina. Abnormalities of joint angles may partially explain how deformities occur and how compensatory movements may relate to deformity.

Relatively little data is available for upper extremity evaluation, with the exception of the hand. Hand dynamometry has been useful in evaluating grip strength and forces generated during prehensile patterns.[20]

Gait deviations can cause instability and energy inefficient postures and may potentiate muscle contracture or stretching. Inequality of leg length greater than 0.5 inch will result in a significant gait deviation, with excessive dipping of the shoulder on the shorter side; increased hip, knee, and ankle flexion on the longer side; and an excessive rise on the toes of the shorter side to permit the long leg to clear the floor properly. These observations suggest that there should be concern for the metatarso-phalangeal joints of the short side, for the vertebral column, and possibly for the hip and knee joints of the longer leg, all of which may be subject to increased loads and stress and may be at risk in the development of osteoarthritis.[21]

Flexion contracture of the knee creates a short leg, as described above, but also stretches the quadriceps and causes contracture of hamstrings, significantly limiting stability. A stiff knee, while stable, creates a long leg and increases energy expenditure considerably.[22] Flexion contracture of the hip produces a short leg and a forwardly displaced torso. With an ankylosed hip, there is compensatory exaggerated lumbar spine activity and increased movement in the other hip. Muscle weakness also produces gait deviations. Hip flexor weakness results in a backward thrust of the trunk and pelvis to lift the leg off the ground. With quadriceps weakness, the knee may buckle as the foot strikes the floor; with gastroc-soleus weakness, the heel does not rise, and there is no push off from the sole of the foot. With weak foot dorsiflexors, the foot slaps down, and the toe does not clear without excessive knee and hip flexion.

The body can frequently compensate for the loss of one major joint or muscle group. The price, however, as mentioned, may be increased caloric expenditure or stress on other joints, a price too high to pay in some patients with rheumatic disease. When several contiguous joints or muscle groups are affected, stability and/or strength are usually so significantly compromised that ambulation and self-care become impaired.

Loss of more than one joint or muscle group cannot be compensated for without external support, adaptive gait aids, or surgical correction. Specific corrective devices are discussed under Management of Chronic Problems, below.

Functional Assessment. Function has been a most difficult entity to measure. Functional assessments have traditionally measured mobility and activities of daily living, (feeding, dressing, grooming, and so on). Function is multifaceted and describes a global assessment of how the patient is doing. Factors that influence function are physiological, biomechanical, psychological, environmental, and socioeconomic. When rheumatologists ask about function, they wish to know about mobility, self-care, pain, and change in life role.[23-26]

Functional assessments, as any instrument used in scientific study, should be standardized, quantifiable, reliable, valid, and sensitive enough to distinguish change in those areas being studied. Several formalized assessments have been used for patients with arthritis. The Convery polyarticular disability index is a self-report about mobility and activities of daily living.[23] The Keitel index measures functional limitation based on observed performance.[24] Both lack measures of pain, satisfaction, or precise indicators that can be linked to specific diseases.

Partly to address these shortcomings and partly because of the availability of instruments used in the social sciences, new assessments have been generated. The Arthritis Impact Measurements Scale (AIMS)[27] and the Health Assessment Questionnaire (HAQ)[28] and the functional capacity evaluation[29] are standardized and evaluate mobility, level of physical activity, social activity and role, activities of self-care, pain, anxiety, and depression; none of these addresses motivation or compliance.

Recently another approach has been taken to assess function. This model, the Occupational Behavior Model,[30,31] looks at the question of function from a behavioral point of view. It asks what the patient's values are (personal goals, standards, expectation of success); what her habits and roles in life are; and what her performance skills (musculoskeletal, neurologic and cognitive) are that support activity. Through this evaluation one can obtain a dynamic view of function and also partially determine level of satisfaction in life roles or quality of life as subjectively reported.

Often the best method for evaluating function is to ask the patient to keep a daily log of activities and ask her to rate level of satisfaction, fatigue, and frustration.

This is most helpful when the rehabilitation team can follow events over time and it provides good comparative data. Often, questions about sleep can identify depression (e.g., early morning awakening) or anxiety (easy arousability).[32]

TREATMENT

Compliance. Patient participation and cooperation in treatment plans are dependent in part on the ability of the patient to understand the nature of the disease and how it may affect her life. Further, the intervention must be seen as helpful and valuable to the patient.[33] Patient education has been demonstrated to be beneficial in increasing compliance.[34,35] A positive relationship between patient and physician or therapist is likely to increase compliance.[36]

In managing a treatment plan, the patient needs to receive clear instructions, usually in written form, about what regimen to follow. A limited number of activities should be prescribed, beginning with those interventions likely to produce results that are valued by the patient.[37] One study has shown that compliance with an exercise program for arthritics was correlated with patients' understanding of their disease, and that housewives were more compliant than people employed outside the home or nonworkers.[38] Another has indicated that compliant arthritics were likely to have experienced less time waiting to see the physician, and emphasized the importance of the amount of time spent with the physician, and of effective communication between patient and doctor.[39]

Exercise. Exercise is an important therapeutic intervention for patients with rheumatic disease. There are several types of exercise (Table 111–1). It may be passive, during which the therapist moves the extremity for the patient and the patient does not perform an active contraction; active exercise, during which the patient performs all motions and actively contracts the muscle; assistive exercise, during which the patient makes maximal effort and is partially assisted by the therapist; and resistive exercise, during which an active contraction against resistance, either mechanical or manual, is performed.

Passive exercise is not frequently used for patients with arthritis, but those with severe muscle weakness due to polymyositis or neuropathic disease associated with vasculitis and stroke or peripheral neuropathy can benefit by passive exercise. The purpose of the exercise is to provide range of motion (ROM) to joints that are incapable of moving and are at risk of developing contracture, to provide some stretch and compression to muscles and to act as a pump to enhance venous return.

Active exercise is generally recommended for patients with rheumatic diseases. There are three different types of active muscle contraction. (1) A static or isometric contraction produces minimal shortening, and there is no joint motion with this type of contraction. It is ideally suited for maintaining muscle strength in patients with inflammatory arthropathy because maximal tension is generated with minimal joint stress, and only a few maximal contractions per day are necessary to maintain or increase muscle strength. There is some evidence that strength increases made with isometric training are not transferable to isotonic performance, and vice versa.[40] (2) An isotonic or dynamic contraction is associated with shortening (concentric) or lengthening (eccentric) of muscle. The limb is moved and the joint is stressed through range. (3) Isokinetic contraction is associated with the generation of a maximum torque using a preset rate-limiting device. This type of exercise is rarely prescribed in inflammatory arthropathy.

Muscle strengthening and maintaining strength are important in supporting the patient's ability to perform daily activities. In rheumatoid arthritis and osteoarthritis, loss of muscle strength and function frequently occur.[41] A muscle can lose 30 percent of its bulk in a week[42] and can lose 3 percent of its function per day when maintained at strict rest.[43]

Table 111–1. Guide to Selection of Therapeutic Exercise for Patients with Rheumatic Disease

Goal	Associated Disease(s)	Passive	Isometric	Active Isotonic	Assistive	Frequency
Preventive						
a. Disuse atrophy	RA, OA, scleroderma, psoriatic arthritis		++		+	Daily
Restorative						
a. Increase endurance	Polymyositis, SLE, RA		++	+	++	Daily
b. Muscle re-education	Postoperative neuropathy			+*	++	Daily
c. Increase ROM	Capsulitis, RA, scleroderma, OA, psoriatic arthritis, spondyloarthropathies	+		+	++	Several times daily
d. Increase strength	Inflammatory arthropathies,		++	+		Daily
	noninflammatory arthropathies		+	++		Daily

*With progressive increase in resistance

For the arthritic, isometric contraction, in which relatively little fatigue and little repetitive joint motion are produced, is the treatment of choice. It causes the least possible joint inflammation and least amount of intra-articular pressure and juxta-articular bone destruction.[44-46] The benefit of isometric quadriceps exercise and short-term physical training in rheumatoid arthritis has been documented.[4] Recently the results of long-term training (4 to 8 years) using bicycle ergometry and a variety of sports demonstrated less progression of x-ray changes in arthritis, more improvement in hamstring strength, and less sick leave taken by the exercised group.[47] Another comparison study also demonstrated improvement in activities of daily living (ADL) in the exercised group.[48] The patient with arthritis can benefit from isotonic exercise to tolerance. Indications of excessive exercise include significant, persistent fatigue or pain, increased weakness, joint pain, or swelling.

Evidence is accumulating that bone mineralization is in part dependent upon muscle contraction. Conversely, bed rest results in a decrease in lean body mass and total body potassium and calcium depletion.[49,50] Exercises for post-menopausal women have demonstrated positive effects on bone mineralization,[51] and bone mineralization, as determined by densitometry, is increased in athletes.[52] It is likely that exercise can increase bone mass and may be useful in the management of senile osteoporosis. There is little data to support one form of active exercise over another, but most studies employed isotonic and some resistive exercise.[52] We know that patients with rheumatic diseases develop osteopenia, possibly from disuse, medication, or abnormalities of calcium and collagen metabolism.[53]

Stretching is often coupled with the use of heat, cold, whirlpool, or medication to control pain and edema. The technique is to apply a gentle but steady force on the limb that lacks full range of motion. Clinical judgment needs to be used in grading the amount of force necessary to attain the goal, and in working within the range of pain tolerance of the patient. Passive ROM is used to decrease limb edema, maintain functional positions, or to prepare the limb for active exercise. It is frequently used when weakness or pain limits active motion, or when assistance is needed to break up capsular adhesions. Active and active assistive stretching is used when the patient is able to initiate muscle contraction, and is the preferred form of stretching for maintenance.

Occasionally devices are used to aid in stretching. Serial casting has been used to stretch out knee flexion contractures with success in RA[54] and in hemophiliac arthropathy.[55] For management of hand stiffness and contractures, casting and dynamic splinting to provide a constant tension have been used.[56,57] Traction and overhead pulleys have been used with some success in the management of frozen shoulders.[58]

For many patients with RA the following muscle groups deserve special attention: strengthening of the intrinsic muscles of the feet and stretching the long toe extensors, peronei, and gastrocnemius; strengthening the quadriceps and stretching the hamstrings, hip flexors, and iliotibial band; and strengthening finger and wrist extensors and stretching the intrinsics. While these exercises will not restore bony architecture, preservation of muscle balance will maximize the possibility of preserving or restoring normal function.

Positioning. Contracture often occurs from improper positioning and poor posture. Improper posture can result in abnormal joint positions and contracture even in joints that are not primarily involved with the disease process. The use of pillows under the knees and other body props to relieve pain often result in limb malpositioning and contracture. Prone lying to minimize hip and knee flexion contractures is useful, and the bed should have a firm mattress with a small soft pillow for the head. Patients with ankylosing spondylitis should use no pillow.

Standing posture should consist of keeping the head in the midline with chin slightly retracted; shoulders at a neutral position (neither elevated nor protracted); abdomen pulled in; a minimal lumbar lordosis; and the knees, hips, and ankles at neutral. Upper extremity motions most critical for preservation of function include external rotation of the shoulder, supination of the forearm, extension of the wrist and MCP, and flexion of the PIP.[59] In the lower extremity critical motions include extension and abduction of the hip, extension of the knee, and dorsiflexion of the ankle.[60] Information about positions for optimal function in the lower extremity and critical ranges of motion have been determined from methodical gait analysis.[14] Those for upper extremity function have been determined from clinical experience.

When range of motion can be preserved, the critical ranges are the following: hip, from 0 degrees of extension to 30 degrees of flexion; knee, from neutral to 60 degrees of flexion; and ankle, from 20 degrees of plantar to 10 degrees of dorsiflexion. A critical range of motion for upper extremity function is not universally agreed upon. In the hand, loss of full finger extension usually does not seriously interfere with function. Loss of flexion of the distal interphalangeal joints rarely limits function. However, loss of even a few degrees of metacarpophalangeal joint flexion (especially in the little and ring fingers) may be significant. The proximal interphalangeal joints should be able to flex more than 50 degrees to preserve adequate function.[61] The thumb primarily requires joint stability, but without 30 degrees of internal rotation at the carpometacarpal joint, normal apposition is not possible. The elbow requires 90 degrees of flexion to approximate hand and mouth. Shoulder range should include a minimum of 45 degrees of flexion, 90 degrees of abduction, and 20 degrees of external rotation.

When motion cannot be preserved, positioning of joints for optimal function is as follows: hip, 5 to 10 degrees of flexion and in neutral with respect to rotation; knee, 5 to 10 degrees of flexion; ankle, neutral; shoulder, 30 to 45 degrees of flexion, 10 degrees of internal rotation; elbow, 70 to 80 degrees of flexion with 10 to 15 degrees of supination in the forearm; wrist, 5 to 10 degrees of dorsiflexion; hand, 30 degrees of metacarpophalangeal flexion and thumb abduction; jaw, at least 1 inch open; head position, upright and looking forward.

Rest. Strict bed rest over a protracted period of time is contraindicated in inflammatory arthropathies because of the potential for muscle atrophy,[42] increased osteoporosis,[49] joint contracture or ankylosis, and deleterious effects on articular contracture or cartilage.[62] Punctuating the day with rest periods, however, may be energy conserving and may be an effective way to reduce pain and inflammation.[63,64] Recumbency is a time when near-normal body mechanics can be restored and joints supported to reduce stress. Finally, rest periods may provide psychological rest and be of benefit to patients.[65]

Local rest is universally accepted as clinically valuable in the management of inflammatory arthropathies.[66] There is even some evidence that the inflamed joint that is immobilized undergoes a more rapid resolution of the problem than the nonsplinted joint.[66]

The purposes of splinting are to reduce inflammation, to support the extremity in optimal functional position, to maintain alignment postoperatively, to provide stretch to tight tendons and ligaments, and to increase function. There is no consensus that splinting corrects deformities or even slows their progression.[67] Splinting and bracing may lead to decreased strength, a reversible problem, to joint contracture, which is reversible when immobilization is less than four weeks,[65] and possibly to osteoporosis.

Certain caveats need to be invoked when a splint is prescribed. Clearly, compliance is important, and those factors that influence compliance should be maximized. For example, the splint should be lightweight and easy to put on, adjust, and take off (preferably by the patient without any assistance). It should not limit function, and care to align the splint properly must be taken so that deformity is not induced. This last point cannot be overemphasized. Often, a stock splint is provided that limits thumb opposition, limits MCP flexion, and puts the wrist in extension. The patient returns complaining that the splint does not permit reasonable activity, and occasionally a child will come in with the wrist in an extension contracture.

Modalities. Instruments or devices used to deliver heat, cold, sound, and electricity are used primarily to control pain, to reduce swelling and local inflammation, and to aid in stabilization of joints and strengthening of muscles.

The therapeutic effects of heat and cold are both local (increased local circulation or decreased local circulation) and systemic, mediated by reflex responses.[68]

Heat produces sedation and analgesia,[69] probably by acting on free nerve endings[70] and gamma fibers of the muscle spindles.[68] There is some evidence that it has a positive effect on viscoelastic properties of collagen, such that when tension is applied, an effective stretch can be performed.[71,72] It can be delivered in a variety of forms and to a variety of depths, using a variety of methods (Table 111–2). Selection depends upon personal preference, ease of application, expense, and availability.

Table 111–2. Varieties of Heat

Type of Heat	Mechanism of Heating
Superficial Heat	
1. Hot pack	
a. moist	
b. dry	Conduction
2. Whirlpool	
3. Paraffin	
4. Infrared	Radiation
5. Sauna	Convection
Deep Heat (Diathermy)	
1. Short wave	
2. Microwave	
3. Ultrasound	

Superficial heat rarely penetrates more then a few millimeters, and therefore it does not raise intra-articular temperatures. Superficial heat causes demonstrable increases in peripheral circulation and has been shown to raise skin temperature to 40 to 44° C and core body temperature by a few degrees.[73] This increases metabolic rate, causes arteriolar dilatation, and may cause edema. The cardiovascular system must be adequate to respond and dissipate the increased heat. While superficial heat does increase skin temperature and peripheral circulation, and is in widespread clinical use, its causal relationship to pain relief and muscle relaxation is far from clear.[74] Superficial heating is often used for minor aches and pains, to produce relaxation and sedation prior to muscle stretching and exercise and to increase range of motion, especially in adhesive capsulitis, scleroderma, and low back and neck pain. It should not be used in patients with impaired circulation or sensation.

There are three types of diathermy modalities: shortwave, microwave, and ultrasound. Shortwave utilizes high frequency current to transmit energy. Microwave uses electromagnetic waves with higher frequencies and shorter wavelengths than radiowaves, and ultrasound uses frequencies of acoustic vibration higher than can be perceived by the human ear.

A thorough discussion of the biophysics and designs of each modality is available for review.[75] As a brief guide for the appropriate modality selection, evidence indicates that shortwave is best at heating the superficial musculature.[76] It probably does not penetrate to deep joints, such as the hip. Its chief use is in the treatment of muscle spasm. Microwave available for clinical use at frequencies of 2456 and 915 MHz is used for heating the superficial and deeper musculature. It should not be applied to the eye, for it has been demonstrated to induce cataract formation,[77] and it should be used with caution over bony prominences, metallic implants, or abscesses because of their selective absorption of energy.[75] Microwave is the modality of choice in heating the deeper musculature.

The depth of penetration of ultrasound is greater than shortwave or microwave. It is selectively absorbed by bone and is a particularly good modality for heating joints and periarticular structures. Energy exposures are 0.5 to 4.0 watts per square centimeter for 5 to 10 minutes. It is a safe modality, and its use has been beneficial as an adjunct for the relief of joint contractures, regardless of cause. Ultrasound has been demonstrated to be superior to microwave in the treatment of periarthritis of the shoulder when given in conjunction with standard physical therapy.[78] It is the treatment modality of choice for heating joints and can be safely used with surgical implants.[75]

The general contraindications to the use of heat apply to diathermy as well. One should not heat areas that are ischemic or have impaired sensation. The eye should not be heated. Areas with hemorrhage, edema, severe inflammation, or tumor probably should not receive diathermy treatment. Shortwave and microwave must not be used in patients with cardiac pacemakers.

A large literature and a sizeable body of clinical observations have supported the use of heat for the relief of joint pain.[75,76] These are not controlled clinical trials, nor are they physiologic studies designed to determine efficacy of modalities, mechanism of action, or guidelines for treatment. In fact, there is some doubt that deep heating should be used in treating articular problems at all.[79] Joints are closed systems, subject to mechanical and metabolic stresses, about whose heat-dissipating mechanisms we know little. In fact, there is evidence that the normal intra-articular temperature is lower than body temperature,[80] and, further, that an increase of 5° C increases enzymatic lysis of human cartilage by rheumatoid synovial collagenase, suggesting that increased temperature may accelerate cartilage destruction. The use of deep heat has also been associated with increased leukocytosis and inflammation in urate crystal–induced synovitis.[81] Clearly, there is a mounting controversy about whether diathermy is a safe and effective tool in the treatment of acute arthritis. We await better studies that will place the use of these treatments on a firmer scientific basis, help in proper selection, and explain mechanisms of action.

Common applications for heating modalities include frozen shoulder, subacute tendinitis, scleroderma (often subaqua), and the working out of contractures and muscle spasm and stiffness. The results are often temporary, and one is unable to affect the progression of disease using these treatments.[82]

Cold has been demonstrated to be an effective analgesic and can induce surgical anesthesia;[83] it is often used for acute strains, sprains, and edema as well as in treating hemarthroses because of induced vasoconstriction.[84] Cold is useful in treating muscle spasm and spasticity; the mechanism of action is by direct effect on the muscle spindle.[85] Application of cold to rheumatoid joints may inhibit collagenase activity in rheumatoid synovia.[86] Cold has been demonstrated to raise the threshold for pain in the normal shoulder[87] but seems to have no effect on the development of chronic synovitis.[81] Ice has been shown to be as effective as heat in the treatment of frozen shoulder.[88] Cold is usually administered in the form of ice cubes or ice packs, ice massage, or coolant spray (ethylchloride or fluoromethane).[89,90]

Hydrotherapy, while it is a convenient mode of delivering warmth to a body part, also provides a near stressless medium in which to move joints and exercise.[91] Tanks are available for upper extremity, lower extremity, and total body submersion. Immersion is associated with local peripheral vasodilatation and often with a reflex vasodilatory effect at a site remote from the warmth.[92] Body or Hubbard tank should be kept at 32 to 38° C. and optimal treatment time is 20 minutes. Prolonged exposure or temperatures in excess of 40° C can result in circulatory compromise.

A therapeutic pool can facilitate general reconditioning and can be useful in postoperative joint replacement rehabilitation[93] and as an aid to progressive ambulation and increased joint range of motion. There are no data to support any increased benefit from the agitators, though the patient usually experiences the water movement as very comfortable.

Other Modalities to Control Pain. Electrical stimulation of muscle (galvanic stimulation) has been used to relieve muscle spasm with some success, although no controlled trials have been reported.[94] It has also been used as an adjunct to help stretch out contractures in patients with spasticity and in an attempt to maintain muscle bulk and strength in denervation. Recently, electrical stimulation has been used to heal cutaneous ulcers.[95]

Another form of electricity used in managing pain in connective tissue diseases has been the transcutaneous electrical nerve stimulator (TENS). It consists of a battery pack with electrodes that can be attached to limb or trunk. Rationale for its use is based upon the gate control theory, which claims that by stimulating large-diameter cutaneous fibers one blocks the noxious stimuli released from the small bore fibers, thereby inhibiting transmission of painful stimuli to the spinal cord.[96] This technique is easy and safe to use. Usually the electrodes are applied with a coupling agent to areas that bracket a painful joint or dermatomes. Success has been reported in treatment of rheumatoid neuropathy[97,98] and fractures associated with linear scleroderma,[99] and relief of pain has been reported in patients with rheumatoid arthritis.[100]

Aids and Appliances. Aids and appliances are used to promote independence for patients with rheumatic diseases. Included in this category are assistive devices for activities of daily living, orthotics and splints, corsets, and ambulation devices.

There are many assistive devices available commercially[101-104] that may be of use. Before prescribing them, a number of issues that may influence patient compliance need to be considered. First, the device must be affordable; second, it needs to offer the patient something that improves his or her lifestyle and that the patient values, that is, something that he or she wants; and third, the item must be reliable and simple to use.

Mobility is an important function for most people. Support might include use of cane, crutch, or walker, occasionally with a molded handpiece or platform for specific needs of patients with RA. If the functional deficit is balance, a cane is the appropriate device. If a limb needs to be unweighted by more than 50 percent, as in avascular necrosis or postoperatively, or with a painful hip or knee, a crutch or walker is appropriate. The cane or single crutch is best used on the side opposite that which is most symptomatic. Biomechanically, it has been demonstrated that the cane can unweight up to 50 percent of body weight.[105] A Loftstrand or long arm cane is often easier to use. Two crutches using a toe-touch gait are the best at unweighting the lower extremity.[106] The platform crutch is useful for patients with wrist involvement because it distributes weight on the forearm, reducing the need for wrist extension. Crutch and cane fitting require attention to detail, as does gait training.[106] If the problem is endurance and strength, consider a wheelchair as a reasonable way of preserving mobility.[107] A small motorized chair such as the Amigo is appropriate and easily fits in the trunk of a car. Adaptive equipment for the car may be essential for patients with osteoarthritis, rheumatoid arthritis, or scleroderma. These include a car door opener, an ignition adaptive piece, and an overhead strap or sliding board to help with transfers. A lamb's wool seat and steering wheel covers may help patients with Raynaud's disease. Portable car seats are useful for patients with low back pain.

Toileting, dressing, and feeding are important self-care activities that most people would rather do for themselves. Arising from toilets and baths is often difficult for patients with pelvic girdle weakness, as in myositis or inadequate hip range, or pain, as in osteoarthritis or rheumatoid arthritis. A commode chair, elevated toilet seat, or tub seat can increase safety and independence, as can grab bars placed around tubs and toilets. Specific aids can be used to help wipe and cleanse the perineum and to reach the head and face.[108]

Dressing and undressing may be one of the more time- and energy-consuming tasks for arthritics. Adaptive aids such as long-handled reachers, shoe horns, brushes, and button and zipper hooks are useful. Perhaps more beneficial for patients with limited range of motion is clothing that is designed to accommodate the handicap, which will facilitate comfort, enhance self-esteem, and reduce time required for dressing. The patient with chronic disease is concerned with cost, weight of clothing, ease of care, and appearance, as well as function. Fabrics made of natural fibers are absorbent and when blended with synthetics are more durable, retain their shape, resist wrinkles, and are easy to clean. Mohair and alpaca are warm and lightweight. Smooth linings facilitate donning and doffing garments. Open weave fabrics tend to catch and run the fabrics and so are less practical than tightly knit fabrics. Small buttons, hooks, and zipper tabs are difficult to manipulate with stiff, weak, or arthritic fingers. Adaptations using large, textured buttons, zipper rings, velcro, and other fusible and binding fabrics are available in most variety stores. A long towel with a small hook may be attached to the zipper at the back of a garment before putting the garment on and will facilitate pulling up the zipper. Stretch straps and waists are generally easier to use than hooked or belted waists. Garments with raglan sleeves and gussets increase maneuverability in pulling garments over the head. Outerwear such as capes, ponchos, and down jackets are also easy to don and are warm and lightweight.

Eating and preparing food occupy a significant proportion of one's day. Nutritional status is in part determined by how easy it is for patients to prepare and eat meals as well as by their knowledge of appropriate diets. Most kitchens can be designed to minimize the need to reach and bend by placing more shelves at counter level and designing cabinets with pull-out drawers. Useful kitchen devices include food processors, long-handled reachers, built-up handles on utensils, electric knife and mounted wedge-shaped jar openers. Lightweight aluminum pans are durable, and some are made with compartments to permit cooking different things in the same pan. Lining pans with aluminum foil saves scrubbing. One of the most valuable suggestions one can provide patients is to encourage them to make weekly meal plans in order to minimize trips to the stores and possibly to cook double portions, which may be used at future times.

Splints and Orthotics. Orthoses, splints and casts, are frequently used in the management of patients with rheumatic diseases. They are used for unweighting joints and for decreasing joint motion or stabilizing joints. Splints are also useful for preserving extremities in the most functional positions and help to improve patterns of motion, and must be designed to incorporate positions that achieve maximum function (see Positioning, above). Splinting is a safe procedure when used properly and will not produce joint contractures even if the joint is immobilized, provided the length of immobilization does not exceed 4 weeks.[66] Despite the frequent use of splints, no objective data are available that demonstrate efficacy in the prevention of deformity. In fact, with the exception of postoperative management, splints do not reverse deformity.[109]

Prefabricated splints often inadequately immobilize the intended joint or impede movement of adjacent joints. The physician must decide if the availability of the splint is the critical factor and outweighs its drawbacks.

Traditionally plaster and elastic wraps have been used to fabricate splints and orthotics. The former is inexpensive and rigid; but it is also heavy, chips and cracks, and cannot be washed. Elastic compresses soft tissues but does not effectively immobilize a joint. Plastics have become essential to the fabrication of custom orthotics. These materials are lightweight, durable, and washable and can be molded with ease. They are commercially available under the names of Orthoplast and Aquaplast, are heat labile at 160° F, and are used for hand splints; polyethylene, which requires heating to 375° F and must be vacuum formed, is used primarily for ankle-foot and longer leg orthotics. Microcellular rubber (tradename: Spenco) and polyurethane heat-bondable materials (tradenames: Aliplast and Plastazote) are frequently used for fabrication of soft shoe inserts (Fig. 111–1).[110]

Lower Extremity Orthotics. Foot problems are almost

Figure 111–1. Shoe inserts. *Top*, Plastic UCB; *bottom*, Spenco and heat molded combinations of Aliplast and Plastazote.

universal in our population. Clinically significant foot problems occur most frequently in patients with rheumatoid arthritis, juvenile rheumatoid arthritis, osteoarthritis, and psoriatic arthritis. It is estimated that 80 percent of patients with rheumatoid arthritis[111] and 50 percent of those with osteoarthritis[112] have significant foot problems. Rheumatoid foot problems that frequently require intervention include forefoot with subluxed MTP and painful callus, cock toes, and hallux valgus; hindfoot problems with significant pronation and loss of the medial arch and loss of subtalar movement; and some ankle or tibiotalar limitation of motion and pain.

The treatment of forefoot problems includes a shoe that is wide enough and deep enough to accommodate the hallux and clear the cock toes. It should have a soft Neoprene crepe sole to permit some cushioning of the metatarsal callus and a low (less than 1½ inch) heel. Preferably the shoe should be made of leather or canvas to permit some stretching and breathing of the material. Inserted metatarsal pads or externally placed metatarsal bars are helpful in unweighting the metatarsal heads. In general, inserting the pad provides better and more lasting control than using an external bar, which is harder to properly place and wears down. Additional softness can be added using Spenco or Plastazote, provided the shoe is deep enough to accommodate the insert.

Management of hindfoot problems is a bit more complicated, partially because successful management requires careful biomechanical evaluation and the ability to measure outcome. The physician must be sure that the problem seen is a foot problem and not compensation for a more proximal problem, e.g., rotation of the tibia or hip. The treatment for pronation of the foot is to try to balance the foot and bring the calcaneus perpendicular to the floor while keeping the forefoot parallel to the floor. This usually requires an orthotic of soft material, but occasionally a rigid insert may be needed and will be improved by lining it with Spenco

or Plastazote. The shoe must have a sturdy heel counter and must be adequately sized to accommodate the insert. Often a scaphoid pad may be added to support the arch and an extension of softness under the 1st ray may be needed to assure it makes contact during gait.

Heel modifications are frequently very useful. They can be used for foot problems such as heel cushions for calcaneal spurs or for ankle problems. The solid ankle cushion heel (SACH) or beveled heel that makes a 20-degree angle with the floor will compensate for tibiotalar or dorsiplantar movement of the ankle and hence decrease motion at the joint. These heel modifications can also help decrease knee flexion, promoting a more stable, extended knee.[113] A lift should be added to the shoe when there is more than a 1-cm leg length discrepancy, to equalize the pelvis and avoid back strain and scoliosis, especially in the growing child, but also to spare the hip of the longer leg undue stress. This has been referred to as the long-leg syndrome and has been implicated in producing osteoarthritis of that hip.[114]

Control of instability and pain in the knee can be successfully managed in some patients using an orthotic. A Swedish knee cage, or Lerman type brace, offers some support along the medial and lateral borders of the knee and can limit full flexion and extension (Fig. 111–2). Better medial/lateral support comes from a Lenox Hill brace or a long leg brace.[115] The latter is quite cumbersome, and the former is frequently associated with significant quadriceps atrophy. In general, immobilizing the knee should be used with caution in arthritics.

Since the rise of popularity of total knee arthroplasty, serial casting of the knee to reduce flexion contractures

Figure 111–2. Hinged knee brace.

is less frequently performed. It can be a useful treatment, however, and is one that is safe and can be done on an outpatient basis. Gains in knee extension are facilitated by either recasting or advancing a turnbuckle 1 to 2 degrees every day.[54] The process must be slow to avoid undue stretch to the peroneal nerve, skin tearing, subluxation of the tibia, or fracture of an often osteoporotic bone. Goals of serial casting should be full extension if possible; if it is not possible to reduce the contracture to less than −15 degrees, a surgical procedure may be necessary. We have used this procedure to manage arthritis in children with monoarticular arthritis.

Upper Extremity Orthotics. In patients with rheumatoid arthritis, daily activities such as grasping, writing, and needle work may produce deforming forces that potentiate ulnar deviation and boutonnière deformities.[116,117] In osteoarthritis, the muscular balance of the hand seems to be unaffected by the deformities. To what degree daily hand function produces or accentuates these deformities has been addressed in a study comparing arthritic changes in left and right hands of textile mill workers, and determining which hand performed which function.[118] The dominant hand clearly had more arthritic changes, suggesting that patterns of use were related to development of arthritic changes.

Orthotic management of the upper extremity includes resting hand splints, functional wrist splints, thumb post splint, ring splints, and dynamic splints (Fig. 111–3). The resting hand splint significantly limits function, as it immobilizes the wrist and all phalanges, and is best worn at night. The functional wrist splint stops at the midpalmar crease and permits finger motion.

Resting and functional splints of the upper extremity are designed to support the wrist (Figs. 111–4 and 111–5), thereby reducing chronic synovitis and providing support for wrist ligaments. As soon as the ligaments relax, the carpal bones slip in a volar direction on the radius. If the extensor carpi ulnaris is displaced laterally, it will act as a wrist flexor and compound the subluxation. If the radioulnar ligament becomes lax and is not supported, the wrist deviates in a radial direction, potentiating the ulnar drift at the phalanges. Adding a restraining bar at the ulnar carpal joint or an ulnar deviation splint with struts along the ulnar border of the fingers can provide a resistance to this deviation and substitute for an ineffective metacarpoglenoidal ligament (Fig. 111–6).

The swan neck orthosis (ring or Bunnell-type splint) is designed to minimize extension at the proximal interphalangeal joint. This not only helps to reduce synovial proliferation secondary to movement and to stabilize the lax proximal interphalangeal volar capsule, but also helps to relax intrinsic muscle spasm and contracture. The boutonnière orthosis is the swan neck splint rotated 180 degrees. It supports the transverse fibers, permitting the interossei and lumbricals to extend the proximal interphalangeal joint. It supports the dorsal capsule so that the extensor mechanism is not overly stretched. These ring splints should be worn during normal daily activity (Fig. 111–7).

Functional wrist splints are used for relieving painful wrists and treating carpal tunnel syndrome. For extensor tendinitis (DeQuervain's) the thumb needs to be immobilized and a thumb post splint similar to the one used for CMC joint pain is desirable.

Dynamic splints are frequently used postoperatively or to stretch out a contracture. The indication for dynamic splinting is to provide gentle stretch through limited range while supporting the wrist and MCPs in a fixed position (Fig. 111–8).

Rarely, elbow contractures are treated with serial plaster casts. It is important to remember that elbow

Anatomical Site	Problem	Splint
Wrist	Swelling Pain Carpal tunnel	Functional wrist splint " " " " " "
Hand	Swelling Pain	Resting hand splint " " " "
	Swan neck Boutonnière	Finger ring splint
Thumb	Carpometacarpal pain Metacarpophalangeal pain Metacarpophalangeal instability	Thumb post splint " " " " " "

Figure 111–3. Schematic drawing of hand splint application.

Figure 111–4. Resting hand splint.

Figure 111–5. Functional wrist splint.

Figure 111–7. Ring splints, on index finger for swan neck deformity and on middle finger for boutonnière deformity.

flexion is the function that needs to be preserved, and rarely is there an extension contracture.

The design and the execution of splints require care. The wrist must be in functional position, which is in neutral or a few degrees of extension; the fingers and thumb must be free to maintain normal prehensile pinch and grasp. It is important to instruct the patient in the proper use of the splint, which includes taking it off periodically and putting the joint through range of motion exercises. Alignment needs to be checked periodically to make sure deformity does not progress and that detrimental compensatory motion is not substituted.

There are manuals that are available to guide the professional in the fabrication and use of splints.[119-121]

Spinal Orthotics. Spinal orthotics are used primarily for relief of pain, for stabilization of the spine, and for partial unloading of the vertebral column. The cervical spine is frequently involved in rheumatoid arthritis and osteoarthritis, and usually involved in the spondyloarthropathies. A soft cervical collar is comfortable and useful for pain relief, and only minimally limits motion. A Philadelphia collar offers more support, but a four-poster would be needed to appreciably limit flexion/ extension.[122,123] None is adequate to control C1-2 instability. Occasionally, patients with ankylosing spondylitis may require cervical collars to maintain their heads in enough extension to look straight ahead. Rigid collars are often used following cervical fusions and especially while riding in a car or on an airplane.[126]

The thoracic or lumbar spinal brace is prescribed for symptomatic back pain unresponsive to bed rest, analgesia, or anti-inflammatory medication. Often this is due to strain, disc, or compression fracture. Its mechanism of action is by partially limiting motion and supporting the spine, hence reducing lordosis, reinforcing abdominal muscles, and permitting inflamed tissues to quiet down.[127,128] The orthotic of choice for lumbosacral problems is the L-S corset, which is well tolerated and easy

Figure 111–6. Ulnar deviation splint.

Figure 111–8. Dynamic splint.

to don. The orthotic of choice for the thoracic spine depends upon which thoracic level is involved and what degree of immobilization is required. The Knight-Taylor brace and body jacket are effective immobilizers but are uncomfortable and compliance with use is low. Both thoracic and L-S orthotics provide a 3-point pressure system consisting of posteriorly directed forces from axillary and chest straps in the former, and the pelvic and abdominal supports in the latter; and anteriorly directed forces from posterior uprights in the former, and paraspinal bars and pelvic and thoracic bands in the latter.[129]

A lumbosacral cynch acts more like a girdle. It does not use a 3-point design, nor does it limit movement. It basically provides abdominal support.

Corsets are often prescribed to assist in postoperative stabilization; they are used for relief of pain associated with osteoarthritis and rheumatoid arthritis and for osteoporosis and vertebral body collapse. In general osteoporosis and continued weakening of abdominal musculature occur with use of orthotics and may even be accelerated. Therefore, prescription should be time limited when possible and should be accompanied by abdominal muscle strengthening. A weaning process with progressively longer amounts of time out of the brace is a safe and effective way of tapering its use.

Traction. Traction is an accepted form of therapy in relieving contractures,[130] especially in the knee, as well as in relieving pain of the extremities and axial spine. The mechanism of pain relief in the axial spine is thought to be stretching of tight and stiff muscles. It is questionable, however, whether or not traction physically separates vertebrae and increases intervertebral space, permitting material to retract back into the center of the annulus or permitting more normal alignment to occur. The lumbar spine traction required to cause intervertebral separation would need to be in excess of 200 pounds[131] for 30 minutes; the customary pelvic traction force is 50 pounds (beginning at 25 pounds and increasing); continuous bed traction rarely exceeds 25 pounds. Hence, it is unlikely that pelvic traction works by vertebral distraction. Many believe it is effective because it keeps people in bed.

The efficacy of cervical traction has not been scientifically proved;[132] yet its use for neck pain and particularly radiculopathy is widespread. The mechanism of action is probably similar to that of lumbar traction employing stretch on spinal structures, but there is more evidence that even 30 pounds of distractive force can increase intervetebral space.[133] The usual amount of force applied to the cervical spine is 15 to 25 pounds. Extreme caution should be taken for patients with cerebral vascular disease, because the amount of distraction may occlude vessels.[134] In addition, it should not be used in patients with C1-2 instability.

Counseling. The real magnitude of the impact of chronic illness on the socioeconomic functioning of patients with rheumatic diseases is just being reported.[135,136] In terms of earning power, those hit by rheumatoid arthritis are frequently subsisting at or just above the poverty level.[136] Young mothers, a particularly high-risk group for the rheumatic diseases, are usually least well protected, for often they have never worked; hence, they are not eligible for Social Security disability and the family cannot afford full-time help to substitute for mother.

The practicing rheumatologist is in an excellent position to assist patients and their families in their plight. First, questions must be asked to determine that a socioeconomic problem exists. Referrals to social workers and rehabilitation counselors are often helpful. Next the physician should determine if the patient should continue in the present work situation. Frank discussion about vocational rehabilitation or a new career direction may be appropriate. While each state has different statutes pertaining to vocational rehabilitation and qualifications for Medicaid, anyone with disability is eligible for vocational rehabilitation, even with no work history. The Social Security Administration establishes listings for those medical conditions eligible for disability. Disability from work is the inability to maintain gainful employment (earnings of less than $300 per month). The disability is compensable if it is caused by the job (e.g., black lung) or is aggravated by the job (asthmatic attacks induced by working in high dust area) or if the disability is not work related but interferes with ability to work. This latter group must correspond to medical listings that are accepted by the Social Security Administration as medically definable impairments. Many of the musculoskeletal diseases are listed as medically defined impairments. A discussion of the legal aspects of disability is available.[137] A brief outline is presented in Appendix I at the end of this chapter along with appropriate resource material.

MANAGEMENT OF SPECIFIC DISEASES

Osteoarthritis. Osteoarthritis (OA) is the most commonly occurring form of arthritis and probably has the greatest socioeconomic impact of all the rheumatic conditions. The most frequently affected joints include neck, CMC, DIPs, hips, knees, and 1st MTP. Fatigue is not a frequent major complaint. Often the patient leads an active and near normal life except for one or two activities (e.g., climbing stairs, opening jars, or holding a pencil). A gel phenomenon is particularly bothersome to those with knee involvement.

Evaluation of the patient will include range of motion (ROM) and strength assessment of all joints and muscles and a determination of functional level, including vocational and avocational activity. A gait analysis should be done.

Treatment is directed at maintaining strength and critical ROM to preserve function. A program of quadriceps isometric exercise twice daily, gentle ROM daily to the knee to assure extension, and rotation and extension of the hip are important. A hinged knee cage can offer support for a stiff, moderately painful knee. A very unstable knee may benefit from use of a Lenox Hill brace. The use of a cane or crutch is often suggested to help unload the hip or knee and offer pain relief.

The CMC joints are usually tender, and often prehension is limited in that tip pinch and thumb opposition are weak or cannot be performed. Treatment is aimed at stabilizing the thumb in an abducted position, one that is functional and permits IP flexion so that the 2nd digit can effect tip pinch. The splint should be worn continously while functional activity is performed. Little can be done about DIP involvement except local heat and anti-inflammatory or analgesic medication.

Management of neck pain usually includes discussion of posture so as to identify risk factors, such as bifocals, driving, and typing, that tend to produce neck extension and aggravate symptoms; recommendation of soft, but not foam rubber pillows; and instructions in neck retraction exercises. Intermittent traction should be set at 15 pounds for 15 minutes if there is radiculopathy without C1-2 instability or cerebrovascular disease. Heat, including deep heat, ice, and traction are useful adjunctive therapies and should be tried for at least 2 weeks before being abandoned.

Soft, wide crepe-soled shoes are often recommended for patients with 1st MTP arthritis and for those with knee or hip involvement. These shoes may also decrease the progression of hallux valgus. The softness may absorb some of the ground reactive forces and decrease stress on the knee. A beveled heel can decrease the amount of force transmitted as well.

Patients need to be educated about the disease process, its course, and its nonsystemic nature. There are some known stresses, including obesity (the hip experiences a load three times body weight during walking and more during running) and hard surfaces (e.g., hard tennis courts versus clay courts). Since some vocational activities correlate with the development of osteoarthritis,[118] counseling and educating the patient may be useful.

Rheumatoid Arthritis. The rehabilitation problems of patients with rheumatoid arthritis (RA) often require a comprehensive approach that addresses problems of fatigue, depression, and change in self-image as well as specific problems of joint pain, strength, and range of motion. Often the patient with RA is a young homemaker and mother, often post partum, and has problems with coping with motherhood and a severe illness. Management centers around an attempt to control inflammation in order to reduce synovitis while preserving function. Instruction in joint protection and energy conservation techniques may be useful in helping the patient pace herself throughout the day.

Initially the patient is provided with wrist splints to support her wrists in a functional position while keeping them immobile if synovitis is a problem. If median nerve compression due to carpal tunnel is a problem, the splint should also be worn at night. Often there is fusiform swelling of the PIPs and synovitis of the MCPs, which should be treated twice daily with a gentle ROM program with hands submerged in cool or warm water to

tolerance. Exercise should include wrist flexion and extension and flattening out PIPs and MCPs on a firm surface.

Lower extremities are usually involved in RA, with MTP tenderness and ankle, knee, and hip pain. The feet are best managed with soft-soled, deep shoes with a wide forefoot. Often an MTP pad can relieve pressure on the MTPs, and an added soft liner made of Pelite, Plastazote, or Spenco can be inserted into the shoe. A cane or crutch may be useful in unweighting an extremity. A knee cage or Ace wrap is also useful in providing some support to the knees. Other adaptive equipment might include grab bars for the toilet and tub area to assist with lift-off or a raised toilet seat to aid in arising. A tub or shower seat can provide a stable surface upon which to sit while bathing. Exercises should include ROM to knees to preserve full extension, if possible, and at least 30 degrees of flexion. Hip range should be maintained from 0 to 30 degrees of flexion. Ankle motion should be maintained from 10 degrees of plantar flexion to 10 degrees of dorsiflexion. Strengthening of quadriceps, using isometric contractions, should be done twice daily.

An expanded ROM program can be introduced as the disease progresses, to include preservation of glenohumeral motion in the shoulder (internal and external rotation) and elbow flexion. It is best not to add all exercises at the same time.

Exercise should be performed at an optimal time for the patient and about 1 hour after medication has been taken. The application of cold or heat just prior to exercise may be helpful.

A series of instructional sessions with the physiatrist and the occupational therapist must be instituted at this time. The physiatrist checks the progress of splinting and shoeing, decides if other modalities of heat or cold need to be initiated, and evaluates compliance and level of depression, sleeping patterns, and level of activity.

After performing an assessment of function (ADL, pain, and level of satisfaction with current status), the occupational therapist should ask the patient to fill out an activities monitor that demonstrates a typical day's activity, hour by hour. The therapist and physician review this jointly to determine level and appropriateness of activity and counsel the patient about rest, the need for help, and organization of the day's events. A general satisfaction score can be useful as a guide to response to treatment. Rest, in half-hour allotments, punctuating normal activity, is urged. Review of methods of picking up a baby, if relevant, and other household activities in order to assess energy-draining postures and stressful joint behavior is often done. Behavior modification to correct inappropriate activity is attempted. Every effort is made to include husband and family members, in order to educate them about the nature of this chronic illness and the importance of support for the patient and the therapeutic program. Help for the patient and his or her partner will be needed to adapt a specific physical disability to techniques for facilitating healthy sexual function (see Chapter 34).

If the patient is planning to return to the work force, and now cannot, a review of her prior work record is made and consideration of application for disability is raised. If the number of quarters worked is inadequate for Social Security, the patient may still be eligible if the disability lasts for 1 year or more. Discussion of this problem is often best left until the patient has visited the rehabilitation department at least a few times.

Scleroderma. Progressive systemic sclerosis and its variants, CREST and MCTD, are particularly difficult to treat. The inexorable persistent skin tightness and progressive loss in ROM make maintenance the most reasonable goal for rehabilitation.

Problems presented to the rehabilitation team include difficulty in mouth opening, fine motor coordination of the hands, Raynaud's phenomenon with digital ulceration, pleuritic chest pain, and ambulation difficulties due to tightness of the skin.

The rehabilitation approach is directed at increasing ROM, and the focus is on lubricating and stretching soft tissues, including the skin. Paraffin, cocoa butter, and other natural oils are used. Range of motion, using an active-assistive technique with prolonged stretch is recommended and should be performed twice daily. This is most important for the hands, in which one hand can apply overpressure to PIPs and MCPs in order to increase extension. Most patients find that warmth enhances stretch and do exercises in warm water or after paraffin. We have used ultrasound sub aqua with good results. Swimming and/or Hubbard tank therapy permits total body submersion, enhances a sense of relaxation, and is a good medium in which to perform exercises.

Raynaud's phenomenon and digital ulcers can be of significant concern. The first step in management is to explain the physiology of the problem and to encourage the patient to keep the hands as warm as possible. Recommendations of down mittens and electric warmers are made. Other management techniques include using topical nitroglycerine paste to the hands; making large circles with the arms, to drive blood to the digits;[138] and using relaxation techniques or temperature biofeedback to control attacks of Raynaud's phenomenon.[139] Wound care and hygiene of the ulcerated fingertips must be discussed. When pregangrenous areas are present it is essential to apply direct heat as a modality to the hands and fingers. In these cases, heat should be applied proximally.

Mouth opening must be preserved if eating solid foods is to be possible. Jaw opening should be done frequently during the day, and mandibular forward and lateral thrusting should also be done. The use of deep heat modalities to facial skin may enhance the efficacy of exercise. A passive stretch, using fingers or a soft wedge between the jaws, provided there is minimal pressure on the teeth, is also recommended.

Psoriatic Arthritis. Rehabilitation management of these patients if often a challenge because of the rapidity with which fixed contractures can occur. The use of functional wrist splints and ring splints is indicated and should be coupled with twice daily ROM of affected joints. Muscle atrophy occurs, and hence a maintenance exercise program to those involved muscles should be initiated. Careful attention to joint positioning, to maximize function, must be made.

Back and neck care must start with education about posture and sitting in a chair that provides good back support and comes up to the scapulae. Use of a soft cervical collar intermittently during the day and a Wal-Pil-O (a well designed pillow with a soft center and firmer border) are recommended for pain relief. Traction is often beneficial, especially for radicular symptoms. For spondylitics, bed positioning is crucial. No pillow, or a baby pillow, is used to minimize neck flexion. Periodic prone lying is encouraged to reduce hip flexion. Shoulder ROM must be preserved, using flexion, abduction, and external and internal rotation. Chest expansion using deep breathing techniques is taught. Adaptive equipment is frequently necessary for spondylitics. Specifically, double mirrors, one on each side of the car, aid in visualization; and reachers and elastic laces assist in dressing the lower extremities. Kitchen aids and adaptive writing instruments can be very useful. Management of the feet usually includes the use of soft, deep shoes with metatarsal pads and a heel cushion.

Juvenile Arthritis. The child with polyarthritis has special rehabilitation needs.[140] Not only is there pain, swelling, and stiffness, and limitation of function, but growth retardation and the inability to participate fully in daily events may set the child apart from his peers and socially isolate him.

The rehabilitation approach incorporates techniques to minimize acute synovitis; to preserve range of motion; to minimize joint contracture, which can occur very quickly in this population; and to support age-appropriate behavior. Because compliance can often be a problem, early alliance with parents in re-inforcing the goals of treatment and educating them to enhance their commitment to the program are top priorities.

Continued movement is critical to the well-being and proper development of children. Although competitive sports are usually discouraged, exercise should be maintained, with, for example, biking and exercise using pool therapy. If bed rest is indicated, it should be only for short periods of time, and careful attention must be given to limb position and range of motion. Pillows must not be used under knees, and side-lying knee-chest positions must be discouraged. Heel cord tightness frequently develops if dorsiflexion is not done or if splints maintaining the foot in neutral position are not placed. Knee flexion contractures should be treated with serial casting, a procedure well tolerated by even young children.

Splinting must be done with great care, because fixed deformity occurs quickly. Positions in which anatomic parts are placed must be functional and should be accompanied by a ROM program.

Education of parents and the child about the nature of the disease and its natural history should be undertaken. This information should also be communicated to the school. An occupational therapist can help evaluate the patient's level of performance, given his age.

Systemic Lupus Erythematosus (SLE). Because the patient with lupus is confronted with a myriad of symptoms whose severity and duration are unpredictable, planning and completing tasks and coping with the frustration are most difficult. The occupational therapist is equipped to evaluate the impact of lupus on daily functioning and help the patient organize the day in a format likely to result in task completion and satisfaction. Using an activity analysis, instruction in techniques of energy conservation and rest breaks and identification of support systems and how they can be mobilized can be established. The therapist can help the patient organize her life to meet the challenge of coping with this chronic disease.

Musculoskeletal complaints are frequent in SLE patients. The usual problems are transient hand arthralgias, mild functional problems (such as opening jars), and deformities that are usually reducible and not fixed (ulnar deviation of the phalanges and swan neck deformities of the fingers). The patient with MCTD, however, does have fixed deformities and a stiff hand. Other problems seen in patients with SLE include lax joints, often of the knees, associated with recurvatum and painless effusion of the knees. Tendinitis and rupture occur in Achilles and quadriceps tendons, which are often treated with nonoperative means and subsequently referred for physical therapy.[141]

Hand splinting is used to control ulnar deviation (Fig. 111–6) and swan neck deformities. An ankle-foot orthotic may be used to control hyperextension at the knee. Usually plaster casts (leg for Achilles tendon and thigh length for patellar tendon) are provided for repair of tendon ruptures.

Patients with neurologic manifestations may require stroke rehabilitation aimed at helping the patient become ambulatory and independent in self-care. Speech therapy is offered for aphasia. Patients with SLE may have cognitive impairment, with complaints of memory deficits and decreased attention span.[142] There are some techniques (practice drills and hints about list making and cuing) that may be helpful in improving performance in this area.

The hip and femoral condyle, followed by shoulder, are often involved by avascular necrosis. Rehabilitation management includes unweighting the extremity with the use of a cane or crutch, gentle range of motion exercise to preserve range, and isometrics in an attempt to preserve muscle strength. Occasionally, bed rest is recommended, to completely unweight a limb for a limited period of time.

Raynaud's phenomenon is common in lupus patients and the use of relaxation tapes and temperature biofeedback may be helpful in controlling these problems. The relaxation tapes may be generally useful in the reduction of stress and anxiety in this often anxious group of patients, who frequently have sleep disorders.[142]

Shoulder-Hand Syndrome. This entity, which is poorly understood, is characterized by a painful shoulder that has limited ROM and associated pain and swelling in the hand, usually the dorsum of the wrist. There is usually restriction of motion of PIPs, but not always. The hand is cool and sweaty, but pulses are intact. If the syndrome is not treated, the hand and shoulder become less functional, and often the patient undergoes a significant personality change as a result of chronic pain.

Rehabilitation techniques are aimed at restoring shoulder ROM, and often this is done by trying to control pain with the aid of ice, heat, TENS, or ultrasound. A gentle stretching program is initiated when the patient can tolerate it. The hand is also put through a gentle stretching program. An Isotoner glove is sometimes prescribed to control swelling, and a resting night splint is prescribed for those who demonstrate increasing contractures. Reports of the use of TENS indicate success in several case reports.[143,144]

When the above is inadequate to control symptoms and regain range, a series of lidocaine injections into the sympathetic chain in the neck is begun.[145] This is very effective in controlling the hand swelling and sweating and often helps with the shoulder pain. Once these injections are given, a more vigorous range of motion program can be started.

Fibrositis. The rehabilitation intervention for management of this problem often includes injections into painful trigger points and the use of relaxation tapes to assist patients in relieving anxiety and helping to normalize sleep patterns; general exercise, including swimming and light conditioning exercises, may be useful.[12A]

References

1. Krusen, F.H.: The scope of physical medicine and rehabilitation. In Krusen, F.H., Kottke, F.J., and Ellwood, P.M. (eds.): Handbook of Physical Medicine and Rehabilitation, Philadelphia, W. B. Saunders Co., 1971.
2. Robinson, H.S., Haldeman, J., Imrie, J., et al.: Evaluation of a province-wide physiotherapy monitoring service in an arthritis control program. J. Rheum. 7:387, 1980.
3. Machover, S., and Sapecky, A.J.: Effect of isometric exercises on the quadriceps muscle in patients with rheumatoid arthritis. Arch. Phys. Med. Rehabil. 47:737, 1966.
4. Ekblom, B.: Effect of short-term physical training on patients with rheumatoid arthritis. Scand. J. Rheum. 4:80, 1975.
5. Moll, J.M.H., and Wright, V.: Measurement of joint motion. Clin. Rheum. Dis. 2:3, 1976.
6. Radin, E.L.: Mechanical aspects of osteoarthrosis. Bull. Rheum. Dis. 26:862, 1976.
7. Favreau, J.C., and Laurin, C.A.: Joint effusions and flexion deformities. Can. Med. Assoc. J. 88:757, 1963.
8. Jayson, M.I., and Dixon, A.S.: Intra-articular pressure in rheumatoid arthritis of the knee. 3. Pressure changes during joint use. Ann. Rheum. Dis. 29:401, 1970.
9. Finsterbush, A., and Friedman, B.: Early changes in immobilized rabbits' knee joints. Clin. Orthop. 92:305, 1972.
10. Bigland, B., and Lippold, O.C.J.: Motor unit activity in the voluntary contraction of human muscle. J. Physiol. 125:322, 1954.
11. Gollnick, P.D., Armstrong, R.B., Saltin, B., et al.: Effect of training on enzyme activity and fiber composition of human skeletal muscle. J. Appl. Physiol. 34:10, 1972.
12. Barnard, J., Edgerton, V.R., and Peter, J.B.: Contractile properties of muscle. J. Appl. Physiol. 28:767, 1970.
12A. Melzack, R.: Myofacial trigger points: Relation to acupuncture and mechanisms of pain. Arch. Phys. Med. Rehabil. 62:114, 1981.

13. Huskisson, E.C.: Measurement of pain. Lancet 2:1127, 1974.
14. Perry, J.: Normal and pathological gait. Syllabus. Pathokinesiology Service and Physical Therapy Department. Rancho Los Amigos Hospital, Downey, California, 1981.
15. Mazin, J.M., Schwartz, E., and Simon, S.R.: Ankle arthrodesis: Long-term follow-up with gait analysis. J. Bone Joint Surg. 61A:964, 1979.
16. Marshal, R.N., Myers, D.B., and Palmer, D.G.: Disturbance of gait due to rheumatoid disease. J. Rheum. 7:617, 1980.
17. Dhanendran, M., Hutton, W.C., Klenerman, L., Witemeyer, A., and Ansell, B.M.: Foot function in juvenile chronic arthritis. Rheum. Rehab. 19:20, 1980.
18. Inman, V.T., Ralston, H.J., and Todd, F.: Human Walking. Baltimore, William & Wilkins, 1981.
19. Ralston, H.J.: Energy-speed relation and optimal speed during level walking. Int. Z. Agnew. Physiol. 17:177, 1958.
20. Pearson, R., MacKinnon, M.J., Meek, A.P., Myers, D.B., and Palmer, D.G.: Diurnal and sequential grip functions in normal subjects and effects of temperature change and exercise of the forearm on grip function in patients with rheumatoid arthritis and in normal controls. Scand. J. Rheum. 11:113, 1982.
21. Radin, E.L.: Aetiology of osteoarthrosis. Clin. Rheum. Dis. 2:509, 1976.
22. Saunders, J.B., Inman, V.T., and Eberhart, H.D.: The major determinants in normal and pathological gait. J. Bone Joint Surg. 35A:543, 1953.
23. Convery, R.F., Minteer, M.A., Amiel, D., et al.: Polyarticular disability: A functional assessment. Arch. Phys. Med. Rehab. 58:494, 1977.
24. Eberl, D.R., Fasching, V., Rahlfs, V., Schleyer, I., and Wolf, R.: Repeatability and objectivity of various measurements in rheumatoid arthritis. Arthritis Rheum. 19:1278, 1976.
25. Katz, S., Downs, T.D., and Cash, H.R.: Progress in development of an index of ADL. Gerontologist 10:20, 1970.
26. Bombardier, C., Tugwell, P., Sinclair, A., Dole, C., Anderson, G., and Buchanan, G.W.: Conference on outcome measures in rheumatological clinical trials. J. Rheum. 9:798, 1982.
27. Meenan, R.F., Gertman, P.M., and Mason, J.H.: Measuring health status in arthritis: The arthritis impact measurement scales. Arthritis Rheum. 23:146, 1980.
28. Fries, J.F., Spitz, P., Kraines, R.G., and Holman, H.R.: Measurement of patient outcome in arthritis. Arthritis Rheum. 23:137, 1980.
29. Jette, A.M.: Functional capacity evaluation: An empirical approach. Arch. Phys. Med. Rehab. 61:85, 1980.
30. Kielhofner, G., and Burke, J.P.: A model of human occupation. Part 1. Conceptual framework and content. Am. J. Occup. Ther. 34:578, 1980.
31. Kielhofner, G.: A model of human occupation. Part 2. Ontogenesis from the perspective of temporal adaptation. Am. J. Occup. Ther. 34:657, 1980.
32. Muldofsky, H.: Rheumatic pain modulation syndrome: The interrelationships between sleep, central nervous system serotonin and pain. Adv. Neurol. 33:51, 1982.
33. Fordyce, W.E.: Research on influence of level of patient participation in the rehabilitation process. Selected Research Topics in Spinal Cord Injury. Rehabilitation, 1975, pp. 55–69.
34. Fordyce, W.E.: Behavioral Methods in Chronic Pain and Illness. St. Louis, C. V. Mosby Company, 1976, p. 236.
35. Vignos, P.J., Parker, W.T., and Thompson, H.M.: Evaluation of a clinic education program for patients with rheumatoid arthritis. J. Rheumatol. 3:155, 1976.
36. Haynes, R.B., Sackett, D.L., Gibson, E.S., Taylor, D.W., Hackett, B.C., Roberts, R.S., and Johnson, A.L.: Improvement of medication compliance in uncontrolled hypertension. Lancet 1:1265, 1976.
37. Haynes, R.B.: A critical review of the 'determinants' of patient compliance with therapeutic regimens. In Sackett, L., and Hayes, R.B. (eds.): Compliance with Therapeutic Regimens. Baltimore, Johns Hopkins University Press, 1976.
38. Carpenter, J.O., and Davis, L.D.: Medical recommendations—Followed or ignored? Factors influencing compliance in arthritis. Arch. Phys. Med. Rehab. 57:241, 1976.
39. Geersten, H.R., Gray, R.M., and Ward, J.R.: Patient non-compliance within the context of seeking medical care for arthritis. J. Chron. Dis. 26:689, 1973.
40. DeLateur, B.J., Lehmann, J., Stonebridge, T., et al.: Isotonic versus isometric exercise: Double-shift transfer of training study. Arch. Phys. Med. Rehab. 53:212, 1972.
41. Downey, J.A.: The physiatrist in arthritis management. In Ehrlich, G.E. (ed.): Rehabilitation Management of Rheumatic Conditions. Baltimore, Williams and Wilkins Co., 1980, pp. 31–32.
42. Muller, E.A.: Influence of training and inactivity on muscle strength. Arch. Phys. Med. 51:449, 1970.
43. Kottke, F.: The effects of limitation of activity upon the human body. JAMA 196:117, 1966.
44. Castello, B.A., El Sallab, R.A., and Scott, J.T.: Physical activity, cystic erosion, and osteoporosis in rheumatoid arthritis. Ann. Rheum. Dis. 24:522, 1965.
45. Jayson, M.I.V., Rubenstein, D., and Dixon, A.S.: Intra-articular pressure and rheumatoid geodes (bone cysts). Ann. Rheum. Dis. 29:496, 1970.
46. Jayson, M.I.V., and Dixon, A.S.J.: Intra-articular pressure in rheumatoid arthritis of the knee III: Pressure changes during joint use. Ann. Rheum. Dis. 29:401, 1970.
47. Nordemar, R., Ekblom, B., Zachrisson, L., and Lundquist, K.: Physical training in rheumatoid arthritis: A controlled long term study I. Scand. J. Rheum. 10:17, 1981.
48. Nordemar, R.: Physical training in rheumatoid arthritis: A controlled long-term study. II: Functional capacity and general attitude. Scand. J. Rheum. 10:25, 1981.
49. Donaldson, C.L., Hulley, S.B., Vogel, J.M., Hattner, R.S., Boyers, J.H., and MacMillan, D.E.: Effect of prolonged bed rest on bone mineral. Metabolism 19:1071, 1971.
50. Kazarian, L.E., and Vangreibl, H.E.: Bone loss as a result of immobilization and chelation. Clin. Orthop. Rel. Res. 65:67, 1969.
51. Aloia, J.F., Cohn, S.H., Ostuni, J.A., Cane, R., and Ellis, K.: Prevention of involutional bone loss by exercise. Ann. Intern. Med. 89:356, 1978.
52. Aloia, J.F., Cohn, S.H., Babu, T., Abesamis, C., Alici, N., and Ellis, K.: Skeletal mass and body composition in marathon runners. Metabolism 27:1793, 1976.
53. Hahn, T.J., and Hahn, B.H.: Osteopenia in patients with rheumatic diseases: Principles and diagnosis of therapy. Semin. Arthritis Rheum. 6:165, 1976.
54. Fried, D.M.: Splints for arthritis. In Lieht, S. (ed): Arthritis and Physical Medicine. New Haven, E. Licht, Publisher, 1969, pp. 185–314.
55. Stein, H., and Kickson, R.A.: Reversed dynamic slings for knee flexion contractures in the hemophiliac. Bone Joint Surg. 51A:282, 1975.
56. Adamson, J.E.: Treatment of the stiff hand. Orthop. Clin. North Am. 1:467, 1970.
57. Flatt, A.E.: Non-operative Treatment in the Care of the Rheumatoid Hand. 3rd ed. St. Louis, C. V. Mosby Co. 1947, p. 33.
58. Rizik, I.E., Christopher, R.P., Pinals, R.S., Higgins, A.C., and Frix, R.: Adhesive capsulitis (frozen shoulder): A new approach to its management. Arch. Phys. Med. Rehabil. 64:29, 1983.
59. Potter, T.: Prevention of deformities from arthritis. In Hollander, J.L., and McCarty, D.J. (eds.): Arthritis and Allied Conditions. 8th ed. Philadelphia Lea & Febiger, 1972.
60. Swezey, R.L.: Arthritis. In McCarty, D.J. (ed.): Arthritis and Allied Conditions. 9th ed. Philadelphia, Lea & Febiger, 1979, p. 525.
61. Brewerton, D.A., and Lettin, A.W.F.: The rheumatoid hand and its management. In Parry, C.B.W. (ed.): Rehabilitation of the Hand. Boston, Butterworth & Co, 1973, p. 300.
62. Palmoski, M.J., Colyer, R.A., and Brandt, K.D.: Joint motion in the absence of normal loading does not maintain normal articular cartilage. Arthritis Rheum. 23:325, 1980.
63. Lee, P., Kennedy, A.C., Anderson, J., and Buchanan, J.W.: Benefits of hospitalization in rheumatoid arthritis. Quart. J. Med. 170:205, 1974.
64. Mills, J.A., Pinals, R.S., Ropes, M.W., et al.: The value of bedrest in patients with rheumatoid arthritis. N. Engl. J. Med. 284:453, 1971.
65. Partridge, R.E.H. and Duthie, J.J.R.: Controlled trial of the effect of complete immobilization of the joints in rheumatoid arthritis. Ann. Rheum. Dis. 22:91, 1963.
66. Gault, S.J., and Spyker, J.M.: Beneficial effect of immobilization of joints in rheumatoid arthritis and related arthritides. Arthritis Rheum. 12:34, 1969.
67. Van Brocklin, J.D.: Splinting the rheumatoid hand. Arch. Phys. Med. Rehab. 47:262, 1966.
68. Fischer, E., and Solomon, S.: Physiological responses to heat and cold. In Licht, S. and Kamenetz, H.L. (eds.): Therapeutic Heat and Cold. 2nd ed. New Haven, E. Licht, Publisher, 1965, pp. 126–169.
69. Benson, T.B. and Copp, E.P.: Effects of therapeutic forms of heat and ice on pain threshold of normal shoulder. Rheumatology 13:101, 1974.
70. Lehmann, J.F., Brunner, A.D., and Stowe, R.W.: Pain threshold measurements after therapeutic application of ultrasound microwaves and infra red. Arch. Phys. Med. Rehab. 39:560, 1958.
71. Lehmann, J.F., Masock, A.J., Warren, C.G., and Koblanski, J.N.: Effect of therpeutic temperatures on tendon extensibility. Arch. Phys. Med. Rehab. 51:481, 1970.
72. Warren, C.G., Lehmann, J.F., and Koblanski, J.N.: Heat and stretch procedures: Evaluation using rat tail tendon. Arch. Phys. Med. Rehab. 57:122, 1976.
73. Davis, F.A.: The hot bath test in the diagnosis of multiple sclerosis. J. M. Sinai Hosp. N.Y. 33:280, 1966.
74. Swezey, R.L.: Arthritis: Rational Therapy and Rehabilitation. Philadelphia, W. B. Saunders Co., 1978, p. 136.
75. Lehmann, J.F.: Diatheramy. In Krusen, F.H., Kottke, F., and Elwood, P.M. (eds.): Handbook of Physical Medicine and Rehabilitation. 2nd ed. Philadelphia, W. B. Saunders Co., 1971, pp. 273–345.
76. Lehmann, J.F., Warren, C.G., and Scham, S.M.: Therapeutic heat and cold. Clin. Orthop. 99:207, 1974.
77. Kramer, P.O., Emery, A.F., Guy, A.W., and Lin, J.C.: Ocular effects of

microwave on hypothermic rabbits: Study of microwave cataractogenic mechanism. Ann. N.Y. Acad. Sci. 247:155, 1975.

78. Lehmann, J.F., Erickson, D.J., Martin, G.M., and Krusen, F.H.: The present value of ultrasonic diathermy. JAMA 147:996, 1955.

79. Feibel, A., and Fast, A.: Deep heating of joints: A reconsideration. Arch. Phys. Med. Rehab. 57:513, 1976.

80. Hollander, J.L., Stoner, E.K., Brown, E.M., et al.: Joint temperature measurement in evaluation of anti-arthritic agents. J. Clin. Invest. 30:701, 1951.

81. Dorwart, B.B., Hansell, J.R., Schumacher, H.R., Jr.: Effects of cold and heat on urate crystal-induced synovitis in the dog. Arthritis Rheum. 17:563, 1974.

82. Mainardi, C.L., Walter, C.M., Spiegel, J.K., Goldkamp, O.G., and Harris, E.D., Jr.: Rheumatoid arthritis: Failure of daily heat to affect its progression. Arch Phys. Med. Rehab. 60:390, 1979.

83. Crossman, L.W., Ruggiero, W.F., Hurley, V., and Allen, F.M.: Reduced temperature in surgery: Amputations for peripheral vascular disease. Arch. Surg. 44:139, 1942.

84. Stillwell, G.K.: Therapeutic heat and cold. In Krusen, F.H., Kottke, F., and Elwood, P.M. (eds.): Handbook of Physical Medicine and Rehabilitation. 2nd ed. Philadelphia, W. B., Saunders Co., 1971, pp. 265–267.

85. Miglietta, O.: Action of cold on spasticity. Am. J. Phys. Med. 52:198, 1973.

86. Harris, E.D., Jr., and McCroskery, J.A.: Influence of temperature and fibril stability on degradation of cartilage collagen by rheumatoid synovial collagenase. N. Engl. J. Med. 290:1, 1974.

87. Benson, T.B., and Copp, E.P.: The effects of therapeutic forms of heat and ice on the pain threshold of the normal shoulder. Rheum. Rehab. 13:101, 1974.

88. Hamer, J., and Kirk, J.A.: Physiotherapy and the frozen shoulder: A comparative trial of ice and ultrasonic therapy. N.Z. Med. J. 83:191, 1976.

89. Kangliaski, J.: "Baggie therapy" simple pain relief for arthritic knees (Neuro) JAMA 246:317, 1981.

90. Travell, J.: Ethylchloride spray for painful muscle spasm. Arch. Phys. Med. Rehab. 33:291, 1952.

91. Zislis, J.M.: Hydrotherapy. In Krusen, F.H., Kottke, F., and Elwood, P.M. (eds.): Handbook of Physical Medicine and Rehabilitation. 2nd ed. Philadelphia, W. B. Saunders Co, 1971, p. 346.

92. Behrend, H.J.: Hydrotherapy. In Licht, E. (ed.): Medical Hydrology. New Haven, E. Licht, 1963, p. 133.

93. Harris, R.: Therapeutic pools. In Licht, S. (ed.): Medical Hydrology. New Haven, E. Licht, 1963, p. 189.

94. Stillwell, G.T.: Clinical electrical stimulation. In Licht, E. (ed.): Therapeutic Electricity and Ultraviolet Radiation. New Haven, E. Licht, 1965, p. 133.

95. Ersek, R.A.: Transcutaneous electrical neurostimulation: A new therapeutic modality for controlling pain. Clin. Orthop. Rel. Res. 128:314, 1977.

96. Melzach, R., and Wall, P.D.: Psychophysiology of pain. Int. Anesthesiol. Clin. 8:3, 1970.

97. Duncan, M.E.: Transcutaneous nerve stimulation in rheumatoid neuropathy. Rheum. Rehabil. 21:187, 1982.

98. Mannheimer, C., Lund, S., and Carlsson, C.A.: The effect of transcutaneous electrical nerve stimulation (TENS) on joint pain in patients with rheumatoid arthritis. Scand. J. Rheum. 7:13, 1978.

99. Rizk, T.G., and Park, S.J.: TENS and extension splinting in linear scleroderma knee contracture. Arch. Phys. Med. Rehabil. 62:86, 1981.

100. Mannheimer, C., and Carlsson, C.A.: The analgesic effect of TENS in patients with rheumatoid arthritis: A comparative study of different pulse patterns. Pain 6:329, 1979.

101. Self-Help Manual for Arthritis Patients (prepared by Judith Lannefeld Klinger). Allied Health Professions, Section of Arthritis Foundation, 1974, Home Care Programs in Arthritis, 1969.

102. Sources of Information on Self-help Devices for the Handicapped. National Easter Seal Society for Crippled Children and Adults. Chicago, Education and Information Services, 1972.

103. Hale, G. (ed.): Source Book for the Disabled, Philadelphia, W. B. Saunders Company, 1979.

104. Kreisler, N., and Kreisler, T.: Catalog of Aids for the Disabled. New York, McGraw-Hill, 1982.

105. Blount, W.P.: Don't throw away the cane. J. Bone Joint Surg. 38A:695, 1968.

106. Sorenson, L., and Ulrich, P.G.: Ambulation: A manual for nurses. Minneapolis, American Rehabilitation Foundation, 1966.

107. Pamphlets available: Medical Equipment Distributors, Everest & Jennings, and The Amigo Co.

108. Chamberlain, M.A.: Aids and equipment for the arthritic. Practitioner. 224:73, 1980.

109. Bennett, R.: Orthotic devices to prevent deformities of the hand in rheumatoid arthritis. Arthritis Rheum. 18:100, 1976.

110. Demopoulos, J.T.: Orthotic and prosthetic management of foot disorders. In Jahss, M.H. (ed.): Disorders of the Foot. Philadelphia, W. B. Saunders Company, 1982, p. 1785.

111. Vainio, K.: The rheumatoid foot: A clinical study with pathological and roentgenological comments. Ann. Chir. Gynecol. Suppl. 1, 1956, p. 45.

112. Seder, J.I.: Management of foot problems in arthritis. Clev. Clin. Quart. 37:111, 1970.

113. Weist, D.R., Waters, R.L., Bontrager, E.L., et al.: The influence of heel design on a rigid ankle foot orthosis. Orthotics-Prosthetics 33:3, 1979.

114. Gofton, J.P., and Trueman, G.E.: Studies in osteoarthritis of the hip II: Osteoarthritis of the hip and leg length disparity. Can. Med. Assoc. J. 104:791, 1971.

115. Smith, E.M., Juvinoll, R.C., Corell, E.B., et al.: Bracing the unstable anthritic knee. Arch. Phys. Med. Rehabil. 51:22, 1970.

116. Swanson, A.B., and Swanson, G.DeG.: Pathogenesis and pathomechanics of rheumatoid deformities in the hand and wrist. Orthop. Clin. North Am. 4:1085, 1973.

117. Flatt, A.: The pathomechanics of ulnar drift. Washington, D.C., Social and Rehabilitation Services, 1971.

118. Hadler, N.M., Gillings, D.B., Imbus, H.R., Levitin, P.M., Makuc, D., Utsinger, P.D., Yount, W.J., Slusser, D., and Moskovitz, N.: Hand structure and function in an industrial setting. Arthritis Rheum. 21:210, 1978.

119. Malick, M.H.: Manual on Static Hand Splinting. Pittsburgh, Harmarville Rehabilitation Center, 1973.

120. Malick, M.H.: Manual on Dynamic Splinting of the Hand. Pittsburgh, Harmarville Rehabilitation Center, 1973.

121. Melvin, J.L.: Rheumatic Disease: Occupational Therapy and Rehabilitation. Philadelphia, F. A. Davis, 1977.

122. Colachis, S.C., Jr., Strohm, B.A., and Ganter, E.L.: Cervical spine motion in normal women: A radiographic study of the effect of cervical collars. Arch. Phys. Med. Rehabil. 54:161, 1973.

123. Morris, J.M., Lucas, D.B., and Bresler, B.: Role of the trunk in the stability of the spine. J. Bone Joint Surg. 43A:327, 1961.

124. Fisher, S.V.: Cervical orthoses effect on cervical spine motion: Roentgenographic and goniometric method of study. Arch. Phys. Med. Rehabil. 58:109, 1977.

125. Smith, P.H., Sharp, J., and Kellgren, J.A.: Natural history of rheumatoid cervical subluxations. Ann. Rheum. Dis. 31:222, 1972.

126. Swezey, R.L.: Arthritis: Rational Therapy and Rehabilitation. Philadelphia, W.B. Saunders Company, 1978, p. 120.

127. Stillwell, G.K.: The law of Laplace: Some clinical applications. Mayo Clin. Proc. 48:863, 1973.

128. Norton, P.L., and Brown, T.: The immobilizing efficiency of back braces. J. Bone Joint Surg. 39A:111, 1957.

129. Bunch, W.H., and Keagy, R.D.: The Spine. In Bunch, W.H., and Keagy, R.D. (eds.): Principles of Orthotic Treatment. St. Louis, C. V. Mosby, 1976, pp. 84–90.

130. Karten, I., Koatz, A.V., and McEwen, C.: Treatment of contractures of the knee in rheumatoid arthritis. Bull. N.Y. Acad. Med. 44:763, 1968.

131. Lawson, G.A., and Godfrey, C.M.: A report on studies of spinal traction. Med. Serv. J. Can. 14:762, 1958.

132. Brewerton, D.A., et al.: Pain in the neck and arm: A multicenter trial of the effects of physiotherapy. Br. Med. J. 1:253, 1966.

133. Colachis, S.C.J., Jr., and Strohm, B.R.: A study of tractive forces and angle of pull on vertebral interspaces in the cervical spine. Arch. Phys. Med. Rehabil. 46:820, 1965.

134. Bland, J.H.: Rheumatoid arthritis of the cervical spine. Bull. Rheum. Dis. 18:471, 1967.

135. Meenan, R.F., Yelin, E.H., Nevitt, M., and Epstein, W.V.: The impact of chronic disease: A sociomedical profile of rheumatoid arthritis. Arthritis Rheum. 24:544, 1981.

136. Meenan, R.F., Yelin, E.H., Henke, C.J., Curtis, D.L., and Epstein, W.V.: The costs of rheumatoid arthritis: A patient oriented study of chronic costs. Arthritis Rheum. 12:827, 1978.

137. Meenan, R.F., Liang, M.H., and Hadler, N.M.: Social Security disability and the arthritis patient. Bull. Rheum. Dis. 33:1, 1983.

138. McIntyre, D.R.: A maneuver to reverse Raynaud's phenomenon of the fingers. JAMA 240:2760, 1978.

139. Gerber, L.H., Smith, C., Novick, A., et al.: Autogenic training in the treatment of Raynaud's phenomenon. Arch. Phys. Med. Rehabil. 59:522, 1978.

140. Ansell, B.M.: Rehabilitation in juvenile chronic arthritis. Rheum. Rehabil. Suppl. 1979, pp. 74–76.

141. Twining, R.H., Marcus, W.Y., and Garey, J.L.: Tendon rupture in SLE. JAMA 189:377, 1964.

142. Bresnehan, B., Holimeister, R., Cutting, J., Travers, R.L., Waldburger, M., Black, C., Jones, T., and Hughes, G.R.V.: The neuropsychiatric disorder in SLE: Evidence for both vascular and immune mechanism. Ann. Rheum. Dis. 38:301, 1979.

143. Meyer, G.A., and Fields, H.L.: Causalgia treated by selective large fiber stimulation of peripheral nerve. Brain 95:163, 1972.
144. Stilz, R.J., Cowan, H., and Sanders, D.B.: Reflex sympathetic dystrophy in a 6-year old: Successful treatment by transcutaneous nerve stimulation. Anesth. Analg. 56:438, 1977.
145. Thompson, J.E.: The diagnosis and management of post-traumatic pain syndrome. Aust. N. Z. J. Surg. 49:299, 1979.

APPENDIX I: FINANCIAL AND VOCATIONAL RESOURCES FOR HANDICAPPED PERSONS

I. Financial Assistance
  A. Social Security Office: to qualify, has to meet one of the following specifications:
    1. Disabled
    2. Blind
    3. Over 65
  B. Department of Social Services (on county level)
    1. Welfare
    2. Medicaid
    3. Food stamps
    4. Aid to dependent children
    5. Shelter for homeless
II. Vocational
  A. State Department of Vocational Rehabilitation
    1. Vocational assessment
    2. Education/training
    3. Job placement
    4. Follow up
    5. Vocational counseling
    6. Several other services are provided to assist person with a handicap returning to work.
  B. Workmen's Compensation (if patient is injured on job)
III. Resources (sources of financial and vocational assistance throughout the country for patient with handicap)
  A. The National Rehabilitation Information Center (maintains an accurate national listing of agencies) (202) 635-5826; TDD (202) 635-5884
  B. Arthritis Information Clearing House (lists sources of funding, sources of general information, and agencies) P.O. Box 7782; Arlington, VA; (703) 558-8250
  C. Directory of National Information Sources on Handicapping Conditions and Related Services (Government Printing Office Document #E-82-2207) Superintendent of Documents U.S. Government Printing Office, Washington, D.C. 20402 Price: $8.00 (subject to change); check made to Superintendent of Documents
IV. Books for Handicapped Persons
  1. Lorig, K., and Fries, J.K.: The Arthritis Helpbook: What you can do for your arthritis. Reading, Massachusetts, Addison Wesley Publishing Company, 1980, $6.95.
  2. Toohey, P., and Larson, C.W.: Range of Motion Exercise: Key to Joint Mobility. Minneapolis, Minnesota, Sister Kenny Institute 977.
  3. Wiggins, P., Freeman, L., Collier, M.: Arthritis: Fighting The Wear and Tear—A Patient Guide to Self-Management. Charleston, South Carolina, Multipurpose Arthritis Center.
  4. Bland, J.H.: Arthritis Medical Treatment and Home Care. London, Collier-Macmillan, 1960.
  5. Kraus, Hans, M.D., The Cause, Prevention and Treatment of Backache, Stress and Tension. New York, Simon & Schuster, 1965.

Section XXIV
Reconstructive Surgery

Chapter 112
Introduction to the Surgical Management of Arthritis

Clement B. Sledge

INTRODUCTION

The various forms of arthritis produce similar consequences in the involved joints: pain, loss of function, progressive damage, and deformity. Reconstructive surgery may be indicated to *relieve* any or all of these disabilities. In selected situations, surgery may be indicated to *prevent* these consequences.

Although the general consequences of arthritic damage to the joint are similar, there are significant differences between osteoarthritis and rheumatoid arthritis; indeed, there are unique surgical aspects to many of the "rheumatoid variants." In some instances these unique features place the patient at risk from surgery, and in others they jeopardize the eventual result. These features will be discussed under the heading Preoperative Evaluation and serve to emphasize two philosophical points: (1) the surgeon who operates on arthritic patients, especially rheumatoid patients, should be familiar with the special technical aspects necessitated by the unusual requirements of the patient with multiple joint involvement, and (2) he or she should be part of a team, composed of rheumatologists, nurses, therapists, social workers, and—most important–the patient. At first glance it may seem foolish to list the patient as part of the team. To do so emphasizes the fact that the surgical patient with rheumatoid arthritis is frequently weak and discouraged and must look forward to a series of operations before reasonable functional independence is achieved. Often the patient has excessive expectations regarding the outcome of surgery.[1] By participating in the planning and staging of the surgical events, the patient can better understand the duration of treatment, necessity of prolonged physical therapy, and the ultimate realistic goal of the procedure or procedures.

Since relief of pain is the most consistent feature of reconstructive surgery, pain is the primary indication for operative intervention. Restoration of motion and function, distinct from relief of pain, are less predictable and require careful assessment of each patient's disability before improvement can be offered. Some surgical procedures in rheumatoid arthritis are as much prophylactic as therapeutic (e.g., synovectomy, fusion of the first and second cervical vertebrae, fusion of the base of the thumb). The patient should understand the preventive aspects so that there will not be disappointment when the therapeutic result does not seem to justify the pain and inconvenience of surgery.[1]

Finally, the goals of society must be considered. The surgical patient with rheumatoid arthritis has an average length of hospitalization of about 18 days and may require two to six or more major procedures. The economic costs are considerable even when everything proceeds without complication. If a deep infection occurs after a hip replacement, the costs may be as much as $100,000. Most patients coming to multiple joint replacement surgeries have either left the work force because of disability or postponed surgery until they are ready for retirement. The majority are women who have not worked outside the home. These factors make calculation of a cost-benefit ratio difficult. Without putting a dollar value on "the quality of life," can such extensive procedures be justified by society? One recent study of 16 patients undergoing bilateral hip and knee replacement showed that none of those patients returned to work after this expensive series of operations involving an average of 3 months of hospitalization.[2] Precise data are not yet available, but preliminary studies strongly suggest that society does benefit in terms of decreased need for home help, home modifications, hospitalization or confinement to an institution because of loss of independent functional capacity, and release of the spouse from his or her helping role allowing return to the working force. For many individual patients, however, the goal must be relief of pain, restoration of functional independence, and a qualitative improvement in their existence without the hope of pure economic justification.[3] Part of the difficulty in assessing the potential benefit of a surgical procedure, to the patient or to society, is the lack of uniform measures of functional assessment before and after surgery.[3a,3b] Few studies have reported critical assessment of the outcome of patients with rheumatoid arthritis following joint replacement[3c]; further studies await adoption and general application of uniform criteria of assessment.

Certainly the major single advance in the care of patients with arthritis was the development of the concept of total joint replacement by Sir John Charnley nearly 20 years ago.[4] The concepts initially involved in replacement of the arthritic hip have now been expanded to cover most of the other joints. In patients with osteoarthritis, there are numerous alternatives to joint replacement, many of which are preferable, especially in younger patients. In patients with rheumatoid arthritis, procedures such as arthrodesis, synovectomy, repair of ruptured tendons, and other "nonprosthetic" procedures still play an important role. For predictable relief of pain and restoration in function, however, joint replacement surgery has revolutionized the outlook for patients with multiple joint involvement. Subsequent chapters of this book will therefore emphasize joint replacement surgery in patients with rheumatoid arthritis and its variants, but, when appropriate, alternative procedures will be mentioned, as will certain features pertinent to the patient with osteoarthritis.[5]

PREOPERATIVE EVALUATION

The first consideration is whether a painful joint in a patient with rheumatoid arthritis requires surgery or not. If synovitis is the cause of the patient's pain and disability, continued medical management with drugs and physical modalities is appropriate. If it can be determined that structural damage to the joint is the problem, then it is unrealistic to expect that medication will be sufficient. A trial of anti-inflammatory medication and physical therapy is appropriate, particularly for the weight-bearing joints where the use of crutches may allow the acute disabling symptoms to subside to an acceptable level, even in the presence of structural damage. If these measures fail and structural damage can be demonstrated on physical examination or by radiographic examination, arthrodesis or arthroplasty can be considered. It is better to perform surgery on each joint as it becomes structurally destroyed than to wait until the patient has multiple destroyed joints requiring prolonged hospitalization, multiple anesthetics, and a series of debilitating surgical procedures. General operative risk should be assessed, especially from the point of view of the systemic manifestations of the rheumatic diseases. The patient should be in optimal medical condition and, when on steroids, should be on the lowest possible maintenance dose. Obvious sources of infection should be identified and eradicated to prevent postoperative hematogenous seeding of the operative site. Carious teeth should be extracted before surgery on the joints, and urinary tract infections should be identified and treated. Many female patients have asymptomatic bacteriuria, and urine culture before surgery is an absolute requirement. In males, prostatic hypertrophy, if severe, should be treated before surgery to avoid post-operative catheterization with its attendant risk of infection and bacterial seeding. It is useful to determine if the patient is able to void in the supine position. Frequently, preoperative practice at supine voiding will facilitate recovery in the postoperative period. Most difficult to evaluate is the patient's motivation and ability to participate meaningfully in the postoperative program. Patients should be evaluated by physical and occupational therapists, both to assess their ability to participate in the program and to determine what special requirements might present in the postoperative period. Instruction in crutch ambulation before surgery shortens the postoperative instruction period. If multiple procedures are envisioned, it is often useful to perform a simple procedure first so that the ability of the patient to follow the postoperative program can be assessed. If both hips and knees require surgery, the hip can be used for this assessment. The relief of pain and improvement in function following hip arthroplasty are essentially independent of the patient's cooperation. The postoperative period is characterized by minimal pain. If the patient is unable to cooperate with a therapy program following hip replacement, it is unlikely that he or she will be able to participate in the postoperative program following a more painful arthroplasty, which requires maximal patient cooperation.

The patient with rheumatoid arthritis or its variants poses certain special problems that bear on the results and risks of surgery. The patient with rheumatoid arthritis frequently has multiple joints involved, each interfering with the function of the others. The rheumatoid patient undergoing surgery averages 10 years younger than patients with osteoarthritis undergoing similar procedures and therefore has longer to live with a prosthetic joint than does his or her osteoarthritic counterpart.[6] This means that there will be more time for complications to appear such as delayed infection, late loosening, and wear of the component parts. Much as been written of the increased susceptibility to infection in patients with rheumatoid arthritis,[7,8] and we have recently documented that the patient undergoing total hip replacement in rheumatoid arthritis does have a significantly increased risk of late hematogenous seeding of the prosthetic joint (see Chapter 120). Approximately 10 percent of patients coming to surgery at our institution are on maintenance steroids, and this has been shown in some studies to increase the risk of infection.[9] Aspirin, used by almost all patients, may produce difficulties with intraoperative and postoperative bleeding. Careful assessment of bleeding and clotting times is useful, but platelet transfusions are occasionally required. Some patients are on chronic immunosuppressive treatment, and the effect of these drugs on postoperative infection must be considered.[10,11] Although there is controversy regarding the relationship between penicillamine treatment and wound healing,[12-14] it is the opinion of most surgeons with experience in the field that there is a definite delay in wound healing in patients on penicillamine. This may delay the postoperative rehabilitation program until satisfactory wound healing is achieved.

There is both clinical and laboratory evidence to suggest that the rheumatoid process is perpetuated in a given joint by retention of articular cartilage.[15,16] Whether this is because of sequestered antigen-antibody complexes, the continued release of cartilage breakdown products producing synovial inflammation, or undiscovered factors is unknown. It has been a frequent observation, however, that patients undergoing total knee replacement in whom the patellar cartilage is retained will have involvement of the prosthetic joint in systemic flare-ups, whereas patients in whom all cartilage has been removed will not experience involvement of the prosthetic knee in such "flare-ups." The quality of bone in patients with rheumatoid arthritis is frequently poor. This may be because of direct involvement of the subchondral trabecular bone by rheumatoid granulation tissue, or may be related to the catabolic effects of chronic steroid use, the bone resorption related to excessive production of prostaglandins by rheumatoid synovium,[17] or an excess of parathyroid-like activity in these patients.[18,19] Regardless of the cause, the quality of bone is of great concern with regard to the long-term fixation of prosthetic components to bone. Many prosthetic devices transfer the enormous joint reactive forces directly to the bone-cement interface, which may be unable to withstand these forces over a long period of time. For this reason, it is desirable to use prosthetic devices that are minimally constrained and to transfer forces away from the bone-cement interface into the more compliant and forgiving soft tissues.

The patient with juvenile rheumatoid arthritis presents certain unique features that bear directly upon the results to be expected from surgical intervention. As in patients with ankylosing spondylitis, there appears to be a much greater involvement of the soft tissues surrounding the joint, with the result that the ultimate range of motion achieved after joint arthroplasty is less than would be predicted from the range achieved at surgery.[20] Following arthroplasty, there is a progressive loss of motion in these patients, and the effect of this loss on ultimate functional capacity must be anticipated.[21] The young age at which patients with juvenile rheumatoid arthritis undergo arthroplasty exposes their prosthetic joints both to greater functional demands and a longer period of exposure to late complications such as infection and loosening.[22] In addition, these patients often have severe micrognathia, which may make intubation difficult and/or produce postoperative respiratory problems (see Chapter 119).[23]

The patient with ankylosing spondylitis has diminished chest excursion and is therefore at greater risk for postoperative pulmonary problems and requires chest physical therapy to minimize these problems. Because of rigidity of the cervical spine, intubation is extremely difficult, sometimes requiring preoperative tracheostomy before an anesthetic agent can be delivered. Ossification in the spinal ligaments can produce great difficulty in carrying out spinal anesthesia; careful assessment of the patient by the anesthesiologist is useful in choosing the appropriate type and route of anesthetic and in antici-pating difficulties. Following total hip replacement, the patient with ankylosing spondylitis frequently fails to achieve the same range of motion that patients with rheumatoid arthritis or osteoarthritis achieve.[24] This is due not only to the increased involvement of the periarticular soft tissues seen in this disease but also to an increased incidence of heterotopic ossification in the muscles and capsules surrounding the hip joint.[25] Although the range of motion achieved may be only 65 degrees of hip flexion, this often makes a significant improvement in the patient's function and independence.[26] If warned of this preoperatively, the patient can make a more informed decision regarding the desirability of surgery and is less likely to experience disappointment in the postoperative period.

Patients with gout, either as their primary diagnosis or as a secondary diagnosis, often experience painful postoperative flares that require skillful management, as these attacks of gouty arthritis are more difficult to treat in this period than the usual spontaneous gouty attack.

Patients with psoriatic arthritis sometimes have involvement of the skin in the area of the proposed surgical incision. Several papers report the frequent contamination of psoriatic skin with microorganisms and suggest an increased risk of infection following incision through such skin.[27-29] Although we have not experienced this complication, it is desirable to clear up the skin in the operative site by appropriate local therapy before surgery.

The arthropathies related to inflammatory bowel disease pose a special threat of postoperative infection because of both late hematogenous seeding from a focus of infection in the bowel and the occasional source of contamination from a colostomy in proximity to the incision for hip replacement.

Systemic lupus erythematosus presents a very difficult problem for both the patient and the physician. The patients are often young and on large doses of steroids, and may have a near-normal life expectancy when they develop osteonecrosis.[30] To implant a prosthetic joint in a young patient invites the long-term failures related to wear and loosening; to do so in a patient on long-term steroid treatment adds the further risk of infection. The presence of renal involvement in these patients may have implications with regard to their life expectancy. In the young patient with a limited life expectancy, prosthetic replacement may well be justified to relieve pain and improve the quality of life for the remaining years. On the other hand, in the patient with a normal life expectancy, there will almost certainly be late problems following joint replacement in the third and fourth decades. These patients often present with avascular necrosis of a femoral condyle with pain, deformity, and functional loss. It may be better to accept the lesser result produced by a high tibial osteotomy than to carry out joint replacement surgery with the high probability of eventual complication.

Patients with Reiter's syndrome (see Chapter 65), as well as those with ankylosing spondylitis (see Chapter 64), have a significant incidence of cardiac involvement.

Careful preoperative cardiac assessment should be carried out in such patients.

In addition to the systemic problems presented by the patients with rheumatoid arthritis, the involvement of multiple joints presents special problems. Since the patient will require crutches after lower extremity surgery, it is essential preoperatively to evaluate the ability of the patient to use crutches. If there is extensive involvement of the shoulder, elbow, or wrist, axillary crutches may not be appropriate. Forearm crutches will sometimes be a suitable alternative, particularly if involvement of the wrist or elbow makes the use of axillary crutches painful. Occasionally, it will be necessary to carry out arthrodesis or arthroplasty of the wrist before surgery on the lower extremities so that the patient will be able to use forearm crutches in the postoperative period (see Chapter 114).[31] In addition, patients who do not have 110 degrees of knee flexion find it difficult to arise from a seated position without applying major force to the upper extremity. If the upper extremities are unable to cope with these forces, special attention must be directed to obtaining maximal hip and knee flexion after surgery in order to minimize the need for upper extremity assistance.[2] The major joints of the upper extremity, the elbow and shoulder, require arthroplasty less often than the weight-bearing joints of the lower extremity. Indeed, relieving the patient of the need to use crutches by performing arthroplasties of the hips and knees often diminishes shoulder pain to a tolerable level. In a few patients, pain or lack of motion with the attendant difficulty in placing the hand in a functional position requires surgical treatment. In the elbow, synovectomy (with or without radial head excision) may be adequate.[32] If pain relief is not adequate following synovectomy, or if motion is inadequate, elbow replacement is appropriate (see Chapter 115).[33-35] The shoulder achieves great compensatory motion by virtue of the mobile scapula. Unremitting pain, however, may suggest shoulder arthroplasty (see Chapter 116).

Patients with rheumatoid arthritis usually have involvement of both hips even though only one may require arthroplasty. Involvement of the contralateral hip will handicap the patient's postoperative recovery and may diminish the ultimate range of motion achieved in the operated hip. If it is obvious that both hips will require arthroplasty, it is preferable to carry out both during the same hospitalization to facilitate functional recovery. Except under unusual circumstances, such as extremely difficult and hazardous intubation, it is perhaps not justifiable to carry out bilateral total hip replacements during the same anesthetic,[36] although several studies report no decrease in quality of outcome or increase in complications with simultaneous procedures.[37]

Patients undergoing hip or knee arthroplasty are sometimes disappointed to find that painful foot deformities prevent comfortable ambulation after their extensive surgical procedures. In addition, the plantar surface of the feet and dorsum of the toes are subject to skin breakdown because of rheumatoid deformities.

These may become sources of bacterial contamination following arthroplasty to more proximal joints. These areas of skin breakdown should be healed before surgery on proximal joints to prevent proximal spread of infection. This can often be achieved by satisfactory shoe modifications and protective footwear (see Chapter 31) but may require surgical correction (see Chapter 118). Such surgery should be carried out before hip and knee arthroplasty so that problems of skin breakdown and infection, frequent after foot surgery, will not compromise the results of arthroplasties of the proximal joints. The temporomandibular joint is frequently involved in patients with juvenile rheumatoid arthritis as well as adult rheumatoid arthritis. In the juvenile, involvement of the temporomandibular joint combined with micrognathia may produce difficulties with intubation and respiration following extubation.[23] Careful preoperative analysis by the anesthesiologist will prevent some of these difficulties, and fiberoptic intubation will minimize trauma and postoperative laryngeal edema.

The cervical spine is significantly involved in 30 to 40 percent of patients with rheumatoid arthritis.[38-40] Usually this is asymptomatic and unknown by the patient, but it should be sought in the preoperative evaluation to avoid the potentially disastrous consequences of excessive manipulation of the neck during intubation. The patient with marked C1-2 instability may sustain damage to the medullary respiratory center and long spinal tracts when the neck is manipulated during intubation. While carrying out spinal anesthesia, the patient is often asked to "curl up" to facilitate insertion of the spinal needle. Flexion of the cervical spine in the presence of C1-2 instability should be avoided during this maneuver.

In addition to these general considerations, there are specific interactions between adjacent joints that may jeopardize the technical aspects of surgery. For example, involvement of the ipsilateral hip and knee usually leads to the performance of hip arthroplasty first. The position of the flexed knee is used as a guide for insertion of the femoral component in the hip arthroplasty. In the presence of severe knee instability and/or valgus deformity, proper placement of the hip component will be compromised.[41] If the component is placed in retroversion, postoperative dislocation of the hip becomes more frequent. Similarly, if the hip has been arthrodesed, the position of knee components must be suitably altered, depending upon the degree of abduction or adduction of the arthrodesed hip.

CHOICE OF PROCEDURE—OPERATIVE VERSUS NONOPERATIVE TREATMENT

In some instances, advanced age, increased risk factors, lack of patient motivation, or relatively minor pain will suggest that the patient should accept limited function rather than undergo a complex and potentially dangerous surgical procedure. In the upper extremity, the wrist is a good example of this dilemma. Three options are available: splinting, arthrodesis, or arthroplasty. Arthrodesis provides a stable, painless wrist but jeopardizes function to some extent, particularly in the performance of personal hygienic chores.[42] For that reason, patients with bilateral involvement are often advised to have a wrist arthroplasty, using some form of prosthetic implant.[43] Such prostheses carry the obvious risk of breakage, loosening, and infection. For some patients prostheses or fusion is indicated, but others would be better served by the use of a wrist splint, worn at night and during work but removed when flexibility is required.[44] Similarly, in the lower extremity, painful foot and ankle deformities are often best managed by special shoes and inserts to minimize pressure points or an orthosis to splint the ankle and correct heel valgus (see Chapter 31).

POSTOPERATIVE MANAGEMENT

The role of physical therapy in the postoperative management of patients undergoing joint replacement surgery has not been clearly defined. Controlled prospective studies are notably lacking. In their place is the nearly universal acceptance of the importance of postoperative physical therapy, an acceptance based on personal experience. The requirements for such therapy appear to vary from joint to joint. For example, Charnley does not advocate postoperative physical therapy for patients undergoing hip replacements.[4] His early and late follow-up studies suggest that physical therapy may play a minimal role in the rehabilitation of these patients. At the other extreme is the clear-cut advantage of careful and prolonged therapy following surgery of the hand.[45] Regardless of the lack of scientific evidence, essentially all surgeons with experience in the field of joint replacement surgery are convinced that the active participation of both the patient and the physical therapist in a postoperative exercise program will improve muscle strength, increase motion, and educate the patient in proper protection of the operated joint.

Orthoses are frequently useful following reconstructive surgery of the upper extremity where they may function either as static devices to maintain position and prevent deformity or as dynamic devices to aid in the restoration of motion and strength.[45] In the lower extremity, the most frequently used orthotic device is the crutch.[44] Its function is to protect weakened muscles until they become strong, prevent falls as the patient learns to function with a new prosthetic joint, and protect the bone-cement interface until healing can occur, ideally minimizing the complication of late loosening.

Radiographic evaluation, critical in the preoperative assessment of the need for surgery and proper technical approach, is the mainstay of postoperative evaluation (see Chapter 122). Parameters to be assessed are the alignment of the prosthetic components, adequacy of cement fixation, restoration of joint alignment, and detection of postoperative loosening as indicated by the development of a radiolucent zone between the methacrylate cement and the bone. Studies of prosthetic

placement in the hip have indicated the undesirability of a varus configuration to the femoral component as well as increased incidence of loosening in patients with incomplete filling of the proximal femur with methacrylate, voids in the methacrylate, and increased rates of dislocation with retroverted femoral components or excessively abducted acetabular components.[46] In the knee, late loosening has been correlated with faulty alignment of the prosthetic components,[47] and the early development of a radiolucent line, particularly at the bone-cement interface on the tibial side, has given early warning that certain prosthetic designs are inappropriate[48] (see Chapter 117).

Since loosening is a time-related complication and infection may make its appearance late,[46] prolonged follow-up of patients undergoing joint arthroplasty is necessary. If early signs of loosening develop, decrease in joint loading by appropriate use of crutches and avoidance of strenuous activities may prevent or slow the progress of such loosening. Because of evidence that patients with artificial joints continue to be at some increased risk for hematogenous infection,[49,50] careful attention must be devoted to the prevention of infection anywhere in the body and its prompt recognition and treatment. We recommend that patients utilize prophylactic antibiotics before dental or urologic procedures and that they be aware of the potential danger of untreated infections and seek early medical attention.[51]

CONCLUSION

In spite of the dramatic advances in joint replacement surgery in the last two decades, all such procedures must still be considered evolutionary. Changes in design, surgical technique, and materials continue, with improvements coming rapidly in some joints and more slowly in other joints such as the hip. For this reason, such surgery should be delayed as long as possible in patients who continue to function at a satisfactory level with tolerable discomfort. The old and reliable procedures such as fusion and osteotomy should be utilized when appropriate, especially in younger patients. One clear lesson gained from experience with joint replacements is that the more anatomical the replacement, the greater its long-term success is likely to be. The other clear lesson is that there is a close and obvious relationship between the technical expertise with which an arthroplasty is performed and its immediate and ultimate functional result. New materials for prosthetic replacement and for the fixation of prosthetic devices to bone will certainly be developed. Clearer understanding of normal joint anatomy and function will result in improved anatomical designs with greater life expectancy. Functional analysis of large numbers of patients who have undergone arthroplasty will determine the appropriate indications for surgery and choice of prosthetic designs, but medical judgment in selecting patients for surgery with precise surgical technique in carrying out the operation will remain the dominant aspects in the surgical management of arthritis.

References

1. Burton, K.E., Wright, V., and Richards, J.: Patient's expectations in relation to outcome of total hip replacement surgery. Ann. Rheum. Dis. 38:471, 1979.
2. Jergesen, H.E., Poss, R., and Sledge, C.B.: Bilateral total hip and knee replacement in adults with rheumatoid arthritis. An evaluation of function. Clin. Orthop. 137:120, 1978.
3. Johnson, K.A.: Arthroplasty of both hips and both knees in rheumatoid arthritis. J. Bone Joint Surg. 57A:901, 1975.
4. Charnley, J.: Low Friction Arthroplasty of the Hip. Theory and Practice. Berlin, Springer-Verlag, 1979.
5. Poss, R., and Sledge, C.B.: Symposium on Rheumatoid Disease. Philadelphia, J.B. Lippincott Co., 1984.
6. Poss, R., Ewald, F.C., Thomas, W.H., and Sledge, C.B.: Complications of total hip replacement arthroplasty in patients with rheumatoid arthritis. J. Bone Joint Surg. 58A:1130, 1976.
7. Gristina, A.G., Rovere, G.D., and Shoji, H.: Spontaneous septic arthritis complicating rheumatoid arthritis. J. Bone Joint Surg. 56A:1180, 1974.
8. Kellgren, J.H., Ball, J., Fairbrother, R.W., and Barnes, K.L.: Suppurative arthritis complicating rheumatoid arthritis. Br. J. Med. 1:1193, 1958.
9. Garner, R.W., Mowat, A.G., and Hazleman, B.L.: Wound healing after operations on patients with rheumatoid arthritis. J. Bone Joint Surg. 55B:134, 1973.
10. Foker, J.E., Schwartz, R., Smith, D.C., and Matas, A.: Surgical problems in immunodeficient and immunosuppressed children. Surg. Clin. North Am. 59:213, 1979.
11. O'Loughlin, J.M.: Infections in the immunosuppressed patient. Med. Clin. North Am. 59:495, 1975.
12. Burry, H.C.: Penicillamine and wound healing—a potential hazard? Postgrad. Med. J. August Supplement:75, 1974.
13. Deshmukh, K., and Nimni, M.E.: A defect in the intramolecular and intermolecular cross-linking of collagen caused by penicillamine. J. Biol. Chem. 244:1787, 1969.
14. Schorn, D., and Mowat, A.G.: Penicillamine in rheumatoid arthritis: Wound healing, skin thickness and osteoporosis. Rheumatol. Rehabil. 16:223, 1977.
15. Cooke, T.D., Richer, S., and Hurd, E.: Localization of antigen-antibody complexes in intra-articular collagenous tissues. Ann. N. Y. Acad. Sci. 256:10, 1975.
16. Ohno, O., and Cooke, T.D.: Electron microscopic morphology of immunoglobulin aggregates and their interactions in rheumatoid articular collagenous tissues. Arthritis Rheum. 21:516, 1978.
17. Robinson, D.R., Tashjian, A.H., Jr., and Levine, L.: A possible mechanism for bone destruction in rheumatoid arthritis. J. Clin. Invest. 56:1181, 1975.
18. Kennedy, A.C., Allam, B.F., Boyle, I.T., Nuki, C., Rooney, P.J., and Buchanan, W.W.: Abnormalities in mineral metabolism suggestive of parathyroid over-activity in rheumatoid arthritis. Curr. Med. Res. Opin. 3:345, 1975.
19. Kennedy, A.C., Allam, B.F., Rooney, P.J., Watson, M.E., Fairney, A., Buchanan, K.D., and Hillyard, C.J.: Hypercalcaemia in rheumatoid arthritis: Investigation of its causes and implications. Ann Rheum. Dis. 38:401, 1979.
20. Bisla, R.S., Inglis, A.E., and Ranawat, C.S.: Joint replacement surgery in patients under thirty. J. Bone Joint Surg. 58A:1098, 1976.
21. Singsen, B.H., Isaacson, A.S., Burnstein, B.H., Patzakis, M.J., Kornreich, H.K., King, K.K., and Hanson, V.: Total hip replacement in children with arthritis. Arthritis Rheum. 21:401, 1978.
22. Sledge, C.B.: Joint replacement surgery in juvenile rheumatoid arthritis. Arthritis Rheum. 20:567, 1977.
23. Conway, W., Bauer, G., and Barns, M.: Hypersomnolence and intermittent upper airway obstruction. Occurrence caused by micrognathia. JAMA 237:2740, 1977.
24. Bryan, R.S., Scott, W.T., and Bickel, W.H.: Results of surgical management of the hip in patients with rheumatoid arthritis or rheumatoid spondylitis. In Cruess, R.L., and Mitchell, N.W. (eds.): Surgery of Rheumatoid Arthritis. Philadelphia, J. B. Lippincott Company, 1971, p. 63.
25. Ritter, M.A., and Vaughan, R.B.: Ectopic ossification after total hip arthroplasty: Predisposing factors, frequency, and effect on results. J. Bone Joint Surg. 59A:345, 1977.
26. Williams, E., Taylor, A.R., Arden, G.P., and Edwards, D.H.: Arthroplasty of the hip in ankylosing spondylitis. J. Bone Joint Surg. 59B:393, 1977.
27. Aly, R., Maibach, H.I., and Mandel, A.: Bacterial flora in psoriasis. Br. J. Dermatol. 95:603, 1976.
28. Lambert, J.R., and Wright, V.: Surgery in patients with psoriasis and arthritis. Rheumatol. Rehabil. 18:35, 1979.
29. Marples, R.R., Heaton, C.L., and Kligman, A.M.: Staphylococcus aureus in psoriasis. Arch. Dermatol. 107:568, 1973.
30. Griffiths, I.D., Maini, R.N., and Scott, J.T.: Clinical and radiological features of osteonecrosis in systemic lupus erythematosus. Ann. Rheum. Dis. 38:413, 1979.
31. Beckenbaugh, R.D.: Implant arthroplasty in the rheumatoid hand and wrist: Current state of the art in the United States. J. Hand Surg. 8:675, 1983.
32. Copeland, S.A., and Taylor, J.G.: Synovectomy of the elbow in rheumatoid arthritis. Arthritis Rheum. 61:69, 1979.
33. Ewald, F.C., Scheinberg, R.D., Poss, R., Thomas, W.H., Scott, R.D., and Sledge, C.B.: Capitellocondylar total elbow arthroplasty. J. Bone Joint Surg. 62A:1259, 1980.
34. Morrey, B.F., Bryan, R.S., Dobyns, J.H., and Linscheid, R.L.: Total elbow arthroplasty: A five-year experience at the Mayo Clinic. J. Bone Joint Surg. 63A:1050, 1981.
35. Ewald, F.C., and Jacobs, M.A.: Total elbow arthroplasty. Clin. Orthop. 182:137, 1984.
36. Head, W.C., and Paradies, L.H.: Ipsi-lateral hip and knee replacements as a single surgical procedure. J. Bone Joint Surg. 59A:352, 1977.
37. Hardaker, W.T., Jr., Ogden, W.S., Musgrave, R.E., and Goldner, J.L.: Simultaneous and staged bilateral total knee arthroplasty. J. Bone Joint Surg. 60A:247, 1978.
38. Nakano, K.K.: Neurologic complications of rheumatoid arthritis. Orthop. Clin. North Am. 6:861, 1975.
39. Rana, N.A., Hancock, D.O., Taylor, A.R., and Hill, A.G.S.: Upward translocation of the dens in rheumatoid arthritis. J. Bone Joint Surg. 55B:471, 1973.
40. Rana, N.A., Hancock, D.O., Taylor, A.R., and Hill, A.G.S.: Atlantoaxial subluxation in rheumatoid arthritis. J. Bone Joint Surg. 55B:458, 1973.
41. Poss, R.: Total hip replacement in the patient with rheumatoid arthritis. American Academy of Orthopedic Surgeons Instructional Course Lecture XXVIII:298, 1979.
42. Millender, L.H., and Nalebuff, E.A.: Arthrodesis of the rheumatoid wrist. An evaluation of sixty patients and a description of a different surgical technique. J. Bone Joint Surg. 55A:1026, 1973.
43. Volz, R.G.: Total wrist arthroplasty: A new approach to wrist disability. Clin. Orthop. 128:180, 1977.
44. Convery, F.R., and Minteer, M.A.: The use of orthoses in the management of rheumatoid arthritis. Clin. Orthop. 102:118, 1974.
45. Melvin, J.L.: Rheumatic Disease: Occupational Therapy and Rehabilitation. Philadelphia, F. A. Davis Company, 1977.
46. Coventry, M.B., Beckenbaugh, R.D., Nolan, D.R., and Ilstrup, D.M.: Hip arthroplasties: A study of postoperative course and early complications. J. Bone Joint Surg. 56A:273, 1974.
47. Lotke, P.A., and Ecker, M.L.: Influence of positioning of prosthesis in total knee replacement. J. Bone Joint Surg. 59A:77, 1977.
48. Statistics of total knee replacement. Clin. Orthop. 120:1976 (entire volume).
49. D'Ambrosia, R.D., Shoji, H., and Heater, R.: Secondarily infected total joint replacements by hematogenous spread. J. Bone Joint Surg. 58A:450, 1976.
50. Poss, R., Thornhill, T.S., Ewald, F.C., Thomas, W.H., Batte, N.J., and Sledge, C.B.: Factors influencing the incidence and outcome of infection following total joint arthroplasty. Clin. Orthop. 182:117, 1984.
51. Lattimer, G.L., Keblish, P.A., Dickson, T.B., Jr., Vernick, C.G., and Finnegan, W.J.: Hematogenous infection in total joint replacement. Recommendations for prophylactic antibiotics. JAMA 237:1463, 1977.

Chapter 113
Synovectomy

Norbert Gschwend

HISTORICAL

It appears that Volkmann,[1] in 1877, was the first surgeon to recommend surgical removal of inflamed soft tissues for tuberculous knee joints. Schüller[2] (1887) extended the indication to chronic joint diseases, particularly chronic rheumatic inflammation. Other German surgeons[3–12] performed synovectomies more or less routinely in the first decade of this century. W. Müller[13] from Aachen, however, may be credited as the first to perform the operation for a rheumatoid arthritic knee.

The term "synovectomy" was introduced by the Frenchman, Mignon,[14] in 1899. In the USA, Goldwaith[15] reported in 1904 on synovectomy for nontuberculous arthritis. In the years that followed, the operation seems to have fallen into a state of oblivion, at least until Murphy[16] appeared on the scene in 1916 with his description of two patients suffering from hypertrophic villous synovitis, on whom he performed synovectomy. His efforts led to a certain amount of popularity for the operation in the USA,[17] but it was hardly practiced in Europe at the time owing to the fear of secondary infection. In fact not until after World War II was synovectomy reintroduced, initially for tuberculous joints. Its successful use was reported by Wilkinson[18] in England during 1953.

Authorities such as Aidem and Baker,[19] Vainio,[20] and Vaughan-Jackson,[21] as well as many others, deserve credit for developing synovectomy into a routine operation for rheumatoid arthritis.

THEORETICAL BASIS

If synovectomy, irrespective of whether it is conducted operatively or as chemical or radioisotope therapy, has now established itself in the treatment program for rheumatoid arthritis, it is for two principal reasons, one being rheumatologic and the other surgical.

From the rheumatologic standpoint rheumatoid arthritis must be regarded as a systemic illness. Its focus is in the synovium, which is looked upon as the immunocompetent tissue. According to Hollander,[22] its removal is comparable to the elimination of a secreting lymphoma, with the hope that temporary or even permanent quiescence of the inflammatory process will result, at least locally. As a consequence, the destructive process should be stopped or, at least, arrested. Even though this formulation implies a well-founded skepticism as to the healing effect of synovectomy, it expresses all the more the hope of winning time. The latter, however, is linked with the possibility of discovering the actual cause of the disease and thus a curative therapy on the one hand and the provision of improved reconstructive possibilities for destroyed joints on the other.

From the standpoint of the rheumatoid surgeon, synovectomy—even if not curative—is at least a pathogenetically effective procedure that enables the integrity of the joint or tendon to be restored in the best manner and, through the elimination of mechanical obstacles, facilitates normal function. Early synovectomy, the possible total and atraumatic elimination of the diseased synovium, careful after-treatment, and the inclusion of the operation in a medically balanced treatment plan have brought this procedure increasingly back into the foreground during the last 15 to 20 years. Long-term studies conducted by orthopedic surgeons (see below) with large series of synovectomies (under constant conditions, particularly in respect to the operative technique and after-treatment) confirm the efficiency of the operation for a high percentage of patients.

Like the positive clinical results, the experimental investigations conducted with synovectomized joints[23] and the histopathologic and serologic findings before and after the operation[25,114] appear to us to support this procedure. For this discussion only the investigations made by Goldie[23] have been selected. He measured temperature, pH value, and the presence of rheumatoid factors in the synovial fluid before and after synovectomy. He showed quite clearly that inflammation—assessed on the basis of the direct and indirect temperature measurements, as well as an increase in the pH value—was reduced significantly after synovectomy. There was no clinical or radiological evidence to show that additional structural damage was reduced.

The question of recurring disease of the regenerated synovium, however, warrants a reply of its own (see below).

INDICATIONS AND CONTRAINDICATIONS FOR SYNOVECTOMY

Although in individual cases opinions differ with regard to the indications for synovectomy, there is unity as far as the following general formulation is concerned: Synovectomy, performed operatively or as chemical or radioisotope synovectomy, must be seriously considered if conservative measures, generally regarded as effective, are not able to eliminate pain associated with chronic swelling of a polyarthritic joint or the tendon sheaths within a reasonable period of time.

Differences in opinions largely arise with regard to the optimal type of conservative therapy and its duration before deciding in favor of synovectomy. At two of the world's leading hospitals for patients suffering from rheumatic diseases, which are exclusively engaged in the handling of inflammatory rheumatic complaints (Heinola, Finland, and Warsaw, Poland), the operation is contemplated if a classic basic therapy such as gold salts or a course of antimalarial or salicylate is not able to eliminate the swelling. Penicillamine or immunosuppressives—but not cortisone preparations with which a recession of swelling does not indicate any actual healing effect—may also be used instead of gold.

Nevertheless, in practice the inflammation and pain associated with rheumatoid arthritis are frequently of a fluctuating character, and swelling can recede without disappearing. When is synovectomy indicated in such cases? We tend to respect the views of Jakubowski and Pongowska,[28] who base the decision for operation on the expected prognosis without operation. Using the analysis of 333 polyarthritic patients as a basis, these authors recommended synovectomy for patients in whom erosions appear in the radiographs after a period of 24 to 30 months, because otherwise the disease would inevitably continue to progress. The same applies to patients with more than six positive ARA criteria—in particular, those who are seropositive and develop rheumatic nodules. However, patients with fewer than six positive ARA criteria (morning stiffness, pain when walking or in the muscles or a joint, inflammation of a joint, swelling of another joint, symmetrical inflammation of the joints) should not be operated upon until the clear failure of conservative therapy or radiologic evidence of further deterioration have been established. Admittedly, in the case of the latter group this means that early synovectomies are hardly ever performed, but with the former group the progress of the destruction of individual joints is an indication that other swollen joints should be operated upon before it is too late.

A glance at the world's pertinent literature[29-36] reveals that so-called *early synovectomy* (synovectomy at a time when only the synovial layer is the seat of the disease)[37] is an exception, and that *late synovectomies* are usually performed in stages 2 and 3 (ARA criteria). The differences in success, based on residual symptoms and radiological deterioration in the years that follow the operation, are not extensive and will be the subject of further discussion (see below). Without doubt, however, such practice has an erroneous assessment of the chances of success for synovectomy, and thus favors an all too common "wait and see" attitude. The "image" of synovectomy can hardly be improved if one decides to give it a chance only at the last minute.

These reflections concerning the indications for synovectomy are based chiefly on immunological considerations, which make the removal of the synovial layer largely dependent on the degree of activity or degree of immunocompetence. The still insufficient amount of knowledge in this sector and a greatly varying optimism concerning the drugs available today explain the differences with regard to the indications for synovectomy. At the same time, we must be fully conscious of the fact that these drugs do not have any direct therapeutic effect, but, in the majority of cases, only a symptomatic effect. In a number of cases, the orthopedic surgeon has to offer a *biomechanical indication* for synovectomy instead of invoking theoretical, unproved immunologic reasons. This is valid for some joint synovectomies and for almost all tenosynovectomies. This indication is also the reason for a number of successes that were not necessarily expected from the immunologic standpoint. Severe villonodular proliferating synovial swellings and those associated with massive fibrin production frequently lead to a plugging of the joint and a partial loss of mobility. Apart from inhibiting flexion, they often cause a lack of extension in the knee joint. Since, in contrast to simple effusion, they cannot be punctured, their operative elimination remains the only effective action.

In such cases, the chances of success with *chemical and radioisotope synovectomy* are reduced (see below). Wherever the destructive process has already reached an advanced stage, intra-articular structures (e.g., menisci) and para-articular formations (e.g., finger extensor tendons) are damaged, with the result that additional biochemical disturbances occur; here, conservative measures and chemical or radioisotope synovectomy can no longer help. Operative synovectomy, in combination with joint debridement and reconstructive measures (e.g., meniscectomy, recentering of the extensor mechanism) will not only eliminate or greatly reduce the pain and swelling but also, through restoration of the best possible mechanical conditions, protect the joint against any rapidly progressing destruction. A pronounced biomechanical consideration constitutes the basis for the indication of *tenosynovectomy*. This arises from the topographical anatomy of the tendon sheaths, which are the center of the swelling. Tendon sheaths are present only in narrow places and at bending points over osseous pivots. In such locations we already must contend with difficult working conditions for the sliding mechanism of the tendons, for which the tendon sheaths are provided. Any process that allows this physiologic "bottleneck" to become an absolute one makes continued function problematic. We have only to recall the consequences of synovitis in the flexor compartment, where all transitions from painful restriction of flexion to the rapid and almost complete blocking of movement can be observed. This is in addition to the nerve compression problem in the carpal tunnel and the spontaneous ruptures that may be experienced there and not only in the back of the hand.

This biomechanical indication has probably been accorded too little attention, particularly from rheumatologists. It deserves more attention, because irrespective of the immunological situation the results of many joint synovectomies and particularly of tenosynovectomy are favorable over many years in the majority of cases, and noteworthy recurrences may be looked upon as an exception (see below).

A final indication for synovectomy is particularly applicable for joints and explains why astonishing results in elimination of pain can be attained even with advanced changes—i.e., carried out as late synovectomy in Stage 3 and on joints, such as wrist joints, where purely anatomically synovectomy is far from being complete. I refer to the *denervation effect* of synovectomy, which is to be expected not only when single branches leading to the joint are deliberately severed (e.g., interosseus dorsalis nerve in the hand), but also incidental to the incision or partial excision of the fibrosis joint capsule, which eliminates some nerve branches. The pros and cons of chemical and radioisotope synovectomy also warrant consideration from this standpoint.

CONTRAINDICATIONS

Synovectomy is not an operation that is vital to life. Accordingly, general surgical contraindications such as a poor general condition and advanced age have increased validity here. In this connection, however, it should be mentioned that currently available regional anesthesia (plexus and intravenous regional anesthesia for the upper limb and sciatic and femoral cutaneous nerve block and spinal and epidural anesthesia for the lower extremity) can reduce the patient's stress appreciably, so that nowadays with good local indications we can decide to operate much more safely than in the past. A high degree of activity of the disease does not represent a contraindication, although most authors suggest refraining from operation when a pronounced flare-up is observed. Restraint should also be exercised in the case of polyarticular joint swelling with pain in all the joints, a situation in which we do not know where to start and finish the operation. Here, it is especially important to do the utmost to dampen the activity with currently available drugs, so that an operation can be undertaken on the joints exhibiting the largest swelling. Similar considerations are valid for collagen diseases for which the overall prognosis is unfavorable. Nevertheless, we do not shun synovectomy here either, as long as the indications are substantiated in the main by biomechanical considerations (see above). Perhaps the most important contraindication is lack of motivation on the part of the patient. After all, any synovectomy can be successful only if the patient agrees to it and is willing to participate intensively in the after-treatment phase. It is better not to perform the operation if the patient is lacking in understanding, will, or cooperation.

The *local contraindications* are of particular importance. Infectious skin changes, interdigital mycoses, or other rashes on the skin should be healed before any operation is undertaken. Particular attention should be given to rheumatoid nodules that lie very close to the surface and are covered with crusts. Quite often they are the source of a latent infection, which, when located in the vicinity of a more extensive operation, can manifest itself by formation of a hematoma. On the other hand, in our experience the thin "cigarette-paper skin,"

often with petechial spots, seen in patients on steroids heals without any special problems. We merely avoided the application of tight bandages before inflating the tourniquet, because otherwise the cutis becomes detached from the subcutis, and extensive, deep necrosis may result.

Although there is agreement on the aforementioned contraindications, opinions vary as to the stage of local destruction at which synovectomy should no longer be performed (see above). According to our experience, synovectomy is not contraindicated until Stage IV destruction with dislocation of the joint components or severe limitation of movement is present and cannot be remedied by means of combined reconstructive measures such as recentering, reconstruction, or transfer of tendons (on the metacarpophalangeal or proximal interphalangeal joints). In Stage III, there are cases in which, in all good faith, various opinions can be held but no actual contraindication formulated. In the European countries the appraisal of the radiologic stages has been done in the last few years more according to the 6 stages (0–5) of Larsen.[38,39]

JOINT SYNOVECTOMIES ON THE LOWER EXTREMITY

Knee Synovectomy

It would appear that the first synovectomies were carried out on the knee joint. This joint is still one of the most frequently indicated areas for synovectomy. This is because of its frequent involvement and because the operation can eliminate a large immune-competent tissue in one procedure, and is thus most likely to influence the overall process. If it is to be given preference over other methods, knee synovectomy must fulfill two conditions:

1. It must be radical, particularly where the synovial membrane performs its destructive work—namely, at the edge of the cartilage and on the cartilage-free bony sections covered by the synovial membrane, especially in the pouches underneath the ligaments and menisci.

2. An atraumatic technique and systematic postoperative treatment must ensure more or less normal function of the joint within the space of a few weeks.

According to the experience gained by orthopedic surgeons active in this special field, especially in the case of early synovectomy, these conditions can largely be fulfilled.

Indications. With regard to indications and contraindications, the remarks made above apply here. In stage III disease (ARA or at stage III according to Larsen-Dahle-Eek), the decision must be made from case to case, according to the personal experience of the surgeon, the psychological attitude of the patient, and the number and degree of involvement of the other joints. Numerous reports have been made of the favorable results obtained with elimination of pain and swelling even in advanced stages and with a relatively long follow-up.[40–48] Other publications reflect more scepticism,[49,50] particularly when ROM and functions are concerned. With increased experience, there is a tendency for the indications to be extended rather than diminished. On the other hand, it is better to correct a flexion contracture in a conservative manner (by serial plaster casts) prior to the synovectomy, and to dispense with the latter if flexion does not exceed an angle of 90 degrees.

Preoperative Treatment. To facilitate a complete synovectomy, no intra-articular injection of steroids should be given at least 6 weeks prior to the planned operation, since it is easier to remove completely a thickened, readily visible synovial membrane.

Technique. The operation is always performed under tourniquet, because this is the only way to ensure a clear view, completeness of the synovectomy in critical areas, and atraumatic work. Certain authors proceed from a large parapatellar incision on the joint.[51,52] The author has long been using two parapatellar incisions, as suggested by Mori. He has, however, as of a few years ago, converted to employing a long, slightly laterally curved incision, for the following reason. The long-term results of late synovectomies (the majority of cases) have shown that in a considerable number of cases an arthroplasty of the knee joint proved necessary at a later date. This operation, however, is most simply performed through a long midline incision. Two lateral incisions compromise healing and favor the development of marginal necroses in the wound, whereby the risk of infection becomes increased. Conversely, a central incision—with the knee joint flexed—offers the additional advantage of approaching the dorsal portion of the joint in its so-called soft spot. In this way it is possible to perform a complete synovectomy and, if desired, a reconstruction of the overstretched dorsal capsuloligamentous apparatus.

On the fascia we proceed by two parapatellar incisions.[41] The insertion of the vastus musculature is only partly incised, and the fibrous capsule is split in the direction of the incision until its synovial lining shimmers bluishly through. The author starts by dissecting off the upper recess with large scissors before he opens the joint itself; this facilitates its exposure, especially in the presence of an effusion. According to the suggestion of Mori, the synovial sac is split laterally by a transverse incision, approximately at the level of the middle of the patella. In this way, the proximal chief portion of the synovial sac is separated from its distal portion. Sparing the fatty tissue anterior to the femur and the extensor apparatus, the operator dissects the synovial sac free from the lateral to the medial side; this can be done most easily with the knee joint slightly hyperextended. Thus, the synovial sac is detached from the surrounding structures as far as the midportion of the joint to facilitate the procedure through the smaller medial incision where, what is more, the vastus medialis extends farther distally.

Now, the distal sac, which has been split vertically, is pulled down with a strong clamp; frequently it can be detached like a membrane, from the osteocartilaginous border of the femoral condyle. The joint is opened, and its contents are sucked out. Any synovial tissue is removed from the cartilaginous border of the femur, the tibia, and the patella, using a Luer's forceps or a raspatory. The distal portion of the synovial sac situated anterior to the collateral ligament is resected in toto, together with part of Hoffa's fat pad. With the knee joint flexed, the collateral ligaments can be readily exposed. The recesses of the collateral ligaments should be cleaned with special care. Using a fine Hohmann rectractor covered with a rubber tube, it is also possible to inspect the internal aspect of the opposite femoral condyle and the cruciate ligaments inserting there. For synovectomy of the intercondylar space, the author makes use of a rongeur, which is commonly employed in laminectomy.

Subsequently, the menisci are inspected; when abnormally loose and movable or ruptured, they are removed or an incision is made parallel to the anterior insertion of the meniscus. Thereby, the osseochondral border of the tibial condyles can be adequately exposed; in this place one often encounters numerous finely honeycombed erosions, which undermine the cartilaginous border. With the knee strongly flexed, the operator also enters the dorsal portion of the joint, with a separate incision in the so-called soft spot posterior to the collateral ligament, where he can perform a rather extensive synovectomy when villous synovium is encountered.

Now the joint is thoroughly irrigated with Ringer's solution, the tourniquet is removed, and careful hemostasis is performed. The wound is closed in layers and without tension; heed is paid to solid suturing of the nicked insertion of the vastus muscle. Two tubes for suction drainage are inserted over the sutures capsule and, through a small gap in the capsule, are introduced into the joint. A solid pressure dressing with unglued cotton and a ventral foam rubber cushion ensure continuing hemostasis. The operator is advised to place on record the damage established in the cartilage and the interior structures, which is of importance to after-treatment and prognosis. A considerable discrepancy between the roentgen findings and the actual damage can be ascertained in almost all cases.

Postoperative Treatment. We place the operated leg on a rectangular splint at an angle of about 80 to 90 degrees of flexion of the hip and knee joint. Particular attention must be given to the blood supply of the skin. On the day after the operation, the knee is stretched passively to the full extent but then is placed on the splint again for 2 hours. This manipulation is repeated twice daily in the first week, and the patient is encouraged to assist actively shortly after removal of the suction drain (48 hours postoperative). We allow the patient to sit on the side of the bed the very first day. During the day, the leg is held in the flexed position for two 2-hour periods and in the extended position for the remaining time. Instead of a simple static splint, we have made increasing use of the new electrodynamic splint (Kinetec). The patient should perform isometric exercises with the quadriceps every hour. He is allowed to get up and walk with elbow crutches after 10 days, or earlier if his condition warrants. Treatment, however, is not complete when the patient is released from hospital. Compensation for already damaged ligaments and thus protection of the joint against further damage can be realized only through daily exercises over several months. These strengthen the knee extensor apparatus (particularly the vastus musculature for the final 20 to 30 degrees of extension) and are designed to eliminate pronounced atrophy of the muscles. We attach particular importance to the mobility of the patella, especially in the vertical direction, which is undertaken passively by the physiotherapist using both hands. Increased patellar mobility is a precondition for preventing active extension lag and thus for averting secondary flexion contracture. For a similar reason, extensive effusions should be aspirated if persistent.

With bilaterally affected knee joints, it is possible to synovectomize the two joints simultaneously. However, we feel it is advisable to perform the operation at intervals and to wait until the first operated extremity is functional again.

In cases in which mobility of 90 degrees or more is not attained within a period of 2 weeks, it is advisable to perform a manipulation under general anesthesia no later than 14 days after the operation. The subsequent placing of the knee joint in flexion, daily exercises, the administration of analgesics and anti-inflammatory drugs, and occasional local doses of steroid ensure continuous good mobility. The results of knee synovectomy are dealt with on 14-25.

Synovectomy of the Hip Joint

Early synovectomy, which is so beneficial and promising in the hand and knee, is seldom mentioned in connection with the hip joint. The reason for this is not only the difficulty of access but also the danger of disturbing the blood supply of the femoral head with secondary necrosis in the event of a too radical procedure on the dorsal side of the neck of the femur. Furthermore, without dislocation it is also impossible to perform a synovectomy in the depths of the acetabulum, where we frequently find a synovial pannus extending out of the incisura acetabuli in the direction of the fovea capitis. Nevertheless, we believe synovectomy should be considered much more than it has in the past. For example, Meuli[54] reported good results when the operation was performed early and with younger patients. We have performed synovectomies successfully in individual patients mostly in combination with an osteotomy. We feel that this is all the more justified, because access is provided without any great difficulty with an intertrochanteric osteotomy, which also facilitates the undertaking of a synovectomy in the ventral, caudal, and cranial areas.

In ten patients, five of whom suffered from rheumatoid arthritis, three from osteochondromatosis, and two from synovitis of uncertain cause, we have performed total synovectomy with temporary and careful dislo-

cation. Up to now, more than 4 years on average after surgery, there has been no sign of disturbance to the blood supply of the femoral head. Our results with synovectomy of the hip joint were good in the case of mono- and oligoarticular involvement of the hip joint in young patients. Six patients had few or no complaints at all. Up to now, there has been no indication of progressive destruction in any of the patients. Because of simultaneous coxa valga, in single cases we combined varus osteotomy with the synovectomy. With these hip joints, we took the opportunity of obtaining a biopsy of the hip joint capsule when removing the metal plate. There were no signs of recurrent synovitis 2 years after the synovectomy.

Quite frequently, cases of rheumatic coxitis are referred to the orthopedic surgeon (e.g., for the exclusion of tuberculous synovitis) for biopsy. In such cases and in the presence of a confirmed synovitis, we take the opportunity of carrying out a substantial synovectomy.

Ankle Synovectomy

Synovectomy of the ankle joint has been performed frequently in the last 10 years.[55-60] Amazingly there has been no mention of it in major treatises concerned exclusively with operative treatment of rheumatoid feet.[61-62]

The ankle joint is undoubtedly readily accessible for a substantial synovectomy. The swelling has mostly a clear external appearance as a doughy bulge in front of and behind the malleoli.

At the same time, we frequently encounter a painful synovitis, especially in the peroneal tendons or the posterior tibial tendon. From time to time, we also see a pronounced tenosynovitis of the toe extensors. The hourglass shape of the swelling, owing to the constriction caused by the retinacular ligament, usually allows it to be differentiated without difficulty from synovitis of the ankle joint. The synovectomy can be performed just as easily and as successfully. Attention should also be paid to inflammatory changes in the vicinity of the Achilles tendon. For example, painful bursitis and erosive bony changes in the attachment area of the Achilles tendon are not so rare. The fact that infiltration of synovial tissue in a tendon can weaken it and lead to spontaneous rupture has already been discussed in detail. Even bilateral Achilles tendon ruptures are not uncommon in rheumatoid arthritis. We have found that when the tendon sheaths are affected to a marked extent, frequently there is no or only slight participation of the joints. In other words, there appear to be pronounced tendinous and pronounced articular types of rheumatoid arthritis. For those intending to perform a synovectomy of the ankle joint, this means that a systematic search should be carried out for possible participation of the tendons surrounding the ankle joint, because synovectomy of the joint and the tendons is possible in the same operation. Arner and associates,[63] den Herder,[64] and Hansson[65] have been able to prove a connection between the tendon sheaths of the flexor hallucis and the posterior joint recess in about 30 percent of cases. Not so frequent is the connection between the ankle joint and the tendon sheaths of the posterior tibial or peroneal tendons.

Technique. The operation can be performed either with a transverse incision in front of the ankle joint[66] or with a longitudinal incision in front of the tibial or fibular malleolus. With a view to sparing the longitudinal structures, in particular the veins, we prefer a longitudinal incision in front of the lateral malleolus. From here we obtain a good view of both the medial and lateral front joint parts and can also inspect the tibiofibular pouch. From the same incision it is possible to clean the sinus tarsi and part of the subtalar joint from hypertrophic synovial tissue. A second posterolateral incision gives free access to both, the posterior part of ankle and subtalar joint underneath the Achilles tendon. Moreover, it allows for tenosynovectomy if the peroneal tendons are involved. Synovectomy of the medial retromalleolar tendons is performed, if necessary, from a separate incision.[67] Our results with synovectomy of the ankle joint are satisfactory and can be compared with those of the major reports, e.g., Jakubowski.[68] In 80 to 90 percent of the cases, pain and swelling can be relieved completely or largely for years. In the last years, synoviorthesis has become more and more an alternative to operative synovectomy, particularly in the earlier cases. Seventy percent of very good and good results are reported for the first 2 to 3 years. They deteriorate as time progresses.[69]

If there are paresthetic phenomena in the plantar aspect of the foot and the toes or disturbances of sensation, we must consider the possibility of a *tarsal tunnel syndrome.* An electromyogram or nerve conduction study will confirm the diagnosis. After exposure of the tibial nerve, following splitting of the retinacular ligament of the flexor tendons, synovectomy of the tendons and decompression of the nerve will result in speedy relief.

Synovectomy of Other Joints of the Foot

Synovectomy of the subtalar joint and the Chopart joint are advocated by Mori (personal communication). He has performed these successfully in individual cases, using a lateral and medial skin incision. We have not come across any analogous reports in the literature, and we have synovectomized the subtalar joint on few occasions as a rule in combination with ankle synovectomy.

JOINT SYNOVECTOMIES OF THE UPPER EXTREMITY

Synovectomy of the Metacarpophalangeal Joints

Specific Aspects at the Metacarpophalangeal Joint Level. The indication includes not only the specific biomechanical considerations valid for every synovectomy

but also those relevant to this particular area. In other words, it is not just an immunological problem or a case of eliminating inflammation and pain; rather, it is a question of preventing the finely adjusted balance from being ultimately destroyed through overstretching of the capsule and ligaments and tendons in the immediate vicinity. However, disturbances of balance are inevitable with synovitis of longer duration, and can never be eliminated completely even with the most subtle operative techniques. In practice, this means that in the event of chronic overstretching—especially of the fibers inserting on the proximal phalanx—the extensor tendon is insufficient; further, because of overstretching of the collateral ligament, the anular ligament, which is not fixed to the metacarpal, slips in the direction of the palm. As a result this enables the flexors to have a stronger effect on the metacarpophalangeal joint. Retraction of the interossei, whose pivot has also slipped toward the palm owing to overstretching of the extensor hood, finally fixes the deformity (Fig. 113–1). Because of overstretching of the normally longer radial collateral ligament, the finger is subject to additional ulnar drift, which increases as a result of the increased ulnar position of the extensor and flexor tendons and the radially acting forces of everyday life. Following slippage of the finger extensors into the ulnar interdigital space, the deformity becomes fixed.

This explains why, as shown in the results, late synovectomies cannot prevent progressive deformity over a long period of time even with the best technique.

On the other hand, this supports the need for early synovectomy, and suggests that late synovectomy should be restricted to cases in which the deformity, in particular the ulnar drift, can be corrected passively, easily, and completely, and in which irreparable damage to the joints, with severe subluxation of dislocation, has not been established either radiologically or operatively. Such cases require reconstructive procedures, not synovectomy. Consequently, special radiograms of the finger joints, such as the ball-catching x-rays made by Norgaard[70] or, even better, the x-ray techniques em-

Stretching of the collateral ligaments

Capsular stretching

Contracture of intrinsic muscles

Volar subluxation of phalanx with enhanced volar pull of flexor tendon

Figure 113–1. Pathogenesis of volar subluxation of the proximal phalanx of the metacarpophalangeal joint. Persistent synovitis and effusion produce capsular laxity, stretching of the collateral ligaments and extensor mechanism, and contracture of the interossei. A fixed flexion deformity with volar subluxation in the proximal phalanx results.

ployed by Brewerton,[71] which provide us with information on conditions in the pouches of the collateral ligaments, should be regarded as a constituent part of the preoperative assessment.

Swelling of the metacarpophalangeal joints is a frequent and early phenomenon in rheumatoid arthritis. Since such hands are frequently *emaciated,* one cannot fail to notice them.

If it is not possible to bring about complete regression of the inflammation by means of conservative treatment (generally or locally administered drugs), possibly also through the injection of erbium, then we must expect progressive destruction of the joint and the appearance of irreversible deformities. In the first place, the inflamed synovial layer damages the joint pouches not covered by the cartilage, especially the insertions of the collateral ligaments,[72] and also leads finally to the formation of a vascular pannus with undermining of the cartilage to its destruction. Following destruction of the cartilage, the atrophic bones cannot withstand the increased pressure of the finger flexors on the palmar aspect so that they break, especially if they have been weakened by erosions, and increase the palmar subluxation or dislocation of the proximal phalanx. In extreme cases, the fingers displace themselves in the direction of the palm, and the abnormal protruding metacarpal heads take on a characteristic appearance.

Synovial inflammation also influences the finger extensor mechanism at the level of the metacarpophalangeal joint. Whereas the flexor tendons are separated from the metacarpophalangeal joint by a rigid, cartilaginous volar plate and thus protected, the extensor apparatus—i.e., the tendon of the long finger extensor, the interosseus muscles, and the transverse lamina, which are in closest relationship with the joint capsule—will be overstretched.

Knowledge of these relationships again supports the call for synovectomy of the metacarpophalangeal joints.

Indications and contraindications for synovectomy of the metacarpophalangeal joints are based on the considerations put forward earlier in this chapter.

Like Kenesi,[73] we feel that indication for synovectomy exists when the inflammation continues between the flare-up phases and in spite of basic therapy, because then the fear of progressive destruction is completely justified.

Vaughan-Jackson[74] indicates with emphasis that in the initial stage there is still no periarthritis and still no damaging pannus, but only a swollen synovial membrane which has to be removed to prevent further damage. For him, the objectives of the operation are the hope that (1) destruction can be halted, (2) pain can be relieved, and (3) mechanical disturbance can be corrected.

In stages I and II of the disease (corresponding to the stages 0 to 2 of Larsen), the success justified the decision of the surgeon in the majority of cases. In stage IV (or stage 4 and 5 of Larsen), with subluxation of the joints, synovectomy may only be performed together with a reconstruction of the joint. As far as indications

are concerned, difficulties are encountered only in stage III. The joint cartilage is already badly damaged, the collateral ligament is overstretched, the finger has frequently already drifted quite distinctly to the ulnar side, the patient complains of pain while mobility is still good, and function, thanks to clever adaptation, is sufficient for daily needs. Although theoretically synovectomy would offer the best prospects, experience frequently shows that the porotic bone of the joint, robbed of its cartilage, is not strong enough to withstand the pressure once the synovium—acting as a fluid coating—has been removed, with the result that it collapses.[75] Pain and deformity are the consequences. On the other hand, an arthroplasty at this stage would appear premature to the surgeon, because it is usually not possible to guarantee retention of the preoperative extent of movement. The surgeon runs the risk of having an unsatisfied patient and discredit of an operation which, in itself, was good. In such cases, the surgeon should recommend an operation in Stage III only if the patient, exhausted by continuous pain, agrees to it, knowing full well that the success of the operation may be judged less on preoperative function than on function expected in the future. Otherwise, the patient must be allowed to mature psychologically. Vaughan-Jackson[74] put it succinctly when he said "How often have we hesitated with an operation in stage III only to regret our actions bitterly a few years later."

Technique of Synovectomy of the Metacarpophalangeal Joint of the Long Fingers. In operating on three or four metacarpophalangeal joints, a transverse incision is made over the knuckles; in operating on one or two metacarpophalangeal joints, the skin incision is longitudinal and slightly curved at the level of the metacarpophalangeal joint. The longitudinally running veins are spared. The extensor hood is divided parallel to the tendon down to the synovium, 1 to 2 mm radially to the long extensor tendon. An important item is the division of the fibrous joint capsule. The synovial pouch, which in most cases protrudes markedly, is dissected free proximal to the metacarpal head, where, similarly to the knee joint, an outpouching is encountered. At the border of the cartilage and in the recesses of the collateral ligaments, which become plainly visible on flexion of the fingers, the synovial tissue is curetted with particular care.

After the set of ligaments has been sufficiently loosened, it is mostly easy to gain access to the volar pouch. Often, however, it is preferable to follow the suggestion of Stellbrink[106] in flexing the finger at the metacarpophalangeal joint and lifting the metacarpal head with a fine sharp hook. By alternating radial and ulnar abduction, the operator not only gains a good view of the recesses of the collateral ligaments but also can reach the volar pouch with a fine curved forceps for synovectomy. It is of utmost importance to preserve the fibers running from the extensor tendon to the base of the first phalanx, in order to prevent any volar displacement of the finger. The suturing of the fibrous capsule serves the same purpose; moreover it helps prevent adhesion formation between the tendon and the underlying metacarpal bone.

The connecting fibers of the extensor mechanism, which have been divided on the radial side, are sutured with moderate reefing of their borders. This is the best means of counteracting the tendency for the extensor tendon to deviate toward the ulnar side. A suction drain is inserted, followed by suture of the skin, and application of a pressure dressing with plenty of cotton, foam rubber pad, and elastic bandage, and elevation of the hand. Synovectomy of the metacarpophalangeal joints can be combined with other operations on the same hand (synovectomy of individual proximal interphalangeal joints, caput ulnae syndrome, carpal tunnel syndrome).

Postoperative Treatment. Early mobilization, which we start after removing the compression bandage 2 to 3 days after the operation, is critical as long as tendon transplants or arthroplasties have not been combined with the synovectomy. The mobilization is primarily active. Passive assistance should be provided only if progress in mobility is slight or nonexistent. In order not to endanger the sutures, one should not try to force things at all during the first few days. With the metacarpophalangeal joints of the fourth and fifth fingers, postoperative restriction of mobility is relatively common if we ignore the fact that the fourth and fifth carpometacarpal joints (as opposed to the second and third) are readily movable. These two joints also participate in the closing of the fist and allow the mobility of the ring and little fingers to appear more extensive than it actually is. During exercises, the physiotherapist should therefore fix the fourth and fifth metacarpals and exercise flexion only in the metacarpophalangeal joint. This is all the more important, because normally flexion in the fourth and fifth metacarpophalangeals is more extensive than with the second and third. Additional *occupational therapy* is introduced once the wound has healed up. To prevent ulnar drift, we use special grips for the various therapeutic tools.[76] It is only on rare occasions that splints—to stretch the fingers—are considered necessary for the night. We contemplate their use only if full extension is not attained during the first 2 weeks. Knuckle bender splints may be used if flexion of 90 degrees is not obtained during the same period.

Results. The results of synovectomy of the metacarpophalangeal joints of the fingers are considered promising by most authors who performed synovectomies with the necessary care and when no significant cartilage and ligament damage existed.[77-87]

According to earlier publications.[88-90] about two thirds of the results are expected to be good. However, Ellison and associates are more skeptical following an observation period of some 4½ years, in which only 43 per cent of the operated joints could be regarded as excellent and good, and recurrent synovitis was observed in 14.4 per cent of the cases. Nevertheless, 50 per cent were completely free of pain, and mobility improved in nearly half the patients. Our results shall be discussed in more detail on pages 1807 and 1810. There is no doubt that the results are very much dependent on the stage of destruction found at operation. The late outcome is largely determined by the grade of general activity of the disease. On the other hand there exists a remarkable discrepancy between the late x-ray findings, which may show severe alterations, and a positive assessment of the result by the patient. The pain-relieving effect of the capsulosynovectomy of the finger joints by denervation should not be underestimated.

Synovectomy of the Metacarpophalangeal Joint of the Thumb. Technically, synovectomy of the metacarpophalangeal joint of the thumb is more or less similar to synovectomy of the other metacarpophalangeal joints. From a dorsal, slightly ulnar-convex curved incision we approach the joint between the tendon of the long and short thumb extensor. When the collateral ligaments are elongated, it is not too difficult to remove the synovium from the volar aspect. We hesitate to sever (as Lipscomb[91] advocated) one of the collateral ligaments at the first metacarpophalangeal level. It would require a fixation with a K-wire for 2 to 3 weeks.

Careful handling of the attachments of the tendon to the proximal phalanx and, in the event of overstretching of the extensor pollicis brevis, reefing or reinsertion of the tendon on the proximal phalanx ensure the best possible postoperative function. If the collateral ligaments are insufficient, it is advisable to reef them by suture. In these cases and when the short extensor has been reinserted, it is advisable to fix the joint for 2 weeks in extension with a K-wire and to protect the joint thereafter with a splint. In such cases we expect a reduction in mobility, but this is generally unimportant considering that many people already have a remarkably reduced range of motion at this level.

Synovectomy of the Proximal Interphalangeal Joints, the Distal Interphalangeal Joints of the Fingers, and the Interphalangeal Joint of the Thumb

Indications. The statements made with regard to synovectomy of metacarpophalangeal joints also apply here. The indication for synovectomy in the PIP joints is even more extensive than in the MP joints as far as late synovectomy is concerned. It may include stage III (ARA and Larsen-Dale-Eek). This may be particularly important before considering an MP-arthroplasty, the results of which are very dependent on the good and painfree mobility of the PIP joints. If a boutonnière deformity is already present, the surgeon and the patient must know that the deformity cannot be totally eliminated (see below), and that success to a certain degree should not be judged on the basis of the normal condition, but in relation to the deterioration which is to be expected if the operation is not performed.

Technique. Although for a long time surgeons contented themselves with removing about 75 per cent of the synovial mass, it is now generally agreed that only a near-complete synovectomy is the basis for prolonged success. An essential premise is meticulous cleaning of the borders of bone and cartilage as well as the recesses of the collateral ligaments. In our experience, this can best be accomplished in the following manner: A straight or curved longitudinal dorsal skin incision with the convexity to the ulnar aspect exposes the extensor mechanism. Two longitudinal incisions are made on both sides of the central slip of the extensor tendon; following this, the dorsal outpouching of the synovial sac is first detached on one side and then withdrawn to the other. In this way it can be totally removed. With the proximal interphalangeal joint flexed, both recesses of the collateral ligaments can be readily exposed and are cleaned gently, without injuring bones and ligaments, using a fine sharp curet or our special forceps. With the same instruments, the adhering synovium is stripped from the borders of bone and cartilage. As in the knee joint, any loose gliding tissue adjacent to the bone is spared so as to prevent the postoperative formation of major adhesions.

In recent years, unilateral temporary division of the collateral ligament, which originally was performed by Lipscomb[91] alone, has found an increasing number of supporters because it allows performance of a near-complete synovectomy of the volar recess of the joint. In so doing, we follow the suggestion of Pahle,[92] who, in operating on the second, third, and fourth fingers, divides the ulnar collateral ligament (on the fifth finger, the radial ligament near its origin) and separates the joint surfaces, using the nonsevered ligament as a hinge. In this way, the entire volar pouch is exposed and can be cleaned of synovial tissue with a fine forceps. Upon completion of the operation, the ligament is fastened to its origin with two to three atraumatic sutures. Originally, Lipscomb felt that 3 to 4 weeks of fixation of the joint with a Kirschner wire was necessary to ensure uneventful healing of the collateral ligament, and this was certainly the principal reason why few other surgeons adopted the technique. In contrast, we and many other workers have learned from personal experience that a simple suture also permits institution of active mobilization on the third or fourth postoperative day without running any risk. Only passive strain on the operated finger through abduction, e.g., by supporting the body, should be avoided; for this reason, in the little finger, not the ulnar but the radial collateral ligament is divided. Unlike us, Pahle,[92] Stellbrink,[106] Vainio,[86] and other workers do not approach the joint through two longitudinal incisions between the lateral and the central slip of the extensor but by splitting the ligament of Landsmeer (transverse retinacular ligament). Stellbrink and Vainio also leave the collateral ligament intact and open the volar pouch proximally to the collateral ligament. Exposure by this procedure is less satisfactory than by division of the collateral ligament. Upon completion of the operation, the connecting fibers between the central and the lateral slip of the extensors are carefully sutured with moderate reefing of their borders. This procedure is of decisive importance in preventing a bou-

tonnière deformity. In the latter instances, reconstruction of the extensor apparatus should be attempted by a different technique. Synovectomy of individual proximal interphalangeal joints can be combined with other operations on the same hand (synovectomy of metacarpophalangeal joints, operations for the caput ulnae syndrome or the carpal tunnel syndrome).

Postoperative Care. A pressure dressing suffices for the fixation of the fingers during the first 3 days; then purely active mobilization is started. After healing of the wound, i.e., about 10 days after the operation, mobilization is intensified; occupational therapy and hourly exercises (kneading a silicone mass and paraffin baths) are beneficial measures. Passive assistance should be given only when stiffness of the joint threatens or when the patient is unable to make a firm fist. The follow-up therapy should be continued until the preoperative range of motion has been reached, which will be the case in a few weeks, provided that the operative indication had been correctly established. The use of splints, especially so-called lively splints proposed by Bunnell,[93] is recommended if flexion or extension is still incomplete after 2 to 3 weeks. To promote flexion one can employ the knuckle-bender splint, and to promote extension the so-called reversed knuckle-bender or the Capener splint. The splint should be worn intermittently several times a day and, if well tolerated, also overnight. In the presence of marked boutonniere deformity, the aftertreatment will be modified.

The *distal interphalangeal joints* are affected much less frequently by rheumatoid arthritis (exceptions are juvenile and psoriatic polyarthritis and arthritis mutilans). However, McCarty and Gatter[94] hold the view that distal interphalangeal joints are affected much more than is generally assumed. In one third of their examined polyarthritic patients, they observed an average of three painful distal interphalangeal joints (distal interphalangeal tenderness). The indication for synovectomy is the same as for the other finger joints. It is best not to wait until a hammer finger (caused by overstretching of the extensor mechanism) or a swan-neck deformity at the proximal interphalangeal level (reflecting a disturbance in the balance of the extensor mechanism) occurs. As long as the lateral stability of the distal interphalangeal joint is maintained, the chances for permanent functional improvement are also more favorable.

Synovectomy of the *interphalangeal joint of the thumb* is all the more worthwhile, because the operation can be undertaken, as in the DIP joint, from an L-shaped or oblique incision without any great difficulty, even if not so totally as is the case with the PIP joint. Maintenance of joint stability through preservation of the collateral ligaments against further destruction and protection of the insertion of the long thumb extensor are important for the function of the thumb and thus the hand. Here, temporary detachment of the lateral ligament is worth considering if the volar pocket appears to contain large synovial masses. The results of finger joint synovectomies are discussed on pages 1807 and 1808.

Synovectomy of the Wrist

Synovectomy of the wrist with swelling at the back of the hand has to be considered frequently. Since the ligaments are weaker on the dorsal than on the palmar aspect, overstretching is easier and therefore swelling appears earlier.

As long as the joint surfaces are preserved, synovectomy must be considered if the inflammatory changes with pain and functional impairment persist, and when the resistance of the disease cannot be broken through consistently applied measures over a long period of time.

Opinions differ widely as to the value of synovectomy for the wrist. Flatt,[95] who rejected synovectomy of the wrist because of his unsatisfactory early results, now regards it as being of limited value, i.e., for relieving pain and retarding the destructive process. He sees the main difficulty as being the anatomical impossibility of total synovectomy. Most authors[95-97] do not perform synovectomy as an isolated procedure, but only in combination with resection of a dorsally projecting ulnar head or as part of synovectomy of the extensor tendons. Fernandez-Palazzi and Vainio[98] and Mori[99] strongly advocate early synovectomy of the wrist. Vaughan-Jackson[100] feels the operation can be delayed because an arthrodesis is always possible.

Although it is technically more difficult than with other joints and cannot be complete, most authors see in the resection of sensitive nerve endings (amply present in the capsule) a possibility for the simultaneous elimination of pain that leads to flexor spasm and deformity.[101] Besides the dorsal synovectomy, Mori undertakes a palmar synovectomy from a separate incision in the more difficult cases. He also devotes attention to the radical removal of the synovial membrane which penetrates into the cavities of the metacarpal and intercarpal bones or protrudes between the carpal bones. As a result of jamming, they lead to pain and flexion deformity. Our extremely satisfactory results appear to justify more frequent application of this technique. Proceeding from the experience that every total synovectomy of the wrist leads to restriction of movement, we support Savill and Duthie's advice[102] to be cautious in performing synovectomy in the early stage, when movement is still practically normal.

Isolated wrist synovectomy, therefore, is considered primarily with persisting painful swelling of the wrist joint and where signs of a progressive radiological deterioration are visible. Using the stages 0 to 5 by Larsen-Dahle-Eek, we advocate particularly synovectomy of the wrist in the stages 2 and 3. With persistent swelling of the extensor tendons, the danger of spontaneous rupture is high. Here, the success with extensor tendon synovectomy must be noted (see Chapter 114). If a simultaneous swelling of the wrist and extensor teno-synovium exists, we have become much more liberal in the last few years with regard to synovectomy of the wrist. Our indications for wrist synovectomy are as follows:

1. When dorsal tenosynovitis—despite basic therapy—exists for more than 6 months, and when swelling of the wrist joint is established at the same time.

2. With caput ulnae syndrome, when it is found necessary to resect the distal ulnar end, and synovitis of the wrist is also established.

3. With therapy-resistant pain primarily limited to the radiocarpal area, radiographic evidence of destruction not exceeding stage 3 (Larsen-Dahle-Eek), no signs of subluxation, and clinically sufficient movement (at least 50 percent of the normal range of movement). Wrist synovectomy may also be justified with far advanced destruction (without subluxation) for the purpose of gaining time, provided that there is evidence of pronounced and definitely localized pain in the radiocarpal and intercarpal joints, combined with swelling of the capsule, and that there is no reason to consider the possibility of performing arthrodesis or arthroplasty.

The *technique* is shown in Figure 113–2.

Our *results* covering more than 50 cases[103] conform largely to those of the 47 wrist synovectomies performed by Fernandez-Palazzi and Vainio,[98] even if the synovectomy was not so complete pain was reduced in 85 percent and inflammation in 71 percent of the cases. An

Figure 113–2. Steps in synovectomy of the wrist joint. *A,* Through a straight dorsal incision, the retinacular ligament is reflected with a radial base. Extensor tendons are reflected to the radial side and the dorsal capsule is elevated. *B,* Exuberant synovium between the radius and carpus as well as between the carpal bones can be removed with a rongeur. *C,* The capsule is closed and the dorsal retinaculum has been placed deep to the extensor tendons to protect them from continued erosion by recurrent synovium or rough bony surfaces.

increase in strength was observed in 63 percent of the patients. The dorsal flexion decreased by some 37 percent and the volar flexion by 55 percent. These results, and those cited, support the conclusion that synovectomy is worthwhile.

Synovectomy of the Elbow Joint

In the last few years, the number of authors who have carried out routine synovectomy of the elbow joint has risen continually. The reason for this is not just the likelihood of success, but also new techniques (see below) which permit practically total synovectomy.

The *indications* for elbow joint synovectomy are as follows:

1. Swelling, which is resistant to conservative therapy (excluding steroid treatment), with pain and restriction of movement.

2. Only minimal radiologic changes of the ulnar component of the articulation, suggesting that the surfaces of the joint are still smooth and congruent.

3. Resection of the radial head indicated in the presence of radiographic evidence of incongruency.

4. Signs of a compression-irritation of the ulnar nerve at the level of the elbow. With impaired nerve conduction, the indication is absolute.

5. Signs of compression of the deep branch of the radial nerve (interosseus posterior) (see below), with impairment or paralysis of the extensor carpi ulnaris and the finger extensors.[104,105]

It is not easy to lay down the limits for synovectomy, because—as Stellbrink[106] was able to show and we have confirmed—late synovectomy in combination with debridement (see below) still produces a relatively high percentage of satisfactory results even in the presence of advanced destruction of the humeroradial joint, since it may allow one to avoid arthroplasty.

Technique (Fig. 113–3). Using a dorsoradial incision, the extensor carpi radialis brevis is nicked. The origins of the extensor digitorum and carpi ulnaris with the underlying collateral ligament are left intact. Blunt separation of the fibers is performed between the extensor carpi radialis brevis and digitorum anteriorly and at the dorsal edge of the extensor carpi ulnaris. By flexing the elbow and detaching the anconeus muscle from its origin in the humerus, the ventral as well as the dorsal segment and the bulging synovium can be adequately inspected. In the flexed position, the entire ventral synovial sac is isolated and detached from its humeral, radial, and ulnar attachments. With the elbow stretched, the distal radial fibers of the triceps are held back with a retractor, and the anconeus is turned back; now the dorsal synovial pouch at the olecranon fossa and the radial portion of the ulnar articular surface can be adequately inspected.

The fibers of the extensor digitorum longus muscle are separated anteriorly and the extensor carpi ulnaris posteriorly by blunt dissection as far as 3 cm distally to the head of the radius. Following exposure of the synovial layer of the elbow joint, the elbow is flexed, the musculature lying anteriorly to the incision is lifted with an angular hook, and the synovial sac is exposed anteriorly and to the ulnar side as far as possible; then this sac is detached by sharp dissection from its attachment to the humerus, the anular ligament is partly severed, and the synovial sac is resected from the neck of the radius. The edge of the cartilage and especially the "pouch" on the head of the radius are carefully "cleaned" with a Luer forceps and a sharp curet. As a rule, synovectomy of the entire ventral segment, including the radioulnar recess, can be readily performed. Only when there are indications of compression of the ulnar nerve by underlying masses of synovium is an additional incision made over the medial ulnar nerve groove; the floor of the groove is then incised and the ulnar segment

Figure 113–3. Author's technique of synovectomy of the elbow joint. *A,* Dorsoradial incision. *B,* Half of the extensor carpi radialis longus origin and the whole origin of extensor carpi radialis brevis are detached from the humerus. The joint is entered at the anterior border of the extensor digitorum longus and the posterior border of the extensor carpi ulnaris. *C,* By flexing the elbow and detaching the anconeus muscle from its origin in the humerus, the ventral as well as the dorsal segment and the bulging synovium can be adequately inspected. (The major portion of the set of ligaments is left intact underneath the origin of the extensor digitorum and carpi ulnaris muscles.) In the flexed position, the entire ventral synovial sac is isolated and detached from its humeral, radial, and ulnar attachments.

of the joint is synovectomized. In such exceptional instances it is customary to displace the ulnar nerve ven-
trally. Synovectomy of the dorsal segment of the joint
is done through the radial incision, which is carried
dorsally. The anconeus muscle is detached from the
humerus, the elbow is extended, and the distal radial
part of the triceps fibers that run in the same direction
is retracted dorsally with an angular hook. Now, thorough inspection of the olecranon fossa becomes possible.
As in the case of the ventral synovial sac, the dorsal
sac-like structure is removed, if possible in its entirety.
Resection of the head of the radius should be done only
when the cartilage shows major lesions or when the
preoperative radiogram shows that flexion against resistance reveals a tendency to subluxation. Resection of
the head of the radius is by no means an absolute prerequisite for synovectomy, although it facilitates this
operation.

In recent years, performing late synovectomies, we
have regularly replaced the head of the radius with a
Silastic prosthesis so as to achieve an improved distribution of pressure in the entire joint and especially to
take weight from its humeroulnar segment, which has
suffered damage. Spontaneous fractures of the implant
after a few years prove the enormous stresses to which
any implant at this level is exposed and raise the question
of the suitability of Silastic prostheses for radial head
replacement.

Upon completion of the operation, the wound is irrigated. The anular ligament is sutured, and the detached
musculature is carefully reinserted. The principal portion
of the radial set of collateral ligaments remains intact,
the bony insertions of the extensor carpi ulnaris are
entirely retained, and most of the insertions of the extensor digitorum communis are left in situ.

Suction drainage is instituted, the anconeus muscle is
reinserted, and the wound is closed in layers. A thick
compression dressing is usually sufficient. Many patients, however, feel more at ease with a radiodorsal
plaster splint applied for a couple of days.

Postoperative Treatment. We commence with active
and assisted exercises 3 days after the operation. Occupational therapy is started after 1 week (flexion/ex-
tension exercises on the Fletcher loom with different
material with regard to resistance; wood-work: sawing,
filing, grinding of different materials). The preoperative
degree of movement is nearly always attained after 10
to 14 days; frequently we obtain a markedly better degree of movement because of the rapid decrease in pain
and the absence of the constriction phenomenon of the
synovial masses in the olecranon fossa.

Results. Certainly the largest series of elbow joint
synovectomies (about 500 in number) has been analyzed
in Heinola. The results for 123 patients with 154 elbow
synovectomies have been evaluated by Vainio et al. and
published by Raunio and Pätiälä.[107] A single lateral approach was chosen in 62 of the 154 operated elbows,
while a medial incision with displacement of the ulnar
nerve was added in 92 cases. After a period of 1 to 6

years, 71 percent of the results were assessed as being
good and 29 percent were found to be unsatisfactory.
In most of the patients with residual complaints, the
medial side of the joint had not been opened. Resynov-
ectomy or arthroplasty was necessary on six and five
occasions, respectively.

Movement improved in one of five, deteriorated in
one of five, and remained about the same in three of
five of the patients. The duration of the observation
period, age of the patients, length of illness, sedimentation rate, and number of preoperative erosions did not
appear to influence the outcome to any noteworthy degree. Our results in almost 50 cases agree more or less
with those contained in the Finnish report.[103] Since we
began routinely using our new approach (see Fig. 113–
3), the results have definitely improved; in the great
majority of the patients the range of motion has significantly increased postoperatively, especially in late synovectomies. The improvement of mobility in more than
80 percent of our cases[25] and the absence of ulnar nerve
problems led us to the conclusion that the described
approach to the elbow joint may be responsible for the
progress made even in late synovectomies.

In 1972, Ehrlich[108] reported so-called *antecubital cysts*
on the elbow for the first time. As in the case with
popliteal cysts, overpressure in the joint—caused by synovitis and joint effusion, as well as the need for the
patient to support himself completely on the diseased
elbow on rising from a sitting position—leads to an
anterior rupture of the capsule. The resultant cyst fills
itself with joint fluid, while a valve mechanism usually
prevents any backward discharge. Irritation of the ulnar
aspect may result. As in the case of the knee, elimination
of elbow joint synovitis is equally as important as the
extirpation of the cyst to prevent possible recurrence.

In conclusion, elbow synovectomy resembles wrist
synovectomy in that it may produce satisfactory results
even in the presence of radiographic evidence of advanced destruction.

Synovectomy of the Shoulder Joint

This was hardly mentioned in the world literature
until just a few years ago. The difficulty of approach
for a subtotal synovectomy, the predominant importance of periarticular changes, and the resultant danger
of a secondary frozen shoulder explain the apprehension.
For a long time, partial synovectomy was associated
only with cases in which the joint had to be opened up
in the course of another shoulder operation (synovectomie partielle).[109] In 1969, Ansell and Arden[110] reported
good results following the removal of large cystic swellings in the shoulder areas of four of five patients. The
operation should be carried out as early as possible.

In recent years, there has been more interest with
regard to the shoulder joint. Admittedly, most reports
actually relate to bursectomy. However, since the subdeltoid bursa is in the immediate vicinity of the joint

cavity (and may possibly connect when synovitis occurs), inspection of the joint cavity should be a requirement with bursectomy. In view of the large number of patients that he has synovectomized and the favorable results, the report of Pahle[111] is worthy of note among the small number of publications on this subject. We have employed his technique for our patients, together with an anteromedial skin incision and temporary detachment of the clavicular portion of the deltoid. We have encountered spontaneous rupture of the long biceps tendon on frequent occasions. This should be firmly sutured in the sulcus intertubercularis. The further operative procedure is dependent on the presence or absence of defects in the rotator cuff. We found that almost all patients presenting with large swellings of the bursae around the shoulder joint had defects in the rotator cuff. If a defect is found, a repair according to one of the well known methods,[112,113] depending on the size of the defect, is carried out. Otherwise, the rotator cuff is incised between the insertion of the supra- and infraspinatus tendon, because this simplifies cleansing of the joint as well as repair of the rotator cuff. With the best possible internal rotation of the humerus, such an incision enables the head of the humerus to be dislocated partially from the glenoid in the dorsal direction, thus facilitating good access to the rim erosions on the anatomical neck. A radical synovectomy can then be performed. Debridement of the joint is carried out when necessary.

Postoperative Treatment. On completion of the operation, the arm is placed in an abduction splint in about 70 degrees abduction, 30 degrees flexion, and slight external rotation for 14 days until fixation of the muscle is sufficiently secure. During this period the deltoid muscle can be treated with isometric tension exercises. What is most important, however, are exercises for internal and external rotation; strengthening of the external rotators is particularly vital for a full elevation of the arm. The arm can rest freely on the abduction splint during the day.

It is important to instruct the patient carefully in the preoperative period, so that he realizes the purposes of these exercises. Depending on mobility, the abduction splint is replaced after 2 or 3 weeks by a sling, and active movement exercises are introduced. If mobilization under general anesthesia is deemed necessary, it should be done within the first 3 weeks after the operation.

Results. In the series of results published by Pahle,[111] which cover an observation period of 2 to 9 years, and in which only 5 of 29 synovectomies could be classified as early, it was observed that shoulder synovectomy gave good results even in advanced cases. The relief of pain was significant and an important increase in the range of motion, particularly internal rotation and abduction, was noted. Clinically there has been no recurrence of swelling or of other clinical signs. Radiologic deterioration was found as well, as in other late synovectomies. The best results were obtained in early cases. Our experiences in a smaller series are very similar.

RESULTS OF JOINT SYNOVECTOMY

It is very difficult to survey the flood of publications that have been written on the subject of synovectomy over the last 15 to 20 years. Nevertheless, between the lines both optimism and pessimism are reflected constantly. Is the effort worthwhile for the operated joint or the operated tendon sheath? Is the pathological process influenced in any way? These are only two of the most important questions that have still not been answered definitely.

There is general agreement in most of the papers on synovectomy concerning the following points (Table 113-1):

1. It has a favorable effect on pain and thus usually a positive influence on function.

2. It enables us to eliminate or reduce the swelling.

3. It has, with the exception of late synovectomies of the elbow and shoulder joint, no appreciable influence on the mobility of the operated joint.

4. The result depends on the degree of preoperative destruction, and therefore we find relatively frequent deterioration of the radiographic picture after the operation.

5. There is a gradual deterioration in the clinical result as time goes on after the operation, and so an increase of recurrent synovitis in the years following the operation is to be expected.

On the other hand, opinions are divided as to how far synovectomy, particularly in the case of a larger joint, is able to influence the entire process—i.e., the activity of the disease, and thus the progress on the other nonoperated joints. Most notable is the lack of comparable studies dealing with the progress of the disease in operated and nonoperated joints. Some studies purport to use a symmetrically involved contralateral joint as a control, but this is clearly a crude clinical selection in view of the tremendous variability of synovitic involvement. Serious ethical and psychological questions must accompany the withholding of an operation which has been found to be successful on one side, if the patient requests it on the second side. Not only is the prognosis of the entire rheumatoid process highly variable from patient to patient, but there are often capricious differences in the course of the disease in various joints of the same individual. Given the tremendous number of variables involved, it is surprising that the reported results of synovectomy are at all uniform. Critical variables that should be addressed in reviewing the reported statistics on synovectomy include the following:

1. The groups of patients on which the statistics are based are nonuniform (a) according to size; (b) according to age; (c) according to profession (depending on the physical strain on the operated joints, we must expect different results); (d) according to the duration of the disease; (e) according to the number of affected joints; (f) according to the immunologic parameters; (g) according to the stage of illness (a rough classification into early and late synovectomy is not fair, particularly to

Table 113-1. Knee Synovectomy—Results by Various Authors

Authors	Year of Publication	Number Cases	Number Knees	Follow-up	Stage	Surgical Procedure	Results Excellent	Good	Fair	Poor	Complications	Recurrence
Staf Geens et al.	1972	23	31	7–49 months (23 months)	Mostly III ARA	Synovectomy and debridement	7 42.5%	6	7 23%	11 35.5%		5 cases (biopsy confirmed 2 cases)
Ranawat et al.	1972	46	60	1–8 years (31 months)	II/III ARA	Patellectomy 24 and synovectomy 22	1 37%	21	22 37.5%	16 27%	Valgus 4, flexion contracture 5, repeat surgery 16	7 cases
Tillmann	1972		82	6 months–3 years	10 early, 72 late synovectomy	In late synovectomy, also meniscectomy (30), removal of osteophytes (34), band replacement (8)	Early 6 90% Late 33 85%	3 28	1 10% 7 9.5%	0 4 5.5%	Ligament slackening (7) after additional surgery	2 cases
Taylor et al.	1969	78	110	6 months–6 years	II/III/IV ARA	Patellectomy 11	60.8%		26.8%	37%		
Jakubowski	1972	102	150	2.5–7 years	Mostly late synovectomy	Simple synovectomy 91; synovectomy + debridement, perhaps patellectomy 59		56 37%	38 26%	56 37%	Repeat surgery (24) after poor results	
Behnke and Holland	1973	21	32	3 months–3 years (1.7 years)	III (Steinbrocker)	Debridement 24	9 68.5%	14	3 10.5%	6 21%	Ossification of distal quadriceps muscle (1)	
Mohing	1973	140		1–7 years	Mostly early synovectomy	Mori operation		86.8%	8.7%	4.5%		
Goldie	1974	29	32	7 years	Mostly II/III	Synovectomy and sometimes debridement		24 75%		8 25%	Stiffening after synovectomy (4)	
Laurin et al.	1974	49	66	7.5 years	Mostly II/III ARA		20 63%	18	13 21.5%	9 15.5%		

the last group, in which the degree of destruction varies to a considerable extent) (h) according to the time after the operation (although it would be possible to make a comparison of sufficiently large groups over analogous periods of time, only a few of the data known to us pursue one and the same case over periods of months and years); (i) according to the histological picture; and (j) according to the disease activity at the time of the re-examination.

2. There is no consideration of the drug therapy used prior to, during, and after operation.

3. In the various reports we find different surgical and postoperative treatment techniques.

4. There is no uniform follow-up examination.

5. Various criteria are used for the follow-up.

The rating of the success with the attributes *very good, good, satisfactory,* and *poor,* or their equivalent, is justified in such cases in which a subjective assessment of the patients is desired. The objective measurement of the effectiveness of synovectomy—as was applied in many of the studies—is associated with a decisive disadvantage—namely, that it tends to compare the postoperative state with the normal condition instead of considering individually the gain or loss in comparison with the preoperative condition of an individual joint.

Considering these objections, therefore, it seems desirable to summarize the results of an extensive study conducted by us together with Böni[114] and his coworkers. In order to remain as objective as possible, the evaluation was not undertaken by the surgeon responsible for the operation, but by rheumatologists using easily reproducible evaluation criteria and a point system. For the latter, a rating of 0 for the normal condition and 3 for the poorest state was employed for the evaluation of the clinical parameters: pain, swelling, mobility, stability, and deformity. The radiographs were assessed

according to an 18-point system by two independent physicians. Over a period of 5 years, the graphic representation of the various parameters (Figs. 113–4 to 113–8) discloses the following characteristics: (1) High initial value for the summation of all parameter—easily understandable when we consider that four out of five cases were late synovectomies. (2) Very positive influence, particularly on pain and swelling, which improve sharply in the direction of normality; slight influence only on mobility; slow but progressive deterioration in subsequent years, during which the initial result is not maintained.

This pattern for 100 knee synovectomies corresponds to a major extent with that obtained for 370 finger synovectomies (Fig. 113–5). There was a difference, however, in that the renewed clinical deterioration with finger synovectomy is chiefly attributable to an increase in the number of deformities. But is this remarkable when we consider that over 80 percent of the cases were late synovectomies? Is it not also a completely sufficient explanation for the deterioration in the radiographs in about 30 percent of the cases, most of which exhibited degenerative and not inflammatory characteristics? The definitely better progress with early synovectomy and mono- as well as pauciarticular cases may be seen quite clearly in the comparable curves. We have followed up these cases for nearly 13 years (average, 8 years) and find that good results have been obtained in two thirds of the cases, with pain and swelling absent or present only to a minor degree. Figure 113–9 shows the synovectomized left knee joint just before synovectomy, just after synovectomy, and 7 years later. Figure 113–10 shows radiographs of both hands prior to and 5 years after synovectomy of the metacarpophalangeal joints of the left hand. The synovectomized joints still look much better than the nonsynovectomized. As a subtotal syn-

Figure 113–4. Results of synovectomy in 100 knees followed over a period of 5 years. The joints were assessed using a grading system which assigned a grade of 0 for the normal joint and 3 for the worst changes. The immediate improvement seen at 3, 6, and 12 months diminishes only slowly with time.

Figure 113–5. Results of 370 finger synovectomies followed for 5 years. Immediate improvement in the overall rating is primarily due to decreased swelling, whereas the long-term deterioration of results is primarily due to progressive deformity.

Figure 113–7. Radiographic assessment of 86 knee synovectomies followed for 2 years. The graph shows the marked difference in results between early and late synovectomy, while the histogram shows the cumulative radiographic assessment at 2 years. Radiographic deterioration was described as due to either increased rheumatoid arthritic changes or onset of secondary degenerative changes. The most common cause of deterioration assessed radiographically 2 years after surgery was progressive secondary degenerative change with loss of joint space and sclerotic subchondral bone changes.

ovectomy of a finger joint in advanced cases (late synovectomies) inevitably removes some bone from the erosions, the postoperative radiographs will always show more destructive lesions than the preoperative radiographs.

On the basis of the reduction of the sedimentation rate and the decrease in titer of the latex test, we were able to show a positive influence on the general disease activity only in some of the cases and only for a period of 1 to 2 years.

Somewhat different results concerning the value of synovectomy of the finger joints have been reported independently by British and American controlled studies;[117] the British study[115] was undertaken by the Arthritis and Rheumatism Council and the British Orthopaedic Association, and the American study by McEwen and O'Brian[116] of the Arthritis Foundation (1974). Both were so-called controlled studies, comparing operated joints clinically and roentgenologically with joints treated by conservative means during a 3-year period. The British study was concerned with knee joints (weight-bearing) and metacarpophalangeal joints (non-

weight-bearing). The American Study also included proximal interphalangeal joints.

Regarding the finger joints (metacarpophalangeal joints), the British study came to the conclusion that the result of surgical treatment was disappointing because comparison with the nonoperated joints revealed no improvement by clinical and radiographic criteria. However, the writers were impressed by the fact that almost all the patients spoke highly of the results, and, in the same circumstances, would be willing to undergo the operation again. The American study, 3 years after the operation, found nothing to recommend surgical management. In contrast to synovectomy of the metacarpophalangeal joints, the British study definitely revealed better results of synovectomy of the knee joint with regard to pain, swelling, and radiographic changes. The American study, on the other hand, established that synovectomy of the joint had improved only swelling.

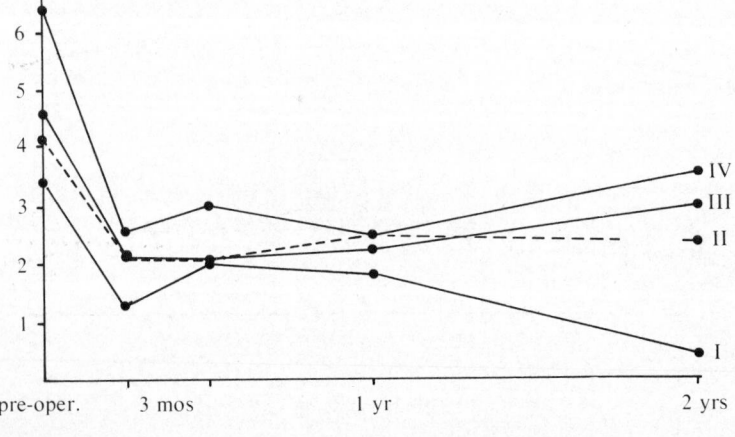

Figure 113–6. The relationship between preoperative disease stage and clinical result. The most significant improvement seen at 2 years is in Stage I disease.

Figure 113–8. Radiographic classification of modes of failure following knee synovectomy. Radiographic changes were described as rheumatoid arthritic, osteoarthritic, both, or indeterminate.

What factors could be invoked to explain the remarkable differences in evaluating operative success between these two studies and all the others, especially those by Pahle, Raunio, and the present author? Most important is the small number of cases; the British study, for instance, included no more than 22 knee joints with

Figure 113–9. *A*, Before synovectomy of left knee. *B*, Immediately after surgery. *C*, Seven years after surgery. The right knee, which has not been synovectomized, shows a significant deterioration in contrast to the operated knee.

Figure 113–10. Radiographs of both hands prior to (*A*) and 5 years after (*B*) synovectomy of the metacarpophalangeal joints.

11 controls and 41 metacarpophalangeal joints in 13 patients with 28 control joints in 9 patients. In addition, despite all the calculations of statistical significance of the values encountered, the conclusions are questionable because the small number of cases was derived from no less than 12 different centers. These centers, in turn, provided an unequal number of cases for evaluation. The present author feels that the value of a controlled study becomes doubtful when there is a difference between the essential factors influencing such a study—namely, uniform evaluation of the criteria of investigation and uniform technique of operation as well as of postoperative management. How could one otherwise explain the study performed in 1973 by Thompson, Douglas, and Davison,[118] which also included control cases and came to entirely different conclusions regarding the value of synovectomy of the metacarpophalangeal joints? The writers mentioned encountered, 2 years after operation, significant improvement regarding swelling, muscle power, pain, and subjective evaluation by the patient.

In addition, a further reason can be advanced to explain why in the British study the synovectomies of the knee fared better than those of the metacarpophalangeal joints. In evaluating the usefulness of synovectomy on the basis of radiographs, it should be realized that in the knee joint erosions must have attained a considerable degree of severity to become demonstrable. In the finger joints there is also a striking discrepancy between the preoperative picture and the findings at operation. At surgery, lesions are revealed which are not visible in the radiograph. In performing as nearly a total synovectomy as possible, special care is taken to remove synovial proliferations in the recesses of the joint and the collateral ligaments, and to eradicate erosions. It goes without saying that during this procedure portions of bone are liable to be concomitantly removed. It must therefore be expected that lesions which were barely visible preoperatively are more clearly visualized in the postoperative radiograph. The author, in his analysis, has also observed and discussed this deterioration of the radiographs which, despite clinical improvement, occurs in a relatively large percentage of cases. It is easily understood that in the knee joint, owing to the far greater thickness of its layers, the curetting of erosions does not have such an adverse effect. In this joint osteoarthritic changes usually develop after a late synovectomy (hence, in the majority of cases), which, on comparing the pre- and postoperatie radiographs, could lead to misinterpretation of the usefulness of synovectomy. The author is therefore of the opinion that long-term studies of the largest possible number of patients subjected to uniform surgery, after treatment and evaluation, have greater value than any calculations of statistical significance in small-scale studies without uniform control.

Our analysis of 55 patients who had undergone 74 knee synovectomies (70 percent late) on average 8 years before showed that about two thirds were without noticeable pain, and over 70 percent of them still found their condition better than before the operation. More than two thirds of the operated knee joints exhibited minimal swelling after the synovectomy.

The ERASS (European Rheumatoid Arthritis Surgical Society)[119] has undertaken a multicenter study on the long-term results (more than 10 years) of synovectomy of various joints. All X-rays have been evaluated carefully on the operated and nonoperated side according to Larsen-Dahle-Eek. The clinical situation was registered in all patients and compared with the preoperative state as well as the functional class according to the ARA criteria. Without entering into details, the following conclusions could be drawn: (1) The general disease progress (ARA functional classes) has not been influenced significantly. (2) The operated joint has mostly not or only partly contributed to the deterioration of the functional class. The x-ray appearance was mostly the same in the operated and nonoperated joints irrespective of the starting point. It seems that the endpoint was determined by the type of disease and its degree of activity. In contrast to this, pain and swelling have diminished remarkably on the operated side. The patients accessment on the effect of the synovectomy was positive in the great majority of cases.

RECURRENT SYNOVITIS

As far as we know there has not yet been any satisfactory answer to the question of recurrent synovitis, mainly with regard to its frequency. The reasons are evident.

1. No unanimous views have been stated about the definition of recurrent synovitis or as to which and how many histologic criteria are required in the light-microscopic examination to diagnose a recurrent synovitis. Which of those criteria shall be allotted specific characteristics and to which extent? Moreover, there are Hirohata's and Morimoto's statements that the regenerated synovium is qualitatively very similar to the removed pathologic synovium in the ultra-microscopic picture, with mostly just quantitative differences.

2. In view of the fact that the majority of synovectomies are late ones, a rather considerable rate of recurrent swelling can also be explained as irritative effusion, for example, in case of reduced joint stability or chondromalacia. Only routine biopsies at several sites of the joint would lead to progress in the question of recurrent synovitis.

We were able to re-examine 11 patients with swelling by means of arthroscopy. Biopsies taken during arthroscopy were examined by means of light microscopy, and the joint fluid withdrawn was assessed immunologically.

The results may be summarized as follows:

1. Arthroscopically, there were more or less extensive adhesions and increased scar formation in the new synovial membrane.

2. Microscopically, there was increased fibrosis in comparison with the findings at the first operation.

3. Our assumption that swelling after synovectomy is not necessarily due to a polyarthritic recurrence is confirmed by the histological findings. An extensive recurrent rheumatoid synovitis was diagnosed only once. In three more cases a moderate rheumatoid synovitis was found.

4. The joint fluid analyses indicated five definite recurrences.

5. The comparison made between the histologic findings and joint fluid analysis also showed general agreement in the assessments.

CHEMICAL AND RADIOISOTOPE SYNOVECTOMY

To an increasing degree, in selected cases, chemical and radioisotope synovectomy (synoviorthesis) constitute effective alternatives to operative synovectomy. Since there are few references to the subject in the literature and any discussion of results with operative synovectomy calls for knowledge of the possibilities with synoviorthesis, we shall deal with this procedure in more detail.

When we consider the temporal and financial efforts

involved, the physical and psychological stress placed on the patient with every operation or even a number of operations, as is frequently the case with rheumatoid arthritis, not to mention the possibility of complications and the uncertainty of the long-term result, we can well understand the efforts that have been made for a long time to eliminate the diseased synovium through intra-articular injection of certain obliterating substances or radioisotopes.

The first tests with chemical synovectomy and osmic acid can be traced to Von Reis and Swensson[120] in 1951; radioactive colloids were used by Ansell, Crook, Mallard, and Bywaters[142] in 1963, and by Makin and Robin[122] in 1964. The following agents have been used for chemical synovectomy: thio-tepa,[123-127] osmic acid,[120,128-133] Varicocid,[134] and gold.[135]

None of these agents had a truly selective effect on the synovial layer. Frequently all the articular structures were more or less affected. This was reflected in a considerably painful reaction, which induced a number of authors[131,132,136] to inject cortisone and a local anesthetic at the same time. On the other hand, when osmic acid was used, the cartilage underwent a massive brown coloration, which allows one a certain amount of skepticism with regard to assurances that no actual damage to the cartilage is produced.[120,129,133,137] A further interesting factor is the finding of Piattier-Piketty and associates[138] during tests with rabbits, that cartilage damage is much more dependent on the age of the rabbit than on the dose of the osmic acid.

The success rates for the various methods differ to a considerable extent. With thio-tepa[123-127] the short duration of the positive results (6 to 9 months) and their rather small number (25 percent, according to Gross[126]) are particularly noticeable.

With osmic acid we find larger discrepancies, from an unusually high success rate of 90 to 95 percent[139] to only about 50 percent 1 year after treatment in other reports.[129,130,133]

In the case of Varicocid,[134,140] the numbers are too small to prove any superiority of this method over the others (80 percent improvement with an observation period of 1 to 27 months). This same criticism applies to the intra-articular gold injections employed with success by Delbarre and associates[135] and Lewis and Ziff.[141]

Added attention, however, should be given to radioisotope synoviorthesis with which English,[142,143] French,[130,135] Austrian,[148,154] and Scandinavian authors[133,150] have been able to gather positive experience.

The following radioactive substances are available: ^{198}Au, ^{90}Y citrate, ^{90}Y resin, rhenium-186, erbium-169, ^{90}Y ferric hydroxide, radium-224, and ^{32}P-chromic phosphate. A common feature associated with them is the application of locally effective β-rays, absence of α-rays, and relative lack of γ-rays.

The *indications* for the application of the various radioisotopes depend on the β-ray energy and various penetration depths. Accordingly, the particularly deeply penetrating yttrium-90 is selected as the substance for knee and hip joints, admittedly only for patients of over 50 years of age.[133,135,143,151] For younger patients, osmic acid[129,130,133] is preferred. For finger and interphalangeal joints, the use of erbium is recommended[130,135] for analogous reasons. Compared with Au 198, more and more interest has been shown recently in rhenium-186, because of reduced radiation and a more favorable effect, particularly in the case of medium-sized joints (e.g., elbows, wrists).[130,135]

The injection techniques are described in more detail in the references cited. Apart from the exact adherence to the dose, the secure intra-articular position of the needle (image amplifier control) is important, as well as the simultaneous injection of a local anesthetic with steroid additive. The last measure helps to reduce the pain considerably. Immobilization for at least 48 hours helps to prevent unwanted leakage of the isotope to the distant parts of the body.[130,133,152,153]

Generally speaking, the results obtained with radioisotope synoviorthesis appear to be superior to those attained with chemical synovectomy.[130,133,135] Concerning the effectiveness of synoviorthesis, opinions still differ remarkably. Whereas Gumpel and associates[144] considered synoviorthesis as being as effective as operative synovectomy after 2 years and Onetti and associates[145] even after a follow-up of 1 to 10 years, Yates and associates[146] in a double-blind trial cast doubt on the benefit of radioactive yttrium. In an editorial Lee[149] criticized the lack of control series in most studies. From the few controlled studies he drew the conclusion that ^{90}Y resin was no more effective than saline in preventing radiologic evidence of disease progression. There is a similar controversy among various authors concerning operative synovectomy, and these controversies will remain until more representative controlled studies are available.

Controversial opinions are also found in the literature concerning eventual damage to the cartilage. Whereas Ingrand,[147] using autoradiographs, showed that the cartilaginous surface was not usually affected, Kerschbaumer and associates[148] reported significant degenerative changes in human chondrocytes with cartilage necrosis. Similarly controversial conclusions were reached by different research groups concerning the risks of chromosomal aberrations in circulating lymphocytes.[152,153,155,156] So far no cases of leukemia or other malignant tumors have been reported. Prediction of those cases most likely to respond is still unsatisfactory. There is almost agreement that patients with marked articular damage are unlikely to respond, whereas cases showing radiologic grades I and II are associated with a better response. Using ^{99m}Tc-pertechnetate for measuring the uptake of yttrium-90 in knee joints, Kyle and associates[156] were able to show a varying distribution within the knee joint, the uptake reflecting uneven disease activity. Technetium uptake was useful in confirming inflammation and improvement after treatment but allowed no prediction of which cases would respond.

The mode of action of synoviorthesis has been discussed by Onetti and associates[145] for ^{32}P-colloidal chromic phosphate, a radionuclide with maximum therapeutic benefit (pure beta emitter without gamma radiation, longer half-life) and minimum side effects (the large diameter of the colloidal particles makes it difficult for them to leak from the joint cavity into the lymphatic system).

The changes of the type "A" cells suggest an alteration of some metabolic activities and an increase of their phagocytic properties. In type "B" cells the alteration suggest a reduction of their synthetic properties. Relief of the inflammatory signs could be the result of the reduction of the polynuclear cell infiltration and the living cells, whose functions are probably altered by the beta-radiation. Moreover, the reduction of the mononuclear infiltration (lymphocytes and plasma cells) suggests that the immunologic events at the synovial level are suppressed.

When we compare the results of chemical and radioisotope synovectomy with those of operative synovectomy, the former should perhaps be considered more frequently in early disease.

The clear advantages of synoviorthesis are as follows: (1) simple technique, (2) reduced period of time in hospital, (3) no narcotics, (4) low costs, (5) simple mobilization, and (6) the possibility of resorting to operative synovectomy in the event of failure.

On the other hand, we should not forget the disadvantages of synoviorthesis in comparison with operative synovectomy; (1) no application in the case of tenosynovitis, (2) limited effect with multiloculated joints (e.g., wrist joints) and with pronounced hypertrophic villous synovitis, (3) no reconstructive possibilities, and (4) side effects, resulting from leakage, which have not been completely assessed.

Although it is too early to establish definite boundaries between synoviorthesis and operative synovectomy, the indications for the application of radioisotope synovectomy may be outlined as follows: early cases of mono- or oligoarticular synovitis without evidence of a severe hypertrophic, villous synovitis; psoriatic arthritis; Reiter's syndrome; nonspecific arthritis; villonodular synovitis; degenerative arthropathies with large effusions; hemophilia; and ankylosing spondylitis.

The superiority of operative synovectomy remains undisputed in the case of tenosynovectomy and for late synovectomies of joint, in which, with the removal of the synovium, reconstructive measures can be performed (e.g., recentering of the extensor mechanism on the fingers, excision of the softened patellar cartilage, resection of a torn meniscus, suturing of overstretched ligaments in the knee). The operative approach is also superior in multiloculated joints (wrist joint), where the entire joint cannot be reached by the injected substance, and with severe fibrin-producing hypertrophic synovitis, in which the injected substance may lose part of its effectiveness. It is conceivable that the remaining fibrin and necrotic tissue may have an unfavorable effect, which is also supported by the positive effect of arthroclysis (joint washings).[130,157-160] However, only comparable observa-

tions of analogous series over a longer time will show us the safest boundary between the two methods.

TREATMENT OF TENOSYNOVITIS

Tenosynovitis of the tendon sheaths disturbs function in several ways: through pain with every movement, restricted mobility, painful friction with temporary locking (trigger finger), and spontaneous rupture. However, the joints are also affected by this, because every disturbance to the finely adjusted muscle balance inevitably leads to deformities. Mention has already been made of the significance of tenosynovitis on the carpal tunnel. Damage can be avoided only through early recognition and early treatment. If conservative measures do not lead to disappearance of inflammatory symptoms in a short while, then synovectomy is indicated. With tenosynovitis, there is little to lose but much to gain with an early synovectomy.[161]

Synovectomy of the Finger Flexor Tendons

This corresponds with the treatment of the carpal tunnel syndrome (see above). Decompression of the median nerve is realized after severing of the transverse carpal ligament through careful excision of the synovial tissue around the flexor tendons, from the muscle belly to the lumbrical tunnel. Any scar that may have formed in the vicinity of the median nerve must be excised. The number of those suggesting simultaneous inspection of the flexor tendon sheath located distally to the lumbrical tunnel is on the increase.[102,162] In actual fact, we have repeatedly been able to confirm the presence of a trigger finger or painful thickening of the synovial sheet within the finger canal during flexor tendon synovectomy of the carpal tunnel.

A simple examination, by which the soft tissues over the base phalanx can be tested, enables a swift diagnosis to be made as to involvement of the tendon sheaths in the finger tunnel (pinch test according to Savill).[166] Normally a fold of skin can be lifted without difficulty, but with pathological thickening of the flexor tendons in the finger channel the palpating fingers detect an actual tumor, which is usually painful and frequently visible. In contrast to trigger finger, the patient can extend the finger actively, but cannot flex it completely if the flexor tendons in the finger channel are thickened to any marked degree. On the other hand, passive flexion may be full, provided the finger joints are not severely involved. A simple test proves the disturbed course of the tendon in its sheath: if the metacarpophalangeal joint is held flexed and the proximal interphalangeal joint extended, the distal interphalangeal joint cannot be actively flexed. In such cases, it is advisable to undertake synovectomy in the finger tunnel. The operation is best performed from a zig-zag incision,[167] which facilitates a better view than the earlier, conventional lateral incision.

When possible, the thickened synovium should be removed completely, but without injuring the surface of the tendon. If severe adhesions are found between the sublimis and profundus tendons, it is advisable to resect the sublimis tendon or one slip of it.[103,123,163] When severe changes to the profundus tendon rule out the possibility of reconstruction, we prefer to resect the tendon and to perform an arthrodesis of the distal interphalangeal joint or a tenodesis of the distal profundus stump. Simple trigger fingers are best relieved with a transverse incision in the distal palmar crease.

Synovectomy of the Finger Extensor Tendons

Externally, the swelling is easily recognized, and the retinacular ligament frequently causes a typical hour-glass-shaped constriction. However, occasionally this ligament is infiltrated and destroyed by synovial tissue. Differential diagnosis enables tenosynovitis to be distinguished from synovitis of the wrist joint; with inflammatory swelling of the tendon sheaths, active extension of the finger causes a bulging at the distal rim of the retinacular ligament, whereas with wrist synovitis uniform swelling persists in the wrist region. The swelling of the finger extensor tendons rarely extends beyond the middle of the metacarpals (exception: the extensor pollicis longus). Tenosynovitis of the tendon of the extensor carpi ulnaris is particularly frequent and makes itself apparent externally only when the swelling is especially severe. For this reason, it is advisable to undertake systematic examination of this tendon, which is of particular importance for wrist stability.

Technique. We prefer a straight central skin incision extending as far as the middle of the third metacarpal. The retinacular ligament is detached on the ulnar side and turned back radially. Following synovectomy of each individual tendon, the ligament is then drawn under the extensor tendons to protect the latter against the frequently roughened carpal bones, and then sutured again to its original place. In view of the relationship between the tendon of the extensor carpi ulnaris and the ulna, it is important for the retinacular ligament to be sutured over and not under this tendon. In this way, we also prevent any unesthetic drawing-in of the skin and abnormal tapering of the carpal region. If necessary, according to a suggestion made by Swanson,[164] the retinaculum can also be cut into two flaps. The distal one with a radial base embraces and lifts up the tendon of the extensor carpi ulnaris, and the proximal flap, with an ulnar base, is drawn under the tendon of the extensor carpi ulnaris, thus covering the resection site of the distal ulna so as to provide a reinforcement for the distal radioulnar ligament. With early synovectomy of the extensor carpi ulnaris, there may be a possibility of preventing the progression of a caput ulnae syndrome. When this is already present, it is advisable to resect the head of the ulna. We have frequently synovectomized the wrist simultaneously (see above). In general, synovectomy of the tendons is thus rarely isolated, but is usually undertaken in combination with other operations.

We were able to confirm uniformly good results with tenosynovectomies of over 100 hands.[165] Recurrences were rare. In the early stage, when the tendon was not infiltrated by the diseased tissue, detachment of the tendon sheath can be effected without difficulty and the danger of secondary adhesion is much less. The lack of adhesions induced Savill[166] to propose simple decompression of the extensor tendons through detachment of the retinacular ligament, which is then drawn under the extensor tendons (see above).

Results of Tenosynovectomy. We have been able to re-examine 60 patients (113 hands) for whom tenosynovectomy was performed on an average of 6 years before. Fifty-six were extensor tendon synovectomies, 12 at the level of the carpal tunnel, 39 at the distal crease of the palm, and 45 in the finger tunnel.

The assessment of results for tenosynovectomy is not easy, because the joints moved by the operated tendons are nearly always affected at the same time. Pain or a loss of function through reduced mobility or strength can be attributed correspondingly just as much to the progressive destruction of the joint. In order to obtain clear-cut results, we have therefore restricted ourselves to only the specific signs of tenosynovitis—namely, swelling and free gliding of the tendons, the latter being assessed on the basis of a difference between active and passive flexion.

Subjective Results. Compared with joint synovectomy, the judgement of the patient as to the success of the tenosynovectomy was extremely high. Only one of 60 patients was dissatisfied with the result. In her case, the disease was highly active and showed recurrent synovitis. Two patients were undecided because they thought that nothing had been gained through the operation.

Recurrent Swelling of Extensor Tendons. The follow-up of 56 hands having undergone synovectomy of the extensor tendons showed recurrent swelling in five cases. On the basis of the history, we had to assume in two further cases that a swelling had occurred temporarily in the postoperative period but was no longer detectable at the time of the follow-up check. Such recurrent swellings affected the extensor carpi ulnaris on two occasions, and the extensor carpi radialis, extensor pollicis longus, and finger extensors once each. In each case, it was established during the operation that the tendons had been infiltrated to a marked degree by the synovial tissue. Accordingly, radical synovectomy was not possible.

The low rate of recurrence may be explained by the translocation of these tendons that is performed simultaneously with the drawing of the retinacular ligament under the extensor tendons. On the other hand, the occasional recurrent swelling of the extensor carpi ulnaris may be explained by the fact that here we relocate the tendon in a closed compartment at the end of the operation, with the intent of restoring the normal anatomical relationship between this important tendon and the ulna, as well as the wrist.

Owing to the soft tissue cover, it is more difficult to detect recurrent swellings in the flexor compartment. We were able to detect this on only one occasion. In a series of 96 operated hands, we found two with triggering, one with swelling, one with pain, eight with crepitation, and three with active flexion deficit; we found no instances of paresthesia.

Residual crepitation may be explained by irreparable damage of the tendon surface. The scar may provoke crepitations under the partly retained anular ligament during to and fro movement. An analysis of the cause of the active flexion deficiency (three cases) showed that in each case it was a question of extensive lesions of one or both flexor tendons in the finger canal which led to adhesions after synovectomy. Several approaches to minimize this complication are suggested: extremely atraumatic operative technique, active movement therapy introduced immediately after the operation, and resection of the more severely affected tendon, usually the sublimis tendon.

Synovectomy of the flexor tendons may also be recommended for children with juvenile rheumatoid arthritis, because here misinterpretation of the genesis of the inability to make a fist must inevitably result in permanent deformity of the fingers, instead of complete restoration of function by means of tenosynovectomy.

No evidence of recurrence and/or the repetition of paresthesia was observed in any of the patients in whom the carpal tunnel was synovectomized.

To sum up, it may be said that tenosynovectomy is one of the most rewarding operations for rheumatoid arthritis. It quickly relieves pain and eliminates functional disturbances, and also effectively prevents rupture of the tendons. It is also characterized by its long-term effect, which might correspond to active local healing in the majority of cases.

SYNOVECTOMY IN NONRHEUMATIC CONDITIONS

As already stated, the first synovectomy was performed more than 100 years ago, apparently for a tuberculous knee joint. Nowadays, the operation is still undertaken for various conditions, admittedly with different degrees of success. The following are worthy of note: synovectomy for (1) inflammatory diseases such as purulent arthritis or tuberculosis, (2) post-traumatic conditions, (3) osteoarthritis, (4) hemophilia, (5) synovial chondromatosis, and (6) pigmented villonodular synovitis.

In *purulent arthritis*, synovectomy represents a logical therapeutic procedure if the synovial membrane becomes necrotic as a result of delayed application of an effective therapy (antibiotics, drainage), if pockets with retained pus form, and if conservative measures are incapable of coping with the infection. Depending on the state of the joint structures, the synovectomy must be combined with debridement (removal of destroyed menisci, frayed cartilage, necrotic portions of the patellar fat pad, re-

section of adhesions, etc.). Owing to the increased risk of stiffening, particular importance is paid to early mobilization. In case of unsatisfactory mobility we may have to do a manipulation under general anesthesia within the first 2 weeks. The results of this traditional method of treatment for purulent arthritis[168] are satisfactory,[168,169] despite a negative selection of patients being operated upon.

As already stated, *synovectomy in tuberculous joints* would appear to have been the first indication for synovectomy. As long as the process did not originate from the bone or had not already affected the bone, the actual focus of the disease was eliminated by the operation. Even today, when the antibiotic therapy of tuberculosis helps reduce the frequency of the disease to a major extent, synovectomy in combination with drug therapy is one of the most important therapeutic weapons. Particularly with children, in whom the chances of cartilage survival are better than with adults, the results are predominantly good, including restoration of function.[170,171] As long-term studies show, however, secondary arthrotic changes are to be expected in practically every case.[172] Warnings are also expressed[172] with regard to overly optimistic expectations that the disease has been permanently healed by removal of the synovial membrane. When a lesion of the bone is encountered at the same time, efforts to cure must be made through curettage and removal of all the necrotic tissues and abscess pockets, possibly in combination with cancellous bone graft.[171]

Post-traumatic synovitis (e.g., of the knee) is usually associated with recognizable causes: torn menisci, extensive cartilage degeneration, or ligament insufficiencies. The synovitis, which produces a painful effusion, is only a secondary phenomenon and is not the actual cause of the disturbance. Hence, it follows that synovectomy is unable to solve the actual problem. Consequently, long-term improvement cannot be expected unless it is possible to overcome the usual mechanical causes. If, however, an appreciable improvement is realized through synovectomy in a certain percentage of cases,[173] then we are faced with a similar situation to that of synovectomy for osteoarthritis (see below). A significant proportion of the reduction in pain may be attributed to the denervation effect.

Painful swellings in connection with osteoarthritis may be observed in practically every joint. Above all, they are clearly visible externally on the knee and finger joints (proximal interphalangeal—Bouchard osteoarthritis; distal interphalangeal—Heberden osteoarthritis), and occasionally on the elbow joint as well. Based on the satisfactory results obtained with synovectomy in connection with inflammatory arthritis, repeated efforts have recently been made to adapt this procedure for the treatment of osteoarthritis as well. It should be observed, however, that the favorable results are not so frequent as with rheumatoid arthritis and with simple synovectomy they are of only short duration in the majority of cases. For example, the follow-up checks made by Schulitz[174] 3 years after the operation reveal that improvement was observed in only one-fifth of the patients, and that there was a recurrence of pain in the majority of patients within the first year. Only extended debridement, in which synovectomy was accompanied by the removal of osteophytes and free joint bodies, drilling of eburnated bony surfaces, and removal of badly degenerated menisci, yielded a higher success rate.[175-177] In osteoarthritis, synovectomy will not be as successful as it is with rheumatoid arthritis, because with rheumatoid arthritis the main center of the disease is removed by the synovectomy and it is possible that the new articular capsule will exhibit practically normal function.[178] With osteoarthritis, it is different because the disease is primary in the articular cartilage and the synovium is only secondarily involved.

On the basis of our experience, we feel that synovectomy is indicated in osteoarthritis only in exceptional cases, namely, when the synovial membrane is very hyperplastic and inflamed and when a debridement is performed at the same time.

With *hemophilia*, synovectomy has gained increased significance over the last few years, since the risk of bleeding has been shown to be reduced appreciably through specific substitution therapy (see Chapter 99).

According to Storti and associates[179] synovectomy enables two goals to be reached: (1) treatment of already existing hemophilic arthropathy, and (2) prevention of recurrent bleeding. Removal of the hypertrophic synovial tissue improves the hemostatic equilibrium, since synovial tissue is a major source of plasminogen's tissue activators. Clinically, the pain largely disappears and mobility and the ability to walk are improved. Some authors[180,181] advocate an active procedure and recommend synovectomy after two or three hemorrhages in the same joint; others perform repeated aspiration before the operation. Those of us who have had the opportunity to observe extremely hypertrophic tissue, which is repeatedly the source of hemorrhage, will certainly favor early synovectomy.

Synovectomy is particularly indicated as actual therapy when the synovial tissue is of neoplastic, tumor-like character and has a marked tendency toward joint destruction, whether it be attributable to infiltration or mechanical and osteoarthritic joint destruction. This is the case with *pigmented villonodular synovitis* and synovial chondromatosis. With villonodular synovitis, it is the diffuse (in contrast to the nodular, more localized) form for which total synovectomy is now recommended.[182] Whereas both the extra- and intra-articular nodular forms can be excised locally without a recurrence risk in practically every case, the diffuse intra-articular form—despite even radical excision—shows a strong inclination toward recurrence. Since radiotherapy carries some risk of malignant degeneration, there is a trend toward operative removal of the capsule in most cases.

With *synovial chondromatosis*, which primarily affects the knee joint (40 to 60 percent), elbow joint (35 percent), and hip joint (about 10 percent), the latest view[183] with regard to synovectomy is to differentiate the chondromatosis into its respective stages of development. Synovectomy appears to be logical only in the early stage and stage I, in which the pure intrasynovial process has not produced any free joint bodies. Characteristic for this is the swelling of the joint with active intrasynovial proliferation of the cartilage, which occurs repeatedly over a number of years. The value of synovectomy in stage II of intrasynovial affection with the formation of free joint bodies is disputed, whereas in the third and no longer active stage there does not appear to be any justification for synovectomy because the synovial membrane is not productive any more. It may then be the task of the surgeon to remove any existing free joint bodies.

Since the majority of authors do not consider this stage differentiation in their indications, it is difficult to prove numerically to what extent synovectomy is superior to the simple removal of free joint bodies.[184] Because of the frequent osteoarthritic degeneration of the affected joint, early synovectomy is now recommended in conformity with the relevant stage. With this, very good or good results may be obtained in 80 percent of the cases.[185,186] However, with the hip joint, total synovectomy is accomplished only by means of temporary dislocation.[184] On the basis of our experience, this could be effected with an atraumatic procedure without any disadvantage to the blood supply to the femoral head.

References

1. Volkmann, R. von: Cited by Hoffmann, R.: Die Synovektomie unter besonderer Berücksichtigung der an der Erlanger Chirurgischen Universitätsklinik erzielten Erfolge. Dissertation, Erlangen, 1952.
2. Schüller, M.: Cited by Wehner, E.: Die chirurgische Behand-lung der chronischen (nicht spezifischen) Gelenkerkran-kungen. Kapitel 9: Die operative Behandlung der chron-ischen Arthritis (chronischer Gelenkrheumatismus). Köln, 1926.
3. Payr, E.: Erweiterung der Anzeigenstellung für blutige Mobili-sierung versteifter Gelenke. Zentralbl. Chir. 37:746, 1919.
4. Nieny, K.: Zur Behandlung der chronischen Arthritis. Zen-tralbl. Chir. 50:3218, 1927.
5. Jaroschy, W.: Zur Frage der operativen Behandlung der chron-ischen, nicht spezifischen Gelenkerkrankungen. Med. Klin. 32:1214, 1927.
6. Hellner, H.: Die nicht tuberkulöse, chronische Kniegelenks-entzündung und ihre Folgen. Arch. Klin. Chir. 188:251, 1937.
7. Benkovich, G. von: Die chronische zottenbildende Gelenkhautentzündung. Zentralbl. Chir. 34:1572, 1940.
8. Fründ, A.: Binnenerkrankungen des Kniegelenkes. Zentralbl. Chir. 25:1417, 1937.
9. Rostock, P.: Indikationen zur Eröffnung des Kniegelenkes. (64. Tagung der Deutschen Gesellschaft Für Chirurgie.) Zentralbl. Chir. 19:878, 1940.
10. Läwen, A.: Zur Frage der Synovektomie bei chronischen, nicht spezifischen Kniegelenkserkrankungen, Beitr. Klin. Chir. 156:153, 1932.
11. Hoffheinz, S.: Pathologie und Therapie der Gelenkerkrankungen. Zentralbl. Chir. 32:2078, 1931.
12. Erb, V.: Weitere Erfahrungen über die operative Behandlung unspezifischer Kniegelenkserkrankungen. Bruns' Beitr. Klin. Chir. 153:737, 1931.
13. Müller, W.: Zur Frage der operativen Behandlung der Arthritis deformans und des chronischen Gelenkrheumatismus. Langenbecks Arch. Klin. Chir. 47, 1894.
14. Mignon, M.A.: Synovectomie du genou. Bull. Soc. Chir. Paris 26:113, 1900.
15. Goldwaith, J.E.: Infectious arthritis. Boston Med. Surg. J. 150:363, 1904.
16. Murphy, J.B.: Hypertrophic villous synovitis of the knee joint in synovial capsulectomy. Surg. Chir. Murphy 5, 1916.
17. Swett, P.P.: Synovectomy in chronic infectious arthritis. J. Bone Joint Surg. 6:800, 1924.
18. Wilkinson, M.C.: Synovectomy and curettage in treatment of tuberculosis of joints. J. Bone Joint Surg. 35B:209, 1953.

19. Aidem, H.P., and Baker, L.D.: Synovectomy of the knee joint in rheumatoid arthritis. JAMA 187:4, 1964.

20. Vainio, K.: Indications and contraindications for surgery in rheumatoid arthritis. Rheumatism 22:10, 1966.

21. Vaughan-Jackson, O.J.: Le rôle de la chirurgie dan le traitement de la main rhumatismale. Méd. Hyg. (Genève) 24:618, 1966.

22. Hollander, J.L.: Arthritis and Allied Conditions. Philadelphia, Lea & Febiger, 1966.

23. Goldie, J., Göteborg, Sweden: Theoretical aspects on synovectomy of the rheumatoid joint. Personal communication, 1978.

24. Gschwend, N.: Die operative Behandlung der chronischen Polyarthritis. 2nd ed. Stuttgart, Thieme, 1977.

25. Gschwend, N.: Surgical Treatment of Rheumatoid Arthritis. Stuttgart, Thieme, 1980; Philadelphia, W. B. Saunders Company, 1980.

26. Fassbender, H.G.: Pathologie Rheumatischer Erkrankungen. Berlin, Springer, 1975.

27. Fehr, K.: Pathogenese der progredient-chronischen Polyarthritis (pcP). Bern/Stuttgart, Hans Huber Verlag, 1972.

28. Jakubowski, S., and Pongowska, J.: Indikationen zur Synovektomie bei pcP. Orthopäde 2:6, 1973.

29. Gschwend, N.: Die operative Behandlung der chronischen Polyarthritis, 2nd ed. Stuttgart, Thieme, 1977, p. 216.

30. Gschwend, N.: Surgical Treatment of Rheumatoid Arthritis. Stuttgart, Thieme, 1980; Philadelphia, W. B. Saunders Company, 1980.

31. Barbier, M.: Die Synovektomie in der Behandlung der pcP.Z. Rheumaforsch. 32:89, 1973.

32. Flatt, A.: The care of the Rheumatoid Hand. 2nd ed. St. II Louis, C. V. Mosby, 1968.

33. Marmor, L.: Surgery of Rheumatoid Arthritis. Philadelphia, Lea & Febiger, 1967.

34. Benjamin, A., and Helal, B.: Surgical Repair and Reconstruction in Rheumatoid Disease. London, Macmillan Press, 1980.

35. Goldie, I.F. (ed.): Surgery in Rheumatoid Arthritis. Basel, Karger, 1981.

36. Gay, R.: Les synovéctomies dans le traitement de la polyarthrite rhumatoide. Conférence d'enseignement SOFCOT 1971. L'expansion éditeur.

37. Hijmans, W.D.P., and Herschel, H.: Early Synovectomy in Rheumatoid Arthritis. Amsterdam, Excerpta Medica Foundation, 1969.

38. Larsen, A.: A radiological method for grading the severity of rheumatoid arthritis. Thesis, Helsinki, 1974.

39. Dahle, K., and Eek, M.: Preliminary experiences with Larsen's radiological method for grading rheumatoid arthritis. Scand. J. Rheumatol. 4(Suppl. 8):27–28, 1975.

40. Jakubowski, S.: Frühzeitige Synovektomie der Kniegelenke bei primär chronischen Polyarthritis. Beitr. Orthop. Traum. 12:680, 1965.

41. Mori, M.: Anterior capsulectomy in the treatment of rheumatoid arthritis of the knee joint. Arthritis Rheum. 8:130, 1963.

42. Vainio, K.: Synovectomie de genou dans les arthrites rhumatismales. Méd. Hyg. (Genève) 24:616, 1966.

43. Gschwend, N., Winer, J., and Böni, A.: Indikation und Ergebnisse der Synovektomie. Ther. Umsch. 31:475, 1974.

44. Gschwend, N., Winer, J., Böni, A., Busse, W., Dybowski, R., and Zippel, J.: Die operative Synovektomie. Z. Rheumaforsch. 35:32, 1976.

45. Laurin, C.A., Desmarchais, J., Daziano, L., Gariépy, R., and Derome, A.: Long-term results of synovectomy of the knee in rheumatoid patients. J. Bone Joint Surg. 56A:521, 1974.

46. Patiäla, H.: Follow-up study of synovectomy of the knee joint in patients suffering from rheumatoid arthritis. Scand. J. Rheumatol. 5:167, 1967.

47. Mohing, W., and Richter, R.: Die Kniegelenkssynovektomie bei chron. Polyarthritis. Therapiewoche 27:5262, 1977.

48. Lebarbier, P.: Synovéctomie du genou dans la maladie rhumatoide. Résultats à long terme. Thèse 445, 1977.

49. Ranawat, C.S., Ecker, M.L., Straub, L.R.: Synovectomy and debridement of the knees in rheumatoid arthritis. Arthritis Rheum. 15:571, 1972.

50. Taylor, A.R., and Harbison, J.S.: Synovectomy of the knee in RA. Longterm results. Ann. Rheum. Dis. 29:564, 1970.

51. Kuhns, J.G., and Potter, P.A.: Nylon arthroplasty of the knee joints in chronic arthritis. Surg. Gynecol. Obstet. 91:351, 1950.

52. Milch, R.A.: Rationale and technique for radical surgical débridement in the treatment of chronic arthritis of the knee joint. Minerva Med. 52:1514, 1961.

53. Marmor, L.: Surgical treatment of chronic arthritis. Mod. Treat. 1:1313, 1964.

54. Meuli, H.C.: Zur operativen Behandlung der polyarthritischen Hüfte. Deutsch. Med. Wschr. 91:1779, 1966.

55. Jakubowski, S.: Discussion of Symposium on Early Synovectomy in Rheumatoid Arthritis. Amsterdam, 1967.

56. Jakubowski, S.: Synovektomie des obern Sprunggelenkes. Orthopäde 2:79, 1973.

57. Vainio, K.: The Role of Surgery on the Rehabilitation of Rheumatoid Arthritis Patients. Proc. IV European Rheum. Congress. Instanbul Press, Istanbul, 1959.

58. Gschwend, N., Dubs, L., and Humbert, J.-L.: La cheville rhumatoide. Collection de pathologie locomotrice. Paris, Masson, 1982.

59. Tillmann, K.: Der rheumatische Fuss und seine Behandlung. Stuttgart, Thieme, 1977.

60. Vahvanen, V.: Synovectomy of the talo-crural joint in rheumatoid arthritis. Ann. Chir. et Gyn. Fenniae 57, 1968.

61. Clayton, M.L.: Surgery of the lower extremity in rheumatoid arthritis. J. Bone Joint Surg. 45A:1517, 1963.

62. Marmor, L.: The rheumatoid foot. Geriatrics 21:132, 1966.

63. Arner, O., Ekengren, K., Hulting, B., and Linholm, A.: Arthrography of the talo-crural joint. Acta Chir. Scand. 113:253, 1957.

64. Herder, J.W.: De Arthrografie van Net Enkelgewricht. Amsterdam, Soc. Verzekeringsbank, 1961.

65. Hansson, C.J.: Arthrographic studies on the ankle joint. Acta Radiol. 22:281, 1941.

66. Vainio, K.: The rheumatoid foot. Ann. Chir. Gynaec. Fenn. (Suppl. 1):45, 1956.

67. Gschwend, N., Dubs, L., and Humbert, J.-L.: Oberes Sprunggelenk und Polyarthritis. Akt. Rheumatol. 7:199, 1982.

68. Jakubowski, S.: Synovektomie des oberen Sprunggelenks. Orthopäde 2:79, 1973.

69. Roux, H., and Dobbels, E.: Synoviorthèses de la cheville dans la polyarthrite rhumatoide. In Simon, L., et Rodineau, J.: Cheville et médecine de rééducation. Paris, Masson, 1982.

70. Norgaard, F.: Earliest roentgenological changes in polyarthritis of the rheumatoid type: Rheumatoid arthritis. Radiology 85:325, 1965.

71. Brewerton, D.A.: The rheumatoid hand. In Dixon, A. St. J. (ed.): Progress in Clinical Rheumatology. London, Churchill, 1964.

72. Martel, W., Hayes, J.T., and Duff, I.F.: The pattern of bone erosion in the hand and wrist in rheumatoid arthritis, Radiology 84:204, 1965.

73. Kénesi, C.: Traitement chirurgical de la main rhumatismale. L'articulation métacarpophalangienne. Rev. Rhum. 38:307, 1971.

74. Vaughan-Jackson, O.J.: Le rôle de la chirurgie dans le traitement de la main rhumatismale. Méd. Hyg. (Genève) 24:618, 1966.

75. Gschwend, N.: Synovectomy of the finger joint. In Orthopaedic Surgery and Traumatology. 12th SICOT Congress, Tel Aviv, 1972.

76. Gschwend, N., Ehrensperger, E., and Moser, D.: Occupational Therapy in Rheumatoid Arthritis. Occupational Therapy Today and Tomorrow. Proc. 5th Int. Congr. WFOT, Zürick, 1970. Basel, Karger, 1971.

77. Clayton, M.L.: Surgery of the rheumatoid hand. Chir. Orthop. 36:47, 1964.

78. Flatt, A.E.: The Care of the Rheumatoid Hand. 3rd ed. St. Louis, C. V. Mosby Company, 1974.

79. Fowler, S.B.: The hand in rheumatoid arthritis. Am. J. Surg. 29:6, 1963.

80. Henderson, E.D., and Lipscomb, P.R.: Surgical treatment of rheumatoid hand. JAMA 175:341, 1961.

81. Jakubowski, S., Dybowski, W.R., and Bazylczuk, L.: Prophylaktische Chirurgie der Gelenke und Sehnenscheiden bei pcP. Orthop. Traum. 11:806, 1966.

82. Linscheid, R.L., and Lipscomb, P.R.: Advances in surgical treatment of the rheumatoid hand. Minn. Med. 45:273, 1962.

83. Marmor, L.: The rheumatoid hand. Am. Acad. Gen. Pract. 27:120, 1963.

84. Pulvertaft, G.: Surgery in the treatment of the rheumatoid hand. Postgrad. Med. J. 35:113, 1964.

85. Straub, L.R.: Surgical rehabilitation of the hand and upper extremity in rheumatoid arthritis. Bull. Rheum. Dis. 12:265, 1962.

86. Vainio, K.: Synovectomies of the hand and wrist in rheumatoid arthritis. In La Main Rhumatismale. Paris, Expansion Scientifique Francaise, 1966.

87. Vaughan-Jackson, O.J.: Le rôle de la chirurgie dans le traitement de la main rhumatismale. Méd. Hyg. (Genève) 24:618, 1966.

88. Ellison, M.R., Kelly, K.J., and Flatt, A.E.: The results of surgical synovectomy of the digital joints in rheumatoid disease. J. Bone Surg. 52A:1041, 1971.

89. Kénesi, C.: Traitement chirugical de la main rhumatismale. L'articulation métacarpophalangienne. Rev. Rhum. 38:307, 1971.

90. Stellbrink, G., and Tillmann, K.: Resection Arthroplasty of the Wrist in Rheumatoid Arthritis. Vortrag 12. Tel Aviv, SICOT-Kongress, 1972.

91. Lipscomb, P.R.: Synovectomy of the distal two joints of the thumb and fingers in rheumatoid arthritis. J. Bone Joint Surg. 49A:1135, 1967.

92. Pahle, J.: Die Synovektomie der proximalen Interphalangealgelenke. Orthopäde 28:13, 1973.

93. Bunnell, S.: Active splinting of the hand. J. Bone Joint Surg. 28:732, 1946.

94. McCarty, D.J., and Gatter, R.A.: A study of distal interphalangeal joint tenderness in rheumatoid arthritis. Arthritis Rheum. 9:325, 1966.

95. Flatt, A.E.: The Care of the Rheumatoid Hand. St. Louis, C. V. Mosby Company, 1966.

96. Bäckdahl, M.: The caput ulnae syndrome in rheumatoid arthritis. Acta Rheum. Scand. (Suppl. 5), 1963.

97. Lipscomb, P.R.: Tenosynovitis, of the hand and the wrist, carpal tunnel syndrome. De Quervain's disease. Trigger digit. Clin. Orthop. 13:1964, 1959.

98. Fernandez-Palazzi, F., and Vainio, K.: Synovectomy of the carpal joints in rheumatoid arthritis. A report of 47 cases. A. J. R. Arch. Interam. Rheum. (Rio de J.) 8:249, 1965.

99. Mori, M.: Wrist. In Milch, R.A. (ed.): Surgery of Arthritis. Baltimore, Williams & Wilkins Company, 1964.

100. Vaughan-Jackson, O.J.: Le rôle de chirurgie dans le traitement de la main rhumatismale. Méd. Hyg. (Genève) 24:618, 1966.

101. Goldie, J.: Cited by Fernandez-Palazzi and Vainio, Reference 98.

102. Savill, D.L., and Duthie, J.J.R.: Synovectomy of the wrist. In Symposium on Early Synovectomy in Rheumatoid Arthritis. Amsterdam, 1967.

103. Gschwend, N.: Die operative Behandlung der chronischen Polyarthritis. 2nd ed. Stuttgart, Thieme, 1977, p. 83.

104. Popelka, S., and Vainio, K.: Compression of the deep branch of the radial nerve in patients with rheumatoid arthritis. Acta Chir. Orthop. Traum. Cech. 38:195, 1971.

105. Raunio, P., and Jakob, R.: Die Ellbogenarthroplastik in der rheumatoiden Arthritis. Orthopäde 2:102, 1973.

106. Stellbrink, G.: Synovektomie an der oberen Extremität, Indikation und Ergebnisse. Beitr. Orthop. Traum. 18:117, 1971.

107. Raunio, P., and Pätiälä, H.: Synovektomie des Ellbogengelenks. Orthopäde 2:68, 1973.

108. Ehrlich, E.E.: Antecubital cyst in rheumatoid arthritis. A corollary to popliteal (Baker's) cyst. J. Bone Joint Surg. 54A:165, 1972.

109. Michotte, L.J.: La chirurgie de la main et du pied dans la polyarthrite rhumatoide. J. Belge Méd. Phys, Rhum. 18:307, 1963.

110. Ansell, B.M., and Arden, G.P.: Synovectomy of the shoulder. In Early Synovectomy in Rheumatoid Arthritis. Amsterdam, Excerpta Medica Foundation, 1969.

111. Pahle, J.A.: The shoulder joint in rheumatoid arthritis: Synovectomy. Reconstr. Surg. Traumat. 18:33, 1981.

112. McLaughlin, H.L.: Trauma. Philadelphia, W. B. Saunders Company, 1959.

113. Debeyre, J., Patte, D., and Elmelik, E.: Repair of ruptures of the rotator cuff of the shoulder. J. Bone Joint Surg. 47B:35, 1965.

114. Gschwend, N., Winer, J., and Böni, A.: Clinical Results of Synovectomy in Rheumatoid Arthritis. Darmstadt, D. Steinkopff Verlag, 1977.

115. Arthritis and Rheumatism Council and British Orthopaedic Association: Controlled trial of synovectomy of knee and metacarpophalangeal joints in rheumatoid arthritis. Ann. Rheum. Dis. 35:437, 1976.

116. McEwen, C., and O'Brian, W.B.: A multi-center evaluation of early synovectomy in the treatment of rheumatoid arthritis. J. Rheumatol. Suppl. 1:107, 1974.

117. Arthritis Foundation Committee on Evaluation of Synovectomy: Multicenter evaluation of synovectomy in the treatment of rheumatoid arthritis. Arthritis Rheum. 20:765, 1977.

118. Thompson, M., Douglas, G., and Davison, E.P.: Evaluation of synovectomy in rheumatoid arthritis. Proc. Roy. Soc. Med. 66:197, 1973.

119. ERASS (European Rheumatoid Arthritis Surgical Society): Late (more than 10 years) results of synovectomy. Multicenter study. 2nd Congress ERASS, Moskau, 1983.

120. Von Reis, G., and Swensson, A.: Intra-articular injections of osmic acid in painful joint affections. Acta Med. Scand. Suppl. 259, 27, 1951.

121. Ansell, B.M., and Bywaters, E.G.: Rheumatoid arthritis (Still's disease). Pediat. Clin. North Am. 10:921, 1963.

122. Makin, M., and Robin, G.C.: Chronic synovial effusions treated with intra-articular radioactive gold. JAMA 188:725, 1964.

123. Flatt, A.E.: Intra-articular thio-tepa in rheumatoid disease of the hands. Rheumatism 18:70, 1962.

124. Fearnley, M.E.: Intra-articular thio-tepa therapy in rheumatoid arthritis. Ann. Phys. Med. 7:294, 1963.

125. Zuckner, J., et al.: Evaluation of intra-articular thio-tepa in rheumatoid arthritis. Ann. Rheum. Dis. 25:178, 1966.

126. Gross, D.: Chemische Synovektomie mit Senfgas bei primär chronischer Polyarthritis. Z. Rheumaforsch. 22:456, 1963.

127. Mondragon Kalb, M.: Thiotepa en al tratamiento de la arthritis rhumatoide. Medicina 15:82, 1965.

128. Berglöf, F.E.: Further studies on the use of osmic acid in the treatment of arthritis. Acta Rheum. Scand. 10:92, 1964.

129. Martio, J., Isomäki, H., Heikkola, T., and Laine, V.: Intra-articular osmic acid in juvenile rheumatoid arthritis. Scand. J. Rheumatol. 1:5, 1972.

130. Menkes, C.J., Allain, J.P., Genil, C., Witvoet, H., Tak-Tak, H., Simon, F., and Delbarre, F.: La synoviorthèse à l'acide osmique chez l'hémophile. Rev. Rhum. 40:255, 1973.

131. Brattström, H., and Brattström, M.: Kombinierte chemische und operative Synovektomie des Kniegelenks. Orthopäde 2:73, 1973.

132. Jakubowski, S., and Pongowska, J.: Indikationen zur Synovektomie bei pcP. Orthopäde 2:6, 1973.

133. Oka, M., Rekonen, A., and Ruotsi, A.: The fate and distribution of intra-articularly injected osmium tetraoxide. Acta Rheum. Scand. 16:271, 1970.

134. Tillmann, K.: Chemische Synovektomie. Orthopäde 2:10, 1973.

135. Delbarre, F., Menkes, C.J., Aignan, M., Ingrand, J., Lego, A., and Ron-cayrol, R.C.: La synoviorthèse par les radio-isotopes à la main et au poignet. Rev. Rhum. 40:205, 1973.

136. Laine, V.A.I., and Vainio, K.: Möglichkeiten, Begrenzungen und Aussichten der chirurgischen Behandlung des entzündlichen Rheumatismus. Z. Rheumaforsch. 24:81, 1965.

137. Fellinger, K., and Thumb, N.: Résultats du traitement intra-articulaire par l'or radioactif. Rhumat. 2:81, 1972.

138. Piattier-Piketty, Menkes, C.J., Juckman, J., and Delbarre, F.: Effets des injections articulaires d'acide osmique chez le lapin. Rhumat. 3:65, 1973.

139. Boussina, I., Kuzmanovic, J., Esselinck, F.W., and Fallet, G.H.: Résultats thérapeutiques de la synoviorthèse à l'acide osmique. Schweiz. Med. Wschr. 104:693, 1974.

140. Niculescu, N., et al.: Chemische Synovektomie durch Natriumsalze and Fettsäuren. Z. Rheumaforsch. 29:27, 1970.

141. Lewis, D.C., and Ziff, M.: Intra-articular administration of gold salts. Arthritis Rheum. 9:682, 1966.

142. Ansell, B.M., Crook, A., Mallard, J.R., and Bywaters, G.L.E.: Evaluation of intra-articular colloidal gold Au-198 in the treatment of persistent knee effusions. Ann. Rheum. Dis. 22:435, 1963.

143. Gumpel, J.M., Farrar, H.E., and Williams, E.D.: Use of yttrium in persistent synovitis of the knee. Ann Rheum. Dis. 33:126, 1974.

144. Gumpel, J.M., and Roles, N.C.: A controlled trial of intra-articular radiocolloids versus surgical synovectomy in persistent synovitis. Lancet 1:488, 1975.

145. Onetti, C., Gutiérrez, E., Hliba, E., and Aguirre, C.R.: Synoviorthesis with ^{32}P colloidal chromic phosphate in rheumatoid arthritis: Clinical, histophathologic and arthrographic changes. J. Rheumatol. 9:229, 1982.

146. Yates, D.B., Scott, J.T., and Ramsey, N.: Double-blind trial of yttrium 90 for chronic inflammatory synovitis of the knee. Ann. Rheum. Dis. 36:481, 1977.

147. Ingrand, J.: Characteristics of radioisotopes for intra-articular therapy. Ann. Rheum. Dis. 32(Suppl.):3, 1973.

148. Kerschbaumer, F., Falser, N., and Bauer, R.: Synoviorthesis: Therapeutic value, side effects on human cartilage. International Congress of Rheumatology, San Francisco, Abstract No. 610.

149. Lee, P.: Editorial. J. Rheumatol. 9:2, 1982.

150. Virkunen, M., Krusius, E.E., Heiskanen, F.: Experiences of intra-articular administration of radioactive gold. Acta Rheum. Scand. 13:81, 1967.

151. Kalliomäki, J.L., Jalava, S., and Möttönen, M.: On the development of adjuvant arthritis in the joint intra-articularly irradiated by radioactive yttrium 90Y resin. Scand. J. Rheumatol. 3:25, 1974.

152. De la Chapelle, A., Oka, M., Rekonen, A., and Ruotsi, A.: Chromosome damage after intra-articular injections of radioactive yttrium. Ann. Rheum. Dis. 31:508, 1972.

153. Roberts, S.D., and Gillespie, P.J.: Effect of immobilisation on retention of 90Y. Ann. Rheum. Dis. 32:46, 1973.

154. Bauer, R., and Jürger, J.: Die Behandlung der chronischen Arthritis mit radioaktiven Isotopen. Verh. Dtsch. Ges. Orthop. Traum. 57:78, 1971.

155. Stevenson, A.C.: Chromosomal damage in human lymphocytes from radioisotope therapy. Ann. Rheum. Dis. 32:19, 1973.

156. Kyle, V., Hazelman, B.L., and Wraight, E.P.: Yttrium-90 therapy and ^{99m}Tc pertechnetate knee uptake measurements in the management of rheumatoid arthritis. Ann. Rheum. Dis. 42:132, 1983.

157. Guiraudon, D.: Les modifications histologiques de la synoviale après synoviorthèse, Rhumat. 2(Suppl. 1):153, 1972.

158. Isomäki, A.M., Inoué, H., and Oka, M.: Uptake of 90Y resin colloid by synovial membrane in rheumatoid arthritis. Scand. J. Rheumatol. 1:53, 1972.

159. Collan, Y., Lorincz, G., and Laine, V.: Deposition of osmium in rheumatoid synovial tissue after intra-articular injection of osmic acid. Scand. J. Rheumatol. 1:27, 1972.

160. Aignan, M., and Millet-Tesson, M.C.: Aspect macroscopique arthroscopique de la synoviale après synoviorthèse. Rhumat. 2:149, 1972.

161. Howard, L.D.: Surgical treatment of rheumatic tenosynovitis. Am. J. Surg. 89:1163, 1955.

162. Jakubowski, S., Dybowski, W.R., and Bazylczuk, L.: Prophylaktische Chirurgie der Gelenke und Sehnenscheiden bei pcP. Orthop. Traum. 11:806, 1966.

163. Vainio, K.: Die Behandlung rheumatischer Kontrakturen unter besonderer Berücksichtigung von Hand und Finger. Vortr. Kongress der Nordwestdtsch. Orthop. Ges. Marburg a. L., 1965.

164. Swanson, A.B.: Flexible Implant Resection Arthroplasty in the Hand and Extremities. St. Louis, C. V. Mosby Company, 1973.

165. Gschwend, N.: Die Tenosynovektomie bei chronischer Polyarthritis. Sonderheft der Zeitschrift für Orthop. und ihre Grenzgebiete. Stuttgart. Ferdinand Enke Verlag, 1978.

166. Savill, D.L.: Some aspects of rheumatoid hand surgery. In La Main Rhumatismale. Paris, Expansion Scientifique Francaise, 1966.

167. Bruner, I.M.: The selective treatment of Dupuytren's complications and indications for treatment. Edinburgh, Livingstone, 1960.

168. Ballard, A., Burkhalter, W.E., Mayfield, G.W., Dehne. E., and Brown,

P.W.: The functional treatment of pyogenic arthritis of the adult knee. J. Bone Joint Surg. 57A:8, 1975.

169. Kelly, P.J., Martin, W.J., and Coventry, M.B.: Bacterial (suppurative) arthritis in the adult. J. Bone Joint Surg. 57A:1595, 1970.

170. Mortens, J.: Tuberculosis of the Knee Joint. London H.K. Levis & Company Ltd., 1948.

171. Wilkinson, M.C.: Synovectomy and curettage in the treatment of tuberculosis of joints. J. Bone Joint Surg. 35B:209, 1953.

172. Zvantseva, V.A.: Remote results of subtotal synovectomy of the knee joint in adults with tuberculous synovitis. Probl. Tuberk. 53:46, 1975.

173. Lindholm, S. and Pylkkänen, P.: Recurrent effusion in the synovectomized knee joint. Scand. J. Rheumatol. 6:11, 1977.

174. Schulitz, K.P.: Der Wert der Synovektomie bei der Gonarthrose (klinische und experimentelle Ergebnisse). Z. Orthop. 111:537, 1973.

175. Insall, J.: Intra-articular surgery for degenerative arthritis of the knee. J. Bone Joint Surg. 49B:211, 1967.

176. Van der Linden, A.J.: Débridement in case of gonarthrosis. Acta Orthop. Belg. Tome 42:Fasc. 4, 1976.

177. Isserlin, B.: Joint débridement for osteoarthritis of the knee. J. Bone Joint Surg. 32B:302, 1950.

178. Goldie, J.: Theoretical aspects on synovectomy of the rheumatoid joint. Vortrag 1978 Kongress International Rehabilitation Medicine Association. III, Basel.

179. Storti, E., Traldi, A., Tosatti, E., and Davoli, P.G.: Synovectomy in haemophilic arthropathy. Schweiz. Med. Wschr. 100:2005, 1970.

180. Schwägerl, W., Niessner, H., Novotny, C., Thaler, E., and Lechner, K.: Synovektomie bei Blutern. Orthopäde 6:44, 1977.

181. Duthie, R.B., Matthews, J.M., Rizza, C.R., and Steel, W.M.: The management of musculo-skeletal problems in the haemophilias. Oxford, Blackwell, 1972.

182. Martens, M., Tanghe, W., Mulier, J.C., and Willems, D.: Pigmented villonodular synovitis of joints, tendons and bursae. Acta Orthop. Belg. 38:2, 1972.

183. Milgram, J.M.: Synovial osteochondromatosis—a histopathological study of thirty cases. J. Bone Joint Surg. 59A:6, 1977.

184. Christensen, J.H., and Poulsen, J.O.: Synovial chondromatosis. Acta Orthop. Scand. 46:919, 1975.

185. Murphy, S.P., Dahlin, D.C., and Sullivan, C.R.: Articular synovial chondromatosis. J. Bone Joint Surg. 44A:77, 1962.

186. Simon, L., Claustre, J., and Blotman, F.: L'ostéochondromatose synoviale de la hanche. Réunion de l'Académie des Sciences Médicales de Catalogne et des Baléares et de la Société des Sciences Médicales et Biologiques de Montpellier, Barcelona, April 20, 1974.

Chapter 114

Reconstructive Surgery and Rehabilitation of the Hand

Edward A. Nalebuff and Lewis H. Millender

INTRODUCTION

Evaluating the patient with rheumatoid hand deformities and developing a rational plan of treatment can be among the more difficult aspects of rheumatoid surgery, especially considering the great number of joints and tendons which may become involved, the complexity and severity of the deformities, and the functional disabilities which can occur. In addition, patients are seen during various stages of the disease, and the progress and severity of disease will vary with different patients. A clear knowledge of the pathogenesis of the hand deformities, tendon involvements, and interrelationships of the different joints in the hand permits prediction of the types of deformity that may develop and treatment before serious joint destruction develops. For example, when it becomes apparent that a boutonnière deformity or a thumb deformity is occurring, better results can be obtained if surgery is carried out before loss of bone stock and destruction of soft tissue occur. At later stages, more extensive surgical procedures are required.

Because of the progressive nature of the rheumatoid process, it is helpful to consider the treatment in different categories: nonsurgical treatment, preventive or therapeutic surgery, and reconstructive or salvage surgery for specific hand deformities.

NONSURGICAL TREATMENT

Although one often thinks of rest and exercise, splinting, and steroid injections early in the management of rheumatoid hand involvement, these modalities are important during all stages of the disease.[1,2]

Rest and Exercise. The patient with rheumatoid arthritis should understand the principles of rest and exercise and their practical application. Diseased joints require exercise to prevent stiffness and maintain motion; active motion exercise is needed to maintain strong muscles. Conversely, inflamed, painful, swollen joints require rest to decrease acute synovitis. Therefore, when a joint is warm, painful, and inflamed, exercise must be reduced and rest increased. As the inflammatory process subsides, exercise can be increased. Short, frequent periods of exercise are more beneficial than long, vigorous ones, which can activate the synovial inflammation.

One should teach the patient to decide how much exercise and activity she can carry out. She must learn to titer her activity. If after any activity, such as working in the garden, hands become more swollen, more painful, or stiff, then the activity has been too strenuous and it should be altered.

Splinting. Resting and dynamic splints alleviate pain, prevent deformity during the active stages of the disease, and aid in postoperative management. Resting splints can be especially effective for wrist pain and can be fabricated to allow patients to use the hand while wearing the splint.[2] Thumb splints and total hand splints also alleviate pain and rest joints. Various types of dynamic splints are used to stretch out fixed deformities, such as boutonnière deformities. Dynamic splinting is also very important after reconstructive surgery, such as metacarpophalangeal joint arthroplasty.[3–5]

Steroid Injections. The judicious use of local injections of steroids often reduces active synovitis and tenosynovitis. They can be used for symptomatic carpal tunnel syndrome, flexor tenosynovitis, and dorsal tenosynovitis. Frequent and repeated administration to the same area may cause tendon ruptures and steroid-induced arthropathies. One should probably not inject one joint or one tendon sheath more than three times a year.[2] If there is persistence or increase of the local disease after this time, surgical intervention is indicated.[6]

PREVENTIVE AND THERAPEUTIC SURGERY

Dorsal Tenosynovitis. Dorsal tenosynovitis is a frequent manifestation of rheumatoid hand disease, resulting from a proliferation of the tenosynovium which surrounds the extensor tendons over the dorsum of the wrist.[6–8] Dorsal tenosynovitis may be the presenting sign in rheumatoid arthritis, and rheumatoid arthritis must be the primary diagnosis to rule out when dorsal tenosynovitis is present. It produces a soft, nonpainful mass which may be located along any or all of the extensor compartments, and accompanying pain should alert one to underlying radiocarpal or radioulnar involvement.[6,8]

Dorsal tenosynovitis is significant because it may lead to extensor tendon ruptures, either from attrition or from infiltrative disease. Although one cannot predict which patients will rupture tendons, there are certain guidelines which we have found helpful to predict who might rupture. Patients with progressive disease who have not responded to medical therapy rupture tendons more frequently. Patients who have had a previous tendon rupture are more prone to rupture another tendon if they develop tenosynovitis. Patients with a rapidly enlarging synovial mass tend to rupture more frequently.[6,9]

Tenosynovectomy is recommended for patients with persistent tenosynovitis who have not responded to a 4- to 6-month period of conservative therapy. Earlier tenosynovectomy is indicated for patients who are more prone to tendon ruptures.[1,6–10]

The surgical technique is safe and effective and the morbidity is low. The procedure can be carried out under regional anesthesia and the hospital stay is generally only 3 days. Postoperative immobilization is short, and therefore patients generally have little problem regaining their range of motion. Dorsal tenosynovectomy can be carried out in conjunction with other rheumatoid hand surgical procedures, such as distal ulnar excision and wrist synovectomy, which would be carried out through

the same incision or other procedures on the hand and digits. Recurrence after dorsal tenosynovectomy is low, being 5 to 6 percent in 73 patients we reviewed.[11] Tendon rupture after dorsal tenosynovectomy is rare.

Dorsal Tenosynovitis with Extensor Tendon Rupture. The complication of dorsal tenosynovitis is tendon rupture, which occurs secondary to infiltrative tenosynovitis or attrition on a bony spur, such as the distal ulna or Lister's tubercle.[12–14] The most frequent tendons to rupture are the extensors to the ring and small fingers and the long extensor of the thumb. In severe destructive disease, multiple digital extensor tendons rupture. Even the wrist extensor tendons can rupture with a resultant severe flexion deformity of the wrist.[15]

Single extensor tendon ruptures may cause a slight extension lag because of cross-connections between the tendons. A rupture of the extensor digiti quinti tendon may even cause a minimal extensor lag because its function is shared with the common digital extensor. When more than one tendon is ruptured, the extension lag and functional loss become obvious. When patients are examined for extensor tendon function, the extensor digiti quinti should be tested independently, especially when there is a prominent distal ulna which will frequently lead to this tendon rupture.

Because the results of tendon transfer are inversely proportional to the number of tendon ruptures, prompt diagnosis and early treatment are important. In addition, a single rupture frequently is followed by a second and even third rupture. Therefore, an extensor tendon rupture is an indication for prompt surgery to correct the loss and to prevent further complications.[6,11,16,17]

The technique for extensor tendon repair is not complicated. Dorsal tenosynovectomy is carried out and distal ulnar excision is performed if indicated. Also, any bony spicule of the carpus is carefully rongeured away. Wrist joint synovectomy also may be carried out. Either adjacent tendon suture or tendon transfer using extensor indicis proprius is generally used for single and double ruptures (Fig. 114–1). For more complicated ruptures, wrist extensor tendons or flexor digitorum superficialis tendons are utilized.[17,18] In the presence of multiple ruptures with a painful subluxed wrist joint, wrist fusion is carried out in conjunction with tendon transfer. In this situation, the wrist extensor tendons can be utilized to replace the ruptured digital extensors.

The morbidity and the results are directly proportional to the number of tendons ruptured plus the status of the adjacent joints. Because much of the hand must be immobilized for 4 weeks after surgery to allow for tendon healing, joint stiffness may develop, and therefore rehabilitation requires more time plus additional therapy. Because of this, both patients and physicians should be alerted to the complications of dorsal tenosynovitis. Ideally, early tenosynovectomy should be carried out before tendon rupture occurs.

Flexor Tenosynovitis. Flexor tenosynovitis is due to a proliferation of tenosynovium which normally lines the flexor tendons. The signs and symptoms of flexor tenosynovitis are related to the anatomical differences

Figure 114–1. Example of patient with dorsal tenosynovitis and tendon rupture. *A,* Dorsal tenosynovitis with double tendon rupture. *B,* Dorsal tenosynovectomy. Note tenosynovium held by forceps. *C,* Dorsal tenosynovectomy. Note tenosynovium excised prior to transfer. *D,* Tendon transfer completed. Extensor indicis proprius has been transferred to ruptured extensor tendon of fifth digit and ruptured fourth extensor tendon transferred to intact third extensor tendon.

and can be categorized as wrist, palmar, and digital flexor tenosynovitis. As with dorsal tenosynovitis, early diagnosis and prompt treatment of flexor tenosynovitis will prevent the complications of tendon rupture and permanent damage secondary to median nerve compression.[6,9,19]

Wrist Flexor Tenosynovitis. Wrist flexor tenosynovitis presents with signs and symptoms of carpal tunnel syndrome secondary to tenosynovitis within the carpal tunnel, causing compression of the median nerve. Some patients may present with limited active digital flexion owing to impairment of flexor tendon excursion. On physical examination, unless there is limited active range of motion, the signs will be minimal. Because the flexor tendons are covered by thick fascia, wrist flexor tenosynovitis does not bulge, and therefore, in contrast to dorsal tenosynovitis, is much less apparent. If the volar surface of the wrist is observed carefully, loss of skin wrinkles and lack of venous markings can sometimes be

observed. Additionally, evidence of thenar muscle atrophy will sometimes be noted, especially with longstanding median nerve compression.

The treatment for early wrist flexor tenosynovitis is steroid injection, wrist splinting, and medical management. For persistent wrist flexor tenosynovitis, carpal tunnel release and tenosynovectomy should be carried out early to prevent permanent median nerve damage, to restore active digital flexion, and to prevent tendon rupture.[6,9] (Fig. 114–2).

Palmar Flexor Tenosynovitis. Tenosynovitis proliferating within the proximal portion of the palm will result in snapping and locking as the tendon slides within the tendon sheath. Patients will usually be able to flex the digit fully, but as the digit extends the nodule catches on the proximal edge of the tendon sheath and the digit snaps into extension. Sometimes the digit will become acutely locked in flexion and cannot be extended actively. A painful snap occurs as the digit is passively

Figure 114–1 *Continued. E* and *F*, Range of motion demonstrated 3 months postoperatively.

extended. On examination, the flexor tendon nodule can be palpated and one can feel a grating as the patient actively flexes and extends his digit.[6,9]

Digital Flexor Tenosynovitis. In contrast to palmar flexor tenosynovitis, digital flexor tenosynovitis is due to proliferation of tenosynovium within the digit. The most common finding in this condition is loss of active digital flexion with preserved passive digital flexion. This is due to impairment of tendon excursion within the narrow tendon sheath. Additionally, grating and locking can be seen as the tendon nodule slides within the sheath, and a fullness can sometimes be felt and observed over the volar surface of the digit.[6,9]

A less common but important manifestation of digital flexor tenosynovitis is stiffness of the proximal interphalangeal joints. In some rheumatoid patients, especially those with proximal interphalangeal joint synovitis associated with pain, limited active flexion associated with digital flexor tenosynovitis can lead to proximal interphalangeal joint stiffness. This occurs because the patients are unable to flex the digits actively, and this, plus the associated proximal interphalangeal joint synovitis with pain, will lead to proximal interphalangeal joint stiffness. The diagnosis is established by obtaining a history of flexor tenosynovitis (previous locking, snapping, or limited active range of motion prior to stiffness) and from noting proximal interphalangeal joint stiffness

with minimally involved joints by x-ray. In addition, some digits may show only loss of active motion with preserved passive range of motion which will help to establish the diagnosis.

The treatment for early palmar and digital flexor tenosynovitis is steroid injection and medical therapy. However, palmar and digital flexor tenosynovectomy should be carried out for persistent flexor tenosynovitis that does not respond to conservative therapy. For proximal interphalangeal joint stiffness secondary to this condition, tenosynovectomy plus proximal interphalangeal joint manipulation and a vigorous postoperative hand therapy program can often restore a considerable range of motion.[6,9]

Flexor Tendon Rupture. Flexor tendon rupture can occur within the carpal tunnel, palm, or digit. Fortunately, it is not common, because the results of treatment for multiple palmar and digital flexor tendon ruptures are not as good as their extensor counterpart.

At the wrist, attrition ruptures of the flexor pollicus longus and/or the flexors of the index finger are caused by a bony spur of the scaphoid which protrudes volarly. Additionally, flexor tendon rupture within the carpal tunnel can occur from infiltrative flexor tenosynovitis.[6,9]

Within the palm and digit, flexor tendon ruptures are less common because there are no bony spurs which lead to attrition ruptures and also because the symptoms

Figure 114–2. Patient with flexor tenosynovitis. *A*, Patient presents with symptoms of carpal tunnel syndrome. Note limited active digital flexion. *B*, Passive digital flexion preserved. *C*, Flexor tenosynovectomy. Note median nerve retracted with Penrose drain. Also note flexor tendons bound with flexor tenosynovium which prevents active digital flexion. *D*, Flexor tenosynovectomy. Note flexor tenosynovium being excised from tendons. *E*, Flexor tenosynovectomy completed. Note specimen demonstrated on 4 × 4 sponge. Also note that all flexor tendons are intact and show little evidence of infiltration or damage.

of locking and snapping will cause the patient to seek earlier medical treatment, which will result in earlier diagnosis and treatment.[6,9]

Flexor tendon rupture in the wrist is treated with tenosynovectomy, removal of the scaphoid spur, and often a bridge graft or tendon graft for the ruptured flexor pollicis longus and a side-to-side suture of the ruptured flexor digitorum profundus (Fig. 114-3). If a single rupture is diagnosed within the digit or palm, prompt flexor tenosynovectomy is advisable to prevent a rupture of the remaining intact tendon.[6,9] If flexor digitorum profundus rupture occurs, tenodesis or arthrodesis of the distal interphalangeal joint is indicated. For flexor digitorum sublimis rupture, only tenosyno-

vectomy is indicated to protect the intact flexor digitorum profundus.

The difficult problem arises when both flexor digitorum profundus and flexor digitorum sublimis ruptures occur within the same digit, thereby eliminating both distal interphalangeal and proximal interphalangeal joint flexion. The results of tendon grafts, either primary or secondary to a tendon rod, are often disappointing. Therefore, in older patients or those with severe joint involvement, the best approach has generally been to carry out proximal interphalangeal and distal interphalangeal joint arthrodeses in an acceptable position of function. Active motion of the metacarpophalangeal joints will still be possible because of the intact intrinsic

Figure 114–3. Flexor pollicis longus rupture. *A,* Roentgenogram of patient with ruptured flexor pollicis longus. Note erosion of the scaphoid which caused attrition rupture of the flexor pollicis longus. *B,* Another patient with ruptured flexor pollicis longus. Flexor tendons exposed. Ruptured flexor pollicis longus held with forceps. Synovium from scaphotrapezial joint can be seen (arrow). Sharp spur on scaphoid can be palpated adjacent to this capsular tear. Also, note ruptured proximal tendon plus intact digital flexors. *C,* Flexor tendon graft attached by pull-out wire prior to proximal anastomosis. *D* and *E,* Range of motion of interphalangeal joint of thumb 4 months postoperatively.

muscles. One can also suture one of the ruptured long flexor tendons into the base of the proximal phalanx to increase strength of metacarpophalangeal joint flexion.

Synovectomy (see also Chapter 113). In contrast to tenosynovectomy, which is an established surgical procedure, the case for synovectomy in the small joints of the wrist and hand is certainly less well established. The reason for this is that no good data have been presented to show that synovectomy will appreciably alter the natural course of the disease. Even though we cannot predictably state the long-term results of synovectomy, the procedure does have some definite, although limited, indications in the hand.[2,8]

The primary indications for synovectomy of the wrist or digital joints are for the small group of patients with smoldering, slowly progressive disease who are responding to systemic medication but who continue to show synovitis in one or more joints. Typically, this patient has responded to three steroid injections over a 6- to 12-month period, but continues to develop recurrent synovitis, sometimes with pain. Roentgenograms show minimal involvement with little evidence of progression. Synovectomy will alleviate pain in this patient and, ideally, delay or prevent further joint destruction. In contrast to this patient with mild disease, when synovectomy is attempted in patients who show a more destructive progressive type of disease, it is less frequently successful in preventing further joint destruction and further progression of the disease and is often followed by a loss of joint motion.

Synovectomy can be carried out in almost any joint of the hand or wrist. On our service, it is more frequently carried out in the wrist to relieve pain. Synovectomy is also useful in the proximal interphalangeal joints, especially to prevent progressive boutonnière deformities, which are difficult to treat in the advanced stages.[20]

Synovectomy is less frequently indicated in the digital metacarpophalangeal joints.[21] Because of the many factors working to cause volar and ulnar deformity, progression of the deformity is frequently not altered by this procedure. Even though there is little articular cartilage or bony joint destruction within the metacarpophalangeal joints, if there is early subluxation or a moderate amount of ulnar drift, we have been reluctant to carry out synovectomy even when associated with intrinsic release and extensor tendon relocation. In these conditions, we would either carry out arthroplasty or wait until there was more deformity, and then resort to arthroplasty.

RECONSTRUCTIVE AND SALVAGE SURGERY

In spite of early recognition, splinting, and "prophylactic surgery," the natural progression of rheumatoid arthritis often leads to destructive changes in the joints of the hand and wrist. The late effects of this disease include loss of articular cartilage, stretching of the joints' supporting structures, and actual bone loss. The clinical aspects of these changes include pain, instability, and deformity with subsequent loss of function. Once these changes have occurred, it is no longer possible to restore the joint to its former state. The surgeon must then resort to "salvage" surgery to relieve pain and provide stability and motion. No joint of the hand is immune to these destructive changes. The surgeon in reality has only two choices in the management of destroyed joints—fusion or arthroplasty. Each of these procedures has pluses and minuses and therefore represents a compromise with full function. The surgical choice between these two operations takes judgment and experience.

Many factors must be considered in making the choice between fusion and arthroplasty. The most important factor to consider is which joint is involved. Other factors that must be taken into account at each joint level will be discussed in more detail.

Metacarpophalangeal Joints. The metacarpophalangeal joints of the hand are single condylar joints allowing 70 to 80 degrees of flexion as well as rotary and lateral motions. They play a very important role in positioning the fingers; if fixed in poor position, they will greatly reduce hand function. Unfortunately, metacarpophalangeal joint involvement is common in rheumatoid arthritis. The capsule laxity which gives the joints varied mobility makes subluxation and dislocation common late sequelae of synovitis. The extensor tendons pass precariously across the joints and, with stretching of the supporting attachments, often deviate ulnarward and then slip between the metacarpal heads. Once this has occurred, all extensor force is lost and progressive flexion of the metacarpophalangeal joints occurs. As the patient tries to extend the joints, they deviate ulnarward instead. There is often a stretching of the radial collateral ligaments and subsequent shortening of the ulnar collateral ligaments and intrinsic muscles. The end result may appear as dislocated metacarpophalangeal joints with the fingers fixed in flexion or severely deviated ulnarward. The net result is a significant loss of hand function—for example, the ability to grasp large objects if the fingers are fixed in flexion. With ulnar deviation, the fingers are beyond the reach of the thumb, and precision activities requiring thumb-digit apposition are lost.

In order to restore function, we feel that arthroplasty is the treatment of choice at the metacarpophalangeal level. Although fusion of the metacarpophalangeal joints can be obtained with the finger realigned, the presence of metacarpophalangeal joint motion greatly enhances overall gripping ability. With the arthroplasty techniques now available, this can be achieved in a predictable way. Arthroplasties to correct deformity and relieve pain while maintaining motion are best exemplified at the metacarpophalangeal joint level. It was here that arthroplasties of rheumatoid hands were first attempted, and the surgical lessons learned were later used at the proximal interphalangeal joint levels.

The initial attempts to correct metacarpophalangeal deformities while maintaining motion were made 20 years ago by Riordan and Fowler.[22] Their resection-type arthroplasty consisted of resecting enough of the metacarpal heads to allow digital realignment. The fingers were then held in place with Kirschner wires for approximately a month, after which motion was allowed, using dynamic splinting to maintain alignment as motion was regained. In order to support the resected joint surfaces, local soft tissue structures such as the extensor tendons were sutured to the bases of the proximal phalanges. Vaino,[23] in Finland, and Tupper,[24] in this country, modified the resection arthroplasty using the volar plate as a supporting structure interposed between the metacarpal and proximal phalanges. Although these techniques are still being used today, most surgeons utilize an implant to help maintain digital alignment and motion. The search for the ideal implant is a continuing process. Initial attempts to improve upon resection arthroplasty using a prosthetic replacement were made by Flatt,[1] who designed a hinged metallic device with double prong stems, inserted into the medullary canals of the metacarpal and proximal phalanges. These first generation joint replacements were utilized during the early 1960s but lost popularity as a result of the frequent complications, such as implant fracture, bone resorption, and perforation of the rigid metallic stems of the prostheses. In the latter 1960s, Swanson[5,25,26] and Neibauer[27] independently developed a "second generation" prosthesis made of silicone rubber. In both designs, the prosthesis acts as a flexible implant or spacer between the resected bone ends. The design of each implant differs, in that the stems of the Neibauer implant are Dacron coated to allow bone ingrowth into the prosthesis. The Swanson implant does not have a Dacron covering, and does not become fixed to the intramedullary canals. The implant depends for support upon the encapsulation which surrounds it. Motion is achieved both by implant flex and by a sliding action along the implant stem. We prefer the Swanson-type implant arthroplasty, and in this chapter use of the term "arthroplasty" at the metacarpophalangeal and proximal interphalangeal joints is to be construed by the readers as this type (Fig. 114-4D).

"Third generation" prostheses have been developed, in which miniature total joint replacements, made of metal and plastic portions cemented into the intramedullary canal of the resected joints, are used. There are numberous designs of these prostheses. As yet, none has replaced the flexible implant arthroplasty's popularity.

Figure 114–4. Arthroplasty of the metacarpophalangeal joints—indications. *A,* Even with severe finger deformities this patient maintains significant hand function. She demonstrates ability to manipulate delicate electronic components. Arthroplasty was delayed until function decreased. *B,* This patient has dislocated metacarpophalangeal joints limiting extension and ability to grasp large objects. Metacarpophalangeal arthroplasties are indicated. *C,* A common indication for arthroplasty is severe fixed ulnar deviation as seen in the patient's middle, ring, and small fingers. *D,* Preferred arthroplasty is the Swanson flexible hinge implant shown here.

The newer designed prostheses are more difficult to insert, have more potential complications, and do not provide better motion or alignment than the flexible silicone rubber implants.

Results of Arthroplasty. With the flexible implant arthroplasty, the surgeon can, in most cases, correct metacarpophalangeal joint subluxation, dislocations, and ulnar deviation of the fingers (Fig. 114-5). There are numerous factors which affect the ultimate result, including the condition of the surrounding soft tissues, the strength and mobility of the controlling muscles, the status of the adjacent joints, the use of the postoperative splinting and exercises,[7] and, last but not least, the motivation of the patient. With proper surgical technique, and barring complications, the surgeon should expect to realign the digit, relieve pain originating at the metacarpophalangeal level, and maintain between 30 and 75 degrees of motion.

The complications of implant arthroplasty include recurrent ulnar drift, limited motion, implant fracture, dislocation, and infection.[28] Recurrent ulnar drift is seen with insufficient soft tissue repairs on the radial side of the joint or failure to adequately release the right, shortened ulnar structures. Failure to utilize postoperative splinting also can lead to this problem. However, if sufficient soft tissue release and bone resection are obtained at surgery and then followed by postoperative splinting, this complication is unlikely to occur. In some patients, realignment of the fingers and relief of pain are obtained but the range of motion is less than anticipated. Inadequate surgical release of contracted soft tissues may be a factor, but this complication often occurs if the patient has limited excursion and strength of the flexor muscles and tendons. Postoperative exercises play a very important role in determining the range of motion achieved.[7] If inadequate motion is obtained, revision of the arthroplasty is possible and can restore motion. Implant fracture can also occur, but its frequency is low (less than 5 percent) with the high performance "silicone rubber" used today. In fact, implant fracture is often

Figure 114–5. Example of metacarpophalangeal arthroplasty to improve joint function and appearance of rheumatoid hand deformity. *A*, Preoperative digital extension. Note metacarpophalangeal joint subluxations with associated boutonniere deformity of middle finger. *B*, Preoperative radiograph shows advanced wrist involvement in addition to metacarpophalangeal and proximal interphalangeal joint deformities. *C*, Note improved function and appearance of hand and wrist following second stage wrist fusion and metacarpophalangeal arthroplasties. *D*, Excellent postoperative digital flexion.

asymptomatic and noted only by x-ray. Several months following implant insertion, encapsulation has already taken place. Once this has occurred, implant fracture may not significantly affect the result. Dislocations of the implant are rare and usually occur at the time of surgery or shortly thereafter. When this complication occurs, replacement is usually needed to restore proper digital alignment.

Infections around the implant occur in fewer than 1 percent of the joints inserted.[28] Usually an isolated joint is involved, and removal of the implant combined with appropriate antibiotic coverage is sufficient to control the infection. Removal of the implant converts the arthroplasty to a resection type, and some loss of motion is anticipated.

Proximal Interphalangeal Joints. The proximal interphalangeal joints, like their distal counterparts, are hinge joints allowing flexion and extension. The range of motion at this level is normally full extension to 110 degrees of flexion. This mobility, although only slightly greater than that at the distal joint, is far more important in bringing the fingertip toward the palm. Its flexion combined with 70 or 80 degrees of metacarpophalangeal joint motion is all that is required for the fingertips to reach the distal palmar crease without any additional help from the distal joints. For this reason, loss of motion at the proximal interphalangeal level is more of a hardship for the patient, and attempts to preserve it are more frequently indicated (Fig. 114–6). The need for lateral stability is still important. However, it is technically easier to restore collateral ligament support, and in the middle digits (ring and long fingers) the adjacent finger provides a measure of lateral support when the patient makes a fist. This lack of adjacent digital support is particularly noted in the index finger and makes fusion of the proximal interphalangeal joint more frequently indicated in this finger (Fig. 114–7). Unlike the distal joints, in which fusion is the procedure of choice in salvage conditions, the surgeon has a choice between a fusion or flexible implant arthroplasty at this level. Factors to consider in making this decision include the type or severity of deformity, which digit is involved, the condition of adjacent joints, and the status of the extensor and flexor apparatus.

The deformities at the proximal interphalangeal joint are flexion, hyperextension, and lateral deformities. Flexion deformities are usually secondary to a lack of extensor support at the proximal interphalangeal joint. The central slip of the extensor mechanism attaches to the base of the middle phalanx and is essential in maintaining or providing active extension. Unfortunately, synovitis of the proximal interphalangeal joints stretches out this thin structure, and the ability to extend the proximal interphalangeal joint actively is lost. As the joint slips into flexion, secondary changes occur. The lateral bands of the extensor mechanism are displaced volarly, and, as they contract in this position, they lead to distal joint hyperextension. At first, this "boutonnière deformity" is passively correctible, but later the accessory collateral ligaments and volar plates shorten and

the deformity becomes fixed. As the fixed deformity increases in degree, the surgical ability to restore extension becomes less. Beyond a certain point (70 to 80 degrees of fixed flexion), it is usually not possible to restore full extension at the proximal interphalangeal level even by a resection of bone, and one must choose fusion as a salvage procedure of choice.

Hyperextension deformities of the proximal interphalangeal joint can be primary or secondary. Stretching out of the volar plate by synovitis or rupture of the superficial flexor tendon can lead to primary proximal interphalangeal joint hyperextension. A mallet deformity distally or a metacarpophalangeal flexion deformity with intrinsic tightness can also lead to secondary proximal interphalangeal joint hyperextension followed by a distal joint flexion. The combined proximal interphalangeal joint hyperextension and distal joint flexion is called a "swan neck deformity." If the proximal interphalangeal joint surfaces are intact and nonpainful, correction of the deformity and restoration of motion can be achieved by various soft tissue procedures. However, in the late stages with irregular joint surfaces, the surgeon again must resort to either fusion or arthroplasty to correct the deformity and eliminate pain. If mobility is also desired, the arthroplasty must be selected as the surgical procedure. At this point, the surgeon must weigh the other factors to be considered in making this choice, including which finger is involved.

The ability to flex the proximal interphalangeal joints becomes increasingly important as one moves from the index to the small digit. The index finger is used in picking up objects or performing delicate tasks in opposition with the thumb. It is particularly important in lateral pinch, in which the thumb presses against this radial surface. Most of these functions are carried out with the proximal interphalangeal joint in slight to moderate flexion. For this reason, fusion of the index finger proximal interphalangeal joint is less of a handicap than fusion of the more ulnar digits used in grasp. In the ring and small fingers, acute flexion of the PIP joint is needed to grasp small objects firmly. For this reason, we are apt to choose arthroplasty over fusion in these digits, and, if fusion is selected because of other factors, the position chosen to stabilize the joint is in more flexion than that chosen for the index finger.

The condition of the adjacent joints must be taken into account in making the choice between proximal interphalangeal joint fusion or arthroplasty. If the distal joints have already been or must be fused, this increases the indication for arthroplasty at the proximal interphalangeal level. On the other hand, if one anticipates arthroplasties at the metacarpophalangeal joint level, the surgeon may decide on fusion for the proximal interphalangeal joints. If the intramedullary canals are of sufficient size and the extensor flexor tendons are functioning well, it is possible and even desirable to perform arthroplasties at both the proximal interphalangeal and metacarpophalangeal levels, particularly for the ulnar digits, in order to allow grasping of small objects. In order for an implant arthroplasty to function, it is nec-

Figure 114–6. Example of proximal interphalangeal joint arthroplasties for severe deformities. *A,* Preoperative views of hand with fingers in extension. Note severe lateral deformities of proximal interphalangeal joints. *B,* Patient's fingers overlap on attempted flexion. Grasping ability is poor. *C,* Postoperative extension following proximal interphalangeal arthroplasties. *D,* Postoperative flexion.

essary that the tendon muscle units controlling motion of the joints have sufficient power and amplitude. It is foolhardy to insert a joint prosthesis, unless the extensor and flexor tendons are functioning or can be restored. This is particularly important with the flexor tendons. If the flexor tendons are ruptured, it is probably wiser to fuse a destroyed proximal interphalangeal joint than to try to obtain motion. On the other hand, flexor tendons with limited excursion secondary to adhesions and/or nodular tenosynovitis can usually be restored by ten-

osynovectomy and tenolysis. This type of tendon involvement is, therefore, not a contraindication to arthroplasty.

Distal Interphalangeal Joints. The distal interphalangeal joints of the digits, like the proximal interphalangeal joints, are hinge joints, normally allowing 70 to 80 degrees of flexion from a fully extended position. With intact collateral ligaments, the joints are quite stable against lateral stresses. The volar support is provided by a thickened capsule (volar plate) which with

Figure 114–7. Proximal interphalangeal fusion of index finger for fixed flexion deformity. *A*, Note poor pinch posture because of severe flexion contracture of index proximal interphalangeal joint. *B*, Improved function obtained by fusion of proximal interphalangeal joint in 25-degree flexion.

an intact flexor digitorum profundus tendon resists hyperextension forces. Normal extension is provided by an intact extensor mechanism attached to the base of the distal phalanges. This extensor mechanism is activated by both the digital extensor muscles and the intrinsics (lumbrical and interossei muscles) of the hand. As a result of rheumatoid arthritis, the cartilaginous joint surfaces can be destroyed, which results in pain and limitation of motion. The loss of bone substance or collateral ligament support can lead to lateral deformities. Attenuation or rupture of the distal extensor attachment is followed by a "mallet" deformity, while stretching out of the volar plate or rupture of the long flexor tendon can result in distal joint hyperextension. As a result of these changes, either singularly or in combination, the patient develops an unsightly deformity which not only is painful but also results in decreased function.

Unfortunately, it is not possible to restore a damaged joint to its former state, and the surgeon must then aim his sight at a somewhat lower target—relief of pain, correction of deformity, and restoration of useful function. Of the two salvage procedures, fusion or arthroplasty, fusion is the preferred treatment at the distal joint level. There are two main reasons for this approach: (1) the difficulty involved in restoring active motion and joint stability; and (2) the relative unimportance of mobility in the distal joints. Although it is technically possible to insert a joint prosthesis, repair the extensor mechanism, reconstruct the collateral ligaments, and even restore flexor tendon function, the potential gain is not worth the inherent risks, except in highly selected

cases. Actually, the loss of motion in the distal joint is not particularly disabling if the joint is stable in good position. The best position of the distal joint is either full extension or, at most, 5 to 10 degrees of flexion. In this position, the digit has a normal appearance with the fingers extended. When the patient makes a fist, the lack of distal joint motion is not obvious and of little functional significance. Picking up or holding objects between the thumb and the involved digit is not compromised, with the distal joint being almost straight. This position enhances "pulp to pulp" pinch, which is more useful than "tip pinch," which requires distal joint mobility.

Fusion of the distal joints not only achieves a beneficial effect at the operative site but can help function at the more proximal joint level. For example, a distal joint fusion in neutral position balances the extensor and flexor forces. This can be helpful in correcting a mild swan neck deformity (proximal interphalangeal hyperextension) that was secondary to a distal joint mallet deformity.[20,21,29] In addition, fusion in the distal joint simplifies and strengthens extensor or flexor forces at the proximal interphalangeal joint level, where active motion is more important than at the distal joint.

The Wrist. The wrist is the foundation upon which hand function is built. A painful unstable wrist will reduce hand function without digital involvement and, in fact, may be a primary factor in producing digital deformities. Deformities of the wrist result from several factors. Early synovial involvement occurs between the carpal bones, with the scaphoid-lunate being the most common area of early synovitis. Stretching of the intercarpal and radiocarpal ligaments by synovitis leads to a disruption and subsequent shifting of the carpal bones in relationship to the radius. The carpus can shift ulnarward or volarward in relationship to the radius. With volar shift, the carpus can dislocate and displace proximally. A secondary phenomenon that occurs is attrition ruptures of the wrist extensor tendons, further aggravating the dislocation and leading to severe flexion deformity of the wrist. With ulnar shift of the carpus, there is often a radial rotation of the wrist. Stretching of the extensor carpi ulnaris tendon or rupture of this stabilizing force is also thought to be a significant factor in this deformity. With radial rotation of the carpus, the metacarpals become angulated radially in relationship to the radius, and this in turn is followed by ulnar deviation of the digits at the metacarpophalangeal joints.[30] Patients who have this "zigzag" deformity are poor candidates for metacarpophalangeal arthroplasties to correct the ulnar deviation until the wrist alignment has been restored. Chronic synovitis of the distal radioulnar joint stretches the supporting ligaments, maintaining proper alignment between the radius and ulna. Dorsal displacement of the ulna follows, and, if bony erosions have occurred, the rough edge which protrudes dorsally can wear away the adjacent extensor tendons to the fingers.

In advanced cases, surgical attempts to realign the wrist and alleviate pain include total or partial fusion and arthroplastsy. The choice between these procedures depends upon many factors, including the condition of the wrist extensors, the amount of bone resorbed in the carpus, and the status of the hand, the opposite wrist, and even the lower extremities. Total wrist fusion accomplishes several things. It eliminates pain, provides stability for hand function, and corrects alignment.[31–35] Although the patient gives up flexion and extension motions, supination and pronation are preserved. The position of fusion is important. At one time, it was felt that the dorsiflexed position was best, as grip strength was enhanced in this position. However, experience with many patients having undergone surgical or spontaneous wrist fusion has shown that the preferred position is with the wrist in neutral or slightly flexed.[35] This puts the wrist in a natural position from which it is easy to carry out personal hygiene and other activities of daily living. The great advantage in a solid wrist fusion is stability and dependability. Disease is arrested at this site, and it no longer is a source of pain. Progression or recurrence of deformity is now halted. If the patient has lower extremity problems which require a cane or crutch support, the fused wrist provides the necessary support. The benefits of a single fused wrist far outweigh the disadvantages of the loss of flexion and extension, and in the young vigorous patient this is a reliable solution to the problem of a destroyed wrist joint.

Although total wrist fusion has been an accepted treatment for the severely involved wrist, there are many patients in whom the major changes are limited to the radiocarpal joints with the midcarpal area still preserved. In those patients with ulnar shift of the lunate (usually associated with rotary subluxation of the scaphoid) the articulations about the capitate are preserved. We feel the preferred treatment in these patients is partial wrist fusion. This implies radiolunate fusion, which stops ulnar translocation of the carpus and usually includes radioscaphoid fusion as well. Those patients undergoing partial (radiocarpal) wrist fusion maintain about 50 percent of normal wrist motion.

Since this disease is usually symmetrical in its distribution, the loss of bilateral wrist motion can create a functional loss for the patient. In those patients whose major difficulty with the wrist is pain and in whom a significant range of motion is still present an alternative treatment, arthroplasty, is available. Attempts to preserve motion at the wrist have paralleled those in the digits. Initial arthroplasties relied upon the wrist capsule and surgical alterations of the shape of the distal radius to form a shelf.[36] Swanson introduced a flexible wrist implant shaped like the digital implant.[5] In this arthroplasty, the lunate and scaphoid are removed, and the stems of the implant are inserted into the radius proximally and the capitate and third metacarpal shaft distally. The early results of this implant have been excellent, relieving pain, restoring alignment, and allowing some motion. In our early series of 60 Swanson implants, an average range of motion of over 60 degrees was obtained. Our results have shown that patients with implants obtained relief from pain with grip strengths equal to the fused side. Therefore, if there is good bone stock, an adequate-sized intramedullary canal in the third metacarpal, functioning extensor tendons, and involvement of the opposite wrist, we are more likely to perform a wrist arthroplasty than a total wrist fusion.

With the popularity and success of total joint replacements at the hip and knee, it was inevitable that total wrist joints would be developed. In order to insert most of the presently available total wrist joint prostheses, considerable bone must be resected and the prostheses are usually cemented into place. At present, we are reluctant to utilize this technique because of the added risks and seriousness of the potential complications.

Disabilities of the distal radiocarpal joint are treated by limited resection of the distal ulna. If adequate soft tissues are preserved, the ulna does not subluxate with rotation. By removing irregular bone ends and covering the resected end of the distal ulna with the dorsal retinaculum, the risk of extensor tendon rupture is minimized. Swanson has developed a distal ulnar prosthesis which provides a cap over the distal ulna.[37] The prosthesis restores some length to the ulna, and also reduces the risk of tendon rupture.

The Thumb. The thumb of the rheumatoid patient deserves special comment. Its importance to hand function is well recognized. Unfortunately, it is frequently involved with rheumatoid arthritis and can, as a result of muscular imbalance and/or joint destruction, assume bizarre deformities.[38] The most common deformity seen originates at the metacarpophalangeal joint, which assumes a flexed position secondary to stretching out or loss of the extensor force. As sequelae of this, the distal joint assumes a hyperextended position, and the patient tends to adduct the first metacarpal to substitute for the lack of extension. This thumb deformity is made worse with each pinch force of the thumb against the other digits. The reverse deformity with metacarpophalangeal joint hyperextension is usually secondary to changes at the carpometacarpal joint level with synovitis. The carpometacarpal joint subluxes and the first metacarpal adducts. The patient then hyperextends the metacarpophalangeal joint to substitute for the lost abduction. With the tendon imbalance produced, the distal joint often assumes a flexed position. Other deformities can occur as a result of collateral ligament or tendon ruptures occurring in combination with joint changes.

How does one treat the advanced thumb deformity? The distal joint of the thumb is treated in similar fashion to the distal joints of the other digits—by fusion. It is usually fused in the straight or slightly flexed position to restore a stable pinch (Fig. 114–8). At the thumb metacarpophalangeal joint level, as at the digital proximal interphalangeal joints, one can choose between fusion or arthroplasty. With isolated metacarpophalangeal

joint disease, a fusion in 15 degrees of flexion gives excellent results with little functional loss. However, with associated interphalangeal joint disease we would prefer an arthroplasty at the metacarpophalangeal level in order to avoid fusion of two adjacent joints. At the carpometacarpal joint level it is important to maintain motion. A fusion here could become quite disabling if the patient developed subsequent instability and required fusions distally. Because of the loss of bone stock in the carpus, the trapezium implants found to be successful in degenerative arthritis have tended to sublux in rheumatoid arthritic patients. For this reason, the resection type arthroplasty has been preferred, in which the trapezium is removed, allowing the metacarpal to be realigned properly. We now use a modified arthroplasty in which the base of the metacarpal is resected and a Swanson toe implant inserted as a space maintainer between the metacarpal base and the remaining portion of the trapezium or carpus.

In summary, much can be done for the rheumatoid patient with hand involvement. Early prophylactic surgery, splinting, and exercises can slow but not stop the

Figure 114–8. Unstable distal joint treated by fusion with bone graft. *A,* Clinical appearance of the thumb with collapse of interphalangeal joint. *B,* Radiograph shows significant absorption of the distal end of the proximal phalanx. *C,* Postoperative radiograph shows use of bone graft to restore length and facilitate joint fusion. *D,* Note stable pulp pinch between lengthened thumb and index finger. Distal joint fused in slight flexion.

progression of deformity. Therapeutic operations on the tendons and nerves can restore lost function, and salvage surgery such as fusion can correct deformities and eliminate pain where motion is not essential. Arthroplasties have also been developed which make it possible to maintain mobility in those joints that must move in order to maintain significant function.

OSTEOARTHRITIS

Osteoarthritis of the hand is characterized not by synovial hypertrophy but by a gradual loss of articular cartilage. This condition is most prevalent in postmenopausal females but can appear at a younger age in men, in whom previous joint trauma is thought to be a positive factor. The onset of this condition is slow, with pain being the chief symptom. X-ray examination of the involved joints initially shows a loss of joint space followed by the appearance of osteophytes. Sclerosis of adjacent bone is also seen. With loss of collateral ligament support or as a result of stretching of the extensor mechanism, these joints become deformed with decreased functional capacity. Although any joints in the hand or wrist can be the site of rheumatoid arthritis, there are three sites where osteoarthritis is frequently seen: the distal interphalangeal and proximal interphalangeal joints and the carpometacarpal joint of the thumb.

Distal joint arthritis is the most common location of osteoarthritis. The typical patient with symptomatic involvement at this level is the postmenopausal female. These patients seek medical attention because of pain and/or unhappiness with the appearance of the distal joints of their fingers. Osteophyte formation at the margins of the joints (Heberden's nodes) are typical physical findings. There is a loss of joint motion noted on clinical examination, but this is seldom of concern to the patient. In fact, as the joint loses motion, pain decreases. These patients with distal joint arthritis may develop a small cystic mass on the dorsal aspect of the distal phalanx. These mucous cysts gradually enlarge and stretch the overlying skin. Although they originate from the joint, they may appear at the base of the fingernail, where pressure against the nail root causes irregular nail growth (Fig. 114–9).

The treatment of distal joint arthritis includes splinting, analgesics for mild pain, and arthrodesis with spur removal for unstable and unsightly joints. The preferred position for fusion is essentially full extension. Bothersome mucous cysts are treated with local excision of the cyst and removal of any underlying bony spurs which are thought to be contributing factors to their development. If the skin over the mucous cyst is very thin, it may have to be removed and the resultant defect closed with either a small skin graft or a local rotation flap. Recurrence of mucous cysts is occasionally seen and can be eliminated by joint fusion. When distal joint fusion is contemplated in these patients, one should also carefully evaluate the proximal interphalangeal joint. The fusion of the distal joint puts an additional strain on

Figure 114–9. Mucous cyst associated with distal joint osteoarthritis. Note alteration in nail growth.

the proximal interphalangeal joint, and the patient may develop increased symptoms in this area.

Proximal interphalangeal joint arthritis is the second common site of involvement. At this level the gradual loss of joint motion assumes major significance, with the patient finding it difficult to grasp small objects. The joints enlarge with spur formation (Bouchard's nodes) and become unsightly. Pain may also be noted with loss of joint articular cartilage. Lateral deformities of this joint are common with stretching of the collateral ligaments. This leads to overlapping of the fingers and considerable loss of functional ability. The pain at this level can be controlled by splinting, but restoration of motion can be achieved only by arthroplasty. The use of flexible implants has been worthwhile in this regard in those patients who have less than 50 degrees of active motion. Although some patients regain 70 to 80 degrees of motion with arthroplasties, one cannot expect to achieve more than an average of 60 degrees with this procedure. When patients are being considered for proximal interphalangeal joint arthroplasties because of osteoarthritis, attention should be directed toward the distal joints. If there is distal joint involvement, it is advisable to combine fusion of the distal joint with the arthroplasty of the proximal interphalangeal joint. This eliminates pain distally and concentrates all the flexor and extensor force to the proximal interphalangeal joint.

The third area of the common hand involvement in osteoarthritis is the carpometacarpal joint of the thumb. These patients present with increasing pain at the base of the thumb. The joint space between the first metacarpal and trapezium narrows with loss of articular cartilage. Rotary motions of the joint are particularly painful. With a gradual lateral subluxation of the joint the typical patient develops a "shoulder" or a prominence at the base of the thumb. With the first metacarpal adducted there is a gradual development of metacarpophalangeal joint hyperextension. These patients have increasing difficulty applying pressure with the thumb.

Simple activities such as opening a car door become difficult and painful. With increased adduction of the first metacarpal the patient had difficulty grasping large objects as the first web space between the thumb and index finger narrows.

Increased use and exercise cause a flare-up of pain and should be avoided. Resting and splinting are frequently helpful in relieving pain and certainly should be tried before any surgery is contemplated. Many of these patients respond to a conservative approach with relief of pain that is long lasting in spite of advanced radiographic findings. In those patients who do not respond to conservative treatment, arthroplasty affords an excellent solution. Two surgical approaches are commonly used. In one the trapezium is simply removed (resection arthroplasty), and in the other it is replaced with a trapezium prosthesis.

The resection arthroplasty gives predictable relief of pain with some loss of pinch power. In order to prevent or minimize proximal migration of the first metacarpal, a portion of rolled-up tendon "anchovy" is commonly utilized. The advantage of this technique is simplicity of surgery and a consistency of satisfactory results.

Trapezium replacement arthroplasties can also be used to maintain space and thumb alignment. The results of this technique have been excellent in relieving pain and restoring motion and strength to a level close to normal. However, this approach requires close attention to surgical technique to prevent prosthetic subluxation, which is the major complication encountered. With any carpometacarpal joint arthroplasty it is important to correct any metacarpophalangeal joint hyperextension deformity which may be present. This can be accomplished by fusion in fixed deformities and by volar capsular repair in patients with flexible joints.

Finally carpometacarpal fusion can be successful in restoring stability and relieving pain in these patients but should be utilized only in those patients who have localized carpometacarpal joint involvement and in whom metacarpophalangeal flexion is maintained. This procedure requires 10 to 12 weeks of postoperative casting and has become less used since the introduction of replacement prostheses.

LUPUS ERYTHEMATOSUS

Systemic lupus erythematosus is a multisystem connective tissue disease which often has musculoskeletal involvement.[39] This includes muscle pain and atrophy as well as various articular complaints.[40] The latter are some of the most frequent clinical manifestations of the disease.[41] The most common joints involved are the knees, but the smaller joints of the hands and the wrists are also frequently involved.[42,43] The most typical pattern of involvement is one of migratory arthralgias.

The hand involvement in lupus is generally more benign than is seen in rheumatoid arthritis. Bleifield and Inglis reported that there was some hand involvement in 86 percent of 50 randomly examined lupus patients.[44]

Most patients reported evanescent arthralgias, although some described definitive evidence of swelling and synovitis. The most common cause of symptoms in the hand is Raynaud's phenomenon, occurring in 50 percent of patients. Definite hand deformities have been reported in as many as 35 percent of lupus patients. These deformities can affect any joint in the hand and can cause any of the rheumatoid-like deformities (Fig. 114-10).

In contrast to rheumatoid or osteoarthritis, the articular cartilage in lupus is not involved, and, unless there is a secondary degenerative type of arthritis from the ligamentous laxity, the articular cartilage will be completely normal (Fig. 114-10). However, because of the ligamentous laxity, some of the most severe unstable digital deformities can be seen in these patients. Because of this, early reconstructive surgery prior to severe dislocations and severe fixed deformities is indicated.

Wrist. Wrist involvement is a frequent radiologic manifestation of the lupus hand but usually is asymptomatic. The most common findings are those of ligamentous laxity. This results in dorsal subluxation of the distal ulna which can result in pain and limited rotation. Ulnar translocation of the carpus is common, and intercarpal dissociation manifested by an increased scapholunate gap and rotation of the lunate is also seen. These generally are asymptomatic, and even in the more significant collapse patterns pain is unusual.

Digital Deformities. The digital deformities seen in systemic lupus erythematosus are secondary to subluxation of the extensor tendons at the metacarpophalangeal joint resulting in flexion deformities. Initially, these deformities are passively correctible, but eventually they become fixed. In contrast to rheumatoid arthritis, ulnar drift of the digits is less common.

The deformities seen at the proximal interphalangeal joints are often swan neck deformities, but boutonnière deformities and lateral deformities also occur. Initially these deformities are supple, but with time they become fixed and develop secondary degenerative changes.

Surgery for lupus deformities should be carried out prior to that for destructive changes and fixed deformities. For passively correctible metacarpophalangeal joint deformities, soft tissue surgery, including relocation of the extensor tendon, is advised. When this is carried out, a portion of the extensor tendon should be tenodesed to the proximal phalanx. Prolonged splinting is necessary to prevent recurrence of the deformity. In a group of our patients in whom only soft tissue surgery was carried out with no attempts to tenodese the tendon to the proximal phalanx, there was a significant recurrence rate.

For recurrent metacarpophalangeal joint deformities or for fixed deformities, metacarpophalangeal joint arthroplasty is indicated. In our experience better results were obtained when surgery was performed prior to the development of fixed deformities (Fig. 114-11).

Surgery for proximal interphalangeal joint deformities should be done in conjunction with metacarpophalangeal surgery. Lateral deformities can be repaired by collateral ligament reconstruction, and boutonnière de-

Figure 114–10. Hand deformities seen with lupus erythematosus. *A,* Severe dislocated metacarpophalangeal joints with fixed deformities. Also note dislocated carpometacarpal joint. *B,* Severe skin maceration associated with fixed metacarpophalangeal joint dislocations and poor skin hygiene. *C,* Radiograph showing dislocated metacarpophalangeal joints and severe thumb deformity with dislocation of carpometacarpal joint of thumb. *D,* Metacarpophalangeal joints exposed at surgery. Note minimal loss of cartilage and no evidence of any bony erosions or bony destruction.

Figure 114–11. Metacarpophalangeal joint involvement in lupus erythematosus. *A*, Subluxed metacarpophalangeal joints with supple swan neck deformities. Also note recent arthrodesis of carpometacarpal joint of the thumb. *B*, Same patient after metacarpophalangeal joint arthroplasty of digits 2 to 5. *C* and *D*, Extension and flexion 4 years after metacarpophalangeal joint arthroplasties.

formities can also be repaired. For supple swan neck deformities sublimis tenodesis is indicated. Four to 5 weeks of Kirschner wire fixation to allow good soft tissue healing is indicated after this surgery. Using this program in the face of a joint with good articular cartilage, a good functional range of motion can be restored with restoration of alignment and stability.

Thumb. The lupus thumb deformity most commonly results from involvement in all three joints. Initially, one will see an extension lag at the metacarpophalangeal joint, with hyperextension at the interphalangeal joint. Even at this early stage, one will note an early laxity at the carpometacarpal joint. As the laxity increases to dorsal radial subluxation and ultimately dislocation, the thumb deformity abruptly changes to one with adduction of the first metacarpal and hyperextension of the metacarpophalangeal joint and flexion at the interphalangeal joint (Fig. 114-12).

As in other areas surgery is most effective when carried out early. Carpometacarpal ligamentous stabilization, using a portion of the flexor carpi radialis, has been successful in maintaining stabilization of the joint. Reinforcement of the metacarpophalangeal joint with a rerouted extensor pollicis longus for supple flexion de-

Figure 114–12. Advanced lupus erythematosus thumb deformity. *A,* Dislocated carpometacarpal joint with adduction deformity of metacarpal and hyperextension deformity of metacarpophalangeal joint. *B,* Radiograph of patient in *A.* Also note collapsed deformity of wrist, dislocation of metacarpophalangeal joints, and lateral dislocation of index proximal interphalangeal joint. *C,* Postoperative status: hemiarthroplasty of carpometacarpal joint and soft tissue reconstruction of metacarpophalangeal joint. *D,* Radiograph demonstrating hemiarthroplasty utilizing silicon prosthesis, with K-wire used for temporary prosthetic fixation.

formity is helpful. For dislocated carpometacarpal joints or carpometacarpal joints with articular changes, arthrodesis or arthroplasty is carried out. As discussed previously, appropriate distal surgery such as metacarpophalangeal ligamentous stabilization or fusion must be included. Interphalangeal fusion is frequently needed for marked instability of the interphalangeal joint.

References

1. Flatt, A.E.: The Care of the Rheumatoid Hand. St. Louis, C. V. Mosby Company, 1963.
2. Millender, L.H., and Nalebuff, E.A.: Evaluation and treatment of early rheumatoid hand involvement. Orthop. Clin. North Am. 6:697, 1975.
3. Millender, L.H., and Nalebuff, E.A.: Metacarpophalangeal joint arthroplasty utilizing the silicone rubber prosthesis. Orthop. Clin. North Am. 4:349, 1973.
4. Nalebuff, E.A.: Metacarpophalangeal surgery in rheumatoid arthritis. Surg. Clin. North Am. 49:823, 1969.
5. Swanson, A.B.: Flexible Implant Resection Arthroplasty in the Hand and Extremities. St. Louis, C. V. Mosby Company, 1973.
6. Millender, L.H., and Nalebuff, E.A.: Preventive surgery—tenosynovectomy and synovectomy. Orthop. Clin. North Am. 6:765, 1975.
7. Kessler, L., and Vainio, K.: Posterior (dorsal) synovectomy for rheumatoid involvement of the hand and wrist. A follow-up study of sixty-six procedures. J. Bone Joint Surg. 48:1048, 1966.
8. Linscheild, R.L.: Surgery for rheumatoid arthritis—timing and techniques: The upper extremity. J. Bone Joint Surg. 50A:605, 1968.
9. Nalebuff, E.A., and Potter, T.A.: Rheumatoid involvement of tendons and tendon sheaths in the hand. Clin. Orthop. 59:147, 1968.
10. Lipscomb, P.R.: Surgery for rheumatoid arthritis—timing and techniques: Summary. J. Bone Joint Surg. 50A:614, 1968.
11. Millender, L.H., Nalebuff, E.A., Albin, R., Ream, J., and Gordon, M.: Dorsal tenosynovectomy and tendon transfer in the rheumatoid hand. J. Bone Joint Surg. 56A:601, 1974.
12. Cracchiolo, A., III, and Marmor, L.: Resection of the distal ulna in rheumatoid arthritis. Arthritis Rheum. 12:415, 1969.
13. Vaughan-Jackson, O.J.: Attrition ruptures of tendons in the rheumatoid hand. In Proceedings of the Joint Meeting of the Orthopaedic Association of the English-Speaking World. J. Bone Joint Surg. 40A:1431, 1958.
14. Vaughan-Jackson, O.J.: Rupture of extensor tendons by attrition at the inferior radioulnar joint. Reports of two cases. J. Bone Joint Surg. 30B:528, 1948.
15. Straub, L.R., and Wilson, E.H., Jr.: Spontaneous rupture of extensor tendons in the hand associated with rheumatoid arthritis. J. Bone Joint Surg. 38A:1208, 1956.
16. Nalebuff, E.A.: Surgical treatment of finger deformities in the rheumatoid hand. Surg. Clin. North Am. 49:833, 1969.
17. Nalebuff, E.A.: Surgical treatment of tendon rupture in the rheumatoid hand. Surg. Clin. North Am. 49:811, 1969.
18. Nalebuff, E.A., and Patel, M.R.: Flexor digitorum sublimis transfer for multiple extensor tendon ruptures in rheumatoid arthritis. Plast. Reconstr. Surg. 52:530, 1973.
19. Nalebuff, E.A.: Surgical treatment of rheumatoid tenosynovitis in the hand. Surg. Clin. North Am. 49:799, 1969.
20. Nalebuff, E.A., and Millender, L.H.: Surgical treatment of the boutonnière deformity in rheumatoid arthritis. Orthop. Clin. North Am. 6:753, 1975.
21. Millender, L.H., and Nalebuff, E.A.: Reconstructive surgery in the rheumatoid hand. Orthop. Clin. North Am. 6:709, 1975.
22. Riordan, D.C., and Fowler, S.B.: Surgical treatment of rheumatoid deformities of the hand. J. Bone Joint Surg. 40A:1431, 1958.
23. Vaino, K.: Arthrodeses and arthroplasties in the treatment of the rheumatoid hand. In La Main Rheumatismale, Paris, 1966, Expansion Scientifique Francaise, 30–35.
24. Tupper, J.W.: Personal communication.
25. Swanson, A.B.: Silicone rubber implants for replacement of arthritic or destroyed joints in the hand. Surg. Clin. North Am. 48:1113, 1968.
26. Swanson, A.B.: Flexible implant arthroplasty for arthritic finger joints. J. Bone Joint Surg. 54A:435, 1972.
27. Neibauer, J.J.: Dacron-silicone prosthesis for the metacarpophalangeal and interphalangeal joints. In Cramer, L.H., and Chase, R.A. (eds.): Symposium on the Hand, Vol. 3. St. Louis, C. V. Mosby Company, 1971, pp. 96–105.
28. Millender, L.H., Nalebuff, E.A., Hawkins, R.B., and Ennis, R.: Infection After Silicone Prosthetic Arthroplasty in the Hand. J. Bone Joint Surg. 57A:825, 1975.
29. Nalebuff, E.A., and millender, L.H.: Surgical treatment of swan neck deformity in rheumatoid arthritis. Orthop. Clin. North Am. 6:733, 975.
30. Pahle, J.A., and Raunio, P.: The influence of wrist position on finger deviation in the rheumatoid hand. A clinical and radiological study. J. Bone Joint Surg. 51B:664, 1969.
31. Carroll, R.E., and Dick, H.M.: Arthrodesis of the wrist for rheumatoid arthritis. J. Bone Joint Surg. 53A:1365, 1971.
32. Clayton, M.L.: Surgical treatment at the wrist in rheumatoid arthritis. A review of thirty-seven patients. J. Bone Joint Surg. 47A:741, 1965.
33. Dupont, M., and Vainio, K.: Arthrodesis of the wrist in rheumatoid arthritis. A study of 140 cases. Ann. Chir. Gynec. Fenn. 57:513, 1968.
34. Mannerfelt, L., and Malmsten, M.: Arthrodesis of the wrist in rheumatoid arthritis. A technique without external fixation. Scand. J. Plast. Reconstr. Surg. 5:124, 1971.
35. Millender, L.H., and Nalebuff, E.A.: Arthrodesis of the rheumatoid wrist. An evaluation of sixty patients and a description of a different surgical technique. J. Bone Joint Surg. 55A:1026, 1973.
36. Albright, J.A., and Chase, R.A.: Palmar-shelf arthroplasty of the wrist in rheumatoid arthritis. A report of nine cases. J. Bone Joint Surg. 52A:89, 1970.
37. Swanson, A.B.: Implant arthroplasty for disabilities of the distal radioulnar joint. Use of a silicone rubber capping implant following resection of the ulnar head. Orthop. Clin. North Am. 4:373, 1973.
38. Nalebuff, E.A.: Diagnosis, classification and management of rheumatoid thumb deformities. Bull. Hosp. Joint Dis. 29:119, 1968.
39. Ropes, M.W.: Systemic Lupus Erythematosus. Cambridge, Mass., Harvard University Press, 1976, pp. 12–74.
40. Labowitz, R., and Schumaker, H.R., Jr.: Articular manifestations of systemic lupus erythematosus. Ann. Intern. Med. 74:911, 1971.
41. Dubois, E.L.: Lupus Erythematosus: A Review of the Current Status of Discoid and Systemic Lupus Erythematosus and Their Variants. 2nd ed. Los Angeles, University of Southern California Press, 1974, pp. 40–42, 58–61, 70–71, 232–437, 464–475, 525–536.
42. Green, N., and Osmer, J.C.: Small bone changes secondary to systemic lupus erythematosus. Radiology 90:118, 1968.
43. Weisman, B.N., Rappaport, M.B.B., Sosman, J.L., and Schur, P.H.: Radiographic findings in the hands in patients with systemic lupus erythematosus. Radiology 126:313, 1978.
44. Bleifield, C.J., and Inglis, A.E.: The hand in systemic lupus erythematosus. J. Bone Joint Surg. 56A:1207, 1974.

Chapter 115

Reconstructive Surgery and Rehabilitation of the Elbow

Frederick C. Ewald

FUNCTION AND DISEASE

The elbow joint complex consists of three separate articulations that allow the hand to move through an arc of 160 degrees in the lateral plane and rotate 180 degrees around the longitudinal axis of the forearm. Combining these motions with those of the shoulder and wrist allows the hand to be placed anywhere in space in the frontal and lateral planes of the body with the hand in a position of useful function. These combinations of motions are often selectively affected by disease, and a major goal of reconstructive surgery of the upper extremity is to restore function of the hand. The usual pattern of pain, deformity, and motion is different for rheumatoid arthritis, traumatic arthritis, and osteoarthritis.

Rheumatoid Arthritis. The most complicated problems occur in the rheumatoid patient, who often has joint destruction in the hand, wrist, elbow, and shoulder. Timing and sequence of indicated reconstructive procedures in the upper extremity of these patients become very important, and the patient as a whole must be considered. For instance, crutch walking for lower extremity problems may influence the timing of upper extremity reconstruction. However, reconstruction of the hand may proceed independently of the elbow and shoulder, provided there is adequate motion in these joints to place the hand in a functional position. The hand, despite severe deformity and pain, is never completely useless, because it is always a valuable tactile organ provided it can be placed where desired. However, the hand becomes completely useless when shoulder and/or elbow pain completely immobilizes the entire upper extremity. These are the prime indications for reconstructive surgery of the elbow and shoulder—to relieve intractable pain in the radiographically destroyed joint and restore mobility to the hand in space. The shoulder usually presents with the most pain compared to the elbow and wrist, but since a large range of motion of the shoulder for usual activities of living is not necessary, hand function can often be restored merely by relieving shoulder pain. The elbow is the most important joint for positioning of the hand. For instance, if a patient has a fused shoulder or wrist, the functional loss is usually accepted. If the elbow is fused at any angle, the functional loss is great, and the frustration of being unable to place the hand in space is intolerable to most patients. Elbow fusion is not recommended in rheumatoid arthritis but may often occur spontaneously in the juvenile rheumatoid patient. The goal of elbow re-

construction is to restore painless motion. The destroyed rheumatoid elbow often has adequate motion, but there is usually intractable pain whenever the joint moves a few degrees. If the patient can be given a painless arch of motion from (−)30 degrees of extension to 135 degrees of flexion with 80 degrees of pronation of the forearm, good function will be restored. Therefore, except for the case of intractable shoulder pain, the elbow joint becomes the key to restoring hand function in the rheumatoid patient when the entire upper extremity is involved.

Post-traumatic Arthritis. In post-traumatic arthritis there is usually limited motion associated with pain. The problem is less complicated, because the joints above and below the elbow are normal. Limited motion may vary from a 90-degree arc to solid fusion. Severe flexion deformities are common. The usual clinical picture is a disrupted painful joint with excessive new bone formation and 10 to 15 degrees of motion. The ultimate problem in treatment of the post-traumatic elbow is restoration of motion.

Osteoarthritis. Osteoarthritis or primary degenerative arthritis of the elbow is rare. The osteoarthritis may be secondary to avascular necrosis associated with renal transplantation, lupus erythematosus, or cortisone therapy, or may be secondary to old sepsis. This group usually maintains motion with pain without new bone formation. The joints above and below are usually unaffected, so attention can be directed to relieving elbow pain.

BIOMECHANICS

Center of Rotation. Elbow motion has been recently studied by Morrey and Chao,[1] Walker,[2] and London,[3] and each, after measuring two cadaver elbows, concluded that the elbow was essentially a uniaxial articulation moving about a single axis of rotation. Additional radiographic studies in living patients[4-7] showed movement of the center between full extension and full flexion. However, it is difficult to control positioning when taking multiple radiographs in a living patient, and this method has a high degree of inherent error. Nonetheless, the elbow is uniaxial in unloaded joints except at full extension and full flexion.[3]

Carrying Angle. The carrying angle in full extension has been reported at 10 to 15 degrees of valgus with a range of 5 to 25 degrees.[1,8,9] This cubitus valgus increases slightly with age[9] and decreases with increasing flexion[1,8] to a reversal into 3 to 6 degrees of varus in full flexion.[1,8] Several investigators[1,2] have noted that the forearm rotates along its transverse axis first internally at the beginning of elbow flexion and then externally at the end of flexion.

In addition to these movements in cadaver specimens, the elbow joint may have other changing relationships (center of rotation, ulnar shift) when moved by normal musculature. Ray and colleagues[8] looked at the rotation of the forearm in living subjects and found that the ulna transcribes a transverse arc of 9 degrees between full supination and pronation. This was not observed by Morrey and Chao when they studied motion in the cadaver elbow.[1]

Joint Reactive Forces. The forces across the elbow have been studied by free body analysis,[2,9,10] and most of the forces have been estimated in one plane only. Nicol and associates[8] have calculated the elbow joint reactive forces for some routine activities of daily living and have taken into account torque and dynamic forces. These forces are listed in Table 115-1. The static free body analyses[2,10,11] in the lateral plane show maximal joint reactive forces in order of magnitude of 10 to 22 times the weight held in the hand. This assumes that the maximal force is generated with the elbow at 90 degrees of flexion, and that the average weight of the forearm along with the major flexors and their moments are considered. For instance, in this oversimplified system, an individual holding a 5-pound weight in the hand will generate 50 to 60 pounds of joint reactive force in the elbow and with 50 pounds in the hand will generate 500 to 600 pounds in the elbow. These estimates of forces are crude but helpful and necessary for the design of elbow replacement or resurfacing prostheses.

Function of Radial Head and Interosseous Membrane. Walker has published an elegant study of the forces across the radial-capitellar joint.[2] He applied longitudinal forces across the distal radius of eight fresh specimens and recorded a load-deflection curve. At forces up to 22 lbs (10 kgf), 70 percent of the load was carried by the interosseous membrane and transmitted to the ulna and ultimately to the humerus through the ulnar-trochlear articulation. However, when the load exceeded 22 lbs, 40 percent of the load was carried by the membrane and most (60 percent) was transmitted to the radial-capitellar joint. Therefore, under modest pushing loads, the radial head bears little force, but when the loads become heavy, the radial head comes into play and bears the majority of the force. These load-deflection experiments are confirmed by clinical observation in which fractures of the lateral column of the elbow joint (radial head and capitellum) after a fall on the outstretched arm are more common than fractures of the medial side of the joint (trochlea).[12,13]

ARTHROPLASTY

Resection

Synovectomy and Radial Head Excision. The first recorded synovectomy for rheumatoid arthritis of the knee was by Shuller in 1887.[15] The first American report was in 1900 by Goldtwait,[16] who listed 38 knee joint procedures for "non-tubercular conditions." Synovectomy for major rheumatoid joints has been recommended, along with appropriate systematic medical therapy.[17,18] (For a complete historical review of synovectomies, the reader is referred to an excellent paper by Geens in 1969[19] and to Chapter 113 of this volume.)

Historically, radial head excision in rheumatoid arthritis was first recommended by Smith-Petersen and associates in 1943.[20] Elbow joint synovectomy has usually been accompanied by radial head resection. Indication for elbow synovectomy with or without radial head resection has been primarily to relieve intractable pain and recurrent swelling. Synovectomy and radial head resection have not consistently improved elbow motion, and if there is limited motion or ankylosis, then arthroplasty is indicated. There are numerous recent reports in the literature (Table 115-2), with follow-up of 6 months to 8 years. Most of the series average 2 to 3 years postoperative at time of review. Listed in Table 115-2 are the number of good or satisfactory results according to the reported criteria for each series. All the authors used different criteria for the evaluation of results, but most took into account relief of pain and improved function and joint motion. Adding all the reports together, over 70 percent of the procedures resulted in a satisfactory outcome at an average follow-up of 2.6 years.

Porter and colleagues[28] reviewed the radiographic appearance of the elbow joint after synovectomy and noted progressive deterioration of the joint. When the radiographic findings were added to the review, the satisfactory results dropped to 55 percent. The results of a 16-center prospective evaluation of synovectomy in rheumatoid arthritis have recently been published[31] and confirm the findings of Porter and colleagues.[28] Synovectomy is useful in relieving pain and recurrent effusion at 1 year postoperative but will not necessarily prevent progression of radiographic joint destruction at 3 years. The concept of synovectomy for prophylaxis on a long-term basis is therefore questionable.

Elbow synovectomy may also be indicated for painful, tense antecubital cysts, which have been compared to popliteal cysts in rheumatoid arthritis.[32] Posterior synovectomy has been suggested[17] to relieve the anterior mass, and the author has performed one such procedure with relief of pain, pressure, and swelling at 1 year

Table 115–1. Biomechanical Analysis of Elbow Joint Function*

Activity	Joint Reactive Force	
	Newtons	Pounds
Dressing and eating	300	67
Assisted seat rise	340	76

*From Nicol, A.C., et al.: *In* Joint Replacement of the Upper Limb. London, Mechanical Engineering Publications Ltd., 1977.

Table 115–2. Elbow Synovectomy and Radial Head Resection in Rheumatoid Arthritis

Author	Year Reported	Number Elbows/ Patients	Follow-up (Years), Min.-Max.	Radial Head Resection (%)	Excellent- Good Result (No. elbows)	Poor Result (No. elbows)	Complications	Comment	Surgical Approach
Wilkinson and Lowry[21]	1965	7/7	Average 3½	Not reported	5	2	Not reported	"Severely affected joint selected"	Not reported
Laine and Vainio[22]	1969	92/82	Average 1	100	80%	Not reported	Not reported	80% "benefited" from procedure	Medial and lateral
Torgerson and Leach[23]	1970	5/5	1½–2½; average 2	100	5	0	0	One joint—early involvement	Lateral
Inglis et al.[24]	1971	28/26	1–6; average 3½	100	25	3	1 nerve palsy; 2 nonunited, olecranon	All Class III and IV rheumatoid patients	Posterior-lateral and trans-olecranon osteotomy
Peterson and Jones[25]	1971	22/22	1–4	59	17	2	0	7 patients had <85% of tissue removed	4 patients had only radial head resection
Marmor[26]	1972	25/19	0.6–7; average 3½	100	23	2	0	6 had simultaneous ulnar head resection	Posterior-lateral
Wilson et al.[27]	1973	57/48	0.8–4; average 1.5	50	45	12	1 infection; 1 delayed healing	Radial head resected if damaged	Medial and lateral
Porter et al.[28]	1974	154/123	1–6	100	97	57	1 infection; 1 nerve palsy	When x-rays considered, only 54% had satisfactory result	Medial and lateral
Taylor et al.[29]	1976	44/38	0.5–8; average 5	100	35	6	Not reported	Synovectomy not performed in every case	Lateral
Ferlic et al.[30]	1976	43/43	Average 2½	100	40	3	0	0	Lateral

postoperative. The antecubital rheumatoid cyst communicated with the elbow joint via a soft tissue "ball" or "flap" valve as demonstrated by preoperative posterior arthrography.

One group of authors[29] feels that radial head resection is more important than synovectomy and performs a synovectomy only if the humeroradial joint appears intact.

Distal Humerus and Proximal Ulna. In the late 1800s, arthroplasty of the elbow was used to provide motion in elbows with ankylosis secondary to old tuberculosis. More recently Hurri and associates[33] reported a series of 76 elbows with rheumatoid arthritis in which 51 underwent a resection arthroplasty as described by Herbert.[34] This procedure is a radical resection of the capitellum, trochlea, radial head, and most of the olecranon down to the insertion of the triceps tendon with no interpositional material used. This group was compared with an additional 22 cases in the same report of those who underwent a Hass procedure, which is a resection arthroplasty with skin (cutis) added as an interpositional membrane around the distal humerus. The Hass procedure[35] is interesting, because instead of trying to maximize bony contact between the resected ends of the arthroplasty, the distal humerus is shaped to a point to minimize contact between the distal humerus and the proximal ulna. This would greatly increase unit loading, but the good part about the Hass resection is preservation of the olecranon as a stabilizer compared to almost complete resection in the Herbert operation.[34] Most of the procedures were performed for bony fibrous ankylosis (59 out of 76). The results of the two groups showed the final arc of motion to be 104 degrees in the simple resection group and 78 degrees in the interposition group. Complete relief of pain was attained in 64 percent of the simple resection group and 40 percent in the skin interposition group. Twelve elbows (15 percent) were considered failures because of either limited motion (six) or constant pain (six). The authors concluded the results at an average of 3.6 years postoperative were better after simple resection than after Hass type resection with cutis interposition. More recently, Dickson and associates[36] reported the results of ten excision arthroplasties in rheumatoid arthritis performed to relieve severe elbow pain. Mean follow-up age was 9½ years, with a range of 6 months to 30 years. Half the elbows had complete pain relief, while two elbows had no pain relief. Improvement in range of motion was equivocal, with half gaining and half losing. Seven out of ten were unstable after surgery. The authors concluded that the procedure can give good pain relief, but instability will be a problem if the patient has to use crutches, and bilateral procedures should not be performed.

Distraction-Resection. In a 1975 report Volkov and Oganesian[37] presented a distraction technique that they used for obtaining elbow motion in 13 patients after excisional arthroplasty, 11 patients with contractures or fibrous ankylosis, 2 with nonunited supracondylar fractures of the humerus, and 2 with old unreduced dislocations. The device is unique, because distraction of the joint surfaces can be maintained while a functional range of motion is pursued postoperatively by physical therapy. All the patients in this report were post-traumatic, and the 13 arthroplasties were performed by radial head excision and shaping congruent surfaces on the humerus and ulna. No interpositional material was used. The remaining elbows were treated closed; in the cases of old unreduced dislocations, distraction was slowly applied until the joint surfaces were aligned, and then the force was reduced. In the closed elbows with fibrous ankylosis, slow distraction was applied until the joint surfaces separated and then motion was started. The key to the apparatus is the use of small Kirschner wires under tension via traction clevis, and the center of rotation of the apparatus is at the wire that goes through the center of the trochlea in the sagittal plane. This is the approximate center of rotation of the elbow joint.

The results at 4 to 6 years postoperative showed the following arcs of motion for those with previous arthroplasty: 80 to 120 degrees, seven patients; 50 to 70 degrees, five patients; 40 degrees, one patient. Eleven out of 13 arthroplasty patients returned to their previous work, and two who had pain changed jobs.

Arc of motion for patients who had flexion deformities and fibrous ankylosis was as follows: 70 to 120 degrees, six patients; 50 to 60 degrees, four patients; 40 degrees, one patient. These patients were treated closed and nine returned to previous work, although three had pain after use. The two other patients changed jobs.

In two patients with old dislocation, the flexion arcs were 55 to 100 degrees and 0 to 140 degrees. The two patients with nonunited supracondylar fractures ended with 0 to 140 degree and 15 to 100 degree arcs of motion. The average arc of motion for all patients was 43 degrees, and the best result was in the smallest group of nonunited fractures and old dislocations. It is not known how a rheumatoid elbow would respond to such an arthroplasty, but the bone could not be osteoporotic; otherwise the Kirschner wires would loosen or wear through.

Although the following paragraphs deal with the more popular interpositional arthroplasties, simple resection arthroplasties have great current significance, since after removal of a failed total elbow arthroplasty prosthesis, one is left with a resection arthroplasty. This fact should influence current total elbow design so that reasonable salvage is possible in case of failure of the implant from loosening, dislocation, sepsis, breakage, wear, limited motion, or intractable pain.

Interpositional Arthroplasty

Fascia. In 1921 MacAusland[38] published a classic monograph on fascial arthroplasty with an excellent historical review of interpositional materials. The variety of such materials used in the past is endless and includes ivory pegs, magnesium sheets, wood, celluloid, gutta-percha, temporary gauze packing, mixture of yellow wax and lanolin, periosteal flaps, rib cartilage, transplanted joints, muscle, and fascia. He noted that except for excisional arthroplasty, interpositional fascial arthroplasty had exceeded all others in popularity at that time. He also eloquently pointed out that the elbow is a unique joint, and that unlike the knee, wrist, or shoulder where painless stability may be functional, no position of ankylosis of the elbow is functional or cosmetic. The following year Campbell[39] reported his technique of arthroplasty, using triceps muscle and periosteum as interpositional material. Two cases were reviewed with short follow-up. In 1947 MacAusland[40] again published his technique of fascial arthroplasty and noted that over 100 elbows had been mobilized with excellent results regarding motion and stability. Among the cases of infectious etiology, he felt that those patients with old gonorrheal sepsis had the best prognosis, and that old tuberculosis was a contraindication to the procedure. In 1952, Knight and Van Zandt[41] reviewed their experience in fascial arthroplasty at the Campbell clinic. They reported 45 cases with follow-up of 3 to 30 years, with 91 percent followed 6 or more years. Ten cases were reviewed 21 to 30 years postoperative. This report has the longest follow-up in the literature. The results were classified as 56 percent good, 22 percent fair, 2 percent poor, and 20 percent failures. Their contraindications for fascial arthroplasty included a patient returning to heavy labor, tuberculosis, osteomyelitis, extra-articular ankylosis, and extreme muscle weakness (as seen with "atrophic arthritis"). Silva,[42] in 1967, also confirmed that fascial arthroplasty has contraindications in patients performing heavy labor. The range of postoperative motion in his 11 patients with old fractures or unreduced dislocation was unsatisfactory. The average arc of motion was only 18 degrees, with a range of motion of 30 degrees to less than 15 degrees. His results regarding motion were better with open reduction, acrylic arthroplasty, and Teflon prosthesis arthroplasty. The most recent report,[30] with an average follow-up of 2½ years, lists five elbows with rheumatoid arthritis as having a satisfactory result after fascial arthroplasty.

Cutis Arthroplasty. First reported by Gui[43] in 1953, cutis arthroplasties were reviewed in 1964 by Hurri and associates.[33] These authors performed resection arthroplasties with cutis interpositions around the distal humerus. Twenty cases were reported, with an average follow-up of 3.6 years. Complete relief of pain was seen in eight patients (40 percent), pain at certain positions or after strenuous work in eight patients (40 percent), and constant pain in four patients (20 percent). The arc of motion was 78 degrees. The authors concluded that the results from simple resection arthroplasty were superior. More recently, Fromison and colleagues[42] recorded results after cutis arthroplasty in five patients, with an average follow-up of 3½ years. Three of the patients were post-traumatic, one had a birth injury and one had rheumatoid arthritis. This small series of patients represents extraordinary medium-term results, because only one had slight pain (20 percent), and the average postoperative arc of flexion was 105 degrees, compared to an average preoperative arc of 20 degrees. Stability was rated as good in three, fair in one, and

poor in one. One of the patients who had no pain preoperatively was the one who had slight pain postoperatively.

Fat and Sponge Arthroplasty. One series[45] used fat as interpositional material and reported 19 cases with five unsatisfactory results. Another report[46] listed two cases of Ivalon sponge interpositional arthroplasty.

Hemiarthroplasty

Acrylic, Teflon. Prosthetic hemiarthroplasty of the elbow has been performed in small numbers since 1927 when the distal humerus was replaced by a rubber-covered metal prosthesis.[47] Silva,[42] in 1967, reported the results of 21 cases of acrylic replacement of the distal humerus in post-traumatic injuries among Ceylonese workers. He concluded that the results were superior to those obtained in 11 cases of fascial arthroplasty. One additional case of acrylic replacement of the distal humerus appeared in 1952,[46] for a total of 26 cases in the world literature. MacAusland, however, was the exception and reported four cases of replacement of the distal humerus with a nylon prosthesis.[49] As better materials have become available, these procedures have been supplanted.

Metal. *Humeral Replacement.* In the mid 1950's, metal prostheses for replacing all or part of the distal humerus were introduced with one report in 1952,[50] two case reports in 1957,[51] and one in 1958.[52]

Barr. In 1965, Barr and Eaton[53] reported a 4-year follow-up of a patient who had replacement of the distal humerus with a chrome-cobalt-molybdenum prosthesis. The 32-year-old patient had been using the elbow in manual labor, and after strenuous work aching developed, forcing him to quit each job after 3 months. On follow-up at 4 years, the arc of motion was 95 degrees and the patient was symptom free, working at a less strenuous job. Stress x-rays and fluoroscopy showed no loosening, but there was some resorption at the distal humerus.

Stevens-Street. In 1974, Street and Stevens[54] reported the results of a metal replacement for the distal humeral articular surface. The prosthesis resurfaces the trochlea and capitellum with no methacrylate or medullary canal stem fixation. Ten procedures were reported, with follow-up of 1 to 7 years. Five elbows were post-traumatic, three had rheumatoid arthritis, and two had ankylosis secondary to hemophilia. Overall results were assessed as unpredictable or poor in rheumatoid arthritis or hemophilia. However, four out of five of the post-traumatic elbows ended with a stable, painless elbow with functional range of motion (average arc, 65 degrees). The fifth post-traumatic case ended with an elbow fusion. In 1977,[55] when the series was updated, one of the early implants had to be removed for pain. At the last report[56] 22 cases were listed with follow-up from 9 months to 11 years, with an average of 3 years. Fifteen had improved motion, and six were unchanged. Two patients had residual joint pain, and four had nerve pain. Three patients had subluxation and one dislocated.

Ulnar Replacement. All the hemiarthroplasties reviewed here have replaced the humeral side of the elbow joint. The first published case in the English literature of ulnar replacement of the elbow was in 1970.[57] The patient, who sustained a shotgun injury, achieved a good result with minimal pain at 13-year follow-up. The patient had a 40 degree arc of motion and continued his work as a farmer. Radiographic examination revealed erosion of the distal humerus with posterior subluxation of the ulna. Peterson and Jones, in 1971,[25] mentioned two cases of replacement of the trochlear notch of the ulna with a chrome-cobalt-molybdenum "saddle" prosthesis. At a mean follow-up of 2½ years one case was rated excellent and the other fair.

Total Replacement of the Elbow Joint

Fully Constrained Metal Hinges. In 1942, Boerema and deWaard[58] reported for the first time implantation of two stainless steel hinge total elbow arthroplasties fixed with screws and wires. This was, of course, in the pre-methacrylate era, and follow-up was only 1 year. Another case report[59] of a metal hinge replacement for the elbow appeared in 1958. This metal hinge was implanted for extensive post-traumatic loss of the distal humerus. More recently Chatzidakis[60] reported implantation of three chrome-cobalt elbow hinge prostheses. Roentgenograms taken 2 to 5 years postoperative showed a satisfactory result. No comment was made regarding loosening or radiolucent lines.

Dee, McKee. The addition of methyl methacrylate led to an explosion of activity in total joint replacement in the 1970's, and Dee[61] was one of the first to report on a total elbow replacement metal hinge prosthesis (Fig. 115-1) fixed with methacrylate. Dee initially reported 12 cases with maximum follow-up of 2 years, and ten were rated as an excellent result, one fair, and one poor. Average arc of motion was 108 degrees. In a follow-up article the next year, 1973, Dee[62] reported the results of 30 arthroplasties with follow-up of 6 months to 3 years. Twenty-five were rated excellent, two fair, and three poor. In this article, Dee raised the problem of a fully

constrained hinge joint transmitting torque normally developed at the elbow joint directly to the bone-cement interface. Souter in the same volume[63] listed his experience with the McKee and Dee prosthesis. The McKee prosthesis is a metal to metal single center hinge joint replacement. Follow-up was from 4 months to 2½ years. Twenty McKee and five Dee prostheses were implanted. Sixteen elbows rated good to excellent and eight fair. One elbow failed because of sepsis. There were a number of complications, including fracture, 3; wound hematoma, 6; pressure sore over tip of olecranon, 4; possible bone reaction to cement, 2; and loosening of humeral components, 5 (two symptomatic). The author concluded that the early results of hinge arthroplasty were promising, but felt that the concept should be approached with caution and raised doubt about long-term results because of loosening of the humeral component with the passage of time. One other report,[64] in 1974, listed 12 Dee replacements in short-term follow-up, with ten excellent results and two fair results after secondary surgery.

In 1977 Dee[65] reported long-term results of 40 elbow hinge arthroplasties. Follow-up was from 2 to 5 years; 35 patients had rheumatoid arthritis, and five were post-traumatic. The major complication was loosening. Eleven prostheses were loose, and eight were reoperated, with the remaining three not symptomatic enough for revisional surgery. He concluded that this hinge was obsolete with an unacceptable loosening rate, and noted that salvage for the failed implants was difficult.

GSB Hinge. In 1972 Gschwend also reported[66,67] the initial results of a metal to metal single center hinge prosthesis fixed with methacrylate (Fig. 115-2). The GSB prosthesis offered the advantage of minimal bone resection, which made resection arthroplasty a viable alternative if the prosthesis had to be removed. Twelve cases with minimum follow-up of 6 months were studied and good results reported.[67] The next report[68] listed 17 prostheses with good results and no evidence of loosening. The only complication was an infection. In 1975, 31 cases were reviewed,[69] with an average follow-up of 35 months (range 12 to 50 months). The major problem

Figure 115–1. Dee hinge prosthesis.

Figure 115–2. GSB hinge prosthesis, lateral view.

was loosening in 10 cases. These 10 prostheses were all designs that did not have an antirotation pin on the humeral or ulnar components. Gschwend reported the 5-year follow-up of the fixed single center metal to metal hinge in 1977.[70] The average time since operation of the 39 cases was 37 months, with a range of 12 to 60 months. There was good pain relief and good restoration of motion postoperatively. The main complication continued to be loosening. Twelve prostheses were loose, 7 at the humerus, 2 at the ulna, and 3 at both. The two loose prostheses at the ulnar side had an antirotation pin on the humeral component, so the loosening rotational forces were apparently directed to the ulna. The prosthesis has been redesigned and will be discussed below.

In a preliminary report[6] of our results with the GSB metal hinge elbow prosthesis, 13 elbows in 11 patients were followed 10 to 21 months. The early failure or revision rate was 23 percent (3 of 13), resulting from loosening of the ulnar component, loosening of both components, and inadequate motion in one post-traumatic case in the series. In 1977 the GSB hinge series was reviewed in detail and reported by Garrett[71] with a 3- to 4-year follow-up on 12 replacements in 10 patients with rheumatoid arthritis. Loosening occurred in five replacements at 5 to 15 months postoperative and was preceded by pain in every case. Two of the loosenings were reoperated, two are under observation, and the patient with the fifth requires narcotics for pain.

Fully Constrained Metal to Plastic Hinge. *Stanmore.* In 1977, the group from the Royal National Orthopedic Hospital presented their results with the Stanmore hinged elbow prosthesis.[72] The design is a hinge with a slotted polyethylene brushing on the humeral component to facilitate assembly at time of operation. Fourteen implants were reviewed with follow-up from 16 months to 6 years. Two patients were lost to follow-up, two implants were revised for loosening, and ten were reported having a satisfactory result. Twelve patients have rheumatoid arthritis, one has old tuberculosis, and one is post-trauma. No comment was made on radiographic appearance at time of review.

Semi-constrained Metal to Plastic Hinge. These elbow prostheses were all developed in the United States,

with one exception, as opposed to the preceding designs, which are all European in origin. A semi-constrained hinge means that the humeral and ulnar components are linked together with a loose metal to plastic bearing that has varying degrees of play or laxity. The theory of the developers is that the "loose" hinge will allow the soft tissue to absorb high moments and other forces instead of direct transmission to the bone-cement interface via a rigid hinge.

Flexible Elbow Joint Replacement. Pritchard[73,74] reported the results of a metal to plastic loose hinge prosthesis that has 5 degrees of axial rotation and 8 degrees of medial-lateral laxity. The humeral component is all polyethylene and the ulnar component cobalt-chrome-molybdenum (Fig. 115–3). Twenty-five patients were listed with follow-up of 2 to 3 years.[73] Twenty-three of the implants were rated good to excellent and two rated poor. The two poor implants were caused by a fracture of the distal polyethylene component owing to insufficient bony support. As a result of this experience, a long stem metal humeral component with polyethylene bushings was designed to be used in patients with deficient bone in the distal humerus (Fig. 115–4).

Radiographs reviewed[73] at 18 to 24 months postoperative showed no evidence of loosening. In addition, Pritchard[75] has had no subsequent radiographic or clin-

Figure 115–3. Flexible hinge Mark I. All polyethylene humeral component.

Figure 115–4. Flexible hinge Mark II. Metal humeral component.

ical loosening of the prosthesis in his personal series at 5 years postoperative.

Coonrad. The Coonrad elbow prosthesis[76] is a metal to plastic hinge with 2 to 3 degrees of toggle or laxity and relatively long triangular stems for the humeral and ulnar canals (Fig. 115–5). Cubitus valgus is built into the prosthesis, and the center of rotation is anterior in the anatomic location. From a multicenter review, 150 implants have been followed from 1 to over 4 years. This represents the largest series of total elbow replacements that have been reviewed in detail and reported. The overall rating results at 4 years were 67 percent good, 25 percent fair, four elbows poor, and six elbows failed. Looking at the 87 rheumatoid elbow replacements only, the ratings were 70 percent good, 24 percent fair, and one elbow poor. The rating system categories were established, using the following criteria: good, 90 to 135

degrees of motion without significant pain; fair, 45 to 90 degrees of motion and no significant pain; poor, less than 45 degrees or significant pain. The biggest single problem was loosening of the prosthesis either suspected by radiographic appearance or proved at the time of revisional surgery (11 percent). The author concluded that the results were better in the rheumatoid patient than in the post-traumatic patient (70 percent good versus 59 percent good), and that the procedure is indicated for salvage only. The addition of longer humeral fixation stems is important in resisting torque and should reduce the incidence of loosening.

In 1981, the Mayo clinic reported a 2- to 6½-year follow-up of 33 Coonrad prostheses. Twenty-five (75 percent) were rated good to fair; and 8 (24 percent) poor. Five patients underwent revisional surgery for a loose humeral component.[80]

Tri-axial. Since 1975 the tri-axial elbow arthroplasty prosthesis (Fig. 115-6) has been used at The Hospital for Special Surgery. The prosthesis is a loose, flexible metal to plastic hinge with long intramedullary fixation stems. The hinge mechanism itself has more laxity than the Pritchard-Walker prosthesis, which was used from 1974 to 1975.[76] The combined series of these two prostheses was published in 1980[77] and included 36 implants in 31 patients. The average follow-up was 2½ years, and 23 elbows were followed 2 years or longer. Nineteen patients had rheumatoid arthritis, 9 post-traumatic, and 3 juvenile rheumatoid arthritis. Age range was 18 to 79. Results based on a predetermined rating system showed that the rheumatoid group achieved the

Figure 115–5. Coonrad prosthesis.

Figure 115–6. Tri-axial prosthesis.

greatest postoperative gains, while the post-traumatic group failed to show significant gains. Pre- and postoperative ratings for each of the diagnostic groups were rheumatoid arthritis, 35 to 85 percent; post-traumatic, 40 to 80 percent; and juvenile rheumatoid arthritis, 30 to 80 percent. Overall complication rate was 50 percent, and 19 percent underwent reoperation (seven cases). The reoperations were for hematoma evacuation (two), humeral fracture, triceps rupture, "cementophyte" loose body, deep sepsis, and broken axle. All patients with revisions are reported doing well except for persistent drainage in the deep sepsis. Two of the Pritchard-Walker prostheses are radiographically loose with radiographic lines greater than 2 cm on the ulnar side. The author concluded that this total elbow replacement gives excellent results in carefully selected patients.

Semi-constrained Metal to Plastic. *Dee*[79] (Fig. 115–7) *Mayo*[80] (Fig. 115–8). The Mayo total elbow prosthesis is a metal to plastic semi-constrained design with a snap-fit articulation (Fig. 115–8). There is laxity or play in the articulation, allowing forces to be taken up by soft tissues. The radial head can be replaced and will articulate with the capitellar portion of the metal humeral component. The Mayo Clinic has had extensive experience with total elbow arthroplasty and has reviewed their results.[80] Forty-seven Mayo total elbow arthro-

plasties were reviewed, and follow-up was 2 to 6½ years, with an average of 4.1 years. Forty-four of the patients had rheumatoid arthritis, and three had post-traumatic arthritis. Thirty-six elbows were rated fair to good; and 11, poor. Six prostheses required revisional surgery, five for loosening of the humeral component and one for loosening of the ulnar component.

Nonconstrained Metal to Plastic. *Kudo.* In 1980, Kudo published the results of 24 implants (Fig. 115–9) in rheumatoid arthritis with a minimum follow-up of 2 years and an average follow-up of 3.8 years. Fourteen (58 percent) elbows were rated excellent, seven (30 percent) fair, and three (12 percent) poor. There were no revisions for loosening of the components in bone, but one humeral component migrated proximally, and one elbow had persistent subluxation and instability.[81]

Souter. In 1977, Souter[82] reported a new resurfacing type of elbow prosthesis that replaces the trochlear articulation. The two piece metal to plastic unit has a short stem for fixation on the ulnar plastic side and three very short fixation lugs for the metal humeral component

Figure 115–7. Dee semi-constrained prosthesis.

Figure 115–8. Mayo elbow prosthesis.

Figure 115–9. Kudo total elbow prosthesis.

(Fig. 115–10). The surfaces of the prosthesis closely follow normal anatomy, and inherent stability is obtained by a rider-in-the-saddle effect. The ligaments and capsule about the elbow function normally. A personal communication from Dr. Souter dated November 8, 1978, revealed that 22 arthroplasties had been performed and that the average follow-up was 11 months, with a range of 6 to 18 months. Pain relief had been excellent. The mean preoperative flexion was 126 degrees (S.D., 16 degrees) and postoperative, 143 degrees. Gains were also noted in forearm rotation, but no significant change in extension was achieved.

London. London,[83] in 1978, reported a series of 16 patients with rheumatoid arthritis that had received a metal to plastic resurfacing prosthesis. The original components had no medullary stem fixation and simulated normal anatomy. Average follow-up was 15 months (6 to 26 months). Pain relief was excellent, and elbow motion and strength were increased by a factor of two. Two complications were listed: one patient had continued unexplained pain, and one ulnar component was loose. Fixation stems have subsequently been added to both the humeral and ulnar components (Fig. 115–11) as an option.

Capitello-Condylar Elbow Arthroplasty. In July 1974, the first capitello-condylar prosthesis (Fig. 115–12) was implanted in a patient with rheumatoid arthritis. This prosthesis was designed to resurface the joint, and there is three point fixation for both the plastic ulnar and metal humeral components. Bench testing has included wear testing in a simulator, which provided 50 pounds of constant joint reactive force, a flexion arc of 50 degrees, and distilled water lubrication. The simulator was cycled 3 million times, and the estimated combined wear and cold flow of the plastic component was 0.4 mm. Loaded rotational laxity was also measured in both fresh cadavers and the prosthesis. They were placed in an Instron apparatus with flexion fixed at 30 degrees, and

Figure 115–10. Souter elbow prosthesis.

Figure 115–11. London elbow prosthesis.

axial loads with varying normal torques were applied. This is summarized in Table 115–3 and shows that the prosthesis has more loaded rotational laxity than an intact cadaver elbow. Maximum loaded rotational laxity measured was 23 degrees in the metal ulnar stem model (Table 115–3). Varus-valgus laxity was not tested, but in the unloaded state it would be unlimited because there is no linkage or constraint between the components. Stability and location of the prosthetic joint has to be maintained by the capsule and ligaments.

The initial clinical results of the capitello-condylar elbow arthroplasty have been reported[6] and recently updated[10,85,86] for the all-plastic ulnar component. In 1978, 69 implants in 64 patients, all with rheumatoid arthritis, were reported.[86] Maximum follow-up was 4 years and minimum, 1 year. Average age was 58, with a range of 18 to 80. This represents a complete series because the all-plastic ulnar component (Fig. 115–12) was replaced by a metal boat with a medullary stem (Fig. 115–13) to enhance fixation and make the ulnar component more rigid to resist twisting of the plastic during torque loading. Using a prospective elbow rating system,[6] 59 (85 percent) of the cases were rated good to excellent postoperatively. Two elbows rated fair and eight poor or failed. However, three of the poor elbows after reoperation rated excellent. Postoperative elbow motion is seen in Table 115–4 and demonstrates that significant gain can be expected in flexion and pronation but not necessarily in extension or supination. Complications are listed in Table 115–5 and indicate the im-

portance of soft tissue handling in this procedure (dislocations, sepsis, and ulnar nerve palsy in early cases). Two of the three fractures were of the olecranon, one after major trauma. Loosening of the ulnar component with bone resorption may have weakened the bone in the area of the fractures. The third fracture occurred intraoperatively, and the split medial epicondyle healed spontaneously. Examination of the bone-cement interface revealed no evidence of loosening or radiolucent lines in the metal humeral component. The plastic ulnar boat component revealed four cases with asymptomatic radiolucent lines less than 1 mm in width. One additional elbow had an ulnar radiolucent line greater than 1 mm in width that was also asymptomatic.

In March of 1978, implantation was resumed, using the metal ulnar boat (Fig. 115–14) with a plastic liner that had been reduced 0.5 mm in width to increase loaded rotatory laxity (Table 115–3).

Thirty-one additional arthroplasties were performed in the 1978 and 1979 period using a metal ulnar boat and the standard Campbell[39] surgical approach to the elbow joint. At the end of 1979, the surgical approached was changed to an expanded lateral exposure as originally described by Kocher.[87] It was felt that the lateral approach would reduce the incidence of sepsis, postoperative dislocations, ulnar nerve palsies, wound hematomas, and triceps rupture. A recent review[88] compared 54 elbow replacements operated through a lateral approach to the previous series.[86] Although soft tissue complications still occur, the lateral approach is preferred.

From 1974 through 1982, 198 capitello-condylar elbow arthroplasties have been performed for rheumatoid arthritis at our institution. These cases were reviewed to test the viability of the nonconstrained concept for total elbow arthroplasty in long term. The major question to be answered was whether a resurfacing, unlinked type of prosthesis would protect the bone-cement interface and prevent failure through loosening. The average age of the patients was 56, and 80 percent were female. Eighty-eight percent were rated good to excellent in follow-up postoperatively. Average postoperative flexion was 133 degrees, extension (−)33 degrees. Major complications requiring revisional surgery were dislocations, 5 percent; deep sepsis, 2.5 percent; olecranon fracture, 0.5 percent; and ulnar component loosening, 0.5 percent. The other significant complication was a 4 percent incidence of partial permanent ulnar nerve palsy. Radiographic review of the prosthetic bone-cement interface showed a 12 percent incidence of less than 1 mm, mostly incomplete, nonprogressive radiolucent lines, which were considered nonsignificant.

The reviewers concluded that nonconstrained elbow arthroplasty will provide lasting bone-cement fixation without loosening but carries an increased risk for perioperative dislocation, sepsis, and ulnar nerve palsy. These complications have been recently reduced by a change to a lateral surgical approach and by the availability of variously sized prosthetic components to aid restoration of soft tissue length.

Figure 115–12. Capitello-condylar elbow prosthesis. Ulnar component is all plastic.

SURGICAL TECHNIQUE

The skin incision is longitudinal, running between the tip of the olecranon and lateral epicondyle (Fig. 115–15). A plastic incision drape is used, and tourniquet pressure is kept low (250 mm Hg) and monitored with end reading. The fascia is incised in line with the skin incision and the anconeus is separated distally from the extensor carpi ulnaris; proximally the triceps is separated from the brachioradialis (Fig. 115–16). The insertion of the anconeus is incised and the muscle is reflected as a flap towards its origin on the ulna. The underlying joint capsule is incised longitudinally, and this flap is dissected to the ulna. A subperiosteal reflection of all tissue is

Figure 115–13. Capitello-condylar prosthesis with metal ulnar boat and stem. Right and left components are seen with variable heights of plastic lines of ulnar component (3 mm, 6 mm, 9 mm). Fifteen percent oversize components are seen at the left; regular size components are seen at the right.

Table 115–3. Rotatory-loaded Laxity
in Elbow and Prosthesis

| Torque (kgf-cm) | Force (kgf) | Laxity of Rotation in Degrees | | |
		Cadaver	Plastic Stem	Metal Stem
42.5	62	5.3, 1.6	3.5	10.4
	124	2.0, 0.5	0.6	3.1
85	62	16.7, 4.6	7.6	23.6
	124	10.2, 2.0	3.6	19.3

Table 115–4. Range of Elbow Motion in Degrees

	Flexion	Extension	Pronation	Supination
Preoperative	122 ± 16	$(-)\ 34 \pm 15$	53 ± 25	54 ± 4
Postoperative	135 ± 11	$(-)\ 29 \pm 14$	71 ± 17	62 ± 24
p value	<0.0005	<0.15	<0.0025	<0.10

performed proximally to the tip of the olecranon. This sleeve of tissue contains the capsule, anconeus, and triceps tendon. The fat pad is dissected out of the olecranon fossa of the humerus.

Attention is then directed to the lateral epicondyle, and all structures are sharply reflected subperiosteally from the lateral epicondyle. This lateral tissue flap contains capsule, extensor origin, and lateral collateral ligament origin.

A synovectomy and joint debridement with removal of scar will enhance dislocation of the joint laterally, hinging on the medial capsule and ulnar nerve (Fig. 115–17). If ulnar entrapment or compression is suspected, then the nerve can be dissected free and carefully retracted. Whenever possible throughout the procedure, the elbow should be reduced to avoid constant pinching or "kinking" of the ulnar nerve. The radial head is amputated proximal to the annular ligament, and the deep branch of the radial nerve is protected with baby Bennett retractors.

Exposure can be increased by further sharp dissection of the triceps tendon from the tip of the olecranon. Osteophytes on the margins of the olecranon are debrided. The capitellum and trochlea are debrided back to healthy bone and rounded to fit the humeral component. The anterior portion of the distal humerus is freed of scarring with an elevator.

The trial humeral component stem is aligned on the shaft (Fig. 115–18), centered between the epicondyles, marked with methylene blue, and cut out down to the apex of the olecranon fossa with a rongeur or small saw (Fig. 115–19). The bone removed here is cut in half, shaped, and used later as a cement plug for the humeral and ulnar canals. To prepare the humerus an awl is used first, followed by a broach and then a larger reamer. The humerus is supported to minimize fracture while

reaming by hand. The humeral component trials have valgus fixation stem angles of 5, 10, and 15 degrees. A 5-degree stem is most commonly used. The remaining portions of both the trochlea and capitellum are rongeured anteriorly and posteriorly so the metal humeral component will seat on bone. Proper rotational alignment can be achieved by viewing the end of the humerus and using an imaginary line between the center of rotation of the capitellum and trochlea. This line should bisect the metal humeral component when it is seated on bone (Fig. 115–20).

The awl is directed 18 degrees laterally to penetrate the ulnar canal (Fig. 115–21). The fixation hole for the ulnar component is progressively enlarged with reamers. To a large extent the ulnar canal is self-aligning for the ulnar component fixation stem. In the lateral plane, the canal runs at an angle of 55 degrees from the joint line (Figs. 115–22 and 115–23).

The trochlear notch of the ulna is debrided with a rongeur, and a dental burr is used to shape the notch to the metal tray of the ulnar component. This close bony fit is important because it provides rotatory control for the ulnar component. The ulnar component is available in varying sizes and thicknesses. X-ray templates can assist in size selection. A trial reduction of the com-

Table 115–5. Complications in First 69 Total Elbow Replacements (RA)

Complications	Number	Treatment
Sepsis, deep	3	2 removed
Dislocations, recurrent	5	2 converted to flexible 1 septic 2 salvaged
Loose ulnar component	1	Revised to metal boat
Loose humeral component	0	
Fractures	3	None
Ruptured triceps tendon	1	None
Dislocation, single	1	Reduced
Ulnar nerve palsy, permanent	5	None
Ulnar nerve palsy, transient	6	None

Figure 115–14. Capitello-condylar prosthesis with anteroposterior and lateral x-rays five years after operation. Note intact bone–cement interface.

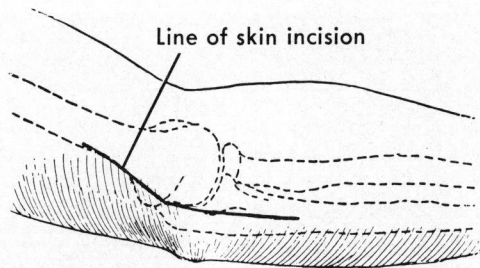

Figure 115–15. Lateral approach for elbow replacement.

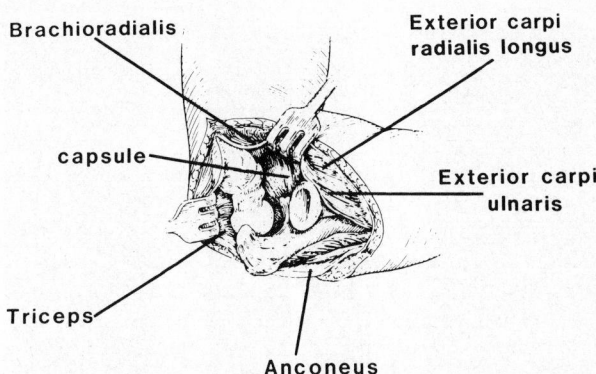

Figure 115–17. Lateral dislocation of elbow during replacement.

ponents is performed. Range of motion, stability, and a lack of toggle of the components are checked. If the elbow dislocates in a rotatory manner, then the soft tissues may be too tight medially and more bone will have to be resected from the medial bony column. If the lateral or capitellar side of the joint is loose, then a more valgus stem should be tried. With the elbow at 90 degrees of flexion, distraction is tested to determine tissue tension. The prosthetic components should not distract more than 1 to 2 mm. If the prosthesis is symmetrically too loose, then thicker plastic components should be tried. The large-size humeral and ulnar components are most appropriate for large males. A small amount of bone may have to be removed from the olecranon fossa to avoid extension block by the prosthesis. No attempt should be made to obtain full extension at surgery unless it existed preoperatively. Likewise, osteophytes may have to be debrided from the coronoid process to gain full flexion.

The bone-cement plugs are inserted into the humeral and ulnar canals by using the medullary canal reamer to drive the bone plug to a position that is distal to the stem tip. Trial components should be inserted again to assure proper positioning of the plugs.

The bone is cleaned with pulsatile lavage, and the canals are packed with dry sponges. Methacrylate is injected into the canals with a syringe and packed with digital pressure. The ulnar component is pressed into place first, followed by the humeral component, which has had cement added to the undersurface of the trochlea and capitellum. The prostheses are tapped into place, cement cleared, and the elbow held in firm extension to provide force across the joint to drive the methacrylate

into the bony interstices. The prosthetic joint should then be dislocated and cement cleared from the medial capsule and collateral ligament prior to the exotherm reaction to prevent thermal injury to the ulnar nerve. The components should be held firmly in place during final polymerization. Excess cured cement is then removed.

The wound is again irrigated, the tourniquet deflated, and bleeding points cauterized. Bleeding can be expected in the lateral extensor mass, branches of the recurrent interosseous artery distally, and the articular branch of the profunda brachii artery proximally.

Closure is in layers, starting with deep capsular tissue, using absorbable interrupted sutures. The next layer to be closed is the anconeus with its fascia to the extensor mass, which is extensor tendon, lateral collateral ligament, and extensor muscle fascia. Suction drainage is placed in the radial head space and led out subcuta-

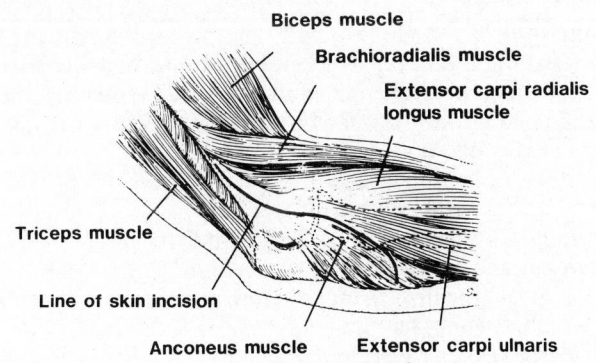

Figure 115–16. Lateral dissection for elbow replacement.

Figure 115–18. Humeral component centered over distal humerus.

Figure 115–19. *A*, Bone resection marked for insertion of humeral component. *B*, Bone resected.

neously. The superficial fascia is then closed. Integrity of the deep repair is tested by elbow flexion and the repair completed. The subcutaneous tissue is closed and interrupted nylon skin sutures are used.

Important. If the capitello-condylar trial components do not track properly and maintain reduction of the joint, then a more constrained total elbow prosthesis should be used. This will avoid the most common postoperative complication of subluxation or dislocation of the elbow.

All of the elbow replacements to date have been for rheumatoid arthritis. This elbow prosthesis is not indicated in patients with previous sepsis, previous fascial

Figure 115–21. Anterior view of ulna with proximal medullary canal marked by 18-degree offset line.

arthroplasty, deficient trochlear notch of the ulna, excessive loss of bone, as in giant rheumatoid cysts, and previous hinge-type arthroplasty. The older post-traumatic or osteoarthritic patient may be a candidate, provided a relatively low activity level is anticipated.

TEAM APPROACH TO POSTOPERATIVE REHABILITATION

The following protocol is a summary of the activities of the "team" and its approach to postoperative rehabilitation of the elbow joint. The protocol is directed toward total joint replacement but can be used after any elbow reconstructive procedure. The team represents the combined efforts of nursing, physical therapy, occupational therapy, and surgery.

Physical therapy goals:

1. Progression to full anatomical range of motion, limited only by prosthetic design and the patient's motivation and potential.

2. Strengthening of musculature associated with normal elbow function.

Physical therapy precautions:

1. Protection of triceps repair in the early postoperative regimen.

Figure 115–20. Distal humerus seen end-on with metal component in place. Note difference between center of rotation of metal humeral component and line connecting the epicondyles.

Figure 115–22. Lateral view of ulna with proximal medullary canal and prosthetic fixation stem marked.

Figure 115–23. Anterior view of ulna with medullary canal reaming for fixation stem marked.

2. Protection of prosthetic placement by allowing permitted activities only with upper arm in adducted position for a period of 6 weeks (until capsular healing is complete).

Occupational therapy goals:

1. To maximize the patient's ability to perform self-care during the postoperative program.

2. To facilitate optimal discharge planning through assessment of home situation.

After appropriate preoperative evaluation and instruction by the hospital team, surgery is performed 2 days after admission. Postoperatively the patient's arm is placed in a commercial posterior Velcro-fastened splint and sling. Neurologic and vascular status are monitored frequently in the immediate postoperative period. Radiographic check for location is performed in the recovery room. The elbow is elevated on pillows. On the first postoperative day, suction drainage is removed, and hand and wrist motion is started. The dressing is changed on the second postoperative day. By the fourth postoperative day, if the wound appears benign and the drainage has stopped, active assisted range of motion exercises are started with the elbow held at the side. These include flexion, extension, and forearm rotation.

The exercises are performed twice daily out of the sling and splint. At 7 to 10 days postoperative, occupational therapy starts instruction in activities of daily living with the elbow held at the side. At this point the sling is used only during the day and the splint at night. The patient is usually discharged 2 weeks postoperative on a program of home physical therapy. The sling during the day and the splint at night are continued for an additional 2 weeks and then discarded. The patient is cautioned not to reach out away from the body to pick up anything for a total of 6 weeks postoperative to allow for capsular healing and to prevent dislocation. After total elbow arthroplasty, the patient cannot return to racket sports, golf, baseball, other competitive athletics, or heavy labor.

SURGICAL INDICATIONS FOR VARIOUS PROCEDURES

Intractable pain is the major indication for elbow surgery in rheumatoid arthritis in all cases at our institution except for bilaterally fused elbows, which are usually painless. In these cases the dominant elbow is resurfaced to restore function. If the elbow has normal range of motion with intact subchondral bone plates and possibly some remaining articular cartilage, a radial head excision and synovectomy is recommended. If there is significant limitation of motion but good bony stock, then resurfacing is the procedure of chioce. If there is loss of bony stock or gross bony destruction, then one of the "loose" metal to plastic hinges is preferred.

References

1. Morrey, B.F., and Chao, E.Y.S.: Passive motion of the elbow joint. A biomechanical analysis. J. Bone Joint Surg. 58A:501, 1976.
2. Walker, P.S.: Human Joints and Their Artificial Replacements. Springfield, Ill., Charles C Thomas, 1977.
3. London, J.T.: Kinematics of the elbow. J. Bone Joint Surg. 63A:529, 1981.
4. Fick, R.: Spezielle Gelenk und Muskelmechanik, Mechanik des Kniegelenkes. Jena, G. Fisher, III:521, 1911.
5. Frankel, V.H., and Burstein, A.H.: Orthopedic Biomechanics. Philadelphia, Lea & Febiger, 1970.
6. Ewald, F.C.: Total elbow replacement. Orthop. Clin. North Am. 6:685, 1975.
7. Sledge, C.B.: Unpublished study. Personal communication, 1977.
8. Ray, R.D., Johnson, R.J., and Jameson, R.M.: Rotation of the forearm. J. Bone Joint Surg. 33A:993, 1951.
9. Nicol, A.C., Berme, N.N., and Paul, J.P.: A biomechanical analysis of elbow joint function. In Joint Replacement in the Upper Limb. London, Mechanical Engineering Publications Limited, 1977.
10. Ewald, F.C., Thomas, W.H., Sledge, C.B., and Poss, R.: Non-constrained metal to plastic elbow arthroplasty in rheumatoid arthritis. In Joint Replacement in the Upper Limb. London, Mechanical Engineering Publications Ltd., 1977.
11. Asher, M.A., and Lilber, S.: Biomechanics of the elbow and forearm. A.A.O.S. Postgraduate Course in Elbow, Wrist and Forearm. Kansas City, Oct. 13, 1973.
12. Blount, W.P.: Fractures in Children. Baltimore, Williams & Wilkins Company, 1955.
13. Cave, E.F., Burke, J.F., and Boyd, R.J.: Trauma Management. Chicago, Year Book Medical Publishers, 1974.
14. Rockwood, C.A., and Green, D.P.: Fractures. Philadelphia, J. B. Lippincott Company, 1975.
15. Schuller, M.: Die Pathologie und Therapie des Gelenkentzundunger. Vienna, Urban and Schwarzenberg, 1887.
16. Goldtwait, J.E.: Knee joint surgery for non-tubercular conditions. A report of thirty-eight operations for synovial fringes, injured semilunar cartilage, loose cartilage, coagula, exploratory incision, etc. Boston Med. Surg. J. 143:286, 1900.
17. Hijmans, W., Paul, W.D., and Herschel, H. (eds.): Early Synovectomy in Rheumatoid Arthritis. Proceedings of the Symposium on early synovectomy in rheumatoid arthritis. Amsterdam. 12-15 April, 1967. Amsterdam, Excerpta Medica Foundation, 1969.
18. Wilkinson, M.C.: Synovectomy for rheumatoid arthritis. Clin. Orthop. Rel. Res. 100:125, 1974.
19. Geens, S.: Synovectomy and debridement of the knee in rheumatoid arthritis. Part I. Historical review. J. Bone Joint Surg. 51A:617, 1969.
20. Smith-Petersen, M.N., Aufranc, O.E., and Larson, C.B.: Useful surgical procedures for rheumatoid arthritis involving joints of the upper extremity. Arch. Surg. 46:764, 1943.
21. Wilkinson, M.C., and Lowry, J.H.: Synovectomy for rheumatoid arthritis. J. Bone Joint Surg. 47B:482, 1965.
22. Laine, V., and Vainio, K.: Synovectomy of the elbow. In Hijmans, W., Paul, W.D., and Herschel, H. (eds.): Early Synovectomy in Rheumatoid Arthritis. Amsterdam, Excerpta Medica Foundation, 1969.
23. Torgerson, W.R., and Leach, R.E.: Synovectomy of the elbow in rheumatoid arthritis. J. Bone Joint Surg. 52A:371, 1970.
24. Inglis, A.E., Ranawat, C.S., and Straub, L.R.: Synovectomy and debridement of the elbow in rheumatoid arthritis. J. Bone Joint Surg. 53A:652, 1971.
25. Peterson, L.F.A., and Jones, J.M.: Surgery of rheumatoid elbow. Orthop. Clin. North Am. 2:667, 1971.
26. Marmor, L.: Surgery of the rheumatoid elbow. J. Bone Joint Surg. 54A:573, 1972.
27. Wilson, D.W., Arden, G.P., and Ansell, B.M.: Surgery of the elbow in rheumatoid arthritis. J. Bone Joint Surg. 55B:106, 1973.
28. Porter, B.B., Richardson, C., and Vainio, K.: Rheumatoid arthritis of the elbow: The results of synovectomy. J. Bone Joint Surg. 56B:427, 1974.
29. Taylor, A.R., Mukerjea, S.K., and Rana, N.A.: Excision of the head of the radius in rheumatoid arthritis. J. Bone Joint Surg. 58B:485, 1976.
30. Ferlic, D.C., Clayton, M.L., and Parr, P.L.: Surgery of the elbow in rheumatoid arthritis. J. Bone Joint Surg. 58A:726, 1976.
31. Arthritis Foundation Committee on Evaluation of Synovectomy: Multi-

32. Ehrlich, G.E.: Antecubital cysts in rheumatoid arthritis—a corollary to popliteal (Baker's) cysts. J. Bone Joint Surg. 54A:165, 1972.
33. Hurri, L., Pulkki, T., and Vainio, K.: Arthroplasty of the elbow in rheumatoid arthritis. Acta Chir. Scand. 127:459, 1964.
34. Herbert, J.J.: Traitement des ankyloses du coude dans le rheumatisme. Rev. Chir. Orthop. 44:87, 1958.
35. Hass, J.: Functional arthroplasty. J. Bone Joint Surg. 26:297, 1944.
36. Dickson, R.A., Stein, H., and Bentley, G.: Excision arthroplasty of the elbow in rheumatoid disease. J. Bone Joint Surg. 58B:227, 1976.
37. Volkov, M.V., and Oganesian, O.V.: Restoration of function in the knee and elbow with a hinge-distractor apparatus. J. Bone Joint Surg. 57A:591, 1975.
38. MacAusland, W.R.: Mobilization of the elbow by free fascia transplantation with report of thirty-one cases. Surg. Gynecol. Obstet. 23:223, 1921.
39. Campbell, W.C.: Arthroplasty of the elbow. Ann. Surg. 76:615, 1922.
40. Mac Ausland, W.R.: Arthroplasty of the elbow. New Engl. J. Med. 236:97, 1947.
41. Knight, R.A., and Van Zandt, I.L.: Arthroplasty of the elbow. An end result study. J. Bone Joint Surg. 34A:610, 1952.
42. Silva, F.J.: Arthroplasty of the elbow. Singapore Med. J. 8:222, 1967.
43. Gui, L.: La cura chirurgica delle rigidita post-traumatiche del gomito e del ginocchio. Arch. Putti. 3:390, 1953.
44. Fromison, A.J., Silva, J.E., and Richey, D.G.: Cutis arthroplasty of the elbow joint. J. Bone Joint Surg. 58A:863, 1976.
45. Unander-Scharin, L., and Karlholm, S.: Experience of arthroplasty of the elbow. Acta Orthop. Scand. 36:54, 1965.
46. Cobey, M.: Arthroplasties using compressed Ivalon sponge. Clin. Orthop. Rel. Res. 54:139, 1967.
47. Robineau, R.: Contribution a l'étude des prostheses osseuses. Bull. Mim. Soc. Nat. Chir. 53:886. 1927.
48. Tessarolo, G.: Endoprotesi acrilica articolare per il girnito. Minerva Ortop. 3:308, 1952.
49. MacAusland, W.R.: Replacement of the lower end of the humerus with a prosthesis. A report of four cases. West. J. Surg. Gynecol. Obstet. 62:557, 1954.
50. Venable, C.S.: An elbow and elbow prosthesis. Case of complete loss of the lower third of the humerus. Am. J. Surg. 83:271, 1952.
51. Jakobsson, A.: Fracture of the capitellum of the humerus in adults. Treatment with intra-articular chrome-cobalt-molybdenum prosthesis. Acta Orthop. Scand. 26:184, 1957.
52. Lenggenhager, V.: Zur Frage des künstlichen Ellbogengelenkes. Helv. Chir. Acta 25:338, 1958.
53. Barr, J.S., and Eaton, R.G.: Elbow reconstruction with a new prosthesis to replace the distal end of the humerus. A case report. J. Bone Joint Surg. 47A:1408, 1965.
54. Street, D.M., and Stevens, P.S.: A humeral replacement prosthesis for the elbow. J. Bone Joint Surg. 56A:1147, 1974.
55. Stevens, P.S.: Distal humeral prosthesis for the elbow. In Joint Replacement in the Upper Limb. London. Mechanical Engineering Publications Ltd., 1977.
56. Stevens, P.S.: Arthroplasty of the elbow with Stevens-Street prosthesis. Orthop. Trans. 2:217, 1978.
57. Johnson, E.W., and Schlein, A.P.: Vitallium prosthesis for the olecranon and proximal part of the ulna. J. Bone Joint Surg. 52A:721, 1970.
58. Boerema, I., and deWaard, D.J.: Osteoplastische Verakening von Metallprosthesen bei Pseudarthrose und bei Orthoplastik. Acta Chir. Scand. 86:511, 1942.
59. Lenggenhager, V.K.: Zur Frage des Künstlichen Ellbogengelenkes. Helv. Chir. Acta. 25:338, 1958.
60. Chatzidakis, C.: Arthroplasty of the elbow joint using a vitallican prosthesis. Joint Surg. 53:119, 1970.
61. Dee, R.: Total replacement arthroplasty of the elbow for rheumatoid arthritis. J. Bone Joint Surg. 54B:88, 1972.
62. Dee, R.: Total replacement of the elbow joint. Orthop. Clin. North Am. 4:415, 1973.
63. Souter, W.A.: Arthroplasty of the elbow with reference to metallic hinge arthroplasty in rheumatoid patients. Orthop. Clin. North Am. 4:335, 1973.
64. Dunn, H.K., and Carson, R.W.: Total replacement of the elbow. J. Bone Joint Surg. 56A:196, 1974.
65. Dee, R.: Five year experience with total replacement of the elbow. In Joint Replacement in the Upper Limb. London, Mechanical Engineering Publications Ltd., 1977.
66. Gschwend, N., Scheier, H., and Bähler, A: Die GSB-Ellbogen-Endoprothese. Arch. Orthop. Unfall-Chir. 73:316, 1972.
67. Gschwend, N.: Arthroplasty of the Elbow Using the GSB Prosthesis. Proceedings of the 12th Congress of the International Society of Orthopedic Surgery and Traumatology. Tel Aviv, Oct. 9-12, 1972. Amsterdam, Excerpta Medica.

68. Gschwend, N., and Scheier, H.: Elbow-arthroplasty with the new GSB-prosthesis. Scand. J. Rheumatol. (submitted for publication).
69. Gschwend, N.: Our experience of elbow arthroplasty with the GSB prosthesis. Acta Orthop. Belg. 41:470, 1975.
70. Gschwend, N., Scheier, H., and Bähler, A.: GSB elbow, wrist and PIP joints. In Joint Replacement in the Upper Limb. London, Mechanical Engineering Publications Ltd., 1977.
71. Garrett, J.C., Ewald, F.C., Thomas, W.H., and Sledge, C.B.: Loosening associated with G.S.B. hinge total elbow replacements in patients with rheumatoid arthritis. Clin. Orthop. Rel. Res. 127:170, 1977.
72. Scales, J.T., Lettin, A.W.F., and Bailey, J.: The evolution of the Stanmore hinged total elbow replacement. In Joint Replacement in the Upper Limb. London, Mechanical Engineering Publications Ltd., 1977.
73. Pritchard, R.W.: Flexible elbow joint replacement. In Joint Replacement in the Upper Limb. London, Mechanical Engineering Publications, Ltd., 1977.
74. Pritchard, R.W.: Flexible elbow joint replacement. Orthop. Trans. 1:109, 1977.
75. Pritchard, R.W.: Personal communication, September 14, 1978.
76. Coonrad, R.W.: Coonrad total elbow replacement. Am. Orthop. Assn. Mtg. June 27, 1978.
77. Inglis, A.E., and Pellicci, P.M.: Total elbow replacement. J. Bone Joint Surg. 62A:1252, 1980.
78. Attenborough, C.G.: Joint replacement in the upper limb. In Joint Replacement in the Upper Limb. London, Mechanical Engineering Publications Ltd., 1977.
79. Dee, R.: Personal communication, November 24, 1978.
80. Morrey, B.F., Bryan, R.S., Dobyns, J.H., and Lindscheid, R.H.: Total elbow arthroplasty. J. Bone Joint Surg. 63A:1050, 1981.
81. Kudo, H., Iwano, K., and Watanabe, S.: Total replacement of the rheumatoid elbow with a hingeless prosthesis. J. Bone Joint Surg. 62A:277, 1980.
82. Souter, W.A.: Total replacement arthroplasty of the elbow. In Joint Replacement in the Upper Limb. London, Mechanical Engineering Publications Ltd., 1977.
83. London, J.T.: Resurfacing total elbow arthroplasty. Orthop. Trans. 2:217, 1978.
84. Ishizuki, M.: Biomechanical analysis of the elbow joint preliminary report of hingeless total elbow arthroplasty. Personal communication. September 18, 1978.
85. Ewald, F.C.: Non-constrained metal to plastic total elbow replacement. Orthop. Trans. 1:110, 1977.
86. Ewald, F.C.: Total elbow replacement. American Orthopedic Association Meeting, June 27, 1978.
87. Kocher, T.: Textbook of Operative Surgery. 3rd ed. (H.J. Stiles and C.B. Paul, translators) London, A.C. Black, 1911.
88. Ewald, F.C., and Jacobs, M.A.: Total Elbow Arthroplasty. Clin. Orthop. Rel. Res., 182:137, 1984

Chapter 116

Reconstructive Surgery and Rehabilitation of the Shoulder

Charles S. Neer II

HOW THE SHOULDER IS UNIQUE

Four Joints. The arthritic diseases may involve one or all of four joints: the glenohumeral joint, the acromioclavicular joint, the sternoclavicular joint, or the scapulothoracic bursa, which functions as the fourth joint. These articulations normally move synchronously and simultaneously. The glenohumeral joint moves twice as rapidly as the scapula. The sum of the motion of the two joints at the end of the clavicle equals the movement of the scapula. Disability in any one of them reduces the efficiency of the others. A frozen glenohumeral joint causes additional strain on the scapular muscle and often results in scapular pain. The result of a perfect glenohumeral arthroplasty can be spoiled by a painful acromioclavicular joint. In rheumatoid patients with shoulder pain, all four of these structures should be evaluated repeatedly, and all must be treated as the need arises.

Rotator Cuff. The normal glenohumeral joint has more motion than any other joint in the body. To allow this motion, the glenoid is relatively flat and is only about one quarter the size of the head. There is no bony socket as in the hip. Furthermore, to allow this motion, the ligaments are loose. They do not provide stability as in the knee. Stability is dependent in large part upon the rotator cuff. The components of the rotator cuff function as active ligaments. The supraspinatus contracts synchronously with the middle deltoid to snub up the head against ascent.[1] This function is aided by the inferior parts of the infraspinatus and subscapularis as well as the teres minor and long head of the biceps. Excessive rotation is controlled by the internal and external rotators.

Not only does the rotator cuff provide stability; it also moves the joint. The most important function of the glenohumeral joint is rotation. This points the hand in the direction needed when the elbow is moved. The elbow flexes and extends while the shoulder rotates, and the two function as a unit (see The Upper Extremity Unit, below). It is important in shoulder reconstruction to appreciate that while there are a number of muscles outside the rotator cuff that internally rotate the shoulder (e.g., teres major, pectoralis, latissimus), on the other hand, the only effective external rotators are rotator cuff muscles (e.g., the infraspinatus and teres minor). A large tear of the rotator cuff that includes the infraspinatus weakens the power of external rotation to such an extent that the hand cannot be used effectively away from the side or above the horizontal. Sufficient cuff muscles to depress the head of the humerus against the force of the deltoid and to provide external rotation are of key importance. Muscle repair and rehabilitation are more demanding in shoulder surgery than in other joints.

Anterior Deltoid. It is now appreciated[2] that the usual arc of shoulder elevation is forward, not lateral. The anterior deltoid is the most important part of this muscle in shoulder reconstruction. In planning approaches one should retain all possible attachments of deltoid origin, especially the anterior part. Without the anterior deltoid overhead function is impossible.

Biceps Long Head. The long head of the biceps stabilizes the humeral head against riding upward. It tends to reduce subacromial impingement.[3,4] In doing reconstructive procedures we believe it should be preserved if possible. Rheumatoid synovitis involving the long head of the biceps is not a separate entity but is an extension of the underlying glenohumeral synovitis. Synovectomy of the sheath and tenodesis of the long head are inadequate and may increase the problem of subacromial impingement.[3]

"Subacromial Mechanism" and Bursa. The subacromial space functions as a second joint space. Rehabilitation following shoulder surgery is more demanding than in other joints because it is necessary to re-establish this second space as well as the large glenohumeral joint space itself. Persistent thickening of the bursa caused by rheumatoid granulation, rice bodies, and scar can interfere with shoulder function. Rheumatoid involvement of the bursa can also interfere with shoulder function. Rheumatoid involvement of the bursa can also interfere with the nutrition of the rotator cuff and lead to attrition of these tendons. A "cuff tear" in a rheumatoid shoulder is usually due to tendon invasion by the inflammatory process with attrition rather than trauma and impingement. However, when the stabilizing effect of the rotator cuff is weakened, the head tends to ride up, impingement develops, and wear from impingement may contribute to the rupture of rotator tendons. We believe that when this type of impingement lesion is seen at surgery, an anterior acromioplasty should be performed to minimize this secondary factor of wear.

Complex Muscle Couplings. In the rheumatoid patient muscle disease can preclude recovery of function following even the most perfect arthroplasty. Nearly all the muscles in the upper half of the body are involved in the process of moving the four shoulder joints. This includes the muscles that rotate and stabilize the scapula and those that attach to the humerus as well as the biceps. It should be anticipated that the rate of recovery following surgery will be slower than in an osteoarthritic or trauma patient in whom the muscles are normal and simple disuse atrophy can easily be overcome.

Influence of Cervical Spine Disease. Involvement of the cervical roots can interfere with a successful shoulder reconstruction. It can account not only for pain but also for weakness in the deltoid and rotator cuff muscles.[5] The fifth and sixth cervical levels are the most critical. Higher roots may cause scapular pain. Electromyographic examination is of great help in assessing these muscles and should be done preoperatively when in doubt.

The "Upper Extremity Unit." Shoulder rotation and elbow flexion form a unit. The two act together to place the hand where it is needed for heavy as well as light activities, e.g., throwing, pushing, lifting, or reaching the face. The painful shoulder assumes the "protective position" against unwanted movement. The arm is held close to the side in internal rotation, the elbow is flexed,

the wrist falls into ulnar deviation, and the fingers tend to drift ulnarward. Thus, the painful shoulder enhances the development of deformities throughout the length of the extremity. Eliminating pain and freeing up the shoulder, either by conservative measures or surgically, has a beneficial effect on both the hand and elbow (see Conservative Treatment, below). The "shoulder-hand syndrome" and pain referred to the elbow are removed. Eliminating shoulder pain also has a beneficial effect upon painful scapular muscles that have been under strain by attempts to compensate for lost glenohumeral motion with scapular motion.

CLINICAL ASPECTS OF THE RHEUMATOID SHOULDER

Insidious Onset. The onset of shoulder arthritis is variable but initially tends to be subacute and transitory rather than constant and destructive. With each rheumatoid attack the painful shoulder is splinted by holding the arm tightly against the chest in the "protective position," and the inactivity has a deleterious effect beyond that of the rheumatoid disease (see Conservative Treatment, below). It is important to recognize the stiffness early and, if possible, to reverse this process by conservative measures before irreversible changes have developed.

Identifying Shoulder Arthritis. The shoulder is a frequent site of rheumatoid arthritis, but it is too often ignored by the physician. There are a number of reasons for this. Shoulders are covered with clothing and less conspicuous than the hands and other parts of the body. They attract less attention. Shoulder pain is often referred distally, causing patients to misunderstand the source of the pain. In addition, the attitude of the patient has at times been a barrier to the early diagnosis of shoulder problems. Many have found that their physician is less interested in the shoulder than in other joints such as the hip, knee, hand, or foot. They have been told that there is not much to be done about shoulders, and they have become complacent regarding their shoulder pain. For these reasons the rheumatologist must seek out shoulder involvement if an early diagnosis is to be made. A systematic physical examination is important.

System for Examination. The initial part of the examination is done with the patient sitting with both shoulders exposed. A good system is to begin at the cervical spine and scapular areas. Referred pain and neurological involvement from the neck are considered, followed by the acromioclavicular and sternoclavicular joints and supraclavicular region, and finally the glenohumeral joint. This is followed by an examination of the elbows, wrists, and hands. The glenohumeral joint is palpated for swelling, thickened tissue, and heat, as well as tenderness. Motion, measured with the patient supine and sitting as described in the following paragraph, strength of the rotators and deltoid, and level of function are recorded. Tenderness along the posterior joint line is the most important sign for arthritic involvement of the glenohumeral joint.

Recording Motion. The earliest evidence of shoulder involvement is usually loss of glenohumeral motion. An efficient method of recording this range of motion is of great importance. In the past, this has been too casual and inconsistent. Glenohumeral rotation is greatest when the arm is at the side and diminishes as the arm is raised. Therefore it is logical to measure internal and external rotation with the arm at the side. Forward elevation is done without rotation, but abduction is a combination of both elevation and rotation. Therefore it seems logical to record "total elevation" rather than abduction.[6] Attempts to measure shoulder motion with the patient standing are just as futile as measuring hip motion with the patient standing. The spine and knees compensate and make accurate measurements impossible. External rotation and total passive elevation are measured with the patient supine. Internal rotation (reaching up the back) and total active elevation are measured with the patient sitting. Recordings of these four measurements give a simple and reproducible way of following clinical progress.

Roentgen Examination. The routine examination is made in the anteroposterior view with the arm in internal and external rotation, and in the true axillary view. The glenohumeral joint space can be evaluated better if the anteroposterior views are made in the scapular plane (with the x-ray beam angled 15 degrees lateral to the coronal plane). The earliest roentgen evidence of disease includes osteoporosis of the bone and erosion of the joint margin. Erosion of the glenoid and subluxation of the head are best seen in the axillary view (see Fig. 116–5), and this finding favors operative intervention. For optimal visualization of the acromioclavicular joint, less exposure is used than for the glenohumeral joint. Tomograms may be helpful for visualizing the sternoclavicular joints.

Patterns of Involvement. *Low Grade, Intermediate, and Severe.* It is helpful to the clinician to classify patients as having low grade, intermediate, or severe disease. The nature of shoulder involvement varies widely and may be mild and intermittent or severe and destructive. Rehabilitation of the muscles in patients with low grade involvement is more difficult than in patients with osteoarthritis but is much easier than in those with intermediate and severe rheumatoid disease. It is a common misconception that all shoulders involved with rheumatoid arthritis have tears of the rotator cuff; actually, while most patients with severe involvement do have cuff tears, the cuff has been found intact in 70 percent of the rheumatoid shoulders I have operated upon.[7] Others have had a similar experience.[8,9]

Dry, Wet, and Resorptive. Three types of involvement are seen: dry, wet, and resorptive (Figs. 116–1 and 116–2). In the dry form (Fig. 116–1*A*) there is marked tendency for stiffness and loss of joint space with sclerosis and areas of cystification in the bone. Minimal marginal erosion is seen, and eventually marginal osteophytes may form similar to those in osteoarthritis. Clinically these patients have much more stiffness and weakness than those with osteoarthritis. In the wet form (Fig. 116–1*B*)

there are exuberant granulations and marginal erosions causing the end of the bone to become pointed. There is progressive intrusion of the humeral head into the glenoid (Fig. 116–1*C*). In the resorptive type (Fig. 116–1*D*), destruction and resorption of the bone is the outstanding feature. In the dry type there is good bone stock for reconstruction, but in the others the bone is usually soft and easily fractured.

Syndrome. Through the years we have repeatedly seen a condition we have referred to as "the syndrome"[10] (Fig. 116–2). It consists of dry, low-grade rheumatoid involvement of the shoulders, usually bilateral, that spares most other joints. There is progressive loss of the joint space and areas of sclerosis mixed with cystification of the head and eventually marginal osteophytes. This is seen more often in women, and the patients are between 35 and 55 years of age. The serology is usually positive for the rheumatoid factor, and they are eventually diagnosed as having rheumatoid arthritis by the rheumatologist. These patients can develop an extremely painful disability, and if so they are ideal candidates for reconstructive surgery.

Bursal Type. Huge enlargements of the subacromial and subdeltoid bursa are occasionally seen in the absence of glenohumeral involvement[8,11,12] (Fig. 116–3). The bursa is filled with rice bodies and with much less fluid than would be expected. The dearth of fluid may cause a dry tap on attempts at aspiration and cause the physician to suspect a solid neoplasm. The acromioclavicular joint is usually diseased in these patients.

Differential Diagnosis. *Osteoarthritis.* Osteoarthritis of the glenohumeral joint is less common than that of the hip or knee, but it is not rare. It is, however, infrequent enough that most clinicians are unfamiliar with it. The roentgen appearance is constant and characteristic and is distinctly different from that of rheumatoid arthritis[13,14] (Fig. 116–4). An area of sclerosis, perhaps with a subchondral cyst, forms on the upper part of the head. This area of head is in contact with the glenoid when the arm is held in an abducted position. In the abducted position there is the maximal joint reaction force, and the weight of the arm is brought against the head with a leverage force of about ten to one. Sclerosis forms at this point on the head where there is maximal pressure. Osteophytes form where there is less pressure and are consistently more prominent inferiorly. The glenoid tends to be eroded more posteriorly than anteriorly (Fig. 116–5). It is of clinical importance to know that the alterations seen in osteoarthritis require great pressure, and this implies an intact rotator cuff. We believe that it is extremely rare to find a tear of the rotator cuff in a shoulder with the typical and classic roentgen appearance of primary osteoarthritis. I have seen only one such patient in over 100 primary osteoarthritic shoulders treated surgically in my personal series,[14] and that patient had sustained an injury after the development of osteoarthritis. In contrast, patients with tears of the rotator cuff do not develop head changes until very late, and these changes are quite different, as described under Impingement Lesions, below. This information is im-

Figure 116–1. Anteroposterior films depicting the variations in rheumatoid arthritis of the shoulder. *A*, The "dry" form, which begins with marked stiffness, loss of joint space, and sclerosis mixed with cystification, as in Figure 116–2. Later marginal osteophytes appear as seen in osteoarthritis, and at this stage it has been referred to as "mixed arthritis." *B*, The "wet" form with sloppy tissue and marginal erosion of the humeral head, glenoid, and acromioclavicular joint. *C*, Late stage of a severe wet form with marked intrusion into the glenoid, acromion, and clavicle. The arrow indicates where the coracoid process has been eroded halfway through. There is a massive tear of the rotator cuff, and the upper humerus resembles the upper femur. It is impossible to properly orient the standard glenoid prosthesis in this type of shoulder, and special glenoid components are being developed for this problem (see Fig. 116–8). *D*, Rheumatoid vasculitis with marked destruction and resorption of bone. There was a massive detachment of the rotator cuff, and the remains of the humeral head were lying out in the subdeltoid bursa. Nevertheless this shoulder was rendered pain free and stable with an unconstrained, resurfacing total shoulder, as in Figure 116–7.

portant in planning shoulder reconstruction. Although fusion has been advised by some[15,16] as the treatment for osteoarthritis, we have found that since the muscles are normal in this condition, it is most ideal for prosthetic replacement arthroplasty.[5,13,14,17-19]

Secondary Osteoarthritis. A number of conditions can cause articular surface damage that may ultimately lead to a picture resembling primary osteoarthritis[13,14] (Fig. 116–4). The list includes metabolic disorders (gout and

ochronosis), inactive suppurative arthritis, infarctional diseases (sickle cell, lupus, and Gaucher's), and articular surface trauma (fractures and dislocations with or without previous operative treatment). Some of them can be confused with rheumatoid arthritis. In addition it appears that some low-grade rheumatoid patients may have "burned-out" disease that can come to resemble osteoarthritis, and this is sometimes referred to as "mixed arthritis."

Figure 116–2. A clinical "syndrome" of low-grade, atypical rheumatoid arthritis that involves the shoulders almost exclusively and spares most other joints. The serology is usually positive for the rheumatoid factor. This anteroposterior view was made in the scapular plane and shows the complete loss of joint space that occurred over a 3-year period. Both shoulders are usually involved. Marginal osteophytes form later, as illustrated in Figure 116–1*A*.

Impingement Lesions. The rotator cuff functions like the acetabulum in the hip; therefore, degenerative and traumatic *lesions of the rotator cuff* are nearly as common as osteoarthritis of the hip. Tears of the complete thickness of the tendon have been found in from 5.0%,[20] 9.3%,[21] and 12.9%[22] of cadavers in the anatomy laboratory. The rotator cuff is not seen in roentgenograms; this makes cuff lesions much harder to diagnose, and they must be differentiated from other types of "arthritis."[2,23-25] We now recognize three impingement lesions: Grade I is edema and swelling, Grade II is fibrosis and thickening, and Grade III is bone reaction and tendon rupture. We believe that over 90 percent of cuff tears are due to subacromial impingement and wear, with trauma playing only a secondary role.[2,17,18,20,23,24,45] They are seen in women almost as frequently as in men, and about half of the patients recall no significant trauma.[2,23,24] Evidences of longstanding impingement (excrescences or eburnation at the greater tuberosity[4] or acromion[2]) are usually seen in radiographs or at surgery. Thinning of the distance from the humerus to the acromion is present in patients with larger tears. Some of these roentgen features may be seen in rheumatoid shoulders, but only after attenuation and weakness of the cuff has allowed the head to ride up against the acromion, leading to subacromial impingement as a secondary phenomenon (see "Subacromial Mechanism" and Bursa, above). Arthrography is the most reliable method for proving the presence of a cuff tear.[25] When there is an incomplete thickness tear, the arthrogram is usually negative. The "impingement test" (pain relief following a subacromial lidocaine injection) is helpful in detecting impingement lesions.[20] Posterior joint-line tenderness,

Figure 116–3. The bursal type of rheumatoid involvement. *A,* Huge enlargement of the subacromial bursa and involvement of the acromioclavicular joint. The glenohumeral joint is almost completely spared. *B,* Contents of the bursa seen after its removal. It was filled with rice bodies and contained very little fluid. The dearth of fluid causes a dry tap on attempts to aspirate and may cause the physician to suspect a solid neoplasm.

Figure 116–4. Anteroposterior view showing the typical, characteristic roentgen appearance of primary osteoarthritis of the glenohumeral joint. There is eburnation and wear on that part of the head that is in contact with the glenoid when the arm is abducted 60 to 100 degrees, as well as marginal osteophytes, which are largest inferiorly where they cover the calcar, and sclerosis with marginal excrescences of the glenoid that cause the glenoid to appear enlarged. These radiographic features are constant and are distinctly different from those of rheumatoid arthritis (see Figs. 116–1 and 116–2).

thickening of the joint, and stiffness are seen in the rheumatoid shoulder to help differentiate it from an impingement lesion.

Biceps lesions may be caused by subacromial impingement[3,20,26] or by irregularities of the bicipital groove. This includes both biceps tenosynovitis and biceps rupture. Rheumatoid involvement of the sheath of the long head can be differentiated because it is associated with involvement of the underlying joint as well.

"Cuff tear arthropathy" is a term I have used since 1975 to describe the condition that is seen with some longstanding tears of the rotator cuff.[7,28-30] An irregular, pebble stone appearance of the articular cartilage of the humeral head develops, and the underlying bone softens and collapses. These changes in the articular

Figure 116–5. True axillary view showing posterior erosion of the glenoid and posterior subluxation of the head in a 55-year-old woman with osteoarthritis. Posterior migration of the head tends to occur in all types of glenohumeral arthritis.

cartilage are probably due to inactivity and malnutrition of the cartilage. In some cases, but not in all, there have been steroid injections that might have contributed to the problem. Massive tears permit dislocations and subluxations of the glenohumeral joint, which inflict abnormal trauma to the articular surfaces and are thought to play an important role in the collapse of the head. It seems important to consider "cuff tear arthropathy" as a separate entity, because its reconstruction is especially difficult. Certainly it is not like osteoarthritis (in which the cuff is intact), not like steroid arthropathy (in which the cuff is intact), and not like rheumatoid arthritis (in which the joint is eroded and the cuff is often intact).[30] Cuff-tear arthropathy is thought to be the same condition that has more recently been referred to as "Milwaukee shoulder."[31]

Aseptic Necrosis. In steroid arthropathy and aseptic necrosis and in infarctional disease (see Secondary Osteoarthritis, above), the rotator cuff remains completely normal and, at least in the early stages, the glenoid is normal.[27] Pain is usually most intense at the period while the head is collapsing. Irregularities of the head may later erode the glenoid. Tomograms can clarify the extent of head involvement. In some cases fragments of bone are engulfed by the synovium, and the picture then resembles a neurotrophic joint.

Neurologic Problems. Cervical spine disease can produce pain and muscle weakness that can mimic rheumatoid involvement of the shoulder. Thoracic outlet syndromes (cervical rib, scalenus anticus syndrome, and hyperabduction syndrome) may also produce pain in the shoulder and arm. Early Charcot shoulders have been confused with rheumatoid involvement because neurotropic shoulders are more frequently painful than other neurotropic joints. Radiographs of the cervical spine and careful neurological examination should be routine in evaluating rheumatoid shoulders. Electromyograms, arteriograms, and neurosurgical and vascular consultations may be needed to identify some of these problems.[5]

CONSERVATIVE TREATMENT

Adverse Effects of Frozen Shoulder. Painful shoulders assume the "protective position" to guard against movement. The arm is clasped to the chest in internal rotation. The shoulder is more prone to "freezing" with inactivity than are other joints because it normally has more motion and, in proportion, has larger bursal and joint spaces. As the joint stiffens in the protective position, external rotation and elevation become progressively more and more restricted. Stiffness is associated with pain of a second type beyond that of the rheumatoid arthritis. This pain occurs at the extremes of motion because of tension on the contracted capsule, ligaments, and muscles, and this causes the patient to avoid movement into the extremes of the excursion. A vicious cycle results with more restriction and more disinclination on the part of the patient to move. Eventually the joint may become completely ankylosed in this position. Immobility has bad side effects. First, a shoulder frozen in the protective position enhances the development of contractures at the elbow, wrist, and fingers as well as stiffening of the scapular muscles and has an adverse effect on the function of the entire "upper extremity unit" (see above). Second, since the nutrition of the articular surfaces is dependent upon joint fluid and the pumping action of motion and activity, disuse impairs the nutrition of the cartilage and produces a deleterious effect on the joint surfaces beyond that of the rheumatoid disease. Conservative treatment should aim at early detection and treatment of shoulder stiffness prior to the stage at which the deleterious side effects of inactivity have become irreversible.

Team Approach. Several disciplines are needed to accomplish the goals of conservative shoulder treatment just outlined. Medication is needed to minimize the activity of the rheumatoid arthritis and control pain. Physical therapy is needed for optimal restoration of motion and strength. Orthopedic surgery is needed to evaluate specific problem joints for special procedures such as injections, manipulation, or surgical reconstruction. A feeling of team play and mutual respect should prevail, with the common goal of controlling pain and re-establishing function by the safest and least harmful method available.

Exercise Regimens.

Regaining Motion. Low heat, analgesia, and assistive exercises (done four or five times a day) form the basis for recovering motion. In the assistive exercise program

the patient should supply the power and monitor the excursion so that the exercises can be done several times each day in a relaxed way. It helps to precede the exercises with gentle heat. Emphasis is placed on regaining external rotation and elevation. When the shoulder is sensitive, supine exercises are especially valuable and a stick is used for assistive external rotation and the good arm for assistive overhead elevation. It has been helpful to work for external rotation and total elevation first before starting work on abduction. When the patient achieves 140 degrees of elevation and 40 degrees of external rotation, complete abduction can be done without pain by having the patient place the hands behind the head and spread the elbows. When both shoulders are involved, the pulley is used for overhead elevation. Later, as the pain subsides, stretching exercises are added.[6] Motion is recorded to depict progress.

Recovering Strength. Active motion that is done during the painful stage when the joint is acutely inflamed or while it is too stiff may be irritating to the joint and very painful for the patient. Isometric exercises can be used during this period to maintain strength. As the pain subsides, active-assistive, active, and later resistive exercises are added.

Special Problems. *Braces.* Patients with bilateral shoulder involvement or with a marked tendency to stiffen may be helped by an abduction-external rotation brace to maintain the arm out of the "protective position" between exercise periods. Braces are also helpful in getting air into the axilla to help clear fungus infection or maceration of the axilla prior to surgery. Assistive exercises are done from the brace. Elevation can be done with the patient in the supine position with the help of the therapist or members of the family, and in addition the patient can use the pulley (when erect) to lift the arm off the brace.

Role of Manipulation. Intra-articular and subacromial injection of lidocaine (Xylocaine), followed by gentle manipulation and stretching, may be helpful for stubborn cases. On the other hand, we see no place for manipulation under general anesthesia in the treatment of the rheumatoid shoulder. The osteoporotic bone may fracture. If adequate conservative measures fail, open release is preferable.

INDICATIONS FOR SURGERY

Glenohumeral Joint. Surgery is considered when the disease has altered the joint, either by proliferation of tissue and thickening of the synovium (Fig. 116–3) or by destruction of the articular surfaces (Figs. 116–1 and 116–2) to the extent that is not possible to control pain and re-establish function by conservative measures without resorting to harmful medication. It is to be remembered that some medications are more radical than properly selected surgical procedures. The overview of the patient is foremost in the decision, and in patients with severe disease the surgical procedures should be limited to those that are most needed to control pain and make the patient independent. The most critical functions of the upper extremity in day-to-day living include perineal and rectal care, cleansing under the axilla, eating, doing the hair, and sleeping. Pain is the primary indication for shoulder surgery. However, there are a few rheumatoid patients with relatively painless bilateral ankylosed shoulders in whom replacements can be considered with the goal of making it possible for them to be independent for these critical activities of daily living, as illustrated in Figure 116–6.

The most frequent procedure now done in our center for rheumatoid arthritis of the glenohumeral joint is a *total joint replacement,*[14,28,30,32,33] in which both sides of the joint are resurfaced (Fig. 116–7). *Humeral head replacement*[14,34,35] alone is now less often done for rheumatoid patients in our center because the glenoid is usually diseased (Fig. 116–1) and also because the stability afforded by the conforming surfaces of the total replacement seems to aid in the rehabilitation of rheumatoid muscles. The glenoid component is used even

Figure 116–6. A severe rheumatoid patient with involvement of both shoulders who is unable to perform day-to-day functions. She is seen attempting to reach under the axillae. Beyond this she is unable to reach to the anal region or in front to the perineum for personal hygiene, and is unable to feed herself, wash her face, brush her teeth, or comb her hair. She is unable to sleep without interruption because of shoulder pain. The primary goal of shoulder replacement is relief of pain, but it is also tremendously important to some patients to restore shoulder rotation so they can independently perform the activities of daily living.

when bone grafting is required to support the prosthesis. The glenoid component is omitted, however, in a few, very severe neglected rheumatoid shoulders with complete destruction of the glenoid, which precludes bone grafting. *Fixed fulcrum*[18,28,36-43] prostheses (one or more hinges) have not been widely used. It was hoped that they might solve the problem of extensive deficits of the rotator cuff and deltoid, but unfortunately they do not supply active power and they invite mechanical failure.[19,28] Few have been used in rheumatoid patients, and the soft bone in this condition does not lend itself to fixed fulcrum implants. A *subacromial spacer,* between the acromion and humeral head, once used by Macnab and also by Clayton[12] in a few patients who had severely destroyed cuff muscles, is of historic interest but is not used now. Macnab and English[44] designed a glenoid component with an overhang to provide more stability for extensively destroyed shoulders. The relative lack of constraint frees it from many of the risks of mechanical failure that are inherently present in a fixed fulcrum implant. We have recently developed three sizes of acetabular-like glenoid components to be used developmentally in those few special cases in which the muscles are of such poor quality that they cannot function (Fig. 116–8). These acetabular-like glenoids are narrow in the anteroposterior width to facilitate reattaching the subscapularis and external rotators, and they have a longer overhang than that of the Macnab design.

The results of synovectomy and joint debridement without replacement have too often been disappointing, and the technique is no longer used if there is any involvement of the articular surfaces.

Bursectomy, release, and synovectomy (see below) is done for the less common "bursal type" of shoulder involvement (Fig. 116–3) and in patients with intractable frozen shoulders in which the articular surfaces of the glenohumeral joint are essentially spared.

Glenohumeral arthrodesis is not done in rheumatoid patients because it eliminates the rotary motion of the shoulder that is so important in personal hygiene and because the immobilization required postoperatively for the fusion has a deleterious effect on the elbow and wrist. Obviously, bilateral shoulder ankylosis is unacceptable because it precludes reaching in back or to the top of the head with either hand.[45]

Humeral head resection[45] is not used because it renders the joint flail and cannot be relied upon to relieve pain.[34]

Glenoidectomy[47,48] is not done in our center because it precludes the better functional result that should be obtainable with prosthetic replacement.

Osteotomies of the proximal humerus and glenoid ("double osteotomy") have been advocated in England but are, in the author's opinion, unable to give nearly as good functional results as prosthetic replacement.

Acromioplasty. In the discussion of the subacromial mechanism, it was stated that rheumatoid disease may weaken the muscles of the rotator cuff so that the humeral head may ride up, producing impingement against the undersurface of the acromion. This impingement may contribute to the formation of a cuff tear (See

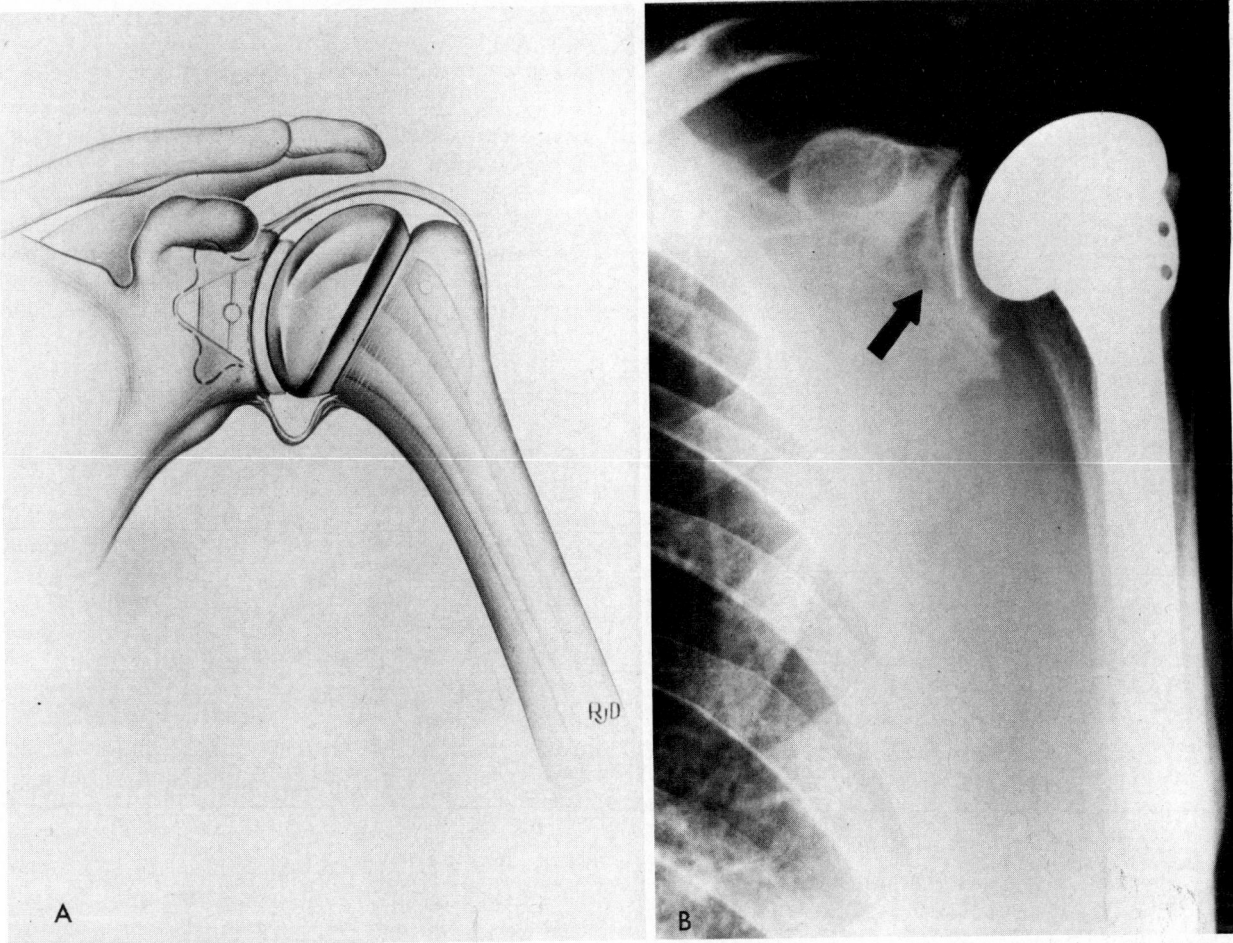

Figure 116–7. Drawing (*A*) and x-ray film (*B*) to show the standard long head total shoulder resurfacing unit. The polyethylene glenoid component is anchored with acrylic cement, and the arrow points to this in the x-ray film. The metal (Mediloy™1) humeral component is made with two lengths of head, three diameters of stem, and three lengths of stem. Half-size replicas of the humeral and "AJ10" glenoid component have been made for Dr. Robert H. Cofield for use in juvenile rheumatoid arthritis, and these are available from the instrument maker.

Impingement Lesions, above). When this condition exists, anterior acromioplasty (to free the cuff from continuing wear) is logical. It is not done as an isolated procedure in rheumatoid patients but may be done at the time of bursectomy, release, and synovectomy and may be done at the time of glenohumeral replacement (see under Surgical Technique, below). Anterior acromioplasty removes only the anterior edge and bevels the anterior third of the undersurface of the acromion. We usually leave part of the coracoacromial ligament intact in rheumatoid patients. The leverage afforded the deltoid muscle by the acromion is preserved. Radical acromionectomy[49] has been used for rheumatoid patients in the past, but it weakens the deltoid and makes the patient worse. It should not be used in rheumatoid patients and, for that matter, should be abandoned in shoulder surgery.[2]

Acromioclavicular Joint. Tenderness, swelling, and pain on adduction of the arm across the chest are the signs of arthritis of this joint. Roentgenographic changes confirm involvement. Lidocaine injection into the joint may be used to make sure of the source of pain. If the discomfort cannot be controlled by steroid injections and medical therapy, acromioclavicular arthroplasty is indicated. This procedure may also be indicated concomitantly with other soft tissue operations or replacement.

Sternoclavicular Joint. Normally there is 40 degrees of motion in this joint, and on rare occasions it becomes symptomatic. Sleeping on that side may be unbearable, and the pain may lead to a frozen shoulder. The pain is usually controlled by steroid injections and reasonable medical treatment. If these fail, sternoclavicular arthroplasty (see below) may be considered.

Shoulder Syndromes. *Biceps tenosynovitis* is not seen as a separate problem in rheumatoid arthritis and, for reasons discussed above, synovectomy of the tendon sheath and tenodesis of the long head are not done as isolated procedures.

Tenderness and pain at the scapula resulting from inflammation of the bursa between the scapula and ribs are referred to as the *scapulothoracic (scapulocostal) syndrome.* A local lidocaine injection into the bursa relieves the pain and differentiates the condition from the re-

200 %

Figure 116–8 *A*, Anteroposterior view in the scapular plane to show a special metal-backed, acetabular-like, polyethylene-lined glenoid component that offers 600 percent more coverage of the long humeral component than the standard glenoid component. However, this large glenoid component is no longer used because it requires a long head humeral component and has so much overhang it precludes closure of the supraspinatus. It also causes greater mechanical leverage on the holding device in the scapula. *B*, A 200% (AJ11) glenoid component (lower part *B*) continues to be used developmentally in selected rheumatoids. It can be used with short head humeral component (which facilitates cuff repair), and it does not preclude closure of the supraspinatus tendon. In two of our rheumatoid patients the destruction of the glenoid by granulation made it impossible to use a glenoid component even with bone grafts, and they were treated satisfactorily with a long head humeral component without a glenoid component. In these cases "centralization" of the humerus due to deep loss of glenoid places the greater tuberosity more medially so that repair of the rotator cuff can be surprisingly easy.

ferred pain that results from overuse of the scapular muscles when a glenohumeral derangement is present. No operative treatment, other than injections, is indicated for this condition in rheumatoids.

Disuse atrophy and vasomotor instability in the upper extremity may develop in patients with chronic shoulder pain, producing the *shoulder-hand syndrome*. The hand becomes puffy, stiffens, and may be wet and pale. Although sympathectomy has been advocated for this condition, it is more beneficial to the entire "upper extremity unit" (see above) to correct the underlying shoulder problem and re-establish motion in the extremity.

Contraindications to Arthroplasty. The only absolute contraindication to an arthroplasty is active infection. Rheumatoid shoulders have often had many injections or previous surgery, and either may introduce low grade infection. Rheumatoid patients have less resistance to infection, especially those on steroids. Steroids may mask the usual warning signs of infection. If anything suspicious is seen at the time of surgery, smears and

frozen sections should be obtained to indicate whether the operation should be discontinued. Wound cultures during surgery should be routine.

Muscle deficits of the cuff and deltoid do not pose a contraindication to replacement arthroplasty, and unconstrained prostheses have not had the problem of instability that was expected by some.[7,19,28] As previously stated, only 30 percent of our rheumatoid patients have complete thickness tears and most of these have been easy to repair and usually rheumatoid patients have often, in our experience, come to function adequately, although the recovery is especially slow in rheumatoid patients. However, in the most severely involved, less than 10 percent of rheumatoid patients, the muscles are so frail and of such poor quality that they do not hold sutures well and do not function after repair. For this special group it is thought that a replacement with more inherent constraint is needed, as discussed under Glenohumeral Joint and as shown in Figure 116–8.

Previous radical acromionectomy weakens the deltoid

to such an extent that active elevation is very limited, but this does not contraindicate surgery and joint replacement may be indicated to relieve intense pain.

Cervical radiculopathy may result in weakness of the deltoid or spinati muscles and cause electromyographic changes. This does not pose an absolute contraindication to replacement, but the cervical problem demands concomitant treatment.

Order of Multiple Procedures in the Upper Extremity. Priorities for planning multiple surgical procedures in the upper extremity should be based upon pain and functional importance of the various joints in the activities of daily living. The functional importance of the shoulder is very great when one considers how much it can interfere with sleeping and personal hygiene (Fig. 116–6). Shoulder pain tends to be made worse whether lying on the good side, on the back, or on the bad side, and the pain is worse at night. Elimination of this pain has a beneficial effect on the entire "upper extremity unit" (see above). It is logical that shoulder replacement should have priority over hand and wrist procedures that are done for relatively asymptomatic conditions. I prefer, in general, to do the shoulder replacement before elbow replacements when both of these joints are involved because this reduces the rotary stress on the elbow (by establishing rotation at the shoulder) and may stop a large portion of the elbow pain by relieving the referred pain from the shoulder to the elbow. Occasionally elbow pain and instability are so great that it would interfere with rehabilitation of the shoulder, and in this case the elbow is replaced first and shoulder replacement is deferred until the elbow is well healed (usually 6 weeks). When there is severe involvement of both shoulders (Fig. 116–9), bilateral replacement is done usually with a 2- to 6-week interval between procedures.

SURGICAL TECHNIQUE

Bursectomy, Release, and Synovectomy. This procedure is limited to patients with bursal-type involvement or unyielding contractures without destruction of the articular surfaces of the glenohumeral joint (see above). It is important to explain to the patient that the postoperative exercise program will continue for at least 6 months and in rheumatoid patients begins from a brace. The patient is taught the exercises preoperatively. The anterior deltoid splitting approach (Fig. 116–10) is used because the acromioclavicular joint is often diseased, requiring concomitant acromioclavicular arthroplasty, and because an anterior acromioplasty may be indicated. It is possible to do this procedure through this relatively small (9.0- or 10.0-cm) incision with minimal deltoid detachment provided the arm is draped completely free so that the humerus can be rotated in all directions. It is important to remember that the humerus must be moved in the incision rather than trying to retract the incision around the humerus.

The patient is placed high on the operating table with a head rest (to avoid hyperextension of the neck) and

Figure 116–9. An early result of bilateral total shoulder replacements seen 4 months after the first operation, in a 52-year-old man who had an intermediate grade of rheumatoid arthritis. Both shoulders had been so extremely painful that the operations were done 3 weeks apart. He is free of shoulder pain and has near normal motion, but at this stage he was expected to continue heat and stretching exercises at least twice daily, and, since his rheumatoid muscles were weak, he was advised to continue strengthening exercises until his muscles approached normal. The rehabilitation of rheumatoid shoulders is always slower because of the concomitant muscle disease, but those with mild and intermediate grades can achieve very excellent results.

with the point of the affected shoulder protruding over the corner of the table. The upper part of the table is raised 30 degrees, and the knee gatch is raised sufficiently to prevent the patient from sliding down. Intratracheal anesthesia is used so that the anesthesiologist is draped from the field. The arm is wrapped so that it can be moved in all directions without interference.

A 9.0-cm incision is made from just lateral to the acromion to just lateral to the coracoid, in Langer's lines. The deep fascia is incised and the deltoid is split 5 cm from above downward (Fig. 116–10). Further splitting jeopardizes the axillary nerve. In rheumatoid patients a stay suture is placed deep within the deltoid at the lower end of the split to prevent extending the split by subsequent retraction of the soft muscle. By sharp dissection, anticipating cutting the acromial branch of the thoracoacromial artery, two flaps of deltoid are raised. A 1.5-cm lateral flap is detached from the anterior edge of the acromion, leaving soft tissue on top of the acromion for later repair, and a 2.0-cm flap of the acromioclavicular joint capsule is raised with the attached

Figure 116-10. The anterior deltoid splitting approach with minimal detachment of deltoid that is used for bursectomy, capsular release, and synovectomy. The deltoid is split 5.0 cm from above downward, and a stay suture prevents extending the split. It is possible to do this procedure quite well through this small opening, provided that the humerus is moved in the incision rather than retracting the incision around the humerus. The tendinous origin of the anterior deltoid on the anterior acromion and the attachment of the deltoid to the acromioclavicular joint capsule are retained with the deltoid that is detached so that a strong repair of the deltoid can be obtained. (Modified from Neer, C.S., II: J. Bone Joint. Surg. 54A:41, 1972.)

deltoid exposing the outer clavicle for excision. The corners of these two flaps are marked with stay sutures to facilitate repair. When the acromioclavicular joint is involved, the distal 2.0 cm of clavicle is removed as described under Glenohumeral Replacement Arthoplasty, below. The clavipectoral fascia, extending laterally from the coracoclavicular ligament, is divided, and an elevator is placed under the acromion. With traction on the arm the rotator cuff is inspected, and the anterior process of the acromion is palpated for sharp edges or traction spurs in the coracoacromial ligament.[2] If an impingement lesion is present, an anterior acromioplasty is performed (removing the anterior edge and beveling the undersurface of the anterior third of the acromion with a thin 19-mm osteotome). Anterior acromioplasty removes an anterior acromial spur if present in the ligament, but it is thought beneficial in rheumatoid patients to leave part of this ligament intact for what stability it might offer.

This approach places the greater tuberosity in the center of the field where, because of the slope of the acromion, the entire rotator cuff may be seen by moving the humerus. The enlarged bursa is then excised by sharp and blunt dissection, avoiding the axillary nerve posteriorly. With flexion and external rotation the subscapularis is exposed and detached 2.0 cm medial to the biceps groove. Some subscapularis tendon remains on the lesser tuberosity to facilitate repair and to allow lengthening if later desired. The inferior capsule is released while a blunt elevator guards the axillary nerve. Synovectomy of the glenohumeral joint and sheath of the long head of the biceps is then completed.

The subscapularis is reattached but is lengthened by a Z-plasty in the coronal plane when contracted. The

capsule is left open. A good deltoid repair is extremely important.

Patients who had stiffness of the glenohumeral joint preoperatively are placed in an abduction brace with slight external rotation, and when wound healing permits, usually in 1 week, passive exercises are given to maintain external rotation and elevation. These are continued until there is essentially full assistive overhead motion. Pendulum exercises can also be made from the brace. The arm is lowered from the brace when the tendency for stiffness seems to have abated, usually within 3 weeks. Early exercises should be assistive (for range of motion) and are preceded by low heat when possible.[6] Appropriate analgesia is given with each meal. Isometrics are begun within 2 weeks, but active and resistive exercises are not added until the muscles have had time to reattach and the patient has regained a good range of motion.

Glenohumeral Replacement Arthroplasty (Total and Humeral Head). Unfortunately glenohumeral replacement is a very demanding procedure and requires a surgeon especially skilled in shoulder surgery for optimal results. The glenoid component is usually used in patients with rheumatoid arthritis, and the patient is required to sign a "new design" permit because at this time a number of the glenoid components we use are considered developmental. The technique for total glenohumeral replacement is the same as that for humeral head replacement except for the additional step of inserting the glenoid component. Both demand meticulous repair and rehabilitation of the muscles and precise technique for inserting the implant. After the humeral head has been removed, it becomes possible to do an acromioclavicular arthroplasty and anterior acromioplasty from below (without detaching deltoid), provided a long deltopectoral incision is used. This approach is now preferred for all replacements.[7]

The humeral components (Fig. 116–7) are made of metal (Mediloy 1) in two lengths of head, 23 mm and 15 mm, each with three different diameters of stem, 6.3 mm, 9.5 mm, and 12.7 mm. Half length stems are also available. The long head provides better leverage for the rotator muscles. The short head facilitates repair of massive cuff lesions and is better for small patients. The stems fit drilling and reaming specifications and are slightly tapered with the thicker portion proximally to enhance a press fit or offer greater ease of removal when used with acrylic cement. The diameter of the head is 44 mm, which approximates the average size of the human head,[35] and, since the arc of the articular surface of the normal glenoid does not match the arc of the normal head, it is thought that these humeral components are suitable for use without the glenoid component, when the scapular side of the joint is spared. The AJ10 glenoid component (Fig. 116–7) is made of high density polyethylene and is anchored with acrylic cement. The anchoring device for this component has been changed from the original design,[14] and several types of metal-backed glenoid components with polyethylene lin-ers are now being made developmentally in the standard size as well as developmental designs that are 200 percent, 400 percent, and 600 percent larger than the standard size for use in very special cases (Fig. 116–8).

The patient is given iron, vitamins, and calcium while awaiting surgery and for 1 week prior to the operation uses antiseptic soap in the axilla to reduce the bacterial count of the skin. Preoperatively instruction is given in the exercise program, which is individualized depending on the condition of the muscles. Prophylactic antibiotics are given on the night before surgery and during the procedure and are continued at least until the wound cultures have been received and longer to patients who have been on steroids.

The patient is positioned high on the table with a head rest to avoid hyperextension of the neck. The arm is draped free so that it can be moved without interference off the side of the table. The point of the shoulder protrudes over the corner of the table. Folded towels are placed under the scapula to hold it forward. A well-padded short arm board is placed at the top of the table so that the arm can be rested upon it in an abducted and externally rotated position while working on the glenoid. The table is adjusted to the beachchair position.

A 17.0-cm skin incision extends over the deltopectoral groove from the clavicle to near the deltoid insertion. The anterior fibers of the deltoid insertion are divided to release tension from retraction on this muscle, but the origin of the deltoid is meticulously left intact. The cephalic vein is ligated. The deltoid is retracted laterally as the arm is abducted 25 degrees, and the clavipectoral fascia, extending downward from the coracoclavicular ligament, is divided. A broad elevator is placed beneath the acromion as a retractor. The shoulder is flexed and externally rotated to facilitate division of the subcapularis tendon at a point 2.0 cm medial to the biceps groove. The subscapularis is tagged with stay sutures. The capsule is then released anteriorly and inferiorly while a blunt elevator prevents injury to the axillary nerve. The long head of the biceps, if intact, is left attached to the glenoid. When there is a cuff tear, the tear is used for exposure and less subscapularis is detached. The humeral head is delivered into the wound by external rotation and extension of the shoulder.

After debriding synovia and bursa, the humeral head is detached with a broad osteotome at the level of the former margins of its articular surface. A surprisingly small amount of bone is removed. It is important to maintain the former angle of retroversion (usually 30 to 40 degrees). The long head of the biceps, if present, is left intact, but osteophytes and rheumatoid granulation tissue are trimmed from its groove. The medullary canal of the humerus is reamed or drilled to the appropriate size to receive the stem of a prosthesis. Drill points that match the three sizes of stems and reach at least 15 cm down the medullary canal are used. Hand reamers to match the flare of the stems are also available. With the humerus extended and pushed upward into the field, a trial prosthesis is inserted. The prosthesis is then reduced

for final check on the angle of retroversion and length of the neck of prosthesis. The trial prosthesis is then removed.

The glenoid is inspected and the decision is made as to whether it needs to be altered or resurfaced. If the glenoid requires revision, it is exposed by retracting the upper humerus backward with a Fukuda ring retractor.[55] A Darrach elevator is placed in front of it to provide better exposure and protection for the axillary nerve. Special care is needed to avoid fracturing the soft bone. A bolster is placed under the elbow to prevent extension at the shoulder, and the humerus is abducted and externally rotated on the armboard in the position that offers the best view. The glenoid labrum is excised and the surface of the glenoid prepared with a power drill, small curettes, and a metal guide. After inserting a trial glenoid component (and after testing it with the humeral component in place), the glenoid component is anchored with acrylic cement, using a syringe. Meticulous care is needed to remove blood from the depth of the glenoid just prior to injecting the cement. Some rheumatoid glenoids have been so completely eroded by granulations that they require the use of metal cement retainers and bone grafts. The erosion occasionally extends halfway through the coracoid (Fig. 116–1C), making it impossible to properly orient the standard glenoid component, and some rheumatoid patients have sloppy, weak rotator tendons that do not hold sutures. For these two specific problems the deep acetabular-like glenoid component (Fig. 116–8) is considered. The 600 percent (AJ12) glenoid component requires a long head humeral component, precludes reconstruction of the supraspinatus, causes more constraint, and has not been used in recent years. The 200 percent (Fig. 116–8B) glenoid component can be used with a short head humeral component (which facilitates cuff repair), does not overhang so much as to preclude cuff repair, and continues to be used developmentally in selected rheumatoid patients. Granulation destruction of the glenoid can make it unwise to use a more constrained component or make it impossible to install it. In two rheumatoid patients with the very worst destruction of the glenoid, a long head humeral component was used without a glenoid component.

Prior to inserting the humeral component, anterior acromioplasty and acromioclavicular arthroplasty are done if indicated. The rotator cuff should be mobilized at this time prior to inserting the head. The tendons are released as necessary not only superficially but also at the base of the coracoid and from the joint capsule. Drill holes are made at the greater tuberosity, and these are threaded with nylon sutures in preparation for later reattachment of the rotator cuff.

The humeral component (previously selected) is then inserted. The sum of the retroversion of both components should be 30 to 40 degrees. The humeral component is anchored with acrylic cement if a good press fit is not obtained.

The soft tissue repair around the implant is of equal

importance to the orientation and seating of the prosthetic components. Mobilization of the tendons should have been completed prior to inserting the head component. It should now be possible to reattach the cuff to the greater tuberosity without tension when the arm is at the side; otherwise, further mobilization is required. The long head of the biceps is left free to run in its groove if it is intact and of adequate shape. The subscapularis is repaired, but the capsule is not sutured. If the subscapularis is short and restricts external rotation, a coronal plane Z-plasty is done. Suction drainage tubes are inserted between the deltoid and cuff, and the deltopectoral interval is closed.

Postoperative exercise regimens must be individualized, depending on the condition of the rotator cuff, but are similar to that for bursectomy, capsular release, and synovectomy (see above). Passive exercises are usually begun within 4 days, with emphasis on external rotation and total elevation. If the shoulder is very stiff, the arm is placed in an abduction brace continuously several weeks and passive elevation done from the brace. We are now beginning to use the continuous motion machine developmentally in selected rheumatoid patients who are stiff and unable to help with the other arm. Since the deltoid is not incised if the rotator cuff was intact, active exercises can be started in 2 weeks. The rehabilitation goal is near normal for the milder and intermediate grades of rheumatoid arthritis (Fig. 116–9). Stretching exercises with low heat are done at least twice a day so long as there is significant restriction of motion, and progressive resistive exercises (with weights or an elastic exerciser) are valuable to strengthen the atrophied and diseased muscles.[6]

Acromioclavicular Arthroplasty. As described above, this may be done at the time of bursectomy or replacement arthroplasty. It also may be done as a separate procedure. When doing this alone, a 5.0-cm incision is made obliquely over the outer end of the clavicle in Langer's lines. The capsule is dissected off the clavicle until a Darrach elevator can be placed under the clavicle and against the coracoclavicular ligaments. When the outer 2.0 cm of the clavicle has been freed of soft tissue, it is cut off with a rib cutter and then shaped with a large rongeur. More bone is removed posteriorly than anteriorly and more superiorly than inferiorly. It is important to preserve the coracoclavicular ligaments. A synovectomy is then performed. The trapezius is sutured to the deltoid to avoid a dead space and forms a muscle envelope over the distal clavicle. The skin closure permits the escape of blood, and exercises are deferred a few days to minimize hematoma formation.

Sternoclavicular Arthroplasty. An 8.0-cm incision is made below the prominence of the clavicle and is retracted upward so that the clavicle can be stripped of soft tissue to a point just lateral to the joint capsule. Throughout this operation scrupulous attention must be given to avoid tearing the great veins. When blunt elevators can be passed both from beneath and from above, the clavicle is cut across about 2.0 cm from the joint line, leaving the distal fragment attached to the costoclavicular ligament. While traction is being applied to the inner fragment, the capsule is divided and this fragment is removed. The clavicular head of the sternocleidomastoid muscle is detached from the clavicle and sutured to fill the dead space. The skin closure permits the escape of blood to minimize hematoma formation.

RESULT TO BE EXPECTED

Acromioclavicular arthroplasty and sternoclavicular arthroplasty in patients who had complete temporary relief after xylocaine injection of these joints and with disease limited to those joints can be expected to give completely satisfactory results and have a beneficial effect on eliminating contractures elsewhere in the extremity. Synovectomy is rarely indicated but has given gratifying and lasting results when done with bursectomy and acromioclavicular arthroplasty in seven of our patients who were free of articular surface involvement. It failed in six patients who had erosion or attritional changes of the articular cartilage.[10]

Results of humeral head replacement in 26 rheumatoid patients were described in 1971.[10] The functional result was usually good in those with low grade disease, but the range of motion was limited in those with severe disease. Pain relief was generally good. The results of this procedure have been much better since the deltoid origin has been left intact.

Reports on the results of the total glenohumeral resurfacing procedure described above that were made to The American Orthopaedic Association[28] and The Canadian Orthopaedic Association[50] in 1977 included 61 rheumatoid shoulders. This implant was first used in 1973. The rotator cuff was found to be intact (with or without attenuation) in 43, moderate tears in seven, and massive tears in ten. Complications included fracture through soft bone, misalignment of the glenoid, and five failures because of riding up of the head that was due to poor cuff function. Lucent lines around the cement in the glenoid were present in one third of the patients and were thought to be due to blood locally at the time of cementing rather than mechanical loosening; however, there has been insufficient time to evaluate loosening. Only one patient required further surgery. Twenty-eight had been followed for 1 or more years. A rating of *excellent* was given when the patient was enthusiastic about the operation and had no significant pain, full use of the shoulder, strength approaching normal, elevation to within 25 degrees of the normal side, and 90 percent rotation (Fig. 116–9). In a *satisfactory* result the patient was satisfied with the operation and had no more than occasional fleeting pain or bad weather ache, good use of the shoulder for daily functions, 30 percent strength, at least 90 degrees of elevation, and 50 percent rotation. In an *unsatisfactory* result these criteria were not met. The results were graded 13 excellent, 7 satisfactory, and 8 unsatisfactory. The unsatisfactory ratings were because of weakness of the muscles rather than pain.

Later studies have been reported. The results of Neer, Watson and Stanton[7] were published in 1982. Of 69 shoulders in 56 patients, 50 shoulders were followed more than 2 years. Seven patients (all with massive cuff tears) were successfully treated on a limited goal basis for less motion and more stability with satisfactory relief of pain and use for the activities of daily living. Five of these had standard glenoid components and two had deep cup glenoid components. The remaining 43 were given the full exercise program, and the results were rated as 28 excellent, 12 satisfactory, and 3 unsatisfactory. Of the 43, 14 had complete cuff tears, and two had been previously operated upon elsewhere. The 3 ratings of "failure" were given for weak muscles and inability to elevate the arm above the horizontal rather than pain or failure of the implant. Lucent lines were present at the bone-cement interface in x-ray films of 30 percent, but there was no clinical loosening. This study has now been extended to over 100 rheumatoid shoulders with 5 years average follow-up. Many of their results approach normal function (Fig. 116–9). Results reported from other clinics in 1983 by Thornhill, Batte, Thomas, and Sledge;[51] Bade, Warren, Ranawat, and Inglis;[52] Wilde;[53] and Cofield[54] also indicate that good pain relief and function are dependent on the preservation or reconstruction of the rotator cuff and deltoid muscles and their rehabilitation. To date I have heard of only two cases of clinical loosening of the glenoid component requiring reinsertion. The bone at the rheumatoid glenoid, however, is often eroded by granulation tissue, requiring careful cement technique and occasionally bone grafting. All of these studies emphasize the need for attention to the details of technique during surgery and aftercare if optimum results are to be achieved.

It is now thought that the criteria for a satisfactory rating for the really severe rheumatoid patients should be different from that for patients with other conditions because the diseased muscles precluded full active motion and strength regardless of the type of fulcrum. The severe rheumatoid patients in this study who received unsatisfactory ratings were actually delighted to be free of shoulder pain and to have independent function for the activities of daily living. It seems inappropriate that their results be graded unsatisfactory because they were unable to elevate 90 degrees when shoulder and elbow motion combined placed the hand where it was needed. For this most severe group the new acetabular-like glenoid component has been designed in the hope of giving more strength and stability but without risk of mechanical failure that is inherent in a fixed fulcrum prosthesis. Two thirds of the rheumatoid patients who came to glenohumeral replacement had an essentially intact rotator cuff, and their results have been good by any standard. The approach described above in which the deltoid origin remains intact has been used consistently only during the past year and has made a marked improvement in the speed of recovery and strength. It is thought that shoulder replacement is not behind other joint replacements, but it is recognized that it is more difficult. In the hip only bone stability is required. In the knee, ligaments are needed. But in the shoulder neither the bone nor the ligaments provide stability, and the level of function depends upon the muscles. The surgeon must have the ability to repair and rehabilitate the muscle for optimal results.

References

1. Inmann, V.T., Saunders, J.B., and Abbott, L.C.: Observations on the shoulder joint. J. Bone Joint Surg. 26:1, 1944.
2. Neer, C.S., II: Anterior acromioplasty for the chronic impingement syndrome in the shoulder. A preliminary report. J. Bone Joint Surg. 54A:41, 1972.
3. Neer, C.S., II, Bigliani, L.U., and Hawkins, R.J.: Rupture of the long head of the biceps related to subacromial impingement. Orthopaedic Transactions by J. Bone Joint Surg. 1:111, 1977.
4. Codman, E.A.: The Shoulder. Rupture of the Supraspinatus Tendon and Other Lesions in or about the Subacromial Bursa. 2nd ed. Boston, Thomas Todd Company, 1934.
5. Bateman, J.E.: The Shoulder and Neck. Philadelphia, W. B. Saunders Company, 1972.
6. Hughes, M.A., and Neer, C.S., II: Glenohumeral joint replacement and postoperative rehabilitation. Phys. Ther. 55:85, 1975.
7. Neer, C.S., II, Watson, K.C., and Stanton, F.J.: Recent experience in total shoulder replacement. J. Bone Joint Surg. 64A:319, 1982.
8. Preston, L.: The Surgical Management of Rheumatoid Arthritis. Philadelphia, W. B. Saunders Company, 1968.
9. Cofield, R.H.: Joint Replacement in Rheumatoid Arthritis. Instructional Course. American Academy Orthopaedic Surgeons Annual Meeting, Las Vegas, 1981.
10. Cruess, R.L., and Mitchell, N.S.: Surgery of Rheumatoid Arthritis. Philadelphia, J. B. Lippincott Company, 1971, Chapter 17.
11. Marmor, L.: Arthritis Surgery. Philadelphia, Lea & Febiger, 1976.
12. Clayton, M.L., and Ferlic, D.C.: Surgery of the shoulder in rheumatoid arthritis. A report of nineteen patients. Clin. Orthop. 106:166, 1974.
13. Neer, C.S., II: Degenerative lesions of the proximal humeral articular surface. Clin. Orthop. 20:116, 1961.
14. Neer, C.S., II: Replacement arthroplasty for glenohumeral osteoarthritis. J. Bone Joint Surg. 56A:1, 1974.
15. Barton, N.J.: Arthrodesis of the shoulder for degenerative conditions. J. Bone Joint Surg. 54A:1759, 1972.
16. Straub, L.R.: An overview of surgical procedures in arthritis. In Hollander, J.L. (ed.): The Arthritis Handbook. West Point, Pa., Merck & Company, 1974, Chapter 8.
17. DePalma, A.F.: Surgery of the Shoulder. 2nd ed. Philadelphia, J. B. Lippincott Company, 1973.
18. Moseley, H.F.: Shoulder Lesions. 3rd ed. Edinburgh and London, E and S Livingstone Ltd., 1969.
19. Cofield, R.H.: Status of total shoulder arthroplasty. Arch. Surg. 112:1088, 1977.
20. Neer, C.S., II: Impingement lesions. Clin. Orthop. 173:70, 1983.
21. DePalma, A.F.: Surgery of the Shoulder. 2nd ed. Philadelphia and Toronto, J. B. Lippincott Co., 1973.
22. Pettersson, C.: Supraspinatus tendon ruptures: A morphological analysis. Presented to Swedish Orthopaedic Association, Gavle, Sweden, May, 1983.
23. McLaughlin, H.L.: Lesions of the musculotendinous cuff of the shoulder. J. Bone Joint Surg. 26:31, 1944.
24. McLaughlin, H.L., and Asherman, E.G.: The lesions of the musculotendinous cuff of the shoulder. J. Bone Joint Surg., 33A:76, 1951.
25. Lindblom, K., and Palmar, I.: Ruptures of the tendon aponeurosis of the shoulder joint—the so-called supraspinatus ruptures. Acta Chir. Scand. 82:133, 1939.
26. Meyer, A.W.: Further observations upon use-destruction in joints. J. Bone Joint Surg. 4:491, 1922.
27. Cruess, R.L.: Steroid-induced avascular necrosis of the head of the humerus. J. Bone Joint Surg. 58B:313, 1976.
28. Neer, C.S., II, Cruess, R.L., Sledge, C.B., and Wilde, A.H.: Total shoulder replacement. A preliminary report. Orthopaedic Transactions by J. Bone Joint Surg. 1:244, 1977.
29. Neer, C.S., II, Craig, E.V., and Fukuda, H.: Cuff-tear arthropathy. Ortho. Trans. 5:477, 1981.
30. Neer, C.S., II, Craig, E.V., and Fukuda, H.: Cuff-tear arthropathy. J. Bone Joint Surg. 65A:1232, 1983.
31. McCarty, D.J., Halverson, P.B., Guillerino, F.C., Brewer, B.J., and Kozin, F.: "Milwaukee shoulder." Association of microspheroids containing hydroxyapatite crystals, active collagenase, and neutral protease with rotator cuff defects. Arthritis Rheum. 24:464, 1981.
32. Zippel, J.: Vollstandiger Schultergelenksersatz ans Kunststoff und Metall. Biomed. Technik 17:87, 1972.

33. Kenmore, P.I.: A Simple Shoulder Replacement. Read at Clemson University Biomaterials Symposium, 1973.

34. Neer, C.S., II, Brown, T.H., Jr., and McLaughlin, H.L.: Fracture of the neck of the humerus with dislocation of the head fragment. Am. J. Surg. 85:252, 1953.

35. Neer, C.S., II: Articular replacement of the humeral head. J. Bone Joint Surg. 37A:215, 1955.

36. Letten, A.W.F., and Scales, J.T.: Total replacement of the shoulder joint (Two cases). Proc. R. Soc. Med. 65:373, 1972.

37. Letten, A.W.F., and Scales, J.T.: Total replacement arthroplasty of the shoulder in rheumatoid arthritis (abstract). J. Bone Joint Surg. 55B:217, 1973.

38. Zippel, J.: Luxationssichere Schulterendoprothese Modell BME. J. Orthop. 113:454, 1975.

39. Romano, R.L., and Burgess, E.M.: Total shoulder replacement (abstract). J. Bone Joint Surg. 57A:1033, 1975.

40. Fenlin, J.M., Jr.: Total glenohumeral joint replacement. Orthop. Clin. North Am. 6:565, 1975.

41. Post, M., Haskell, S.S., and Finder, J.G.: Total shoulder replacement (abstract). J. Bone Joint Surg. 57A:1171, 1975.

42. Gristina, A.G., and Forte, M.R.: The trispherical total shoulder prosthesis—biomechanical, anatomical and surgical considerations. In Trans. Soc. for Biomaterials Symposium, Paper 121, New Orleans, 1977.

43. Buechel, F., Pappas, M.J., and DePalma, A.F.: "Floating socket" total shoulder replacement: Anatomical, biomechanical and surgical rationale. J. Biomed. Mat. Res. 12:89, 1978.

44. Macnab, I., and English, E.: Development of a glenohumeral arthroplasty for a severely destroyed shoulder (abstract). J. Bone Joint Surg. 58B:137, 1976.

45. Neer, C.S., II, and Hawkins, R.J.: A functional analysis of shoulder fusions (abstract). J. Bone Joint Surg. 59B:508, 1977.

46. Jones, L.: The shoulder joint; observations on the anatomy and physiology with an analysis of a reconstructive operation following extensive injury. Surg. Gynecol. Obstet. 75:433, 1942.

47. Wainwright, D.: Glenoidectomy in the treatment of the painful arthritic shoulder (abstract). J. Bone Joint Surg. 58B:377, 1976.

48. Gariepy, R.: Glenoidectomy in the repair of the rheumatoid shoulder (abstract). J. Bone Joint Surg. 59B:122, 1977.

49. Hutchins, W.C.: In Campbell's Operative Orthopaedics. 5th ed. St. Louis, C. V. Mosby Company, 1971, p. 101.

50. Cruess, R.L.: Neer's arthroplasty of the shoulder—preliminary report (abstract). J. Bone Joint Surg. 59B:508, 1977.

51. Thornhill, T.S., Batte, N.J., Thomas, W.H., and Sledge, C.B.: Total shoulder arthroplasty: The Brigham experience. Presented at the American Academy of Orthopaedic Surgeons, Annual Meeting, Anaheim, March, 1983.

52. Bade, H.A., III, Warren, R.F., Ranawat, C.S., and Inglis, A.E.: Long-term results of Neet total shoulder replacement. Presented at the American Academy of Orthopaedic Surgeons, Annual Meeting, Anaheim, March, 1983.

53. Wilde, A.H.: Experience with the Neer total shoulder replacement. Presented at the Second International Conference on Surgery of the Shoulder, Toronto, May, 1983.

54. Cofield, R.H.: A long-term review of total shoulder arthroplasty. Presented at the Second International Conference on Surgery of the Shoulder, Toronto, May, 1983.

55. Fukada, H., Mikasa, M., and Ogawa, K.: Ring retractor. A new humeral head retractor. J. Bone Joint Surg. 64A:289, 1982.

Chapter 117

Reconstructive Surgery and Rehabilitation of the Knee

John N. Insall

INTRODUCTION

Campbell[1] reported the successful use of a metallic interposition femoral mold in 1940. A similar type of femoral mold prosthesis was designed at the Massachusetts General Hospital in 1953. McKeever[2] in 1960 and MacIntosh[3] in 1966 reported on the use of metal tibial plateau replacements, and their methods gained considerable popularity in the 1960s, particularly in rheumatoid arthritis.

Interposition arthroplasty of whatever type requires the preservation of ligamentous support to provide the necessary stability. An alternative approach to knee arthroplasty sacrifices the knee ligaments by using a prosthesis which assumes the function of providing both stability and mobility. In 1951, Walldius[4] first inserted the prosthesis that bears his name, and similar hinge type prostheses were developed by Shiers[5] and most recently by the Guepar[6] group in Paris.

Significant advance in knee arthroplasty was made by Gunston.[7,8] This original design was of four separate pieces, and the polycentric arthroplasty was the first attempt to apply to the knee the prosthetic components of high-density polyethylene articulating against metal (either stainless steel or chrome cobalt alloy) bonded to bone by methyl methacrylate cement, which has proved so successful in total hip replacement.

Many implants for knee replacement have since appeared. Metal hinges have lost favor, and most interest is now focused on metal and polyethylene surface replacements.

INDICATIONS

Most knee implants have dished tibial components with an upward concavity that traps debris and therefore may wear more rapidly than total hip prostheses.[9,10]

Polyethylene wear particles become widely distributed, and autopsy studies on dogs after total hip replacement have demonstrated polyethylene in many organs of the body.[11] There is no evidence that the presence of these particles is harmful, but to a cautious person there must be some concern.

Therefore, an important factor involved in the decision to replace the knee joint is the age of the patient. At present, most surgeons hesitate to implant a knee prosthesis in a patient under age 65 if there are reasonable alternatives.

The alternatives must be considered separately for rheumatoid and osteoarthritis.

Figure 117–1. *A,* Radiographs of a patient's knees taken prior to synovectomy. *B,* Similar anteroposterior radiographs of the same patient taken 12 years after bilateral synovectomies. Some advance in arthritic change can be seen, but these changes are minimal, and the patient's symptoms are similarly mild.

Rheumatoid Arthritis. Synovectomy[12,13] may temporarily relieve pain and swelling, but has little effect on the progression of arthritis and is of no value when cartilage erosion has already occurred (see Chapter 113). Synovectomy may defer the need for total replacement in young patients, however, when symptoms are primarily due to persistent effusion (Fig. 117–1*A* and *B*).

Hemiarthroplasty seldom gives results that compare with total replacement, and there is rarely ever an indication for arthrodesis in rheumatoid arthritis except for the salvage of infected cases.

Medical management should be continued as long as possible, perhaps advising synovectomy in very selected cases. When surgical intervention is required to keep the patient walking because of lack of a reasonable alternative, the knee is replaced regardless of age. It is important to use only metal on polyethylene designs and to avoid metal hinges. The techniques required to avoid constraint in prosthetic design will be discussed.

Osteoarthritis. The selection of suitable patients for total replacement becomes more difficult. Multiple joint involvement is less common, and the patients are often healthy and vigorous so that increased activity following relief of pain may put severe stress on the prosthetic components. Patients are also frequently obese. However, there are several alternative procedures that can be considered, and age assumes a more critical importance.

Arthrodesis. It is realistic to consider arthrodesis in a young active man with post-traumatic arthritis of one knee. In such a case the ability to stand and walk for long periods without pain can more than outweigh the awkwardness created by knee stiffness. Nonetheless it is true that even in ideal circumstances it is becoming increasingly difficult to gain patient acceptance for arthrodesis. In fact some patients who have a satisfactory and painless arthrodesis request an arthroplasty to return mobility to the knee. This is seldom advisable.

Debridement (Pridie).[14,15] Removal of degenerated menisci and osteophytes, shaving of degenerated articular cartilage, and drilling of eburnated bone after the method popularized by Pridie remains the best approach for young or middle-aged patients with panarthritis of the kind that may follow athletic ligament injuries. These patients usually retain an interest in sports and wish to participate in some kind of recreational activity; for them an arthrodesis would be unacceptable. The Pridie procedure is successful in about two thirds of patients and can be of long-lasting benefit. There has been renewed interest in débridement done arthoscopically, and good results have been reported. Significant angular deformity is the most important contraindication.

Osteotomy.[16-18] Primary osteoarthritis of the knee is usually compartmental and associated with angular deformity (most frequently a varus angulation). In some cases bowing of the legs may have been present since childhood. Correction of varus malalignment by osteotomy through the upper tibia is a proved and satisfactory operation. The most successful results are obtained in patients who have a relatively small angulation (not more than 10 degrees of varus) and stable knees. Provided that correct postoperative alignment in approximately 10 degrees valgus is obtained, the results are satisfactory in about 90 percent of cases (Fig. 117–2). In knees with more severe deformity, usually associated with instability, the results are much less satisfactory because obtaining correct postoperative alignment is

more difficult and the ligament instability tends to cause either overcorrection or recurrence of the original varus deformity. The effect of osteotomy is explained by the shifting of weight-bearing stress to the uninvolved lateral compartment and is purely mechanical. When good results are not achieved because of either ligamentous instability or incorrect technique, pain is not relieved.

Tibial osteotomy for the correction of the less common valgus deformity is less satisfactory.[19] Most valgus knees by the time advice is sought have a considerable deformity which if corrected in the tibia results in a marked obliquity of the knee joint. Obliquity causes medial subluxation of the femur and the development of late varus deformity. For this reason it is generally preferable to correct valgus knees by lower femoral osteotomy which preserves a horizontal joint axis, although femoral osteotomy is associated with higher morbidity, more frequent nonunion, and sometimes knee stiffness.

However, high tibial osteotomy is satisfactory for valgus deformity (1) when the projected obliquity after osteotomy will not exceed 15 degrees and (2) when the joint is initially stable (before the medial ligament has been stretched by the stress of weight bearing). The best results are obtained in post-traumatic osteoarthritis caused by depressed fractures of the lateral tibial plateau.

In summary, the indications for total replacement of the knee in osteoarthritis are pain and limitation of function of sufficient degree to warrant acceptance of the possibility of arthrodesis because this may be the outcome if the arthroplasty fails. Arthroplasty is the procedure of choice for those over age 65, but should not be selected for patients under this age if a suitable alternative exists. Replacement arthroplasty is also not suitable for individuals who wish to engage in sports.

PATHOLOGY

There are certain aspects concerning the pathologic anatomy of the arthritic knee that relate to the surgical technique of knee replacement and are thus extremely important to understand. Rheumatoid arthritis may be best described as a panarthritis in that the medial, lateral, and patellofemoral compartments are involved equally from the early stages of the inflammatory condition so that cartilage and bone erosion occur more or less symmetrically. Apparent instability in the earlier stages of rheumatoid arthritis is not due to any changes in the ligaments themselves, which retain original length, but is caused by loss of cartilage and bone between the ligament attachments (Fig. 117–3). In these cases stability can be easily restored by recreating substance (the prosthetic components). However, in the later stages of rheumatoid arthritis, varus or valgus deformities occur as a result of asymmetric erosion or collapse, and it is only then that adaptive and secondary changes take place in the collateral ligaments. For example, the most characteristic deformity in longstanding rheumatoid arthritis is valgus angulation with external rotation and

Figure 117–2. Radiograph of a knee with medial compartment osteoarthritis and good ligament stability. This knee is suitable for high tibial osteotomy.

Figure 117–3. Radiograph of a knee in a patient with rheumatoid arthritis. The alignment and bony contours are preserved. This type of knee is technically the easiest for the surgeon to replace.

lateral subluxation of the tibia on the femur. The iliotibial band, lateral ligament, and lateral capsular structures shorten and contract. Over the same period the medial ligament and medial capsule are stretched by weight bearing and as a result become longer and looser. There now exists what may be described as *asymmetric instability* (Fig. 117–4) in that there is a permanent alteration in the length of the ligaments. It is obvious that in such a knee the spacing effect of the prosthetic components cannot compensate for instability even when deformity is corrected because the collateral ligaments remain at different lengths.

Whereas varus angulation is relatively uncommon in rheumatoid arthritis, this type of deformity is characteristically found in osteoarthritis, which, from the beginning, is a focal compartmental disorder. The lateral compartment is initially fairly normal and becomes involved only in very severe and longstanding cases. There is therefore a fundamental difference between rheumatoid and osteoarthritis: in the former, the whole joint is involved early and angulation and asymmetry appear late; in the latter, initially one compartment only is involved, and there is early angulation and associated ligament asymmetry.

The secondary adaptive changes in the collateral ligaments commonly associated with angular deformity create perhaps the most important technical problem that must be solved.

There are other noteworthy alterations that occur in the knee joint as a result of rheumatoid arthritis (although seldom or never in osteoarthritis). Fixed flexion deformities are common, and contractures of 90 degrees or more may be seen in some patients who have taken to a wheelchair. The flexion attitude initially arises because the swollen joint is more comfortable in this position, but after a time fixed deformity develops because of secondary contracture of the posterior capsule. In a determined patient who continues to walk in spite of pain, the flexion deformity seldom exceeds 20 or 30 degrees and does not present a problem. On the other hand, a wheelchair-bound patient who has not walked for some time and has developed very severe contractures presents a considerable technical challenge because the posterior capsule is shortened, the collateral ligaments retain original length, and the quadriceps mechanism is weakened by disuse and often stretched by prolonged swelling. Correction of flexion deformity by removal of extra bone from the femur and tibia therefore results in excessive laxity of the collateral ligaments and relative lengthening of the already insufficient quadriceps mechanism.

Another important and related abnormality in rheumatoid arthritis is excessive loss of cartilage and bone from the posterior femoral condyles so that the shape of the lower femur resembles a drumstick or chicken leg. Consequently there is greater instability of the knee in flexion than in extension; paradoxically this is most frequently found in knees that also have a fixed flexion deformity.

An intact posterior cruciate ligament will often prevent correction of deformity and interfere with the tensioning of collateral ligaments when restoring stability by the insertion of components. In these circumstances the cruciate ligaments must be excised. Goodfellow and O'Connor[20] state that the posterior cruciate ligament causes the femoral condyles, particularly the lateral, to glide backward (posteriorly) as the knee flexes. In the normal knee the shape of the tibial plateau does not restrain this rolling motion, and the laxity of the meniscal attachments permits the menisci to move with the femur. This anatomic function influences prosthetic design; if the cruciate ligaments are retained, the tibial

Figure 117–4. *A,* Photograph of a patient with osteoarthritis. There is a valgus deformity of the right knee and a varus deformity of the left knee. Invariably there is ligament asymmetry with longstanding deformities. *B,* In the right valgus knee the lateral ligament is shorter than the medial. Symmetry is restored by a progressive release of the lateral capsule and iliotibial band from the femur.

components must be flat because otherwise posterior impingement will occur.

In favor of posterior cruciate retention[22] are the following arguments: (1) more motion with greater flexion is permitted; (2) posterior subluxation cannot occur; and (3) stresses at the bone-cement interface are relieved because force is dissipated by the intact posterior cruciate ligament. The arguments against posterior cruciate retention[21] are the following: (1) the increased technical difficulties presented to the surgeon who now must balance not only the collateral ligaments but the posterior cruciate ligament as well to ensure proper function; and (2) the possibility of improper insertion of a cruciate-retaining design, which may then exhibit medial-lateral instability or inadequate flexion. In some instances an overly tight posterior cruciate ligament (Fig. 117–5) may actually increase the stress on the bone-cement interface. The technical difficulties increase with the preoperative deformity of the knee, and posterior cruciate retention is not always possible even in the most skilled hands. In these cases a cruciate-substituting design such as the posterior stabilized condylar knee (Fig. 117–6*A* and *B*) is indicated, and this latter model may be the best choice for routine use in the hands of relatively inexperienced knee surgeons. Finally, it must be emphasized that design concepts must not be mixed; that is to say, the posterior cruciate ligament must not be preserved in a model intended for cruciate excision because a kinematic conflict will occur between the geometry of the prosthesis and the tension in the ligament.

TYPES OF PROSTHESES

It seems unnecessary to advocate an elaborate system of classification. Prostheses can be divided into two categories, surface replacements and constrained protheses, each with subdivisions.

Surface Replacements

Unicompartmental Replacement. Unicompartmental replacement[23-25] of the osteoarthritic knee is widely used in both the United States and Europe. The concept has been recommended because only the abnormal joint surfaces are removed and the total amount of bone excised in minimal. The amount of foreign material used (metal, polyethylene, and cement) is also quantitatively mini-

Figure 117–5. The posterior cruciate ligament was preserved in this knee and because of excessive tightness has assumed a vertical orientation, forcing the tibia to sublux anteriorly. This phenomenon illustrates one of the technical difficulties of preserving the posterior cruciate ligament in total knee arthroplasty.

mal. Finally, it has been claimed that the operative time and complications are less.

Unicompartmental designs include the polycentric,[26] the unicondylar,[27] the modular, the St. Georg, Manchester,[28] and the most recent version of the Freeman. All are similar in concept and are intended to replace osteoarthritic knees in which one compartment alone is involved. The ligaments, including the cruciates, must all be present and relatively normal; therefore, the prosthesis cannot be used in severely involved arthritic knees with a large deformity, severe instability, or significant flexion contracture. Likewise, the procedure has no place in the treatment of rheumatoid panarthritis. The indications for unicompartmental replacement in varus gonarthrosis are essentially the same as for high tibial osteotomy. For lateral compartment arthritis an alternative is lower femoral osteotomy.

The unicondylar prosthesis (Fig. 117–7) consists of a metallic femoral replacement of approximately anatomic design: the sagittal curvature increases posteriorly, and in the frontal plane the curvature mimics the median half of the femoral condyles. As a result, two mirror image femoral components are required with a central peg and anterior flange for fixation and alignment. The components are available in various sizes. The polyethylene tibial component is flat in the sagittal plane and curved in the frontal plane to conform with the femoral component. The deep surface is dovetailed for cement fixation, and the component is available in several thicknesses.

Unicompartmental replacements are tricky to insert and require much precision. The surgical technique may therefore play an important part in the ultimate success of the device.

Bicondylar Replacements. *The Duopatellar Prosthesis.* The duopatellar prosthesis[29] is a cruciate-retaining design intended to preserve the posterior cruciate ligament. The prosthesis has recently been modified and is now known as the Brigham knee. The general shape of the tibial runners is anatomic in the sagittal plane, and coronally the condyles are flat with a median curvature. The femoral flange is inclined 7 degrees laterally so that right and left components are required. The tibial components are dished anteriorly but flat posteriorly to allow for femoral rollback. They are joined anteriorly with a posterior cutout to accommodate the posterior cruciate ligament. There is a median curvature to prevent translocation. The deep surface of the prosthesis has a metal plate with a central fixation peg. A dome-shaped patellar component is provided.

The Total Condylar Prosthesis. The total condylar prosthesis (TCP)[30] (Fig. 117–8) is one of the earliest examples of a cruciate-excising prosthesis that is still widely used in its original form. Although coined as the name of a specific prosthesis, the term total condylar prosthesis has recently acquired a generic meaning describing a whole range of surface prostheses that share general characteristics with the original. The salient features of the design are the following:

(1) The femoral component is made of cobalt chrome alloy and contains a symmetrically grooved anterior flange separated posteriorly into two symmetric con-

Figure 117–6. *A,* A diagram showing the post and cam of the posterior stabilized condylar knee. Articulation between the post of the tibial component and the cam of the femoral component substitutes for the function of the posterior cruciate ligament. *B,* Photograph of the articulated posterior stabilized condylar knee.

Figure 117–7. Photograph of the unicondylar prosthesis.

dyles, each of decreasing radius posteriorly and having a symmetric convex curvature in the coronal plane.

(2) The tibial component is made of high-density polyethylene and is in one piece with two separate biconcave tibial plateaus that articulate precisely with the femoral condyles in extension, thus permitting no rotation in this position. In flexion the fit ceases to be exact, and rotation and gliding motions are possible. The symmetric tibial plateaus are separated by an intercondylar eminence designed to prevent translocation or sideways sliding movements. The peripheral margin of the articular concavities is of an even height both anteriorly and posteriorly. The deeper bony surface of the component now has a metal plate with a central fixation peg 35 mm in length and 12.5 mm in width. The anterior margin of the peg is vertical, but the posterior margin is oblique to conform with the posterior cortex of the tibia.

(3) The patellar component is made of high-density polyethylene and is dome shaped on its articular surface, conforming closely to the curvature of the femoral flange. A dome was selected because this shape does not require rotary alignment like an anatomic prosthesis. The bony surface of the prosthesis has a central fixation lug.

The Posterior Stabilized Condylar Knee. The posterior stabilized condylar knee[31] is a cruciate-substituting design and was developed from the total condylar model. The TCP provides anteroposterior stability in part by the dished shape of the tibial articulation, which, acting together with tension in the collateral ligaments, prevents subluxation of the components, because in order to separate they must run uphill upon one another. The posterior stabilized condylar knee provides more active and concrete posterior cruciate substitution. This function is assumed by a central spine, which articulates against a transverse cam on the femoral component. The cam engages with the femur at 75 degrees, and thereafter with further flexion the cam imposes a progressive rollback of the femoral condyles to prevent posterior impingement (Fig. 117–9). The standard version is designed to reach 120 degrees, but a version designed to fulfill local cultural needs in Asia allows 140 degrees of flexion. In extension the spine does not engage the femur anteriorly until the knee is in 20 degrees of hyperextension, a position that should never be reached. The cam mechanism permits an increasing amount of rotation as the knee is flexed up to a maximum of 20 degrees at right angle flexion. No varus-valgus stability is provided, and the two components disengage freely if stressed in these directions; therefore, varus-valgus stability depends entirely on the integrity of the collateral ligaments.

Compared with the total condylar prosthesis, some minor modifications were made in the curvatures of the femoral component, and the tibial articulation was inclined posteriorly at an angle of 10 degrees so that the

Figure 117–8. The total condylar knee prosthesis. The patella is replaced with a polyethylene button or dome.

Figure 117–9. Diagram of a posterior stabilized condylar knee in flexion. Beyond 75 degrees the post and cam engage, imposing a rollback of the femur on the tibia. The resultant vector of these forces is one of compression at the bone-cement interface. (Courtesy of J. Bone and Joint Surg.)

Figure 117–10. Photograph of four early prosthetic designs, which are now largely obsolete. The Guepar hinge prosthesis is shown at the upper left. The other prostheses in a clockwise direction are the unicondylar, duocondylar, and geometric models. (Courtesy of J. Bone and Joint Surg.)

anterior lip of the articulation is approximately 5 mm higher than the posterior lip. As the intercondylar recess now dovetails into the femur, the fixation lugs were removed from the medial and lateral condyle, which preserves important bone stock in these areas. The fixation peg on the tibial component remains the same as in the total condylar prosthesis, and the patellar buttons are unchanged.

Constrained Prostheses

These prostheses provide all the required stability for the knee joint and therefore both cruciate and collateral ligaments may be excised or absent. Most experience has been with metal-to-metal hinges (Walldius, Shiers, and Guepar) (Fig. 117–10). There is a considerable literature devoted to these specific prosthetic designs, and infection and loosening have been major problems. Consequently their use has now been largely abandoned, and some newer designs have evolved with metal-on-polyethylene articulations, which allow some rotary and gliding movements while continuing to provide the necessary stability. Examples include the total condylar prosthesis III and the spherocentric,[32] Attenborough[33] and Sheehan prostheses.[34]

While the mainstream of prosthetic replacement undoubtedly lies with surface replacement, full constraint is occasionally required for revision surgery and for a few primary cases. As far as the latter group is concerned, it is estimated that between 90 and 99 percent are replaceable using a surface prosthesis, the exact proportion being dependent on the experience and technical skill of the surgeon. It is preferable for the patient to leave the operating table with a stable arthroplasty, even if this means the use of a constrained design, rather than an unsatisfactory and unstable surface replacement that is doomed to failure from the outset. The constrained prosthesis should therefore be kept as a back-up "in the cupboard"; the presence of this security also encourages a neophyte surgeon to perform boldly the necessary soft-tissue releases, which are the key to successful surface replacement arthroplasty.

TCP III. The total condylar prosthesis III (Fig. 117–11) evolved from the total condylar and stabilocondylar designs. Stability is provided by a rectangular tibial post that fits snugly within a recess in the femoral component. Stems are provided on both components because of the increased stresses of the articular linkage.

The TCP III is used by us mainly as a back-up prosthesis that is available as an intraoperative choice for revisions or in cases of technical error in which, for example, a collateral ligament is inadvertently divided. The prosthesis is also occasionally used as a primary prosthesis for knees with severe valgus or flexion deformities in which it is judged that stretching will cause a postoperative peroneal nerve palsy.

The Spherocentric Prosthesis. The spherocentric knee is a nonhinged, intrinsically stable knee joint prosthesis that permits controlled triaxial rotation and is designed specifically for use in severely deformed or unstable knees. There are three surfaces bearing metal on high-density polyethylene: a ball-and-socket joint located within the femoral component and two runner and track joints between the femoral and tibial condyles. The ball-and-socket joint is composed of a central metal sphere on top of a column rising from the tibial component,

Figure 117–11. A total condylar prosthesis III design substitutes for the collateral ligaments as well as the posterior cruciate ligament. This substitution is by means of the rectangular peg on the tibial component engaging within a similarly shaped recess of the femoral component.

which in the articulated prosthesis is contained within a polyethylene socket within the femoral component. The ball-and-socket joint formed permits triaxial rotation, but dislocation is not possible in any direction. The center of the sphere lies above the joint surfaces and posterior to the long axis of the femur, thus approximating the location of the average flexion axis of the normal knee. The location, dimensions, and contour of the metal femoral runners and their mated tibial polyethylene tracks serve to guide and control flexion, varus-valgus movement, and torsion and to increase the total weight-bearing surface of the joint. As the knee approaches full extension, the anterior surfaces of the femoral condylar runners with their larger radius of curvature bear increasingly on the plastic tibial tracks, thereby unloading the top of the central sphere. As the prosthesis flexes, the femoral condylar surfaces slowly lift off the plastic tracks, gradually transferring all of the load to the dome of the sphere. At a maximum flexion of 120 degrees the prosthesis permits up to 30 degrees of tibial rotation and up to 5 degrees of varus-valgus motion.

INDICATIONS FOR TOTAL KNEE REPLACEMENT

It goes without saying that only severe symptoms and disability justify knee joint replacement. While it is no longer true that a patient should consent to an arthro-

desis before undergoing an arthroplasty, a frank discussion with the patient concerning the consequences of failure is essential. Medical management should be continued as long as possible, and alternative techniques, such as tibial osteotomy, selected when feasible. In the presence of severe and unremitting symptomatology, total knee arthroplasty is indicated in the following circumstances:

(1) Rheumatoid panarthritis.

(2) Osteoarthritis of the knee. The age of the patient, occupation, level of activity, sex, and weight are all factors that must be considered. In general terms an arthroplasty should be avoided in patients under 65 years of age, in manual laborers, in athletes, and in those who are grossly overweight.

(3) Post-traumatic osteoarthritis. There may rarely be an indication for knee replacement in the younger patient following intra-articular fractures or other traumatic injuries to the joint.

(4) Failure of high tibial osteotomy. When high tibial osteotomy has failed to relieve symptoms or when symptoms recur after an interval due to progressive arthritis, total knee replacement can be performed without difficulty (Fig. 117–12A, B, and C).

(5) Patellofemoral osteoarthritis. In most cases patellofemoral osteoarthritis is not an indication for total replacement of the joint, and the condition is better managed by another technique. Femorotibial narrowing on a weight-bearing radiograph is therefore usually a prerequisite for joint replacement, but occasionally an elderly patient will present with very severe patellofemoral arthrosis without significant femorotibial narrowing, despite a finding of patchy articular degeneration throughout the joint at arthrotomy. This type of case, although rare, does better with total joint replacement than with any other method.

(6) The neuropathic joint. Joint replacement in neuropathic states is controversial and represents a technical challenge, as instability and deformity are often extreme (Fig. 117–13A). We believe that knee replacement is feasible provided that a surface replacement can be used, the joint is thoroughly debrided, and correct alignment and stability are achieved. Metal-backed components with longer than usual stem fixation are desirable (Fig. 117–13B).

CONTRAINDICATIONS TO KNEE REPLACEMENT

The following are contradictions to knee replacement:

(1) A sound, painless arthrodesis in good position should not be converted to a knee arthroplasty. The prospects of a successful arthroplasty are not good, and a constrained prosthesis is usually required. Should the arthroplasty fail, rearthrodesis of the knee may not succeed.

(2) Genu recurvatum associated with muscular weakness and paralysis is likely to recur after a surface replacement, and the stresses imposed on a constrained prosthesis will probably loosen it.

Figure 117–12. *A*, Radiograph of a knee with medial compartment osteoarthritis, taken shortly after high tibial osteotomy. *B*, A radiograph of the same knee taken 5 years later, showing recurrence of varus deformity with some stretching of the lateral ligaments. *C*, This knee was replaced using a total condylar prosthesis. There were no unusual technical difficulties.

Figure 117–13. *A*, A radiograph of a neuropathic joint. Radiograph 2 years after replacement with a metal-backed medial wedge tibial component and a posterior stabilized condylar articulation. No instability is present. The knee is without effusion and is asymptomatic, and there is no evidence of component loosening.

(3) Gross quadriceps weakness.

(4) Active sepsis. When infection is caused by a susceptible organism, thorough debridement and appropriate antibiotic therapy may be followed by a later replacement after eradication of infection. Tuberculous joints can be managed in a similar manner. When the infecting organism cannot be adequately treated because of the potential toxicity of the necessary antibiotic therapy, arthrodesis is a better choice.

SURGICAL TECHNIQUE

The success of any total knee replacement depends on the following four factors: patient selection, prosthetic design, prosthetic materials and surgical technique.[35]

Prosthetic design has evolved to the point where little improvement of results can be expected from continued refinement in design. Current prostheses possess many basic similarities and, if correctly inserted, will give satisfactory results. However, whereas total hip arthroplasty is relatively forgiving of surgical error, total knee replacement is not. Component malposition of 5, 10, or even 20 degrees may not affect the outcome in arthroplasty of the hip; in knee replacement, an error of 5 degrees is significant, and one of 10 degrees is often catastrophic. Furthermore, even when the components themselves are correctly positioned, the adjustment of tension in the soft tissues must also be exactly right for the arthroplasty to function. In the hip, for instance, a loose fit between the components is not in itself of great consequence. Shifting the greater trochanter downwards will often compensate; and provided the hip is prevented from dislocating during the early postoperative phase, the soft tissues, aided by the muscles acting across the joint, will adjust and contract, ending with a stable arthroplasty and, at worst, slight shortening of the leg.

In contrast, the knee surgeon must consider not only the overall soft-tissue tension but the relative tightness both medially and laterally and in the positions of flexion and extension. All must be correct at the end of the operation. Prolonged immobilization does not usually improve inadequate soft-tissue balance, and muscle development will not prevent subluxation or dislocation of the components. Therefore, in the knee, the component placement and overall alignment must be correct within narrow tolerance limits, and the soft tissues must be adjusted while the patient is in the operating theater. When these requirements are not met, the arthroplasty will, at best, be suboptimal and often will be a total failure.

Principles of Surgical Technique. Most prostheses have femoral components which are available in various sizes and tibial components of various thicknesses so that component size can be adjusted to the dimensions of the knee. Attempting to replace the knee with components that are grossly mismatched in size is likely to be difficult, so that an adequate inventory of component parts is essential.

The simplest knee to replace is one in which only the articular cartilage is damaged, so that normal alignment is retained, the ligaments are unaltered, and there are no bone defects. The following description applies to a knee of this kind, and it is assumed that the tibial component is in one piece and that the femoral component has the deep surface shaped to fit right angle bone cuts.

The bone ends must be reshaped (Fig. 117–14) in order that they may be capped by the components, which must fit so that the new prosthetic geometry will be compatible with existing ligament lengths throughout the range of motion.

The femoral condyles are measured using templates, and a prosthesis is selected that roughly approximates the original size of the femur, particularly in its anteroposterior dimensions (Fig. 117–15). The anterior femoral groove is cut flush with the anterior surface of the metaphysis of the femur. The posterior femoral condyles are removed symmetrically. Approximately 5 mm of bone is removed from the upper surface of the tibia; thus a gap is created between the femur and tibia with the knee flexed that must be filled by the combined bulk of the femoral and tibial components. If this space is too small to permit the use of the thinnest available tibial component, the gap must be enlarged by selecting a smaller femoral prosthesis and removing more bone from the posterior femoral condyles. To enlarge the gap by resecting more tibial bone results in the exposure of weaker cancellous bone, which may predispose to tibial loosening because the strength of the cancellous bone of the tibia decreases rapidly with distance from the subchondral bone plate (Fig. 117–16).

The size of the flexion gap is assessed by using a spacer which selects the thickness of tibial component needed (Fig. 117–17A). The knee is then extended, and with traction applied, sufficient bone is removed from the distal femur to produce an extension gap that will admit the same spacer used in the flexion gap (Fig. 117–17B). Once these steps have been completed, the basic operation is complete, and it only remains to shape the bone ends to accept the prosthetic components.

Instrumentation. Whereas the skilled surgeon may be able to replace the knee consistently by eye, most will need the aid of instruments. Just as there has been a convergence of prosthetic design in recent years, most

Figure 117–14. Diagram showing sculpting of the bone ends so that the femur may be "capped" by the femoral component.

Figure 117–15. Diagram showing the use of templates to select the correct size of the femoral component.

Figure 117–17. *A,* The spacer and aligning rod are used to check the fit in flexion. This is done between stages two and three. *B,* The spacer and aligning rod are used to check the fit in alignment in extension. This is done after stage three. The distal end of the aligning rod should pass through the center of the ankle joint, and the proximal end of the rod through the hip joint (approximately 1 inch medial to the anterior superior iliac spine).

instrument systems also have a basic similarity and are based upon concepts originally elaborated by Freeman.[36,37] Templates or cutting blocks are positioned upon the bones to guide an oscillating saw, making possible the necessary accuracy in the bone cuts. Alignment and ligament tension are assessed in extension by an instrument called the Tenser (Fig. 117–18), which mechanically distracts the knee and allows precise positioning before the distal end of the femur is resected. The overall alignment of the leg should be such that the mechanical axis[38] is restored. The mechanical axis (Fig. 117–19) refers to a line drawn through the head of the femur, center of the knee, and center of the ankle and corresponds approximately to a femorotibial angle of 7 to 9 degrees.

Figure 117–16. The upper tibia is resected at right angles to the shaft of the bone, always at the same level regardless of bony defects. The amount of bony resection should be approximately 5 mm.

Figure 117–18. Diagram of a Tenser, showing its ability to distract the medial and lateral compartments of the joint separately.

Figure 117–19. After adjusting the Tenser, the alignment rod should lie in the mechanical axis of the limb (center of hip, center of knee, and center of ankle), with the soft tissues on the medial and lateral sides possessing equal tension.

MANAGEMENT OF INSTABILITY, DEFORMITY, AND CONTRACTURE

The technique described applies only to knees with normal anatomy, and, of course, such joints rarely require replacement. In most cases some degree of instability, deformity, contracture, or a combination of these elements will be found. Moreover, even in knees without an initial deformity, some change in alignment may be required to restore the correct mechanical axis (for example, in the patient who is habitually bowlegged). While some minor degree of postoperative ligament asymmetry or laxity may be tolerated, it is better to obtain near-perfect stability through surgical technique. Some workers use a constrained prosthesis for unstable or deformed knees. Kaufer and Matthews[32] have stated that optimal results are not achieved with a resurfacing knee prosthesis when there is greater than 20 degrees of fixed varus or valgus deformity, greater than 30 degrees of fixed flexion deformity, or gross preoperative instability with incompetence of two or more of the major knee ligaments. For this group of patients they recommend a constrained prosthesis (the spherocentric).

It has been our experience that such prostheses are very rarely required for a primary knee arthroplasty, although they may be needed in occasional revision cases. Essentially, use of the resurfacing knee prosthesis is possible only when the nature of the underlying pathology is recognized and when the surgeon is versed in the soft-tissue techniques necessary for correction.

Bone Deficiency. Bone deficiency is often asymmetric, involving one side of the joint more than the other. In varus knees the defect is usually tibial, and after making the tibial cut 5 mm beneath the articular surface on the lateral side, a sloping defect of varying size will be present in the medial tibia. In the femur the defect is usually in the lateral femoral condyle, which may mean that only the medial femoral condyle needs resection. Rather than removing a greater amount of bone to establish a flat surface, the surgeon should build up the tibia or femur. Small defects can be managed with cement; larger ones require reinforcement with screws or wire mesh or correction by an asymmetric, custom-shaped prosthesis (Fig. 117–20). Alternatively, the defect can be corrected by a bone graft (Fig. 117–21).

Ligamentous Instability and Asymmetry. Ligament laxity may be merely the result of bone deficiency, and if no other adaptive changes have occurred in the soft tissues, the management is as described previously, and the instability is corrected by removing less bone. However, in long-standing arthritis, secondary adaptive changes take place in the ligaments. The commonly encountered situations are (1) varus deformity, (2) valgus deformity, sometimes with external rotation of the tibia on the femur, and (3) flexion contracture.

Figure 117–20. A method of compensating for asymmetric bony defects is by the use of wedge shaped tibial components.

Figure 117–21. Radiograph showing an alternative method of filling a medial defect of the tibia by the use of a bone graft.

Figure 117–22. Photograph showing the typical varus deformity of osteoarthritis of the knee.

Varus Deformity. Varus deformity is most common in osteoarthritis (Fig. 117–22), and its elements are medial bone deficiency, contracture of the medial ligament, and stretching of the lateral soft tissues.

To correct a varus deformity, the contracted medial ligament is released by removing all osteophytes and the protruding medial border of the tibia and then stripping the soft tissues progressively from the medial upper tibia (Fig. 117–23). The deep portion of the medial collateral ligament is divided at the margin of the bone, and often part of the posterior capsule and semimembranous insertion is divided as well. Cruciate excision is a necessary part of this release. The objective is not merely to bring the leg into the mechanical axis but also to equalize the medial and lateral soft tissues; and if those on the lateral side are stretched, overlengthening of the contracted medial ligament is needed.

Ligament balance is monitored by inserting spreaders in the joint. If varus still persists when both compartments are stretched, the release is inadequate. In this situation the distal insertion of the superficial medial collateral ligament is stripped from the tibia in a subperiosteal manner. The tension in the medial laminar spreader is then increased, causing the distal insertion to gradually give way and allow correction of the deformity. The mechanism is one of shredding rather than transection, and as the release occurs distal to the incision, it often cannot be seen. The release may be per-

Figure 117–23. Diagram of a varus release. The structures released are the pes anserinus, periosteum, and deep medial collateral ligament. Sometimes the superficial medial ligament will require a distal release.

formed after making the tibial resection but must be done before any of the other bone cuts are made.

Valgus Deformity. Valgus deformity is found in both osteoarthritis and rheumatoid arthritis, although pronounced external rotation in association with valgus is typically a rheumatoid deformity. Valgus release follows the same principles as the corresponding medial procedure except that the soft tissues are separated from the femur (Fig. 117–24).

The lateral capsule, lateral ligament, popliteus tendon, lateral posterior capsule, and part of the lateral origin of gastrocnemius are divided at their origin. Laminar spreaders are inserted, and the joint is distracted. Cruciate excision is required to permit the necessary distraction, and again it is not enough to passively correct the deformity. The medial and lateral tissues must be in balance, and depending upon the degree of medial stretching, this means overlengthening on the lateral side.

If necessary, further release is effected by dividing the iliotibial band and lateral intramuscular septum from "inside out." Usually a lateral patellar release is needed, and the lower fibers of vastus lateralis are divided, providing access to the iliotibial band. Naturally, when correcting this type of deformity, stretching and compression of the peroneal nerve are likely and some risk of foot drop exists.

Figure 117–24. Diagram of a valgus release, which is done in this case from the femur. The structures divided are the iliotibial tract, lateral collateral ligament, lateral capsule, and popliteus tendon.

Flexion Contracture. A flexion contracture of minor degree can be corrected by removing more bone than usual from the distal femur. When the contracture is pronounced in rheumatoid arthritis, a posterior capsulotomy is necessary; when associated with valgus deformity, the release described above is continued around the back of the knee, crossing the midline and dividing the medial posterior capsule. Posterior neurovascular structures can be protected because the capsulotomy is fully visualized.

Soft-tissue release techniques are designed to restore normal alignment and motion and to preserve sufficient ligamentous integrity to enable the use of the surface knee joint replacement (Fig. 117–25). The techniques usually require cruciate ligament excision, so that anteroposterior stability after the arthroplasty is dependent upon the surface geometry of the prosthesis, which must possess some degree of cupping. It is our judgment that the posterior stabilized condylar knee is the best choice of prostheses after ligamentous release.

The alternative to soft-tissue release techniques is to obtain correction of deformity by additional bone resection; a constrained prosthesis that assumes ligament function is then required. However, constrained prostheses (Fig. 117–26) have higher rates of loosening, breakage, and infection, so that their use should be limited to as few cases as possible. With experience, soft-tissue release techniques make it possible to correct most deformities and permit the use of a surface replacement prosthesis.

The Patella. Routine resurfacing is recommended whenever this is practical (the patella must be of sufficient size and thickness to accept a prosthesis). Resection of the articular surfaces is judged by eye, holding the patella everted. A small fixation hole is made centrally. At the time of the trial fit, patellar tracking should be carefully observed; and if the patella tends to sublux with flexion of the knee, a lateral patellar release should be performed.

Most surgeons advocate routine patellar resurfacing, although some practice a selective resurfacing in osteoarthritis (Fig. 117–27), preserving patellae that appear more or less normal, with a good surface of articular cartilage. In rheumatoid arthritis there is an argument for always resurfacing the patella, so that all articular cartilage (which may be the source of synovitis) is removed from the articulation.[21]

Fixation. Provided that correct alignment and stability are achieved at the time of the arthroplasty, the long-term fixation of modern prosthetic designs of the total condylar type has been very good (Fig. 117–28*A* and *B*). In fact, present evidence suggests that the durability of knee prostheses is likely to prove better than that of total hip prostheses. There have been some recent advances that may further improve the fixation of the components to bone using methyl methacrylate cement. Cleansing of the exposed cancellous bone surfaces with a pulsatile water lavage system is recommended to remove blood, marrow, and fat. The bone should be thor-

Figure 117–25. *A*, Radiograph of an osteoarthritic knee with severe valgus deformity. *B*, Radiograph after correction by lateral release and insertion of TCP. This is a recovery room radiograph.

oughly dried before applying cement to the exposed cancellous surfaces. With standard cementing techniques, penetration of 2 to 3 mm into the cancellous bone can be obtained. Miller[39] has devised a delivery system that allows the use of low-viscosity cement which can be applied to the bone and pressurized using special equipment. With this method even greater penetration can be achieved. If the prosthesis itself is coated with a porous material such as titanium wire mesh or sintered cobalt chrome beads, a very firm interlock among the prosthesis, cement, and bone can be obtained.

There has also been recent interest in cementless fixation of knee implants. In 1977, Freeman[40] began to use a modification of his original prosthesis without cement. The tibial component incorporated two polyethylene pegs with a series of protruding flanges, which, on insertion into tibial drill holes, deformed and interlocked to give immediate mechanical fixation of the device. By 1982, Freeman was able to report on more than 50 knees without mechanical loosening.

In 1980, Hungerford and his associates[41] began to use a knee prosthesis of anatomic configuration intended for biologic fixation. The design incorporates a relatively coarse porous coat on tibial, femoral, and patellar components. Primary mechanical fixation of the tibial component is achieved with two short angled pegs and a screw introduced into an expandable plastic sleeve placed in the bone beneath the implant. The femoral component is immobilized by press fit augmented by two studs. The patella depends entirely on two very short porous pegs for its initial fixation. The early reports are enthusiastic, but data regarding the effectiveness of fixation by bony ingrowth must be considered preliminary at this time.

Aftercare of Total Knee Arthroplasty Patients. Intravenous antibiotics (usually oxacillin or cephalosporin) are administered immediately preoperatively and for 48 hours postoperatively. No further antibiotic prophylaxis is recommended. We do recommend that antibiotic coverage be given afterwards when there is a known infection elsewhere in the body or for dental manipulations, genitourinary tract instrumentations, or other major surgery in which there is a possibility of bacteremia.

The prevention of thrombophlebitis and pulmonary embolism[42] should be a major goal of every orthopedic surgeon who performs total knee arthroplasty. In a recent study of patients undergoing total knee arthroplasty at The Hospital for Special Surgery,[43] 64 percent were

Figure 117–26. Radiograph of a Guepar with a broken femoral stem. Mechanical failure, loosening, and a high rate of infection are drawbacks to this type of prosthesis.

found to have evidence of thrombophlebitis as indicated by a positive venogram on the fifth postoperative day. This result occurred despite all types of prophylactic anticoagulation, including aspirin, dextran, and mini-

heparin. All patients also had a preoperative lung scan and a postoperative lung scan on day 6. There was an 11 percent incidence of postoperative lung scan changes consistent with small pulmonary emboli, although only a few of these patients had clinical symptoms or signs of pulmonary embolism. As with other investigators, we found the clinical diagnosis of deep vein thrombosis to be totally unreliable, with numerous examples of both false-negative and false-positive findings. Most patients with clinical or scintigraphic evidence of pulmonary embolism also had positive venography, suggesting that the positive venogram, although not itself associated with local symptoms, is of clinical significance. Patients with a positive venogram or lung scan are therefore anticoagulated for 2 to 3 months unless there are also correlating clinical symptoms and signs of pulmonary embolism, in which case the anticoagulation is continued for 6 months. Anticoagulation is accomplished using sodium warfarin (Coumadin). We do not recommend the use of heparin in therapeutic doses except in life-threatening situations, because of the considerable risk of hemarthrosis in the knee. Early in our total knee experience and before this regimen of venography and prophylactic anticoagulation, three patients had fatal pulmonary emboli from silent deep vein thrombosis.

Total knee patients are allowed to walk on the third or fourth postoperative day using a walker or crutches with weight bearing as tolerated. The compressive dressing is removed on the fifth postoperative day, and active assisted flexion exercises are begun. More recently, early motion in the recovery room using a continuous passive motion machine has been employed with encouraging early results. Muscle strengthening exercises are not begun in the first few weeks because of the risk of capsular disruption. We also recommend against the lifting of weights at any time in the rehabilitation process. Upon discharge from the hospital, patients should be walking independently with a cane, should be able to climb stairs, and should have 90 degrees of flexion. The use of the static bicycle is a great aid in gaining flexion.

Figure 117–27. Radiograph showing a Merchant or skyline view of the patellae 5 years after replacement. In this case it was elected not to replace the patellar surface. This particular patient is doing well and is asymptomatic. When the patella is not resurfaced, some patients will complain of anterior knee pain, particularly when climbing stairs. However, the complication of patellar bone fracture is avoided. There is a case for not resurfacing the patella in obese or particularly active patients, who are those most likely to sustain a fatigue fracture.

Figure 117–28. *A*, Anteroposterior standing radiograph of a patient 9 years after total condylar knee replacement. This patient has a stable bone-cement interface, and it has remained unchanged for many years. This is typical of the majority of properly implanted knee prostheses of the total condylar type. Clinical and radiographic evidence suggests that the longevity of the joint after total knee replacement may ultimately prove better than total hip replacement. *B*, Patellar view of the same patient.

COMPLICATIONS OF KNEE REPLACEMENT

General Complications. Despite the advanced age of most patients and the frequency of associated medical conditions, the general complications of knee replacement are relatively few. At The Hospital for Special Surgery in a consecutive series of 1500 arthroplasties, there were no intraoperative deaths, although one patient undergoing placement of bilateral sequential Guepar prostheses died of fat embolism in the recovery room.[44] Six patients suffered a cerebral vascular accident within 2 days of surgery, one of which was fatal. Three patients died of pulmonary embolism in the third postoperative week in the first group of 400 arthroplasties performed before any form of thromboembolic prophylaxis was used. Two patients died of myocardial infarction during the postoperative period. Two of the early patients died from septicemia secondary to an infected prosthesis; this was approximately 1 year after operation. Urinary retention and urinary tract infections occurred with some frequency, especially in bilateral cases (21 percent). All cases eventually responded to conservative measures and appropriate antibiotic therapy. The organism most frequently recovered was *Escherichia coli*. In none of these was the postoperative urinary tract infection related to the development of a deep wound infection in the operated knee.

Local Complications. *Nerve Palsy.* Most nerve palsies involve the peroneal nerve[45] and are related to the correction of valgus or flexion deformity. Twenty-three peroneal nerve palsies were identified in a total of 2626 total knee anthroplasties performed at The Hospital for Special Surgery between January, 1974, and December, 1980. The time of appearance was variable and ranged from discovery in the recovery room to the sixth postoperative day. The treatment rendered on discovery of these findings varied according to the discretion of the surgeon involved. The most frequent therapeutic measure was to loosen the compression dressing and place the knee in a more flexed position. In two cases this maneuver brought immediate improvement of both motor and sensory deficits. At the follow-up examination a residual deficit was found in all 18 patients in whom a sensory deficit had been present at the beginning. Motor power was clinically normal in 6 of the patients; the remaining 16 patients had motor power clinically assessed in the good to poor range.

The following factors contribute to the development of peroneal nerve palsy: (1) stretching of the nerve in valgus and flexion contractures: (2) fascial compression of the nerve and its vascular supply; and (3) direct pressure from the dressing. There are rare idiopathic cases in which none of the above mechanisms seem to apply.

Patellar Complications. *Subluxation and Dislocation.* Subluxation and dislocation are usually caused by incorrect patellar tracking, which should be recognized and corrected at the time of surgery.

Patellar Fractures. Patellar fractures[46] can occur with and without patellar resurfacing, although they are more common when a patellar implant has been used. The fractures can be either traumatic, occurring as the result of a fall, or, more commonly, of the fatigue type, which occur spontaneously without significant trauma. The fatigue fractures are of three types.

(1) *Horizontal fractures* in which the patella separates horizontally, the portion containing the patellar implant remaining centralized while the other fragment subluxes laterally. The mechanism of fracture is improper patellar tracking and is akin to a patellar dislocation.

(2) *Vertical fractures*, often with separation of the fragments. The presentation may be one of transient mild pain and swelling, but at times the fracture is entirely asymptomatic.

(3) *Comminuted and displaced fractures* are the most common type and are a combination of types 1 and 2. The presentation is nearly always asymptomatic, and the fracture is often found on routine follow-up.

In a sense, patellar fractures are a complication of success, as they are seen in the most active patients with the greatest range of motion, who tend to use the knee arthroplasty in a normal manner for stair climbing, arising from a chair, and other stressful activities. The fracture can usually be treated conservatively unless the patellar button is loosened, in which case the button requires removal.

Inadequate Motion. The range of motion obtained after arthroplasty is dependent on several factors, including body habitus, patient motivation, adequacy of physical therapy, and prosthetic design. However, probably the most important determinant is the range of motion that existed before the arthroplasty.

It has been our policy to manipulate knees postoperatively if motion is not rapidly regained, and usually this is done at the end of the second postoperative week when flexion is not 75 degrees or more by this time. A general anesthetic with full muscular relaxation is needed, as the purpose of the manipulation is to overcome articular adhesions, which can be done with less force when the quadriceps resistance is eliminated.

Some of our patients may not have needed a manipulation and might have regained motion if left alone to continue physical therapy. Fox and Poss[47] studied 343 total knee replacements performed in a 12-month period in which 81 (23 percent) were manipulated. Manipulation did not increase the ultimate flexion of the knee when compared with a larger group of knees that were not manipulated at all. However, their study did not address the critical question of whether the knees chosen for manipulation would have done just as well without. Some patients do not easily regain flexion of the knee after arthroplasty, and in some, restriction of motion may be permanent. A selective manipulation is done for the following reasons: (1) It improves the immediate course by allowing more normal function, and (2) it prevents permanent restriction of motion in certain patients who are not easily identified until it is too late for manipulation to be effective.

Instability, Subluxation, and Dislocation. Instability after knee arthroplasty is usually the result of an error at the time of surgery either in the soft-tissue balancing and tensioning or in the overall alignment of the limb. A revision of the arthroplasty is usually required.

Loosening. Component loosening, usually of the tibial component, was the most frequent cause of failure with hinged prostheses and early surface replacements. The results of hinges often appeared deceptively good when the follow-up time was short,[48] because loosening was a time-related phenomenon usually heralded by the development of a complete radiolucency at the bone-cement interface. On the other hand, with surface replacements, most component loosening occurs within the first 2 years. Therefore, a 2-year follow-up examination of a surface replacement model serves as a good indication of the security of fixation, while similar data for a constrained prosthesis may be misleading.

There is now reason to believe that the high failure rate due to tibial component loosening represented a design problem. High rates of loosening have been reported with polycentric,[26] geometric,[49] and early Freeman-Swanson[50] designs. Modifications to the tibial component in more recent models[51] have resulted in a marked decrease in loosening. For example, the total condylar prosthesis has a one-piece tibial component with a central fixation peg, and only two cases of tibial component loosening were identified in 100 osteoarthritic knees followed from 5 to 9 years, and one of these was caused by malposition and malalignment (Fig. 117-29A and B). Metal backing of the tibial component, which increases the rigidity of the polyethylene, and improved cement techniques should in the future reduce component loosening to almost zero in technically correct arthroplasties.

Infection. Persistent symptoms following total knee replacement in the absence of a clear mechanical explanation should alert the surgeon to the possibility of infection.[52] Although diagnosing acute severe infection with local and general symptoms poses no particular problem, occasionally latent infections can manifest themselves, mainly by knee pain, with mild or no general symptomatology. The wound can be benign, and the usual laboratory tests and radiologic findings may prove negative.

Incidence of Infection. It is well known that joint infection occurs more frequently in patients with rheumatoid arthritis, who are often immunologically deficient.[53] In addition, frequently these patients have had previous operations, and sometimes the placement of previous incisions may predispose to skin necrosis that can lead by extension to a deep prosthetic infection.

The surgeon can influence the ultimate infection rate not only by his technique but also by his selection of prostheses. For example, with surface replacements such as the duocondylar, duopatellar, or total condylar prostheses, the overall infection rate is less than 1 percent. On the other hand, with the metal-on-metal constrained hinged prostheses such as the Guepar the infection rate may approach 15 percent, with many of these infections occurring late, sometimes years after implantation.[54] The reason for this very high incidence of infection is not altogether clear but is probably related to the amount of metallic debris, which in turn causes a sac containing fluid and debris to form around the prosthesis.[55]

Wound drainage defined as leakage from the incision

Figure 117–29. *A,* This osteoarthritic knee was positioned after the arthroplasty in slight varus. After one year there was a pronounced radiolucent line beneath the medial part of the tibial component. *B,* There was progressive medial subsidence until this 5-year standing radiograph showed a considerable increase in the varus attitude with medial sinkage and bending of the polyethylene. At this point a revision was performed, and the tibial component was found to be loose. (Courtesy of J. Bone and Joint Surg.)

is quite frequent and requires no modification of the postoperative regimen except cessation of physical therapy until the leakage ceases. Antibiotics should usually not be given, since latent deep infection might be masked.

Deep Infection. Deep or periprosthetic infection may be either early, defined as within 3 months of surgery, or late, occurring after this ime.

Early Infection. An early infection, provided that its course is not modified by injudicious use of antibiotics, is usually not difficult to recognize. The clinical course is abnormal, with prolonged pain, swelling, inflammation, and fever. The white cell count and sedimentation rate remain elevated. The recommended procedure for establishing the presence of infection is a knee aspiration performed under strict aseptic conditions. The fluid aspirated is sent immediately to the laboratory for direct smear, Gram stain, and anaerobic microbacterial and fungal cultures and sensitivities. Occasionally the infecting organism can be an indolent type of bacteria. In order to increase the chance of bacterial growth, the aspirate should be inoculated as soon as possible into the appropriate broth and culture medium. At times an open biopsy is indicated. At surgery a thorough débridement is done; frozen tissue sections, complete Gram stains, cultures of the tissues, and the macroscopic appearance of the wound should also provide diagnostic information. In early infections of this type, the prosthetic components should be left in situ, and after débridement the wound should be closed over wide-bore suction drains. These drains are removed at 36 hours, and we do not favor closed suction irrigation, owing to the risk of exogenous superinfection.

Intravenous antibiotic therapy is begun under the supervision of an infectious disease specialist and subsequently modified if necessary according to the sensitivities of the organism. Antibiotic blood levels are monitored against cultures of the infecting organism, with the objective of maintaining mean inhibitory concentrations at a minimum eightfold dilution.

The wound is inspected after 2 weeks, and the wound is reaspirated under strict aseptic conditions. When the wound is benign and the cultures are negative, antibiotic therapy is continued for a further 4 weeks. When this is not the case, reoperation with removal of the prosthetic components and all cement is performed. It is our belief that infections complicating total knee replacement should not be treated with antibiotic therapy alone. This treatment might suppress the symptoms of infection transiently and may be indicated only as a temporary measure if surgery is contraindicated for medical reasons or if the patient does not accept it.

We also condemn procrastination and the prolonged use of oral antibiotics, particularly when the infection is only suspected and not confirmed by bacteriologic evidence. The end result of this course is likely to be an indolent subclinical infection and a painful prosthesis. In addition, it may make subsequent culture of the organism very difficult even after the components have been removed, so that proper and appropriate antibiotic therapy is impossible and ultimate salvage of the arthroplasty by reimplantation of another prosthesis becomes much less likely.

Late Infection. Late infection is more common, and the diagnosis is usually straightforward unless antibiotics have been previously given. The usual presentation is acute pain and swelling in the knee in a previously satisfactory arthroplasty. Aspiration will usually provide the diagnosis, although the diagnosis may be much more difficult in patients who have received antibiotics. We believe that any painful prosthesis for which a cause is not readily apparent should be assumed infected until proven otherwise.

The treatment for proven or suspected late deep infection is incision, drainage, thorough débridement of the involved tissues, and removal of the prosthetic components along with the acrylic cement. This course should be followed even in suspected cases because only cultures obtained from the bone-cement interface may be positive.

Adequate preoperative planning is necessary, and the availability of special instruments is recommended. Removal of the prosthetic components and acrylic cement can be a difficult task, particularly if the septic process has not loosened the components. The removal of hinged total knee replacements with intramedullary stems can prove rather difficult. For these, special cement osteotomes and a high-speed, low-torque cement drill are helpful. A custom-made sliding hammer with a special attachment to lock onto the prosthesis is also available.

All scarred, inflamed, and devitalized tissue should be thoroughly excised, leaving viable, healthy, well-perfused tissues.

Primary wound closure can usually be performed over closed suction tubes, which are removed after 24 to 48 hours. The knee is immobilized in a bulky Robert Jones dressing with plaster splints. Unless there are clinical signs that suggest problems, we prefer to leave this dressing untouched for several weeks. We do not advise skeletal traction and prefer to leave the bone ends in contact to reduce dead space.

When the cultures and sensitivities are finally available, a subsequent course is planned. When the diagnosis of infection is erroneous and all cultures are negative, a new prosthesis can be reimplanted as soon as primary wound healing has occurred. When the infecting organism is resistant to antibiotic therapy, or when adequate blood levels cannot be obtained without undue risk of toxicity, secondary arthrodesis is performed by inserting multiple transfixion pins and applying an external compression apparatus. Usually this can be done without reopening the wound. Arthrodesis is most likely needed when the infecting organism is gram negative.

When the organism is susceptible, the wound is inspected after completion of 6 weeks of intravenous therapy with the appropriate antibiotic. If the wound is completely benign and the patient has had an uneventful postoperative period, we would consider reinsertion of another total knee prosthesis provided the patient accepts and understands the increased risk of recurrence of infection. Frozen tissue sections as well as Gram-stained tissue cultures are obtained at the time of surgery to assess tissue inflammation. The macroscopic appearance of the wound should be completely benign; all scarred and devitalized tissue is then excised, leaving only viable, well-irrigated, healthy tissues. Exposure can sometimes be difficult after prolonged immobilization.

In such a case a modification of the Coonse and Adams quadriceps turn-down exposure is used by making an oblique incision across the tip of the quadriceps tendon into the vastus lateralis muscle.

Again, preoperative planning is essential in order to have on hand adequate prosthetic components for a satisfactory biomechanical reconstruction. When there is bone stock deficiency, a special custom-designed prosthesis might be necessary. Alternatively, bone defects can be made good by using screws, titanium mesh, or bone graft. In most cases, proper alignment can be re-established with adequate soft-tissue tension. Excision of the patella has proved helpful in cases in which the skin closure was too tight. Normally reconstruction can be achieved using standard total condylar components or variants thereof, even when the removed prosthesis is a hinged or other more constrained design. The soft-tissue capsule that forms around the knee provides an excellent substitute for the collateral ligaments, and after adequate spacing with the prosthetic components, both alignment and stability can be restored.

Sometimes the use of constrained components is unavoidable. When this is so, we select the TCP III, which has intramedullary stems on both components and restricts varus-valgus, anteroposterior, and rotary motions by means of a centrally positioned peg. However, stemmed components should be avoided whenever possible because of the risk of recurrent infection.

Postoperative management after reimplantation is the same as for a primary arthroplasty unless a quadriceps turn-down was done for exposure. On the assumption that the knee was sterile at the time of reimplantation, we do not believe that there is a need for prolonged antibiotic therapy.

Since 1976, twenty-four cases of septic failure have been managed and in eighteen a reimplantation was done.[56] Reimplantation was not done in some cases for a variety of reasons, for example, the age and general condition of the patient, infections caused by mixed organisms making antibiotic therapy difficult, or refusal by the patient to undergo surgery. Four of these cases were treated by incision and drainage and prolonged antibiotic therapy. The result was suppression of the infection in two and persistent infection in the other two. Two patients had the prosthesis removed and a fusion attempted, arthrodesis being obtained in one.

The remaining 18 patients had a removal of the prosthesis followed by reimplantation 6 weeks to 3 months later (Fig. 117–30A to D). With a follow-up time ranging from 3 months to 5 years, all have remained free of infection. Ten of the cases have been followed for more than 2 years after reimplantation, and the quality of the arthroplasty has been generally good, even approaching that of a primary operation. However, three cases have extensor mechanism weakness and an extension lag.

Revision of Total Knee Arthroplasty.[57,58] Component loosening was by far the major cause of failure with early prosthetic designs. This is not the case with later models such as the total condylar prosthesis. In a recent study of both our own patients and those referred to us, failure was caused by malposition, loosening, infec-

Figure 117–30. *A,* This patient presented with an infected knee prosthesis with multiple draining sinuses along the incision. *Staphylococcus aureus* was cultured. *B,* Lateral radiograph of this patient showing a Shiers prosthesis, which was not loose. The patella had been excised. The Shiers prosthesis was removed; the patient was treated with intravenous antibiotic therapy, and after 6 weeks a new total condylar III prosthesis was reimplanted. *C,* Radiograph taken 21 months after reimplantation, at which time the patient had a good knee rating. There was an extension lag related to the previous patellectomy. *D,* The appearance of the skin incision with the knee flexed 3 years after reimplantation. The knee was cool, and there was no evidence of inflammation or recurrence of infection. (Courtesy J. Bone and Joint Surg.)

tion, and subluxation in about equal numbers. Both malposition and subluxation are mostly attributable to errors in surgical technique and hence avoidable.

The technical principles of the revision surgery are much the same as those described for revision prompted by infection, although immediate exchange of the components is done when the case is aseptic. Bone loss of either the femur or the tibia is the major technical problem, and various means of building up bony deficits are required. Custom components have been our most frequently used approach. The posterior stabilized condylar prosthesis is the recommended prosthesis for most revision procedures. The results of revision are not quite as good as those of primary operation, and the complete pain relief normally found after knee replacement is not so often obtained in revision cases. Restricted motion has not been a difficulty, and the average range of motion after revision is almost the same as occurs after the primary operation. Radiographic evaluation has revealed that radiolucent lines are much more frequent in revision cases. These lines are often visible soon after surgery and in some cases reflect the difficulty of cleaning the bone ends after removing the previous component.

RESULTS OF TOTAL KNEE ARTHROPLASTY

The earlier designs for knee replacement did not provide for the patellofemoral articulation, usually preserved the cruciate ligaments, and relied on small fins for tibial fixation or even in some cases a bony surface that was flat, e.g., the duocondylar. Examples of early prostheses were the duocondylar, geometric, UCI, and the Guepar. The results with these designs were not encouraging, and because of this the reputation of knee arthroplasty has suffered even to this day. The major problem with the earlier prostheses was component loosening, usually because of either excessive constraint or poor design of components.

The current generation of resurfacing prostheses began with such designs as the total condylar and Townley prostheses, which have now been in use for 10 years. It has become evident that the results with these prostheses, properly implanted, are much better and in fact may be superior to the results obtained with total hip arthroplasty.

The total condylar prosthesis has been in use at The Hospital for Special Surgery since January 1974. The first 100 consecutive patients to have the prosthesis implanted for gonarthrosis on the Knee Service were recently studied.[59] The diagnosis in all patients was osteoarthritis. They are generally the most active patients and will give the best assessment of problems related to long-term prosthetic viability. The minimum follow-up period was 6 years and the maximum 9 years. The average age was 68.2 years and the average weight 76.6 kg. Patellar replacement was used in all but 9 knees.

At follow-up, 70 knees (70 percent) were rated excellent, 23 knees (23 percent) good, 2 knees (2 percent) fair, and 5 knees (5 percent) poor. The average postoperative range of motion was 96 degrees (range, 75 to 120 degrees). Patients with excellent and good results had no pain and were not limited functionally in their everyday activities by the knee itself.

The two fair results were attributable to unexplained pain in one case and a patellar tendon avulsion with subsequent quadriceps weakness in the other. The five poor ratings were due to loosening in two knees, posterior subluxation in one knee, component malposition in one knee, and sepsis in one knee.

In the two cases with tibial loosening, the result was rated after 2 years as good in one knee and fair in the other. The initially good result was correctly positioned, but 3 years after operation a complete and progressive radiolucent line developed around the tibial component. Thereafter, increasing pain was felt, and a revision was performed because of pain at 5 years. The component was loose, as the radiograph suggested. The other patient who initially had a fair result was malpositioned in varus at the time of surgery, and the knee was always painful on the medial side. Over the follow-up period the varus deformity increased and subsidence of the medial tibial component was noticed and was associated with bending of the polyethylene (see Fig. 117–29B). At reoperation after 5 years, the component was found to be loose, with considerable bone necrosis of the medial tibia. The other case of malposition was somewhat similar in that the knee was positioned in varus at the time of surgery. This patient also complained of pain from the beginning, but no change in position of the tibial component was observed. The knee was explored after 3 years and no obvious cause for the pain was found. However, because of the malposition and deformity, the tibial component was removed and a new component inserted correctly with the knee in 7 degrees of valgus. This patient has subsequently been free of pain. It seems, therefore, that either malposition or malalignment may cause pain in the absence of loosening, perhaps due to excessive stress on bone.

The radiolucent lines at the bone-cement interface were studied on serial radiographs. Thirty-one percent of the knees had a radiolucency present on some prosthetic surface at 1 year, increasing to 39 percent after 5 years. Thus, eight knees that initially had no radiolucencies subsequently developed one. The most common locations for a radiolucency were the medial and lateral plateaus of the tibial component. With the one exception noted, no knee prosthesis had a complete circumferential radiolucency, and in a few knees an initially prominent radiolucency became less pronounced with time. Measurements of the polyethylene thickness were made to determine if any wear of the polyethylene was taking place. We were unable to demonstrate unequivocally in any case significant polyethylene wear using this method.

It seems from this study that modern designs of surface knee replacement are proving acceptably durable. There is no evidence that either component loosening or polyethylene wear is likely to prove to be a major problem, and projecting from our results, we believe that for patients over the age of 65 years, a knee prosthesis will last for the remainder of life in most cases.

For younger patients, who are likely to be more active, current data are inadequate to form an opinion concerning the durability of the implants. We do believe that the technical skill of the surgeon performing the arthroplasty and the overall balance and alignment of the leg are the most important determinants of a successful and long-lasting result. Most modern prosthetic designs will give a good result provided they are properly inserted into the knee.

The use of unicompartmental replacement remains controversial, and the published results of these prostheses are conflicting. Insall and Aglietti[60] reported on 22 unicondylar knee replacements with a 5 to 7 year follow-up. Although the results of the unicondylar arthroplasties were initially considered good, they subsequently showed a marked deterioration. At the time of review, one knee was rated excellent, seven knees good, four knees fair, and ten knees poor. Seven knees (28 percent) were revised to a total condylar prosthesis. Lateral replacements did much better than the medial ones. Perhaps to some extent the poor showing of this prosthesis could be attributed to incorrect selection of patients and deficiencies in surgical technique. Also, more than one-half of this series had a concomitant patellectomy, and in retrospect the decision to remove the patella seems unwise. In both the medial and lateral replacements, knees with a patellectomy did worse. However, the major reason for failure was progressive degeneration in the unreplaced compartments, and at revision acrylic cement and polyethylene debris were observed in all knees and a metallic synovitis was also present in two.

Laskin, reporting on 37 Marmor modular prostheses, also found the results inferior to bicompartmental replacement, particularly for medial osteoarthritis.[23]

However, Marmor[24] himself has reported better results with a minimum follow-up of 4 years on 59 knees with unicompartmental replacement. The results were good to excellent in 75 percent of the patients, with no difference between those with medial and those with lateral disease. Poor results were usually associated with the use of a thin tibial component that was prone to bend and loosen. Scott and Santori[25] reported on 100 knees in 86 patients with osteoarthritis followed for 2 to 6 years. These workers used the same unicondylar prosthesis as that used by Insall and Aglietti, but their clincial results were much better. Pain relief was satisfactory in 92 of the 100 knees, the average range of motion was 114 degrees, and 49 percent of the knees had at least 120 degrees of flexion. On the basis of their findings, Scott and Santori continue to recommend unicompartmental replacement for elderly patients with unicompartmental osteoarthritis as confirmed by thorough exploration of the knee at arthrotomy.

With regard to constrained prostheses, metal-hinged-type prostheses should no longer be used. Hui and Fitzgerald[61] report a 23 percent incidence of major complications. The incidence of infection rate was 11.7 percent. There seems to be a consensus of opinion that with hinged prostheses (1) there is higher incidence of complications; (2) the procedure is technically easy and by

virtue of the stems the prosthesis is largely self-aligning; (3) the short-term results are often good; but (4) results deteriorate rapidly with time largely as a result of late infection and loosening.

We have no specific data on the TCP III design, in part because of the small numbers done, most of which were used in revision cases. However, we have formed the impression that loosening with the TCP III is higher than would be expected with the total condylar or posterior stabilized models. Kaufer and Matthews have more information on the spherocentric prosthesis.[62] Reviewing 82 consecutive spherocentric arthroplasties with an average follow-up of 4 years, they report an infection rate of 4 percent and a 10 percent incidence of aseptic loosening. Convery and associates[63] report 8 cases of confirmed or suspected loosening in 36 spherocentric arthroplasties followed for an average of 3 years. Because of this loosening, they propose a long-stem modification of the prosthesis and believe that the short stem of the original version may have been a factor in the "unacceptable rate of revision" (22 percent). Modified constrained prostheses such as the spherocentric seem to occupy an intermediate position between fixed-axis hinges and surface replacements in their rates of infection and loosening.

With regard to surface designs that retain the cruciate ligaments, Sledge and his co-workers[64] have reported 92 percent clearly satisfactory results with the kinematic model. The average range of motion was 106 degrees. The posterior stabilized cruciate substituting knee prosthesis has in our hands proved most satisfactory, with 96 percent of the results being in the good to excellent category, which is a higher proportion than with any other prosthesis that we have used. The average range of motion in this series was 115 degrees (Fig. 117–31),

Figure 117–31. Lateral radiograph of a posterior stabilized condylar knee taken at 125 degrees of flexion. (Courtesy J. Bone and Joint Surg.)

Figure 117–32. Anteroposterior radiograph 5 years after implantation of a posterior stabilized condylar prosthesis to illustrate the bone-cement interface, which in every respect resembles the total condylar prosthesis with respect to the extent and degree of radiolucencies observed.

A

B

Figure 117–33. Anteroposterior (*A*) and lateral (*B*) radiographs of a total condylar prosthesis in "ideal" position. Balance is crucial to the function of the arthroplasty, which can be expected to last indefinitely provided the prosthesis is correctly implanted. With total condylar type prostheses, the surgical technique has a greater influence on the outcome than the variant of the prosthesis selected.

and 76 percent of the patients had normal function in stair climbing activities. Fixation appears comparable to the total condylar prosthesis. (Fig. 117–32)

SUMMARY

We believe that further developments in prosthetic design, such as refinement of the articular surfaces into more anatomic shapes with perhaps left and right femoral and tibial components, will provide only marginal improvement over those already being obtained with current designs, such as the latest kinematic prosthesis and the posterior stabilized condylar knee. We believe that cruciate retention, when possible, or alternatively cruciate substitution in the prosthetic design is probably desirable, although definitive data are still lacking in long-term follow-up reports.

Fixation of the components with conventional cementing techniques has set a standard that will be hard to improve upon, with very low rates of component loosening over long periods of time. However, Freeman and Hungerford are experimenting with cementless techniques, the latter worker using a prosthesis intended for biologic fixation by bone ingrowth.

It is our view that by far the most important determinant of the clinical result lies in the area of surgical technique, and most failures can be traced to inadequate positioning and alignment (Fig. 117–33A and B) or poor fixation techniques. More sophisticated instrument systems are becoming available to aid the surgeon in this respect. However, total knee replacement remains a technically demanding procedure, and the unavoidable technical difficulties make the operation unsuitable for those surgeons who perform it infrequently. A measure of continuing experience is necessary, and although it is hard to define exactly what this should be, the operation should probably be performed not less than once or twice a month to maintain competence. Otherwise the patient would be better served by referral to a more experienced surgeon or alternatively by a simpler operation, such as an osteotomy in cases of osteoarthritis.

References

1. Campbell, W.C.: Interposition of vitallium plates in arthroplasties of the knee. Preliminary report. Am. J. Surg. 47:639, 1940.
2. McKeever, D.C.: Tibial plateau prosthesis. Clin. Orthop. 18:86, 1960.
3. MacIntosh, D.L.: Arthroplasty of the knee in rheumatoid arthritis. J. Bone Joint Surg. 48B:179, 1966.
4. Walldius, B.: Arthroplasty of the knee joint using endoprosthesis. Acta Orthop. Scand. (Suppl.) 24:19, 1957.
5. Shiers, L.G.P.: Arthroplasty of the knee. Preliminary report of a new method. J. Bone Joint Surg. 36B:553, 1954.
6. Deburge, A., and G.U.E.P.A.R.: Guepar hinge prosthesis. Complications and results with two years' follow-up. Clin. Orthop. 120:47, 1976.
7. Gunston, F.H.: Polycentric knee arthroplasty. Prosthetic simulation of normal knee movement. J. Bone Joint Surg. 53B:272, 1971.
8. Gunston, F.H., and MacKenzie, R.I.: Complications of polycentric knee arthroplasty. Clin. Orthop. 120:11, 1976.
9. Shoji, H., D'Ambrosia, R.D., and Lipscomb, P.R.: Failed polycentric total knee protheses. J. Bone Joint Surg. 58A:773, 1976.
10. Bullough, P.G., Insall, J., and Ranawat, C.S.: Wear and tissue reaction in failed knee arthroplasty. J. Bone Joint Surg. 58A:754, 1976.
11. Mendes, D.G., Figarola, F., Bullough, P.G., and Loudis, P.: High density polyethylene prosthetic femoral head replacement in the dog. Clin. Orthop. 111:274, 1975.
12. Ranawat, C.S., Ecker, M.L., and Straub, L.R.: Synovectomy and debridement of the knee in rheumatoid arthritis. Arthritis Rheum. 15:571, 1972.
13. Geens, S., Clayton, M.L., Leidholdt, J.D., Smyth, C.J., and Bartholomew, B.A.: Synovectomy and debridement of the knee in rheumatoid arthritis. J. Bone Joint Surg. 51A:626, 1969.
14. Insall, J.: Intra-articular surgery for degenerative arthritis of the knee. A report of the work of the late K.H. Pridie. J. Bone Joint Surg. 49B:211, 1967.
15. Insall, J.: The Pridie debridement operation for osteoarthritis of the knee. Clin Orthop. 101:61, 1974.
16. Coventry, M.B.: Osteotomy of the upper portion of the tibia for degenerative arthritis of the knee. A preliminary report. J. Bone Joint Surg. 47A:984, 1965.
17. Insall, J., Bauer, G.C., and Koshino, T.: Tibial osteotomy in gonarthritis (osteoarthritis of the knee). J. Bone Joint Surg. 51A:1545, 1969.
18. Insall, J., Shoji, H., and Mayer, V.: High tibial osteotomy. A five year evaluation. J. Bone Joint Surg. 56A:1397, 1974.
19. Insall, J., and Shoji, H.: High tibial osteotomy for osteoarthritis of the knee with valgus deformity. J. Bone Joint Surg. 55A:963, 1973.
20. Goodfellow, J., and O'Connor, J.: Kinematics of the knee and the prosthetic design. J. Bone Joint Surg. 59B:119, 1977.
21. Sledge, C.B., and Ewald, F.C.: Total knee arthroplasty experience at the Robert Breck Brigham Hospital. Clin. Orthop. 145:78, 1979.
22. Freeman, M.A.R., Insall, J., Besser, W., Walker, P.S., and Hallel, T.: Excision of the cruciate ligaments in total knee replacement. Clin. Orthop. 126:209, 1977.
23. Laskin, R.S.: Unicompartmental tibiofemoral resurfacing arthroplasty. J. Bone Joint Surg. 60A:182, 1978.
24. Marmor, L.: Marmor modular knee in unicompartmental disease. Minimum four-year follow-up. J. Bone Joint Surg. 61A:347, 1979.
25. Scott, R.D., and Santore, R.F.: Unicondylar unicompartmental replacement for osteoarthritis of the knee. J. Bone Joint Surg. 63A:536, 1981.
26. Bryan, R.S., and Peterson, L.F.A.: Polycentric total knee arthroplasty: A prognostic assessment. Clin. Orthop. 145:23, 1979.
27. Insall, J., and Aglietti, P.: A five- to seven-year follow-up of unicondylar arthroplasty. J. Bone Joint Surg. 62A:1329, 1980.
28. Manchester knee arthroplasty, editorial. J. Bone Joint Surg. 61B:225, 1979.
29. Ewald, F.C., Thomas, W.H., Poss, R., Scott, R.D., and Sledge, C.B.: Duopatella total knee arthroplasty in rheumatoid arthritis. Orthop. Trans. 2:202, 1978.
30. Insall, J., Scott, W.N., and Ranawat, C.S.: The total condylar knee prosthesis: A report of 220 cases. J. Bone Joint Surg. 61A:173, 1979.
31. Insall, J.N., Lachiewicz, P.F., and Burstein, A.H.: The posterior stabilized condylar prosthesis: A modification of the total condylar design. Two- to four-year clinical experience. J. Bone Joint Surg. 64A:1317, 1982.
32. Kaufer, H., and Matthews, L.S.: Spherocentric arthroplasty of the knee. J. Bone Joint Surg. 63A:545, 1981.
33. Attenborough, C.G.: The Attenborough total knee replacement. J. Bone Joint Surg. 60B:320, 1978.
34. Sheehan, J.M.: Arthroplasty of the knee. J. Bone Joint Surg. 60B:333, 1978.
35. Insall, J.N.: Technique of total knee replacement. In Instructional Course Lectures, The American Academy of Orthopaedic Surgeons, Vol. 30. St. Louis, C.V. Mosby, 1981, p. 324.
36. Freeman, M.A.R., Swanson, S.A.V., and Todd, R.C.: Total replacement of the knee using the Freeman-Swanson knee prosthesis. Clin. Orthop. 94:153, 1973.
37. Freeman, M.A.R., and Insall, J.: Tibio-femoral replacement using two unlinked components and cruciate resection. (The ICLH and total condylar prosthesis.) In Freeman, M.A.R. (ed.): Arthritis of the Knee. Clinical Features and Surgical Management. New York, Springer-Verlag. 1980, p. 254.
38. Johnson, F., Leitl, S., and Waugh, W.: The distribution of load across the knee. J. Bone Joint Surg. 62B:346, 1980.
39. Miller, J.: Improved fixation in total hip arthroplasty using L.V.C. Surgical Technique Brochure. Warsaw, Ind., Zimmer, 1980.
40. Blaha, J.D., Insler, H.P., and Freeman, M.A.R., et al.: The fixation of a proximal tibial polyethylene prosthesis without cement. J. Bone Joint Surg. 64B:326, 1982.
41. Hungerford, D.S., Kenna, R.V., and Krackow, K.A.: The porous-coated anatomic total knee. In Scott, W.N. (ed.): Symposium on Total Knee Arthroplasty. Orthop. Clin. North Am. 13:103, 1982.
42. Harris, W.H., Salzman, E.W., and DeSanctis, R.W.: The prevention of thromboembolic disease by prophylactic anticoagulation: A controlled study in elective hip surgery. J. Bone Joint Surg. 49A:81, 1967.
43. Stulberg, B.N., Insall, J.N., and Williams, G.: Deep vein thrombosis following total knee replacement: An analysis of 643 arthroplasties. Presented at the Annual Meeting of the American Academy of Orthopaedic Surgeons, Anaheim, California, March 1983.
44. Bisla, R.S., Inglis, A.E., and Lewis, R.J.: Fat embolism following bilateral total knee replacement with the Guepar prosthesis: A case report. Clin. Orthop. 115:195, 1975.

45. Rose, H.A., Hood, R.W., Otis, J.C., et al.: Peroneal nerve palsy following total knee arthroplasty: A review of the Hospital for Special Surgery experience. J. Bone Joint Surg. 64A:347, 1982.

46. Thompson, F.M., Hood, R.W., and Insall, J.: Patellar fractures in total knee arthroplasty. Orthop. Trans. 5:490, 1981.

47. Fox, J.L., and Poss, R.: The role of manipulation following total knee replacement. J. Bone Joint Surg. 63A:357, 1981.

48. Insall, J.N., Ranawat, C.S., Aglietti, P., et al.: A comparison of four models of total knee replacement prostheses. J. Bone Joint Surg. 58A:754, 1976.

49. Ilstrup, D.M., Coventry, M.B., and Skolnick, M.D.: A statistical evaluation of geometric total knee arthroplasties. Clin. Orthop. 120:27, 1976.

50. Goldberg, V.M., and Henderson, B.T.: The Freeman-Swanson ICLH total knee arthroplasty. Complications and problems. J. Bone Joint Surg. 62A:1338, 1980.

51. Walker, P.S., Greene, D., Reilly, D., et al.: Fixation of tibial components of knee prostheses. J. Bone Joint Surg. 63A:258, 1981.

52. Salvati, E.A., Brause, B.D., Chekofsky, K.M., et al.: Reimplantation in infected total joint arthroplasty. Orthop. Trans. 5:449, 1981.

53. Garner, R.W., Mowat, A.G., and Hazleman, B.L.: Wound healing after operations on patients with rheumatoid arthritis. J. Bone Joint Surg. 55B:134, 1973.

54. Jones, E.C., Insall, J.N., Inglis, A.E., et al.: GUEPAR knee arthroplasty results and late complications. Clin. Orthop. 140:145, 1979.

55. Shurman, D.J., Johnson, B.L., Jr., and Amstutz, H.C.: Knee joint infections with Staphylococcus aureus and Micrococcus species: Influence of antibiotics, metal debris, bacteremia, blood, and steroids, in a rabbit model. J. Bone Joint Surg. 57A:40, 1975.

56. Insall, J.N., Thompson, F.M., and Brause, B.D.: Two-stage reimplantation for the salvage of infected total knee arthroplasty. J. Bone Joint Surg. 65A:1091, 1983.

57. Hood, R.W., and Insall, J.N.: Total knee revision arthroplasty: Indications, surgical techniques and results. Orthop. Trans. 5:412, 1981.

58. Insall, J.N., and Dethmers, D.A.: Revision of total knee arthroplasty. Clin. Orthop., 170:123, 1982.

59. Insall, J.N., Hood, R.W., Flawn, L.B., and Sullivan, D.J.: The total condylar knee prosthesis in gonarthrosis: A five- to nine-year follow-up of the first one hundred consecutive replacements. J. Bone Joint Surg. 65A:619, 1983.

60. Hood, R.W., Wright, T.M., Burstein, A.H., et al.: Retrieval analysis of 70 total condylar knee prostheses. Orthop. Trans. 5:319, 1981.

61. Hui, F.C., and Fitzgerald, R.H., Jr.: Hinged total knee arthroplasty. J. Bone Joint Surg. 62A:513, 1980.

62. Mathews L.S. and Kauter, H.: The spherocentric knee: a perspective on seven years of clinical experience. Orthop. Clin. North Am. 13:173, 1982.

63. Convery, F.R., Minteer-Convery, M., and Malcom, L.L.: The spherocentric knee: A re-evaluation and modification. J. Bone Joint Surg. 62A:320, 1980.

64. Sledge, C.B., and Walker, P.S.: Total knee replacement in rheumatoid arthritis. In Insall, J.N. (ed.): Surgery of the Knee. New York, Churchill Livingstone, 1984, pp. 697–715.

Chapter 118

Reconstructive Surgery and Rehabilitation of the Ankle and Foot

William H. Thomas

ANKLE

Incidence. Primary osteoarthritis of the ankle is exceedingly rare, but the vulnerability of the joint to a wide variety of bony and ligamentous injuries commonly results in early or late secondary arthritic changes. In rheumatoid arthritis the ankle is the initial joint to be involved in only 4 percent of cases,[1] but in a review of 104 consecutive admissions to a rheumatoid unit, 48 percent of the patients indicated that "ankle" pain was contributing to their disability.[2] Twenty-six percent of the symptomatic patients had radiographic findings confirming arthritic changes in the tibiotalar articulation. Nearly half of the symptomatic patients had misinterpreted inflammation of adjacent soft tissues or involvement of neighboring hindfoot joints as involvement of their "ankle."

Physical Examination. Examination of the ankle should include inspection for evidence of swelling of the joint capsule, which is most easily observed anteriorly when the ankle is in a dorsiflexed position. The three major tendon groups—the posterior tibial, the peroneal, and the ankle dorsiflexors—should be examined for evidence of tenosynovitis. Active and passive motion of the ankle should be recorded for dorsiflexion and plantar flexion. If dorsiflexion is limited when the knee is in the extended position, the measurement should be repeated with the knee in a flexed position to eliminate the influence of a contracted gastrocnemius–heel cord complex.

Varus and valgus stress should be applied to assess stability of the joint; if instability is suspected, roentgenograms should be obtained, stressing the medial and lateral ligaments. The joint should be moved through its full range with both varus and valgus stress applied, palpating the joint to assess the quality of the articular cartilage on both the medial and lateral sides of the tibial surface. If a dry, bony type of crepitus is noted during these stress maneuvers, a total loss of cartilage in some part of the articular surfaces is assumed. Symptoms and crepitus noted with valgus stress should raise the possibility of impingement of the tip of the fibular malleolus against the lateral aspect of the calcaneus.[3]

Standard anteroposterior and lateral roentgenograms should be obtained to complete the evaluation of the ankle (Fig. 118–1), and varus and valgus stress views should be added if indicated by physical examination. If standard views of the ankle are inconsistent with the physical findings, anteroposterior radiographs of the ankle bearing full weight may be of value. The roentgen-

Figure 118–1. Lateral radiograph of a rheumatoid ankle showing loss of cartilage in tibiotalar and talonavicular articulations.

ograms should be carefully evaluated not only for evidence of narrowing of the tibiotalar joint but also for involvement of the joints of the hindfoot, which may have been misinterpreted by the patient as "ankle" involvement.

To complete the physical examination of the ankle, the patient should be observed walking both with and without footwear to evaluate alignment and stability of the ankle-hindfoot complex, noting the position of the ankle when symptoms are encountered and any compensatory mechanisms the patient utilizes to minimize the symptoms.

Conservative Management. Special shoes and braces that diminish the forces across the ankle and limit its motion should be tried before any operative procedures are considered (see Chapter 31). The alignment of the entire lower limb should be evaluated, with the ultimate goal being a plantigrade foot. If there is significant varus or valgus deformity in the hip or knee, surgery to the ankle should probably be deferred until the other joints have been corrected because an ankle and hindfoot that were optimally aligned and fused when the knee was in valgus could become malaligned if the valgus knee is corrected.

Deformity and motion of the hindfoot and midfoot joints should be carefully assessed because the presence of deformity or limitation of motion in the hindfoot will influence the choice of the procedure to be performed on the tibiotalar joint. If symptoms persist in the tibio-

talar joint in spite of conservative measures after the other joints of the limb are optimally aligned, then surgical treatment of the ankle should be considered.

Choice of Procedure. With the subject supine a normal ankle dorsiflexes 12.2 degrees $\pm$ 4.4 degrees and plantar flexes 56.2 degrees $\pm$ 6.1 degrees.[4] An arc of approximately 25 degrees is utilized in level gait by normal subjects; for stair climbing 36 degrees of ankle motion is required to ascend and 56 degrees to descend stairs in a normal fashion.[5] Twenty-five to 35 degrees of dorsiflexion is utilized by the normal subject to rise from a chair.

Until recent years the only procedure available for treatment of the arthritic ankle was arthrodesis. Most studies of ankle arthrodeses have noted nearly normal function in patients whose ankles were solidly fused in optimal position. Even with critical gait analysis utilizing instrumented walk ways and photographic goniometric analysis, Mazur and associates[6] found nearly normal gait in patients whose ankles were solidly fused in 0 to 5 degrees of plantar flexion and 0 to 5 degrees of hindfoot valgus. In studies that have evaluated subtalar motion before and after ankle arthrodesis, none has shown an increase in subtalar motion following ankle fusion, but they have shown an increase in motion in the other hindfoot joints and the joints of the midfoot. A patient can anticipate a satisfactory result from ankle fusion if the pain is relieved as the arthrodesis becomes solid and the mid- and hindfoot joints can provide the 25 degree arc of motion needed for normal level gait.[7]

If all ankle fusions could lead to painless unlimited function, there would be no need to consider alternative forms of therapy. Unfortunately, in spite of 100 years of experience with ankle fusion, there is still no single method that guarantees a successful result. More than 30 different methods have been described and advocated as the optimal procedure. Compression arthrodesis seems to offer a slightly higher percentage of satisfactory unions,[8,9] but no series of over 25 cases has a 100 percent rate of union. A review of 380 attempted ankle arthrodeses using various methods reveals a pseudoarthrosis rate of 17.1 percent (15 to 23 percent), and an additional 1.6 percent required amputation to salvage complications associated with attempted arthrodesis.[7,9-11]

The period of immobilization required to achieve a solid arthrodesis may be as short as 10 weeks, but an average of 17.5 weeks is required, with many cases requiring more than 20 weeks. To many patients this prolonged period of immobilization may not be detrimental other than the aggravation of the cast, but to some older patients and many patients with rheumatoid arthritis the addition of even a short leg walking cast can seriously curtail the patient's level of activity. Prolonged immobilization of the rheumatoid foot and ankle can lead to limitation of motion and even ankylosis of the joints of the hindfoot and midfoot that are needed to provide satisfactory function after the ankle fusion has become solidly united.

Even when the tibiotalar joint is solidly united, most

series indicate an 8 to 20 percent rate of residual discomfort. In an unpublished series reported by Stauffer, the percentage of patients with residual discomfort rose to 33 percent when the patients were followed for an average of 16 years.[12]

Feet that have spontaneous or surgical fusion of joints in the midfoot and hindfoot cannot be expected to compensate for the loss of motion that results from ankle fusion. Rheumatoid patients, in particular, are liable to develop symptoms necessitating arthrodesis of the hindfoot joints either before or after ankle fusion, and their function following arthrodesis can be severely compromised.

In the early 1970s, several total ankle prostheses were developed both in the United States and abroad. The goal of prosthetic replacement was relief of pain and preservation or improvement in motion and function. None of these prostheses has had sufficient follow-up to prove its superiority over another. A review of 250 total ankle replacements from the literature[5,13-17] reveals satisfactory results in 75 percent, unsatisfactory results being attributed to infection in 3.5 percent and loosening in 6.7 percent, with 15 percent requiring revision either to another total ankle (10 percent) or fusion (5 percent). Our own experience with 60 total ankle replacements[18] in the past 5 years, utilizing six different prostheses, nearly parallels the published results. Gait analysis of patients with total ankle replacement showed significantly decreased walking velocity when compared to normal or even arthrodesed ankles. Careful scrutiny of radiographs of 22 total ankles at a minimal follow-up of at least 2 years reveals that 10 percent have gross loosening and 88 percent have radiolucent lines at the bone-cement interface, suggesting that excessive forces were being transmitted to this level of fixation (Fig. 118–2).

Greenwald and colleagues have recently tested ten different total ankle prostheses in cadaver bone, loading the joint with physiologic forces and testing for displacement in rotation and when physiologic medial-lateral and anteroposterior forces were applied.[19] None of the prostheses matched the biomechanics of the normal ankle joint, but utilizing this information old prostheses can be modified or new prostheses can be developed to more closely approximate normal ankle function and reduce the incidence of mechanical failure of the devices.

At the time of this writing arthrodesis is the procedure of choice for the osteoarthritic patient whose vocation or avocation will place high demands on his limb. For older osteoarthritic patients who desire only the ability to walk short distances, some consideration of total ankle replacement should be given if there is associated arthritis, ankylosis, or previous surgical fusion of joints in the hindfoot and midfoot. For the rheumatoid patient with multiple joint involvement whose ankle is stable and whose hindfoot deformity is not severe, total ankle replacement is the procedure of choice. Those rheumatoid patients with moderate to severe hindfoot deformity will require surgical correction of the hindfoot deformity before the total ankle replacement is per-

Figure 118–2. Lateral radiograph of ankle pictured in Figure 118-1, 3 years after total ankle replacement and talonavicular arthrodesis. Note radiolucent lines along the bone-cement interface of tibial component. The ankle has 15 degrees of dorsiflexion and 30 degrees of plantar flexion and is asymptomatic.

formed. Patients with gross instability of the ankle or marked uncorrectable hindfoot deformity should be managed by arthrodesis.

Technique for Arthrodesis. The Charnley compression arthrodesis,[8] modifying the anterior approach to spare the tendons, arteries, and nerves, offers the best opportunity for solid union. The approach is made through an anterior vertical incision just lateral to the neurovascular bundle, retracting the artery, nerve, extensor hallucis longus, and anterior tibial tendon medially and the extensor communis tendons laterally. Transverse saw cuts are then made in the distal tibia perpendicular to the long axis of the tibia in both the sagittal and coronal planes. A similar saw cut is then made in the talus parallel with the plantar surface of the foot. This usually involves a resection of approximately ¼ inch of bone. If less than ¼ inch of bone is resected, the malleoli may be left intact, but this is seldom the case. When more than ¼ inch of bone is resected, impingement of the medial or lateral malleolus against the sides of the talus and os calcis may interfere with adequate contact of the tibiotalar surface or position the malleoli too close to the plantar surface of the foot. Complete or partial resection of the malleoli will often be necessary to avoid contact with the counter of the shoe. Compression pins are inserted parallel to each other in the coronal plane of the tibia and the talus, making certain that the talar pin is slightly anterior to the tibia to balance the forces of the Achilles tendon. Intraoperative anteroposterior and lateral radiographs of the ankle must be obtained after the compression has been applied to assure optimal alignment and bony contact. The compression apparatus with plaster supplement should be continued for 6 weeks, at which time the compression apparatus and pins are removed and a short leg walking cast is applied and continued until healing is complete.

Technique for Total Ankle Replacement. The surgical approach for total ankle replacement has utilized a vertical anterior incision between the extensor hallucis longus and the anterior tibial tendons. Care should be taken to avoid division of either the superficial or deep peroneal nerves as the extensor retinaculae are divided and the extensor hallucis longus and neurovascular bundle are retracted laterally. Dissection of the subcutaneous tissue should be held to a minimum to preserve the thickness of the skin flaps and assure their healing. Self-retaining retractors should be avoided, and special care should be taken to avoid excessive retraction on either skin flap as dissection is developed medially and laterally to expose the anterior ankle joint. A vertical incision is made in the anterior periosteum over the tibia, through the capsule, down to the neck of the talus. Exuberant synovium is removed with a rongeur, but the capsule is retained intact with the periosteum. A thin osteotome is used to make a vertical cut just lateral to the medial malleolus, and an oscillating saw is used to resect the distal tibia perpendicular to its long axis. Injury to the posterior structures can be avoided by first removing the anterior portion of the distal tibial surface, followed by excision of the dome of the talus. Once this portion of the talus has been removed, the posterior aspect of the tibial cut can be completed under direct vision. The cut through the dome of the talus should be parallel to the plantar surface of the foot. After the articular surfaces of the tibia and talus have been resected, tension should be placed on the medial and lateral collateral ligaments to make certain that the bony surfaces are parallel. The largest prosthesis that will fit between the malleoli should be selected in an effort to maximize the stability and minimize the unit loading of the prosthetic surfaces. The tibial component will be aligned with the tibial tubercle, and the talar prosthesis between the second and third metatarsals. Methyl methacrylate is prepared and inserted first on the tibial surface, with care taken to remove excess cement posteriorly, and then the talar component is inserted with the foot in plantar flexion to avoid pushing excess cement into the posterior aspect of the joint. Small curved curettes are used to remove any excess cement that can be seen, and prior to setting of the cement the foot should be plantar flexed to make certain that any remaining posterior cement will not impinge on the posterior aspect of the com-

ponents. After the cement has hardened, the wound should be irrigated and any residual bone or cement fragments removed. The capsule and periosteum are reapproximated with interrupted sutures, and special care is exercised to repair the extensor retinaculae to avoid "bow stringing" of the tendons. The subcutaneous tissues and skin are closed in a meticulous fashion with fine suture material, the ankle is placed in a posterior splint in the neutral position, and the foot is elevated until edema subsides enough to permit active and passive range of motion, which generally takes place by the third to fifth day. Ambulation is permitted shortly thereafter, but dependency of the foot for long periods is avoided until the swelling subsides and wound healing is assured. If equinus deformity was present prior to surgery, a night cast is used until the patient is able to stretch out the heel cord and the posterior capsule. Weight bearing is permitted as tolerated, and efforts to gain motion and strength with active and passive motion to the ankle are encouraged for several months postoperatively. Partial weight-bearing crutch support is continued until the patient has regained sufficient strength to ensure stability.

HINDFOOT

Incidence. In patients with rheumatoid arthritis, symptoms of hindfoot involvement are frequently confused with ankle symptoms and the incidence of arthritic involvement of the hindfoot joints is nearly equal to the incidence of ankle involvement.[1] Forty-eight percent of patients admitted to a rheumatology unit with complaints of "ankle" pain had physical findings and radiographic evidence of involvement of joints in the hindfoot with normal findings in the ankle.[2] Varus deformities of the hindfoot are common in patients with juvenile rheumatoid arthritis, but in rheumatoid patients whose symptoms develop during their adult years, valgus deformities are generally noted. A recent study of 120 ankles and hindfeet randomly selected from a rheumatoid outpatient clinic revealed that hindfoot symptoms were the primary cause of disability in 16 percent of patients, and in 42 percent of patients some hindfoot symptoms were noted.[3] In this study all the patients with valgus deformity had symptoms in the lateral side of the foot, and many demonstrated impingement of the fibula against the lateral aspect of the calcaneus.

Physical Examination. If physical examination of the ankle has been performed and found to be within normal limits, careful attention should be directed to the alignment of the hindfoot. Hindfoot alignment is best observed by standing behind the patient and noting the angle between the heel and the tibia during barefooted stance. This angle should normally not exceed 5 degrees of valgus. When the patient is seated with the feet dangling free of the floor in front of the examiner, brisk inversion of the forefoot may elicit spasm in the peroneal muscles and the patient will note discomfort in the region of either the subtalar or talonavicular joint (Fig.

Figure 118–3. Test for peroneal spasm is performed by gently but rapidly inverting the foot and observing for spasm of the peroneal tendons. Discomfort in the region of the sinus tarsi and/or the talonavicular joint will be noticed by patients who have arthritic involvement of the hind foot.

118–3). The presence of peroneal spasm is convincing evidence of involvement of the joints of the hindfoot.

The examiner should then test to see if the deformity of the hindfoot is fixed or if it can be corrected passively. With the hindfoot held in a corrected position, the forefoot should be observed to make certain that sufficient midfoot motion is present to permit the metatarsal heads to make even contact with the floor.

Routine anteroposterior and lateral radiographs of the foot will generally identify the areas of involvement of the hindfoot (Fig. 118–4), but occasionally lateral weight-bearing views will show a marked plantar displacement of the head of the talus, indicating erosion of the supporting process of the os calcis known as the sustentaculum tali.

Conservative Management (see also Chapter 31). Arch pads and inner heel wedges may be sufficient to relieve symptoms in the milder correctable deformities, and these devices are easily accommodated in most shoes. Individually molded plastic heel cups will offer better support of the hindfoot, but these devices often require a wider than normal heel area in the shoe. Female patients may manage nicely in shoes made on a wider male shoe last, but male patients frequently require extra wide or specially made shoes to accommodate the orthosis. The device that is most likely to relieve hindfoot symptoms is an individually molded posterior plastic orthosis which extends from the calf to just proximal to the metatarsal heads. The use of this orthosis will require a larger than normal size shoe, and frequently an "extra depth" type of shoe is necessary. Prolonged use of these devices may lead to a painless ankylosis of the involved joint and obviate the need for surgery or the further use of the device. If the symptoms persist in spite of the use of orthotic devices, surgical correction should be considered.

Figure 118–4. Lateral radiograph of foot and ankle of rheumatoid patient who complained of disability as a result of "ankle" pain. Note the preservation of cartilage in the ankle and the marked destruction of the talonavicular articulation.

Surgical Management. *Triple Arthrodesis.* If the hindfoot deformity is uncorrectable passively, a triple arthrodesis, removing appropriate wedges of bone from the respective joints, will be required.[20] This is also the procedure of choice for the correctable hindfoot associated with rigidity of the midfoot that would not permit an even distribution of forces beneath the metatarsal heads if the hindfoot became fused in a corrected position.

Technique. Triple arthrodeses can be quite difficult in the rheumatoid hindfoot because of the softness of the bone and the typical valgus hindfoot and abducted forefoot. Correction of these deformities may be accomplished either by resecting a medially based wedge of bone between the talus and os calcis[21,22] or by inserting a laterally based bicortical graft of autogenous bone from the iliac crest, which is similar to the procedure described by Grice.[23] If the forefoot is abducted or malrotated following correction of the subtalar component of the deformity, a medially based wedge of bone is excised, including both the talonavicular and calcaneocuboid joints. To obviate the need for a long leg cast that would have a deleterious effect on knee function, metallic staples should be used to help maintain fixation in the corrected position. Intraoperative radiographs of the foot in both the anteroposterior and lateral planes should be taken to make certain that optimal placement of the staple and correction of the deformity have been obtained. A posterior plaster splint should be applied prior to awakening the patient from anesthesia.

After several days of bedrest with the foot elevated, the surgical dressings are changed and, if the wounds are satisfactory, a well-molded short leg plaster is applied. Minimal weight-bearing ambulation with crutches is permitted for the first 6 weeks following surgery. Thereafter, weight bearing is progressed to full weight bearing if the increase in weight bearing is not associated with increased discomfort. Twelve weeks of cast immobilization should be anticipated for the fusion to become solid and immobilization can be discontinued when radiographs show incorporation of the fusions. Moderate swelling and the need to reinstitute the use of crutches should be expected for several weeks following the removal of the cast. A custom-molded arch support will facilitate the transition to full unsupported weight bearing.

Talonavicular Arthrodesis. If the hindfoot deformity is passively correctable, arthrodesis of the single involved joint will usually relieve the symptoms and prevent further deformity. Arthrodesis of the talonavicular joint has been commonly used at the Robert B. Brigham Hospital, and a review of the first 104 cases revealed that over 95 percent had a marked reduction in symptoms and improvement of function.[24,25]

Technique. Talonavicular arthrodesis is performed through a medial longitudinal incision over the tuberosity of the navicular between the anterior tibial and the posterior tibial tendons (Fig. 118–5). The tuberosity of the navicular is excised and set aside for use as a bone graft. The joint is identified; if there is any question

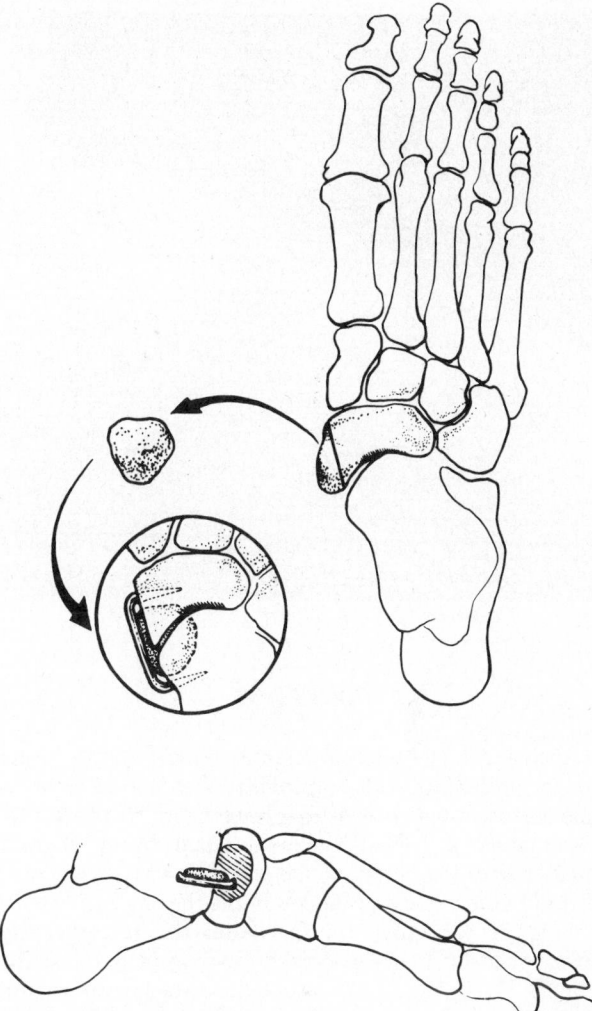

Figure 118–5. Diagram of technique used to perform talonavicular arthrodesis utilizing navicular tubercle as a bone graft across the joint with staple fixation.

about the identification of the joint, this is verified by intraoperative radiographic examination. Any residual cartilage over the articular surface is removed along with bony osteophytes if present, and the eburnated articular surface is excised to expose the underlying cancellous bone, which will offer a suitable surface for fusion. While the foot is held in a corrected position, a slot is fashioned perpendicular to the joint surfaces, and the bone graft is then inserted in this slot and held in position with a firm metal staple. Following closure of the overlying soft tissues and skin, a posterior splint is applied and the foot is held in an elevated position for several days until swelling has subsided. When wound healing seems well assured, a short leg plaster cast is applied, and the patient is allowed to ambulate, bearing weight as symptoms will permit. Ten to 12 weeks of immobilization is generally sufficient to produce solid union (Fig. 118–6); if the patient has used a posterior plastic orthosis preoperatively, this device may be used in lieu of a cast after 6 to 8 weeks of plaster immobilization.

Figure 118–6. Lateral radiograph of foot pictured in Figure 118–4, 4 years after talonavicular arthrodesis. This foot and ankle have remained totally asymptomatic after surgery.

FOREFOOT

Incidence. The forefoot is an extremely common site for the presentation of symptoms of rheumatoid arthritis and is the initial area of involvement in 16 percent of rheumatoid patients,[1] which is equal to or slightly greater than the initial incidence of hand involvement.[26] Careful examination of the feet in the rheumatoid patient should be performed routinely, but this is frequently overlooked by many examiners, owing, in part, to the added time required to remove the patient's shoes and stockings, but mostly because many physicians are not familiar with the examination of the foot.

The foot should be examined in stance and while walking both with and without shoes to detect static malalignment and biomechanical abnormalities of gait. The footwear should be inspected for adequacy of fit and uneven wear on the heel and sole. In well-worn shoes the leather of the toe box will frequently reflect deformities of the underlying toes. The bare foot should be inspected for alignment, swelling, erythema, and adaptive changes in the skin. Adequacy of circulation should be assessed by palpation of pulses and the temperature and color of the skin. Sensory deficits should be carefully recorded. Areas of tenderness should be palpated to detect underlying bursae and nodules as well as to evaluate the thickness of the subcutaneous tissues and the prominence of the underlying bones. The active and passive range of motion of the toes should be recorded if limitations are noted.

Physical Findings. The physical findings associated with rheumatoid involvement of the forefoot include (1) tenderness to metatarsal compression; (2) synovitis; (3) tenosynovitis; (4) bursitis; (5) dorsal subluxation of the proximal phalanx; (6) flexion contractures of the proximal interphalangeal joints; (7) thinning of the plantar fat pad; (8) prominence of the metatarsal heads;

(9) rheumatoid nodules; (10) plantar keratoses; (11) hallux valgus; and (12) involvement of the interphalangeal joint of the great toe.

The physical findings listed above may be present alone or in association with one or all of the additional findings, depending on the severity of the disease. These findings represent a natural progression of deformity of the forefoot afflicted with rheumatoid arthritis.

Rheumatoid involvement of the forefoot begins with synovitis and swelling in the metatarsophalangeal joints and may be so diffuse that it is easily overlooked unless the metatarsal heads are compressed. Tenderness to metatarsal compression applied just proximal to the metatarsophalangeal joints, although not absolutely diagnostic, is a strong supporting sign in making the diagnosis of rheumatoid disease even in the absence of confirmatory laboratory studies.[23] When the metatarsal compression test has been positive early in the disease, evaluation of this finding can serve as a useful gauge in assessing the patient's response to medical therapy.

Tenderness to metatarsal compression is also noted in patients who have plantar neuromas (Morton's toe),[28-30] but neuroma pain can usually be differentiated from rheumatoid synovitis by increased sensitivity to dorsal-plantar compression of the distal intermetatarsal space. Plantar neuromas are classically, though not exclusively, located between the third and fourth intermetatarsal spaces, and compression of the involved interspace produces marked discomfort. Other common causes for pain with metatarsal compression include stress fractures and osteochondritis of the head of the second metatarsal (Freiberg's disease), but these causes are readily identified by routine radiographs.

On rare occasions a synovial protrusion from one or two metatarsophalangeal joints may be so pronounced that a soft tissue mass can be observed on the dorsum of the foot. If these protrusions cause persistent symptoms, aspiration and injection of steroids are indicated;

should steroid injection fail, surgical removal of the synovium should be considered.

The extensor and the flexor tendons of the foot can develop swelling along the tendon sheath similar to those associated with the hand. Aspiration and steroid injection will frequently be sufficient to control the swelling, but on occasion surgical resection is indicated. The flexor tendon sheath is prone to tenosynovitis which decompresses itself through the skin at the flexor creases, forming a fistulous tract that can lead to a chronic low-grade infection. These should be treated by surgical excision and appropriate antibiotics.

Bursae between or beneath the metatarsal heads can become inflamed in rheumatoid arthritis, mimicking synovial proliferation. Although these usually respond to medical management of the disease or steroid injections, persistent painful bursae may have to be excised surgically.

Progress of Deformity. If the disease process remains active and synovitis of the metatarsophalangeal joint persists with distention of the joint capsule and loss of the articular cartilage, a dorsal subluxation of the proximal phalanx will be noted (Fig. 118–7). Plantar subluxations have been noted on rare occasions, usually in the feet of patients who are no longer ambulatory. The normal active contraction of the long toe extensors, which is present through 65 percent of the gait cycle, and the passive extension of the metatarsophalangeal joint during the remaining part of the stance phase of gait favor a dorsal direction for subluxation in the ambulatory patient. Once dorsal subluxation begins, it usually progresses. With further capsular distention the flexor and intrinsic tendons dislocate into the valleys between the metatarsal heads and become extensors of the metatarsophalangeal joint, perpetuating the dorsal subluxation of the joint (Fig. 118–8). The unopposed flexion of the interphalangeal joints of the toe produces a claw or hammer toe deformity. The plantar fat pad is anatomically attached to the plantar capsule and moves distally with dorsiflexion of the proximal phalanx, so the dorsally located proximal phalanx creates a relative diminution of the padding beneath the metatarsal heads.

Figure 118–8. Diagram of rheumatoid toe in a shoe, showing flexor tendons dislocated in the "valleys" between the metatarsal heads, leading to fixed dorsal subluxation of the metatarsophalangeal joint with resultant pressure over the proximal interphalangeal joint and the area beneath the metatarsal head. Note that the plantar fat pad has followed the proximal phalanx and now lies distal to the metatarsal, contributing to apparent thinning of subcutaneous tissues beneath the metatarsal head.

With the proximal phalanx now in a more vertical position, the toe box of a normal shoe exerts pressure beneath the metatarsal head, promoting the formation of rheumatoid nodules in the subcutaneous tissues and calluses or keratoses on the plantar surface.

Rheumatoid nodules generally form over bony prominences and initially are a firm mass of fibrous tissue. They can break down to form a thick-walled cyst containing fluid and fibrin deposits. The nodules may disappear spontaneously, but if they are persistent and painful, they should be injected with steroids or surgically removed. Chronic low-grade infections in rheumatoid nodules may develop either from hematogenous dissemination or via fistulous tracts through the plantar surface of the skin.

Subluxation also occurs in the first metatarsophalangeal joint, but the action of the muscles of the big toe favors a lateral deviation of the great toe, producing a hallux valgus deformity. The lateral force of the great toe is sufficient to cause lateral displacement of the minor toes unless the second and third toes overlap the displaced hallux.

The rheumatoid process may lead to limitation of motion of the great toe metatarsophalangeal joint, creating a hallux limitus or hallux rigidus without an associated valgus deformity. When this occurs, additional stress is exerted at the interphalangeal joint of the great toe, leading to disruption of the joint and dorsal angulation of the distal phalanx. As long as the disease process remains active, the progression of these deformities will continue, and any surgery that is considered should anticipate the tendency for this process to worsen even if treated well by appropriate surgical procedures.

Treatment. *Conservative.* The goals of treatment should be to make the patient as comfortable and the foot as functional as possible. Comfort and function can

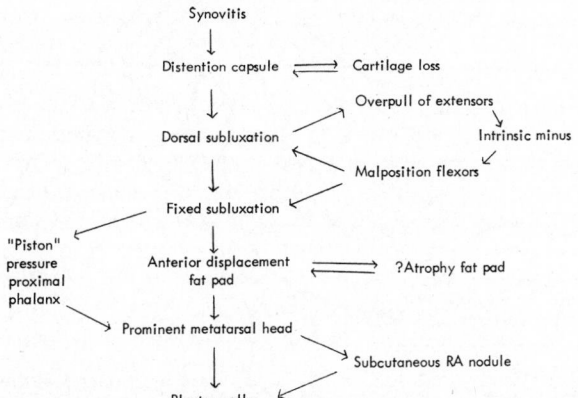

Figure 118–7. Pattern of progression of deformity of rheumatoid forefoot.

often be restored by having the patient fitted to a shoe that is wide enough in the forefoot to prevent compression of the metatarsal heads and high enough in the toe box to avoid contact with the proximal interphalangeal joint. Forty percent of patients treated in one rheumatologic clinic were noted to have ill-fitted or improper footwear.[2] Exercises to gain plantar flexion of the metatarsophalangeal joints should be encouraged to prevent dorsal subluxation of the less severely involved toes. Clinically inflamed bursae or rheumatoid nodules over bony prominences can occasionally respond to steroid injections, but these will surely recur unless pressure from the footwear is relieved. Sandals are particularly useful in avoiding problems related to contact areas on the dorsum and sides of the foot, and a material called Plastizote, which distributes pressures evenly over the plantar surface, has been particularly effective as an insole for either sandals or shoes (Fig. 118–9). Adding an insole of sufficient thickness (¼ to ⅜ inch) to offer relief for the plantar prominences is usually incompatible with insertion into a regular shoe owing to the limited height of the toe box. Specially constructed extra-depth shoes are available commercially at reasonable cost and can accommodate moderately severe deformities. Individually molded shoes that are fashioned from a plaster impression of the foot may be required for more severely deformed feet, but these shoes have the disadvantages of being noncompliant and expensive and requiring replacement if the deformities progress (see also Chapter 31).

As mentioned above, it is best not to recommend surgery while the deformities are progressing rapidly, owing to the likelihood of deformity occurring in adjacent toes, which would require similar surgery some months later. For those patients whose disease is relatively inactive, pain and disability related to joint destruction and deformity can be diminished by appropriate surgical procedures.

Metatarsal Osteotomy. Indications. When a painful callus occurs over a prominent metatarsal that is not fixed in dorsal subluxation at the metatarsophalangeal joint, a very simple osteotomy of the neck of the metatarsal can provide significant relief. The "push test," as described by Kelikian,[31] will determine whether or not the subluxation is "reducible" or "fixed" (Fig. 118–10). Digital pressure is applied to the plantar surface of the metatarsal just proximal to the metatarsal head. If the toe is thereby extended to a normal relationship to the metatarsal, the subluxation is "reducible." If the proximal phalanx fails to assume a normal extended relationship to the metatarsal, the subluxation is considered to be "fixed." A number of different types of metatarsal osteotomy of varying degrees of complexity have been recommended,[32-34] but the ultimate goal is to produce shortening and dorsal displacement of the prominent metatarsal head. A simple oblique osteotomy of the metatarsal neck, as originally described by Meisenbach (Fig. 118–11), is effective in over 80 percent of the cases and produces minimal morbidity.[35]

Procedure. The osteotomy is performed via a dorsal transverse or longitudinal incision over the neck of the metatarsal. The dorsal capsule and the extensor brevis tendon are routinely divided, and the metatarsal neck is exposed. An oblique osteotomy of the neck of the metatarsal just proximal to the head is performed with an osteotome or small rongeur, and the distal metatarsal shaft is inspected to ensure a smooth plantar surface. The metatarsal head is manually displaced dorsally, and, if the proximal phalanx continues to rest in a dorsiflexed position, the extensor longus tendon is divided. Routine skin closure completes the procedure.

If the fifth metatarsal is the offender, the osteotomy should be performed obliquely in the sagittal plane to encourage medial as well as some dorsal displacement of the distal fragment.[36] When osteotomy of the most prominent metatarsal has been completed, the surgeon should carefully examine the adjacent metatarsals to be certain that the osteotomy has not produced excessive prominence of the adjacent metatarsal heads. Osteotomy of one or two additional metatarsals adds little morbidity to the procedure.

Figure 118–9. Schematic diagram of foot on a sandal with Plastizote immediately beneath the plantar surface of the foot. Note that the Plastizote deforms over the areas of pressure to distribute forces more evenly.

Figure 118–10. "Push test," which is performed by plantar pressure proximal to the metatarsal head, will reduce the metatarsophalangeal joint to normal alignment if dorsal subluxation has not become "fixed."

Figure 118–11. Osteotomy of metatarsal just proximal to metatarsal head will produce some shortening of the metatarsal and slight dorsal displacement of the metatarsal head. If dorsal subluxation of the proximal phalanx has not become fixed, some correction of cock-up deformity can also be achieved.

Postoperative Management. Many patients will note an immediate decrease in the discomfort they felt preoperatively, and ambulation may be permitted as tolerated. It is important to discard any previously used foot molds or pads, as they would lessen the tendency for the osteotomy to heal in its new dorsally displaced position. Postoperative plaster casts are to be particularly avoided, and no attempt is made to reduce the plantar callus, as it will disappear with the passage of time. Roentgenographic evidence of healing may not be present for 6 to 10 weeks, but only minimal discomfort will be perceived by the patient as the osteotomy progresses to solid bony union.

Metatarsal Head Excision (Single) or Condylectomy. *Indications.* If the symptomatic metatarsal is associated with a dorsal subluxation that has become "fixed" so that active and passive flexion fail to reduce the joint to normal alignment, excision of the symptomatic metatarsal head or condyle is indicated.[37] Condylectomy is usually reserved for the milder deformities, because excision of a portion of the proximal phalanx is required if the toe does not lie in a normal position following the condylectomy. Proximal phalangectomy leads to excessive instability of the toe unless a surgical syndactyly to the adjacent toes is performed;[31] even with syndactyly almost all toe function is lost following proximal phalangectomy. Toe function is also diminished when the metatarsal head is excised, but stability of the toe is preserved and the need for syndactyly is eliminated. For these reasons we prefer the simpler metatarsal head excision to any form of proximal phalangectomy.

Procedure. Metatarsal head excision is performed through a dorsal approach similar to that described for metatarsal osteotomy. Special care should be exercised to ensure that the entire head has been removed and the distal end of the metatarsal is smooth.

Condylectomy[38] utilizes a similar dorsal approach, dividing both extensor tendons and the dorsal capsule of the metatarsophalangeal joint, but only the plantar

aspect of the metatarsal head is excised to reduce the plantar prominence. As mentioned above, if deformity or prominence of the metatarsal persists following condylectomy, we prefer excision of the entire metatarsal head.

After the condylectomy or metatarsal head excision has been completed, the surgeon must re-evaluate the plantar surface of the foot to make certain that adjacent metatarsals have not become so prominent that osteotomy, condylectomy, or excision is indicated. If the excision of three metatarsals is indicated, it is probably best to excise all four of the lesser metatarsal heads.

Postoperative Management. Excision or condylectomy of one or two metatarsal heads produces only slightly more disability than metatarsal osteotomy, and most patients are able to ambulate within 2 days following surgery, using support only as necessitated by involvement of the other joints of the lower extremity.

Metatarsal Head Excision (Multiple). *Indications.* Excision of four or more metatarsal heads should be performed only on severely involved feet and will usually be required on both feet at the same time. Some shortening of the foot should be anticipated following multiple metatarsal head resections, and if only one foot is treated, the patient would be subjected to the unnecessary expense of buying mismated shoes. The length of hospitalization is only 1 or 2 days longer for bilateral head resections than for single foot surgery, and the 2- to 3-month period from surgery to complete subsidence of postoperative swelling is the same for both bilateral and unilateral procedures. If anesthesia time is a concern, simultaneous procedures can be performed, using two surgical teams. Excision of all the metatarsal heads has been quite effective in correcting severe deformity and reducing discomfort, but rarely can these results be considered "excellent," since very few will regain normal pushoff of the toes.[39] Approximately 25 percent of patients will continue to require some minor modification of conventional footwear to permit comfortable ambulation, and a small percentage of the more severely deformed feet may continue to need custom-molded shoes.[40-44] Ten to 20 percent of feet will later require minor revision owing to inadequate removal of bone at the time of surgery or the growth of bony spurs at the site of resection.

The decision to excise the first metatarsal should be based on the degree of deformity of the great toe, the length of the first metatarsal, and the relationship of the first metatarsal to the lateral metatarsals after the heads have been excised. The aim is to produce a smooth curved metatarsal arc that distributes forces uniformly and avoids any single prominent metatarsal.

Procedure. Several different surgical approaches have been described for the performance of multiple metatarsal head resections. Hoffman[45] was the first to advocate excision of the metatarsal heads; he used a plantar approach, excising the callused skin beneath the metatarsal heads. Kates, Kessel, and Kay[46] modified this approach by excising a more proximal ellipse of the plantar skin. Larmon in 1951[47] and Fowler in 1959[48] recommended the use of three separate longitudinal incisions. In the early 1960s, both Aufranc[49] and Clayton[39] advocated the use of a dorsal transverse incision. Either of these incisions is adequate to perform the procedure, and the selection is based on the extent of deformity, scars from previous surgery, and the surgeon's familiarity with the approach. In general, the thicker, desquamated epithelium of the plantar skin heals a little more slowly than a dorsal incision, and dorsal longitudinal incisions tend to produce contracting scars that favor recurrence of the cock-up deformity of the proximal phalanges. Transverse incisions are favored for the less severely involved feet, but the surgeon must be certain to remove sufficient bone to permit closure of the skin without tension on the suture line. Complete exposure of the metatarsal head is necessary to prevent a bony spur forming from an incompletely removed fragment. Plantar incisions, because of their complete exposure of the metatarsal head, are favored for complete removal of the head. By excision of an ellipse of skin, the plantar fat pad is relocated beneath the end of the metatarsal. The plantar approach is therefore preferred for the more severely contracted deformities.

The second metatarsal head should be excised first, and each successive metatarsal should be trimmed slightly more proximally to form a smooth arc tapering proximally as the surgeon progresses laterally to the fifth metatarsal (Fig. 118–12). Surgery to the great toe should be performed last, with the first metatarsal resected at the same level as the second. A dorsomedial approach to the great toe is preferred regardless of the approach used for the lesser toes.

When excision of all the metatarsal heads has been completed, the contracted lesser toes are manually straightened; if the cock-up deformity persists, thin in-

Figure 118–12. When multiple metatarsal head resections are indicated, the decision regarding excision of the first metatarsal should be based on the length of the first metatarsal relative to the length of the second metatarsal after the second metatarsal head has been removed.

tramedullary Kirschner wires are inserted in the toes for 2 to 3 weeks. After all the metatarsal heads have been excised, the toes should lie in normal alignment with the metatarsal ends as the wound edges are held together. If this is not the case and a cock-up deformity persists, the extensor tendons should be divided and consideration given to excising more of the metatarsal or possibly the proximal end of the proximal phalanx. Excision of the proximal end of the proximal phalanx as recommended by Clayton[39] and Larmon[47] can lead to excessive floppiness of the toes unless Kirschner wires are used to maintain the toes in proper relationship to their respective metatarsals. An intraoperative radiograph should be taken prior to skin closure to make certain that optimal resection of the heads has been achieved and that no fragments of bone have been left in the depths of the wound.

If the plantar approach has been used, an elliptical piece of plantar skin, including the thickened plantar calluses, is excised. The wound edges are approximated with interrupted sutures, avoiding tension on the suture line, without need for subcutaneous stitches.

The postoperative dressing must be applied carefully to maintain proper alignment of the toes without producing necrosis of the thin rheumatoid skin over bony prominences of the toes. Sterile Webril cut in thin strips offers an ideal soft dressing to apply over the gauze dressings that are placed directly over the suture line. A loosely wrapped elastic bandage is then applied, and the feet are elevated on pillows.

Postoperative Management. The patient is kept at complete bed rest with the feet elevated for 3 or 4 days until brief periods of dangling fail to produce an exacerbation of symptoms. The feet are then fitted to open toe wooden sandals, and the patient is allowed to ambulate, using support only as necessitated by involvement of other joints in the lower extremity.

Unless the patient's clinical postoperative course demands an earlier inspection, the initial postoperative dressing remains intact for approximately 1 week when a similar light compressive dressing is reapplied. The patient is usually able to be discharged by the tenth postoperative day, but prolonged weight bearing and dependency are discouraged. Sutures are removed at 2 to 3 weeks, and an elastic wrapping is encouraged for several additional weeks until the swelling has subsided. Throughout this period the patient continues to use the postoperative wooden sandals unless Plastizote sandals or other loose-fitting footwear was used preoperatively. Some slight swelling will persist for 2 to 3 months, so the purchase of conventional footwear should be postponed until all swelling has subsided.

Surgical Correction of Hallux Valgus. Treatment of hallux valgus has received a great deal of attention as exemplified by the plethora of procedures designed to correct it. Valgus deformity of the great toe is almost always associated with some varus deformity of the first metatarsal, and any attempt to correct the valgus deformity the great toe should incorporate some correction of the metatarsal if this deformity is present. The Keller procedure has been widely recommended and extensively used and involves a resection of the proximal third of the proximal phalanx and removal of the medial prominence of the first metatarsal. This procedure, as originally described, does not alter the alignment of the first metatarsal and is associated with some loss of the weight-bearing function of the great toe, especially if more than 1 cm of the proximal phalanx is excised. There is a strong correlation between the reduced weight-bearing function of the great toe and the development of metatarsalgia in adjacent toes. One review of patients having Keller procedures noted that over 40 percent had increased metatarsalgia if the great toe did not bear weight.[50] Fusion of the great toe in slight dorsiflexion and a few degrees of valgus will maintain the weight-bearing function of the great toe and eliminate the tendency for the valgus deformity to recur.[37,51,52] Fusion is frequently difficult to achieve in the rheumatoid patient owing to the softness of the bone and the difficulty of maintaining adequate fixation until fusion can occur, but arthrodesis of the first metatarsophalangeal joint should be strongly considered when the hallux valgus deformity exceeds 90 degrees or the environs of the great toe have been associated with chronic or recurrent infections.

Fusion. When performing an arthrodesis of the great toe metatarsophalangeal joint in the rheumatoid foot, either as an isolated procedure or in conjunction with excision of the lateral metatarsal heads, special attention should be given to the interphalangeal joint of the great toe and the length of the first metatarsal. If the interphalangeal joint is nearly normal, the proximal one third of the proximal phalanx is excised and the proximal phalanx is fused in 10 to 15 degrees of dorsiflexion relative to the plantar surface of the foot (25 to 40 degrees of dorsiflexion relative to the metatarsal). The proximal phalanx should not be so dorsiflexed that the pulp of the distal phalanx fails to bear weight on a flat surface. The proximal phalanx should be aligned with the lesser toes in the sagittal plane or in 10 to 20 degrees of valgus relative to the first metatarsal, depending on the degree of metatarsus varus. A lateral dorsal spicule of the distal first metatarsal should be preserved to act as an intramedullary projection into the medullary canal of the proximal phalanx. Two intramedullary Kirschner wires or small staples are used to maintain alignment until the fusion is solid.

If the interphalangeal joint of the great toe is unstable, it should be stabilized by fusion either as a separate procedure or in conjunction with other forefoot surgery. If the interphalangeal joint is ankylosed either by surgery or as a result of arthritic involvement, then strong consideration should be given to restoring motion to the metatarsophalangeal joint by using a double-stemmed intramedullary silicone rubber prosthesis. When chronic or recurrent infections obviate the use of a prosthesis, arthrodesis of the metatarsophalangeal joint should be performed, but the toe should be further shortened by resecting at least half of the proximal phalanx. The additional shortening is necessary to minimize the pressure

on the toe by reducing the lever arm of the great toe as the patient reaches the toe-off phase of the gait cycle.

A metatarsus varus deformity usually accompanies a chronic hallux valgus condition, and reduction of the varus malalignment should be attempted at the time of forefoot reconstruction.[53] A lateral closing wedge or medial opening wedge osteotomy of the base of the first metatarsal may be required for the more severe deformities, but some correction of the metatarsus varus may be achieved by suturing the stump of the adductor hallucis tendon to the distal end of the first metatarsal while it is held in maximal lateral deviation.

Prosthetic Arthroplasty. When the integrity of the skin permits the insertion of an intramedullary silicone prosthesis, this is the procedure of choice for hallux valgus in the rheumatoid foot, because it restores stability, alignment, and motion to the great toe.[52,54,55] The restoration of weight-bearing function to the great toe by the use of this prosthesis, whether used as an isolated procedure or in conjunction with resection of the lesser metatarsal heads, has provided some of our most gratifying results (Fig. 118–13). The tendency for rheumatoid patients to develop infections in bursae and calluses around the foot must be considered when implanting any foreign material that could provide a focus for later infection.

The prosthesis is inserted through a dorsomedial approach, preserving the integrity of the extensor hallucis longus tendon. The distal end of the first metatarsal is excised in proper relationship to the metatarsal heads or the distal end of the second metatarsal if performed in conjunction with excision of the lesser metatarsal heads. The medullary canal of the metatarsal is reamed to accept the largest possible prosthesis after excision of the medial osteophyte of the distal metatarsal. The proximal end of the proximal phalanx is excised to provide ample space for the insertion of the prosthesis and easy correction of the deformity by reefing of the medial capsule. Once adequate reaming has been achieved, the distal stump of the adductor hallucis is sutured to the distal metatarsal while lateral compression is maintained. The prosthesis is inserted with the U-shaped spaces directed dorsally, opposite to the direction of insertion of similar prostheses when used in the hand. The medial capsule is then repaired to maintain the toe in neutral alignment, and the skin closure is performed in routine fashion. The postoperative dressing should relieve tension on the medial capsule repair. After the dressing is changed on the fourth or fifth postoperative day, a hallux valgus splint is worn continuously for 3 weeks except when removed for active assistive exercises, which can be initiated as soon as the integrity of the wound is assured. The splint is used at night for an additional 3 weeks, by which time the medial capsule repair should be healed. Throughout the first 6 weeks the patient should use an open toe wooden sandal for ambulation. Sandals are the ideal type of footwear to use until swelling has subsided sufficiently to permit the use of more conventional shoes.

Surgical Correction of Hallux Rigidus. *General Con-*

Figure 118–13. *A*, Anteroposterior radiograph of rheumatoid foot requiring excision of all metatarsal heads. *B*, Anteroposterior radiograph of foot shown in *A*, 10 months after resection of all five metatarsal heads with introduction of an intramedullary Silastic prosthesis in the first metatarsophalangeal joint.

siderations. Hallux rigidus or limitus is a term applied to reduced dorsiflexion of the metatarsophalangeal joint of the great toe without accompanying valgus deformity. This condition is more commonly associated with osteoarthritis than with rheumatoid disease, but it occurs in both conditions, producing pain as the dorsal spurs of the proximal phalanx impinge against similar spurs on the dorsal aspect of the first metatarsal. Lack of metatarsophalangeal motion produces increased forces beneath the interphalangeal joint of the great toe. In the rheumatoid foot, limited metatarsophalangeal motion may be associated with the formation of painful rheumatoid nodules beneath the interphalangeal joint.

Arthroplasty. For the youthful osteoarthritic patient who desires to remain active in athletics, a dorsal approach should be used to remove spurs and debride the joint, as recommended by DuVries.[56]

Prosthetic Replacement. For the rheumatoid and the older osteoarthritic patient who will not place high demands on the joint surfaces, more certain restoration of motion and relief of symptoms can be achieved by replacing the articular surface of the proximal phalanx with a silicone rubber prosthesis.[57] The prosthesis is held in place by inserting the stem of the prosthesis down the medullary canal of the proximal phalanx. The spurs around the periphery of the metatarsal head are excised, and the proximal phalanx is excised sufficiently to accommodate the prosthesis and provide adequate restoration of motion. The insertion of the short flexors on the plantar aspect of the proximal phalanx should be

retained or reattached to the base of the proximal phalanx to increase flexor power.

Active assistive exercises are encouraged as soon as symptoms permit so that maximal motion can be achieved. No splints or restriction of activity is required other than those imposed by the patient's symptoms.

Cock-up Deformities. Contractures of the interphalangeal joints of the toes can result from muscular imbalance, arthritic involvement of the joints, or a combination of both. When the contracture involves the plantar aspect of the proximal interphalangeal joint with some dorsal subluxation of the metatarsophalangeal joint, the condition is referred to as a cock-up deformity, and this is the condition most frequently associated with rheumatoid arthritis. When the proximal interphalangeal joint is plantar flexed without subluxation of the metatarsophalangeal joint, the condition is referred to as a hammer toe, and this situation can occur without any associated arthritic involvement. Claw toes are most often the result of neuropathy and muscle imbalance and are identified by flexion contractures of both the proximal and distal interphalangeal joints. The term mallet toe is generally reserved for those toes that have plantar or lateral deformities involving only the distal interphalangeal joint.

Symptoms related to any of these conditions are usually the result of pressure by shoes, with painful calluses being noted over the dorsum of the proximal joint, the tip of the toe, or both.

Fusion of the involved joint, using the peg-in-hole

Figure 118–14. When cock-up deformities produce pain over the proximal interphalangeal joint with associated metatarsalgia, resection of the distal portion of the proximal phalanx and dorsal capsulotomy of the metatarsophalangeal joint will relieve symptoms and partially correct the deformity.

technique, offers the simplest method of correction for those toes not associated with dorsal subluxation of the metatarsophalangeal joint. In the rheumatoid foot, there will always be a tendency toward dorsal subluxation of the metatarsophalangeal joint, so fusion of the interphalangeal joints is rarely indicated.

Cock-up deformities of rheumatoid toes which are not associated with metatarsalgia are best treated by excision of the distal third of the proximal phalanx, as recommended by Key[58] and popularized by DuVries[56] (Fig. 118–14). This procedure relieves the fixed deformity, restores some motion to the interphalangeal joint, and reduces the prominence over the distal end of the proximal phalanx even in the event that dorsal subluxation of the metatarsophalangeal joint should occur or become more pronounced. Giannestras[59] has advocated resection of the proximal end of the proximal phalanx for cockup deformities, but this procedure can result in aggravating instability of the toe. Kelikian[31] has recommended a surgical syndactyly of the toe to adjacent toes to counteract the instability associated with partial proximal phalangectomy, but although effective, this procedure is far more technically demanding than excision of the distal portion of the proximal phalanx and offers no added advantages.

CONCLUSION

Relieving pain in the rheumatoid foot, whether by conservative or operative methods, can be just as effective in restoring function to the patient as the more glamorous total replacement of other lower extremity joints. The feet of the rheumatoid patient should be included in the routine examination of the patient, not only to assess the patient's response to medical therapy but also to discover minor disabilities that could be corrected by simple conservative or surgical procedures.

It should be emphasized that the deformities described above will tend to progress as long as the disease process remains active, and any contemplated surgical procedure should include consideration of this tendency so that the patient can be informed of both the short- and long-term benefits of any corrective therapy.

References

1. Clayton, M.L.: Surgical treatment of the rheumatoid foot. *In* Giannestras, N.J. (ed.): Foot Disorders, Medical and Surgical Treatment. Philadelphia, Lea & Febiger, 1967.
2. Vidigal, E., Jacoby, R.K., Dixon, A. St. J., Ratliff, A.H., and Kirkup, J.: The foot in chronic rheumatoid arthritis. Ann. Rheum. Dis. 34:292, 1975.
3. King, J., Burke, D., and Freeman, M.A.R.: The incidence of pain in the rheumatoid hindfoot and the significance of calcaneo-fibular impingement. Int. Orthop. 2:255, 1978.
4. Boone, D.C., and Azen, S.D.: Normal range of motion of joints in male subjects. J. Bone Joint Surg. 61A:756, 1979.
5. Stauffer, R.N.: Total joint arthroplasty, the ankle. Mayo Clin. Proc. 54:570, 1979.
6. Mazur, J.M., Schwartz, E., and Simon, S.R.: Ankle arthrodesis. Long term follow-up with gait analysis. J. Bone Joint Surg. 61A:964, 1979.
7. Said, E., Houka, L., and Siller, T.N.: Where ankle fusion stands today. J. Bone Joint Surg. 60A:211, 1978.
8. Charnley, J.: Compression arthrodesis of the ankle and shoulder. J. Bone Joint Surg. 33B:180, 1951.
9. Thomas, F.B.: Arthrodesis of the ankle. J. Bone Joint Surg. 51B:53, 1969.
10. Johnson, E.W., Jr., and Boseker, E.H.: Arthrodesis of the ankle. Arch. Surg. 97:766, 1968.
11. Lance, E.M., Pavel, A., Patterson, R.L., Fries, I., and Larsen, I.J.: Arthrodesis of the ankle. J. Bone Joint Surg. 53A:1030, 1971.
12. Stauffer, R.N.: Personal communication.
13. Scholz, K.C.: Total ankle replacement arthroplasty. *In* Bateman, J.E. (ed.): Foot Science. W. B. Saunders Company, 1976, pp. 106–135.
14. Evanski, P.M., and Waugh, T.R.: Management of arthritis of the ankle. Clin. Orthop. 122:110, 1977.
15. Buckholz, H.W., Engelbrecht, E., and Siegel, A.: Totale sprunggelenksendoprosthese Modell "St. Georg." Chirurg 44:241, 1973.
16. Freeman, M.A.R., Kempson, G.E., Tuke, M.D., and Samuelson, K.M.: Total replacement of the ankle with the ICLH prosthesis. Int. Orthop. 2:327, 1979.
17. Newton, S.E.: Total ankle replacement. J. Bone Joint Surg. 57B:1033, 1975.
18. Demottaz, J.B., Mazur, J.M., Thomas, W.H., Sledge, C.B., and Simon, S.R.: Clinical study of total ankle replacement with gait analysis. J. Bone Joint Surg. 61A:976, 1979.
19. Greenwald, A.S., Matijczyk, M.B., and Black, J.D.: Ankle implant systems: Laboratory evaluation and clinical correlation. Orthop. Trans. 3:199, 1979.
20. Adam, W., and Ranawat, C.: Arthrodesis of the hindfoot in rheumatoid arthritis. Orthop. Clin. North Am. 7:827, 1976.
21. Hoke, M.: An operation for the correction of extremely relaxed flat feet. J. Bone Joint Surg. 13:773, 1931.
22. Ryerson, E.W.: Arthrodesing operations on the foot. J. Bone Joint Surg. 21:3, 1923.
23. Grice, D.B.: An extra-articular arthrodesis of the subastragalar joint for correction of paralytic flat feet in children. J. Bone Joint Surg. 34A:927, 1952.
24. Dalziel, R., Thornhill, T.S., and Thomas, W.H.: Isolated talonavicular fusion for hindfoot arthritis. Orthop. Trans. 6:34, 1982.
25. Elboar, J.E., Thomas, W.H., Weinfeld, M.S., and Potter, T.A.: Talonavicular arthrodesis for rheumatoid arthritis of the hindfoot. Orthop. Clin. North Am. 7:821, 1976.
26. Murray, W.R., and Inman, V.T.: Vascular and metabolic disorders affecting the foot. *In* DuVries, H.L. (ed.): Surgery of the Foot. St. Louis, C. V. Mosby Company, 1973, Chapter 10.
27. Bayles, T.B.: Personal communication.
28. Morton, T.G.: A peculiar and painful affection of the fourth metatarsophalangeal articulation. Am. J. Med. Sci. 71:37, 1876.
29. Gauthier, G.: Thomas Morton's disease: A nerve entrapment syndrome. Clin. Orthop. 142:90, 1979.
30. Vainio, K.: Morton's metatarsalgia in rheumatoid arthritis. Clin. Orthop. 142:85, 1979.
31. Kelikian, H.: Hallux Valgus, Allied Deformities of the Forefoot and Metatarsalgia. Philadelphia, W. B. Saunders Company, 1965.

32. Mau, C.: Eine Operation des kontrakten Spreizfusses. Zbl. Chir. 67:667, 1940.

33. Borggreve, J.: Zur operativen Behandlung des kontrakten Spreizfusses, Zeitsch. Orthop. Grenzgh. 78:581, 1949.

34. Giannestras, N.J.: Shortening of the metatarsal shaft in the treatment of plantar keratosis. J. Bone Joint Surg. 40:61, 1958.

35. Meisenbach, R.O.: Metatarsal osteotomy. Am. J. Orthop. Surg. 14:206, 1916.

36. Helal, B.: Metatarsal osteotomy for metatarsalgia. J. Bone Joint Surg. 57B:187, 1975.

37. Lipscomb, P.R., Benson, G.M., and Sonnes, D.A.: Resection of proximal phalanges and metatarsal condyles for deformities of the forefoot due to rheumatoid arthritis. Clin. Orthop. 82:24, 1972.

38. Mann, R.A., and DuVries, H.L.: Intractable plantar keratosis. Orthop. Clin. North Am. 4:67, 1973.

39. Clayton, M.L.: Surgery of the lower extremity in rheumatoid arthritis. J. Bone Joint Surg. 45A:1517, 1963.

40. Brattstrom, M., and Brattstrom, H.: Metatarsophalangeal joints in rheumatoid arthritis. J. Bone Joint Surg. 50B:221, 1968.

41. Anathakrishnan, C.V., and Wiedel, J.D.: Forefoot resection in rheumatoid arthritis. Orthop. Trans. 2:243, 1978.

42. Barton, N.J.: Arthroplasty of the forefoot in rheumatoid arthritis. J. Bone Joint Surg. 55B:126, 1973.

43. Amuso, S.J., Wissinger, H.A., Margolis, H.M., Eisenbeis, C.H., and Stolzer, B.L.: Metatarsal head resection in the treatment of rheumatoid arthritis. Clin. Orthop. 74:94, 1971.

44. Watson, M.S.: A long-term follow-up of forefoot arthroplasty. J. Bone Joint Surg. 56B:527, 1974.

45. Hoffman, P.: An operation for severe grades of contracted or clawed toes. Am. J. Orthop. Surg. 9:441, 1912.

46. Kates, A., Kessel, L., and Kay, A.: Arthroplasty of the forefoot. J. Bone Joint Surg. 49B:552, 1967.

47. Larmon, W.: Surgical treatment of deformities of rheumatoid arthritis of the forefoot and toes. Quart. Bull. Northwestern Univ. Med. School 25:37, 1951.

48. Fowler, A.W.: A method of forefoot reconstruction. J. Bone Joint Surg. 41B:507, 1959.

49. Aufranc, O.: Reconstructive surgery of the lower extremity in rheumatoid arthritis. AAOS Instructional Course, Miami, 1961.

50. Henry, A.P.J., and Waugh, W.: The use of footprints in assessing the results of operations for hallux valgus. J. Bone Joint Surg. 57B:478, 1975.

51. Moynihan, F.J.: Arthrodesis of the metatarsophalangeal joint of the great toe. J. Bone Joint Surg. 49B:544, 1967.

52. Raymakers, R., and Waugh, W.: The treatment of metatarsalgia with hallux valgus. J. Bone Joint Surg. 53B:684, 1971.

53. Gould, N.: Surgery of the forepart of the foot in rheumatoid arthritis. Foot Ankle 3:173, 1982.

54. Whalley, R.C., and Wenger, R.J.J.: Total replacement of the first metatarsophalangeal joint. J. Bone Joint Surg. 57B:398, 1975.

55. Kampner, S.L.: Total joint replacement in bunion surgery. Orthopedics 1:275, 1978.

56. DuVries, H.L. (ed): Surgery of the Foot. St. Louis, C. V. Mosby Company, 1973.

57. Swanson, A.B., Lumsden, R.M., and Swanson, G. deG.: Silicone implant arthroplasty of the great toe. Clin. Orthop. 142:30, 1979.

58. Key, J.A.: Surgical revision of arthritic feet. Am. J. Surg. 79:667, 1950.

59. Giannestras, N.J. (ed.): Foot Disorders, Medical and Surgical Treatment. Philadelphia, Lea & Febiger, 1967.

Chapter 119

The Surgery of Juvenile Rheumatoid Arthritis

Richard D. Scott and Clement B. Sledge

INTRODUCTION

The deformity and functional loss produced by juvenile rheumatoid arthritis (JRA) have a devastating effect on the physical and emotional development of the child. The physical handicap often evokes cruel comments from peers, condescension from adults, and overprotection from parents. The efforts of physicians, nurses, and therapists should be a coordinated attempt to normalize function and thereby facilitate emotional development. In many instances, anti-inflammatory treatment (see Chapter 80) combined with physical therapy and splinting (see Chapter 111) will maintain function and prevent deformity. Occasionally contractures develop which require surgical release, or chronic synovitis threatens the joint and requires synovectomy. Rarely, joint destruction is so severe that replacement surgery is necessary, bearing in mind the disastrous effect of complications (such as sepsis) and lack of long-term assessments of such procedures. In spite of these concerns, however, most patients (and their parents) will opt for surgery which restores near-normal function during the important formative years when the pressure of education, spouse-seeking, and career demand maximal effort.

The surgery of rheumatoid arthritis in children presents some problems unique from those encountered in the adult patient. In the adult patient with rheumatoid arthritis, pain is usually the primary indication for surgery. The child often denies pain and accepts contracture, so that restoration of function is the primary goal. The adult patient has usually been "normal" for much of his life, and the surgery attempts to return him toward this normal state. The young child with severe rheumatoid arthritis has never been normal, and often suffers from retarded psychological and social development. Surgery attempts to bring him toward a normal state with which he is totally unfamiliar. There are frequent significant adjustment problems at home and at school. The extreme importance of a continuous vigorous physical therapy program is not appreciated by the child. Poor patient cooperation can lead to stiffness and contracture that require surgical therapy, and later that same lack of cooperation can compromise the potential benefits gained from surgery. The child with rheumatoid arthritis has small bones that need special prostheses for joint replacement. Finally, the effect *of* growth and the effect *on* growth must be carefully considered with any surgical procedure in the child.

The surgical procedures most frequently required in

the patient with JRA include synovectomy, epiphysiodesis for leg length discrepancy, and arthroplasty of the hip and knee. Isolated soft tissue release for severe disabling contracture about the hip, knee, or ankle is occasionally indicated if there is no significant intraarticular disease and the nonsurgical methods have failed (physical therapy, casting, traction). Arthrodesis is rarely indicated in JRA except in the hand (see Chapter 114) and foot (see Chapter 118) when there is advanced disease and splinting fails to relieve symptoms. Osteotomy is sometimes necessary to correct significant angular or torsional deformities about the hip and knee.

Figure 119–1. The incidence of severe wrist involvement in JRA increases dramatically as the patient grows older. (Courtesy of Dr. E. A. Nalebuff.)

SYNOVECTOMY

The indications for synovectomy in the child are similar to those in the adult: persistent synovitis which has not responded to medical management in a joint with adequate articular cartilage. In the adult, 6 months is an acceptable period of time to wait for a medically induced or spontaneous remission. In the child, since spontaneous remissions are more common, some rheumatologists recommend waiting 18 months as long as the joint space is well preserved.[1] On the other hand, if joint destruction and loss of motion are occurring rapidly in the face of active disease, synovectomy may offer the only chance to prevent complete joint destruction and permanent contracture. In reported series, the most frequent joints that required synovectomy were the wrists and metacarpophalangeal joints in the upper extremity and the knee in the lower extremity.[1-4] The tendency today is to avoid synovectomy in the wrists and to treat the patients with vigorous physical therapy and appropriate splinting.[5] Even if the wrist stiffens, it will be quite functional if it has been held in proper position. Many pediatricians may carry the false impression that upper extremity surgery is rarely necessary in the patient with JRA. This is because most of these patients do not require the surgery until they are adults. In a series of 184 juvenile rheumatoid arthritics whose average onset of disease was at 8 years, surgery was performed an average of 12 years later.[6] The most common procedures were wrist fusion, digital fusions, and metacarpophalangeal arthroplasties. Although wrist fusion was surgically necessary in some patients, the incidence of spontaneous fusion was 11 percent for the entire group whose average age was 19 years at follow-up. The incidence of severe wrist involvement increased dramatically as the patients grew older (Fig. 119–1). This tendency stresses the importance of prolonged, adequate splinting to maintain functional position of the wrist as spontaneous fusion occurs.

The knee is the joint most likely to require synovectomy in the child. This is probably because it is a weight-bearing joint where contracture causes marked dysfunction. The best results of synovectomy are obtained in the older child (over 7 years) with chronic monarticular or oligoarticular disease and a good joint space.[2,4] In the younger child, poor patient cooperation

will hamper the results and the disease tends to be more malignant. Synovectomy of the hip in JRA has not been reported frequently, and the results do not appear to be encouraging.[7]

EPIPHYSIODESIS

Leg length inequality can develop in juvenile rheumatoid arthritis, and may require epiphyseal arrest of the lower extremity for correction. The effects of the disease on growth, however, are unpredictable, and skeletal measurements at 6- to 12-month intervals are often necessary to determine accurately the need and timing of surgery. We know that the proximal femoral epiphysis contributes approximately 3 mm of growth per year to the lower extremity. The distal femoral epiphysis, the proximal tibial epiphysis, and the distal tibial epiphysis contribute 12 mm, 9 mm and 6 mm, respectively, each year.[8] Put another way, there are 3 mm of growth per year at the hip joint, 21 mm at the knee joint, and 6 mm at the ankle joint. Unilateral disease at the knee, therefore, is most likely to produce leg length discrepancy. The greatest reported leg length discrepancy resulting from JRA is 5.7 cm.[9] The synovitis appears to stimulate growth in the younger child, but growth retardation is more often seen in the older child. Children with onset of disease before age 5 often have the affected leg grow longer. Factors such as the chronicity of the synovitis, the weight-bearing status of the limb, and the effect of surgery all make the overall results on growth difficult to predict. In our experience, only 15 percent of the patients with early detected leg length discrepancies fail to stabilize or correct their discrepancy and require surgery.[10]

The growth plate can be surgically arrested by a number of methods. Some techniques produce immediate and permanent growth arrest.[11] Stapling across the plate produces delayed arrest which is reversible, if necessary, within several years. If there is an accompanying angular

Figure 119–2. *A,* Preoperative x-ray of a patient with JRA who requires total hip replacement. The bones are small and osteoporotic. The pelvis is lordotic, reflecting the bilateral hip flexion contractures. *B,* The same patient following bilateral total hip replacement. Custom miniature prostheses have been used. Trochanteric osteotomy was not necessary.

deformity to the knee on the longer side, it may be treated by asymmetric stapling of the epiphysis.[12]

ARTHROPLASTY OF THE HIP AND KNEE

We are now in the era of total joint replacement arthroplasty for joints with permanent structural damage and significant pain or deformity. Metal-to-plastic total joint prostheses are now available for use in the hip and knee as well as the shoulder, elbow, and ankle.

Prosthetic joint replacement in young patients remains a controversial issue centering on questions of prosthetic fixation to bone, wear characteristics, fatigue properties of materials, and the effects of skeletal growth. The literature contains relatively little work detailing the experience of total joint arthroplasty in young patients. Some of these series contain young people with many different diagnoses. JRA is a unique disease and the results of arthroplasty in this group must be considered separately.

Between 1971 and 1981, 55 patients with JRA underwent a total of 64 hip replacements and 48 knee re-

Figure 119–3. *A* and *B*, Preoperative x-ray of a patient with JRA who requires bilateral total knee replacement. The bones are small and osteoporotic. There are severe flexion contractures. *C* and *D*, Same patient following bilateral total knee replacement with custom miniature prostheses.

placements at the Robert Breck Brigham Hospital or Brigham and Women's Hospital in Boston, Massachusetts.[17] The youngest patient undergoing hip replacement was 11 years old at the time of surgery, and the youngest patient undergoing knee replacement was 12 years of age.

In our experience, preoperative pain was usually not the primary indication for hip or knee replacement surgery. Functional impairment and deformity were the chief indications in the majority of cases. Skeletal immaturity was considered only a relative contraindication to surgery. Clearly, there are advantages to waiting until the epiphyses are closed, the bones are larger, and the patient is older and more able to cooperate fully with the rehabilitation program. Once the patient becomes nonambulatory or fixed contractures occur, however, further delay may worsen the chance for successful restoration of the involved joint.

Alternative surgical treatment was always considered in our patients prior to joint replacement. Osteotomy, soft tissue release, synovectomy, traction, serial cast application, and vigorous physical therapy will usually yield only transient improvement in the patient with advanced joint destruction. We no longer consider cup arthroplasty in a JRA patient because the results in this group are usually poor and inconstant. In the knee, we will still occasionally perform McKeever metallic hemiarthroplasty in a select group of JRA patients showing complete loss of joint space with good stability, minimal angular deformity, flexion of at least 80 degrees, and flexion contracture less than 15 degrees. We do not normally consider hip or knee fusion as a primary procedure in JRA because it will not sufficiently relieve functional disability in the patient with multiple joint involvement.

When total hip and knee replacements were both indicated in the same patient, the hip arthroplasty was performed first for several reasons. It is possible to rehabilitate the hip joint in the presence of a stiff contracted knee joint but very difficult to rehabilitate the knee in the presence of a painful contracted ipsilateral hip. Manipulation and casting to gain extension in the contracted knee can be performed during the anesthetic administered for hip replacement. By operating on the

Figure 119–4. *A*, Preoperative lateral x-ray of a patient with a 90 degree flexion contracture and deformity secondary to an old supracondylar femoral fracture. *B* and *C*, Anteroposterior and lateral x-rays of the same patient following a preoperative program of physical therapy, traction, and serial casts. Longstanding contractures usually do not respond to this program and must be corrected at surgery.

hip prior to the knee, any pain that had been referred from the ipsilateral hip could be resolved. Finally it seems beneficial to resolve the tensioning of muscles that cross both the hip and knee joint prior to any knee surgery by operating first on the hip.

Careful preoperative planning is mandatory in these patients. Custom or special mini-sized prostheses were required in 50 percent of the hip arthroplasties (Fig. 119–2) and 40 percent of the knee arthroplasties (Fig. 119–3). During hip surgery, we found trochanteric osteotomy to be necessary in approximately 40 percent of the patients in order to provide adequate exposure. This is in contrast to the use of trochanteric osteotomy in only 5 percent of our patients with other diseases. In patients with ankylosing spondylitis and a fused hip, however, it might be advisable to avoid trochanteric osteotomy in order to diminish the incidence of heterotopic bone.[17] In most JRA patients, complete capsulectomy will usually be necessary to relieve a flexion contracture and provide exposure. A psoas tenotomy was required in 16 percent of our patients to help correct the flexion contracture. It must be remembered that with the release of contractures and improvement in range of motion comes the potential for increased morbidity in terms of sciatic or femoral nerve palsy. Transient incomplete nerve palsies were seen in 4 percent of patients, and permanent partial palsies were seen in an additional 4 percent.

For the knee patients, the preoperative management of flexion deformity can reduce the magnitude of soft tissue release required at surgery.[18] We found the preoperative use of traction, physical therapy, and serial casting to be valuable adjuncts to surgical management (Fig 119–4).

The improvement in functional status of JRA patients undergoing total hip and knee replacement has been gratifying. Most patients were able to return to school and complete their education. All but 2 of the surviving 52 patients in our series were limited or full community ambulators at long-term follow-up.[17] For the optimum result, a team approach involving the rheumatologist, surgeon, physical therapist, psychiatrist, social worker, and the patient's entire family is essential. Many children come from broken homes, magnifying their adjustment problems.[20]

The long-term concerns we have in these young people with prosthetic joint replacement are the prevention of failure by late metatastic infection, wear, or loosening. The patient, his family, medical physician, and his dentist must all be educated about the need for rapid intervention with therapeutic use of antibiotics in the treatment of any infectious disease and the judicious use of prophylatic antibiotics when appropriate. Component wear has not been a problem in most series addressing this issue, and some long-term clinical studies suggest that 25 to 30 years might be expected before significant component wear would occur.[19] The small size of our patients and their relatively low activity level would make them even less likely to wear our their joint surface compared with the normal population. The most likely complication leading to failure is component loosening. This has been shown in virtually all series of total hip replacements in young people. The occurrence of component loosening is particulary related to high activity level, heavy patients, and patients with monoarticular disease. The JRA group may well be protected from this complication by their small size and the restraints imposed by their polyarticular disease. Loosening, however, was responsible for all failures to date in our hip replacements (7 percent). In our knee replacement patients, there have been no revisions for loosening. In the knees there was a high rate (18 percent) of reoperation of patellofemoral pain when the patella had not been resurfaced at the time of original arthroplasty. We now perform patellar resurfacing during knee arthroplasty in all patients with JRA.

Total shoulder replacements, total elbow replacements, and total ankle replacements are occasionally necessary to relieve pain in the adult but are rarely necessary in the child. Experience, therefore, is limited, but appropriate prostheses are available for each joint and have been used with success.

Anesthesia poses potential complications in the child with JRA. Cervical spine and temporomandibular joint disease can make intubation difficult and hazardous. Regional anesthesia has become the anesthetic choice for JRA patients at our institution. If regional anesthesia fails or is contraindicated, the fiberoptic laryngoscope is a useful tool to facilitate intubation in difficult cases. We prefer to use the same anesthesiologist in each of the patient's successive procedures. Both the doctor and the patient benefit from familiarity with one another. We use spinal or epidural anesthesia for lower extremity procedures and regional block with intravenous lidocaine for upper extremity operations.

REFERENCES

1. Eyring, E.J., Longert, A., and Bass, J.C.: Synovectomy in juvenile rheumatoid arthritis. J. Bone Joint Surg. 53A:638, 1971.
2. Arden, G.P., and Ansell, B.M.: Surgical management of juvenile chronic polyarthritis. J. Bone Joint Surg. 54B:16, 1972.
3. Garrett, A.L., and Campbell, C.: Synovectomy in children. *In* Cruess, R.L., and Mitchell, N. (eds.): Surgery of Rheumatoid Arthritis. Philadelphia, J. B. Lippincott Company, 1971, pp. 111-116.
4. Kampner, S.L., and Ferguson, A.B., Jr.: Efficacy of synovectomy in juvenile rheumatoid arthritis. Clin. Orthop. 88:94, 1972.
5. Granberry, W.M., and Mangum, G.L.: The hand in the child with juvenile rheumatoid arthritis. J. Hand Surg. 5:105, 1980.
6. Nalebuff, E.: Unpublished data.
7. Albright, J.A., Albright, J.P., and Ogden, J.A.: Synovectomy of the hip in juvenile rheumatoid arthritis. Clin. Orthop. 106:48, 1975.
8. Green, W.T., and Anderson, M.: Epiphyseal arrest for the correction of discrepancies in length of the lower extremities. J. Bone Joint Surg. 39A:853, 1957.
9. Kuhns, J.G., and Swaim, L.T.: Disturbances of growth in chronic arthritis in children. Am. J. Dis. Child. 43:1118, 1932.
10. Simon, S., Whiffen, J., and Shapiro, F.: Leg-length discrepancies in monoarticular and pauciarticular juvenile rheumatoid arthritis. J. Bone Joint Surg. 63A:209, 1981.
11. Phemister, D.B.: Operative arrestment of longitudual growth of bones in the treatment of deformities. J. Bone Joint Surg. 15:1, 1933.

12. Blount, W.P., and Clar, G.R.: Control of bone growth by epiphyseal stapling. J. Bone Joint Surg. 31A:454, 1949.
13. Singsen, B.H., Issaacson, A.S., Bernstein, B.H., Patzakis, M.J., Kornreich, H.K., King, K.K., and Hanson, V.: Total hip replacement in children with arthritis. Arthritis Rheum. 21:401, 1978.
14. Arden, G.P., Ansell, B.M., and Hunter, M.J.: Total hip replacement in juvenile chronic polyarthritis and ankylosing spondylitis. Clin. Orthop. 84:130, 1972.
15. Crowe, W., Hauselman, C., Shear, E., Miller, E.H., Baly, G.P., and Levinson, J.E.: Total hip arthroplasty in children with juvenile rheumatoid arthritis. Proceedings of the 43rd Annual Meeting of the American Rheumatism Association. Arthritis Rheum. 22:602, 1979.
16. Sledge, C.B.: Joint replacement surgery in juvenile rheumatoid arthritis. Arthritis Rheum. 20:567, 1977.
17. Scott, R.D., Sarokhan, A., and Dalziel, R.: Arthroplasty of the hip and knee in juvenile rheumatoid arthritis. Clin. Orthop. 182:90, 1984.
18. Sarokhan, A., Scott, R.D., Thomas, W.H., Ewald, F.C., Sledge, C.B., and Cloos, D.W.: Total knee replacement in juvenile rheumatoid arthritis. J. Bone Joint Surg. 65A:1071, 1983.
19. Charnley, J., and Cupic, Z.: The nine and ten year results of the low friction arthroplasty of the hip. Clin. Orthop. 95:9, 1973.
20. Henoch, J.J., Batson, J.W., and Baum, J.: Psychosocial factors in juvenile rheumatoid arthritis. Arthritis Rheum. 21:229, 1978.

Chapter 120
Surgery of the Hip in Rheumatoid Arthritis and Ankylosing Spondylitis

Robert Poss and Clement B. Sledge

INTRODUCTION

Total hip arthroplasty has revolutionized the treatment of advanced hip disease. Today, it is still the treatment of choice for the patient with rheumatoid arthritis, but doubts about its longevity and concerns regarding the seriousness of complications persist. The frequency of major hip involvement in the patient with rheumatoid arthritis is difficult to estimate. In two series of total hip replacement reported from large referral centers, only 5.8 percent of 2012[1] hips and 15 percent of 1975[2] hip arthroplasties were performed on patients with rheumatoid arthritis. At our hospital, 38 percent of total hip replacements are performed on patients with rheumatoid arthritis. In contrast, 50 percent of the knee arthroplasties we perform are on patients with rheumatoid arthritis.

In this chapter we will discuss the unique problems presented by the rheumatoid patient as a candidate for total hip replacement; alternative surgical therapies, which had been found wanting prior to the era of total hip replacement; the rationale of total hip replacement and its results and complications in rheumatoid arthritis and ankylosing spondylitis; and finally some modes of surgical intervention to be considered in the treatment of the patient with osteoarthritis but not advocated for the patient with rheumatoid arthritis.

EVALUATION OF THE PATIENT WITH A PAINFUL HIP

The history and physical examination, including roentgenograms, will help the physician decide on the proper course of treatment for the patient with hip disease.

History. The duration of symptoms and their increasing severity are important determinants. The patient with a long history of hip discomfort that has not changed in quality and that limits certain activities, but not sleep or personal hygiene, is less a candidate for surgery than the patient with increasing pain over a few months who requires pain medication to sleep. The distribution of pain is not of prognostic help. In the patient with rheumatoid arthritis knee pain may be referred pain from the hip or may actually represent involvement of the knee. The physician should attempt to assess the degree of pain and the limitations of function imposed by the diseased hip. i.e., support required, distance walked, ability to climb stairs, ability to reach the feet to put on socks or shoes, and ability to sit for periods of time. Toward this end a number of rating systems have been devised to quantify the degree of limitation imposed on a patient by pain and limitation of motion.[3,4]

Physical Examination. The patient will limp, favoring the affected side. This antalgic limp is characterized by a decreased stance time on the painful side, a lurching of the trunk *toward* the affected side, and a drooping of the pelvis *away* from the affected hip. The reasons for the patient's assuming this gait are discussed below. The range of motion may be limited by either muscle spasm or structural deformity. Eliciting bony crepitus on motion implies loss of articular cartilage. To assess the true degree of flexion contracture the hips should be flexed on a firm examining table, thus fixing the pelvis; then one hip at a time is extended and the angle the thigh makes with the examining table is recorded as the flexion contracture (Thomas test).

Assessment of the patient's ability to perform personal

hygiene can be made by measuring the combined abduction (or lack of it) of the hips. Inability to sit or reach the foot is caused by lack of flexion or rotation, respectively. Because of limited motion or actual loss of bone and cartilage, the patient may have a true or apparent leg length discrepancy. True leg lengths are measured from the anterior superior iliac spine to the ipsilateral medial malleolus; apparent leg length is measured from the umbilicus to the medial malleolus. A thorough discussion of the examination of the hip and pelvis is beyond the scope of this chapter.[5]

Roentgenograms. The patient whose symptoms and limitations are severe enough to suggest surgical treatment will usually have radiographs showing complete loss of articular cartilage with varying degrees of bone loss (see Chapter 39).

NONSURGICAL THERAPY

If on the basis of the aforementioned investigations the patient is felt not to be a surgical candidate, there are modalities that should help alleviate the degree of his symptoms.

Crutches or Cane. Relief of weight bearing will reduce pain in the inflamed hip. Using two crutches, the patient can be trained to walk so that only the weight of the affected extremity touches the ground (touchdown gait). This is a more comfortable gait than is "non–weight bearing," which, because of the force of muscle contraction, actually loads the hip to a greater degree and is impractical in a patient who has other joint involvement. The rheumatoid patient with shoulder or elbow involvement may find platform crutches more comfortable and useful than axillary or Lofstrand crutches (Fig. 120–1).

A cane held in the opposite hand is of great help in unloading the involved hip. By applying 20 pounds to a cane with the left hand, an involved right hip can be relieved of more than 150 pounds of force[6] (see below for explanation).

Physical Therapy. Range of motion exercises are individualized. Much of the limitation of motion imposed by pain can be reversed by a program of active, active-assisted, and passive exercises once pain has been controlled. In particular, prone lying will help stretch out flexion deformities, while a stationary bicycle will increase flexion. Muscle strengthening, particularly of the hip abductors, is helpful in diminishing the fatiguing effects of an abductor lurch.

Traction. We have found no benefit from bed rest and traction except for the patient with acute severe pain who requires short-term immobilization for relief of muscle spasm secondary to synovitis.

THE RHEUMATOID PATIENT AS A CANDIDATE FOR SURGERY

Progressive pain, despite adequate medical and physical therapy, is the prime indication for surgery. Functional limitations caused partly by pain and partly by restricted motion of the hip are considered in the context of the patient's needs and goals.

An important task for the rheumatologic team is to set reasonable goals for the patient. A patient who is bedridden with structural damage to four lower extremity joints, foot deformities, and weak upper extremities stands a poor chance of becoming an independent walker in spite of numerous operations, but might be a better sitter after bilateral hip arthroplasties. A patient with a destroyed hip joint and early loss of articular cartilage in the knees would be better served by immediate hip arthroplasty than by waiting until three major joints

Figure 120–1. Platform crutches. *A,* A patient with weak or unstable elbows or shoulders can still bear weight with the upper extremities by using platform crutches. *B,* Rheumatoid hand deformities do not preclude the use of platform crutches (see text).

required arthroplasty consecutively. In a recent review of the results of arthroplasty of both knees and hips, 14 of 16 patients had improved functional ratings postoperatively.[7] Factors that predisposed to a lesser functional improvement were older age at initial surgery, longer duration of disease, and severe upper extremity involvement. If the patient requires both hip and knee arthroplasties as well as surgery to other joints, we will generally perform surgery on the most painful joint first. If pain is not the determining factor, we prefer to perform hip arthroplasty first for the reason that hip arthroplasty provides the patient with almost immediate pain relief. The postoperative physical therapy program is not rigorous compared with that for the knee, and the patient will achieve functional improvement with relatively little personal effort.

Following total hip replacement the rheumatologic team has the chance to reassess the patient's commitment to further surgery as a means of reaching the goals set preoperatively. The patient who will not work at the physical therapy program following hip arthroplasty is a poor candidate for knee or elbow arthroplasty. The almost certain pain relief obtained following total hip arthroplasty provides a great psychological boost to a patient depressed by pain and functional loss, facing prolonged hospitalization and multiple operations.

If bilateral hip arthroplasty is required, we perform these procedures 2 weeks apart. Bilateral hip arthroplasty should be performed if the hips have equal involvement and significant flexion deformities. If the interval between hip arthroplasties is excessive (longer than 2 months), the prosthetic hip will lose motion because the patient yields to the flexion contractures of the unoperated hip.

For the patient in whom administration of anesthesia is a formidable task, simultaneous knee arthroplasties[8] or ipsilateral hip and knee arthroplasties[9] and simultaneous hip arthroplasties[10] have been reported.

ASSESSMENT OF STATUS OF OTHER JOINTS

Rheumatoid involvement of certain joints may compromise the results of total hip replacement or be the cause of unforeseen complications.

Cervical Spine. Between 30 and 40 percent of rheumatoid patients admitted to the hospital have roentgenographic evidence of cervical spine subluxation, usually C1 on C2.[11] Between 2 and 5 percent of these patients have demonstrable long tract signs. It is therefore important that the anesthesiologist be aware of this situation and avoid maneuvers which cause hyperflexion of the cervical spine.

Temporomandibular Arthritis. Limitation of mandibular motion because of temporomandibular arthritis should be assessed preoperatively. Such limitation may require alternatives to endotracheal intubation.

Feet. Often the source of pain because of metatarsal head prominence of talonavicular arthritis, the feet are sources of skin breakdown and indolent infections secondary to toe and foot deformities. It is of obvious importance to heal these areas prior to embarking on surgery of the ipsilateral hip.

Ipsilateral Knee. With the involvement of the hip producing a flexion-adduction contracture, degenerative changes in the ipsilateral knee may be accelerated as it is thrown into more valgus with weight bearing. Conversely, at surgery a valgus knee can cause the surgeon to estimate true femoral anteversion incorrectly and place the femoral component in malposition. In patients with a knee ankylosed in extension, manipulations of the hip at the time of surgery can cause sciatic stretch with resultant neuropraxia.

PROFILE OF PATIENTS WITH RHEUMATOID ARTHRITIS UNDERGOING TOTAL HIP ARTHROPLASTY

The median age decade for patients undergoing total hip replacement at our hospital is 61 to 70. Osteoarthritics have a mean age of 66, while the rheumatoid patient averages 56 years. Approximately 15 percent are on maintenance steroids, usually 5 to 15 mg of prednisone every other day. Ideally a surgical candidate should not be obese, but the limitations of function imposed by the disease make attempts at any significant loss of weight impractical. We prefer to perform total hip replacement on patients no younger than 60, but the absence of an acceptable alternative procedure in the rheumatoid patient has forced us to lower this age requirement and offer this procedure to patients with juvenile rheumatoid arthritis in their late teens and twenties.

The patient should be in optimal medical condition. Particular attention should be paid to the urinary tract as a source of potential infection. Many females have asymptomatic bacteriuria; elderly males with symptoms of prostatism may be unable to void postoperatively and require repeated catheterizations, which may predispose to metastatic infection. We would prefer, if feasible, that an appropriate urologic procedure be performed some months prior to hip arthroplasty to obviate the need for catheterizations.

PREVIOUS SURGICAL ALTERNATIVES TO TOTAL HIP REPLACEMENT

Prior to the advent of total hip replacement, many procedures had been advocated for treatment of the rheumatoid hip. None of these procedures offers the reliable pain relief and functional improvement of total hip arthroplasty. Their use, particularly in the rheumatoid patient, is limited. These procedures are listed below:

Hip Arthrodesis. There is a definite place for this procedure in the patient who is young with a normal back and ipsilateral knee, or the patient with previous septic arthritis. Furthermore, successful conversion of arthrodesis to total hip replacement can be done, even after many years. The rheumatoid patient, however, often has ipsilateral knee involvement; a hip arthrodesis would throw additional strain on the knee and low back. Furthermore, hip involvement is often bilateral in the rheumatoid patient; bilateral hip arthrodeses would be incompatible with independent function.

Cup Arthroplasty. This operation is performed rarely today. Its principal indication would be in the patient who is felt to be too young for total hip replacement, or in the patient with previous sepsis of the hip.[12] In 1957, Aufranc reported the results of 1000 consecutive cup arthroplasties performed at the Massachusetts General Hospital.[13] The clinical follow-up varied from 4 to 15 years. Twenty-two percent of patients reported no pain and 31 percent reported slight pain. Eight percent had pain at all times. The revision surgery rate was high: 22.5 percent of the entire series required reoperation, while 30 percent of the rheumatoid patients were reoperated. The incidence of postoperative infection was 4.3 percent overall, and 3.7 percent in the rheumatoids. Twenty-seven percent of patients with unilateral arthroplasties required cane or crutches at all times. Bryan and associates[14] in reviewing the Mayo Clinic experience, reported that initial results were good; 73 percent of patients with rheumatoid arthritis had good or very good hips at 5 years; however, the percentage of good results had diminished to 50 percent by 10 years. The results of total hip replacement to date would favor it as a more definitive procedure.

Hemiarthroplasty. While still popular for treating intracapsular fracture of the femur, hemiarthroplasty has no role as a reconstructive procedure in the patient with rheumatoid arthritis. At the Mayo Clinic,[14] of 36 hips receiving Austin Moore prostheses, 56 percent had good or very good motion at 1 to 5 years. This figure had decreased to 24 percent good motion at follow-up longer than 5 years. Salvati and colleagues[15] followed patients with hemiarthroplasty for longer than 5 years. They found that the patients who had normal acetabula, i.e., postfracture or avascular necrosis, achieved better results than patients with arthritis. In 1964, Barr and associates[16] reported long-term results of Austin Moore hemiarthroplasties done for a variety of diagnoses. They concluded that hemiarthroplasty was not the procedure of choice in arthritic hips and was unlikely to achieve the results obtained by arthroplasty.

Occasionally a patient with rheumatoid arthritis will sustain a fracture of the femoral neck. An endoprosthesis may be used if the joint is felt to be normal, but if there is loss of articular cartilage by roentgenogram, we would prefer to perform a primary total hip replacement.

Synovectomy. A few reports advocate synovectomy for the rheumatoid hip. Lipscomb[17] suggested that this procedure might be of use early in the course of hip involvement and did not feel that there was an increased chance of avascular necrosis secondary to hip dislocation. Cruess[18] felt that the indications for hip synovectomy are similar to those for the knee, i.e., persistent pain and synovitis which does not respond to medical therapy and has not yet resulted in loss of articular cartilage. He felt that under these circumstances synovectomy could be considered. We have no experience with this procedure in the hip. Freeman and Sturrock[19] reported discouraging results in three patients and did not recommend use of this procedure.

A number of other procedures advocated for the patient with degenerative arthritis have had limited or no application in the rheumatoid patient.

BIOMECHANICS OF THE HIP
(Fig. 120–2)

Abnormalities of gait in the patient with hip disease, the rationale for use of a cane, and the technical goals of total hip replacement can best be understood by an appreciation of the forces exerted on the hip joint. Definitive studies of this subject may be found elsewhere.[6,20,21]

The femoral head may be thought of as a fulcrum about which opposing forces must balance. If the patient is envisioned as standing on one lower extremity with the other raised off the ground and the pelvis held level, an equilibrium exists which is achieved by balancing body weight on one side of the fulcrum and the pull of the hip abductors on the other. Each of these forces acts through a lever arm. Body weight is seen from the hip at a distance approximately three times that from which the abductors exert their pull.[21] Therefore, to achieve the equilibrium described above, the hip abductors must exert a force three times body weight. The compressive force on the hip in this example is approximately four times body weight (three times body weight exerted by the abductors, plus one times body weight at the center of gravity).

Rydell[22] studied the forces about the hip joint by inserting specially designed hip endoprostheses containing strain gauges into two patients. He found that the greatest *static* load is applied to the hip in one-legged stance (2.6 times body weight). With slow walking the forces are approximately 1.6 times body weight in stance and 1.0 times body weight in swing phase. These forces increase to 2.8 times body weight with fast walking, up to 5 times body weight in stance phase, and 3 times body weight in swing phase while running. Of particular interest is the fact that forces generated by hip flexion and extension while the patient is at bed rest are *greater* than those generated in slow walking or using crutches. From this analysis certain conclusions become evident:

1. Weight loss is of great benefit because every pound lost results in at least 3 fewer pounds "seen" by the hip.[23]

2. The patient with a painful hip lurches toward the affected hip to reduce the length of body weight lever arm. Thus the force generated by the hip abductors to balance body weight is reduced and the hip is relatively unweighted.

Figure 120–2. Hip biomechanics demonstrated diagrammatically (*left*) and experimentally (*right*). *A,* Normal. The stick figure is now in stance phase on the right lower extremity. For the pelvis to remain level, the forces about the hip must be in equilibrium; i.e., the lever arm of body weight exerted through a distance of approximately 3 inches (circled B) must be balanced by the force of contraction of the hip abductors exerted through a lever arm of approximately 1 inch (circled A). Note that in the actual experiment, body weight (central block) to the right of the hip is balanced by three times the body weight exerted through one third the distance to the left of the hip. That these forces are in equilibrium is demonstrated by the observation that there is no weight on the scale to the reader's right. Note that in stance phase the hip "sees" four times body weight (the sum of the patient's weight and the force of contraction of the hip abductors).

B, Antalgic gait. The patient with a painful hip will limp *toward* the affected side. By doing so the lever arm through which body weight is exerted is diminished. Thus less abductor force is required to stabilize the pelvis, and the hip effectively "sees" less force. In the experimental model, the same body weight shown in *A* is now exerted nearer the hip. Now only two times body weight is exerted by the hip abductors, and the hip "sees" three rather than four times body weight. By decreasing forces across the hip, it should be less painful.

C, A more effective way to unload a painful hip is to use a cane in the opposite hand. In the illustration, the figure is holding a cane at a distance of 18 inches from the affected hip. By exerting force on the cane—i.e., by the ground pushing up on the cane—at such a great distance from the hip, the force of the contraction required by the hip abductors to balance the pelvis is dramatically reduced. In the experiment, body weight is exerted at its normal distance from the hip. Note that a force of approximately 15 percent body weight in the right hand scale exerted at 18 inches from the hip reduces the hip abductor force to one time body weight. Thus the hip now sees only a total of two times body weight (see text).

3. Pushing down with a cane in the opposite hand reduces the effective body weight "seen" by the hip.[6] Because this force acts through a long lever arm, moderate force exerted on the cane results in a large reduction of compressive force on the hip. Exertion of approximately 30 pounds on a cane can reduce the force on the opposite hip by a factor of almost twice body weight.[23]

4. In total hip arthroplasty the technical goals are to *medialize* the acetabular component, thus reducing the body weight lever arm; and to restore the greater trochanter to its normal lateral and distal position in relation to the femoral head, thereby restoring the ab-

ductor lever arm. Failure to achieve either of these goals results in excessive forces on the prosthetic hip and may accelerate the possibility of loosening.

5. The forces on the normal or prosthetic hip are in multiples of body weight for activities considered *routine* in daily living. Any activities requiring increased muscular force, e.g., running or athletics, probably place excessive forces on the prosthetic system. These activities should not be one of the goals of the patient undergoing total hip replacement.

TOTAL HIP REPLACEMENT (LOW FRICTION ARTHROPLASTY)

The present era of total joint replacement was forecast in 1960, when Charnley reported successful implantation of femoral head prostheses, using cold curing acrylic cement to achieve firm fixation.[24] He felt that use of cement would provide a more equal distribution of forces to the bone and obviate the problems of loosening associated with a prosthesis that contacts bone in a few areas of high pressure. In 1961, Charnley reported on the first 97 hip arthroplasties performed using a metal femoral prosthesis articulating with an acetabulum made of Teflon, and fixation of both components in bone with acrylic cement (polymethyl-methacrylate).[25] By reducing the size of the femoral head to 22 mm, he was able to achieve a joint with low friction between metal and plastic, thereby decreasing loosening forces between the socket and acetabular bone. In 1966, McKee and Watson-Farrar reported on their 10-year experience with metal femoral and acetabular components.[26] In 1968, Ring described his metal to metal system which did not require acrylic cement.[27] In 1970, Muller described the total hip replacement system he had evolved during 10 years of experimentation.[28]

Of these variations, the Charnley system has emerged as the most popular. Virtually all total hip replacements performed in the United States are variations of the metal-plastic "low friction" system, using acrylic cement to secure fixation (Fig. 120–3).

Total hip replacement was first performed in this country in 1968 and 1969. Today an estimated 75,000 to 80,000 total hip replacements are performed in the United States annually.[29,30,50]

Technical Aspects. The surgical technique of total hip replacement has been described.[1,25,26,28,31] There is no essential difference in technique when the patient is one with rheumatoid arthritis, but certain additional precautions must be taken. Because of osteopenic bone in the rheumatoid patient, great care must be used during the surgical preparation. Holding the extended extremity by the foot or ankle is sufficient to cause fracture of the femur. Particular gentleness should be used in dislocating the femoral head to avoid fracture.

The question of trochanteric osteotomy persists. Some feel that it is an essential part of the technique of total hip replacement,[32-34] while others contend that the same or improved results are assured without trochanteric osteotomy while complications such as nonunion of the

trochanter and broken wires are avoided.[35,36] Two recent studies suggest that the hip without trochanteric osteotomy has better biomechanics[37] and that there is less patient morbidity.[36] We recommend total hip replacement without trochanteric osteotomy unless exposure is compromised or trochanteric advancement is necessary to re-establish proper abductor tension. We believe it prudent to perform trochanteric osteotomy in all revision surgery.

Pre- and Postoperative Program. The patient is admitted to the hospital 48 hours prior to surgery. During this time the final preoperative medical and anesthetic evaluations are performed. Physical and occupational evaluation is begun, and the patient becomes acquainted with crutch gait and exercises performed in bed. Twice-a-day pHisoHex scrubs to the thigh and leg are begun. Patients taking salicylates continue to take them until the night before surgery. We use prophylactic antibiotics, usually cephalothin sodium (Keflin), 1.0 gram intravenously 1 hour before incision and then 1.0 gram intravenously every 4 hours for 24 hours. Surgical shave and prep are performed in the operating room on the morning of surgery. Postoperatively, anticoagulation is achieved in the rheumatoid patient by resumption of the preoperative salicylate dose.[38] In patients with a prior history of thromboembolic disease, warfarin is used.

After surgery the patient is placed in pillow suspension and Buck's traction for 48 hours. Range-of-motion exercises are begun on the second postoperative day. The patient sits on the side of the bed at approximately day 4 to 5, stands and begins walking on day 6 to 8, and usually is independent on crutches by day 12 to 14. If bilateral hip arthroplasty is to be done, these procedures are performed 2 weeks apart. During the convalescent period particular attention is devoted to aids the patient will require for activities of daily living, for example, long-handled shoe horns, elastic shoe laces, and elevated toilet seats. We encourage the use of a stationary bicycle at home as a means of maintaining motion.

Long-Term Results. A survey of the orthopedic liturature demonstrates that most authors have achieved greater than 85 percent complete or almost complete pain relief using a variety of total hip replacement systems.[39] A Swiss multicenter study found that while 96 percent of patients had severe pain preoperatively, 96 percent had minor or no pain postoperatively.[39] Furthermore, overall function was improved. Forty percent of patients regained their full working capacity after 6 months; after 1 year 66 percent had resumed work.[40]

Similar encouraging results have been reported in two large series of rheumatoid patients. Welch and Charnley reported 95 percent complete pain relief in 307 hips, with an average follow-up of 32.3 months.[41] Poss and associates reported 96 percent pain relief in 275 rheumatoid hips followed for an average of 3.5 years.[42]

Initial enthusiasm about the high rate of success achieved with total hip replacement has been tempered somewhat by the increasing incidence of late complications. Loosening of components with time has emerged as the most serious technical problem.

Figure 120–3. *A*, This patient with advanced rheumatoid arthritis has complete loss of articular cartilage of the right hip. *B*, Contemporary total hip arthroplasty emphasizes proper component placement and improved cement pressurization to maximize cement and bone interlock. The acetabular component is placed into the anatomic socket. Subchondral bone is retained and cement fixation enhanced by the use of multiple small fixation holes. Modern femoral components fill a greater volume of the proximal femur and have rounded surfaces to diminish stresses on the cement.

A number of published studies that report the results of total hip replacement at longer than 10 years postoperatively are now available.[43-49] The results of these studies may be summarized as follows:

1. The incidence of femoral component loosening, as judged by radiographic changes may be as high as 25 percent of total hip replacements at 5 years postoperatively. At 10 years postoperatively, the rate of increase is nonlinear and appears to diminish with time.[44,45,48] While the radiographic incidence of loosening is high at 10 years (30 to 40 percent), the number of hips requiring revision because of failed femoral components is approximately 6 percent.[50]

2. With time, the incidence of acetabular component loosening increases. Charnley[47] found that at 10 years the incidence of severe demarcation (impending failure) about the acetabular component was 9.2 percent. At 15 years, severe demarcation was seen in 25 percent of acetabular components. In the American literature, radiographic evidence of acetabular loosening at 10 years ranged from 11 percent[43,45] to 29 percent.[44]

3. The incidence of failure of total hip replacement is higher in younger, active, heavier patients.[44] In one study, 57 percent of patients under 30 years of age who had undergone total hip replacement had actual or potential loosening of at least one component.[51]

A number of points should be stressed. These results are based on total hip replacements done 10 or more years ago with what now are considered to be obsolete prosthetic designs and inadequate cementing techniques. Recognition of the importance of certain factors listed below[46] should confer improved long-term results on the current generation of hip arthroplasties:

1. Optimum preparation of bony surfaces for cementing by the use of pulsatile lavage.

2. Pressurization of cement to achieve maximum cement interlock.

3. Improved femoral component designs that minimize stress on cement.

4. Retention of acetabular subchondral bone to distribute transmitted load more physiologically.

5. Use of acetabular bone graft to augment deficient bony coverage.

6. Avoidance of varus position of the femoral component.

We have reviewed our long-term results of total hip

replacement in patients with rheumatoid arthritis and have found that despite the low functional demands of this group of patients, the incidence of mechanical loosening appears to be increasing with time.[52] While 96 percent of patients were clinically improved as a result of total hip replacement at 6 to 11 years postoperatively, radiographic analysis suggests that mechanical failure will increase with time. The combined incidence of femoral component subsidence and/or calcar resorption was 40 percent.

Approximately 30 percent of rheumatoid patients have some degree of protrusio acetabuli. In this situation the acetabular component may fracture into the pelvis.[53] In our recent review, acetabular component migration and loosening were seen in 14 percent of hips. Nine of 10 hips with significant preoperative protrusio were seen to migrate with time. Improved surgical technique and component design, as well as the recognition of the importance of bone graft and/or protrusio shells[54-58] to augment deficient bone stock in protrusio, and the importance of restoring the acetabulum to its anatomic position,[52,57] should reduce the incidence of femoral and acetabular failure in this group of patients (Fig. 120–4).

COMPLICATIONS

Infection. Charnley definitively showed that adherence to meticulous sterile surgical technique augmented by effective air changes in the operating room could result in dramatically lower infection rates. His early infection rate of 6.6 percent[59] was reduced to less than 0.5 percent.[60] in this manner. Subsequent reports have shown that similar low infection rates can be achieved by using ultraviolet lights and prophylactic antibiotics.[31] Equally impressive results have been reported from surgeons who perform total hip replacement in conventional operating rooms[61] and in community hospitals.[62] One can surmise from these results that the joint replacement era has reminded the surgeon that scrupulous adherence to sterile technique is of primary importance in avoiding sepsis.

In the United States, the incidence of deep infection following total hip arthroplasty is approximately 1 percent.[50] About 40 percent of infections present in the early postoperative period, 45 percent have delayed onset (2 to 24 months), and 15 percent are thought to be the result of hematogenous spread and may present in the previously well patient at any time after surgery.[50] The groups with delayed hematogenous spread underscore the importance of prolonged follow-up of patients. Patient education is mandatory. Patients should notify physicians and dentists of their prosthetic joint when a potentially bacteria-contaminating procedure is to be done (dental extraction, urologic procedure) and should be given prophylactic antibiotics.

The rheumatoid arthritic patient is at an increased risk for the development of infection following total joint replacement.[59,63-66] In our 6- to 11-year follow-up of total hip replacement,[52] the rheumatoid patient was 1.8 times

more likely to become infected than an osteoarthritic counterpart. Of particular importance, all infections that presented over 3 years postoperatively were in rheumatoid patients and were felt to be of hematogenous origin. The rheumatoid arthritic patient often has multiple sites of skin breakdown and is vulnerable to bacterial infections. This group of patients must be closely managed indefinitely following total hip replacement. Many authors have noted that the incidence of infection increases when total hip replacement is performed as a revision of a previous procedure. Dupont and Charnley reported that the rate of late infection increased twofold when they compared a group of patients who had a revision with those who had primary total hip replacement.[67,68] Murray reported an incidence of infection of 3.1 percent in revision cases compared with 0.7 percent in primary cases.[69] Poss and associates[42] found a 13-fold difference in infection rates when a revision group was compared with patients having a primary procedure.

We recommend that patients undergoing total hip replacement as a revision of some other procedure be informed that they are at higher risk for development of postoperative infection. Preoperative aspiration of the involved hip and anaerobic and aerobic culture of joint fluid obtained may disclose indolent sepsis. An arthogram performed as part of the aspiration procedure provides assurance that the needle is in the hip joint and may detect abnormal sinus tracts. If the suspicion of sepsis is high, hardware may be removed at a preliminary procedure, at which time tissue specimens may be obtained for bacteriologic and histologic examination.

Although the incidence of infection is now considered acceptably low, the patient who becomes infected is seriously jeopardized. The seriousness of the problem presented by an infected total hip is portrayed in the report of Canadian patients with this complication.[70] Of 135 infected patients, 23 died; only one of these patients had a painless hip implant and a healed wound at the time of death. Only 17 patients retained their prosthesis without further wound infection. The remainder had their prosthesis removed, and most had dry wounds.

We have found that early (24 to 48 hours after presentation) surgical intervention with thorough debridement and appropriate antibiotics in large doses may arrest the infection and allow the patient to retain the prosthesis. For established infection, the prothesis and cement must be removed as part of the surgical debridement. Wilson and colleagues treated 19 patients with subacute or recently arrested sepsis with massive doses of antibiotics and reimplantation of the prostheses.[71] At two years they had no recurrence of infection in 17 of the 19 patients.

The use of antibiotic-impregnated bone cement has gained in popularity in Europe and is considered by some the method of choice in treating previously infected total joints.[72] Its use in the United States has not yet been approved by the Food and Drug Administration.

The treatment of established infection about a cemented prosthesis is controversial and must await longer follow-up. Salvati and associates[73] have reviewed the

Figure 120–4. *A*, Advanced rheumatoid arthritis with protrusio. Note that axial migration of the socket has occurred. *B*, Acetabular reconstruction has been achieved. The prosthetic socket has been returned to its anatomic position by being brought laterally and distally. The deficient medial wall has been augmented with bone graft (the patient's femoral head) and peripheral rim support obtained by the use of a metal shell.

results of the reimplantation following infection. They compared the published results of a variety of techniques that used either one- or two-stage reimplantations, with or without antibiotic-impregnated cement, and found an overall success rate of 80 to 90 percent. They concluded that a good result was somewhat more likely following two-stage reimplantation.

Regardless of the method used, the following principles must be observed:

1. Diagnosis must be established by clinical, bacteriologic, histologic, and radiographic evidence and the organism(s) identified.

2. Adequate surgical debridement and prosthetic removal along with all cement are mandatory.

3. Determination of bacterial sensitivity must be made by modern bacteriologic assays, including monitoring of the patient's serum bactericidal levels during the course of intravenous antibiotic therapy.

4. Gram-negative infections, particularly those caused by Pseudomonas are particularly difficult to eradicate, but determination of an organism's "sensitivity" is best made by bacteriologic assay rather than by its generic family.

Wear. The durability of high-density polyethylene has been extraordinary. Charnley calculated an average rate of wear of 0.15 mm per year in his 9- and 10-year follow-up.[59,74] Wear of more than 2.5 mm was seen in 15 percent of these patients.[74] Surprisingly, weight or activity did not correlate with the degree of wear. If one assumes that the socket should be changed once there is 5 mm of wear, the average patient should expect 33 years of service from the acetabular component.

Stem Breakage. Charnley has reported 17 femoral component fractures in 6500 hip operations with longer than 3½ years' follow-up.[75] The overall fracture rate was 0.23 percent, but the rate for heavy males was 6.0 percent.[75] Reports of failed stems in other series[76-78] may be summarized as follows:

1. Improved position of the prosthetic components (i.e., avoidance of varus), better cement technique, and restoration of favorable mechanical lever arms will diminish the risk of this complication.

2. The larger, more vigorous patient is at greater risk for these complications.

3. Loosening almost always precedes femoral component fracture. With loss of the cement buttress, the proximal portion of the prosthesis is not well supported, while the distal end may be well fixed in the femoral canal. This may lead to fatigue fracture of the component.

4. In recent years, femoral component design has evolved toward larger dimensions and stronger metal-

lurgic compositions and fabrications. These improved qualities, along with improved surgical techniques, should diminish the incidence of stem breakage in the future.

Heterotopic Bone Formation. Heterotopic bone may be seen on radiographs in up to 40 percent of patients.[50] Fewer than 2 percent of patients suffer limitation of motion because of this phenomenon.[50] Certain patients, however, are at high risk to develop heterotopic bone, e.g., patients who have developed heterotopic bone about the hip following a previous hip operation or injury or those who had heterotopic bone in the contralateral hip following total hip replacement. Recently, two groups have reported successful inhibition of heterotopic bone formation in high-risk patients using radiation therapy (2000 rads) over a 10-day period postoperatively.[79,80]

Overall Complication Rates of Primary Total Hip Replacement. Three series, including both rheumatoid and osteoarthritic patients, report a complication rate of approximately 7 to 8 percent for technically related problems (dislocation, loosening, fractures, infection) and approximately 20 percent incidence of related medical complications (e.g., cardiopulmonary, urogenital).[1,32,69]

RESULTS OF REVISION TOTAL HIP REPLACEMENT

Revision hip arthroplasty is associated with an increased rate of complications. A recent review of 110 hips (at a mean follow-up of 3 to 4 years post revision) following failed aseptic mechanical loosening found an infection rate of 3.8 percent, failure of trochanteric union in 13 percent, recurrent mechanical failure in 14 percent, and progressive radiolucent zones in 26 percent.[81] Sixty percent of the group were good to excellent at the time of follow-up.

Prolonged operating time, difficult exposure, loss of bone stock, and inadequate cement penetration into sclerotic bone—all militate against the long-term success of revision surgery. Clearly, definitive primary surgery is preferable; therefore, proper patient selection assumes even greater importance.

TOTAL HIP REPLACEMENT IN ANKYLOSING SPONDYLITIS

As candidates for total hip replacement arthroplasty, patients with ankylosing spondylitis differ from rheumatoid arthritics in several important respects. They tend to be younger and more active. Joint involvement is usually limited to the spine and hips, so that the knees, ankles, feet, and upper extremities are spared. Limitation of motion of the lumbar and thoracic spine imposes increased mechanical demands upon the hip joints. These factors suggest that the long-term results of total hip arthroplasty in this group may show an increased rate of mechanical loosening with time.

The presenting complaints in these patients more often include stiffness, poor posture, and limitation of motion rather than pain. Because the primary goal of total hip replacement in this group is often the improvement of a functional range of motion, rather than pain relief, published results are of interest. Resnick and colleagues[82] reviewed the results of 21 total hip arthroplasties in 11 patients with definite ankylosing spondylitis. Fifty-six percent had reankylosis by radiographic criteria, and 30 percent had reankylosis by clinical criteria. Wilde and associates[83] reported reankylosis in a patient who underwent total hip arthroplasty as a revision of ankylosed cup arthroplasties. Bisla and colleagues[84] found an average of 150-degree gain in total hip motion in patients with preoperative fibrous ankylosis; and a 96-degree gain in total hip motion in patients with preoperative bony ankylosis. It is of interest that while extensive myositis ossificans occurred in 9 of 34 hips overall, it was seen in 6 of 7 patients who had bony ankylosis preoperatively. In contrast to these reports, a number of authors[85-87] report no ankylosis following total hip arthroplasty in this group of patients. Review of the cumulative results of these three series finds no reankylosis in 67 total hip arthroplasties followed for as long as 83 months postoperatively. A number of conclusions may be drawn from this review. (1) Patients with a painful arc of motion can expect pain relief and generally no decreased range of motion following total hip arthroplasty.[84] (2) Hip arthroplasty in this generally young, active group of patients may be at increased risk of early mechanical failure. (3) Previous hip surgery, and bony ankylosis preoperatively, may predispose the patient to extensive postoperative myositis ossificans. These high-risk groups might be considered candidates for procedures designed to decrease the chances of heterotopic bone formation.[79,80]

CURRENT SURGICAL ALTERNATIVES TO CONVENTIONAL TOTAL HIP REPLACEMENT

Total Surface Replacement Arthroplasty. Surface replacement differs from conventional total hip replacement by conserving the femoral head and neck and capping the head with a prosthetic cup, usually made of metal (Fig. 120–5). Because the femoral head is retained, the acetabulum must be enlarged to accept a plastic cup that is larger and thinner than the components used in total hip replacement.

The following two factors contributed to the early appeal of surface replacement:

1. A basic principle of orthopedic surgery dictates the necessity of preserving bone stock when possible. Retaining the proximal femoral bone stock in surface replacement theoretically results in a more physiologic dissemination of transmitted forces via the normal trabecular architecture. In conventional total hip replacement, replacement of bone by a prosthetic stem and cement results in abnormal stress concentrations directed primarily at the distal portion of the stem.

Figure 120–5. *A* and *B*, Model and postoperative roentgenogram of surface replacement arthroplasty components. *C*, Conventional total hip components shown for comparison. Note that the larger acetabular component necessitated by surface replacement arthroplasty will require increased reaming of acetabular bone.

2. With the realization that loosening of components is the most prevalent long-term complication of conventional total hip replacement, surface replacement offers a theoretical means for obviating the problems of loosening on the femoral side. Therefore, in younger patients requiring hip arthroplasty, for example, juvenile rheumatoid arthritics, the theoretical advantage of retaining the femoral head and neck is inviting.

Ironically, Charnley designed and implanted the first surface replacement prior to 1961.[25] The components were made of Teflon, and initial results at 3 months were encouraging. However, the operations failed because of recurrence of pain as a result of ischemic necrosis of the femoral head under the Teflon cup. Charnley felt that in this instance the preservation of bone stock resulted in technical failure. He went on to design the total hip replacement system as we now know it. Modern surface arthroplasty was introduced independently by Trentani in Italy and by Furuya in Japan in

1971. There are approximately ten designs now being used worldwide. The early results for many of these designs have recently been reported.[88,89]

Surface replacement is a technically demanding procedure and requires expertise to avoid certain pitfalls, most notably, fracture of the femoral neck and ischemic necrosis of the femoral head. Preparation of the bony stock follows the principles advocated by Smith-Peterson and Aufranc in performing cup arthroplasty. Advocates of the procedure state that early results are similar to those obtained with conventional total hip replacement.[90] Because bony stock is preserved, revision to conventional total hip replacement, should surface replacement fail, is possible.

The following disadvantages of surface replacement must be considered:

1. Any previous operation renders conventional total hip replacement technically more difficult and increases the incidence of complications. Therefore, the use of

surface replacement as an interim procedure delaying the need for eventual conventional total hip replacement may carry with it an increased incidence of complications that primary total hip replacement would avoid. Recent improvements in cement technique and advanced prosthetic design should result in a decreased incidence of loosening in conventional total hip replacement.

2. It is now generally agreed that retention of subchondral acetabular bone provides more physiologic stress transmission and reduces the likelihood of component loosening in conventional total hip arthroplasty. Because of the size of components used in surface replacement arthroplasty, increased resection of the acetabulum is more likely. Most surgeons would agree that the problem of salvaging lost stock in the acetabular side is more formidable than dealing with loss of stock in the femoral side. Since long-term results of conventional total hip arthroplasty suggest that acetabular loosening increases with time, the theoretical advantages of a procedure that requires increased sacrifice of acetabular bone stock must be carefully considered.

3. The incidence of loosening of the thin acetabular component has not been established. In their short-term follow-up of the first 100 patients undergoing surface replacement arthroplasty followed for 4 to 32 months, Amstutz and colleagues reported that on roentgenographic examination, 88 of 135 hips demonstrated radiolucent zones at the acetabular cement–bone interface.[90]

4. The fate of the femoral head under the cup is unknown. Only long-term follow-up can establish whether ischemic necrosis will lead to the ultimate failure of this type of procedure, or whether with reaming and better load distribution afforded by cementing the cup to the head, the proximal femur will remain viable. In Wagner's series,[91] loosening of components was seen only in patients with "inflammatory arthritis." He considered rheumatoid arthritis to be a relative contraindication to surface replacement.

Osteotomy. Since McMurray[92] and Malkin[93] presented favorable results of treatment of osteoarthritis by osteotomy in 1935 and 1936, the procedure has gained acceptance, especially in Europe. Particular interest in medial displacement intertrochanteric osteotomy as a treatment for early symptomatic osteoarthritis was generated in this country by the report of Harris and Kirwan in 1964.[94] The procedure achieved some popularity in the United States in the late 1960s because it was technically straightforward and offered good symptomatic relief in selected patients.[95] At that time, however, the era of total hip replacement had just begun in the United States, and further use and development of this technique were generally abandoned.

In contrast, the development of osteotomy as a treatment for all stages of osteoarthritis continued in Europe. Pauwels[21] viewed the osteoarthritic process as one of mechanical overload. Therefore, angulation osteotomy combined with muscle releases could diminish the excessive unit load and arrest, if not reverse, the pathogenesis of the disease. Results of angulation osteotomy

from many European centers demonstrate that in appropriately selected patients, more than 80 percent achieve good to excellent *long-term* results.[96-99]

Today, osteotomy is performed in Europe as a primary treatment for osteoarthritis in appropriate patients, whereas in the United States the symptomatic osteoarthritic hip is generally treated by some form of replacement arthroplasty. While osteotomy is feasible for patients with osteoarthritis, it has no role in the treatment of rheumatoid arthritis, in which joint destruction is uniform and thus precludes realignment of cartilage-bearing surfaces.

CURRENT STATE OF SURGERY OF THE HIP FOR ARTHRITIS

Total hip replacement has revolutionized the treatment of advanced arthritis of the hip joint. Long-term results indicate that loosening of components is the complication most frequently associated with failure. In the past few years, improved cement technique and prosthetic design have resulted in technically improved total hip replacement surgery. Ideally this improved technique will be reflected in an even lower incidence of long-term component loosening.

Long-term results of total hip replacement in rheumatoid arthritic patients demonstrate that even in this group of "low demand" patients adherence to modern technical principles is mandatory. Disease progression, osteopenia, and protrusio militate against a good result unless proper surgical technique is used.

Total surface replacement offers a theoretically attractive alternative to conventional total hip replacement. However, good results are short-term and seem to deteriorate with time.[89] The place of total hip surface replacement will be clarified with continued clinical experience.

Osteotomy for osteoarthritis is advocated by the European school. By altering the forces across the hip, it may achieve biologic improvement and preclude prosthetic replacement. For the younger, active patient with osteoarthritis, osteotomy performed by an experienced surgeon would seem the most conservative and biologically sound procedure. For the older patient with osteoarthritis or for the patient with rheumatoid arthritis, conventional total hip replacement has stood the test of time for a period now approaching 15 to 20 years.

References

1. Coventry, M.D., Beckenbaugh, R.D., Nolan, D.R., and Ilstrup, D.M.: 2012 total hip arthroplasties: A study of postoperative course and early complications. J. Bone Joint Surg. 56A:273, 1974.

2. Welch, R.B., and Charnley, J.: Low friction arthroplasty of the hip in rheumatoid arthritis and ankylosing spondylitis. Clin. Orthop. 72:22, 1970.

3. Harris, W.H.: Traumatic arthritis of the hip after dislocation and acetabular fractures: Treatment by mold arthroplasty. J. Bone Joint Surg. 51A:737, 1969.

4. D'Aubigne, R.M., and Postel, M.: Functional results of hip arthroplasty with acrylic prosthesis. J. Bone Joint Surg. 36A:451, 1954.

5. Hoppenfeld, S.: Physical Examination of the Spine and Extremities. New York, Appleton-Century-Crofts, 1976.

6. Blount, W.P.: Don't throw away the cane. J. Bone Joint Surg. 38A:695, 1956.
7. Jergesen, H.E., Poss, R., and Sledge, C.B.: Bilateral total hip and knee replacement in adults with rheumatoid arthritis: An evaluation of function. Clin. Orthop. 137:118, 1978.
8. Hardaker, W.T., Ogden, W.S., Musgrave, M.D., and Goldner, J.D.: Simultaneous and staged bilateral total knee arthroplasty. J. Bone Joint Surg. 60A:247, 1978.
9. Head, W.D., and Paradies, L.H.: Ipsilateral hip and knee replacements as a single surgical procedure. J. Bone Surg. 59A:352, 1977.
10. Salvati, E.A., Hughes, P., and Lachiewicz, P.: Bilateral total hip replacement arthroplasty in one stage. J. Bone Joint Surg. 60A:640, 1978.
11. Nakano, K.K.: Neurologic complications of rheumatoid arthritis. Orthop. Clin. North Am. 6:861, 1975.
12. Harris, W.H.: The role of cup arthroplasty in contemporary reconstructive surgery of the hip: A reappraisal in surgical management of degenerative arthritis of the lower limb. In Cruess, R.L., and Mitchell, N. (eds.): Philadelphia, Lea & Febiger, 1975, p. 79.
13. Aufranc, O.E.: Constructive hip surgery with the vitallium mold (a report on 1,000 cases of arthroplasty of the hip over a 15 year period). J. Bone Joint Surg. 39A:237, 1957.
14. Bryan, R.S., Scott, W.T., and Bickel, W.H.: Results of surgical management of the hip in patients with rheumatoid arthritis or rheumatoid spondylitis. In Cruess, R.L., and Mitchell, N.W. (eds.): Surgery of Rheumatoid Arthritis. Philadelphia, J.B. Lippincott Company, 1971, p. 63.
15. Salvati, E.A., and Wilson, P.D., Jr.: Long-term results of femoral head replacements. J. Bone Joint Surg. 55A:516, 1973.
16. Barr, J.S., Donovan, J.F., and Florence, D.W.: Arthroplasty of the hip. J. Bone Joint Surg. 46A:249, 1964.
17. Lipscomb, P.R.: Surgery for rheumatoid arthritis—timing and techniques: Summary. J. Bone Joint Surg. 50A:614, 1968.
18. Cruess, R.L.: Synovectomy of the hip in rheumatoid arthritis. In Cruess, R.L., and Mitchell, N.S. (eds.): Surgery of Rheumatoid Arthritis. Philadelphia, J.B. Lippincott Company, 1971, p. 59.
19. Freeman, P.A., and Sturrock, R.D.: Surgery of the weight bearing joints in rheumatoid arthritis. In Buchanan, W.W., and Dick, W.C. (eds.): Recent Advances in Rheumatology. Edinburgh, Churchill Livingstone, 1976, p. 138.
20. Inman, V.T.: Functional aspects of the abductor muscles of the hip. J. Bone Joint Surg. 29:607, 1947.
21. Pauwels, F.: Biomechanics of the Normal and Diseased Hip. Berlin, Springer-Verlag, 1976.
22. Rydell, N.: Intra-vital measurements of forces acting on the hip joint. In Evans, F.G. (ed.): Studies on the Anatomy and Function of Bone and Joints. New York, Springer-Verlag, 1966, p. 52.
23. Greenwald, A.S., and Nelson, C.L.: Biomechanics of the reconstructed hip. Orthop. Clin. North Am. 4:435, 1973.
24. Charnley, J.: Anchorage of the femoral head prosthesis to the shaft of the femur. J. Bone Joint Surg. 42B:28, 1960.
25. Charnley, J.: Arthroplasty of the hip: A new operation. Lancet 1:1129, 1961.
26. McKee, G.K., and Watson-Farrar, J.: Replacement of arthritic hips by the McKee-Farrar prosthesis. J. Bone Joint Surg. 48B:245, 1966.
27. Ring, P.A.: Complete replacement arthroplasty of the hip by the ring prosthesis. J. Bone Joint Surg. 50B:720, 1968.
28. Muller, M.D.: Total hip prosthesis. Clin. Orthop. 72:46, 1970.
29. Hori, R.Y., Lewis, J.L., Zimmerman, J.R., and Compere, C.L.: The number of total joint replacements in the United States. Clin. Orthop. 132:46, 1978.
30. Harris, W.H.: Total joint replacement N. Engl. J. Med. 297:650, 1977.
31. Poss, R.: Total hip replacement. Orthop. Clin. North Am. 6:801, 1975.
32. Charnley, J.: Low friction arthroplasty. Clin. Orthop. 72:7, 1970.
33. Lazansky, M.G.: Trochanteric osteotomy in total hip replacement. In Harris, W.H. (ed.): The Hip: Proceedings of the Second Open Scientific Meeting of the Hip Society, 1974. St. Louis, C.V. Mosby Company, 1974, p. 237.
34. Thompson, R.C., and Culver, J.E.: The role of trochanteric osteotomy in total hip replacement. Clin. Orthop. 106:102, 1975.
35. Muller, M.E.: Total hip replacement without trochanteric osteotomy. In Harris, W.H. (ed.): The Hip: Proceedings of the Second Scientific Meeting of the Hip Society, 1974. St. Louis, C.V. Mosby Company, 1974, p. 231.
36. Parker, H.G., Wiesman, H.J., Ewald, F.C., Thomas, W.H., and Sledge, C.B.: Comparison of pre-operative, intraoperative and early post-operative total hip replacements with and without trochanteric osteotomy. Clin. Orthop. 121:44, 1976.
37. Wiesman, H.J., Simon, S.R., Ewald, F.C., Thomas, W.H., and Sledge, C.B.: Total hip replacement with and without osteotomy of the greater trochanter. Clinical and biomechanical comparisons in the same patient. J. Bone Joint Surg. 60A:203, 1978.
38. Harris, W.H., Salzman, E.W., Athanasoulis, C., Waltman, A.C., Baum, S., and DeSanctis, R.W.: Comparison of warfarin, low-molecular-weight dextran, aspirin, and subcutaneous heparin in prevention of venous thromboembolism following total hip replacement. J. Bone Joint Surg. 56A:1552, 1974.
39. Debrunner, H.U., and Izadpanah, M.: The effect of total prosthesis operation on pain. In Gschwend, N., and Debrunner, H.U. (eds.): Total Hip Prosthesis. Baltimore, Williams & Wilkins Company, 1976, p. 27.
40. Gartenmann, W.P., and Gschwend, N.: The influence of the hip arthroplasty on the profession of the patient, on his rehabilitation time and on his sex life. In Gschwend, N., and Debrunner, H.U. (eds.): Total Hip Prosthesis. Baltimore, Williams and Wilkins Company, 1976.
41. Welch, R.N., and Charnley, J.: Low friction arthroplasty of the hip in rheumatoid arthritis and ankylosing spondylitis. Clin. Orthop. 72:22, 1970.
42. Poss, R., Ewald, F.C., Thomas, W.H., and Sledge, C.B.: Complications of total hip replacement arthoplasty in patients with rheumatoid arthritis. J. Bone Joint Surg. 58A:1130, 1976.
43. Stauffer, R.N.: Ten year follow-up study of total hip replacement. J. Bone Joint Surg. 64A:983, 1982.
44. Sutherland, C.J., Wilde, A.H., Borden, L.S., and Marks, K.E.: A ten-year follow-up of one hundred consecutive Muller curved-stem total hip replacement arthroplasties. J. Bone Joint Surg. 64A:970, 1982.
45. Salvati, E.A., Wilson, P.D., Jr., Jolley, M.N., Vakili, F., Aglietti, P., and Brown, G.D.: A ten-year follow-up study of our first one hundred consecutive Charnley total hip replacements. J. Bone Joint Surg. 63A:753, 1981.
46. Pellicci, P., Salvati, E.A., and Robinson, H.J.: Mechanical failures in total hip replacement requiring reoperation. J. Bone Joint Surg. 61A:28, 1979.
47. Charnley, J.: Low Friction Arthroplasty of the Hip. Theory and Practice. Berlin, Springer-Verlag, 1979.
48. Moreland, J.F., Gruen, T.A., Mai, L., and Amstutz, H.C.: Aseptic loosening of total hip replacement: Incidence and significance. In The Hip: Proceedings of the Eighth Open Scientific Meeting of the Hip Society, 1980. St. Louis, C.V. Mosby, 1980.
49. Muller, M.E.: Results 12 years and over. Orthop. Trans. 5:349, 1981.
50. N.I.H. Consensus Conference on Total Hip Replacement in the United States. JAMA 248:1817, 1982.
51. Chandler, H.P., Reineck, F.T., Wixson, R.L., and McCarthy, J.C.: Total hip replacement in patients younger than thirty years old. J. Bone Joint Surg. 63A:1426, 1981.
52. Poss, R., Maloney, J.P., Ewald, F.C., Thomas, W.H., Batte, N.J., and Sledge, C.B.: Six- to eleven-year results of total hip replacement in rheumatoid arthritis. Clin. Orthop. 182:109, 1984.
53. Salvati, E.A., Bullough, P., and Wilson, P.D., Jr.: Intrapelvic protrusion of the acetabular component following total hip replacement. Clin. Orthop. 111:212, 1975.
54. Eichler, J.: Ein Vorschlag zur operativen Behandlung der protrusio Acetabuli. Arch. Orthop. Unfallchir. 75:76, 1973.
55. McCollum, D.E., Nunley, J.A., and Harrelson, J.M.: Bone grafting in total hip replacement for acetabular protrusion. J. Bone Joint Surg. 62A:1065, 1980.
56. Oh, I., and Harris, W.H.: Protrusio acetabuli and total hip replacement: Bone grafting and use of protrusio shell. Orthop. Trans. 3:275, 1979.
57. Ranawat, C.S., Dorr, L.D., and Inglis, A.E.: Total hip arthroplasty in protrusio acetabuli of rheumatoid arthritis. J. Bone Joint Surg. 62A:1059, 1980.
58. Salvati, E.A., Bullough, P., and Wilson, P.D., Jr.: Intrapelvic protrusion of the acetabular component following total hip replacement. Clin. Orthop. 111:212, 1975.
59. Charnley, J., and Cupic, F.: The nine and ten year results of the low friction arthroplasty of the hip. Clin. Orthop. 95:9, 1973.
60. Charnley, J.: Post-operative infection after total hip replacement with special reference to air contamination in the operating room. Clin. Orthop. 87:167, 1972.
61. Collis, D.K., and Steinhaus, K.: Total hip replacement without deep infection in a standard operating room. J. Bone Joint Surg. 58A:446, 1976.
62. Mallory, T.H., Meyer, T.L., and Bombach, J.D.: Six hundred ninety total hip replacements: A comparative study. Ohio State Med. J. 74:23, 1978.
63. Arden, G.P., Taylor, A.R., and Ansell, B.M.: Total hip replacement using McKee-Farrar prostheses in rheumatoid arthritis, Still's disease, and ankylosing spondylitis. Ann. Rheum. Dis. 29:1, 1970.
64. Freeman, P.A., Lee, P., and Bryson, T.W.: Total hip replacement in osteoarthrosis and polyarthritis: A statistical study of the result. Clin. Orthop. 95:224, 1973.
65. Harris, J., Lighttowler, C.D.R., and Todd, R.C.: Total hip replacement in inflammatory disease using the Charnley prosthesis. Br. Med. J. 2:750, 1972.
66. Todd, R.C., Lightowler, C.D.R., and Harris, J.: Total hip replacement in osteoarthrosis using the Charnley prosthesis. Br. Med. J. 2:752, 1972.
67. Charnley, J.: The long-term results of low friction arthroplasty of the hip performed as a primary intervention. J. Bone Joint Surg. 54B:61, 1972.
68. Dupont, J.A., and Charnley, J.: Low friction arthroplasty of the hip for the failures of previous operations. J. Bone Joint Surg. 54B:77, 1972.

69. Murray, W.R.: Results in patients with total hip replacement arthroplasty. Clin. Orthop. 95:80, 1973.
70. Hunter, G., and Dandy, D.: The natural history of the patient with an infected total hip replacement. J. Bone Joint Surg. 59B:293, 1977.
71. Wilson, P.D., Jr., Aglietti, P., and Salvati, E.A.: Subacute sepsis of the hip treated by antibiotics and cemented prosthesis. J. Bone Joint Surg. 56A:879, 1974.
72. Ganz, R., and Meyer, P.: Late infection after total hip replacement. *In* Gschwend, N., and Debrunner, H.U. (eds.): Total hip prosthesis. Baltimore, Williams & Wilkins Company, 1976, p. 97.
73. Salvati, E.A., Chekofsky, K.M., Brause, B.D., and Wilson, P.D., Jr.: Reimplantation in infection: A 12-year experience. Clin. Orthop. 170:62, 1982.
74. Charnley, J., and Halley, D.K.: Rate of wear in total hip replacement. Clin. Orthop. 112:17D, 1975.
75. Charnley, J.: Fracture of femoral prostheses in total hip replacement. Clin. Orthop. 111:105, 1975.
76. Collis, D.K.: Femoral stem failure in total hip replacement. J. Bone Joint Surg. 59A:1033, 1977.
77. Galante, J.O., Rostoker, W., and Doyle, J.M.: Failed femoral stems in total hip prosthesis. J. Bone Joint Surg. 57A:230, 1975.
78. Carlsson, A.S., Gentz, C.F., and Stenport, J.: Fracture of the femoral prosthesis in total hip replacement according to Charnley. Acta Orthop. Scand. 48:650, 1977.
79. Coventry, M.: Heterotopic bone in total hip arthroplasty. Orthop. Trans. 5:362, 1981.
80. Parkinson, J.R., Evarts, C.M., and Hubbard, L.F.: Radiation therapy in the prevention of heterotopic ossification after total hip arthroplasty. Orthop. Trans. 61:441, 1982.
81. Pellicci, P.M., Wilson, P.D., Jr., Sledge, C.B., Salvati, E.A., Ranawat, C.S., and Poss, R.: Revision total hip arthroplasty. Clin. Orthop. 170:34, 1982.
82. Resnick, D., Dwosh, I.L., Goergen, T.G., et al.: Clinical and radiographic "reankylosis" following hip surgery in ankylosing spondylitis. Am. J. Roentgenol. 126:1181, 1976.
83. Wilde, A.H., Collins, H.R., and Mackenzie, A.H.: Reankylosis of the hip joint in ankylosing spondylitis after total hip replacement. Arthritis Rheum. 15:493, 1972.
84. Bisla, R.S., Ranawat, C.S., and Inglis, E.A.: Total hip replacement in patients with ankylosing spondylitis with involvement of the hip. J. Bone Joint Surg. 58A:233, 1976.
85. Baldursson, H., Brattstrom, H., and Olsson, T.H.: Total hip replacement in ankylosing spondylitis. Acta Orthop. Scand. 48:499, 1977.
86. Welch, R.B., and Charnley, J.: Low function arthroplasty of the hip in rheumatoid arthritis and ankylosing spondylitis. Clin. Orthop. 72:22, 1970.
87. Shannon, W.R., Jr., Kaprove, R.E., Major, P.A., Hunter, T., and Baragar, F.D.: Assessment of long-term benefit of total hip replacement in patients with ankylosing spondylitis. J. Rheumatol. 9:101, 1982.
88. Freeman, M.A.R. (ed.): Total surface replacement hip arthroplasty. Clin. Orthop. 134:2, 1978.
89. Steinberg, M.E. (ed.): Surface replacement arthroplasty of the hip. Orthop. Clin. North Am. 13:661, 1982.
90. Amstutz, H.C., Graff-Radford, A., Gruen, T.A., and Clarke, I.C.: Tharies surface replacements: A review of the first 100 cases. Clin. Orthop. 134:87, 1978.
91. Wagner, H.: Surface replacement arthroplasty of the hip. Clin. Orthop. 134:102, 1978.
92. McMurray, T.P.: Osteoarthritis of the hip. Br. J. Surg. 22:716, 1935.
93. Malkin, S.A.S.: Femoral osteotomy in treatment of osteoarthritis of the hip. Br. Med. J. 1:304, 1936.
94. Harris, N.H., and Kirwan, E.: The results of osteotomy for early primary osteoarthritis of the hip. J. Bone Joint Surg. 46B:477, 1964.
95. Harris, W.H.: Role of intertrochanteric osteotomy in the treatment of arthritis of the hip. Orthop. Clin. North Am. 49:775, 1969.
96. Bombelli, R.: Osteoarthritis of the Hip. 2nd ed. Berlin, Springer-Verlag, 1982.
97. Langlais, F., Roure, J.L., and Maquet, P.: Valgus osteotomy in severe osteoarthritis of the hip. J. Bone Joint Surg. 61B:424, 1979.
98. Morscher, E.W.: Intertrochanteric osteotomy in osteoarthritis of the hip. *In* The Hip. Proceedings of the Eighth Open Scientific Meeting of the Hip Society, 1980. St. Louis, C.V. Mosby Company, 1980.
99. Muller, M.E.: Intertrochanteric osteotomies in adults: Planning and operating technique. *In* Cruess, R.L., and Mitchell, N.S. (eds.): Surgical management of degenerative arthritis in the lower limb. Philadelphia, Lea and Febiger, 1975.

Chapter 121

Surgery for Arthritis of the Cervical Spine

J. William Fielding and A.G. Björkengren

INTRODUCTION

The neck, and particularly the atlantoaxial joint, is a common target for rheumatoid arthritis and is the most frequent area of spinal involvement. Berens gives Walton credit for first describing cervical vertebral subluxations in America in 1889.[1]

Various studies attest to its frequency. It was mentioned as early as 1890 by Garrod, reporting neck involvement in 178 of 500 cases.[2] His observations, as well as those of Walton, are thought provoking, since they were made well before the introduction of radiology by Roentgen in 1896.

In a retrospective study of 845 patients with rheumatoid arthritis, Conlon, Isdale, and Rose found 60 percent had neck involvement varying from mild to severe.[3] Bland and associates in 1963 noted that 86 percent of 100 patients with definite or classic rheumatoid arthritis had radiologic signs of cervical spine involvement.[4]

Atlantoaxial Involvement. The most common cause of atlantoaxial subluxation is rheumatoid arthritis; it is perhaps the most helpful and easily identifiable radiologic sign of this disease in the neck. Mathews,[5] as well as Meikle and Wilkinson,[6] have noted it early in the disease process (Fig. 121–1).

Even though Bell[7] first described C1-2 displacement in 1830, it was not until 1951 that Davis and Markley[8] first reported that rheumatoid arthritis could produce atlantoaxial subluxation and death from medullary compression. Various observers have attempted to elucidate its frequency in rheumatoid arthritis, most using 3 mm. as the upper limit of normal motion between the odontoid and ring of C1.

Isdale and Conlon, in a prospective study of 333 consecutive hospital admissions, showed atlantoaxial sub-

Figure 121–1. Rheumatoid arthritis with forward displacement of the atlas. The odontoid process is in the center of the C1 ring. (Figures 121–1, 121–2, 121–5, 121–6, and 121–7 through 121–13, from Fielding, J. William: Rheumatoid athritis of the cervical spine. *In* The American Academy of Orthopaedic Surgeons: Instructional course lectures. Vol. XXXII. St. Louis, The C.V. Mosby Co., 1983.)

luxation in 25 percent, in one fourth of these, it was greater than 5 mm. Six years later, 171 of the 333 cases were available for further study, and these showed a marked increase in the rheumatoid features, but surprisingly there was no instance of serious neurologic complication. Fifty-nine of the original 333 died, 17 of whom had atlantoaxial subluxation, but in no case was death known to be due to this anomaly. The authors concluded that in the absence of neurologic vascular complications, surgery seemed unnecessary.[9]

In 1969, Mathews,[5] using 3 mm or more as abnormal, found atlantoaxial subluxation in 25 percent of 76 consecutive out-patients. In 1961, Martel,[10] using lateral tomograms in flexion, found subluxation in 24 of 34 patients with neck discomfort or severe progressive·disease. The same author examined 100 unselected clinic cases and found 34 instances of atlantoaxial subluxation.

In 1961, Sharp and Purser noted that atlantoaxial subluxation varied with the severity of the disease, being approximately 1 in 30 in those with minimal evidence of rheumatoid arthritis, 1 in 15 in those with clinical evidence, and 1 in 5 in those with disease sufficiently severe to require hospitalization.[11]

Conlon and associates in 1966 reported a correlation between vertebral luxations and widespread peripheral destructive lesions but indicated no correlation with the use of oral corticosteroids or disease duration.[3] In 1969 Mathews[5] and Meikle and Wilkinson,[6] however, found that subluxation was related to disease duration and corticosteroid therapy.

Pathology. Unlike osteoarthritis, rheumatoid arthritis of the neck is a demineralizing, destructive process. Osteopenia results in decreased bony density, often causing difficult radiologic assessment. Unlike degenerative spondylosis, it mainly affects the upper cervical segments, and in the typical case there is little osteophyte formation and sclerosis at the vertebral endplates. In degenerative spondylosis, the cervical spine becomes stif-

fer, while in rheumatoid arthritis it subluxates at multiple levels and may become unstable.

No bony interlocking occurs at occiput, C1 and C2; joint strength is dependent upon ligaments. These articulations are surrounded by synovial tissue, rendering them prone to the synovial inflammatory process.

The synovial joints between the transverse ligament and odontoid posteriorly and the anterior arch of C1 anteriorly are close to the synovial joints between the lateral masses of the occiput and C1, and C1 and C2. Therefore, the upper cervical spine, the C1-2 articulation in particular, is very vulnerable.

The cervicomedullary portion of the spinal cord lies at the C1-2 level, where the potential for displacement is greatest. The vertebral arteries course through the foramen transversarium of C1 and C2 and can be compromised by abnormal atlantoaxial displacement. About 50 percent of cervical rotation takes place at C1-2, the canal of C1 rotating on the eccentric odontoid, causing physiologic narrowing. To allow for this, the canal of the axis is large, approximately 3 cm in diameter, occupied equally by cord, odontoid, and free space—1 cm each.[12,13] Hence, some pathologic forward displacement of C1 is possible without cord compromise as the cord moves into the free space.

Suboccipital Involvement. In the suboccipital area, some bony interlocking occurs at the facet joints, reducing the degree of displacement. Since the occiput-C1-C2 complex is a series of synovial joints, destruction of the occipital condyles, lateral masses of C1, and the upper facets of C2 can cause the skull to settle downward, with resultant upward translocation of the dens. This was described by Davis and Markley in 1951 in a patient who died from medullary compression.[8] Others have also recorded it as a cause of death[14-16] (Figs. 121–2 and 121–3).

In 1973, Rana and associates presented 8 cases of upward translocation of the dens without platybasia.[17]

Figure 121–2. *A,* The atlas "settled" on the axis. The anterior arch of C1 is opposite the upper portion of the body of C2, and the odontoid process is abnormally high, occupying space in the foramen magnum. The posterior arch of C1 is markedly thin, and there is over 50 percent anterior displacement of C4 on C5. *B,* Advanced destruction of the atlantoaxial articulation and odontoid process with lateral displacement of the atlas on the axis. *C,* Advanced destruction of the atlantoaxial articulation with upward displacement of the odontoid. (Courtesy of Harvey L. Barish, M.D.)

Figure 121–3. Stages in destruction of the atlantoaxial articulation with resultant settling of the skull and upward displacement of the odontoid process into the foramen magnum. Fischgold and Metzger's line (a line drawn between the two digastric grooves on the antero-posterior laminogram of the skull) will pass well above the odontoid tip (10.7 mm). It can be used to determine the degree of upper displacement of the odontoid process. (From Fischgold, H., and Metzger, J.: Etude radiotomographique de l'impression basilaire. Rev. Rhum. Mal. Osteoartic. 19:261, 1952.)

Normally, the tip of the odontoid process should be no more than 4.5 mm above McGregor's line (a line from the upper surface of the posterior edge of the hard palate to the most caudal point of the occipital curve)[18] (Fig. 121–4). All of Rana's 8 cases had the tip of the odontoid process 10 mm or more above this line. Two of the 8 required surgery for acute neurologic problems from the forward C1 shift in association with upper displacement of the odontoid, which competes with the cord for space in the foramen magnum.

Involvement of the odontoid process may lead to bony erosion and notching of the posterior aspect of the odontoid at the area of contact with the transverse ligament. The odontoid may be reduced to a narrow peg with little or no strength to anchor ligaments and protect the atlantoaxial joint (Figs. 121–5 and 121–6). This is compounded by the pathologic laxity of the transverse, alar, and capsular ligaments, with decalcification and weakening at the fibro-osseous junction.

The disease process is compounded by osteopenia, which may be further compounded by the use of steroids and by inactivity, often leaving the vertebra the same density as the soft tissues, increasing the problems of

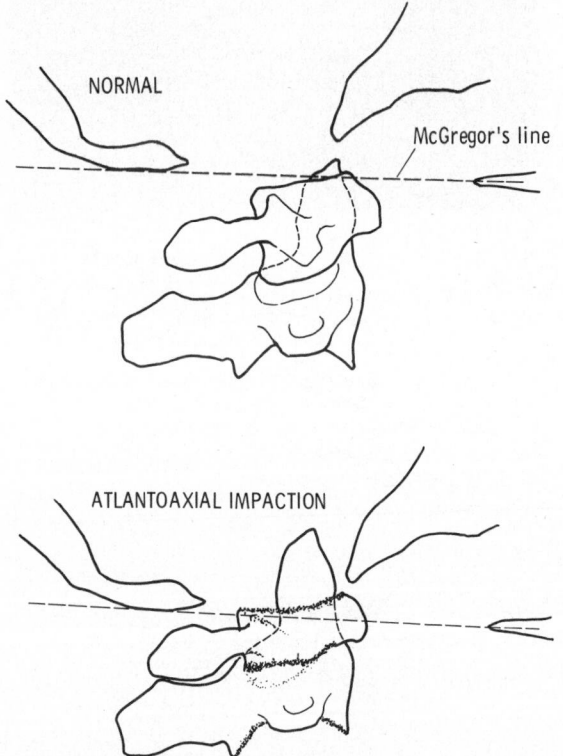

Figure 121–4. Schematic representation of the normal relationship of the odontoid to the base of the skull and upward displacement of the odontoid incident to destruction of the atlantoaxial articulation. McGregor's line can be used for routine screening. Normally, the tip of the odontoid process should be no more than 4.5 mm above McGregor's line, which is drawn from the upper surface of the posterior edge of the hard palate to the most caudal portion of the occipital curve of the skull. (From McGregor, M.: The significance of certain measurements of the skull in the diagnosis of basilar impression. Br. J. Radiol. 23:171, 1948.)

roentgen diagnosis. The posterior arch of C1 may be sclerotic or markedly thinned and unable to support an atlanto-axial fusion (Fig. 121–2).

Subaxial Involvement. In the subaxial area, the apophyseal joints are narrowed and eroded. The spinous processes tend to become sharp rather than "squareended." The synovial process may involve the joints of Luschka between the bodies of adjacent vertebrae. The intervertebral disc is involved by the same synovial process, and the disc space narrows without associated vertebral endplate sclerosis. One vertebra tends to "jigsaw" into its neighbor (Fig. 121–7). Later, multiple luxations at one, two, or more levels, sometimes in "stepladder fashion," result from bony destruction and loss of ligament stability. Characteristically, these are rarely more than 3.5 mm and are more frequent in the upper regions of the spine (Fig. 121–8).

Meikle and Wilkinson, in a study of 118 rheumatoid patients, found subaxial dislocation of greater than 1 mm in 26.3 percent, endplate erosions in 15.3 percent of patients, and narrowed discs in 72.9 percent.[6]

Park notes that 50 percent of loss of total height of the cervical spine is possible in patients with advanced rheumatoid arthritis.[19]

Neurologic Complications. Compromise of the medullary cord by bony pressure from atlantoaxial subluxation may be compounded by pressure from the mass of inflammatory tissue in the synovial joint between the transverse ligament and the odontoid projecting backward against the cord.[20-24]

Involvement of the vertebral arteries may also cause neurologic signs. Crellin and associates[20] reported two such cases. In one, the right vertebral artery was smaller than the left and was kinked at the level of the foramen transversarium of C4 and the axis.

An inflammatory arachnoiditis has been described in rheumatoid arthritis.[22] Dural fibrosis compressing the cord has been noted, as well as vertebral artery thrombosis at the atlantoaxial level with compromise of the cervicomedullary blood supply.

Clinical Signs. The spinal cord tolerates gradual pressure better than acute compression. A narrowed cord may continue to function, and the patient may be unaware of neurologic symptoms because of their gradual onset. Such a cord may be even more susceptible to trauma and may cease to function following a trivial injury (Fig. 121–9). Surprisingly, it is not always possible to correlate the degree of C1 displacement with either the presence or the severity of neurologic findings, and this suggests that factors other than the subluxation may cause neurologic difficulties and that the onset of these problems may be difficult to predict.[5,24]

Weissman and associates studied 194 patients with rheumatoid arthritis and atlantoaxial subluxation and settling of the skull and C1 on to C2. They noted that 24 percent of patients with 9 mm or more atlantoaxial subluxation developed spinal cord compression compared with only 2 percent with lesser amounts. Those patients with additional settling of the skull and C1 on to C2 had approximately a 20 percent chance of devel-

Figure 121–5. *A*, Advanced destruction of the odontoid and lateral masses of C1. Only the base of the odontoid is visible. The anterior arch of C1 is opposite the body of C2, and there is destruction of the posterior arch of C1. There is no visible bony continuity between the base of the skull and the first and second cervical vertebrae. *B*, Advanced destruction of odontoid and lateral C1 masses of the anterior arch of C1 opposite the body of the second cervical vertebra. *C*, Advanced erosion of the odontoid process. *D*, Complete destruction of the odontoid.

oping spinal cord compression compared with 7.3 percent without. Neurologic sequelae were more prevalent in men (24 percent) than women (7.5 percent).[25]

In contrast to the usual gradual onset of symptoms, minor trauma to an already weakened and unstable atlantoaxial articulation may produce sudden and alarming symptoms (Fig. 121–9).

Atlantoaxial displacement may vary from extreme mobility to relative fixation. In the latter instance, the gradual glacier-like slip of the atlas on the axis may be overlooked, leading to the erroneous conclusion that the displacement is "fixed," whereas it actually increases year by year. If there is spinal cord compromise, increased displacement may lead to weakness that may be mistakenly attributed to the crippling arthritic process in the peripheral areas. The disease produces weakness and painful, deformed, and contracted joints, making range of motion and strength evaluation difficult. Weakness may be a function of pain rather than neurologic damage. A dislocated and contracted great toe may not respond to the plantar reflex. Reflexes may be difficult to evaluate or even impossible to obtain, especially with joint stiffness. Other conditions found in the rheumatoid patient, such as a carpal tunnel syndrome, may mislead the examiner into believing that the patient has a cervical nerve root involvement when the fingers are numb.

In 1973, Rana and associates[17] stated that the neurologic picture confronting the clinician may be complex: progressive loss of reflexes suggests peripheral neuropathy; loss of consciousness on neck movement implies vertebral artery insufficiency; palatal weakness, deafness, tinnitus, vertigo, and facial parasthesias indicate intrinsic pontine vascular disease; and urinary urgency suggests parapyramidal tract involvement.

TYPE 1
up to ⅓ erosion

TYPE 2
⅓ to ⅔ erosion

TYPE 3
⅔ erosion to
complete absence

Figure 121–6. Schematic representation of three stages of odontoid destruction. Type 1—destruction of one third or less; Type 2—destruction of one third to two thirds; and Type 3—destruction of more than two thirds.

Figure 121–8. Subaxial involvement. The disc spaces are markedly narrowed without significant scleroris. The endplates tend to "jigsaw" one into the other, and the vertebral spines are thinned and "sharpened." Subluxation from C3 to C6 has occurred in "stepladder" fashion.

Neurologic problems can be produced by compression of the spinal cord, brainstem or vertebral arteries either by vertebral displacement and/or inflammatory masses. The neurologic picture varies with the site and extent of compression.

The following neurologic signs may be present:

1. Signs of spinothalmic tract involvement (decreased pain sensation).

2. Signs of the first two divisions of trigeminal nerve involvement (facial numbness, depressed or absent corneal reflex). This is due to the fact that the spinal nucleus of this nerve is at the level of C2.

3. Signs of pyramidal tract involvement (hyperactive reflexes, spasticity and weakness).

4. Pontine signs such as palatal weakness.

5. Fasiculation due to involvement of the anterior horn cells.

6. Signs of brainstem ischemia from vertebral artery occlusion or stenosis.

7. Signs of urinary tract difficulty due to parapyramidal tract involvement.

There are few reports of impaired position sense, indicating that the cord and brainstem damage is anterior and does not involve the posterior columns.

In addition to the neurologic problems, patients with rheumatoid arthritis usually complain of varying degrees of neck pain, limited motion, and crepitation.

If the atlantoaxial joint is involved and/or displaced, the patient may complain of the following:

1. Neck pain radiating to the occiput.

2. When the neck is flexed, the patient may feel that his head is "slipping off" as C1 shifts forward on C2. This causes prominence of the spine of C2 in the posterior neck and difficulty looking upward, with associated flattening of the occipitocervical curve.

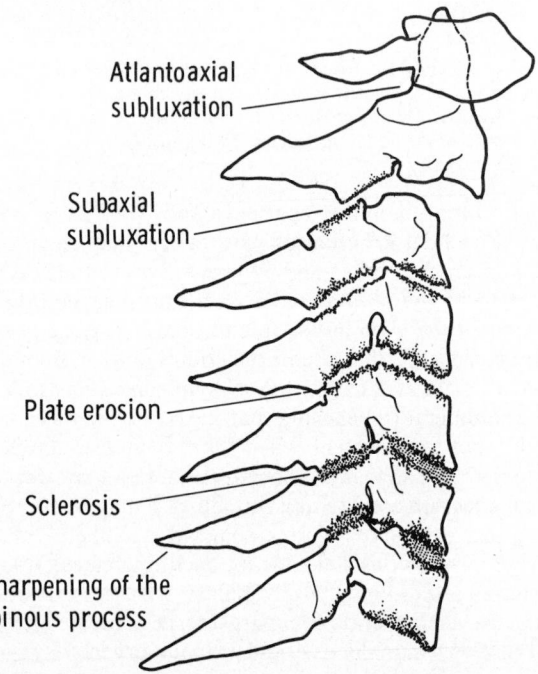

Atlantoaxial
subluxation

Subaxial
subluxation

Plate erosion

Sclerosis

Sharpening of the
spinous process

Figure 121–7. Schematic representation of the effects of the rheumatoid process on the cervical spine. (Courtesy of William Park.)

Figure 121–9. *A,* Posterior displacement of C1 and C2 due to destruction of the atlantoaxial joint and odontoid. *B,* Marked anterior displacement of C1 and C2 with quadraparesis and marked narrowing of the space available for the cord (the distance between the posterior aspect of the odontoid and anterior aspect of the posterior ring of C1).

Treatment. Surgery is rarely necessary for atlantoaxial or subaxial subluxation in the patient with rheumatoid arthritis[9] (Fig. 121–10). It is generally difficult to draw firm conclusions from the infrequent reports of surgical management. It is the consensus that nonoperative treatment is preferred. Smith and associates gave strong support to this concept,[26] and Isdale and Conlon[9] stated that in the absence of neurologic or vascular complications, operative intervention was unwarranted. Ranawat and associates[27] noted that fusion was infrequently needed and performed in only 0.7 percent of a clinic population of nearly 2897. Ferlic and colleagues[21] reported only 12 cervical fusion operations in 1975. Others, however, have strongly advocated surgery.[27] Between these two extremes lie the majority of patients, for whom judgment plays the major role.

Conservative management generally consists of analgesia and soft or hard collars that restrict motion depending upon their degree of rigidity. Collars do not prevent or correct progressive subluxation or neurologic problems and may be poorly tolerated by some patients irrespective of their neck pain.[26] The same can be said of halter traction.

If the patient's condition will permit, surgery may be indicated in cases of the following: (1) intractable pain associated with vertebral luxation and unrelieved by conservative treatment; (2) significant vertebral artery compromise; (3) significant spinal cord or brainstem compression, especially when progressive; and (4) progressive instability associated with pain and or neurologic involvement.

Surgical procedures generally take one of two forms—fusion or decompression of neural or vascular structures. If decompression produces instability, it may be combined with fusion. Anterior fusion may be associated with graft collapse into the soft osteoporotic bone and is generally reserved for instability following laminectomy when posterior arthrodesis cannot be carried out. Posterior arthrodesis is generally preferable and may be done in the occiput–C1-2 area, the subaxial region, or both.

Complications and pseudarthrosis rates are high, partly the result of the generalized rheumatoid process, bony demineralization, and destruction of bony structure in the area to be fused. These patients tolerate postoperative fixation devices poorly, and the rate of fusion is low compared with that in other patients. Only 6 of Ferlic's 12 patients had solid union.[21] The fatality rate after surgery is high. Ranawat[27] reported 27 percent; Cregan,[28] 33 percent, Crellin and associates,[20] 27 percent, and Meijers and associates,[23] 42 percent.

Prior to surgery, attempts to reduce displacement and maintain reduction include skull tong traction and/or halo devices. Atlantoaxial fusion is generally carried out utilizing bone graft and wire fixation, as described by Gallie. Indications to include the occiput include absence or deficiency of the posterior C1 arch and/or atlantoaxial impaction. In the subaxial area, fusion is performed by the standard midline technique with or without wire fixation. Internal stabilization has been enhanced by the use of wires or wire mesh incorporated in methylmethacrylate to avoid or minimize the hazards of external fixation. In a series of 11 patients for whom this was used, the pseudarthrosis rate was 18 percent and complications included wound dehiscence and late instability below the fusion mass.[29]

ANKYLOSING SPONDYLITIS

Unlike rheumatoid arthritis, which results in joint destruction, ankylosing spondylitis results in joint fusion. In the cervical region, this often produces ankylosis from occiput downward (Fig. 121–11).

Figure 121–10. *A,* Advanced destruction of the odontoid, anterior arch, and lateral masses of C1. There is separation of C1 from C2, and the posterior arch of C1 "floating free" without bony connection to its anterior components. *B,* Posterior fusion had to be carried out from the skull to the lower cervical vertebra, since it was impossible to obtain bony fusion from the "free floating" posterior cervical arch.

Pathology. Post-mortem studies have suggested an initial inflammation followed by ossification of joint capsule and articular cartilage resulting in ankylosis.[1] In the spine, the vertebral bodies tend to become "square"; ossification of ligaments and disc tissue follows.

Clinical Signs. The onset is insidious and is usually associated with morning stiffness, decreasing during the day and recurring in the evening, and unremitting low back pain. The sacroiliac joints are usually involved early in the disease, explaining the initial area of symptoms. In the cervical region, the pain, stiffness, and limitation of motion associated with a flexion deformity usually cause patients to seek medical advice. To compensate for this, they may simultaneously flex hips and knees to obtain a horizontal "line of sight." O'Driscoll and as-

Figure 121–11. Ankylosis from the skull downward in ankylosing spondylitis.

sociates report that lateral flexion is the movement most commonly restricted; further restriction is proportional to the degree of ankylosis.[30]

Surgical Management. If the patient's head position is satisfactory, and the cervical spine completely fused, there is little that surgery can offer. Surgical intervention may be necessary in unacceptable cervical flexion deformities, in fractures, and in threatening atlantoaxial displacements.

Fixed Flexion Deformity. Probably the most common complication of this disease is unacceptable fixed cervical flexion. Cervical osteotomy, as described by Mason, Cozen, and Addelstein,[31] Urist,[32] and Simmons,[33] has been found to provide satisfactory correction. Simmons recommends that the procedure be performed under local anesthesia, with the patient in the sitting position and a halo ring and halo jacket applied. A laminectomy is performed at the C7 level, extending upward into C6 and downward into D1 with appropriate local resection of the C7-D1 facets. The spine is then manually fractured at the C7-D1 level under temporary general anesthesia by backward pressure on the head and correction obtained. The halo ring is then fastened to the body jacket. Osteotomy of the C7-D1 level is recommended because the vertebral canal is wider in this region and also because the vertebral arteries enter the foramen transversarium at C6, above the osteotomy site. The neurologic and other hazards of this operation should be known to the patient prior to operation to aid in the surgical decision.

Fractures. The rigidity of the spondylitic cervical spine, unprotected by ribs or normal musculature, renders it particularly vulnerable to trauma. The force of a blow cannot be absorbed by mobile cervical segments, and the ankylosed spine may behave in a manner similar to a long bone. Since there is a degree of osteoporosis, the spine may fracture easily with minimal pain and the patient may not recall the injury. The fractures are usually transverse, occur at the level of a disc space, and are generally at the midportion of the neck. Woodruff and Dewing in 1963 reported 20 cases; 5 were above C5 and 15 below.[34]

Simmons has noted the significance of minor injuries in patients with severe flexion deformities. In 40 cases presenting for cervical osteotomy with unacceptable flexion deformity, 36 percent had evidence of previous fractures, and in 31 percent of these 40 the fracture contributed significantly to the deformity.[35] Such fractures may go unnoticed for a variety of reasons. First, the fracture may spontaneously reduce without displacement; secondly, the patient may not recall the incident; and third, the fracture may be difficult to detect, particularly in the lower portions of the cervical spine in an individual in whom x-ray positioning is difficult. Hudson reported correcting a flexion deformity at the site of a fresh fracture dislocation between C5 and C6 in a patient without significant neurologic or vascular injury.[36]

Not all fractures of the ankylosed cervical spine are benign; some present a very poor prognosis. The normal flexibility of the neck is eliminated by the ankylosing process. Therefore, all motion takes place at the fracture site. This is in close proximity to the vulnerable vertebral arteries and spinal cord as described by Taylor and Blackwood.[37] (Fig. 121–12).

In 1979, Bohlman[38] presented 8 fractures in patients with ankylosing spondylitis. Three were above C5, and 5 were at C5 or below. All had cord lesions, and 5 died. Others have also noted problems with these injuries.[39-41]Woodruff and Dewing presented 20 cases of ankylosing spondylitis with fracture. They made four observations:[33]

1. Fractures may be caused by relatively slight trauma, since the fused rigid spine compounded by osteoporosis cannot give the stress. In none of their cases was the blow considered severe, and in one the weight of the head alone was thought to cause the fracture.

2. The ankylosed spine breaks like a solid long bone. Vertebral body compression is not a feature, since the line runs transversely; hence, every fracture is complete, and the chance of dislocation and spinal cord injury is high.

3. Mortality is high. Of their 20 cases, 9 died within a short period of time. Generally, the degree of displacement correlated with the severity of the spinal cord injury. They also noted that there can be gross malalignment with minimal or no cord impairment.

4. Treatment will vary with the clinical situation. They recommended "neutral traction."

Atlantoaxial Displacement. Jefferys reports that the incidence of this complication in the literature is as high as 90 percent, cautioning that this high percentage may reflect the severity of the disease in patients referred to the hospital. He indicates that in his own experience atlantoaxial subluxation in ankylosing spondylitis is un-

Figure 121–12. Cervical spine fracture in ankylosing spondylitis.

common, an opinion shared by this author.[42] This complication would suggest that either this joint is unfused, particularly prone to trauma, or both (Fig. 121–13).

Surgical arthrodesis is probably the safest method of management, although it will sacrifice rotary motion at the atlantoaxial joint.

Figure 121–13. The spine is fused from C2 downward owing to ankylosing spondylitis.C1-C2 has been displaced forward with marked narrowing of the space available for the cord.

References

1. Berens, D.: Roentgen Diagnosis of Rheumatoid Arthritis, Springfield, Ill., Charles C Thomas, 1969.
2. Short, C.L.: The antiquity of rheumatoid arthritis. Arthritis Rheum. 17:193, 1974.
3. Conlon, P.W., Isdale, I.C., and Rose, B.S.: Rheumatoid arthritis of the cervical spine: An analysis of 333 cases. Ann. Rheum. Dis. 25:120, 1966.
4. Bland, J.H., Davis, B.H., London, M.G., van Buskirk, F.W., and Duarte, C.G.: Rheumatoid arthritis of the cervical spine. Arch. Intern. Med. 112, 892, 130, 1963.
5. Mathews, J.A.: Atlanto-axial subluxation in rheumatoid arthritis. Ann. Rheum. Dis. 28:260, 1969.
6. Meikle, J.A.K., and Wilkinson, M.: Rheumatoid involvement of the cervical spine: Radiological assessment. Ann. Rheum. Dis. 30:154, 1971.
7. Bell, Sir Charles: The Nervous System of the Human Body. London, 1830.
8. Davis, F.W., Jr., and Markley, H.E.: Rheumatoid arthritis with death from medullary compression. Ann. Intern. Med. 35:451, 1951.
9. Isdale, I.C., and Conlon, P.W.: Atlanto-axial subluxation—a six-year follow-up report. Ann. Rheum. Dis. 30:387, 1971.
10. Martel, W.: The occipito-axial joint in rheumatoid arthritis and ankylosing spondylitis. Am. J. Roentgenol. Rad. Ther. Nucl. Med. 86:223, 1961.
11. Sharp, J., and Purser, D.W.: Spontaneous atlanto-axial dislocation in ankylosing spondylitis and rheumatoid arthritis. Ann. Rheum. Dis. 20:47, 1961.
12. Fielding, J.W.: Cineradiography of the normal cervical spine. J. Bone Joint Surgery 39A:1280, 1957.
13. Steele, H.H.: Anatomical and mechanical considerations of the atlanto-axial articulation (abstract). J. Bone Joint Surg. 50A:1481, 1968.
14. Martel, W., and Abell, M.R.: Fatal atlanto-axial luxation in rheumatoid arthritis. Arthritis Rheum. 6:224, 1963.
15. Storey, G.: Changes in the cervical spine in rheumatoid arthritis with compression of the cord. Ann. Phys. Med. 4:216, 1958.
16. Webb, F.W.S., Hickman, J.A., and Brew, D.S.J.: Death from vertebral artery thrombosis in rheumatoid arthritis. Br. Med. J. 2:537, 1968.
17. Rana, N.H., Hancock, D.O., and Hill, A.G.S.: Upward translocation of the dens in rheumatoid arthritis. J. Bone Joint Surg. 55B:471, 1973.
18. McGregor, M.: The significance of certain measurements of the skull in the diagnosis of basilar impression. Br. J. Radiol. 21:171, 1948.
19. Dr. William M. Park: Personal communication.
20. Crellin, R.Q., Maccabe, J.J., and Hamilton, F.B.D.: Severe subluxation of the cervical spine in rheumatoid arthritis. J. Bone Joint Surg. 52B:244, 1970.
21. Ferlic, D.C., Clayton, M.L., Leidholt, J.D., and Gamble, W.E.: Surgical treatment of the symptomatic unstable cervical spine in rheumatoid arthritis. J. Bone Joint Surg. 57A:349, 1975.
22. Hauge, T.: Chronic rheumatoid polyarthritis and spondylarthritis associated with neurogenic symptoms and signs occasionally simulating an intraspinal expansive process. Acta Chir. Scand. 120:395, 1961.
23. Meijers, K.A.E., Van Beusekom, G.Th., Luyendijk, W., and Duijfjes, F.: Dislocation of the cervical spine with cord compression in rheumatoid arthritis. J. Bone Joint Surg. 56B:668, 1974.
24. Rana, N.A., Hancock, D.O., Taylor, A.R., and Hill, A.G.S.: Atlanto-axial subluxation in rheumatoid arthritis. J. Bone Joint Surg. 55B:458, 1973.
25. Weissman, B.N.W., Aliabadi, P., Weinfeld, M.S., Thomas, W.H., and Sosman, J.L.: Prognostic features of atlanto-axial subluxation in rheumatoid arthritis patients. Radiology 144:745, 1982.
26. Smith, P.H., Benn, R.T., and Sharp, J.: Natural history of rheumatoid cervical luxations. Ann. Rheum. Dis. 31:431, 1972.
27. Ranawat, C.S., O'Leary, P., Pellicci, P., Tsairis, P., Marchisello, P., and Dorr, L.: Cervical spine fusion in rheumatoid arthritis. J. Bone Joint Surg. 61A:1003, 1979.
28. Cregan, J.C.F.: Internal fixation of the unstable rheumatoid cervical spine. Ann. Rheum. Dis. 25:242, 1966.
29. Bryan, W.J., Inglis, A.E., Sculco, T.P., et al.: Methyl-methacrylate stabilization for enhancement of posterior cervical arthrodesis in rheumatoid arthritis. J. Bone Joint Surg. 64A:1045, 1982.
30. O'Driscoll, S.L., Jayson, M.I.V., and Badley, H.: Neck movements in ankylosing spondylitis. Ann. Rheum. Dis. 37:64, 1978.
31. Mason, C., Cozen, L., and Addelstein, L.: Surgical correction of flexion deformity of the cervical spine. Calif. Med. 79:244, 1963.
32. Urist, M.R.: Osteotomy of the cervical spine. Report of case of ankylosing rheumatoid spondylitis. J. Bone Joint Surg. 40A:833, 1958.
33. Simmons, E.H.: The surgical correction of flexion deformity of the cervical spine in ankylosing spondylitis. Clin. Orthop. Rel. Res. 86:132, 1972.
34. Woodruff, F.V., and Dewing, S.B.: Fracture of the cervical spine in patients with ankylosing spondylitis. Radiology 80:17, 1963.
35. Simmons, E.H.: Personal communication.
36. Hudson, C.P.: Cervical osteotomy for severe flexion. J. Bone Joint Surg. 54B:202, 1972.
37. Taylor, A.R., and Blackwood, W.: Paraplegia in hyperextension in cervical injuries. J. Bone Joint Surg. 30B:245, 1948.
38. Bohlman, H.: Acute fractures and dislocations of the cervical spine. J. Bone Joint Surg. 61A:1119, 1979.
39. Bergmann, E.W.: Fractures of the ankylosed spine. J. Bone Joint Surg. 45B:21, 1963.
40. Harris, L.S., and Adelson, L.: "Spinal injury" and sudden infant death: A second look. Am. J. Clin. Pathol. 52:289, 1969.
41. Hollin, S.A., Gross, S.W., and Levin, P.: Fracture of the cervical spine in patients with rheumatoid spondylitis. Am. Surg. 31:532, 1965.
42. Jeffreys, E.: Disorders of the Cervical Spine. London, Butterworths, 1980.

Chapter 122

Radiographic Evaluation of Total Joint Replacement

Barbara N. W. Weissman

INTRODUCTION

The remarkable success of total hip replacement (THR) has led to the performance of an estimated 75,000 such operations in this country annually[1] and the development of a large number of prosthetic devices for most other major joints. Radiographic examination contributes to the care of patients with joint disease by helping establish a diagnosis, evaluate and follow articular damage, and assess the results of surgical treatment, including total joint replacement. Evaluation of postoperative radiographs is becoming an increasing part of many radiographic practices. In this chapter, the "normal" radiographic appearances of some of the frequently used prosthetic devices and the radiographic evaluation of complications of total joint replacement will be discussed.

TOTAL HIP JOINT REPLACEMENT

Types of Prostheses, Normal Appearances. Total hip prostheses can be categorized by the composition of the acetabular and femoral components into plastic-to-metal, metal-to-metal, and combination types.

In the plastic-metal type, the acetabular component is made of either high-density or ultrahigh-density polyethylene plastic and the femoral component of stainless steel, a chromium-cobalt-molybdenum alloy (Vitallium), or titanium.[2] The Charnley, Charnley-Muller, trapezoidal-28, and Aufranc-Turner prostheses are of this type.

In young patients and in patients with good bone stock who have damage limited to the joint surfaces, "conservative total hip replacement" may de done. This entails reaming and reshaping the acetabulum and the femoral head and inserting a high-density polyethylene acetabular liner and a metallic femoral cup. Both components are cemented in place.[3] The radiographic appearances will differ from those of a cup arthroplasty in that the immediate postoperative films will show the 4- to 5-mm thickness of the acetabular component rather than the very thin joint space that is seen after cup arthroplasty. Careful inspection will reveal cement around the acetabular component (Fig. 122–1).

Metal-metal prostheses consist of metal acetabular and femoral components and include the McKee-Farrar, Ring, and Stanmore prostheses.[2] The acetabular component may be fixed to the acetabulum with methyl methacrylate, screws, or spikes (Fig. 122–2).

The third type of total hip prosthesis *combines metallic and polyethylene components.* It usually consists of three parts: fixed metallic acetabular and femoral components and a third piece, either a high density polyethylene acetabular liner (Harris prosthesis, Sbarbaro) or a separate high density polyethylene femoral head (Tronzo and Weber prostheses).[2]

In the bipolar endoprostheses (i.e., Giliberty, Bateman) the metallic acetabular component is not fixed and can move within the acetabular socket.[4] A polyethylene acetabular liner is present. The femoral component consists of a Muller or Aufranc device fixed with cement or a Moore femoral component which is not cemented (Fig. 122–3).

Figure 122–2. Ring metal-to-metal prosthesis. The acetabular component is fixed into the ilium by a long screw. The femoral component is press fitted into the femur. Some bone resorption has occurred around the acetabular screw and the femoral stem.

Bipolar endoprostheses are used in some institutions in place of conventional hemiarthroplasty (Thompson, Austin-Moore) in patients with minimal or no acetabular abnormality, including those with displaced subcapital fractures, avascular necrosis of the femoral head, or osteoarthritis with minimal acetabular involvement.[4] It is thought that because motion occurs preferentially between the femoral and acetabular components (rather than between the metallic cup and the acetabulum), degenerative change in the acetabulum will be less pronounced than with conventional hemiarthroplasty. If these changes do occur, the acetabular component can be replaced with a cemented acetabular socket.

Radiographic examination should show most motion occuring between the femoral component and the acetabular liner,[4] although some movement does occur at the outer articulation, particularly at the extremes of motion.[5] Acetabular changes, including cartilage space narrowing and acetabular sclerosis, should theoretically be minimal. Because the metallic cup overlies the femoral component, no radiographic estimation of the integrity of the liner can be made except by indirect evaluation of femoral-acetabular motion.

Positioning of Components. Postoperative radio-

Figure 122–1. Conservative total hip replacement. The thickness of the acetabular component is shown by the separation between the metallic femoral component and the opaque cement.

Figure 122–3. Bateman total hip prosthesis. *A*, Anteroposterior view. *B*, Frog lateral view. The acetabular component is not fixed to the ilium. Although most motion occurs between the femoral component and the polyethylene acetabular liner, some motion will be noted between the acetabular component and the acetabulum. The polyethylene liner cannot be seen.

graphs allow assessment of the positions of the acetabular and femoral components.

Acetabular Component. In each of these prostheses, the acetabular component is placed so that the base of the cup is at a particular angle to the horizontal (i.e., 45 degrees for the Charnley and Charnley-Muller prostheses, 42 degrees for the trapezoidal-28, and 30 degrees for the Aufranc-Turner prosthesis) in an effort to provide as much motion as possible without too great

a hazard of dislocation.[2,6] The acetabular angle is measured by drawing a line through the medial and lateral poles of the equatorial marker wire and another line through the most inferior aspect of each ischial tuberosity (Fig. 122–4).

Frontal and lateral views centered on the acetabulum are necessary for accurate evaluation. The immediate "portable" postoperative film may suggest that the acetabular cup is in too much anteversion (or retroversion),

Figure 122–4. Reference lines for evaluating the position of total hip replacements. The ischial tuberosity line (ITL) and the midline (MID) are shown. The acetabular angle (curved arrow) is measured between the ITL and a line through the long axis of the acetabular marker wire. Differences in limb length can be assessed by comparing the distance (D) from the top of the lesser trochanter to the ITL on each side when the femora are identically positioned. (Modified from Gore et al.)

but the appearances are often due to the slightly flexed position that is maintained postoperatively. Subsequent films centered on the acetabulum demonstrate the true tilt of the acetabular component.

The orifice of the acetabular component is placed in slight anteversion (tipped anteriorly) or in neutral position (Fig. 122–5*A*).[2,7] The degree of acetabular anteversion is measured on a true lateral film. When only frontal views are available, however, the equatorial marker wires should form a thin ellipse if the prosthesis is in slight anteversion. With increasing anteversion (or retroversion) the wire marker assumes a more circular shape.[8] Quantitation of the degree of acetabular anteversion from frontal views can be done by dividing the maximal diameter of the acetabular ring by the minimal diameter and comparing this quotient to a standard reference table.[9]

Two points should be emphasized when determining the degree of acetabular anteversion from frontal views alone. The first is that although anteversion is usually assumed, retroversion cannot be excluded. The second is that the apparent degree of acetabular anteversion varies considerably, depending on the location of the central ray of the x-ray beam. Films should be centered over the acetabulum.[10]

The change in acetabular appearance with differences in centering of the x-ray beam can be used to determine the degree and direction of acetabular version. Two AP views are taken, one with the x-ray beam centered on the pubic symphysis, and the other with it centered on the acetabulum.[11,12] When the ring appears wider (more circular) on the film centered on the acetabulum than on the one centered on the symphysis, the component is anteverted. When it is more circular in appearance on the film centered on the pubic symphysis, the component is retroverted. The angle of version (β) can then be derived from the following formula: $\sin\beta = d2/D2$ Where d2 is the short diameter and D2 is the long diameter of the acetabular marker wire as projected on the film centered over the acetabulum (Fig. 122–5*B*).

Fluoroscopy has also been used to determine the angle of anteversion.[13] As the fluoroscopic tube is angled either toward the feet or toward the head, the degree and direction of angulation are noted at which the anterior and posterior rims of the acetabular marker wire are superimposed. The component is anteverted if the tube is angled toward the head and retroverted if it is directed toward the feet. Using a reference table, correction can be made for the degree of inclination of the component, since this influences the observed angle of anteversion.

Femoral Component. On the frontal view, the prosthetic femoral stem should be in the center of the medullary cavity or in slight valgus position.[6] Valgus or varus position of the stem refers to the angle between the long axis of the stem and the long axis of the femoral shaft.[14] When the tip of the stem is near the lateral femoral cortex, the prosthesis is said to be in varus; when near the medial cortex, the prosthesis is in valgus. On true lateral views, the femoral head should be in about 10 degrees of anteversion or in neutral position.[6,7,15]

Multiple reference lines have been constructed to compare the position of a total hip prosthesis to the normal contralateral side (Fig. 122–4).[16] Some of these are applicable following bilateral joint replacement. A view of the pelvis with the hips in neutral position can be used to determine differences in limb length by comparing the distance on each side from the proximal end of the lesser trochanter to a line through the most inferior portions of each ischial tuberosity.

Methyl Methacrylate. Methyl methacrylate has no adhesive properties when applied to wet bone.[17] It bonds to bone through a mechanical interlocking of surface irregularities and functions to distribute transmitted stresses evenly from the prothesis to bone.[21,22] It is prepared by mixing a liquid monomer with a powdered polymerized material. The surfaces of the pearls of polymerized material are dissolved by the monomer, and within minutes a single block is formed by polymerization of the monomer.

The surgical procedure of total hip arthroplasty includes cleaning the acetabulum of cartilage and ebur-

Figure 122–5. *A*, Acetabular anteversion. The degree of tilt of the acetabular orifice can be measured on true lateral views (arrow). *B*, On this film, the angle of version (β) may be derived from the formula $\sin \beta = d2/D2$. An estimation of d2 must be made, owing to the opacity of the femoral head.

nated bone, enlarging the acetabulum if necessary, and drilling ½-inch diameter holes into the ischium, ilium, and pubis.[17] When the methyl methacrylate cement reaches a doughy consistency, it is pressed into the acetabulum and the prepared holes. The acetabular component is then inserted and held in position.

Methyl methacrylate is also placed into the medullary canal of the femur after the cancellous bone is removed. Cement should fill the medullary cavity medially and laterally along the distal two thirds of the shaft and should extend 2 cm distal to the tip of the prosthesis.[6,18] According to Amstutz and colleagues inadequate cement fixation is suggested by radiolucent zones at the cement–bone or cement–metal junctions, or by the presence of voids and laminations within the cement.[19] Beckenbaugh and Ilstrup found loosening of the femoral component to be inversely related to the degree of extension of cement past the prosthetic tip.[18]

Currently a Silastic or cement plug is often inserted into the femoral canal distal to the expected position of the tip of the femoral stem. This plugging allows higher intrusion pressure and better filling of the femoral canal to be achieved, and when the plug is correctly positioned, it ensures a cement filling at least 2 cm beyond the tip of prosthesis.[20]

Histologic examination has shown a reaction of bone to methacrylate that may be divided into three phases: necrosis, repair, and a steady state.[23] Within the first 3 weeks after surgery, a zone of necrotic tissue and fibrin is noted extending up to 3 mm in depth from the cement–bone interface. The cause of this necrosis remains uncertain, but possibilities include toxic effects from remaining nonpolymerized monomer or thermal injury related to the polymerization of methyl methacrylate (an exothermic reaction).[24] From 3 weeks to 2 years postoperatively, repair of tissue damage occurs and, in most cases, leads to the development of a fibrous layer along the cement–bone interface. A stable appearance is usually reached in 2 years with a 0.1 to 1.5 mm connective tissue membrane formed around the cement.[23]

Radiologic evaluation of the cement–bone interface can be accomplished only when the methacrylate is made opaque, usually by the addition of barium sulfate. If a radiolucent line is present at the cement–bone interface, it will be made apparent on radiographs by its contrast to the adjacent opaque cement on one side and a thin sclerotic line on the other side. When such a radiolucent line is present in the immediate postoperative period, it may represent residual cartilage, soft tissue, or blood within the prosthetic bed. Later, the lucency may correspond to the histologically demonstrable fibrous tissue layer.

Radiolucent zones at the cement–bone interface are very frequent around the acetabular component and less frequent around the femoral component. A summary of the data relating to this lucency is shown in Table 122–1. These zones are usually established by 6 months postoperatively but may occasionally begin later.[25] Lucencies of more than 2 mm or progressive lucency suggest the possibility of loosening or infection and correlate on histologic examination with the presence of a synovial lining capable of producing substances that stimulate bone resorption.[26]

Trochanteric Osteotomy. Trochanteric osteotomy may be done to facilitate surgical exposure. The trochanter is reattached using heavy wire sutures, usually in the anatomical position or to a more distal location, depending on mechanical considerations. In over 95 percent of cases, bony union between the trochanter and the femur is evident on radiographic examination within 6 to 12 weeks postoperatively.[6,14] If bony union is not seen at 3 months but the trochanter remains unchanged in position, it is likely that fibrous union has occurred, especially if the wire sutures remain intact.[6] Clinical results appear to be as satisfactory with fibrous union as with bony union,[27] and fibrous union may progress to bony union.[28] Separation of the greater trochanter was present in 2.7 percent of hips followed for 9 to 10 years by Charnley, and all these patients were classified as having excellent clinical results.[28] Separation of the greater trochanter may be of clinical significance, since this is occasionally associated with pain, limp, and a tendency to develop an adduction contracture.[29] Bergstrom and colleagues noted that displacement of the greater trochanter of 5 to 20 mm (44 cases) did not impair the functional result, whereas 2 of 4 patients with more than 2 cm of displacement required reoperation.[30]

Fracture of the wires holding the greater trochanter occurs in up to one third of cases and is of very little significance unless it is associated with proximal migration of the trochanter. Wire breakage can occur owing to metal fatigue even after there is solid bony union between the trochanter and femur. Occasionally, symptoms result from irritation of the overlying soft tissues. Rarely a metal fragment can migrate to an intra-articular location.

Wire Mesh. Chrome cobalt metal (Vitallium) mesh may be used to reinforce the medial acetabular wall in cases in which this area is deficient (i.e., protrusio acetabuli or excessive removal of bone at the time of surgery). According to Harris and Jones,[31] half of the methacrylate is inserted into the prepared acetabulum, and then the wire mesh is pressed into this. The remaining cement is then added on top of the mesh, and the acetabular component is positioned as usual. The wire mesh projections are bent around the edges of the hardened cement and the acetabular rim.

These authors also describe the use of wire mesh to cap an osteoporotic greater trochanter at the time of initial surgery or at the time of repair of a migrated osteoporotic trochanter. The trochanteric wires are brought through the mesh and tied over it to distribute the load across the trochanter.

Measuring Wear. Theoretically, wear can be assessed by measuring changes in the distance from the metallic femoral head to the metallic wire on the surface of the acetabular cup. Two methods have been used to assess wear.[28,32] In the first, the width of the narrowest part of the socket in the weight-bearing area is subtracted from the width of the widest part in a non-weight-bearing

Table 122–1. Cement–Bone Lucency

	DeLee and Charnley, 1976[25]	Bergstrom et al., 1973[30]	Beckenbaugh and Ilstrup, 1978[18]	Salvati et al., 1976[14]	Amstutz et al., 1976[19]
Acetabular component					
Number of hips with lucent zones	98/141 (70%) (13 loose)	15/15 (100%) control patients	252/255 (99%) without symptoms of loosening	93/93 (100%)	300/389 (77%)
Percentage of circumference involved	—	—	87.5% incomplete	Widest and most frequent laterally	13% completely around acetabular cement
Thickness	>1.5 mm in 3/85 without motion and in 9/13 with motion	<1 mm lucency in 100% of controls	≤1 mm in 87.5%; >1 mm in 6.5%	≤1 mm in 63/93 (68%); 1–2 mm in 29/93 (31%)	—
Time to appearance	17% immediate; 71% within first year; 5.3% after 3 years postoperative	100% before 6 months	—	—	—
Femoral component					
Number of hips involved	—	10/15 (67%) of control patients	—	55/93 (59%)	43/389 (11%)
Thickness	—	<1.5 mm in controls	—	≤1 mm in 36/55; 1–2 mm in 19/55	Most frequent proximally and medially

area and the result halved. In the second method, the thickness of the acetabular component in the latest radiograph is compared with the thickness determined on the immediate postoperative radiograph. Correction for magnification is done by comparison with the known diameter of the femoral head. Using the second method, in 72 hips with 9- to 10-year follow-up, Charnley and Halley found that total wear ranged from 0 to 4.5 mm and averaged 1.5 mm. Patient weight and physical activity did not seem to influence the rate of wear, and the rate of wear appeared to decrease with time.[32]

Clarke and colleagues assessed both methods of measuring wear in vitro, using a total hip prosthesis mounted on a Plexiglas orientation apparatus.[33] Although the technique of comparison of early and later films at first seemed more accurate, assessment of wear by clinicians, even when shown the approximate area of wear, yielded errors so large that it was "impossible to make any valid wear assessments; . . . it was concluded that wear measurements could not be made from clinical radiographs."[33]

Resorption of the Medial Femoral Neck. Three or 4 mm of resorption of the medial femoral neck (apparently resulting from ischemic necrosis) occurs in almost 20 percent of patients when the femoral prosthesis is fixed with cement.[7,28] Resorption does not usually occur in the absence of cement fixation.[7] Generally this bone loss does not progress and is not significantly related to loosening.[44] Bechtol, however, has suggested that this represents an early stage in a sequence of findings that eventually lead to bending or fracture of the femoral stem[34] (see also Development or Widening of a Metal–Cement Lucency, and Femoral Stem Fracture, below).

Complications of Total Hip Replacement. *Dislocation.* Dislocation is most frequent in the immediate postoperative period, presumably as a consequence of laxity of para-articular soft tissues, combined with improper handling of the patient during transfer from the operating room or poor positioning of the leg in bed.[35,36] Improper placement or selection of the prosthesis may also be responsible for early dislocation.[37]

Dislocation occurring later than 3 months postoperatively is most often the result of malpositioning of components[35] but may be due to failure to develop adequate muscle control or to the patient's developing a range of motion that exceeds the limits of the prosthesis.[37]

Radiographic examination confirms the presence of dislocation, helps define any associated malposition of the prosthetic components, and aids in identification of associated complications. Anteroposterior and true lateral radiographs will best define the type of dislocation present. Daffner and colleagues described the "Saturn-ring sign," useful in detecting subtle dislocation when only a frontal radiograph is available.[38] This sign is based on the observation that when the femoral head is in the center of the acetabular component, distances measured medially and laterally from the femoral head to the poles of the acetabular wires will be equal (Fig. 122-6). When the femoral head is dislocated, these measurements will be unequal. This sign is of value only for prostheses in which the femoral head is centrally located (i.e., Charnley and Charnley-Muller prostheses). With others, such as the Aufranc-Turner prosthesis, the acetabular component is thicker along the superolateral aspect to provide extra durability in the weight-bearing area. The femoral component of these prostheses will normally appear eccentrically located, with the lateral measurement about twice the medial one. In fact, equal measurement may indicate dislocation[39,40] in these cases (Fig. 122-6).

Malposition of the acetabular and/or femoral com-

Figure 122–6. "Saturn-ring sign." *A*, Normally, as in this Charnley-Muller THR, the femoral head is centrally located within the acetabular component and distances B-C and D-E are equal. *B*, Dislocation of the femoral head will be associated with unequal measurements—the "Saturn-ring sign." *C* and *D*, The acetabular component of the Aufranc-Turner prosthesis is thicker superolaterally, giving an erroneously positive "Saturn-ring sign." *C*, Photograph. *D*, Radiograph. *E*, Ligamentous laxity in a recent postoperative patient has resulted in widening of the distance between the femoral head and the surface acetabular marker wire but no true dislocation.

ponents is a frequent predisposing factor in prosthetic hip dislocation. Fackler and Poss, for example, noted component malposition (defined as acetabular or femoral component retroversion or acetabular anteversion of more than 25 degrees) to be present in 44 percent of patients with dislocated prostheses as compared with only 6 percent of control patients.[12] Excessive anteversion of the acetabular component favors anterior dislocation with the hip in extension, retroversion may lead to posterior dislocation with the hip in flexion, and excessive vertical tilt favors dislocation with adduction of the leg. Excess bone or cement around the acetabular rim may lever the femoral head out of the acetabulum. Eleven of 13 dislocations in a series studied by Beckenbaugh and Ilstrup occurred with the hip in flexion with internal rotation or adduction or both.[18]

Detachment of the greater trochanter may accompany posterior dislocations.[36] Rarely, displacement of a fragment of cement or wire into the joint will block attempts at successful closed reduction of a dislocated total hip prosthesis.[41] These intra-articular foreign bodies may be visable on plain films or on arthrography.

Loosening and Infection. Two of the most frequent postoperative complications leading to failure of the total hip replacement are loosening and infection.[42] Loosening may involve one or both components and may be due to inadequate fixation at the time of surgery[19] or to infection. Recent improvements in surgical technique including better filling of the medullary canal by cement and the use of larger femoral stems with rounding of their medial margins has markedly decreased the incidence of femoral component loosening.[20]

Plain film findings that suggest loosening and/or infection include a large cement-bone interface, widening of the cement-bone interface, migration of prosthetic components, cement fractures, periosteal reaction, motion demonstrated on stress views, or evidence of osteomyelitis (Table 122-2).

Cement–Bone Lucency Greater Than 2 mm or Widening of the Cement–Bone Lucent Zone. A lucency of 2 mm or more at the cement-bone interface suggests loosening (Fig. 122-7). This finding correlated with motion of prosthetic components with manual stress at surgical exploration in 16 of the 18 patients (89 percent) in whom this lucency was observed.[43] Lucency around both the femoral and acetabular components was associated with an increased incidence of infection. Similarly, progressive widening of the cement–bone lucency suggests loosening and/or infection. The significance of wide or increasing cement bone lucent zones is more certain if they occur on the femoral rather than on the acetabular side. In one study of the efficacy of the plain film in the diagnosis of loosening, no false-positive or false-negative results were found on the femoral side (using the criteria of a wide cement–bone or metal–cement lucency, change in component position or the presence of an irregular, wide zone of bone resorption as evidence of loosening). In contrast, of 50 acetabular components embedded in opaque cement, there were 5 false positive and 1 false negative case.[45] Patients with clear radiographic evidence

Table 122–2. Radiographic Findings Suggesting Loosening and/or Infection of Total Hip Prostheses

Plain film findings
1. Cement-bone lucency of 2 mm or more
2. Widening of the cement-bone lucency
3. Migration of prosthetic components
4. Development or widening of metal-cement lucency
5. Cement fracture
6. Periosteal reaction
7. Motion of components demonstrable on stress views or fluoroscopy
8. Bone destruction

Arthrographic findings
1. Extension of contrast between the cement and bone or between the prosthesis and bone
2. Filling of irregular para-articular cavities or fistulous tracts

Scintigraphic findings
1. Increased activity in the acetabular and/or femoral shaft regions after 6 to 10 months postoperatively
2. Focal uptake around the femoral component suggests loosening without infection
3. Diffuse uptake, especially around both components suggests infection
4. Increased gallium uptake in comparison to bone agent uptake suggests infection

of loosening may be asymptomatic. In these cases, however, careful follow-up is suggested, since radiographic evidence of loosening may precede clinical symptoms (Fig. 122-8).[43] It is noteworthy that the diagnosis of infection cannot be reliably made from standard radiographs.

Change in Position of Prosthetic Components. Motion resulting in a change in position of a component may occur between the cement and bone or between the prosthesis and the cement. Four patterns of femoral component loosening have been described. (Fig. 122–9).

In the first and most common, there is pistoning of either the prosthesis within the acrylic cement or the prosthesis and cement within the bone. Loosening of the stem within the cement may be due to weak support at the proximal medial femoral neck and is seen as medial migration of the prosthesis with lucency at the cement-metal interface, usually along the lateral aspect. A crack in the cement at the tip of the prosthesis may be seen. When the loosening occurs between the cement and the bone, a lucency wider than 2 mm or an increasing zone of lucency is noted.

The second mode of failure, termed the medial midstem pivot mode, results from poor support medially at the calcar, as well as distally, and is seen as medial migration of the proximal stem, lateral migration of the distal stem, and a fracture of the acrylic cement in the midstem region.

The third category of femoral loosening consists of pivoting of the distal stem on the calcar, resulting from poor fixation distally. This is uncommon.

The fourth type of loosening results from poor support medially and proximally but good fixation of the distal stem. Medial migration of the proximal stem may occur, and fracture of the stem may result.

Figure 122–7. Loosening of femoral component. *A*, Examination 1 week postoperatively shows no lucency at the cement-bone interface of the femoral component and minimal lucency around the acetabular cement. *B*, Four and one-half years later, a lucent zone has developed at the cement-bone interface (arrow) of the femoral component, and the component has shifted to a more varus position. The lucent zone around the acetabular component has increased also, suggesting loosening. The patient was symptomatic.

Acetabular component loosening may occur at the cement–bone interface or between the component and the cement. A change in the orientation of the acetabular component on serial examinations may be noted (Fig. 122–10).

Development or Widening of a Metal–Cement Lucency. Separation between the femoral prosthesis and the cement is most frequently seen along the proximal lateral aspect of the femoral stem (Fig. 122-11). Although Beabout states that there should be "intimate contact between the acrylic cement and the femoral prosthesis,"[6] lucencies in this area are noted in the immediate postoperative period and on follow-up examination in 3.6[46] to 24 percent[18] of patients. When seen early in the postoperative period, it is likely that the cement did not remain in contact with that portion of the femoral component (owing to motion of the component while the methacrylate was setting)[19] or that the cement was eccentrically placed along a portion of the stem. In these cases, loosening should not be suggested. Some cases of

stable 1- to 2-mm lucent zones at the cement-metal interface have been shown to be due to the Mach effect,[47] a visual phenomenon in which accentuation of high contrast borders of objects occurs as a result of lateral inhibition produced by the neural networks in the eye.[48]

Later development of lucency between the femoral component and the adjacent cement has been referred to as "subsidence,"[49] The prosthesis sinks inferiorly and medially and, at least, according to Charnley, a new point of stability is reached.[18,49] This view is in concert with the findings of DeSmet and colleagues in which a metal–cement lucency was present along the lateral aspect of 23 of 101 Charnley-Muller total hip prostheses, although only 4 of these hips had clinical evidence of infection or loosening.[47] Weber and Charnley studied a group of patients with cement fracture and also noted that patients with subsidence of up to 3.5 mm generally had good or excellent clinical results.[49] Even progressive widening of this lucency may be seen in patients without clinical evidence of loosening.[47] However, Beckenbaugh

Figure 122–8. Asymptomatic loosening. *A*, 1973 examination shows a thin zone of lucency around the left acetabular component. *B*, Two years later cement-bone lucent zones have developed around both components on the right (arrows) and there is marked widening of the lucent zone around the left acetabular component (solid arrow). Bone resorption of the medial femoral neck (arrowhead) is noted. The patient has remained asymptomatic.

and Ilstrup noted a higher incidence of pain in patients with more than 2 mm of drift,[18] and the long-term effects of this finding are unknown.

Subsidence may be associated with radiographically demonstrable cement fracture (20 of 61 patients with subsidence studied by Beckenbaugh and Ilstrup),[18] but presumably all cases have cement fracture or breakdown as the underlying mechanism. Beckenbaugh and Ilstrup noted that subsidence occurred least often when all the cancellous bone is removed medially at the level of the lesser trochanter and more than 0.5 cm of cement is present and when the cancellous bone is removed along the lateral aspect of the distal two thirds of the shaft and the canal filled with cement to a level of greater than 2 cm past the tip of the femoral component.[18]

Cement Fracture. A transverse fracture through the opaque cement was noted near the tip of the femoral component in 1.5 percent of 6649 hips studied.[49] In most cases, the fracture was demonstrable within the first postoperative year (Fig. 122-12). Most (70 percent, Weber and Charnley) patients with distal cement fracture show medial migration of the proximal femoral stem ("subsidence"), thought to result from weak support by methacrylate along the proximal medial portion of the femoral stem[18,19] (see above). Cement fracture may also occur in the midstem region when there is poor support distally as well as proximally.[19] As with other findings of loosening, however, the majority of patients with cement fracture are asymptomatic.[49]

Periosteal Reaction. Cortical thickening and periosteal

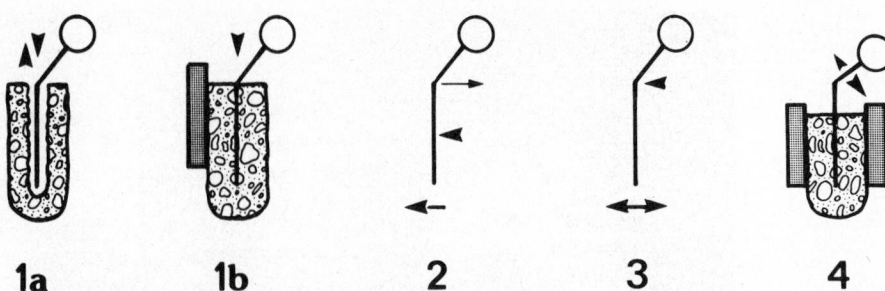

Figure 122–9. Modes of loosening. Four modes of loosening have been distinguished by Gruen, McNeice, and Amstutz. In type 1 there is pistoning of either the metal stem within the cement (*1a*) or the cement within the bone (*1b*). In type 2, there is medial migration of the proximal stem and lateral migration of the tip of the stem. Type 3 is characterized by poor support distally, the prosthesis pivoting on the medial femoral cortex. In type 4, there is poor support proximally with medial migration of the proximal stem while the distal stem remains fixed. The stem may subsequently bend or break.

reaction may occur with or without infection or loosening. Salvati and colleagues noted that in four hips with periosteal reaction near the tip of the femoral component, cortical thickening occured laterally when the stem was in varus and both medially and laterally when the stem was in neutral position.[14] Dussault et al. suggest that periosteal reaction tends to be thicker and more uniform in cases of loosening alone and moore lamellar when associated with infection.[43]

Visible Motion of Components on Radiographic Examination. Stress views (push, pull, adduction, or abduction) or fluoroscopy may demonstrate motion of one or both components (Fig. 122–13). Usually such examination is done at the time of fluoroscopy for joint aspiration and arthrography.

Osteomyelitis. Radiographic evidence of osteomyelitis, including bone destruction, sclerosis, and irregular cortical thickening is occasionally seen.[29]

Myositis Ossificans. Some studies have suggested a higher incidence of infection in patients with ectopic bone.

Arthrography. Hip aspiration and arthrography are usually indicated prior to total joint replacement when there is a history of sepsis or previous surgery and after total hip replacement if pain continues.,[42] Contrast injection permits confirmation of the intra-articular position of the needle tip as well as assessment of local anatomy. Arthrography may demonstrate loosening of prosthetic components or irregular para-articular cavities virtually diagnostic of infection.

The arthrographic technique followed at the Brigham and Women's Hospital is similar to the originally described by Salvati and colleagues,[50] except that provision is made by subtraction when this is thought to be necessary. Preliminary anteroposterior and frog lateral films that include the entire prosthesis and adjacent cement are reviewed.

The patient is placed supine on the table and, after

Figure 122–10. Loose acetabular component. *A*, Five months after THR. *B*, Five years later. Note the change in orientation of the acetabular component and fragmentation of the marker wire.

Figure 122–11. Metal-cement lucency. The femoral component has settled into a varus position with development of lucency at the metal-cement interface superolaterally (small arrows), remodeling of the lateral femoral cortex, and fracture of the distal cement (large arrow).

preparing and draping the area, 1 percent lidocaine is injected into the skin and subcutaneous tissue lateral to the femoral artery and distal to the inguinal ligament. A 20-gauge disposable, short beveled spinal needle is inserted and directed toward the neck of the prosthesis. If joint fluid can be aspirated, a sample is removed and sent for bacteriological study. If no fluid can be aspirated, sterile isotonic saline (not bacteriostatic saline or lidocaine) is injected and reaspirated in an effort to obtain material for culture. Whether or not joint fluid is aspirated, contrast is always injected. The stylet is removed, and a syringe and extension tubing with about 15 ml of Renografin-60* is attached to the needle. A few drops of contrast are then injected. If the needle is within the joint capsule, the contrast will flow away from the needle tip. A radiograph is then taken to be used for subtraction, and the patient is instructed to remain motionless. If the tip of the needle is extra-articular, the small amount of injected contrast will

remain at the tip of the needle. The needle is then repositioned.

When satisfactory needle placement is confirmed, contrast is injected under fluoroscopic monitoring until the joint appears to be full, the patient complains of pain, or there is resistance to injection. A radiograph is then taken and the needle withdrawn. Usually less than 15 ml of contrast is sufficient to fill the joint, but considerably more may be necessary. Underfilling may lead to failure to demonstrate abnormal collections of contrast or loosening of components. Once the needle has been removed, the hip is exercised and repeat anteroposterior and lateral views are taken. Anteroposterior films with traction applied to the leg may also be done. The patient is then instructed to walk around the room, and anteroposterior and lateral radiographs are repeated with additional views if necessary. Traction films[50] and films after walking[51] have, on occasion, shown evidence of loosening not demonstrable on standard views.

Subtraction technique refers to a photographic method used to eliminate densities present on both the preliminary and postinjection films so that the injected contrast will be more easily seen. Photographic subtraction is done by making a negative of the film prior to contrast injection (the "subtraction mask") and superimposing this negative on the film obtained after contrast injection.[52] This is of greatest value in patients with opaque cement around the components of total hip replacements,[50,53-55] since the injected contrast and opaque cement are of similar density (Fig. 122–14). Subtraction technique requires strict patient immobilization, and this is often difficult to maintain. In order to minimize the possibility of motion, both pre- and postinjection films to be used for subtraction are exposed after the needle has been correctly positioned.

Recently a color subtraction technique has become available. This technique utilizes filters of two opposite primary colors. The film prior to contrast injection and that following contrast injection are placed behind each of the filters, and a single superimposed image is achieved by means of a beam-splitting mirror. Objects that are identical on both films will appear gray. The injected contrast will appear in the color of the filter in front of that film. The advantages to photographic subtraction are said to be the immediate viewing of the subtracted image and decreased cost. No permanent record is made.

A normal postoperative arthrogram demonstrates filling of a small smooth "pseudojoint" space that forms within 4 to 5 months postoperatively.[6,55] Contrast parallels the neck of the prosthesis and flares out proximally under the acetabular component and distally along and sometimes under the flanges of the femoral component. In a normal postoperative arthrogram, contrast is not present between the cement and the bone. Aside from contrast just under the femoral flanges, contrast should not flow between the component and the adjacent cement.

Abnormal arthrographic findings include extension of contrast along the cement-bone or prosthesis-cement

*Renografin-60—meglumine diatrizoate. E.R. Squibb and Sons, Princeton, New Jersey.

Figure 122–12. Cement fracture. *A,* Two weeks after total hip replacement. *B,* Follow-up examination 3 years later shows medial settling of the femoral component and slight shift of the femoral stem laterally associated with cement fracture (arrow). There is bone loss from the medial femoral neck.

interface, filling of irregular cavities, and lymphatic filling (Table 122–2).[42,43,50,55,57-59]

Extension of Contrast Along the Cement–Bone or Metal–Cement Interface. Arthrography for the evaluation of patients with persistent pain after total hip replacement was introduced by Salvati, Freiberger, and Wilson in 1971.[50] Surgical or clinical confirmation of their arthrographic findings in 30 hips (31 arthrograms) revealed only one case in which a loose femoral component was not demonstrated by arthrography. The appearance of contrast material between the acrylic cement and bone seemed to be conclusive proof of loosening (Fig. 122–15). They concluded that although "a normal arthrogram does not definitely rule out the presence of a complication, a positive arthrogram appears to be diagnostic."[50]

Subsequent studies have compared arthrographic evidence of loosening (contrast at the cement–bone or metal–cement interface) with evidence of motion of components following manual stress at the time of surgical re-exploration. The results are not as optimistic as this first report suggested (Table 122–3). The study by Murray and Rodrigo in 1975 is of particular interest, since

the conclusion reached was that "arthrographic evidence of loosening may not identify the cause of pain after total hip replacement."[51] These investigators compared the arthrographic findings in 53 asymptomatic total hip prostheses (42 patients) with those in 25 painful total hip prostheses (21 patients). Arthrographic evidence of loosening of the acetabular component was noted in 22.6 percent of asymptomatic hips. No asymptomatic patients demonstrated loosening of the femoral component. Twelve patients with pain underwent reoperation. In seven patients, loosening demonstrated by arthrography was confirmed at surgery (true positive rate 78 percent).* There were three patients in whom loosening of the acetabular component was demonstrated at arthrography but not at surgery and two patients with normal arthrograms but loosening demonstrated at surgery. Thus, acetabular loosening may be asymptomatic, and loosening demonstrated on arthrography may not correlate with loosening demonstrated at the time of surgery.

---

*The authors' stated true positive rate of 58 percent is not calculated in the standard manner.

Figure 122–13. Stress views. *A*, A radiograph 2 weeks postoperatively shows a total hip prosthesis with nonopaque cement around the components. *B* and *C*, Radiographs 7½ years postoperatively show increasing lucency, particularly around the distal stem of the femoral component. "Push" (*C*) and "pull" (*B*) films confirm motion of the femoral component, most easily seen by noting the change in the distance between the flange of the prosthesis and the lesser trochanter and the change in position of the tip of the stem within the medullary canal.

Figure 122–14. Subtraction technique. *A,* Arthrogram showing lymphatic filling (arrow). Because of the opaque cement around the components, contrast around the cement or components is difficult to see. *B,* Photographic subtraction (same patient as in *A*) allows differentiation between injected contrast and opaque cement. There is no arthrographic evidence of loosening.

The accuracy of the arthrogram in demonstrating loosening is complicated by ambiguity in the term "loosening." According to Amstutz and colleagues loosening can be defined (1) in a mechanical sense, when there is inadequate bonding between materials of different elasticity; (2) radiographically, when there is a crack in methyl methacrylate or development of lucency at the metal-cement or cement-bone interface; or (3) as motion of prosthetic components, demonstrated by applying force to these components at the time of initial surgery or at reoperation.[19]

Logic suggests that contrast along the cement–bone or metal–cement interface denotes poor bonding between these materials, and in this sense they are loose. The long-term consequence of such an abnormality is still unknown. Pending the outcome of such long-term studies correlating arthrographic finding with clinical outcome, it seems prudent to carefully evaluate each arthrogram for evidence of "loosening" and to consider the arthrographic findings only in light of the patient's clinical symptoms. Demonstration of contrast at the cement–bone interface of the femoral component seems more reliable than similar findings on the acetabular side.

Filling of Irregular Para-Articular Cavities or Fistulous Tracts. These findings are considerably less controversial. The filling of irregular para-articular cavities or fistulas indicates infection. Infection was found in all five patients reviewed by Dussault and colleagues, who demonstrated filling of such cavities.[43] It should be noted, however, that infection may be present in the absence of abnormal radiographic findings (i.e., cavities, fistulas or loosening).

Lymphatic Opacification. This was seen in 12 patients studied by Dussault and colleagues. Four had no loosening or infection, three had both loosening and infection, and five had loosening only.[43] As discussed by Coren, Curtis, and Dalinka,[57] resorption of injected contrast material from normal joints occurs through venous and lymphatic channels. Lymphatic visualization may

Figure 122–15. Loosening of femoral and acetabular components. *A,* Examination 3 years after surgery shows irregular lucency around the femoral component, which was wider than that attributable to the nonopaque cement present previously. A thin zone is noted around the opaque cement of the acetabular component. *B,* Arthrography confirms loosening of both components with contrast at the cement-bone interface of each component (arrows). Note the difficulty in visualizing the contrast around the opaque acetabular cement.

Table 122–3. Correlation of Arthrographic Evidence of Loosening (With or Without Infection) With Clinical or Surgical Findings (Total Hip Replacement)

	Patients	True Positive Rate	False Positive Rate
Salvati et al., 1971[50]	29 (30 hips) 8 not loose 7 loose 9 loose and infected 2 infected not loose 3 miscellaneous conditions	16/17	0/13
Selby Brown and Knickerbocker, 1973[58]	16 surgically proved cases	13/14	1/2
Murray and Rodrigo, 1975[51]	12 with pain and reoperation	7/9	3/3
McLaughlin and Whitehill, 1977[42]	5 with acetabular loosening and re-operation	5/5	
Gelman et al., 1978[59]	9 with painful total hip replacements and surgical evidence of 14 loose components	14/14	1/4
Weighted average		55/59 = 90%	5/22 = 23%

be noted when the resorption rate is increased, apparently resulting from increased permeability of the synovial lining and hyperplasia of the lymphatic system. Although lymphatic visualization is usually associated with rheumatoid arthritis, these workers suggest that it is a nonspecific sign of inflammation.

Arthrography following total hip prostheses may also demonstrate filling of the trochanteric bursa suggesting trochanteric bursitis, occult fracture of the femoral stem,[42] nonunion of the greater trochanter,[55] and postoperative hematoma preventing reduction of a dislocated femoral component.[55]

Scintigraphy. Bone scanning has evolved as a reliable technique for the evaluation of patients with pain following total hip arthroplasty. Campeau, Hall, and Miale performed serial[99m] technetium bone scans on patients undergoing total hip replacement[60] and found increased isotopic activity in the acetabular and femoral shaft regions in all patients during the first 3 months. By 6 months the activity returned to normal levels in patients without complication. Patients with increased activity 6 months or more postoperatively all had loosening and/or infection, and often the routine radiographs were normal. No patient with a proved complication had a normal scan. Similarly, Feith and colleagues used [87m]strontium scans to evaluate patients with pain following total hip arthroplasty and showed that patients with positive scans generally went on to require surgery while patients with normal scans responded to conservative therapy with gradual diminution in symptoms.[61] Thus, a negative scan virtually excludes the presence of significant loosening or infection.[62,63] A few false-negative studies, are, however, reported, particularly on the acetabular side.[45,59,63]

The distribution of abnormal isotopic activity may help distinguish between infection and aseptic loosening.[64] Focal uptake at the proximal and distal ends of the femoral component suggests aseptic loosening with high reliability. In contrast, diffuse uptake around the femoral component or diffuse activity around both the femoral and acetabular components suggests infection.[64] In one series, this diffuse uptake pattern about both components correctly identified all infected prostheses.[45] Teranzedeh and colleagues, therefore, suggest that evaluation for pain following total joint replacement consists of standard radiographs followed by bone scanning.[45] Joint aspiration and arthrography are then suggested only in cases in which diffuse isotopic uptake is present, raising the possibility of infection.

Gallium accumulation in inflammatory conditions is largely due to uptake by leukocytes, although uptake by various bacteria has also been demonstrated. [67]Gallium scans must be correlated with the [99m]technetium bone scan, since the factors that increase the uptake of bone tracer will also increase the uptake of gallium. When an "incongruent" distribution of gallium with relation to the technetium bone scan (that is, gallium uptake in areas that are not "hot" on bone scan) or intense uptake of gallium as well as technetium phosphate complexes is present, infection is suggested. Thus,

a study of patients with different types of orthopedic hardware using both [67]gallium and [99m]technetium methylene diphosphonate scans allowed three groups to be distinguished.[65] In the first group, the gallium image was negative and the technetium bone scan was positive or negative; none of these patients had inflammatory disease. In the second group, the gallium scan was positive but its distribution was similar to the uptake on bone scan. Fifteen of these 16 patients had no inflammatory disease and the sixteenth had a sterile bursitis. In the third group, the gallium scan was positive in an "incongruent" spatial distribution in comparison with the technetium bone scan; all 18 patients had inflammatory disorders, including osteomyelitis, cellulitis, and nonseptic synovitis. Similarly, Reing and colleagues noted positive gallium citrate scans in 18 of 19 patients subsequently proven at surgery to be infected.[66] There were no false-positive gallium scans.

[111]*Indium*-labeled leukocytes have been used with some success to identify infection following total hip replacement.[67] In comparison with [67]gallium citrate, [111]indium-labeled white cells have better imaging characteristics and a higher ratio of abscess to blood activity.

Femoral Stem Fractures. Fractures of the femoral component usually are fatigue fractures, resulting from poor support of the femoral stem. As summarized by Bechtol,[34] poor blood supply to the medial femoral neck results in loosening of the cement-bone bond and bone resorption of the proximal femur medially. The resulting stress placed on the unsupported cement may lead to cement fracture and medial and/or distal migration of the femoral stem and cement ("subsidence"). Subsequent fracture of the cement near the tip or the neck of the femoral component may result in further shift of the prosthesis and additional stress on the femoral stem. Over months or years there is widening of the cement–metal lucency along the lateral aspect of the femoral component. The end result of continued unsupported weight bearing by the femoral component may be bending or fracture of the femoral stem.

Several radiographic findings document the aforementioned sequence of events and should suggest the need for careful follow-up examination and the search for small defects in the continuity of the femoral component. Thus, early breakage of trochanter wires, resorption of bone along the medial femoral neck, the appearance of a metal–cement lucency along the proximal femoral component laterally, widening of the cement–bone lucency laterally, and cement fracture may all precede fracture of the femoral stem. The actual fracture may be very difficult to demonstrate, however (Fig. 122–16).

Factors thought to be associated with increased risk of stem fracture[34,68,69] include lack of valgus position of the femoral component, inadequate cement support, metallurgical imperfections in the prosthesis, and increased patient height and/or weight.

Femoral and Pelvic Fractures. Femoral fractures may occur intraoperatively and are occasionally difficult to recognize on the anteroposterior examination done with

Figure 122–16. Femoral stem fracture. *A*, A metal-cement lucency is present due to settling of the femoral component. The stem fracture (arrow) is difficult to see and was missed on initial evaluation. *B*, The stem fracture is now obvious (arrow).

a mobile x-ray unit. Opaque cement in the soft tissue adjacent to the femoral shaft indicates the presence of a fracture and suggests the need for additional views. Penetration of the femoral cortex by the tip of the prosthesis may also be associated with methyl methacrylate in the soft tissues and may result in apparent foreshortening of the stem of the femoral component on frontal radiographs.

Defects in the inner wall of the acetabulum occurring during preparation of the acetabular bed are identified on postoperative x-rays by visualization of a mass of opaque cement in the pelvic cavity (Fig. 122–17). Usually this extravasation is asymptomatic; however, cases of sciatic nerve entrapment,[70] femoral artery damage[71] or occlusion,[72] defects in the sigmoid colon associated with transient abdominal cramps and bloody diarrhea,[73] bladder fistula,[74] and dyspareunia[75] have been reported in association with extravasation of methyl methacrylate into the pelvis. Of particular note are four patients, reported by Greenspan and Norman, who developed gross hematuria and dysuria 1 to 2 weeks following total hip replacement.[76] These patients had extravasation of cement into the pelvis and urographic examination confirming extrinsic impression on the urinary bladder by

the mass of methyl methacrylate. Symptoms were thought to be related to inflammatory changes in the bladder owing to local temperature increases associated with the polymerization of methyl methacrylate. The symptoms disappeared rapidly with conservative therapy.

Postoperative fractures have been divided into three categories by McElfresh and Coventry:[77] stress fractures, fractures caused by stress raisers in the femoral shaft, and fractures caused by severe trauma.

Stress fractures occur in patients with severe osteopenia, such as those with longstanding rheumatoid arthritis.[78] These fractures appear to be related to the increased activity made possible by joint replacement, and, as such, they should probably be termed "insufficiency" fractures, since they are the result of normal stresses applied to abnormal bone.

The second type of fracture results from local factors that increase stress at a particular point. For example, fractures may occur following relatively minor trauma if there is any defect in the femoral cortex, such as might be produced during reaming of the femur in an osteoporotic patient, or by prior surgery (i.e., a screwhole). McElfresh and Coventry recommend having methyl

Figure 122–17. Cement extravasation into the pelvis. This is an unusual example of massive extravasation of cement into the pelvis. The medial lucent zone within the cement appears to be bone graft.

methacrylate around the tip of the prosthesis and extending at least 2 cm distally in order to prevent undue stress concentration at the tip of the prosthesis.

The third category of fracture occurs following trauma sufficient to fracture a normal limb. Since the endosteal blood supply has been compromised by the surgical procedure, fractures occuring near a femoral component are often treated with closed reduction if adequate alignment and apposition of fracture fragments can be achieved. Open reduction with stripping of the periosteum may jeopardize the blood supply to the proximal fragment.[77] Methyl methacrylate does not appear to interfere with fracture healing.

Para-Articular Ossification. Bone develops within para-articular soft tissues in up to 39 percent of patients following total hip replacement.[14] Although in most instances this appears to be of little clinical consequence, Beckenbaugh and Ilstrup have noted lower hip scores in these patients.[18] In a few patients, surgical intervention is necessary to remove ectopic bone if it significantly interferes with joint motion.

The cause of this bone formation is obscure. It is histologically similar to that resulting from other causes of ectopic bone (i.e., myositis ossificans progressiva or the para-osteoarthropathy seen in patients with paraplegia) and trabecular bone eventually develops. Radiologic examination shows irregular, poorly defined densities developing 2 to 3 weeks postoperatively, primarily in the region of the abductor muscles[79] (Fig. 122–18). Progression to complete bony bridging may occur in about 12 weeks. The amount of ectopic bone that is present has been graded on the basis of standard radiographs as:[80]

Class 1: Islands of bone within the soft tissues

Class 2: Bony projections from the pelvis or proximal femur with 1 cm between bony margins

Class 3: Less than 1 cm remaining between opposing bony surfaces

Class 4: Apparent bony ankylosis

Bone scanning has been shown to demonstrate para-articular ossification prior to its appearance on radiographs.[81] Tanaka and colleagues performed serial ^{99m}technetium polyphosphate bone scans on quadriplegic and paraplegic patients with para-articular ossification in an effort to gauge the maturity of the heterotopic bone.[82] Isotopic uptake in the area of heterotopic bone was compared to a control area (i.e., spine, sacrum, or ilium), and this ratio was followed with time. It was suggested that surgical removal of ectopic bone should be done after 2 to 3 months of steady uptake in order to decrease the incidence of recurrent ossification. No assessment of bone maturity could be made from a single examination. Application of these data to patients with total joint replacement has not been reported.

TOTAL KNEE REPLACEMENT

The aim of total knee joint replacement is to create a painless and stable joint which allows both rotatory and flexion-extension motion.[83] Normal knee motion is complex, including flexion-extension motion with a changing center of rotation, abduction-adduction motion, and axial rotation with the tibia rotating externally on the femur on extension ("screw home mechanism").[84,85] The difficult problem of duplicating such complex motion and maintaining stability using a prosthetic joint has led to the development of many different prostheses and ongoing investigation in the field.

Three major types of total knee prostheses (TKP) may be distinguished by the degree of stability they provide.[85] In the first group, the prosthesis provides no constraint (stability) or minimal constraint to knee motion (e.g., polycentric and modular prostheses). Joint stability will depend on ligamentous and capsular structures. The second group of prostheses produces partial constraint (geometric, UCI, Freeman-Swanson). With these prostheses the fit of the prosthetic surfaces to each other provides some stability. In the third group of prostheses, stability is provided totally by the prosthesis rather than the patient's ligamentous or capsular structures. This group includes the hinge prostheses (Guepar, Walldius, and Shiers hinge prostheses) and the spherocentric knee.

Unconstrained or Partially Constrained Prostheses. The unconstrained or partially constrained prostheses are made of stainless steel or chrome-cobalt–nickel alloy femoral components and high density polyethylene tibial components. "Total knee arthroplasties" may or may not include revision of the patellofemoral joint. If the patellofemoral joint is replaced (such as in the total condylar prosthesis), a polyethylene button is used to replace the articular surface of the patella and the femoral groove is an extension of the femoral prosthesis.

Geometric TKP. According to Lotke and Ecker,[86] a perfectly positioned geometric prosthesis has overall knee alignment of 3 to 7 degrees of valgus, with the

Figure 122–18. Ectopic ossification. *A*, A radiograph at 3 weeks shows early calcification within soft tissues. *B*, Examination 1 year postoperatively shows mature bone.

tibial component perfectly horizontal in both anteroposterior and lateral planes, the femoral component in 4 to 6 degrees of valgus, and the femoral and tibial components centered in the midline of the joint. On the lateral view the prosthetic femoral condyles should lie posterior to a line drawn down the anterior cortex of the femur,[87] and the flat portion of the femoral unit should form an angle of 60 degrees with the longitudinal axis of the femur (Fig. 122–19).[88]

Polycentric TKP. The polycentric prosthesis attempts to recreate normal knee motion. The modified polycentric prosthesis consists of two-chrome-cobalt semicircular runners and two ultrahigh molecular weight polyethylene tracks. The medial femoral component is placed as close to the intercondylar notch as possible, and the anterior portion is positioned more medially than the posterior portion. The lateral femoral component is centered in the lateral condyle.[87] On the lateral view the femoral components should not extend past the anterior surface of the condyle, and there should be an angle of approximately 40 degrees between the flat (nonarticular) surface of the component and the femoral shaft.

The tibial components of the polycentric total knee

prosthesis can be differentiated on the lateral radiograph, since one of them has a straight wire embedded longitudinally and the other has a curved wire located perpendicular to the long axis of the prosthesis at its midpoint. The medial tibial component is set farther posteriorly than the lateral one. Varus or valgus deformities can be corrected by using larger or smaller components or by removing more or less bone before insertion.

Newer TKPs. At present, several other prostheses are being used at the Brigham and Women's Hospital, most frequently the RBBH and kinematic. With these prostheses, as with most other newer models (Figs. 122–20 and 122–21), several radiographic features should be noted. Standing frontal radiographs should show the overall knee alignment to be about 7 degrees of valgus, and this should not change on serial examinations with weight bearing. Most of the valgus is due to valgus positioning of the femoral component. The tibial components should be parallel to the ground on anteroposterior view and parallel or sloping backward up to 10 degrees in the lateral view. Alignment of the knee in relation to the hip and ankle can best be appreciated on

Figure 122–19. Geometric total knee prosthesis. The tibial component is tipped more anteriorly than usual as documented by its greater than 90 degree angle with the tibial shaft. There is marked patellofemoral cartilage space narrowing. *A*, Anteroposterior. *B*, Lateral projection.

3-foot long films taken at a 72-inch tube-film distance.[89] The center of the knee should be in line with the centers of the femoral head and ankle. The tibial component should be perpendicular to this axis (Fig. 122–22). The positions of the components should remain unchanged on serial examinations. Tangential patellar views should be routinely obtained and should show a fairly good fit

Figure 122–20. Duopatellar total knee prosthesis. An extension of the prosthesis is present to articulate with the patella. Single or separate (shown) polyethylene tibial components may be used. The tibial components in this case are tipped centrally. A patellar prosthesis is present, and its articular surface shows the decreased radiographic density of high density polyethylene in comparison to the adjacent soft tissues.

of the patella into the femoral groove with a thin cartilage space remaining.

Thin cement bone lucent zones occur fairly often along parts of the tibial cement–bone interface but usually do not involve its entire length (Table 122–4). Cement–bone lucencies are considerably less frequent around the femoral component.[90,91]

Complications of Total Knee Replacement. *Loosening* (Table 122–5). Gradual or abrupt loosening of prosthetic components accounts for the largest number of failures of total knee replacement.[85] Loosening usually involves the tibial components and usually occurs at the cement–bone interface. As in patients with total hip replacements, a thin lucency may develop at the cement–bone interface in asymptomatic individuals. Ducheyne and colleagues studied 100 patients with UCI total knee replacements and noted the development of lucency at the cement–bone interface greater than 2mm in thickness in 14 patients with satisfactory clinical results[89] and in all seven patients requiring revision for loose tibial components. The seven patients with loose tibial prostheses had an increase in the width and length of this lucent zone with time, with a thickness of 2 to 3 mm present at the time of revision. As in patients with total hip replacement, a cement-bone lucency may be present on the immediate postoperative examination. Ducheyne and associates noted this to be a more frequent finding in patients who go on to loosening than in control patients.[92]

In addition to widening of the cement-bone lucency,

Figure 122–21. Total knee prosthesis. *A*, Kinematic. (Left, anteroposterior; right, lateral.) *B*, Stabilocondylar. (Left, anteroposterior; right, lateral.)

Figure 122–22. The mechanical axis. The components of the total knee prosthesis should be perpendicular to the mechanical axis of the leg, drawn from the epicenter of the femoral head to the midpoint of the tibial plafond. This line should fall at the center of the knee.

Table 122–5. Findings Suggesting Loosening of Total Knee Prostheses

Plain films
1. Cement-bone lucency > 2 mm
2. Increasing cement-bone lucency
3. Collapse of underlying trabecular bone or cement
4. Change in position of a component
5. Change in the varus or valgus angle
6. Development of metal–cement lucency

Arthrography
   Contrast along the cement–bone interface

Scintigraphy
   Increased isotopic uptake (?after 6 months)

nation is preferred (i.e., Renografin-60 or -76) and no attempt is made to remove all the joint fluid. Instead, a sample of joint fluid is aspirated and sent to the laboratory for culture, and contrast is then injected until the suprapatellar pouch is full (at least 15 ml).[93] The needle is then removed. If subtraction is to be done, anteroposterior films are taken immediately before and after contrast injection. The knee is flexed and extended several times and films are taken in the anteroposterior projection with and without traction, in both oblique projections, and in the flexed and extended lateral positions. Additional films after walking are obtained if no abnormality is detected on the first films. Contrast filling the cement-bone lucency indicates an abnormal bond at this interface (Fig. 122–25). In patients with draining sinus tracts, it has been noted that contrast injection directly into the tract usually, but not always, demonstrates any communication with the joint. In cases in which such a communication is suspected, and in which the sinogram reveals no communication, arthrography is also indicated.[89]

Bone scanning with ^{99m}Tc phosphate complex can also demonstrate loosening or infection. Since the cement–bone interface of the femoral component may be difficult to see radiographically, isotope study seems particularly valuable in this area.[59] Increased isotopic uptake over the femoral component on anterior scans may be due to patellar damage, and a lateral scan should be done to confirm the location of such increased activity. According to Schneider and colleagues mild to moderate increase in isotopic uptake may persist for years after total knee arthroplasty even without apparent complication.[89] Such increased uptake is, therefore, nondiagnostic. A normal scan is, however, good evidence that neither loosening nor infection is present.

Infection. Deep sepsis is the second most frequent cause of failure of total knee replacements and, as in total hip replacements, may be immediate or delayed. Radiographic evidence of loosening and soft tissue swelling may indicate infection.

Separation of Marker Wires. Posterior displacement of a radiographic wire marker from the undersurface of a tibial plateau component of a geometric total knee replacement has been reported.[94] The prothesis itself was not loose. The design of the marker wires has since been changed to avoid this.

collapse of underlying trabecular bone, fragmentation of underlying cement, change in the position of a component (Fig. 122–23), and change in the degree of varus or valgus position on weight-bearing views are radiographic features suggesting loosening. Medial or lateral tilt of the tibial component was a more frequent finding in patients who went on to develop loosening.[92] Occasionally loosening may occur at the metal-cement interface of the femoral component, as seen in the patient in Figure 122–24.

Preliminary investigation has shown both arthrography and scintigraphy to be useful in documenting loosening or infection.[93] In contrast to arthrography done for the study of meniscal tears, single contrast exami-

Table 122–4. Incidence of Radiolucent Lines at The Cement–Bone Interface*

	Tibial Lucency > 2 mm (percent)	Femoral Lucency (percent)
Anametric	28	14
Total Condylar	41	8.6
Duopatellar	24[†]	
Variable Axis	74	
Spherocentric	42.5	10

*From references 90 and 91.

[†]Three other patients with lucencies > 1 mm.

Figure 122–23. Loose tibial component of duopatellar total knee prosthesis. The medial tibial component has dislocated posteriorly. The lateral component is tipped slightly medially, a more frequent finding in patients who go on to loosening. *A*, Anteroposterior view. *B*, Lateral projection.

Patellar Complications. Following total knee replacements with or without resurfacing of the femoral aspect of the patellofemoral joint, tangential patellar views should show the patella to fit fairly well within the femoral articular groove. Follow-up examination has shown several complications related to the patellofemoral joint, including progressive damage to the articular surface and subchondral bone of the patella, patellar dislocation, and catching of the patella on an overhanging shelf of anterior femoral condyle[88] or on an anteriorly positioned femoral component. Replacement of the articular surface of the patella may be complicated by fracture near or loosening of the prosthesis (Fig. 122–26). Decreased patellar blood flow after extensive lateral release has been documented by scanning and is felt to contribute to the development of postoperative patellar stress fracture.[91]

Fractures. Fractures related to trauma, osteoporotic bone, or abnormal localization of applied stress (such as at the ends of intramedullary rods).[91] may all be seen in patients with total knee replacements. Subtle change in the position of one of the components may be the only sign of fracture.

Component Fracture. Component fracture is very uncommon. Deformation of the tibial component did occur, however, in 11 percent of cases in one series[91] and may be asymptomatic or associated with loosening or angular deformity. Metal backing of the tibial component is expected to decrease the incidence of this complication.

Hinge Total Knee Protheses. Hinge prostheses (e.g., Walldius, Shiers, and Guepar) both resurface the joint and provide stability. Since these units are rigid and do not duplicate normal knee motion, they are subjected to considerable stress that may loosen the prosthesis or fracture adjacent bone. Hinge prostheses are therefore used only in patients with limited activity demands and marked instability or as a salvage procedure following other types of knee replacement.[95]

Radiographic examination should show the hinge to be parallel to the ground on weight-bearing views. Sclerosis of the weight-bearing bone adjacent to the femoral and tibial components is a usual finding on long-term follow-up examination.[96] Settling of the components into the femur and/or tibia also occurs frequently in uncemented prostheses; if this is asymmetrical, gradually increasing deformity may result.

Complications include loosening, infection, metal synovitis, fracture of bone or prosthesis, patellar subluxation or damage, and tendon rupture. A 2- to 3-mm lucent zone (indicating loosening) is routinely seen around the stems of uncemented Walldius prostheses followed 5 years or longer.[96,97] According to Merryweather and Jones, this loosening is not only the rule but is "necessary for a hinge prosthesis to destress itself."[97] More motion than this should be evaluated clinically, since it may be associated with symptoms and require reoperation. Components fixed with cement should not demonstrate any evidence of motion. As in total hip replacement with opaque cement, a wide lucency at the cement–bone interface or widening of a thin lucent zone is suspicious. Stress films may help demonstrate gross motion of components, and in some cases arthrography is useful. Evidence of loosening or continued synovitis should raise

Figure 122–24. Loose femoral component of a duopatellar total knee prosthesis. *A,* Examination at 1 week postoperatively shows good position of components with no evidence of loosening. *B,* At 2 years postoperatively there is beginning separation of the retropatellar flange from the underlying cement. *C,* At 3 years this separation is obvious and there is rotation of the femoral component posteriorly. Severe changes have occurred in the articular surface of the patella.

Figure 122–25. Loose tibial component of lateral total knee replacement. *A,* There is an abnormally wide lucency at the cement-bone interface of the tibial component. *B,* The lucent zone fills with contrast at arthrography (arrow).

Figure 122–26. Patellar fracture. A fracture has occurred just above the patellar prosthesis (arrow).

the possibility of infection. Scott noted a 2 percent incidence of infection that increased to about 12 percent on continued follow-up.[91]

Fractures may occur intraoperatively or postoperatively. When the Walldius prosthesis is inserted, fracture of the anterior-medial femoral cortex may occur since the knee is often in valgus but the prosthesis is straight. According to Wilson,[96] this complication does not adversely affect the clinical outcome. Stress fractures (insufficiency fractures) may occur as a consequence of increased mobility in an osteoporotic patient. Post-traumatic fractures in patients with uncemented prostheses may occur near the tips of the prosthesis owing to transmission of stress along the stem.[93]

Quadriceps and patellar tendon ruptures have been seen in association with hinge prostheses (Fig. 122–27). A localized soft tissue mass with obliteration of adjacent fat lines and change in the position of the patella may be noted. The normal tendon shadow is not seen. Calcification within the tendon, such as has been noted in post-traumatic rupture of the quadriceps tendon, is occasionally seen.[98]

McKeever and MacIntosh Hemiarthroplasty. Prior to the current generation of metal-to-plastic total knee prostheses, several attempts at joint resurfacing were made. Tibial resurfacing with McKeever or MacIntosh prostheses is still occasionally done, particularly in patients with osteoarthritis with failed osteotomy or contraindications to osteotomy and those too young or too heavy for total joint replacement.[91] Therefore, a brief description of these prostheses is in order. The more frequently used McKeever prosthesis consists of a semicircular Vitallium disc with a smooth concave upper

Figure 122–27. Patellar tendon rupture. A cemented Guepar prosthesis is in place. There is calcification of the patellar tendon (arrow) and marked elevation of the patella as compared to earlier radiographs.

surface and a T-shaped fin projecting from the inferior surface (Fig. 122–28). Several thicknesses of the prosthesis are available to allow correction of varus or valgus deformity. The MacIntosh prosthesis has a flat inferior surface with multiple serrations. The prosthesis is made in several thicknesses and in different sizes to cover the surfaces of the tibial plateau and correct angular deformity. Methyl methacrylate is not routinely used in the insertion of these prostheses.

Both prostheses are placed so that they "toe-in" at approximately 10 degrees to the sagittal plane, and, therefore, frontal views will not show these devices exactly in profile. Both types of prostheses are theoretically inserted so that they are horizontal to the ground on both the frontal and lateral projections. They should not extend medially or laterally beyond the margins of the tibial condyles. On lateral view, the McKeever prostheses should extend to or slightly beyond the anterior margins of the tibial plateaus. Flexion and extension lateral views can allow measurement of the shift in the relative positions of the two prostheses. Kay and Martins described the radiological findings following MacIntosh prostheses and noted that some motion (less than 10 percent) occurred in "most" patients.[99] Follow-up examinations in patients with McKeever arthroplasties often show a thin lucency under the prosthesis and the fin of the prosthesis with a subjacent thin zone of sclerosis. Sclerosis, irregularity, and loss of volume of the femoral condyles may be noted. Such collapse of the femoral condyles or collapse of the bone supporting the prostheses has been noted by Anderson et al. to be associated with a poor result following MacIntosh hemiarthroplasty.[100]

TOTAL SHOULDER REPLACEMENT

Total shoulder replacement is a relatively recent technique used primarily in patients with incapacitating pain and secondarily for improvement in function. Normally, the stability of the glenohumeral joint is provided largely by the joint capsule and rotator cuff.[101] Since some of the diseases treated with these prostheses (e.g., rheumatoid arthritis) have associated damage to these structures, they must either be repaired or their functions replaced or augmented by the prosthesis. Cofield has categorized the currently available prostheses into three groups:[101] (1) prostheses that replace the articular surfaces of the joint (e.g., Neer II); (2) prostheses that replace the articular surfaces and provide some additional stability; and (3) prostheses that replace the articular surface and replace the constraining functions of the soft tissue (i.e., the Stanmore and Michael Reese prostheses).

The Neer prosthesis is the one most frequently used at the Brigham and Women's Hospital. It consists of a chromium-cobalt humeral component (the revised humeral component used in hemiarthroplasty) and a dish-shaped high density polyethylene glenoid component which is fixed into the glenoid with methyl methacrylate. Osteotomy of the greater tuberosity may rarely be required.

Postoperative radiographic examination should include a posterior oblique view (approximately 45 degrees) to evaluate the components in profile, as well as an internal rotation and axillary view. Usually, the inferior aspect of the humeral component is aligned to the inferior edge of the glenoid component. The humeral component is placed as in a hemiarthroplasty so that the edge of the head of the prosthesis is parallel to the cut surface of the neck and the mesh holes are well seated in cancellous bone (Fig. 122–29).[102]

Complications that may be detected radiographically include dislocation, upward subluxation of the humeral component (especially frequent in patients with rheumatoid arthritis), heterotopic bone formation, and widening of the cement-bone lucency around the glenoid component indicative of loosening or infection (Fig. 122–30).

Figure 122–28. McKeever tibial plateau prosthesis. Some roughening, sclerosis, and volume loss of the femoral condyles have occurred. *A*, Anteroposterior view. *B*, Lateral view.

TOTAL ELBOW PROSTHESES

Total elbow prostheses are currently being developed for use in patients with severe sequelae of rheumatoid arthritis or post-traumatic arthritis. Most total elbow prostheses are of the hinge type. The early models (e.g.,

Figure 122–29. Total shoulder prosthesis. The posterior oblique view shows each component in profile. There is a thin lucency at the cement-bone interface of the glenoid component. Severe changes of rheumatoid arthritis are present in the clavicle and acromion.

Dee, Shiers, and McKee) are metal-to-metal hinge protheses which are fixed to bone using methyl methacrylate.[103,104] Later hinge prostheses include the Mayo,[105] which replaces both the humeroulnar and radiohumeral joints; the Coonrad; the Schlein metal-to-polyethylene hinge; and the GSB metal-to-metal hinge. Long-term results are still not available, but the primary cause of failure appears to be loosening, seen on radiographs as widening of the cement-bone lucency (Fig. 122–31).

The Pritchard-Walker humeroulnar hinge prosthesis has a metal-to-polyethylene interface and looseness built into the hinge to lessen the possibility of component loosening.[106] The Ewald capitellocondylar prosthesis is a nonconstrained prosthesis consisting of separate metallic humeral and high density polyethylene ulnar components (Fig. 122–32). This type of prosthesis does have a lower rate of loosening than do constrained prostheses[107] (Fig. 122–33). Dislocation of the components may occur, however and fractures of the olecranon process are also seen (Fig. 122–34).[106]

TOTAL ANKLE PROSTHESES

Normally, the tibiotalar, subtalar, and midtarsal joints function together to allow motion in three planes.[108] The tibiotalar articulation itself provides only flexion and extension motion. Ten degrees of extension (dorsiflexion) and 25 degrees of flexion (plantar flexion) are said to be necessary for normal gait.[109]

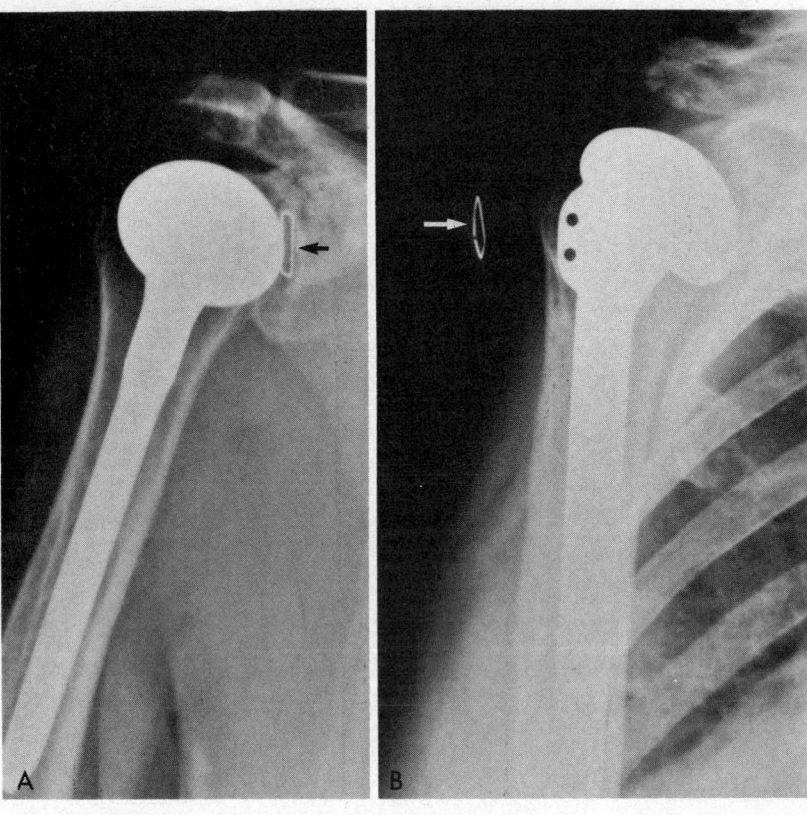

Figure 122–30. Loose, displaced glenoid component. *A*, Postoperative film shows no apparent complication. The glenoid marker wire is seen (arrow). *B*, Routine follow-up examination shows displacement of the glenoid component (arrow) so that it now lies within the lateral soft tissues (most likely within the subdeltoid bursa).

As summarized by Demottaz and colleagues, two main types of total ankle replacement are available.[110] The first type, a multiaxis joint, allows rotation of the tibial component in any of the three major axes and unrestricted rotation (Waugh, Smith). The second type of prosthesis (a single-axis joint) allows only flexion-extension motion (Mayo, TPR, Bucholz, Oregon).

Some of the prostheses in use currently are shown in Figures 122–35 and 122–36. The tibial component is inserted so that it is perpendicular to the long axis of the tibia with the foot in neutral position.[111] The talar component is then positioned parallel to the tibial component. Complications include loosening (usually at the cement–bone interface), infection, impingement between

Figure 122–31. Loose hinge total elbow prosthesis. There is marked resorption of bone at the cement-bone interface. *A*, Lateral projection. *B*, Anteroposterior projection.

Figure 122–32. Ewald total elbow prosthesis. The medial portion of the metallic humeral component articulates with the high density polyethylene ulnar component. Opaque cement fixes the components and makes the nonopaque stem of the ulnar component easily visible. *A*, Anteroposterior view. *B*, Lateral view.

A

B

A

B

Figure 122–33. Loose Ewald prosthesis. *A*, There is a wide lucency around the cement of the ulnar component. *B*, Arthrography confirms loosening of the ulnar component. The humeral component is not loose.

Figure 122–34. Olecranon fracture. The fracture through the olecranon process (arrow) has resulted in a change in the orientation of the olecranon component with dislocation of the humeral component anteriorly.

the talus and the lateral malleolus, fracture of the medial malleolus at the time of surgery, and instability.

HAND PROSTHESES

Silicone rubber prostheses are used primarily in the hand and wrist to replace damaged carpal, metacarpophalangeal, or interphalangeal joints. The metacarpophalangeal joints are the most frequently replaced, and the Swanson and Niebauer prostheses are the most frequently used prostheses.

The Swanson silicone rubber prosthesis (Fig. 122–37) consists of a single Silastic component with a central curved section and a stem on each end. Joint motion results both from the hinge action of the central portion of the prosthesis and from pistoning of the stem within the bone.[112] Eventually a joint capsule develops around the prosthesis so that stability can be maintained following implant removal or fracture.

The stems of the Niebauer prosthesis are coated with Dacron mesh, which is gradually infiltrated by bone. Since the stems become fixed within the medullary canal, all finger motion will be the result of the hinge action of the mid-portion of the prosthesis.

Postoperative radiographs will demonstrate the degree of correction of deformity, the positions of the components, and most complications. Silicone rubber is only slightly more dense than soft tissue and will be quite difficult to see. On the frontal view, the hinge portion of the prosthesis appears rectangular and the long axis

Figure 122–35. Mayo total ankle prosthesis. There is a thin lucent zone under the tibial component on the anteroposterior (*A*) radiograph.

Figure 122–36. Loosening of Smith total ankle prosthesis. *A*, Immediate postoperative film. *B*, Nine months postoperatively there is loosening of the tibial component. *C* and *D*, Replacement with Waugh prosthesis. The metallic tibial component has a polyethylene articular surface.

Figure 122–37. Swanson metacarpophalangeal prosthesis. *A,* Lateral view. *B,* Anterior surface. *C,* Posterior surface.

Figure 122–38. Dislocation of the stems of metacarpophalangeal prostheses. The stems of several of the Swanson prostheses have pulled out of the intramedullary canals (arrows).

Figure 122–39. Infected metacarpophalangeal prosthesis. *A,* Periosteal reaction, bone destruction, and development of a sequestrum are noted around the middle finger metacarpophalangeal prosthesis. *B,* There is evidence of healing following removal of the prosthesis.

of the rectangle is parallel to the resection margin of the metacarpal. The dense band is located proximally. The lateral view shows that the concavity of the hinge is directed anteriorly, and the proximal portion of the stem protrudes 1 to 2 mm from the cut surface of the bone. In our experience, a very thin periosteal reaction may develop along the metacarpals close to the resection margin without any other radiographic evidence of infection.

Complications include loss of correction of deformity, development of rotational deformity, subluxation or dislocation, fracture of the prosthesis, slipping of a stem out of the medullary canal (Fig. 122–38), and infection.[112,113] Fracture usually occurs at the base of the distal stem and may be associated with the development of instability and subluxation or dislocation. Satisfactory function may continue after fracture of a prosthesis, particularly with the Swanson prosthesis, which functions as a "dynamic spacer" rather than as a fixed hinge.

Infection is an uncommon complication (<1 percent)[113,114] and is suggested on radiographs by increasing soft tissue swelling, osteoporosis, periosteal reaction, and bone destruction (Fig. 122–39).

References

1. Harris, W.H.: Total joint replacement. N. Engl. J. Med. 297:650, 1977.
2. Gilula, L.A., and Staple, T.W.: Miniature atlas of total hip prostheses. Radiol. Clin. North Am. 13:21, 1975.
3. Symposium on Surface Replacement Arthroplasty of the Hip. Steinberg, M.E. (ed.) Orthop. Clin. North Am. Philadelphia, W.B. Saunders Co., 1982.
4. Giliberty, R.P.: Low friction bipolar hip endoprosthesis, Int. Surg. 62:38, 1977.
5. Drinker, H., and Mall, J.C.: Radiologic aspects of the new universal proximal femoral hip prosthesis. Am. J. Roentgenol. 129:531, 1977.
6. Beabout, J.W.: Radiology of total hip arthroplasty. Radiol. Clin. North Am. 13:3, 1975.
7. Matisonn, A., and Weber, F.A.: Radiological assessment of the Charnley total hip arthroplasty. S. Afr. Med. J. 49:1299, 1975.
8. Pepper, H.W., and Noonan, C.D.: Radiographic evaluation of total hip arthroplasty. Radiology 108:23, 1973.
9. McLaren, R.H.: Prosthetic hip angulation. Radiology 107:705, 1973.
10. Goergen, T.G., and Resnick, D.: Evaluation of acetabular anteversion following total hip arthroplasty: Necessity of proper centring. Br. J. Radiol. 48:259, 1975.
11. Pettersson, H., Gentz, C.-F., Lindberg, H.O., and Carlsson, A.S.: Radiologic evaluation of the position of the acetabular component of the total hip prosthesis. Acta Radiol. Diag. 23:259, 1982.
12. Fackler, C.D., and Poss, R.: Dislocation in total hip arthroplasties. Clin. Orthop. Rel. Res. 151:169, 1980.
13. Ghelman, B.: Radiographic localization of the acetabular component of a hip prosthesis. Radiology 130:540, 1979.
14. Salvati, E.A., Im, V.C., Aglietti, P., and Wilson, P.D., Jr.: Radiology of total hip replacements. Clin. Orthop. 121:74, 1976.
15. Magilligan, D.J.: Calculation of the angle of anteversion by means of horizontal lateral roentgenography. J. Bone Joint Surg. 38A:1231, 1956.
16. Gore, D.R., Murray, M.P., Gardner, G.M., and Sepic, S.B.: Roentgenographic measurements after Muller total hip replacement. J. Bone Joint Surg. 59A:948, 1977.
17. Riley, L.H., Jr., and Hughes, J.L.: Total replacement of the hip joint. Surg. Ann. 5:157, 1973.
18. Beckenbaugh, R.D., and Ilstrup, D.M.: Total hip arthroplasty. A review of 333 cases with long follow-up. J. Bone joint Surg. 60A:306, 1978.
19. Amstutz, H.C., Markolf, K.L., McNeice, G.M., and Gruen, T.A.: Loosening of total hip components: Cause and prevention. Proceedings, fourth open scientific meeting of the Hip Society, 1976, p. 102.
20. Harris, W.H., McCarthy, J.C., Jr., and O'Neill, D.A.: Femoral component loosening using contemporary techniques of femoral cement fixation. J. Bone Joint Surg. 64A:1063, 1982.
21. Freitag, T.A., and Cannon, S.L.: Fracture characteristics of acrylic bone cements. I. Fracture toughness. J. Biomed. Mater. Res. 10:805, 1976.
22. Radin, E.L., Paul, I.L., Rose, R.M., et al.: Wear and loosening of total replacements. Acta Orthop. Belg. 40:831, 1974.
23. Willert, H.G., Ludwig, J., and Semlitsch, M.: Reaction of bone to methacrylate after hip arthroplasty. J. Bone Joint Surg. 56A:1368, 1974.
24. Reckling, F.W., and Dillon, W.L.: The bone-cement interface temperature during total joint replacement. J. Bone Joint Surg. 59A:80, 1977.
25. DeLee, J.G., and Charnley, J.: Radiological demarcation of cemented sockets in total hip replacement. Clin. Orthop. 121:20, 1976.
26. Goldring, S.R., Schiller, A.L., Roelke, M., Rourke, C.M., O'Neill, D.A., and Harris, W.H.: The synovial-like membrane at the bone-cement interface in loose total hip replacements and its proposed role in bone lysis. J. Bone Joint Surg. 65A:575, 1983.
27. Eftekhar, N.: Low-friction arthroplasty. JAMA. 218:705, 1971.
28. Charnley, J., and Cupic, Z.: The nine and ten year results of the low-friction arthroplasty of the hip. Clin. Orthop. 95:9, 1973.
29. Dolinskas, C., Campbell, R.E., and Rothman, R.H.: The painful Charnley total hip replacement. Am. J. Roentgenol. 121:61, 1974.
30. Bergstrom, B., Lindberg, L., Fersson, B.M., and Onnerfalt, R.: Complications after total hip arthroplasty according to Charnley in a Swedish series of cases. Clin. Orthop. 95:91, 1973.
31. Harris, W.H., and Jones, W.N.: The rise of wire mesh in total hip replacement surgery. Clin. Orthop. 106:117, 1975.
32. Charnley, J., and Halley, D.K.: Rate of wear in total hip replacement. Clin. Orthop. 112:170, 1975.
33. Clarke, I.C., Black, K., Rennic, C., and Amstutz, H.C.: Can wear in total hip arthroplasties be assessed from radiographs? Clin. Orthop. 121:126, 1976.
34. Bechtol, C.O.: Failure of femoral implant components in total hip replacement operations. Orthop. Rev. 4:23, 1975.
35. Green, D.L.: Complications of total hip replacement. South. Med. J. 69:1559, 1976.
36. Mullins, M.F., Sutton, R.N., and Lodwick, G.S.: Complications of total hip replacement. A roentgen evaluation. Am. J. Roentgenol. 121:55, 1974.
37. Murray, W.R.: Total joint prosthesis: Complications with emphasis on hips. *In* Symposium on Osteoarthritis. St. Louis, C.V. Mosby Company, 1974.
38. Daffner, R.H., Carden, T.S., Jr., and Gehweiler, J.A.: Complication of unrecognized dislocation of Charnley-Muller hip prosthesis. Importance of early roentgen diagnosis. Radiology 108:323, 1973.
39. Goodman, L., and McGee, J.W.: Eccentric femoral heads in total hip prosthesis. Radiology 111:235, 1974.
40. Jackson, D.M.: Total hip prosthesis: Real and apparent dislocation. Clin. Radiol. 26:63, 1975.
41. Campbell, R.E., and Marvel, J.P., Jr.: Concomitant dislocation and intra-articular foreign body: A rare complication of the Charnley total hip arthroplasty. Am. J. Roentgenol. 126:1059, 1976.
42. McLaughlin, R.E., and Whitehill, R.: Evaluation of the painful hip by aspiration and arthrography. Surg. Gynecol. Obstet. 144:381, 1977.
43. Dussault, R.G., Goldman, A.B., and Ghelman, B.: Radiologic diagnosis of loosening and infection in hip prostheses. J. Can. Assoc. Radiol. 23:119, 1977.
44. Stauffer, R.N.: Ten-year follow-up study of total hip replacement: With particular reference to roentgenographic loosening of the components. J. Bone Joint Surg. 64A:983, 1982.
45. Tehranzadeh, J., Schneider, R., and Freiberger, R.H.: Radiological evaluation of painful total hip replacement. Radiology 141:355, 1981.
46. Nicholson, O.R.: Total hip replacement: An evaluation of the results and techniques, 1967-1972. Clin. Orthop. 95:217, 1973.
47. DeSmet, A.A., Kramer, D., and Martel, W.: The metal-cement interface in total hip prostheses. Am. J. Roentgenol. 129:279, 1977.
48. Lane, E.J., Proto, A.V., and Phillips, T.W.: Mach bands and density perception. Radiology 121:9, 1976.
49. Weber, F.A., and Charnley, J.: A radiological study of fractures of acrylic cement in relation to the stem of a femoral head prosthesis. J. Bone Joint Surg. 57B:297, 1975.
50. Salvati, E.A., Freiberger, R.H., and Wilson, P.D., Jr.: Arthrography for complications of total hip replacement. A review of thirty-one arthrograms. J. Bone Joint Surg. 53A:701, 1971.
51. Murray, W.R., and Rodrigo, J.J.: Arthrography for the assessment of pain after total hip replacement. J. Bone Joint Surg. 57A:1060, 1975.
52. Christensen, E.E., Curray, T.S., III, and Nunnally, J.: An Introduction to the Physics of Diagnostic Radiology. Philadelphia, Lea & Febiger, 1972.
53. Firooznia, H., Baruch, H., Seliger, G., and Weathers, R.: The value of subtraction in hip arthrography after total hip replacement. Bull. Hosp. Joint Dis. 35:36, 1974.
54. Anderson, L.S., and Staple, T.W.: Arthrography of total hip replacement using subtraction technique. Radiology 109:470, 1973.
55. Gelman, M.J.: Arthrography in total hip prosthesis complications. Am. J. Roentgenol. 126:743, 1976.
56. Drinker, H., Turner, R.H., McKenzie, J.D., Bierbaum, B.E., and Laws-

ing, J.F., III: Color subtraction arthrography in the diagnosis of component loosening in hip arthroplasty. Orthopedics 1:224, 1978.

57. Coren, G.S., Curtis, J., and Dalinka, M.: Lymphatic visualization during hip arthrography. Radiology 115:621, 1975.

58. Selby Brown, C., and Knickerbocker, W.J.: Radiologic studies in the investigation of the causes of total hip replacement failures. J. Can. Assoc. Radiol. 24:245, 1973.

59. Gelman, M.I., Coleman, R.E., Stevens, P.M., and Davey, B.W.: Radiography, radionuclide imaging, and arthrography in the evaluation of total hip and knee replacement. Radiology 128:677, 1978.

60. Campeau, R.J., Hall, M.F., and Miale, A., Jr.: Detection of total hip arthroplasty complications with Tc-99m pyrophosphate. J. Nucl. Med. 17:526, 1976.

61. Feith, R., Slooff, T.J.J.H., Karem, I., and van Rens, T.J.G.: Strontium [87m]Sr bone scanning for the evaluation of total hip replacement. J. Bone Joint Surg. 58B:79, 1976.

62. McInerney, D.P., and Hyde, I.D.: Technetium 99 Tcm pyrophosphate scanning in the assessment of the painful hip prosthesis. Clin. Radiol. 29:513, 1978.

63. Weiss, P.E., Mall, J.C., Hoffer, P.B., et al.: 99m Tc-methylene diphosphonate bone imaging in the evaluation of total hip prostheses. Radiology 133:727, 1979.

64. Williamson, B.R.J., McLaughlin, R.E., Wang, G.J., et al.: Radionuclide bone imaging as a means of differentiating loosening and infection in patients with a painful total hip proshtesis. Radiology 133:723, 1979.

65. Rosenthall, L., Lisbona, R., Hernandez, M., et al.: 99m Tc-PP and 67-Ga imaging following insertion of orthopedic devices. Radiology 133:717, 1979.

66. Reing, C.M., Richin, P.F., and Kenmore, P.L.: Differential bone-scanning in the evaluation of a painful total joint replacement. J. Bone Joint Surg. 61A:933, 1979.

67. Mountford, P.J., Hall, F.M., Coakley, A.J., and Wells, C.P.: Assessment of the painful hip prosthesis with in-labelled leucocyte scans. Br. J. Radiol. 55:378, 1982.

67a. Resnick, D., and Guerra, J., Jr.: Stress fractures of the inferior public ramus following hip surgery. Radiology 137:335, 1980.

68. Martens, M., Hernoudt, E., DeMeester, P., et al.: Factors in the mechanical failure of the femoral component in total hip prosthesis. Acta Orthop. Scand. 45:693, 1974.

69. Collis, D.K.: Femoral stem failure in total hip replacement. J. Bone Joint Surg. 59A:1033, 1977.

70. Casagrande, P.A., and Danahy, P.R.: Delayed sciatic-nerve entrapment following the use of self-curing acrylic. J. Bone Joint Surg. 53A:167, 1971.

71. Dorr, L.D., Conaty, J.P., Kohl, R., and Harvey, J.P.: False aneurysm of the femoral artery following total hip surgery. J. Bone Joint Surg. 56A:1059, 1974.

72. Hirsch, S., Robertson, H., and Gorniowsky, M.: Arterial occlusion secondary to methylmethacrylate use. Arch. Surg. 111:204, 1976.

73. Switzer, P.J., Cooperberg, P.L., and Knickerbocker, W.J.: Defects in the sigmoid colon caused by placement of a left hip prosthesis. J. Can. Assoc. Radiol. 25:151, 1974.

74. Lowell, J.D., Davies, J.A.K., and Bennett, A.H.: Bladder fistula following total hip replacement using self-curing acrylic. Clin. Orthop. 111:131, 1975.

75. Evanski, P.M., Waugh, T.R., and Orofino, C.F.: Total hip replacement with the Charnley prosthesis. Clin. Orthop. 95:69, 1973.

76. Greenspan, A., and Norman, A.: Gross hematuria: A complication of intrapelvic cement intrusion in total hip replacement. Am. J. Roentgenol. 130:327, 1978.

77. McElfresh, E.C., and Coventry, M.B.: Femoral and pelvic fractures after total hip arthroplasty. J. Bone Joint Surg. 56A-483, 1974.

78. Schneider, R., and Kaye, J.J.: Insufficiency and stress fractures of the long bones occurring in patients with rheumatoid arthritis. Radiology 116:595, 1975.

79. Nollen, A.J.G., and Slooff, T.J.J.H.: Para-articular ossification after total hip replacement. Acta Orthop. Scand. 44:230, 1973.

80. Brooker, A.F., Bowerman, J.W., Robinson, R.A., et al.: Ectopic ossification following total hip replacement: Incidence and a method of classification. J. Bone Joint Surg. 55A:1629, 1973.

81. Suzuki, Y., Hisada, K., and Takeda, M.: Demonstration of myositis ossificans by ^{99m}Tc pyrophosphate bone scanning. Radiology 111:663, 1974.

82. Tanaka, T., Rossier, A.B., Hussey, R.W., et al.: Quantitative assessment of para-osteo-arthropathy and its maturation on serial radionuclide bone images. Radiology 123:217, 1977.

83. Chand, K.: The knee joint in rheumatoid arthritis. IV. Treatment by nonhinged total knee prosthetic replacement. Int. Surg. 60:11, 1975.

84. Radin, E.L.: Biomechanics of the knee joint. Its implications in the design of replacements. Orthop. Clin. North. Am. 4:539, 1973.

85. Peterson, L.F.A.: Current status of total knee arthroplasty. Arch. Surg. 112:1099, 1977.

86. Lotke, P.A., and Ecker, M.L.: Influence of positioning of prosthesis in total knee replacement. J. Bone Joint Surg. 59A:77, 1977.

87. Gilula, L.A., and Staple, T.W.: Radiology of recently developed total knee prostheses. Radiol. Clin. North. Am. 13:57, 1975.

88. Goergen, T.G., and Resnick, D.: Radiology of total knee replacement. J. Can. Assoc. Radiol. 27:178, 1976.

89. Schneider, R., Hood, R.W., and Ranawat, C.S.: Radiologic evaluation of knee arthroplasty. Orthop. Clin. North Am. 13:225, 1982.

90. Insall, J.N., Hood, R.W., Flawn, L.B., and Sullivan, D.J.: The total condylar knee prosthesis in gonarthrosis. J. Bone Joint Surg. 65A:619, 1983.

91. Symposium on Total Knee Arthroplasty. Orthop. Clin. North Am. 13 (entire volume), 1982.

92. Ducheyne, P., Kagan, A., II, and Lacey, J.A.: Failure of total knee arthroplasty due to loosening and deformation of the tibial component. J. Bone Joint Surg. 60A:384, 1978.

93. Gelman, M.I., and Dunn, H.K.: Radiology of knee joint replacement. Am. Roentgenol. 127:447, 1976.

94. Mains, D.B.: Marking pin dislocation in total knee arthroplasty. Clin. Orthop. 99:137, 1974.

95. Thomas, W.H.: Total knee replacement with hinged prostheses. Orthop. Clin. N. Am. 6:823, 1975.

96. Wilson, F.C.: Total replacement of the knee in rheumatoid arthritis. A prospective study of the results of treatment with the Walldius prosthesis. J. Bone Joint Surg. 54A:1429, 1972.

97. Merryweather, R., and Jones, G.B.: Total knee replacement. Orthop. Clin. N. Am. 4:585, 1974.

98. Newberg, A., and Wales, L.: Radiographic diagnosis of quadriceps tendon rupture. Radiology 125:367, 1977.

99. Kay, N.R.M., and Martins, H.D.: The MacIntosh tibial plateau hemi-prosthesis for the rheumatoid knee. J. Bone Joint Surg. 54B:256, 1972.

100. Anderson, G.B.J., Jessop, J., Freeman, M.A.R., and Mason, R.M.: MacIntosh arthroplasty in rheumatoid arthritis. Acta Orthop. Scand. 45:245, 1974.

101. Cofield, R.H.: Status of total shoulder arthroplasty. Arch. Surg. 112:1088, 1977.

102. Neer, C.S., II: Replacement arthroplasty for glenohumeral osteoarthritis. J. Bone Joint Surg. 56A:1, 1974.

103. Dee R.: Total elbow replacement. J. Bone Joint Surg. 56A:233, 1974.

104. Dee, R.: Total replacement arthroplasty of the elbow for rheumatoid arthritis. J. Bone Joint Surg. 54B:88, 1972.

105. Bryan, R.S., Dobyns, J.H., Linscheid, R.L., and Peterson, L.F.A.: Preliminary experience with total elbow arthroplasty. In Symposium on Osteoarthritis. St. Louis, C.V. Mosby Company, 1974.

106. Bryan, R.S.: Total replacement of the elbow joint. Arch Surg. 112:1092, 1977.

107. Ewald, F.C., Scheinberg, R.D., Poss, R., et al.: Capitellocondylar total elbow arthroplasty. J. Bone Joint Surg. 62A:1259, 1980.

108. Stauffer, R.N.: Total ankle joint replacement. Arch. Surg. 112:1105, 1977.

109. Murray, M.P., Drought, A.B., and Kory, R.C.: Walking patterns in normal men. J. Bone Joint Surg. 46A:335, 1964.

110. Demottaz, J.D., Maxur, J.M., Thomas, W.H., et al.: Clinical study of total ankle replacement with gait analysis: A preliminary report. J. Bone Joint Surg. 61A:976, 1979.

111. Scholz, K.C.: Total ankle replacement arthroplasty. In Bateman, J.E. (ed.): Foot Science. Philadelphia, W.B. Saunders Company, 1976.

112. Calenoff, L., and Stromberg, W.B.: Silicone rubber arthroplasties of the hand. Radiology 107:29, 1973.

113. Beckenbaugh, R.D., Dobyns, J.H., Linscheid, R.L., and Bryan, R.S.: Review and analysis of silicone-rubber metacarpophalangeal implants. J. Bone Joint Surg. 58A:483, 1976.

114. Millender, L.H., Nalebuff, E.A., Hawkins, R.B., and Ennis, R.: Infection after silicone prosthetic arthroplasty in the hand. J. Bone Joint Surg. 57A:825, 1975.

INDEX

Note: Page numbers in *italics* refer to illustrations; page numbers followed by t refer to tables.

AA protein, 1472–1473
Abdominal pain, in polyarteritis, 1144
   in rheumatic fever, 1284
   in systemic lupus erythematosus,
      1081–1082
Abdominal skin reflex, 428t
Accessory nerve, tests of, 420t
Acetaminophen, aspirin interaction with, 733
   in juvenile rheumatoid arthritis, 1266
N-Acetylhexosaminidase, 245
Achilles bursitis, corticosteroid in, 552
Achilles tendinitis, 471, 1748–1749
   corticosteroid in, 552–553, 559
Achilles tendon, disorders of, 388
   in rheumatoid arthritis, 936
   tophi of, *1365*
Acid hydrolase, macrophage secretion of,
   155–156
Acid maltase deficiency, adult, polymyositis
   vs., 1234
Acquired immune deficiency syndrome,
   1332–1333, *1333*
   in hemophilia, 1569
Acromegaly, *1588–1589*, 1588–1590,
   1590t
   osteoarthritis in, 1445
   radiography in, 602–604, *603*
Acromioclavicular joint, arthritis in, 442
   arthroplasty of, 1868
   examination of, 373
   injection into, 554
   rehabilitation and reconstruction of, 1863
   separation of, 1735, *1735*
Acromioplasty, in rotator cuff lesion,
   1862–1863
Acropachy, thyroid, 1586, *1586*, 1598
ACTH test, for hypothalamic-pituitary-adrenal function, 824–825, 824t
ACTH therapy, glucocorticoids vs., 828
Actin, 287–288, *288*
   fibronectin and, 232
Actinomycosis, 1534
   in spine, 463
Action potential, mechanism of, 300–303,
   303–304
Acute phase protein, 653, 654t
Acute phase reactant, 653–664
   clinical value of, 659–661
   in rheumatic fever, 1286
   mechanisms, teleology, and clinical use-
      fulness of, 654
   stimuli of, 653

Adductor reflex, 428t
Adenine, chemical structure of, *337*
Adenine phosphoribosyltransferase, 340–341
   deficiency in, 1390, *1390*
Adenosine, chemical structure of, *338*
Adenosine deaminase deficiency, 1321–1322
Adenosine kinase, 341
Adenovirus, 1551
Adenylic acid, biosynthesis of, 340
Adhesive capsulitis, in shoulder, 445, 627,
   628
Adhesive radiculitis, 462
Adson test, 426
AE protein, 1473
AF protein, 1473
African histoplasmosis, 1535
Agammaglobulinemia, adult-acquired,
   1327–1328
   Swiss-type, 1320–1323
   X-linked, 22, 1324–1326
Agarose well assay, 116
AIDS, 1332–1333, *1333*
   in hemophilia, 1569
AL protein, 1471–1472
Albers-Schönberg's disease, 1673–1674,
   1674
Albright's hereditary osteodystrophy, 1584
Alcohol ingestion, in gout, 1388
Alcoholism, avascular necrosis in,
   1692–1693
   septic arthritis in, 1507
Aldamine crosslink, in collagen, *221*, 222
Aldol crosslink, in collagen, 222, *222*
   in elastin, *222*, 229
Alkaline phosphatase, serum, in metabolic
   bone disease, 1646
Alkaptonuria, radiography in, 600
Alkylating agents, 838–841
Allele, 38
Allergic granulomatous angiitis, 1137, 1138,
   1153–1155, 1309
Allergic vasculitis, 1138, 1149–1153, *1308*,
   1308–1309
Allergy, aspirin, 735–736, 763
   drug, in Sjögren's syndrome, 964
Allopurinol, 861–867
   biological effects of, 862–864
   clinical use of, *864*, 864–865, 865t
   complications of, 865–866
   drug interaction with, 864
   in hyperuricemia, 1387–1388, 1387t
   inhibition of drug metabolism by, 720

Allopurinol *(Continued)*
   maintenance dose of, 865t
   metabolic effects of, 863t
   pharmacokinetics and metabolism of, 862,
      862
   toxicity of, 866–867
Allotype, 40
Allysine, in collagen, 221, *221*
Alopecia, in systemic lupus erythematosus,
   538, 1077, 1101
Alpha heavy-chain disease, 1342
Alphavirus, 1547–1548
Alveolitis, cryptogenic fibrosing, 1217
Alymphoplasia, thymic, 1320–1323
Alzheimer's dementia, amyloid deposits in,
   1473
American Rheumatism Association Criteria,
   in rheumatoid arthritis, 916t
   in systemic lupus erythematosus, 1072t
Amidophosphoribosyltransferase, inhibition
   of, 342, *342*
Amine, platelet interaction with, 175–176,
   176
Amino acid, in elastin, tropoelastin, and fibronectin, 228t
AMP deaminase deficiency, polymyositis
   vs., 1234
Amphotericin B, 1537, 1537t
Amyloid deposits, 1470–1473
   characteristics of, 1470t
   electron microscopy of, 1470–1471,
      1470–1471
   glomerular, 1481, *1481*
   in endocrine disease, 1473
   light microscopy of, 1470
   of light chain immunoglobulin origin,
      1471–1472
   of protein origin, 1472–1473
   senile, 1473
Amyloidosis, 1469–1487
   arthropathy in, 1478–1479, *1479*
   biopsy in, 1481, *1481*
   cardiomyopathy in, 1480
   classification of, 1474–1475, 1475t
   cutaneous, 542, 1478, *1478*
   definition of, 1469
   diagnosis of, 1481, *1481*
   familial cardiopathic, 1477
   familial nephropathic, 1477
   familial neuropathic, 1476–1477
   gastrointestinal tract in, 1480–1481
   historical, 1469–1470
   in ankylosing spondylitis, 998

Index

Index

x

Erythema infectiosum, 1552–1553
Erythema marginatum, in rheumatic fever, 1284
Erythema nodosum, 1178–1179, *1179*
Erythrocyte sedimentation rate, 654–657, *655*
  clinical significance of, 656
  in ankylosing spondylitis, 660–661
  in giant cell arteritis, 660
  in polymyalgia rheumatica, 660
  in rheumatic fever, 661
  in rheumatoid arthritis, 660
  in systemic lupus erythematosus, 661, 1091
  mechanisms governing, 655, *655*
  methods for determination of, 656
  plasma protein abnormalities and, 655
  shape and size abnormalities and, drugs and, 655–656
Erythromycin, in Lyme disease, 1563
Esophagus, in amyloidosis of, 1480
  in scleroderma, 1185, 1191, 1199
Estrogen deficiency, rheumatic manifestations in, 1591
Ethambutol, 1531t
Ewald total elbow prosthesis, *1967*
Examination of patient, 371–372, *372*
  crepitation in, 371
  deformity in, 371
  instability in, 371
  motion limitation in, 371
  recording of, 371–372, *372*
  swelling in, 371
Excitation-contraction coupling, 292
Exercise. See also *Physical therapy.*
  for hand, 1818
  for shoulder, 1861
  in rheumatoid arthritis, 983–984
  therapeutic, 1772–1773, 1772t
    active vs passive, 1772
    bone mineralization and, 1773
    important muscle groups in, 1773
    isometric, 1773
    stretching as, 1773
Extensor tendon, rupture of, in dorsal tenosynovitis, 1819, *1820*
Extra Depth Shoe, 477, *478*
Eye symptoms. See *Ocular manifestations.*

Fabere test, 452
Facet block, in low back pain, 458
Facioscapulohumeral muscular dystrophy, polymyositis vs, 1234
Factor, coagulation, macrophage secretion of, 154
Factor VIII replacement, 1568–1569
Factor IX replacement, 1569–1570
Factor XI, 105–106
  activation of, 105–106
  inhibition of, 108
  interactions of, 96–97, *97*
Familial arthropathy, synovial biopsy in, 652
Fanconi syndrome, osteomalacia in, 1669
Fasciitis, eosinophilic, 1195–1196
  malignancy and, 1613–1614
  plantar, 389

Fat pad sign, 574
Fatigue, in patient history, 370
  in systemic lupus erythematosus, 1071, 1101
Fatty acid, as nutritional intervention, 359
  long-chain, metabolism of, *294*
Feet, 469–481
  anatomy of, 386, *387*
  Charcot's joint in, 471
  corticosteroid in, 552–553, 559
  examination of, 386–390
  flat, 388
  forefoot, in diabetes mellitus, 1581, *1583*
    in rheumatoid arthritis, 477–478
    orthotics for, 1777
    reconstructive surgery for, 1902–1909, *1903–1909*
  gout in, 470, *470*
  heel pain in, 470–471
  hindfoot, in rheumatoid arthritis, 480
    orthotics for, 1777
    reconstructive surgery for, 1899–1901, *1900–1902*
  march, 390
  muscles in, 389
  neuropathic arthropathy in, 471
  normal, 469
  orthotics for, 1776–1777
  osteoarthritis in, 469–471
    radiography in, 590
    treatment of, 1456
  osteoporosis of, 390
  preoperative evaluation of, 1790
  psoriatic arthritis in, radiography in, 582, *582*
  reflex sympathetic dystrophy of, 390
  Reiter's syndrome in, radiography in, 583–584, *584*
  rheumatoid arthritis in, 471–480, 936–938, *938*
    conservative management in, 477–480
    footwear in, 477, *478–479*
    forefoot in, 477–478
    general principles of, 477
    injections in, 479–480
    orthoses in, 478
    rearfoot in, 480
    shoe modifications in, 479
    deformities in, 472, *473*
    evaluation in, 472–473, *473*
    Harris Mat imprint in, 474, *474*
    history in, 472
    juvenile, 480
    nail care in, 476
    palpation in, 473–474, *474*
    radiography in, 476, 574–575, *574–575*
    range of motion in, 473, *473*
    rearfoot and midfoot involvement in, 476–477
    skin changes in, 475–476
    tenderness in, 474–475, *475*
    varus deformity in, *937*
Felty's syndrome, 950–955
  clinical features of, 950–952, *951*, 951t
  hematologic features of, 952
  pathogenesis of, 952–954, *953*

Felty's syndrome, pathogenesis of *(Continued)*
    impaired granulocyte production in, 953–954
    increased granulocyte removal in, 952–953
  serologic features of, 952, 952t
  splenectomy in, 954
  vasculitis in, 1148
Femoral capital epiphysis, slipped, osteoarthritis in, 1440
Femoral head, avascular necrosis of, 1697–1698
  in hyperuricemia, 491
Femoral nerve, 1766–1767
  course and distribution of, *1765*
  entrapment of, 1766–1767, *1767*
Fenoprofen, 766, *766*
  in gouty arthritis, 1384
  in juvenile rheumatoid arthritis, 1266
Ferritin, in hemochromatosis, 1495, 1498
Fever, in dermatomyositis in children, 1298
  in inflammatory bowel disease, 408
  in juvenile rheumatoid arthritis, 408, 1251–1252, *1252*
  in mixed connective tissue disease, 1120, *1120*
  in polyarticular arthritis, 407–408
  in rheumatic fever, 1284
  in rheumatoid arthritis, 407
  in systemic lupus erythematosus, 1071, 1101
Fibrillation, of cartilage, 265, 1434–1435, *1436*
Fibrillogenesis, collagen, 219–220
Fibrin formation, in synovial fluid, 893
Fibrinogen, fibronectin and, 232
Fibrinoid degeneration, in rheumatic heart disease, 1280
Fibrinolysis, in synovial fluid, 893
  intrinsic coagulation pathway in, 106–107, *107*
Fibroblast, 1211–1215
  adherence of, 1213
  biosynthesis, processing, deposition of connective tissue by, 1213
  inflammatory cell modulation of, 1215
  migration and chemoattraction of, 1211–1212, 1212t
  platelet interaction with, 177–179
  proliferation of, 1212–1213
Fibroblast growth factor, 1212
Fibroendothelioma, synovial, 1719
Fibrogenesis imperfecta ossium, osteomalacia in, 1670
Fibroma, of tendon sheath, 1724
Fibronectin, 230–234
  actin and, 232
  amino acid composition of, 228t
  bacteria and, 232–233
  biologic function and significance of, 234
  cell adhesion to, 232, *232*
  cell origin and tissue distribution of, 233–234
  chemical properties of, 231
  collagen and, 231–232
  fibrinogen and, 232
  glycosaminoglycan and, 232
  heparin and, 232
  molecular binding sites on, 233, *233*
  molecular interactions of, 231t
  structural model for, *231*